Principles and Practice of Hospital Medicine

NOTICE

Medicine is an ever-changing science. As new research and clinical experience broaden our knowledge, changes in treatment and drug therapy are required. The authors and the publisher of this work have checked with sources believed to be reliable in their efforts to provide information that is complete and generally in accord with the standards accepted at the time of publication. However, in view of the possibility of human error or changes in medical sciences, neither the authors nor the publisher nor any other party who has been involved in the preparation or publication of this work warrants that the information contained herein is in every respect accurate or complete, and they disclaim all responsibility for any errors or omissions or for the results obtained from use of the information contained in this work. Readers are encouraged to confirm the information contained herein with other sources. For example, and in particular, readers are advised to check the product information sheet included in the package of each drug they plan to administer to be certain that the information contained in this work is accurate and that changes have not been made in the recommended dose or in the contraindications for administration. This recommendation is of particular importance in connection with new or infrequently used drugs.

Principles and Practice of Hospital Medicine

Second Edition

Editors

Sylvia C. McKean, MD, SFHM, FACP
Deputy Editor for Editorial Projects, UpToDate
Formerly:
Leave of absence:
Associate Professor of Medicine,
Harvard Medical School
Hospitalist
Brigham and Women's Hospital
Boston, Massachusetts

John J. Ross, MD, CM, FIDSA
Assistant Professor of Medicine
Harvard Medical School
Hospitalist Service
Brigham and Women's Hospital
Boston, Massachusetts

Daniel D. Dressler, MD, MSc, SFHM, FACP
Professor of Medicine
Director, Internal Medicine Teaching Services
Emory University Hospital
Associate Program Director
J. Willis Hurst Internal Medicine Residency Program
Co-Director, Semmelweis Society
Emory University School of Medicine
Atlanta, Georgia

Danielle B. Scheurer, MD, MSCR, SFHM
Chief Quality Officer and Hospitalist
Associate Professor of Medicine
Medical University of South Carolina
Charleston, South Carolina

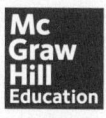
Mc
Graw
Hill
Education

New York   Chicago   San Francisco   Athens   London   Madrid   Mexico City
Milan   New Delhi   Singapore   Sydney   Toronto

Principles and Practice of Hospital Medicine, Second Edition

4 5 6 7 8 9   LWI   21 20

ISBN 978-0-07-184313-3
MHID 0-07-184313-2

This book was set in Myriad pro by Cenveo® Publisher Services.
The editors were Amanda Fielding and Kim J. Davis.
The production supervisor was Richard Ruzycka.
Project management was provided by Vastavikta Sharma, Cenveo Publisher Services.
The designer was Alan Barnett; the cover designer was Dreamit, Inc.

LSC Communications was printer and binder.

Library of Congress Cataloging-in-Publication Data

Names: McKean, Sylvia C., editor. | Ross, John J. (John James), 1966-editor.
   | Dressler, Daniel D., editor. | Scheurer, Danielle, editor.
Title: Principles and practice of hospital medicine / editors, Sylvia C.
   McKean, John J. Ross, Daniel D. Dressler, Danielle B. Scheurer.
Description: Second edition. | New York . McGraw-Hill Education Medical, [2017]
   | Includes bibliographical references and index.
Identifiers: LCCN 2016022668 (print) | LCCN 2016023825 (ebook)
   | ISBN 9780071843133 (hardcover : alk. paper) | ISBN 0071843132 (hardcover :
   alk. paper) | ISBN 9780071843140 (ebook)
Subjects: | MESH: Hospital Medicine—methods | Hospitalization | Inpatients |
   Hospitalists Classification: LCC RA972 (print) | LCC RA972 (ebook) | NLM WX 21 |
   DDC 362.11—dc23
LC record available at https://lccn.loc.gov/2016022668

CONTENTS

PART I: THE SPECIALTY OF HOSPITAL MEDICINE AND SYSTEMS OF CARE

SECTION 1 The Value and Values of Hospital Medicine

SECTION 2 Critical Decision Making at the Point of Care

SECTION 3 Transitions of Care

SECTION 4 Patient Safety and Quality Improvement

SECTION 5 Practice Management

SECTION 6 Billing, Coding, and Clinical Documentation

SECTION 7 Principles of Medical Ethics and Medical-Legal Concepts

SECTION 8 Professional Development

CONTENTS

CONTENTS

SECTION 16   Rheumatology

SECTION 17   Toxicology and Addiction

SECTION 18   Vascular Medicine

Online Chapters

EDITORS

Sylvia C. McKean, MD, SFHM, FACP

John J. Ross, MD, CM, FIDSA

Daniel D. Dressler, MD, MSc, SFHM, FACP

Danielle B. Scheurer, MD, MSCR, SFHM

CONTRIBUTORS

Numbers in brackets refer to the chapters written or co-written by the contributor.

Samer Abdel-Aziz, MD
Pain Medicine Fellowship
Medical College of Wisconsin
Milwaukee, Wisconsin [99]

Meredith C. B. Adams, MD, MS
Assistant Professor of Anesthesiology and Pain Medicine
Director
Pain Medicine Fellowship
Medical College of Wisconsin
Milwaukee, Wisconsin [99]

Aaron W. Aday, MD
Division of Cardiovascular Medicine
Department of Medicine
Brigham and Women's Hospital
Boston, Massachusetts [255]

Bhavin Adhyaru, MD
Emory University School of Medicine
Atlanta, Georgia [10]

Kush Agrawal, MD
Advanced Endovascular and Structural Interventional Fellow
VIVA Physicians
El Camino Hospital
Mountain View, California [101]

Mikhail Akbashev, MD
Assistant Professor of Medicine
Emory University School of Medicine
Atlanta, Georgia [11]

Afsaneh Alavi, MD, MSc, FRCPC
Department of Medicine (Dermatology)
University of Toronto
Toronto, Ontario, Canada [148]

G. Caleb Alexander, MD, MS
Associate Professor of Epidemiology and Medicine
Bloomberg School of Public Health
Johns Hopkins University
Baltimore, Maryland [e3]

Anne E. Allan, MD
Miraca Life Sciences
Irving, Texas [146]

Ashwin Ananthakrishnan, MD
Attending Physician
Massachusetts General Hospital
Instructor in Medicine, Harvard Medical School
Boston, Massachusetts [183]

Daniel A. Anaya, MD
Associate Professor of Surgery
Division of Surgical Oncology
Michael E. DeBakey Department of Surgery
Research Scientist
The Houston Center for Quality of Care & Utilization Studies
Director
Liver Tumor Program, Michael E. DeBakey VAMC
Baylor College of Medicine
Houston, Texas [55]

Douglas S. Ander, MD
Professor of Emergency Medicine
Emory University School of Medicine
Atlanta, Georgia [121]

Eddy Ang, MD
Instructor in Medicine
Harvard Medical School
Division of Gerontology
Beth Israel Deaconess Medical Center
Boston, Massachusetts
Department of Medicine, Hebrew SeniorLife
Roslindale, Massachusetts [68]

Kelly Armstrong, PhD
Senior Clinical Ethicist
Memorial Health System
Adjunct Assistant Professor
Department of Medical Humanities
SIU School of Medicine
Springfield, Illinois [34]

Vineet M. Arora, MD, MAPP
Associate Professor and Assistant Dean for Scholarship and Discovery
Director
GME Clinical Learning Environment Innovation
Pritzker School of Medicine
University of Chicago
Chicago, Illinois [13]

Cameron Ashbaugh, MD
Assistant Professor
Harvard Medical School
Division of Infectious Diseases
Brigham and Women's Hospital
Boston, Massachusetts [196]

Saima Aslam, MD, MS
Assistant Professor
Director
Solid Organ Transplant Infectious Diseases service
Division of Infectious Diseases
University of California, San Diego
San Diego, California [188]

Mark J. Ault, MD
Professor of Medicine
University of California
Los Angeles School of Medicine
Department of Medicine
Cedars-Sinai Medical Center
Los Angeles, California [125]

Patrick Avila, MD, MPhil, MPH
Internal Medicine Resident Physician
Brigham and Women's Hospital
Boston, Massachusetts [160]

Vasilis C. Babaliaros, MD
Professor of Medicine and Surgery
Co-Director
Emory Structural Heart and Valve Center
Emory University Hospital
Atlanta, Georgia [131]

Lindsey R. Baden, MD
Associate Professor
Harvard Medical School
Infectious Diseases Division
Brigham and Women's Hospital and Dana-Farber Cancer Institute
Boston, Massachusetts [204]

Meridale V. Baggett, MD
Assistant Professor of Medicine
Harvard Medical School
Inpatient Clinician Educator Service
Department of Medicine
Massachusetts General Hospital
Boston, Massachusetts [78]

James L. Bailey, MD
Professor
Emory University School of Medicine
Atlanta, Georgia [241]

Stephen J. Balevic, MD
Adult and Pediatric Rheumatology Fellow
Duke University Medical Center
Durham, North Carolina [248]

Peter A. Banks, MD
Professor of Medicine
Harvard Medical School
Director of the Center for Pancreatic Disease
Division of Gastroenterology, Hepatology and Endoscopy
Department of Medicine
Brigham and Women's Hospital
Boston, Massachusetts [157]

Aditya Bardia, MD, MPH
Assistant Professor
Harvard Medical School
Attending Physician
Massachusetts General Hospital Cancer Center
Boston, Massachusetts [177, 183]

Maria F. Barile, MD
Clinical Instructor in Radiology
Harvard Medical School
Thoracic Radiologist,
Brigham and Women's Hospital
Boston, Massachusetts [114, 115]

Robert B. Baron, MD, MS
Professor of Medicine
Associate Dean for Graduate and Continuing Medical Education
Vice Chief, Division of General Internal Medicine
University of California
San Francisco School of Medicine
San Francisco, California [36]

Tom Baudendistel, MD, FACP
Internal Medicine Residency Program Director
Kaiser Permanente
Oakland, California [39]

Mihaela H. Bazalakova, MD, PhD
Assistant Professor
Department of Neurology
Center for Sleep Medicine and Sleep Research
University of Wisconsin-Madison
Madison, Wisconsin [96]

Joshua A. Beckman, MD, MSc
Section of Vascular Medicine
Cardiovascular Division
Vanderbilt University Medical Center
Nashville, Tennessee [255]

Nicole M. Bedi, RD, CNSC
Birmingham, Michigan [58]

Laurence Beer, MD, SFHM
Emory University School of Medicine
Atlanta, Georgia [8]

Michael Belkin, MD
Division of Vascular Surgery
Brigham and Women's Hospital
Boston, Massachusetts [256]

Elie F. Berbari, MD
Professor of Medicine
Mayo Clinic College of Medicine
Rochester, Minnesota [194]

Colm Bergin, MD, FRCPI, FRCP, FIDSA
Clinical Professor of Medicine
Trinity College Dublin
Consultant Physician in Infectious Diseases
Associate Director
Wellcome-Health Research Board Clinical Research Facility
St. James's Hospital
Dublin, Ireland [195]

Aaron L. Berkowitz, MD, PhD
Department of Neurology
Brigham and Women's Hospital
Harvard Medical School
Boston, Massachusetts [98]

Rachelle E. Bernacki, MD, MS
Assistant Professor of Medicine
Harvard Medical School
Director of Quality Initiatives
Palliative Care
Dana-Farber Cancer Institute
Brigham and Women's Hospital
Ariadne Labs
Boston, Massachusetts [105, 214]

Robert A. Bessler, MD
CEO
Sound Physicians
Tacoma, Washington [23, 25]

John P. Bilezikian, MD
Dorothy L. and Daniel H. Silberberg Professor of Medicine
Professor of Pharmacology
Columbia University Medical College
Chief, Division of Endocrinology
Director
Metabolic Bone Diseases Program
Columbia University Medical Center
New York, New York [240]

Courtney Bilodeau, MD, FACP
Assistant Professor
The Warren Alpert Medical School of Brown University
Department of Obstetric Medicine, Women's Medicine
Collaborative
Miriam Hospital
Providence, Rhode Island [222]

Kenneth D. Bishop, MD, PhD
Assistant Professor of Medicine
Division of Hematology/Oncology
Rhode Island Hospital
The Warren Alpert Medical School of Brown University
Providence, Rhode Island [176]

Ioannis A. Bliziotis, MD, PhD, MSc
Internal Medicine and Infectious Diseases Specialist
Senior Researcher
Alfa Institute of Biomedical Sciences
Athens, Greece [184]

Arline D. Bohannon, MD
Associate Professor of Internal Medicine
Virginia Commonwealth University
Richmond, Virginia [103]

Peter A. Boling, MD
Professor of Internal Medicine
Virginia Commonwealth University Health System
Richmond, Virginia [103]

Marcy B. Bolster, MD
Associate Professor
Harvard Medical School
Director
Rheumatology Fellowship Training Program
Massachusetts General Hospital
Boston, Massachusetts [248, 249]

Diego F. Bonilla Arcos, MD
Pulmonary Critical Care
Boston University
Pulmonary Center
Boston Medical Center
Boston, Massachusetts [237]

Joanna M. Bonsall, MD, PhD
Assistant Professor of Medicine
Division of Hospital Medicine
Emory University School of Medicine
Atlanta, Georgia [12]

Ghada Bourjeily, MD
Associate Professor of Medicine
The Warren Alpert Medical School of Brown University
The Miriam Hospital
Pulmonary, Critical Care, Obstetric Medicine
Department of Medicine
Providence, Rhode Island [220]

John M. Braver, MD
Assistant Professor
Harvard Medical School
Director
Gastrointestinal Radiology
Brigham and Women's Hospital
Boston, Massachusetts [116, 117]

Ursula C. Brewster, MD
Associate Professor of Medicine
Section of Nephrology
Yale University School of Medicine
New Haven, Connecticut [245]

Joseph Brito, MD
Division of Urology
The Warren Alpert Medical School of Brown University
Providence, Rhode Island [180]

Jared R. Brosch, MD, MS
Assistant Professor of Neurology
Indiana University School of Medicine
Indianapolis, Indiana [192]

Katherine L. Brown, MD, MPH
Suncoast Dermatology
Orlando, Florida [148]

Tod A. Brown, MD
Assistant Professor
Anesthesia and Perioperative Medicine
Medical University of South Carolina
Charleston, South Carolina [62]

Avery L. Buchholz, MD, MPH
Department of Neurosurgery
Medical University of South Carolina
Charleston, South Carolina [64]

Tina Budnitz, MPH, MHM
Senior Advisor
Society Hospital Medicine
Philadelphia, Pennsylvania [e4]

Robert Burakoff, MD, MPH
Associate Professor of Medicine
Division of Gastroenterology, Hepatology, and Endoscopy
Brigham and Women's Hospital
Harvard Medical School
Boston, Massachusetts [155]

T. Karl Byrne, MD, FACS
Professor of Surgery
Director
Bariatric Surgery Program
Medical University of South Carolina
Charleston, South Carolina [63]

Amanda Caissie, MD, PhD, FRCPC
Department of Radiation Oncology
Dalhousie University
Saint John Regional Hospital
Saint John, New Brunswick, Canada [215]

Evelyn Cantillo, MD, MPH
Clinical Instructor of Obstetrics and Gynecology
Program in Women's Oncology
Women & Infants' Hospital of Rhode Island
The Warren Alpert Medical School of Brown University
Providence, Rhode Island [178]

Stephanie M. Cantu, MD
Department of Medicine
Brigham and Women's Hospital
Boston, Massachusetts [109]

Mitchell S. Cappell, MD, PhD
Professor of Medicine
Oakland University William Beaumont School of Medicine
Chief, Division of Gastroenterology and Hepatology
Department of Medicine
William Beaumont Hospital
Royal Oak, Michigan [163]

Alexander R. Carbo, MD, FACP, SFHM
Assistant Professor of Medicine
Harvard Medical School
Hospitalist
Beth Israel Deaconess Medical Center
Boston, Massachusetts [15]

Teresa L. Carman, MD
Assistant Professor of Medicine
Case Western Reserve University School of Medicine
Director
Vascular Medicine
University Hospitals Case Medical Center
Cleveland, Ohio [86]

Patrick J. Cawley, MD, MHM
CEO
MUSC Health
Vice President for Health Affairs
Medical University of South Carolina
Charleston, South Carolina [1]

Laura K. Certain, MD, PhD
Instructor in Medicine
Harvard Medical School
Division of Infectious Diseases
Massachusetts General Hospital
Boston, Massachusetts [193]

Matthew E. Certain, MD
Interventional and Peripheral Cardiologist
Southeast Georgia Health Systems
Brunswick, Georgia [130]

Sukit Chaiyachati, MD
Assistant Professor of Medicine
Division of Hospital Medicine
Emory University School of Medicine
Atlanta, Georgia [90]

Olga S. Chajewski, MD
Department of Pathology and Laboratory Medicine
Medical University of South Carolina
Charleston, South Carolina [57]

Walter W. Chan, MD, MPH
Assistant Professor of Medicine
Division of Gastroenterology, Hepatology, and Endoscopy
Harvard Medical School
Brigham and Women's Hospital
Boston, Massachusetts [155]

Arjun S. Chanmugam, MD, MBA
Associate Professor of Emergency Medicine
Johns Hopkins University School of Medicine
Baltimore, Maryland [79]

Helen Chen, MD
Assistant Professor of Medicine
Harvard Medical School
Division of Gerontology
Beth Israel Deaconess Medical Center
Chief Medical Officer
Hebrew SeniorLife
Boston, Massachusetts [73]

Kenneth K. Chen, MD, FRACP
Assistant Professor of Medicine and OB/GYN
Division of Obstetric and Consultative Medicine
The Warren Alpert Medical School of Brown University
Providence, Rhode Island [221]

Steven T. Chen, MD, MPH
Instructor in Dermatology
Harvard Medical School
Massachusetts General Hospital
Boston, Massachusetts [145]

Xi Chen, MD, PhD
Neurology Department
Atrius Health
Boston, Massachusetts [96]

Nishay Chitkara, MD
Assistant Professor of Medicine
NYU Langone Medical Center/Bellevue Hospital
Department of Medicine
Division of Pulmonary
Critical Care and Sleep Medicine
New York, New York [143]

Louisa W. Chiu, MD
Assistant Professor of Surgery
Michael E. DeBakey Department of Surgery
Baylor College of Medicine
Houston, Texas [55]

Elbert B. Chun, MD
Assistant Professor
Division of Hospital Medicine
Department of Internal Medicine
Emory University School of Medicine
Emory University Hospital
Atlanta, Georgia [132]

Roger P. Clark, DO
Assistant Professor of Medicine
Division of Geographic Medicine and Infectious Diseases
Tufts Medical Center
Consultant, Infectious Diseases
Brigham and Women's Faulkner Hospital
Boston, Massachusetts [199]

John O. Clarke, MD
Associate Professor of Medicine
Division of Gastroenterology & Hepatology
Johns Hopkins University
Baltimore, Maryland [97]

Stephen D. Clements, Jr., MD
Professor of Medicine (Cardiology)
R. Harold Harrison Chair in Cardiology
Division of Cardiology
Department of Medicine
Emory University School of Medicine
Atlanta, Georgia [130]

Steven L. Cohn, MD, FACP, SFHM
Professor of Clinical Medicine
University of Miami Miller School of Medicine
Medical Director
UHealth Preoperative Assessment Center
Director
Medical Consultation Services
University of Miami Hospital and Jackson Memorial Hospital
Miami, Florida [49, 50]

Lauren Colbert, MD
Fellow
Radiation Oncology
MD Anderson Cancer Center
Houston, Texas [182]

Alexandra Columbus, MD
Resident
General Surgery
Brigham and Women's Hospital
Boston, Massachusetts [45]

Jose F. Condado, MD, MS
Cardiology Research Fellow
Structural Heart and Valve Center
Division of Cardiology
Emory University School of Medicine
Atlanta, Georgia [131]

Nicholas J. Connors, MD
Assistant Professor of Medicine
Medical University of South Carolina
Division of Emergency Medicine
Section of Medical Toxicology
Charleston, South Carolina [100]

Darin J. Correll, MD
Assistant Professor of Anesthesia
Harvard Medical School
Director
Postoperative Pain Management Service
Department of Anesthesiology, Perioperative, and Pain Medicine
Chair, Acute Pain Committee
Brigham and Women's Hospital
Boston, Massachusetts [48]

Frank E. Corrigan, III, MD
Cardiology Fellow
Emory University School of Medicine
Atlanta, Georgia [101]

Dominique L. Cosco, MD, FACP
Assistant Professor of Medicine
Associate Program Director
Grady Memorial Hospital
J. Willis Hurst Internal Medicine Residency Program
Emory University School of Medicine
Atlanta, Georgia [230]

Douglas B. Coursin, MD, FCCP
Professor of Anesthesiology and Medicine
University of Wisconsin School of Medicine and Public Health
Madison, Wisconsin [153]

Lisa Criscione-Schreiber, MD, MEd
Associate Professor of Medicine
Rheumatology Training Program Director
Duke University Medical Center
Duke University School of Medicine
Durham, North Carolina [248, 249]

Yvette M. Cua, MD
Associate Professor of Medicine
Department of Medicine
Associate Vice Chair for Clinical Affairs
Department of Medicine
University of Louisville
Louisville, Kentucky [28-30, 32]

Randall Czajkowski, MS, RRA, RT(R)(CT)
Lead Clinical CT Technologist
Brigham and Women's Hospital
Boston, Massachusetts [119]

Sonye K. Danoff, MD, PhD
Associate Professor of Medicine
Department of Medicine
Division of Pulmonary and Critical Care Medicine
Johns Hopkins University School of Medicine
Baltimore, Maryland [233]

Jatin K. Dave, MD, MPH
Part-Time Instructor, Harvard Medical School
Division of Aging, Brigham and Women's Hospital
Boston, Massachusetts
Medical Director
Geriatrics and Senior Care Options
Tufts Health Plan
Watertown, Massachusetts [68, 73]

David B. De Lurgio, MD
Professor
Clinical Cardiac Electrophysiology
Emory Saint Joseph's Hospital
Atlanta, Georgia [136]

Steven B. Deitelzweig, MD, MMM, SFHM, FACP
Ochsner Health System
Medical Director of Regional Business Development
System Chairman, Hospital Medicine
Associate Professor of Medicine-Ochsner Clinical School [24]

Paul F. Dellaripa, MD
Associate Professor
Harvard Medical School
Division of Rheumatology
Brigham and Women's Hospital
Boston, Massachusetts [246]

E. Patchen Dellinger, MD
Professor and Vice Chair
Department of Surgery
University of Washington
Seattle, Washington [55]

Harry A. Demos, MD
Associate Professor
Department of Orthopedics
Medical University of South Carolina
Charleston, South Carolina [65]

Rebecca Dezube, MD
Postdoctoral Fellow
Johns Hopkins University
Pulmonary and Critical Care Medicine
Baltimore, Maryland [95]

Lorenzo Di Francesco, MD, FACP, FHM
Professor of Medicine
Division of General Medicine & Geriatrics
Program Director
J. Willis Hurst Internal Medicine Residency Program
Assistant Chief of Medicine, Grady Memorial Hospital
Emory University School of Medicine
Atlanta, Georgia [93]

Shira Doron, MD, FIDSA
Antimicrobial Steward
Associate Hospital Epidemiologist
Division of Geographic Medicine and Infectious Diseases
Tufts Medical Center
Boston, Massachusetts [191]

Michael Dougan, MD, PhD
Gastroenterology Fellow
Massachusetts General Hospital
Boston, Massachusetts [183]

James D. Douketis, MD, FRCP(C), FACP, FCCP
Professor of Medicine
McMaster University
Hospitalist Service
St. Joseph's Healthcare Hamilton
Hamilton, Ontario, Canada [56, 252]

Aeron A. D. Doyle, MD, CM, FRCPC
Assistant Professor of Anesthesiology
University of British Columbia
Department of Anesthesiology, Perioperative Medicine, and Pain
Management
Providence Health Care
Vancouver, British Columbia, Canada [47]

Tracy J. Doyle, MD, MPH
Instructor in Medicine
Harvard Medical School
Pulmonary and Critical Care Medicine
Brigham and Women's Hospital
Boston, Massachusetts [85]

Daniel D. Dressler, MD, MSc, SFHM, FACP
Professor of Medicine
Director
Internal Medicine Teaching Services
Emory University Hospital
Associate Program Director
J. Willis Hurst Internal Medicine Residency Program
Co-Director
Semmelweis Society
Emory University School of Medicine
Atlanta, Georgia [101]

Jacob M. Drew, MD
Assistant Professor
Department of Orthopedics
Medical University of South Carolina
Charleston, South Carolina [65]

Catherine E. DuBeau, MD
Professor of Medicine
Family Medicine and Community Health, and Obstetrics and
Gynecology
Clinical Chief of Geriatrics
University of Massachusetts Medical School
Worcester, Massachusetts [71]

Jennifer Duff, MD
Assistant Professor of Medicine
Division of Hematology and Oncology
Department of Medicine
University of Florida College of Medicine
Hematology and Oncology Section
NF/SG Veterans Affairs Medical Center
Gainesville, Florida [175]

Liam Durcan, MD, FRCPC
Assistant Professor
Department of Neurology and Neurosurgery
McGill University
Consultant Neurologist
McGill University Health Centre
Montreal, Quebec, Canada [207]

Kent Russell Edwards, Jr., MD
Urology Research Assistant
University of South Carolina School of Medicine
Columbia, South Carolina [67]

Mikhael F. El-Chami, MD, FACC, FHRS
Associate Professor of Medicine
Division of Cardiology-Section of Electrophysiology
Emory University
Atlanta, Georgia [134]

Elwaleed A. Elhassan, MD, FACP, FASN
Assistant Professor of Medicine
Division of Nephrology and Hypertension
Wayne State University School of Medicine
Detroit, Michigan [242]

William J. Elliott, MD, PhD
Chair
Department of Biomedical Sciences
Chief, Division of Pharmacology
Professor of Preventative Medicine, Internal Medicine, Pharmacology
Pacific Northwest University of Health Sciences
Yakima, Washington [244]

John M. Embil, MD, FRCPC, FACP
Professor of Internal Medicine and Medical Microbiology
University of Manitoba
Director
Infection Prevention and Control Unit, Health Sciences Centre
Winnipeg, Manitoba, Canada [147, 202]

Scott F. Enderby, DO, MMM, SFHM, FACP
CEO/Medical Director
Bay Area Hospitalist Associates, Inc.
San Francisco, California [25]

Jeannine Z. Engel, MD
Associate Professor of Medicine
Internal Medicine, Huntsman Cancer Hospital
Physician Advisor, Billing Compliance
Compliance Services
University of Utah Health Sciences
Salt Lake City, Utah [31]

Joseph C. English, III, MD
Professor of Dermatology
University of Pittsburgh Department of Dermatology
Pittsburgh, Pennsylvania [144]

Mary Eno, MD, MPH
Regional Chief of Addiction Medicine
Southern California Permanente Medical Group
Los Angeles, California [251]

Andrew S. Epstein, MD
Assistant Attending
Memorial Sloan Kettering Cancer Center
Gastrointestinal Oncology Service
New York, New York [182]

Evert A. Eriksson, MD, FACS, FCCP
Associate Professor of Surgery
Department of Surgery
Medical University of South Carolina
Charleston, South Carolina [46]

Samir M. Fakhry, MD, FACS
Charles F. Crews Professor of Surgery
Chief, Division of General Surgery
Department of Surgery
Medical University of South Carolina
Charleston, South Carolina [46]

Matthew E. Falagas, MD, MSc, DSc
Adjunct Associate Professor of Medicine
Tufts University School of Medicine
Boston, Massachusetts
Director
Alfa Institute of Biomedical Sciences
Director
Department of Internal Medicine and Infectious Diseases
Iaso General Hospital
Athens, Greece [184]

Kenneth R. Falchuk, MD
Associate Clinical Professor of Medicine
Harvard Medical School
Co-Director
Inflammatory Bowel Disease Center
Department of Medicine, Division of Gastroenterology
Beth Israel Deaconess Medical Center
Boston, Massachusetts [164]

James C. Fang, MD, FACC, FAHA
Chief
Cardiovascular Division
Professor of Medicine
John and June B. Hartman Presidential Endowed Chair
Executive Director
Cardiovascular Service Line
University of Utah Health Sciences Center
Salt Lake City, Utah [129]

John Fanikos, RPh, MBA
Department of Pharmacy Services
Brigham and Women's Hospital
Boston, Massachusetts [254]

Harrison W. Farber, MD
Professor of Medicine
Boston University School of Medicine
Director
Pulmonary Hypertension Center
Boston Medical Center
Boston, Massachusetts [237]

Claire E. Farel, MD, MPH
Clinical Assistant Professor of Medicine
University of North Carolina School of Medicine
Medical Director
UNC Infectious Diseases Clinic
UNC Institute for Global Health and Infectious Diseases
Chapel Hill, North Carolina [203]

Dimitrios Farmakiotis, MD
Assistant Professor of Medicine
New York University School of Medicine
Division of Infectious Diseases and Immunology, NYU Langone
Medical Center
New York, New York [201]

Jeanne M. Farnan, MD, MHPE
Associate Professor
Section of Hospital Medicine
Assistant Dean, Curricular Development and Evaluation
Pritzker School of Medicine
University of Chicago
Chicago, Illinois [13]

Grace Farris, MD
Beth Israel Deaconess Medical Center
Boston, Massachusetts [168]

Kevin Felner, MD
Associate Professor
Division of Pulmonary and Critical Care
New York University School of Medicine
Harbor VA Medical Center
New York, New York [141]

Andrew Z. Fenves, MD, FACP, FASN
Associate Professor of Medicine
Harvard Medical School
Clinician Educator Service
Massachusetts General Hospital
Boston, Massachusetts [38]

Joseph D. Feuerstein, MD
Assistant Professor of Medicine
Harvard Medical School
Attending in Gastroenterology
Center for Inflammatory Bowel Disease
Beth Israel Deaconess Medical Center
Boston, Massachusetts [164]

Joseph J. Fins, MD, MACP
The E. William Davis, Jr., MD Professor of Medical Ethics and
Professor of Medicine
Weill Cornell Medical College
Director
Medical Ethics and Attending Physician
New York Presbyterian Hospital-Weill Cornell Medical Center
New York, New York [33]

Leslie A. Flores, MHA, SFHM
Nelson Flores Hospital Medicine Consultants
La Quinta, California [26]

John A. Flynn, MD, MBA, MEd, FACP, FACR
Medical Director
Spondyloarthritis Program
Associate Dean and Executive Director
Clinical Practice Association
Vice President, Office of Johns Hopkins Physicians
Johns Hopkins University
Baltimore, Maryland [76]

Ryan M. Ford, MD
Assistant Professor of Medicine
Director of Viral Hepatitis
Emory Transplant Center
Transplant Hepatologist
Emory University Hospital
Atlanta, Georgia [159]

Vance G. Fowler Jr., MD, MHS
Division of Infectious Diseases
Duke University Medical Center
Durham, North Carolina [189]

Gil Freitas, MD
Division of Trauma, Burn, and Surgical Critical Care
Harvard Medical School
Fellow, Metabolic Support Service
Brigham and Women's Hospital
Boston, Massachusetts [42]

Joseph M. Furman, MD, PhD
Professor
Departments of Otolaryngology
Neurology, Bioengineering and Physical Therapy
University of Pittsburgh School of Medicine
Director
Divisions of Balance Disorders
Pittsburgh, Pennsylvania [84]

Julia M. Gallagher, MD
Medical Director
MGH Home Based Palliative Care Program
Division of Palliative Care
Massachusetts General Hospital
Boston, Massachusetts [74]

Michael Gardam, MD, MSc, FRCPC
Associate Professor of Medicine
University of Toronto
Director
Infection Prevention and Control
University Health Network
Medical Director
Tuberculosis Clinic
Toronto Western Hospital
Toronto, Ontario, Canada [200]

Brian T. Garibaldi, MD
Assistant Professor of Medicine
Johns Hopkins University School of Medicine
Department of Medicine
Division of Pulmonary and Critical Care Medicine
Baltimore, Maryland [233]

Steven Garlow, MD, PhD
Associate Professor
Chief of Psychiatry
Emory University Hospital
Atlanta, Georgia [223]

Germán E. Giese, MD
Assistant Professor of Medicine
University of Miami Miller School of Medicine
Attending, Division of Hospital Medicine
University of Miami Hospital
Miami, Florida [37]

Richard S. Gitomer, MD, MBA, FACP
Assistant Professor
Emory University School of Medicine
President and Chief Quality Officer
Emory Healthcare Network
Atlanta, Georgia [18]

Jeffrey J. Glasheen, MD, SFHM
Chief Quality Officer
University of Colorado Hospital
Associate Dean for Clinical Affairs, Quality and Safety Education
Director
Institute for Healthcare Quality, Safety and Efficiency
Professor
Division of General Internal Medicine
University of Colorado School of Medicine
Aurora, Colorado [59]

Dragan Golijanin, MD
Associate Professor of Surgery
Director
Genitourinary Oncology
The Warren Alpert Medical School of Brown University
Providence, Rhode Island [180]

Lucas Golub, MD
Emory University School of Medicine
Atlanta, Georgia [8]

Steven M. Gorbatkin, MD, PhD
Associate Professor
Emory University School of Medicine
Nephrologist, Atlanta VA Medical Center
Decatur, Georgia [241]

Norman D. Grace, MD
Lecturer on Medicine
Harvard Medical School
Professor of Medicine
Tufts University School of Medicine
Staff Physician
Division of Gastroenterology, Hepatology, and Endoscopy
Department of Medicine
Brigham and Women's Hospital
Boston, Massachusetts [53, 160]

Yonatan H. Grad, MD, PhD
Assistant Professor
Harvard T. H. Chan School of Public Health
Division of Infectious Diseases
Brigham and Women's Hospital
Boston, Massachusetts [193]

Charles S. Greenberg, MD
Department of Medicine
Division of Hematology/Oncology
Medical University of South Carolina
Charleston, South Carolina [54]

Stephen B. Greenberg, MD, MACP
Distinguished Service Professor, Herman Brown Teaching
Professor
Baylor College of Medicine
Vice Chief of Staff, Chief of Medicine
Ben Taub Hospital
Houston, Texas [198]

Norton J. Greenberger, MD, MACP
Clinical Professor of Medicine
Harvard Medical School
Senior Physician
Brigham and Women's Hospital
Boston, Massachusetts [75]

Anne F. Gross, MD
Assistant Professor of Psychiatry
Associate Residency Training Director
Oregon Health & Science University
Portland, Oregon [229]

Angela S. Guarda, MD
Associate Professor of Psychiatry and Behavioral Sciences
Johns Hopkins School of Medicine
Director
Eating Disorders Program
The Johns Hopkins Hospital
Baltimore, Maryland [226]

Navin R. Gupta, MD
Department of Medicine
Renal Division
Brigham and Women's Hospital
Boston, Massachusetts [243]

Sarah P. Hammond, MD
Assistant Professor of Medicine
Harvard Medical School
Division of Infectious Diseases
Brigham and Women's Hospital
Boston, Massachusetts [204]

Caroline N. Harada, MD
Associate Professor of Medicine
Assistant Dean for Community-Engaged Scholarship
University of Alabama School of Medicine
Division of Gerontology, Geriatrics, and Palliative Care
Birmingham, Alabama [166]

Nikroo Hashemi, MD, MPH
Instructor of Medicine
Harvard Medical School
Brigham and Women's Hospital
Division of Gastroenterology and Hepatology
Boston, Massachusetts [109]

Joaquim M. Havens, MD
Assistant Professor of Surgery
Harvard Medical School
Division of Trauma, Burn, and Surgical Critical Care
Brigham and Women's Hospital
Boston, Massachusetts [45]

Meghan Hayes, MD, FACP
Department of Internal Medicine
Sutter Medical Group
Clinical Instructor
University of California
Davis Medical Center
Sacramento, California [218, 220]

Catherine P. M. Hayward, MD, PhD, FRCPC
Professor
Pathology and Molecular Medicine/Medicine McMaster University
Head, Coagulation
Hamilton Regional Laboratory Medicine Program
West Hamilton, Ontario, Canada [172]

Galen V. Henderson, MD
Director
Neurocritical Care and Neuroscience Intensive Care Unit
Brigham and Women's Hospital
Assistant Professor, Harvard Medical School
Boston, Massachusetts [209]

Kathie L. Hermayer, MD, MS, FACE, FACP
Professor of Medicine
Medical Director for Diabetes Management Services at MUSC
Division of Endocrinology, Diabetes, and Medical Genetics
Medical University of South Carolina
Chair, Diabetes Task Force
Ralph H. Johnson Veteran's Affairs Medical Center
Charleston, South Carolina [52]

Heather Herrington, MD
Associate Professor of Medicine
Division of Gerontology, Geriatrics, and Palliative Care
University of Alabama at Birmingham
Birmingham, Alabama [166]

Stacy Higgins, MD, FACP
Associate Professor of Medicine
Division of General Medicine and Geriatrics
Emory University School of Medicine
Atlanta, Georgia [12]

Keiki Hinami, MD, MS
Collaborative Research Unit
Cook County Health & Hospitals System
Chicago, Illinois [41]

Ashley B. Hink, MD, MPH
General Surgery Resident
Medical University of South Carolina
Department of General Surgery
Charleston, South Carolina [63]

Kerstin Hogg, MD, MBChB, MSc
Assistant Professor
Department of Medicine
McMaster University
East Hamilton, Ontario, Canada [253]

Fernando Holguin, MD, MPH
Associate Professor of Medicine and Pediatrics
Asthma Institute
Division of Pulmonary
Allergy and Critical Care Medicine
University of Pittsburgh
Pittsburgh, Pennsylvania [231]

Anthony N. Hollenberg, MD
Professor of Medicine
Harvard Medical School
Chief, Division of Endocrinology, Diabetes, and Metabolism
Beth Israel Deaconess Medical Center
Boston, Massachusetts [152]

Elizabeth H. Holt, MD, PhD
Associate Professor
Yale School of Medicine
Yale Endocrinology
Yale Endocrine Oncology Program
New Haven, Connecticut [240]

Michael H. Hoskins, MD
Assistant Professor
Clinical Cardiac Electrophysiology
Emory University Hospital
Atlanta, Georgia [133, 136]

Susy Hota, MD, MSc, FRCPC
Assistant Professor of Medicine
University of Toronto
Hospital Epidemiologist and Infectious Diseases Specialist
University Health Network
Toronto, Ontario, Canada [200]

Liangge Hsu, MD
Assistant Professor of Radiology
Division of Neuroradiology
Brigham and Women's Hospital
Harvard Medical School
Boston, Massachusetts [118]

Margo S. Hudson, MD
Assistant Professor of Medicine
Harvard Medical School
Diabetes Management Service
Brigham and Women's Hospital
Boston, Massachusetts [150]

Jeff C. Huffman, MD
Associate Professor of Psychiatry
Harvard Medical School
Medical Director
Inpatient Psychiatry
Massachusetts General Hospital
Boston, Massachusetts [229]

John T. Huggins, MD
Associate Professor of Medicine
Division of Pulmonary and Critical Care
Medical University of South Carolina
Charleston, South Carolina [236]

Daniel P. Hunt, MD
Professor of Medicine
Director
Emory Division of Hospital Medicine
Department of Medicine
Emory University School of Medicine
Atlanta, Georgia [78]

William R. Hunt, MD
Assistant Professor of Medicine
Division of Pulmonary, Allergy, Critical Care, and Sleep Medicine
Department of Medicine
Emory-Children's Center for Cystic Fibrosis
McKelvey Lung Transplant Center
Emory University School of Medicine
Atlanta, Georgia [234]

Aubrey Ingraham, MD
Department of Internal Medicine
Kaiser Permanente
Oakland, California [39]

Bertrand L. Jaber, MD, MS
Associate Professor of Medicine
Tufts University School of Medicine
Vice Chair for Clinical Affairs
Department of Medicine
Caritas St. Elizabeth's Medical Center
Boston, Massachusetts [243]

Claire S. Jacobs, MD, PhD
Department of Neurology
Brigham and Women's Hospital
Boston, Massachusetts [211]

Francine L. Jacobson, MD, MPH
Thoracic Radiologist at Brigham and Women's Hospital
Assistant Professor
Department of Radiology
Harvard Medical School
Boston, Massachusetts [107, 112-119]

Shilpa H. Jain, MD
Clinical Assistant Professor (Affiliated)
Division of Endocrinology, Gerontology, and Metabolism
Stanford University School of Medicine
Veterans Affairs Palo Alto Health Care System
Palo Alto, California [154]

Kunal Jajoo, MD
Assistant Professor
Harvard Medical School
Associate Physician
Brigham and Women's Hospital
Boston, Massachusetts [158]

Edward C. Jauch, MD, MS
Professor
Director
Division of Emergency Medicine
Professor, Department of Neurosciences
Vice Chair, Research, Department of Medicine
Professor, Department of Bioengineering (Adjunct)
Clemson University
Medical University of South Carolina
Charleston, South Carolina [100]

Brent Jewett, MD
Clinical Instructor of Surgery
Department of Surgery
Medical University of South Carolina
Charleston, South Carolina [46]

Danielle Jones, MD, FACP
Associate Professor of Medicine
Division of General Medicine and Geriatrics
Emory University School of Medicine
Atlanta, Georgia [93]

J. Ryan Jordan, MD
Cardiovascular Disease and Clinical Cardiac Electrophysiology
South Denver Cardiology Associates, PC
Littleton, Colorado [135]

S. Andrew Josephson, MD
Vice President
Neurohospitalist Society
Carmen Castro-Franceschi and Gladyne K. Mitchell Distinguished
Neurohospitalist Professorship
Vice Chairman, Parnassus Programs Director, Neurohospitalist
Program
Department of Neurology
University of California, San Francisco
San Francisco, California [104]

Brian W. Kaebnick, MD
Structural Cardiology Fellow
Department of Cardiology
Emory University Hospital
Atlanta, Georgia [131]

Stephen P. Kalhorn, MD
Assistant Professor Neurosurgery
Medical University of South Carolina
Charleston, South Carolina [64]

Jameela Kari, MD
Pediatric Nephrology Unit
Department of Pediatrics
King Abdulaziz University
Jeddah, Kingdom of Saudi Arabia [239]

Laurence Katznelson, MD
Associate Dean of Graduate Medical Education
Professor of Neurosurgery and Medicine (Endocrinology and
Metabolism)
Medical Director
Pituitary Center
Stanford University School of Medicine
Stanford, California [154]

Clive Kearon, MB, MRCPI, FRCPC, PhD
Jack Hirsh Professorship in Thromboembolism
Department of Medicine
McMaster University
Juravinski Hospital
Hamilton, Ontario, Canada [253]

Robert T. Keenan, MD, MPH
Assistant Professor of Medicine
Director
Duke Gout and Crystal Arthropathy Clinic
Duke University School of Medicine
Durham, North Carolina [247]

Corey D. Kershaw, MD
Associate Professor of Medicine
Division of Pulmonary & Critical Care Medicine
University of Texas Southwestern Medical Center
Medical Director, MICU
William P. Clements Jr. University Hospital
Dallas, Texas [142]

Adeel M. Khan, MD, MPH
Taussig Cancer Institute
Cleveland Clinic Foundation
Cleveland, Ohio [181]

Claude Killu, MD
Intensive Care
Los Angeles Medical Center
Los Angeles, California [125]

Emmanuel S. King, MD, FHM, FACP
Associate Professor of Clinical Medicine
Perelman School of Medicine
University of Pennsylvania
Director of Clinical Operations
Section of Hospital Medicine
Division of General Internal Medicine
Hospital of the University of Pennsylvania
Philadelphia, Pennsylvania [21]

Joyce E. King, MD
Assistant Professor
Georgetown University School of Medicine
Washington, DC
Clinical Instructor
University of Maryland Medical School
Director Inpatient Medicine
Family Medicine Residency
Medstar Franklin Square Medical Center
Baltimore, Maryland [228]

Emad Kishi, MD
Assistant Professor of Surgery
Division of Abdominal Transplant
Department of Surgery
Medical University of South Carolina
Charleston, South Carolina [66]

Joshua P. Klein, MD, PhD
Associate Professor of Neurology and Radiology
Harvard Medical School
Chief, Division of Hospital Neurology
Department of Neurology
Brigham and Women's Hospital
Boston, Massachusetts [106]

Michael Klompas, MD, MPH
Associate Professor
Department of Population Medicine
Harvard Medical School
Division of Infectious Diseases
Brigham and Women's Hospital
Boston, Massachusetts [187]

Christopher Knudson, MD
Instructor of Medicine
Division of Hospital Medicine
Emory University School of Medicine
Atlanta, Georgia [90]

Serena Koenig, MD, MPH
Assistant Professor
Harvard Medical School
Division of Global Health Equity
Division of Infectious Diseases
Brigham and Women's Hospital
Boston, Massachusetts [205]

Sophia Koo, MD
Assistant Professor of Medicine
Harvard Medical School
Division of Infectious Diseases
Brigham and Women's Hospital
Boston, Massachusetts [201]

Makeida B. Koyi, MD
Deputy Director of Adult Inpatient Consultation Service
Clinical Instructor
Community Psychiatry Program
Department of Psychiatry and Behavioral Sciences
Johns Hopkins Bayview Medical Center
Baltimore, Maryland [81]

Svetlana Krasnokutsky, MD, MS
Assistant Professor of Medicine
Co-Director
NYU Crystal Diseases Study Group
New York University School of Medicine
New York, New York [247]

Harold Kudler, MD
Adjunct Associate Professor
Department of Psychiatry and Behavioral Sciences
Duke University Medical Center
Durham, North Carolina [224]

Carlos E. Kummerfeldt, MD
Staff Pulmonologist
TJ Samson Community Hospital
Glasgow, Kentucky [236]

Mark S. Lachs, MD, MPH
Irene and Roy Psaty Distinguished Professor of Medicine
Co-Chief of Geriatrics and Palliative Medicine
Weill Cornell Medicine
Director of Geriatrics
New York Presbyterian Health System
New York, New York [167]

Victoria D. Lackey, MD
Duke University School of Medicine
Division of Rheumatology and Immunology
Duke University Medical Center
Durham, North Carolina [249]

Joshua R. Lakin, MD
Harvard Medical School
Dana-Farber Cancer Institute
Boston, Massachusetts [105]

Albert Q. Lam, MD
Associate Physician
Division of Renal Medicine
Brigham and Women's Hospital
Harvard Medical School
Boston, Massachusetts [61]

Lindy H. Landzaat, DO, FAAHPM
Assistant Professor
Division of Palliative Medicine
University of Kansas Medical Center
Kansas City, Kansas [217]

Vijay H. Lapsia, MD, MBBS
Assistant Professor of Medicine
Mount Sinai School of Medicine
New York, New York [238]

Lucia Larson, MD, FACP
Associate Professor of Medicine
Director
Division of Obstetric Medicine
Women's Medicine Collaborative
The Alpert Medical School of Brown University
Providence, Rhode Island [218]

Jodi Layton, MD
Assistant Professor of Medicine
The Warren Alpert Medical School of Brown University
Hematology and Oncology
Rhode Island Hospital Comprehensive Cancer Center
Providence, Rhode Island [180]

Brian Leber, MDCM, FRCPC
Professor of Medicine
McMaster University
Attending Physician
Hamilton Health Sciences/Juravinski Hospital and Cancer Centre
Hamilton, Ontario, Canada [170]

Noah Lechtzin, MD, MHS, FCCP
Assistant Professor
Director
Johns Hopkins Adult Cystic Fibrosis Program
Pulmonary Director
Johns Hopkins Amyotrophic Lateral Sclerosis Clinic
Pulmonary and Critical Care Medicine
Johns Hopkins University
Baltimore, Maryland [95]

CONTRIBUTORS

Ji Yeon Lee, MD
Pulmonary/Critical Care Fellow
Emory University School of Medicine
Division of Pulmonary, Allergy, Critical Care & Sleep Medicine
Atlanta, Georgia [235]

Linda A. Lee, MD
Clinical Director
Division of Gastroenterology and Hepatology
Johns Hopkins University School of Medicine
Director of Endoscopy
Johns Hopkins Hospital
Director
Johns Hopkins Integrative Medicine & Digestive Center
Lutherville, Maryland [80]

Linda S. Lee, MD
Assistant Professor of Medicine
Harvard Medical School
Director
Endoscopic Education and Women's Health in GI
Co-Director
Pancreas Center
Brigham and Women's Hospital
Boston, Massachusetts [161]

Blair J. N. Leonard, MD, PhD, FRCP
Senior Hematology Fellow
McMaster University
Hamilton, Ontario, Canada [170]

William I. Levin, MD
Associate Professor of Medicine
Division of General Internal Medicine
University of Pittsburgh School of Medicine
Pittsburgh, Pennsylvania [60]

Katherine Lewis, MD, MSCR
Assistant Professor of Medicine and Pediatrics
The Medical University of South Carolina
Charleston, South Carolina [52]

Cindy Lien, MD
Assistant Professor of Medicine
Harvard Medical School
Palliative Care Physician
Internal Medicine Hospitalist
Beth Israel Deaconess Medical Center
Boston, Massachusetts [216]

Elaine Chiewlin Liew, MD, FRCA
Assistant Professor of Anesthesiology
Department of Anesthesiology and Perioperative Medicine
David Geffen School of Medicine
University of California, Los Angeles (UCLA)
Ronald Reagan UCLA Medical Center
Los Angeles, California [153]

David J. Likosky, MD, SFHM, FAHA, FACP
President
Neurohospitalist Society
Medical Director
EvergreenHealth Neuroscience Institute
Clinical Assistant Professor
University of Washington
EvergreenHealth
Kirkland, Washington [104]

Ming Y. Lim, MB BChir
Department of Medicine
Division of Hematology/Oncology
Medical University of South Carolina
Charleston, South Carolina [54]

Walter Limehouse, MD, MA, FACEP
Associate Professor of Emergency Medicine
Medical University of South Carolina
Charleston, South Carolina [33]

Lori-Ann Linkins, MD, MSc (Clin Epi), FRCPC
Associate Professor
Department of Medicine
Division of Hematology & Thromboembolism
McMaster University
Juravinski Thromboembolism Service
MF1 Director/MF1 Hematology Subunit Planner
Michael G. DeGroote School of Medicine
Thrombosis & Atherosclerosis Research Institute
Hamilton, Ontario, Canada [253]

Rafael H. Llinas, MD
Associate Professor of Medicine
Associate Professor of Neurology
Chairman of Neurology
Johns Hopkins Bayview Medical Center
Baltimore, Maryland [89]

Hermioni N. Lokko, MD, MPP
Clinical Fellow of Psychiatry
Harvard Medical School
Administrative Chief Resident
Massachusetts General Hospital
Boston, Massachusetts [229]

Lenny López, MD, MPH, MDiv
Associate Professor of Medicine
Chief of Hospital Medicine
San Francisco VA Medical Center
University of California
San Francisco, California [3]

David J. Lucier, Jr., MD, MBA, MPH
Instructor of Medicine
Harvard Medical School
Director of Quality and Patient Safety
Hospital Medicine Group
Assistant in Medicine
Division of General Internal Medicine
Massachusetts General Hospital
Boston, Massachusetts [15]

Courtney H. Lyder, ND, ScD(Hon), FAAN
Professor of Nursing, Geriatric Medicine, and Public Health
Dean Emeritus
School of Nursing
University of California
Los Angeles, California [72]

William L. Lyons, MD
Professor
Division of Geriatrics and Gerontology
Department of Internal Medicine
University of Nebraska Medical Center
Omaha, Nebraska [165]

Elizabeth H. Mack, MD, MS
Pediatric Critical Care
Medical University of South Carolina
Charleston, South Carolina [19]

James H. Maguire, MD, MPH
Professor of Medicine
Harvard Medical School
Senior Physician
Division of Infectious Diseases
Brigham and Women's Hospital
Boston, Massachusetts [205]

Rahul Maheshwari, MD
Gastroenterology Fellow
Division of Digestive Diseases
Emory University School of Medicine
Atlanta, Georgia [159]

Scott Manaker, MD, PhD
Associate Professor of Medicine, Pulmonary, Allergy, and Critical Care Division
Vice Chair for Regulatory Affairs
Department of Medicine
Perelman School of Medicine, University of Pennsylvania
Philadelphia, Pennsylvania [27]

Efrén Manjarrez, MD, SFHM
Chief, Division of Hospital Medicine
Associate Professor of Clinical Medicine
Miller School of Medicine
University of Miami
Miami, Florida [37]

Kimberly D. Manning, MD, FACP, FAAP
Associate Professor of Medicine
Director
Distinction in Teaching and Leadership
J. Willis Hurst Internal Medicine Residency Program
Department of Medicine
Division of General Medicine and Geriatrics
Emory University School of Medicine
Atlanta, Georgia [5]

Michael Manogue, MD
Fellow in Cardiovascular Disease
Emory University School of Medicine
Atlanta, Georgia [133, 135]

Gary Margolias, MD
Assistant Professor of Anesthesiology
Emory University School of Medicine
Atlanta, Georgia [139]

Merry Jennifer Markham, MD
Associate Professor of Medicine
Division of Hematology and Oncology
Department of Medicine
University of Florida College of Medicine
Gainesville, Florida [175]

Alayne D. Markland, DO, MSc
Associate Professor of Medicine
Division of Gerontology, Geriatrics, and Palliative Care
University of Alabama at Birmingham
Birmingham, Alabama [71]

Greg S. Martin, MD, MSc, FACP, FCCP, FCCM
Professor and Associate Division Director for Critical Care
Division of Pulmonary, Allergy, and Critical Care
Emory University School of Medicine
Director of Research
Emory Critical Care Center
Section Chief, Grady Memorial Hospital
Atlanta, Georgia [142]

R. Kirk Mathews, MBA
Partner, Schmidt
Mathews LLC
Providing Executive Search and Leadership
Development Services [24]

Melissa Mattison, MD, SFHM, FACP
Assistant Professor of Medicine
Harvard Medical School
Chief, Hospital Medicine Unit
Massachusetts General Hospital
Boston, Massachusetts [168]

Saverio M. Maviglia, MD, MSc
Assistant Professor of Medicine
Harvard Medical School
Hospitalist Service
Brigham and Women's Hospital
Boston, Massachusetts [22]

Laura K. Max, BA
Clinical Research Assistant
Johns Hopkins School of Medicine
Anesthesiology and Critical Care Medicine
Johns Hopkins Hospital
Baltimore, Maryland [81]

Matthew W. McCarthy, MD
Assistant Professor of Medicine
Weill Cornell Medicine
Assistant Attending Physician
NewYork-Presbyterian Hospital
New York, New York [33]

Michael McDaniel, MD, FSCAI
Assistant Professor of Medicine
Emory University School of Medicine
Director
Cardiac Catheterization Lab
Grady Health Systems
Atlanta, Georgia [128]

Timothy B. McDonald, MD, JD
Professor, Anesthesiology and Pediatrics
Chief Safety and Risk Officer for Health Affairs
University of Illinois
Chicago, Illinois [20]

Andrew McFarlane, MLT, ART, FCSMLS(D)
Technical Specialist
Molecular Hematology and Red Cell Disorders
Lecturer McMaster University
Department of Medicine
McMaster University Medical Centre
Hamilton, Ontario, Canada [169]

John W. McGillicuddy, MD, FACS
Associate Professor of Surgery
Medical University of South Carolina
Charleston, South Carolina [66]

Gerard Michael McGorisk, MD, FACC, MRCPI
Assistant Professor of Medicine
Emory University
Atlanta, Georgia [132]

Sylvia C. McKean, MD, SFHM, FACP
Deputy Editor for Editorial Projects, UpToDate
Boston, Massachusetts [107, 112, 116, 123, 124, e4]

Graham T. McMahon, MD, MMSc
Adjunct Professor
Northwestern University
Feinberg School of Medicine
President and Chief Executive Officer
Accreditation Council for Continuing Medical Education
Chicago, Illinois [150]

Julia McNabb-Baltar, MD
Instructor of Medicine
Harvard Medical School
Center for Pancreatic Disease
Division of Gastroenterology, Hepatology, and Endoscopy
Department of Medicine
Brigham and Women's Hospital
Boston, Massachusetts [157]

Thomas E. McNalley, MD
Associate Professor
University of Washington School of Medicine
Department of Rehabilitation Medicine
Seattle Children's Hospital
University of Washington Medical Center
Seattle, Washington [69]

Jakob I. McSparron, MD
Instructor in Medicine
Harvard Medical School
Division of Pulmonary, Critical Care, and Sleep Medicine
Beth Israel Deaconess Medical Center
Boston, Massachusetts [85]

Niharika D. Mehta, MD
Assistant Professor of Medicine
The Warren Alpert Medical School of Brown University
Director of Ambulatory services
Division of Obstetric and Consultative Medicine
Women and Infants Hospital of Rhode Island
Providence, Rhode Island [221]

Karina Meijer, MD, PhD
Division of Haemostasis and Thrombosis
Department of Haematology
University Medical Centre Groningen
Groningen, The Netherlands [173]

David Meltzer, MD, PhD
Fanny L. Pritzker Professor of Medicine
Economics and Public Policy Chief
Section of Hospital Medicine
Director, Center for Health and The Social Science
The University of Chicago
Chicago, Illinois [e2]

Peter A. Merkel, MD, MPH
Chief, Division of Rheumatology
Professor of Medicine and Epidemiology
University of Pennsylvania
Philadelphia, Pennsylvania [257]

Joseph J. Miaskiewicz, Jr., MD, FCCP, SFHM
Assistant Clinical Professor
Tufts Medical School
Chief of Utilization Review and Clinical Documentation
Hospitalist
North Shore Medical Center
Salem, Massachusetts [110, 122]

Chad S. Miller, MD, FACP, FHM
Associate Professor
Division Director
General Internal Medicine
Saint Louis University School of Medicine
St. Louis, Missouri [92, 94]

Tracey A. Milligan, MD, MS, FAAN
Assistant Professor of Medicine
Harvard Medical School
Vice Chair for Education
Department of Neurology
Brigham and Women's Hospital
Boston, Massachusetts [211]

Elinor Mody, MD
Division of Rheumatology
Brigham and Women's Hospital
Boston, Massachusetts [127]

Daniel L. Molloy, Jr., MD
Division of Cardiology
Emory University
Atlanta, Georgia [130]

Paul A. Monach, MD, PhD
Chief, Rheumatology Section
VA Boston Healthcare System
Associate Professor
Section of Rheumatology
Boston University School of Medicine
Boston, Massachusetts [257]

Carmen Monzon, MD
Clinical Assistant Professor of Psychiatry and Human Behavior
The Warren Alpert Medical School of Brown University
Women's Behavioral Medicine, Women's Medicine Collaborative
Miriam Hospital
Providence, Rhode Island [221]

Luis Fernando Mora, MD
The Arrhythmia Center of South Florida
Delray Beach, Florida [134]

CoLette Morgan, MD, FHM, CCDS, CDIP
Assistant Professor
Division of Hospital Medicine
Department of Medicine
Emory University School of Medicine
Atlanta, Georgia [32]

Christopher Moriates, MD
Assistant Clinical Professor
Division of Hospital Medicine
University of California at San Francisco
Director of Caring Wisely Program
UCSF Center for Healthcare Value
San Francisco, California
Director of Implementation Initiatives
Costs of Care, Inc.
Boston, Massachusetts [2]

Ala Moshiri, MD, PhD
Assistant Professor of Ophthalmology
Eye Center
University of California, Davis
Sacramento, California [83]

John E. Moss, MD
Assistant Professor of Medicine
Department of Critical Care Medicine
Mayo Clinic Florida
Jacksonville, Florida [137]

Srinivasan Mukundan, MD, PhD
Associate Professor of Radiology
Brigham and Women's Hospital
Boston, Massachusetts [113]

L. Silvia Munoz-Price, MD, PhD
Associate Professor of Clinical Medicine
Institute for Health and Society
Medical College of Wisconsin
Enterprise Epidemiologist
Froedtert Health System
Milwaukee, Wisconsin [185]

Mandakolathur R. Murali, MD
Director of Clinical Immunology Laboratory
Massachusetts General Hospital
Harvard Medical School
Boston, Massachusetts [230]

Ernest Murray, MD
Hospital Medicine Section
General Internal Medicine and Geriatrics
Medical University of South Carolina
Charleston, South Carolina [250]

Daniel M. Musher, MD
Distinguished Service Professor of Medicine
Professor of Molecular Virology and Microbiology
Chief Emeritus, Infectious Disease Section
Michael E. DeBakey VA Medical Center
Houston, Texas [186]

Jennifer S. Myers, MD, FACP, FHM
Associate Professor of Clinical Medicine
Department of Medicine
Division of General Internal Medicine
Section of Hospital Medicine
Perelman School of Medicine
University of Pennsylvania
Philadelphia, Pennsylvania [21]

Satish N. Nadig, MD, PhD, FACS
Assistant Professor
Surgery, Microbiology, and Immunology
Medical University of South Carolina
Transplant Surgery
Charleston, South Carolina [66]

Amulya Nagarur, MD
Instructor in Medicine
Harvard Medical School
Hospital Medicine Group
Massachusetts General Hospital
Boston, Massachusetts [38]

Peter Najjar, MD
Resident
Department of Surgery
Brigham and Women's Hospital
Harvard Medical School
Boston, Massachusetts [44]

Dale M. Needham, MD, PhD, FCPA
Professor
Division of Pulmonary & Critical Care Medicine
Department of Physical Medicine & Rehabilitation
School of Medicine, Johns Hopkins University
Baltimore, Maryland [81]

John Nelson, MD, MHM
Overlake Medical Center
Nelson Flores Hospital Medicine Consultants
Bellevue, Washington [24]

Karin J. Neufeld, MD, MPH
Clinical Director of Psychiatry
Johns Hopkins Bayview Medical Center
Associate Professor
Johns Hopkins University School of Medicine
Department of Psychiatry and Behavioral Sciences
Baltimore, Maryland [81]

Tobenna Nwizu, MD
Taussig Cancer Institute
Cleveland Clinic Foundation
Cleveland, Ohio [181]

Christopher D. Ochoa, MD
Fellow
Pulmonary and Critical Care Medicine
Emory University School of Medicine
Atlanta, Georgia [232]

Victor M. Orellana, MD
Department of Medicine
Rhode Island Hospital
Providence, Rhode Island [174]

Karin Ouchida, MD
Assistant Professor of Medicine
Weill Cornell Medical College
New York Presbyterian Hospital
New York, New York [167]

Thomas A. Owens, MD
Vice President for Medical Affairs
Chief Medical Officer
Duke University Health System
Associate Professor of Medicine and Pediatrics
Duke University School of Medicine
Durham, North Carolina [189]

David A. Oxman, MD, FACP
Assistant Professor of Medicine
Sidney Kimmel Medical College
Medical Intensive Care Unit
Thomas Jefferson University Hospital
Philadelphia, Pennsylvania [206]

Menaka Pai, MD, MSc, FRCPC
Associate Professor
Department of Medicine
Associate Member, Department of Pathology and Molecular
Medicine
McMaster University
Transfusion Medicine Quality Lead and Consultant Laboratory
Hematologist
Hamilton Regional Laboratory Medicine Program
Hamilton, Ontario, Canada [56, 252]

Sumanta K. Pal, MD
Assistant Professor and Co-Director
Kidney Cancer Program
Department of Medical Oncology & Experimental Therapeutics
City of Hope Comprehensive Cancer Center
Duarte, California [179]

Robert M. Palmer, MD
Director
Glennan Center for Geriatrics and Gerontology
Eastern Virginia Medical School
Norfolk, Virginia [87]

Anand K. Pandurangi, MD, MBBS, DABPN
Professor of Psychiatry and Adjunct Professor of Radiology
Vice Chair, Department of Psychiatry and Chair, Division of
Inpatient Psychiatry
Virginia Commonwealth University (VCU)
Medical Director
Inpatient Psychiatry
VCU Health System
Richmond, Virginia [225]

Jonathan B. Parr, MD, MPH
University of North Carolina School of Medicine
Division of Infectious Disease
Chapel Hill, North Carolina [203]

Jennifer C. Passini, MD
Clinical Assistant Professor
Hospital Medicine
University of Wisconsin Department of Medicine
Madison, Wisconsin [153]

Nicholas J. Pastis, MD
Assistant Professor of Medicine
Division of Pulmonary and Critical Care
Medical University of South Carolina
Charleston, South Carolina [236]

Vihas Patel, MD
Instructor
Department of Surgery
Director
Metabolic Support Service
Brigham and Women's Hospital
Division of Trauma, Burn, and Surgical Critical Care
Harvard Medical School
Boston, Massachusetts [42]

Timothy J. Patton, DO
Assistant Professor of Dermatology
University of Pittsburgh
Pittsburgh, Pennsylvania [144]

Jill M. Paulson, MD
Assistant Professor of Endocrinology
George Washington University School of Medicine.
George Washington Medical Faculty Associates
Washington, DC [152]

Allan B. Peetz, MD
Instructor
Department of Surgery
Brigham and Women's Hospital
Division of Trauma, Burn, and Surgical Critical Care
Harvard Medical School
Boston, Massachusetts [42-45]

Vincent D. Pellegrini, Jr., MD
John A. Siegling Professor and Chair
Department of Orthopedics
Medical University of South Carolina
Charleston, South Carolina [65]

Jason Persoff, MD, SFHM
University of Colorado School of Medicine
Hospital Medicine Group
Aurora, Colorado [137]

Brent G. Petty, MD
The Johns Hopkins Hospital
Baltimore, Maryland [9]

Kurt Pfeifer, MD, FACP, FHM
Professor of Medicine
General Internal Medicine
Medical College of Wisconsin
Milwaukee, Wisconsin [51]

Tania J. Phillips, MD
Professor of Dermatology
Boston University School of Medicine
Boston, Massachusetts [148]

Edward F. Pilkington, III, MD
Instructor of Medicine
Hospitalist Service
Brigham and Women's Hospital
Boston, Massachusetts [189]

Michael H. Pillinger, MD
Professor of Medicine and Biochemistry and Molecular
Pharmacology
Co-Director
NYU Crystal Diseases Study Group
New York University School of Medicine
Rheumatology Section Chief
VA New York Harbor Health Care System, New York Campus
New York, New York [247]

J. Richard Pittman, Jr., MD, FACP
Assistant Professor of Medicine
Division of General Medicine and Geriatrics
Department of Medicine
Emory University School of Medicine
Atlanta, Georgia [11, 101]

Carol Pohlig, RN, BSN, CPC
Senior Coding and Education Specialist
Office of Clinical Documentation
Department of Medicine
Hospital of the University of Pennsylvania
Philadelphia, Pennsylvania [27]

Timothy J. Poterucha, MD
Resident Physician and Clinical Fellow
Harvard Medical School
Department of Medicine
Brigham and Women's Hospital
Boston, Massachusetts [108]

Raymond O. Powrie, MD, FRCP, FACP
Professor of Obstetrics, Gynecology, and Medicine
Alpert School of Medicine of Brown University
Chief Medical Quality Officer
Care New England
SVP for Population Health
Chief of Medicine
Women & Infants Hospital of Rhode Island
Providence, Rhode Island [219]

Michaella Maloney Prasad, MD
Assistant Professor of Urology and Pediatrics
Medical University of South Carolina
Charleston, South Carolina [67]

Alicia Privette, MD
Assistant Professor of Surgery
Medical University of South Carolina
Department of Surgery
Charleston, South Carolina [46]

Alberto Puig, MD, PhD, FACP
Associate Professor of Medicine
Harvard Medical School
Director
Clinician Educator Service
Massachusetts General Hospital
Boston, Massachusetts [38]

Rana C. Pullatt, MD, MS, MRCS, FACS, FASMBS
Diplomate in Obesity Medicine
Associate Professor of Surgery
Director Robotic Surgery
Director Bariatric Surgery VISN-7
Medical University of South Carolina
Charleston, South Carolina [63]

Amir A. Qamar, MD
Assistant Professor of Medicine
Tufts University School of Medicine
Boston, Massachusetts Senior Staff Hepatologist
Lahey Hospital and Medical Center
Burlington, Massachusetts [53]

Susan Y. Quan, MD [97]
Clinical Assistant Professor (Affiliated)
Stanford University School of Medicine
Division of Gastroenterology and Hepatology
Veterans Affairs Palo Alto Healthcare System
Palo Alto, California

Timothy R. Quinn, MD, CM
Medical Director of Dermatopathology
Dermpath Diagnostics New England
Marlborough, Massachusetts [146]

Talat H. Raja, MD
Instructor
Hospital Medicine
Division of General Internal Medicine and Geriatrics
Medical University of South Carolina
Charleston, South Carolina [82]

Graham W. Redgrave, MD
Assistant Professor of Psychiatry and Behavioral Sciences
Director for Residency Education
Johns Hopkins School of Medicine
Assistant Director
Eating Disorders Program
The Johns Hopkins Hospital
Baltimore, Maryland [226]

John J. Reilly, Jr., MD
Vice Chancellor for Health Affairs
Dean for School of Medicine
University of Colorado School of Medicine
Aurora, Colorado [60]

Kerry Reynolds, MD
Instructor in Medicine
Harvard Medical School
Attending Physician
Massachusetts General Hospital Cancer Center
Boston, Massachusetts [177, 183]

Joseph Rhatigan, MD
Associate Professor of Medicine
Harvard Medical School
Division of Global Health Equity
Brigham and Women's Hospital
Boston, Massachusetts [e1]

Jessica Rimsans, PharmD, BCPS
Senior Clinical Pharmacist
Hemostatic and Antithrombotic Stewardship Pharmacist
Brigham and Women's Hospital
Boston, Massachusetts [254]

Tina Rizack, MD, MPH
Assistant Professor of Medicine and Obstetrics and Gynecology
The Warren Alpert Medical School of Brown University
Hematology/Oncology
Program in Women's Oncology
Women & Infants Hospital
Providence, Rhode Island [176]

Malcolm K. Robinson, MD
Assistant Professor of Surgery
Harvard Medical School
Director
Nutrition Support Service
Brigham and Women's Hospital
Boston, Massachusetts [58]

Katina Robison, MD
Assistant Professor of Obstetrics and Gynecology
Program in Women's Oncology
Department of Obstetrics and Gynecology, Women &
Infants' Hospital of Rhode Island
The Warren Alpert Medical School of Brown University
Providence, Rhode Island [178]

Thomas P. Rocco, MD
Associate Chief of Cardiology
VA Boston Healthcare System
West Roxbury, Massachusetts
Associate Professor of Medicine
Harvard Medical School
Boston, Massachusetts [108]

Clare Rock, MD, MS, MRCPI
Department of Medicine
Division of Infectious Diseases
Johns Hopkins University
Baltimore, Maryland [195]

Sarahi Rodríguez-Pérez, MD
Director of Clinical Operations
Assistant Professor of Clinical Medicine
Miller School of Medicine
Division of Hospital Medicine
University of Miami Hospital
Miami, Florida [37]

Vinayak S. Rohan, MD
Department of Surgery
Medical University of South Carolina
Charleston, South Carolina [66]

Karen L. Roos, MD
John and Nancy Nelson Professor of Neurology
Professor of Neurological Surgery
Indiana University School of Medicine
Indianapolis, Indiana [192]

Alexander E. Ropper, MD
Assistant Professor
Department of Neurosurgery
Baylor College of Medicine
Houston, Texas [208]

Allan H. Ropper, MD, FRCP
Professor of Neurology
Harvard Medical School
Executive Vice Chair of Neurology
Brigham and Women's Hospital
Boston, Massachusetts [208, 212]

Bradley T. Rosen, MD, MBA, FHM
Medical Director
ISP Hospitalist Service
Medical Director
Supportive Care Medicine (Palliative Care)
Director
Care Transitions and Complex Medical Management
Associate Professor, Cedars-Sinai Medical Center
Associate Professor, UCLA School of Medicine
Cedars-Sinai Health System
Los Angeles, California [120]

Karen Rosene-Montella, MD, FACP
Senior Vice President
Vice Chair of Medicine for Quality/Outcomes
Division Chief Obstetric Medicine
Professor of Medicine and Obstetrics and Gynecology
The Warren Alpert Medical School at Brown University
Providence, Rhode Island [219, 221, 222]

John J. Ross, MD, CM, FIDSA
Assistant Professor of Medicine
Harvard Medical School
Hospitalist Service
Brigham and Women's Hospital
Boston, Massachusetts [197, 201, 212]

Stephen R. Rotman, MD
Gastroenterology Fellow
Brigham and Women's Hospital
Boston, Massachusetts [156]

Joseph Rudolph, MD
Department of Neurology
Cleveland Clinic
Cleveland, Ohio [210]

Matthew L. Russell, MD, MSc
Medical Director
Rehabilitation Service Units
Hebrew Rehabilitation Center
Hebrew Senior Life
Boston, Massachusetts [73]

Daniel F. Ruthven, MD
Clinical Associate of Psychiatry and Behavioral Sciences
Johns Hopkins University School of Medicine
Baltimore, Maryland [226]

Arturo P. Saavedra, MD, PhD
Assistant Professor
Harvard Medical School
Medical Director
Medical Dermatology
Massachusetts General Hospital
Boston, Massachusetts [145]

Michel J. Sabbagh, MD
Assistant Professor
Anesthesia and Perioperative Medicine
Medical University of South Carolina
Charleston, South Carolina [62]

Cheryl A. Sadow, MD
Assistant Professor of Radiology
Harvard Medical School
Division of Abdominal Imaging and Intervention
Brigham and Women's Hospital
Boston, Massachusetts [117]

Bisan A. Salhi, MD, MA
Assistant Professor of Emergency Medicine
Emory University
Department of Emergency Medicine
Atlanta, Georgia [121]

John R. Saltzman, MD, FACP, FACG, FASGE, AGAF
Associate Professor of Medicine
Harvard Medical School
Director of Endoscopy
Brigham and Women's Hospital
Boston, Massachusetts [156, 162]

Kenneth Sands, MD, MPH
Associate Professor of Medicine
Harvard Medical School
Senior Vice President, Health Care Quality
Beth Israel Deaconess Medical Center
Boston, Massachusetts [16]

Milda Saunders, MD, MPH
Assistant Professor
Section of Hospital Medicine and MacLean Center for Clinical
Medical Ethics
Department of Medicine
University of Chicago
Chicago, Illinois [e3]

Marianne E. Savastano, MS, CCC-SLP
Speech/Language Pathology Practice Leader
Stroke and Spinal Cord Injury Programs
Spaulding Rehabilitation Hospital
Boston, Massachusetts [70]

Paul E. Sax, MD
Professor of Medicine
Harvard Medical School
Brigham and Women's Hospital
Division of Infectious Diseases
Boston, Massachusetts [203]

Adam C. Schaffer, MD
Instructor in Medicine
Harvard Medical School
Hospital Medicine Unit
Brigham and Women's Hospital
Boston, Massachusetts [35, 111]

Danielle B. Scheurer, MD, MSCR, SFHM
Chief Quality Officer and Hospitalist
Associate Professor of Medicine
Medical University of South Carolina
Charleston, South Carolina [82, 190]

Lynn Schlanger, MD
Associate Professor
Emory University School of Medicine
Atlanta, Georgia [241]

Robert K. Schneider, MD, FACP
Associate Professor
Departments of Psychiatry, Internal Medicine, and Family Medicine
Virginia Commonwealth University
Director of Mental Health and Primary Care Integration
McGuire VA Medical Center
Richmond, Virginia [227]

Jeffrey L. Schnipper, MD, MPH, FHM
Associate Professor of Medicine
Harvard Medical School
Director of Clinical Research, Hospitalist Service
Brigham and Women's Hospital
Boston, Massachusetts [40, 151]

Robert W. Schrier, MD, MACP
Professor Emeritus of Medicine
University of Colorado School of Medicine
Division of Renal Diseases and Hypertension
University of Colorado Hospital
Aurora, Colorado [242]

Allison R. Schulman, MD
Gastroenterology Fellow
Brigham and Women's Hospital
Boston, Massachusetts [158]

David A. Schulman, MD, MPH, FCCP
Associate Professor of Medicine
Division of Pulmonary, Allergy Critical Care, and Sleep Medicine
Emory University School of Medicine
Atlanta, Georgia [235]

Sam Schulman, MD, PhD
Thrombosis Service, McMaster Clinic
Hamilton Health Sciences-General Hospital
Hamilton, Ontario, Canada [173]

Richard M. Schwartzstein, MD
Gordon Professor of Medicine and Medical Education
Harvard Medical School
Associate Chief, Division of Pulmonary, Critical Care, and
Sleep Medicine
Beth Israel Deaconess Medical Center
Boston, Massachusetts [85]

Julian L. Seifter, MD
Harvard Medical School
Senior Nephrologist and the James Haidas Family Master Clinician
Brigham and Women's Hospital
Boston, Massachusetts [61]

Samir K. Shah, MD
Division of Vascular Surgery
Brigham and Women's Hospital
Boston, Massachusetts [256]

Daniel S. Shapiro, MD
Professor of Internal Medicine
University of Nevada School of Medicine
Reno, Nevada [e5]

Ann M. Sheehy, MD, MS
Associate Professor and Division Head, Hospital Medicine
Department of Medicine
University of Wisconsin
Madison, Wisconsin [153]

Eugenie Shieh, MD
Clinical Fellow
Johns Hopkins Medicine
Division of Gastroenterology
Baltimore, Maryland [80]

Deborah M. Siegal, MD, MSc, FRCPC
Division of Hematology and Thromboembolism
Department of Medicine
McMaster University
Hamilton, Ontario, Canada [77]

Eric M. Siegal, MD, SFHM
Clinical Associate Professor of Medicine (Adjunct)
University of Wisconsin School of Medicine and Public Health
Medical Director
Aurora Critical Care Service
Aurora St Luke's Medical Center
Milwaukee, Wisconsin [138]

Mark Siegler, MD
Lindy Bergman Distinguished Service Professor
Professor, Departments of Medicine and Surgery
Director
MacLean Center for Clinical Medical Ethics
University of Chicago Medical Center
Chicago, Illinois [e3]

Ross D. Silverman, JD, MPH
Professor of Health Policy and Management
Indiana University Richard M. Fairbanks School of Public Health
Professor of Public Health and Law
Indiana University Robert H. McKinney School of Law
Indianapolis, Indiana [34]

Christian T. Sinclair, MD, FAAHPM
Assistant Professor
Division of Palliative Medicine
University of Kansas Medical Center
Kansas City, Kansas [217]

Ajay K. Singh, MBBS, MBA, FRCP
Renal Division
Brigham and Women's Hospital
Boston, Massachusetts [239]

Anika T. Singh
Renal Division
Brigham and Women's Hospital
Boston, Massachusetts [239]

Mousumi Sircar, MD
Geriatrics Fellow
Harvard Medical School
Department of Gerontology
Beth Israel Deaconess Medical Center
Boston, Massachusetts [73]

Gerald W. Smetana, MD, FACP
Professor of Medicine
Harvard Medical School
Division of General Medicine and Primary Care
Beth Israel Deaconess Medical Center
Boston, Massachusetts [51]

Dustin T. Smith, MD
Emory University School of Medicine
Atlanta, Georgia [8, 10]

Robert L. Smith, MD
Associate Professor
Division of Pulmonary and Critical Care
New York University School of Medicine
Harbor VA Medical Center
New York, New York [141]

Scot T. Smith, MD
Chief Medical Officer
Sound Physicians
Denver, Colorado [25]

Diana L. Snow, MA, CCS, CPC, CHC
Director of Revenue Integrity & Quality
University of Utah Healthcare
University of Utah School of Medicine
Salt Lake City, Utah [31]

David R. Snydman, MD, FACP, FIDSA
Professor
Tufts University School of Medicine
Chief, Division of Geographic Medicine and Infectious Diseases
Hospital Epidemiologist
Tufts Medical Center
Boston, Massachusetts [191]

Society of Hospital Medicine Key Characteristics Workgroup [24]
Members of the Society of Hospital Medicine Key Characteristics Workgroup are Patrick Cawley, MD, Steven Deitelzweig, MD, Leslie Flores, MHA, Joseph Miller, MS, John Nelson, MD, Scott Rissmiller, MD, Laurence Wellikson, MD, and Winthrop Whitcomb, MD

Aaron Sodickson, MD, PhD
Associate Professor of Radiology
Harvard Medical School
Section Chief of Emergency Radiology
Medical Director of CT
Brigham and Women's Hospital
Boston, Massachusetts [113]

Lauge Sokol-Hessner, MD
Instructor in Medicine
Harvard Medical School
Associate Director of Inpatient Quality
Attending Hospitalist
Beth Israel Deaconess Medical Center
Boston, Massachusetts [16]

Margarita Sotelo, MD
Associate Clinical Professor
Divisions of Geriatrics and Hospital Medicine
San Francisco General Hospital
San Francisco, California [165]

Geoffrey L. Southmayd, MD
Instructor of Medicine
Emory University School of Medicine
Chief Medical Resident, Emory University Hospital
J. Willis Hurst Internal Medicine Residency Program
Atlanta, Georgia [102]

Nathan Spell, MD
Associate Professor of Medicine
Emory University School of Medicine
Chief Quality Officer
Emory University Hospital
Atlanta, Georgia [17]

Kelly Cunningham Sponsler, MD, SFHM
Assistant Professor of Medicine
Section of Hospital Medicine
Vanderbilt University Medical Center
Nashville, Tennessee [14]

Jerry E. Squires, MD, PhD
Department of Pathology and Laboratory Medicine
Medical University of South Carolina
Charleston, South Carolina [57]

Christopher J. Standaert, MD
Clinical Associate Professor
Rehabilitation Medicine, Neurological Surgery, and Orthopedics
and Sports Medicine
University of Washington School of Medicine
University of Washington Medicine Sports and Spine Physicians
Clinic
Harborview Medical Center
Seattle, Washington [69]

Gerald W. Staton, MD
Professor of Medicine
Division of Pulmonary and
Critical Care Medicine
Department of Medicine
Emory University School of Medicine
Atlanta, Georgia [232]

Arlene Stecenko, MD
Associate Professor of Pediatrics and Medicine
Chief, Division of Pulmonary, Allergy and Immunology,
Cystic Fibrosis and Sleep
Department of Pediatrics
Director
Emory-Children's Center for Cystic Fibrosis
Associate Director
Emory-Children's Center for Cystic Fibrosis and Airways
Disease Research
Emory University School of Medicine
Atlanta, Georgia [234]

Daniel I. Steinberg, MD
Mount Sinai Beth Israel
New York, New York [7]

Michael Sterling, MD
Assistant Professor of Medicine
Division of Pulmonary, Allergy and Critical Care Medicine
Emory University School of Medicine
Atlanta, Georgia [139]

Theodore A. Stern, MD
Ned H. Cassem Professor of Psychiatry in the field of
Psychosomatic Medicine/Consultation
Harvard Medical School
Chief, Avery D. Weisman Psychiatry Consultation Service
Massachusetts General Hospital
Director
Office for Clinical Careers
Massachusetts General Hospital
Boston, Massachusetts [229]

Melissa B. Stevens, MD
Assistant Professor of Medicine
Division of Hospital Medicine
Emory University School of Medicine
Atlanta, Georgia
Atlanta VA Medical Center
Decatur, Georgia [12]

Ashley Stuckey, MD
Assistant Professor of Obstetrics and Gynecology
Program in Women's Oncology
The Warren Alpert Medical School of Brown University
Department of Obstetrics and Gynecology
Women & Infants' Hospital of Rhode Island
Providence, Rhode Island [178]

Prem S. Subramanian, MD, PhD
Professor of Ophthalmology, Neurology, and Neurosurgery
Vice Chair for Academic Affairs, Department of Ophthalmology
University of Colorado School of Medicine
Aurora, Colorado [83]

Ram M. Subramanian, MD
Associate Professor of Medicine and Surgery
Hepatology and Critical Care
Emory University School of Medicine
Atlanta, Georgia [159]

Katelyn W. Sylvester, PharmD, BCPS, CACP
Pharmacy Manager
Clinical Pharmacy Specialist
Brigham and Women's Hospital
Boston, Massachusetts [254]

Jeffrey A. Tabas, MD
Professor of Emergency Medicine
Director of Outcomes and Innovations
Office of Continuing Medical Education
University of California
San Francisco School of Medicine
San Francisco, California [36]

Jennifer K. Tan, MD
Associate Physician
Northstar Dermatology
Fort Worth, Texas [149]

Todd A. Taylor, MD
Assistant Professor of Emergency Medicine
Emory University
Atlanta, Georgia [121]

Tracy J. Tipton, MD
Urology Resident
Medical University of South Carolina
Charleston, South Carolina [67]

Catherine Dawson Tobin, MD
Assistant Professor
Anesthesia and Perioperative Medicine
Medical University of South Carolina
Charleston, South Carolina [62]

Derrick J. Todd, MD, PhD
Instructor in Medicine
Harvard Medical School
Division of Rheumatology
Brigham and Women's Hospital
Boston, Massachusetts [246]

David Tong, MD, MPH
Assistant Professor of Hospital Medicine
Department of Medicine
Emory University School of Medicine
Atlanta, Georgia [234]

Anne C. Travis, MD, MSc
Department of Medicine
Division of Gastroenterology, Hepatology and Endoscopy
Brigham and Women's Hospital
Boston, Massachusetts [162]

Glenn J. Treisman, MD, PhD
Eugene Meyer, III Professor of Psychiatry and Medicine
Departments of Psychiatry and Behavioral Sciences and
Internal Medicine
Johns Hopkins University School of Medicine
Baltimore, Maryland [228]

Elly Trepman, MD
Department of Medical Microbiology
University of Manitoba
Winnipeg, Manitoba, Canada [147]

Geoffrey Tsaras, MB, ChB, MPH
Clinical Assistant Professor of Medicine
University of Illinois College of Medicine at Rockford
Rockford, Illinois [194]

Jeffrey Turner, MD
Assistant Professor of Medicine
Section of Nephrology
Yale University School of Medicine
New Haven, Connecticut [245]

Amit Uppal, MD
Assistant Program Director
Director of MICU
Bellevue Hospital
Division of Pulmonary, Critical Care, and Sleep Medicine
New York University Medical Center
New York, New York [140]

W. Alexander Vandergrift, III, MD
Associate Professor Neurosurgery
Medical University of South Carolina
Charleston, South Carolina [64]

Joseph Varon, MD, FACP, FCCP, FCCM, FRSM
Chief of Critical Care Services
University General Hospital
Professor
Department of Acute and Continuing Care
University of Texas Health Science Center at Houston
Clinical Professor of Medicine
University of Texas Medical Branch at Galveston
Professor of Medicine and Surgery UDEM, UNE, UABC, UAT,
Anahuac, UACH, USON, UPAEP – Mexico [91]

Alvaro Velasquez, MD
Assistant Professor of Medicine
Division of Critical Care and Respiratory Medicine
Emory University School of Medicine
Atlanta, Georgia [90]

Nicole F. Velez, MD
Westmoreland Dermatology Associates
University of Pittsburgh Medical Center East
Pittsburgh, Pennsylvania [145]

Madeleine Verhovsek, MD, FRCPC
Assistant Professor
Division of Hematology and Thromboembolism
McMaster University
Consultant Laboratory Hematologist, Red Cell Disorders Laboratory,
Hamilton Regional
Laboratory Medicine Program
Hamilton, Ontario, Canada [77, 169]

Donald C. Vinh, MD, FRCPC, FACP
Assistant Professor
Faculty of Medicine
McGill University
Division of Infectious Diseases, Department of Medicine
McGill University Health Centre
Montreal, Quebec, Canada [202]

Kittane S. Vishnupriya, MBBS
Assistant Professor of Medicine
Johns Hopkins University School of Medicine
Baltimore, Maryland [79]

Ruth Ann Vleugels, MD, MPH
Associate Professor of Medicine
Harvard Medical School
Director
Autoimmune Skin Disease Program
Department of Dermatology
Brigham and Women's Hospital
Boston, Massachusetts [149]

Megan Ann Waldrop, MD
Pediatric Neurology Fellow
University of California, Irvine
Children's Hospital of Orange County
Orange, California [213]

Ruth H. Walker, MB, ChB, PhD
Departments of Neurology
James J. Peters Veterans Affairs Medical Center, Bronx, NY
Mount Sinai School of Medicine
New York, New York [210]

Leon Walthall, MD
Hospital Medicine Section
General Internal Medicine and Geriatrics
Medical University of South Carolina
Charleston, South Carolina [250]

David A. Walton, MD, MPH
Division of Global Health
Brigham and Women's Hospital
Boston, Massachusetts [e1]

John Scott Walton, MD
Associate Professor
Anesthesia and Perioperative Medicine
Medical University of South Carolina
Charleston, South Carolina [62]

Annabel Kim Wang, MD
Associate Professor (Neurology)
University of California, Irvine
Orange, California
Staff Neurologist
VA Long Beach Healthcare System
Long Beach, California [213]

Sally Wang, MD
Instructor
Harvard Medical School
Hospitalist
Brigham and Women's Hospital
Boston, Massachusetts [126]

Martha C. Ward, MD
Assistant Professor
Department of Psychiatry and Behavioral Sciences
Department of Medicine
Society Advisor, Osler Society
Assistant Course Director
Essentials of Patient Care Course
Emory University School of Medicine
Atlanta, Georgia [223]

Theodore E. Warkentin, MD, FRCP(C), FACP, FRCP(Edin)
Professor
Department of Pathology and Molecular Medicine and Department of Medicine Michael G. DeGroote School of Medicine
McMaster University
Transfusion Medicine, Hamilton Regional Laboratory Medicine Program
Service of Clinical Hematology,
Hamilton General Hospital
Hamilton, Ontario, Canada [171]

Kathryn Webert, MD, MSc, FRCPC
Associate Professor
Department of Pathology and Molecular Medicine
McMaster University
Medical Director, Utilization
Canadian Blood Services
Hamilton, Ontario, Canada [172]

Steven Weinberger, MD, FACP
Executive Vice President and CEO
American College of Physicians
Adjunct Professor of Medicine
University of Pennsylvania
Philadelphia, Pennsylvania
Senior Lecturer on Medicine
Harvard Medical School
Boston, Massachusetts [6]

Saul N. Weingart, MD, PhD
Chief Medical Officer and Senior VP Medical Affairs
Tufts Medical Center
Professor of Medicine
Tufts University School of Medicine
Boston, Massachusetts [15]

Stacy Westerman, MD, MPH
Fellow, Cardiovascular Disease
Department of Medicine, Division of Cardiology
Emory University School of Medicine
Atlanta, Georgia [133]

Tosha B. Wetterneck, MD, MS
Department of Medicine
School of Medicine and Public Health
Center for Quality and Productivity Improvement
University of Wisconsin Madison
Madison, Wisconsin [41]

Omar Wever-Pinzon, MD
Assistant Professor of Medicine
University of Utah School of Medicine
Department of Medicine, Cardiology Division,
Heart Failure Section
University of Utah Health Science Center
Salt Lake City, Utah [129]

Christopher M. Whinney, MD, FACP, FHM
Clinical Assistant Professor of Medicine
Cleveland Clinic Lerner College of Medicine
Chairman, Department of Hospital Medicine
Cleveland Clinic
Cleveland, Ohio [4]

I. David Wiener, MD
Professor of Medicine and Physiology and Functional Genomics
University of Florida College of Medicine
Chief, Nephrology and Hypertension Section
Gainesville VA Medical Center
Gainesville, Florida [238]

Jeffrey G. Wiese, MD, FACP, FSM, SFHM
Professor of Medicine
Tulane University
Associate Chairman, Department of Medicine
Senior Associate Dean for Graduate Medical Education
Director
Tulane Internal Medicine Program
Tulane University Health Sciences Center
New Orleans, Louisiana [92, 94]

B. Robinson Williams, III, MD
Assistant Professor of Medicine
Program Director
Cardiovascular Disease Fellowship
Emory University School of Medicine
Atlanta, Georgia [135]

Neil H. Winawer, MD, SFHM
Professor of Medicine
Emory University School of Medicine
Director
Hospital Medicine Unit
Grady Memorial Hospital
Atlanta, Georgia [230]

Eric S. Winer, MD
Division of Hematology/Oncology
Rhode Island Hospital
Providence, Rhode Island [174]

Kristin R. Wise, MD, FHM
Assistant Professor of Medicine
Hospital Medicine Section, General Internal Medicine and Geriatrics
Medical University of South Carolina
Charleston, South Carolina [250]

Karl D. Wittnebel, MD, MPH
Medical Director
Pre-Operative Pain Program
Department of Medicine
Cedars-Sinai Medical Center
Hospitalist
Division of General Internal Medicine
Cedars-Sinai Medical Center
Los Angeles, California [120]

Brian D. Wolfe, MD
Assistant Professor of Medicine
Hospital Medicine Section
University of Colorado Denver
University of Colorado Hospital
Aurora, Colorado [59]

Kenneth E. Wood, DO, FCCP
Chief Medical Officer
Geisinger Medical Center
Director
Center for Systems Re-engineering in Healthcare, Geisinger
Health System
Clinical Professor of Medicine
Temple University School of Medicine
Geisinger Medical Center
Danville, Pennsylvania [153]

Rollin Wright, MD
Division of Geriatric Medicine and Gerontology
University of Pittsburgh
Pittsburgh, Pennsylvania [87]

Irene M. Yeh, MD, MPH
Division of Adult Palliative Care
Dana-Farber Cancer Institute
Brigham and Women's Hospital
Harvard Medical School
Boston, Massachusetts [214]

Brian K. Yorkgitis, DO
Assistant Professor
Department of Surgery
University of Florida College of Medicine-Jacksonville
Jacksonville, Florida [43]

Bishoy Zakhary, MD
Pulmonary and Critical Care Fellow
Department of Pulmonary, Critical Care, and Sleep Medicine
New York University Medical Center
New York, New York [140]

Shanta M. Zimmer, MD
Associate Professor of Medicine
University of Pittsburgh
Director
Internal Medicine Residency Training Program
University of Pittsburgh Medical Center
Pittsburgh, Pennsylvania [88]

Camilla Zimmermann, MD, PhD, FRCPC
Head, Palliative Care Program
University Health Network
Director of Research
Lederman Palliative Care Centre
Princess Margaret Hospital
Associate Professor of Medicine
University of Toronto
Toronto, Ontario, Canada [215]

SECTION REVIEWERS

Joanna M. Bonsall, MD, PhD
Assistant Professor of Medicine
Division of Hospital Medicine
Emory University School of Medicine
Atlanta, Georgia
Part I, Section 3

Yvette M. Cua, MD
Associate Professor of Medicine
Department of Medicine
Associate Vice Chair for Clinical Affairs
Department of Medicine
University of Louisville
Louisville, Kentucky
Part I, Section 6

Jatin K. Dave, MD, MPH
Part-Time Instructor
Harvard Medical School
Division of Aging, Brigham and Women's Hospital
Boston, Massachusetts
Medical Director
Geriatrics and Senior Care Options
Tufts Health Plan
Watertown, Massachusetts
Part III

Steven B. Deitelzweig, MD, MMM, SFHM, FACP
Ochsner Health System
Medical Director of Regional Business Development
System Chairman, Hospital Medicine
Associate Professor of Medicine-Ochsner Clinical School
Part I, Section 5

Don S. Dizon, MD, FACP
Associate Professor of Medicine
Harvard Medical School
Clinical Co-Director, Gynecologic Oncology
Director
The Oncology Sexual Health Clinic
Massachusetts General Hospital Cancer Center
Boston, Massachusetts
Part VI, Section 7

Francine L. Jacobson, MD, MPH
Thoracic Radiologist at Brigham and Women's Hospital
Assistant Professor
Department of Radiology
Harvard Medical School
Boston, Massachusetts
Part V, Section 2

Tina Rizack, MD, MPH
Assistant Professor of Medicine and Obstetrics and Gynecology
The Warren Alpert Medical School of Brown University
Hematology/Oncology
Program in Women's Oncology
Women & Infants Hospital
Providence, Rhode Island
Part VI, Section 7

Karen Rosene-Montella, MD, FACP
Senior Vice President
Women's Services and Clinical Integration, Lifespan
Vice Chair of Medicine for Quality/Outcomes
Division Chief Obstetric Medicine
Professor of Medicine and Obstetrics and Gynecology
The Warren Alpert Medical School at Brown University
Providence, Rhode Island
Part VI, Section 12

Dustin T. Smith, MD
Emory University School of Medicine
Atlanta, Georgia
Part I, Section 2

FOREWORD

I well remember reading the landmark article by Wachter and Goldman entitled "The emerging role of 'hospitalists' in the American health care system," published in the *New England Journal of Medicine* in 1996.[1] In this article, the authors recognized the need for "a new breed of physicians … specialists in inpatient medicine" and coined the term "hospitalist" to refer to this new type of physician specialist. Since then, the specialty of hospital medicine has become an increasingly popular and successful career pathway, and has expanded beyond its roots in internal medicine to other disciplines, such as pediatrics, family practice, and obstetrics. The Society of Hospital Medicine estimated there were approximately 44,000 hospitalists in the United States in 2014, and predicted that number will continue to grow.[2]

When hospital medicine started, the expertise of hospitalists was focused on the clinical issues surrounding care of the hospitalized patient. More recently, there has been increasing emphasis on the hospitalist's role in designing and improving the systems of care in the hospital. These added responsibilities have necessitated an expansion of the hospitalist's skills set beyond just a clinical knowledge base to an understanding of such topics as teamwork, transitions of care, quality metrics and improvement, and patient safety, among many others. A consequence of this proliferation of specific competencies has been the creation of an optional pathway for internal medicine hospitalists to maintain their certification with the American Board of Internal Medicine, officially referred to as Focused Practice in Hospital Medicine.

In the first edition of *Principles and Practice of Hospital Medicine*, McKean and her co-editors took on the herculean task of assembling an outstanding group of contributing authors and putting together a superb, comprehensive textbook of hospital medicine that was published in 2012. In this second edition, the editors have not only updated content but have also added a number of important topics in both clinical and nonclinical areas, ranging from value-based medicine to transplant surgery consultation. The section on billing, coding, and clinical documentation has been greatly expanded, as has coverage of a wide host of malignancies. Because of the importance of the recovery period and transitions to a variety of settings after hospital discharge, a welcome new section on rehabilitation and skilled nursing care has also been added.

The editors and authors are to be congratulated on again having made a major contribution to the care of hospitalized patients and to those physicians, whether or not they formally identify themselves as hospitalists, who care for these patients. Given the breadth and the depth of this text, there are few questions that clinicians will not be able to answer or guidance that they will not be able to obtain about how to provide the best care for the wide spectrum of their hospitalized patients.

Steven E. Weinberger, MD, MACP, FRCP
Executive Vice President and Chief Executive Officer
American College of Physicians
Adjunct Professor of Medicine
Perelman School of Medicine at the University of Pennsylvania
Senior Lecturer on Medicine
Harvard Medical School

REFERENCES

1. Wachter RM, Goldman L. The emerging role of "hospitalists" in the American health care system. *N Engl J Med.* 1996;335:514-517.

2. Bureau of Labor Statistics. http://www.bls.gov/careeroutlook/2015/youre-a-what/hospitalist.htm. Accessed April 12, 2016.

PREFACE

Since its initial publication in 2012, *Principles and Practice of Hospital Medicine* has become established as a leading resource for the specialty of hospital medicine. More than 200 renowned generalists and specialists contributed to make this book comprehensive and authoritative, but as practical as possible. Clinical chapters presented questions that commonly arise in the course of practice and emphasized core concepts with well-illustrated subject matter, radiology, clinical images and quick-view decision trees. The scope of content defined most of the field of hospital medicine as it existed in 2012, and the format of the text itself was enhanced both with an online edition available through the widely used AccessMedicine.com, and an app version for use on iPad.

Since the publication of the first edition, the field of hospital medicine has continued to evolve into areas beyond evidence-based general medical care into the practice of co-management of surgical and medical subspecialties, rehabilitation medicine, and palliative care. Driven by quality improvement efforts, as well as reimbursement models such as bundled payments, the last few years have seen an increased emphasis on coordination of care between acute care hospitals and other settings, including skilled nursing facilities, rehabilitation facilities, and long-term acute care facilities. The rapid growth of the field has been accompanied by an emerging cadre of outstanding clinicians and leaders, both at the local, national, and international level, and this book is the product of their collective efforts.

The second edition of *Principles and Practice of Hospital Medicine* provides tools to address the unique set of challenges hospitalists face in a healthcare system that ought to be safer and more effective. It comprehensively covers topics not included in any other print or online textbook. For example, this edition has new sections and chapters on the value and values of hospital medicine; practical, specialty information relating to what consulting hospitalists need to know as they co-manage patients from other services; key information in rehabilitation and skilled nursing care pertinent to patient safety and quality; expanded content on the approach to the patient at the bedside and clinical conditions in the inpatient setting. Using the basic format of the first edition, all content has been updated to incorporate new medical knowledge relevant to the practice of hospital medicine.

The second edition has six major parts, covering issues of importance to hospitalists everywhere:

Part I: The Specialty of Hospital Medicine and Systems of Care. The authors of this section represent some of the most knowledgeable and forward-thinking people in the areas of value based medicine, critical decision making at the point of care, transitions of care, patient safety and quality improvement, practice management, ethics and professional development. This part emphasizes the multidisciplinary approach, teamwork, prevention of hospital-acquired complications, and patient-centered communication to ensure safe and efficient care transitions and handoffs.

Part II: Medical Consultation. This part explains the traditional role of the medical consultant and updates preoperative cardiac and pulmonary risk assessment and risk reduction. Chapters that reflect the evolving role of hospitalists in co-management of surgical patients include general principles of surgery and anesthesia, perioperative pain management, and management of common complications in noncardiac surgery. The surgical specialties section concentrates on what the consulting hospitalist needs to know when consulting on patients undergoing bariatric surgery, neurosurgery, orthopedic surgery, transplant surgery and urologic procedures. All chapters focus on problems commonly encountered in the hospital setting, such as assessment and management of the diabetic patient, risk assessment and risk reduction for patients with end-stage liver disease, and preoperative assessment of patients with hematologic disorders.

Part III: Rehabilitation and Skilled Nursing Care. This new part, written primarily by experts in rehabilitation medicine, provides key information that hospitalists need to consider as they work to ensure safe transitions from the inpatient setting to extended care facilities. Individual chapters address rehabilitation options, physical and occupation therapy, common issues such as bowel and bladder incontinence, dysphagia, pressure ulcers, care of surgical wounds and pressure ulcers. The chapter on patient safety and quality improvement emphasizes core concepts embraced by hospitalists—the multidisciplinary approach, prevention of complications, and patient-centered communication in the transition of patients to and from the post-acute setting. The chapter on hospice focuses on common issues that clinicians need to address as they shift toward palliative care and consider the best setting for their patients.

Part IV: Approach to the Patient at the Bedside. These chapters provide detailed guidance for the initial inpatient evaluation, diagnostic testing, and management of patients with common presenting complaints that may be encountered at the time of admission or in the middle of the night. Each disorder is addressed from the perspective of hospital care, which in many cases differs significantly from initial outpatient care for the same complaint. Even experienced clinicians will find value in reviewing an initial, sometimes algorithmic, approach to common problems such as anemia, falls, delirium, dizziness and vertigo, insomnia, numbness, and weakness (how to localize the problem). Many of the chapters refer to subsequent chapters in Part VI, which covers the diagnosis and management of specific diagnoses.

Part V: Diagnostic Testing and Procedures. Efficiency of care, reduced cost, especially length of stay, coupled with high quality begins with clinical problem solving at the time of admission. This part explains how to interpret common admission tests, such as liver biochemical tests or arterial blood gas reports, and how to avoid wasteful, unnecessary medical tests and treatments. The radiology section reviews indications of radiology studies typically ordered in the hospital setting, a general approach to interpretation, patient safety issues in imaging and procedures performed by interventional radiologists. A comprehensive textbook in hospital medicine would not be complete without a section on procedures. The procedures' section provides some standardization of procedure performance, highlights indications, initial assessment, prevention of complications, and interpretation of results with links to video online resources that provide additional instruction, not possible in a text format. This section includes the core set of procedures most likely to be performed or supervised by hospitalists and acknowledges local and regional variations in the role of hospitalists performing or supervising these procedures.

Part VI: Clinical Conditions in the Inpatient Setting. Updated clinical content across the breadth of hospital medicine includes major disciplines in internal medicine such as cardiology, gastroenterology, and infectious diseases as well as sections with special relevance to hospital medicine, such as geriatrics, palliative care, psychiatry, toxicology, and addiction. In response to the evolving role of hospitalists on oncology inpatient services, the section covering hematology and oncology has been substantially expanded.

Electronic chapters (available on AccessMedicine.com) cover hospital medicine aspects of global health and hospital medicine, the core competencies of hospital medicine, the economics of health care, principles of medical ethics, and bioterrorism.

In summary, the second edition of *Principles and Practice of Hospital Medicine* takes into account how the field and practice of hospital medicine has evolved and the skills required of hospitalists so that they can provide exceptional patient care and clinical care leadership. We thank the American College of Physicians for its collaborative publishing arrangement with McGraw-Hill that included input into the editors, contributors, and overall scope for this new edition. Through its engagement in this book, the college advances it mission to enhance the quality and effectiveness of health care.

Sylvia C. McKean, MD, FACP, SFHM

ACKNOWLEDGMENTS

The editors of *Principles and Practice of Hospital Medicine* would like to acknowledge and thank our publisher McGraw-Hill, specifically, James Shanahan, publisher; Amanda Fielding, editor; Kim Davis, managing editor; Laura Libretti, administrative assistant; Richard Ruzycka, production manager; and the numerous people assisting them to complete this effort. We also express our gratitude to the many contributors who worked diligently to create a comprehensive resource for our readers and all the people who supported us, including family and friends. Finally, we wish to recognize physicians who took the time out of their busy schedules to review chapters and/or sections of the book that clearly benefited from their valuable expertise.

Sylvia C. McKean, MD, FACP, SFHM, FACP

John J. Ross, MD, CM, FIDSA

Daniel D. Dressler, MD, MSc, SFHM, FACP

Danielle B. Scheurer, MD, MSCR, SFHM

PART I

The Specialty of Hospital Medicine and Systems of Care

SECTION 1
The Value and Values of Hospital Medicine

CHAPTER 1

The Face of Health Care: Emerging Issues for Hospitalists

Patrick J. Cawley, MD, MHM

INTRODUCTION

Hospital medicine is entering its third decade since the term "hospitalist" was first created by Wachter and Goldman. There are now approximately 40,000 hospitalists and the number is likely to reach 50,000 in the next decade. The specialty has emerged from vigorous early debate about whether there was sufficient evidence to justify the role of hospitalists to a point where hospital medicine programs are hard-wired and indispensable in the majority of US hospitals. Early leaders and pioneers in hospital medicine were frequently two to three physician programs with heavy call burdens. Current hospital medicine groups, particularly in larger hospitals, average approximately 15 clinicians and have complicated alternating schedules with clear time off. Early hospitalists often served in hospital leadership roles with no dedicated time. They were often the only source of quality and safety leadership across the hospital. Today, hospitalists frequently have committed time to serve in quality and safety positions as well as other medical leadership roles. Most hospitals now have numerous staff that oversee various quality functions and ably assist these hospitalist leaders. While some aspects have greatly advanced for hospital medicine, two things have not changed:

- *Pressure to care for sick patients requiring hospitalization*—In many hospitals, the severity of illness across the patients cared for by hospitalists continues to rise. The number of patients covered by hospitalists grows in most hospitals and it is not unheard of for all medical inpatients to be cared for by hospitalists.
- *Juggling time between clinical care and hospital leadership*—While there are greater numbers of hospitalists and more hospital staff focused on quality and safety, the need for clinician leadership has never been more necessary. The vacuum caused by physicians no longer seeking hospital staff privileges as well as the overall urgent need for a new paradigm in health care to increase quality and decrease the cost of care has only resulted in greater need for hospitalists and physician leadership. Hospitalists are quickly expected to assume formal leader roles as well as clinical team leaders.

The need for inpatient care will not go away but how we care for the acutely ill may change. The demand for physician leadership does not diminish, but our focus on certain issues will vary. So what are the issues facing hospitalists in the next decade? Based on careful study of patients, families, hospitalists, hospitals, and health systems, we can predict the likely emerging issues.

"VALUE"

Similar to history, certain issues in health care predominate during a particular era because of timing related to unique discovery, emerging evidence, or simply greater knowledge by the masses of a problem. In the late 1990s, quality began its emergence as the principal concern in health care. This started in the 1980s with early studies examining inconsistency and errors as well as problems associated with overuse, misuse, and underuse of health care services. The Institute of Medicine released reports about the quality of health care in the United States in 1994, 1999, and 2001. Each of these had a slightly different focus, and over the next decade, improving quality became a common theme in health care. American hospitals, health systems, and clinicians responded, albeit slowly and deliberately, but by 2010, no area of medicine had failed to grasp the fundamentals of the quality movement and make changes for the better. During this same decade, another concept gained broad consensus—improved quality is usually less expensive. This first began as outcomes that were seen alongside quality improvement, but steadily it became clearer and today there is wide spread evidence that quality and cost are closely interconnected. The best quality is often the least expensive. As the linkage grew, the focus on value in clinical care emerged to a significant degree among the large numbers of leaders in health care. The value equation (value = quality/cost) in health care is certainly not new. One can go back decades and read numerous references in the health care literature. There have been many proposed versions of the value equation depending largely on how one defines quality. The early concept of value was mainly in reference to the health care system and the overall approach to strategically improving health care. Today, after almost two decades of quality improvement along with the more recently acceptance of cost containment as an independent quality measure, the concept of value is rapidly approaching majority acceptance by physicians and health care leaders. The next decade will see value broadly and deeply pushed into the health care system. Forward thinking hospitalists and hospital medicine groups will be ready for the emergence of value as an outcome by which they will be measured.

PRACTICE POINT

- Hospitalists, by virtue of their unique role in the health care system, will be expected to embrace the concept of value (value = quality/cost) and drive its use into everyday clinical practice. Quality is defined as safe, effective, efficient, equitable, patient centered, and timely care. Cost is defined as the unit cost of care delivery by the hospitalists. Each of these should be defined, measured, and incrementally improved by the hospital medicine team.

HIGH RELIABILITY

As quality and safety improvement has been embraced by health care, it has become abundantly clear that more radical transformation is necessary in order to accomplish a greater magnitude of error reduction and quality consistency. This need for transformation led health care to an examination of how other industries such as nuclear power and aviation have achieved a higher degree of reliability resulting in safety improvement and avoidance of potentially catastrophic events. Subsequent research revealed that successful organizations in high-risk industries achieve high reliability by maintaining a cultural mindfulness that allows them to continually reinvent themselves in the face of highly complex environments.

As high-reliability organizations (HRO) were studied, it became clear that there are common challenges across organizations pursuing high reliability:

- Hypercomplex environment
- Tight coupling teams where members depend on tasks performed across their team
- Extreme hierarchical differentiation
- Multiple decision makers in a complex communication network
- Need for frequent, immediate feedback
- Compressed time constraints

Many of these challenges exist in hospitals, and as a result the concept of high-reliability organizations in health care has been broadly embraced as potentially the transforming approach needed to vastly improve quality and safety.

As health care incorporates the methodology of HRO, it is important to study the work of Weick and Sutcliffe who have identified five organizing characteristics that need to guide the thinking of people in a high-reliable organization:

- *Preoccupation with failure*—Everyone in the organization is focused on errors and near-misses in order to learn from them and figure out how to prevent recurrence. Finding and fixing problems is everyone's responsibility. Leaders support and encourage this approach.
- *Reluctance to simplify interpretations*—Everyone in the organization is driven to ask why something happens and do not rely on the first or easiest explanation.
- *Sensitivity to operations*—Everyone in the organization is focused on ways their work processes might break down and are then encouraged to share potential failures and create best practices. Situational awareness is part of the organizational culture.
- *Commitment to resilience*—Everyone in the organization works quickly to contain errors that do occur in order to minimize potential harm. Additionally, errors do not disable the organization. The organization responds robustly and looks for new solutions to prevent catastrophes.
- *Deference to expertise*—Everyone in the organization listens to people who have the most developed knowledge of the task at hand and empowers them to make decisions in order to quickly mitigate harm. Sometimes, those individuals might not have the most seniority, but they are still encouraged to voice their concerns, ideas, and input—regardless of hierarchy.

These organizing processes are essential to the development of a highly reliable organization and all leaders and physicians in an organization attempting to achieve high reliability should understand the theory and application of each characteristic.

PRACTICE POINT

- Hospitalists are key to the development of an HRO because of their central role in hospital operations. Hospitals on the HRO journey will rely heavily on hospitalists to successfully navigate the process. Hospitalists should study the science of high reliability as it holds great promise to transform hospital medicine and health care in general.

PATIENT-CENTERED CARE/CONSUMERISM

The word "consumer" turns off many physicians, but the movement cannot be underestimated in how it is changing health care. The most strident opponents to the word frequently become some of the most vocal advocates for a more patient-centric approach when they become users of the health care system.

The history of patient-centered care can be directly traced to the civil and human rights activism in the 1960s. In 1978, Angelica Thieriot started the Planetree organization after a series of upsetting personal health care experiences. The organization "vowed to reclaim for patients the holistic, patient-centered focus that medicine had lost." Harvey Picker founded the Picker Institute in 1986 for similar reasons and then teamed up with the Commonwealth Fund to research a patient-centric approach. The term "patient centered" was coined and then later changed to "patient and family centered" by the Institute for Family Centered Care which was founded in 1992, subsequently becoming the Institute for Patient and Family Centered Care in 2010. Through the Picker/Commonwealth Fund research, we began to see differences in what patients noted as important versus physicians. Surveying patients about patient experience with the health care system started. This led to the Institute of Medicine emphasizing the concept of patient-centered care in its reports on quality care in the United States. Patient-centered care was defined as providing care that is respectful of and responsive to individual patient preferences, needs, and values and ensuring that patient values guide all clinical decisions.

In addition to patient-centered care, two additional notions are important to understand. Both are subsets of patient-centered care, which as an expression has come to mean a lot of different things, and it is important to differentiate.

Patient experience is the sum of all interactions, shaped by an organization's culture, that influence patient perceptions across a continuum of care. It is measured by patient surveys. For hospitalists, the most frequent measurement method is the HCAHPS (Hospital Consumer Assessment of Healthcare Providers and Systems) survey which is used for adult inpatients and measures patients perceptions about communication with nurses, communication about medicines, communication with doctors, pain management, cleanliness and quietness of the hospital environment, responsiveness of hospital staff, discharge information, and the overall rating of the hospital. Patient experience and satisfaction surveys are common to all hospitals and are important as a method of understanding the patient viewpoint. They are used as quality measure to be continuously improved, but they are only one element of patient-centered care and should be understood as that.

Patient engagement are actions taken by individuals to obtain the greatest benefit from the health care services available to them. Patient engagement occurs when patients feel empowered to move to a state of active participation and self-efficacy in managing their health. This does not mean just obeying directives from health care providers, but rather moving to a higher plain of involvement, interest, and self-awareness.

Why is patient engagement so important? Engaged patients have better health outcomes, incur less costs, and enjoy greatest value (quality/cost) from health care system. A patient can conceivably be satisfied with their health care experience while having minimal engagement.

In order to optimize patient engagement, there are key patient concepts to understand and incorporate into the health care experience such as literacy level, readiness to learn, readiness to change, learning style, and patient activation.

PRACTICE POINT

- Hospitalists should embrace the concepts of patient-centered care, patient satisfaction, and patient engagement. Each of these concepts overlaps, yet differs in meaningful ways and should be used in the right context.

TRANSITIONS OF CARE

Since the dawn of hospital medicine, there has been a focus on care transitions, which are the movement patients make between health care practitioners during the course of a chronic or acute illness. Early in the hospital medicine movement, this time period was often referred to as the "voltage drop." Because of the discontinuity introduced when a patient's outpatient physician is different than their inpatient physician, the importance of care transition in terms of patient quality and safety is paramount. One of the professional organizations of hospital medicine, the Society of Hospital Medicine, was an early adopter in promulgating the study of transitions and the determination of best practices by hospitalists and hospitals. Many potential models have been developed to improve hospital to home transitions including BOOST, Care Transition Intervention, Project Red, and the Naylor Model. Health care payers are developing financial incentives for hospitalists as well primary care physicians to focus on care transitions. The wider use of electronic health records (EHR) by physicians and hospitals holds great promise as a tactic to improve information transfer as patients move between providers. However, EHR issues such as how information is displayed as well as the lack of linkage between different EHR systems limit the effectiveness of EHRs in fully improving the knowledge "voltage drop."

In the last several years, the focus on thirty-day hospital readmission rates has become a significant driver of the emphasis on care transitions. This is largely driven by the Centers for Medicare and Medicaid penalties to hospitals with poor performance effective October 1, 2012. Readmission rates are seen as a potential outcome measure for poor care transitioning. There is increasing evidence that socioeconomic factors play a large role in determining readmission rates, so one should be care in completely linking readmission rates to poor transition efforts by hospitals and hospitalists. As the link to socioeconomic factors is further understood, this will likely require hospitals and health systems to work closely with community programs and governments to address these factors if more transformative improvement is to be made in readmission rates.

PRACTICE POINT

- Health care will remain fragmented, but the advent of electronic health records and formal transition of care programs offer potential for lessening the dangers to patients during this time. All hospitalists and hospital medicine groups should have an active transition of care program.

TELEHEALTH/TELEMEDICINE

Telehealth is a broad term used to refer to the process of providing health care services at a distance. It is increasingly performed via synchronous or asynchronous video connection. Telemedicine is a component of telehealth and refers to the delivery of clinical services to patients in other locations. Examples of telemedicine include video consultations with physicians, digital transmission of medical imaging, and remote monitoring of intensive care unit patients.

The delivery of clinical care via video is rapidly improving. Early issues such as network availability, capability, and delivery cost continue to progress on an annual basis. Open, secure software platforms are replacing closed proprietary systems. This brings in an era of ease of use as well as significant cost decrease. Patients are increasingly accepting telehealth visits. The growing use of smartphones and tablets by patients and families present a potential platform for the provision of enhanced communication and clinical care.

Regulators of the practice of medicine such as state boards of medicine have been slow to fully accept and grant unrestricted licensure, but public demands for telehealth are likely to pressure regulators to relax constraints. Similarly, 2015 was a landmark year for telemedicine in that over half of the states now require health plans to cover and reimburse for telemedicine in the same manner and at the same rate as in-person services. Telehealth parity in the remaining states or via federal mandate is only a matter of time.

Provider acceptance has been limited at first and mainly related to early adopters and innovators trialing new methods and systems. As telehealth visits have increased, the need for more dedicated provider time and systems to schedule, record, and follow-up visits has increased.

PRACTICE POINT

- Telehealth is rapidly growing and likely to impact the practice of hospital medicine over the next decade in many potential ways. Examples include the care of patients by hospitalists remotely, enhanced availability of specialists in many hospitals, and tele-critical care monitoring.

TRANSPARENCY

There are multiple major approaches to improving quality and safety in health including adherence to a quality improvement methodology, outcomes transparency or public reporting, financial incentives, regulation or accreditation, and competition. Outcomes transparency is the one which most physicians and organizations have the least expertise, but it is very high on the list of importance for patients and families. There is not a long history of transparency in health care and one of the earliest was the publication of hospital mortality rates and outliers by the Healthcare Financing Administration (HCFA) in the 1980s. This resulted in backlash from hospital executives who when surveyed overwhelmingly found the data of little use. Since then, there has been persistent and increasing outcomes transparency including severity adjusted mortality rates for coronary artery bypass grafts survey in New York and Pennsylvania in the late 1980s and early 1990s, and National Committee for Quality Assurance reporting in 1993 of managed care plans and Healthcare Effectiveness Data and Information Set (HEDIS) indicators. In 2002, the Joint Commission began reporting outcomes and the National Quality Foundation developed the serious reportable events classification. By the mid-2000, many companies such as HealthGrades and Consumer Report as well as multiple states were releasing a variety of health care outcome reports on a regular basis. Price transparency in health care also began to rise. In 2006, President Bush signed a Transparency Executive Order, which further opened avenues for pricing and quality transparency. In 2015, the Robert Wood Johnson Foundation held its second transparency summit with the following conclusions:

1. Transparency may not be ubiquitous, but it is now a permanent feature of the health care landscape.
2. For all the progress made in transparency, there is much more work to be done.
3. There is a paradox: The more transparency we have in health care, the more we expose how little we actually know or understand.

Health care transparency is part of a larger transparency trend due to the rise in global market economics and its resultant demand for data, an increase in communication technology which facilities transparency, and an "internet culture" which demands a more open interaction. Health care transparency is clearly growing and not a fad. The OpenNotes project, in which patients are able to see their doctors' visit notes, found that patients become more engaged with such access. This is likely to become routine in the near future. While transparency in health care is largely viewed positively, for patients to achieve optimal engagement from transparency will require better design principles into public reports.

PRACTICE POINT

- Hospitalist and hospital medicine group should prepare for greater transparency and expect probable full access by patients and families in the future to the medical record as well as quality and pricing data.
- We should not underestimate the patients and families ability to assimilate the information in public transparency reports!

GENOMICS/GENETICS

The past two decades has birthed a dizzying array of genomic technologies that ranges from rapid genome sequencing to the ability to evaluate genomes across large populations to the discovery of genetic basis of certain diseases as well drug responsiveness. The combination of these genomic technologies is resulting in new types of genetic testing which will increasingly result in clinical relevance. In addition, genetic tests are now directly marketing to the consumer who comes to the physician seeking additional knowledge.

The combination of genomic technologies and the electronic health record holds great promise for medical care to become more precise and individualized, however many record systems are often lacking core data to optimize this connection. To fully permeate these technologies into medical care, health care leaders and physicians must ensure that electronic health records are built to obtain appropriate information, such as demographics, medications, diagnosis, vital signs, and other information.

Pioneers of learning health care systems have established streamlined consenting processes and data warehouses. However, systems are not consistently incentivized to build these capacities. Health leaders want evidence before investing resources, yet without those investments such evidence is hard to gather.

PRACTICE POINT

- Hospitalists should prepare for the coming clinical relevance in genetic testing, particularly in the patient's individual potential response to drug therapy.
- Hospitalist leaders should work with their hospital information technology team to ensure that the hospital electronic health record is optimized to link genomic and patient information.

TEAMWORK TRANSFORMATION

The acceptance and rapid growth of hospitalists, based on personal observation, in many hospitals and health systems is tied to the team approach by early hospitalists. These hospitalists were available to hospital personnel to a great degree than nonhospitalists and this often resulted in close relationships and greater teamwork. Studies of nursing satisfaction showed higher results in hospitals with hospitalists. Today, many hospitalist leaders have typically been trained in the mechanics of teamwork and advocate for greater interaction and voice across the hospital medicine team.

The focus on value in the coming decade will force a reexamination of the hospital medicine team. The typical hospitalist is likely to assume the care of much greater numbers of patients on a daily basis and this will only be achieved through a transformation of the hospital medicine team. To alter the present system will require first and foremost a willingness of both hospitalists and hospital leaders to modify it. This is not an easy task as significant change management skills are required as well as a commitment to a higher level of team reliance, communication, and trust. There will need to be a diligent focus on patient satisfaction, each team member's satisfaction, and clinical outcomes. It can be achieved faster if there is payer flexibility in professional and hospital reimbursement.

PRACTICE POINT

- Hospitalists should continue to focus on teamwork and continue to advocate for an interprofessional multidisciplinary approach. Forward thinking hospitalists should trial the use of nonphysician providers, such as nurses, pharmacists, advanced practice providers, nutritionists, and others in innovative ways in order to achieve greater value to the patients.

HOSPITALIST/PHYSICIAN STRESS

The health care system is undergoing tremendous change and because of the central role in the health care system physicians will experience significant change. In addition, there are professional reimbursement challenges, increased scrutiny in terms of quality outcomes, cultural transparency, and increasing demands for physician time and presence. Incorporating new electronic health records into the daily work of physicians requires retraining and optimization. Medical knowledge and techniques advance requiring constant relearning. Administrative burdens related to reimbursement continue to rise. There are simply many pressure points on the individual physician. For hospitalists, who interact with patients and families at a very stressful time—acute illness requiring hospitalization, this can lead to tense and demanding interactions and communications. On the leadership side, there is pressure for hospitals to deliver greater value and all hospital leaders, including hospitalists, will experience great demands to develop and lead innovations. The list of stress points seems endless and overwhelming on the individual hospitalist.

However, the ability to positively impact patients and families has never been greater in the history of medicine. Hospitalists should recognize that despite the numerous stressors as well as ambiguity of the future, the ability to help patients and families is tremendously satisfying and professionally fulfilling.

Professional dissatisfaction and burnout is treatable if recognized and managed appropriately. There are personal and organizational approaches to prevent physician distress as well as optimize physical, emotional, and psychological wellness. Hospitalists and particularly hospital medicine leaders should fully understand the signs and symptoms of distress and have options for referral.

PRACTICE POINT

- All hospitalists should be aware of high burnout and professional dissatisfaction potential and understand the signs and symptoms in order to appropriately intervene to treat physician distress. Hospital medicine group leaders need to activity manage high physician stress levels and institute physician wellness programs.

LEADERSHIP

The need for hospital medicine leadership has never been greater. It was there at the dawn of hospital medicine and it will not wane in the coming years. The demand spans from clinical team leadership to program leadership to hospital and health system senior executive levels. If you have been a user of the health care system, you understand the need immediately. We can do great things in medicine, but it can be undone by some of the most trivial issues. To rectify this, particularly in the hospital setting, requires focus and leadership as well as the right emotional commitment by hospitalists. William Welch, the first dean of the Johns Hopkins School of Medicine, said it eloquently in his reference to a new approach to medical training—"*I can think of but one motive which might influence you to come here with us and that is …our ideals and our future…This will not appeal to the great mass of the public, not even to the medical public, for a considerable time. What we shall consider success, the mass of doctors will not consider a success.*"

As hospitalists, we should keep the patient in our focus at all times and continue to lead the transformation in quality and safety across health care.

PRACTICE POINT

- Hospitalists and hospital medicine groups should focus on ensuring high functioning leadership and leadership succession planning within the hospital medicine group at all times. Hospital medicine groups can enhance their effectiveness and should implement high-performance strategy.

SUGGESTED READINGS

Berwick DM, Wald DL. Hospital leaders' opinions of the HCFA mortality data. *JAMA*. 1990;263(2):247-249.

Cawley PJ, Deitelzweig S, Flores L, et al. The key principles and characteristics of an effective hospital medicine group: an assessment guide for hospitals and hospitalists. *J Hosp Med*. 2014;9:123-128.

Coleman EA. Falling through the cracks: challenges and opportunities for improving transitional care for persons with continuous complex care needs. *J Am Geriatr Soc*. 2003;51(4):549-555.

Hansen LO, Greenwald JL, Budnitz T, et al. Project BOOST: effectiveness of a multihospital effort to reduce rehospitalization. *J Hosp Med*. 2013;8:421-427.

Institute of Medicine. *America's Health in Transition: Protecting and Improving Quality*. Washington, DC: National Academies Press; 1994.

Institute of Medicine. *Crossing the Quality Chasm: A New Health System for the 21st Century*. Washington, DC: National Academy Press; 2001.

Institute of Medicine. *To Err Is Human: Building a Safer Health System*. Washington, DC: National Academy Press; 1999.

Jack BW, Chetty VK, Anthony D, et al. A reengineered hospital discharge program to decrease rehospitalization: a randomized trial. *Ann Intern Med*. 2009;150(3):178-187.

Naylor MD, Aiken H, Kurtzman ET, Olds DM, Hirschman KB. The importance of transitional care in achieving health reform. *Health Aff (Millwood)*. 2011;30(4):746-754.

Roberts KH, Rousseau DM. Research in nearly failure-free, high-reliability organizations: having the bubble. *IEEE Trans Eng Manage*. 1989;36(2):132-139.

Wachter RM, Goldman L. The emerging role of "hospitalists" in the American health care system. *N Engl J Med*. 1996;335:514-517.

Weick KE, Sutcliffe KM. *Managing the Unexpected: Assuring High Performance in an Age of Complexity*. San Francisco, CA: Jossey-Bass; 2001.

Wolf JA, Niederhauser V, Marshburn D, LaVela SL. Defining patient experience. *Patient Exp J*. 2014;1:7-19.

ONLINE RESOURCES

Center for Advancing Health. 2010. A New Definition of Patient Engagement: What Is Engagement and Why Is It Important. http://www.cfah.org/pdfs/CFAH_Engagement_Behavior_Framework_current.pdf. Accessed December 19, 2015.

Weiss A, Dantzler S. 2015. Three Key Lessons from the Healthcare Transparency Summit. Robert Wood Johnson Foundation. http://www.rwjf.org/en/culture-of-health/2015/04/3_key_lessons_fromt.html. Accessed December 19, 2015.

CHAPTER 2

Value-Based Health Care for Hospitalists

Christopher Moriates, MD

The field of hospital medicine was built on the premise that hospitalists would promote and deliver more efficient, safer, and higher-quality inpatient care. Indeed, over the past decade hospitalist care has led to shorter lengths of stay and relatively lower hospital costs. However, as national health care costs have continued to rise unabated, on track to consume approximately 20% of the United States gross domestic product by 2020, the government, payers, and the public have all focused renewed efforts on improving health care value—commonly defined as

$$\text{Value} = \frac{\text{Quality of care (including outcomes and patient experience)}}{\text{Costs}}$$

Hospital costs represent the single largest segment of the nearly $3 trillion annual US health care expenditure. Thus, hospitalists are vital to any effort to rein in health care costs. This chapter reviews concepts and strategies critical for hospitalists to understand in the emerging world of value-based health care.

HOSPITAL COSTS IN THE NATIONAL SPOTLIGHT

In February 2013, *Time* magazine published an expose on health care costs, "Bitter Pill: Why Medical Bills Are Killing Us," which was trumpeted across popular media and helped the hospital "chargemaster" become nearly a household term. The chargemaster (also known as the charge description master or "CDM") is the list of prices for the tens of thousands of billable items at a given hospital. Shortly following the *Time* article, the Centers for Medicare and Medicaid Services (CMS) publicly released a database of how hospitals billed Medicare for the 100 most common inpatient procedures, revealing in stark relief the baffling amount of variation in charges and reimbursements for the same procedures between similar hospitals. Later that same year, the *New York Times* published a front-page article with the headline, "As Hospital Prices Soar, a Stitch Tops $500," continuing to shine a bright national spotlight on the issue of hospital costs. As the "Bitter Pill" and the "$500 stitch" highlighted, charges found on hospital bills usually appear arbitrary and grossly inflated.

Despite the pressures to increase transparency, health care costs have largely remained hidden from the public and medical professionals. As a result, hospitalists are generally not aware of the costs associated with their care. In addition, most clinicians find the concepts of "charge," "price," "cost," and "reimbursement" confusing (**Table 2-1**). In most medical centers, the majority of health care transactions occur between the organization and large payer organizations, such as insurance companies or Medicare. The price or charge refers to the amount reported on the bill to each of these payers. The cost depends on perspective; providers, payers, and patients each evaluate costs differently:

- To providers, costs are the expense incurred to deliver health care services to patients.
- To payers, costs are the amount payable to the provider for services rendered.
- To patients, costs are the amount payable out-of-pocket for health care services.

The chargemaster is theoretically meant to relate to both costs and payments, but since there is tremendous inexplicable variation in prices between similar organizations and because the prices are highly inflated, the chargemaster routinely fails at this function. Instead, the

TABLE 2-1 Costs, Charges, Reimbursements, and Prices in Health Care

Term	Definition
Cost	Account of the true cost of providing health services, defined from a specific stakeholder perspective (provider, patient, payer, society)
Charge	Amount asked by a provider for delivering a service (typically more than reimbursement, used as a starting point for negotiation)
Reimbursement	Amount paid to the provider for delivering a service
Price	Amount paid by the patient for receiving a service

Source: Moriates C, Arora V, Shah N. *Understanding Value-Based Healthcare.* New York: McGraw-Hill; 2015.

chargemaster is generally used as a starting point for closed-door bargaining with different payers. While insurance companies pay a relatively small fraction of the charge on the chargemaster, uninsured patients have often been stuck with full chargemaster prices.

The Affordable Care Act (ACA) now formally requires all providers to publish their chargemasters, and some states are requiring hospitals to also disclose the "allowed amount" (contractually agreed amount paid by a private insurance company) to any patient who asks. In California, health care providers cannot bill uninsured patients an amount greater than the reimbursement the hospital would receive from a government payer.

Newer methods for determining more accurate measurements of actual costs are now increasingly being applied in health care. For example, Michael Porter and Robert Kaplan from Harvard Business School have advocated for the use of time-driven activity-based costing (TDABC). With TDABC, the costs of space, nonconsumable equipment, and administrative overhead are all assigned minute-to-minute cost rates that are relevant to specific processes of care. The care that is delivered over an entire episode of care is broken down into discrete activities or process steps, such as check-in, vitals and intake, physician evaluation, nursing care, and so on. A cost is assigned to each step by tracking who is doing the activity, what resources they use, which space they are in, and how long it takes them. Each item (personnel, resources, and space) is assigned a per-minute cost rate by bundling together all costs (fixed and variable) and then dividing by the total amount available for patient care. For a more detailed explanation of TDABC, one can refer to "How to Solve the Cost Crisis in Health Care" by Kaplan and Porter in the *Harvard Business Review* (2011). Using TDABC, some progressive medical centers have begun to establish a true "cost-master" to replace the controversial charge-master.

> **PRACTICE POINT**
>
> - Most hospitalists do not set the prices on the chargemaster or on hospital bills, but hospitalists can advocate for a more rational health care pricing system and for increased price and data transparency at their hospitals.

■ THE EFFECT OF PRICE TRANSPARENCY ON HOSPITALIST ORDERING PRACTICES

One seemingly obvious solution to hospitalists' lack of knowledge about costs is to provide diagnostic test prices at the point of ordering. After all, many have remarked that when ordering off a menu

without prices, it is easy to unwittingly order the filet mignon every time. So, why not just put the prices back on the menu?

Initial studies on this strategy showed mixed results, and the conventional wisdom evolved that displaying price information had limited effect, with prices often becoming "white noise" and being quickly disregarded. More recent studies, however, including a controlled trial at Johns Hopkins suggest that, perhaps due to the recent global attention to the importance of health care costs, clinicians are now more likely to react to price information. Displaying the Medicare Allowable Rates of lab tests to hospital physicians led to substantial decreases in certain higher-cost lab tests and resulted in a more than $400,000 net cost reduction over the course of a 6-month intervention period. It is not clear if this effect too will abate over time.

Similarly, a study using dollar signs ($-$$$$) to translate relative costs of antibiotics on culture and susceptibility testing reports resulted in a significant decrease in prescriptions for high-cost antibiotics.

Taken as a whole, a 2015 systematic review on the topic of providing price information for diagnostic testing concluded that "charge information changed ordering and prescribing behavior" in the majority of studies.

Remaining challenges include determining which price to display (the charge, the Medicare allowable fee, the estimated marginal cost, or some other measure), as well as whether prices should be displayed for all orders or rather be limited to only specific orders that may be ordered frequently or that are associated with high cost or marginal benefit.

> **PRACTICE POINT**
>
> - Recent research suggests that displaying price information at the point of care may help clinicians and patients make high-value care decisions.

HOSPITAL PAYMENTS SHIFTING FROM VOLUME TO VALUE

If there is one thing that most policymakers can agree on, it is that the payment system, which currently rewards volume of services delivered, should be realigned to compel the delivery of value. Not all policymakers, however, agree exactly how to best do that.

Medicare's Value-Based Purchasing (VBP) program has already tied a percentage of hospital payments to metrics of quality, patient satisfaction, and cost. In addition, with the proliferation of accountable care organizations (ACOs) and other bundled payment models, hospitals will continue to have an increasing share of reimbursement at risk related to the value of care that they deliver. According to the US Health and Human Services Secretary, Medicare aims to have at least 50% of all payments tied to quality or value through alternative payment models by the end of 2018.

■ MEDICARE'S HOSPITAL VALUE-BASED PURCHASING PROGRAM

The federal government introduced their hospital VBP program in 2012, initially with 1% of Medicare hospital payments based on some measures of quality. This percentage will continue to rise. The first quality indicators included process measures for pneumonia, acute myocardial infarction, congestive heart failure, health care-associated infections, and patient experience (largely based on patient survey responses to the Hospital Consumer Assessment of Healthcare Providers and Systems Hospital survey [HCAHPS]). Subsequently, risk-adjusted mortality, hospital-acquired conditions, and patient safety were added. The 2016 VBP metrics include eight clinical process of care measures, eight patient experience dimensions, three 30-day mortality outcome measures, one Agency for

TABLE 2-2 Medicare's Hospital Value-Based Purchasing Metrics for Fiscal Year 2016

Domain	Weight	Measures
Clinical process of care	10%	Fibrinolytic therapy received within 30 min of hospital arrival in patients with acute myocardial infarction
		Influenza immunization
		Initial antibiotic selection for community acquired pneumonia in immunocompetent patient
		Surgery patient on a beta blocker prior to arrival that received a beta blocker during perioperative period
		Prophylactic antibiotic selection for surgical patients
		Prophylactic antibiotics discontinued within 24 h after surgery ends
		Postoperative urinary catheter removal on postoperative day 1 or 2
		Surgery patient who received appropriate venous thromboembolism prophylaxis within 24 h prior to surgery to 24 h after surgery
Patient experience of care	25%	Communication with nurses
		Communication with doctors
		Responsiveness of hospital staff
		Pain management
		Communication about medicines
		Cleanliness and quietness of hospital environment
		Discharge information
		Overall rating of hospital
Outcome	40%	Acute myocardial infarction 30-d mortality rate
		Heart failure 30-d mortality rate
		Pneumonia 30-d mortality rate
		Complication/patient safety indicators (AHRQ PSI-90 composite score)
		Catheter-associated urinary tract infection
		Central line-associated bloodstream infection
		Surgical site infections in colon surgery and abdominal hysterectomy
Efficiency	25%	Medicare spending per beneficiary

Source: Data from www.medicare.gov. Accessed May 8, 2015.
AHRQ: Agency for Healthcare Research and Quality. AHRQ PSI-90 is a composite score consisting of eight weighted component patient safety indicator measures: pressure ulcers, iatrogenic pneumothorax, central venous catheter-related bloodstream infections, postoperative hip fracture, postoperative pulmonary embolism or deep vein thrombosis, postoperative sepsis, postoperative wound dehiscence, and accidental puncture or laceration.

Healthcare Research and Quality composite score, four health care-associated infection rates, and one efficiency measure based on Medicare spending per beneficiary (**Table 2-2**).

Payment for achieving higher-quality metrics seems to be a step in the right direction for our health care system, but there are criticisms that the current mechanism will unfairly punish safety net hospitals and clinicians caring for the most vulnerable populations.

■ HOSPITAL COMPARE

CMS hopes to also drive value through better public transparency of quality and cost data via their Hospital Compare website (www.medicare.gov/hospitalcompare). Hospital Compare provides data on a large number of metrics and even allows the public to select up to three hospitals at a time to compare head to head. In an effort to make the website more user-friendly for public consumers, CMS recently borrowed a strategy from the vast majority of popular rating websites and added a "star rating." The star rating, from one to five stars, is initially based on validated patient experience metrics.

■ BUNDLED PAYMENTS AND ACCOUNTABLE CARE ORGANIZATIONS

Whereas the VBP program is based on annual rewards and penalties, other payment models including bundled payments aim to more directly incentivize quality and efficiency. Strategies for payments exist on a spectrum from straight fee-for-service to fixed global budgets. If we consider reimbursements to a hospital, a payer may pay a specific amount for every service delivered (fee-for-service), for each day in the hospital (Per Diem), for each episode of hospitalization (eg, Diagnosis Related Groups [DRGs]), or for each patient in their community considered to be under their care (Capitation). Alternatively, the hospital could be given a fixed fee for all services performed on every patient during a full year (Global Budget). Currently, the majority of payments are still primarily based on fee-for-service, but this is projected to rapidly change (**Figure 2-1**).

Bundled payments could theoretically encourage improved efficiency and reductions in hospital-acquired complications as these would lead to increased costs, length of stay, and spent resources. For example, a hospital could be paid one fee for pneumonia, regardless of the number and type of interventions or resources used. CMS has used a prospective flat fee per inpatient episode of care, based on a diagnosis-related group (DRG) system, since 1983. CMS sets the base payment amounts "for the operating and capital costs that efficient facilities would be expected to incur in furnishing covered inpatient services." This rate is then weighted by DRG (which accounts for relative severity of a given condition), and then adjusted according to an algorithm that accounts for a number of factors such as the regional cost of labor, and whether the hospital

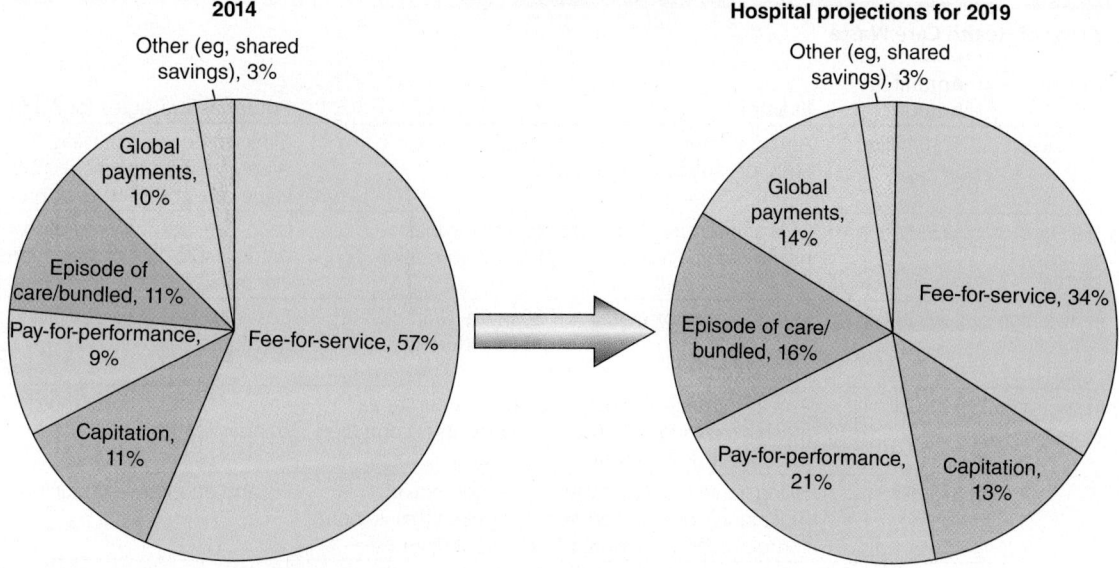

2014

Other (eg, shared savings), 3%

Global payments, 10%

Episode of care/bundled, 11%

Pay-for-performance, 9%

Fee-for-service, 57%

Capitation, 11%

Hospital projections for 2019

Other (eg, shared savings), 3%

Global payments, 14%

Episode of care/bundled, 16%

Fee-for-service, 34%

Pay-for-performance, 21%

Capitation, 13%

Figure 2-1 *Hospital or hospital system reimbursements.* (The State of Value-Based Reimbursement and the Transition from Volume to Value in 2014. McKesson Health Solutions, 2014.)

is a teaching facility. Medicare also provides higher payments for patients with "complicating or comorbid conditions," or with "major complicating or comorbid conditions." For particularly complex patients, Medicare provides "outlier payments" that are calculated based on an imprecise ratio of costs to charges.

Global or bundle payments could potentially combine payments across different providers and settings, encouraging better coordination and communication between hospitals, postacute care facilities (eg, a skilled nursing facility [SNF]), and outpatient providers. This is some of the logic behind the emergence of ACOs, which were included as part of the ACA to provide an experiment in global payments and shared risk. According to the CMS definition, ACOs are "groups of doctors, hospitals, and other health care providers, who come together voluntarily to give coordinated high quality care to their Medicare patients." When an ACO delivers high quality care at low costs, the organization shares in the savings that the ACO achieves.

Interpretations of the early results of ACOs have been mixed. The pilot Pioneer ACO program, which included 32 medical care organizations, was estimated to save 1.2% of health care spending, translating to about $400 million, over the first 2 years. Critics point out that the pilot programs were highly selected and unlikely to represent the abilities of the rest of the health care system once the model is more widely deployed. Moreover, 13 of the 32 pilot programs had dropped out due to not achieving savings in the first year or because they felt that the program was too complex with too many quality metrics to track. While we await additional research evidence on the true potential impact of ACOs, their premise in improving efficiency and coordinated care is strong, and their numbers will likely expand in the near future.

HEALTH CARE WASTE

The Institute of Medicine (IOM) estimated that over $750 billion annually spent on health care does not make anyone healthier, and thus is considered waste. This represents up to more than 30 cents on every health care dollar spent. Although there are many contributors to health care waste including prices that are excessively high, unwarranted administrative costs, fraud, and inefficiencies due to system errors and failures of coordination, the largest component is *unnecessary services*, which includes overuse, discretionary

use beyond benchmarks, and unnecessary choice of higher-cost services (**Table 2-3**). Unnecessary services account for $210 billion of waste annually. This is the area of waste that individual hospitalists have the most direct control over.

■ OVERUSE IS A PATIENT SAFETY PROBLEM

The 1998 IOM National Roundtable on Healthcare Quality classified three types of health care quality problems: underuse, overuse, and misuse. However, the following decade of the patient safety movement focused nearly exclusively on preventable complications related to misuse. Only recently has overuse of medical care—which refers to providing care in circumstances where the potential for harm exceeds the potential benefits—gained attention as an important patient safety hazard.

Overuse of medical care is a widespread problem in the US health care system. According to a 2011 study, nearly half of primary care physicians in the United States believe that their patients are receiving too much care. Overuse of medical care can directly lead to patient harm as a result of the known risks or adverse effects of the provided test, procedure, or medication. There are numerous frequently cited instances of overuse, including inappropriate imaging, laboratory tests, antibiotics, and catheter usage (**Table 2-4**). For example, despite evidence and clear guidelines that suggest imaging is unhelpful for patients with acute low back pain who lack specific clinical findings, routine diagnostic imaging is frequently obtained for these patients. This places patients at risk for excessive radiation, costs, and substantial downstream effects, including ineffective spine operations and perceptions of lessened overall health status.

Antibiotic prescribing is another area rife with overuse, which has led to the emergence of a number of antibiotic-resistant pathogens, making infections more difficult to treat. When prescribed incorrectly, antibiotics pose serious risks to both individual patients and the public health at large. Antibiotic overuse can place patients at risk for allergic reactions, antibiotic-associated diarrhea, and other dangerous adverse effects.

More medical care may also lead to overdiagnosis and overtreatment, which may result in a cascade effect of potential harms, including adverse events, mistakes, anxiety and disability, and additional unnecessary treatments. With patients bearing more

TABLE 2-3 Areas of Health Care Waste

Areas of Waste in Healthcare	Annual Amount	Examples	Potential Strategies for Addressing
Unnecessary services	$210 billion	Antibiotics for nonbacterial infections or MRIs for routine low back pain	Clinician decision making, "Choosing Wisely," appropriateness criteria, high-value care committees or programs
Inefficiently delivered services	$130 billion	Lack of interoperability between electronic health records resulting in missing information	Lean, care pathway redesign, accountable care organizations, electronic health record coordination
Prices that are too high	$105 billion	MRIs cost approximately $1080 in the United States and $280 in France, mostly due to differences in price setting	Cost transparency, regulatory measures
Excess administrative costs	$190 billion	American medical providers spend four times as much interacting with insurance companies compared to Canadians (who have a single payer system)	Payment reform, insurance form standardizations
Fraud	$75 billion	Billing for services that were not rendered, or "upcoding" for a procedure or diagnosis that is more complex than the actual procedure or diagnosis	FBI and other law enforcement
Missed prevention opportunities	$55 billion	Failing to provide appropriate immunizations or counseling	Improved access to primary care, decision support systems, accountable care organizations
TOTAL	$750 billion		

FBI, Federal Bureau of Investigation; MRI, magnetic resonance imaging.

and more of the cost of care themselves, some have further argued that clinicians should also consider the potential financial harm to individual patients due to excessive medical evaluations and subsequent overtreatments.

The many drivers of overuse include medical culture, fee-for-service payments, patient expectations, and fear of malpractice litigation.

TABLE 2-4 Common Examples of Overuse in Medical Care

Some Common Areas of Overuse	Examples
Antibiotics for nonbacterial illnesses	• 70% of patients with acute bronchitis are prescribed antibiotics, a rate that has been increasing over time • Antibiotic prescribing could potentially be improved in 37% of common inpatient prescription scenarios, according to the Centers for Disease Control and Prevention
Diagnostic imaging	• An estimated 3.8 million Americans receive routine imaging for low back pain each year • One-third of imaging performed in the emergency department for suspected pulmonary embolism may be avoidable
Laboratory testing	• Approximately 20% of lab testing may represent overutilization • Daily blood tests are routinely drawn in many patients in the hospital, which can contribute to hospital-acquired anemia
Urinary and central venous catheters	• Between 21% and 63% of urinary catheters are placed in patients who do not have an appropriate indication • According to one study, hospitalists felt 10%-25% of peripherally inserted central catheters (PICCs) placed at their facility were inappropriate or avoidable

A survey study using clinical vignettes of common hospital clinical situations revealed a large amount of overuse of testing among practicing hospitalists, with 52% to 65% of respondents requesting unnecessary testing in a preoperative evaluation scenario, and 82% to 85% in a syncope work-up scenario. The majority of physicians reported that they knew the testing was not clinically indicated based on evidence or guidelines, but were ordering the test due to a desire to reassure the patients or themselves. This finding suggests efforts to decrease overuse will need to engage clinicians and patients in ways that help overcome the attitude that more testing is required to provide reassurance.

STRATEGIES FOR HOSPITALISTS TO PROVIDE HIGH-VALUE CARE

As payment systems and health care organizations shift toward rewarding and supporting a focus on value, individual hospitalists can help deliver higher value care for their patients through: (1) providing appropriate care, (2) ensuring care coordination, (3) considering patient affordability in customizing treatment plans, and (4) leading local value improvement initiatives.

■ PROVIDING APPROPRIATE CARE

Hospitalists should address the problem of overuse by directly practicing appropriate care for their patients. Emerging resources for identifying specific targets of common overuse include the Choosing Wisely lists, guidelines, and appropriateness criteria. The Choosing Wisely campaign (www.choosingwisely.org) is an effort organized by the ABIM Foundation to engage specialty societies in identifying lists of commonly overused medical services "that physicians and patients should question." In 2013, the Society of Hospital Medicine published an initial Choosing Wisely list for both adult and pediatric hospital medicine (**Table 2-5**), and many other professional organizations' Choosing Wisely lists (eg, American College of Physicians, American Academy of Neurology, etc) have components that apply directly or indirectly to hospital medicine practice.

One strategy for encouraging and communicating appropriate care is to create a cognitive forcing function by explicitly documenting these types of decisions in daily progress notes. For example,

TABLE 2-5 Society of Hospital Medicine Choosing Wisely Lists

Adult Hospital Medicine Recommendations	Pediatric Hospital Medicine Recommendations
1. Do not place, or leave in place, urinary catheters for incontinence or convenience, or monitoring of output for noncritically ill patients (acceptable indications: critical illness, obstruction, hospice, perioperatively for <2 d or urologic procedures; use weights instead to monitor diuresis).	1. Do not order chest radiographs in children with uncomplicated asthma or bronchiolitis.
2. Do not prescribe medications for stress ulcer prophylaxis to medical inpatients unless at high risk for GI complication.	2. Do not routinely use bronchodilators in children with bronchiolitis.
3. Avoid transfusing red blood cells just because hemoglobin levels are below arbitrary thresholds such as 10, 9, or even 8 mg/dL in the absence of symptoms.	3. Do not use systemic corticosteroids in children under 2 y of age with an uncomplicated lower respiratory tract infection.
4. Avoid overuse/unnecessary use of telemetry monitoring in the hospital, particularly for patients at low risk for adverse cardiac outcomes.	4. Do not treat gastroesophageal reflux in infants routinely with acid suppression therapy.
5. Do not perform repetitive CBC and chemistry testing in the face of clinical and lab stability.	5. Do not use continuous pulse oximetry routinely in children with acute respiratory illness unless they are on supplemental oxygen.

Source: Adapted from the Society of Hospital Medicine's adult and pediatric hospital medicine Choosing Wisely® recommendations. www.choosingwisely.org. Accessed May 8, 2015.

hospitalists Drs Scott Flanders and Sanjay Saint recommend including the indication, day of administration, and expected duration of therapy for all antimicrobial therapies in all progress notes and sign-outs, as an approach for curbing inpatient antibiotic overuse. Likewise, hospitalists may eliminate use of routine labs, telemetry, continuous pulse oximetry, or other recurrent interventions or monitoring by documenting daily the patient needs and reasons for continued use or ordering.

PRACTICE POINT

- Avoiding overuse is the simplest way to simultaneously enhance patient safety and decrease costs. Common areas of potential overuse in hospitalized patients include antibiotics, telemetry and monitoring, imaging, and routine labs.

■ THE IMPORTANCE OF CARE COORDINATION

The typical hospital patient is handed off from one physician to another more than 15 times during a single 5-day hospital stay, a rate that has been increasing with new duty hour restrictions and hospitalist staffing models. Not surprisingly, studies show the majority of hospital patients are unable to identify the clinician in charge of their care. Hospital physician discontinuity may lead to increased resource utilization and lower patient satisfaction. Coordinating structured handoffs between inpatient providers and with outpatient providers during transitions in care is critical to delivering high-value care.

Currently, about one-fifth of Medicare patients are readmitted within 30 days of hospitalization, and more than half of these patients do not see any outpatient health care provider between these visits. This population of frequently readmitted patients is particularly important for hospitalists. Some care coordination programs have been experimenting with the use of hospitalists that care for a subset of the highest risk patients both during hospitalization and following discharge, either in a high-risk clinic or at postacute care facilities such as skilled nursing facilities. These physicians are increasingly becoming known as "extensivists." The early data on the cost-effectiveness of these types of programs have been mixed, but, much like ACOs, it may be too early to draw conclusions.

■ CONSIDERING PATIENT AFFORDABILITY

More Americans than ever before are on high-deductible insurance plans, making them responsible for an increasing share of health care costs. As "financial harms" for individual patients become increasingly recognized, and more patients forgo recommended medical treatments due to out-of-pocket costs, hospitalists must customize care plans to help patients afford their care.

Hospitalists may be able to improve their prescribing practices, particularly at the time of discharge. Nearly one-quarter of hospitalized adults in a survey reported cost-related underuse in the year prior to admission, and only 16% of patients knew how much their prescribed medications at discharge would cost them. Virtually nobody had spoken to their inpatient providers about the cost of the newly prescribed drugs.

Discussing drug costs with patients has been shown to be strongly associated with providing individualized lower-cost medication options. Health care professionals and patients can rely on an increasing number of freely available resources that provide price information and cheaper alternatives for most medications (**Table 2-6**). High-value prescribing has been defined as "providing the simplest medication regimen that minimizes physical and financial risk to the patient while achieving the best outcome."

PRACTICE POINT

- Hospital staff can help screen patients for financial concerns, particularly related to prescribed discharge medications. An increasing number of tools are available to help determine the most cost-effective medication for a given patient's condition and insurance coverage (Table 2-6).

■ IMPLEMENTING VALUE-BASED INITIATIVES

Hospitalists across the country have largely taken the lead on designing value improvement pilots, programs, and groups within hospitals. Although value improvement projects may be built upon the established structures and techniques for quality improvement (see Section IV: Patient Safety and Quality Improvement, Chapter 21: Quality Improvement Methodologies), importantly these programs should include expertise in cost analyses. Furthermore, some traditional quality improvement programs have failed to result in actual cost savings; thus it is not enough to simply re-brand quality improvement with a banner of "value." Value improvement efforts must overcome the cultural hurdle of "more care as better care," as well as pay careful attention to the diplomacy required with value

TABLE 2-6 Some Resources That Provide Price Information for Medications

Websites	Consumer reports best buy drugs	http://www.consumerreports.org/cro/health/prescription-drugs/best-buy-drugs/index.htm
	GoodRx	www.goodrx.com
Mobile applications	Epocrates	http://www.epocrates.com
	Lowestmed	http://www.lowestmed.com
	GoodRx	http://www.goodrx.com
$4 Generic drug lists	Walmart	http://www.walmart.com/cp/4-Prescriptions/1078664
	Target	http://www.target.com/pharmacy/generics
	Sam's Club	http://resources.samsclub.com/health-and-wellness/pharmacy-and-health/Extra-Value-Drug-List.aspx
	Krogers	http://www.kroger.com/topic/save-on-generic-prescriptions

improvement since reducing costs may result in decreased revenue for certain departments or even decreases in individuals' wages.

The national nonprofit group Costs of Care has proposed a "COST" framework to guide value improvement project design. COST stands for **c**ulture, **o**versight accountability, **s**ystem support, and **t**raining. This approach leverages principles from implementation science to ensure that value improvement projects successfully provide multipronged tactics for overcoming the many barriers to high-value care delivery.

PRACTICE POINT

- Hospitalists are uniquely positioned to identify potentially wasteful or inefficient practices within medical centers and to lead value improvement initiatives. Value improvement work requires the inclusion of expertise in health care cost accounting, as well as thoughtful diplomacy, and the design of multipronged efforts that explicitly target **c**ulture, **o**versight, **s**ystems, and **t**raining (**COST**).

■ APPLYING LEAN AND REDESIGNING CARE PATHWAYS

On a health system level, methods for ensuring better value may focus on techniques to improve efficiency and decrease "defects." To achieve this goal, an increasing number of hospitals are now adopting lean methodologies and systems. Lean principles stem from the Toyota Production System developed by the automaker in Japan to focus on improving quality while reducing waste. In 2002, Virginia Mason Medical Center in Seattle famously began applying to health care the five general principles of lean: (1) define value from the customer's perspective, (2) identify the value stream and remove any waste, (3) make value flow without interruption, (4) help customers pull value, and (5) pursue perfection.

Some lean tools have quickly been adapted to health care, including value stream maps that depict all of the individual steps in a process from beginning to end, and provides a graphical tool for identifying any non–value-added steps, delays, waiting times, and inefficiencies, as well as the commitment to rapid improvement cycles that are built around "small tests of change." Lean

programs have led to remarkable improvements in hospital processes and outcomes across the country from safety net hospitals like Denver Health to Veteran's Affairs hospitals to the University of Michigan.

Similar in concept to lean are efforts to design and hone specific care pathways for certain patients and conditions. For example, many joint-replacement programs have created care pathways that standardize when patients will have catheters removed, mobilize with physical therapy, and be discharged to a specific disposition. Hospitalists are increasingly creating similar models for patients with pneumonia, chronic obstructive pulmonary disease (COPD) exacerbations, syncope, or other common clinical conditions. Intermountain Healthcare in Utah has applied evidence-based protocols to more than 60 clinical processes, re-engineering roughly 80% of all care that they deliver. Cincinnati Children's Hospital partnered with local physicians to create large-scale improvements in the care of children with asthma, resulting in 92% adherence to best practices for asthma care, which has yielded many avoided hospital admissions and emergency department visits. These types of care redesigns and standardization promise to provide better, more efficient, and often safer care for more patients.

CONCLUSION

Hospitalists are now faced with the massive responsibility of providing better health care value. Based on the history of the hospitalist movement, we are up to the task. Value is defined as providing the highest quality care at lower costs, and should include components of patient outcomes, safety, and experience. To achieve this goal, measuring and understanding metrics related to quality and costs will be vitally important. There is an inexorable trend toward greater transparency in health care and it is likely soon that true health care costs will be publicly accessible across the country. Evidence is mounting that providing some cost information at the point-of-care may help support behavior changes and decrease unnecessarily expensive test ordering.

The most potent strategy for simultaneously improving care and decreasing costs is to reduce waste and overuse, which accounts for more than $200 billion in health care costs annually in the United States and causes significant patient harms. There are many common areas of overuse in hospital care, including the use of antibiotics, telemetry monitoring, transfusions, imaging, catheter usage, and routine lab draws. Many of these are highlighted in Choosing Wisely lists and other emerging appropriateness criteria.

Hospitalists can deliver high-value care to their patients by specifically considering appropriateness of care, care coordination, patient affordability, and value-based initiatives and care pathways.

SUGGESTED READINGS

Conway PH. Value-driven health care: implications for hospitals and hospitalists. *J Hosp Med.* 2009;4(8):507-511.

Feldman LS, Shihab HM, Thiemann D, et al. Impact of providing fee data on laboratory test ordering: a controlled clinical trial. *JAMA Intern Med.* 2013;173(10):903-908.

Flanders SA, Saint S. Why does antimicrobial overuse in hospitalized patients persist? *JAMA Intern Med.* 2014;174(5):661-662.

Goetz C, Rotman SR, Hartoularos G, Bishop TF. The effect of charge display on cost of care and physician practice behaviors: a systematic review. *J Gen Intern Med.* 2015;30(6):835-842.

Institute of Medicine. *Best Care at Lower Cost: The Path to Continuously Learning Health Care in America.* Washington, DC: National Academies Press; 2012.

Kachalia A, Berg A, Fagerlin A, et al. Overuse of testing in preoperative evaluation and syncope: a survey of hospitalists. *Ann Intern Med*. 2015;162(2):100-108.

Kaplan RS, Porter ME. How to solve the cost crisis in health care. *Harvard Business Review*. 2011;89(9):46-52, 54, 56-61 passim.

Moriates C, Arora V, Shah N. *Understanding Value-Based Healthcare*. New York: McGraw-Hill; 2015.

Moriates C, Mourad M, Novelero M, Wachter RM. Development of a hospital-based program focused on improving healthcare value. *J Hosp Med*. 2014;9(10):671-677.

Owens DK, Qaseem A, Chou R, Shekelle P. High-value, cost-conscious health care: concepts for clinicians to evaluate the benefits, harms, and costs of medical interventions. *Ann Intern Med*. 2011;154(3):174-180.

CHAPTER 3

Racial/Ethnic Disparities in Hospital Care

Lenny López, MD, MPH, MDiv

Racial and ethnic disparities in care have been consistently documented in the treatment and outcomes of many common clinical diseases. The 2003 Institute of Medicine (IOM) report, "Unequal Treatment: Confronting Racial and Ethnic Disparities in Health Care," defines disparities as differences in the treatment that are not directly attributable to access-related factors, clinical needs, patient preferences, or appropriateness of intervention (**Figure 3-1**). The elimination of health care disparities is a high priority for the federal government and several academic organizations.

Documented disparities of disease prevention and treatment include rates of vaccination, cancer screening, secondary prevention of myocardial infarction (MI), transplant surgery, curative surgery, and angioplasty. Disparities in health outcomes include cardiovascular disease, HIV/AIDS, diabetes, cancer, asthma, pregnancy outcomes, mental health, and hospitalization.

Specific examples include the following (**Table 3-1**):

- A higher risk of stroke, heart failure, and renal failure associated with hypertension (African Americans)
- A higher rate of complications from diabetes (African Americans and Native Americans)
- Later-stage colon, breast, and prostate cancer at presentation (African Americans)
- Less aggressive evaluation and treatment: curative lung cancer resection, cardiac catheterization, peripheral angioplasty, and renal transplantation (African Americans)
- Diabetic more likely to receive amputations (African Americans)
- Higher death rates per 1000 hospital admissions in low-mortality diagnosis-related groups (African Americans, Hispanics, and the uninsured)

The observed racial/ethnic health care disparities have multifactorial etiologies. Patients face multiple barriers as they engage the health care system: (1) personal and family; (2) access to the health care system (structural, financial, types of services); and (3) the quality of the available providers (**Figure 3-2**). These barriers can occur individually or in combination to have an additive effect on health outcomes.

PRACTICE POINT

- Disparities in health outcomes include the following: cardiovascular disease, HIV/AIDS, diabetes, cancer, asthma, pregnancy outcomes, mental health, and hospitalization. Hospitalists may significantly influence the health status of African American and Latino patients if they comprehend their health care needs, communicate effectively, and advocate for additional local and institutional resources to ensure optimal discharge back to the community.

Historically, disparities in hospital care originated in the policy of hospital segregation during the first 66 years of the 20th century. Before the creation of Medicare, the Hospital Survey and Construction Act of 1946, commonly known as "Hill-Burton," was the largest federal grant program in health care. This law was intended to increase the number of hospital beds throughout the country. However, this was the only federal legislation in the 20th century that explicitly permitted use of federal funds to provide racially

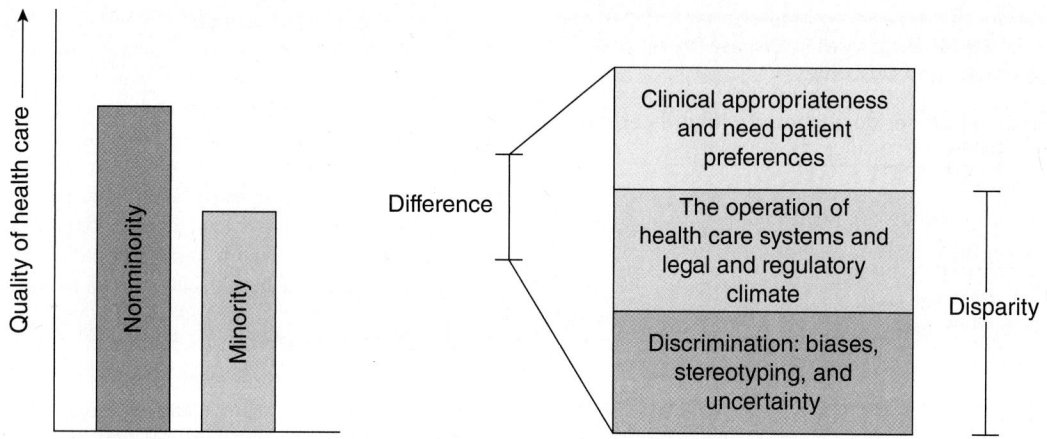

Figure 3-1 *Defining differences, disparities, and discrimination in populations with equal access to health care.* (Reproduced, with permission, from Smedley BD, Stith AY, Nelson AR. *Unequal Treatment. Confronting Racial and Ethnic Disparities in Health Care.* Washington, DC: National Academies Press; 2002.)

exclusionary services ("separate but equal") thus augmenting the wide divide in poor-quality hospital services and facilities for African Americans. Hospital segregation ended with President Johnson signing into law the Medicare bill on July 9, 1965. The Medicare bill was tied to Title VI of the Civil Rights Act of 1964, which banned discrimination in any activities that used federal funds for training, employment, or construction. Because of this legal requirement, more than 95% of hospitals desegregated their facilities by the first day Medicare was implemented on July 1, 1966, in order to receive Medicare reimbursement.

The elimination of health care disparities is a high priority for the federal government, and many academic organizations are beginning to take steps to educate physicians about this problem. To date, existing data suggest that the type of hospital facility and its location explain some of the observed racial and ethnic disparities in health care services; less is known, however, about disparities in hospital care. This chapter reviews the racial disparities in hospital care that can be impacted by hospitalists and proposes directions for future research.

MECHANISMS AND ETIOLOGY

■ INTERINSTITUTIONAL AND INTRAINSTITUTIONAL VARIATIONS IN CARE

Although where patients receive care likely explains some of the observed racial and ethnic disparities in health care service, prior studies suggest that hospital-level factors may play an important role in creating disparities in care. In addition, minorities live disproportionally in parts of the country that have lower-quality hospitals and fewer primary care physicians.

Safety-net hospitals predominantly serve poor and underserved patients and provide care for a disproportionate number of racial and ethnic minorities in the United States. Multiple studies have shown that these hospitals often provide a lower quality of care. This decreased quality is likely due to shortages of resources, nurse staff, technical support such as health information systems, and capital to make improvements. These hospitals have increased post-MI mortality rates and decreased performance measure scores for acute MI, lower performance on national quality process indicators for acute myocardial infarction (AMI), congestive heart failure (CHF), and pneumonia, and higher postoperative colon cancer mortality rates. In addition, they tend to have smaller gains over time on process measures for AMI, CHF, and pneumonia, and are less likely to achieve high-performing status.

A large proportion of minority patients receive their care in a small number of hospitals and these facilities seem to provide a lower

quality of care for common medical and surgical conditions. One study demonstrated that 90% of Hispanic and black Medicare beneficiaries receive their care at 25% of the 4500 acute care hospitals in the United States. Another study found significant racial/ethnic disparities in clinical processes for AMI, CHF, and pneumonia explained primarily by hospital factors and not individual patient characteristics. They also found that lower-performing hospitals tended to serve a larger proportion of minority patients. Similar findings have been demonstrated using national Hospital Quality Alliance (HQA) patient-level data. Other national studies demonstrate that African Americans go to hospitals that have lower rates of evidence-based medical treatments and worse risk-adjusted mortality after AMI, are less likely to receive optimal care for pneumonia as measured by national HQA measures, and have higher operative mortality risks for eight different procedures because the hospitals they attend have higher mortality rates for all patients.

In addition to differences in quality of care based on institution, data suggest that among patients hospitalized in the same institutions, racial and ethnic disparities in care often exist. Several studies have demonstrated significant racial and ethnic differences in utilization of cardiovascular procedures for patients hospitalized within the same institutions. For example, African Americans have a lower rate of coronary artery bypass procedures than whites, even with similar presentation and clinical features.

■ DIFFERENTIAL UTILIZATION OF MEDICAL PROCEDURES AND TECHNOLOGY AVAILABILITY

Racial differences in the utilization of medical procedures are well documented, especially for "referral-sensitive" procedures and invasive, costly procedures such as coronary revascularization. The reasons for these differences are complex and may reflect differences in clinical presentation, medical decision making, differential access to providers and institutions providing procedures, and differential care at hospitals.

Studies have demonstrated that Caucasian patients more often receive renal transplantation, cardiac surgical procedures, total joint replacement, and other procedures than do African Americans. African Americans are less likely to receive coronary revascularization compared to whites, even in hospitals with revascularization services. Additionally, African Americans are less likely to be transferred from hospitals without revascularization services to those with these cardiac services, and, even when they are transferred, they are still less likely to receive revascularization as compared to Caucasians. These differences in procedure use have been associated with increased African American mortality rates. Finally,

TABLE 3-1 Racial/Ethnic Disparities in Disease Prevention, Treatment, and Outcomes*

Conditions where minorities documented with greater rates compared with whites

Cardiovascular disease:
- Hypertension, stroke, congestive heart failure

Incidence and mortality from HIV

Type 2 diabetes:
- Prevalence
- Amputations
- Hospitalizations

Malignancy:
- Advanced-stage breast cancer
- Advanced-stage colon cancer
- Advanced-stage prostate cancer

Pregnancy outcomes:
- Infant mortality
- Low birth weight
- Maternal mortality

End-stage renal disease

Preventable hospitalizations

Conditions where minorities documented with lower rates compared with whites

Cardiovascular procedures:
- Cardiac catheterization
- Peripheral artery angioplasty
- Implantable cardiac defibrillators

Adult vaccinations

Solid organ transplantations

Secondary prevention for myocardial infarction

Conditions where minorities documented with greater rates compared with whites

Curative surgery for lung cancer

Inadequate hemodialysis

Renal transplantation

Receipt of recommended care for acute myocardial infarction

Receipt of recommended care for pneumonia

Receipt of recommended care for congestive heart failure

Receipt of recommended care for type 2 diabetes

Satisfaction with hospital care

Age-adjusted life expectancy

*Adapted from Unequal Treatment and Agency for Healthcare Research and Quality. *National Healthcare Disparities Report 2009.* Agency for Healthcare Research and Quality, US Department of Health and Human Services.

procedure volume has been shown to be a proxy for quality of care. African Americans and Hispanics tend to get care at low-procedure-volume hospitals with low-volume surgeons and cardiologists. A study of coronary artery bypass surgery (CABG) surgery outcomes in New York State found that African Americans and Asians were more likely to receive care from surgeons with higher risk-adjusted mortality. African Americans at low-volume hospitals have greater risk-adjusted mortality than Caucasian patients after elective aortic abdominal aneurysm (AAA) repair, CABG, and carotid endarterectomy (CEA).

Technology availability likely contributes to low performance. Hospitals with a high proportion of African American inpatients may have lower rates of adoption of new technologies. In general, safety-net providers are slower to adopt new technologies than non–safety-net providers. Providers and hospitals that invest in technology score higher on standard quality measures. However, national studies have demonstrated that providers who cared for uninsured and Medicaid African American and Hispanic patients are less likely to use electronic health records. These differences underscore the need to provide higher funding of public and other safety-net hospitals in order to reduce disparities in health care by ensuring the delivery of high-quality care for all patients.

PATIENT EXPERIENCES

Perceived provider attitude (both physicians and nonphysicians), including perceptions of provider prejudice, by minority patients has been shown to have a direct relationship to patient decision making and perceived quality and satisfaction. Reports of patient experiences with health care are therefore important correlates with quality. There are significant differences in hospitalized patients' self-reported experiences among different groups. African American and Latino patients are less satisfied with their hospital care, particularly in the dimension of having their preferences respected consistent with prior studies demonstrating racial/ethnic differences in satisfaction with provider communication and management. Both African American and Hispanic patients report that perceived attitudes of social workers and nursing staff have an important direct relationship with their perceived satisfaction and quality. Hispanic patients correlate high satisfaction with care when well-qualified medical interpreters are available.

These findings have several important implications for prioritizing quality improvement efforts in improving patient satisfaction with care. First, physicians and hospital staff should strive to better understand and address the expectations of African American and Latino patients. Second, hospital administrators should include allied health professionals and social workers in addition to nurses and physicians in training on patient-centered and culturally appropriate counseling techniques and communication. All clinicians should use medical interpreters when English is not the first language. Finally, hospitals should collect satisfaction data stratified by race and ethnicity in order to better tailor quality improvement (QI) efforts.

ROLE OF HOSPITALISTS

Hospitalists are specialists in the general medical care of hospitalized patients. Their activities include patient care, teaching, research, and leadership related to inpatient care. The number of hospitalists continues to grow significantly across the nation; as a result, this specialty will care for increasing numbers of hospitalized underserved patients. Existing literature has demonstrated that hospitalists are associated with lower inpatient costs and shorter lengths of stay compared to general internists and family physicians, and such savings did not have a detrimental effect on rates of death or readmission. Importantly, hospitalists are associated with providing higher-quality inpatient care because of closer adherence to treatment guidelines and better post discharge follow-up. A recent national study has demonstrated that hospitals with hospitalists were associated with better performance on quality indicators for AMI, pneumonia, and the composite domains of disease treatment, diagnosis, counseling, and prevention controlling for hospital characteristics such as size, location, ownership type, and staffing availability. There are, however, no data reported on the performance of hospitalists compared to other providers relating to their care of different ethnic groups.

Previous research using national quality measures has found substantial variability and room for improvement in the care of hospitalized patients across medical conditions. With the continued growth

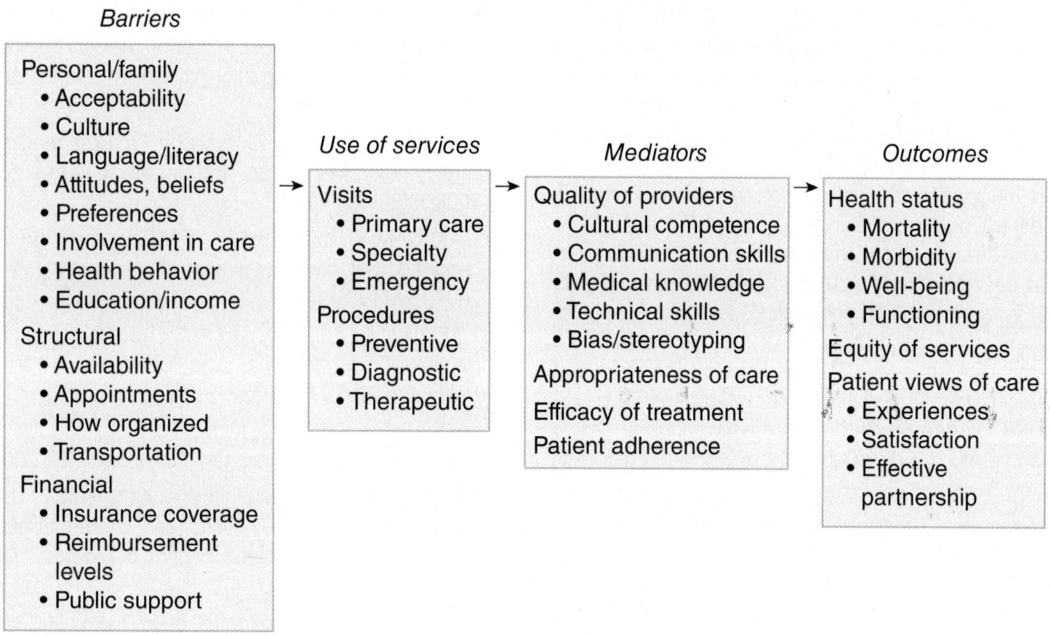

Barriers

Personal/family
- Acceptability
- Culture
- Language/literacy
- Attitudes, beliefs
- Preferences
- Involvement in care
- Health behavior
- Education/income

Structural
- Availability
- Appointments
- How organized
- Transportation

Financial
- Insurance coverage
- Reimbursement levels
- Public support

Use of services

Visits
- Primary care
- Specialty
- Emergency

Procedures
- Preventive
- Diagnostic
- Therapeutic

Mediators

Quality of providers
- Cultural competence
- Communication skills
- Medical knowledge
- Technical skills
- Bias/stereotyping

Appropriateness of care

Efficacy of treatment

Patient adherence

Outcomes

Health status
- Mortality
- Morbidity
- Well-being
- Functioning

Equity of services

Patient views of care
- Experiences
- Satisfaction
- Effective partnership

Figure 3-2 *Barriers and mediators of racial/ethnic health care disparities.* (Adapted, with permission, from Cooper LA, Hill MN, Power NR. Designing and evaluating interventions to eliminate racial and ethnic disparities in health care. *J Gen Intern Med.* 2002;17:477-486. Copyright 2002 Society of General Internal Medicine.)

of the hospitalist inpatient care model, further research is needed to delineate the specific hospitalist model characteristics associated with improved quality and outcomes of care. The hospitalist model of inpatient care should be considered an essential component of quality improvement for hospitals seeking to improve inpatient care. This is especially true for public/municipal hospitals and smaller hospitals, which have been shown to be consistently associated with lower quality and provide care for the disproportionate number of racial/ethnic minority patients.

■ HOSPITALISTS AND THE USE OF INTERPRETERS IN THE CLINICAL ENCOUNTER

In 2011, over 25 million Americans rated themselves as speaking English less than "very well," and as a result, health care providers increasingly encounter patients with limited English proficiency (LEP). The use of professional medical interpreters is associated with increased patient satisfaction, quality of care, and improved disease-specific process measures and outcomes. The Institute of Medicine report *Crossing the Quality Chasm* states that the use of an interpreter is not only a quality but also a patient safety imperative. Patients with communication problems due to language barriers are at high risk for preventable adverse events. Recent research has documented that patient safety events affecting hospitalized LEP patients are more severe and more frequently due to communication errors compared to English-speaking patients. Similarly, drug complications in outpatients are more common in patients who speak a primary language other than English. Hospitals should stratify their adverse events data by language in order to improve patient safety.

Although Federal law, the Institute of Medicine, and hospital guidelines, including the Joint Commission standards, all recommend the routine use of professional interpreters during clinical encounters, many LEP patients do not have access to interpreters and some clinicians continue to "get by" without using interpreters consistently. In addition, nonprofessional interpreters cause an increase in interpretation errors that may potentially harm the patient through the misinterpretation of information and alteration of key patient details. Language barriers between patients and their

clinical providers are not only an inconvenience to workflow but are also a patient safety hazard.

Inpatient care is a continuum of clinical care encounters with both clinical and nonclinical staff. All patient interactions with clinical providers should document whether an interpreter or a bilingual clinician was used in order to allow quality assessment both in real time and retrospectively. It is likely not enough to have interpreter use only at the time of admission or possibly only at discharge given that the clinical care received by patients' change may change rapidly during admission. Increasing the availability and use of professional interpreters throughout the hospital stay is essential. This will also require educating physicians about the quality of available interpretation modalities. Recent studies have demonstrated that remote telephone or video conferencing modes are as effective as in-person interpretation as measured by communication quality and patient satisfaction. Use of these non–in-person methods should be encouraged in the hospital setting where in-person interpretation may not be readily available throughout the 24-hour hospital continuum of care.

PRACTICE POINT

- To ensure high quality and maximize patient safety, always use certified interpreters in any clinical encounter with patients who have limited English proficiency. Hospitals should stratify their adverse events data by language in order to improve patient safety.

CONCLUSION

Racial/ethnic disparities in hospital care and outcomes are based in a tradition of hospital segregation that has residual, significant, and persistent effects. A growing body of literature has demonstrated disparities in processes of care, utilization of procedures, clinical outcomes, and patients' experiences. These disparities are due in large part to differences in access to higher-quality hospitals; however, variation in intrainstitutional care has also been documented.

A small number of hospitals nationwide serve a high number of minorities. Ameliorating health care disparities includes improving hospital quality of care. The hospitalist model of inpatient care provides a vehicle for driving high quality by engaging hospitalists as quality improvement and patient safety leaders. All clinicians should strive to improve quality and patient safety through the consistent use of certified interpreters during clinical encounters involving patients with limited English proficiency.

It is incumbent among policy makers, hospital administrators, and clinicians to develop strategies to achieve racial/ethnic equity in care. These strategies should include (1) examining within-institution differences in care, outcomes, and patient experience based on patients' race/ethnicity; (2) improving infrastructure and quality within largely minority-servicing institutions; and (3) developing QI initiatives focused on cultural competency and targeting high-risk racial and ethnic groups such as those with limited English proficiency.

SUGGESTED READINGS

Agency for Healthcare Research and Quality. *National Healthcare Disparities Report 2013*. http://nhqrnet.ahrq.gov/inhqrdr/reports/nhdr. Accessed April 30, 2015.

Divi C, Koss RG, Schmaltz SP, Loeb JM. Language proficiency and adverse events in US hospitals: a pilot study. *Intl J Qual Health Care*. 2006;18:383-388.

Groeneveld PW, Laufer SB, Garber AM. Technology diffusion, hospital variation, and racial disparities among elderly Medicare beneficiaries 1989–2000. *Med Care*. 2005;43:320-329.

Hasnain-Wynia R, Baker DW, Nerenz D, et al. Disparities in health care are driven by where minority patients seek care. Examination of the Hospital Quality Alliance Measures. *Arch Intern Med*. 2007;167:1233-1239.

Hicks LS, Tovar DA, Orav EJ, Johnson PA. Experiences with hospital care: perspectives of black and Hispanic patients. *J Gen Intern Med*. 2008;23(8):1234-1240.

Jha AK, Orav EJ, Li Z, Epstein AM. Concentration and quality of hospitals that care for elderly black patients. *Arch Intern Med*. 2007;167:1177-1182.

Jha AK, Orav EJ, Li Z, Epstein AM. The characteristics and performance of hospitals that care for elderly Hispanic Americans. *Health Aff*. 2008;27:528-537.

López L, Hicks L, Cohen AP, McKean S, Weissman JS. Hospitalists and the quality of care in hospitals. *Arch Intern Med*. 2009;169:1-6.

López L, Huerta D, Soukup J, Rodriguez F, Hicks L. Use of interpreters by physicians for hospitalized limited English proficiency patients and its impact on patient outcomes. *J Gen Intern Med*. 2015;30(6):783-789.

Trivedi AN, Nsa W, Hausmann LR, et al. Quality and equity of care in U.S. hospitals. *N Engl J Med*. 2014;371(24):2298-2308.

Werner RM, Goldman LE, Dudley RA. Comparison of change in quality of care between safety-net and non-safety-net hospitals. *JAMA*. 2008;299:2180-2187.

CHAPTER 4

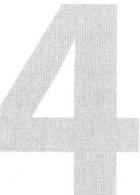

Comanagement of Orthopedic Patients

Christopher M. Whinney, MD, FACP, FHM

INTRODUCTION

From the beginning of the hospitalist movement, hospitalists have filled a collaborative role in assuming care of primary care physicians' patients in the hospital. Just as primary care physicians (PCPs) cannot feasibly be in two places at once (the office and the hospital), surgeons and medical subspecialists cannot simultaneously manage complex inpatients and perform procedures and other specialty services. The limited surgical availability with restricted surgical resident work hours creates added pressure on surgical residents to maximize operating room time. Likewise, medical subspecialties face similar pressures with limited fellow work hours. The active involvement of a medical comanager may make practical and economic sense if it is planned well and actively managed. In addition, co-management may improve the quality of care by having a generalist on site to anticipate and address common problems that arise during hospitalization without the delays that may occur with traditional medical consultation.

Comanagement is now a prominent practice pattern as an integrated part of hospitalist practice. Comanagement practices have now been described in collaboration with orthopedic surgery, neurosurgery, vascular surgery, otolaryngology, hepatology, and pediatrics. Thus, in all likelihood, the practice of comanagement by hospitalists will not wane, and both surgeons and medical subspecialists will call on hospitalists in this collaborative spirit. Some authors express concerns for exacerbating the workforce shortage of internists by increasing overall workload with comanagement and increasing the "silo" delineations in medicine. However, comanagement may provide value if there is a clear delineation of roles and responsibilities and the value equation is articulated for all parties—hospitalists, surgeons, patients, and hospital leadership. Based on the author's experience with orthopedic comanagement and on other hospitalists' successful collaborations, this chapter will suggest specific steps that can be taken to initiate a potential comanagement effort and avoid common pitfalls.

ANTICIPATE THE GROWTH OF THE SPECIALTY IN THE HOSPITAL SETTING

Musculoskeletal disorders and diseases are the leading cause of disability in the United States and account for more than one-half of all chronic conditions in people over 50 years of age in developed countries. One in two Americans has a musculoskeletal condition requiring medical attention, twice the rate of chronic heart and lung conditions. Annual direct and indirect costs for bone and joint health are $874 billion, 5.7% of the gross domestic product.

Based on these data, it is little wonder that orthopedic surgeons will have increasing volumes of patient visits and operative interventions in the coming years, especially in the setting of an aging population with increasing expectations for functional recovery and quality of life. The challenge associated with this growth will be the increasing number of medical comorbidities in these older patients and the need for systematic evaluation of these comorbidities to optimize the perioperative course. It is estimated that surgery-related costs will rise 50% and surgical complications 100% in the United States in the next two decades.

REVIEW AVAILABLE LITERATURE ON COMANAGEMENT

Early literature on orthopedic comanagement focused on geriatrician collaboration with surgeons. Despite inconsistent data on length of hospital stay and mortality, these studies and more recent ones demonstrate that systematic geriatric evaluation and management can decrease the incidence of common postoperative medical complications such as congestive heart failure, arrhythmias, venous thromboembolism (VTE), and delirium, and improve compliance with antiosteoporotic therapy and VTE prophylaxis. More recent literature has focused on hospitalist collaboration with orthopedics and has shown lower adjusted length of hospital stay and decreased complication rates in some studies, although mortality and readmission rates were not changed. In one study of hip fracture patients, delirium was diagnosed more often in the comanagement group, and this was associated with an earlier discharge after surgery. This may reflect greater attention to the presence of delirium, better documentation, and more prompt treatment. A single-center retrospective cohort study of 501 patients who experienced at least one postoperative complication found that comanagement was associated with a lower mortality rate and a shorter length of stay, suggesting that this was a "rescue" phenomenon of the medically complex surgical patient.

ASK KEY QUESTIONS SPECIFIC TO YOUR HOSPITAL

Comanagement of surgical (and medical subspecialty) patients has rapidly evolved with much initial enthusiasm. However, when proposals do not clearly delineate the nature of these relationships, great potential for confusion of roles, miscommunication, suboptimal patient care, and dissatisfaction of both parties can result as the service expands and staffing becomes more of an issue. Institutional support for this activity is paramount and the medical administration should be involved in these initial meetings from the outset.

Initially, ask the following questions:

1. Why are we doing this?

    To start out, it is best to explicitly clarify the motivation for starting such a program: Are the surgeons stretched thin between operating room time and patient care responsibilities on the floors and in the office? Are orthopedic residents more limited by duty hour restrictions and therefore less able to focus on patient care on the floors? Are there concerns with care quality within the standard structure of medical subspecialty consultation? Are nursing and ancillary staff having issues with access to practitioners for patient medical needs and issues? Do they want someone to take on the role and responsibility of completing histories and physicals and discharge notes and summaries? These are just a few questions that might help to focus the expectations of the proposing surgeons.

2. Is the hospitalist service the best solution to this problem?

    Once it becomes clear what your surgical or medical colleagues desire, then clarify how hospitalist services and skills can (or should) address these issues. Is a hospitalist the best solution to this problem? Certainly hospitalists are adept at addressing medical issues in hospitalized patients as medical consultants, but to what degree should they assume the detailed minutia of patient care (ie, acetaminophen orders, renewing intravenous fluids)? This presents the potential to become a "glorified resident" in the care of these patients, which many hospitalists abhor. In addition, expectations for surgical wound care and drain management may be tasked to hospitalists despite concerns that this may extend outside the scope of practice of their internal medicine training. Similar concerns have been raised when hospitalists assume primary responsibility for patients with intracranial bleeds for neurosurgeons.

3. What other options have been considered?

    If the first call from nursing for a problem traditionally has gone to orthopedic residents and/or staff who now are tied up elsewhere, is the hospitalist the next logical call in an equitable "comanagement" relationship? Some newer hospitalists or hospitalist groups may accept this as part of their growth and cultivation of their practice, whereas others fear the mission creep to becoming a "glorified resident" as described previously. In our institution, nurses channel most first calls for a variety of issues to one nurse practitioner (NP) and one physician's assistant (PA), both stationed on the dedicated orthopedic ward. If relevant medical issues arise that require hospitalist involvement, they will find us on the ward and relay the information to us. This allows us as hospitalists to focus on the more sophisticated medical issues that are more consistent with our scope of practice; in addition, we can also serve as the gatekeeper to further subspecialty consultation when needed, avoiding superfluous consultations and testing.

4. How would a comanagement service affect other relationships? For example, consultants or other medical groups who traditionally round on their own patients may lose revenue as a result of this service.

5. Does the hospitalist service have adequate staffing to expand services? Initially, comanagement may be limited to certain groups who admit to the hospitalist service, or to specific diagnoses, or time of day.

ANALYZE THE CURRENT STRUCTURE

Analysis of the current structure of care delivery in surgical or medical subspecialty services serves a useful measurement both as a baseline and after the intervention. In our analysis at the Cleveland Clinic, we found that there were significant differences in the delivery of care on medical services and orthopedic services due to the following factors:

- Limited supervision of medical care provided by the NP and PA.
- Competing responsibilities of orthopedic residents providing backup for other providers or assisting in the operating room.
- Lack of internal medicine training of orthopedic residents to address complicated medical issues.
- Significant medical comorbidities of patients requiring routine medical surveillance to prevent, detect, and intervene during their hospitalization.
- Limitations of general medical consultation service that typically "reacts" to consultation requests when problems have already been identified and lacks the capacity to prospectively affirm or develop a medical plan of care for high-risk or complicated medical patients.

CLARIFY ROLES AND EXPECTATIONS

At this point clarifying and documenting roles and expectations may avoid the potential for confusion and divisiveness. **Table 4-1** outlines our expectations for our hospitalist roles and responsibilities and the ongoing orthopedic roles and responsibilities. **Table 4-2** lists the conditions that should trigger referral to the hospitalist comanagement service.

These are not firm and inflexible rules; other comanagement relationships may opt to take on some of the responsibilities listed above in the orthopedic section, such as blood and fluid management, pain management, and communication with patients and families regarding medical issues, all of which are in a reasonable scope of hospitalist practice. However, it is critical to delineate who will take on these tasks and to have a mechanism for resolution of disagreements. Some hospitalists may wish to "specialize" in comanagement and become more familiar with the specialty. See Part II (Medical Consultation), Section V (Specialty Consultation: What the Consulting Hospitalist Needs to Know).

TABLE 4-1 Delineation of Hospitalist versus Orthopedics Roles and Responsibilities

Hospitalist	Orthopedics
Confer each morning with orthopedic providers and review outpatient preoperative assessment (done in our hospitalist-run preoperative clinic) or the medical comorbidities of nonelective admissions to identify suitable patients for comanagement	Retain the appropriate clinical support infrastructure including residents and current physician's assistant and nurse practitioner positions
Promptly evaluate and document findings on comanaged patients, and enter orders on these patients	Perform daily rounding, assessments, and progress notes and orders for routine and stable medical issues including postoperative orders
Follow-up on tests and studies ordered by the comanager	Address the "first call" from nurses for questions and patient assessments, perform full and appropriate patient assessments prior to calling medical physicians for further support
Provide formal and informal preoperative and postoperative medical consultation as requested	Remain as primary service for patients without substantial medical complexity
Provide teaching to orthopedic surgery service providers on medical issues	Provide night, weekend, and holiday coverage of orthopedic patients with support by the medicine consult resident
Participate in daily multidisciplinary rounds with nursing, nonphysician providers, and case management to identify patients with ongoing medical needs not otherwise captured by the mechanisms above	Follow-up on studies and tests ordered by the orthopedic service
	Address routine postoperative management orders including:
	Initiate and comply with orthopedic protocols
	Manage blood and fluids
	Manage pain and routine prn medications
	Order DVT prophylaxis and medications
	Assess and care for wounds and order perioperative antibiotics
	Admit and plan discharge, prepare forms, and provide discharge prescriptions
	Communicate with families and facilitate discharge planning

Periodic meetings between hospitalist and orthopedic champions as well as nursing, other members of the comanagement team, and administration should review program functioning and processes of care; address specific problems in direct patient care; and further define roles and expectations. In addition, this group may assess the impact of the comanagement service on teaching of medical and surgical trainees and explore future directions. Our medicine residents rotate with our hospitalist comanager as part of their medical consultation experience, and our relationship provides opportunities for creating academic value such as the potential for publication of outcomes data, collaboration in research, and orthopedic quality improvement projects. **Table 4-3** delineates the development timeline of our comanagement service.

PATIENT SELECTION AND TRIAGE

Decisions about which patients should be followed by the comanager should be based on patient needs and provider capacity. Patients with minimal or no medical comorbidities rarely benefit from hospitalist input and may only serve to direct clinician efforts away from the patients that need more intensive medical attention. Patients with acutely decompensated problems and/or multiple chronic comorbidities will more likely benefit from comanagement attention; in some circumstances, admission to a medical service with orthopedic consultation may be the most appropriate path. **Figure 4-1** delineates the decision process for triage at our institution.

ROLE OF A PREOPERATIVE ASSESSMENT CLINIC

Some institutions (including ours) have an internist- or hospitalist-run preoperative assessment clinic that works in conjunction with the surgeon and anesthesiologist to provide a broad systematic evaluation of readiness for surgery and to facilitate optimization of key medical conditions. Instead of being seen in the hospital or by the patient's primary care provider, clinicians with more concentrated expertise in assessing and preparing patients for surgery see the patient in advance and then communicate their findings and recommendations to the surgeon and anesthesiologist. In our case, we also communicate with the orthopedic comanager via e-mail, page, or shared EMR (electronic medical record) patient list about planned admissions of surgical patients with relevant comorbidities. The preoperative clinic model may reduce cancellation rates and may identify decompensated medical problems that might lead to increased perioperative morbidity and mortality, as well as identify conditions that could easily decompensate if not scrutinized (eg, excessive intravenous fluids postoperatively in a patient with systolic heart failure).

MEASURING SUCCESS

Defining what constitutes success of the program in measurable terms is an essential piece of the puzzle, as it may provide information about practice changes, variability of practice patterns, outcome changes, and financial benefits or risks of the relationship.

Table 4-4 lists some suggested metrics to consider at the outset. It would also help to obtain data on these metrics prior to the initiation of comanagement to determine the influence of the program.

Especially challenging for the modern orthopedic surgeon is that since August 2008 the U.S. Centers for Medicare and Medicaid Services (CMS) has included deep venous thrombosis and pulmonary embolism after total knee arthroplasty and total hip arthroplasty on the list of nonreimbursed Hospital Acquired Conditions.

TABLE 4-2 Conditions Triggering Referral to Comanagement Service

Chronic Medical Conditions

- Stable or known coronary artery disease (chest pain, shortness of breath [SOB], electrocardiogram [ECG] changes)
- Congestive heart failure (SOB, pulmonary edema, edema, oxygen desaturation)
- Hypertension (especially if blood pressure > 160 systolic blood pressure or > 100 diastolic blood pressure)
- History of stroke
- Moderate/severe peripheral vascular disease
- Mild-moderate chronic obstructive pulmonary disease (COPD) (SOB, wheezing, oxygen desaturation)
- Mild-moderate/stable asthma (SOB, wheezing, oxygen desaturation)
- Current antibiotic treatment for pneumonia/acute bronchitis
- History of upper/lower GI bleed in the last 3 mo (drop in Hgb/Hct, concern for active bleeding)
- Patients on chronic enteral tube feedings or hyperalimentation/total parenteral nutrition (TPN) (in addition to nutrition team/TPN consult)
- Diabetes mellitus type 1 or 2
- Stable psychiatric illnesses including affective disorders, dementias, bipolar disorder, schizophrenia (with additional psychiatry consultation for medication concerns or decompensation of psychiatric illness)
- Chronic anticoagulation (comanagement consultation on all patients)
- Recent anticoagulation for deep vein thrombosis (DVT) or pulmonary embolism (PE) within the last 6 mo (comanagement consultation on all patients and possibly vascular medicine consultation)
- Chronic immunosuppression (prednisone, cyclosporine, methotrexate, FK 506, azathioprine, TNF-alpha blockers, etc)
- Physiologic glucocorticoid treatment within the last year (≥ 7.5 mg/d of prednisone, or the equivalent, for ≥ 2 wks)
- Medical issues that require medical evaluation, monitoring, or treatment:
  - Atypical chest pain without evidence of an acute coronary syndrome
  - Shortness of breath
  - Acute DVT or PE
  - Baseline anemia or postoperative anemia
  - Urinary tract infection with indwelling Foley catheter
  - Acute delirium
  - Electrolyte disorders
  - Hyperglycemia without evidence of diabetic ketoacidosis (DKA) or nonketotic/hyperosmolar state
  - Acute renal failure
  - Others

A portion of the payment made by CMS to hospitals is withheld if a patient experiences deep venous thrombosis or pulmonary embolism following one of these procedures. While this decision has been criticized because prophylaxis is neither perfect nor risk free, it is a reality of practice, and the hospitalist comanager must be aware of this and engage the orthopedist regarding appropriate evidence-based prophylaxis methods.

One must keep in mind that not all metrics can be expected to improve in a "positive" way; in the study described previously about hip fractures, the rates of delirium were increased, which traditionally would be perceived as a negative result. However, this was due to increased recognition, documentation, and treatment of delirium by physicians, which many would agree is a beneficial intervention. Also, these individual metrics are not in a vacuum; an increase in

TABLE 4-3 CCF Program Timeline

December 2007	Presentation of the concept of the "embedded consultant" with a mini white paper summarizing the literature regarding benefits of comanagement by the department of orthopedics to the chairs of the Medicine Institute and department of Hospital Medicine
December 2007–March 2008	Draft proposal resulting from outreach to existing programs and internal multidisciplinary planning
March 2008	Acceptance of pilot program by departments of Hospital Medicine and orthopedics
March 2008	Presentation of proposed pilot to hospital operations committee and approval of the hiring of two additional full-time equivalent (FTE) for the program
April 2008–July 2008	Recruitment and finalization of pilot protocols with NPs
August 2008	Kickoff
Ongoing	Oversight with orthopedic champion
	Metrics collection
	Creation of a link with IMPACT (preoperative clinic)

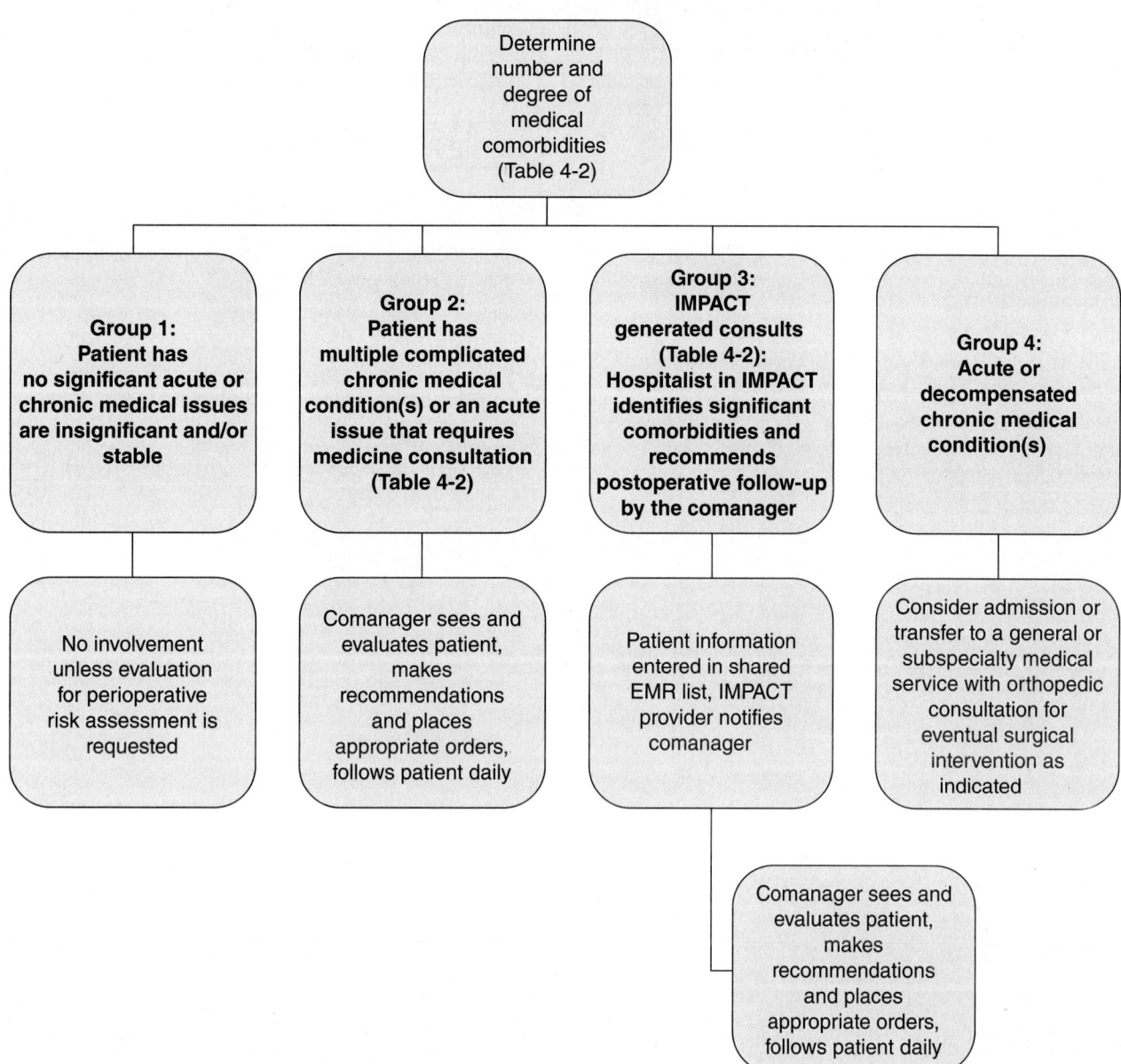

Figure 4-1 *Cleveland Clinic orthopedic comanagement triage algorithm.*

length of hospital stay coupled with decreased readmission rates might reflect the hospitalist taking an extra half to full day to optimize certain medical conditions, which results in fewer readmissions for decompensation.

Early results revealed that our program provided a net cost savings to the orthopedic department in terms of reduced surgical cancellations and improved patient satisfaction with care delivery.

CONCLUSION

Comanagement of specialty patients provides a novel diversity of practice to hospitalists and may be professional rewarding with improved collegiality with surgical specialties, opportunities for leadership, and quality improvement research. Engaging in a new comanagement relationship requires forethought and planning, and clarifying expectations, responsibilities, and metrics of success. However, when designed and managed well, a comanagement service can benefit hospitalists, surgeons, and, most importantly, the patients who trust us with their care.

TABLE 4-4 Proposed Program Metrics

Volume data
Case mix
Patient satisfaction
Length of stay
OR cancellation rates
Hospital cost and ancillary utilization
Productivity measures (RVUs and billing)
Provider satisfaction (hospitalist, orthopedist, nursing, residents)
Mortality
Unplanned ICU or medical service transfers
Readmission rates
Quality/patient safety metrics
JCAHO core measures

SUGGESTED READINGS

Fisher AA, Davis MW, Rubenach SE, et al. Outcomes for older patients with hip fractures: the impact of orthopedic and geriatric medicine cocare. *J Orthopaed Trauma.* 2006;20(3):172-178; discussion 9-80.

Jaffer A, Michota F. Why perioperative medicine matters more than ever. *Clev Clin J Med.* 2006:73(Suppl 1);2006:S1.

Marcantonio ER, Flacker JM, Wright RJ, et al. Reducing delirium after hip fracture: a randomized trial. *J Am Geriatr Soc.* 2001; 49(5):516-522.

Sharma G, Kuo Y, Freeman J, et al. Comanagement of hospitalized surgical patients by medicine physicians in the United States. *Arch Intern Med.* 2010;170(4):363-368.

Streiff MB, Haut ER. The CMS ruling on venous thromboembolism after total knee or hip arthroplasty: weighing risks and benefits. *JAMA.* 2009;301(10):1063-1065.

Zuckerman JD, Sakales SR, Fabian DR, et al. Hip fractures in geriatric patients. Results of an interdisciplinary hospital care program. *Clin Orthopaed Relat Res.* 1992;274:213-225.

ONLINE RESOURCES

American Academy of Orthopedic Surgeons. *The Burden of Musculoskeletal Diseases in the United States: Prevalence, Societal and Economic Cost;* 2012. http://www.boneandjointburden.org/. Accessed September 13, 2015.

Hospital Acquired Conditions (Present on Admission Indicator). http://www.cms.gov/HospitalAcqCond. Accessed September 13, 2015.

Society of Hospital Medicine. *Measuring Hospitalist Performance: Metrics, Reports and Dashboards;* 2006. http://www.hospitalmedicine.org/AM/Template.cfm?Section=White_Papers&Template=/CM/HTMLDisplay.cfm&ContentID=14632. Accessed March 10, 2010.

CHAPTER 5

Professionalism in Hospital Medicine

Kimberly D. Manning, MD, FACP, FAAP

Professionalism in medicine has long focused on the tenets of patient welfare, patient autonomy and social justice. As health care has evolved, our definitions and value statements have broadened. Evidence-based medicine, quality improvement, access to care, cost-effective practices, and conflicts of interest are now at the forefront of these discussions—all of which are salient in hospital medicine.

The 2002 jointly published *Medical Professionalism in the New Millennium: A Physician Charter* articulated fundamental principles and responsibilities to which all physicians should aim to maintain. The ABIM Foundation, The European Federation of Internal Medicine, and the ACP Foundation worked together to develop a charter that reconciled the selfless expectations of the physician with the ever-changing landscape of health care delivery. The American Academy of Pediatrics' Committee on Bioethics followed with their policy statement on professionalism in pediatrics, which addressed some of the unique considerations for those caring for children.

Hospitalists are trusted with the well being of some of the most vulnerable patients. This distinctive contract with society calls for some variation in our emphasis when discussing professionalism. Here we will define professionalism in hospital medicine, clarify concepts most applicable to those caring for hospitalized patients, and translate this into clinical practice. These concepts apply to all clinicians at all levels, team members, and hospital systems caring for patients admitted to the hospital.

WHAT DOES "PROFESSIONALISM" MEAN IN HOSPITAL MEDICINE?

Members of any profession are expected to have acquired a body of knowledge and skills specific to their chosen field. Through a shared commitment, there is self-regulation and a contract with society to judiciously apply skills and expertise. Hospitalists, like all physicians, have made an agreement to heal. This pact requires an establishment of trust and a willingness to place patient needs above all other considerations. Self-regulation is administered through state medical boards, clinical leadership, and ethical codes. Professionalism is what binds this treaty to our profession.

The high stakes and lack of predictability in caring for inpatients creates unique challenges for hospitalists. Beyond the standard definitions of medical professionalism, special emphasis on patient safety, provider interdependency and communication, financial reimbursement and patient satisfaction reshape our understanding and must always be considered. Finally, with a substantial component of undergraduate, graduate and interprofessional training taking place in the hospital setting, the impact of hidden curricula in medical education is arguably greatest in hospital medicine. Given this, the ripple effects of our behaviors are far reaching. Professionalism for the hospitalist translates to more than outcomes for patients—it has the potential to define generational culture in medicine.

PROFESSIONALISM AND PATIENT SAFETY

Safety for hospitalized patient relies upon a collaborative work climate, teamwork, and effective communication. Intimidating and disruptive behaviors have been linked to increases in medical errors, poor patient satisfaction, cost of care and higher rates of attrition for staff. Behaviors that threaten the performance of the health care team create significant barriers to quality.

In 2008, the Joint Commission released a sentinel event alert addressing behaviors that undermine a culture of safety. From this came new requirements:

1. Every hospital or patient care organization should have a code of conduct defining acceptable and disruptive behaviors.
2. Hospital leadership must have processes in place for managing inappropriate or disruptive behaviors.

Disruptive behaviors have been described as a spectrum of actions such as egregious verbal and physical actions to subtle refusals to cooperate within a system. Specifically, this could manifest as reluctance to answer phone calls or pages, condescending intonation with nurses, colleagues and patients and impatience with queries. These behaviors are not rare in health care organizations. In a survey conducted by the Institution of Safe Medication Practices on intimidation, as many as 40% of clinicians reported keeping quiet or remaining passive rather than confront an intimidating person. Other surveys have revealed that such behaviors are not limited to one gender or a specific discipline. In hospital medicine, which relies upon frequent transitions of care and heavy collaboration with nurses and colleagues, this can pose significant threats to patients.

The standard in hospital organizations should also include (but are not limited to) these additional recommendations from the Joint Commission:

1. Education of all team members defined by the organization's code of conduct with particular emphasis on respect.
2. Accountability of all team members to model desirable behaviors regardless of hierarchal rank with equitable consequences and reinforcement.
3. "Zero tolerance" for intimidating and/or disruptive behaviors with incorporation of specific verbiage into by-laws and employee agreements.
4. Protection of those who report witnessing or experiencing disruptive behaviors through nonretaliation clauses in policy statements.
5. Timely and thorough responses to all patients and/or families with emphasis on acknowledgement, empathy, and apology.
6. Development of organizational processes that solicit input from a broad representation of team members when addressing intimidating and disruptive behaviors including encouragement of ongoing interprofessional dialogue.
7. Offering training for all leaders and managers of hospital groups to build skills in team building, conflict resolution, and feedback on unprofessional behavior.
8. Assessment of the working climate to assess perceptions of unprofessional behaviors and risk of harm to patients.
9. Provision of anonymous and confidential surveillance and reporting systems for detecting unprofessional behavior.
10. Clear documentation of all attempts to address intimidating and disruptive behaviors with outcomes.

PROFESSIONALISM ISSUES AMONG HOSPITALISTS

Hospitalists strive to provide uninterrupted care to hospitalized patients. Given this, transitions of care and responsibility are dependent upon respectful interactions between providers. Provider interdependency also plays a role in patient satisfaction, burnout risk, and quality. Healthy relationships and working climates are essential though challenging to maintain.

In a study published in the Journal of Hospital Medicine, Reddy and colleagues looked at participation in unprofessional behaviors among internal medicine hospitalists. They found that factors most likely to underlie such behaviors were: making fun of others, learning environment, workload management and time pressure.

Additionally, from this study we glean that certain job and provider characteristics increased this likelihood.

Hospitalists with less clinical time were more likely to make fun of other colleagues. It is postulated that those with heavier clinical loads have more opportunities to form relationships and are thus more apt to avoid unflattering commentary of others. Moreover, more clinical time could also cause hospitalists to be less easily influenced by the opinions of others. Night work and age also seemed to be factors in unprofessional behaviors. Those working at night felt more pressure to wrap up work. Hasty handovers and celebration of intercepted admissions are just a few things that could happen as a result.

Given the understanding that unique characteristics increase the incidence of unprofessional behaviors, special attention should be given to more junior hospitalists as well as those with night shifts, limited clinical duties due to competing priorities, and at sites known for heavier workloads. Efforts to better understand the reasons for participating in these behaviors should continue to be explored.

PROFESSIONALISM AND PATIENT SATISFACTION

Patient satisfaction is linked to reimbursements and is a key factor in determining quality of care. Interestingly, the technical dimensions of quality of care are rarely called into question with regards to hospitalized patients. Instead, perception of quality for patients is most connected to what is personally valued by patients and their families. Among those things being treated with respect and dignity coupled with clear communication around treatment decisions are areas that have been identified to be of paramount importance to patients. Professional behaviors are generally the defining features of these perceptions.

Surveys have been developed to best ascertain patient satisfaction in hospitals. The Hospital Consumer Assessment of Healthcare Provider and Systems (HCAHPS) is now the core metric against which health care systems are evaluated. As the first national, standardized and publicly reported survey of patients' viewpoints on hospital care, HCAHPS now serves as a tool for valid comparisons between hospitals locally, regionally and nationally.

A random sample of patients receives this survey between 48 hours and 6 weeks after discharge. Among the 32 questions about their hospitalization, patients are asked to recall their perceptions of physician and nurse communication, responsiveness of hospital staff, communication about medications and care transition. Though HCAHPS data are not limited to hospitalists, as the "face" of the hospitalization for many patients their impact can be substantial. Special attention to communication skills training, strategic planning around availability to patients and enhanced discharge paperwork and medication reconciliation are just a few measures that have been shown to improve potential areas of weakness. Other simple tips have been offered to enhance patient satisfaction and experience include:

- Make a positive patient experience a part of the culture.
- Adopt patient-centered, multidisciplinary rounds with transparent discussions that include patients.
- Avoid giving off cues of indifference or uncaring (eg, rushing, lack of eye contact, standing instead of sitting).
- Encourage every employee to think about purpose and people, not just tasks.
- Equip every team member with skills for handling patient or family member complaints.
- Recognize that system inadequacies can be responsible for individual lapses in professionalism. Unreasonable scheduling algorithms and workloads are examples of system issues that can undermine professional behavior.
- Collect and act on data related to patient satisfaction.

Hospitalists are poised to have great impact in all of these areas through their continuum of contact throughout the hospitalization. Intentional approaches to both individual behaviors and the systems in which hospitalists work are essential.

PROFESSIONALISM AND THE ACADEMIC ENVIRONMENT

The Accreditation Council of Graduate Medical Education (ACGME) and the Liaison Committee on Medical Education (LCME) have identified professionalism as a crucial competency for developing physicians and have labored to build program requirements around this expectation. For example, the LCME uses this verbiage in their accreditation data collection tools for medical schools:

A medical school ensures that the learning environment of its medical education program is conducive to the ongoing development of explicit and appropriate professional behaviors in its medical students, faculty, and staff at all locations and is one in which all individuals are treated with respect. The medical school and its clinical affiliates share the responsibility for periodic evaluation of the learning environment in order to identify positive and negative influences on the maintenance of professional standards, develop and conduct appropriate strategies to enhance positive and mitigate negative influences, and identify and promptly correct violations of professional standards.

The hospital setting accounts for a substantial proportion of learning environments in undergraduate and graduate medical education. Given this fact, the importance of professionalism must be emphasized for hospitalists through institutional efforts and programs.

Medical education literature informs us that learners report that values exhibited by their teachers and institutions directly impact their own professionalism. Regrettably, a majority of medical students endorse witnessing peers and supervising physicians speaking of patients and/or other health care professionals in unflattering, cynical or derogatory ways. Multiple studies have shown that the humanistic attitudes essential to patient-centered care unravel during medical school and residency, increasing the risk of burnout and depression.

Hospital medicine provides much of the backdrop for this "hidden curriculum," originally described by Hafferty as *"a set of influences that function at the level of organizational structure and culture."* There can be profound dichotomy between the negative behaviors exhibited by some physician role models and the desired attributes described in formal curricula. The insidious nature of a hidden curriculum is powerful enough to become institutional culture. Newer mandates through accreditation organizations call for more honest appraisals of the informal influences on learners. They also charge institutions with building ongoing strategies to reshape and mitigate their untoward effects.

NEW CONSIDERATIONS

■ PROFESSIONALISM AND DIRECT PHARMACEUTICAL MARKETING

The interaction between physicians and the pharmaceutical industry and its sales representatives remains controversial. Though lessening in frequency, direct marketing (usually trade name drugs) promoted to providers and groups through gifts, sponsored meals and lectures, travel and symposia are not foreign to most physicians. Though clinicians do not typically report that such interactions influence their prescribing practices, evidence supports otherwise. A large meta-analysis of over 500 studies revealed that attending sponsored CME events, accepting funding for travel, and participating in pharmaceutical sponsored lectures were associated with

certain prescribing and professional behavior. Institutional policies are in place at many hospitals regarding disclosure of conflicts of interest. This continues to be an important discussion at the level of policy and education, as well as among professional organizations such as Society of Hospital Medicine (SHM), American College of Physicians (ACP), and Society of General Internal Medicine (SGIM).

■ PROFESSIONALISM AND SOCIAL MEDIA

Social media has redefined the interface between physicians, patients, learners, and the public. The once passive viewing of content on early iterations of the websites has exploded over the last decade to include interactive exchanging, sharing and communication in real time. Facebook, Twitter, Instagram, and LinkedIn are among the most widely used social media platforms, all made even more accessible by recent advances in mobile smartphone technology and their near universal use by the public. As of 2014, it was estimated that more than 1 billion people were on Facebook and, of these individuals, nearly 400 million only log in using mobile smartphones. Tablets, Internet ready televisions and even smart watches, all with capability to access these same social media platforms, have also emerged in very recent years. These developments, along with more unrestricted Wi-Fi "hotspots" (even in most hospitals) and robust search engines using collective intelligence tools, have closed the gaps that once stood between the professional and private personas of physicians.

Though social media presents new challenges to the landscape of medical professionalism, it also presents opportunities. Specific health information can be quickly disseminated to large groups of individuals in moments. Platforms aimed toward health professionals such as Doximity offer encrypted, HIPAA compliant privacy settings for idea sharing, consultation, and collaboration in ways previously unforeseen. Moreover, Twitter use at professional meetings keeps attendees and allows those unable to leave the hospital to stay abreast of ongoing activities as they are happening. In less than half of a decade this culture of "tweeting" professional meetings in real time has become not only a welcomed feature but an expected one as well.

A growing number of academic institutions and organizations have begun to develop policies about judicious use of social media, most of which emphasize confidentiality. Professional development centered on social media is becoming more frequent on meeting agendas. From concrete tips on privacy settings to abstract ways to seize collaborative opportunities, hospitalists and other health care providers should all gain some proficiency with social media and its potential impact on the care of patients.

CONCLUSION

Hospitalists, with their large imprint in medical education and contract to care for a diverse and vulnerable patient population, must approach professionalism with intentionality. New considerations such as direct pharmaceutical marketing and social media have shifted prior understandings of what it means to be a medical professional. Thoughtful consideration of professional behaviors along with their impact on patient safety, patient satisfaction, and the hidden curriculum should guide ongoing individual, institutional and organizational development.

SUGGESTED READINGS

Gholami-Kordkheili F, Wild V, Strech D. The impact of social media on medical professionalism: asystemic qualitative review of challenges and opportunities. *J Med Internet Res.* 2013;15(8):e184.

Hafferty FW. Beyond curriculum reform: confronting medicine's hidden curriculum. *Acad Med.* 1998;73(4):403-407.

Joint Commission: Behaviors that undermine a culture of safety. *Sentinel Event Alert*. vol. 40. http://www.jointcommission.org/sentinel_event_alert_issue_40_behaviors_that_undermine_a_culture_of_safety/. Accessed July 9, 2008.

Kirk LM. Professionalism in medicine: definitions and considerations for teaching. *Proc (Bayl Univ Med Cent)*. 2007;20(1):13-16.

Project of the ABIM Foundation, ACP–ASIM Foundation, and European Federation of Internal Medicine. Medical professionalism in the new millennium: a physician charter. *Ann Intern Med*. 2002;136:243-246.

Rosenstein AH, O'Daniel M. A survey of the impact of disruptive behavior and communication defects on patient safety. *Joint Comm J Qual Patient Saf*. 2008;34(8):464-471.

Swick HM. Toward a normative definition of medical professionalism. *Acad Med*. 2000;75(6):612-616.

CHAPTER 6

Principles of Leadership

Steven Weinberger, MD, FACP

Physicians are frequently called upon to take on leadership roles. These roles can come in various forms, ranging from academic leadership roles (eg, division or department chief or chair) to educational leadership roles (eg, clerkship or residency program director) to leadership roles in a practice setting (eg, director of a practice group). Although some of the desired skills and competencies for the leader may be specific to particular roles and responsibilities, others are more generic and applicable to any of these leadership positions. This chapter concentrates initially on the generic aspects of leadership and concludes by discussing some of the challenges that are more specific to hospitalists and to the hospital environment. In addition, instead of trying to review the voluminous leadership literature, presented here will be a personal perspective, based upon experiences in a variety of leadership positions over many years. Discussion of leadership will be divided into four primary components: the *personal attributes* that a leader should demonstrate, the *skills* that should be acquired, a suggested *approach to reach a goal*, and *leadership challenges* for hospitalists in the hospital environment.

LEADERS VERSUS MANAGERS

Before considering the important attributes of a leader, it is worthwhile to understand the distinction between a *leader* and a *manager*. Much has been written about these differences, which can be readily summarized and understood by any of several descriptions or aphorisms:

- Leaders have followers; managers have subordinates. Individuals voluntarily follow a leader because of the qualities of the leader; subordinates work for managers because of the reporting relationship and the organizational authority vested in the manager.
- Leaders lead people; managers manage tasks.
- Leadership is doing the right thing; management is doing things right.
- Managers focus on tactics and tasks; leaders focus on strategy and direction.

In fact, however, these distinctions often blur in the setting of actual roles and responsibilities in the workplace. The individuals who are most successful in assuming roles with greater authority and responsibility are those who are both effective leaders and effective managers. A leader who does not have good management skills can generate visionary ideas but will be unable to implement or operationalize them. A manager who does not have good leadership skills will be unable to mobilize and motivate a supportive team.

Some activities and responsibilities of a physician leading a group of hospitalists can readily illustrate the differences between leadership and management. "Managing" the group means assuring that the patients are covered, that transitions of care are effectively handled, that chart and billing documentation is complete and accurate, and that teaching responsibilities are assigned and well integrated with patient care responsibilities. In contrast, "leading" the group means exploring and developing ideas for improving the system and its productivity, improving quality of care, developing the skills of the team, and facilitating the professional development of the team members.

For the purposes of this chapter, I will primarily use the terms "leadership" and "leadership skills," recognizing, however, that we are really considering both leadership and management skills. In the medical leadership positions that are likely to be assumed by readers of this chapter, success will hinge upon both leadership and managerial qualities and the importance of each in reinforcing the other. Therefore, the approach here to discussing leadership and management qualities will be one of lumping rather than splitting.

DESIRABLE ATTRIBUTES OF THE LEADER

A leader must demonstrate professional integrity, including honesty. High standards of integrity and honesty are a prerequisite for obtaining the respect of colleagues, superiors, and subordinates. The leader sets the model of behavior for the rest of the team, and lack of professional integrity exhibited by the leader will soon be mirrored by cracks in professionalism among others.

The leader needs to be an effective communicator; openness and transparency in communicating to all constituencies assure that everyone is on the same page. A commonly held perception of a talented leader is often someone who can communicate both values and vision, including a set of goals and how those goals might be achieved. However, that is only part of the communication equation, which also involves establishing and transmitting expectations for others. It is critical that subordinates, trainees, and team members understand the expectations being placed on them, including how and on what basis they are being judged.

Communication must also occur on a two-way street, that is, the leader must be an excellent listener as well. If the leader is unable or unwilling to hear what others have to say, he or she will be doomed to failure. Without ideas and feedback from others, the leader will invariably make mistakes of both commission and omission that can be avoided by hearing the ideas and opinions of others and considering all perspectives when making important decisions.

Another important aspect of communication relates to feedback. The effective leader provides feedback in a constructive, professional manner. This feedback must be based on established expectations, not on the subordinate's or trainee's ability to read the leader's mind and guess what s/he wants. In addition, the feedback should be done in a way that is formative, that is, giving the receiver of the feedback an opportunity to, and advice on how to improve performance. Providing only summative feedback at the end of a responsibility or task allows no room for improvement and often proves frustrating to the person receiving the feedback.

An effective leader remembers that success is determined by the contributions or development of the people s/he leads or trains. The leader must acknowledge the contributions of others and not always take credit for success. Nothing is as demoralizing to a team member as the feeling that his contributions are not being recognized and that someone else is taking credit for his work or accomplishments. At the same time, a successful leader is cognizant of, and aims to promote the professional development of the individuals for which she is responsible. For example, true success for an academic leader is often determined as much by the ultimate careers of the individuals trained by the leader, as it is by the academic contributions of the leader himself. Supporting the professional development of one's trainees is one of the most important and enduring legacies that a leader can leave to the profession.

Finally, an intangible but critical quality of a successful leader is the ability to create and maintain a positive work environment. The leader needs to establish a workplace tone that is positive, in which people feel they are supported and a "can do" attitude prevails. Productivity of the individuals for whom a leader is responsible is dependent upon their interest in, and commitment to the team and to the shared goals and vision that have been defined by the leader. A setting in which individuals are competitive with each other, where back-biting is common, and people feel they do not respect and share the values of their colleagues and the leader, is not an enjoyable workplace. It is also one that will never reach its true potential.

LEADERSHIP SKILLS

An important prerequisite for a successful leader is a high level of competence in the particular field related to the leadership role. For example, an educational leader must be accomplished as a teacher and educator in order to command the necessary respect of trainees and other educational colleagues. Similarly, a clinical leader must be highly regarded as an excellent clinician in order to have credibility with other clinicians.

Another important skill that leaders must acquire is the ability to negotiate effectively. This topic is covered extensively in a later chapter (Chapter 26, Negotiation and Conflict Resolution), but it is important to stress that leaders must exercise their negotiation skills in many settings—when dealing with superiors, dealing with subordinates, or dealing with third parties with whom there is no reporting relationship. Physicians typically have not been trained in negotiation, but fortunately a number of excellent and readily accessible resources can provide valuable guidance to the previously untrained leader.

Many leaders have responsibility for budgets, and a working familiarity with balance sheets and with revenue and expense statements is therefore useful. Although providing such financial training is beyond the scope of this chapter, a valuable resource that can provide basic training in the principles of accounting is a short, easy to read, programmed text used in many business schools.

Finally, the responsibility of running meetings often accompanies leadership roles. Everyone has participated in meetings that run effectively, where the participants feel they have not wasted their time, and they leave the meeting with a well-defined action plan. On the other hand, everyone has also participated in meetings that are poorly organized, do not make best use of participants' time, and do not have a well-defined purpose or outcome. Several important aspects of well-designed meetings include:

- **Sending an advance agenda to the participants,** so that they can prepare appropriately.
- **Starting on time and finishing on time (or early).** Time is an incredibly valuable commodity, and meeting participants become distracted and resentful when time is wasted at the beginning of a meeting or when a meeting runs overtime and potentially affects their subsequent commitments.
- **Assuring that the meeting is interactive and makes good use of the participants' time and expertise.** A successful meeting is not a monologue provided by the meeting coordinator. Rather, it involves active engagement and participation by all attendees, so that the participants feel they have contributed to the meeting and have not just been wasting their time.
- **Wrapping up the meeting with a summary and a well-defined action plan.** Everyone should understand the outcome of the meeting and the expected action plan, including the *assignments* that have been meted out to individuals and the *timeline* according to which they should be completed.

REACHING A GOAL

In trying to generate ideas and complete desired tasks necessary to reach a goal, the successful leader may find it helpful to use a set of principles: (1) establish the goal, (2) identify and include stakeholders, (3) assemble a team, (4) engage all team members to generate ideas, (5) accept ideas from outside the team or organization, (6) delegate responsibility, and (7) assess interim outcomes and reassess the plan.

At the outset, the leader needs to *establish the goal* and communicate it to others. In other words, the leader must define the destination before anyone can plot the route of how to get there. Success in achieving a goal depends critically upon the process of engaging others at least as much as the goal itself. This process involves *identifying stakeholders* who are either impacted by the goal, or who will feel disenfranchised if they have not been included in developing or working to achieve the goal. For example, if a residency program director needs to restructure a schedule for the residents based upon changing regulatory requirements, s/he is much more likely to be successful when including residents in developing the new model, rather than imposing it upon them without their input. No matter how sound an idea or plan, its acceptance and implementation can be obstructed by those who were not included or engaged—but feel they should have been—in its generation and development.

In making plans for a project or reaching a goal, the leader often needs to *establish a team* of individuals who can work together. Assembling the right people is critical for a successful outcome. Team members need to be chosen based upon their skills, their interest in and enthusiasm for the project, their ability to work well with others on the team, and their openness in providing ideas and feedback about how things are going.

Once the goal is established, stakeholders are identified, and the team is assembled, the leader must recognize that s/he does not need to generate all the ideas. Great work is typically done in teams in which everyone is encouraged to *share ideas*, no matter how crazy or far-fetched they may initially seem. In addition, not all good ideas need to come from within the team. One can adopt and build upon ideas and successful initiatives that have been developed by individuals outside the organization. The "not invented here" attitude often precludes an open mind to accepting ideas that have worked successfully in other settings.

The ideas necessary to reach a goal are often not grand and sweeping ones. A series of small steps, each of which can be judged and modified as necessary based upon the outcome achieved, is often more successful than a single, revolutionary idea that does not allow for opportunities to provide mid-course assessment and correction.

In making the best use of the team members, the leader must be willing to *delegate responsibility* appropriately. From the time of their training, physicians are often used to feeling that they need to take full responsibility for a patient, and this attitude of individual responsibility and accountability should often be modified when one assumes leadership responsibilities. Members of a team work best when they feel that responsibility has been bestowed upon them. Delegating responsibility is not a sign of weakness; rather, appropriate delegation demonstrates an understanding of how to share responsibility, engage others, make best use of available resources, and capitalize on each person's strengths.

As a project progresses, the leader must critically *assess interim outcomes*. Based upon these outcomes, the leader must be willing to *reassess the plan* and adjust accordingly. The leader and the team members should also recognize that not all plans will be successful. A plan that does not succeed should not necessarily be viewed as a failure. Important lessons are often learned and new ideas generated based upon unanticipated problems or unexpected results.

LEADERSHIP CHALLENGES IN THE HOSPITAL ENVIRONMENT

Hospitalists who are in leadership positions or who are expected to effect change are often confronted with challenges that arise specifically from working in the hospital environment. Besides dealing with physicians, hospitalists are constantly working with nonphysician personnel and administrators whose management and reporting structure is quite independent of the physicians at the institution. A hospitalist leader who is trying to effect change but is not part of the hospital's administrative hierarchy may have difficulty shaping opinions and getting buy-in from a group of nursing leaders or from nonphysician hospital administrators. Even among physician leaders at the hospital, challenges arise often centered around a competition for resources, so that the interpersonal relationships become adversarial rather than cooperative.

An additional challenge confronted by hospitalists stems from their basic demographic characteristics. Age, gender and even race could impact abilities to break into a hospital hierarchy that tends to be older, male, and Caucasian. A young physician who goes on staff as a hospitalist at the institution where s/he completed residency may find it difficult to shake the image of being a resident rather than a staff member and colleague. On the other hand, a young hospitalist who takes a position at an institution where s/he did not train may find it difficult to parachute in as a newcomer unfamiliar with a particular hospital's culture and personalities.

Although there are no proven methods to overcome such challenges, some strategies may be helpful. First, it is extremely valuable to obtain the trust and support of a more senior, well-respected person, ideally a current physician leader at the institution. Such an individual not only can serve as a mentor and advisor to guide the hospitalist in charting a path through unfamiliar territory, but s/he can also smooth the way for the young hospitalist to become accepted by the more established hospital hierarchy. For example, the support and trust from a well-respected division chief or department chair can be invaluable in easing the way for a hospitalist to deal with an older, potentially intimidating chief of surgery or hospital's chief operating officer.

Second, as mentioned earlier in this chapter, it is critical for any clinician leader, particularly a hospitalist leader, to be viewed by both physician and nonphysician staff as an outstanding clinician. It is very difficult to have credibility in the hospital environment, particularly from physician colleagues and from nursing staff, if one is viewed as a "clinical lightweight." The hospitalist's conscientiousness, clinical skills, decision-making ability, communications skills, and professionalism all contribute to the individual's reputation and ability to command respect from others at the institution.

Third, when trying to effect change and garner support from both physician and nonphysician staff, the hospitalist leaders must initially establish, promote, and focus on the principles underlying any proposed plan. Although it is easy for a hospital administrator to argue with a specific proposal, it is much more difficult to take a position against an ultimate goal of improving the quality and safety of patient care, improving hospital systems and efficiency, or improving the financial performance of the hospital.

Finally, it is important for the hospitalist to seek out defined leadership roles. Such roles can obviously be within the hospital community, for example, by serving on committees. However, establishing a presence and reputation outside the institution, for example, through involvement at regional and national levels, can only help the hospitalist's reputation and credibility within her own hospital setting.

FINAL WORDS

The concept of being a "born leader" has clearly given way to a philosophy that leadership skills can be learned. It is perhaps based on this premise that so many books and articles have been written about every possible aspect of leadership. Yet, it is fair to say that many personal qualities and aspects of personality do have an impact on potential success as a leader. When placed in a position with leadership responsibilities, it is valuable to take some time to self-reflect upon personality traits and how they will likely influence leadership style. In addition, one should try to assess what additional skills s/he needs to acquire to be an effective leader. Even though physicians are often placed in either clinical or academic leadership positions, they have not typically received leadership training. Recognizing the interplay between personal style and leadership skills, and acknowledging the importance of self-reflection on successes and failures as a leader will serve to make one an increasingly effective leader over time.

REFERENCES

Breitner LK, Anthony RN. *Essentials of Accounting*. 11th ed. Upper Saddle River, NJ, Prentice Hall, 2012.

Fisher R, Ury W, Patton B. *Getting to Yes: Negotiating Agreement without Giving*. New York, NY: Penguin Books; 2011. Updated and revised ed.

Shell GR. *Bargaining for Advantage: Negotiation Strategies for Reasonable People*. 2nd ed. New York, NY: Penguin Books; 2006.

SECTION 2

Critical Decision Making at the Point of Care

CHAPTER 7

Principles of Evidence-Based Medicine and Quality of Evidence

Daniel I. Steinberg, MD

A BRIEF HISTORY

The March 1, 1981 issue of the *Canadian Medical Association Journal* included a landmark article titled "How to read clinical journals: I. Why to read them and how to start reading them critically." Written by David Sackett, MD (1934–2015) of McMaster University, it introduced a series of articles that highlighted the importance of critical appraisal of the literature. Starting in 1993, a set of articles in the *Journal of the American Medical Association* titled "Users' guides to the medical literature" reprised and expanded on the earlier series. These works, and other efforts by their authors, made critical appraisal of the literature accessible to the masses and laid the groundwork for evidence-based medicine (EBM).

Gordon Guyatt, MD, coined the term "evidence-based medicine" in the early 1990s, while he served as the internal medicine residency program director at McMaster University. Dr. Guyatt and colleagues had incorporated critical appraisal of the literature into the residency program curriculum, and Dr. Guyatt wanted a term to describe and advertise their efforts.

EBM caught on quickly over subsequent years as practicing physicians and training programs embraced and taught its methods, with dissemination greatly fueled by the rise of the Internet.

ROLE OF CLINICAL JUDGMENT AND PATIENT PREFERENCES IN EBM

An early criticism of EBM, which some still harbor, was that it did not properly acknowledge the importance of clinical judgment or patient preferences. In an updated framework for evidence-based practice by R. Brian Haynes, P.J. Devereaux, and Gordon Guyatt in 2002, evidence-based decisions are based on four cardinal elements: (1) the research evidence, (2) the patient's clinical state and circumstances, (3) the patient's preferences, and (4) the clinician's judgment and expertise.

> **PRACTICE POINT**
>
> - Clinical judgment and expertise are essential to the practice of EBM. These skills facilitate optimal decision making by allowing the clinician to properly weigh the research evidence in the context of the patient's individual clinical circumstances and preferences. Decisions should never be based on the evidence alone.

Practicing EBM may appear to be a straightforward affair with its methodical approaches to clinical question construction and to searching and critically appraising the literature. However, hospitalists should not confuse process with content, and they will often find that EBM tends to highlight clinical uncertainty and gaps in the medical literature. High-quality evidence does not exist to guide all clinical decisions, and extrapolation from lower quality evidence is often necessary. Bayesian diagnostic decision making often relies on clinical judgment to formulate pretest probabilities or to deal with the uncertainty that accompanies inconclusive post-test probabilities. Learning to deal with uncertainty is a core competency of EBM, which draws heavily on clinical judgment and experience.

■ PUSH INFORMATION RESOURCES

Few clinicians have the time to consistently read medical journals, identify relevant new research and critically appraise new studies to determine if they should be incorporated into one's practice. "Push" information resources are resources that send content out to their users on a regular basis. "Pull" information resources are databases that clinicians search in order to answer a clinical question. Pull resources are discussed later in this chapter. **Table 7-1** lists selected high-quality push and pull information resources.

McMaster PLUS (Premium Literature Service) continuously searches over 120 medical journals and selects evidence for critical appraisal. Articles that pass the critical appraisal process and are also rated as clinically relevant and newsworthy by their team of reviewers are then transferred to the PLUS database. The PLUS database contributes content to evidence-based summary resources such as EvidenceUpdates, ACP JournalWise, DynaMed, and ClinicalEvidence. These resources all offer e-mail alerts to users. ACP Journal Club and NEJM Journal Watch critically appraise and produce synopses of high-quality evidence accompanied by expert commentary. PubMed, through its free account service "My NCBI," allows users to receive the results of literature search strategies they either design or select (via the "Clinical Queries" feature) by e-mail on a regular basis.

TABLE 7-1 High-Quality Push and Pull Resources

Push Resources	Pull Resources
Resources that automatically send new, high-quality evidence to users via e-mail or RSS feed aggregator	Databases that are searched as needed to answer clinical questions
ACP JournalWise http://journalwise.acponline.org	ACP Journal Club http://annals.org/journalclub.aspx
BMJ Clinical Evidence http://clinicalevidence.bmj.com	BMJ Clinical Evidence http://clinicalevidence.bmj.com
DynaMed https://www.dynamed.com	Cochrane Collaboration http://www.cochrane.org
Evidence Updates https://plus.mcmaster.ca/evidenceupdates	DynaMed https://www.dynamed.com
NEJM Journal Watch http://www.jwatch.org	NEJM Journal Watch http://www.jwatch.org
PubMed (using an My NCBI account and search strategies created by the user, see text) http://www.ncbi.nlm.nih.gov/pubmed	Practice Guidelines from professional societies, eg, AHRQ National Guideline Clearing House http://www.guideline.gov PubMed http://www.ncbi.nlm.nih.gov/pubmed Trip Database https://www.tripdatabase.com

- Hospitalists should strongly consider using an e-mail-based alerting service or RSS (Rich Site Summary) feed aggregator from a high-quality evidence-based summary push resource to effectively stay up to date on the literature.
- Hospitalists can pair a virtual file cabinet with these resources to form an effective information management system that will make evidence readily available at the point of care.

■ KEEPING INFORMATION AT HAND: THE VIRTUAL FILE CABINET

Although the traditional way of storing articles for later reference is to use a physical file cabinet, this approach has a number of disadvantages. File cabinets are not mobile, they cannot be quickly searched or updated, and determining how to best file something for easy retrieval can be confusing. A clinician might ask himself/herself in frustration: "Did I file that great article on pulmonary manifestations of HIV under 'HIV,' or 'infectious disease,' or 'pulmonary'?" They do not offer a way to electronically add content to them or electronically share content with others, making them incompatible with modern communication methods such as e-mail.

The virtual file cabinet (VFC) is an Internet cloud-based electronic document storage system that synchronizes across multiple electronic devices (eg, smartphone, tablet, laptop computer). A VFC is an effective way for hospitalists to electronically file articles they receive from a push information resource as described above for easy retrieval at the point of care. Box, Dropbox, Evernote, and Google Drive are some examples of the commercial products that currently exist that can be used as a virtual file cabinet. Products such as these also offer easy options for electronically sharing content with others.

THE EBM PROCESS: ASKING AND ANSWERING CLINICAL QUESTIONS

Practicing EBM often involves asking and answering questions that arise during the care of patients. There are four steps in this process: (1) asking a focused clinical question, (2) searching the literature for the best available evidence, (3) critically appraising the literature, and (4) applying the literature to an individual patient. This chapter explores the basic principles of EBM as they relate to these four steps.

■ STEP 1: ASKING A FOCUSED CLINICAL QUESTION

Clinical questions fall into two general groups: background or foreground questions. Background questions ask about general knowledge, pathophysiology, epidemiology, and broad aspects of diagnosis and treatment. "What are the treatments for epilepsy?" is an example of a background question. Junior learners often ask background questions, and answers can often be found in textbooks. Foreground questions are more focused, address specific clinical situations, and facilitate the delivery of the most up-to-date, evidence-based care. Experienced clinicians ask foreground questions, with answers residing more in the medical literature. Hospitalists should always aim to construct focused foreground questions. These are further discussed below.

Most hospitalists would recognize the question, "Should patients with heart disease receive regular vaccinations?" as one that is overly broad. Not all heart diseases are the same, nor are all vaccinations, and the specific benefits patients might reap from vaccination are not specified by the question. Clinical questions need to be focused in order to be answerable. In addition to clinical questions about therapy, clinicians can ask focused clinical questions about diagnostic tests, about the harm an intervention might cause, about prognosis, or about differential diagnosis.

Clinical questions should be constructed using the "P-I-C-O" format. "P" stands for "population" and describes the patient the question is about in proper detail. "I" stands for "intervention" and refers to the therapy or diagnostic test in question. "C" stands for "comparison" and describes either an alternative treatment or standard of care (for questions about therapy) or the gold standard test (for questions about diagnostic tests). "O" stands for "outcome," which should be clinically important and patient-centered. Surrogate markers of clinically important outcomes are acceptable.

An example of a well-built clinical question about therapy is: "In patients admitted to the hospital with non-ST elevation myocardial infarction (P), what is the effect of influenza vaccination at discharge (I) as compared to no vaccination (C) on recurrent acute coronary syndrome or mortality (O)?"

An example of a properly designed clinical question about a diagnostic test is: "In patients presenting to the emergency department with suspected infection (P), how accurate is a history of shaking chills (I), as compared a gold standard of blood cultures (C) in diagnosing bacteremia (O)?"

When clinical questions do not perfectly fit into the P-I-C-O format, clinicians should follow as many of the above principles as possible.

PRACTICE POINT

- Clinical questions must be focused to be answerable. Hospitalists should use the widely accepted "Population–Intervention–Comparison–Outcome" (P-I-C-O) format to construct focused clinical questions.

■ STEP 2: SEARCHING THE LITERATURE

Pull information resources

With a properly constructed clinical question in hand, the hospitalist can now search the literature to find the answer. The first step is to select an information resource that is appropriate for the clinical question and the amount of time available. Databases that are searched in an on-demand way in order to answer a clinical question are called pull resources.

In many cases, and especially when time is limited, one should first consult a high-quality summary pull resource. Summary resources that are frequently updated assess the quality of the evidence presented and are user-friendly and preferable. Examples include BMJ Clinical Evidence, ACP Journal Club, DynaMed, the Cochrane Collaboration, NEJM Journal Watch, UpToDate, and practice guidelines from professional societies. All are highly useful. Each has its strengths and weaknesses. UpToDate is fast to use, comprehensive, and provides expert guidance in an easy to digest, narrative format, but it is not as rigorously constructed as the others. ACP Journal Club provides excellent summaries of highly selected literature deemed valid and relevant to clinical practice, but as a result its database is not comprehensive. DynaMed is rigorously constructed and presents a lot of primary data from clinical trials, often in an outline format. The Cochrane Collaboration produces high-quality systematic reviews of the evidence. Practice guidelines are excellent resources that offer clear recommendations, but their quality can vary, update intervals can be long, and users must pay close attention to the level of evidence and strength of recommendations in published practice guidelines.

If one has more time, or if a deeper dive is needed after consulting a summary resource, the primary literature can be searched via PubMed (preferably using "Clinical Queries" option for clinical questions) or Trip Database (preferably using "PICO search" option for clinical questions). For certain questions, a content-specific resource can be best. JAMAEvidence catalogs evidence on the accuracy of history and physical exam findings. The Cochrane Collaboration focuses on systematic reviews. No single resource is perfect and clinicians should adopt a "toolbox" approach by becoming familiar with a few resources.

PRACTICE POINT

- Pull resources are databases that are searched in an on-demand way to answer a clinical question. Pull resources have different and often complementary roles. None are perfect, and hospitalists should adopt a "toolbox" approach in which they become familiar with a few resources. The type of question and the amount of time available to answer the question should help determine which resource the hospitalist consults.

■ THE HIERARCHY OF EVIDENCE

Hospitalists should know which types of clinical trials will best answer different types of clinical questions, and which study designs will provide the most powerful results. The randomized controlled trial (RCT) is the gold standard for determining the effect of a therapeutic intervention.

Determining the accuracy of a diagnostic test requires a prospective design in which the test is studied in the same clinical setting it will be used, and is compared against an acceptable gold standard. The effect of a diagnostic test on clinical outcomes can be determined by a randomized controlled trial, in which the test in question is treated as the intervention and another diagnostic approach (preferably a gold standard if available) is considered the comparison.

A systematic review is a summary of the evidence on a topic in which the literature search and selection of evidence has been performed in a rigorous, transparent, and reproducible way. The most valuable systematic reviews will also include a meta-analysis. In a meta-analysis, the results of multiple similar types of studies (RCTs, observational studies, or studies of diagnostic tests) are statistically combined to offer more powerful results. What a meta-analysis gains in power, it can sometimes lose in applicability and focus if too much clinical heterogeneity exists among the patients included from individual studies. With that caveat, a high-quality systematic review that includes a meta-analysis is considered to be the highest level of evidence. **Table 7-2** describes the hierarchy of evidence for different types of clinical questions.

■ STEP 3: CRITICALLY APPRAISING THE LITERATURE

Although summary resources that appraise the medical literature have risen in quality and are an essential resource for clinicians, they will not always provide the answer to a clinical question. In addition, hospitalists may participate in discussions around particular studies, attend "journal club" conferences, or teach junior learners about evidence-based medicine. Hospitalists must have solid critical appraisal skills. The *Users' Guides to the Medical Literature* (McGraw-Hill, 2014) is the benchmark textbook for learning how to practice EBM. It proposes an effective method for critical appraisal that has been widely adopted. The principles and approach it endorses are discussed further in this chapter.

In appraising any type of study, three broad questions must be answered:

1. Are the results valid?
2. What are the results?
3. How can I apply the results to patient care?

The critical appraisal process asks these three questions of each type of study, including those about therapy, diagnosis,

TABLE 7-2 Hierarchy of Evidence for Different Types of Clinical Questions

Type of Clinical Question	Best Types of Articles (Listed in Decreasing Level of Evidence)
Therapy or harm	1. Systematic review/meta-analysis of randomized controlled trials
	2. Randomized controlled trial
	3. Cohort study
	4. Case-control study
	5. Case series
	6. Case reports
	7. Expert opinion
Accuracy of a diagnostic test	1. Systematic review/meta-analysis
	2. Prospective comparison against gold standard conducted in setting diagnostic test will be used in practice
Prognosis	1. Systematic review/meta-analysis
	2. Prospective cohort study of a representative, homologous patient group with appropriate follow-up and objective outcomes.
	3. Retrospective case-controlled study
Differential diagnosis of a condition	1. Systematic review/meta-analysis
	2. Prospective evaluation of a representative sample that includes definitive diagnostic evaluation, performed in a setting similar to actual practice

TABLE 7-3 Critical Appraisal Questions for an Article About Therapy

Main Question	Supplemental Questions
1. Is the study valid?	a. Were patients randomized?
	b. Was group allocation concealed?
	c. Were patients in the study groups similar with respect to prognostic variables?
	d. To what extent was the study blinded?
	e. Was follow-up complete?
	f. Were patients analyzed in the groups to which they were first assigned (ie, intention to treat)?
	g. Was the trial stopped early?
2. What are the results?	a. How large was the treatment effect? (What were the RRR and the ARR?)
	b. How precise were the results? (What were the confidence intervals?)
3. How can I apply the results to patient care?	a. Were the study patients similar to my patients?
	b. Were all clinically important outcomes considered?
	c. Are the likely treatment benefits worth the potential harm and costs? (eg, what is the number needed to treat? What is the number needed to harm?)

Adapted from Guyatt G, et al., eds. *Users' Guides to the Medical Literature: A Manual for Evidence-Based Clinical Practice*, 3rd ed. New York, NY: McGraw-Hill Education; 2014.

harm, prognosis, and systematic reviews. Each of the three major questions is answered through a subset of critical appraisal questions that are specific to each study type. The critical appraisal questions help determine if a study used proper methods to prevent bias, if the results are large enough to be meaningful, and whether the results can be applied to a particular patient or population.

PRACTICE POINT

- Critical appraisal focuses on answering three broad questions: Are the results valid? What are the results? How can I apply the results to patient care? The *Users' Guides to the Medical Literature* offers a methodical approach to answering these questions for studies about therapy, diagnosis, harm, and prognosis, and for systematic reviews.

In recent years, a new type of evidence, the results of quality improvement studies, has risen in prominence. As hospitalists often are involved in quality improvement efforts, they should have a working knowledge of how to critically appraise this type of evidence. The *Users' Guides to the Medical Literature* offers further instruction in this area.

This chapter will illustrate the critical appraisal process through analysis of an article about therapy, as randomized controlled trials and prospective cohort studies are among the most common types of evidence encountered in practice. **Table 7-3** outlines the critical appraisal questions, which are discussed in detail below. Clinicians should refer to the *Users' Guides to the Medical Literature* for a complete list of critical appraisal questions for different types of research studies.

CRITICAL APPRAISAL OF AN ARTICLE ABOUT THERAPY

To critically appraise an article about therapy, the clinician should answer the following set of questions.

Are the results valid

Were patients randomized? Randomization will best ensure that the intervention and control groups are equal at the start of the trial, except for the intervention being tested. In observational studies, investigators must take special steps to ensure experimental and comparison cohorts are evenly matched. Randomization does much of this automatically.

Was group allocation concealed? When allocation concealment is present, those enrolling patients into the study during randomization are blinded to what group (ie, intervention or control) the patients are being assigned. Without allocation concealment, for example, a patient being enrolled but who is viewed as likely having a bad outcome might be steered into the comparison group, potentially improving the results in the intervention group.

Were patients in the study groups similar with respect to known prognostic variables? This is necessary to isolate the effect of the intervention and minimize confounders. Proper randomization will ensure this. In the absence of randomization, clinicians should look to see that the intervention and comparison groups were carefully matched so as to be equal for all possible confounders. This is often difficult to do, which is why randomization is preferred.

To what extent was the study blinded? The term "double-blind" does not describe all parties that should be blinded in an RCT. For maximum validity, multiple groups should be blinded, including those selecting patients for randomization (ie, allocation concealment), the patients, those administering the intervention, the data collectors/analysts, and the outcome assessors. When patients or those administering the intervention cannot be blinded (as in trials of certain surgeries or procedures), allocation concealment, as well as blinding of data analysts and outcome assessors, is essential.

Was the follow-up complete? Studies should track the outcomes of all participants. Patients may be lost to follow-up if they suffer a negative outcome or find the intervention too difficult to comply with. Both of these reasons would be highly relevant to the results of a study.

Were patients analyzed in the groups to which they were first assigned (ie, intention to treat)? The principle of "intention to treat" highlights that in a clinical trial, the offering of an intervention to participants is being tested as much as the other effects of the intervention. If for instance participants do not like the taste of a pill or find a study protocol too hard to comply with and drop out of a trial or asked to be switched to the other arm as a result, these consequences must be recorded as part of the results of the study. Outcomes must be attributed to the group to which participants were initially assigned. A trial that follows the intention to treat principle will give the best estimate of what will happen if a therapy is offered to a population. In a "per protocol analysis," the study results represent only what happened to those who actually accept the intervention and complete the trial. This type of analysis can inform what effect a therapy would have if taken properly by a highly compliant patient.

Was the trial stopped early? Follow-up must be an appropriate length for the outcome measured. For example, 3 days might be an appropriate follow-up period for an intervention to reduce acute pain, but it would likely be too short for an intervention designed to reduce LDL cholesterol or to improve functional status. Randomized controlled trials that are stopped early because of benefit may overestimate the effect of an intervention. A large benefit observed early in a trial may be due chance, and may be greater that what would be observed if the trial were allowed to run to completion.

What are the results

How large was the treatment effect (ie, what were the relative risk reduction and absolute risk reduction?)? Clinicians should consider results of a study using the absolute risk reduction (ARR), where the ARR% = event rate in comparison group – event rate in experimental group. The relative risk reduction (RRR) is calculated as RRR% = event rate in comparison group – event rate in experimental group/event rate in comparison group. The RRR allows one to determine the effect of a therapy on an individual patient according to their baseline risk.

Consider the study by Sharma et al., published in the *American Journal of Gastroenterology* in 2013, that randomized 120 hospitalized patients with cirrhosis and overt hepatic encephalopathy to rifaximin versus placebo. In-hospital death occurred in 24% of the rifaximin group and in 49% of the placebo group. Here the ARR is 25% (49% – 24%) and the RRR is 51% (49% – 24%/49%).

Clinicians can use the RRR to estimate the effect a therapy will have on individual patients they treat that may be more or less sick than the average patient in a study. For example, if a patient is estimated to have a baseline risk of dying of 60%, rifaximin will reduce this patient's risk of dying to 30.6% (60% × 0.51). In this case the ARR will be 60%-30.6% = 29.4% which is higher than what the rifaximin group as a whole experienced in the trial. In a similar way, lower baseline risk will result in lower absolute risk reduction.

PRACTICE POINT

- A randomized controlled trial describes the average effect of an intervention across the group of patients studied. The effect an intervention will have on any individual patient can be determined by combining that patient's baseline risk with the relative risk reduction (RRR) reported in the trial. Clinicians can estimate their patient's baseline risk by comparing them to the clinical characteristics and comorbidities of patients in a trial, and by using their clinical judgment and expertise.

■ HOW PRECISE WAS THE ESTIMATE OF THE TREATMENT EFFECT? (WHAT WERE THE CONFIDENCE INTERVALS?)

Confidence intervals provide more information than *P*-values alone, giving an estimate of the range of possible results. Some high-quality evidence-based summary resources, such as ACP Journal Club, emphasize confidence intervals and the helpful picture they paint of the results.

In the study of rifaximin described above, the RRR = 51% (95% CI, 20-71). In "plain English," this 95% confidence interval tells us that rifaximin most likely reduces in-hospital death by 51% (the "point estimate") but it may reduce in death by as little as 20%, or by as much as 71%. There is a 95% chance that the true effect is between 20% and 71%, a 2.5% chance the true effect is below 20%, and a 2.5% chance it is above 71%.

In order to determine whether a trial has found two therapies to be equivalent, clinicians should examine the upper and lower limits of the 95% confidence interval. If either would be clinically significant if true, the two therapies studied cannot be called equivalent, and further research is needed. A 2014 study by Regimbeau et al. published in the *Journal of the American Medical Association* found that in patients undergoing cholecystectomy for acute calculous cholecystitis, postoperative antibiotics reduced infection by an absolute risk reduction of 1.9% (95% CI, −9.0-5.1, *P* < 0.05). The confidence interval indicates that antibiotics most likely reduce infection by 1.9%, but may reduce infection by as much as 5.1% (in which case most clinicians would prescribe them), or may increase infection by as much as 9% (in which case most clinicians would not prescribe them). In this study, the true effect of antibiotics on postoperative infection could not be determined as they could be either beneficial or harmful, and further study is needed. A common misinterpretation of these results, which could occur if the confidence intervals are not noted, would be: "the *P*-value is greater than 0.05 so there is no difference between antibiotics and placebo and the two are equivalent."

Two factors affect the width of a confidence interval: the number of patients and the frequency of the outcome in a study. In our example of the Regimbeau trial, further studies that enroll larger numbers of patients or measure more postoperative infections could result in a narrower confidence interval as well as a different point estimate.

PRACTICE POINT

- Confidence intervals are preferable to *P*-values when considering the results of a clinical trial, as they give more information about the range of possible results, including the best and worst case scenarios.

How can I apply the results to patient care

Were the study patients similar to my patients? The more a patient meets the inclusion criteria, and the less they meet the exclusion criteria, the more confidently the results of a study can be applied to them. Clinicians should consider the setting of a study as well as whether those who administered the intervention had specialized expertise that is not available locally.

Were all clinically important outcomes considered? The "grandmother test" can help determine if an outcome is clinically relevant. Outcomes that would be valued by the average person (eg, someone's grandmother) are clinically important; outcomes that would not be valued are not clinically relevant and should not be measured by clinical trials. For example, outcomes such as a reduction in pain, an increase in survival, or a reduction hospital admission are likely to be meaningful to patients, while biochemical, laboratory, or purely hemodynamic outcomes are not. An exception is when nonclinical outcomes are established surrogate markers for clinically important outcomes. Composite outcomes of clinical endpoints are valid, but if possible studies should make clear how much each individual endpoint is driving the composite result.

PRACTICE POINT

- Hospitalists should value studies that measure clinically important endpoints (or surrogate markers of these) over those that measure physiologic or biochemical endpoints.

◼ ARE THE LIKELY TREATMENT BENEFITS WORTH THE POTENTIAL HARM AND COSTS? (WHAT IS THE NUMBER NEEDED TO TREAT? WHAT IS THE NUMBER NEEDED TO HARM?)

The number needed to treat (NNT) describes how many patients must be treated with an intervention to produce one positive outcome or prevent one negative outcome. The NNT allows clinicians to compare the effects of different therapies, and is calculated as NNT = 100/ARR%. In the study by Sharma et al. discussed above, in-hospital death occurred in 24% of the rifaximin group and in 49% of the placebo group. Here the ARR is 25% (49% − 24%) and the NNT is 4 (100/25). In other words, we need to give four patients rifaximin to prevent one patient from dying in the hospital.

In order to best inform risk/benefit discussions about a therapy, studies should measure important adverse effects. The number needed to harm (NNH) describes how many patients must be treated for one to experience a particular adverse effect. These two numbers can be compared for an intervention and a particular adverse effect to determine the net benefit or harm. In addition to the likelihood of adverse events and their morbidity, the level of concern a patient has about particular side effects must be considered. Many studies do not assess cost, and those that do often determine cost-effectiveness at the population level, which is less relevant to the individual patient. The extent to which a therapy is covered by insurance is highly relevant to patients and should always be considered.

◼ STEP 4: APPLYING THE LITERATURE TO AN INDIVIDUAL PATIENT

For the findings of a study to be useful in clinical care, the critical appraisal process must yield a satisfactory answer to each of the three broad questions discussed above: a study must be valid, it must report important results, and it must be applicable to the patient at hand. If any of these three elements is missing, the study findings may not be appropriate for implementation into practice.

When a study has used valid methods, has reported highly important results, and has enrolled patients clearly similar to the patient in question, the hospitalist can confidently apply its findings. But conducting clinical studies is often difficult work, and few studies are perfect in every way. Clinicians need to learn which validity or applicability issues represent fatal flaws, and which ones still allow the results of a study to be considered. This is a skill that comes with experience.

The hospitalist must remember that best evidence-based decisions incorporate not only the evidence, but also the individual clinical circumstances and preferences of patients. In most cases, patient values and preferences are more important than the other factors.

CONCLUSION

This chapter has focused on skills such as the construction of focused clinical questions and how to search and critically appraise the literature. These skills are necessary but not sufficient for the practice of EBM. The hospitalist's knowledge of the patient is at the heart of evidence-based practice. The right clinical questions cannot be asked unless the hospitalist first has a clear understanding of the patient's clinical issues, and the literature cannot be applied to a patient without knowledge of their values and preferences. Communication skills, history and physical examination skills, illness scripts, problem representation, and clinical reasoning skills are some of the ways hospitalists come to know their patients. To be a top-notch practitioner of EBM really starts and ends with being an outstanding clinical doctor.

SUGGESTED READINGS

Devereaux PJ, et al. Double blind, you are the weakest link—goodbye! *Evidence-Based Med.* 2002;7:14-15.

Guyatt G, et al., eds. *Users' Guides to the Medical Literature: A Manual for Evidence-Based Clinical Practice*, 3rd ed. New York, NY: McGraw-Hill Education; 2014.

Haynes RB, et al. Clinical expertise in the era of evidence-based medicine and patient choice. *ACP Journal Club.* 2002; March/April: A11-A14.

Regimbeau JM, et al. FRENCH Study Group. Effect of postoperative antibiotic administration on postoperative infection following cholecystectomy for acute calculous cholecystitis: a randomized clinical trial. *JAMA.* 2014;312:145-154.

Sharma BC, et al. A randomized, double-blind, controlled trial comparing rifaximin plus lactulose with lactulose alone in treatment of overt hepatic encephalopathy. *Am J Gastroenterol.* 2013;108:1458-1463.

Diagnostic Reasoning and Decision Making

Laurence Beer, MD, SFHM
Lucas Golub, MD
Dustin T. Smith, MD

INTRODUCTION

Diagnosis is the art of identifying a disease by the signs, symptoms, and test results of a patient. Diagnosis stems from the Greek word, *diagignoskein*, which means to distinguish or discern. Indeed, the ability to distinguish or discern a patient's underlying illness is critical to being an effective clinician as a hospital medicine provider. In many cases, hospitalized patients may be quite complicated with multiple competing possible reasons to explain their underlying signs or symptoms. Patients do not always read textbook (ie, they may not always describe their symptoms or have findings on exam that are pathognomonic or as classically described). Therefore, diagnostic reasoning and diagnostic decision making are crucial skills for hospital medicine providers. In addition, cognitive biases exist and diagnostic errors occur when there is any mistake or failure in the diagnostic process that leads to a misdiagnosis, a missed diagnosis, or a delayed diagnosis. This chapter will discuss diagnostic reasoning and diagnostic decision making.

DIAGNOSTIC REASONING

■ CLINICAL REASONING

Clinical reasoning is the process where a clinician applies reasoning in combination with the clinician's knowledge and skills (**Figure 8-1**). Clinical reasoning is a constant process that does not end when the diagnosis has been made. It may be considered complete upon autopsy or when a gold standard has confirmed a diagnosis, but it is important to acknowledge that in many instances the gold standard is not 100% accurate. In the hospital setting clinicians are operating under a running diagnosis until the diagnosis has been confirmed and/or until the patient has improved both subjectively and objectively. Sometimes patients do not improve when a treatment strategy is implemented; thus, it is important that providers continuously use clinical reasoning skills as information is collected in an attempt to verify the diagnosis. Once a treatment or workup plan has been implemented, it is crucial to reassess the patient's response to this to further confirm if the correct diagnosis or treatment strategy has been made (**Figure 8-2**). If the diagnosis does not appear correct or the treatment strategy is failing, the clinician must review the information and data collected and reconsider the other possible diagnoses to explain a patient's presenting signs and symptoms. Hence, a clinician's ability to successfully reason and diagnose is in some ways anchored by that clinician's ability to create an adequate differential diagnosis.

■ DIFFERENTIAL DIAGNOSIS

A differential diagnosis is more than just a list of illnesses that potentially explain why a particular sign, symptom, and/or diagnostic test result exists. Rather, the clinician uses the differential diagnosis to distinguish a disease or condition from others that present with similar signs, symptoms, or diagnostic test results. Initially start with a broad list of diagnoses until further information or data is obtained. A clinician must consider the prevalence of disease and other factors, which make up a provider's patient population, when formulating a differential. It is more often the case where a common disease presents in an atypical fashion rather than a rare or exotic disease actually being present.

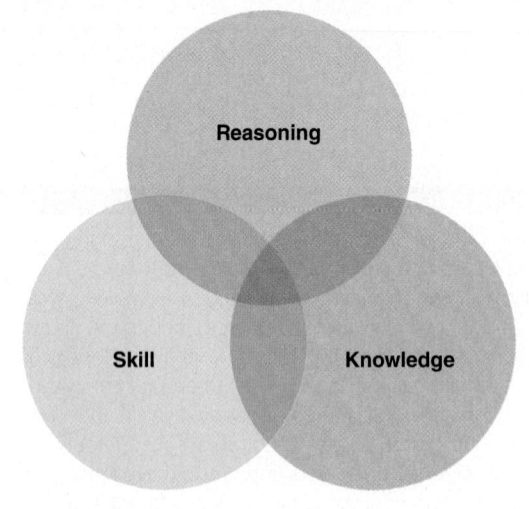

Figure 8-1 *Clinical reasoning.*

List your top diagnosis first followed by other potential diagnoses for a specific problem but keep it problem oriented until you have the actual diagnosis (eg, chest pain differential diagnosis: most likely acute coronary syndrome but consider heart failure, pneumonia, pneumothorax, pulmonary embolism, and musculoskeletal pain). Aggressively prioritize workup of the most likely and most harmful (ie, life threatening) diagnoses under consideration. Prioritize the workup of acute and reversible diseases followed by chronic and irreversible diseases (eg, delirium due to a medical cause versus chronic, progressive dementia). As information or data that effectively rules out a particular diagnosis for a chief complaint becomes available, remove that diagnosis from your list and focus your attention on remaining possibilities. Clinicians should always keep a broad differential until the top diagnosis has been confirmed but also have a plan for workup of other alternate diagnosis if the top diagnosis

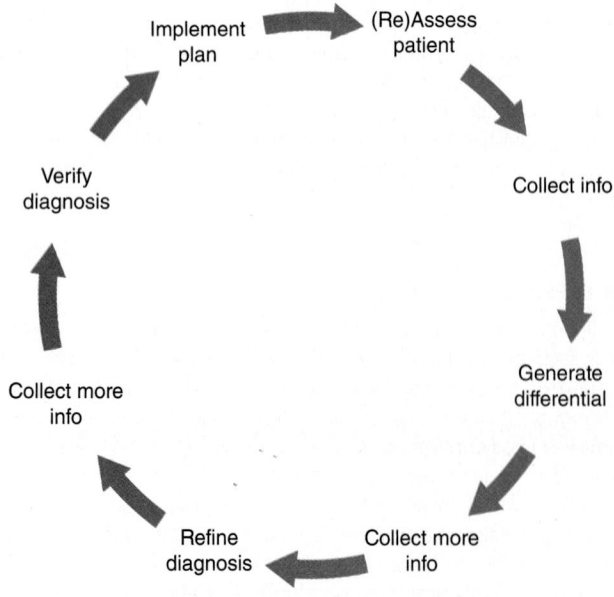

Figure 8-2 *The process of clinical reasoning.*

is excluded. Once a diagnosis has been confirmed, the problem list should be diagnosis-oriented rather than problem-oriented. Should a patient not respond to a treatment plan for a diagnosis where a clear and obvious benefit is expected, the clinician should then re-evaluate the patient, review the data obtained, and finally provide a summary of key data to ensure that the diagnosis is indeed correct.

■ ILLNESS SCRIPTS

Illness scripts are made up of key risk factors, pathophysiology, and clinical presentations that summarize a specific clinical problem or syndrome. An illness script can be a very powerful tool for clinicians. The number of illness scripts an individual clinician has increases with time and experience. Illness scripts may also diminish if a provider's site of practice, specialty, or patient population becomes limited (eg, a clinician whose only site of practice is in a private hospital setting for adult hospitalized patients). An example of some commonly agreed upon illness scripts may be found in **Table 8-1**.

■ REASONING PROCESSES

The dual-process theory of reasoning consists of two systems of reasoning, which clinicians can utilize to correctly arrive at a diagnosis (**Figure 8-3**). The first system is intuitive while the second system is analytical. A careful balance of these two systems is necessary to ensure efficient and effective clinical reasoning.

System 1 (intuitive)

The first system of the dual-process theory is intuitive, implicit or automatic. Often an unconscious or subconscious process involving pattern recognition or matching against illness scripts markedly affects the clinician's judgment; the clinician's past clinical experience and clinical expertise weighs heavily on this system. Heuristics, or mental shortcuts, are also utilized in this system.

TABLE 8-1 Examples of Illness Scripts

Key Risk Factors	Pathophysiology	Clinical Presentation	Diagnosis
• Usually 1-3 mo old infants • Rare after 12 wks of age • 4:1-6:1 male:female • First born son • Maternal smoking increases the risk	• Pyloric muscular hypertrophy • Pyloric canal narrows • Near-complete obstruction	✓ Nonbilious projective vomiting ✓ Infant demands to be refed soon afterwards ✓ No diarrhea ✓ Severe weight loss ✓ Emaciated with "olive-like" mass on abdominal exam ✓ Hypochloremic metabolic alkalosis ✓ Hypokalemia	➤ Pyloric stenosis
• Usually idiopathic • Common disorder among adults • More frequent in women • Involved in activities that involve flexing or extending of wrist repeatedly (eg, typing a book chapter)	• Repetitive actions of the hand or wrist • Increased pressure in the intracarpal canal • Median nerve compression • Ischemia and mechanical disruption of nerve	✓ Pain and parasthesia in the medial nerve distribution ✓ Worse at night ✓ Changes in hand posture or shaking the hand mitigates symptoms ✓ + Phalen maneuver and Tinel test	➤ Carpal tunnel syndrome
• Uncommon event • Most common predisposing factor is hypertension • Typically occurs in 60- to 80-y-old men	• Tear in the aortic intima • Degeneration of the aortic media • Hemorrhage into the media • Creation of a false lumen • Propagation of dissection both distal and proximal to initial tear involving branch vessels, aortic valve, and/or pericardial space • Ischemia, aoritic regurgitation, and/or cardiac tamponade	✓ Severe, "tearing" chest pain radiating to the back ✓ Blood pressure not equal in both arms ✓ Widened mediastinum on chest radiography ✓ Acute hemodynamic compromise	➤ Aortic dissection
• Most common indication for emergent abdominal surgery in childhood • More common in older children and adolescents • More common in boys	• Obstruction of the vestigial vermiform appendix • Inflammation of the appendiceal wall • Localized ischemia, perforation, and the development of a contained abscess or generalized appendicitis	✓ Abdominal pain, typically beginning in the periumbilical region and migrating to the right lower quadrant ✓ Anorexia ✓ Nausea or vomiting ✓ Low-grade fever ✓ Peritoneal signs on abdominal examination ✓ +McBurney's point tenderness, Rovsing's sign, ilopsoas sign, and/or obturator sign ✓ Mild leukocytosis	➤ Acute appendicitis in children
• Most common cause of acute abdomen • Occurs most frequently in second and third decades of life • 1.4:1 male:female	• Obstruction of the vestigial vermiform appendix • Inflammation of the appendiceal wall • Localized ischemia, perforation, and the development of a contained abscess or generalized appendicitis	✓ Abdominal pain, typically right lower quadrant ✓ Anorexia ✓ Nausea or vomiting ✓ Low-grade fever ✓ Peritoneal signs on abdominal examination ✓ +McBurney's point tenderness, Rovsing's sign, psoas sign, and/or obturator sign	➤ Acute appendicitis in adults

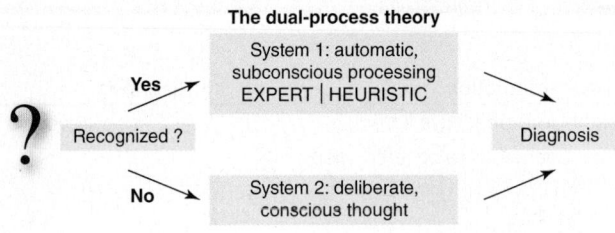

Figure 8-3 *The dual-process theory of reasoning.*

System 2 (analytic)

The second system of the dual-process theory is the analytic, conscious and deliberate type of reasoning. The clinician uses rational and careful analysis when evaluating a differential diagnosis for a specific problem. This system involves hypothesis testing as a tool for clinical reasoning (Figure 8-3).

■ PITFALLS AND STRATEGIES TO AVOID PITFALLS

Numerous pitfalls exist in clinical reasoning and practice. Clinicians may overly rely on heuristics, or mental shortcuts. Cognitive biases may alter a clinician's judgment and clinical reasoning. In the modern era of clinical practice, information overload and overreliance on diagnostic tests may lead to excessive testing or "overdiagnosis," or the diagnosis of a "disease" that will never cause a patient symptoms or death. Certain diagnoses prompt treatments and interventions which may cause harm, especially if the alternative is best managed by watchful waiting regarding the identification of an incidental finding or very early stage disease.

PRACTICE POINT

- In the modern era of clinical practice, information overload is another pitfall as is overreliance on diagnostic tests, which may lead to overtesting or "overdiagnosis" (ie, the diagnosis of a "disease" that will never cause a patient symptoms or death).

Strategies to avoid pitfalls exist include:

- Always begin by defining the problem a patient faces or reports.
- Deliberate and gather key information, as opposed to gathering large amounts of information.
- Perform a summary of key elements in abstract terms to provide a discriminatory and useful overview of the patient's clinical case when faced with large amounts of clinical information. This is often referred to as problem representation.
- Utilize illness scripts which summarize a specific clinical problem.
- Pay particular mind to not prioritize exotic or rare diseases initially for aggressive work-up (see base-rate neglect below).
- Always consider the diagnostic testing and treatment thresholds for the diagnoses he/she is considering in the differential.
- Nonanalytic and analytic reasoning must be balanced, especially when a clinical pattern does not fit a known illness script.
- Be cognizant of biases in clinical reasoning and avoid them at all costs.
- Always keep in mind that patients "do not always read the textbook."

■ COGNITIVE HEURISTICS AND BIASES

The worse heuristic comes from the Greek word, *heuriskein*, meaning to find or discover. Diagnostic decision making is ultimately a path toward discovery, requiring deliberate, systematic thought. There are many avenues of systematic approach to a common question, each with unique issues and pitfalls. A summary of cognitive heuristics and biases with examples given can be found in **Table 8-2**.

■ ANCHORING

Anchoring bias arises when undue importance is placed on information that is received early in the diagnostic evaluation. The clinician does not adjust the differential diagnosis commiserate with the totality of information as new, possibly contradictory data, emerges. The inverse of anchoring is known as the "order effects" bias, where recent information is given more weight in the decision process.

TABLE 8-2 Description of Cognitive Biases or Heuristics with Examples

Bias or Heuristic	Description	Example
Anchoring	Undue focus on a case's starting point, without adequate adjustment for new information	Patient with chronic obstructive pulmonary disease presents for dyspnea, does not improve with medical therapy, and is later found to have a pulmonary embolism
Availability (recall)	Overestimation of diagnostic likelihood based on vivid or easily recalled events	Suspicion of pheochromocytoma in a patient with chronic, resistant hypertension
Base-rate neglect	Impression that two diseases which present similarly are equally likely	Overestimation of the probability of aortic dissection in chest pain
Commission	Preference for intervention over inaction	Thrombolysis for submassive pulmonary embolus
Confirmation	Attempting to confirm a diagnosis rather than testing other possibilities	Leading (non open-ended) questions aimed at eliciting history which confirms a suspected diagnosis
Hindsight	Clinical decisions judged by the result rather than the logic of the choices	Use of bilevel ventilation is judged to be beneficial because the patient survived severe hypoxia
Omission	Iatrogenesis is perceived to be worse than naturally occurring adverse events	Surgery not pursued for appendicitis and overwhelming sepsis because operative mortality is judged to be too high
Premature closure	Early cessation of investigative thought once a presumed diagnosis has been made	Altered mental status and fever are attributed to alcohol withdrawal, but aspiration pneumonia is also present
Representativeness	Patients do not read textbooks and pathology will not always present as expected	Cholecystitis dismissed because Murphy's sign is negative
Search satisfying	An end to information gathering once something has been found	Rib fractures are not identified on a chest radiograph with infiltrate

AVAILABILITY

Availability bias, also referred to as recall bias, involves the overestimation of the likelihood of disease, creating a false sense of prevalence. Largely driven by the clinician's personal experience, diseases that have been encountered either recently or vividly may be given too much credence.

BASE-RATE NEGLECT

Base-rate neglect occurs when true prevalence is distorted. The similar presentation of two different diseases creates a false sense that the rare disease is equally likely compared to its true prevalence.

COMMISSION BIAS

This popular saying provides a good representation of commission bias: "when you are a hammer, everything looks like a nail." Commission bias speaks to the clinician's preference for active intervention over passive inaction.

CONFIRMATION BIAS

Confirmation bias is the inclination to seek information that confirms the current clinical assessment rather than delving into alternative hypotheses. Confirmation bias may aggravate anchoring and thereby cause a vicious cycle that hampers diagnostic momentum.

HINDSIGHT BIAS

Hindsight bias or outcome bias may produce misguided positive feedback if inappropriate testing occurred but a positive clinical outcome resulted or negative feedback despite appropriate management if an adverse or unexpected outcome transpired. Knowledge of a case's outcome may influence perception of preceding events.

OMISSION BIAS

Primum non nocere (first do no harm). Omission bias occurs when clinicians do not therapeutically intervene because an adverse event resulting from treatment is perceived to be worse than one due to inaction, even if the likelihood is exactly the same in both scenarios. Excessive emphasis is placed on avoiding iatrogenic harm.

PREMATURE CLOSURE

Deliberate diagnostic consideration may be curtailed hastily if a presumed diagnosis is accepted before it has been completely established. Premature closure may occur either when a patient has multiple comorbid processes and the clinician fixes on one or when the wrong diagnosis is made in the first place.

REPRESENTATIVENESS

Many diseases have a prototypical or "classic" presentation, and the probability of disease is often assessed according to how closely a specific patient's case mirrors that ingrained portrait of the disease in question. This search for representative presentations will miss atypical variants of common disease. It also predisposes clinicians to dismiss diagnostic possibilities because a cardinal feature is absent, even if that feature is not necessarily present in all cases.

SEARCH SATISFYING

Search satisfying describes the cessation of information acquisition once something has been found. This heuristic is different from premature closure in that it applies to features beyond the primary diagnosis. With clinical focus on this, other subtle features may be missed including additional comorbidities, subtle lab abnormalities, and radiologic findings that do not fit with the reason for presentation.

> ### PRACTICE POINT
>
> - A clinician should be cognizant of cognitive biases in clinical reasoning and avoid them at all costs.
> - Remember that patients "do not always read the textbook."

IMPROVING DIAGNOSTIC REASONING

Both individual skills can be developed and systems-based practices can be instituted to minimize diagnostic error and improve diagnostic reasoning. Individual skills that may be taught include situational awareness, deliberate practice, and metacognition. Systems-based solutions include creating a process for providing individual feedback, developing a nonpunitive error reporting culture, the use of electronic medical records, and furnishing computer-based decision support tools. A summary of cognitive debiasing strategies can be found in **Table 8-3**.

SITUATIONAL AWARENESS

Health care safety and quality researchers have borrowed concepts from other high-risk industries like the military, aviation, and nuclear power generation that have proven successful at minimizing adverse outcomes. Situational awareness refers to having a keen awareness of the multitude of environmental factors that influence decision making in complex, dynamic situations. Having broad situational awareness facilitates understanding of what is happening, why it is happening, and anticipating what is likely to happen next, making it easier to identify problems at an early stage, before they become catastrophic.

The concept of situational awareness may be used to mitigate the types of errors engendered by both the limitations and complexity of hospital medicine and by the complex organizational and systems structures that define modern hospitals. Sources of error due to the nature of hospitalist work include lack of long term relationships with their patients and knowledge of their prior level of functioning, incomplete medical histories, large volumes of rapidly changing and sometimes conflicting data, polypharmacy, and misperception of disease prevalence due to a particular hospital's demographics. Systems-based sources of error, which in one study are present in two-thirds of all errors, include discontinuities in care, lapses in communication, and lack of coordination between departments. Explicit acknowledgement of and extra attention to both sources of error can elucidate ways in which the individual clinician and the institution as a whole may decrease error.

Increasingly, hospitalists are working on wards organized as Accountable Care Units (ACUs). ACUs by definition are structured around shared missions and goals, and are ideal organizations for the implementation of group-based situational awareness techniques. In this formulation, team members are expected to operate from the same script, share a common knowledge base and language, anticipate the needs of other team members, and be

---

TABLE 8-3 Cognitive Debiasing Strategies to Improve Clinical Reasoning

Situational awareness
Error reporting and accountability
Deliberate practice
Feedback
Decision support tools and other electronic-based systems
Metacognition

able to adapt to tasks as they arise. All team members, regardless of role on the team, are taught to recognize "red flags" such as feeling confused, having a gut instinct that something is wrong, sensing that other team members are overlooking important information, or observing improper procedures. They are then empowered to bring these concerns to the attention of the rest of the team without fear of reprimand.

■ ERROR REPORTING AND ACCOUNTABILITY

In order to learn from medical errors clinicians must first and foremost be encouraged to report them. Accomplishing this requires the careful cultivation of a nonpunitive culture in which team members are freed from fear of reprisal. In order to further de-stigmatize medical error and create a climate of transparency clinicians are now being encouraged and in many institutions required to report medical errors to their patients. These progressive views of error do not mean that clinicians should not be held accountable for their errors, but rather that examination of errors should be for the purposes of quality improvement rather than punishment. Since many errors are at least in part due to flawed systems or a breakdown of multiple processes, an appropriate apportionment of responsibility between the hospital, clinician, and ancillary staff is warranted. In fact, due to their presence throughout the hospital, hospitalists are uniquely positioned to encounter, understand, and report on systems-based errors.

To get the most information about medical errors hospitals should not only employ anonymous error-reporting systems, but should actively solicit cases of medical error from their staff. If these errors are not obvious because no substantial harm was caused or because the patient nonetheless recovered, they might not otherwise be reported. Even the reporting of "near-misses," in which a potential error is identified before it is actually committed, should also be encouraged.

■ DELIBERATE PRACTICE

Rote practice (ie, expertise in any field requires a minimum of 10,000 hours of practice) is not sufficient. Instead, goal-directed, carefully measured, deliberate practice (ie, reflective practice) is also required. Without deliberate practice the mere accumulation of experience leads to a plateauing of clinical skills and in some cases even a decline as previously acquired knowledge is forgotten.

Deliberate practice is a training method that follows the iterative cycle of planning, performance, and reflection. The planning phase consists of goal setting, self-motivation, and orientation toward learning. The performance stage consists of time-management, careful record-keeping, benchmarking, and seeking out expert assistance and direction. The reflective phase consists of self-evaluation and studying shortcomings and failures.

One review of research on deliberate practice found that trainees should be given tasks with clearly defined goals, motivated to improve, provided feedback as soon as practically possible, and given numerous opportunities to refine their skills. Experts engaged in deliberate practice consciously seek out clinical challenges just beyond the current skill level of trainees. Properly modeling such habits for trainees allows them to become more self-motivated, self-critical, and able to engage in life-long improvement.

■ FEEDBACK

Without feedback, it is impossible for clinicians to properly calibrate their sense of diagnostic accuracy leading to both over- and underconfidence. Overconfidence has been identified as a frequent cause of diagnostic error. Feedback should be real time, specific, and coupled with corrective instruction.

Web-based morbidity and mortality conferences, interactive medical cases, clinical conundrums, and other real-time tools have largely replaced feedback from autopsies and morbidity and mortality conferences. Case simulations and standardized patients, a now common feature of medical training programs, also present opportunities for trainees to receive real-time feedback.

■ DECISION SUPPORT TOOLS AND OTHER ELECTRONIC-BASED SYSTEMS

Electronic decision support tools (DSTs) include order sets, electronic health record (EHR) embedded alerts and reminders, quality metric dashboards, web-based differential diagnosis engines (eg, ISABEL and DXplain), and clinically oriented literature review resources such as UpToDate and Epocrates. All of these have the potential of guiding physician behavior toward evidence-based practice (and away from anecdotal, bias-driven practice). Data regarding the effectiveness of DSTs, except in very specific domains such as medication dosing, or in institution-specific applications, is mixed. One meta-analysis found that DSTs modestly improve morbidity but have no effect on adverse events or mortality. Conversely, DSTs did seem to improve adherence to preventative care guidelines and ordering clinical studies. There are no rigorous examinations of the potential negative effects of using DSTs. Nonetheless, DSTs provide a resource that is more free from the cognitive biases that influence much of physician clinical practice and may provide the occasion for a clinical "time-out" (Table 8-2).

EHRs themselves are an oft-overlooked form of DST. By collating and organizing large volumes of data, well-designed EHRs facilitate diagnostic reflection, enhance collaboration, and provide a means for receiving feedback. Increasingly, EHRs are also including elements of data analysis such as the ability to graph lab values over time.

■ METACOGNITION

Metacognition is defined as "thinking about thinking." It involves self-questioning and reflecting on personal biases and assumptions. It implies an active, rather than an automatic, control of the thinking process. Examples of metacognition include planning how to approach a cognitive task (eg, diagnosis) and how to evaluate progress in that task. Several authors have suggested the use of a diagnostic checklist (Figure 8-7) to prompt metacognition.

DIAGNOSTIC DECISION MAKING

■ BEDSIDE DIAGNOSIS

Bedside diagnosis with a comprehensive history and physical exam continue to form the bedrock of clinical medicine despite the astronomical technical innovations of modern medicine. It is impossible to fully interpret even the best diagnostic testing without a thorough prior knowledge of the patient. The adage that "ninety percent of the diagnosis is in the history" remains true, even in the 21st century. For example, the differentiation of stable and unstable angina (not to mention cardiac from noncardiac causes of chest pain) requires a skilled clinician at the bedside and carries dramatic therapeutic implications.

■ DIAGNOSTIC TESTS AND INTERVENTIONS

Some diagnostic tests are better screening tests for disease whereas others are better confirmatory tests. Some diagnostic tests are powerful enough to screen and confirm disease. Many laboratory tests do not simply report a positive (presence of disease) and negative (absence of disease) but rather a range requiring application of the result to specific patients. For example, a very low brain or B-type natriuretic peptide (BNP) level (eg, <50 pg/mL) is excellent at excluding heart failure in a patient presenting with a chief complaint of dyspnea. Raising the cutoff to either 100 pg/mL or 200 pg/mL is still good for the exclusion of heart failure but not as powerful as when using a lower cutoff. Additionally, research has shown that patients with a history of left ventricular dysfunction who present with dyspnea due to noncardiac causes often have a higher baseline BNP level than those patients without a history of left ventricular dysfunction.

Consider the laboratory threshold cutoffs used to report a test as abnormal. For example, a D-dimer assay cutoff level 500 ng/mL performs very well as a rule out test in patients unlikely to have acute venous thrombosis and/or pulmonary embolism. Lowering the cutoff level to 250 ng/mL improves the ability of the D-dimer test to exclude acute venous thromboembolism (VTE) with more certainty; however, a lower cutoff will increase false positive results compared with the traditional assay cutoff level of 500 ng/mL.

■ BAYES' THEOREM

Bayes' theorem quantifies how new evidence changes the probability that an existing belief is correct. Bayes' theorem may be applied to any new clinical information such as a historical finding, physical exam finding, test result, or outcome following an intervention. Bayesian reasoning or analysis refers to the pretest probability or odds combined with the test result to the posttest probability or odds. Bayesian analysis offers a simple construct for incorporating new lab, radiology, and other clinical information, as it arises, into our existing diagnostic hypotheses. For interested clinicians many free online calculators exist for doing quite sophisticated Bayesian analysis. A simplified version of Bayes' theorem states that the pretest odds multiplied times likelihood ratio equals the posttest odds.

Sidebar 8-1

The simplified Bayes' theorem and likelihood ratios deal with odds. Disease prevalence is quoted as a probability. To apply Bayes' theorem one must be able to convert between the two. Odds = Probability/1 – Probability and Probability = Odds/1 + Odds. Consider a 43-year-old male with flank pain presenting to the emergency department. For such patients the prevalence of kidney stones is 20%. He undergoes renal ultrasound, which identifies a stone. Renal ultrasound has a likelihood ratio (LR) of 12 if a stone is identified.

Step 1: Find the pretest probability (prevalence) of the disease: 20%
Step 2: Find the LR of the Test: 12
Step 3: Convert pretest probability to pretest odds:

odds = probability/1 – probability = .2/.8 = .25

Step 4: Multiply pretest odds by the LR to obtain the posttest odds:
.25 × 12 = 3

Step 5: Convert the posttest odds back to probability:

Probability = odds/1 + odds = 3/4 = .75 or 75%

This method may be cumbersome, especially without a calculator. As an alternative, some have suggested memorizing the "Rule of 15's" (Table 8-5) or keeping a nomogram (Figure 8-5) handy to estimate the change in the posttest probability from the pretest probability based on the LR for a test.

If data on prevalence is unknown and a clinician's best guess is the only starting point, Bayesian analysis may still be applied. Not as accurate as if you had prevalence data, but more accurate than your starting assumption. As you obtain more information, you may continue to incorporate this information and refine your posttest probability using your knowledge to that point as the pretest probability.

■ PRETEST PROBABILITY

Pretest probability percentage represents the probability of a specific pathology for a patient prior to initiating further diagnostic testing. Pretest probability may be the prevalence of the disease in question in the population. At any point in the diagnostic workup, the clinician may pause and estimate the prevalence or pretest probability of disease in light of what information is known about the patient. The pretest probability of clinical gestalt is frequently delineated as low, intermediate, and high probability for simplicity.

■ SENSITIVITY

A sensitive test correctly identifies patients who have the disease in question. To calculate sensitivity the number of patients who have the disease and test positive (ie, true positives or "TP") is divided by all who have the disease, including those who falsely test negative (ie, false negatives or "FN"). Tests with high sensitivity are ideal screening tests to discover as many patients as possible with the disease, frequently with a tradeoff of increased false positive results. Confirmatory testing may require a more specific test.

$$\frac{TP}{TP + FN}$$

■ SPECIFICITY

Specificity refers to the ability of testing to recognize patients who do not have the disease. To calculate specificity, the number of patients who test negative and do not have the disease (ie, true negatives or "TN") is divided by the total number without the disease, including those who falsely test positive (ie, false positives or "FP").

$$\frac{TN}{TN + FP}$$

For example, D-dimer has high sensitivity and will be positive in most cases of pulmonary embolism; however this comes at the cost of a high false positive rate due to low specificity. A confirmatory, more specific, imaging test may be required to make the diagnosis.

■ "SPIN" AND "SNOUT"

SPecific tests rule IN disease ("SPIN") while SeNsitive tests rule OUT disease. ("SNOUT").

■ POSITIVE PREDICTIVE VALUE

Positive predictive value reports the probability that a patient has the disease after testing positive for it. Positive predictive value is markedly dependent on the prevalence of the disease in question.

$$\frac{TP}{TP + FP}$$

■ NEGATIVE PREDICTIVE VALUE

Negative predictive value describes the probability that a patient does not have the disease following a negative test result. Both positive and negative predictive values are dependent on the prevalence or pretest probability prior to testing.

$$\frac{TN}{TN+FN}$$

■ ACCURACY

Accuracy is the proportion of all test results, whether positive or negative, which are correct. It assesses whether a test actually measures what it claims to measure (**Figure 8-4**).

■ LIKELIHOOD RATIOS

Likelihood ratios are more helpful to make clinical decisions than sensitivity and specificity. For a given diagnostic test, positive likelihood ratios apply to positive results; negative likelihood ratios apply to negative results.

• POSITIVE LIKELIHOOD RATIO

The positive likelihood ratio is the likelihood that a patient with the disease tests positive compared to the likelihood that a patient without the disease tests positive. If a test result is positive and the positive likelihood is greater than 1, then it is more likely than chance that the patient has the disease. However if the likelihood ratio for that test is less than 1, then it is less likely the patient has this disease.

$$\frac{sensitivity}{1-specificity} = \frac{\%TP}{\%FP} = \frac{\left(\dfrac{TP}{total\ with\ disease}\right)}{\left(\dfrac{FP}{total\ without\ disease}\right)}$$

• NEGATIVE LIKELIHOOD RATIO

The negative likelihood ratio is the likelihood that a patient with the disease tests negative compared to the likelihood that a patient without the disease tests negative.

$$\frac{1-sensitivity}{specificity} = \frac{\%FN}{\%TN} = \frac{\left(\dfrac{FN}{total\ with\ disease}\right)}{\left(\dfrac{TN}{total\ without\ disease}\right)}$$

	Patient has disease	Patient does not have disease
Positive test result	True Positive (TP)	False Positive (FP)
Negative test result	False Negative (FN)	True Negative (TN)

Figure 8-4 The 2 × 2 table.

TABLE 8-4 Using Likelihood Ratios to Calculate Posttest Probability

Step 1	Convert pretest probability to pretest odds
	$\dfrac{pretest\ probability}{1-pretest\ probability} = pretest\ odds$
Step 2	Multiply pretest odds by the likelihood ratio to obtain posttest odds
	$pretest\ odds \times likelihood\ ratio = posttest\ odds$
Step 3	Convert posttest odds to posttest probability
	$\dfrac{posttest\ odds}{1+posttest\ odds} = posttest\ probability$

■ POSTTEST PROBABILITY

Diagnosis depends on achieving or accepting a high posttest probability. Each diagnostic test may bring you closer to a diagnosis, but there can rarely be 100% certainty. A posttest probability may be calculated for any disease if two things are known: the pretest probability of disease for the patient and the pertinent likelihood ratio for the diagnostic test performed depending on whether the test is positive or negative (**Table 8-4**).

The likelihood nomogram facilitates application of these calculations to clinical care, but it may not be helpful in clinical practice to approach clinical problem-solving with such clinical precision (**Figure 8-5**).

The "Rule of 15's" is an easily remembered rule of thumb for adjusting pretest probability based on likelihood ratio. The sequence of numbers 1, 2, 5, and 10 corresponds to positive likelihood ratio values. For each progression in the sequence, the pretest probability increases by an additional 15% to arrive at a posttest probability. A positive likelihood ratio of 1 for a positive test does not change the

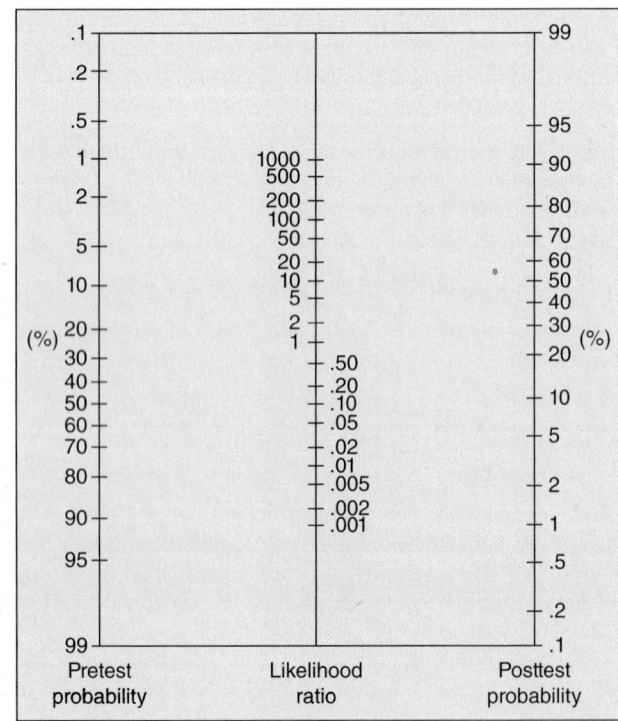

Figure 8-5 Nomogram.

TABLE 8-5 The Rule of 15's

Likelihood Ratio	Change in Probability
0.1	−45%
0.2	−30%
0.5	−15%
1	No change
2	+15%
5	+30%
10	+45%

probability of disease (ie, pretest = posttest). Similar adjustments for negative likelihood ratios may be conducted by taking the inverse of the corresponding positive likelihood ratios. The inverse of 2 is 0.5, which decreases probability by 15% (**Table 8-5**). Estimating the change in probability for values that fall between these notable numbers is easy for positive likelihood ratios between 2 and 6, as there is a 5% change for each single digit (ie, 2 = 15%, 3 = 20%, 4 = 25%, 5 = 30%, 6 = 35%). This simple sequence breaks down at higher values.

> **PRACTICE POINT**
> - Utilize the "rule of 15's" to quickly calculate posttest probability for a disease if the likelihood ratios are known for the diagnostic test performed.

DIAGNOSTIC TESTING AND TREATMENT THRESHOLDS

Answering the question of whether to pursue further diagnostic testing requires an understanding of testing and treatment thresholds. The testing threshold is a pretest probability which is high enough to warrant further diagnostic testing, while the treatment threshold is a pretest probability which is high enough forgo any more testing and warrants intervention for the presumed pathology (**Figure 8-6**).

These thresholds will vary depending on any number of factors including the patient, the disease in question, and the clinician. For example, highly morbid disease processes, especially so-called cannot miss diagnoses, will have lower diagnostic and treatment thresholds. At what pretest probability should the clinician

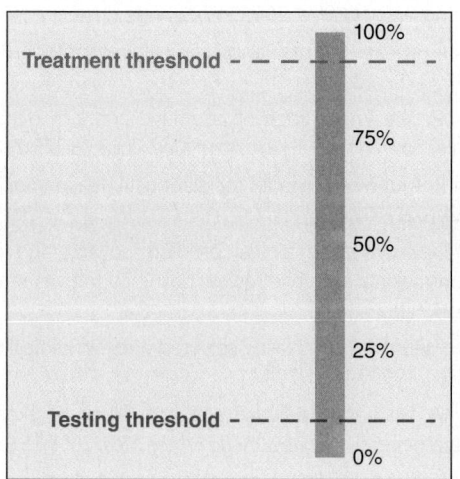

Figure 8-6 *Arbitrary diagnostic testing and treatment thresholds.*

feel comfortable not ordering an abdominal CT for questionable appendicitis: 5%, 1%, or less than 1%? Lower testing and treatment thresholds will find and treat more disease, but at the cost of more false positives, adverse outcomes from some ultimately unnecessary interventions, radiation and contrast exposure, and increased cost burden for our already overburdened health care system, to name a few. Ideally, any such threshold would be the point at which benefits of either testing or treatment outweigh the risks; however this remains a judgment call, and the real numbers behind these decisions remain unknowable.

> **PRACTICE POINT**
> - It is important to know the diagnostic testing and treatment thresholds for certain patients and specific illnesses being considered.

CLINICAL EXPERIENCE AND EXPERTISE

Expertise in medicine may be defined as reliably superior performance through highly developed perceptual and cognitive skills. In medicine this is manifest as an organized and efficient approach to hypothesis generation and testing. Experts at medical diagnosis share the following attributes:

- Accurate calibration: match between observed and objectively measured diagnostic skills.
- Use of intuitive type I reasoning for common problems or limited time and analytic type II reasoning for less common problems, double-checking type I conclusions, or when time more readily available.
- Extensive internal database of "illness scripts," previously acquired collections of signs, symptoms, and patient characteristics, to which a new patient presentation can be compared.

DIAGNOSTIC ERROR

In 1999, the landmark Institute of Medicine report *To Err is Human: Building a Safer Health System* identified medical error as the fifth leading cause of death in the United States. Diagnostic error includes incorrect diagnosis, missed diagnosis, and materially delayed diagnosis. It may proceed from any cognitive failure in the diagnostic process including failure take an adequate history, perform an adequate exam, formulate or prioritize a differential diagnosis, create and enact a diagnostic plan, correctly interpret test results, or seek specialist opinion. While many diagnostic errors are inconsequential, in several studies in the United States and abroad, diagnostic errors accounted for roughly 10% to 20% of all adverse events.

> **PRACTICE POINT**
> - A diagnostic error occurs when there is any mistake or failure in the diagnostic process that leads to a misdiagnosis, a missed diagnosis, or a delayed diagnosis.

Across many studies the diagnostic error rate, at least for clinical specialties like internal medicine, has consistently been around 15%. This consistency, however, belies the inherent difficulty in studying diagnostic error. Diagnostic error is a process measure rather than an easily measured endpoint. Diagnostic error is a concept built on reference to a gold standard such as a confirmatory test, clinical outcome, second opinion, consensus review, or autopsy that not infrequently do not exist or do exist but are not readily available. Error reporting systems have historically been underutilized and

A checklist for diagnosis

Obtain your own, complete medical history.

Perform a focused and purposeful physical examination.

Generate some initial hypotheses and differentiate these with appropriate additional questions, physical examination, or diagnostic tests.

Pause to reflect—Take a diagnostic time-out:

- Was I comprehensive?
- Did I consider the inherent flaws of heuristic thinking?
- Was my judgment affected by any other biases?
- Do I need to make the diagnosis NOW, or can I wait?
- What's the worst-case scenario? What are the "do not miss" entities?

Embark on a plan, but acknowledge uncertainty and ensure a pathway for follow-up.

Figure 8-7 *A checklist for diagnosis.*

even when employed often lack, within their schema, a category for diagnostic error. There is no evidence base on which to rest conclusions about when a diagnosis should or could have been made and whether a more accurate or timely diagnosis would have affected outcomes.

CONCLUSION

Numerous authors have suggested clinicians should use a diagnostic checklist to help avoid or mitigate diagnostic error. An example of a checklist for diagnosis can be found in **Figure 8-7**.

PRACTICE POINT

- A differential diagnosis is the ability to distinguish a disease or condition from others that present with similar signs, symptoms, or diagnostic test results.
- List the top diagnosis first but keep it problem oriented until the diagnosis has been made.
- Aggressively prioritize most likely then most harmful in clinical workups.
- Exclude what diseases can easily be excluded and then remove those from differential diagnosis.
- Keep a broad differential until the top diagnosis has been confirmed and always plan for workup of other alternate diagnoses if the top diagnosis is excluded.
- When presented with a clinical conundrum, begin by defining the problem, be deliberate and gather key information, and then finally summarize the case when faced with large amounts of information.
- Utilize illness scripts, which can be very powerful tools for clinicians and aid in diagnosis.
- Perform the dual-process theory of reasoning and make sure to balance the intuitive and analytical components to maintain highly efficient and effective clinical reasoning.
- A clinician should be cognizant of cognitive biases in clinical reasoning and avoid them at all costs.
- Remember that patients do not always read the textbook."
- Recognize that bedside diagnosis (ie, history and physical), diagnostic tests, and interventions all carry diagnostic power

and often times have been studied with published data on measures of diagnosis (eg, sensitivity and specificity) that can be utilized when performing Bayesian reasoning in clinical practice.
- In the modern era of clinical practice, information overload is another pitfall as is overreliance on diagnostic tests, which may lead to overtesting or "overdiagnosis" (ie, the diagnosis of a "disease" that will never cause a patient symptoms or death).
- It is important to know the diagnostic testing and treatment thresholds for certain patients and specific illnesses being considered.
- Utilize the "rule of 15's" to quickly calculate posttest probability for a disease if the likelihood ratios are known for the diagnostic test performed.
- A diagnostic error occurs when there is any mistake or failure in the diagnostic process that leads to a misdiagnosis, a missed diagnosis, or a delayed diagnosis.

SUGGESTED READINGS

Bowen JL. Educational strategies to promote clinical diagnostic reasoning. *N Engl J Med.* 2006;255:2217-2225.

Charlin B, et al. Scripts and clinical reasoning. *Med Educ.* 2007;41:1178-1184.

Croskerry P. The importance of cognitive errors in diagnosis and strategies to minimize them. *Acad Med.* 2003;78:775-780.

Croskerry P. A universal model for diagnostic reasoning. *Acad Med.* 2009;84:1022-1028.

Elstein AS, Schwartz A. Clinical problem solving and diagnostic decision-making: selective review of the cognitive literature. *BMJ* 2002;324:729-732.

Elstein AS. Heuristics and biases: selected errors in clinical reasoning. *Acad Med.* 1999;74:791-794.

Ericsson KA. Deliberate practice and acquisition of expert performance: a general overview. *Acad Emerg Med.* 2008;15:988-994.

Graber ML, et al. Cognitive interventions to reduce diagnostic error: a narrative review. *BMJ Qual Saf.* 2011;21:535-557.

Marcum JA. An integrated model of clinical reasoning: dual-process theory of cognition and metacognition. *J Eval Clin Pract.* 2012;18:954-961.

McGhee S. *Evidence-Based Physical Diagnosis,* 3rd ed. St. Louis, MO: Saunders; 2012.

Norman GR, Eva KW. Diagnostic error and clinical reasoning. *Med Educ.* 2010;44:94-100.

ONLINE RESOURCE

Journal of the American Medical Association Collection. *The Rational Clinical Exam.* http://jama.jamanetwork.com

CHAPTER 9

Principles of Evidence-Based Prescribing

Brent G. Petty, MD

INTRODUCTION

Medications are the principal tools doctors use to maintain health, reverse illness, and extend patients' survival, hopefully with good quality of life. Yet medications may also cause serious illness and fail to have the desired effect if they are used improperly. Medications may be extraordinarily expensive, and the cost to individual patients, to hospitals, and to our health system has become almost prohibitive. Thus, the proper use of medications and prescribing of medications is critically important.

PRINCIPLES OF RATIONAL THERAPEUTICS

"It's not likely to be harmful" is no justification for trying something without demonstrated efficacy for the patient's problem, unless the intervention is in the setting of a clinical trial or the patient is informed of off-label use without evidence of benefit.

PRACTICE POINT

- Before any medication is ordered in a hospital or prescribed for an outpatient, the prescriber needs to consider the (1) efficacy, (2) safety, and (3) cost of the medication, in that order of importance. Without efficacy for the condition being treated, no medication should be given. There is a risk of toxicity with virtually all medications, so there must be a consideration of risk and benefit before starting or continuing medications.

EVIDENCE FOR EFFICACY

The quality of medical studies supporting the use of medications varies widely. In recent years, the quality of data has been graded by the groups reviewing the literature and making recommendations, such as the *Chest* guidelines for anticoagulation (**Table 9-1**). These grading systems consider the methodologies of the studies as well as the strength of the results.

Among the difficult issues with clinical trials is whether they can be extrapolated for all drugs in the same class. In general, extrapolation across a class is somewhat hazardous, as drug formulation, absorption, duration of effect, and sometimes drug interactions differ among drugs in the same class. Even with HMG-CoA reductase inhibitors, whose effects on LDL cholesterol are mostly affected by drug potency and can often be equated through adjustment of dose, the efficacy related to clinical outcomes and adverse effects may vary. What is true for one drug in a certain class may not be true for other drugs in the same class.

Another issue regarding the validity of clinical trials is the use of "surrogate markers" in place of "hard clinical end points." An example is a reduction of human immunodeficiency virus (HIV) RNA levels as a surrogate for medication efficacy instead of extended survival in patients with acquired immune deficiency syndrome (AIDS). Some surrogate markers have been demonstrated through rigorous clinical studies to be closely associated with hard clinical end points, providing assurance that they may be trusted as substitutes. Other surrogate markers have less data to justify their use as substitutes. The hazard of using surrogate markers is exemplified in a study of interleukin-2 therapy in patients with HIV infection, which showed a substantial and sustained elevation of CD4+ cell count over a period of 7 to 8 years average follow-up, but demonstrated no improvement in survival or the incidence of opportunistic infections.

TABLE 9-1 Strength of Recommendations Grading System

Grade of Recommendation	Benefits vs Risks and Burdens	Methodological Strength of Supporting Evidence	Implications
Strong recommendation, high-quality evidence (1A)	Benefits clearly outweigh risk and burdens or vice versa	Consistent evidence from randomized controlled trials without important limitations or exceptionally strong evidence form observational studies.	Recommendation can apply to most patients in certain circumstances. Further research is very unlikely to change our confidence in the estimate of effect.
Strong recommendation, moderate-quality evidence (1B)	Benefits clearly outweigh risk and burdens or vice versa	Evidence from randomized controlled trials with important limitations (inconsistent results, methodological flaws, indirect or imprecise) or very strong evidence from observational studies.	Recommendation can apply to most patients in certain circumstances. Higher-quality research may well have an important impact on our confidence in the estimate of effect and may change the estimate.
Strong recommendation, low or very low-quality evidence (1C)	Benefits clearly outweigh risk and burdens or vice versa	Evidence for at least one critical outcome from observational studies, case series, or randomized controlled trials, with serious flaws or indirect evidence.	Recommendation can apply to most patients in certain circumstances. Higher-quality research is likely to have an important impact on our confidence in the estimate of effect and may well change the estimate.
Weak recommendation, high-quality evidence (2A)	Benefits closely balanced with risk and burdens	Consistent evidence from randomized controlled trials without important limitations or exceptionally strong evidence form observational studies.	The best action may differ depending on circumstances or patient or societal values. Further research is very unlikely to change our confidence in the estimate of effect.
Weak recommendation, moderate-quality evidence (2B)	Benefits closely balanced with risk and burdens	Evidence from randomized controlled trials with important limitations (inconsistent results, methodological flaws, indirect or imprecise) or very strong evidence form observational studies.	Best action may differ depending on circumstances or patient or societal values. Higher-quality research may well have an important impact on our confidence in the estimate of effect and may change the estimate.
Weak recommendation, low- or very low-quality evidence (2C)	Uncertainty in the estimates of benefits, risks and burden; benefits, risk and burden may be closely balanced	Evidence for at least one critical outcome from observational studies, case series, or randomized controlled trials, with serious flaws or indirect evidence.	Other alternatives may be equally reasonable. Higher-quality research is likely to have an important impact on our confidence in the estimate of effect and may well change the estimate.

Another common outcome strategy in clinical trials is the use of "composite end points," combining as an "event" any one of several conditions, such as cardiac death, nonfatal myocardial infarction, and admission to a hospital for unstable angina. Obviously, all of these conditions are defensible as outcomes in patients with coronary artery disease, but they are decreasingly reliable as "hard clinical end points" for an intervention intended to influence the course of coronary artery disease. Especially when one of the three conditions contributing to the composite end point is the result of variable clinician judgment (eg, when to admit a patient for unstable angina), the reliability of the composite end point decreases.

All three of these problems with assessing efficacy of medications relate to how physicians evaluate and utilize randomized clinical trials (RCTs) for making clinical decisions in their practices. The application of results from an RCT to a specific patient ideally depends on assuring that the patient is similar to those described as subjects for the study and that the intervention being tested will be provided in the same way described in the RCT. Both of these elements (similarity to the subjects and following the intervention described in the study) require a careful review of the "Methods" section of the paper, not just the "Abstract" and/or "Conclusions" section.

SAFETY

Throughout all phases of drug development before drug approval (phases I, II, and III), safety is assessed, but at best these studies involve only a few thousand study subjects for the vast majority of drugs. With this number of patients, only side effects of moderate frequency

(around 1-10 per thousand) will be identified. More rare (and often more serious) side effects may only become recognized with much more extensive use, involving tens of thousands of people. The experience with drugs such as troglitazone emphasizes the importance of postmarketing reporting of toxicities associated with newly approved medications to MedWatch (the FDA Safety Information and Adverse Event Reporting Program) and/or to the manufacturer.

There is a risk of toxicity with virtually all medications, so there must be a consideration of risk and benefit before starting or continuing medications. In many cases, the toxicity emerges without warning ("idiosyncratic"), such as rashes in response to sulfa drugs. These "adverse drug events" are usually unpredictable and are not considered "medication errors." In other cases, the possible toxicities of medications can be identified and treated before they become clinically dangerous (eg, hypokalemia with loop diuretics or hyperkalemia with angiotensin-converting-enzyme [ACE] inhibitors). These adverse drug events are not medication errors either, unless the patient is not monitored appropriately with occasional serum potassium measurements.

COST

The cost of medical care is staggering, partly fueled by the cost of medications. The contribution of medication cost to overall health care expenses more than doubled from 4.7% in 1982 to 10.5% in 2002. Interestingly, while drug costs continued going up thereafter, the rate of increase in the cost of prescription drugs generally decreased over the years from 1998 to 2008 and leveled off to around 4% in the years from 2007 to 2011. In 2012, there was actually a 1% decline in total dollars spent on medications in the United States, then the expenditures rebounded to a 3.2% increase in 2013 and then to a whopping 13% increase in 2014, the largest increase since 2001. This large increase was driven by the largest number of new molecular entities launched in more than a decade (numbering 42), by reduced patent expirations, and by increased price and volume of drugs ordered to treat patients with hepatitis C virus (HCV). The high cost of medications affects patients as individuals, who sometimes find that they are unable to afford their medications, and as a result these patients often go without them. This "economic noncompliance" increases during difficult economic periods or when people have fixed incomes and must choose between paying for these medications or for their food or mortgage for instance. The high cost of medicine also affects hospitals and health systems. If hospitals and health systems would pay less for their medications, they would have more funds available for capital improvements or expanded personnel services.

Clinical trials have increasingly been including assessment of the quality of life saved, not just the survival rate. The measure of quality-adjusted life years (QALYs) is a standard and internationally recognized method to assess the relative benefit of medical interventions. It combines duration of survival and the quality of life during each year of life. Although one treatment might help patients live longer, it might also have serious side effects (eg, it might make them feel sick or put them at risk for other illnesses). Another treatment might not extend survival but it may improve quality of life (eg, by reducing pain or other symptoms of disease). The quality of life rating can range from 0 (ie, worst possible health) to 1 (ie, best possible health). Having the QALY measurement allows one to consider cost effectiveness (ie, how much the drug or treatment costs per QALY). This is the cost of providing a year of the best quality of life available, which could be one person receiving one QALY, but is more likely to be a number of people receiving a portion of a QALY (eg, four people receiving 0.25 QALY). In this example, cost effectiveness is expressed as dollars per QALY.

Cost effectiveness analysis is another increasingly popular approach to assess the impact of interventions that may have financial benefit. For example, aspirin's cost is much lower than the cost of caring for the number of heart attacks and strokes it prevents. Sometimes the benefit is secondary or indirect. For example, acetylcholinesterase inhibitors are reported to cause a temporary delay in the cognitive decline of patients with dementia. If this delay in cognitive decline can prevent a patient from requiring institutionalization or full-time care at home for a period of months or years, the costs of such care may be much more than the cost of the medication and so the medication would then be deemed cost effective. Policymakers, including governmental bodies, payers, and influential foundations, are interested in maximizing cost effectiveness. They are convinced, with some justification that many practices and interventions might well be replaced with less costly approaches, without diminishing the quality of the care and the benefit our patients derive. "Choosing Wisely," an initiative of the American Board of Internal Medicine (ABIM) Foundation and Consumer Reports, is a good example.

OTHER FACTORS INFLUENCING MEDICATION SELECTION

PATIENT PREFERENCES AND VALUES

With rare exception, prescribers have a number of possible medications for managing diseases, and each may cause likely responses, either good or bad, in addition to the intended response. In all cases, the patient's inclination to accept the proposed therapy should be considered.

The very choice of initiating medication treatment or not should be weighed. It is always an option in medicine to do nothing (ie, offer no treatment), and sometimes no treatment is the best option. For example, in a patient with an acute inferior wall myocardial infarction who develops second-degree atrioventricular block,

Mobitz type I (aka Wenkebach), the occasional missed beat is of no clinical consequence, creates no risk for the patient, and almost always resolves without intervention. Treating such a patient with atropine or a pacemaker would be a mistake, introducing some risk of toxicity or complication for no clinical benefit, so no treatment is the best approach in this case.

The prescriber should also consider coexisting medical conditions that might likewise benefit from the same therapy, as this may magnify the benefit of the medication without adding additional risk of toxicity. For example, in a patient with hypertension who also suffers from frequent migraine headaches, a beta blocker or calcium channel blocker such as verapamil might be favored over other medications because they may reduce the frequency and/or severity of the migraine episodes at the same time the blood pressure is being reduced.

Patients with potentially life-threatening conditions (eg, metastatic cancer) are often treated with potent medications with the potential of side effects that are not only miserable but may also be life-threatening. When treatments are similar in efficacy but differ in types of toxicities, the patients' preferences are important, since hair loss may be more adverse for some patients than risk of infection or incidence of diarrhea. Tailoring the medications used in such cases preserves the patient's autonomy and properly respects his or her right to choose among reasonable options. This is an example of the important principle of shared decision making.

PRACTICE POINT

- When treatments are similar in efficacy but differ in types of toxicities, the patients' preferences are important. Tailoring the medications used in such cases preserves the patient's autonomy and properly respects his or her right to choose among reasonable options.

INDIVIDUAL RISK

Sometimes patient characteristics create special susceptibility to adverse events. For example, the toxicity seen with the nucleoside reverse-transcriptase inhibitor abacavir causes a hypersensitivity reaction in about 5% to 10% of patients. This reaction usually occurs in the first 2 months of treatment and is sufficiently severe enough that it requires discontinuation of the drug. The manifestations include fever, rash, and respiratory, gastrointestinal, and constitutional symptoms. The reaction was found to be associated with the HLA-B*5701 gene variant. Investigators in Australia have demonstrated that screening with genotyping before instituting abacavir therapy is effective in reducing the number of such reactions. In fact, there were no hypersensitivity reactions in the HLA-B*5701-negative patients. This exemplifies the value of pharmacogenomic biomarkers to enhance the treatment of patients with medications.

Patients age 65 or over constitute about 15% of the US population, but they consume around 30% of the medications prescribed. The natural deterioration of both renal and hepatic function with age makes older patients more susceptible to toxicity from the regular use of medications. **Figure 9-1** demonstrates the altered pharmacokinetics after an intravenous dose of verapamil in an 82-year-old man as compared to a 23-year-old man. Elimination is delayed and the peak blood concentration of verapamil is higher in the older man, perhaps related to a modest change in volume of distribution. **Figure 9-2** shows the relationship of age and intravenous diazepam dose needed to achieve adequate sedation for a procedure. As predicted by pharmacokinetics, the dose needed for an older adult is less than that needed for a younger patient. **Figure 9-3** shows the relationship of age and serum concentration of diazepam needed to achieve adequate sedation for a procedure. Note that the concentration required diminishes

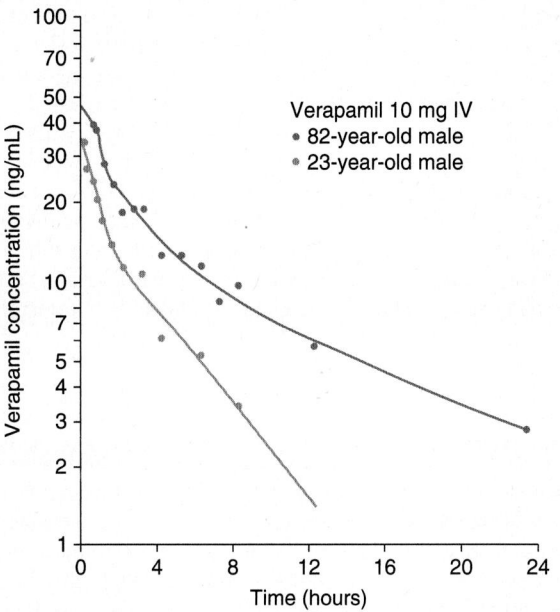

Figure 9-1 *Altered pharmacokinetics in the elderly.* (Reproduced, with permission, from Schwartz JB. Clinical pharmacology. In: Hazzard WR, et al., eds. *Principles of Geriatric Medicine and Geronotology,* 3rd ed. New York, NY: McGraw-Hill; 1994.)

steadily with advancing age, demonstrating that older adults are more sensitive to diazepam than younger patients. So for both of these reasons (delayed elimination and increased sensitivity to the medication), dosing diazepam is best accomplished with particular caution in older adults. While this relationship between medication concentration and age is not seen with all benzodiazepines, starting at low doses and increasing slowly, according to individual patient response, is an especially good principle when prescribing medications for older adults.

ASSESSING THE EVIDENCE

Well-designed, randomized, controlled, "blinded" or "masked," and prospective clinical trials provide the strongest evidence to direct medical practice. Each of these elements increases the likelihood that the results of the study can be accepted rather than be the result of chance. The study question is ideally framed as a null hypothesis, which is often not what the investigators actually expect

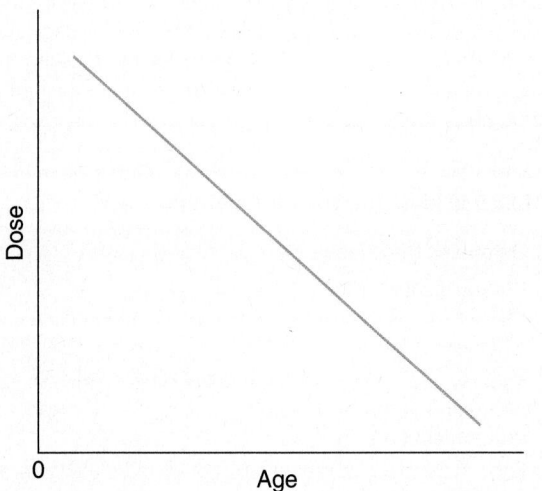

Figure 9-2 *Relationship of age and dose required to achieve a desired effect.*

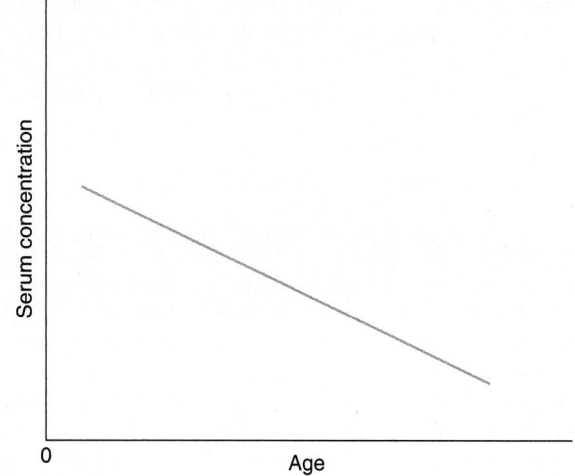

Figure 9-3 *Relationship of age and serum concentration required to achieve a desired effect.*

to find. In fact, most investigators begin with the expectation of showing a difference between the test compound and either standard treatment or inactive treatment (ie, placebo). For example, if one were comparing the effect of two HMG-CoA reductase inhibitors (aka statins) on serum cholesterol, a null hypothesis could be: "There is no difference between atorvastatin and rosuvastatin in patients with hypercholesterolemia and symptomatic coronary artery disease." The study requires a sufficient sample size to attempt to disprove the null hypothesis with a certainty of at least 95% that the degree of difference between the response to the two drugs is a true difference and not just the result of chance (alpha or type I error = 0.05). Investigators may expect that there will not be a significant difference between the two arms and employ what is called a non-inferiority study. Confirming that two medications are equivalent or that one is noninferior requires a larger sample size than needed for confirming that medications are different. The beta, or type II, error is normally set at 0.2, but when investigators want more certainty that the observed similarity is more likely to be true than just the result of chance, the beta error may be reduced to 0.1.

Once the study is completed with the intended sample size, the results are analyzed. The most balanced approach is to assume that either of the two groups could be superior to the other, which leads to a two-tailed statistical test. It is especially interesting to see how each arm performed compared to the predicted response. The analysis can determine whether one group had a more favorable outcome than the other, and by how much they differed. The difference is statistically significant if it is less likely than 5% to have reached that difference through chance alone. The 5% threshold is, of course, arbitrary as a level to embrace an observation with absolute conviction versus 6% to discount the difference as nothing very meaningful. In fact, when the difference reaches a 6% degree of certainty for being beyond a chance finding, it seems inappropriate to say that the performance of the groups was "not different." The truth is that the groups' performance was different, but that difference did not reach the accepted level of statistical significance. In such cases, one often hears the term "trend" used to describe the difference, and the difference would likely have reached statistical significance if the study's sample size were larger and the proportional responses continued to occur with the same frequency in additional subjects.

Too often readers ignore the "Methods" section of published papers, giving their limited time and attention instead to the "Abstract," a few figures or tables in the "Results" section, and the highlights of the "Discussion" section. This approach may save time, but it ignores the critical information about characteristics of the study population recruited, what kinds of patients were excluded, how other medications were managed, and many other aspects that ultimately determine whether the results of the study are valid and whether they can be applied to any other population/patient group besides those enrolled in the study. The paper rises or falls on its methods, so results or conclusions are not valid if the procedures involved with conducting the study are seriously flawed.

THE HOSPITAL FORMULARY

Decisions about which specific drugs are included in a hospital's formulary are usually made by a multidisciplinary formulary committee, which includes physicians and other prescribers, nurses, pharmacists, and others. This group reviews the available data on efficacy, safety, and cost of products proposed to be added to or removed from the hospital formulary. To be an effective member of such a committee, an individual would need to understand the importance of efficacy, safety, and cost as they relate to the population of patients served by the hospital. Clear thinking is especially important as the committee members consider the hospital's welfare in addition to advocacy for individual patients or a small group of patients. Workflow issues for all members of the care team are important. Likewise, the incremental cost of one medication compared to another may ultimately influence whether sufficient money is available for other hospital priorities, such as hiring or maintaining staff members. It is the balance of these multiple issues that makes the work of the formulary committee interesting and important.

During a hospitalization, the patient may receive a different drug than what he or she was taking at home before admission. This may be the result of provider preference or formulary restriction. Hospital formularies are either open or closed, and may have additional restrictions. Open formularies allow prescribers to order any marketed product, and the patient will get whatever specific product was ordered. Closed formularies limit the selection of medications to a small number of products within either a chemical class or an indication class. For example, rather than having all H2 receptor antagonists and proton pump inhibitors on the hospital's formulary, the hospital may restrict the choice to famotidine and pantoprazole. These determinations are generally made based on the assumptions of (1) equal, or at least adequate, efficacy, (2) no worse toxicity profile for the selected product, and (3) substantial cost savings.

MEDICATION RECONCILIATION

When the history, physical examination, and relevant laboratory data have been obtained, treatment begins. The treatment may be either specific (ie, based on the establishment of a specific diagnosis) or empiric (ie, based on the best guess of diagnosis using the available evidence and considering the usual etiology responsible for the condition, such as the most likely bacterial pathogens for a community-acquired pneumonia). The initiation of new medication in the hospital or in the outpatient setting must be framed on the background of the medication(s) that the patient previously had taken. Medication reconciliation refers to the cognitive process of considering the immediate previous medications (eg, the patient's "home medications") when ordering new treatment. Medication reconciliation is not simply duplicating the patient's "home medications" (eg, outpatient medications) into the hospital's order system, but rather a thoughtful consideration of the value and appropriateness of providing each medication in light of the patient's new medical situation. There should be a conscious decision, for each and every medication, whether to stop, continue, or modify administration of the drug.

At the time of transfer to a new service or level of care and at the end of the patient's hospitalization, another medication reconciliation should occur. This process differs from the one at the time of admission because the consideration of medications to prescribe upon transfer or at discharge should take into account not only the medications the patient was taking in the hospital just before transfer or discharge, but also the patient's "home medications." The purpose of this dual consideration is to avoid costly and potentially hazardous duplication of medications. As already explained, a patient may receive one proton pump inhibitor while in the hospital (eg, pantoprazole), which is different than the one taken at home (eg, omeprazole) or one that could be prescribed at discharge (eg, lansoprazole). Patients have been known to be taking supplies of both warfarin and "Coumadin" following hospital discharge because one had been provided by prescription from the family doctor and the other was prescribed by the hospital doctor(s). Since generic and brand products may look different, it is not hard to understand how patients may not recognize a hazardous duplication.

THERAPEUTIC DRUG MONITORING

Treatment of any patient should follow the "ideal therapeutic algorithm" (**Table 9-2**). First, the prescriber should have a therapeutic goal in mind, whether it is to lower the blood pressure to a certain point, reduce the hemoglobin A1c below a certain threshold, or drive the LDL cholesterol down under 100 mg/dL. With the goal in mind, an appropriate agent is selected, and then an appropriate dose of the agent is chosen. When relevant patient characteristics or concomitant medications are known, the dose may be individualized somewhat. After allowing a sufficient period of time for the intervention to reach a substantial or peak effect, which may be days or weeks, a repeat measurement is performed and is compared to the pretreatment reading and the therapeutic goal. Then, whatever the starting dose may have been, adjustments in the dose may well be needed to achieve the therapeutic goal. After the response to the new dose is observed, another adjustment in dose, or adding or substituting another medication, can be considered. All the while there is monitoring for evidence of adverse effects.

"Therapeutic drug monitoring" is a term that usually implies the measurement in some body fluid of a substance that is either the medication that is being monitored or a related substance. Therapeutic drug monitoring is best employed when certain criteria can be met (**Table 9-3**). If measuring a physiological result (eg, prothrombin time) or if a drug concentration is part of the monitoring (eg, phenytoin serum level), one must be confident that the laboratory to be used can measure the item accurately and in a timely fashion. Then, it must be known that the efficacy of the drug is enhanced or the toxicity of the drug is reduced by adjusting the dose of the medication. We should avoid the temptation to measure drug concentrations just because we can. Achieving and maintaining results in a "therapeutic range" should reduce the risk of toxicity or improve efficacy, or ideally both. If the efficacy or toxicity of a medication cannot reliably be improved by adjusting the dose to achieve a result in the therapeutic range, then therapeutic drug monitoring is not of value.

TABLE 9-2 Ideal Therapeutic Algorithm

1. Determine the therapeutic goal.

2. Choose an appropriate agent.

3. Choose the appropriate dose, individualizing for each patient when possible.

4. Know when/how to monitor for effectiveness and safety, including the essential criteria for appropriate therapeutic drug monitoring.

5. Know how to adjust the therapy (eg, increase the dose, add another medication, switch to another agent etc) to attain the therapeutic goal and avoid toxicity.

TABLE 9-3 Criteria for Appropriate Therapeutic Drug Monitoring

1. Medication concentration or effects can be measured reliably and accurately.

   AND

2. The efficacy of medication treatment can be enhanced by achieving a certain concentration or effect range.

   AND/OR

3. The toxicity of medication treatment can be reduced by maintaining a certain concentration or effect range.

Measuring drug concentrations in plasma or serum establishes individual patient pharmacokinetics. One well-done drug concentration is more valuable than any algorithm that seeks to predict concentration or effect using patient characteristics, comorbidities, or other factors. Poorly done therapeutic monitoring may produce results that are misleading, and in this way are worse than having no testing at all. The duration of an infusion and the correct timing of the sample after the infusion are critical to having results that can be assessed in light of published data and guidelines. Especially hazardous is drawing blood samples for drug concentrations too soon after an intravenous dose of a drug, which may put the sample in the period of the alpha half-life or distribution phase rather than in the beta half-life or elimination phase, which is a more predictable and interpretable portion of the drug elimination curve. On the other hand, especially with oral medications, checking drug concentrations after too few doses are given to have the concentrations at or near steady state may lead to an underestimation of the adequacy of a dose, and a premature increase to a higher dose may lead to serious toxicity when the drug concentration does achieve steady state at a level too high for safety.

ROLE OF PHARMACISTS IN ASSISTING WITH MEDICATION ORDERING

More hospitals are employing pharmacists to assist prescribers in their management of patients. These trained professionals are especially knowledgeable about medication issues, including indications for medications, their doses (in both normal and physiologically impaired patients), drug-drug and drug-food interactions, and other important matters in medication use. They are familiar with resources that help identify medications, including foreign and generic products. Some pharmacists serve on hospital policy-making committees because of their perspectives related to drug dispensing and monitoring. In some hospitals, they see patients with conditions such as hypertension and evaluate the propriety of the patients' medications, the patients' knowledge of their medications and how to use them, and the most likely adverse events that the patients may encounter. Pharmacists round with care teams and provide information on medications during the discussions about the patients. In some states, pharmacists may be granted ordering authority by the hospital, and pharmacists may staff anticoagulation monitoring clinics. Pharmacists, like nurses, are the physicians' compatriots and can help physicians avoid making serious errors. As important team members, they should be heeded, respected, and appreciated.

MANAGEMENT OF DRUG SAMPLES

The topic of drug samples is only a portion of the larger topic of the relationship of prescribers and hospitals to the pharmaceutical industry. Whether to allow samples in a practice or hospital at all can be very controversial. At balance is the advantage of "free" medication for those patients who cannot afford it versus the clear marketing motivation of the suppliers of the samples. Samples may be allowed in the offices of individual practitioners or in the clinical space of a multidisciplinary group. Some hospitals have centralized samples into the pharmacy to be dispensed to the medically indigent with special prescriptions, while other hospitals have forbidden drug samples altogether. There are justifications on all sides of this issue, but if samples are allowed in an office, practice, or hospital, their use should be documented in each case they are dispensed, the patient should be supplied with product information (eg, from a pharmacy), and expiration and recalls should be monitored.

Samples are not the only strategy used by industry to influence prescribing and medication-ordering habits. Direct-to-consumer advertising, gifts, grants, support of clinical investigation, journal advertising, and even unrestricted donations to hospitals and medical schools have the potential to introduce a sense of obligation and indebtedness in those who influence the specific medications that patients receive. The issue is complicated, but we should institute measures to minimize our biases or their effects. We must act as objectively as possible for the benefit of our patients.

"Academic detailing" is a concept that has been proposed to help reduce undue influence from industry. Academic detailing involves the distribution of knowledge from trusted medical personnel, often the leaders of academic departments or divisions, government advisers (eg, from the U.S. Food and Drug Administration, Centers for Disease Control and Prevention, or National Institutes of Health), or other external experts who can be invited into hospitals to educate the hospitals' medical staffs on the pros and cons of various medications. Leaders and other members of the hospital's formulary committee, as well as leaders and members of the hospitalist group at the hospital, may be considered for academic detailing if they have appropriate knowledge about the medications under discussion and are free from conflicts of interest that would potentially affect their opinions.

SUGGESTED READINGS

Guyatt GH, Norris SL, Schullman S, et al. Methodology for the development of antithrombotic therapy and prevention of thrombosis guidelines: antithrombotic therapy and prevention of thrombosis. *Chest*. 2012;141:53S-70S.

IMS Institute for Healthcare Informatics, Press Releases, IMS Health Study. 2014 A Record-Setting Year for U.S. Medicines. http://www.us.imshealth.com. Accessed May 9, 2015.

INSIGHT-ESPRIT Study Group and SILCAAT Scientific Committee. Interleukin-2 therapy in patients with HIV infection. *N Engl J Med*. 2009;361:1548-1559.

Mallal S, Phillips E, Carcosi G, et al. HLA-B*5701 screening for hypersensitivity to abacavir. *N Engl J Med*. 2008;358:568-579.

Petty BG. Trends in medication use: implications for medication errors. *J Pharmacist Fin Econ Pol*. 2006;15:137-174.

Reidenberg MM, Levy M, Warner H, et al. Relationship between diazepam dose, plasma level, age, and central nervous system depression. *Clin Pharm Ther*. 1978;23:371-374.

Schumock GT, Li EC, Suda KJ, et al. National trends in prescription drug expenditures and projections for 2015. *Am J Health Syst Pharm*. 2015;72:717-736.

ONLINE RESOURCES

- Choosing Wisely. An initiative of the ABIM Foundation. http://www.choosingwisely.org/
- MedWatch. The FDA Safety Information and Adverse Event Reporting Program. http://www.fda.gov/Saftey/MedWatch/

10

Summary Literature: Practice Guidelines and Systematic Reviews

Dustin T. Smith, MD
Bhavin Adhyaru, MD

INTRODUCTION

Summary literature represents the highest quality of evidence and the top portion of the evidence-based medicine pyramid. In this chapter, summary literature refers specifically to practice guidelines and systematic reviews. If done properly, authors will have performed a comprehensive systematic review of the literature available as well as summarized findings from the available literature for both of these types of manuscripts. For practice guidelines, the summary typically exists in the form of graded recommendations. For systematic reviews, the summary comes in the form of a meta-analysis where a quantitative statistical analysis is conducted of pooled data from several separate but similar studies. Although articles featuring literature reviews (ie, narrative review, aka "review articles") by authors exist for many clinical topics in medicine, the methods used for reviewing the literature in these articles are not necessarily systematic or comprehensive and it is typically left to the authors' discretion for which data and studies to include. **Table 10-1** offers a comparison of narrative reviews, systematic reviews, meta-analysis, and guidelines.

PRACTICE GUIDELINES

■ INTRODUCTION

Hospitalists face the challenging task of managing patients with a diverse array of important and sometimes complicated medical conditions. Clinical practice guidelines exist and are designed to assist both health care providers and patients in making appropriate decisions regarding clinical care for the prevention, diagnosis, and treatment of health care conditions. Practice guidelines are systematically developed statements summarizing available medical literature for a specific clinical circumstance. The summary for practice guidelines usually comes in the form of graded recommendations based on the amount of data and quality of evidence that exists for a specific clinical circumstance. Ideally, practice guidelines should be presented in a user-friendly format that allows hospitalists the ability to deliver the best medical care possible.

■ BENEFITS

Medical practice guidelines facilitate consistency, efficiency, and effectiveness to improve health care outcomes. Good clinical practice guidelines have been compared to receiving good recommendations from a consultant. Practice guidelines should provide clear recommendations, discuss alternatives, acknowledge biases, and consider extenuating circumstances for a specific clinical case.

■ BARRIERS

Physician adherence to guidelines has been demonstrated to be surprisingly low at times. Guidelines have been shown to have had a limited effect on changing physicians' practices and behaviors despite widespread implementation. Incorporating guidelines into the daily practice face numerous barriers, including both internal (eg, provider awareness or familiarity) and external (eg, environmental-related or systems-related factors). Some physician perceived barriers to using guidelines include concerns for reduced autonomy and/or loss of the patient-physician relationship when following an oversimplification or "cookbook" approach to medicine or that they may not be practical or easy to use. Practice guidelines may not be applicable to a clinician's patient and/or practice population

TABLE 10-1 Comparison and Contrast of Overview Article Types

	Narrative Review	Systematic Review	Meta-Analysis	Guideline
Focused Clinical Question	Not generally	Yes	Yes	Yes (Multiple questions addressed)
Structured Search Strategy	No	Yes	Yes	Yes
Selection of Included Articles	Dependent on author	Systematic	Systematic	Systematic
Quality Assessment of included articles	No	Yes	Yes	Yes
Qualitative or Quantitative result	Qualitative	Qualitative	Quantitative	Qualitative and Quantitative
Sources/Example	UptoDate or Dynamed	Cochrane Review	Cochrane Review	http://www.guideline.gov

(eg, outpatient management guidelines when a providers' sole form of practice is the inpatient setting). Concerns regarding the credibility of a guideline may have existed in the past; however, numerous professional groups have worked to improve the standards and credibility of practice guidelines.

STANDARDS TO IMPROVE CREDIBILITY

In 2012, the Guidelines International Network (G-I-N) proposed standards for clinical practice guidelines. This global network comprises numerous organizations and individual members from countries represented on all continents of the world to support evidence-based health care and improved health outcomes by reducing inappropriate variation throughout the world. Their published mission is to lead, strengthen, and support collaboration and work within the guideline development, adaptation, and implementation community. The G-I-N addressed the key components of high quality and trustworthy guidelines, that is, composition of guideline development group, decision-making process, conflicts of interests, scope of a guideline, methods, evidence reviews, guideline recommendations, rating of evidence of and recommendations, peer review and stakeholder consultations, guideline expiration and updating, and financial support and sponsoring organization. The G-I-N also houses the world's largest international guideline library.

The Appraisal of Guidelines for Research and Evaluation Enterprise (AGREE) is another group that has worked to address the variability in practice guideline quality by creating the AGREE Instrument. The AGREE Instrument is a tool that assesses methodological rigor and transparency in guideline development and use. The AGREE II is comprised of 23 items and organized into six quality domains for practice guidelines: scope and purpose, stakeholder involvement, rigor of development, clarity of presentation, applicability, and editorial independence. A modified framework in both interpretation and assessment of the quality of clinical practice guidelines is divided into three general domains: validity, results, and applicability.

VALIDITY

The credibility of clinical practice guidelines is markedly swayed by the validity in which guideline developers gathered, appraised, and combined evidence to formulate recommendations. Clinicians should consider the following components that determine the validity of a guideline: scope and purpose, group composition, conflicts of interests, literature review, group processes, external review and endorsements, editorial independence, and current guidelines.

SCOPE AND PURPOSE (AKA PRIORITY SETTING)

Well-written clinical practice guidelines should begin by describing the scope and purpose of the guidelines. The scope and purpose often include the target patient population including but not limited to parameters for age, gender, ethnicity, and disease type/subtypes.

GROUP COMPOSITION

The validity of clinical practice guidelines is markedly impacted by the composition of the developers. Selection of a multidisciplinary team to review data and generate the guidelines should decrease the chance for bias. A guideline that is developed by only one group of medical subspecialists may be biased to likely recommend an intervention that falls within their realm of practice. The multidisciplinary team should include both generalists and specialists, providers from both medicine and surgery if applicable, as well as experts from other allied health professions such as nursing, pharmacy, and therapy fields (eg, respiratory therapy if applicable). Members should have expertise in the scope of practice the guideline is trying to address and may have extensive research backgrounds in the general or specific field of medicine for which the guideline is being developed. Many professional medical societies sponsor guideline development so often times the group is comprised of members from the actual organization sponsoring the guideline. Additionally, many well-formed groups who develop clinical practice guidelines will include an expert in statistics, evidence-based medicine, and/or grading recommendations.

CONFLICTS OF INTERESTS

As for any publication, authors must report any conflicts of interests somewhere in the text for each individual. Any and all relevant financial relationships with any commercial interests related, directly or indirectly, to the subject of the clinical practice guideline must be addressed in the guideline. If members of the group comprising the guideline do have any significant conflicts of interests, this may affect the validity of the guideline in a negative way. The role of the sponsoring organization in formulating the guidelines should also be made clear in the text of the guidelines.

LITERATURE REVIEW

The validity of a clinical practice guideline is markedly affected by the completeness of the search strategy and review of literature used to formulate recommendations. The search strategy should be reported after the introduction but before the recommendations in the guideline similar to a "methods" section in a research manuscript. The review typically follows the protocol of a valid systematic review and meta-analysis. The search for relevant studies includes electronic databases (eg, National Center for Biotechnology Information PubMed), conference abstracts/symposia, and references provided by the identified studies. In some instances, researchers of previous studies may need to be contacted in order to gather final or complete results if they have not been published and in order to avoid publication bias. The search terms, synonyms, different spellings (eg, anemia and anaemia), and Boolean Operators used are also important to ensure an exhaustive search and provide evidence of validity for the guidelines. The criteria for including and excluding studies used to formulate the guidelines should be defined and reported within the text. The process of reviewing included studies for quality should be elucidated within the text. Additionally, other limits for the search strategy and literature review such as by language (eg, articles published in English only), date of publication, demographics, or subgroups should be reported and considered when assessing the validity of guidelines. Some of this may be clear in the scope and purpose of the clinical practice guideline but an explicit description of the literature review used to collect data in formulating the clinical practice guideline is crucial in determining the validity of the guideline.

■ GROUP PROCESSES

The process used by the group developing the guidelines should be made clear in the text of the guidelines. Numerous group processes exist which have been validated (eg, Delphi method) but a particular clinical practice guideline may be distinctive and require a unique process. The process should be defined, systematic, and fair while still allowing members of the group to equally contribute to the decision making and the recommendations developed therein the clinical practice guideline.

■ EXTERNAL REVIEW AND ENDORSEMENTS

Valid clinical practice guidelines must undergo an external review by another group of experts or a separate medical profession society or organization that did not sponsor or participate in the initial development of the guidelines. One or more societies or organizations may have reviewed the guidelines prior to publication and also provided their endorsement for the guidelines. Two or more organizations may formulate joint guidelines, a process which increases the validity of the guidelines as long as they adhered to proper group processes. For example, societies representing both interventional cardiologists and cardiothoracic surgeons may jointly formulate a clinical practice guideline on coronary revascularization.

■ EDITORIAL INDEPENDENCE

The authors developing clinical practice guidelines should have editorial independence, both from any relevant conflicts of interests as well as the sponsoring organization. This may markedly affect the validity of the guidelines if complete independence is not maintained. For many sponsoring organizations, there may exist a guideline development committee to ensure accurate and consistent guidelines, both in content, development, and structure. It should be explicitly stated that the actual group of authors who comprised the guidelines had editorial independence throughout the process.

■ CURRENT GUIDELINES

Valid clinical practice guidelines should reflect current research to accurately address the scope and purpose of the intended guideline. The time it takes to develop a guideline is considerable and puts the guideline at risk of being out of date at the time of publication if current research is not included. Approximately 7% of guidelines are out of date at the time of publication and the median survival of guidelines of is approximately 5.5 years. There are three important timelines to consider in the assessment of whether a guideline reflects current practice:

1. The date of publication for the guideline for which the final recommendations were given.
2. The dates of the literature reviewed in formulating the guidelines to determine if recent evidence was utilized.
3. The date and the procedure for updating the guideline.

In some instances there may ongoing studies in progress during the guideline development that may change the recommendations

of the guideline. If this is the case, guideline developers should explain which evidence was considered or not considered in making the final recommendations.

■ RESULTS

The results of clinical practice guidelines differ from that of an observational study, clinical trial, or meta-analysis. Whereas these publications typically report results in statistical and numerical terms, practice guidelines provide results in the form of recommendations as both the results of the systematic review and conclusions made by the guideline developers. Practice guidelines that are summarized appropriately should involve graded recommendations (ie, the recommendation receives an assigned grade by the experts involved in developing the guidelines). There are numerous grading systems in place for recommendations and many guideline developers adopt a system that is endorsed or created by either the sponsoring organization or professional society representing the guideline. Some have called for the adoption of a standard approach to grading recommendations for all guidelines. The unifying principle for most grading systems is that both the strength of a recommendation (eg, effect size and/or risk-benefit ratio) and level of evidence supporting a recommendation are considered when assigning a grade.

The Grading of Recommendations Assessment, Development and Evaluation (GRADE) Working Group came together in 2000 with the goal of developing a common, sensible, and transient approach for grading quality of evidence and strength of recommendations. The GRADE system classifies quality of evidence into one of four levels: high, moderate, low, or very low. With the GRADE system, evidence that is based on randomized controlled trials begins as high-quality evidence but may be lowered if any of the following are present: study limitations, inconsistency of results, indirectness of evidence, imprecision, or reporting bias. Observational studies start as low quality but may be graded up if the size of the treatment affect is very large, if a dose-response relation is present, or if all possible biases would decrease the size of the treatment affect. In the GRADE system, high-quality evidence is where further research is very unlikely to change the confidence in the estimate of effect for an intervention. Moderate quality is when further research is likely to have an impact and may change the estimate. Low quality is when further research is very likely to have an impact and likely change the estimate. Very low quality is when any estimate of effect is very uncertain. The GRADE system offers two grades for the strength of a recommendation: strong or weak. A strong recommendation is assigned if the beneficial effects of an intervention clearly outweigh the risks or clearly do not. A weak recommendation is assigned if there is a concern either because of the quality of the evidence, uncertainty in benefit-risk ratio for an intervention, uncertainty or variability in values and preferences, or uncertainty about whether an intervention represents a wise use of resources. An example of a grading system for Clinical Practice Guideline recommendations is provided in **Table 10-2**.

Clinicians should familiarize themselves with the grading system used to grade the recommendations when reviewing practice guidelines. The grading process should be explicit and well defined. The concepts of strength of recommendation and level of evidence supporting a recommendation will be further elucidated below.

■ STRENGTH OF RECOMMENDATIONS

The strength of a recommendation, sometimes referred to as the class of a recommendation (eg, Class I), designates whether a treatment or intervention is recommended or not as well as the level of

TABLE 10-2 A Grading System for Evaluating Evidence

Quality of Evidence	Strength of Recommendation	
	1 (Strong)	2 (Weak)
A (High)	1A—Strong recommendation, high-quality evidence.	2A—Weak recommendation, high-quality evidence.
	Consistent evidence for RCTs without important limitations or exceptionally strong evidence from observation studies.	Consistent evidence from RCTs without important limitations or exceptionally strong evidence from observational studies.
B (Moderate)	1B—Strong recommendation, moderate-quality evidence.	2B—Weak recommendation, moderate-quality evidence.
	Evidence from RCTs without important limitations (inconsistent results, methodological flaws, indirect or imprecise), or very strong evidence from observational studies.	Evidence from RCTs without important limitations (inconsistent results, methodological flaws, indirect or imprecise), or very strong evidence from observational studies.
C (Low)	1C—Strong recommendation, low- or very low-quality evidence.	1C—Weak recommendation, low- or very low-quality evidence.
	Evidence for at least one critical outcome from observational studies, case series, or from RCTs with serious flaws or indirect evidence.	Evidence for at least one critical outcome from observational studies, case series, or from RCTs with serious flaws or indirect evidence.

RCT, randomized controlled trial.

certainty behind the recommendation. The strength of a recommendation may be affected by numerous factors but generally is a representation for the size of treatment effect and degree of benefit versus risk for a specific intervention. Some interventions may have an unfavorable risk-benefit profile and thus would receive a recommendation strength denoting the risk is greater than the expected benefit. Some interventions shown to be of no benefit may be classified as such.

LEVEL OF EVIDENCE

The level of evidence surrounding a recommendation is an estimate of the certainty or precision for the treatment effect of a specific intervention. The level of evidence is graded based on the number of different populations studied, the actual number of study participants, and also what types of studies exist for a specific intervention. A higher level of evidence would be assigned to an intervention that has been validated in multiple study populations and with a high number of study participants. A higher level of evidence would also be assigned to an intervention where data has been acquired by randomized controlled trials rather than observational studies. The lowest level of evidence designation is typically assigned to the recommendation when very limited populations were evaluated for a specific intervention and thus only expert opinion, case reports, or previously accepted standard of care exist to support a recommendation. Although there is some relation and overlap between the concepts of strength of recommendation and level of evidence for a recommendation, they may exist exclusively. The strength of a recommendation for treatment based on a study demonstrating a very large treatment effect would be considered to be high; however, the level of evidence would be considered low if based on a single observational study until additional studies involving either more populations and/or higher quality studies (eg, randomized, controlled trial) are completed. For example, the American Heart Association and American College of Cardiology in 2013 grades the use of diuretics for symptom relief in patients with heart failure and volume overload as a "Class I" recommendation, indicating the benefit of this therapy is much greater than the risk (ie, benefit >>> risk); the

evaluation of very limited patient populations resulted in only a "C" grade for level of evidence. Likewise, a recommendation may be considered of low strength if the treatment effect or benefit-risk ratio is very small and still considered of high level of evidence if multiple populations have been studied and results have proven to be both certain and precise. Repeated studies are less likely when the following occurs:

- Expected benefits clearly outweigh any undesirable effects of the intervention as highly recommended.
- Desired benefits more closely balanced with any undesirable effects, given only marginal benefit upon initial study.

APPLICABILITY

Clinical practice guidelines that are useful must be applicable to a clinical provider's patient population and clinical scope of practice. The practices and recommendations described in guidelines must be able to be replicated by clinical providers in their own practice in order for them to be relevant and worthwhile. Additionally, factors such as disease prevalence, risk factors, comorbidities, and individual patient preferences that differ from the target population from which the guidelines were developed may affect the applicability of the guidelines to different patient populations.

Conflicting guidelines or discordant recommendations may be made by different organizations such a venous thromboembolism prophylaxis in subpopulations (eg, orthopedic surgery). Clinicians may not be able to reconcile discordant recommendations for every occasion.

Tools are available to facilitate guidelines comparisons so that clinicians may determine the quality and applicability of guideline to specific patient populations. One example of a tool that exists to aid clinicians is the "Compare Guidelines" tab that exists at www.guideline.gov sponsored by Agency for Healthcare Research and Quality. The simplest and most appropriate approach should always take into account individual patient risk factors, health care preferences and goals of care. Before offering interventions (including screening) and therapies to patients, always ask the question: "Do these clinical practice guidelines apply to my patient?"

SYSTEMATIC REVIEWS

INTRODUCTION

There are four major overviews, and they include narrative reviews, systematic reviews, meta-analysis, and guidelines. They represent the highest quality of evidence on the quality pyramid as they synthesize evidence from many sources. Narrative reviews elucidate a health context, condition, or intervention. They tend to answer background questions, biologic, or social issues. However, the methods for article inclusion and quality assessment are not structured and the credibility of the review is tied to the reviewer expertise. Systematic reviews and meta-analyses may focus on therapy, diagnosis, or prognosis depending on the clinical question at hand. Table 10-1 highlights the similarities and major differences between the various types of overview articles.

The goals of systematic reviews include answering questions where conflicting data exist and/or where sample sizes of individual trials are small. The ultimate goal of systematic reviews may be to generate hypotheses. Meta-analyses are a type of systematic review that use quantitative methods to combine results from multiple studies to yield a summary estimate of effect and a confidence interval around the estimate. A common source to search for systematic reviews and meta-analyses is the Cochrane Database (http://www.cochranelibrary.com/).

DEFINE THE QUESTION

Whereas in narrative reviews the clinical question tends to be more general, the clinical question in systematic reviews should be focused in a format with a clearly defined patient population, intervention, control, and clear outcomes. An example would be: "What is the risk of bleeding in adult patients with recurrent venous thromboembolism on rivaroxaban as compared to warfarin?"

LITERATURE SEARCH

Because the goal of systematic reviews is to synthesize information from many sources, it is important that a thorough review of the literature is done to prevent missing relevant studies. There should be a discussion of the bibliographic databases searched with the search terms included. The search strategy and included databases will depend on the question being asked. There should be an attempt to locate unpublished studies such as conference abstracts, experts in the field, pharmaceutical companies, and investigators of studies. There should also be consideration to searching in languages besides English based on prevalence of diseases in certain countries. Consideration of these factors can reduce the potential for publication bias, which may produce misleading summary effects.

INCLUSION AND EXCLUSION CRITERIA

In systematic reviews, inclusion and exclusion criteria for articles should be stated and there should be a discussion of the patients included, the exposures or interventions, the outcomes of interest and the methodological standards for study selection (eg, randomized controlled trials, diagnosis cohort, or observational studies). To improve the quality of studies, if randomized controlled trials exist, then these should be used preferentially to minimize bias. There should be specific inclusion and exclusion criteria based on the clinical question such as patient demographics (eg, age, sex, ethnicity, etc).

QUALITY OF STUDIES

There should be an assessment of individual studies that are included in the systematic review. For therapy studies, there should be evaluation for randomization (ie, allocation concealment), blinding (of investigators, patients, data collectors), and loss to follow-up as these can introduce systematic error in the meta-analysis. Ideally, the studies should report intention-to-treat (ie, all patients who underwent allocation are analyzed regardless of how long they stayed in the study) or per protocol (ie, only patients who remained within the protocol for a predetermined period are analyzed). For diagnostic studies, there should be evaluation of the appropriate reference standard.

Typically in systematic reviews, there should be quality assessment by more than one individual and investigator other than the principal investigator of the review. There are several ways to assess for the quality and differences amongst the individuals making the quality assessment. The kappa statistic (κ) represents the inter-reviewer reliability and is a measurement of the agreement between observers beyond chance. The κ-value ranges from -1.0, which is no agreement, to 1.0, which is perfect agreement. For most studies, a κ-value of 0.8 or higher is acceptable and represents excellent agreement and a κ-value of less than 0.4 represents poor agreement. The Jadad score is another structured way of assessing the quality of individual studies. The score is based on upon points for randomization, double blinding, and withdrawals. **Table 10-3** shows the modified Jadad scoring template for randomized controlled trials. The Newcastle-Ottawa score can be used for nonrandomized controlled trials.

META-ANALYSIS

If it seems reasonable and suitable, data from several studies can be combined to give an overall estimate result. The overall results produced from the results of a larger number of patients than individual studies are more accurate and reduce type 2 error (ie, failing to detect a difference that exists between the two groups), which increases the power of the analysis. It is important that the results can be appropriately combined (ie, individual studies have similar interventions, patients, outcome measures); otherwise, it would be like the popular idiom: "combining apples and oranges." Data in meta-analyses are presented as Forest plots. There are various statistical methods used to combine different data types, which will be discussed later in this chapter.

POOLED ESTIMATES AND FOREST PLOT

Figure 10-1 shows an example of a forest plot produced for a meta-analysis. On the left side, the names of the individual studies are listed. The green box represents the individual data from the studies and the risk ratio (with 95% confidence interval) is calculated taking

TABLE 10-3 The Modified Jadad Scoring System for Randomized Controlled Trials

	Score
1. Was the study described as randomized? If yes, score 1 point.	
2. If yes to question 1, was an **appropriate** randomization sequence described and used (eg, table of random numbers, computer generated, etc)? If yes, score 1 point.	
3. If yes to question 1, was an **inappropriate** method to generate the sequence of randomization used (patients were allocated alternately, or according to date of birth, hospital number, etc)? If yes, subtract 1 point.	
4. Was the study described as double blinded? If yes, score 1 point.	
5. If yes to question 4, was an appropriate method of blinding used (eg, identical placebo, active placebo, dummy, etc)? If yes, score 1 point.	
6. If yes to question 4, was an inappropriate method for blinding used (eg, comparison of tablet vs injection with no double dummy)? If yes, subtract 1 point.	
7. Were the withdrawals and dropouts described? If yes, score 1 point.	

into account the weight of the study. The weight (ie, importance in the overall result) is based on the sample size and precision of the results. More weight is given to studies with a larger sample size and a smaller standard deviation.

The orange box shows the pooled data and risk ratio. The absolute risk difference and number needed to treat or harm can also be calculated from this figure. In this example meta-analysis, the total experiment event rate is 0.25 and the control event rate is 0.16. Thus, the approximate risk ratio is 1.57 (favors control), absolute risk increase is 0.09, and the number needed to harm in this case is 11. Whereas many of the individual studies are small and not statistically significant, when pooled together, the overall effect becomes statistically significant with a narrower confidence interval.

The right side of the graph shows the individual mean effect as a dot with the line representing the 95% confidence interval. The larger the dot, the larger the weight it is given to the overall result. The diamond represents the overall effect size, and the size of the diamond is dependent on the 95% confidence intervals. A larger and/or wider diamond implies larger confidence intervals and a low

sample size. The x-axis represents the net effect or risk ratio either favoring control or experimental with the baseline at 1.0, which would indicate no effect. If the line or diamond width cross 1.0, then the result is not statistically significant. If the result is on the left side of the plot, it favors experimental. If the result is on the right side of the plot, then it favors the control.

■ HETEROGENEITY

When the results are pooled in a meta-analysis, determine that the data being pooled are appropriate without significant differences between study results (ie, "we are not comparing apples and oranges"). This is done using various tests for heterogeneity. The null hypothesis of the test for heterogeneity is that the underlying effect is the same in each study so that all of the variability between studies is just due to chance alone. A visual inspection for heterogeneity can be done. Random error (ie, chance) is a plausible explanation for the differences in the point estimates if the confidence intervals overlap widely (**Figure 10-2A**). Random chance cannot explain the differences in the apparent treatment effect if the confidence intervals do not overlap (**Figure 10-2B**). The P-value is a statistical test of significance for heterogeneity or difference between study results. In most instances, there is no heterogeneity if the P-value is greater than 0.05 (this is set based on type I error), as this represents the null hypothesis holding true. Random chance alone cannot explain the differences between studies and there is heterogeneity between the study results if the P-value is less than 0.05.

Another test for the magnitude of heterogeneity is the I^2 statistic, a percentage from 0% to 100%. Zero percent represents no heterogeneity and 100% represents significant heterogeneity. Ideally for a meta-analysis, there should be minimal heterogeneity, typically with I^2 values of less than 40%. The higher the I^2 statistic, the more cautious we should be in interpreting the treatment effects. Significant heterogeneity may be related to significant differences in patient populations, interventions, and/or outcomes being measured.

■ PUBLICATION BIAS AND FUNNEL PLOTS

In meta-analyses, publication bias may often be present. Results with significant positive findings are more likely to be submitted and accepted for publication. This phenomenon leads to an overestimate of treatment effects. Publication bias may be evident from comparing results from published versus registered trials, published studies versus doctoral dissertations, and randomized trials versus observational studies. Studies with significant positive results are likely to generate multiple publications, hence propagating the bias. Researchers from countries where English is not the major spoken language may tend to submit nonsignificant results to their own respective domestic journals. Searching for articles published only

Study or subgroup	Experimental Events	Total	Control Events	Total	Weight	Risk ratio M–H, Fixed 95%CI	Risk ratio M–H, Fixed 95%CI
Black 2004	3	25	2	23	4.1%	1.38 [0.25, 7.53]	
Dolittle 1999	6	26	5	22	10.8%	1.02 [0.36, 2.88]	
Finlay 1999	15	56	10	54	20.2%	1.45 [0.71, 2.93]	
Higgins 2001	4	44	5	42	10.2%	0.76 [0.22, 2.65]	
Lector 2000	24	75	12	71	24.5%	1.89 [1.03, 3.49]	
Strangelove 2005	17	54	10	52	20.2%	1.64 [0.83, 3.24]	
Watson 2005	12	43	5	42	10.0%	2.34 [0.90, 6.04]	
Total (95% CI)		323		306	100.0%	1.57 [1.14, 2.15]	
Total events	81		49				

Heterogeneity: Chi^2 = 3.09, df = 6 (P = 0.80); I^2 = 0%
Test for overall effect: Z = 2.78 (P = 0.005)

0.01   0.1   1   10   100
Favours experimental   Favours control

Figure 10-1 *Example of a forest plot in a meta-analysis.*

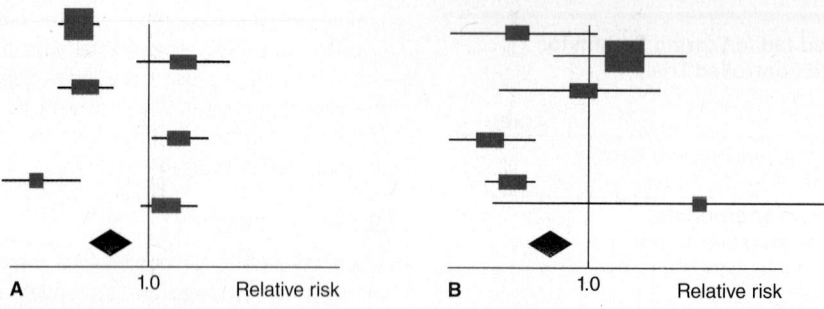

Figure 10-2 *Two plots demonstrating heterogeneity in meta-analysis. Plot (A) by visual inspection shows minimal heterogeneity (I^2 0, P-value > 0.05) and plot (B) demonstrates significant heterogeneity (I^2 > 40%, P-value < 0.05).*

in English adds to publication bias. A funnel plot is used to assess for the presence of publication bias in a meta-analysis. As shown in **Figure 10-3A**, a plot of the sample size (or standard error) versus the effect size (relative risk or risk ratio) is made. Each dot represents the overall effect from one randomized controlled trial. The larger the sample size is (or smaller the error), then the higher the dot on the graph is placed. The dotted red line shows the overall estimate and if there are no missing studies, then the results should be located in a symmetric, triangular area centered on the overall effect of all studies. If there are missing studies as in seen **Figure 10-3B**, then they will appear as a gap in the portion of the funnel plot where one would expect to find negative studies. The unopposed positive studies will shift the apparent treatment effect (blue line) toward a larger size than it really is.

FIXED-EFFECTS MODEL VERSUS RANDOM-EFFECTS MODEL

There are two statistical models used to combine the results from multiple studies in a meta-analysis: the fixed-effects model and the random-effects model. Each model has advantages that influence interpretation of results.

A fixed-effects model assumes there is a single true value underlying all of the study results. All the studies should give identical estimates of the effect if all of the studies addressing the same question are large and free of bias. Variance in this model is derived only from within-study variance and does not incorporate between-study variance (ie, heterogeneity). A fixed-effects model generally gives more weight to larger studies with narrower confidence intervals. This model may be reasonable when there are a small number of studies

included for a meta-analysis or when one large study may be more trustworthy than smaller studies with differing results.

A random-effects model assumes that the studies include a random sample of the population of studies that address the question in the meta-analysis. Because there are differences in patients, interventions, and outcomes in the studies, each study estimates a difference underlying true effect that has a normal distribution. The pooled effect in the random-effects model is not a single effect but a mean effect across populations, interventions, and outcomes. This model takes into account both within-study variance as well as between-study variance (ie, heterogeneity). In the random-effects model, large studies with wider confidence intervals have more weight. The random-effects model is generally considered the more reliable approach of the two models.

Figure 10-4 highlights some of the differences in these two models. In Figure 10-4A, both models yield a similar net estimate when there is no heterogeneity. However, the fixed-effects model yields tighter confidence intervals compared to the random-effects model, which is a more conservative estimate of the overall effect, when there is similar sample size in each study but variability between studies as in Figure 10-4B.

SUBGROUP AND SENSITIVITY ANALYSIS

Subgroup analyses are often presented in systematic reviews to determine if certain groups of patients may respond to treatment as compared to other groups (eg, patients more or certain comorbidities versus patients with less or no comorbidities). While these subgroup analyses may help individualize treatment, they must be interpreted with caution. A few principles or critical questions

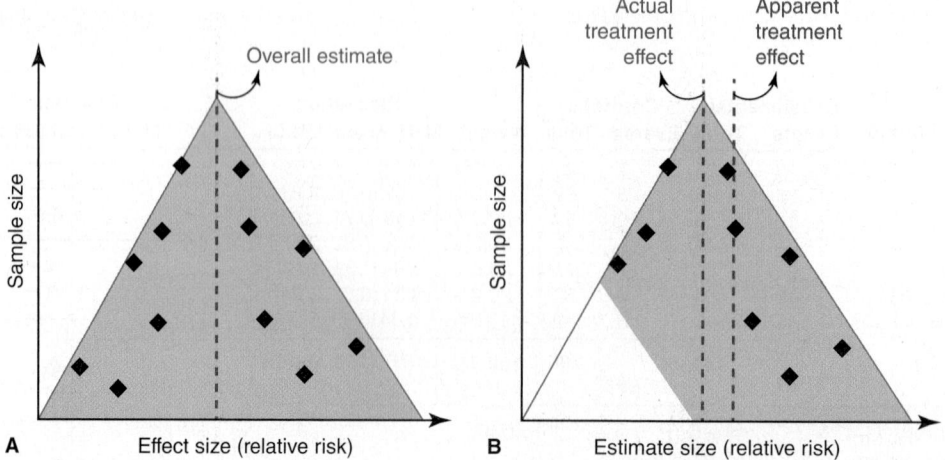

Figure 10-3 *Funnel plot for assessment of publication bias. Plot (A) shows a normal funnel plot and plot (B) shows an example of how missing studies shift the treatment effect.*

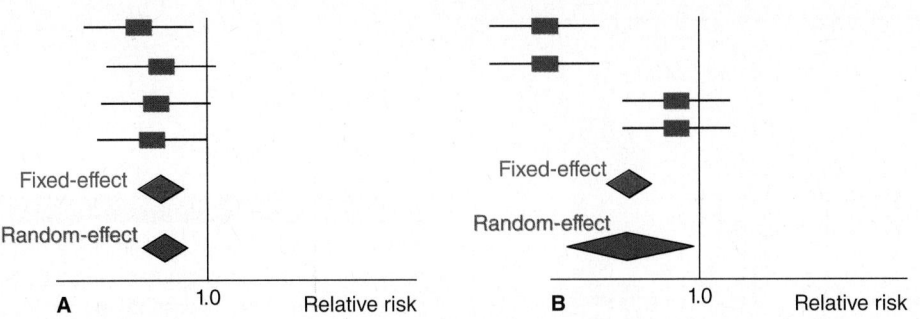

Figure 10-4 *Example of a random-effects model and a fixed-effects model on overall effect with (A) minimal variability between study results and (B) significant variability between study results.*

to help guide in determining the credibility of subgroup analysis include:

(1) Does chance explain the subgroup difference?
(2) Is the subgroup consistent across studies?
(3) Is there a biologic plausibility supporting the subgroup effect?
(4) Is the subgroup difference suggested by meta-analysis comparisons within rather than between studies?

A sensitivity study may also be performed in a meta-analysis if there are relatively lower quality data used. It may refer to a comparison of analyses using the random-effects model versus fixed-effects model. Alternatively, it may refer to the use of quality scores of included trials to modify the impact of lower quality studies to the overall result of the analysis. Although this may reduce the contribution of lower quality studies, there may be bias because it allows authors to somewhat arbitrarily reduce the effects or dismiss the effects of studies they may not like.

■ APPLICABILITY

The next question asks if the results may be applied to a specific patient and/or patient population now that it has been determined that the systematic review and meta-analysis answers the original clinical question, that there was an appropriate search for the evidence and an assessment of the quality of the evidence, and that the study results were appropriate to combine. This step requires consideration of all clinical outcomes as well as the benefits versus the harms and costs. Evidence-based medicine relies not only on the best evidence available but also clinical expertise, clinical experience, and patient preferences. Clinical experience improves the efficiency of diagnosis and treatment, expands the ability to determine the applicability of research data to the individual patients, and allows for the consideration of patient preferences. First ask the question: "Do these results apply to my patient?" whenever considering offering interventions and therapies to patients based on data from systematic reviews and meta-analyses.

PRACTICE POINT

- Meta-analysis provides a quantitative, pooled estimate of a treatment effect. Key advantages of a meta-analysis are that it can pool smaller studies yielding a larger sample size as well as summarize disparate data.
- Systematic reviews and meta-analyses are subject to publication bias, which can lead to some studies being missed and thus not included in the analysis. Bias in individual studies will lead to bias in the systematic review and meta-analysis.
- The final conclusion should be based on the evidence, rather than personal opinion.

SUGGESTED READINGS

Atkins D, Best D, Briss PA, et al. Grading quality of evidence and strength of recommendations. *BMJ.* 2004;328:1490.

Brouwers MC, Kho ME, Browman GP, et al. Development of AGREE II, part 1: performance, usefulness and areas for improvement. *CMAJ.* 2010;182:1045-1052.

Brouwers MC, Kho ME, Browman GP, et al. Development of AGREE II, part 2: assessment of validity of items and tools to support application. *CMAJ.* 2010;182:E472-E478.

Guyatt GH, Oxman AD, Kunz R, et al. GRADE: an emerging consensus on rating quality of evidence and strength of recommendations. *BMJ.* 2008;336:924-926.

Irwig L, Tosteson AN, Gastonis C, et al. Guidelines for meta-analyses evaluating diagnostic tests. *Ann Intern Med.* 1994;120:667-676.

Jadad AR, Moore RA, Carroll D, et al. Assessing the quality of reports of randomized clinical trials: is blinding necessary? *Controlled Clin Trials.* 1996;17:1-12.

Moher D, Cook DJ, Eastwood S, et al. Improving the quality of reports of meta-analyses of randomized controlled trials: the QUOROM statement. Quality of Reporting Meta-analyses. *Lancet.* 1999;354:1896-1900.

Murad M, Montori VM, Ioannidis JA, et al. Understanding and applying the results of a systematic review and meta-analysis. In: Guyatt G, Rennie D, Meade MO, Cook DJ, eds. *Users' Guides to the Medical Literature.* 3rd ed. New York, NY: McGraw-Hill; 2014;471-490.

Neumann I, Aki EA, Vandvik PO, et al. How to use a patient management recommendation: clinical practice guidelines and decision analysis. In: Guyatt G, Rennie D, Meade MO, Cook DJ, eds. *Users' Guides to the Medical Literature.* 3rd ed. New York, NY: McGraw-Hill; 2014;547-560.

Qaseem A, Forland F, Macbeth F, et al. Guidelines International Network: toward international standards for clinical practice guidelines. *Ann Intern Med.* 2012;156:525-531.

ONLINE RESOURCES

- Agency for Healthcare Research and Quality (AHRQ) National Guideline Clearing House. http://www.guideline.gov.
- American Medical Association, JAMAevidence. http://jamaevidence.mhmedical.com.
- Cochrane Collaboration, Cochrane Library. http://www.cochranelibrary.com.
- Guidelines International Network (G-I-N). http://www.g-i-n.net.
- The Appraisal of Guidelines for Research and Evaluation Enterprise. http://www.agreetrust.org.
- The Grading of Recommendations Assessment, Development and Evaluation (GRADE) Working Group. www.gradeworkinggroup.com.

CHAPTER 11

Practical Considerations of Incorporating Evidence into Clinical Practice

J. Richard Pittman, Jr., MD

Mikhail Akbashev, MD

INTRODUCTION

With over 21.5 million unique articles and more than 1 million randomized controlled trials indexed in MEDLINE as of 2014 and more than 1 million new publications published and indexed annually, clinicians now must process a vast volume of medical literature. Many clinicians feel like they are drowning in information. Hospitalists must balance the need to find relevant and accurate answers to their clinical questions with the need for efficiency in finding those answers to immediately guide high-quality care to multiple acutely ill patients. Formulating and answering questions efficiently and effectively will improve care and reduce the rates of consultation, testing, and potential errors.

The volume of data and limited time for searching for answers compound each other. A recent systematic review examining clinical questions raised by clinicians at the point of care found approximately one clinical question arises for every two patient encounters. Clinicians only pursued 51% of the questions raised and found answers to only 78% of those questions pursued. Studies reported the main barriers to seeking information included a clinician's lack of time and a doubt that a useful answer existed. The state of relying on information already known prevails when the energy required to get a new answer outweighs the perceived benefit. Clinical inertia may be illustrated by considering the gap between the potential benefits of evidenced-based care and actual rates of implementation as in the treatment of heart failure with reduced ejection fraction (HFrEF). Optimal implementation of strong evidence-based therapies for HFrEF could save an estimated 35,000 to 117,000 thousand lives per year. See Chapter 129 (Heart Failure).

In an ideal practice setting, the majority of clinical questions would have a readily accessible, evidence-based answer. Clinicians would have current knowledge of guideline-based therapy and could apply pertinent point-of-care reminders from the electronic medical record for best practice for every patient under their care. As a result, patients would yield maximal benefit from clinical trials and guideline-driven information. This ideal state may not be attainable; however, clinicians may take steps toward better utilizing the evidence-based answers currently available to meaningfully impact clinical practice.

CURRENT CONSEQUENCES AND MOTIVATORS FOR CHANGE

■ PRACTICING WITH OUTDATED INFORMATION

Relying on outdated information for patient care (ie, clinical inertia) may limit potential benefits of current therapies and expose patients to risks of disproven therapies. An example would be practicing based off outdated guidelines for the treatment of blood cholesterol to reduce atherosclerotic cardiovascular disease (ASCVD) risk in adults where a clinician tailors treatment and statin dosing based solely on the low-density lipoprotein cholesterol (LDL-C) levels rather than selecting a moderate- or high-intensity statin strategy based on ASCVD risk, an LDL-C $\geq$ 190 mg/dL, and/or the presence of diabetes as recommended in the current updated guidelines.

■ UTILIZING UNVERIFIED INFORMATION SOURCES

Clinicians may utilize unverified information sources. Examples of possible unverified information sources include seemingly more informed colleagues, television programming/advertisements, popular media, drug company representatives, and searching for "evidence" or answers to clinical questions using search engines that may provide information from unverified sources (eg, "Googling"). Heavy reliance on unverified information sources can significantly limit the quality of information with which a clinician practices and should be avoided if possible.

■ SEARCH SATISFACTION BIAS

Depending on a clinician's comfort level with evidence-based medicine and available search tools and time, a clinician may only read article summaries or conclusions from abstracts. This represents a form of search satisfaction bias. When an answer is found to a clinical question that is frequently encountered in a clinician's scope of practice, the clinician might jump to apply this answer to all subsequent patients without fully assessing the validity and quality of the source or considering the applicability of this information to the individual patient.

■ EVIDENCE-BASED PRACTICE IMPROVES PATIENT OUTCOMES

Perhaps the strongest and most important motivator for change should be the fact that evidence- or guideline-based practice has been shown to improve patient outcomes across a wide spectrum of illnesses.

SOLUTIONS TO INCORPORATE EVIDENCE INTO CLINICAL PRACTICE

Solutions should take into consideration how a clinician might encounter information during the flow of practice. "Keeping up" with the literature is increasingly difficult, and staying abreast of important developments that may not directly relate to patients that the clinician is actively managing. "Keeping up" single-source publications from an area of clinical focus are useful, but they may narrow a clinician's awareness of broader advances across different disciplines. There are numerous methods to "keep up" with the literature that transcend traditional postal mail by utilizing e-mail or designated applications for mobile devices. Users sign up for these "keeping up" resources as reputable and reliable evidence sent to them from trusted sources. These tools may help clinicians keep up with a particular field or topic by organizing information by discipline, relevance to that discipline, and newsworthiness or impact level. This information may be delivered to an e-mail inbox, a website, or to a discrete mobile application. The focus below will be on free resources available or those included with professional society memberships common for most hospital medicine providers.

Advantages of push resources available for most hospital medicine providers include:

- Preset, reliable stream of information lowers the energy required to incorporate new information into clinical practice, leaving a clinician less subject to clinical inertia or anchoring.
- Many of the tools are free and can focus on a specific discipline or a topic.
- The volume of information presented can be adjusted based on clinician desire or tolerance.
- The frequency of the delivery of this information can be customized.
- Article summaries by colleagues trained in evidence-based analysis can be accessed and can raise awareness of potential inclusion biases.

Disadvantages include:

- These streams may become overwhelming if the amount and frequency of content is not properly customized to the individual clinician preferences. There is a risk of attending a conference or reading a publication on mobile resources that may be tempting to clinicians to sign up for too many resources at one time.
- Selection methodology for choosing the articles presented may not always be clear.

Suggestions

1. **Setting up digital resources.** It may be helpful for a clinician to initially take consider what information he or she needs and the areas of knowledge deficiencies (eg, original research manuscripts, clinical updates, and guidelines). Any individual clinician may not be aware of each of her or his personal deficiencies, especially since "blind spots" are by definition not seen. Thoughtful attention to one's knowledge base, deficiencies, and practice gaps may lead to crucial first digital steps for change. In addition, a comparison of professional needs and knowledge gaps should be made with regards to any resources a clinician is actively subscribed. A busy clinician should pay careful attention to cutting down on infrequently used resources prior to subscribing to new ones.

   Consideration should be made for an individual clinician's preferred method of receiving information. Some like information to come straight to their e-mail with a link to a website while others prefer opening a designated application on their device(s). E-mails clutter e-mail inboxes, but most people regularly check e-mail. Mobile applications clutter your devices while also continuing to collect new material unnoticed to the clinician. This can be corrected by removing unused applications that clutter mobile devices while also taking steps to become familiar with how applications work and aggregate information. Most tools discussed in this chapter strive to deliver information in a way that best fits the workflow of different clinicians (**Table 11-1**). The key is for any individual practitioner to identify resources most convenient and reliable for that individual clinician.

   Once an account is setup for the any of the resources, the next step is to select specialty and topic preferences. Once these steps are completed, the information will then be sent either via e-mail or to a mobile application depending on which resource is selected (**Figure 11-1**).

   A critical step is to then monitor the usefulness of information and then after a period of time (eg, a couple of weeks or a month) go back into the tool and adjust the settings or unsubscribe from the resource based on its helpfulness or not.

2. **Schedule time for new reading.** A seemingly simple step, but one that can make a large difference in "keeping up" is to schedule time for new reading. Carrying a paper or virtual file with articles, presentations, and/or books may make a half an hour before rounds, between appointments, or while sitting in carpool lines a lot more productive.

3. **Attend institutional conferences.** Attending institutional conferences (eg, Grand Rounds, noon conferences) is an excellent way for a clinician to acquire new information while also providing the opportunity to spark conversations and clinical questions with colleagues. Volunteering to present a topic at conference promotes expertise acquisition of new and updated clinical knowledge.

4. **Participate in professional societies and their scientific meetings.** Scientific meetings hosted by medical professional societies are designed to help clinicians stay abreast of the ever-changing information and also to offer credit for Continuing Medical Education.

5. **Encourage a culture of learning.** Activities such as journal club, case conference, and clinical updates in hospital medicine at hospitalists' sites of practice can be an effective way to

TABLE 11-1 Example Digital Resources for "Keeping Up"

E-mail/Website-Based	Website Link
BMJ Evidence Updates	https://plus.mcmaster.ca/evidenceupdates/
ACP Journal Club	http://annals.org/journalclub.aspx
NEJM Journal Watch	www.jwatch.org
PubMed—My NCBI	http://www.ncbi.nlm.nih.gov/pubmed/
Application-Based (App)	**Website Link**
Docphin	https://www.docphin.com/
Read by QXMD	http://www.qxmd.com/apps/read-by-qxmd-app
Doximity	https://www.doximity.com/

promote a culture of learning, which can help providers further keep up with the flow of new information.

6. **Utilize the electronic health record.** Perhaps the most pertinent time to receive updated information on any treatment or diagnostic test is at the time of ordering the treatment or test. Recent advances and expansions in electronic health records (EHR) offer a limited opportunity for "just-in time" learning about specific medical concepts. Many EHRs incorporate evidence-based recommendations into order sets, as well as linking users to literature regarding updated recommendations. A recent meta-analysis showed improvement in both efficiency and adherence to guidelines through use of EHR. Similarly, a study of an older computer support tool for antibiotic management found a dramatic decrease in pharmacy antibiotic expenditures and mortality rates over a 6-year period. A systematic review of 68 controlled trials of computer decision support systems found the majority of the trials demonstrated benefit in physician performance and patient outcomes. Multiple health systems have implemented quality improvement projects to adhere to core measures using order sets within the EHRs with great success.

■ QUICK QUESTION

The context is essential for any clinical question. The ideal "quick question" resource would be readily available at the point of care,

pertinent to the patient, with specific, actionable information that is quickly and reliably accessed. Unlike the "keeping up" resources previously discussed, these "quick questions" need to be answered for a real patient right now. That is why using these types of resources is essential in day-to-day patient care. Fortunately, multiple resources exist including current textbooks, database search tools such as Trip Database, popular portable resources such as UpToDate or Dynamed, and large databases like PubMed. These resources have been developed to answer specific, patient-related questions. Hospitalists should check with their institutional subscriptions first and utilize these before personally enrolling in subscriptions that may be expensive.

Developing "quick questions" require clinicians to stop their flow of work and look for an answer. Cumbersome retrieval of information may lead to clinical inertia. Initial searching using summary resources, such as textbooks or review articles, can be efficient and more likely to yield pertinent answers. However, these resources are subject to authorship biases. Important articles could potentially be omitted while smaller studies maybe overly emphasized in recommendations. Summary resources can also be delayed in incorporating the most recent study results, even sometimes those of large pivotal studies. Many clinicians start with a Google search with Wikipedia as the top listed initial resource. This may often be a quick and satisfying way to answer simple medical definition questions such as "what is an antimitochondrial antibody." Mainstream publicly available search engines such as Google or Yahoo can offer fast and free searches but often are less reliable and may not provide a robust and accurate answer to clinical questions as would more rigorously vetted medical resources, such as AccessMedicine, ClincialKey (formerly MD Consult), DynaMed, Medscape (a.k.a. eMedicine), UpToDate and a growing list of other compiled medical summary resources and reviews (**Table 11-2**). These resources have made incorporation of new information a priority.

Suggestions

Despite the apparent limitations, actively and efficiently searching for answers to clinical queries is an essential part of patient care. Overcoming clinical inertia to identify and explore questions is the first step. This may be as simple as an index card with questions for the day or lunches with colleagues to discuss cases. Having identified questions, a clinician needs to formulate the question as specifically as possible and identify an efficient search strategy (**Figure 11-2**).

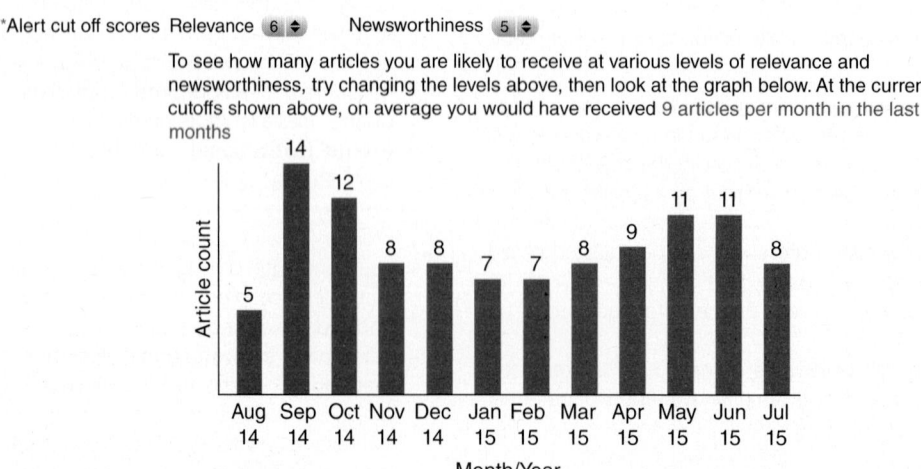

Figure 11-1 *Screenshot of BMJ evidence updates. This is an example of a free online "keeping up" resource which allows users filter paper alerts by topic, relevance and newsworthiness, to narrow to a manageable amount.*

TABLE 11-2 Example Digital Resources for Answering Clinical Questions

Resource (*Publisher*)	Description	CME
AccessMedicine ACCESS Medicine. *Trusted Content. Instant Answers.* *McGraw-Hill*	Compendium of rapidly searchable medical textbooks	Yes
Clinical Key (a.k.a. MDConsult) ClinicalKey® *Elsevier*	Automated evidence search engine, allow users to search the primary medical literature, guidelines and standard textbooks	Yes
Dynamed DynaMed Plus *EBSCO Health*	Collection of evidence-based summary reviews on common clinical topics; presented in bulleted format with specific citations and assessment of evidence quality for recommendations. Systematic rapid inclusion of newly published high-quality evidence, including systematic reviews	Yes
Essential Evidence Plus ESSENTIAL EVIDENCE PLUS *Wiley*	Search engine to browse guidelines and systematic reviews; integrated with other resources such as calculators, coding helper, or decision support tools	Yes
Medscape (a.k.a. eMedicine) Medscape *WebMD*	Compilation of summaries by specialists in the field; includes new article formats	Yes
PubMed Clinical Queries PubMed.gov *NIH*	Indexed database of articles from a multitude of medical journals	No
TRIP Database (Translating Research Into Practice) Trip *TRIP*	Automated evidence search engine of primary studies, guidelines, textbooks and other clinical resources with filters available; scores articles based on how recent, pertinence, and publication source	No
Up-To-Date UpToDate® *Wolters Kluwer*	Evidence-based online textbook. Compendium of expert written invited reviews on a broad array of topics; evidenced based and graded recommendations, primarily prose and directive in nature	Yes

Many hold to dogma and use PubMed as an initial search. This often yields a time-consuming search, with many published articles to sift through, and challenges finding relevant studies efficiently. This also has been shown to take 41% longer (29 vs 17 minutes) than UpToDate searches in a cohort of resident physicians. Furthermore, a study of 54 medical students, residents, and faculty searching multiple methodologies to answer critical-care-related questions showed that users most frequently searched Google first (45% of the time), with Google and UpToDate providing faster answers than PubMed (3.8 vs 3.3 vs 4.4 minutes, respectively). Importantly, Google and UpToDate were more likely to lead to a correct answer than PubMed (60% vs 70% vs 36%, respectively). The highest value first resource is often a compiled resource such as Dynamed or UpToDate, but multiple resources are available from various publishing organizations (Table 11-2).

Regardless of the initial search strategy, there are often clinical situations that require more nuanced answers and specific expertise.

These questions should be very concrete and specific. A standard "PICO" (Patient, Intervention, Comparison, Outcome) format identifies the pertinent parts of a question (eg, "What is the effect of 23-valent pneumococcal polysaccharide vaccine versus placebo on mortality in patients with systolic heart failure exacerbations?" or "What is the relative risk of bleeding with rivaroxaban versus warfarin in patients with venous thromboembolism?"). For questions too specific or narrow to be found in summarized resources, a primary literature search may be preferred. PubMed offers free access to users, and its "Clinical Queries" search option quickly filters results for clinical and systematic review articles. Other electronic resources like TRIP (Translating Research into Practice) database can quickly filter studies indexed in MEDLINE, guidelines and other resources, and it also ranks them on quality and type of study. Guideline searches may be completed through the National Guideline Clearinghouse (http://www.guideline.gov), which is a resource maintained by the U.S. Department of Health and Human Services. This resource

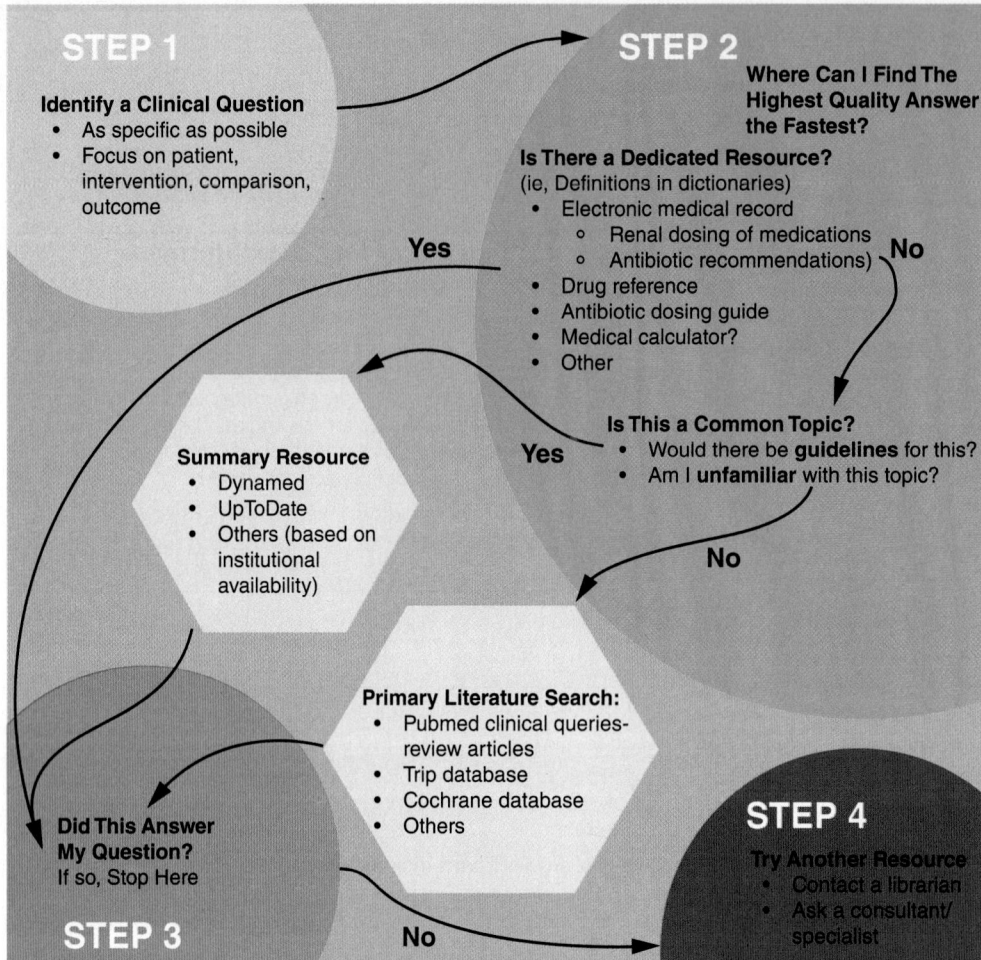

Figure 11-2 *An effective search strategy for answering clinical questions.*

facilitates comparison of guidelines on topics published from different societies (eg, breast cancer screening guidelines from American College of Physicians versus American College of Obstetrics and Gynecology). Although somewhat cumbersome to use initially, it is readily updated. Actively recruiting clinical trials are indexed in the registry ClinicalTrials.gov (https://clinicaltrials.gov), provided by the U.S. National Institutes of Health.

Although there are advantages and disadvantages to the different resources, the least useful resource is the unavailable resource. For this reason, clinicians should find the resources available at their home institutions. Clinicians should identify clinical questions and explore the available resources to find answers. Ideally, a query should obtain a high-quality answer in less than 5 minutes.

■ STORAGE FOR FUTURE REFERENCE

A challenge of the digital and increasingly paperless work environment is how to keep up with the materials that an individual clinician would like to save for future reference. Mobile technology can really help take busy clinicians far beyond the traditional physical file cabinet into a system that can travel on mobile devices with certain ones that can even help create bibliographies if needed.

Many digital storage solutions follow the "freemium" model. "Freemium" is a pricing strategy that refers to an initial free price for the limited use of an application that then tiers to paid subscriptions for heavier use. The real advantage of the digital storage solutions is their use of storing files virtually in the "cloud." The "cloud" refers to the storage of files in a server (ie, high-capacity computer) that

is connected to a clinician's personal computer or mobile device via the Internet. The advantages of this include an online backup and the ability to synchronize files across multiple devices with very little effort. Many of these services allow a clinician to keep a copy of the files on a computer or mobile devices so these files can be accessed even when not connected to the Internet. These systems retrieve information by storing text documents that can be searched using terms that obtain results based not just on the title of the file but also from the text of the document. This allows use of these resources with almost no organization necessary.

With a digital storage solution, the important tactile experience of touching and annotating the original article is lost. The clinician must convert from paper to digital files, name folders, and move documents to the folders that have been created. A similar effort would be required to set up a new file cabinet, but many struggle to invest the time into a similar digital system. Theoretically, this digital storage solution is still a mechanical system that could fail.

Suggestions

1. **Understand the cloud** Many clinicians already have user accounts for cloud-based storage solutions but are simply unaware that they do. Programs such as Dropbox, Google Drive, Box, Evernote, OneDrive, and iCloud all meet the definition for cloud-based storage solutions. If a clinician already has one of these accounts, then it may be best for that clinician to first explore all the features of that solution, before considering others (**Table 11-3**).

TABLE 11-3 Example Cloud-Based Storage Solutions

Platform	Cost/Memory	Pros	Cons
Box.com	Free up to 10 Gb, then $10/mo for 100 Gb	Only solution that advertises HIPAA complaint for enterprise clients; great amount free; can edit documents on web, make comments, and assign tasks to documents	Web editing, commenting, and tagging have some flaws that limit their usefulness
Dropbox	Free up to 2 Gb, $10/mo 1 Terabyte of storage	Established company; cross platform with easy sharing and well-integrated into mobile devices	Small amount of data free
Evernote	Free up to 60 Mb data transfer per mo, then $45/per y for heavier use	Accepts multiple types of inputs including audio, photos, scanned documents, and web clips; advanced organization with notebooks and tagging	Best use requires some organization
Google drive	15 Gb free, paid plans for 100 Gb per mo	Best for working on files with other users, even simultaneously; great if you use Android mobile device(s)	Navigation of the drive is somewhat nonintuitive
Microsoft Onedrive	Free up to 7 Gb	Ideal if heavy user of Microsoft® Office, especially on a windows platform computer	

While the solutions can be accessed through websites using a web browser, most also offer applications that can be downloaded and placed on personal computers and mobile devices that allow for more convenient access of their stored files. The applications work by turning files and folders meant for storage into ones that are automatically synchronized and immediately uploaded to the cloud, which allows them to thereby be available from anywhere.

2. **Use cloud-based storage** After gaining an understanding of the "cloud," clinicians should strongly consider using cloud-based storage in their practice.

   In general, any of these cloud-based storage solutions will work to get started, so once a choice is made regarding which one to use then time must be invested by users in order to learn how to use all of the features. Many have "getting started" videos which can be viewed on their respective websites. Once a clinician is familiar with the tool, time should be set aside for at least an hour or two to allow for some files or articles to be moved over to the cloud folders. Investing time up front will allow a busy clinician to get the most of out of the system and generally be better organized moving forward in clinical practice. Choosing a system-based organization (eg, cardiology, gastroenterology, infectious diseases, and so on.) versus by more specific topic areas (eg, heart failure, cirrhosis, pneumonia, and so on.) depends on the file contents and personal preferences of the individual clinician.

   The next time a clinical question comes up about the topic previously searched and saved in this storage system, the clinician can simply check the system rather than doing another search.

3. **Comply with patient confidentiality** As with any new developments or advances in technology that affects or modifies a clinician's practice, care should be taken to assure the safety and protection of a patient's confidentiality. Most cloud resources are not compliant with the Health Insurance Portability and Accountability Act (HIPAA). As such, patient or personal health information should not be stored on these digital and cloud-based drives. The notable exception is "enterprise services" provided by the digital platform Box, but it should be noted the "personal service" of Box is not HIPAA compliant.

4. **Annotate articles** Some clinicians prefer to read paper articles, which then allows for highlighting or annotating. Digital versions of these articles often allow of highlighting or annotating as well depending on the viewer used on a computer or mobile device. This latter way of reviewing articles allows the clinician to more easily save notes taken right inside the cloud-based storage solution being used. For those who still prefer the paper version to initially review an article, clinicians should consider document scanner to convert the annotated paper version of the article into a digital one which can then be stored in these cloud-based storage platforms. The scanner that uses "Optical Character Recognition" or OCR to turn the documents scanned into a text searchable document after storage provides optimal functionality. At the time of this chapter being drafted, Evernote is the only one of the cloud-based solutions that has annotation (eg, highlighting) or drawing built into its system. Many of these other platforms can integrate easily with software/application viewers or readers (eg, "Portable Document Format" or PDF) which are available on most mobile devices.

■ CULTURAL CHANGE

Fostering a culture of education, accountability for actions, and support for evidence-based, high-quality care can encourage all clinicians to keep learning for better patient care. Although intangible personal attributes contribute greatly to culture, leadership can adjust policy to achieve desired outcomes by nurturing a workplace of collaboration, learning, open feedback, and accountability. A supportive, collaborative environment encourages clinicians to discuss individual studies or publications, treatment decisions on complicated cases, and even to work together on quality improvement and system-based projects. Impediments to collaboration among hospitalist groups include provider scheduling and workload. Seven-day-cycled schedules may isolate providers to those other providers on for the same shifts only. Potential interventions to improve collaboration could include standardized work schedules, physician lounges, physician cafeterias, grouped offices, and consideration of patient census caps.

Open feedback also plays an important role in incorporating evidence and improving patient care. Increasing isolation of physicians and high workload limits the available time to discuss the management of individual patients and/or to follow up on subsequent care while off-service. Handoffs could be an opportunity for colleagues to review care and potentially notify providers of updates in hospital medicine or new literature. In order to be successful, this should be done in a collegial manner with adequate time allotted. Hospitalists should be encouraged to both give and request feedback regularly. Morbidity and mortality conferences may also offer an opportunity to discuss updates in new literature using a pertinent clinical case. "Word of mouth" spread of information is a pertinent and powerful way to share medical information and encourage a culture that strives to keep up with the literature.

CONCLUSION

The volumes of literature and increasing demands on physician time have complicated the process of finding and incorporating evidence into clinical practice. Multiple new methods exist to receive new evidence on pertinent topics in manageable volumes. Compiled review resources are significantly quicker and more reliable initial resources than primary literature searches for most clinical questions. Cloud-based storage options offer the advantages of better search-ability and portability over filing cabinets and stacks of printed manuscripts and journals; most cloud storage options are not HIPAA compliant but are good for storing medical references. Simple steps can be taken to foster a positive learning culture at a hospitalist's respective institution (eg, starting a journal club or scheduling lunchtime discussions of current topics). Some hospitalists may pursue resources to better keep up, while others may inquire at their institution for "quick question" resources. Some clinicians may already be inundated with what they have collected and need to invest in a cloud-based resource to decrease the stress every time they ask, "Where is that article?" Encouraging a work culture shift toward addressing gaps may help clinician scope with information overload. Even the most current or seemingly up-to-date clinicians started one step at a time and invested continued effort.

SUGGESTED READINGS

Banzi R, et al. Speed of updating online evidence based point of care summaries: prospective cohort analysis. *BMJ*. 2011;343:d5856.

Campanella P, et al. The impact of electronic health records on healthcare quality: a systematic review and meta-analysis. *Eur J Public Health*. pii:ckv122 [Epub]; Jun 30, 2015.

Del Fiol G, et al. Clinical questions raised by clinicians at the point of care: a systematic review. *JAMA Intern Med*. 2014;74:710-718.

Elliott DJ, et al. Effect of hospitalist workload on quality and efficiency of care. *JAMA Intern Med*. 2014;174:786-793.

Hunt DL, et al. Effects of computer-based clinical decision support systems on physician performance and patient outcomes: a systematic review. *JAMA*. 1998;280:1339-1346.

Kronenfeld MR, et al. Survey of user preferences from a comparative trial of UpToDate and ClinicalKey. *J Med Libr Assoc*. 2013;101:151-154.

Michtalik HJ, et al. Impact of attending physician workload on patient care: a survey of hospitalists. *JAMA Intern Med*. 2013;173:375-377.

Rangachari P, et al. Awareness of evidence-based practices alone does not translate to implementation: insights from implementation research. *Qual Manag Health Care*. 2013;22:117-125.

Sayyah EL, et al. To compare PubMed Clinical Queries and UpToDate in teaching information mastery to clinical residents: a crossover randomized controlled trial. *PLoS One*. 2011;6:e23487.

Thiele RH, et al. Speed, accuracy, and confidence in Google, Ovid, PubMed, and UpToDate: results of a randomised trial. *Postgrad Med J*. 2010;86:459-465.

ONLINE RESOURCES

- Society of Hospital Medicine's learning portal at https://shmlearningportal.org
- Table 11-1 Digital Resources

SECTION 3
Transitions of Care

CHAPTER 12

Care Transitions into the Hospital: Health Care Centers, Emergency Department, Outside Hospital Transfers

Joanna M. Bonsall, MD, PhD
Stacy Higgins, MD, FACP
Melissa B. Stevens, MD

INTRODUCTION

For patients being admitted into the hospital, hospital admission may be the first and most significant care transition that they will experience in their medical care. The number of inpatients being cared for by their primary care physicians has decreased significantly in the last several years. In a study reported in JAMA in 2009, outpatient to inpatient continuity with a primary care physician decreased from 44.3% in 1996 to 31.9% in 2006, correlating with the growth of hospital medicine during the same time period. As a result, patients are frequently cared for by physicians who are meeting them for for the first time in the hospital, and who are unfamiliar with their medical history, past hospitalizations, or family and social support network. In addition, due to the "shift" structuring of many hospital medicine groups, patients are likely to be cared for by multiple physicians during a single hospital stay, each one having to learn anew the subtleties of their history.

Patients may be admitted to the hospital through the Emergency Department (ED), directly from an outpatient office, or transferred from an outside facility such as another hospital, a Skilled Nursing Facility (SNF) or a Subacute Rehabilitation Facility (SAR). While these transitions have much in common, they also have unique challenges in care transitions that are specific to their sites. We will discuss these challenges as well as potential solutions here.

ADMISSIONS FROM THE EMERGENCY DEPARTMENT

The majority of unscheduled admissions to the hospital come through the Emergency Department. The American College of Emergency Physicians estimates that over the past decade the percent of admissions through the ED has increased from 64% to over 80% while at the same time there was a decline in the percentage of unscheduled admissions from clinics or doctor's offices. Patients admitted through the Emergency Department experience two transitions—the transition into the ED and the transition from the ED into the hospital. As patients' transition from the ED to the hospital the need to not only transfer information but also to clarify who is primarily responsible for the patients' care is critical as there is often a delay between the exchange of information and the physical relocation of patients. Admissions that occur during shift changes may be particularly problematic as they result in multiple transfers of information and responsibility. In the ED, patients may be admitted at a shift change with data pending rather than be signed out to a new ED provider. These transitions can result in ambiguity and conflicting expectations between ED providers and hospitalists specifically regarding patient care responsibilities and can contribute to dropped information, delays in treatment, and other errors that threaten the safety of patients. Strategies to improve the transitions are discussed below and outlined in **Table 12-1**.

■ TRANSITION OF INFORMATION

Hospitalists and ED physicians have varied expectations of the ED to hospital handoff both in terms of the information that should be communicated and the data that should be available at the time of admission. ED physicians and hospitalists have different roles in patient care and different information needs, which may lead to erroneous assumptions and misunderstandings. Understanding the factors that affect care of patients and communication on both sides is crucial. Fatigue and increased workload can impact

TABLE 12-1 Strategies to Improve ED to Hospital Transitions

1. Vital signs should be rechecked at regular intervals while patients are boarded, consistent with protocol for their intended floor location.
2. Orders written in the emergency department (ED) should be readily available for hospitalists to review in the electronic medical record (EMR).
3. Formalized structured feedback should immediately occur when there is an adverse event or handoff miscommunication.
4. Standardized handoff tools including an admission check-list should be used to set expectations.
5. Clearly delineate the responsibility for follow-up of *pending tests results*.
6. Minimize asking EM physicians to order additional tests before patients are accepted for admission or transfer to the floor unless the tests will alter bed acuity level.
7. Clearly identify the clinician of record.
8. Hospitalist changes of shift for boarded patients should be communicated to ED staff expediently.
9. Responsibilities for boarded patients should be specified at the institutional level with written policy.
10. Prioritize getting boarders out of the ED to their inpatient units.

communication and updating of patient information and contribute to unintended outcomes.

In order to improve safety and quality of care and avoid ambiguity hospitalists and ED providers at any facility should clearly identify and mutually agree upon a minimum set of data elements that should be part of the transition. The use of checklists and standardized communications tools are recommended in assisting this process. In keeping with existing guidelines, the *minimum* data set should include a principle diagnosis and problem list, medication list, patient's cognitive status, and test results/pending tests. Information should be communicated between providers in a secure, private and HIPAA compliant manor. Communication of information should be done in person or by phone with an opportunity for both the admitting and receiving provider to ask questions and get clarification and feedback. This last step, while recommended for all handovers, is especially crucial in this type of transition, given the different backgrounds and roles of the providers.

While hospitalists frequently ask for additional information to help with patient management decisions, such requests may lead to a delay in patient transfer. Requests for additional workup prior to admission may be appropriate if this information will affect one of the following: (1) the level of inpatient care (ie, ward vs telemetry unit vs ICU), (2) the admitting service (medicine vs surgery vs other), or (3) time to obtain critical information (ie, the patient may be able to get a CT more rapidly in the ED than once they are admitted to the floor). In the event that additional workup is warranted prior to a patient being accepted for admission, the ED provider and hospitalists should have a protocol for communicating information about the patient at shift change with their colleagues who will be responsible for following up these tests and ultimately admitting these patients.

■ TRANSITION OF RESPONSIBILITY

Unlike other transitions, the exact moment of the transfer of responsibility for patient care may be ambiguous. When patients are admitted from the outpatient clinic setting or skilled nursing facilities, it

is clear that the admitting provider is responsible for the patient while they remain at their facility and once the patient leaves the admitting facility they become the responsibility of the accepting provider. However, patients do not typically leave the ED immediately after they have been accepted for admission by the hospitalist, leading to confusion on the part of patients, nurses and other staff as to who is responsible for the patient's care. The ED provider and hospitalist should identify pending labs and studies and who will be responsible for follow up and communication of results. In the event that patients remain in the ED for any length of time after the communication of information between the ED provider and hospitalist, there should be an established protocol for identifying the responsible provider to be contacted with any new test results, question/concerns, or any change in the patient's clinical condition.

■ PROLONGED ED BOARDING

ED overcrowding and inadequate inpatient capacity lead to prolonged ED boarding and increased risk of harm not only for admitted patients but for ED patients as well. Admitted patients boarded in the ED do not receive the same level of care as they would on an inpatient unit and studies have shown that prolonged ED boarding is associated with an increase in preventable adverse events, length of stay and mortality. Institutions should develop a clear plan for standardized communication and transfer of responsibility of patients with prolonged ED boarding that should include a plan for shift changes and may include standardized order sets to be initiated in the ED prior to transfer to an inpatient unit.

Reducing ED boarding is a challenge at most facilities that requires the input of a multidisciplinary team. Prolonged ED boarding is usually the result of hospital overcrowding and there are many possible strategies to improve patient flow including: using a "full capacity protocol" where the burden of boarding patients is shared between the emergency medicine and hospital medicine department; coordinating discharges as early in the day as possible; moving toward a 24/7 operational culture, active bed management/hiring a "Bed Czar" to match bed needs to resources and utilizing observation units.

■ COMMUNICATION BETWEEN THE PCP AND THE HOSPITALIST

Barriers in communication between the primary care provider (PCP) and the ED physician or admitting hospitalist are similar on admission and discharge. On admission, patients may be in pain, confused, and distressed, providing limited or unreliable histories. The communication with the PCP can provide information on past medical history, past hospitalizations, previous testing done, medication reconciliation, social history, and the baseline medical status of the patient. However, conversations require identification of the PCP by the patient, ability to reach the PCP in a timely fashion, easy access by the PCP to the patient's updated medical record, and a mutually available time for the conversation. System barriers interrupting this communication include inadequate reimbursement to the PCP for the time involved in reviewing the record and the conversation; time shortage in a busy outpatient schedule; and fragmented patient care with an incomplete record. There is also the transition process barrier of the lack of a standardized communication system—successful completion of a single phone call may require multiple calls in each direction as neither party is available at the time of the phone call, and lengthy waits between calls; text pages may not be responded to until records are reviewed and there is time in the schedule; and e-mails may not be secure and do not allow for interactive dialogue.

In cases where the hospitalist and primary care physician share a common electronic health record, communication through the EHR can be secure and timely, with ongoing real time access by both parties. However, this is likely the exception rather than the rule, and it assumes that patients obtain all of their care within a single health system. Where this does not exist, methods such as e-mail and fax are acceptable. With the growth of the Patient Centered Medical Home, it is possible that care coordinators in the health care system can help to facilitate information transfer from the medical home to the admitting physician. Employment of nurse case managers by practices can assist with the barrier of communication coordination, have access to the patient's medical record, and can standardize the transfer of information.

PRACTICE POINT

- The ED-to-hospital admission process can be a high-risk event due to differing backgrounds/roles of providers and ambiguity at the time of admission about transfer of responsibility for patient care. To minimize the risk, ED and hospital medicine groups should develop mutually agreed upon information checklists or standardized templates to aide transfer of information; and should develop clear guidelines around who will assume responsibility for pending test results and changes in patient status in the period after the patient has been accepted by the hospitalist but still remains in the ED.

■ DIRECT ADMISSIONS FROM AMBULATORY HEALTH CARE CENTERS

While fewer patients are being admitted directly from a physician's office to the hospital, there are significant advantages to continuing this practice for appropriate patients. A direct admission means the patient can avoid the potentially long wait in the ED and prolonged ED boarding while also reducing ED overcrowding. The direct admission process also allows the opportunity for the PCP to speak directly to the hospitalist, sharing the patient's medical history as well as providing some anticipatory guidance to the hospitalist, who is not as familiar with the patient. However, as with all transitions, the direct admission has some specific risks that need to be anticipated and managed. First, the patients appropriate for direct admission should be carefully selected, to ensure that they will be admitted to the correct care location and that they are not at risk for deterioration before being seen by the hospitalist. Second, there should be clear communication between the PCP and the hospitalist regarding the patient to be admitted.

■ SELECTION OF APPROPRIATE PATIENTS FOR DIRECT ADMISSION

Advantages to admitting a patient directly to the hospital include convenience to the patient, improved patient satisfaction, reduced crowding of the Emergency Department, and decreased cost to the system. In evaluating who is appropriate for direct admission, there are a few recommendations in the literature:

- The admitting diagnosis is fairly certain and no additional triage is needed.
- The patient is clinically stable in their vital signs and does not require supplemental oxygen, immediate IV fluids, antibiotics or urgent imaging.
- The patient has been seen and evaluated on the day of admission by their primary provider.
- The patient arrives at the hospital early in the day (before 4 PM) to facilitate communication between the admitting physician and the hospital team and before shift changes.

If the admitting hospital team is concerned about the patient's condition or need for more extensive initial workup after getting

signout, they can advise against a direct admission. Familiarity and trust between the outpatient and hospitalist group can help facilitate direct admissions as each learns the other's practice style and comfort.

While a patient may initially be assessed as stable for direct admission, an extensive wait time in patient registration where the patient is unmonitored or may miss scheduled medications may lead to the patient becoming unstable. As the number of inpatient beds is reduced, and the fill rate goes up, patients may have to wait several hours before receiving a bed assignment. Solutions include having a Care Initiation Unit that serves as a transition zone where the patient can check in, have their vital signs checked, and be evaluated by the admitting hospitalist there. This decreases time spent in the ED and catches patients who may need stabilization prior to going to the floor bed. It also allows for continuous monitoring and initiation of orders while awaiting a bed assignment.

■ TRANSFER OF INFORMATION

As with ED-to-hospitalist communications, primary care providers and hospitalists have different patient care roles and perspectives, which may contribute to misunderstandings and missed information. Opportunities to improve care at this transition can likely improve the experience of the hospitalized patient, reduce unnecessary testing, reduce length of stay, and potentially reduce cost to the system. On admission, as with all care transitions, there should be a minimum shared data set that should include the rationale for admission, the working diagnosis, the problem list, key history components and recent changes, relevant laboratory and radiologic results, medication list and allergies, and patient/family preferences and support system. Ideally this information should be shared both verbally and in a written format in a HIPAA compliant manor. Verbal conversations allow the hospitalist opportunities to ask questions and clarify information. As the "accepting" hospitalist may not be the hospitalist who ultimately cares for the patient, the information should also be in an accessible paper or electronic format for future providers to reference. This may be sent with the patient or sent by fax. Alternatively, the receiving hospitalist may fill out an electronic template during or after a phone conversation; however, this may be cumbersome. On initial contact, agreeing upon how, when, and under what circumstances further communication should occur between in and outpatient physicians should be established.

PRACTICE POINT

- A direct admission from the PCP's office to the hospital can save the patient hours of waiting in the ED and can help reduce ED overcrowding. However, patients appropriate for direct admission should be selected carefully, and clear communication between the PCP and hospitalist should occur. Institutions should partner with admitting PCPs to develop a checklist to determine whether a patient is appropriate for direct admission, and standardize what information should be transmitted and how that information should be transmitted.

■ ADMISSIONS/TRANSFERS FROM OUTSIDE HOSPITALS

While transfers from outside hospitals account for a minority of hospital admissions (3%-5%), transferred patients typically have a higher severity of illness and are more medically complex. Additional risks present at time of transfer often include a medical record system that is not shared with the transferring hospital and delays in transfer due to transportation, distance from receiving hospital, bed availability and physician acceptance, resulting in more than two-thirds of patients arriving at the accepting facility at night. While studies

TABLE 12-2 Risks of Interhospital Transfer

Prior to Transfer	During Transfer	After Transfer
Delays in care initiation due to lack of expertise	Decompensation during transfer	Discontinuity of care plan
Delays in care due to delays in finding an accepting facility	Arrival at night	Unnecessary and/or duplicative testing
	Arrival to inappropriate level of care	Medication errors
Inappropriate transfer		Back-end discontinuity

have shown improved outcomes for disease-specific transfers such as myocardial infarctions and trauma, in general, transferred patients have overall higher levels of morbidity and mortality; these differences cannot always be accounted for by severity of illness alone. Therefore, although only a minority of patients go through a transfer, special attention should be paid to this care transition.

Reasons for transfer typically include disease-specific interventions not available at the transferring institution and availability of subspecialty expertise at the receiving institution. However, reasons for transfer can also be less well-defined and include lack of bed availability at the sending institution, patient request, and insurance coverage reasons. Medicaid patients continue to be transferred at a higher rate than those covered by private insurance. Most studies on interhospital transfers have focused on disease-specific reasons for transfer such as patients requiring percutaneous angioplasty for myocardial infarctions, trauma patients, or stroke patients requiring management at a comprehensive stroke center. Other patient populations that have been studied include critically ill patients being transferred to a hospital with greater intensive care capacity. Patients transferred for reasons that fall outside these parameters have been not been studied; thus overall best practices must be inferred from the existing literature.

Challenges that are specific to interhospital transfers can be divided up into risks prior to transfer, during transfer, and after transfer (**Table 12-2**). Prevention of decompensation during travel requires specialized transport and personnel and will not be covered in this chapter.

■ RISKS PRIOR TO TRANSFER

Prior to transfer, the risks and benefits of the transfer should be considered. While patients clearly benefit from appropriate transfer to specialty facilities in the case of stroke, trauma, and acute coronary syndrome requiring percutaneous angioplasty, the benefits of transfer in other cases are less clear. Therefore, a careful review should be done by both the sending and receiving physicians to ensure that the patient is appropriate for transfer and that the benefit of care received at the receiving facility will outweigh the risks of transfer. In the case of the patient requesting the transfer, a thorough conversation should occur to ensure that the patient (a) is not requesting the transfer merely because of poor communication at the sending facility and (b) is not overestimating the impact of quality metrics at the receiving facility. In the case of a patient who is perceived to require specialized care, the sending hospitalist, the sending subspecialist (if available), the receiving subspecialist, and the receiving hospitalist should conference to determine medical necessity and plan of care, both to initiate care and ensure that appropriate care is immediately implemented upon the patient's arrival. Except in cases of urgency, overnight transfers should be avoided as these have been shown to have more negative outcomes.

Another risk inherent to interhospital transfers is in delaying the appropriate care of the patient. Delays in patient care are multifactorial and can be caused by lack of expertise at the transferring facility as well as delays in acceptance at an appropriate facility and arrangement of transportation. Minimizing these delays requires a coordinated effort among administrators, physicians, and medical staff. Transfer centers and rapid transfer protocols at large medical centers have helped facilitate transfers by (a) ensuring that a bed is available at the appropriate level of care; (b) coordinating conversations between the sending and receiving physicians; and (c) in some cases, "triaging" transfers to ensure that those with the most urgent needs have priority. Delays in care initiation can be minimized by the receiving physician making treatment recommendations to the sending physician when applicable. Implementation of the proposed therapy should be up to the discretion of the sending physician. In addition, coordinated efforts can also determine optimal timing and method of transport.

If transfer is delayed by more than a few hours, a repeat verbal conversation should occur between the current sending and receiving physicians to ensure that no changes have occurred and that the physician who is receiving the patient at time of transfer has the opportunity to ask clarifying questions. If at any point a patient has a change of status, this should be communicated to the receiving physician as well.

■ RISKS AFTER TRANSFER

Once the patient has transferred, the main risks are with discontinuity of care plans—both discontinuity of care between the sending and receiving facilities and discontinuity once the patient has been discharged or sent back to the receiving facility. In addition, transferred patients often receive unnecessary repeat imaging or testing, leading to increased charges and radiation doses. To minimize discontinuity, best practice suggests the inclusion of the following in the documentation sent to the receiving hospital: referring physician and contact number, reason for transfer and nature of illness or injury, current and outpatient medications, vital signs and relevant physical findings at time of transfer, results of pertinent diagnostic studies, treatment up until time of transfer, and pending tests (including cultures). Use of a standardized accept form—either by the sending or receiving facility—have been shown to reduce missing information. Another method to minimize discontinuity, particularly for patients being transferred for a single procedure, is to transfer the patient back to the sending facility when appropriate. At time of discharge, care should be taken by the receiving facility to include the relevant hospital course and diagnostic findings from the sending hospital into the discharge information sent to the patient's outpatient physicians.

Failure at any point reduces quality and delays intervention, leads to inappropriate allocation of resources, and increases the financial burden on the patient, hospital, and health care system.

PRACTICE POINT

- Intrahospital transfers are at high risk for dropped patient information and delays in patient care. Risks may be minimized by (a) creating guidelines to ensure that patients are being transferred appropriately; (b) facilitating conversations between the sending and receiving physicians, in addition to any relevant subspecialists; (c) providing treatment recommendations to the sending physicians when appropriate; and (d) creating standardized checklists for documentation required upon transfer and upon discharge. Transfer centers and rapid transfer protocols can help streamline many of these processes.

■ ADMISSIONS FROM SKILLED NURSING FACILITIES

While patients from skilled nursing facilities (SNFs) or subacute rehabilitation facilities (SARs) usually present to the hospital through the ED, they nevertheless represent a significant care transitions challenge for the hospitalist. Not only are they usually medically complex, they also frequently are unable to provide a coherent medical history or describe their medication regimen. In addition, they are less likely to be accompanied by a relative or caregiver than elderly patients who present from their homes. In recent studies, up to 10% are transferred to the ED without any documentation and up to an additional 40% are missing information. Most frequently absent from the documentation are baseline cognitive function, current medications, and advance directive status. Because this population frequently presents with non-specific complaints such as falls, dehydration, or confusion, these omissions resulted in more investigations, particularly head CTs. They are also at risk for medication errors, unnecessary testing, and inappropriate/unwanted care.

While there have been few studies looking at interventions, one study showed that while providing the SNFs/SARs with transfer forms did not result in a significant use of the transfer forms, follow up found that the data transmitted still improved. Therefore, hospital medicine groups should strongly consider partnering with the SNFs/SARs that frequently send patients to their facility.

There is no consensus on information that should be included on transfer forms, but recommendations include reason for ED transfer, past medical history, baseline cognitive function, medication list and mediation allergies, vital signs at time of complaint, advanced directives, contact information for the SNF/SAR's health care provider, and contact information for the patient's next of kin or medical decision maker.

PRACTICE POINT

- Patients transferred from SNFs/SARs are at high risk of medication errors and unnecessary testing and treatment. Providing partnering SNFs/SARs with standardized transfer forms may help improve communication.

SUGGESTED READINGS

Admissions from the ED

Beach C, Cheung D, Apker J, et al. Improving interunit transitions of care between emergency physicians and hospital medicine physicians: a conceptual approach. *Acad Emerg Med.* 2012;19:1188-1195.

Horwitz L, Meredith T, Schuur J, Shah NR, Kulkarni RG, Jeng GY. Dropping the baton: a quality analysis of failures during the transition from emergency department to inpatient care. *Ann Emerg Med.* 2009;53(6):701-710.

Singer A, Thode H, Viccellino P, Pines J. The association between length of emergency department boarding and mortality. *Acad Emerg Med.* 2011;18:1324-1329.

Snow V, Beck D, Budnitz T, et al. Transitions of Care Consensus Policy Statement American College of Physicians-Society of General Internal Medicine-Society of Hospital Medicine-American College of Emergency Physicians-Society of Academic Emergency Medicine. *J Gen Intern Med.* 2009;24(8):971-976.

Admissions from the Ambulatory Health Care Center

Carrier E, Yee T, Holzwart RA. Coordination between Emergency and Primary Care Physicians. National Institute for Health Care Reform Research Brief Number 3; February 2011.

Eichner JE, Cooley WC. Coordinating the Medical Home with Hospitalist Care. *Hospital Pediatrics Online.* 2012;2(2):105-108. Available at http://hosppeds.aapublications.org. Accessed May 18, 2015.

Van Blarcom JR, Srivastava R, Colling D, Maloney CG. The development and implementation of a direct admission system at a tertiary care hospital. *Hosp Pediatr.* 2014;4(2):69-77.

Transfers from Other Hospitals

Hernandez-Boussard T, Davies S, McDonald K, Wang N. Interhospital facility transfers in the United States: a nationwide outcomes study. *J Patient Saf.* 2014 [epub]:Nov 13

Iwashyna T. The incomplete infrastructure for interhospital patient transfer. *Crit Care Med.* 2012;40:2470-2478.

Admissions from Skilled Nursing Facilities

Griffiths D, Morphet J, Innes K, Crawford K, Williams A. Communication between residential aged care facilities and the emergency department: a review of the literature. *Int J Nurs Stud.* 2014;51:1517-1523.

CHAPTER 13

Care Transitions within the Hospital: The Hand-Off

Vineet M. Arora, MD, MAPP
Jeanne M. Farnan, MD, MHPE

INTRODUCTION

In-hospital care has suffered as a result of the increased fragmentation in the delivery of care, specifically secondary to new clinical models such as the rise of hospitalist care in the United States, and the move toward cutting hours for residency trainees in teaching hospitals. This fragmentation has resulted in a greater need for care coordination and a focus on transitions, particularly for the hospitalized elderly population. For example, for a typical patient, a member of the patient's primary team is present in the hospital only 50% of the time. Hospitalized patients are passed between doctors an average of 15 times during a single 5-day hospitalization.

In addition to the focus on end-of-shift changes that are germane to hospital medicine, there is increasing recognition that the focus on handoff behaviors needs to extend to cover the vulnerable "service change," which represents a more permanent change in primary hospital care provider. While the current literature has focused on strategies for to effectively "give" information during the handoff, recent literature has also highlighted the need to examine the critical role of the receiver.

The handoff is

> a fluid, dynamic exchange that is subject to distraction, interruptions, fluctuates on aptitude of and confidence in off-going and on-coming clinician and is contingent on the on-coming clinician's confidence in the quality, completeness of the information.
>
> *Cook et al (2000)*

While the scope of Cook's definition refers primarily to shift change, the term *handoffs* has taken on a life of its own, with the term being used synonymously with a broader set of care transitions, such as admission, discharge, and even communication between outpatient physicians. In this chapter, we will focus on the skills that are essentially to those handoffs which permeate the in-hospital setting for hospitalists, with a special focus on shift and service change, as well as introduce assessment strategies to ensure the safety and efficacy of these handoffs.

TYPES OF INTRAHOSPITAL HANDOFFS

■ SHIFT CHANGE

Shift change is the transfer of content and professional responsibility from one clinician to another at the end of the shift. One important distinction among shift changes is whether the outgoing clinician is returning to assume ongoing care of this patient or the handoff is just a temporary coverage for emergencies until the primary team returns. In the case of the latter, the covering physician is often accepting a handoff only to manage overnight emergencies, but planning and execution of care are largely on hold.

- *Signout:* A type of shift change that often preferentially refers to a primary team who is assuming care of the patient and transfers care temporarily to another clinician and that primary team member will return to assume care of patient. Can also refer to the written document used to transfer information. It can also refer to the time period when people are actively handing over patients to another group of providers.
- *Cross-coverage:* The care that a clinician provides when "covering" a patient whose daily responsibility is assumed by another clinician or team.

■ SERVICE CHANGE

A service change is a permanent transfer of content and professional responsibility at the end of one's on-service time or rotation to a new physician or team of providers who will assume ongoing care of the patients. This service handoff is often more extensive and includes description of the initial reason for the patient's need for hospitalization, hospital course to date, current status, and anticipated plan of care, including discharge. The timing of the service change is driven by the duration of the rotation and can happen as frequently as weekly to as long as monthly. Service changes may not always include face-to-face opportunities for discussion and are frequently supplemented with a written account of the patients' hospital course, often referred to as an "off-service note."

■ SERVICE TRANSFER

Service transfer is the change of service of a patient from care of one group of clinicians to an entirely different group of clinicians, usually from a different specialty or ward, to receive a different service that is unique to the receiver's specialty or ward. This could include an "escalation of care" due to worsening patient illness (transfer to the intensive care unit) or transfer to a subspecialty service for a specific management issue (transfer from medicine team to surgical team for procedure and postoperative care). As with the service change, the service transfer is accompanied by a verbal exchange of patient information as well as a comprehensive transfer summary which includes a written documentation of the patient's reason for transfer and detailed information about their hospital course.

RISK STRATIFICATION OF HANDOFFS

In considering the various risks associated with these handoffs, a white paper from University Health System Consortium suggests that the following three questions can be used to triage risk to patients during handoffs: (1) Is the patient physically moving? (2) Is the handoff permanent (more than just a few hours or a night)? (3) Is the patient unstable? If the answer to any of these questions is a yes, then the risk is inherently higher. Therefore, the highest risk transitions may be a service transfer to the ICU or emergent surgery—since the patient is unstable, moving, and it is a "permanent handoff," meaning more than just a few hours. Another example certainly includes the service change, in which the handoff is permanent and the clinician is likely not returning to assume care of the patient.

In addition to these questions to stratify risk during handoffs, another philosophy that has emerged is the concept of "common ground"—or rather how much knowledge do the incoming and outgoing clinicians already share about the patient? When a receiver may not know a patient at all, the handoff may be at greater risk due to the high degree of uncertainty that can cloud the initial evaluation of a patient. This is not only true during service and shift handoffs, but other transfers of care, such as a patient being admitted from the emergency department to the hospitalist on the floor. Uncertainty is a definite risk for patients and has been demonstrated to lead to patient harm or near misses and inefficient work in both resident signouts and hospitalist service changes. In addition, uncertainty can also lead to rework, including procedures and testing, which may also negatively impact the patient's overall care. Therefore, handoffs are inherently risky when the receiver does not have any a prior knowledge of the patient (**Table 13-1**).

CORE COMPONENTS OF HANDOFFS

Regardless of the type of in-hospital transition involved, handoffs have the common goal of creating a shared mental model between the sender and the receiver in order to ensure that surrogate

---

TABLE 13-1 Questions to Risk Stratify Handoffs—If Yes, to Any, Inherently Higher Risk

(1) Is the patient physically moving?

(2) Is the handoff permanent (more than just a few hours or a night)?

(3) Is the patient unstable?

(4) Is this the first time the receiver is hearing about a patient?

---

decisions and judgments. Certain core elements of handoffs include the following:

■ VERBAL COMMUNICATION

A handoff typically, and ideally, has some element of verbal communication, either face-to-face or over the phone. The goal of verbal communication is often to build a shared mental model for a patient, with a focus on anticipatory guidance and tasks to be done and the rationale which accompanies those tasks, as well as their priority. Verbal communication also allows for other critical actions such as questioning and reading back information relayed and received. One key feature of verbal communication is that it should not "rehash" what is already available in printed or electronic records. It is important to strike the right balance between too much and too little information, particularly to focus on what the receiver really needs to know. While verbal face-to-face communication is not always possible, it is certainly the ideal as it provides for these opportunities. During shift change in hospitals, this process is often called *"signing out."* During an admission, this could take the form of a report given over the phone between the emergency room physician and the hospital-based physician.

■ WRITTEN COMMUNICATION

There is usually some form of a written communication (or "transition record") that supplements the verbal handoff with additional information that could become important at a moment's notice, such as the patient's primary care physician or code status. The written handoff document generally either is a user-created document that is computer-based, is auto-generated by the electronic medical record (EMR), or is a hybrid of these. Often, this written communication is used as a peripheral guide for the conversation during the verbal handoff of information. During shift change in many academic teaching hospitals, this written communication is known as the signout.

■ TRANSFER OF PROFESSIONAL RESPONSIBILITY

A handoff is more than just the transfer of information; it is also the transfer of professional responsibility. Acknowledgment of the accountability for a patient's care is an important feature of successful handoffs. Given the need for frequent shift handover in the current hospital systems, this is a critically important step in the process. Prior work has indeed demonstrated that the being cared for by a cross-covering physician is associated with an increased risk of preventable adverse events. The etiology of this risk is multifactorial. Not only do covering physicians lack the primary knowledge regarding a patient they are caring for, but they could also lack of professional ownership of patients who they did not directly admit or care for a on a more routine basis. While improving the process of handoffs can increase the knowledge a covering physician, efforts to improve professional responsibility are equally important. In essence, a high-performing team culture that functions such that "every patient is our patient" is what is needed to support the necessary professional responsibility.

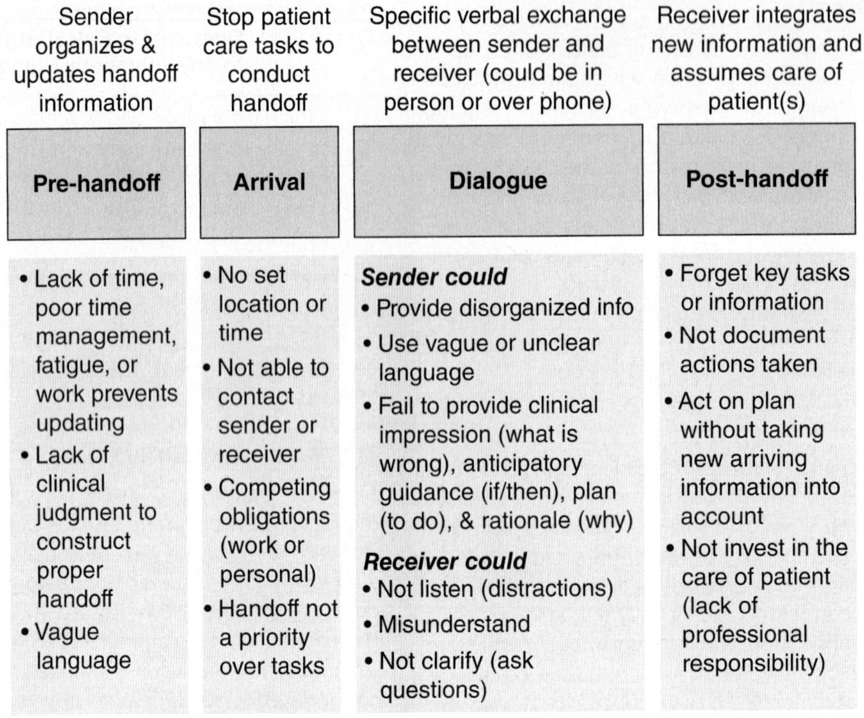

Sender organizes & updates handoff information	Stop patient care tasks to conduct handoff	Specific verbal exchange between sender and receiver (could be in person or over phone)	Receiver integrates new information and assumes care of patient(s)
Pre-handoff	**Arrival**	**Dialogue**	**Post-handoff**
• Lack of time, poor time management, fatigue, or work prevents updating • Lack of clinical judgment to construct proper handoff • Vague language	• No set location or time • Not able to contact sender or receiver • Competing obligations (work or personal) • Handoff not a priority over tasks	***Sender could*** • Provide disorganized info • Use vague or unclear language • Fail to provide clinical impression (what is wrong), anticipatory guidance (if/then), plan (to do), & rationale (why) ***Receiver could*** • Not listen (distractions) • Misunderstand • Not clarify (ask questions)	• Forget key tasks or information • Not document actions taken • Act on plan without taking new arriving information into account • Not invest in the care of patient (lack of professional responsibility)

Figure 13-1 *Phases of the hand-off.*

CORE STEPS TO THE HANDOFF PROCESS

In addition to the core components of a handoff, it is important to consider the core steps to the process of handoffs. In thinking about handoffs as a process, one can conceptualize four basic phases to the process. Modified from a consensus paper for Emergency Medicine handoffs, these four phases would include the following (**Figure 13-1**):

1. *Pre-handoff:* Sender organizes and updates written information for handoff. This often critical step will be discussed further in handoff failures, as this is where many errors can occur.
2. *Arrival:* Sender completes patient care tasks to conduct handoff (or participate in "signing out"). This step also includes the negotiation between sender and receiver for time and meeting place for the handoff.
3. *Dialogue:* A specific verbal exchange that takes place between sender(s) and receiver(s). This verbal exchange could either be face-to-face (often preferred) or over the phone in cases when an in-person handoff is not possible.
4. *Post-handoff:* Receiver integrates new information and assumes ongoing care of patient(s).

DIFFERENTIAL DIAGNOSIS OF FAILED HANDOFFS

Understanding the content and process of handoffs is essential to understanding how handoffs may fail. Each step in the process of handoffs is prone to failure as outlined here.

◼ PRE-HANDOFF FAILURES

Since the focus of the pre-handoff phase is to create and update the written communication for the handoff, failures in this phase lead to errors in the transition record. Often the inability to carry out the pre-handoff phase is due to lack of time, ineffective time management, workload, or forgetting to do so. Systems issues can contribute to the inability to update the written information, including not scheduling protected time near the end of a shift to ensure

information transferred is up-to-date, or more cultural issues such as a lack of priority for the signout process itself.

Failing to update the written communication can result in either omissions (information not present) or commissions (information provided is incorrect). For example, in one study of written signouts, 80% contained at least one medication omission and 40% one commission. Over half had the potential to cause significant harm to a patient. Although omissions were more common, commissions, such as including medications that were not actively being used in the patient's care, were more serious. Examples included anticoagulants, intravenous (IV) antibiotics, narcotics, and hypoglycemics (insulin, etc). While the advent of EMR, and the ability to autofill certain fields, including medications, has helped to minimize the medication omission and commission errors, prior data has established that technological solutions alone are not robust enough to prevent handoff related errors such as these.

For these reasons, written communication that is linked to the electronic health record is often preferred although care must be taken to ensure the written section is updated daily as well. In addition to omissions and commissions in the written communication, the use of vague language such as "today," "tomorrow," or "yesterday" can result in confusion as can the use of nonstandard abbreviations that either are not understood or can be mistaken for something else (eg, HL for hyperlipidemia, which is often perceived as Hodgkin lymphoma). Written communication can be plagued by the TMI (too much information) phenomenon, in which extraneous and nonessential information are included in the written signout which do not provide information useful for those covering the patient during a shift handoff and can serve to clutter the existing, useful information. Finally, cutting and pasting information into the written signout document can also serve to perpetuate inaccurate information.

◼ ARRIVAL FAILURES

Arrival failures include not arranging a specific location or time to meet for a handoff. Even with a telephone handoff, if a time is not specified, the sender or receiver may fail to make contact at the handoff time. Moreover, experienced hospitalists may make an assumption that they do not "need" a verbal handoff, since their experience will be enough to guide them on what to do. It is equally possible that the high workloads night hospitalists face may hinder verbal handoffs, because the night hospitalist is covering too many patients for a meaningful verbal handoff to occur. Likewise, other work demands (competing clinical work, unstable patient, etc) or personal issues (late to work or having to leave work early due to family illness) can also compromise the arrival phase of a handoff. Systems issues can also contribute to arrival failure, with shifts that start and end at the same time, requiring either one individual stay late or one arrive early, in order to provide adequate time to effectively transition patients. This is especially likely if the handoff does not take explicit priority over other clinical tasks. For example, the sender could be ready to arrive to the handoff but the receiver could be in the operating room. For service changes, this is especially problematic as residents and faculty are often transitioning from other rotations, such as vacations or elective time, and so may not be physically present in the same city, or have access to the EHR or even e-mail. Identifying a time to turn over a service also requires that the individual handing off is aware of the identity of their replacement, and in some systems this can pose a challenge.

When the transfer of content is separated in time and space from the transfer of professional responsibility, arrival failures can often arise. For example, during service transfers, such as from the ICU to the floor, it is possible that due to timing of bed availability a different team may receive the patient than originally received the transfer handoff. This is often exacerbated during times of bed shortages, since days may elapse from when a transfer is initiated to when a patient actually receives a bed.

DIALOGUE FAILURES

Similar to arrival, the dialogue phase of handoffs could result in failure on the part of either the sender or the receiver. For example, the sender could provide disorganized information; use vague or unclear language; or fail to provide enough clinical background to enable future decision making. On the other hand, receivers could fail to listen due to either inattention or external distractions. They could also misunderstand the information or fail to clarify any items they misunderstood through the use of questions. Both senders and receivers have a responsibility to focus on the process, and are both critical actors in the transfer of information.

Data from routine studies of human communication suggest that senders often overestimate how well receivers will understand the information that they are transferring. Interestingly, this worsens the more familiar two people are with one another. This "egocentric heuristic" can lead to communication errors due to the use of vague language. For example, a husband may tell a wife, "Meet me there after work" but not clarify where "there" is or whether he means after her workday ends or after his workday ends. In his mind, he understood what he was trying to say, but he did not effectively communicate it. This same problem applies in handoffs. A study of pediatric handoffs in optimal conditions (dedicated room, time, limited interruptions) demonstrates that 60% of the time, the most important piece of information about a patient was not communicated despite the sender believing it had been. In addition, the rationale for to-do actions was often not provided. A common example reported was that the covering intern was told to "check the CBC (complete blood count)" but not given any reason for doing so or what to do with abnormal results. This study occurred with optimal physical conditions and a dedicated time for the handoff process, and still communication failures and

over-estimation of effectiveness occurred. One way to mitigate the trap of the egocentric heuristic is to improve the "common ground" or the a priori knowledge that senders and receivers have about the patient. For example, if the night hospitalist has covered the patient before, they have some "common ground" with the day hospitalist in the sense that they both have had some knowledge and interaction with the patient from which the verbal handoff can build. Improving common ground is a design problem—a key question is can you enhance the structure of the team or the schedule such that the receiver shares more a priori knowledge with the sender?

In addition to failures on the part of senders and receivers, information transmission can be hampered due to noisy, distracting settings that discourage conversation, the hierarchal nature of medicine (which can discourage open discussion between providers), language barriers, lack of face-to-face communication, and time pressures that lead to a hurried dialogue. Using this framework, service transfers could be especially prone to communication failures due to dialogue failures if the services are from different disciplines (eg, emergency medicine and hospital medicine) since the sender and receiver may have very different expectations of the level of detail or type of content to be reviewed. In this setting, the lack of a "shared mental model" for the handoff is missing, and therefore it is likely that the handoff may be unsatisfactory to one or both parties.

POST-HANDOFF FAILURES

Post-handoff failures can take many forms, and one of the most common is the diminished professional responsibility toward patients of receivers who are "just covering the patient." One key question is, "does the incoming clinician have the same investment in the patient care as the outgoing clinician?" It is often very clear when this is not the case. For example, night moonlighters or nocturnists may adopt an attitude that the patients they are caring for are "not their patients" and that their job is just to hold down the fort until the day team arrives. In these instances, the default could be to do as little workup as possible for any acute patient issues and defer to the primary team. While in many cases this "temporizing approach" may not result in any harm to a patient, there are clearly time when delays in clinical decisions could harm the patient. For example, a patient who is meeting sepsis criteria may not receive antibiotics because the night physician could be deferring the choice to the primary hospitalist. Likewise, in service changes, it is also possible that the physician who is leaving the service may no longer be invested in the ongoing care of the patient or patients, especially those who have been passed from physician to physician in multiple service changes. Post-handoff failures in service transfers could manifest in the receiving service never "learning the patient" or expediting discharge for a patient without fully addressing their issues because of a relative lack of professional responsibility.

STRATEGIES FOR IMPROVEMENT

In the effort to improve in-hospital handoffs, The Joint Commission made standardized handoff communications the subject of a 2006 national patient safety goal requiring institutions to "implement a standardized approach to handoff communication, including an opportunity to ask and respond to questions." Critical elements in this standardized model should include an interactive, timely process that contains up-to-date information with minimal interruptions. Evidence for these goals emerges from the experience of other industries, trials of technological solutions, or communication practices in health care.

■ STANDARDIZED OR STRUCTURED TEMPLATES FOR WRITTEN HANDOFF INFORMATION

The importance of the implementation of a standardized strategy is critical for both the verbal and the written component of the intrahospital handoff. The use of standardized language during the verbal handoff helps to ensure transmission of consistent information and allows for interactivity in the handoff. One popular model is the Situation Briefing model (SBAR), which is a technique that originated in the U.S. Navy to ensure the relay of critical information. SBAR has been used successfully by allied health professionals, such as in nursing. Other mnemonics that have been used include SIGNOUT?, ANTICipate, HANDOFF, and IPASS. A prior systematic review of handoff mnemonics yielded 46 articles detailing 24 handoff mnemonics; few were evaluated or validated in research settings.

Several institutions have successfully used structured templates, such as computer-aided and electronic health record (EHR)-aided signouts, to ensure the transmission of accurate and updated information in the written component of the handoff. In fact, Petersen and colleagues demonstrated a trend toward reduction of preventable adverse events after the implementation of a computerized signout system over 20 years ago! Lee and colleagues demonstrated in a randomized, controlled trial that a standard signout guide that ensured the inclusion of critical content resulted in improved written signout quality. However, using a standardized template for communication does not mean it is updated and has the correct or most pertinent information for the covering physician. Not only is it critical to ensure that the information included in the written signout is accurate, it is equally important to ensure adequate time to perform this update. Technological solutions, when combined with systems changes, can yield the best results.

■ FACE-TO-FACE VERBAL UPDATE WITH INTERACTIVE QUESTIONING

Studies of shift Changes in other industries highlight that the use of face-to-face (in person) verbal update with interactive questioning is critical in conducting an effective handoff. Studies of health care professionals demonstrate general agreement with this principle. Moreover, face-to-face verbal update is often suggested as a recommendation for inpatient handoffs.

PRACTICE POINT

- Major strategies to improve intrahospital handoffs include standardized or structured templates, face-to-face verbal update with interactive questioning, an emphasis on anticipatory guidance and tasks to be done, and use of read-back.

■ EMPHASIZE ANTICIPATORY GUIDANCE AND TASKS TO BE DONE

Receivers of intrahospital handoffs often state that they need only the pertinent information—what may happen and what to do about it. Unfortunately, the actual practice is often that the sender provides too much information or too little information. As a result, emphasis on these items can be especially helpful to hone receiver understanding of the patient. Indeed, one study shows that after the receipt of an intrahospital handoff, receivers are more likely to remember "if/then" items or "to-do" items more than general knowledge items about a patient. Moreover, the Society of Hospital Medicine Handoffs Task Force recommends that "insight on what to anticipate and what to do is the focus of the verbal exchange" and that "anticipated events are clearly labeled" and "tasks to be done are highlighted" for incoming hospitalists. Avoiding editorializing and extraneous information allows the handoff to be a streamlined flow of clinically useful information that is pertinent for the covering (receiving) physician and allows the sender to create a picture for their shared mental model.

■ USE OF READ-BACK

Read-back allows the physician receiving the handoff to check the information received from the sender. The use of read-back is also a Joint Commission requirement for receipt of critical lab tests. Use of read-back has been shown to reduce the number of laboratory reporting errors during requested read-back of lab results. Although performing a read-back of the entire verbal handoff could be cumbersome and undesirable, the use of focused read-back can enhance memory for the high-priority items of a verbal handoff, namely tasks to do, and to clarify anticipatory guidance as already highlighted. One misconception about read-back is that it does not need to occur for every patient on the handoff, but can occur as a part of a synthesis for a 'chunk' of patients, or for an entire handoff.

■ IMPROVING PROFESSIONAL RESPONSIBILITY DURING HANDOFFS

While it is hard to imagine telling people to be more "professional" during handoffs, it is worth noting that some organizational cultures and systems do a better job of promoting this shared responsibility, or what has been described as "continuity-enhanced" handoffs. For example, systems in which the sender and receiver both meet the patient first hand since they function on the same team are likely more effective at promoting common ground and professional responsibility than a system in which the receiver is a "hired gun" that is "just covering." While this type of system is not technically feasible or essential for all patients, it may be beneficial for the sickest patients, such as those that are in an ICU setting, who depend on a high degree of primary knowledge regarding their hospital course.

Another model for improving professional responsibility during the post-handoff period that falls short of having the sender and receiver both "know the patient" is to ensure a structure of repeated interaction between the sender and receiver such that trust is built between both parties. This could be accomplished in multiple ways, including a system that schedules hospitalists for blocks and avoids having a new clinician each night or day. This could improve professional responsibility for a good handoff and post-handoff care since both the sender and receiver will face each other again in the future and have an opportunity to receive follow-up or updates on any clinical questions that were outstanding at the time of the initial handoff.

EDUCATION, EVALUATION, AND SIMULATION

Given recent regulatory, accreditation and education requirements, several educational curricula geared toward teaching trainees and faculty effective handoff strategies have been piloted and evaluated. In fact, educators have encouraged framing the approach to handoff education as one would any other entrustable professional activity, in a milestone-directed fashion tied to the measurement of competency. One large multisite study in pediatric teaching hospitals tested the effectiveness of the IPASS initiative, a handoff improvement "bundle" which includes a mnemonic to standardize oral and written handoffs, handoff communication training, patient safety culture training, and faculty development in handoff observation and a sustainability campaign. The evaluation of this educational bundle was shown to decrease the rate of preventable adverse events in the postintervention period, as well as significant reduction in error rates and a significant increase in the quality of handoffs. While this curriculum holds great promise, understanding what parts of the bundle worked most effectively as well as why it did not work in all sites is important. Several other curricular bundles exist within the literature, based upon specialty focus area and program need. In addition, longitudinal approach to handoff education, beginning in medical school, predicts improved performance on standardized measures, and comfort with handoffs as an early trainee. However, the education needed is not just at the student or resident level. Faculty-based education is required in order to ensure the efficacy and quality of observed trainee handoffs. Work done at the University of Chicago has demonstrated that the use of video-based scenarios in a faculty development program led to valid reliable rating instrument, the mini Handoff CEX.

While several validated instruments exist for measuring *in vivo* handoff behaviors, the development of standardized, objectives clinical encounters (OSCEs) to measure handoff quality, are only beginning to be recognized as a method of evaluation. Prior work has demonstrated that a simulation-based exercise for students, in which a mock, or standardized handoff was performed, improved confidence and self-efficacy when performed at the transitional time period in the fourth year.

Finally, although most educational and evaluation modules focus on the communication skills of the sender, we are just now realizing the need for training on how to be an effective receiver. As we have discussed, handoffs are often plagued by interruptions, both clinical and otherwise, as well as reluctance to question colleagues, and competing demands on our attention. Work done within hospital medicine has demonstrated that the longer the handoff, and the more patients signed over, the higher the likelihood of interruption. In addition, this work has generated the HEAR checklist, an observation-based instrument which allows for the evaluation of the receivers listening behaviors.

CONCLUSION

Ensuring safe and effective handoffs is critical to patient safety and the delivery of quality care. These handoffs occur during times of patient care transition in the hospital setting. To ensure the continued provision of safe care during these transitions, providers should be aware of the types of transitions and the ways in which these transitions represent vulnerability for patients and their safety. With this knowledge, employing strategies to ensure effective communication is critical to the delivery of safe patient care during transitions.

SUGGESTED READINGS

Arora VM, Berhie S, Horwitz LI, Saathoff M, Staisiunas P, Farnan JM. Using standardized videos to validate a measure of handoff quality: the handoff mini-clinical examination exercise. *J Hosp Med.* 2014; 9(7):441-446.

Arora VM, Manjarrez E, Dressler DD, et al. Hospitalist handoffs: a systematic review and task force recommendations. *J Hosp Med.* 2009;4(7):433-440.

Chang VY, Arora VM, Lev-Ari S, D'Arcy M, Keysar B. Interns overestimate the effectiveness of their hand-off communication. *Pediatrics.* 2010;125:491-496.

Cheung DS, Kelly JJ, Beach C, et al. Improving handoffs in the emergency department. *Ann Emerg Med.* 2010;55(2):171-180.

Greenstein EA, Arora VM, Staisiunas PG, Banerjee SS, Farnan JM. Characterising physician listening behaviour during hospitalist handoffs using the HEAR checklist. *BMJ Qual Saf.* 2013;22(3):203-209.

Hinami K, Farnan JM, Meltzer DO, et al. Understanding communication during hospitalist service changes: a mixed methods study. *J Hosp Med.* 2009;4(9):535-540.

Riesenberg LA, Leitzsch J, Little BW. Systematic review of handoff mnemonics literature. *Am J Med Qual.* 2009;24(3):196-204.

Starmer AJ, Spector ND, Srivastava R, et al. Changes in medical errors after implementation of a handoff program. *N Engl J Med.* 2014;371:1803-1812.

UHC Best Practice Recommendation: Patient Hand Off Communication White Paper. University Health System Consortium; May 2006.

CHAPTER 14

Care Transitions at Hospital Discharge

Kelly Cunningham Sponsler, MD, SFHM

INTRODUCTION

Hospital discharge is a critically important care transition. Due to the complexity and potential for errors inherent in the discharge process, this care transition continues to be an area of focus for many patient safety organizations, regulatory agencies, and quality improvement initiatives.

The discharge transition represents a vulnerable time for patients for several reasons. There is a shift of responsibility from the inpatient care team to the outpatient or postacute care providers, and with that comes great risk for breakdown in communication. Medications and other treatment plans are often adjusted in the hospital, and patients and caregivers are challenged with new self-care tasks and follow-up responsibilities at hospital discharge. Adverse outcomes are common in the postdischarge period, with studies showing that about one-half of patients experience a medical error and approximately one in five patients suffer an adverse event. These adverse events, which include adverse drug events and increased health care utilization such as unscheduled hospital readmissions and emergency department visits, are often judged to have been preventable. **Table 14-1** outlines some of the patient, clinician, and system factors that contribute to unsuccessful discharge transitions.

RISK STRATIFICATION

Due to the complexity of care transitions, all patients are potentially at risk for an unsuccessful hospital discharge. However, certain patient populations may be at higher risk than others. Most studies of discharge interventions have targeted geriatric patients or patients with specific disease processes, such as congestive heart failure, as these populations are known to have high rates of hospital readmission, upward of 20% within 30 days. Other patient-specific characteristics, such as low health literacy, low socioeconomic status, and psychiatric comorbidity are also associated with worse outcomes after discharge. While it is important to have standardized care processes in place that facilitate safe transitions for all types of patients, it is advantageous to have strategies for identifying patients who may benefit from more intensive care transitions interventions.

There have been several tools and models developed to identify patients who are at highest risk for readmission. However, these models are not able to fully and reliably predict hospital readmission, and many incorporate administrative data that can be burdensome to collect. Thus, having a process to easily flag patients with certain high-risk disease processes, psychosocial factors, and/or frequent health care utilization, is optimal.

A few of the more commonly used scoring systems are listed in **Table 14-2**. The LACE index incorporates hospital length of stay, acuity of the admission, comorbidity measured with the Charlson score, and emergency department visits in the previous 6 months to predict the rate of readmission or death within 30 days. The 8P risk scale, part of Project BOOST (Better Outcomes by Optimizing Safe Transitions), accounts for prior hospitalizations, problem medications, psychiatric problems, principal diagnosis, polypharmacy, poor health literacy, patient support, and unmet palliative needs. The HOSPITAL score was more recently published and was designed to predict potentially avoidable readmissions. Variables include discharge hemoglobin <12 g/dL, oncology as the discharging service, discharge sodium level <135 mEq/L, performance of any procedure during index hospitalization, being admitted on a nonelective basis, number of admissions in the last 12 months, and hospital length of stay ≥5 days.

TABLE 14-1 Factors Contributing to Unsuccessful Discharge Transitions

- Premature discharge
- Inappropriate discharge setting
- Unrecognized medical, functional, social needs
- Specific clinical conditions
  - Congestive heart failure
  - Psychiatric comorbidities
- Poor social support
- Low health literacy
- Inadequate handoffs
  - Pending tests
  - Additional work-up
  - Incomplete or unreceived discharge summary
- Delayed or unscheduled follow-up
- Lack of advanced care planning
- Failure to ensure comprehension
  - Disease-specific education
  - Discharge instructions
- Medication-related problems
  - Adverse drug events
  - Failure to obtain necessary medications
  - Therapeutic duplication
  - Poor adherence
- Preventable complications from hospitalization

While these existing tools are not perfect, they may help providers identify many of the highest risk patients and could serve as a trigger for more robust discharge planning interventions. Medical judgment, or "gut check," remains a critical part of the risk assessment and should supplement any objective scores.

A STANDARDIZED APPROACH TO DISCHARGE PLANNING

Hospital-based providers typically care for a heterogeneous patient population characterized by a wide range of medical and psychosocial needs. As such, it is essential to have a standardized approach to discharge planning that starts early during hospitalization and involves collaboration with a multidisciplinary team. Key elements of discharge care coordination include identification of the appropriate discharge destination, proactive scheduling of follow-up appointments, careful medication reconciliation, and engagement of patients and caregivers.

CHOOSING A DISCHARGE DESTINATION

Discharge planning should begin at admission and continue throughout hospitalization in parallel to the medical evaluation and treatment plan. Once hospitalized patients are medically ready for discharge, they may be transitioned to a number of locations and levels of care. Discharge to a site that cannot meet a patient's medical, functional and social needs can lead to adverse events, so it is important to identify these needs and match them to available services and support. The most common discharge locations include home with or without caregivers, home with home health services, inpatient rehabilitation facilities, skilled nursing facilities, long-term acute care hospitals, and extended care facilities. Patients may also be transitioned to hospice care that can be provided in the home, in nursing facilities, or in dedicated inpatient palliative care units.

The Centers for Medicare and Medicaid Services categorize health care facilities into different groups based on the acuity and intensity

TABLE 14-2 Select Tools for Assessing Readmission Risk

Name	Elements	Comments
LACE index	- **L**ength of stay - **A**cuity of admission - **C**omorbidity (Charlson score) - **E**mergency department visits in the previous 6 mo	Predicts rate of unplanned readmission or death within 30 d; scores range from 0-19 with a fair discriminative index (C statistic 0.684)
The 8P screening tool	- **P**roblems with medications (polypharmacy, high-risk medications) - **P**sychological (depression) - **P**rincipal diagnosis (cancer, stroke, DM, COPD, heart failure) - **P**oor health literacy - **P**atient support (absent or insufficient) - **P**rior hospitalization (in last 6 mo) - **P**alliative care (advanced illness, life expectancy < 1 y)	From the Project BOOST toolkit; has not been rigorously validated
HOSPITAL	- **H**emoglobin < 12 g/dL at discharge - **O**ncology as the discharging service - **S**odium level < 135 mEq/L at discharge - **P**rocedure performed during hospitalization - Index admission **t**ype (nonelective) - Number of **a**dmissions in last 12 mo - **L**ength of stay ≥ 5 d	Predicts 30-d potentially avoidable readmissions with fair discriminatory power (C statistic 0.71)

TABLE 14-3 Available Services and Requirements for Common Postacute Care Sites

	Specific Certification or Medicare Requirements	Nursing Services	Physician Services	Rehabilitation Services	Diagnostic, Ancillary Services
Skilled nursing facilities (SNF)	"Qualifying event" of 3-night inpatient stay; skilled needs >1 h per day, 5 d per week; initial physician visit required within 30 d of admission to facility	2-4 h per patient per day	Physician visit required every 30 d; often utilize nonphysician providers for medically necessary visits	Physical, occupational, speech therapy, approximately 1 h per day	Off-site laboratory and radiology, limited ability to manage unstable patients
Inpatient rehabilitation facilities (IRF)	75% of patients fall into 13 diagnosis categories; require multidisciplinary therapy; >3 h of therapy per day, 5 d per week	5-6 h per patient per day	Face to face visits by a rehabilitation physician at least 3 times per week	Multimodal services, at least 3 h per day	Lab and radiology available, some ability to handle unstable patients
Long term acute care hospitals (LTAC)	Average length of stay ≥25 d; highly complex medical patients (ventilator management, complex wound care)	5-6 h per patient per day	Daily or near-daily physician visits; consultant specialists widely available	Multimodal services	Lab and radiology available, some ability to handle unstable patients
Extended care facilities (ECF)	Long term custodial care; reimbursement through Medicaid	<2 h per patient per day	Physician visits every 30 d	Physical, occupational, speech, recreational therapy	Off-site laboratory and radiology, limited ability to manage unstable patients
Home health	Medicare requires Face to Face Encounter form and physician certification of homebound status	Examples: wound care, IV therapy, medication and disease education	Requires a physician (usually primary care) to oversee plan of care	Physical, occupational, speech therapy	N/A

of care that can be provided, and numerous federal regulations exist regarding the required services and patient eligibility for coverage of these services. **Table 14-3** provides a brief overview of the certification criteria and types of services available. There are two Medicare requirements of which inpatient physicians should be particularly aware. First is the need for a "qualifying event" of a preceding 3-night inpatient hospitalization for Medicare patients who are referred to skilled nursing facilities. Second, for Medicare patients who are referred for home health services, documentation of a face-to-face physician (or nonphysician provider) encounter must be provided, along with evidence that the patient is homebound and has skilled needs that can be met on an intermittent, rather than continuous, basis. See Section III: Rehabilitation and Skilled Nursing Care.

Selecting the appropriate discharge disposition will often require input from several members of the care team, as well as consideration of patient and family preferences. Involving physical and occupational therapy is imperative for those patients who have functional deficits at baseline or who have experienced debility due to acute illness. Physical and occupational therapists can evaluate patients' mobility and ability to perform self-care and will provide expert recommendations regarding the need for skilled services and equipment postdischarge.

Social workers and case managers are also important members of the care team and will assist with identifying and coordinating the most appropriate discharge destination. They are skilled at assessing patients' support systems and identifying social barriers to a successful discharge. They help clinicians and patients understand what services will be covered by the patient's insurance.

Other members of the care team may also provide insight into patients' postdischarge care needs, including but not limited to nurses, pharmacists, respiratory therapists, geriatrics and palliative care consultants, and psychiatrists. Having shared understanding regarding patients' estimated day of discharge and developing a mechanism for

team members to discuss disposition regularly, such as through daily huddles or collaborative rounds, will help facilitate discharge planning. Implementing a structured format to these discussions and clearly identifying roles and responsibilities will foster communication among team members and further streamline the discharge transition.

> ## PRACTICE POINT
>
> • Utilizing the expertise of a multidisciplinary team, such as social workers, case managers, and physical and occupational therapists, coupled with patient preferences, goals of care and skilled needs, will facilitate timely referral to the appropriate level of postdischarge care.

■ SCHEDULING FOLLOW-UP APPOINTMENTS

Discharged patients typically have ongoing medical issues and require continued examination, medication adjustment and reassessment of their treatment plan to ensure that they continue to recover from the acute illness that precipitated hospitalization. Thus, timely follow-up with a primary care provider (or a specialist or facility-based physician, if appropriate) is essential in order to provide ongoing evaluation and management of medical conditions, to identify barriers to recovery, and to troubleshoot problems that arise after discharge. Studies have shown that lack of follow-up is associated with hospital readmission, though the evidence is mixed regarding the degree to which follow-up impacts patient outcomes. In a large analysis of Medicare claims data, 50% of the patients who were rehospitalized within 30 days after discharge to the community had no associated bill for an outpatient visit during that time frame, suggesting an opportunity to improve the timeliness and reliability of posthospital follow-up.

Identification of a patient's primary care physician should be done at the time of hospital admission. Although the inpatient team should confirm that each patient has a follow-up provider and communicate with this clinician as medically appropriate, the actual task of identifying and documenting the name and contact information for the provider may be assigned to administrative personnel. Equally important is early identification of patients who do not have a primary care physician. Institutions and hospital-based providers should have a process for assigning primary care providers to patients who are not already established with outpatient care.

For patients who are transitioning to facilities, a medical director (and often other facility-based physicians and physician extenders) will oversee general acute and chronic medical needs in the postdischarge period. The medical director will typically serve as a primary care physician for patients residing in long-term care settings, but it is important to recognize that patients who are receiving short-term postacute care in skilled nursing facilities or inpatient rehabilitation will still need to have a primary care provider identified for later follow-up needs. Outpatient follow-up care with specialists may also be indicated.

It is recommended that follow-up appointments be made by the hospital-based team before the patient leaves the hospital, so that there is clarity among care team members and the patient regarding the follow-up plan. This is preferred over delegating the responsibility to patients to schedule their own appointments after discharge. Case managers may be most knowledgeable about community resources that provide medical care for uninsured or underinsured patients.

Several factors impact timing of follow-up appointments, including severity of the patient's acute illness, pre-existing comorbidities, the patient's ability to manage medications and self-care needs, social issues such as transportation and caregiver support, and physician availability. For most patients, postdischarge follow-up within 7 to 14 days is reasonable, provided they are given sufficient instructions at discharge regarding "red flag" symptoms and who to contact with questions and concerns. For patients who are at high risk for readmission and adverse drug events, follow-up as early as 48 to 72 hours following discharge may be preferable. Follow-up phone calls and home visits may be utilized, especially for high risk patients.

PRACTICE POINT

- Patients need timely follow-up with a primary care provider following hospital discharge, with high risk patients being seen earlier, ie, within 7 days of discharge. Appointments should be made before the patient leaves the hospital to ensure access to follow-up care.

■ MEDICATION RECONCILIATION

Medication errors are common during transitions of care, with hospital discharge being particularly hazardous. During hospitalization, preadmission medications are often changed or discontinued, and new agents added. Fifty percent of patients experience a clinically significant medication error, ie, and adverse drug event or a medication discrepancy with the potential to cause harm, in the 30 days following hospital discharge.

Medication reconciliation, the process by which a patient's medication list is obtained, compared, and clarified across different sites of care, is a strategy for decreasing medication errors during transitions. Medication reconciliation is a care process supported by national and international organizations including the Joint Commission, the Institute for Healthcare Improvement and the World Health Organization. Studies have consistently shown that medication reconciliation is associated with reductions in medication discrepancies and adverse drug events; there is less evidence regarding the role of medication reconciliation in decreasing readmissions and emergency department visits. Existing literature suggests that involving clinical pharmacists in medication reconciliation and targeting high risk patients, for example, those taking more than 10 medications or high alert medications such as anticoagulants and insulin, are associated with more favorable outcomes.

Medication reconciliation is also an opportunity to evaluate polypharmacy, screen for high alert drugs and potentially inappropriate medications, and identify drug-drug or drug-disease interactions, all of which can contribute to postdischarge adverse drug events. Clinicians should assess medication adherence, address barriers to adherence, such as inability to afford medications or complex dosing regimens, and communicate the updated medication list to the patient and follow-up provider. The medication list should include explicit notation of which medications have been added, discontinued, or changed during hospitalization to minimize the potential for confusion and patient harm. See Chapter 9: Principles of Evidence-Based Prescribing and Chapter 73: Patient Safety and Quality Improvement.

■ PATIENT ENGAGEMENT AND EDUCATION

Patient and family engagement is a fundamental component of the discharge planning process and may help bridge the discontinuity inherent between inpatient and outpatient settings. Many factors contribute to observations that patients leave the hospital unprepared, including both provider barriers (time constraints, competing priorities, failure to utilize patient-friendly language or to confirm comprehension of information delivered) and patient barriers (low health literacy, cognitive impairment, reluctance to ask questions).

Evidence suggests that engaged patients have higher levels of satisfaction and improved health outcomes. Thus, health care organizations such as the Institute of Medicine, Agency for Healthcare Research and Quality, National Quality Forum, and the Joint Commission prioritize patient engagement and the principles of patient-centered care and shared decision making. Initiatives have focused on encouraging patients to ask questions of their health care providers, enabling patient access to medical information, supporting communication with care providers, and facilitating self-management of illnesses. As patients and their caregivers may be the only continuity across care settings, it is particularly important to reinforce these behaviors during the vulnerable periods of care transitions.

There are several approaches that may help patients understand their disease processes, treatment plans and discharge instructions. Patients recall and comprehend only about half of the information provided in a medical encounter; thus, patient education should occur in small sessions throughout hospitalization and main points should be reiterated. Health information technology applications are being increasingly incorporated. Patients should be encouraged to ask questions and should be provided with disease-specific education materials that are easily understandable with regard to language, font and reading level.

Discharge instructions may be confusing, especially when they contain excess content and are given just as the patient is leaving the hospital. Steps should be taken to create patient-centered instructions that are clear, tailored to patient language and literacy, and focused on critical details of self-management. Patients should be given the following information:

- Reason for hospitalization, treatment received, names of clinicians involved in care if questions arise postdischarge.
- Pertinent test results as well as pending test results.
- Diet and activity.

- Medications, including any changes in regimen and potential side effects.
- Follow-up appointments.
- Identification of the person to contact with questions or concerns.
- List of concerning symptoms and how to respond.

Patient education and discharge instructions must be reviewed with the goal of ensuring comprehension of the material. Teach back is one method for assessing patient understanding, whereby the provider relays the material then asks the patient to explain the concept or directions in his own words. This approach allows the provider to identify any misunderstandings and address them before the patient leaves the hospital.

PRACTICE POINT

- Discharge instructions should highlight information the patient needs to understand and manage medical conditions after discharge and should be confirmed using teach back.

THE DISCHARGE HANDOFF

A systematic review of studies investigating communication between hospital-based and primary care physicians revealed that direct communication occurred infrequently (3%-20% of hospital discharges) and that the availability of the discharge summary was low (12%-34% at the time of the first postdischarge appointment). The timeliness, accuracy, completeness, and quality of the discharge handoff can have significant impact on patient care, and as such, is an important part of the discharge transition.

■ DISCHARGE SUMMARY

The hallmark of the discharge handoff is the discharge summary, which is a written transition record documenting a patient's diagnostic findings, hospital management, and postdischarge follow-up arrangements. This document is frequently the only form of communication that occurs between the inpatient team and the follow-up providers. Unfortunately, existing literature suggests that discharge summaries frequently lack important information, including diagnostic test results, hospital course, pending tests at discharge, discharge medications, follow-up plans, and patient counseling.

Several organizations, including the Joint Commission and the Society of Hospital Medicine, as well as expert panels, such as representatives convened through the Transitions of Care Consensus Conference, offer expectations and recommendations for discharge summary communication. At minimum, the discharge summary should include diagnoses; important test results; pending results; recommendations regarding additional work-up; patient's condition at discharge; the reconciled medication list; follow-up arrangements; and identification and contact information for the sending and receiving providers. **Table 14-4** lists the suggested elements of the discharge summary, including those which some may consider to be optional.

The format, timeliness, and availability of the discharge summary are just as integral as the content. The use of structured templates with subheadings is recommended to facilitate inclusion of information that will be valuable to follow-up providers, organized in a way that highlights the information most pertinent to posthospital care. Prompt completion of the discharge summary, preferably on the day of discharge, is necessary to ensure that follow-up clinicians and other care team members are aware of the hospital course and treatment plan. The summary should then be forwarded to the appropriate follow-up providers via fax or secure electronic

---

TABLE 14-4 Recommended Components of the Discharge Summary

- Primary and secondary diagnoses
- Important test results
- Pending results and responsible party
- Recommendations regarding additional work-up or treatment plan
- Patient's condition at discharge (including cognitive and functional status and abnormal exam findings)
- Complete list of reconciled medications
- Follow-up arrangements
- Identification and contact information for the sending and receiving providers
- Resuscitation status
- Documentation of patient education

---

communication; mail may lead to delays in information transfer. With electronic medical records becoming more widely implemented, the ability to leverage health information technology has the potential to improve the accuracy and efficiency with which discharge summaries are generated and communicated.

PRACTICE POINT

- The discharge summary is the primary method of communication between the hospital care team and the follow-up provider. To ensure effective communication, the discharge summary content and format should be standardized, and reliable processes should be developed to ensure timely generation of the summary and prompt transfer to the receiving provider.

■ VERBAL COMMUNICATION

Verbal communication is considered an important component of hospital-based handoffs, however it is uncommonly utilized at hospital discharge. A "warm handoff," that is, direct communication between the discharging and receiving provider with an opportunity for the receiving provider to ask questions, may be a valuable supplement to the written discharge summary in certain situations. Verbal communication should focus on anticipatory guidance and tasks to be done. For a discharged patient, this conversation may emphasize pending tests, recommended outpatient work-up, or proposed medication adjustments during the follow-up visit.

■ MANAGEMENT OF PENDING TESTS

Patients are commonly discharged from the hospital with test results still pending, and results that return after discharge sometimes require a change in care plan. This presents a potential patient safety issue, as failure to follow-up these results may lead to delays in diagnosis or appropriate therapy, excess testing, and patient harm. Approximately one-third of patients have pending laboratory results, most frequently microbiology such as blood cultures that have not been finalized, and reference laboratory tests. As previously mentioned, discharge summaries often lack this information and the critical guidance regarding follow-up. Moreover, studies have shown that physicians are often unaware of test results returning after discharge. In one study of patients discharged from the hospitalist services of two academic hospitals, 41% had pending radiology or laboratory results at discharge, and nearly one in 10 of these results were judged to be actionable. In subsequent survey of the inpatient or primary care physicians for these patients with actionable results, physicians had been unaware of 61% of results.

Electronic systems may be able to automate inclusion of pending tests in the discharge summary, but explicit designation of the responsible party is needed, along with a way to acknowledge and address the results. A few studies have investigated systems designed to improve notification of pending results, but more work is needed.

PRACTICE POINT

- Test results that are pending at hospital discharge present a patient safety concern, as a subset of these results require action. Pending results should be identified by the discharging provider and communicated to the receiving provider via discharge summary as an explicit part of the discharge handoff.

BUNDLED INTERVENTIONS

Patient safety, a health care climate where hospitalized patients are being discharged "quicker and sicker," and increasing accountability of institutions and providers for high quality, cost-conscious care have prompted interventions that may improve the safety of the discharge transition. Many studies of discharge interventions have focused on parts of the discharge process, such as medication reconciliation or follow-up appointments. However, there are a few well-known discharge programs that have been shown to facilitate smooth transitions and decrease readmissions. Several of the most well-known and successful have consisted of multifaceted interventions that include both in-hospital and postdischarge elements. Facilitation by a dedicated transition provider, usually a trained nurse, is another component common to many successful interventions.

■ PROJECT BOOST

The Better Outcomes by Optimizing Safe Transitions program, also known as Project BOOST, was developed by a panel of nationally recognized experts in care transitions, hospital medicine, and quality and patient safety, with input from key stakeholders including payers, regulatory agencies, professional societies and patient advocates. BOOST encompasses a comprehensive discharge intervention, supplemented by a step-by-step implementation guide and toolkit. These materials are designed to provide a framework for quality improvement (eg, forming a team, setting aims, defining measurement strategies) while supporting evidence-based interventions (eg, scripts for follow-up telephone calls, training videos for teach-back, discharge checklists). A unique aspect of Project BOOST is its mentored implementation program that coaches participating sites through the planning and implementation process and enables them to tailor best practices to their local settings. Among an 11-site cohort of both academic and nonacademic hospitals that participated in the mentored implementation program, hospital units that implemented BOOST tools were found to have reductions in average rates of 30-day hospitalization.

■ PROJECT RED

Reengineered discharge, also known as RED, is a discharge intervention that was developed and implemented at Boston Medical Center. With this intervention, nurse discharge advocates work closely with patients to deliver a 10-component discharge package, consisting of individualized patient education, coordination of follow-up appointments, review of pending tests, reconciliation of medications, counseling on postdischarge problems, transmission of the discharge summary, and creation of a written after-hospital care plan. These 10 in-hospital interventions are supplemented by a pharmacist post-discharge telephone component to reinforce the discharge plan, review medications and address questions and concerns. In a randomized controlled trial of general medicine patients, the group who received the RED process had a lower rate of 30-day combined emergency department visits and hospital readmissions. Because the elements were bundled, the investigators were unable to clearly determine which components contributed to the reduction in hospital utilization, and to what degree. Many institutions have subsequently modeled their discharge programs based on Project RED.

■ CARE TRANSITIONS INTERVENTION

The Care Transitions Intervention is a patient-centered program which is designed to empower patients and their caregivers to take an active role in the discharge transition. This bundled intervention utilizes a series of tools and a nurse transition coach and consists of both in-hospital and postdischarge components. The four core elements, referred to as pillars, include medication self-management skills, creation of a patient-owned personal health record, scheduling and completion of timely follow-up, and knowledge of "red flag" indications that suggest a worsening condition, with an accompanying response plan. These pillars are realized through the coaching of an advanced practice nurse transition coach who meets with the patient in the hospital, during a follow-up home visit, and through a series of follow-up phone calls. In a randomized controlled trial of community-dwelling, cognitively intact patients aged 65 years and older who were admitted to a hospital in Colorado, Coleman and colleagues found that intervention patients had lower readmission rates at 30 days and at 90 days compared to patients receiving usual care.

■ TRANSITIONAL CARE MODEL

The transitional care model is an advanced practice nurse-directed discharge planning and home follow-up intervention which has been well-studied in a number of patient populations. Developed by Naylor and colleagues at the University of Pennsylvania, this comprehensive intervention relies heavily on the advance practice nurse to perform in-hospital assessments and collaborate with care team members to design an individualized discharge plan for each patient. Additionally, the nurse supports clinical care, provides patient and caregiver education, and coordinates home services and supplies. Following discharge, the nurse conducts a series of home visits and is available by phone 7 days per week to address medication-related problems, symptom management, follow-up appointments, and other individual patient needs. Randomized controlled studies of this model in a geriatric medical and surgical population as well as in geriatric heart failure patients demonstrated reductions in hospital readmissions, decreased health care costs and longer periods of time between discharge and first readmission compared to routine care.

DISCHARGES TO POSTACUTE CARE FACILITIES

The majority of discharge transition studies examine interventions between hospital and home, but many of the best practices can also be applied to patients who discharge to post-acute care facilities. In general, the discharge process should emphasize the importance of medication reconciliation, timely completion of and communication of discharge summaries with key information, management of pending studies, and patient education. However, since this patient population typically is older with more functional impairment at baseline, there may be a greater emphasis on advanced care planning with the patient and family, functional status, and anticipatory guidance to the receiving provider. Physician Orders for Scope of Treatment (POST) forms, which are physician-signed order forms that communicate treatment preferences for patients with serious illnesses who are transferring across care settings, are often completed when patients are discharged to postacute care. A full set of transfer orders also must accompany patients who are being transferred to facilities. When writing these orders, discharging providers should be mindful that daily physician visits are not expected at most postacute care facilities; therefore, physicians should be very specific when communicating patient needs for wound care, laboratory follow-up, and medication titration. See Section III: Rehabilitation and Skilled Nursing Care.

CONCLUSION

Hospital discharge is a complex process that can be associated with adverse events such as medication errors, missed diagnoses and hospital readmissions. The discharge process should be made safer by implementing standardized approaches to risk stratification, discharge planning, the discharge handoff, and patient education.

SUGGESTED READINGS

Coleman EA, Parry C, Chalmers S, Min S. The Care Transitions Intervention: results of a randomized controlled trial. *Arch Intern Med.* 2006;166:1822-1828.

Forster AJ, Murff HJ, Peterson JF, Gandhi TK, Bates DW. The incidence and severity of adverse events affecting patient after discharge from the hospital. *Ann Intern Med.* 2003;138:161-167.

Halasyamani L, Kripalani S, Coleman E, et al. Transition of care for hospitalized elderly patients—development of a discharge checklist for hospitalists. *J Hosp Med.* 2006;1:354-360.

Jack BW, Chetty VK, Anthony D, et al. A reengineered hospital discharge program to decrease rehospitalization. *Ann Intern Med.* 2009;150:178-187.

Kripalani S, Jackson AT, Schnipper JL, Coleman EA. Promoting effective transitions of care at hospital discharge: a review of key issues for hospitalists. *J Hosp Med.* 2007;2:314-323.

Kripalani S, LeFevre F, Phillips CO, Williams MV, Basaviah P, Baker DW. Deficits in communication and information transfer between hospital-based and primary care physicians. *JAMA.* 2007;297:831-841.

Naylor MD, Brooten DA, Campbell RL, Maislin G, McCauley KM, Schwartz JS. Transitional care of older adults hospitalized with heart failure: a randomized, controlled trial. *J Am Geriatr Soc.* 2004;52:675-684.

Roy CL, Poon EG, Karson AS, et al. Patient safety concerns arising from test results that return after hospital discharge. *Ann Intern Med.* 2005;143:121-128.

SECTION 4
Patient Safety and Quality Improvement

CHAPTER 15

Principles of Patient Safety: Intentional Design and Culture

David J. Lucier, Jr., MD, MBA, MPH

Alexander R. Carbo, MD, SFHM

Saul N. Weingart, MD, PhD

In the last 15 years, Quality Improvement and Patient Safety have emerged as major focus areas for health care systems around the world. The landmark 1999 report, *To Err is Human*, defined Patient Safety as freedom from accidental medical injury, which is often the result of error. Errors are defined as failures of execution or planning. Unplanned events that arise from medical care, whether due to human or systems-based errors, are further classified into near-misses or adverse medical events; a near-miss (or "close call") is an event that causes no harm but had the potential to do so, while an adverse medical event causes patient harm.

Identifying adverse medical events as a source of human suffering, the World Health Organization in 2002 recognized that the need to improve Patient Safety as a fundamental principle of all health systems. The concept of Patient Safety offers a positive spin on the more emotionally laden concept of medical error. Traditionally regarded as the result of incompetence, poor preparation or lack of motivation, medical error is now understood as a product of poorly designed systems of care that contribute to harm. The modern view of medical error is that Patient Safety can be produced only in organizations that take a systems-based approach to the problem, recognizing the inherent limits of human performance and the need to engineer the care delivery process in a way that is based on scientific principles. Nowhere is this issue more pressing than in the acute care hospital.

■ DEFINING THE PROBLEM

Patient Safety emerged as a public health problem following the November 1999 release of *To Err Is Human* by the Institute of Medicine (IOM). This report described the epidemic of medical errors in the United States, accounting for as many as 98,000 unnecessary deaths per year. The IOM report described an approach to understanding this problem that relied on developments in human factors engineering and cognitive psychology. By focusing on methods to diagnose and improve systems of care, the report pointed to a novel approach for addressing this epidemic.

The IOM report provoked a broad response. The President of the United States directed the Federal health care agencies to review and implement the recommendations outlined in the report. The predecessor of the Agency for Healthcare Research and Quality (AHRQ) issued $50 million in research grants. Accreditation agencies such as The Joint Commission and the Accreditation Council for Graduate Medical Education developed standards and goals related to Quality Improvement and Patient Safety that are required of hospitals as well as residency and fellowship programs. A group of Fortune 500 companies organized themselves into a consortium called the Leapfrog Group in order to encourage large businesses to purchase health care from organizations that met high standards for Patient Safety. Advocacy groups such as the Institute for Healthcare Improvement and the National Patient Safety Foundation created campaigns and collaborative partnerships to spread Patient Safety-related improvements. Local, regional, state, and national government organizations banded together to develop and cooperate on initiatives to reduce medical errors. In short, the *To Err Is Human* report helped to crystallize a movement in the United States and abroad that brought a new intensity of purpose to enhancing Patient Safety and reducing medical errors.

■ HOSPITALIZED PATIENTS

Much of the early work on Patient Safety focused on hospitalized patients. This occurred for several reasons. Inpatients were judged to be particularly vulnerable by virtue of their acute illness, comorbidities, and the intensity of the interventions delivered. Hospitalized patients were more accessible to investigators for study. Improvements that affected the system of care were more readily developed and deployed in the hospital compared to settings such as ambulatory care, with fewer centralized resources to support measurement and improvement initiatives. While Patient Safety in ambulatory and chronic care settings is an area of increasing importance, inpatient acute care services remain the mainstay of safety study and intervention.

Given the central role of the acute care hospital in efforts to study and improve Patient Safety, hospitalists are particularly well positioned to serve as Patient Safety champions in their organizations. Hospitalists are directly responsible for health care delivery, giving them firsthand knowledge about how errors and injuries occur. They understand how current systems may play a role in contributing to harm. Most importantly, they are likely to have an informed perspective about the types and methods of improvement that are both feasible and effective. Frontline provider involvement is a critical component of successful improvement projects, and hospitalists are well equipped to participate in a meaningful way.

SCOPE OF THE PROBLEM

■ EPIDEMIOLOGY OF MEDICAL ERROR

Medical error was long regarded as a rare phenomenon. In the 1980s and 1990s, however, sentinel cases brought widespread attention to this problem. Among the most widely publicized was the case of Libby Zion, a young woman who died at a New York Hospital in 1984 after she was prescribed meperidine and a monoamine oxidase inhibitor—a fatal combination. Ten years later, Betsy Lehman, a young mother and *Boston Globe* reporter, died of an accidental chemotherapy overdose due to an ambiguous medication order.

A series of subsequent studies found that errors were common, especially among patients admitted to the hospital through the emergency department. The first large, epidemiologic study of medical errors was reported in the *New England Journal of Medicine* in 1991. The Harvard Medical Practice study examined over 30,000 medical records of patients hospitalized in New York State in 1984.

Investigators learned that 3.7% of patients had an adverse event, defined as an injury due to medical care. These patients had serious adverse events, including those that extended the patient's hospitalization, or resulted in death or disability. These medical injuries resulted from surgical and medical care at similar rates, though the events that occurred on the medical service were more often judged to be preventable. Indeed, about one in four events was found to be the result of negligence: care that fell below community standards of medical care.

The Medical Practice Study was an affront to the concept that medical injuries are rare events. Although critics challenged the results, the findings have proven robust. Replications of the Medical Practice Study in Colorado and Utah (in the United States), Canada, United Kingdom, Australia, Spain, and France all show substantially similar results. Five to 25% of hospitalized patients experience an adverse event due to medical care during their hospitalizations, and many are preventable. Researchers extrapolated the Colorado and Utah study results to calculate the 44,000 to 98,000 excess deaths reported in the IOM's *To Err Is Human* report.

■ VULNERABLE PATIENTS

Although all hospitalized patients are at risk of medical errors, certain groups seem to be at particularly increased risk. Both extremes of age are particularly vulnerable, perhaps due to their reduced physiological reserve. An error affecting a sick, elderly person may be more likely to result in injury than in a younger person with fewer comorbidities. The same is true for young children. The need to calculate weight-based medication doses confers on children an increased risk due to medication errors. Other patients at high risk include those undergoing neuro, thoracic, or vascular surgery. These are inherently risky procedures and often performed on individuals with multiple or serious underlying comorbidities. Patients admitted urgently are at higher risk than elective admissions. In addition, the number of interventions a patient experiences increases the opportunities for a mishap. In the Adverse Drug Event Prevention study, Bates and colleagues reported that the highest rates of adverse drug events were among patients in the medical intensive care unit. This was due to the greater number of medications and doses these patients received. Medication-related errors and adverse drug events are an area of special interest to researchers and practitioners, since these events account for the greatest proportion of adverse events among admissions to the medical service. Studies that examined adverse drug events among hospitalized patients identified a consistent list of medications that account for a disproportionate share of serious incidents: anticoagulants, antibiotics, chemotherapy agents, narcotics and sedatives, and insulin.

■ EMERGING AREAS OF RISK

Adverse drug events have been a particularly fruitful area of work in Patient Safety, resulting in the dissemination of improvements in electronic order-entry systems, pharmacy safe practices, and guidelines for use of high-alert medications. Researchers have been tackling the problem of diagnostic error as well, driven in part by the prominence of missed or delayed cancer diagnoses and miscommunication with outpatient providers. Research has focused on the development of methods to understand lapses in critical processes of care, such as communicating and interpreting critical test results, and ensuring timely completion of referrals. Other thought leaders have focused attention on how doctors think. Can we train clinicians to avoid premature closure of diagnostic options by maintaining a broad differential diagnosis? How can we help them to avoid common mistakes, such as confirmation bias or premature conclusions?

Hospitalists are well suited to study and address the risks associated with handoffs and transitions of care. Hospital medicine practice is rife with opportunities to transition patient care to other hospitalists at the end of the shift or the week, to coordinate care with subspecialists and with colleagues in nursing and pharmacy, and to interact with the referring community practitioner. Research shows that hospital discharge is a particularly vulnerable time for patients, and a time when errors may occur for a variety of reasons. Failure to reconcile mediations at discharge may lead to confusion on the part of patients, reducing outpatient medication adherence rates or increasing the risk of adverse drug events, in turn increasing readmissions. Handoffs to community physicians may fail to occur if the hospital discharge summary is delayed, incomplete, or if there is no system in place to transmit information efficiently. Recommended tests and procedures following discharge are often missed. Promising approaches that hospitalists can utilize to address these problems include standardization of handoffs through the use of templated signout forms, electronic communication with referring providers, and hospitalist-staffed postdischarge clinics designed to support high-risk patients closely after discharge but before their primary care follow-up appointment. Communication and coordination between hospitalists and outpatient providers is increasingly identified as a risk area, and future collaboration between providers in different care settings will be necessary to address it.

As health care moves toward value-based payment and delivery systems, overtreatment and overutilization are increasingly identified as areas contributing to Patient Safety risk. In the decade after *To Err is Human*, underuse has improved while overutilization has not. Overutilization of inappropriately broad spectrum antibiotics can lead to bacterial resistance or opportunistic infections, as in the case of carbapenem-resistant *Enterobateriaceae* or *Clostridium difficile*; hospitalists have an opportunity to become champions of antibiotic stewardship. Medical care can also cause indirect harm: excessive or unnecessary CT scans expose patients to radiation and reveal "incidentalomas"—findings of benign or uncertain significance that would otherwise have gone undetected, but that prompt repeat imaging, laboratory studies, or biopsy. Hospitalists must also be aware of incidentalomas that are missed when transitioning to the outpatient setting, and ultimately can cause delays in diagnosis of malignancy. More diagnoses, more testing, and more treatments increase the potential for patient harm.

The advent of Meaningful Use legislation provided incentives to adopt qualifying electronic health records (EHRs) rapidly, creating new Patient Safety vulnerabilities in many hospital and health systems. While technological innovations like Computerized Physician Order Entry (CPOE) systems can improve efficiency and safe care, Health Information Technology (HIT) may have unintended consequences. After implementing CPOE, one institution found that the adjusted mortality rate in their pediatric population increased from 2.8% to 6.3%. Newly described errors are being recognized, such as the right order being placed on the wrong patient through a CPOE system. Other examples of risk include fragmentation in EHRs, lack of HIT interoperability, and poorly-designed user interfaces. Implementation of a new HIT system is a particularly vulnerable time for patients, and must be monitored closely to mitigate patient harm. During new HIT implementation, hospitalists can have a large impact on patient safety by identifying malfunctioning systems and bringing these glitches to attention.

Creating effective interventions relies on a solid understanding of the nature of error in health care, the methods to assess risk in health care organizations, and the tools that are used to develop Patient Safety improvements. These topics are the focus of the remainder of this chapter.

THE NATURE OF ERROR IN HEALTH CARE

■ HUMAN BASED

Human error is a complex phenomenon, but one that has come into better focus. Students of human error have argued that both human and systems factors contribute to error. By "human factors" we mean the environmental, work conditions, organizational, and individual characteristics that influence work performance. Experts conceive of human performance in several categories: skills, rule-based actions, and performance that rely on novel problem solving. When skills, knowledge, and rules break down or are misapplied, errors occur. These so-called active failures can further be subdivided into errors of execution and errors of planning.

Skills are stereotyped behaviors that require little conscious thought. When the appropriate skill is chosen but carried out incorrectly, the error is classified as a *slip*. For example, choosing an antibiotic to treat infection but inadvertently setting the wrong rate on the infusion pump would be an example of a *slip*. Similar to a *slip*, a *lapse* is when the appropriate action is omitted or not carried out, rather than being carried out incorrectly. When facing an unfamiliar scenario where one cannot readily apply an automatic or routine skill, knowledge-based and rules-based cognition takes over. *Mistakes* can be knowledge- or rules-based, and result when an individual did what they intended, but it did not work as planned. For example, recognizing the infection but choosing to treat with a diuretic would be a mistake.

Everyone is prone to *slips*, *lapses*, and *mistakes*. We can reduce the frequency of these errors through education and training. However, no one is infallible, and therefore, no one is immune from error. In fact, certain conditions can increase the risk of harm. Workers are more likely to make slips and mistakes when they are tired or overworked, bored, distracted, intoxicated, or ill.

Skills, rules and knowledge-based cognitive errors are often unavoidable, and therefore clinicians should not be held accountable for these innocent errors. In contrast, individual actors should be accountable for *at-risk behaviors*, which occur when an individual is unaware of the hazard associated with a behavior that deviates from the standard, and *reckless behaviors*, which occur when an individual knowingly acts dangerously. These behaviors are rare and may merit disciplinary action.

■ SYSTEMS BASED

Although all humans err, the impact of mistakes is more serious for individuals whose decisions and behaviors have a consequential effect on others. Military and commercial aviation, nuclear power, and health care are examples of industries where error can be catastrophic. In these settings, researchers and organizational leaders have begun to focus on the systems in which individuals work in order to design defenses that identify, intercept, and prevent errors before they result in harm.

A system is defined as a set of interdependent processes designed to accomplish a common aim. Certain characteristics of systems can allow or facilitate individuals' performance of unsafe acts. These characteristics are often called latent conditions or latent factors. Examples of latent factors include poor training, duty schedules that provide little time for sleep, lack of adequate supervision, lack of sufficient supplies, and a culture that discourages cooperation and teamwork. Analysts often focus on latent factors that represent design flaws for a particular process and that, in turn, allow unsafe acts to result in harm.

Consider the case of a physician who failed to follow-up on a radiology report showing a new lung nodule. The unsafe act must be understood in the context of the latent factors that contributed to the error. Was the physician overworked, covering for vacationing colleagues? Was there a consistent approach in place for the practice for follow-up of test results? Did a radiologist attempt to contact the ordering clinician unsuccessfully? Multiple latent factors typically contribute to an accident—and few are apparent until after an accident occurs. When a series of latent failures align, harm can result. This model of organizational failure has been described by British psychologist James Reason as the "Swiss cheese model."

Errors in medicine can be classified in other ways, into categories such as diagnostic errors, medication errors, and communication and transition errors. It is important to examine the underlying contributions of human and systems factors to each of these categories. These issues will be addressed in subsequent chapters.

EFFECTIVE PATIENT SAFETY PROGRAM DESIGN AND CULTURE

No single model has emerged for an "ideal" Patient Safety program in hospitals. There are, however, several key components of effective programs. Effective programs must have methods to *detect errors*, *analyze events*, and *implement improvements*. In addition, effective programs *build a safety culture* in the organization that fosters an environment where reporting, analyses, and improvement initiatives can flourish. *Buy-in* from senior leadership and physician engagement is a particularly important ingredient of the mix. Effective Patient Safety programs are resourced adequately to fulfill their mission. Many hospitals appoint and support Patient Safety officers, risk managers, and data analysts, data managers, and process improvement specialists. These professionals and their activities are usually housed in a Department of Healthcare Quality, although the specific arrangements will vary from organization to organization.

■ MEASUREMENT AND ANALYSIS

Hospitals use a variety of tools and techniques to measure Patient Safety. Most hospitals have voluntary systems for reporting near-misses and adverse medical events. This approach is in widespread use, in part because of government and accreditation agency requirements. Certain serious events must be reviewed internally and reported to the appropriate external oversight agency. Most hospital pharmacy departments use a similar approach, reporting "interventions" that pharmacists perform when they clarify or correct a clinician's order. Pharmacy interventions and safety incidents together represent an important source of data about errors and injuries, but these methods are subject to reporting bias. Busy clinicians often do not have time to complete these reports and may be less likely to report their own errors than those performed by colleagues upstream in the care process. In addition, clinicians tend to report very few adverse events compared to nurses or other hospital staff, but those that they do report tend to be more serious. In some organizations, an increasing number of incident reports is interpreted appropriately as a sign that safety is taken seriously by frontline clinicians. Hospitalists should consider reporting adverse events, particularly life-threatening ones, as part of their duty to patient care.

Given the limitations of incident reporting and pharmacy interventions, hospital leaders and Patient Safety researchers have examined a variety of alternative approaches. Direct observation of clinicians at the point of care is a fruitful strategy but requires a tremendous amount of time and effort to maintain. Chart review methods are also well established but potentially resource intensive. Since not all errors result in harm, recent measurement tools have been developed to focus on harm events. The Institute for Healthcare Improvement Global Trigger Tool allows for the identification of adverse events, based on clues seen in the medical record.

Some organizations have access to sophisticated tools that can screen electronic medical records for possible errors or adverse events. These tools examine medication records for events—such as an order for antidote drugs like diphenhydramine, naloxone, and epinephrine—that may signal the presence of an adverse event. AHRQ has developed a set of Patient Safety Indicators (PSIs) that screen administrative records for adverse events based on diagnosis and procedure codes.

Once a critical incident or set of incidents has been identified, health care organizations need to cull the lessons that can be learned from these events. Traditionally, this has been the subject of the Morbidity and Mortality Conference, though the focus of M&Ms has often been on individual performance rather than systems factors that contributed to errors. In contrast, root cause analysis is a systematic and structured approach to identify the latent conditions that contributed to an error. Root cause analyses, performed properly, help organizations to learn about the causes of errors and injuries and, in turn, to develop initiatives that prevent these errors from happening again.

■ IMPROVEMENT IMPLEMENTATION

It is not enough to measure and analyze adverse events and near misses; effective Patient Safety programs integrate quality improvement techniques and personnel to implement interventions designed to prevent harm. Near-misses are particularly important, as they signal weakness in the care delivery process that have not yet resulted in harm but might do so if left unaddressed.

After an event is analyzed, the processes of care leading to that event must be elucidated in order to design an effective intervention. This step is critical. When the processes are mapped, examined, and understood, appropriate interventions can be designed.

Improvement interventions vary from changing one step in a provider's workflow to redesigning entire care delivery processes. The scale and scope dictates the resources and method of implementation necessary to produce reliable, durable changes. Hospitalists not only have opportunity to review adverse events via root cause analyses, they also can aid quality improvement personnel in understanding frontline provider workflows.

■ FOSTERING A CULTURE OF SAFETY—LEADERSHIP AND FRONTLINE PROVIDER ENGAGEMENT

Other high-risk industries, like aviation and nuclear power, recognized long ago that organizational leadership shapes culture. Obtaining buy-in from hospital boards and executive leadership for Patient Safety programs is essential to securing the engagement of front line providers.

The Institute for Healthcare Improvement (IHI), in their 5 Million Lives campaign, recommended "Getting Boards on Board," in an effort to "fully engage the governance leadership in quality and safety." Hospital boards can drive safe care by using the following approaches:

- "Setting aims: Set a specific aim to reduce harm. Make an explicit, public commitment to measurable quality improvements.
- Getting data and hearing stories: Select and review progress toward safer care… at every board meeting, grounded in transparency.
- Establishing and monitoring system-level measures: Identify a small group of organization-wide 'roll-up' measures of Patient Safety that are continually updated and are made transparent to the entire organization and its customers.
- Changing the environment, policies, and culture: Commit to establish and maintain an environment that is respectful, fair, and just.
- Learning, starting with the board: Develop the board's capability and learn about how 'best in the world' boards work with executive and medical staff leaders to reduce harm.
- Establishing executive accountability: Oversee the effective execution of a plan to achieve aims to reduce harm, including executive team accountability for clear quality improvement targets."

While many institutions strive to establish a nonpunitive environment, as of 2014 up to 50% of employees still worry about negative repercussions from reporting. Emphasizing a nonpunitive environment for adverse event and error analysis can help to establish a culture of safety, where all employees feel comfortable disclosing errors knowing that their disclosure will lead to improvement. The importance of front-line provider engagement is essential, and hospitalists play a critical role.

Hospitalists understand the systems and processes of care within their local environment. They can identify potential safety risks, escalate their concerns, advocate for improvements, and evaluate improvement designs critically. Hospitalists can weigh the feasibility of implementation plans and become local champions for process or cultural changes.

QUALITY IMPROVEMENT

Although Patient Safety is a cornerstone of medical care, the notion of "quality" in health care includes several other important components. The IOM has defined six dimensions by which quality in health care can be evaluated:

- Safe: avoiding injuries to patients from the care that is intended to help them.
- Effective: providing services based on scientific knowledge to all who could benefit, and refraining from providing services to those not likely to benefit.

- Patient-centered: providing care that is respectful of and responsive to individual patient preferences, needs, and values, and ensuring that patient values guide all clinical decisions.
- Timely: reducing waits and sometimes harmful delays for both those who receive and those who give care.
- Efficient: avoiding waste, including waste of equipment, supplies, ideas, and energy.
- Equitable: providing care that does not vary in quality because of personal characteristics such as gender, ethnicity, geographic location, and socioeconomic status.

In this formulation, safety is one of several components of high quality care.

IMPROVEMENT METHODS

How does a health system improve its performance in one or more of these domains? Many organizations rely on the Model for Improvement, a well-described approach used to promote organizational change. The basic steps in the Model for Improvement include the following:

- Setting aims
- Establishing measures
- Selecting changes
- Small tests of change, as in Deming's plan-do-study-act (PDSA) model
- Implementing changes
- Spreading changes

After setting aims, measures must be established to determine whether improvement results from the changes that have been implemented. There are three fundamental types of measures:

- Outcome measures: evaluate the end result of a given system or process.
- Process measures: evaluate the steps involved in a process.
- Balancing measures: evaluate whether changes in one area result in (unintended) changes elsewhere.

Unlike measurement in research, measurement in quality improvement is used to bring new knowledge into daily practice. It consists of small tests of change, with many sequential tests, and just enough data gathered in each round of testing to assess if change results in improvement. The process is then continued with the implementation and spread of change.

Another improvement method that was developed originally for industry uses a detailed study of production processes to improve efficiency by eliminating various forms of waste. The Toyota Production System is an example of this management philosophy, which has become known generically as the Lean production system. Lean methodologies have made their way into health care, with a focus on improving quality and reducing cost by streamlining the complex care delivery process. Reducing complexity and waste reduces resources and risk. A care process that takes 50 steps and 10 people to accomplish is more expensive and potentially riskier than a 10-step process involving two people. While Lean is not engineered to improve Patient Safety, it may do so indirectly by eliminating inefficiencies that increase the potential for error and harm.

QUALITY IMPROVEMENT AND SAFETY RESEARCH

Quality Improvement and Patient Safety have intersected in recent years, as quality improvement methods have been applied to solve Patient Safety problems. For example, health leaders used the PDSA model to develop medication safety improvements

for anticoagulants and other high-alert medications. Rapid-cycle improvements have led to innovation in communication of critical test results and handoff communication. As researchers understood the value of human factors principles and system-based design, Patient Safety leaders have embraced and promulgated "best practice" interventions that rely on these concepts. Key principles include the concepts of standardization and reliability, appropriate redundancy, use of communication, and teamwork tools. Best practice recommendations have been incorporated into recommendations and standards put forth by The Joint Commission and the National Quality Forum. Recognizing that there are limits to human performance, researchers have investigated the use of forcing functions as prompts. Attention has also been focused on the limits of human performance during times of fatigue, with efforts to reduce these effects. Each of these concepts will be expanded upon in subsequent chapters.

CONCLUSION

Recognizing the need to mitigate patient harm from preventable adverse medical events, Patient Safety has become an organizational priority of many health care institutions across the world. The epicenter of work in the area continues in hospital care, given the multiple interventions delivered there and the vulnerability of the patient population. New areas of Patient Safety risk are identified regularly and become the focus of scholarly research and improvement initiatives. Effective Patient Safety programs are built on the understanding that medical errors are the result of human factors and systems issues, obtain executive, board, and frontline provider engagement, and establish a culture of safety by reinforcing a nonpunitive environment. The leaders of these programs design systems that identify errors and learn from them, build interventions to prevent errors and mitigate harm, and disseminate their work as best practices to the greater medical community. Organizations that do these things well create safer, more effective patient care.

SUGGESTED READINGS

Bates DW, Cullen DJ, Laird N, et al. Incidence of adverse drug events and potential adverse drug events. Implications for prevention. ADE Prevention Study Group. *JAMA*. 1995;274:29-34.

Brennan TA, Leape LL, Laird NM, et al. Incidence of adverse events and negligence in hospitalized patients. Results of the Harvard Medical Practice Study I. *N Engl J Med*. 1991;324:370-376.

Conway J. 5 Million Lives Campaign: getting boards on board: engaging governing boards in quality and safety. *Jt Comm J Qual Patient Saf*. 2008;34:214-220.

Institute of Medicine, Committee on Healthcare in America. *Crossing the Quality Chasm: A New Health System for the 21st Century*. Washington, DC: National Academies Press; 2001.

Kohn LT, Corrigan J, Donaldson MS, eds. *To Err Is Human: Building a Safer Health System. Report of the Committee on Quality of Health Care in America*. Washington, DC: National Academy Press; 2000.

Langley GL, Nolan KM, Nolan TW, et al. *The Improvement Guide: A Practical Approach to Enhancing Organizational Performance*. San Francisco, CA: Jossey-Bass; 1996.

Reason J. Human error: models and management. *BMJ*. 2000;320:768-770.

Weingart SN, Wilson RM, Gibberd RW, et al. Epidemiology of medical error. *BMJ*. 2000;320:774-777.

CHAPTER 16

Patient-Centered Care

Kenneth Sands, MD, MPH
Lauge Sokol-Hessner, MD

"Patient-centered care" is a core principle in health care, and the concept continues to move from innovation to expectation and in some cases, even regulation. But what exactly does it mean to provide patient-centered care, and how does one achieve this, at either the individual or institutional level? This chapter explores the term *patient-centered*, and current thinking about how to strengthen the partnership between patients and providers in the delivery of care. Throughout, emphasis is given to those innovations most relevant to the hospitalized patient.

DEFINING PATIENT-CENTERED CARE

While the term *patient centered* now appears commonly in both medical literature and lay media, one may encounter a variety of definitions for this phrase. Perhaps the most "official" definition is the one proposed by the Institute of Medicine (IOM) in the landmark 2001 document *Crossing the Quality Chasm*. It describes patient-centered care as "…care that is respectful of and responsive to individual patient preferences, needs, and values, and ensuring that patient values guide all clinical decisions." The IOM goes on to describe patient-centered care as one of the six key "aims for improvement" for quality of care. As such it is presented as an intrinsic value, fundamental and irrefutable, as opposed to a system property with a known association with better outcomes. The concept has been advanced in the form of slogans such as "Nothing about me without me," "Every patient is the only patient," "You're a person before you're a patient," and "Human First." At its core, patient-centered care can be described as treating each patient with the respect and dignity that every human being inherently deserves.

Overlapping terms appear in the both the lay and medical literature, including *patient partnering* and *family-centered care*. In this chapter, the term "patient-centered" will be used to encompass the general concept of making care delivery more responsive to the needs and wishes of the individual patient and his or her family. Family can be defined broadly as all the individuals whom the patient wants involved in his or her care regardless of whether they are related biologically, legally, or otherwise. From this definition, it follows that if a patient has any family, patient-centered care must include them.

The construct presumes that care delivery under current models is not adequately patient-centered. The IOM "Chasm" report conceptualizes the health care delivery system as in evolution, from a clinician-centric, poorly coordinated and non–evidence-based model to a patient-centric, integrated system that consistently applies scientifically supported interventions. In "clinician-centric" models, the patient plays a passive role in decision making regarding choice, timing, and settings of care delivery; these are the exclusive domain of the providers, and those same providers decide what information reaches the patient. Stories abound in the lay and medical literature of patients feeling at the mercy of the medical system, unable to exert control over their own care. However, it is hard to find a quantitative assessment of the current state of patient-centered care (or lack thereof) in the US health care system. Some insights can be gleaned from national results of the Hospital Consumer Assessment of Health Care Providers and Systems inpatient survey distributed by the Centers for Medicare and Medicaid Services (CMS). Although scores have been improving, 18% of patients still report "never or sometimes" receiving communication about new medications and their side effects, and 9% answer similarly to questions about the responsiveness of hospital staff (composite scores, July 2012-June 2013 data).

The IOM describes the fully evolved stage of organizational development as characterized by the patient and family being part of the health care team, with full access to information and the ability to exercise as much control over care as desired. What specific actions can institutions and providers take to advance toward this model? These can be divided into three key properties: (1) free flow of information, (2) partnering around individual patient needs, and (3) involving patients in system design.

FREE FLOW OF INFORMATION

Patients are not truly partners in their own care if information, either about themselves or the care they are receiving, is only selectively available. The IOM suggests two "rules for redesign" to achieve transparency:

- Knowledge is shared and information flows freely.
- Transparency is necessary.

The first rule recognizes that patients should have the ability to receive complete and understandable information about their condition, in real time. The second "rule" establishes that patients are entitled to information about the care itself, including the performance of the health care system and its providers, as well as the approach to care and its justification. While these concepts may seem self-evident, the health care system has not traditionally been aligned with these rules. Prior to passage of The Health Insurance Portability and Accountability Act (HIPAA), exchange of medical documentation sometimes required that a patient obtain a subpoena. Today, care still remains far from transparent: published reports suggest the majority of hospitalized patients are unable to easily determine the name of the physician in charge of their care, let alone the details of the care plan. Fortunately, recent innovations are improving information exchange with patients and changing longstanding traditions of care delivery.

■ OPEN COMMUNICATION OF THE PLAN OF CARE

Typically, the discussion, development, and implementation of a hospitalized patient's plan of care occur without the patient's involvement. Communication of the plan of care is a separate responsibility of the physician, occurring most often as an unstructured verbal communication. There is thus no system that guarantees that the patient understands the plan, or has had the chance to ask questions. Approaches that provide structure to these exchanges, and thus more reliable sharing of information, are appearing in the interest of both patient-centered care and patient safety. For example, the Veterans Health Administration introduced "The Daily Plan," a structured document reviewed with the patient each day of his or her hospitalization. It contains information such as medications, scheduled procedures, and diet, reviewed with the patient each day of his or her hospitalization. The expectation is this kind of intervention could improve provider-patient information exchange in both directions, provide an opportunity for patients to ask questions and share concerns, and identify problems that might cause risks to safety or make the provider's plan ineffective or infeasible. Reported experience shows that the large majority of patients receiving such a plan perceive a better understanding of their hospitalization, have a better ability to ask questions, and a higher level of comfort with their hospital stay. Similar positive findings have been seen by introducing structured patient involvement with hospital discharge planning. A key element of these new models is some mechanism for "closed loop communication," meaning there is verification that the communication has been received, understood, and any remaining questions have been answered.

Several hospitals have actually embedded communication with patients into the work model by adapting bedside "rounds" to include the patient and/or family member. In a typical format, the patient and/or family member is oriented to the process of rounds and is given the option to participate. On rounds, the patient/family member is introduced to the members of the team, hears the presentation of the clinical situation and is invited to participate in developing the plan. Teaching, including discussion of the condition and demonstration of physical findings, occurs with the patient's permission. For patients, such programs have been associated with higher satisfaction, better clinical outcomes, and shorter lengths of stay. Health care workers, in turn, have reported higher satisfaction with work and with the quality of some aspects of teaching in academic medical centers, but have also identified challenges that have inhibited widespread adoption of such processes.

■ COMMUNICATION AND RESOLUTION IN SETTING OF ADVERSE EVENTS

Flow of information should not stop if care does not go as planned. Patients who experience an adverse event are ethically entitled to receive information about that event, and typically respond favorably to "I'm sorry" in those situations where apology is indeed appropriate. Unfortunately, open communication with patients about medical error has been inhibited by a conventional wisdom, held for decades, that open disclosure and apology would increase risk of litigation. There is a growing body of evidence that this is a false premise, and that open communication following error is not only ethically correct, but is likely to decrease malpractice costs since it provides an opportunity to bring issues to resolution without involving the court system. A growing number of institutions are now implementing a systematized approach to harm events that involves open communication, root cause analysis, and early resolution if the analysis determines that the harm was preventable. Many of these programs are now reporting a coincident improvement in malpractice costs. Such programs are also more patient-centered in that time to resolution is quicker, and nonmonetary elements can be part of the resolution. For example, patients suffering harm often look for an institutional commitment to decrease risk of a similar harm event occurring in the future.

Remaining patient-centered in the context of adverse events requires that an institution establish an unambiguous position on the topic, and communicate that position to the workforce. Mechanisms must be put in place to educate and support clinicians in the process of disclosure and apology, which is often an ongoing event, requiring multiple communications as facts become available. For any given clinician, personal involvement in disclosing an error to a patient will be a rare event, so systems for "just in time" support and training must be available. Many institutions address this by creating a resource group with specific interest and training in best practice for communication, empathy, and apology (where appropriate). Physicians, nurses, social workers, patient safety professionals could all potentially serve in such a role. In the setting of an adverse event, the expert resource can support the clinicians involved and help determine the best timing, setting and participants for communicating the event (see Chapter 20: Preventing and Managing Adverse Patient Events).

■ ACCESS TO MEDICAL DOCUMENTATION

Medical documentation has traditionally been the purview of the clinicians and not the patient. The passage of HIPAA in 1996 established that patients must be permitted to review and amend their medical records, but access to the record is still largely based on an exception process, the record being provided when there is an active request by the patient, which in practice occurs rarely. On the other hand, surveys show that when given the option to view the clinical record, the large majority of patients will accept. Many institutions have responded with systems that allow patients to directly access elements of clinical documentation electronically. This is often limited to objective content such as problem lists, medication lists, and test results.

Ready access to clinician documentation is now gaining momentum. A formal, multi-institutional trial of "OpenNotes," a system for electronically sharing outpatient clinical documentation, demonstrated that more than two-thirds of patients reported better understanding of their medical conditions, and felt more in control of their care. At the same time, only 3% of physicians reported spending more time answering patient questions outside of visits. The clinical impact of more open access to documentation is now getting more attention. For example, physicians in the OpenNotes trial report they are more attentive to the accuracy of their documentation, and the approach to documentation of sensitive conditions such as cancer, mental health, and substance abuse. Results of the OpenNotes trial were compelling enough that all three participating institutions have adopted the program as standard practice throughout their ambulatory operations. More research is needed in areas such as the potential for open sharing of clinical documentation to better identify medical error, and/or to improve clinical outcomes.

■ PATIENT-GENERATED HEALTH DATA

Patient-generated health data (PGHD) include biometric data (eg, home blood pressure readings), medical history, symptoms, and administrative information (eg, the name of a surrogate medical decision maker). They are recorded by patients, as opposed to providers, and the growth of Internet-enabled devices has encouraged a movement to collect more PGHD. Proponents of PGHD hope that it will engage patients more in their care and believe that it could shift some of the burden of data collection from providers during time-limited encounters to patients outside of such encounters, freeing patients and providers to spend their time together in more valuable ways, such as more deeply engaging in the shared decision-making process. However, there are many challenges. Information technology professionals must ensure that PGHD interfaces are user friendly, facilitate high-quality data collection, and maintain appropriate privacy. Simultaneously, it is important to ensure maximal interoperability between different electronic medical record systems. Frontline clinicians must be involved in the design of PGHD systems so that the new streams of data will fit into their busy workflows. And all parties must develop ways of reviewing PGHD, especially prior to including them in patients' medical records.

■ PATIENT-REPORTED OUTCOMES

Current standards for assessment of clinical outcomes are based largely on objective measures and rarely include the patient's perspective. For example, outcome of a joint replacement surgery might be evaluated on the basis of range of motion or occurrence of a complication, without formal capture of what the patient has experienced in terms of pain relief or ability to pursue daily activities. For some time, evaluation of clinical outcomes in the research domain has included such patient-reported outcomes (PROs). Now, attention to PROs is growing as part of routine clinical practice, spurred in part by provisions in the US Patient Protection and Affordable Care Act, which specifies a focus on PROs and launched the Patient-Centered Outcomes Research Institute. At the same time, the increasing presence of electronic formats for collecting and storing survey data is fueling the ability to collect PROs.

PROs might include information about which outcomes matter most to patients as well as actual measures of symptoms, functional status, or quality of life. Collection of such outcomes is especially relevant to conditions involving longitudinal care such as cancer, heart disease, mental illness, or arthritis. There is growing interest in developing standardized instruments for collecting PROs, and formal guidance from the National Quality Forum on valid design of PRO-performance measures has been issued. Some of the best examples of broad implementation of PROs in clinical practice come from outside the United States. The National Health Service in the

United Kingdom, for example, collects information on symptoms and functional status for all patients undergoing certain elective surgeries.

■ ACCESS TO INFORMATION ON CLINICAL PERFORMANCE

There is a slow but undeniable trend toward sharing more information about clinical performance with the lay community. Health care institutions have resisted this trend, on the basis that clinical performance data are too difficult to correctly interpret, cannot be adequately risk adjusted, and/or will perversely impact clinician behavior. Thus, much of the initial effort to make performance data public has been involuntary, driven by regulators, creditors, or insurers, each of which may have its own unique requirements for public reporting of clinical performance. As a result, clinical information available in the public domain can vary dramatically from state to state. At a federal level, the patient can find a growing list of measures of hospital performance disseminated by CMS via their website, http://www.medicare.gov/hospitalcompare/search.html.

Simultaneously, many institutions are now choosing to voluntarily share information on clinical performance (**Figure 16-1**). This trend is most readily apparent as a component of hospital websites, but some hospitals are also choosing to share information in the form of mailings or posted material within the facility (illustration). Reasons to pursue this strategy likely vary by institution, but might include (1) the ability to provide context and explanation to information already being shared elsewhere, (2) the ability to determine and expand the portfolio of information being shared, (3) the belief that sharing clinical performance information is a good business strategy, (4) the belief that sharing clinical performance information is consistent with institutional values. The result is that a current survey of hospital websites will demonstrate a broad range of approaches to transparency: some provide a great breadth of information on performance, others almost none. Some hospitals provide metrics with a minimal amount of explanatory information, while others appear to go to great lengths to make the information accessible and available to a lay audience.

Few data are available regarding the degree to which patients use clinical performance data to make decisions regarding their own care. The data that do exist suggest that public opinion strongly favors the concept of public sharing of performance data, even though few consumers currently direct their care on the basis of objective, publicly reported metrics.

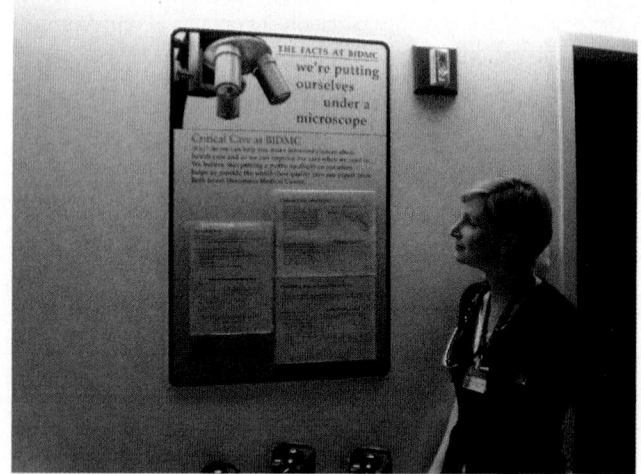

Figure 16-1 *Public display of performance on several clinical outcomes outside of an Intensive Care Unit. The format allows for the information to be continuously updated. (Courtesy of Beth Israel Deaconess Medical Center, Boston, MA.)*

PARTNERING AROUND INDIVIDUAL PATIENT NEEDS

Assuming the first ideal has been met and there is complete transparency and flow of information; how much control does the patient have over the plan of care, or the ways in which that plan is carried out? Patients often encounter systems that are unresponsive to their individual needs. Truly patient-centered care requires institutions to have the capability to fully elicit individual patient preferences, and the capacity to reliably customize care in response to those preferences.

■ APPRECIATION OF INDIVIDUAL NEEDS

At one level, the system can be made more responsive to the patient simply by ensuring that the clinicians have a complete understanding of individual preferences. Unfortunately, despite the central role of interpersonal communication in almost every aspect of care delivery, evidence suggests that clinician-patient communication is often imperfect, and communication skills have only relatively recently been recognized as a core competency by entities such as the Accreditation Council for Graduate Medical Education and The National Board of Medical Examiners. Training can in fact lead to improved communication skills, allowing the clinician to better identify the unique needs and values of the patient, while simultaneously improving patient understanding of his or her clinical situation.

Since needs and preferences may be linked to individual ethnic and religious traditions, patient-centered care requires that providers have an appreciation for this context. Cultural competence refers to the provider's ability to bridge cultural differences in the provider-patient relationship, through understanding and respect of the patient's beliefs and awareness of one's own biases. Cultural competency is most often discussed as a strategy for decreasing the persistent inferior clinical outcomes among minority populations (see Chapter 37: Cultural Competency in Healthcare), but it is equally clear that cultural competency is an essential component of patient-centered care. Like communication, cultural competency is teachable; training programs in cultural competency are on the increase, and in fact are mandated for physicians in many states. In addition, institutions with significant numbers of patients from specific ethnic communities should look for ways to partner with those communities to develop both a shared appreciation of specific needs and preferences as well as appropriate institutional supports.

■ CAPACITY TO PREPARE FOR AND RESPOND TO INDIVIDUAL NEEDS

Full appreciation of the unique needs of the individual is only meaningful if the system can customize care in response to those needs. The concept of partnering with patients is one way to think about the process of customizing care. Helping patients understand the reasons underlying their care is likely to make them engaged participants rather than passive recipients, and therefore more likely to lead to patient-centered care. For instance, imagine a patient who just had a hip replacement and is asking to leave the hospital as soon as possible. One approach would be to tell her she cannot yet leave, and that the health care team will decide when she is ready to be discharged. A partnering approach would start by asking about her concerns (Patient: "I am worried about getting a hospital-acquired infection"), align with those (Hospitalist: "We do not want you to get an infection or stay in the hospital any longer than is necessary"), help her understand the events that need to occur before it is safe for her to leave the hospital (Hospitalist: "In order for you to be able to function when you leave the hospital, we feel it's important that you be able to…"), and finish by asking if the team has addressed her concerns (Hospitalist: "How does that sound to you? What questions do you have?"), thereby making her a more active participant in her care.

In some cases, customizing care requires some preparation. For example, encouraging patients to legally designate a surrogate medical decision maker is a critical part of advance care planning; without that information, by the time the patient loses capacity to make their own medical decisions, it may be too late to determine what their preferences are and who they would prefer to speak on their behalf. Other examples include reliably recording who the patient wants involved—and who they do not want involved—in their care, as well as how he or she prefers to be addressed, and which language is best for him or her. Customized patient-centered care then means consistently using that information when speaking with the patient and family, as well as arranging any necessary interpreter services in advance of an encounter. Electronic medical record systems must be designed to support busy clinicians by making it easy to record such information, and then ensuring it is easily retrieved at the point of care.

Being responsive to individual needs also requires ceding some control to the patient. For example, many hospitals are eliminating restrictions on visiting hours in favor of open access for the patient's family. Family presence during invasive procedures and resuscitation events is endorsed by several professional societies. Programs that allow patients or family members to activate rapid response teams are now well described. Sometimes called "Condition H" or "Code Help," the concept was initially advanced for the pediatric setting, where serious adverse events have occurred in the presence of a concerned parent who was unable to bring immediate assistance to the bedside. The same principal has now been extended to the adult setting. A typical response team will include both a physician and nurse, and in some models may include critical care specialists, social workers, chaplains, and/or patient representatives. It is not unusual for clinicians to initially express resistance to the concept, citing concerns that patients and family members will overuse "code help" for inappropriate, nonurgent issues. However, the experience of institutions that have implemented response teams is that the option is used prudently, and allows earlier interception of potential adverse events as well as other important issues such as inadequate pain control or communication problems. Successful implementation of a "code help" program requires patient and family education about its purpose, a well-structured activation mechanism, and a predefined set of individual responders. Protocols that define the mechanism for recording the incident, and debriefing with the patient and family, should also be established.

Partnering around individual needs becomes particularly important when treatment options carry significant risks or consequences to the patient. Conditions with multiple potential approaches to management such as chronic back pain, depression, cancer, or organ failure, are all examples of conditions where patient preference plays a major role in determining the best plan of care. Such situations call for informed, shared decision making, a term for the process of communicating with the patient about what matters most to him or her in the context of the medical situation, with the ultimate goal of making patient-centered medical decisions. Shared decision making and partnering with patients replace two inappropriate alternatives: telling patients what to do without their input, and asking them to make choices from a list of options without any guidance or advice. Education about shared decision making may help clinicians and patients navigate this complex process and find the right balance.

The first step is to ensure the patient understands his or her condition, the prognosis, and the treatment options, to the degree they desire. This can be accomplished using established communication techniques such as "Ask-Tell-Ask": (1) "ask" the patient how much they would like to know, how involved they would like to be in decision making, and what they understand; (2) "tell" them about what they do not yet understand in patient-centered language; (3) "ask" them how they feel about that information, what questions they have and to reiterate their understanding to ensure everyone has a shared understanding.

Before discussing treatment options, it is important for clinicians to understand what matters most to the patient, in the context of the medical situation. Although it is a seemingly vague construct, understanding "what matters most" becomes increasingly important as the stakes of the medical decisions rise. Asking about the patient's hopes, goals, fears, and worries, and about any tradeoffs they are willing to make in order to reach their goals, brings clarity to what matters most to a patient, and provides invaluable information for the next step in shared decision making.

Discussion of treatment options must include information about the anticipated benefits and risks of each option, and should include a recommendation from the clinician based on knowledge of what matters most to the patient. Without such knowledge, the clinician risks suggesting options that will not actually benefit the patient. For instance, recommending an aggressive chemotherapy regimen may be inappropriate for a patient who prefers to maximize quality of life and minimize time spent in health care settings, even if that means they may die sooner than they would if they received that regimen. Informed shared decision making can be supported by decision aids, that is, structured materials such as a videotape or printed algorithm that help to illustrate treatment options and associated risks and benefits.

PRACTICE POINT

Hospitalists can better meet patients individualized needs by taking the following steps:

- Acquire and maintain communication skills and cultural competency.
- Identify who the patient does and does not want involved in his or her care, including his or her surrogate decision maker.
- Communicate in the patient's native language.
- Encourage and empower family presence.
- Confirm that the patient-family understand information presented to them, via techniques such as "Ask-Tell-Ask," and decision aids to illustrate difficult concepts (such as a videotape or printed algorithms).

INVOLVING PATIENTS IN SYSTEM DESIGN

Systems of care delivery have largely evolved in response to the needs of providers and the design of the payment system. The patient thus encounters a care delivery model that is confusing to navigate, inconvenient, and severely fractured between care delivery settings. Improved coordination of care for a patient can help (see the section in this volume about "Transitions of Care") but

more broadly, the concept of patient-centered care extends beyond the approach to the individual patient, and includes as a tenet that patients have a voice in the design of the care delivery system itself. In what might be described as a traditional model for hospital administration, the patient is seen as a consumer of services, without any formal role as part of hospital operations. Consequently, despite the patient's experiences with the institution, he or she has little or no ability to advocate for change, and the institution lacks the voice of the patient in the design of care processes. This is beginning to change as hospitals move to involve patients in operational activities, either by creating positions for patients or family members on existing hospital committees, and/or creating a separate "Patient/Family Advisory Council" (PFAC) function. Indeed the presence of a PFAC is now mandated by regulation in some states. An institution may have a single PFAC or multiple PFACs based on a desire for specific patient involvement in discreet service lines.

A role for patient/family participation has been described for a myriad of institutional processes, including strategic planning, facility redesign, research oversight, ethics, care coordination, education, finance, credentialing, leadership search, information technology, process improvement, patient safety, service excellence, and personnel practices. **Table 16-1** demonstrates the range of involvement possible for patient-family advisors. Whether the plan is to involve patients on existing operational committees and/or to create one or more PFACs, a successful model for patient involvement in the design of care should begin with a vision and a plan that addresses a number of key issues:

- What are the goals for including a patient in this design process?
- What is the organizational model for patient involvement?
- Who from the organization will manage patient involvement?
- What criteria will be used for selecting patient participants?
- What are the expectations of the patient participants?
- What is the selection process?
- How long is a term of service, and are there term limits?
- What is the orientation process for patients to a hospital administrative role?
- What are the expectations for attendance?
- What criteria will be used to assess the performance of patient participants, and/or the PFAC committee itself?

An up-front strategy to define these issues is likely to be rewarded with a smooth functioning program for patient involvement in hospital operations.

FRONTIERS IN PATIENT-CENTERED CARE

How will we know if we are becoming more patient-centered? Developing measures of patient-centered care is an important step. One approach is to assess whether a hospital has the elements of patient-centered systems described in this chapter. A self-assessment tool created through a partnership of the Institute for Patient-Centered and Family-Centered Care and the American Hospital Association is available for this purpose (http://www.aha.org/aha/content/2005/pdf/assessment.pdf). But having the capability to be patient-centered is not sufficient; a system must also reliably deliver patient-centered care for each patient.

What does it mean to be patient-centered on an individual level? Certainly one can imagine situations where it is clear whether or not the care was patient-centered: for example, failure to use an interpreter when it was requested by the patient would demonstrate a failure to be patient-centered, whereas eliciting and honoring end-of-life care preferences would be a great example of patient-centered care. But in many situations, it may not be clear how to assess whether or not care has been patient-centered. Imagine a patient is admitted to the hospital for a viral illness. Despite its etiology, the

TABLE 16-1 Patient-Family Advisor Involvement at Beth Israel Deaconess Medical Center, Boston, MA

Committees with Patient-Family Advisors	Projects with Patient-Family Advisor Involvement
Patient Care Assessment Committee of the Board of Directors (quality and safety)	Communication apology and resolution program improvements
Patient Care Committee of the Board of Directors	Patient rights and responsibilities update
Ethics Advisory Committee	Information, security and privacy policy
Medication Safety Subcommittee	OpenNotes project
Drug Shortage Task Force	PatientSite (patient portal) design
Critical Care Executive Committee	Health care proxy material redesign
Critical Care Experience Task Force	Improving the discharge experience through better educational materials
Conversation Ready Initiative (End-of-Life Planning)	Communication before, during and after surgery
Moore Foundation Grant Committee	Nurse competency training curriculum
Respect and Dignity Workgroup	MOLST (Medical Orders for Life-Sustaining Treatment) educational material development
OpenNotes Workgroups	Hospital room design
Service Excellence Steering committee	Diversity planning group

patient requests an antibiotic for his illness, saying he believes it will help him improve. But instead of prescribing the antibiotic, the doctor listens to the patient's concerns, tries to ensure he feels heard, respectfully counsels him about the risks of antibiotics, prescribes other medications for the patient's symptoms, and reassures him that his symptoms will improve soon. In this situation, who is the judge of whether the care was "patient-centered"? Although most readers would agree that the doctor provided excellent medical care, the patient may feel that his care was not "patient-centered" because his request was not honored.

Measures of patient-centered care should be defined based on both what matters most to patients *and* what is consistent with acceptable medical practice. As a starting point, future work could begin to define and measure specific elements of patient-centered care, and through collaboration with patients and providers could identify elements around which there is strong consensus. Applying these measures to populations could reveal the degree to which a system delivers patient-centered care. Such information could reveal the opportunities for improvement and drive innovation by patients, providers, and institutional leaders.

Much work remains to fully define best practice in patient-centered care, and the known steps to achieving optimally patient-centered care are numerous and complex. Yet in spite of these challenges, as providers, it is our responsibility to prioritize patient-centered care. As a historical figure once said: "It is not incumbent upon you to complete the work, but neither are you at liberty to desist from it." [Avot 2:21, attributed to Rabbi Tarfon.]

ACKNOWLEDGMENTS

Thank you to the following Beth Israel Deaconess Medical Center Patient/Family Advisors for their insightful and formative comments on this chapter: Terri Payne Butler, Peter Tarsa, and Nicola Truppin.

SUGGESTED READINGS

Berwick DM. What "patient-centered" should mean: confessions of an extremist. *Health Aff (Millwood)*. 2009;28(4):w555-w565.

Delbanco T, Walker J, Bell SK, et al. Inviting patients to read their doctors' notes: a quasi-experimental study and a look ahead. *Ann Intern Med*. 2012;157:461-470.

Gerteis M, Edgman-Levitan S, Daley J, et al. *Through the Patient's Eyes. Picker/Commonwealth Program for Patient Centered Care*. San Francisco, CA: Jossey-Bass; 1993.

Johnson B, Abraham M, Conway J, et al. *Partnering with Patients and Families to Design a Patient- and Family-Centered Health Care System: Recommendations and Promising Practices*. Bethesda, MD: Institute for Family-Centered Care and the Institute for Healthcare Improvement; 2008.

Lazare A. Apology in medical practice: an emerging clinical skill. *JAMA*. 2006;296:1401-1404.

Peto R, Tenerowicz LM, Benjamin EM, et al. One system's journey in creating a disclosure and apology program. *Jt Comm J Qual and Patient Saf*. 2009;35(10):487-492.

Teutsch C. Patient-doctor communication. *Med Clin N Am*. 2003;87:1115-1145.

CHAPTER 17

Harnessing Data to Make Quality Improvement Decisions: Measurement and Measures

Nathan Spell, MD

Assessing and improving quality depends upon good measurement. This chapter will discuss basic principles of measuring quality in medical practice and how data can be used to identify opportunities for improvement and support improvement efforts.

ASSESSING QUALITY THROUGH MEASUREMENT

■ PERFORMANCE ASSESSMENT FOR EXTERNAL COMPARISON

At all levels of the health care industry, from national to local and from health systems to individual practitioners, performance assessment is now routine. Care is assessed in multiple domains, such as clinical outcomes, adherence to standards, the patient experience of care, and the cost of care. Through external comparison, or "benchmarking," payers, the government, the public, and others attempt to judge the quality of health care providers and organizations. Performance measurement is more and more being tied to payment in the form of value-based contracts, with financial risks for performance shifting toward the providers of care, behooving us to understand how performance is assessed and improved. In order for external comparisons to be meaningful, several criteria need to be met:

- The measure should be accurately and reliably recorded across sites. As an example, length of stay for an emergency department visit will have defined starting and ending times that are routinely captured, recorded, and reported. If the standard definitions and practices are followed across all emergency departments, then length of stay comparisons should be meaningful.
- The measure should be valid and meaningfully reflect an important outcome or process. Mortality is an example of an outcome measure that has face validity, but how it is defined will affect its meaningfulness. If mortality is measured only during the inpatient stay, it will appear better for hospitals that are effective at transferring patients to other settings prior to death. Measuring mortality over a longer term, such as 30 days, 6 months, or 1 year, may be more meaningful.

Measures like mortality, patient functional status, and unintended hospital readmissions are examples of outcome measures. Outcome measures tend to be the most salient to patients, the public, and to health care providers. When using outcome measures for external comparison, however, the validity of comparison often requires adjusting for influences on the outcome that are not determined by the quality of care provided. Factors such as age, comorbid illness, and social support often impact outcomes. Some of these factors can be identified from the available data sources and included in risk adjustment algorithms. The degree to which an algorithm can truly adjust for risk depends upon the quality of the data available for the adjustment model and the power of the model itself to reflect these influences.

Process measures reflect the steps in clinical care provided to patients. Common examples of process measures used to assess hospital performance are the CMS core measures. Generally, process measures do not have to be adjusted for clinical or demographic factors, as it is assumed that these factors have little influence on our ability to carry out the processes. To be valid for assessment, process measures must also reflect meaningful clinical care. Measurement of medication reconciliation upon admission to the hospital is an example of a performance measure of questionable validity. A provider may achieve credit for performing medication reconciliation by use of an electronic tool embedded in the health record, but if an accurate list of home medications has not been obtained, the act of medication reconciliation may not be clinically meaningful.

LOCAL QUALITY ASSESSMENT AND IMPROVEMENT

External performance measures assess only a small portion of the care provided by individual health professionals and organizations. What is measured locally should reflect the priorities of the organization and the needs of patients. Accrediting bodies, such as The Joint Commission, require that hospitals routinely assess and improve care for patients. Individuals and hospitals may be less able to perform risk adjustment on internal data compared to data submitted to external organizations, yet tracking clinical outcomes against past performance can be a valid and useful way to assess quality.

SOURCES OF DATA FOR MEASUREMENT AND IMPROVEMENT

ADMINISTRATIVE OR "BILLING" DATA

Administrative data are one of the oldest sources of data on hospital performance. To bill an external payer, hospitals must accurately identify the patient, principle and secondary diagnoses, procedures, and any supply items charged. These data are generally obtained from the hospital registration system, financial system, and medical record. Names of physicians involved in care (attending physician, admitting physician, discharging physician, procedural physician, consulting physician) are generally recorded. Administrative data will include the nature of the patient's admission (elective, urgent, or emergent), the source of admission (physician office, emergency department, transfer from other hospital or facility, etc) and the patient's disposition at discharge (alive or dead, discharged to home or other facility, etc). Limitations of administrative data are that it is an incomplete reflection of the clinical information, is dependent upon the thoroughness and accuracy of provider documentation, and is subject to interpretation by trained chart coders and abstractors. Despite these limitations, much of the data for external performance measures originate in administrative data sets, as these data have been available for many years in standard formats across the health care industry.

CLINICAL DATA

The source of most clinical data for quality assessment and improvement is via an electronic health record (EHR). The EHR brings together patient demographics, orders, provider documentation, pharmacy data, laboratory results, radiology reports, and any clinical information documented by nurses and other health professionals. Often the EHR is interfaced with data from separate electronic systems for patient registration, pharmacy, laboratory, and radiology. Since EHRs are designed primarily to support clinical care and patient interaction, they often do not contain all of the important operational details about patient care. For instance, movement of patients within the hospital is not well reflected in most EHRs; the hospital may have a separate electronic bed management system that can be an important source of data for projects related to patient flow.

A limitation of many EHRs is that the architecture supports the care of individual patients but may not include an easy way to view aggregate data across patient populations and time. The hospital or health system may have a clinical data warehouse which holds data from the EHR and other supporting electronic systems. Data warehouses are structured to allow for more sophisticated reporting and analysis of aggregate data, and may therefore be a better source of data for local improvement than the EHR itself.

COST DATA

Costs of care can be challenging to identify, obtain, and understand. Detailed accounting of actual costs to provide individual components of a given patient's care is not available in many hospitals. Charges may be available, but charges do not have a direct relationship to actual costs to provide care, and serve primarily for negotiating contracts and generating bills with payers. If costs are of interest in an improvement project, the hospital finance office can often provide guidance on how to generate close estimates, or how to impute costs based on utilization of resources.

CLINICAL REGISTRIES

The hospital or clinical practices may participate in collecting data for registries of specific diseases, conditions, or procedures. Professional organizations such as the American Heart Association, American College of Cardiology, and American College of Surgeons sponsor registries where clinical data from patient care at one site can be aggregated and compared to data from other sites. Often, these data are more clinically detailed and rich than data extracted from a data warehouse or an EHR since they usually reflect the skilled interpretation of trained clinical abstractors who are able to read the charts and make judgments about the care, which is more detailed than what is usually recorded in discrete data fields in the EHR.

USING DATA TO IDENTIFY OPPORTUNITIES FOR IMPROVEMENT

Benchmarking against other organizations or established targets can elucidate opportunities for performance improvement. A hospital or health system will have identified quality targets from external benchmarking or through opportunities identified internally to improve care or value to patients. Where gaps exist between current and desired performance, there are often opportunities for quality improvement (QI) projects. Aligning QI work with these identified system priorities has many advantages. Access to data, project facilitation, change management assistance, and leadership support will be easier to obtain.

Another useful approach to identifying opportunities is to develop reports from the electronic data systems or data warehouse to assess how closely the care provided matches professional standards or best practice. For example, recommended management of diabetes and hyperglycemia for most inpatients includes basal insulin with or without corrective dosing of short acting insulin. A data report showing the rate at which patients receiving short acting insulin are also given basal insulin can be useful to assess an opportunity to improve management.

Unnecessary variation in clinical practice is now a recognized problem in health care delivery. The Dartmouth Atlas project has demonstrated this phenomenon. The greater the ambiguity in care practices, the greater the likelihood exists for variation between providers. Data reports displaying variation in costs, treatment, or diagnostic approaches between providers for the same condition may highlight opportunities for improvement.

CHOOSING MEASURES FOR A QUALITY IMPROVEMENT PROJECT

USEFULNESS

Though grounded in the scientific method of hypothesis testing, quality improvement techniques differ from research methods by attempting to improve processes and outcomes in the local environment, as distinct from the intent to prove an underlying generalizable truth. The measures chosen should be useful enough for the local improvement work and should not require the degree of rigor necessary in research projects. To be useful, measures should be easily obtained and checked frequently enough to guide the improvement work. Performance should be shared with the improvement team and others in real time, whereas research methods may call for blinding the involved clinicians to reduce bias in the results.

■ A BALANCED SET OF MEASURES

For most quality improvement projects, there is a clear intended measurable goal. Readmissions to the hospital within 30 days of discharge, wound infection rates, and length of stay are good examples. Achieving progress on such measured goals, however, requires complex interventions occurring within the ecosystems of hospitals and other clinical environments; as such, it is frequently useful to measure other aspects of the complex systems when making changes, and create a "balanced set" of measures. A useful framework is the Clinical Value Compass (CVC), which consists of four domains: clinical outcomes, functional status or outcomes, experience or satisfaction, and costs. Not every project will have potential measures in each of these domains, yet the CVC prompts consideration of perspectives beyond the main focus, which is often on the clinical outcome of interest. Building on the example of reducing readmissions to the hospital within 30 days of discharge, one may choose to measure the combined costs of the principal and readmission stay. Patient satisfaction with the discharge process and overall care is relevant. If feasible, a measure of patient functional status at 30 days or longer may be a good complement to the clinical outcome measure of the readmission rate. If a balanced set of measures has been chosen, it is also more likely that the team will detect unintended consequences of their improvement efforts. For example, if readmissions decrease, does the principal admission length of stay increase? The outcome measure may also be remote in time and not directly connected to day-to-day work. For example, 30-day readmissions are influenced by many factors and, by definition, at least 30 days following discharge must pass to judge the effect of any intervention on the readmission rate. Adding process measures that are relevant may be very useful, such as follow-up appointments scheduled prior to discharge, transmission of discharge information to the primary physician, and confirmation of patient learning through a "teach back" method.

A GOOD MEASUREMENT PLAN

After project measures are selected, a measurement plan is necessary to make the measures available for improvement work.

■ MAKING MEASURES OPERATIONAL

Measures begin at the conceptual level. An example of a conceptual measure is "the rate at which patients discharged from the hospital medicine service have a follow-up appointment scheduled prior to discharge." To make a measure operational is to define it in such a way that different people assessing the measure would come to the same answer. To express this measure as an equation, the denominator could be defined as all patients discharged from the hospital medicine service, regardless of the recommendations for postdischarge appointments or where the patients will be seen. The numerator could be defined as only those patients discharged from the service whose follow-up appointments are within 30 days of discharge and that are present on the discharge instructions

with a specific date and time. With the operational definitions in hand, measures then need a specific measurement plan. If reports can be generated out of the electronic data systems, the measurement plan would include setting up those reports and validating their accuracy by comparing to the chart documentation. A simpler method in many cases is to measure a random sample. A measurement plan for sampling might include creating a work sheet for data gathering and outlining the sampling strategy, such as a convenience sample of 10 consecutive charts, or two random discharges each day of the week.

■ BUILD MEASUREMENT INTO THE WORKFLOW

For measures that cannot be easily pulled from electronic systems, the measurement plan must identify the collection method. Even enthusiastic improvement team members do not relish extra work. Assigning cases for retrospective chart review may meet more resistance than building measurement into the routine work of team members. Consider whether there are tools already in use that can be modified to collect the additional data. In the readmission example, does the team already work from a daily patient list on which they could record whether discharged patients have had appointments scheduled? Does an assistant already print discharge paperwork from which the follow-up appointment status can be recorded into a daily log?

■ TEST THE MEASUREMENT PLAN

Because measurement is key for success and should not be taken for granted, testing the measurement plan on a small scale is a useful step early in the project. The electronic report should be generated and validated early in the project (doing so allows you to trust future electronic reports). For manual data collection, test the collection tool on a few patients to verify that all abstractors interpret the operational definitions the way they were intended. The measurement plan should also ensure timeliness of the data. The pace at which the team can judge the results of improvement efforts will be limited by the frequency of measurement. When feasible, measuring on a daily or weekly basis allows the team to make progress quickly, compared to a monthly or quarterly measurement cycle.

■ DISPLAYING THE DATA

Optimally, data for improvement work are available frequently and are used to drive change. Creating a run chart, which is a line graph of the data over time, visually demonstrates variability, trends, and, when annotated with changes to the process, the success or failure of those changes. Regularly updating and sharing these results with team members and other stakeholders helps maintain momentum of the project.

SUGGESTED READINGS

Berwick DM, James B, Coye MJ. Connections between quality measurement and improvement. *Med Care*. 2003;41:I-30-I-38.

Donabedian A. Evaluating the quality of medical care. *Milbank Q*. 1966;44:166-203.

Nelson EC, Splaine ME, Batalden PB, Plume SK. Building measurement and data collection into medical practice. *Ann Int Med*. 1998;128:460-466.

Pronovost PJ, Nolan T, Zeger S, Miller M, Rubin H. How can clinicians measure safety and quality in acute care? *Lancet*. 2004;363:1061-1067.

CHAPTER 18

Standardization and Reliability

Richard S. Gitomer, MD, MBA, FACP

CASE 18-1

Midway through a wound debridement, the scrub nurse noted that the sterilization indicators had not changed colors (indicating an inadequate sterilization process). A subsequent root cause analysis revealed that the sterile processing technician, at the end of his shift, forgot to push the button to start the autoclave. The next arriving technician did not notice that the sterilization indicator on the cart had not changed color, so he took the cart with the unsterile trays, and placed them on the shelf for use.

INTRODUCTION

In 1999, the Institute of Medicine (IOM) highlighted two studies from the 1980s, which suggested that between 44,000 and 98,000 patients die every year due to preventable medical errors. The subsequent IOM report, Crossing the Quality Chasm, noted, "The current systems cannot do the job. Changing systems of care will." The report went on further to describe the six aims of safety, effectiveness, efficiency, patient-centeredness, timeliness, and equity. With these aims, the IOM has defined the ultimate vision for the US health care system.

The limitations of the current health care system were further highlighted by Elizabeth McGlynn's study in 2003, which demonstrated that patients only received 55% of the care warranted by medical evidence. Furthermore, they found that the likelihood that an individual patient would receive all appropriate care was only 2.5%.

HUMAN FACTORS

■ THE INDIVIDUAL

A main contributor to the performance shortfall is the limitation of human performance. **Table 18-1** illustrates expected human error rates in conditions of no undue time pressure or stress. Note that "under very high stress when dangerous activities are occurring rapidly," the error rate can be as high as one in four (25%). Therefore, system designs that depend on perfect human performance are destined to fail at a very high rate. Furthermore, systems designed to function in conditions of high stress with frequent dangerous activities have a higher burden in order to ensure a favorable outcome.

As defined by the Federal Aviation Administration "human factors entails a multidisciplinary effort to generate and compile information about human capabilities and limitations, and apply that information to equipment, systems, facilities, procedures, jobs, environments, training, staffing, and personnel management for safe, comfortable, and effective human performance." When considering human factors, it is helpful to consider the impact of the human and the impact of the system separately. Reliable systems must compensate for the limitations of human performance. In addition, organizational characteristics can negatively or positively impact human performance. When redesigning systems to improve performance, it is helpful to understand the factors that may negatively impact human performance, so that the design can account for the expected vulnerability.

It is helpful to understand typical human limitations, which allow for and encourage the creation of systems that may accommodate for such limitations. The first is human memory; on average, a typical human is only able to keep 7 ± 2 elements in their short-term

TABLE 18-1 Nominal Human Error Rates for Selected Activities

Activity (Assume no Undue Time Pressure or Stresses)	Rate
Error of commission, eg, misreading a label	.003
Error of omission without reminders	.01
Error of omission when item is embedded in a procedure	.003
Simple arithmetic errors with self-checking	.03
Monitor or inspector fails to recognize an error	.1
Personnel on different shifts fail to check the condition of hardware unless directed by a checklist	.1
Error rate under very high stress when dangerous activities are occurring rapidly	.25

Adapted from Park K. Human error. In: Salvendy G, ed. *Handbook of Human Factors and Ergonomics*. New York, NY: John Wiley & Sons, Inc.; 1997:163.

memory. Systems that rely on human memory, therefore, are inherently imperfect. Reliable systems provide key information at the time when it is needed, rather than relying on memory. Humans also naturally cut corners or create "workarounds" when feeling rushed. Over time, repeated short cuts or workarounds result in a narrowing safety margin. This is described as "normalization of deviance." The natural tendency to cut corners and the lack of detectable consequences falsely reassures the individual that they remain within an appropriate level of safety, or reliability, which reinforces future unsafe behaviors. Diane Vaughan first coined this term in describing the root cause of the 1986 shuttle Challenger explosion 72 seconds after lift-off. The cause was a failed "O-ring" on one of the fuel cells. The Report of the "Presidential Commission on the Space Shuttle Challenger Accident" described how normalization of deviance led to the disaster. "NASA and Thiokol accepted escalating risk apparently because they 'got away with it last time.'" As Commissioner Feynman observed, the decision making was "a kind of Russian roulette… (The Shuttle) flies (with O-ring erosion) and nothing happens. Then it is suggested, therefore, that the risk is no longer so high for the next flights. We can lower our standards a little bit because we got away with it last time… You got away with it, but it should not be done over and over again like that." Normalization of deviance occurs because of the natural human tendency to slip into believing that in spite of the short cuts, adequate safety or reliability margins remain. In health care, normalization of deviance is often a barrier when trying to implement and sustain basic and quality and safety interventions, such as the "Universal Protocol" or central line insertion bundles. Over time, as strict adherence to the protocols wane, and "nothing bad is happening," then further slippage and workarounds ensue.

Stress also significantly impacts human performance by causing tunnel vision and filtering. This causes a loss of pattern recognition that humans use to rapidly discern complex situations. Fatigue negatively impacts human performance by impacting both short-term and long-term memory. The impact of fatigue is similar to having a blood alcohol level of 0.1%. Other significant factors that impact health care worker performance include multitasking, interruptions, and environmental factors (such a poor lighting, noise, distractions, etc). All of these natural human limitations must be factored into any system design (or redesign) intended to improve quality or safety.

■ THE ORGANIZATION

James Reason described characteristics that impact an organization's capacity to support or impede an individual's ability to function reliably. Human error can be addressed from an organizational perspective with a "person approach" or a "system approach." The person approach focuses on the actions of the frontline staff who commit errors. The errors, it is believed, are due to flawed mental processes that can be voluntarily corrected, with enough motivation, attention, and vigilance. The institutional response is focused on correcting the variation in human behavior. Frequently, the responses focus on engendering fear (disciplinary measures, threat of litigation, retraining, naming, blaming, and shaming), so that the individual will focus more intently on the task at hand and not make a similar error. Often, new policies and procedures are written to ensure the correct behavior. In short, the person approach implicitly assumes that bad things happen to bad people.

In the system approach, however, human fallibility is a fundamental premise; human errors are to be expected. The errors are seen as consequences of inadequate system design. It is believed that most errors occur because system barriers and defenses that are "upstream" to the event, lead to the undesired outcome. The fundamental premise for countermeasures in the system approach focuses on changing the conditions under which humans work, rather than changing the human condition. When an error occurs, the focus is on how the defenses failed.

The person approach is somewhat appealing on at least two levels. It is emotionally satisfying to blame an individual for an adverse event. In addition, divorcing the unsafe act from the organization may be perceived as being in the best interest of the organizational leaders. But, these benefits come at a great cost. In 90% of aviation maintenance mishaps, the worker is found blameless. In order to improve it is important to perform detailed analysis of incidents, near-misses, and unsafe conditions. Within a "blame and shame" culture, the information is not voluntary reported, out of fear of retribution.

Conversely, the system approach recognizes human fallibility and system designs are successful in spite of human error. In reliable organizations, admission of errors and near-misses is encouraged and rewarded. Leadership in reliable organizations realizes that early detection of latent conditions that promote human error is essential to creating reliable systems.

As such, most organizations now create barriers and defenses to prevent the errors when designing systems of care. However, each barrier and defense is not perfect and has unique vulnerabilities. Reason describes this as a slice of Swiss cheese. However, these vulnerabilities are dynamic. Sometimes the holes are larger; sometimes they are located in a different place. For example, if one of the barriers is a second nurse checking the dose of insulin, this step may be less reliable on a specific day if the checking nurse was sleep deprived or distracted.

In well-designed systems, when one barrier fails, a second is able to catch the defect and the outcome is not compromised. In Reason's model, the defect may pass through one slice of Swiss cheese, but is caught by the next slice. However, there are times when all the holes of multiple slices of Swiss cheese line up and the outcome is compromised … the patient is harmed or the process is not executed reliably.

Implicit in Reason's system approach to human error is the importance of culture. Reason notes that high-reliability organizations have a reporting culture. It is essential for the staff to feel safe surfacing errors and near-misses. In high-reliability organizations, leadership accepts the accountability to create safe environments that facilitate successful outcomes. The staff member is accountable to make safe choices by following the processes that they helped to create. The staff is also accountable for surfacing existing and potential opportunities for defects. If all live up to these accountabilities, the leadership response to error is supportive of the staff, with a focus on identifying the source of the defect and developing a remedy to prevent its occurrence in the future.

RELIABILITY

As suggested in Crossing the Quality Chasm, new systems of care are required to achieve the level of reliability necessary to ensure that all patients receive the care they deserve. The new systems of care will necessarily need to account for human factors on the organizational level, as well as at the individual process level.

■ THE ORGANIZATION

The health care industry has a level of complexity that matches, if not exceeds other industries. Challenging the reliability of the system is that humans execute most key processes. The complex systems, the dynamic environment, and the human involved with process execution are major reasons for the reliability gap described at the beginning of this chapter. Principles gleaned from other complex organizations can help overcome the reliability gap.

Karl Weick described key organizational characteristics evident in highly reliable complex organizations. The organizations studied include, nuclear power plants, nuclear aircraft carriers, and commercial airlines. He describes those organizations as having mindfulness or "a rich awareness of discriminatory detail." Individuals functioning in high-reliability organizations are aware of context, can discriminate details, and how the current situation differs from expectations. The five principles of mindfulness include:

- preoccupation with failure,
- reluctance to simplify interpretations,
- sensitivity to operations,
- commitment to resilience,
- deference to expertise.

Preoccupation with failure is a relentless focus on potential failure modes and how they can be prevented. An example in health care might be a detailed examination of an order set looking for ambiguities or potential error traps. A preoccupation with failure helps overcome the natural tendency to drift into unsafe behaviors that result in normalization of deviance.

Mindful organizations resist the tendency to normalize unwanted occurrences into expected events. This *reluctance to simplify* interpretations helps to maintain margins of safety and process reliability. Inappropriate simplification of the causes of adverse events, or a lack of focus on these events, over time, can result in major problems that might have been avoided if the initial interpretation had been more rigorous. For example, resisting attributing a medication error to a nurse failing to use the "five rights" because she did not focus (right patient, right medication, right dose, right route, right time). A mindful organization might ask if the process for executing the "five rights" is robust, and if there are adequate protections to ensure completion of the "five rights."

Sensitivity to operations reflects a deep understanding of the processes at a frontline level. This reflects knowing what really happens in the messy world of reality, not what is policy, or what is supposed to happen. In response to low pneumococcal vaccine rates, leaders in a mindful organization do not assume that the nurses are not doing their job, but examine the process and appreciate that the cause is an overly complex screening tool.

Highly-reliable organizations realize that all systems can fail. But, these organizations have a relentless focus on not allowing that failure to compromise performance. A key element of the *commitment to resilience* is that the specifics are not anticipated. A preoccupation with failure might result in the development of a medical rapid response team to attend to deteriorating patients before they arrest. This team's capabilities can be further enhanced through simulation exercises that expose the team to diverse scenarios. The simulations help reduce complexity by allowing team roles to be defined ahead of time rather than in the chaos of the acute event.

In highly reliable organizations, decision-making authority seamlessly flows to the person with the best information to make the decision. The *deference to expertise* might be exhibited on an aircraft carrier where a seaman can stop the activities on the flight deck because he sees a condition that might be unsafe for the landing planes. In the ICU, a nurse might "stop the line" if she does not see all elements of the central line insertion bundle, regardless of who is the central line insertion practitioner.

Other organizations may not have all the complexities of health care, but the five principles of mindfulness are directly applicable to health care. Organizations that exhibit these characteristics have a culture that promotes reliability.

■ THE RELIABILITY GAP

Karl Weick paints a compelling picture of what reliability looks like at the level of the organization. But, what does reliability look like at the level of the process? Reliability is intentional, and there are principles that guide that work. The lack of reliability in health care is multifactorial. Understanding these causes helps shape the interventions. While not exhaustive, the following three explanations highlight key barriers to process reliability.

1. While readily acknowledging human fallibility in others, many health care providers expect perfection of themselves. In addition, there is often a feeling that the only way to ensure reliability is to rely on no one else. From this high standard comes an over-reliance on vigilance and hard work. The reality of human factors, however, prevents the individual from performing reliably.

2. Individual providers tend to look at their personal delivery of health care one patient at a time. Ideally, the provider customizes a plan for the individual patient based on personal experience and the medical evidence. However, due to the limitations of human factors, and the paucity of high-level evidence for much of the care of the average practitioner, there is high variation in how patients are treated from one to the next. While understandable, this lack of standardization comes at a cost … complexity. It is no longer possible for an individual to deliver the full spectrum of reliable care to their patient. Teams are essential for the delivery of reliable care. The more variation from patient to patient in a care plan, the greater the level of complexity for the rest of the care team. The consequence of this unwarranted variation and increased complexity is lower reliability. This is not to say that standardization in a "cookie cutter" approach is required to reduce complexity. Rather, standardize what is "standardizable." This relieves the care provider of the mundane and allows focus on those parts of the care plan that does require additional focus or expertise. For the rest of the care team, their work is less complex because of the reduced unwarranted variation and they are in a better position to plan and anticipate.

3. A third reason for the reliability gap is that many current processes fail to account for human factors. Process design based on human infallibility is inherently unreliable. The following section describes an approach to process design that facilitates accounting for human factors.

■ MEASUREMENT

The framework in **Table 18-2** describes specific interventions associated with predictable levels of reliability. Interventions that result in 10^{-1} reliability rely on vigilance and hard work. Examples of these interventions include:

1) Common equipment, standard order sheets, multiple choice protocols, and written policies/procedures,

TABLE 18-2 Levels of Reliability in Typical Processes Infrastructure

Level of Reliability	Typical Processes Infrastructure
<80% >2 defects in 10	Chaos
10-1 (80%) 2 defects in 10	No articulated common process Reliance on training and reminders
10-2 (95%) 1-5 defects in 100	Intentionally designed Utilizes principles of human factors engineering
10-3 (99.5%) 1-5 defects in 1000	Well-designed system with attention to process, structure, and outcomes

2) Personal checklists,
3) Feedback of information on compliance,
4) Suggestions of working harder next time,
5) Awareness and training.

Processes that result in 10^{-2} reliability use principles based on human factors and reliability science. These interventions tend to be more resource intensive. They include:

1) Decision aids and reminders built into the system,
2) Desired action the default (scientific evidence),
3) Redundant processes utilized,
4) Scheduling used in design development,
5) Habits and patterns known and taken advantage of in the design,
6) Standardization of process, based on clear specification and articulation.

■ THE PROCESS

The reliability design strategy was described by a group at the Institute for Healthcare Improvement (IHI). It consists of four steps:

1) Segmentation,
2) Standardization,
3) Detection and mitigation,
4) Redesign the process based on the defects identified.

1. Segmentation: When embarking on an improvement project it is often helpful to divide the population into smaller groups in order to simplify the tests of change. Process improvement is taking general knowledge or procedures and making them relevant in the local context. Unlike research, it is not possible to remove confounding variables. However, with segmentation the confounding variables can be controlled until the appropriate time.

   To illustrate the power of segmentation, consider implementation of congestive heart failure (CHF) discharge instructions. The improvement team might consider segments based on familiarity of the medical and nursing staff with the care of CHF patients. Clearly, there is a greater level of comfort on the cardiology floor than on the orthopedic floor. One might consider a continuum of comfort as follows: cardiology floor, general medicine floor, general surgery floor, and orthopedic floor. Segmenting this way, and choosing to start the work on the cardiology floor allows the team to focus on the process of delivering the discharge instructions without having to manage the barriers of knowledge deficit and comfort with the medications. Once the process for delivering the instructions is well defined and operational, the team can move on to the other floors and directly address the barriers unique to the other floors, rather than trying to address the barriers while also determining the correct process for delivering the instructions. The segments should have the following qualities:

   - Be based on a design theme that helps simplify the improvement activity (eg, knowledge, geography, willingness to participate, patient characteristics, etc).
   - Contain a reasonable volume, so there are enough opportunities to do tests of change.
   - Have clear-cut defined boundaries so there is no confusion about the population of patients being addressed.

2. Standardization: Standardization yields several key benefits. First, it improves reliability by reducing complexity, as described above. Second, it helps provide an infrastructure where roles and responsibilities are clearly defined. A standard infrastructure also allows for simplification of training, and competency testing. Standardizing key processes allows consistent implementation of evidence-based medicine. Lastly, it simplifies identification of defects that can be analyzed for redesign, and facilitates performing tests of change. The standardization step should be refined by serial tests of change. The reliability goal for the standardization step is 80%. If the step is less than 80% reliable, the defects will overwhelm the detection and mitigation step, which tends to be more resource intensive.

3. Detection and mitigation: The value of the detection and mitigation step is that it helps reduce the complexity of the standardization step. Since the standardization step need only capture 80% of the opportunities, it is not necessary to develop contingencies for lower frequency occurrences. If the standardization step had to include those contingencies, it would be too complex and therefore less reliable. The detection and mitigation step includes two processes. The first process reliably identifies the defects from the standardization step utilizing 10^{-2} level interventions. The second process mitigates the defect, using 10^{-1} level interventions. An example might be detecting failures by running an electronic report daily for all patients who have not been screened for administration of the pneumococcal vaccine. Those failures would then be mitigated by a supervisor contacting the nurses caring for the patients who experienced the process failure.

4. Process redesign based on defects identified: In pursuit of continuous improvement, the fourth step in the reliability design strategy is to examine the defects identified in the previous step and feed the learning back into the design of the standardization and detection and mitigation steps. Once the processes in the first segment achieve an acceptable level of reliability, the team should move on to the next easiest segment. Now that the processes have been defined and tested, work in the next segment can focus on the barriers unique to the new segment. Attacking the segments from easiest to hardest allows the team to gain experience and further refine the process, which simplifies the work in even the most difficult segment.

CONCLUSION

As highlighted by the IOM reports and McGlynn's work, patients are regularly experiencing preventable harm and are not receiving all of the care that is intended. Closing that reliability gap requires focused multidisciplinary team involvement to develop and oversee the process redesign. Understanding human factors and having a structured model for increased reliability is essential. Reliable process design, regardless of the improvement methodology, is an effective approach to closing the reliability gap.

SUGGESTED READINGS

McGlynn EA, Asch SM, Adams J, et al. The quality of health care delivered to adults in the United States. *N Engl J Med*. 2003;348:2635.

Nolan T, Resar R, Haraden C, Griffin FA. *Improving the Reliability of Health Care. IHI Innovation Series White Paper*. Boston, MA: Institute for Healthcare Improvement; 2004.

Reason J. Human error: models and management. *BMJ*. 2000;320:768.

Vaughan D. *The Challenger Launch Decision: Risky Technology, Culture, and Deviance at NASA*. Chicago, IL: University of Chicago Press; 1996.

Weick KE, Sutcliffe KM. *Managing the Unexpected: Resilient Performance in an Age of Uncertainty*. 2nd ed. San Francisco, CA: Jossey-Bass; 2007.

ONLINE RESOURCES

Crossing the Quality Chasm. http://iom.nationalacademies.org/~/media/Files/Report%20Files/2001/Crossing-the-Quality-Chasm/Quality%20Chasm%202001%20%20report%20brief.ashx

IHI Reliability Online Resources. http://www.ihi.org/IHI/Topics/Reliability/ReliabilityGeneral/EmergingContent/SegmentPresentationandDesignTable.htm

Just Culture Resources. https://www.justculture.org/tag/david-marx/

Resar RK. Practical Applications of Reliability Theory. http://high-reliability.org/Practical_Reliability_Resar.pdf

To Err is Human. http://www.nap.edu/read/9728/chapter/1

CHAPTER 19

Tools to Identify Problems and Reduce Risks

Elizabeth H. Mack, MD, MS

INTRODUCTION

Every organization needs a structure and a tool kit to support employee and patient safety and continuous quality improvement. Since what cannot be seen cannot be fixed, robust identification of adverse events and latent safety threats (risk to patients, families, and employees) should be a priority of every hospital. Here, we discuss structures and tools to identify adverse events and risk. Once identified, the hospital and staff must then prioritize efforts and determine which techniques will be applied to reduce adverse events and risk. Risk reduction efforts may focus on error prevention or on harm prevention, and both approaches are key to risk reduction. **Table 19-1** reviews definitions for the key terms used throughout the chapter.

THE ROLE OF THE CULTURE OF SAFETY IN IDENTIFYING RISK

In organizations with a robust culture of safety, it is evident to all involved that safety is the top priority. People working in the area focus on safe practices and support one another in delivering safe care. Individuals in a mature culture of safety exhibit the principles of a highly reliable organization, including "preoccupation with failure" as described by Weick and Sutcliffe, such that there is a constant obsession with mitigation of risk. Instead of ignoring small, nagging concerns, workers share those concerns with others, and team members rally to help resolve the concerns. When the culture of safety is strong, people report concerns without fears of retaliation. Employees respond supportively to concerns about risks to patient safety and do not seek to blame individuals when an error occurs. When safety is a priority, leaders routinely inquire about safety concerns and take the time to listen, seek to understand root causes, demonstrate their commitment to safety through action, and communicate back to staff on the organizational response to adverse events and concerns. An organization's culture of safety can be measured by the Agency for Healthcare Research's survey on patient safety culture. The scores of this survey have been correlated with patient outcomes in multiple studies and can assist an organization with monitoring their culture over time. Specific questions may also be useful to assess the effect of culture on identifying problems (**Table 19-2**).

RISK IDENTIFICATION AS PART OF A SAFETY PROGRAM

Identification of patient safety risks requires an intentional multifaceted approach. The National Quality Forum identifies and promotes safe practices in health care (see http://qualityforum.org). Among these best practices is the presence of leadership structures and systems to ensure organizational awareness of safety failures and performance gaps that need attention. Government and commercial health care purchasers, insurance providers, and hospital accreditation organizations provide strong incentives for hospitals to invest in infrastructure supporting the identification, analysis, and correction of risk. Less obvious sources of harm, including deviations from generally accepted practice standards such as evidence-based guidelines of care, are also important to detect. For example, identifying variation within a subspecialty of blood product ordering, compliance with tonsillectomy guidelines, or ordering of computed tomography scans for suspected appendicitis is likely to lead to institutional cost savings and improved quality of care. Because information about errors and risks comes from many potential sources,

TABLE 19-1 Common Terms Used to Describe Errors and Harm

Term	Explanation
Adverse event	Harm resulting from medical care
Preventable adverse events	Harm due to medical care that could have been avoided
Latent safety threat	Factors that make error more likely but are not directly visible; also called blunt error
Near miss	Error occurs but does not reach the patient
Sentinel event	Unexpected death or serious harm or risk thereof
Adverse medication event	Error resulting from medication-related interventions
Slip	Failure of execution in which the technical action is observable
Lapse	Failure of execution typically due to memory failure

hospitals face challenges to bringing this disparate information together, investigating and mitigating risk, and providing feedback to employees about actions taken in a meaningful way.

One major challenge is that only a small fraction of preventable harm is detected by most methods, especially those based on voluntary human reporting. Computerized data mining methods tend to greatly increase the number of potential errors identified, but the specificity can be low. For example, a rule to identify nephrotoxicity from medications may look for a rise in the serum creatinine during hospitalization. Most of the cases identified will not result from an adverse drug event, and additional resources will be required to further investigate each case.

TABLE 19-2 The Effect of Culture on Identifying Problems

Questions to Assess the Culture of Safety

Are people comfortable reporting errors they witness?

Are people willing to report their own errors?

Do staff members freely discuss their concerns about patient safety?

Are supervisors receptive to these concerns?

Do people fear retribution for reporting or fear being blamed for adverse events?

Do staff members feel that leaders care about patient and staff safety?

Can people give examples of actions to improve safety that resulted from reports of adverse events or concerns?

Questions to Assess Leaders' Commitment to Safety

Are leaders visible where patient care is delivered, asking staff about their concerns for safety?

Do leaders ensure that staff members do not suffer retribution for reporting?

Is there an identified patient safety officer who reports to system leaders or to the board?

Is safety regularly on the agenda at meetings of hospital departments, medical staff, and leaders?

Are adequate resources applied to identification and analysis of adverse events and risks?

Knowing that the detected errors are but a sample of true preventable adverse events, hospital safety leaders must decide whether there is value to applying additional resources to enhance detection. Bringing together the multiple sources of information allows for a broader view, and this effort benefits from having a central safety committee or safety officer to whom the information funnels.

METHODS OF IDENTIFYING ADVERSE EVENTS AND ERRORS

Some methods are reactive and retrospective, being generated in response to specific events that come to attention. In contrast, systematic methods tend to identify latent or hidden errors or risk points, and are often both reactive and proactive. Both types of approaches are necessary in the overall strategy to identify risks. Certainly, there are some errors that will never come to the attention of leadership, either because they are not recognized as errors or because employees do not feel comfortable reporting them.

■ REACTIVE METHODS

Event-reporting systems

Voluntary event-reporting systems rely on employees to take time to report a concern, trusting that action will be taken by leaders, and that retaliation will not occur. In a healthy culture of safety, employees report freely and openly, with few barriers. Employees do not fail to report events that seem to represent temporary or minor areas of potential harm, because they are aware that these are important opportunities to learn. Indeed, a robust reporting system will collect a significant number of system failures or errors that were successfully intercepted or that did not result in harm, known as near misses. Near misses are golden opportunities to identify risk-prone conditions or processes and to intervene before harm results. The ideal state would involve occurrence of near misses only, and no incidents of preventable harm. An effective reporting system enhances the engagement of frontline staff in patient safety by providing an identified channel for their observations. To be effective, employees must be aware that the reporting system exists, reporting must be user-friendly, and it must be known that leaders place value on the reports. Timely acknowledgment, expressions of appreciation, and feedback regarding actions taken reinforce the desired reporting behaviors.

Ease of reporting is key to maintaining a low reporting threshold. Paper reports and verbal reports via telephone recording have advantages of speed, though the information has to be transcribed and aggregated separately. Lengthy written or electronic reporting systems with a large number of required fields are not likely to be used widely. Electronic reporting systems may prompt for more precise and complete information from each report and may produce structured reports from which data are more easily analyzed. Electronic systems may also enable immediate notification of appropriate personnel. For instance, an event reported as causing significant patient harm may generate an automated communication to a risk manager, safety officer, or hospital leader, facilitating a timely response to the event. Of note, most states provide legal protection for event reporting such that the information contained with the reports is not discoverable.

How leaders and managers respond to aggregate data from event-reporting systems will send strong signals to employees. Because event reports are dependent on willingness to report and are unlikely to reflect true incident rates, leaders and managers should exercise caution in inferring that a high number of events reported represents worse safety in one area versus another. In fact, the number of reports may be more indicative of the culture of safety than of safety itself. However, it is human nature to conclude that higher numbers of reports indicate an area of unsafe conditions. Managers may worry that reports reflect poorly on their performance and discourage use of the reporting system. Leadership, particularly of the "C-suite" and the board of directors, should pay attention to the use of data for learning rather than for judging in order for the reporting system to be effective.

The options for reporter identity protection deserve intentional thought when designing an event-reporting system. An open system makes no attempt to protect the reporter's identity, so colleagues and supervisors may identify the reporter. This kind of system may work in organizations where the culture of safety is strong enough that there is no retribution for reporting and, in fact, reporting is rewarded, whether by peer appreciation or formal recognition. It is worth noting most health care organizations are not yet at this point in their safety culture journey. If reporters face criticism or retaliation in even a few instances, willingness to report may be severely affected.

A confidential reporting system allows identification of the reporter only to responsible system administrators who will follow up on the event with the reporter. Confidential reporting may overcome reluctance of some people to report and enhance detection of sensitive issues. For example, a person reporting inappropriate sexual comments or behavior may be reluctant to have his or her identity known to the person whose behavior is being reported.

Anonymous reporting serves to fully protect the reporter's identity and thus may expand reporting of sensitive events and reporting in work areas where a climate of fear exists. If inadequate information was submitted to identify the event, however, further investigation and learning are severely hampered. To the other extreme, if the reporter gave full information in a detailed report and few people are fully aware of the event, it may be impossible to maintain anonymity. Regardless of whether reporting system is open or confidential, it is important in most health care organizations to allow for the option to report anonymously. Where necessary to provide for anonymous reporting, efforts to improve the culture of safety will ideally allow movement toward a more open reporting system.

PATIENT COMPLAINTS AND CONCERNS

Patient complaints and concerns are another source of reports, whether submitted by patients or families or by employees on behalf of them. The perspective of patients and families may be very valuable and complementary to the insights of staff members. These reports are more likely to reflect the level of service, compassion, communication, and partnering with patients and families. The reports are not likely to be anonymous and bring with them a duty to respond back to the patient or family. As with reports from staff members, treating the information as a learning opportunity may shape how frontline workers respond to complaints. While the volume and content of patient complaints and concerns may predict the likelihood of legal action, it may be difficult to draw actual conclusions about patient safety from rates of complaints.

CLAIMS ANALYSIS

Analysis of medicolegal claims may be a tempting source of information, but it is less likely to generate useful ideas about how to improve patient safety, compared to other methods. Since the vast majority of patients harmed through medical care do not bring claims, this subset is idiosyncratic. Deep understanding of any given event degrades rapidly with time, and investigation of an event should have occurred long before a claim is filed.

■ SYSTEMATIC METHODS
Patient safety walk rounds

Scheduled rounding in patient care areas by leaders may be an effective method to accomplish several goals, including promotion

of a culture of safety. As described by Frankel et al, structuring the content of rounds and recording the comments and concerns of staff members may yield valuable insights. Past events deserving of investigation and concerns about ongoing risks can be heard directly by the leadership team. These reports stimulated by the visit of leaders may not have been collected through other means. It is important to provide feedback to employees on items discussed in safety rounds. If possible, it is useful to develop a rotating schedule to include all shifts and all areas.

MORBIDITY AND MORTALITY CONFERENCES

Morbidity and mortality (M&M) conferences are a time-honored tradition in medicine. Discussion of patient deaths, complications, or harms resulting from care provides a learning opportunity for the attendees. Too often, perhaps due to the confidential nature of many conferences, the learning stops at the door, and feedback to the larger system does not happen. Traditional M&M often involves individual blame rather than a systems-based approach. Additionally, the discussion of failures may be inhibited if the culture is not open, and the lack of a structured process of case review may lead to wide variation in the conclusions drawn from case review.

Structuring case reviews, identifying underlying causes of failures, involving organizational quality and risk leaders, and assigning responsibility for making system changes can make the M&M conference benefit the larger system.

TRIGGER TOOLS

Adverse events and errors that surface through reporting systems and complaints poorly represent the rate at which such problems actually occur. Structured reviews of medical records can identify problems that have not been reported and provide a rate estimate. One such method has been developed by the Institute for Health Care Improvement. Triggers are explicit criteria or clues to the presence of an adverse event, stimulating a deeper review of the record. For example, administration of naloxone as a trigger is likely to detect some causes of nonpreventable harm as well as preventable harm. Errors in warfarin management may be identified among patients in whom vitamin K is administered. Most commonly trigger tools are used to detect adverse drug events, but they can also be used to detect other causes of potential preventable harm. Applying the tool to a random sample of hospital discharges can give an estimate of the rates of common sources of harm to patients. These rates can be tracked over time, and the information obtained may be used by the hospital to set improvement priorities.

■ MONITORING OF HIGH-RISK PROCESSES

Some processes of care are inherently risky, such as provision of sedation, performing invasive procedures, and responding to cardiopulmonary arrests. Particularly concerning are the low-frequency, high-risk events. Monitoring the processes of care and the outcomes may identify deviations from standard practice that may pose undue risks and point to opportunities for improvement. Using the example of cardiopulmonary resuscitation (CPR), the hospital may have a mechanism to review that the right complement of personnel responded to the emergency, that the team was alerted in a timely fashion, that a team leader was identified and roles assigned, that the patient was correctly assessed, that the correct resuscitation algorithms were followed, and that the medications and other therapies were correctly administered. The results of CPR reviews and the outcomes of the resuscitation attempts are then reported to the appropriate hospital representative or committee. Debriefing immediately after such events is likely to yield discovery of areas for improvement.

In a hospital with a robust culture of safety, the insights from monitoring are shared and lead to actions to address deficiencies.

Suppose, for example, resuscitation monitoring identifies that patients with difficult airways are not managed as well late at night as during the daytime hours when an anesthesiologist is available. This insight should be reviewed by hospital leaders who determine the actions needed to provide better airway management at night. One solution may be to train and certify hospitalist physicians to manage difficult airways. Additionally, processes may be monitored using open auditing such as observing the surgical safety checklist preoperatively or using secret shoppers posing as family members to audit hand-hygiene practices. Health care processes must be monitored using multiple different methods to assure compliance.

■ *IN SITU* SIMULATION

Both Institute of Medicine reports, *To err is human* and *Crossing the Quality Chasm*, suggested that health care utilizes both crew resource management and simulation to improve patient safety. *In situ* simulation involves practicing team-based care on actual patient care units and this form of training provides a method to identify latent safety threats.

■ MINING ELECTRONIC DATA

Health care facilities are rich in electronic data that can be mined for possible adverse events. Every hospital has administrative systems to support billing. Among the diagnosis codes are those that may indicate safety problems, such as codes for accidental puncture or laceration of an organ and for foreign body left in during a procedure. Since October 2008, hospitals routinely indicate whether conditions were present on admission. Reviewing diagnoses such as pressure ulcers and deep vein thromboses that were not present on admission may identify opportunities for improvement.

Electronic laboratory and pharmacy systems can be used to identify potential adverse events for further review. Acute renal failure occurring after admission to the hospital may be identified by searching the laboratory data for patients in whom the serum creatinine has risen significantly. Practically, however, often the needed data are available within the electronic health record, but there are not enough resources available to satisfy the many demands for data throughout the system.

■ FAILURE MODES AND EFFECTS ANALYSIS

Failure modes and effects analysis (FMEA) is a prospective technique to anticipate the ways in which a process may fail and to prioritize the efforts to prevent failures. With roots in the military, FMEA is widely used in manufacturing and more recently is being applied to health care delivery. While there are a number of models, including health care failure modes and effects analysis used in the Veterans Health Administration, FMEA generally follows these steps.

1. **Choose the target for analysis.** Because conducting FMEA requires expertise and the commitment of significant time and resources, a hospital must select where to apply the technique. A frequent consideration is to focus where prior problems have occurred. For example, an institution might use FMEA to identify and prevent errors in the placement and use of nasogastric tubes. FMEA can help a hospital safely implement a new technology such as bar coding the steps of medication preparation, distribution, and administration.

2. **Assemble the team.** To understand the process in fine detail, it is critical to identify and involve team members with expertise from all disciplines that use, interact with, or maintain the process. A trained facilitator should be part of the team, as FMEA has a specific structure.

3. **Describe the process to be analyzed in detail.** This is best done graphically, beginning with a high-level flow diagram that serves as a framework for analysis. The flow diagram allows team members to share a mental model of the process steps. From the high-level diagram, the team can develop a detailed understanding of the different steps and supporting processes. When important gaps in the process cannot be filled in by team members, additional information is sought.

4. **Identify the ways that failure may occur (failure modes).** Drawing upon the expertise of team members and upon data where available, the team identifies vulnerabilities and underlying causes among the process steps. Failure modes may occur under normal conditions or when the system is stressed.

5. **Prioritize the failure modes.** The team must decide where to focus attention for improvement or process redesign among the failure modes found in the previous step. To prioritize, most FMEA models apply a grading scale (eg, 1-10) to several aspects of each failure mode and its causes:

   Severity: The effect of each failure is described and assigned a grade. A low grade indicates a failure that would have minor consequences or is easily recoverable; a high-grade failure effect is catastrophic (would cause grave harm and cannot be stopped once the failure occurs).

   Frequency: The probability of occurrence of the failure mode or its causes is also graded. Low-grade frequency suggests a very rare event and high grades suggest more frequent events.

   Risk of escaping detection: Failures that are immediately obvious allow for early detection and the opportunity to recover or to mitigate the effects. Easily detected failures receive a low score for risk of escaping detection. Other failures may be detected through routine inspection some time after occurrence. The highest score goes to failures that are not detected until the outcome (failure effect) has happened.

   Multiplying the grades of severity, frequency, and risk of escaping detection for each failure mode produces a risk priority number. The failure modes can then be ranked, with the highest risk priority numbers indicating where the team should focus attention. Because this ranking process is imprecise, the results provide a guide rather than a prescription for the next steps.

6. **Determine the action steps.** If the FMEA leads the team to the conclusion that the process is far too unsafe to continue, a complete redesign may be necessary. Or, the team may conclude that bringing in a new piece of equipment is unjustified given the associated risks. More commonly, the team will identify ways to eliminate causes of failures, to provide earlier warning of failures, or to mitigate the effects of failures in service of improving overall safety.

■ RETROSPECTIVE INVESTIGATION OF EVENTS ROOT CAUSE ANALYSIS

Root cause analysis (RCA) is complementary to FMEA. It is a retrospective technique that provides a robust structure to review an adverse event or near miss. RCA is reactive; FMEA is proactive. But, the ultimate goal of each technique is to identify ways to prevent future adverse events. See **Table 19-3** for a comparison of these two techniques.

Effective RCA requires a detailed, intimate understanding of the event being studied and necessitates the participation or interview of people directly involved in the event. Because RCA is usually performed in response to a recent adverse event, emotions of people involved may be fragile. A poorly performed RCA that permits blaming of individuals can seriously undermine the culture of safety. RCA done well results in learning the underlying (root) causes of human failures, process failures, or equipment failures. Focus on correcting the root causes of failure fosters safer care of patients and a safer work environment for employees.

TABLE 19-3 Comparison of FMEA and RCA

Failure Modes and Effects Analysis (FMEA)	Root Cause Analysis (RCA)
Prospective technique to predict the ways a process or equipment may fail and to plan prevention efforts	Retrospective technique to analyze an incident for the underlying causes of failure and to identify potential solutions
Steps:	Steps:
1. Choose target for analysis	1. Assemble the team
2. Assemble the team	2. Set the atmosphere
3. Describe the process in detail	3. Describe the events in detail
4. Identify the failure modes	4. Identify root causes
5. Prioritize the failure modes	5. Identify solutions to prevent recurrences
6. Determine the action steps	6. Report findings and recommendations to leaders

Conducting RCA requires a trained facilitator and an investment of time and resources. Hospitals will have to select where to focus this tool. Serious adverse events, such as the unexpected death of a patient related to an error, are obvious targets for RCA. However, near misses that reveal a potentially serious process failure should also be considered for RCA. A patient who recognizes that his chemotherapy has been mixed incorrectly because it is the wrong color may have prevented a serious medication error. RCA of this error may reveal weaknesses in the chemotherapy mixing process that need to be fixed. The Just Culture algorithm would encourage us to handle investigation of events independent of the outcome that resulted. Failure in duty to follow a procedural rule would result in the same treatment of the employee whether the patient died or caused no harm. Root cause analysis will generally follow these steps:

1. **Assemble the team.** Some hospitals have an existing team for conducting RCAs. This team rarely has firsthand knowledge of the event being reviewed and will probably not have an intimate understanding of the focused work processes and environment of those involved in the event. The team will add members with such knowledge or will gain that knowledge through extensive interviews. More commonly, a team is brought together specifically for the RCA. In addition to the trained facilitator, the team should be interdisciplinary and involve people who work closely with the processes being evaluated. Some experts advise against including people directly involved with the event as team members because of their potential difficulty with being objective and open in such a forum. If those with direct involvement are invited to join the RCA team, the facilitator must be sensitive to this conflict and create an atmosphere conducive to openness. If employees who were directly involved in the event do not participate in the RCA, they should be interviewed in depth in order to understand the processes, culture, and root causes. Hospital leaders, when possible, can strengthen team function by participating and supporting improvement opportunities that result from the RCA. If a leader does not participate directly, knowing that a leader will closely focus on the team recommendations can also lend weight to the RCA.

2. **Set the atmosphere.** In teams brought together for the RCA, the leader or facilitator may be the only person formally trained or experienced in the technique. Setting the atmosphere by providing an orientation to the process and laying out ground rules for the conduct of the RCA can be critical to success. Among the ground rules should be a prohibition against finger-pointing and personal attacks. While humans may have erred, directing blame at an individual stifles learning. Rather, for every failure point, ask "why" and "what conditions existed to permit this failure?" Human error alone should not be an acceptable root cause. Another useful ground rule is to avoid speculation. Where gaps in understanding occur, the team should seek additional information. It is also important to discuss up front whether peer review statues will protect the information discussed, and whether or not the information will be discoverable.

3. **Describe the events.** Create a detailed flow diagram or a timeline of the sequence of events. The team seeks additional information to fill in gaps in understanding.

4. **Identify root causes.** Using structured questions as in the triggering and triage questions of the VA National Center for Patient Safety (see http://www4.va.gov/NCPS/rca.html) creates a more complete analysis by prompting consideration of categories of causes, including environmental conditions, equipment function, policies and procedures, training, communication, and fatigue. Again, digging deeper with each question and not accepting human error or procedural violation as a root cause are essential to identifying preventable causes.

5. **Identify solutions to prevent recurrences.** Using standardization and reliability science will create more robust actions. Consider where similar vulnerabilities exist in the organization and generalize the learning where possible.

6. **Report findings and recommendations to leaders.** This step will help secure leadership support for actions needed.

7. **Follow-up.** It is important to complete the action items discussed in the RCA within a specified time period. Teams may consider stressing the system using *in situ* simulation to determine if the same vulnerabilities still exist or if the solutions implemented have closed the gaps.

INCIDENT INVESTIGATIONS

Most adverse events and near misses will not be investigated with an RCA, simply because the hospital is not capable of responding to all with this level of investigation. Still, the personnel performing the investigations should be seeking root causes of problems, detecting trends, identifying solutions, and generalizing to other areas. The results of incident investigations should feed back into the safety structure of the hospital through the safety committee or safety officer so that further action may be taken. Providing feedback to reporters is a key.

PEER REVIEW

Peer review processes are intended to adjudicate the competence and professionalism of health care providers. As such, peer review is fundamentally different from the investigations already described. This approach focuses not on problems in the health care system, but on individual performance. Peer review usually occurs as a physician or other provider is newly hired or granted specific hospital privileges to confirm competence or in response to some concern raised about performance. Concerns may arise in response to a particular incident or in response to data compiled over time. For instance, an unexpectedly high rate of procedural complications or resource utilization compared with peers may prompt closer review. Using a construct such as Just Culture may facilitate a fair treatment when the temptation is to punish the employee in the face of a bad outcome.

Peer review may generate insights about an error-prone process or other system problems that can be fed into the hospital safety or quality improvement structure. Judgments about the professional competence of individuals are managed through hospital medical staff governance structures.

As a strategy for reducing errors, peer review follows a "person approach" that is weak to the extent it assumes that human competence and behavior are responsible for most errors. Reliance on human perfection flies in the face of what is known about human performance in a variety of tasks, and the personal approach to error reduction undermines a culture of safety when individuals are blamed for errors and outcomes. The goal of peer review should be to ensure that health professionals are able to function on a level commensurate with the specific privileges granted. A "system approach" to error reduction assumes that most errors result from flaws in the system in which people work. The focus turns to creating a system that recognizes human fallibility, discourages and does not facilitate workarounds, and prevents harm to patients.

Peer review also encompasses the behavioral norms expected of health professionals. Behavior that is disruptive to safe patient care or that threatens the safety of employees, such as verbal abuse of employees, lying about events in the care of patients, throwing public temper tantrums directed at others, or making unwanted sexual advances, must be dealt with by leaders. Failing to do so contributes to fear among employees and distrust of leaders, undermining the culture of safety.

RESPONDING TO IDENTIFIED ERRORS AND RISK POINTS

■ PRIORITIZATION

Health care delivery is an inherently complex and dangerous field. Patients enter hospitals with conditions that may be either known or unclear. The methods we apply to diagnosis and treat patients involve sharp objects, ionizing radiation, and toxins, delivered in a team setting where we must plan and communicate clearly across professional disciplines and across multiple handoffs. The challenge then lies in deciding which problems to tackle first and which problems to set aside. When creating new processes or introducing new equipment, leaders must take the opportunity to apply FMEA or other strategic safeguards so the number of potentially chaotic and unsafe processes does not continue to rise exponentially.

Frontline employees bring their expertise about the risks they encounter. They should collaborate with the safety officer or committee that has a broader view of the problem areas in the hospital. The broader view comes from formal assessments of high-risk areas or processes, as with the FMEA technique, and from the accumulated experiences of risks and errors collected from the reporting system and other methods already discussed. When appropriate, local problems can be addressed with local solutions by the people who do the work. The hospital safety officer or committee will decide where and how to apply the more resource-intensive efforts to improve safety.

■ AVOIDING OVERREACTION AND UNINTENDED CONSEQUENCES

In the face of an adverse event, it can be tempting to apply intense focus and impose a quick solution. Indeed, when a serious continuing risk of harm is found, an immediate safeguard is appropriate.

Reacting quickly to every danger, though, may cause loss of focus on higher-priority risks. Ill-considered solutions can overburden employees to the point of paralysis or can introduce additional harms. As an example, computerized order entry systems permit checking for drug-drug interactions as a safety feature. System administrators can select the level of interaction (severe, moderate, minor) at which an alert interrupts the prescribing process. If, in response to an adverse drug event, the level is set to include all potential interactions, the number of interruptions may overwhelm prescribers, creating alert fatigue. As a result, cognitive errors may increase and prescribers may ignore more serious drug alerts. The net effect may well be to increase risks.

CONCLUSION

A robust safety program helps to manage the complex and dangerous inpatient hospital environment. It sets strategies and tactics for engendering a safe culture, identifying and investigating harms and risks, and prioritizing improvement efforts. The tools described in this chapter support the execution of such a robust and comprehensive safety program.

ACKNOWLEDGMENT

The author would like to acknowledge Nathan Spell, MD, for his contribution to the first edition chapter.

SUGGESTED READINGS

Berenholtz SM, Hartsell TL, Pronovost PJ. Learning from defects to enhance morbidity and mortality conferences. *Am J Med Qual.* 2009;24:192-195.

DeRosier J, Stalhandske E, Bagian JP, et al. Using health care failure mode and effect analysis: the VA National Center for Patient Safety's prospective analysis system. *Jt Comm J Qual Saf.* 2002;27(5):248-267.

Frankel A, Graydon-Baker E, Neppl C, et al. Patient safety leadership walkrounds. *Jt Comm J Qual Saf.* 2003;29(1):16-26.

Griffin FA, Resar RK. *IHI Global Trigger Tool for Measuring Adverse Events.* 2nd ed. IHI Innovation Series White Paper. Cambridge, MA: Institute for Healthcare Improvement; 2009.

Kohn LT, Corrigan JM, Donaldson MS, eds. *To Err is Human: Building a Safer Health System.* Washington, DC: National Academies Press; 2000.

Reason J. Human error: models and management. *BMJ* 2000;320:768-770.

Root Cause Analysis page. VA National Center for Patient Safety website. http://www.patientsafety.va.gov/media/rca.asp. Accessed October 10, 2015.

Weick KE, Sutcliffe KM. *Managing the Unexpected: Assuring High Performance in an Age of Complexity.* San Francisco, CA: Jossey-Bass; 2001.

Wheeler DS, Geis G, Mack EH, LeMaster T, Patterson MD. High reliability emergency response teams in the hospital: improving quality and safety using *in situ* simulation training. *BMJ Qual Saf.* 2013;22:507-514.

CHAPTER 20

Preventing and Managing Adverse Patient Events: Patient Safety and the Hospitalist

Timothy B. McDonald, MD, JD

INTRODUCTION

In November 1999, the Institute of Medicine (IOM) issued the report *To Err is Human*, detailing a problem of preventable medical errors that were killing as many as 98,000 inpatients per year. Subsequent publications have estimated it may be as high as 400,000 per year. Specific types of medical errors highlighted in the IOM report include error in the administration of treatment, failure to order and follow-up on indicated diagnostic exams, and avoidable delays in care and treatment. Many years later problems still exist: nearly 2 million patients a year develop infections during their hospitalizations, and 90,000 to 100,000 of those infected die, while hand-hygiene rates range from 30% to 70% at most acute care facilities. The IOM report also estimated that medical errors cost the US $17 billion to $29 billion a year, and called for sweeping changes to the health care system to improve patient safety.

Improvements in patient safety have focused on addressing the root causes of these preventable patient harm events, specifically events related to poor communication, lack of teamwork, fragmentation of care, and a lack of leadership from the medical community. In addition, patient safety experts have also implored physicians and hospitals to approach patient harm events with transparent, open, and honest communication between caregivers and patients and families in order to learn from mistakes and poorly designed systems.

This chapter reviews ways in which hospitalists may actively participate in the prevention of patient harm and provide appropriate management and assistance when patient harm does occur.

PREVENTING ADVERSE PATIENT EVENTS

Most patient safety experts would agree that the areas of highest priority to proactively maximize patient safety fit into three broad domains: communication, teamwork, and leadership. Within each of these domains lie critical concepts and issues about which the highly reliable and safe-practicing physician must remain mindful.

■ COMMUNICATION

No chapter on the prevention of patient harm is complete without a major focus on the role communication—or lack thereof—plays in serious patient safety events. The most common types of communication of high priority in patient safety are listed in **Table 20-1**.

Handoffs

Year after year The Joint Commission (TJC) publishes data showing 65% to 70% of all sentinel events are rooted in communication breakdowns. It appears that since the implementation of the Accreditation Council for Graduate Medical Education resident physician work hour limitations the communication problems have increased, especially in the area of **handoffs**, when the responsibility of care is passed from one provider to the next. With this limitation of resident physician work hours, the need and demand for hospitalists to "fill the gaps" in patient care has increased substantially. Associated with that increase in demand, hospitalists in particular have recognized the imperative of a standardized, user-friendly, and reliable method of handing off care from one provider to the next.

The content and process for handing off in the inpatient setting has evolved as practitioners try to meet regulatory requirements while maintaining simplicity, efficiency, and usability of the various

TABLE 20-1 Preventing Patient Safety Events

Communication
Handoff within and between services
Document in the electronic health record
Manage critical test results

Teamwork
Multidisciplinary rounds
Infection prevention
Patient triage
Rapid response teams

Leadership
Hospital/Medical Center Committees
Safety culture

handoff tools that are available. Various pneumonic tools, such as **S**ituation, **B**ackground, **A**ssessment, and **R**ecommendation have been devised to assist in the handoff process but have come and gone from institutional policies and guidelines as providers struggle with a reliable way to meet this important imperative. Hospitalists must play a role in designing and implementing a best practice handoff process appropriate for the context in which they work.

Vendors of electronic health records (EHRs) have also entered the arena with EHR-based tools to facilitate the often onerous process of handing off care of large numbers of patients. Regardless of the chosen method, all hospitalists must employ a reliable process to transmit necessary patient information from physician to physician. Defective or unreliable handoffs substantially increase risk of patient harm and the associated liability.

Documentation in the electronic health record (EHR)

With the passage of the 2010 Health Care Reform Act, it has become increasingly clear that the use of electronic health records will become much more ubiquitous in the coming years. While patient safety benefits of EHRs are well documented, only recently have informatics experts been publishing the unintended, unsafe consequences related to their use.

One of the most glaring examples of an unintended, unsafe consequence to EHR implementation is the abuse of "cut and paste" or "copy and paste" functionality, the process by which entire sections of nursing or physician documentation are copied and pasted from past to present notes. Numerous published reports demonstrate cases in which erroneous information has propagated, almost "virally," throughout a patient's EHR through the use of copy and paste. This process creates unsafe conditions for the patient such as in the example of the erroneous propagation of a "faux" allergy to an important medication. Serious medical-legal consequences can result for those who continue to misrepresent medical information through subsequent "copies" of the erroneous information or for those who act upon this unreliable information. The credibility of physicians comes into question when they are forced to defend misinformation they have propagated throughout the medical record, such as a temperature of 1101.5°F or a blood pressure of 1180/60.

While the "copy and paste" functionality provides useful efficiencies for documentation of long lists of medications or past surgical procedures, hospitalists must be aware of the deleterious consequences of the inappropriate use of this functionality and they should serve as positive role models and mentors throughout the organization for others who document in the EHR. From a patient safety and legal perspective, it is also incumbent upon the hospitalist to facilitate the correction of erroneous information encountered in the EHR.

MANAGEMENT OF CRITICAL TEST RESULTS

Critical test results management cuts to the heart of the health care business. US hospitals complete approximately 12 billion diagnostic tests every year. Most test results are within normal range and do not require follow-up by the clinician. However, a small but important number of test results, approximately1% to 5% of a hospital's test volume, are abnormal or critical. Hospitals and hospitalists have a professional, legal, and ethical obligation to ensure that these results are communicated to the responsible physician and appropriate action is taken.

Traditional systems to communicate and manage critical results are full of potential points of failure. In many hospitals, especially for hospitalists, contact information changes on a regular basis. Radiology departments and the pathology lab may not have the correct contact information for the responsible physician. Faxes can be equally problematic as the receiving machine might be off or out of paper. And once communicated, the right person might not receive the information. Unfortunately, radiologists and laboratory technicians may spend hours or days trying to track down the appropriate physician for results communication. Not surprising, miscommunication of critical findings have been identified as the causative factor in 85% of radiology lawsuits. Appropriately, The Joint Commission has deemed the management of critical test results as a national patient safety priority and requires hospitals and health care professionals to improve processes involved in such results. To improve the safety and quality of care their patients receive, hospitalists must play an integral role in the design and implementation of systems and processes to manage critical test results. At a minimum, in the hospital setting they must actively participate in a process to ensure the proper identification of responsible physicians and an efficient means for involving those responsible physicians in the communication and action based upon these results.

◼ TEAMWORK

MULTIDISCIPLINARY ROUNDS

Data abounds on the value teamwork brings to the safe and effective delivery of health care. The days of a single physician effectively micromanaging a patient's entire hospital stay are long gone. Research has shown that physicians can mitigate the negative effects of the necessary fragmentation of health care delivery by participating in multidisciplinary rounds during which physicians, nurses, pharmacists, and other allied health professionals discuss the daily plan for the patient and coordinate the transition of care to the outpatient setting. Inclusion of the patient and family in these rounds also provides benefit.

Especially for complicated patients, multidisciplinary rounds have been demonstrated to reduce length of stay, decrease the incidence of medication errors, prevent hospital readmissions, and improve overall patient and family satisfaction related to the hospital stay. As health care reimbursement models transition to a "pay for performance" or "pay for quality" metric, hospitals and hospitalists will find multidisciplinary rounds fundamental to the business model of health care.

INFECTION PREVENTION

All patient safety and quality organizations as well as health care regulators have identified health-care-associated infections (HAIs) as a top priority. The human and financial toll of HAIs accounts for a large portion of preventable harm in the United States. Therefore, the elimination of any significant proportion of HAIs is paramount to control health care costs and preventing patient harm. The role of the hospitalist as an essential, active member of the health care team is central to the efforts to reduce HAIs.

Three easily identifiable areas of quality improvement related to prevention of HAIs include (1) hand hygiene, (2) prevention of catheter-associated urinary tract infections (CAUTIs), and (3) prevention of intravenous line-associated blood stream infections, especially those related to central lines (CLABSIs). With observed hand-hygiene rates in most hospitals hovering around an abysmal 40% to 50%, administrators struggle to find solutions. Many leaders have found the solution to the hand-hygiene dilemma in the active engagement of hospitalists in their institution-wide efforts. Numerous success stories show that hospitalist engagement, by actively promoting hand-hygiene within their team, has taken 40% to 50% compliance rates to a sustainable 90% or higher. From the patient perspective, these increases in hand-hygiene rates translate into substantial reductions in methicillin-resistant staph infections and other HAIs.

The involvement of hospitalists on daily rounds in which they are able to order the removal of nonessential Foley catheters substantially reduces the incidence of CAUTIs. The same holds true for CLABSIs, in which the reduction in the days of use for invasive intravenous lines is also associated with a heath care-associated infection. With all these efforts, hospitalists are ideally situated to affect safety outcomes for their patients and others on their teams and in the institutions where they practice.

▪ PATIENT TRIAGE AND RAPID RESPONSE TEAMS (RRT)

As the frontline physicians accepting or coordinating inpatient hospital admissions, the hospitalist has an affirmative obligation to make certain newly admitted patients are placed on units and into beds that are appropriate for the level of care they need. Nonetheless, patients on appropriate wards or units will still deteriorate faster than the care professionals anticipate. When that happens, in the interest of patient safety, hospitals must have a process for rapidly summoning a team of professionals to assess the patient's current state of deterioration and to assist in a "retriaging" process.

Whether activated by other physicians, nurses, patients, or family members, hospitalists play an important role in the response to the deteriorating patient in many institutions. Effective and valuable physician members of a rapid response team, or any team assigned to respond to the clinically deteriorating patient, possess certain necessary attitudes and skills. As a leader of the team, the hospitalist must approach each "call for help" with a high degree of "mindfulness" in order to avoid premature closure based upon selective information provided to them by the care professionals previously caring for the patient. Regardless of whether the "call for help" or activation of the RRT seems appropriate after the initial response and investigation, it remains critical that the physician leader of the response team supports those who trigger the activation and helps prevent ridicule or criticism of those who asked for help.

Hospitalists must remain open minded while gathering all potentially important information that might be useful for arriving at solutions or treatments to reverse the deteriorating trend in condition. While carefully listening to other team members and caregivers, the leader of the team must be able to synthesize an approach that considers all the relevant factors, especially unexpected findings, and avoid the temptation to disregard information that might be inconsistent with their preliminary diagnosis—the concept of premature closure. They must remain cognizant of their own confirmation biases and strive to keep them in check. Not all chest pain is a myocardial infarction and not all wheezing is asthma!

From the skills perspective, a successful hospitalist RRT team leader must demonstrate competence in basic airway skills, use of emergency medications, and the ability to interpret electrocardiograms. The most important skill, however, rests in the ability of the hospitalist to function as an effective team leader with an ability to communicate clearly, concisely, and calmly and demonstrate a capacity to coordinate the activities of other care professionals they might be meeting for the first time.

Hospitalists also add value by actively participating in hospital-wide committees that review the outcomes of rapid response team actions and other emergency cardiac care activities. Only then can they facilitate change in the processes the hospital puts in place for recognizing and responding to the patient with unexpected changes in clinical condition.

▪ LEADERSHIP

Medical staff or hospital-wide committees

In recent years, The Joint Commission, the National Quality Forum, and the Centers for Medicare and Medicaid (CMS) have built standards and endorsed safe practices around medical staff and medical center leadership's responsibility and accountability for the safety and quality within their organizations. This focus provides the hospitalist with important opportunities to take leadership roles on medical staff and hospital committees, working groups, and task forces that focus on safety and quality. As physicians who concentrate wholly on hospital-based care, no group is better positioned to influence outcomes than hospitalists. They should work as solution seekers for the best ways to standardize handoffs, design the electronic health record, improve infection control practices, create accountabilities for the CMS Core Measures, and oversee team building and rapid response teams throughout the entire organization. Failure to engage in these efforts represents significant lost opportunities.

Safety culture

As hospitalists are clearly some of the most visible physicians in any organization, they bear a unique role and responsibility for promoting a robust "safety culture" within the organization and specifically in the units where they focus their practice. The Agency for Healthcare Research and Quality identifies key features of a "safety culture" that includes the willingness of hospital staff to openly communicate concerns about patient care on their units. Units where staff express comfort when questioning physicians or other authority figures when they disagree or have concerns are considered units with a "safer" culture. Other positive attributes of "safe" units are those in which mistakes are openly discussed and those discussions focus on "systems" issues instead of blaming specific individuals.

The difference between the culture of one unit to that of another in the same hospital often correlates with the difference between the middle management communication styles of the associated units. Units with nursing managers and physician leaders who focus on open, honest, effective, and nonpunitive communication related to adverse patient events score higher on safety culture surveys than others. In addition, there are data to suggest that those units with positive safety culture survey results have a lower incidence of adverse patient events when compared to units with less positive surveys. To that end, the hospitalist is uniquely situated to foster a culture of curiosity, inquiry, and appropriate challenging of authority through role modeling and mentoring. By setting positive examples for other physicians and staff, the hospitalist can lead in the efforts to ensure all of the units in which they work strive toward a safe, patient-centered approach to medical care.

■ THE PRINCIPLED APPROACH

Even when hospitalists do their best to proactively maximize the safety of their patients, unintentional harm still occurs. Importantly, the integrity of the individual physician or institution rests on the response to patient harm as much as it does to prevention. When harm occurs there is a choice to deny, minimize, rationalize, and blame others, including the patient, or to approach each harm event with a commitment to an open inquiry and honest communication following harm—the "principled approach." The hospitalist is constantly presented with this choice.

It is well recognized that there are a multitude of barriers to honest communication following harm that include fear of litigation, humiliation, lost income, reputational damage, risk to privileges and license, and the uncertainty of outcome. Nonetheless, the "deny and defend" approach to patient harm and the delegation of managing harm to the legal community has arguably not prevented any of those feared outcomes and instead has damaged the reputation of the medical profession and prevented any learning following patient harm events. The "principled approach" to patient harm is arguably the smarter approach because it effectively addresses many of the reasons that patients sue (lack of communication, need for explanation, sense of dishonesty or "hiding something") and provides a forum for learning and improving patient safety.

The principled approach to patient harm relies heavily on the hospitalist in at least six specific areas: (1) the immediate response, (2) reporting of harm, (3) communication, initially and in follow-up, (4) investigation, (5) identification of process and performance improvement opportunities, and (6) the necessary follow-up. See **Table 20-2**.

Responding and reporting

Responding to and the reporting of patient safety events are the first step in any principled process to patient harm (**Table 20-3**).

Reporting triggers the institutional response process, while the health care team responds to the immediate medical needs of the patient. Most hospitals encourage care professionals, especially physicians, to report any patient safety incident to its Safety and/or Risk Management Department. Reports are often made by telephone, handwritten, online, and in person. Hospitals are mandated by the Centers for Medicare and Medicaid and The Joint Commission to provide for a reporting process for patient harm events.

It is incumbent upon the hospitalist to understand and appreciate the reporting process used in any hospital where they work. Importantly, the hospitalist needs to recognize the importance of their role in taking care of the patient when harm occurs and ensuring that neither the patient nor the family is abandoned during this critical time.

Benefits of reporting

The benefits of rapid institutional reporting of patient safety events within the organization provide substantial incentive for all

hospitalists to report and encourage reporting harm events. These benefits include (1) the activation of the internal patient safety and risk management processes including a crisis management plan, if indicated, (2) the preservation of data and information, (3) the opportunity to trigger immediate support for patient, family, and care professional, (4) the initiation of a "quality committee" investigation and the "legal privilege" most states afford such investigations, and (5) the establishment of a communication link with the harmed patient and his or her family.

As with documentation in the medical record, when reporting a patient safety event, hospitalists should take care to provide only the necessary factual information to commence an investigation. They should avoid documenting speculation, hasty conclusions with incomplete facts, or "finger-pointing" in the report.

Investigation

As advocates for quality medical care and patient safety, hospitalists possess special skills for participating in the investigation of serious adverse outcomes (see **Table 20-4**). Patients and families want and deserve the "facts" after a harm event. An appropriate investigatory process is needed to provide them with the necessary information. The hospitalist should commit to participating in any institutional root cause analysis or other investigatory process following a serious harm event. Such investigations should try to avoid the traditional "shame and blame" approach to adverse events and instead focus on system-based issues and identification of possible areas of improvement.

Nonetheless, prior to knowing all the facts, patients and families are still entitled to effective communication in the early aftermath of a harm event.

Communication

Once harm occurs, honest and effective communication helps maintain trust between the patient and family and care professionals. With their easy availability, often 24 hours a day, the hospitalist is uniquely positioned to facilitate such communication. After all, for the patient who has experienced an unexpected outcome, every hour that goes by without effective communication constitutes more harm.

TABLE 20-3 Immediate Response

Address current needs of patient and family
Contact risk management or patient safety hotline
Identify care professionals for ongoing care
Identify key persons for patient/family communication
Preserve data, equipment, etc
Document "just the facts" in medical record or risk management report

---

TABLE 20-2 Principled Response to Patient Harm Events

Respond immediately
Report
Investigate
Communicate
Performance improvement
Follow-up

TABLE 20-4 Investigation

Perform within context of authorized quality improvement process
Involve interprofessional personnel as indicated
Utilize a validated root cause analysis (RCA) process or tool
Incorporate organizational quality and patient safety personnel
Consider involving patients and families in RCA process

Honest and effective communication after a harmful adverse event is not just the right thing to do, but the smart thing to do as well. Patients and families sue, in large part, because they perceive a lack of transparency, abandonment, or "cover-up." A transparent process with open lines of communication and disclosure of all pertinent information can mitigate those patient and family perceptions.

Disclosure of any actual error associated with the harm is a multifaceted process that requires careful planning, preparation, and coordination by physicians and hospital administrators. Given its complexity, physicians understandably fear that an inadequate or poorly executed disclosure of medical errors will only serve to frustrate frontline practitioners, ruin the reputation of the organization and individual practitioners involved in the incident, and encourage lawsuits.

Successful adverse event response programs that include "full disclosure" rely heavily upon integration between the clinical departments and hospital risk management. This integration ensures that the various stakeholders are "on board" or at least aware of the plan for communication after adverse events. The stakeholder list must include the medical malpractice insurance carriers for the various parties who might be affected. In order to provide a consistent approach to adverse events for providers, patients, and families, all of the steps involved in the response to harm should be preapproved by all appropriate stakeholders, before implementation.

The process of communication after harm occurs generally falls in three phases: immediate, intermediate, and final or follow-up phase (**Table 20-5**). The extent of hospitalist involvement in this type of communication will depend upon the relationship of the hospitalist with the patient and his or her family. Long-term close physician-patient relationships are conducive to multiple meetings and discussions wherein the hospitalist will quickly discover that "disclosure" is a process and not an event.

A liaison for the family should be identified and appropriate empathy and assurance of nonabandonment is expressed at each

visit. It is critical for the hospitalist to understand the difference between "empathy" and "apology." Empathy is the understanding or sharing of another person's emotions and feelings whereas an "apology" is admitting a mistake that caused harm. In medicine, there is an ethical imperative to express empathy when patients suffer harm but apologies should be reserved for situations when it is clear mistakes or errors have caused the harm. Therefore, apologies should only be offered when the facts are clear and agreed upon by the stakeholders with knowledge of the event.

Example of expression of empathy: "I am sorry your pneumonia has progressed to the point where despite our best efforts we now need to put a breathing tube in your windpipe to help you breathe."

Example of apology: "I am sorry I did not check your abnormally low blood sugar result this morning. If I had seen the result, I could have given you some extra sugar to prevent your seizure this morning."

PROCESS IMPROVEMENTS

The value in a principled, transparent approach to adverse patient events lies in the ability to learn from mistakes within a rigorous, reflective environment that promotes performance improvement efforts designed to significantly improve the delivery of care. To be effective, hospitalists must play a role in these performance improvement efforts that follow suboptimal care. Patients and families involved in adverse events caused by inappropriate care are intensely interested in learning the ways in which similar events are less likely to occur. Discussing these quality improvement measures with them also helps to maintain the trust and bond between patient and provider.

CONCLUSION

The evidence for abundant opportunities to improve patient care and prevent patient harm has become indisputable. Earlier estimates on the annual number of preventable deaths in hospitals far underestimated the actual number of deaths that could be prevented, especially from health-care-associated infections. Moving forward it has become clear the mantra "no outcome, no income" or "no pay for low-quality performance" is going to apply to a significant number of episodes of care. To that end, hospitalists are ideally situated to positively influence issues in quality of care outcomes through their active engagement on performance improvement efforts, their communication skills, and their ability to lead multidisciplinary efforts.

In addition, hospitalists can take a lead in providing honest, open, and effective communication to patients and families after unexpected adverse event outcomes. This transparent approach can be the catalyst, for the transformation of an organization's culture for effectively responding to the needs of patients, providers, and the health care system. Adopting a policy and practice of transparency related to harm events represents a major shift in organizational focus and will need the full support of hospitalists to fully implement. This approach will require strong and persistent endorsement by the kind of leadership that hospitalists can provide their organizations. The added value of transparency is found in the opportunity to rapidly learn from, respond to, and modify practices based on harm investigation with these now transparent events.

TABLE 20-5 Communication

Immediate
Express empathy
Do not make promises you cannot keep
Disclose "known" facts
Assure nonabandonment
Identify persons (liaison) for follow-up
Intermediate
Ensure liaison presence
Continue to express empathy
Disclose facts discovered during investigation
Ask and answer clarifying questions
Apologize if consensus exists about error or substandard care causing harm
Explain plan for prevention of future harm
Offer ongoing contact and communication
Final or follow-up phase
Ensure liaison presence
Answer additional questions
Express empathy, apology, if indicated
Discuss performance improvement measures
Offer ongoing contact and support

SUGGESTED READINGS

Boothman RC, Blackwell AC, Campbell DA Jr, Commiskey E, Anderson S. A better approach to malpractice claims? The University of Michigan Experience. *J Health Life Sci Law.* 2009;2(2):125-159.

Hickson GB, Federspeil CF, Pichert JW, Miller CS, Gauld-Jaeger J, Bost P. Patient complaints and malpractice risk. *JAMA*. 2002;287(22):2951-2957.

Institute of Medicine. *To Err Is Human: Building a Safer Health System*. In: Kohn LT, Corrigan JM, Donaldson MS, eds. Washington, DC: National Academy Press; 2000.

Leape LL, Berwick DM. Five years after to err is human: what have we learned? *JAMA*. 2005;293(19):2384-2389.

McDonald T. Error disclosure within a principled approach to adverse events. *ASA Newsletter*. 2009;73(5):20-22.

McDonald TB, Helmchen LA, Smith KM, et al. Responding to patient safety incidents: the seven pillars. *Qual Saf Health Care*. 2010;19(6):e11.

National Quality Forum. *Safe Practices for Better Healthcare–2010 Update: A Consensus Report*. Washington, DC: NQF; 2010.

C H A P T E R 21

Principles and Models of Quality Improvement: Plan-Do-Study-Act

Emmanuel S. King, MD, FHM
Jennifer S. Myers, MD, FHM

Achieving better health outcomes for patients and populations requires a focus on continuous quality improvement (QI). While physicians pride themselves on being subject matter experts in their focused area of medical practice, such knowledge alone is insufficient to produce fundamental changes in the delivery of health care. Physicians who practice in complex hospital and health care systems must acquire another kind of knowledge in order to develop and execute change.

W. Edwards Deming, an American statistician and professor who is widely credited with improvement in manufacturing in the United States and Japan, has described this knowledge as a "system of profound knowledge" (**Figure 21-1**). This knowledge is composed of the following items: appreciation for a system, understanding variation, building knowledge, and the human side of change. These concepts are just beginning to be taught to health care professionals and are essential for anyone who wishes to improve the health care delivery system.

All hospitalists have witnessed changes that did not result in fundamental improvements within their hospital systems: the computerized order set that was successfully implemented but never revised based on prescribers' feedback, the paper checklist for medication reconciliation that never gets filled out, or the new rounding system that worked for the first few weeks but then failed to become a standard part of practice due to physician variation or lack of commitment. These are all examples of *first-order changes*—changes that ultimately returned the system to the normal level of performance. In quality improvement work, individuals must strive for *second-order changes*, which are changes that truly alter the system and result in a higher level of system performance. Such changes impact how work is done, produce visible, positive differences in results relative to historical norms, and have a lasting impact. Although the model for improvement described below may seem simple, it is actually quite demanding when used properly; and the process is essential to both learning and ultimately changing complex systems.

PLAN-DO-STUDY-ACT AS A TOOL FOR QUALITY IMPROVEMENT

The Plan-Do-Study-Act (PDSA) model is a commonly used method in quality improvement. Shewart and Deming described the model many years ago when they studied quality in other industries. This model first appeared in health care when Berwick described how the tools could be applied using an iterative approach to change. Using a "test-and-learn approach" in which a hypothesis is tested, retested, and refined, the PDSA cycle allows for controlled change experiments on a small scale before expansion to a larger system. The four repetitive steps of PDSA—plan, do, study, and act—are carried out until fundamental improvement, which can be exponentially larger than the original hypothesis, takes place (**Figure 21-2**).

PRACTICE POINT

- Use a "test-and-learn approach" to solve quality problems. The PDSA—plan, do, study, and act—framework is one popular model to organize your approach to quality improvement work.

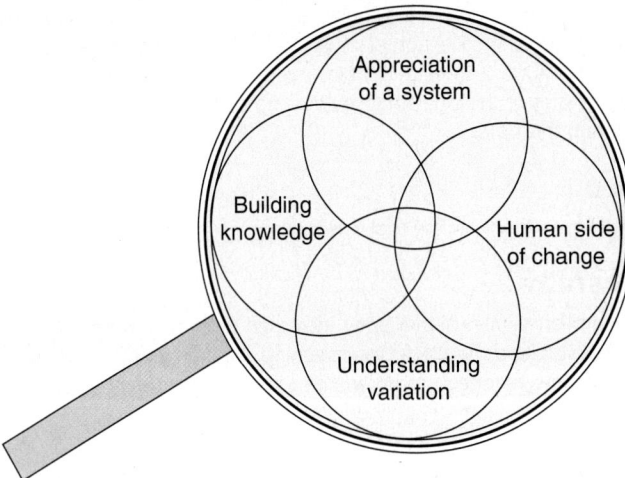

Figure 21-1 *Deming's System of Profound Knowledge.* (Reproduced, with permission, from Langley GJ, et al. *The Improvement Guide: A Practical Approach to Enhancing Organization Performance,* 2nd ed. San Francisco, CA: Jossey-Bass; 2009.)

PLAN

During the Plan phase, the team generates broad questions, hypotheses, and a data collection plan. It is critically important during this period to define expectations and assign tasks and accountability to every team member. In the planning phase of the PDSA cycle, it is prudent to invest significant time and develop a well-framed question by reviewing related research and local projects and defining meaningful process and outcome measurements. Broad questions at the outset of a PDSA cycle can include "What are we trying to accomplish?" and "What changes can we make that will result in an improvement?" The ideal data collection tool answers the question: "How will we know that a change is an improvement?" It is also helpful for the team to generate predictions of the answers to questions early on. This aids in framing the plan more completely,

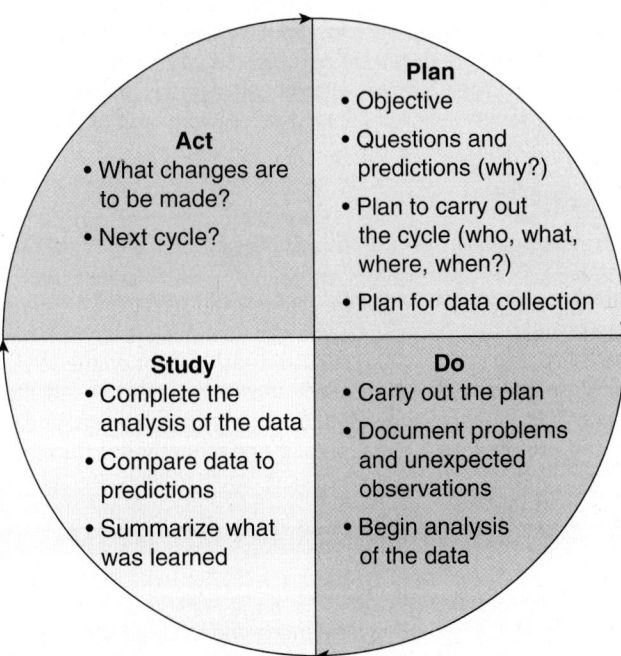

Figure 21-2 *The Plan-Do-Study-Act Cycle.* (Reproduced, with permission, from Langley GJ, et al. *The Improvement Guide: A Practical Approach to Enhancing Organization Performance,* 2nd ed. San Francisco, CA: Jossey-Bass; 2009.)

to uncover underlying assumptions or biases before any testing, and to enhance learning in the Study phase by providing a baseline point of comparison.

Teams new to QI frequently will struggle with the question, "How do we measure improvement?" Defining discrete process measures is a good starting point when using PDSA. Process measures are used to assess whether the cycle is being carried out as planned. This is in contrast to outcome measures, which are used to track success or failure and focus on the specific outcome that the team is trying to achieve.

DO

The Do phase in PDSA is a period of active implementation. It involves feedback on the new process from end users and rigorous data collection. An overarching goal of this phase is to capture and document not only compliance with the new process, but also deviations, defects, or barriers in the process. There are always aspects of quality improvement projects that do not go as planned, and flexibility and open-mindedness are critical to maximize learning from improvement. The quality of the Do phase is intimately related to the quality of the Plan phase. A pitfall for many novice QI teams is to give in to the temptation to jump straight to implementing change without spending a significant amount of time planning. A poorly conceptualized improvement plan, an absence of a sound data collection model, or unclear accountabilities can have adverse effects on the implementation or "do" phase of a new initiative.

STUDY

Analysis of available process and outcome metrics and a qualitative appraisal of the process are the key activities in the Study phase. Time should be set aside to perform a critical review of the data collected and compare it to historical data (when available) and baseline predictions. Close attention should be paid to possible defects in any element of the process, including the data collection plan. If such issues are uncovered, the team may need to revise the initial data collection tools and overall plan. Thoughtful review of all trials, even those that were clearly unsuccessful based on metrics, is a critical and valuable process for the team. In fact, the "failures" in a PDSA cycle can yield unanticipated and improved directions. As the Study phase progresses, time should be spent considering if a follow-up PDSA cycle is planned and exactly what elements to include in that cycle.

ACT

The final component in a PDSA cycle is Act. The team should convene for a feedback and action planning session. Frontline workers in the system that is being changed should be included for honest input. A team approach rather than a "top-down" approach facilitates an open review of successes and failures. An action plan that encompasses lessons learned in the first three steps should then be put into motion. During this stage decisions are made about repeating certain test cycles after improvements are made or "spinning off" new test cycles based on the original one.

RAPID CYCLE, CONTINUOUS, AND SEQUENTIAL PDSA

In its most basic form, the PDSA model described above can be applied to change a single process. However, teams in health care often confront problems that require multiple changes, in parallel or succession, in order for improvement to happen. Caution is advised when initiating several PDSA cycles simultaneously, especially if there are significantly different data collection plans or if the team is inexperienced in QI methods. An alternative is a sequential PDSA model in which one PDSA cycle feeds into the next. This approach, in which teams continually change and refine their processes based on data evaluation and feedback, is called "continuous quality improvement." Experienced QI teams strive to utilize this approach. Rapid cycle PDSA is a continuous QI process that lends itself well to projects that are focused on relatively small-scale changes. It is typically used by seasoned QI teams who are familiar with the PDSA model and who wish to implement rapid change.

AN EXAMPLE OF PDSA IN ACTION

To illustrate the PDSA model for improvement, a real QI project is presented here from start to finish. A hospitalist group sought to implement a new discharge planning toolkit aimed at improving transitions in care through risk assessment at the time of hospital admission. A QI team was formed with representatives from health care professionals involved in the discharge planning process. While their ultimate goal was to reduce unplanned readmissions, their first team goal involved creating a new process to coordinate and request risk-specific interventions from other teams (eg, nurse educators, pharmacists, a nurse for postdischarge follow-up phone calls) for patients deemed "high risk for hospital re-admission or transition in care problems" by a screening tool. In preparation for the project, the QI team also performed a stakeholder analysis, which is a tool that QI teams can use to identify all of the individuals and groups with a "stake" in the process being discussed.

CYCLE 1

■ PLAN

The initial PDSA cycle involved piloting a readmission risk screening tool. A weekly meeting was convened that included representative users of the tool and assigned specific responsibilities and tasks with due dates to each team member. At baseline, the biggest barriers to overcome were the perception that the new tool was extra work, introducing a paper-based tool in a largely electronic health care environment, and lack of a tight infrastructure tying the requests to existing risk-specific interventions. Based on these concerns, the team reduced the number of interventions on the initial tool. A data collection plan was started and included both quantitative process metrics (eg, compliance rates with the tool, frequency of risk factors identified on the tool) and qualitative data from the users of the tool.

■ DO

The new tool was piloted for 2 weeks, during which time data was collected and feedback was solicited from the frontline team.

■ STUDY

After 2 weeks, the data showed that overall compliance with the tool was moderately high, but that two risk factors, health literacy and depression, had unexpectedly low percentages. On further inquiry, members of the team admitted that when they performed the risk screen, they paused on those two questions and frequently left them blank, concerned that it might take too much time during the admission process and frustrate new users of the tool.

■ ACT

The team decided to make another edit to the tool before the second PDSA cycle. The health literacy and depression screening questions were removed based on feedback, with a plan to reintroduce them when the tool was more embedded in the hospital admission workflow.

CYCLE 2

■ PLAN

The second PDSA cycle focused on follow-up data collection with the health literacy and depression screening questions removed

from the tool, to test the theory that this would improve compliance. The data collection plan was to track overall compliance with the tool for a 2-week period. In order to isolate any improvement as a result of this one small change, no other changes were made during this time.

■ DO

The new version of the tool was implemented.

■ STUDY

Compliance rates significantly increased from moderately high to very high, and the risk factor screening data remained unchanged. Qualitative feedback from frontline users was that the risk screening process was more streamlined and acceptable.

■ ACT

A brief but successful cycle 2 ended with a plan to add an intervention checklist to the tool in the next phase.

CYCLE 3

■ PLAN

The goal of cycle 3 was to associate risk-specific interventions (education, follow-up phone calls, and social work interventions) with a patient's individual risk factor profile. To meet this goal, the team implemented a new version of the tool that included the risk-specific intervention requests and tracked request type and volume. A 2-week cycle was planned with continued weekly meetings during this time.

■ DO

The team implemented a tool that allowed for interventions to be requested at the time of risk factor screening.

■ STUDY

After 2 weeks, the data showed stable high compliance with the form, stable risk factor data, but very low utilization of intervention requests. At feedback meetings, frontline users stated that at the time of admission, they were not ready to place a request for an intervention. They felt that intervention requests should be discussed in a multidisciplinary team on a follow-up hospital day when more information was available.

■ ACT

Discharge planners on the team suggested that the intervention request process be integrated into daily discharge planning rounds, during which the entire patient care team (physician, nurse practitioner, registered nurse, discharge planners, patient service representative, and social worker) discussed each patient on the service. A nurse practitioner and patient service representative drafted paper forms that could be used to communicate requests for each of the interventions to the appropriate personnel and to document completion of the task. The next phase would trial this new process.

CYCLE 4

■ PLAN

Cycle 4 was focused on implementing and studying the new discharge rounds process to request risk-specific interventions. The frequency of intervention requests in each category was added to the existing process metrics. Since this was a more substantial change than before and involved more than just one team of frontline users, a 4-week cycle duration was chosen.

DO

Clinicians continued to screen patients using the risk screening tool, intervention request forms were kept on hand during discharge rounds, and the patient service representative and discharge planners prompted the teams to request interventions based on patient risk factors. The requests were forwarded to the appropriate personnel (registered nurse, pharmacist, nurse educator), who then documented completion of the intervention on the form.

STUDY

Compliance rates and risk factor data remained steady, but there was a significant increase in intervention requests in all categories. However, documentation of completion of the intervention was low. It was determined that the documentation requirements were unfamiliar to the intervention teams, which was an oversight.

ACT

For the next cycle further improvements in documentation of intervention completion and a reintroduction of the health literacy and depression screening questions was planned.

LESSONS LEARNED

This example illustrates several important points for successful use of the PDSA model. First, the engagement and involvement of the end users of new QI tools and processes is critical to the success of any improvement project. These users are experts in the process who often know what should be tested next, and perfect champions when changes are disseminated on a larger scale. While it may be impossible to address or fix every problem that they identify, hearing their input, implementing changes based on their suggestions, and giving praise for their involvement and patience is an important skill for leaders of QI. Second, flexibility and creative thinking, skills that are used frequently in clinical care, are also essential in QI. In the case study, several barriers were identified such as: concerns about paper forms, perception that certain risk factors would halt the risk screening process, and lack of infrastructure around the systematic documentation of interventions. As these barriers became apparent, the team remained flexible and changed a part of the new process without compromising the integrity and team goals of the project.

PRACTICE POINT

Critical to the success of any quality improvement project:

- Performing a stakeholder analysis to help identify all individuals and teams that have a "stake" in the quality problem that is being addressed.
  - Engagement and involvement of the "end" users of new QI tools and processes.
  - Small tests of change that include data collection followed by data analysis and decisions on how to proceed.

ALTERNATIVE MODELS OF QUALITY IMPROVEMENT

In addition to the PDSA model described above, there are other frameworks that have been used to design and execute quality improvement projects. Adopting one specific framework (as opposed to adopting several) allows an organization to learn a common language and approach to improvement. Six Sigma and Lean are two common frameworks that will be briefly described.

Six Sigma was developed by Motorola in the mid-1980s and is focused on reducing variations in a process. Six Sigma is a popular performance improvement methodology which uses a five-phase approach to problem solving, called DMAIC (Define, Measure, Analyze, Improve, and Control). This framework guides users to define their QI goals, measure the current process, analyze root causes of the quality problem, improve the process on the basis of the previous steps, and finally control the process to ensure that variances are corrected before they result in defects and the new process becomes standard work.

Lean manufacturing (or just "Lean") was adapted from the Toyota Production Systems and is focused on continuously reducing waste in operations and enhancing the value proposition to customers. The Lean approach is based on a few key principles: defining the problem from the customer perspective, identifying the activities required to provide the customer with a product or service, producing the products or services only when needed by customers, and pursuing perfection in the process.

CONCLUSION

Plan-Do-Study-Act has remained a fundamental tool for continuous quality improvement. Once comfortable applying this iterative approach, hospitalists can affect both small- and large-scale changes in their health care systems. Other QI frameworks that hospitalists should be aware of include Six Sigma and Lean methodologies. Adopting one specific framework (as opposed to adopting several) allows hospitalists and organizations to learn a common language and approach to improvement.

SUGGESTED READINGS

Berwick D. Developing and testing changes in delivery of care. *Ann Intern Med*. 1998;128:651-656.

Langley GJ, Moen RD, Nolan KM, Nolan TW, Norman CL, Provost LP. *The Improvement Guide: A Practical Approach to Enhancing Organizational Performance*. 2nd ed. San Francisco, CA: Jossey-Bass; 2009.

Varkey P, Reller K, Resar R. Basics of quality improvement in health care. *Mayo Clin Proc*. 2007;82(6):735-739.

CHAPTER 22

The Role of Information Technology in Hospital Quality and Safety

Saverio M. Maviglia, MD, MSc

INTRODUCTION

The practice of medicine is at heart an exercise of collecting, filtering, summarizing, managing, analyzing, and acting upon information. This information comes directly from the patient's narrative history, but also from family and caretakers, and other providers. It is also derived from diagnostic interventions, including the physical examination, laboratory tests, radiologic exams, and procedures. Combined with reference knowledge about physiology, pathology, pharmacology, and other basic science disciplines, the physician makes an expert assessment of the patient's conditions and risks, and then recommends an action plan. Information about this plan must be communicated and coordinated with a larger team and with the patient and their family, executed, and then information about how the patient responds fed back, in order to make adjustments over time. If this flow of information is compromised or hampered at any point in this cycle, then the potential for quality and safety problems emerges. Given this intense information-rich environment that the clinician must navigate, especially in the inpatient setting, it is clear that the judicious application of information technology (IT) can greatly empower the hospitalist in providing high quality and safe patient care; and conversely, that injudicious application of IT can promote errors and adverse outcomes.

Information technologies that impact patient safety and quality of care can be grouped into three major categories. First, there are the interventions that impact care as it is delivered in real time—this class is generally called *decision support* because it involves clinicians while they are making diagnostic and therapeutic decisions. The second class of information technologies, broadly known as *surveillance*, monitors the immediate downstream care processes to detect anomalies and unintended consequences so that effective corrective action may be taken quickly. The last general category of IT for safety and quality is *data mining*, or retrospective analysis of large repositories of data, such as patient registries, electronic health records (EHRs), and administrative databases in order to detect meaningful patterns and signals that may help inform ways to improve one or more health care delivery processes. Data mining overlaps with classical epidemiological health services outcomes research.

DECISION SUPPORT

As defined above, decision support is any type of information system that intends to direct, guide, or alter medical decision making as it occurs in real time. This may occur via passive delivery of knowledge, such as quick access to online digital references, drug compendia, clinical calculators, or differential diagnosis tools. In this case, the user must voluntarily choose to activate the service. This type of decision support is usually well received by busy clinicians, because the clinician is motivated to get a question answered. However, passive decision support does not address latent information needs, or knowledge deficits unknown to the clinician.

Decision support may also occur via active knowledge delivery, such as alerts to avoid unsafe or undesired behavior, or reminders to promote desired behavior; the service is activated automatically. Usually, the intended behavior is evidence based, such as avoiding drug combinations that have been shown to result in adverse effects; but it can also be policy driven, such as to promote some medications over others based on formulary or insurance criteria. As active decision support is often interruptive, clinician acceptance of this information is variable, depending upon the perceived usefulness of the information provided and the manner in which it is displayed.

There are certain decision support systems which fall somewhere between active and passive, which facilitate workflow. Examples include messaging systems such as signout applications and secure e-mail or text paging, electronic medication reconciliation applications, and results management programs. Also in this category is the organized presentation, or summarization, of patient data that lowers cognitive burden.

The ideal decision support intervention simultaneously facilitates the desired workflow(s) while impeding the undesired workflow(s). In other words, the most effective decision support interventions make it "easy" to do the right thing, and "hard" to do the wrong thing. For example, compare two ways to implement decision support for optimal drug dosing. The first, more common approach is to analyze medication orders after they are entered; compare them to rules that assess patient factors such as age, gender, and comorbidities such as renal dysfunction; and then display a series of corrective alerts. The second approach does as much of the patient-specific calculations as possible up front, so that only the most reasonable medication alternatives for a given indication are offered in the first place, with default dose and frequency precalculated to match the patient's condition. Only the prescriber who chooses to override the defaults is interrupted to provide an override reason. Of course, the more sophisticated consultative approach to delivering decision support requires more data in computable form about a patient, as well as more complicated and nuanced rules, than the typical critical approach.

Evidence suggests that decision support can successfully influence provider behavior, improve process measures, increase quality of care, and reduce errors and adverse events. However, the way decision support is implemented can dramatically affect effectiveness. For example, when influenza vaccination reminders were first implemented at one inpatient site, the effect was minimal; but when the alert was changed to a complete prewritten order, and the default was set to "accept" instead of to "decline," the inpatient vaccination rate increased from 1% to 51%.

PRACTICE POINT

- Evidence suggests that decision support can successfully influence provider behavior, improve process measures, increase quality of care, and reduce errors and adverse events. However, the way decision support is implemented can dramatically affect effectiveness; poorly implemented systems can have unintended adverse consequences on health care providers or promote error.

More problematic is the growing recognition that poorly implemented systems can have unintended adverse consequences on health care providers, to the point of inciting clinician revolt, such as occurred at Cedars-Sinai Medical Center in Los Angeles in 2003. Worse yet, computerized provider order entry, coupled with decision support, can potentially promote errors. Therefore, the behavior of such systems must be continually scrutinized, and the information they provide must never be accepted blindly.

SURVEILLANCE

Surveillance IT is analogous to secondary prevention or care—it is meant to detect complications of care early so that the consequences can be prevented or ameliorated. The most prevalent example, which is still relatively rarely implemented in practice, is adverse event detection. This requires an electronic monitoring

system that oversees all digital transactions in a health information system, such as new orders, new lab results, and new patient encounter records; a repository of rules that define potential events and the actions that should be taken; and a variety of effector systems to carryout the actions, such as texting or e-mail alerting. Collectively, these components form what is commonly known as an event engine. As an example, the monitoring system registers all new lab results, including an individual patient's falling platelet level. A rule in the repository defines a clinically significant rapid rate of decline (eg, an absolute drop of 50,000 or a relative drop of 30% over 2 days, or of 75,000 or 50% over 3 days) in the right clinical context (the patient has a current active order for a heparin-containing medication), to generate a response (alert the responsible clinician the next time she logs into the system, or text page a backup clinician if this does not occur within 24 hours). It is clear from this example that the effectiveness of this surveillance system is only as good as the breadth of events that can be monitored, the granularity with which rules can be authored to define clinically significant events, and the breadth of interventions available for actions.

Surveillance systems can collect and analyze quality-related data, as well as safety data. Such systems, sometimes called profiling or detailing systems, have been long utilized by pharmaceutical companies to direct and tailor marketing efforts, but they can also be used to track how often a hospitalist utilizes nonformulary medications; or how well a provider is achieving quality of care metric goals, such as percentage of their patients who have a Foley catheter for over 48 hours; or rates of resource utilization, such as magnetic resonance imaging for headaches. This information can be shared with just the relevant provider, or with an entire practice, either deidentified or not. The most sophisticated profiling systems present the data in a quality dashboard that the provider can query dynamically in real time and link the data to relevant actions, such as e-mailing patients, flagging them for callback appointments, or automatically referring patients to a disease management program.

In addition to patient-specific and provider-specific event engines, surveillance systems have also been developed to work at the population level. For example, there are monitoring systems that track aggregated data about visits to regional emergency rooms, including chief complaints, to detect early signals of disease outbreaks such as from influenza or bioterrorism.

DATA MINING

The final class of IT that can be brought to bear on quality and safety is the retrospective analysis of large datasets to look for trends and patterns and their relationship or association with significant events, interventions, or behaviors. This traditionally has been called health services research, and can focus on either health care outcomes (mortality, morbidity, readmissions, adverse event rates) or their process-based proxies (frequency of deep vein thrombosis [DVT] prophylaxis measures, rate of compliance with recommended guidelines, or proportion of completed discharge summaries within 24 hours). Both are valid indicators of quality and safety effectiveness, though hard outcomes are often preferred, but usually more difficult to measure and influence. For example, measuring the effect of an intervention on incidence of DVT would be ideal, but in practice would require significant manual data collection by chart abstraction, and may be too infrequent an event in the time window allowed for study to make statistically sound conclusions. Instead, measuring how the intervention impacts the number of orders for subcutaneous heparin, especially where such orders are placed via computer-based provider order entry (CPOE), is much easier and a more common event.

The newest direction this type of research has taken is the combination of large datasets from different disciplines, to look for new and sometimes unanticipated or counterintuitive associations. Because of the increasing likelihood of chance alone being responsible for observing such relationships between data when multiple statistical tests are performed with the same data, this type of knowledge discovery requires large collections of data, runs the risk of uncovering statistically significant but clinically irrelevant patterns, and should always be considered hypothesis generating rather than confirming or refuting. A simplistic example is that if one were to measure how frequently lung cancer patients carry matches compared to patients without lung cancer, one might be tempted to conclude that carrying matches is a very dangerous activity. Another example is that since test results are typically defined to be in the normal range when they lie within the 95th percentile of results from a healthy population, then a battery panel of 20 tests will have at least one false positive result almost two-third of the time.

MEANINGFUL USE

In the United States, a recent potent driver of health IT efforts has been Meaningful Use (MU). Through the Health Information Technology for Economic and Clinical Health Act, up to $27 billion (or over $60,000 per clinician) over 10 years is set aside to promote not just the adoption, but the "meaningful use" of Electronic Health Records in order to achieve improved patient outcomes. This is being pursued incrementally via three stages enacted over time.

- Stage 1 (2011-2013): Capture health information electronically in a structured format; use that information to track key clinical conditions and coordinate care; implement clinical decision support tools; use EHRs to engage patients and families and report clinical quality measures and public health information.
- Stage 2 (2014-2016): Encourage the use of health IT for continuous quality improvement at the point of care and the exchange of information in the most structured format possible.
- Stage 3 (starting 2017): Promote improvements in quality, safety and efficiency leading to improved health outcomes by focusing on decision support, patient access to self-management tools, access to comprehensive patient data and improving population health.

Compliance with the initial stages is incentivized with bonus payments from Medicare and Medicaid to both eligible providers and to hospitals. These payments decrease over time and eventually disappear, to be replaced by payment penalties starting in 2015 for noncompliant providers and hospitals.

There are growing data to support the claim that MU Stages 1 and 2 have had a major impact on the use of EHRs and clinical decision support (CDS) in the United States. For example, a longitudinal study of 493 nonfederal hospital IT budgets from 2009 to 2011 found increases in the percentage of hospital annual operating budgets allocated to IT in the years leading up to these federal incentives. Adoption of EHRs by US hospitals has increased dramatically since the MU program was implemented. In 2011, 833 hospitals and 57,652 professionals attested for MU. The following year, an additional 1726 hospitals and 132,395 professionals attested. According to CMS data presented in April 2013, over 77% of eligible hospitals and approximately 53% of eligible providers qualified to earn the bonus. The data also indicate major increases in CDS use compared to 2008 baseline.

On the other hand, data suggesting that the MU program actually has improved health IT is mixed. For example, 60% of hospitals responding to a survey reported that their EHRs did not contain all features essential for high-quality care. And data that MU has positively impacted patients are indirect and inconclusive.

THE HOSPITALIST'S ROLE

There is great opportunity for clinicians such as hospitalists, who are often experts in workflow and systems thinking (whether by formal training or simply by experience), to help guide implementations of decision support interventions within their practice sites in order to increase the chance of success. Even after successful implementation of information technologies, there is ongoing need for clinicians to provide feedback about what works, what does not, and what could be done to improve the system. A higher level of involvement of hospitalists is to provide subject matter expertise to tweak rules and author new ones to make the decision support more specific, relevant, and effective. This never-ending work to keep the content of rules in line with ever changing knowledge has emerged as a new field of its own, called knowledge management.

PRACTICE POINT

- Knowledge management requires keeping the content of rules in line with ever-changing knowledge, and creating new ones to make decision support more specific, relevant, and effective. Even after successful implementation of information technologies, there is ongoing need for clinicians to provide feedback about what works, what does not, and what could be done to improve the system.

SUGGESTED READINGS

Ash JS, Berg M, Coiera E. Some unintended consequences of information technology in health care: the nature of patient care information system-related errors. *J Am Med Inform Assoc.* 2004;11(2):104-112.

Bates DW, Cohen M, Leape LL, Overhage JM, Shabot MM, Sheridan T. Reducing the frequency of errors in medicine using information technology. *J Am Med Inform Assoc.* 2001;8(4):299-308.

Fieschi M, Dufour JC, Staccini P, Gouvernet J, Bouhaddou O. Medical decision support systems: old dilemmas and new paradigms? *Methods Inf Med.* 2003;42(3):190-198.

Jung E, Li Q, Mangalampalli A, et al. Report central: quality reporting tool in an electronic health record. *AMIA Annu Symp Proc.* 2006:971.

Kaushal R, Shojania KG, Bates DW. Effects of computerized physician order entry and clinical decision support systems on medication safety: a systematic review. *Arch Intern Med.* 2003;163(12):1409-1416.

Schedlbauer A, Prasad V, Mulvaney C, et al. What evidence supports the use of computerized alerts and prompts to improve clinicians' prescribing behavior? *J Am Med Inform Assoc.* 2009;16(4):531-538.

Sittig DF, Wright A, Simonaitis L, et al. The state of the art in clinical knowledge management: an inventory of tools and techniques. *Int J Med Inform.* 2010;79(1):44-57.

The Joint Commission. Safely implementing health information and converging technologies. Sentinel Event Alert, Issue 42; 2008.

Weiner JP, et al. "e-Iatrogenesis": The most critical unintended consequence of CPOE and other HIT. *J Am Med Inform Assoc.* 2007;14(3):387-388.

SECTION 5
Practice Management

CHAPTER 23

Building, Growing and Managing a Hospitalist Practice

Robert A. Bessler, MD

According to the Society of Hospital Medicine, the number of hospitalists has increased from approximately 5,000 hospitalists in 2005 to more than 44,000 hospitalists in 2015. Despite this explosive growth and the fact that the majority of hospitals now have hospitalist programs, not all of them have been successful in establishing a thriving organization that becomes part of the fabric of the hospital. The supply-demand imbalance for hospitalists continues. The etiology for the imbalance is multifactorial. Contributing factors include the small number of medical school graduates pursing hospital medicine continues to be below the market needs and the relative ease of moving from one hospitalist team to another. Couple these factors with the increased level of physician stress secondary to understaffed programs and a continued push on scope of practice with physicians who are younger than those in other specialties and these factors together perpetuate the supply-demand imbalance in the market today. The issues experienced by hospitalists are not unique; other specialties including emergency medicine and critical care have similar challenges with turnover, recruiting physicians and temporary workers.

More emphasis is now placed on the patient experience of care with the introduction of value-based purchasing. There has been a focus on educating patients about the role of hospitalists yet many patients and their families continue to express confusion about the role. It is still common for patients to misconstrue the term "hospitalists" for "hospice." Too often, hospitalists assume patients understand their presence at the bedside. More effort in explaining the role of the hospitalist as the internal medicine physician or family medicine physician who is responsible for patient care while the patient is in the hospital is essential. Once patients understand that the hospitalist is the physician assuming responsibility for everything from admission to discharge, including making patient rounds and ordering all needed tests and procedures it helps them understand why the hospitalist is caring for them. An important component of the dialog is that the patient understands that their primary care provider (PCP) is informed of their progress and resumes care for the patient postdischarge.

With the Centers for Medicare and Medicaid Services moving from a fee-for-service to a fee-for-value payor, the hospitalist takes on an important role in coordination of care with a focus on population health. Today there is a deeper understanding of the importance of managing population health to drive the health of the community that a *health system* serves. Central to this movement is the need for robust measurement systems that enable us to concentrate on the outcomes of a population instead of individual silos within the delivery system. Hospitalists are in unique position to deliver on the Institute of Medicine's "Triple Aim," targeting better health for the population, better quality and patient experience of care while lowering the cost of care. With more than 50% of all health care spending generated from the acute care admission through the 90-day postacute period, the hospitalists team is ideally suited to manage care from the emergency department (ED) to postacute care.

The highest performing hospitalist groups can bring value to the populations they serve through predictable outcomes. Hospitals would benefit from bringing hospitalists into the discussion about population health and overall performance improvement in acute and postacute care management. Many hospital Accountable Care Organizations (ACOs) have not focused on a postacute care strategy, where much of the variability and costs occur in the 90-day period following discharge nor have they recognized the role hospitalists can play in tackling this issue. Improving performance across the acute episode of care is best achieved with a comprehensive hospitalist infrastructure that incorporates physician development, leadership support and incorporation of evidence-based data to measure performance and drive continuous quality improvement. High-performing hospitalist teams that hardwire these elements into their practice will drive performance improvements and grow their practice.

This chapter explores the specific components essential to building, growing, and managing a thriving hospitalist practice with staying power in light of the new fee-for-value environment.

STRATEGIC PLANNING

It is important to have a strategic plan for the practice around growth and the types of hospitals and programs best aligned with agreed upon goals and objectives. For example, strategic planning may require not aligning with all groups requesting support of the hospitalist team. If a group does not fit your strategic profile or geography, it may be best to decline the opportunity to manage a program. Depending on the goals of the practice, certain approaches may not promote patient satisfaction or continuity of care goals. For example, when a hospital simply wants your team to cover admissions during the "off hours" that residents are not covering patients and then transfer patients back to residents or surgeons during "peak hours". These practices work against the goals of improving the patient experience of care and can erode coordination of care. Obstacles of geographic distance requiring a day of travel of the core management team present an additional burden that may make it best to pass up the opportunity to service a hospital if key management team members cannot be present on a regular basis. Each hospitalist group should critically evaluate whether the growth in a new hospital makes sense based on the values and goals of the hospitalist practice, in addition to the hospital seeking hospitalist services.

STRATEGIC PLANNING PROCESS

Before starting a hospitalist practice, determine factors that predict the success or failure. Identify the business and financial motivators required to build, expand, and manage a hospitalist service. These factors should incorporate the needs of the hospital and community the practice it serves.

PRACTICE POINT

The hospitalist practice must start with a strategic planning process.

- *What are the goals of the practice?*
- *What are the needs of the hospital?*
- *How feasible is it to recruit to the location?*
- *What outcomes and metrics are expected by the hospital?*
- *Can the practice commit to the hospital's performance expectations?*

In order to **build** a hospitalist practice, hospital leaders should:

- Define the scope of services.
- Articulate the vision, mission, values, and key value drivers (KVDs) of the practice.
- Establish the employment model and compensation strategy to drive performance.
- Determine the size and cost of the program.

TABLE 23-1 Building a Hospitalist Program: Key Factors to Consider

Characteristics	Examples
Recruiting	• Is the location conducive to recruiting hospitalists? Do they need to recruit a leader?
Compensation plan	• What is the market rate?
Number of encounters/physician	• What is the number of patients at 7 AM census?
	• What total number of patient encounters will physicians manage per day?
	• What is the acuity of patients in the mix?
Schedule	• Is a traditional block schedule feasible?
	• Do you offer additional vacation days?
Management support	• What local support is required?
	• What regional support is required?
Tools to support communications, charge capture, scheduling, metrics	• How will hospitalists record charges?
	• Is there a convenient method to communicate to PCPs?
	• How will you demonstrate improvement in performance?
	• How will the group demonstrate quality?
Clinical processes development	• What best practices does the group adopt?
	• How do the processes impact care?

After a program is up and running, successful practices may be faced with unprecedented **growth**. Hospital leaders will need to:

- Set expectations and priorities for growth.
- Define key stakeholders.
- Plan for growth.
- Assess the evolving needs of the service, such as using advance practitioner providers (NPs and PAs).
- Determine the skills in a hospitalist practice and the need for additional provider training.
- Determine whether the requested skill set of providers by hospital administration coincides with the ability to recruit to the program.
- Reassess the compensation model as the needs of the service change. For example, hospitalists with the skills to provide ICU procedures will cost more per shift than general medical hospitalists.

From the building stage forward, there is a constant need for outstanding **management** to ensure a hospitalist practice thrives by using the steps provided in the following tables: (**Tables 23-1, 23-2,** and **23-3**)

- Define the right leadership and structure.
- Create an ownership mentality.
- Setting up the right processes.
- Tracking and reporting actionable data.
- Provider education focused on leadership excellence and performance management.
- Promoting outreach to the physician community and facilitating transitions of care.

BUILDING A HOSPITALIST PRACTICE

Building a hospitalist practice starts with defining the prospective hospital partner's needs for a hospitalist program. In many community hospitals, a hospitalist program is created to care for

TABLE 23-2 Growing a Hospitalist Program: Core Values and Goals

Characteristics	Examples
Quality	• Measure length of stay • Measure readmissions rate • Measure CMS core measures • Measure time of discharge • Measure case mix index
Satisfaction	• Measure patient satisfaction • Measure nursing satisfaction • Measure PCP satisfaction • Measure specialist satisfaction • Measure administrative staff satisfaction
Efficiency	• Determine how to improve admission and discharge efficiency
Innovation	• What tools can be developed to support the team's core values?
Teamwork	• Determine how the team interacts with monthly and quarterly meetings. • How do you organize in teams? • What is the role of advance practice providers?
Leadership	• Is there a leadership development training path? • Is there a medical director or chief hospitalist on the site? • Are there regional leaders for clinical and business operations?
Financial	• Does the group charge a fee for services? • What are the overhead costs to manage the practice? • Is there a clear return on investment for the hospital to retain services of the group?
Integrity	• What guidance does the team provide to the physicians in the group? • How do we manage the impact of actions, values, methods, measures, principles, expectations, and outcomes of the team? • What criteria are used to assess integrity of candidates?
Research	• Is the group involved in research? • Is there support for data collection and analysis? • What funding is available to the group to support research?
PCP satisfaction	• How does the group measure PCP satisfaction? • Does the group reach out to the PCPs? • How does the group track referrals from PCPs?
Nursing satisfaction	• How does the group measure nursing satisfaction? • Does the group interface with nursing? • How does the group track nursing impact on outcomes?
Specialist satisfaction	• How does the group measure specialist satisfaction? • Does the group reach out to the specialist? • How does the group track referrals from specialists?

TABLE 23-3 Managing a Hospitalist Program: Key Strategies for Effective Management

Characteristics	Examples
Recruiting	• How does the group identify new hires? • Does the group use a recruiting agency?
Overhead	• What percentage of revenue is allocated to support programs (overhead)? • Do costs incorporate utilization of advance practice professionals, nurses, support staff, and locum tenens?
Training	• What allocation of resources does the group have for CME training? • How are new group members trained? • How are leaders mentored?
Growth	• Does the group want to expand? • Is the group capable of taking on additional patients at the primary site?
Service lines	• Does the group focus on acute care contracts with traditional hospitalists? • Does the group provide intensivists services? • Are there other service lines to consider: surgicalists, laborists, academic hospitalists, post-acute care/transitional care?
Improvement strategies	• Where is the group's focus on quality? Efficiency? Satisfaction?

the unassigned patient population. But even the definition of an unassigned patient is subject to much interpretation. For example, at many hospitals in the Puget Sound region of Washington State, an unassigned patient is any patient showing up in the emergency department and requiring admission who does not have a primary care doctor that admits patients at the hospital. In contrast, in Orlando, Florida, an unassigned patient is only defined as a patient who has no primary care doctor. In Orlando, if a patient has a primary care provider but that doctor does not have admitting privileges, it is standard practice to call the primary care provider to identify who will care for the patient in the hospital.

PRACTICE POINT

The *needs assessment*, from the perspective of the hospital might include:

- PCP and/or surgical dissatisfaction
- Admission and management of unassigned patients
- Admission and management of overflow patients due to American College of Graduate Medical Education (ACGME) work hour restrictions
- High inpatient census and long average length of stay (ALOS)
- Low reported performance measures
- External regulation (rapid response teams, code teams, etc)

In addition to covering the unassigned patient population, many hospitalist services cover those primary care providers who do not want the responsibility of admitting their own patients. There are two main forms of coverage relationships: coverage arrangements for 24 hours per day, 7 days per week; and coverage which is more like a house staff model in which the hospitalist admits the patients but then turns the care back over to the PCP the next day. These latter models continue to decline in numbers because of difficulty with

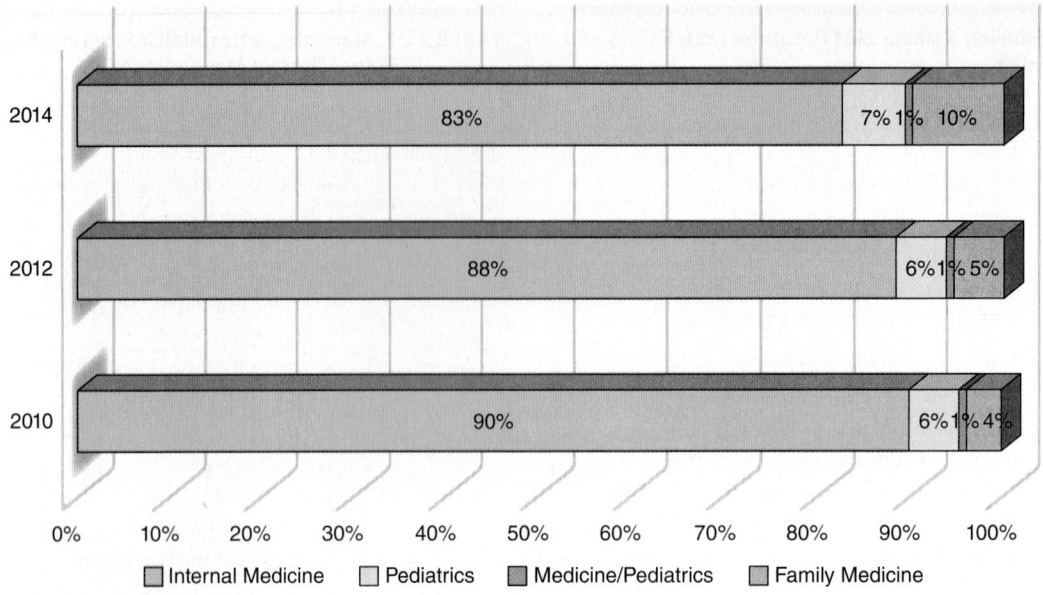

Figure 23-1 *Specialty composition of survey respondents. (Source: 2014 State of Hospital Medicine Report. Reprinted with permission from the Society of Hospital Medicine.)*

recruitment of high-quality providers motivated to build a meaningful career with a resident-type model.

Hospitalist programs may also be created to manage medical specialty and surgical patients, usually after establishment of the initial hospitalist program.

It is essential to determine which patients the hospitalist group will manage, the scope of services, and whether additional training for some of the program members will be required. According to the Medical Group Management Association and Society of Hospital Medicine 2014 State of Hospital Medicine Report ($n = 4867$) (see **Figure 23-1**).

Eighty-three percent of practicing hospitalists are trained in internal medicine, 10% in family medicine, 7% in pediatrics, and 1% in med/peds. Data from the American Medical Group Association ($n = 3700$) report hospitalist training to represent 89% internal medicine, 6% family medicine, 5% pediatrics (did not ask about med/peds). When looking at the combined MGMA (community hospitals) and AMGA (academic hospitals) data, the distribution represents training spanning 80% internal medicine, 8.5% family medicine, 10% peds and 1% med/peds. The general trend represents and increased in hospitalists with family medicine training.

In most community hospitals today, hospitalists manage ICU patients. While there are just over 10,000 intensivist physicians in the United States, there is an increasing demand for critical care services to serve the aging population and extended life expectancy. Although the number of critical care physicians in training has been growing, it will be difficult to meet the patient demand with the rapidly aging population. Research indicates the increased demand creates a shortfall of intensivists equal to 35% by 2020, requiring hospitalists to step in to fill some of the demand. In general, the larger the hospital the less ICU medicine a hospitalist performs. Many hospitals have mandatory ICU consults after a set number of days or hours in the ICU or they provide specific guidelines on managing ventilated patients. The most popular model may be a hybrid arrangement in which access to a critical care physician occurs during the day and for emergencies but in-house at night. In such cases the hospitalist commonly does the work around admissions and daily visits with a consult and a follow-up visit by the pulmonary critical care physicians.

With the labor shortage being even more severe for critical care, hybrid models, along with the advent of telemedicine, are likely to take on even more ICU coverage responsibilities in the future. In general, leapfrog compliance guidelines drive a dedicated intensivist model, typically mandated in regional and tertiary hospitals.

"Code coverage" also defines the scope of the hospitalist practice. Many hospitals provide a separate code team, made up of the emergency medicine physician or in-house intensivist plus respiratory therapy, nurses, technicians, and pharmacists. Increasingly, hospitalists are being asked to partake in responding to the code process and arranging patient transfers to the ICU. In general, emergency physicians have more training and chances to keep their skills sharp around the procedures of a code, including intubation, starting central lines, and transvenous pacing. Typically, while an emergency medicine physician may respond first, a hospitalist with advanced cardiac life support training assumes leadership of the code.

Whether the hospitalist scheduled for the night shift is actually in the hospital or at home on call for emergencies also defines the scope of practice. Hospital-employed and hospital-contracted models tend to have in-house coverage while physicians who are part of a private fee-for-service group without a hospital contract tend to be available as an on-call physician available from home. Variables that impact the decision beyond economics include the volume of cross-coverage patients, the number of admissions per night, coexisting resident coverage, and the response time of the physician, if on call from home.

■ DEFINING THE TYPE OF EMPLOYMENT MODEL

There are several common employment models for hospitalist practices: employed by a private practice, by a hospital, by a multispecialty group, by a health plan/HMO, or a multisite or national practice. Among the multisite or national practice subgroups there are staffing solutions that specialize in emergency medicine, anesthesia, and a host of other physician specialists. Some of these multisite specialty practices will hire hospitalists who work as independent contractors alongside the specialist. Among the national hospitalist groups there is a wide spectrum of employment arrangements ranging from those offering ownership and partnership to those that operate solely with independent contractors.

■ DEFINING THE VISION, MISSION, VALUES, AND KEY VALUE DRIVERS OF YOUR PRACTICE

It is critically important to define the vision, mission and values of the practice from its inception. The leaders and hospitalists should take this task seriously. Schedule time to discuss and debate what is important to the group and leadership. The process of constructing your program's mission and vision statement should not be taken lightly. This process can take weeks to develop. Start by establishing dedicated time and secure an environment that is conducive to having uninterrupted, frank discussions. Enlist the input of all team members.

A **mission statement** explains the overall purpose of the hospitalist practice. The mission statement articulates what the organization does right now, in the most general sense. In this way, the mission also sets parameters for what the organization, through omission, does not do. Example of a mission statement: "The Hospitalist Group of Hilltop builds healthy relationships between St. John's Hospital and primary care providers in the community through public education and direct assistance services."

By comparison, the **vision statement** articulates the future of the organization and the community that it serves. The vision statement, when compared with the current reality of the organization or the community, implies the work still needs to be accomplished. In this way, it lends credibility and motivation to the mission statement. Example of a vision statement: "The Hospitalist Group envisions a group practice that drives improvements in patient outcomes including evidence that reflects our value to hospitals in our community."

On a yearly basis the practice should define key value drivers that articulate the focus of the organization and those areas that require organizational focus in order for the business to grow. Key value drivers (KVDs) should be set by the leaders with input from the entire team. KVDs must be easy to remember, measurable, and achievable. The behaviors that support the key values should also be clearly defined. In doing so, those in the practice will have a clear understanding of expectations even prior to joining the practice. These behaviors should be reinforced through the compensation and promotion practices of the group to make the practice values meaningful and alive on a daily basis. Typically teams evaluate progress on KVDs monthly or quarterly.

■ ESTABLISHING METRICS AND SETTING NEW GOALS FOR PERFORMANCE AND OUTCOMES

Standard outcome metrics including average length of stay, core measures, case mix index, cost per case, and discharge efficiency are expected by hospital administration from the hospitalist group. It is essential to meet with the hospital and obtain agreement on which initiatives the hospitalist team will focus. Establish a data collection and reporting mechanism and the frequency of assessments. Practice metrics that are becoming increasingly important to hospitals include the Healthcare Cost and Utilization Project (called "H-CUP"). HCUP is a set of health care databases, software tools, and products developed through a Federal-State-Industry partnership and sponsored by the Agency for Healthcare Research and Quality. Using the HCUP databases collates data collection from State organizations, hospital associations, private data organizations, and the Federal government creating a national data benchmark.

HCUP databases include the largest collection of longitudinal hospital care data in the United States, with all-payer, encounter-level information going back to 1988. These databases enable evaluation of cost and quality of health services, medical practice patterns, access to health care, and outcomes of treatments at the national, State, and local levels.

In addition to the standard outcome measures and HCUP data, it is useful to track and report other practice related trends, including PCP referral volume and referral patterns, patient satisfaction, physician recruiting efficiency, physician retention and 30-day same diagnosis readmission rates (**Figure 23-2**).

■ MARKETING YOUR HOSPITALIST SERVICES

The best marketing generates word-of-mouth public relations based on how satisfied your patients are as well as the nursing and other hospital staff. An effective campaign requires all hospitalists on the team to be fully engaged with the practice's vision, mission and values.

In addition to the passive marketing that comes from word-of-mouth marketing, it is important to develop a marketing plan. A typical marketing plan for a practice includes initiatives that drive patient satisfaction to generating awareness in the community through PCP outreach. Create a budget that supports the plan.

PRACTICE POINT

Your marketing plan should include segments that target the following areas:

- Identify your target markets: *Decide which target markets you want to canvas. You can either target referrals in specific geographic areas or by targeting outreach to specialists.*
- Develop a public relations plan: *Launch a new program with press releases, open house events, or broadcast the addition to new physicians through flyers or direct mail campaigns.*
- Create a promotion/awareness plan: *You can develop practice-branded written articles on a variety of topics that convey answers to patients' questions using topics such as What is a Hospitalist? or Improving Patient's Health Literacy. Use these in a mailing to your community or have the hospital place your articles in their newsletter. Develop a social media campaign to highlight the culture of your practice to support recruiting and growth efforts.*
- Develop patient satisfaction tools: *Create large, oversized business cards with photos of physicians, hospitalist brochures with photos of engaged, friendly physicians; consider web-based information to share with patients.*
- Create recruiting advertisements for physicians: *Provide your recruiters with materials about the opportunity or special information about the location and hospital. Place them in hospitalist journals as print advertisements and classified ads.*
- Conduct market research: *Conduct market research in your local area to be sure you know what the local market is paying for hospitalists and places they practice and who might be interested in joining your practice in the area.*
- Profile your team: *Utilize a website and direct mail with photography of your team or host an open house or educational event.*
- Develop a social media strategy: *Share the culture of your team to encourage prospective referrals for service and for recruiting.*

■ DESIGNING THE MODEL

It is essential to determine the size of the practice needed. The volume of patients who will be seen on a daily, nightly, and monthly basis determines the size of the practice. Next, assess the number of physicians required to meet the needs of the practice based on that estimated patient volume. The number of physicians depends on what is considered an acceptable workload of patients to manage per day, per night, and per month. To determine the number of patients, define the average number of admissions per day. If the emergency department uses a tracking tool, review the data to project the number of unassigned patients based on historical data. In many hospitals, these data are not accessible prior to initiating a program. Historically, the ward clerks simply entered the admitting physician's name in the hospital information system without mention of the fact that the patient did not have a primary care physician. It is essential to have a way to track the types of patients by referral type (eg, by PCP, unassigned, or consultations) when the hospitalist program begins operation.

Standard Outcome Metrics Site Report

1234—Hospital A
Quarters Range: 2014:Q2 - 2015:Q2

Adjusted LOS % for Medicare, Medical, Regular Patients

2014:Q2 - 2015:Q2					
Target : 95%	2014:Q2	2014:Q3	2014:Q4	2015:Q1	2015:Q2
ALOS Ratio (% HCUP)	72.6%	66.5%	73.3%	72.4%	72.2%
Actual ALOS (days)	2.90	2.77	2.94	3.17	3.08
Expected ALOS (days)	3.99	4.17	4.01	4.38	4.27
Discharges (Regular Inpatient)	107	102	93	136	118

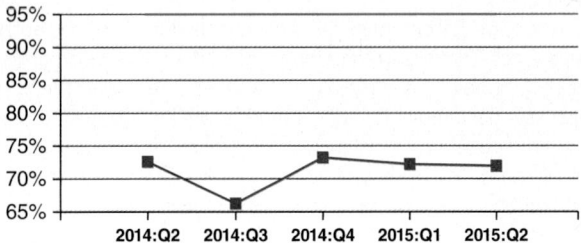

Adjusted CMI % for Medicare, Medical, Regular Patients

2014:Q2 - 2015:Q2					
Target : 102%	2014:Q2	2014:Q3	2014:Q4	2015:Q1	2015:Q2
CMI Ratio (% HCUP)	98.8%	101.5%	100.8%	105.0%	105.8%
Actual CMI	1.01	1.16	1.09	1.16	1.18
Expected CMI	1.02	1.14	1.08	1.11	1.11
Discharges (Regular Inpatient)	107	102	93	136	118

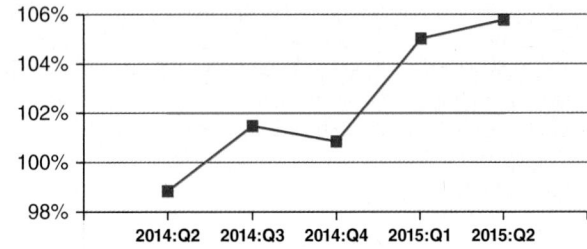

Observation Length of Stay (Hours)

2014:Q2 - 2015:Q2					
	2014:Q2	2014:Q3	2014:Q4	2015:Q1	2015:Q2
Average LOS (Hours)	24.67	19.04	20.81	24.43	28.85
Observation Hours	2911	2171	2705	2981	3318
Discharges (Observation)	118	114	130	122	115

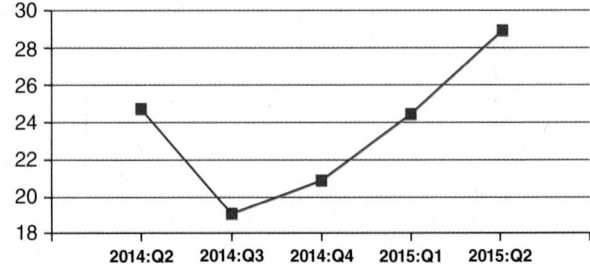

Percentage of Patients with Observation Status

2014:Q2 - 2015:Q2					
	2014:Q2	2014:Q3	2014:Q4	2015:Q1	2015:Q2
Percent	39.5%	41.3%	47.1%	39.7%	37.3%
Observation Discharges	118	114	130	122	115
Discharges (Inpatient and Observation)	299	276	276	307	308

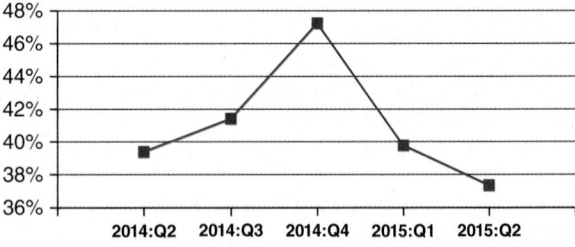

Figure 23-2 *A dashboard of standard outcome metrics organized by volume of patients, quality, utilization, satisfaction trend, and market data indicators including evaluating performance to HCUP data.*

In addition to determining the volume of unassigned patients, estimate the number of PCPs interested in turning over care. The only risk of double counting is if no hospitalist program existed before a new program starting up. Typically, in that scenario, the primary care provider was also likely cover unassigned patients.

After determining the number of admissions per year, divide the admissions by 365 days per year to obtain a rough estimate of the number of physicians required. Then take the average length of stay for the patients and add 1 extra for the day of discharge. Take this number and multiply it by the number of admissions per day to determine the 7:00 AM census. For example, if there are five admissions per day with an average 4-day length of stay, the 7:00 AM census would be calculated as 5 × (4 ALOS + 1) = 25 patients at 7:00 AM. With the 7:00 AM

census determined, calculate the number of the physicians per morning required for the hospitalist program.

There is much debate over the most appropriate census for the physician who begins rounding at 7:00 AM. In general, based on a typical mix of a few ICU patients and the balance of the load being medical patients, a hospitalist can manage 15 patients safely and efficiently. This number varies considerably due to the different agendas, acuity of patients, concomitant responsibilities such as rapid response teams, code teams, teaching, and goals of practices. To achieve the objectives of early discharge, multiple visits a day and a considerable amount of committee involvement, hospitalists can maintain a census in the range of 14 to 15 patients. If the goal is productivity, and in some cases the use of advanced practitioner providers (APPs), the

Standard Outcome Metrics Site Report

1234—Hospital A
Quarters Range: 2014:Q2 - 2015:Q2

Readmission Rate for Medicare, Medical, Regular Patients

2014:Q2 - 2015:Q2					
Target : 9.5%	2014:Q2	2014:Q3	2014:Q4	2015:Q1	2015:Q2
Achieved	15.9%	9.8%	9.7%	5.9%	5.9%
Discharges (Regular Inpatient)	107	102	93	136	118

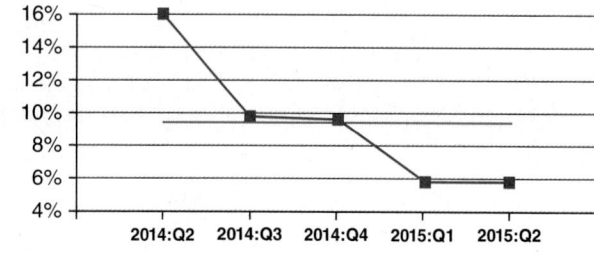

Adjusted Mortality Rate for Medicare, Medical, Regular Patients (Rolling Avg)

2014:Q2 - 2015:Q2					
Target : 90%	2014:Q2	2014:Q3	2014:Q4	2015:Q1	2015:Q2
Mortality Ratio (% HCUP)	54.3%	46.3%	35.6%	13.5%	25.2%
Actual Mortality	1.21	1.20	0.93	0.46	0.89
Expected Mortality	2.23	2.59	2.62	3.39	3.54
Discharges (Regular Inpatient)	330	418	430	438	449

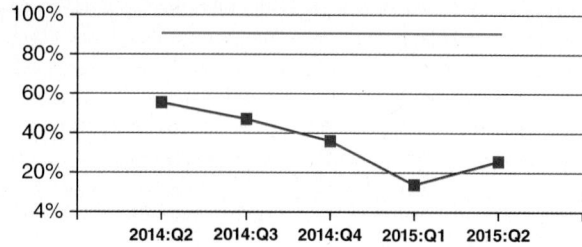

Quality Measures

2014:Q2 - 2015:Q2					
Target : 100%	2014:Q2	2014:Q3	2014:Q4	2015:Q1	2015:Q2
Achieved	ND	98.7%	100.0%	100.0%	100.0%
Total Responses	ND	154	78	55	43

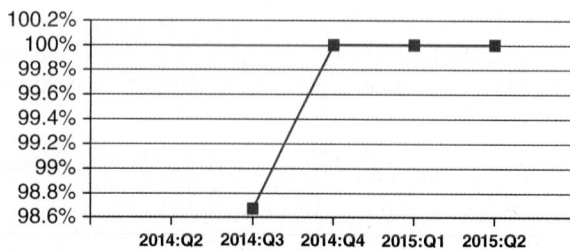

HCAHPS Physician Communication TOP Box %

2014:Q2 - 2015:Q2					
Target : 80%	2014:Q2	2014:Q3	2014:Q4	2015:Q1	2015:Q2
Achieved	82.0%	73.1%	78.6%	79.2%	83.3%
Total Responses	167	78	28	48	48

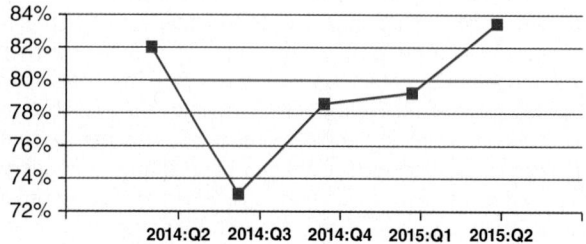

Figure 23-2 *(Continued)*

volume per hospitalist may be as high as 20 patients per day. Some practices define the census as the number of encounters per day, which include new admissions as well as discharges.

In a pure productivity-driven private practice model, the night shifts are often covered from home (eg, only coming back to the hospital for emergencies). This typically also means that the day-shift doctors might share night call, even after working all day. In many practices today, the night shift is covered by a separate physician, a nocturnist, due to the volume of admissions at night and the volume of cross-cover work needed.

In general, the billing revenue of a nocturnist hospitalist is lower than a day-shift hospitalist.

A highly prevalent hospital-employed and national group practice model includes a schedule in which the hospitalist physician is on duty for 12 hours, 7 days a week and the following week the

physicians is off for 7 days. There are also hybrid arrangements in which the physician works about the same total number of hours per month but with shorter periods of time on duty. In such a model, a 7:00 AM census of 25 to 30 patients would likely have six full-time physicians. In contrast, a private group model may take every fourth night of call from home, which could be managed with four full-time physicians on the team. The marketplace supply and demand for physicians and goals of various clients (eg, a hospital, HMO, or payor) often dictates the type of model required.

■ DETERMINING THE COST AND DIRECT COST OF THE HOSPITALIST PROGRAM

Calculating the cost of a hospitalist program includes direct labor costs: salaries of the providers, benefits cost, malpractice coverage, and billing costs. The volume of patient visits, the payer mix, and the distribution of CPT codes reported determine the direct patient care revenues of the practice. The medical director who typically has responsibility for driving hospital outcomes determines any additional revenues. According to a survey conducted by the Society of Hospital Medicine in 2014, 89.3% of hospitalist programs required a subsidy or fee to help with the payer mix of the unassigned patients, night call coverage in-house, and for those organizations that focus on driving performance through service offerings. The ranges of fees hospitals pay range from $0 per year to $250,000 per physician annually. Fees are typically based on scope of work and payer mix.

■ SETTING THE COMPENSATION MODEL

In conjunction with determining the cost of the program, a compensation model must be established. In the past decade, two significant challenges drove hospitalist compensation: an imbalance of supply and demand, coupled with the rapid rise of salaries that began escalating in 2001. This phenomenon has created a significant compression in salaries. Often the least experienced physician's compensation is closely aligned with the most experienced physicians in the practice. This compensation compression creates a dichotomy in the reward system on physician skill and experience levels creating challenging team dynamics. There are two primary models: a productivity model or a salary model. Many salary models also include a component of compensation focused on productivity and quality metrics as well as outcomes.

Recruiting a team of physicians and hiring a leader is a critical core competency for every hospitalist practice as discussed in Chapter 25. Acquiring effective recruiting techniques is an area of investment that should not be minimized or overlooked in the development of a strong hospitalist practice.

GROWING A HOSPITALIST PRACTICE

■ SETTING PRIORITIES FOR GROWTH

Once the practice launches, priorities must be established for the growth of the hospitalist program. If the unassigned patients are already covered in the practice, the next step could be a myriad of other opportunities, including contracting with PCP practices. It is essential to understand the scope of growth and prepare in advance of the patients' arrival. Many practices have failed or imploded by taking on more growth than they could handle. If there is a desire to handle 15 more patients per day with a 7 days on/7 days off model, it might be as simple as figuring out the need to hire two more physicians. However, if the program is already quite busy and adding three to four new admissions per day is in the growth plan, adding an admitting shift may be called for as well.

PRACTICE POINT

Use these common areas of practice management and determine whether you are prepared to grow.

Reflect about your hospitalist practice:

- What are your priorities?
- What are your goals and core values?
- What effort can you invest to grow?

What are the expectations of external interests?

- Performance measures.
- Satisfaction of outside primary care physician groups.
- The Joint Commission requirements.

- ACGME.
- Public performance reporting, obtaining ≥ 90% core measure scores.

What is your work environment saying about the practice?

- Patient safety, quality, satisfaction.
- Efficiency of care.
- Career satisfaction that integrates core values.
- Service excellence and patient safety.
- Continuous quality improvement and innovation.
- Professional growth, leadership, and scholarship.

What are the expectations of hospital management?

- Caring for unassigned/uncompensated patients.
- Reducing ALOS for top 10 DRGs by hospitalist discharge volume.
- 24/7 service demands.
- Reducing practice variation of hospitalists.
- Hospitalist training on palliative care, end-of-life, and other medical specialties.
- Development of a comanagement consulting service or a preoperative testing center.
- Improvement of patient ED to floor times.
- Care of admitted patients in the ED.
- Managing the chest pain unit or rapid admission team.
- Improvement of chart documentation for core measures (such as smoking cessation counseling).
- Improvement of billing for services provided.
- Leadership of rapid response teams for ill inpatients.
- Development of a transitional care program to address continuity of care in postacute facilities or providing care in the patient's home.

Does the practice have these evaluations and measurements in place?

- Report card for hospitalists.
- Primary care physician survey.
- Multiyear strategic planning, quarterly reports.
- Hospitalist career satisfaction survey.
- Hospitalist annual retreat with management to establish goals.
- Develop a 3-year plan for a hospitalist service that mirrors the hospital's multiyear plan.
- Create a meaningful, motivating, and achievable blueprint for clinical enterprise.
- Proactively support mission of patient care, quality improvement, and patient-centered care.

■ DEFINING KEY STAKEHOLDERS

The key stakeholders in the practice need to be clearly defined. Certainly, the doctors and advanced practice team members in the practice are key stakeholders, but in many practices the hospital administration is also a key stakeholder. Identifying priorities is much like a game of chess. For example, if you choose to help solve another primary care group's needs before helping the orthopedic group with comanagement needs there may be repercussions. You should expect that the hospital administrator want to weigh in on how this decision impacts the hospital and its development plans.

■ INCORPORATING ADVANCED PRACTITIONER PROVIDERS

Another key decision for program growth is how to incorporate advanced practice providers in the practice. While this topic is covered in the literature, there are plenty of mixed opinions on the use of advanced practice providers in the inpatient setting. We have found two main areas of optimal benefit in our practices.

The first benefit for incorporating nurse practitioners (NPs) and physician assistants (PAs) is in very small programs of four full-time physicians with a daily census that can have dramatic swings around the average. The cost of an NP or PA provider is about one-half the labor cost of a physician, and this can be a cost-effective way to leverage the existing physician coverage.

There is also a benefit from the use of advanced practice providers (APPs) in very large programs, particularly in the management of surgical patients for their comorbid conditions. Many practices have incorporated APPs due to the physician shortage and a failure to recruit and retain high-quality physicians. One unique challenge is that many APP's value comes from their experience. An APP practicing in the acute care setting for 10 years is much more likely to be able to function as a hospitalist than a new graduate APP. For hospitalist physicians, there is clearly value and competency in new a physician starting to work directly upon completing their training. It is crucial to understand both the state and hospital-specific by-laws associated with the use of NPs and PAs. Without such understanding, the proposed program plan could be rejected by the hospital. For example, if the rules state that the NPs' work must be signed off and reviewed by a hospitalist it does not create the same workforce multiplier as a site where on the right patients, the NP can operate relatively independently.

▪ TYPES OF PHYSICIANS IN THE PRACTICE

Another area of importance in growing a hospitalist practice involves the types of physicians utilized. It is becoming more common to have family medicine-trained hospitalists practicing alongside internal medicine hospitalists in the same practice. Much has been debated on this topic and today nearly 10% of hospitalists nationwide are family medicine trained. Factors that go into the determination to hire them include their comfort level with ICU patients and their experience managing the higher-level acuity patients. Another challenge is their ability to navigate the local politics associated with an internal medicine outpatient practice referring its inpatient practice to a family medicine physician. We have found that the experience of the provider trumps all board certification. There are plenty of internal medicine physicians unqualified to practice as hospitalists as well.

▪ THE PROS AND CONS OF CAPS ON SERVICES

During the hospitalist practice growth phase, the group must be able to handle all of the new patients it agreed to accept or have a Plan B. Plan B might include a floodgate that closes in the form of a cap. This has been achieved at some hospitals to maintain safe and effective volumes. Two types of caps exist including those requiring a backup system. The backup system can be the existing hospitalists at a very high labor cost to a hospital or the new group of primary care physicians who have asked for coverage; this group may need to agree to provide occasional coverage at the hospital. The latter group of physicians tends to be a short-term patch; they can quickly lose their skills and credentialing in the inpatient setting. Ideally, if the hospitalist group has agreed to accept a new group of patients, they need to have the capacity 24 hours per day, 7 days per week. A "sick call" rotation to cover anticipated maternity and paternity leaves as well as unexpected absences may have the benefit of allowing hospitalists to focus on career development, especially quality improvement initiatives when they are not seeing patients, and not overwhelming them with service obligations.

MANAGING THE HOSPITALIST PRACTICE

▪ SELECTING THE RIGHT LEADERSHIP AND STRUCTURE

There is a shortage of high-quality physician leaders in the United States. To properly manage the practice, it is critical to appoint the most capable physician leader and establish an effective practice structure. The hospitalist leaders' roles are complex; they not only serve the hospitalists' team but also play significant roles within the hospital. In these roles, hospitalist directors are the most connected to how things work on a daily basis. Strong hospitalist physician leaders must lead by example. They must have effective organizational skills, be great communicators, and seek win-win situations for the hospitalist team, medical staff, and hospital. Hospitalist leaders also need to be aware of the professional goals of their members and delegate some responsibilities so that each member can also flourish and find a professional niche within the organization. Hospitalist directors may become isolated in their role, so it is important to ensure that they have advocates or mentors who can promote their agendas as well as provide counseling related to hospital politics. See Chapter 6: Leadership.

Many hospitalist programs include a version of shift work. This type of schedule combined with the Generation Y culture in medical school today, *centered on work hours and patient volume restrictions,* have led to a unique challenge in hospital medicine. Many physicians seek direct employment models. They place a very high level of value for time off. This can make it challenging to engage them in what matters to make a practice successful. Ensuring the right fit begins with the initial interview when performance expectations are clearly articulated.

▪ CREATING AN OWNERSHIP MENTALITY

Like any small business, an ownership mentality is essential to the success of the hospitalist practice. It is ideal to introduce the importance of the ownership mentality expected during the hiring process. Those applicants who give solid examples of times in their career where they got involved, highlight scenarios when they did things because they thought no one else could do it better, and are passionate about those experiences is telling of their potential. These are typically indicators that the physician is the type of hospitalist who can make the practice excel. Defining the behaviors that support the values of the practice and then evaluating and rewarding those behaviors goes a long way to reinforcing what is important. For example, if participating in hospitalist committees is important and it can be rewarded as part of how the productivity dollars are allotted. Leading a hospital committee or playing a leadership role within the medical staff could be rewarded to an even greater extent.

▪ SETTING UP THE RIGHT PROCESSES

Part of managing the practice is ensuring that the right processes are in place. Processes should be established for physician scheduling and daily case management meetings. Hospitalist processes should be highly sophisticated to drive improvements in utilization, documentation, discharge planning, and prospective quality metric monitoring. All of these processes require a tremendous amount of time, energy, and in many cases, technology and infrastructure to drive clinical and financial performance for the hospital and hospitalist practice. The scope of processes is beyond the scope of this chapter, but this is a core competency that should not be overlooked in the management of an effective hospitalist program. Hospitalist leaders can promote simple solutions that make it easy for clinicians to communicate at transition points such as setting up dedicated phone lines in primary care practices so that the hospitalists do not waste valuable time trying to reach PCPs. Delegating postdischarge phone calls to hospitalist nurses, APPs or case managers helps create capacity for the hospitalist team.

■ THE VALUE OF DATA TRACKING AND REPORTING

The well-known saying "you can't manage what you don't measure" is quite true in hospital medicine. It is essential to define what is relevant to the practice and measure outcomes that matter most. Many hospitalist teams require sophisticated technology solutions and partnerships with the hospital to obtain data. Benchmarking performance and then creating an action plan to improve upon areas is an effective approach. Evaluating performance on a monthly and quarterly basis is a best practice.

Metrics that matter on the revenue side of the equation include:

- Volume
- Work RVUs total
- Work RVU/CPT code
- Payer mix
- Collections per encounter (accrued)
- Charges
- Collections per month
- Readmissions

On the labor cost side of the equation, there are a myriad of labor cost metrics. However, cost per shift is a commonly used metric that helps to manage the performance of the practice, inclusive of benefits for the providers.

Outside of financial performance of the practice, there exist three main areas of performance monitoring: quality, utilization, and satisfaction.

For quality, most practices manage core measure performance and readmission rates. In 2016, most hospitals face 30-day readmissions penalties. According to Modern Healthcare's analysis of the CMS data, 38 out of 3,400 hospitals will be subject to the maximum 3% reduction in reimbursement. This requires added focus and processes to address the issues, as the etiology surrounding readmissions is so multifactorial. Mortality and complication rates have an added importance in the years ahead as well.

Utilization is a challenge for the average practice without a deep investment in infrastructure. Discharge order time by physician and utilization of the follow-up CPT codes to discharge codes are other significant measures of throughput for the average hospitalist. The more follow-up visits a doctor has within a group compared to the same number of discharges of his or her peers could indicate the physician holds on to patients longer. Clearly, to be statistically valid, a large enough sample size will be needed to compare to peers. Other important metrics include cost per case by major DRG group.

The third pillar of a high-quality hospitalist program is to measure satisfaction. Patient, PCP, nurse, and hospital administration satisfaction are key areas to track. Surveys and call centers are effective tools to monitor and analyze performance and test the effectiveness of improvement initiatives.

By identifying the parameters for measurement, any hospitalist service can develop a hospitalist scorecard to clarify the vision and strategy of the service by gaining consensus regarding what will be measured and reported. The scorecard requires setting targets, aligning strategic initiatives, allocating resources, and establishing milestones. Once these goals are set, a process of communication and education of the members of the service must take place about the goals and linking rewards to performance measures. There are pitfalls relating compensation to quality of care if the candidate measure is not attainable or if the performance measure link to flawed data. Computer-generated data is much easier to obtain

than chart review but is often based on the discharging physician, which may or may not reflect an individual's performance. Supplemented with primary care satisfaction data and chart review of key quality indicators (eg, transfers to intensive care units and/or readmissions) the hospitalist service can initiate rapid cycle improvements and educational initiatives. The impact of initiatives may be tracked over time.

■ PHYSICIAN OUTREACH TO THE COMMUNITY OF PHYSICIANS

A successful practice ideally includes the community of physicians raving about the hospitalist group they partner with for their inpatient coverage. Many practices have imploded by not building relationships with the community of primary care providers and specialists. An outreach plan and daily communication on shared patients are essential to building the bridges necessary to the medical staff. Nothing is more important to this communication than a phone call at discharge linking the patient back to the community physician and, as a bonus, having the opportunity for the hospitalist to let the community doctor know what a great job he or she did for the patient during the hospitalization. Faxing, electronic messaging through an EMR, or e-mailing in an HIPAA-compliant way all of the necessary information on discharge is also an essential element to this process.

■ TRANSITIONS OF CARE BACK TO THE COMMUNITY

With the advent of the focus on transitions in care in the bundled payment care improvement program from CMS, it is now essential to link the inpatient hospitalization to the continuum of care in the postacute environment—including home care for those patients at highest risk for readmissions. Many successful practices are already on the forefront of this by placing partner physicians in these facilities on the same hospitalist platform as their acute care partners. It is essential to have clear and deliberate handoff plans and processes in place, especially if the patient's next site of care is not home. The goal is to get patients home and stay home for as long as possible.

■ INTEGRATION TO THE POSTACUTE PHYSICIAN

Finally, for those patients discharged from the hospital back to their home, it is essential that the hospitalist ensures a smooth transition. The window of time from when patients are discharged from acute care until they have a follow-up visit with their PCP is an especially risky timeframe for adverse outcomes and readmissions. Instituting a patient callback program or having a team that has a plan to check on patients postdischarge, having a way to track this data and teams that communicate along the care pathway is a necessary and essential part of care for a high-quality hospitalist program.

CONCLUSION

The creation of new hospitalist practices is likely to continue in the coming decade with the changes forthcoming in our health care delivery system. Building, growing, and managing a successful and thriving hospitalist practice is possible by focusing on the essential elements outlined in this chapter.

SUGGESTED READINGS

Dye CF. *Leadership in Healthcare: Essential Values and Skills*. Chicago, IL: Health Administration Press; 2010.

Kaufman KP. *Best Practice Financial Management: Six Key Concepts for Healthcare Leaders*. Chicago, IL: Health Administration Press; 2006.

Lee BD, Herring JW. *Growing Leaders in Healthcare: Lessons from the Corporate World*. Health Administration Press. Chicago, IL: Health Administration Press; 2009.

Levoy B. *222 Secrets of Hiring, Managing, and Retaining Great Employees in Healthcare Practices*. Sudbury, MA: Jones and Bartlett Publishers; 2006.

Maccoby M. *Leaders We Need: And What Makes Us Follow*. Boston, MA: Harvard Business School Publishing; 2007.

Murphy S. *Building and Rewarding Your Team: A How-To Guide for Medical Practices*. Englewood, CO: MGMA; 2008.

Nemeth C. *Improving Healthcare Team Communication*. Burlington, VT: Ashgate Publishing; 2008.

Simone KG. *Hospitalist Recruitment and Retention: Building a Hospital Medicine Program*. Hoboken, NJ: Wiley-Blackwell; 2009.

Zahaluk DW. *The Ultimate Practice Building Book: How To Regain Control Of Your Practice, Achieve A Competitive Advantage In Your Local Market, And Reconnect With The Joy Of Medicine In The New Healthcare Economy*. Bloomington, IN: Trafford Publishing; 2007.

ONLINE RESOURCES

Gummadi S, Geyer C, Rossi C. *Employment Opportunities for Hospitalists Trained in Family Medicine [abstract]. J Hosp Med.* 2014;9(suppl 2). http://www.shmabstracts.com/abstract/employment-opportunities-for-hospitalists-trained-in-family-medicine/. Accessed June 1, 2015.

ICU staffing shortages linked to aging population. ATS Bulletin. http://ats-365.ascendeventmedia.com/highlight.aspx?id=1135&p=45. Accessed December 1, 2011.

US Department of Health and Human Services, Health Resources and Services Administration Report to Congress. *The Critical Care Workforce: A Study of the Supply and Demand for Critical Care Physicians*. http://bhpr.hrsa.gov/healthworkforce/reports/studycriticalcarephys.pdf. Accessed May, 2006.

CHAPTER 24

Best Practices in Physician Recruitment and Retention

Steven B. Deitelzweig, MD, MMM
R. Kirk Mathews, MBA
John Nelson, MD, MHM
Society of Hospital Medicine Key
Characteristics Workgroup[1]

According to the Society of Hospital Medicine (SHM), more than 44,000 clinicians have chosen hospital medicine for their career, approximately 40% of hospitalists are employed directly by hospitals, and the practice of hospital medicine is the fastest growing medical specialty, growing at a rate of 5% to 10% annually.

Because of the strong demand for hospitalists, recruiting competition is fierce. Consequently, hospitalist practices must view recruiting and retention as core competencies. This chapter provides best practices and key principles for recruiting and retaining qualified hospitalists.

In addition to updated information provided by Kirk Mathews and Dr. John Nelson, this chapter includes information from the 10 Key Principles and Characteristics of an Effective Hospital Medicine Group developed by the SHM Key Characteristics Workgroup. The 10 key principles are effective leadership, engaged hospitalists, adequate resources, effective planning and management infrastructure, alignment with hospital and/or health system, support of care coordination across the care setting, taking a leadership role in clinical issues, scope of clinical activities, a patient/family-centered, team-based model, and recruitment and retention of qualified clinicians. While all of these principles are important aspects of a successful group, this chapter focuses primarily on the 10 characteristics that support Principle 10—recruitment and retention: sourcing and recruiting candidates who are committed to a career in hospital medicine and who are board certified or board eligible, developing a good orientation program, providing resources for professional growth, paying competitive compensation, ensuring that employment agreements are valid and fair, measuring job satisfaction, and monitoring clinical competency and professionalism.

SOURCING AND RECRUITING CANDIDATES

The sourcing and recruitment process consists of seven steps:

1. Preparing a job description
2. Defining the profile of a quality candidate
3. Finding candidates
4. Managing the application process
5. Interviewing candidates
6. Making selection decisions
7. Extending job offers

■ 1. PREPARING A JOB DESCRIPTION

A good job description can help attract the right candidates, create appropriate expectations, assist in evaluating employee performance, and more. A well-written job description will contain the following elements:

- Position title
- Department
- Reports to
- Overall responsibility
- Key areas of responsibility
- Terms of employment
- Qualifications and credentials

[1]Members of the Society of Hospital Medicine Key Characteristics Workgroup are Patrick Cawley, MD, Steven Deitelzweig, MD, Leslie Flores, MHA, Joseph Miller, MS, John Nelson, MD, Scott Rissmiller, MD, Laurence Wellikson, MD, and Winthrop Whitcomb, MD.

When preparing a job description, it can also be useful to reflect upon the group's culture and include candidate characteristics that are compatible with that culture in the qualifications section. For example, if the group functions in a very team-oriented manner, an otherwise "perfect" candidate who strongly prefers to work autonomously and avoid team meetings would not be a good fit.

A good job description is not just a laundry list of responsibilities. It should reflect the culture, mission, and priorities of the group. It should be reviewed and updated for each hire so it reflects the group's current situation and goals.

Finally, the job description must avoid any reference to race, color, religion, age, gender, national origin, nationality, or physical or mental disability as such references are illegal.

2. DEFINING THE PROFILE OF A QUALITY CANDIDATE

Every good candidate sourcing strategy begins with the establishment of candidate parameters, including training requirements (MD, DO, internal medicine, family practice, etc), board certification, and a commitment to a career in hospital medicine.

- **Training Requirements:** Practice leaders must have a good understanding of their customers—the referring physicians—when establishing candidate training requirements. For example, the decision to hire family practice physicians as hospitalists should only be made with the approval of the referring medical staff.
- **Board Certification:** All full-time and regular part-time hospitalists should be board certified or board eligible in an applicable medical specialty or subspecialty. Certification by a medical specialty board has become an accepted structural measure of physician quality and competence. In the United States, 24 medical specialty boards certify physicians in various specialties and subspecialties. To become board certified, a physician must receive supervised, in-practice training for several years after medical school. In addition, specialty boards require passage of a written exam. The exams are intended to assess medical knowledge and clinical judgment.

  Medical board certifications are time limited, typically for 10 years. Doctors whose certificates are time limited must successfully complete recertification requirements under a program called Maintenance of Certification (MOC). The policy of the American Board of Medical Specialties states that "maintenance of competence should be demonstrated throughout the physician's career by evidence of lifelong learning and ongoing improvement of practice." Each specialty board is implementing this policy in its own way, but all are committed to a program that requires that the physician to do the following:

  - Maintain a license in good standing with state licensing boards
  - Periodically do surveys of patients and of peers
  - Periodically show evidence of knowledge and judgment
  - Show evidence of a commitment to lifelong learning and involvement in a periodic self-assessment process
  - Periodically show evidence of self-evaluation of performance in practice

- **Commitment to Hospital Medicine:** To maintain the stability of the practice, a significant proportion of the full-time hospitalists in the group should demonstrate a commitment to a career in hospital medicine. A hospitalist can demonstrate a commitment to a career in the specialty in several ways:

  - Participate in specialty professional activities. The SHM is the professional society for hospitalists. A hospitalist can join SHM and take advantage of the educational programs, resources, and meetings and/or seek a leadership role at SHM through participation in committees, task forces, and/or the board of directors. Alternatively, a hospitalist could participate in other regional or national activities in which there is interaction with hospitalist peers on issues/topics relevant to the specialty.
  - Become a Fellow in Hospital Medicine. SHM established the Fellowship in Hospital Medicine program to recognize hospitalists who have committed to the specialty. The three levels of recognition are Fellows, Senior Fellows, and Masters. Criteria include 5 years as a practicing hospitalist, no disciplinary action that resulted in the suspension/revocation of credentials or license, and endorsement by two active SHM members. Additional criteria are the demonstration of personal dedication in any or all of the following: teamwork, quality improvement, and leadership.
  - Earn the Focused Practice in Hospital Medicine MOC Credits. The American Board of Internal Medicine and the American Board of Family Medicine established the Focused Practice in Hospital Medicine (FPHM) program as part of their MOC processes. The FPHM program "assesses, recognizes and sets standards for the specific knowledge, skills and attitudes of general internists who focus their practice in the care of hospitalized patients." The FPHM MOC program does not result in a subspecialty designation; it recognizes internal medicine and family medicine physicians who practice as hospitalists.

3. FINDING CANDIDATES

One of the most important recruiting principles is to ensure that the group's hospitalists are actively engaged in sourcing and recruiting new group members. Involving the staff hospitalists with the sourcing and recruitment of new physicians can be valuable for several reasons:

- They might be able to identify good sources of candidates.
- The common identity and engagement of the group's hospitalists are reinforced as they seek to identify and recruit physicians who would be a good fit with their practice.
- Physician candidates are well informed about the position because they meet their potential colleagues in person and can get an honest perspective on what it would be like to work in the group.
- Both parties, the hospitalists in the group and the physician candidates, can make informed decisions.

A candidate sourcing plan is similar to an investment portfolio—diversity is good. In addition to recommendations from staff hospitalists, the following recruitment strategies and tools can help practices identify candidates.

- **Existing Medical Staff:** Asking medical staff leadership to suggest staff physicians who might be good candidates could yield good results. Leaders are likely to know which physicians are the best clinicians and who might be thinking about changing their practice situation.
- **Medical Staff Referrals:** Newly trained physicians will be aware of physicians behind them in the next graduating class, and recently relocated experienced physicians will know former colleagues who might be good candidates. Some employers offer a financial incentive for candidates hired as a result of a medical staff referral.
- **Residency Program Relationships:** Establishing relationships with the program directors of residency programs within 200 miles can yield outstanding low-cost results. Offering to provide a noon lecture or some other resource to the program director can be an excellent way to begin to develop the relationship and to gain exposure to the residents. This exposure—even exposure to first- and second-year residents—is valuable for future recruiting.

- **Other Local/Regional Hospitals:** Recruiting physicians from other local hospitals can be effective because these physicians have already decided to live in the area. If the hospital is a friendly competitor or a patient referral source, political and/or business caution is advised.
- **Online Hospitalist Job Boards:** Because candidates do most of their job investigations online, online job boards are an important recruiting tool. The SHM Career Center (www.hospitalmedicine.org/careercenter) is an excellent candidate sourcing tool. Other popular job boards are hospitalistjobs.com, practicelink.com, jobs.todayshospitalist.com, nejmcareer-center.org, and jama.careers.adicio.com.
- **Journal Advertising:** Journal ads should be eye-catching and brief and should prompt the candidate to take action—either place a phone call or visit a website to learn more. Many medical journals also offer online job boards.
- **Direct Mail:** Because direct mail campaigns usually generate a very low return, an inexpensive and colorful postcard is the most cost-effective tool, and purchasing a very targeted mailing list is necessary.
- **Career Fairs:** Career fairs are designed to give second- and third-year residents exposure to various employers and to give employers the opportunity to begin recruiting relationships with candidates. Career fairs are most effective if they are within relatively close geographic proximity of the practice.

PRACTICE POINT

- One of the most important recruiting principles is to ensure that the group's hospitalists are actively engaged in sourcing and recruiting new group members.

- **Recruitment Firms:** Some groups use recruitment firms to extend their reach on difficult-to-fill searches. Contingency-based companies only charge a fee if they are successful. Although using a contingency-based company is a risk-free approach, contingency recruiters may shop marketable candidates to a variety of potential employers with no real obligation to any of those employers. Retained recruiting firms typically charge a monthly fee in return for their efforts to fill a position. However, retained firms rarely offer a guarantee of success, so the employer takes the risk of making a significant investment without successfully hiring a candidate. Both types of firms can and do produce results, but before signing a contract, employers thinking of using a recruitment firm should first establish a relationship with the recruiter who would be assigned to their search and make sure they have an acceptable level of comfort with the recruiter's approach.

■ 4. MANAGING THE APPLICATION PROCESS

PRACTICE POINT

- The most important aspect of managing the application process is to make every effort to thoroughly assess key aspects of each candidate prior to extending an invitation for an onsite visit.

Because onsite interviews are time consuming and expensive, properly managing the application process is imperative. The most important aspect of managing the process is to make every effort to thoroughly assess key aspects of each candidate prior to an onsite

visit. Performing this kind of in-depth assessment before extending an interview invitation will minimize the possibility of learning something about the candidate during the onsite interview that will eliminate him/her from consideration.

This approach to recruiting is foreign to most employers but is best illustrated by considering how major universities recruit their star athletes. College coaches never invite athletes to visit their campus for official recruiting visits before they thoroughly assess them. College coaches watch hours of game films of the prospective recruit. They interview the candidate by phone. They interview the recruit's high school coach, guidance counselor, and sometimes even the girlfriend or boyfriend! Only after they are convinced the athlete is someone they want to recruit do they invite him/her to campus for the official visit. During the visit, the recruit will briefly visit face to face with the head coach, and the rest of the visit is organized to convince the athlete that his/her athletic and academic goals can be achieved at that university.

To bring this same level of thoroughness to the hiring process for a hospitalist, here are the aspects of each candidate that must be assessed prior to an onsite visit:

- **Training and Clinical Skills:** Identify and question any gaps in the candidate's training. Most candidates will be able to provide a thorough explanation for gaps in their training and/or work history without difficulty, but employers should verify the candidate's explanation whenever possible. Also verify that the candidate has the skills (including any procedural skills) required for the practice.
- **Prior Work Experience:** Discuss all prior work experiences with the candidate. Asking the candidate about the reasons for terminating each employment relationship can uncover a pattern of discontent or employer dissatisfaction.
- **Communication Skills:** Good verbal communication skills are critical for a hospitalist. Many employers make the mistake of talking too much when assessing a candidate. Set the stage with a question and then allow the candidate to speak as long as s/he wishes.
- **Work Ethic and Workplace Attitude:** The following questions can help determine a candidate's work ethic and workplace attitude:
  - How many patients do you feel you can comfortably see in one day?
  - Describe a situation where you felt overworked.
  - How hard do you like to work?
  - When do you typically begin your workday?
  - Describe a time when you were asked to work overtime without compensation.
  - Describe any volunteer work that you have performed including outside the field of medicine.
  - What personal gratification do you get from your work?
- **References:** The process of checking references has become less valuable because employers and program directors fear legal recourse if they provide a negative report. However, because checking references is a required element of any recruitment, here are tips to enhance the process:
  - Ask for specific references. Employers should always ask to speak with the candidate's supervisor or residency program director. Other potentially valuable references are hospital administrators, referring physicians, unit nurses, and ED physicians who have worked with the candidate.
  - Speak directly with the reference whenever possible. Much can be gained from listening carefully when the reference is questioned. Pregnant pauses and voice inflections can speak volumes about what that person believes about the candidate.

- Describe the practice. Employers should describe their practice and ask how the candidate might perform in such a practice. Attempt to engage the reference in a meaningful dialogue about the candidate's strengths and weaknesses.

■ 5. INTERVIEWING CANDIDATES

The purpose of the face-to-face interview is to confirm an evaluation that has already been conducted. This approach allows the employer to focus on what should be the real goal of the onsite visit—convincing the candidate that s/he wants the job!

When a physician candidate has passed the preinterview assessment and the likelihood is high that s/he will receive an offer during the onsite visit, the candidate should then be invited to an onsite visit that includes the following elements:

- **Ice-Breaker Event:** Often a meal, coffee, or an open-house type of event is best for an ice breaker. The event should be casual and informal with plenty of opportunity for discussion and social interaction.
- **Business Discussion:** This is the time to review the financial elements of the position, including a review of the employment agreement. The employer should make sure the candidate has the opportunity to ask any questions about the financial arrangements including income, benefits, and vacation.
- **Community Introduction:** The community tour should include introductions to key people in the community who might play a role in the candidate's life after relocation. For example, if the candidate has children of school age, a drive by the school would be nice, but making an appointment for the candidate to meet the school principal is better.
- **Time with Future Colleagues:** Every onsite visit should provide time for the candidate to communicate with other physicians in the practice about how the practice functions. The candidate should be encouraged to ask any questions about practice operations.
- **Hospital Tour:** A hospital tour should include time with both physician and nonphysician hospital leaders. For example, even a brief hello and handshake with the hospital CEO can convey a valuable message to the candidate that the hospitalist program is important to the hospital.
- **Wrapup Discussion:** The wrapup discussion is the time to ask for the candidate's initial feedback on the visit, correct any false impressions, and ask the candidate if s/he wants the job.

PRACTICE POINT

- Many employers make the mistake of talking too much when assessing a candidate. Set the stage with a question and then allow the candidate to speak as long as s/he wishes.

Here are tips to keep in mind when planning a candidate visit.

- **Be Honest.** No practice is perfect and no community is utopia, so employers should not try to hide deficiencies from the candidate. However, take care not to overemphasize any potential concerns. This can happen inadvertently when every person who speaks with the candidate mentions a negative aspect of the community. They are doing so with the candidate's best interest in mind, but repetition might give more weight to the concern than is warranted. One way to avoid this problem is to assign one person to mention the concern and make sure the entire interview team understands who has received the assignment.

- **Control the Agenda.** The interview team should be composed of the very best the practice has to offer, and they should be well prepared for their role. The employer should hand-select this team, bypassing chronic complainers.
- **Invite the Candidate's Spouse.** Practices recruit an entire family, not just the physician. Often the spouse represents *more* than 50% of the decision to accept or decline an offer, so every effort should be made to set a date for the visit when the spouse will be able to attend.
- **Do Not Invite the Candidate's Children.** Encourage the candidate to leave children at home if possible. Parents are likely to be distracted if the children attend. If the candidate insists in bringing the children, arrange for child care during portions of the visit.
- **Plan for One Onsite Visit.** If the preinterview assessment and the onsite visit are well structured and thorough, the employer should be prepared to make a decision after the visit. Some employers think that if they like the candidate on the first interview, they can bring him/her back for a second visit. In the current recruiting environment, they may not get a chance at a second trip. It is important the interview be structured to ensure both the candidate and the group leaders obtain all the information required to make a decision about moving forward—or not.
- **Remember that Time Kills All Deals.** Because recruiting competition is strong, employers must act with a sense of urgency, responding to candidate questions immediately, providing a sample agreement during the interview, and sending an executable agreement immediately following the visit. Every candidate should receive a follow-up phone call within a day or two of the visit.
- **Expect the Unexpected.** Employers should be flexible enough to allow for unexpected and unavoidable changes to the interview agenda.

■ 6-7. MAKING SELECTION DECISIONS AND EXTENDING JOB OFFERS

As already stated, it is critically important for employers to respond to candidates' questions and concerns in a timely manner following the onsite visit. Negotiations will be simplified if the practice has valid and comprehensive employment/independent contractor agreements. A formal contract is important to both the hospitalist and the employer. A contractual relationship requires the parties to think clearly about their expectations and obligations. The contracting process should allow the parties to articulate what they want out of the arrangement and to discuss important practical issues. Furthermore, even the best of relationships may change. The parties may change their minds about the type of contract terms to which they wish to be bound. A formal contract ensures that even during periods of disharmony, the parties will be required to abide by the agreed-upon contract terms.

In 2011, the American Medical Association published the *Annotated Model Physician-Hospital Employment Agreement* that suggests physician-hospital agreements address the following topics:

1. Preliminary considerations and basic agreements
2. Term
3. Duties of the physician
4. Employer's obligations
5. Physician compensation
6. Reimbursement of expenses
7. Employer-paid benefits and time off
8. Loyalty and confidentiality covenants
9. Termination
10. Disability or death
11. Remedies
12. Miscellaneous

When a candidate wants to negotiate one or more elements of the contract, the employer should implement "big picture negotiations." Both parties are best served when each considers specific contract requests in light of all requested contract concessions. The employer should inform the candidate of this policy and instruct him/her to thoroughly review the employment agreement and present all concerns/requests at one time. This approach will protect the employer from making a significant concession without knowing if another significant request will follow. If the candidate presents a long list of contract requests, the employer should ask which, if any, of the requests are deal breakers and address these first to avoid the frustration of working through a long list of relatively minor concerns only to see the deal fall apart at the end. These negotiations should always be conducted in an unemotional, businesslike manner. Such conduct will have the added benefit of giving the candidate confidence that the practice leaders handle difficult issues with professionalism.

COMPENSATION

To attract and retain qualified hospitalists, compensation must be market competitive. According to *The State of Hospital Medicine in 2014* report prepared by the SHM, median compensation for adult hospitalists increased 8.2%—from $233,855 to $252,996—since the 2012 report.

When a practice hires a new hospitalist or performs an annual review, the level of compensation can set the tone for long-term satisfaction or disappointment. If the practice pays below market compensation, it runs the risk of losing good talent and/or creating resentment. If the practice pays above market compensation, it can create an entitlement mentality among some hospitalists, generate unnecessary expenses for the practice, and create potential compliance issues.

An effective practice has a compensation philosophy that reflects the values of the practice, conducts sufficient research to ensure that the compensation program is market competitive, has a compensation communication strategy, and explains individual compensation decisions credibly.

ATTRIBUTES OF A WELL-DESIGNED COMPENSATION PLAN

Groups should compute the value of **total** compensation to the hospitalists: a summary of salary, benefits, and other costs required to retain, train, support, and reward a hospitalist. Although the amounts and methods of hospitalist compensation have evolved, the characteristics of a desirable compensation plan have not changed. These characteristics are as follows:

- **Is Easy to Understand:** Any compensation plan should be simple enough that the hospitalist can explain it from memory. Complicated formulas used as the basis for paying a quality bonus or end-of-year profit distribution are problematic if the hospitalists do not fully understand them. Disputes and resentment may arise when a doctor has misunderstood the formula and anticipated a larger bonus than the one that was paid.
- **Is Easy to Defend in Public:** Despite efforts to keep the details of a compensation plan private, the information can become public through members of the practice or during a malpractice suit. Avoid incentives that could be embarrassing or damaging. For example, a financial reward for reducing length of stay could be interpreted as an incentive to send patients home before they are ready.
- **Complies with All Laws and Regulations:** Because the regulations governing physician compensation and the financial relationships between doctors and hospitals or other entities are complex and always changing, compensation plans should be always reviewed by personnel knowledgeable in these

areas to ensure that the plan does not inadvertently violate any legal requirements.
- **Can Be Modified over Time:** Practices often evolve to the point that the compensation plan is not a good match with the current situation and may even inhibit the ability of the practice to make adjustments in scheduling and other areas. For example, compensating hospitalists at a set dollar amount per shift worked may be reasonable today, but in the future the schedule may need to change so shifts are longer or shorter and no longer match the single shift rate in the compensation plan. Because it is typically difficult and time consuming to make significant changes to a compensation plan, a practice might decide to simply keep the compensation plan as it is and forgo making the needed scheduling changes. In this case, the compensation plan is an impediment to effective practice operations. In many practices, a compensation plan based on hours of work or productivity will be easier to adjust in response to changes in scheduling and patient volume.
- **Rewards Good Work:** Ideally, a compensation plan should encourage and reward the performance and behaviors that the practice desires. A portion of total compensation may be tied to the doctor's citizenship in the practice or to performance on quality measures or other domains. The amount of money at stake and the thresholds that trigger payment must be planned carefully to ensure that they influence behavior and are not viewed as too easy or too difficult to reach.

PRACTICE POINT

- When a practice hires a new hospitalist or performs an annual review, the level of compensation may set the tone for long-term satisfaction or disappointment. If the practice pays below market compensation, it runs the risk of losing good talent and/or creating resentment. If the practice pays above market compensation, it may create an entitlement mentality among some hospitalists, generate unnecessary expenses for the practice, and create potential compliance issues.

METHODS OF HOSPITALIST COMPENSATION

A reasonable way to think about the various methods or formulas used to compensate hospitalists is to think of them as consisting of up to three distinct elements. These three elements can be combined in varying proportions to create a compensation method.

- **A Fixed Component, Often Called a Base Salary:** A fixed salary has the advantages of being known to all parties in advance, eliminating uncertainty in budgeting and providing certainty for the hospitalist. However, a fixed salary model alone is not a good choice for most practices because it does not reward or encourage good performance. Hospitalist compensation surveys show a fixed salary was the most common method in use in 1997, but since then its popularity has steadily declined in favor of a combination of fixed and variable elements based on production, performance, or both.
- **A Productivity Component Based on Patient Care Workload or Production:** Here is a sample compensation plan formula based entirely on production: (*collected professional fees + other support [if any]) – overhead*. The "other support" in the formula is most commonly money paid by the hospital in which the hospitalists see patients. Production compensation has the advantages of allowing each doctor to work more or less than others in the group, and it encourages everyone in the group to be attentive to optimal staffing and scheduling and to business practices such as proper current procedural terminology

(CPT) coding. A significant weakness in compensating hospitalists solely on production is that it incentivizes volume and not quality. Potential consequences are the occasional hospitalist who takes on an unreasonable and unsafe workload and providing financial rewards for increased lengths of stay.

- **A Performance-Based Component:** Compensation elements related to performance may be based on quality targets such as patient and/or referring physician satisfaction, proper CPT coding, committee participation, and meeting attendance. An effective plan requires that a meaningful dollar amount of salary be at risk, and careful choices of metrics and thresholds on which payment is based must be made. Good metrics include those that hospitals are already required to measure and report, such as performance on quality measures and patient satisfaction. The number of metrics should be small enough that the dollar amount of payment available for each remains significant. Consequently, no more than three or four metrics should be part of performance compensation. Changing the metrics in the plan every year or so is reasonable. For thresholds that trigger payment, if achieving the threshold is too easy, there will be little or no effect on behavior. If it is too difficult, the doctors may ignore it. Setting a single performance threshold that triggers payment of all available dollars often causes problems. Instead, a predetermined scale—from no payment to the maximum amount available—is a better, more equitable approach. For example, if patient satisfaction for hospitalist patients is currently 70% and the goal is 75%, the portion of dollars paid could be determined by subtracting the baseline (70% in this example) from actual performance (assume it is 73.8%). In this example, patient satisfaction improved 76% ([3.8 ÷ 5] × 100), so 76% of the available dollars would be paid as a measure of percentage of improvement toward the goal.

SOURCES OF DATA ON HOSPITALIST COMPENSATION AND WORKLOAD

The Medical Group Management Association conducts the largest survey of hospitalist compensation, productivity, and professional fee collections each year; results are published each summer based on data collected at the end of the prior calendar year. The SHM *State of Hospital Medicine Survey* is published in the summer on even years and includes detailed data on hospitalist schedules, incentive compensation metrics, scope of clinical services, advanced practice clinician (NP and PA) staffing, and other topics.

PRACTICE POINT

- An effective practice has a compensation philosophy that reflects the values of the practice, conducts sufficient research to ensure that the compensation program is market competitive, has a compensation communication strategy, and explains individual compensation decisions credibly.

RETENTION

Physician turnover is expensive and disruptive, underscoring the critical importance of good recruiting. Every practice should work hard during the recruitment phase to ensure the candidate is a good fit for the practice. However, the work does not end once the new hire is brought on board. Retention is an ongoing process with elements directed to brand-new hires and to seasoned veterans alike. Important components of a retention strategy are an orientation process for new staff, resources for professional growth and development, job satisfaction monitoring, and a documented method for monitoring clinical competency and professionalism.

ORIENTATION FOR NEW STAFF

An effective orientation program will make a positive first impression on new clinicians, facilitate more rapid assimilation, contribute to job satisfaction and retention, and reflect feedback from hospitalists who have participated in the program.

An orientation program provides an opportunity to welcome the new clinician; introduce him/her to colleagues and key support staff; convey the group's vision, mission, and values; clarify job expectations and responsibilities; familiarize the new clinician with the work environment; and mentor recent graduates of training programs. Potential topics to address in a hospitalist orientation program include the following:

- History and philosophy of the practice
- Policies and procedures
- Hospitalist job description
- Compensation program, including incentives
- Medical record standards
- The hospital's EMR system
- Key members of the medical and hospital staff
- Coding/documentation

Good practices are to pair the new clinician with an established hospitalist for a period of shadowing and to conduct an orientation tour that includes the following:

- Hospital departments (emergency department, pharmacy, nursing, case management, etc)
- Hospital administration
- Key referring physicians (PCPs)

Other best-practice elements of a hospitalist orientation are the following:

- A welcome meeting
- An announcement in the local newspaper
- An update of the practice website and brochure
- Printed business cards
- Assignment of a mentor for 60 to 90 days

EDUCATIONAL OPPORTUNITIES

Professional education and development are a formal requirement of the profession of medicine, as specified by the American Medical Association (AMA), the various specialty boards, state licensing agencies, and the Accreditation Council for Continuing Medical Education (ACCME). To maintain their licenses and/or specialty accreditations, physicians must obtain a sufficient number of continuing medical education (CME) credits during a specified period. ACCME and the AMA define CME as "educational activities that serve to maintain, develop, or increase the knowledge, skills, and professional performance and relationships that a physician uses to provide services for patients, the public, or the profession."

The *AMA PRA (Physician's Recognition Award) Category 1 Credit*™ system has become the CME standard for licensing boards and specialty organizations nationwide and is recognized by all US jurisdictions. For an activity to be designated for *AMA PRA Category 1 Credit*, it must be certified by an accredited CME provider.

An effective practice provides its hospitalists with resources for professional growth and enhancement, including access to CME. A wide variety of educational activities qualify for CME certification, including lectures and meetings and activities based on recorded or published content.

The practice should have a policy for encouraging and financially supporting the continuing education and professional development of its hospitalists, including CME credits, and should have a procedure for confirming that all hospitalists in the group have participated in the CME program.

HOSPITALIST JOB SATISFACTION

One of the most important aspects of retention is to measure, monitor, and foster hospitalists' job satisfaction, well-being, and professional development.

Job stress and dissatisfaction among physicians can lead to burnout and a range of undesirable outcomes, including unplanned turnover, absenteeism, judgment/action errors, and conflicts/alienation from professional colleagues. Furthermore, the potential for more tangible adverse outcomes such as accidents, litigation, and increased worker compensation cases may exist. Research has documented that work stress and dissatisfaction also can lead to physical illness. Finally, job stress and dissatisfaction may lead to a poor balance between work and personal life and the reliance on maladaptive coping strategies such as drug and alcohol abuse and dependence. Therefore, it is important that the group leadership assume responsibility for addressing the job satisfaction of the hospitalists in the practice.

The SHM publication *A Challenge for a New Specialty: A White Paper on Hospitalist Career Satisfaction* outlines the following job stresses and dissatisfactions that hospitalists face:

Nature of the Work	Nature of the Work Environment	External Influences
• High acuity/complexity of illness/lack of predictability	• Volume of work	• Impact of ACGME work rules on patient care/teaching
• Life and death implications of clinical decisions	• Time pressure	• Legal and regulatory concerns
• Provider interdependency and communication	• Night and weekend coverage responsibilities	• Financial pressures from payers
• Limited patient information	• High census conditions	**Career/organizational issues**
• Administrative and documentation requirements	• Intermittent demand (beeper always going off)	• Reimbursement based on office model
• Medical legal risk	• Workplace conflicts and interruptions	• No established track for promotion
• Potential hostility from patient's family	• Workplace discrimination	• Little control over key issues (workload, schedule, case types)
Personal issues	• Lack of understanding of the role of the hospitalist by hospital administrators	• Conflict between service mission and other equally important responsibilities
• Professional advancement	• Hospitalists working on a temporary basis while waiting to pursue other career plans	• Limited professional recognition and funding for scholarly activities
• Financial pressures	• Medical staff conflicts	• Leadership structure within the hospital (not "at the table")
• Pressures from spouse/family	• Ergonomics (poorly designed work space and/or equipment)	
• Unrealistic job expectations	• Limited workspace	
• Inability to say "no"		

Effective groups will systematically—at least yearly—monitor job satisfaction and well-being through meetings with individual hospitalists and/or anonymous surveys. Practice leaders should also routinely communicate examples of initiatives undertaken to address hospitalist job stress, dissatisfaction, and/or burnout.

Here are additional strategies for enhancing job satisfaction:

- Create a work/life/compensation balance that makes sense and do everything possible to keep it in balance. If any one element of this three-sided scale is significantly out of balance with the other two for an extended period of time, turnover is inevitable.
- Provide a physician feedback forum of some kind. Frustration will build when physicians feel that their issues are not being heard. They may not always get the answers they wanted, but fair-minded physicians will understand if they are at least allowed such a forum.
- Use team-building exercises or events, such as social events and professional retreats, to keep individuals from feeling isolated within the group.

CLINICAL COMPETENCY AND PROFESSIONALISM

Patients and the public in general expect their health care providers to be clinically competent and to act professionally. The group leadership is accountable for the care delivered by the physicians and other providers in the practice. Clinicians can make one or more significant errors, exhibit poor judgment, behave poorly with patients or other clinicians, or demonstrate a pattern of poor or unsafe care. A documented, structured process for identifying and addressing such issues will not only prevent the well-functioning members of the practice from becoming resentful of a practice that allows a colleague to get away with providing poor care but can also, in many cases, remediate the troublesome clinician.

Clinician competency and professionalism should be addressed at two points in time: when the clinician applies for privileges and is initially credentialed and when a deficiency is identified related to current clinical competence, practice behavior, or the ability to perform a procedure. Practice leadership should monitor clinicians to identify deficiencies in care and implement appropriate remedies for health care providers found to be deficient such as remedial training, proctoring, reassignment, and, if remedial actions fail, termination from the practice.

PRACTICE POINT

- One of the most important aspects of retention is to measure, monitor, and foster hospitalists' job satisfaction, well-being, and professional development.

CONCLUSION

An understaffed hospitalist program or one with a number of dissatisfied clinicians will quickly become unstable, resulting in significant clinical and financial consequences. It is imperative that hospitalist program leaders become proficient in recruiting and retaining the physicians they need to provide the outstanding care their patients deserve.

CHAPTER 25

Teamwork in Leadership and Practice-Based Management

Scot T. Smith, MD
Scott F. Enderby, DO, SFHM
Robert A. Bessler, MD

INTRODUCTION

Multidisciplinary care refers to the active collaboration between various members in the health care system to deliver optimal care for every hospitalized patient. Successful teamwork is a core competency that can be taught and incorporated into patient care processes. The Association of American Medical Colleges (AAMC), the Accreditation Council for Graduate Medical Education (ACGME), and the Society of Hospital Medicine (SHM) require specific teamwork-related competencies for medical students, residents, and hospitalists. Hospitalists can improve multidisciplinary care of hospitalized patients by demonstrating group dynamic skills, conducting effective multidisciplinary team rounds, evaluating performance, providing feedback, teaching about error and how teamwork and communication can reduce error, and by leading quality improvement initiatives.

The US health care system is a highly organized and complex system. Over the last three decades of the public safety movement there have been landmark studies and published reports about individual and systemic failures that have not only cost lives but wasted billions of US dollars while delivering unsafe care. Although different solutions may be debated, it is clear that the US health care system will need to be redesigned to deliver the highest quality of care possible while being ever mindful of ways to improve efficiencies and reducing the cost of care delivery. Sweeping change requires effective teamwork on every level: hospital networks, hospital, hospitalist service, skilled nursing, and home care—a more comprehensive approach to multidisciplinary patient care.

In general, most physicians have little formal training relating to complex hospital systems or human error and lack insight into their own limitations during conditions of stress, lack of sleep, or conflicting demands. Strong hierarchy, power differentials, lack of clarity requiring specific tasks and roles, and lack of coordination are common teamwork and communication failures in health care. Lessons learned from the aviation industry can be applied to the delivery of hospital care, and hospitalists can take steps to reduce the likelihood of (1) individual error resulting from physiological and psychological limitations of human beings and (2) team errors resulting from failure to act or deviation from established standards. Although it is not possible to eliminate individual error, systems can be designed that reduce the likelihood of error and make hospitals a safer environment for patients. Working in teams and serving as the hub of communication network in the hospital, hospitalists are ideally poised to change the culture of "how we do things around here" by serving as clinical role models and as leaders of patient safety on the multidisciplinary care team and truly coordinating care throughout the acute episode of care. Without effective teamwork and medical leadership, however, these complex systems have been shown to be less effective in producing quality outcomes.

THE MULTIDISCIPLINARY HEALTH CARE TEAM

The hospitalist team is a unit of professionals that directly provides care and so most directly impacts the patient experience and the quality of care. Composition of the team varies, but a team typically may include hospitalists, consulting physician(s), advanced care practitioners, nurses, case managers, social workers, and pharmacists, amongst others.

Individuals have particular tasks based on their particular specialties, but the hospitalist team depends on each other for situational awareness and goal success strategies. Situational awareness is a common, accurate understanding of the patient's condition, needs, clinical trajectory, and feelings based on the multiple perspectives of team members. The team only obtains situational awareness when these perspectives are communicated within the team. Without the perspectives of team members, no individual—including the hospitalist—truly has situational awareness. High-quality, coordinated care is compromised when decisions are made, orders written and even discussions with patients and their families occur without the perspective of other members of the care delivery team. It is vital to quality, patient-centered care that a single message is delivered from everyone on the team. The hospitalist is the hub of communications and transitions in care and leads the health care team to ensure the patient is at the center of decisions.

PRACTICE POINT

Limit your blind spots and those of your team

Unless you must, do not deliver care without situational awareness.

Create workflow scenarios that allow multiple team members' perspectives before making decisions, writing orders, and interacting with the patient.

At a minimum, round with the patient's nurse before you see the patient.

Communicate your perspective to the team. The team relies on the hospitalist for clinical perspective. At a minimum ask:

What problems are being addressed and is each problem getting better or worse?

- What is being done for the patient (tests, evaluation by consultants, interventions, medication changes, etc) and why?
- What does the patient need to be safer?
- What does the patient need to feel better?
- What does the patient need for safe, timely discharge?
- What is the next site of care and how is this being coordinated postdischarge?
- What are the risks of readmission? How can we work together as a team to reduce avoidable readmissions to the hospital?

Goal success is an optimal patient experience. The team relies on each member to provide best practice care by limiting unnecessary variation in practice, enhancing patient satisfaction with the hospitalization experience, effective communications throughout the team, and discharging the patient as safely and as soon as possible. Reducing performance variability of the team ultimately helps to address the patient's problems and ensures better outcomes. By using evidence-based protocols, order sets, checklists and other institutional-specific processes, the team can help standardize performance.

PRACTICE POINT

Limit unnecessary variation in practice

Reliable systems make improved quality more likely:

If there isn't clear evidence supporting a particular choice, the team should consistently use institutional therapeutic choices (eg, antibiotic choices, VTE prophylaxis, etc).

- Set consistent times for rounds.
- Use institutional order sets.

PRACTICE POINT

Provide care that satisfies the patient

- Improve the patient's perception of your team. Patients often feel that their care team is not coordinated or that various members are not talking to one other.
- Specifically, address your coordination with nurses, other physicians on your team and specialists, pharmacists, therapists, etc.
- Let patients know that you are aware of and approve of what others on the team are doing.

Limiting the risks associated with prolonged unnecessary hospitalization should be a stated goal of the hospitalist team. In support of that goal, each team member—*as they round on their patients and decide whether to discharge now or not*—must determine whether the benefits of continued hospitalization outweigh the inherent risks of continued hospitalization. Each team member should be encouraged to articulate the rationale for their decision to the rest of the care team.

PRACTICE POINT

Discharge the patient safely and as soon as possible

Hospitalization exposes patients to a host of physical and psychological risks including:

- Blood stream infections
- Respiratory infections
- Urinary infections
- Adverse drug events
- Pressure ulcers
- Falls
- Functional decline
- Anxiety

A hospitalist typically leads the inpatient care team and is increasing more involved in postdischarge care coordination, particularly with Accountable Care Organizations (ACOs) and CMS' Bundled Payment Care Improvement (BPCI) initiative. As the leader, the hospitalist is responsible for goal clarity, role clarity, communication, and team cohesiveness. Effective teamwork requires the willingness of the team members to work toward a shared goal. Goal clarity requires explicitly stating what defines success for the team and a quality outcome for the patient. And, now with ACOs and BPCI the hospitalist team has an important role to help reduce readmissions by coordinating transitions in care and ensuring that the risks that could bring the patient back to the hospital are identified and mitigated.

- What medical conditions are or are not being treated as an inpatient?
- What is the goal of treatment?
- What is the endpoint of hospitalization?
- What is the reason for each test, intervention, change?
- What care coordination is required postdischarge to limit avoidable readmissions?

PRACTICE POINT

Be explicit about goals

Write the goal in the patient chart. For example:

- "Chest pain: The patient has multivessel CAD and demand ischemia. He declines intervention other than medication changes. I am titrating nitrates and beta-blockers. My goal for discharge: pain free at rest and while walking slowly in room, tolerating medication without orthostatic symptoms."

Role clarity requires explicitly identifying who will do what on the team.

- Who on the care team is responsible for which aspects of care?
- Who is discussing which issues with the patient?
- Which consultant is managing which problem?
- Who is writing orders for what?

Effective communication requires sharing essential information across the hospitalist team and in this new environment of pay for quality; hospitalist teams are also leading change in the postcharge care strategies and communications. The team leader is responsible for demonstrating techniques that encourage specific teamwork, modeling behaviors that ensure that roles are clearly defined, sharing information in a timely and accurate fashion, discussing and mutually agreeing to plans of care. Effective teamwork can reduce the number of medical errors and avoidable readmissions through improved communication and better coordination of care.

- What method will the team use to communicate? Examples may include reading each other's chart notes or discussing face-to-face or by phone.
- How often will members communicate? Will this occur once a day or throughout the day? Will there be consistent expectations for communication such as during daily rounds, prior to the end of the day or only on an as-needed basis?
- How can tone and language be used effectively to decrease barriers and misunderstandings?

PRACTICE POINT

Structure your communication

Make team communication more reliable by:
- Using checklists
- Setting predictable rounding times
- Using agreed-upon care protocols
- Using structured communication such as SBAR

Situation: the specific problem:
"Mrs. Johnson has a headache and is hypotensive."

Background: the specific history that may relate to the current situation:
"She fell last night and did not have a CT of her head; she does take anticoagulants."

Assessment: the analysis of the problem:
"I believe she has a bleed in her head."

Recommendation/Request: the team member makes a recommendation and request of another:
"Dr. Smith, please see her immediately."

Cohesiveness requires recognition of a shared purpose, defined roles, and task interdependence. As the facilitator of optimal team function, the leader limits disruption and fragmentation of the team that can occur with any dynamic and complex process. This requires active listening and frequent communication with all members of the team, sharing decision-making responsibilities, and proactively providing opportunities for everyone to contribute according to their abilities, including patients and families.

- How do we help each other succeed?
- How do we eliminate what pulls us apart?

TEAM COMMUNICATION WITH PRIMARY CARE PROVIDERS, POSTACUTE PROVIDERS, PATIENTS, AND FAMILIES IS A BIDIRECTIONAL PROCESS

Hospitalists generally define themselves as specialists of the medical care of hospitalized patients. Mistakenly, however, hospitalists may believe that they do not need either the input of the outpatient practitioner(s) or to partner with them. This is another silo mentality that neither fosters high-quality care nor patient satisfaction. In this new era of accountable care, the hospitalist has an opportunity to set the patient up for success by having a strategy for postacute care following discharge. From a patient perspective, care does not begin with admission and end with discharge, and many patients wish that their practitioners had an ongoing role in their care during hospitalization and today many do have ways to extend care following discharge. Many hospitalist teams are now partnering with a postacute care providers who manage transitions in care that occurs in skilled nursing or rehab centers and even a team of home health providers who check-in on high-risk patients after discharge. Ensuring that primary care and postacute providers are involved at various points in the continuum of care is a major quality issue that is being addressed increasingly by hospitalist teams.

Based on experience, we know that the quality of communication from the hospitalist to the community physician is paramount. The inpatient health care team must understand and synthesize outpatient goals into the initial hospital care plan and then proactively communicate with the outpatient team as the hospitalization proceeds. The hospitalist-leader should focus the inpatient team on processes in the transition of patients to other settings, ensure accuracy, thoroughness and timeliness of documentation, and optimize communication before discharge actually takes place to increase the likelihood that discharge orders are carried out as intended.

The first step in understanding outpatient goals is identifying the leader of outpatient care and to ensure that those at high risk for readmission have a specific plan to minimize this risk. This simple act can be challenging. Some patients have established primary care providers; some have multiple specialists; many have no outpatient care providers. The hospitalist team must develop a discharge plan that supports outpatient goals to the greatest extent possible; then communicate that plan to the patient's outpatient and postacute care teams.

PRACTICE POINT

Outpatient and postacute care goals

On admission ask, actively listen, and communicate key information:
- Talk to the patient. Who is the primary provider? What are the patient's own goals of care? If they require postdischarge care, what is the most appropriate next site of care for the patient, if it is not home?
- Talk directly to the outpatient or postacute team and confirm the goals.
- Talk to the patient's support team (eg, family, friends, etc) identified and authorized by the patient. What are their goals?
- Are the patient's long-term goals identified and documented in an advanced directive or POLST form? The hospitalization offers an opportunity to approach the subject of life choices and should be part of the dialog for all patients, and especially for those who may benefit from palliative or hospice care.

Transitions in care are inherently risky events and effective discharge planning begins on the day of admission. Inadequate preparation can compromise care, contribute to medication errors, and create a sense of discontinuity for the patient and those who provide their longitudinal care. Hospitalists must focus on improving not only the substance of transitions, but also the experience of the transition for patients, their families, primary care physicians and postacute providers. From day one of hospitalization, communicate with family, advanced practitioners, nurses, primary care providers, and others who will provide longitudinal care of the patient during and after hospitalization. The hospitalist should determine, with the receiving community provider, how communication should take place, (telephone, e-mail, page, or fax); how often; by whom; what communication should occur; and determine the level of involvement of the outpatient practitioner in discharge decisions rather than simply relying only on discharge summaries to transfer information.

Importantly, the hospitalist-led team must also communicate to patients and their families in clear next steps with regard to their continued diagnosis, treatment, timing of anticipated discharge, and care beyond the hospital. To do this effectively, the team should have a shared understanding about all of the issues impacting the patient, diagnostic findings, and management plans. The patient's primary care nurse should not be overlooked as a key communicator of information to patients and families. The team leader should include the patient's nurse in rounds and update that nurse regularly. Likewise, patients and families are important members of the care team and should be informed and actually have an opportunity to ask questions and give consent to treatment. Patients should not receive conflicting information from doctors, nurses, consultants, and other members of the team. The information provided should be structured in straightforward simple language in accordance with the patient's literacy, utilizing interpreters when English is not the primary language.

Patient satisfaction surveys provide information that can be used to improve team performance. Using feedback from Hospital Consumer Assessment of Healthcare Providers and Systems (HCAHPS) survey results, physicians can better understand how patients perceive the quality of communication coming from their hospital physician. Whether it be how well the patient felt their doctor listened to them, how well the doctor explained things in a manner that they could comprehend, or whether they felt their doctor treated them with courtesy and respect, we all benefit from understanding how we are *perceived* by our patients. This type of direct feedback can be used in educating hospitalists on the importance of providing patient-centered care. It also enables leaders to mentor team members and to set expectations for the desired performance, educating the service on how to effectively provide patient-centered care, and mentoring hospitalists who have lower scores.

PRACTICE POINT

Consistent, understandable patient education

On admission identify the patient-authorized family contact and make sure to update him or her daily as well as the patient, if appropriate, of:

- Provisional diagnosis
- Areas of uncertainty
- Planned diagnostic workup, consultation
- Management plan
- Anticipated date and time of discharge and to what setting
- What to do if something goes wrong and patient does not respond as anticipated
- How to avoid readmissions—things to do and what to look for in the immediate postdischarge period that may be signs that the patient needs medical attention

Answer any questions and confirm that the patient's family contact understands what you have said.

On a daily basis, make sure multidisciplinary team rounds include a review of:

- Provisional diagnosis
- Planned diagnostic work
- Management plan
- Anticipated date and time of discharge and to what setting
- What to do if something goes wrong

Answer any questions and confirm understanding and consensus.

Continuously update the primary nurse and other members of the team when:

- There is a change in plan
- There are results of a diagnostic workup
- There are new diagnoses
- There is a new complication
- There is a postdischarge plan to a site other than home

Listen to concerns and address them.

On the day of discharge summarize prior conversations:

- Medication changes and the reasons for changes
- New medications
- Diagnostic studies, the results and pending results
- Consultations performed during hospitalization and specific ongoing recommendations postdischarge
- Who to contact if there is an unexpected problem

Provide written materials to complement verbal instructions that the patient should bring with him or her to the primary care provider's office or ensure the postacute care facility has the appropriate information to transition the patient's care.

THE ROLE OF THE DIRECTOR OF A HOSPITALIST SERVICE

Typically a hospitalist team is led by a chief hospitalist or medical director who provides daily clinical management of the team. In this role, the chief hospitalist is also the liaison to the hospital administration. The chief hospitalist has responsibility for the performance of the hospitalist service, provides administrative support for the service, develops schedules for hospitalists that reflect manageable workloads, and typically serves on hospital committees including pharmacy and therapy, critical care, safety, utilization review, The Joint Commission, HCAHPS Survey, and compliance review boards to name a few.

The comprehensive hospitalist service is a team of physicians, advanced care practitioners, and business managers. Depending on the institution, the hospitalist team may be employed by the hospital or part of an independent group of hospitalists, a member of a large multispecialty group practice, or affiliated with a larger regional or nationally-based hospitalist organization. A small percentage of hospitalists are *locum tenens* physicians who fill an important temporary role when teams require temporary staffing.

Hospitalist leaders have the opportunity to set clinically appropriate and standardized care. As a result, teams of hospitalists have the ability to improve the quality of care of a larger group of hospitalized patients by delivering measurable and consistent quality care. To be effective, hospitalist leaders should:

- ***Set Clear Expectations.*** Effective leaders provide teams with clear performance expectations. When the team understands how the leader measures excellence, they know what is expected of them.

  In addition to their clinical responsibilities, all hospitalists should understand the hospital's key initiatives and the areas in which the hospitalist team is going to be accountable to key hospital administrators including the chief executive officer (CEO), chief financial officer (CFO), chief medical officer (CMO), and chief nursing officer (CNO). Using metrics provides an objective method for communicating consistently on team performance measured against team goals. Hospitalist leaders should focus their hospitalist teams on delivering measurable quality improvements by reducing practice variability.

- **Delegate Responsibility.** The hospitalist leader delegates responsibilities to team members and establishes open lines of communication. When teams have a clear understanding of expectations, there is no room for ambiguity. Establishing open and honest communication encourages teamwork and collaboration. Unfortunately, many hospitalist programs are carried on the back of the medical director. This model is destined to fail as it usually is the result of a lack of overall physician engagement within the group. Even with limited clinical responsibilities, the medical director must have superb delegation skills to reduce the potential for burnout.

- **Empower Team Members.** Excellent leaders empower hospitalist team members to get involved. When teams feel supported to make decisions they become more effective as a group. This also helps to develop future leaders by providing them the opportunity to learn decision-making skills within the framework of the team.

- **Deal with Conflicts Swiftly.** Effective leaders must be capable of dealing with conflicts immediately and removing roadblocks that can impair the effectiveness of the team. Train team members in how to engage in difficult conversations using an approach or methodology that is common to the team, such as the program outlined in the book "Crucial Conversations," by Joseph Grenny, Kerry Patterson, and Ron McMillan. Having a common framework and language helps the team deal with conflicts.

- **Ensure Resources Are Available.** Leaders ensure their teams have the necessary resources to do their work effectively. In Hospital Medicine the leader has to compete with the other hospital priorities and resources. The successful leader can navigate competing priorities without the emotion that often overtakes individual members of the team in the desire to help change a process.

- **Recognize the Impact of Workload on Quality.** When the hospitalist workload is based on manageable encounters, hospitalists are more apt to deliver very consistent, high-quality care. There is no national body of evidence that supports the ideal workload. The right workload depends on a myriad of factors including the following:

    Does the physician already know the patients on his or her rounding list? How many new patients are there?
    What kind of support staff is available to help the physicians? What administrative duties does the physician have during the work day? Is there specialty backup coverage?
    Does the physician have to do the procedures?
    How efficiently does the hospital run?

    For the average hospitalist starting their day at 7:00 AM, a workload of 14-15 patients and admitting or consulting on a few more patients during the remainder of the day is ideal. The hospitalist's appropriate workload must also take into account the acuity of the patients and the wRVUs represented in the care of patients. In the case of a workload that does not include new patients, it is often easy for an individual provider to manage a higher volume of patients. In a smaller hospital with no ICU coverage or a lack of specialty support, that same volume typically takes much more effort and time. A well-managed workload optimizes the provider's ability to coordinate care with the entire team, make additional visits with patients when

necessary and ultimately be more effective directors of the patients' care. Providers need adequate time to communicate with the various stakeholders in a thorough fashion, focus on the accuracy of documentation and deliver high-quality, efficient care. When hospitalists have a well-managed workload, it results in better work-life balance and a more sustainable and rewarding career.

- **Commit to Develop Team Members.** Hospitalist leaders provide professional development opportunities for their team members. Effective teams benefit from growth and advancement and from group incentives that drive performance excellence. Most physicians lack formal leadership training. Providing didactic skill development opportunities, access to professional coaches, and an ongoing support network are keys to successful professional growth for all team members, including the leader. Providing 360° reviews of the chief hospitalist are also essential to help the leader understand their blind spots and opportunities for improvement as well. These evaluations and important to conduct annually as the team composition can change and new members have an opportunities for feedback. It can also be an opportunity for the leader to assess improvement year over year.

- **Embrace Diversity of Teams.** Today's hospitalist teams are diverse and require leaders who recognize and embrace different points of view. With a variety of cultural backgrounds, skill levels, training and team roles, it is important that the leader promote acceptance and openness when dealing with different situations. Team leaders can also help diverse teams with communication skills, especially where English may not be the provider's first language. There are a number of support programs available to give providers the coaching and training needed to be as effective as possible in their communications and pronunciation when talking with each other and their patients.

- **Measure and Recognize Performance.** Measuring performance and providing objective feedback to team members drives continuous improvement. Effective leaders provide training and coaching to team members. They also find ways to recognize and reward performance excellence and improvement for both the team and individuals. Most physicians feel they have "arrived" after medical school and residency. Most are not used to a performance evaluation as part of being on a physician team. Tools, such as an annual evaluation can be a great opportunity for the leader of the team to provide feedback on specific areas that will make the individual and the team more effective. The hospitalist should be presented the metrics that matter to the patient and to the institution consistently.

- **Recruit the Right People to Your Hospitalist Service.** Recruiting the right team is another important factor in developing an effective hospitalist team. Taking time to evaluate candidates for both clinical and technical competency, as well as chemistry with the team, is critical for ensuring the success of effective teams. Evaluate the candidate's communication style and skills of the rest of the team. A well orchestrated interview agenda allows all team members to have time to interact with the candidate. It is important to have a cross-section of data points to assess compatibility of the candidate with the existing team. Finally, be sure to reach out to individuals who worked with the candidate previously to get a comprehensive picture of the candidate you are considering.

- **Solicit Feedback from Members of the Team to Improve Operations.** A strong sense of team has been associated with higher retention.

Physicians have many allegiances, including their outside interests and families, their hospital, their medical group, and their team. If a team is functioning well, members want to stay and make the team stronger.

According to the 2015 salary survey by Today's Hospitalist, the mean age of hospitalists is now 44 years of age [http://www.todayshospitalist.com/survey/15_salary_survey/e03.php], an advancement of nearly a year older. There continues to be a significant need to develop leaders and not wait for leaders to evolve. A respected and effective hospitalist leader is a prerequisite to achieving a highly functioning hospitalist team. The field of Hospital Medicine has recognized this need and the Society of Hospital Medicine (SHM) recently established the Fellow in Hospital Medicine with three levels (Fellow, Senior Fellow, and Master Fellow) recognition. While specific traits are identified in the FHM, SFHM and MHM charters, they are typically skills acquired by hospitalists who have benefited from mentors or coaches and/or completed additional training. SHM also provides additional certification in leadership in Hospital Medicine (leadership fundamentals and advanced leadership).

The effective hospitalist leader must inherently be an effective manager. Managing a team includes allocating resources skillfully, meeting deadlines and obligations, and serving multiple stakeholders. It also requires effective communication, conflict management, and deft delegation ability. Masters-degree-level work, such as a Masters in Medical Management (MMM), Masters in Business Administration (MBA) or Masters in Healthcare Administration (MHA) can help hone these skills. Alternatively, SHM advanced leadership courses offer strategies and tools for personal leadership excellence and for developing a winning team and strengthening your organization.

ALIGNING HOSPITALISTS WITH HOSPITAL GOALS

The successful hospitalist service has teams assigned to drive performance that are aligned with hospitals goals and report on the results to hospital administration regularly. The most common hospital initiatives are in the areas of quality, operations, satisfaction, and financial performance. The hospitalist teams that survive and thrive in the next decade must master the role of managing effective hospitalist teams that drive real value and measurable results for their hospital partner.

To improve outcomes, it is necessary for hospitalists to have clear and functional processes that incorporate utilization of best practices. They should be encouraged to identify ways to reduce variables in patient care, and importantly, they must be good stewards of their time and resources and focus on what matters most. Effective prioritization and time management are critical for driving improvements in all outcomes, whether clinical, satisfaction, or financial performance.

Each hospitalist service should determine benchmark performance expectations for their hospitalist team around admissions, discharge planning, processes for signing off care between shifts, and creating and managing care pathways. While there are a plethora of data sets that can be measured to drive performance, it is essential for hospitalist service teams to identify metrics that can be used to drive performance improvement and consistently measure them. Whether measuring continuous quality improvements, satisfaction, efficiency or readmissions data, hospitalist teams cannot improve unless performance is measured. Once the performance is measured, it can be managed. Performance measurements also can be used to provide reward systems to reinforce the behaviors.

The Hospital Consumer Assessment of Healthcare Providers and Systems (HCAHPS) survey developed by the Centers for Medicare and Medicaid Services (CMS) asks questions directed largely at the patient's experiences in the hospital. The survey probes efficacy of the health care team's communication with patients, instruction about medications, quality of nursing services, adequacy of planning for discharge, and pain management. Responses are reported in six composite domains, largely focused on the effectiveness of communication. The HCAHPS score is meant to reflect the patient's perception of the quality of the care they received in the hands of the doctors, nurses, and by the hospital. The following three broad goals shaped the HCAHPS instrument to produce data about patients' perspectives of care that allow:

1. objective and meaningful comparisons of hospitals on topics that are important to consumers,
2. the creation of new incentives for hospitals to improve quality of care, and
3. accountability in health care by increasing the transparency of the quality of hospital care provided in return for the public investment.

The average scores reflect the entire hospital experience, but the hospitalist team can significantly influence HCAHPS survey results and improve patient satisfaction scores. The 2008 *New England Journal of Medicine* article, "Patients' Perception of Hospital Care in the United States," by Ashish K. Jha, et al. concludes that the current level of communication and care leaves plenty of room for improvement. In this study, 63% of hospitals received a rating of 9 or 10 from patients, and 89% scored their experience at 7 or better. The quality of hospital care continues to be highly variable, signaling an opportunity for the hospitalist team to take the leadership role in driving quality improvements and ratings that reach 90% or more consistently.

While the objectives of the CMS' HCAHPS instrument were carefully considered and the tool skillfully designed, the results pose challenges in interpretation. Many consider the HCAHPS data to be flawed due to the multivariate nature of the patient's course of care. Nevertheless, tracking and communicating data on clinical performance, however flawed, is a starting point and has previously prompted improvements in the quality of clinical care in hospitals.

When the hospitalist actively participates in the patient's transition of care from hospital to home or to a skilled nursing facility, data shows that satisfaction scores skyrocket. In addition, typically the family, case manager, nursing staff, and primary care physicians' satisfaction scores also increase. There also should be expectations set for hospitalist relations and assessments with critical partners including emergency physicians, primary care providers, and specialists. These relationships must be monitored on a regular basis to ensure cooperative integration is achieved.

With bundling of payments and more scrutiny on readmissions, hospitals may prioritize resources to reduce readmission rates. Hospitalist leaders can develop communication standards to reduce practice variation, identify patients at increased risk for readmission, and work with other hospital leaders to redesign the systems in place that do not promote safe transitions. For example, the University of Pennsylvania attributed a drop in readmissions from a high of 15% to 5% in the short period from the fall of 2008 to February 2009 to the implementation of tools from the SHM Project BOOST, including the "7P" checklist. The checklist tool simplifies the major modifiable risk factors to consider for readmission to the hospital. There are seven risk factors tied to suggested interventions for problem medications, principal diagnosis, depression, polypharmacy, poor health literacy, patient support, and prior hospitalization.

PROJECT BOOST

Project BOOST (Better Outcomes for Older adults through Safe Transitions) is one effort to improve the care of older patients as they transition from inpatient care to an outpatient facility or home. The SHM, working with Blue Cross and Blue Shield of Michigan and the

University of Michigan, is launching a multisite implementation of the program seeking to:

- Avoid unplanned or preventable hospital readmissions and emergency department visits within 30 days of hospital discharge.
- Improve facility patient satisfaction scores.
- Improve patient satisfaction associated with discharge.
- Improve communication between inpatient and outpatient providers.
- Improve patient and family education about disease management and risk issues.
- Identify patients at high risk and mitigate that risk with multi-disciplinary risk mitigation tools and strategies; including

> *Discharge coordination/communication with follow-on providers*
> *Patient and caretaker disease and disease management education including a "teach-back" strategy to ensure comprehension*
> *Medication reconciliation including a review of interactions between discharge medications and previously prescribed medications interactions*
> *Essential team members include nurses, case managers, patient educators, hospitalists*

To be effective, Project BOOST requires multidisciplinary teamwork, coordinating seamless transitions of care by utilizing the combined expertise of team members. This has significant economic and quality implications. In a study by Cauwels, Jensen and Winterton a hospitalist group highlights progress made in reducing readmissions rates through Project BOOST. In this report, case managers implemented BOOST, working with hospitalist teams. They achieved statistically significant decreases in readmissions in 30 days for all patients regardless of treating specialty or reason for admission.

Hospitalist teams must be integrated into these processes. When the team is evaluated as part of the process, individual outliers are identified and receive the necessary training and mentoring to improve individual performance. Equally as important, the hospitalist can help improve institutional performance. High-performing teams are indispensable to high-performance hospitals. Examples include the following:

- **A High-Functioning Team Becomes the Lifeblood of the Hospital.** Hospitalists who improve the quality of the hospital, improve the quality of patient care. Physicians who work in such hospitals are involved in everything from the dietary needs of patients, to the workflow, to access to CT results 24 hours per day. Many hospital CEOs cannot imagine life without a hospitalist team helping to carry their hospital forward.
- **An Effective Team Builds the Brand of the Hospital.** An engaged and committed team is essential in advancing the hospital's brand. By reaching out to local providers, improving referrals, and making surgeons want to practice at their hospital, the hospitalist contributes significantly to the overall brand value of the hospital in the community. It is often the hospitalist

whom the family and patient see more than specialists or other hospital staff. It is incumbent on the hospitalist to ensure that the hospital's success is largely dependent on the hospitalist and his or her interaction with others.
- **Employing a Service-Focused Mindset.** Hospitalists are one of the most visible groups in the hospital. The team that is service-oriented and prioritizes quality patient care and communication high on the list will be a sought-after change agent in the hospital. The hospitalist team that can demonstrate effective communications and satisfaction as well as a commitment to patient education is an invaluable resource to the hospital.

CONCLUSION

By virtue of their presence, hospitalist teams have changed the system of health care delivery in the United States. Hospital Medicine is now a major cost center in the US health care system. Although the variety of impending solutions to remedy our nation's health care ills range from insurance reform to health care IT solutions, one common important resource has emerged, namely, the active leadership of hospitalists engaged to design and implement sweeping improvements in the quality, satisfaction, and efficiency of care delivered for hospitalized patients. Today, hospitalist teams play a more significant role in recognizing the needs of patients and their families and have developed ways to demonstrate accountability. Hospitalists impact the majority of clinical decisions made on behalf of hospitalized patients and therefore directly determine how medical resources are utilized and drive health outcomes and costs on medical care collectively.

SUGGESTED READINGS

Bohmer R. *Designing Care: Aligning the Nature and Management of Health Care.* Boston, MA: Harvard Business Review Press; 2009.

Cauwels JM, Jensen BJ, Winterton TL. Giving readmissions numbers a boost. *SD Med.* 2013;66(12):505-507, 509.

Jha A, Orav J, Zheng J, et al. Patients' Perception of Hospital Care in the United States. *N Engl J Med.* 2008;359:1921-1931.

Khatri N, Baveja A, Boren SA, Mammo A. Medical Errors and Quality of Care: From Control to Commitment. *California Management Rev.* 2006;48(3):115-141.

Lee TH. Turning Doctors into Leaders. *Harvard Business Rev.* 2010:50-58.

Lee TH, Mongan JJ. *Chaos and Organization in Health Care.* Cambridge, MA: MIT Press; 2009.

Patterson K, Grenny J, McMillan R, Switzler A. *Crucial Conversations.* 2nd ed. New York, NY: McGraw-Hill; 2012.

Sehgal NL, Green A, Vidyarthi AR, Blegen M, Wachter R. Patient whiteboards as a communication tool in the hospital setting: a Survey of practices and recommendations. *J Hosp Med.* 2010;5(4):234-239.

What Makes a Leader? *Harvard Business Rev.* 2004:43-52.

CHAPTER 26

Negotiation and Conflict Resolution

Leslie A. Flores, MHA

Hospitalists face the potential for conflict every day. They work in highly complex organizations and in order to be successful they must interact effectively with a wide variety of individuals in what is often a challenging, emotionally charged environment. Hospitalists must learn to navigate not only the formal organizational bureaucracy of rules, systems, and processes, but also the informal political hierarchy that influences power and decision making. Often, they must do so with little or no formal training in conflict management at an early stage in their medical careers. In addition, they may encounter conflicts between what others would like them to accomplish and their own workload demands and professional expectations.

Hospital Medicine is also a young, evolving specialty that has enjoyed unprecedented growth by serving the needs of multiple competing stakeholders. Although the specialty is maturing, it is still populated by a high proportion of recent residency graduates and early-career clinicians who may not have a complete understanding of the specialty or even have career advancement on their radar screen. The potential exists for the service obligations—both clinical and in the area of institutional performance improvement—of hospitalists to overwhelm opportunities for professional development, and this may promote career dissatisfaction, turnover, and symptoms of burnout. Leaders of hospitalist services may find themselves isolated as they advocate for the professional development and job satisfaction of group members while meeting the service expectations of their employers or supervisors. The professional medical society for hospitalists, the Society of Hospital Medicine, is rapidly developing flexible support resources for hospitalists relating to business and clinical practice, engagement and career satisfaction, core competencies, and role expectations. Until these standards become widely disseminated and health care services become better designed and hence less prone to error, hospitalists will continue to work in a hospital environment where they will increasingly be expected to perform as change agents at a time when change may not be welcomed by their hospitalist colleagues or others at their institutions.

For the purposes of this chapter, it will be important to distinguish between *disagreements* and *conflicts*. Disagreements happen regularly in human interactions, and occur whenever two or more individuals have differing opinions about something. A disagreement need not devolve into a conflict, and many do not. Conflicts arise when a party perceives that another party has negatively affected or will negatively affect agendas that the first party cares about. Conflicts are defined as processes that occur when tensions develop, that is, the emotions associated with a disagreement become so elevated that they impede the ability of the parties to interact with each other effectively.

Almost all conflict is a result of unmet expectations. For hospitalists, this commonly arises when there is a lack of understanding or a difference in expectations about their role. Hospitalists may assume that primary care physicians have explained to patients that someone else will be seeing them in the hospital. Patients and families, however, may not understand why their primary care physician is not present in the hospital and directing their care. Emergency Medicine physicians may expect the hospitalist to respond promptly to take a complicated social admission off their hands whereas hospitalists may feel that it is the role of the emergency room physicians to discharge patients who do not require admission. Emergency Medicine physicians and staff may expect for patients be triaged to hospital floors (to reduce emergency department length of stay) before critical information is available, or may expect hospitalists to care for patients in the emergency department when no beds are available. Meanwhile, floor nurses may expect hospitalists to be immediately available to address nonurgent requests. There may be differences of opinion among specialists and generalists regarding diagnosis, workup, and treatment or the role of the hospitalists in comanagement of specialty patients. All physicians expect to be treated professionally, to have some autonomy over clinical decision making, and to have a reasonable work-life balance. Hospital administrators and employers, however, may demand that hospitalists to perform nonphysician tasks or solve problems for other physician groups without taking into account the perspectives of the hospitalists or staffing needs for time-consuming tasks. When such expectations go unmet, people get frustrated or angry. They often respond in ways that then heighten frustration or anger on the part of others. Emotions on both sides become elevated, and the stage is set for a conflict.

PRACTICE POINT

- Almost all conflict is a result of unmet expectations. For hospitalists this commonly arises when there is a lack of understanding or a difference in expectations about their role.

The most common reasons that expectations go unmet include:

- **Lack of *Clarity* About What is Expected, or About How the Expectation Will Be Met.** It is easy to assume that because one's expectations are clearly understood by oneself, they are clear to others as well. Hospitalists may assume a patient understands the proposed treatment plan, but the patient or family member may fail to understand the implications for likely discharge plans. Even when expectations are carefully explained, the other party may hear or interpret them differently than the speaker intends. The other party may also react more to the emotional aspect of the discussion or who is doing the talking rather than to the content.
- **Lack of *Agreement* About What is Expected Or How to Achieve It.** The high degree of complexity in error prone health care systems, stress and pressure, and the need for rapid change are important sources of potential conflict. Sometimes each party's expectations are clearly understood by the other party, but they simply disagree with each other about the desired outcome, the method of achieving it, or both. This can occur if the parties have competing needs or interests. For example, although resident work hour restrictions are clearly delineated in the academic setting, stress and pressure develop for hospitalists when the increased service obligations resulting from such restrictions conflict with their expectation for professional advancement. All parties may agree on the importance of improving patient flow from the Emergency Department to the inpatient floor, but may disagree about the specific methods to be employed by Emergency Medicine physicians, hospitalists, and others to achieve this goal. Changing hospital processes to promote improved quality or greater efficiency often demand changes to hospitalist work flow that are stressful for the hospitalists.

In addition, age, gender, and cultural differences may play a role in the development and management of conflict. A generational gap may result in differences in work expectations, a paternalistic view of who is actually in charge, or resistance to changing to new work requirements. Men and women may have different expectations of their work, and often have different ways of responding to stress, emotion, and conflict. In the United States, men often tend to use a competing or forcing style when faced with conflict, whereas women often tend to use compromising, accommodating, and avoiding.

A key aspect of cultural differences is the degree to which a person tends to identify most strongly with the group of which he or she is a part (a "collectivist culture") as opposed to identifying with the self (an "individualistic culture"). Individualistic cultures, which are the dominant cultures found in North America and Western Europe, value autonomy, creativity, and personal initiative. Much of the rest of the world is composed of collectivist cultures, which instead value conformity and harmony. A meta-analysis of studies on culture and conflict resolution styles found that people in individualistic cultures tend to choose forcing as a conflict style more often and people who come from collectivistic cultures tend to choose withdrawing, compromising, or problem-solving styles instead.

THE POTENTIAL BENEFITS OF CONFLICT

Conflicts are inevitable in human interactions. The increasingly complex and collaborative nature of the work that hospitalists do as team-based care models have emerged increases the risk that interpersonal conflicts may arise. The increasing cost pressures and competition for scarce resources that exist in an era of national health care reform have increased stress and opportunities for conflict for all health care professionals. These conflicts can be destructive if not effectively managed. But a healthy approach to conflict management acknowledges that not all conflict is entirely negative. There are potential benefits that may be derived from conflicts under certain circumstances. DeChurch and Marks (2001) reported that the ways in which groups handle conflict help to determine whether or not benefits were realized, noting that "the relationship between task conflict and group performance was positive when conflict was actively managed and negative when it was passively managed." This suggests that Hospital Medicine physicians will be well served to develop effective conflict management skills that can help them increase the likelihood that the conflicts they will inevitably face may yield positive results. In order to do so, it will be important for hospitalists to think strategically about how one may extract the maximum benefit from conflicts that do occur. Some of the potential benefits of appropriately managed conflict include:

- **Catalyst for Change.** Conflicts can force needed change by surfacing problems that otherwise might not be recognized, and by elevating latent issues to a level that demands attention. This can be especially valuable in tradition-bound, change-resistant organizations.
- **Improved Outcomes.** Similarly, conflicts can ultimately yield improved outcomes when they facilitate learning in the search for better solutions and bring to the forefront useful information and emotions that lie below the surface.
- **Balance.** Healthy conflict helps to ensure that balance is maintained among competing needs and perspectives.
- **Increased Accountability.** Because conflicts involve strong emotions, healthy conflict resolution usually involves careful articulation of what the parties have agreed to do to resolve it, and a significant degree of accountability to ensure that the agreements are followed through.
- **Improved Relationships.** When people skillfully manage a conflict in healthy, respectful ways, it can actually serve to strengthen their relationship going forward. They end up understanding each other better, and building greater trust because they have demonstrated that they can overcome differences.

TABLE 26-1 Five Key Principles of Effective Conflict Management

1. Commit to *confronting*
2. Attend to the *conditions*
3. Identify one's personal *contribution*
4. *Consider* what is underlying others' behavior
5. *Clarify*

KEY PRINCIPLES IN CONFLICT MANAGEMENT

This chapter offers five key principles that represent a good start for those who wish to build better conflict management skills (**Table 26-1**). However, more detailed treatments of all of these principles and others are contained in the references at the end of this chapter.

1. **Commit to *Confronting.*** Most people tend to shy away from conflict. It is tempting to believe that the problem will go away by itself if left alone; that others will soften their positions, forget about the issue, or change their minds, if given enough time. But when pressed, most people will acknowledge this is simply a convenient excuse for avoiding a confrontation that they fear could become uncomfortable or out-and-out unpleasant. Another important reason that people avoid conflict is their fear that openly confronting the situation will make things worse, rather than better. They may worry about handling the confrontation badly and unintentionally causing the situation to deteriorate, or they may fear that the conflict is intractable and that no matter how carefully and skillfully the situation is handled, the outcome will be negative.

In fact, conflicts cannot be resolved if they are not confronted. They may be glossed over or pushed into the background, but not truly resolved. And such conflicts are likely to surface again, often in unanticipated and damaging ways. Thus, a willingness to acknowledge the existence of a conflict and to step up and confront it is a precondition to effectively managing the conflict.

> ## PRACTICE POINT
> - A willingness to acknowledge the existence of a conflict and to step up and confront it is a precondition to effectively managing the conflict. This requires an open and honest discussion of the issue, usually face to face, with the goal of understanding the root causes (the unmet expectations) that led to the conflict and addressing them.

In this context, the term "confrontation" is not intended to mean an angry, emotional exchange of verbal attacks. Instead, "confrontation" refers here to an open and honest discussion of the issue, usually face to face, with the goal of understanding the root causes (the unmet expectations) that led to the conflict and addressing them. The remaining principles in this secion are intended to assist the confronter, once the decision to confront has been made, to carefully plan the confrontation (when time permits), and to handle it successfully.

2. **Attend to the *Conditions.*** Patterson et al (2002) note that there are two components to every successful crucial conversation: the actual ***content*** of the conversation, and the ***conditions*** under which the conversation occurs. Most people, when planning to confront or actually engage in a confrontation (a "crucial conversation"), think primarily about the content of the conversation: "What is this conflict about? What steps will resolve it? What points do I need to be sure to make? What will I say to get my points across? What will the other person say?"

People skilled in conflict management realize that the conditions matter just as much as—in fact, maybe more than—the content does. What types of conditions matter? The physical conditions matter a great deal. Is the conversation taking place in a private place instead of in public? Are the people involved in the conversation sitting or standing so they can engage each other at eye level, or is one person sitting with the other standing over him? Is there a desk or other impediment between the participants? Is the room too large or too small, too hot or too cold to be comfortable?

Psychological conditions matter even more. The hospitalist who wishes to be skilled at conflict management must learn to pay attention to what the other person or people involved in the conflict are experiencing emotionally. Are they feeling attacked or are they feeling safe? Do they feel that the hospitalist respects them and has their best interests at heart, or do they feel that their interests will be ignored or belittled? Do they sense that the hospitalist is going to push her agenda or opinion and ignore theirs, or do they believe the hospitalist is willing to listen and take their point of view into consideration? Do they feel that the hospitalist's opinion matters, or that dialogue should occur at a "higher level" with senior physician leaders to the exclusion of hospitalists?

Before the actual content—what the conflict is about and how it should be resolved—can be effectively addressed, the skilled conflict manager must take steps to set up conditions that allow all parties to feel comfortable, safe, and heard. The necessary steps to creating these positive conditions involve ensuring mutual respect among the parties, and identifying or creating a mutual purpose. In other words, do others believe the hospitalist sees them as individuals worthy of the respect and consideration due to every human being, and do they believe that the hospitalist is mindful of their interests as well as his own in seeking an acceptable resolution?

> ## PRACTICE POINT
> - Before the actual content—what the conflict is about and how it should be resolved—can be effectively addressed, the skilled conflict manager must take steps to set up conditions that allow all parties to feel comfortable, safe, and heard. The necessary steps to creating these positive conditions involve ensuring mutual respect among the parties and identifying or creating a mutual purpose.

3. **Identify One's Personal *Contribution.*** Conflicts occur when emotions get in the way of resolving disagreements. This is true not only of others with whom a hospitalist may come in conflict, but of the hospitalist himself. Another important competency for skilled conflict managers is the ability to step back from their own emotions and assess their personal contribution to the situation; in other words, what impact are their own biases, assumptions, emotions, and actions having on the conflict itself, and on their approach to managing it? Do they truly intend to seek mutually acceptable solutions or do they just want to win?

For example, the person seeking to manage a conflict must pay attention not only to what others are experiencing emotionally but also to what he is experiencing emotionally himself. He needs to ask, "Am I feeling safe or am I under attack? Do I believe the others involved in this conflict will listen to me and take my interests into consideration, or not?" However, simply identifying one's own emotional state is not adequate. Effective conflict managers should also have the self-awareness to understand how their emotions will tend to influence their behavior in the confrontation. These tendencies are described as a person's "style under stress."

The Style Under Stress Inventory[3] in **Table 26-2** is based on the concept of *conversational safety*, and will assist individuals in assessing their own personal style under stress. In completing the questions, one should answer "T" for true or "F" for false, based on one's most common tendencies when in conflict situations in the work setting. People feel safe in a crucial conversation if they believe that they will be listened to respectfully and if they do not feel attacked or ignored. They feel that the other parties have their interests at heart, or at least that others' interests and their own are not diametrically opposed without room for finding common ground. The inventory is designed to help people understand how they tend to behave when they do not feel safe in a crucial conversation.

Individuals responding "true" for several of the first six questions are said to be *going to silence* when under the stress of a challenging conflict situation. This means they will tend to try to downplay or sugarcoat an issue, or even avoid it outright by changing the subject or disengaging when they do not feel safe. In such cases, they may believe that they have raised an issue and articulated their concerns,

but others may be left confused or unaware of how strongly the person feels about the issue because of his *silence* tendencies. On the other hand, answering "true" to some or all of questions 7 through 12 means the person tends to *go to violence* when feeling unsafe in a conversation. These people will often try to force their opinion on others by controlling the conversation and either prevent others from speaking or belittle their contributions when they do.

Both silence and violence can be extremely damaging, when the goal of the conversation is to confront disagreements and work toward mutually acceptable solutions. When people understand their own silence or violence tendencies, they can begin to pay attention to how they are responding during conflict situations. They can look for evidence that they are not feeling safe and then step back to assess the impact their silence or violence is having on the conversation and adjust their interactions accordingly. As awareness of these tendencies grows over time, people can begin to anticipate situations in which safety may be at risk and to proactively develop plans to manage their own tendencies to go to silence or violence.

When thinking about one's personal contribution to a conflict situation, one should also be cognizant of individual assumptions and biases about others involved in the conflict, and especially one's beliefs about others' intentions. For example, it is usually helpful to consider the problem of *intent* versus *impact*. When analyzing a conflict, one should consider asking, "Is it the *impact* (ie, the outcome) of the other person's behavior that is bothering me so much, or is it what I believe about the person's *intentions*?"

This distinction is important because humans tend to overemphasize dispositional factors such as personality type or motives, and to discount situational factors such as external stressors, when interpreting the behavior of others; this phenomenon is known by psychologists as *the fundamental attribution error* or *correspondence bias*. Because of this bias, the emotions a person experiences about a disagreement, and thus the level of conflict that ensues, may be heightened as a result of presumed negative intentions on the part of others ("that surgeon is just lazy") and discounting the circumstantial factors that may be influencing others' behavior ("that surgeon is under real pressure to produce good outcomes, and does not have the training or experience to manage these complex medication regimens").

The fundamental attribution error may be exacerbated by a related tendency known as *the actor-observer bias* in which one tends to attribute others' behavior to their dispositions but to attribute one's own behavior to the circumstances ("that family member lost her temper because she's a demanding jerk, but I only lost my temper because she pushed me over the edge"). Self-awareness is critical for effective conflict management, especially awareness of one's own assumptions and biases.

TABLE 26-2 Style Under Stress Test

1. Rather than tell people exactly what I think, sometimes I rely on jokes, sarcasm, or snide remarks to let them know I'm frustrated.	T	F
2. When I have got something tough to bring up, sometimes I offer weak or insincere compliments to soften the blow.	T	F
3. Sometimes when people bring up a touchy or awkward issue I try to change the subject.	T	F
4. When it comes to dealing with awkward or stressful subjects, sometimes I hold back rather than give my full and candid opinion.	T	F
5. At times I avoid situations that might bring me into contact with people I'm having problems with.	T	F
6. I have put off returning phone calls or e-mails because I simply did not want to deal with the person who sent them.	T	F
7. In order to get my point across, I sometimes exaggerate my side of the argument.	T	F
8. If I seem to be losing control of a conversation, I might cut people off or change the subject in order to bring it back to where I think it should be.	T	F
9. When others make points that seem stupid to me, I sometimes let them know it without holding back at all.	T	F
10. When I'm stunned by a comment, sometimes I say things that others might take as forceful or attacking, comments such as "give me a break!" or "that's ridiculous!"	T	F
11. Sometimes when things get heated I move from arguing against others' points to saying things that might hurt them personally.	T	F
12. If I get into a heated discussion, I've been known to be tough on the other person. In fact, they might feel a bit insulted or hurt.	T	F

Excerpted with permission from Patterson K, Grenny J, McMillan R, et al. *Crucial Conversations: Tools for Talking When Stakes are High.* New York, NY: McGraw-Hill; 2002.

PRACTICE POINT

- Self-awareness is critical for effective conflict management, especially awareness of one's own assumptions and biases.

---

4. ***Consider* What is Underlying Others' Behavior.** One of the keys to effective conflict management is the ability to analyze why others respond the way they do in conflict situations (taking into account both dispositional factors and situational factors), and to modify one's interactions accordingly. The concept of conversational safety applies to the other parties involved in a conflict situation, as well as to oneself. Skilled conflict managers become adept at not only reading and adjusting their own behaviors, but also at looking for signs that others are not feeling safe. Hospitalists may become more accepting

of the anger expressed by patients' families, the critical comments from other medical staff members, or the sugar-coated change of subject by the hospital executive when they realize that these behaviors often result from others' fear(s) that they will be treated with disrespect, attacked, or ignored. If they can then work to address those underlying fears (part of paying attention to conditions) before launching into the content of the conversation, they will be more successful.

PRACTICE POINT

- One of the keys to effective conflict management is the ability to analyze why others respond the way they do in conflict situations (taking into account both dispositional factors and situational factors), and to modify interactions accordingly. When someone acts in ways that contribute to a heightened level of conflict, it is worth considering whether that person has underlying human needs that are going unmet and that are contributing to his or her challenging behavior.

Another way of thinking about this issue is to anticipate that the more significant the conflict, the greater the chance that people will respond to it emotionally rather than logically. While it is not a clinically accurate model, it may be useful to think of peoples' brains as having a logical core, surrounded by a layer of emotion (**Figure 26-1**). Every interaction a person has, no matter how logical it is, passes through this emotional filter on its way in or out.

For most people and under normal circumstances, the layer of emotion surrounding the logical core is relatively thin and the information from the interaction passes through it in both directions, informed by the emotion but not substantially altered by it. In a conflict situation, however, the emotional layer surrounding the logical core inflates like a balloon. In this situation, the expanded emotional layer takes over and prevents logical conversation and data from passing through. The person is responding from her or his emotion, rather than from logic. A hospitalist may be attempting to have a very logical conversation with a family member, assuming that she is addressing the family member's logical core. But the hospitalist's logical words cannot get through the family member's inflated emotional layer. The hospitalist is talking logic, and the family members are responding from emotion; so no wonder they are unable to relate to each other. In such situations, it is necessary to let some air out of the balloon—to give the emotional layer a chance to deflate—before it will be possible to re-engage the logical core in problem solving or conflict resolution. Sometimes this requires stepping away from the conversation for a while and coming back to it later.

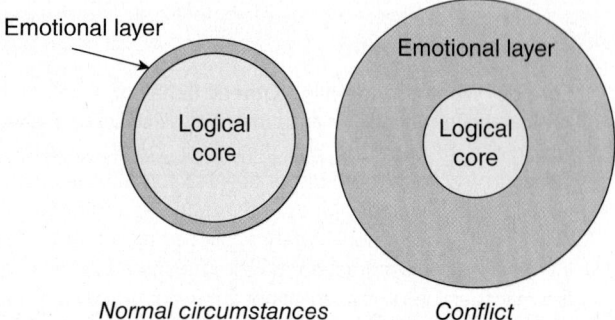

Figure 26-1 *Logic and emotion diagram.*

In addition to the overwhelming influence of emotion on how others respond to conflict situations, Heifetz and Linsky (2002) have argued that there are powerful and universal human needs that influence behavior, sometimes in dysfunctional or disruptive ways:

> Every human being needs some degree of power and control, affirmation and importance, as well as intimacy and delight…. We all have hungers, which are expressions of our normal human needs. But sometimes those hungers disrupt our capacity to act wisely or purposefully. Perhaps one of our needs is too great and renders us vulnerable. Perhaps the setting in which we operate exaggerates our normal level of need, amplifying our desires and overwhelming our usual self-controls. Or, our hungers might be unchecked simply because our human needs are not being met in our personal lives.

When someone acts in ways that contribute to a heightened level of conflict, it is worth considering whether that person has underlying human needs that are going unmet, and that are contributing to his or her challenging behavior.

5. **Clarify.** When confronting another person about a conflict situation, effective communication skills are essential. It is important to clarify what one is attempting to convey; it is also important to clarify the other person's point of view. Important communication skills include

- *Setting the stage.* Keeping in mind the principles of mutual respect and mutual purpose, it may be valuable to start out by communicating one's own positive intentions to the other person(s) in a way that builds toward these goals.
- *Managing expectations.* Hospitalists should clearly communicate what their own expectations were in the situation that gave rise to the conflict, and seek to understand what the other person's expectations were. This will create a foundation for further dialogue about the differences between what each party expected and what actually occurred.
- *Active listening.* Active listening skills involve not just hearing what the other person says, but also
  - actively engaging the other person with eye contact and body language;
  - working to enable the other person to feel comfortable sharing potentially difficult information;
  - listening "between the lines" for what *is not* being said, as well as what *is* being said;
  - acknowledging the reality and legitimacy of the other person's emotions;
  - paraphrasing and reframing to ensure understanding of the other person's perspective;
  - asking questions and probing to understand root causes;
  - staying focused on the other person, rather than one's own planned response.
- *Joint problem solving.* Engaging all parties to the conflict in joint problem solving will help to clarify what needs to happen to resolve the conflict, and what the alternatives are for moving forward out of conflict. It will also help build mutual support of and commitment to the agreed-upon approach.
- *Articulating next steps.* Establishing a clear path of next steps and assigning responsibilities are vital components of a clear and effective communication process. It is worth talking both about the expected outcome, and about the method or process by which the outcome will be achieved: it is not uncommon for new conflicts to arise inadvertently when two parties believe they understand *what* will happen, only to clash over *how* it will be accomplished.

STRATEGIES FOR EFFECTIVE CONFLICT MANAGEMENT: CONFLICT RESOLUTION AND NEGOTIATION

1. **The Talking Stick.** Stephen Covey (1989) highlighted the importance of empathetic communication in describing the principle, "Seek first to understand, then to be understood." Covey (2004) further described the use among Native American cultures of the Talking Stick as a tool to help people resolve differences by creating greater mutual understanding and respect.[5] The Talking Stick is passed from one person to another, and only the person who is holding the Talking Stick is allowed to present her or his perspective. This ensures that only one person talks at a time, and increases the ability of others to listen because they are not permitted to argue or make their own points until the person holding the Talking Stick has finished.

The most powerful aspect of the Talking Stick, however, is that the person holding it does not relinquish it until she is satisfied that she has been fully understood by the others. It is the responsibility of the listeners to listen carefully and with empathy, and to ensure that the speaker feels understood—not necessarily agreed with—just understood. Once the speaker is satisfied that others understand him, she passes the Talking Stick on and assumes the responsibility to listen and make the next speaker feel understood. Covey describes the value of the Talking Stick as follows:

> This way, all of the parties involved take responsibility for one hundred percent of the communication, both speaking and listening. Once each of the parties feels understood, an amazing thing usually happens. Negative energy dissipates, contention evaporates, mutual respect grows, and people become creative. New ideas emerge. Third alternatives appear.

One does not need to use a physical Talking Stick to gain these benefits. It is possible to establish a framework for interacting in which the parties agree that they will alternate the responsibilities of talking and listening until both feel fully understood. This process can be very effective in facilitating the resolution of conflicts between hospitalists and other specialists regarding scope and service issues. Some parties may be able to do this independently, while others may benefit from facilitation by a third party mediator.

2. **Unhappy Patients and Families: Take the HEAT.** Some of the most challenging conflicts that hospitalists must manage are those that involve the unmet expectations of patients and families. Keeping in mind the role of emotion in conflict, Byham (1993) recommends the following approach for those who are responsible for addressing the needs of unhappy patients and families, as summarized by the acronym "Take the HEAT":
   - *Hear them out.* Active listening without interrupting, disagreeing, or defending is the crucial first step. Angry patients and family members need to be able to express their emotions in order to let some of the air out of the emotional balloon.
   - *Empathize.* As with Covey's Talking Stick example, patients and families need to feel understood. It is not necessary to agree with them, but it is important to acknowledge their feelings and to attempt to understand the issue from their perspective.
   - *Apologize.* Byham points out that even if one does not wish to admit fault, it is important to apologize for the situation, and for the fact that the patient's expectations were not met.
   - *Take responsibility for action.* Once the emotional balloon has been deflated, it is often possible to re-engage the patient or family member on a logical basis. A good way to make this transition is to take some concrete action, either to resolve the problem on the spot or to demonstrate a desire to improve the situation.

3. **Principles of Effective Negotiation.** Hospitalists frequently find themselves in potential conflict situations in which negotiation is an effective strategy for addressing the issue. These may include formal negotiations such as the development of professional service agreements, employment contracts, or incentive compensation metrics, or they may be less formal interactions such as working with specialists to define admitting responsibilities or co-management services. Strong negotiation skills are also valuable for hospitalists working on medical staff committees or quality improvement projects when the diverse interests of many parties must be reconciled.

In traditional negotiations, each party stakes out a formal position and then proceeds to bargain from that position, using various tactics to "win" points that bring the final compromise outcome closer to this position. By contrast, the Principled Negotiation model developed by Fisher and Ury (1981) focuses on understanding all the parties' underlying interests and on identifying objective, fair options that can satisfy everyone. The four tenets of Principled Negotiation are as follows:

- *Separate the people from the problem.* This principle addresses the role of emotions and relationships in influencing one's perceptions about the negotiation. The authors suggest that negotiators seek to identify when relationships (either as friends or adversaries) may be getting in the way of seeking the best outcome, and that negotiators address these emotional aspects directly and openly with the goal of moving beyond them into objective and collaborative problem solving.
- *Focus on interests, not positions.* It is crucial to look beyond the formal stance a person has taken and attempt to understand his underlying interests, the "root causes" of his position. By understanding all parties' basic interests (both one's own and the other person's), one increases the chances of identifying new perspectives or solutions that will meet both parties' interests.
- *Invent options for mutual gain.* The authors argue that once emotional and relationship issues have been separated from the substantive problem, and all parties' underlying interests are understood, the role of the parties is to invent better options. The steps in this process are: separating the identification of options from the act of judging them, looking for many options rather than a single answer, focusing on options that result in mutual gains, and then coming up with ways to make the decisions easy.
- *Insist on using objective criteria.* Finally, Fisher and Ury acknowledge that despite one's best efforts, negotiators will sometimes face situations in which interests are truly in intractable conflict and mutually acceptable options may not be available. In these cases, effective negotiators will insist that decisions be made using objective, usually externally validated, criteria.

In addition to the tenets of Principled Negotiation outlined above, it is important to recognize that when the issues are complex, even the best and most carefully documented negotiation will probably fail to anticipate every nuance that may arise going forward. For example, when hospitalists negotiate and memorialize a "service agreement" with a group of specialists to define who will admit which types of patients, invariably a patient will present who does not fit neatly into any of the categories specified in the service agreement. If the potential for this to occur is not acknowledged and planned for up front, additional conflicts may arise despite the parties' careful efforts. The most valuable asset in such situations is a strong underlying relationship of mutual trust and respect that will enable the parties to resolve these issues on a case-by-case basis. The bottom line is that even the best negotiation skills and most clearly drafted documents cannot substitute for strong relationships.

CONCLUSION

Conflict is inevitable in human interactions, and the potential for serious conflict will grow as the complexity of interactions increases. The extremely challenging milieus in which hospitalists practice are rife with misunderstandings, disagreements, and unmet expectations, placing hospitalists at risk for conflict on a daily basis. Therefore, the ability to understand and effectively manage conflict should be a core competency for all hospitalists. The first step in building effective conflict management skills is to understand the causes and potential benefits of conflict. Next, hospitalists should learn and apply key principles of conflict management; and finally, hospitalists need to develop competence and confidence in implementing useful strategies for managing different types of conflict.

SUGGESTED READINGS

Covey SR. *The 7 Habits of Highly Effective People*. New York, NY: Simon and Schuster; 1989:235-260.

DeChurch LA, Marks MA. Maximizing the benefits of task conflict: the role of conflict management. *Int J Conflict Manag*. 2001;12:4-22.

Gilbert DT, Malone PS. The correspondence bias. *Psychol Bull*. 1995;117:21-38.

Holt JL, DeVore CJ. Culture, gender, organizational role, and styles of conflict resolution: a meta-analysis. *Int J Intercult Relat*. 2005;29:165-196.

Jones EE, Nisbett RE. *The Actor and the Observer: Divergent Perceptions of the Causes of Behavior*. New York, NY: General Learning Press; 1971.

Patterson K, Grenny J, McMillan R, et al. *Crucial Conversations: Tools for Talking when Stakes are High*. New York, NY: McGraw Hill; 2002.

Ross L. The intuitive psychologist and his shortcomings: distortions in the attribution process. In: Berkowitz L, ed. *Advances in Experimental Social Psychology*. vol. 10. Orlando, FL: Academic Press; 1977:173-240.

Thomas KW, Thomas GF, Shaubhut N. Conflict styles of men and women at six organization levels. *Int J Conflict Manage*. 2008;19:148-166.

Triandis HC. *Individualism and Collectivism*. Boulder, CO: Westview Press; 1995.

REFERENCES

1. Patterson K, Grenny J, et al. *Crucial Conversations: Tools for Talking when Stakes are High*. New York, NY: McGraw Hill; 2002:45-51 and 68-74.

2. Patterson K, Grenny J, et al. *Crucial Conversations: Tools for Talking when Stakes are High*. New York, NY: McGraw Hill; 2002:32-34 and 51-62.

3. The authors provide a free expanded version of the Style Under Stress Inventory online at https://www.vitalsmarts.com/styleunderstress.aspx, along with additional guidance on interpreting the results.

4. Heifetz RA, Linsky M. *Leadership on the Line: Staying Alive through the Dangers of Leading*. Boston, MA: Harvard Business School Publishing; 2002:164.

5. Covey SR. *The 8th Habit*. New York, NY: Simon and Schuster; 2004:197-201.

6. Byham WC. *Zapp! Empowerment in Health Care*. New York, NY: Random House; 1993:145-146.

7. Fisher R, Ury W. *Getting to Yes: Negotiating Agreement Without Giving In*. Boston, MA: Houghton Mifflin; 1981:16-98.

SECTION 6
Billing, Coding, and Clinical Documentation

CHAPTER 27

Professional Coding and Billing Guidelines for Clinical Documentation

Carol Pohlig, RN, BSN, CPC
Scott Manaker, MD, PhD

The medical record of an individual patient serves numerous functions. Ideally, the record should provide a comprehensive historical vehicle promoting excellence in care delivery to a patient, transcending communication barriers, and facilitating care coordination among multiple disparate providers and facilities (such as hospitals). However, the medical record also serves as the basis for a variety of financial, legal, and administrative functions including the documentation for both professional and facility fee reimbursement, quality and safety assessments (including pay for performance), malpractice litigation and disability determinations, and community-based care and public health initiatives.

Currently, the medical record of an individual patient is fragmented, with various pieces shared only sometimes among numerous providers. Hospitalists typically provide episodic, facility-based care. Fortunately, the proliferation, adoption, and increasing interoperability of electronic medical records (EMRs), and their evolution into personalized health records, still holds promise for consolidation and availability of all relevant clinical information to each provider participating in the care of a single patient.

■ SOME GENERAL PRINCIPLES

This chapter focuses upon the documentation requirements incumbent upon hospitalists for professional fee billing of their clinical services. Some general principles of clinical documentation warrant discussion despite this focus, and apply to both paper and EMRs.

The documentation of professional services should always comprise the essential components of a patient's chief complaint, history, physical examination (PE), and medical decision making (MDM). The concerns of both patient and provider should be clearly recorded, including expectations (realistic or not) and satisfaction (and dissatisfaction). All diagnostic test orders and results should reside in the chart, as well as documentation of various specific services (eg, physical, occupational, speech, or rehabilitation therapy; home health services, durable medical equipment needs, and social work evaluations).

PRACTICE POINT

- The clinical documentation of professional services should always comprise the essential components of a patient's chief complaint, history, physical examination, and medical decision making. The concerns of both the patient and provider should be clearly recorded, including expectations (realistic or not) and satisfaction (dissatisfaction).

Corrections

At some point in time, every medical record requires a correction. In a paper document, draw a single line through the inaccurate portion and write a correction nearby, dating and signing the revision. The original entry thereby remains legible for future reference. For example, consider misidentification of a right swollen knee joint, when actually it is on the left: when the physician recognizes the mistaken documentation, the *right* side should have a single line drawn through it (ie, overstrike text appearing as ~~right~~) and a note written nearby indicating that the *left* side is the accurate side. Sign and date these changes on the day of correction. Methods and appearances of corrections and amendments in EMRs continue to evolve, but all incorporate password-protected signatures with electronic date- and time-stamped entries.

Late-entry documentation

Like corrections, addenda or late entries can be made at any time and labeled as such, with a currently dated and timed signature. Also, explain why the entry was made late and not contemporaneously. For example, following a hospital visit, a hospitalist responds to a rapid response call and neglects to document the visit in the hospital medical record. When recognized the next day, document the hospital visit as a late entry and specify that the care was delivered the previous day.

■ AN OVERVIEW OF HOSPITAL INPATIENT PAYMENT SYSTEMS

As the most prominent payer in the United States, Medicare payment systems are of paramount importance to understand. Fortunately, Medicare policies are established by the Centers for Medicare and Medicaid Services (CMS) and available online through the CMS On-Line Manual System, so that everyone can in principle understand how claims are processed and payments are made. Medicare policies are largely consistent across the United States, and many private payers follow CMS's lead. However, remember that regional Medicare Administrative Contractors develop local coverage determinations from CMS payment policy, and can create idiosyncratic interpretations of the documentation guidelines for evaluation and management (E/M) services. One such example would be the nuanced medical allowances for a detailed exam (see *Physical Exam* section) implemented by Novitas Solutions. Similarly, various third party payers have the right, as allowable under their contract with physician groups, to create unique documentation mandates and payment policies. Facilities also generate requirements, such as a required history and physical before a procedure, which do not comprise medically necessary, billable physician services.

Medicare pays hospitals for inpatient services using an inpatient prospective payment system (IPPS), which relies primarily on the diagnosis in order to group the services delivered to an inpatient into a Medicare severity-adjusted diagnosis related group (MS-DRG). Many diagnostic categories have two or three severity levels, differentiated by the presence or absence of a specified set of complications and comorbidities (CCs) or major complications and comorbidities (MCCs). Hospitals and other facilities frequently request hospitalists to clarify, expand, or specify their clinical documentation to ensure the assignment of a hospitalization to the proper MS-DRG. This single MS-DRG payment covers all facility services during the inpatient stay. Many payers have adopted a similar mechanism of providing a single, fixed payment for an entire hospitalization, often referred to as a case rate.

Some non-Medicare payers still reimburse hospitals and facilities with a fixed payment for each day, commonly described as a per diem rate. The daily payment potentially varies depending upon the types of services provided to the patient (eg, intensive care versus skilled nursing care). Other payment models continue to emerge as a result of health care reform, including the evolution of accountable care organizations and the proliferation of patient-centered medical homes.

■ AN OVERVIEW OF PHYSICIAN PAYMENT SYSTEMS

Physician services are typically reported using the American Medical Association (AMA) *Current Procedural Terminology* (CPT), fourth edition, which lists descriptive terms and identifying codes to report medical services and procedures. CPT provides a uniform language to accurately describe all medical, surgical, and diagnostic services and procedures. Even physicians receiving capitated payments or participating in various advanced payment models still typically report CPT codes for their services.

Hospitalists predominantly report E/M codes (CPT 99201-99499), which for Medicare exceed $32 billion annually and account for more than 40% of the Medicare physician fee schedule allowed charges. Other bedside procedures and diagnostic testing, sometimes performed by hospitalists, are also found in CPT. In selecting the proper E/M code, the site and nature of service determine the *visit category*; and the key components of history, physical examination, and MDM determine the specific level of CPT code within a visit category.

Many payers are now adopting Medicare's recognition and regulation of nurse practitioners and physician assistants as advanced practice providers, independently able to provide, document, and bill for E/M services. The number of advanced practice providers performing hospitalist services is rapidly increasing. Therefore, when we refer to *providers* throughout this chapter, we include both physicians and these qualified advanced practice providers functioning in an independent billing role.

THE KEY COMPONENTS OF PHYSICIAN E/M DOCUMENTATION

Selection of an E/M level focuses upon the content of the three key components: history, PE, and MDM. Time is considered a fourth key component, but only affects the E/M level when counseling and/or coordination of care dominate more than 50% of the physician's total visit time (see below). When counseling and/or coordination of care involves less than 50% of the physician's total visit time, time is only considered a contributory factor and does not determine the E/M level.

Two sets of documentation guidelines have been elaborated by Medicare and largely adopted by other payers. The earlier 1995 guidelines are the most widespread, and generally applicable to hospitalists along with most medical and surgical specialists. The later 1997 guidelines elaborate specialty-specific physical examinations, as well as clearly articulate detailed physical examination requirements lacking in the 1995 guidelines. An added variation also exists between the two guidelines in aspects of history. The 1995 guidelines will be described in detail throughout this section, and the 1997 guidelines are highlighted below in a separate section for completeness.

■ HISTORY

The elements of history include the chief complaint (CC), history of present illness (HPI), review of systems (ROS), and the past, family, and social histories (PFSHs). A chart note may not segregate these elements into unique subtitled areas, but rather the information may be interspersed amid the written, typed, or even dictated narrative.

Chief complaint (CC)

Typically, the reason for the visit is often quoted from the patient's own words as a sign or symptom, such as, "my belly hurts." Always document a CC in the progress note, even absent an acute complaint, such as, "pneumonia follow-up." Avoid statements lacking a specific clinical reference (eg, "post-op visit Day #3").

History of present illness (HPI)

The HPI conveys information about the CC, from either the origin (at an initial encounter) or the interval between sequential patient encounters. This information is arbitrarily allocated into eight elements: location, quality, severity, duration, timing, context, modifying factors, and associated signs/symptoms. The HPI is then quantified as *brief* (one to three elements) or *extended* (four or more elements). For example, consider this extended HPI: "Patient complains of increased (severity) pedal (location) edema that began 2 days ago (duration). Less able to walk. No chest pain (associated signs/symptoms)."

Review of systems (ROS)

The ROS refers to signs or symptoms experienced in conjunction with the CC. Fourteen systems are recognized: constitutional, eyes, ears/nose/mouth/throat, cardiovascular, respiratory, gastrointestinal, genitourinary, musculoskeletal, integumentary (which includes the breast), neurologic, psychiatric, endocrine, hematologic/lymphatic, and allergic/immunologic. Medical necessity, as deemed by the treating provider in light of the patient's current or previous conditions, determines the number of systems required for review.

A ROS may be problem pertinent, extended, or complete. A *problem-pertinent* ROS documents one system directly related to the CC. An *extended* ROS requires documentation of two to nine systems, that is, the system that is directly related to the CC, along with one or more additional systems. A complete ROS documents 10 or more individual systems. When obtaining a complete ROS, to decrease the amount of time spent listing each system individually, both the 1995 and 1997 (see below) E/M documentation guidelines allow the physician to comment on the positive and pertinent negative systems, with an additional comment that the "remainder is negative." However, insurers may not accept alternative phrases, and Medicare (and some non-Medicare) contractors seek individual documentation of each system when less than 14 systems are reviewed.

Past, family, and social histories (PFSHs)

The past history includes documentation of previous illnesses, hospitalizations, surgeries, medications, allergies, and immunizations. The family history provides information regarding potential hereditary illnesses. The social history may list details of the patient's substance use (tobacco/alcohol/illicit drugs), sexual history, employment status, level of education, marital status, or living arrangements.

A *pertinent* PFSH includes a comment in any one of the three histories (ie, past, family, or social). Full credit for a *complete* PFSH requires a comment in each history (ie, past, family, and social) when reporting initial hospital, observation, or nursing facility care, consultations, and new office, home, and domiciliary visits. In contradistinction, emergency department (ED) services or established patient visits in the home, domiciliary, office, or other outpatient area require one comment in two of the three histories for credit as a *complete* PFSH.

Providers may review and comment that the "family history is noncontributory" and still receive credit for the family history from some insurers. Certain Medicare contractors, such as Palmetto GBA, prohibit this terminology and require specific documentation regardless of clinical relevance (eg, "family history negative for liver disease"). Also note that with subsequent services, both for hospital care and nursing facility visits, only an "interval history" is required and redocumentation of the PFSH is unnecessary from a billing perspective.

Determination of history level

The number of historical elements present in the chart note determines the level of history (**Table 27-1**). If all of the requirements are not met for a given level of history, select the level associated with the *deficient* element. For example, a comprehensive history requires documentation of the CC, ≥4 HPI elements, ≥10 ROS, and a complete PFSH. If the ROS only includes documentation for nine systems, a comprehensive history cannot be selected; report a service that requires only a detailed history: CC, ≥4 HPI elements, 2-9 ROS, and a pertinent PFSH.

Other circumstances

A PFSH obtained during an earlier encounter does not need to be rerecorded if the provider documents review and updating of the previous information. Update the history by describing any new information or noting the absence of change, along with the date and location of the earlier PFSH; this earlier PFSH must be contained in a printable area of the medical record. CPT requires only an *interval* history for subsequent hospital or subsequent nursing facility visits, and it is usually unnecessary to record information about the PFSH, which is unlikely to change in these settings.

Most auditors disallow a single statement as both an HPI element and ROS element. The ROS and/or PFSH may be recorded by ancillary staff, or on a form completed by the patient. The provider must document review and confirmation of this information recorded by others, either by a reference to the history form in the progress note or by initialing and dating the form, making any necessary annotations, additions, or corrections.

If unable to obtain history from the patient, the record should describe the patient's condition or the circumstance that precludes obtaining a history, and what attempts the provider made to obtain the information. For example, "… patient sedated and paralyzed, unable to obtain additional history. Family currently unavailable to contact; information obtained from the staff and available medical records." However, reviewers expect providers to incorporate historic information to the extent possible, from all reasonably available sources (eg, old records, emergency medical services documents, other provider documentation, or conversations).

Finally, although the physician may collect all of the information required for a complete ROS, the most common underdocumentation error is failure to document at least 10 systems. The second most common mistake is a missing family history or social history.

■ PHYSICAL EXAMINATION (PE)

Individual PE elements will be assigned to body areas (head and face, neck, chest, abdomen, genitalia/groin/buttocks, back/spine, and each extremity) or organ systems (constitutional, eyes, ears/nose/mouth/throat, cardiovascular, respiratory, gastrointestinal, genitourinary, musculoskeletal, integumentary, neurologic, psychiatric, and hematologic/lymphatic/immunologic). Providers may document specific findings (eg, "abdomen soft") or make a generalized comment (eg, "HEENT normal"). Abnormal findings must be

TABLE 27-1 Levels of History

History Level	HPI	ROS	PFSH
Problem-focused	Brief (≤3)	None	None
Expanded problem-focused	Brief (≤3)	Problem pertinent (1)	None
Detailed	Extended (≥4)	Extended (2-9)	Pertinent (1)
Comprehensive	Extended (≥4)	Complete (≥10)	Complete (2 or 3)*

*All three for new patient encounters; two of three for subsequent or ED encounters.

specifically documented, such as "S₃"; however, a comment indicating "abnormal" without elaboration is insufficient.

The PE documented in the medical record is categorized as problem-focused, expanded problem-focused, detailed, or comprehensive. One comment in one area constitutes a *problem-focused exam*. The distinction between the expanded problem-focused and detailed examination under the 1995 Guidelines is the greatest ambiguity in physical examination documentation. Both the *expanded problem-focused* and *detailed* exams require documentation of two to seven systems. However, "detailed" is defined as an extended examination of the affected body area or organ system, in addition to other symptomatic or related organ systems. The number of required comments regarding the affected body area or organ system to consider the examination detailed has never been defined by either CPT or Medicare. Attempting to decrease ambiguity and variability among auditors, Novitas Solutions scores a detailed exam using the "4 × 4" rule: four elements examined in four body areas or four organ systems (totaling 16 documentation elements). In contrast, other contractors suggest using the 1997 guidelines (discussed later) for detailed exam requirements.

The *comprehensive* examination is a general multisystem examination or a complete examination of a single organ system. Medicare requires the minimum documentation for the general multisystem examination to include one comment in each of eight systems; of course, additional comments in each system and more than eight systems may be described, as clinically indicated. For example, a comprehensive examination may be documented as follows: "P = 76, BP = 120/80, RR = 12 (constitutional); HEENT normal (eyes and ENMT); neck supple (musculoskeletal); regular rate and rhythm (cardiovascular); lungs clear (respiratory); normal bowel sounds (gastrointestinal); no rashes (integumentary), normal gait (neurological)." The requirements for a comprehensive single organ system still remain undefined for use with these 1995 guidelines.

■ MEDICAL DECISION MAKING (MDM)

The complexity of MDM drives selection of a level of service. MDM is categorized as *straightforward, low, moderate,* or *high*. Three categories must be considered to determine the level of MDM complexity: the number of diagnoses, the amount and complexity of data, and the risk to the patient.

Number of diagnoses considered

This first category identifies the number of diagnoses and/or management options considered in the encounter, based upon the documentation. Up to four points are assigned to each problem, with more points assigned for new problems than for established problems, and a new problem requiring additional workup (ie, diagnostic testing) given the maximum four points. Established problems identified as worsening receive a higher value than stable or improving problems. A self-limited or minor problem (eg, sunburn) receives minimal credit as these issues typically do not warrant a defined plan of care (**Table 27-2**).

New problems require initiation of a care plan, while established problems may require modification or continuation of a care plan. An *established* problem has been previously considered by the physician or provider group (to allow for cross coverage and handoffs between same specialty providers in the same group) in the strictest of interpretations of the guidelines. Note that credit is also given for a problem considered, although not primarily under treatment by the physician. For example, in a patient receiving steroids for an inflammatory disease, the hospitalist receives credit for noting the potential adverse consequence upon serum lipids, even if a cardiologist is primarily treating the dyslipidemia. Notice, a chronic condition such as diabetes, cared for by an endocrinologist,

TABLE 27-2 Valuation of Diagnostic and Treatment Options

Number of Diagnoses/Treatment Options	Points per Problem
Self-limited/minor problem (stable, improved, or worsening)	1 (max = 2 problems)
Established problem (stable or improving)	1
Established problem (worsening)	2
New problem, without additional workup	3 (max = 1 problem)
New problem, with additional workup planned	4

is categorized as a *new* problem to the hospitalist newly treating the patient during an admission for ketoacidosis.

Established patients may also have *new* problems. For example, an asthmatic with a resolving flare may experience heartburn. This additional new complaint of heartburn may be considered *new* if commented upon in the progress note and no prior care plan by the hospitalist team for gastroesophageal reflux exists.

Physicians receive credit only for issues considered in the care plan. Diagnoses merely listed in the assessment and plan without elaboration of the care, or simply ascribing the care to others (eg, "diabetes—per endocrinologist") are considered part of the patient's *problem list* in the PFSH and do not add to the complexity of MDM. Additionally, new hospitalizations warrant new care plan development, and physicians can receive *new problem* credit even if the patient has been previously hospitalized by the same group. This is a nuance of inpatient and observation care only.

Data considered

The second category of determining the MDM complexity is the amount and/or complexity of data reviewed or ordered by the provider during the patient encounter. Both the type and source of information considered are valued (**Table 27-3**).

Ordering and/or reviewing of pathology/laboratory, radiology, and medicine data each provide separate but equal credit. Irrespective of the test volume in each category, only one point is allocated

TABLE 27-3 Valuation of Data Considered

Amount and/or Complexity of Data Ordered/Reviewed	Points
Review and/or order of clinical test(s)	1
Review and/or order of test(s) in the pathology/laboratory section of CPT	1
Review and/or order of test(s) in the radiology section of CPT	1
Review and/or order of test(s) in the medicine section of CPT	1
Decision to obtain old records and/or obtain history from someone (nonhealth care provider) other than the patient	1
Review and summarize old records, obtain additional history, or discuss the case with another health care provider	2
Independent visualization of actual image, tracing, or specimen	2

per category (ie, pathology/laboratory, radiology, or medicine) for the encounter. For example, the provider ordering a dozen serologic collagen vascular studies in the morning may also review the three results received in the afternoon; nonetheless, only one point is granted for this care. A single, separate point may be assigned each to pathology/laboratory, radiology, and medicine data, respectively, are cumulative in nature, and the chart note should refer to all the data reviewed or ordered to capture all of the provider work. In other words, if the chart note comments upon a radiology result (one point) and an echocardiogram order (one point), two points may be awarded for the amount of data in that encounter. Independently visualizing images, tracings, or specimens is considered separately, and additional to reviewing the formal interpretation, as long as the chart note clearly documents this occurrence (ie, "…my review of the EKG tracings showed…"). Without such specific reference distinguishing personal review of the images and of the formal interpretation, an auditor only provides minimal credit for merely reviewing the report. A reference to data review without a comment about the result (eg, "CXR reviewed…") will yield no credit; therefore, be sure to include a comment on the findings (eg, "CXR reveals cardiomegaly…").

Providers also receive credit for the additional effort of obtaining historical information from sources other than the patient, such as records from previous encounters or hospitalizations, and conversations with other health care professionals or family members. The chart note should specifically mention the source, along with the information reviewed (eg, "…spouse confirms loud snoring").

Risk to the patient

The third MDM category assesses the *patient's* risk of complications, morbidity, or mortality, with respect to the presenting problem, diagnostic procedures ordered, or management options chosen. Four levels of patient risk exist (minimal, low, moderate, and high), with examples of each risk type included in Medicare's "Table of Risk" (**Table 27-4**). The limited number of examples serves as an illustrative reference for common clinical scenarios, but not as a comprehensive list.

When determining the level of risk, consider comorbidities as well as the plan of care in assessing a patient's risk, thereby potentially increasing the complexity of MDM. Similarly, diagnostic studies or alternatively, procedures under consideration or excluded based upon excessive risk, impact the complexity of MDM (eg, "…will defer MRI, as potential morbidity of transport to magnet exceeds risks of empiric treatment"). Although many bulleted items on the table may pertain to a particular chart note, the single bulleted item in any risk category associated with the highest risk determines the patient's risk level. For example, a note documenting the monitoring of liver function tests for potential hepatotoxicity, or blood counts for possible cytopenias, comprises high risk (drug therapy requiring frequent monitoring for toxicity). However, remember risk does not equal complexity: risk is but one category (among three) of MDM and not the sole contributor to complexity.

Assigning MDM complexity

Based upon the chart note, points are assigned for diagnoses managed and data considered, and patient risk is assessed. The final result of MDM complexity hinges on the two highest valued categories. In other words, *two of the three categories must meet or exceed the requirements assigned to a specific level of complexity* to select that level, as illustrated in **Table 27-5**.

To illustrate the assignment of MDM complexity, consider the following example. The chart note considers three stable established diagnoses (three points), several blood tests (one point), and high patient risk. The lowest of the three categories (data

considered) is eliminated, and the lower of the two remaining categories (number of diagnoses) determines the moderate MDM complexity for the note. While most contractors utilize standardized concepts when assigning points, beware of contractors and other auditing programs who may impose different standards.

■ 1997 GUIDELINES

Medicare issued a second set of revised documentation guidelines for E/M services in 1997. MDM and the level categories remained unchanged from the prior 1995 documentation guidelines, as detailed above. While ambiguity plagues many aspects of the 1995 guidelines, excessive proscription limits the 1997 guidelines. The 1997 guidelines made a single minor revision to the history, while the physical examination content received extensive modification. The requirements for each level of physical examination were heavily revised, and specialty-specific single organ system examinations defined. In response to widespread complaints from the physician community, CMS allowed physicians to document using either the 1995 or 1997 guidelines, according to their individual preference, and directed auditors to review the physician documentation based on the set of guidelines most favorable to the physician for the E/M code reported for the encounter. Most physicians, including hospitalists, find the 1995 guidelines most applicable.

History

The 1997 guidelines do not limit the provider to identifying individual factors associated with the CC (eg, duration, timing, and context). Rather, a provider may document the status of one or more chronic conditions; this option is most useful for subsequent hospital visits. A brief HPI documents one or two conditions, while an extended HPI documents a minimum of three conditions. Some reviewers allow this option only if applying the 1997 guidelines to the entire note. However, beginning with dates of service September 10, 2013, Medicare gives credit for the status of chronic conditions from the 1997 guideline and the physical examination from the 1995 guideline mixed within the same note.

Physical examination

The 1997 guidelines allow a provider to select either a general multisystem examination or any one of the single organ system examinations. Hospitalists typically utilize the general examination, which specifies examination elements to perform and document. *Negative* or *normal* comments remain acceptable for the 1997 guidelines, along with the mandate to specify comments on any abnormal findings. Documentation in the medical record of 1 to 5 specified (referred to as *bulleted*) physical examination elements comprises a *problem-focused* examination; 6 to 11 bulleted elements defines the *expanded problem-focused* examination; and a *detailed* examination requires 12 or more bulleted items.

For the 1997 *comprehensive* general multisystem examination (**Tables 27-6** and **27-7**), the provider must perform all the elements specified in at least nine organ systems or body areas but only needs to document a minimum of two elements from each of those nine systems or areas. For single organ system exams, all bullets must be performed; however all bullets in all shaded boxes and at least one bullet in each unshaded box must be documented.

■ DETERMINING LEVEL OF SERVICE

For both the 1995 and 1997 guidelines, assign a specific level to each of the three key components. Rate history and examination each as either problem-focused, expanded problem-focused, detailed, or comprehensive. Rate the complexity of MDM as either straightforward, low, moderate, or high. CPT correlates specific levels of the key components with certain levels of most E/M services.

TABLE 27-4 Table of Risk

Level of Risk	Presenting Problem(s)	Diagnostic Procedure(s) Ordered	Management Options Selected
Minimal	• One self-limited or minor problem (eg, cold, insect bite, tinea corporis)	• Laboratory tests requiring venipuncture • Chest x-rays • ECG/EEG • Urinalysis • Ultrasound (such as echocardiography) • KOH prep	• Rest • Gargles • Elastic bandages • Superficial dressings
Low	• Two or more self-limited or minor problems • One stable chronic illness (eg, well-controlled hypertension, noninsulin dependent diabetes, cataract, BPH) • Acute uncomplicated illness or injury, (eg, cystitis, allergic rhinitis, simple sprain)	• Physiologic tests not under stress (eg, pulmonary function tests) • Noncardiovascular imaging studies with contrast (such as chest or abdominal CT) • Superficial needle biopsies • Clinical laboratory tests requiring arterial puncture • Skin biopsies	• Over-the-counter drugs • Minor surgery with no identified risk factors • Physical therapy • Occupational therapy • IV fluids without additives
Moderate	• One or more chronic illnesses with mild exacerbation, progression, or side effects of treatment • Two or more stable chronic illnesses • Undiagnosed new problem with uncertain prognosis (eg, lump in breast) • Acute illness with systemic symptoms (eg, pyelonephritis, pneumonitis, colitis) • Acute complicated injury (eg, head injury with brief loss of consciousness)	• Physiologic tests under stress (such as cardiac stress test, fetal contraction stress test) • Diagnostic endoscopies with no identified risk factors • Deep needle or incisional biopsy • Cardiovascular imaging studies with contrast and no identified risk factors (eg, arteriogram, cardiac catheterization) • Obtain fluid from body cavity (such as lumbar puncture, thoracentesis, paracentesis)	• Minor surgery with identified risk factors • Elective major surgery (open, percutaneous, or endoscopic) with no identified risk factors • Prescription drug management • Therapeutic nuclear medicine • IV fluids with additives • Closed treatment of fracture or dislocation without manipulation
High	• One or more chronic illnesses with severe exacerbation, progression, or side effects of treatment • Acute or chronic illnesses or injuries that pose a threat to life or bodily function (such as multiple trauma, acute MI, pulmonary embolus, severe respiratory distress, progressive severe rheumatoid arthritis, psychiatric illness with potential threat to self or others, peritonitis, acute renal failure) • An abrupt change in neurologic status (eg, seizure, TIA, weakness, sensory loss)	• Cardiovascular imaging studies with contrast with identified risk factors • Cardiac electrophysiological tests • Diagnostic endoscopies with identified risk factors • Discography	• Elective major surgery (open, percutaneous, or endoscopic) with identified risk factors • Emergency major surgery (open, percutaneous, or endoscopic) • Parenteral controlled substances • Drug therapy requiring intensive monitoring for toxicity • Decision not to resuscitate or to de-escalate care because of poor prognosis

TABLE 27-5 Levels of Medical Decision Making

Complexity	Diagnosis or Treatment Option Points	Data Points	Risk Level
Problem-focused	≤1 (minimal)	≤1 (minimal)	Minimal
Low	2 (limited)	2 (limited)	Low
Moderate	3 (multiple)	3 (multiple)	Moderate
High	4 (extensive)	4 (extensive)	High

Initial patient encounters (initial hospital care, CPT 99221-99223; initial and subsequent observation care, CPT 99218-99220 and 99234-6; consultations, CPT 99241-99245 and 99251-99255; and new office visits CPT 99201-5) require consideration of all three key components. Consider only two of the key components for subsequent hospital (CPT 99231-99233), observation visits (CPT 99224-99226), or established outpatient (CPT 99211-5). The lowest component of the two or three key components required determines the visit level. For example, a level three initial hospital service (CPT 99223) includes a comprehensive history, comprehensive exam, and high-complexity decision making (**Table 27-8**). If the documentation merely supports a detailed level of history, yet meets the requirements for a

TABLE 27-6 **1997 General Multisystem Physical Examination**

System/Body Area	Elements of Examination
Constitutional	• Measurement of *any three of the following seven* vital signs: (1) sitting or standing blood pressure, (2) supine blood pressure, (3) pulse rate and regularity, (4) respiration, (5) temperature, (6) height, (7) weight (may be measured and recorded by ancillary staff) • General appearance of patient (eg, development, nutrition, body habitus, deformities, attention to grooming)
Eyes	• Inspection of conjunctivae and lids • Examination of pupils and irises (eg, reaction to light and accommodation, size, and symmetry) • Ophthalmoscopic examination of optic discs (eg, size, C/D ratio, appearance) and posterior segments (vessel changes, exudates, hemorrhages)
Ears, nose, mouth, and throat	• External inspection of ears and nose (overall appearance, scars, lesions, masses) • Otoscopic examination of external auditory canals and tympanic membranes • Assessment of hearing (eg, whispered voice, finger rub, tuning fork) • Inspection of nasal mucosa, septum, and turbinates • Inspection of lips, teeth, and gums • Examination of oropharynx: oral mucosa, salivary glands, hard and soft palates, tongue, tonsils, and posterior pharynx
Neck	• Examination of neck (masses, overall appearance, symmetry, tracheal position, crepitus) • Examination of thyroid (enlargement, tenderness, mass)
Respiratory	• Assessment of respiratory effort (eg, intercostal retractions, use of accessory muscles, diaphragmatic movement) • Percussion of chest (dullness, flatness, hyperresonance) • Palpation of chest (tactile fremitus) • Auscultation of lungs (breath sounds, adventitious sounds, rubs)
Cardiovascular	• Palpation of heart (location, size, thrills) • Auscultation of heart with notation of abnormal sounds and murmurs Examination of: • carotid arteries (pulse amplitude, bruits) • abdominal aorta (size, bruits) • femoral arteries (pulse amplitude, bruits) • pedal pulses (pulse amplitude) • extremities for edema and/or varicosities
Chest (breasts)	• Inspection of breasts (symmetry, nipple discharge) • Palpation of breasts and axillae (masses or lumps, tenderness)
Gastrointestinal (abdomen)	• Examination of abdomen with notation of presence of masses or tenderness • Examination of liver and spleen • Examination for presence or absence of hernia • Examination of anus, perineum, and rectum, including sphincter tone, presence of hemorrhoids, rectal masses • Obtain stool sample for occult blood test when indicated
Genitourinary	Male: • Examination of the scrotal contents (hydrocele, spermatocele, tenderness of cord, testicular mass) • Examination of the penis • Digital rectal examination of prostate gland (size, symmetry, nodularity, tenderness) Female: Pelvic examination (with or without specimen collection for smears and cultures), including • Examination of external genitalia (general appearance, hair distribution, lesions) and vagina (eg, general appearance, estrogen effect, discharge, lesions, pelvic support, cystocele, rectocele) • Examination of urethra (masses, tenderness, scarring) • Uterus (size, contour, position, mobility, tenderness, consistency, descent or support) • Adnexa/parametria (masses, tenderness, organomegaly, nodularity) • Examination of bladder (eg, fullness, masses, tenderness) • Cervix (general appearance, lesions, discharge) • Uterus (size, contour, position, mobility, tenderness, consistency, descent or support) • Adnexa/parametria (masses, tenderness, organomegaly, nodularity)

(Continued)

TABLE 27-6 **1997 General Multisystem Physical Examination (Continued)**

System/Body Area	Elements of Examination
Lymphatic	Palpation of lymph nodes in two or more areas: • Neck • Axillae • Groin • Other
Musculoskeletal	• Examination of gait and station • Inspection and/or palpation of digits and nails (clubbing, cyanosis, inflammatory conditions, petechiae, ischemia, infections, nodes) Examination of joints, bones, and muscles of one or more of the following six areas: (1) head and neck; (2) spine, ribs, and pelvis; (3) right upper extremity; (4) left upper extremity; (5) right lower extremity; and (6) left lower extremity. The examination of a given area includes: • Inspection and/or palpation with notation of presence of any misalignment, asymmetry, crepitation, defects, tenderness, masses, or effusions • Assessment of range of motion with notation of any pain, crepitation or contracture • Assessment of stability with notation of any dislocation (luxation), subluxation, or laxity • Assessment of muscle strength and tone (flaccid, cog wheel, spastic) with notation of any atrophy or abnormal movements
Skin	• Inspection of skin and subcutaneous tissue (rashes, lesions, ulcers) • Palpation of skin and subcutaneous tissue (induration, subcutaneous nodules, tightening)
Neurologic	• Test cranial nerves with notation of any deficits • Examination of deep tendon reflexes with notation of pathological reflexes (eg, Babinski) • Examination of sensation (by touch, pin, vibration, proprioception)
Psychiatric	• Description of patient's judgment and insight Brief assessment of mental status including: • Orientation to time, place, and person • Recent and remote memory • Mood and affect (depression, anxiety, agitation)

TABLE 27-7 **Levels of 1997 Physical Examination**

Level of Exam	Performance and Documentation
Problem-focused	*1 to 5* elements identified by a bullet.
Expanded problem-focused	*At least 6* elements identified by a bullet.
Detailed	*At least 2* elements identified by a bullet from *each of 6 areas/systems* OR *at least 12* elements identified by a bullet in *2 or more areas/systems*.
Comprehensive	Perform *all elements* identified by a bullet in *at least 9* organ systems or body areas and document *at least 2* elements identified by a bullet from *each of 9 areas/systems*.

TABLE 27-8 **Levels of Initial Hospital Care**

Initial Hospital Care	History	Examination	MDM	Time
99221	Detailed or comprehensive	Detailed or comprehensive	Straightforward or low	30 min
99222	Comprehensive	Comprehensive	Moderate	50 min
99223	Comprehensive	Comprehensive	High	70 min

TABLE 27-9 Levels of Subsequent Hospital Care

Subsequent Hospital Care	History	Examination	MDM	Time
99231	Problem-focused	Problem-focused	Straightforward or low	15 min
99232	Expanded	Expanded	Moderate	25 min
99233	Detailed	Detailed	High	35 min

comprehensive examination and high-complexity decision making, report only a level one initial hospital service (CPT 99221). In contrast, if a subsequent hospital visit note contains a complete examination and high-complexity MDM, then report CPT 99233 and history need not even be considered (**Table 27-9**). When selecting visit levels for services that only consider two key components, MDM should be one of those two key components. While not stated in the documentation guidelines, medical necessity underlies every physician service and is most appropriately demonstrated through MDM. Reporting subsequent services with MDM as a key component thereby precludes the allegation of an unwarranted high-level subsequent encounter based upon merely a comprehensive, but medically unnecessary, history and examination for management of the presenting problem (eg, common cold).

■ TIME COUNSELING/COORDINATING CARE

CPT assigns most E/M codes a *typical* time to render a service, but importantly, the service duration need not last that length. For inpatient services, time accrues as unit or floor time in addition to face-to-face time. When more than 50% of the total service time involves counseling and/or coordination of care, the provider may select a code reflecting the total time spent with the patient, rather than the three key components. Time and the corresponding counseling details must be documented in the medical record when selecting the E/M code on the basis of time (eg, "25 of 35 minutes spent urging the patient to undergo a diagnostic biopsy"). Of course, record patient responses to counseling and all relevant history, examination, and MDM as necessary for good patient care. A subsequent hospital service involving 35 minutes spent by the provider permits selection of 99233 (Table 27-9).

TEMPLATED NOTES

Templated chart notes, whether formatted as preprinted paper progress notes with check boxes or electronically constructed as combinations of macros and click-boxes, are common, appropriate documentation tools. Such tools enhance legibility and facilitate efficient documentation in accord with the E/M guidelines. Unfortunately electronic notes often become the source for increasingly prevalent "cut-and-paste" errors, highlighting the need to balance efficiency with accuracy in providing safe, efficient care to complex patients. Make each note specific to the patient on that encounter date. Modify information and language brought forward from any previous encounters so the current documentation demonstrates the distinct clinical service of today. Do not include excessive data or repetitious information that is not relevant to the current service; such content is often misconstrued as being included merely to increase the billing level.

■ AUDIT TOOLS

Audit tools are useful adjuncts to ensuring adherence to E/M billing guidelines, patient safety and quality initiatives, and other process assessments. Such tools are often custom designed in the context of chart reviews and institutional initiatives, or implementing coding and billing audits associated with practice compliance plans. CMS has not developed or endorsed any formal audit tool for E/M services, although virtually all Medicare and non-Medicare contractors (eg, Novitas and First Coast Service Options, Inc) make their E/M score sheets available to assist providers in adhering to documentation guidelines.

SUGGESTED READINGS

American Medical Association. *Current Procedural Terminology (CPT) 2016*. Chicago, IL: American Medical Association; 2015.

Centers for Medicare & Medicaid Services. *Evaluation and Management Services guide*; November 2014. Available at http://www.cms.gov/Outreach-and-Education/Medicare-Learning-Network-MLN/MLNProducts/downloads//eval_mgmt_serv_guide-ICN006764.pdf.

Centers for Medicare and Medicaid Services. *Medicare Claims Processing Manual*. Bethesda, MA: Department of Health and Human Services; 2014. Available online at www.cms.hhs.gov/manuals/downloads/clm104c12.pdf.

Kuhn T, Basch P, Barr M, et al. Clinical documentation in the 21st century: executive summary of a policy position paper from the American College of Physicians. *Ann Intern Med*. 2015;162:301-303.

Levinson DR. *Coding Trends of Medicare Evaluation and Management Services*. Office of the Inspector General, Department of Health and Human Services; 2012. Available at http://oig.hhs.gov/oei/reports/oei-04-10-00180.pdf.

Levinson DR. *Improper Payments for Evaluation and Management Services Cost Medicare Billions in 2010*. Office of the Inspector General, Department of Health and Human Services; 2014. Available at http://oig.hhs.gov/oei/reports/oei-04-10-00181.pdf.

Manaker S, Merlino D, Pohlig CA. *Coding for Chest Medicine 2016: Pulmonary, Critical Care and Sleep*. Northbrook, IL: American College of Chest Physicians; 2015.

Novitas Solutions, Inc. *Novitas Solutions: Specialty Exam Scoresheets*. Available online at http://www.novitas-solutions.com/webcenter/faces/oracle/webcenter/page/scopedMD/sad60252a_5537_4c5d_9350_ca405e36e159/Page133.jspx?contentId=00024402&_afrLoop=475344439251000#!%40%40%3F_afrLoop%3D475344439251000%26contentId%3D00024402%26_adf.ctrl-state%3D141uivweue_335.

Siegler EL, Adelman R. Copy and paste: a remediable hazard of electronic health records. *Am J Med*. 2009;122:495.

Siegler EL. The evolving medical record. *Ann Intern Med*. 2010;153:671-677.

Siegler JE, Patel N, Dine CJ. Prioritizing paperwork over patient care: why can't we do both? *J Grad Medical Educ*. 2015;7:16-18.

CHAPTER 28

Consultation, Comanagement, Time-Based, and Palliative Care Billing

Yvette M. Cua, MD

■ INTRODUCTION

Medicare stopped paying for the consult codes [99241-99245, 99251-99255] January 1, 2010. The consult codes paid more than their corresponding inpatient follow-up [99231-99233] and outpatient visit [99201-99215] alternatives, but came with very specific, but strict and confusing, situational and documentation criteria to allow for their reimbursement. Although Medicare stopped paying for the consult codes, they did not stop paying for consult services. The concept of needing the expertise of another provider is still essential to the practice of medicine. What has changed is how those services need to be reported for reimbursement to Medicare. Some private payors still reimburse for the consult codes, using the old Medicare situational and documentation guidelines, but these numbers are decreasing. Until 100% of insurers stop paying for the consult codes [99241-99255], two different payment systems for consults exist. Thus, the same work provided to two identical patients may be reimbursed differently depending on the patient's insurer.

■ MEDICARE PATIENTS AND THOSE INSURERS FOLLOWING MEDICARE CONSULT RULES

The set of codes submitted for a consult to a Medicare patient is based on several variables: inpatient versus outpatient status, disposition after being seen in an emergency room (eventual admission vs observation status vs discharge home), and whether a patient is new or established to the physician specialty and billing group. (See **Figure 28-1**.)

■ INPATIENTS

Initial consults for patients in acute care hospitals and skilled nursing facilities (SNF) are billed with the same initial inpatient visit codes used for admissions [99221-99223 (initial inpatient visit), 99304-99306 (initial SNF visit)]. All subsequent consult visits are billed using the subsequent inpatient or SNF visit codes respectively [99231-99233, 99307-99310]. The final day seeing the patient as a consultant will still be billed using the subsequent inpatient and SNF codes, even if the consultant is contributing to or fully providing the patient's discharge management. Only the admitting physician/billing group can bill for discharge management services [99238-99239]. Medicare will only pay for medically necessary visits and not just daily "routine" visits because the patient is still in the inpatient hospital or SNF.

If a new problem or question surfaces, or the consultant is reconsulted during the *same* inpatient admission, with or without a time lapse since the last consultant visit, a subsequent inpatient/SNF visit code [99231-99233, 99307-99310] would be submitted for this service.

If a consultant is asked to see a patient whom they provided a consult on during a previous admission, even with the same problem(s) as last admission, the consultant would still bill an initial inpatient/SNF visit code [99221-99223, 99304-99306] for this work.

In the event that the documentation for the initial consult does not meet the minimum documentation criteria for the lowest level of initial inpatient service [99221], Medicare will allow this work to be reported with subsequent inpatient visit codes [99231-99232]. The documentation criteria for these services parallels those of the

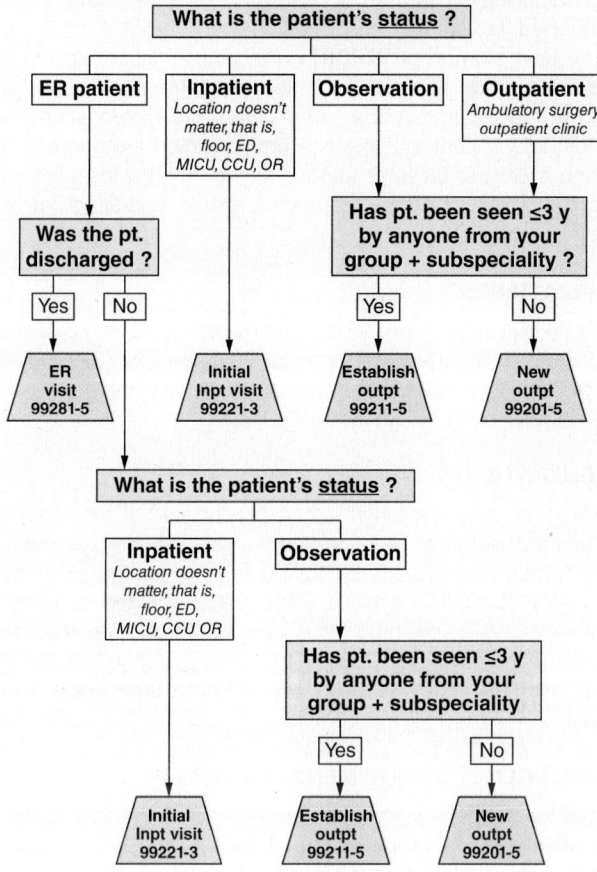

Algorithm for selecting the proper CPT code set for mediCARE consults in a hospital setting

What is the patient's <u>status</u> ?

- **ER patient**
- **Inpatient** *Location doesn't matter, that is, floor, ED, MICU, CCU, OR*
- **Observation**
- **Outpatient** *Ambulatory surgery outpatient clinic*

Was the pt. discharged ?
Yes / No

Has pt. been seen ≤3 y by anyone from your group + subspeciality ?
Yes / No

- **ER visit 99281-5**
- **Initial Inpt visit 99221-3**
- **Establish outpt 99211-5**
- **New outpt 99201-5**

What is the patient's <u>status</u> ?

- **Inpatient** *Location doesn't matter, that is, floor, ED, MICU, CCU OR*
- **Observation**

Has pt. been seen ≤3 y by anyone from your group + subspeciality
Yes / No

- **Initial Inpt visit 99221-3**
- **Establish outpt 99211-5**
- **New outpt 99201-5**

Figure 28-1 *Algorithm for selecting the proper CPT code set for medi-CARE consults in a hospital setting. (Copyright 2010, Yvette M. Cua, MD. Used with permission.)*

lowest two levels of consult service for the old code set [99251-99252], which explains the rationale for this practice. Keep in mind that the ability to submit an initial consult service with a subsequent inpatient visit code *does not hold true for admissions*. For an initial inpatient visit (ie, admission) reported by the primary attending of record, if the documentation for this service does not meet the minimum criteria for the lowest level of service [99221], subsequent inpatient visit codes *cannot* be submitted for this work. This work would be reported with E/M code 99499 which means that the documentation for the service does not meet criteria for recognized E/M services. This would fall under manual review and be left up to the Medicare contractor to determine what if any payment would be given. Check with local Medicare intermediaries for deviation from this rule. At least one carrier, Noridian, as of the time of publication of this chapter, *will* allow use of subsequent inpatient visit codes [99231-99232] for this admission scenario.

Since more than one physician will now be submitting an initial inpatient/SNF code, the primary attending of record for the patient needs to attach modifier –AI (A "eye," not A "one" or A "el") to their initial inpatient/SNF service. Consultants should not use this modifier.

■ OUTPATIENTS

Occasionally, hospitalists are consulted on patients in an outpatient unit of the hospital, such as the ambulatory surgery center. Also, observation status patients are considered outpatients even though

they may occupy a hospital bed in the same room as an inpatient. Initial consults for these patients are billed using outpatient visit codes [99201-99215]. Initial observation visit codes [99218-99220, 99234-99236] should not be submitted for this work. Within the outpatient set of codes are *new* patient [99201-99205] and *established* patient [99211-99215] codes. A consultant now needs to determine if a patient is *"new"* versus *"established"* to select the correct code set to use. A patient is considered "new" to an individual physician if they have not received any E/M services from any member of that physician's billing group and specific (sub)specialty within the past 3 years, regardless of the location of the service. Note that billing for the professional component of a service, or writing an order on a patient does not affect the "new" or "established" status of a patient.

Below are some common examples to illustrate nuances with this definition.

1. An internal medicine consultant evaluates a Medicare observation patient on the neurology service. The consultant has never seen the patient before, but the patient was seen in the emergency room by an internal medicine partner in their billing group, moonlighting 2 years ago. This consult would be reported with an *established* outpatient code [99212-99215].

2. A hospitalist evaluates a patient in observation status at the request of the ENT service. This patient has a history of monthly admissions to the hospital medicine service for severe chronic obstructive lung disease (COPD) although not recently. The initial medicine consult would be billed using the *new* outpatient code set [99201-99205].

3. A patient, seen routinely by an endocrinologist in a multispecialty practice for years, is placed in observation status on the general surgery service with a consult request to an internal medicine hospitalist in the same multispecialty group as the endocrinologist. The patient has never been seen by the internal medicine group in the past. This consult would be reported with a *new* outpatient code [99201-99205].

4. A cardiologist read an electrocardiogram (ECG) on a patient last week and billed for the formal ECG report, but has never seen the patient before, and no one in their group has ever provided an E/M service to this patient. Subsequently, the cardiologist evaluates this patient who is being observed on the internal medicine service. The cardiologist would bill their initial consult using the *new* outpatient codes [99201-99205].

If a follow-up consultant visit is necessary, even on discharge day, all of these patients are now established patients, and this work would be billed using the established outpatient visit codes [99212-99215].

■ EMERGENCY DEPARTMENT PATIENTS

For consults on patients seen in the emergency department, *the patient's ultimate disposition* will determine which set of codes to use to bill for the consult.

Admission to an inpatient service. Only one CPT code will be submitted for an evaluation by a consultant in the emergency department, followed by admission to the inpatient service, an initial inpatient visit [99221-99223]. If that patient is admitted to a different subspecialty's inpatient service, an initial inpatient visit code [99221-99223] is still reported for this work.

Placement into observation status. If the above patient is eventually placed into observation status on the consultant's service, only one CPT code will be submitted for both the work of the consult and the placement into observation, an initial observation visit code [99218-99220, 99234-99236]. If the patient is placed into observation status on a different subspecialty's service, this work will now be reported with an outpatient visit code [99201-99215] based on whether they are "new" or "established" to the consultant's billing group and subspecialty. *Discharged home.* Finally, if the emergency room patient is eventually discharged home, an emergency room visit code [99281-99285] will be submitted for the work of the consult.

■ PAYORS WHO STILL RECOGNIZE THE OLD CONSULT CODES

For individual state Medicaid programs and for private insurers, check with plan representatives to see if they follow the new Medicare rules, or if they still pay for the consult codes [99241-99255]. For those that still recognize consult codes, check with the individual payors as well as your compliance office to see if they follow the old Medicare consult situational and documentation guidelines or if they have their own internal set of requirements.

In order to bill for a consult based on the old Medicare guidelines, several criteria have to be met. The Mnemonic "The 3 R's" refer to these criteria. The consult has to be **REQUESTED** by another provider who wants the consultant to **RENDER** their *opinion* about (a) specific question(s), and the ensuing recommendations must be **REPORT**ed back in writing to the requesting provider. The essence of a consult in this system, is that *another provider* seeks the *opinion* of a consultant with expertise above and beyond his own for a particular problem or set of problems. The concept of a "REQUEST for opinion" is stressed for three reasons (1) to distinguish it from a self-referral by the patient, which cannot be reimbursed as a consult (2) to distinguish it from a transfer of care, and (3) to prevent improper payment for "protocol" care that may not have adequate medical necessity documented in the chart. For example, if a hospital mandates that 100% of patients admitted for surgery or to a psychiatry ward must have a medicine consult, this could lead to nonbillable work. In these situations, a preprinted admission form requesting a medicine consult per "hospital policy" without documented medical necessity for each individual patient situation, would lead to nonbillable work. If a 25-year-old healthy female is admitted to general surgery for complications after an elective cholecystectomy, but has no other medical issues, there is no medical necessity for a medicine consultant to see the patient. The surgeon does not consciously request this service or have a particular question for the medicine consultant to answer, and does not need the internist's expertise to manage the postoperative issues. A hospital mandated task is therefore not reimbursable through the patient's insurance.

Because the consult codes reimburse higher level per level, than their subsequent follow-up counterparts, there is a big push to ensure that an *opinion* was requested, and not a *transfer of care.* This is the essence of a consult for those insurers that still follow these guidelines. For example, medical consultation request for an opinion regarding selection of anti-hypertensive medication in a pregnant inpatient would meet criteria for allowing a consult [99251-99255] to be billed, even if the recommendations include continued concurrent care of the hypertension by the internist. On the other hand, if the obstetrician is not comfortable managing hypertension at all, and wants the care of that problem to be totally managed by the internist, the essence of the request for help is no longer for an "opinion" about management. The request is for the internal medicine consultant to take over the care of the hypertension while the obstetrician continues to manage the other aspects of the patient's care is referred to as a "transfer of care." If the patient remains on the obstetrician's service and the internist provides concurrent care, managing hypertension, this work cannot be reported with the "transfer of the patient to another service" consult codes [99251-99255]. In this concurrent care situation, the internal medicine consultant would report this work with a subsequent inpatient visit code [99231-99233]. For those payors who do not follow the

new Medicare rules, only one initial inpatient visit [99221-99223] can be reported and reimbursed per patient per admission, thus the reimbursement for this work is substantially lower than if it were reimbursed through the consult codes [99251-99255].

The final criterion of **REPORT**ing recommendations speaks to good medical documentation. Although a consultant may opt to call the requesting physician with urgent recommendations for good quality patient care, these recommendations need to exist in writing, accessible by the requesting physician. In the inpatient setting, the consultant note entered into a shared medical record will satisfy this criterion.

■ INPATIENTS

Initial consult visits to inpatients in both acute care settings as well as SNFs are billed using inpatient consult codes [99251-99255]. All subsequent visits are billed using inpatient/SNF follow-up codes respectively [99231-99233, 99307-99310].

■ OUTPATIENTS

Consults to patients seen in an outpatient area of the hospital, including observation status patients, are billed with the outpatient consult codes [99241-99245]. If a follow-up consultation visit is needed, it would be billed using the established outpatient visit codes [99212-99215]. Check with individual state Medicaid programs and private payors to see if they require the subsequent observation visit codes [99224-99226] instead, for observation status patients.

■ EMERGENCY DEPARTMENT PATIENTS

Just as for Medicare patients, the physical location of the patient is not what determines the selection of codes to use for billing consults. It is the patient's "status."

Admission to an inpatient service. For patients located in the emergency department who have already been admitted to an inpatient service, use the inpatient consult codes [99251-99255]. If the consultant admits the patient to their inpatient service on the same date as the consult, only one CPT code for the work of both the consult and the admission should be submitted—an initial inpatient admission code [99221-99223]. *Observation status.* If the patient in the emergency department is assigned observation status on a different service from the consultant's, the consult will be billed using the outpatient consult codes [99241-99245]. If the consultant places the patient into observation status on his own service on the same calendar date, only one CPT code should be submitted for all of this work—an initial observation visit [99218-99220, 99234-99236]. *Discharge to home.* If the patient is only under the care of an emergency room physician, and is eventually discharged home, report this work with outpatient consult codes [99241-99245].

■ CRITICAL ILLNESS

If the patient is critically ill during the initial consult visit and >30 minutes of critical care is provided by the consultant, only critical care [99291, 99292] and no other consult code set would be reported for that day. In the event that a consult is completed and at a later time on that calendar date, the consultant provides >30 minutes of critical care to the patient, both the consult and critical care service can be paid. The consult work would be reported using the rules above to select the appropriate code set.

■ SPLIT/SHARED VISITS

Although previous guidance from Medicare has stated that a consult cannot be provided as a split/shared service, those rules only applied to consults reported with CPT codes 99241-99255. With Medicare consults now reported using different code sets, the rules for split/shared visits for Medicare patients now default to the rules for whichever set of codes are being reported for the consult. Thus, for inpatient consults reported with initial inpatient visit codes [99221-99223], these services can be provided and billed as split/shared visits. Check with individual nonmedicare payors for their rules regarding this situation.

COMANAGEMENT

The terms "comanagement" and "concurrent care" are often used interchangeably. **Concurrent care** is the situation when two physicians are managing different aspects of the patient's care on the same calendar date on a more extensive basis than a one-time consultation, usually discussed in reference to two physicians submitting claims for inpatient follow-up services [99231-99233]. Two initial inpatient services [99221-99223] submitted on the same calendar date will be interpreted as consultation care and not fall under this discussion. The Medicare manual clearly states that the work of both physicians is reimbursable as long as the documentation reflects the medical necessity for each physician to provide their service. Although the two physicians are usually from different subspecialties, in the event that both are from the same specialty but one has documented expertise above and beyond the other, both services may be paid. An example of this could be an internal medicine hospitalist who is managing a patient with a COPD exacerbation, but elicits the help of another internal medicine hospitalist with expertise in pain management, to take over the daily care of the patient's severe refractory chest pain from lung cancer. The medical necessity of each physician's care should not only be reflected in the medical record, but also by each claim being submitted with different ICD-10 codes, showing the different aspects of care each provider is managing on that particular date. If both providers submit their service with the same primary ICD-10 code, only the first claim received by Medicare will be reimbursed. The second one will be denied.

Comanagement, defined by the Society of Hospital Medicine (SHM) and its Advisory Panel, is the "shared responsibility, authority, and accountability for the care of a hospitalized patient." By convention, this term is used when a more formal arrangement is made between two physicians providing concurrent care. In the common situation involving a surgeon and medicine provider, the surgeon manages surgery related issues and the medicine hospitalist manages the patient's medical conditions *on an ongoing basis*, often for the entire duration of the admission, and usually with the formal arrangement outlining each specialty's responsibilities. From the start, the patient will be admitted to one service, with an order for the other subspecialty physician to see the patient. Just as in the example in the consult section above, the documentation must support the medical necessity for the second physician to be involved, not just for the initial visit, but also for each daily visit. Situations will arise where each physician in a comanagement arrangement may not need to see the patient every single day of the admission. No billing should be submitted for these days, even if the patient is physically seen by the physician, based on a mandated hospital protocol. Without documented medical necessity, this work is not reimbursable.

TIME-BASED BILLING

Several E/M services can be billed based on time (**Table 28-1**), with different billing nuances for each code set. In certain situations, the rules allowing reimbursement for these services differ between the CPT and Medicare manuals. When billing based on time, the only time that can be counted toward reimbursement of a service, is the billing provider's time, not time spent on patient care by the resident, student, social worker, or nursing staff. For hospital based services, in addition to face-to-face time, the majority of E/M services also allow inclusion of time spent by the provider on the patient's floor or in their unit ("unit/floor time") providing patient care, toward billable time. In general, time is added up from 12:01 AM to 11:59 PM, not over a 24-hour period, and does not need to be continuous. One exception to this is in the event that a time-based service is started before midnight, continuously provided, but not completed until after midnight. The CPT handbook advises if this should occur, to add up time that the service was provided continuously, and to bill for it on the date the service began.

■ COUNSELING AND COORDINATION OF CARE

When counseling and/or coordinating care (CCC) is the dominant feature of certain E/M visits, that is, when more than 50% of the total visit time (face to face and/or unit/floor), is spent counseling the patient and or coordinating their care, the level of service provided may be determined by the total visit time rather than by quantification of the documented history, physical, and medical decision making (MDM). The typical total visit times associated with these services are shown below.

For example, if a patient is seen for inpatient follow up of a pulmonary embolism (PE) and a compliant level 2 [99232] visit is documented based on history, physical, and MDM, but it is also documented that >50% of a 35-minute face-to-face visit is spent counseling the patient on risk factors for a PE, evaluation, and treatment, time is now the controlling factor and a level 3 [99233] visit can be billed even though the history, physical, and MDM only amount to a level 2. Medicare will only allow time-based billing for CCC for inpatient admissions and follow-ups [99221-99233], SNF admissions and follow-ups [99304-99318], new outpatient visits [99201-99205], established outpatient visits [99212-99215], and other home services [99324-99350]. Medicaid and other insurers who follow the CPT handbook may also allow time-based billing for CCC for observation services [99218-99236] and consults [99241-99255] as well.

The Medicare Claims Processing Manual Chapter 12 states that the amount of CCC time may be estimated. In addition, the CPT manual instructs the provider to round the total visit time to the closest "average" total visit time. Thus in the example above, if 32 minutes were spent with the patient, 32 is closer to 35 minutes (average visit time for a level 3 follow-up [99233]) than it is to 25 minutes (average visit time for a level 2 follow-up [99232]), and a level 3 service would be billed. This differs from the rules governing prolonged service total time determination below.

Tasks that count toward counseling the patient include but are not limited to discussions of the plan, evaluation, procedures, prognosis, treatment options, risk factor reduction, and patient and family education.

In order to bill for these services, **two different amounts of time** must be documented: the total visit time, and the portion of that total visit time that was spent CCC. Check with insurers and local compliance offices to see if the term *">50% of the total visit time was spent counseling the patient"* is acceptable or if the specific number of minutes spent CCC needs to be explicitly documented. Neither the Medicare manual nor the CPT handbook list this as a documentation requirement. The most common documentation pitfall in successfully getting reimbursed for CCC time, is reporting only one time amount, thus making it impossible to determine that >50% of the total visit time was spent CCC. In addition, lack of a brief description of what was discussed during that time will cause a denial; the medical necessity for investing that time into the visit may not be obvious.

TABLE 28-1 Average Visit Times for E/M Services Billed as Counseling/Coordination Services and Threshold Times for Prolonged Services

Medicare allows billing for counseling/coordination time and prolonged service only for services in bold below. The CPT manual allows both for all services in the table.

CPT Code	Threshold to Visit Type	Level	Visit Time	(Minutes) Average Bill 99356	Threshold to Bill 99357
99218	105	Initial observation	(1)	30	60
99219		(2)	50	80	125
99220		(3)	70	100	145
99221	**Initial inpatient**	**(1)**	**30**	**60**	**105**
99222		**(2)**	**50**	**80**	**125**
99223		**(3)**	**70**	**100**	**145**
99224	Observation follow-up	(1)	15	45	90
99225		(2)	25	55	100
99226		(3)	35	65	110
99231	**Inpatient follow-up**	**(1)**	**15**	**45**	**90**
99232		**(2)**	**25**	**55**	**100**
99233		**(3)**	**35**	**65**	**110**
99234	Observation same day discharge	(1)	40	70	115
99235		(2)	50	80	125
99236		(3)	55	85	130
99251	Inpatient consult	(1)	20	50	95
99252		(2)	40	70	115
99253		(3)	55	85	130
99254		(4)	80	110	155
99255		(5)	110	140	185
99304	**Initial SNF**	**(1)**	**25**	**55**	**100**
99305		**(2)**	**35**	**65**	**110**
99306		**(3)**	**45**	**75**	**120**
99307	**SNF follow-up**	**(1)**	**10**	**40**	**85**
99308		**(2)**	**15**	**45**	**90**
99309		**(3)**	**25**	**55**	**100**
99310		**(4)**	**35**	**65**	**110**
99318	**Annual NF assessment**		**30**	**60**	**105**

CPT Code	Visit Type	Level	Average Visit Time	(Minutes) Threshold to Bill 99354	Threshold to Bill 99355
99201	**New outpatient**	**(1)**	**10**	**40**	**85**
99202		**(2)**	**20**	**50**	**95**
99203		**(3)**	**30**	**60**	**105**
99204		**(4)**	**45**	**75**	**120**
99205		**(5)**	**60**	**90**	**135**
99212	**Established outpatient**	**(2)**	**10**	**40**	**85**
99213		**(3)**	**15**	**45**	**90**
99214		**(4)**	**25**	**55**	**100**
99215		**(5)**	**40**	**70**	**115**
99241	Outpatient consult	(1)	10	40	85
99242		(2)	20	50	95
99243		(3)	30	60	105
99244		(4)	45	75	120
99245		(5)	60	90	135

CPT codes 99324-99350 not included in the chart above as not used in hospital medicine.

Examples of minimally acceptable reporting of time for billing the visit based on CCC:

1. I spent 20 minutes out of a 25-minute visit face-to-face and unit/floor time, counseling the patient on the safe use of home oxygen, and coordinating care with social work, setting up home oxygen, home nursing, and pulmonary rehab *(level 2 inpatient follow-up visit [99232]).*

2. I spent 35 minutes face to face with the patient today. Twenty-five of those minutes were spent counseling the patient on her new diagnosis of breast cancer, the next steps in work-up, and possible treatment options including chemotherapy and XRT *(level 3 inpatient follow-up visit [99233]).*

3. I spent 75 minutes with Mr X face-to-face and unit/floor time. More than fifty percent of that time was spent counseling the patient. The patient has very low health literacy and needed extensive counseling regarding acute renal failure, necessary inpatient work-up, and possible need for dialysis *(level 3 inpatient admission [99223]).*

4. I spent 40 minutes face to face with the patient. One hundred percent of the time was spent counseling the patient on hospice and the grave prognosis for his metastatic lung cancer *(level 3 inpatient follow-up visit [99233]).*

Examples of unacceptable reporting of CCC time for billing:

1. I spent 25 minutes counseling the patient on new diagnosis of lung cancer.

2. I spent 15 minutes face to face with the patient discussing the hospital course for his pneumonia.

3. I spent 10 minutes out of a 30-minute visit counseling the patient on what CHF is, low salt diet, and decreased fluid intake (10 minutes is less than 50% of the total visit time). This visit cannot be billed based on time; the documentation of history, physical, and MDM would be used to determine the level of service. Specifically, even though 10 minutes is >50% of a level 1 inpatient follow-up average visit time (15 minutes), this statement cannot be used in lieu of documenting the history, physical, and MDM to bill for the service.

4. I spent today's entire visit counseling the patient on the differential diagnosis of his diarrhea and the planned work-up. (An auditor cannot try to determine how much time you spent with the patient based on the time orders were written, or the note was entered in the EMR. This service cannot be billed based on time.)

▇ PROLONGED SERVICES

Prolonged service codes [99354-99359] are add on codes used when more than 30 minutes of care is provided beyond the typical or average visit time for the E/M service. They can never be billed alone, without their companion code—the primary E/M service. Time can be added up over the course of the calendar date not only by the provider, but also by their covering partners, including involvement by a nocturnist; the time each provider spent over the calendar date can be aggregated to determine to level of service provided. In this situation, the prolonged service would be reported under the NPI of the provider who is billing for the primary E/M service. Relative value units (RVUs) between the two providers would need to be adjusted internally for productivity purposes. Both physicians and nonphysician providers (NPPs) can bill for prolonged services. Finally, prolonged services may be provided and billed for as a split/shared visit. No restrictions are identified in either the CPT or Medicare manuals on how much time the physician must spend on the service relative to the NPP, in order to bill a split/shared visit. The documentation must clearly reflect that each provider performed a substantive portion of the service.

There are several differences between Medicare and CPT manuals' rules governing how and when prolonged services may be provided and how they must be documented. Medicare only allows prolonged services to be billed when the primary E/M visit is an inpatient admission or follow-up [99221-99233], SNF admission or follow-up [99304-99318], new outpatient visit [99201-99205], established outpatient visit [99212-99215], or home or domiciliary visit [99324-99350]. Medicare does not allow prolonged services to be billed with observation admissions and follow-ups [99218-99236], however, the CPT manual *does* allow prolonged service billing with these observation services as well as with the consults codes [99241-99255]. For all payors including Medicare, prolonged services can never be billed with discharge management services [99238-99239, 99217], critical care [99291-99292], or procedures. In general, the direct patient contact services 99356-99357 are added on to inpatient and observation services, and 99354-99355 are added on to outpatient services (Table 28-1). 99358-99359 are prolonged services without direct patient contact, that is, without a face to face, and are not reimbursed by Medicare. These codes are usually used when extensive time is spent in chart review. Payment for these services varies among private insurers.

99354, 99356, and 99358 are billed for the "first hour" of prolonged service provided. These services can be billed once 30 minutes of prolonged service has been provided; the rules governing prolonged service care allow for each unit of service to be billed once 50% of the service time in the description has been met. 99355, 99357, and 99359 are billed for each additional "half hour" of prolonged service after the first hour of prolonged care. These services cannot be billed unless 99354, 99356, or 99358 has already been billed with the primary E/M. Again, once half of the time in the description is met, that is, 15 minutes, these services can be billed. Thus, in the inpatient setting, if 105 minutes of prolonged service has been provided beyond the typical visit time for the primary E/M visit, the first hour of prolonged care may be billed, *PLUS* the next half hour of care, *PLUS* another half hour of care. In addition to the primary E/M service, 99356 and 99357 × 2 would be submitted in this example. No modifiers are needed for billing these services. Medicare requires the service to "meet or exceed" the threshold time to allow reimbursement for prolonged services (Table 28-1). Note that this is different from the instruction to "round" to the nearest average visit time when billing for CCC. Thus if a level 2 inpatient visit is performed (typical visit time 25 minutes) and 52 minutes of face-to-face care was provided, the 55-minute threshold needed to bill for the first hour of prolonged service [99356] has not been met, and the additional 27 minutes of care provided in this example is not reimbursable; only the level 2 inpatient follow-up [99232] would be submitted for this care. **Table 28-2** shows the cut off times needed to bill each unit of prolonged service.

The rest of the discussion will focus only on services with direct patient contact [99354-99357]. Medicare only allows face-to-face time with the patient to be counted toward prolonged service billing, both in the outpatient as well as the inpatient setting [99354-99357]. Notice that this is different from Medicare's rules for CCC, discharge management services, and critical care which all allow unit/floor time to be included as well. The CPT manual defines "direct patient contact" to mean only face-to-face time in the outpatient setting [99354-99355] but also time spent on the patient's floor or in their unit for inpatient services [99356-99357]. This has a large impact on how prolonged services may be billed.

Prolonged services may be provided in addition to any level of service within the code sets above as long as >50% of the prolonged service time was not spent counseling the patient or coordinating their care. In the situation where CCC is the key feature of the visit, the highest level of service in the E/M code set must be used as the primary E/M before determining if any prolonged service time is

TABLE 28-2 Prolonged Service Billing

Minutes of Prolonged Service	Outpatient	CPT Codes Submitted Inpatient and Observation	No Direct Patient Care
0-29	Only primary E/M	Only primary E/M	Only primary E/M
30-74	99354	99356	99358
75-104	99354 + 99355	99356 + 99357	99358 + 99359
105-134	99354 + 99355 × 2	99356 + 99357 × 2	99358 + 99359 × 2
135-164	99354 + 99355 × 3	99356 + 99357 × 3	99358 + 99359 × 3
165-194	99354 + 99355 × 4	99356 + 99357 × 4	99358 + 99359 × 4
195+	- - - - - - - - - - - - - - - - - - follow the pattern above - - - - - - - - - - - - - - - - - -		

billable. If less than 30 minutes of prolonged services are provided, that work is not separately reimbursable.

Example 1: A patient is seen with a new diagnosis of colon cancer and a fully compliant level 2 inpatient follow-up visit [99232] is documented, based on history, physical, and MDM. Seventy-five minutes of face-to-face plus unit/floor time care (total visit time) is provided to the patient. Only 60 minutes of that time was face-to-face time, and >50% of the total visit time was spent counseling the patient regarding the new diagnosis, further necessary testing, treatment options, and plans for consultants. Although only a level 2 visit is documented, since CCC is the key feature of the service, the visit can be billed based on time. The highest level of inpatient follow-up service is a level 3 [99233] which is associated with an average visit time of 35 minutes. In Medicare patients, only face-to-face time can be used when determining if prolonged service time is separately reimbursable. Only 60 minutes of the total visit time was face to face. This means that 25 minutes of prolonged service care was provided (60 minutes total face-to-face time minus 35 minutes typical visit time for a level 3 follow-up). In this scenario, those 25 minutes are not separately reimbursable. This service for a Medicare patient would be reported as a level 3 inpatient follow-up [99233].

Reimbursement would be different if this patient does not have Medicare, and the insurer follows the CPT manual. The total visit time would now be 75 minutes, adding in time spent providing care on the patient's floor or in their unit. Now in addition to the level 3 inpatient follow-up visit, there are 40 minutes of prolonged service (75 minutes direct patient care time minus 35 minutes typical visit time for a level 3 inpatient follow-up). This service would now be reported as a level 3 inpatient follow-up [99233] PLUS the first hour of prolonged service [99356] which would result on average in ~$95 additional income.

Example 2: A non-English-speaking patient with an asthma exacerbation and lots of anxiety continues to call nursing several times during the day with shortness of breath, requiring repeated history taking, physical exam, and reassessment after each albuterol nebulizer treatment. In addition, each interaction with the patient requires the assistance of an interpreter. A compliant level 2 inpatient follow-up visit [99232] is documented. Sixty minutes of face-to-face care is provided intermittently over the course of the day. The typical visit time for 99232 is 25 minutes. Thirty-five minutes of prolonged service that is not dominated by counseling or coordination of care is best reflected by 99232 PLUS 99356.

For Medicare, start and stop times for prolonged services and the indication for the prolonged time need to be documented along with a brief summary of what was done during that time in addition to the total face-to-face time providing care on that calendar date. The CPT handbook does not include a requirement for documenting start and stop times to bill for this service. There may be variable requirements among state Medicaid and private payors.

■ CRITICAL CARE

Critical care is defined in the Medicare Claims Processing Manual, Chapter 12, Section 30.6.12, as a physician's direct delivery of medical care of a high-complexity MDM, to a critically ill or injured patient to prevent or stop imminent or active acute organ failure. A **critical illness** or injury *acutely* impairs one or more vital organ systems so that there is high probability of imminent or life threatening deterioration in the patient's condition. Some examples of critical illness from the Medicare manual include circulatory failure, shock; renal, hepatic, or respiratory failure. *Chronic* organ failure management does not meet criteria for critical care services. Examples of this include chronic vent management and routine hemodialysis.

For a service to qualify as critical care, all four criteria must be met and adequately documented:

1. The *medical necessity* refers to a statement about the patient's illness. The Medicare manual states "…*The failure to initiate these interventions on an urgent basis would likely result in sudden, clinically significant or life threatening deterioration in the patient's condition*…."
2. The service meets criteria for *high-complexity medical decision making*, and the high-complexity MDM is adequately documented in the chart.
3. The care is *directly* furnished by the physician, not by the resident, and not by a NPP in a split/shared situation. Critical care cannot be performed and billed as a split/shared visit.
4. The patient has a critical condition as defined above. Since critical care encompasses not only the "treatment of organ failure" but also the "prevention of further deterioration in the patient's condition," it is not a requirement that the person have an emergency or crisis situation to bill for critical care. The physician's documented clinical judgment that the patient is at high risk of impending organ failure, or further deterioration in clinical condition, will support this criteria.

Seeing a critically ill patient does not automatically allow critical care billing. For example, an ophthalmologist seeing a septic patient on pressors, for glaucoma treatment, cannot bill for critical care.

There is no restriction to where critical care can be provided. It is not uncommon to provide critical care to a patient in a regular medical ward with an acute change in clinical status, while awaiting transfer to an intensive care unit. A patient is in the intensive care unit does not automatically allow for a critical care service to be billed. For example, a patient admitted to the ICU for acute respiratory failure 7 days ago, unable to wean off the ventilator, but stable for 3 days on their current vent settings, awaiting tracheostomy, no longer meets critical illness criteria. Neither does a patient who is in the ICU due to increased nursing needs such as a patient in diabetic ketoacidosis who needs glucose finger checks every hour, and the high nurse to patient ratio on the general ward, makes this level of care impossible or unsafe. Critical care billing is not warranted on a patient in an ICU bed only because the hospital policy requires it for their treatment, such as an insulin drip.

Critical care is a time-based service that follows the general rules of time-based coding. Both face-to-face and unit/floor time can be counted toward billable critical care time as long as the physician is in close proximity to the patient to immediately intervene for the minutes of reported critical care. If the physician is reviewing lab data on the patient's floor but the patient is on a different floor getting a test done, in this scenario, the unit/floor time cannot be counted toward critical care time. For time reported as critical care time, the physician must provide their entire attention to management of the critically ill patient. For example, if the physician is at the critically ill patient's bedside while an ECG is being performed, and while waiting, he is multitasking and looking up labs on *another* patient, this time cannot be counted toward critical care time. A minimum of 30 minutes of critical care must be provided to bill for critical care services. Twenty nine minutes or less of critical care would be billed with an E/M code that best reflects the service provided, such as an admission code [99221-99223] or inpatient follow-up code [99231-99233]. Once 30 minutes of critical care is provided, the first hour of critical care [99291] can be billed. Each additional half hour of critical care [99292] can be billed for thereafter (**Table 28-3**).

In addition to time spent face to face with the patient taking a history and performing a physical exam, other activities that count toward critical care time include the following:

1. Time spent reviewing test results while on the patient's floor or in their unit, and does not fall into the pitfall situation above. Time spent personally viewing a chest x-ray in the radiology suite on a different floor or looking at a peripheral smear in the hematology lab cannot be counted toward critical care time.
2. Time spent discussing the care plan with nursing staff or other consultants.
3. Discussions with family members or surrogates when both of these criteria are met (a) the patient lacks capacity or unable to participate in their own care and (b) the discussion directly impacts decision making. These discussions will count toward critical care time even if they occur via phone on the patient's floor or in their unit. However, time spent on routine updates to family cannot be counted toward critical care services, and is not separately reimbursable.
4. Time spent performing procedures that are bundled into critical care (**Table 28-4**).

Activities that cannot *count* toward billable critical care time include work that does not directly contribute to the patient's care, even if performed at the patient's bedside:

1. Time teaching
2. Time looking up literature
3. Family updates, even if at the request of the patient
4. Time performing separately reimbursed procedures

TABLE 28-3 Critical Care Billing

Minutes of Critical Care	CPT Codes Submitted
0-29	Submit appropriate E/M
30-74	99291
75-104	99291 + 99292
105-134	99291 + 99292 × 2
135-164	99291 + 99292 × 3
165-194	99291 + 99292 × 4
195+	- - - - follow the pattern above - - - -

TABLE 28-4 Procedures Bundled into Critical Care

Procedure	CPT
IV placement	36000
Arterial blood gas	36600
Blood draws, physician skill needed	36410, 36415, 36591
NG tube placement (+fluoro, +lavage)	43752, 91105
Chest x-ray, professional component	71010-26, 71015-26, 71020-26
Temporary transcutaneous pacing	92953
Interpretation of cardiac output indices	93561, 93562
Ventilator management	94002-94004, 94660, 94662
Pulse-oximetry	94760, 94761, 94762
Data analysis from a computer	99090

Certain procedures when performed on the same date as a critical care service and by the same provider, are bundled into the reimbursement for critical care and cannot be billed for separately. (Table 28-4). Any medically necessary procedure not included in this table can be billed separately from critical care, such as central line placement, cardiopulmonary resuscitation, and intubation to name a few. The documentation should clearly state that the time performing these unbundled procedures is not included in the reported critical care time.

When critical care is provided by the same physician/billing group on the same date that another E/M service such as an inpatient admission, follow-up, or consult was provided earlier in the day when the patient was not critically ill, both the earlier E/M and the critical care service can be reimbursed. The exception to this rule is when the other E/M service is an emergency room visit [99281-99285]. An emergency room service cannot be paid on the same date as a critical care service by the same physician/billing group.

In a coverage situation, such as a change in shifts where a partner in the same billing group continues to provide critical care on the same calendar date, critical care time can be aggregated as long as the initial physician provided at least 30 minutes of critical care. For example, if Dr A provides 40 minutes of critical care at 6 PM and then Dr B takes over and provides an additional 35 minutes of critical care at 7 PM, the critical care time can be aggregated. A total of 75 minutes of critical care was provided; the first hour of critical care [99291] would be submitted by Dr A and an additional half hour of critical care [99292] would be submitted by Dr B. However, if Dr A had only provided 25 minutes of critical care and Dr B provided 50 minutes, although they still provided a total of 75 minutes of critical care, Dr A did not provide at least 30 minutes before going off shift. They cannot aggregate their critical care time. Dr A would bill an appropriate E/M code that best represents their work such as an inpatient admission or follow-up, and Dr B would bill for the first hour of critical care [99291].

■ CONCURRENT CARE

Two different physicians from different specialties can both receive payment for critical care services on the same calendar date if there is medical necessity for each of them to provide this level of care; however, two physicians cannot get paid for the same exact same minutes of critical care. For example, if Dr A, an internal medicine hospitalist, provides 30 minutes of critical care from 9 to 10 AM stabilizing a patient with impending respiratory failure, and Dr B, the intensive care physician, provides critical care between 10 and 11 AM, each physician would submit a claim for the first hour of critical care [99291]. In the event that both physicians provide care at the same time, only one physician will get paid for critical care. The other physician should submit an E/M code that best represents their work.

Having different subspecialty designations does not automatically allow each physician to submit a claim for the first hour of critical care. In the event that a member cross covering a patient happens to have a different subspecialty designation, but their role is to continue the care started by the previous physician, the work of the two physicians would be aggregated. For example, in a hospital medicine group, if Dr A is an internist and provides critical care for 30 minutes and then their partner Dr B, a cardiologist, comes on to cover the night shift and provides an additional 30 minutes of critical care, even if the patient's critical illness happened to be a cardiac problem, in this situation, the two physicians would aggregate their work. A total of 60 minutes of critical care was provided, which is only enough to bill for the first hour of critical care. Only 99291 can be submitted in this scenario.

When providing critical care in tandem with a resident, the only time that the physician can count toward critical care billing, is the time they personally provide critical care, or time they are physically present while the resident provides critical care. For documentation, the resident's note can help support the high complexity of MDM. In addition to meeting all teaching physician (TP) presence and documentation criteria, and writing a valid attestation statement linking the TP's note to the resident's note, the TP must personally document the following to bill for critical care.

1. The patient was critically ill at the time the TP was physically present and provided the service.
2. What the critical illness is. ICD-10 codes for a critical illness must be used, or the claim will be at high risk of initial denial.
3. The nature of the treatment and management they personally provided.
4. The number of minutes of critical care that they personally provided.

Documentation of the above by the resident is insufficient for billing. An example from the Medicare manual of minimally acceptable TP documentation for critical care: "Patient developed hypotension and hypoxia; I spent 45 minutes while the patient was in this condition, providing fluids, pressor drugs, and oxygen. I reviewed the resident's documentation and I agree with the resident's assessment and plan of care."

■ DISCHARGE MANAGEMENT SERVICES

Discharge management services can only be billed by the primary attending of record, or a partner covering that day. All other consultants should bill an inpatient follow-up visit [99231-99233] or an established outpatient visit [99212-99215] based on the patient's inpatient versus observation status as well as payor rules for observation services. For inpatient discharge management, there are two levels of service: <30 minutes [99238] or >30 minutes [99239]. Both face-to-face and unit/floor time spent in discharge activities count, including but not limited to taking a history, the final physical exam, counseling the patient and family, reviewing data, writing prescriptions, and ordering follow-up appointments.

The only required documentation to bill for discharge management services is a statement attesting to having a face-to-face visit with the patient on the date of discharge management services. For legal, ethical, and high-quality patient care reasons, further documentation of the details of that visit would be prudent. When providing the higher level of inpatient discharge management [99239], documentation must explicitly state how much time was spent on discharge management as well as a brief summary of what was done during that time. Lack of this statement will prevent

reimbursement for the higher level of care [99239]. No time amount needs to be documented when billing the lower level of care [99238]. If extensive amounts of time over 30 minutes are spent on discharge management, there is no additional reimbursement for this care. Prolonged services cannot be billed with any discharge management code. There is only one level of discharge management for observation services regardless of the amount of time spent on care.

One of the most common documentation errors preventing reimbursement for the higher level of inpatient discharge is the statement "I spent 30 minutes on discharge management." As opposed to other time-based services where 30 minutes is the minimum amount needed to bill a unit of service (ie, prolonged service, critical care), **more than 30 minutes** must be spent in discharge management to allow reimbursement for the 99239. This author suggests documenting the actual amount of time spent, in minutes.

PALLIATIVE CARE

Although palliative care has had its own subspecialty designation (17) since October 2009, many internal medicine hospitalists (subspecialty 11) have developed expertise in this field without formally changing their subspecialty designation from 11 to 17. When functioning as a consultant providing concurrent care to patients under the care of a colleague in the same subspecialty, there are several "best practices" to be aware of to minimize claims denials.

■ SUBSPECIALTY DESIGNATION

When providing concurrent care, one of the first pieces of evidence that medical necessity exists for two physicians to manage a patient on the same calendar date, is different subspecialty designations. A physician can go into the Medicare Provider Enrollment, Chain and Ownership System (PECOS) at any time and change their primary and secondary subspecialty designations. The physician should have evidence of expertise in their primary subspecialty designation; this does not have to be completion of an accredited fellowship program in that field. Recognition at the local, regional, or national level of expertise via activities such as publications, public speaking engagements, or development of institutional protocols or curricula, would satisfy this criteria. Documentation of constant and updated Continued Medical Education (CME) credit in that field would also count. Many physicians list their primary subspecialty designation as the field that they provide >50% of their services in. For internal medicine palliative care hospitalists, the percent of services provided as an internist may often outweigh that of their palliative care services; symptom-driven ICD-10 coding, complete descriptive documentation, and vigilant claims tracking are key to ensure appropriate reimbursement for these services.

■ SYMPTOM-DRIVEN ICD-10 CODING

Palliative care providers are often consulted to assist with maximizing quality of life and minimizing suffering for the time a patient has left. In doing so, the goals of care often center around symptom control and not disease management. This may differ from the primary attending's care plan, which may employ palliative services, but which are still overall managing a disease state. Use of ICD-10 codes for symptoms being managed, not only better reflects the work of the palliative care provider, but also ensures that different ICD-10 codes will be submitted from the primary physician's claim. For example, a patient with end-stage COPD is admitted for the eighth time this year with a COPD exacerbation, contemplating hospice care, and most bothered by dyspnea and fatigue. The palliative care provider's documentation and plan will focus on control of the symptoms of dyspnea and fatigue, while the primary hospitalist's note will focus on appropriate management of COPD. Claims for these services will be submitted with the ICD-10 codes for dyspnea [R06.0] and fatigue [R53.83], and COPD [J44.1] respectively.

■ COMPLETE AND DESCRIPTIVE DOCUMENTATION

Palliative care providers often spend enormous amounts of time counseling patients, and may bill a significant percent of their visits based on CCC. More detailed descriptions of the clinical situation will better support the medical necessity to spend these larger amounts of time with the patient. Adjectives may make a huge difference. A statement such as *"patient extremely distraught over their terminal condition and required intense counseling regarding goals of end of life care"* paints a much better picture for the need for 90 minutes of counseling than a statement like *"Patient upset over terminal diagnosis. I counseled the patient on goals of care."*

■ TRACK CLAIMS AND CLAIM DENIALS

The best way to prevent future denials is to determine the reason for denial of a medically necessary visit, and use information learned from that encounter to prevent a denial for similar services. For example, a private insurer who sees two inpatient follow-up services [99231-99233] from the same subspecialty group on the same calendar date, even with different ICD-10's, may deny it upfront simply because they require modifier –25 to be attached to one of the services. Another provider may require documentation to be submitted upfront for all situations where two inpatient follow-up visits are submitted on the same date. Lessons learned from these two denials alone may prevent hundreds more.

One way to help track these services internally would be to remember to submit ICD-10 code [Z51.5] for "encounter for palliative care services" with 100% of these services. This code should never be the primary diagnosis. Its use will not alter the amount of reimbursement for the visit; however its presence on a claim may alert an insurer that this service is separate and distinct from another E/M submitted by the same billing group, and prevent an upfront denial. At minimum, it will allow a physician to more easily search for these encounters in their data base to monitor payment for these services.

SUGGESTED READINGS

CPT 2015: Current Procedural Terminology. *Cpt/Current Procedural Terminology Professional Edition*. American Medical Association Press.

Lustbader Dr, Nelson JE, Weissman DE, et al. Physician reimbursement for critical care services integrating palliative care for patients who are critically Ill. *Chest*. 2012;141(3):787-792.

ONLINE RESOURCE

Centers for Medicare and Medicaid Services. *Medicare Claims Processing Manual: Section 30.6.1.C; Section 30.6.10, Section 30.6.12, Section 30.6.15.1* (Chapter 12). CMS Web Site. Available at www.cms.hhsgov/manuals/downloads/clm104c12.pdf. Accessed December 14, 2015.

CHAPTER 29

Billing for Procedures and Use of Modifiers in Inpatient Practice

Yvette M. Cua, MD

■ INTRODUCTION

Procedures are commonplace in hospital medicine; more and more hospitalists have invested additional educational time in becoming proficient in performing them. Understanding the documentation requirements necessary to ensure proper payment of procedures, including adequate documentation of the medical necessity to perform them, is crucial. In addition, making sure that the Current Procedural Terminology (CPT) code is correctly linked to the proper International Classification of Diseases, 10th Revision (ICD-10) code(s) will further prevent claim denials.

Details regarding the service requirements of each procedure are outlined in the CPT Handbook, published by the American Medical Association. The Medicare Claims Processing Manuel discusses nuances in Medicare guidelines regarding situational and documentation requirements for reimbursement. Procedures may be described as "minor" or "major." These terms have caused significant confusion in the literature. There are actually two different ways in which the terms "minor" and "major" procedures are used within the Medicare manual.

■ MINOR VERSUS MAJOR PROCEDURES

Surgeries and global packages

Within the Medicare Processing Manual, procedures are referred to as "surgeries" or "surgical procedures." When discussing payment for the medically necessary care provided immediately before and after the procedure, one must be aware of the global period associated with the service. Services with global periods of 90 days are defined as "major *surgeries*" or "major *procedures*." These terms are used interchangeably in the manual. Services with global periods of 0 or 10 days are described as "minor surgeries" or "minor procedures." Endoscopies are included in this category. Most procedures performed by nonsurgical specialties fall into the "minor" procedure category.

One example of the importance of this distinction is use of modifier −57 (decision to perform surgery). Modifier −57 is only used when deciding to perform major and not minor procedures. Reimbursement for all care related to the surgery, by the surgeon performing the procedure, occurring 1 day before the procedure and for the ensuing 90-day global period, is bundled into the reimbursement for the surgery's CPT code. One exception is the reimbursement for the E/M visit at which time the decision to operate is made if it occurs 1 day prior to surgery or on the day of surgery. Modifier −57 attached to that E/M code will allow for its reimbursement in addition to the reimbursement for the major procedure. For the situation where the decision to perform a minor procedure is made at an E/M visit the same day of the procedure, modifier −25 should be attached to that E/M code to show that it was medically necessary work, separate from the usual history and physical needed to safely perform the procedure.

Teaching physician procedural billing

With regard to teaching physician (TP) rules for procedural billing, a "minor" procedure is defined as taking <5 minutes to perform, and the TP must be present for the entire procedure to bill for it. A "major" procedure takes >5 minutes. The TP must be present for the critical or key portion(s) of the procedure and must be immediately available for the entire procedure, in order to bill for it. The definition of "major" and "minor" in this context is based on the usual total procedure time. Examples of minor procedures include drainage of a subungal hematoma [11740], or a skin punch biopsy [11100]. Most inpatient procedures hospitalists perform, are considered "major" procedures, such as central line placement [36555-36556], thoracentesis [32554, 32555], or lumbar puncture [66270, 66272].

■ DESCRIPTION OF SELECTED PROCEDURES

Below are nuances of some common procedures performed in hospital medicine.

Central venous access procedures

Central venous access can be achieved through various locations and processes, and with various apparatuses. Different CPT codes exist based on the following key pieces of information: (1) location of access—central, peripheral; (2) method of placement—tunneled, nontunneled; (3) apparatus—catheter, port, pump; (4) number of access sites in the apparatus; and (5) age of the patient. Each of these factors plays a role in determining the usual amount of work needed to perform the service, which directly ties into graded reimbursement amounts. For example, tunneled catheters require more expertise and take longer to place than nontunneled lines; centrally placed lines are more challenging than their peripherally placed counterparts; and a device with a port takes more work to place than a catheter without one. There are separate codes for repair, replacement, and removal of these apparatuses as well (**Table 29-1**). These central venous catheters (CVC), also called "central lines," and central venous access devices (CVAD), like "ports," have tips that

terminate in either the subclavian, brachiocephalic, innominate or iliac veins, or where one of these joins with the superior or inferior vena cava. Medical documentation should include these key pieces of information not only to select the correct CPT code, but also to adequately support reimbursement for these services. This information is usually found in a procedure note.

"Placing a central line" at bedside, by convention, has become synonymous with "placing a nontunneled catheter in a central location" such as the internal jugular vein or the subclavian vein. This corresponds to CPT codes [36555, 36556] which differ only by the age of the patient. In this example, to ensure accurate CPT code selection, at minimum, the body of the procedure note should include reference to insertion of a nontunneled catheter (such as a triple lumen) into a central vessel (such as the right subclavian). In addition, postprocedure chest x-ray results verifying tip location should be documented. The CPT codes for peripherally inserted central catheter (PICC) placement [36568, 36569] only differ by age of the patient.

Use of ultrasound guidance [76937] or fluoroscopy [77001] for placement, is reimbursed through an additional code and is not bundled into the reimbursement for central line placement. Billing for imaging used to guide line placement requires very specific documentation. Ultrasound guidance for central vascular access [76937] is only reimbursable when used with a "dynamic" technique and not a "static" technique. A dynamic technique implies that the ultrasound is used throughout the entire procedure, not only to identify the target vessel, but to watch successful entrance of the needle into it. "Static" use of the ultrasound purely identifies the vessel and its patency, and is not reimbursable.

TABLE 29-1 CPT Codes for Central Venous Access Procedures

Centrally Placed

Method	Type	Age	Insert	Repair	Partial Replace	Total Replace	Remove
Nontunneled	CVC	<5 y old	36555	36575	*	36580	*
		≥5 y old	36556	36575	*	36580	*
Tunneled	CVC	<5 y old	36557	36575	*	36581	36589
		≥5 y old	36558	36575	*	36581	36589
	CVAD (port)	<5 y old	36560	36576	36578	36582	36590
		≥5 y old	36561	36576	36578	36582	36590
	CVAD (pump)		36563	36576		36578	36583
2-Tunneled cath	CVC		36565	36575 × 2	*	36581 × 2	36589
	CVAD (port)		36566	36576 × 2	36578 × 2	36582 × 2	36590 × 2

Peripherally Placed

Method	Type	Age	Insert	Repair	Partial Replace	Total Replace	Remove
Nontunneled	PICC	<5 y old	36568	36575	*	36584	*
		≥5 y old	36569	36575	*	36584	*
Tunneled	CVAD (port)	<5 y old	36570	36576	36578	36585	36590
		≥5 y old	36571	36576	36578	36585	36590

Imaging guidance	CPT
Ultrasound guidance for vascular access	76937
Fluoroscopic guidance for vascular access	77001

* Not separately reimbursable.
Insertion = placement for catheter in newly established site.
Repair = fixing device without replacing any component of it.
Partial replacement = replacing only the catheter portion of a CVAD, not a port or pump.
Total replacement = replacing entire device through the same access site. If a new access site is established, submit CPT for insertion, not replacement.

TABLE 29-2 CPT Codes for Pleural Access Procedures

Service	Description	Imaging Guidance	CPT
Chest tube placement	Tube thoracostomy with or without connection to waterseal	add **75989**	**32551**
Thoracentesis	Needle/catheter aspiration of pleural space	without imaging	**32554**
		with imaging	**32555**
Pigtail catheter placement	Percutaneous pleural drainage with placement of indwelling catheter	without imaging	**32556**
		with imaging	**32557**

At minimum, documentation needs to include a description of potential access sites, patency of the vessel selected, and successful entry of the seeker needle into the target vessel in order to bill for ultrasound guidance for central vascular access [76937]. In addition, permanent visual recording in the form of a printed image, digital image, or video must be captured and available in an audit. The CPT manual implies that at least an image of the patent target vessel is sufficient. Attempting to shift focus away from the procedure to try to capture an image of the actual seeker needle in the vessel may pose a risk to the patient. A postprocedural image of the catheter sitting in the target vessel would be a safer and acceptable way to meet these criteria. When submitting the claim, remember to attach modifier –26 to the CPT code since the technical component of the service is not separately reimbursable in a facility setting. Placement of a nontunneled Quinton triple lumen catheter into the right subclavian vein of a 45-year-old patient using dynamic real-time ultrasound guidance, would be reported using CPT codes 36556 PLUS 76937-26.

There is no reimbursement for repositioning or removing a nontunneled catheter at bedside. However, changing a nontunneled central line over a wire (central location [36580], PICC [36584]) is separately reimbursable. If a second line needs to be placed on the same day as the first (ie, the patient pulls the first one out completely, or the patient had a dialysis catheter placed on the same day as a triple lumen CVC), the CPT code for the procedure would be reported twice with the appropriate modifier (–76, –77) appended to the second procedure.

Thoracentesis and chest tube placement

The CPT codes for accessing the pleural space [32554-32557] were updated in 2013 to better reflect a change in practice with improved technology. At that time, over 75% of thoracenteses with or without catheter placement were being done with ultrasound guidance. This new set of CPT codes contains *bundled codes*, such that a separate CPT code for the use of imaging (ultrasound [76942], fluoroscopy [77002]) to identify a pocket of fluid, should no longer be submitted with the appropriate pleural access code; reimbursement for the use of imaging is already included in the payment for the primary procedure code [32555, 32557]. Documentation for a thoracentesis ("puncture and aspiration of the pleural cavity") needs to specifically identify if ultrasound guidance was used [32555] or not [32554]. No adjustment in reimbursement is made for a diagnostic versus therapeutic procedure. Similarly, placement of a pigtail catheter ("percutaneous pleural drainage with insertion of indwelling catheter") with ultrasound guidance [32557] reimburses higher than the blind placement [32556] (**Table 29-2**).

For chest tube placement [32551], if imaging guidance is used (ultrasound, fluoroscopy, computed tomography), a separate CPT code [75989] must still be submitted for reimbursement of imaging. The reason for higher reimbursement than pigtail catheter placement is that this open procedure requires cutdown and

dissection. The procedure entails moderate sedation which is not separately reimbursable. Chest tube insertion is not separately reimbursable if placed intraoperatively during another cardiac or thoracic procedure.

There is no separate reimbursement for removal of chest tubes or pigtail catheters. If any of these procedures is done bilaterally, modifier –50 should be used.

Paracentesis

Just as for a thoracentesis, paracentesis codes [49082, 49083] were revised in 2012 to reflect the increased use of imaging guidance. The intent to do a diagnostic versus therapeutic procedure, the difference between small and large volume taps, and performing the initial versus subsequent tap, do not play a role in determining the level of reimbursement. For the higher level of reimbursement, documentation must clearly state that imaging was used, otherwise the reimbursement will default to the lower reimbursing service done without imaging [49082]. [49083] is a bundled code reimbursing for both the work of the procedure as well as the imaging. A separate CPT code such as 76942 (ultrasound guidance) should not be used with it (**Table 29-3**).

Incision and drainage

The selection of the correct CPT code for incision and drainage (I&D) procedures is based on the location of the lesion, on the type of lesion being treated, the complexity of the procedure, and if it occurred in the postoperative period. Certain locations have unique CPT codes for I&D such as an abscess of the eyelid [67700] or external ear [69000, 69005]. I&D of the majority of abscesses are reported using CPT codes 10060 (simple) and 10061 (complex or multiple). There is no universal definition of "complex"; the CPT manual states that it is left up to the clinical judgment of the provider and substantiated by their documentation. Complex I&D procedures include (1) large lesions, though "large" is also not universally defined; (2) significant packing or placement of a drain; (3) disintegration of loculations; (4) incision and drainage of multiple lesions. I&Ds of hematomas are reported with CPT code 10040 (**Table 29-4**).

TABLE 29-3 CPT Codes for Paracentesis and Peritoneal Lavage

Service	Imaging Guidance	CPT
Paracentesis	Without imaging	**49082**
	With imaging	**49083**
Peritoneal lavage	Includes reimbursement for imaging	**49084**
	Even if not used	

TABLE 29-4 CPT Codes for Incision and Drainage Procedures

CPT Code	Description
10060	I&D of cutaneous or subcutaneous abscess, cyst, or paronychia; simple or single
10061	I&D of cutaneous or subcutaneous abscess, cyst, or paronychia; complicated or multiple
10080	I&D of pilonidal cyst; simple
10081	I&D of pilonidal cyst; complicated
10120	Incision and removal of foreign body, subcutaneous tissues; simple
10121	Incision and removal of foreign body, subcutaneous tissues; complicated
10140	I&D of hematoma, seroma or fluid collection
10160	Puncture aspiration of abscess, hematoma, bulla, or cyst
10180	I&D, complex, post-op wound infection

MODIFIERS

A modifier is a two character alpha numeric code, attached to a CPT code, to further describe a service or to signify that a service has been altered by a specific circumstance without changing the description/definition of the service. Some situations require more than one modifier to be used with a CPT code. There are two levels of modifiers. Level 1 modifiers, also called CPT modifiers, are numeric, and updated by the American Medical Association. Level 2 modifiers, also called HCPCS modifiers, begin with a letter followed by either a number or another letter, and are updated by CMS.

There are hundreds of modifiers. Some directly impact reimbursement amounts; some directly enable payment for a service, while others are for informational purposes alone. Below are some of the more common ones needed for proper claims processing in Hospital Medicine.

■ MODIFIER –25: SIGNIFICANT AND SEPARATELY IDENTIFIABLE E/M SERVICE BY THE SAME PROVIDER ON THE SAME DAY AS A PROCEDURE OR OTHER SERVICE

This may only be attached to an E/M code and not to a procedure code. On occasion, it is necessary for a provider and/or covering member of their billing group, to provide more than one medically necessary service to a patient on the same calendar date.

E//M and procedure

The most common scenario would be a medically necessary E/M visit plus a procedure on the same calendar date. Modifier –25 should be attached to the E/M code to signify that it is a separately identifiable service, distinct from the routine pre- and postwork needed for the procedure. For example, a hospitalist admits a patient with altered mental status and fever, determines that a lumbar puncture (LP) is needed, and performs it on the same date as the admission. The hospital may receive payment for BOTH the initial inpatient visit [99221-99223] PLUS the LP [62270]. Modifier –25 should be attached to the initial inpatient visit CPT code [99221-99223] to show that the cognitive work of that visit is separate and above and beyond that necessary for just safely performing the LP. In contrast, a neurologist may only bill for the LP and not for an E/M visit, if his or her role is one of proceduralist and not consultant. A proceduralist should take and appropriately document a brief history and perform a brief physical preprocedure to ensure the safety

and necessity of performing the procedure. A consultant is asked for and provides an opinion on diagnosis, evaluation, and treatment. A consultant can be reimbursed for both the consult that generated the decision to perform an LP plus the procedure.

Two E/M services

A modifier –25 may be needed when two medically necessary E/M services are provided on the same calendar date. Only one primary E/M code should be submitted for all E/M work done from 12:01 AM to 11:59 PM by one physician and/or multiple physicians in a billing group functioning as coverage/continuance of care for each other. However, a few exceptions to this rule exist. One exception is when an E/M service such as an inpatient admission or inpatient follow-up visit is completed and followed later that same day by a critical care service by the same provider and/or billing group. The provider may be compensated for both services. Some insurers may require modifier –25 to be attached to the CPT code for the noncritical care service to show that it was separate and distinct from the critical care service. Medical necessity and complete documentation for both services must exist in the medical record.

■ MODIFIER –26: BILLING FOR THE PROFESSIONAL COMPONENT OF A PROCEDURE

Many procedures such as chest x-rays and ultrasounds have reimbursement that is divided into a technical component (TC) and a professional component (PC). Reimbursement for the TC covers the cost of purchasing or leasing equipment, and for maintenance. The reimbursement for the PC covers the supervision/performance of a test, and its formal written interpretation. When billing for the professional component of a service, attach modifier –26.

For example, many hospitalists read their own chest x-rays (CXR) to make immediate management decisions for their patients, and document their findings in their progress notes, followed by a formal or official radiology report some time later. This work counts toward their level of medical decision making for the E/M service and is not separately reimbursable. However, some institutions do not have radiologists immediately available after hours and may have a system in place whereby hospitalists or emergency department providers are responsible for producing the official written reports, not a radiologist the next day. In this situation, with a valid written report generated, this work is separately reimbursable by the hospitalist or emergency department provider. The TC of the global fee (total reimbursement) for the procedure, is not separately reimbursable in this setting. Modifier –26 should be added to the procedure's CPT code for reimbursement of the PC. For the CXR above, 71020-26 would be submitted for reimbursement for the work of viewing and interpreting the film, and creating the official report. The provider cannot count that work toward the complexity of his medical decision making for any associated E/M service to the patient if receiving separate reimbursement for CXR interpretation. Minus one situation, in the erroneous event that both the hospitalist and a radiologist submit 71020-26 for reimbursement for the same film, only the first bill received with be reimbursed. A system needs to be in place to ensure that this situation does not occur.

There are some procedures that do not have a global fee divided into a TC and PC. Instead, there are separate CPT codes for billing for TC + PC, TC alone, or PC alone. For example, EKGs: CPT 93000 is for TC + PC, 93005 is for TC alone, and 93010 is for the PC alone.

■ MODIFIER –76: SAME EXACT PROCEDURE PERFORMED BY THE SAME PROVIDER ON THE SAME DATE

A procedural CPT code and never an E/M code is used when the same exact procedure is done twice on a patient on the same calendar date and/or during the procedure's global period. For example, a hospitalist places a central line on a patient in the morning, the patient pulls it out, and the hospitalist places another one later that day. The central line CPT code [36556] would be reported twice, attaching modifier –76 to the second one. Likewise, you would report cardiopulmonary resuscitation CPR [92950] twice attaching modifier –76 to the second CPR billing code if a patient requires CPR at two different times in the day. Reimbursement for two procedures requires appropriate documentation of each procedure (ie, two notes with the time each procedure was performed).

A left knee arthrocentesis and a right shoulder arthrocentesis would not be coded using this modifier. Although an arthocentesis was performed in both locations, it is not the exact same procedure—one is of the knee and the other is of the shoulder. This would be coded using modifier –XE instead.

■ MODIFIER –77: SAME EXACT PROCEDURE PERFORMED ON THE SAME DATE BY A DIFFERENT PROVIDER

This modifier is used exactly like modifier –76 except when the same exact procedure is performed by a different provider on the same date.

■ MODIFIER –AI: PRINCIPAL ATTENDING PHYSICIAN OF RECORD

This modifier is used to identify the principal physician of record for the patient, ie the main physician overseeing care. Medicare stopped paying for inpatient consult codes [99251-99255] on January 1, 2010. All consultants seeing inpatients now bill their consult with the same initial inpatient visit codes [99221-99223] and initial skilled nursing facility codes [99304-99306] that the admitting attending uses. The –AI modifier (letter I, not number 1) will distinguish the admitting attending from all other consultants, but will not change the amount of reimbursement for the visit. By attaching it to the initial inpatient or skilled nursing visit code, it also aids CMS with identifying which physician will bill for discharge management services. Only attach it to the initial inpatient [99221-99223] or initial skilled nursing facility [99304-99306] visit codes. Do not attach it to any other CPT codes such as subsequent visits [99231-99233, 99307-99310], discharges [99238-99239, 99315-99316], or observation services [99217-99220; 99224-99226].

■ MODIFIER –GC: CARE PROVIDED IN PART BY A RESIDENT, SUPERVISED BY A TP

Attached modifier –GC to all services performed in conjunction with a resident (including interns and fellows) in a teaching situation, provided that the TP was present and personally participated in the critical or key component(s) of the encounter. It is not appropriate to attach to services performed in supervision of medical students.

■ MODIFIER –GV: CARE RELATED TO THE TERMINAL ILLNESS

The –GV modifier can only be attached to services rendered by a hospice patient's primary attending if (1) the attending is not employed or paid by the hospice under any agreement and is not a volunteer, and (2) the care is for the patient's terminal illness. This modifier is used to submit claims to Medicare Part B for reimbursement. It cannot be used by consultants, nor can it be used by the patient's primary attending for care unrelated to the terminal illness.

■ MODIFIER –GW: CARE UNRELATED TO THE TERMINAL ILLNESS

Attach modifier –GW to services provided to a hospice patient when care is unrelated to the terminal illness.

■ MODIFIER –Q5: RECIPROCAL BILLING

Attach modifier –Q5 to services provided in a reciprocal billing arrangement. A reciprocal billing situation exists when two or more physicians from different billing entities agree to cover for each other in one's absence. This agreement does not need to be in writing, but clearly understood between parties. The criteria for reciprocal billing are (1) the regular physician is unavailable; (2) the patient is seeking care from the regular physician; (3) the substitute physician does not cover for more than 60 consecutive days. The substitute physician, with one exception, is *not a member* of the regular physician's billing group. These services are actually billed under the *regular* physician's National Provider Identifier (NPI) number, attaching modifier –Q5 to each CPT service code. The reimbursement will go to the *regular* physician. Ideally, when the substitute physician needs time off, the regular physician will return the favor, and in the long run, reimbursement evens out. This arrangement is commonly used by solo practitioners, but may also be used by group practices who acquire coverage from a physician outside their billing group. Notice that the usual scenario: partners in a billing group and subspecialty cover for each other on weekends, holidays, and vacations, does not fit the definition of a reciprocal billing arrangement. In this scenario, the physician providing the service would simply submit charges under their own NPI number.

The hospice setting is an exception from the situation where the substitute physician is actually from *the same billing group*. Hospice patients select or are assigned a primary attending who oversees their care. Unlike the role of principal attending of record for other hospital inpatients, the role of primary hospice attending is specific to an *individual provider*, not to a billing group/subspecialty. In the event that the hospice attendings require coverage, such as weekend coverage, and one of their partners covers these patients, this is also considered a reciprocal billing arrangement. These services, provided by a partner in the same billing group, will be billed under the regular hospice attending's NPI number with modifier –Q5 attached to each CPT code. Thus in a group practice, Dr Sub may be covering for Dr Hospice for the weekend. All services provided by Dr Sub to Dr Hospice's *regular inpatients* will be billed under Dr Sub's own NPI; however, those services provided by Dr Sub to *hospice patients* will be billed under Dr Hospice's NPI, attaching modifier –Q5.

■ MODIFIER –Q6

Modifier –Q6 is attached to all services performed by a locum tenens provider (LT), with claims submitted under the regular physician's NPI. Reimbursement will go to the regular physician. A LT has no practice of their own, and functions as an independent contractor, receiving payment on a fixed per diem or fee-for-time basis. They can only provide coverage for any individual physician for a consecutive *not* cumulative 60-day period, even if not providing care on all of those days. The 60-day period starts to the first day the LT provides services. If a physician returns to work for a period of time and needs to leave again, the locum tenens may provide coverage for another 60-day period. The only exception to the 60-day time period for Medicare patients is for coverage of a physician called to active duty—coverage time is unlimited. If a second physician in a group practice needs time off, the LT can provide a separate 60 days of coverage for that physician as well, regardless of the number of days of coverage they already served for the first physician.

Common reasons a physician may not be available, include pregnancy, illness, continuing medical education, and vacation. In a group practice setting, a physician may need to leave the practice, and the practice may employ a LT for up to 60 days while finding a replacement. The purpose of a LT is to provide temporary coverage for an *existing* physician. They cannot be used as temporary help to fill a newly created position while growing a practice.

LT is an attractive short term coverage option. They do not have to be enrolled in Medicare to provide services since the billing is under the regular physician's NPI. LT can only be employed to substitute for an absent *physician*. They cannot be hired to cover an absent *nonphysician provider (NPP)*. Also, they cannot be employed to cover an absent physician if the reason for absence is death. NPI numbers are deactivated upon death.

LT guidelines were created by Medicare, but private insurers and Medicaid may differ. For example, Texas Medicaid and Healthcare Partners has a 90 consecutive day LT limit. Some private insurers do not recognize LT services and require LTs to be credentialed through the normal new member process. It is imperative for this and all billing situations, to check with individual payors for deviations from the Medicare guidelines.

ONLINE RESOURCES

Centers for Medicare and Medicaid Services. *Medicare Claims Processing Manual: Section 40* Chap 12. CMS Web site. www.cms.hhs.gov/manuals/downloads/clm104c12.pdf. Accessed December 14, 2015.

Centers for Medicare and Medicaid Services. *Medicare Claims Processing Manual: Section 100.1.2.* Chap 12. CMS Web site. www.cms.hhs.gov/manuals/downloads/clm104c12.pdf. Accessed December 14, 2015.

2012 Coding Updates, American Gastroenterology Association. http://www.gastro.org/journals-publications/aga-edigest/Tri-Society_Coding_Sheet.pdf.

Noridian healthcare Solutions. https://med.noridianmedicare.com/web/jeb/topics/modifiers.

Billing for Procedures and Use of Modifiers in Inpatient Practice

CHAPTER 30

Billing in the Teaching Setting and Billing with Advanced Practice Providers

Yvette M. Cua, MD

TEACHING PHYSICIAN GUIDELINES

■ INTRODUCTION

Teaching physician (TP) guidelines date back to 1969 with the publication of Intermediary Letter 372, but did not come under serious scrutiny until 1995 when the results of the Office of the Inspector General's (OIG) first physicians at teaching hospitals (PATH) audit resulted in a $30 million dollar settlement by the University of Pennsylvania. The audit revealed that there was insufficient documentation in the medical record that the TP was physically present and actively participated in the critical portions of the services billed. This index case prompted a nationwide PATH audit initiative, and on December 8, 1995, the Health Care Financing Administration (HCFA), now the Centers for Medicare and Medicaid Services (CMS), published in the Final Rule, more detailed instructions for documenting and billing for services in a teaching setting. The rules officially went into effect July 1, 1996 and were added to the Medicare Claims Processing Manual, Chapter 12, Section 100. These rules have had modifications and clarifications over the years, last in 2011. Although state Medicaid programs and private insurers often follow Medicare, there are individual differences among these programs, especially in regards to requirements for TP presence and TP documentation. This author suggests using this chapter as a starting point, but checking with local payers for deviation from these guidelines.

DEFINITIONS

The term "**resident**" in the Medicare Processing Manual refers to "… an individual who participates in an approved graduate medical education (GME) program or a physician who is not in an approved GME program but who is authorized to practice only in a hospital setting …." Of note, receiving a faculty or staff appointment, or being included in a hospital's full time equivalency (FTE) count, in and of itself does not alter a resident's status. For billing purposes, and for this chapter, *the term "resident" includes interns and fellows, but not students.*

A **student** is someone in an accredited educational program like a medical school, dental school, or school of osteopathy that is not an approved GME program. Medicare does not pay for student services.

A **TP** is a physician who is not another resident, who provides care to patients in conjunction with a resident. A TP does not need to have a faculty appointment, thus these regulations are also applicable to private practice physicians who work with residents. Finally, these guidelines are specifically for physicians, and are not applicable to nonphysician providers (NPP), discussed separately in the second part of this chapter.

PAYMENT FOR PHYSICIAN SERVICES PROVIDED IN A TEACHING SETTING

The reason that medical and surgical services provided only by residents, within the scope of their training program, cannot be reimbursed through the Medicare Physician Fee Schedule (MPFS), is because Medicare Part A already pays for resident services upfront through direct graduate medical education (DGME) and indirect medical education (IME) payments. In a teaching setting, these services may be reimbursed through the MPFS if the TP personally performs or is physically present while a resident performs the critical or key portions of the service, assuming that the documentation clearly reflects this.

EVALUATIONS AND MANAGEMENT SERVICES

Teaching physician presence

There are several common scenarios in which the TP provides services in tandem with a resident. The key feature in all of these is that the TP is physically present and has a face to face encounter with the patient on the date of service, personally performing all of the service or at minimum, the critical or key portions to allow for billing, regardless of the extent of care the resident provided.

1. *The TP personally provides the service.* There may be situations when a resident has a day off, or the TP has completed a service before the resident has seen a patient and/or has discussed it with the TP. The TP would document the service as they would in a nonteaching setting as there is no resident note to link to. In absence of a resident's note, attempting to write an attestation alone without personally documenting elements of the history, physical, and medical decision making, is insufficient to support reimbursement for the service provided.

2. *The TP personally provides the service at a different time on the same calendar date as the resident.* An example of this situation would be when a resident sees a patient and provides a service like a subsequent inpatient visit [99231-99233], and later on the same date, the TP sees the patient and personally performs the service. Notice that the *personal performance* and not the *personal documentation* of the entire service is the main feature that allows the TP to bill for this service. If the documentation by the resident earlier in the day contains the same information that the TP personally obtained later, the TP does not have to redocument any of it. The TP needs to document a valid attestation statement linked to the resident's note, plus any additional findings, discrepancies, or changes in clinical condition.

3. *The resident performs the entire service, or at minimum the critical or key components in the physical presence of the TP*, and the TP personally documents that he or she was present for the critical or key portions of the service. The clinical judgment of the TP determines the critical or key portion(s) of a service, based on standards of care, specifics of the service, and individual patients' situational factors.

DOCUMENTATION REQUIREMENTS

For E/M services (excluding outpatient Primary Care Exception situations), at a minimum, TPs must personally document:

1. *The TP was present.* All E/M services in the context of hospital medicine require a face to face encounter with the billing TP on the date of service. If something prevents the TP from seeing the patient, such as the patient being in the operating room all day, or at a procedure during the only time frame that the TP is available that day, even though the TP may have invested the time in complete data review, discussion with consultants, and care plan development with the resident, the service cannot be billed or reimbursed.

2. *The TP personally performed the service or was present for the critical or key portions performed by a resident.*

3. *The TP participated in the management of the patient.* In a teaching setting, the TP's management of the patient is often not the direct writing of orders or calling of consultants. Instead, care plan development and supervision of proper execution or orders are commonplace: review of the resident's documented assessment and plan for accuracy, discussion with the resident of the details of the plan, including any deviances from their documentation, and vigilant follow-up to ensure timely and correct follow-through of the plan. Documentation of these activities will satisfy these criteria.

These three criteria are often documented in a sentence called an "attestation statement." This statement must always be written by the TP. *The resident's documentation of the presence and participation of the TP is insufficient to support reimbursement for the service.* An acceptable attestation correctly linking the TP's note to the resident's note will allow for the combination of the resident's and the TP's documentation to determine the level of service provided.

Medicare manual examples of unacceptable attestation statements that do **not** meet the above criteria include the following statements which do **not** make it possible to determine if the TP was actually present, evaluated the patient, and/or participated in the plan of care.

1. "Agree with above." followed by valid authentication (ie, legible signature or electronic password protected signature).
2. "Rounded, Reviewed, Agree." followed by valid authentication.
3. "Discussed with resident. Agree." followed by valid authentication.
4. "Seen and agree." followed by valid authentication.
5. "Patient seen and evaluated." followed by valid authentication.
6. Valid authentication alone.

In addition, a TP's attestation statement referencing a resident's note but written and signed before the resident's note is written will not allow linkage to the resident's documentation, and thus not allow the resident's documentation to be used to determine the level of service provided. *You cannot attest to reviewing and agreeing with documentation that has yet to be written.*

Examples from the Medicare manual of *minimally acceptable attestations* include:

1. "Hospital Day #3. I saw and evaluated the patient. I agree with the findings and the plan of care as documented in the resident's note."
2. "I saw the patient with the resident and agree with the resident's findings and plan."
3. "See resident's note for details. I saw and evaluated the patient and agree with the resident's findings and plan as written."

Although not specifically stated in the Medicare manual as a requirement, the use of the word "I" at the beginning of the attestation is the best way to document that you personally performed the service.

In addition to the attestation statement, the TP should document any information that the resident forgot to document, new information or changes in clinical picture since the time of the resident's note, as well as any discrepancies or disagreements with the resident's findings, thoughts, or plans. This not only helps support billing, but more importantly, high-quality patient care as well. Below are a couple examples of this from the Medicare manual:

1. "Hospital Day #5. I saw and examined the patient. I agree with the resident's note except the heart murmur is louder, so I will obtain an echo to evaluate."
2. "I saw and evaluated the patient. I reviewed the resident's note and agree, except that picture is more consistent with pericarditis than myocardial ischemia. Will begin NSAIDs."

In fact, this additional documentation, individualizing the documentation to each patient, is better verification of the TP personal participation in the case.

■ STUDENT E/M DOCUMENTATION

The only parts of a student's documentation that may be referred to and used to determine the level of E/M service provided, are the review of systems (ROS) and past medical history, family history, and social history (PFSH). The TP note must document their review and agreement with the information. No matter how accurate and complete a student's documentation of the history of present illness (HPI), physical exam (PE), and medical decision making (MDM), reference to it without the TP personally verifying and redocumenting it, will not allow it to contribute to a billable service.

■ LATE NIGHT ADMISSIONS

In all of the above examples, the understanding is that the TP and resident performed a service jointly on the same calendar date. The TP can only link their attestation to the resident's documentation from the same calendar date, and thus use it to determine their level of service. There is one special *exception* to this rule. In the teaching setting, it is not uncommon for a resident to admit a patient late at night when there is no TP in the facility to immediately provide the initial inpatient service. In 2010, the author of this chapter worked directly with CMS to augment the Medicare manual to include this scenario. In 2011, this scenario was added to the Medicare manual allowing a TP to link their attestation statement to the resident's documentation of the initial inpatient visit the night before, allowing that documentation to be used to determine the level of service, provided that the TP also documents any additional information or significant changes since the time of the resident's note. *The date of the service for claim submission should be the date that the TP actually had their initial face to face visit, even if it is different from the patient's admission date.*

■ PROCEDURES

There is some confusion and controversy over TP documentation requirements for procedures due to the way the Medicare manual is worded. In addition, with the wide variability in state Medicaid and private insurer regulations, many compliance offices opt for more defendable approaches than what seems to be required in the Medicare manual, to ensure documentation meets any entity's strictest regulations. The Medicare manual uses the terms "procedure" and "surgery" interchangeably at times, making the guidelines for TP documentation in certain circumstances, left up to interpretation. For all "surgical procedures," the manual is clear that the TP must be present for the critical or key components of the procedure, but no blanket statement is made regarding TP documentation requirements.

Single surgeries

In order to bill for these services, a TP must be physically present for the critical or key components, plus for the noncritical portions, the TP must be immediately available to return if needed. If the TP is unavailable for the noncritical components, they need to make arrangements for another qualified physician to be available. If the

TP is present for the entire procedure, the resident or operating room nurse may document the TP's presence without need for the TP to personally document it. The manual does not elaborate on the TP documentation requirements if the TP is only present for the critical or key components of a single surgery. In this situation, check with institutional compliance office regulations regarding if the TP needs to personally document their presence versus having the resident or operating nurse's documentation of their presence satisfy billing criteria.

Two overlapping surgeries

In order to bill for each of two overlapping surgeries, the TP must be physically present for the critical or key components of each surgery. Thus, the critical or key components cannot overlap. They must also be immediately available to intervene for the noncritical components of each surgery. They must arrange for another qualified physician to be available for the noncritical components of the other surgery if they are not available for the noncritical components of one surgery (ie, they are in the second surgery during its critical or key components). The TP must personally document that they were present for the critical or key components of each surgery to bill for them.

Three or more overlapping surgeries

If a TP is involved in three or more overlapping surgeries, they cannot bill for any of those services.

Minor versus major

In the context of discussions about extent of TP participation in a procedure, one must determine if the procedure is "minor" or "major." In this context, a "minor" procedure is defined as taking <5 minutes to perform. By default, a major procedure takes >5 minutes to perform. The vast majority of Hospital Medicine procedures are major. For minor procedures, the TP must be present for the entire procedure to allow for reimbursement. For major procedures, the TP needs to be present for the critical or key portions to bill for the service. Although the procedure note may be written by the resident, the TP must personally attest to their presence for the entire procedure or for the critical or key portions of the procedure, for minor and major procedures respectively. The resident's reference to their presence is insufficient.

■ ENDOSCOPIES

The TP must be physically present for the entire viewing time (insertion of endoscope until removal of endoscope) to bill for endoscopic procedures. Viewing the procedure from a monitor in a different room does not meet criteria for TP physical presence. Because endoscopies are discussed in the Medicare manual in the same section as single surgeries, it is unclear if they follow the guidelines for single surgeries, meaning that it is not explicitly stated that the resident or the operating room nurse may document the TP's presence in lieu of the TP personally documenting it. This is another situation to clarify with the institution's compliance office.

■ TIME-BASED SERVICES

When a resident is involved in a service that is billed based on time, to meet minimum time requirements, the TP can only count their personal time spent, not the resident's time spent. For example, if a resident spends 25 minutes on discharge management services for an inpatient, and the TP spends another 10 minutes, the TP cannot aggregate their documentation of time with the resident's time to achieve 35 minutes of time, enough for the higher level of discharge service [99239]. The TP can only bill for the 10 minutes of time they personally spent on the encounter and thus only bill for the <30 minutes discharge service [99238].

CRITICAL CARE

When providing critical care services in conjunction with a resident, just as in other time-based services, the TP may only count personal time spent providing critical care to the patient, and not time spent by the resident. Time spent rounding and teaching, but not in direct patient care also cannot be counted toward critical care time. In addition, the TP can only bill for critical care services if the patient was critically ill during the time the TP was physically present and managing the patient. For example, if the patient is critically ill, going into impending respiratory failure, and the TP is not physically at the hospital, but assists the resident over the telephone in deciding to initiate noninvasive ventilation, order blood gases, and consult the intensive care unit, this time cannot be counted toward critical care, as the TP was not physically present providing the critical care service. More importantly, if the patient is off noninvasive ventilation and oxygen, breathing normally, and clinically no longer at risk of impending organ failure at the time the TP finally has their face to face visit, the TP still cannot bill for critical care since the patient did not require critical cares services at the time of the TP's physical presence.

Although the resident's documentation of the patient's critical condition and their details of the history, physical, and high complexity of medical decision making all greatly support the medical necessity for critical care billing, in addition to a valid TP attestation statement, the TP must personally document their physical presence while the patient was critically ill, the amount of time they personally spent providing critical care, and a brief summary of their activities. The *resident's documentation of the TP's presence and participation is insufficient to support billing for critical care services.*

MODIFIER –GC

Attach **modifier –GC** to all services' CPT codes when performed in conjunction with a trainee. By attaching modifier –GC, the TP is attesting to meeting all physical presence and documentation requirements to bill for these services.

MIDLEVEL PROVIDERS

INTRODUCTION

Advanced practice providers (APPs) including physicians are trained, licensed clinicians who can provide medical services. Some nonphysician providers (NPPs) may work and bill independently, such as nurse practitioners (NP) and physical therapists (PT). Others may only work under the direct supervision of a physician, such as physician assistants (PA). Other health care workers that fall under the term NPP include: certified registered nurse anesthetists (CRNA), certified nurse midwives (CNM), clinical nurse specialists (CNS), clinical psychologists (PhD), nonclinical psychologists, occupational therapists, and speech pathologists. Medicare has very specific rules that govern how services involving an NPP can be provided and how they can be reimbursed. However, each state's Medicaid program, and private insurers have their own regulations which may differ from Medicare. For example, some private insurers such as Aetna will only allow PAs to bill incident to a physician, not under their own license. This chapter will discuss NPP billing with regard to Medicare guidelines. Clinicians should check with individual state Medicaid programs and private payers for deviations from the information below.

NPPs must have their own National Provider Identification (NPI) number in order to bill Medicare. When NPPs bill under their own license, Medicare reimbursement is at 85% of the MPFS rate. *Certain NPPs, including NPs, PAs, and CNSs, can provide evaluation and management (E/M) services in tandem with a physician, billing under the* physician's license, and allowing 100% MPFS reimbursement, in two very specific ways.

NPP REQUIREMENTS

In addition to meeting state licensing and credentialing requirements, in order to allow NPPs to bill under the supervising physician's license, these two criteria need to be fully satisfied.

1. *The NPP must be a financial responsibility to the billing physician and/or their group.* Often the NPPs and the physicians are employed and paid by the same financial entity; they are members of the same group practice. Sometimes a physician group may directly hire an NPP or NPP group to work with them as an employee or as an independent contractor. *In the event that the NPP is not the financial responsibility of the physician they are working with, this criteria will not be satisfied.* An example of this type of relationship would be a private hospitalist group working with an NPP directly employed by the hospital. The hospital would usually report the NPP's salary and benefits on their cost report. In this situation, the work of the NPP is not separately reimbursable, and thus any contribution by the NPP to a service performed with a physician, cannot be aggregated with the physician's work to determine the level of service provided.

2. *The service being provided by the NPP must be within the scope of their practice* as defined by laws of the state they are practicing in, and in accordance with the Collaborate Billing Agreement with their supervising physician(s). These agreements are usually reviewed and signed annually, based on state regulations.

E/M SERVICES PROVIDED IN CONJUNCTION WITH A PHYSICIAN

SPLIT/SHARED BILLING

Service requirements

When an NPP and a physician each provide a "substantive" face to face portion of an E/M service on the same calendar date, the service may be billed under either the NPP or the physician's NPI. Medicare does not define what exactly constitutes a "substantive" portion of the visit. It is expected however that a "substantive" portion will include all or some portion of history, physical, and/or medical decision making. There is no required percentage of the service that has to be provided and documented by the physician versus the NPP in order to bill under the physician's NPI. The NPP and the physician must each personally document their portion of the E/M service in the medical record, and sign it. The level of service will be determined by the aggregate of their documented work.

Documentation requirements

The medical record needs to clearly reflect that both the NPP and the physician each had a face to face encounter with the patient on the date of service. Both NPP and physician must personally document their work in the medical record, both must be identified in the chart and provide valid signatures, and the two documentation entries must be linked to show that the aggregate of the documentation will be used to determine the level of service provided.

There are two key features to the billing physician's documentation to ensure proper support for billing under their NPI in a split/shared situation.

1. *The billing physician's documentation should reflect that the physician had a face to face visit with the patient on the date of service,* unlike "incident to" services which may be billed without the physician having a face to face visit. The physician's personal entry in the medical record of their work, plus a valid signature constitute evidence of the face to face visit.

2. *The billing physician's documentation should reflect the medically necessary and unique contribution to the patient's evaluation and care plan development.* In contradistinction to visits in conjunction with a resident, where the billing TP must personally perform the critical and key portions of the service, in a split/shared service, the billing physician does not need to perform or attest to performing the critical and key portions of the service. Instead, *the billing physician needs to personally document exactly what they obtained for history and physical, and their thoughts related to medical decision making.* Examples of *insufficient* documentation of a substantive portion of work being done by the physician include:

a. A notation by the NPP of the physician's involvement.

b. A simple cosignature of the NPP's note.

c. The billing physician's documentation should not look like a TP attestation statement. Although the billing physician does play a supervisory role in their relationship with the NPP, and from an institutional policy, may need to make comment about reviewing the NPP's work for legal purposes, the billing physician's documentation should not look like they did nothing more than review and agree with the NPP's work and documentation.

In the above three documentation scenarios, the service may only be billed under the NPP's NPI.

The roles of the NPP and physician should be complementary; the relationship between a billing physician and an NPP in a split/shared visit is similar to two colleagues covering for each other, seeing a patient sequentially on a given day. There will inevitably be overlap in the historical, physical exam, and decision-making information obtained and documented; however, the documentation needs to clearly reflect that the NPP and physician each contributed unique and medically necessary care. Specifically, the physician documentation needs to reflect their independent contribution to the care of the patient outside the work of the NPP. When the physician sees the patient earlier in the day and documents their encounter before the NPP, their contribution to the service is more easily discerned. In the scenario where the NPP sees the patient and documents their encounter first, by remembering to document additional historical information, physical exam findings, new information since the NPP's visit, changes in clinical status, and additional medical decision making not reflected in the NPP's note, the medical necessity of the physician's role in the service is better supported.

Split/shared services can only be provided in the hospital inpatient, hospital outpatient (Place of Service, POS 22), hospital observation, emergency room, and nonhospital based (private) office settings. In order for split/shared services to be performed in a private office setting (POS 11), "incident to" criteria must be met, thus new patient visits [99201-99205] in the private office setting can never be billed as split/shared visits (see section "Incident to"). Note that new patient visits *can* be billed in a hospital based clinic since "incident to" rules do not apply to hospital settings and are thus not a requirement for these services in *that* setting. Below is a summary of services that can and cannot be performed with split/shared billing (see **Table 30-1**).

The aggregate work in a split/shared service follows CPT E/M rules such that work is added up from 12:01 AM to 11:59 PM, and not over a 24-hour period. If the NPP sees a patient at 10 PM, for example and performs the work of admission, but the physician does not see the patient until 8 AM the next morning, the physician cannot aggregate his work the next calendar date with the NPP's from the night before to submit a claim as a split/shared service. The TP rules for late night admissions do not hold true for split/shared services. The NPP would bill the admission (initial inpatient visit [99221-99223]) under her or his own NPI, not the physician's NPI, on calendar date 1, and

TABLE 30-1 Split/Shared Billing

Services Eligible for Split/Shared Billing	CPT Code
Initial inpatient visits (admissions)	99221-99223
Subsequent inpatient visits (follow-up)	99231-99233
Inpatient discharge management services	99238-99239
Observation same day discharge services	99234-99236
Initial observation visits	99218-99220
Subsequent observation visits (follow-up)	99224-99226
Observation discharge management services	99217
Emergency room services	99281-99285
Hospital-based clinic: new and established outpatient visits*	99201-99215
Nonhospital based (private) office: established outpatient visits*	99211-99215
Prolonged services	99254-99357
Services Ineligible for Split/Shared Billing	**CPT Code**
Nonhospital based (private) office: new outpatient visits	99201-99205
Consults	99241-99255
Prolonged services	99291-99292
Skilled nursing facility and nursing home services Procedures	99304-99316

* Only if "incident to" criteria are met. If not, then bill under NPP.

physician's work the next morning will go toward determining the level of E/M service on day 2, such as a subsequent inpatient visit [99231-99233].

■ CONSULTS

Although Medicare's guidelines do not allow consult services to be billed as split/shared visits, since January 1, 2010 Medicare no longer recognizes or reimburses for consult codes [99241-99255]. Medicare however still pays for consult services, just through different code sets [99221-99223; 99231-99232; 99201-99215; 99281-99285]. All of these code sets may be billed as split/shared services. So now for Medicare patients, even though the intent of the service is to provide a consult, when submitted with one of these services codes, the care may now be provided as a split/shared visit. Clinicians should check with Medicaid and private insurers for how these services should be billed.

■ INCIDENT TO

"Incident to" services are defined as medically necessary services that are provided incident to a physician's professional services, but are an integral part of the plan of care. "Incident to" services can only be provided in a nonhospital based (private) office (POS 11) or patient's home, but never in a hospital setting. Several criteria must hold true to allow for this billing.

1. The care by the NPP is provided under the direct supervision of the physician. The physician must have had an initial face to face visit with the patient at some previous point in time to establish a plan of care, with the intent of the NPP carrying out the plan of care at (a) subsequent visit(s). Thus "incident to" services can never be provided to new *patients* or to established patients with a new *problem*. If a patient presents for planned follow-up with the NPP, and in the course of the visit, in addition to the expected problem with an established plan of care, the NPP uncovers a new problem, the NPP must now bill the entire encounter under their own NPI.

2. The physician must stay active in the patient's care. Usually this is satisfied by the physician seeing the patient at intervals to review, revise, or update the plan of care. The interval of time between physician visits is left up to the clinical judgment of the physician, the specific patient needs, and standards of care.

3. The physician must be physically present in the office or suite and be immediately available during the time the NPP provides the service. The physician does not have to be physically present inside the individual treatment room with the NPP and patient. It is helpful to keep records of physician schedules in the event of an audit to aid in supporting their presence. If however the physician must leave the office while the NPP is providing a planned "incident to" service, if the physician's partner is physically present in the office and immediately available to cover, the visit can still be submitted under the physician as an "incident to" service. Otherwise, the visit must be billed under the NPP's NPI.

Incident to services do not require the billing physician to have a face to face visit with the patient on the date of service. In addition, for billing purposes, "incident to" services do not require the supervising physician to document anything in the medical record. However, based on physician comfort level, and certain state or individual institution internal policies, the supervising physician may need to sign each note. No modifier is necessary for submitting these claims.

SCRIBES

Occasionally practices employ NPPs as scribes. A scribe's role is to document an encounter for a physician, in the medical record. Scribing is not reimbursable. Scribes are not allowed to enhance or alter documentation to improve billing, nor can they add their opinions or personal observations. When using a scribe, the documentation must be very clear that the scribe "A" is functioning purely to document physician "B's" findings and plans. Practices that employ NPPs as scribes need to be very careful to have protocols in place to ensure that the documentation clearly reflects the physician's work, and not the clinical work of the NPP while serving as scribe. Physician B needs to attest that the documentation of history, physical and decision making reflects his own personal work.

ONLINE RESOURCES

Centers for Medicare and Medicaid Services. *Medicare Claims Processing Manual: Section 100*. Chap 12. CMS Web site. Available at: www.cms.hhs.gov/manuals/downloads/clm104c12.pdf. Accessed December 14, 2015.

Centers for Medicare and Medicaid Services. *Medicare Claims Processing Manual: Section 30.6.1.B*. Chap 12. CMS Web site. Available at: www.cms.hhs.gov/manuals/downloads/clm104c12.pdf. Accessed December 14, 2015.

Medicare Learning Network. Available at: https://www.cms.gov/Outreach-and-Education/Medicare-Learning-Network-MLN/MLNProducts/Downloads/Teaching-Physicians-Fact-Sheet-ICN006437.pdf.

CHAPTER 31

Hospital-Driven Documentation

Jeannine Z. Engel, MD
Diana L. Snow, MA, CCS, CPC, CHC

The documentation of the inpatient episode of care follows the general principles outlined in Chapter 27: Professional Billing and Coding, and is primarily a record of the patient's clinical experience. A number of regulatory changes in the payment for hospital facility care have occurred over the past decades which subtly change the documentation requirements and may lead to increased interactions of hospitalists with others in the hospital systems such as clinical documentation improvement (CDI) and utilization review (UR) personnel. A better understanding of these regulatory changes and their impact on both facility reimbursement and patient financial liability will help the hospitalist document care more completely. In addition, there will be fewer interruptions and queries, less back-end work for facilities and fewer surprises for the patients when their hospital bills arrive.

■ DIAGNOSTIC RELATED GROUPS AND PAYMENT FOR HOSPITAL SERVICES

Predetermined payment based on diagnosis

Medicare pays hospitals for inpatient services using the inpatient prospective payment system (IPPS). Although IPPS is only applicable to Medicare, the concept of prospective payment for inpatient stays has been adopted by most third party payers. The primary driver of payment in the inpatient setting is a grouping methodology, called a diagnostic related group (DRG).

The basic premise of a DRG system is prospective payment, or a predetermined, fixed amount. The original DRG system began in the early 1980s in some states, with congress implementing the IPPS for Medicare services in 1983. Prior to the introduction of the DRG system, hospital reimbursement was made on a percentage of costs, and hospitals billed for the actual costs for an inpatient admission and received a true "fee for service."

Each DRG payment is based upon an analysis of prior claims data in regard to how much it costs, and how many resources are required on average, to treat patients of that type. There are modifications to this payment amount for hospitals based on location, the percentage of low income patients treated, teaching hospital status, and whether or not the specific case was "unusually costly." DRGs are three digit numerical assignments which are divided into categories, called major diagnostic categories (MDCs) based upon the patient's symptoms, comorbidities, whether the care provided was medical or surgical, the organ system affected, age, and discharge status. Each DRG was intended to be a reflection of the resources required to care for patients in specific categories, and is designed to make one single payment to cover all of the services provided by the facility during the inpatient stay.

Modification of the DRG system

There were initially many limitations to the DRG system, as it was developed for use with a Medicare population and had limited applicability to other populations of patients, most notably children and expectant mothers. As a result, many private payers began using a modification of the DRG system called the All Patient Refined DRG system, or an APR-DRG. This was the first introduction of adjustments for patient severity of illness and the intensity of resources needed to care for specific patients who had multiple conditions which represent significant comorbidities and thus intensified resource requirements.

On October 1, 2008, the Centers for Medicare and Medicaid Services (CMS) followed suit and introduced the MS-DRG system: the Medicare Severity DRG. Upon initial implementation, the MS-DRG system changed the number of available code assignments from 500 to 746. The increase in the number of possible code assignments was a reflection of the introduction of major complications or comorbidities (MCCs), complications or comorbidities (CCs), or noncomplications or comorbidities (non-CCs).

ICD-9/ICD-10 codes

Each year, CMS produces lists of ICD-9/ICD-10 codes which are designated as major comorbid conditions (MCCs) or comorbid conditions (CCs) which impact the severity and increase the payment of a DRG. Frequently, physician education is centered around these concepts to ensure that physicians are adequately documenting these diagnostic categories so the hospital can be paid appropriately for services they have provided to patients and the hospital is able to report the most appropriate DRG on the claim.

Although the concept of DRG coding sounds simple, it may be very tricky for patients with multiple, complicated conditions. Documentation by the treating physicians is the key to understanding the principal diagnosis. The medical record must contain sufficient clarity for a coder to determine which diagnosis is principal. Frequently, a physician may not know what the principal diagnosis is, especially at the beginning of an admission when a patient presents with undefined symptoms. It is also common for a patient to be discharged without a definitive diagnosis, in which case the symptom treated becomes the principal diagnosis.

Coders determine the DRG code. The coder abstracts, or reads the medical record, and determines which diagnosis was the principal diagnosis for the hospitalization. According to the Official Guidelines for Coding and Reporting, the Principal Diagnosis is the "condition, after study, which occasioned the admission to the hospital." This principal diagnosis assists the coder in determining the category of the MS-DRG code. The other two main factors in determining the proper DRG assignment are (1) whether or not a surgical procedure was completed during the stay, and (2) whether or not there are complicating or comorbid conditions present. When a coder is unclear about what the documentation is attempting to convey, he/she will submit a query to the physician. Many physicians have expressed consternation at the lack of clarity in coder queries; specifically that it is unclear what the coders are asking of the physicians. Because it could be financially advantageous to the facility for a physician to document a specific diagnosis, there are professional standards regarding the wording of queries which are not "leading" the physician to answer a certain way. For example:

> Documentation states, "Obtunded patient admitted with 3-day history of nausea and vomiting. CXR revealed right lower lobe (RLL) pneumonia. Clindamycin ordered."
> Inappropriate Query, "Is the patient's pneumonia due to aspiration?"
> Appropriate Query, "Can you specify the etiology of the patient's pneumonia? It is noted in the admitting H&P this obtunded patient had a history of nausea and vomiting prior to admission. If the etiology of the pneumonia can be further specified, please document the type/etiology of the pneumonia in the progress note."

Hospital payment is directly tied to the quality of the clinical documentation provided by the practitioners treating the patient. In the inpatient setting, there are many coding rules regarding what documentation can be utilized, and although there are exceptions to this rule, in general, the patient's attending documentation carries the final weight if there are inconsistencies or contradictions regarding the patient's diagnosis from residents, consultants or specialists.

■ OBSERVATION STATUS

Short hospital stays

Observation status applies to conditions that do not meet criteria as an inpatient, but it is otherwise inappropriate to send the patient home. Observation is considered an outpatient stay in the hospital and is reimbursed under Medicare Part B. This distinction means that a patient will have to pay a coinsurance, which is generally 20% for Medicare patients. Out of pocket costs can go up significantly when they are paying a percentage of Medicare approved charges. Additionally, patients who are classified as outpatients are not eligible for coverage for a Skilled Nursing Facility (SNF) by Medicare.

Hospitals began using observation services almost immediately after the IPPS was introduced in 1983. A problem with a capitated system of inpatient hospital payment began to surface, specifically what to do with cases which were short stays and did not approach the median length of stay for a particular DRG, but still fell into that DRG. Patients and their hospital care began to fall into the gap between what was expected as an inpatient admission and what was expected as an outpatient service. As part of this, there became three distinct categories for patients: Inpatient, Outpatient, and Observation.

Review of observation status

In the late 1980s and early 1990s, organizations called Peer Review Organizations, or PROs, reviewed admission decisions by providers and questioned the validity of the provider's decision. This resulted in providers keeping patients in observation status for weeks at a time rather than risk admitting a patient who did not quite meet inpatient criteria. This resulted in excessive charges to Medicare and to the Medicare beneficiary, as outpatient stays for Medicare are billed as a coinsurance (20%, copay for instance) while the beneficiary charges for an inpatient stay are a set amount called the deductible ($1260 deductible in 2015). As a response CMS implemented a 48-hour target for observation services stating that it would be "unusual" for a patient to stay in observation longer. Currently, the CMS manuals state, "Observation care is a well-defined set of specific, clinically appropriate services, which include ongoing short-term treatment, assessment, and reassessment, that are furnished while a decision is being made regarding whether patients will require further treatment as hospital inpatients or if they are able to be discharged from the hospital."

Issues with observation status

Observation status has been problematic for many hospitals from both operational and payment perspectives. CMS has issued additional instruction on the use of observation services almost every year for the past 20 years. Each year, they have changed the rules and the payment modeling slightly. For a period of time in the early 2000s, hospitals could only receive additional observation payments for patients who had congestive heart failure, chest pain, or asthma, as CMS had recognized that those were the categories most likely to require a longer assessment than an Emergency Room visit, but a shorter visit than the average inpatient admission for those conditions. Several years later, CMS reversed this policy and implemented different policies allowing any patient with any condition to be treated under observation, but they would only pay the hospital if the stay lasted at least 8 hours.

■ RECOVERY AUDIT CONTRACTORS

Further changes in the payment and definition of inpatient services for Medicare beneficiaries were largely shaped by the actions of and reactions to the Recovery Audit Contractor program.

Congress created the Recovery Audit Contractors (RACs) in 2003 as part of the Medicare Modernization Act (MMA) to recover underpayments and discover overpayments to the Medicare Trust Fund. The RAC program began as a demonstration project in selected states (NY, FL, SC, CA, MA, and AZ). From 2005 to 2008, the program recovered nearly $38 million in overpayments to the Medicare Trust fund, although these numbers may not include claims that were appealed. In 2006, Congress wrote into law (Tax Relief and Health Care Act of 2006) a permanent and national Recovery Audit Program to recoup overpayments associated with services made under part A or B of title XVIII of the Social Security Act (Medicare payments). While the RACs reviewed a number of areas of potential overpayments, the largest area by dollar amount was short-stay (1-3 days) inpatient hospitalizations. The records for these hospitalizations were reviewed, and the DRG payments denied and recouped, with the rationale "inpatient stay not reasonable and necessary, services could have been provided in an outpatient or observation setting." The full payment amount was recouped, and the facilities had no mechanism for recovering a portion or the entire payment amount except to appeal inpatient denial. Even if the facility agreed that the patient could have received the service as an outpatient, or in observation status, to agree to this meant forfeiting all of the DRG payment. This lead to an unprecedented number of appeals by facilities around the country, and the federal appeal system was overwhelmed. The result was a backlog of appeals being processed, and millions of dollars tied up in the appeal system.

In March 2013, CMS issued an interim ruling which allowed facilities to rebill Part A claims which were denied by a CMS contractor for the inpatient admission deemed "not reasonable and necessary," to Part B. In addition, they released a proposed rule defining which services could be rebilled under Part B. This proposed rule increased the number of services that could be rebilled for Part B payments, making this "Part B rebill" an attractive option in certain circumstances. In essence, the rule allowed facilities to rebill the denied inpatient claim as if the services had originally been provided in an outpatient setting/status. Later in 2013, the IPPS (IPPS) proposed and then Final Rules (1599-F) wrote into law a new definition of "inpatient" for Medicare Beneficiaries, and the "two Midnight Rule" was born.

■ TWO MIDNIGHT RULE AND PROBE AND EDUCATE AUDITS

On October 1, 2013, the two midnight (2MN) rule took effect for Medicare Beneficiaries, and the RAC audits for short stays were placed on temporary hold. The definition of an inpatient changed from a subjective one of potential risk and intensity of service, to a mostly objective time-based payment model. Per CMS: If a Medicare beneficiary requires medically necessary hospital services for two or more midnights, then the facility may bill for the services under Part A, as a DRG. If the patient is expected to require only 1MN of services, the provider should place the patient in observation, and the facility should bill for the stay under Part B. The only statutory exception is a patient receiving a procedure on the Medicare inpatient-only list. These patients must receive their care as an inpatient in order for the facility to receive payment for the surgical procedure.

There are certainly nuances to this rule. The most straightforward are the exceptions to the 2MN timeframe. These include: patients who leave Against Medical Advice (AMA) prior to the second MN; patients who die unexpectedly; patients who are discharged to hospice unexpectedly; patients requiring new, unexpected mechanical ventilation; and patients who have an unexpected clinical improvement and are discharged prior to the second MN. CMS is clear that these exceptions should be rare, and that documentation would need to support the Part A billing of 1MN stays in these circumstances.

Another change was start time for the 2MN. The clock starts at the time the patient begins to receive care at the facility, regardless of the time of the inpatient order. For instance, time in the emergency department, in observation, in the clinics, in the operating room or other procedures all count toward to the 2MN. In addition, if a patient is transferred from an outside facility, the accepting facility can count the time spent in the outside facility's ED toward the 2MNs. One example: if a patient is originally placed in observation because he is not expected to require 2MN of care, but does not recover as expected and requires an additional night of medically necessary hospital services, the order can be changed to inpatient on hospital day #2, and the entire stay can be billed under Part A because the patient stayed in the facility for a total of 3 days and 2MN. However, to qualify for skilled nursing facility care, the beneficiary must still have a three midnight inpatient hospitalization, specifically, three midnights after an inpatient admission order. In the example above, only one midnight was spent in the facility after the inpatient order was written, therefore only one midnight would count toward the SNF qualifying stay.

The 2MN rule defined several new terms, the 2MN presumption, the 2MN expectation and the 2MN benchmark. The presumption essentially states that medical reviewers (auditors), in the absence of evidence of gaming, should not review claims for patients who receive 2MN of hospital care after the inpatient order, as it will be presumed that the inpatient admission was reasonable and necessary. The 2MN expectation and 2MN benchmark are used interchangeably. These terms define the premise under which the admitting provider makes the decision to write an admission order, using the information available **at the time of admission**. That is, physicians and other providers should generally admit as *inpatients* the Medicare beneficiaries they expect will require two or more midnights of hospital services, and should treat most other beneficiaries on an outpatient or *observation* basis.

The 2MN rule was and is a departure from the previous method of determining inpatient status, which involved screening criteria of severity of illness and intensity of service. And, this rule applies to Medicare beneficiaries only, not other payers. In order to help providers and facilities understand the rule, and allow CMS to determine the need for more education, they immediately instituted a "probe and educate" period for all facilities. CMS instructed the Medicare Administrative Contractors (MACs) to review a small sample of Medicare Part A inpatient hospital claims spanning 0 or 1 midnight after formal inpatient admission to determine the medical necessity of the inpatient status in accordance with the 2MN benchmark. Each facility then received feedback, and if required, a second sampling of 1MN stays. This process required more time than originally expected, and the probe and educate period was extended, from March 2014 to September 2014, then March 2015, April 2015, and most recently to September 2015. During this period, the RAC audits for medical necessity related to inpatient status were placed on hold, and all admissions during this period are prohibited from future review related to inpatient status by the Recovery Audit Contractors.

■ CERTIFICATION REQUIREMENTS

In addition to the 2MN rule, the 2014 IPPS final rule (1599-F) outlined new certification requirements for all inpatient hospitalizations. While certification was not a new concept, it had been in place primarily for long stays and payment outliers. For 14 months, until most of the Certification requirements for all inpatient admissions were removed in January 2015, many hospitals and providers scrambled to understand and comply with the certification requirements. As of January 1, 2015, the only portion of these short-lived requirements which remained for all inpatient hospitalizations was the inpatient order requirement. CMS defined the admission order requirements in the Code of Federal Regulations, making this a condition of payment in federal law under Medicare Part A. The inpatient admission order must be present in the medical record, and supported by admission and progress notes. The order must be "furnished by a qualified and licensed practitioner who has admitting privileges at the hospital as permitted by state law." Other requirements include familiarity with the patient's case, and the timing of the order should be at or before the time of inpatient admission. The regulations specifically state that the admitting practitioner cannot delegate the order to another individual who does not meet the criteria, but subregulatory guidance does address trainees and verbal admission orders. The expectation is that any inpatient admission order placed by a resident, mid-level provider (without admitting privileges) or verbal inpatient admission orders will be signed by an authorized provider prior to the patient's discharge from the hospital. The requirement to have delegated inpatient orders signed prior to discharge has been challenging to successfully implement for facilities around the country, especially for short stays. Process choices have included close tracking with e-mail or other reminder notifications, hard stops on D/C orders or actual discharges, and back-end rebilling for IP stays that do not meet this requirement.

It may be helpful for Hospitalists to view the 2MN rule and the inpatient order requirements as a payment policy as opposed to one which defines the care provided to the patient. CMS and its contractors are not making judgments about the need for or the quality of care provided to Medicare Beneficiaries. They are defining the parameters under which they will pay for this care. Under certain parameters (signed admission order and greater than 2MN stay or one of the exceptions), the care will be paid under Part A, as a DRG. Failing these parameters, the care will be paid through Medicare Part B as an outpatient hospitalization.

ROLE OF UTILIZATION REVIEW

Getting the patient status correct is not always obvious, and it is a single action (the admission order) embedded in a very busy sequence of evaluating and starting the course of care for a new hospitalized patient. Most facilities have a team of nurse reviewers who are looking at the admission information, and helping the admitting team make this decision. These professionals, generally named UR nurses, have the training and expertise to understand the nuances of admission status for all payers. Some facilities have divided Case Management and UR, while other facilities may have the same team members performing both of these tasks. UR teams have been trained to use screening criteria such as Milliman or InterQual to determine if a patient meets inpatient or observation status. These criteria are based in medical literature, but also are clear that they are guidelines, and are not meant to overrule the provider's medical judgment. Interestingly, the Medicare Conditions of Participation (COP) require that facilities employ some type of screening criteria, but do not designate which one. With the implementation of the 2MN rule, the use of screening criteria became essentially moot for Medicare patients, as they now defined inpatient in terms of hospital care and time, not intensity of service and severity of illness. However, the COP for UR did not change, and screening criteria are still required. In addition, many commercial payers, and some state Medicaids still rely on these screening criteria to determine inpatient versus outpatient status.

The interaction of the hospitalist with the UR nurses often involves a conversation around the expected length of stay of a Medicare patient on hospital day two. If the patient has an order for observation, and it appears the patient will stay an additional MN, the UR nurse will suggest that the patient have an IP order written. If the patient has an IP order, and it appears that the patient will be discharged, the UR nurse will discuss whether or not the status should be down-graded to Observation, which will require a process called condition-code 44 (CC44). Any of these interactions may involve an additional physician for secondary review (usually the

physician director of CM/UR), particularly if the hospitalist does not respond, or is not moving in the direction that seems appropriate to the UR nurse.

Because the downgrading of a Medicare patient from inpatient status to outpatient status involves potential increased financial impact for the beneficiary, CMS requires that the facility follow certain specific steps if they change a patient from IP to OP (observation) while the patient is still hospitalized. This process is called CC44. The basic steps include notifying the patient, and providing financial counseling, in addition to actually changing the order. Upgrading status from Observation to Inpatient only requires the written order.

The 2014 IPPS final rule also allowed facilities to change the billing status of inpatient hospital stays which are internally audited, as long as the billing change occurs within 1 year of the date of service (timely filing). This regulatory change allowed facilities to put in place back-end review processes for 1MN inpatient stays and decide whether to leave the billing under Part A (DRG) or change the billing to Part B, if the documented care did not fulfill the 2MN expectation/benchmark. Facilities must follow the Utilization Review Conditions of Participation, which require notification of the patient and the attending provider within 2 days of the decision to change the billing from IP (Part A) to OP (Part B). The primary reason to change the billing status to Part B is that the patient received care in the facility for only 1MN, there was a signed inpatient order, but there was no documentation to support that 2MN of medically necessary hospital care was expected at the time of admission.

INPATIENT DOCUMENTATION OF CARE: NUTS AND BOLTS

Adding to the confusion created by an onslaught of regulatory changes is the multitude of payers and their differing rules for status decisions and payment. Clinicians could spend all of their time thinking about these issues, and lose sight of the patient and their care. For inpatient hospital care, the documentation requirements include a history and physical exam (admission note), daily progress notes and a discharge day note. These notes are used for professional billing. For the hospital to bill for the inpatient care, a signed inpatient admission order is also required, as well as a discharge summary.

PRACTICE POINT

Medicare patients

- Facility Inpatient Part A billing = signed inpatient order and two midnight medically necessary hospital care.

The best documentation of hospital care tells the patient's story, and the provider's plan for care. There are three levels of services for initial hospital care, CPT codes 99221, 99222, and 99223.

The only significant difference in documentation requirements between the three service levels is the medical decision making (**Table 31-1**). While the lowest admission service may be billed with a lower level history and examination, in general, when a patient is sick enough to require inpatient admission, there is usually medical necessity to document a comprehensive history and physical examination. In order to demonstrate the medical decision making and cognitive work performed, any personal work should be documented, including personal review of ECGs, x-rays, or other tests, conversations with consultants, pertinent history obtained from family members, and any review and summary of old records. This work is counted in the "data" section of medical decision making, along with tests ordered and reviewed. Risk to the patient may be indicated by presenting problems, the diagnostic procedures

TABLE 31-1 Documentation Requirements for Hospital-based Professional Billing (All Three Elements Needed: History, Exam, and MDM)

Inpatient Admit	99221	99222	99223
Observation	99218	99219	99220
Observation/same day D/C	99234	99235	99236
History: CC and	4 HPI	4	4
	2 ROS	10	10
	1 PFSH	3	3
	(DET)	(COMP)	(COMP)
Exam	5 (DET)	8 (COMP)	8 (COMP)
Medical decision making (MDM)	Straight-forward/low	Moderate	High
Time (admit only)	30	50	70

ordered, or management options selected. The risk table which most coders and auditors use as a reference does not include all disease processes, so the documentation of risk to the patient, whether through literature references (eg, high PESI or PSI scores) or your expert opinion is a reasonable part of the admission and subsequent hospital day documentation. Notations such as "stable on pressors" can be misinterpreted by nonclinical personnel. The admission note should include all of the patient's problems which are being addressed or treated, including chronic medical conditions, if prescribing chronic medications, or the condition affects the patient's current reason for hospitalization, include it in the assessment.

The authors favor problem-based notes, following the pattern of: problem, attribution, and plan. Each problem should include the provider's clinical reasoning or a differential diagnosis (attribution), and some indication of the patient's short-term risks and severity of illness. What makes this particular patient need to be in the hospital? Why is this illness particularly risky for this patient? The proposed plan of care with an expectation of length of stay should be stated outright, or implied. Instead of stating "IV cefepime," include an expected length of treatment: "IV cefepime for 2 to 3 days, or until afebrile for 24 hours." When cosigning or attesting after residents, students or advanced practice clinicians, the responsible physician should include additional information to augment the documentation, particularly if these providers downplay the severity of a patient's presentation, or do not have the knowledge or experience to recognize the significance of certain clinical scenarios.

Daily progress notes should include all of the problems from the admission note until resolved, and any new problems. Hospitalists should be aware of information carried forward via a macro to be sure that the documentation is accurate and makes sense for the date of service. Resolved problems should be deleted (eg, that hypokalemia from 3 days ago, now resolved). Daily progress notes which include pages of radiographic and laboratory data from the past week will often be ignored by a reader due to their prohibitive length. Consider referring to laboratory test and x-rays as ordered or reviewed and only include pertinent details in your notes. Linking your orders with a statement in your notes "see my orders for any additional plans," also adds all of your orders to the daily plan and medical decision making.

A "quality" note generally has the following attributes: concise, clear, current, organized, prioritized, and trustworthy. If a Medicare patient is discharged earlier than expected, especially after 1MN of care, the provider should include a statement in the discharge

day note or discharge summary outlining the clinical course and unexpected recovery, if this occurred. Again, the goal is to tell the patient's story: this patient looked very ill when they arrived; we expected 2 to 3 days of IV antibiotics so we wrote an IP order, but they recovered more quickly than we expected, and we were able to send them home after 1MN of outstanding care.

Inpatient facility billing requires a discharge summary (both Medicare Conditions of Participation, and most accreditation bodies such as The Joint Commission), and it is a useful tool for summarizing the story of a patient's hospitalization. Professional billing allows for a discharge day note (99238, 99239) which is time based. The documentation requirements are slightly different, but it is simple to combine these two documents into a single note, saving time and duplication of effort. Both require a discussion of the hospital stay, discharge instructions including medications and plans for follow-up, as well as the attending provider's signature. The discharge day note requires a face-to-face service from the billing provider, a final examination, and some notation of time spent. The Joint Commission standards also include procedures and treatments provided and the patient's discharge condition. The authors suggest that hospitalists discuss the expectations of the discharge summary with their facility, and work to make a discharge day template which includes all of the required elements for both the professional day of discharge service and the discharge summary into a single note. To prevent scrutiny of the discharge day service payment, the documentation needs to clearly reflect that a face-to-face visit occurred on discharge day. If residents are documenting this service, then only the billing provider's time can be counted toward the discharge day time. Mid-level provider time may be combined with attending MD time and billed as a split-shared service. This time may be discontinuous, and you can count time that is spent in the days prior to discharge, as long as you only "count" this time once. And, if your partner spends time on discharge on Sunday, and you are the actual discharging provider on Monday, then your partner's time is combined with your time, and all billed together on Monday, as there can only be a single discharge day service billed per hospitalization. If no documentation of time is included in the discharge day note, then 99238 will be billed. In order for 99239 to be billed, the provider must document that he or she spent greater than 30 minutes coordinating the patient's discharge.

Observation documentation of care

Observation documentation requires an admission note (initial observation services 99218-20), updates in the patient's clinical condition at some appropriate interval by providers or nursing staff, and a discharge note (observation care discharge, 99217). If the observation services occur within a single calendar day, the services must span greater than 8 hours to be billed to Medicare as the combined observation admission/discharge on the same date (99234-36). Documentation that reflects less than 8 hours of observation services on a calendar date may only be billed as initial observation services (99218-20) with the reimbursement for the discharge work bundled into that payment for Medicare billing; however, this 8-hour rule for observation billing does not necessarily apply to private insurance providers. These time-based requirements may vary among private payers and Medicaid. There is no requirement for a discharge summary in order for the facility to bill observation services. The decision to require a discharge summary for observation stays should be local and facility-based, and is often related to having a concise summary of the patient's hospitalization. The basic documentation requirements for initial observation care are identical to those for initial inpatient care (Table 31-1). In order for the facility to bill for observation services, an order for observation is also required.

The uncertain future (a last minute update)

CMS has issued the Calendar Year 2016 Outpatient Prospective Payment (OPPS) Proposed Rule (CMS-1633-P) which adds another wrinkle to the payment of short stay inpatient hospital services. The proposed changes include allowing for Part A payment on a case by case basis based on the judgment of the admitting physician, despite the expectation of less than 2MN stay at the time of admission. In addition, the task of reviewing short hospital stays will now fall to the Quality Improvement Organizations (QIOs) with referral to the Recovery Audit Contractors for facilities that have "high" error rates. The details of the review process have not yet been defined at this time. The CY16 OPPS Final Rule will be published around November 1, 2015 for implementation on January 1, 2016.

CONCLUSION

Documentation of a patient's hospital care has become increasingly complex as the regulations surrounding facility billing for inpatient and observation care have changed, and continue to evolve. Every year, the Center for Medicare and Medicaid Services publishes new rules which alter the billing regulations for both professional and facility services. Commercial payers may have slightly different interpretations. All of these services use provider's notes and orders to explain and justify the medical necessity for the services rendered. Some knowledge of these billing regulations will allow the hospitalist to comprehensively document the patient's story and the provider's medical decision making, while decreasing the back-end work and queries. The classic admission note, daily progress notes and discharge summary that we all learned in medical school are still the backbone of hospital documentation.

SUGGESTED READINGS

CFR § 412.3 Admissions.

CMS, 2013. *Medicare Learning Network: Acute Care Hospital Inpatient Prospective Payment System*; 2013. http://www.cms.gov/Outreach-and-Education/Medicare-Learning-Network-MLN/MLNProducts/downloads/AcutePaymtSysfctsht.pdf.

CMS 1455-P Proposed Rule. Medicare Program: Part B. Inpatient Billing in Hospitals. *Q&A Related to Patient Status Reviews*. http://www.cms.gov/Research-Statistics-Data-and-Systems/Monitoring-Programs/Medicare-FFS-Compliance-Programs/Medical-Review/Downloads/Questions_andAnswersRelatingtoPatientStatusReviewsforPosting_31214.pdf.

CMS 1633-P Proposed Rule. https://www.cms.gov/Medicare/Medicare-Fee-for-Service-Payment/HospitalOutpatientPPS/Hospital-Outpatient-Regulations-and-Notices-Items/CMS-1633-P.html.

CMS 1455-R Interim ruling, March 13, 2013 (18 pages).

CHAPTER 32

Taming the ICD-10 Monster

CoLette Morgan, MD, FHM, CCDS, CDIP
Yvette M. Cua, MD

INTRODUCTION

The transition from ICD-9 to ICD-10 and to future ICD revisions is challenging but also provides unique opportunities to improve health care and disease/procedure tracking and data. This transition will better support current technology and health care reform initiatives including the Centers for Medicare & Medicaid Services (CMS) value-based purchasing and pay-for-performance programs; coordinated care models such as accountable care organizations and patient-centered medical homes; the government's Physician Quality Reporting System; and the move toward adoption of electronic health record systems. In addition, it affords great potential to decrease audit risk since ICD-10 codes allow the physician's documentation to be translated into a more accurate clinical picture, thereby reducing the chance of misinterpretation by third parties, auditors (eg, recovery audit contractors—RAC), and attorneys.

With improved specificity, ICD-10 codes help health care providers submit highly specific codes for the care they provide, and better reflect severity of illness and support medical necessity. This will hopefully reflect in a physician's profiling on national registries, consumer health sites, and also with health care entity's quality reporting.

HISTORY

Classifying illnesses to document disease prevalence and causes of death is not a new concept. The first attempts were made as far back as the 1600s. Initially, it was nothing more than a crude and inconsistent nomenclature with little reliable data. However, during the 1800s, an earnest effort began to create a uniformed system. Medical statisticians were commissioned to embark upon this enormous task. They began their work by using the Bertillion Classification of Causes of Death developed by the French statistician, Jacques Bertillion.

In 1893, the first international classification of diseases (ICD) was adopted by the International Statistical Institute. The United States did not utilize a formal disease classification system until 1898, when the American Public Health Association recommended all of North America adopt this system, and recommended it be updated every 10 years.

Each revision made the ICD more detailed. In 1948, the World Health Organization assumed responsibility for the ICD and published the sixth version, which incorporated morbidity for the first time. At this time, they decided to make ICD the official means of collecting international data for epidemiological surveillance and for health management. The WHO Nomenclature Regulations, adopted in 1967, stipulated that Member States use the most current ICD revision for mortality and morbidity statistics. In 1979, the United States adopted ICD-9, and in 1983 the Inpatient Prospective Payment System in the US required ICD-9 codes to be linked to diagnosis related groups (DRGs) for reimbursement. ICD-9 quickly became antiquated, running out of room for new codes for new diseases and new technology. The 43rd World Health Assembly endorsed ICD-10 in May 1990, however, the United States did not adopt it until October 1, 2015. ICD-10 is dramatically more robust and allows for many more codes than any previous edition, including ICD-9 which has been used in the United States since 1979 (**Table 32-1**). The 11th revision process is underway and the final ICD-11 will be released in 2017.

TABLE 32-1 Differences Between ICD-9 and ICD-10 Code Sets

	ICD-9-CM	ICD-10 Code Sets
Procedure Codes	3284 Codes	71,924 Codes
Diagnoses	14,025 Codes	69,823 Codes
	Old	New
Diagnosis structure	ICD-9-CM • 3-5 characters • First character is numeric or alpha • Characters 2-5 are numeric	ICD-10-CM • 3-7 characters • Character 1 is alpha • Character 2 is numeric • Characters 3-7 may be alpha or numeric
Procedure structure	ICD-9-CM • 3-4 characters • All characters are numeric • All codes have at least three characters	ICD-10-PCS (only used in the inpatient hospital setting) • ICD-10-PCS has seven characters • Each can be either alpha or numeric • Numbers 0-9; letters A-H, J-N, P-Z

TABLE 32-2 Unusual ICD-10 Codes and Their Analogous ICD-9 Codes

ICD-10	ICD-9
Accidental injury due to paintball discharge W34.011	Accident caused by paintball gun, E922.5
Hurt/fall walking into a lamppost, initial encounter—W2202XA	Activities involving walking, marching and hiking, E001.0 Other fall, E888.8 (required two codes)
Burn due to water-skis on fire, initial encounter—V9107XA	E831 Accident to watercraft causing other injury
Problems in relationship with in-laws—Z63.1	Conflict family V61.9

any additional encounters with the provider for this same condition would code to T75.82XD.

There are not yet ICD-10 codes for "injured while texting," or "distracted by cell phone while driving." However, with the ability ICD-10 has to expand, one would expect such codes to be added soon.

BENEFITS AND USES OF ICD

- The ICD is the global health information standard for codes to allow comparison of mortality and morbidity statistics. This system helps to monitor death and disease rates worldwide and measure progress toward the Millennium Development Goals.
- About 70% of the world's health expenditures (USD 3.5 billion) are allocated using ICD for reimbursement and resource allocation.
- It is the diagnostic classification standard for all clinical and research purposes. These include monitoring of the incidence and prevalence of diseases, observing reimbursements and resource allocation trends, and keeping track of safety and quality guidelines. It allows the counting of deaths as well as diseases, injuries, symptoms, reasons for encounter, factors that influence health status, and external causes of disease.

The United States was one of the last industrialized nations to adopt ICD-10. They actually use considerably more codes, about 90,000 of those in ICD-10, than most other nations. They use ICD-10 codes in the outpatient setting, and are one of the few countries that use ICD codes for billing. These factors played a major role in the huge monetary investment health care entities made in switching from ICD-9 to ICD-10, and are speculated to have led to the numerous delays in implementation.

WHY DOES ICD-10 HAVE SO MANY UNUSUAL CODES?

ICD was developed to track diseases and procedures for morbidity and mortality data, not for billing. Many ICD-10 codes are quoted as unusual, however were present in ICD-9, just less specific and rarely used (**Table 32-2**). An example is the ICD-10 code X52.XXXA which is "prolonged stay in weightlessness environment." ICD-9 has the code E928.0 which is "effects of weightlessness in spacecraft."

Another point that comes up when comparing ICD-10 to ICD-9 is that ICD-10 has codes for initial and subsequent encounters. It is often asked, "do we really need a code for 'getting hit by a spacecraft' the first time and then another code for 'getting hit by a spacecraft' a second time?" The "initial" and "subsequent" terms actually refer to the care the provider gives, not the condition itself. So, the first encounter with this patient would code to T75.82XA and

SOME CLINICALLY NOTABLE CHANGES IN ICD-10

- Acute MI codes changed from 8 weeks duration to <4 weeks (28 days) duration.
- New terminology for asthma from worldallergy.org.
- Additional codes need to be used to identify resistance to antimicrobial drugs (Z16-), whenever infection with resistance is documented (V09 was used for all in ICD-9).
- A new code Z91.120- was created for "under dosing due to financial hardships."
- Injuries grouped by body part, rather than category of injury (eg, femur fracture will be under femur rather than fracture).
- Three different categories for pathologic fractures (due to neoplastic disease, due to osteonecrosis, and due to other specified disease).

ICD-10 IMPACT ON SOME COMMON HOSPITAL DIAGNOSES

HYPERTENSION

- Some of the specificity of hypertension has been eliminated—there is only one code (I10) for benign, accelerated, malignant, hypertensive urgency, hypertensive emergency, and hypertensive crisis. Despite lumping of these hypertension types, it is still important to describe hypertension completely to show severity of illness.
- There are still different specific hypertension codes if it is secondary to heart (I11), kidney (I15), or both diseases combined (I13).

ACUTE RENAL FAILURE

- Documenting Acute Renal Insufficiency and "prerenal azotemia" are vague and nonspecific and usually result in incorrect coding.
- ARF and AKI both code to N17.9 and is a CC.
- ATN codes to N17.0 and is a MCC, "vasomotor nephropathy" and "toxic nephropathy" also code to ATN (N17.0).

SEPSIS

- ICD-10 does not offer much clarification regarding the use of the diagnosis sepsis.

- Sepsis replaces the term "septicemia" that was used in ICD-9.
- SIRS diagnosis use has changed from a coding standpoint—only use for noninfectious origin (eg, DKA, trauma, burn) SIRS w/ organ dysfunction (R65.11) and SIRS if w/o organ dysfunction (R65.10).
- If SIRS leads to an infection resulting in "sepsis" or "severe sepsis," sepsis supersedes SIRS. So, a noninfectious SIRS leading to an infection resulting in severe sepsis is coded as "severe sepsis" (R65.2-), not SIRS (R65.1-).
- Sepsis must be specifically diagnosed under ICD-10 coding since there is not a code for "SIRS due to infection" as there is in ICD-9.

■ CLINICAL IMPORTANCE OF ICD-10 TO MS-DRG SELECTION

Clinical documentation is paramount to code selection not only for the provider's professional fee, but also for the hospital's MS-DRG reimbursement. The medical record must clearly document the primary diagnosis, and each actively managed condition, contributing comorbidity, and differential diagnosis to the highest specificity known.

■ DEFINITIONS

Medical Severity Diagnosis Related Groups (**MS-DRG**) is a classification system that bases hospital reimbursement for inpatient admissions on similar resource use for the identified principal diagnosis and contributing complications or comorbidities. The majority of principal admitting diagnoses have three levels of reimbursement based on the presence or absence of complications or comorbidities (CC) or major complications or comorbidities (MCC). Each MS-DRG is assigned a relative weight (RW). Each facility is assigned a base rate (BR) which is the dollar value of a RW of 1. The hospital's reimbursement for an admission is calculated by multiplying the RW × BR. Thus, the MS-DRG is the key determinant of the hospital's reimbursement for an admission.

Complications or comorbidities (CC) and major complications and comorbidities (MCC) are conditions known to increase necessary resources and length of stay (LOS) for a given primary admitting diagnosis. This translates into increased hospital reimbursement when they are present. A list of CCs and MCCs can be found at the CMS website: https://www.cms.gov/icd10manual/fullcode_cms/P0370.html.

■ KEY PRINCIPLES OF DOCUMENTATION

The selection of MS-DRG's is based entirely on ICD-10 combinations. The ICD-10 codes are chosen based on documentation in the medical record. Although a more specific diagnosis may actually exist clinically, without adequate documentation to alert a coder or auditor of its presence, the optimal code cannot be submitted.

Three key features of ideal documentation necessary to empower optimal hospital reimbursement are:

1. *Clear identification of the primary diagnosis whenever possible.* The patient's physician, is in the best position to determine the principal and secondary diagnoses. Coders and auditors who review the medical record at a later time may never appreciate the clinical picture as well as the provider. Thus, it is crucial for the provider to document their medical judgment regarding all aspects of care, including principal diagnosis. The usual scenario is that ancillary documentation will support these statements, and even make it possible for a coder to come to the same conclusion as the provider; however, sometimes that is not the case. Often there may be more than one diagnosis responsible for the admission. In this circumstance, ICD rules allow for the provider or the coder to select the principal

diagnosis that is most beneficial for reimbursement, but that selection must be supported by documentation in the chart. For example, if a patient is admitted with both a COPD and CHF exacerbation *without any other conditions that qualify as a CC or MCC*, the provider can choose to list COPD exacerbation as the principal diagnosis with acute on chronic LV systolic dysfunction as the secondary diagnosis, which reimburses higher than if the acute on chronic LV systolic dysfunction was listed as principal with COPD exacerbation as secondary.

COPD exacerbation with acute on chronic LV systolic CHF as an MCC, maps to MS-DRG 190 with a RW = 1.1743 ($5000 × 1.1743 = $5871.50). Acute on chronic LV CHF with COPD, only a CC, maps to MS-DRG 292 with a RW = 0.9824 ($5000 × 0.9824 = $4912.00). Assuming a BR ~ $5000, failing to correctly label principal and secondary diagnoses would result in ~$1000 lost revenue for the institution.

Notice that if the patient had a metabolic encephalopathy from concurrent hyponatremia, this is an MCC. Now listing acute on chronic LV systolic CHF as the principal diagnosis with metabolic encephalopathy as a MCC, mapping to MS-DRG 291 (RW = 1.5097, ~$7,548.50) will reimburse higher than COPD exacerbation with an MCC, MS-DRG 190 (RW = 1.1743, $5871.50). If a patient has more than one MCC, no additional reimbursement is given. It also does not matter which condition is counted as the MCC.

2. *Documentation should reflect the highest level of specificity.* In the example above, if COPD exacerbation is the principal diagnosis but only "CHF" is listed in the chart without further specifying it as "acute on chronic," this is a nonspecific term which does not count as either a CC or MCC; the MS-DRG would now change to COPD without MCC/CC, which is MS-DRG 192 (RW = 0.7190, $3595), and result in a $2276 loss in deserved hospital revenue.

3. *Complete differential diagnosis and listing of correctly labeled comorbid conditions.* Many patients with COPD exacerbations are found to have hyponatremia. A significant number of these present with an altered mental status from the hyponatremia, also called metabolic encephalopathy. However, often neither a comment about the sodium, nor mention of a metabolic encephalopathy ever enters the chart clinical documentation by the clinician within the history and physical or progress notes. With lack of any comment on comorbid conditions, COPD, MS-DRG 192 would only reimburse $3595. With hyponatremia listed, a CC, the MS-DRG would change to 191, reimbursing at $4685, and finally with the documentation of metabolic encephalopathy, a MCC, the MS-DRG would change to 192, worth $5871.50.

The medical record should always represent the patient's true complete medical status. These examples are meant to illustrate common documentation pitfalls resulting in unnecessary revenue loss, but should not be misconstrued or used to falsify the clinical picture to "up-code."

■ SUMMARY

The transition from ICD-9 to ICD-10 presents challenges to clinicians and hospitals, but also offers unique opportunities to improve health care and disease/procedure tracking and data. A few notable possible benefits of ICD-10 include:

- Addressing technology and health care reform initiatives—CMS value-based purchasing, pay-for-performance programs; coordinated care models such as accountable care organizations and patient-centered medical homes; the government's Physician Quality Reporting System; and the move toward adoption of electronic health record systems.

- Decreasing audit risk—ICD-10 codes allow the physician's documentation to be translated into a more accurate clinical picture, thereby reducing the chance of misinterpretation by third parties, auditors (eg, recovery audit contractor—RAC), and attorneys.
- Improving care from improved disease tracking—ICD-10 codes will generate more detailed health care data and a greater flow of that data to improve medical communication, which can potentially lead to advances in disease management and clinical pathways.
- Improve accurate reimbursement—ICD-10 codes help health care providers submit highly specific codes for the care they provide.
- Better determine severity of illness and prove medical necessity—ICD-10 codes better describe the extent and comorbidities involved in a patient's illness, which in turn facilitates validation of a patient's condition in support of utilization of goods, services and complex procedures. Correct utilization of ICD-10 should translate into more accurate severity of illness and risk of mortality for patients, resulting in a likely more accurate reflection of a physician's profiling on national registries, on consumer health sites and with health care entity's quality reporting.

As of October 1, 2015, the ICD-10 coding classification became the new baseline for clinical data, clinical documentation, claims processing, and public health reporting in the United States. While the outcomes and potential benefits (or risks) of transition to ICD-10 remain to be realized, hospitalists and all clinicians will need to practice within this new documentation environment to optimize clinical care and the accurate representation of patients' diseases and clinical conditions.

ONLINE RESOURCES

CMS ICD-10 information guide. https://www.cms.gov/medicare/coding/icd10/downloads/032310_icd10_slides.pdf.

CMS website: History of ICD-10. https://www.cms.gov/Medicare/Medicare-Contracting/ContractorLearningResources/downloads/ICD-10_Overview_Presentation.pdf.

Complete MCC and CC tables. https://www.cms.gov/Medicare/Medicare-Fee-for-Service-Payment/AcuteInpatientPPS/FY2015-IPPS-Final-Rule-Home-Page-Items/FY2015-Final-Rule-Tables.html. Tables 6I and 6K.

MS-DRG Relative weight files. https://www.cms.gov/Medicare/Medicare-Fee-for-Service-Payment/AcuteInpatientPPS/FY2015-IPPS-Final-Rule-Home-Page-Items/FY2015-Final-Rule-Tables.html. Table 5.

SECTION 7

Principles of Medical Ethics and Medical-Legal Concepts

CHAPTER 33

Common Indications for Ethics Consultation

Joseph J. Fins, MD, MACP
Matthew W. McCarthy, MD
Walter Limehouse, MD, MA, FACEP

INTRODUCTION

Nearly 2500 years ago, the Hippocratic writers decreed in the Epidemics, Bk. I, Sect. XI, "Declare the past, diagnose the present, foretell the future; practice these acts. As to diseases, make a habit of two things—to help, or at least to do no harm." The basic tenets of ethics apply to all medical specialties. The hospitalist-patient relationship depends upon a long-standing tradition of practices and manifestations of professionalism in which the physician places the interests of the patient above his or her own, and practices with competence, integrity, and beneficence. The context of care determines the application of ethical principles; however the ethical issues encountered in Hospital Medicine share with other forms of medical practice a rich history in bioethics, social movements, and landmark court cases.

The nature of the doctor-patient relationship and the new dichotomy of the inpatient and outpatient settings continue to evolve as specialized care becomes more localized to geographic areas such as the emergency room, intensive care unit, most recently, general medical units, and in the future, the medical home. This fragmentation of the clinical encounter into a unit of hospitalization represents a departure from the time-honored, and almost mythic, longitudinal doctor-patient relationship of general practice and primary care.

Unlike the classic doctor-patient relationship, decision making in the hospital is generally more harried and of a more critical nature. This may jeopardize the doctor-patient relationship if patients do not understand the role of hospitalists, perceive that their primary care physicians have abandoned them, or have questions of trust due to cultural differences or other factors. Dedication to ethical practice preserves stability in a "crisis" and promotes a culture of trust necessary for advocacy and a sound doctor-patient relationship.

Ethics, expertise, and availability of the hospitalist may help balance patient-centered obligations with the need to efficiently manage interventions. Hospitalists should not make initial assumptions about their patients' priorities without first evaluating each patient with a fresh perspective. Communication with the patient's outpatient provider, familiarization with the medical record, and meetings with patients and their family or friends who may have essential information to share during the patient's illness are both good clinical care and congruent with ethical practice.

PRACTICE POINT

- Having a longitudinal perspective from an outpatient colleague may mitigate diagnostic and prognostic errors that may occur when the object of one's practice is hospitalized patients. Consultation with an outpatient physician builds a trusting hospitalist-patient relationship. Patients may suspect potential conflicts of interest or dual agency between hospitalists and the patient needs.

The ethical mandate to optimize cooperation, or comanagement, between doctors and other members of the health care team is an essential element of the hospitalist model. In hospitals different professional specialties have traditionally functioned, often in isolation. Hampered care coordination—and the splitting of the clinical team—potentially compromises the therapeutic relationship. However, the hospitalist's appropriate use of consultants, awareness of

TABLE 33-1 Decision-making Capacity and Competence

- Ability to communicate a choice
- Understand the nature and consequences of the choice
- Manipulate rationally the information necessary to make the choice
- Reason consistently with previously expressed values and goals

one's sphere of practice, and appreciation for continuity of care sustains trust. Being transparent and sharing the results of consultations with patients and their families promotes a trusting and effective doctor-patient relationship.

This chapter will review key ethical concepts and standards in the context of Hospital Medicine and explain the role of ethics consultation to facilitate patient care.

HOSPITAL ETHICS COMMITTEES AND ETHICS CASE CONSULTATION

The Joint Commission requires that hospitals develop and implement a process to handle ethical issues in patient care, but it does not specify how this should be done. Typically, an ethics consultant—alone or as a small team—or the full ethics committee may conduct consults. Ethics committees consist of physicians, nurses, social workers, attorneys, theologians, and others representative of the immediate community that the hospital serves. Ideally, the committee should have specific members capable of ethics mediation. Importantly, the role of ethics committees is advisory. Through mediation, ethics consultants usually make recommendations rather than prescribe solutions to resolve conflict. Ethics committees consult on a range of issues across the life cycle helping patients, families, and staff grapple with challenging questions that require expert assistance.

COMMON INDICATIONS FOR ETHICS CONSULTATION

■ INFORMED CONSENT AND REFUSAL

Informed consent is the ethical lynchpin of modern medical ethics in which the dialogue between the patient and physician preserves the patient's voice in directing care. Respect for persons grounds this doctrine. Informed consent promotes autonomy and patient self-determination as an interpersonal process between physicians and patients to select an appropriate course of medical care, with the patient critically assessing his or her own values and preferences (**Table 33-1**).

Once a patient has made a choice, ongoing consent maintains the moral warrant permitting clinicians to infringe upon the patient's zone of privacy. Patients who provide consent retain the ability to revise that decision and withdraw it.

PRACTICE POINT

Indications for ethics consultation

Ethical Issues

- Advance directive
- Brain death
- Capacity/informed consent
- Confidentiality
- Futility (demands for medically ineffective treatment)

- Discharge/placement
- Do Not Resuscitate (or Allow Natural Death) orders
- Isolated incapacitated patient
- Maternal/fetal conflict
- Medical error
- Pain management
- Refusal of recommended treatment
- Research ethics
- Resource allocation
- Surrogate decision making
- Transplant issues
- Truth telling
- Withdrawal of ventilator
- Withdrawal of other life sustaining therapy
- Withdrawal or withholding artificial nutrition and hydration
- Withholding of other life-sustaining therapy

Contextual Issues

- Cultural/ethnic/religious
- Communication
- Dispute/conflict
  - Intrafamily
  - Intrastaff
  - Staff-family
  - Staff-patient
  - Patient or family in denial
  - Physician attitude toward treatment
- Quality of life

Data from Nilson EG, Acres CA, Tamerin NG and Fins JJ. Clinical Ethics and the Quality Initiative: A pilot study for the empirical evaluation of ethics case consultation. *Am J Med Qual.* 2008;23(5): 356-364.

PRACTICE POINT

- Medical decision-making capacity does not reflect global cognitive ability or intelligence, but rather a discrete capability of understanding the consequences of specific choices offered and made. This capability for a patient may change during the course of an illness. Determining medical decision-making capacity is a clinical judgment. A court presumes competence but may determine its absence. Moreover, for a person to be competent legally, he or she must possess both decision-making capacity necessary to make a specific choice and be of age or an emancipated minor.

Informed consent imposes responsibilities on both the patient and the hospitalist but also creates opportunity to build a trusting doctor-patient relationship. A properly executed informed consent depends upon mutual respect, good communication (involving adequate, accurate, and relevant information provided in a form and language the patient can understand), and shared agreement about the course of medical care. A relationship forged through the informed consent process can facilitate realistic patient expectations and help prevent disputes. Barriers to the informed consent process include:

- **Poor Care Coordination.** Mixed communication, or even contradictory information to the patient and/or family, may cause confusion and undermine care decisions.
- **Fragmentation of Care.** Lack of clarity about one's overall condition may also encumber the patient's ability to make informed choices.
- **Adaptation to the New Set of Potentially Limited Choices.** Prolonged hospitalization or progressive illness may displace the patient's sense of autonomous decision making; it requires both the patience and compassion of the hospitalist to help the patient understand how the experience of hospitalization might influence the response to illness.

A clinician claiming to have "consented the patient" mistakenly prizes outcome (agreement to a proposed procedure) over process (a clear and informed decision whether that choice resulted in the acceptance or refusal of a treatment). The importance of the informed consent process is the act of deliberation in making a sound medical choice (**Table 33-2**).

PRACTICE POINT

- Informed consent is not a recitation of facts by the physician, nor is it the placement of a signature on a document. Instead, informed consent provides the patient with decisional capacity or surrogate decision maker, either to accept or refuse a medical intervention. This process requires adequate disclosure in clear language of the nature and purpose of the contemplated procedure and associated risks and benefits. The decision must be voluntary without coercion, and the patient or surrogate must be offered any available alternatives to the proposed intervention.

Concern about patient decision-making capacity typically occurs with refusal rather than with agreement of a proposed therapy. A clinician may equate treatment refusal with loss of decision-making capacity because the decision challenges the doctor's expert recommendation. However, under the rubric of self-determination, patients retain the right to refuse treatments and physicians have a corollary obligation to ascertain that the patient understands the consequences of that choice. Mere refusal of a recommendation does not mean a patient lacks capacity for decision making.

The philosopher James Drane developed a tool to assess a patient's capacity for making choices. Invoking a "sliding scale of competence," Drane linked the increasing gravity of a patient's

decision with a progressive degree of explication. If a patient were to refuse life-sustaining therapy, he would have to more fully demonstrate his reasons, rationale, and appreciation of the consequences than if he were refusing an elective procedure. The level of decision-making capacity should be in accordance with the risks and benefits of the decision to be made. These reasons can be founded on personal, religious, or cultural beliefs. The stringency of the standard of capacity at each level correlates with the dangerousness of the treatment decision. Refusal of care by a capacitated patient who is well informed needs to be respected, even if that refusal would lead to serious harm. This is ethically supported by the principle of autonomy and legally by the patient's right to privacy and dominion over one's self.

Every effort should be made to discern the patient's rationale for refusal of recommended treatment and counter any misinformation with appropriate facts. Ethics consultation may help resolve ethical issues when treatment refusals are made by a surrogate, on behalf of an incapacitated patient.

■ TRUTH TELLING AND SHARING BAD NEWS

In our pluralistic society, some patients may prefer nondisclosure of medical information. In traditional Japanese culture, withholding of medical information is the norm founded upon *ishin denshin*, the Japanese term for the nonverbal communication of the truth. Many Islamic societies operate with less doctor-patient dialogue and a greater reliance on cultural and contextual clues in order to implicitly, versus explicitly, communicate information to the patient. In such contexts of overt nondisclosure, patients eventually deduce their status because they observe the nature of their treatments and the reactions of those around them (**Table 33-3**).

Part of the art in doctor-patient communication is titrating generic advice to the particular patient's willingness to know and use information. The burdens and benefits of "truth telling" and breaking bad news are weighed against the information necessary to make an informed treatment choice.

Approach the patient by stating that in this country standard practice requires sharing all medical information with the patient, unless he decides to delegate the dialogue and the implicit authority to make choices using that information to a surrogate as the health care agent.

If a patient requires emergent treatment, physicians can provide care to a patient who is unable to provide consent when no surrogate is available to provide authorization. The ethical foundation for this provision of care is grounded in the legal notion of the "emergency presumption" first articulated by Benjamin Cardozo when he was chief judge of the New York State Court of Appeals in *Schloendorff versus the Society of the New York Hospital* in 1914. In this landmark decision, Cardozo articulates and anticipates the modern notion of informed consent and opines that urgent and necessary treatment can occur in the absence of consent by a patient when such treatment is necessary. If the patients recovers and regains

---

TABLE 33-2 Informed Consent and Refusal

- Informed consent is a patient right
- Not all patients retain this right, predicated on the ability to be self-determining, which requires capacity
- Patients must have decision-making capacity to participate in informed consent
- Patients without capacity need a surrogate decision maker
- Urgent care can be provided when appropriate under the emergency presumption

---

TABLE 33-3 Truth Telling and Sharing Bad News

- The physician must communicate to the patient specific information necessary for making informed and deliberate choices
- No precise metric determines what patients need to know to make choices; however, most physicians adhere to a "reasonable person" standard by providing the amount of information that an "average" person would need to make an informed choice
- Full medical disclosure is the norm for most Western people

capacity or if surrogates become available, physicians should disclose the rationale and nature of the emergent treatment. These discussions should not impede the urgent provision of care.

■ THERAPEUTIC EXCEPTION OR PRIVILEGE

On that rare occasion when the risks associated with disclosure outweigh the benefits, practitioners can deliberately withhold information counter to the patient's self-determination and right to know. Typically, such a deviation from standard practice, referred to as "therapeutic exception" or "privilege," would involve a severely depressed patient who might become suicidal with grievous news. We recommend that a psychiatrist and the local ethics committee participate in determining the need to limit disclosure.

■ ADVANCE DIRECTIVES

Seventy percent of seriously ill patients are unable to decide treatment options at the end of life. The majority of these patients do not have advance directives at the time of hospitalization. By taking on discussions at the onset of care, practitioners can establish a doctor-patient/family relationship and mitigate many ethical dilemmas that could ensue should the patient deteriorate. These discussions should occur ideally within a framework that prospective planning can be emotionally fraught. To guide these discussions it is best to first identify goals of care and then determine the desirability of specific diagnostic and therapeutic interventions.

Advance directives allow the patient the opportunity to specify preferences in advance of incapacity through a living will and/or designate a surrogate to speak on his behalf as a "durable power of attorney" or "health care agent" or "proxy." With an advance directive, an incapacitated patient can be treated in accordance with his prior wishes. Such advance care planning can decrease speculation about what the patient would have wanted and decrease the moral angst associated with the proxy role, a burden that is often understated (**Table 33-4**).

When there is no surrogate (a health care agent appointed by the patient or a guardian appointed by a court), ethical norms and the law assign standing to these surrogates:

1. The patient's spouse (and in many jurisdictions to domestic partners)
2. Thereafter, a relative such as an adult child, parent, sibling
3. Finally, in some jurisdictions, a close friend

Each state has its own hierarchy for this prioritization. We recommend the use of a health care agent over a living will, when the patient can identify a trusted surrogate. In the living will, an adult with capacity sets forth directions regarding medical interventions and other actions that should or should not be taken in circumstances if he becomes incapacitated. A living will document may contain inherent contradictions and fail to anticipate possible scenarios. In contrast to a living will, a designated surrogate through a health care proxy or durable power of attorney allows for more

dynamic decision making and provides an individual who can interpret the patient's prior wishes in light of evolving circumstances and the patient-proxy covenant.

All 50 states recognize an advance directive as an extension of the patient's voice under the Patient Self-Determination Act (PSDA) of 1990, which requires health care institutions that participate in Medicare and Medicaid programs to ask patients whether they have an advance directive, inform patients of their right to complete an advance directive, and incorporate advance directives into the medical record.

Surrogates make decisions for incapacitated patients according to three distinct decision-making standards: patients' expressed wishes, substituted judgments, and best interests. When invoking substituted judgment, the surrogate places themselves in the shoes of the patient and tries to make a decision as the patient would. When neither knowledge of expressed wishes nor inference of substituted wishes exist, the surrogate makes a decision based on what a reasonable person would make, balancing benefits, and burdens.

Even when surrogates consider the patient's values, the stress of the surrogate role coupled with family dynamics and imprecise prior patient wishes can lead to morally ambiguous situations. Conflicts can also arise between surrogates of equal standing, such as two sisters who cannot agree on their mother's care. A rigid hierarchical approach to surrogate decision-making oversimplifies a process that is complex, dynamic, and personal. When two surrogates disagree, ask them to set aside their own preferences and articulate what each believes is in the patient's best interest. This minimizes potential conflicts of interest and may lead to a concordance of views. When this approach fails, hospitalists may give ethical—if not legal—precedence to that surrogate who has been assuming more of the care responsibilities.

Sometimes the conflict about goals of care arises from an incongruity between a written directive and an oral one. Given the objective reality of documentation, deference will more likely be given to a previous written rather than verbal directive, even if more contemporaneous verbal preferences emerge—which ethically would take precedence. Hence, all practitioners should clearly document, *in the medical record*, any and all expressed preferences on the part of the patient. The discharge summary should include documentation of advance care planning as a guide to future care.

Physician Orders for Life-Sustaining Treatment where available also provide means of expressing patient near end-of-life treatment choices. Patients and their clinicians complete and together sign this order set when the patient has a 1-year life expectancy with understanding of the patient's current clinical condition and potential complications. These medical orders are valid across treatment locations, from home/nursing home/hospice to emergency medical services to hospital emergency/inpatient units. The orders address whether to attempt resuscitation in the event of cardiopulmonary arrest, and how aggressively to manage intercurrent illness or disease progression, such as, medical interventions including intensive care with invasive monitoring, aggressive intervention short of intensive care (especially mechanical ventilation), or care directed toward hospice; orders may also include whether to use feeding tubes or antibiotics. Some states give POLST order the statutory authority of an advance directive. Regardless, the orders provide direct expression of patient choices to guide treatment when a patient lacks capacity, until so confirmed with the surrogate or the recapacitated patient.

While POLST orders can be useful, like living wills they can contain contradictions. Our preference for advance care planning is through the use of a designated surrogate decision maker, when available, to allow maximal responsiveness to real time challenges in the care of the decisionally incapacitated patient.

TABLE 33-4 Standards for Surrogate Decision Making

- Adhere to the explicit wishes of the patient
- If unknown, determine what decision the patient probably would have made based on the patient's values, beliefs, and past decisions as interpreted by the surrogate
- When neither knowledge of expressed wishes nor inference of substituted wishes exists, make a "best-interests" judgment based on what a generic patient would want in a given circumstance

ETHICS CONSULTATION AT THE END OF LIFE

Establishing clear goals of care and having a working awareness of the inherent conflicts and biases that may arise at life's end can help prevent conflict and enhance patient care at a time when comfort and tranquility are at a premium. Decisions to accept or refuse life-sustaining therapy are all predicated upon the aforementioned principle of self-determination as exercised through a process of informed consent or refusal. Clinicians need to distinguish responsibility and culpability when considering their role in helping patients die comfortably.

WITHHOLDING LIFE-SUSTAINING THERAPY: DO NOT RESUSCITATE ORDERS OR ALLOW NATURAL DEATH

Causality is least complex in cases where a decision is made to withhold life-sustaining therapy (LST). By withholding LST, we mean a decision not to institute an intervention that could prevent death or prolong a dying process. The prototypic example of withholding LST is a do-not-resuscitate (DNR) order, which, in the hospital setting, means the forgoing of cardiopulmonary resuscitation (CPR) or basic cardiac life support (BCLS) as well as advanced cardiac life support (ACLS) to patients who have sustained a cardiopulmonary arrest. When a patient, health care agent, or other surrogate consents to a DNR order, an intervention will not interrupt the natural course of events. In such cases, the cause of death is clearly the underlying disease process.

Unlike other interventions, to *withhold* CPR requires consent, based on the *emergency presumption* of providing care if consent cannot be obtained. Traditionally, physicians are obligated to perform CPR unless the patient has agreed to or requested a DNR order, which constitutes an informed refusal.

Essentially, all patients who undergo cardiopulmonary arrest receive CPR unless the patient or their surrogate consents to a DNR order. When a patient or surrogate provides consent, the order should be clearly placed into the medical record and the medical and nursing teams informed in a standard manner. The patient's DNR status should travel with the patient when he or she goes off the floor and be readily available for consultation should an event occur. A DNR order should be reviewed periodically and may be reversed by the patient at any time and by the surrogate decision maker if the decision does not undermine a patient's decision while capacitated.

Seventy to 80% of deaths occur with DNR orders in place for hospitalized dying patients. In the modern hospital, DNR orders take many forms, ensconcing the patient's *negative right to be left alone*. Despite the prevalence and resonance of a dying patient with DNR orders on a general medical ward, DNR orders do not preclude other treatments or interventions. DNR solely applies to decisions about cardiopulmonary arrest. Ethically, patients with DNR orders may receive care in the intensive care unit (ICU) or in the operating room. DNR status should be honored across specialties and not impede access to appropriate palliative care if it can only be offered through an intensive care or operative intervention. Indeed, some assert that to condition appropriate care upon the presence or absence of a DNR order is patently unethical.

In practice, institutions vary in their triage of patients with a DNR order regarding ICU or surgical care or other interventions requiring intubation such as endoscopy. The Task Force of the American College of Critical Care Medicine and the Society of Critical Care Medicine argues against ICU admissions, for example, noting that: "ICU admissions should be reserved for patients with reversible medical conditions who have a reasonable prospect of substantial recovery."

Significant variation may relate to how to precisely identify patients who have a "reasonable prospect of substantial recovery." Moreover, if allocation or scarce resources (eg, ICU beds) or cost containment motivates triage decisions, adherence for individual clinicians creates ethical conflicts because of their primary fiduciary obligation to the patient. Existing data suggests that the presence of a DNR order at the time of MICU consultation was significantly associated with the decision to refuse a patient to the MICU.

Because any arrest during surgery could be considered reversible, secondary to the procedure, physicians, patients, and/or surrogates should discuss DNR status prior to surgery. We echo the recommendation of the American College of Surgeons for a process of "required reconsideration" of the preexisting DNR order as part of the informed consent process for surgery. If the patient or surrogate rescinds the DNR order perioperatively, a decision is made to reinstitute it upon arrival in the recovery room or at a specified time interval after surgery.

If the patient, or surrogate, wants to maintain a DNR status during the procedure, this must be documented in the preoperative consent. If the patient dies in the OR, it is considered an "expected death" under the rubric that DNR situations result in the patient's demise. In some institutions, the physicians may find honoring an intraoperative DNR order to be against their conscience. In these cases, there should be a provision of conscientious objection and removal from the case, so long as the primary physician responsibility of nonabandonment is not breached.

Both decisions to treat patients with a DNR order in the ICU or in the surgical suite ultimately hinges on achieving clarity about the goals of care. In each care decision, a conflict may exist between a negative right to be left alone (the DNR order *not* to resuscitate) and the positive right to needed care. This balance of negative and positive engagement makes sense when the goals cohere, such as in the example of a palliative colostomy for an obstructing colon cancer. In that case, the surgical diversion is meant to provide comfort to a dying patient who had a DNR order, an ethically balanced plan of care.

In summary, the choice to forgo cardiopulmonary resuscitation supports the patients' right to refuse medical care even if this refusal leads to death. Notably, surrogate decision makers make approximately 80% of DNR requests. Hospitalists and primary care physicians are encouraged to initiate DNR discussion with the patient or proxy as soon as possible, preferably not when patients are immediately faced with cardiopulmonary cessation and imminent death.

THE DO-NOT-INTUBATE (DNI) CONUNDRUM

Do-Not-Intubate (DNI) or partial DNR orders compromise the integrity of practitioners because they imply resuscitation without intubation as a medically efficacious intervention despite the marginal effectiveness of comprehensive cardiopulmonary resuscitation itself. Most patients who have asystole or a ventricular tachyarrhythmia requiring cardioversion and/or chest compressions will also need intubation. Restoration of a viable cardiac rhythm places clinicians in the untenable position of being unable to fully complete resuscitation efforts.

In our experience, a DNI decision suggests ambivalence about goals of care, that is, a desire to survive without remaining on a ventilator for a protracted period of time. We recommend that these patients be fully resuscitated and also complete an advance directive that would allow a withdrawal of the ventilator if they were to linger beyond an aforementioned time limit.

Some patients or their surrogates would choose to be DNR but desire intubation in nonarrest situations in order to "pull through an illness." This might occur in the management of a COPD exacerbation, acute congestive heart failure, or pneumonia. Analogous to patients who are DNR in the OR, such patients want to be palliated (as per the aforementioned, diverting colostomy for obstructive colon cancer) or treated for potentially reversible conditions (sepsis) while setting limits on resuscitation should they deteriorate and sustain a cardiac arrest or complete respiratory failure. Intubation of patients with DNR orders might be regarded as a time trial.

WITHDRAWING LIFE-SUSTAINING THERAPY

Accepted as a norm, dating from the blue-ribbon President's Commission for the Study of Ethical Problems in Medicine and Biomedical and Behavioral Research, no ethical distinction exists between withholding and withdrawing treatment. The statement that the removal of LST device *causes* a patient to die, especially if the death is closely related temporally, is a *misconstrual* of causality. Withdrawal of LST simply removes an impediment to death. The intent is freedom from interventions that are perceived as burdensome. Death after refusal or withdrawal of an intervention results from the underlying disease. A decision to withdraw life-sustaining therapies may be challenging due to:

- Transference and counter transference often embedded in end-of-life decisions
- Physicians reluctance due to a misconstrued view that there is an ethical, and certainly psychological, difference between withholding and withdrawal of LST
- A sense of failure or sense of culpability
- Uncertainty about prognostication
- Inadequate communication with patients and/or surrogates about goals of care
- Differences between how physicians and lay people view these decisions

State and federal law regulate who is entitled to authorize the plan when the patient cannot speak for himself regarding a decision to withdraw LST. In the wake of the US Supreme Court decision in the *Cruzan* case and the federalism of the aforementioned Patient Self-Determination Act, each state can set an evidentiary standard about the amount of evidence from the patient's prior wishes or values, if known, necessary to permit a surrogate to authorize withdrawal of LST. Although the Supreme Court in *Cruzan* observed that there is no difference between the withdrawal of artificial nutrition and hydration and the withdrawal of a ventilator, some religious traditions view the provision of food and water as normative obligations that require a higher degree of foreknowledge of the patient's wishes.

MEDICAL DEVICES AT LIFE'S END

The philosophical and legal status of implantable medical devices has been a source of confusion in clinical practice amongst hospitalists. These devices, which include automated implanted cardioverter defibrillators (AICDs) and permanent pacemakers (PPMs) may engender ambivalence in the clinician. They can be viewed as a treatment, comparable with external medical devices like dialysis machines or ventilators, or they may considered similar to a biologic transplant, like a liver or lung transplant. The distinction, if not properly understood can lead to the perception that neither physician nor patient has the ability to withhold or withdraw the effects of the device. It is critical to appreciate that the patient—or in the setting of decision incapacity, the surrogate—retains the ability to deactivate or remove these devices under the rubric of informed refusal.

When AICDs and PPMs only provide standby interventions, we view deactivation of their resuscitative role as withholding of care. In contrast, when a patient is paced continuously by a permanent pacemaker, either in a PPM or as a function of the AICD, or uses a left ventricular assist device, deactivation is defined as a withdrawal of LST. Deactivation decisions should adhere to evidentiary decision-making standards as consistent with applicable state law, and ethics consultation may provide expert guidance. In our view, consider disabling the AICD and/or the episodic functions of the PPM when a

patient or surrogate consents to a DNR, given the similarity between internal and external defibrillation.

RELIEF OF SUFFERING AND PALLIATIVE SEDATION

Suffering is defined as an existential threat to the self and distinct from pain. Palliative sedation is defined as the use of specific sedating medications to relieve intolerable pain and suffering from refractory symptoms, even at the risk of death. Palliative sedation aims to control symptoms rather than to end life; archaic, misleading terminology such as "terminal sedation" should be avoided. Palliative sedation provides different levels:

1. Ordinary sedation (for relief of heightened anxiety or stress without reduction of consciousness)
2. Proportionate sedation (for reduction of patient's awareness of distressing symptoms with the minimum dose necessary to promote the patient's ability to engage with his family and his immediate environment)
3. Palliative sedation to unconsciousness (when less extreme measures have not relieved suffering)

The initiation of palliative sedation to unconsciousness often invokes ethical dilemmas due to confusion about physician-assisted suicide or euthanasia. The doctrine of double effect, originating from Catholic theology, refers to the doctrine where a physician uses a treatment, or gives a medication, for an intended effect where the potential outcome is good (eg, relief of a symptom), knowing that there could be an undesired secondary effect (such as death). Double effect distinguishes between the ethically mandated goal of treating intolerable patient suffering from hastening death by engaging in physician-assisted suicide or euthanasia. In all circumstances, the degree of sedation must be proportional to the severity of suffering and is given only after the patient and or surrogate have completed the informed consent process and agree. Having noted the importance of disclosure and shared decision making, we do not believe that surrogates have the moral authority to limit the provision of analgesia, including the provision of palliative sedation or general anesthesia, if they are the only means by which to ensure the patient's comfort. We assert that the right to pain management is a basic human right that can not be abridged by surrogate intervention. When there is a disagreement on the scope and level of pain management it is best to involve the expertise of the ethics committee and palliative care consultants.

MEDICAL INEFFECTIVENESS (FUTILITY)

Broadly defined, medical futility can be broken down into several domains:

- Physiologic futility (when it is absolutely—or to a reasonable degree of medical certainty—impossible to achieve a physiologic effect such as CPR in the setting of persistent acidosis)
- Qualitative futility (when the patient's physiology may improve, but there is no patient-centered benefit)
- Quantitative futility (when the intervention has not worked in similar patients within an accepted confidence interval)

Disagreement about the effectiveness of ongoing care may evoke strong emotions on the part of patients, families, and physicians entrusted to provide care. Multiple prior admissions when the patient "pulled through" despite negative odds, many clinicians with disparate views about aggressiveness of care at the end of life, communication failures, and cultural differences all contribute to a family's view of the patient's overall condition, prognosis, and how they would want him to spend the end of his life. Clinicians should try to prevent these disputes through ongoing communication during the course of the illness, to be reflective about the implicit force of one's countertransference and avoid mixed messages from different physicians by ensuring coherent comanagement.

The best way to overcome fragmentation is to have a meeting including all key clinicians involved (physicians, social work, nursing, etc), significant others designated by the patient, and family members. The aim of the discussion is to create a comprehensive factual understanding of patient's condition and prognosis. Then, after achieving a broad understanding of the medical facts, a fruitful discussion regarding both family and clinician expectations can ensue over the course of multiple meetings.

Ultimately, the imperative for members of the health care team rests on exploring the intricacy of their patient's history and values and appreciate that many surrogates may be reluctant to immediately accept a physician's prediction of medical futility. In these circumstances, clinicians should ask the surrogate to make judgments believed to be in the patient's best interest and to articulate goals of care. On many occasions a surrogate may desire something that is unachievable through the provision of care. Having the surrogate articulate these goals provides an opportunity for reality testing and an occasion to redirect a beneficent impulse, so long as practitioners appreciate why they are so potentially distressed by family demands for interventions perceived by the treating team as medically ineffective.

The increasing complexity of medical decision making often necessitates the assistance of an ethical consultant (or consulting committee). These consultations tend to be utilized by physicians who believe in shared decision making. Providers who do not utilize these services tend to believe that it is their responsibility to resolve issues with patients and families and that they are already proficient in ethics. These self-assessments may not reflect the physician's knowledge, skills or ability to mediate ethical disputes in clinical practice and thus practitioners need to cultivate a reflective stance toward the utility of ethics consults in order to best serve patients and their families.

CONCLUSION

The hospitalist model was founded on the premise that it could improve inpatient medical care. Ensuring that a model founded on efficiency and cost-effectiveness does not in any way compromise the primacy of the patient requires a familiarity with bioethics and legal precedent as well as a willingness to call upon clinical ethics consultants and hospital ethics committees when their role in the institution places them in a potentially integrity-compromising situation. These conflicts can be best understood and managed through interdisciplinary consultation and collaboration.

At the epicenter of inpatient care, hospitalists should maintain clarity, mediate misunderstandings about the diagnosis, prognosis, or goals of care, and minimize the opportunity for conflict to arise by organizing the medical team, without dominating it—all in the service of patient-centered care. Hospital ethics consultants and committees stand ready to provide assistance and remind us of the centrality of patient beneficence in all its many forms.

ACKNOWLEDGMENT

The authors acknowledge the coauthorship of Heather X. Cereste, MD, FACP of this chapter in the prior edition of this text.

SUGGESTED READINGS

Berger JT, DeRenzo EG, Schwartz J. Surrogate decision making: reconciling ethical theory and clinical practice. *Ann Intern Med*. 2008;149(1):48-53.

Bosslet GT, Pope TM, Rubenfeld GD, et al. An official ATS/AACN/ACCP/ESICM/SCCM policy statement: responding to requests for potentially inappropriate treatments in intensive care units. *Am J Resp Crit Care Med*. 2015;191(11):1318-1330.

Drane JF. Competency to give an informed consent. A model for making clinical assessments. *J Am Med Assoc*. 1984;252(7):925-927.

Etchells E. Bioethics for clinicians. 3. Capacity. *Can Med Assoc J*. 1996;155:657-661.

Fins JJ. *A Palliative Ethic of Care: Clinical Wisdom at Life's End*. Sudbury, MA: Jones & Bartlett; 2006.

Guidelines for intensive care unit admission, discharge, and triage. Task Force of the American College of Critical Care Medicine, Society of Critical Care Medicine. *Crit Care Med*. 1999;27(3):633-638.

Institute of Medicine. Committee on approaching death: addressing key end of life issues. Model advance care planning initiatives. In: *Dying in America: Improving Quality & Honoring Individual Preferences Near the End of Life*; 2015:172-192.

Limehouse WE, Feeser VR, Bookman KJ, et al. A model for emergency department end-of-life communications after acute devastating events. Part I. Decision-making capacity, surrogates, and advance directives. *Acad Emerg Med*. 2012;19(9):E1068-E1072.

Orlowski JP, Hein S, Christensen JA, et al. Why doctors use or do not use ethics consultation. *J Med Ethics*. 2006;32(9):499-502.

Rosenbloom AH, Jotkowitz A. The ethics of the hospitalist model. *J Hosp Med*. 2010;5(3):183-188.

Satyanarayana Rao KH. Informed consent: an ethical obligation or legal compulsion? *J Cutan Aesthet Surg*. 2008;1(1):33-35.

Truog RD, Campbell ML, Curtis JR, et al. Recommendations for end-of-life care in the intensive care unit: a consensus statement by the American College of Critical Care Medicine. *Crit Care Med*. 2008;36:953-963.

ONLINE RESOURCE

Aid to Capacity Evaluation (ACE). http://jcb.utoronto.ca/tools/documents/ace.pdf. Accessed May 31, 2016.

CHAPTER 34

Medical-Legal Concepts: Advance Directives and Surrogate Decision Making

Kelly Armstrong, PhD
Ross D. Silverman, JD, MPH

INTRODUCTION

Advance directives, such as living wills, health care powers of attorney, do-not-resuscitate orders, and mental health care directives, are written legal documents that offer patients the opportunity to reflect upon and provide direction for their future medical care. They are important and useful tools to facilitate discussions between patients, family members, and physicians about end-of-life care choices, and they provide guidance and legal protection in those situations when a patient is no longer capable of declaring care preferences, when critical and difficult treatment decisions need to be made. Following an advance directive facilitates making end-of-life care decisions at the patient's bedside rather than through contentious court proceedings. More importantly, advance directives are legal mechanisms that reinforce the fundamental professional and moral responsibility of health care providers and institutions to promote and protect patient autonomy, welfare, and dignity.

PRACTICE POINT

- Advance directives are legal mechanisms that reinforce fundamental professional and moral responsibilities of health care providers and institutions to promote and protect patient autonomy, welfare, and dignity. Advance directives are best thought of as the result and documentation of a patient-centered process aimed at extending the rights of patients to guide their medical care, even through periods when they are no longer able to directly participate in decisions about their own care.

This chapter offers an introduction to advance directives, examining the general structure of the various types of advance directives, when they may be triggered, what clinical circumstances and decisions they may cover, and the relative strengths and weaknesses of the different advance directive instruments. Every state has laws describing the types of advance directives available in its jurisdiction, the processes by which such documents may be created and triggered, how and where they can be employed, and the legal protections afforded to care providers and health care facilities that carry out care decisions when guided by such documents. These laws may be supplemented by policies and procedures adopted by your local hospital or health care facility to direct the use of advance directives in your particular setting. Given the unique idiosyncrasies found in different state laws and different facility policies, hospitalists should note that not all varieties of advance directive instruments may be available locally, and the processes used to carry out a particular advance directive may diverge from what is described in this chapter.

CONCEPTUAL FOUNDATIONS

The 1960s and 1970s saw a movement toward greater patient participation in health care that resulted in new ways to ensure shared decision making between patients and their physicians. During this time, dramatic medical and technological advances underscored the importance of recognizing and incorporating the goals and values of all patients, while ethicists, the courts, and others came to a consensus that a decisionally capable patient has the right to accept or refuse any type of medical care. However, many persons feared a loss of control may occur if they became incapacitated and unable to make their own medical decisions. As a result, patients and potential patients became increasingly aware of the need to make provisions for their own future medical treatment.

■ PATIENT SELF-DETERMINATION ACT

In 1990, the US Supreme Court heard the case of Nancy Cruzan, a 33-year-old woman diagnosed in a persistent vegetative state after a car accident in 1983. In the case of *Cruzan v. Commissioner, Missouri Department of Health*, 497 US 261 (1990), Nancy's parents sought to have the feeding tube removed and allow Nancy to die. The Court found that decisionally capable patients have the right to refuse life-sustaining therapies, including nutrition and hydration. However, the Court also indicated that states could require third parties acting on behalf of patients who are no longer decisionally capable to submit evidence of the patient's wishes before granting a request to withdraw life-sustaining treatment.

Partly in response to the Cruzan decision, Congress passed the Patient Self-Determination Act in 1990. This law attempts to make it clear that patients have the right to make decisions regarding their medical care. This includes the right to accept or refuse treatment and the right to complete an advance directive as evidence of their wishes. The law requires any health care provider participating in Medicare or Medicaid to provide all persons over the age of 18 with written information regarding the patient's right to accept or refuse treatment and right to complete an advance directive. Providers include hospitals, nursing homes, home health care providers, hospices, and health maintenance organizations, but not outpatient-service providers or emergency medical personnel. The Patient Self-Determination Act also requires health care providers to document whether patients have advance directives, establish policies to implement advance directives, and educate their staff and the community about advance directives. Patients should also be informed that having an advance directive is not required to receive medical care.

■ UNIFORM HEALTH CARE DECISIONS ACT

After the Cruzan decision, significant changes occurred in state laws across the United States regarding health care decision making. While every state passed legislation authorizing the use of at least one form of advance directive, there was very little uniformity between the laws. By 1993, state laws regarding health care decision making were often fragmented, incomplete, and sometimes inconsistent. Statutes in one state frequently conflicted both with other statutes from the same state, and with statutes from other states. With this confusion in mind, the Uniform Health care Decisions Act (UHCDA) was drafted in 1993. Under the UHCDA, any adult or emancipated minor may execute or provide an "advance health care directive," which refers to either a "power of attorney for health care" or other "individual instruction." If an individual fails to execute a power of attorney for health care or if the agent is not available, the UHCDA authorizes health care decisions to be made by a "surrogate" to be selected from a priority list. The Act also recognizes an individual's authority to define the scope of any instruction or agency as broadly or as narrowly as the individual chooses.

ADVANCE DIRECTIVES

Advance directives empower individuals to make their goals, values, and treatment preferences known before a loss of decisional capacity may occur. The term *advance directives* refers to oral or written instructions about a person's medical care that provide guidance regarding medical treatment to health care professionals if and when the patient becomes unconscious or otherwise unable to make his or her own decisions. All 50 states, either through statute or case law, have provisions for honoring advance directives. Despite this, different jurisdictions utilize different standards, terminology, and limitations of authority. Physicians should become familiar with the local requirements for completing and honoring a legal advance directive.

The legal requirements for a valid advance directive vary from state to state, but in general any adult or emancipated minor with decisional capacity can execute an advance directive. In some rare instances an advance directive may have an expiration date, however, in general an advance directive remains in effect until such time as the patient revokes it. Different states have different requirements for validly revoking an advance directive, but most recognize a decisionally capable person may revoke an advance directive at any time simply by making the intention to revoke clear to a lawyer or health care provider, either verbally or in writing.

Because of the additional effort required to complete a written directive, the written directive is generally held to have more power than oral statements; however, this should be evaluated on a case-by-case basis.

■ NONCONFORMING DOCUMENTS

While many state statutes contain standard or recommended language for advance directives, people are introduced to advance directives from a variety of sources, including financial planners, senior organizations, national agencies, and religious organizations, not to mention the Internet. Most state statutes explicitly acknowledge that versions of advance directives that do not contain the recommended statutory language, as well as some oral statements, may also be valid. Such nonconforming directives cannot be dismissed just because they do not contain the language recommended by statute. Evaluating directives that do not conform to the recommended language found in state statutes requires physicians to determine, with the assistance of the ethics committee or legal counsel if necessary, whether a nonconforming directive meets the state's standard of reliability. In other words, is it clear that the patient intended to document his or her wishes with the intention that such documentation would be relied upon and followed by the health care team? Such seriousness of purpose can be demonstrated by a variety of means including if the document contains the patient's signature, if the document is witnessed, if the document was presented to the physician by the patient as an advance directive, or if the patient discussed the document with family members as evidence of the patient's wishes.

■ ADVANCE CARE PLANNING

When advance directives first came into existence, they were viewed as legal documents offering legal protection from unwanted treatment at the end of life. As the practice of medicine has become more patient centered, a greater focus has emerged on ensuring all medical decisions are not only clinically sound, but also based on the patient's personal goals for care. Advance directives are best thought of as the result and documentation of a patient-centered process aimed at extending the rights of patients to guide their medical care, even through periods when they are no longer able to directly participate in decisions about their own care.

Optimally, before completing an advance directive, individuals will have the opportunity to have a structured discussion with their physician or other clinician about their health care wishes and goals. Ideally, these conversations are held before the patient becomes ill, even though physicians cannot discuss with specificity every scenario that may occur. Advance directives may simply contain general preferences, or they may contain specific instructions about particular treatments. Those that contain only general preferences can be less helpful in guiding care than those with specific instructions because general preferences can require more interpretation in light of the current medical evidence. For example, a patient's statement "I don't want to live hooked up to machines," may mean the patient's does not want CPR, or it may mean the patient wants all aggressive therapies until such time as those therapies fail to restore the patient to an acceptable quality of life. A comprehensive process of advance care planning includes a discussion of possible or likely scenarios based on the patient's unique medical situation, a discussion of the patient's values and goals, documentation of the patient's values and goals, and a way to ensure that this information is available to present and future care providers. The advance directive as a document provides a legally recognized way to record this discussion.

TYPES OF ADVANCE DIRECTIVES

Although state statutes vary, there are three basic types of advance directives: instructional, such as living wills; proxy, such as a power of attorney for health care; and combination directives, which provide both instructions for care and name a proxy to make decisions.

■ INSTRUCTIONAL ADVANCE DIRECTIVES

Instructional directives provide consent or refusal for specific treatments that may need to be utilized when the patient is unable to make the decision, traditionally at the end of life (**Table 34-1**).

Living wills

Living wills are the most common instructional directive. A living will directs physicians to withhold or withdraw life-sustaining measures and to provide only comfort care if the patient has a terminal illness and life-sustaining measures are prolonging the dying process without a chance for recovery. The living will thus addresses only a small subset of medical situations and critics cite the typically vague language and difficulty physicians have predicting with certainty when a patient is at the end of life as primary reasons that the document has fallen out of favor in terms of utility. Nevertheless, the document can be helpful as a starting point for further discussion, and it serves as evidence of a patient's values, specifically that there are certain outcomes the patient would not wish to pursue. The living will is also a useful document for persons who do not have a designated agent or proxy since it speaks directly to the physician and does not require the consent of a designated agent or proxy in order for the physician to take action.

Some jurisdictions have placed restrictions on how the living will may be invoked. For example, Illinois and Missouri do not permit the withdrawal of artificial nutrition and hydration if the withdrawal would be the proximate cause of death (rather than the patient's terminal condition). Most states also have provisions invalidating the document if the patient is pregnant, and some states dictate that the power granted to a designated agent such as a power of attorney for health care takes precedence over the power provided in the living will. Physicians should refer to the specific statutes in their state for guidance.

As the first widely known advance directive, the living will is the most well known and physicians should be aware that many patients refer to all advance directives by the name "living will," and others may confuse the living will with a last will and testament. Care should be taken to verify the exact type of directive(s) the patient may have.

Do-not-resuscitate orders

Do-not-resuscitate (DNR) orders have become increasingly common in the care of the dying patient. The decision whether to resuscitate a patient who suffers a cardiac or respiratory arrest involves consideration not only of the potential clinical outcomes, but also the patient's preferences regarding the intervention and if the likely outcome is one that would be desired by the patient. In order to streamline care from the inpatient to outpatient setting, a majority of states now have legislation permitting the use of out-of-hospital DNR orders. These DNR orders are physician orders that direct health care professionals across all emergency, living, or health care settings to withhold or withdraw (if treatment has already begun in absence of the form) specific types of life-sustaining treatment, such as CPR or defibrillation, in the event of a respiratory or cardiac arrest.

Physician's orders for life-sustaining treatment (POLST)

POLST stands for physician's orders for life-sustaining treatment, and the POLST form has been adopted by several states (some states such as New York use the acronym MOLST for medical orders for life-sustaining treatment). POLST addresses the desire some persons may have, particularly those persons who are experiencing a chronic or life-limiting illness, to avoid unwanted emergency medical care like CPR or a transfer to the hospital. POLST takes advance directives a step further by not only documenting a patient's treatment preferences, but also providing emergency and other medical personnel with clear physician orders to follow in the case of an emergency. Depending on the state, the POLST form has three or four sections outlining the patient's desire to have or refuse CPR, whether the patient would like to be taken to a hospital, and the types of medical interventions desired by the patient, including the provision of comfort care, antibiotics, or artificially administered

TABLE 34-1 Types of Advance Directives

Advance Directive	Type	Covered Activity
Living will	Instructional	End-of-life document for patients with a terminal illness who wish to forgo death-delaying procedures
Physician's orders for life-sustaining treatment/medical orders for life-sustaining treatment	Instructional	Portable physician orders for life-sustaining treatment that apply across all emergency and care settings
Power of attorney for health care	Proxy	Appoints a person over the age of 18 to make decisions on behalf of the patient
Psychiatric advance directive	Combination	Allows patient to preauthorize certain types of mental health treatment in the event of acute psychiatric illness; also allows the patient to appoint someone to make mental health treatment decisions
"Five wishes"	Combination	Combines a living will, power of attorney for health care, and instructions for comfort care and personal matters

nutrition. In those states that have adopted the POLST paradigm, the orders are valid in all emergency, living, and health care settings. If a patient presents the POLST document in a state that has not adopted the POLST paradigm, the document should be interpreted as strong and reliable evidence of the patient's known wishes regarding treatment.

Other types of instructional directives

Other types of instructional directives allow individuals to refuse specific therapies, such as blood transfusion or dialysis, for persons who have specific desires to refuse those types of therapy. For example, many Jehovah's Witnesses do want blood or blood products administered under any circumstances, even though death may be an outcome of the refusal. The instructional directive provides evidence of the patient's wishes, and many will specifically release the physician from any liability for following the directive.

■ PROXY ADVANCE DIRECTIVES

Proxy advance directives such as the power of attorney for health care allow a patient to appoint another person over the age of 18 to make health care decisions in circumstances when the patient is unable to make those decisions for himself or herself. The proxy advance directive is not limited to end-of-life decisions and is therefore a more useful document for the vast number of decisions that can be encountered throughout the lifespan. The only requirement before the instrument takes effect is the patient must lack decisional capacity regarding the decision at hand. Physicians should note that because decisional capacity is decision specific, a patient may have the capacity to make some decisions, but require assistance to make other types of decisions.

The person appointed by a power of attorney for health care is called a power of attorney or an "agent." Because a power of attorney has been directly appointed by the patient, a power of attorney typically has broad authority to make the same kinds of decisions as the patient unless that authority has been limited by the patient or by statute. Thus, in most states, a power of attorney can accept or refuse any type of treatment. Because the power of attorney can execute a broad range of powers, health care professionals and others should ensure the appointment of a power of attorney is executed without coercion or duress. Some states require the power of attorney to accept the agency in writing, while others restrict agency to a single individual in order to minimize the chances that disagreement or differences of opinion between two or more agents stall medical decisions. Physicians should refer to the specific statutes in their state for guidance.

■ COMBINATION ADVANCE DIRECTIVES

There is a growing trend in advance directives toward allowing persons to combine instructions regarding treatment preferences with appointing a decision maker to make proxy decisions. Many state forms now allow persons completing an instructional form to also specify or appoint a power of attorney at the same time. It is important to note that while many combination forms grant the proxy decision maker broad powers of decision making, the document may also contain a limitations or exclusions section that limits the types of decisions that the proxy decision maker can make on behalf of the patient.

Psychiatric advance directives

Psychiatric advance directives allow persons with mental illnesses to engage in advance planning with their physicians regarding potential future care. Persons with mental illnesses retain the right to refuse treatment, as long as they do not pose a serious risk of harm to themselves or others. However, during an acute episode of psychiatric illness an individual may become unable to make or communicate decisions about treatment. A psychiatric advance directive allows currently competent patients who may experience an acute episode of psychiatric illness in the future, to agree in advance to treatment they may refuse later when ill. Unlike many other types of advance directives that focus on empowering the patient to refuse unwanted interventions, psychiatric advance directives are generally "opt-in" documents where the patient may preconsent to inpatient hospitalization, medication, or other helpful treatment modalities. In addition to offering a clear written statement of an individual's treatment preferences, the psychiatric advance directive can also be used to assign decision-making authority to another person while the individual is incapacitated. Correctly executed and implemented directives not only promote individual autonomy and empowerment, they can eliminate the need for court involvement and assist in recovery by communicating to the physician and others the types of treatments that have or have not worked for the person in the past.

"Five wishes"

"Five wishes" is a combination advance directive introduced in 1996 that has become popular because of its easy-to-read language. It introduces the subjects of a living will, power of attorney, comfort care, spirituality, and other personal matters such as forgiveness and memorial plans in the form of five distinct but overlapping "wishes." The first two wishes—"the person I want to make care decisions for me when I can't" and "the kind of medical treatment I want or don't want"—are intended to serve as legal documentation fulfilling the requirements of many states' living will and power of attorney statutes.

HONORING ADVANCE DIRECTIVES

Today's health care providers, and physicians in particular, have the simultaneous responsibility of respecting patients' autonomous choices while protecting from harm those patients who are incapable of making an authentic or informed decision. For patients with variable or fluctuating capacity, circumstances may arise where the patient is capable of being involved in some, but not all, decisions. The minimum standard for decisional capacity is directly related to the risk involved in the decision. Thus, a patient may legitimately consent to a low-risk procedure such as a blood draw or CT scan, but need assistance with more complex decisions such as whether to have surgery. The presumption is that a coherent care plan should be established around the patient's known wishes whenever possible.

■ INFORMED CONSENT

Informed consent is, with rare exceptions, required before treatment can be provided to a patient. In order for consent to be valid, it must be given voluntarily in light of accurate and relevant information—in a language intelligible to the recipient—regarding the risks, benefits, and alternatives of the proposed interventions. In addition to providing information that the average reasonable person might desire, it is important that patients receive sufficient information within the priorities that have the most meaning for them. For instance, some religious belief systems require or preclude certain forms of medical treatment. Other patients may want to know how incapacitated they may be after a surgery, or how long they must wait before driving. Valid consent also requires the person giving consent to have sufficient decisional capacity to make the decision at hand.

■ DECISIONAL CAPACITY

There are relatively few guidelines informing physicians and others when to conduct and document an explicit assessment of an individual's decisional capacity. However, assessments of decisional capacity should be ongoing and not restricted to instances where the patient disagrees with a physician's recommendation for treatment. Assessment and documentation may be warranted whenever the individual consents to complex or high-risk interventions, when the patient makes choices that do not appear prudent or when the decision is outside the patient's norms, or when the patient has marked cognitive deficits or other risk factors for impaired decisional capacity.

It is important to note that because capacity may fluctuate over time, physicians may be dealing with a proxy decision maker for some aspects of treatment, and directly with the patient for other aspects. When reasonable, important decisions should wait until the patient regains decisional capacity (if expected), and decisions made by others should be reviewed with the patient if and when he or she regains capacity. The presumption is that patients can make their own decisions until they demonstrate otherwise. Therefore, each decision should be put before the patient and if the patient concretely demonstrates that he or she is unable to make the particular decision at hand, this should be carefully documented in the patient's medical record. Many jurisdictions also require documentation of the reason for the patient's incapacity and its expected duration.

Decisional capacity is functionally defined in light of a specific decision. As the risk of a proposed intervention increases, so too does the threshold standard for decisional capacity. For instance, the capacity needed to consent to routine labs would be lower than the capacity required for consent to open heart surgery. Grisso and Appelbaum have put forward the most frequently used model for assessing decisional capacity standards 1 to 4 in **Table 34-2**.

Some commentators have also indicated that under certain circumstances it may be prudent to add the fifth criterion, particularly if the decision being made by the patient represents a radical or abrupt change in treatment goals, or does not conform to what is known about the patient values or other decisions.

■ COMPETENCE AND DECISIONAL CAPACITY.

Decisional capacity and competence are not synonymous. Competence is a legal designation that must be made by a court, whereas decisional capacity is determined by a physician or other clinician. Not all patients with a developmental, cognitive, or mental illness have impaired decisional capacity, even if they have been declared

TABLE 34-2 Standards for Assessing Decisional Capacity

Assessing Decisional Capacity

1. The patient can make and communicate a choice
2. The patient demonstrates understanding of his or her medical condition, prognosis, and the risks and benefits of the available treatment options
3. The patient has the capacity for reasoned decision making
4. The patient is able to apply his or her own values to the decision at hand
5. The patient's decision remains stable over time (if the situation allows), or the patient can make a reasoned explanation why the decision is not consistent with the patient's previously known wishes

incompetent or have been appointed a guardian. On the contrary, there is significant variability in the decisional capacity among these patients. The examining clinician should evaluate each patient's capacity in light of the particular decision at hand.

PROXY DECISION MAKING

Physicians respect a patient's autonomy by recognizing that the patient's right to accept or refuse treatment remains even after he or she loses decision-making capacity. Patients who have lost decisional capacity may continue to communicate through their advance directives, or through a power of attorney or surrogate who interprets what the patient would choose in a given situation.

When medical decisions need to be made for a patient who lacks decisional capacity, physicians should first inquire whether the patient has documented any wishes in a written advance directive such as a POLST form or a durable power of attorney for health care. Optimally, the patient will have documented preferences that directly relate to the proposed treatment. However, this rarely happens. More commonly, a third party is necessary to represent the patient's interests and interpret the patient's known wishes and values in light of the current medical situation. If the patient has designated a decision maker in an advance directive such as a power of attorney for health care, the designated agent should be relied upon to make decisions. If the patient does not have a power of attorney or some other document that directs care, such as a POLST form or living will (or those documents exist but do not apply to the situation at hand), a surrogate should be appointed.

■ SURROGATE DECISION MAKING IN THE ABSENCE OF ADVANCE DIRECTIVES

Many states have established protocols for identifying a legal third-party decision maker in the absence of a documented advance directive. This third-party decision maker may be called a proxy or a surrogate, depending on the state. Most patients have not completed an advance directive and there should be no presumption inferred from the fact that an advance directive has not been executed. The guiding principle in appointing any surrogate is to find the person, or group of persons, who best know the patient's values and health care goals. This person or persons should be able to effectively communicate with the health care team, and be willing to make choices the patient would most likely make if he or she could speak for himself or herself.

Where they exist, state statutes generally indicate the family of the patient should be responsible for making medical decisions. The order of priority for appointing a surrogate is listed in **Table 34-3**. While "family" is generally recognized as a biological or legal relationship, most states have not specifically addressed more complicated

TABLE 34-3 Priority Hierarchy for Appointing a Surrogate

Typical Order of Priority for Appointing a Surrogate in Absence of Applicable Advance Directive (Check Local Jurisdiction)
1. Court-appointed guardian
2. Spouse or domestic partner (where legally recognized)
3. Adult children
4. Either parent
5. Adult siblings
6. Other family members
7. A close friend of the patient

relational ties such as when the patient has full siblings, half siblings, and step siblings who all consider themselves to be close relatives of the patient on the same level of the surrogate hierarchy. If more than one person has the same level of priority (such as several adult children), consensus is preferred, but many states allow for a majority decision when consensus cannot be reached. The disagreeing party then has the option of turning to the court to assist in resolving the dispute. In states that do not appoint surrogates by statute, case law may offer guidance, or the physician or ethics committee can nominate the decision maker according to the standards of the institution.

Guiding standards

Two basic principles should guide treatment decisions for decisionally incapable patients: respecting and promoting the patient's autonomy, and fostering the patient's well-being. All surrogates and care providers have an obligation to follow the informed verbal or written wishes of the patient and to act in the person's best interests. They should also take into account the person's values and goals if those are known. Three legal and ethical standards have been established to guide such decisions: (1) The highest standard is a directly relevant autonomous directive where the patient's wishes in regard to the decision at hand are known, either through documentation or discussion. (2) The most common standard used is substituted judgment where the proxy decision maker is tasked with making the decision he or she believes the patient would have made in this situation based on what is known about the patient's wishes, personal values and preference, and goals. (3) In the best interest standard, the patient's wishes are unknown or have never been known (such as cases involving infants), and the proxy decision maker must weigh the risks and benefits of all of the alternatives and make a decision that achieves the greatest net benefit from the perspective of the patient.

Confidentiality and HIPAA

Although medical care has always included the need to keep patients' medical information confidential, the Health Insurance Portability and Accountability Act (HIPAA) has further specified and codified the responsibility of health care providers. In order to make effective decisions, proxy decision makers need information about the patient's medical history and care. HIPAA regulations recognize this and entitle duly documented proxy decision makers to the same medical information as the patient in regard to the decision at hand. However, physicians should disclose only that information needed by the proxy to make an informed choice regarding the decision at hand. If possible and/or when directed by the patient, physicians should avoid discussing highly personal information such as sexually transmitted diseases, HIV status, chemical dependency, mental illness, or any history of sexual or physical abuse, unless such information is absolutely necessary in order for the proxy to make appropriate and informed decisions.

Scope of authority

The exact scope of a surrogate's decision-making authority varies by state. Patients may also document certain limits on the kinds of decisions that may be made by their surrogate. For example, some living wills state the surrogate decision maker cannot override specific instructions such as a request not to receive CPR. Some state laws also suggest the patient must assent to, or minimally not refuse, decisions made by the surrogate. This offers a layer of protection to those patients who may not reach the threshold for decisional capacity with respect to the decision at hand, but who are still aware of and engaged with what is happening to them. When there is disagreement between the patient and surrogate, and a clinically appropriate compromise that is acceptable to both parties cannot be found, it is advisable to contact the hospital's ethics committee.

Because the surrogate is often an individual whom the patient has not explicitly appointed to the role of decision maker, many states place restrictions on the types of end-of-life decisions that can be made by the surrogate. Broadly speaking, these restrictions may require the attending physician and one additional physician to document that the patient has a "qualifying condition," such as a terminal illness or permanent unconsciousness, before honoring a request by the surrogate to withhold or withdraw life-sustaining treatment.

Generally, a proxy decision maker for a decisionally incapable patient may conduct routine medical affairs for the patient including consulting with the patient's health care providers, providing verbal or written consent for medical procedures, applying for public benefits such as Medicare or Medicaid, authorizing the release of information and clinical records needed for continued care, and authorizing the transfer of the patient to or from health care facilities. Care should be taken that such activities are warranted by the patient's clinical condition, do not conflict with the patient's known wishes, and that they are undertaken by the proxy only when it is not expected that the patient will be returned to a decisionally capable state in the time necessary to assure continuity of care.

Conflicts

Occasionally, situations arise in which a surrogate makes a decision or requests an intervention that conflicts with either the patient's advance directive or other instructions the patient provided to the care team while the patient was still decisionally capable. For instance, it is not uncommon for a patient's child to request CPR be provided even when the patient has specifically requested a DNR order. Plans and treatment goals previously established between the patient and the physician should not be changed without concrete evidence that those decisions were made due to factual, conceptual, or clinical error. The primary responsibility of the physician is to the patient, and decisions made after the patient loses decisional capacity should further the continued interests of the patient. Additionally, surrogates are morally and legally required to make decisions that conform as closely as possible to those the patient would choose for himself or herself. Physicians thus are not obligated to follow requests by surrogates that do not comply with the patient's known wishes. If the physician is unable to resolve the conflict, it may be helpful to involve a third party to help mediate the situation such as an ethics consultant or committee, or hospital legal counsel. If an ethically, legally, and clinically sound agreement cannot be reached, court review may be necessary.

■ SPECIAL CASES

Implied consent

In health care, the principle of implied consent is sometimes colloquially referred to as "emergency consent" since it is most commonly invoked when the following conditions are met: (1) there is an emergency circumstance where the patient is unable to participate in the informed consent process (usually because the patient is unconscious), and there is no available evidence of the patient's wishes not to receive the therapy; (2) no other proxy decision maker is available to make decisions for the patient; and (3) the physician is compelled to immediately provide necessary treatment without which serious or irreversible harm to the patient's life or health may result. Thus, implied consent is presumed when a person needs help and cannot explicitly provide consent. Implied consent also refers to situations where the patient does not expressly state, either verbally or in writing that a procedure may be done, but his or her actions imply consent. A common example is when the patient extends an arm after being told that the physician wants to draw blood for laboratory analysis. Implied consent is legally accepted and provides a defense against claims of battery, but not against claims of negligence. Physicians should follow their institutions' documentation standards when relying on implied consent in the context of a medical emergency, and clearly identify why emergency treatment was necessary as well as the nature and immediacy of the threat.

Minors

The rights of minors to make decisions about their medical care have expanded over the past decade. While in general, a parent or legal guardian of a minor has to provide consent for treatment, some jurisdictions are granting older minors, especially those over the age of 16, broad leeway to make decisions about their medical treatment. Nearly all jurisdictions allow legally emancipated minors and minors who are pregnant or parents themselves to make medical decisions for their care and their own minor children. However, some states now have statutes or case law that allow mature minors to provide consent to procedures if they can demonstrate that they are mature enough to understand and appreciate the nature and consequences of a proposed medical procedure or treatment. Rather than reliance on an "all-or-none" phenomenon, the mature minor doctrine allows for individual assessment of the stability of the minor patient's value system along with their emotional and intellectual development. This approach recognizes that decisional capacity in a minor is a gradual process affected by personal characteristics and environment. The laws concerning the extent minors are allowed to make their own medical decisions vary from jurisdiction to jurisdiction, and most jurisdictions are reluctant to allow minors to refuse potentially life-sustaining treatment without involvement of the court. It is therefore advisable that each physician be familiar with the local statutes.

Artificial nutrition and hydration

Medical and legal issues abound when it comes to the use of artificial nutrition and hydration (ANH), particularly in the dying or permanently unconscious patient. The US Supreme Court made it clear in its 1990 Cruzan decision that ANH is a medical treatment and a decisionally capable patient may refuse any and all types of medical treatment, including ANH and other types of life-sustaining treatment. Patients may also execute a specific instructional directive that references ANH and clearly communicates the patient's refusal of ANH. However, state laws are highly variable in regard to proxy decision-maker requests to withhold or withdraw ANH, and many living will laws expressly forbid the withholding or withdrawal of ANH as a means to shorten the dying process. Some states require "clear and convincing" evidence of the patient's wishes to forgo

administration of ANH before a proxy request may be honored. Clear and convincing evidence would require either a written directive or evidence of a serious, reflective discussion with the patient on the subject. Other states have lesser evidentiary standards, and some include ANH within the parameters of life-sustaining treatment that may be terminated upon request of a proxy decision maker whenever the standards are met for withdrawal of life-sustaining treatment. Physicians should refer to the specific statutes in their state for guidance.

Physician-assisted suicide

The US Supreme Court ruled in 1997 that states may maintain laws that prohibit or allow euthanasia and assisted suicide. A few states now allow terminally ill adult patients, who are decisionally capable and able to communicate their wishes, to end their lives through the voluntary self-administration of a lethal dose of medication prescribed by a licensed physician expressly for that purpose. In Oregon and Washington, the statutes are called the Death with Dignity Act. Patients must fulfill several requirements before receiving the medication, including initiating verbal and written requests, undergoing a second opinion consultation, receiving psychiatric intervention if the patient is perceived to be depressed, and undergoing a 15-day waiting period. This process is sometimes called "physician-assisted suicide" because patients self-administer the medication at a time of their choosing with the intention of ending their life. Because the patient actively takes steps to end his or her life, this is different than withholding or withdrawing medical treatment where barriers to the dying process are removed. This is also different than voluntary active euthanasia where the physician acts upon the voluntary request of a decisionally capable patient and the physician intentionally administers medications or other interventions to cause the patients death. In states that allow it, patients must request and self-administer the lethal medication. No state allows the medications to be administered or requested by a proxy decision maker, even where there is clear evidence of the patient's wishes.

SUGGESTED READINGS

Appelbaum PS. Assessment of patients' competence to consent to treatment. *N Engl J Med*. 2007;357:1834-1840.

Burns JP, Edwards J, Johnson J, et al. Do-not-resuscitate order after 25 years. *Crit Care Med*. 2003;31(5):1543-1550.

Johnstone MJ, Kanitsaki O. Ethics and advance care planning in a culturally diverse society. *J Transcult Nurs*. 2009;20(4):405-416.

Jonsen AR, Siegler M, Winslade WJ. *Clinical Ethics: A Practical Approach to Ethical Decisions in Clinical Medicine*, 7th ed. New York: McGraw-Hill; 2010.

Scheyett AM, Kim MM, Swanson JW, et al. Psychiatric advance directives: a tool for consumer empowerment and recovery. *Psychiatr Rehabil J*. 2007;31(1):70-75.

Siegel MD. End-of-life decision-making in the ICU. *Clin Chest Med*. 2009;30:181-194.

Valvano TJ. Legal issues in sexual and reproductive health care for adolescents. *Clin Pediatr Emerg Med*. 2009;10:60-65.

Von Gunten CF, Ferris FD, Emanuel LL. The patient-physician relationship. Ensuring competency in end-of-life care: communication and relational skills. *JAMA* 2000;284(23):3051-3057.

CHAPTER 35

Medical Malpractice

Adam C. Schaffer, MD

Medical malpractice is a serious concern for many physicians and a topic that often prompts intense debate. In this chapter, we review the elements of medical malpractice, as well as data about the frequency of both negligent medical care and actual claims of medical malpractice. We will also review how well the malpractice system achieves its purpose of deterring negligent medical care and compensating patients who are harmed by such negligence. We also discuss malpractice issues that are of particular concern to hospitalists, and what can be done to reduce the risk of being the subject of a medical malpractice claim.

THE ELEMENTS OF MEDICAL MALPRACTICE

Medical malpractice is a form of negligence that applies to health care providers including doctors, nurses, and institutional medical care providers like hospitals. At the core of negligence-based liability is the notion that individuals committing unintentional but reasonably avoidable acts that cause injury should be required to compensate the victims of those acts. To determine whether negligence is present in a given situation, courts require plaintiffs to prove four elements through a preponderance of the evidence: duty, breach, causation, and harm.

> ### PRACTICE POINT
>
> - To determine whether negligence is present in a given situation, courts require plaintiffs to prove four elements through a preponderance of the evidence: duty, breach, causation, and harm.
> - In the hospital setting, physicians have a duty to provide care with the same skill and diligence as a reasonably competent physician in the same specialty or field of practice would under similar circumstances.
> - The question of whether a physician breached the duty of care, then, often hinges on competing testimony provided by expert witnesses as to the applicable standard of care and whether the conduct in question failed to meet that standard.
> - To establish legal causation, the plaintiff must show that the breach was both the "cause in fact" and the "proximate cause" of the injury.

The duty of care in negligence claims is a hypothetical standard by which the court judges the conduct of the defendant to determine whether he or she had an obligation to act differently. In the hospital setting, physicians have a duty to provide care with the same skill and diligence as a reasonably competent physician in the same specialty or field of practice would under similar circumstances. Failure to meet this standard constitutes a breach of the physician's duty of care. In most cases, for this duty to exist, a physician-patient relationship must have been established.

In order to determine whether a physician has breached the duty of care, an expert witness must testify as to the applicable standard in court. In the majority of states, physicians are judged by a national standard of care that all physicians in the same specialty would be expected to follow. However, in a significant number of states, physicians are judged by what other physicians in the same specialty and in the same geographic area would have done in a particular situation. In either case, the relevant testimony must come from expert witnesses who have the education, training, or other credentials that would make them familiar with the applicable standard of care. The question of whether a physician breached the duty of care then, often hinges on competing testimony provided by expert witnesses as to the applicable standard of care and whether the conduct in question failed to meet that standard.

Even if a physician breaches this duty by failing to adhere to the standard of care, the plaintiff in a case cannot establish liability unless that breach is the actual cause of the injury. To establish legal causation, the plaintiff must show that the breach was both the "cause in fact" and the "proximate cause" of the injury. As a breach of the duty of care is the "cause in fact" of damages if the plaintiff can establish that the presence of the breach was the "deciding factor" in determining whether the damage would have occurred. Put differently, a breach of the duty of care would not be the "cause in fact" of harm if the harm would have occurred despite the negligent care of a physician. In addition to being the cause in fact of harm, a breach of the duty of care must also be the proximate cause in order to satisfy the causation element of negligence. To be the proximate cause of harm, the harm must be, by its nature, a foreseeable or direct consequence of a breach of the duty of care. Some courts require an additional or alternative finding that the breach was a "substantial factor" in causing the injury, especially when two or more parties may be responsible.

If the court or jury finds that a physician has breached a duty by failing to adhere to the applicable standard of care and that the breach is the cause in fact and proximate cause of a patient's injury, then the physician will be liable for damages. The measure of such damages is often highly dependent on the facts and circumstances surrounding the particular incident. Generally, a claimant can recover compensatory damages for both economic and noneconomic harm. Economic damages include the specific costs associated with treating the injury, such as medical bills and drug expenses, as well as current and future loss of earnings. Economic damages also include the costs of living with the injury such as modifications to the home to accommodate a wheelchair. Noneconomic damages most often include pain and suffering (physical and emotional) from the injury. In addition, courts may order punitive damages for injuries that are the result of malicious conduct or a willful disregard of patient safety. However, such instances are rare.

Medical malpractice claims usually involve numerous medical personnel involved in every stage of the patient's care. Malpractice plaintiffs cast a wide net when filing suit for a number of reasons. First, it is often cost prohibitive to file an individual suit against each defendant because of the increased costs of legal discovery. Second, because most states employ a comparative negligence standard (meaning that total damages are calculated and then allocated to defendants based on their percentage of contribution of fault), it is difficult to allocate damages among separate claims. It is also more likely that naming multiple defendants will help the plaintiff narrow down which of the defendants was actually at fault (if any). Third, joining multiple defendants in the same suit allows plaintiffs to use the defendants' own knowledge and testimony to establish standards of care, cutting down on the costs of hiring independent expert witnesses. Finally, there may be jurisdictional rules that prohibit separate claims and require naming all the responsible parties in a single claim if a failure to do so would result in an unfair outcome or an increased burden on the judicial system.

THE EPIDEMIOLOGY OF MEDICAL MALPRACTICE

Up until relatively recently, little data existed about liability environment for hospitalists specifically. However, data recently published by Schaffer et al, looked at claims rates for hospitalists, based on data from a medical liability insurer, covering physicians in the New England region. This study showed that the claims rate against hospitalists (0.52 claims per 100 physician coverage years [PCYs]) was significantly lower than that for nonhospitalist internal medicine physicians (1.91 claims per 100 PCYs), and emergency medicine physicians (3.50 claims per 100 PCYs). Among the claims filed against hospitalists, 32% resulted in payment, with a mean payment of $384,617. The severity of injury to the patient in the claims against hospitalists was high, with 50% of the claims involving the death of the patient.

Some studies have analyzed the epidemiology of medical injury in specific states. Examining more than 30,000 records of patients hospitalized in New York State in 1984, the Harvard Medical Practice Study is the largest study to assess the rate of medical malpractice injuries and claims. This study showed that adverse events occurred in 3.7% of hospitalizations; of these adverse events, 27.6% were determined to be due to negligence. In a further analysis of the Harvard Medical Practice Study by Localio et al, the overall rate of malpractice claims per discharge was 0.13%. In this study, the vast majority of adverse events did not result in a malpractice claim. Of the adverse events due to negligence that were identified, remarkably only about 2% resulted in malpractice claims. The estimated ratio of negligence to claims was 7.6 to 1.

Testing the generalizability of the results of the Harvard Medical Practice Study, a subsequent, methodologically similar study by Thomas et al, examined 15,000 hospital records from Utah and Colorado. In this study, which yielded comparable results to the Harvard Medical Practice Study, 2.9% of hospitalizations in each state involved adverse events. Of these adverse events, 32.6% were a result of negligence in Utah, and 27.4% were a result of negligence in Colorado. Additional analysis of these data by Studdert et al in 2000 showed that only about 3% of those patients who suffered a negligent injury filed a malpractice claim. Characteristics more common among patients who suffered negligence but did not file a malpractice claim include low income, uninsured, insured by Medicare or Medicaid, and age ≥75 years. Of those malpractice claims identified during the study period, 78% were made despite the absence of negligence and 56% were made despite the absence of an adverse event. The ratio of negligent adverse events to claims was 5.1 to 1 in Utah and 6.7 to 1 in Colorado.

The two main purposes of the medical malpractice system are to compensate patients who suffered injuries resulting from negligence, and to deter negligent behavior by imposing costs on physicians who practice negligently. These data call into question whether the medical malpractice system is achieving these objectives. Given the large number of adverse events due to negligence not leading to a malpractice claim, the medical malpractice system is not efficient at holding negligent physicians accountable, and many patients who have been injured as a result of malpractice are not receiving compensation. One implication of these data is that the rate of claims is a problematic metric to use in assessing quality of care, since most episodes of negligence do not lead to malpractice claims, and a significant number of malpractice claims are filed in the absence of negligence or injury.

A somewhat different picture emerges when the outcomes of claims are analyzed, rather than simply the filing of claims. Studdert et al in 2006 evaluated 1452 closed malpractice claims in which objective assessments were made by reviewers as to whether there were medical errors resulting in injury. Of those claims filed involving injuries, 63% were determined to be a result of error. In cases in which there was injury due to error, compensation was paid 73% of the time. In cases in which there were no errors, no compensation was paid 72% of the time. The authors of the study concluded that, although the malpractice system does a reasonable job of providing compensation only when there is injury as a result of a medical error, the process has significant shortcomings. Namely, cases take a long time to come to resolution (5 years, on average, from injury to disposition) and the monetary costs of litigating the claims are steep (54% of the compensation paid).

Thus the data show a very limited correlation between malpractice claims made and acts of actual malpractice. Based on the 2006 data from Studdert et al looking at the outcomes of claims, it appears that the majority of claims with merit result in compensation and the majority of meritless claims are denied compensation. However, the system of determining which claims have merit is protracted and expensive.

AREAS OF MEDICAL MALPRACTICE OF SPECIAL CONCERN TO HOSPITALISTS

■ INTRODUCTION

One analysis of 272 malpractice claims made against hospitalists found that the most common contributing factor underlying the cases was a problem with clinical judgment, such as failing to order an indicated diagnostic test or having too narrow a diagnostic focus. The second most common contributing factor was a breakdown in communication—either between the providers and the patient/family or among providers (**Table 35-1**).

Many of the areas of malpractice risk of specific concern to hospitalists relate to communication issues. The discontinuity between inpatient and outpatient care that is inherent to hospital medicine, as well as the multiple handoffs of patient care that can occur when hospitalists work shifts, both increase the risk of a communications breakdown that could result in injury due to negligence. Examples of areas of liability concern for hospitalists related to inadequate communication include failure to follow up on incidental findings (Case 35-1) and appropriately addressing test results that may be pending at the time of discharge.

CASE 35-1

FAILURE TO FOLLOW UP ON AN INCIDENTAL FINDING

A 62-year-old male with a significant smoking history presented to the emergency department (ED) in November 1999 after a fall resulting in a left shoulder injury. The ED physician took x-rays of the chest and left shoulder, read them as showing no fracture, and discharged the patient home. Four days later, the attending radiologist read the x-ray as showing a left lung nodule, and a report of the x-ray was sent to the ED physician and primary care physician (PCP). The radiologist did not call either the ED physician or the PCP. The patient saw his PCP twice in December 2000 for back and shoulder pain and was sent for physical therapy. The patient presented to the ED in August 2001 with chest and shoulder pain. A chest x-ray was obtained, which the ED attending read as normal, but the radiologist noted a large mass in the left lung. This information was not conveyed to the patient's PCP. After another visit to his PCP in September 2001, the patient presented to the ED again in October 2001 with back and chest pain, and a chest x-ray showed a mass occupying the majority of his left lung. The patient died of metastatic disease soon thereafter. The patient's children filed suit against the PCP, ED physician, and radiologist, and the suit was settled for more than $500,000.

Adapted from Wright J, McCormack P. Failure to act on incidental finding. CRICO Forum 2007;25:6-7.

The preceding case illustrates the liability pitfalls that can result from inadequate communication among the physician ordering a radiologic study (the ED physician), the physician interpreting the study (the radiologist), and the physician who is best suited to follow

TABLE 35-1 Contributing Factors in Hospitalist Medical Malpractice Cases (*n* = 272)*

Contributing Factor	# of Cases	% of Cases (95% CI)	Definition or Example
Clinical judgment	**148**	**54.4% (48.3%-60.4%)**	Problems with patient assessment or choice of therapy; failure/delay in obtaining consult/referral
Failure or delay in ordering a diagnostic test	36	13.2% (9.4%-17.8%)	
Failure or delay in obtaining a consult or referral	35	12.9% (9.1%-17.4%)	
Having too narrow a diagnostic focus	34	12.5% (8.8%-17.0%)	
Communication	**99**	**36.4% (30.7%-42.4%)**	Issues with communication among clinicians or between the clinicians and the patient or family
Inadequate communication among providers regarding the patient's condition	61	22.4% (17.6%-27.9%)	
Poor rapport with/lack of sympathy toward and patient and/or family	15	5.5% (3.1%-8.9%)	
Insufficient education of the patient and/or family regarding the risks of medications	9	3.3% (1.5%-6.2%)	
Documentation	**53**	**19.5% (14.9%-24.7%)**	Insufficient or lack of documentation
Administrative	**47**	**17.3% (13.0%-22.3%)**	Problems with staffing or hospital policies and protocols
Clinical systems	**44**	**16.2% (12.0%-21.1%)**	Failure or delay in scheduling a recommended test or failure to identify the provider coordinating care
Behavior related	**28**	**10.3% (7.0%-14.5%)**	Patient not following provider recommendations; seeking other providers due to dissatisfaction with care

*An individual case may have multiple contributing factors. Categories including <10% of cases are not reported. Nonsubstantive categories, such as inadequate information available, are excluded. Where subcategories are specified, only the top three subcategories are reported.
Adapted from Schaffer AC, Puopolo AL, Raman S, Kachalia A. Liability impact of the hospitalist model of care. *J Hosp Med.* 2014;9(12):750-755.

up on the abnormal results (the primary care physician). This case had features that are common in ED cases leading to malpractice claims, including the misreading of plain radiographs, the involvement of multiple individual failures, and process breakdowns.

■ PENDING TESTS AND INCIDENTAL FINDINGS

Hospitalists frequently find themselves in the same position as the ED physician in the above case, ordering a study of which the final results may not come back until after the patient has been discharged. The same problem applies to laboratory tests. One study by Roy et al encompassing the hospitalist services at two academic medical centers found that 41% of patients had laboratory or radiology results pending at the time of discharge and in 9.4% of cases the results of these studies were considered potentially actionable. Seventy percent of the inpatient physicians and 45.8% of the outpatient physicians were unaware of these potentially actionable results.

The problem of pending test results at the time of discharge is best addressed at a systems level—for example, through a mechanism that automatically notifies the ordering provider of the final results of such tests. However, such systems are not widely in place and even when they are, physicians still often fail to follow up on clinically significant results. Consequently, physicians need to take responsibility for following up on the final results of the tests that they order.

Physicians may also be held responsible for responding to test results ordered by another physician when these results come back while that physician is on duty, as was held in *Siggers v. Barlow* (906 F.2d 241). Responding to these test results often means communicating with the patient's PCP about what additional follow-up needs to occur, such as serial imaging for an incidentally discovered pulmonary nodule. Discharge summaries, while important, are generally not adequate as the only means of communicating important findings that need to be followed up by the PCP. Kripalani et al and Pantilat et al identified a number of potential deficiencies in the discharge summary as the sole means of communicating with the PCP. These deficiencies include the possibility that the discharge summary does not reach the correct PCP (occurring 25% of the time), failure to include tests pending at discharge (occurring 65% of the time), and the PCP not receiving the discharge summary prior to follow-up (occurring 67% of the time). Therefore, hospitalists should contact PCPs directly regarding important test results or other matters that need to be followed up, by phone and/or letter, and this communication should be documented in the patient's chart.

■ COORDINATION OF CONSULTANT CARE

Another potential area of malpractice liability is the use and coordination of consultants. Hospitalists list active coordination of consulting specialists as one of the benefits they bring to patient care. However, with this responsibility for coordination of specialists, and in their role of the attending physician of record for the patient, hospitalists are at risk of incurring malpractice liability based on the actions of the consulting specialists (see Case 35-2).

CASE 35-2

DOMBY V. MORITZ (2008 CAL. APP. UNPUB. LEXIS 1856)

A 67-year-old female with a history of hypertension checked her own blood pressure, found that it was elevated, and contacted her PCP. As instructed by her PCP, the patient took an extra dose of atenolol, after which she had an episode of syncope. She presented to the hospital, where she was bradycardic and so the ED physician gave the patient atropine and glucagon to reverse

the effects of the atenolol. A partner of the patient's cardiologist was contacted and advised to put an external pacemaker on the patient, but the cardiologist did not see the patient. The patient was admitted to the ICU by a hospitalist. In anticipation that an internal pacemaker might be needed, the hospitalist reversed the patient's warfarin with fresh frozen plasma. The ICU nurses called the cardiologist to report that the patient was bradycardic and feeling unwell. The cardiologist never placed an internal pacemaker. The hospitalist was next contacted by the ICU nurses once the patient was in cardiac arrest. The patient's family filed suit against both the cardiologist and the hospitalist. The court ultimately found in favor of the hospitalist.

Domby v. Moritz (2008 Cal. App. Unpub. LEXIS 1856) illustrates this risk. In filing suit against both the cardiologist and the hospitalist, the family of the patient asserted that the hospitalist should have ensured that the cardiologist physically came in to evaluate the patient. Although the court ultimately found in favor of the hospitalist, this case shows that hospitalists have to take an active role in discussing the treatment plan with consultants and in clearly delineating who has responsibility for which aspects of the patient's care. It may be legally hazardous to consider a clinical decision "not my call" and exclusively within the purview of a specialist, because the hospitalist, as the attending physician of record, may face litigation based on the decisions made by the consulting specialists.

RISK FACTORS FOR MEDICAL MALPRACTICE CLAIMS AND STRATEGIES TO REDUCE THIS RISK

In considering ways to reduce the risk of facing a medical malpractice claim, a key question to ask is why patients decide to file claims, given that the vast majority of patients who are injured due to medical errors do not initiate a malpractice action. One study, by Beckman et al examined 45 plaintiff depositions in medical malpractice cases and found that in 71% of cases there were significant relationship issues between the plaintiff and the defendant physician. The most common issue was the feeling by the patient of having been deserted by the physician. Examples include abandonment, and the physician being unavailable and sending associates such as residents in the place of the attending physician. Other relationship issues that were present in the examined depositions included: devaluing the patient (such as by discounting the patients' illness or pain); delivering information poorly (including failure to explain what was occurring); and failing to understand the patient's or family's perspective (such as by not asking for the patients' opinion).

The behavior of consulting specialists who are brought in after an adverse event has occurred may also influence whether a malpractice claim is filed. In 54.8% of cases, health care professionals raised questions about the care the patient had received, and in 70.6% of these cases, the health care professional who cast doubt on the quality of the care that had been provided by the defendant physician was a consultant who saw the patient after the adverse event. In a couple of cases, it was an acquaintance—who happened to be a health care professional but was not directly involved in the case—who suggested that the care received was substandard. Therefore, consultants seeing a patient after an adverse event need to be mindful that even an offhand remark on the care the patient has received may affect whether the patient pursues a malpractice claim.

These data suggest specific measures that may be taken to reduce the risk of a malpractice claim being filed. It is important to avoid those physician behaviors, such as creating conditions in which the patient may feel abandoned and not fully acknowledging the patient's concerns or discomfort. Given the possibility that having associates such as residents or physician assistants see the patient runs the risk of the patient feeling abandoned, the attending physician should explain the expected involvement of associates up front. It may also be helpful to frame the care to the patient as being provided by a team, so the patient does not feel connected only to the attending physician. It is also important to ensure that patient expectations about the outcome of a procedure or treatment are realistic. The informed consent process is an opportune occasion to address the patient's expectations.

Strong communication skills are also important. Supporting the benefit of good communication skills in reducing litigation, another study by Lester et al found that physicians, who exhibited "positive communication behaviors" such as making eye contact, acknowledging what the patient says, and spending more time with the patient, elicited reduced litigious feelings in observers. Hickson et al in 1994 showed that the patients of obstetricians with a high frequency of malpractice claims complained about these physicians' communication skills, including these physicians not listening and not providing information. The rate of these complaints about poor communication was significantly higher for physicians with a history of a high frequency of medical malpractice claims than for physicians with a better claims record.

On a systems level, it may be possible to identify physicians within an organization who are at increased risk of a malpractice claim. Physicians with an increased number of patient complaints have more risk management episodes, defined as both malpractice claims that are filed and incidents reported by staff members to the risk management department. One study by Hickson et al from 2002 retrospectively examined a cohort of 645 physicians, looking for an association between the number of unsolicited patient complaints and the number of risk management episodes. A small number of physicians generated a markedly disproportionate number of patient complaints, with 9% of the physicians garnering more than 50% of the complaints. There was a significant positive correlation between the number of complaints received and both the total number of risk management episodes and the number of lawsuits.

Similarly, another study by Stelfox et al found that scores from a commonly used hospital satisfaction survey were significantly associated with risk management episodes, which included both malpractice lawsuits and incidents identified by risk management as having the potential to result in a malpractice claim. The survey instrument included five questions asking patients to rank their inpatient attending physician in different areas, using a scale of 1 to 5 for each question, with a score of 5 denoting the highest rating. Each 1-point decrement on the survey correlated with a 5% increase in the rate of risk management episodes. The specific questions on the survey that had the strongest correlation with risk management episodes were those regarding the time the physician spent with the patient and the concern the physician showed for the patient's qualms. No significant correlation was found between the responses to questions on how satisfied the patient was with the physician's skill and the rate of risk management episodes. There was also a positive correlation between the rate of patient complaints and the rate of risk management episodes. Notably, a breakdown of complaints against physicians again suggested the crucial importance of good communication with the patient. Of the 483 complaints analyzed in the study, 75% of them concerned communication issues and 25% of them related to patient care matters. These two studies by Hickson et al and Stelfox et al show that by using data that are commonly collected by hospitals—number of complaints and the results of patient satisfaction surveys—it may be possible to identify physicians who are at elevated risk of being named in a malpractice action.

CASE 35-3

COMPLAINTS AGAINST DOCTOR A

Dr A is a physician who joined the hospitalist service 4 years ago. During his time as a member of the hospitalist group, his scores on patient satisfaction surveys have been in the lowest decile of physicians at the hospital. As the director of the hospitalist service, you receive a call from a manager in the patient relations department saying that Dr A has been the subject of two complaints within the past 6 months. The patient relations manager says both complaints are very similar, and the complaints describe Dr A as being unwilling to fully discuss his patients' medical conditions. The complaints further state that it seems like Dr A is always trying to get out of the patients' rooms as quickly as possible and that he appears annoyed when the patients ask questions. One of the patients who complained wrote: "Dr A just did not seem like he really cared about me or my many medical problems. I would not want him to take care of me again or any members of my family."

When you, as the director of the hospitalist service, meet with Dr A about these issues, he seems irritated and explains that every physician has at least a few disgruntled patients and that is part of practicing medicine. Dr A says he wants to make sure he sees all his patients and completes his billing forms promptly, and so he cannot be expected to linger in patients' rooms. Dr A further explains that if a patient asks a question that he deems important, then he makes sure to answer that question fully.

If it is possible to recognize physicians at increased risk of malpractice suits, such as Dr A in the preceding case, then potentially actions may be taken to mitigate this risk. For example, physicians who receive a high number of complaints or with particularly low satisfaction ratings could undergo educational programs aimed at enhancing their patient-communication skills. One approach, advocated by Moore et al consists of a tiered intervention system. Initially, a physician who has been identified as being at high risk is approached by a peer to discuss the issue. If that is not effective in improving the physician's complaint rate, then a plan for improvement is developed in conjunction with someone in authority, such as the department chair. If these efforts are still unsuccessful, meetings can be held with senior officials in hospital management, with the possibility of discipline or dismissal. Components of the plan to reduce the complaint rate (and so potentially also the risk of facing a malpractice action) can include enhancements to the management of the physician's practice, continuing medical education on the physician-patient relationship, and/or mental health evaluation.

DISCLOSING ERRORS TO PATIENTS

Physicians understandably are often conflicted about whether to disclose medical errors. Historically, physicians have been hesitant to disclose mistakes for fear of inviting litigation over an error that may otherwise have gone unnoticed by the patient, and in order to avoid possible censure over having made a mistake. An opposing view holds that disclosing errors will help avoid the strain in the patient-physician relationship and the breakdown in communication that may occur after a mistake, and so may decrease the risk of litigation, or at least lead to smaller awards.

The empirical evidence is inadequate to clearly answer what effect disclosure of medical errors will have on the likelihood of malpractice litigation. Policy changes regarding notification of patients about medical errors implemented by some medical centers do provide examples of the possible consequences of disclosure policies. In 1987, the Lexington, Kentucky, Veterans Affairs Medical Center (VAMC), in reaction to two large malpractice payouts, decided to put into place a policy of proactively identifying and investigating cases of possible medical negligence. If medical negligence was found, the representatives from the Lexington VAMC would have a face-to-face meeting with the patient or next of kin. At this meeting, hospital representatives would explain the situation, answer any questions, and offer restitution—the amount of which was based on a determination of actual loss. Claims assistance was also offered. Reviewing 15 years of experience with this full disclosure policy at the Lexington VAMC, Kraman et al concluded that this approach appeared to reduce the amount of overall malpractice payouts. Although the Lexington VAMC had an increased number of payouts, the average amount of these payouts was relatively small, at $14,500. This compares to a mean pretrial settlement amount of $98,000 for all medical centers in the VA system. Despite the Lexington VAMC being in the top quarter of all VAMCs in the number of tort claims filed, it was in the bottom quarter of all VAMCs in terms of total malpractice payouts. This VAMC experience has major limitations regarding its generalizability, because physicians in VAMCs do not pay individual malpractice premiums and, as federal government entities, VAMCs are not subject to punitive damages.

Several hospital systems and liability insurers have instituted programs that couple disclosure of unanticipated care outcomes with rapid offers of compensation in appropriate cases. The most widely published program is the one implemented by the University of Michigan Health System (UMHS) in 2002. In this program, unanticipated outcomes are promptly disclosed and investigated. The three principles the UMHS cites as defining their risk management approach are: (1) rapid offers of compensation when "unreasonable" care was the cause of the injury; (2) forceful defense of claims in which the care provided was reasonable; and (3) use of knowledge gained from the incidents to prevent future injuries and claims. With this policy in effect, the UMHS saw a decrease in monthly liability costs, in the rates of new claims, and in the time to resolution of claims. As with the VAMC program, questions exist about the generalizability of the UMHS program, especially since UMHS as an institution could assume legal responsibility when the outcome was due to systems-level problem. As a result of how tort laws are structured in some states, claims in those states are usually filed against individual physicians, rather than institutions, which might make some physicians hesitant to accept settlements, with the accompanying requirement of reporting the payment to the National Practitioner Data Bank.

Despite the encouraging reports from organizations implementing disclosure-and-offer programs, some uncertainty remains about disclosure as a risk management strategy, particularly when disclosures are not made in the context of compensation programs. A major legal concern about disclosure in the absence of some mechanism for awarding rapid and modest compensation is that, because most medical errors do not result in malpractice claims, aggressive disclosure of medical errors may prompt claims that would otherwise not have been filed. A theoretical modeling of this issue by Studdert et al in 2007 concluded that routine disclosure would have a 94% likelihood of increasing malpractice compensation costs. Regulatory protections that exist, such as state "apology laws" designed to allow physicians to apologize without having it used against them, may provide only very limited protection. These laws may prevent expressions of regret from being used against the physician, but not ancillary information surrounding that expression of regret, such as information about causation or fault.

Ultimately, one may expect to see progressively wider implementation of policies encouraging or even requiring error disclosure. The basis for this expectation is independent of the effect of error disclosure policies on malpractice costs, but is instead based on regulatory, public policy, and ethical considerations. Some states and accreditation organizations, such as The Joint Commission,

are increasingly implementing standards requiring error disclosure. Error disclosure, with the accompanying ability to gather data on what types of mistakes are recurring, also supports the public policy goal of improving systems so as to reduce future errors.

Disclosure of medical errors is generally considered the ethically appropriate course. Honesty is necessary to maintain a strong physician-patient relationship, and informed consent requires that patients be fully aware of the circumstances surrounding their treatment so they can decide about further care. Demonstrating this trend toward increasing disclosure of medical errors, a consensus statement from the Harvard-affiliated hospitals in 2006 expressed a commitment to full disclosure of medical errors in order "to change our systems to prevent future error" and because "it is the right thing to do."

PRACTICE POINT

- Disclosure of medical errors is generally considered the ethically appropriate course. Honesty is necessary to maintain a strong physician-patient relationship, and informed consent requires that patients be fully aware of the circumstances surrounding their treatment so they can decide about further care.

DEFENSIVE MEDICINE

Defensive medicine, as defined by a 1994 Office of Technology Assessment report, is "when doctors order tests, procedures, or visits, or avoid high-risk patients or procedures, primarily (but not necessarily solely) to reduce their exposure to malpractice liability." Defensive medicine may be categorized by whether it is positive, such as ordering of extra tests to try to forestall a malpractice claim, or negative, such as avoiding patients perceived as representing an increased malpractice risk. Some authors prefer the term "assurance behavior" in place of positive defensive medicine, and "avoidance behavior" in place of negative defensive medicine, so as to avoid the suggestion of approval or disapproval about defensive medicine.

Particularly in environments of high-liability stress, defensive medicine appears to be very common. A 2005 study by Studdert et al surveyed physicians in litigation-prone specialties (emergency medicine, general surgery, orthopedic surgery, neurosurgery, obstetrics/gynecology, and radiology) in Pennsylvania, which had experienced rapidly increasing malpractice premiums. Of the physicians who responded to the survey, 93% had engaged in defensive medicine and 42% were limiting the scope of their practice because of fear of liability. The most common type of defensive medicine in the survey was ordering extra tests, which 59% of physicians reported doing. This was especially common among emergency physicians, 70% of whom reported ordering extra tests. Physicians concerned about whether their malpractice insurance coverage was adequate and those who felt their insurance premiums were particularly onerous were especially likely to engage in defensive medicine. Common negative defensive medicine practices included avoiding high-risk patients, reported by 39% of physicians, and avoiding high-risk procedures, reported by 32% of physicians. Positive and negative defensive medicine practices have differing implications for the health care system. Positive defensive medicine has the potential to increase costs while offering modest, if any, benefits to patients. In contrast, negative defensive medicine may limit patients' access to certain medical services viewed as high risk, such as obstetrics.

Not only is defensive medicine common, but it is also expensive. Estimates of the costs of defensive medicine vary and are fraught with methodological limitations. One estimate is that approximately

5% to 9% of health care spending can be labeled as defensive. A concern is that if defensive medical practice becomes common enough, it may become the standard of care, which could force all physicians to practice in a defensive manner.

Overall, there is no clear empirical evidence that defensive medicine affects patient outcomes. There are some theoretical arguments against the practice of defensive medicine. Patients who perceive that their physician is ordering a test or procedure for a defensive reason may react negatively to this and be more likely to file a claim in the event of an adverse outcome. Some forms of defensive medicine involve physical risk to the patient—for example, ordering unnecessary biopsies and other invasive procedures. Particularly for these cases, services ordered primarily to serve the desire of the physician for minimizing risk and not the medical needs of the patient are ethically suspect. However, if fear of malpractice causes physicians to lower their tolerance for the possibility that a significant finding, such as a cancer, could be missed, then this effect is not necessarily deleterious. Indeed, some tests ordered primarily or solely to benefit the physician (by reducing medicolegal risk) end up having clear benefit to the patient. In the aggregate, though, defensive medical practices are likely cost ineffective.

ADDITIONAL STRATEGIES TO REDUCE THE RISK OF A MALPRACTICE CLAIM

A number of different strategies can be employed to potentially reduce the risk of a malpractice action. As discussed above, good communication practices with patients and their families are crucially important. Feelings on the part of patients that the physician is unavailable or dismissive of the patients' concerns may increase the risk of a malpractice claim. Delegating important communication tasks should be avoided. Residents and other trainees may not provide complete information to patients, may not convey information in a sensitive manner, and may not carefully document the communications they do have with patients.

A 2007 case decided by the Massachusetts Supreme Judicial Court highlighted the importance of informing patients about the potential side effects of their medications. The case, *Coombes v. Florio* (450 Mass. 182), concerned a 72-year-old patient on multiple medications (including oxycodone, tamsulosin, and oxazepam) who was driving and fatally struck a 10-year-old boy. The boy's mother sued both the driver of the car and the driver's physician, Dr Roland J. Florio. The Massachusetts court ruled that this was not a medical malpractice case, because the boy who was killed and his mother had no physician-patient relationship with Dr Florio. Nonetheless, the court held that Dr Florio could still be subject to a negligence claim, because he did have a duty to make the patient aware of the side effects of the medications the patient was taking so that the patient could make an informed decision about whether it was safe to drive. The court reasoned that if it was not safe for the patient to drive, then an accident, which might result in harm to parties other than the patient, was a foreseeable consequence. The court drew an analogy with a bar owner being found negligent when someone becomes inebriated at the bar and then drives and becomes involved in a fatal collision.

Inadequate communication among physicians, both between hospitalists, and between hospitalists and PCPs, is a significant liability concern for hospitalists. These communications should be standardized whenever possible. Handoffs of patient care between hospitalists should use a standardized form so that crucial information, such as diagnostic uncertainties and the status of communication with the PCP, is not overlooked. Although the discharge summary is not in and of itself adequate as the only means to communicate important information to a patient's PCP, it can be designed to help make sure the PCP receives important information arising from the hospitalization. For instance, the discharge summary can have standardized sections dedicated to tests pending at the time of discharge and issues requiring outpatient follow-up. Having these sections in all discharge summaries ensures that the person preparing the discharge summary addresses these areas and also gets PCPs accustomed to looking for this information in the discharge summaries. Even with standardized discharge forms, important issues requiring outpatient follow-up should still be directly communicated to the PCP, so as to minimize the chance that these matters get overlooked.

Checklists have been found to reduce complications and mortality in the surgical setting, and the benefits of checklists also extend to the medical setting. Checklists in Hospital Medicine have the potential to reduce errors that could give rise to a malpractice claim, such as the failure to use appropriate deep vein thrombosis (DVT) prophylaxis in a patient who subsequently develops a pulmonary embolus while in the hospital, or leaving a central venous catheter in a patient who then develops a catheter-related bloodstream infection. Checklists could also improve efficiency, such as by making sure a patient who needs a physical therapy evaluation receives one promptly. To enhance the effectiveness of a checklist in Hospital Medicine, other members of the care team, such as the nurses, should be involved in ensuring the components of the checklist have been met, and are empowered to raise the issue when the components of the checklist have not been met.

Informal "curbside" consultations is a potentially legally perilous practice. Questions to consultants about a specific patient should generally be made as a formal request for consultation, not an informal "curbside" consultation. When consultants provide "curbside" consultations, they are usually not seeing the patient and evaluating all the data, so their assessment may be based on incomplete information. Moreover, a "curbside" consultation does not result in a note from the consultant in the chart, so the basis for the consultant's recommendations will not be part of the medical record. A consultant who formally sees the patient will also usually be able to continue to follow the patient as an outpatient, which can help with the transition of care to the outpatient setting and provide a resource to whom the patient's PCP can turn for assistance. If the name of a consultant who provides a "curbside" consultation is placed in the chart, then if a malpractice claim arises, it is likely that the consultant will be named in the claim. **Table 35-2** summarizes strategies designed to reduce the risk of a malpractice claim.

COPING WITH A MALPRACTICE CLAIM

Being the subject of a malpractice claim is usually intensely stressful. Common reactions to being sued include anger, depressed mood, frustration, irritability, and insomnia. Samkoff and Gable have even compared physicians' reaction to a lawsuit with the five Kübler-Ross stages of grief: denial, anger, bargaining, depression, and then acceptance. Physicians are at risk of personalizing the claim and considering it an attack on their competence and character. The process of adjudicating is commonly protracted, often taking 4 to 5 years from the time of the adverse event to resolution of the case, thereby adding to the stress of a malpractice claim.

Approaches that may help physicians cope with the stress of a malpractice claim include discussing the stress with trusted friends, family, and colleagues. Discussions of specific details of the case should occur only in settings where privilege applies, such as with one's lawyer or with a therapist with whom one has a formal patient-clinician relationship. Open discussion with family about the accompanying stress may be especially helpful, since the stress of the malpractice claim is likely to affect family members. Colleagues should express support when they know an associate is facing a malpractice action. Some professional societies also offer specific counseling resources or referrals for physicians trying to deal with the stress of a malpractice action.

TABLE 35-2 Strategies to Reduce the Risk of a Medical Malpractice Claim

Strategy	Explanation
Maintain open and empathetic communication with patients and their families	Inadequate or insensitive communication from the physician is commonly cited as a reason that patients file a malpractice claim. Good communication with the patient may reduce the likelihood that a malpractice claim is filed, especially in the event of an unexpected outcome
Be careful about delegating communication	Delegating important communication tasks to trainees runs the risk of the information being conveyed in an insensitive manner, the communication not being well documented in the chart, and the patient taking offense that the attending physician did not care enough to come in person
Standardize handoffs	Standardizing handoffs, such as by having predesigned handoff forms, helps ensure that important information, such as pending tests requiring follow-up, are communicated to the incoming physician
Standardize discharge summaries	One way to make sure that the discharge summary contains crucial items, such as tests pending at the time of discharge and issues that require outpatient follow-up, is to have a standardized discharge template with sections prompting the inclusion of this information
Directly communicate with PCPs	Important items requiring outpatient follow-up, such as an incidentally discovered lung nodule, should be communicated directly to the PCP by letter or telephone call, and this communication should be documented in the chart. A discharge summary alone is not adequate to communicate important follow-up matters
Use checklists	Checklists can ensure that routine measures required for most patients, such as DVT prophylaxis, are not overlooked. Implementation of checklists should involve the entire care team
Avoid "curbside" consultations	Consultants who provide "curbside" consultations make recommendations based on what may be incomplete information and there is no record of the consultation in the chart
Recognize that hospitalists can be held responsible for consultants' decisions	When a consultant is negligent, the hospitalist, as the attending of record, is likely to be named in the claim. When a hospitalist has concerns about the decisions of a consultant, this should be discussed with the consultant. The responsibilities of the consultant should be clearly defined
Collect and provide feedback to physicians	Negative feedback from patients about a physician, particularly about the physician's communication skills, can signal that this physician is at elevated risk of a malpractice claim. This feedback should be conveyed to the physician, and a plan to remedy the identified deficiencies should be made

One of the reasons malpractice claims can be so stressful for physicians is that so much of their own identity revolves around their profession. Realizing this, the physician should attempt to depersonalize the claim. Most claimants have as their primary objective obtaining compensation, not vilifying the physician. Physicians dealing with a malpractice suit should use it as an occasion to assess whether they have appropriate balance between their professional lives and their leisure time. Spending time engaged in vocational pursuits, such as hobbies and time with friends, is important. Physicians should also have the lawyer representing them explain what the process of adjudicating the claim will entail, so that the process is demystified and surprises are minimized. The facts surrounding the case should be examined to see if there is a systems-level issue that can be addressed to help prevent future claims—for example, designing a system for reviewing incoming radiology studies if a radiographic finding was missed.

There are some specific pitfalls that must be avoided during the stress of malpractice litigation. Physicians facing a malpractice claim who do not have a formal PCP should obtain one, as a PCP can be helpful with medication for symptoms and referrals for counseling. Self-medication should be avoided. Insomnia is a common symptom arising from the stress of a malpractice claim, and physicians who feel medication is needed to treat insomnia should discuss this with their own physician, and should not self-prescribe or obtain medication from a colleague informally. One action that should never be taken is going back and altering any documents in an effort to assist one's defense. Not only is this unethical and potentially criminal, but also by the time a physician is aware that a malpractice claim may be filed, the filing party almost certainly has copies of the medical records and related documents.

When a claim results in payment on behalf of an individual physician, there are reporting requirements. Information about this payment must be reported to the National Practitioner Data Bank (NPDB), which was established by the Health Care Quality Improvement Act of 1986. The Act was intended to improve the quality of medical care, in part by requiring the submission of malpractice payments to the NPDB, which can then be queried by health care institutions when making hiring decisions. Patients and individuals do not have access to reports of physician malpractice payments made to the NPDB, although physicians can request their own NPDB files. Some states, however, have web sites that allow patients to look up individual physicians and find out information about their malpractice histories.

CONCLUSION

Popular perceptions notwithstanding, the medical malpractice system appears to do a reasonable job of awarding compensation primarily in cases that actually involve an injury due to negligence. Nevertheless, the system is inefficient and expensive. In addition, most adverse events resulting from negligence never lead to claims or compensation, and meritless malpractice claims also remain a problem.

PRACTICE POINT

- In seeking to avoid malpractice claims, physicians need to be conscientious about communicating with the patient, so that the patient does not feel abandoned or devalued. Although medical liability experience involving hospitalists specifically is limited, issues hospitalists need to be careful about include coordinating the actions of consulting specialists, following up on pending tests, and communicating with PCPs about issues that require outpatient follow-up.

Legal citations

Domby v. *Moritz*, 2008 Cal. App. Unpub. LEXIS 1856

Coombes v. *Florio*, 450 *Mass*. 182 (2007)

Siggers v. *Barlow*, 906 F.2d 241 (1990)

Beilke v. *Coryell*, 524 N.W.2d 607, 610 (N.D. 1994)

Hill v. *Medlantic Health Care Group*, 933 A.2d 314, 325 (D.C. App. 2007)

Kent v. *Pioneer Valley Hospital*, 930 P.2d 904, 906 (Ut. App. 1997)

Palandjian v. *Foster*, 842 N.E.2d 916, 921-22 (Mass. 2006)

Polozie v. *United States,* 835 F. Supp. 68, 72-74 (D. Conn. 1993)

Health Care Quality Improvement Act of 1986, Pub. L. No. 99-660, 100 Stat. 3743 (codified as amended in scattered sections of 42 U.S.C.).

ACKNOWLEDGMENT

The author would like to thank Prof. Michelle M. Mello for her review of the manuscript and Nicholas Beshara, JD, MPH for his contribution to the previous edition's chapter.

SUGGESTED READINGS

Beckman HB, Markakis KM, Suchman AL, et al. The doctor-patient relationship and malpractice. Lessons from plaintiff depositions. *Arch Intern Med*. 1994;154:1365-1370.

Brennan TA, Leape LL, Laird NM, et al. Incidence of adverse events and negligence in hospitalized patients. Results of the Harvard Medical Practice Study I. *N Engl J Med*. 1991;324:370-376.

Schaffer AC, Puopolo AL, Raman S, et al. Liability impact of the hospitalist model of care. *J Hosp Med*. 2014;9(12):750-755.

Stelfox HT, Gandhi TK, Orav EJ, et al. The relation of patient satisfaction with complaints against physicians and malpractice lawsuits. *Am J Med*. 2005;118:1126-1133.

Studdert DM, Mello MM, Brennan TA. Medical malpractice. *N Engl J Med*. 2004;350(3):283-292.

Studdert DM, Mello MM, Gawande AA, et al. Claims, errors, and compensation payments in medical malpractice litigation. *N Engl J Med*. 2006;354:2024-2033.

SECTION 8
Professional Development

C H A P T E R 36

Principles of Adult Learning and Continuing Medical Education

Jeffrey A. Tabas, MD
Robert B. Baron, MD, MS

INTRODUCTION

Most physicians learn through informal approaches, including reading, point-of-care learning, and consulting colleagues. More formal adult learning occurs mainly through continuing medical education (CME). The approach to physician learning through CME is changing and hospitalists are poised to play a crucial role in its development. Hospitalists are increasingly the primary teachers in the hospital setting and play a major role in performance improvement. Modern CME integrates these two processes. In this chapter, we discuss principles of adult learning, the changing landscape of CME, and the resultant responsibilities and opportunities for hospitalists.

ADULT LEARNING

Adult learning is complex. Understanding the framework of adult learning theory can help inform curricular design, teaching, and evaluation. Of the many theories of adult learning, three are most influential: the behaviorist, cognitivist, and constructivist theories. No single theory fits the learning style of all adult learners, and most educators use elements from each.

- Behaviorism, popularized by B.F. Skinner, focuses on using consequences to shape behavior. A desired behavior is rewarded with positive reinforcement, while undesired behavior is discouraged with negative reinforcement. This theory emphasizes that feedback is critical to learning.
- Cognitivism tries to explain learning through information-processing models and minimizes the focus on the behavioral response. It highlights the importance of information that is appropriately organized by the educator and the development of problem-solving skills by the learner.
- Constructivism, popularized by Jean Piaget, teaches that learners construct new knowledge from experiences they integrate into their own existing framework of understanding when the experience is consistent with that framework. When the experience is inconsistent with that framework, they either change their perceptions of the experience or reframe their internal model of understanding. This theory emphasizes the educator's role as facilitator instead of didactic teacher and the learner's need for a social and active learning process.

Together, these theories suggest that adults learn most effectively when they (1) perceive the relevance of educational material, (2) are actively engaged, (3) have input into choosing educational experiences and directing their own learning, and (4) have the chance to step back and reflect on their learning.

Moore has proposed that adult learning involves a five-stage process. These are: (1) recognizing an opportunity for learning; (2) searching for resources for learning; (3) engaging in learning to address an opportunity for improvement; (4) trying out what was learned; and (5) incorporating what was learned. Learning occurs not as a linear progression through these stages, but as a dynamic process with complex interactions that include revisiting and concurrence of various stages. CME may stimulate the first stage by providing the recognition that the opportunity for learning exists ("I did not know that continuous positive airway pressure [CPAP] decreases intubation in patients with congestive heart failure [CHF]") or the third stage by providing the learning needed to address the opportunity for improvement ("I developed the competence to appropriately select candidates for CPAP and the steps to implement it").

As described above, learners most readily progress through stages when they see relevance ("ICU beds are limited and I can save hospital resources by avoiding intubation"), are actively engaged ("The CME presentation used dynamic learning approaches such as case presentations, question and answer, or audience response systems"), have chosen the subject ("I want to learn how to implement CPAP"), and reflect on their learning experience ("Is this something that would work in my institution and do I need more learning to effectively implement this?").

CME EFFECTIVENESS

The best available evidence suggests that CME is effective in achieving and maintaining knowledge, competence, and procedural skills, as well as improving physician performance and patient health outcomes, if the activity is planned and implemented according to recommended approaches. Assessments show that interventions using live educational strategies are more effective than print, that multimedia are more effective than single media, and that multiple exposures are more effective than a single exposure. Simulation methods in medical education seem effective in disseminating psychomotor and procedural skills.

THE ROLE OF THE HOSPITALIST IN CONTINUING EDUCATION

Research reveals significant gaps between the medical care that patients actually receive and the care they should be getting. Hospitals that have hospitalists provide care closer to the ideal—their care is associated with better performance measures, such as improved diagnosis, treatment, counseling, and prevention, as well as decreased length of stays and hospital costs. The hospitalist plays an essential role in closing the quality gaps through implementing guidelines and reporting and implementing quality measures. Much of that role involves changing physician behaviors, which is the essence of CME. Given that many nationally reported quality measures—heart failure, acute myocardial infarction, pneumonia, asthma, venous thromboembolism, and stroke care, among others—fall within the purview of the hospitalist, the hospitalist must be versed in the theory of CME and be prepared to deliver such activities.

THE CHANGING LANDSCAPE OF CME

Continuing medical education has traditionally used didactic lectures and reading followed by testing to confirm knowledge, with little heed paid to the importance of physician practice behaviors. The focus of modern CME has evolved from increasing knowledge to improving physician competence, physician performance, and patient outcomes. This is reflected in the drive to incorporate practice-based learning and improvement into all aspects of continuing education and accreditation. Driven by the link to quality in patient safety, the American Board of Medical Specialties has mandated that all specialty boards adopt practice performance assessment as the fourth component in maintaining certification. The American Board of Internal Medicine was one of the first specialty boards to adopt this requirement. The Federation of State Medical Boards has also discussed the value of performance improvement in maintaining licensure. As a result of this changing focus, the Accreditation Council for Continuing Medical Education (ACCME) has incorporated self-directed physician improvement and change as a desired outcome of CME activities. ACCME has developed the following systematic approach to ensure appropriate planning, implementation, and assessment of each CME activity:

1. Identify the professional practice gap—the difference between current practice and optimal performance—appropriate to learners of this activity. Current practice can be identified through auditing individual physicians or practice groups, or from reported hospital, regional, or national data involving registries or national quality measures. Performance can reflect patient outcomes, such as mortality or readmission rates, or process measures, such as counseling for smoking cessation in patients with pneumonia. Optimal performance can be determined through assessing practice guidelines, medical literature, national benchmarks, and the like. The difference between the two is the practice gap. Professional practice gaps are not limited to patient care but can also involve other areas, such as research or administrative practice.

2. Identify the educational needs—improved knowledge, competence, or performance—that should be addressed to close the practice gap. These can be determined by surveying learners, interviewing thought leaders in the content area, or reviewing literature.

3. Identify which outcomes the activity is designed to improve—competence (strategies to apply knowledge), performance (what is done in practice), or patient outcomes—and how they will be measured (for example by looking at changes in hospital quality measures). Improved knowledge alone, which may be an educational need, is not an adequate outcome. For example, the educational need may be a lack of knowledge of the indications for CPAP in patients with CHF, but the outcome should be the ability to apply that knowledge to appropriately select the patients that might benefit from the therapy when presented with several case scenarios.

4. Select an appropriate educational format to encourage this change (for example, a case-based lecture with spaced learning using follow-up e-mail reminders).

5. Identify the potential barriers to change, and describe how to address them.

6. Identify ways to cooperate and collaborate outside of the CME activity to help facilitate change, such as interaction with the quality department or other organizations.

Educators who thoroughly understand and apply this approach will be better able to provide the quality learning needed to effect the desired improvements.

OTHER FORMS OF CME

Point of Care CME (PoCCME) is CME developed by an accredited provider that includes self-directed online learning. A physician answers a clinical patient question in real time using an evidence-based source and then documents the question, the sources consulted, and the resultant application to practice. For example, a physician needs to know the parameters used to determine when a patient with CHF can be weaned off CPAP. Working with an accredited provider, she goes online to determine the criteria for weaning, and then documents her question, sources, and how she will use the information. That physician can then receive PoCCME credit.

Performance Improvement CME (PICME) is awarded when a physician or group of physicians performs a three-step process in which they (1) learn how to measure performance and then assess their practice, (2) develop an intervention based on best practice, and (3) remeasure performance and then reflect on the impact of the intervention. PICME typically involves longer-term interventions and activities that require chart review or data collection. These activities may address the structure, process, or outcome of a physician's practice with direct implications for patient care. The goal is for CME to be an active process that occurs within the clinical care setting, as opposed to a more passive process in a nonclinical setting. It acknowledges that some process changes require systems-level change. Objectives include learning the performance improvement process, taking an active role in learning and change, and attempting to directly improve patient care processes and outcomes through an educational activity.

For example, a hospitalist group identifies a gap between the observed Central Line-Associated Bloodstream Infection (CLASBI) rate and the desired rate, based on national guidelines. They develop a tool to self-report compliance with the central catheter insertion "bundle" and measure the rate of compliance. The group then implements a training activity and monitors the self-reported rate of compliance or subsequent CLASBI infection rates. If rates have not improved, they analyze their approach again, looking for other needs that can be addressed to improve these outcomes. While drawbacks to this approach are the prolonged effort and time required, these may not be any greater than the effort, time, and cost of traveling to a several-day live meeting, and may yield significantly greater improvements in care. With their established track record in patient safety and quality and the advent of PICME, hospitalists are a natural resource for implementing this form of CME.

The American Board of Medical Specialties (ABMS) released updated standards in 2015 for maintenance of certification part 4 activities—Improvement in Medical Practice. These require the physician to demonstrate competence in systematic measurement and improvement in patient care. Such activities can also meet the requirements for PICME, thereby allowing multiple forms of credit for activities that are integrated into the normal workflow of practice to improve patient care.

PRACTICAL IMPACT OF THE HOSPITALIST ON CME

The role of hospitalists in CME continues to expand. Programs have been developed for hospitalists as agents of change in venues ranging from university CME programs, to the Society of Hospital Medicine, to the Agency for Healthcare Research and Quality (AHRQ). Hospitalists should incorporate the principles described above into the CME planning and education process. This would include close collaboration and communication between educators and the institutional staff responsible for quality and safety initiatives. Approaches to planning internal CME such as grand rounds might include comparing hospital-quality data to national guidelines to identify gaps and then surveying physicians to identify needs related to those gaps. An example of a planned activity after identification of a practice gap and learning needs, such as for CLASBI rates, might include hands-on skills workshops with trainers to improve techniques (performance) in central line insertion practices. CME activity assessment could include before-and-after surveys to determine whether the activity's content relates to their practice and how it has changed that practice. More robust assessment would include measuring changes in process or patient outcomes in conjunction with the hospital quality department.

CONCLUSION

Hospitalists are poised to play a major role in the future of CME. This will include use of interactive case-based learning, simulation, and other learning formats, in the same way we teach students and residents. It will also include defining practice gaps, providing process and outcomes data as a basis for self-assessment, teaching performance improvement principles as a template for educational interventions, and incorporating point-of-care learning and teaching into their practice.

SUGGESTED READINGS

Accreditation Council for Continuing Medical Education (ACCME). Proposal for New Criteria for Accreditation with Commendation. http://www.accme.org/requirements/accreditation-requirements-cme-providers/proposal-new-criteria-accreditation-commendation. April 23, 2014. Accessed October 1, 2015.

Cervero RM, Gaines J. The impact of CME on physician performance and patient health outcomes. *J Contin Educ Health Prof.* 2015;35(2):131-137.

Combes JR, Arespacochaga E. Continuing Medical Education as a Strategic Resource. http://www.ahaphysicianforum.org/resources/leadership-development/CME/index.shtml. September 2014. Accessed October 1, 2015.

Iglehart JK, Baron RB. Maintenance of certification. *N Engl J Med.* 2013;368(13):1262-1263.

Institute of Medicine (IOM). Measuring the Impact of Interprofessional Education and Collaborative Practice and Patient Outcomes. http://www.iom.edu/Reports/2015/Impact-of-IPE.aspx. April 22, 2015. Accessed October 1, 2015.

McMahon GT. Advancing continuing medical education. *JAMA.* 2015;314(6):561-562.

O'Leary KJ, Afsar-Manesh N, Budnitz T, et al. Hospital quality and patient safety competencies: development, description, and recommendations for use. *J Hosp Med.* 2011;6(9):530-536.

Rosenbluth G, Tabas JA, Baron RB. What's in it for me? Maintenance of certification as an incentive for faculty supervision of resident quality improvement projects. *Acad Med.* 2016;91(1):56-59.

Tabas JA, Baron RB. Commercial funding of accredited continuing medical education. *BMJ.* 2012;344:e810.

CHAPTER 37

Cultural Competence

Germán E. Giese, MD

Sarahi Rodríguez-Pérez, MD

Efrén Manjarrez, MD, SFHM

INTRODUCTION AND NEEDS ASSESSMENT

During the last 25 years cultural diversity has increased dramatically due to global migration. The 2013 International Migration Report from the Department of Economic and Social Affairs of the United Nations revealed that the United States has six times as many immigrants as all of Latin America. The United States also resettles the largest number of migrants in the world and provides more benefits and welfare than any other nation. The United States hosts about 20% of the world's global migrants.

In 2013, about 39% of the US population identified themselves as members of minority groups. Hispanic and African American groups were the largest minority groups, accounting for 17% and 13% of the population, respectively. By 2050, it is projected that minority groups will account for almost half of the US population (**Figure 37-1**).

While African Americans and Hispanics are the largest minority groups in the United States, they are also the most underrepresented minorities in medicine. Only 6% of practicing physicians come from these groups (**Figure 37-2**). These physicians often carry the responsibility of providing health care for these minority communities. Although the number of minority students entering medical school is increasing, it is not increasing at a rate to ensure a culturally competent physician workforce (**Table 37-1**). The racial and ethnic disparities are an ongoing phenomenon in both medical school enrollment and graduating physicians from US medical schools (**Table 37-2**). The inclusion of International Medical Graduates (IMGs) into residency programs in different specialties might mitigate some of these disparities. However, the proportion of residency positions filled with IMGs is still small compared to the number filled by US graduates (**Table 37-3**).

IMPACT OF CULTURAL COMPETENCE AND DISPARITIES ON HEALTH CARE QUALITY

The National Quality Forum (NQF) defines cultural competency as the "ongoing capacity of health care systems, organizations, and professionals to provide for diverse patient populations high-quality care that is safe, patient and family centered, evidence based, and equitable." Cultural competency may be achieved through "policies, learning processes, and structures by which organizations and individuals develop the attitudes, behaviors, and systems that are needed for effective cross-cultural interactions." When caring for different cultural groups, physicians should ideally have awareness and appreciation of the specific traditions, and cultural and religious values of their patients, as these factors greatly influence human behavior and decision making.

Differences in ethnicity and traditions may impact the patient-provider relationship, specifically when there is discordance between provider and patient ethnicity or language, and impact effective delivery of quality health care. Health care systems need to be able to understand and accommodate multicultural population needs. In addition to this being "the right thing to do," understanding and accommodating diverse patient populations will also affect health care system reimbursement. For example, the Physician Quality Reporting System (PQRS, formerly known as the Physician Quality Reporting Initiative), is a health care quality improvement incentive program that was initiated by the Centers for Medicare and Medicaid Services (CMS) in 2006; it constitutes an example of a "pay for performance" program that financially rewards providers

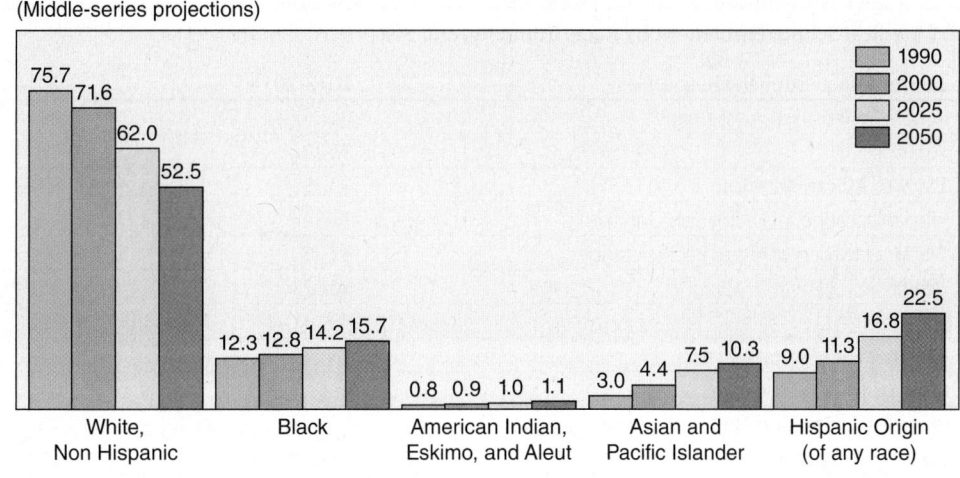

(Middle-series projections)

Figure 37-1 *Percent of US population by race and Hispanic origin: 1990, 2000, 2025, 2050.*

for reporting health care quality data to CMS. Beginning in 2015, the program will apply a negative payment adjustment to practices which do not satisfactorily report data on quality measures. The PQRS program includes 254 quality measures further grouped into six main health care quality domains, one of which is related to patient satisfaction. The same is true of the hospital Value-Based Purchasing program; hospitals can gain or lose up to 2% of their CMS funding based on their performance in the program, of which 25% rests on patient satisfaction scores. Meeting a patient's needs with cultural competence (and therefore ensuring their satisfaction) is now necessary to be financially viable in many value-based purchasing programs.

The 2001 Institute of Medicine (IOM) report, *Crossing the Quality Chasm*, identified a significant gap between the quality of health

care people should receive, and the quality of care they actually receive. Another influential IOM report, *Unequal Treatment: Confronting Racial and Ethnic Disparities in Health Care* (2002), concluded that people of color often receive lower-quality care than their white counterparts—even when insurance and socioeconomic status, comorbidities, stage of presentation, and other factors are taken into account.

Health disparities at any level pose a significant threat to patient safety and therefore represent an opportunity to implement institutional quality improvement strategies to mitigate the disparities. For example, improving patient–provider communication via interventions such as the appropriate use of interpreters should decrease the risk of misdiagnosis, decrease unnecessary procedures and diagnostic testing, and increase the participation of patients

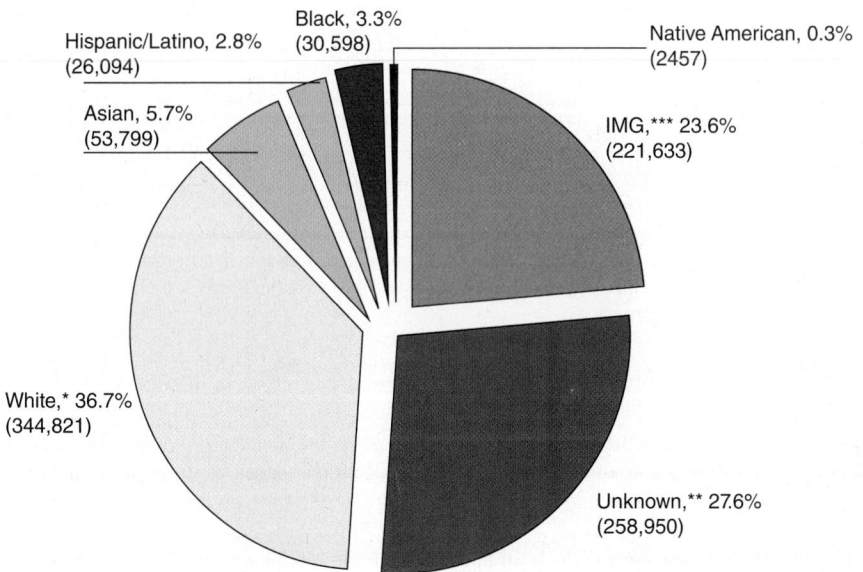

Note: Asian includes Chinese, Filipino, Korean, Japanese, Vietnamese, Indian/Pakistani, Other Asian;
Hispanic/Latino Includes Mexican American, C'Wealth Puerto Rican, Mainland Puerto Rican, Other Hispanic;
Native American includes American Indian/Alaska Native, and as of 1996, Native Hawaiians.
*These data mainly represent White physicians who graduated from U.S. allopathic medical schools from 1978 to 2004.
**Includes physicians who graduated from Canadian medical schools, doctors of osteopathic medicine, and most likely Whites who graduated prior to 1978.
***International Medical Graduates.

Data Source: AAMC Data Warehouse: Minority Physician Database, Applicant-Matriculant file, and AMA Physician Masterfile, as of March 16, 2006.

Figure 37-2 *2004 US physicians by race/ethnicity.*

TABLE 37-1 Total US Medical School Enrollment by Race, Ethnicity, and Sex

	Student Race/Ethnicity Responses[1]	2013-2014	2014-2015
Women[2]	American Indian or Alaska native	94	97
	Asian	8,329	8,511
	Black or African American	3,185	3,188
	Hispanic, Latino, or of Spanish Origin	11,527	1,615
	Native Hawaiian or Other Pacific Islander	47	56
	White	20,623	20,895
	Other	402	529
	Multiple Race/Ethnicity	3,447	3,560
	Unknown Race/Ethnicity	494	648
	Non-U.S. Citizen and Non-Permanent Resident[3]	762	789
	Total For Women	*38,910*	*39,888*
Men[2]	American Indian or Alaska Native	89	108
	Asian	8,818	8,885
	Black or African American	2,043	2,147
	Hispanic, Latino, or of Spanish Origin	1,630	1,829
	Native Hawaiian or Other Pacific Islander	46	61
	White	*26,371*	*26,497*
	Other	507	635
	Multiple Race/Ethnicity	3,469	3,559
	Unkown Race/Ethnicity	655	799
	Non-U.S. Citizen and Non-Permanent Resident[3]	853	852
	Total for Men	*44,481*	*45,372*
All	American Indian or Alaska Native	183	205
	Asian	17,147	17,396
	Black or African American	5,228	5,335
	Hispanic, Latino, or of Spanish Origin	3,157	3,444
	Native Hawaiian or Other Pacific Islander	93	117
	White	46,994	47,392
	Other	909	1,164
	Multiple Race/Ethnicity	6,916	7,119
	Unknown Race/Ethnicity	1,149	1,447
	Non-U.S. Citizen and Non-Permanent Resident[3]	1,615	1,641
	Total	*83,391*	*85,260*

[1]In 2013, the methodology for acquiring race/ethnicity information was updated. Rather than one question asking an applicant's Hispanic origin and a second question asking the applicant's race, the Hispanich origin and race response options are now listed together under a single question about how applicants self-identity, Applicants could select multiple response options.
[2]Four applicants in 2013 and six applicants in 2014 who declined to resport gender are not reflected.
[3]The "Non-U.S. Citizen and Non-Permanent Resident" Category may include students with unknown citizenship.

and families in clinical decision making. Utilizing providers that are familiar with the social and cultural traditions of patients is an effective strategy to improve their health care outcomes. For example, a study performed at a rural clinic in Canada treating an aboriginal community found that the introduction of culturally sensitive programs was associated with increased appointment attendance (from 25% before the program to 85% after the program). Involvement of aboriginal nurses, inclusion of culturally sensitive activities, and participation in spiritual ceremonies were also associated with higher patient satisfaction, higher trust toward the health care team, and better communication amongst participants.

STANDARDS FOR CULTURAL COMPETENCE

Unfortunately, cultural competence is a vague concept for front line health care providers. That is one of the reasons why specific strategies to improve it are still lacking across the board. The majority of physicians and health care providers are unable to articulate approaches or culturally sensitive strategies to practice in a culturally competent way, and there is an historical lack of standardized training nationally. This is consistent with the literature, which suggests that although "cultural competence" is broadly supported, consensus definition, detailed understanding, and standardized training frameworks are lacking.

Facing this reality, the US Department of Health and Human Services' Office of Minority Health published in 2000 the first *National Standards for Culturally and Linguistically Appropriate Services in Health Care* (National CLAS Standards), which provided a framework for all health care organizations to best serve the nation's increasingly diverse communities (later updated between 2010 and 2013). The CLAS Standards are divided into a "principal standard," plus 14 other standards grouped into three domains which are (1) Governance, Leadership, and Workforce, (2) Communication and Language

TABLE 37-2 Total US Medical School Graduate Race/Ethnicity and Sex, 2012-2013 and 2013-2014

	Graduate Race/Ethnicity Responses[1]	Class of 2013	Class of 2014
Women[2]	American indian or Alaska Native	11	16
	Asian	1,837	1,829
	Black or African American	656	675
	Hispanic, Latino, or of Spanish Origin	446	479
	Native Hawaiian or Other pacific Islander	3	3
	White	4,816	4,674
	Other	132	126
	Multiple Race/Ethnicity	634	587
	Unknown Race/Ethnicity	5	18
	Non-U.S. Citizen and Non-permanent Resident[3]	180	172
	Total for Women	*8,720*	*8,579*
Men[2]	American Indian or Alaska Native	14	11
	Asian	1,809	1,872
	Black or African American	336	377
	Hispanic, Latino, or of Spanish Origin	429	449
	Native Hawaiian or Other pacific Islander	2	1
	White	5,947	5,784
	Other	166	174
	Multiple Race/Ethnicity	556	581
	Unknown Race/Ethnicity	5	57
	Non-U.S. Citizen and Non-permanent Resident[3]	170	193
	Total for Men	*9,434*	*9,499*
All	American Indian or Alaska Native	25	27
	Asian	3,646	3,701
	Black or African American	992	1,052
	Hispanic, Latino, or of Spanish origin	875	928
	Native Hawaiian or Other pacific Islander	5	4
	White	10,763	10,458
	Other	298	300
	Multiple Race/Ethnicity	1,190	1,168
	Unknown Race/Ethnicity	10	75
	Non-U.S. Citizen and Non-permanent Resident[3]	350	365
	Total	*18,154*	*18,078*

[1]In 2013, the methodology for acquiring race/ethnicity information was updated. Rather than one question asking an applicant's Hispanic origin and a second question asking the applicant's race, the Hispanich origin and race response options are now listed together under a single question about how applicants self-identity, Applicants could select multiple response options.

[2]Four applicants in 2013 and six applicants in 2014 who declined to resort gender are not reflected.

[3]The "Non-U.S. Citizen and Non-Permanent Resident" Category may include students with unknown citizenship.

Assistance, and (3) Engagement, Continuous Improvement, and Accountability. The principal standard is "to provide effective, equitable, understandable and respectful quality care, and services that are responsive to diverse cultural health beliefs and practices, preferred languages, health literacy, and other communication needs."

IDENTIFYING AND OVERCOMING BARRIERS OF CULTURAL COMPETENCE

Cultural and social differences represent imaginary lines separating multicultural health care providers and patients, predisposing and contributing to stereotyping, xenophobic, and discriminatory behaviors. For example, the 1932 US Public Health Service Tuskegee Syphilis Study on Untreated Syphilis in the Negro Male was a federally funded trial that withheld available treatment from African American men with syphilis. Research has demonstrated that African Americans' knowledge of this history of racial discrimination is associated with reluctance to participate in medical research, and may be associated with low rates of trust (and subsequent adherence to treatment). Patterns of trust in different components of our health care system (physicians vs hospitals vs insurance companies) also differ by race. Differences in trust may reflect different cultural experiences and expectations for care.

One major barrier in mutual cultural understanding is the lack of intercultural care training within the health care workforce. Hiring translators or translation services can easily overcome a language barrier, but it will not overcome cultural and social barriers. Most health care organizations have not implemented formal training programs to enhance culture competence among their workforce.

Health care institutions and provider groups should promote hiring ethnically diverse physicians and professional staff, as working in a culturally diverse environment allows prejudice and stereotypes to be contrasted with reality through awareness and understanding.

TABLE 37-3 Matches by Applicant Type, 2015

Specialty	Number of Positions	Number Filled	U.S. Senior	U.S. Grad	Osteo	Canadian	5th Pathway	U.S. IMG	Non-U.S. IMG	Number Unfilled
PGY-1 Positions										
Anesthesiology	1094	1,066	799	19	137	1	0	58	52	28
Child Neurology	104	95	73	0	10	0	0	5	7	9
Dermatology	22	22	20	2	0	0	0	0	0	0
Emergency Medicine	1,821	1,813	1,438	60	203	1	0	75	36	8
Emergency Med-Family Med	4	4	1	0	1	0	0	2	0	0
Family Medicine	3,195	3,039	1,405	139	446	3	0	680	366	156
Family Med-Preventive Med	5	5	5	0	0	0	0	0	0	0
Iternal Medicine (Categorical)	66,770	6,698	3,317	101	511	5	1	894	1,869	72
Medicine-Anesthesiology	6	6	4	1	0	0	0	1	0	0
Medicine-Dermatology	6	6	6	0	0	0	0	0	0	0
Medicine-Emergency Med	28	27	23	0	3	0	0	1	0	1
Medicine-Family Medicine	2	2	1	0	0	0	0	1	0	0
Medicine-Medical Genetics	4	4	2	0	0	0	0	1	1	0
Medicine-Neurology	1	0	0	0	0	0	0	0	0	1
Medicine-Pediatrics	380	379	319	2	34	0	0	15	9	1
Medicine-Preliminary (PGY-1 Only)	1,928	1,805	1,388	27	119	0	0	125	146	123
Medicine-Preventive Med	7	7	4	0	0	0	0	0	3	0
Medicine-Primary	341	339	206	3	16	0	0	38	76	2
Medicine-Psychiatry	21	21	13	0	1	0	0	2	5	0
Neurodevelopmental Disabilities	1	1	0	0	0	0	0	0	1	0
Neurological Surgery	210	208	188	4	0	1	0	1	14	2
Neurology	404	396	222	7	37	0	0	27	103	8
Obstetrics-Gynecology	1,255	1,255	1,002	17	121	0	0	65	50	0
OB/GYN-Preliminary (PGY-1 Only)	21	14	3	0	1	0	0	3	7	7
Orthopedic Surgery	703	703	663	24	3	0	0	10	3	0
Otolaryngology	299	298	283	13	2	0	0	0	0	1
Pathology	605	568	282	23	44	1	0	55	163	37
Pediatrics (Categorical)	2,668	2,654	1,889	32	303	2	0	174	254	14
Pediatrics-Anesthesiology	9	9	9	0	0	0	0	0	0	0
Pediatrics-Emergency Med	9	9	8	0	0	0	0	1	0	0
Pediatrics-Medical Genetics	15	15	12	0	0	0	0	0	3	0
Pediatrics-PM&R	1	1	0	0	1	0	0	0	0	0
Pediatrics-Prelim (PGY-1 Only)	36	30	21	0	2	0	0	3	4	6
Pediatrics-Primary	74	74	26	2	8	0	0	17	21	0
Peds/Psych/Child Psych	19	19	18	0	0	0	0	1	0	0
Physical Medicine & Rehab	107	107	65	4	29	0	0	7	2	0
Plastic Surgery (Integrated)	148	144	136	3	1	0	0	1	3	4
Psychiatry (Categorical)	1,353	1,339	774	39	183	1	0	178	164	14
Psychiatry-Family Medicine	10	10	10	0	0	0	0	0	0	0
Psychiatry-Neurology	3	2	0	0	1	0	0	0	1	1
Radiation Oncology	17	15	14	1	0	0	0	0	0	2
Radiology-Diagnostic	133	120	67	7	19	0	0	12	15	13
Surgery (Categorical)	1,224	1,222	979	86	36	0	0	71	50	2
Surgery-Preliminary (PGY-1 Only)	1,296	821	476	37	24	1	0	104	179	475
Thoracic Surgery	35	35	28	3	2	0	0	0	2	0
Transitional (PGY-1 Only)	842	790	685	5	39	1	0	30	30	52
Vascular Surgery	57	55	48	1	2	0	0	2	2	2
Total PGY-1	**27,293**	**26,252**	**16,932**	**662**	**2,339**	**17**	**1**	**2,660**	**3,641**	**1,041**

Another major barrier in mutual cultural understanding is the lack of ethnically diverse health care leaders. Health care institutions should also prioritize mentoring and promoting physician and professional staff leaders from underrepresented ethnic and minority groups, to ensure future diversity in leadership to drive health care policy.

EDUCATING HEALTH CARE PROVIDERS IN CULTURAL COMPETENCE

Despite increased awareness about health care disparities and the need for a diverse workforce, there is still a ubiquitous lack of appropriate cultural competence training for providers. Most medical schools have cultural competency lectures embedded within larger courses in the preclinical years, but those usually occur when medical students do not get to reinforce these concepts within their clinical training. Some also have cultural immersion programs either locally or in foreign locations, but most student do not get this exposure. Most residency programs completely lack structured or formal training programs in cultural competence, and most teaching faculty do not have the skills to teach cultural competence, due to lack of training themselves and/or having trained in an era when the patient population was much less diverse.

Improving intercultural communication skills of health care providers is key to a culturally competent health care system. One way of improving these communication skills among physicians is to implement courses during the medical school clinical years and/or residency training, and continue throughout practice; these courses should focus on the cognitive, emotional and behavioral components of communication, targeted to the ethno cultural groups most prominent in the local community. This way, providers can become more knowledgeable about local cultures and alternative ways they may experience health and disease processes.

The Association of American Medical Colleges (AAMC), supported by a Commonwealth Fund grant, has developed a self-administered assessment tool, the TACCT (Tool for Assessing Cultural Competence Training). The aim of the TACCT is to help medical schools in meeting two of the accreditation standards from the LCME (Liaison Committee on Medical Education) (ED-21 and ED-22). It also can be used as a guide to develop cultural competence curriculum, as well as to examine all components of the entire curriculum to identify the extent to which cultural competent care is currently taught. The AAMC has identified six core domains needed for effective cultural competence training: health disparities, bias and stereotyping, community strategies, cross-cultural communication skills, working with interpreters, and the culture of medicine. Hospitalists and trainees should ensure they are receiving some training in these six domains, and they should strive to improve self-directed learning if a core curriculum does not currently exist.

Betancourt and colleagues have outlined three different but complementary conceptual approaches for cross-cultural education:

1. "Cultural sensitivity-awareness approach" is focused on improving *attitudes* central to professionalism such as humility, empathy, curiosity, respect, sensitivity and awareness of all outside influences on the patient. This approach uses exercises designed to promote self-reflection and to detect biases and tendencies to stereotype or appreciate the values of other cultures.
2. "Multicultural-categorical approach" is focused on improving *knowledge* about the attitudes, values, beliefs and behaviors of different cultural groups.
3. "Cross-cultural approach" is focused on improving communication *skills*, training learners to be able to detect certain cross-cutting cultural/social/health issues, and improving their skills to deal with issues, once detected. The aim is for the provider to be able to encourage the patient to provide facts of his/her understanding of their illnesses, their rationale for decision making, and the role and influence of their family and their opinions about available treatments and complementary medicine. Also, the provider should be able to create an environment that is comfortable for the patient to express opinions, concerns, sources of mistrust, prejudice, etc.

Multiple teaching and evaluation strategies have been evaluated in different settings, including standard surveys, structured interviews, presentation of clinical cases, and OSCEs (Objective Structures Clinical Exam). Of those, the OSCE is the only one that is able to effectively teach and evaluate the three conceptual approaches to cross cultural education. OSCEs provide a hands-on, real-time practical training that enhances participation in a case-based learning environment. Trainees can be exposed to multiple clinical scenarios and situations from a wide array of patients with very diverse cultural, social, racial, economic and religious backgrounds.

The AAMC developed the Cultural Competence Education and Training Assessment Inventory (CCETAI). The CEETAI is a pool of 35 peer-reviewed research studies evaluating the impact of cultural competence education and training in the medical profession. They present the educational goals addressed in each study, the educational activity/tool, and the outcome assessment method used. Each also presents the target learners (eg, residents, medical students of different years) and allows for comparisons of the studies by curricular goals as categorized by the TACCT.

Ideally, a cultural competence curriculum should be an integral part of any medical school and residency curriculum, and should involve case-based, hands-on learning with real life scenarios. For such a curriculum to be successful, there must be full support from institution leadership, faculty, and students; there also much be adequate institutional and community resources committed, with a clearly defined evaluation process.

POTENTIAL STRATEGIES TO IMPROVE CULTURAL COMPETENCE

In addition to structured and longitudinal education, here are some strategies that hospital medicine groups can employ to improve cultural competence. The American Hospital Association suggests the following:

- Conduct an assessment to understand staff knowledge on local cultures
- Use the resources above to create a curriculum with multiple methods of training, including case studies (and OSCE) with real patients, which should be repeated at regular intervals
- Track data from patient satisfaction scores to detect areas of concern
- Track your local health care disparities from your organization by race, ethnicity or language proficiency

We also suggest the following to enhance culture competence within hospital medicine groups:

- Actively recruit physicians that are of the same ethnicity and/or speak the same language as the local population.
- Educate your staff on mistrust in the health care system from African American patients, and reinforce the legitimate historical basis for it; actively employ shared decision-making strategies to gain their trust.
- Create more effective patient-physician communication practices for your Limited English Proficiency (LEP) patients (eg, by a better use of interpreters).
- Target patients with limited health literacy and/or alternative health beliefs by the appropriate use of resources such as pastoral care, social workers, and case managers.

- Create and use instructional materials provided in multiple languages specific to the community being served, at least for the most common admission diagnoses.
- Create interventions to reduce such disparities where they current exist in your organization.

The ultimate goals in enhancing cultural competence are to avoid misdiagnosis, enhance patient safety, improve adherence to treatment plans, reduce inpatient and post discharge mortality and readmissions, improve outpatient follow-up, and decrease medico-legal liabilities for all of your patients.

CONCLUSION

The United States has rapidly become a racially diverse country. Different ethnic groups have different beliefs when it comes to experiencing health care, and health care disparities continue to exist. Government accrediting agencies and funders have taken notice. With the advent of value-based payment models, there is a financial imperative for health care organizations to provide patient-centered, high-quality care to all patients. The need to develop cultural competence of health care practitioners is now more important than ever. More research is needed to evaluate the impact that provider cultural competence has on patient outcomes, but improving cultural competence should improve patient satisfaction, as well as promote social harmony and cultural respect.

SUGGESTED READINGS

Berger G, Conroy S, Peerson A, et al. Clinical supervisors and cultural competence. *Clin Teach*. 2014;11:370-374.

Betancourt JR. Cross-cultural medical education: conceptual approaches and frameworks for evaluation. *Acad Med*. 2003;78: 560-569.

Boulware LE, Cooper LA, Ratner LE, et al. Race and trust in the health care system. *Public Health Rep*. 2003;118(4):358-365.

Lie D, Boker J, Cleveland E. Using the Tool for Assessing Cultural Competence Training (TACCT) to measure faculty and medical student perceptions of cultural competence instruction in the first three years of the curriculum. *Acad Med*. 2006;81:557-564.

Weech-Maldonado R. Moving towards culturally competent health systems: organizational and market factors. *Soc Sci Med*. 2012;75(5):815-822.

ONLINE RESOURCES

American Hospital Association. Becoming a Culturally Competent Health Care Organization. http://www.hpoe.org/Reports HPOE/becoming_culturally_competent_health_care_organization.PDF.

Association of American Medical Colleges Enrollment, Graduates, and MD/PhD Data. Available online at https://www.aamc.org/data/facts/enrollmentgraduate/.

Association of American of Medical Colleges. Assessing change: evaluating cultural competence education and training. Position paper, March 2015. https://members.aamc.org/eweb/upload/Assessing%20Change%20-%20Evaluating%20Cultural%20Competence%20Education%20and%20Training.pdf.

National Resident Matching Program, Results and Data: 2015 Main Residency Match. National Resident Matching Program, Washington, DC. 2015. http://www.nrmp.org/wp-content/uploads/2015/05/Main-Match-Results-and-Data-2015_final.pdf.

US Department of Health and Human Services' Office of Minority Health: National Standards for Culturally and Linguistically Appropriate Services in Health and Health Care (The National CLAS Standards). http://minorityhealth.hhs.gov/omh/browse.aspx?lvl=2&lvlid=53.

CHAPTER 38

Career Design and Development in Academic and Community Settings

Amulya Nagarur, MD
Andrew Z. Fenves, MD, FACP, FASN
Alberto Puig, MD, PhD, FACP

INTRODUCTION

The rapid growth of the hospitalist movement has dramatically changed the delivery of inpatient care in the United States over the last two decades. Hospital medicine has an increasing presence within general internal medicine in academic and community hospitals.

Historically, the hospitalist movement attracted a number of recent internal medicine residency graduates who were seeking a transitional period before entering subspecialty fellowship training. With the growing financial burden of medical school education, several physicians also entered into short-term hospitalist practices to help repay debt prior to further training. Consequently, in its infancy, a substantial percentage of hospital medicine was populated with this transient physician population, leading to a paucity of investment in hospitalist career development and leadership. Excessive patient workloads, long hours, a shortage of mentorship and other factors have led to high attrition rates and significant physician burnout. See Chapter 41: For the Individual: Career Sustainability and Avoiding Burnout.

The site where hospitalists practice defines their area of expertise. Distinguishing between academic and community hospitalists is often based on the type of institution in which they practice (academic medical centers vs community hospitals). This definition may lead to an oversimplification of the differences between these physicians, as some hospitalists in the community do have academic responsibilities in addition to clinical care. Academic hospitalists typically hold a faculty appointment conferred by a hospital-affiliated university. When community hospitals become affiliated with universities, or merge with academic medical centers, the role of their staff may change accordingly to include an academic component. In addition to community and academic hospitals providing salary support, companies have been developed to outsource hospitalists and related services to multiple hospitals. In any of these settings, hospitalists have opportunities to acquire additional skills and leadership that will provide them with the option of transitioning from one setting into another. This chapter offers strategies for professional development for early-career hospitalists.

THE ACADEMIC SETTING

Achieving traditional academic success in hospital medicine has many challenges. Increasing demands of clinical work is due to a number of factors, including:

- Expansion of patient care into specialty areas
- Increased on-site coverage (nights, weekends)
- Lack of funding for protected time to pursue scholarly activities
- Restricted resident work hours and availability

Many academic clinicians build careers that follow a classic triad of clinical care, research, and teaching in the inpatient setting. In the inpatient setting career-hospitalists may specialize in acute general medicine, one of the medical specialties, general medical consultation, or comanage a specialty such as orthopedic surgery and neurosurgery. Each of these clinical areas provides opportunities for hospitalists, including acquiring new skills, leading a program, performing quality improvement, and education. In addition, some hospitalists may expand their clinical duties to involve some outpatient care.

Many hospitalists cite higher job satisfaction when able to complement inpatient clinical duties with other nonclinical activities (**Table 38-1**).

TABLE 38-1 Nonclinical Roles in the Hospital Setting

Research	• Clinical studies of commonly encountered medical problems
Teaching	Primary teaching attending responsible for • Conducting rounds • Observing clinical skills • Supervising procedures
Mentorship	• Trainees and junior hospitalists • Nurse practitioners and physician assistants
Scholarship	Local Level • Discussants at trainee conferences • Development of new curricula for trainees • Interdepartmental educational efforts (medical consultation, comanagement) Regional, national, and international level • Speaking engagement at society meetings • Publication: articles, chapters, books, studies of the process of teaching and learning • Curriculum development
Leadership	Leadership of: • Hospitalist programs • Medicine divisions or departments • Administrative officers of medical centers • Medical consultative service • General medical service • Comanagement services • Hospital committees • Medical student core clerkships • Residency programs
Hospital systems improvement (patient safety and quality improvement)	• VTE prophylaxis • Management of diabetes • Transitions and hand-offs • Utilization review
Health information technology	• Design and implementation of electronic health records • Physician order entry • Clinical decision support • Databases for research
Community outreach	• Community education • Referral networks

Federal funding sources such as K-series and R-series grants remain limited for the type of quality and safety research that many academic hospitalists pursue; therefore, many hospitalists will need to seek out alternative sources of funding within their institutions. Fellowship opportunities and grants are available on local and national levels. Improving processes and outcomes in a cost-effective manner requires meaningful use of data and information via health information technology (IT). For clinicians interested in the

health IT sector, there may be funding through their local hospital. Regional and national societies are supportive of both health IT training and innovation.

Physicians with academic careers refer to the guidance of a mentor as having the most positive influence on academic productivity and professional satisfaction. Mentored faculty at all levels in their careers are more successful at producing peer-reviewed publications and procuring grant support, and have higher confidence in their career trajectory. Institutions also benefit from their faculty having rich mentoring opportunities. Mentorship has been most successfully associated with clinician-scientists as this group of physicians has a more objective means for measuring academic productivity. Many junior faculty choosing careers as clinician educators have had exposure to master clinicians; however, mentorship is often difficult to find or identify. Typically, clinician-educators have a career trajectory that follows a natural pattern: at the start of their careers, educators are entry-level teachers who are still refining their clinical and teaching skills. Over time, they develop more robust content and teaching skills. Some clinician-educators move on to direct clerkships and residency programs. The highest level of faculty participation in education involves those who study the process and outcomes of teaching and learning or delve into curriculum development. See Chapter 39: Mentorship of Peers and Trainees.

THE COMMUNITY SETTING

The early hospitalist movement originated in the community setting, and many hospitalists choose to practice exclusively in this setting. The lack of structured pathways for the early-career hospitalists has made career development difficult to navigate. Community hospitalists cite numerous reasons for requesting formal mentorship. Institution-based mentoring programs for hospitalists engaged in full-time community practice have shown to strengthen professional satisfaction.

The clinical responsibilities of hospitalists who practice in a community setting overlap with those of academic hospitalists. Community hospitalists provide medical ward care, medical consult services, emergency medicine triage, intensive care unit and surgical unit care, and at times coordinated subspecialty care. These physicians require expertise and skill managing the breadth and depth of resources available at their institutions and must also safely negotiate transfers to higher-care facilities when needed. Operationally, community hospitals have expanded the roles of their hospitalists as they have become essential to the productivity and mission of local health centers. Some community hospitalists oversee treatment in postacute care facilities such as long-term acute care, rehabilitation, skilled nursing, and hospice centers.

Regardless of hospital size and type, hospital medicine programs benefit medical centers and communities by virtue of expertise in hospital medicine and quality improvement, availability for admissions and efficiency associated with cost-savings. Many community hospitals develop academic affiliations over time, and their hospitalist faculty may assume academic roles teaching medical students and residents as well as serving as discussants at resident reports, lectures and conferences. Hospitalists in the community collaborate, educate and mentor nurse practitioners and physician's assistants, and supervise many of these advanced practice clinicians on medical services.

Increasingly, community hospitalists are accountable for implementing community support systems for their patients that include robust social work, case management, pharmacy, and educational supports in order to decrease readmissions and improve compliance postdischarge. Most hospital medicine groups in the community settings are actively engaged in quality and process improvement and focus on patient safety, resource allocation, and hospital efficiency. Multidisciplinary hospital committees often include or are led by staff hospitalists. Hospitalist groups encourage their staff to take on operational and administrative duties such as utilization review, as these are locally valuable to the hospital system. Ranging from hospital medicine group administrators to chief operating officers and chief executive officers, hospitalists may participate or lead initiatives in hospital operations, recruitment, policy development, financial affairs, and compliance.

In addition to hospital work, community hospitalists may assume expanded roles as community educators on local, regional, and national levels. Some partake in grassroots activities, educating their local communities on various health care issues. Others may direct efforts to educate local or national policymakers to affect more widespread legislative change in hospital medicine, community health, or hospital administration.

PROFESSIONAL DEVELOPMENT PLAN

■ SELF-EVALUATION

Achieving success in both settings requires developing a personal professional plan. This process begins with self-evaluation:

- Strengths: What are your key strengths and how may you highlight your strengths?
- Development needs: What are one or two areas that need improvement?
- Career aspirations: What do you like to do? What are your goals over the next one to 2 years? What are your goals over the next 3 to 5 years (ie, longer term milestones)?
- Periodic reassessment of goals: Do you feel that you are reaching your goals? Do you need to revise your goals? Do you need to take additional steps to achieve your goals?

■ SELECTING A HOSPITALIST POSITION

Your selection of a hospitalist position hinges on your core values and priorities. Your priorities may change over time depending on your stage of life and needs:

- Financial priorities: Nocturnist salaries are usually higher than daytime work, and community hospitals may be more competitive than academic hospitals. There are also regional variations.
- Work-life balance: Is the hospitalist service chronically understaffed with high turnover? Is it possible to work part time?
- Professional development: Is there a dedicated faculty development program with a robust structured mentor focus? Is there protected time for professional development?

Does the hospital invest in career development or is the focus solely on clinical responsibilities?

- Clinical interests: Does the hospital provide opportunities in your area of focus: quality improvement, teaching, medical informatics, or clinical research?

Strong faculty development programs, mentorship, and transparent promotions criteria are critical to the success of career hospitalists and job satisfaction.

■ EARLY MILESTONES (FIRST 1 TO 2 YEARS)

Networking

Exposure to other hospitalists is crucial for career development. The Society of Hospital Medicine (SHM), the American College of Physicians (ACP), the Society of General Internal Medicine (SGIM), and the Association of Chiefs and Leaders of General Medicine (ACLGIM) sponsor leadership and mentorship retreats as well as interest-specific workshops. The annual Academic Hospital Academy is an intensive multi-day workshop for junior academic hospitalists that provide essential skills for succeeding in academic medicine,

including teaching effectively, producing scholarly work, and understanding the promotion process and the business of health care. Attending such meetings fosters collaboration, allows for networking, and in many cases ignites rich mentoring relationships.

Participation and leadership in local hospital initiatives

From an individual and departmental perspective, hospitalists should take advantage of opportunities to increase their presence by leading hospital-based committees, quality improvement initiatives, and comanagement. SHM, ACP, SGIM, and ACLGIM offer training opportunities that teach leadership, evaluation, communication skills, and hospital metric derivations that drive leadership decisions. SHM offers a Certificate of Leadership in Hospital Medicine (CLHM) through which candidates complete a leadership project and build skills for successful executive leadership positions. In addition, many academic centers offer training in leadership through their Centers for Faculty Development.

Most medical centers have strong ties to local organizations, including health advocacy groups, legislative entities, outpatient community health centers, and schools. Both early and late career community hospitalists with specific areas of interest (clinical or nonclinical) may advance their careers by developing durable relationships with such groups.

Promotion process

Many hospitalists find the promotions process difficult to navigate due to their heavy clinical workload, lack of mentorship, and participation in nontraditional academic activities (such as QI and education). Criteria for promotion vary widely across various institutions, and hospitalists should become familiar with this process. In a cross-sectional survey published in the *Journal of Hospital Medicine*, successfully promoted academic hospitalists considered peer-reviewed publications to be the most important activity in achieving promotion. Promotion within community hospitals may involve an opportunity to manage a hospital committee, lead the local hospital unit, or serve as the clinical director of a specific clinical activity.

Because many hospitalists engage in QI projects that do not fit the traditional triad of academia (clinical care, teaching, and research), it is important to establish a portfolio to showcase QI endeavors. The SGIM Academic Hospital taskforce created the Quality Portfolio, a structured accompaniment to a promotions package that documents and organizes QI work. Similarly, the Educator Portfolio documents teaching, awards, and educational scholarship for clinician-educators. Templates and resources for developing Quality and Educator portfolios are available online.

Strategic professional plan

A strategic professional plan begins with:

- Mentorship: regular meetings with faculty mentors so that hospitalists may take advantage of leadership, research, speaking, and teaching opportunities that are instrumental in promotion.
- Networking: participation in local, regional, and national meetings.
- Participation in skill building sessions: local, regional and national workshops in peer-observation, educational, leadership, competency in manuscript writing, grant writing and procurement, oral presentation, study design and execution.
- Additional training: formal degree-granting programs in public health, public policy, finance and operations management, health care administration, QI, education, health care informatics, courses in biostatistics, study design, epidemiology.
- Scholarship: identification of an area of special interest or expertise with eventual goal of becoming an institutional,

regional, and national expert and pursue foundational opportunities with a built-in curriculum, such as the various Robert Wood Johnson Foundation Scholars programs.

- Documentation of portfolio of progress: case reports, evaluation of QI projects, development and assessment of education curricula, and participation in inpatient clinical studies. This documentation will be required for academic promotion.
- Education about the promotion process from the beginning of career: focus on the best avenue to achieve goals.
- Review the process for achieving Society of Hospital Medicine fellowship and senior fellowship for planning purposes as well as that of other professional societies such as the American College of Physicians.

Hospital medicine as a specialty: future directions

Currently, the American Board of Family Medicine and the American Board of Internal Medicine (ABIM) offer a Recognition of Focused Practice in Hospital Medicine (RFPHM) program. As hospital medicine continues to expand and leaders rise in both the academic and community sectors, the field will likely develop into an independent subspecialty with its own board certification.

Several clinical training programs have introduced careers in hospital medicine as part of medical student and residency education. The SHM has a comprehensive guide to residency hospitalist tracks as well as hospital medicine fellowships for those seeking more formal training early in their careers. Building such pathways and standardizing curricula for hospitalist career development will need to become a focus in hospital medicine. Creating a framework for assessment and evaluation of the hospitalist will allow for specialized tracks for promotion purposes within academic and community settings.

In 2001, the Institute of Medicine called for an overhaul of the US health care system for the 21st century that prioritizes efficient patient-centered teams. In response to this call for redesign, the Accreditation Council for Graduate Medical Education included aptitude for working in multidisciplinary teams as part of its core competencies. Medical students and residents will increasingly be expected to learn and work collaboratively alongside other health care providers such as nurses, physical therapists, and occupational therapists. The cadre of career-hospitalists will remain invaluable participants and leaders in these movements, and will need to acquire and teach the skills for successful multidisciplinary collaboration.

ACKNOWLEDGMENT

We are indebted to Dr. Sue Williams from Baylor University Medical Center, Dallas, Texas, for her revision of the manuscript, input on sections regarding Community Hospital Careers and invaluable advice on the chapter.

SUGGESTED READINGS

Farrell SE, Digioia NM, Broderick KB, et al. Mentoring for clinician-educators. *Acad Emerg Med.* 2004;11(12):1346-1350.

Flanders SA, Centor B, Weber V, et al. Challenges and opportunities in academic hospital medicine: report from the Academic Hospital Medicine Summit. *J Hosp Med.* 2009;4(4):240-246.

Harrison R, Hunter AJ, Sharpe B, et al. Survey of US academic hospital leaders about mentorship and academic activities in hospital groups. *J Hosp Med.* 2011;6(1):5-9.

Leykum LK, Parekh VI, Sharpe B, et al. Tried and true: a survey of successfully promoted academic hospitals. *J Hosp Med.* 2011;6(7):411-415.

Mookherjee S, Monash B, Wentworth KL, et al. Faculty development for hospitals: structured peer observation of teaching. *J Hosp Med.* 2014;9(4):244-250.

Reid MB, Misky GJ, Harrison RA, et al. Mentorship, productivity, and promotion among academic hospitals. *J Gen Intern Med.* 2012;27(1):23-27.

Sehgal NL, Sharpe BA, Auerbach AA, et al. Investing in the future: building an academic hospital faculty development program. *J Hosp Med.* 2011;6(3):161-166.

Tietjen P, Griner PF. Mentoring of physicians at a community-based health system: preliminary findings. *J Hosp Med.* 2013;8(11):642-643.

ONLINE RESOURCES

Niebuhr V, Johnson R, Mendias E, et al. *Educator Portfolios. MedEdPORTAL Publications*; 2013. Available at: https://www.mededportal.org/publication/9355.

Society of General Internal Medicince (SGIM) Quality Portfolio—Template and Instructions. Available at: http://www.sgim.org/File%20Library/ACLGIM/Tools%20and%20Resources/QualityPortfolioTemplate.pdf.

39

Mentorship of Peers and Trainees

Tom Baudendistel, MD, FACP

Aubrey Ingraham, MD

INTRODUCTION

The word "mentor" comes from Homer's *Odyssey*, in which Odysseus entrusts his young son to the care of his close friend, Mentor. A transitional figure in the youth's growth, Mentor acts as the son's guardian and wise advisor, and through their mutual relationship the son develops his own identity. Good mentors have played key roles in the history of medicine and discovery, in the development of young doctors, and in the institutions that train physicians.

Today's health care leaders underscore the importance of mentoring on career choice as well as on career advancement and productivity. Yet, the available evidence shows that a minority of medical students and faculty have mentors. Because Hospital Medicine is a young specialty, peer mentorship is crucial to the success of the specialty.

PRACTICE POINT

Benefits of mentorship include:

- Mentoring is a powerful predictor of academic advancement
- Academic advancement and productivity promote the specialty of Hospital Medicine
- Mentoring of medical students, trainees, and junior faculty facilitates recruitment and retention of hospitalists
- Faculty members derive personal and professional satisfaction from mentoring trainees

THE VALUE OF MENTORING IN MEDICINE

Surveys of faculty and health care leaders and a systematic review identified several potential benefits of mentoring in medicine. Mentoring influences career choice, including medical students' specialty selections; promotes career advancement; increases scholarly productivity; develops physicians' leadership skills; shapes professional ethics; fosters development of academic departments, institutions, and professional societies; and increases career satisfaction. Clinician-educators view mentoring as an important determinant of promotion and development, and are more likely to remain in academia if they are mentored.

While most studies have focused on the benefits to the mentee, potential benefits to the mentor should not be underestimated. Faculty members derive personal and professional satisfaction from mentoring residents, and mentoring may facilitate promotion, result in special awards, and increase scholarly productivity (**Table 39-1**).

BARRIERS TO MENTORING FOR HOSPITALISTS

The absence of mentoring is a powerful predictor of delayed academic advancement. Despite consistent reports of the benefits of mentoring—and the disadvantages faced by those without mentors—fewer than 20% of faculty members have a mentor. Clinician-educators are less likely than clinician-scientists to identify a mentor and also less likely to serve as mentors. Faculty cite competing time pressures, inadequate faculty development around mentoring, and lack of recognition of mentoring by promotions committees as factors dampening their willingness to mentor.

TABLE 39-1 Benefits of Mentoring

Benefits to the Mentee

- Increased advocacy for career development
- High-level career advice from experienced senior person
- Enhanced access to opportunities beyond the current level of the mentee, including:
  - research (grants, editing, publications, collaborations)
  - promotions
  - new job openings (within or outside the institution)
  - committee membership
  - roles in professional organizations
  - networking with key thought leaders
- Valuable, nonthreatening, feedback from "third party" who is separate from the employer-employee relationship
- Access to a role model of professionalism, ethics, and values
- More directed and formal timeline and framework for career success

Benefits to the Mentor

- Renewed sense of excitement for career brought about by revisiting own history of professional growth; participating in the professional and personal development of a colleague; and continuing professional legacy of shaping "the next generation" of physicians
- Enhanced recognition among peers and junior staff
- Cultivation of specific interpersonal skills (active listening, effective communication, modeling)
- Exposure to new ideas and opportunities, often leading to increased creativity and productivity (including publications and projects)
- Pride in a mentee's successes
- Enhanced personal growth
- Broadened network via mentee's collaboration and connection to other personnel, including cross-discipline and cross-department interactions
- Discussion and exploration of mentor's values with others
- An accurate perspective on barriers experienced by current junior staff
- Credit toward career advancement as a result of mentoring

Benefits to the Department

- Bolstered staff morale, motivation, institutional dedication, and career satisfaction
- Enhancement of productivity and creativity
- Discovery and development of personnel talent
- Insurances of department's future survival through development of leadership
- Communication and demonstration of the department's values, goals, and expected personal and professional standards
- Reinvigoration of senior faculty
- Development of cross-departmental, national, and international networks

Junior hospitalist clinician-educators often spend their early faculty years learning to master the many aspects of the inpatient arena, including patient safety, quality improvement, transitions of care, surgical comanagement, and ward teaching. Such jack-of-all-trades hospitalists, while valuable to their groups, can be perceived by promotions committees as "masters of none." A second tension inherent in hospitalist careers exacerbates the problem. Hospitalist clinician-educators often cannot generate enough revenue from clinical duties to support unfunded nonclinical work, making it hard to secure protected time and financial compensation to develop expertise in education, scholarly activity, or administration. Without time or expertise, hospitalists find it challenging to advance academically and feel underqualified to serve as mentors.

OVERCOMING THE BARRIERS: STRATEGIES FOR SUCCESSFULLY MENTORING

To become more promotable, hospitalist clinician-educators must ramp up their productivity during nonclinical time. The traditional clinician-educator paradigm—periods of intense clinical work interspersed with more relaxing nonclinical time—must be rethought. To paraphrase one department chair, just as diastole is now recognized as an active time of the cardiac cycle, so too must clinician-educators view their nonclinical periods.

Overarching goals in mentoring clinician-educators include personal and career satisfaction and professional advancement. To achieve this, successful mentors can help mentees optimize their nonclinical "diastolic" time. In some instances, clinical and nonclinical duties may overlap and provide a "two-for-one" opportunity. During a ward attending block, for example, a hospitalist may be encouraged to pilot a quality improvement initiative or a novel patient-centered multidisciplinary bedside rounding structure. A mentor might help identify the opportunities, suggest local leaders to contact, determine what metrics to analyze to demonstrate success, and recommend a forum for disseminating the results locally or extramurally.

Ultimately, without protected time or funding clinician-educators may struggle to advance. Resources to support the nonclinical work of junior hospitalists is often limited, but mentors can steer mentees to education research grants, administrative roles with associated support, or medical school work which includes remuneration. When these resources fall short, mentors and mentees often turn to their division leaders for support. A strong hospitalist leader successfully lobbies leadership to support nonclinical hospitalist work. In these negotiations, hospitalist leaders can highlight favorable return-on-investment by demonstrating the impact of hospitalists on: length of stay; readmission rates; bed availability for more profitable surgical cases; patient satisfaction scores; hospital-acquired infection rates; satisfaction of referring primary care, emergency, and consulting physicians; physician retention; teaching evaluations; and committee contributions.

Creative mentors can also facilitate career advancement and promotion by developing focused areas of mastery within mentees. Hospitalist duties have expanded far beyond general medicine wards to include comanagement of patients under the care of other specialties and protected time for peer review, quality improvement and safety, teamwork, and leadership. Each of these areas represents a potential locus of expertise and leadership for a junior hospitalist. A successful mentor can guide the mentee to become the local institutional champion, and then map a strategy for demonstrating quantitatively the impact of the mentee's work in this area. Eventually, the mentor can suggest strategies for disseminating the mentee's successes at professional society meetings and via publication in peer-reviewed journals, society newsletters or blogs, and other social media.

Specific behaviors associated with successful mentoring for clinician-educators differ at each step in the mentoring relationship: preparing for mentoring, approaching a mentor for the first time, ongoing mentoring, and ending the mentorship. Novice mentors and junior faculty should receive structured faculty development to learn a core set of mentoring skills. **Table 39-2** elaborates further on key elements for success at each phase of mentorship.

PRACTICE POINT

- Successful mentoring requires self-reflection, a key means by which both participants initiate personal, relationship, and practice improvements.

TABLE 39-2 Best-Practice Behaviors for Successful Mentoring

	Mentee	Mentor
Preparing for mentoring	• Assess your competencies in the roles you currently hold (preparation of clinician-educator portfolio may facilitate this) • Define specific career goals and steps required to achieve them • List specific activities and experiences you seek* • Identify specific questions pertaining to the kinds of help you think you need • Determine the key personal and professional qualities you desire or value in a mentor • Consider seeking a mentor 1 level above your current career level and a more senior mentor	• Make a realistic assessment of your availability to commit to a new mentee • Consider requesting and reviewing an updated CV from your prospective mentee prior to meeting • Enumerate the particular areas in which you might be of value to a mentee*
First meeting	• Explain your current academic role, how your goals may be aligned with the mentor's work, and what you think you might need in terms of advice and guidance • Recognize a potential mentor's time and energy • Ensure you have the mentor's updated contact information and ask which method of communication he or she prefers • Consider sending a thank you note after your first meeting	• Befriend the mentee to diffuse the power dynamic • Start with open-ended questions (eg, "What do you hope to gain from our work together?") • Recognize your limitations and provide alternative resources to those whom you cannot effectively mentor • Summarize and confirm (eg, "It sounds like I could best help you now by…Is this true?") • Ensure you have the mentee's updated contact information and ask which method of communication he or she prefers
Ongoing mentoring	• Determine the structure of meetings (eg, e-mail, in person, telephone) • Take the initiative, when in doubt • Prepare and set the agenda for mentoring meetings • Schedule meetings at regular intervals • Inform your mentor of changes in goals, barriers, and progress in reaching your goals • Seek and accept challenges and feedback • Clarify realistic expectations of the mentee-mentor relationship • Consider creating and following a written checklist or timeline to track progress	• Assist mentee in establishing goals • Listen to your mentee actively and patiently • Refine mentee's specific goals, and push mentee for his or her "dreams" (what may seem unobtainable to mentee may seem achievable to you) • Hold mentee to high but obtainable standards • Advocate for mentee • Inform the mentee about new opportunities and suggest alternate resources for information about academic opportunities, political culture, and networking • Protect the mentee from possible threats • Use your experience, clout, and influence to serve as a champion for the mentee • When you are unable to meet mentee's needs, refer mentee to another mentor • Foster mentee development • Commit your time and energy on a regular, ongoing, and flexible basis • Recognize different mentee learning styles and tailor your approach: some mentees may need direct, task-oriented assistance, while others need help with problem solving or articulating ideas • Assist in the mentee's identity development; consider how you will "wean" the mentee • Collaborate with mentee if this helps promote mentee's agenda, not yours • Credit the mentee for his or her diligence and creative output (includes authorship or grants) • Provide honest feedback in a constructive and caring manner • Serve as role model and confidante • Exhibit high professional and moral character • Be responsive and available • Follow through on promises • Maintain confidentiality (except in rare circumstances as required by law, such as harassment, danger to self/others, professional misconduct) • Seek out feedback from mentee • Accept personal differences with sensitivity and do not judge gender, culture, or age-related differences • Share personal knowledge (medical and nonmedical), including failures, so that the mentee feels comfortable seeking guidance

(Continued)

TABLE 39-2 Best-Practice Behaviors for Successful Mentoring (*Continued*)

	Mentee	Mentor
Ending the mentoring relationship	• Talk about when the relationship should end (eg, a certain time point, or once certain goals are achieved) • Ask for advice on future advisors or mentors • Thank your mentor	• Talk about when the relationship should end • Offer suggestions for future mentors or directions of interest • Thank your mentee

*Common mentoring goals include: assistance with grant-writing or manuscript preparation, advice for promotion and advancement (including advice unique to women and minorities), building a network, research collaboration, teaching skills, negotiation, enhancing educator portfolio, improving understanding of organization politics, oral presentation skills, and work-life balance.

• The goal of self-reflection is to identify specific short- and long-term goals to aid future career development. To achieve this, the mentor needs to guide the mentee so the mentee can articulate personal strengths and weaknesses and then transform the self-assessments into concrete goals for future career development.

• Role modeling self-reflection and actively promoting self-reflection may cause the mentee to internalize an important skill of a self-directed lifelong learner.

A mentor would first lead the mentee to recognize these areas of relative strength and weakness. Then, the mentor might suggest specific ways for the mentee to improve didactic teaching skill, or may encourage the mentee to seek experiences that maximize the mentee's strengths and minimize exposure to areas of weakness. Importantly, the mentor should periodically request the mentee to evaluate the quality and effectiveness of the mentoring relationship.

PRACTICE POINT

Key questions for junior hospitalists to consider include:

• What do I perceive as my strengths and weaknesses?

• How do these strengths and weaknesses compare with how others have evaluated me?

• What activities provide me the greatest source of career satisfaction?

• What activities would I like to do more or less of?

• Which senior faculty member's career path do I want to emulate?

• What specific roles do I see myself in within the next 3 to 5 years? 5 to 10 years?

• What obstacles stand in the way of my career goals?

• What skills or knowledge do I need to acquire to address my weaknesses or to be able to realize my career goals?

• What are the goals and vision of my supervisor (eg, chairperson) and do my interests and strengths align with these goals? If not, how can I demonstrate my value to the division or group?

CHOOSING WISELY: SELECTING THE RIGHT MENTOR-MENTEE RELATIONSHIP

Mentoring is a protected relationship occurring between a more advanced career incumbent (mentor) and a younger novice (mentee). An effective mentoring relationship: focuses on achievement or acquisition of expertise through direct assistance with career development and role modeling; includes emotional and psychological support; involves direct personal direct interaction; utilizes the mentor's greater experience and influence within an organization or field; and is reciprocal, designed to enrich the professional and personal lives of both mentor and mentee. While most interactions occur within the workplace, many find that meals, social events, shared hobbies, and professional meetings provide additional opportunities for career guidance. The effective mentoring relationship assumes an always professional and nonsexual focus. Failures in mentoring derive from inadequate communication, commitment, or experience; personality differences, and perceived (or real) competition. **Table 39-3** illustrates the key qualities of a good mentor.

The best way to pair mentors with mentees is unknown. Mandatory mentor assignments offer the advantage of engaging all mentees in some form of advising. On the other hand, independently sought out mentee-mentor relationships may be more effective and enduring.

TABLE 39-3 A Good Mentor

• Maintains confidentiality

• Is knowledgeable and respected in his or her field

• Encourages independent behavior with an approachable, nonthreatening, accessible, facilitative, empowering style of communication

• Challenges and debates mentee in a constructive way

• Employs a careful and dynamic balance between compassion and empathy, and impartiality and honesty

• Shows genuine interest and investment in a mentee's concerns, well-being, and future

• Asks questions that provoke critical thinking, reasoning, analysis, and contemplation

• Recognizes and admits limitations, then guides mentee to appropriate resource

• Acknowledges importance of work-life balance in professional success

• Demonstrates confidence in a mentee

• Possesses strong interpersonal and negotiation skills

• Listens actively and communicates clearly

• Avoids abuse of his or her influence or position

• Provides frequent and detailed feedback

• Seeks opportunities for a mentee to assist with his or her own projects (if appropriate and relevant to mentee's goals)

• Expects and tolerates expressions of emotion from mentees at times of significant anxiety or frustration

■ MENTORING MODELS

Although most discussions focus on the traditional model of mentorship as a one-to-one relationship at one institution, junior hospitalists should be aware of other models which may enhance their career development, such as collaborative group mentoring, mentorship between one mentee and multiple mentors, integrated peer mentoring, networking at annual society meetings, or from a distance (telementoring), and combinations thereof. **Table 39-4** reviews mentoring models and the strengths and weaknesses of each.

Peer mentoring can serve important advising and networking functions. The nonhierarchical nature of peer mentoring addresses problematic issues in senior-junior mentoring relationships such as power, dominance, dependency, and transference. Peer mentors also may be more readily available and provide a way to gain different perspectives and current information on diverse opportunities, especially in a young specialty such as Hospital Medicine, which has relatively few practicing senior hospitalists.

DOCUMENTING ACCOMPLISHMENTS: THE CLINICIAN-EDUCATOR PORTFOLIO

The clinician-educator "portfolio" enumerates and organizes a faculty member's educational activities and achievements for the purposes of academic promotion and self-reflection. Traditionally, decisions regarding academic promotion were based on information summarized in a *curriculum vitae* (CV) and letters of recommendation. The educator portfolio adds several elements: a novel structure to capture all clinician-educator activities, including those elements not traditionally captured in a CV; demonstration of the impact of the educator's activities on trainees, peers, the organization, and the field as a whole; and self-reflection.

The concept of the clinician-educator "portfolio" is analogous to an architect's or artist's portfolio. The educator portfolio includes faculty member's educational achievements, which have expanded from classic "teaching" duties to include a broader array of hospitalist activities: clinical duties, teaching and curriculum development, mentoring, scholarly productivity, leadership, and administration

TABLE 39-4 Mentoring Models

	Description	Advantages	Disadvantages	Best Uses
Closed Models				
Assignment model	Assigns mentors to new trainees based on professional interests, gender, minority status	Guarantees mentee engagement with a senior person	Risks pairing participants who have little natural or mutual affinity Mentee receives only one mentor's perspective	Provides mentorship within the first several months of early in career
Choice model	Requires new resident or junior faculty to choose a more senior faculty to serve as a mentor within several months of beginning employment	Allows some self-selection between participants, which may be especially important for women and minority mentees	Risks leaving a mentee without a mentor during an often stressful transition	Facilitates seeking a confidante for a mentee with issues of a sensitive or confidential nature
Open Models				
Multiple mentor model	Encourages new resident or junior faculty to actively seek multiple mentors from different places, career levels, or career paths	Provides flexibility and broad expertise for the mentee	Risks creating many "diluted" relationships with less continuity, no central senior overseer Relies heavily on the mentee's level of self-motivation and management	Provides advice from senior faculty in multiple domains/departments
Layered model	Assigns new trainees to a group of similar-experienced peers, all of whom share one mentor Schedules periodic meetings (attended by all mentees) Provides reference to individual faculty for specific advising	Allows some guided peer-to-peer mentoring and provides a flexible and broad network of potential senior advisors Safe environment for idea sharing	Provides less individually tailored and private counsel Risks diminishing mentor advocacy for individual mentee Relies heavily on the mentee's level of self-motivation and management	Provides networking opportunities and general advice to mentee with undifferentiated career focus Involves mentee in peer groups and projects spanning many disciplines
Facilitated group/ Collaborative mentoring model	Assigns trainees to structured group forums facilitated by senior faculty (such as skill development, career planning, scholarly writing, role play, videotaping, group discussion, peer and facilitator feedback, narrative writing, and self-reflection)	Facilitates relevant education across broad content areas Provides a broad network of potential senior advisors	Provides less individually tailored and private counsel overseeing mentee, and lacks content and scheduling flexibility Relies heavily on the mentee's level of self-motivation and management	Provides opportunity to junior faculty seeking to strengthen fundamental skills in teaching, research, and publication

TABLE 39-5 Elements of a Clinician-Educator Portfolio

Category	Examples to Support This
Clinical activities	List of clinical duties and average time per week spent on each
Direct teaching	List of teaching activities (ward or ICU teaching, lectures, small group facilitation, resident report, clinic precepting, visiting professorships)
	Summary of evaluations from ward rotation, ideally with comparison to peer averages
	Teaching awards
Curricular design • Instructional development	Revision or implementation of new course, rotation, or program (eg, procedural simulation training, journal club curriculum, homeless clinic rotation) and how participation in course was evaluated
	Outcome assessments (eg, evaluations from course participants; end-of-course test scores or observed procedural competence)
Mentoring • Interns and residents • Medical students • Junior faculty • Peers	List of mentee names by academic year, with hours spent mentoring each and outcomes of mentoring (eg, implemented global health rotation in residency; nominated mentee for regional award; helped determine career choice, etc)
	Collaborations with mentees: manuscripts, curricular change, research
	Participation in formal mentoring program locally, regionally, or nationally
	Formal evaluations by mentees, of the clinician-educator's mentoring abilities
Educational administration and leadership	Admissions committees (for residency or medical school), including interviewing activity
	Course or clerkship director
	Education or curriculum design and oversight committees
	Dean's office or student affairs position
	Evaluation committee
	Program directing
	Elected positions and committee involvement in professional societies for medical education activity (eg, Association of Program Directors or Clerkship Directors in Internal Medicine; education committee work within professional society, such as Society of Hospital Medicine)
	Faculty development leader (eg, taught small group of faculty on ultrasound-guided central venous catheter insertion)
Educational scholarly activity	Grants for education research or education activity (eg, funding to design new curriculum)
	Publications (peer-reviewed publications, book chapters, editorials, opinion pieces, letters)
	Editing and peer reviewing of grants or manuscripts related to education research
	Test question writer (eg, for American Board of Internal Medicine or In Training Exam)
	Posters or oral presentations involving educational topics at society meetings
	Workshop moderator or presenter at society meeting (eg, promoting quality improvement activity in residency)
Hospital administration	Committee work: role on committee (eg, member, chairperson) and specific activities for that committee
	Quality improvement activities
	Patient safety activities (eg, peer review committee, root cause analyses)
	IT development

including quality improvement and patient safety (**Table 39-5**). Importantly, the portfolio often serves as the basis for professional review, academic promotion, as a "body of work" when meeting prospective employers, and as the basis for self-reflection. Ideally, the portfolio's format aligns directly with institutional promotion criteria, thus allowing chairpersons and promotion committees (members of which may not be clinicians) to appreciate the value of distinct activities.

The portfolio is intended to complement, not replace, the curriculum vitae. Whereas the curriculum vitae serves as a detailed outline, the portfolio goes further to exhibit the quality and breadth of accomplishments. For example, an effective portfolio often contains the actual curricula that a clinician-educator developed, manuscripts and miniaturized poster presentations that a faculty coauthored with mentees, a summary of numerical evaluations of the faculty by trainees, and detailed information on mentee outcomes resulting from the faculty member's mentorship. Commonly, a narrative

on the faculty member's medical education philosophy and career goals is included. Continuous maintenance of a portfolio ensures that important activities are captured as they occur. To emphasize the most significant accomplishments, we suggest a limit of 10 pages without attachments.

SPECIAL MENTORING RELATIONSHIPS IN ACADEMIC MEDICINE: TRAINEES, WOMEN AND MINORITIES

■ MENTORING TRAINEES

From the perspective of trainees, ideal mentor attributes include maintaining confidentiality; being approachable, accessible, and nonjudgmental; getting to know the mentee on a personal level; promoting the mentee's goals over the mentor's; opening doors for the mentee; and encouraging self-reflection. See **Table 39-6** ingredients for successful resident mentoring.

TABLE 39-6 Strategies to Promote Successful Mentoring of Trainees

- Formal assignments of faculty mentors that takes into consideration the needs of women and minorities
- Dedicated time for trainees and mentors to meet: formal meetings at least twice annually with readily available access to mentor at other times
- Buy-in from department chairperson:
  - Ensure protected faculty time for mentoring
  - Establish bonuses or awards for successful mentoring
  - Explicitly recognize mentoring as criteria for faculty promotion
- Faculty development to augment mentoring skills around the following common topics for house staff mentees:
  - Helping residents apply for jobs after residency:
    - Preparing a curriculum vitae
    - Focusing the job search
    - Interviewing skills
    - Communication with potential employers
    - Negotiating strategies
    - Timeline
  - Assisting residents with the fellowship application process:
    - Advantages to applying during second- vs third-year of residency
    - Fellowship match through ERAS (how the process works, key deadlines)
    - Selecting faculty to write letters of recommendation
    - Preparing personal statements and curriculum vitae
    - Selecting programs to apply to (reputation, location, unique program aspects, when to consider programs outside the match)
    - Elements sought by fellowship directors
    - Interviewing skills
    - Lifestyle considerations in the specialty
  - Mentoring resident scholarly activity:
    - Preparing a clinical vignette abstract, poster, or case report
    - Giving oral presentations and speaking publicly
    - Establishing a quality improvement project
    - Writing effective review articles
    - Providing potential networking opportunities locally, regionally, nationally
    - Involving residents in professional societies
    - Submitting to the institutional review board
    - Providing resources for statistical support
    - Optimizing clinical and professional development:
    - Selection of elective rotations
    - Ethics, integrity, and professionalism
    - Interpersonal skills with physicians, nurses, and staff
    - Time management, organization, and efficiency
- Providing resources for handling difficult situations (burnout, psychiatric illness, substance abuse, interpersonal conflicts, family/social stressors, career angst, financial stress, and medical errors)

MENTORING WOMEN AND MINORITIES

A recent systematic review highlights the existing evidence gap in mentoring programs for women and minorities and also serves as a call to action to reduce disparities in student and faculty recruitment, retention, and promotion of women and minorities. **Table 39-7** highlights strategies specific to this problem.

CONCLUSION

No single mentoring model is superior, so the mentoring pair should use one that best meets the mentee's specific goals. Clinician-educator mentees should be encouraged to assemble

TABLE 39-7 Strategies to Promote Successful Mentoring of Underrepresented Minorities

URM mentoring programs should emphasize the following areas in addition to characteristics common to any successful mentoring relationship:

- Skills development in:
  - Cross-cultural communication
  - Socializaion into the field of medicine
  - Networking
  - Career advancement: specific guidance in faculty promotion, especially as URM faculty are more likely to engage in activities such as community-based endeavors and pipeline development which have less clearly established path for promotion
  - Negotiating
  - Research: grant writing, navigating the IRB, manuscript preparation, editing
- Leadership development
- Creation of a welcoming environment to reduce feelings of isolation
- Assignment of mentees with mentors who share race, culture, ethnicity, language, or gender
- Introduction of mentees to national URM leaders
- Partnership with the affiliated medical center to ensure the mission of the medical center includes promotion of diversity and reduction of disparities in order to achieve a successful and sustainable URM mentoring program

their activities and achievements into an educator portfolio, a tool designed to enhance their chances of promotion at academic medical centers. Resident mentoring should focus on career planning and preparedness, networking, identifying opportunities for scholarly activity, role modeling of work-life balance, and supporting the resident.

SUGGESTED READINGS

Beech BM, Calles-Escandon J, Hairston KG, et al. Mentoring programs for underrepresented minority faculty in academic medical centers: a systematic review of the literature. *Acad Med.* 2013;88:541-549.

Daley SP, Palermo AG, Nivet M, et al. Diversity in academic medicine no. 6. Successful programs in minority faculty development: ingredients of success. *Mt Sinai J Med.* 2008;75:533-551.

Farrell SE, Digioia NM, Broderick KB, et al. Mentoring for clinical-educators. *Acad Emerg Med.* 2004;11:1346-1350.

Ramanan R, Phillips R, Davis RB, et al. Mentoring in medicine: keys to satisfaction. *Am J Med.* 2002;112:336-341.

Ramani S, Gruppen L, Kachur EK. Twelve tips for developing effective mentors. *Med Teacher.* 2006;28:404-408.

Sambunjak D, Straus SE, Marusic A. Mentoring in academic medicine: a systematic review. *JAMA.* 2006;296:1103-1115.

Straus SE, Johnson MO, Marquez C, et al. Characteristics of successful and failed mentoring relationships: a qualitative study across two academic health centers. *Acad Med.* 2013;88:82-89.

Tsen LC, Borus JF, Nadelson CC, et al. The development, implementation, and assessment of an innovative faculty mentoring leadership program. *Acad Med.* 2012;87:1757-1761.

Zerzan JT, Hess R, Schur E, et al. Making the most of mentors: a guide for mentees. *Acad Med.* 2009;84:140-144.

CHAPTER 40

Research in the Hospital

Jeffrey L. Schnipper, MD, MPH, FHM

Hospitalists are often asked to participate in or lead quality improvement (QI) and research initiatives, locally and nationally. Because data collection and feedback are part of any QI effort, and because the results of these efforts are often published, the hospitalists who lead these efforts often ask (or are asked by others) the question: "Is this research?" The short answer is that QI research is different from standard QI efforts in many respects. In this chapter, we will address the differences between standard QI efforts and research, some reasons to do QI research, the appropriate time to do QI research (for you and for the scientific question at hand), how "rigorously" to conduct QI research, getting started with the process, the ingredients for a successful project, and issues related to study design and methods that are either unique to or are particularly relevant to QI research.

This chapter will address both "quality improvement" and "patient safety" research. The two terms are often used interchangeably, and often the line between them is gray. For example, is an effort to increase β-blocker use to prevent a second myocardial infarction an issue of QI or safety? That said, "safety" is often used in the context of rare incidents where there is a strong link between an error and its associated outcome (eg, wrong-site surgery). The issues regarding both types of research are often the same. This chapter will review additional issues unique to patient safety research that take account of the rarity of many safety events.

PRACTICE POINT

- Collecting, analyzing, and reporting data does not turn a QI project into research. The important characteristic of QI research, as opposed to standard QI efforts, is that the question to be answered is not "can we improve care here?" but "does this intervention work in general?" If the goal is to design and test a novel intervention to improve care (or to test an established intervention in a novel setting), to establish whether a particular intervention works in a wide variety of settings such that it might become a new standard of care, and/or to learn generalizable lessons about how to successfully implement such an intervention, then it is research.

OVERVIEW OF QI RESEARCH

QI VERSUS QI RESEARCH

QI research is not just writing up the results of a QI project. In fact, writing up the results should be part of almost all QI efforts so that other institutions may learn from your experience and you may earn "academic credit" for having done the work. The SQUIRE Guidelines (http://www.squire-statement.org/) provide detailed advice on how to write up such results. Content unique to these reports (as opposed to conventional research manuscripts) include:

- Introduction: description of the local problem and the intended improvement
- Methods: discussion of any ethical issues, planning the intervention, and planning the study of the intervention
- Results: description of the environmental context, a timeline of the intervention, degree of success in implementation, how and why the plan evolved, and lessons learned from that evolution

- Discussion: issues of maintaining improvement over time, causal mechanisms regarding the specific components of the intervention, and how environmental context played a role in the success (or failure) of the intervention and its implementation

In a standard QI project, results over time may be displayed using run charts with statistical process control limits, with results plotted over time, a central line at the mean, and limit lines at three standard deviations (SD) above and below the mean. In a chart with 25 data points, the chance of a point being outside the 3SD lines, indicating "special cause variation," is 6.5%, similar to the 0.05 threshold for statistical significance in standard statistical tests. Such charts allow participants in a QI effort to see whether their interventions are working, whether the improvements seen are likely to be due to chance, and to help guide further improvements to the intervention.

The important characteristic of QI research, as opposed to standard QI efforts, is that the question to be answered is not "can we improve care here?" but "does this intervention work in general?" Human subject research is defined as "a systematic investigation, including research, development, testing, and evaluation designed to develop or contribute to generalizable knowledge." "Generalizable knowledge" may be further defined as "enduring knowledge about the nature and function of human beings." If the only goal of a QI effort is to improve local compliance with currently recognized best practices (or a safety effort designed to reduce medical errors) using recognized procedures, without adding to existing knowledge about the general nature and function of human beings, then it is not research. On the other hand, if the goal is to design and test a novel intervention to improve care (or to test an established intervention in a novel setting), to establish whether a particular intervention works in a wide variety of settings such that it might become a new standard of care, and/or to learn generalizable lessons about how to successfully implement such an intervention, then it is research.

WHY AND WHEN TO CONDUCT QI RESEARCH

Are the reasons to conduct QI research enough to motivate you to do the work required?

Reasons to conduct QI research include general reasons, such as expanding the body of medical knowledge and helping your patients; local reasons, such as answering a burning question important for your institution or your practice; and personal reasons, such as professional satisfaction or to provide balance to your clinical duties. QI research requires a great deal of work and, especially at the beginning of a research career, may come as an addition to an already full clinical schedule. The rewards can be considerable if you are motivated.

Is it the right time scientifically to conduct QI research?

In phase 1 of QI, the question is usually, "Can this intervention work in at least one place?" We could think about this phase using the analogy of drug trials, where early research and development work in a pharmaceutical company and phase I/II clinical trials look for safety and efficacy in a limited number of carefully selected patients. In this phase, interventions are often not well defined. The best approach in this phase is to do standard QI work, iterative refinement of the intervention using Plan-Do-Study-Act cycles, and to monitor improvement using run charts. In other words, it is not time to do QI research yet. However, some of the groundwork for later research may be done at this time. In addition to optimizing the intervention itself, measures of process and outcome may be developed, and measures of environmental context and intervention fidelity may also be developed.

In phase 2, the primary questions are the following:

- Does this intervention work outside of its original location?
- Does it require refinement?
- How likely is it to work?

- What is the magnitude of benefit?
- Is it cost-effective?
- Should this intervention be spread widely?

The time to do rigorous QI research is during phase 2 of an intervention, analogous to phase III drug trials (often randomized controlled trials) needed for FDA approval. The intervention should be studied as rigorously as possible, especially more novel, expensive, or risky interventions, in order to know whether the benefits truly outweigh the risks and costs.

> ### PRACTICE POINT
>
> - In "Phase I" of quality improvement, the question is usually "can this intervention work in at least one place?"
> - In "Phase 2," a more rigorous evaluation is required to answer the question of whether an intervention that might work is ready for widespread use. This is time for QI research.
> - In "Phase 3," QI interventions proven effective in Phase 2 are disseminated widely.

Once an intervention has been proven to work, the goal is to spread the intervention widely. Phase 3 usually requires adaptation to each local environment, ideally using lessons learned from prior work (eg, the most effective components of the intervention and how to optimize implementation). Standard QI methods are now focused on local adaptation of the intervention and making the micro- and macro-environment more conducive to effective implementation. Lessons about how, why, and where an intervention works should have already been answered in prior QI research to help guide this process.

SHOULD QI RESEARCH BE CONDUCTED RIGOROUSLY?

The best ways to think about and conduct QI research are not without controversy. There are some, such as Dr Donald Berwick, former head of the Institute for Health Care Improvement, who would argue that all QI efforts are local. Inherently complex behavioral interventions need different approaches than just testing a pill. Randomized controlled trials purposefully control for environmental context in the name of unbiased outcome assessment. And yet, it is precisely the context and the process that are most important to evaluate, because they reveal how, why, and where an intervention is successful. Proponents of this approach argue for more case studies and "formative evaluation" to better study these issues.

However, ignoring stronger study designs may lead to gross overestimation of treatment effects. Observational before-after studies are inherently confounded by temporal trends (ie, general improvement over time), cointerventions (other interventions that may affect the outcome), and biased by the Hawthorne effect (improvement that comes when people know they are being watched). And studies that compare those who volunteer to implement an intervention early to those who do not may be completely confounded by inherent differences between implementation and control sites. QI research does not differ from biomedical research in requiring some estimate about how likely an intervention will be successful before institutions invest time, money, and resources in their implementation. For example, a very successful intervention at one hospital, but not successful in the next 10 hospitals studied, is very different from a successful intervention in 75% of the hospitals in which it is evaluated.

We therefore advocate for strong study designs when appropriate and possible, but we also advocate complementing this work with "mixed methods" (ie, quantitative and qualitative research) that look carefully at contextual factors, intervention fidelity (ie, how faithfully an intervention is implemented as designed), and barriers and facilitators to successful implementation. Not every study can (or should be) a randomized controlled trial.

CONCEPTUAL MODEL OF QI RESEARCH

Celia Brown and Richard Lilford wrote a series of articles in 2008 describing an approach for rigorously evaluating patient safety interventions based on the recommendations of a network sponsored by the Medical Research Council, United Kingdom that echoes this sentiment. Their conceptual framework is shown in **Figure 40-1**. It is based on the Donabedian "structure-process-outcome" model and provides additional detail for studies of patient safety interventions. They note that such interventions may be aimed at *management processes*, such as nurse to patient ratios and time allocated to professional development, and/or *clinical processes*, such as washing hands between patients. The effectiveness of an intervention should be observed at all points to the right of the intervention. *Patient outcomes* may be "hard" (such as hospital readmission or patient mortality), which are clearly relevant but may be relatively insensitive to change. Surrogate outcomes, process measures, and error rates are more sensitive to change and should complement hard outcome measurement.

Observations at the point of intervention should be used to assess the *fidelity* with which the intervention was implemented and how it has been adapted over time. If an intervention is not implemented with high fidelity, it is unlikely to cause improvements in outcomes, even if they are observed. And when improvement is not seen, low fidelity may explain those findings even if the intervention were theoretically efficacious.

Observations to the left of the intervention provide information about environmental *context* and may explain differences among sites. Organizational *structure* may influence management processes, which in turn affect *intervening variables* such as morale, safety culture, teamwork, and provider knowledge and beliefs. These variables then influence clinical processes. If an intervention, implemented with high fidelity, improves all downstream processes and outcomes (even if some are not statistically significant), then it increases the likelihood that the intervention itself was really the cause of the improvement.

GETTING STARTED

■ ASKING THE RIGHT QUESTION

The most important first step is choosing the right research question, ie, the uncertainty about something in the population that the investigator wants to resolve by making measurements on his or her study population. Good research questions are indeed everywhere and may be provoked by your clinical experience, by the advent of new technologies, by acknowledging the need to improve, and/or by maintaining a healthy skepticism about prevailing beliefs. Initial challenges to beginning a QI research project may include psychological (getting over the fact that you are not a "researcher"), scientific (developing a good research question), and logistical (choosing study designs that are feasible). Developing questions is an iterative process, and we recommend consulting early and often with advisors and colleagues.

A good research question has the following attributes:

1. The study that can answer the question is feasible: adequate number of subjects, availability of adequate technical expertise, affordable in time and money.
2. The question is interesting: it confirms, extends, or refutes previous findings (this implies that you have done the background reading on the subject).
3. The question is relevant: it has implications for clinical knowledge, practice, or policy.
4. The question can be answered ethically.

Research questions often start out vague (eg, "Are fewer nurses bad for patients?"). To carry out a study, these questions need to be refined so that they become measurable. The hypothesis needs to be testable by getting specific about three elements: the patient population, the intervention, and the outcome. Using the above example, a refined research question might be "for medical inpatients, is there an association between the patient-to-nurse ratio and in-hospital mortality?"

■ PLANNING YOUR RESEARCH

Once a research question has been refined, the next steps are to develop a specific aim (or aims) and a hypothesis. The specific aim is

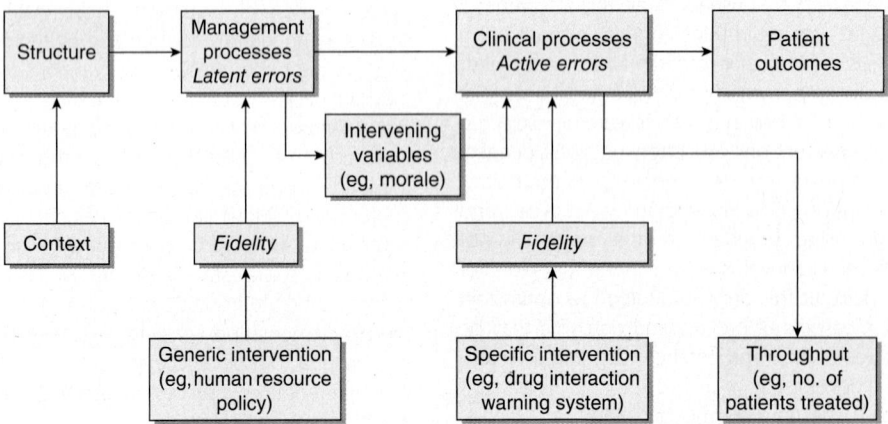

Figure 40-1 *Conceptual framework for evaluating patient safety interventions. Observations can be made at all points in the chain to provide information on context, fidelity, and quality and safety outcomes.* (From Brown C, Lilford R. *BMJ* 2008;337:a2764, with permission from BMJ Publishing Group Ltd.)

TABLE 40-1 Outline of a Research Proposal

Research Speak	English Translation
Research question	What questions will the study address?
Background and significance	Why are these questions important?
	What do we already know about them?
Aims and hypothesis	What do you plan to do?
	What do you expect to happen?
Subjects:	Who will you study?
Inclusion/exclusion criteria	How will they agree to participate?
Consent	
Design	How will you actually do the study?
	What is your "protocol"?
Data sources	Where will you get your data?
	What do you plan to collect?
Outcome variables	Which data are key to your question (or hypothesis)?
Predictor variables (covariates)	Which will confuse (or confound) the issue?
Statistical issues	How large is the study and how will it be analyzed?
Human subjects	How will you maintain ethical standards?
	How will you protect patients' rights?

what (exactly) you want to do. For example, "Determine the effects of an enoxaparin guideline on the appropriate use of enoxaparin." The hypothesis is the a priori, testable expectation for what you think is going to happen (or has happened). For example, "implementing an enoxaparin guideline will increase appropriate use of enoxaparin."

The next step is to develop a study proposal. Writing everything down in a standardized way serves several purposes: it forces you to address all the issues that may come up with a study's design and execution; it provides a convenient way for you to explain your study to others, get feedback, and refine your methods; and it is necessary for Institutional Review Board (IRB) approval and to obtain funding if needed (but we recommend developing a study proposal even if you do not intend to apply for funding). **Table 40-1** provides a list of the elements of a research proposal, both in "research speak" and their English translations.

INGREDIENTS FOR A SUCCESSFUL RESEARCH PROJECT

Once you have a good research idea, what else do you need to turn it into a successful project? The basic components are data, research training or experience, time, funding, a research team, IRB approval, and a plan for dissemination of the results.

DATA SOURCES

Data may come from a wide variety of sources, including institutional data, publicly available data, data from collaborators, and data you collect yourself. Every institution collects data for billing, public reporting, and other purposes. Find out who leads this effort, whether and how you can access these data, and how clean they are (eg, whether the owners have already taken care of issues like missing or erroneous data, misspellings, and other features that make research quality analyses possible). Publicly available data have obvious advantages, but it may sometimes be time consuming and/or expensive to obtain, and data sets can be large and unwieldy, requiring a certain level of statistical expertise. Data you

collect yourself is obviously under your complete control and may be designed to answer your exact question but takes time and resources to collect. Data from collaborators is sometimes the best of all worlds if such opportunities are available and you are interested in the questions the data can answer.

RESEARCH TRAINING AND EXPERIENCE

You *can* do research, but it helps to have some background. This background may take many forms, from mentors and collaborators, short-term programs, all the way to degree programs and fellowships. In our experience, a summer-long program in research methods (such as those at the Harvard School of Public Health and at the University of California, San Francisco School of Medicine), followed by a research project done in close collaboration with an experienced mentor, is often enough to pave the way for further collaborative research projects and/or small independent projects.

TIME

One of the most challenging ingredients to obtain is time. Unless you have protected time built into your schedule or you have negotiated for protected time up front, the short-term solution is often an investment of your own time. If you can prove your ability to successfully conduct projects, especially QI and safety projects of inherent value to the institution, then protected time can often be negotiated the second time around. An important early step is to estimate the time needed to complete a research project. We recommend designing a timeline as part of your initial proposal (**Figure 40-2**). You should consult early with someone else to make sure the timeline is feasible. Almost all studies take more time than you initially anticipate!

FUNDING

The degree of funding required, if any, will depend on the project. Be sure to consider the opportunity costs of you and your collaborators (ie, time taken away from other activities) in addition to direct costs. Direct costs might include the paid effort of research assistants and statisticians, office supplies and incidentals. As with a timeline, it is never too early to design a preliminary budget and share it with others for refinement (**Table 40-2**). Line items include personnel costs (salary and fringe for employee effort, hourly or daily fees for consultants), equipment, travel, and miscellaneous costs like office supplies, software, computer hardware, and photocopying.

Potential sources of funding depend on the scale of the project and the purpose of the study. For most QI and safety projects, begin with your institution, especially if the costs are modest ($50,000-$100,000). If you can link your research question to financial and performance priorities of your hospital, internal funding becomes more likely. Internal sources include division or department funds, hospital-wide research grants, funding from the risk management organization at the hospital, and charitable giving. For questions less closely linked to hospital priorities or for larger projects, external funding is often required. Sources include foundations such as the National Patient Safety Foundation, the Commonwealth Fund (US), and the Robert Wood Johnson Foundation; governmental sources such as Veterans Affairs, Agency for Health Care Research and Quality, and National Institutes of Health; statewide or national QI or safety initiatives; the Patient-Centered Outcomes Research Institute (PCORI, a nonprofit nongovernmental organization authorized by Congress in 2010); and industry, including pharmaceutical companies and device makers. Relationships between physicians and industry are under more scrutiny than in the past, but some companies are still willing to fund investigator-initiated projects if priorities are closely aligned.

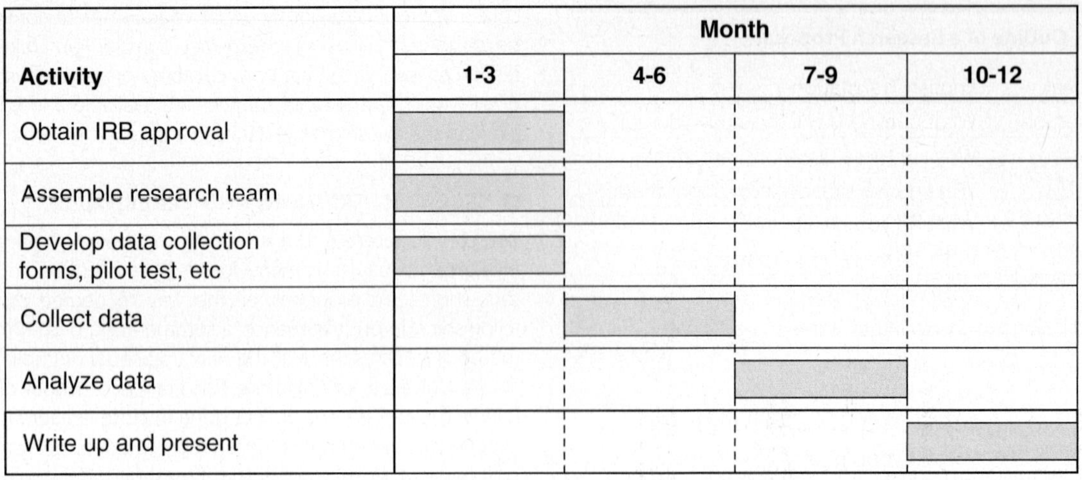

Activity	Month			
	1-3	4-6	7-9	10-12
Obtain IRB approval	▭			
Assemble research team	▭			
Develop data collection forms, pilot test, etc	▭			
Collect data		▭		
Analyze data			▭	
Write up and present				▭

Figure 40-2 *Sample timeline.*

■ RESEARCH TEAM

The research team should be multidisciplinary, as is true of QI teams in general. One economical way to find collaborators is to work with medical students and residents, as long as the work can be done around their busy schedules (as for example, retrospective chart review). Paid research assistants are often required for daily, prospective data collection. It is never too early to involve a statistician to help determine sample size (and therefore costs and feasibility of the study) and identify other methodologic issues before they become problems.

■ IRB APPROVAL

Institutional Review Board approval is often the source of much angst and controversy. To complicate matters, there is yet to be consensus on when IRB approval is needed. Some recent clarity was provided by Lynn et al. in a 2007 article in *Annals of Internal Medicine*, "The ethics of using QI methods in health care." They note the characteristics of activities that are likely to be both QI and human subjects research, such as

1. Issues that go beyond current best practice
2. Allocation of patients to different treatments
3. Deliberately delayed feedback of data to avoid bias
4. Key involvement of researchers without commitment to ongoing QI at that site
5. Funding by parties outside the clinical setting

TABLE 40-2 Sample Budget

Item	Description	% Time	Amount
Principal investigator	Oversees project	20%	$30,000
Coinvestigator	Research collaborator	10%	$15,000
Consultant	Specialized assistance	5%	$5000
Research assistant	Collects data	50%	$15,000
Statistician	Cleans, analyzes data	10%	$10,000
Travel to SHM	Presentation of findings		$1500
Office supplies	Copying, faxes, etc		$500
Total			$77,000

SHM, Society of Hospital Medicine.

For our purposes, QI research (as opposed to QI efforts alone) is human subjects research and requires IRB approval. However, in many cases, it is possible to obtain expedited approval with waiver of patient consent on the grounds that the studies are of minimal risk, that patient confidentiality will be rigorously protected, that the study could not be practically done if patient consent were required, and that the rights of patients will not be adversely affected by waiver of consent and authorization. As with your research proposal, begin the IRB application process early and have others with experience look through it (human research committees often have consultants who can help with this). Interview forms and consent forms will need to be created as part of this process. Do not worry if these are not finalized—amendments can always be submitted later. Lastly, as part of the IRB approval process, study staff must complete training in the ethical treatment of research subjects. Each institution has its own specific requirements.

■ DISSEMINATION PLAN

A successful research project should include a dissemination plan. Research in a vacuum is not useful. You have a responsibility to let others know the results of your study, positive or negative. Besides manuscripts, other study products might include detailed descriptions of your interventions, software specifications, data collection instruments (surveys and interview guides). Outlets for dissemination include not only peer-reviewed journals but presentations at your own institution and professional society meetings, reports to your funders, and press releases.

STUDY DESIGN ISSUES IN QI AND SAFETY RESEARCH

■ INTERNAL AND EXTERNAL VALIDITY

Two attributes make a research study useful to others: (1) internal validity, meaning that the results of the study reflect reality and can be believed; and (2) external validity, or generalizability, meaning that the results can be applied to other patients or settings. Without internal validity, generalizability is a moot point, so in a sense internal validity is the more important of the two attributes.

■ THREATS TO INTERNAL VALIDITY

Chance

There are three main threats to the internal validity of a study: chance, confounding, and bias. Chance means that the results were simply due to the "luck of the draw." Type 1 error is when the null hypothesis is rejected due to chance when in fact it is true (for example, drug A is found to be better than drug B when in fact the two are equal). This can be thought of as a false-positive study. By convention, the threshold for type 1 error in most studies (known as alpha) is set at 0.05. When the *P* value from a statistical test is below this threshold, we call the difference statistically significant. Another way to think of this is to say that for every 20 studies that find a statistically significant difference, one of those studies is wrong simply due to chance.

Type 2 error results in accepting the null hypothesis when in fact it is false (eg, concluding that drug A and drug B are no different from each other when in fact drug A is better). The threshold, called beta, is typically set at 0.10 for definitive studies and 0.20 for preliminary studies—two to four times higher than alpha. In other words, the medical scientific community has implicitly decided that it is more acceptable to have a false-negative study than a false-positive study. This makes sense for drug trials when the consequence of a positive study is FDA approval. It is less clear whether this argument holds for QI research. Statistical *power* is 1—*β*. So, a study with 90% power means there is a 10% chance that it will not find a difference when in fact one exists, simply due to chance.

Confounding

A confounder is a third factor (ie, not the exposure or the outcome), associated with the exposure of interest (like the QI intervention you are studying) that independently causes the outcome of interest. For example, the earliest work in the epidemiology of lung cancer found a strong association with alcohol consumption. The confounder, of course, was cigarette smoking: something associated with alcohol use (people smoke in bars) that causes the outcome of interest (lung cancer). Confounding has to do with the science of what is being studied. Managing confounding requires knowledge of what factors could cause the outcome(s) you are studying. In QI research, major confounders include temporal trends (ie, general improvement with time, a problem with before-after studies), cointerventions (ie, other interventions that affect your outcome, implemented at the same time but apart from your intervention), and "indication" (ie, in nonrandomized studies, the reasons why sites choose to implement an intervention that may be strongly related to the outcomes being studied).

Bias

In general terms, bias is error in a study that results in an incorrect estimate of the association between the exposure and the outcome. There are two broad categories: selection bias, which is an error in the process of identifying the study populations; and, much more common, observation or information bias, which is an error in measurement of the exposure and/or the outcome. There are many types of information bias, each with its own story: recall bias, interviewer bias, loss to follow-up, misclassification. Unlike confounding, bias has more to do with human nature and how the study is conducted. In QI research, one major bias is the Hawthorne effect, or changes in measurement caused by participants' knowledge that they are being observed. Another potential bias arises when the intervention itself affects measurement. For example, in early studies of rapid response teams (RRTs), patients whose status was Do Not Resuscitate (DNR) were often excluded from the outcome of in-hospital mortality. When RRTs approached patients in extremis, one common activity was verifying code status. In several cases, patients and their caregivers decided to change code status to DNR. These patients were therefore excluded from the outcome. But before the advent the RRTs, these patients would have been included in outcome assessment because no one verified their code status at that time. A before-after study could find a difference in mortality simply because the intervention altered who was in the denominator for outcome assessment.

■ MANAGING THREATS TO INTERNAL VALIDITY

Table 40-3 provides ways to manage the threats to internal validity while the study is being designed (ie, before data are collected) and/or while the study is being analyzed (after data are collected). For example, during the study design phase, chance is managed using power and sample size calculations. If alpha and beta are chosen and the effect size can be estimated (ie, how beneficial the intervention will be), then the sample size can be calculated. Effect size may be estimated from preliminary studies, or more conservatively, may be chosen as the smallest effect that would be considered "clinically significant" by clinical experts. Conversely, if the sample size is fixed (eg, the ward has a known daily census and the study must be completed in 6 weeks), then statistical power to detect different effect sizes can be calculated. Once a study is completed, the effect of chance is derived using tests of statistical significance (ie, calculation of *P* values).

During the study design phase, confounding can be managed most effectively through randomization (confounding cannot exist if the confounder is evenly distributed among those who do and do not receive the intervention). Anything short of randomization is going to be less effective at managing confounding, but attempts may still be made to pick patient populations that are as comparable as possible (eg, medical wards from medium-sized, nonteaching community hospitals in the suburbs). During the data analysis phase, confounding can be managed with stratification (eg, looking at the effect of alcohol on lung cancer in smokers separately from the effect in nonsmokers). This is very effective if there are only one or two major confounders, but is impractical when the list of confounders is large (*N* confounders means 2^N subgroups to analyze, each with a very small sample size). The purpose of multivariable (sometimes called multivariate) analysis is to simultaneously "adjust" for multiple confounders at once. But keep in mind that confounding can still exist, either because of incomplete adjustment, inaccurate measurement of the confounder, or existence of other unmeasured confounders.

During the study design phase, bias can be minimized by employing principles of sound study design: blinding to intervention status (not just "double-blind," but as many people involved in the study as possible: patients, research assistants, outcome assessors, statisticians), prospective data collection, valid data collection instruments such as previously validated surveys and questionnaires, and thorough follow-up for all endpoints. Once the study has been conducted, bias cannot be "adjusted for" during the data analysis phase, although sometimes its direction and magnitude may be estimated. For example, to estimate the impact of loss-to-follow-up, some experts recommend assuming that everyone who received the intervention and was lost to follow-up did poorly, while everyone who received usual care and was lost to follow-up

TABLE 40-3 Managing Threats to Internal Validity

Threat to Validity	Study Design (Before)	Analysis (After)
Chance	Power calculations	Statistics
Confounding	Randomization	Stratification
	Picking comparable groups	Multivariable regression
Bias	Blinding, prospective data collection, valid instruments, thorough follow-up	Unable to manage (although sometimes direction and magnitude can be estimated)

did well. Even large effect sizes can crumble under the weight of such assumptions if the loss to follow-up rate is large. On the other hand, poor data collection instruments often create noise and bias "toward the null" (ie, finding no difference). Therefore, if a difference is found, it is probably not the result of such bias. Because bias cannot really be adjusted for after the fact, it is important to manage study design issues up front, before any data are collected.

■ IMPROVING GENERALIZABILITY

Guidelines for improving the generalizability of a study include the following: (1) describe your patient population well, so that others can determine whether their patient populations are comparable; (2) describe your interventions well, so that others can determine what they would need to do to replicate your experience; and (3) describe your environmental context well, so others can determine whether a comparable intervention could be implemented in their settings. A common question related to generalizability is whether interventions should be maximally customized to the particular site where it is being studied. Such an approach increases the chances of success, but it may come at the price of generalizability. The answer should depend on which aspects of the study site are unique. Ideally, during phase 1 work, exactly which features need to be customized (and how) has already been determined; and these customizations can then be specified in advance.

■ TYPES OF STUDIES USED IN QI RESEARCH

Study designs appropriate for QI and safety research include randomized controlled trials (with randomization at either the individual patient level or "clustered" by physician, ward, service, or hospital), before-after studies, interrupted time series, "stepped wedge," and observational cohort studies (prospective and retrospective). Each has its advantages and disadvantages. Not all QI research needs to be a randomized controlled trial to provide valid information.

Randomized controlled trials

A randomized controlled trial (RCT) minimizes confounding by ensuring that potential confounders are equally distributed in the different arms of the study. This is true regardless of whether the confounders are known or can be measured. To the extent that RCTs require prospective data collection and at least allow the possibility of some blinding, they minimize bias as well, as long as there are valid data collection instruments and thorough follow-up. And these studies still require adequate sample size to deal with chance. Note that the outcome may be measured at one point in time (after the intervention has been implemented in those sites randomized to receive it) or as relative improvement over time (preintervention to postintervention). The latter may be preferred if you suspect large variation in baseline performance and especially if the same patients are going to be followed for the entire study period. All RCTs should be analyzed on an "intention-to-treat" basis, meaning that outcomes are measured according to the original intent of the randomization, regardless of what treatment (if any) was actually received. This preserves the sanctity of the randomization and is particularly important in QI studies, where the factors that lead to successful implementation or compliance with an intervention may independently predict positive outcomes. However, RCTs may not always be feasible or ethical. You may have limited control over who receives a QI intervention or you may be required (eg, for regulatory reasons) to provide it to everyone. It is often not ethical to study potentially harmful interventions with an RCT. And for outcomes that are rare or take a long time to develop, RCTs may be prohibitively expensive to conduct. Rare outcomes are particularly an issue with safety (as opposed to QI) studies. The best times to use an RCT are when an

intervention can be randomized; there is particularly big concern for temporal trends, cointerventions, and other confounders that may not be known or cannot be measured; when the costs or potential risks of the intervention is high (such that they need to be balanced against a precise estimate of benefits); the target outcome is of high value (such as mortality); many settings will be affected by the results (eg, possible incorporation into a regulatory requirement); and any other situation that requires a precise estimate of effects and costs.

Cluster randomization

Cluster randomized trials are a type of RCT in which the unit of randomization is larger than the individual patient. For example, in a recent trial of a medication reconciliation intervention, we randomized by both medical team and floor so that we had clean separation of both nurses and doctors in the two arms of the study. This avoids treatment group "contamination" (ie, clinicians who change their behavior even with control patients because they have been exposed to or know about the intervention), it facilitates implementation of the intervention (eg, service-wide educational efforts), and administrative convenience. The major disadvantage is loss of statistical power. When patients of one physician, for example, are treated similarly to each other but different from the patients of another physician, this results in "intraclass correlation." This reduces the effective sample size, depending on the degree of the correlation and the size of the clusters (eg, the number of patients per physician). This correlation therefore needs to be anticipated and estimated in advance and used when making estimates of required sample size. Nevertheless, this is the preferred study design in many cases, especially when there are big advantages to training and implementation, the threat of contamination is high, the intervention requires it, the cluster size is small, and/or when the advantages are otherwise worth the loss in power.

RCTs, whether clustered or not, may suffer from issues of generalizability in that not every patient or health care setting may be willing to participate in one. In general, this is a sacrifice worth making in the name of internal validity, if feasible and appropriate to do so. Describing your patients, intervention, and environment well goes a long way toward alleviating these concerns.

Stepped wedge

The stepped wedge refers to a study design in which an intervention is sequentially rolled out to different groups at different times, such as different floors of a hospital (**Figure 40-3**). The order of the rollout is randomized to avoid confounding by indication (ie, those most ready for the intervention get it first). Each group serves a different amount of time in the usual care and intervention arms. This

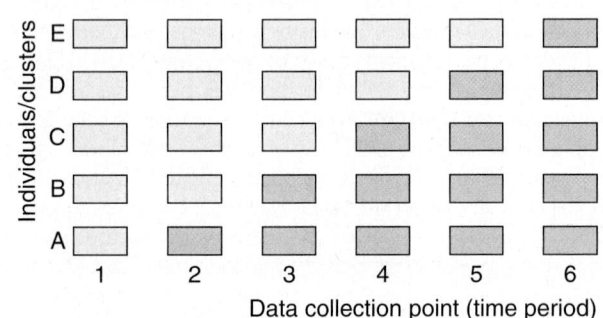

Figure 40-3 *Stepped wedge study design. The intervention is rolled out to individuals or clusters sequentially over time, from blank cells (usual care) to shaded cells (intervention). (From Brown C, Lilford R. BMJ 2008;337:a2764, with permission from BMJ Publishing Group Ltd.)*

approach allows adjustment for temporal trends and also minimizes confounding because each group serves as its own control. Thus, the stepped wedge provides the advantages of a control group but is more practical than an RCT, especially if the intervention requires a gradual rollout anyway. The disadvantages are practical constraints regarding implementation, logistical challenges, and the risk of contamination (eg, colleagues hearing about the intervention occurring on a different floor).

Time series

Before-after studies and interrupted time series may be more feasible than RCTs when you have limited control over who receives the intervention and when they receive it. In a simple before-after study, outcomes are measured at one point before the intervention and one point after the intervention (eg, use of measures to prevent venous thromboembolism before and after a mass e-mail reminder is sent out). This is probably the most common QI research study design, but unfortunately is one of the worst. It is very sensitive to temporal trends and to cointerventions. Much preferred is an interrupted time series (ITS), in which repeated observations (at least 3) are made prior to and after the intervention is implemented. The effect of the intervention can then be measured over and above temporal trends (although it still does not adjust for cointerventions). ITS is useful if the intervention needs to be given to everyone, all at once. Because there is no control group, one disadvantage is lack of generalizability, especially if the study site is particularly enthusiastic and well equipped to conduct the intervention. Another disadvantage is that the analysis assumes that the intervention is implemented once and does not change over time. However, newer sophisticated analytical techniques, such as random effects models with nonlinear time-by-intervention effects, can take into account such phenomena as continuous improvement over time (eg, as the intervention is refined) and/or reaching a plateau due to a ceiling effect (inability to improve further because quality is already so high).

Cohort studies

A word of caution is in order about observational cohort studies, in which sites that choose to implement an intervention are compared with sites that choose not to. Because of potentially large differences in baseline rates of quality, the analysis should never be a simple comparison of outcomes at one point in time (eg, after

implementation in the intervention arm). However, even if the analysis incorporates baseline rates by comparing improvement over time, these types of studies are potentially flawed. Those sites that are "early adopters" are often very different from those that are not in terms of culture of quality and safety, leadership, organizational structure, etc. These confounders may have large effects on the ability to implement and improve outcomes in response to an intervention. These confounders are also pervasive, potentially unknown, and difficult to measure. This confounding may be a fatal flaw to internal validity. A better approach is to deliver the intervention to as many groups as possible (to improve generalizability) and do an ITS.

Summary of study design issues

In conclusion, the optimal study design for a QI or safety study depends on answers to several questions.

1. Is it feasible and ethical to have a control group?
2. Do you have control over who gets the intervention and when?
3. Does the intervention need to be implemented all at once or gradually?
4. Can/should the intervention be delivered to individual patients, or does it make more sense to deliver it to a higher level (eg, physician, floor, service)?
5. Are the outcomes rare or do they take a long time to develop?
6. Are the costs and risks of the intervention low?
7. Will the results be used to promote widespread adoption of this intervention?

Table 40-4 illustrates how the answers to these questions may influence your choice of study design.

■ ADVANCED TOPICS AND CONTROVERSIES IN QI RESEARCH

Should the interventions be held fixed while they are being studied? On the one hand, such an approach allows for better description of the intervention, makes it clear "what" is being studied, and makes analyses easier to conduct. On the other hand, this approach does not allow for standard continuous QI methods and may therefore limit the effectiveness of the intervention. The answer may depend on how much customization is considered necessary for a given intervention. In a phase 2 study, an intervention may already be optimized and it may be appropriate to hold it fixed. But even under these circumstances, we would still recommend a long pilot period

TABLE 40-4 Questions that Influence Choice of Study Design

Question	Preferred Study Designs	
	If Yes	If No
Is it feasible and ethical to have a control group?	RCT or clustered RCT	ITS Stepped wedge
Do you have control over who gets the intervention and when?	RCT or clustered RCT Stepped Wedge	ITS
Does the intervention need to be implemented all at once?	RCT or clustered RCT ITS	Stepped wedge
Can/should the intervention be delivered to individual patients?	RCT (randomization by patient)	Clustered RCT
Are the outcomes rare or do they take a long time to develop?	Multicenter ITS	RCT or clustered RCT
Are the costs and risks of the intervention low?	ITS Before-after studies	RCT or clustered RCT
Will the results be used to generate a requirement for adoption of this intervention?	RCT or clustered RCT	ITS Before-after studies

ITS, interrupted time series; RCT, randomized controlled trial.

that allows for continuous QI methods and/or a multiphase study in which improvements to an intervention are planned for at periodic intervals. For example, a study of a novel software application should likely be conducted as a multiphase study; changes to software often take a while and "version 1" of software is almost never ideal.

Can an intervention be different at each site? Under some circumstances it may be desirable to standardize the goals and functions of the intervention rather than the exact form and structure. This allows for flexibility and maximizes the chances of success at each site. Such an approach may be preferred when the intervention is complex and when baseline achievement and environment are very different from site to site. Hawe et al. recommend this approach. For a recently conducted multisite study of medication reconciliation, we chose to standardize the components of the intervention along functional lines (eg, "improve access to sources of preadmission medication information"). This was necessary because each site was different in terms of its current processes, its local strengths and weaknesses, and its environment. On the other hand, it makes the description of the intervention and the analysis more difficult.

One way to improve the analytic approach to both these issues (continuous improvement over time and different interventions at each site) is to break down an intervention into its component parts and quantify the effects on outcomes when each component is implemented at each site, adjusting for site and other potential confounders. Using the above multicenter medication reconciliation QI study as an example, such an approach, using time-varying covariates, allowed us to determine which intervention components were most (and least) effective in lowering medication discrepancy rates.

CONCLUSION

Regarding study design, chance, confounding, and bias are the major threats to the internal validity of a study. It is far better to minimize these when designing your study than to deal with them later at the analysis phase. Different study designs address these issues to different degrees. More formal study designs, such as cluster-randomized controlled trials, are preferred (if possible and ethical) when the benefits of the intervention are not self-evident or the intervention is costly and not without risk. But other study designs, such as stepped wedge and interrupted time series, are also excellent study designs depending on the situation.

It always makes sense to have adequate sample size to adequately answer your study question, to describe your interventions well, use unbiased measurement tools to collect data, look at both processes and outcomes, look at potential unintended consequences of your intervention, and examine environmental context and intervention fidelity. Studies are most successful when study design issues are anticipated and managed early, well before data are collected. Therefore, get the help of experts in study design and statistics as soon as your study question has been refined.

Interesting research questions are everywhere and hospitalists are in an ideal position to recognize these questions. Choose the right time to do research, both personally and for the research question. Plan your study in advance and get the help and training you need. Do not be afraid of the IRB: they can actually help you with your proposal, but allow enough time for the approval process to occur. You *can* do QI research, and by getting started, you may find that the rewards and the potential impact of your work on large patient populations are well worth the effort.

SUGGESTED READINGS

Benneyan JC, Lloyd RC, Plsek PE. Statistical process control as a tool for research and healthcare improvement. *Qual Saf Health Care.* 2003;12(6):458-464.

Brown C, Hofer T, Johal A, et al. An epistemology of patient safety research: a framework for study design and interpretation. Parts 1–4. *Qual Saf Health Care.* 2008;17(3):158-181.

Brown C, Lilford R. Evaluating service delivery interventions to enhance patient safety. *BMJ.* 2008;337:a2764.

Donabedian A. Explorations in quality assessment and monitoring. In: Griffith JR, ed. *The Definition of Quality and Approaches to it Assessment.* Washington, DC: Health Administration Press; 1980:4-163.

Dumas JE, Lynch AM, Laughlin JE, et al. Promoting intervention fidelity. Conceptual issues, methods, and preliminary results from the EARLY ALLIANCE prevention trial. *Am J Prev Med.* 2001; 20(1 Suppl):38-47.

Hawe P, Shiell A, Riley T. Complex interventions: how "out of control" can a randomised controlled trial be? *BMJ.* 2004;328(7455):1561-1563.

Lynn J, Baily MA, Bottrell M, et al. The ethics of using quality improvement methods in health care. *Ann Intern Med.* 2007;146(9): 666-673.

Ogrinc G, Mooney SE, Estrada C, et al. The SQUIRE (Standards for QUality Improvement Reporting Excellence) guidelines for quality improvement reporting: explanation and elaboration. *Qual Saf Health Care.* 2008;17(Suppl 1):i13-i32.

Pawson R, Tilley N. *Realistic Evaluation.* London: Sage Publications, Ltd; 1997.

Salanitro AH, Kripalani S, Resnic J, et al. Rationale and design of the Multicenter Medication Reconciliation Quality Improvement Study (MARQUIS). *BMC Health Serv Res.* 2013;13:230.

Schnipper JL, Stein JM, Wetterneck TB, et al. What are the best ways to improve medication reconciliation? Paper presented at: An on-treatment analysis of the MARQUIS study. Plenary session, Society of General Internal Medicine Annual Meeting; 2015; Toronto, ON.

Stetler CB, Legro MW, Wallace CM, et al. The role of formative evaluation in implementation research and the QUERI experience. *J Gen Intern Med.* 2006;21(Suppl 2):S1-S8.

CHAPTER 41

For Individuals and Practices: Career Sustainability and Avoiding Burnout

Keiki Hinami, MD, MS
Tosha B. Wetterneck, MD, MS

INTRODUCTION

Anywhere from a quarter to half of physicians worldwide are estimated to experience job burnout. General internal medicine and family medicine—the specialties for most adult hospitalists—claim some of the highest rates of physician burnout in the United States. Within the adult generalist fields, several studies suggest clinic-based primary care physicians report burnout more frequently than their inpatient peers, but hospitalists remain among the physicians most susceptible to job burnout.

The unique work-life challenges of hospital medicine practice include demands on hospitalists to serve several contemporary physician roles as boundary spanners, communicators, nonleader team members, quality enhancers, and caregivers. Even as hospitalists have become permanent fixtures in most hospitals, role conflicts remain common with the competing demands of patients, other clinicians, administrators, and employers. Shiftwork with day/night schedule changes and sleep deprivation causes physiologic stress. Productivity and efficiency demands are pervasive in modern health care organizations and a driver of high workload. Pay uncertainties with health care reform and capitated care, and the pressures to standardize care which lead to loss of autonomy and intense scrutiny of performance contribute to conditions under which job burnout is expected to remain a concern for the discipline.

WHAT IS BURNOUT?

Burnout is a psychological syndrome leading to a worker's erosion of engagement with their job due to long-term exposure to emotionally demanding work. It is a condition observed predominantly among those in the helping professions, like health and social services where direct, frequent, and intense interactions with people are common and where the outcomes of work are not fully dependent on worker actions. Burnout is commonly conceptualized as having three constitutive dimensions. The first, *emotional exhaustion* is a literal depletion of worker energy due to work demands. It may manifest in hospitalists as "compassion fatigue" or the tendency to distance themselves—cognitively and emotionally—from their work as they realize they cannot continue to give of themselves to patients and coworkers. In essence, it is a coping response to work overload. The second is *depersonalization*, marked by a detached emotional callousness or cynicism that manifests as indifference or dysfunctional attitudes and behaviors toward patients. It is often a protective response to emotional exhaustion. The final component of burnout, *diminished personal accomplishment*, is the erosion of a worker's sense of personal effectiveness, which brings on a feeling of powerlessness and the tendency to negatively evaluate oneself. This may manifest as a hospitalist not completing assigned tasks or as worsening professional self-esteem. Emotional exhaustion is usually considered necessary for burnout to be diagnosed, the other components may occur in parallel, sequentially, or not at all.

Burnout is distinct from related concepts like stress, depression, and dissatisfaction. The definitions of each have been established empirically and while they overlap significantly, burnout is specific to the context of the workplace as an ongoing emotional response to chronic demands and interpersonal stressors. Job dissatisfaction is a predictor of burnout; workers who are dissatisfied are more likely to be burned out. However, it is not fully clear whether dissatisfaction always precedes burnout or is a result of burnout (or other workplace conditions that also produce burnout). Individuals who are depression-prone have higher rates of burnout and even though burnout is specific to the workplace it can also affect home-life. Job stress can be conceptualized by two models: the demand-control-support model and the effort-reward imbalance model. In the first model, job stress is more likely when there are high job demands (workload; time pressure), low control over job (autonomy in decision making; power over outcomes) and low support (from colleagues, supervisor, organization; inadequate resources). Given the high job demands inherent in the medical profession, control and support are important mediators. With effort-reward imbalance, there is a discrepancy between the demands and obligations of the job (effort) and the rewards offered like salary, career opportunities, esteem, and job security. For workers who are committed to their jobs, this imbalance leads to job stress. Again, given the high demands associated with hospitalist jobs and the professional commitment displayed by most physicians, rewards are very important to mediate stress.

WHY IS BURNOUT IMPORTANT TO HOSPITALISTS?

Across a wide variety of professions, burnout has been associated with negative work outcomes including decreasing work hours or job turnover, decreased work effectiveness and productivity, reduced job and organizational commitment, and stress-related health outcomes such as substance abuse and depression. In addition, the negative attitudes and actions of burned out workers can negatively impact others in and out of the workplace. These outcomes and the impact on Hospital Medicine are considered in depth in the proceeding section.

■ PHYSICIAN BURNOUT AND JOB PERFORMANCE

Burnout predicts poor physician job performance. For example, providers who are happy with their work are known to increase patients' satisfaction, adherence to physician advice, trust, and confidence. On the other hand, patients of depersonalized physicians have been shown to take longer to recover from their illness. Physicians in the United Kingdom reported providing lower standards of care, being angry and sometimes abusive with patients as a result of chronic stress. Similarly, burned out general internists and medicine residents reported engaging in suboptimal patient care such as making errors not due to a lack of knowledge or inexperience. There appears to be a reciprocal relationship between burnout and perception of committing medical errors. In a longitudinal study, residents who were burned out subsequently reported more perceived errors than those who were not burned out and those who had more perceived errors initially were more likely to report burnout in the future. A recent systematic review of the relevant literature demonstrated burnout's potential impact, also, on nontrainee physician productivity through self-perceived "insufficient" work ability and job retention measures.

Although the mechanisms connecting burnout to poor-quality and poor-quantity patient care have not been empirically proven, one proposed causal pathway involves the providers' emotional state. One measure of emotions—positive affect—is associated with enhanced decision making and problem solving as well as higher levels of patient centeredness in health care providers. Therefore, burned out hospitalists may be less cognitively vigilant and less likely to put forth the extra effort necessary to deliver the highest quality, patient-centered care.

■ REDUCED ORGANIZATIONAL COMMITMENT AND JOB TURNOVER

Virtually all hospitalists work in organizations or are direct employees of hospitals and health systems. Therefore, employers depend on hospitalists' commitment to advance patient care, quality

improvement, and their specific organizational mission and character. Organizational commitment refers to employee identification with and involvement in a particular community. Higher levels of commitment are reflected in lower rates of attrition and better job performance. Burnout is associated with decreased worker organizational commitment in health care professionals. In addition, being around burned out workers and having negative interactions with them may impact other workers' organizational commitment.

Although burnout is not the only or even the dominant reason for physicians leaving their jobs, the 2009 Hospitalist Physician Satisfaction Survey found 65% of hospitalists at risk of burnout (compared to 31% without burnout risk) reported their intent to leave their current practice within 2 years. Moreover, 68% of hospitalists at risk of burnout (compared to 45% without burnout risk) reported their intent to leave the hospital medicine specialty within 5 years. The cost of replacing a hospitalist may be comparable to the 250,000 US dollars estimated turnover cost of an outpatient-based generalist. The cost of physician burnout in all of Canada was estimated to be over 200 million Canadian dollars, of which two-thirds were from early retirement. Given the high cost of turnover and recruitment, it is essential that burnout be minimized to ensure that experienced hospitalists remain clinically active in the profession to train the future workforce.

■ STRESS-RELATED HEALTH PROBLEMS AMONG PHYSICIANS

Like all health care providers, physicians experience high levels of job stress. A study in the Netherlands found a correspondingly high proportion of hospital-based physicians suffering work-related fatigue (42%), depression (29%), anxiety (24%), and posttraumatic stress complaints (15%). Burnout was the term originally coined by Herbert Freudenberger in the context of alcoholism and drug abuse in the 1970s, and it remains a feature of the 8% to 12% of health professionals who develop a substance-related disorder at some point in their lives. Suicide is another disturbing problem for health care providers. According to the Psychiatric Clinics of North America, male physicians are two times more likely to commit suicide than the average American, and female physicians are three times more likely. Although only a few studies have tied job burnout to the profound psychological and spiritual dislocation that predispose physicians to self-destructive behavior, the traditional lack of self-care among physicians, scarcity of resources for physician support, and burnout are understood to be related aspects of the same stress-related problem.

WHAT LEADS TO BURNOUT IN HOSPITALISTS?

The key features of hospitalist work and individual characteristics that are associated with burnout are summarized in **Table 41-1** and discussed in detail below.

■ WORKLOAD

Excessive workload is confirmed as the overriding source of burnout in physicians. Cost and time pressures pose additional job demands on the typical hospitalist. Irregular night shifts, extended work weeks, and other nontraditional work patterns can predispose hospitalists to physical and mental exhaustion. Some hospitalists engaged in nonclinical responsibilities spend additional time on administrative work, education, and research. The average number of daily patient encounters by a hospitalist in 2009 was 15, but depending on practice type this number ranged from 13 in typical academic groups to 17 in private practice groups. Variability in workload across practice types was also apparent in the number of clinical shifts per month for full time hospitalists (15 shifts in academic groups compared to 19 shifts in local hospitalist-only groups), and hours of nonclinical

TABLE 41-1 Characteristics Associated with Job Burnout

Job Characteristics	Individual Characteristics
Job demands: workload, time pressure, complex patients	Early career
Role conflict and role ambiguity	Male gender
Lack of job control/autonomy	Not married
Lack of support or good relationships with colleagues and supervisors	Lack of social support outside of work
Lack of reciprocity from patients	Personality factors: external locus of control, low hardiness, low self-esteem
Lack of resources to do the job	
Lack of organizational commitment to hospitalist groups or individuals	

work per month (19 vs 17 hours in multistate hospitalist groups vs academic groups, respectively). A big data study from the Christiana Care Health System demonstrated a J-shaped increase in hospital length of stay and costs with increasing workload, suggesting that hospitalists are routinely stretched to manage clinical loads large enough to impinge on efficiency.

Both qualitative and quantitative work overload contribute to exhaustion by depleting the capacity of physicians to meet job demands. Numerous studies, including the Physician Worklife Study (PWS) of US generalists and specialists, demonstrated the unfavorable effects of overload, time pressure, and resource scarcity on physician stress, burnout, and dissatisfaction. Workload is perceived variably by individuals and cannot be measured simply by the number of hours worked. Another study found that work hours only indirectly predicted quality of care through perceived overload, suggesting other considerations mitigate the effects of physician work hours. One consideration is the protective effect of recovery time. Acute fatigue resulting from an especially demanding event at work does not necessarily lead to burnout, given recovery during restful periods at work or at home. When work overload is persistent, as opposed to sporadic, there is little opportunity to rest and restore balance. A sustainable workload or work-life balance, in contrast, may provide opportunities to refine coping skills to draw energy from other restorative aspects of daily life.

■ WORK ROLE AND AUTONOMY

The demand-control model of occupational stress offers a framework in which control of the work environment mitigates stress created by ongoing work demands. According to the 1999 national survey of hospitalists, 97% of hospitalists reported being "highly autonomous" or "autonomous" in their clinical role. Since that time, the role of some hospitalists may have evolved in ways that diminish control over their work. This is reflected in the fraction of hospitalists in 2009 who indicated having "much" or "very much" influence over the following aspects of their work: quality of work, 83%; order of tasks to perform, 69%; pace of work, 50%; schedule, 33%; amount of work, 13%.

In addition to workload described above, the perceived decline in autonomy may be related to growing administrative oversight over hospitalists in the form of performance assessments, volume-based reimbursements, privacy rules, patient safety evaluations, resource stewardship, and malpractice litigations. While requirements for billing or service documentation are aimed at eliminating excessive

variations in care, these efforts contribute to a sense of reduced clinical autonomy. Much of the drivers of care standardization is now written into the Affordable Care Act, and the negative impact of quality incentives on physicians' sense of autonomy has been empirically demonstrated.

Physician autonomy is also reduced when their role is uncertain or unpredictable. This is often the case in hospitalist work where the work demands rise and fall erratically. A potential for role conflict exists, in theory, when hospitalists are required to reconcile their responsibilities as advocates both for the hospital and for the patient. Primary or comanagement of patients typically cared for by surgeons or specialists, also introduce the potential for role ambiguity and decreased autonomy.

■ INTERPERSONAL CONTACTS

The typical hospitalist routinely interacts with many individuals at work. Whether patients, colleagues, administrative leaders, or any number of coworkers on an interdisciplinary team, hospitalists are expected to communicate well and seamlessly coordinate care with other stakeholders. A central proposition of social exchange theory is that individuals pursue reciprocity in interpersonal relationships, and those who find themselves participating in an unreciprocated relationship will become distressed. Physicians who do not receive the intrinsically sought-after positive feedback from patients and coworkers are more likely to manifest signs of burnout.

A study by Bakker and colleagues examined the relationships between general practitioners and patients over a period of 5 years, and found that emotional exhaustion evoked negative attitudes toward patients. In turn, physicians who attempted to gain emotional distance from their patients as a way of coping with exhaustion were found to engender the demanding patient behaviors that they sought to avoid. Additional research establishes burnout's association with a greater exposure to patients with poor prognosis. Unlike traditional practitioners with whom patients have longitudinal relationships, clinical encounters with hospitalists are relatively brief. The difficulty of rapidly establishing rewarding relationships with patients may pose a unique risk for burnout among hospitalists. Hoff and colleagues found that favorable patient-related interactions, more than peer relations, predicted hospitalists' intent to stay in the career.

Coworker support augments the personal accomplishment dimension of burnout, reflecting the value physicians place on expert evaluation by peers. Hinami and colleagues demonstrated hospitalist job longevity proportionate to more favorable organizational climate and relationship with nonphysician staff. The PWS showed that support from colleagues has a significant protective effect against stress. To highlight the importance of coworker support, solo practitioners were found to be particularly susceptible to stress. Furthermore, Hoff and colleagues show that burnout in hospitalists is more closely associated with less favorable social relations involving colleagues and coworkers than negative experiences related to the economically induced pressures of the job, such as reduced autonomy and the use of financial incentives. Shanafelt and colleagues found that physicians and scientists' negative relationship with their leaders is a strong predictor of burnout.

■ ORGANIZATIONAL CHARACTERISTICS

Hospitalist practice models are as diverse as the number of practices that exist in the United States. Although, hospitalist groups are unified in the goals of containing cost while improving quality of care, the organizational culture, incentive structures, hierarchies, and operating rules that govern job demands vary widely. All of these factors can influence individual hospitalists' fit with their organization. Additional negative impact on burnout can surface when organizations violate basic expectations of fairness and equity.

Various studies demonstrate how economic pressures adversely affect attitudes related to physician career quality and longevity. For instance, job satisfaction is negatively impacted by more restrictive forms of reimbursement such as capitation, less time available to spend with patients, and the use of financial incentives related to productivity. These findings help to anticipate the potential impact of bundled payment models on hospitalist work-life.

The lack of fit between a hospitalist and his or her job is another determinant of burnout. Hospitalists have been shown to vote with their feet to find jobs that align with their personal goals. A study by Shanafelt and colleagues found that physicians in an academic department of internal medicine were less likely to show burnout when they spent more time engaged in the activities—patient care, research, education, or administration—they found most meaningful. The practice of Hospital Medicine offers ample opportunities for physicians to pursue customized careers in unconventional areas of medicine like management and advocacy. While some hospitalists find the variety of activities to be satisfying, others risk mismatch when they commit to jobs to which they are not well suited.

Fairness refers to the extent to which work decisions are perceived to be just. When organizational policies are fair, emotional exhaustion correlates with job performance but when they are consistently unfair, poor job performance is prevalent even where employees show no signs of burnout. Hospitalists may perceive injustice through differential treatment of physician groups by hospitals. Disproportionate distribution of responsibilities or rewards among members of a hospitalist group can breed resentment that can affect quality of care and burnout status. The earnings disparity that disadvantages women in hospital medicine as they do in the rest of society is another example of organizational injustice that persists.

■ PERSONAL CHARACTERISTICS

Hospitalist jobs usually do not require special training beyond the typical hospital-based residency experience. As a result, it is an attractive career opportunity for young physicians who can feel proficient immediately out of residency training. However, studies consistently show that younger individuals are more susceptible to burnout compared with more experienced counterparts. The reason for this has not been studied thoroughly but one possible explanation is that young physicians are closer to their training experiences that reward perfectionism and denial of personal vulnerability, while being surrounded by peers accustomed to delayed gratification. Young workers with high expectations of a work environment and a desire to express their skills and abilities can become burned out when expectations are unmet.

Unmarried workers, especially men, seem to be more prone to burnout; and single workers seem to experience higher burnout levels than those who are divorced. Family can be protective of stress and burnout, presumably because social support can buffer the pathologic influences of stressful events. Social support, especially from informal contacts, is positively related to good health and efficacy, irrespective of the presence or absence of work stressors.

Individuals with certain psychological dispositions are more prone to burnout. Traits like compulsiveness, guilt, and self-denial may confer short-term advantages to physicians, but often fuel feelings of inadequacy over the long term making individuals with these traits less resilient to external pressures. Those with an internal locus of control attribute daily events to personal effort while those with an external locus of control attribute them to outside forces or chance. Not surprisingly, burnout is higher among individuals with an external locus of control. Persons with low self-esteem and low levels of resilience or hardiness are associated with higher burnout due to not being open to change and feelings of not being in control.

HOW CAN BURNOUT IN HOSPITALISTS BE ADDRESSED?
■ FOCUS ON THE JOB AND THE INDIVIDUAL

Considerable evidence supports the fact that organizational and job factors play a greater role in burnout than individual worker characteristics and may be more remediable. It can be said that the organization acts upon the physician, whose personality, coping style, early experiences, skills, and competencies filter or exacerbate its effects. Solutions to the burnout problem, therefore, should be addressed primarily at the level of the job or organization. The goal should be to balance the demands of the job with the control, reward, and support needs of the worker. This may not be an easy task; most burnout interventions in the past have focused on individuals rather than jobs or organizations because it is perceived to be easier and less expensive to change people. Nevertheless, given the evolving nature of hospitalist programs and their relationships with organizations, job design should be a primary focus. An expert in generalist physician work-life, Mark Linzer, advocates for a process improvement approach to addressing physician burnout through his "10 Bold Steps to Prevent Burnout in General Internal Medicine" (Table 41-2). This requires systematically measuring the known predictors and outcomes of burnout and using them for continuous feedback. Four of his 10 steps focus on work conditions: ensure adequate resources, plan rather than react to reductions in FTE from predictable life events, resist thoughtless efforts to standardize processes by allowing physician flexibility, and control workload. Additionally, he endorses cultivating "career fit" to allow physicians to engage in meaningful career development. These, in addition, to self-care through resilience building are advocated to nurture a renewed professionalism. Many of these recommendations have been incorporated into publicly available online resources offered by the STEPS Forward program of the American Medical Association (www.stepsforward.org). Resources for monitoring burnout and other work-life parameters are also available from the AMA and the Society of Hospital Medicine through its Hospital Medicine Engagement Benchmarking Program.

■ OPTIMIZE WORK LOAD, FLOW, AND FIT

The strongest evidence to reduce burnout supports controlling job demands: workload and time pressure. But as stated above, simply

TABLE 41-2 Ten Steps to Prevent Physician Burnout for Hospital Medicine Practices

Institutional Metrics
1. Make clinician satisfaction and wellbeing quality indicators
2. Incorporate mindfulness and teamwork into practice
3. Decrease stress from electronic health records

Work Conditions
4. Allocate needed resources to reduce health care disparities
5. Hire physician floats to cover predictable life events
6. Promote physician control of the work environment
7. Maintain manageable workload

Career Development
8. Preserve physician "career fit"
9. Promote flexibility of work schedule

Self-Care
10. Make self-care a part of medical professionalism

Adapted from Linzer M, Levine R, Meltzer D, Poplau S, Warde C, West CP. 10 Bold steps to prevent burnout in general internal medicine. *J Gen Intern Med.* 2013;29(1):18-20. With permission of Springer.

reducing work hours or patient encounters does not alleviate the consequence of burnout and high demands are inherent to the medical profession. The Healthy Work Place Study was a cluster randomized trial of an intervention that was primarily designed to improve workflow in the outpatient setting. Some specific modifications to existing workflow included off-loading administrative tasks to nonphysician assistants, removing bottlenecks of care at the bedside, extending visit times, and scheduling standing meetings dedicated to addressing management issues. Sites with improved workflow exhibited odds of improving their physician burnout rate by 5.9 (95% confidence interval: 1.4, 24.6) compared to controls. Adapting these interventions to the inpatient setting may involve employing administrators to handle nonclinical tasks, making the workload more predictable on a day by day or a week by week if not an hourly basis, adjusting patient census, using electronic resources ergonomically, and addressing system flaws that restrict flexibility for individual hospitalists.

Addressing job fit in mismatched areas may be an alternative strategy. For example, although early-career hospitalists are known to switch jobs to successfully align personal and organizational goals, hospitalists established in a practice have been shown to tailor their jobs to their strengths. As a result, some hospitalists diversify their responsibilities across clinical, administrative, and academic domains while others choose to work in settings that allow them to handle larger than average work load for commensurate control and rewards. Hospitalists, in general, are likely to tolerate greater workload if they have control over the work they do, value the work they are doing, and feel they are doing something important, or if they feel well rewarded for their efforts. Creative scheduling may decrease perceived workload by introducing necessary time for recovery. This is particularly important given evidence linking burnout and health problems with nonstandard work shifts (nights and weekends) in workers of almost every industry. Providing hospitalists with skills to care for nonmedical patients and to form better relationships with consultants may relieve the demands of comanagement.

■ CULTIVATE A SUPPORTIVE CULTURE

Hospitalists are also social creatures, thus focusing on relationships are important. Fostering a mutually supportive organizational culture focused on common goals, mutual respect, and implementing systems to facilitate rewarding interpersonal interactions are likely to minimize burnout. Hospitalists who feel they are working as part of a cohesive team, supported and appreciated by those around them (other hospitalists, nurses, consultants, primary care providers, practice leaders, etc), and who feel positively recognized by patients and families will have less burn out. The most important relationships that impact hospitalist work-life are with patients. Satisfaction with one's ability to deliver the highest quality of care is consistently the strongest driver of job satisfaction for hospitalists and other specialists, alike. Strengthening the patient-doctor relationship is an effective strategy to enhance physicians' personal accomplishments, as proven by palliative care specialists and pediatricians whose examples should inform the practices of adult hospitalists. These and other interventions may be particularly important in supporting younger hospitalists who are more vulnerable to emotional exhaustion.

■ RECLAIM RESILIENCE

At the individual level, numerous studies have found the benefits of mindfulness training and other stress reduction interventions to reduce burnout rates. Courses in Mind Body Stress Reduction (MBSR) are proliferating as a result. But where burnout is an aftermath of chronic stress from modifiable work conditions, simply asking physicians to better tolerate stress neglects root causes and MBSR should not be considered a sufficient work-life intervention on its own.

According to self-determination theory, people are growth-oriented and predisposed to using their capacities fully to connect with others and integrate their experiences in a relative unity. The theory proposes that intrinsic motivations autonomously facilitate this growth orientation while extrinsic motivations compel behaviors for its instrumental value. Individuals are more vulnerable to burnout under conditions dominated by extrinsically motivated behaviors. Consequently, cultivating the sources of hospitalists' intrinsic motivations may potentially protect them from burnout. Professional coaching is a strategy used by athletes and business leaders and recently being adopted by physicians to amplify internal locus of control, self-efficacy, and self-determination. By challenging fixed thoughts and circumstances, coaches empower clients to reclaim control and innate resilience. Hospitalists can learn coping skills for stress in a number of other ways. Evidence suggests that skills to improve relaxation, time management, assertiveness, and social skills can be learned. Recruiting resilient individuals with interpersonal skills and favorable personality profiles may be a strategy for organizations. Although medical schools and training programs routinely select based on characteristics like personality traits, an exclusionary approach to burnout prevention may sacrifice diversity in the hospitalist workforce without addressing the underlying systems problems. The most durable and feasible interventions may involve tailoring practice models to individual needs, but evidence to guide such interventions is still sparse. The fit of the job to the worker is key to job satisfaction and avoiding burnout.

CONCLUSION

The work of typical hospitalists is characterized by high work demands, decreased autonomy, and potentially difficult interpersonal interactions that puts them at risk for burnout. The consequences of burned-out hospitalists include poor job performance, dissatisfaction, turnover, and various health-related problems like depression and substance abuse. Evidence to guide efforts to prevent or minimize the impact of burnout is emerging. More studies examining the work-life impact of organizational processes and material incentives are necessary to guide ongoing health care reform. Organizational efforts to protect work-life balance and support vulnerable individuals from destructive behavior are worthwhile.

SUGGESTED READINGS

Bakker AB, Schaufeli WB, Sixma HJ, Bosveld W, Van Dierendonck D. Patient demands, lack of reciprocity, and burnout: a five-year longitudinal study among general practitioners. *J Organ Behav.* 2000;21:425-441.

Elliott DJ, Young RS, Brice J, Aguiar R, Kolm P. Effect of hospitalist workload on the quality and efficiency of care. *JAMA Intern Med.* 2014;174(5):786-793.

Hinami K, Whelan CT, Miller JA, Wolosin RJ, Wetterneck TB. Job characteristics, satisfaction, and burnout across hospitalist practice models. *J Hosp Med.* 2012;7(5):402-410.

Hoff T, Whitcomb WF, Nelson JR. Thriving and surviving in a new medical career: the case of hospitalist physicians. *J Health Soc Behav.* 2002;43:72-91.

Lindenauer PK, Pantilat SZ, Katz PP, Wachter RM. Hospitalists and the practice of inpatient medicine: results of a survey of the National Association of Inpatient Physicians. *Ann Intern Med.* 1999;30:343-349.

Linzer M, Levine R, Meltzer D, Poplau S, Warde C, West CP. 10 bold steps to prevent burnout in general internal medicine. *J Gen Intern Med*. 2013;29(1):18-20.

Linzer M, Poplau S, Grossman E, et al. A cluster randomized trial of interventions to improve work conditions and clinician burnout in primary care: results from the Healthy Work Place (HWP) study. *J Gen Intern Med*. 2015;30(8):1105-1111.

Maslach C, Leiter MP. Early predictors of job burnout and engagement. *J Appl Psychol*. 2008;93:498-512.

Shanafelt TD, Boone S, Tan L, et al. Burnout and satisfaction with work-life balance among US physicians relative to the general US population. *Arch Intern Med*. 2012;172(18):1377-1385.

West CP, Huschka MH, Novotny PJ, et al. Association of perceived medical errors with resident distress and empathy: a prospective longitudinal study. *J Am Med Assoc*. 2006;296(9): 1071-1078.

PART II

Medical Consultation

SECTION 1
Surgery

CHAPTER 42

Physiologic Response to Surgery

Gil Freitas, MD
Vihas Patel, MD
Allan B. Peetz, MD

INTRODUCTION

A Scottish physician and metabolism researcher named Dr David Cuthbertson first reported on the metabolic consequences of surgery in 1932 when he coined the term "ebbs and flows" when studying the effects of lower limb injury. Since that time scientific study has added a great deal more to what we know about the physiological response to surgery, and understanding this response lends itself to more effective management, including mitigating risks of the surgical patient.

This chapter outlines the primary physiologic responses to surgery, and their impact on the management of the postoperative patient, including the typical surgical stress response, effects on fluids and electrolytes, and common organ-specific effects.

SURGICAL STRESS RESPONSE

The surgical stress response has three key physiologic components:

- Sympathetic nervous system activation
- Endocrinologic activation
- Immunologic activation with the production of cytokines and acute phase reactants, and resultant neutrophil release and demargination, and lymphocyte proliferation

■ SYMPATHETIC NERVOUS SYSTEM ACTIVATION

Surgical stress stimulates the hypothalamic-pituitary-adrenal (HPA) axis and leads to sympathetic nerve activation, which triggers the release of catecholamines. In addition to their cardiovascular affects (tachycardia, hypertension), these hormones also affect the liver, kidneys, and pancreas.

■ ENDOCRINOLOGIC ACTIVATION

Surgical stress results in a variety of changes in serum levels of endocrinologic hormones (**Table 42-1**).

These endocrine responses are normal after surgery, but can sometimes result in clinically significant complications. For example, increased cortisol can lead to hyperglycemia, which is associated with surgical complications and poorer outcomes. Cortisol also stimulates protein catabolism, whereby both skeletal and visceral muscle are broken down to release amino acids for energy or to be used by the liver to form new protein including the acute phase reactants. This process can result in weight loss, muscle wasting, and impaired healing. Arginine vasopressin can result in free water retention, which can result in hypervolemia and hyponatremia.

■ IMMUNOLOGIC ACTIVATION

Surgical stress also results in a variety of immunological changes. Such activation is essential for recovery and wound healing, but can also have untoward physiologic effects (such as fever). White blood cells and endothelial cells produce interleukins and interferons, which contribute to an inflammatory cascade. Interleukin-1 (IL-1), tumor necrosis factor-α (TNF-α), and IL-6 are the primary cytokines released after surgery. Increased IL-6 production after surgery activates acute phase proteins such as C-reactive proteins (CRP), fibrinogen, and α-2 macroglobulin, which act as inflammatory mediators and scavengers in tissue repair. CRP levels rise approximately 4 to 12 hours after surgery, peak at 24 to 72 hours, and are elevated for approximately 2 weeks. D-dimer protein, a fibrin degradation

TABLE 42-1 Principal Hormonal Responses to Surgery

Endocrine Gland	Hormone	Change in Secretion
Anterior pituitary	ACTH	Increases
	Growth hormone	Increases
	TSH	May increase or decrease
	FSH and LH	May increase or decrease
Posterior pituitary	AVP	Increases
Adrenal cortex	Cortisol	Increases
	Aldosterone	Increases
Pancreas	Insulin	Often decreases
	Glucagon	Usually small increases
Thyroid	Thyroxine	Decrease

product, also increases in the postoperative period, and may remain elevated for several weeks. This normal inflammatory state response to surgery is thought to be the cause for the mild fevers and leukocytosis commonly seen in the first 48 hours after surgery.

FLUIDS AND ELECTROLYTES

■ FLUIDS

Fluid balance is a key element for perioperative management. Many surgical patients fast for 12+ hours prior to surgery. This preoperative fast, in combination with intraoperative blood loss and evaporative losses, can lead to significant fluid deficits. Postoperative redistribution of fluids, or third spacing, may also contribute to intravascular hypovolemia. Patients in the perioperative period should be continuously monitored for volume status, as under- or overcorrection are both problematic. Signs and symptoms of hyper- and hypovolemia are outlined in **Table 42-2**.

If the patient is hypovolemic and needs fluid resuscitation, crystalloids are preferable to colloids; most surgeons prefer Lactated Ringer's solution for resuscitation. Maintenance fluids should be D5$\frac{1}{2}$NS + 20 mEq/L K$^+$ at an appropriate rate based on patient weight. The purpose of the dextrose component is it maintains tonicity, and prevents catabolism, ketosis, and hypoglycemia (a liter of 5% dextrose solution provides about 170 kcal). Typical IVF composition rates are outlined in **Table 42-3**.

TABLE 42-2 Signs and Symptoms of Volume Disturbances

System	Volume Deficit	Volume Excess
Generalized	Weight loss	Weight gain
	Decreased skin turgor	Peripheral edema
Cardiac	Tachycardia	Increased cardiac output
	Orthostasis/ hypotension	Increased central venous pressure
	Collapsed neck veins	Distended neck veins
Renal	Oliguria	Polyuria
	Azotemia	
GI	Ileus	Bowel edema
Pulmonary	–	Pulmonary edema

TABLE 42-3 Intravenous Crystalloid Fluids Commonly Used in the Perioperative Period

Type of Fluid	Indications	Composition per Liter
Lactated Ringer's (LR)	Typically used for the first 48 h postoperatively; replacement fluids	130 mEq Na, 109 mEq Cl, 4 mEq K, 3 mEq Ca, 28 mEq lactate, pH 6.4, 273 mOsm
D5$\frac{1}{2}$NS+20K	Hypotonic maintenance fluids used after initial fluid resuscitation completed	50 g dextrose; 77 mEq Na, 77 mEq Cl, 20 mEq K; pH 5.7, 452 mOsm
Normal saline (NS)	Alternative to LR; watch for hyperchloremic metabolic acidosis	154 mEq Na, 154 mEq Cl, pH 5.7, 308 mOsm
$\frac{1}{2}$ NS	Hypotonic maintenance solution	77 mEq Na, 77 mEq Cl, pH 5.7
3% NS	Used with neurosurgical or neurology teams to treat cerebral swelling	513 mEq Na, 513 mEq Cl, pH 5.7, 1027 mOsm
D5Water	Free water; no role in resuscitation	50 g dextrose, 278 mOsm
Human plasma		140 mEq Na, 103 mEq Cl, 4 mEq K, 5 mEq Ca, 2 mEq Mg, 25 mEq HCO3, pH 7.4, osmolality 290 mOsm

PRACTICE POINT

- Perioperative fluid replacement:

- Intraoperative fluid losses are typically isotonic.

Lactated Ringer's (LR) solution is typically the intravenous crystalloid of choice for fluid resuscitation in the first 48 hours after surgery.

- Ongoing fluid losses are typically hypotonic.

D5$\frac{1}{2}$NS + 20 mEq/L of K$^+$ is typically the intravenous crystalloid of choice for fluid maintenance, after the 48 hours after surgery.

■ ELECTROLYTES

Electrolyte and acid-base imbalances are common in the perioperative period, and are exacerbated by being NPO, and by fluid-electrolyte losses from tubes, drains, or fistulas.

Sodium

High-output nasogastric tubes, emesis, or enteric fistulas may result in a hyponatremic, hyperchloremic metabolic alkalosis. Leakage from large wounds may also deplete extracellular water and sodium. ADH secretion from surgical stress and resuscitation with large volumes of LR may also contribute to postoperative hyponatremia.

Potassium

Hypokalemia is common in the surgical patient, and can be exacerbated by diarrhea, fistula, or vomiting losses. Most patients are asymptomatic until plasma K$^+$ falls below 3.5 mEq/L. Symptoms of hypokalemia are primarily related to failure of normal contractility of muscle fibers, and present as ileus, constipation, fatigue, weakness, or cardiac arrest. Potassium replacement therapy is most safely administered orally; intravenous replacement should be reserved for patients unable to tolerate oral administration, and rate of intravenous infusion should not exceed 20 mEq/h.

Magnesium

Magnesium levels should also be monitored perioperatively and supplemented if low. Hypermagnesemia perioperatively is unusual and is usually spurious. Symptoms of hypomagnesemia include hyperactive reflexes, muscle tremors, and tetany. Magnesium should be aggressively replaced to restore potassium or calcium homeostasis when hypokalemia or hypocalcemia are concomitant with hypomagnesemia. Hypomagnesemia can be repleted orally with 50 to 100 mEq, but if it results in diarrhea, intravenous replacement is preferable.

Calcium

Calcium is another important electrolyte that frequently becomes out of balance in the perioperative period and needs to be closely monitored. Hypocalcemia is defined as a serum calcium level below 8.5 mEq/L, or an ionized calcium level below 4.2 mg/dL (which is more physiologically important). Symptoms include tetany, Chvostek's sign, Trousseau's sign, laryngospasm (stridor), and confusion. Transient hypocalcemia commonly occurs after removal of a parathyroid adenoma, due to atrophy of the remaining glands and avid bone remineralization, and may require high doses of supplementation. Symptomatic hypocalcemia is best corrected with intravenous calcium gluconate or calcium chloride.

COMMON ORGAN-SPECIFIC RESPONSES TO SURGERY
■ NEUROLOGIC AND PSYCHIATRIC

See Chapter 62 (Neurologic and Psychiatric Complications) and Chapter 81 (Delirium).

■ CARDIOVASCULAR

Preoperatively patients should be assessed for cardiac risk and monitored for cardiac complications. See Chapter 50 (Preoperative Cardiac Risk Assessment and Risk Reduction) and Chapter 59 (Cardiac Complications).

■ PULMONARY

Surgical patients are susceptible to a myriad of postoperative pulmonary complications. See Chapter 51 (Perioperative Pulmonary Risk Assessment and Management).

■ GASTROINTESTINAL

Paralytic ileus, the temporary disruption of normal peristalsis, is common in surgical patients. The symptoms of ileus may include bloating, abdominal distention, inability to pass flatus and intolerance to an oral diet. Although the underlying mechanism for postoperative ileus is not well understood, catecholamine surges, electrolyte changes, and fluid shifts are likely contributors. Ileus is particularly common after gastrointestinal surgery and is potentially related to bowel manipulation and inhibiting spinal reflex arcs via adrenoreceptors. Other contributors include metabolic abnormalities such as hypokalemia or hypomagnesemia.

Although postoperative ileus is usually self-limited, it can impede enteric feeding and therefore significantly slow normal recovery from surgery. Postoperative ileus is also associated with impaired wound healing, prolonged hospital stays, and overall postoperative morbidity. Treatment is supportive and includes adequate hydration, correction of electrolyte imbalances (especially potassium and magnesium), use of epidurals during and after surgery, and limiting perioperative opiate use (by using multimodal pain regimens). Early ambulation is highly encouraged and can significantly improve both the symptoms and the duration of the ileus. Promotility medications such as metoclopramide and erythromycin do not improve the symptoms or duration of an ileus and can have side effects, so should not be routinely prescribed.

TABLE 42-4 Surgical and Medical Conditions Predisposing to Perioperative Acute Renal Failure

Trauma	Vascular disease
Cardiopulmonary bypass	Hypotension
Underlying renal disease	Hypovolemia
Renal transplantation	Liver failure
Urologic surgery	Sepsis
Pigment nephropathy	Contrast agents
Drugs (eg, aminoglycosides)	

■ RENAL

Postoperative renal failure is uncommon but significantly increases perioperative morbidity and mortality. Risk factors for postoperative renal failure are outlined in **Table 42-4**. Perioperative acute renal failure is often initiated by perioperative hemodilution (from aggressive fluid resuscitation) and hypovolemia (from hemorrhage or inadequate volume replacement); this reduces the viscosity of capillary blood flow, and redistributes blood from the renal medulla to the renal cortex, subjecting the medulla to ischemia. Ischemic kidney injury can also be incited by the constriction of the afferent and efferent arterioles by circulating catecholamines in response to surgical stress. Renal tubular injury, or acute tubular necrosis, is another common cause of perioperative acute renal failure. Once tubular damage occurs, a number of factors contribute to ongoing tubular damage, including intraluminal obstruction from cell swelling and sloughing, persistent vasoconstriction, back-leakage of luminal fluid across damaged tubular epithelium, and decreased glomerular capillary membrane permeability.

Perioperative management should include close monitoring of urine output and electrolytes, daily weights, avoidance of all nephrotoxic medications, and appropriate adjustment of all renally cleared medications. For patients that become oliguric, management includes the placement of a bladder catheter, and an isotonic fluid challenge (500 mL of normal saline or Ringer's lactate). A urinalysis should be evaluated for specific gravity, casts, or evidence of infection, a fractional excretion of sodium should be calculated, and nephrology should be consulted.

CONCLUSION

Surgical stress is associated with predictable metabolic and hormonal changes and affects nearly every organ system. Understanding these physiologic changes that result from surgery are critical for appropriately managing perioperative patients.

SUGGESTED READINGS

Jamieson RA, Ledigham I, Kay AW, MacKay C. *Jamieson and Kay's Textbook of Surgical Physiology*, 4th ed. Philadelphia, PA: Churchill Livingstone; 1988.

Kanani M, Elliott M. *Applied Surgical Physiology Vivas*. London: Greenwich-Medical; 2004.

Morgan GE, Mikhail MS, Murray MJ. *Clinical Anesthesiology* (Lange Series), 4th ed. New York: McGraw-Hill; 2002.

Townsend CM, Beauchamp D, Evers MB, Mattox KJ, eds. *Sabiston Textbook of Surgery: The Biologic Basis of Modern Surgical Practice*, 18th ed. Philadelphia, PA: Saunders; 2007.

CHAPTER 43

Perioperative Hemostasis

Brian K. Yorkgitis, DO
Allan B. Peetz, MD

INTRODUCTION

Perioperative bleeding is a dreaded surgical complication. More often than not you will hear, "It was dry when we closed..." as your surgical colleagues struggle to identify the source. Hospitalists are often involved in managing patients before and after surgery, hence they need a good working knowledge of how to predict, evaluate, and manage perioperative bleeding. This chapter will focus on the preoperative evaluation of bleeding risk, intraoperative risk factors for bleeding, typical presentations of postoperative bleeding, and how a hospitalist needs to evaluate and manage the bleeding.

PREOPERATIVE EVALUATION OF BLEEDING RISK

To identify patients at increased risk of perioperative bleeding complications, inquire about any history of bleeding problems, such as a known bleeding diathesis, excessive bleeding from minor trauma, menorrhagia, gingival bleeding, hemarthoses, excessive bruising, petechiae, liver, or renal disease. Review medications that can affect normal coagulation, such as antiplatelet agents and anticoagulants, and review the risks and benefits of stopping these agents with the surgeon. All patients identified with risk factors for bleeding should have preoperative laboratory evaluations including a complete blood count, liver function tests, chemistry panel, prothrombin time (PT), activated partial prothrombin time (aPTT), and international normalized ratio (INR). The laboratory test results should be interpreted based on the information in **Table 43-1**.

INTRAOPERATIVE RISK FACTORS FOR BLEEDING

Ideally, hemostasis is achieved before the patient leaves the operating room. In cases of minimally invasive surgery, it may be difficult for the surgeon to appreciate injury to vascular structures from trocar insertion, such as retroperitoneal vascular structures or superficial vessels such as the epigastric vessels. In pelvic and retroperitoneal surgery, it can be difficult for the surgeon to obtain hemostasis due to loss of anatomical planes and rich blood supplies.

Patients who receive anticoagulation during surgery, experience large-volume blood loss (>500 cc) during surgery, or require >10 units of blood have a significant risk for postoperative bleeding. Certain procedures are also associated with higher risk of postoperative bleeding, including vascular surgery, cardiac surgery, any surgery with cardio-pulmonary bypass (CPB), orthopedic surgeries with muscle and bone bleeding, liver surgeries, oncologic tumor resections, prostate surgery (due to the location and release of urokinase), and obstetrical cases (due to the rich vascular supply to the pelvic organs). Any bleeding associated with surgeries of the neck, oropharynx and upper respiratory tract can compromise the patient's airway and needs immediate evaluation. Emergency surgery is associated with higher blood loss compared to elective operations, due to frequent coagulopathy and hypothermia that often accompany emergency surgery.

TABLE 43-1 Expected Laboratory Results by Type of Bleeding Disorder

Bleeding Disorder	CBC	Platelet Count	PT*	aPTT	TT	Reptilase	Fibrinogen**	Clotting Time	Comment
Antiplatelet agents	Normal	Normal	Normal	Normal	Normal			Prolonged	Skin hemorrhage, bleeding at sites of surgery, trauma
Renal failure		Qualitatively abnormal	Normal	Normal	Normal			Prolonged	
Myeloproliferative disorders		Usually high, qualitatively abnormal	Normal	Normal	Normal			Prolonged	Bleeding and/or thrombosis
Liver failure (+/− vitamin K deficiency, thrombocytopenia, fibrinolysis, DIC)	+/− MAHA with schistocytes, helmet cells	Low in liver disease due to splenic sequestration and TPO deficiency	Prolonged (lack of procoagulant and anticoagulant proteins in unpredictable ratios)	Prolonged (lack of procoagulant and anticoagulant proteins in unpredictable ratios)	Prolonged		Low due to abnormal fibrinogen, increased fibrinolysis, DIC	Variable	Transient correction of prolonged INR with administration of Vit K and FFP
DIC	MAHA with schistocytes, helmet cells	Low	Prolonged due to consumption of coagulation factors	Prolonged due to consumption of coagulation factors	Prolonged		Low due to increased fibrinolysis		Oozing from sites of trauma, catheters, or drains & petechiae, ecchymoses
Vitamin K deficiency, warfarin therapy, argatroban, oral direct thrombin and factor Xa inhibitors		Normal	Prolonged due to predominant effect on factor VII	Normal if mild, prolonged if severe					Due to poor nutrition, prolonged use of broad spectrum antibiotics and other drugs
Deficiency or inhibition of factors VII, X, II (prothrombin), V, or fibrinogen		Normal	Prolonged	Normal	Prolonged				Rarely, acquired prothrombin deficiency in antiphospholipid syndrome
Combined UFH and warfarin, fibrinolytic agents (tPA) Direct factor Xa inhibitors, fondaparinux (slight)		Normal	Prolonged	Prolonged					
Heparin, Dabigatran, Argatroban		May be low (UFH)	Normal	Prolonged	Prolonged	Normal			
Deficiency of factors VIII, IX, or XI		Normal	Normal	Prolonged					aPTT can miss mild deficiencies of common pathway factors and fibrinogen

(Continued)

TABLE 43-1 Expected Laboratory Results by Type of Bleeding Disorder (Continued)

Bleeding Disorder	CBC	Platelet Count	PT*	aPTT	TT	Reptilase	Fibrinogen**	Clotting Time	Comment
VWD		Normal except in some patients with type 2V VWD	Normal	Prolonged if low fibrinogen; normal if Factor VIII activity >40%	Normal		If fibrinogen <30%		
Lupus anticoagulant		Normal, or low if in association with SLE	Normal	Prolonged					
Inhibitors of factors VIII, IX, XI, or XII		Normal	Normal	Prolonged					
Inhibitors of PT, fibrinogen, factors V or X, primary amyloidosis associated factor X deficiency		Normal	Prolonged	Prolonged					

aPTT, activated partial thromboplastin time; DIC, disseminated intravascular coagulopathy; direct factor Xa inhibitors, rivaroxaban, apixaban, edoxaban; MAHA, microangiopathic hemolytic anemia; PT, prothrombin time; tPA, recombinant tissue-type plasminogen activator; TPO, thrombopoietin; TT, thromboplastin time; UFH, unfractionated heparinp; VWD, von Willebrand's disease.

*More sensitive to deficiencies of common pathway factors, fibrinogen than aPTT.

**Fibrinogen has to fall <100 mg/dL before PT prolongs, even lower before aPTT prolongs.

Hospitalists should know a patient's intraoperative factors that increase the risk of postoperative bleeding, including:

- Type of surgery
- Use of anticoagulants
- Blood loss >500 cc
- >10 units of blood administration

Any bleeding with surgeries of the neck, oropharynx, or upper respiratory tract can compromise the airway and needs immediate evaluation.

PRESENTATION OF PERIOPERATIVE BLEEDING

Nonsurgical bleeding—commonly called "medical bleeding"—usually results from dysfunction in coagulation and clot formation. The presentation is typically slow oozing, particularly capillary bleeding from traumatized surfaces. This often presents after many hours or days postoperatively, although more rapid blood loss can occur (depending on the type and degree of the dysfunction).

Surgical bleeding usually results from a blood vessel that the surgeon was unable to adequately identify and/or control. This often presents within hours postoperatively and is more brisk and robust than medical bleeding. Physical exam may reveal signs of hypovolemic shock due to loss of circulating volume (**Table 43-2**).

Patients with drains in the surgical bed may have bloody output. If the bleeding is intra-abdominal, the patient may have increasing abdominal girth or a tense/tender abdomen. A tense abdomen with impaired renal function and ventilation may be signs of abdominal compartment syndrome. Patients with a retroperitoneal hematoma may have weakness of hip flexion and knee extension due to a femoral neuropathy.

Extremity bleeding may be external (ie, on the dressing, floor, or in the bed) or may present with tense compartments or symptoms of compartment syndrome. Cardiac and thoracic patients may present with bleeding into a chest tube, or signs-symptoms of a hemothorax (shortness of breath, cough, hypoxia, diminished breath sounds). Retroperitoneal bleeding poses a special problem because its presentation is often nonspecific—sometimes the only sign is a decreasing hemoglobin/hematocrit without any obvious source. Because retroperitoneal bleeding can be an insidious source of significant hemorrhage, a high index of suspicion should be maintained especially when the patient has recently undergone aortic, kidney, or prostate surgery. Likewise, obese patients' bleeding may be subtle, since there is more subcutaneous tissue that can allow blood to accumulate, and the abdominal examination can be compromised by their body habitus. Diffuse oozing and petechiae may be signs of disseminated intravascular coagulopathy (DIC).

No matter the potential source, the operating surgeon should be notified immediately about any change in the patient's condition or possibility of postoperative bleeding.

EVALUATION AND MANAGEMENT OF PERIOPERATIVE BLEEDING

■ EVALUATION

In evaluating a patient with suspected perioperative bleeding, the hospitalist should quickly review the history and physical exam, including the operative note. Key points to evaluate in the operative note should include type of procedure, use intraoperative anticoagulants, volume of blood loss and/or blood products administered, and if the patient had any hypotension or reduced urine output during the surgery (**Table 43-3**). **Figure 43-1** provides management assistance when postoperative bleeding is encountered.

The physical exam should focus on vital signs (hypotension, tachycardia, hypoxia), any external signs of bleeding (including from any surgical drains), or any internal signs of bleeding (such as abdominal fullness or tenderness). The evaluation of the patient should be rapid, and resuscitation should begin simultaneous to the evaluation.

Postoperative bleeding should be suspected in any postoperative patient with hypotension, low urine output, tachycardia, or other signs of shock.

- Surgical bleeding is usually from a blood vessel that the surgeon was unable to adequately identify and/or control and commonly occurs in the early postoperative period.
- Medical bleeding is usually more insidious is associated with coagulation dysfunction due to medications, medical conditions, or large volume resuscitations with resultant coagulation factor depletion.
- Resuscitation should occur **simultaneously** with the evaluation of suspected bleeding to prevent hemodynamic collapse.

■ MEDICAL MANAGEMENT

Resuscitation of the patient should begin simultaneous with the evaluation. The patient needs secure IV access (with two large bore IVs or central venous access) and circulatory volume should be maintained with isotonic IV fluid or blood products. To accurately monitor fluid resuscitation, a Foley catheter should be inserted. The patient should be made nil per os (NPO) in the event there is a need to return to the operating room or undergo other invasive procedures, and the patient should be considered for the need for ICU monitoring.

TABLE 43-2 Classifications of Hemorrhagic Shock and Associated Findings

Class	I	II	III	IV
Blood loss (mL)	<750	750-150	1500-2000	>2000
Blood loss (% body volume)	<15	15-30	30-40	>40
Pulse rate (per min)	<100	100-120	120-140	>140
Blood pressure	Normal	Normal	Decreased	Decreased
Pulse pressure	Normal or increased	Decreased	Decreased	Decreased
Respiratory rate (per min)	14-20	20-30	30-40	>40
Urine output (mL/h)	>30	15-30	5-15	<5
Mental status	Slightly anxious	Mildly anxious	Anxious, confused	Confused, lethargic

TABLE 43-3 Procedure-Related Risk Factors for Perioperative Bleeding

Intraoperative blood loss >500 cc

Blood products administered >10 units

Procedure type

- Trauma surgery
- Emergency surgery
- Vascular, cardiac surgery, cardiopulmonary bypass
- Obstetrical
- Orthopedic surgery
- Liver surgery
- Prostate
- Tonsillectomy

Perioperative medications

- Antiplatelet agents
- Anticoagulants

Hypothermia ($T < 35°C$)

The degree of resuscitation in the bleeding patient depends on the suspected pace of the bleeding and degree of end organ effect. Therapy should be guided by physiologic endpoints such as heart rate, blood pressure, urine output, oxygen saturation, end-organ perfusion, and electrocardiography. More advanced monitoring including echocardiography and invasive hemodynamic measurements may be needed if the patient is not responding or is clinically unstable.

Hypothermia can exacerbate and complicate surgical bleeding due to the enzymatic reactions of coagulation inhibition by low temperatures. The patient should be made normothermic through the use of warm IV fluids, warming blankets, or warming devices. Additionally, any electrolytes should be corrected, particularly calcium and acidosis, to maintain an optimal milieu for coagulation reactions to occur.

Additional interventions should be undertaken based on the results of coagulation studies (Table 43-1), and blood products should be administered in conjunction with clinical assessment and based on the American Society of Anesthesia (ASA) guidelines for perioperative bleeding (**Table 43-4**).

Patients with qualitative platelet dysfunction (who have been taking antiplatelet agents or have uremia) may require desmopressin, which can partially reverse the platelet dysfunction. Tranexamic acid (TXA) is an agent with some utility in ameliorating perioperative

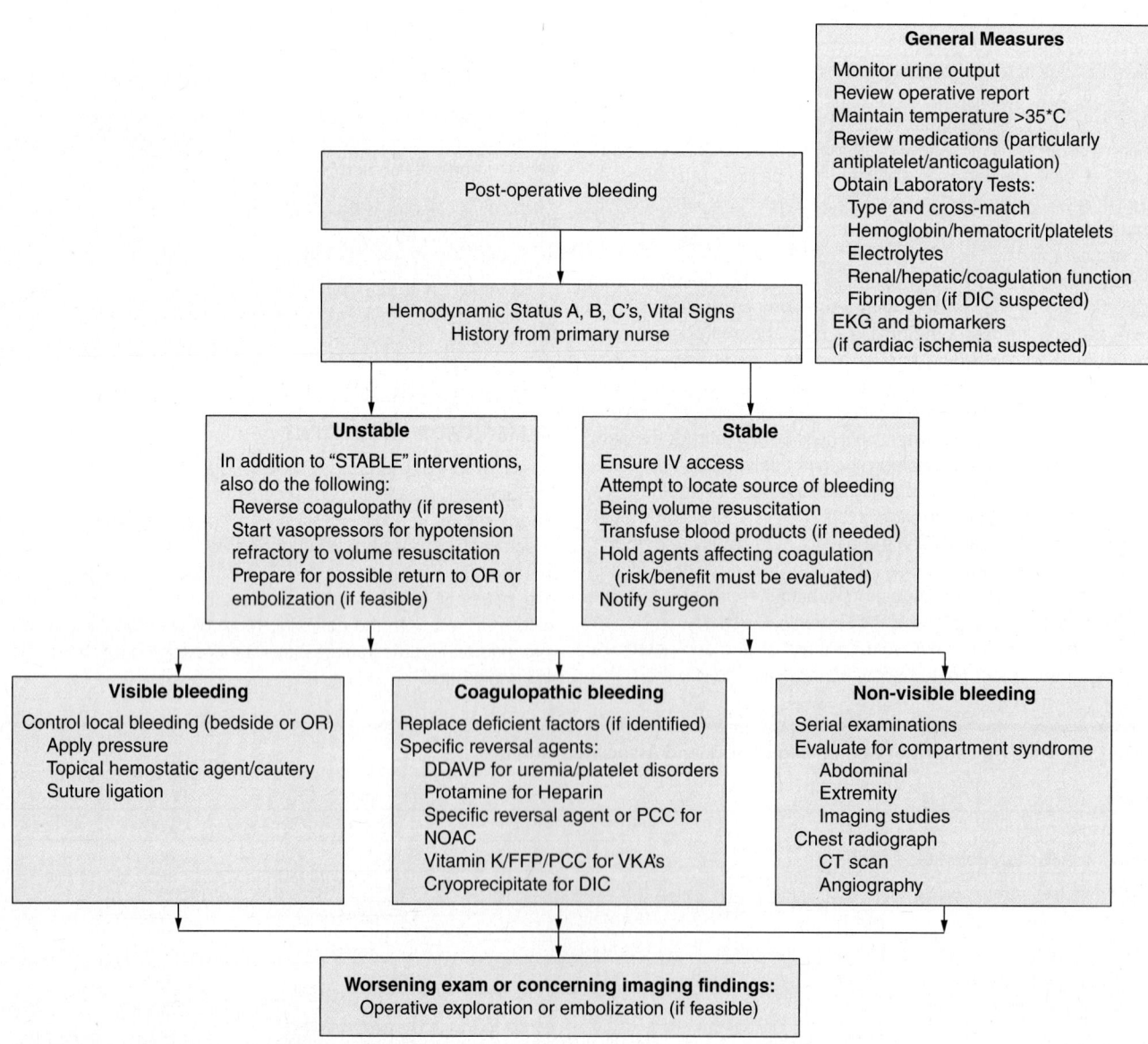

Figure 43-1 *Approach to managing postoperative bleeding.*

TABLE 43-4 American Society of Anesthesiologists (ASA) Guidelines for Perioperative Transfusion in Excessive Bleeding

Therapy	Laboratory Value Indicates need for Transfusion	Laboratory Value Exceeds Indication for Transfusion
Packed red blood cells	Hemoglobin ≤6 g/dL	Hemoglobin ≥10 g/dL
Platelets	≤50,000 cells/mm³*	≥100,000 cells/mm³
Fresh frozen plasma	INR ≥ 2.0*	Normal values
Cryoprecipitate	Fibrinogen ≤80-100 mg/dL	Fibrinogen ≥150 mg/dL

*Central nervous system surgeries: platelets <100,000 and INR >1.5.

bleeding; however, it is associated with the risk of thrombosis, and its use should be decided upon in conjunction with the surgeon.

For patients who have received intraoperative unfractionated heparin (UFH) administration within 6 to 12 hours of the bleeding, it should be reversed with the use of protamine, and the activated clotting time (ACT) can guide the appropriate dosage. Protamine can also reverse the effects of low-molecular weight heparins, but it is less effective than it is for UFH.

Coagulopathy from warfarin should be reversed with fresh frozen plasma and/or vitamin K. Prothrombin concentrate complex (PCC) contains vitamin K-dependent clotting factors and can be used for urgent correction of bleeding associated with acquired coagulation factor deficiency. Recombinant factor VII can also be effective in ameliorating bleeding associated with acquired coagulation factor deficiency; however, it is very expensive and is associated with a risk of thrombosis. Its use should be decided upon in conjunction with the surgeon.

The newer oral direct factor inhibitors include factor Xa inhibitors and direct thrombin inhibitors. They pose challenges due to lack of routine laboratory testing to monitor their effect on coagulation, and lack of specific reversal agents; as such, these drugs should be stopped 3 to 5 days prior to major surgery. If bleeding does occur on these agents, traditional measures to control bleeding locally should be employed such as direct pressure, topical hemostatic agents, cuatery, or embolization. Due to their short half-lives, stopping the agent and providing expectant support is usually sufficient in minor bleeding. In cases of more severe hemorrhage; specific or non-specific reversal agent should be employed to abate bleeding. See Chapter 78 "Bleeding and Coagulopathy" and Chapter 57, "Postoperative Blood Transfusion."

■ **SURGICAL MANAGEMENT**

Visible bleeding from a surgical wound itself may represent a small "skin bleeder" that can be managed with a stitch, by holding direct pressure, or with bedside cautery. Gauze applied to the bleeding wound with constant, continuous pressure maintained for 10 minutes is usually effective. After 10 minutes, pressure can be released and the wound reassessed—if bleeding has not stopped then pressure should be reapplied and the surgeon should be notified.

Deep surgical bleeding requires prompt evaluation by a surgeon so that exploration and definitive control of the culprit blood vessel can be established. Invasive interventions are likely required in cases of postoperative hemodynamic instability, hemothorax, hemoperitoneum and compartment syndromes.

CONCLUSION

Postoperative bleeding is a serious surgical complication. Preoperative evaluation can help determine which patients present the highest risk of suffering this complication. Bleeding should be considered in any postoperative patients with tachycardia, hypotension, oliguria, or evidence of shock. Postoperative bleeding may be medical, surgical, or both. Physical exam and laboratory tests should guide a focused management of the problem, and resuscitation should be initiated immediately. The surgical team should be involved in the work-up and decision making as soon as postoperative bleeding is suspected.

SUGGESTED READINGS

Bougle A, Harrois A, Duranteay J. Resuscitative strategies in traumatic hemorrhagic shock. *Ann Intensive Care.* 2013;3(1):1.

Hammond KL, Margolin DA. Surgical hemorrhage, damage control, and the abdominal compartment syndrome. *Clin Colon Rectal Surg.* 2006;19:188-194.

Hunt BJ. Bleeding and coagulopathies in critical care. *N Engl J Med.* 2014;370:847-859.

Ker K, Prieto-Merino D, Roberts I. Systematic review, meta-analysis and meta-regression on the effect of tranexamic acid on surgical blood loss. *Br J Surg.* 2013;100:1271-1279.

Levy JH, Faraoni D, Spring JL. Managing new oral anticoagulants in the perioperative and intensive care unit setting. *Anesthesiology.* 2013;118:1466-1474.

Practice Guidelines for Perioperative Blood Management. An updated report by the American Society of Anesthesiologists Task Force on perioperative blood management. *Anesthesiology.* 2015;122:241-300.

Phillips LE, Zatta AJ, Schembri NL, Noone AK, Isbister J. Uncontrolled bleeding in surgical patients: the role of recombinant activated factor VIIa. *Curr Drug Targets.* 2009;10(8):744-770.

Shah A, Stanworth SJ, McKenchnie S. Evidence and triggers for the transfusion of blood and blood products. *Anaesthesia.* 2015;70(Suppl 1):10-19.

Spinella PC, Holcomb JB. Resuscitation and transfusion principles for traumatic hemorrhagic shock. *Blood Rev.* 2009;23(6):231-240.

C H A P T E R 44

Postoperative Complications

Peter Najjar, MD
Allan B. Peetz, MD

INTRODUCTION

Postoperative complications are common and costly. Recent studies suggest that, on average, each avoidable surgical complication costs payers >$10,000. Their incidence, risk factors, and impact on patient outcomes are as varied as the field of surgery itself. Surgical site infections (SSIs) alone affect >500,000 patients annually and are associated a 2 to 11 times increase in the risk of postoperative mortality. Good communication among all providers caring for surgical patients is fundamental to both the prevention and management of surgical complications. Hospitalists caring for surgical patients should, accordingly, understand what surgical procedure was performed, the indication for the procedure, and any perioperative concerns from the operating surgeon, based on the circumstances of that particular patient or procedure. This chapter will review some of the more common postoperative complications that a hospitalist needs to recognize and manage. Each section will review the risk factors of the complication, how to mitigate those risks in the perioperative period, and how the hospitalist should identify and manage such complications.

Elective procedures provide more of an opportunity to identify and mitigate risk factors before surgery, although an attempt should take place before any surgery (even urgent or emergent). A thorough history and physical examination should aim to identify risks outlined in this chapter, and optimize the risk-benefit profile of the procedure. For example, when deciding whether to hold antiplatelet or anticoagulation medications in patients with cardiac indications, the risk of cardiac complications is weighed against the risk of bleeding. This decision making should occur in concert with the surgeon, and with the patient, to ensure all parties have a common understanding of the risks and the benefits of the surgery.

PRACTICE POINT

- Prevention of postoperative complications begins in the preoperative period.
- Surgical complications are common and costly; interdisciplinary teams must work together on their prevention and management.

COMMON COMPLICATIONS WITHIN THE POST ANESTHESIA CARE UNIT (PACU)

After surgery, patients usually stay in a postanesthesia care unit (PACU) for close monitoring while they recover from the effects of anesthesia. Common problems managed in the PACU include postoperative pain, hyper- and hypotension, respiratory insufficiency, and nausea and vomiting.

■ POSTOPERATIVE PAIN

Patients in this phase of care are often unable to verbalize pain due to effects of anesthesia; accordingly, pain assessments are often based on other objective assessments such as blood pressure, heart rate, respiratory rate and signs of agitation. See Chapter 48 (Perioperative Pain Management).

POSTOPERATIVE HYPER- AND HYPOTENSION

Pain and elevated catecholamines can contribute to hypertension and tachycardia. β-blockers should be continued in the perioperative setting for patients who took them preoperatively.

Hypertension in the PACU is most commonly caused by pain and/or a history of hypertension. Certain procedures, such as carotid endarterectomy, require immediate and aggressive control of systolic blood pressure regardless of etiology to avoid catastrophic vascular, cardiac, or neurologic complications. Invasive monitoring with an arterial line may be necessary for such patients. Clear communication with the surgical team regarding target blood pressure is essential and hemodynamic agents including vasodilators and negative chrono- and inotropes are frequently used as first-line agents in these settings. Absent an indication for strict hemodynamic control, the patient should be assessed for pain and treated appropriately before treating blood pressure directly. For patients with pre-existing hypertension requiring medication, it is generally most appropriate to gradually reintroduce the preoperative antihypertensive regimen with the exception of diuretics in the immediate postoperative period.

Hypotension in the PACU is usually due to hypovolemia, narcotic and benzodiazepine administration, or epidural anesthesia; postoperative bleeding must also be considered. Markers for hypovolemia include low urine output, signs of shock, and altered mental status, which can be masked by the residual effects of anesthesia. Invasive monitoring with a urinary catheter, central line, or arterial line should be utilized if a patient remains hypotensive despite initial resuscitation with crystalloid. Epidural anesthesia can cause hypotension by blunting sympathetic tone and decreasing vascular resistance. In the absence of hypovolemia, however, epidurals do not usually cause hypotension. Treatment of epidural-related hypotension should include administration of a fluid bolus; temporarily holding the anesthetic infusion can also be helpful until euvolemia is obtained.

POSTOPERATIVE RESPIRATORY INSUFFICIENCY

Although most patients will require some supplemental oxygen immediately after surgery, dyspnea, tachypnea, wheezing, and signs of respiratory distress are not normal postoperative signs and symptoms, and need to be addressed in the PACU. The causes and degree of risk of postoperative respiratory insufficiency are complex and patient specific, but all patients recovering from anesthesia require close monitoring of their respiratory status, with personnel and equipment for reintubation readily available. The primary factors that contribute to postoperative respiratory insufficiency include use of general anesthesia, upper abdominal and thoracic surgeries, longer duration surgeries, use of endotracheal intubation, and use of narcotics. Significant pain also puts patients at increased risk, as pain impairs respiratory function by limiting vital capacity and can result in hypoxia and dyspnea.

Pulmonary edema is a common etiology for respiratory distress in the postoperative period, often secondary to the effects of fluid shifts and sometimes overload from intraoperative resuscitation. Initial evaluation of pulmonary edema should include physical exam and chest x-ray; some patients may need further work-up or evaluation by a cardiologist. Pneumothorax should be considered in patients with a central line recently placed, and should also be evaluated with a Chest x-ray. For patients with a postoperative chest tube (usually cardiac or thoracic surgery patients) a poorly functioning chest tube or residual pneumothorax can also cause or exacerbate respiratory distress. This can be detected by physical exam and confirmed with a chest x-ray followed by prompt contact with the operating surgeon to relay the concern.

PRACTICE POINT

Low urine output in the immediate postoperative setting

- Intravascular volume depletion may occur concurrently with pulmonary edema due to increased vascular permeability associated with perioperative inflammation; administration of diuretics for postoperative pulmonary edema can exacerbate intravascular depletion, hypotension, and inadequate end-organ perfusion.
- Postoperative oliguria (less than the equivalent of 0.5 cc/kg/h) requires urgent evaluation.

POSTOPERATIVE NAUSEA AND VOMITING

Postoperative nausea and vomiting (PONV) is also common in the PACU, the causes of which are multifactorial. Prior history is the most significant risk factor; other risk factors include longer duration procedures, use of volatile anesthetics (such as isoflurane), and procedures involving the inner ear, eye, and abdominal viscera. Patients at moderate to high risk of PONV benefit from prophylactic antiemetics, motility agents, or a scopolamine patch before emerging from anesthesia.

POSTOPERATIVE FEVER

Low-grade fevers in the first 48 hours after surgery are a normal sequelae of inflammation, atelectasis, or hematoma absorption following surgery, and usually not from an infectious process. In the absence of any localizing signs or symptoms, self-limited fever within the first 48 hours postoperatively usually does not need infectious work-up. After 48 hours, temperatures greater than 38.5°C should prompt a complete fever workup. In the postoperative patient, the surgical wound and site of venous access are potential sources of infection and need to be carefully examined. See Chapter 206 (Undiagnosed Fever in Hospitalized Patients).

SURGICAL SITE INFECTIONS

Surgical site infections (SSIs) account for approximately 30% of nosocomial infections and are the most common infections after surgery. They are associated with a 7-day increased length of stay and cost ~$400 for a superficial SSI and ~$30,000 for organ space SSIs.

SSIs are classified as superficial, deep, or organ space infections. Superficial infections are wound infections involving the skin and subcutaneous tissues. Deep infections involve the fascia or muscle below. Organ space infections involve organs below the cutaneous and muscular layers (**Figure 44-1**).

PRACTICE POINT

Wound infections

- Despite the most rigorous aseptic technique, all wounds are contaminated to some degree and have some risk of infection. Even "clean" wounds have a 1.5% risk of infection (**Table 44-1**).
- Wound infections commonly occur between 5 and 10 days after an operation.
- Antibiotics are not necessary for simple wounds that have been drained.
- Deep space infections usually require drainage; antibiotics alone are insufficient.

Risk factors for wound infection are patient and operation dependent. Patient related risk factors include large body habitus,

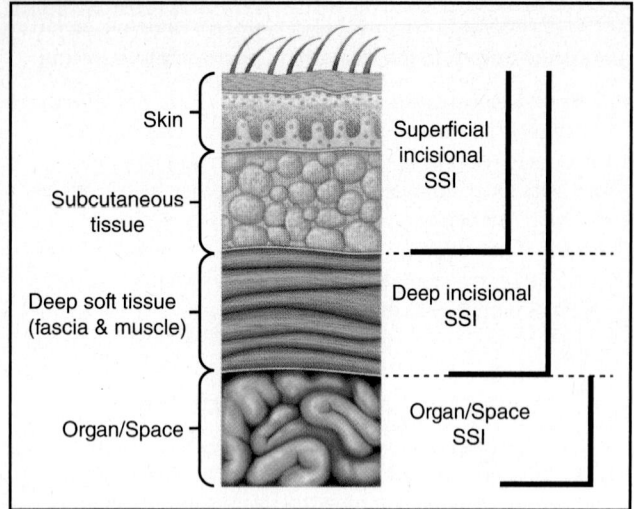

Figure 44-1 *Categories of surgical site infections.*

diabetes, disability, immunosuppression, malnutrition, and smoking. Certain operations, such as those involving the colon or small bowel, are higher risk than others. Other operative risk factors include operating room conditions, surgical technique (eg, laparoscopic or open), administration of antibiotic prophylaxis, and hypoxia or hypotension during the procedure.

Prophylactic antibiotics are very effective at reducing the risk of SSIs; they should be administered within 1 hour of incision and continued for no more than 24 hours after surgery. In the event of significant contamination in the OR, wounds may be left open and managed with delayed primary closure or wet to dry dressings.

The hallmarks of a wound infection are fever, pain, tenderness, or purulent drainage. The typical presentation is between 5 and 10 days postoperatively. Some infections can present earlier; clostridial necrotizing wound infection should be suspected when a patient has a very high fever in the immediate postoperative period; these require immediate surgical evaluation and drainage.

TABLE 44-1 Surgical Wound Classification

Wound Classification	Infection Risk	Procedure Type
Clean	1.5%	Vascular surgery
No infection or inflammation		
Respiratory, gastrointestinal, biliary, and urinary tracts not entered		
Clean contaminated	10%	Appendectomy
Entry into respiratory, biliary, gastrointestinal, urinary tracts with minimal spillage No evidence of infection or major break in aseptic technique		
Contaminated	20%	Foreign body in a wound
Inflammation, gross spillage from GI tract, break in technique		
Fresh traumatic wound		
Dirty or infected	40%	Abscess, perforated viscous
Purulent drainage, fecal contamination, perforated viscous, delayed or contaminated traumatic wound, presence of devitalized tissue		

Deep space infections occur in enclosed spaces with some degree of isolation from blood supply, making them relatively impervious to antibiotics. Such infections usually require drainage either percutaneously or in the operating room. Anastomotic leaks typically occur between postoperative days 5 and 7 and should be suspected in surgical patients with tachycardia, abdominal pain, fever, and elevated white count. This constellation of symptoms after an enteric anastomosis should prompt a CT scan. These leaks can often be managed with percutaneous drainage, but inability to control the infection may require operative drainage.

WOUND DEHISCENCE, HEMATOMAS, SEROMAS

Wounds typically heal to a maximum of 80% of the tensile strength within ~6 weeks among healthy, well-nourished patients. Because of this, most surgeons restrict postoperative activities to avoid stress on the wound for 4 to 6 weeks. Wounds that have been closed primarily should be kept clean, dry, and covered for a minimum of 48 hours after surgery. Dry, sterile operative dressings may be kept in place until postoperative day 2; thereafter, patients can usually shower without submerging the wound.

Wound dehiscence is disruption of any layer of the surgical wound. This rare complication results from increased pressure on the wound and can arise for a variety of reasons. Suspected dehiscence should be promptly evaluated by a surgeon and may require a return to the operating room. Poor wound healing often leads to dehiscence. Malnutrition, liver disease, diabetes, immunosuppression, and chronic steroid use inhibit normal wound healing and are risk factors.

The most common layers involved are the skin and fascia. Sudden output of serosanguinous fluid from the wound is usually the first sign of dehiscence. Therefore, daily evaluation by multiple team members (including surgeons, hospitalists, and nurses) may help identify subtle changes that may be harbingers of dehiscence.

The management of postoperative wound dehiscence depends on the size and location of the wound as well as the patient's condition. Fascial dehiscence—separation of the deepest layer of the abdominal wall—typically requires urgent closure in the operating room. In the most severe of cases, dehiscence leads to extrusion of intra-abdominal contents (eg, evisceration). Evisceration is a surgical emergency that requires immediate return to operating room.

Hematomas are more common, and can be caused either by inadequate hemostasis during surgery or disruption of hemostasis postoperatively; risk factors for hematomas include bleeding disorders and anticoagulant use. A hematoma can result in wound elevation, pressure, pain, dehiscence, and infection. The surgeon should always be alerted if there is a suspected hematoma; depending on the size and location, treatment can vary from watchful waiting to re-exploration in the OR. Hematomas following neck exploration may rapidly compromise the airway in the postoperative period. Precipitating factors include abrupt increases in intrathoracic pressure from coughing, emesis, or Valsalva maneuvers. Treatment involves emergent evacuation of the hematoma prior to reintubation.

Seromas are collections of serous fluid that form after procedures involving disrupted lymphatic flow and raised skin flaps. They are generally the result of a normal physiologic response to anatomic dead space, and their incidence is dependent on the anatomic location of the wound. Examples of procedures commonly associated with seromas include inguinal hernia repair, groin exploration, and mastectomy. Suction drains may be left in place at the end of the procedure to increase tissue apposition and remove fluid. Compression dressings can also reduce the risk of seroma formation. Seromas may increase the risk for wound disruption and infection but are usually nothing more than a nuisance. Management may be expectant or include serial aspirations. Rarely, return to the OR is indicated to ligate contributing lymphatics.

PULMONARY AND CARDIAC COMPLICATIONS

See Chapters 60 (Pulmonary Complications) and 59 (Cardiac Complications).

GASTROINTESTINAL COMPLICATIONS

Postoperative ileus is expected after gastrointestinal surgery but is also common after other procedures, usually due to narcotic use and/or immobility. Ileus usually presents with abdominal distention, nausea, belching, and inability to pass flatus. Resolution of the symptoms usually occurs within 5 days of surgery but can be longer, particularly in debilitated patients or those with significant narcotic use. Classically, an ileus on plain abdominal x-ray is associated with uniform distribution of air throughout the bowel, but this finding is not specific. Abdominal CT scan with enteric contrast has close to 100% sensitivity and specificity in distinguishing postoperative obstruction from ileus.

Colonic pseudo-obstruction is a rare postoperative complication, and most likely occurs in older patients with prolonged immobility, preoperative institutionalization and functional limitation. It more commonly occurs after orthopedic surgeries than other types of surgeries. Patients present with signs of an ileus, and radiographs demonstrate a decompressed small bowel and uniformly dilated colon. Treatment involves hydration, bowel rest, and decompression (distally with rectal tube placement and proximally with nasogastric tube placement if there is evidence of gastric distension). In refractory cases, neostigmine is an option but can be associated with bradycardia. If the cecum is dilated >11 cm, additional measures should be undertaken to avoid perforation, such as a cecostomy tube or a cecal resection. General surgeons should be engaged early in the management of suspected postoperative colonic pseudo-obstruction.

DELIRIUM

Postoperative delirium is most common in patients with advanced age, a history of sensitivity to narcotics or anesthetics, heavy alcohol use, dementia or prior delirium. Delirium can occur after any surgical procedure, but is most common after cardiovascular and thoracic surgery. The causes are multifactorial, including a myriad of medications, loss of environmental cues, insomnia, and recovery from cardiopulmonary bypass.

Delirium presents with waxing and waning severity with periods of lucidity, recurrent confusion, agitation, hallucination, and confabulations. These patients may present a risk to themselves and others by trying to get out of bed without assistance, or trying to remove tubes and drains. Prevention is the best strategy and entails maintaining a regular sleep-wake cycle, restoring environmental cues (such as daylight and clocks), and removing extraneous environmental stressors (minimizing bright lights and loud noises). Some patients will respond well to reassurance and emotional support. If at risk for self-harm, low-dose antipsychotics are first line agents. It is best to start at low doses and titrate up as needed, as these medications can be sedating, may worsen delirium at higher doses, and may interfere with pulmonary function and physical therapy. These pharmacologic treatments may provide symptom control but do not treat the underlying causes of delirium and at times can exacerbate delirium. When managing patients with postoperative delirium it is also important to rule out other organic disease triggers such as sepsis, stroke, or metabolic derangements. See Chapter 81 (Delirium).

DEEP VENOUS THROMBOSIS AND PULMONARY EMBOLUS

Venous thromboembolism (VTE) is a leading cause of preventable death in the postoperative setting. Surgical patients are at high risk for VTE due to the surgical procedure itself as well as induction of general anesthesia, which results in prolonged immobility, hypercoagulability, and endothelial damage. Patients with known hypercoaguable states, prior VTE, and malignancy are at especially high risk. High-risk surgical procedures include orthopedic surgery, trauma, and neurosurgical treatment of head injury and brain tumors. Prophylaxis starts before surgery with the application of pneumatic compression devices and subcutaneous heparin 2 hours prior to anesthetic induction. In the absence of procedure- or patient-specific concerns, pharmaceutical prophylaxis should not be held preoperatively. Unless there are clear contraindications, such as increased bleeding risk, patients should receive pharmacologic prophylaxis and pneumatic boots throughout and perioperative period. See Chapter 56 (VTE Prophylaxis for Patients Requiring Non-Orthopedic Surgery).

Pulmonary embolus (PE) still causes considerable mortality in hospitalized patients. PE should be suspected in all surgical patients presenting with symptoms of dyspnea, tachycardia, and hypoxemia. The decision to start anticoagulation should be made with the operating surgeon, while pending further diagnostic testing. See Chapter 253 (Diagnosis and Treatment of VTE).

URINARY TRACT INFECTIONS (UTI)

Urinary tract infections (UTI) are most common after vaginal or urologic surgery and any surgery with the use of indwelling catheters. Women and obese patients are at highest risk. The most common pathogens are *Escherichia coli*, *Staphylococcus saprophyticus*, and *Proteus mirabilis*. However, hospitalized and immunosuppressed patients are also susceptible to *Klebsiella*, *Proteus vulgaris*, *Candida albicans*, and *Pseudomonas*. The standard for prevention is the removal of indwelling catheters within 48 hours of insertion. The need for continued urinary catheterization should be assessed at least daily to prevent needless prolongation of catheter placement and increased risk of catheter-associated UTI. Criteria for diagnosis and treatment are the same as for UTIs in the nonpostoperative period. See Chapter 197 (Urinary Tract Infection and Pyelonephritis).

POSTOPERATIVE URINARY RETENTION

Postoperative is common but rarely prolonged. Common risk factors for postoperative urinary retention include male sex, prostatic enlargement, epidural/spinal/prolonged anesthesia, use of antihistamines or narcotics, and pelvic/perineal procedures. An overdistended bladder (>500 mL) and disruption of the neural pathways that control voiding impairs urinary contraction and micturition. Prophylactic catheterization in the operating room is recommended for any procedure lasting more than 3 hours, or when interruption of the sacral plexus is anticipated (eg, abdominoperineal resection). If a catheter is not present, patients should be encouraged to void soon after the procedure. If the patient has not voided for more than 6 hours, it is appropriate to evaluate retention with a bedside ultrasound; alternatively, an in-out catheter may be used to determine the extent of retention. The treatment for bladder distention is intermittent catheterization along with mitigation of any contributing factors. Some patients may have prolonged urinary retention in the postoperative period (>48 hours). In this scenario, appropriate pharmacologic treatment should be initiated and an indwelling Foley catheter should be placed. Some may require subsequent outpatient urologic follow-up for a void trial after discharge. See Chapter 67 (Urology).

CONCLUSION

Postoperative complications are associated with significant morbidity, prolonged length of stay, and hospital costs. Hospitalists should know how to identify and manage the most common postoperative complications. Comprehensive assessment preoperatively, attention to surgical technique and anesthetic management, and a multidisciplinary approach to medication management, infection control, and patient mobility can reduce the risk of surgical complications.

SUGGESTED READINGS

Arozullah AM, Khuri SF, Henderson WG, et al. Development and validation of a Multifactorial risk index for predicting postoperative pneumonia after major noncardiac surgery. *Ann Intern Med.* 2001;135:847-857.

Güldner A, Pelosi P, De abreu MG. Nonventilatory strategies to prevent postoperative pulmonary complications. *Curr Opin Anaesthesiol.* 2013;26(2):141-151.

Mattei P, Rombeau JL. Review of the pathophysiology and management of postoperative ileus. *World J Surg.* 2006;30(8):1382-1391.

Najjar PA, Smink DS. Prophylactic antibiotics and prevention of surgical site infections. *Surg Clin North Am.* 2015;95(2):269-283.

CHAPTER 45

Surgical Tubes and Drains

Alexandra Columbus, MD
Joaquim M. Havens, MD
Allan B. Peetz, MD

Surgical drains are used to monitor for postoperative leaks or abscesses, collect normal physiologic fluid, or to minimize dead space. **Table 45-1** lists various types of drains, with their indications for use. This chapter will review the most common types of surgical drains, and the basic care of these drains from a hospitalist perspective.

PRACTICE POINT

- Hospitalists should know the location and purpose of all surgical drains in their patients, but should not manipulate these drains without input from the surgeon who placed them.

CHEST TUBES

Chest tubes are placed in the pleural space to evacuate air or fluid. They can be as thin as 20 French or as thick as 40 French (for adults). Chest tubes are typically placed between the fourth and fifth intercostal spaces in the anterior axillary or mid-axillary line, however, location may vary according to the indication for placement. The tubes can be straight or angled.

The tubes are connected to a collecting system with a three-way chamber. The water chamber holds a column of water which prevents air from being sucked into the pleural space with inhalation. The suction chamber can be attached to continuous wall suction to remove air or fluid, or it can be placed on "water seal" with no active suction mechanism. The third chamber is the collection chamber for fluid drainage.

Indications for a chest tube include pneumothorax, hemothorax, or a persistent or large pleural effusion. Pneumothorax and hemothorax usually require immediate chest tube placement. Chest tubes are also commonly placed at the end of thoracic surgeries, to allow for appropriate re-expansion of the lung tissue.

A chest x-ray should be obtained after any chest tube insertion to ensure appropriate location. Chest tubes are equipped with a radiopaque line along the longitudinal axis, which should be visible on x-ray. Respiratory variation in the fluid in the collecting tube, called "tidling," should also be seen in a correctly placed chest tube, and should be monitored at the bedside to reassure continued appropriate location. The interventional radiologist or surgeon who placed the tube should determine the subsequent frequency of serial chest x-rays required to monitor the location of the chest tube.

If the patient has a pneumothorax, air bubbles will be visible in the water chamber (called an "air leak") which is often more apparent when the patient coughs. The chest tube should initially be set to continuous suction at −20 mm Hg to evacuate the air. Once the "air leak" has stopped, the chest tube should be placed on water seal to confirm the pneumothorax is resolved (water seal mimics normal physiology). If the pneumothorax is not resolved, the chest tube should be placed back on continuous suction. A chest x-ray should be obtained anytime the chest tube is changed from suction to water seal or vice versa.

If the patient experiences ongoing or worsening pain, fever, or inadequate drainage, a chest computed tomographic (CT) scan may be warranted to identify inappropriate positioning or other complications, such as occlusion or effusion, of the tube. Chest tubes may become clogged by blood or other debris; the surgical team may be able to evacuate the tube with suction tubing at the bedside. If unsuccessful, the tube may need to be removed and reinserted.

TABLE 45-1 Surgical Tubes and Drains

Type	Location	Clinical Indication	Clinical Scenario
Chest tube	Pleural space Mediastinal space	Pneumothorax Hemothorax Pleural effusion	Trauma, cardiac surgery, thoracic surgery, malignant effusion, empyema
Nasogastric tube	Stomach	Intestinal decompression, gastric feeding	Small bowel obstruction, ileus, temporary dysphagia
Gastric tube (gastrostomy)	Stomach	Prolonged enteral access, gastric decompression	Prolonged mechanical ventilation, gastric outlet obstruction
Jejunal tube (jejunostomy)	Jejunum	Prolonged postgastric feeding, gastric outlet obstruction, high aspiration risk	Prolonged mechanical ventilation, malignant gastric outlet obstruction, recurrent aspiration pneumonia
Duodenal tube	Duodenum	Postgastric feeding, gastric outlet obstruction, high aspiration risk	Mechanical ventilation, dysphagia, acute aspiration risk
Penrose drain	Peritoneal space, small surgical space	Used to maintain surgical tract for adequate drainage	
Closed suction drain (eg, Jackson Pratt, Hemovac)	Surgical space	Evacuate serous fluid or blood, prevent seroma formation, tissue apposition to improve wound healing, drain GI secretions	Mastectomy, ventral hernia repair, plastic surgery flaps, gastrointestinal anastomoses, orthopedic surgery

The team that placed the tube should help the hospitalist determine the timing of the chest tube removal. If the patient has a pleural effusion, the chest tube can usually be removed when the output is less than 100 to 200 mL per day, and the lung is expanded. The tube should usually be taken off suction and placed on water seal (to rule out pneumothorax) prior to tube removal.

PRACTICE POINT

Chest tubes

- Contact the team who placed the chest tube if it needs adjustment or removal.
- Never advance a chest tube into the pleural space, due to the risk of introducing infection.
- Do not clamp a tube when pneumothorax is suspected, due to the risk of precipitating a tension pneumothorax.

PENROSE DRAINS

Penrose drains are often used to drain fluid or to keep a space open for drainage. Surgeons may anchor penrose drains to skin with sutures. Common indications include:

- Ventral hernia repair
- Debridement of infected pancreatitis
- Drainage of superficial abscess cavities

Penrose drains are simple, flexible tubes open at both ends; in contrast to closed drains, they permit ingress as well as egress, facilitating colonization.

CLOSED SUCTION DRAINS

Closed suction drains with a plastic bulb attachment (ie, Jackson-Pratt, Blake, Hemovac) are used to collect fluid from a postoperative cavity. Common indications include:

- Postmastectomy to drain subcutaneous fluid
- Abdominal surgery

- Plastic surgery to prevent seroma formation and to promote tissue apposition
- Cholecystectomy to drain bile
- Inadvertent postoperative leakage following a difficult rectal anastomosis
- Post pancreatic surgery

Typically, closed suction drains will be left in place until the drainage is less than 20 mL per day. These drains can be left in for weeks if necessary and will often be removed upon the patient's scheduled surgical follow-up. Rare complications include erosion into surrounding tissues and inadvertent suturing of the drain in place such that re-exploration is required to remove it. If a closed suction drain becomes occluded, contact the team who placed the drain for further recommendations on adjustment, replacement, or removal.

PRACTICE POINT

Penrose and closed suction drains

- Always check with the surgeon who placed the drain before readjustment or removal.
- Notify the surgeon if a patient has bloody drainage and/or a falling hematocrit.

NASOGASTRIC AND DUODENAL TUBES

Nasogastric tubes (NGTs) are often used in the nonoperative management of small bowel obstruction or ileus. NGTs should be placed in the most dependent portion of the gastric lumen, and confirmed by chest or abdominal x-ray. NGTs are sump pumps and have a double lumen, which includes an air port to assure flow. The air port should be patent for optimal functioning. The tube may be connected to continuous wall suction or intermittent suction, set to low (<60 mm Hg) to avoid mucosal avulsion.

NGT output should decrease during the resolution of obstruction or ileus, and symptoms of nausea, vomiting, and abdominal distention should concomitantly improve. Persistently high output in a patient with other indicators of bowel function (eg, flatus) may suggest postpyloric placement (and placement should be checked by an x-ray). A gastric fluid loss can cause electrolyte disturbances, a daily electrolyte panel should be checked and repleted as needed. The timing of NGT removal depends on resumption of bowel function. NGTs may also be helpful in gastric lavage and in diagnosing the source of gastrointestinal bleeding. Bloody output indicates an upper bleed, proximal to the ligament of Treitz, whereas clear or bilious output suggests a lower gastrointestinal bleed.

Duodenal tubes are small-bore tubes used when postpyloric feeding is desired. Like NGT's, small-bore duodenal tubes are placed through the nares. They are very narrow caliber and require a long wire for insertion. The wire should be removed as soon as placement is confirmed by x-ray. They are very soft and flexible, but the wire used for placement is very stiff, increasing the risk of inadvertent insertion into the airway. Therefore, placement by an experienced operator is particularly important. In patients who are intubated or who have undergone tracheostomy placement, nasoenteric feeding tubes should be placed under bronchoscopic or fluoroscopic guidance to ensure that the tube is properly positioned.

PRACTICE POINT

Nasogastric tube removal in the management of abdominal ileus or obstruction

- The NGT can likely be removed if the patient is having flatus and/or bowel movements.
- Place the NGT to gravity and check the aspirate after 4 hours; NGT output less than 100 cc indicates passage of gastric contents through the GI tract.
- Recurrence of nausea, abdominal distention, or pain prior to the 4 hours indicates ongoing ileus or obstruction, and NGT suction should continue.

GASTROSTOMY AND JEJUNOSTOMY TUBES

Gastrostomy tubes are most commonly used for feeding but may also be used for decompression of functional or anatomic gastric outlet obstruction. They are indicated when patients need prolonged enteral access (such as prolonged mechanical ventilation or head and neck pathology that prohibits oral feeding). They are also rarely used for gastropexy, to tack an atonic or patulous stomach to the abdominal wall or to prevent recurrence of paraesophageal hernias. These tubes can be placed percutaneously by interventional radiologists, endoscopically by surgeons and gastroenterologists, or via laparoscopy or laparotomy by surgeons. This last option is often reserved for patients with difficult anatomy or who are having laparotomy for another reason.

Because of the stomach's generous lumen, gastrostomy tubes rarely clog. In the event that they do get clogged, carbonated liquids, meat tenderizer, or enzymes may help dissolve the obstruction. If a gastrostomy tube is left to drainage, this can result in significant fluid and electrolyte losses; a daily electrolyte panel should be checked and repleted as needed.

Jejunostomy tubes are used exclusively for feeding and are usually placed 10 to 20 cm distal to the ligament of Treitz. These tubes are indicated in patients who require distal feedings, due to gastric dysfunction or following a surgery in which a proximal anastamosis requires time to heal. These tubes are more apt to clog and can be more difficult to manage because the lumen of the small bowel is smaller than the stomach. Some prefer not to put pills down the tube to mitigate this risk. Routine flushes (30 mL every 4-6 hours) with water or saline are also helpful in mitigating the risk of clogging. In the event that they do get clogged, similar to gastrostomy tubes, carbonated liquids, meat tenderizer, or enzymes can help dissolve the obstruction.

Percutaneous tube sites should be examined frequently for signs of infection. Though gastrostomy and jejunostomy tubes are typically well secured intra-abdominally, it is possible for them to become dislodged. If a gastrostomy or jejunostomy tube has been in place for more than 2 weeks, it can easily be replaced at the bedside with a tube of comparable caliber by a member of the surgical team or by an experienced hospitalist. If the tube has been in place less than 2 weeks, it requires replacement with radiographic guidance, as the risk of creating a false lumen is high. Over time, tubes can become loose and fall out. If they need replacement, the preceding guidelines apply.

PRACTICE POINT

Gastrostomy and jejunostomy tubes

- Notify the surgeon if a gastrostomy or jejunostomy tube becomes dislodged.
- Correct positioning of these tubes should be confirmed radiographically before use.

CONCLUSION

There are several types of tubes and drains used for a variety of indications in surgical patients. Hospitalists should know the location and purpose of all surgical drains, but should not manipulate these drains without input from the team who placed them. Drain output should be closely monitored; if unexpected changes in the quantity or quality of the output are observed, the team who placed the tube or drain should be notified immediately.

SUGGESTED READINGS

Brunicandi FC, Andersen DK, Billiar TR, et al. *Schwartz's Principles of Surgery*, 10th ed. New York: McGraw-Hill; 2014.

Sugarbaker D, Bueno R, Krasna M, et al. *Adult Chest Surgery*. New York: McGraw Hill; 2009.

Wiley W, Souba MP, Fink GJ, et al. *ACS Surgery: Principles and Practice*. WebMD; 2006.

CHAPTER 46

Surgical Critical Care

Evert A. Eriksson, MD, FACS, FCCP
Alicia Privette, MD
Brent Jewett, MD
Samir M. Fakhry, MD, FACS

INTRODUCTION

Caring for critically ill patients began through recognizing the unique needs of the acutely injured and postoperative patient. In the 1850s during the Crimean War, Florence Nightingale placed the most seriously ill patients in beds near the nursing station. This stressed the importance of a separate geographic location for critically ill and injured patients. Dr Walter E. Dandy, in 1923, at the Johns Hopkins Hospital created a three bed postoperative unit for neurosurgical patients and staffed the unit with specially trained nurses to manage and monitor these patients. The Second World War brought about the creation of specialized shock units to provide resuscitation for the large number of critically injured soldiers. The 1950s experienced the widespread development of shock units and postoperative recovery units. In addition, respiratory units were created due to the large number of polio patients requiring mechanical ventilation. In 1986, the American Board of Medical Specialties approved certification in Critical Care for the four primary boards: anesthesiology, internal medicine, pediatrics, and surgery.

Surgical Critical Care is a core competency of surgical training and relates to the care of patients with acute, life-threatening or potentially life-threatening surgical conditions. Surgical Critical Care brings together the art of critical care management of severely ill patients with the science of surgical procedures targeted at improving their altered physiology. These surgeons are well versed in the pre and postoperative management of patients after undergoing surgical procedures from any surgical discipline and of any age group. While much of the knowledge base is shared with other critical care specialists, fellowship training provides the surgical critical care specialist with specific expertise relating to the interactions between the patients disease process and the pathophysiologic response to infections, inflammation, ischemia, trauma, burns, and operations. Given the rising rate of Hospitalist comanagement of surgical patients, this chapter will cover the most common surgical critical care patient types, and the management of the most common surgical conditions encountered among these patients for the Hospitalist.

SURGICAL CRITICAL CARE ADMIT TYPES

SURGICAL ICU ADMITS

Patients may be admitted to the ICU from the Emergency Department, preoperatively, immediately postoperatively, or postoperatively after initial admission to the postanesthesia care unit or the ward. Preoperative admission may be required for resuscitation in the event of preoperative respiratory failure, shock, or sepsis. ICU admission may also be required for patients who need invasive monitoring for hemodynamic optimization prior to undergoing surgical procedures.

Postoperatively, patients may be admitted to the ICU for respiratory failure, hemodynamic instability, or close monitoring for complications such as bleeding or other physiologic derangements. Patients may also require admission to the ICU due to exacerbation of underlying comorbidities or after procedures with significant blood loss or massive fluid shifts. Some patients need prolonged mechanical ventilation due to the effects of general anesthesia, airway edema, dysfunctional pulmonary mechanics, acute lung injury, traumatic injury to the respiratory tract, cardiovascular disease, or volume overload. Patients with preoperative renal, hepatic, or pulmonary insufficiency may also benefit from elective postoperative ICU admission, as they may be more susceptible to the adverse effects of narcotics and less likely to tolerate hemodynamic fluctuations.

■ TRAUMA ICU ADMITS

In the United States, injury is the most common cause of death up to the age of 44 years and the fourth most common cause of death overall based on data from the Centers for Disease Control and Prevention. Three million people were hospitalized for injury in 2013 and many of these patients required admission to a critical care unit. While most severely injured trauma patients are managed at Trauma Centers with comprehensive resources, some will receive at least part of their care at hospitals that are not trauma centers. In most trauma systems, severely injured patients are identified in the field and taken to a Level 1 trauma center because there is an approximately 25% improvement in survival at such centers. Once a trauma patient arrives at a trauma center, they undergo a highly standardized resuscitation process using the Advanced Trauma Life Support (ATLS) program.

The modern day care of trauma patients frequently involves critical care admission. Trauma patients may require ICU admission for many reasons such as observation and management for severe and/or multiple trauma, management of acute respiratory failure, resuscitation of hemorrhagic shock, medical management of traumatic brain injury, and pain control. Patients with multiple injuries frequently require ICU care for both management of their injuries and control of pain, agitation, and delirium. Management of specific injuries requires experience and training in trauma care. When a trauma surgeon is not available, a general surgeon can provide needed expertise as the principles of trauma care are part of general surgery training.

The management of pain and agitation is important for all ICU patients but especially injured patients. Consensus guidelines for the management of pain, agitation, and delirium are available and apply to trauma patients with little if any modification (see suggested readings). Because they have high requirements for pain medication with its attendant risks of respiratory depression and altered sensorium, trauma patients requiring moderate to large doses of analgesia and/or sedation are best managed in an ICU setting to optimize outcomes and minimize complications.

Since traumatic brain injury (TBI) accounts for one third of injury deaths, TBI is a frequent indication for ICU admission. In addition, nearly all trauma patients undergoing acute neurosurgical intervention will require ICU admission for postoperative care. In general, TBI patients need admission to the ICU if they require intubation and mechanical ventilation, if they need frequent (more than every 4 hours) neurologic examination and if they have severe TBI requiring modern-day care. The principles of severe TBI management are best outlined in the consensus guidelines developed by the Brain Trauma Foundation. In addition to emphasizing adequate oxygenation and brain perfusion, the guidelines describe the role of many ICU interventions in the care of patients with severe TBI.

■ BURN ICU ADMITS

As with any critically injured patient assessment of burn patients begins with the ABCs (airway, breathing, and circulation). Airway compromise must be considered in any burn patient. Signs of airway compromise may not be immediately obvious but may progress rapidly. Supportive measures for potential airway injury should be initiated and early intubation should be considered if signs of airway compromise are present. Clinical signs of potential inhalational injury include: face and/or neck burns, singeing of the eyebrows and nasal vibrissae, carbon deposits, and acute inflammatory changes in the oropharynx, carbonaceous sputum, hoarseness,

history of impaired mentation, and/ or confinement in a burning environment, explosion with burns to head and torso, and carboxyhemoglobin level greater than 10%. Stridor or circumferential burns to the neck are absolute indications for endotracheal intubation.

Breathing and oxygenation issues arise from several possible injuries after burns. Direct thermal injury results in upper airway edema and obstruction. Inhalation of combustion products and toxic fumes can cause a chemical tracheobronchitis, edema, and predispose patients to develop pneumonia. Carbon monoxide (CO) poisoning should be considered in any burn patient from an enclosed area. Patients' with CO levels of less than 20% usually do not exhibit symptoms. CO levels of 20% to 30% result in headache and nausea, 30% to 40% confusion, 40% to 60% coma, and more than 60% death. The classically described cherry-red skin is rare. CO displaces the oxyhemoglobin dissociation curve to the left and as a result hemoglobin has an increased affinity for hemoglobin. The half-life for dissociation is approximately 4 hours at room air but decreases to 40 minutes for patients breathing 100% oxygen. High-flow oxygen should be initiated immediately if CO poisoning is suspected. Inhalational injuries often require bronchoscopy if intubation is needed. An adequately sized endotracheal tube should be used to allow subsequent bronchoscopy. If intubation is delayed until respiratory distress begins intubation is often not possible and a surgical airway must be established.

Blood pressure may be difficult to measure in patients with burn injuries and endovascular volume is often difficult to assess. Often patients are hypovolemic and require large volumes of crystalloid to normalize hemodynamic parameters. For patients with more than 10% BSA burns, fluid requirements for initial resuscitation can be estimated using the Parkland formula. The Parkland formula is calculated by multiplying four times the patient's weight in kilograms times the percent total body surface area involved in second and third degree burns. This volume of fluid should be administered over the first 24 hours after the burn. Half of the total volume should be administered in the first 8 hours after the burn. The remaining half should be administered over the following 16 hours. The goal urinary output is 1 mL/kg/h for adult patients. In the experience of the authors, this formula effectively approximates the fluid needs for patients with burns between 10 and 40% of total body surface area. Patients with burns larger than 40% often need additional fluid to maintain adequate urine output and hourly urine production should be carefully monitored.

In evaluating the degree of injury, the amount of body surface injured must be evaluated. First degree burns are erythematous skin that is moderately painful to touch without blistering. Partial thickness burns, or second degree burns consist of blistered or broken skin that has a red appearance, is very painful and has wet weeping surfaces. Full thickness burns, or third degree burns are often white or pale and leathery in consistency without pain to pinprick evaluation and are dry on the surface. As a rule of thumb, the area of the palm of the hand with the fingers extended represents 1% body surface area for each person. This can be used as a gauge to determine the total burn area. For calculating initial resuscitation fluids, only the surface of second and third degree burns are used for the calculation. Some clinicians find **Figure 46-1** useful in estimating total body surface area burned helpful in evaluating these patients. In adults, a reasonable system for calculating the percentage of body surface burned is the "rule of nines": Each arm equals 9%, the head equals 9%, the anterior and posterior trunk each equal 18%, and each leg equals 18%; the sum of these percentages is 99%. 1% is made up of the perineum.

Patients should receive adequate supplementary oxygen and endovascular volume replacement. Pain control is extremely important in these patients as well. Second degree burns are extremely sensitive to air-flow so patients should be covered with clean

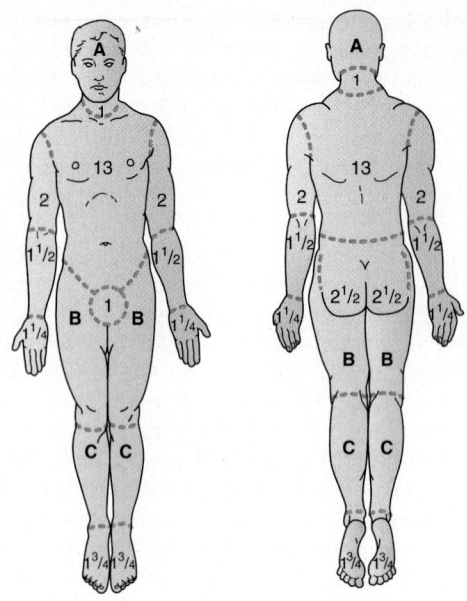

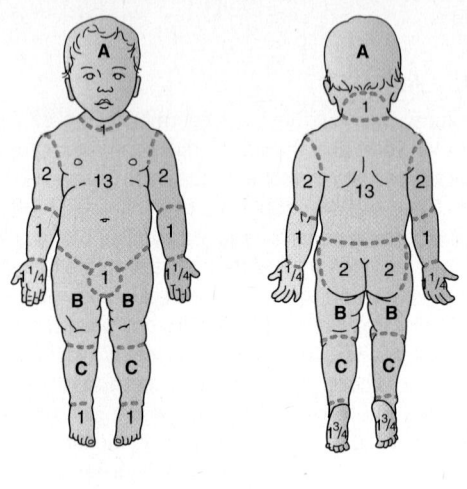

Relative percentages of areas affected by growth

Area	Age		
	10	15	Adult
A = half of head	5 1/2	4 1/2	3 1/2
B = half of one thigh	4 1/4	4 1/2	4 3/4
C = half of one leg	3	3 1/4	3 1/2

Relative percentages of areas affected by growth

Area	Age		
	0	1	5
A = half of head	9 1/2	8 1/2	6 1/2
B = half of one thigh	2 3/4	3 1/4	4
C = half of one leg	2 1/2	2 1/2	2 3/4

Figure 46-1 *Estimating extent of burns.* (From Demling RH. Burns & other thermal injuries. In Doherty GM, ed. *Current Diagnosis & Treatment: Surgery,* 14th ed. New York: McGraw-Hill; 2015:227-240.)

linens or nonadherent dressings to decrease the flow of air across the wounds. Blisters should not be purposefully ruptured and cold packs should not be applied to burned skin. Systemic antibiotics are not indicated. Tetanus status should be evaluated and vaccination given if needed. Criteria for transfer are presented in **Table 46-1**.

TABLE 46-1 Criteria for Transfer of Burn Patients

Burn injuries that should be referred to a burn center include:

1. Partial thickness burns greater than 10% total body surface area (TBSA).

2. Burns that involve the face, hands, feet, genitalia, perineum, or major joints.

3. Third degree burns in any age group.

4. Electrical burns, including lightning injury.

5. Chemical burns.

6. Inhalation injury.

7. Burn injury in patients with preexisting medical disorders that could complicate management, prolong recovery, or affect mortality.

8. Any patient with burns and concomitant trauma (such as fractures) in which the burn injury poses the greatest risk of morbidity or mortality. In such cases, if the trauma poses the greater immediate risk, the patient may be initially stabilized in a trauma center before being transferred to a burn unit. Physician judgment will be necessary in such situations and should be in concert with the regional medical control plan and triage protocols.

9. Burned children in hospitals without qualified personnel or equipment for the care of children.

10. Burn injury in patients who will require special social, emotional, or rehabilitative intervention.

CLINICAL MANAGEMENT OF SELECTED CONDITIONS IN THE SURGICAL ICU

■ RIB FRACTURES

Rib fractures are a commonly encountered traumatic injury across many medical disciplines. The overall mortality of rib fractures is approximately 10%, with mortality increasing with each additional rib fracture and worsening prognosis among patients older than 55 years old. Patients with limited pulmonary reserve at baseline or due to lung contusion are at higher risk for adverse outcome. Flail chest deformity, commonly defined as three or more consecutive ribs fractured at two or more locations results in impaired pulmonary physiology. This impairment can also be produced when ribs are fractured on each side of the sternum. These fracture patterns result in paradoxical chest wall movement which limits the ability of patients to comfortably breathe. Morbidity is increased in this patient population from short and long term disability and disease related complications, with up to 60% of patients remaining disabled. Common complications include prolonged mechanical ventilation, pneumonia and acute respiratory distress syndrome. Epidural anesthesia has been shown to decrease need for mechanical ventilation and retain baseline pulmonary status. Despite aggressive analgesia and excellent pulmonary hygiene, up to 60% of patients inevitably require prolonged mechanical ventilation. The duration of this ventilation on average is 13 days. Surgical rib fixation has recently grown in popularity due to recent data showing that this procedure may decrease the length of mechanical ventilation. Surgical rib fixation has also been described as a salvage therapy to decrease the duration of mechanical ventilation after failing medical management for flail chest.

■ POSTOPERATIVE BLEEDING

Early recognition of postoperative bleeding and initiation of appropriate therapy is imperative as patients can progress quickly to life-threatening hemorrhagic shock. In the immediate postoperative period (<24 hours), the presence of hypotension and tachycardia should constitute a presumptive diagnosis of bleeding until another cause is clearly identified. The patient should be examined immediately for signs of hemorrhage from surgical incisions, drains, tubes, or intravenous lines. If significant (>100-200 mL) or ongoing drainage is noted, the surgical team should be notified immediately. The patient should also be examined for evidence of ecchymosis, soft tissue swelling, and abdominal distension. In the case of trauma patients, missed external (ie, lacerations) or internal (solid organ) injuries may also be present and need to be rapidly identified. A large volume of blood can be sequestered within the chest, abdomen, retroperitoneal, and thigh compartments. Hemorrhage into these areas may be difficult to identify and often require advanced imaging such as x-ray, bedside ultrasound, or CT scan. Imaging studies that can be performed in the ICU should be used preferentially and transporting the patient should be avoided unless they have been appropriately stabilized. If a patient is stable enough to undergo a CT scan, it should be performed with IV contrast as this will demonstrate both old hematoma and the presence of active bleeding.

Postoperative bleeding can be the result of bleeding from the surgical site or surrounding tissues, diffuse coagulopathy, or a combination of these factors. Coagulopathic, or "nonsurgical," bleeding is often propagated by factors such as hypothermia and acidosis. Hypothermia causes platelet dysfunction via decreased platelet adhesion and aggregation and acidosis decreases thrombin generation, factors which combine to significantly impair the clotting cascade. Bleeding also propagates coagulopathy through the ongoing loss and consumption of clotting of factors as well as dilutional coagulopathy from resuscitation. Hypothermia should be addressed immediately by administering warmed intravenous fluids, applying warmed blankets or forced-air rewarming units, and increasing the ambient room temperature. Acidosis can be addressed with volume resuscitation to improve tissue perfusion, mechanical ventilatory adjustments, and correction of the underlying source (bleeding, infection, etc).

As noted above, postoperative coagulopathy is often multifactorial. The patient's history should be reviewed for the presence of known congenital bleeding disorders, such as Von Willebrand disease or hemophilia A or B, and these should be addressed as indicated. In the setting of suspected ongoing bleeding, serial laboratory tests (CBC, PT, PT, INR, fibrinogen) should be drawn every 4 to 6 hours. Platelets should be administered in order to maintain a level more than 50,000. Cryoprecipitate should be given in the setting of consumptive coagulopathy to maintain a fibrinogen level more than 100 g/L. An INR of ≤1.5 should be achieved using fresh frozen plasma (FFP), which contains all of the clotting factors, or prothrombin complex concentrate (PCC). PCC contains the vitamin K-dependent coagulation factors (II, VII, IX, and X) and stored as a lyophilized powder following extraction from large donor-pooled plasma. PCC can be used to rapidly reverse warfarin-induced coagulopathy with a significantly lower volume of administration as compared to FFP. In addition, there is some data to suggest it is also effective for hemorrhage or trauma induced coagulopathy.

■ BLOOD TRANSFUSION—MASSIVE TRANSFUSION

The use of blood transfusion in the ICU is extremely common, with as many as half of all ICU patients receiving at least one transfusion during their stay. In nonbleeding postsurgical patients, the criteria for blood transfusion may vary widely among individual surgeons. Historically, many patients were managed using a liberal transfusion strategy in order to achieve hemoglobin of 10 g/dL. However, recent data suggests that the use of liberal transfusion criteria actually has

negative consequences for patients. As a result, hemoglobin of 7 g/dL in nonbleeding patients without evidence of cardiovascular disease is used routinely as a transfusion trigger. (See Chapter 57: Blood Products in the Postoperative Period.)

Massive transfusion is most commonly defined as the administration of 10 or more units of packed red blood cells within a 24-hour period. The need for massive transfusion is most commonly associated with gastrointestinal bleeding and severe traumatic injuries. These patients often receive large volumes of crystalloid in addition to packed red blood cells which can result in a dilutional coagulopathy. In addition, as many as 25% of trauma patients arrive at the hospital already coagulopathic and are at an increased risk of mortality. The presence of coagulopathy needs to be addressed early among patients requiring massive transfusion with the addition of FFP and platelets in a balanced ratio. Over the last 10 years, data from the military experience in Iraq and Afghanistan has suggested improved outcomes with the early use of a 1:1:1 ratio of plasma to red blood cells to platelets in patients at high risk for needing massive transfusion. This ratio was selected in order to more closely mimic the composition of the whole blood lost by the patient. Subsequent analysis in civilian trauma centers has demonstrated a 3- to 4-fold decrease in early mortality with the administration of a 1:1:1 ratio within the first 6 hours although overall mortality was not affected. Thus, the early use of a balanced blood product transfusion ratio should be considered in massively bleeding patients.

In order to effectively administer blood products in emergent situations, many institutions have developed a protocol for massive transfusion in order to streamline rapid delivery. The protocol is activated following clinical evaluation, frequently without waiting for laboratory confirmation, as this can lead to unacceptable delays. As part of the protocol, the blood bank has blood products available that can be delivered rapidly in large quantities and in predefined ratios. The ideal ratio and the quantity of blood products are determined by individual institutions. A typical protocol may consist of an initial container containing 10 units of PRBCS, 10 units of plasma, and two to four packs of platelets. Subsequent containers may contain smaller quantities of these components. Blood products continue to be delivered until the protocol is discontinued by the ICU team, ideally once hemostasis has been achieved. The use of a massive transfusion protocol has demonstrated improved patient survival and reduced rates of organ failure. The development of a massive transfusion protocol requires institutional support and cooperation among multiple services (physicians, nurses, transfusion services, and laboratory) in order to be successful.

■ DAMAGE CONTROL SURGERY AND THE OPEN ABDOMEN

Critically ill surgical patients and trauma patients often require emergent life-saving surgery. These patients may have extensive injuries that necessitate time-consuming and complex repairs. Historically, a definitive repair of these injuries was attempted during the initial operation despite prolonged operative times. Unfortunately, many of these patients deteriorated intraoperatively or in the acute postoperative period due to the detrimental physiological effects of long operative time combined with extensive comorbidities and traumatic injuries. Therefore, surgical management of these patients shifted from prolonged definitive repair to damage control techniques to avoid further physiological derangement.

In 1993, Rotondo et al are credited with modernizing the techniques of damage control surgery for trauma patients. Damage control surgery is defined as the use of surgical techniques to rapidly control hemorrhage and contamination and defer definitive repair in an effort to temporize the patient and leave the operating room expeditiously to initiate aggressive resuscitation in the intensive care unit postoperatively. Definitive repair is deferred to avoid the lethal triad, which consists of hypothermia, acidosis, and coagulopathy.

Prolonged time in the operating room inevitably leads to progressive hypothermia which leads to dysfunctional coagulation. As the coagulation cascade begins to fail, the patient will lose more blood which leads to further hypothermia and increased acidosis secondary to inadequate perfusion. Acidosis further uncouples the coagulation cascade leading to more hemorrhage. By employing damage control surgery, bleeding and contamination is rapidly controlled to avoid the inevitable death spiral of the lethal triad.

Preoperative identification of patients who would benefit from damage control surgery is paramount to fully mobilize the essential personnel and equipment to prepare for these critically ill patients. Therefore, current recommendations for a trauma patient in which damage control surgery should be considered include patients arriving from the emergency department with a revised trauma score 5 or greater, patients requiring greater than 2 L of crystalloid or 2 units of blood for resuscitation, or have a pH less than 7.2. For nontrauma patients, indications for damage control surgery include uncontrolled hemorrhage for elective general surgery, complications during complex duodenal ulcer operations, generalized peritonitis, and other forms of severe intra-abdominal sepsis.

Intraoperative indications to abort a traditional definitive operative procedure and transition to damage control surgery include patients who require more than 10 units of blood or more than 12 L of resuscitation, continued acidosis of less than 7.2 and hypothermia of less than 34, major inaccessible venous bleeding, refractory oozing from coagulopathy, need to reassess intra-abdominal contents postoperatively, and the concern for likely abdominal compartment syndrome if the abdomen was closed.

Once the decision has been made to proceed with damage control surgery, the intraoperative goals are appropriately narrowed to expeditiously restore hemostasis and leave the operating room as quickly as possible. Therefore, after opening the patient's abdomen, the first step is to control hemorrhage. This is initially accomplished with packing to tamponade bleeding followed by various rapid maneuvers such as splenectomy, blood vessel isolation, liver packing, etc. Once bleeding has been temporarily controlled, this provides a crucial window for the anesthesia team to "catch up" and try to replace lost intravascular volume and blood products. Following hemorrhage control, the next step in damage control surgery is to stop enteric contamination. Often, this means removing portions of damaged or necrotic bowel, stapling off the ends, and leaving the intestine in discontinuity. Taking additional time to reconnect the remaining intestine would only add unnecessary time to the operation and have a high chance of anastomotic failure.

With bleeding and enteric contamination controlled, the abdominal fascia is left open with the plan of returning to the operating room in 24 to 48 hours for definitive repair once the patient can be adequately resuscitated in the intensive care. In general, most surgeons temporarily cover the visceral contents of the abdomen with a vacuum assisted dressing (**Figure 46-2**). This aids in keeping abdominal domain and preventing desiccation of the intra-abdominal contents. If the intestine is edematous secondary to the massive resuscitation required in these critically ill patients, several return trips to the operating room are often necessary for abdominal washout and replacement of temporizing dressings. Ideally, the abdomen should be closed within 7 days of the initial surgery because complications of fascial closure rise dramatically after this timeframe. If this is not achieved, the abdomen sometimes has to remain without fascial closure and be allowed to granulate over time. The bowel must not become dry and wound care is extremely important. These patients are at high risk for gastrointestinal atmospheric fistula formation (**Figure 46-3**).

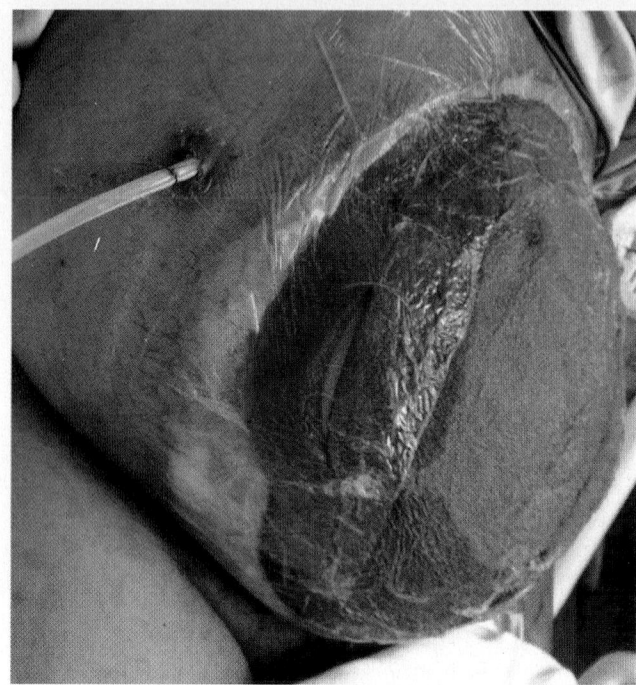

Figure 46-2 *An open abdomen covered with a vacuum assisted closure device.*

■ PREVENTION AND MANAGEMENT OF STRESS GASTRITIS

Patients admitted to critical care units are at risk for developing stress-related mucosal damage (SRMD) leading to stress gastropathy. Approximately 1.5% of critically ill patients develop SRMD as a result of severe physiologic stress. The cause of SRMD is splanchnic hypoperfusion and mesenteric ischemia making SRMD a form of organ-failure. With hypoperfusion, gastric mucosal cells cannot neutralize acid, perpetuating cellular toxicity. Stress gastropathy may occur as a result leading to gastrointestinal bleeding which may be severe leading to hemodynamic instability and, in severe cases, death. Stress gastropathy should therefore be distinguished from peptic ulcer disease where increased acid production is the norm. Most patients with stress gastropathy are actually achlorhydric.

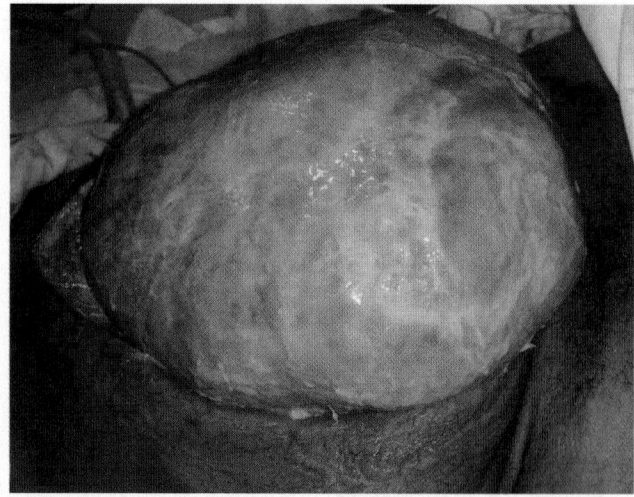

Figure 46-3 *An open abdomen due to severe abdominal edema; granulation tissue and fibrous exudate can be seen over this abdomen. Over time the wound will contract and re-epithelize if fistulas do not form.*

The currently accepted risk factors for SRMD in ICU patients are mechanical ventilation for at least 48 hours and primary coagulopathies. Other variables that have been associated with increased risk include the use of high dose glucocorticoids, severe head trauma, extensive thermal burn injury, organ transplantation and severe liver dysfunction. Although now uncommon, gastrointestinal bleeding secondary to stress gastropathy is associated with a fourfold increase in ICU.

Stress gastritis prophylaxis reduces SRMD and is indicated in ICU patients who are on mechanical ventilation or in those with coagulopathy or one of the other risk factors described above. The most commonly employed prophylaxis is pharmacologic, and both histamine type 2 receptor antagonists and proton pump inhibitors are utilized. Other options for prophylaxis include antacids administered every 4 hours and titrated to an alkaline gastric pH, and sucralfate, an orally administered cytoprotective agent that coats the gastric mucosa providing protection against damage. There are data to suggest that once a patient is tolerating enteral feedings, they likely do not need stress gastritis prophylaxis. It is important to emphasize that stress gastritis prophylaxis is not indicated in patients who are NPO or have an NG tube, unless they are on mechanical ventilation or have one of the other recognized risk factors. As a result, stress gastritis prophylaxis should very rarely be used outside the ICU.

CONCLUSION

With the rising rate of hospitalist comanagement of surgical patients, many hospitalists will need to be able to manage patients in and out of the surgical ICU. The most commonly encountered types of surgical critical care patients are postoperative, trauma, and burn patients. Effective comanagement requires the hospitalist to know how to recognize and manage common conditions and complications in these patient populations.

SUGGESTED READINGS

Advanced trauma life support (ATLS(R)): the ninth edition. *J Trauma Acute Care Surg*. 2013;74:1363-1366.

Alexander RH, Proctor HJ, American College of Surgeons. Committee on Trauma. *Advanced Trauma Life Support Program for Physicians: ATLS*, 5th ed. Chicago, IL: American College of Surgeons; 1993.

American College of Surgeons. Committee on Trauma. Resources for optimal care of the injured patient. Chicago, IL: American College of Surgeons, Committee on Trauma; 2006.

Barr J, Fraser GL, Puntillo K, et al. Clinical practice guidelines for the management of pain, agitation, and delirium in adult patients in the intensive care unit. *Crit Care Med*. 2013;41:263-306.

Guidelines for the management of severe traumatic brain injury. *J Neurotrauma*. 2007;24(Suppl 1):S1-S106.

MacKenzie EJ, Rivara FP, Jurkovich GJ, et al. A national evaluation of the effect of trauma-center care on mortality. *N Engl J Med*. 2006;354:366-378.

Vincent JL. Critical care—where have we been and where are we going? *Crit Care*. 2013;17(Suppl 1):S2.

SECTION 2
Anesthesia

CHAPTER 47

Anesthesia: Choices and Complications

Aeron A. D. Doyle, MD, CM, FRCPC

Hospitalists are often involved in perioperative patient care and should be familiar with techniques and complications of anesthesia, as well as preoperative and postoperative considerations. Current modalities include general anesthetics, neuraxial techniques (spinal and epidural), regional anesthetics (nerve blocks), and monitored anesthetic care (MAC), or so-called conscious sedation. Each mode of anesthesia has benefits and risks that must be weighed in view of the operative procedure and the condition and comorbidities of each patient. The administration of regional or local anesthetics does not preclude the necessity for general anesthesia in the event of unforeseen events or complications. Therefore, patients undergoing all but the most minor procedures should be assessed as potential candidates for general anesthesia.

PRACTICE POINT

Cardiovascular and psychiatric medications in the perioperative period

- Beta-blockers, calcium channel blockers, and amiodarone should be continued in the perioperative period. Patients who receive perioperative angiotensin-converting enzyme inhibitors and angiotensin receptor blockers may be at greater risk of intraoperative hypotension. Some authorities recommend holding these drugs on the day of surgery, particularly for operations with significant fluid shifts or using techniques associated with systemic inflammatory responses, such as cardiopulmonary bypass. It is traditionally recommended to stop monoamine oxidase inhibitors (MAOIs) 2 weeks prior to surgery. Patients who take MAOIs perioperatively are at risk of serotonergic toxicity and hypertension, especially with vasopressor use, as well as excessive sedation from inhibition of opioid metabolism by MAOIs. Some anesthesiologists continue MAOIs perioperatively, avoiding indirect-acting sympathomimetics such as ephedrine, and using narcotics such as morphine with lesser degrees of interaction with MAOIs, instead of meperidine. Tricyclic antidepressants (TCAs) and selective serotonin reuptake inhibitors (SSRIs) may be continued perioperatively. TCAs have rarely been associated with intraoperative hypotension, requiring norepinephrine for reversal. SSRIs are occasionally implicated in perioperative serotonin syndrome, particularly when given with serotonin 5-HT$_3$ receptor antagonists such as ondansetron, and phenylpiperidine opioids such as fentanyl.

GENERAL ANESTHESIA

General anesthesia is usually induced with a short-acting intravenous agent such as propofol and maintained with inhaled halogenated ethers or intravenous propofol. The mechanism of action of inhalational anesthetics remains unclear and may be a membrane effect, a receptor effect, or both. These agents may be used in conjunction with narcotics and muscle relaxants to achieve balanced anesthesia and may also be supplemented with inhaled nitrous oxide. Airway protection may be obtained by endotracheal intubation; airway patency, but not protection, may be ensured with a laryngeal mask airway, or oropharyngeal airway with mask.

Complications of general anesthesia include postoperative nausea and vomiting (PONV); aspiration; complications of intubation, such as dental, mucosal, or laryngeal trauma; atelectasis and complications of positive pressure ventilation, such as barotrauma; complications of positioning during surgery; and allergic or idiosyncratic reactions to anesthetic agents. Additionally, ischemic or thromboembolic events may occur perioperatively because of physiologic stresses from surgery or anesthesia.

PRACTICE POINT

Side effects of anesthesia induction

- Propofol is the most commonly used agent for anesthesia induction. A common side effect is hypotension from vasodilation and decreased cardiac output, which occurs in up to 16% of patients. Barbiturates such as methohexital and thiopental sodium are occasionally used for anesthesia induction but also have cardiovascular depressant effects. Etomidate and ketamine are sometimes used for anesthesia induction in patients at higher risk of hypotension from propofol, such as the elderly. Etomidate rarely has significant cardiovascular side effects, but it does inhibit 11-β-hydroxylase, an enzyme involved in steroid synthesis, thus attenuating the adrenal stress response and potentially leading to postoperative hypotension. This effect may persist for up to 24 hours in elderly patients after a single dose for anesthesia induction. Ketamine does not depress respiratory drive, unlike most anesthetic agents, and it actually has bronchodilator effects that make its use attractive in patients with reactive airway disease. However, ketamine has side effects that make its use in elderly patients problematic, including increases in heart rate and blood pressure, myocardial depression that is masked by its sympathomimetic effects, postoperative delirium and hallucinations, and neurodegenerative apoptosis in animal models.

■ POSTOPERATIVE NAUSEA AND VOMITING

PONV occurs after approximately 10% of surgeries. Risk factors include younger age; female gender; intra-abdominal, ophthalmic, or ear, nose, and throat (ENT) surgery; past history of PONV or motion sickness; and being a nonsmoker. Strategies to lower the risk of PONV include avoidance of general anesthesia in favor of regional anesthesia, use of propofol, avoidance of nitrous oxide and volatile anesthetics, minimization of opioids, and adequate hydration. Intraoperative prophylaxis and postoperative treatment may include central dopaminergic antagonists such as prochlorperazine, peripheral dopaminergic antagonists such as metoclopramide, serotonin 5-HT$_3$ receptor antagonists such as ondansetron, and corticosteroids such as dexamethasone. These agents may also be used as rescue agents after emesis to prevent further symptoms. PONV usually abates in 24 to 48 hours. The examination of a patient with presumed PONV should assess for bowel sounds and the presence or absence of abdominal distention to avoid missing a diagnosis of postoperative ileus.

■ ASPIRATION

Aspiration is the entry of gastric contents into the trachea and lower airways. It may occur prior to or during induction of anesthesia, intraoperatively if the airway is unprotected, or during emergence from anesthesia and postoperatively. A chemical pneumonitis usually results with severity increasing with lower pH or particulates. Risk factors include a full stomach, preexisting gastroesophageal

reflux disease (GERD), obesity, intra-abdominal obstruction or other pathology, pregnancy, and trauma. American Society of Anesthesiologists guidelines for nil per os (NPO) status preoperatively recommend 2 hours for clear fluids, 6 hours for a light meal (essentially toast and clear fluids), and 8 hours for full meals. These guidelines are for healthy elective patients with no GERD or other risks. Routine antireflux prophylaxis is not recommended, but in patients with GERD, histamine H$_2$-receptor antagonists, proton pump inhibitors, physical antacids, or promotility agents such as metoclopramide may be indicated. Patients on these medications should have them ordered preoperatively.

■ COMPLICATIONS OF INTUBATION AND AIRWAY MAINTENANCE

In closed claim studies, the most common awards for anesthetic complications are those for dental trauma (approximately 1 in 5000). Laryngeal injury may have an incidence as high as 6% in general anesthesia but is usually minor and self-limiting, such as sore throat or vocal cord hematoma. Hoarseness lasting longer than 7 days should be evaluated by an otolaryngologist. Mucosal lacerations have an incidence of 1 in 1000, but again are usually self-limiting.

■ ATELECTASIS

Atelectasis, alveolar collapse generally in dependent areas of the lung, is common with general anesthesia, particularly in surgery involving the upper abdomen. Postoperative fever and hypoxia due to physiologic intrapulmonary shunt are typical manifestations. Mobilization is the most effective treatment, with chest physiotherapy and incentive spirometry generally having disappointing results. Continuous or bilevel positive airway pressure (CPAP or BiPAP) devices may be beneficial if tolerated by the patient.

■ POSITIONING COMPLICATIONS

Nerve injuries may occur as a complication of various positions under anesthesia. Ulnar neuropathies are the most common, with an incidence varying from 4 to 50/10,000 patients. Risk factors include male gender, extremes of body weight, and prolonged hospitalization. The common peroneal nerve may be injured by pressure at the fibular head in the lithotomy position (feet in stirrups). Brachial plexus injuries may occur from sternotomy and retraction of the chest wall during coronary bypass surgery. Compartment syndrome in the extremities may occur if tissue swelling causes obstruction of venous and lymphatic drainage, with failure of capillary perfusion and cell death. This may result from improper positioning, or more often from extensive and prolonged surgery. It presents as intractable pain, with examination revealing an absence of pulses. Surgical fasciotomies are required to decrease tissue pressure.

■ EYE INJURY

Eye injury is reported in up to 0.05% of patients postoperatively. The majority of cases are corneal abrasions. These resolve within days with topical antibiotics and rarely cause permanent visual impairment. Rarely, patients develop ischemic optic neuropathy or central retinal artery occlusion. Risk factors include prone or lateral position, prolonged surgery, hypotension, spine surgery, and anemia. Unfortunately, the prognosis for recovery is poor in these instances.

■ ALLERGIC AND OTHER REACTIONS

Anaphylactic reactions under anesthesia are rare but potentially life threatening. As many medications are given in the perioperative period, it may be difficult to determine the causal agent, which may include antibiotics, muscle relaxants, or latex. Opioids cause histamine release, resulting in redness and itching, but rarely anaphylaxis.

Malignant hyperthermia (MH) is a rare reaction triggered by inhalational anesthetics (except nitrous oxide) or succinylcholine (a depolarizing muscle relaxant). It generally presents with increased metabolic rate, acidosis, and finally rhabdomyolysis. Treatment consists of discontinuing triggering agents, the administration of dantrolene, and supportive care in an intensive care setting. MH is an autosomal dominant disorder, so patients with relatives with suspected or confirmed MH should receive nontriggering anesthetics.

Abnormalities of the enzyme pseudocholinesterase may result in the prolongation of action of the muscle relaxant succinylcholine, leading to postoperative weakness or paralysis. Heterozygous individuals may have mild prolongation, lasting 20 to 30 minutes, whereas homozygous individuals may require sedation and ventilation support for hours, depending on the dosage initially given. Succinylcholine should be avoided in these patients if possible.

ACUTE RENAL FAILURE

Acute renal failure, defined as a fall in creatinine clearance to 50 mL/min or less, occurs within the first week after major noncardiac surgery in approximately 0.8% of patients with previously normal renal function, with 0.1% of patients requiring renal replacement therapy. The development of postoperative acute kidney injury (AKI) is an independent predictor for hospital mortality. Preoperative predictors of AKI in various studies have included age, emergent surgery, liver disease, diabetes mellitus, an elevated body mass index, high-risk surgery, congestive heart failure, ischemic heart disease, peripheral vascular occlusive disease, and chronic obstructive pulmonary disease necessitating chronic bronchodilator therapy. Intraoperative strategies to minimize the risk of AKI include maintenance of euvolemia, avoidance of nephrotoxins, and maintenance of optimal blood pressures.

PERIOPERATIVE MYOCARDIAL INFARCTION

Myocardial infarction occurs in two distinct clinical settings in the perioperative period. Patients may develop an acute coronary syndrome related to plaque rupture. Major contributing factors are physiologic stress and high levels of catecholamines leading to tachycardia, hypertension, and coronary thrombosis, coupled with increased coagulability because of tissue trauma and cessation of antiplatelet agents. The other scenario is the patient with severe but stable coronary disease who develops subendocardial ischemia because of an imbalance between myocardial oxygen supply and demand. Causative factors may include tachycardia, hypotension or hypertension, anemia, and hypoxemia. In this latter setting, anesthesia may be a contributing factor, leading to hypotension and decreased cardiac output.

STROKE

Perioperative stroke has many contributing factors, including hypercoagulability from tissue trauma, emboli from vascular manipulation, temporary cessation of antiplatelet and anticoagulant drugs, and hypotension from bleeding or anesthetic agents. The risk of stroke is highest in vascular surgery: 1.4% to 3.8% in patients undergoing coronary artery bypass grafting (CABG), 7.4% in combined CABG and valve replacement, and 9.7% in multiple valve replacement. The risk of stroke in patients undergoing general surgery ranges from 0.08% to 0.7%. Atrial fibrillation, valvular disease, renal disease, and prior stroke are the most robust predictors of perioperative stroke in general surgery patients. Most perioperative strokes are embolic in origin, with only 9% being related to hypoperfusion. The risk of perioperative stroke may be increased when high doses of beta-blockers are begun just prior to surgery in patients who have not taken β-blockers previously. Chronic β-blocker use does not appear to increase the risk of perioperative stroke.

NEURAXIAL ANESTHESIA

Neuraxial anesthesia techniques include the introduction of medications, usually local anesthetics or opioids, into the subarachnoid space (spinal fluid) or epidural space. In the epidural space, a catheter may be inserted for injections or infusions. Local anesthetics then act on the spinal cord and nerve roots to inhibit sodium channel conduction and block nerve impulses. Opioids act directly on spinal cord receptors, as well as having varying degrees of rostral and systemic spread. The benefits of neuraxial anesthesia may include preemptive analgesia (the prevention of establishment of pain pathways), decreased sympathetic activation, hypercoagulability and inflammation caused by the stress of surgery, and potential avoidance of airway manipulation. Although there are short-term benefits of postoperative analgesia through an indwelling epidural catheter inserted just before surgery, there are conflicting mortality and morbidity benefits. Contraindications to neuraxial anesthesia include untreated sepsis, bacteremia, infection at the injection site, bleeding diatheses, increased intracranial pressure, and patient refusal.

Relative contraindications include preexisting neurological deficit, hypovolemia, left ventricular outflow obstruction such as aortic stenosis, and lack of cooperation or communication. Complications of neuraxial anesthesia include pain at insertion site, dural puncture headache, hypotension, high level of block, epidural or spinal hematoma or abscess, and pruritis from opioids.

DURAL PUNCTURE HEADACHE

Dural puncture headache results from persistent leakage of cerebrospinal fluid (CSF) following spinal anesthesia or inadvertent dural puncture during epidural anesthesia. It is typically positional and severe. Rates following spinal anesthesia are about 1 in 400. The risk is reduced by use of a smaller-gauge needle with a pencil-point tip, rather than a cutting tip. The risk also decreases with patient age. Dural puncture after epidural is operator dependent; a rate of 1 in 200 is usually quoted. Treatment includes bed rest, hydration, caffeine, and epidural blood patch if headache persists despite conservative therapy. Epidural blood patch involves injecting the patient's own blood into the epidural space to occlude and clot the CSF leak, with about 70% lasting success the first time performed. The procedure may be repeated if initial results are not satisfactory.

HYPOTENSION AND HIGH BLOCK

Hypotension occurs secondary to loss of vascular tone. It may be mitigated by preprocedural fluid loading and treated with vasopressors and fluid after it develops. In epidural anesthesia, incremental dosing may also limit hypotension, particularly in patients with a fixed cardiac output. High block occurs when nerve conduction is lost at a higher level than intended. It may result in perceived respiratory distress due to loss of chest wall proprioception, loss of diaphragm function at midcervical levels, and unconsciousness if the brain stem level is reached. Shock may ensue from profound vasodilation accompanied by block of cardioaccelerator sympathetic fibers. Treatment includes physiologic support and sedation until the block recedes.

HEMATOMA OR ABSCESS

Spinal hematoma or abscess may cause nerve root or spinal cord compression and constitutes a medical emergency, as decompression must occur within 8 hours for reasonable chance of recovery. The overall rate of hematoma is 1:220,000 for spinals and 1:150,000 for epidurals but is higher in certain groups of patients and procedures. Half of all cases of epidural hematoma result in devastating, preventable, and permanent neurologic injury, even after prompt

TABLE 47-1 Timing of Cessation of Antiplatelet Drugs and Thromboprophylaxis in Patients Receiving Spinal or Epidural Anesthesia

Drug	Perioperative Management
Aspirin	Stop 6 d prior to procedure in patients taking for primary prophylaxis; platelet rebound phenomenon may occur in patients taking aspirin for secondary prophylaxis, requiring individualized assessment and risk stratification
Nonsteroidal anti-inflammatory drugs	Should be stopped 5 half-lives prior to procedure
Clopidogrel	Stop 7 d before neuraxial block
Prasugrel	Stop 7-10 d before neuraxial block
Glycoprotein (GP) IIb/IIIa inhibitors	Stop 8-24 h (eptifibatide, tirofiban) to 2-5 d (abciximab) before neuraxial block
Warfarin	Stop 4-5 d before procedure; document normal INR before initiation of neuraxial block
Subcutaneous heparin	Stop 8-10 h before procedure
Intravenous heparin	Stop 2-4 h prior to procedure
Low-molecular-weight heparin (LMWH)	Stop 24 h prior to procedure
Fondaparinux	Stop 4 d before procedure
Dabigatran	Stop 4-5 d before procedure (6 d if impaired renal function)
Rivaroxaban	Stop 3 d before procedure
Apixaban	Stop 3-5 d before procedure

Data from Narouze S, Benzon HT, Provenzano DA, et al. *Reg Anesth Pain Med*. 2015;40:182-212.

surgical intervention. As mentioned, bleeding diatheses are a contraindication to neuraxial anesthetics, but if time permits, a bleeding tendency may be corrected preoperatively with plasma or specific coagulation factors. The use of anticoagulant drugs significantly increases the risk of spinal hematoma. Unfractionated heparin may be reversed with protamine, but low-molecular-weight heparin must be held for 24 hours preprocedure. Platelet inhibitors should be held preoperatively, though low-dose aspirin is not contraindicated if no other anticoagulant is present. Specific perioperative anticoagulant therapy guidelines are published by the American Society of Regional Anesthesia and Pain Medicine (**Table 47-1**).

REGIONAL ANESTHESIA

In regional anesthesia, specific nerves or a nerve plexus is blocked to create a discrete area of anesthesia. These techniques may be utilized alone or in combination with sedation or general anesthesia

and may involve a single injection of local anesthetic or the placement of a catheter to provide for multiple injections or infusions for postoperative analgesia. Traditionally, injections were guided by anatomical landmarks with or without electrical nerve stimulation to confirm proximity to the nerve. With the advent of ultrasound-guided techniques, the success rate of regional nerve blocks can be improved, and the risk of nerve injury lessened. Contraindications include infection at the injection site or patient refusal or inability to cooperate. Preexisting nerve injury or progressive neuropathies may also be contraindications. Certain block techniques may have specific contraindications, such as interscalene block and respiratory failure, as hemidiaphragm paralysis results. Complications of regional blocks include direct injury to nerve fibers by injection needles or local anesthetics, systemic anesthetic toxicity, and hematoma or abscess at the injection site. Anticoagulant guidelines are similar to those for neuraxial techniques.

MONITORED ANESTHETIC CARE

MAC, also referred to as conscious sedation or local-combined anesthesia, refers to the use of periprocedural sedation, with or without local, regional, or neuraxial anesthesia. Medications are the same as those used for induction of general anesthesia, including narcotics, benzodiazepines, and propofol. In some cases, only the dosage of sedative agents or the absence of airway maintenance distinguishes this from general anesthesia. Therefore, full monitoring, airway equipment, and resuscitative medications should be available. MAC does not preclude the need to sometimes progress to general anesthesia, and preoperatively should be treated similarly with regard to NPO status, medications, or resuscitation.

SUGGESTED READINGS

Bateman BT, Schumacher HC, Wang S, Shaefi S, Berman MF. Perioperative acute ischemic stroke in noncardiac and nonvascular surgery: incidence, risk factors, and outcomes. *Anesthesiology*. 2009;110:231-238.

Blessberger H, Kammler J, Domanovits H, et al. Perioperative beta-blockers for preventing surgery-related mortality and morbidity. *Cochrane Database Syst Rev*. 2014;18;9:CD004476.

Green L, Machin SJ. Managing anticoagulated patients during neuraxial anaesthesia. *Br J Anaesth*. 2010;149:195-208.

Kheterpal S, Tremper KK, Englesbe MJ, et al. Predictors of postoperative acute renal failure after noncardiac surgery in patients with previously normal renal function. *Anesthesiology*. 2007;107:892-902.

Landesberg G, Beattie WS, Mosseri M, et al. Perioperative myocardial infarction. *Circulation*. 2009;119:2936-2944.

Narouze S, Benzon HT, Provenzano DA, et al. Interventional spine and pain procedures in patients on antiplatelet and anticoagulant medications. *Reg Anesth Pain Med*. 2015;40:182-212.

Selim M. Perioperative stroke. *N Engl J Med*. 2007;356:706-713.

CHAPTER 48

Perioperative Pain Management

Darin J. Correll, MD

INTRODUCTION

Pain is the most common presenting symptom of disease. It is defined as an unpleasant sensory and emotional experience, associated with actual or potential tissue damage. There are sound medical and legal reasons to treat pain aggressively in hospitalized patients. The Joint Commission, which certifies health care institutions in the United States, mandates that all patients have the right to adequate pain assessment and management (**Table 48-1**).

In the inpatient setting, patients may be more concerned about pain relief than the outcome of their underlying illness. Poor pain control has adverse physiologic consequences that lead to worse outcomes (**Table 48-2**).

In postoperative patients, better analgesia improves cardiovascular, respiratory, endocrine, immunologic, gastrointestinal, and hematologic status. Following many common surgeries, acute pain that is not satisfactorily treated may become persistent.

PATHOPHYSIOLOGY: NOCICEPTIVE AND ANTI-NOCICEPTIVE PATHWAYS

Nociception, the perception of noxious stimuli, is a preconscious neural activity that is normally necessary, but not sufficient, for pain. It is more accurate to refer to nociceptive pathways, rather than pain pathways. The peripheral nerve fibers acting as nociceptors are lightly myelinated A-delta and unmyelinated C fibers, which are triggered or sensitized (peripheral sensitization) by several substances, including adenosine triphosphate (ATP), prostanoids, bradykinin, serotonin, histamine, and hydrogen ions. Heat, pressure, or nerve damage also results in activation.

The primary nociceptors synapse in the dorsal horn of the spinal cord (**Figure 48-1**), where the excitatory amino acids glutamate and aspartate and peptides such as substance P serve as neurotransmitters. Noxious impulses ascend in the lateral spinothalamic tract to the medial and lateral thalamus and spread to sensory regions of the cerebral cortex. Parts of the limbic system are also activated; most likely, this is where nociception is associated with emotion and arousal and is then perceived as pain.

The nociceptive system has built-in positive and negative feedback loops. Prolonged firing of nociceptors enhances synaptic transmission to dorsal horn neurons. This process of *central* sensitization involves glutamine and a host of other mediators. Central sensitization is an adaptive response that prevents further injury during a vulnerable period of tissue healing. This heightened sensitivity generally returns to baseline over time. However, if central sensitization is prolonged beyond the healing phase, chronic pain may result.

Substance P–mediated nociception is antagonized by local production of endogenous opiates, such as enkephalins and endorphins, in the dorsal horn and the brain stem. Binding of opioids to opiate receptors in these locations may account for the analgesic effects of these drugs. As well, powerful top-down, endogenous mechanisms of pain modulation originate in the cortex and travel through brain stem and midbrain structures en route to the spinal cord. These descending pain control pathways are mediated by nor-adrenergic and serotonergic transmission, as well as endogenous opiates.

CHARACTERIZING PAIN INTENSITY

The most commonly used measures of pain intensity in the acute setting are single-dimension scales (**Table 48-3**). A numerical rating scale has the numbers 0 to 10 spaced evenly across a page,

TABLE 48-1 Joint Commission Pain Assessment and Management Standards for Hospitals

1. The hospital respects the patient's right to pain management.

2. The hospital educates all licensed independent practitioners on assessing and managing pain.

3. The hospital assesses and manages the patient's pain. The hospital conducts a comprehensive pain assessment that is consistent with its scope of care, treatment, and services and the patient's condition.

4. The hospital uses methods to assess pain that are consistent with the patient's age, condition, and ability to understand.

5. The hospital assesses and reassesses its patients. The hospital defines, in writing, criteria that identify when additional, specialized, or more in-depth assessments are performed for pain.

6. Based on the patient's condition and assessed needs, the education and training provided to the patient by the hospital include any of the following: discussion of pain, the risk for pain, the importance of effective pain management, the pain assessment process, and methods for pain management.

where 0 is "no pain at all" and 10 is "the worst pain imaginable." Patients are instructed to circle the number that represents the amount of pain they are currently experiencing. A common variation is the verbal numeric scale, where patients are asked to verbally state a number between 0 and 10 to correspond to their present pain intensity. Some people prefer to use words to describe the intensity of their pain; these are termed verbal descriptor scales. Another variant that may be useful in the elderly or cognitively impaired are scales with drawings of faces, ranging from a contented smiling face to a distressed-looking face.

Single-dimensional scales are quick and simple to use, an important benefit in the acute setting when repeated measures are needed over a brief period of time. One disadvantage is that they attempt to assign a single value to a complex, multidimensional experience. Another is that patients can never know if the present experience is the "worst." If a value of "10" is chosen and the pain worsens, the patient has no official means to express this; in practice many patients state a number over 10.

Several multidimensional scales exist that attempt to assess various aspects of the patient's pain experience (eg, McGill Pain

TABLE 48-2 Physiologic Consequences of Uncontrolled Pain

Cardiovascular	Tachycardia, hypertension, increased cardiac workload
Pulmonary	Hypoxia, hypercarbia, atelectasis, decreased cough
Gastrointestinal	Decreased gastric emptying, nausea/vomiting, ileus
Renal	Urinary retention
Endocrine	Increased adrenergic activity, catabolic state, sodium/water retention
Immunologic	Impairment, slowed wound healing
Musculoskeletal	Splinting, contractures, decreased mobility (deep vein thrombosis)
Hematological	Increased coagulability
Neurological	Anxiety, fear, anger, fatigue, delirium

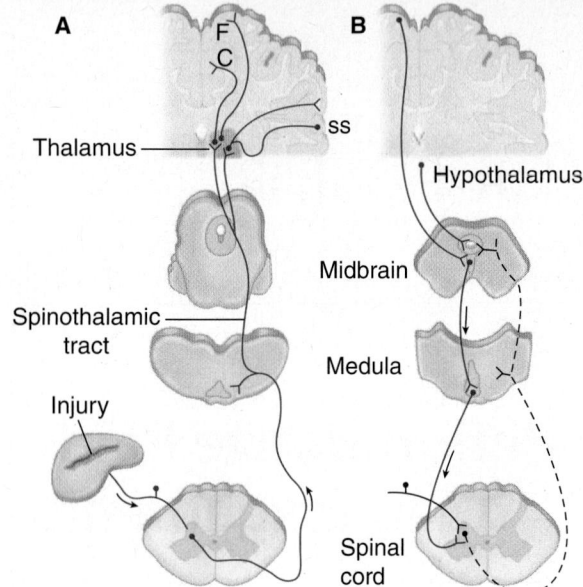

Figure 48-1 *Nociception transmission and pain modulatory pathways. (A) Transmission system for nociceptive messages. Noxious stimuli activate the sensitive peripheral ending of the primary afferent nociceptor by the process of transduction. The message is then transmitted over the peripheral nerve to the spinal cord, where it synapses with cells of origin of the major ascending pain pathway, the spinothalamic tract. The message is relayed in the thalamus to the anterior cingulate (C), frontal insular (F), and somatosensory cortex (SS). (B) Pain-modulation network. Inputs from frontal cortex and hypothalamus activate cells in the midbrain that control spinal pain-transmission cells via cells in the medulla.* (Reproduced with permission from Fauci AS, Braunwald E, Kasper DL, et al. *Harrison's Principles of Internal Medicine,* 17th ed. New York: McGraw-Hill; 2008, Fig. 12-4.)

Questionnaire, Brief Pain Inventory). These multidimensional scales attempt to take into account the complex nature of pain. However, in the inpatient setting, they are too time consuming for rapid or repeated use. One compromise is to address a limited number of the dimensions of pain, using a few single-dimensional scales to address issues that are important to hospitalized patients—for example pain, anxiety, depression, anger, fear, and interference with physical activity.

DIAGNOSIS

■ HISTORY

The history of the patient in pain includes the pain's *location* and the presence, or absence, of *radiation* from the primary site. *Intensity* should be determined using appropriate scales, as already described. The patient should describe the pain's *character* (eg, aching, burning, dull, electric-like, sharp, shooting, stabbing, tender, and throbbing). This may provide clues to help diagnose the generator of the pain which aides in deciding the correct therapy (**Table 48-4**). Does the pain have a *pattern* (constant, intermittent, or better or worse at certain times of day) and *aggravating and alleviating factors*? Does the pain have an *impact on functional status*? Are the patient's activities of daily living affected as an outpatient, or is it hampering their ability to cough, get out of bed, and ambulate while in the hospital? The patient's *prior analgesic history*, in particular, what therapies have either worked or not worked in the past, helps to decide what agents may be effective now. Exact doses of *ongoing analgesics* should also be determined.

TABLE 48-3 Single-Dimension Pain Scales

Numerical Rating Scale

0	1	2	3	4	5	6	7	8	9	10

Verbal Descriptor Scales

No pain	None	Mild	Moderate	Severe	Worst pain imaginable

0	2	4	6	8	10

The Faces Pain Scale—Revised. From Pain 2001;93:173-183. Used with permission from IASP.

PAST MEDICAL HISTORY

The patient's medical history should be obtained. Medical conditions that cause pain include cancer, diabetes, osteoarthritis, rheumatoid arthritis, herpes zoster (shingles), and spinal cord injury. Psychological conditions may adversely impact a patient's pain experience and need appropriate diagnosis and therapy. These include anxiety (especially in acute pain states), depression (most prevalent in persistent pain states), fear, catastrophizing (assuming the worst-case scenario), and personality disorders. A family history that is positive for substance abuse in the patient's relatives is a risk factor for addiction in the patient. A social history positive for alcohol, tobacco, or other drugs may indicate a need to prescribe agents to prevent withdrawal (ie, benzodiazepines or nicotine patches). Even patients with a history of addiction still need to be appropriately treated for pain in the acute setting. In this setting, it may be useful to enlist the help of a psychiatrist or psychologist trained in addiction management.

PHYSICAL EXAMINATION

A directed *physical examination* of the painful site, and a generalized physical exam of the patient as appropriate, should be performed. Pain (especially acute) may be associated with tachycardia, hypertension, diaphoresis, and tachypnea. However, since sympathetic activation is a common and nonspecific finding in hospitalized patients, it offers little help in the diagnosis and treatment of pain in an awake, competent patient. These measures may be used as surrogates in patients who cannot express their pain experience.

PRACTICE POINT

- Patients may not exhibit any alterations in vital signs despite significant levels of pain, especially patients who have persistent pain.

DIAGNOSTIC TESTING

Diagnostic tests to determine the etiology of pain may be useful in some situations (eg, radiographs to assess for fracture, magnetic resonance imaging [MRI] to diagnose nerve impingement in the spinal cord, or electromyography [EMG] to diagnose a neuropathy). However, normal test results should not be used to discount a patient's report of pain.

CARDINAL PRINCIPLES OF PAIN MANAGEMENT

Pain is a subjective phenomenon, resulting from the processing, filtering and modulating of nociceptive input through the affective (limbic system) and cognitive processes unique to each individual.

TABLE 48-4 Determining the Mechanism and Treatment of Pain

Pain Mechanism	Character	Examples	Treatment Options
Somatic	Usually well localized and constant Aching, sharp, stabbing	• Laceration • Fracture • Burn • Abrasion • Localized infection or inflammation	• Heat/cold • Acetaminophen • NSAIDs • Opioids • Local anesthetics (topical or infiltration)
Visceral	Not well localized—constant or intermittent Generalized ache, pressure or cramping, can be sharp	• Muscles/spasm • Colic or obstruction (gastrointestinal or renal) • Sickle cell • Internal organ infection or inflammation	• NSAIDs • Opioids • Muscle relaxants • Local anesthetics (nerve blocks)
Neuropathic	Can be localized (ie, dermatomal) or radiating, can also be generalized and not well localized Burning, tingling, electric shock, lancinating	• Trigeminal • Postherpetic • Postamputation • Peripheral neuropathy • Nerve infiltration	• Anticonvulsants • Tricyclic antidepressants • Muscle relaxants • NMDA antagonists • Neural/neuraxial blockade

NMDA, *N*-methyl-ᴅ-aspartate; NSAIDs, nonsteroidal anti-inflammatory drugs.

The patient's report of pain must be respected and believed. As pain is an affective and cognitive experience, the placebo response to analgesics is real and may be helpful. However, using the placebo response does not mean misleading patients, or administering an inactive substance to determine whether they are lying or to punish them. Rather, the placebo effect in contemporary medicine is that patient belief in a particular therapy makes it more likely to work. Physician attempts to truthfully "talk up" genuine attempts at analgesia are thus likely to enhance the effects. The reverse is also true. If a patient states that a particular therapy "never works for them," it is less likely to be effective.

The patient's pain level and degree of pain relief should be assessed appropriately and regularly. Pain should be treated quickly. Therapy should not be withheld while the diagnosis is unclear; pain treatment does not impede the ability to diagnose disease. A comprehensive plan should be used that addresses the multidimensional aspects of pain. This may require an interdisciplinary team approach (eg, hospitalist, pain specialist, anesthesiologist, surgeon, psychiatrist or psychologist, and physical therapist), especially for patients with persistent pain.

The analgesic plan should be discussed with the patient and, when appropriate, the patient's family. The patient's expectations for pain management should be understood, and patients should be offered reasonable goals for the outcomes of therapy.

PRACTICE POINT

- A multimodal approach for managing pain, employing both pharmacologic and nonpharmacologic measures, is better than using just one modality. This approach allows for optimal analgesia with the lowest incidence of side effects. In the absence of a contraindication, all patients in pain should be prescribed a nonopioid analgesic. Clinicians should be familiar with several agents within each class of analgesics, including possible side effects, because individual responses vary greatly.

If pain is present most of the time or expected to last for an extended period of time (eg, more than a few weeks), long-acting agents or round-the-clock dosing of short-acting agents should be used. When long-acting drugs are used, immediate-release agents will also be needed for breakthrough pain. When pain is intermittent or expected to be of brief duration (eg, less than a few weeks), then as-needed dosing of immediate release agents can be used alone.

TREATMENT

Pharmacologic and nonpharmacologic treatment measures are often used together. Pain medication falls into three categories: nonopioid analgesics, opioids, and adjuvant analgesics. Therapy should be individualized in a multimodal, stepwise approach, adding or changing agents when pain control is inadequate, and withdrawing agents as pain resolves (**Table 48-5**).

■ NONPHARMACOLOGIC MEASURES

Although scientific data on nonpharmacologic measures are limited, most have little risk. At a minimum, they may have placebo benefit, due to the cognitive and affective influence on pain. Application of cold (to reduce inflammation) or heat (to reduce spasms) to muscles or joints are commonly used, but the evidence for an analgesic benefit is mixed. Hypnosis has been shown to reduce pain associated with procedures. However, it requires specific training and time to administer. In the acute setting, the results with transcutaneous electrical nerve stimulation (TENS) are conflicting, with somewhat better evidence of effectiveness in the setting of

chronic pain, particularly painful diabetic neuropathy. Relaxation and guided imagery have shown little benefit in the acute setting. Attention techniques can be complicated in that one needs to determine which approach is better for a particular patient. Some patients do better when instructed to shift attention away from the pain, whereas others do better if instructed to attend to a particular portion of the pain (eg, the sensory component, as opposed to the emotional component). Acupuncture and electroacupuncture have been shown to be beneficial in the acute setting, reducing both pain and common side effects from opioid analgesics. However, these are labor intensive, and specific training is required. The use of virtual reality has been shown to reduce levels of pain and unpleasantness for burn care procedures, common painful cancer procedures and treatments, and routine medical procedures. The major hindrance to its use is the cost and availability of the equipment.

■ NONOPIOID ANALGESICS

In the absence of a contraindication, all patients in pain should be prescribed a nonopioid analgesic. These agents have analgesic effects and are opioid sparing, leading to decreased side effects. They are the primary analgesics for low-intensity pain associated with headache or musculoskeletal disorders and are useful adjuncts in moderate to severe pain. These agents have a plateau effect, such that doses beyond the recommended range increase the incidence of side effects but do not improve analgesia.

Acetaminophen does not inhibit peripheral prostaglandin synthesis. This explains its lack of side effects on gastric mucosa and platelets, but it also means that it is not active at peripheral sites of inflammation. In diseases where inflammation plays a major role in generating pain (eg, rheumatoid arthritis), acetaminophen is of minimal benefit. The analgesic mechanism of acetaminophen is not well characterized but may involve facilitation of central antinociceptive pathways via serotonin, increasing levels of endogenous cannabinoids, or inhibition of nitric oxide synthesis in the spinal cord, which may interfere with substance P–related nociception.

The nonacetylated salicylates (eg, choline magnesium trisalicylate) have a relatively low incidence of gastrointestinal bleeding, perhaps related to their lack of inhibition of platelet aggregation. The nonselective nonsteroidal anti-inflammatory drugs (NSAIDs) are potent anti-inflammatory analgesics with significant risk for gastrointestinal bleeding and renal insufficiency. No single NSAID appears to be more effective as an analgesic than any other, but as there is great interpatient variability in response, thus changing agents may be of benefit if one does not seem to be effective. The COX-2 selective NSAIDs have a reduced risk of peptic ulceration compared to nonselective NSAIDs, but an equivalent chance of renal toxicity. Celecoxib is currently the only COX-2 selective NSAID available in the United States. It should not be considered a first-line agent given it's cost, and should not be used long term at high doses, as it increases the risk of major cardiovascular events. **Table 48-6** lists the dosing regimens and adverse effects of selected nonopioid analgesics.

■ OPIOIDS: TERMINOLOGY

Tolerance is the diminished response to a drug over time, such that, in order to maintain the same effect, the drug dose needs to be increased. *Dependence* is a state of physiologic adaptation that develops with continued use of a drug, presenting as a withdrawal syndrome if the drug is abruptly stopped, the dose is dramatically reduced, or an antagonist is given. *Addiction* is a primary, chronic, neurobiologic disease with many factors influencing its development. It manifests as drug-seeking behaviors, impaired control over the drug, and continued use despite negative effects. Tolerance to and dependence on opioids do not equal addiction!

TABLE 48-5 Suggested Pain Management Schemes

The World Health Organization devised the analgesic ladder for the treatment of cancer pain. The concepts behind its use are helpful in the management of all types of pain, both persistent and acute.

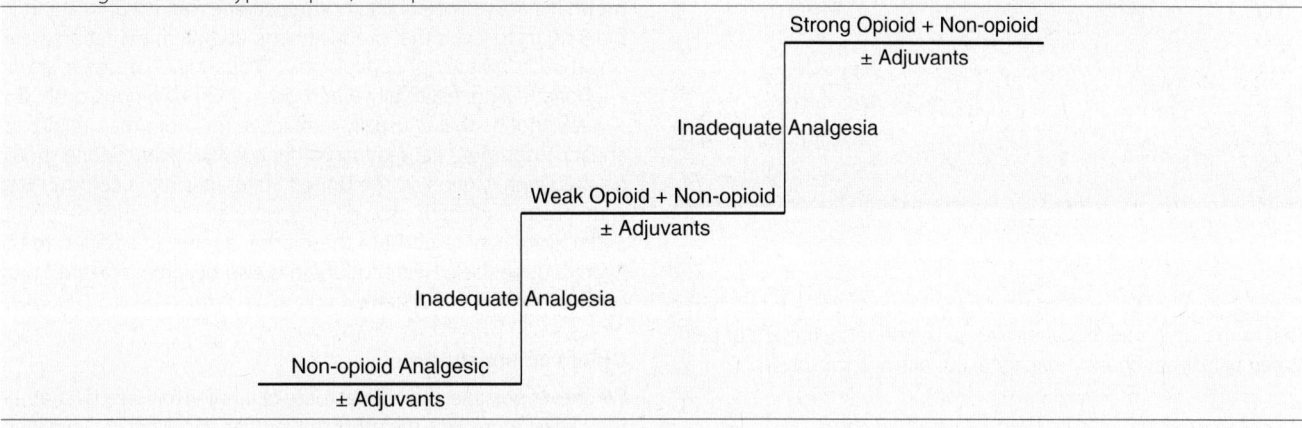

The World Federation of Societies of Anesthesiologists devised another analgesic ladder to use for the treatment of acute/postoperative pain.

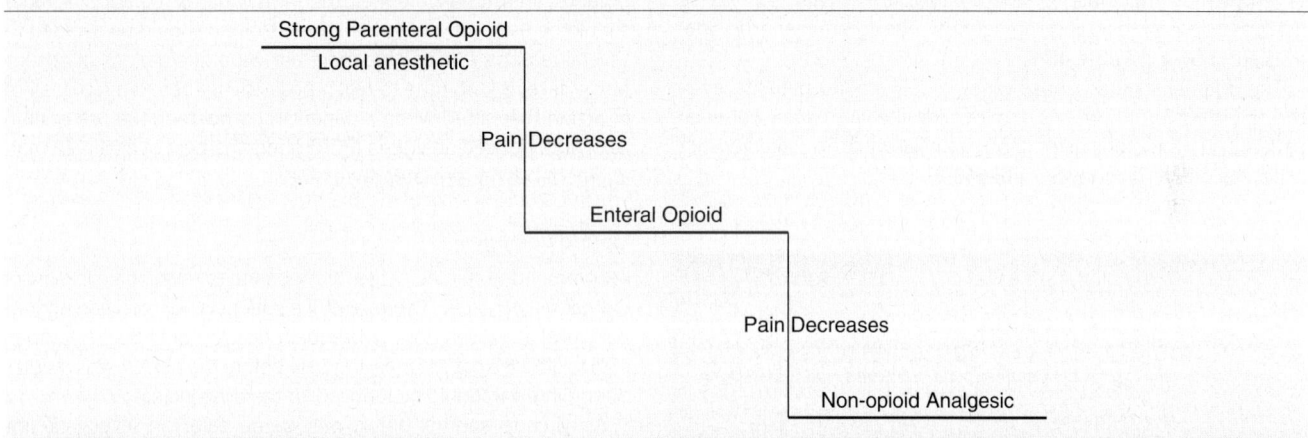

Data from World Health Organization. *Cancer Pain Relief*. Geneva, Switzerland: World Health Organization; 1986 and Data from *Charlton JE. WFSA Update in Anesthesia*. 1997;7:2-17.

TABLE 48-6 Select Nonopioid Analgesics

Agent	Adult Dosing	Maximum Daily Dose	Comments
Acetaminophen	650-1000 mg every 6 h	4000 mg	Single doses above 1000 mg do not improve analgesia
Choline magnesium trisalicylate	1000-1500 mg twice a day	3000 mg	Caution in liver disease, avoid in severe liver disease
Diclofenac	50 mg twice a day-four times a day	200 mg	Low GI effect incidence, but possible increased renal effects, recent data suggest increased negative CV effects
Etodalac	200-400 mg every 6-8 h	1000 mg	Low GI and renal effect incidence, safest NSAID in liver disease
Ibuprofen	400-600 mg every 4-6 h	3000 mg	<1500 mg daily has low risk of GI effects, possible increased renal effects, inhibits CV benefits of aspirin when given concomitantly
Ketorolac	30 mg every 6 h	120 mg	High risk of renal and GI complications; use for no more than 5 d; 15 mg every 6 h in renal impairment, age >65, weight <50 kg
Nabumetone	750-1500 mg daily or twice a day	1500 mg	Low GI effect incidence
Naproxen	250-500 mg every 6-12 h	1500 mg	Possible increased liver and renal effects, probably least negative CV effects
Celecoxib	100-200 mg daily	200 mg	Use 100 mg dose if possible; long-term use has increased negative CV effects

CV, cardiovascular; GI, gastrointestinal.

TABLE 48-7 Opioid Classification

Not Recommended	Weak	Strong
Meperidine	Codeine	Fentanyl
	Hydrocodone	Hydromorphone
	Tramadol	Methadone
		Morphine
		Oxycodone
		Oxymorphone

Pseudoaddiction denotes iatrogenically induced patient behaviors that mimic drug seeking, due solely to the under treatment of pain. When pain is adequately managed, the behaviors resolve.

Opioid therapy basics

When treating moderate to severe pain, pure agonists should be used, as opposed to agonist/antagonists. The commonly used agonists are shown in **Table 48-7**.

The optimal analgesic dose varies widely among patients, even the opioid naïve. Side effects from opioids also vary widely between patients. It is, therefore, helpful to be familiar with the characteristics of several different agonists (**Table 48-8**).

PRACTICE POINT

Opioids

- Patients should be asked which opioids have worked or not worked in the past, or have given them intolerable side effects.
- Whenever possible, the enteral route of administration is best, as it is the easiest route with the most stable pharmacokinetics. If a patient cannot take anything by mouth or adequate analgesia cannot be obtained in a timely manner, then intravenous (IV) administration should be used. Intramuscular administration should be avoided.
- If pain is present most of the time or expected to last for an extended period of time (ie, more than a few weeks), long-acting agents or round-the-clock dosing of short-acting agents should be used. When long-acting drugs are used, immediate-release agents will also be needed for breakthrough pain.
- Patients should be monitored closely for effectiveness and adverse events whenever there is a change of agent or route of administration.
- When pain is intermittent or expected to be of brief duration (eg, less than a few weeks), then as-needed dosing of immediate release agents can be used alone.
- When a patient is competent, the use of an IV patient-controlled analgesia (PCA) offers the best overall pain management option for postoperative hospitalized patients.

Selecting an opioid

Codeine is not a good first choice due to the fact that 10% to 20% of the population lacks an active form of the enzyme (cytochrome P450 2D6) necessary to convert codeine into an active drug in the body (ie, morphine). All opioids should be used with caution in patients with renal or hepatic insufficiency; lower doses or longer dosing intervals are wise in this setting. Morphine is relatively contraindicated in patients with severe renal insufficiency due to the

accumulation of the metabolite, morphine-6-glucuronide, which can lead to sedation and respiratory depression.

Meperidine (Demerol) is not recommended for pain management. Its active metabolite, normeperidine, can accumulate in 24 to 48 hours to levels that produce nervous system excitation (tremors, muscle twitching, convulsions). Meperidine causes a strong euphoric feeling, especially when given by intravenous push. It is a weak agonist that is usually ineffective for more than mild pain, and it causes more nausea than other agents. Hydrocodone should be used with caution. In the United States, it is often coformulated with acetaminophen, aspirin, or ibuprofen, and adverse events and toxicity may result from these other agents, in addition to the hydrocodone itself. Hydrocodone has also become a favored drug of abuse in the United States.

Opioid administration

Whenever possible, the enteral route of administration is best, as it is the easiest route with the most stable pharmacokinetics. If a patient cannot take anything by mouth or adequate analgesia cannot be obtained in a timely manner, then intravenous (IV) administration should be used. Intramuscular administration should be avoided for several reasons: It is painful; there are wide fluctuations in absorption; it takes a long time to reach peak effect; there is a rapid fall-off of action thereafter. When a patient is competent, the use of an IV patient-controlled analgesia (PCA) offers the best overall pain management option (see later discussion).

Opioid dosing

Recommended starting doses for moderate to severe pain in the opioid-naïve are listed in **Table 48-9**. If a patient is not receiving enough pain relief at a given dose, subsequent doses should be increased by 25% to 50%. If a patient is having pain before the next dose is due, the dosing interval should be reduced, or the dose increased.

A switch to another opioid may be necessary in several circumstances. First, patients on therapeutic opioid doses who are not receiving any pain relief may not have a receptor population at which that particular opioid is effective. A different opioid may provide better analgesia. Second, if a patient is having intolerable side effects, rotation to a different opioid may provide relief. In this case, the patient's receptor population may bind a particular opioid in regions that cause side effects. Third, if a particular opioid cannot be given by the route of administration required, then changing to another opioid will be necessary. Finally, if a patient has been on an opioid for a long time and has developed tolerance, rotation to a different opioid may provide better analgesia, usually at less than the expected equianalgesic dose. A similar effect may also be seen in patients on long-term opioid therapy for chronic pain who have an episode of acute pain; better analgesia may also be experienced in this setting with a switch to a different opioid.

Equianalgesic-dosing charts (see Table 48-8) are based on the relative potency of opioid agonists, as determined by single-dose clinical studies and experience. These calculations are estimates only, and clinical judgment is always required for use. Incomplete cross-tolerance exists between the various opioids. This means patients will not be as tolerant to a new opioid agonist as they are to the one they were on previously. Thus, when converting between opioids, the calculated equianalgesic dose of the new agent must be reduced by 25% to 75% to prevent over sedation and respiratory depression. **Table 48-10** shows an example of opioid conversion.

Sustained-release or long-acting opioids

Episodic pain or pain expected to be of a brief duration should be treated with immediate-release agents alone. Sustained-release

TABLE 48-8 Opioid Characteristics

Agonist	Route	Equianalgesic Dose (mg)	Onset (min)	Peak Effect (min)	Duration of Effect (h)
Morphine	IV	10	5-10	10-30	3-5
	Oral	30	15-60	60-120	4-6
	Oral CR	–	30-120	180-240	8-12
	Oral SR	–	30-120	480-600	8-24
Codeine	IM	120	10-30	90-120	4-6
	Oral	200	30-45	60	3-4
Hydromorphone	IV	1.5	5-20	15-30	3-4
	Oral	7.5	15-30	90-120	4-6
Oxycodone	Oral	20	15-30	30-60	4-6
	Oral CR	–	30-60	90-180	8-12
Methadone	IV	10*	10-20	60-120	4-6
	Oral	20*	30-60	90-120	4-12
Fentanyl	IV	0.1	<1	5-7	0.75-2+
	TD	(see Table 48-11)	720-1080	1440-4320	48-72
Oxymorphone	IV	1	5-10	30-60	3-6
	Oral	10	"meaningful relief" = 60		4-6

CR, controlled release; IM, intramuscular; IV, intravenous; SR, sustained release; TD, transdermal.

*These doses are based on single administrations and should only be used to convert between oral and IV methadone. If converting a patient who has been on a different opioid, use the following table that takes into account the dose-dependent potency changes seen with methadone:

Equianalgesic Conversion to Methadone§		
Oral Morphine Equivalent That Patient Is Taking	Oral Methadone (mg)	Oral Morphine (mg)
< 100 mg/d	1	4
101-300 mg/d	1	8
301-600 mg/d	1	10
601-800 mg/d	1	12
801-1000 mg/d	1	15
> 1000 mg/d	1	20

To determine the starting dose of oral methadone:
- Convert the patient's daily opioid dose into oral morphine equivalents.
- Convert the daily oral morphine equivalents to a daily oral methadone dose using the table.
- Reduce the calculated daily oral methadone dose by 33%-50%.
- Divide the resulting reduced daily dose by 3.
- Prescribe this dose of oral methadone (in mg) every 8 h.

§This table is not meant to be used to convert from methadone to other opioids. There is limited data on the conversion from methadone to other agents, and inadequate analgesia often results. Thus, if it is necessary to convert from methadone to another opioid agonist, it is best performed in stages, with close monitoring of the patient for effectiveness (eg, introduce the new agent over a 3-d period as the methadone dose is tapered by one-third each day).

TABLE 48-9 Recommended Starting Doses of Opioids for Adults Over 50 kg

Agonist	Oral	IV
Codeine	15-60 mg every 3-4 h	n/a
Hydrocodone	5-10 mg every 3-6 h*	n/a
Tramadol	50-100 mg every 4-6 h†	n/a
Oxycodone	5-10 mg every 3-4 h	n/a
Morphine	10-30 mg every 3-4 h	5-10 mg every 2-4 h
Hydromorphone	2-6 mg every 3-4 h	1-1.5 mg every 3-4 h
Oxymorphone	10-20 mg every 4-6 h	1 mg every 3-4 h

*Daily dose limited by acetaminophen component in available preparations.
†Maximum recommended 24-h dose: 400 mg in adults < 75 y old; 300 mg in adults > 75 y old.

formulations should be initiated in the acute setting if pain is present most of the time, and pain is expected to last for an extended period of time (2-3 weeks or more). When using a sustained-release opioid, an immediate-release opioid equivalent to 10% to 15% of the 24-hour total every few hours on an as-needed basis should also be prescribed. If more than four to five rescue doses of immediate-release opioid are needed in 24 hours, the dose of sustained-release agent should be increased by 50% to 100% of the total 24-hour breakthrough dose used.

Transdermal fentanyl is not appropriate to treat acute pain, especially in the opioid-naïve. Its use in the acute setting may lead to severe respiratory depression from the delayed peak effect of the drug. It should only be used in patients already tolerant to opioids of comparable potency. **Table 48-11** gives recommendations for conversion from other opioids to transdermal fentanyl.

Methadone is also not appropriate as a first-line agent in the acute setting, especially in the opioid-naïve. Its use requires an

TABLE 48-10 Example of Opioid Conversion

1. Patient used 15 mg of IV hydromorphone in the past 24 h.
2. According to the equianalgesic table:

   1.5 mg of IV hydromorphone = 20 mg of oral oxycodone

   $$\frac{1.5\,mg\,of\,IV\,hydromorphone}{20\,mg\,of\,oral\,oxycodone} = \frac{1.5\,mg\,of\,IV\,hydromorphone}{X}$$

   X = 200 mg of oral oxycodone/d
3. Taking into account incomplete cross-tolerance, decrease the total daily opioid dose by 25%-75%:

   200 − (0.25 × 200) = 150 mg of oral oxycodone/d

   200 − (0.75 × 200) = 50 mg of oral oxycodone/d
4. Dose initially every 4 h:

   150/6 ≅ 25 mg oxycodone every 4 h

   50/6 ≅ 8 mg oxycodone every 4 h

Therefore, order: oxycodone 10-25 mg every 4 h as needed for pain.

---

understanding of the unique pharmacology of the drug, especially its extended duration of action and its dose-dependent potency. Also, as it takes several days to reach a stable plasma concentration, patients need to be monitored closely for efficacy and side effects. As methadone is a racemic mixture of a mu agonist and an N-methyl-D-aspartate (NMDA) antagonist (see later discussion), patients develop less analgesic tolerance. Patients must be made aware of the long duration of action of methadone, be warned not to take extra doses or mix it with other medications, and be familiar with signs of overdose.

■ PATIENT-CONTROLLED ANALGESIA BASICS

PCA is intended as maintenance therapy. If the patient is in moderate to severe pain when it is begun, IV loading doses must be given

TABLE 48-11 Dose Conversion Guidelines from Another Opioid to Transdermal Fentanyl

24-h Oral Morphine Equivalent Dose (mg/d)*	Transdermal Fentanyl Initial Dose (mcg/h)
60-134	25
135-224	50
225-314	75
315-404	100
405-494	125
495-584	150
585-674	175
675-764	200
765-854	225
855-944	250
945-1034	275
1035-1124	300

*Convert other opioid to oral morphine equivalents using an equianalgesic dose table.

This table should not be used to convert from transdermal fentanyl to another opioid because the conversion to transdermal fentanyl in this table is conservative. Therefore, use of this table to convert from transdermal fentanyl to another opioid can overestimate the amount of the new agent, resulting in overdosage and respiratory depression.

---

to achieve comfort, because the incremental dosing of the PCA will not be effective in a reasonable period of time. The use of a PCA helps overcome the wide interpatient variation in opioid requirements by allowing the patient to control the dosing regimen. Morphine is the most common first-line agent. It is not the best choice in patients with renal insufficiency, due to accumulation of the active metabolite. Fentanyl has a quicker onset and shorter duration of action than morphine. This decreases the likelihood of oversedation, but the patient must activate the PCA more often, making it difficult for some patients to sleep at night. Hydromorphone is generally more effective in opioid-tolerant patients and given its pharmacokinetics is an excellent choice for use in PCAs. Recommended starting doses in the opioid-naïve patient are listed in **Table 48-12**, along with suggestions for dose titration.

The lockout interval, or minimum time between doses, is typically set at 5 to 10 minutes. Even though the time to peak effect may be longer than this, in practice no major differences are seen with longer lockouts. There have also been no good studies to suggest that a particular lockout interval is better than any other.

A basal rate on the PCA may be needed in opioid-tolerant patients or in patients receiving fentanyl, given its short half-life. Basal rates are not recommended in the opioid-naïve, elderly, or patients with obstructive sleep apnea or morbid obesity. Some people advocate use of basal rates at night however this is not recommended as there is no data that basal rates help patients get more sleep at night, pain scores are not improved and the risk of respiratory depression is increased. Basal rates should be decreased or discontinued if a patient is not activating the PCA, or if the patient is becoming excessively sedated.

■ COMPLICATIONS/OPIOID-INDUCED SIDE EFFECTS

Nausea, vomiting, pruritus, constipation, sedation, and respiratory depression are common opioid-related side effects. They occur more often in opioid-naïve patients, as tolerance eventually develops to all these effects, except constipation. Adverse effects can be ameliorated by changing the drug dose or schedule, switching to a different agent (side effects of different opioid agonists vary among patients), using specific therapy to counteract the side effect, or adding another analgesic or adjuvant to allow a lower opioid dose.

Constipation should always be expected with opioids. Prophylactic use of stool softeners, such as docusate, and stimulant laxatives, such as senna preparations, is recommended. Nausea and vomiting can be treated with any of the available agents (eg, prochlorperazine, ondansetron, metoclopramide, and promethazine), as none has been shown to be more or less effective. Metoclopramide is a promotility agent with limited antinausea effects and is most effective if there is vomiting. Promethazine or possibly a scopolamine patch (especially if used before the symptoms onset) may be effective if the patient has a history of motion sickness, or if nausea is provoked by movement, as opioids sensitize the inner ear labyrinthine system. Extreme caution must be used with promethazine because of its possibility to cause severe tissue damage if extravasation occurs. Pruritus is thought to be a central mu opioid receptor-related phenomenon. Diphenhydramine is only effective if the

TABLE 48-12 Suggested Starting Patient-Controlled Analgesia Dose and Dose Changes

	Morphine	Hydromorphone	Fentanyl
Staring PCA dose	1.0-1.5 mg	0.2 mg	20-25 mcg
PCA dose change	0.5 mg	0.1 mg	5-10 mcg

TABLE 48-13 Treatment of Suspected Opioid-Induced Respiratory Depression

Suggested definition of respiratory depression

- Oxygen saturation below 90% or decrease of more than 5% from baseline in patients with baseline oxygen saturation of <90%.

    AND

- Respiratory rate less than 8 breaths per minute.

Primary, nonpharmacologic treatments of respiratory depression

- If patient is taking effective breaths but at a rate of <8 per minute:
    - Tactile and verbal stimulation, naloxone administration may not be essential.
- If patient is taking ineffective breaths and/or with a respiratory rate <4 per minute:
    - May require ventilatory assist with bag-valve mask and supplemental oxygen. This should be instituted while diluting and administering naloxone.

Naloxone should only be considered in the following situations

- Patient is unarousable or minimally arousable to tactile/verbal stimulation.
- Patient is requiring ventilatory assistance.

Proper naloxone dilution and dosing

- 1 ampule (0.4 mg) of naloxone must be diluted with 9 mL saline to yield 0.04 mg/mL.
- Administer to patient in 1-2 mL increments (0.04-0.08 mg) at 2-3 min intervals until response.
- If no change in respiratory depression after 0.4 mg naloxone has been titrated, consider another etiology other than opioid induced.
- If there is some, but not enough, improvement after 0.4 mg of naloxone has been titrated, continue titration.
- Naloxone's half-life is less than most of the opioid agonists, so be aware that rebound respiratory depression may recur. Therefore, be prepared for the need to readminister naloxone boluses or consider use of a naloxone infusion.

etiology is definitely due to histamine release, which is usually only the case for large doses of morphine given quickly, or a true allergic reaction. Nalbuphine 5 mg IV every 4 hours as needed is more effective in that it treats the cause, by antagonism of the central mu receptors. Sedation may be a troublesome side effect, particularly when using opiates to alleviate persistent pain in terminal illness. The proper treatment of respiratory depression from opioid agonists is described in **Table 48-13**.

■ ADJUVANT ANALGESICS

Adjunctive agents are useful for additional analgesia especially in opioid-tolerant patients, and have a particular role in the treatment of neuropathic symptoms and chronic pain. Examples of adjuvant analgesics with dosing guidelines and common side effects are listed in **Table 48-14**.

The most commonly used antiepileptic agents are gabapentin and pregabalin. They are effective for neuropathic pain and may have benefits in the acute setting as well. Antidepressants are also effective in neuropathic pain. Analgesic doses are lower than those for depression treatment, and the onset of analgesia is faster (days)

than the antidepressant effects (weeks). Skeletal muscle relaxants are useful for muscle injury or spasms. The antispasmodic baclofen is useful for the treatment of pain with a spastic component or in certain neuropathic pain states. Antagonism of the NMDA receptor has no primary analgesic effect, but it has opioid-sparing, opioid tolerance-reversing, and antihyperalgesic effects. Ketamine, in addition to being an NMDA antagonist, interacts with opioid and other receptors, and thus it has true analgesic properties in addition to the NMDA class effects. Ketamine use improves pain scores and has an opioid-sparing effect of up to 50% although there are equivocal benefits in reduction of opioid side effects. The alpha-2 agonist, clonidine, has analgesic and opioid-sparing effects. Dexmedetomidine has documented opioid-sparing effects when given by IV infusion. It may have analgesic effects as well, although this effect may only occur at sedating doses, restricting its use to sedated intensive care patients. Glucocorticoids are used in cancer pain management to reduce inflammation from tumor invasion of nerves.

Benzodiazepines may reduce the insomnia and anxiety that often accompany acute pain. However, these agents do *not* have analgesic properties. They must be used with extreme caution in acute pain, especially when high doses of opioids are required, as significant sedation and respiratory depression can occur in the benzodiazepine-naïve patient. In the anxious patient with pain, adequate titration with analgesics should occur before the addition of a benzodiazepine.

■ ACUTE PAIN IN THE OPIOID TOLERANT

When opioid-tolerant patients experience an event resulting in pain escalation, opioid use is expected to be higher than mere replacement of what the patient was receiving before. The additional doses of opioids required may be much higher than in opioid-naïve patients. More complaints of pain and high pain scores should be expected. Discussion of reasonable goals and expectations of analgesic therapy with the patient is crucial. Multimodal therapy in this patient population is helpful to achieve the best pain control, and have the least escalation of home opioid dose as possible.

CONSULTATION

Involvement of a pain specialist may be appropriate in the patient with severe pain that remains uncontrolled after several escalations of drug doses and use of multiple classes of agents. Concomitant psychiatric illness may warrant input from a psychiatrist or psychologist. Certain diagnostic tests, such as diagnostic epidural injections, require an interventional pain physician. Physical therapy, surgery, complementary therapies, or invasive treatment modalities, such as epidural injections, intrathecal pumps, and spinal cord stimulators, will require referral to the appropriate provider.

DISCHARGE CONSIDERATIONS

Communication with the patient's primary care provider about the discharge analgesic plan is essential, especially if the prior analgesic regimen has been changed. Follow-up should be arranged to ensure effectiveness of the analgesic regimen, monitor for side effects after discharge, and taper the patient off analgesics, or reduce doses to baseline if the patient was on chronic analgesics before.

■ WEANING OPIOIDS

If the cause of pain is gone, patients need discontinuation of opioids in a manner that prevents the occurrence of withdrawal symptoms, such as abdominal pain, diarrhea, tachycardia, vomiting, diaphoresis, runny nose, muscle cramps, piloerection, anxiety, and irritability. When weaning a patient from long-acting agents, the

TABLE 48-14 Select Adjuvant Analgesics

Class	Agent	Adult Dosing	Side Effects/Comments
Antiepileptics	Gabapentin	Start with 300 mg orally every 8 h, increase by 300 mg daily after a few days to a max of 3600 mg/d in divided doses	Dizziness and somnolence; do not stop abruptly
	Pregabalin	Start with 50 mg orally every 8 h or 75 mg orally every 12 h; in 1 wk increase to max of 300 mg/d in divided doses	
Tricyclic antidepressants	Amitriptyline Nortriptyline	25 mg orally every night at bed time; increase to max of 150 mg/d in a single or divided doses	Anticholinergic symptoms (eg, dry mouth, confusion, sedation, and hypotension)
Local anesthetics	Lidocaine 2.5% and prilocaine 2.5% cream	2-2.5 g per 10-25 cm² skin for 1-2 h before procedure	Localized skin reactions; rare cardiovascular and/or CNS toxicity; prilocaine may contribute to methemoglobinemia in patients treated with other agents known to cause this
	Lidocaine patch 5%	Up to three patches for up to 12 h within a 24-h period	Localized skin reactions; rare cardiovascular and/or CNS toxicity; only FDA indication is for treatment of postherpetic neuralgia
Glucocorticoids	Dexamethasone	4-8 mg orally every 8-12 h	Typical steroid-induced side effects from long-term use (>2-3 mo) usually outweigh benefits; concomitant use with NSAIDs not recommended
Skeletal muscle relaxants	Cyclobenzaprine	5-10 mg orally every 8 h	Long-term use can lead to the development of dependence
	Tizanidine	4-8 mg orally every 6-24 h	
	Orphenadrine	100 mg orally every 12 h 60 mg IV every 12 h	
Antispasmodic	Baclofen	10 mg orally every 8 h, titrate slowly to max of 80 mg/d in divided doses	Drowsiness; may impair renal function; abrupt discontinuation may cause seizures
NMDA antagonists	Ketamine	0.1-0.2 mg/kg/h IV	Sedation, dreams, and hallucinations possible but infrequent at analgesic (low) dose, treat with the addition of benzodiazepine or dose-reduction
	Dextromethorphan	Start with 30-90 mg orally every 8 h, increase to max of 360 mg/d in divided doses	Best dose and regimen not well defined
Alpha-2 agonist	Clonidine	0.2 mg/d via a transdermal patch, left on for 1 wk	Hypotension and sedation; monitor for rebound hypertension on discontinuation if used for >1 wk

CNS, central nervous system; FDA, US Food and Drug Administration; NSAID, nonsteroidal anti-inflammatory drug.

dose of the long-acting agent should be decreased by 25% to 50% every 2 days. Once the patient is off the sustained-release form, the immediate-release agent can also be weaned. In weaning a patient from immediate-release agents, the opioid dose should be reduced by 50% for 2 days, and then reduced by 25% every 2 days thereafter until the total dose in oral morphine equivalents is 30 mg/d. The drug may be discontinued after 2 days on the 30 mg/d dose.

QUALITY IMPROVEMENT

Data on pain management quality should be collected periodically to assess the quality of care, to establish baseline data, and to identify areas in which care can be improved. The American Pain Society has proposed the following six quality indicators for hospital-based pain management: (1) pain intensity is documented with a numeric or descriptive rating scale; (2) pain intensity is documented frequently; (3) pain is treated by a route other than intramuscular; (4) pain is treated with regularly administered analgesics, and whenever possible, a multimodal approach is used; (5) pain is prevented and controlled to a degree that facilitates function and quality of life; and (6) patients are involved in the treatment plan and are informed and knowledgeable about pain management.

SUGGESTED READINGS

American Pain Society. *Principles of Analgesic Use in the Treatment of Acute Pain and Cancer Pain*, 6th ed. Glenview, IL: American Pain Society; 2008.

Australian National Health and Medical Research Council's Acute pain management: scientific evidence website. https://www.nhmrc.gov.au/guidelines-publications/cp104. Accessed May 26, 2015.

Gordon DB, Dahl JL, Miaskowski C, et al. American Pain Society recommendations for improving the quality of acute and cancer pain management. *Arch Intern Med*. 2005;165:1574-1580.

Gruener D, Lande SD, eds. *Pain Control in the Primary Care Setting*. Glenview, IL: American Pain Society; 2006.

Morrison RS, Meier DE, Fischberg D, et al. Improving the management of pain in hospitalized adults. *Arch Intern Med*. 2006;166:1033-1039.

United States Food and Drug Administration/Center for Drug Evaluation and Research website. http://www.fda.gov/Drugs/. Accessed May 26, 2015.

Whelan CT, Jin L, Meltzer D. Pain and satisfaction with pain control in hospitalized medical patients. *Arch Intern Med*. 2004;164:175-180.

SECTION 3

Perioperative Risk Assessment and Management

CHAPTER 49

Role of the Medical Consultant

Steven L. Cohn, MD, FACP, SFHM

Medical consultation has become an important component of Hospital Medicine. These consultations include preoperative evaluation, perioperative management, and medical care of patients on various nonmedical services. Previous surveys found that many primary care physicians and hospitalists felt inadequately trained in perioperative medicine, and as a result, this area received additional emphasis as part of the core competencies for Hospital Medicine. With the growth of the hospitalist movement, the role of the consultant has evolved from providing evaluation and advice to include comanagement of the patient in certain settings. The goal of this chapter is to review the role and responsibilities of the medical consultant, focusing on the principles of consultation and techniques to improve effectiveness.

GENERAL PRINCIPLES OF CONSULTATION

More than 25 years ago, Goldman and colleagues described the concepts for performing medical consultations. His "Ten Commandments" for effective consultation included the following:

1. Determine the question.
2. Establish urgency.
3. Look for yourself.
4. Be as brief as appropriate.
5. Be specific and concise.
6. Provide contingency plans.
7. Honor thy turf.
8. Teach with tact.
9. Talk is cheap and effective.
10. Follow-up.

These concepts, which incorporated many of the ethical principles described by the American Medical Association (AMA), are important and remain valid for the traditional consultation. However, some modifications are necessary to cover the new role of hospitalists as comanagers.

■ TYPES OF CONSULTATION

The traditional or standard medical consultation consisted of a formal request from the requesting physician to evaluate a patient and answer a specific question (**Table 49-1**). The consultant was expected to address the question and to provide advice and recommendations, but not to write orders or bring in other consultants; the requesting physician remained in control and responsible for the patient's overall care and treatment. The consultant also focused on the specific problem rather than looking for and addressing other issues. Consultations were requested only when necessary and not for routine management. The follow-up period was usually brief and did not involve daily visits for the duration of hospitalization.

This traditional role of the consultant has been changing over the past 5 to 10 years. A survey by Salerno and colleagues revealed that many surgeons wanted the medical consultant to assume more of a comanagement role. Specifically, they wanted the consultant to address all medical issues as necessary as well as to write orders and continue to follow the patient. Comanagement arrangements have most often been with orthopedic surgeons and more recently with neurosurgeons. Comanagement has potential advantages of

TABLE 49-1 Roles and Responsibilities of Different Types on Consultations

	Traditional	Comanagement	Curbside
MD in charge overall	Requesting physician	Shared responsibility	Requesting physician
Primary care of medical problems	Requesting physician	Medical consultant Surgical—requesting physician	Requesting physician
Question addressed	Specific	Broader issues—other medical problems	Should not address either but offer to do formal consult or give only general advice
Order writing	No	Yes	No
Follow-up	Limited-as needed	Daily until discharge	No—no formal relationship

decreasing length of stay and reducing complications. Surgeons and nurses often prefer comanagement; however, one possible disadvantage is that the comanaging consultant may feel subservient to the surgeon and may be asked to assume responsibilities outside his area of training.

Yet another type of consultation is the so-called curbside or informal consult in which the consultant is asked to provide an opinion or advice without personally seeing the patient. Although these should be avoided from a medicolegal standpoint, they occur frequently. Ideally the consultant should offer to perform a formal consult but if any advice is given, it should be generic and simple. The requesting physician should not refer to the consultant in the medical record if he has not seen the patient, and if he has had any contact with the patient, the consultant should write a note in the chart.

PRACTICE POINT

If the consultant is asked to provide an opinion or advice without personally seeing the patient (the "curbside consult"), the consultant should:

- Offer to perform a formal consult.
- Provide only generic and simple advice.
- Document any patient encounter in the chart.

The requesting physician should not refer to the consultant in the medical record if the consultant has not seen the patient.

■ **DETERMINING THE QUESTION**

In view of the multiple types of consultations, it is imperative that the requesting physician specify exactly what is being requested, and if there is any uncertainty, the consultant should clarify this question by communicating directly with the requesting physician. In addition to specifying the role of the consultant, the requesting physician should be specific as to the question being asked of the consultant. For example, a request for preoperative consultation may be for surgical risk assessment, a "green light" to proceed with anesthesia and surgery, a diagnostic or management issue, reassurance, or documentation for medicolegal purposes. As obvious as this may be, disagreement regarding the primary purpose for the consult still occurs between the requesting physician and the consultant. Several studies noted that the consult requests were vague and nonspecific (eg, clearance or evaluation), or did not even ask a question. Without clarifying the reason for the consult, the consultant may respond in a manner

that fails to answer the question being asked by the requesting physician.

PRACTICE POINT

In view of the multiple types of consultations, it is imperative that the requesting physician specify:

- The expected role of the consultant
- The question to be answered by the consultant

If there is any uncertainty, the consultant should clarify this question by communicating directly with the requesting physician. The consultant should avoid making recommendations about the type of anesthesia and other areas outside his or her area of expertise.

■ **ANSWERING THE QUESTION**

Traditionally, the consultant restricted his or her advice to the specific problem or question. However, more frequently the consultant is addressing other issues noted during the evaluations. Assuming these other findings and recommendations are relevant and important, most surgeons are in favor of this approach. What the requesting physician does not want is a laundry list of things to do for minor problems or issues that do not need to be addressed during the current hospitalization.

If the consultation is for preoperative evaluation, the consultant needs to:

1. Assess the severity and degree of control of the patient's medical problems.
2. Estimate surgical risk.
3. Determine if the patient is in his or her optimal medical condition for surgery.
4. Decide whether further tests or interventions are indicated.
5. Make recommendations regarding the patient's medications and any necessary prophylaxis.

The consultant should avoid making recommendations about the type of anesthesia and other areas outside his or her area of expertise. Also, the consultant should refrain from using the term "cleared for surgery," even if consulted for that reason, as this implies a guarantee that the patient will not have a complication.

■ **OPTIMIZING EFFECTIVENESS**

Factors influencing or improving compliance

Various studies found a number of factors that have been associated with improved compliance with the consultant's recommendations

TABLE 49-2 Factors that Influence or Improve Compliance with Consultant Recommendations

Prompt response (within 24 h)

Limit number of recommendations (≤ 5)

Identify crucial or critical recommendations (vs routine)

Focus on central issues

Make specific relevant recommendations

Use definitive language

Specify drug dosage, route, frequency, duration

Frequent follow-up including progress notes

Direct verbal contact

Therapeutic (vs diagnostic) recommendations

Severity of illness

From Cohn SL, Macpherson DS. Overview of the principles of medical consultation. In: Basow DS, ed. *UpToDate*. Waltham, MA: UpToDate; 2009; with permission.

(**Table 49-2**). In general, following Goldman's Ten Commandments or Salerno's modification (see Salerno SM, Hurst FP, Halvorson S, Mercado DL. Principles of effective consultation: an update for the 21st-century consultant. *Arch Intern Med*. 2007;167(3):271-275) will result in effective consultation.

Determine and clarify the question: As noted, the reason for the consultation needs to be clearly defined by the requesting physician and understood and addressed by the consultant.

Punctual response: The consultant should be available to respond in a timely fashion, depending on the urgency of the consultation. Truly "stat" consults should be answered in less than 30 minutes, and in general, elective consults should be answered within 24 hours, preferably the same day they were requested.

Recommendations:

1. **Prioritize and limit:** The consultant should make specific, precise recommendations that should be listed in order of importance. Crucial or critical recommendations are more likely to be followed, as are those at the top of the list. For this reason, it was previously felt that the number of recommendations should be limited to no more than five, but more recently the feeling is to leave as many recommendations as needed to answer the consult and offer to help with writing and implementing them (comanagement). Therapeutic recommendations are more likely to be followed than diagnostic ones.
2. **Language:** The consultant should use definitive language, be specific with his recommendations, and provide contingency plans. For example, recommendations for medications should specify the drug name, dose, frequency, route of administration, and duration of therapy. The requesting physician should be told what response to expect, how long it will take, as well as how and when to adjust the medication dose if necessary.
3. **Communication:** Direct verbal communication with the requesting physician is crucial and preferable to just leaving a note in the chart. A quick call to the requesting physician will let him know that the consult has been answered, what the recommendations are, and what needs to be done so the orders can be written and the process expedited. It is also important to communicate with other members of the health care team to coordinate care.

4. **Follow-up:** Appropriate follow-up visits will reassess the patient's condition and ensure that recommendations were followed. The consultant should clearly document his findings and update recommendations in the medical record. There is no standard regarding how often the consultant needs to see the patient, but this should be determined by the patient's medical condition, type of surgery, and whether the requesting physician wants comanagement or not. When the patient is medically stable and there is no longer a need for the medical consultant, he should sign off and document this in the chart. Recommendations and arrangements for long-term follow-up can also be noted at this time.

PRACTICE POINT

The consultant should document:

- Specific and precise recommendations listed in order of importance
- Name, initial dose, frequency, route of administration, titration, and duration of recommended therapy

The consultant should provide:

- Prompt service
- Direct verbal communication with the requesting physician upon completion of the initial consult
- Updates and follow-up as appropriate depending on requested role

---

CONCLUSION

The ideal medical consultant will "render a report that informs without patronizing, educates without lecturing, directs without ordering, and solves the problem without making the referring physician appear to be stupid." It is hoped that by following these principles, the medical consultant will be effective in providing useful information and recommendations to the requesting physician who will then implement them in an attempt to improve patient outcome.

SUGGESTED READINGS

Choi JJ. An anesthesiologist's philosophy on "medical clearance" for surgical patients. *Arch Intern Med*. 1987;147(12):2090-2092.

Cohn SL, Macpherson D. Overview of the principles of medical consultation. In: Basow D, ed. *UpToDate*. Waltham, MA: UpToDate; 2015.

Devor M, Renvall M, Ramsdell J. Practice patterns and the adequacy of residency training in consultation medicine. *J Gen Intern Med*. 1993;8(10):554-560.

Goldman L, Lee T, Rudd P. Ten commandments for effective consultations. *Arch Intern Med*. 1983;143(9):1753-1755.

Kleinman B, Czinn E, Shah K, Sobotka PA, Rao TK. The value to the anesthesia-surgical care team of the preoperative cardiac consultation. *J Cardiothorac Anesth*. 1989;3(6):682-687.

Kuo D, Gifford DR, Stein MD. Curbside consultation practices and attitudes among primary care physicians and medical subspecialists. *JAMA*. 1998;280(10):905-909.

Lee T, Pappius EM, Goldman L. Impact of inter-physician communication on the effectiveness of medical consultations. *Am J Med.* 1983;74(1):106-112.

Plauth WH, Pantilat SZ, Wachter RM, Fenton CL. Hospitalists' perceptions of their residency training needs: results of a national survey. *Am J Med.* 2001;111(3):247-254.

Rudd P, Siegler M, Byyny RL. Perioperative diabetic consultation: a plead for improved training. *J Med Educ.* 1978;53(7):590-596.

Salerno SM, Hurst FP, Halvorson S, Mercado DL. Principles of effective consultation: an update for the 21st-century consultant. *Arch Intern Med.* 2007;167(3):271-275.

CHAPTER 50

Preoperative Cardiac Risk Assessment and Perioperative Management

Steven L. Cohn, MD, FACP, SFHM

INTRODUCTION

Hospitalists and internists are frequently called upon to perform preoperative medical consultations, and cardiac risk assessment is what is most often requested. Preoperative evaluation is now part of the core curriculum for Hospital Medicine, but when surveyed a number of years ago, many hospitalists felt inadequately trained to do this.

Preoperative cardiac risk assessment has evolved over the past 40 years from a simple global assessment of a patient's physical status (the ASA classification) to multivariate risk analyses (Goldman, Detsky) to a simplified scoring system (Lee RCRI) to guidelines from the American College of Cardiology/American Heart Association, American College of Physicians (ACC/AHA, ACP). The most current of these is the 2014 ACC/AHA guidelines for perioperative cardiac evaluation and management, which was originally published in 1996 and incorporated the RCRI factors in the 2007 update. Using these guidelines and selective cardiac testing (pharmacologic stress tests), physicians are now better able to provide a more accurate assessment of perioperative risk, and the focus has turned to risk reduction strategies. These include revascularization by coronary artery bypass grafting (CABG) or percutaneous coronary intervention (PCI), medical therapy (β-blockers, α-agonists, statins), and other intraoperative measures (normothermia, anesthetic technique). Although surgical and anesthetic techniques have improved and perioperative cardiac events have decreased, operative mortality and cardiac morbidity remain significant, especially among high-risk patients or high-risk procedures.

This chapter reviews the current state of the art for perioperative risk assessment and risk reduction in patients with cardiac disease.

PREOPERATIVE RISK INDICES

Goldman and colleagues published the first large prospective multivariate analysis of preoperative cardiac risk. They identified nine independent predictors of death or major postoperative cardiac complications. These risk factors were assigned points based on their relative importance, and the event rates were correlated with the point total in this risk index. Detsky and colleagues modified this risk index by expanding the list of risk factors and combining this with the pretest probability of complications based on the risk of the surgery itself. Eagle and colleagues identified five factors—age, diabetes mellitus (DM), angina, myocardial infarction (MI), and heart failure—associated with perioperative cardiac events and used these to stratify risk and decide when to do further cardiac testing.

Lee and colleagues identified and validated six factors associated with increased risk of perioperative complications. These factors were high-risk surgery, coronary artery disease (CAD), heart failure, cerebrovascular disease (stroke or transient ischemic attack), DM requiring insulin, and renal insufficiency (creatinine >2.0 mg/dL). These studies, using simple clinical evaluation (history, physical examination, and basic laboratory studies) found many similar factors predicting increased risk of perioperative cardiac complications and helped refine preoperative risk stratification.

The newest risk calculators were derived from the National Surgical Quality Improvement Program (NSQIP) database. The Gupta calculator (http://www.surgicalriskcalculator.com/miorcardiacarrest) was derived from over 200,000 patients and validated on another

250,000 patients in the database. It estimates risk of MI or cardiac arrest based on five independent predictors: type of surgery, dependent functional status, abnormal creatinine, American Society of Anesthesiologists (ASA) class, and increasing age. The American College of Surgeons (ACS) surgical risk calculator (http://riskcalculator.facs.org) was derived from over 1.4 million patients in the NSQIP database. It is more comprehensive and is based on the CPT code for the surgical procedure and an additional 20 variables. It predicts mortality, serious complication, cardiac complications, and several others and states whether these risks are average, above average, or below average.

CLINICAL RISK FACTORS

A detailed history and focused physical examination are key in clinical risk assessment, and a few basic diagnostic tests may also be helpful. Current risk assessment is usually based on the ACC/AHA guidelines which now include the Lee RCRI and the NSQIP risk calculators.

The 2014 ACC/AHA guideline algorithm is now specifically for evaluation of patients with CAD and therefore removed heart failure, arrhythmias, and valvular disease, recommending that those conditions be evaluated and managed based on current guideline directed medical therapy (GDMT). Of the previous "active cardiac conditions," only the presence of an acute coronary syndrome (ACS) remains in the algorithm.

PROCEDURAL RISK

Independent of the patient's clinical risk factors, the type of surgery has its own inherent risk that needs to be taken into account. This concept was used in Detsky's modified cardiac risk index and is also considered in the ACC algorithm. For example, a patient undergoing cataract surgery, a low-risk operation, is unlikely to have a complication even if the patient's clinical risk is high. Conversely a patient with no clinical risk factors undergoing high-risk surgery, such as a Whipple procedure, is more likely to have a postoperative complication than would have been predicted based on clinical pretest probability alone. Therefore, the risk of the surgery itself may alter management and influence the decision to do further testing. The 2014 ACC guidelines now define surgical risk as either low risk (<1% MACE) or elevated risk (>1% MACE) based on a combined procedural and clinical risk. The 2007 ACC guidelines defined three groups for surgical risk—vascular, intermediate, and low. The previous designation of high risk was changed to vascular surgery to reflect that the preponderance of evidence for cardiac testing was done for patients undergoing aortic and major vascular surgery, and the approach to these patients may be somewhat different than that for nonvascular surgery. The intermediate risk category includes most intrathoracic, intra-abdominal, head and neck, orthopedic, and urologic procedures as well as some lower-risk vascular procedures such as carotid endarterectomy and endovascular abdominal aortic aneurysm repair. Low-risk surgery includes procedures not invading the chest or abdomen such as endoscopic or superficial procedures, eye surgery, and breast surgery. The risk indices recommended by the new ACC/AHA guidelines incorporate the type of surgery and those using the NSQIP database include even more specific data based on procedural risk.

PRACTICE POINT

- The ACC/AHA guidelines now classify perioperative risk as low (<1% complication rate) or elevated (>1%) based on combined clinical and procedural risk. They suggest using either the RCRI or NSQIP calculators to determine risk.

FUNCTIONAL CAPACITY

Goldman and colleagues noted that patients with good exercise capacity, even with mild, stable angina, tend to do well. This follows the concept of the ischemic threshold in which a patient developing ischemia on a stress test at a lower exercise level and with a lower rate-pressure product is at higher risk than someone who can perform 8 to 10 metabolic equivalents (METS) before developing symptoms. Reilly and colleagues found that a patient's self-reported exercise capacity correlated with the risk of postoperative complications, and the ACC guidelines use this in their risk assessment algorithm.

PRACTICE POINT

- Because a patient's self-reported exercise capacity correlates with the risk of postoperative cardiac complications, clinicians should factor functional capacity into their risk assessment.

LABORATORY TESTS

Many preoperative screening blood tests are performed unnecessarily, but a few may be helpful in assessing cardiac risk. These include measures of renal function, blood urea nitrogen (BUN) and creatinine, and glucose (as a screen for diabetes). Unless serum potassium is significantly abnormal (<3.0 or >5.5 mEq), it is unlikely to increase risk or alter management. Anemia has been noted as a risk factor in some studies, but there is no evidence that treating it with transfusions alters risk. An electrocardiogram (ECG) looking for evidence of CAD or conduction defects may be of value in at-risk patients. Other findings can either be identified by clinical exam (arrhythmias) or do not change management (left ventricular hypertrophy [LVH], nonspecific ST-T changes).

2014 ACC/AHA ALGORITHM

The new ACC guidelines use a stepwise approach to preoperative cardiac risk evaluation for patients with CAD or risk factors for it using the information obtained from the history, physical examination, and laboratory tests (**Figure 50-1**). The underlying theme is to minimize testing and not to order a test if the result will not change management. The approach is as follows:

1. Is the surgery *emergent* (or *urgent*, meaning within 24 hours)?

   If it is, time does not permit diagnostic testing or revascularization and the patient will proceed to surgery. In the short time period available, the physician can try to medically optimize the patient's problems.

2. Assuming surgery is not emergent, has the patient had an acute coronary syndrome (ACS) (as opposed to any of the *active cardiac conditions* in the 2007 guidelines)?

   If so, elective surgery should be delayed for further diagnostic workup and therapy. Most patients do not have these conditions.

3. Is the estimated perioperative risk of MACE based on combined clinical/surgical risk low (<1%)?

   If it is, the patient should proceed to surgery without any further testing or intervention because we cannot further reduce risk that is already low (<1%).

4. If elevated risk, does the patient have moderate or greater functional capacity (≥4 METS)?

   If so, for the most part, these patients will do well and do not need to undergo further cardiac testing.

5. If the patient has poor or unknown exercise capacity, the next question is whether or not further testing will impact decision

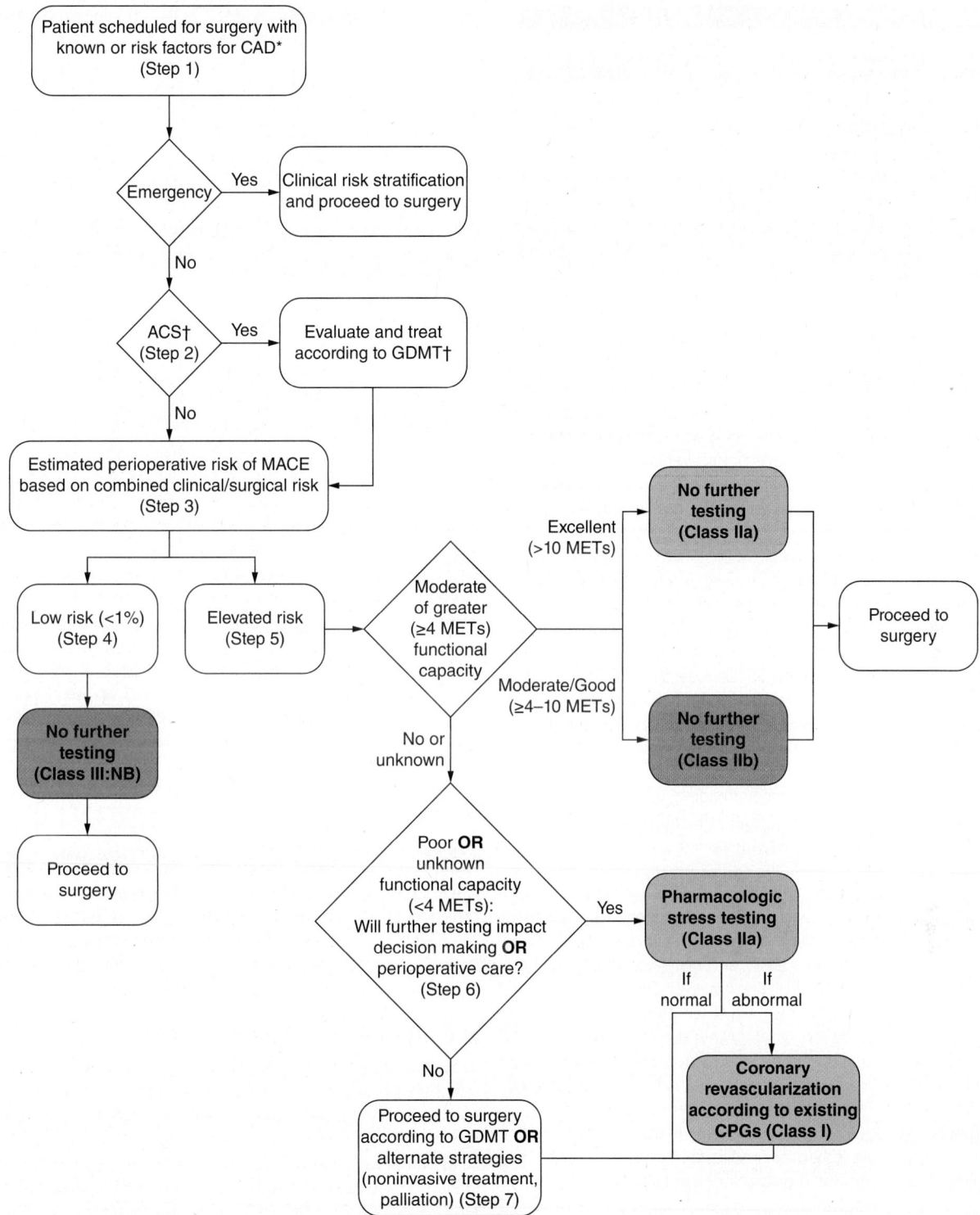

Figure 50-1 *ACC/AHA Stepwise approach to perioperative cardiac assessment for CAD.* (Reproduced, with permission, from Fleisher LA, Fleischmann KE, Auerbach AD, et al. American College of Cardiology; American Heart Association. 2014 ACC/AHA guideline on perioperative cardiovascular evaluation and management of patients undergoing noncardiac surgery: a report of the American College of Cardiology/American Heart Association Task Force on practice guidelines. *J Am Coll Cardiol.* 2014;64(22):e77-e137.)

making or perioperative care. This decision should be based on a discussion with the physician, patient, and perioperative team.

If the answer is yes, then pharmacologic stress testing is indicated. If the stress test is abnormal, coronary angiography and revascularization may be indicated based on the degree of abnormality, and after that, the patient can proceed to surgery following GDMT. Other alternatives include changing to a lesser surgical

procedure, a nonsurgical treatment, or palliation. If the test is normal, proceed to surgery according to GDMT.

6. If further testing will not impact decision making or management, then proceed to surgery according to GDMT or consider alternative as previously mentioned.

These last two steps allow for individualizing management, but are somewhat vague and may lead to significant differences in opinion and approach.

DIAGNOSTIC TESTS

> ### PRACTICE POINT
>
> - The underlying theme of preoperative testing is to minimize unnecessary testing and not to order a test if the result will not change management. A preoperative stress test may be considered for patients with a low functional capacity (<4 METs) undergoing an intermediate-to-high risk procedure, but only if it will change management.

Stress tests were designed to diagnose CAD and myocardial ischemia and not to predict short-term events. Because the pathophysiology of perioperative MIs includes unstable plaque rupture or coronary thrombosis as well as myocardial ischemia related to coronary stenosis and an imbalance of oxygen supply and demand, stress tests are poor at predicting which patients are at increased risk for surgery. Although they are good at identifying a patient with CAD, they have a low positive predictive value (PPV), usually between 15% and 20% for perioperative MI, and most patients, even with an abnormal test, will not have a postoperative cardiac complication. On the other hand, a normal or negative stress test is usually associated with a high negative predictive value (NPV), ranging from 95% to 99%, indicating that there is a low likelihood that these patients will have a perioperative event.

Because many patients with cardiac disease undergoing surgery have suboptimal exercise capacity and would be unable to achieve 85% of their target heart rate on an exercise test, pharmacologic stress testing is usually used. Furthermore, if these patients had adequate exercise capacity, they probably would not be candidates for stress testing in the first place. The tests most commonly used are dobutamine stress echocardiography (DSE) and dipyridamole, adenosine, or regadenoson nuclear imaging (either thallium or technetium). These tests are effective in identifying CAD, but as noted earlier, are poor at identifying patients who will develop postoperative cardiac events and should be used selectively in conjunction with the patient's pretest probability for the results to be meaningful. The test characteristics are influenced by patient selection and pretest probability. In general, results are similar with DSE and dipyridamole thallium (DPT), and test selection should be based on the local expertise available; however, DSE tends to have fewer false-positives except in the case of left bundle branch block (LBBB) where DPT is preferred. On the other hand, DSE is preferred for patients with asthma or chronic obstructive pulmonary disease (COPD) because DPT can cause bronchospasm. The role of cardiac CT or MRI angiography in the perioperative setting is unclear. Resting two-dimensional (2D) echocardiography is not recommended to predict perioperative ischemic complications and should only be used to evaluate valvular heart disease or heart failure.

WHO NEEDS STRESS TESTING BEFORE SURGERY?

The goal of NIT is to further refine clinical judgment and identify patients at significantly increased risk. Bayes theorem can be applied to preoperative evaluation to decide which patients might benefit from stress testing. A patient with a low pretest probability will usually remain at low risk for perioperative complications even if the NIT is positive. Similarly, a patient with high pretest probability will remain at relatively high risk even if the stress test is negative (may represent a false-negative). Therefore, NIT should probably be restricted to intermediate-risk patients where a positive test can move a patient into a higher-risk category and a negative test can reclassify a patient as being at lower risk. The utility of this theoretical approach was supported by L'Italien and colleagues who showed that clinical assessment correlated with outcomes for low- and high-risk patients, and stress test results only changed the probability of complications (confirmed by outcomes) for intermediate-risk patients. Boersma and colleagues also demonstrated that the clinical risk score correlated with outcomes and was rarely changed by stress testing. However, a study by Poldermans and colleagues randomized intermediate risk patients, all of whom were treated with bisoprolol (titrated to a target heart rate of 60 to 65 beats per minute), to preoperative stress testing or no testing. They found no difference in perioperative MI or cardiac death regardless of whether they had a preoperative stress test assuming they were adequately β-blocked. The results of this study beg the question of whether anyone needs NIT if they can be optimally treated medically. However, questions have been raised about the scientific integrity and results of this and other β-blocker studies (DECREASE trials) by the Poldermans group.

WHEN IS PREOPERATIVE CORONARY ANGIOGRAPHY INDICATED?

The ultimate goal of the preoperative evaluation process is to identify the high-risk patient and intervene in some manner to reduce risk of postoperative complications. Assuming stress testing identifies a patient at high risk for postoperative complications, the next step should be to further define risk using cardiac catheterization with a goal of possible revascularization. Otherwise, if the patient is to be treated medically, the stress test was probably unnecessary as it did not change management. Potential candidates for coronary angiography are those high-risk patients with demonstrated ischemia on stress testing or those with unstable coronary syndromes (recent MI, severe angina, or unstable angina) whose clinical risk is high enough to bypass stress testing and who have independent criteria for coronary angiography independent of their need for noncardiac surgery. If coronary angiography demonstrates significant anatomic lesions, a decision must be made regarding revascularization options—PCI or CABG.

RISK REDUCTION STRATEGIES

Once a patient has been identified as being at high risk, either by clinical evaluation or after stress testing or coronary angiography, the next step is to take measures to reduce that risk. The two main options include revascularization or medical therapy or both. The question is whether these therapies are effective.

CORONARY REVASCULARIZATION

Results from the Coronary Artery Surgery Study (CASS) showed that patients who underwent CABG, were symptom free, and then went on to have noncardiac surgery had a lower risk of postoperative mortality and nonfatal MI than similar study patients treated medically. This benefit was only for high-risk surgery, and the protective effect of CABG appeared to last for 4 to 6 years. However, the morbidity and mortality after CABG were not taken into account, and these patients did not have prophylactic CABG in preparation for noncardiac surgery.

These results differ from those of the Coronary Artery Revascularization Prophylaxis (CARP) trial in which patients with stable cardiac symptoms scheduled to undergo elective major vascular surgery were evaluated by NIT, and those with abnormal tests went on to coronary angiography. Patients with suitable anatomy for revascularization were then randomized to medical therapy with or without revascularization (CABG or PCI). Exclusion criteria included >50% stenosis of the left main coronary artery, significant aortic stenosis, or left ventricular ejection fraction (LVEF) less than 20%. Prophylactic revascularization was associated with a mortality of 1.7%, perioperative MI of 5.8%, and reoperation rate of 2.5%. In this particular study, there were no perioperative strokes, but typically this occurs in up to 2%. A subgroup analysis of this study, as well as a recent meta-analysis showed that CABG appeared to be more protective than PCI, possibly because of a more complete revascularization.

Because of the associated morbidity and mortality, prophylactic revascularization would only be expected to benefit patients at high risk undergoing high-risk surgery. However, DECREASE V, a small study of these very high-risk patients (three or more risk factors and extensive stress-induced ischemia on DSE undergoing major vascular surgery) in whom a previous study showed no benefit from perioperative β-blockers, failed to demonstrate improved short- or long-term outcomes with revascularization in addition to optimal medical therapy. Criticisms of these studies raised concerns that the CARP trial patients did not have severe enough CAD, whereas the DECREASE V patients were too sick.

Another trial found a benefit to routine versus selective cardiac catheterization for screening patients before elective aortic surgery. Intention-to-treat analysis showed decreased cardiac mortality and a similar trend in major adverse cardiac events (MACE) in the routine cardiac catheterization group at 30 days and at follow-up 4 years later.

It was felt that prophylactic PCI, with its lower risk for adverse events related to the procedure than CABG, might be better, but there are no studies to confirm this. On the other hand, numerous studies and a meta-analysis reported an increased risk associated with noncardiac surgery soon after PCI. This is related to stent thrombosis in patients who have prematurely discontinued the recommended course of dual antiplatelet therapy (DAPT) and, to a lesser degree, bleeding in patients who were taking aspirin and clopidogrel. The ACC/AHA guidelines recommend delaying elective surgery for at least 2 weeks after balloon angioplasty, 4 to 6 weeks after placement of a bare metal stent (BMS), and 12 months after a drug-eluting stent (DES) in order to complete the course of DAPT. Should surgery be required before these time intervals in a patient who had PCI, the recommended options, in priority order, are to try to perform the surgery on dual antiplatelet therapy if possible, to continue aspirin but discontinue the second antiplatelet agent (discontinue clopidogrel 5 to 7 days before surgery, prasugrel 7 days before, and ticagrelor 5 days before), or to discontinue both antiplatelet drugs 5 to 7 days before surgery. However, the 2014 ACC/AHA guidelines now state that elective noncardiac surgery may be considered with DES after 180 days of DAPT if the risk of surgical delay is greater than the expected risks of ischemia and stent thrombosis (IIb). The antiplatelet therapy should be resumed as soon as possible after surgery, assuming adequate hemostasis has been assured.

PRACTICE POINT

The ACC/AHA guidelines recommend delaying elective surgery for patients with recent stent placement at least:

- Two weeks after balloon angioplasty
- Four to six weeks after placement of a bare metal stent (BMS)
- Twelve months after a drug-eluting stent (DES)* in order to complete the course of dual antiplatelet therapy

*Except if after 6 months, the risk of delaying surgery exceeds expected risks of ischemia and stent thrombosis, surgery may be considered.

■ MEDICAL THERAPY

Beta-blockers

Note: The scientific integrity of the DECREASE trials from the Poldermans group has been questioned but they will be mentioned in the text that follows to illustrate the controversy.

Early studies with prophylactic β-blockers demonstrated beneficial effects. Mangano and colleagues randomized 200 patients undergoing various operations to placebo or atenolol, started immediately preoperatively, titrated to a heart rate of 55 to 65 beats per minute and continued for less than 7 days postoperatively. There was less ischemia in the atenolol-treated group but no reduction in short-term outcomes of death or nonfatal MI. However, surviving patients in the β-blocker group went on to have fewer cardiovascular events by 2 years. Poldermans and colleagues randomized 112 patients with abnormal DSEs undergoing major vascular surgery to placebo or bisoprolol, started at least 7 days preoperatively, titrated to a heart rate between 55 and 65 beats per minute, and continued for at least 30 days postoperatively. The trial was stopped early because the bisoprolol-treated group had a significant reduction in postoperative MI and cardiac death (3% vs 34%). Despite the small numbers of patients in these trials and methodologic criticisms, various agencies and society guidelines began recommending prophylactic β-blockers.

Three subsequent studies involving approximately 1500 patients (POBBLE, DIPOM, MaVS) using metoprolol, started at most 1 day before surgery and not titrated to a specific heart rate, showed no benefit in various cardiovascular outcomes. Lindenauer and colleagues using an administrative database of over 600,000 patients, reported that being on a β-blocker within 2 days of surgery was associated with decreased in-hospital mortality in high- but not low-risk patients (stratified by RCRI score).

The POISE trial was expected to resolve this controversy but instead raised more questions. In this study over 8000 patients with atherosclerotic heart disease (ASHD) or risk factors for it who were scheduled for various surgical procedures were randomized to metoprolol controlled release (CR) or placebo. Patients received the first dose (metoprolol CR 100 mg or placebo) 2 to 6 hours before surgery followed by a second dose (100 mg) within 6 hours after the end of surgery, and then a maintenance dose of 200 mg daily started 12 hours after the postoperative dose. The drug was withheld for heart rate less than 45 beats per minute or systolic blood pressure (BP) less than 100 mm Hg and then restarted at half the dose 12 hours later if BP and pulse improved. Primary outcome, a composite of cardiac death, nonfatal MI, and cardiac arrest, was significantly better in the metoprolol-treated group (see Figure 50-1) but was primarily due to a reduction in nonfatal MIs. However, this benefit came at the expense of a significant increase in stroke and total mortality (two of the secondary outcomes) in the treatment group, in part due to more episodes of hypotension and bradycardia. Mortality was increased in patients with sepsis, and stroke risk appeared to be increased in patients with prior strokes and intraoperative hypotension. This study generated significant commentary and criticism, mainly related to the high dose of metoprolol that was started shortly before surgery in β-blocker-naïve patients, many of whom underwent emergency surgery or had sepsis. This tempered the enthusiasm for prophylactic β-blockers.

The DECREASE IV trial using bisoprolol, started well in advance (median 34 days) of surgery and titrated to a heart rate between 50 and 70 beats per minute reduced cardiac death and nonfatal MI in intermediate risk patients. If β-blockers are to be beneficial based on the positive although controversial trials, it appears that they need to be started more than 1 and probably at least 7 days before surgery and potentially titrated to a heart rate somewhere in the range of 55 to 70 beats per minute to minimize the risk of significant hypotension or bradycardia (although most patients remained on their initial β-blocker dose). Higher-risk patients or those undergoing vascular or higher-risk surgical procedures would be most likely to benefit.

Multiple meta-analyses have come to different conclusions based on the studies included or excluded in the analysis. Although the final answer is not in, the ACC/AHA published a systematic review of randomized controlled trials with perioperative β-blockers analyzing the results with and without inclusion of the DECREASE and POISE trials. Their recommendations were to continue β-blockers in patients taking them chronically, that it may be reasonable to begin them before surgery in patients with ischemia on stress testing or with three or more RCRI factors, and that initiating β-blockers in patients with other indications but no RCRI factors was of uncertain benefit. If initiating β-blockers preoperatively, they should be started far enough in advance to assess safety and tolerability. This should be done more than 1 day before surgery and not started on the day of surgery, which was found to be harmful. Although not specifically recommended in the ACC/AHA guidelines, a cardioselective β-blocker (bisoprolol or atenolol) was recommended over metoprolol by the ESC guidelines.

PRACTICE POINT

The 2014 ACC/AHA recommendations for administration of β-blockers

Class I recommendations:

- Continue β-blockers for patients already on them.

Class IIa recommendations:

- Reasonable for management of β-blockers postoperatively to be guided by clinical circumstances, regardless of when they were started preoperatively.

Class IIb recommendations:

- Reasonable to start β-blockers before surgery in patients with ischemia on stress testing or with three or more RCRI factors.
- Usefulness uncertain for patients with other long-term indications for β-blockers but no RCRI factors.
- Reasonable to initiate β-blockers far enough in advance of surgery to assess safety and tolerability—preferably more than 1 day before surgery.

Class III recommendations (Harm):

- Do not start β-blockers on the day of surgery.

Alpha-2 agonists and aspirin

Although some earlier studies suggested that clonidine might be beneficial in reducing postoperative cardiac complications, the POISE-2 trial, which randomized 10,010 patients to clonidine, aspirin, both, or neither before noncardiac surgery, demonstrated that prophylactic clonidine did not reduce MI or cardiac death but was associated with an increase in nonfatal cardiac arrest and hypotension. The ACC/AHA guidelines state that clonidine is not recommended to prevent perioperative cardiac events. However, in patients already taking clonidine it should be continued to prevent rebound hypertension.

The two aspirin groups—patients already on it and those who were aspirin naïve—also showed no benefit in terms of reducing MI or death but did have an increased risk of bleeding. The earlier the aspirin was started postoperatively, the higher the bleeding risk. Patients with cardiac stents who had not completed their course of antiplatelet therapy, recent strokes, and patients undergoing carotid endarterectomy were excluded. Some controversy exists because there was no subgroup analysis of patients on aspirin for primary versus secondary prevention or for higher versus lower bleeding risk procedures. The ACC/AHA guidelines state that the risk of a cardiovascular event needs to be weighed against the risk of a bleeding event in determining whether or not to continue aspirin in patients already on it (for secondary prevention).

Statins

In addition to lowering cholesterol, statins have a number of so-called pleotropic effects. These include reduced platelet aggregation, improved endothelial function, and reduced inflammation. It is thought that this latter effect in particular may help stabilize plaques and prevent plaque rupture, which might lead to an MI.

Most observational studies report that perioperative statin use is beneficial in reducing postoperative cardiac complications and death in both cardiac and noncardiac surgery. A meta-analysis by Kapoor and colleagues confirmed this benefit; however, there are few randomized controlled trials. The first of these, a small study of 100 patients using atorvastatin 20 mg started 30 days before surgery, demonstrated a beneficial effect on a composite outcome including some weaker end points.

The DECREASE III trial randomized 497 patients to fluvastatin 80 mg extended release or placebo started approximately 1 month before vascular surgery and showed that the statin-treated group had less ischemia and a statistically significant reduction in the composite end point of cardiac death and nonfatal MI. It also demonstrated that statins reduced LDL and total cholesterol, multiple inflammatory markers including C-reactive protein (CRP) and interleukin (IL)-6, but also were safe in that there were no cases of rhabdomyolysis or significant hepatic injury. Although no safety issues were found in a review of statin use in vascular surgery patients, the drug manufacturers still recommend discontinuing statins before major surgery due to these potential safety concerns. However, the ACC/AHA recommends continuing them perioperatively as the potential benefit outweighs the theoretical risk. Based on the DECREASE III trial it appears that patients who are not on a statin but are scheduled for vascular surgery would benefit from starting a statin preoperatively. However, the fluvastatin arm of the DECREASE IV trial in intermediate risk patients only showed a trend toward decreased MI and death that was not statistically significant. The ACC/AHA also states that preoperative initiation of statin therapy is reasonable in patients undergoing vascular surgery and may be considered in patients with clinical indications (CAD, DM, peripheral arterial disease (PAD), hyperlipidemia) undergoing elevated risk surgery. Unanswered questions regarding perioperative statin use are whether this is a class effect, what dose should be used, how long in advance to start it prophylactically for it to be effective, and which patients are most likely to benefit from them.

OTHER CARDIOVASCULAR CONDITIONS

■ HYPERTENSION

Hypertension is at best a minor risk factor. Although various recommendations mention blood pressures (diastolic BP > 110 mm Hg or systolic BP > 180 mm Hg) when cancellation of elective surgery should be considered or which might be associated with increased risk, there is no hard evidence to support them. Hypertensive patients are more likely to have more labile blood pressure perioperatively and intraoperative hypotension. The etiology of the hypertension, and presence of end organ damage are more likely to be associated with any cardiac morbidity than the preoperative blood pressure itself.

Most antihypertensive medications should be continued, including on the morning of surgery, with the possible exceptions of diuretics and angiotensin-converting enzyme (ACE) inhibitors or angiotensin receptor blockers (ARBs). Of note, the 2014 ACC/AHA guidelines state that continuation of ACEIs or ARBs is reasonable perioperatively although many anesthesiologists recommend stopping them at least 10 hours before surgery due to concerns for potential hypotension with induction of anesthesia. If they are stopped, they should be restarted as soon as safe postoperatively.

■ ARRHYTHMIAS

Hemodynamically significant arrhythmias including tachyarrhythmias (rapid atrial fibrillation (AF), supraventricular tachycardia (SVT), ventricular tachycardia (VT)) as well as bradyarrhythmias (symptomatic sinus bradycardia, high-degree atrioventricular (AV) block) should be evaluated and treated as per GDMT before elective surgery.

■ HEART FAILURE

Heart failure is a predictor of postoperative MACE. Systolic and symptomatic heart failure carry a greater risk than diastolic or asymptomatic dysfunction. Decompensated heart failure requires further evaluation and treatment as per GDMT before proceeding with elective surgery. Beta-blockers should not be started preoperatively in these patients, and in a subgroup analysis of the CIBIS II study, patients with heart failure had little benefit from β-blockers.

■ VALVULAR HEART DISEASE

Patients with valvular heart disease should be evaluated and treated as per GDMT. The lesion most likely to be associated with perioperative cardiac complications is symptomatic, severe aortic stenosis (AS). Patients with a systolic murmur suggestive of AS, particularly if they have chest pain, dyspnea, or syncope, should have a 2D echocardiogram performed. If they have symptomatic severe AS and the planned noncardiac surgery is elective, the recommendation is for valve replacement. Should the patient refuse or if the surgery is more urgent, it has been possible to get most of these patients through surgery successfully using medical therapy and intraoperative monitoring. Patients with asymptomatic aortic stenosis tend to tolerate surgery much better than those with symptoms and comparable severity of stenosis. Mitral stenosis, when associated with atrial fibrillation and heart failure, may also increase risk, but most of the other valvular lesions do not require surgical intervention before noncardiac surgery. The ACC/AHA guidelines state that it is reasonable to perform elevated risk elective noncardiac surgery in patients with asymptomatic valvular disease (even if severe) with appropriate intraoperative and postoperative monitoring. Pulmonary hypertension is now being recognized as a risk factor as well, but studies are limited.

Endocarditis prophylaxis is only indicated for patients undergoing dental and upper respiratory procedures who have a prosthetic valve, previous endocarditis, complex congenital heart disease that has not been repaired (or was repaired in the past 6 months), or valvular disease in a transplanted heart.

BIOMARKERS

Elevated natriuretic peptides (BNP, NT-proBNP) preoperatively and postoperatively have been associated with MACE. These tests have been used in conjunction with the RCRI and may provide incremental value in risk assessment. However, which test to use, when to obtain it, what cutoff is best, and what to do with the results are not known, and at this time their role, if any, in preoperative risk assessment is unclear.

Most postoperative myocardial infarctions are not associated with chest pain, which raises the question of whether patients should be screened postoperatively with troponins or EKGs. An entity termed MINS—myocardial injury after noncardiac surgery—defined as an elevated troponin presumed to be of ischemic etiology but not requiring diagnostic criteria for an MI, is associated with adverse outcomes. However, it is unclear what to do in these situations and whether or not any treatment is beneficial or harmful. For these reasons the ACC/

AHA did not recommend routine postoperative screening in patients without signs or symptoms of myocardial ischemia.

CONCLUSION

Using the ACC guidelines and risk calculators, the patient can be classified as low versus elevated risk based on combined clinical and surgical risk. The physician can then decide not only whether further testing is indicated but also whether it is likely to change management. Prophylactic revascularization is rarely necessary just to get a patient through surgery, and the majority of the patients will be managed medically. It is important for future studies to determine optimal use of β-blockers, statins, and other therapies in order to have patients in their optimal medical condition prior to elective noncardiac surgery to reduce postoperative complications.

SUGGESTED READINGS

Bilimoria KY, Liu Y, Paruch JL, et al. Development and evaluation of the universal ACS NSQIP surgical risk calculator: a decision aid and informed consent tool for patients and surgeons. *J Am Coll Surg.* 2013;217(5):833-842.

Fleisher LA, Fleischmann KE, Auerbach AD, et al. American College of Cardiology; American Heart Association. 2014 ACC/AHA guideline on perioperative cardiovascular evaluation and management of patients undergoing noncardiac surgery: a report of the American College of Cardiology/American Heart Association Task Force on practice guidelines. *J Am Coll Cardiol.* 2014;64(22):e77-e137.

Grines CL, Bonow RO, Casey DE Jr, et al. Prevention of premature discontinuation of dual antiplatelet therapy in patients with coronary artery stents: a science advisory from the American Heart Association, American College of Cardiology, Society for Cardiovascular Angiography and Interventions, American College of Surgeons, and American Dental Association, with representation from the American College of Physicians. *J Am Coll Cardiol.* 2007;49(6):734-739.

Gupta PK, Gupta H, Sundaram A, et al. Development and validation of a risk calculator for prediction of cardiac risk after surgery. *Circulation.* 2011;124(4):381-387.

Kristensen SD, Knuuti J, Saraste A, et al. 2014 ESC/ESA Guidelines on non-cardiac surgery: cardiovascular assessment and management: the Joint Task Force on non-cardiac surgery: cardiovascular assessment and management of the European Society of Cardiology (ESC) and the European Society of Anaesthesiology (ESA). *Eur Heart J.* 2014;35(35):2383-2431.

L'Italien GJ, Paul SD, Hendel RC, et al. Development and validation of a Bayesian model for perioperative cardiac risk assessment in a cohort of 1,081 vascular surgical candidates. *J Am Coll Cardiol.* 1996;27(4):779-786.

Nuttall GA, Brown MJ, Stombaugh JW, et al. Time and cardiac risk of surgery after bare-metal stent percutaneous coronary intervention. *Anesthesiology.* 2008;109(4):588-595.

Rabbitts JA, Nuttall GA, Brown MJ, et al. Cardiac risk of noncardiac surgery after percutaneous coronary intervention with drug-eluting stents. *Anesthesiology.* 2008;109(4):596-604.

Wilson W, Taubert KA, Gewitz M, et al. Prevention of infective endocarditis: guidelines from the American Heart Association: a guideline from the American Heart Association Rheumatic Fever, Endocarditis, and Kawasaki Disease Committee, Council on Cardiovascular Disease in the Young, and the Council on Clinical Cardiology, Council on Cardiovascular Surgery and Anesthesia, and the Quality of Care and Outcomes Research Interdisciplinary Working Group. *Circulation.* 2007;116(15):1736-1754.

Perioperative Pulmonary Risk Assessment and Management

Kurt Pfeifer, MD, FACP, FHM
Gerald W. Smetana, MD, FACP

Key Clinical Questions

1. What risk factors predict postoperative pulmonary complications?
2. What role does diagnostic testing play in the evaluation of perioperative pulmonary risk?
3. What objective tools are available for performing a preoperative pulmonary risk assessment?
4. What strategies are effective to reduce and manage postoperative pulmonary risk?

INTRODUCTION

A comprehensive preoperative evaluation must include assessment of the risk of postoperative pulmonary complications. While few would argue this point, pulmonary risk is often underappreciated as clinicians typically focus the majority of their energy on the preoperative cardiac evaluation and preventing venous thromboembolic complications. Highlighting the risk of this approach, postoperative respiratory problems occur with similar frequency and greater morbidity than cardiovascular complications.

Pulmonary complications following anesthesia and surgery result from central nervous system suppression and altered respiratory dynamics. Administration of sedating agents and neuromuscular blockade exposes the patient to the risk of aspiration. Furthermore, regardless of the type of anesthetic technique utilized, patients will experience a reduction in lung volumes perioperatively. Reduction in lung volumes is the primary mechanism that may lead to atelectasis and predispose a patient to the additional complications of pneumonia and respiratory failure. This reduction in lung volumes is greatest for patients undergoing thoracic and upper abdominal surgery. **Table 51-1** lists specific postoperative pulmonary complications and diagnostic considerations for each.

RISK STRATIFICATION

Clinicians intuitively recognize several risk factors for pulmonary complications, but some predictors of postoperative respiratory problems are not obvious. Additionally, clinicians may struggle with the appropriate utilization of preoperative pulmonary diagnostic testing. Recently published risk indices and practice guidelines provide valuable assistance in the identification of risk factors and the performance of evidence-based preoperative evaluation.

■ PATIENT-SPECIFIC RISK FACTORS

Several different patient characteristics increase postoperative pulmonary risk (**Table 51-2**). While most of these patient-specific factors are nonmodifiable, their identification is important for providing patients, surgeons and anesthesiologists with an accurate assessment of perioperative risk and to identify patients for whom one should employ risk reduction strategies.

Chronic lung disease

Multiple studies have identified chronic obstructive pulmonary disease (COPD) as a significant risk factor for postoperative respiratory problems. However, the risk attributable to COPD is lower than several other patient-related risk factors, including total functional dependence, obstructive sleep apnea and age 70 years or greater. The impact of other forms of chronic lung disease on perioperative pulmonary risk has been much less studied, but at least one retrospective review of interstitial lung disease patients found them to have rates of postoperative pneumonia higher than the general population. Additionally, pulmonary hypertension has recently been shown to increase the risk of postoperative pulmonary complications as well as perioperative mortality and cardiac complications.

Advanced age

Advanced age is a major independent predictor of pulmonary complications. Contrary to previous belief, this risk is not a result of the cumulative morbidities associated with aging. Elevated risk begins

TABLE 51-1 Common Postoperative Pulmonary Complications

Condition	Diagnostic Considerations
Atelectasis	• Potential cause of *mild* hypoxia • Generally not a cause of postoperative fever or moderate to severe hypoxia
Pneumonia	• Diagnostic criteria vary—utilize same as nosocomial pneumonia • Often polymicrobial—common pathogens include *Pseudomonas, Staphylococcus aureus, Streptococcus pneumoniae* and enteric Gram-negative bacilli • Though aspiration of secretions is a likely contributor to development, anaerobic bacteria rarely cause postoperative pneumonia
Respiratory failure	• Inability to wean off ventilator support within 48 h of surgery or unplanned reintubation • Typically, a combination of hypoxic and hypercapnic respiratory failure
COPD exacerbation	• Diagnostic criteria and assessment same as in nonoperative population

COPD, chronic obstructive pulmonary disease.

at age 50 and is especially high in patients aged 70 years and older (adjusted odds ratio of 3). Recognition that age, even in the absence of other comorbidities, is an important source of pulmonary risk is critical as the population ages and more elderly patients undergo surgical procedures. The consequence of these observations is that even healthy older patients are at risk for postoperative pulmonary complications.

Smoking

Cigarette smoking is associated with increased postoperative pulmonary complications, but the degree of risk elevation is actually

TABLE 51-2 Patient-Specific Risk Factors for Postoperative Pulmonary Complications

Chronic obstructive pulmonary disease
Advanced age (age >50)
Functional dependence
Comorbid disease (ASA class ≥2)
Smoking
Obstructive sleep apnea
Pulmonary hypertension
Congestive heart failure
Impaired sensorium
Respiratory infection within past month
Preoperative anemia and/or transfusion
Preoperative sepsis
Preoperative hypoxemia
Consumption of >2 alcoholic drinks per day within 2 wk
Preoperative transfusion of >4 units of packed red blood cells
Chronic corticosteroid use
Weight loss of >10% within 6 mo
History of stroke

ASA, American Society of Anesthesiologists.

less than that from most other patient-specific factors including COPD. The adjusted odds ratio (OR) for pulmonary complications in smokers is 1.3, and the risk is greatest among active smokers and recent (<4 weeks) quitters. Patients who have abstained from smoking for at least 2 months have similar rates of postoperative pulmonary complications as nonsmokers. Clinicians should consider a recent history of cigarette smoking to be a moderate predictor of pulmonary complications.

Medical comorbidities

As the number of comorbid illnesses increases, so does the risk of perioperative complications. The American Society of Anesthesiologists (ASA) classification system is easy-to-use and predicts the risk of postoperative respiratory problems, as well as overall morbidity and mortality. Compared to ASA class I patients (no comorbidities), patients with an ASA class of II or greater have a nearly five-fold increase in the rate of postoperative pulmonary complications. The risk increases with each higher ASA class.

Functional status

Large multivariate studies have also identified dependence on others for assistance with activities of daily living as a significant risk factor for postoperative pulmonary complications. The contribution of functional dependence to perioperative pulmonary risk is greater than cigarette smoking and chronic lung disease. For patients with a completely dependent functional status, the adjusted OR for respiratory complications is greater than 4, and for partial functional dependence the adjusted OR is approximately 2.

Congestive heart failure

Congestive heart failure (CHF) is not only an obvious risk factor for perioperative cardiac complications but also a predictor of postoperative respiratory failure. Although the cause of respiratory failure may be CHF-related pulmonary edema, a history of heart failure is nonetheless an independent risk factor for pulmonary complications that confers a relative risk of approximately 6 in the geriatric population.

Obstructive sleep apnea

For years, clinicians have presumed that obstructive sleep apnea (OSA) increases the risk of postoperative complications. Only recently have high-quality studies established this to be true. In several studies OSA patients have increased rates of postoperative pulmonary complications as well as statistically significant increases in cardiac complications and unplanned ICU admissions. This risk extends not only to airway compromise in the immediate postoperative period, but also traditional postoperative pulmonary complications including pneumonia and respiratory failure. Other recent studies also suggest that patients who screen positive for OSA but do not yet carry the diagnosis have an increased risk of postoperative complications. For example, patients with at least two clinical features of OSA (snoring, crowded oropharynx, daytime somnolence, or witnessed apneas) who have abnormal overnight oximetry are more likely to develop postoperative hypoxemia or airway management problems than patients without these features. Whether formally diagnosed or suspected based on clinical features, OSA should be considered at least a moderate risk factor for perioperative respiratory problems.

Other risk factors

In addition to the previously described risk factors, several other patient characteristics have been less consistently linked to postoperative pulmonary complications. For instance, one large study found consumption of more than two alcoholic drinks per day within 2 weeks of surgery, recent weight loss exceeding 10% of total body weight, chronic corticosteroid use, preoperative transfusion of more than 4 units of blood, acute alteration of mental status, and a history of stroke to be modest risk factors for postoperative pneumonia. More recent risk models have not identified these as independent predictors but demonstrated that respiratory infection within a month prior to surgery as well as preoperative sepsis, hypoxemia and anemia significantly contribute to the risk of postoperative pulmonary complications.

Factors not associated with increased pulmonary risk

Notably absent from the described risk factors are four conditions often mistaken as predictors of postoperative pulmonary complications: well-controlled asthma, obesity, diabetes mellitus and immunosuppression. Although a potential relationship between perioperative pulmonary risk and morbid obesity and/or asthma has been assumed by some clinicians, multivariate investigations have consistently found no such correlation. The current literature provides little data on the contributions of immunosuppression and diabetes mellitus to pulmonary surgical complications.

■ PROCEDURE-SPECIFIC RISK FACTORS

Patient characteristics impact perioperative pulmonary risk significantly, but procedure-specific factors are even greater predictors of postoperative pneumonia and respiratory failure (**Table 51-3**). Unlike the majority of patient-specific risk factors, some of these surgery-related factors may be modifiable.

Surgery type

The type of surgery is the most important determinant of postsurgical pulmonary risk. As expected, intrathoracic procedures and surgeries in close proximity to the diaphragm carry the highest risk of postoperative pulmonary complications. Head and neck operations are high-risk procedures due in part to impairment of the upper airway. Restriction of diaphragmatic motion by pain from abdominal procedures leads to reduced lung volumes, the precursor of pulmonary complications. Particularly high risks are esophageal and aortic surgeries.

Anesthetic technique

Several studies have identified general endotracheal anesthesia (GETA) as an independent predictor of postoperative pulmonary complications. In some analyses, neuraxial blockade (spinal and epidural anesthesia), either alone or in combination with GETA, has been associated with lower rates of postoperative morbidity and mortality compared to GETA alone. However, randomized controlled trials (RCTs) have not consistently identified GETA as a risk factor. While these data suggest general anesthesia may contribute to pulmonary risk, selection of anesthetic technique is the primary responsibility of the anesthesiologist and is dependent on multiple other factors outside the purview of the hospitalist. The medical consultant should share his or her risk assessment with the anesthesiologist so they can incorporate this into anesthesia planning, but in general should defer the selection of anesthetic type to the anesthesiologist.

Other risk factors

Regardless of the surgical site or anesthetic technique, procedures performed on an emergent basis carry a higher risk of respiratory complications. Surgeries with duration greater than 2 to 3 hours are also associated with an increased risk for postoperative pneumonia and respiratory failure. There is probably no difference in risk between laparoscopic versus open surgeries; decisions regarding

TABLE 51-3 Procedure-Specific Risk Factors for Postoperative Pulmonary Complications

Surgery type	Head and neck
	Thoracic, including esophageal
	Abdominal
	Abdominal aortic aneurysm repair
	Neurosurgical
	Vascular
General anesthesia	
Nasogastric intubation	
Emergency surgery	
Prolonged surgery (>2-3 h)	

the surgical approach should be made by the surgeon based on other factors.

PRACTICE POINT

Strongest Predictors of Postoperative Pulmonary Complications

The strongest predictors of postoperative pulmonary complications are:

- **Surgery type**: A location anywhere from the mouth to upper abdomen disrupts the airway and/or normal respiratory dynamics.
- **Advanced age**: Beginning at age 50, perioperative pulmonary risk begins to increase and becomes particularly high in patients over the age of 70 years.
- **Obstructive sleep apnea**: Known or presumed OSA, based on a positive screen, is an important risk factor.
- **Functional dependence**: Reliance upon others for assistance with activities of daily living increases the risk of multiple complications, including postoperative respiratory problems.

■ DIAGNOSTIC STUDIES

A thorough history and physical examination are the cornerstones of the preoperative evaluation. In most instances, diagnostic testing adds little to the risk assessment as established by clinical evaluation. Testing has a role when the risk is uncertain after history and physical examination.

Chest radiography

Chest radiography is part of many clinicians' routine preoperative evaluation despite evidence that chest x-ray results rarely change perioperative management. Abnormalities on preoperative chest radiography are relatively common, occurring on 10% to 20% of x-rays. However, a minority of these findings are unexpected based on the clinician's physical assessment and history, and an even smaller number influence perioperative care. Clinicians should reserve chest imaging for the same indications as in the nonoperative setting: evaluation of new or changed cardiopulmonary symptoms. As part of the American Board of Internal Medicine's Choosing Wisely initiative, three different professional societies have specifically recommended not obtaining preoperative chest radiographs in patients without clinical findings suggestive of pulmonary abnormalities.

Arterial blood gas analysis

Early studies of preoperative arterial blood gas (ABG) analysis suggested that hypercarbia and hypoxemia predicted postoperative pulmonary complications. Subsequent reviews concluded that clinical assessment was equally accurate in predicting postsurgical respiratory problems. Taking into account that no arterial CO_2 or O_2 value is an absolute contraindication to surgery, clinicians should perform ABG analysis only if the results will significantly influence perioperative management (eg, excluding hypercarbia and respiratory acidosis in a patient with COPD and increased shortness of breath).

Pulmonary function testing

Formal pulmonary function testing has an established role in the preoperative evaluation of patients before lung resection, but its role in nonthoracic surgery is questionable. Analogous to ABG analysis, initial studies of preoperative spirometry suggested it was useful for predicting postoperative morbidity, but later data comparing spirometry to history and physical examination showed no clear incremental benefit from pulmonary function testing. Further, no spirometric values are a prohibitory threshold for noncardiothoracic surgery. Indications for pulmonary function testing are the same as in the general setting: evaluation of unexplained respiratory symptoms and characterization of lung disease when it is unclear if a patient's airflow obstruction is optimally reduced.

PRACTICE POINT

Diagnostic Testing for Perioperative Pulmonary Risk

- Diagnostic testing rarely adds value to perioperative pulmonary risk assessment in noncardiothoracic surgery. A thorough history and physical examination is sufficient in almost all cases.

▪ RISK ASSESSMENT TOOLS

In recent years, the scientific community has paid more attention to the importance of postoperative pulmonary complications. The result has been the generation of practical risk assessment tools.

In 2006, the American College of Physicians developed clinical guidelines for perioperative pulmonary risk assessment and reduction for patients undergoing noncardiothoracic surgery. This systematic review provides a valuable resource for performing an evidence-based preoperative evaluation. Several perioperative pulmonary risk prediction models have also been developed to assist clinical risk stratification. Most of these are restricted to either specific types of surgery or unique respiratory complications (eg, acute respiratory distress syndrome), but three recent models show promise for being fairly generalizable.

Using data from the American College of Surgeons National Surgical Quality Improvement Program, Gupta and colleagues developed separate models for prediction of postoperative respiratory failure and pneumonia. Predictive risk factors for postoperative respiratory failure were: site of surgery, emergency surgery, ASA classification, sepsis and functional status (ie, ability to perform activities of daily living). The pneumonia risk model used the same variables except that age, COPD and smoking were included and emergent surgery was not. Both models were incorporated into risk calculators that are freely available online (www.surgicalriskcalculator.com). The Gupta postoperative pulmonary risk calculators performed very well in their initial study but have not been externally validated.

In 2010, Canet and colleagues developed the ARISCAT index for predicting postsurgical pulmonary complications. This model uses seven predictive factors, each with a weighted score based on its risk contribution (**Table 51-4**). Tallying the score in this model the

TABLE 51-4 ARISCAT Index for Predicting Postoperative Pulmonary Complications

Risk Factor		Risk Score
Age (y)	51-80	3
	>80	16
Preoperative SpO2 (%)	91-95	8
	<91	24
Respiratory infection in past month		17
Location of surgery	Upper abdominal	15
	Thoracic	24
Duration of surgery (h)	>2-3	16
	>3	23
Emergency surgery		8
Preoperative hemoglobin ≤10 g/dL		11

Risk Class	Risk Score	Postoperative Pulmonary Complications (%)
Low	<26	1.6-3.4
Intermediate	26-44	13-13.3
High	>44	38-42.1

Used with permission from Canet J, Gallart L, Gomar C, et al. *Anesthesiology.* 2010;113(6):1338-1350.

clinician can determine which of three different risk classes a patient fits into. The ARISCAT index was originally derived and validated from a geographically localized population but has subsequently been validated in a sample of patients from across Europe.

Although the above risk indices are helpful for estimating risk in the general population, they do not account for risks associated with obstructive sleep apnea. The ASA recommends screening all surgical patients for OSA. Several tools for this purpose are available, including the STOP-BANG, Berlin and Flemons surveys. The STOP-BANG questionnaire accurately identifies patients at risk for moderate to severe OSA and postoperative complications (**Table 51-5**). A score of 5 or higher (of eight possible points) increases the likelihood of moderate to severe OSA, as well as rates of perioperative complications.

TABLE 51-5 STOP-BANG Screening for Obstructive Sleep Apnea

S	**Snoring**: Do you **snore loudly** (loud enough to be heard through closed doors or your bed-partner elbows you for snoring at night)?
T	**Tired**: Do you often feel **tired**, **fatigued** or **sleepy** during the daytime (such as falling asleep during driving)?
O	**Observed**: Has anyone **observed** you **stop breathing** or **choking/gasping** during your sleep?
P	**Pressure**: Do you have or are being treated for **high blood pressure**?
B	**BMI > 35 kg/m²?**
A	**Age older than 50 y?**
N	**Neck size large?** For male, shirt collar ≥17 in/43 cm; for female, shirt collar ≥16 in/41 cm?
G	**Gender = male**

Used with permission from University Health Network.

RISK REDUCTION STRATEGIES

Many pulmonary risk factors are nonmodifiable, but for patients with elevated perioperative risk several evidence-based risk reduction methods exist. Although some of these strategies are outside the scope of hospitalists, medical consultants should be aware of all potential risk reduction interventions. For all patients with increased pulmonary risk, special consideration should be given to the patient's postoperative triage (home vs general hospital admission vs intensive care unit placement), and the hospitalist should incorporate the patient's preoperative pulmonary risk assessment into postoperative care decision making. For instance, more aggressive work-up of postoperative fever or hypoxia may be initiated in the patient who was preoperatively assessed to be at increased risk for respiratory failure or pneumonia.

■ PREOPERATIVE SMOKING CESSATION

The role of smoking cessation in perioperative risk reduction remains an area of debate. Some studies have shown that preoperative smoking cessation decreases the risk of postsurgical respiratory complications, while others have demonstrated similar pulmonary morbidity between smokers and nonsmokers. An older study actually suggested an increase in postoperative pulmonary complications if smoking cessation occurred shortly before surgery. Recent meta-analyses of preoperative smoking cessation have identified no statistically significant increase in risk for patients who quit smoking less than 4 to 8 weeks before surgery. Patients who stop smoking more than 4 weeks prior to surgery have a significant decrease in postoperative pulmonary complications. Randomized controlled trials have confirmed that smoking cessation interventions started at least 1 month before surgery lower the incidence of overall complications. The greatest benefit occurs with durations of cessation of at least 8 weeks before surgery. Preoperative smoking cessation interventions (including the use of tobacco cessation pharmacotherapy) cause no harm, and increase rates of long-term abstinence. For any hospitalized surgical patient, clinicians should advise smoking cessation.

■ ANESTHETIC TECHNIQUES

Anesthesia considerations are the responsibility of the anesthesiologist, but it is important for hospital medicine practitioners to understand potential risk reduction strategies related to anesthetic techniques. Previous studies have shown that avoidance of long-acting neuromuscular blockade medications (pancuronium) can reduce the risk of postoperative pulmonary complications. This results from less residual neuromuscular blockade and resultant hypoventilation after surgery. Data supporting the use of neuraxial (epidural or spinal) anesthesia as a risk reduction modality has been mixed as well. However, a 2012 Cochrane review determined that neuraxial (spinal or epidural) anesthesia either alone or when added to general anesthesia significantly reduced the risk of postoperative pneumonia.

■ ANALGESIC TECHNIQUES

Sedating analgesics (including opioids and some adjunctive agents) increase the risk of hypoventilation which can lead to atelectasis and other respiratory complications. Thus, limitation of systemic opioids through epidural or regional analgesia or patient-controlled analgesia (PCA) offers the potential for pulmonary risk reduction. Neuraxial analgesia offers more risk reduction than PCA. In addition to less potential for hypoventilation, these strategies reduce postoperative pain, and increase the ability to take deep breaths and increase lung volumes after surgery. Meta-analyses of abdominal aortic and cardiac surgery patients have demonstrated reduced postsurgical respiratory problems with the use of thoracic epidural analgesia. However, evidence of benefit from other regional analgesia is scant. Administration of intravenous opioids through PCA reduces the risk of pulmonary complications when compared to intermittent intravenous administration on a PRN basis.

■ LUNG EXPANSION TECHNIQUES

The largest body of evidence for a perioperative pulmonary risk reduction strategy is for lung expansion techniques. Incentive spirometry, intermittent positive pressure breathing, deep breathing exercises and continuous positive airway pressure each reduce the risk of postoperative pulmonary complications. None of these strategies has been shown to be superior to another. Given the minimal risk associated with these techniques, the American College of Physicians recommends that incentive spirometry or deep breathing exercises be used for all patients at risk for pulmonary complications. Furthermore, a number of studies have demonstrated the value of lung expansion techniques or cardiopulmonary conditioning therapy started 1 to 2 weeks prior to surgery. This strategy reduces rates of pneumonia and all pulmonary complications by approximately one-half. Preoperative initiation of lung expansion or cardiopulmonary physiotherapy should be considered for patients with elevated pulmonary risk.

■ SELECTIVE NASOGASTRIC DECOMPRESSION

The American College of Physicians also recommends use of nasogastric tubes only as needed for postoperative nausea or vomiting, oral intake intolerance or symptomatic abdominal distention. This recommendation results from observations that routine, rather than selective, nasogastric decompression following abdominal surgery led to increased rates of pneumonia and atelectasis.

■ LUNG-PROTECTIVE VENTILATION

A growing body of evidence also supports the use of lung-protective ventilation (lower tidal volume, higher levels of positive end-expiratory pressure [PEEP] and lung recruitment maneuvers) in patients who require perioperative mechanical ventilation. This approach has long been utilized in patients with acute respiratory distress syndrome to reduce ventilator-associated lung injury. More recently, studies and meta-analyses have also shown reduced postoperative pulmonary complications in patients ventilated with tidal volumes of 6 to 8 cc/kg and PEEP of 5 to 10 cm of water pressure (cwp). Data from a 2014 randomized controlled trial indicates that use of lower tidal volume (8 cc/kg) with PEEP levels more than 10 cwp results in an increased risk of hypotension. Therefore, multiple factors influence the selection of an optimal postoperative ventilation strategy (eg, risk of hypotension).

■ OBSTRUCTIVE SLEEP APNEA MANAGEMENT

As the impact of OSA on perioperative risk is now well established, experts have developed a number of strategies to reduce the risk of sleep apnea-related postoperative complications. Most of these interventions were not derived from RCTs, but prospective studies of patients screened as high risk for OSA provide some evidence of their efficacy. High-risk patients in whom such OSA-targeted interventions were employed have complication rates similar to patients at low risk for OSA. The 2014 ASA practice advisory for perioperative OSA management suggests several strategies for mitigating sleep apnea-related risks (**Table 51-6**). For patients likely to have severe OSA, empiric use of positive airway pressure (PAP) ventilation is recommended if signs of severe hypoxia or airway obstruction are evident. At least one recent RCT demonstrated no reduction in postoperative pulmonary complications from empiric PAP initiation postoperatively (ie, without signs or symptoms of hypoxemia or

TABLE 51-6 ASA Recommendations for Postoperative Management of Patients with Known or Suspected Sleep Apnea

Elevate head of bed (unless contraindicated by surgical requirements)	
Continuous pulse oximetry (with centralized monitoring)	
Use adjunctive analgesics (eg, NSAIDs) to reduce systemic opioid needs	
Minimize use of nonopioid sedatives	
PAP therapy	*Previously on home PAP:* have patient use home PAP device whenever sleeping
	No previous PAP: initiate PAP for frequent or severe airway obstruction or hypoxemia

ASA, American Society of Anesthesiologists; NSAIDs, nonsteroidal anti-inflammatory drugs; PAP, positive airway pressure.

airway obstruction). When possible, surgery should be delayed for preoperative evaluation and management of OSA for patients likely to have severe sleep apnea and are undergoing major surgery. Retrospective studies suggest that patients who are formally diagnosed and started on appropriate PAP therapy preoperatively have lower rates of postoperative complications compared to those who were diagnosed and treated after surgery.

CONCLUSION

Postoperative pulmonary complications are an under-recognized source of significant surgical morbidity and mortality. Estimation of pulmonary risk is an essential part of the preoperative evaluation and includes assessment of both patient- and procedure-related risk factors. Most risk factors are not modifiable, but the preoperative pulmonary evaluation provides an accurate estimation of risk for patients and physicians that improves informed decision making. Moreover, identification of high-risk patients can heighten postoperative vigilance for respiratory failure and pneumonia and lead to the use of those strategies proven to reduce risk.

PRACTICE POINT

Why Preoperative Pulmonary Evaluation Matters

Pulmonary evaluation has been traditionally undervalued for a number of reasons:

- Most of the risk factors for postoperative pulmonary complications are nonmodifiable.
- Many of the available risk reduction strategies are either beyond the responsibility of the primary care physician/hospitalist (choice of anesthesia and surgical approach) or routinely utilized (incentive spirometry and deep breathing exercises).

However, identification of patients at increased pulmonary risk remains critical for the following reasons:

- Communication of increased pulmonary risk to the anesthesiologist and surgical team prompts consideration of risk reduction strategies under their control.
- Modification of the postoperative care unit team's triage decisions. For example, after a surgery that would usually be done as an outpatient, a high-risk patient may be admitted for extended observation.
- Heightened postoperative vigilance for respiratory problems. Specific examples of effects on management include:
  - Lower threshold for initiating workup for pneumonia in setting of postoperative fever (which might otherwise be attributed to benign causes)
  - Admission to unit specializing in respiratory care or mobilization of respiratory therapy resources beyond traditional scope
  - Lower threshold for treatment of postoperative pneumonia when chest radiographs are equivocal

SUGGESTED READINGS

American Society of Anesthesiologists Task Force on Perioperative Management of patients with obstructive sleep apnea. Practice guidelines for the perioperative management of patients with obstructive sleep apnea: an updated report by the American Society of Anesthesiologists Task Force on Perioperative Management of patients with obstructive sleep apnea. *Anesthesiology.* 2014;120:268.

Chung F, et al. High STOP-Bang score indicates a high probability of obstructive sleep apnea. *Br J Anaesth.* 2012;108:768.

Gupta H, et al. Development and validation of a risk calculator predicting postoperative respiratory failure. *Chest.* 2011;140:1207.

Gupta H, et al. Development and validation of a risk calculator for predicting postoperative pneumonia. *Mayo Clin Proc.* 2013;88:1241.

Mazo V, et al. Prospective external validation of a predictive score for postoperative pulmonary complications. *Anesthesiology.* 2014;121:219.

Minai OA, et al. Perioperative risk and management in patients with pulmonary hypertension. *Chest.* 2013;144:329.

Qaseem A, et al. Risk assessment for and strategies to reduce perioperative pulmonary complications for patients undergoing noncardiothoracic surgery: a guideline from the American College of Physicians. *Ann Intern Med.* 2006;144:581.

Wong J, et al. Short-term preoperative smoking cessation and postoperative complications: a systematic review and meta-analysis. *Can J Anaesth.* 2012;59:268.

CHAPTER 52

Perioperative Risk Assessment and Management of the Diabetic Patient

Katherine Lewis, MD
Kathie L. Hermayer, MD

INTRODUCTION

About 21 million adults have diabetes in the United States, and 5.5 million hospital discharges include diabetes as one of the listed diagnoses. Annual inpatient health care costs directly related to diabetes were estimated at $76 billion in 2012. People with diabetes have a higher lifetime probability of requiring surgery compared to the general population due to increased cardiovascular, ophthalmic, renal, and neuropathic complications from their disease. Diabetes mellitus itself may complicate surgical wound healing and recovery. Surgical site infections may be twice as high in patients with diabetes, potentially from small vessel disease impairing oxygen and nutrient delivery to tissues, impaired leukocyte and monocyte function due to hyperglycemia, and decreased release of neuropeptides in those with peripheral neuropathy. Patients with diabetes also have higher postoperative in-hospital mortality compared to those without diabetes. Patients with higher postoperative blood sugars after coronary bypass surgery have an increased rate of complications. Surgery and anesthesia provoke release of counter-regulatory hormones, which cause hyperglycemia and increased catabolism. Care for the surgical patient with diabetes should focus on avoidance of marked hyperglycemia, which can alter wound healing and disrupt fluid balance, while also avoiding hypoglycemia, which can cause cardiac stress. Perioperative evaluation for patients with diabetes allows for the development of an individualized plan to reduce perioperative complications and to determine a safe and effective diabetes discharge plan.

PREOPERATIVE EVALUATION

A thorough history remains a key component in the preoperative evaluation of the patient with diabetes. A history of comorbidities and complications associated with diabetes may provide additional insight into surgical risk, and therefore perioperative management. For example, elective surgery should be delayed in patients with diabetes after a recent cardiac event (see Chapter 50: Preoperative Cardiac Risk Assessment and Perioperative Management). Patients with concomitant renal disease need to be monitored carefully, with precautions to avoid contrast materials and other nephrotoxic agents. Diabetic autonomic neuropathy may predispose patients to perioperative hypotension. Gastroparesis with impaired gastric emptying may predispose patients to aspiration during intubation and extubation.

Clarification of the patient's home diabetes regimen and assessment of their home glycemic control and adherence will help guide perioperative management. Ideally, patients will have good glycemic control prior to undergoing elective surgery, but this will not always be possible. Some experts advocate delaying elective surgery if the patients HbA1C is >8.5%, but there is no good literature to support or negate this practice. In addition, the management plan should take into consideration the patients' typical diet and activity, which may change drastically in the perioperative period. The type and duration of surgery is also important to consider, as longer surgeries and recovery times (including ICU admission or prolonged NPO status) will affect the perioperative glycemic management plan.

Specific physical exam components for patients with diabetes should include inspection of injection sites or insulin pump infusion sites (if applicable) for evidence of lipohypertrophy, which may affect insulin absorption. Evaluation for signs and symptoms of peripheral neuropathy will help plan for fall prevention tactics during the hospital stay. Inspection for associated wounds will help plan for wound prevention and care during the stay. In addition, obtaining orthostatic blood pressures may identify patients who may have a component of autonomic neuropathy, which should be taken into account for blood pressure management during and after surgery.

An inpatient HbA1C measurement is recommended if not obtained within the last 3 months. The HbA1C correlates with the risk for complications, perioperative hyperglycemia, and increased length of stay. More importantly, it may guide both perioperative and discharge diabetes management. Clinicians must be aware of the limitations of HbA1C accuracy, such as in the settings of recent transfusion, anemia, and hemoglobin variants.

Immediate preoperative glucose values predict postoperative glucose and may lead to an alteration of management plan in cases of extreme hyperglycemia or hypoglycemia. A comprehensive chemistry should be checked preoperatively, and will provide information on renal function, liver function, electrolytes, and bicarbonate status; impaired renal function reduces insulin clearance and increases a patient's risk for hypoglycemia, and impaired liver function increases the risk of hypoglycemia. Correcting hypokalemia is important for patients receiving insulin, as insulin treatment lowers plasma potassium levels. Patients in diabetic ketoacidosis will have an increased anion gap with decreased bicarbonate and hyperglycemia; this should be corrected prior to any surgical procedure.

PREOPERATIVE RECOMMENDATIONS FOR PATIENTS

In addition to receiving recommendations from their surgical team, patients need guidance as to what to do with their home diabetes regimen prior to surgery. In general, oral diabetic agents and other noninsulin diabetic medications should be held prior to surgery (**Table 52-1**). However, some controversy in the literature exists for certain medications.

- **Metformin**: It is generally recommended that metformin be held up to 48 hours before surgery and restarted 48 hours after surgery, due to risk of lactic acidosis; however, in diabetic cardiac surgery patients, one study showed better outcomes in patients who inadvertently took metformin. These patients had a lower incidence of prolonged intubation, lower risk of infections, and lower overall morbidity compared to matched patients not taking metformin. While these findings are interesting, routine use of preoperative metformin is not recommended, but this information is reassuring should metformin inadvertently be taken preoperatively.
- **Glucagon-like receptor 1 (GLP-1) agonists**: These agents are generally held prior to surgery due to the gastric emptying delays and nausea seen with these agents; however, some studies have shown better glucose control with (compared to without) these agents in cardiac and noncardiac surgery patients. A current study may help clarify the potential role for these agents in perioperative management in patients undergoing noncardiac surgery. Several formulations of GLP-1 agonists are dosed once weekly; therefore, it may not be possible to effectively hold these medications given their long half-lives.
- **Dipeptidyl peptidase-4 (DPP- IV) inhibitors**: These agents are often held perioperatively, though one study of sitaglipitan showed it was safe and effective in selective medical-surgical hospitalized patients (without significant renal disease, liver disease or high degree of insulin resistance).

For patients on insulin, basal insulin in many cases can be given at the regular dose or slightly reduced doses for short procedures. In patients with Type 1 diabetes, basal insulin should not be held due to the risk of diabetic ketoacidosis. A reduction in basal insulin may be needed if the patient gives a history of frequent snacking in his or her normal routine, or if they endorse fasting hypoglycemia on their home regimen. In one study, use of 80% of the basal dose was safe and effective in patients with both Type 1 and Type 2 diabetes undergoing noncardiac surgery. **Table 52-2** lists commonly used insulin formulations, approach to preoperative dosing, and recommendations for when and how to resume insulin regimens postoperatively and at the time of discharge.

PREOPERATIVE RECOMMENDATIONS FOR THE CARE TEAM

Once a preoperative diabetes plan has been devised and communicated with the patient, the plan should be relayed to the rest of the patient care team, including the surgical team and anesthesiologists. Type of diabetes, duration of diabetes, and complications related to diabetes should also be relayed to the surgical care team, and well documented in the medical record.

Given the limitations of oral diabetic agents in the perioperative setting, insulin management is preferred. Patients with Type 1 diabetes must continue with some form of basal insulin to prevent diabetic ketoacidosis. Basal insulin may be in the form of long acting insulins such as once a day glargine, detemir, or twice daily NPH. Rapid acting insulin analogs (lispro, aspart, and glulisine) act over several hours and are used for prandial insulin and for supplemental (correction) insulin. Regular insulin given subcutaneously can also be used for prandial and supplemental insulin.

Basal bolus regimens have been recommended for the majority of noncritically ill-diabetic patients. This consists of basal insulin + prandial insulin + supplemental insulin. Basal bolus regimens are superior to sliding scale insulin alone (which is not recommended). Basal bolus regimens confer better glycemic control and reduced complications such as wound infection, renal failure, pneumonia, respiratory failure, and bacteremia. In patients with Type 2 diabetes on home oral agents and/or relatively low insulin, basal insulin + supplemental insulin only is comparable to basal bolus insulin, and is a reasonable regimen for these patients.

MONITORING AND GLYCEMIC TARGETS FOR NONCRITICALLY ILL

During surgery, glucose should be monitored hourly for procedures lasting >60 minutes. Glycemic targets for noncritically ill patients on insulin should be <140 mg/dL before a meal and <180 mg/dL randomly. Dose reductions should be considered for any blood glucose levels of <100 mg/dL to prevent hypoglycemia, and dose reductions should be mandatory for any blood glucose levels of <70 mg/dL (unless the event is easily explained by an identified preventable factors). In-patient point-of-care monitoring should be performed four or more times a day, including before meals and at bedtime. For patients who are not eating, monitoring should occur every 4 to 6 hours (around the clock). A plan for preventing hypoglycemia, and a protocol for treating hypoglycemia, should be in place; any episode of hypoglycemia should be documented in the medical record.

■ INSULIN PUMP THERAPY

Continuous subcutaneous insulin infusion (CSII, eg, insulin pump therapy) has become much more commonly used among patients with diabetes. It provides flexibility, convenience, and ease of adjustments in insulin-treated patients. Often it is associated with less glycemic variability and improved glycemic control. It is often recommended that CSII be discontinued during inpatient hospital stays if the patient is not able to self-manage their pump; however, use during surgery has been less clear. For patients admitted for same day surgery for procedures of <120 minutes, CSII appears to be safe when used with a protocol that allows for the addition of IV insulin by anesthesiology for glucose >250 mg/dL or any extension of surgery

TABLE 52-1 Recommendations for Oral Diabetic Agents and Other Noninsulin Diabetic Therapies in the Perioperative Setting

Medication	Mechanism of Action	Perioperative Recommendation	Explanation	When to Resume
Sulfonylureas Glipizide (Half-life 2-5 h) Glyburide (Half-life 10 h) Glimeperide (Half-life 9.2 h) Tolazamide (Half-life 7 h) Tolbutamide (Half-life 4.5-6.5 h) Chlorpropamide (Half-life 36 h)	Increases insulin secretion	Hold medication day of surgery and during hospitalization May need to hold chlorpropamide the day before surgery as well due to long half-life	Risk of hypoglycemia Possible adverse cardiovascular effects	At time of discharge when oral intake is back to normal
Meglitinides Repaglinide (Half-life 1 h) Nateglinide (Half-life 1.5 h)	Increases insulin secretion (given at time of a meal)	Hold medication day of surgery and during hospitalization	Risk of hypoglycemia with fasting	At time of discharge when oral intake is normal
Biguanides Metformin	Sensitizes tissues to insulin	Hold medication for surgery and prior to contrast administration (up to 48 h in advance) and during hospitalization	Risk of lactic acidosis, particularly in the setting of renal insufficiency	At time of discharge if fluid status and renal function are reasonable (hold for Cr >1.4 in female and >1.5 in male)
Alpha-glucosidase inhibitors Acarbose Miglitol	Reduces oligo- and disaccaridoses in intestinal brush border	Hold medication day of surgery and during hospitalization	No role in fasting patient	At time of discharge when oral intake is normal Caution in renal insufficiency
Thiazolidinediones Rosiglitazone Pioglitazone	Sensitizes tissues to insulin	Hold medication day of surgery and during hospitalization	May cause additional fluid retention Concern for heart failure and MI increased risk	At time of discharge if no heart failure concern Caution in hepatic impairment
Dipeptidyl peptidase-4 inhibitors Sitagliptan Saxagliptan Linagliptan Alogliptan	Work in glucose dependent fashion to increase insulin	Hold medication day of surgery and during hospitalization	Limited role in fasting patient There is one small study of safety and efficacy in selective hospitalized patients when used with basal insulin	With resumption of oral intake
GLP-1 agonists Exenatide Exenatide QW (Half-life 2 wk) Liraglutide Albiglutide (Half-life 5-8 d) Dulaglutide (Half-life 4-7 d)	Increases insulin secretion, decreases glucagon secretion, delays gastric emptying	Hold medication day of surgery for formulations given daily or twice daily Hold once weekly medications in the days leading up to surgery Hold medications during hospitalization (May not be possible to effectively hold once weekly formulations given long half-life of these formulations)	Delay of gastric emptying Recommendations may change in future: One study of benefit using IV form Ongoing study looking at role in post-surgical patients	At time of discharge when oral intake is normal
Sodium glucose cotransporter-2 inhibitors Canagliflozin Empagliflozin Dapagliflozin	Increase glucose excretion in the urine	Hold medication up to several days in advance	Reported cases of euglycemic DKA in post-operative patients Fluid loss from increased urine output	At time of discharge when oral intake is normal

(Continued)

TABLE 52-1 Recommendations for Oral Diabetic Agents and Other Noninsulin Diabetic Therapies in the Perioperative Setting (Continued)

Medication	Mechanism of Action	Perioperative Recommendation	Explanation	When to Resume
Bromocriptine-QR (quick release)	Short-acting dopamine agonist which lowers postprandial blood sugars; given in morning to reset circadian rhythms of hypothalamic dopamine and serotonin resulting in reduced insulin resistance; reduced cardiovascular events in Type 2 diabetes compared to placebo	Hold medication day of surgery and during hospitalization	Short half-life of just a few hours with low risk of hypoglycemia Causes modest blood pressure lowering May cause nausea	At time of discharge

TABLE 52-2 Recommendations for Insulin Regimens in the Perioperative Setting

Insulins	Onset and Duration of Action	Preoperative Adjustment of Home Dose	Perioperative Management in the Hospital	Discharge Dosing
Long-acting basalinsulins				
Glargine	Onset 1 h, duration 24 h	Consider reduction by 20% of dose prior to surgery	Basal regimen preferred over sliding scale alone	Consider dosing based on preoperative A1C:
Detimir	Onset 1 h, duration 6-24 h	Do not hold basal insulin for patients with Type 1 diabetes	Dosing 0.15-0.3 units/kg/d Little known about degludec in perioperative setting	A1C <7%: home insulin regimen and home oral agents
Degludec	Half-life of 24 h, duration of >42 h			A1C 7-9%: home oral agents with addition of 50% of inpatient basal insulin A1C >9%: home oral agents plus 80% inpatient basal insulin plus 80% inpatient prandial insulin
Intermediate-acting basal insulins				
NPH	Onset 1-2 h, peak 4-14 h, duration 10-24 h	Consider full evening dose (or slight reduction) and half morning dose on day of surgery	May be used as basal insulin dosed twice daily Twice daily dosing allows for more frequent dose adjustments	Consider similar dosing to long-acting basal noted above
Mixed insulins: Combined NPH with rapid-acting analogs or regular insulin				
70/30	See separate components: given with meals, typically twice daily	Give full evening meal dose the day before surgery Consider giving half morning dose on day of surgery	Recommend substituting separate basal and prandial insulin for increased flexibility of dosing	Consider inpatient insulin needs, home regimen, oral intake, degree of post-operative stress and A1C
75/25	NPH is acting as basal insulin	Consider providing NPH only on day of surgery		Consider using 50%-80% of total daily inpatient insulin dose converting to twice daily regimen of mixed insulin regimen with home oral agents
50/50	Other components are prandial insulin			Consider discharge instead on basal bolus regimen Patient should be eating meals to resume mixed insulin

(Continued)

TABLE 52-2 Recommendations for Insulin Regimens in the Perioperative Setting (Continued)

Insulins	Onset and Duration of Action	Preoperative Adjustment of Home Dose	Perioperative Management in the Hospital	Discharge Dosing
Concentrated insulins				
Glargine (300 units/mL) *U-500*	Onset 6 h, duration 24-36 h Onset 30 min, peak 1-3 h, duration 8 h	Consider 20% reduction of concentrated glargine the dose prior to surgery For U-500 insulin, consider converting to a U-100 basal since this insulin has a long half-life and acts as both a basal and prandial insulin	Consider using alternate basal insulin Consider perioperative insulin infusion because of degree of baseline insulin resistance If using U-500 in the hospital because of extreme insulin resistance, take special precautions to avoid dosing errors	Concentrated glargine: consider dosing strategy similar to standard basal therapy U-500: Consider inpatient needs and oral intake and dosing at 80% of inpatient needs; take special precautions to clarify dosing as dosing errors are common
Rapid-acting insulin analogs				
Aspart	Onset 0.25 h, peak 1-3 h, duration 3-5 h	Hold prandial dosing while npo for surgery	Used for prandial and supplemental insulin in addition to basal insulin Prandial insulin dosing: 0.1 unit/kg/meal (adjust for renal insufficiency and poor oral intake) OR 0.15-0.25 units/kg/d divided over 3 meals	Consider home regimen, A1C, inpatient needs and oral intake If A1C >9%, consider adding to home regimen at 80% of prandial inpatient dosing
Lispro	Onset <0.5 h, peak 0.5-1.5 h, duration <6 h			
Glulisine	Onset <0.5 h, peak 0.5-1.5 h, duration <6 h			
Regular insulin		Hold prandial dosing while npo for surgery	Used in IV insulin infusions for perioperative management May use as prandial insulin instead of rapid acting analogs but has slower onset and longer duration	Consider home regimen, A1C, inpatient needs and oral intake and dose similar to rapid-acting analogs Consider using rapid-acting analogs as alternative to regular for prandial insulin

beyond 2 hours. Patients with insulin pumps should be instructed to place a fresh infusion set in an area not affected by surgery. A retrospective review of CSII patients found similar control between perioperative CSII versus conversion to perioperative IV insulin drip.

<h3>MONITORING AND GLYCEMIC TARGETS FOR CRITICALLY ILL</h3>

The American College of Physicians endorses a blood glucose target of 140 to 200 mg/dL in surgical and medical intensive care unit (ICU) patients. The American Diabetes Association and American Association of Clinical Endocrinologists endorse a blood glucose target of 140 to 180 mg/dL for most ICU patients. A target of <110 mg/dL is never recommended, due to increased hypoglycemia and mortality seen with the NICE-Sugar trial. See **Table 52-3** for further recommendations for glycemic targets for critically ill.

In a review of patients undergoing cardiac surgery treated with IV insulin infusion postoperatively with a lower glycemic target (80-110 mg/dL) compared with those treated using a higher target (110-140 mg/dL), patients in the higher target group experienced similar mean glucose values, no significant differences in 30-day morbidity and mortality (with the possible exception of increased reintubation), and less hypoglycemia than the lower target group. Similarly, in a study of cardiac patients treated with IV insulin infusion to a target of 110 to 140 versus 140 to 180, there were no significant differences in morbidity or mortality between the groups. Therefore lower targets have been essentially abandoned for ICU patients.

<h3>■ IV INSULIN INFUSION THERAPY</h3>

In critically ill patients, glycemic management with an IV insulin infusion is recommended for the majority of patients; it should be initiated at a threshold of 180, with target blood sugars between 140 and 180. The use of insulin protocols are highly recommended, to reduce variability and increase the amount of time within target.

<h3>DISCHARGE PLANNING</h3>

Discharge planning should begin shortly after admission, so that very clear instructions are provided to the patient at time of discharge. Preoperative HbA1C can be a valuable tool in devising a discharge diabetes regimen. Umpierrez et al demonstrated improved HbA1C at 4 and 12 weeks postdischarge with the use of a discharge protocol based on initial HbA1C in surgical and medical patients with Type 2 diabetes. Follow-up included nursing phone calls every 2 weeks for the first 2 months and visits at 1 and 3 months:

- Patients with HbA1C <7% were discharged on their home regimen (oral agents or insulin).
- Patients with HbA1C between 7% and 9% were discharged on their home oral agents as well as basal insulin at 50% of the inpatient hospital regimen.
- Patients with HbA1C >9% were discharged on their home oral agents as well as 80% of inpatient basal insulin or basal bolus therapy (using 80% basal insulin and 80% prandial insulin used in the hospital).

TABLE 52-3 Summary of the Most Current Professional Society Guidelines for Glycemic Control

Organization	Year	Patient Population	Rx Threshold (mg/dL)	Target Glucose (mg/dL)
American Diabetes Association	2015	ICU patients	180	140-180; 110-140, select pts
Surviving Sepsis Campaign	2009	ICU patients	180	<180
Inst.Healthcare Improvement	2009	ICU patients	180	<180
American Heart Association	2009	ICU patients with ACS	180	90-140
European Society of Cardiology	2009	Patients after major noncardiac surgery	180	140-180
American College Physicians	2014	ICU patients	180	140-200
Societyof Thoracic Surgeons	2009	ICU patients after	180	<180
		Adult cardiac surgery		<150 if requires > 3 days ICU care for ventilatory, inotrophic Ormechanical support, Renalin sufficiency, on antiarrhythmics

CONCLUSION

High-quality perioperative care of diabetic patients can reduce morbidity, mortality, and cost. A thorough preoperative diabetes evaluation along with clear communication with all members of the surgical care team remains necessary for the development and implementation of an individualized perioperative care plan. Hospitalists have the opportunity to collaborate and coordinate care for these patients throughout the perioperative process. Hospitalists can play a key role in identifying areas of need and collaborating with surgical teams and diabetologists in improving perioperative and inpatient care.

SUGGESTED READINGS

Barker P, Creasey PE, Dhatariya K, et al. Peri-operative management of the surgical patient with diabetes 2015: Association of Anaesthetists of Great Britain and Ireland. *Anaesthesia*. 2015. online early release. doi: 10.1111/anae.13233.

Bock M, Johansson T, Fritsch G, et al. The impact of preoperative testing for blood glucose concentration and haemoglobin A1c on mortality, changes in management and complications in noncardiac elective surgery: a systematic review. *Eur J Anaesth*. 2015;32(3):152-159.

Evans AS, Hosseinian L, Mechanick JI. Emerging paradigms on glucose managemnt in the intensive care unit. *Minerva Endocrinol*. 2014;39:261-273.

Fleisher LA, Fleischmann KE, Auerbach AD, et al. 2014 ACC/AHA guideline on perioperative cardiovascular evaluation and management of patients undergoing noncardiac surgery: a report of the American College of Cardiology/American Heart Association Task Force on Practice Guidelines. *Circulation* 2014;130(24): e278-e333.

Handelsman Y, Bloomgarden ZT, Grunberger G, et al. American association of clinical endocrinologists and american college of endocrinology—clinical practice guidelines for developing a diabetes mellitus comprehensive care plan. *Endoc Prac*. 2015; 21(Suppl 1):1-87.

Qaseem A, Chou R, Humphrey LL, Shekelle P. Inpatient glycemic control: best practice advice from the Clinical Guidelines Committee of the American College of Physicians. *Am J Med Qual*. 2014;29(2):95-98.

Udovcic M, Castro JC, Apsey HA, Stearns JD, Schlinkert RT, Cook CB. Guidelines to improve perioperative management of diabetes mellitus: assessment of the impact of change across time. *Endoc Prac*. 2015;21(9):1026-1034.

Underwood P, Seiden J, Carbone K, et al. Early Identification of Individuals with Poorly Controlled Diabetes Undergoing Elective Surgery: improving A1C testing in the preoperative period. *Endoc Prac*. 2015;21(3):231-236.

Umpierrez GE, Reyes D, Smiley D, et al. Hospital discharge algorithm based on admission HbA1c for the management of patients with type 2 diabetes. *Diabetes Care*. 2014;37(11):2934-2939.

CHAPTER 53

Preoperative Evaluation of Liver Disease

Amir A. Qamar, MD
Norman D. Grace, MD

INTRODUCTION

Many hospitalists will be asked to assess the operative risk of patients who have acute or chronic liver disease. The following chapter outlines an assessment plan and a basis for predicting operative morbidity and mortality. Evaluation of patients with liver disease prior to surgery is crucial to estimate perioperative morbidity and mortality. The operative risk of liver disease can be related to the rapid changes in liver function that can occur in acute hepatitis, or can be related to chronic complications of portal hypertension and parenchymal liver disease in patients with cirrhosis. Therefore, establishment of a risk profile should be based on the etiology of the underlying liver disease, the degree of hepatic decompensation associated with the presence of cirrhosis and portal hypertension, and the type of surgery the patient is undergoing.

FACTORS THAT AFFECT PERIOPERATIVE OUTCOMES IN LIVER DISEASE PATIENTS

■ CHANGES IN HEPATIC BLOOD FLOW

The liver receives dual blood supply from the portal vein and the hepatic artery. Unlike most other organs, the majority of hepatic oxygen supply in normal individuals is venous, via the portal vein. Administration of anesthesia and surgery influences both portal and hepatic blood flow; usually, when flow through the portal vein is reduced, the hepatic artery vasodilates to increase oxygen supply to the liver. This compensatory vasodilatation is reduced in patients with altered hepatic architecture (such as fibrosis and nodular formation associated with cirrhosis). Due to intraoperative decreases in blood pressure and cardiac output, blood flow in patients with cirrhosis is decreased in the portal vein, splanchnic vessels, and hepatic artery; anesthetics also reduce the hepatic artery's ability to vasodilate in response to these changes in portal blood flow.

These changes in hepatic blood flow may lead to hepatic ischemia and necrosis. The release of inflammatory mediators may result in multiorgan system failure. In a study of 733 cirrhosis patients undergoing surgery, Ziser et al found an 11.6% mortality rate. Intraoperative hypotension correlated strongly with perioperative complications and decreased survival.

■ TYPE OF SURGERY

Postoperative morbidity and mortality in patients with cirrhosis is also influenced by the type of surgery.

Abdominal surgery

During abdominal surgery, direct trauma due to surgical retraction can lead to hepatic injury. Manipulation of the splachnic and portal vasculature may also reduce portal or hepatic flow leading to ischemic injury. In particular, patients with Child-Pugh class C cirrhosis who undergo abdominal surgery have a 75% perioperative mortality.

Cardiovascular surgery

Cardiovascular surgery, due to effects on portal and hepatic artery blood flow, is also associated with high perioperative morbidity and mortality. The need for perioperative pressor support and prolonged cardiopulmonary bypass are factors that strongly correlate with hepatic injury.

Emergency Surgery

Many patients who require emergency surgery may be hemody-namically unstable from systemic vasodilation (eg, sepsis) or hypo-tensive due to hemorrhage (eg, trauma, abdominal surgery), and their outcome is often poor regardless of underlying conditions. In a study by Demetriades and colleagues of 46 patients with cirrhosis who underwent emergency laparotomy, the postoperative mortal-ity rate was 45%, which was significantly greater than noncirrhotic control patients.

Orthopedic surgery

There is little information in the literature regarding specific opera-tive risks for patients with cirrhosis who undergo orthopedic surgery. Hsieh et al reviewed 38 patients who underwent hip arthroplasty over a 20-year period and found the 30-day complication rate was 27%. Advanced cirrhosis, age, elevated serum creatinine, low serum albumin, low platelet count, ascites, hepatic encephalopathy, and high operative blood loss correlated with the high complication rate.

■ TYPE OF ANESTHETIC

Anesthetic agents may reduce hepatic blood flow by reducing car-diac output. Even spinal and epidural anesthesia, by reducing the mean arterial pressure, may affect hepatic blood flow. In patients with liver disease, effects on hepatic metabolism may lead to pro-longed action of anesthetic agents or production of toxic radicals resulting in increased morbidity and mortality.

■ CAUSE AND SEVERITY OF LIVER DISEASE

Perioperative morbidity and mortality is highly influenced by the etiology and severity of the patient's liver disease. The presence of cirrhosis or acute hepatitis at the time of surgery adversely influ-ences surgical outcomes. Generally, patients with chronic hepatitis from any etiology, without features of hepatic decompensation, do very well with surgery and specific precautions are not necessary. However, in patients with acute liver disease or cirrhosis, it is critical to assess their perioperative risk as part of informed consent. Acute hepatitis, especially alcoholic hepatitis, or decompensated cirrhosis are relative contraindications to elective surgery. A number of scor-ing and staging systems are useful in assessing the perioperative risk, the most common of which are the Child Pugh Score and the MELD score. Measurement of the hepatic venous pressure gradient (HVPG) has excellent prognostic value but its use is confined to a limited number of medical centers. A recent study showed that patients with compensated cirrhosis with clinically significant portal hypertension, defined by a HVPG ≥10 mm Hg, were at significant risk of developing clinical decompensation defined as the occurrence of jaundice, ascites, variceal bleeding, or hepatic encephalopathy.

Child Pugh Score

The Child-Pugh Score combines a subjective and objective assess-ment of liver function (**Table 53-1**). In a recent study of 33 patients

TABLE 53-2 Operative Mortality Rates in Patients Undergoing Abdominal Surgery Based on Child-Pugh Class

Child-Pugh Class	Risk of Operative Mortality
A	10%
B	30%
C	80%

Adapted from Garrison RN, Cryer HM, Howard DA, et al. Clarification of risk factors for abdominal operations in patients with hepatic cirrhosis. *Ann Surg.* 1984;199(6):648-655 and Mansour A, Watson W,; Shayani V, et al. Abdominal operations in patients with cirrhosis: still a major surgical challenge. *Surgery.* 1997;122(4):730-735.

with cirrhosis, compared to 31 age- and sex-matched control patients, the Child-Pugh score accurately predicted morbidity after cholecystectomy. In another study of 44 patients with cirrhosis who underwent cardiac surgery, a preoperative Child-Pugh score ≥8 was predictive of postoperative mortality. **Table 53-2** summarizes the operative mortality risk of patients with different Child-Pugh scores who undergo abdominal surgery.

MELD score

The Model for End Stage Liver Disease (MELD) score predicts short term mortality in patients with cirrhosis. The scoring system uses serum bilirubin, creatinine, and prothrombin time (international nor-malized ratio) to assess hepatic function. Recent data also suggests the presence of hyponatremia further increases the risk of mortality.

Teh et al assessed 772 patients with cirrhosis who underwent major digestive, cardiac or orthopedic surgery. They found that the 30-day mortality ranged from 5.7% for MELD score <8 to 50% for a MELD score >20. **Table 53-3** summarizes the mortality risk for surgi-cal patients with different preoperative MELD scores.

PREOPERATIVE MANAGEMENT

The preoperative management of patients with cirrhosis should involve aggressive treatment of portal hypertension and hepatic insufficiency to reduce operative morbidity and mortality. Depend-ing on the specific etiology of the liver disease, certain preoperative changes in management may be considered (more below).

■ DIAGNOSTIC STUDIES

Table 53-4 lists laboratory and radiology studies that should be considered in the preoperative assessment of a patient with liver disease to ascertain their perioperative risk.

■ COAGULOPATHY

Hepatic insufficiency leads to inadequate production of factors II, V, VII, and IX resulting in the development of coagulopathy with an increased risk of perioperative bleeding. Thrombocytopenia

TABLE 53-1 Child Pugh Scoring System

	1	2	3
Bilirubin	<2.0 mg/dL	2.0-3.0 mg/dL	>3.0 mg/dL
Albumin	>3.5 g/dL	3.5-2.8 g/dL	<2.8 g/dL
PT	<4 s greater than control	4-6 s greater than control	>6 s greater than control
Ascites	Absent	Mild-Moderate	Moderate-Severe
Encephalopathy	Absent	Mild (Grade I-II)	Severe (Grade III-IV)

Score 5-6: Child Class A; 7-9: Child Class B; ≥10: Child Class C.

TABLE 53-3 Preoperative MELD Scores and 7-day and 30-day Mortality Rates

MELD Score	7 d	30 d
0-7 (n = 351)	1.9 (314)	5.7 (301)
8-11 (n = 257)	3.3 (236)	10.3 (219)
12-15 (n = 106)	7.7 (94)	25.4 (78)
16-20 (n = 35)	14.6 (29)	44.0 (19)
21-25 (n = 13)	23.0 (7)	53.8 (4)
≥26 (n = 10)	30.0 (6)	90.0 (1)

MELD, Model for End-stage Liver Disease.
With permission from Teh SH, Nagorney DM, Stevens SR, et al. Risk factors for mortality after surgery in patients with cirrhosis. *Gastroenterology.* 2007;132(4):1261-1269. With permission from Elsevier.

in liver disease is multifactorial, including portal hypertension-induced sequestration of platelets, which further increases the risk of bleeding. Administration of platelets, fresh frozen plasma and cryoprecipitate should be administered prior to surgery to reduce the risk of bleeding during and after surgery. There has been interest in the use of recombinant factor VIIa in situations of emergency uncontrollable bleeding in cirrhotic patients. However, studies have not shown any improved outcomes with the use of this factor in patients undergoing hepatic resection, liver transplantation, and upper gastrointestinal bleeding. This agent should be used with caution due to an increased risk of arteriothromboembolic events including myocardial ischemia, myocardial infarction, cerebral ischemia, and cerebral infarction.

■ VARICES

The risk of bleeding in patients with cirrhosis who have esophageal varices is approximately 8% per year. Once variceal bleeding occurs, there is a 20% mortality associated with the bleeding event. Preventive therapies include the use of nonselective beta blockers and endoscopic variceal ligation. There are no specific treatments to reduce the risk of perioperative variceal bleeding. Preventing "over transfusion" with a target hematocrit of no more than 25 is recommended. In patients who do experience postoperative gastrointestinal bleeding, the use of antibiotics is recommended to reduce the risk of mortality from spontaneous bacterial peritonitis (SBP).

■ ASCITES AND SPONTANEOUS BACTERIAL PERITONITIS

Ascites is the most frequent and generally the first event to occur in patients with cirrhosis and hepatic decompensation. Treatment includes salt restriction, the use of diuretics (including furosemide

TABLE 53-4 Laboratory and Radiologic Testing to Be Considered for Preoperative Risk Assessment in the Patient with Liver Disease

Liver chemistries

Complete blood count

Prothrombin time and international normalized ratio

Electrolytes and renal function

Abdominal ultrasound and Doppler study of hepatic vasculature

CT scan or MRI of liver

Hepatic venography for hepatic venous pressure gradient (HVPG)

TABLE 53-5 Risks Factors for Morbidity and Mortality in Patients with Biliary Obstruction

- Hct < 30
- Bilirubin > 11 mg/dL
- BUN > 90
- Creatinine > 1.4 mg/dL
- Albumin < 3.0 g/dL
- Age > 65 y
- AST > 90
- Malignancy

and spironolactone) and paracentesis. Transjugular intrahepatic portosystemic shunting (TIPS) in the management of ascites prior to surgery is *not* recommended except for patients who may be undergoing liver transplantation. For patients with hypoalbuminemia, ascites or edema, perioperative fluid management should include the use of colloids such as albumin. In patients without third space accumulation of fluids, crystalloids (ie, saline) are appropriate.

■ TRANSJUGULAR INTRAHEPATIC PORTOSYSTEMIC SHUNT PRIOR TO SURGERY

Transjugular intrahepatic portosystemic shunts are effective in reducing the complications of portal hypertension (such as variceal hemorrhage and ascites). Preoperative placement of a TIPS may reduce the risk of portal hypertensive complications in patients with cirrhosis, but data regarding its effectiveness is limited.

■ BILIARY OBSTRUCTION

Biliary obstruction preoperatively is associated with increased morbidity and mortality and should be treated with decompression prior to surgery. Specific factors that increase operative risk are noted in **Table 53-5**.

■ HEPATIC ENCEPHALOPATHY

Hepatic encephalopathy is provoked by a number of factors listed in Table 53-3. The risk of hepatic encephalopathy after surgery can be reduced by avoiding specific precipitants (**Table 53-6**).

■ ADRENAL INSUFFICIENCY

Adrenal insufficiency can be found in 33% of patients with fulminant hepatic failure and 66% of patients with cirrhosis. In patients with decompensated cirrhosis or acute liver failure who develop

TABLE 53-6 Precipitants of Hepatic Encephalopathy

- Gastrointestinal bleeding
- Hypovolemia
- Renal failure
- Use of sedating agents
- Hypokalemia
- Alkalosis
- Trauma
- Infection
- Constipation
- Colon surgery

TABLE 53-7 Etiology-Specific Perioperative Management

Etiology of Liver Disease	Perioperative Management
Alcoholic liver disease	Should be abstinent ≥3 mo preoperative (if possible)
	Should be assessed for alcohol dependence preoperative
	If evidence of alcoholic hepatitis, surgery should be delayed
Hepatitis B and C	Treatment with nucleoside/nucleotide analogues or direct antiviral agents should continue perioperative
	All new perioperative medications should be reviewed for interactions with Hepatitis B and C drugs
	Interferon should be held perioperative
Autoimmune hepatitis	Treatment with prednisone or azathioprine should continue perioperative (stress dose steroids if warranted)
α-1 antitrypsin deficiency	Should be evaluated for underlying lung disease
Hemochromatosis	Should be evaluated for underlying cardiomyopathy
Wilson's disease	Treatment with penicillamine should continue, but at reduced dose perioperative
	Treatment with zinc or trientene should continue perioperative

signs of adrenal insufficiency (including hypotension and hypoglycemia after surgery), treatment with stress dose steroids should be considered.

ETIOLOGY-SPECIFIC MANAGEMENT

Perioperative management by liver disease etiology is outlined in **Table 53-7**.

CONCLUSION

It is important to identify the operative risk of patients with liver disease based on the acuity, etiology and severity of the liver disease and the urgency and type of surgery. Generally, patients with mild liver enzyme abnormalities (without cirrhosis) and most compensated Child-Pugh Class A patients can safely undergo surgery. For all other patients, a careful assessment of the benefits of surgical intervention must be weighed against the risk of hepatic decompensation and mortality. These risks should be enumerated as part of the informed consent process.

SUGGESTED READINGS

Angeli P, Gines P, Wong F, et al. Diagnosis and management of acute kidney injury in patients with cirrhosis: revised consensus recommendations of the International Club of Ascites. *J Hepatol*. 2015;62:968-974.

Garcia-Tsao G. Current management of the complications of cirrhosis and portal hypertension: variceal hemorrhage, ascites, and spontaneous bacterial peritonitis. *Gastroenterology*. 2001;120(3):726-748.

Garcia-Tsao G, Sanyal AJ, Grace ND, et al. Prevention and management of gastroesophageal varices and variceal hemorrhage in cirrhosis. *Hepatology*. 2007;46(3):922-938.

Gustot T, Fernandez J, Garcia E, et al. Clinical course of acute-on-chronic liver failure syndrome and effects on prognosis. *Hepatology*. 2015;62(1):243-252.

Mansour A, Watson W, Shayani V, et al. Abdominal operations in patients with cirrhosis: still a major surgical challenge. *Surgery*. 1997;122(4):730-735.

Qamar AA, Grace ND. Abnormal hematological indices in cirrhosis. *Can J Gastroenterol*. 2009;23(6):441-445.

Surman A, Barnes DS, Zein NN, et al. Predicting out after cardiac surgery in patients with cirrhosis: a comparison of Child-Pugh and MELD score. *Clin Gastroetnerol Hepatol*. 2004;(8):719-723.

Teh SH, Nagorney DM, Stevens SR, et al. Risk factors for mortality after surgery in patients with cirrhosis. *Gastroenterology*. 2007;132(4):1261-1269.

Ziser A, Plevak DJ, Wiesner RH, et al. Morbidity and mortality in cirrhotic patients undergoing anesthesia and surgery. *Anesthesiology*. 1999;90(1):42-53.

CHAPTER 54

Preoperative Assessment of Patients with Hematologic Disorders

Ming Y. Lim, MB BChir
Charles S. Greenberg, MD

INTRODUCTION

Hematologic disorders are diseases of circulating blood cells and plasma proteins that play a role in oxygen delivery, inflammation, infection control, hemostasis, and thrombosis. Given that surgery can result in bleeding and induce hemostatic changes that promote thrombosis, it is not surprising that patients with hematologic disorders present serious preoperative management challenges. The ability of hospitalists to manage diseases associated with blood disorders, and hemostatic and thrombotic risks associated with surgery is vital to the welfare of these patients. This chapter will discuss preoperative assessment of patients with hematologic disorders, and review the risk of perioperative hematologic complications and specific management strategies to reduce perioperative risks in this vulnerable patient population.

PREOPERATIVE ASSESSMENT OF PATIENTS WITH HEMATOLOGIC DISORDERS

■ HISTORY AND PHYSICAL EXAMINATION

The most important aspect in the preoperative assessment of patients with a hematologic disorder is a thorough history. This is especially true for patients with hemostatic disorders (**Table 54-1**). Though the patient may have a known hemostatic diagnosis, the clinical phenotype of these patients may vary considerably. Occasionally, a patient may report an unexpected personal and/or family history of bleeding or thrombosis, or a hematologic diagnosis as a child with no subsequent follow-up. Depending on the severity of the presumed diagnosis, these subjective accounts may need to be confirmed objectively. The physical examination is rarely helpful in such situations. However, the presence of petechiae, purpura, ecchymoses, jaundice, ascites, and splenomegaly may alert one to the presence of potential hematologic disorder.

Similarly, given the high perioperative complications in patients with sickle cell disease (SCD), a careful history is critical to ensure optimal surgical outcomes. Specific questions include recent cough, wheezing, dyspnea on exertion, fever, ankle edema, right upper quadrant pain, change in stool or urine color, hematuria, or dysuria. In addition, details on past SCD-related complications should be documented, including acute chest syndrome, frequency of pain episodes, strokes, hyperhemolytic crisis, pulmonary hypertension, aplastic crisis, transfusion reactions, and alloimmunization.

In addition to the specific questions above, all patients with hematologic disorders should have the following documented: alcohol use, smoking history, past anesthesia history, current medications (including vitamins, supplements, and herbal preparations), and allergies. Herbal remedies are often self-administered by patients and can modify hemostasis. These medications should be stopped prior to surgery.

■ DIAGNOSTIC STUDIES

It has been established by multiple prospective studies that the use of routine preoperative coagulation testing is not helpful in the absence of a bleeding history. In contrast, a preoperative complete blood count and coagulation testing is essential in patients with known hematologic disorders. **Table 54-2** list laboratory and radiology studies that should be considered in the preoperative assessment of these patients.

TABLE 54-1 Recommended Questions to Ask in Patients with Known or Suspected Hemostatic Disorders

- Have you or anyone in your family ever been labeled a "bleeder"? Has someone in the family ever experienced abnormal bleeding?
- Have you ever bled with surgery or following childbirth? What surgical procedures have you had, including major surgery, minor surgery, biopsies, and dental extractions?
- Did a surgeon or dentist ever have to re-explore the wound site or did you ever have to return to the operative suite for hemorrhagic control?
- Have you ever had excessive menstrual periods? How long do your periods last? How many pads or tampons are needed each day? Have you ever required iron supplementation for anemia due to a menstrual blood loss?
- Do you bruise excessively? Are these bruises multiple? Are they confined only to the outer thighs or other areas that are subject to trauma? Are any of these bruises palpable (ie, are they true hematomas) or are they level with the surface of the skin?
- Do you have nosebleeds now or was there ever a time in your life when you did have spontaneous nosebleeds?
- Have you ever required a blood or plasma transfusion and, if so, why?
- Have you ever bruised or experienced hemorrhage following trauma, car accidents, falls, organized or unorganized sports, altercations, or any acts of violence?

Reproduced, with permission, from Kitchens CS, Kessler CM, Konkle BA, eds. *Consultative Hemostasis and Thrombosis*. 3rd ed. Philadelphia: Elsevier Saunders; 2013.

TABLE 54-2 Laboratory and Radiology Studies

All patients with hematologic disorders
- Complete blood count with differential
- Coagulation testing (PT, aPTT)
- Biochemistry profile
- Liver function tests
- Type and cross

Hemostatic disorders*
- Platelet function tests
- von Willebrand antigen and ristocetin cofactor
- Factor assay (eg, factor V, factor VIII, factor IX, factor XI, factor XII)

Hemolytic anemias
- Peripheral blood smear
- Reticulocyte count
- Iron studies and ferritin
- Vitamin B12 and folate levels
- Lactate dehydrogenase (LDH)

Sickle cell disease
- Same as in patients with hemolytic anemia
- Hemoglobin electrophoresis
- Chest radiograph

*Order based on their specific hemostatic disorder.
aPTT, activated partial thromboplastin time; PT, prothrombin time.

PERIOPERATIVE RISK ASSESSMENT AND MANAGEMENT FOR HEMATOLOGIC DISORDERS

Patients with hematologic disorders are at increased risk for complications related to changes in blood cells and plasma factors initiated by surgery. The magnitude of the risk may vary considerably with the underlying hematologic disorder, nature of the surgery, age of the patient and other comorbidities. These disorders may require specific treatment and consultation with hematologists to ensure an accurate assessment of risk of perioperative complications and to improve outcomes. This involves understanding the nature and severity of the hematologic disorders with the goal to minimize the risk of intraoperative bleeding and postoperative complications including bleeding, infection, thrombosis, and abnormal wound healing. This section discusses several common hematologic disorders that hospitalists may encounter, the nature of the perioperative risk and specific perioperative management.

■ DISORDERS OF RED BLOOD CELLS

Anemia is a very common abnormality in patients undergoing surgery and is even more common in patients with active hematologic disorders due to treatment, marrow involvement by the disease, bleeding, renal failure, inflammation, or advanced age. Adequate red cell mass is needed to promote tissue oxygen delivery and is a vital factor to aide wound healing and prevent myocardial and central nervous system injury in surgical patients. Red cells can also promote hemostasis and play an important role in postoperative recovery.

Given the importance of red cells, the presence of anemia needs to be recognized preoperatively and corrected if surgery is not emergent. Previously, transfusion of red cells was considered a desirable intervention. However, the administration of red cells was discovered to adversely affect the morbidity and mortality of hospitalized patients in a wide variety of clinical settings. Preoperative anemia has to some extent been a silent risk factor for adverse clinical outcomes due to unnecessary transfusion of red cells that can increase perioperative complications. On the other hand, excess number of red cells may cause hyperviscosity and lead to thrombosis. For instance, patients with polycythemia may need preoperative phlebotomy to reduce the risk, especially when it is caused by polycythemia vera. Common hematologic disorders that can cause anemia and polycythemia will be reviewed.

Nutritional anemias

Patients with iron deficiency anemia should have their anemia corrected preoperatively with oral iron if there is sufficient time, or with intravenous iron if a more urgent response is required. The cause of iron malabsorption or loss should be identified and any possible source of bleeding identified. Folic acid and vitamin B12 are nutrients required to promote proliferation of marrow cells to produce red cells, as well as white cells and platelets. Once these nutrients are replete, it may take several days to start to see a reticulocyte response and several weeks to restore the blood count to normal.

More commonly, some patients do not have a single factor contributing to anemia and correction is often difficult due to diseases associated with renal insufficiency and chronic inflammation that can adversely affect iron utilization, resulting in reduced red cell production. In such circumstances, red cell transfusion may be required to maintain adequate tissue oxygen delivery during surgery.

Hemolytic anemias

Anemia due to production of IgG or IgM autoantibodies is challenging and may require pre- and postoperative interventions. Patients with autoimmune-mediated hemolytic anemia (AIHA) usually have positive Coombs tests, with pan-agglutination of their plasma with donor red cells. The presence of warm IgG autoantibodies results in hemolysis of both the native and transfused red cells making it difficult to provide "crossmatch" compatible blood for surgery. Despite this, when medically necessary, serologically incompatible but type-specific red cells should be transfused if the patient's hemoglobin levels are causing hypotension and organ dysfunction. Acutely decompensating patients with AIHA who received serologically incompatible blood transfusion do not experience transfusion-related alloimmunization or an increase in hemolysis. Thus, life-saving red cell transfusion should not be denied due to serologically incompatible blood.

Patients with cold agglutinin disease produce IgM antibodies that react in the cold and fix complement to the red cells, promoting extravascular clearance by the reticuloendothelial system. Cold agglutinin disease can occur in response to mycoplasma infection, autoimmune disease and in lymphoproliferative disorders, such as Waldenstrom's macroglobulinemia. These antibodies can be detected with a positive Coombs test that is complement-mediated. Blood transfusion in patients with cold agglutinin disease should be infused via a blood warmer. If the antibodies are actively promoting hemolysis at room temperature, the patient should be kept warm to prevent hemolysis by increasing the room thermostat.

Many patients with antibody-mediated hemolytic anemia may have had a surgical splenectomy as treatment for their hematologic disorder. Splenectomized patients are at increased risk for both bacterial infection and thromboembolism, both of which can affect perioperative morbidity and mortality. All splenectomized patients should receive immunization against the following organisms: *Streptococcus pneumoniae*, *Haemophilus influenzae* type B, and *Neisseria meningitidis*. These vaccinations should be given at least 14 days prior to elective splenectomy or immediately after an emergent splenectomy. In addition, splenectomized patients are at increased risk for venous thromboembolism (VTE) and should receive adequate VTE prophylaxis in the immediate postoperative period.

Patients with atypical hemolytic-uremic syndrome (aHUS) or paroxysmal nocturnal hemoglobinuria (PNH) experience hemolysis due to defects in complement regulation. These patients may be receiving treatment with the complement inhibitor, eculizumab. Since this drug inhibits complement activation, a major mechanism to fight infection, these patients are prone to meningococcemia. A raised awareness of the possibility of meningococcal infection is warranted in these patients.

Patients with hemolytic disorders should receive folic acid, vitamin B12 and iron supplementation to promote hemoglobin synthesis and red cell production. These nutrients should be replete prior to any elective surgery. Patients with coexisting renal failure or chronic inflammation may not produce adequate erythropoietin to promote accelerated erythropoiesis in response to anemia. These patients typically have red cell half-lives that are reduced at least 8-fold and require reticulocyte levels >10% to maintain normal levels of red blood cells. Exogenous erythropoietin injections may be required to compensate for the shortened red cell survival.

Sickle cell disease and other hemoglobinopathies

There exists a substantial degree of variability in the clinical severity of all molecular forms of sickle cell disease. This is due to a wide variety of abnormalities in the hemoglobin molecule. The most common form of sickle cell disease is due to a homozygous point mutation in the beta chain of hemoglobin that leads to the intracellular polymerization of soluble hemoglobin. The cells undergo a change in their shape and forms cells that can be seen on blood smears as irreversible sickle cells. Sickle cell disease presents major challenges to the hospitalist during the pre- and perioperative care.

There can be variable degrees of anemia and end organ damage in sickle cell disease. Some patients experience mild anemia and limited pain crisis while others can have severe hemolytic anemia complicated by pulmonary hypertension, liver disease, renal insufficiency and osteonecrosis of hip and other bones. Strategies for risk reduction require a multidisciplinary approach with surgery, anesthesia and medicine developing a customized care plan for the patient based on surgical risk and severity of sickle cell disease. During the perioperative period, patients with sickle cell disease are at increased risk of painful crisis, acute chest syndrome, and cerebrovascular accidents as surgical procedures may be complicated by hypoxia, hypothermia or acidosis; all of which promotes red cell sickling. The surgical and anesthesia team need to pay special attention to perioperative hydration, oxygenation status and underlying pulmonary, and cardiovascular disease. If the surgery involves general anesthesia, it is strongly recommended that red blood cells be transfused (either through simple or exchange transfusion) in patients with sickle cell anemia (Hb SS) to bring the hemoglobin level to 10 g/dL as this has been shown to reduce perioperative mortality and complications. In patients who already have a hemoglobin level higher than 8.5 g/dL without transfusion, are on chronic hydroxyurea therapy or require high-risk surgery (eg, neurosurgery, prolonged anesthesia, cardiac bypass), a hematologist with experience in sickle cell disease management should be consulted for guidance on appropriate transfusion methods.

As these patients are at high-risk for red blood cell (RBC) alloimmunization, a presurgery type and screen is sent to Blood Bank ahead of time to identify and characterize RBC antibodies (if any), which can be a laborious effort. If no antibodies are found, typically leukocyte-reduced RBC units, which are phenotypically matched for C, E, and Kell as well as ABO and D antigens, are transfused. If antibodies are present, finding compatible phenotypic match units can be time-consuming, hence the need to plan ahead.

Postoperatively, if the patient has a history of acute chest syndrome, admission to the intensive care unit should be considered for close respiratory monitoring. Regardless of location, the primary team should pay particular attention to hydration and oxygenation status. Dehydration and low oxygen levels can precipitate erythrocyte sickling, leading to vaso-occlusive crisis. For management of postoperative surgical pain, patients with chronic pain may have opioid tolerance and require higher doses of narcotics. Reports of pain should be treated accordingly and narcotics should not be withheld for fear of addiction as stress from acute pain can trigger the onset of a vaso-occlusive crisis. On the other hand, overhydration and excessive narcotic use can lead to pulmonary edema and respiratory depression, respectively. Hence, these patients require strict monitoring of hydration and oxygenation status. An incentive spirometer should be prescribed to all patients with sickle cell disease postoperatively as this has been shown to reduce pulmonary complications. Patients with sickle cell disease are also at increased risk of venous thromboembolism (VTE). Given that surgery is a known transient risk factor for VTE, appropriate VTE prophylaxis (either mechanical and/or pharmacological) should be prescribed.

Hemolytic anemia can also occur due to metabolic defects in red cells. Red cell membrane proteins are prone to oxidative damage. The red cells must be capable of reducing oxidatively damaged cells or they will be removed from the body, resulting in hemolysis. Glucose-6-phoshate dehydrogenase deficiency is a common X-linked metabolic disorder that can lead to hemolytic anemia. Patients with this disorder are usually well compensated but will become symptomatic when exposed to drugs that lead to oxidative stress. These patients must not be exposed to specific drugs that can lead to a major hemolytic crisis. The list of drugs that causes hemolysis is published online at: http://g6pd.org/en/G6PD-Deficiency/SafeUnsafe/DaEvitare_ISS-it and should be reviewed to minimize the hemolytic risk to these patients preoperatively.

DISORDERS OF STEM CELLS: MYELODYSPLASTIC SYNDROME AND MYELOPROLIFERATIVE DISORDERS

There are several hematologic disorders that can alter white blood cell counts and qualitative function that may lead to serious complication for patients should they require surgical intervention. There are a growing number of individuals over 60 years of age with myelodysplastic syndrome (MDS). This disease syndrome represents a wide variety of defects in the bone marrow stem cells that can cause abnormalities in the production of red cells, white cells and/or platelets. These patients may have varying degrees of blood cell production abnormalities and be at risk for bleeding, infection or thrombosis and cardiopulmonary compromise due to anemia. They may require support with red cells because they are severely anemic and have a low reticulocyte count. Some patients with MDS are responsive to exogenous erythropoietin but others require transfusion support. The hematologist caring for these patients should assist in providing guidance regarding marrow function.

In patients with myeloproliferative disorders, such as polycythemia vera (PV) and essential thrombocythemia (ET), there is an increased perioperative thrombohemorrhagic risk. A high proportion of these surgeries are complicated by vascular occlusion or by major hemorrhage. Uncontrolled PV leads to marked increase in blood viscosity and stasis, reduced capillary blood flow, and subsequently tissue hypoxia. The risk of cardiovascular death and major thrombosis is reduced in patients with PV when the hematocrit is maintained at less than 45% with the use of phlebotomy, with or without cytotoxic chemotherapy. However, it is unclear if an acute reduction in hematocrit results in a decrease in perioperative thrombohemorrhagic risk. A large retrospective study of patients with myeloproliferative disorders undergoing surgery found that despite adequate control of blood count with phlebotomy and administration of standard VTE prophylaxis, these patients had increased bleeding risk (7.3%) and high rates of symptomatic VTE (7.7%) after surgery.

In patients with ET, the uncontrolled production of platelets and megakaryocyte proliferation can often lead to a dramatic increase in platelet count over one million. Platelet function may also be abnormal with defects in both adhesion and/or aggregation responses. The bleeding risk seen in patients with ET can be attributable to either dysfunctional platelets or acquired von Willebrand disease. Patients with acquired von Willebrand disease and ET are more likely to suffer from hemorrhagic events than thrombotic events. The risk of both thrombosis and hemorrhage is higher in older patients and in those who have had prior events. Lowering of hematocrit and platelet count should ideally be done over several weeks to months. Elective surgery should be delayed to allow the hematologist to treat the elevated platelet count or increased red cell mass. If surgery is imminent, repetitive phlebotomy in PV patients to lower the red cell count or platelet pheresis to rapidly lower platelet count in ET are also therapeutic options.

DISORDERS OF WHITE BLOOD CELLS: BENIGN AND HEMATOLOGIC MALIGNANCIES

Hospitalists sometimes encounter a patient that has a low neutrophil count but is not symptomatic and no history of recurrent infections. Benign ethnic neutropenia is due to a polymorphism seen in several ethnic groups of African and Middle East descent. These patients usually do not have an increased risk of infection and no specific intervention is required perioperatively. In contrast, patients with severe congenital neutropenia are prone to infections and have a much lower absolute neutrophil count, usually <500/mm³. About half of all cases of severe congenital neutropenia are caused by mutations in the ELANE gene. These patients may require granulocyte-colony stimulating factor (G-CSF), which increases the neutrophil count and decreases the severity and frequency of infections.

Patients with acute hematologic malignancies (acute myeloid or lymphocytic leukemia) are often anemic, leukopenic and/or thrombocytopenic. They are at a high perioperative risk for bleeding and infection risk. These cytopenias can occur as a clinical manifestation of the underlying hematologic disorder or from bone marrow suppression from treatment with antineoplastic agents. If a patient receiving treatment for a hematologic malignancy requires surgery, the cytopenias secondary to antineoplastic agents or radiation therapy usually recovers 14 to 21 days after exposure to these marrow suppressive agents. It may be prudent to delay elective surgery to allow for bone marrow recovery to minimize both bleeding and infection risk. If surgery is imminent, red cells and platelet transfusion may be required along with aggressive antimicrobial therapy. The use of G-CSF may also be considered to promote leukocyte recovery.

In addition, these patients are often deconditioned with poor functional status from the effects of chemotherapy and prolonged hospitalization, placing them at higher risk for postoperative complications. Antineoplastic agents can also result in poor wound healing. Postoperatively, careful attention should be paid to their nutritional status and rehabilitation to minimize these risks.

DISORDERS OF PLATELETS: CONGENITAL PLATELET DISORDERS AND THROMBOCYTOPENIA

For patients with congenital platelet disorders with a known bleeding history, transfusion of single-donor platelets is usually recommended prior to surgery. The most common platelet disorder is storage pool disease, but there are several other abnormalities that affect platelet aggregation. Postoperatively, depending on the type of surgery, additional platelet transfusion maybe recommended prophylactically or if clinically indicated to manage postoperative bleeding. In patients in whom platelet transfusion is ineffective due to alloantibody development, recombinant factor VIIa (rFVII) has also been used with some success. In certain individuals with mild bleeding phenotype, the consulting hematologist may recommend the use of desmopressin (DDAVP). This is given daily or twice daily for about 3 days before it becomes ineffective due to tachyphylaxis. DDAVP is known to cause fluid retention leading to hyponatremia, thus strict fluid balance is required to avoid electrolyte imbalances postsurgery.

Another common acquired hemostatic disorder is thrombocytopenia, which can be due to decreased production (eg, bone marrow suppression from hematologic malignancies) or increased platelet destruction (eg, immune thrombocytopenia). With the availability of platelet transfusion, even high-risk surgeries can be performed in the severely thrombocytopenic patients. A platelet count of >100,000/μL is usually adequate for all surgical procedures, including high-risk procedures (eg, neurosurgical or spinal surgery). For low- to moderate-risk surgical procedures, transfusion to increase the platelet count to >50,000/μL is usually recommended. Serial monitoring of the platelet count is important during the postoperative period as platelet survival is usually shortened and additional platelet support may be needed. In cases of coexisting liver disease due to cirrhosis or other disease process, the patient may have an enlarged spleen that will sequester platelets, resulting in variable degrees of thrombocytopenia. Furthermore, patients with hepatitis C and cirrhosis may have low thrombopoietin (TPO) levels. These patients may respond to TPO-mimetic agents (romiplostim and eltrombopag) and can be treated for a short duration if needed to optimize management. There is a thrombotic risk with the use of TPO-mimetic agents and this treatment should only be considered when other approaches have failed and bleeding risk is high.

In patients with immune thrombocytopenia (ITP), prophylactic platelet transfusion prior to surgery is usually ineffective. Instead, glucocorticoids and/or intravenous γ-globulin are prescribed to increase the platelet count. Since prednisone and other glucocorticoids can interfere with wound healing, other regimens are preferred in the patient that needs surgery. Other options include RhoGAM (anti-Rh therapy if the patient is Rh antigen positive) and TPO-mimetic agents to increase the platelet count. This can take several days to weeks to observe a response.

■ DISORDERS OF HEMOSTASIS

Patients with inherited disorders of coagulation (eg, hemophilia A, hemophilia B) are at increased risk of intra and postoperative bleeding. These patients often have an established outpatient hematologist that can define the severity of the patient's disease and risk for bleeding. The risk should not be underestimated as bleeding into deep tissues, vital organs or along tissue planes can lead to severe hypotension, organ damage and death. A wide variety of hemostatic agents are available to reduce bleeding risk. Issues that assist in defining the dose of hemostatic agent depend upon baseline clotting factor level, nature of surgery and prior clinical response to treatments.

Specific guidelines have been published for management of defects in coagulation factors. All patients should have a treatment plan defining the nature of the product to be used to correct the defect, how the treatment should be monitored and the duration of therapy. Elective surgery should not be performed at an institution that does not have the availability to monitor and infuse the recommended coagulation factor replacement. Perioperative recommendations should be detailed in the medical chart prior to surgery. In the event of an emergent surgery where no recommendations are available, a hematologist should be consulted. In cases of an emergency, it is recommended to infuse either fresh frozen plasma (FFP) or cryoprecipitate to stabilize the patient and transfer to a tertiary center that can manage these patients. FFP can be used in cases of factor IX or XI deficiency. Cryoprecipitate is enriched in vWF, factor VIII, and fibrinogen and can be used in cases of hemophilia A or von Willebrand disease.

Generally, in patients with hemophilia A, B, or von Willebrand disease, specific factor levels should be maintained as high and for as long as clinically indicated based on published guidelines and clinical response to surgery. The prescribed factor is usually infused as a bolus in the morning prior to surgery, with specific factor levels measured before anesthesia induction to confirm that the factor has been administered and the appropriate factor level achieved. Failure to achieve an adequate factor level may be a sign of an inhibitor or inadequate dosing which may require that the surgery be postponed. If the patient has developed an inhibitor the patient may need to be transferred to a center with significant experience in managing inhibitor patients.

Postoperatively, the duration of maintenance therapy depends on the type of surgery performed, ranging from a few days for fairly minor surgical procedures (dental work, simple biopsies) to 2 weeks for more invasive surgery such as abdominal or orthopedic surgery. Factor levels are monitored daily for the first few days and can usually be lowered once surgical hemostasis is achieved (usually by the fourth or fifth day). Once the patient is safe to discharge from a surgical standpoint, it is important to ensure that these patients have an adequate care plan in place for home factor infusion (central line placement, factor delivered to home, self-infusion vs home health nurse infusion) as they will likely require additional days of factor infusion. If a care plan is not in place or not feasible, the patient should remain in the hospital until completion of factor maintenance therapy. Inadequate factor replacement therapy is one of the main risk factor for surgical readmissions due to postoperative bleeding and wound dehiscence in these patients.

TABLE 54-3 Treatment Options for Coagulation Factor Deficiencies

Deficiency	Treatment Options
Fibrinogen	Fibrinogen concentrate, cryoprecipitate, FFP
Factor II	PCC, FFP
Factor V	FFP, platelets (contains factor V)
Factor VII	rFVIIa, PCC containing factor VII, FFP
Factor X	PCC, FFP
Factor XI	FFP, factor XI concentrate*
Factor XIII	Factor XIII concentrate, FFP, cryoprecipitate

*Not available in the United States. FFP, fresh frozen plasma; PCC, prothrombin complex concentrates; rFVIIa, recombinant VIIa concentrate.

Similar principles apply for patients with rare factor deficiencies (fibrinogen, factor II, factor V, factor VII, factor X, factor XI, and factor XIII). **Table 54-3** lists the type of factor deficiencies and their treatment options.

The wound healing process is dependent upon a provisional matrix composed of fibrin. Hemostatic defects that limit the formation of a fibrin matrix may lead to wound healing defects resulting in delayed bleeding or reduced rate of wound closure. Patients with hemophilia or other congenital bleeding disorders display delayed bleeding after trauma or surgery if the initial clot that forms is not stable and resistant to breakdown. Furthermore, wound healing is a dynamic process. The initial clot is subsequently remodeled and the ability to reform fibrin must be maintained until the initial fibrin matrix is replaced by the synthesis of extracellular matrix.

Antifibrinolytics such as aminocaproic acid and tranexamic acid are often prescribed as adjunct therapy postsurgery in patients with congenital hemostatic disorders. These agents inhibit tissue fibrinolysis, leading to clot stabilization. The prophylactic use of antifibrinolytics has been shown to reduce postoperative bleeding in cardiac, orthopedic and liver transplant surgery. In patients with hematuria of upper urinary tract origin, antifibrinolytics are not recommended as it can cause intrarenal or ureteral obstruction through clot formation. Of note, there have been case reports of thrombotic complications associated with the use of antifibrinolytics in patients that have chronic DIC syndrome and cancer. Judicious use of these agents is recommended in patients who are known to be prothrombotic (eg, recent thrombotic events, known coronary artery disease, or cancer patients).

The lupus anticoagulant represents a common preoperative issue that generates significant confusion and often leads to delays in surgery. These patients will have an abnormal aPTT and no history of bleeding, assuming there is no other defect reported. The lupus anticoagulant is a misnomer because patients that have this laboratory abnormality do not bleed and are in fact at an increased risk of thrombosis. Lupus anticoagulants are likely to be detected in routine pre-op screening of patients that do not have any bleeding history. Laboratory testing will often document a prolongation of the aPTT. A mixing study of the patient's plasma with normal plasma will not correct the defect after incubating the plasma for 60 minutes. The only caveat that warrants further consideration is the lupus anticoagulant patient that has a bleeding history or a very prolonged PT. These patients may have a coexisting factor inhibitor or very low prothrombin levels due to the presence of antiprothrombin antibodies that promote the clearance of prothrombin. Consultation with a hematologist will be needed to further define the lab abnormality and provide medical clearance for surgery.

TABLE 54-4 Established Risk Factors for Perioperative Hematologic Complications

Patient specific
- Advanced age
- Other comorbidities
  - Liver disease
  - Kidney disease
  - Cardiovascular disease

Procedure specific
- Type of surgery
- Choice of anesthesia

■ FACTORS THAT INCREASE RISK OF HEMATOLOGIC COMPLICATIONS

There are several patient-specific and procedure-specific risk factors that are known to increase hematologic complications with surgery (**Table 54-4**).

■ PATIENT-SPECIFIC RISK FACTORS

Advanced age

Hematologic complications are greatly influenced by advanced age. The incidence of venous thromboembolism increases sharply with age. In individuals in the 25 to 30 years age group, the incidence is approximately 1 per 10,000 person-years. In contrast, the incidence increases about 80-fold with nearly 8 per 1000 person-year in the 85 years and older age group. Advanced age is also a risk factor for bleeding. The IMPROVE bleeding risk model which provides an estimate of in-hospital bleeding from the time of admission up to 14 days following admission for an acute medical illness demonstrated that the probability of major in-hospital bleeding for men was 0.1% in the <40 years, 0.2% in the 40 to 84 years, and 0.5% in the ≥85 years. The probability of a clinically important in-hospital bleeding was 0.5%, 1.1%, and 2.2%, respectively.

The prevalence of anemia, a known risk factor for postoperative mortality, also increases with advancing age, especially after the fifth decade of life and exceeds 20% in those 85 years and older. Anemia in the elderly may be due to decreased red cell production from age-related decline in normal bone marrow function, nutritional deficiencies (iron, B12 or folate) from poor dietary intake or decreased erythropoietin production from chronic kidney disease. Inflammatory response related to chronic disease conditions can also causes anemia of chronic inflammation, a disorder mediated by an increase in hepcidin production. Preoperative anemia can result in increased morbidity and mortality, particularly in elderly patients, as the surgery itself stresses the cardiovascular system, resulting in tissue hypoxia from reduced cardiac output and underlying atherosclerosis. This risk can be minimized through the correction of anemia using iron to correct the anemia or through exogenous erythropoietin injection. However, many elderly patients may have a primary marrow defect and not be responsive to such therapy. Underlying MDS or other changes that influence marrow response may affect the elderly and the threshold for providing transfusion support is dependent on the magnitude and extend of other organ dysfunction such as pulmonary, cardiac, vascular, or neurologic problems.

Other comorbidities

The presence of other comorbidities such as liver and kidney disease also increases the risk of perioperative hematologic complications.

Patients with liver disease are often coagulopathic from decreased hepatic synthesis of procoagulant and anticoagulant clotting factors, impaired hepatic clearance of fibrinolytics, malabsorption of vitamin K from impaired bile salt recirculation, dysfibrinogenemia, thrombocytopenia from hypersplenism and impaired thrombopoietin production, and platelet dysfunction. As both procoagulant and anticoagulant activities are affected, these patients are not "autoanti-coagulated." Instead, these patients remain in a balanced hemostatic state, albeit a more tenuous state, which is easily disturbed by any external stressors, such as surgery. As a result, patients with liver disease are at increased perioperative risk of bleeding and thrombosis.

For patients with mild liver disease (prolongation of INR <2.0) undergoing low- or moderate risk surgery, prophylactic intervention is usually not required. For high-risk surgery or severe liver disease, the correction of factors that are severely depressed may aide hemostasis. However, aggressive therapy with FFP to correct the INR is not feasible and will lead to volume overload in these patients. Recent studies using thromboelastograms to guide therapy have demonstrated that correction of the INR can be replaced by an approach that attempts to correct low fibrinogen, low platelet count and low coagulation factor levels. These patients are often undernourished or exposed to antibiotics. As these patients may be vitamin K deficient, vitamin K replacement therapy can be given to see if this helps to correct the coagulopathy.

Chronic kidney disease is associated with increased perioperative morbidity from impaired hemostasis secondary to acquired platelet dysfunction, leading to uremic bleeding. Both DDAVP and conjugated estrogen have been used, either alone or concurrently, as prophylaxis prior to surgery or for treatment of acute bleeding. As DDAVP has a limited clinical effect due to tachyphylaxis, it is more commonly used prior to minor surgical procedures (eg, biopsies and endoscopies) whereas conjugated estrogen, which has a longer duration of action of up to 10 days, can be used for elective surgery. Depending on the severity of the platelet dysfunction, platelet transfusion may be indicated. Patients with chronic kidney disease are also frequently anemic from reduced erythropoietin production. Besides tissue hypoxia, anemia can also cause platelet dysfunction by several possible mechanisms. Thus, a decrease in hematocrit may further enhance risk for bleeding and should be corrected prior to surgery. Correction of anemia by use of erythropoietin or transfusion may improve platelet function and is an additional strategy to aide hemostasis in uremic patients.

Given the rising incidence of cardiovascular disease, majority of the population are on aspirin and other antiplatelet agents, including GPIIb/IIIa antagonists, which cause defects in platelet aggregation. The concomitant use of antiplatelet and anticoagulant agents increase the risk of bleeding perioperatively. Prior to surgery, these drugs should be discontinued or avoided in the perioperative period, if safe to do so from a cardiovascular perspective. If needed, platelet transfusion may be indicated prior to surgery or in the case of excessive bleeding.

■ PROCEDURE-SPECIFIC RISK FACTORS

Type of surgery

The postoperative risk of bleeding, which is the highest contributor to morbidity and mortality in patients with malignant or nonmalignant hematologic disease, is greatly influenced by the type of surgery. A bleeding risk stratification based on the type of surgical or invasive procedures helps predict postoperative risk of bleeding and guide preoperative management (**Table 54-5**).

Choice of anesthesia

The choice of anesthesia can influence perioperative morbidity and mortality. General anesthesia may reduce myocardial contractility

TABLE 54-5 **Risk for Bleeding with Surgical or Invasive Procedures**

Risk	Type of Procedure	Examples
Low	Nonvital organs involved, exposed surgical site, limited dissection	Lymph node biopsy, dental extraction, cataract extraction, most cutaneous surgery, laparoscopic procedures, coronary angiography
Moderate	Vital organs involved, deep, or extensive dissection	Laparotomy, thoracotomy, mastectomy, major orthopedic surgery, pacemaker insertion
High	Bleeding likely to compromise surgical result, bleeding complications frequent	Neurosurgery, ophthalmic surgery, cardiopulmonary bypass, prostatectomy or bladder surgery, major vascular surgery, renal biopsy, bowel polypectomy

Reprinted with permission from Reding MT, Key NS. Hematologic problems in the surgical patient: bleeding and thrombosis. In: Hoffman R, Benz RJ, Shattil S, et al, eds. *Hematology: Basic Principles and Practice*, 6th ed. Philadelphia: Churchill Livingstone; 2013.

and cardiac output. This further decreases tissue oxygen-delivery in elderly patients with borderline anemia, and may potentially lead to acute cardiac decompensation, resulting in myocardial ischemia, infarction and/or stroke. Certain inhalational general anesthetic agents can also inhibit the enzymatic activity of glucose-6-phosphate dehydrogenase (G6PD) activity, which leads to acute hemolysis in patients with G6PD deficiency. An awareness of this diagnosis should be communicated to the surgical and anesthetic team and placed in the chart to avoid the use of drugs known to precipitate hemolysis.

CONCLUSION

As the risk of perioperative complications can vary considerably depending on the underlying hematologic disorder, it is important to identify the disorder and its severity. A careful assessment of the benefits of surgery against the risk of perioperative complications is essential. With appropriate perioperative evaluation and management strategies, these patients should be able to undergo the majority of surgeries with risk reduced by managing known risk factors.

SUGGESTED READINGS

Feely MA, Collins CS, Daniels PR, Kebede EB, Jatoi A, Mauck KF. Preoperative testing before noncardiac surgery: guidelines and recommendations. *Am Fam Physician*. 2013;87(6):414-418.

Fellin FM. Perioperative evaluation of patients with hematologic disorders. In: Merli F, Weitz H, eds. *Medical Management of the Surgical Patient*. Saunders Elsevier, Philadelphia 2008.

Kitchens CS, Lawson JW. Surgery and hemostasis. In: Kitchens CS, Kessler CM, Konkle BA, eds. *Consultative Hemostasis and Thrombosis*, 3rd ed. Philadelphia: Elsevier Saunders; 2013.

Reding MT, Key NS. Hematologic problems in the surgical patient: bleeding and thrombosis. In: Hoffman R, Benz RJ, Shattil S, et al, eds. *Hematology: Basic Principles and Practice*, 6th ed. Philadelphia: Churchill Livingstone; 2013.

Prevention, Assessment, and Management of Common Complications in Noncardiac Surgery

CHAPTER 55

Antimicrobial Prophylaxis in Surgery

Louisa W. Chiu, MD
E. Patchen Dellinger, MD
Daniel A. Anaya, MD

It is estimated that over 40 million surgical procedures are performed every year in the United States. Surgical site infections (**Table 55-1**) complicate approximately 2% to 5% of these procedures, representing 38% of nosocomial infections occurring in surgical patients. Risk factors for surgical site infections (SSIs) can be classified as either patient-related factors or surgical factors, and can be stratified into modifiable, potentially modifiable, and nonmodifiable risk factors. Modifiable risk factors include elective operations in the presence of associated infections, prolonged preoperative hospital stays, seromas, dead space, foreign bodies, and routine drain use, among others, and can be improved with the use of good surgical practice and specific preventive strategies. Nonmodifiable risk factors are most commonly patient-related and have an important effect on the incidence of SSI for each individual patient. The wound class (**Table 55-2**) is a relatively good predictor of SSI and has traditionally been used to estimate the risk of SSI and as a benchmark for comparisons between institutions. However, with the better recent understanding of SSI and its multifactorial risk factors, more sophisticated predictive scores, such as the National Nosocomial Infection Surveillance (NNIS) score, have been developed to better estimate the risk of SSI for each individual patient, after considering the interaction between different risk factors (**Table 55-3**). Specific preventive measures have been identified and are used to decrease the risk of SSI. These include minimizing the presence of microorganisms with prophylactic antibiotics and optimizing the patient's ability to fight those still present at the surgical site during the perioperative period.

PRACTICE POINT

- Patient risk factors for surgical site infections may include obesity, diabetes mellitus, older age, malnutrition, prolonged hospital stay prior to surgery, active infection at another site, cancer, immunosuppression, and tissue ischemia due to irradiation or vascular disease. Although some of these risk factors may not be reversible, hospitalists taking care of preoperative patients should optimize glycemic control and nutritional status, and encourage smoking cessation.

IMPACT OF SURGICAL SITE INFECTION

SSIs are associated with several adverse outcomes. Patients with SSI are more likely to develop additional complications, including wound dehiscence, hernias, and necrotizing soft tissue infections. Multiple large, single-center, multicenter, and population-level analyses have revealed at least a twofold increased risk of postoperative mortality in patients with SSI. Additionally, SSI is associated with longer hospital stays (10-12 excess days), a higher risk of intensive care unit (ICU) admission, and a fivefold higher risk of hospital readmission. Similarly, the treatment of patients with SSI results in excess costs of over $5000 per patient, representing a US national cost between $130 and $845 million per year. Given the availability of multiple preventive measures, SSI is used as a health care quality indicator.

TABLE 55-1 Criteria for SSI

Classification	Definition

Superficial incisional	• Within 30 d postoperatively
	• Involves skin or subcutaneous tissue of the incision and at least one of the following:
	    Purulent drainage from the superficial incision
	    Organism isolated from an aseptically obtained culture of fluid or tissue from the superficial incision
	    At least one of the following signs or symptoms of infection: pain or tenderness, localized swelling, redness, or heat and incision is deliberately opened by surgeon and is culture-positive or not cultured
	    Diagnosis by surgeon or attending physician

Deep incisional	• Within 30 d if no implant in place; within 1 y if implant
	• Involves deep soft tissues and at least 1 of the following:
	    Purulent drainage from the deep incision but not from the organ/space component
	    Deep incision spontaneously dehisces or is deliberately opened and is culture-positive or not cultured and has at least one of the following: fever or localized pain or tenderness
	    An abscess or other evidence of infection found on direct examination, during reoperation, or by histopathologic or radiologic examination
	    Diagnosis by surgeon or attending physician

Organ/space	• Within 30 d if no implant in place; within 1 y if implant
	• Involves any part of the body, excluding the skin incision, fascia, or muscle layers, that is opened or manipulated during the operative procedure
	• Has at least one of the following:
	    Purulent drainage from a drain that is placed through a stab wound into the organ/space
	    Organisms isolated from an aseptically obtained culture of fluid or tissue
	    An abscess or other evidence of infection found on direct examination, during reoperation, or by histopathologic or radiologic examination
	    Diagnosis by surgeon or attending physician

RATIONALE FOR ANTIMICROBIAL PROPHYLAXIS

Antimicrobial prophylaxis is used when infection *is not present* but the risk of postoperative SSI *is present*. The goal of prophylaxis is not necessarily to sterilize the surgical site, but to reduce microbial colonization of the wound to levels that the patient's immune system is able to handle. The absolute benefit of antibiotic prophylaxis and the number needed to treat to prevent an SSI varies by the baseline risk of infection for each procedure. The decision to use prophylaxis should be based on an assessment of the risk of infection and the cost and morbidity of the infections that might occur for that procedure, balanced against the cost of prophylaxis and its potential for adverse effects, including allergies, superinfections, and the generation of bacterial resistance by overuse.

INDICATIONS FOR ANTIBIOTIC PROPHYLAXIS

John Burke first demonstrated the value of prophylactic antimicrobials in the 1950s with animal studies. Since then, many retrospective studies, prospective randomized trials, systematic reviews, and meta-analyses have confirmed the efficacy of prophylactic antimicrobials in decreasing the risk of SSI and established the basic principles. The magnitude of this protective effect relates directly to the magnitude of the risk of SSI. The majority of studies have focused on evaluating the efficacy of prophylactic antibiotics when used for specific operations. This has resulted in high-level data supporting their use for clean-contaminated and contaminated operations, and more controversial data for their use in operations classified as clean. However, the risk of SSI can vary significantly between patients

TABLE 55-2 Surgical Wound Classification Based on Degree of Potential Contamination According to the Centers for Disease Control and Prevention (CDC) Guidelines

Classification	Description
Clean	• An uninfected operative wound in which no inflammation is encountered and the respiratory, alimentary, genital, or uninfected urinary tract is not entered. • Operative incisional wounds that follow nonpenetrating (blunt) trauma should be included in this category if they meet criteria.
Clean contaminated	• An operative wound in which the respiratory, alimentary, genital, or urinary tracts are entered under controlled conditions and without unusual contamination. • Specifically, operations involving the biliary tract, appendix, vagina, and oropharynx are included in this category, provided no evidence of infection or major break in technique is encountered.
Contaminated	• Open, fresh, accidental wounds • Operations with major breaks in sterile technique (eg, open cardiac massage) or gross spillage from the gastrointestinal tract • Incisions in which acute, nonpurulent inflammation is encountered are included in this category
Dirty	• Old traumatic wounds with retained devitalized tissue • Involve existing clinical infection or perforated viscera • This definition suggests that the organisms causing postoperative infection were present in the operative field before the operation

TABLE 55-3 National Nosocomial Infection Surveillance (NNIS) System Classification for Determining the Risk of Surgical Site Infection

Risk Factors	Points
Procedure duration ≥ 75th percentile of duration for that specific operation	1
Contaminated or dirty wound	1
American Society of Anesthesiology score III-V	1

Final Score	Risk of Surgical Site Infection
0	1.5%
1	2.9%
2	6.8%
3	13.0%

undergoing similar surgical procedures. Various studies have shown that using a more comprehensive predictive tool (such as the NNIS score), the risk of SSI can in fact be higher for some patients with less contaminated wounds, depending on the presence of other risk factors. This has been supported by randomized trials and meta-analyses demonstrating a clinical benefit of using prophylactic antibiotics for breast, cardiac, orthopedic, and vascular surgery, as well as other clean operations. Antimicrobial prophylaxis may be reasonable for some clean operations, especially when the potential consequences of SSI may be dire, as after prosthetic joint replacement or a coronary artery bypass grafting (CABG).

Based on existing data and the foregoing considerations, prophylactic antibiotics are indicated for the following:

- Clean-contaminated and contaminated operations
- Clean operations with a high risk of SSI
  - NNIS score ≥ 1 +/– other associated important risk factors
  - Immunocompromised host
  - Other clean operations with known increased risk of SSI, such as groin incisions and mastectomy
- Clean operations for which SSI has significant clinical consequences
  - Examples: craniotomy, cardiac and vascular operations, and operations involving placement of prosthetic material, such as joint replacements and mesh hernia repairs

---

PRACTICE POINT

- Antimicrobial prophylaxis is indicated for contaminated procedures, such as laparotomy for bowel perforation, and clean-contaminated procedures, such as elective intestinal resection, lung resection, or vaginal hysterectomy. It is indicated for clean procedures only in procedures with a significant inherent infection risk, such as mastectomy or operations with groin incisions, or when the consequences of SSI are severe, as in prosthetic joint replacement, craniotomy, and cardiac surgery.

SELECTION OF ANTIMICROBIAL AGENT

The characteristics of the ideal agent for effective antibiotic prophylaxis include (1) bactericidal effect on microorganisms expected to be present at the surgical site, (2) adequate biodistribution in the surgical site, (3) low risk of potential side effects (allergic reactions,

Clostridium difficile colitis, change in resistance patterns), and (4) low cost. The majority of guidelines helping to choose the appropriate agent are based on randomized trials in which a specific antibiotic regimen has been tested for a specific procedure. We support the use of this evidence-based decision making. However, the vast majority of procedures are prone to SSI with similar species of bacteria, and similar types of antibiotics have been tested. If clinical trial data are not available for a specific procedure, it is reasonable to generalize from trial data on procedures with comparable bacterial flora and risk.

The first consideration is to determine the class of wound and the most common bacteria causing SSI in each case. For clean wounds, gram-positive skin flora, including *Staphylococcus aureus* and coagulase-negative staphylococci, are the most common pathogens causing SSI. For these operations, cefazolin is the most commonly used antibiotic, following the four main principles already outlined. Alternatives include other first- or second-generation cephalosporins, oxacillin, and clindamycin. For patients with documented and clinically relevant beta-lactam allergies, clindamycin or vancomycin is an adequate alternative. Most clean-contaminated and contaminated operations are expected to result in exposure to gram negative and anaerobic bacteria. Appropriate regimens in this setting include ertapenem, cefotetan, and cefoxitin as single agents, or multiple-agent regimens such as an aminoglycoside or a quinolone plus clindamycin or metronidazole (**Table 55-4**). Antimicrobials agents with the narrowest spectrum of activity required for efficacy in preventing infection are recommended.

PRACTICE POINT

Selection of antimicrobial agent

1. Determine the class of wound and the most common bacteria causing SSI in each case.
2. Consider local resistance data from your hospital's surveillance systems.
   - A specific agent may be recommended for an operation based on national guidelines. However, if microbiologic data derived from local surveillance programs reveal that expected flora have a high resistance rate to that agent, another antibiotic must be used.
   - Trending patterns of resistance to the different agents used can help identify emergence of resistance early and can guide local protocols.

Recent concern in the media regarding methicillin-resistant *Staphylococcus aureus* (MRSA) infections has led to calls to use vancomycin routinely as a prophylactic agent for clean operations. Per 2013 ASHP/IDSA guidelines, routine use of vancomycin prophylaxis is not recommended for any procedure. However, it may be included in the regimen of choice when cluster cases are detected at an institution, for patients with known MRSA colonization or at high risk for colonization. One recent study randomized cardiac patients to vancomycin versus cefazolin in a hospital with a high rate of MRSA, and found more MRSA infections in the cefazolin arm but more methicillin-sensitive *Staphylococcus aureus* (MSSA) infections in the vancomycin arm, with no difference in overall rates between the two groups. Thus, the use of vancomycin alone may decrease the risk of MRSA SSI, but does not convey protection against other common gram positive bacteria (including MSSA); its routine use may simply result in a shift from MRSA to MSSA SSI, without a significant impact on the overall reduction of SSI. These observations have led to use of two-drug regimens, with vancomycin combined with cefazolin to cover both MRSA and MSSA.

TABLE 55-4 Recommended Antibiotic Prophylaxis Regimens for Different Types of Surgical Procedures Based on Published Guidelines and Most Current Available Data

Type of Surgical Procedure	Recommended Antibiotic Regimen	Alternative Regimens for β-Lactam Allergies
Cardiac procedures	Cefazolin	Clindamycin
	Cefuroxime	Vancomycin
Thoracic procedures	Cefazolin	Clindamycin
	Ampicillin-sulbactam	Vancomycin
Vascular operations	Cefazolin	Clindamycin
		Vancomycin
Gastrointestinal clean procedures and those involving entry into the upper gastrointestinal tract	Cefazolin	Clindamycin
		Vancomycin + ciprofloxacin or aztreonam or aminoglycoside
Small intestine obstruction	Cefazolin + metronidazole	Metronidazole + aminoglycoside or fluoroquinolone
	Cefoxitin	
	Cefotetan	
Biliary tract operations	Cefazolin	Clindamycin
	Ampicillin/sulbactam	Vancomycin + ciprofloxacin or aztreonam or aminoglycoside
	Cefotetan	
	Cefoxitin	Metronidazole + aminoglycoside or ciprofloxacin
	Ceftriaxone	
Appendectomy	Cefoxitin	Ciprofloxacin or an aminoglycoside + metronidazole or clindamycin
	Cefotetan	
	Ampicillin/sulbactam	
	Cefazolin + metronidazole	
	Piperacillin/tazobactam	
	Ertapenem	
	Ciprofloxacin or an aminoglycoside + metronidazole or clindamycin	
Colorectal	Ertapenem	Ciprofloxacin or an aminoglycoside + metronidazole or clindamycin
	Cefoxitin	
	Cefotetan	
	Cefazolin + metronidazole	
	Ciprofloxacin or an aminoglycoside + metronidazole or clindamycin	
	Ampicillin-sulbactam	
In conjunction with mechanical bowel prep	Oral neomycin + erythromycin or oral metronidazole	
Hip or knee arthroplasty	Cefazolin	Clindamycin
		Vancomycin
Hysterectomy	Cefazolin	Ciprofloxacin or an aminoglycoside + metronidazole or clindamycin
	Cefotetan	
	Cefoxitin	
	Cefuroxime	
	Ampicillin-sulbactam	
Head and neck operations	Cefazolin ± metronidazole	Clindamycin
	Cefuroxime + metronidazole	
	Ampicillin-sulbactam	
Urologic operations	Cefazolin	Ciprofloxacin
Neurosurgery	Cefazolin	Vancomycin
		Clindamycin
Liver transplantation	Piperacillin-tazobactam	Clindamycin or vancomycin + aminoglycoside or aztreonam or fluoroquinolone
	Cefotaxime + ampicillin	
Plastic surgery	Cefazolin	Clindamycin
	Ampicillin-sulbactam	Vancomycin

Indications may vary based on the specific operation and standard principles of prophylaxis.

Another approach is to screen for MRSA preoperatively, as MRSA colonization may increase the risk of SSI by 2- to 14-fold. This allows for targeted use of vancomycin (and double coverage when indicated) for patients at risk. Some data also exist to support the use of mupirocin nasal ointment and chlorhexidine baths before surgery to eradicate staphylococcal colonization. Further studies are needed to define the role of routine or selective vancomycin prophylaxis, and measures to eradicate the MRSA carrier state.

Although still controversial, recent studies have shown that for colorectal operations, mechanical bowel preparation (MBP) accompanied by oral prophylactic antibiotics decreased the incidence of SSI. Oral regimens typically include a combination of neomycin sulfate plus erythromycin or metronidazole, and should be given in addition to standard preoperative IV prophylaxis. The oral antimicrobials should be given as three doses over approximately 10 hours, starting the afternoon and evening before the operation and after the MBP.

ANTIBIOTIC TIMING

PRACTICE POINT

Timing, dosage, and duration of prophylactic antibiotics

1. Administer antibiotics within 1 hour prior to incision time.
2. The chosen dose should accomplish adequate tissue levels throughout the whole operation.
   - Higher than standard doses are recommended for obese patients.
   - Current guidelines recommend redosing of antibiotics for procedures lasting two or more half-lives of the specific agent used.
3. No studies have shown the superior efficacy of longer courses of prophylactic antibiotics in the postoperative period.
   - Specifically, for patients undergoing colorectal, other abdominal and gastrointestinal procedures, vascular, cardiac, gyn0ecologic, urologic, orthopedic, and head and neck operations, there is evidence to support the use of short (<12-24 hours) regimens over longer ones, and in the majority of cases, significant evidence to recommend a single-dose strategy.
   - Prolonged courses of prophylactic antibiotics are not associated with clinical benefit and may be attended with significant harms, such as an increased risk of *C. difficile* colitis and the acquisition of antibiotic-resistant pathogens.

The importance of antibiotic administration before incision was the first key fact determined about prophylaxis. John Burke first described the direct relation between timing of prophylaxis (in relation to incision time) and effectiveness, and identified the decisive period to be as close to the incision time as possible. More recently, other investigators have corroborated these findings, showing a linear increase in the rate of SSI as the time of prophylaxis administration gets further from the incision time. All studies show a dramatic rise in SSI when antibiotics are first given after incision. This probably results from both the serum and the tissue antibiotic levels at the time of operation, with the best and most persistent levels achieved when the antibiotic is given close to the incision time. Based on these principles, current guidelines recommend administering prophylactic antibiotics within *1 hour* prior to incision time. This is a more specific time frame than the previously recommended time "at induction of anesthesia." The exceptions are

vancomycin or fluoroquinolones, which both require slow infusion and have longish half-lives. Infusion of these agents may begin 2 hours prior to the incision time, to avoid undesired antibiotic-related side effects. In addition, when the operation involves placement of a proximal tourniquet, the antibiotic infusion must be completed before the tourniquet is inflated, to allow for adequate tissue levels at the surgical site. If a patient was previously receiving therapeutic antimicrobials for an infection before surgery, an extra dose should be given in the 60 minutes prior to incision.

ANTIBIOTIC DOSING

The dose of antibiotic should achieve adequate tissue levels throughout the whole operation. The most accurate way to assure this is to use doses based on body weight. Most weight-based recommendations are derived from the pediatric literature, making this approach somewhat cumbersome, and hence standard doses that fit within recommended parameters are commonly used for the majority of adult patients. However, weight-based recommendations are particularly helpful when using prophylactic antibiotics in patients with extreme body weights. Specifically, the standard dose may need to be decreased to avoid antibiotic toxicity in extremely thin or pediatric patients, particularly when using antibiotics with a narrow therapeutic window. More frequently, however, appropriate doses must be selected to achieve adequate tissue levels in obese patients. Forse and colleagues demonstrated that in obese patients undergoing bariatric surgery, a dose of cefazolin twice the standard dose (2 g vs 1 g) was necessary to achieve adequate serum and tissue levels, and was associated with a lower rate of surgical site infection. Based on this study and others, higher than standard doses are recommended for obese patients. Given the low cost and favorable safety profile of cefazolin, it is reasonable to increase the dose to 2 g for patients weighing more than 80 kg, and to 3 g for those weighing over 120 kg.

In prolonged operations, it may be necessary to repeat the antibiotic dose, given the need for adequate antibiotic tissue levels throughout the whole operation. Randomized trials, large single- and multiple-institution analysis, and the NNIS score have repeatedly identified duration of operation as an important independent risk factor for SSI. The specific mechanisms behind this have not been completely clarified. However, subtherapeutic antibiotic tissue levels at the end of long operations can at least partially explain this association. Studies evaluating redosing of antibiotics for cardiac and gastrointestinal procedures longer than 3 to 4 hours have shown a lower incidence of SSI when following this practice. Given variation in the pharmacokinetic properties of different antibiotics, current guidelines recommend redosing of antibiotics for procedures lasting two or more half-lives of the specific agent used, or if there is excessive blood loss (>1500 mL). Adjustments to this rule need to be considered for patients with renal insufficiency, in which the half-life of most antibiotics is prolonged (**Table 55-5**).

DURATION OF ANTIBIOTIC PROPHYLAXIS

Although adequate intraoperative antibiotic tissue levels are necessary to decrease the risk of SSI, the same is not true for the postoperative period. Despite an extensive body of evidence supporting the use of a single preoperative dose (and intraoperative redosing when indicated) over a multiple-dose strategy (ie, one preoperative dose with subsequent postoperative doses), this is perhaps one of the most difficult principles to translate into real-life practice. A recent analysis demonstrated that in current practice, antibiotics are continued for over 24 hours after the operation in over 50% of patients. Multiple studies in different populations of patients have evaluated the role of single- versus multiple-dose prophylaxis. Specifically, for

TABLE 55-5 Characteristics of Selected Antibiotics More Commonly Used for Surgical Site Infection Prophylaxis

Antibiotic	Recommended Weight-Based Dose	Standard Recommended Dose	Half-Life* (in Hours)	Recommended Redose Interval (in Hours)
Ampicillin-sulbactam	50 mg/kg	3 g	0.8-1.3	2
Cefazolin	20-30 mg/kg	1-2 g	1.2 2.5	2-5
		3 g if > 120 kg		
Cefoxitin	1-2 g	20-40 mg/kg	0.5-1.1	2-3
Cefotetan	1-2 g	20-40 mg	2.8-4.6	3-6
Cefuroxime	50 mg/kg	1.5 g	1-2	3-4
Cefotaxime	50 mg/kg	1 g	0.9-1.7	3
Cefepime	-	1-2 g	2.2	4
Ceftriaxone	50-75 mg/kg	2 g	5.4-10.9	NA
Ciprofloxacin	400 mg	400 mg	3.5-5	4-10
Clindamycin	3-6 mg/kg	600-900 mg	2-5.1	3-6
Ertapenem	-	1 g	4	8
Fluconazole	6 mg/kg	400 mg	30	NA
Gentamicin	3-5 mg/kg	300 mg	2-3	6
Levofloxacin	10 mg/kg	500 mg	6-8	NA
Metronidazole	15 mg/kg	500-1000 mg	6-14	12
Piperacillin/tazobactam		3.375 g	0.7-1.2	2-4
Vancomycin	10-15 mg/kg	1 g	4-6	6-12
Oral antibiotics for colorectal surgery in conjunction with mechanical bowel prep				
Erythromycin base	20 mg/kg	1 g	0.8-3	NA
Metronidazole	15 mg/kg	1 g	6-10	NA
Neomycin	15 mg/kg	1 g	2-3	NA

Reported values applicable to adults.
*Half-life calculated for normal renal function.

patients undergoing colorectal, other abdominal and gastrointestinal, vascular, cardiac, gynecologic, urologic, orthopedic, and head and neck operations, evidence supports the use of shorter (<12-24 hours) regimens over longer ones, and in the majority of cases, significant evidence to recommend a single-dose strategy. There are no studies demonstrating superior efficacy of longer courses of prophylactic antibiotics. McDonald and colleagues reported results of a systematic review based on 28 randomized trials totaling over 9000 patients and reported no difference in the overall rate of SSI with either approach. Based on these findings, the authors recommended the use of a single-dose practice and emphasized the equivalent benefit and decreased cost of this strategy, with the additional benefit of decreasing the emergence of infections caused by resistant pathogens. There are no data to support the continuation of antimicrobial prophylaxis until all indwelling drains and intravascular catheters are removed.

SPECIFIC PROCEDURES

Different single- and multiple-antibiotic regimens have been evaluated for various procedures. Based on these data, the expected microorganisms at the surgical site of each specific procedure, and the similar pharmacologic characteristics of these regimens, different alternatives are recommended. Table 55-4 lists some of these alternatives by surgical type. While this is a helpful guideline for choosing antibiotics, the decision of which antibiotic to use is dynamic, and should also incorporate local and system-related aspects such as cost and antibiotic resistance data.

IMPLEMENTATION PRACTICES/QUALITY IMPROVEMENT

Given the relative high incidence of SSI, its clinical impact, and the significant burden to the health care system, preventive strategies have been receiving more attention by physicians, health care institutions, and policymakers. One strategy to focus efforts on the effective delivery of known preventive strategies is to classify all SSIs as *potentially preventable* (not all prevention measures used or used incorrectly) or *not apparently preventable* (all known preventive measures used appropriately). Several local and national guidelines, specific implementation strategies, and collaborative group approaches have been recently developed with the objective of improving current practice targeted to minimize the number of potentially preventable SSIs. In 2002, the Centers for Medicare and Medicaid Services (CMS) and the Centers for Disease Control and Prevention (CDC) implemented the National Surgical Infection Prevention (SIP) project, with the aim of decreasing undesired outcomes and costs derived from potentially preventable SSIs. The appropriate use of prophylactic antibiotics was identified as a crucial measure in preventing SSI, and three practice performance measures were developed: (1) antibiotic dose given within 60 minutes of incision time, (2) appropriate selection of antibiotic, based on national guidelines, and (3) discontinuation of antibiotics within 24 hours of the end of the procedure.

An examination of over 11,000 operations performed on Medicare patients around the United States revealed that only 56% had antibiotic prophylaxis given within 1 hour of incision time, and only 40% had the antibiotic discontinued within 24 hours after the operation ended. Multiple efforts have focused on improving practice patterns for the use of prophylactic antibiotics. Overall, practice patterns have improved over time, with more recent assessments revealing better—although still inadequate—compliance with the three SIP performance measures. Various interventions have been used to help improve substandard practice and generally focus on education/feedback interventions and detailed changes in the process of care. A recent study led by the CMS and the SIP collaborative group, involving 56 different hospitals, demonstrated that an intervention based on educational/feedback sessions, models of improvement, and methods of implementing and measuring changes resulted in significant improvement in the timing and duration of antibiotics as well as improved performance with other nonpharmacologic preventive measures, and led to a 27% drop in the rate of SSI when comparing the before and after study periods. Other studies implementing educational and process-of-care interventions have shown similar findings, emphasizing the importance of information dissemination and culture change. Some investigators have focused on more specific interventions, such as shifting the responsibility of providing the antibiotic from the preoperative nurse to the anesthesiologist, developing checklists and standardized printed preoperative prophylaxis orders, and using automated systems to improve practice of this strategy. All such interventions have resulted in equivalent success.

Gagliardi and colleagues recently published a systematic review assessing the factors likely to influence appropriate antibiotic prophylaxis. Their results support the implementation of interventions such as development of multidisciplinary pathways focused on influencing individual physicians' knowledge, attitudes, and beliefs, enhancing team communication, and promoting the use of written and computerized order sets. However, they also emphasize the need for further research to better characterize the benefit of these strategies. These future efforts should ideally be carried on within a framework of regional or national collaborative groups, which have the advantage of overcoming difficulties in translating knowledge to practice at a single-institution level.

CONCLUSION

Surgical site infection is the most common complication following surgical procedures. It is associated with significant impact on patient outcomes and health care resource utilization. The use of prophylactic antibiotics is a proven strategy to reduce this risk. Current guidelines for the appropriate use of antibiotic prophylaxis are well supported by level I data. Although different antibiotics are recommended for different operations, general principles for the use of prophylaxis can help guide the use of this preventive measure. Prophylactic antibiotics are indicated when there is a significant risk

of SSI such as in clean-contaminated and contaminated operations, as well as for selected clean operations, based on the presence of other risk factors and the impact of SSI for each specific patient population. With few exceptions, antibiotics must be given within 1 hour prior to incision, using generous (but safe) doses, redosed for longer operations (usually at two to three half-lives), and should be discontinued within 24 hours of the end of the operation, if not at the end of the operation. When compliance with these principles improves, the incidence of SSI decreases.

SUGGESTED READINGS

Bowater RJ, Stirling SA, Lilford R. Is antibiotic prophylaxis in surgery a generally effective intervention? Testing a generic hypothesis over a set of meta-analyses. *Ann Surg*. 2009;249:551-556.

Bratzler DW, Houck PM, Richards C, et al. Use of antimicrobial prophylaxis for major surgery: baseline results from the National Surgical Infection Prevention Project. *Arch Surg*. 2005;140:174-182.

Bull AL, Worth LJ, Richards MJ. Impact of vancomycin surgical antibiotic prophylaxis on the development of methicillin-sensitive staphylococcus aureus surgical site infections: report from Australian Surveillance Data (VICNISS). *Ann Surg*. 2012;256:1089-1092.

Bratzler DW, Dellinger EP, Olsen KM, et al. Clinical practice guidelines for antimicrobial prophylaxis in surgery: from the American Society of Health-System Pharmacists, the Infectious Diseases Society of America, the Surgical Infection Society, and the Society of Health Care Epidemiology of America. *Surg Infect*. 2013;14:73-156.

Forse RA, Karam B, MacLean LD, Christou NV. Antibiotic prophylaxis for surgery in morbidly obese patients. *Surgery*. 1989;106:750-756.

Gagliardi A, Fenech D, Eskicioglu C, Nathens AB, McLeod R. Factors influencing antibiotic prophylaxis for surgical site infection prevention in general surgery: a review of the literature. *Can J Surg*. 2009;52:481-489.

Kirkland KB, Briggs JP, Trivette SL, Wilkinson WE, Sexton DJ. The impact of surgical-site infections in the 1990s: attributable mortality, excess length of hospitalization, and extra costs. *Infect Control Hosp Epidemiol*. 1999;20:725-730.

McDonald M, Grabsch E, Marshall C, Forbes A. Single- versus multiple-dose antimicrobial prophylaxis for major surgery: a systematic review. *Aust N Z J Surg*. 1998;68:388-396.

Steinberg JP, Braun BI, Hellinger WC, et al. Timing of antimicrobial prophylaxis and the risk of surgical site infections: results from the trial to reduce antimicrobial prophylaxis errors. *Ann Surg*. 2009;250:10-16.

CHAPTER 56

Venous Thromboembolism (VTE) Prophylaxis for Nonorthopedic Surgery

Menaka Pai, MD, MSc, FRCPC
James D. Douketis, MD, FRCP(C), FACP, FCCP

WHAT IS THE RISK FOR VENOUS THROMBOEMBOLISM IN PATIENTS REQUIRING NONORTHOPEDIC SURGERY?

■ EPIDEMIOLOGY

Each year, surgeons in the United States perform more than 51 million inpatient surgeries, the majority of which are nonorthopedic surgeries. Patients undergoing nonorthopedic surgeries are a heterogeneous group in terms of surgery type, comorbidities, and associated risk for venous thromboembolism (VTE), which comprises deep vein thrombosis (DVT), and pulmonary embolism (PE). There have been a number of risk stratification models proposed to guide VTE prophylaxis in surgical patients; they are limited by complexity, and lack of rigorous prospective validation. However, in general, patients are considered to be at very low risk for VTE if they undergo minor surgical procedures lasting <30 minutes, have no medical comorbidities, and are immediately mobile following surgery. Their estimated baseline risk of VTE, if no prophylaxis is given, is estimated to be <0.5%. All other surgical patients are considered to be at moderate or high risk for VTE and merit some consideration for prophylaxis. VTE in the patient undergoing nonorthopedic surgery can cause significant morbidity and mortality and is a common cause of readmission to the hospital.

■ PATHOPHYSIOLOGY

Many factors contribute to VTE after nonorthopedic surgery (**Table 56-1**).

Trauma and surgery both contribute to venous injury and activation of the coagulation system. Postoperatively, patients may have persistently reduced mobility, which causes stasis of blood flow in the deep venous system. Patients undergoing certain types of surgery may also have independent risk factors for VTE, such as obesity in the bariatric surgical patient.

As in the orthopedic surgery setting, most episodes of postoperative DVT in nonorthopedic surgery are clinically silent. These unnoticed clots usually resolve spontaneously without administration of antithrombotic therapy. However, 25% to 50% extend and cause symptomatic DVT or PE.

WHICH PATIENTS UNDERGOING NONORTHOPEDIC SURGERY NEED VTE PROPHYLAXIS?

■ DOES THIS PATIENT UNDERGOING GENERAL SURGERY NEED VTE PROPHYLAXIS?

CASE 56-1

A 32-year-old mother of two comes to the emergency room with abdominal pain and nausea. An ultrasound confirms acute appendicitis, and the general surgeon at your center feels this patient should have an appendectomy within the next 6 hours. He feels she is at low operative risk, since she has no past medical history and is taking no medications, apart from an oral contraceptive pill. The general surgery resident phones you to ask if the patient needs VTE prophylaxis.

Data from studies done more than 20 years ago involving patients who did not routinely receive VTE prophylaxis found that rates of asymptomatic DVT in patients having general surgical procedures were between 15% and 30%, while fatal PE occurred

TABLE 56-1 Factors that Increase Risk for Venous Thromboembolism in Surgical Patients

Surgical Factors

Antecedent trauma (as reason for surgery)

General anesthesia (compared with regional/local anesthesia)

Arthroplasty

Abdominal surgical approach (compared with vaginal approach)

Open surgical approach (compared with laparoscopic approach)

Use of the lithotomy position intraoperatively

Extrinsic venous compression intraoperatively

Extended duration of surgery (>1 h)

Postoperative infection

Central venous catheterization

Postoperative immobility (confined to bed, needing assistance to ambulate)

Nonsurgical Factors

Increasing age

Pregnancy and the puerperium

Comorbid medical illness (eg, congestive heart failure, obstructive lung disease, acute myocardial infarction, inflammatory bowel disease)

Recent ischemic stroke

Cancer (active or occult)

Sepsis

Previous VTE

Prior pelvic radiation

Inherited or acquired thrombophilia

Obesity (BMI > 25 kg/m²)

Drugs (eg, chemotherapy, hormonal therapy, erythropoeisis stimulating agents)

---

in 0.2% to 0.9% of patients. Current surgical practices, including better perioperative care, rapid postoperative mobilization, and greater use of regional anesthesia have likely reduced these figures. However, general surgery patients are still considered to be at moderate to high risk of VTE. Numerous randomized clinical trials and meta-analyses have shown that VTE prophylaxis with low dose unfractionated heparin (LDUH) or low molecular weight heparin (LMWH) reduces the risk of symptomatic VTE by 40% to 70% in these patients. However, both of these agents—and others currently used for VTE prophylaxis—can increase the risk of postoperative bleeding.

PRACTICE POINT

The risk of thrombosis

- The type of surgery and the type of anaesthesia are the primary determinants of VTE risk in nonorthopedic surgical patients.

  - The approximate DVT risk without prophylaxis is based on objectively confirmed rates of DVT in asymptomatic patients who did not receive prophylaxis.

  - There is a range of DVT risk of approximately 10% to 40% in general surgical patients, depending on the specific procedure, complications, and traditional risk factors.

- General anesthesia poses a greater risk of VTE than spinal or epidural anesthesia and the duration of anesthesia irrespective of the type of anesthesia influences VTE risk, with >3.5 hours associated with the highest risk.

- Postoperative complications may further increase the risk.

Patients at very low risk of VTE do not require any specific VTE prophylaxis, but should be mobilized postoperatively. All other patients should be evaluated for VTE prophylaxis. Patients at a low risk for bleeding should receive pharmacologic prophylaxis with LDUH, LMWH, or fondaparinux. There have been no trials that directly compare the two most popular dosing regimens of subcutaneous LDUH, 5000 units every 8 hours and 5000 units every 12 hours. A meta-analysis of 51 randomized controlled trials compared LMWH and LDUH in general and abdominal surgery patients, and found that the risk of clinically evident VTE was ~30% lower in the LMWH group. However, this difference disappeared when the analysis was restricted to high-quality (blinded, placebo-controlled) trials. The meta-analysis also failed to show any difference in PE, death from any cause, major bleeding, or wound hematoma between the LMWH and LDUH groups. Our practice is to use the lowest recommended dose of heparin for prophylaxis, to minimize bleeding complications, and reduce the number of injections that a patient must receive. Further, we prefer LMWH as it carries a lower risk of heparin induced thrombocytopenia than LDUH. Parental anticoagulants can be given at various points in the patient's hospitalization: 0 to 2 hour preop (if the patient does not receive an epidural and does not undergo a very high bleed risk procedure, such as liver resection); the evening of the day of surgery; or the morning after surgery. Timing of administration is dependent on bleeding concerns, and should be a shared decision between all of the patient's health care providers.

The selective factor Xa inhibitor fondaparinux has also been evaluated for major abdominal surgery. There does not appear to be any significant difference in PE, or nonfatal symptomatic VTE, or death when fondaparinux is compared with LMWH. There was a trend to increased nonfatal major bleeding in the fondaparinux, but there was no demonstrable increase in fatal bleeding or bleeding requiring reoperation.

Direct-acting oral anticoagulants (eg, rivaroxaban and apixaban, factor Xa inhibitors, and dabigatran etexilate, a factor IIa inhibitor) have shown efficacy in VTE prophylaxis as well. These agents are appealing to clinicians and patients, as they are ingested orally, in a fixed dosing schedule. They have not yet been approved for use after nonorthopedic surgery in the United States.

Mechanical VTE prophylaxis is an option in patients with a high risk of bleeding. However, graduated compression stockings (GCS) and intermittent pneumatic compression devices (IPC) are not as effective as pharmacologic prophylaxis, and do not appear to reduce the risk of proximal DVT or symptomatic PE. Though many use them as an "add-on intervention" in general surgery patients who are at particularly high risk of VTE, such as those with cancer, there is little evidence that they add to the protective effect of pharmacologic prophylaxis. If mechanical VTE prophylaxis is used, bleeding risk should be reassessed regularly, and pharmacologic VTE prophylaxis should be started as soon as it is acceptably low.

The risk of VTE appears to be elevated for at least 12 weeks following inpatient surgery. However, the evidence for extended VTE prophylaxis in general surgery is not as robust as in orthopedic surgery. A multicenter, randomized, blinded, placebo-controlled trial studied extended 21-day prophylaxis with bemiparin (a LMWH) in patients who underwent abdominal or pelvic surgery for cancer. The primary outcome was a composite of any DVT (including asymptomatic and distal events), nonfatal PE, and death from any cause. Though the bemiparin group's had a 24% lower risk of the composite outcome and an 88% lower risk of proximal DVT than the placebo group, neither group had and symptomatic, nonfatal VTE events. The results also showed no difference in bleeding. At this time, it is not recommended that all general surgery patients receive extended VTE prophylaxis. However, cancer patients who are at particularly high risk of VTE should be considered for post discharge prophylaxis for 4 weeks.

PRACTICE POINT

A risk assessment does not have to be complicated

- The number of risk factors determines whether a patient is low, moderate, or high risk, not just the surgical procedure itself.
- Once a patient exceeds two risk factors, the patient is at least moderate risk.

■ DOES THIS PATIENT UNDERGOING GYNECOLOGIC OR UROLOGIC SURGERY NEED VTE PROPHYLAXIS?

CASE 56-2

A 78-year-old man is undergoing a radical prostatectomy for prostate cancer. His past medical history is significant for type 2 diabetes mellitus, peripheral neuropathy, and a below-knee amputation performed 10 years ago. He has no history of bleeding. The urologist asks you if you are aware of any intraoperative or postoperative strategies to reduce this patient's VTE risk.

There are fewer randomized clinical trials of VTE prophylaxis in gynecologic or urologic surgery. Existing risk assessment models have also not been validated specifically in these patients. However, the rates of DVT, PE, and fatal PE in major gynecologic surgery are similar to those in general surgery. For this reason, VTE prophylaxis recommendations are similar. There is data that cancer, use of hormones and the pregnancy state are associated significantly with thrombosis in gynecologic surgery, and must be considered in risk assessment.

VTE is an important problem in major urologic surgery, with rates of postoperative symptomatic VTE between 1% and 5%. However, there has been only one methodologically rigorous randomized clinical trial in the last 20 years in this area. Again, VTE prophylaxis recommendations are similar to those in general surgery. It is known that open procedures (vs transurethral procedures) and the use of the lithotomy position are associated with increased VTE risk. Communication with the surgeon and the anesthetist can modify these intraoperative factors and help reduce the patient's VTE risk.

■ DOES THIS PATIENT UNDERGOING CARDIAC OR VASCULAR SURGERY NEED VTE PROPHYLAXIS?

CASE 56-3

An 82-year-old woman is undergoing femorodistal bypass for longstanding peripheral arterial disease. She is an ex-smoker, and has a history of hypertension and hyperlipidemia. The patient is currently on aspirin and has been told that she will receive additional blood thinners at the time of her operation to keep her arteries from getting blocked. She has read about deep vein thrombosis, and wonders if she should receive any extra care to prevent this complication of surgery.

There is limited evidence for VTE prophylaxis in vascular surgery patients, with few well-designed randomized clinical trials in this area. Studies have not shown a clear benefit for prophylaxis, with no significant difference in rates of DVT detected by routine ultrasound screening or rates of major bleeding. Why does VTE prophylaxis not appear to have a benefit in vascular surgery patients? One potential reason is that vascular surgery patients frequently receive antithrombotic agents such as intravenous heparin, and antiplatelet agents such as aspirin and clopidogrel, to prevent arterial occlusion after vascular reconstruction. These agents lower the risk of VTE, making routine use of additional anticoagulants redundant (and possibly harmful). However, the methodologic limitations of existing evidence are also a concern; vascular surgery patients do have an increased risk of VTE postoperatively, and these patients were included in validation studies of surgical risk assessment models. At this time, it is recommended that vascular surgery patients should receive pharmacologic VTE prophylaxis in a similar fashion to general surgery patients. Caution should be used with mechanical prophylaxis; GCS and IPC are relatively contraindicated in vascular surgery patients undergoing lower limb bypass.

There is also limited evidence for VTE prophylaxis in cardiac surgery patients. Like vascular surgery patients, these individuals commonly receive antithrombotic agents such as intravenous heparin, and antiplatelet agents such as aspirin and clopidogrel. Patients who undergo cardiac valve replacement generally receive full-dose anticoagulation postoperatively, making pharmacologic VTE prophylaxis redundant. The incidence of symptomatic VTE after cardiac surgery is thought to range from 0.5% to 1.1%. Patients at highest risk are those on prolonged bed rest, those with prolonged hospitalization before surgery, those with postoperative complications, and those with congestive heart failure. Coronary artery bypass grafting (particularly if done off-pump) carries a higher risk of VTE than valve surgery. The risk of heparin-induced thrombocytopenia (HIT) also influences decision making regarding VTE prophylaxis. Approximately 20% of patients undergoing coronary artery bypass grafting (CABG) who develop a PE are diagnosed with HIT. HIT has been shown to be more common when LDUH is used, versus LMWH. It is uncertain if VTE prophylaxis should be administered

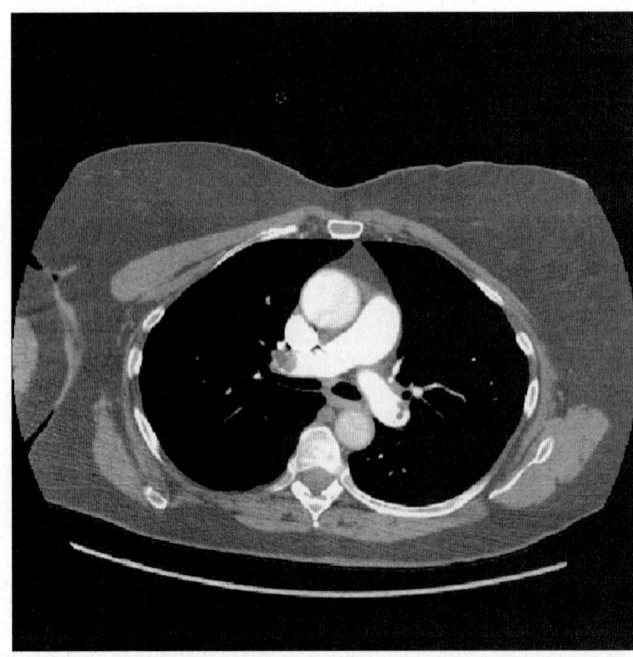

Figure 56-1 *Computed tomography pulmonary angiography showing emboli in both pulmonary arteries.*

to all cardiac surgery patients; however, in CABG patients who do not receive full-dose therapeutic anticoagulation postoperatively most physicians elect to use prophylactic-dose heparin or bilateral mechanical VTE prophylaxis (if the patient has not had saphenous vein grafting). Because the risk of HIT is high in cardiac surgery, LMWH is preferred over LDUH. Attention must, however, be paid to bleeding risk; this risk goes up with concomitant antiplatelet use, older age, renal insufficiency, and longer bypass time. If bleeding is a concern, mechanical VTE prophylaxis is preferred over pharmacologic VTE prophylaxis.

◼ DOES THIS PATIENT UNDERGOING NEUROSURGERY NEED VTE PROPHYLAXIS?

Patients undergoing major neurosurgery are at a moderate risk for VTE, with rates of proximal DVT as high as 5% postoperatively. Those with malignant brain tumors are at particularly high risk. One prospective study of more than 250 patients with gliomas showed that 31% had symptomatic, venographically confirmed DVT within 5 weeks of their surgery. However, a major barrier to optimal VTE prophylaxis in neurosurgery patients is their risk of bleeding. Intracranial bleeding can have devastating clinical consequences, and for this reason, preoperative and early postoperative pharmacologic prophylaxis should be used with caution in craniotomy patients. Rates of intracranial hemorrhage appear to double when postoperative LMWH is compared to mechanical or no VTE prophylaxis (approximately 2%-6% vs 1%-3%). Most of these bleeds occur within the first 2 days after surgery. A reasonable approach that balances the risks of bleeding and thrombosis is to start mechanical VTE prophylaxis with properly fitted IPC at the time of neurosurgery. Perioperative use of IPC is highly effective, reducing the risk of VTE by more than two-thirds. If a careful clinical assessment is stable and postoperative CT scan does not show bleeding at 24 to 48 hours, LMWH or LDUH can be added to further protect the patient from VTE. There is no evidence for extended prophylaxis in neurosurgery patients.

◼ DOES THIS PATIENT UNDERGOING LAPAROSCOPIC OR BARIATRIC SURGERY NEED VTE PROPHYLAXIS?

Laparoscopic surgery is becoming an increasingly popular alternative to conventional open surgical procedures, due to decreased tissue trauma and faster recovery times. However, there are some unique features of laparoscopic surgery that increase thrombosis risk, including longer intraoperative time, the reverse Trendelenburg position, and pneumoperitoneum (which creates venous stasis in the lower extremities). Nevertheless, rates of symptomatic VTE following laparoscopic surgery are lower than in general surgery, less than 0.5% in most series. Rates of asymptomatic VTE are thought to be lower than 1%. For this reason, routine VTE prophylaxis is not recommended in laparoscopic surgery.

Bariatric surgery, which includes Roux-en-Y gastric bypass, gastric banding, vertical-banded gastroplasty, and biliopancreatic diversion, is also a growing field. More than 100,000 bariatric surgeries for morbid obesity are performed in the United States every year. Obesity is a known risk factor for VTE and puts bariatric surgery patients in a unique risk group. Rates of symptomatic VTE vary depending on the study quoted, anywhere from 0.8% to 2.4%. However, there is still insufficient high-quality evidence to make clear recommendations regarding VTE prophylaxis in bariatric surgery. Early ambulation and mechanical prophylaxis (either IPC or GCS) are widely accepted components of postoperative care in bariatric surgery patients. The American College of Chest Physicians' most recent guidelines also recommend LMWH, LDUH, or fondaparinux be routinely used. Consultation with a pharmacist is important, as patients who are obese who may require higher drug doses.

TABLE 56-2 Contraindications to VTE Prophylaxis with Anticoagulants

Excessive active bleeding (beyond that expected after surgery)

High risk for bleeding that precludes anticoagulants (eg, brain lesion)

Recent serious bleeding (within 1 mo)

Coagulopathy (eg, INR > 1.5, aPTT > 40)

Thrombocytopenia (platelets < 75 × 10^9/L)

WHAT PHARMACOLOGIC AND NONPHARMACOLOGIC STRATEGIES SHOULD BE USED FOR VTE PROPHYLAXIS?

Physicians have a number of options available when choosing the type of VTE prophylaxis in nonorthopedic surgery. Mechanical methods of prophylaxis, which include graduated compression stockings and intermittent pneumatic compression devices, are a safe option in patients with an increased bleeding risk (**Table 56-2**). However, they are inferior to pharmacologic prophylaxis and are insufficient protection against VTE in patients at high risk of thrombosis. All patients with an increased risk for bleeding should be reassessed regularly so pharmacologic prophylaxis can be started when the bleeding risk decreases to an acceptable level.

Pharmacologic prophylaxis should be the thromboprophylaxis strategy of choice in nonorthopedic surgery. Refer to **Table 56-3** for the recommended dose regimens. Note that these doses may be inadequate in the bariatric surgery population, and that LMWH dosing in obese patients remains controversial. Two studies have shown that enoxaparin 40 mg every 12 hours subcutaneously (for bariatric surgery patients with BMI ≤50 kg/m^2) or 60 mg every 12 hours (for BMI >50 kg/m^2) appears to be an effective VTE prophylaxis strategy.

PRACTICE POINT

- Pharmacologic prophylaxis should be the thromboprophylaxis strategy of choice in nonorthopedic surgery.
- Mechanical methods of prophylaxis, which include graduated compression stockings and intermittent pneumatic compression devices, are a safe option in patients with an increased bleeding risk.
- However, they are inferior to pharmacologic prophylaxis, and are insufficient protection against VTE in patients at high risk of thrombosis.

Other studies have tried to address this issue by using anti-Xa levels as a primary outcome instead of clinical events. Prospective nonrandomized studies have questioned the validity of a "maximum LMWH dose" by showing that increasing the total daily dose

TABLE 56-3 Pharmacologic Prophylaxis Options in Nonorthopedic Surgery

Fondaparinux (Arixtra) 2.5 mg SC once daily

Dalteparin (Fragmin) 2500 units or 5000 units SC once daily

Enoxaparin (Lovenox) 40 mg SC once daily or 30 mg SC every 12 h

Nadroparin (Fraxiparine) 1900-3800 anti-Xa units SC once daily

Tinzaparin (Innohep) 3500 or 4500 anti-Xa units SC once daily

Heparin 5000 units SC every 12 h or every 8 h

of LMWH by 50% for patients with a BMI >50 kg/m² can effectively increase patients' anti-Xa levels to the target prophylactic range (0.2-0.4 IU/mL). However, these studies were not all sufficiently powered to detect clinically relevant bleeding. Higher doses of anticoagulant do seem necessary to achieve an appropriate level of prophylaxis for obese patients, though physicians must be cautious of bleeding complications as they increase LMWH dosing. Anti-Xa levels, though not a surrogate marker for bleeding risk, can provide a useful adjunct to close clinical monitoring.

WHAT ARE SOME PRACTICAL MANAGEMENT ISSUES FOR THE HOSPITALIST IN VTE PROPHYLAXIS?

■ CONSIDERATIONS UPON DISCHARGE FROM HOSPITAL

There is no evidence that patients undergoing nonorthopedic surgery benefit from routine DVT screening using Doppler ultrasound or venography. This strategy may pick up asymptomatic venous thrombosis in a small number of patients, but does not appear to reduce the rates of clinically significant events. There is also no robust evidence that VTE prophylaxis should be extended after hospital discharge. Patients at particularly high risk of thrombosis (eg, major abdominal or pelvic surgery, cancer surgery, prolonged immobility, and multiple other risk factors), may be candidates for extended prophylaxis for four additional weeks, generally with parenteral anticoagulants. The hospitalist can facilitate this transition by arranging nursing care at home, instructing the patient (or a caregiver) on injection technique and safe disposal of used needles, and clarifying who to call if bleeding develops. All patients should be educated about the signs and symptoms of VTE during their hospital stay and at the time of discharge.

■ QUALITY IMPROVEMENT INITIATIVES TO OPTIMIZE VTE PROPHYLAXIS

VTE prophylaxis in nonorthopedic surgery patients is a critical public health issue. In 2009, the US Surgeon General cited VTE as one of the most preventable hospital-acquired illnesses, and issued a call to action to optimize its prevention. Though VTE prophylaxis in nonorthopedic surgery is based on scientific evidence, the quality and number of trials is limited compared to the orthopedic surgery population. There is also significant room for improvement in compliance rates with the American College of Chest Physicians' guidelines for in-hospital VTE prophylaxis. Concerted system-wide and local efforts must be made to increase the appropriate use of VTE prophylaxis in nonorthopedic surgery.

SUGGESTED READINGS

Agnelli G, Bergqvist D, Cohen AT, et al. Randomized clinical trial of postoperative fondaparinux versus perioperative dalteparin for prevention of venous thromboembolism in high-risk abdominal surgery. *Br J Surg.* 2005;92:1212-1220.

Bergqvist D, Agnelli G, Cohen AT, et al. Duration of prophylaxis against venous thromboembolism with enoxaparin after surgery for cancer. *N Engl J Med.* 2002;346:975-980.

Borkgren-Okonek MJ, Hart RW, Pantano JE, et al. Enoxaparin thromboprophylaxis in gastric bypass patients: Extended duration, dose stratification, and antifactor Xa activity. *Surg Obes Relat Dis.* 2008;4(5):625.

Caprini JA. Risk assessment as a guide for the prevention of the many faces of venous thromboembolism. *Am J Surg.* 2010;199:S3.

Clagett GP, Reisch JS. Prevention of venous thromboembolism in general surgical patient: results of meta-analysis. *Ann Surg.* 1988;208:227-240.

Collins R, Scrimgeour A, Yusuf S. Reduction in fatal pulmonary embolism and venous thrombosis by perioperative administration of subcutaneous heparin: Overview of results of randomized trials in general, orthopedic, and urologic surgery. *N Engl J Med.* 1988;318:1162-1173.

Goldhaber SZ, Schoepf UJ. Pulmonary embolism after coronary artery bypass grafting. *Circulation.* 2004;109:2712-2715.

Gould MK, Garcia DA, Wren SM, et al. *Prevention of VTE in* nonorthopedic surgical patients: Antithrombotic therapy and prevention of thrombosis, 9th ed. American College of Chest Physicians evidence-based clinical practical guidelines. *Chest.* 2012;141:e227S.

Mismetti P, Laporte S, Darmon JY, Buchmüller A, Decousus H. Meta-analysis of low molecular weight heparin in the prevention of venous thromboembolism in general surgery. *Br J Surg.* 2001;88(7):913-930.

Scholten DJ, Hoedema RM, Scholten SE. A comparison of two different prophylactic dose regimens of low molecular weight heparin in bariatric surgery. *Obes Surg.* 2002;12(1):19.

Simone EP, Madan AK, Tichansky DS, et al. Comparison of two low-molecular-weight heparin dosing regimens for patients undergoing laparoscopic bariatric surgery. *Surg Endosc.* 2008;22(11):2392-2395.

CHAPTER 57

Postoperative Blood Transfusion

Olga S. Chajewski, MD
Jerry E. Squires, MD, PhD

INTRODUCTION

Over 13.8 million units of red blood cells are transfused to over 5 million patients in the United States in 2011; blood transfusion is one of the most common procedure codes recorded at discharge for hospitalized patients. It is estimated that 60% to 70% of these transfusions occur in relation to surgical procedures. For over 40 years it was generally assumed that patients benefitted from transfusions whenever the hemoglobin fell below 10 g/dL or if the hematocrit fell below 30% (the so-called "10/30 rule"). Controversy remains regarding the appropriate selection of patients requiring transfusion, as well as the recognition and management of adverse transfusion reactions.

POSTOPERATIVE ANEMIA

Transfusion in the postoperative period generally occurs due to anemia. The prevalence of postoperative anemia is difficult to assess accurately, but it is undoubtedly common, particularly in critically ill patients. Hemoglobin concentrations on admission to the intensive care unit (ICU) are on average 11.0 to 11.3 g/dL in two large studies, with overall transfusion prevalence rates of 37% to 44%. Postoperative anemia can result from several factors, but acute and chronic blood loss is most frequently cited. While intraoperative or traumatic blood loss is generally replaced during the surgical procedure, a significant number of patients still leave surgery with some degree of anemia. Patients admitted to the ICU following surgery on average have hemoglobin levels ranging from 10.8 to 11.5 g/dL. Perhaps more insidious is the chronic blood loss that can occur during the postoperative period itself. Causes for this include ongoing bleeding from the surgical site (eg, chest tube drainage) and repeated blood collections for laboratory testing. It has been suggested that 40 to 60 mL of blood is routinely collected from ICU patients daily. While this daily blood loss may seem minimal, it is aggravated by the decreased production of erythropoietin (EPO), resistance to the effects of EPO, and an inability to utilize iron in red cell production, all of which have been documented in the postoperative period. In patients who display symptoms of anemia in the postoperative period, there are limited alternatives to transfusion. EPO and iron therapy are often ineffective in the postoperative period and are of little use in the patient with an acute need for blood.

PRACTICE POINT

Arguments in favor of conservative management of postoperative anemia without the use of blood products include:

- Risks associated with blood transfusion.
- Accumulating evidence that transfusion can negative impact patient outcomes.

Steps that may be taken include:

- Minimize blood draws to tests that would influence management.
- Assess the clinical need for transfusion in each individual patient and only transfusing patients likely to benefit from transfusion (ie, generally those with a hemoglobin <7 g/dL or those who are hemodynamically unstable with a hemoglobin <10.0 g/dL).

POSTOPERATIVE TRANSFUSION

Several well-documented randomized controlled trials have demonstrated that a hemoglobin of 7.0 g/dL, when used as a trigger for the transfusion of red blood cells, is at least as safe (noninferior) as a hemoglobin of 10.0 g/dL. Transfusion has also been associated, in a number of reports, with increased risk of infection, morbidity, mortality, length of hospital stay, and length of ICU stay. A number of professional organizations, such as the College of American Pathologists, American Society of Anesthesiologists, and the American College of Physicians, have published guidelines for the transfusion of red blood cells in nonbleeding anemic patients. In general, each of these sets of guidelines recommend that at hemoglobin levels less than 7.0 g/dL red blood cell transfusion will be necessary, while at hemoglobin levels greater than 10.0 g/dL transfusion is rarely required. These guidelines all stress the priority of assessing the clinical need for transfusion in each individual patient. These guidelines suggest that a slightly higher hemoglobin transfusion threshold of 8.0 g/dL may be more appropriate for patients with acute coronary syndrome. A red blood cell transfusion practice guideline from the American Association of Blood Banks (AABB) makes four recommendations as outlined in **Table 57-1**. Patients with evidence of poor tissue perfusion (eg, hypotension, tachypnea, tachycardia, chest pain) may require a red blood cell transfusion despite a hemoglobin value above the trigger threshold of 7 g/dL. In adult patients with anemia who are not actively bleeding, each unit of red blood cells should increase the hemoglobin level by approximately 1.0 g/dL.

ADVERSE TRANSFUSION OUTCOMES

Many adverse outcomes are preventable. One national hemovigilance program reported adverse reactions occur at a rate of 10/100,000 components transfused, and ~70% of these events are "preventable."

NONINFECTIOUS ACUTE TRANSFUSION REACTIONS

Transfusion reactions are often classified as either acute (occur within 24 hours of transfusion) or delayed. The prompt recognition and management of acute reactions is critical to the patient's care.

TABLE 57-1 American Association of Blood Banks (AABB) Red Blood Cell Transfusion Practice Guidelines

Recommendation	Evidence/Grade
Clinicians should adhere to a restrictive transfusion strategy (ie, hemoglobin 7-8 g/dL) in hospitalized, stable patients	Strong recommendation; high-quality evidence
Clinicians might consider a slightly higher transfusion threshold trigger (ie, hemoglobin 8 g/dL) in hospitalized patients with pre-existing cardiovascular disease	Weak recommendation; moderate-quality evidence
Recommendations cannot be made for or against a liberal or restrictive transfusion threshold for hospitalized, hemodynamically stable patients with acute coronary syndrome	Uncertain recommendation; very low-quality evidence
Transfusion decisions should be influenced by symptoms as well as hemoglobin concentration	Weak recommendation; low-quality evidence

All transfusion reactions should be promptly reported to the blood bank or transfusion service, as additional testing may be required; it may also affect the management of other blood components collected from the donor of the implicated product. Acute transfusion reactions are listed in **Table 57-2**.

PRACTICE POINT

- It is critical that transfusion reactions be promptly recognized so that appropriate management of the patient and investigation of other blood components from the implicated donor can be initiated.

TRANSFUSION-TRANSMITTED INFECTIONS (TTI)

The current risk for transfusion transmitted infection is low. See **Table 57-3**.

In addition, with the recent FDA approval of *pathogen-reduction* technology for platelet and plasma components, these risks (and the risks associated with new pathogens in the blood supply) will be further reduced.

PATIENTS REQUIRING BLOOD PRODUCT IRRADIATION

Certain patients, usually those who are immunocompromised, require cellular blood products (red blood cells, platelets, white blood cells) that are irradiated in order to prevent transfusion-associated graft versus host disease (GvHD). See **Table 57-4**.

PATIENTS REQUIRING CYTOMEGALOVIRUS (CMV) NEGATIVE BLOOD

While CMV infections for most individuals cause mild, if any, symptoms, some patients require the transfusion of "CMV-safe" blood products. Leukoreduced blood products are considered to be CMV-safe and provide a more readily alternative to the use of blood products collected from CMV seronegative donors.

FILTERS

All blood products, including red blood cells, platelets, plasma, and cryoprecipitate, must be transfused through a filter. The standard blood filter has a pore size of 170 to 260 microns.

INFUSION TIME

Blood product infusions must be completed with 4 hours of the product being dispensed from the blood bank. In general, a red blood cell transfusion should be started slowly (approximately 2 mL/min) and the patient monitored for the first 15 minutes. Most serious reactions occur within the first 10 to 15 minutes of the transfusion. After the initial 15 minutes the rate of transfusion can be increased to approximately 4 mL/min.

No medications or solutions other than 0.9% sodium chloride should be infused with blood components. Solutions containing dextrose have caused lysis of red blood cells and solutions containing calcium, such as Lactated Ringer's solution, can cause clotting of the blood component. There are a limited numbers of other products that are compatible with blood, but the package insert should be consulted to insure that that have been approved to be compatible with blood or blood components.

TABLE 57-2 Acute Transfusion Reactions

Risk	Incidence	Etiology	Signs/Symptoms	Management
Allergic (urticarial) reactions	1:100-1:33	Antibody in recipient to donor plasma protein	Urticaria Flushing Itching	SUSPEND transfusion Administer antihistamines Report to blood bank
Anaphylactic reactions	1:20,000-1:50,000	Antibody to donor plasma proteins (often anti-IgA in IgA deficient recipient)	Hypotension Urticaria Bronchospasm Local edema	STOP transfusion Maintain blood pressure Report to blood bank
Febrile reactions	1:100	Antibody to donor white blood cells or presence of cytokines in blood product	Fever Chills	STOP transfusion Administer antipyretics Report to blood bank
Acute hemolytic reactions	1:76,000	Red cell incompatibility (often ABO incompatibility)	Fever Chills/rigors Hypotension Back/flank pain Pain at injection site Hemoglobinemia Hemoglobinuria Renal failure/oliguria Disseminated intravascular coagulation	STOP transfusion Manage hypotension Maintain renal perfusion Report to blood bank
Transfusion-related acute lung injury (TRALI)	1:5000	Donor HLA or white cell antibodies	Respiratory distress Fever Tachycardia Hypotension Chest x-ray with bilateral infiltrates	STOP transfusion Provide respiratory support *Mechanical ventilation*
Transfusion-associated circulatory overload (TACO)	1:100	Excess volume	Respiratory distress Orthopnea Cough Hypertension	STOP transfusion Diuretic therapy Respiratory support
Bacterial contamination	RBC: 2.6:100,000 Plts: 1:75,000	Bacterial contamination of blood product	Fever Chills/rigors Hypotension Nausea/vomiting	STOP transfusion Maintain blood pressure Administer antibiotics Obtain blood cultures Report to blood bank

TABLE 57-3 Most Common Transfusion-Transmitted Viral Infections

Agent	Estimated Risk with Test-Negative Blood Product
Human Immunodeficiency Virus (HIV)	1:2135,000
Hepatitis C Virus (HCV)	1:1935,000
Hepatitis B Virus (HBV)	1:205,000-488,000

TABLE 57-4 Patients Requiring Irradiation of Cellular Blood Products

Well-Documented	Intrauterine transfusions
	Low-birth-weight premature infants
	Congenital immunodeficiencies
	Hematologic malignancies
	Peripheral blood or marrow transplantation
	Fludarabine therapy
	Granulocyte products
	HLA-matched platelet products
	Blood components donated by blood relatives
Potential Indications	Malignancies treated with cytotoxic agents
Generally NOT Indicated	Patients with human immunodeficiency virus
	Full-term infants
	Nonimmunosuppressed patients

SUGGESTED READINGS

Carson JL, Terrin ML, Noveck H, et al. Liberal or restrictive transfusion in high-risk patients after hip surgery. *N Engl J Med.* 2011;365:2453-2462.

Hebert PC, Wells G, Blajchmann MA, et al. A multicenter randomized, controlled clinical trial of transfusion requirements in critical care. *N Engl J Med.* 1999;340:409-417.

Liumbruno GM, Bennardello F, Lattanzio A, et al. Recommendations for the transfusion management of patients in the perioperative period. III. The post-operative period. *Blood Transfus.* 2011;9:320-335.

Murphy GJ, Reeves BC, Rogers CA, et al. Increased mortality, postoperative morbidity, and cost after red blood cell transfusion in patients having cardiac surgery. *Circulation.* 2007;107:2544-2552.

Stramer SL. Current risks of transfusion-transmitted agents. *Arch Pathol Lab Med.* 2007;131:702-707.

CHAPTER 58

Nutrition and Metabolic Support

Nicole M. Bedi, RD, CNSC
Malcolm K. Robinson, MD

INTRODUCTION

The importance of providing adequate nutrition as an adjunct to medical care was identified as early as the era of Hippocrates. The prevalence of malnutrition in the hospitalized patient was largely ignored until 1974 when Butterworth published his landmark paper entitled "The Skeleton in the Hospital Closet." 30% to 50% of hospitalized patients are malnourished upon admission, and they tend not to improve nutritionally, and frequently worsen, while hospitalized.

Malnutrition is associated with increased infection rates, longer hospital length of stay, increased hospital costs, and mortality. Therefore, the nutritional status of most patients should be assessed throughout their hospitalizations.

This chapter will provide the hospitalist with a framework for assessing nutritional status, identifying patients at increased risk of malnutrition, and determining the most appropriate nutritional prescription. This chapter will not cover nutrition at the end of life. See Chapter 216 (Palliation of Common Symptoms).

NUTRITION EVALUATION AND SCREENING

Usually a dietitian or nurse uses a nutrition screening questionnaire to assess patients for malnutrition at the time of admission. The assessment process includes a combination of anthropometric measurements, and the history and physical examination. Most validated nutrition screening tools evaluate a combination of body mass index (BMI), recent unintentional changes in weight, recent changes to oral intake, and severity of present illness.

Nutritional screening may identify patients who are underweight and therefore at significant risk for developing nutritionally related complications during treatment of acute illness. However, nutritional screening may fail to identify other patients at increased risk based simply on weight. Patients admitted with volume overload due to heart failure, cirrhosis, or renal insufficiency may have their true dry weight masked by excessive fluid retention. Acutely ill patients who have received aggressive fluid resuscitation gain several kilograms above their true dry weight. Patients whose dry weight is in the obese range may have malnutrition due to protein degradation and loss of lean body mass from rapid weight loss during acute illness.

■ ANTHROPOMETRIC MEASUREMENTS AND PHYSICAL ASSESSMENT

Anthropometric measurements are a set of noninvasive, quantitative techniques for determining an individual's body fat composition by measuring specific dimensions of the body, such as height and weight, triceps skin-fold thickness, mid-upper arm circumference, and bodily circumference at the waist, hip, and chest. If such measurements fall below standard norms then one is considered malnourished. For example, health care professionals can compare a patient's weight to the ideal body weight (IBW) found in tables from various sources, such as the 1952 Metropolitan Life tables. Alternatively, one can use the Hamwi "rule of thumb," which was developed from the Metropolitan table.

Every patient should have a nutrition assessment when admitted to the hospital.

One assessment is the Hamwi "rule of thumb," which can be used to compare a patient's IBW to actual body weight:

- IBW for a woman is 100 pounds for the first 5 feet plus an additional 5 pounds for every inch over 5 feet.
- IBW for a man is 106 pounds for the first 5 feet plus an additional 6 pounds for every inch over 5 feet.

Another assessment is the body mass index (BMI):

- Underweight is a BMI less than 18 kg/m^2
- Overweight is a BMI greater than 25 kg/m^2
- Obese is a BMI greater than 30 kg/m^2

Pitfalls to relying on body weight as an indicator of nutritional status include

- Fluid overload states, which falsely elevate weight in a malnourished patient.
- Obesity, which may mask the relevance of recent weight loss.

BMI is independent of gender and body frame size. However, those who meet the BMI criteria for overweight and obese may still have significant depletion of nutrient stores, particularly when acutely ill. Thus, the BMI alone is insufficient to classify an individual as nutrient replete. Highly trained and muscular athletes with disproportionately high lean body mass may not have a high body fat percent despite a BMI in the overweight or obese category.

In 2012, the Academy of Nutrition and Dietetics (AND) and the American Society for Parenteral and Enteral Nutrition (ASPEN) produced a consensus statement for standardizing diagnostic criteria of malnutrition. As no single parameter is definitive for adult malnutrition, the identification of two or more of the following six characteristics is recommended for diagnosis:

- Insufficient caloric (energy) intake (estimated from dietary recall)
- Weight loss (based on objective measurement of weight)
- Loss of muscle mass (temporal/interosseus muscle wasting; clavicular prominence)
- Loss of subcutaneous fat (cheeks/orbital area, or space between thumb and forefinger)
- Localized or generalized fluid accumulation, that may mask weight loss (pitting edema)
- Diminished functional status (assessed by handgrip strength with a dynamometer)

Additional nutrition related physical assessment should include evaluation of skin, hair, mouth, and nails for signs of nutrient deficiencies. Dry skin or rash, dry hair or hair loss, poor skin turgor, night blindness, glossitis, and muscle weakness may also point to vitamin, mineral, or fatty acid deficiencies.

■ LABORATORY DATA

There is no reliable laboratory marker to determine the presence of malnutrition, or the response to adequate feeding in acutely ill, hospitalized patients. Serum proteins, most frequently albumin (but also prealbumin, retinol binding protein, and transferrin) were historically used for this purpose; however, these proteins are all acute phase reactants. The liver decreases their production during acute illness or following surgery. Hyper- or hypovolemia, steroid administration, alcoholism, liver, and renal failure can also alter circulating nutrition protein levels, independent of nutritional status. A decreased albumin is more accurately a marker of inflammation in the acute setting.

- Unintentional weight loss has consistently been shown to be a reliable measure of malnutrition, especially in older adults. A loss of greater than 5% of one's usual body weight (UBW) in 1 month or 7.5% of UBW over 3 months is considered clinically significant, even if one is initially obese.

Typically, albumin and prealbumin rise as patients recover from their inflammatory insult. However, during ongoing inflammatory illness (eg, cancer, wound infection, abscess, and necrotic tissue), albumin and prealbumin will be persistently low despite adequate nutrition.

Many non-nutritional factors may alter the level of circulating nutritional proteins used to monitor nutritional status. C-reactive protein (CRP), an acute phase reactant, will usually be elevated due to the presence of inflammation. If the CRP is normal and the prealbumin is low, this likely represents malnourishment. If the CRP is high and the prealbumin is low, one will not be able to reliably distinguish between malnourishment and inflammation. Although such levels should be monitored, physicians must use caution when interpreting these markers.

THE NUTRITION PRESCRIPTION

Patients who are well nourished and are not at risk for malnourishment on admission do not need a plan, but should be reassessed every 3 to 5 days. All patients who are malnourished on admission, or who are at risk of developing malnutrition, should have a formal nutrition plan developed.

■ DETERMINATION OF NUTRIENT REQUIREMENTS

Both under- and overfeeding calories is detrimental. Excess carbohydrate administration can result in hyperglycemia, and excess carbon dioxide production, which is of particular concern in patients with lung disease (who may retain CO_2 and have difficulty weaning from the ventilator). Long-term overfeeding may lead to hepatic steatosis, ureagenesis, and immunosuppression (especially overfeeding of lipids). The goal is to determine nutrient needs precisely, and to avoid both under- and overfeeding.

The "gold standard" for determination of caloric requirements is indirect calorimetry, or a "metabolic cart" study. The metabolic cart measures oxygen consumption and carbon dioxide production and then calculates resting energy expenditure (REE) through utilization of the Weir equation. Indirect calorimetry provides a result which already includes the additional caloric expenditure related to disease stress, but not the caloric expenditure related to activity. Hence, the results of the metabolic cart study are increased by an activity factor to calculate the final daily caloric expenditure. Typically, activity factors range from 0% to 5% in intubated patients to as high as 30% in ambulatory patients.

Metabolic cart testing remains the most reliable way to determine caloric requirements for patients with a very low or high BMI, for those with amputations, and for those who have severe illness or injury such as multiple traumas or burns. Use of predictive equations to estimate caloric requirements in such patients can lead to highly inaccurate results.

However, the use of predictive equations is the most common method for determining caloric requirements because metabolic cart studies are usually impractical (requires trained personnel and expensive equipment).

- The Harris-Benedict equation (HBE) is based on studies of healthy volunteers; *it is the oldest and most widely used equation* for determining basal metabolic rate (BMR).

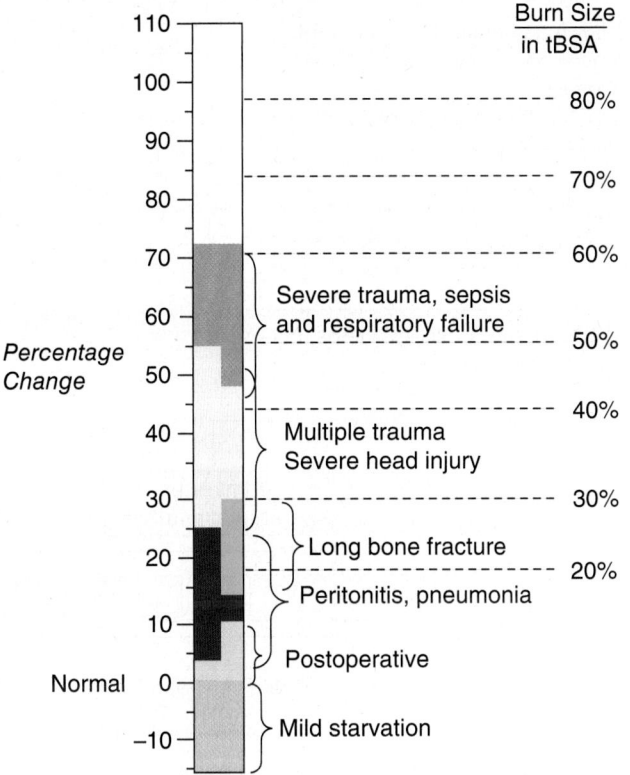

Figure 58-1 *Percent change in metabolic rate due to injury.*

- The Mifflin-St. Jeor equation may be more accurate than the HBE for determining caloric needs (when compared to indirect calorimetry). *This equation is recommended for obese noncritically ill patients* (although precision goes down with increasing obesity).
- Penn State equation is the Mifflin-St. Jeor equation modified with age, body temperature, and minute ventilation for eucaloric feeding. *This equation is recommended for obese critically ill patients.*

No equations factor in the increased caloric expenditure related to disease. Hence, once the BMR is determined, an estimate of the additional caloric expenditure from activity *and* metabolic stress (from disease or acute illness) is factored in to determine the overall daily caloric requirement. Stress factors can range from 10% in routine patients to 100% in severe burn patients (**Figure 58-1**).

The actual body weight (ABW) is generally used for caloric assessment. In patients >120% of their ideal weight, IBW is recommended. Some nutrition professionals will use an "adjusted weight" for obesity, although no routine standardized adjustment has been published (**Figure 58-2**).

For obese patients, "permissive underfeeding" aims to feed the patient at a target goal of 50% to 70% of estimated calorie requirements, providing an abundance of protein to preserve lean body mass. With this, patients with a BMI 30 to 50 kg/m^2 should receive 11 to 14 kcal/kg/d using ABW and those with a BMI >50 kg/m^2 should receive 22 to 25 kcal/kg/d using IBW.

In addition to a caloric prescription, providers should determine their patients' protein goals. Generally, hospitalized patients require between 1.2 and 1.5 g/kg/d, with burn patients requiring up to 2.0 g/kg/d. In critically ill obese patients, up to 2.5 g/kg/d (IBW) is recommended.

PRACTICE POINT

A quick "rule of thumb" for most hospitalized patients caloric and protein needs (IBW):

- 25 to 30 calories/kg/d
- 1.2 protein g/kg/d

ROUTE OF FEEDING

The next component of the nutrition prescription is determining the route of feeding (**Figure 58-3**). Oral nutrition is preferred. Specialized nutritional support must be considered when patients cannot safely or adequately meet their nutrient requirements through oral diet alone.

ENTERAL NUTRITION

For the purpose of this discussion, *enteral nutrition* will refer to feeding of patients via enteric tubes placed in the stomach or small bowel. The old adage "if the gut works, use it" guides decision making for specialized nutritional support.

Provision of nutrients into the GI tract preserves structural and functional integrity and maintains gut-associated lymphoid tissue. Relative and absolute contraindications to enteral feeding include major GI hemorrhage, peritonitis, severe ileus, bowel obstruction or fistulae distal to enteral access site, intestinal ischemia, and malabsorptive disorders with high-volume diarrhea (eg, short bowel syndrome, radiation enteritis, graft vs host disease of the GI tract).

Harris Benedict Equation

Men: [13.75 x weight (kg)] + [5.00 x height (cm)] – [6.78 x age (y)] + 66.5
Women: [9.56 x weight (kg)] + [1.85 x height (cm)] – [4.68 x age (y)] + 655.1

Mifflin-St. Jeor Equation

Men: (9.99 x weight) + (6.25 x height) – (4.92 x age) + 5
Women: (9.99 x weight) + (6.25 x height) – (4.92 x age) – 161

Example: A 45-year-old man presents a diverticular abscess with ileus. He is 6 ft tall (182.9 cm) and 176 lbs (80 kg).

BMR (using Mifflin-St. Jeor) = [9.99 x 80] + [6.25 x 182.9] – [4.92 x 45] + 5 = 1726
Calorie Requirement = 1726 (BMR) x 1.25 (ie, 25% activity factor) x 1.10 (ie,10% stress factor) = 2473 calories/d

Figure 58-2 *Equations for determining basal metabolic rate.*

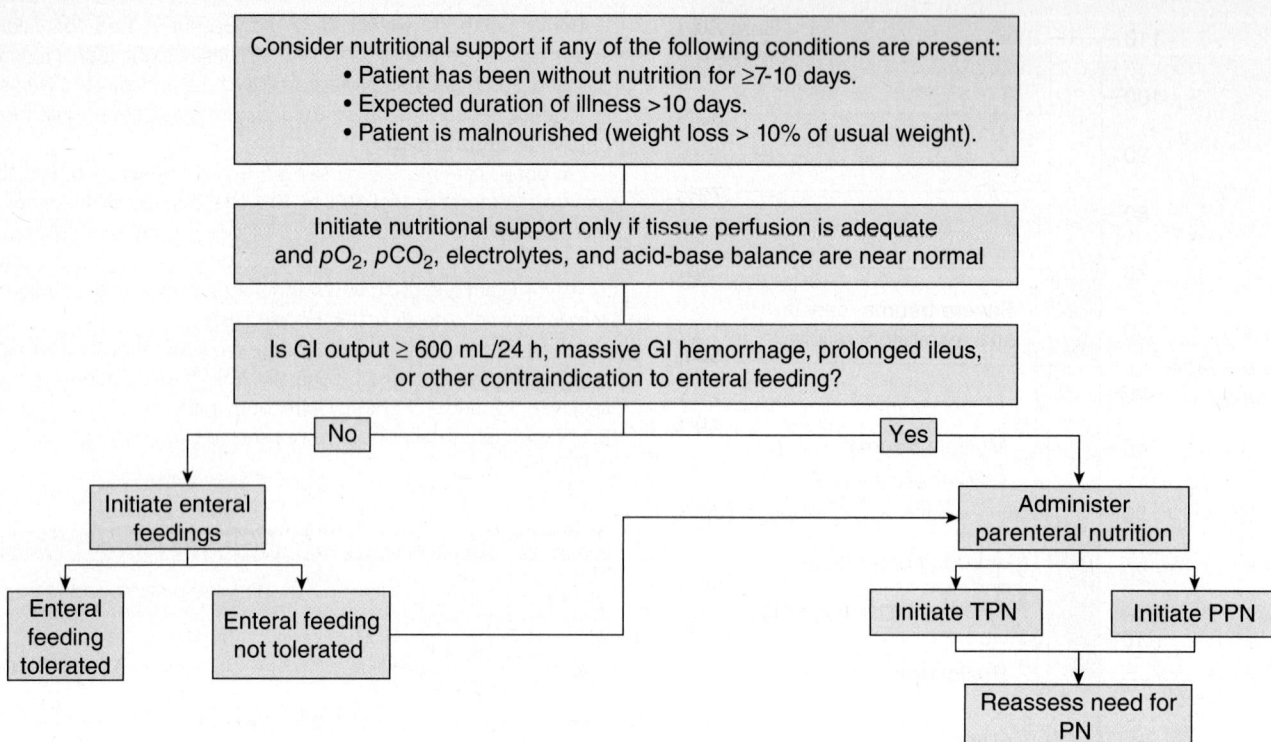

Figure 58-3 *Determining route of nutritional support.*

■ **ENTERAL ACCESS**

The physician must determine the most appropriate access route based on two major factors: (1) whether the patient requires short- or long-term feeding, and (2) whether the gastric status is normal. Refer to Chapter 45 (Surgical Tubes and Drains) on inserting and maintaining enteral tubes.

■ **ENTERAL FORMULAS**

Standard and specialized enteral formulas can be used to provide nutrition. Since all of these formulas have fixed macronutrient content, it may not be possible to deliver sufficient protein without overfeeding calories. Hence, one usually delivers the feedings at a rate to provide appropriate calories and then supplements protein with a protein modular. **Table 58-1** describes typical enteric formulas. Specialty formulas for a variety of disease states such as pulmonary, renal, and liver dysfunction and diabetes should be selected with caution due to increased cost and low benefit to risk profiles.

■ **MONITORING ENTERAL FEEDING TOLERANCE**

Feedings are typically started at a low rate, and gradually advanced to the infusion goal over a period of 24 to 48 hours.

Patients are evaluated for other symptoms such as nausea, vomiting, diarrhea, abdominal pain, and bloating. Diarrhea commonly occurs due to gastrointestinal pathogens, bowel edema or inflammation, malabsorptive disorders, and medications (**Figure 58-4**). Also see Chapter 82 (Diarrhea) for more on the assessment and management of hospitalized patients with diarrhea.

If signs and symptoms of intolerance develop, the feedings are held until resolution. Persistent intolerance requires an alternative plan. Patients receiving gastric feedings should be considered for postpyloric feeding as this may improve most symptoms of intolerance with the exception of diarrhea.

Checking gastric residuals has traditionally been the hallmark for monitoring tube feeding tolerance and avoiding tube-feed-associated aspiration. However, several well-designed studies have failed to demonstrate a significant link to gastric residual volume (GRV) and aspiration risk. Routine monitoring of gastric residuals interrupts tube feeding with questionable proven benefit.

TABLE 58-1 Typical Enteric Formulas

Type	Composition	Indications	Side Effects
Polymeric (1.0, 1.2, 1.5, and 2.0 cal/mL)	Intact protein, fats, carbohydrates	To meet daily requirements: for most patients 1-1.5 L/d Concentrated feeding best if patient is volume restricted	Concentrated feeding may cause diarrhea and may require free water supplementation
Elemental or Semi-elemental	Peptide-based amino-acids or di- or tri-peptides and simple sugars	Maximizes absorption in patients with malabsorption disorders	May cause diarrhea
Immune enhancing diets	Fortified with arginine, glutamine, omega-3 fatty acids and/or antioxidants	May reduce infection risk in surgical patients	Unclear benefit in medical patients

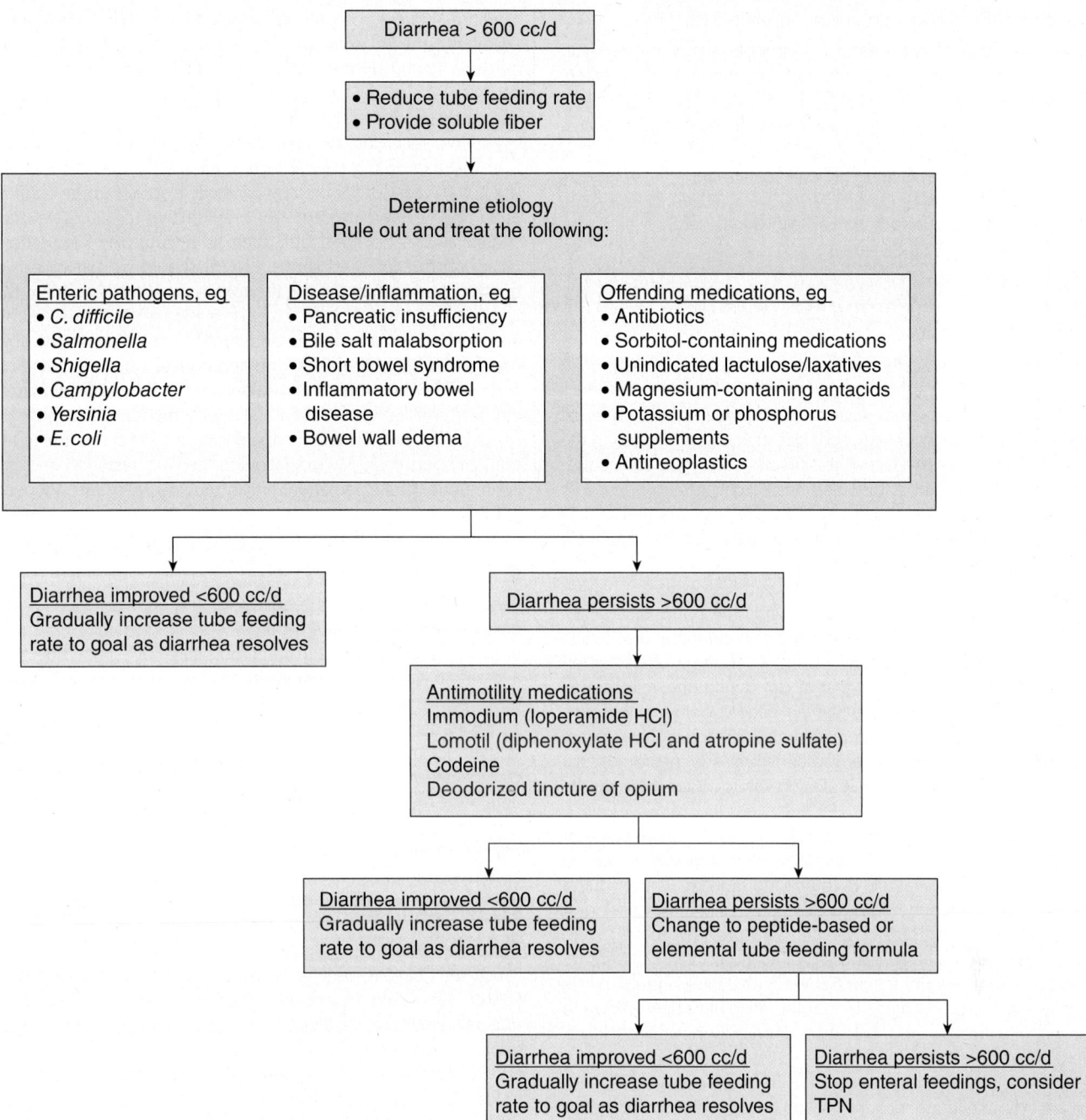

Figure 58-4 *Management of diarrhea in tube-fed patients.*

The American Society for Parenteral and Enteral Nutrition (A.S.P.E.N.) recommends monitoring of gastric residual volume (GRV) for the first 48 hours of enteral nutrition initiation.

● If the GRV is greater than 250 mL on two residual checks, the physician should consider a motility agent such as metoclopromide or erythromycin.
● If the gastric residual is greater than 500 mL, the feedings should be held and the patient evaluated by a physician for abdominal distention, glycemic control, adequacy of motility agents if not already ordered, or consideration of small bowel feeding access.

Patients who cannot tolerate EN should be considered for parenteral nutrition (PN). PN is associated with higher rates of infectious and metabolic complications such as volume overload, hyperglycemia, and electrolyte abnormalities compared to EN. The risk of nutritionally related complication rates increases beyond 10 to 14 days of inadequate enteral feeding in well-nourished individuals. The decision of when to initiate TPN depends on the nutritional status of the patient, the acute illness, the patient's prognosis, and the estimated duration of inadequate enteral feeding. ASPEN recommendations suggest around 7 days as an appropriate starting point for PN. PN is only justified if the need is anticipated for a minimum of 5 days.

Indications for PN include, but are not limited to:

- Severe malabsorptive disorders (short bowel syndrome, graft vs host disease of the GI tract, radiation enteritis, inflammatory bowel disease)
- High-output enterocutaneous fistulae if distal feeding access is not feasible
- Pancreatitis with enteral feeding intolerance
- Bowel obstruction
- Uncontrolled anastomotic leak following GI surgery
- Prolonged postoperative ileus

PARENTERAL NUTRITION PRESCRIPTION AND MONITORING

PN solutions contain carbohydrate in the form of dextrose, protein as crystalline amino acids, and lipids from polyunsaturated long-chain triglycerides such as soybean oil or a safflower/soybean oil mixture. Vitamins, electrolytes, and trace elements are added to the formulation as needed. Electrolytes and other additives (eg, medications) must be added at the appropriate concentrations to avoid "cracking" of lipid-containing PN. If cracking occurs, precipitates form in the solution, and the lipid emulsion separates into layers, making it unsafe for administration.

Physicians must carefully monitor patients for metabolic changes such as hyperglycemia or refeeding syndrome upon initiation of PN. Hyperglycemia may increase infectious complications, hospital length of stay, and cost. Refeeding syndrome is characterized by electrolyte abnormalities that occur during the reinstitution of carbohydrate calories to a starved patient. Serum phosphate, magnesium, and potassium depletion may develop and precipitate potentially life-threatening cardiac arrhythmias or neuromuscular complications. See Chapter 226 (Eating Disorders for more on the refeeding syndrome).

PN prescriptions typically provide from 1 to 3 liters of fluid per day depending on the physician's assessment of maintenance fluid requirements. A general rule of thumb is 30 mL/kg. Carbohydrates generally make up about 50% to 60% of the caloric prescription, at 3.4 calories/g of dextrose. Protein generally provides about 15% to 25% of the calories at 4.0 calories/g of amino acid. The current US Food and Drug Administration (FDA)-approved lipid emulsions are primarily made up of omega-6-rich oils, which have been shown to be proinflammatory and potentially immunosuppressive. Hence, lipid provision should be limited to 20% to 25% of calories (at 10 calories/g of IV lipid). Novel IV lipids made up of olive oils or fish oil are available in other countries, and are currently under consideration by the FDA.

It is advisable to start with a lower volume and concentration of dextrose when initiating PN to avoid metabolic complications. One liter of a 10% dextrose solution is a good starting point. Subsequently the volume, and dextrose, lipid, and protein concentrations are increased as needed in the metabolically stable patient to the eventual goal caloric and fluid provision (**Figure 58-5**). Blood sugar levels should be closely monitored and maintained below 180 mg/deciliter (dL), and abnormal electrolyte levels should be corrected, especially potassium, phosphate, and magnesium, before starting or advancing to the goal solution. Additionally, any patient who is at high risk for refeeding syndrome should receive IV thiamine replacement prior to initiation of total parenteral nutrition (TPN) to prevent development of Wernicke's encephalopathy. Traditionally, patients affected with alcohol use were the hallmark high-risk patient for Wernicke's. However, those recovering from weight loss surgery (eg, gastric bypass) with prolonged nausea and vomiting is a newly recognized group of patients who are at risk for this complication. The solutions should be administered using a volumetric pump set at a constant rate. In general, PN lipid infusion should not exceed

1 g/kg/d, and dextrose infusion should be less than 5 mg/kg/min. Eventually, the PN solution can be cycled nocturnally (generally between 10 and 16 hours) in long-term PN patients, once glycemic control is achieved. Once stable, patients can have lab monitoring decreased to once or twice weekly.

Patients receiving *long-term* PN may develop PN-associated liver dysfunction (PNALD). However, alterations that occur within the first 2 weeks of PN therapy generally resolve despite continuation of TPN. Alternate causes of liver function test (LFT) elevation should always be ruled out, such as hepatotoxic medications, biliary obstruction, and sepsis. PNALD should be a diagnosis of exclusion rather than the first thought in the acutely ill patient that has just been started on PN. Excess provision of IV dextrose or lipid, and deficiencies of carnitine and choline may increase the likelihood of PNALD. Provision of the appropriate amount of dextrose and carbohydrate, repleting carnitine and choline, and administering even small amounts of enteral nourishment may decrease the risk of developing PNALD. Finally, decreasing PN cycle time to less than 24 hours each day may allow for hepatic "rest" and decrease continuous insulin secretion, which may decrease fatty deposits in the liver.

PARENTERAL ACCESS

Central venous access is required for the administration of TPN because TPN solutions are hyperosmolar. Peripheral PN (PPN) solutions, which are available in some hospitals, have limited dextrose and amino acid concentrations in order to keep osmolarity lower; this improves tolerance of PN delivery via a peripheral vein, but lowers caloric density. PPN is generally not a good long-term (>3-5 days) solution for most patients and only useful for those patients who can tolerate high volumes of fluid daily. The physician must also determine the most appropriate access device for PN. See Chapter 120 (Vascular Access, for more information about types and indications of catheters).

SPECIAL CONSIDERATIONS

PANCREATITIS

Pancreatitis patients require no nutritional intervention in 80% to 90% of cases as most will resume an oral diet within 7 days of admission. EN remains the preferred route of nutritional support for the remaining patients because it is associated with a significant reduction in infectious morbidity, length of stay, and mortality compared to PN. EN can be appropriately achieved by feeding into the stomach or jejunum depending on gastric emptying. Of note, patients who are fed within the first 24 to 48 hours of admission may tolerate enteral feeding better than those who start feeding later, and such early feeding is associated with substantial outcome benefits. These benefits diminish in patients who start feeding as late as day 4.

PN should be considered in severe pancreatitis patients who cannot receive enteral feeding for prolonged periods. PN may exacerbate the inflammatory response to pancreatitis if initiated too early; ASPEN guidelines suggest not starting PN for 5 days in those with severe pancreatitis, even if enteral feeding is not possible.

RENAL DISEASE

Dialysis patients often have poor oral intake, increased nutrient losses in their dialysates, and increased catabolic stress. Thus malnutrition is common in this patient population. The Kidney Disease Outcomes Quality Initiative (K/DOQI) guidelines recommend protein restriction for *outpatient* dialysis patients, but notably recommend that dialysis patients receive 1.2 to 1.3 g/kg of protein when hospitalized for acute illnesses. Many nutrition experts also believe that acutely ill patients who are "predialysis" should still

Patient is a 45-year-old man with diverticular abscess, as in Figure 58-2. Advancement to an oral diet has been unsuccessful for 10 days, and TPN is required.

A. Estimate nutrient requirements:

Calorie requirement: 2373 calories/d (see Figure 58-2)

Protein requirement: 1.5 g/kg/d = 80 x 1.5 = 120 g/d

Fluid requirement: 30 mL/kg body weight = 80 x 30 = 2400 mL

B. Determine the solution

1. Protein content

120 g protein ÷ 2.4 L fluid = 50 g/L

50 g = 5% amino acids per liter

4 calories/g of amino acids x 120 g = 480 kcals of protein

2. Lipid content (*approximately 20%-25% of nonprotein kcals*)

2373 total calories – 480 protein calories from protein = 1893 nonprotein kcals

20% of 1893 calories = 380 fat calories

Round to nearest 100 = 400 kcals lipid/d

2 kcals/mL of 20% lipid solution = 200 mL of 20% lipid

3. Carbohydrate (CHO) content (*approximately 50%-60% of nonprotein calories*)

2373 total calories – 480 protein calories – 400 fat calories = 1493 CHO kcals

1493 CHO kcals ÷ 3.4 kcals/g of dextrose = 439 g dextrose

439 g dextrose ÷ 2.4 L = 183 g dextrose/L

183 g dextrose = 18% dextrose per liter

4. Final solution*

2.4 liters of 18% dextrose, 5% amino acids, with 400 calories (40 g) lipid/day.

*This assumes a triple mix (ie, mix of carbohydrate, lipid, and amino acids in one bag). Some institutions will hang lipid separately. Other institutions do not allow for customized solutions and have a limited selection of solutions from which the clinician chooses to get close to the calorie and protein needs of the patient.

Figure 58-5 *Parenteral nutrition calculation.*

receive 1.2 to 1.5 g/kg/d of protein, even if this precipitates the need for dialysis.

■ HEPATIC DISEASE

Malnutrition is also highly prevalent among patients with liver disease. Laboratory markers of nutrition status may be more reflective of diminished hepatic synthetic capacity rather than nutrition. In addition, anthropometric measurements maybe altered by fluid status. Previous thoughts regarding the benefits of protein restriction in those with hepatic encephalopathy have not been supported by more recent studies. For example, Cordoba and colleagues found no differences in outcomes of encephalopathy between those on normal and protein restricted diets, and that low protein diets in fact caused breakdown of lean body mass. Although much research has been devoted to the evaluation of diets supplemented with branch chain amino acids (BCAAs), the routine use of BCAA-enhanced formulas is only recommended for those with encephalopathy refractory to luminal-acting antibiotics and lactulose therapy.

■ PREOPERATIVE NUTRITION SUPPORT

Several papers indicate that malnourished patients suffer more postoperative complications than those who are adequately nourished. Weight loss of greater than 10% of body weight most consistently predicts adverse outcomes. Buzby and colleagues developed a measure of perioperative complication risk, which they termed "nutrition risk index" (NRI) and is calculated as follows:

$$\text{NRI}: 1.519 \times \text{the serum albumin level (in g/L)} + 0.417$$
$$\times \text{(current weight/usual weight} \times 100)$$

Patients were classified as borderline, mildly, or severely malnourished. The patients who met criteria for severe risk with an NRI <83.5 benefited from preoperative feeding with TPN because they had fewer noninfectious surgical complications (wound dehiscence, pressure ulcers, GI bleeding, cardiac arrest, renal failure) compared to controls. Mildly malnourished patients did not experience the same benefit; rather they suffered additional infectious complications related to TPN. Hence, one can conclude that the malnourished patient may benefit from preoperative feeding, while the well-nourished individual may be adversely affected by this type of nutritional intervention.

Less is known about forced enteral feeding (eg, tube feeds) in a preoperative patient. EN may be considered in patients who have some degree of malnutrition but do not meet NRI criteria for preoperative feeding. Nutrition support should be administered for a minimum of 10 to 14 days prior to surgery to provide optimal benefit. Close consultation with the surgeon is required to determine both the optimal route of feeding and the timing of the operation.

CONCLUSION

Malnutrition is prevalent in a significant number of hospitalized patients. Because of the adverse effects of malnutrition on the host, appropriate nutrition intervention may improve outcomes, decrease cost, and speed recovery. All patients should be screened for malnutrition, have nutrition plans put in place to prevent deterioration of nutritional status, and be treated for malnutrition when identified. EN is the feeding route of choice, but parenteral nutrition is appropriate in those who cannot receive adequate nutrition by the enteral route for prolonged periods.

SUGGESTED READINGS

Bankhead R, Boullata J, Brantley S, et al. Enteral nutrition practice recommendations. *JPEN J Parenter Enteral Nutr*. 2009;33:122-167.

Choban P, Dickerson R, Malone A, et al. A.S.P.E.N. Clinical guidelines: nutrition support of hospitalized adult patients with obesity. *JPEN J Parenter Enteral Nutr*. 2013;37:714-744.

Clinical practice guidelines for nutrition in chronic renal failure. K/DOQI, National Kidney Foundation. *Am J Kidney Dis*. 2000;35:S1-S140.

Correia MI, Waitzberg DL. The impact of malnutrition on morbidity, mortality, length of hospital stay and costs evaluated through a multivariate model analysis. *Clin Nutr*. 2003;22:235-239.

Gramlich L, Kichian K, Pinilla J, Rodych NJ, Dhaliwal R, Heyland DK. Does enteral nutrition compared to parenteral nutrition result in better outcomes in critically ill adult patients? A systematic review of the literature. *Nutrition*. 2004;20:843-848.

McClave SA, Chang WK, Dhaliwal R, Heyland DK. Nutrition support in acute pancreatitis: A systematic review of the literature. *JPEN J Parenter Enteral Nutr*. 2006;30:143-156.

McClave SA, Martindale RG, Vanek VW, et al. Guidelines for the provision and assessment of nutrition support therapy in the adult critically ill patient: Society of Critical Care Medicine (SCCM) and American Society for Parenteral and Enteral Nutrition (A.S.P.E.N.). *JPEN J Parenter Enteral Nutr*. 2009;33:277-316.

Mogensen K, Andrew B, Corona J, Robinson M. Validation of the Society of Critical Care Medicine and American Society for Parenteral and Enteral Nutrition Recommendations for caloric provision to critically ill obese patients. *JPEN J Parenter Enter Nutr*. 2015 [epub Apr 20, 2015].

Perioperative total parenteral nutrition in surgical patients. The Veterans Affairs Total Parenteral Nutrition Cooperative Study Group. *N Engl J Med*. 1991;325:525-532.

Pittiruti M, Hamilton H, Biffi R, MacFie J, Pertkiewicz M. A.S.P.E.N. Guidelines on parenteral nutrition: Central venous catheters (access, care, diagnosis and therapy of complications). *Clin Nutr*. 2009;28:365-377.

White J, Jensen G, Schofield M, et al. Consensus statement: Academy of Nutrition and Dietetics and American Society for Parenteral and Enteral Nutrition: characteristics recommended for the identification and documentation of adult malnutrition (undernutrition). *JPEN J Parenter Enteral Nutr*. 2012;36:275-283.

CHAPTER 59

Cardiac Complications after Noncardiac Surgery

Brian D. Wolfe, MD

Jeffrey J. Glasheen, MD

INTRODUCTION

Over the past two decades, much had been learned about perioperative cardiac issues and the resultant short- and long-term complications. This chapter addresses their demographics, risk factors, and management. It is divided into sections of the most commonly encountered postoperative cardiac complications; postoperative myocardial infarction, congestive heart failure, atrial fibrillation, and ventricular arrhythmias.

POSTOPERATIVE MYOCARDIAL INFARCTION

■ BACKGROUND

Postoperative myocardial infarction (PMI) is a distinct clinical entity from nonpostoperative myocardial infarction (MI). Compared with patients presenting to emergency departments with MI, patients with PMI die nearly twice as often. The incidence of PMI is dependent upon patient risk factors and the type of surgery and the technique used. Reported rates of PMI and associated mortality have varied widely in the literature because of differences in patient selection, changes over time in surgical and anesthetic techniques, differences in screening strategies and definitions of PMI, and the ever-increasing sensitivity of biomarkers for myocardial necrosis. Nonetheless, PMI remains a common and devastatingly morbid postoperative complication.

■ PATHOPHYSIOLOGY

There are three major conditions associated with the rise of cardiac biomarkers in the perioperative period. Two of these are defined by Third Universal Definition of Myocardial Infarction Consensus, published in 2012, which describes Type I PMI as infarction secondary to plaque rupture and intracoronary thrombus formation and Type II PMI as an infarction secondary to a mismatch between the supply of oxygen and the metabolic demands of the myocardium. The third cause of biomarker rise has generated several names, most recently described as nonischemic myocardial injury with necrosis.

Type 1 PMI

Traditional MIs result from an acute coronary syndrome (ACS). More to the point, a vulnerable plaque experiences a spontaneous rupture, fissuring, erosion, or other event leading to intracoronary thrombus and downstream infarction. In the perioperative period, a number of contributing mechanisms exist including an increase in inflammation with an associated hypercoagulable state and an increase catecholamine secretion leading to increase shear stress on preexistent coronary plaques. The end result is intracoronary plaque rupture, which initiates the coagulation cascade, leading to thrombus and infarction. Electrocardiographically there may be ST segment elevations, Q waves, or less specific ST segment depressions or T-wave changes.

Type 2 PMI

Type 2 PMI is associated with myocardial oxygen supply and demand imbalances and occurs in operative and nonoperative settings. The main driver for type 2 PMI is tachycardia secondary to factors such as increased adrenergic tone, postoperative pain, systemic vasodilation, hypovolemia, anemia, and the withholding of chronic β-receptor blocking medications. Patients with fixed coronary disease and increased left ventricular mass possess increased risk for this mechanism of injury. Electrocardiographically this presents with ST-depression, nonspecific T-wave changes or even a normal electrocardiogram (ECG) much more commonly than ST-segment elevation.

Nonischemic myocardial injury with necrosis

This clinical entity is defined by the presence of elevated cardiac-specific biomarkers without evidence of ischemia. It occurs in a variety of clinical syndromes including sepsis, kidney failure, heart failure and other conditions. One proposed mechanism of this myonecrosis is from circulating inflammatory mediators such as tumor necrosis factor.

■ DIAGNOSIS AND PROGNOSIS

Perioperative MI can be difficult to diagnose as the key symptom of chest pain is often masked at least partially by anesthesia, analgesia, and sedation. Several studies agree that approximately two-thirds of patients with PMI have no ischemic symptoms. Importantly, in one study mortality was unchanged by the presence or absence of ischemic symptoms. Beyond symptoms, the role for ECG in the diagnosis of PMI remains unclear due to its low sensitivity, especially in the more common Type 2 PMI described above. In addition, the association between ECG findings with important outcomes has recently been questioned.

As a result, PMI rates and prognosis depends heavily on how the disease is defined and how aggressively patients are screened for this entity. In most studies, PMI is defined as evidence of myocardial necrosis plus symptoms consistent with infarction, ECG changes or hemodynamic alterations or complications.

In the PeriOperative ISchemic Evaluation (POISE) trial cohort, postoperative biomarker measurements and ECGs were obtained in all patients as a screening test, and found an incidence of PMI of 5% with an attendant 30-day mortality of 12%. While in the large National Surgical Quality Improvement Program (NSQIP) cohort, there were no specific screening recommendations and only 0.65% of the patients were found to have a PMI, likely due to these physicians ordering testing in only symptomatic patients; however, their 30-day mortality rate was 61%. Interestingly, though these cohorts were different in size and in inclusion/exclusion criteria, relatively similar amounts of absolute patients (six per one thousand patients vs four per one thousand patients) died at 30 days with the diagnosis of PMI in POISE versus NSQIP patient cohorts, respectively. This begs the question of whether categorizing nearly eight times as many people with an aggressive screening strategy as having a PMI was beneficial.

Differentiating between the previously described pathophysiological entities can be quite challenging, though this is a critical distinction as it heavily impacts complex treatment decisions. In general, Type 1 PMI has the highest elevation in troponin values and is most clearly characterized by ST-segment elevation. It typically presents later in the postoperative course than Type 2 PMI. Multiple studies show that most Type 2 PMI events occur in the first 24 to 48 hours postoperatively while Type 1 PMI events are more equally distributed over the first two postoperative weeks. Type 2 PMI mismatch events are felt to occur in at least four out of five perioperative MI cases; however, there are two small postoperative autopsy trials completed over the last 30 years that would indicate Type 1 PMI-indicative intracoronary thrombosis occurs in nearly 50% of PMI patients. These data highlight our incomplete understanding of what pathophysiological mechanism predominates during the perioperative period.

Differentiating Type 2 PMI from nonischemic myocardial injury with necrosis is particularly difficult as both can be associated with tachycardia, fever, changes in blood pressures and modest

troponin rises. This issue is further complicated by the advent of ever more sensitive troponin assays, which certainly increases the number of patients meeting the PMI definition and others with asymptomatic troponin elevations. While it is tempting to disregard these "troponin leak syndromes," even mild elevations in these ultra-sensitive assays are associated with poor outcomes as shown in the Vascular Events in Noncardiac Surgery Patients Cohort Evaluation (VISION) study.

PRACTICE POINT

- Postoperative MI usually occur within 48 hours of surgery but a small percentage may occur as late as 2 weeks postoperatively.
- 30-day mortality of PMI is higher than that of patients with MI without recent surgery, but varies widely dependent on whether screening strategy is employed.
- The underlying pathology determines optimal management.
- Type 1 PMI with true ST-elevation MI is generally treated as a traditional ACS. Risks of management (increased surgical site bleeding) and benefits (of restoring coronary blood flow) need to be carefully weighed with the surgical team prior to initiation of therapy.
- Type 2 PMI is best treated by restoring the oxygen supply-demand balance. Optimizing hemodynamics is the primary goal in these patients.
- Recognition and treatment includes management of arrhythmias, volume resuscitation, and transfusion.

■ MANAGEMENT

The management of PMI should reflect its presumed pathophysiology; however, the differentiation between these entities is challenging and is not always possible. Type 1 PMI with true ST-elevation MI is relatively uncommon; when it occurs it necessitates a traditional approach to ACS with the goal of restoring flow in an acutely thrombosed artery, similar to the nonpostoperative setting. This management is complicated by increased risks of surgical site bleeding but generally involves anticoagulation and antiplatelet therapy along with coronary revascularization. These risks and benefits need to be carefully weighed with the surgical team prior to initiation of therapy. β-blockers and statin medications are also indicated.

Type 2 PMI is best treated by relieving the oxygen supply-demand imbalance. This includes reducing the adrenergic drive and associated tachycardia through correction of hypo- or hypervolemia, treatment of heart failure, aggressive pain control, and treatment of fever. Other traditional therapies such as aspirin, β-blockers, and statins require consideration on a case by case basis. In the POISE cohort, patients with PMI that were given aspirin had better outcomes than those not given antiplatelets. However, in the POISE 2 trial when perioperative patients were randomized to aspirin or placebo, there was no difference in mortality or other important endpoints associated with PMI. Thus, the following recommendations for Type 2 PMI are consistent with expert guidelines but lack trial data support.

Treatment of nonischemic myocardial injury with necrosis is focused not upon the cardiac issue, but instead upon the sepsis, renal failure or other disease to which the necrosis was attributed. As mentioned earlier, the differentiation between these entities is difficult at times. Moreover, there are no interventional trials to support a specific treatment regimen. Postoperative hypotension and associated tachycardia due to a combination of volume depletion and anesthetic effect are commonly associated with demand ischemia and Type 2 PMI. This can be treated with isotonic fluids. Hypertension-induced Type 2 PMI should be treated with antihypertensives and diuretics as needed. Volume overload is an underrecognized cause of hypertension and thereby increased myocardial demand and should be addressed aggressively. Primary tachyarrhythmias such as atrial fibrillation with rapid ventricular response should be rate controlled or cardioverted as the situation dictates. Initiation of β-blockers in the setting of Type 2 PMI is thought to be appropriate when demand ischemia is due to hypertension and nonhypovolemic tachycardic syndromes (eg, fever). However, β-blockers should be held in the setting of hypotension and anemia-induced ischemia as they will likely worsen these processes and clinical outcomes.

Postoperative anemia management to prevent and treat PMI is controversial as both postoperative anemia and liberal transfusion have been shown to worsen outcomes. For example, a retrospective study found preoperative hemoglobin (hgb) <13 g/dL were associated with increased cardiac complications and mortality. The Functional Outcomes in Cardiovascular Patients Undergoing Surgical Hip Fracture Repair (FOCUS) trial evaluated transfusion cutoffs of 10 g/dL versus 8 g/dL or symptomatic. The trial clearly showed that the lower cutoff was superior and not associated with provoking higher rates of myocardial ischemia; however, in that trial nearly one-half of the transfusions in the restrictive strategy group were given for hypotension, tachycardia and chest pain. Until more evidence is forthcoming using a transfusion threshold of 8 g/dL appears reasonable with close consideration of volume status and other hemodynamic indicators.

■ SURVEILLANCE

There are few data to guide the use of perioperative surveillance for PMI. Due to the relatively asymptomatic nature of PMI, screening with troponins and ECG greatly enhances the detection of PMI. Given the predominance and accepted pathophysiology of Type 2 PMI, it follows that early intervention to improve supply and decrease demand could alter outcomes; however, there are no data to support this interventional approach. Moreover, there are concerns about the potential negative impacts of some interventions such as antiplatelet or anticoagulant medication administration and revascularization procedures. The ACC/AHA guidelines have evolved over time now calling into question any surveillance ECG or troponin strategy in asymptomatic patients. Other authors and societies recommend the screening of high-risk patients, as defined by severe underlying coronary disease or active cardiac symptoms. All agree that ischemic symptoms should prompt ECG and troponin assessment, but as outlined previously this represents the minority of patients. Hopefully, interventional trials will be forthcoming to aid in the management of these complex issues.

■ CONCLUSION

Postoperative MI is common, driven by the increasing frequency of surgical procedures in an aging, comorbid population. Despite prudent preoperative assessment, PMI still occurs and is often masked by the operative state. PMI more often occurs from oxygen supply-demand imbalances than ACS and as such is most often treated with a return to homeostasis.

POSTOPERATIVE HEART FAILURE

■ BACKGROUND

Heart failure (HF) following noncardiac surgery is a common postoperative cardiac complication. The incidence depends on the patient population because it occurs after less than 5% of major surgeries but as frequently as 25% in patients with known cardiac disease. In a single-center series, the incidence of postoperative pulmonary edema was 7.6% with a mortality rate of almost 12%. Many of the landmark perioperative cardiac outcomes trials such as the POISE

Trial do not include postoperative HF in their combined cardiac endpoint. Nonetheless, it is an important postoperative complication that leads to increased morbidity, mortality, length of stay, and cost.

■ DEFINITION AND DIAGNOSIS

There is no formal definition of postoperative HF. However, in trials that have included HF as a major adverse cardiac event, it is defined as pulmonary edema. This is a reasonable definition because pulmonary edema, with its resulting dyspnea and hypoxemia, is the most common presenting syndrome. That said, all postoperative pulmonary edema is not HF. Noncardiac causes of airspace disease, including aspiration, acute respiratory distress syndrome (ARDS), and pneumonia should also be considered. Once airspace disease has been identified, the evaluation should focus on volume status, including the amount of fluid infused in the perioperative period, examination of the neck veins for distension, and nonpulmonary edema, particularly in the sacrum for patients who have been bedridden. A patient with pulmonary edema and such signs of volume overload likely has postoperative HF.

Risk factors for postoperative HF include preexisting cardiac disease, particularly recent MI or unstable angina, diabetes, significant intraoperative hemodynamic changes (mean arterial pressure increase or decrease >40 mm Hg from preoperative baseline), and abdominal aortic aneurysm repair. A case series of fatal postoperative pulmonary edema in largely healthy patients found that the average positive fluid balance was 67 mL/kg/d positive, or about 5 liters in a 70-kg patient. Interestingly, another prospective evaluation of the risk of development of postoperative HF found that lower volumes of administered fluid and negative net fluid balance were associated with higher rates of postoperative HF. These findings may be explained by the lower use of intravenous fluids in patients with a history of cardiac disease. Certainly, the amount of fluids given in the perioperative period is an important historical fact, and despite these counterintuitive findings, it is reasonable to consider more intraoperative IV fluids to be a risk factor for postoperative pulmonary edema.

■ EVALUATION AND MANAGEMENT

Once it has been determined that a patient has HF, initial evaluation should focus on early identification of myocardial ischemia. While all postoperative HF is not ischemic in nature, postoperative MIs often have atypical presentations requiring a high degree of suspicion. Therefore, electrocardiography, cardiac monitoring, and serial cardiac enzymes are prudent in the workup of postoperative HF. Interestingly, patients with ischemia-induced postoperative HF have increased risk of subsequent cardiac events, whereas those with nonischemic postoperative HF do not. Patients with ischemia-induced postoperative HF should be managed according to ACC/AHA guidelines (refer to the section on PMI).

Postoperative HF typically occurs within the first 36 hours after surgery. Pulmonary edema occurring immediately after extubation, particularly in the postanesthesia care unit, could be a result of "negative pressure pulmonary edema." This is a poorly characterized clinical syndrome associated with postextubation laryngospasm. This leads to increased use of accessory muscles and greater negative intrathoracic pressures, which in turn causes pulmonary edema. The classic patient is a young healthy male undergoing surgery of the aerodigestive tract. Treatment is supportive, with diuretics, oxygen, continuous positive airway pressure (CPAP) and, occasionally, reintubation. Although one series revealed that nearly half of the patients with this entity required reintubation, the prognosis for a complete recovery is excellent.

Nonischemic postoperative HF warrants further evaluation. ACC/AHA guidelines recommend, at a minimum, a complete history and physical as well as laboratory, ECG, chest radiography, and transthoracic echocardiography (TTE). Consideration for noninvasive or invasive coronary angiography should be reserved for patients presenting with ischemic HF. While these guidelines are not specific to the postoperative setting, it is reasonable to apply them to this scenario.

Historical information should include preoperative symptoms of heart failure or angina, use of stimulant drugs and alcohol, as well as chemotherapeutic agents that increase the risk of development of HF. Laboratory evaluation should include assessment of hepatic, thyroid, and renal function as well as complete blood counts, glycohemoglobin, and lipid testing. An exhaustive search for less common causes of HF such as amyloidosis should be reserved for those in which the clinical scenario is suggestive of such an etiology.

Initial management of postoperative pulmonary edema consists of diuresis and discontinuation of IV fluids coupled with fluid and sodium restriction. Supplemental oxygen can be used as needed. If left ventricular systolic dysfunction is discovered during the workup, patients should be managed similarly to those in a nonoperative setting. This includes initiation of an angiotensin-converting enzyme inhibitor, β-blocker medication among others. Statin medications are indicated in most of these patients irrespective of their lipid levels based on 10-year estimations of cardiac risk. Aspirin as secondary prevention of ischemic events is indicated, although surgical hemostasis needs to be considered in the timing of antiplatelet initiation.

In summary, HF is a relatively common and serious postoperative cardiac complication that is best defined as cardiogenic pulmonary edema. Risk factors are preexisting cardiac disease, diabetes, kidney disease and intraoperative hemodynamic changes. Large amounts of perioperative IV fluids most likely present an additional risk factor, although data are discordant on this issue, and "threshold" levels for the development of pulmonary edema are not well established. Ischemic and nonischemic HF should be distinguished because this differentiation has the largest impact on subsequent management and prognosis. Ischemic HF should be managed per current societal guidelines, weighing the benefits of anticoagulation and antiplatelet agents against the risks of surgical site bleeding. The evaluation and management of nonischemic postoperative HF is similar to those encountered in other clinical settings and should follow current guidelines.

POSTOPERATIVE ATRIAL FIBRILLATION
■ INCIDENCE, RISK FACTORS, AND PREVENTION

Atrial fibrillation (AF) is the most common atrial arrhythmia following surgery. While it is a well-known complication of cardiac surgery, affecting as many as 40% of coronary artery bypass procedures, it is also common following noncardiac surgery with an aggregate incidence of about 3%, though much higher after thoracic surgery.

PRACTICE POINT

Peak incidence of postoperative atrial fibrillation occurs on postoperative day 2 and it typically lasts 1 to 4 days.
- In 20% to 30% of cases it resolves without specific intervention and less than 20% of patients will remain in AF at the time of discharge.
- While the need for cardioversion is rare, most patients will require rate control. Initial rate control is best achieved via parenteral medications that slow conduction through the atrioventricular (AV) node.
- First-line agents include nondihydropyridine calcium channel blockers or β-blockers.

- For patients with a known or suspected accessory pathway or heart failure, amiodarone is the first-line agent.
- For those patients who do not have resolution of their arrhythmia, they will need basic cardiac evaluation according to the American College of Cardiology/American Heart Association (ACC/AHA) guidelines for atrial fibrillation.
- Stroke prophylaxis with anticoagulation hinges on balancing the risk of stroke and risk reduction from anticoagulation against the risk and consequences of surgical bleeding.

The risk factors for postoperative AF are similar to those following cardiac surgery. Patient-specific risk factors include advanced age, male sex, premature atrial contractions on preoperative ECG, valvular heart disease, American Society of Anesthesiologists class III or IV, CHF, hypertension, and preoperative hypokalemia. Abdominal aortic aneurysm repair, thoracic surgery, and abdominal surgery all carry increased risk of postoperative AF in comparison to orthopedic and other surgeries.

Preoperative statin use prior to noncardiac thoracic surgery has been shown to reduce the risk of postoperative AF, an effect that has been attributed to the pleiotrophic or anti-inflammatory effect of statins. Perioperative β-blocker use is associated with an increased risk of death in low-risk patients and an increased risk of death and stroke when started immediately preoperatively in moderate- to high-risk patients and is therefore not recommended solely for prophylaxis of postoperative AF (see Chapter 50: Preoperative Cardiac Risk Assessment and Perioperative Management). Amiodarone has been shown in some thoracic surgery studies to reduce postoperative atrial fibrillation rates, but it remains unclear that this improves outcomes or is worth the risks that accompany amiodarone administration.

■ EVALUATION AND MANAGEMENT

The initial step in management of atrial arrhythmias is to verify the specific diagnosis by ECG. AF is characterized by the absence of p waves and an irregularly irregular R-R interval. Initial management depends on the clinical status of the patient. Hemodynamically unstable patients, characterized by hypotension or signs of poor perfusion such as loss of consciousness, need immediate direct current electrical cardioversion. This is an uncommon clinical scenario, and this management should be reserved for life-threatening hemodynamic collapse.

While the need for cardioversion is rare, most patients will require rate control. Initial rate control is best achieved via parenteral medications that slow conduction through the atrioventricular (AV) node. First-line agents include nondihydropyridine calcium channel blockers or β-blockers. For patients with a known or suspected accessory pathway, AV blocking agents can lead to faster ventricular response and are thus contraindicated. In these cases, amiodarone is the first-line agent. Likewise for patients with concomitant heart failure, amiodarone is the preferred agent. While postoperative AF may convert spontaneously or following initial rate control, patients with AF that persists beyond a few minutes will likely need long-acting oral medications. It is reasonable to use the oral equivalent of the agent that was successful with the initial rate control. It is important to remember that AF is often a manifestation of an underlying perturbation such as infection or venous thromboembolism (VTE), and these diagnoses should be considered before escalating AV nodal blockade.

Anticoagulation is challenging in postsurgical patients with new onset AF where the risk of stroke and risk reduction from anticoagulation must be balanced against the risk and consequences of surgical bleeding. In patients with atrial fibrillation it is recommended to use the $CHADS_2$ or CHA_2DS_2-VAS_c risk scoring systems to decide

upon the long-term risk of thromboembolism and whether antico-agulation would be beneficial. There are no specific guidelines for the timing or method of starting a new anticoagulant in the postoperative setting. Many experts would use warfarin without a heparin/low-molecular-weight heparin run-in phase to avoid raising the risk for postoperative bleeding. Others would recommend heparin or low-molecular-weight heparin to prevent the exceedingly rare skin necrosis that can occur in patients with protein C deficiency. In either case, the surgical site, risk of bleeding and other co-morbidities must be considered. Most protocols would recommend starting warfarin 24 to 72 hours after hemostasis has been achieved; however, there are no randomized data to support this approach.

More than 80% of new postoperative AF will resolve by discharge. Patients who do not have resolution of their arrhythmia will need basic cardiac evaluation. The American College of Cardiology/American Heart Association (ACC/AHA) guidelines for AF list the minimum initial evaluation to include history and physical, ECG, Transthoracic Echocardiogram (TTE), and laboratory tests of thyroid, renal, and hepatic function. The goal of this evaluation is to deline-ate whether this is paroxysmal AF has been present in the past or is likely to recur in the future. The TTE is helpful for determining left ventricular function, atrial size, and valvular function—factors that will help guide decisions regarding stroke prophylaxis.

If a patient's symptoms resolve with rate control, the employed strategy should be continued. In this approach, no attempt is made at restoration of sinus rhythm, and the patient's ventricular rate is controlled with AV nodal blockade alone. Rhythm control strategy is aimed at restoration of sinus rhythm and can be accomplished via chemical or electrical cardioversion and subsequent antiarrhythmic medications. The rhythm control strategy mandates anticoagulation such that patients whose surgery precludes therapeutic anticoagu-lation are not candidates for cardioversion. Despite the theoretical benefit of rhythm control, it is not associated with lower rates of stroke and death, and there are inconsistent reports of improved quality of life. (See Chapter 132 [Supraventricular Tachyarrythmias].)

■ ASSOCIATED CONDITIONS

Postoperative AF may occur in isolation or be associated with underlying systemic conditions. More than half of patients with AF after noncardiac surgery have a major underlying condition, with infection having the strongest association. For example, patients with postoperative AF have a relative risk of 7.4 for bacterial pneu-monia and 6.2 for sepsis compared to those without arrhythmia. For patients in the surgical intensive care unit (ICU), the leading cause of death in patients with new-onset AF is sepsis. In general, the inci-dence of sepsis in patients with new postoperative arrhythmias is 20% to 30%, although this figure is primarily from surgical ICU data.

Primary cardiac events are less commonly antecedent to new AF. The relative risk of MI in patients with a new arrhythmia is 4.2. In colorectal surgery patients, both pulmonary edema and overall complications are more common in patients with new arrhythmias. Other postoperative complications associated with new-onset AF include pulmonary embolism, gastrointestinal bleed, cerebrovascu-lar accident, hypokalemia, and anastomotic leakage.

Given the frequency of serious underlying etiologies, new AF following noncardiac surgery should be regarded as a possible harbinger of life-threatening postoperative complications. Thus, appropriate evaluation of new postoperative arrhythmia warrants a complete evaluation of the patient with consideration of infectious, cardiac, and thrombotic complications.

■ SUMMARY

AF is the most common arrhythmia following noncardiac surgery, with patient-specific risk factors similar to those for AF in the general population. It typically occurs early in the postoperative course. Preoperative statin therapy is associated with a lower risk of developing AF in some surgical populations, but there are insuf-ficient data to recommend this practice routinely, particularly in lower-risk patients. β-blockers are not recommended solely for prophylaxis of postoperative AF. Initial management of postopera-tive AF commences with verification of the diagnosis with an ECG. Hemodynamically unstable patients require emergent cardioversion. Patients with rapid ventricular responses require IV administration of nodal blocking agents followed by an oral equivalent. The decision to anticoagulate must balance stroke risk in the acute setting with the risk of operative bleeding. Patients with persistent AF will need adequate rate control and, should they remain symptomatic, consid-eration of cardioversion and subsequent rhythm control. A CHADS2 score of 2 or greater is an indication for chronic anticoagulation in most patients with persistent AF at the time of discharge.

POSTOPERATIVE VENTRICULAR ARRHYTHMIAS

Ventricular arrhythmias are uncommon following noncardiac sur-gery. Because of this, data are sparse regarding risk factors and outcomes. In the thoracic surgery population, one study found the incidence of nonsustained ventricular tachycardia (NSVT) to be 15%, but there were no episodes of sustained ventricular arrhythmias, nor did any of these episodes lead to hemodynamic instability. Impor-tantly, nonischemic ventricular tachycardia (VT) following noncar-diac surgery is not associated with worse long-term outcomes.

The most common scenario described in the literature for serious ventricular arrhythmias is following postoperative MI in patients with underlying heart disease. Fatal ventricular arrhythmias are included in the outcomes of major trials such as CARP and DECREASE-V, but the contribution of ventricular arrhythmias to the endpoint is not reported.

When confronted with a ventricular arrhythmia, the first decision point is to ascertain the patient's hemodynamic status. Unstable patients, defined as having hypotension or loss of consciousness, need emergent treatment as described in Advanced Cardiac Life Support (ACLS) protocols. Hemodynamically stable patients with ventricular arrhythmias need urgent evaluation for acute ischemia including 12-lead ECG and serial cardiac enzymes. Should this workup reveal myocardial ischemia, treatment according to pub-lished guidelines should commence. Significant electrolyte abnor-malities, notably hypokalemia and hypomagnesemia, are reversible causes of ventricular arrhythmias and thus warrant prompt evalu-ation and repletion. In the setting of torsades de pointes, or poly-morphic ventricular tachycardia with prolonged QT interval, empiric magnesium should be given. As QT prolongation is often a result of medication use, the patient's medication list should be reviewed and potentially offending medications discontinued. Hemodynami-cally stable but sustained VT requires antiarrhythmic drugs.

In summary, postoperative ventricular arrhythmias are an uncom-mon cardiac complication, but with potentially serious conse-quences. Hemodynamically unstable patients will need emergent defibrillation. Patients with ventricular arrhythmias need urgent evaluation for cardiac ischemia. Fortunately, nonischemic VT does not appear to negatively impact long-term prognosis.

SUGGESTED READINGS

Amar D. Prevention and management of perioperative arrhyth-mias in the thoracic surgical population. *Anesthesiology Clinics.* 2008;26:325-335.

Amar D, Zhang H, Heerdt PM, et al. Statin use is associated with a reduction in atrial fibrillation after non-cardiac thoracic surgery independent of C-reactive protein. *Chest.* 2005;128:3421-3427.

Botto F, et al. Myocardial injury after noncardiac surgery: a large, international, prospective cohort study establishing diagnostic criteria, characteristics, predictors, and 30-day outcomes. *Anesthesiology*. 2014;120:564-578.

Carson JL, et al. Liberal or restrictive transfusion in high-risk patients after hip surgery. *N Engl J Med*. 2011;365:2453-2462.

Devereaux PJ, Yang H, Yusuf S, et al. Effects of extended-release metoprolol succinate in patients undergoing non-cardiac surgery (POISE trial): a randomized controlled trial. *Lancet*. 2008;371:1839-1847.

Fleisher LA, Fleischmann KE, et al. ACC/AHA 2014 guidelines on perioperative cardiovascular evaluation and management of patients undergoing noncardiac surgery. *JACC*. 2014;64:e77-e137.

Fuster V, Rydén LE, Cannom DS, et al. ACC/AHA/ESC 2006 guidelines for the management of patients with atrial fibrillation. *Circulation*. 2006;114:700-752.

Go AS, Hylek EM, Chang Y, et al. Anticoagulation therapy for stroke prevention in atrial fibrillation. *JAMA*. 2003;290:2685-2692.

Gupta PK, et al. Development and validation of a risk calculator for prediction of cardiac risk after surgery. *Circulation*. 2011;124:381-387.

Landesberg G, Beattie WS, Mosseri M, Jaffe AS, Alpert JS. Perioperative myocardial infarction. *Circulation*. 2009;119:2936-2944.

CHAPTER 60

Management of Postoperative Pulmonary Complications

William I. Levin, MD

John J. Reilly, Jr., MD

INTRODUCTION

Hospitalists are frequently called upon to provide perioperative care to a broad spectrum of surgical patients, in either a consultative or a comanagement role. Although historically much emphasis has been placed on postoperative cardiac complications, postoperative pulmonary complications are known to occur with equal or greater frequency and contribute substantially to morbidity, mortality, and health care costs. Broadly defined, postoperative pulmonary complications are conditions affecting the respiratory tract that adversely influence the clinical course of patients after surgery. The Confederate general, Thomas "Stonewall" Jackson, wounded in the Battle of Chancellorsville in 1863, was perhaps the earliest recorded victim of a postoperative pulmonary complication, dying of pneumonia 8 days after the successful amputation of his left arm. It is estimated that over 1 million patients undergoing nonthoracic surgery in the United States annually experience postoperative pulmonary complications. Pulmonary complications produce the highest attributable costs among common categories of postoperative complications and can result in a fivefold increase in the median cost of an operation. The presence of pulmonary complications after major surgery increased 30-day mortality from 2% to 22%, and 1-year mortality from 8.7% to 45.9% based on data from the National Surgical Quality Improvement Program (NSQIP). The most important postoperative pulmonary complications are atelectasis, pneumonia, respiratory failure, and exacerbation of underlying chronic lung disease, although earlier studies have also included transient and self-limited clinical findings. A general principle is that the closer the operative site is to the diaphragm, the higher the likelihood of postoperative pulmonary complications. Interventions to reduce the incidence of these complications depend on the aggressive application of preventive measures to high-risk patients. Obstructive sleep apnea in particular has received greater recognition as a frequently undiagnosed and prevalent condition in surgical patients that increases pulmonary risk. Programs such as the NSQIP allow institutions to track their performance and engage in quality improvement in this area. Anticipation, early diagnosis and prompt effective therapies form the next line of defense in treating postsurgical complications once they occur. Studies of hospital mortality associated with inpatient surgery suggest the variation between institutions is explained more by their ability to "rescue" patients from complications when they occur rather than differences in incidence. This chapter focuses on the pathogenesis, early recognition, and evidence-based treatment of common postoperative pulmonary complications.

PRACTICE POINT

- A general principle to predicting the risk of postoperative pulmonary complications is that the closer the operative site is to the diaphragm, the higher the likelihood of complications.

ATELECTASIS

Atelectasis, or reversible alveolar collapse, is a common perioperative phenomenon and occurs in 90% of patients receiving general anesthesia. Computed tomographic (CT) studies have demonstrated collapse of 15% to 20% of the lung volume near the diaphragm. Dr William Pasteur, a Swiss physician practicing in England in the early part of the last century, wrote extensively on the postoperative lung and noted, "when the true history of postoperative lung complications comes to be written, active collapse of the lung from deficiency of inspiratory power will be found to occupy an important position among determining causes." Most atelectasis appearing during general anesthesia resolves within 24 hours after surgery in normal subjects and is of little clinical significance. Atelectasis can persist for 2 days or longer after major surgery, including abdominal and thoracic surgery, and is thought to represent the starting point in a cascade of events that leads to the more serious complications of pneumonia and acute respiratory failure.

■ PATHOPHYSIOLOGY

The formation of perioperative atelectasis can be understood by considering the effect of surgery on normal respiratory mechanics as well as the mechanisms involved in alveolar collapse. The induction of anesthesia alters the distribution and timing of neural drive to the respiratory muscles, interfering with coordination of activity. The supine position and use of positive pressure ventilation alter the distribution of ventilation and lead to hypoventilation of dependent areas. Surgical trauma can produce reflex inhibition of the phrenic nerve from stimulation of the viscera, mechanical disruption of the intercostal or abdominal respiratory muscles, and voluntary limitation of respiratory motion from postoperative pain. The characteristic postoperative mechanical abnormality is a restrictive pattern with severely reduced inspiratory capacity, vital capacity (VC), and functional residual capacity (FRC), clinically demonstrated by rapid shallow respirations.

Pulmonary atelectasis occurs by three mechanisms: compression atelectasis, absorption (resorption) atelectasis, and loss of surfactant. Compression atelectasis results when the transmural pressure distending the alveolus is reduced, allowing the alveolus to collapse. During anesthesia, change in diaphragmatic function and chest geometry causes pressure from the abdomen to be transmitted into the thorax, resulting in compression of lung tissue. Resorption atelectasis describes collapse of alveoli related to absorption of gas from occluded or hypoventilated areas of the lung. Since oxygen is absorbed more rapidly than nitrogen, air with high inspired FiO_2 will be absorbed more rapidly, resulting in collapse. Surfactant function, important in stabilizing the alveoli, may be disrupted by anesthesia and mechanical ventilation. The physiologic consequence is ventilation-perfusion (V/Q) mismatch resulting in hypoxemia.

There is strong interest in refining anesthetic technique to ideally deliver a patient with no atelectasis and open lungs to the post anesthesia care unit. Key areas of investigation include modulation of FiO_2 to optimize oxygen delivery but minimize resorption atelectasis, use of recruitment maneuvers, PEEP, and CPAP during the course of the patient's perioperative care.

■ DIAGNOSIS—DOES THIS PATIENT HAVE ATELECTASIS?

Atelectasis is recognized by the finding of persistent postoperative hypoxemia in the absence of other plausible diagnoses. The patient demonstrates dyspnea or tachypnea, and physical findings can include basilar rales and decreased breath sounds in the affected area. Atelectasis is often cited as a cause of postoperative fevers, but studies have demonstrated no association between atelectasis and fever and suggest that early postoperative fevers are more likely due to the inflammatory response to surgery. Atelectasis is detected radiographically by opacification of a lobe or lobar segment and evidence of volume loss. The most reliable sign is displacement of the interlobar fissure, but other signs include elevation of the hemidiaphragm, mediastinal shift, and compensatory overinflation of adjacent aerated segments. There may be linear opacities ("plate-like") in the parenchyma in dependent portions of the lungs. Silhouette

sign can be positive, with obliteration of adjacent boundaries. Posteroanterior (PA) and lateral images of the chest are preferred, and the ability of plain radiographs to detect atelectasis in recumbent critically ill patients is less certain. CT is sensitive in detecting areas of collapse, and may also reveal other pathology. MRI and bedside ultrasound can also be useful.

■ TREATMENT

Treatment of postoperative atelectasis centers on lung expansion techniques, shifting from supine position when possible, and adequate postoperative analgesia. The FRC has been identified as the single most important postoperative lung volume parameter, and efforts to restore normal pulmonary mechanics are beneficial. A simple posture change from supine to seated will increase FRC by 0.5 to 1.0 liters. Standing and early ambulation are also helpful when tolerated.

The goal of lung expansion maneuvers is to produce a large and sustained increase in transpulmonary pressure that distends the lung and re-expands the collapsed lung units. Techniques include incentive spirometry, deep breathing exercises, chest physical therapy, intermittent positive-pressure breathing (IPPB), and continuous positive airway pressure (CPAP). A systematic review found that for patients undergoing abdominal surgery, any type of lung expansion intervention improved outcome, with no one modality being superior. Incentive spirometry was the least labor intensive. IPPB is the most costly and was associated with unacceptable abdominal distension in a significant number of cases. Low-quality evidence suggests that use of incentive spirometry does not improve outcome, but it has been included in preventative care bundles. Another systematic review also found evidence that use of CPAP in patients who underwent abdominal surgery led to lower rates of postoperative atelectasis and pneumonia.

The effect of different types of analgesia in decreasing postoperative atelectasis has been examined. Studies have been heterogeneous and small, but a recent meta-analysis found a trend toward decreased postoperative atelectasis and pneumonia with the use of postoperative epidural analgesia in patients undergoing abdominal surgery. Postoperative epidural and patient-controlled intravenous analgesia both seem superior to on-demand delivery of opioids in preventing postoperative pulmonary complications. The potential benefit of epidural anesthesia must be weighed against bleeding risk from deep vein thrombosis (DVT) prophylaxis.

■ COMPLICATIONS

Mild hypoxemia from atelectasis is usually well tolerated, but more severe hypoxemia can affect end organs. Atelectrauma refers to the mechanism by which atelectasis can trigger acute lung injury, and includes overexpansion of adjacent aerated lung tissue along with repetitive sheer forces from the opening and closing of alveoli that results in the release of local inflammatory cytokines. Left untreated, atelectasis likely predisposes to the development of pneumonia and respiratory failure, including acute respiratory distress syndrome.

POSTOPERATIVE PNEUMONIA

Pneumonia ranks as the third most common postoperative infection behind urinary tract infection (UTI) and wound infection. The incidence of pneumonia following major abdominal surgery ranges between 2% and 19% and is a principal factor in increased mortality. Development of hospital-acquired pneumonia is associated with a 30% to 50% increased risk of developing acute respiratory failure requiring mechanical ventilation and increases hospital stays by an average of 7 to 9 days at an excess cost of $40,000 per patient.

Postoperative pneumonia is a subset of hospital-acquired pneumonia (HAP), which is pneumonia occurring 48 hours or more after

TABLE 60-1 Risk Factors for Multidrug-Resistant Pathogens

Antimicrobial therapy in the preceding 90 d

Current hospitalization of 5 d or more

High frequency of antibiotic resistance in the community

Presence of risk factors for health-care-associated pneumonia (HCAP)

    Hospitalization for 2 d or more in the preceding 90 d

    Residence in a nursing home or extended care facility

    Home infusion therapy

    Chronic dialysis within 30 d

    Home wound care

    Family member with multidrug-resistant pathogen

Immunosuppressive disease and/or therapy

TABLE 60-2 Early-Onset Hospital-Acquired Pneumonia without MDR Risk Factors

Potential Pathogen	Recommended Antibiotic
Streptococcus pneumoniae	Ceftriaxone
Haemophilus influenzae	or
Methicillin-sensitive *Staphylococcus aureus*	Levofloxacin, moxifloxacin, or ciprofloxacin
Antibiotic-sensitive enteric Gram-negative bacilli	or
Escherichia coli	Ampicillin/sulbactam
Klebsiella pneumoniae	or
Enterobacter species	Ertapenem
Proteus species	
Serratia marcescens	

admission and not incubating at the time of admission. The major early management goal for postoperative pneumonia is to provide appropriate antibiotics in adequate doses based on the best prediction of suspected pathogens and resistance pattern.

The timing of onset of HAP is an important epidemiologic variable. Early-onset HAP, less than 5 days into admission, is more likely to be caused by antibiotic-sensitive bacteria unless other risk factors for multidrug-resistant (MDR) pathogens are present. Late-onset HAP, 5 or more days after admission, is more likely to be associated with MDR pathogens. Additional risk factors for MDR pathogens are included in **Table 60-1**. Hospital- and unit-specific microbiologic data are also very important in selecting appropriate treatment.

The 2005 American Thoracic Society/Infectious Diseases Society of America (ATS/IDSA) guideline emphasizes ventilator-associated pneumonia (VAP) because it is more readily studied, but suggests it is reasonable to extrapolate the conclusions regarding risk factors for infection with specific pathogens to nonintubated, nonventilated HAP patients.

■ PATHOPHYSIOLOGY

The sequence of events in HAP begins with colonization of the oropharynx with pathogens, which can occur within 48 hours of admission. Sources of pathogens include contaminated health care devices, the environment, and transfer from other patients or staff. These pathogens must be aspirated from the oropharynx into the lower respiratory tract, and then overwhelm the natural host defense mechanisms. Microaspiration is known to occur in up to 45% of healthy subjects during sleep and can be worsened in postsurgical patients by decreased gag reflex, ineffective coughing, sedation, supine posture, especially during enteral feeds, and routine (rather than selective) use of nasogastric (NG) tubes. The host defenses are also affected in multiple ways by general anesthesia, including mechanical impairment of normal mucociliary transport and interference with function of alveolar inflammatory cells, including polymorphonuclear leukocytes, macrophages, lymphocytes, cytokines, antibodies, and complement.

The microbiology of early-onset HAP without MDR risk factors tends to mirror community-acquired pneumonia and includes *Streptococcus pneumoniae*, *Haemophilus influenzae*, methicillin-sensitive *Staphylococcus aureus*, and antibiotic-sensitive Enterobacteriaceae (**Table 60-2**). Pathogens in late-onset HAP or the presence of MDR risk factors also include methicillin-resistant *S. aureus* (MRSA), *Pseudomonas aeruginosa*, extended-spectrum β-lactamase (ESBL)-producing *Klebsiella*, and *Acinetobacter baumannii* (**Table 60-3**).

■ DIAGNOSIS—DOES THIS PATIENT HAVE POSTOPERATIVE PNEUMONIA?

The goal of diagnosis is to identify which patients have a pulmonary infection so that antibiotics are not delayed but that patients with noninfectious etiologies are not exposed unnecessarily to the antibiotics. All patients should undergo a comprehensive history and physical exam, chest x-ray (preferably PA and lateral), measurement of arterial O_2 saturation, complete blood count (CBC), electrolytes, liver function tests, and blood cultures. All ventilated patients should have lower respiratory cultures obtained, ideally prior to starting antibiotics, to guide de-escalation of therapy. Other processes that produce similar symptoms including congestive heart failure, atelectasis, pulmonary thromboembolism, drug reactions, pulmonary hemorrhage, and acute respiratory distress syndrome (ARDS) need to be considered.

The Centers for Disease Control and Prevention (CDC) criteria for diagnosis of nosocomial pneumonia in adults require radiologic as

TABLE 60-3 Late-Onset Hospital-Acquired Pneumonia or HAP with MDR Risk Factors

Potential Pathogens	Recommended Antibiotic Combination
Streptococcus pneumoniae	Antipseudomonal cephalosporin (cefepime, ceftazidime)
Haemophilus influenzae	
Methicillin-sensitive *Staphylococcus aureus*	or
Antibiotic-sensitive enteric Gram-negative bacilli	Antipseudomonal carbapenem (imipenem or meropenem)
Escherichia coli	or
Klebsiella pneumoniae	β-lactam/β-lactamase inhibitor (piperacillin-tazobactam)
Enterobacter species	
Proteus species	plus
Serratia marcescens	Antipseudomonal fluoroquinolone (ciprofloxacin or levofloxacin)
Plus	
Pseudomonas aeruginosa	or
Klebsiella pneumoniae (ESBL)	Aminoglycoside (Amikacin, gentamicin, or tobramycin)
Acinetobacter species	
Methicillin-resistant *Staphylococcus aureus*	plus
	Linezolid or vancomycin

TABLE 60-4 Centers for Disease Control and Prevention Criteria for Diagnosis of Nosocomial Pneumonia

Radiology	Signs/Symptoms/Laboratory
Two or more serial chest x-rays with at least one of the following: New or progressive infiltrate Consolidation Cavitation	At least one of the following: Fever (>38°C) with no other source Leukopenia (<4000 WBC/μL) or leukocytosis (>12,000 WBC/μL) Mental status changes with no other cause in adult >70-y old And at least two of the following: New onset of purulent sputum New-onset cough, dyspnea, tachycardia Rales or bronchial breath sounds (BS) Worsening gas exchange

well as clinical and laboratory findings (**Table 60-4**). The ATS/IDSA guideline describes two diagnostic approaches to HAP: clinical and bacteriologic. The clinical approach bases the diagnosis on a new infiltrate on chest x-ray plus clinical evidence of infection. The bacteriologic strategy is based on lower respiratory tract samples and is more suited to ventilated patients where there is ready access to the lower respiratory tract. The presence of a new or progressive radiographic infiltrate plus two of three clinical features (fever, leukopenia or leukocytosis, and purulent secretions) yields a sensitivity of 69% with specificity of 75% and represents the most accurate clinical criteria for starting antibiotics.

■ TREATMENT

Treatment strategies seek to balance the need to provide early, appropriate empiric antibiotic therapy with avoidance of excessive antibiotic exposure in both spectrum and duration. Delay in initiating appropriate antibiotics in VAP patients with severe sepsis has been shown to increase mortality, and initial inadequate drug selection, even when later adjusted, is also associated with worse outcome. Aggressive early therapy combined with de-escalation of initial antibiotics based on clinical or microbiologic data is encouraged. Empiric drug selection takes into account the epidemiologic timing and presence of MDR risk factors, previous antibiotic exposure, and the institution-/unit-specific antibiogram.

For early-onset HAP without MDR risk factors, single-agent therapy is reasonable (Table 60-2). For early-onset HAP with MDR risk factors or late-onset HAP, a three-drug regimen is recommended (see Table 60-3). Considerations in antibiotic selection might also include pharmacodynamic properties and mechanism of action. Fluoroquinolones and linezolid achieve high concentration in bronchial secretions. Aminoglycosides and fluoroquinolones are bactericidal in a concentration-dependent fashion, whereas vancomycin and β-lactams are bactericidal in a time-dependent fashion. Aminoglycosides and the quinolones also have a postantibiotic effect and suppress antibiotic growth even after concentrations fall. A number of new antibiotics have become available for treating hospital acquired pneumonia, including doripenem, telvancin, ceftobiprole, and avibactam. The most appropriate use of these alternatives remains to be established. Aerosolized delivery of antibiotics is another mode of treatment that may have benefit for patients who have failed IV therapy or have MDR organisms.

The patient should be reevaluated in 48 to 72 hours, and antibiotics narrowed or discontinued based on culture results and clinical response. Therapy lasting 7 to 8 days has been shown to be equally effective to longer courses in patients receiving an appropriate initial antibiotic regimen with a good clinical response. *Pseudomonas* and MRSA are the exception due to significant rates of recurrence and should still be treated with a longer course of antibiotics.

■ COMPLICATIONS

Patients who fail to respond or worsen should be reevaluated at 48 to 72 hours. Possible reasons for lack of response include the presence of a complication (empyema, lung abscess, drug fever), an alternate site of infection (*Clostridium difficile* colitis, line-related infection), wrong diagnosis (atelectasis, pulmonary embolism (PE), ARDS, pulmonary hemorrhage, neoplasm), or wrong organism (clinically unrecognized immunosuppression).

RESPIRATORY FAILURE

Acute respiratory failure is defined as the requirement for mechanical ventilation longer than 48 hours postoperatively or unplanned reintubation for cardiac or respiratory failure. It can be considered the most severe of the clinically significant postoperative pulmonary complications based on its impact on morbidity, mortality, and cost. Mortality data from the Department of Veterans Affairs National Surgical Quality Improvement Program showed an increase in 30-day mortality from 2.3% to 29.1% in patients with respiratory failure, and an increase in 1-year mortality from 9.3% to 55.9%. Another study found the rate of postoperative respiratory failure in patients undergoing general and vascular surgery to be 3%, with 30-day mortality of 26.5%. Pulmonary complications raised median hospital costs to $62,704 compared to $5015 when the complications were absent, more expensive than thromboembolic, cardiovascular, or infectious complications.

■ PATHOPHYSIOLOGY

Postoperative acute respiratory failure results from the onset over minutes to hours of impaired pulmonary gas exchange severe enough to cause organ dysfunction or to threaten life. Respiratory failure can be broadly categorized as hypoxemic respiratory failure (respiratory insufficiency) or hypercapnic respiratory failure (ventilatory failure), and the two forms may coexist. Mechanisms underlying hypoxemic respiratory failure, defined as an arterial pO_2 of less than 60 mm Hg, include decreased FiO_2, hypoventilation, impaired diffusion, V/Q mismatch, and right-to-left shunt. Most hypoxemic hospitalized patients have some combination of V/Q mismatch and right-to-left shunt. A structural-anatomic classification that localizes the primary pathology to the alveoli, interstitium, cardiopulmonary vasculature, airways, or pleura may be helpful when trying to make a specific diagnosis. In the postoperative patient, the alveoli and interstitium can be affected by pulmonary edema, acute lung injury/ARDS, atelectasis, and pneumonia. The vasculature can be affected by pulmonary embolism or develop pulmonary hypertension due to hypoxic vasoconstriction and/or elevated left atrial pressures. The airways can be affected by exacerbations of COPD, asthma, and mucous plugging, and the pleura may be affected by pneumothorax or pleural effusion.

Hypercapnic respiratory failure, characterized by a pCO_2 greater than 45 mm Hg and respiratory acidosis, can be classified as drive failure or pump failure. Drive failure results when the patient's ventilatory effort is insufficient and can be caused by drug overdoses, general anesthesia, central nervous system (CNS) disease, and obesity hypoventilation syndrome. The most common contributors in the perioperative setting are residual sedation from general anesthesia or the effects of opioid analgesics on respiratory drive and level of consciousness. Pump failure results when ventilatory demand exceeds the patient's capability and can be caused by prolonged effect of neuromuscular blocking agents, underlying neuromuscular disorders, electrolyte abnormalities and metabolic disturbances, pleural disorders, chest wall abnormalities, and respiratory muscle fatigue. It can be aggravated by increased CO_2 production in the setting of a hypermetabolic postoperative state; this is especially true in patients with underlying loss of parenchyma (emphysema) who have a decreased alveolar surface area available for gas exchange.

■ DIAGNOSIS—WHAT IS CAUSING THIS PATIENT'S RESPIRATORY FAILURE?

Diagnostic workup should begin with the ABCs—airway, breathing, and circulation—and treatment initiated concurrently. Supplemental oxygen should be provided and intravenous (IV) access obtained, as well as cardiac monitoring and pulse oximetry. A focused history and physical exam will yield clues to the presence or absence of underlying cardiac and pulmonary disease. The hypoxemic respiratory failure patient will appear tachypneic and tachycardic, perhaps with central cyanosis. The hypercapnic respiratory failure with decreased ventilatory drive will appear hypopnic or apneic, in no respiratory distress. The ventilatory pump failure patient will appear in respiratory distress with rapid shallow ineffective respirations. All patients should receive a chest x-ray, electrocardiogram (ECG), and routine bloodwork including CBC and serum chemistries. An arterial blood gas should be obtained in order to calculate an A—a gradient, establish whether ventilatory failure is present, and determine acid–base status. Further diagnostic workup will be guided by the results of these initial studies. If the etiology is not apparent on initial evaluation, further testing might include CT angiography of the chest and echocardiography.

■ TREATMENT

The goal for management of acute postoperative respiratory failure is to quickly and correctly identify the underlying pathophysiologic process and provide targeted treatment that will avoid the need for intubation and mechanical ventilation. Hypoxemic respiratory failure has a broad differential diagnosis, and initial supportive care should be followed by treatment of the specific disease process identified. Pneumonia or other infection should be treated with prompt initiation of appropriate antibiotics after obtaining cultures. Volume overload and pulmonary edema can be treated with diuretics and additional cardiac evaluation. Bronchospasm should be aggressively treated with inhaled β-agonists and anticholinergics with systemic corticosteroids as indicated. Suspected pulmonary embolism should be expeditiously evaluated and treated as the postoperative conditions allow.

With hypercapnic respiratory failure, the most common cause of insufficient ventilatory drive is medication effect. Opioids are the most potent suppressor of both hypoxic and hypercapnic ventilatory drive, but other sedatives and hypnotics also cause respiratory depression. Unrecognized obstructive sleep apnea may also present as postoperative respiratory depression. CPAP or positive pressure ventilation can be initiated if needed, and precautions can be taken to minimize the use of opioids, patient controlled anesthesia, and sedative hypnotics. Respiratory arrest, inability to protect the airway and severe respiratory acidosis mandate intubation. Noninvasive ventilation (NIV) is an important tool that can be used both to prevent and also to treat postoperative acute respiratory failure. When successful it has been shown to decrease the need for intubation, the rate of complications, and the intensive care unit (ICU) length of stay. NIV is indicated when there is a demonstrated need for ventilatory support and no contraindications (**Table 60-5**). Level 1 evidence

TABLE 60-5 Noninvasive Ventilation—Indications and Contraindications

Indications	Contraindications
Clinical observations	Absolute
• Moderate to severe dyspnea	• Respiratory arrest
• Tachypnea (>24 for hypercapnic, >30 for hypoxemic)	• Unable to fit mask
	Relative
• Accessory muscle use or abdominal paradox	• Medically unstable
Gas exchange	• Unable to protect airway
• Acute ventilatory failure: $PaCO_2 > 45$ mm Hg, pH < 7.35	• Excessive secretions
	• Agitated, uncooperative
• Hypoxemia: $PaO_2/FiO_2 < 200$	• Recent upper gastrointestinal or airway surgery
	• Multiple-organ failure

supports the use of NIV to treat COPD exacerbations, cardiogenic pulmonary edema, and to facilitate weaning from the ventilator in patients with COPD. Level 2 evidence supports its use in postoperative respiratory failure, community-acquired pneumonia with COPD, asthma, extubation failure, and in do-not-intubate-status patients (Table 60-5). Noninvasive ventilation (NIV) should be initiated early when indicated to take advantage of a therapeutic window of opportunity. Improvement is expected over the first one to two hours. If hypoxemia persists, then there may be a concomitant complication such as aspiration or pneumonia. After initial stabilization, a decision should be made regarding appropriate level of care. Determinants of this will include ability to manage the airway, method of oxygen delivery to maintain adequate O_2 status, and the intensity of nursing care required. Intubation should not be delayed in patients who fail an NIV trial.

■ COMPLICATIONS

Complications of postoperative respiratory failure include increased risks related to intubation, ventilator-induced acute lung injury progressing to ARDS, VAP, GI bleeding, and DVT.

COPD EXACERBATION

Patients with COPD have an elevated risk of developing postoperative pulmonary complications, including an exacerbation of obstructive lung disease. Ideally these patients will have had good preoperative risk assessment, with optimization of medical management and initiation of preventive measures such as lung expansion maneuvers and smoking cessation 4 or more weeks prior to the procedure (when applicable). Postoperative management consists of continuing the preventive measures as well as maintenance of home medications. Patients with COPD have a higher prevalence of comorbid conditions such as congestive heart failure and coronary artery disease (CAD), so they must be carefully evaluated should they become short of breath. There is also a high rate of concomitant PE with COPD, up to 20%, so this also needs to be ruled out.

■ PATHOPHYSIOLOGY

A COPD exacerbation is defined as an event in the natural course of the disease characterized by a change in the patient's baseline dyspnea, cough, and/or sputum that is beyond normal day-to-day variations, is acute in onset, and may warrant a change in regular medication. Exacerbations are thought to be an inflammatory event, and the airway manifestations include edema, bronchospasm, and increased sputum production. Exacerbations are heterogeneous events caused by complex interactions between the host, respiratory viruses, airway bacteria, and environmental pollution, but in approximately one-third no cause is identified. Hyperinflation and bronchospasm lead to increased work of breathing. Progressive hypoxemia develops, producing a downward spiral that can progress to acute ventilatory failure when the respiratory muscles fatigue. COPD is associated with other comorbid conditions, including ischemic heart disease (HD), pneumonia, and diabetes mellitus (DM), as well as venous thromboembolism (VTE), and one of these can contribute.

■ DIAGNOSIS—DOES THIS PATIENT HAVE A POSTOPERATIVE EXACERBATION OF COPD?

Typical symptoms include increased breathlessness accompanied by wheezing and chest tightness, increased cough and sputum production, change in color and tenacity of sputum, and fever. Routine evaluation should include chest x-ray, routine labs, arterial blood gas, and ECG to differentiate COPD from other causes given the frequent comorbidities.

■ TREATMENT

Treatment of postoperative COPD exacerbation does not differ from typical treatment, except that other medical complications prevalent in the postoperative period, including PE and congestive heart failure, need to be carefully considered. Lung function can be optimized with inhaled short-acting β-adrenergic and anticholinergic agents along with systemic glucocorticoids. A short course of antibiotics may decrease duration of exacerbation. There is currently no role for methylxanthines or chest physical therapy (PT). NIV is the preferred method of ventilatory support and has been shown to improve outcomes in COPD exacerbations. Invasive mechanical ventilation is reserved for patients who have not responded to NIV.

■ COMPLICATIONS

Complications of COPD exacerbation include pneumonia, progression to acute respiratory failure, and pneumothorax.

POSTACUTE CARE

Postoperative pulmonary complications continue to lurk even beyond hospital discharge. Among Medicare beneficiaries who were rehospitalized within 30 days after a surgical discharge, 70.5% were rehospitalized with a medical condition, and pneumonia was the second most frequent reason after heart failure. Specific risk factors for readmission with pulmonary complications have not been studied, but risk is likely to be reduced by effective care transitions that include adequate patient education on continuing preventive measures at home as well as adequacy of postdischarge follow-up. The I COUGH trial described a multidisciplinary intervention that aimed to decrease the incidence of postoperative pneumonia by standardizing use of a "bundle" of simple postoperative interventions. These included

Incentive spirometry, Coughing and deep breathing, Oral care, Understanding (patient and family education), Getting out of bed, and Head of bed elevation. The intervention resulted in a decrease in the number of cases of pneumonia and also of unplanned intubations, and served to illustrate the benefit of a multidisciplinary effort. Patient and family education were featured prominently in the bundle, and encouragement to continue the intervention post discharge could certainly produce some additional benefit. Hospitalists can also help assure adequate discharge planning for follow-up of medical problems as well as communication with primary care to minimize the risks of readmission.

SUGGESTED READINGS

American Thoracic Society. Guidelines for the management of adults with hospital-acquired, ventilator-associated, and healthcare-associated pneumonia. *Am J Respir Crit Care Med*. 2005;171: 388-416.

Cassidy MR, et al. I COUGH: Reducing postoperative pulmonary complications with a multidisciplinary patient care program. *JAMA Surg*. 2013;148(8):740-745.

Duggan M, Kavanagh BP. Pulmonary atelectasis: a pathogenic perioperative entity. *Anesthesiology*. 2005;102:838-854.

Ferreyra G, Long Y, Ranieri VM. Respiratory complications after major surgery. *Curr Opin Crit Care*. 2009;15:342-348.

Global strategy for the diagnosis, management, and prevention of chronic obstructive pulmonary disease. GOLD Executive Summary. *Am J Respir Crit Care Med*. 2013;187:347-365.

Johnson RG, Arozullah AM, Neumayer L, Henderson WG, Hosokawa P, Khuri SF. Multi-variable predictors of postoperative respiratory failure after general and vascular surgery: results from the patient's safety in surgery study. *J Am Coll Surg*. 2007;204:1188-1198.

Lawrence VA, Cornell JE, Smetana GW. American College of Physicians. Strategies to reduce postoperative pulmonary complications after non-cardiothoracic surgery: systematic review for the American College of Physicians. *Ann Intern Med*. 2006;144:596-608.

Liapikou A, et al. Pharmacotherapy for hospital-acquired pneumonia. *Expert Opin Pharmacother*. 2014;15(6):775-786.

Nava S, Hill N. Non-invasive ventilation in acute respiratory failure. *Lancet*. 2009;374:250-259.

Qaseem A, Snow V, Fitterman N, et al. Clinical Efficacy Assessment Subcommittee of the American College of Physicians. Risk assessment for and strategies to reduce perioperative pulmonary complications for patients undergoing noncardiothoracic surgery: a guideline from the American College of Physicians. *Ann Intern Med*. 2006;144:575-580.

Restrepo RD, Braverman J. Current challenges in the recognition, prevention, and treatment of perioperative pulmonary atelectasis. *Expert Rev Respir Med*. 2015;9(1):97-107.

CHAPTER 61

Assessment and Management of Patients with Renal Disease

Albert Q. Lam, MD

Julian L. Seifter, MD

The kidneys are responsible for several vital homeostatic processes, including the excretion of nitrogenous waste products, the regulation of fluid volume and electrolytes, acid–base balance, and the production of hormones important for blood pressure regulation, erythropoiesis, and bone metabolism. They are frequently affected by disease, both acute (occurring over days to weeks) and chronic (occurring over months to years). Acute kidney injury (AKI), formerly known as acute renal failure, has become an increasingly common cause of hospitalization, with an incidence of 5% to 7% among hospitalized patients. Chronic kidney disease (CKD) reportedly affects 13% of adults in the United States, and is associated with significant morbidity, mortality, and expense. The recent advent of automatic reporting of estimated glomerular filtration rate (eGFR) with serum creatinine by hospital laboratories has resulted in more patients being identified as having impaired renal function. In order to provide the highest level of care for patients presenting with acute or CKD, the clinician should have a strong understanding of the fundamental issues relevant to their evaluation and management.

EVALUATION OF THE RENAL PATIENT

■ HISTORY AND PHYSICAL EXAMINATION

The evaluation of the patient with kidney disease begins with a thorough history and physical examination. The clinician should identify whether the renal disease is acute or chronic. If the patient's previous medical records are available, this can be determined by quickly reviewing prior laboratory testing, with particular attention given to serum creatinine, blood urea nitrogen, and urinalyses. Patients who present with AKI should be questioned about recent symptoms (eg, vomiting, diarrhea, edema, difficulty voiding, decreased appetite, weight changes) and events (eg, changes in oral intake, new medications, nonsteroidal anti-inflammatory drug [NSAID] use, intravenous contrast administration, recent colonoscopy) that may help narrow the differential diagnosis of AKI. Symptoms such as fever, rashes, arthralgias, epistaxis, and hemoptysis suggest an underlying inflammatory condition such as vasculitis. For patients who develop AKI during their hospitalization, recent hospital events—including episodes of hypotension, recent diagnostic and therapeutic procedures, and initiation of new medications—should be reviewed. All patients presenting with AKI or CKD should be questioned about symptoms associated with uremia, including fatigue, nausea, vomiting, pruritus, metallic taste, lethargy, and confusion, since these symptoms may indicate the need for dialysis.

Patients should be asked whether they have a prior history of kidney disease or other relevant systemic diseases, such as diabetes and hypertension. In patients with CKD, who may or may not be presenting with an acute kidney-related problem, the clinician should establish the chronicity, severity, and cause of the underlying kidney disease. In patients with end-stage renal disease (ESRD), information about the patient's nephrologist, outpatient dialysis unit, and regular dialysis schedule (including the timing of the last dialysis session) should be obtained and conveyed to the clinicians and other health care providers who will be facilitating the patient's dialysis during the hospitalization. The clinician should also obtain a complete and current list of the patient's medications, including prescription medications as well as all over-the-counter medications, herbal remedies, and supplements. A family history of kidney disease or other systemic illnesses should also be documented.

The physical examination starts with a review of the patient's vital signs. While fever should always raise suspicion for an infection, particularly in dialysis patients or immunosuppressed patients, it can also be observed in the setting of acute glomerulonephritis, vasculitis, and allergic interstitial nephritis. Blood pressure may be elevated (eg, in acute nephritic syndrome, malignant hypertension, scleroderma, long-standing kidney disease), normal, or low (eg, in volume depletion, sepsis, cirrhosis, heart failure). Fluid intake and output should be reviewed to help determine volume status and the need for fluid repletion, diuresis, or dialysis.

Key aspects of the exam include the bedside determination of volume status and a search for physical signs associated with specific kidney diseases and uremia. Assessment of volume status is essential for the diagnosis and management of most renal diseases. In prerenal acute kidney injury, the presence of hypervolemia (eg, elevated jugular venous pressure, pulmonary congestion, peripheral edema) suggests decreased renal perfusion from congestive heart failure or cirrhosis, whereas hypovolemia (postural pulse increase >30 beats/min, severe postural dizziness, dry axilla or mucous membranes) would be more consistent with volume depletion from bleeding or gastrointestinal losses. To best assess the jugular venous pulsation, the patient should be reclined with the head elevated at 30° to 45°, and the elevation of the right internal jugular vein above the sternal angle should be measured. Certain physical findings are associated with specific renal diseases (**Table 61-1**). Palpable purpura may be observed in vasculitic processes such as

TABLE 61-1 History and Physical Examination Findings in Renal Disease

Renal Disease	History	Physical Exam Findings
Prerenal acute kidney injury	• Volume depletion (hemorrhage, vomiting, diarrhea, diuretics, burns) • Heart failure • Cirrhosis • Medications (NSAIDs, ACE inhibitors/ARBs, cyclosporine, tacrolimus) • Radiocontrast exposure	• Orthostatic hypotension, dry mucous membranes and axillae • Elevated JVP, +S3, lung rales, edema (heart failure) • Jaundice, ascites, edema (cirrhosis)
Intrarenal acute kidney injury Glomerular	• Gross hematuria or cola-colored urine • Cough and hemoptysis (Goodpasture syndrome) • Epistaxis, sinusitis, hemoptysis, arthralgias, (Wegener, Churg-Strauss) • Rash, arthralgias (systemic lupus erythematosus)	• Fever, palpable purpura, arthritis (vasculitis) • Saddle-nose deformity (Wegener) • Oral ulcers, rash, arthritis, pericardial rub (SLE)
Interstitial	• Recent respiratory infection (postinfectious glomerulonephritis, IgA nephropathy) • Fever, arthralgias, rash	
ATN	• Medications (NSAIDs, antibiotics) • Episode of hypotension	• Fever, skin rash
Vascular	• Medications (aminoglycosides, amphotericin B, cisplatin) • Trauma, muscle necrosis (rhabdomyolysis) • History of multiple myeloma • History of atherosclerosis • Recent vascular intervention • Anticoagulation • Flank pain (renal vein thrombosis)	• Hypotension • Warm (early sepsis) or cold extremities (late sepsis) • Elevated BP • Livedo reticularis, ischemic extremities
Postrenal acute kidney injury	• Urinary urgency, hesitancy, oliguria or anuria • Gross hematuria • Flank pain, renal colic • History of nephrolithiasis • Medications (acyclovir, indinavir, anticholinergics)	• Distended bladder • Enlarged prostate • Palpable abdominal or pelvic masses
Nephrotic syndrome	• Weight gain • Foamy urine • Medications (NSAIDs, gold, penicillamine)	• Anasarca, ascites, edema
Uremia	• Fatigue, lethargy, confusion, seizures • Anorexia, nausea, vomiting • Pruritus, metallic taste, bleeding	• Asterixis • Pericardial or pleural friction rub • Half-and-half nails • Dry and atrophic skin, pallor, hyperpigmentation, ecchymoses, uremic frost

ACE, angiotensin-converting enzyme; ARB, angiotensin receptor blocker; BP, blood pressure; JVP, jugular venous pressure; NSAID, nonsteroidal anti-inflammatory drug; SLE, systemic lupus erythematosus.

granulomatosis with polyangiitis (formerly known as Wegener's granulomatosis), microscopic polyangiitis, Churg-Strauss syndrome, or Henoch-Schönlein purpura. Abdominal bruits with refractory hypertension and progressive renal failure are suggestive of renovascular disease. Funduscopic examination can reveal arteriolar narrowing, hemorrhages, exudates, or papilledema—findings consistent with chronic hypertension.

PRACTICE POINT

Key aspects of the physical examination include:
- Determination of the patient's volume status;
- Identification of physical manifestations that suggest specific renal disease conditions;
- Search for signs of uremia.

The physical findings of uremia are highly variable. Uremic pericarditis or pleuritis may be present, as manifested by a pericardial or pleural friction rub, respectively. The pericardial friction rub classically has three components, one systolic and two diastolic, and a scratchy or grating quality. Skin and nail changes may include uremic frost (the fine residue of excreted urea on the surface of the skin), skin hyperpigmentation, or half-and-half nails (sharp demarcation between proximal and distal nail halves). Patients with fluid retention may have pulmonary congestion or peripheral edema. Neurological findings include confusion, coma, asterixis, and sensory deficits. The presence of these physical findings, especially the pericardial friction rub and neurological abnormalities, may indicate the need for dialysis.

■ LABORATORY TESTS

Serum electrolytes

Serum electrolytes are essential to the evaluation of the patient with acute and chronic renal disease. Both hyponatremia and hypernatremia may be seen in patients with kidney disease. Impaired renal function decreases renal potassium excretion, and may lead to potentially life-threatening hyperkalemia in oliguric or anuric patients. The serum potassium concentration may not be an accurate indicator of total body potassium stores, since most of the total body potassium is confined to the intracellular fluid compartment. For example, in diabetic ketoacidosis, patients frequently have elevated serum potassium levels despite diminished total body potassium stores. Serum chloride and bicarbonate levels are useful in the assessment of volume and acid–base status. The serum anion gap, used in the assessment of metabolic acidosis, can be calculated from serum sodium, chloride, and bicarbonate concentrations ($AG = Na^+ - [Cl^- + HCO_3^-]$). Serum calcium, phosphorus, and magnesium levels yield important information about renal tubular function and bone mineral metabolism. Hyperphosphatemia and hypocalcemia are common in patients with acute and chronic renal disease, and contribute to the development of secondary hyperparathyroidism.

Blood urea nitrogen and creatinine

Blood urea nitrogen (BUN) and creatinine are nitrogenous end products of metabolism that rise in the setting of renal disease. Urea is formed from ammonia derived from protein breakdown, while creatinine is a byproduct of muscle creatine metabolism. Urea and creatinine are freely filtered by the kidneys but handled differently in the tubular system. Urea is partly reabsorbed in the proximal tubule and inner medullary collecting duct, while creatinine is secreted to a small extent by the tubules. Despite these confounding effects of tubular handling, BUN and creatinine are still the most commonly used biomarkers of renal function. Neither test is ideal for the

early detection of renal disease. Elevated serum BUN is sometimes attributable to nonrenal factors, such as high-protein intake, upper gastrointestinal tract bleeding, and high catabolism states, such as fever, corticosteroids, and burns. Serum creatinine may also be affected by many factors, including muscle mass and medications that impair tubular creatinine secretion, such as trimethoprim and cimetidine. Though BUN and creatinine are the traditional primary biomarkers of renal injury, their use may decrease in the future in favor of more sensitive and specific biomarkers, including neutrophil gelatinase-associated lipocalin (NGAL), kidney injury molecule-1 (KIM-1), and cystatin C.

Estimated glomerular filtration rate

All patients with kidney disease, both acute and chronic, should have their kidney function assessed by estimation of the glomerular filtration rate (GFR). GFR may be estimated by measuring serum creatinine, calculating the creatinine clearance, or using estimation equations such as the Cockcroft-Gault formula, the Modification of Diet in Renal Disease (MDRD) equation, or the CKD-EPI (Chronic Kidney Disease Epidemiology Collaboration) equation. The normal GFR in a healthy adult is >90 mL/min. GFR decreases with age, at a rate of approximately 1 mL/min/y after age 35. Elderly patients may also have lower-creatinine levels due to decreased muscle mass. Measurement of serum creatinine is the most frequently used surrogate for GFR. As serum creatinine concentrations are affected by muscle mass, dietary protein intake, and certain medications, it is not the most accurate method of estimating GFR. The Cockcroft-Gault, MDRD, and CKD-EPI equations take into account serum creatinine, as well as other defined factors such as age, race, gender, and weight. They were designed to estimate GFR in patients with established CKD, and are most useful for this purpose. While the performance of these equations has been evaluated in a variety of different racial and ethnic populations with and without kidney disease, they should still be interpreted with caution in specific patient populations that have yet to be well validated, including individuals with normal or near-normal renal function, children, and elderly individuals. The CKD-EPI equation may be superior to the MDRD equation in estimating GFR in patients with normal or mildly impaired (GFR >60 mL/min/1.73 m²) renal function. Serum creatinine and the estimation equations should only be used to approximate GFR in patients with *stable* kidney function (unchanging serum creatinine). If the clinician is uncertain about the accuracy of GFR estimation, a 24-hour urine collection can be performed to calculate creatinine clearance.

PRACTICE POINT

Laboratory testing

- Serum creatinine and the estimation equations should only be used to approximate GFR in patients with stable kidney function (unchanging serum creatinine).
- The examination of the urinary sediment by microscopy can provide useful diagnostic information about both acute and chronic kidney disease.
  - Urine particles lyse easily after collection, and therefore urine samples should be examined within 2 to 4 hours of acquisition.
  - The pathognomonic finding of ATN on urinary sediment is the presence of coarse muddy brown granular casts, which represent extensive renal tubular epithelial cell injury.
- In acute kidney injury, a fractional excretion of sodium (FENa) in combination with clinical history and other lab tests may help differentiate between prerenal etiologies and acute tubular necrosis (ATN).

> - While a FENa of <1% in the setting of AKI is generally thought to indicate prerenal azotemia, it can also be seen in contrast-induced nephropathy, rhabdomyolysis, acute glomerulonephritis, hepatorenal syndrome, early urinary obstruction, acute interstitial nephritis, and even ATN.
> - A FENa may be difficult to interpret in the setting of diuretic therapy.
> - If the patient has a nonanion gap metabolic acidosis, the urine anion gap (UAG) may help differentiate between gastrointestinal losses of bicarbonate (eg, diarrhea) and renal tubular acidosis. It is calculated as follows: (urine Na$^+$ + urine K$^+$) – urine Cl$^-$.

Proteinuria

Proteinuria, a hallmark of kidney damage, is most frequently detected qualitatively by urine dipstick, which grades proteinuria on a scale of concentration: trace, 1+ (30 mg/dL), 2+ (100 mg/dL), 3+ (300 mg/dL). Normal urine may test slightly positive if very concentrated. The urine dipstick is only capable of detecting urinary albumin, which is the most abundant protein seen with glomerular proteinuria. The presence of other proteins, such as immunoglobulin light chains, will not be detected by dipstick alone. Proteinuria by dipstick should prompt a more accurate quantification. This is done either by measuring the urine protein and urine creatinine concentrations in a random urine sample to determine the urine protein-to-creatinine ratio, or by a 24-hour urine collection for protein and creatinine excretion rate.

Hematuria

In the absence of gross bleeding, hematuria is most commonly discovered on a urine dipstick (which detects the pseudoperoxidase activity of hemoglobin) or urinalysis. False-positive dipstick results are seen in the setting of hemoglobinuria, myoglobinuria, menstrual blood in the urine, vigorous exercise, and concentrated urine. If significant proteinuria or renal dysfunction is also present, the kidney should be considered the source of hematuria until proven otherwise, and a renal biopsy should be considered to establish a diagnosis. Microscopic hematuria in the absence of proteinuria and renal dysfunction is known as *isolated hematuria*.

The differential diagnosis of isolated microscopic hematuria can be divided into renal (glomerular) or extrarenal (nonglomerular) processes. Immunoglobulin A (IgA) nephropathy, thin basement membrane disease, and Alport syndrome are three of the more common causes of glomerular hematuria. Common etiologies of nonglomerular hematuria include urinary tract infections, kidney stones, urinary tract tumors, trauma, bladder polyps, polycystic kidney disease, medullary cystic disease, and metabolic abnormalities such as hypercalciuria and hyperuricosuria. Hematuria associated with exercise, especially running, is usually a benign condition in which the blood source is likely the renal pelvis.

Hematuria from the glomerulus may or may not be associated with flank pain, while ureteral conditions that obstruct the urinary tract and cause bleeding can produce severe pain and renal colic. Other causes of hematuria are usually painless. In extrarenal hematuria, the red blood cells typically appear normal on urinary sediment, round and uniform, whereas in glomerular hematuria, the red blood cells may appear dysmorphic due to distortion from the passage through the glomerular filtration barrier. Imaging studies are indicated to search for structural causes of hematuria. Detection of persistent extrarenal hematuria should prompt further workup and urologic consultation to identify the source of bleeding. In older individuals, bladder cancer should be considered. In isolated glomerular hematuria, a renal biopsy is not typically indicated, since the pathologic diagnosis rarely has any effect on the management or outcome.

Abnormal urinalysis

The examination of the urinary sediment by microscopy can provide useful diagnostic information about both acute and CKD. Urine particles lyse easily after collection, and therefore urine samples should be examined within 2 to 4 hours of acquisition. White blood cells (pyuria), when greater than 2 per high-power field, can be observed with upper or lower-urinary tract infections, contamination from genital secretions, or renal inflammation, as in interstitial nephritis or acute glomerulonephritis.

Urinary casts are cylindrical aggregates of protein and/or cells that form in the lumen of the distal convoluted tubule or collecting duct. Hyaline casts, the most common type of cast, are acellular and consist primarily of Tamm-Horsfall mucoprotein produced by tubular epithelial cells. They can be seen in the setting of dehydration or vigorous exercise in normal patients who produce concentrated urine, but can be seen in patients with proteinuria. Granular casts, the second most common type of cast, are usually formed from degenerating cellular casts or protein-containing lysosomes, and can appear fine or coarse in texture. Muddy brown granular casts contain degenerating tubular epithelial cells, and are commonly seen in acute tubular injury. Fatty casts are hyaline casts that contain lipid droplets and can be observed in patients with diseases causing lipiduria, such as nephrotic syndrome. The approach to hematuria is described above. When red blood cells leak through the glomerular filtration barrier, they can form red blood cell casts in the tubular lumen, a finding that is consistent with acute glomerulonephritis. White blood cell casts indicate renal inflammation or infection, and can be seen in acute glomerulonephritis, interstitial nephritis, and acute pyelonephritis. Red blood cell casts and white blood cell casts are always pathologic, and should prompt further evaluation of the patient for the clinical entities already mentioned.

Urine chemistries

Measurements of urinary sodium, potassium, chloride, and creatinine can be useful in the evaluation of a number of renal conditions. In acute kidney injury, the fractional excretion of sodium (FENa), combined with clinical history and other lab tests, may help differentiate between prerenal etiologies and acute tubular necrosis (ATN). The FENa can be calculated by the following formula: (urine Na$^+$ × plasma creatinine)/(plasma Na$^+$ × urine creatinine) × 100. A FENa < 1% is commonly seen in prerenal causes of oliguria, and a FENa > 2% is usually indicative of ATN. However, a FENa < % 1 can also be seen in contrast-induced nephropathy, rhabdomyolysis, acute glomerulonephritis, hepatorenal syndrome, early urinary obstruction, acute interstitial nephritis, and even ATN. Furthermore, a FENa may be difficult to interpret in the setting of a patient taking diuretics. In such cases, calculating the fractional excretion of urea (FEUrea) may help to differentiate prerenal AKI (FEUrea < 35%) from ATN (FEUrea 50%-65%).

In nonanion gap metabolic acidosis, one can calculate a urine anion gap (UAG) to help differentiate between gastrointestinal losses of bicarbonate (eg, diarrhea) and renal tubular acidosis using the following formula: (urine Na$^+$ + urine K$^+$) – urine Cl$^-$. A negative UAG is consistent with gastrointestinal losses, whereas a positive UAG is frequently seen with renal tubular acidosis.

Serum enzymes

Serum enzyme levels should be interpreted cautiously in patients with impaired renal function. Cardiac enzymes, including cardiac troponin T (cTnT), cardiac troponin I (cTnI), and the muscle/brain (MB) isoenzyme of creatine kinase (CK-MB), are often elevated in acute or chronic kidney disease, even in the absence of acute myocardial injury. A large percentage of false-positive elevations in cTnT and CK-MB are seen in patients with ESRD when these markers are used to diagnose acute myocardial infarction (MI). The use of cTnI is less likely to be associated with false-positive elevations. Serial measurements of cTnI are currently the most specific marker of myocardial damage in patients with renal failure and suspected acute MI.

Liver and pancreatic enzymes can also be affected in patients with renal failure. Serum aminotransferase levels are frequently found to be in the lower range of normal values in patients with CKD and ESRD. In the absence of liver disease, gammaglutamyl transpeptidase (GGT) levels are most often normal, but may be elevated in a small percentage of patients. Serum alkaline phosphatase levels are often elevated in dialysis patients, usually from coexisting bone disease. An isolated elevation in serum alkaline phosphatase may not correlate well with hepatobiliary disease in ESRD patients; however, if a chronically elevated alkaline phosphatase level is accompanied by an elevation in serum GGT or 5′-nucleotidase, one should be more suspicious of an obstructive or infiltrative hepatobiliary process.

Serum levels of both amylase and lipase can be elevated in patients with CKD and ESRD, even when acute pancreatitis is not present. The levels of these enzymes in ESRD patients are commonly threefold to fivefold higher than baseline, but are typically less than three times the upper limit of normal. The elevations are due primarily to decreased renal clearance, though in the case of serum lipase, the use of heparin during hemodialysis has also been found to contribute to elevated levels.

■ IMAGING STUDIES

Ultrasonography

Ultrasonography is a safe, noninvasive, rapid, and inexpensive diagnostic imaging modality used to study the kidneys. Ultrasonography requires neither ionizing radiation nor a potentially toxic intravenous contrast agent, which makes it a safe initial imaging study, especially for patients with known renal insufficiency. Renal ultrasonography can provide valuable information about kidney size, shape, and gross appearance. Normal adult kidneys are approximately 9 to 13 cm (4-5 in) in length and 5 to 7.5 cm (2-3 in) wide, and should not differ by much more than 1 cm. With chronic injury, the renal parenchyma is replaced with fibrotic tissue and the renal cortex becomes thinner, causing diseased kidneys to shrink. In patients with kidney disease of uncertain duration, the finding of smaller kidneys on ultrasonography suggests longstanding renal disease. Enlarged kidneys may be seen in autosomal dominant polycystic kidney disease, urinary tract obstruction, HIV nephropathy, early diabetic nephropathy, and infiltrative diseases such as amyloidosis or myeloma. Asymmetric kidneys may indicate unilateral kidney disease, and the clinician must determine whether the smaller or larger kidney is abnormal. Increased renal echogenicity is common and nonspecific finding, usually denoting medical renal disease. Renal ultrasonography can also identify the presence of renal cysts, stones, or masses. In patients presenting with acute kidney injury, renal ultrasonography can identify obstructive uropathy, which usually manifests as hydronephrosis, although false-negative results can be seen in patients with early obstruction (<3-4 days), volume depletion, or obstruction due to retroperitoneal fibrosis or compression by retroperitoneal or intraparenchymal tumor or blood.

Doppler ultrasonography

Doppler ultrasonography can provide information about the presence and flow of blood through the vessels of the kidney. High-velocity or disorganized flow patterns can be seen in patients with hemodynamically significant renal artery stenosis. Elevated vascular resistive indices (>0.80) in a stenotic kidney are suggestive of severe parenchymal disease and a low likelihood of response to revascularization. Given the enhanced toxicities of iodinated contrast agents or gadolinium in renal disease, Doppler ultrasonography has become widely used as the initial imaging study to evaluate renal artery stenosis. The sensitivity of Doppler ultrasonography is highly operator dependent, and can be affected by patient anatomy.

Computed tomography

In the evaluation of the patient with suspected renal colic, noncontrast helical CT scanning is currently the gold standard for diagnosing nephrolithiasis and can detect essentially all kidney stones, with the exception of indinavir stones. Noncontrast CT can also detect ureteric obstruction in acute kidney injury, which is particularly helpful when intravenous (IV) contrast should be avoided due to nephrotoxicity.

The drawback to the use of iodinated contrast agents is potential nephrotoxicity, especially in patients with preexisting renal impairment, diabetes, heart failure, or hypovolemia (see below). In patients with ESRD who have residual renal function, administration of contrast dye can induce further tubular damage and lead to loss of the remaining renal function. As preservation of residual renal function in patients with ESRD has been shown to correlate with improved survival even after the initiation of dialysis, the use of contrast in these patients should be avoided if possible. When the risk of nephrotoxicity is not prohibitive, IV iodinated contrast is useful for imaging of the renal parenchyma, facilitating the evaluation and detection of renal mass lesions such as renal cell carcinoma. CT angiography can be used to diagnose suspected renal artery stenosis or aneurysms. CT urography allows imaging of the collecting system and can identify filling defects such as stones, blood clots, and tumors.

Magnetic resonance imaging

The primary role of renal magnetic resonance imaging (MRI) is the evaluation of renal masses. MRI can effectively differentiate benign versus malignant lesions in the kidney, especially when CT scanning with intravenous iodinated contrast is contraindicated or if ultrasonographic and CT scans are nondiagnostic. MR angiography (MRA), which involves the administration of intravenous gadolinium, has become the modality of choice in the evaluation of renovascular disease. According to one meta-analysis, gadolinium-enhanced MRA had a reported sensitivity of 97% and specificity of 85% for the detection of renal artery stenosis. However, the use of gadolinium-based contrast agents in moderate to severe CKD has been associated with the development of nephrogenic systemic fibrosis (NSF), with debilitating fibrosis of the skin, joints, eyes, and other internal organs. Patients with an estimated GFR <30 mL/min or requiring dialysis should not be given gadolinium-based contrast agents. In these patients, Doppler ultrasonography is a safer alternative.

Radionuclide scans

Radionuclide studies may be used to obtain functional information about the kidneys. Static radionuclide scans employ a radiolabeled tracer (eg, technetium 99m-DMSA) that binds to renal parenchymal cells, but is not excreted into the tubules. These studies are useful in quantifying the functional cortical tissue of each kidney and determining the percentage contribution of each kidney to total renal function. Dynamic radionuclide scans use tracers (eg, technetium 99m-DTPA, technetium 99m-MAG3) that are taken up by nephrons and then excreted into the collecting system. A diuretic such as furosemide is often administered just prior to injection of the tracer to ensure high levels of diuresis during the study. Dynamic scans can be used to evaluate potential renal tract obstructions as well as the response to treatment of the obstruction.

ACUTE KIDNEY INJURY

Acute kidney injury (AKI), formerly termed acute renal failure, is a sudden and sustained decline in renal function with the failure to excrete metabolic waste, maintain fluid and electrolyte balance, and regulate acid–base homeostasis. AKI is an increasingly common cause of hospitalization, with 1% of all patients reported to have AKI upon admission to the hospital and 2% to 5% of inpatients subsequently developing AKI during their hospitalization. In spite of advances in intensive care and dialysis support over the last 50 years, the overall mortality rate of AKI remains high, ranging from 20% to 90% depending on illness severity and medical setting. The role of the hospitalist is to diagnose common causes of AKI, to identify and treat reversible factors, to recognize when dialysis is required, and to know when to consult a nephrologist.

Two classification systems, the RIFLE and AKIN criteria, have defined and stratified AKI by stages of severity based on graded increases in serum creatinine and periods of decreased urine output (**Table 61-2**). The more recent AKIN criteria have proposed a definition for AKI that incorporates the prognostic significance associated with small changes in serum creatinine. The diagnosis of AKI can be established by (1) an abrupt (within 48 hours) absolute increase in serum creatinine of ≥0.3 mg/dL from baseline, (2) a percentage increase in serum creatinine of ≥50%, or (3) oliguria of ≤0.5 mL/kg/h for > 6 hours. Although both the RIFLE and AKIN classification systems have been validated in a variety of clinical settings, their utility at this time appears to be greater for research use than for the bedside.

AKI can be divided into three diagnostic categories based on the anatomic location of injury: prerenal, intrarenal, and postrenal (**Table 61-3**). It can be further subdivided into oliguric (urine output < 400 mL/d) and nonoliguric (urine output > 400 mL/d), with patients producing less than 100 mL urine/d considered to be anuric. These distinctions are important, given that epidemiological studies have found that oliguria in the setting of AKI is an independent predictor of mortality. Oliguric AKI is more characteristic of prerenal etiologies and urinary obstruction, while nonoliguric AKI is commonly seen in intrarenal AKI. Anuria is uncommon and is usually associated with complete urinary tract obstruction, bilateral renal infarction, renal vein thrombosis, cortical necrosis, or high-grade ischemic acute tubular necrosis.

■ PRERENAL

Prerenal AKI is defined as a reduction in GFR caused by hypoperfusion of the kidney. In most cases of prerenal AKI, the kidneys are morphologically normal. Prerenal AKI can be divided into conditions that cause volume depletion and conditions that induce renal vasoconstriction. True volume depletion may result from hemorrhage or gastrointestinal, urinary, or cutaneous fluid losses. Effective volume depletion refers to decreased effective circulating volume in the setting of normovolemia or hypervolemia, and can result from marked vasodilatation as seen in the setting of sepsis, heart failure, cirrhosis, and third-spacing. Renal vasoconstriction is most often caused by medications, including angiotensin-converting enzyme (ACE) inhibitors, angiotensin receptor blockers (ARBs), NSAIDs, intravenous iodinated contrast agents, and the immunosuppressant drugs cyclosporine and tacrolimus.

Patients with prerenal AKI usually present with an elevated BUN and creatinine, and the ratio of BUN to creatinine is classically greater than 20:1. Urinalysis often reveals an elevated specific gravity without significant hematuria or proteinuria. The urinary sediment is typically bland but may show hyaline casts. The kidneys, in an appropriate response to the reduction in renal perfusion, maximize sodium and water reabsorption. Urine sodium is typically low, and the FENa and urea are <1% and <35%, respectively. Patients with prerenal AKI often respond favorably to volume resuscitation and discontinuation of any offending therapeutic agents.

Intrarenal

In all cases of intrarenal AKI, the primary abnormality is within the kidney. Intrarenal AKI can be subdivided into four anatomic categories: glomerular disease, interstitial disease, tubular disease, and vascular disease. As in prerenal AKI, patients generally present with an elevated BUN and creatinine, though the ratio is usually normal (<20:1). The FENa may be variable and cannot reliably distinguish between the different causes of intrarenal AKI. The urinalysis is frequently abnormal, and findings on the urinary sediment can provide clues to the location of the kidney injury. In some patients, the clinical presentation and laboratory evaluation are insufficient to establish a diagnosis, and a percutaneous renal biopsy may be indicated to better guide management.

The most common cause of intrarenal AKI is ATN, which is responsible for most cases of AKI in hospitalized patients. ATN may be caused by either ischemic or nephrotoxic injury. Ischemic ATN is often associated with periods of prolonged hypotension and markedly reduced renal perfusion, which can be seen in the setting of heart failure, sepsis, or cardiac surgery. Nephrotoxic ATN can be caused by either endogenous (eg, heme pigments) or exogenous toxins (eg, aminoglycoside antibiotics, amphotericin B, cisplatin, and iodinated contrast agents). While many patients typically experience an oliguric phase (onset within 24 hours of the renal insult and duration of 1-3 weeks) followed by a diuretic phase (increase in urine output that is indicative of renal recovery), some patients remain nonoliguric throughout. The pathognomonic finding on urinary sediment is the presence of coarse muddy brown granular casts, which represent extensive renal tubular epithelial cell injury. Due to impaired tubular sodium reabsorption, the urine sodium is >40 mEq/L and the FENa is usually >2%. Both ischemic and

TABLE 61-2 Definitions and Classification Systems for Acute Kidney Injury

RIFLE Stages	AKIN Stages	RIFLE Increase in Serum Creatinine	AKIN Increase in Serum Creatinine	RIFLE and AKIN Urine Output
Risk (R)	1	≥150%-200%	≥0.3 mg/dL or ≥150%-200%	<0.5 mL/kg/h × >6 h
Injury (I)	2	>200%-300%	>200%-300%	<0.5 mL/kg/h × >12 h
Failure (F)	3	>300%	>300% or acute renal replacement therapy	<0.3 mL/kg/h × ≥24 h
Loss (L)	Complete loss of kidney function for >4 wk			
End-stage kidney disease (E)	Need for renal replacement therapy for >3 mo			

AKIN, Acute Kidney Injury Network; RIFLE, Risk-Injury-Failure-Loss-ESRD.

TABLE 61-3 Etiologies of Acute Kidney Injury

Prerenal	Postrenal
Volume depletion	Prostatic hypertrophy
• True volume depletion	Obstruction
■ GI losses (vomiting, diarrhea)	• Bladder outlet obstruction
■ Renal losses (diuretics, osmotic diuresis)	• Stones
■ Skin losses (burns, sweating)	• Crystals (acyclovir, indinavir)
• Effective volume depletion	• Tumors
■ Congestive heart failure	• Clots
■ Cirrhosis	• Retroperitoneal fibrosis
■ Nephrotic syndrome	
Vasoconstriction	
• NSAIDs	
• ACE inhibitors/ARBs	
• Iodinated contrast agents	
• Cyclosporine and tacrolimus	
Hepatorenal syndrome	
Hypotension	

Intrarenal	
Glomerular	• Nephrotoxic acute tubular necrosis
• Acute glomerulonephritis	■ Aminoglycoside antibiotics
■ ANCA-associated vasculitis (granulomatosis with angiitis, microscopic polyangiitis, Churg-Strauss syndrome)	■ Amphotericin B
	■ Cast nephropathy (myeloma kidney)
	■ Cisplatin
■ Anti-GBM disease (Goodpasture syndrome)	■ Iodinated contrast agents
■ Immune complex disease (lupus nephritis, poststreptococcal glomerulonephritis, cryoglobulinemia, IgA nephropathy)	■ Pigment nephropathy (hemoglobin, myoglobin)
	Vascular
Interstitial	• Large vessel
• Drug-induced (NSAIDs, penicillin analogues and cephalosporins, rifampin, sulfa drugs)	■ Bilateral renal artery stenosis
	■ Renal vein thrombosis
• Autoimmune (SLE, Sjögren syndrome)	■ Renal thromboembolism
• Infections (legionella, leptospirosis, cytomegalovirus, streptococci)	• Small vessel
	■ Thrombotic microangiopathies (HUS, TTP)
Tubular	■ Cholesterol atheroembolism
• Ischemic acute tubular necrosis	■ Malignant hypertension
■ Hypotension	■ Scleroderma renal crisis
■ Sepsis	

ACE, angiotensin-converting enzyme; GI, gastrointestinal; HUS, hemolytic uremic syndrome; NSAID, nonsteroidal anti-inflammatory drug; RB, angiotensin receptor blocker; SLE, systemic lupus erythematosus; TTP, thrombotic thrombocytopenic purpura.

nephrotoxic ATN resolve in most cases, but dialysis is sometimes required when renal injury is severe. A recently reported cause of renal injury is the use of sodium phosphate salts for bowel cleansing prior to colonoscopy, with phosphate precipitation in the kidney in volume-depleted patients or those with CKD.

The glomerular type of AKI involves acute inflammation of the glomeruli or glomerular vessels. Acute glomerulonephritis can be either renal-limited or associated with systemic illnesses such as infections, such as poststreptococcal glomerulonephritis, autoimmune disorders such as systemic lupus erythematosus, or vasculitides such as granulomatosis with angiitis. The urinalysis is always abnormal and classically reveals evidence of damage to the glomerular filtration barrier, with proteinuria, dysmorphic red blood cells, and red blood cell casts. Urine sodium and FENa may be low. The workup of acute glomerulonephritis should include serologic

tests such as complement levels, antistreptococcal antibodies, antibodies against hepatitis B and C, antinuclear antibodies, antineutrophil cytoplasmic antibodies, antiglomerular basement membrane antibodies, and cryoglobulins. Definitive diagnosis usually requires a renal biopsy.

Acute interstitial nephritis (AIN) is defined as inflammation of the renal interstitium that results in AKI. AIN is most often caused by medications, such as antibiotics, NSAIDs, anticonvulsants, and proton pump inhibitors, but can also be associated with infections and autoimmune diseases. Classic symptoms include fever, rash, and arthralgias. However, the classic triad of fever, maculopapular erythematous rash, and eosinophilia is observed in only 10% of cases of AIN. Laboratory testing may reveal a FENa >1%, but this is not always reliable. Urinalysis may show mild proteinuria (<1 g/d), and the urinary sediment may reveal red blood cells, white blood cells, and white blood cell casts. Occasionally, urine eosinophils are observed with a Wright or Hansen stain, but this finding is neither highly sensitive nor specific for the diagnosis of AIN and can be seen in other inflammatory conditions. Definitive diagnosis can be established with a renal biopsy. Treatment of AIN is primarily the identification and cessation of the offending agent.

AKI can also be caused by acute vascular disease affecting either the large or the small renal blood vessels. Large-vessel diseases involve the renal arteries and veins and include bilateral renal artery stenosis, renal thromboembolism, renal artery dissection, and renal vein thrombosis. As a general rule, large-vessel disease must be bilateral in order to cause AKI, with the exception of unilateral disease in the patient with a solitary kidney. Patients may present with symptoms of renal infarction, complaining of acute flank pain and hematuria. Small-vessel diseases that can cause AKI include malignant hypertension, scleroderma renal crisis, and cholesterol atheroembolic disease. Patients with cholesterol atheroembolic disease often have a history of recent aortic instrumentation or surgical intervention or anticoagulation. Physical exam may reveal livedo reticularis on the skin overlying the lower extremities, toe or foot discoloration, or Hollenhorst plaques in the retina. The urinalysis in vascular AKI typically shows microscopic hematuria with or without proteinuria. Eosinophilia, eosinophiluria, and hypocomplementemia can also be seen in cholesterol atheroembolic disease. Imaging (eg, CT, MRI, or radionuclide studies) is often required to confirm the diagnosis of large-vessel disease.

Postrenal

In all patients presenting with AKI, urinary tract obstruction must be ruled out early, since timely intervention often improves or fully restores renal function. Obstruction to the flow of urine commonly occurs at the level of the prostate, particularly in adult men, but can occur at any location along the urinary tract. Upper urinary tract obstruction (ie, at the level of the ureters or renal pelvis) must be bilateral in order to cause AKI; the sole exception is unilateral obstruction in the patient with a solitary kidney. Common causes of postrenal AKI include hypertrophy or cancer of the prostate, obstructing kidney stones, urothelial tumors, and retroperitoneal fibrosis or malignancies. Patients with bilateral obstruction may present with oliguria (partial obstruction), polyuria (a sign of associated nephrogenic diabetes insipidus), or anuria (complete obstruction), and may report symptoms of flank pain, abdominal pain, renal colic, or hematuria. Ultrasonographic imaging usually reveals hydronephrosis, though this may be absent in retroperitoneal or infiltrative diseases that encase the ureters or kidneys. CT and dynamic radionuclide studies can also be used to diagnose urinary obstruction. Treatment of postrenal AKI focuses on relief of the obstruction.

■ MANAGEMENT STRATEGIES

General principles

Management of AKI should be focused on treating and reversing the specific cause of injury. Patients with prerenal AKI, for example, should be given volume resuscitation to restore euvolemia. In postrenal AKI due to urinary obstruction, relief of the obstruction can improve and in many cases fully restore renal function. Currently, there are no effective pharmacologic therapies for the treatment of AKI, and treatment focuses more on supportive management. Basic principles of management in AKI include:

1. **Optimization of volume status and hemodynamic parameters.** Daily weights and intake and output should be monitored closely. Medications that can compromise renal perfusion, including ACE inhibitors, ARBs, NSAIDs, and calcineurin inhibitors, should be discontinued. Patients who are hypovolemic should be given volume accordingly, with either crystalloids, colloids, or blood products. With few exceptions, such as the setting of cirrhosis, the use of colloids has not been proven to be more beneficial than crystalloids in AKI. Vasopressors or inotropes should be considered in patients who remain hypotensive despite volume resuscitation. In patients who are hypervolemic, the role of diuretics in the treatment of AKI is controversial. Although loop diuretics may be useful to treat volume overload in an oliguric patient, conversion of oliguric to nonoliguric AKI with diuretics has not been shown to improve survival or shorten the time to renal recovery. At high doses, loop diuretics may also lead to ototoxicity. Therefore, these medications should be used judiciously in patients with AKI.

2. **Close monitoring and management of renal function, acid–base status, and serum electrolytes.** Serum BUN, creatinine, and electrolytes should be monitored daily. If hyperkalemia is present, medical treatment should be initiated, such as intravenous calcium gluconate, insulin, inhaled albuterol, and sodium polystyrene sulfonate (kayexalate). Specific treatment depends on the severity, urine output, and ECG abnormalities; dialysis may be necessary if electrocardiographic abnormalities are present. Potassium intake via diet, medications, and intravenous fluids should also be eliminated. Hyperphosphatemia can be treated with oral phosphorus binders such as calcium acetate, calcium carbonate, sevelamer hydrochloride, and sevelamer carbonate. Aluminum hydroxide is highly effective at lowering phosphorus levels in severe cases, but its use should be limited to no more than 1 to 2 weeks due to the potential for aluminum toxicity. If acidemia is present, patients can be treated with intravenous fluids containing sodium bicarbonate.

3. **Appropriate adjustment of medication dosing.** All medications should be dosed to reflect the level of renal impairment, based on estimated GFR, or the need for dialysis (**Table 61-4**). Since eGFR can only be calculated when the serum creatinine is stable, a GFR of <10 should be assumed for patients whose serum creatinine is acutely increasing. Narcotics may accumulate in patients with renal impairment and should be used with great caution.

4. **Avoidance of nephrotoxins.** Medications that are nephrotoxic, such as NSAIDs and aminoglycosides, should not be given to patients with AKI. ACE inhibitors or ARBs taken on a chronic basis for hypertension or cardiovascular disease should be stopped until renal function has recovered. Intravenous iodinated contrast agents and gadolinium-containing agents should be avoided.

5. **Management of uremic bleeding.** Patients with severe AKI and uremia may develop bleeding diatheses due to uremic platelet dysfunction. This can be treated with synthetic arginine vasopressin analogues (eg, intravenous DDAVP 0.3 mcg/kg × 1-2 doses). Hemodialysis is the definitive treatment, and should be performed in cases of severe bleeding.

6. **Nutritional support.** Malnutrition is highly prevalent in patients with AKI. It is associated with higher risks of in-hospital mortality, nosocomial complications, and prolonged hospitalization. Appropriate nutritional is thus essential to the management of AKI, and consultation with an experienced dietitian may be beneficial. Hyperkalemia and hyperphosphatemia are common in patients with AKI, and a diet that is low in potassium and phosphorus should be instituted. Critically ill patients with AKI are in a highly catabolic state and at high risk for severe protein energy wasting. Nutritional

TABLE 61-4 Dosing Adjustments for Commonly Prescribed Medications in Patients with Impaired Renal Function

Drug	Usual Dose	GFR > 50 mL/min/1.73 m²	GFR 10-50 mL/min/1.73 m²	GFR < 10 mL/min/1.73 m²
Acyclovir (oral)	200-800 mg every 4-12 h	100%	100%	200 mg every 12 h
Allopurinol	300 mg daily	75%	50%	25%
Ampicillin/ sulbactam (Unasyn)	1.5-3 g IV every 6-8 h	100%	1.5-3 g IV every 12 h (GFR 15-29)	1.5-3g IV every 24 h (GFR 5-14)
Cefazolin (Ancef)	500 mg-1.5 g every 8 h	100%	Every 12 h	50% every 24-48 h
Ceftazidime (Fortaz)	1-2 g every 8-12 h	100%	Every 12-24 h	Every 24-48 h
Ceftriaxone (Rocephin)	1-2 g every 24 h	No adjustment needed		
Ciprofloxacin	400 mg IV or 500-750 mg orally every 12 h	100%	50%-75%	50%
Enoxaparin (Lovenox)	Prophylaxis: 30 mg SC every 12 h	Usual dosage	30 mg SC daily (GFR < 30)	
	DVT treatment: 1 mg/kg SC every 12 h or 1.5 mg/kg SC once daily		1 mg/kg SC every 24 h (GFR < 30)	
Fluconazole (Diflucan)	200-400 mg every 24 h	100%	50%	50%
Gabapentin (Neurontin)	300-600 mg three times daily	Usual dosage	400-1400 mg/d (divided twice daily) (GFR 30-59)	100-300 mg daily
			200-700 mg/d (GFR 15-29)	Not recommended
Levetiracetam (Keppra)	500-1500 mg every 12 h	Usual dosage	250-750 mg every 12 h (GFR 30-50)	
			250-500 mg every 12 h (GFR < 30)	
			Hemodialysis: 500-1000 mg every 24 h, supplemental dose of 250-500 mg recommended after dialysis	
Levofloxacin (Levaquin)	250-750 mg orally/IV daily	Usage dosage	500 mg initial dose, then 250 mg every 24 h	500 mg initial dose, then 250 mg every 48 h
Metformin (Glucophage)	500-1000 mg twice daily	Contraindicated in men with serum creatinine >1.5 mg/dL and women with serum creatinine >1.4 mg/dL or patients with GFR <60		
		Should be temporarily discontinued 24-48 h prior to administration of any radiocontrast agents and not restarted for 48 h afterward due to the risk of developing lactic acidosis		
Metoclopramide (Reglan)	10-15 mg three to four times daily	Usual dosage	50%	25%
Piperacillin/ Tazobactam (Zosyn)	3.375 g IV every 6-8 h	100%	2.25 g IV every 6 h (GFR 20-40)	2.25 g IV every 8 h
			2.25 g IV every 8 h (GFR < 20)	
Simvastatin (Zocor)	10-80 mg daily	Usual dosage	Usual dosage	Start at 5 mg daily
Vancomycin	1 g IV every 12 h	1 g IV every 12 h	Start with 1 g IV every 12 h (GFR 40-60)	
			Start with 1g IV every 24 h (GFR < 40)	
			Determine dose by serum level monitoring	

DVT, deep vein thrombosis; GFR, glomerular filtration rate; IV, intravenous; SC, subcutaneous.

support, parenteral or enteral, is frequently required in order to ensure adequate delivery of protein and energy, prevent further metabolic derangements and complications, improve wound healing, bolster the immune system, and decrease mortality.

It should be noted that, in spite of the available treatment modalities and advances in dialysis technology, mortality in patients with AKI remains high, with a rate of approximately 50% to 80% in critically ill patients.

When to consult a nephrologist

There are a number of common clinical scenarios that are considered nephrologic emergencies, and immediate evaluation by a nephrologist should be requested.

PRACTICE POINT

Indications for emergent nephrology consultation include:
- Volume overload in an oliguric or anuric patient
- Hyperkalemia with serum potassium >5.5 to 6 mEq/L and/or associated with changes on the electrocardiogram and other electrolyte abnormalities, especially in an oligoanuric patient
- Toxic overdoses that can be treated with hemodialysis, including ethylene glycol, methanol, and lithium
- Symptomatic or severe hyponatremia
- Hypertensive crises
- Rapidly progressive glomerulonephritis
- Microangiopathic hemolytic anemias, including thrombotic thrombocytopenic purpura and hemolytic uremic syndrome

Indications for renal biopsy

Percutaneous renal biopsy can be instrumental to the diagnosis of AKI. This procedure is typically performed under ultrasonographic guidance with local anesthesia, although CT-guided biopsy is an alternative in morbidly obese patients. In the setting of AKI, a renal biopsy may be most helpful either when the diagnosis of acute glomerulonephritis is suspected or when the cause of renal failure is unknown. Other common indications for performing a renal biopsy include unexplained glomerular hematuria, significant proteinuria, and nephrotic syndrome. Absolute contraindications to percutaneous renal biopsy include uncontrolled moderate to severe hypertension, uncontrolled bleeding diathesis or severe anemia, an uncooperative patient, and a solitary functional kidney. Relative contraindications include anatomic abnormalities of the kidney that may increase the risk of the procedure, skin infection overlying the biopsy site, active renal or perinephric infection, hydronephrosis, and the presence of multiple renal cysts or a renal tumor. The most common complication following percutaneous renal biopsy is bleeding, which usually occurs within 12 to 24 hours postbiopsy. Other complications include pain, gross hematuria, and infection.

Chronic warfarin anticoagulation is not a contraindication to renal biopsy. However, the need and urgency for biopsy must be weighed against the risk of thrombosis if anticoagulation is stopped. In patients chronically taking aspirin or other antithrombotic agents, these medications should be held as soon as it is known that a biopsy will be performed (ideally 1-2 weeks prior to the procedure) and should not be resumed until 1 to 2 weeks after the procedure. Heparin should be stopped at least 6 hours prior to the biopsy, and held for at least 12 to 24 hours postbiopsy.

Indications for dialysis

Dialysis is initiated to prevent and treat the life-threatening complications and uremic symptoms associated with severe AKI. Generally accepted indications to start dialysis in the setting of AKI include (1) severe metabolic acidosis; (2) hyperkalemia, especially if electrocardiographic abnormalities are present; (3) volume overload refractory to the use of diuretics; and (4) uremic signs and symptoms, such as pericarditis, altered mental status, or seizures. The optimal timing of dialysis initiation has not been well established. Although a few retrospective and nonrandomized trials have found that earlier initiation of dialysis may improve survival, these results have yet to be tested in a large prospective randomized clinical trial.

■ SPECIFIC SYNDROMES

Postoperative renal failure

Postoperative AKI resulting in oliguria and an elevated serum creatinine is one of the most common and serious complications of surgery, representing 18% to 47% of all cases of hospital-acquired AKI. It is associated with a higher risk for serious infections and sepsis, greater costs of hospitalization, and increased mortality following both cardiac and noncardiac surgery. Up to 30% of patients undergoing cardiovascular and thoracic surgeries develop postoperative AKI, and up to 7% of these patients need renal replacement therapy. Furthermore, postoperative AKI that requires dialysis carries an in-hospital mortality rate of 60% to 80%.

The most common cause of postoperative AKI is ischemic ATN resulting from decreased renal perfusion during surgery. Common surgical scenarios for the development of ATN include supra- or infrarenal aortic cross-clamping in vascular surgery and cardiopulmonary bypass during cardiac surgery. Risk factors for the development of postoperative AKI include preexisting renal dysfunction, diabetes mellitus, advanced age (>65), major vascular surgery, cardiopulmonary bypass times greater than 3 hours, and recent exposure to nephrotoxic agents including contrast dyes, NSAIDs, and

aminoglycosides. Patients may present postoperatively with either an acute elevation in serum creatinine or reduced urine output.

A number of principles can guide the evaluation and management of postoperative AKI:

1. **Identification of inciting factors.** Perioperative records and flowsheets should be thoroughly reviewed for evidence of hypotension, significant intraoperative or postoperative fluid losses (eg, blood and intravascular fluid losses, insensible losses, drainage losses, and third-spaced fluid losses), and the administration of potentially nephrotoxic agents (eg, NSAIDs for pain control or hydroxyethyl starches used for volume resuscitation).

2. **Hemodynamic monitoring.** Patients should have close perioperative hemodynamic monitoring, and if necessary, invasive monitoring with intra-arterial, central venous, or pulmonary arterial catheters.

3. **Maintenance of adequate renal perfusion.** Though no optimal mean arterial pressure (MAP) has been established to ensure adequate renal perfusion, maintaining a MAP of at least >65 mm Hg and preferably >75 to 80 mm Hg is recommended.

4. **Optimization of volume status.** Intravenous fluid hydration should be administered to optimize renal perfusion in patients with volume depletion or hemodynamic instability. Patients who develop oliguria are often hypovolemic and should be given a fluid challenge. If they respond favorably with an improvement in urine output or hemodynamic parameters, more fluid challenges can be attempted.

5. **Avoidance of nephrotoxic agents.** Concomitant use of nephrotoxic medications is a risk factor for the development of postoperative AKI. If iodinated contrast agents must be used for diagnostic or therapeutic purposes, the smallest amount of nonionic iso-osmolar volume of contrast should be used. Other drugs such as NSAIDs, aminoglycosides, and amphotericin B should be avoided if possible. Patients who take ACE inhibitors or ARBs on a chronic basis should discontinue these medications prior to surgery, since chronic ACE inhibition reportedly increases the risk of postoperative AKI.

6. **Pharmacologic agents.** Several agents, including dopamine, fenoldapam, atrial natriuretic peptide, mannitol, calcium-channel blockers, and loop diuretics, have been tested for their ability to prevent postoperative AKI. The results of these studies are inconclusive, and there is insufficient evidence to recommend their use at this time.

Hepatorenal syndrome

Hepatorenal syndrome (HRS) is a functional form of AKI that occurs primarily in patients with cirrhosis and ascites. The pathophysiology of HRS is thought to be due to nitric oxide–induced vasodilation of the splanchnic circulation, leading to marked intrarenal arterial vasoconstriction and a reduction in GFR. There are two types of HRS: type 1 HRS is the rapidly progressive form of the disease characterized by a doubling of the initial serum creatinine level to greater than 2.5 mg/dL over a period of less than 2 weeks. The prognosis of patients with type 1 HRS without liver transplantation is generally very poor. Type 2 HRS is a more moderate form of renal failure characterized by serum creatinine levels between 1.5 and 2.5 mg/dL and associated with a more indolent course and improved survival compared to type 1 HRS. Both type 1 and type 2 HRS can occur spontaneously or develop after a precipitating event, most commonly a bacterial infection such as spontaneous bacterial peritonitis (SBP). Diagnostic criteria for HRS were recently revised by the International Ascites Club (IAC) in 2015, taking into account newer definitions of AKI, and now include the following: (1) cirrhosis with ascites; (2) increase in serum creatinine of ≥0.3 mg/dL within 48 hours, or

≥50% increase in serum creatinine from baseline, known or presumed to have occurred within the past 7 days; (3) no response after two consecutive days with diuretic withdrawal and volume expansion with albumin 1 g/kg body weight; (4) absence of shock; (5) no current or recent treatment with nephrotoxic drugs; and (6) no macroscopic signs of structural kidney injury (proteinuria >500 mg/d, microhematuria with >50 red blood cells per high-power field, and/or abnormal renal ultrasonography). With proper medical treatment, HRS is potentially reversible. Type 1 HRS can be treated with vasoconstrictors (eg, terlipressin, midodrine in combination with octreotide, norepinephrine) combined with albumin. Transjugular intrahepatic portal shunt (TIPS) may be considered in patients with type 1 HRS with either partial response (decrease in serum creatinine to ≥0.3 mg/dL above the baseline value) or no response (no regression in AKI) to medication. There is currently no definitive evidence demonstrating a benefit to using vasoconstrictors in patients with type 2 HRS. In patients being treated for SBP, prophylaxis with albumin is indicated, as this has been shown in one randomized clinical trial to lower the incidence of HRS by 66%, with significant reductions in 30-day mortality rates. The suggested dose of albumin is 1.5 mg/kg body weight on the first day, followed by 1 mg/kg body weight on the third day. Liver transplantation remains the treatment of choice for both type 1 and type 2 HRS.

Contrast-induced nephropathy

Contrast-induced nephropathy is one of the most common causes of AKI in the hospital setting, with incidence rates ranging from <5% to >30%. Contrast-induced AKI is commonly defined as an increase in serum creatinine (either an absolute increase of 0.5 mg/dL or a 25% increase from baseline) within the first 24 hours after contrast exposure. The mechanism of injury involves renal vasoconstriction, impaired vasodilation, medullary hypoxia, and direct tubular cell damage. Preexisting renal impairment (eGFR < 60 mL/min) and diabetes mellitus are the most important risk factors for contrast-induced AKI, though heart failure, hypovolemia, nephrotoxic drugs, and hemodynamic instability are also significant risk factors.

A number of preventive strategies have been studied in patients at risk for contrast-induced AKI:

1. **Type of contrast agent.** The choice of contrast agent is important, since higher-osmolar agents are associated with greater nephrotoxicity. In high-risk patients, nonionic iso-osmolar (eg, iodixanol) and low-osmolar (eg, iohexol, ioversol, iopamidol) contrast agents have been shown to have lower nephrotoxicity.

2. **Volume expansion.** Intravenous hydration is clearly beneficial in the prevention of contrast-induced AKI, though the optimal hydration fluid has yet to be determined. The current evidence indicates that isotonic fluids (either normal saline or sodium bicarbonate) are more protective than half-normal saline. Although initial clinical trials showed a benefit to using sodium bicarbonate over normal saline, more recent evidence has not confirmed these findings. The rate and timing of hydration are also unclear. If using normal saline, one possible regimen is 1 mL/kg for 6 to 12 hours before the procedure, followed by 1 mL/kg for 6 to 12 hours after the procedure. Alternatively, if using isotonic sodium bicarbonate (three 50 mL ampules each containing 50 mEq of sodium bicarbonate in 850 mL of 5% dextrose in water), one possible regimen is a bolus of 3 mL/kg for 1 hour prior to the procedure, followed by an infusion of 1 mL/kg for 6 hours after the procedure.

3. **N-Acetylcysteine.** Though frequently used in the prevention of contrast-induced AKI, N-acetylcysteine has had inconsistent results in most clinical studies and meta-analyses. While some trials have reported significant protection, others have shown less substantial or even insignificant benefits. Given its relatively benign side effect profile and low cost, however, N-acetylcysteine is still often recommended as an adjunctive agent to IV hydration. In at-risk patients, it can be administered as 600 or 1200 mg orally twice daily on the day before and the day of the procedure.

4. **Diuretics.** The use of diuretics, particularly mannitol and furosemide, has not shown any benefit and may actually be harmful to patients.

5. **Hemodialysis/hemofiltration.** Although iodinated contrast agents are removable by dialysis, there is currently no definitive evidence to suggest that prophylactic hemodialysis or hemofiltration reduces the incidence of contrast-induced AKI.

Drug toxicity

Therapeutic agents frequently cause AKI in the hospital setting. The clinician should suspect drug toxicity when there is an acute rise in serum creatinine associated with the recent administration of a drug. As with AKI, drug nephrotoxicity can be divided into prerenal, intrarenal, and postrenal mechanisms. The most common mechanisms involve direct renal tubular injury resulting in ATN or renal interstitial inflammation leading to AIN. Other forms of injury include tubular obstruction due to drug precipitation, alterations in intrarenal blood flow, and, less commonly, glomerular disease. Drugs that are commonly associated with nephrotoxicity and their primary mechanisms of toxicity are listed in **Table 61-5**.

TABLE 61-5 Nephrotoxic Drugs in Acute Kidney Injury

Nephrotoxicity	Drugs
Prerenal	ACE inhibitors
	Angiotensin receptor blockers
	Cyclosporine
	IL-2
	Iodinated contrast agents
	NSAIDs
	Tacrolimus
Intrarenal	NSAIDs
• Acute interstitial nephritis	Penicillin analogues (nafcillin, oxacillin)
	Cephalosporins
	Sulfa drugs (sulfamethoxazole, thiazide diuretics)
	Rifampin
	Ciprofloxacin
	Proton-pump inhibitors
	Aminoglycoside antibiotics
	Amphotericin B
• Acute tubular necrosis	Cisplatin
	Iodinated contrast agents
	HIV medications (adefovir, ritonavir, tenofovir)
Postrenal	Acyclovir
	Analgesics
	Indinavir
	Methotrexate

ACE, angiotensin-converting enzyme; HIV, human immunodeficiency virus; IL, interleukin; NSAID, nonsteroidal anti-inflammatory drug.

Drug-induced ATN is seen with the administration of medications that are excreted primarily by the kidneys, including aminoglycoside antibiotics, amphotericin B, and cisplatin. Aminoglycosides, commonly prescribed for the treatment of Gram-negative bacterial infections, cause dose-dependent ATN with a frequency ranging from 10% to 20%. Neomycin causes the greatest nephrotoxicity; gentamicin, tobramycin, and amikacin cause intermediate nephrotoxicity; and streptomycin causes the least nephrotoxicity. It should be recognized that aminoglycoside toxicity may follow oral administration of neomycin in cirrhotics, joint lavage after orthopedic procedures, and skin applications in burn patients. ATN typically develops 5 to 10 days after initiation of aminoglycoside treatment, and is generally nonoliguric. The kidney injury is usually reversible with withdrawal of the drug, but renal replacement therapy may be necessary in some cases.

AIN accounts for 3% to 15% of all drug-induced AKI. The most common offending agents include NSAIDs, penicillins, cephalosporins, sulfonamides, rifampin, ciprofloxacin, and proton-pump inhibitors. While the onset of drug-induced AIN has been reported as early as a few days after a secondary exposure to a medication, it usually occurs 7 to 14 days and as late as weeks to months after a primary exposure. AIN is typically reversible with withdrawal of the drug, though renal recovery may take weeks to months. Treatment of AIN with steroids has an unclear benefit, though some case series suggest that a short course of prednisone (1 mg/kg/d for up to 4 weeks) may increase the rate of recovery.

Drug-induced urinary obstruction generally results from the precipitation of drugs within the renal tubules or ureters. Crystal-induced AKI and nephrolithiasis may occur with acyclovir and indinavir. Certain analgesics containing aspirin, phenacetin, and caffeine may cause renal papillary necrosis, and with sloughing of the necrotic tissue that may lead to acute ureteral obstruction. Patients with drug-induced urinary obstruction may present with symptoms of renal colic and acute urinary tract obstruction. Management involves hydration, pain control, and discontinuation of the medication, although invasive removal of the stones may be required in severe cases.

A number of medications are known to modulate renal hemodynamics and cause a prerenal type of AKI. When renal perfusion is decreased, regulation of GFR involves vasodilation of the afferent arteriole and vasoconstriction of the efferent arteriole. Drugs that inhibit these compensatory mechanisms further impair renal perfusion and lead to AKI. These agents include NSAIDs, ACE inhibitors, ARBs, cyclosporine, tacrolimus, and iodinated contrast agents. NSAIDs inhibit the production of prostaglandins, which mediate afferent arteriolar vasodilation. In patients with normal renal function, this effect is largely inconsequential, but in those whose baseline renal perfusion is already impaired (eg, patients with heart failure or volume depletion), it can significantly reduce intrarenal blood flow and renal function. In contrast, ACE inhibitors and ARBs selectively block angiotensin II-mediated vasoconstriction of the efferent arteriole. An increase in serum creatinine of up to 30% is acceptable with ACE inhibitors and ARBs, given the proven long-term renal protective effects of these medications, but more significant loss of renal function may be observed in patients with decreased renal perfusion or renovascular disease. Cyclosporine and tacrolimus, calcineurin inhibitors widely used as immunosuppressants, cause intense afferent and efferent arteriolar vasoconstriction. Most patients taking these medications experience a reduction in GFR within weeks to months of starting therapy. As this effect is generally reversible and thought to be dose related, cyclosporine-, or tacrolimus-induced AKI can usually be managed with dose reduction.

Chemotherapy-induced nephrotoxicity

Several agents used to treat cancer are toxic to the kidneys and may cause AKI. Intravascular volume depletion, simultaneous administration of other nephrotoxic drugs or iodinated contrast agents, urinary tract obstruction, and underlying renal disease increase the risk of chemotherapy-induced nephrotoxicity. **Cisplatin** can cause dose-related acute tubular necrosis and significant hypomagnesemia due to renal magnesium wasting. AKI may be reversible, though the repeated administration of cisplatin may lead to chronic and irreversible kidney damage. Aggressive hydration with intravenous fluids, particularly isotonic normal saline, can increase urine volume and flow and reduce the risk of cisplatin toxicity. Newer-generation platinum compounds such as carboplatin and oxaliplatin are generally less nephrotoxic, but may also cause acute tubular injury.

Methotrexate is not nephrotoxic at low doses (<0.5-1.0 g/m²) but may have nephrotoxicity at higher doses (1-15 g/m²). Methotrexate may precipitate in the tubules, causing direct tubular injury and urinary obstruction. Prophylaxis with intravenous fluid administration and urinary alkalinization reduces the potential for toxicity. Dosing must be adjusted in patients with preexisting renal impairment.

Alkylating agents such as **cyclophosphamide** and **ifosfamide** are known to cause hemorrhagic cystitis and hyponatremia. Ifosfamide is more nephrotoxic than cyclophosphamide, and can cause significant proximal tubular dysfunction, leading to a Fanconi-like syndrome with renal tubular acidosis and hypophosphatemia, and as well as distal nephron toxicity resulting in nephrogenic diabetes insipidus. **Interleukin-2**, often used to treat renal cell carcinoma and metastatic melanoma, can cause reversible AKI by inducing a capillary leak syndrome that leads to interstitial edema and volume depletion. Treatment is focused on restoring intravascular volume and stabilizing hemodynamic parameters. **Table 61-6** lists several chemotherapeutic agents that commonly cause nephrotoxicity.

Cardiorenal syndrome

Cardiorenal syndrome (CRS) describes a set of acute or chronic conditions involving the heart and the kidney in which dysfunction of one organ leads to dysfunction of the other. Though it was previously thought that primary cardiac disease gave rise to renal dysfunction, evidence now suggests that renal impairment can also lead to cardiac dysfunction. A recently proposed classification system divides CRS into five subtypes: (1) type 1 CRS (acute worsening of cardiac function leads to acute kidney injury), (2) type 2 CRS (chronic abnormalities in cardiac function lead to CKD), (3) type 3 CRS (acute worsening of renal function causes acute cardiac dysfunction), (4) type 4 CRS (CKD contributes to decreased cardiac function, ventricular hypertrophy, diastolic dysfunction, and increased risk of adverse cardiovascular events), and (5) type 5 CRS (a systemic condition causes both cardiac and renal dysfunction). Type 1 CRS,

TABLE 61-6 Chemotherapeutic Agents and Mechanisms of Toxicity

Chemotherapeutic Agent	Mechanism of Toxicity
Alkylating agents	
• Cisplatin, carboplatin, oxaliplatin	Tubular injury, renal magnesium wasting
• Cyclophosphamide	Hemorrhagic cystitis, hyponatremia
• Ifosfamide	Proximal tubular dysfunction
Antimetabolites	
• Methotrexate	• Crystal-induced tubular injury with high-dose treatment
Biological response modifiers	
• Interleukin-2	• Capillary leak syndrome and volume depletion

which is a common occurrence, is most relevant to the discussion of AKI. Patients with type 1 CRS present with acute heart failure that leads to the development of AKI, due to a reduction in renal perfusion. AKI tends to be more severe in patients with acute heart failure with systolic dysfunction compared to those with diastolic dysfunction. The early diagnosis of type 1 CRS is difficult, since at the time when an elevation in serum creatinine is detected, kidney injury has already occurred, and little can be done therapeutically. Often, patients with type 1 CRS develop a decreased responsiveness to diuretic therapy, and the use of higher doses or combinations of diuretics can worsen the AKI. Patients with volume overload who are refractory to diuretics may need fluid removal through ultrafiltration.

Potent vasodilating medications used in heart disease, such as hydralazine and calcium channel blockers, may manifest as edema, decreased urinary salt and water excretion, azotemia, and diuretic resistance. This syndrome occurs primarily in the patient with CKD or renovascular disease and can be thought of as a renal "steal" syndrome. Many drugs used in a cardiac setting are excreted by the kidney and may reach toxic systemic levels in renal disease. These include digoxin, procainamide, and morphine. Blood pressure reduction may have paradoxical effects on cardiac and renal function. For many reasons, management of patients with CRS is challenging, and involvement of a multidisciplinary team consisting of nephrologists, cardiologists, critical care physicians, and cardiac surgeons is recommended.

Rapidly progressive glomerulonephritis

Rapidly progressive glomerulonephritis (RPGN) is characterized by the acute onset of glomerular inflammation and progressive loss of renal function over a short period of time (days to weeks to months). Crescent formation within injured glomeruli is one of the pathologic hallmarks of this disease process. Patients may present with hypertension, azotemia, oliguria, proteinuria, and edema. The urinary sediment is typically active, with dysmorphic red blood cells and red blood cell casts. RPGN is classified into three categories based on the cellular mechanism and immunofluorescence pattern: type 1 (anti-GBM disease, linear pattern of IgG staining), type 2 (immune complex disease, granular pattern of IgG staining), and type 3 (pauci-immune disease, little or no immunofluorescent staining). Serological tests (eg, anti-GBM antibody, antineutrophil cytoplasmic antibodies [ANCAs], antinuclear antibody [ANA], complement levels) should be ordered, though definitive diagnosis frequently requires renal biopsy. The diagnosis of RPGN should be considered a nephrologic emergency, and a nephrology consultation should be requested immediately to assist with renal biopsy and initiate appropriate treatment.

CHRONIC KIDNEY DISEASE

CKD affects approximately 13% of all adults in the United States. The Kidney Disease Outcomes Quality Initiative (K/DOQI) program defines CKD in adults as either (1) evidence of structural or functional kidney abnormalities, such as albuminuria, abnormal urinalyses, abnormal renal imaging, with or without decreased glomerular filtration rate (GFR); or (2) decreased GFR persisting for more than 3 months. The National Kidney Foundation has stratified CKD into five stages of severity (**Table 61-7**). CKD and ESRD are associated with significant complications, including anemia, hypertension, bone disease, and acid–base and electrolyte disturbances, all of which are frequently encountered in the hospital setting.

■ GENERAL INPATIENT MANAGEMENT

The management of a hospitalized patient with CKD or ESRD should be guided by a number of important general principles. First, the patient's nephrologist and dialysis unit, if applicable, should be

TABLE 61-7 Staging of Chronic Kidney Disease

Stage	Description	GFR (mL/min/1.73 m²)
1	Kidney damage with normal or ↑ GFR	≥90
2	Kidney damage with mild ↓ GFR	60-89
3	Moderate ↓ GFR	30-59
4	Severe ↓ GFR	15-30
5	Kidney failure	<15 or dialysis

GFR, glomerular filtration rate.

contacted upon admission and discharge. This promotes communication and facilitates continuity of care, often providing the hospitalist with the most current patient information, including patient history, medication regimen, vascular access history, and baseline parameters such as blood pressure and estimated dry weight. Second, admission orders should take into account the special needs of patients with CKD and ESRD. Vital signs should include regular blood pressure measurements, daily weights, and accurate measurements of intake and output. Unnecessary phlebotomy should be avoided, particularly in patients with anemia, and routine blood tests in dialysis patients can often be drawn at their dialysis sessions just prior to initiation. Third, all measures should be taken to protect the vascular access of ESRD patients who are receiving hemodialysis. Blood pressures and blood draws should be performed in the arm contralateral to the one with the vascular access. If blood must be drawn from the ipsilateral arm, it should be taken from the most distal vein possible, preferably from the dorsum of the hand. Given their increased risk of infection, hemodialysis catheters should be reserved for dialysis use only, and under no circumstances with the exception of life-threatening emergencies should a dialysis catheter be accessed for other purposes.

Patients with CKD frequently have altered drug metabolism due to changes in glomerular flow and filtration, tubular reabsorption and secretion, and renal bioactivation and metabolism. In addition, other factors such as drug absorption, bioavailability, distribution volume, and protein binding may also be altered and can influence the handling of medications. Inappropriate dosing can result in either drug toxicity or ineffectiveness. On hospital admission, the complete medication list should be carefully reviewed, and particular attention should be given to medications that produce long-lasting active metabolites in the setting of reduced renal clearance. All medications, especially those that are initiated during the hospitalization, should be appropriately dosed according to a patient's reduction in GFR.

Nutrition is a vital part of the care of the hospitalized CKD patient. If available in the hospital, a registered renal dietitian can be of tremendous value in providing dietary recommendations during the hospitalization as well as in counseling patients on healthy eating habits following discharge. According to the K/DOQI guidelines, patients with CKD stages 1 to 4 should be on a low-sodium (<2000 mg/d) diet, and potassium and phosphorus intake should be adjusted according to lab values. Provided that urine output is normal, there is no restriction on the amount of fluid in these patients' diets. Patients with ESRD should be placed on a diet that is low in potassium (2000–3000 mg/d), low in phosphorus (800-1000 mg/d), and low in sodium (<2000 mg/d). Fluid intake should be limited to 1.5 to 2 liters daily to prevent large increases in interdialytic weight gain. Certain water-soluble vitamins are lost during hemodialysis and can be replaced with a daily multivitamin such as Diatx ZN (Pamlab, LLC), Dialyvite 3000 (Hillestad Pharmaceuticals),

Nephplex Rx (Nephro-Tech, Inc.), Nephrocaps (Fleming Company), and Nephro-Vite Rx (Watson).

Hypertension

An estimated 50% to 75% of patients with a GFR <60 mL/min/1.73 m² (CKD stages 3-5) have hypertension, and as renal function declines, hypertension becomes increasingly prevalent. Given the higher risk of cardiovascular morbidity and mortality associated with hypertension and CKD, the National Kidney Foundation Clinical Practice Guidelines for Hypertension recommend that in all patients with hypertension and CKD, blood pressure should be targeted to a systolic value of <130 mm Hg and a diastolic value of <80 mm Hg to decrease the risk of cardiovascular events and delay the progression of CKD. ACE inhibitors and ARBs should be considered as first-line therapy for hypertension in CKD, given their antiproteinuric effects and long-term renoprotective effects. Diuretics, particularly loop diuretics, can be particularly useful in optimizing blood pressure. Loop diuretic doses should be titrated upward as tolerated until normalization of blood pressure is achieved or the patient develops symptoms or signs of overly aggressive diuresis (eg, lightheadedness, hypotension, rising BUN and creatinine). The effectiveness of thiazide diuretics decreases in patients with a GFR <30 mL/min; however, these medications can be used synergistically with loop diuretics to improve diuresis in patients with refractory edema. Patients with ESRD on hemodialysis should have their morning doses of blood pressure medications held on dialysis days to prevent intradialytic hypotension and facilitate volume removal during dialysis.

Anemia

Normocytic, normochromic anemia is a common complication of CKD and ESRD. It is primarily due to a deficiency in erythropoietin production by the kidneys, though other contributing factors may include iron deficiency, shortened red blood cell survival, uremic inhibitors of erythropoiesis, hemolysis, bleeding, loss of blood in hemodialysis circuits, and repeated blood draws. Anemia becomes more common as GFR decreases to <60 mL/min/1.73 m². Treatment of anemia in CKD patients improves quality of life and decreases mortality. The K/DOQI guidelines recommend that the hemoglobin target in dialysis and nondialysis patients with CKD is generally in the range of 11.0 to 12.0 g/dL. Treatment with an erythropoiesis-stimulating agent such as erythropoietin or darbepoietin alfa reduces the need for frequent blood transfusions and is recommended in anemic CKD patients. In nondialysis patients, levels above this target should be avoided, due to recent evidence demonstrating that these levels are associated with adverse cardiovascular outcomes. Therefore, the hemoglobin target in dialysis and nondialysis patients with CKD should not be >13.0 g/dL.

To ensure that anemic patients will respond to treatment with erythropoietin or darbepoietin, iron stores should be monitored regularly via the serum ferritin concentration, serum iron concentration, and total iron binding capacity. Iron deficiency in patients with CKD is defined as transferrin saturation (TSAT) <20% or serum ferritin <100 ng/mL. Patients who meet either of these criteria should be given iron supplementation, either orally (eg, ferrous sulfate 325 mg three times daily) or intravenously (eg, iron sucrose, iron gluconate) to maintain a TSAT >20% to 25% and serum ferritin between 200 and 500 ng/mL.

Bone metabolism

Renal phosphorus excretion is decreased in patients with CKD and can result in elevated serum phosphorus levels and lower serum calcium levels due to increased binding of phosphorus. Serum calcium and phosphorus levels should be followed regularly in the inpatient setting. Patients with CKD or ESRD with hyperphosphatemia should be placed on low-phosphorus diets (<800-1000 mg/d) and counseled to limit their intake of foods that are high in phosphorus, such as dairy products, meats, dried beans and peas, and cola drinks. Hyperphosphatemia that cannot be adequately controlled by dietary modification alone should be treated with oral phosphorus-binding agents. Oral aluminum hydroxide, historically the first agent made available to treat hyperphosphatemia, is rarely used these days because of its long-term risk of aluminum toxicity and osteomalacia. It has been largely replaced by the calcium-containing (calcium acetate, calcium carbonate, and calcium citrate) and non–calcium-containing phosphorus binders (sevelamer hydrochloride, sevelamer carbonate, and lanthanum carbonate). When administered with meals, these medications inhibit the gastrointestinal absorption of phosphorus; thus they are not effective at lowering serum phosphorus levels in patients not receiving any dietary intake. Calcium acetate has been demonstrated in a number of studies to be more cost-effective than sevelamer. However, in patients who develop extraskeletal calcifications or recurrent hypercalcemia from calcium-containing phosphorus binders, sevelamer and lanthanum are suitable, though more expensive, alternatives. Calcium-containing phosphorus binders and sevelamer or lanthanum can also be used in combination to treat hyperphosphatemia that is difficult to control with a single agent. Sevelamer hydrochloride has been associated with metabolic acidosis; in these patients, substituting with sevelamer carbonate may be of benefit, as this formulation does not decrease serum bicarbonate levels.

Acid–base and electrolytes

Patients with CKD may have a metabolic acidosis due to impaired acid secretion. Sodium bicarbonate should be administered to patients with serum bicarbonate concentrations <22 mEq/L to prevent the complications of chronic metabolic acidosis, specifically bone disease and loss of lean body mass due to increased breakdown of skeletal muscle. Sodium bicarbonate can be given as oral tablets (650 mg [7 mEq] twice daily with meals) or alternatively in the form of baking soda (1/2 to 1 teaspoon dissolved in water or juice twice daily with meals). Patients may experience some abdominal bloating with bicarbonate treatment. Citrate salts should not be used as alkalinizing agents in CKD, as they may increase aluminum absorption.

Electrolyte disorders are also common in patients with CKD and ESRD. When GFR decreases to <15 to 20 mL/min, renal potassium excretion is impaired and hyperkalemia may occur. In patients who still produce adequate urine output, acute hyperkalemia can usually be managed medically with calcium gluconate (if electrocardiographic changes are present), insulin, inhaled albuterol, potassium-binding resins (eg, sodium polystyrene sulfonate), and loop diuretics. Patients with ESRD and oliguria or anuria will often require dialysis therapy to treat hyperkalemia. Chronic management of hyperkalemia involves dietary potassium restriction. Loop diuretics and potassium-binding resins are usually not necessary but can be useful for long-term control. If resins are used, it should be noted that they can result in hypocalcemia, sodium overload, and malabsorption of other medications. When given as a retention enema, they can cause colonic ulceration. These resins should not be given with aluminum hydroxide gels. Hypokalemia is less common in patients with CKD but can be caused by low-potassium intake, diuretic use, or gastrointestinal losses.

The ability of the kidney to properly concentrate or dilute urine is reduced as renal function is progressively lost, and both hyponatremia and hypernatremia are common in patients with CKD. Hyponatremia may be due to impaired free water clearance or volume depletion through renal or extrarenal sodium losses. A careful assessment of volume status can guide appropriate treatment.

Patients who are euvolemic or hypervolemic will usually benefit from free water restriction and occasionally diuretics, whereas patients who are hypovolemic may require administration of intravenous normal saline. Hypernatremia maybe due to impaired water intake, in patients with poor thirst mechanisms or decreased access to water, or excessive renal or extrarenal water losses. Hypernatremia may also accompany recovery from AKI, during the osmotic diuresis of high levels of urea. Patients should be given free water, either orally or intravenously, to correct the water deficit.

PRACTICE POINT

The management of a hospitalized patient with CKD or ESRD should be guided by the following general principles

- The patient's nephrologist and dialysis unit, if applicable, should be contacted upon admission and discharge.
- Admission orders should take into account the special needs of patients with CKD and ESRD.
- All measures should be taken to protect the vascular access of ESRD patients who are receiving hemodialysis.
- All medications, especially those that are initiated during the hospitalization, should be appropriately dosed according to a patient's reduction in GFR.

PRACTICE POINT

- In ESRD patients with little or no urine production, oral fluid intake should be closely monitored and restricted to 1 to 1.5 L/d. Large interdialytic weight gains (>4-5 kg) due to liberal fluid consumption or administration of intravenous fluids and medications can make volume removal during dialysis more difficult.

SUGGESTED READINGS

Angeli P, Gines P, Wong F, et al. Diagnosis and management of acute kidney injury in patients with cirrhosis: revised consensus recommendations of the International Club of Ascites. *Gut.* 2015;64:531.

Bellomo R, Kellum JA, Ronco C. Acute kidney injury. *Lancet.* 2012;380:756-766.

Coresh J, Selvin E, Stevens LA, et al. Prevalence of chronic kidney disease in the United States. *JAMA.* 2007;298:2038-2047.

Lamiere NH, Bagga A, Cruz D, et al. Acute kidney injury: an increasing global concern. *Lancet.* 2013;382:170-179.

Perazella MA. Onco-nephrology: renal toxicities of chemotherapeutic agents. *Clin J Am Soc Nephrol.* 2012;7:1713-1721.

Ronco C, Di Lullo L. Cardiorenal syndrome. *Heart Fail Clin.* 2014;10:251-280.

Sharp VJ, Barnes KT, Erickson BA. Assessment of asymptomatic microscopic hematuria in adults. *Am Fam Physician.* 2013;88:747-754.

Tan KT, van Beek EJ, Brown PW, et al. Magnetic resonance angiography for the diagnosis of renal artery stenosis: a meta-analysis. *Clin Radiol.* 2002;57:617-624.

CHAPTER 62

Postoperative Neurologic and Psychiatric Complications

Catherine Dawson Tobin, MD

Michel J. Sabbagh, MD

John Scott Walton, MD

Tod A. Brown, MD

INTRODUCTION

Neurologic and psychiatric complications are often encountered in the postoperative period and may be very alarming. Hospitalists must be able to recognize and initiate treatment for many of these postoperative complications. The differential diagnosis of common problems (such as headache) may also be very different in the perioperative period. This chapter will cover common presentations, risk factors and prevention techniques, and management of several postoperative neurologic and psychiatric conditions, including: seizures, delirium, confusion, delayed emergence, muscle weakness by anesthetic drugs, stroke, blindness, awareness under anesthesia, cognitive dysfunction, headache, spinal cord injury, and peripheral nerve injury.

SEIZURES

Seizures in the postoperative are generally rare but require immediate treatment. Dangers of seizures include hypoventilation, hypoxemia, musculoskeletal injury, aspiration, and death.

■ RISK FACTORS

There are many different causes of seizures in the perioperative period, including hypoglycemia from prolonged NPO status, local anesthetic systemic toxicity (LAST) from intravascular injection of local anesthetic such as bupivacaine, and electrolyte abnormalities. Patients with intracranial structural lesions, patients having intracranial surgery, and patients with traumatic brain injury (TBI) are also at risk for seizures.

Most anesthetics drugs are antiepileptic. However, some anesthetic drugs can induce seizure foci or at least cause changes in the EEG while infusing. These include ketamine, methohexital, and meperidine. Of note, methohexital and etomidate are often used as general anesthesia on patients prior to electroconvulsive therapy (ECT) where a seizure is purposely induced.

■ MANAGEMENT

Stopping the seizure is the initial and most important treatment. Airway management and protecting against head or body injuries is also important. Pharmacologic adult intravenous therapy includes benzodiazepines such as midazolam 1 to 5 mg, diazepam 5 to 10 mg, propofol 50 to 100 mg, and phenytoin 500 to 1000 mg (infused slowly). If LAST is the cause, Intralipid (20% fat emulsion) bolus 1.5 mL/kg over 1 minute (about 100 cc) followed by continuous infusion of 0.25/kg/min is the treatment.

PRACTICE POINT

- In patients who have had a peripheral nerve block or who have a continuous nerve catheter for pain management, LAST as the cause of seizure must be considered.
- Intralipid 20% therapy is used to treat LAST.

Electrolyte abnormalities and hypoglycemia must be corrected in the treatment of seizures. Sodium abnormalities leading to seizures are most common in neurosurgical patients, and are most often seen in conjunction with the Syndrome of Inappropriate Antidiuretic Hormone (SIADH), Diabetes Insipidus (DI), or due to hypertonic therapy to treat increased intracranial pressures. Seizures can present in any of those conditions but are more likely when sodium levels are <120 mM or >158 mM.

Management includes ruling out other conditions that are not seizures. If it is unclear if seizure activity is present, an electroencephalogram (EEG) should be obtained in consultation with neurology. Pseudoseizures or psychogenic non epileptic seizures must remain on the differential in the management. Characteristics of pseudoseizures include asynchronous episodes which last about 90 seconds of shaking, forced eye closure, and retained pupil response; autonomic manifestations are usually absent such as urination, defecation, cyanosis, and tachycardia. Pseudoseizures are important to recognize because iatrogenic injury from respiratory depression of antiseizure drugs and unnecessary endotracheal intubation can be harmful. Postoperative shivering can also resemble a seizure; it may be treated with low-dose lorazepam, oxygen therapy and rewarming.

DELIRIUM

Postoperative delirium may affect about 25% to 30% of patients greater than age 65. Two main subtypes of delirium are hypoactive (decreased motor activity and withdrawn behavior) and hyperactive (agitated and possibly aggressive behavior). Patients with delirium often have increased hospital length of stay and are at risk for harm to themselves or others. Postoperative delirium in the elderly is preventable in approximately 40% of cases. Therefore, risk reduction strategies are important.

■ RISK FACTORS AND PREVENTION

Risk factors for postoperative delirium are older age, history of dementia, and prior hearing or visual defects. Other contributing causes include fever, stress of surgery, pain, emesis, sleep deprivation, and loss of regular routine. The incidence can be reduced by using lighter anesthesia, using regional versus general anesthesia, using "fast track" anesthesia (early extubation and ambulation), having good pain control, and avoiding benzodiazepines.

Certain anesthetic drugs are best avoided, especially in the elderly, because they contribute to delirium. These drugs include anticholinergics (promethazine, oxybutynin, scopolamine), antihistamines (diphenhydramine, hydroxyzine, histamine 2 blockers), and meperidine.

Anticholinergics such as atropine (used to treat bradycardia) and scopolamine patches (to prevent postoperative nausea) can cause significant confusion, as both cross the blood brain barrier. Other side effects include dry mouth, tachycardia, pupil dilation, and possible hallucinations. If present, confusion/delirium from these agents can be reversed by the anticholinesterase inhibitor physostigmine at a dose of 0.01 to 0.03 mg/kg (average adult doses range from 1 to 5 mg). Glycopyrrolate is a drug used to treat bradycardia and decrease secretions, and can be used in reversal of neuromuscular drugs along with neostigmine. It does not cross the blood brain barrier and may be a better choice than atropine in an elderly patient.

■ MANAGEMENT

Management of delirium should include an evaluation to rule out an intracranial cause such as a stroke. Brain imaging may be indicated. If hypoactive delirium is seen one must consider oversedation caused by narcotics or benzodiazepines, which can be reversed by naloxone or flumazenil respectively. However, pain control is very important in the postoperative management of delirium so reversal of opioids should be carefully done.

Treatment of delirium should not include benzodiazepines as the first choice. These drugs are commonly requested by nursing staff and education of the care team is often needed. Instead low-dose

antipsychotics are a better choice. Also cholinesterase inhibitors should not be newly prescribed to treat delirium. For more information, see Chapter 81: Delirium.

> ### PRACTICE POINT
>
> - Do not use benzodiazepines as a first line treatment of agitation seen in delirium.
> - Antipsychotics, such as haloperidol, risperidone, or olanzapine, at the lowest effective dose for the shortest amount of time possible should be used if patient is agitated and at risk to harm themselves or others.
> - Cholinesterase inhibitors should not be newly prescribed to treat or prevent postoperative delirium.
> - Pain control is important in treatment and prevention of delirium.

CONFUSION, DELAYED EMERGENCE, AND MUSCLE WEAKNESS BY ANESTHETIC DRUGS

Many anesthetic drugs used in the perioperative period can cause confusion, delayed emergence, and muscle weakness. Although these symptoms can mimic a stroke, they are most likely caused by over sedation and reversal agents should be tried (naloxone for opioids and flumazenil for benzodiazepines).

Ketamine is a dissociate anesthetic which is commonly used in anesthesia. It causes sedation and treats pain, but patient's airway reflexes remain intact and the patient continues breathing. It has properties similar to the drug phencyclidine (PCP). Patients often have emergence delirium or colorful dreams after this drug is used.

Neuromuscular blocking agents are commonly used in during surgery to aid in endotracheal intubation and also to keep a patient still during surgical cases where movement could be dangerous. Normally the degree of neuromuscular blockade can be checked with a peripheral nerve stimulator placed over the ulnar or posterior nerve. A train of four or tetanus can be seen depending on the setting of the device. The depolarizing muscle relaxant succinylcholine is short acting and does not require reversal; however, the use of high-dose succinylcholine can result in a rare condition called a Phase II block where the patient is paralyzed for hours. Additionally, if the patient has a pseudocholinesterase deficiency, succinylcholine can last hours. This condition is also rare and can be tested with a dibucaine test. In these situations, if a prolonged paralyzed state ensues, endotracheal intubation and sedation are needed. More commonly, nondepolarizing blocking agents such as rocuronium, cisatracurium, or vecuronium are used and require reversal with an anticholinesterase inhibitor, such as neostigmine, paired with an anticholinergic such as glycopyrrolate. If reversal drugs are not given or if a full amount is not given, patients are not fully reversed and can have a "floppy fish" appearance; they often are not fully able to move their body, or they try to talk but cannot, and they look in distress. In first hour after surgery it is important to place a peripheral nerve stimulator or make sure the patient has had full pharmacologic reversal of neuromuscular blockers, if they were used.

■ MANAGEMENT

The following treatment algorithm for delayed emergence is recommended:

1. Check vital signs (heart rate, blood pressure, temperature, oxygen saturation)
2. Perform a neurologic exam including pupils and response to pain
3. Check twitches with a peripheral nerve monitor

4. Check finger stick glucose
5. Draw an arterial blood gas with electrolytes
6. Consider pharmacologic reversal with naloxone, flumazenil, and physostigmine
7. Make arrangements for brain imagining (head CT)

STROKE

Stroke is an infrequent but tragic complication of surgery. Perioperative stroke is defined as a cerebral infarction up to 30 days after surgery. Perioperative stroke rates range from 0.1% to 10% depending on how the stoke is diagnosed and the type of surgery. Cardiac, vascular and neurosurgery have the highest rates of neurologic consequence. Covert stroke (defined by MRI) occurs much more frequently than overt stroke (defined by clinical symptoms).

■ RISK FACTORS AND PREVENTION

Traditionally reducing stroke risk has largely focused on maximizing a patient's baseline neurologic health and defining preoperative stroke risk prior to surgery. Risk factors change slightly depending on which studies are cited but, advanced age, previous TIA or stroke and renal failure are consistently associated with increased risk of perioperative stroke. Other associated risk factors are female sex, cardiac disease, atrial fibrillation, hypotension, smoking, recent beta blocker cessation, recent statin cessation, anemia, dehydration, hypercoagulable state, recent MI, and CHF. Modifiable comorbidities should be optimized prior to surgery. For example, patients with recent TIAs should undergo a complete evaluation with an MRI, echocardiogram, carotid scans and neurological consultation, which can appropriately guide therapy during the impending preoperative period. Recent TIA or stroke (within 3 months) likely warrants a delay of *elective* surgery until post infarction/ischemic impairment of cerebral auto regulation improves.

The evaluation of anticoagulation therapy is imperative for patients with atrial fibrillation and a recent TIA/CVA. Certain surgeries (eg, neurosurgery and spine surgery) usually require withholding anticoagulation while others (eg, cataract surgery) are usually safe to remain on normal anticoagulants. Between these two extremes, it is often necessary for the preoperative, neurological and surgical teams to confer in an effort to establish an optimal risk benefit regime of anticoagulation.

Intraoperatively the availability of neuroprotective agents has been elusive; barbiturates, steroids, magnesium, and hypothermia have limited or no proven benefit. Patients do benefit from avoidance of hyperthermia and hyper or hypoglycemia. The maintenance of an adequate perfusion blood pressure is also intuitively reasonable although a strict definition of adequate has not been universally accepted. A commonly agreed upon suggestion is to maintain 20% of the patients baseline blood pressure but the absolute minimums of blood pressure and definitions of baseline pressure have not been adequately defined.

■ MANAGEMENT

Many perioperative strokes (about 92%) do not manifest themselves in the PACU but present over the first few postoperative days. Very few preoperative CVAs are hemorrhagic; rather, most are occlusive from either emboli or thrombus. Diagnosis in the early PACU period is difficult because patients may appear to have neurologic aberrations and even transient focal deficits as they fully emerge from anesthesia. Any suspicion should evoke immediate and ongoing neurologic evaluations. Management requires maintenance of adequate perfusion pressure and possible early therapeutic intervention, such as endovascular techniques shortly after the presentation of symptoms (3-6 hours).

POSTOPERATIVE BLINDNESS

Blindness after surgery is another rare but tragic complication. It occurs in <0.2% of spinal surgeries, and 0.0186% of hip replacement and knee arthroplasty procedures; in other procedures it is exceedingly rare (1/10 to 1/2 this rate). There are three different types of blindness after surgery with some additional rare variations. The most common is ischemic optic neuropathy (ION), which has been described most frequently after prone positioned spine surgery and cardiac surgery. ION appears to be a type of compartment syndrome surrounding the optic nerve as a result of increased venous pressures in the head and neck. This seems to also explain how bilateral radical neck procedures and robotic prostatectomies (performed with steep head down positioning) also can be associated with ION. Another form of blindness is retinal artery thrombosis (retinal vascular occlusion). It is far less common and likely caused by direct pressure on the globe of the eye during surgery. Cortical blindness, which is equivalent to a stroke involving the visual pathways in the brain, is rare and is surprisingly more common in younger patients and children than older adults. Lastly, direct surgical trauma to the visual apparatus can occur in ophthalmic, brain and sinus surgeries.

■ RISK FACTORS AND PREVENTION

ION, which comprises the vast majority of postoperative blindness cases, has the following risk factors in noncardiac surgery: the use of a Wilson frame position head rest (in noncardiac surgery), male gender, obesity, fraction of crystalloid to colloid infused (higher-percentage possibly protective), length of surgery (>6 hours) and high-blood loss (>1 L). Given this, prevention efforts include evaluating the type of table or frame and the height of the head in relation to the heart, and the percent of colloid versus crystalloid infused. Staging cases (two shorter surgeries as opposed to one long surgery) has been proposed as a prevention strategy, but is generally impractical and rarely utilized, but it should at least be considered when the surgery is anticipated to last greater than 6 hours. The use of colloids remains controversial in light of the possible deleterious renal effects in critically ill patients, so is a rarely utilized prevention strategy. The risk of blindness should be part of the informed consent in cases with predictable blood loss greater than 1 liter and length of surgery greater than 6 hours. More research needs to be done in this area but the rare incidence makes this difficult.

■ MANAGEMENT

If blindness is suspected in the PACU, an urgent ophthalmologic consultation should ensue. If the cause is not obvious on ophthalmologic examination, then neuroimaging is often required to clearly define the etiology. At present, there are no good therapies for postoperative blindness like ION. Steroids, mannitol and antiplatelet agents have been utilized, but have not been shown to be beneficial.

AWARENESS UNDER ANESTHESIA

Anesthesia is defined as the presence of muscle relaxation, preserved physiology, analgesia and unconsciousness. Awareness under anesthesia is one of the most feared complications of anesthesia by patients. Although most patients do not have significant complications from it, posttraumatic stress disorder has been described in patients with traumatic experiences, especially those reporting awareness with paralysis. The identification of this complication typically requires systematic follow-up and patient interviews following the anesthetics. Patients often do not understand the difference between a sedation case and a general anesthetic, and most episodes of recall under anesthesia occur under sedation.

Awareness under anesthesia is defined as the recall of specific events during general anesthesia. Incidence varies depending on multiple factors including the method used to identify recall, the definition used for recall, as well as the process (quality assessment versus prospective study). Detection methods during the case include the presence of movement under anesthesia, and EEG (more below). Published studies typically use a question set known as the Brice test postoperatively, at varying intervals ranging from the immediate postoperative period to a month or two following the anesthetic (**Table 62-1**).

The incidence of awareness under anesthesia tends to be higher when reported in study conditions in patients being interviewed using the Brice questions (up to 0.1%), when compared to self-reporting or a quality assurance questionnaire (as low as 0.005%). According to the Fifth National Audit Project (NAP-5) from the United Kingdom published in 2014, recall occurs in roughly 1 in 19,000 anesthetics. High-risk populations, such as patients undergoing cardiac surgery or C-sections under general anesthesia, have a much higher incidence of 0.012% and 0.15%, respectively.

RISK FACTORS AND PREVENTION

Factors associated with awareness include the type of surgery (eg, cardiac surgery and trauma surgery), an intravenous anesthetic

TABLE 62-1 Brice Questions

1. What was the last thing you remember before you went to sleep?
2. What was the first thing you remember after your operation?
3. Can you remember anything in between?
4. Did you dream during your operation?
5. What was the worst thing about your operation?

method (such as used with emergency C-sections), or the use of neuromuscular blockade. There are also patient-specific risk factors, including a history of drug use, significant comorbidities, a history of awareness, or the presence of a difficult airway.

Cardiac and trauma surgery are typically performed on sick and fragile patients who may not tolerate similar levels of anesthetics as their healthier counterparts without the use of vasopressors, volume replacement or both. These lower doses of anesthetics may contribute to the recall. Similarly, C-sections with general anesthesia and the use of total intravenous anesthesia are more prone to inadequate anesthesia (not acknowledging the anesthetic needs or concerns that the patient may not tolerate heavier doses of anesthetics). Neuromuscular blockade, though typically considered to be an integral part of an anesthetic, increases the rates of awareness under anesthesia.

Anesthetic gases are typically titrated to a certain expired concentration of a gas known as an end-tidal value. This type of anesthetic is based on the minimum alveolar concentrations (MAC) of these agents. A MAC of an inhalational anesthetic is defined as the end-tidal concentration of a gas at which 50% of the population will not move in response to a painful stimulus. This value can vary based on age and comorbidities and is adjusted as such. Titration of anesthetics to MAC values has been shown to produce safe anesthetics with low rates of recall.

There are commercially available awareness monitors, the most common of which is the bispectral index (BIS). It is the only device approved by the FDA to monitor intraoperative awareness. This device acquires raw EEG data continuously which is then converted by a proprietary algorithm to a value that can be used to titrate the anesthetic. Studies on this method of monitoring, compared to MAC titration of anesthetics, have varied results and are considered equivocal.

Finally, the use of a balanced anesthetic, which includes other sedative medications such as opioids, benzodiazepines, anticholinergic agents, and even alpha-2 agonists, may decrease MAC requirements by adding to the level of sedation and amnesia, and can reduce the risk of awareness.

POSTOPERATIVE COGNITIVE DYSFUNCTION

Anesthesia alters brain function, which can manifest as changes in attention, memory and reaction time in the immediate postoperative period. These functions return to normal at varying rates following anesthetics. These are due to rates of elimination, length of anesthetics, type of anesthesia, type of surgery, patient characteristics, and any adjuncts used. Postoperative cognitive dysfunction (POCD) is considered separate from postoperative delirium and short-term cognitive disturbance. POCD is described as a change in cognition targeting memory, learning and concentration, ranging from weeks to months. This should be assessed with a preoperative and a postoperative cognition examination. These examinations are often limited or absent due to constraints in the perioperative period. Timing of these examinations is crucial to identifying true cognition changes. The preoperative examination should be thorough enough that a baseline mentation is determined. This examination cannot be so thorough as to lose the interest of the patient or so close to the date of surgery that the patient is overcome by anxiety and stress. Both of these scenarios can significantly alter testing and baseline cognition assessment. Similarly, postoperative examinations should follow similar guidelines, and those performed further out in the postoperative period (at least 4 weeks postoperatively) are more likely to identify persistent and significant mentation changes.

RISK FACTORS AND PREVENTION

Published data associates a 25% incidence of POCD with major noncardiac surgery after 1 week, and 10% after 3 months, compared to 3% in the control group at both time points. Risk factors include advanced age, duration of anesthesia, respiratory complications, second operation, low educational level, and prior stroke. Although anesthetic type has been believed to play a major role in POCD, studies comparing regional to general anesthesia demonstrated a significant difference at 1 week but no difference at 3 months.

POSTOPERATIVE HEADACHE

Postoperative headaches are most commonly due to: postdural puncture headache, caffeine withdrawal headache, pneumocephalus, or hyperperfusion syndrome. Post dural puncture headache (PDPH) is a result of a cerebrospinal fluid (CSF) leak from puncture of the dural membrane. PDPH is defined as a bilateral headache that develops within 7 days (typically 48 hours) of a dural puncture, and is positional (worse when the patient is upright, and better when the patient lies down). Patients typically report a dull or throbbing headache with a stiff neck. There is often some photophobia, nausea, and hearing impairment. Presence of a concomitant subdural hematoma or Chiari malformation may intensify the headache or remove the headache's postural component (pain in all positions). The mechanism is believed to be a compensatory venous hypervolemia and dilation of dural venous sinuses due to low intracranial CSF volume. Risk factors for PDPH include the use of large gauge spinal needles, beveled needles, female gender, pregnancy, age (18-40 years old), and prior PDPH.

Patients with PDPH are typically offered conservative management followed by invasive therapies as needed to improve symptoms. The mainstay of conservative treatment includes bed rest, hydration, prone position, use of an abdominal binder, caffeine, analgesics, and a variety of adjutants including sumatriptan, hydrocortisone and gabapentin. Although hydration does not relieve the headache, dehydration worsens the symptoms. A typical conservative treatment course would include: oral hydration, oral caffeine (300 mg every 6 hours), scheduled anti-inflammatory medication, and as needed narcotic analgesics in severe cases. Invasive management strategies include an intrathecal saline injection, placement of an intrathecal catheter (typically for 24 hours), an epidural saline or morphine injection, or an epidural blood patch. Patients with a known dural puncture with an epidural needle may benefit from the placement of a spinal catheter with a saline infusion for the first 24 hours. This method has been shown to decrease the inflammatory process at the dura, as well supplement any loss in CSF that may have occurred. The epidural blood patch is the gold standard for treatment, with complete symptomatic relief in 65% to 95% of patients in retrospective studies.

Another cause of postoperative headaches is caffeine withdrawal. Oral or intravenous caffeine has been shown to be effective in most cases. A pneumocephalus can also cause a headache, common causes include dural puncture from an epidural needle using a loss-of-resistance to air technique, as well as a result of neurosurgical, ophthalmologic and otolaryngology operations leading to air trapping in the cranial cavity.

Hyperperfusion syndrome following carotid endarterectomy occurs in up to 3% of cases and can cause a headache that is usually one-sided, and may be associated with hypertension, focal neurological deficits and seizures. If left untreated, this may result in cerebral edema, intracerebral hemorrhage, and even death. Treatment is directed toward blood pressure control and regulation of cerebral perfusion pressure.

SPINAL CORD INJURY

■ RISK FACTORS AND PREVENTION

Spinal cord injury related to anesthesia and surgery is a rare occurrence, but there are a few operations that are accompanied with

a significant risk (4%-10%): repair of the descending aorta, correction of kypho-scoliosis, or other major spinal repairs. In the case of descending aortic repair, the arterial blood supply to the spinal cord may be compromised. In the case of spinal corrective surgery multiple mechanisms for spinal cord injury are present. When performing these high-risk operations, the operative team should consider multiple risk reduction strategies and consider intraoperative monitoring of spinal cord integrity. Spinal cord integrity can be monitored intraoperatively using Somatosensory Evoked Potential (SSEP) and Motor Evoked Potential (MEP) monitoring. Both these neurophysiologic monitoring modalities require a devoted neurophysiology technician. Additionally, both SSEP and MEP monitoring are extremely sensitive to anesthetic agents and require careful titration of compatible agents to provide useful monitoring data.

Anesthetic procedures can very rarely cause spinal cord injuries (<0.01%). Spinal block, epidural block, and interscalene block have all been implicated. The mechanism of injury to the spinal cord includes needle trauma, medication toxicity, infection, or hematoma. Spinal and epidural anesthesia are both relatively contraindicated in the presence of coagulopathy or when anticoagulation is planned due to the possibility of compressive hematoma.

Positioning during surgery is another means whereby the spinal cord can be injured. This type of injury is extremely rare and occurs when the patient is placed in a position they would not tolerate when awake. The mechanism of injury in these cases is likely stretch or compression of the vulnerable spinal cord. The spinal cord may be vulnerable in areas of chronic spinal stenosis or spondylosis. Patients who have experienced acute vertebral trauma may be exquisitely vulnerable to cord injury due to movement and positioning for surgery. Finally, intubation of the patient with cervical spine injury can injure the spinal cord. Ideally, the patient should be intubated with no movement of the neck whatsoever with a neurologic exam being performed following the intubation to confirm that no deterioration of neurologic status occurred. Unfortunately the ideal scenario is rarely possible due to the patients' inability to cooperate, altered mental status, acute respiratory failure, hemorrhagic shock or other confounders that require rapid control of the airway.

■ MANAGEMENT

Spinal cord injury following surgery and anesthesia should be rapidly evaluated, treated and documented. With rapid diagnosis some lesions may be corrected and function restored. Neurology and neurosurgical consultation is advisable to speed the evaluation processes and institute treatment quickly. MRI should be performed to determine if a compressive lesion such as a hematoma or unstable fracture is present. Decompression should be performed immediately if compression of the cord is found. If no compression of the cord is noted, therapy usually consists of dexamethasone and management of blood sugar, hematocrit, and blood pressure. The patient will require admission to a neurologic intensive care setting. Long term deficits and the need for rehabilitation are likely.

PERIPHERAL NERVE INJURY

■ RISK FACTORS AND PREVENTION

Peripheral nerve injury during surgery and anesthesia is relatively common. It is such a common complication that the American Society of Anesthesiologists (ASA) maintains a practice recommendation statement on the subject. Each provider involved in operative and perioperative care should become familiar with the recommendations of the ASA regarding peripheral nerve injuries. The most common peripheral nerve injured is the ulnar nerve followed by the brachial plexus, and the lumbosacral nerve roots.

Prevention of perioperative peripheral nerve injury should focus primarily on avoiding surgical positioning that puts traction or compression on any peripheral nerve or plexus. Ample padding is recommended for the ulnar nerve at the elbow and any location where an object may push onto the patient. Objects that may cause inadvertent compression include safety belts, IV tubing and IV tubing connectors, mayo instrument stands, surgical retraction devices, tourniquets, surgical team members, traction devices and traction posts.

Ulnar nerve injury seems to be a particularly vexing problem. It often occurs when guidelines for care are followed, can present in a delayed fashion, and can occur in patients who are awake enough during the surgery to maintain the affected arm in a position of comfort.

The mechanisms for injury to peripheral nerves during anesthesia and surgery are multiple: stretch, compression, surgical trauma, and incidental nerve block procedures. Any position that the patient cannot tolerate due to pain should *not* be used while under anesthesia. Each surgical position conveys unique challenge and risk in positioning the patient. A partial list of named surgical positions include: supine, prone, super-man, jack-knife, decubitus, lithotomy, high lithotomy, sitting, sphinx, with Trendelenberg or other tilt added to each. The supine position with the arms abducted (<90°) on padded armrests is considered the lowest risk position for peripheral nerve injury.

■ MANAGEMENT

When a new peripheral nerve injury is discovered postoperatively it should be evaluated promptly. If there is any compression or stretching of the extremity these should be remedied as soon as possible. Casts, splints, and traction are examples of devices that may cause ongoing injury. Bed rails may also produce injury in a patient unable to feel or move an extremity due to anesthesia block or other factors. The extremity should be examined for adequate perfusion and swelling that may indicate compartment syndrome or compressive hematoma. If there are no obvious explanations for the peripheral nerve deficit, neurology consultation is advisable to document the distribution and extent of the deficit. Steroids are often prescribed along with splinting and range of motion physiotherapy. Rehabilitation therapy to minimize disability should be considered if the deficit does not rapidly resolve.

CONCLUSION

Postoperative neurologic and psychiatric complications require immediate recognition and treatment. Seizures must be treated promptly and with special attention to rule out local anesthetic toxicity (LAST). Delirium is common in elderly patients and avoidance of certain drugs such as anticholinergics, antihistamines, and benzodiazepines can often help prevent this complication. Confusion, delayed emergence, and muscle weakness by anesthetic drugs from pseudo cholinesterase deficiency or residual paralysis must be considered when a patient is not at their baseline state after surgery. Stroke and postoperative blindness must been diagnosed and treated emergently. Awareness under anesthesia is very infrequent

but is seen more with cardiac and trauma surgery, with use of an intravenous anesthetic method (such as used with emergency C-sections), and in cases where paralytic agents were used. Postoperative Cognitive Dysfunction (PCOD) is described as a change in cognition targeting memory, learning and concentration, ranging from weeks to months. Postoperative headache is most commonly due to post dural puncture headache (PDPH), caffeine withdrawal headache, pneumocephalus, or hyperperfusion syndrome. Treatment varies depending on cause. PDPH requires analgesics, caffeine, or an epidural blood patch. Hyperperfusion syndrome is treated with blood pressure and cerebral perfusion pressure (CPP) control. Spinal cord injury from surgery is not common, but most likely with certain surgeries, such as repair of the descending aorta, correction of kypho-scoliosis, or other spine surgeries. Neurology and neurosurgical consultation with MRI are often needed to aid in rapid diagnosis and treatment. Lastly, peripheral nerve injury is a feared complication of surgery, is usually due to positioning; rehabilitation therapy to minimize disability should be considered if the deficit does not rapidly resolve.

SUGGESTED READINGS

The American Geriatrics Society Expert Panel on Postoperative Delirium in Older Adults. American Geriatrics Society abstracted clinical practice guideline for postoperative delirium in older adults. *JAGS*. 2015;63:142-150.

Apfelbaum JL, et al. Practice advisory for the prevention of perioperative peripheral neuropathies. *Anesthesiology*. 2011;114(4):741-754.

Cook TM, et al. 5th National Audit Project (NAP5) on accidental awareness during general anaesthesia: patient experiences, human factors, sedation, consent, and medicolegal issues. *Br J Anaesth*. 2014;113:560.

Horlocker TT, Wedel DJ. Anesthesia for orthopedic surgery. In: Barash PG, et al., eds. *Clinical Anesthesia*, 7th ed. Philadelphia, PA: Lippincott Williams & Wilkins; 2012:1441-1447.

Mashour GA, Woodrum DT, Avidan MS. Neurological complications of surgery and anaesthesia. *Br J Anaesth*. 2015;114(2):194-203.

Ramos JA, Brull SJ. Psychogenic non epileptic seizures in post anesthesia recovery unit. *Rev Bras Anestesiol*. 2014;pii: S0034-7094(13)00127-X.

Rasmussen LS, Stygall J, Newman SP. Cognitive dysfunction and other long-term complications of surgery and anesthesia. In: Miller RD, et al., eds. *Miller's Anesthesia*, 8th ed. Philadelphia, PA: Saunders; 2015:2999-3010.

The Postoperative Visual Loss Study Group. Risk factors associated with ischemic optic neuropathy after spinal fusion surgery. *Anesthesiology*. 2012;116:15-24.

Watson JC, et al. Neurologic evaluation and management of perioperative nerve injury. *Reg Anesth Pain Med*. 2015. http://www.ncbi.nlm.nih.gov/pubmed/26110440.

SECTION 5

Specialty Consultation—What the Consulting Hospitalist Needs to Know

CHAPTER 63

Surgical Management of Obesity

Ashley B. Hink, MD, MPH
T. Karl Byrne, MD
Rana C. Pullatt, MD, MS

INTRODUCTION

Obesity is a global problem and a major contributor to morbidity and mortality in the United States. The World Health Organization (WHO) estimates that 1.9 billion adults worldwide are overweight (BMI > 25 kg/m^2) and 600 million are obese (BMI > 30 kg/m^2). In the United States, 67% of adults are overweight, 35% of adults are considered obese, and 6.4% are morbidly obese (BMI > 40 kg/m^2). While there is increasing knowledge about obesity and efforts to reduce the epidemic in the United States, the prevalence of obesity has remained largely unchanged over the past 10 years. In addition, the number of obese children has more than doubled over the past 3 decades to 17%. The more than 50 million obese Americans are at risk of developing numerous obesity-related health problems, including hypertension, diabetes, and coronary artery disease (**Table 63-1**).

Currently, the annual cost for treating obesity and its related comorbid conditions are estimated at $147 billion and those who are obese have approximately $1400 more in annual medical costs. Obesity accounts for more than 100,000 premature deaths annually and is considered the second most preventable cause of death after cigarette smoking.

To date, surgery is the most effective means of achieving and maintaining long-term weight loss in obese patients. It is also consistently found to be more effective than medical weight loss alone for the improvement or remission of type 2 diabetes and other major comorbid illnesses. In a 2014 Cochrane Review of randomized controlled trials, all seven included trials comparing outcomes of bariatric surgery to nonsurgical interventions found significantly more weight loss in the surgical groups (weight loss is often measured as percentage of excess body weight loss, EBWL, calculated as weight loss/excess weight × 100). Another meta-analysis including more recent trials showed that the mean decrease in BMI for all bariatric surgical procedures was 13.4 kg/m^2 with 55% of EBWL, and 65% of patients experienced remission of diabetes. These outcomes are far superior to medical interventions for obesity and its associated comorbid conditions as long-term maintenance of more than 10% EBWL is uncommon with diet, exercise and other medical interventions alone.

INDICATIONS FOR REFERRAL FOR BARIATRIC SURGERY

Based on the 1991 consensus statement on bariatric surgery for morbid obesity issued by the NIH, it is recommended that patients who have failed lifestyle and medical interventions with a BMI greater than 40 kg/m^2 or 35 kg/m^2 with two or more significant obesity-related comorbidities (Table 63-1) be referred to a bariatric surgeon.

PREOPERATIVE RISK ASSESSMENT SPECIFIC TO BARIATRIC SURGERY

Once a patient has been referred for bariatric surgery, a thorough screening must be conducted by a multidisciplinary team, to determine eligibility for surgical management (**Table 63-2**). Bariatric teams include specialists from bariatric medicine, bariatric surgery, nutrition and behavioral medicine.

Nutrition counseling is extremely important preoperatively to educate the patient about healthy eating habits that lead to long-term success. These habits include regular eating patterns throughout the day (no skipping meals), intake of an adequate amount of protein at each meal so that total protein intake per day is 40 to 60 g,

TABLE 63-1 Obesity-related Comorbidities

Metabolic syndrome

Type 2 diabetes

Hyperlipidemia

    Hypercholesterolemia

    Hypertriglyceridemia

Coronary artery disease

Myocardial infarction

Hypertension

Renal failure

Obstructive sleep apnea

Obesity hypoventilation syndrome

Asthma

Gastroesophageal reflux disease (GERD)

Cholelithiasis

Depression

Pseudotumor cerebri

Cancer

    Colon

    Breast

    Endometrium

    Prostate

Sex hormone anomalies

    Polycystic ovary disease

    Gynecomastia

    Hirsutism

    Infertility

Stress urinary incontinence

Venous stasis disease

Deep venous thrombosis

Degenerative joint disease

NASH

Abdominal wall hernias

Osteoarthritis

Lumbar disc disease

TABLE 63-2 Preoperative Assessment

- History and physical
- ECG
- Cardiac stress test (if indicated by poor exercise tolerance, angina, or history of coronary artery disease)
- Laboratory tests
  - CBC
  - Basic metabolic panel
  - Liver function tests
  - Hemoglobin A1c
  - Albumin
  - Fasting lipid profile
  - Vitamin B12, folate, thiamine levels
  - Pregnancy test
  - ABG
- Abdominal ultrasound to rule out gallstones
- Upper GI series to check for hiatal hernia
- Pulmonary function tests
- Chest x-ray
- Sleep study
- Smoking cessation
- Anesthesia evaluation
- Psychosocial evaluation

binge eating, are screened for since they are associated with poor outcomes after bariatric surgery. Also important is identification of any signs of substance abuse or severe situational stress that would adversely affect the patient after surgery and hinder compliance with strict dietary and lifestyle modifications. Smoking cessation is strongly encouraged for roux-en-y gastric bypass and biliopancreatic diversion and some surgeons will decline performing such procedures if continuing to smoke, as it places patients at a higher risk of ulcer formation at the gastrojeunostomy and GI bleeding. It is important that patients seriously considering bariatric surgery are evaluated to determine whether they would be able to comply with a strict postoperative diet and lifestyle change, whether they have a support system in place, and whether or not long-term follow-up is in place before surgery.

Since morbidly obese patients have had poor results and often-negative experiences with exercise, it is important that physical activity, both aerobic and strength training, be stressed. It is often extremely helpful for patients to be seen by a clinical exercise physiologist to receive advice on implementing an exercise regimen and the benefits of combining cardiovascular activity with strength training. In addition, a clinical exercise physiologist can offer strategies to compensate for weight bearing joint pain during physical activity. These referrals are often quite helpful in reducing barriers to adopting exercise programs, which are necessary for long-term success after any bariatric procedure. Although the help of an exercise physiologist may be quite beneficial, not all bariatric programs have one in their multidisciplinary team, since it is not yet a requirement. When this is the case, it is important for the physician to refer a patient to a clinical exercise physiologist who is certified by the American College of Sports Medicine. Referrals are especially useful for patients with multiple medical problems. Often exercise physiologists working in the cardiac or pulmonary rehabilitation units within the same health care system can be helpful in guiding patients in their exercise regime. When severely overweight

avoidance of high-carbohydrate snack foods that could lead to dumping syndrome after intestinal bypass procedures, and the need for lifetime vitamin supplementation. Patients are also taught that the intense effects of bariatric surgery (such as repression of hunger and decreased appetite) are time-limited to approximately 2 years after surgery. Therefore, long-term success requires permanent lifestyle changes, including modifications in eating habits, dietary changes, and increased exercise and physical activity.

In addition to being seen by a nutritionist, prospective patients are seen by a psychiatrist, psychologist, or social worker during the initial evaluation process to determine the patient's capacity to fully understand the risks and benefits of a life-changing operation. These patients are also counseled on mindful eating; that is, they need to understand whether they are eating to satisfy hunger or to satisfy an emotional need. Counseling may also include addressing the prospective patient's expectations for weight loss, health outcomes, as well as the psychosocial impact of bariatric surgery.

The psychiatrist/psychologist/social worker must also be able to identify if any overt psychoses or mental illnesses are present that would require treatment before surgery. Eating disorders, such as

individuals begin an exercise program, early weight loss is often quite remarkable. This weight loss can be a strong positive reinforcement for an individual. After significant weight loss though, the effect of exercise becomes less impressive.

The remainder of the preoperative assessment focuses on factors that predispose the patient to increased surgical risk such as age, cardiovascular risk factors (coronary artery disease, congestive heart failure, cardiomyopathy, hypertension, pulmonary hypertension), pulmonary risk factors (asthma, obstructive pulmonary disease, obstructive sleep apnea, smoking), and vascular risk factors (venous stasis, hypercoaguable states secondary to obesity, prior deep venous thromboses, use of oral contraceptives). Some imaging studies such as right upper-quadrant ultrasound and contrasted upper GI may be ordered depending on the patient's clinical history of biliary colic or hiatal hernia, for which the patient may benefit from cholecystectomy and repair of the hiatal hernia at the time of surgery.

There are few absolute contraindications for surgery, but severe cardiopulmonary disease based on the preoperative work-up may prohibit bariatric surgery if the operative mortality is deemed significant. Patients who weigh >500 pounds are at an increased risk of complications and death, and may require hospitalization prior to surgery for monitored weight loss. Inability to walk is also a contraindication. There is no defined age cut-off and it may be determined by surgeon preference and assessment of potential longevity to have a meaningful benefit from surgery.

BARIATRIC SURGICAL PROCEDURES

Bariatric surgical procedures are proposed to work in two primary mechanisms—restriction (reduces intake of food) and malabsorption (limits absorption of food); although other physiologic mechanisms have been proposed, they are not entirely understood. Alterations in ghrelin and incretin are also demonstrated, which act to increase satiety and postprandial insulin levels, respectively.

ROUX-EN-Y GASTRIC BYPASS

The Roux-en-Y gastric bypass (RYGB) is currently the most common bariatric procedure performed worldwide and is primarily performed laparoscopically. The procedure consists of creating a small gastric pouch (approximately 30 mL) and creating a gastrojejunal anastomosis with roux-en-y anatomy, leading to bypass of the duodenum of ingested food (**Figure 63-1**). Its efficacy was once thought to be due to its restrictive mechanism, but it is also effective

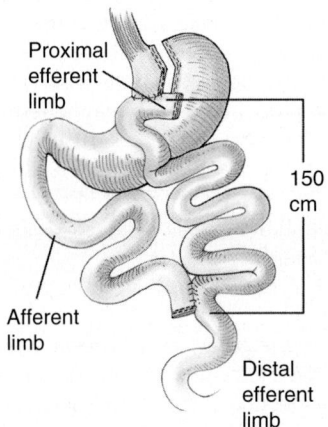

Figure 63-1 *Roux-en-Y gastric bypass anatomy.* (From Zollinger RM, Ellison EC. *Zollinger's Atlas of Surgical Operations, 9th ed.* http://www.accessurgery.com. Copyright © The McGraw-Hill Companies, Inc. All rights reserved.)

due to the exclusion of the first part of the small bowel, decreasing incretin release. Now that most are performed laparoscopically, most patients are discharged in 2 to 3 days postoperatively. The Swedish Obese Subjects Study, the largest study on weight loss surgery to date with the longest follow-up, reports a mean percent weight loss of 32.5% of total body weight (percent of total weight loss is roughly equal to half of EBWL) 1 to 2 years after gastric bypass and 25% 10 years postbypass. A 2004 meta-analysis by Buchwald et al. reported an average weight loss of 46 kg and a mean EBWL of 61.6% after 1 to 2 years, which is comparable to the Swedish Obese Subjects Study.

Roux-en-Y gastric bypass also provides excellent improvement and even remission of comorbid conditions (**Table 63-3**). A meta-analysis showed >80% of patients with diabetes undergoing RYGB had remission of their diabetes and >90% demonstrated improved glycemic control, with remission defined as discontinuation of all diabetes-related medications as well as the ability to maintain blood glucose levels within the normal range.

Roux-en-Y gastric bypass patients also have remission of their hypertension in 65% to 85% of patients. Hyperlipidemia, hypercholesterolemia, and hypertriglyceridemia are also greatly improved in >90% of patients after gastric bypass surgery, with total cholesterol levels decreasing by 0.96 mmol/L, LDL by 0.89 mmol/L, triglycerides by 1.07 mmol/L, and HDL increasing by 0.05 mmol/L. Obstructive sleep apnea is improved or resolved in 80% to 90%, and gastroesophageal reflux disease (GERD) is resolved in 85% of patients after RYGB. Although more difficult to quantify, patients have also reported improvements in depression, joint pain, stress incontinence, infertility, self-esteem, and overall quality of life.

SLEEVE GASTRECTOMY

Laparoscopic sleeve gastrectomy (SG) has recently gained popularity as an operation for weight loss and is now commonly performed. The procedure entails creating an elongated gastric tube that remains in continuity with the pylorus and duodenum, and the resected gastric remnant is removed (**Figure 63-2**). It was initially thought to be a purely restrictive procedure. However, a recent study by Peterli et al. has shown a post-SG impact on incretin secretion similar to post-RYGB and it reduces ghrelin, which increases satiety. Studies show that the weight loss achieved with sleeve gastrectomy is similar to RYGB. In a review series, 24 studies of 1749 patients demonstrated a mean EWL of 46.6% and low complication rate. A recent meta-analysis comparing RYGB to sleeve gastrectomy in 32 studies found that RYGB resulted in greater (but nonsignificant) weight loss and fewer complications/reoperations, but RYGB had significantly better reductions in HTN, cholesterol, GERD, diabetes, and arthritis.

There are occasions in which SG may be the procedure of choice in patients with relative or absolute contraindications for a bypass procedure or a malabsorptive procedure. These include patients with severe pre-existing iron deficiency anemia and other vitamin deficiencies that rely on adequate and specific anatomic small bowel surface area for absorption. Transplant patients and patients with inflammatory bowel disease on chronic steroids, and patients with severe osteoarthritis relying on NSAIDs are better candidates for SG due to the risk of anastomotic leaks and gastrojejunostomy ulceration with NSAID use. Small bowel length should be preserved in patients with inflammatory bowel disease.

LAPAROSCOPIC ADJUSTABLE GASTRIC BANDING

Laparoscopic adjustable gastric banding (LAGB) used to be the most commonly performed bariatric procedure, but has fallen out of favor in recent years due to the demonstrated superiority of other surgical procedures that offer restrictive and metabolic benefits, and due to

TABLE 63-3 Outcomes of Bariatric Surgeries

	Laparoscopic Adjustable Gastric Banding (LAGB)	Roux-en-Y Gastric Bypass (RYGB)	Biliopancreatic Bypass/ Duodenal Switch (BPD/DS)	Sleeve Gastrectomy (SG)
Mean weight loss 1-2 y postoperatively (% EBWL)	40-50	60-94	65-92	49-81
Mortality (%)	0.1	0.5	1.1	0.5
Percentage of patients with diabetes remission	50-80	75-85	95-100	70-75
Percentage of patients with diabetes improvement	60-80	80-95	75-85	70-85
Percentage of patients with hypertension remission	45-70	65-85	80-85	60-65
Percentage of patients with hypertension improvement	60-70	65-85	80-90	60-65
Percentage of patients with hyperlipidemia improvement	58	>90	99	N/A
Percentage of patients with hypercholesterolemia improvement	78	>90	80-90	50%
Percentage of patients with hypertriglyceridemia improvement	77	>90	90-100	N/A
Average change in total cholesterol (mmol/L)	−0.3	−0.96	−1.97	N/A
Average change in HDL (mmol/L)	0.12	0.05	0.07	N/A
Average change in LDL (mmol/L)	−0.11	−0.89	−1.36	N/A
Average change in triglycerides (mmol/L)	−0.76	−1.07	−0.8	N/A
Percentage of patients with obstructive sleep apnea remission	90-95	70-80	70-90	N/A
Percentage of patients with obstructive sleep apnea symptom improvement	90-95	80-95	70-90	80%

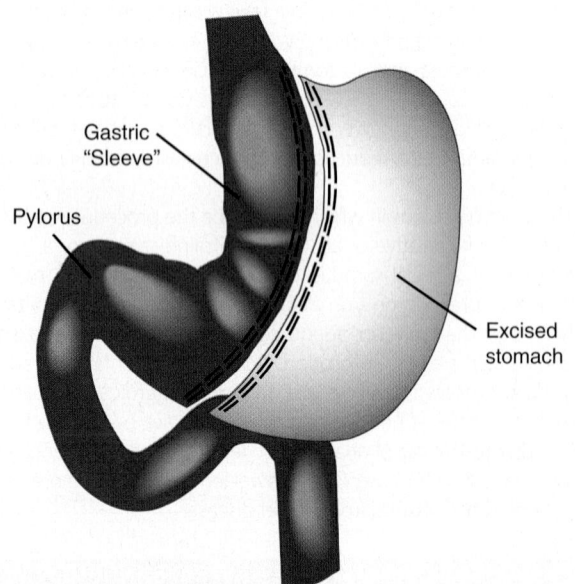

Figure 63-2 *Gastric sleeve anatomy.* (From Greenberger NJ, Blumberg S, Burakoff R. *Current Diagnosis & Treatment: Gastroenterology, Hepatology & Endoscopy,* 3rd ed. www.accessmedicine.com. Copyright © McGraw-Hill Education. All rights reserved.)

the potential long-term complications of banding. The procedure involves placing an inflatable band around the stomach just below the GE junction and an injectable port is anchored below the subcutaneous tissue on the fascia that attaches to the band via a silastic tube. Saline is then injected into the port incrementally to provide increased restriction and limited intake (**Figure 63-3**). Although technically less challenging than RYGB, the LAGB requires frequent clinic visits in order to properly adjust the band with saline injections and maintain the proper amount of gastric restriction to achieve weight loss. Studies have shown good weight loss results with LAGB. The Swedish Obese Subjects Study reports 20% total body weight loss 1 to 2 years after LAGB and 14% 10 years postbanding. Meta-analysis data shows a similar 47.5% EBWL after 1 to 2 years and an average of 34.8 kg.

LAGB may also lead to remission and improvement in comorbidities although less so than the previously described methods because it is purely a restrictive procedure—it does not have physiologic or metabolic effects seen with bypass procedures or sleeve gastrectomy. Multiple studies report remission of diabetes in 50% to 80%, improvement and remission of hypertension in 45% to 70%, and improvement in hyperlipidemia, hypercholesterolemia, and hypertriglyceridemia in 60%, 80%, and 75%. Based on meta-analysis data, total cholesterol, LDL, and triglyceride levels decrease by an average of 0.3, 0.11, and 0.76 mmol/L, respectively, while HDL

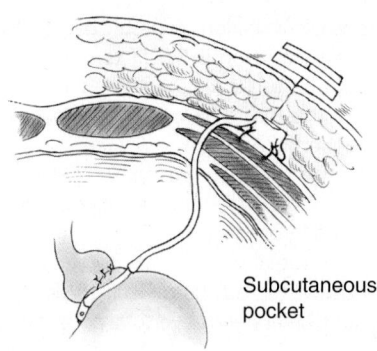

Subcutaneous
pocket

Figure 63-3 *Laparoscopic gastric band anatomy.* (From Zollinger RM, Ellison EC. *Zollinger's Atlas of Surgical Operations,* 9th ed. http://www.accesssurgery.com. Copyright © The McGraw-Hill Companies, Inc. All rights reserved.)

increased by an average of 0.12 mmol/L. Symptoms of sleep apnea improve in 95% of patients, and many also report improvements in menstrual irregularities and GERD after LAGB as well.

MALABSORPTIVE PROCEDURES

Malabsorptive procedures include jejunal-ileal bypass (which is now never performed), and biliopancreatic diversion (BPD) and duodenal switch (DS). In BPD-DS, the stomach is resected from the duodenum (pylorus preserved) and the intestinal tract is reconstructed to allow a short common-channel of small bowel anastomosed with the stomach and ileum just before the ileocecal valve, leaving about 250 cm of small bowel for absorption (**Figure 63-4**). Studies show

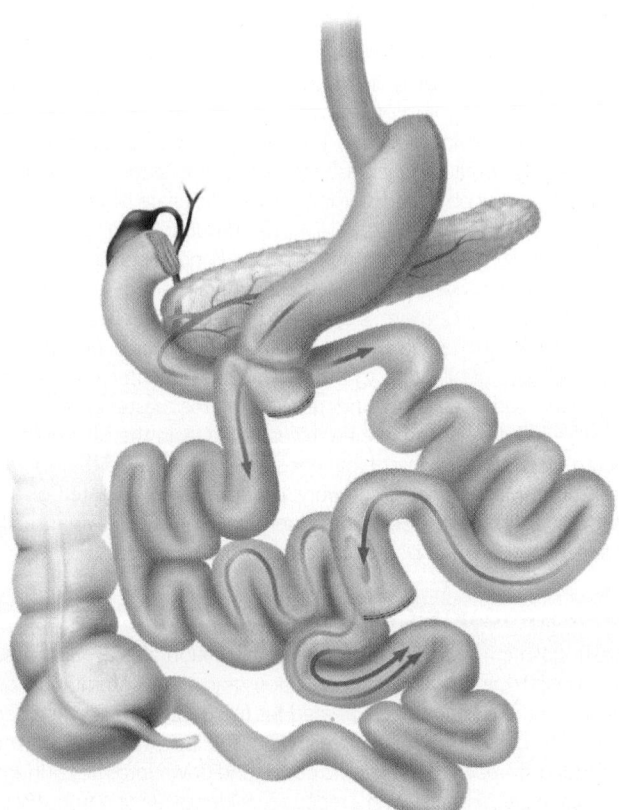

Figure 63-4 *Biliopancreatic diversion—duodenal switch anatomy.* (From Zinner MJ, Ashley SW. *Manigot's Abdominal Operations,* 12th ed. www.accesssurgery.com. Copyright © The McGraw-Hill Companies, Inc. All rights reserved.)

that BPD-DS provides greater early weight loss than RYGB and sleeve gastrectomy, and data show superior weight loss in very obese patients (BMI > 50). A randomized study of 160 morbidly obese adults compared RYGB results to the results of their variation of BPD-DS. After 2 years, 100% of the BPD-DS patients maintained a greater than 50% EBWL while only 88.7% of RYGB patients were able to maintain similar weight loss. A smaller but more recent randomized trial of morbidly obese found after 5 years, total body weight loss was 40% in the BPD/DS group compared to 26.4% in the RYGP group, with the BPD-DS group losing a mean of 25 kg more than the RYGP group.

Although BPD-DS may be a more complex procedure, patients who undergo this procedure appear to have the best outcomes with regard to resolution of comorbidities. A randomized trial found at 2-year follow-up, glucose intolerance, hypercholesterolemia, hypertriglyceridemia, and sleep apnea had completely resolved in both the BPD-DS and RYGB groups; but in the BPD-DS, 100% experienced remission of diabetes (versus 70% of RYGB), 81% of hypertensive patients experienced normalization of blood pressures (versus 63% of RYGB), and changes in total cholesterol, LDL, and HDL in the BPD/DS group were significantly greater than in the RYGB group. Sleep apnea is also greatly improved after BPD-DS in 85% of patients. Additionally, although more difficult to quantify, patients have reported significant improvements in depression, joint pain, stress incontinence, infertility, self-esteem, and overall quality of life.

Although there is great improvement of comorbid conditions, this must be balanced against the increased likelihood for vitamin and nutritional deficiencies, and higher-operative mortality risk (1.1% for BPD/DS, compared to 0.1% for gastric bypass).

POSTOPERATIVE COMPLICATIONS OF BARIATRIC SURGERY

All bariatric surgery patients are at risk of developing the same postoperative complications as patients undergoing general surgery. General late complications from all abdominal surgery may occur including laparoscopic port site hernias or ventral hernias, and intra-abdominal adhesion formation. There are also several potentially life-threatening postoperative complications specific to bariatric surgery that clinicians need to be aware of in order to provide timely diagnosis and treatment.

EARLY POSTOPERATIVE COMPLICATIONS OF GASTRIC BYPASS

■ ANASTOMOTIC LEAK

Anastomotic leak (leak at the gastrojejonostomy or jejunostomy), although rare, is the most feared complication of bariatric surgery. Reported incidence after RYGB ranges from 0.5% to 5% but in most recent literature is often <2%. Risk factors include multiple comorbid conditions, smoking, and poor glycemic control. Smokers are counseled to quit smoking preoperatively and diabetics should keep their HgA1c < 7 preoperatively. Surgical technique risk factors include open gastric bypass technique, retrocolic anastomosis, single layer closure, and surgical revision.

Patients usually present in the first 3 days postoperatively with tachycardia, tachypnea, epigastric pain, and/or fevers. Tachycardia is an early sign, and often times the first and only sign of a leak. Diagnosis varies based on the institution, but usually includes UGI series with gastrografin and/or CT abdomen with oral contrast.

Based on the clinical status of the patient and the radiographic findings, surgeons may opt to treat the anastomotic leak conservatively or with reoperation. Conservative management includes keeping the patient NPO, on intravenous fluids, and antibiotics. If a collection is found on CT scan, this may be drained with CT-guided percutaneous drainage often performed by interventional radiology. Operative intervention is rarely indicated; however, when deemed necessary, many bariatric surgeons recommend placement of a Graham patch over the anastomosis and keeping the patient NPO until the leak heals. Resection and reanastomosis in this urgent setting is usually an extensive operation that is at high risk of releak given the inflamed tissue and contaminated surgical bed. A feeding gastrostomy tube may be placed into the remnant stomach at the time of reoperation if postoperative oral feeding is not anticipated for a prolonged period.

■ GASTROINTESTINAL BLEEDING

Gastrointestinal bleeding (GIB) is another complication that may occur early in the postoperative period. GIB during the first 72 hours is usually due to bleeding from the staple or suture lines. Risk factors include use of anticoagulation or antiplatelet therapy, and thick inflamed tissues, or thin tissues. Diagnosis of GIB in a postoperative RYGB patient is no different than diagnosis in any other patient; however, care must be taken in any invasive diagnostic technique performed, including nasogastric lavage and endoscopy. These procedures can distend the newly created gastric pouch and disrupt the staple or suture line. Most staple and suture line bleeding may be treated nonoperatively by keeping the patient NPO, providing fluid resuscitation, checking frequent hematocrits with administration of blood products as needed, and reversing any anticoagulation.

LATE POSTOPERATIVE COMPLICATIONS OF GASTRIC BYPASS

■ SMALL BOWEL OBSTRUCTION

Although rare, small bowel obstructions may occur after RYGB. The majority of intestinal obstructions after RYGB are due to adhesions, internal hernias resulting from small bowel herniating through one of the mesenteric defects created during the bypass, or kinking of the jejunojejunostomy. Symptoms can be typical of small bowel obstructions: abdominal pain, nausea, vomiting, and/or obstipation. However, they may be subtle with low-grade tachycardia and vague abdominal pain, accompanied by an abdominal exam that is difficult to assess due to body habitus. Clinical and laboratory findings are often nonspecific. Workup should consist of chemistries, complete blood count, radiologic tests including plain abdominal films, and CT scan of the abdomen with PO and IV contrast, which is the gold standard and should be done promptly if a SBO is suspected. If a mesenteric swirl is found on CT scan, an internal hernia—a loop of bowel herniated through an iatrogenic defect in the mesentery—should be suspected. Findings of an obstruction should prompt *urgent* surgical exploration; delay in doing so can lead to necrotic bowel or early perforation.

There should be a low threshold to surgically explore patients with previous RYGB who are suspected of having small bowel obstructions. There is little benefit to nasal-gastric tube placement in these patients. Before an operative intervention is undertaken, however, it is important to have imaging studies as a guide (CT scan is the gold standard). Laparoscopic exploration is feasible in the majority of these patients and a thorough exploration can be conducted to look for internal hernias or kinking of the jejunojejunostomy using this minimally invasive technique. Conversion to open surgery may occasionally be necessary. If an internal hernia or bowel kinking are found at the time of exploration, they can be fixed at that time. A revision of the RYGB can also be carried out as well in that setting if it is deemed necessary by the bariatric surgeon. If adhesions are present, they can be lysed at that time.

■ STOMAL STENOSIS

Stomal stenosis is another potential late complication of RYGB. Stomal stenosis is an anastomotic stricture at the gastrojejunostomy. The reported incidence is between 3% and 15%, making it one of the most common complications of gastric bypass. There is no clear single etiology of stomal stenosis. Risk factors include the method of creation of the anastomosis (circular stapler vs linear stapler vs hand-sewn), ischemia to the anastomosis, and marginal ulcers (discussed later). It most frequently occurs 4 to 6 weeks postoperatively, but may occur later, especially if the patient has developed a marginal ulcer. Symptoms of stomal stenosis include nausea, vomiting, dysphagia, and food intolerance.

The diagnosis of stomal stenosis may sometimes be made with history alone. However, it can be difficult to distinguish between someone who has stomal stenosis versus a patient who is eating too much, too quickly. Tests such as UGI or barium swallow may be of use to diagnose the condition; however, both tests lack sensitivity. Upper endoscopy can be both diagnostic and therapeutic and is a much more sensitive test.

Dilation of the stenosis using endoscopic balloon dilators remains the treatment of choice, and studies report 55% to 80% success. Complications such as perforation are uncommon and can be managed nonoperatively. Surgical repair or revision of the gastrojejunostomy is reserved for those who have complete obstruction or who have failed multiple attempts at endoscopic dilation. This is common when the stricture is due to ischemia or when long-term inflammation has been present, maturing the tissues into scar.

■ MARGINAL ULCER

Marginal ulcer, or ulcer at the gastrojejunostomy anastomosis, is also a potential complication of RYGB with rates ranging from 2% to 4% in recent studies. Marginal ulcers usually occur at the jejunal side of the gastrojejunostomy. These ulcers are thought to be due to exposure of gastric acid to the jejunal mucosa. Risk factors include NSAIDs, tobacco use, ischemia, H. pylori, alcohol, foreign body reaction, large gastric pouch, and gastrogastric fistula. Symptoms usually include unrelenting, severe epigastric pain, and patients may develop GI bleeding with hematemesis or melena. Endoscopy is the diagnostic treatment of choice and can be therapeutic if ongoing bleeding is present.

Treatment begins with acid suppression as well as treatment of the underlying cause, such as eradication of H. pylori, cessation of tobacco and alcohol, and starting an oral sucralfate slurry regimen. Patients must also be in maximal proton-pump inhibitor therapy, and many surgeons have patients on PPIs postoperatively. There is no definitive duration of such therapy, although studies have shown that 6 to 12 months appear to be adequate. Repeat upper endoscopy can help to guide therapy. If symptoms persist or if they become debilitating to the patient, surgical intervention may be warranted. Resection and revision of the gastrojejunostomy may be required to remove the ulcerated area. In the setting of an acute ulcer perforation, the patient should be taken to the operating room. Many bariatric surgeons opt for a Graham patch of the perforation in these cases. More extensive interventions are usually unnecessary and can potentially cause more problems.

■ GASTROGASTRIC FISTULA

Gastrogastric fistula (GGF) is a rare complication after RYGB. These are usually due to staple line disruptions and allow communication between the gastric pouch created for the RYGB and the excluded stomach. This communication allows gastric acid to flow from the excluded stomach to the gastric pouch and down into the jejunum. GGF are extremely rare, with a reported incidence ranging from 1% to 2%. Symptoms include heartburn, epigastric pain, nausea, and weight regain. Several options exist for the treatment of GGF including endoscopic injection of fibrin glue, endoscopic plication/suturing, and endoscopic clipping. Surgical interventions all start with resection of the fistula tract. Some surgeons separate the pouch from the excluded stomach via stapling or oversewing or resection. Others prefer to resect the excluded stomach all together to prevent any future GGF from forming.

POSTOPERATIVE COMPLICATIONS OF SLEEVE GASTRECTOMY

One of the most common early side effects of SG is significant nausea and emesis, occurring more frequently than other bariatric procedures. This can usually be managed with antiemetic agents, and symptoms tend to improve within the first month. Rarely patients may require rehospitalization for IV fluids and IV anti-emetics with gradual return to their diet.

Similar to RYGP, other important early complications include bleeding and leak at the staple line, and are managed the same way. Long-term complications of SG include sleeve stenosis and severe reflux. Stenosis occurs in less than 1% of patients, although the long-term data is limited. Stenosis most often occurs at the incisura angularis, and the clinical presentation includes symptoms of reflux; as the stenosis worsens symptoms include dysphagia and vomiting. It can be easily diagnosed with an upper GI contrast study, and can be managed by endoscopic dilation if identified early, but if presenting with severe symptoms may be operatively managed with conversion to RYGP.

POSTOPERATIVE COMPLICATIONS OF BILIOPANCREATIC DIVERSION-DUODENAL SWITCH (BPD/DS)

Mortality rates after BPD-DS are 0.9% to 1.1%. Similar to RYGP, postoperative risks include anastomotic leaks and marginal ulcers. In two meta-analyses, the leak rates were cited between 0.1% and 1.8%. The clinical symptoms, diagnosis and management are the same as previously mentioned. Marginal ulcer formation has become less common with efforts to preserve the pylorus when dividing the stomach with duodenal switching.

The most common postoperative complications result from malabsorption side effects. Bloating, abdominal pain and diarrhea are not uncommon; BPD-DS causes significantly higher rates of diarrhea compared to RYGP, with 63% reporting significant social limitations secondary to altered bowel function. One of the most common and potentially severe complications of ongoing malabsorption is protein malnutrition, occurring in 11.9% of patients and may require parenteral nutrition. Short term reoperation rate for BPD-DS is 4%, often from protein malnutrition; 44.8% of patients undergoing BPD-DS within 5 years require additional operative interventions related to the initial procedure, some due to severe protein malnutrition. This involves reversal of the BPD completely or lengthening the common channel to allow for more surface area for absorption. A late complication potential is Wernicke's encephalopathy, which may result if the malnutrition is slower and later in onset. Vitamin deficiencies (reviewed later) are a common complication of BPD-DS.

POSTOPERATIVE COMPLICATIONS OF ADJUSTABLE GASTRIC BANDING

Several adjustable gastric band complications are possible and can either occur early or late. The mortality of AGB is <0.1%, but there are a number of potential complications including port or port-site infection, band infection, band slippage or gastric prolapse, hiatal hernia, band erosion and fibrosis. Banding is done less commonly due to its many complications; many now opt to remove the band and convert the patient to a RYGB or sleeve gastrectomy.

■ INFECTION

Port and port-site infections may initially be treated with antibiotics. If these infections occur in the late postoperative period, a prompt upper endoscopy is indicated to exclude a gastric erosion. The intra-abdominal portion of a band may also become infected both in the

early and late postoperative period. Patients may initially present with port or port-site infections that do not resolve despite antibiotic treatment. As the infection progresses patients may develop fever, abdominal pain, abscesses, and peritonitis. Treatment is removal of the infected band. Patients should have intraoperative tests to determine whether there is a leak from the stomach or esophagus. Antibiotics are also warranted for 7 to 10 days postoperatively. Bands can usually be replaced after 3 months.

■ GASTRIC PROLAPSE OR BAND SLIPPAGE

Gastric prolapse or band slippage occurs in approximately 5% of patients, but was as high as 15% for earlier techniques employed for placement in the 1990s. This phenomenon refers to the cephalad herniation of the gastric fundus through the band. Symptoms of band slippage are secondary to a gastric outlet-type obstruction and include nausea, heartburn or reflux, and the inability to swallow liquids. Some patients may complain of erratic function of the band; some days they feel no restriction, whereas other days they are unable to eat anything. These symptoms of gastric prolapse and/or band slippage can sometimes be relieved by removing some of the fluid from the band. In patients with worsening or persistent symptoms and in patients in whom removing fluid from the band does not improve symptoms, urgent surgery is required to either remove the band or move the band to the correct position on the stomach. After reduction of the prolapse, it is important to test the stomach and esophagus for evidence of leak. If uncorrected, a functional stenosis may develop causing distal esophageal dilation.

■ HIATAL HERNIA

Hiatal hernias can be found preoperatively on UGI series. If found preoperatively, these hernias should be repaired at the time of placement of the adjustable gastric banding. Occasionally hiatal hernias are found intraoperatively at the time of the dissection performed to free the right crus. If hiatal hernias are not fixed at the time of band placement or develop after band placement, patients may have symptoms of heartburn and reflux when the band is tightened. These symptoms tend to be alleviated with loosening of the band. If symptoms are persistent or weight loss is suboptimal due to the small amount of fluid in the band, repair of the hernia is indicated. This often requires removal and replacement of the band in addition to repair of the hiatal hernia.

■ BAND EROSION

Erosion of the gastric wall by an adjustable gastric band can occur after the first few weeks of placement or after a prolonged period. Incidence of band erosion is between 0.5% and 1%. Early erosions are thought to be secondary to unrecognized operative trauma to the stomach and may be considered an intraoperative injury more than a true band erosion, but may be secondary to the band being too tight. These patients can present with peritonitis requiring emergent operation; however, the large majority of patients with band erosions have a silent, chronic course that may present with abdominal pain or port-site infection. A typical course of band erosion develops over months to years. As the gastric secretions slowly leak out, the body develops a local inflammatory response. The inflammation eventually tracks out to the subcutaneous port and skin via the tubing that connects the band and the port, leading to local port-site infection. The development of gastric ulcers can also lead to band erosion. Patients with band erosions often do not have overt symptoms; instead they often present with failure of the restrictive properties of the band and/or a nonfunctioning band.

Diagnosis of band erosion is best made with upper endoscopy. Most erosions occur between the gastric fundus anteriorly and the band at the location where the fundus has been plicated over the band. UGI series are rarely useful in diagnosing band erosion.

Treatment is removal of the gastric band and repair of any areas of perforation on the stomach. Intraoperative tests should be conducted to rule out the presence of a leak. If a leak is found, a drain should be placed. Some advocate an UGI series on the first postoperative day to rule out a persistent leak. Diets can usually be resumed after the UGI series, if no abnormalities are found. Most bariatric surgeons do not replace the band during removal of an eroded one given the degree of inflammation and contamination.

LATE COMPLICATIONS OF BARIATRIC SURGERY: NUTRITIONAL DEFICIENCIES

Despite having large stores of energy in the form of excess fat, morbidly obese patients usually have some underlying nutritional deficiencies, even preoperatively, due to poor dietary habits over a prolonged period of time. These deficiencies can be exacerbated postoperatively. The severity of these deficiencies is dependent on several factors: the patient's preoperative nutritional status, the type of bariatric surgery, the patient's compliance to the postoperative diet and vitamin supplement regimen, as well as routine follow-up with the bariatric surgeon, nutritionist, and primary care provider. All bariatric patients are instructed to take a multivitamin daily and undergo routine blood tests to check for any nutritional deficiencies.

Vitamin deficiencies are common after bariatric surgery. Vitamin B12 deficiency is common, especially after a RYGB. The parietal cells that secrete acid and intrinsic factor, and the chief cells that secrete pepsinogen are mainly located in the fundus and body of the stomach, which is excluded from the tiny pouch that is created in the RYGB. There is also no time for the intrinsic factor to mix with the vitamin B12 since the pylorus has been removed and can no longer slow gastric emptying. The small amount of acid secreted by the pouch combined with decreased production of intrinsic factor causes vitamin B12 to remain in the crystalline form, which is not readily absorbed in the terminal ileum. The prevalence of vitamin B12 deficiency is approximately 15% to 30%, and varies depending on compliance with supplementation. Because the body usually has large stores of vitamin B12, levels often do not drop significantly for 2 to 5 years after gastric bypass. For this reason, patients must continue to have vitamin B12 levels monitored long-term on a regular basis and continue with vitamin B12 supplementation. Routine vitamin B12 supplementation can lead to eventual supranormal levels and reduction of the amount of supplementation given.

Calcium deficiency can be seen after procedures such as RYGB and BPD-DS in which the duodenum and proximal intestines are bypassed. Normally calcium absorption occurs in the duodenum. All patients who have undergone RYGB or BPD require a high daily intake of calcium (2 g/d) as well as calcium supplementation (1200-1500 mg calcium/d). A lack of calcium can lead to increased levels of parathyroid hormone (PTH), which can then lead to the release of calcium from bone. Therefore, after RYGB, BPD, or other procedures that bypass the duodenum, patients should have regular tests for serum calcium, ionized calcium, serum phosphorus, alkaline phosphatase, and PTH.

In addition to vitamin B12 and calcium deficiencies, patients who have had a malabsorptive procedure, such as BPD-DS, will have malabsorption of fat-soluble vitamins (A, D, E, K). It is important for these patients to include supplementation of fat-soluble vitamins into their daily regimen and to be monitored for any deficiencies.

Mineral deficiencies are also common in bariatric patients. Iron deficiency and anemia occur frequently in both the preoperative and postoperative bariatric patient. Postoperative causes for iron deficiency include decreased absorption due to bypass of the duodenum, decreased gastric acid, which is needed to reduce iron to its more soluble form, and reduced iron intake. About 20–70% of patients develop iron deficiency after RYGB. Symptoms include fatigue, glossitis, stomatitis, and feeling cold due to impaired temperature regulation. Supplementation of ferrous sulfate 320 mg twice daily is often sufficient. Vitamin C supplementation has been shown to improve absorption of iron.

CONCLUSION

The National Institutes of Health recommend that bariatric surgery be considered in patients with a BMI of ≥40 or if they have a BMI of ≥35 with high-risk comorbid conditions after trying other nonsurgical approaches that augment weight loss. Surgical procedures are superior to alternative approaches in this patient population, and outcomes vary by bariatric procedures. Surgical procedures accomplish weight loss by restriction or by malabsorption, or a combination of the two. Gastric banding is less frequently performed due to long-term risks of band slippage and erosion, and superior weight loss and improvement of comorbid conditions seen with RYGP, SG and BPD-DS. These procedures offer a significant benefit of prolonged weight loss with a high rate of type 2 diabetes remission, better HTN and HLD control, and improvement of other conditions including GERD and OSA. Hospitalists encounter many eligible patients during hospitalization and can play a role in appropriately referring these patients to surgeons after they recover from their illness. As a growing patient population has undergone these procedures, it is imperative that hospitalists also recognize the unique postoperative risks that these patients have both early and late, and how to appropriately initiate the appropriate diagnostic work-up and treatment, and referral to surgical colleagues for management (**Table 63-4**).

TABLE 63-4 Postoperative Complications of Bariatric Surgery

Roux-en-Y Gastric Bypass
- Anastomotic leak
- Marginal ulcer formation at gastro-jejunostomy (GJ) anastomosis
- Small bowel obstruction
- Stomal stenosis (outlet obstruction at GJ anastomosis)
- Gastrogastric fistula

Sleeve Gastrectomy
- Staple line leak
- Sleeve stenosis
- Severe reflux

Biliopancreatic Diversion / Duodenal Switch
- Anastomotic leak
- Marginal ulcer formation
- Severe protein and vitamin malnutrition

Laparoscopic Adjustable gastric banding
- Port infection
- Gastric prolapse/band slippage
- Hiatal hernia
- Band erosion

Nonspecific Complications of all Procedures
- Postoperative bleeding
- Nausea and vomiting, dehydration
- Infection (UTI, pneumonia, surgical site)
- DVT/PE
- Myocardial infarction (variable)
- Vitamin deficiencies
- Cholelithiasis

SUGGESTED READINGS

Buchwald H. Consensus Conference Statement. Bariatric surgery for morbid obesity: health implications for patients, health professionals, and third-party payers. *Surg Obes Rel Dis*. 2005; 371-381.

Fontain KR, Redden DT, Wang C, Westfall AO, Allison DB. Years of life lost due to obesity. *JAMA* 2003;289(2):187-193.

Jones DB, Jones S. *Obesity Surgery: Patient Safety and Best Practices*. Woodbury, CT: Cine-Inc; 2008.

Nguyen NT, DeMaria EJ, Ikramuddin S, Hutter MM. *The SAGES Manual: A Practical Guide to Bariatric Surgery*. New York, NY: Springer; 2008.

Sjostrom L, Lindroos AK, Peltonen M, et al. For the Swedish Obese Subjects Study. Lifestyle, diabetes, and cardiovascular risk factors 10 years after bariatric surgery. *N Engl J Med*. 2004;351(26):2683-2693.

CHAPTER 64

Common Postoperative Complications in Neurosurgery

W. Alexander Vandergrift III, MD
Stephen P. Kalhorn, MD
Avery L. Buchholz, MD, MPH

Neurological surgery is a broad field encompassing a wide range of disorders throughout the body. As with any surgical subspecialty neurosurgery is prone to its own set of unique complications. Some of the more common complications in these patients are often recognized and treated by physicians outside of neurosurgery. The goal of this chapter is to highlight a few of the more common neurosurgical complications and give the hospitalist a better understanding of how to evaluate and treat these patients. This chapter is subdivided into intracranial and spine complications.

INTRACRANIAL COMPLICATIONS

PNEUMOCEPHALUS

The brain is enclosed within the meninges and is not, in the usual situation, communicative with the external environment. Obviously a neurosurgical procedure involving an open craniotomy creates an event in which the brain is exposed to air. At the end of a craniotomy, the closure of the dura, reattachment of the bone flap and reapproximation of the skin unavoidably seals at least a small amount of air inside. In response, the partial pressure differences of gaseous air will cause reabsorption back into the blood and tissues. In the interim, however, the collection of air around the brain can cause dysfunction and even injury. A minor amount of trapped pneumocephalus is usually inconsequential. A voluminous amount of pneumocephalus, however, can cause altered mental status and a depressed level of consciousness. In addition when a passageway to the bony sinuses is inadvertently or purposely created (such as an opening into the frontal sinus with the fashioning of a bone flap), there occurs the possibility of a one-way valve wherein air enters the cranium and is not allowed to escape. Under these situations, pneumocephalus can accumulate over time and occur under pressure hastening and magnifying the neural symptoms even unto coma or death.

Evaluation

Pneumocephalus can occur after any craniotomy or endonasal surgery. Even minor twist drill hole procedures can produce a minor amount of intracranial air (this is almost uniformly benign). Suspicion of this diagnosis should be considered when a postoperative patient does not return to their baseline mentation. An urgent/emergent CT scan is the imaging study of choice and will reveal the amount of air along with the point of entry in the occurrence of "sucking" pneumocephalus from an opened frontal sinus, ethmoid air cell, sphenoid sinus, etc. Severe pneumocephalus produces an "Mt Fuji sign" from the sagging frontal lobes (**Figure 64-1**). When diagnosed and followed, a "brow-up" skull film will demonstrate the bubble of intracranial air quite well and can be compared day to day for proof of improvement (**Figure 64-2**). Use of this imaging study significantly reduces the amount of total radiation exposure over serial CT scans.

Treatment

Supplemental oxygen is the initial treatment of choice for pneumocephalus. This reduces the partial pressure of nitrogen in the blood and helps drive the reabsorption of nitrogen (the main component of atmospheric air) into the CNS parenchyma and blood. A 100% nonrebreather mask is often used for 24 hours, after which the patient is reassessed with imaging if needed. A schedule of on-off administration rotating every 2 hours can also be used when there

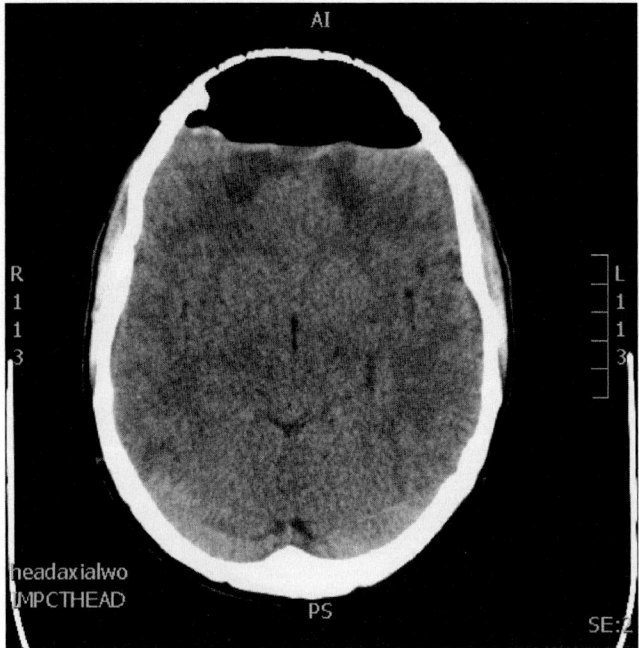

Figure 64-1 *"Mount Fuji Sign." While not classic for the typical peaked pneumocephalus, note the compressive nature of the air collection at the surgical site.*

are concerns for oxygen toxicity. When an opened sinus cavity is the etiology, the leak must be sealed. This is accomplished either via reoperation or temporary CSF diversion via external ventricular drain or lumbar drain.

■ MENINGITIS

As with any surgical procedure, a craniotomy may succumb to a postoperative wound infection. *Staphylococcus* species and Gram-negative rods are the most commonly identified organism. Endonasal surgeries comprise a special circumstance wherein oral and nasal organisms have a higher prevalence.

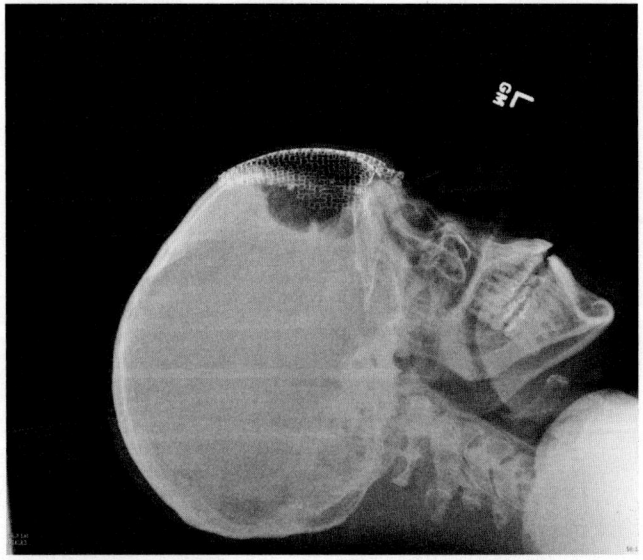

Figure 64-2 *Note the dependent collection of air in this brow up skull film. You can use this radiograph for routine examination and to ensure that the collection is dissipating.*

Evaluation

Classic signs of high fever, chills, rigors, and sweating occur, as well as meningismus, suggested by a positive Kernig's sign (pain with extension of a bent knee) and/or a positive Brudzinski's sign (involuntary bending of the hips and knee with flexion of the head). Laboratory peripheral leukocytosis, raised erythrocyte sedimentation rate and raised C-reactive protein are also usually present. A lumbar puncture may be needed to differentiate sterile aseptic meningitis (chemical meningitis) from bacterial meningitis, as aseptic meningitis can also occur after any craniotomy. In the case of a bacterial infection, the lumbar puncture will show elevated nucleated white cells, decreased glucose, and will usually have a positive Gram stain and culture. Aseptic meningitis may have an elevated white cell count but will usually be lymphocytic predominant and the Gram stain will be negative. Protein counts may be high in both.

Treatment

CSF infection/ventriculitis implies a nonpurulent infection and is treated somewhat differently than purulent drainage of a wound with meningitis. A draining wound with purulence requires operative debridement and usually abandonment of the bone flap. This is followed with broad spectrum antibiotics which are narrowed with direction from final cultures. Initially fourth generation cephalosporins or carbapenems along with vancomycin are used. In the case of nonpurulent ventriculitis, operative intervention is not usually necessary and treatment resides in administration of antibiotics only. Final duration of treatment is determined by clinical response, down trending of laboratory abnormalities but is usually at least 2 weeks, often longer. Imaging is often repeated with purulent infections to ensure walled abscess formation does not occur.

■ POSTOPERATIVE HEMATOMA (EPIDURAL, SUBDURAL, INTRAPARENCHYMAL)

The incidence of postoperative hematoma formation is among patients that are not coagulopathic is low (neurosurgery should always be avoided in patients that are coagulopathic). Unrecognized or undiagnosed coagulopathy may contribute to postoperative clot formation although the most common reasons in elective surgery are lack of intraoperative hemostasis or postoperative hypertensive events. The collection of a significant postoperative clot usually presents within the first 24 hours following surgery.

Evaluation

Postoperative clot formation will produce a local mass effect on the brain tissue with subsequent dysfunction, the characteristics of which reflect the location of the clot. Clots also have the potential for obstruction of the CSF pathways resulting in hydrocephalus. Patients with worsening neurologic defect on postoperative check or over the following 24 hours should raise the concern for clot formation and should be evaluated with an urgent/emergent CT scan. Headache out of proportion is the most common clinical symptom (**Figure 64-3**).

Treatment

Symptomatic clots should prompt a return to the operating room for emergent evacuation, and hydrocephalus should be relieved with CSF diversion usually with an external ventricular drain. The search for an underlying coagulopathy should be concomitantly started via laboratory evaluations and replacement/reversal agents should be administered as indicated.

■ POSTOPERATIVE SEIZURE/STATUS EPILEPTICUS

The incidence of postoperative seizures is roughly 5%. Any variety of seizure may be represented including generalized, complex partial,

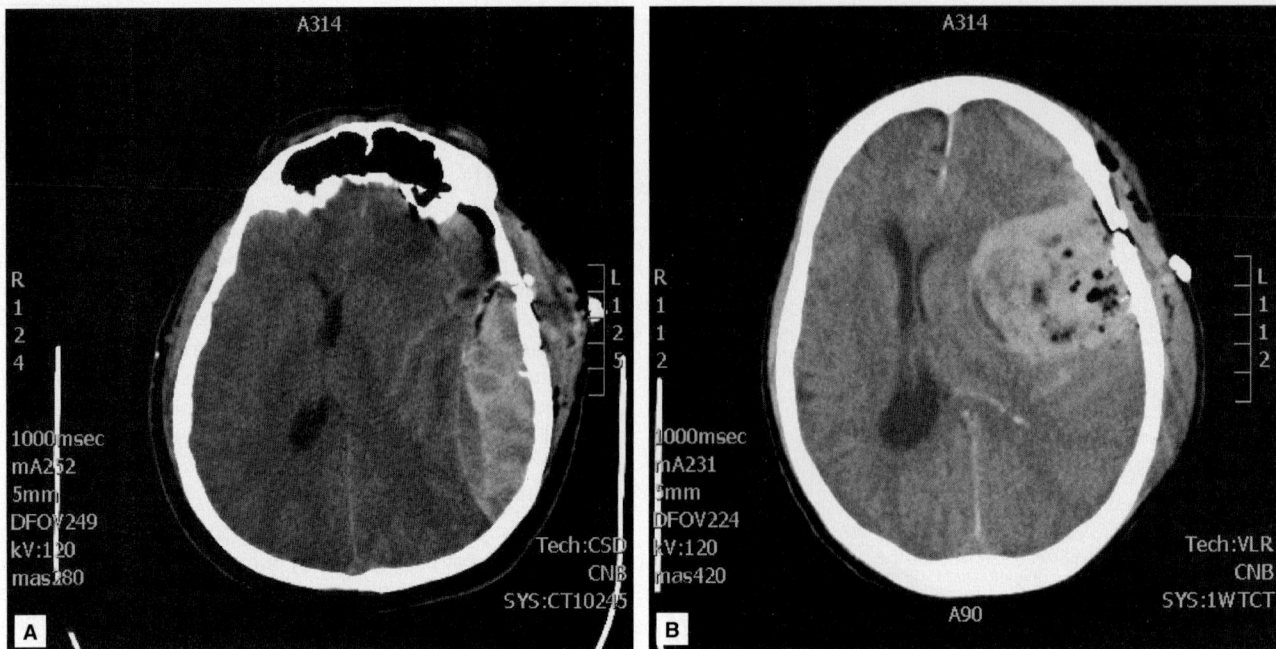

Figure 64-3 *Image A shows a postoperative hematoma in the surgical site. Image B shows a postoperative compressive epidural hematoma despite the drain between the skull and temporalis muscle. Note the degree of midline shift in both images A and B necessitating emergent evacuation.*

and focal motor/sensory. In addition, subclinical status epilepticus should be considered in any patient with persistent altered mental status (it is estimated at 8% incidence in comatose trauma patients). Factors that increase the risk for postoperative seizures include prior seizure disorder (especially with low-antiepileptic medication levels), pathology of the frontal lobe, younger age, malignant pathology, incomplete resection and intraoperative complications.

Evaluation and treatment

Suspicion for seizures should begin with interrogation of those witnessing the event; untrained persons may confuse seizure activity with posturing from brainstem compression. Once suspicion is confirmed, administration of benzodiazepines and antiepileptic's is indicated. For persistent altered mental status or concern for subclinical status epilepticus, patients should be placed on long term EEG monitoring with swift interpretation by an epileptologist so that further medical management may be instituted if necessary. New onset seizure activity after surgery may also herald a brewing intracranial complication such as an infarct or clot, which should be evaluated by a CT scan. In those with significant compromise in their mental status, they may need to be intubated for airway protection.

■ CSF LEAK

Cerebrospinal fluid is made at a volume of roughly 450 mL/d and the intracranial vault and spinal column hold roughly 150 mL thereby resulting in a three times turnover daily. This reabsorption into the bloodstream is driven mainly by the differential pressure between what is most commonly encountered as "opening pressure" on a lumbar puncture and central venous pressure. When a craniotomy is fashioned and then closed, care is taken to reapproximate the dura in at least a semiwatertight nature. Normal intracranial pressures test this seal at a minor level. Pathologic situations that raise the intracranial pressure (ie, postoperative hydrocephalus, aseptic meningitis, etc) can place an even higher stress on healing tissues and result in a spinal fluid leak. Post irradiated wounds, infection, persistent cancer, poor nutrition, surgery of the posterior fossa and poorly closed wounds are at higher risk for

leakage of spinal fluid. The development of a subcutaneous pseudomeningocele implies an "internal" or "contained" spinal fluid leak through the dura (**Figure 64-4**).

Evaluation

Clear fluid drainage from the wound with postural headaches (worse with upright position, better with recumbence) should raise suspicion of a spinal fluid leak. If there is a question of whether the fluid is CSF or more routine serous drainage, the fluid can be sent for a chloride level (which should be higher than serum chloride levels given the high-salt concentration in CSF), or for β-2 transferrin,

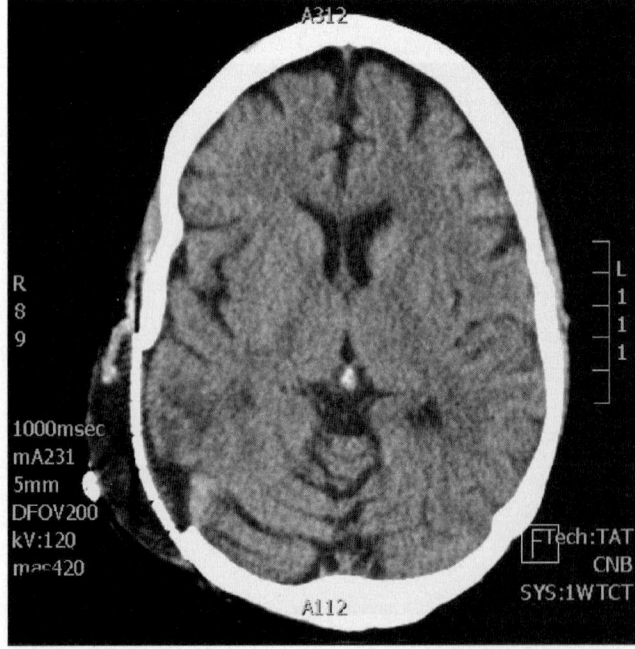

Figure 64-4 *This patient continues to have a cranial pseudomeningocele months after craniotomy for tumor resection.*

a protein only found in CSF. Of note, the chloride test is fast and cheap; β-2 transferrin is a send-out at most hospitals, will take days to come back, and is much more expensive "Haloing" of fluid leaked onto a sheet or pillow or testing for the presence of glucose can give some suspicion but is not diagnostic. On examination, pseudomeningoceles are found to be fluctuant or occasionally firm (when under pressure) fluid pockets under the skin flap used for the craniotomy. They may occasionally regress when upright and recur when lying down. Spinal fluid rhinorrhea can also occur when a craniotomy opens into the mastoid air cells, temporal bone air cells, ethmoid sinus, sphenoid sinus, or frontal sinus. Placing the patient in a nose-down position can usually elicit leakage of fluid from the nose to aid in the diagnosis.

Treatment

The underlying cause for a spinal fluid leak should be sought out and addressed. The most common cause for CSF leakage from a wound is hydrocephalus or infection. These should be treated accordingly (covered elsewhere). Prompt attention to the leak should be taken as its presence opens a pathway in which skin flora may enter the sterile CNS environment. Wounds should be over sewn at the bedside under sterile conditions or taken back to the operating room for repair. CSF diversion in the form of a lumbar drain or external ventricular drain may be necessary to lower the resting intracranial pressure. This provides a pressure-free period of time for the wound to heal. Prophylactic/empiric antibiotics are often administered to prevent meningitis/ventriculitis while the possibility of infection is investigated.

◼ HYDROCEPHALUS

Maintenance of intracranial pressure and stable CSF volumes rely on matched production and reabsorption processes. Imbalance (blockage of CSF pathways, overproduction, or impaired reabsorption) leads to increased CSF volume (and subsequent elevation of pressure) known as hydrocephalus. Hydrocephalus is not uncommon in the neurosurgical patient as is evidenced by the prolific nature of ventriculoperitoneal shunts and external ventricular drains on the neurosurgery service. Left untreated, hydrocephalus in a crescendo nature will ultimately lead to death as intracranial pressure matches blood pressure and cerebral blood flow is halted. Hydrocephalus may occur in the postoperative patient in a variety of ways including blood clot obstruction of the intraventricular system, blood in the CSF causing impaired reabsorption, or edema of the cerebral tissues obstructing CSF pathways. Postoperative patients may demonstrate hydrocephalus through symptoms of headache and signs of vomiting, altered mental status and CSF leak. Papilledema may also be seen although this is not always present in an acute presentation. Surgeries that involve opening of the ventricular cavities, posterior fossa surgery, craniopharyngiomas, epidermoid's, and infectious oriented surgery (cerebral abscess, empyema, etc) pose a higher risk for developing postoperative hydrocephalus.

Evaluation

Patients with suspected hydrocephalus should undergo an urgent/emergent CT scan. This should be compared to a symptom free scan with attention to size of the ventricular system. Comparisons of the width of the third ventricle, intercaudate nucleus distance, evidence of transependymal flow, and presence/size of the temporal horns aid in the diagnosis. In addition, characterization of the lateral, third, and fourth ventricles should be made to pinpoint a possible site of obstruction and differentiate communicative versus noncommunicative hydrocephalus (**Figure 64-5**).

Treatment

Upon the diagnosis of hydrocephalus, neurosurgical consultation is necessary to determine if CSF diversion is necessary. This may be done via lumbar puncture, lumbar drain or external ventricular drain depending on the circumstance. Under no situation should noncommunicative (obstructive) hydrocephalus be treated with a lumbar puncture or lumbar drain as this places the patient at risk for downward herniation. Permanent CSF diversion may ultimately be necessary via a lumbo-peritoneal shunt or ventriculo-peritoneal shunt procedure if temporary measures are unable to be weaned over time.

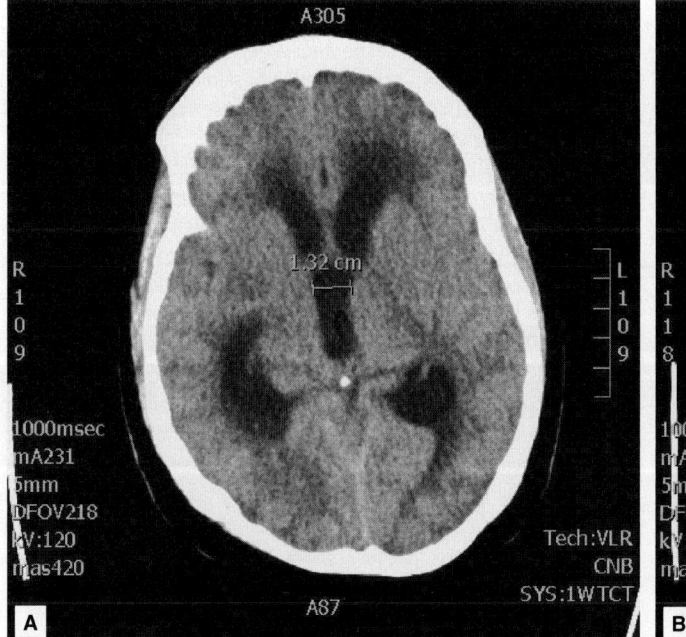
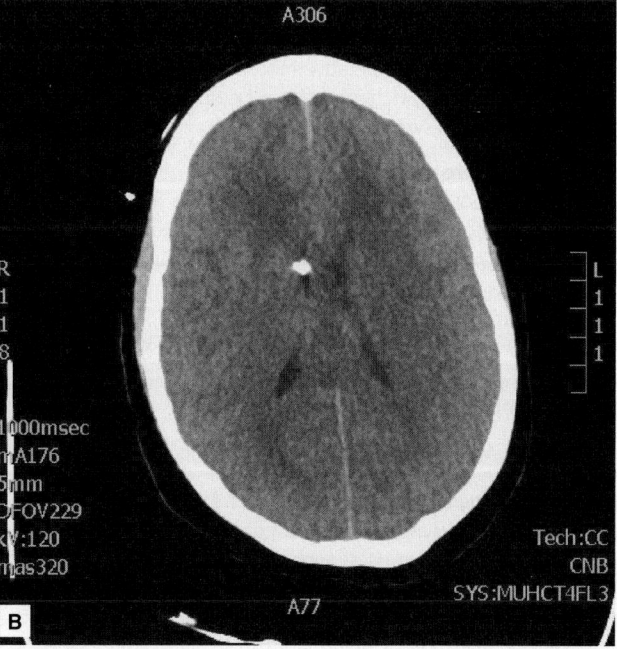

Figure 64-5 *(A) This patient has a classic case of hydrocephalus associated with meningitis. Note the transependymal flow seen in the lateral ventricle as well and prominent temporal horn and widened third ventricle. (B) The second CT is the same patient after placement of an external ventricular drain.*

■ SURGERY SPECIFIC RISKS

Certain surgeries carry particular risks that hospitalists should be aware. These usually revolve around the particular anatomy of the location of the surgery. Three will be mentioned below in more detail:

Facial nerve palsy

While this complication can be seen in any surgery involving the cerebellopontine angle or the course of the facial nerve within the temporal bone, it is best understood in the context of microsurgical removal of vestibular schwannomas (acoustic neuromas). These tumors usually arise from the vestibular nerve but tumors of any significant size will cause the accompanying facial nerve to be quite adherent and stretched upon the tumor capsule. Removal of the tumor has the potential to injury the facial nerve with a subsequent facial palsy, the degree of which can vary from mild to complete. The ramifications of this most immediately include the inability to close the eyelid and poor function of the orbicularis oris muscle making eating and speaking difficult. To prevent a drying injury to the eye, lubrication must be applied intermittently day and night and the eyelid taped shut at night. Implantation of a gold or platinum weight in the upper lid by an oculoplastic surgeon aids in eyelid closure on a more permanent basis and should be considered with complete facial palsies while the patient is still an inpatient after surgery. Speech therapy should be consulted to aid in eating and speaking exercises.

Pituitary insufficiency

This complication may be seen most commonly with pituitary tumor surgery but can also be seen with craniotomies for pathology of the central skull base (meningiomas, craniopharyngiomas, third ventricular tumors, etc). Complete discussion of pituitary hormone function is outside the scope of this chapter but attention to a few points is worthwhile. Injury to the pituitary gland can cause both rapid and slow changes in hormone production. Rapid changes include steroid production under the hypothalamic-pituitary-adrenal axis (adrenal insufficiency) and maintenance of appropriately concentrated urine through the production of vasopressin (diabetes insipidus). The clinician should be watchful for deficiencies of these two hormones as aberrations can produce shock and dehydration quickly. Care should be taken in their replacement however as the post injury underproduction can be a variable thing and dosing can significantly change in the days after surgery. Laboratory evaluation should occur the first postoperative morning and daily sequentially thereafter. More frequent checks should be driven by urine output and clinical signs and symptoms.

Lower cranial nerve palsy

Surgery of the posterior fossa, especially of the jugular foramen region and mid to lower medulla, can produce injury to the lower cranial nerves (CN IX, X, XI). Identification is important as their injury produces a loss of gag reflex and pharyngeal dysmotility that can lead to aspiration. Severe cases may require the placement of a tracheostomy and a percutaneous endoscopic gastrostomy tube. Less severe cases can be managed with close collaboration with speech therapy.

SPINE COMPLICATIONS

Neurosurgeons perform spine surgery to treat a variety of conditions including pain syndromes (back pain, radiculopathies, neurogenic claudication), tumors, degenerative disease, deformity, and instability. Some surgeries allow for patients to be discharged the same day while others require long hospitalizations with extensive rehab and recovery. The average length of stay is around 4 days. Recent literature quotes an 8% complication rate after spine surgery. This includes minor complications (eg, IV site phlebitis, accidental lacerations) and major complications (eg, pulmonary embolus, wound infection, CSF leak). Complication rates are exacerbated by comorbidities such as smoking, obesity, heart disease, advanced age, osteoporosis, and a history of prior spine surgery. For more extensive spinal operations, including deformity surgeries, the complication profile can be much higher (20%-30% or more).

■ PAIN, NAUSEA, CONSTIPATION

The most common postoperative complaint from spine surgery patients is incisional pain. Patients are initially managed with IV opiate medications and transitioned to oral medications as tolerated. Postoperative nausea and vomiting is quite common, limiting this transition to oral medications. The nausea is related to anesthesia and inflammation from surgery. Muscle spasm is also frequent. Short and long acting muscle relaxants will provide significant relief for these patients. Some patients are at a higher risk of developing an ileus, including those undergoing trans-abdominal or retroperitoneal approaches. Neuro-monitoring is frequently used in more complicated cases. This has been implicated in higher rates of postoperative ileus since the anesthetic technique needs to be altered to give no paralytics and high-dose narcotics to allow for motor evoked potentials to be checked during the procedure. Newer medications including methylnaltrexone (Relistor), a mu-opioid antagonist, can be given preoperatively to help reduce this complication in higher-risk patients.

■ INFECTION

Evaluation

The surgical site infection rate from spine surgery is often cited in the literature at 1% or less, however the risk can be much higher in patients with multiple comorbidities and more extensive surgery. Identifying high-risk patients and modifying risk factors such a nicotine use, high-HbA1C levels, obesity, and poor nutrition is mandatory. Proper patient selection is key to keep this very costly complication rate as low as possible.

Some erythema of the skin edges is normal as part of the inflammatory healing process taking place, but significant and/or spreading erythema present weeks to months after spine surgery is rare and an underlying infection should be suspected. A small amount of drainage from the incision in the first days after surgery is expected. If this drainage does not subside or even increases, underlying infection or CSF leak may be suspected. When evaluating an incision be mindful for breakdown or dehiscence of skin edges, purulent drainage, fluctuant masses below the skin (these may also be painful), and spreading erythema.

Occasionally patients with a thin body habitus will have issues with hardware causing pressure points and skin erosion. In all of these cases, it is best to keep the incision clean and covered and consult with the neurosurgeon. Wound care consultation is also useful in those patients with chronic wound breakdown.

Treatment

Imaging is helpful, usually an MRI with and without IV contrast, but plain CT and CT myelogram can be useful in some cases. Inflammatory markers (ESR, CRP), CBC, and blood cultures should be sent. Management ranges from a short course of oral antibiotics for superficial infections to percutaneous IR drainage and in some cases open debridement/washout with a prolonged course of IV antibiotics. Rare and complex cases may even require lifelong oral suppressive antibiotic therapy.

■ HEMORRHAGE

The incidence of acute blood loss anemia requiring intraoperative and postoperative transfusion is highly variable depending on the type of procedure. Noninstrumented surgeries and single level fusions rarely require blood products, but a transfusion for more extensive operations is fairly common and standard for open deformity cases such as scoliosis corrections (even if a cell saver is used to return as many red cells back to the patient intraoperatively). A very rare complication associated with long operative times, high-blood loss, episodes of hypotension, and prone positioning is postoperative blindness from ischemic optic neuropathy. The exact mechanism behind this is not fully known and is likely multifactorial.

Patients will commonly have surgical drains in place postoperatively. The purpose of this is to limit hematoma formation, prevent compression of exposed neural elements such as the spinal cord, and to decrease the rate of surgical site infections. Immediate thought must be given to epidural compression in patients who have a neurologic decline after a spinal decompression surgery. These drains will be monitored for 1 to 3 days in most cases before being removed after the output gradually decreases. Some drains that have persistent drainage will remain in place longer.

Evaluation and treatment

Postoperative patients should be monitored with a CBC on post op day 1 and sooner if needed. Vitals should be monitored for hemodynamic stability. Older patients or those with cardiac dysfunction will have less reserve than others and may need a transfusion at a lower threshold. The transfusion threshold for most postoperative patients is a Hgb of 7, but patient specific factors will influence this and continuing blood loss through drains needs to be taken into consideration by trending the CBC. (See Chapter 57 [Blood Products in the Postoperative Period].) Output of more than 150 cc/d is typically considered significant. The color of the drainage will also change from frank blood to more cool-aid colored drainage termed serosangiunous drainage. This is a mixture of blood and serous fluid that fills the dead space after surgery.

Epidural hematomas can occur and cause weakness, sensory deficit, and/or pain (incisional or radicular). These are fortunately rare. MRI or CT myelogram is the study of choice to evaluate for this. CT myelogram may be needed in cases where there is extensive hardware that would obscure MRI imaging. Surgical evacuation in symptomatic cases is mandatory. Full neurological recovery and elimination of pain is dependent on the timing of clot evacuation, with rather expeditious clot evacuations associated with faster recoveries. Large clots can compress the spinal cord, cause cord contusions, and even with rapid clot removal, some patients can still have residual deficits from sustaining this spinal cord injury (**Figure 64-6**).

■ CSF LEAK

Cerebrospinal fluid (CSF) coats the spinal cord and nerve roots and can be encountered in spine surgery. Iatrogenic CSF leaks are usually identified at the time of the operation, are caused by unintentionally opening the dura and arachnoid, and are either repaired primarily or in some complex cases just contain the fluid below the fascial layer which creates a pseudo-meningocele. These leaks are problematic because they can cause positional headaches similar to postlumbar puncture headaches. The patient is also at risk of developing septic or aseptic meningitis, where inflammatory cells, protein and blood in the CSF can cause headaches and meningeal signs. In addition, they increase the hospital length of stay as the patients are typically kept flat in bed as the dural repair and wound heals. These leaks are also known to increase the rate of other in-hospital complications, particularly in the elderly, who don't tolerate prolonged hospital stays much less kept in the flat in bed. If the fascia is not closed in a water tight fashion, the CSF can leak through the skin, which requires either placement of a lumbar drain to divert CSF until the wound heals or a formal operative repair.

Evaluation and treatment

In most cases, if clear liquid is emanating from the wound, CSF is the culprit. If there is a question of whether the fluid is CSF or more routine serous drainage, the fluid can be sent for a chloride level (which should be higher than serum chloride levels given the high-salt concentration in CSF), or for β-2 transferrin, a protein only found in CSF. Of note, the chloride test is fast and cheap; β-2 transferrin is a send-out at most hospitals, will take days to come back, and is much more expensive. Immediate neurosurgical consultation is recommended.

■ HARDWARE FAILURE

The incidence of a malpositioned screw averages 1% but varies depending on the area of surgery (cervical, thoracic, or lumbar) and type of surgery being performed. Patients may have pain and/or weakness associated with poorly placed hardware. Synthetic grafts may also cause spinal cord of nerve root compression. Over time, a patient's hardware may fail. Screws can come loose and rods may bend or break. In most cases, the instrumentation is only meant to give the patient's spine support while it heals and fuses new bone to compensate. There are early and late hardware failures sometimes seen years after an operation.

Evaluation and treatment

Patients who have worsening pain, pain in a new location, or increased weakness postoperatively should be evaluated with AP and lateral plain film radiographs as an initial evaluation. Further imaging with a CT scan and in some cases an MRI or CT myelogram may be needed but this should be discussed with the operative team in order to coordinate the most useful exam. Not all screws with a cortical breach are problematic and in need of revision. The patient's neurological exam must be compared with the suspected hardware complication. Occasionally flexion/extension or supine/standing radiographs will be needed in order to determine whether the newly implanted hardware is stable and providing support.

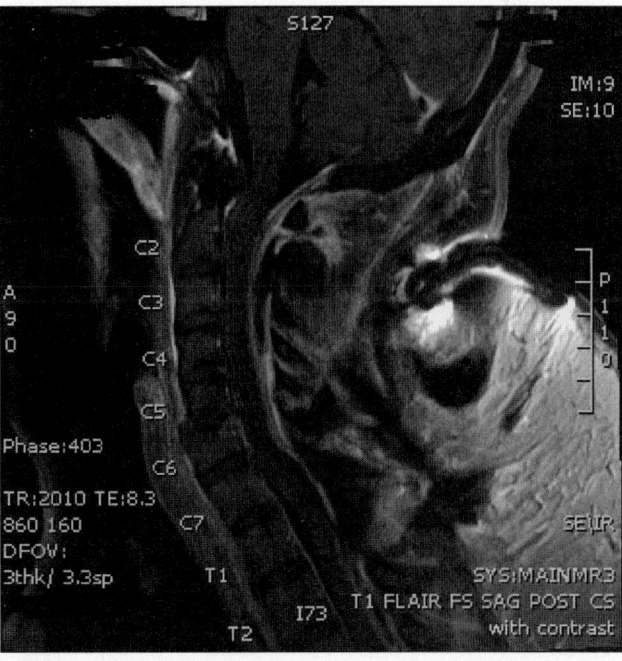

Figure 64-6 *This patient had a postoperative neurologic decline and was found to have a compressive epidural hematoma on emergent MRI. This requires emergent surgical evacuation to prevent permanent loss of motor function.*

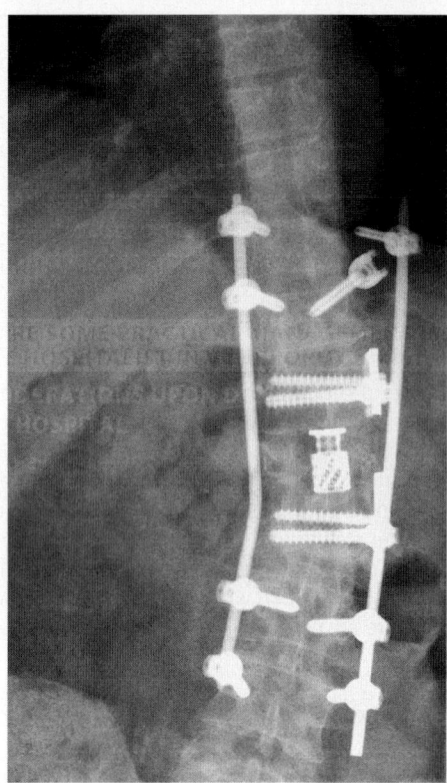

Figure 64-7 *Failure of spinal instrumentation. This patient has instability requiring hardware revision.*

These concerns should be coordinated with the neurosurgical team (**Figures 64-7 and 64-8**).

■ ADDITIONAL COMPLICATIONS

It is not uncommon to see a transient postoperative peripheral neuropathy or an OR positioning-related injury. These patients are commonly in the prone positions for an hour or more and can

suffer from skin tears, bruises, corneal abrasions, ulnar neuropathies, brachial plexus injuries, and meralgia paresthetica to name a few. Most of these issues are minor and resolve on their own without intervention, but some cases can take many months to resolve. It is frustrating for both the patient and surgeon to see this despite careful positioning and padding.

Additional complications seen in spine patients are not unique: this includes postoperative fevers, atelectasis, pneumonia, cardiac abnormalities, urinary tract infections, and thromboembolic events including deep venous thrombosis and pulmonary emboli. In the neurologically compromised population, including myelopathic patients, the DVT and PE rate is significantly higher as they tend to be more immobile from weakness in one or more extremities. Surveillance Dopplers are reasonable in high-risk patients preoperatively. Mechanical prophylaxis with sequential compression devices is standard. Chemical prophylaxis with subcutaneous heparin or lovenox should be initiated postoperative day one, and in high-risk cases, starting this intraoperatively may be wise.

SUGGESTED READINGS

Greenburg MS. *Handbook of Neurosurgery.* 7th ed. New York, NY: Thieme; 2010.

McClelland S, Hall WA. Postoperative central nervous system infection: incidence and associated factors in 2111 neurosurgical procedures. *Clin Infect Dis.* 2007;45(1):55-59.

Nasser R, et al. Complications in spine surgery. *J Neurosurgery Spine.* 2010;13(2):144-157.

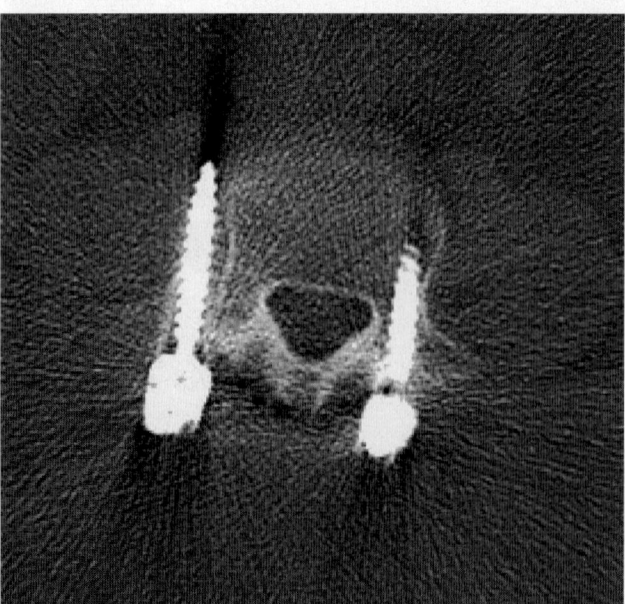

Figure 64-8 *This patient's right sided screw is seen clearly outside the pedicle. While not directly compressing the nerve root it does irritate the lumbosacral plexus at this location and can be a significant source of radicular pain.*

Management of Common Perioperative Complications in Orthopedic Surgery

Jacob M. Drew, MD

Harry A. Demos, MD

Vincent D. Pellegrini, Jr., MD

Key Clinical Questions

① What is the best perioperative volume and blood management in orthopedic patients?

② Which evidence based strategies prevent orthopedic surgical site infections?

③ What are the best strategies for perioperative pain management in these patients?

④ What is the best way to diagnose and manage compartment syndrome?

⑤ What is the best way to recognize fat embolism syndrome?

PERIOPERATIVE VOLUME AND BLOOD MANAGEMENT

■ EPIDEMIOLOGY

Exposed cancellous bone presents a hemostatic challenge, and consequently, nearly all patients undergoing major orthopedic procedures have some degree of acute blood loss anemia. The estimated blood loss for a total hip replacement is approximately 3.2 units or 4.07 g of hemoglobin, while total knee replacement patients may lose 1 to 1.5 L of blood or 3.85 g of hemoglobin. Blood loss after bilateral or revision joint replacement may be significantly more.

Historically, 10% to 38% of total joint-replacement patients received a postoperative blood transfusion, usually 1 to 2 units for primary arthroplasties and 3 to 4 units for revisions. While blood transfusions may restore oxygen-carrying capacity, replace fluid volume, and increase vigor, they expose patients to risks, including transfusion reactions, transfusion-related lung injury, antigen exposure, higher mortality, disease transmission, immunosuppression, and infection, as well as higher costs and length of stay.

■ RISK STRATIFICATION

While the most significant risk factor for acute blood loss anemia is the magnitude of the surgical procedure, several other issues must be considered. Patients on chronic anticoagulation are at high risk for development of postoperative anemia. If possible, medications such as warfarin, rivaroxaban, clopidogrel, aspirin, and even nonsteroidal anti-inflammatory drugs should be stopped preoperatively. Therapeutic anticoagulation should ideally be held postoperatively until adequate hemostasis has been assured and the wound has stabilized. Intraoperative bleeding complications are increased by 1.5 times if preoperative aspirin is not stopped, but discontinuation may increase the risk of postoperative cardiac and vascular complications. Thus, cardioprotective doses of aspirin can be continued for most orthopedic surgery patients who are at increased cardiac risk. Transfusion requirements increase by 50% if clopidogrel is continued perioperatively. Bridging anticoagulant therapy with therapeutic low-molecular-weight heparin is associated with a 92% incidence of bleeding complications, 69% occurrence of hematoma, and 15% development of a prosthetic joint infection; the perioperative use of these drugs in therapeutic doses should therefore be undertaken with caution.

Preoperative anemia should be identified, evaluated, and treated. Anemia is present in 21% of elderly patients who are undergoing elective orthopedic surgery. It is also common in patients with thrombocytopenia, chronic disease, and in menstruating females. Total joint-replacement patients with a preoperative hemoglobin <10 g/dL have a 90% risk of needing a transfusion postoperatively. Of note, preoperative autologous donation (PAD) of blood has declined in popularity because of cost, waste from overcollection, and increased transfusions. Current recommendations for the treatment of preoperative anemia include a thorough hematologic workup, correction of vitamin B12 or iron deficiencies, if present, and evaluation for other sources of ongoing blood loss, such as the gastrointestinal tract.

■ EVALUATION AND MANAGEMENT OF BLOOD LOSS

Intraoperative measures to limit blood loss and resultant anemia include the use of acute normovolemic hemodilution, tourniquets, hypotensive anesthesia, regional anesthesia, avoidance of hypothermia, blood salvage, meticulous hemostasis, topical hemostatic agents, and intravenous antifibrinolytics.

The use of antifibrinolytics has increased dramatically in the past decade. Tranexamic acid and aminocaproic acid are both lysine analogues that inhibit fibrinolysis by reversible competitive blockade of lysine binding sites on plasminogen and plasmin. By impeding conversion of plasminogen to plasmin, which is an enzyme that degrades fibrin clots, and interfering with the action of plasmin, tranexamic acid inhibits clot breakdown and reduces postoperative bleeding. By disturbing the physiologic balance between clot formation and clot dissolution, there is a theoretical concern that these agents may increase the risk of thromboembolic disease but to date the data have not borne out this concern. Numerous studies have demonstrated decreased blood loss, lower incidence of postoperative anemia, and fewer transfusions in total joint, spine, and orthopedic trauma patients. In some of these studies, high-risk patients with ischemic heart disease or previous thromboembolic disease were excluded, but there is increasing evidence that antifibrinolytic therapy does not increase risk of thrombosis in these patients. Nevertheless, rare case reports have documented cerebral thrombosis, arterial thrombosis, ARF, coronary graft occlusion, and PA catheter thrombosis. In our institution, the use of tranexamic acid has decreased the number of patients requiring a transfusion by 44%, with a 55% reduction in the number of units transfused per patient without an increase in thrombotic complications.

Intravenous crystalloid given intraoperatively quickly leaves the pressurized intravascular space and accumulates in the interstitial (or "third") space. Intravascular normovolemia must be maintained perioperatively, but significant postoperative weight gain is a marker of excessive *extravascular* fluid and is frequently a poor prognostic sign. Pathologic interstitial fluid shifts occur with infection, large procedures, major trauma, and inflammation. Isotonic crystalloid for fluid maintenance and replacement decreases the interstitial shift by maintaining an intravascular osmotic gradient. Colloids (hetastarch, dextran, and albumin) are more effective in maintaining this gradient and are preferred to replace blood loss in major surgical procedures. While the majority of blood loss occurs during operation or in the first 24 hours thereafter, decreases in hemoglobin and hematocrit may not stabilize until postoperative day 2 or 3, as interstitial fluid becomes mobilized. Often the decline in lab values is dilutional during this period and does not necessarily indicate ongoing blood loss or create hemodynamic instability. Incremental postoperative blood loss can be reduced by compressive dressings, minimizing phlebotomy, avoidance of continuous passive motion machines, optimized nutrition, and judicious use of chemoprophylaxis for deep vein thrombosis. Therapeutic anticoagulation should be avoided.

Postoperative anemia results in fatigue, decreased vigor, slower recovery, and increased length of stay. More severe cases may lead to impaired cognition, hypotension, tachycardia, dyspnea, and decreased tissue oxygenation. American anesthesia guidelines suggest that transfusions are unnecessary if hemoglobin is >10 mg/dL and is recommended if <6 mg/dL. Decisions about transfusions for hemoglobin values between 6 and 10 should be based on a combination of factors including medical history, symptoms, laboratory studies, and an understanding of operative and ongoing postoperative blood loss. When given, packed red blood cells should be administered on a unit-by-unit basis rather than ordering the historic-standard of two units at a time.

Postoperative anemia substantially recovers between post-op day 7 and 28, but complete recovery may be delayed by iron and nutritional deficiency. Oral iron supplementation is frequently administered, but is of questionable benefit. Gastrointestinal side-effects are frequent, and randomized trials have not shown an increase in hemoglobin recovery in the first 3 weeks of $FeSO_4$ administration, when return to 85% of the pre-op values occurs. There is a statistically-significant improvement of 3% to 3.5% in the next 3 weeks with iron administration, but the clinical importance of this change is questionable.

SURGICAL SITE INFECTION

■ EPIDEMIOLOGY

Surgical site infections are estimated to complicate 0.5% to 2.5% of clean orthopedic cases, including elective joint replacements. Currently, approximately 1 million hip and knee joint-replacement procedures are done in the United States annually. At a rate of 1%, approximately 10,000 post-op joint replacements will become infected annually. At an estimated cost of over $75,000 per case, the cost to the US health care system is approaching $1 billion. In most large centers, infection has replaced aseptic loosening, osteolysis, dislocation, and implant failure as the most frequent cause of revision total joint arthroplasty.

■ RISK STRATIFICATION

The most effective strategy for managing orthopedic infections is *prevention*, making risk stratification and modification essential. Development of a postoperative infection requires introduction of a bacterial load of sufficient quantity and virulence in a favorable environment, which often suggests an immunocompromised host. Knowledge of these factors helps us understand which patients are at risk for development of this serious complication.

There are numerous risk factors associated with the development of postoperative orthopedic infections (**Table 65-1**). These include factors related to the initial contamination of the wound, the patient's intrinsic bacterial flora, the wound environment, and host factors which may limit the patient's ability to eradicate potential contamination.

Assessment of potentially modifiable patient-associated risk factors is an important part of perioperative care of the elective orthopedic patient. It has been shown that 80% of primary total joint replacements and 93% of revision replacements have at least one modifiable risk factor:

- *Diabetes* is a well-established risk factor for SSI. Perioperative hyperglycemia affects the microvascular circulation, impairs oxygen delivery, and inhibits chemotaxis, complement function, and phagocytosis. Each of these factors contribute to problems with wound healing and infection. Uncontrolled perioperative diabetes has been associated with 2.25 times increased risk of wound infection.

TABLE 65-1 Risk Factors for Surgical Site Infection

Risk Factors for Infection	
- Inflammatory Arthritis (2-8%)	- Previous surgeries
- Diabetes (3.1-13.5%)	- Vascular disease
- Immunosuppressed	• Arterial
• HV	• Cardiac
• Transplant (10-15%)	• Venous stasis
• Sickle cell disease	- MRSA Colonization
• Medications	- Obesity (6.7× higher TKA, 42× for THA)
- Malnutrition (3-5× higher)	
- ASE > 3	- Anticoagulation
- Hemophilia (9-13%)	- Atrial fibrillation
- Malignant tumors	- Older patients
- Tobacco use	- Low income
- Renal failure (HD)	- Male gender
- Dental infections/hygiene	- Hospital or surgeon with low volume
- Skin infections	
- Chronic UTI's	- Longer operations (>3 hours)

- There is a strong association of postoperative *urinary tract infections* with prosthetic joint infection, but the significance of preoperative urinary tract infections is unknown. The most important factor is whether patients are symptomatic with obstructive symptoms in the preoperative setting; such patients should have urologic consultation prior to elective surgery. Pre- or postoperative urine cultures demonstrating bacterial counts of >100,000 colonies/mL require treatment even in the asymptomatic patient. Lower-bacterial counts may also warrant treatment in the presence of obstructive or irritative symptoms. Postoperatively, attention toward prevention of bladder distention and stasis is essential, and catheters should be removed as soon as possible to prevent colonization.
- *Malnutrition* is identified by transferrin levels <200 mg/dL, albumin <3.5 g/dL, or a total lymphocyte count <1500 cells/mm^3. Patients that are malnourished have a 5 to 7 times higher risk of major wound complications.
- Patients with *morbid obesity* have a risk of deep infection that is more than twice that of normal controls, and in some cases the risks may outweigh the benefits of surgery.
- Patients with *rheumatoid arthritis* have a 2 to 3 times increased risk of infection compared to patients with osteoarthritis due to a combination of innate autoimmune immunosuppression and the use of immunosuppressive medications. Anti-inflammatories, prednisone, methotrexate, and biologic agents are all associated with wound healing complications and infections. Perioperative cessation of methotrexate and biologic agents is controversial, but frequently recommended. Prednisone has a high association with immunosuppression and perioperative infection, but is not usually stopped because of the risk of disease flares and acute adrenal insufficiency.
- *Smoking* is a frequently occurring modifiable risk factor. Smokers have 3 times the risk of wound healing complications with 3 to 4 times higher rates of nonunion in fractures and spinal fusions. Nicotine-containing products should be stopped 4 to 6 weeks prior to surgery, if possible.

■ EVALUATION AND MANAGEMENT OF SSI

There is no single reliable diagnostic test to rule-in or rule-out *early postoperative infection*, making evaluation difficult. Fever and elevated white cell count in the immediate postoperative period are common and often due to atelectasis and small amounts of embolized fat in patients undergoing orthopedic surgery. Disproportionate pain, prolonged wound drainage, or excessive erythema most commonly occur. Wounds with purulent drainage or a sinus tract should be considered infected. Serologic testing is nonspecific, and therefore only marginally useful in the perioperative period. Both erythrocyte sedimentation rate (ESR) and C-reactive protein (CRP) are typically elevated in the early postoperative setting; the CRP returns to normal in about 3 weeks and ESR in 6 weeks.

Aspiration or biopsy of a suspected orthopedic surgical site infection is the gold standard diagnostic test. Fluid obtained should be sent for cell count with differential, as well as aerobic and anaerobic cultures. In the early postoperative setting, the white blood cell count in a total joint replacement can be as high as 27,000 WBCs/μL, but should be below 3000 in the nonacute setting. A neutrophil count of greater than 89% is highly sensitive and specific for infection even in the first 6 weeks following surgery. Fluid culture has relatively low sensitivity at about 75%, but is 95% specific for infection. False negative cultures are frequently associated with administration of antibiotics, which should be held for at least 2 weeks prior to sending cultures for reliable results.

Treatment of orthopedic surgical site infection requires both operative and medical management. Since there are large amounts

---

TABLE 65-2 Goals of Treatment of Orthopedic Infections*

1. Prevention of life-threatening bacteremia and sepsis.
2. Prevention of local or hematogenous remote extension of the infection.
3. Salvage of the affected extremity and avoidance of potential amputation.
4. Infection suppression to allow for union of fractures or spinal fusion.
5. Preservation of function of the infected prosthesis or hardware.
6. Long-term eradication of the infection and prevention of recurrence.

*In order priority.

---

of surface area around implants that are not exposed to blood and vascularized tissue, antibiotics alone are ineffective in eradicating most hardware associated infections. Moreover, the biofilm layer that forms within days of acute infection and is associated with many bacteria is usually not cleared even with surgical debridement. Most acute postoperative or hematogenous infections warrant a trial of surgical irrigation, debridement, and implant retention followed by IV antibiotic therapy. Chronic infections usually require hardware removal, IV antibiotics, and a staged reconstruction for successful eradication of the infection.

The goals of treatment of orthopedic infections are listed in **Table 65-2**. It is important to realize that management may be variable depending on numerous patient factors, and achieving all of the stated goals may not be possible in all patients. This requires extensive collaboration between the orthopedic surgeon, the hospitalist, and the infectious disease consultants.

Patients should maintain a sterile dressing over the wound until all serous drainage has stopped and the wound has become sealed. Persistent drainage beyond 2 weeks usually warrants operative investigation and debridement for early detection and eradication of a potential infection. Oral antibiotics for erythematous or draining wounds are rarely indicated and may complicate diagnosis via false-negative culture results as a deep infection progresses. Administration of oral antibiotics is associated with poor outcomes if debridement and implant retention is attempted as they often lead to a delay in diagnosis, establishment of a mature biofilm, and development of antibiotic resistance. Fever or an increase in pain or swelling may be the first signs of an infection, and should be thoroughly evaluated.

Long-term protection of previously implanted orthopedic hardware is also important. Patients should be informed of potential risks and understand the importance of prompt treatment of remote infections, particularly of the hands, feet, and mouth. Antibiotic prophylaxis for dental and other procedures is controversial but favored by most orthopedic surgeons.

PERIOPERATIVE PAIN MANAGEMENT
■ EPIDEMIOLOGY

Acute pain following orthopedic surgery remains one of the most vexing challenges impacting patient experience and outcome. Historically, general anesthesia (GA) combined with either oral or parenteral narcotic medications have been the preferred strategies to address postoperative pain in the orthopedic patient. With classic opioid-centric postoperative pain regimens, the incidence of adverse drug events has been reported to be 8.5% among total joint-replacement (TJR) patients. This accounts for greater than half of all postoperative in-hospital complications and contributes to increased length of stay. In recent years, concerns regarding the side-effects of GA combined with high-dose opioids have prompted the evolution and popularity of multimodal analgesic regimens. Multimodal analgesia was first popularized among total joint-replacement patients, but has expanded to orthopedic trauma and spine patients as well.

■ RISK STRATIFICATION

Pain regimens need to be tailored to the individual patient, particularly with respect to opioids in the following situations:

- Elderly patients as well as those with known hepatic or renal dysfunction may have impaired drug clearance, and therefore may be more susceptible to side effects if dosages are not properly adjusted.
- Patients with obstructive sleep apnea have increased rates of cardiopulmonary complications, including arrest, following major surgery. Many analgesics, but most notably opioids, exacerbate hypoxia via reduction of respiratory drive, volume, and alertness, and may cause previously undiagnosed apnea to become clinically relevant in the postoperative setting.
- Patients taking regular doses of opioids preoperatively may develop a tolerance to postoperative narcotic pain medications. These patients are likely to present a challenge in terms of management of acute pain and may require significantly increased doses compared to the opiate-naïve patient.
- Obese patients can require dose adjustments of fat-soluble medications like opioids to avoid sequestration and effective dilution in excess adipose tissue.

■ EVALUATION AND MANAGEMENT OF PAIN

Acute pain that is poorly controlled postoperatively may lead to hypertension, tachycardia, increased tissue oxygen demand, myocardial ischemia, and decreased minute ventilation from respiratory depression with pulmonary complications (including pneumonia). Pain prevents patients from effectively mobilizing and participating in therapy, which may jeopardize the outcome of surgery. Additionally, acute pain affects two of the classic components of Virchow's

triad via indirect inhibition of fibrinolysis as well as limiting mobility and contributing to venous stasis. Safe and effective treatment of acute pain in the postoperative setting is of paramount importance for these reasons and also to improve the overall patient experience.

Now gaining popularity nationwide, the combination of regional plus multimodal anesthesia is replacing the historic strategy of general anesthesia plus opioid-centric analgesia as the new standard of care for orthopedic surgery patients. This concept aims to both prevent and treat acute pain by using a combination of agents with different mechanisms of action in order to maximize the analgesic effects while decreasing undesirable side effects of any single agent (**Figures 65-1 and 65-2**).

One of the principles of multimodal analgesia is the preemptive treatment of acute pain, and therefore medications are initiated prior to surgery and continued postoperatively. Though substantial variability exists between institutions, a typical multimodal protocol will include some combination of opioids, acetaminophen, peripheral as well as central nerve blockade, local anesthetics, steroids, NSAIDs, and anticonvulsants. The synergistic effects of combination agents allows each to be dosed more conservatively than with single medication therapy. Though the severity and likelihood of side effects of any individual agent may be diminished, the spectrum of possible concerns expands with the additional medications.

Regional as opposed to general anesthesia offers advantages including a decreased incidence of postoperative nausea and confusion, improved early postoperative comfort, and facilitates early mobilization. Several potential complications specifically related to neuraxial and peripheral regional anesthesia need to be considered:

- Epidural hematoma is a rare though potentially devastating complication of combined spinal-epidural (CSE) anesthesia, occurring in <1/100,000 patients who receive epidural or spinal anesthesia. Orthopedic patients commonly receive anticoagulants to prevent VTE in the postoperative period, theoretically increasing the risk of hematoma formation.
- Epidural abscess is also rare but can be devastating; it is likely to present with systemic signs of infection, including fever, chills, nausea, and malaise.

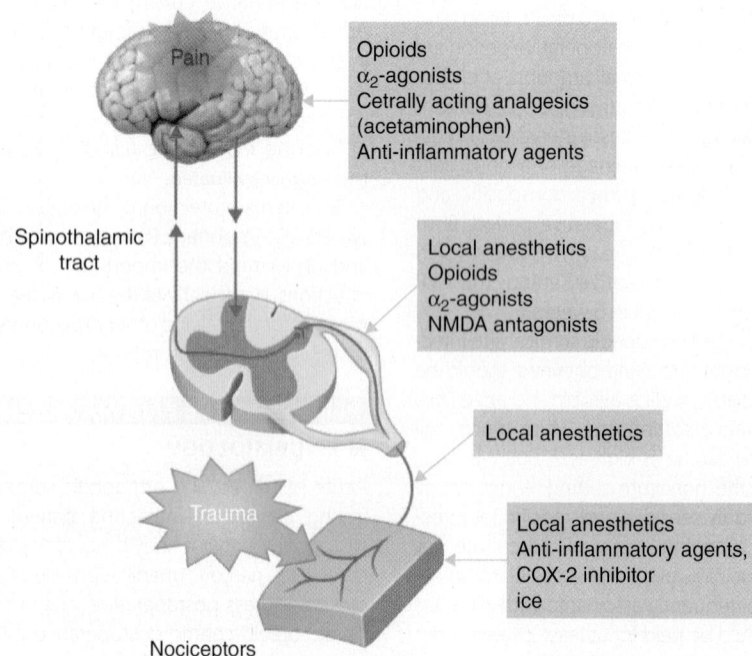

Figure 65-1 *Multimodal analgesia pathways, agents, and targets.* (From Kehlet H, Dahl JB. The value of "multimodal" or "balanced analgesia" in postoperative pain treatment. *Anesth Analg.* 1993;77:1048-1056.)

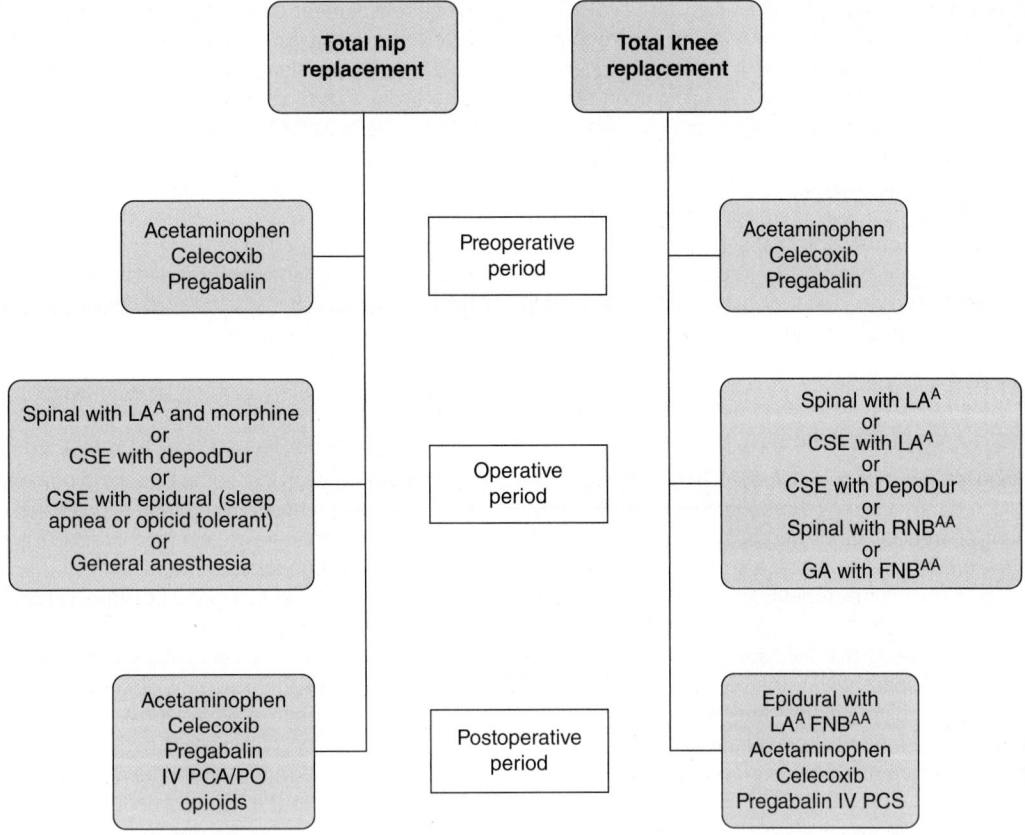

Figure 65-2 *An example of a multimodal analgesia pathway for total joint replacement patients.* CSE, combined spinal-epidural anesthesia; FNB, femoral nerve block; GA, general anesthesia; IV, intravenous; LA, local anesthetic; PCA, patient-controlled analgesia; PO, oral. (From Parvizi J, et al. *J Bone Joint Surg.* 2011;93(11):1075-1084.)

- Abnormal motor blockade in a postoperative CSE patient warrants close monitoring and likely requires further evaluation. Lumbar spine MRI is the most informative and appropriate diagnostic study.
- CSE may be associated with persistent hypotension in the early postoperative period. Anesthetic medications delivered to the lumbar epidural space can affect the lumbosacral sympathetic chain, thereby producing an effective transient sympathectomy. Resulting vasodilation produces hypotension, particularly with the patient erect and standing; it is generally responsive to IV fluid support until the medication wears off.
- Urinary retention is more likely following CSE than after GA; patients receiving CSE may benefit from bladder catheterization postoperatively.

CSE anesthesia is commonly supported by local and/or regional nerve blockade. Local anesthetic toxicity is a particular risk if all three modalities are employed. Depending on the specific type of local anesthetic agent, a mixture of cardiac (hypotension) and neurologic (seizures) symptoms may be present, with bupivacaine being the most common offending agent.

The side-effect profiles of individual components of a multimodal analgesia regimen are well established. A few relevant orthopedic considerations deserve mention here:

- NSAIDs are a mainstay of nonoperative treatment of many orthopedic conditions, but also play an important role in the management of acute postoperative pain. Aside from nephrotoxicity and gastrointestinal effects, animal models and basic science studies suggest interference of NSAIDs with both fracture healing and osseointegration of implants. These biologic pathways are critical not only in the setting of trauma, but also following many joint-replacement procedures, the long-term durability of which often

requires ingrowth of native bone into and around the porous surface of metal prostheses. Though unsupported by clinical trials, most orthopedic surgeons prefer to avoid NSAIDs in the setting of either fracture or cementless arthroplasty despite their analgesic benefits. Similarly, NSAIDs inhibit platelet aggregation and contribute to risk of bleeding complications, particularly in patients who are also receiving prophylactic antithrombotic agents.
- Anticonvulsants such as pregabalin and gabapentin provide effective analgesia and reduce opioid requirements in postoperative orthopedic patients.
- Acetaminophen has long been utilized as an antipyretic as well as a central analgesic agent. Recently, intravenous formulations have been approved for use and proven efficacious as an adjunct for the management of postoperative pain.

COMPARTMENT SYNDROME

■ EPIDEMIOLOGY

Compartment syndrome in the extremities is most commonly encountered in the acute trauma patient. Tibial fracture remains the specific injury most commonly associated with compartment syndrome, and open fractures have a rate of compartment syndrome five times that of closed fractures. Patients with a vascular injury are far more likely to have compartment syndrome than those without. The consequences of unrecognized compartment syndrome may be devastating, including joint contractures, permanent loss of function, loss of limb, and even death.

■ RISK STRATIFICATION

It is important to know which patients are at risk for developing compartment syndrome, as well as those at risk for failure to recognize and diagnose compartment syndrome in a timely fashion. Patients incapable of providing an accurate history secondary to intubation, intoxication, or severe dementia can present a diagnostic dilemma. In these circumstances the clinician must rely solely upon physical examination and objective findings. Similarly, patients who have received a peripheral or central nerve blockade for the purpose of postoperative pain control may be unable to accurately report severity of pain, and this may delay the diagnosis of compartment syndrome. Postoperative orthopedic patients commonly experience swelling and pain, and occasionally neurologic symptoms in the recently operated extremity. Differentiation between expected symptomatology and those concerning for compartment syndrome can be challenging.

■ EVALUATION AND MANAGEMENT

An understanding of the pathophysiology of compartment syndrome is critical to performance of a thorough physical examination and achievement of an accurate diagnosis. Within each anatomic segment of the extremity, the soft tissue contents traversing the limb are contained within compartments bordered and contained by tough, nonexpansile fascial connective tissue. Upon traumatic injury, or other myriad events that increase the fluid content of a compartment, the fixed space within the compartment is unable to accommodate expanding volume and results in increased interstitial pressure. If the interstitial pressure exceeds the capillary perfusion pressure, oxygen-rich arterial blood cannot diffuse to the tissues, and relative hypoxemia occurs. This results in a positive feedback cycle by which the resulting hypoxemia exacerbates local inflammation and increases edema, which again increases volume and raises interstitial pressure, and further impairs oxygen delivery to tissues (**Figure 65-3**).

Once the positive feedback cycle has been established, it is difficult to reverse without operative intervention. Surgery for compartment syndrome entails extensile incisions and complete release of the restrictive fascial boundary of the affected compartment. Upon release, the liberated muscles within the compartment expand, often precluding primary closure of the wound. Open wounds pose risk for secondary infection and necessitate additional surgery for wound closure. Depending on the timeliness of initial diagnosis,

serial debridement of necrotic muscle and soft tissues within the involved compartment(s) may also be necessary.

The goal of evaluation and management of the at-risk patient is to avoid if possible, but at the very least recognize in a timely fashion, the need for surgical treatment of compartment syndrome. This process starts with identification of the at-risk patient. Given the drastic consequences of a missed diagnosis, even low-energy trauma patients with relatively modest symptoms deserve to be screened for compartment syndrome via a careful physical examination. Those patients with more concerning mechanism of injury (high energy, crush injury, delayed discovery), or concerning initial physical exam should be aggressively treated with noninvasive measures to reduce inflammation and swelling in the affected extremity and subjected to serial examinations. Aggressive application of ice along with strict elevation can prevent development of compartment syndrome, yet elevation in the setting of an established or evolving compartment syndrome can exacerbate ischemia. Treatment of concomitant hypotension can maintain capillary perfusion pressure greater than interstitial pressure and ensure continued tissue perfusion.

Other injuries and comorbidities may conspire to conceal the diagnosis of compartment syndrome. A high index of suspicion is necessary to avoid missed diagnoses. Classic medical teaching refers to the six "P's" for the diagnosis of compartment syndrome: pain, pallor, pulselessness, poikilothermia, paralysis, and paresthesias. With the exception of pain and perhaps paresthesias, all are *late* findings of compartment syndrome. If the diagnosis has not been established prior to the development of pulselessness and paralysis, the prognosis becomes dire as tissue necrosis is likely already ongoing.

Pain out of proportion to the injury is the hallmark physical exam finding of compartment syndrome. By definition, compartment syndrome cannot occur without swelling although it may be difficult to appreciate even significant edema contained within the deep posterior compartment in the lower leg. Compartments may be described as, in order of increasing concern, soft, full, tense or firm. The possibility of evolving or early compartment syndrome should be considered in the presence of severe pain despite less worrisome objective exam findings. In such instances, the patient should be reexamined frequently at regular intervals by the same

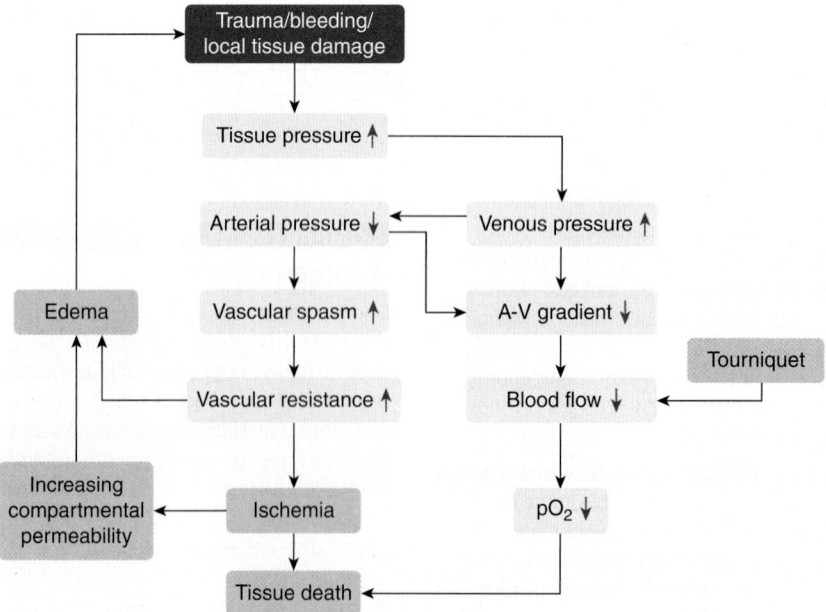

Figure 65-3 *The positive feedback loop and pathophysiology of compartment syndrome.* (From Aguirre JA, et al. Case scenario: compartment syndrome of the forearm in patient with an infraclavicular catheter: breakthrough pain as indicator. *Anesthesiology.* 2013;118:1198-1205.)

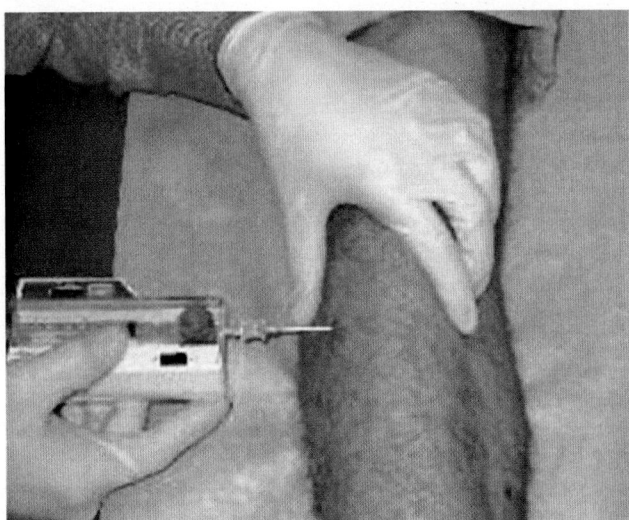

Figure 65-4 *Pressure measurement of the anterior compartment of the lower leg with a commercially available device.*

physician who may therefore recognize trends and changes in serial examinations.

Certainly a worsening examination in a patient at risk for compartment syndrome is concerning and warrants further action. Pain with passive stretch of muscles in the suspect compartment is the most ominous physical finding. Compartment syndrome is a clinical diagnosis, and this scenario would indicate the need for emergent surgical fasciotomies. In instances where the patient and/or the exam is unreliable or equivocal—such as the obtunded or intubated patient—direct measurement of compartment pressures is indicated. This may be accomplished via the use of commercially available devices specifically designed for this purpose, or a modified arterial line setup (**Figure 65-4**). An absolute pressure value >30 mm Hg is consistent with a diagnosis of compartment syndrome. Of more precise diagnostic value is an absolute pressure within 20 mm Hg of the diastolic pressure, that is, the delta (diastolic blood pressure minus compartment pressure). A compartment with a pressure of 30 mm Hg may remain well-perfused in a normotensive patient with a diastolic blood pressure of 70 mm Hg, as opposed to a scenario where that same patient were hypotensive with a diastolic pressure of only 40 mm Hg. Early consultation with orthopedics is advisable if there is any question or concern of compartment syndrome.

VENOUS THROMBOEMBOLIC DISEASE

■ EPIDEMIOLOGY

Venous thromboembolism (VTE), specifically pulmonary embolism (PE), is the most common cause of readmission and death after elective hip and knee replacement. In the absence of prophylaxis, 80% to 85% of THA and TKA patients will develop deep venous thrombosis (DVT), as will patients following hip fracture. Polytraumatized patients are known to be at high risk for DVT; pelvic (60%), femoral (80%) and tibial (77%) shaft fractures, and spinal cord injury (81%) are associated with the highest risk. Compared to patients with head, chest, or abdominal injury, those with isolated femur or tibial shaft fracture have a 5 times greater DVT risk; spinal cord injury imparts an 8.5 times greater DVT risk. Following TKA, in excess of 90% of thrombi occur below the trifurcation of the popliteal vein, and "proximal" clots occur almost exclusively by contiguous extension of primary calf thrombi to the popliteal vein. In contrast, after THA approximately half of thrombi occur primarily in the proximal (popliteal and common femoral) veins, are typically not contiguous with calf clots, and are discontinuous and segmental in nature.

Segmental femoral vein clots after THA typically occur in the region of the lesser trochanter and are thought to result from torsional injury to the intima incurred with positioning of the lower limb. Nearly 20% of postoperative calf clots will extend proximally and, once in the thigh, nearly 50% will embolize to the lung. Accordingly, conventional wisdom holds that patients undergoing THA and hip fracture repair have the greatest risk of PE by virtue of their high frequency of proximal thrombi.

Contemporary prophylaxis against VTE is considered standard of care subsequent to a 1986 NIH consensus conference on the subject. Venographic clot rates with potent new anticoagulants are <5% after THA and <20% after TKA. Reduction in DVT after TKA is relatively more refractory to anticoagulant prophylaxis than after THA; symptomatic VTE is now twice as common in-hospital (1% vs 0.5%) and symptomatic PE is twice as common after discharge (0.27% vs 0.14%) following TKA than THA, respectively. Despite these advancements, fatal PE occurs after 0.1% to 0.5% of total joint replacements, accounting for more than 1000 deaths each year. Appropriately, considerable effort has been directed at identifying the optimal prophylaxis regimen. However, use of potent anticoagulants to mitigate activation of thrombogenesis after orthopedic operations must necessarily be tempered by consideration of the bleeding risk following these procedures, where hemostasis is imperfect in the setting of exposed bony surfaces. It must represent a risk-benefit balance between the fear of fatal PE weighed against the morbidity of persistent wound drainage and hematoma, secondary infection, and reoperation resulting from bleeding associated with perioperative anticoagulant use.

■ RISK STRATIFICATION

Patients who have undergone disruption of the medullary canal of the long bones of the lower limb, either by virtue of traumatic injury or instrumentation for fracture fixation or prosthetic joint replacement, have the highest risk of venous thromboembolism (VTE) of any in the hospital. Intravasation of marrow fat contents is now known to be a potent thrombogenic stimulus and is largely responsible for the peculiar high risk of venous thromboembolism in the orthopedic patient population. Indeed, this risk is appreciated to be so high that all patients undergoing any lower-limb orthopedic procedure are considered "high risk" in the Surgical Care Improvement Project (SCIP) guidelines for VTE risk stratification and all are considered as automatic recipients of directed anticoagulant prophylaxis unless there exist specific contraindications to same. While heritable hypercoagulable conditions such as Factor V Leiden have been shown to account for a majority of spontaneous VTE events in the community, such markers have not been able to identify those among the joint-replacement population at greatest risk for VTE. Neuraxial (spinal or epidural) anesthesia is widely acknowledged to reduce the risk of lower-limb DVT by approximately 50% compared to general anesthesia, independent of the type of anticoagulant VTE prophylaxis employed in the perioperative period.

Orthopedic practitioners typically opt for one of three main regimens for perioperative VTE chemoprophylaxis; aspirin, low-intensity warfarin, or one of the newer anticoagulants such as fractionated heparins or direct factor X or II inhibitors. Choice of anticoagulant is driven by some approach to risk stratification among this group of high-risk patients; most surgeons agree that a past history of VTE warrants more intensive anticoagulation than provided by aspirin alone.

Guideline reconciliation finally occurred between the American Academy of Orthopedic Surgeons and the American College of Chest Physicians in February 2012, largely as a result of agreement that *clinically important* PE and VTE was the relevant endpoint and insufficient data existed to endorse any one specific prophylaxis regimen.

Concurrently, the ACCP placed greater value on avoidance of bleeding events based on acknowledgement of patient preferences and aversion to surgical complications. Likewise, the exhaustive AHRQ Comparative Effectiveness Review on Venous Thromboembolism Prophylaxis in Orthopedic Surgery concluded, "The balance of benefits to harms is favorable for providing prophylaxis … and to extend the period of prophylaxis beyond the standard 7 to 10 days." They noted that "interclass comparisons could not be made due to lack of data, similarities between classes on outcomes, or offsetting effects where benefits on efficacy were tempered by an increased risk of bleeding." In 2014, SCIP added aspirin to its list of acceptable agents for VTE prophylaxis, making the list of appropriate agents uniform and all-inclusive among all groups, with no endorsement of any agent or regimen as best practice.

■ INPATIENT PROPHYLAXIS

Chemoprophylaxis (**Figure 65-5**) can by grouped into three main categories; warfarin, aspirin, and selective heparinoids or direct factor Xa or IIa inhibitors.

Warfarin. Low-intensity warfarin (INR target 2.0), despite its variable dosing and need for monitoring, is a time-honored option for orthopedic thromboprophylaxis, likely because it has an acceptably low-bleeding risk (1%-2%) coupled with efficacy in preventing clinically important PE. In 2008, it was the VTE prophylaxis of choice for nearly 50% of US orthopedic arthroplasty surgeons prior to the release of direct Xa and thrombin inhibitors. Warfarin remains popular in the US, despite the inconvenience and expense of monitoring, because many feel it represents the best available compromise of efficacy in preventing *clinical VTE* and safety in minimizing bleeding.

Critics have been most concerned with its erratic effect, need for monitoring, and associated bleeding. Early studies reported bleeding rates of 10% with a prothrombin time index (PTI) of 1.8 to 2.0, but efficacy is now proven with a PTI of 1.3 to 1.5 (INR 2.0) and reduced bleeding to <2%. Historically, low-intensity warfarin prophylaxis (INR 2.0) results in venographic DVT of 9% to 26% and proximal clot rates of 2% to 5% after THA compared with overall

DVT of 35% to 55% and proximal clot rates of 2% to 14% after TKA performed with general anesthesia. Warfarin preferentially reduces proximal compared with distal DVT after THA and, when combined with epidural anesthesia/analgesia, the residual DVT rate dropped below 10%. Most importantly, *extended* low-intensity warfarin continued for 6 weeks after THA or TKA in 3293 patients was associated with readmission for clinical VTE in 0.3% in THA and 0.2% in TKA with a major bleed rate of 0.1%. In the aggregated THA and TKA groups, 6 weeks of warfarin after hospital discharge *eliminated* the risk of PE, and reduced VTE-related readmissions 0.2% versus 1.6%.

Optimal use of warfarin remains challenging and labor intensive; it ideally begins the night before surgery because of its 48-hour latency to anticoagulant effect. Indeed, this lag in activity is likely responsible for its popular safety margin with low-perioperative bleeding rates.

Aspirin. Aspirin, acetylsalicylic acid, is traditionally considered an arterial drug but has been used in conjunction with mechanical compression devices for *venous* thromboembolism prophylaxis by a consistent minority (10%-20%) of surgeons. Conventional wisdom holds that aspirin reduces arterial thrombosis through inhibition of platelet cyclooxygenase-1, which decreases synthesis of thromboxane A2 (platelet-activating eicosanoid) and related platelet activation, and has demonstrated substantial arterial thrombotic event reduction as well as survival benefit relative to stroke, myocardial infarction, and related deaths in high-risk patients. Conversely, clotting experts often regard aspirin as an inferior and inconsistent agent in mitigating venous thrombosis.

Since 2006, three large observational studies and the British joint-replacement registry have rekindled the notion that aspirin can prevent clinical PE after total joint arthroplasty, especially in conjunction with regional anesthesia. In nearly 10,000 THA and TKA patients managed with neuraxial anesthesia, in-hospital pneumatic compression, and 6 weeks of aspirin (325 mg bid or 150 md qd), overall VTE-related readmission was 3.2% after THA with a clinical PE rate of 0.6% compared with overall VTE-related readmission after TKA of 0.5% with a clinical PE rate of 0.36%. In 2009, National Joint Registry data matched nearly 23,000 patients receiving aspirin or

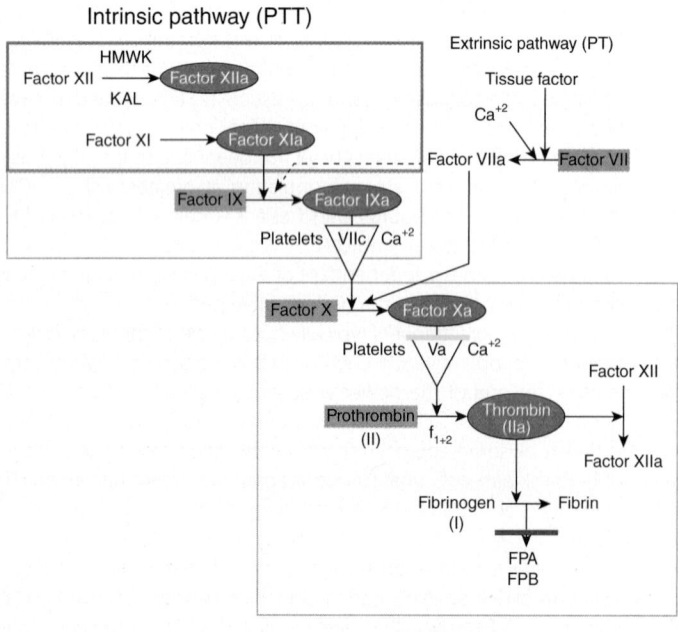

Figure 65-5 *The coagulation cascade.*

LMWH and revealed no difference in 90-day outcomes related to clinical PE (0.7%), DVT (0.95%), stroke or gastrointestinal bleeding (0.75%), or reoperation (0.35%). Yet, patients receiving LMWH had a survival advantage over those receiving aspirin (all-cause mortality 0.49% vs 0.65%; $p = 0.02$).

In two studies of >1200 patients randomized to aspirin or placebo for prevention of *recurrent* VTE after standard therapy, aspirin was associated with a 32% reduction in recurrent VTE and a 34% reduction in major adverse vascular events, without an accompanying increase in bleeding. Given its apparent efficacy without a compromise in safety, the role of aspirin in VTE prophylaxis and prevention of embolization of existing venous thrombi is being reassessed.

Newer Agents. Many new selective anticoagulants have been introduced since the 1986 NIH conference, but the risk of *fatal PE* after THA and TKA has changed very little. Despite venographic clot rates up to 5 times greater than with these newer agents, low-intensity (INR 2.0) warfarin and aspirin offer comparable *clinical* PE rates and two- to three-fold less major bleeding complications.

Low-molecular-weight (fractionated) heparins and pentasaccharide are incrementally smaller sugar molecules with increasing specificity in binding antithrombin III (AT-III) as the critical intermediary prior to deactivating factor X or II (thrombin). Indeed, synthetically derived pentasaccharide exactly corresponds to the five sugar AT-III binding site and enjoys enhanced specificity to bind factor Xa. Due to its more proximal location in the coagulation cascade, this affinity for factor Xa greatly augments the potency of LMW heparins and pentasaccharide. Accordingly, LMWH reduced overall venographic DVT from 44% to 31% after THA compared with unfractionated heparins; DVT reduction was also significant after TKA, but less dramatic. Fondaparinux (pentasaccharide) further reduced venographic DVT by 50% compared with enoxaparin after THA, TKA, and hip fracture. It was the first agent to reduce DVT to <20% after TKA and the most extensively studied agent after hip fracture, but its bleeding rate of 3% to 6% exceeded even that seen with enoxaparin. One meta-analysis demonstrated a two- to three-fold increase in bleeding after THA and TKA with LMWH compared with warfarin prophylaxis.

New direct factor X and II inhibitors require no monitoring and are administered orally. Rivaroxaban, a direct factor Xa inhibitor, has been most extensively studied in two THA and two TKA trials. Compared with enoxaparin, pooled analysis of the four studies demonstrated a 58% reduction in all-cause mortality and *symptomatic* VTE (0.6% vs 1.3%; $p < 0.001$) but aggregate bleeding data revealed an increase in major plus clinically relevant nonmajor bleeding events (3.2% vs 2.6%; $p = 0.039$). Rivaroxaban has enjoyed rapid growth in popularity in the VTE prophylaxis market, but an increase in bleeding events has dampened enthusiasm for its widespread adoption by the orthopedic community. One observational study demonstrated all-cause mortality after total hip and knee replacement in patients who had been given potent anticoagulants was more than twice that in patients receiving aspirin, pneumatic compression, and regional anesthesia. Another report specifically noted the "failure" of low-molecular-weight heparin compared with warfarin prophylaxis; symptomatic DVT (3.8%), nonfatal PE (1.3%), persistent wound drainage resulting in readmission (4.7%) and reoperation (3.4%) all occurred at rates exceeding prior experience with low-intensity warfarin. Finally, one retrospective review of 1048 consecutive THA and TKA reported a two-fold increase in 30-day reoperation for wound complications with rivaroxaban compared with tinzaparin prophylaxis. Not surprisingly, the orthopedic community has been slow to adopt these newer agents in favor of a more balanced strategy that offers less bleeding risk with comparable protection against *clinical* VTED.

■ INPATIENT MANAGEMENT OF ACUTE VENOUS THROMBOEMBOLISM

Management of perioperative DVT requires more vigilant treatment than a spontaneous event in an ambulatory patient. Typically, routine prophylaxis is continued for 35 days after operation and the occurrence of a symptomatic clot may further prolong anticoagulation to mitigate the risk of clot propagation and embolization.

With the advent of multidetector computed tomography for definitive diagnosis of PE, the prevalence of PE has increased 10-fold in the past decade, from 0.2% to >2%, without any explicable change in the operation or perioperative management. It is likely that this increment is largely explained by the recognition of very small peripheral subsegmental filling defects with this more sensitive CT technology. The clinical significance of these lesions has been questioned and it has been proposed that they represent embolization of marrow elements from instrumentation of the medullary canal rather than a conventional PE. When clinically silent hypoxemia is recognized with pulse oximetry, a 10-minute 2 L/min oxygen challenge has been proposed; resolution of hypoxemia has been suggested to indicate the absence of a meaningful PE and no need for further intervention. Persistence of hypoxemia deserves further workup. The observed frequency of PE has returned to less than 1% with this pragmatic clinical protocol.

Acute postoperative PE is conventionally managed with more intensive anticoagulation. There is increasing interest in outpatient management with the newer oral agents, however the substantial risk of bleeding in the early period after hip and knee replacement should temper the enthusiasm for outpatient management of PE within 5 to 10 days of the index operation. Indeed, when initiating therapeutic anticoagulation with an IV heparin bolus for clinically significant PE within 5 days of operation, the risk of major wound hemorrhage is 50% and within 1 week the bleeding rate decreases to 15%. In general, intravenous heparinization should be initiated with a constant continuous infusion without bolus therapy in the first week after total joint replacement.

In general, it is accepted that the risk of VTE after orthopedic surgical procedures extends far beyond the time of operation and hospital discharge. Clinical guidelines endorse 35 days of prophylaxis after THA and 10 to 35 days after TKA.

FAT EMBOLISM SYNDROME

■ EPIDEMIOLOGY

The fat embolism syndrome (FES) was initially described by Zenker in 1861 in a patient following a thoracoabdominal crush injury. It may be practically defined as a complex alteration in coagulation homeostasis that occurs as an infrequent complication of fracture of the pelvis and long bones and is manifest clinically as acute respiratory insufficiency secondary to the filtering function of the lung. The full blown clinical *syndrome* is evident in 0.5% to 2% of patients after isolated long bone fractures and approaching 5% to 10% of patients with multiple fractures and pelvic injuries following polytrauma. In contrast, *fat embolization* occurs as a subclinical event following *all* fractures as well as instrumentation of the medullary canal during total joint replacement. The likelihood that this event results in the clinical manifestations characterized by florid respiratory failure is determined by the quantity of fat intravasated into the systemic circulation and the ability of the patient's cardiopulmonary system to withstand the collection of this material in the lung.

■ RISK STRATIFICATION

Conditions that increase the size and fatty content of the marrow cavity, such as collagen vascular diseases and osteoporosis, increase the risk of FES. Children develop clinical FES nearly 100 times less commonly than adults, secondary to persistence of hematopoietic marrow and a paucity of fatty marrow. Instrumentation of the medullary canal during THA and TKA always results in embolization of marrow fat to the lung; concurrent bilateral TKA under the same anesthetic increases this risk and has been largely curtailed. Whether it is clinically manifest as FES is largely determined by the magnitude of the embolic load, the intrinsic cardiopulmonary reserve, and the ability to maintain oxygenation in the presence of pulmonary capillary occlusion.

■ EVALUATION AND MANAGEMENT

The initial insult after embolic fat to the lungs is characterized by increased right heart pressures and cardiovascular collapse, evidenced by hypotension, hypoxemia, confusion, and bradycardia, and is infrequently clinically evident in humans. It has, however, been reported after cementation of the femoral component during total hip arthroplasty, especially in the elderly osteoporotic patient treated for hip fracture and after intramedullary nailing of the femur for an impending pathologic fracture with concurrent filling of the medullary canal with methylmethacrylate. Autopsy evaluation typically demonstrates embolic marrow elements in the capillary bed of the brain, suggesting a lung filter overloaded with embolic material that leaks into the systemic circulation. Transient aphasia and other central neurologic deficits have been observed after bilateral total knee arthroplasty in patients with a patent foramen ovale; embolic intracerebral events can be seen by magnetic resonance imaging.

The more typical fat embolism syndrome is "delayed" in its appearance; clinical signs and symptoms typically develop in 85% of patients within 48 hours after fracture or instrumentation of the medullary canal. This temporal delay is thought to result from the evolving effects of vasoactive substances in the lung and the resulting decrement in gas exchange. Clinical manifestations are primarily cardiopulmonary in nature and include arterial hypoxemia; oxygen desaturation, sinus tachycardia, and fever comprise the classic triad of early findings. Nonspecific changes of pulmonary congestion may be seen on the chest radiograph and the EKG often exhibits ST segment elevation from ischemia or right heart strain. Alterations in cognition are common and may include lethargy, delirium, and/or seizures secondary to hypoxemia or fat embolization to the brain. Petecchiae develop in more than half of patients and typically occur in the axilla (**Figure 65-6**), over the chest and base of the neck, and

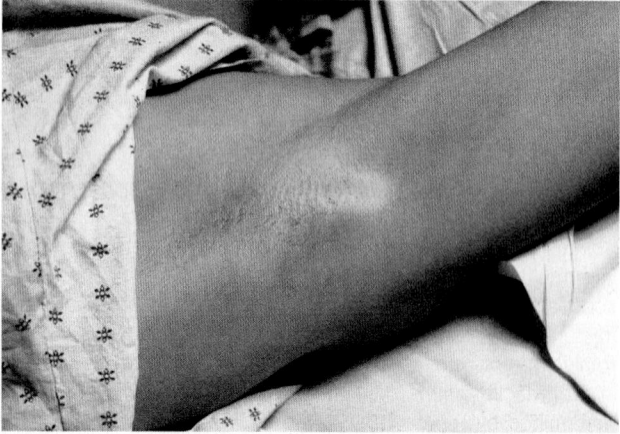

Figure 65-6 *Axillary petechiae in a patient with clinically evident fat embolism syndrome.*

in the conjunctivae; they often appear after a 24- to 48-hour delay and are evanescent in nature. Skin biopsy demonstrates embolic fat in capillaries with local hemorrhage. A variety of laboratory coagulation abnormalities are present but clinical bleeding is rare. While this constellation of findings is uncommon, the mortality rate approaches 10% to 15% after full-blown FES. A high index of suspicion is necessary for early diagnosis and proper treatment.

No specific treatment exists for FES. Rather, acute management is predicated upon provision of supportive pulmonary care, often with intubation, oxygen, and mechanical ventilation with airway pressure support in an effort to mitigate the effects of the adult respiratory distress syndrome. In many circumstances high-dose steroids are empirically utilized as a general measure to blunt the lung reaction, stabilize the pulmonary capillary bed, and improve gas exchange.

SUGGESTED READINGS

Agency for Healthcare Research and Quality. Effective Health Care Program: Venous Thromboembolism Prophylaxis in Orthopaedic Surgery. Comparative Effectiveness Review Number 49. AHRQ Publication No. 12-EHC020-EF, March 2012. Accessed April 4, 2013, at http://effectivehealthcare.ahrq.gov/ehc/products/186/992/CER-49_VTE_20120313.pdf.

Gossling HR, Pellegrini VD Jr. Fat embolism syndrome: a review of the pathophysiology and physiological basis of treatment. *Clin Orthop Rel Res*. 1982;165:68-82.

Hanssen AD, Osmon DR, Nelson CL. Prevention of deep periprosthetic joint infection. *Instr Course Lect*. 1997;46:555-567.

Matar WY, Jafari SM, Restrepo C, Austin M, Purtill JJ, Parvizi J. Preventing infection in total joint arthroplasty. *J Bone Joint Surg Am*. 2010;92(Suppl 2):36-46.

Parvizi J, Bloomfield MR. Multimodal pain management in orthopaedics: implications for joint arthroplasty surgery. *Orthopaedics*. 2013;36(2 Suppl):7-14.

Pellegrini VD Jr. Prophylaxis against venous thromboembolism after total hip and knee arthroplasty: a critical analysis review. *J Bone Joint Surg*. 2015;3(9):e1.

Pruzansky JS, Bronson MJ, Grelsamer RP, Strauss E, Moucha CS. Prevalence of modifiable surgical site infection risk factors in hip and knee joint arthroplasty patients at an urban academic hospital. *J Arthroplasty*. 2014;29(2):272-276.

Raza H, Mahapatra A. Acute compartment syndrome in orthopaedics: causes, diagnosis, and management. *Adv Orthop*. 2015;2015:543412.

Shadgan B, Menon M, O'Brien PJ, Reid WD. Diagnostic techniques in acute compartment syndrome of the leg. *J Orthop Trauma*. 2008;22(8):581-587.

Strunden MS, Heckel K, Goetz AE, Reuter DA. Perioperative fluid and volume management: physiological basis, tools and strategies. *Ann Intensive Care*. 2011;1(1):2.

Tse EY, Cheung WY, Ng KF, Luk KD. Reducing perioperative blood loss and allogeneic transfusion in patients undergoing major spine surgery. *J Bone Joint Surg*. 2011;93A:1268-1277.

Yang ZG, Chen WP, Wu LD. Effectiveness and safety of tranexamic acid in reducing blood loss in total knee arthroplasty: a meta-analysis. *J Bone Joint Surg Am*. 2012;94(13):1153-1159.

C H A P T E R 66

Transplant Surgery

Vinayak S. Rohan, MD
Emad Kishi, MD
John W. McGillicuddy, MD
Satish N. Nadig, MD, PhD

Key Clinical Questions

1 When is renal, pancreas, or liver imaging indicated after transplant?

2 What are the common postoperative complications that arise after liver, kidney, and pancreas transplant?

INTRODUCTION

Organ transplantation is a complex but effective treatment for end-stage organ failure. Since the advent of more potent immunosuppressive medications, the demand for transplantation has far exceeded the supply. Every year in the United States more than 25,000 people undergo organ transplantation, while at the same time more than 100,000 people remain on the waiting list. The combination of complex surgery, immunosuppression, and very ill and debilitated patients make postoperative management very challenging.

Complications related to transplantation are most often divided into early (typically technical in nature) and late (typically related to immunosuppression or other medications). All of the complications associated with less complicated general surgical procedures can also be seen after transplantation. This chapter will focus on the complications that are particular to transplantation and that are most likely to be encountered by Hospitalists.

COMPLICATIONS OF KIDNEY TRANSPLANT (FIGURE 66-1)

■ POSTOPERATIVE OLIGURIA/GRAFT DYSFUNCTION

The causes of early graft dysfunction range from the benign to the truly emergent and include, but are not limited to, thrombus in the Foley catheter, acute tubular necrosis, thrombosis of the renal artery or vein, ureteric leak or stenosis, and rejection. Prompt diagnosis and appropriate management are necessary to salvage the graft.

Low or absent urine output may be attributable to the renal parenchyma (ATN), the renal vasculature, ureteral issues, or Foley catheter obstruction/malfunction. ATN is the most likely cause for poor/delayed graft function and complicates approximately 20% to 30% of kidney transplants. It is more common in the setting of long cold ischemic times, older donors, and highly sensitized recipients. It typically improves spontaneously over the first few weeks posttransplant. Although ATN is the most likely etiology of poor initial function, it is a diagnosis of exclusion, and a rapid and systematic evaluation must occur to rule out the other more worrisome possibilities:

- The Foley catheter should be irrigated to ensure that clot or tissue has not affected its patency.
- The adequacy of resuscitation should be evaluated by reviewing the vital signs, central pressures, and fluid balances; intravascular depletion should be treated with a bolus of an appropriate crystalloid fluid.
- The patency of the renal artery and vein should be evaluated using duplex Doppler ultrasonography. Urgent surgical exploration is indicated when vascular compromise is demonstrated by imaging or when clinical suspicion is high. Renal scintigraphy can be used as a confirmatory test after ultrasound.
- Acute cellular rejection is unlikely early after transplant but must be a part of the differential if the clinical scenario is appropriate (ie, high panel reactive antibodies or PRA, marginal crossmatch, absence of other explanation). When rejection is suspected, either an open renal biopsy (if the patient is post-op day <7) or percutaneous biopsy (if the patient is post-op day >7) is indicated.
- Hyperacute rejection, mediated by preformed antibodies against the donor, is extremely uncommon in the modern era, but leads almost inevitably to graft loss.

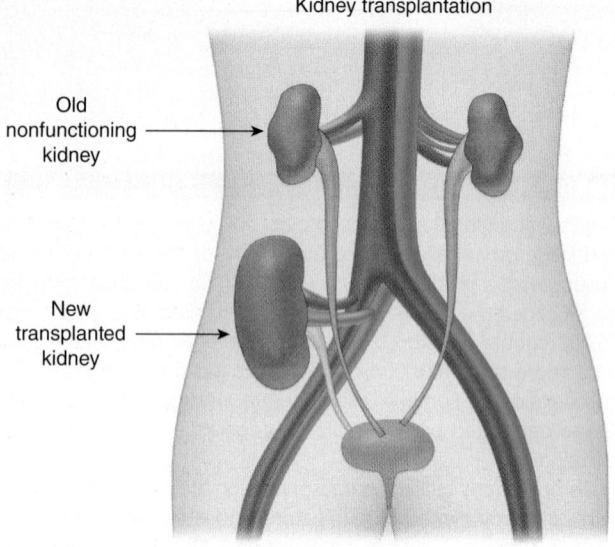

Kidney transplantation

Old nonfunctioning kidney

New transplanted kidney

Figure 66-1 *Kidney transplantation.*

Other common surgical complications after kidney transplant are outlined in **Table 66-1**.

■ OTHER POSTOPERATIVE COMPLICATIONS

Most of the early complications after kidney transplantation may be diagnosed by either ultrasonography or renal scintigraphy. CT scan with IV contrast should be avoided in the posttransplant setting due to the nephrotoxic effects of the contrast. Small perinephric

TABLE 66-1 Surgical Complications After Kidney Transplantation

Vascular complications after kidney transplant:

Early:

- Perinephric Hematoma

- Renal Artery Thrombosis

- Renal Vein Thrombosis

Late:

- Renal Artery Aneurysm (Mycotic Aneurysm)

- Renal Artery stenosis

Urological complications after kidney transplant:

Early:

- Urinary Leak

- Urinary Retention

Late:

- Ureteric stenosis

Lymphatic complications after kidney transplant:

- Lymphocele

Wound Complications:

Early:

- Wound infection

- Subcutaneous Hematoma/Seroma

- Wound dehiscence

Late:

- Incisional Hernia

hematomas are very common, particularly in recipients receiving anticoagulants, antiplatelet agents, thymoglobulin, or plasmapheresis. Most small hematomas will resolve spontaneously and require no intervention. Hematomas with pressure effect on the graft need to be evacuated surgically (percutaneous drainage is almost never sufficient). Thrombosis of the renal artery or vein is uncommon with a cumulative incidence of approximately 2%; when present it is almost invariably due to technical issues (ie, kink, malposition, intimal flap). Such vascular thrombosis typically presents with sudden onset of oliguria/anuria, and in the case of venous thrombosis, frank hematuria and pain over the graft. Confirmation of the diagnosis (best by duplex Doppler ultrasound) requires emergent return to the operating room for exploration. Grafts with venous thrombosis may be salvageable with prompt identification and treatment, but arterial thrombosis is almost universally associated with graft loss.

The most common urological complication following kidney transplantation is hematuria. The source of the bleeding, which is usually minor, is the new anastomosis between the transplanted ureter and the native bladder. In the rare instance that the bleeding does not stop spontaneously, revision of the anastomosis or cystoscopic ablation may be necessary. Care must be taken to avoid (or at least quickly identify) Foley catheter occlusion with clot. Most often gentle irrigation is sufficient to relieve the occlusion, but occasionally Foley replacement is necessary. Urologic consultation is well advised for frank hematuria (after ruling out venous thrombosis) or persistent slow bleeding.

Urine leak, most commonly from the neoureterocystostomy, is a common early postoperative complication, the clinical presentation of which can range from the very subtle to the very obvious. The most obvious presentations typically include an abrupt decrease or cessation of urine output, associated with the development of copious clear wound drainage or drain output. More subtle presentations might include new onset abdominal pain or an unexplained elevation in the serum creatinine. Urine leak should be in the differential diagnosis in the early posttransplant period whenever there is poor urine output, a new fluid collection, new wound drainage, new abdominal pain, or delayed graft function. Any new fluid drainage or aspirated fluid collection should be sent for creatinine measurement and the value checked against the serum value. Diagnostic imaging choices include CT cystogram, contrast cystogram, and renal scintigraphy (the most sensitive test choice).

For small, distal leaks, management typically begins with reinstitution of Foley bladder drainage, placement/replacement of ureteral stent, and percutaneous drainage. Cystoscopic placement of a stent can be challenging due to the ectopic ureteral location and lack of periureteral support. Percutaneous nephrostomy is an option, although this may be technically difficult in the absence of hydronephrosis. If this approach is effective, the catheter should remain in place for at least 2 weeks and a cystogram performed prior to catheter removal. Treatment failure, whether manifest by uncontrolled drainage or persistence of the leak beyond two weeks, suggests ureteral necrosis and is an indication for operative exploration and revision of the neoureterocystostomy.

The development of a lymphocoele after renal transplantation is common and is thought to be related to the disruption of the lymphatics surrounding the iliac vessels. Most collections are small (<100 cc), identified on ultrasound, and clinically silent. Spontaneous resolution of these small collections is the normal course. Larger collections may become apparent clinically and usually do so between 1 week and 6 months after transplantation, with incidence peaking at around 30 days posttransplant. They commonly present with complaints related to nocturnal urinary frequency as a consequence of bladder impingement by the lymphocoele. A sensation of pelvic fullness and ipsilateral painless leg edema are other common complaints. Deteriorating renal function subsequent to ureteral stent removal can be the first presentation of a lympho-cele that is compressing the donor ureter. For symptomatic lym-phoceles, percutaneous drainage is successful in about 50% of the cases. A fraction of the remaining 50% will respond to an attempt at ablation with the instillation of a sclerosant into the cavity. Surgical drainage via creation of a peritoneal window is a last resort and can be done open or laparoscopically.

COMPLICATIONS OF LIVER TRANSPLANT (FIGURE 66-2)

■ INTRAOPERATIVE HEMORRHAGE AND COAGULOPATHY

Patients in need of liver transplantation often have concomitant portal hypertension and coagulopathy as a consequence of their liver disease. This combination results in a tremendously high risk for significant intraoperative blood loss. Additionally, patients with a history of any upper abdominal surgery or past spontaneous bacterial peritonitis (SBP) portends an even greater intraoperative risk, as they are associated with the presence of extensive and heavily collateralized adhesions. As with any procedure associ-ated with massive blood loss, there is a real possibility that the resulting derangements in temperature, fluid homeostasis, and the coagulation cascade will create a vicious cycle that can be extremely difficult, if not impossible, to recover. In these situations, the most prudent action is often to truncate the operation and get the patient off of the operating table and into the ICU as quickly as possible. The transplant can be completed if and when the patient is resuscitated and stabilized.

■ HEPATIC ARTERY THROMBOSIS

The literature suggests that the overall incidence of hepatic artery thrombosis (HAT) is between 1.6% and 8% in adult liver trans-plant recipients. The clinical presentation of HAT ranges from an asymptomatic patient with minimal alterations in liver function to a critically ill-patient with fulminant hepatic necrosis. The most common presentations begin with postoperative biliary com-plications, including leaks, strictures, and ischemic intrahepatic cholangiopathy.

Suspicion of HAT should be raised whenever there is evidence of biliary complication or significant worsening of liver chemistries. Initial investigation is made with duplex ultrasonography. If the duplex is suspicious, further evaluation by visceral angiography or CT angiography is needed, as failure to make a rapid diagnosis can result in hepatic necrosis and graft loss.

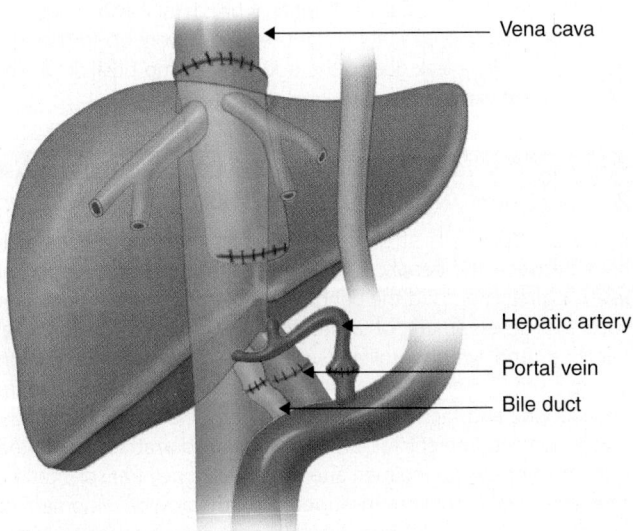

Vena cava

Hepatic artery

Portal vein

Bile duct

Figure 66-2 *Liver transplant.*

The approach to HAT in the early postoperative period, regardless of whether or not symptoms are present, should be an aggressive attempt at the reestablishment of arterial flow to the liver. This often requires urgent operative exploration and revision of the anastomosis or replacement of the artery with conduit (usually a donor iliac artery). Some surgeons attempt to reestablish flow using thrombolytics, but this will be successful only when there are no technical factors contributing to the thrombosis. In most cases of HAT, patients ultimately require retransplantation as a consequence of ischemic biliary cholangiopathy.

■ PORTAL VEIN THROMBOSIS

Portal vein thrombosis after transplantation is an uncommon com-plication in the immediate postoperative period, and is usually the result of a technical issue, such as incomplete recipient portal vein thrombectomy or a mechanical issue with the anastomosis. A high index of suspicion is needed to make the diagnosis, and investiga-tion by duplex Doppler ultrasound is usually initiated with one or more of the following signs: new or persistent ascites, lower-body anasarca, persistent varices, and new or persistent encephalopathy. Early thrombosis is best treated with reoperation, thrombectomy, and anastomotic revision followed by systemic anticoagulation. The treatment of late thrombosis is more controversial as direct repair is technically challenging and not very durable.

■ BILIARY LEAKS

The reported incidence of biliary leaks after liver transplantation varies widely from 10% to 50%. Leaks are observed most com-monly at the site of choledochal anastomosis. Anastomotic leaks encountered in the early postoperative period are most often related to either technical errors (ie, tension, twisting, denuding, malpositioned stitch) or ischemic necrosis following HAT. Signs and symptoms include bilious drainage, abdominal or shoulder pain, increased serum bilirubin, nausea, vomiting, fever, or copious ascites. The diagnosis can be made by HIDA scan, endoscopic retro-grade cholangiography (ERC), or percutaneous transhepatic cholan-giography (PTC). ERC is preferred because it offers an opportunity to treat with endoscopic stent placement without the risk associated with the indwelling transhepatic catheters used during PTC. HIDA is useful very early after transplantation when manipulation of the anastomosis is best avoided in the absence of a confirmed leak. CT scan is useful as an adjunct to identify fluid collections that require percutaneous drainage. Large leaks or leaks associated with ischemic necrosis require surgical intervention, usually with conver-sion to a Roux-en-Y hepaticojejunostomy. The development of early postoperative leaks is associated with late stricture formation and may also be a contributor to late HAT.

■ BILIARY STRICTURE OR OBSTRUCTION

Biliary obstruction occurs in approximately 7% to 15% of patients after liver transplantation. Anastomotic stricture accounts for 50% of obstruction cases and can occur early in the postoperative period secondary to edema, or later, as a result of compromised blood sup-ply. The diagnosis of biliary stricture or obstruction is suggested by an obstructive pattern on routine liver function tests. Commonly, patients present with constitutional symptoms of rigors, fever, head-ache, and fatigue. Occasionally, patients will present with symptoms of cholangitis and sepsis.

After appropriate fluid resuscitation and antibiotic coverage, ERC or PTC is indicated to confirm the diagnosis and to relieve the obstruc-tion by either stenting or proximal drainage. An unpassable stricture or obstruction is indication for surgical revision or, more likely, con-version to Roux-en-Y hepaticojejunosotomy. The rare intrahepatic strictures are best treated with percutaneous balloon dilatation.

■ PRIMARY GRAFT NONFUNCTION

Primary graft nonfunction (PNF) following liver transplantation is an infrequent but life-threatening complication wherein the transplanted liver does not recover function after engraftment. This usually fatal complication occurs in approximately 5% to 6% of cases and is, by definition, without identifiable cause. PNF is usually heralded by severely elevated and rising serum transaminases (often >8000 IU/L) within the first 24 to 48 hours after transplant and a rising PT and INR. The clinical picture also often includes rising serum bilirubin and worsening renal function. PNF is multifactorial and putative causes include all manner of donor, recipient, and procedure-related variables. Patients with PNF require urgent retransplantation, usually within 24 to 72 hours, if mortality is to be avoided. Explantation of the nonfunction liver and creation of a portocaval shunt has some role in patients with PNF and refractory or profound acidemia.

■ RENAL DYSFUNCTION

Renal dysfunction is observed to some degree in nearly every patient who undergoes liver transplantation. In patients with normal preoperative serum creatinine and good initial graft function, the usual mechanism is prerenal azotemia secondary to periods of hypotension and hypovolemia during the operative procedure, as well as the temporary partial occlusion of the inferior vena cava (IVC) that occurs during the implantation. Additionally, the postoperative administration of nephrotoxic agents, especially the calcineurin inhibitors (CNIs) cyclosporine and tacrolimus, contribute to impaired renal function. Management is largely expectant with dialysis as necessary until renal function recovers. Delayed administration of CNIs is prudent in patients at particular risk of renal dysfunction after transplant.

COMPLICATIONS OF PANCREATIC TRANSPLANT

Presently there are more than 1,000,000 individuals with type 1 diabetes in the United States. A successful pancreas transplant will produce a normogylcemic insulin independent state and prevent progression of diabetic nephropathy , stabilize diabetic retinopathy, and potentially reverse diabetic peripheral sensory neuropathy. The vast majority of pancreas transplants are performed as a simultaneous kidney and pancreas transplant (85%-90%) for patients with diabetes and concomitant renal failure. A smaller number are done following a prior successful kidney transplant, and fewer still are done as an isolated transplant for patients with very labile type 1 diabetes complicated by recurrent episodes of hypoglycemic unawareness or diabetic ketoacidosis. When considering isolated pancreas transplantation, it is important to weigh the potential benefits of normoglycemia against the risk of lifelong immunosuppression. In the case of simultaneous kidney and pancreas transplantation or pancreas transplantation following kidney transplant, the risk of the immunosuppression is clearly outweighed by the avoidance of dialysis (**Figure 66-3**).

■ THROMBOSIS

Thrombosis of the donor portal vein is a common complication after pancreas transplantation and is attributable to a the relatively low flow state of the pancreas graft, as compared to normal portal vein flow. Arterial thrombosis is much less common and is usually the result of a technical error at the time of transplantation. Postoperative hyperglycemia suggests the possibility of graft thrombosis and necessitates urgent evaluation with duplex Doppler ultrasound. There is a potential for graft salvage with rapid identification of thrombosis and operative thrombectomy. Approximately 3% to 5 % of the pancreas grafts are lost due to graft thrombosis.

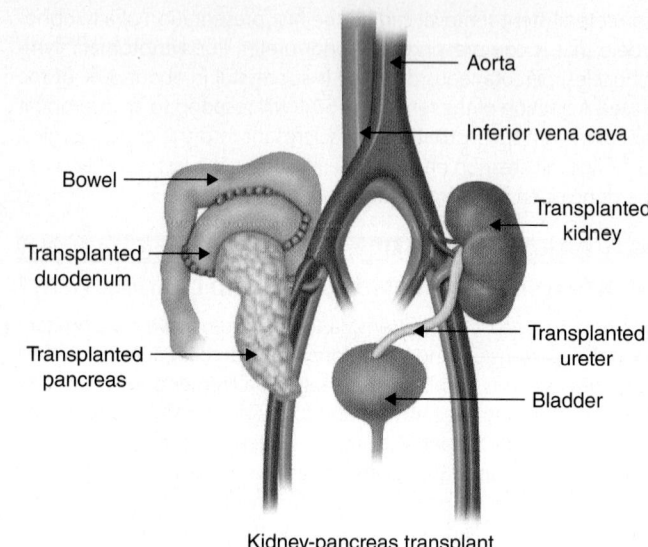

Figure 66-3 *Kidney-pancreas transplant.*

■ PANCREATITIS OF THE GRAFT

Graft pancreatitis is not uncommon and will manifest as elevations in the serum amylase and lipase, usually without associated abdominal pain. Treatment is largely expectant but in some cases the development of phlegmon or abscess will require operative debridement or percutaneous drainage.

■ COMPLICATION OF THE ENTERIC DRAINED TRANSPLANT

Duodenal stump leak or anastomotic leak is one of the most serious complications of a pancreas transplant. Patients present with fever, pain, and a leukocytosis. CT scan is helpful in making the diagnosis. Surgical exploration and repair of the leak is necessary. Removal of the graft might be required if it is not salvageable.

■ COMPLICATIONS SPECIFIC FOR BLADDER DRAINED PANCREAS

There is a greater incidence of urinary infection due to the bicarbonate-rich fluid draining into the bladder. Sterile cystitis, urethritis and balanitis may occur after bladder drainage. Reflux of the urine through the ampulla can result in reflux pancreatitis, which is initially managed by Foley catheterization. Patients might require a work up for bladder dysfunction. Urine leak due to the duodenal stump breakdown will necessitate re-exploration.

GENERAL COMPLICATIONS AFTER TRANSPLANTATION

■ ACUTE IMMUNOSUPPRESSIVE DRUG TOXICITY

Immunosuppression after transplantation must achieve a balance between the beneficial effects of the drugs in preventing or reversing rejection, and the dangers of excess immunosuppression with the development of acute toxicity symptoms, nosocomial infection, and lymphoproliferative disorders. The most common agents used for immunosuppression in liver transplant patients are cyclosporine and tacrolimus (FK506) in combination with steroids. Mycophenolate mofetil has essentially replaced azathioprine in the immunosuppression regimen after liver and kidney transplantation. After the initiation of immunosuppression therapy, development of infection and acute toxicity are usually seen early during treatment, whereas lymphoproliferative disorders and other malignancies are long-term sequelae.

The side-effect profiles of cyclosporine and tacrolimus are similar and include gastrointestinal disturbances, headache, and tremor. Gingival hyperplasia and hirsutism are encountered frequently during cyclosporine and steroid treatment, whereas glucose intolerance is reported more often with tacrolimus treatment than with cyclosporine therapy. Hyperkalemia, hyperuricemia, hypophosphatemia, and hypomagnesemia are manifestations of renal tubular dysfunction and usually can be controlled by adjusting the dose according to drug levels. Nephrotoxicity is the most clinically significant adverse effect of both drugs and is manifested as acute azotemia. This effect is largely reversible after reducing the dose of the drug and providing adequate hydration. Occasionally, progressive chronic renal disease can develop, which is usually irreversible. In such a situation, dialysis or kidney transplantation is required.

■ NEUROPSYCHIATRIC COMPLICATIONS

In addition to the acute neurophysiologic changes associated with fluid and electrolyte shifts during the perioperative period, anxiety and depression are common psychiatric conditions observed in many transplant patients. Seizures, alterations of the levels of consciousness, and infections of the central nervous system are infrequent but are significant causes of morbidity and mortality. Encephalopathy observed after liver transplantation can be related to poor initial graft function, but it is more commonly multifactorial in etiology. Metabolic derangements, hypoxia, sedation, and drug interactions all can contribute.

Neurologic signs and symptoms associated with immunosuppression toxicity related to cyclosporine and tacrolimus include tremors, headaches, and seizures. These can be avoided by close monitoring of drug levels. High-dose steroids can result in emotional liability or mania. Any patients presenting with new neuropsychiatric symptoms should have a cranial CT scan and lumbar puncture to rule out other causes of mental status changes, such as intracerebral bleeding or an infectious etiology. Posterior reversible encephalopthay syndrome (PRES) often manifests in the setting of drug toxicity and hypertension. Clinically, PRESS manifests with headaches, seizures and visual loss. These patients require and urgent MRI and intensive care unit admission and aggressive control of hypertension with minimization of their cyclosporine and tacrolimus.

■ FLUID AND ELECTROLYTE DISTURBANCES

Fluid and electrolyte disturbances and alterations in acid-base status are common after transplantation. Preoperative protein calorie malnutrition and end-stage liver disease lead to derangements in total body water and electrolyte balance that are worsened initially by the metabolic stress of surgery and massive fluid and blood product resuscitation. The rapidity of recovery depends in large part on the patient's renal and liver allograft function postoperatively. For a patient with stable postoperative renal and liver graft function, little metabolic manipulation is required to correct such derangements.

The early development of metabolic alkalosis secondary to metabolism of citrate in blood products is a favorable sign of graft function but can be serious if alkalemia develops. Excess total body water and excess sodium are best treated with gentle diuresis with furosemide. Careful repletion of potassium should be instituted, but it must be monitored closely in the setting of medications such as tacrolimus and cyclosporine, which tend to increase serum potassium levels by afferent arteriolar constriction and direct distal tubular toxicity. Derangements in serum calcium, magnesium, and phosphorus are common and should be repleted to avoid neurologic, skeletal, and cardiac muscle dysfunction.

POSTTRANSPLANT INFECTIONS

Infection risk is determined by a patient's "net state of immunosuppression," a balance contributed to by factors such as the dose, type, and duration of immunosuppressive therapy, the presence of indwelling devices such as catheters, nutritional status, metabolic conditions, certain immunomodulating viral infections, graft function, and underlying diseases. Signs and symptoms of infection are often attenuated in the setting of immunosuppression. The variety of possible pathogens is quite broad but is influenced by the timing of infection in relation to transplantation (**Figure 66-4**). Antimicrobial agents used to treat infections can have important drug interactions with immunosuppressive medications, and consultation with a pharmacist is strongly recommended. Infections in these patients may be more severe and progress more rapidly compared with immunocompetent hosts.

LATE TRANSPLANT COMPLICATIONS

■ HYPERTENSION

Hypertension is common after renal transplantation with nearly 70% of the patients requiring antihypertensive medications. Hypertension can be caused by preexisting disease, medications (tacrolimus, cyclosporin, prednisone) and rarely due to stenosis of the renal artery anastomoses. The treatment of posttransplant hypertension is same as in the nontransplant population.

■ HYPERLIPIDEMIA

Hyperlipidemia is common in the posttransplant patient, and the cause is often multifactorial. Some of the medications used (tacrolimus, cyclosporin, prednisone) are prone to cause hyperlipidemia. The management of these patients should follow the guidelines used to treat general population with dyslipidemias.

■ NEW ONSET DIABETES AFTER TRANSPLANTATION (NODAT)

Exposure to immunosuppressive agents such as tacrolimus, cyclosporin, and steroids can predispose to the development of diabetes after transplantation. The incidence of NODAT can range from 5% to 40%. Tacrolimus has a higher propensity to cause hyperglycemia than cyclosporine. Most of the patients tend to become insulin dependent and the same guidelines used to treat non transplant patients should be used in these patients.

■ SKELETAL COMPLICATIONS

Osteoporosis is common after renal transplantation and seems directly related to amount of steriods used. Treatment involves steroid-free regimens, calcium supplements and bisphosphonates.

■ POSTTRANSPLANT MALIGNANCIES

The incidence of skin cancer, lymphoma and kaposi sarcoma are significantly increased in posttransplant patients. Kaposi's sarcoma is thought to be related to HSV-8 and is generally treated by minimizing immunosuppression. Squamous cell cancers and melanomas appear to be more frequent in the posttransplant population and they tend to have a more aggressive course. Early detection and aggressive management is necessary. Posttransplant patients should minimize sun exposure and should have regular skin examination. Posttransplant lymphoproliferative disorder (PTLD) is a type of B-cell lymphoma related to Epstein Barr virus (EBV) infection. These are most commonly extra nodal in presentation. Treatment of PTLD involves minimizing immunosuppression; some patients will require chemotherapy or radiotherapy.

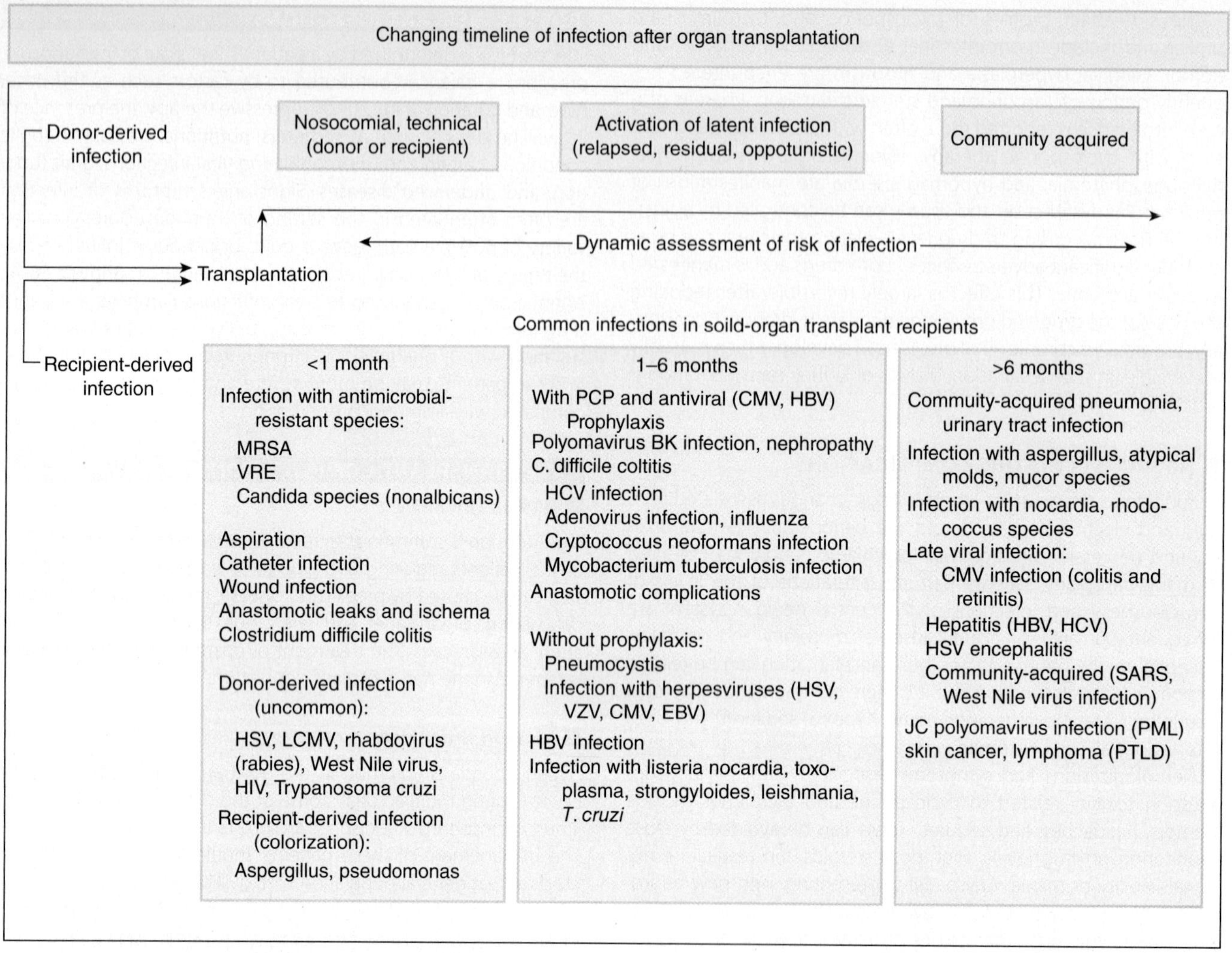

Changing timeline of infection after organ transplantation

Donor-derived
infection

Nosocomial, technical
(donor or recipient)

Activation of latent infection
(relapsed, residual, oppotunistic)

Community acquired

Dynamic assessment of risk of infection

Transplantation

Recipient-derived
infection

Common infections in soild-organ transplant recipients

<1 month	1–6 months	>6 months
Infection with antimicrobial-resistant species: 　MRSA 　VRE 　Candida species (nonalbicans) Aspiration Catheter infection Wound infection Anastomotic leaks and ischema Clostridium difficile colitis Donor-derived infection (uncommon): 　HSV, LCMV, rhabdovirus (rabies), West Nile virus, HIV, Trypanosoma cruzi Recipient-derived infection (colorization): 　Aspergillus, pseudomonas	With PCP and antiviral (CMV, HBV) Prophylaxis Polyomavirus BK infection, nephropathy C. difficile coltitis 　HCV infection 　Adenovirus infection, influenza 　Cryptococcus neoformans infection 　Mycobacterium tuberculosis infection Anastomotic complications Without prophylaxis: 　Pneumocystis 　Infection with herpesviruses (HSV, VZV, CMV, EBV) HBV infection Infection with listeria nocardia, toxoplasma, strongyloides, leishmania, T. cruzi	Commuity-acquired pneumonia, urinary tract infection Infection with aspergillus, atypical molds, mucor species Infection with nocardia, rhodococcus species Late viral infection: 　CMV infection (colitis and retinitis) 　Hepatitis (HBV, HCV) 　HSV encephalitis 　Community-acquired (SARS, West Nile virus infection) JC polyomavirus infection (PML) skin cancer, lymphoma (PTLD)

Figure 66-4 *Changing timeline of infection after organ transplantation.* (From Fishman JA. Infection in solid-organ transplant recipients. *N Engl J Med.* 2007;357:2601-2614. © 2007 Massachusetts Medical Society. Reprinted with permission from Massachusetts Medical Society.)

SUGGESTED READINGS

Danovitch GM, ed. *Handbook of Kidney Transplantation.* 5th ed. Philadelphia, PA: Lippincott Williams & Wilkins; 2010.

Fishman JA. Infection in solid organ recipients. *N Engl J Med.* 2007;357(25):2601-2614.

Humar A, Matas AJ. Surgical complications after kidney transplantation. *Semin Dial.* 2005;18(6):505-510.

Mathew MC, Wendon JA. Perioperative management of liver transplantation patients. *Curr Opin Crit Care.* 2001;7(4):275-280.

Sethi A, Stravitz RT. Medical management of the liver transplant recipient—a primer for non-transplant doctors. *Aliment Pharmacol Ther.* 2007;25(3):229-245.

Silkensen JR. Long-term complications in renal transplantation. *J Am Soc Nephrol.* 2000;11(3):582-588.

Sutherland DE, Gruessner RW, Dunn DL, et al. Lessons learned from more than 1,000 pancreas transplants at a single institution. *Ann Surg.* 2001;233(4):463-501.

CHAPTER 67

Urology

Kent Russell Edwards, Jr., MD

Tracy J. Tipton, MD

Michaella Maloney Prasad, MD

Key Clinical Questions

1. How and when should postoperative urinary retention be further worked up?

2. When does hyponatremia associated with TUR syndrome need intervention?

3. How should postoperative hematuria be managed?

4. What is the approach to managing postoperative urine leak after prostatectomy or partial nephrectomy?

5. How should the postoperative management for adrenalectomy differ based on the type of adrenal tumor removed (pheochromocytoma, aldosteronoma, glucocorticoid-producing tumor)?

Any patient undergoing urology surgery should have a preoperative risk assessment. Obesity significantly contributes to the increased incidence and progression of urologic condition requiring surgery (eg, neoplasms, BPH, stress incontinence, erectile dysfunction, infertility, and urolithiasis); obese patients are also at increased risk for general postoperative complications. Increased peripheral androgen conversion to estrogen and secretion of prothrombin activator inhibitor-1 adipocytes contributes to a hypercoagulable state. Poor wound healing is more common in obese patients because of the proinflammatory state of the body, decreased peripheral perfusion, decreased local angiogenesis, and inhibited cell tissue response. The body habitus of obese patients also predisposes them to complications such as urethral-vesical anastomotic leak (UVAL) due to inadequate surgical exposure.

On the other end of the spectrum, poor preoperative nutritional status has also been well established as a risk factor for developing postoperative complications. Patients with one of four abnormalities in preoperative nutritional parameters have significantly higher-postoperative complication rates as well as longer hospital stays (low body mass index <24, preoperative weight loss >5%, arm muscle circumference <5th percentile, and low-serum albumin [below reference range]).

Risk factors that predispose patients to developing complicated UTIs include older age, external instrumentation, ureteral stent or other foreign body placement, metabolic dysfunction (obesity, diabetes mellitus, poor nutritional status), urinary tract obstruction (anatomic or functional), immunosuppression, and recent antibiotic use.

PRACTICE POINT

- Patients with ureteral stents, indwelling catheters, and urinary ostomies have urine that is chronically colonized with bacteria. These patients should only be treated for a urinary tract infection if they have concomitant symptoms of a urinary tract infection.

- Reflexive antibiotic administration in these patients leads to the development of resistant organisms.

■ URINARY RETENTION

Under normal physiologic conditions, the urgency to void is sensed when the bladder reaches a threshold of approximately 250 to 300 mL. Maximum bladder capacity for the average adult is 400 to 600 mL. Afferent pelvic sensory nerves are stimulated to transmit a signal to the parasympathetic ganglia in the spinal cord. Parasympathetic efferent fibers then fire a signal to the detrusor muscle of the bladder to initiate micturition when socially appropriate. Conversely, if micturition is not desired, afferent fibers will cause activation of the sympathetic nervous system and inhibit contraction of the detrusor muscle and cause contraction of the internal urethral sphincter (visceral efferent) and external sphincter (somatic efferent).

The incidence of postoperative urinary retention (POUR) ranges from 4% to 29%. Factors that contribute to POUR include prior history of urinary retention, the type of surgery performed and whether performed on an emergency basis (anorectal and total knee replacement amongst the highest with incidences of 16% to 20%

TABLE 67-1 Risk Factors for Postoperative Urinary Retention (POUR)

Age	Age > 50
Gender	Male
Type of procedure	Anorectal and lower extremity
Patient comorbidities	Neuropathies, multiple sclerosis, recent stroke, cerebral palsy, spinal lesions, constipation
Medications	Cholinergic medications, beta-blockers, sympathomimetics, opioids
Type of anesthesia	Spinal anesthesia
Duration of procedure	>2 h

and 19% to 70%, respectively), method and duration of anesthesia (>2 hours), emergency surgeries, certain medications (those with anticholinergic properties, opioids), constipation, and inability to ambulate postoperatively (**Table 67-1**).

Evaluation of a patient with suspected POUR includes ultrasound of the bladder, bladder catheterization (when indicated), and post-void ultrasonography of the bladder. Sedated patients may not be able to mount an urgency to void even if their bladder holds an amount of urine that would typically instigate such a sensation. One study found that as many as 61% of patients in the postanesthesia care unit (PACU) did not verbalize that they needed to void despite having 600 mL of urine (confirmed by ultrasound).

If POUR is suspected, an ultrasound is indicated to confirm urinary retention, obtain an approximate amount of retained urine, and to avoid unnecessary catheterizations. Studies have shown good correlation between volumes measured on ultrasound and those determined by catheterization. Ultrasound has been shown to improve detection of POUR at larger volumes in patients who cannot appreciate the need to void. False positive results of bladder scan technology commonly occur in patients with generalized anasarca, gravid uterus or peritoneal dialysis fluid.

Assuming no contraindications, catheterization follows sonography in patients with bladder volumes greater than 250 to 300 mL and the urine is sent to for routine microscopy and culture if indicated. Nurse-driven algorithms (**Figure 67-1**) can help determine the clinical necessity of indwelling catheters and assess for the possibility of early removal.

PRACTICE POINT

Prior to performing catheterization of the bladder, review the medical history for conditions that may make catheterization more difficult, increasing risk for discomfort, urethral trauma, or infection:

- History of benign prostatic hypertrophy, urethral stricture, or hypospadias
- Recent surgery (ie, freshly healing tissue) within the bladder, prostate or urethra

Indications to consider consulting urology for catheter placement include:

- Any history of urologic surgery
- Known history of difficult or complex catheter placement
- Catheter attempt resulting in bleeding or hematuria
- Pelvic trauma with blood at the urethral meatus

Complications of POUR include bladder overdistention leading to hypotonia, renal insufficiency, and infection from urine stagnation. Intermittent catheterization (IC) is justified as an acceptable and appropriate alternative to indwelling catheterization. Both the CDC and the American Urological Association (AUA) recommend clean intermittent catheterization over indwelling catheterization for intermediate and long-term bladder decompression when feasible.

Alpha-adrenergic antagonists, particularly those with favorable affinity for the alpha-1a receptor such as tamsulosin, may reduce the incidence of POUR if initiated preoperatively. If no contraindication to the medication, tamsulosin should be instituted at the time of POUR diagnosis if it was not used prior to surgery. In general, alpha-blockers should be used with caution in patients with hypotension, or a history of cataract or glaucoma surgery. Tamsulosin specifically can stimulate an allergic reaction in someone with a hypersensitivity to sulfonamides.

Although intermittent catheterization is widely accepted for management of POUR for outpatient procedures, the duration of catheterization for inpatient surgeries remains controversial (**Figure 67-2**).

Patients with chronic urinary retention will have a rapid diuresis (>200 mL/h), which usually resolves spontaneously. They need to be closely monitored for dehydration and electrolyte imbalances. If patients have access to water, most can compensate for any deficit. If unable to drink, patients may receive IV fluid supplementation using a hypotonic solution (0.45% normal saline) with replacement of half the urine output every 2 to 4 hours.

■ URETERAL INJURY

Fifty percent of all ureteral injuries occur during gynecologic procedures (with radical hysterectomies and abdominal hysterectomies accounting for 50% and 40% of these, respectively). The injury generally involves the distal one-third of the ureter, where the ureter is in closest proximity to the uterus and associated structures. Risk of injury to the ureter is highest during ligation and division of the cardinal ligaments in abdominal hysterectomies. Other injuries observed intraoperatively include kinking, laceration, burn injury from electrocautery, and insults that compromise the blood supply to the ureter.

Radical prostatectomy, ureterolysis, retroperitoneal lymph node dissection, and female incontinence procedures pose the highest risk of injury amongst the urological procedures. Risk factors for ureteral injury include abnormal anatomy, intraoperative hemorrhage, and failure to recognize the ureter intraoperatively.

Failure to recognize ureteral injury and treat appropriately may result in permanent renal damage and may ultimately result in nephrectomy. Patients with ureteral injury and a urine leak may have fever, ileus secondary to uroperitoneum, abdominal swelling, and flank pain. Laboratory abnormalities include leukocytosis, elevated BUN and creatinine secondary to peritoneal absorption, hematuria and pyuria. Hematuria is absent in 23% to 45% of all ureteral injuries. Imaging may reveal the presence of ascites and pleural effusion. Intraperitoneal drain fluid may be sent for analysis of a creatinine level if there is a higher output than expected. The fluid in the drain contains some urine if the value is much higher than the patient's serum creatinine.

The following tests may diagnose ureteral injury:

- Intraoperative retrograde pyelogram (the gold standard)
- Renal ultrasound to identify urinoma, hydronephrosis
- CT with contrast and delayed images to evaluate function of the kidney ipsilateral to the injury and the integrity of the affected ureter

If a minor ureteral injury is recognized intraoperatively, the surgeon may place a ureteral stent to facilitate the healing process. These stents are typically removed 4 to 6 weeks after the procedure. Ureteral injuries

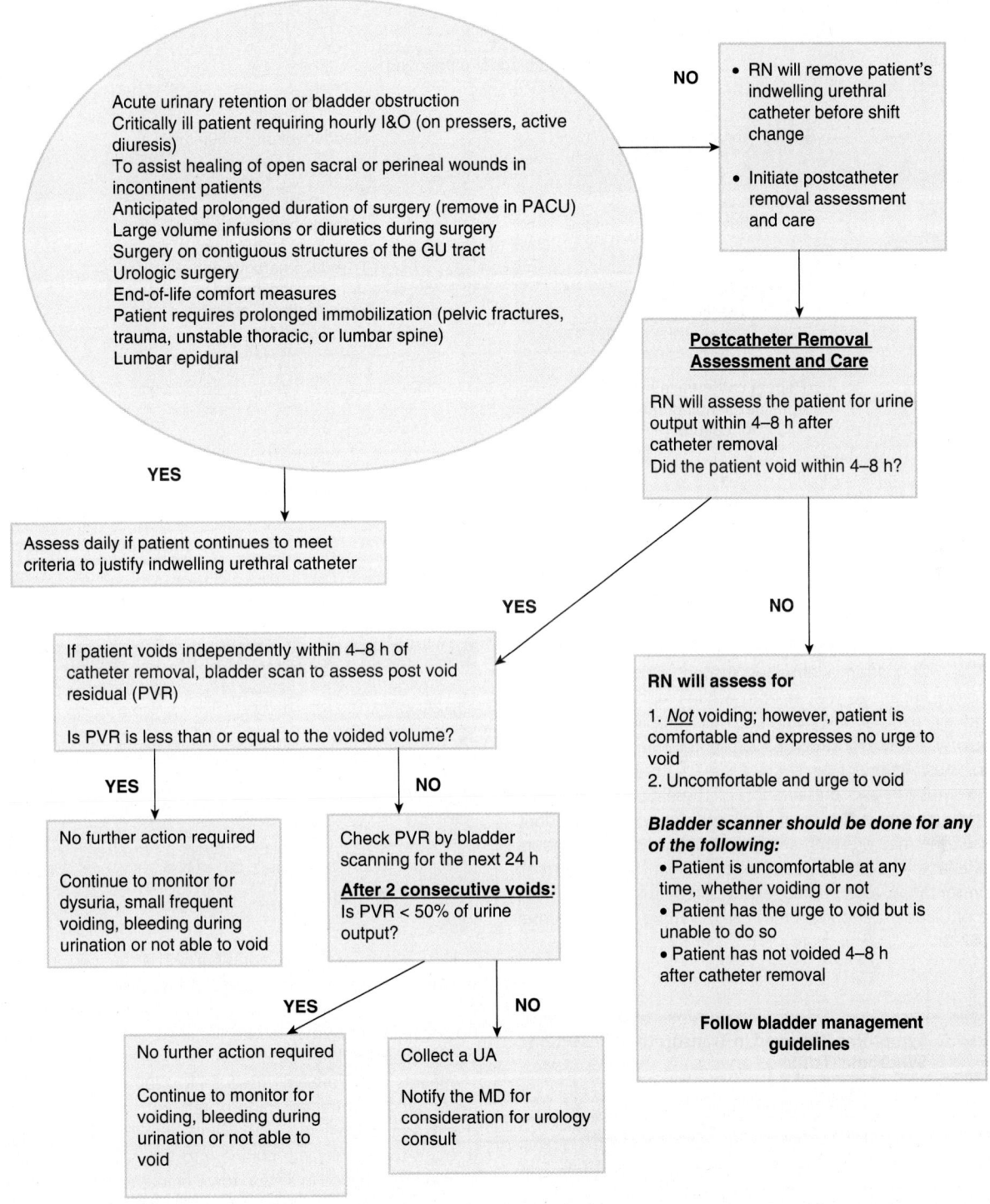

Daily prior to 0600/1800: Nurse (RN) will assess all patients who have an indwelling urethral catheter and physician order for insertion to determine if the patient still meets accepted criteria to justify continuation.

Acute urinary retention or bladder obstruction
Critically ill patient requiring hourly I&O (on pressers, active diuresis)
To assist healing of open sacral or perineal wounds in incontinent patients
Anticipated prolonged duration of surgery (remove in PACU)
Large volume infusions or diuretics during surgery
Surgery on contiguous structures of the GU tract
Urologic surgery
End-of-life comfort measures
Patient requires prolonged immobilization (pelvic fractures, trauma, unstable thoracic, or lumbar spine)
Lumbar epidural

NO

• RN will remove patient's indwelling urethral catheter before shift change

• Initiate postcatheter removal assessment and care

Postcatheter Removal Assessment and Care

RN will assess the patient for urine output within 4–8 h after catheter removal
Did the patient void within 4–8 h?

YES

Assess daily if patient continues to meet criteria to justify indwelling urethral catheter

YES

NO

If patient voids independently within 4–8 h of catheter removal, bladder scan to assess post void residual (PVR)

Is PVR is less than or equal to the voided volume?

RN will assess for

1. *Not* voiding; however, patient is comfortable and expresses no urge to void
2. Uncomfortable and urge to void

Bladder scanner should be done for any of the following:
• Patient is uncomfortable at any time, whether voiding or not
• Patient has the urge to void but is unable to do so
• Patient has not voided 4–8 h after catheter removal

Follow bladder management guidelines

YES

No further action required

Continue to monitor for dysuria, small frequent voiding, bleeding during urination or not able to void

NO

Check PVR by bladder scanning for the next 24 h
After 2 consecutive voids:
Is PVR < 50% of urine output?

YES

No further action required

Continue to monitor for voiding, bleeding during urination or not able to void

NO

Collect a UA

Notify the MD for consideration for urology consult

Figure 67-1 *Nurse driven Foley catheter removal protocol.*

that are not corrected intraoperatively tend to be more complex in nature, require more extensive surgical repairs, and have more associated complications. The vast majority of ureteral injuries will not resolve on their own and require emergent urologic consultation.

■ **TRANSURETHRAL RESECTION SYNDROME**

Transurethral resection syndrome (TURS) is commonly associated with transurethral resection of the prostate (TURP), but

may occur in any endourological procedure using hypotonic solution for mechanical bladder irrigation. After many patients were noted to exhibit extensive hemolysis following irrigation with deionized water, nonelectrolyte hypotonic fluids such as glycine, sorbitol, and mannitol were introduced to decrease this complication.

TURS primarily occurs by direct infusion of the irrigating solution into the venous sinuses of the prostate and by reabsorption of

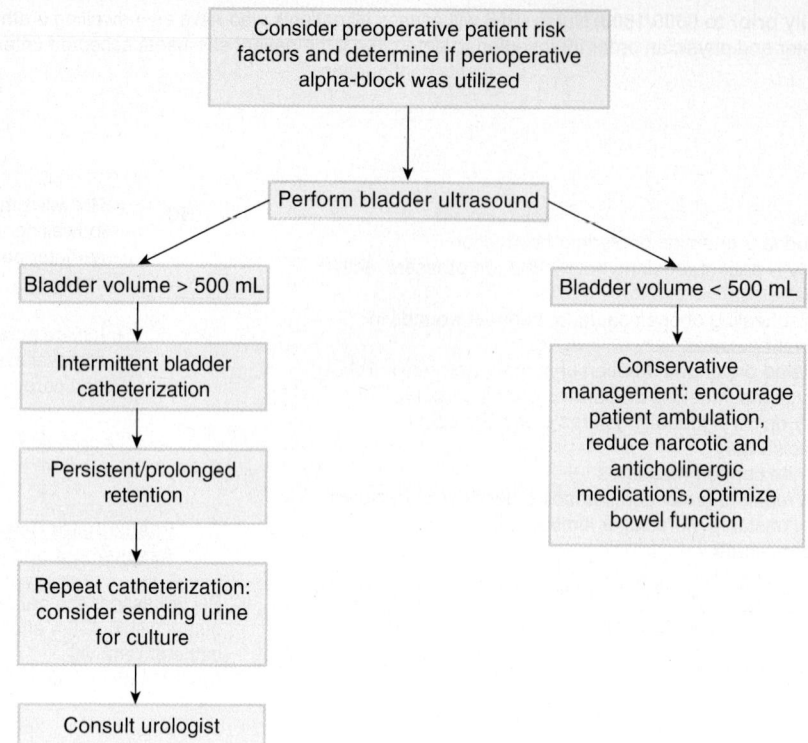

Figure 67-2 *Approach to the patient with suspected postoperative urinary retention.*

extravasated fluid following prostatic capsule and/or bladder wall perforation. Hyponatremia develops secondary to the dilutional effect of the irrigant as well as from a natriuretic response from increased extracellular fluid volume. This complication may be associated with a postobstructive diuresis, following surgical relief of chronic obstruction.

The progression and presentation of these patients depends on the rate, amount, and type of fluid used during the procedure. TUR syndrome may present acutely or insidiously over 24 hours; while direct venous sinus infusion of the irrigant will lead to an acute presentation, resorption of extravasated fluid from prostatic capsule or bladder perforation may cause a more insidious onset (**Table 67-2**).

TABLE 67-2 Symptoms Observed in Transurethral Resection Syndrome (TURS)

Neurologic	Cardiorespiratory	Other
Coma	Labile blood pressure	Abdominal pain
Restlessness/agitation	Hypotension	Thermodysregulation
Altered mental status	Hypertension	Nausea ± vomiting
Headache	Bradycardia	Respiratory depression
Transient visual disturbances (blurry vision and blindness)	Dyspnea	
Seizures	Angina	

PRACTICE POINT

Complications of mechanical irrigation should be suspected when:

- The fluid deficit (ie, the difference between the irrigation instilled and retrieved) is significant.
- Patient develops symptoms of transurethral resection syndrome such as confusion, nausea, vomiting, altered vision, and a decreased sense of consciousness; cardiac symptoms include bradycardia, labile blood pressure, chest pain, shortness of breath.

If risk factors for the development of TURS are present (procedure length >90 minutes, open venous sinuses, high-pressure irrigation, and large volume of resection [>45 g]) and no intraoperative or postoperative sodium level was obtained, serum sodium and serum osmolalities should be ordered immediately.

Patients with TURS will need their volume status stabilized and hyponatremia corrected. Blood pressure may transiently increase due to aggressive fluid replacement; this will resolve as fluid passes through the cellular membrane into the cell. Usually the patient should be managed in a step-down or intensive care unit.

■ HEMATURIA FOLLOWING ENDOSCOPIC SURGERY

With any endourologic resection, the amount of postoperative bleeding will largely depend on the extent of tissue resected. Arterial bleeds typically present with acute onset of hematuria, while venous bleeds will develop gradually. Postoperative bleeds may be due to patient-specific factors such as increased blood pressure as the patient emerges from anesthesia, or a coagulopathic state. A bleeding vessel is compressed with bladder distension during surgery; reinspection with a reduced volume in the bladder will often identify bleeding vessels before the surgery is complete.

A three-way catheter in place following endourological procedures allows for continuous bladder irrigation (CBI), which helps prevent the formation of any blood clots that may obstruct the outflow of urine, and helps to quell the bleeding. Urine return that is light-red to pink in color indicates that the current rate of irrigation is likely sufficient to prevent clot formation.

The lumen of the three-way catheter may become obstructed due to the relatively small size. Any obstruction in the catheter may lead to excessive urine retention and ultimately bladder wall perforation. If CBI is utilized, it should be gravity fed only and never connected to an intravenous pump. If there is any obstruction to the flow of CBI, the catheter should be flushed (by hand) with 60 to 120 mL of saline to remove any blood clots or debris. This is best performed by repeatedly instilling saline with a catheter-tip syringe and withdrawing the fluid present in the bladder, until the majority of clot material is extracted.

The nursing staff should monitor the amount of irrigation and return, to accurately calculate urine output, and should replace the irrigation bag as soon as it is nearly empty. Similarly, the drainage bags can fill up quickly, and need to be emptied frequently so that CBI flow is not reduced (any lull in CBI flow may lead to clot formation). If a clot forms, it needs to be manually extracted before resuming CBI. These patients are at risk for bladder wall perforation, as the wall may be significantly weakened after endourologic procedures, and stretched thin if intravesical pressures are high from obstructed CBI. The use of CBI is contraindicated in patients with confirmed or assumed bladder perforation. CBI should also be avoided or used with extreme caution in patients with fresh anastomoses of the GU tract.

All patients will have some bleeding after a transurethral resection of the prostate (TURP) and are managed postoperatively with a three-way catheter and CBI. The source of bleeding is generally from the venous sinuses of the prostate, so the catheter balloon is inflated to larger volumes than normal (30 mL vs the standard 10 mL) to fill and compress the prostatic fossa or defect left by the TURP. In cases with excessive bleeding, the catheter may be put on gentle traction (with a heavy fabric tape secured to the leg) to force the catheter balloon into the defect. Bed rest is generally necessary during this maneuver to avoid irritation of the bleeding sinus. This traction should be released each morning to reassess the hematuria and release the tension on the tissues. If heavy traction is left for too long, it can result in necrosis of the urethral sphincter muscle or prostate tissue.

Significant and early postoperative hematuria is likely of arterial origin and usually requires a return to the OR for inspection and potentially fulguration. Patients that develop hemodynamic instability nonresponsive to fluid resuscitation may also require re-exploration in the OR. The urologist should be consulted immediately for assessment.

■ URETHRAL-VESICAL ANASTOMOTIC LEAK IN RADICAL PROSTATECTOMY

Urethral-vesical anastomotic leak (UVAL) is one of the most common postoperative complications in radical prostatectomy. UVAL usually occurs early, with the incidence highest in the first 7 to 10 postoperative days. UVAL occurs in 1% to 10% of laparoscopic cases and 2% to 10% of radical retropubic prostatectomy cases. Robotic-assisted laparoscopic prostatectomy has advantages over pure laparoscopic techniques due to better visualization of the surgical field and the ability to perform a running anastomosis. The majority of anastomotic leaks are located in the posterior segment of the anastomosis, which is the site of the initial suture placement.

After surgery, the patients overall clinical condition and surgical drain output should be monitored. Drain output should significantly decrease over the first 24 to 48 hours; continued high output may indicate an injury to the ureter, and the fluid should be sent for a creatinine level. The majority of patients with mild urinary leak will be asymptomatic and the diagnosis is made based on drain output creatinine level (**Figure 67-3**). If symptomatic, the patient may have signs of peritonitis or paralytic ileus, which may indicate extravasation of urine into the peritoneum.

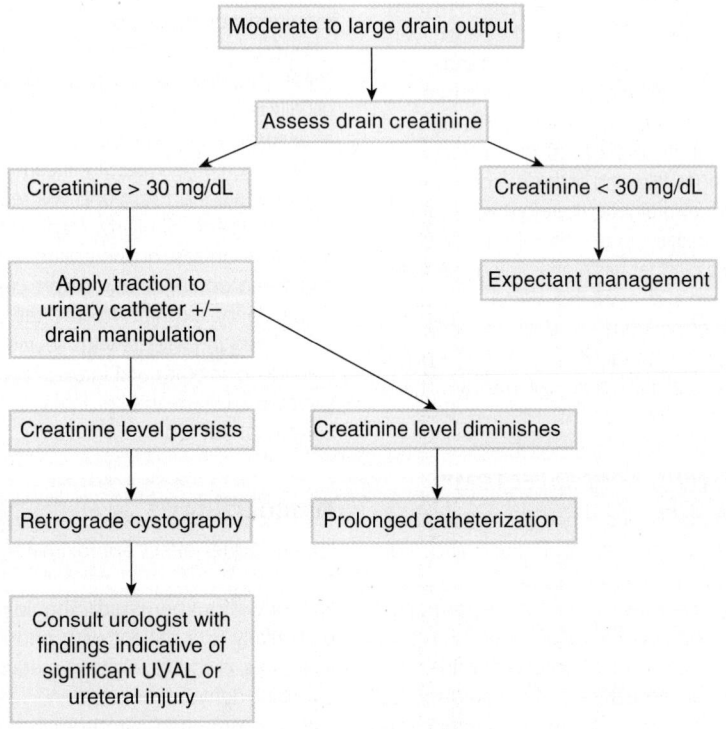

Figure 67-3 *Approach to the patient with suspected urethrovesical anastomotic leak.*

Initial management of a urine leak is conservative; the surgical drain and a transurethral catheter are left in place for a period of time (to aspirate urine from the anastomosis, and decompress the bladder, respectively). The urologist may apply gentle traction or manipulate the transurethral catheter (correct catheter placement can facilitate healing the anastomosis) and may repeatedly switch the surgical drain from active to passive drainage (releasing the pressure of the bulb) and slightly withdrawing the drain over time. If the creatinine content of the drain fluid persists following manipulation of the catheter and drain, a cystogram is indicated to rule out injury to the bladder and/or determine the severity of UVAL (alternative imaging includes CT cystography or retrograde urethrogram). If a ureteral injury is suspected, the best imaging is a CT scan using delayed images or a retrograde study of the ureter in the operating room. Longer term urine leaks are managed with prolonged catheterization, and further interventions may include urinary diversion with a suprapubic catheter or nephrostomy tubes, endoscopic evaluation, or ultimately reoperation.

■ URINE LEAK FOLLOWING PARTIAL NEPHRECTOMY

As partial nephrectomies have become the standard of care for excision of smaller renal parenchymal masses, the incidence of postoperative urinary leak has risen, and currently occurs between 0.5% to 21%, and is more common in excisions that remove endophytic masses involving the collecting system of the kidney.

Urinary leak following partial nephrectomy may present acutely or as a more insidious process. Early leak is typically due to unrecognized insult to the collecting duct system or a defect that was not repaired sufficiently; this should be suspected if drain output exceeds 30 to 40 mL/shift more than 48 hours after surgery. If present, the drain fluid creatinine will be markedly elevated (relative to the serum creatinine). The suspected leak should be evaluated with a noncontrast CT or sonogram to evaluate the drain placement, ensure the kidney is not obstructed (leading to higher pressures in the collecting system thereby perpetuating the leak), and ensure there is no urinoma present.

Delayed urinary leak will present anywhere between 5 and 14 days. The specific etiology of a delayed urine leak is unclear, but it is hypothesized that most are simply unrecognized early leaks. The patient with a delayed urine leak may present with fever, drain site tenderness, flank pain and/or drainage from a port site or incision. The suspected leak should be evaluated with CT with IV contrast (with delayed images to uncover any extravasation of contrast) or sonogram (to identify any perirenal fluid collections). Healing of the leak occurs most rapidly when there is maximal kidney drainage; therefore, a percutaneous drain may be required to evacuate an urinoma if it is impeding kidney drainage. In addition, if the bladder has high voiding pressures, the patient may need a short-term (1-3 days) indwelling catheter to reduce those pressures and allow the kidney to drain properly. The patient can be discharged with the drain and/or the Foley in place; they should be instructed to record daily drain volumes and have close follow-up (within a week) with the surgeon.

■ COMPLICATIONS FOLLOWING ADRENALECTOMY

Adrenalectomies are most commonly performed for the removal of pheochromocytomas, aldosteronomas, and glucocorticoid-producing tumors, and the physician should be able to recognize the symptoms that arise following abrupt removal of the hormones these tumors produce. Pheochromocytoma, aldosteronoma, and glucocorticoid-producing tumors produce norepinephrine/epinephrine, aldosterone, and cortisol, respectively, which predisposes the patient to a relative deficiency of these hormones. Other complications associated with adrenalectomy include postoperative bleeding or pneumothorax. The proximity of the adrenal glands to the liver, spleen and pancreas, as well as the posterior-inferior border of the diaphragm predispose surgical interventions to problems involving these organs.

Patients with a pheochromocytoma are usually on alpha-blockade perioperatively to control hypertension and often have contracted blood volumes due to the chronic exposure to catecholamines (and resulting increase in vascular tone). These patients are very vulnerable to the development of perioperative hypotension due to the abrupt decrease in norepinephrine. Aggressive fluid resuscitation should be started before surgery and continued throughout the procedure; vasopressors may also be required. Hypoglycemia is also a risk, due to a rebound increase in insulin and should be closely monitored.

Patients with an aldosteronoma are at increased risk of developing either hyperkalemia or hypokalemia in the perioperative period. Due to the excess preoperative aldosterone production, hypokalemia is more typical. Alternatively, in some patients the renin-angiotensin-adrenal-axis is down-regulated (due to the chronic hypernatremia associated with primary hyperaldosteronism). Thus, renin production by the renal juxtaglomerular apparatus is suppressed. If the contralateral adrenal gland cannot compensate for the abrupt decrease in aldosterone levels, patients may actually develop a temporary hyperkalemia and salt-wasting. Therefore, close monitoring of electrolytes and blood pressure is needed, and potassium-sparing diuretics should be immediately discontinued postoperatively.

Patients with a glucocorticoid-producing adenoma are at risk for adrenocortical insufficiency (also known as adrenal crisis). Adrenal crisis symptoms include hypoglycemia, hypotension, fever, nausea, vomiting, abdominal pain, hyponatremia, and hyperkalemia. The symptoms are due to the abrupt decrease in serum glucocorticoids from surgical removal, as well as the suppression of the contralateral adrenal gland from negative feedback at the level of the anterior pituitary. Perioperative administration of mineralocorticoids and glucocorticoids can prevent (or at least attenuate) postoperative adrenal crises. Patients who have undergone bilateral adrenalectomy will require long-term steroid replacement therapy. Patients who have had partial or unilateral adrenalectomy may or may not require supplementation.

Due to the anatomy and vascular supply of the adrenal gland, these surgeries have a high risk of hemorrhage; although this is usually recognized intraoperatively, hemodynamic instability shortly after surgery should be considered an unrecognized vascular insult until proven otherwise. Significant bleeding may require exploration in the operating room and will require the immediate notification of the surgeon. Similarly, respiratory difficulties may be related to an unrecognized or increasing pneumothorax, which should be confirmed on chest radiograph. Lastly, pancreatitis can occur from manipulation or injury to the tail of the pancreas, and should be considered in patients with severe back pain, abdominal pain and inability to tolerate oral intake. This finding may be confirmed with elevated amylase and lipase levels and may require bowel rest with parenteral nutrition.

■ UROLITHIASIS

Kidney stones affect approximately 1/11 US adults at some point during their lives. Any patient with unilateral flank or groin pain, with or without hematuria, should raise the suspicion of urolithiasis, particularly in a patient with prior history of stones or known risk factors (ie, diabetes, obesity, metabolic syndrome, gout, Caucasian ethnicity, dehydration, etc).

If an obstructing, symptomatic kidney stone is suspected, imaging should be obtained. Ultrasonography can identify the presence or absence of hydronephrosis, and can often identify stones as well, but the sensitivity is poor and is often inadequate for surgical planning. A low-dose, noncontrasted CT scan of the abdomen and pelvis (CT IVP) is a sensitive and specific modality for determining stone size, location and degree of consequent obstruction, if present. Moreover, it can assess a stone's hardness or composition by noting the Hounsfield Units (HU), which measures the radiodensity relative to distilled water at standard temperature and pressure. An abdominal radiograph of the kidney, ureter and bladder (KUB) can be helpful in patients who can be managed conservatively for stone disease. Additionally, if shock wave lithotripsy is desired, a KUB must be obtained to ensure that the stone is visible prior to scheduling. However, not all stones are visible on KUB, and bowel gas and other artifacts can intermittently obscure the image.

If infection or urosepsis is suspected (based on fever, chills, dysuria, unstable vital signs, leukocytosis, or findings on urinalysis) definitive stone treatment should be delayed and a ureteral stent or percutaneous nephrostomy tube should be placed to relieve the obstruction and allow for decompression of the collecting system. The stent or nephrostomy tube should be left in place while the infection is treated with an appropriate course of antibiotics. After resolution of symptoms and a negative urine culture, the patient can undergo definitive stone treatment.

If the stone is small (generally <6-8 mm), without marked hydro-ureteronephrosis, acute kidney injury, or infection, and the patient is tolerating fluids with adequate pain control on oral medications, it is reasonable to pursue medical expulsive therapy (MET). This consists of 2 to 4 weeks of daily tamsulosin, anti-inflammatory medications (if no contraindication), oral hydration, and pain/nausea control as needed. The hope is the patient passes the stone without surgical intervention. This is most likely in patients with small, distal stones, particularly those who have passed stones from the same ureter previously or who have been treated instrumented for stones previously, as these patients tend to have more dilated ureters. If the patient fails to pass the stone after 2 to 4 weeks on MET, surgical intervention is warranted.

If prior stone analysis data is available, the patient should be educated on proper dieting to avoid stone recurrences. Recommendations vary based on the type of stone, but in general should consist of ample water, low sodium, low oxalate, low animal protein

and normal calcium. Urinary citrate is a known stone inhibitor and is in high concentration in lemon and orange juice. Additional dietary and medical intervention, such as urinary alkalinization or thiazide therapy, is dependent on the type of stone as well as the patient's 24-hour urine collection.

SUGGESTED READINGS

Baldini G, Bagry H, Aprikian A, Carli F. Postoperative urinary retention: anesthetic and perioperative considerations. *Anesthesiology*. 2009;110(5):1139-1157.

Brandes S. Urologic Complications from Pelvic and Vaginal Surgery: How to Diagnose and Manage. http://urology.wustl.edu/en/Patient-Care/ReconstructiveSurgery/Urologic-Complications-from-Surgery. Accessed March 31, 2015.

Gould CV, Umscheid CA, Agarwal RK, Kuntz G, Pegues DA. Guideline for prevention of catheter-associated urinary tract infections. *Infect Control Hosp Epidemiol*. 2010;31(4):319-326.

Litwin MS and Saigal CS. Urologic Diseases in America Project. US Department of Health and Human Services, Public Health Service, National Institutes of Health, National Institute of Diabetes and Digestive and Kidney Diseases. Washington, DC: US Government Printing Office; 2012; NIH Publication No. 12-7865.

Oh BR, Kwon DD, Park KS, Ryu SB, Park YI, and Presti JC. Late presentation of ureteral injury after laparoscopic surgery. *Obstet Gynecol*. 2000;95(3):337-339.

Pearle MS, Asplin JR, Coe FL, Rodgers A, and Worcester EM. Medical management of urolithasis. In: Denstedt J, Khoury S, eds. *Second International Consultation on Stone Disease*. 2008 ed,. Health Publications, Committee 3; 57-84.

Pearle MS, Calhoun EA, Curhan GC. Urologic diseases in America Project: urolithiasis. *J Urol*. 2005;173(3):848.

Taneja SS. *Complications of Urologic Surgery*, 4th ed. Philadelphia, PA: Saunders; 2010.

Tyritzis SI, Katafigiotis I, Constantinides CA. All you need to know about urethrovesical anastomotic urinary leakage following radical prostatectomy. *J Urol*. 2012;188(2):369-376.

PART III
Rehabilitation and Skilled Nursing Care

CHAPTER 68

Postacute Care Rehabilitation Options

Eddy Ang, MD
Jatin K. Dave, MD, MPH

Following acute treatment of injury or illness, many patients require continued medical care, either at home or in a specialized facility. Postacute care refers to a range of such medical, nursing and rehabilitation services that support the individual's continued recuperation and rehabilitation from illnesses or management of a chronic illness or disability.

Medicare's payment to postacute care facilities totaled $59 billion in 2014, more than double since 2001. Also, variation in postacute care is the leading driver for overall Medicare cost. Postacute care providers include three facility based providers: (1) inpatient rehabilitation facilities (IRFs); (2) long-term care hospitals (LTCHs); (3) skilled nursing facilities (SNFs); as well as home based providers, such as home health agencies (HHAs) and hospice. More than 40% of the fee-for-service Medicare beneficiaries received postacute care services after being discharged from an acute care hospital in 2013.

The Medicare Post-Acute Care Transformation (IMPACT) Act of 2014 requires a standardized patient assessment data to be reported by all postacute care providers. In addition, there is significant work accomplished by Medicare policymakers to create a unified postacute care prospective payment system (PAC PPS) due to:

- four separate payment systems for SNFs, IRFs, LTCHs and HHAs;
- similar services provided in all settings with significant payment differences;
- the evidence that placement is driven at times by nonclinical factors such as provider availability;
- significant unexplained variations in postacute care services;
- the paucity of evidence on where the best care is provided.

One of the first steps to site-neutral payment is being implemented in LTCH setting since late 2015. Traditionally, the selection of appropriate postacute care setting and provider was determined by the hospital care managers/discharge planners. However in light of the increasing complexity of patients and rapidly changing postacute care regulations, it is important for hospitalists to be familiar with the options of multiple postacute care sites as well as the capabilities and types of patients different postacute settings care for. Additionally, due to the need for continuity of care and focus on safe transitions, 30% of the hospitalist groups are now practicing in postacute care settings.

The Centers for Medicare & Medicaid has identified 30-day readmission rate as a quality indicator across the nation. There is emerging evidence indicating that the 30-day readmission rates range from 5.8% to 19% among postacute rehabilitation facilities among Medicare beneficiaries. We will describe the different types of rehabilitation/postacute care options (see **Table 68-1** for types of post-acute care options) followed by strategies for selecting the right setting for hospitalized patients (see **Figure 68-1** for a flowchart of post-hospital disposition).

INPATIENT REHABILITATION FACILITIES (IRF OR "ACUTE" REHABILITATION)

Inpatient rehabilitation facilities are designed for the patients requiring intense multidisciplinary rehabilitation. Rehabilitative care typically takes place under the guidance of a physiatrist. Under the guidelines of Centers for Medicare & Medicaid (CMS), there is a requirement that 60% of patient admitted to an IRF meet 1 of following 13 medical diagnoses (**Table 68-2**).

In addition, an interdisciplinary team conference is mandated within 4 days of admission and weekly thereafter. In order to remain

TABLE 68-1 Types of Postacute Care Options

Type	Description	% of FFS Medicare Beneficiaries Discharged after Acute Stay	Case-Mix Adjustment Methodology	Cost Range	Approximate Average Payment/Case in 2013	LOS	Types of Payment	Top 3 Diagnoses	Readmissions during the Stay/within 30 Days of Discharge
LTCH	Facilities providing complex medical care (eg, post-ICU and Ventilator Support)	1%	DRG	1300-1500	$40,070	26.5 d	Hospital payment DRG	Respiratory Failure, Pulmonary Edema, Sepsis	13%
IRF	Facilities providing active rehab to patients who are able to perform at least 3h/d of PT and/or OT	4%	IRF-PAI	1200-1400	$17,995	13 d	Prospective payment per episode	Stroke, Fracture of the lower extremity and Neurological disorder	16%
SNF	Typically nursing homes that provide skilled care (eg, wound care and rehab) Growing need for SuperSNFs providing care to Complex Medical Patients	20%	MDS	350-450	$11,357	27 d	Daily rate (100 d but copayment after 20 d)	Joint Replacement Pneumonia Heart Failure	19%
Hospice/ palliative care	Hospice is intended for those with a life expectancy of <6 mo. Palliative care provides similar service without the restriction of a prognosis of <6 mo	N/A	N/A	150-250	$12,000	71 d	Payment per day	Cancer Dementia Heart Disease	5%
Home health care	Care provided by registered nurses for Medicare-certified conditions	17%	OASIS	100-300	$2674	46 d	Payment per-episode	Diabetes Mellitus Essential Hypertension Heart Failure	26%

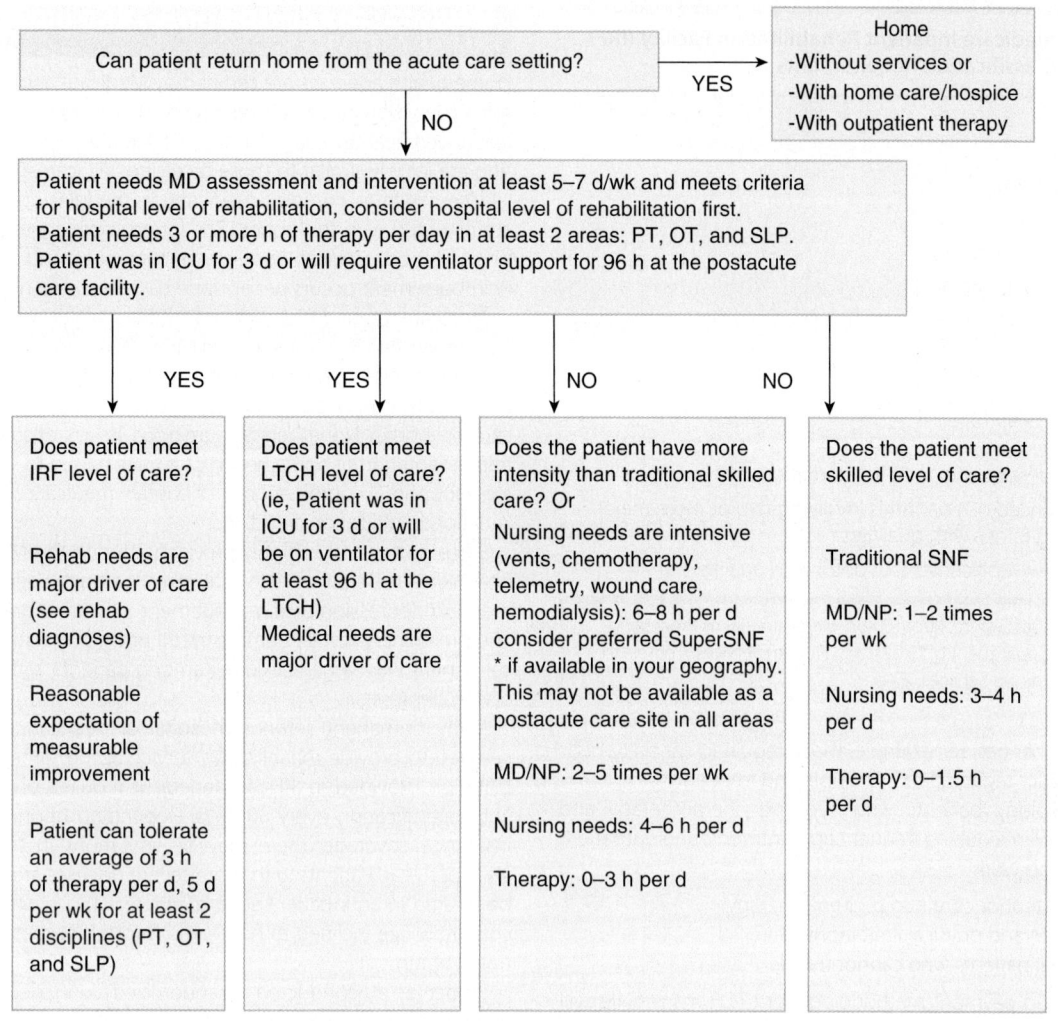

Figure 68-1 *Algorithm for patient disposition.* SuperSNF, SNF with enhanced capabilities such as daily MD/NP/ PA rounds, radiology onsite, ability to manage complex medical patients (eg, with tracheostomy or TPN).

on Medicare coverage, patients must be able to tolerate at least 3 hours a day of physical and occupational therapy and must show signs of progress each week. The costs incurred in this particular setting are relatively high compared to those of other options. Physician coverage is available 24 hours a day, 7 days a week.

LONG-TERM CARE HOSPITALS (LTCHs)

These Medicare-certified facilities provide medically intense care and the care teams are usually led by hospitalists. The vast majority of the patients are severely and chronically ill necessitating continued physician-level care which encompasses, but is not limited to, ventilator/tracheostomy care and weaning, acute dialysis, etc. This type of setting may be the most expensive across the many other postacute care options. Physician coverage is available 24 hours a day. The LTCHs receives discrete payments of more than 5 billion annually from Medicare. In 1997–2006, the average 1-year mortality remains dismal at 50%. During the same period, the number of LTCHs in the United States increased at a rate of 8.8% per year on average.

The average length of stay at the LTCHs approaches 1 month. Traditionally, an LTCH facility has to demonstrate an average length of stay of 25 days or greater in its inchoate demonstration period in order to ensure admissions are appropriate. Nevertheless, the Pathway for SGR Reform Act of 2013 proposed that starting in October 2015, LTCHs will only receive full Medicare payment rate if patients can meet one of the following criteria:

(1) having spent at least 3 days in an intensive care unit (ICU); (2) remaining on a ventilator at LTCH for at least 96 hours. Patient not meeting either of these criteria will be reimbursed at a per diem "site-neutral" payment rate, which is a 50/50 blended rate of the LTCH reimbursement rate and the Inpatient Prospective Payment System (IPPS) rate for a period of 2 years. Beginning in October 2017, admissions not satisfying the criteria will be reimbursed solely at the IPPS rate. Notably, the "25% Rule" remains in place which prohibits LTCHs from accepting more than 25% of its Medicare inpatients from any single hospital. Due to this payment change, other complex patients (who did not require intensive care unit or will be on ventilator for 96 hours at the LTCH) may be transferred to Skilled Nursing Facility requiring increased capabilities. Examples of such complex patients who will not quality for full LTCH payment include:

a. Complex Medical with multiple comorbidities not requiring ICU or ventilator at the LTCH

- Multiple comorbidities
- Complex wound care
- Delirium/sitter
- Frequent transfusions
- Tracheostomy care
- Hemodialysis

b. Complex psychosocial factors impeding discharge

c. Complex wound care requiring extensive dressings and

TABLE 68-2 Medicare Inpatient Rehabilitation Facility (IRF) Classification Requirements

Stroke

Spinal cord injury

Congenital deformity

Amputation

Major multiple trauma

Femur fracture (hip fracture)

Brain injury

Neurological disorders (including multiple sclerosis, muscular dystrophy, Parkinson disease)

Active polyarticular rheumatoid/psoriatic arthritis and seronegative arthritides, with qualifiers

Systemic vasculitides with joint inflammation, with qualifiers

Severe or advanced osteoarthritis involving two or more major weight-bearing joints, with qualifiers

Hip or knee joint replacement, or both, with qualifiers

Source: CMS Manual System. Pub. 100-04, Medicare Claims Processing, Transmittal 347. Department of Health and Human Services, Centers for Medicare and Medicaid Services; 2005.

dressing changes: for example, those requiring specialty beds or antibiotics regime that is multiple and frequent

d. New oncology patients with evolving chemotherapy and radiation plan requiring frequent appointments and outpatient care and lab work

- Intermittent or continuous chemotherapy
- Radiation and physical limitations
- Regional patients who cannot travel

With changing payment methodology for LTCH many SNFs will need to staff and develop capabilities to manage such complex patients. We are calling such advanced SNFs "SuperSNFs."

SKILLED NURSING FACILITY (SNF OR "SUBACUTE" REHAB)

Most of the patients requiring subacute rehabilitative services are discharged to nursing homes that are certified to provide this level of posthospital care. There is a lack of consensus to the term "skilled nursing" and therefore the services provided at the SNFs can vary from one institution to another. However, these facilities are ideal for providing a continuum of care that is typically initiated prior to discharge from a hospital, such as wound care and complex medication schedules. Care usually occurs under the leadership of hospitalists and nurse practitioners. Physician evaluation is mandatory within 2 weeks of admission and every 30 days thereafter.

For the traditional Medicare beneficiaries, there is a 3-night stay rule to the transfer of care from an acute-care hospital to a SNF. This policy has ineluctably led to unnecessary health care spending stemming from patient care that can safely take place in a subacute setting rather than a hospital. Currently, there are some accountable care organizations that can waive this 3-night stay restriction and allow subacute patients to bypass a hospitalization and be directly admitted to a SNF. The savings generated from this waiver could be utilized toward the postacute care for these patients. Some research that analyzed the available quality indicators of a SNF (eg, staffing intensity, the percentages of patients with delirium, pain level, new or worsening pressure ulcers) have concluded that those indicators were not consistently correlated with the adjusted risks of readmission or death.

HOME HEALTH AGENCIES (HHAs) AND OUTPATIENT THERAPY SERVICES

Home health agencies are certified by Medicare and operate under the supervision of registered nurses. It requires physician referral and recertification every 60 days. The patient profiles in this setting are largely similar to those receiving SNF care. Comprehensive services, such as complex medication schedules and wound care, are provided with this option. The interdisciplinary team consists of physical, occupational, and speech therapists, and social workers. Reimbursement occurs per episode based on case mix.

Medicare spent $18.2 billion on home health agencies in 2012 with more than 3.5 million beneficiaries receiving care. Home health care seems effective in bringing support to the struggling patients in the community particularly in the transitions from institutional care to home. Nonetheless, numerous issues ensuing the initial implementation of home health care have begun to surface, including suboptimal coordination with primary medical care, geographic variation in utilization, fraud, etc.

Since depression is highly prevalent among the Medicare home health care recipients, Bruce et al. investigated the efficacy of implementing depression care management in routine practice in 2015. The preliminary results demonstrated promising data but the clinical benefit was rather lackluster among patients with moderate to severe depression.

Many outpatient settings (hospital or free-standing clinic) are certified to provide rehabilitative service at the same level of rehabilitation provided in IRFs. In general, it requires physician referral and recertification every 30 days. Depending upon the individual insurance coverage, there may be limitations in the number of visits per year. Patients with more severe diseases are more likely to be treated in an inpatient setting; whereas those with more stable conditions are inclined to be treated through outpatient rehabilitative programs.

Binder et al. conducted a randomized controlled trial in 2004 comparing the efficacy of extended outpatient rehabilitation with low-intensity home exercise among community-dwelling frail older adults with hip fracture and concluded that the 6 months of extended outpatient rehabilitation not only improved physical function and quality of life, but also reduced disability.

HOSPICE/PALLIATIVE CARE

Hospice care is intended for those who have reached terminal phase of life with expected prognosis of less than 6 months. It commonly takes place at home and is a specific benefit under Medicare. However, some hospitals and nursing homes may have designated hospice units. Comparing Medicare beneficiaries who died in 2000 and those in 2005 and 2009, a declining number of deaths occurred in an acute care hospital. However, patients with limited resources may be more likely to die in a nonhome setting. As shown in a study by Obermeyer et al. in 2014, the patients with poor-prognosis cancer who received hospice care had significantly lower rates of hospitalization and intensive care unit admission. They were also less likely to be subject to invasive procedures at the end of life. The total health care costs were significantly lower during the last year of life among those on hospice care.

Once in the program, patients are allowed to disenroll at any point in time. It is not uncommon that some patients may "graduate" from hospice care and continue to live beyond 6 months. With respect to the prediction of 6-month life expectancy among nursing home residents with advanced dementia, the performance of hospice eligibility guidelines appear somewhat nebulous. A prospective study illustrated that the performance of the Advanced Dementia Prognostic Tool (ADEPT) was slightly superior to hospice eligibility guidelines, though the initiation of hospice care should still be based upon the patient's goals of care as well as their estimated life expectancy.

Hospice Program aims at ameliorating uncomfortable physical symptoms, such as pain, dyspnea, constipation, nausea, excessive mucus production. It also provides emotional and spiritual support for the patients and their family members from the very beginning and continues through the bereavement period. The core staff includes palliative care specialists, chaplains, and social workers. In 2015, Ornstein et al. showed that there was a slight reduction in depressive symptoms among spouses of hospice users compared with spouses of nonhospice users.

In general, hospice use was more common among whites. A study (Givens et al., 2010) that analyzed a national cohort of Medicare beneficiaries with heart failure in 2010 revealed that blacks and Hispanics were less likely to utilize hospice care for heart failure than whites. Interestingly, a survey conducted by Chinn et al. in 2014 explored physicians' preferences for hospice if there terminally ill disclosed that especially female physicians and primary care physicians were more in favor of hospice and thus more likely to discuss the option of hospice care with their patients.

In the Veterans Health Administration (VHA) population, medical patients are more likely to receive either hospice or palliative care in their last 12 months of life compared with surgical patients. Further research is needed to elucidate the disparity of use of hospice care in such cases.

DISCHARGING TO A POSTACUTE CARE SETTING

(1) **Who** requires Postacute care

Patients at high risk for requiring postacute care services include those over the age of 75, with decreased physical or social functioning, patients who were dependent for iADLs but independent of ADLs at baseline, patients with delirium, hospitalization durations greater than 1 week, and patients with previous transfer to a postacute care facility for similar problem.

(2) **When** to Make the Referral to Postacute Care

Referrals should be made early in most patients, once the diagnostic workup is completed and the plan for treatment is in place. Early referrals are beneficial to patients because of the emphasis on rehabilitation, reduced iatrogenesis, improved continuity of care, and increased chances of qualifying for more appropriate and aggressive levels of care. This, in turn, is associated with reduced length of stay and cost savings in the acute care setting.

(3) **Where:** Strategies for selecting appropriate high-value postacute care setting based on patient's needs, postacute care capabilities and current payment model:

The selection of an appropriate postacute care setting is contingent upon the patient's needs (eg, medical, nursing, rehabilitation, etc.) and Postacute Care Setting capabilities (**Table 68-3**). It would also involve the patient's level of motivation and participation. Also, the availability of services may vary significantly among different settings in different geographic locations.

With movement toward value-based payment, creating list of high-value preferred postacute care partners based on quality and clinical criteria is becoming increasing common. Hospitalists can create a scoring system based on their organizational goals and screen available postacute care setting to select preferred postacute care partners. The best practice is to regularly meet and communicate with these preferred providers (home care, SNF or Hospice) to set clear expectation and accountability.

(4) **How:** Barriers to Discharge to Postacute Care

Although early referrals may be made, there are some nonmodifiable and potentially modifiable barriers to early discharge. It is important

for the health care providers to identify those potentially modifiable barriers to early discharge and change the plan accordingly.

Nonmodifiable barriers include lack of bed availability at the postacute care site or if the patient is ineligible by postacute care admission standards.

Modifiable barriers may include:

a. Uncertainty in the clinical trajectory. Health care providers should not get caught up on knowing all the answers or fearing the unknown. Once patients have completed their diagnostic workup and a treatment plan is in place, they can be referred to the postacute care site. If medical complexity is the uncertainty, patients will be better managed at appropriately staffed facility, such as IRF or LTCH.

b. Patient or family reluctance. Many patients and their families do not recognize the term "postacute care." If the health care team is knowledgeable about these different settings and the requirements for each setting, this can alleviate some of the patient's and family's concerns, questions, or uncertainty. Also, it may be helpful to underscore the important fact that many of these postacute care settings are designed to continue care initiated in the hospital with a larger focus on rehabilitation.

c. Loss of involvement with patient's care. This can be improved by continuous communication. The providers at postacute care settings are more than willing to communicate with the acute care physicians about the status of the patient, and likewise, are always appreciative of updates at the time of admission to the postacute care setting. Thorough discharge summaries (at both settings) are key to updating the next health care provider on continuing issues or items that require follow-up.

d. Unawareness and inconsistencies of clinical capabilities of nonacute options. Postacute care facilities do differ from site to site. Many of the social workers or case managers will be able to identify some key differences, but it is important that upon the initiation of screening that physicians and health care providers accurately document in the medical record what services/therapies would be expected at the time of discharge.

e. Poor communication back from facilities.

f. Inadequate documentation of patient's complexity and needs.

(5) Steps to Promote Timely Discharges to Postacute Care

Health care providers should:

a. identify functional needs early and address these with the help of the multidisciplinary team.

b. anticipate which of these medical or functional needs will need to be addressed, if any, at the time of discharge.

c. communicate these needs in the medical record, to the nursing staff, and to the case managers.

d. set clear expectations with the family and the patient about the length of stay and the need for postacute care. The choice of facility at this time of planning is not as important, since this may change and will likely be addressed with the patient and family by the case manager.

e. begin thinking about the discharge process at admission. For example, if discharge to a skilled nursing facility is planned, keep in mind that Medicare patients must be in the hospital under admission status for three midnights to access their SNF benefit. If the plan is to discharge to LTAC or IRF, this does not apply since these are hospital-level facilities.

f. simplify medications and discontinue any unnecessary medications (especially prn medications).

g. complete the discharge summary the day before discharge. By doing so, it can be transmitted to the accepting postacute care facility and medications can be ordered and be ready for the

TABLE 68-3 Criteria Example for Selecting Preferred Postacute Care Partners

Access/geography	Total capacity/occupancy
	Capacity to accept patients during weekend
	Contracted with multiple payers
	Integration with the same Electronic Medical Records
Quality/utilization	Medicare Star Rating
	Department of Public Health Score
	Accreditation
	Length of Stay
	Readmission Rate
Communication	Clear rules of engagement and hand off
	Regular review of outcomes (such as readmissions)
Clinical capabilities	Specialized clinical programs and services, such as heart failure or COPD program
	Responsiveness: See patients within 24-48 h
	Able to handle complex patients via individualized care plan

patient. Any questions or discrepancies can be addressed by the admitting providers before the patient has left the acute care setting.

SUGGESTED READINGS

Feder J. Bundle with care—rethinking Medicare incentives for post-acute care services. *N Engl J Med.* 2013;369:400-401.

Kane, RL. Finding the right level of posthospital care. *JAMA.* 2011; 305(3):284-293.

Medicare Payment Advisory Commission. Medicare's post-acute care: trends and ways to rationalize payments. March 2015 Report to the Congress: Medicare payment policy. Washington, DC: MedPAC.

Mitchell, SL, Miller, SC, Teno, JM, Kiely, DK, Davis, RB, Shaffer, ML. Prediction of 6-month survival of nursing home residents with advanced dementia using ADEPT vs hospice eligibility guidelines. *JAMA.* 2010;304(17):1929-1935.

Neuman, MD, Wirtalla, C, Werner, RM. Association between skilled nursing facility quality indicators and hospital readmissions. *JAMA.* 2014;312(15):1542-1551.

The Society of Hospital Medicine (SHM). 2014 *State of Hospital Medicine* Report.

CHAPTER 69

Physical Therapy and Rehabilitation

Thomas E. McNalley, MD
Christopher J. Standaert, MD

Key Clinical Questions

1. What are the roles of physical and occupational therapy in the inpatient setting?

2. Which patients should be seen by a physical or occupational therapist?

3. What is a physiatrist? What role does he or she play in the care of hospitalized patients, and how does it differ from the role of the hospitalist?

4. How can rehabilitation services assist in discharge planning?

INTRODUCTION

Physical therapists (PTs) and occupational therapists (OTs) address the functional needs of patients through mobilization, conditioning, and training in self-care, and other specific tasks. PTs and OTs practice in many settings, including the hospital, clinic, skilled nursing facility (SNF), long-term care facility, freestanding inpatient intensive rehabilitation center, and home. A smaller number also practice in emergency departments in the assessment and treatment of musculoskeletal injury. Less heralded is the role that PTs and OTs play in minimizing specific in-hospital complications, and optimizing successful transitions to outpatient care. Given the growing economic pressures on hospitals, including nonpayment for some nosocomial complications or for rapid readmission to the hospital after discharge (bounce-backs), PTs and OTs are not only crucial in helping patients regain functional capacity, but are also vital to the financial well-being of inpatient hospitals. Unfortunately, the scope of practice of PTs and OTs often lies beyond the focus of physicians. Medical education often underemphasizes the role of allied health providers and their contributions to restoring health and function. This chapter attempts to correct this underexposure by delineating the roles and responsibilities of these therapists, and indicating their impact on specific diagnoses commonly encountered by the hospitalist.

CASE 69-1

AN ICU TRANSFER TO THE MEDICAL SERVICE AFTER A DEBILITATING MEDICAL ILLNESS

A 53-year-old previously healthy male, with a past medical history of hypertension, developed a febrile illness over several days, and collapsed at his small business. The emergency medical technicians successfully resuscitate him and he is admitted to the intensive care unit. Over a period of 4 weeks he has a complicated course including prolonged intubation necessitating tracheostomy placement due to respiratory failure from community-acquired methicillin-resistant *Staphylococcus aureus* (MRSA) pneumonia, encephalopathy attributed to acute illness delirium, acute kidney injury requiring dialysis, and demand ischemia characterized by an elevated troponin without ECG changes. Ultimately, the patient stabilizes and is transferred to the general medical service after tracheostomy and placement of a percutaneous endoscopic gastrostomy (PEG) tube for nutrition. Communication is difficult due to the tracheostomy. Overnight he becomes agitated and receives haloperidol. He requires suctioning every 1 to 2 hours, and is not yet ready for discharge to a hospital-level rehabilitation facility. On rounds he appears agitated when he requires suctioning. Assessing mental status is difficult due to tracheostomy, and he does not appear to respond to commands optimally.

Although this patient clearly requires acute medical treatment, how can you improve this individual's level of functioning within the framework of his illness? What steps can you take to fast track him to a rehabilitation facility so that he can receive the complex multidisciplinary care he needs to ultimately return home to his family and maybe even return to work?

If available, early consultation with a physiatrist can be instrumental to:

- Reduce the complications that he has already experienced during his hospitalization
- Improve physical and social function

- Identify cognitive and emotional complications of traumatic brain injury (even if not physically apparent by head CT)
- Concentrate coordinated therapy
- Improve the likelihood that this patient may eventually go home

For this patient, physiatry consultation assisted the team in properly diagnosing and treating his agitation, which was initially assumed to be due to a combination of delirium and inability to communicate when he needed suctioning. The physiatrist, however, identified that he had cognitive and emotional complications analogous to patients who had suffered traumatic brain injury while he was in the intensive care unit. The physiatrist made specific pharmacologic recommendations, engaged the family who had not visited him, coordinated the care of physical therapy, occupational therapy, speech therapy, and communicated with a rehabilitation facility best able to meet his complex needs. Due to the physiatrist's intervention, the patient was fast-tracked to a rehabilitation center, which gave him the greatest chance of achieving functional recovery.

PHYSICAL THERAPY

Physical therapists have completed 4 years of postgraduate training, with a focus in musculoskeletal assessment and treating impairments in safety and mobility. Although they most actively provide care for orthopedic and neurosurgical patients, they also clinically assess patients with medical problems such as breathing dysfunction, the need for cardiac rehabilitation, and chronic vertigo. For example, patients with respiratory disease are often readmitted due to exacerbations of their chronic disease. PTs focus on breathing, posture, mobility, range of motion of joints, and strengthening of the respiratory muscles, and they use physical modalities to assist patients with musculoskeletal derangements in the thoracic or rib area. On a busy medical service, PTs can prevent loss of function during long-term hospitalization by improving the patient's ability to move within a bed, and progress from supine to sitting, sitting to standing, and finally to ambulation. PTs review the medical record and the history provided by the patient and family, and perform a focused musculoskeletal examination to identify deformities, atrophy, limitations in range of motion (ROM), weakness, and functional impairments that can be addressed with various interventions. They also provide a wide range of tests and measurements.

Hospitalists find PTs helpful in many areas, but may not request their services until the time of discharge, when the therapist is urgently requested to "assess for home safety." Involving the therapist as early as possible is ideal, since early interventions may decrease the length of hospital stay and increase the likelihood of the patient being discharged directly to home. As well, the patient's mood, appetite, sense of well-being, and general medical condition may all benefit from increased activity.

PT interventions may be educational, such as teaching a patient how to safely roll in bed to allow nursing care. They can also be more complex, including moving from supine to sitting, evaluating and improving sitting balance, and progressing to standing while monitoring for hemodynamic changes. Once upright, the patient may be able to ambulate, and the therapist can recommend assistive devices such as canes or walkers. New gait impairments may require further training, and occasionally lower-extremity bracing with orthoses. If the patient is unable to reliably stand or walk, or lacks adequate endurance, he or she may need a wheelchair. The power wheelchair and the much-promoted power scooter allow greater mobility, with the loss of the aerobic challenge of self-propulsion. In the United States, Medicare will often cover part of the cost of powered mobility devices in patients who meet certain criteria.

A common concern in patients with neuromuscular dysfunction is the risk of joint contractures. Up to 39% of patients who stay in the intensive care unit (ICU) for longer than 2 weeks develop at least one joint contracture. A stay of 8 weeks in the ICU increases the odds ratio of contracture to 7.1, compared with patients staying 2 to 3 weeks. Joint contractures may result in pain, permanent deformity, gait abnormality, and loss of mobility. Contractures also predispose the patient to skin breakdown. Prevention is again best facilitated by early PT consultation. Stretching, strengthening, and protective splints all reduce the likelihood of plantar flexion deformity and other lower-extremity contractures. OTs usually address concerns with the upper extremity, as discussed below.

The PT may help prevent and treat skin injury by ensuring adequate movement to reduce the risk of decubitus ulcers, protect surgical incisions and skin grafts, and reduce discomfort from malpositioning or immobility. The therapist may also instruct the patient about the avoidance of faulty transfer techniques or seating arrangements that may lead to shear injuries to the skin.

Falls, and the fear of falling, contribute to morbidity both in and out of the hospital. In the debilitated elderly, falls may lead to fractures, especially of the hips and forearms, or intracranial pathology, including subdural hematomas. Fear of falls may lead to a downward spiral of immobility and progressive weakness that actually increase the risk of falls. Prevention should begin in the hospital. The PT can assess fall risk using the Berg Balance Scale, and intervene as needed. For some patients, simple reminders and strengthening are adequate protection; for others, an assistive device may suffice. Still others may require intervention in an intensive, interdisciplinary rehabilitation environment. Patients in the latter group usually need evaluation by a physiatrist prior to transfer to in-patient rehabilitation.

OCCUPATIONAL THERAPY

The title *occupational therapist* may confuse both patients and other health care professionals. An occupation is defined as a job or profession, but in OT it is defined as a task or activity fulfilled in daily life. OTs focus on restoring patients to their basic self-care, and ideally to independent living. Like the PT, OTs have completed 4 years of postgraduate training, but with a special focus on assessing, preserving, and restoring upper-extremity strength, function, and ROM. Some undergo additional training to become certified hand therapists. OT interventions include stretching and ROM exercises. Bracing and splinting may be recommended for patients with increased upper-extremity tone from neurologic disease, or scarring from burns that place them at risk for joint contracture. OTs participate in identifying postdischarge needs, and in some hospitals, they perform home-safety evaluations by observing patients in typical tasks done at home, such as cooking a meal. As with physical therapy, the wise clinician will involve OT early in the hospitalization.

SPEECH THERAPY

The ability to swallow or eat affects nutritional status and also quality of life. Many conditions increase the risk of swallow disorders, which are more common in the elderly (**Table 69-1**).

As part of the functional assessment of patients at admission, hospitalists should evaluate for the possibility of a dysphagia disorder. Family members may be the first to suspect a problem. Recurrent pneumonias, malnutrition, and social isolation are important clues (**Table 69-2**).

The role of the speech and language pathologist is to diagnose swallowing disorders, make treatment recommendations, and coordinate an interdisciplinary approach with the health care team, including nurses, respiratory therapists, physical therapists, and nutritionists, as well as educating the patient and family.

TABLE 69-1 Risk Factors for Dysphagia

Complications of Hospitalization

- Intubation
- Deconditioning
- Medications (including anesthesia, opioids, sedatives, some antibiotics, carbidopa-levodopa)
- Delirium

Disorders

- Cancer (especially head and neck)
- Stroke, neurodegenerative
- Burns and trauma
- Diabetes
- Cardiac dysfunction
- Chronic obstructive pulmonary disorder
- Cervical hypertrophic osteoarthropathy (encroachment of osteophytes at the C-6 cricoid cartilage)

Adapted from Brown CJ, Peel C. Rehabilitation. In: *Hazzard's Geriatric Medicine and Gerontology*, 6th ed. New York, NY: McGraw-Hill; 2009.

The speech therapist performs a bedside swallowing assessment unless there are contraindications. Examples that would require postponement of an evaluation include inability to cooperate because of an unstable medical condition such as active gastrointestinal bleeding or respiratory distress, inability to maintain upright or side-lying at 90 degrees, unexplained sudden change in temperature, active ventilator weaning, or altered mental status. If the bedside evaluation is inconclusive, nothing by mouth is recommended until a complete evaluation can be performed under video fluoroscopy. This study examines the oral, pharyngeal, and esophageal stages of ingestion, and should identify if there is aspiration, or significant risk of aspiration, below the level of the vocal cords. It may also evaluate whether the compensatory swallowing techniques are effective in preventing aspiration. Speech and language pathologists may recommend specific techniques to reduce the risk of aspiration such as head posture (chin tuck, turning head to weaker or stronger side, tilting head backward), body posture (upright at 90 degrees, lying on one side between feedings rather than supine), and manner of oral intake (rate, consistency, sizes, liquids by spoon).

PHYSIATRY

A rehabilitation physician, or physiatrist, is a specialist in physical medicine and rehabilitation (PM&R). Physiatry has been recognized as a specialty by the American Medical Association since 1946. The original impetus for growth of the field was the demand for

TABLE 69-2 Indications for Swallowing Evaluation

Any patient with:

- Past medical history of reported dysphagia symptoms
- Observed dysphagia
- Suspected aspiration
- Decreased oral feeding, dehydration, malnutrition
- Parenteral or enteral feeding
- Intubation, tracheostomy, or ventilator weaning
- Vocal cord paresis, paralysis, or laryngospasm
- Deconditioning

TABLE 69-3 Common Indications for Physiatry Consultation

Amputation

Spinal cord injury

Stroke, in conjunction with speech therapists, recreational therapists, physical therapists, and occupational therapists

Traumatic brain injury

Medical patients requiring complex rehabilitation

Musculoskeletal syndromes: low back pain, fibromyalgia

Chronic pain management, in conjunction with psychologists, physical therapists, occupational therapists, chiropractors, and anesthesiologists with expertise in pain management and interventional procedures

sophisticated rehabilitation techniques for the large influx of injured soldiers returning from World War II. Physiatrists concentrate on the ability of patients to function optimally within the limits placed upon them by disease processes which may not be reversible. A team approach to chronic conditions is emphasized to coordinate care by building on and strengthening the resources of the person and family, providing for a facilitating environment, and developing performance goals in that environment.

A PM&R residency includes training in spinal cord injury, brain injury, stroke, neuromuscular disease, and musculoskeletal injury, as well as the performance of electrodiagnostic studies and the assessment of neuromusculoskeletal impairment. A physiatrist can help determine why a patient is weak, distinguishing between critical illness neuromyopathy, steroid myopathy, and other causes of debility. They can evaluate patients with specific impairments and recommend orthoses, bracing, or other assistive devices to improve mobility, and provide recommendations for formal physical or occupational therapy, as well as weight-bearing and fall precautions. Physiatrists work closely with PTs, OTs, speech-language pathologists, and allied providers in the coordinated delivery of multidisciplinary care. They often oversee the rehabilitation process, and work with hospitalists to ensure that care is appropriate for the medical context (**Table 69-3**).

REHABILITATION

The definition of *rehabilitation* by the World Health Organization is "the use of all means aimed at reducing the impact of disabling and handicapping conditions and at enabling people with disabilities to achieve optimal social integration."

Acute rehabilitation refers to treatment that occurs within the first month of illness once the patient has been resuscitated or received definitive care, and by definition involves more acute medical or surgical issues than postacute rehabilitation.

Rehabilitation begins with improving mobility by getting the patient out of bed. Depending on the underlying condition of the patient, this may begin immediately, or be delayed for weeks with patients with spine injuries. Patients with upper extremity injuries will need to learn how to get out of bed without using that arm, and require forearm supports on ambulatory assistive devices. If the lower extremity is affected, the patient must learn how to get out of bed while elevating the injured leg. Walking with a walker or crutches for patients with reduced or no weight-bearing requires 30% to 50% more energy compared with normal walking. For patients with decreased cardiopulmonary reserve, this can be especially challenging. For patients with preexisting impaired mobility, the goal of rehabilitation is to return the patient to functional status prior to the injury. As the patient regains mobility, rehabilitation

471

also addresses affected joints with the goal of regaining range of motion. The next step of rehabilitation is to improve motor control and coordination so that the patient will eventually be able to exercise. Strengthening exercises with progressive resistive exercises can then begin. Finally, rehabilitation helps patients and families adapt to permanent impairments.

Rehabilitation is provided at different levels with a hierarchy of interventions depending on the complexity of the patient's problems and needs. The lowest level of consultation in the hospital setting is a single therapeutic intervention by PT or OT, such as a PT safety assessment for home discharge, or to identify postdischarge needs for PT and OT. Other patients with complex needs may require continued acute hospitalization for active and potentially unstable conditions. Still other patients who have complex disabilities as a consequence of an acute injury, stroke, or medical conditions or an acute event in a patient with prior disabilities, such as multiple sclerosis, benefit from high-level rehabilitation. Complex rehabilitation requires the involvement of at least three specialists such as gait retraining, continence management, and speech therapy.

To qualify for a rehabilitation hospital, patients generally carry a "rehab diagnosis"—stroke or traumatic brain injury or spinal cord injury, among many—and must demonstrate the ability to perform over 3 hours of therapy daily or require complex treatment such as ventilator care, wound care, physical therapy, OT, and speech therapy (**Table 69-4**).

TABLE 69-4 Rehabilitation Providers and Typical Methods Used for Evaluation and Treatment

Provider	Methods of Evaluation and Treatment
Physical therapist	Assessment: • Joint range of motion, muscle strength, motor skills, coordination • Gait and mobility, including ability to perform ADLs • The need for appropriate assistive devices Educational goals: • Relieve discomfort • Regain, maintain, or improve function Treatment: • Active and passive exercise training to increase range of motion, strength, endurance, balance, coordination, and gait • Physical modalities (heat, cold, ultrasound, massage, hydrotherapy, and electrical stimulation)
Occupational therapist	Assessment: • Self-care skills and other activities of daily living • Home environment • The need for assistive technology Education: • Self-care skills training • Training in use of assistive technology Treatment: • Fabrication of splints • Upper extremity deficits
Speech therapist	Assessment: • All aspects of communication • Swallowing disorders Education: • Alteration of diet to reduce aspiration risk • Maneuvers to reduce aspiration risk Treatment: • Communication deficits
Nurse	Assessment: • Self-care skills • Family and home-care factors Education: • Self-care training • Patient and family regarding ADLs, IDLs, medications, underlying medical problems, preventive measures Treatment: • Primary focus on cure of acute medical issues or palliation if patients are terminal • Liaison with community

(Continued)

TABLE 69-4 Rehabilitation Providers and Typical Methods Used for Evaluation and Treatment (*Continued*)

Provider	Methods of Evaluation and Treatment
Social worker	Assessment: • Family and home care factors • Psychosocial factors Education: • Patient and family rights Treatment: • Counseling • Liaison with community
Dietician	• Assess nutritional status • Recommend dietary alterations to maximize nutrition • Monitor TPN
Recreation therapist	• Assess leisure skills and interests • Involve patients in recreational activities to maintain social roles
Prosthetist	• Makes and fits prosthetic limbs
Orthotist	• Makes a variety of orthotics including braces, ankle–foot orthoses, splints, and shoe inserts • Assesses fit of orthotics

Adapted from Brown CJ, Peel C. Rehabilitation. In: *Hazzard's Geriatric Medicine and Gerontology*, 6th ed. New York, NY: McGraw-Hill; 2009.

The term *rehab* is often applied to SNFs that offer therapy services, but do not provide hospital-level or more formal inpatient interdisciplinary rehabilitation. Many elderly patients, in particular, primarily need physical therapy for endurance training so that they can safely perform ADLs and go home. Despite having a "rehab diagnosis," these patients are not candidates for intensive rehabilitation because of low endurance, weight-bearing precautions, or other factors such as inability to participate due to dementia. These patients may be more appropriate for "subacute rehab," often delivered in a SNF, with a less intensive schedule of rehabilitation services. Rehabilitation providers can generally make recommendations for the proper level of intensity in the patient's ongoing recovery, and assist with the process of establishing an appropriate discharge location.

Homebound individuals may qualify for home-health physical or occupational rehabilitative therapies, with an eye toward eventually transitioning to outpatient therapies. In general, patients receive 2 to 3 days of therapy per week in SNFs, outpatient clinics, or at home.

COMMON INPATIENT CONDITIONS THAT BENEFIT FROM REHABILITATION CONSULTATION

■ MUSCULOSKELETAL IMPAIRMENTS

Although rarely the primary cause of a patient's admission, osteoarthritis (OA) and other joint complaints are frequent in hospitalized persons. Joint complaints impair mobility through pain, restricted movement or contracture, and weakness from disuse. Low back pain is a particular source of limitation, and is highly prevalent in older populations. Knee osteoarthritis is also common, particularly in the obese and the elderly. Mobilization frequently requires adequate pain control. Both acetaminophen and nonsteroidal anti-inflammatory drugs (NSAIDs) are effective in osteoarthritis pain, although the risks of bleeding, renal damage, and hypertension limit the use of NSAIDs. For acute flares of joint pain, intra-articular injections may reduce pain and improve mobility and function. Splinting and bracing may also contribute to pain relief and mobility. Opiates are generally reserved for the final stages of OA, and should be used with great restraint.

PTs are of high value to patients with back and knee pain, as they can help to improve gait mechanics, strengthen weak muscles around painful joints, and provide assistive devices for joint protection and stability, and thereby allowing faster mobilization of a hospitalized patient. In the order for physical therapy, the physician should detail specific joints known to be affected. The PT should also know about upper extremity limitations, especially when use of crutches or a walker may be required. OTs are helpful for patients with upper extremity dysfunction related to OA or other causes.

■ JOINT REPLACEMENT

PTs and OTs are an integral component of care for patients undergoing joint-replacement surgery, assisting in tasks ranging from mobilization, education, and self-care to home safety and modifications. Surgeons involve these providers early in the care process to individualize exercises depending on the patient's condition. In the immediate postoperative period, patients are educated about the importance of early mobilization to optimize function of the new joint, movements to avoid to protect the prosthetic joint, exercises to perform to avoid thrombophlebitis, and when to call for assistance. Weight-bearing progresses based on the surgical technique and materials and the patient's ability to participate. PTs facilitate better outcomes, shorter hospital stays, fewer medical complications, and more successful transitions to home or rehabilitative care.

■ OSTEOPOROSIS

Risk factors for osteoporotic fractures include age, female gender, tobacco use, corticosteroid treatment, caffeine intake, low body weight, and inactivity. As inactivity is common in hospitalized patients, early mobilization, strength, and gait training are important strategies to mitigate the risk of worsening osteoporosis, in addition to drug therapies such as calcium and vitamin D supplementation, bisphosphonates, and teriparatide.

■ STROKE

There is now evidence that the best results for functional recovery occur for young patients and when PT and OT are involved early after the stroke occurs. In the early phase of stroke, individuals often have flaccid paralysis and are at high risk for pressure palsies and joint injury. Proper positioning and support are essential at this juncture. The speech-language pathologist has an equally important role. Death from aspiration and pneumonia is common after stroke, and a speech-language pathologist can assess aspiration risk and devise an appropriate diet or approach to feeding.

Loss of bladder control is a troubling complication of stroke that may be aggravated by problems with muscle control, speech, and cognition. Improving mobility, attention, and communication through physical, occupational, and speech therapy interventions can greatly improve bladder management. This may lessen the risk of urinary tract infections during hospitalization and lead to more successful home discharge. Depression is another significant and common complication of stroke; roughly 30% of stroke patients develop clinical depression. In addition to psychological and pharmacologic intervention, the role of rehabilitation services in enhancing recovery may also be helpful in depression.

Although neurologic impairments older than 4 to 6 months are unlikely to be completely reversed by therapy, functional performance may benefit from skilled therapies. Thus, the patient with an older stroke who is readmitted to the hospital may enjoy a better outcome if PTs, OTs, and speech therapists are consulted early in the hospital stay.

■ CRITICAL ILLNESS NEUROMYOPATHY

Persons who have had sepsis, hypotension, or hypoxemia may develop critical illness neuromyopathy. An electrodiagnostic study may clarify the diagnosis and provide prognostic information. Patients with more profound axonal damage generally have a worse outcome. Patients with critical illness neuromyopathy may need weeks to months to recover from their neurologic impairment; some never do. Weakness predisposes the individual to loss of joint movement and contractures. Decubitus ulcers are a threat. These individuals frequently require a high level of care upon discharge. Mobilization with a therapist can improve blood flow, encourage cardiovascular fitness, and contribute to better pulmonary hygiene. With true muscle atrophy (loss of muscle fibers), there is unlikely to be an improvement in muscle bulk through short-term interventions by therapists. However, neuromuscular control and improved recruitment of extant fibers likely contribute to improved performance. Similarly, function can improve with adaptive techniques and equipment provided by therapists.

■ DEBILITY

For deconditioning related to bed rest or inactivity, also known as debility, the loss of strength in healthy young men is about 1% per day, or roughly 10% per week. In elderly patients, this process is accelerated significantly, and the recovery time may exceed the duration of the initial hospitalization. In the general medical inpatient setting, debility can be compounded by medical illness, poor nutrition, orthopedic problems, and contractures. The cardiopulmonary system also declines with inactivity. Ferretti and colleagues found that after 42 days of bed rest, VO_2 max was reduced by 16%, cardiac output by 30%, and oxygen delivery by 40%. Maintenance of muscle strength during immobility can be accomplished by muscle contractions of 30% to 50% of maximal tension for several seconds each day. Studies have shown an improvement in ability to perform activities of daily living in elderly patients who had an exercise program while in the hospital.

■ CARDIAC CONDITIONS

Formal cardiac rehabilitation (CR) programs may benefit a wide range of patients: those recovering from myocardial infarction, those with stable heart failure, and those who have had coronary artery bypass grafting, heart transplantation, valve surgery, angioplasty, and pacemaker placement. Studies have demonstrated the value of CR in reversing coronary artery disease, reducing lipoprotein levels, and increasing physical work capacity. In the hospital setting, CR focuses on the identification of risk factors, previous and current performance status, and referral for outpatient activity. For those recovering from surgeries, this phase of CR also includes education on protecting sternal incisions. Education on safe activities to resume after discharge, risk factor modification, and vocational counseling may complete the acute CR process. Both PTs and OTs should be part of the CR team.

■ PULMONARY REHABILITATION

Rehabilitation programs in patients with chronic obstructive pulmonary disease and other chronic lung diseases have been shown to improve exercise capacity and quality of life, and reduce dyspnea and hospitalization. The main focus of pulmonary rehabilitation is exercise, including strength training for the upper and lower extremities, as well as respiratory muscle-specific training. Patients with chronic sputum production benefit from chest physical therapy. Patients receive education about medications, energy conservation, work simplification, and breathing techniques, such as pursed-lip breathing, posture, and diaphragmatic breathing. Nutritional interventions and psychosocial and emotional support are also provided. Pulmonary rehabilitation may be carried out in inpatient and outpatient settings.

PRACTICE POINT

Strategies to minimize negative consequences of bedrest

- Minimize duration of bedrest
- Avoid strict bedrest
- Allow bathroom privileges
- Have patient stand 30 to 60 seconds when transferring from bed to chair
- Encourage family to ambulate patient, engage patient with meals, and walk to hospital testing
- Encourage daily exercises adapted to individual patient (such as ankle exercises to prevent venous thromboembolism)
- Involve physical therapy, occupational therapy, and nursing to encourage mobilization, optimize feeding, use of protective splinting, and pain management
- Avoid physical or pharmacologic restraints
- Daily reassessment of the need for tethers such as Foley catheter, supplemental oxygen, IVs, and other devices that confine the patient to bed

---

■ OTHER CONDITIONS

Other conditions less commonly seen in the standard inpatient setting require rehabilitation services. These include closed head injury, spinal cord injury or infection, burns, amputation, polytrauma, and the Guillain-Barré syndrome (acute inflammatory demyelinating polyneuropathy). In acute trauma, patients are frequently taken to level I trauma centers where rehabilitation services are ingrained into the provision of health care services. When trauma patients are cared for in settings with less formal infrastructure, it may be helpful to proactively involve PTs, OTs, physiatrists, and other rehabilitation providers in the care process. Many of the same issues of concern described above, such as contractures, immobility, and skin breakdown, are present in these other processes. Additionally, rehabilitation providers may also be particularly aware of the potential for medical complications in specific conditions (eg, heterotopic ossification after burns, autonomic dysreflexia after spinal cord injury, pulmonary aspiration, or bladder dysfunction associated with neurologic injury).

CONCLUSION

Hospitalists can enlist numerous professionals in the acute treatment of impairment and in discharge planning. Involving PTs and OTs early in a patient's hospital course may reduce length of stay, minimize inpatient complications, and lead to a more successful discharge at a higher level of independence. Physiatrists can assist in the diagnosis and management of neurologic and musculoskeletal conditions, and recommend appropriate levels of therapy upon discharge. Other providers, such as speech-language pathologists, psychologists, vocational counselors, and therapeutic recreation specialists, contribute to the restoration of function after illness or injury. Understanding the role of these providers and utilizing their services in an effective and timely manner are essential skills for the hospitalist.

SUGGESTED READINGS

American Physical Therapy Association. *Guide to Physical Therapist Practice 3.0.* Alexandria, VA: American Physical Therapy Association; 2011.

de Morton NA, Keating JL, Jeffs K. Exercise for acutely hospitalised older medical patients. *Cochrane Database Syst Rev.* 2007;(1):CD005955.

Ferretti G, Antonutto G, Denis C, et al. The interplay of central and peripheral factors in limiting maximal O_2 consumption in man after prolonged bed rest. *J Physiol.* 1997;501(Pt 3):677-686.

Hochberg MC, Altman RD, April KT, et al. American College of Rheumatology 2012 recommendations for the use of nonpharmacologic and pharmacologic therapies in osteoarthritis of the hand, hip, and knee. *Arthritis Care Res (Hoboken).* 2012;64:465-474.

Kosse NM, Dutmer AL, Dasenbrock L, Bauer JM, Lamoth CJ. Effectiveness and feasibility of early physical rehabilitation programs for geriatric hospitalized patients: a systematic review. *BMC Geriatr.* 2013;13:107. http://www.biomedcentral.com/1471-2318/13/107.

Mueller E. Influence of training and of inactivity on muscle strength. *Arch Phys Med Rehabil.* 1970;51:449-461.

Siebens H, Aronow H, Edwards D, Ghasemi Z. A randomized controlled trial of exercise to improve outcomes of acute hospitalization in older adults. *J Am Geriatr Soc.* 2000;48:1545-1552.

Uusi-Rasi K, Patil R, Karinkanta S, et al. Exercise and vitamin D in fall prevention among older women: a randomized clinical trial. *JAMA Intern Med.* 2015;175:703-711.

CHAPTER 70

The Role of Speech/Language Pathologists in Dysphagia Management

Marianne E. Savastano, MS, CCC-SLP

INTRODUCTION

The term dysphagia refers to any type of difficulty with moving food and/or liquid from the mouth to the stomach. A wide variety of conditions and circumstances can cause dysphagia. Speech/Language Pathologists (SLPs) typically receive specialized training in the diagnosis and treatment of oropharyngeal dysphagia. However, physicians working in both acute and subacute settings must be able to recognize the signs, symptoms, and possible causes of dysphagia in order to direct a plan of care that maximizes patient safety. This chapter will focus on the differences between normal and disordered swallowing and management of swallowing disorders, with an emphasis on oropharyngeal dysphagia.

EPIDEMIOLOGY

There is a lack of clear data regarding the prevalence of dysphagia in the general population; however, Bhattacharyya (2014) analyzed the 2012 National Health Interview Survey and found that in a single 12-month period, an estimated 9.44 million adults in the United States reported a swallowing problem, which correlates to 1 in 25 adults annually. The survey further revealed that approximately 31% of those with dysphagia reported it to be a moderate problem and approximately 25% of those with dysphagia felt that it was a very large problem. The average number of days that individuals reported being affected by dysphagia was 139 ± 7. While stroke was found to be the most common cause of dysphagia, other neurologic conditions and head and neck cancer were also common etiologies.

Dysphagia may occur at any point throughout the lifespan and it may result from a wide variety of circumstances from acute medical events, to diseases, to normal aging. Neurological events, conditions, and diseases that can be associated with dysphagia include but are not limited to stroke, traumatic brain injury, brain tumor, cerebral palsy, Parkinson's disease, and amyotrophic lateral sclerosis. Many autoimmune diseases and conditions such as multiple sclerosis, myasthenia gravis, Guillain Barre Syndrome, and various forms of myositis may also be associated with dysphagia. Physical changes to the anatomy such as development of a Zenker's diverticulum, cervical osteophyte, Schatzki ring, or damage to the vocal folds may result in dysphagia. Numerous surgical and/or medical interventions such as intubation, anterior cervical spine surgery, carotid endartarectomy, and resections for various forms of head and neck cancer may also be associated dysphagia. A variety of medications used to treat other conditions such as antipsychotics, antidepressants, anticonvulsants, and medications to treat anxiety may actually induce or worsen dysphagia. Finally, prolonged illnesses that require hospitalization may cause muscular deconditioning which may be correlated with the development of dysphagia.

Common, physical complications of dysphagia include, but are not limited to choking, dehydration, malnutrition, respiratory distress, and pneumonia. Additional, but often overlooked, complications of dysphagia are its social and psychological impacts. Since a great deal of the social occasions that people enjoy are centered around preparing and consuming food, individuals who are unable to swallow safely are often embarrassed by their swallowing problem and become isolated when they feel unable to participate in social events that involve food and drink.

NEURAL CONTROL OF THE SWALLOW

Swallowing is a complex activity which involves 26 pairs of muscles and six cranial nerves. In 2008, Mistry and Hamdy published an article on the neural control of feeding and swallowing that contained a useful, detailed description of the roles of various parts of the brain in the process of feeding and swallowing. That information is summarized in the following section, but the reader is directed to the full article for further information.

■ CRANIAL NERVES

The trigeminal nerve (V) conveys sensory information, with the exception of taste, from the anterior two thirds of the tongue. It is also responsible for motor innervation of muscles involved in mastication and posterior bolus propulsion. The facial nerve (VII) conveys information about taste from the anterior two-thirds of the tongue. It also plays a role in motor innervation for facial muscles such as the lips, which help to clear utensils and keep boluses in the oral cavity. The glossopharyngeal nerve (IX) conveys sensory information from the posterior one third of the tongue as well as the palatine tonsils and faucial arches. The glossopharyngeal nerve also works with the vagus nerve (X) to help with the superior and anterior movement of the larynx, which assists with cricopharyngeal relaxation. The vagus nerve assists with velar elevation, works with the glossopharyngeal nerve to innervate the pharyngeal constrictors for bolus propulsion, works with the spinal accessory nerve (XI) to innervate the intrinsic lingual muscles, and innervates the muscles that cause vocal fold adduction during the swallow in addition to those that assist with cricopharyngeal relaxation. Additionally, the superior and recurrent laryngeal nerves (branches of the vagus nerve) convey sensory information from the velum and portions of the pharynx as well as the larynx. The recurrent laryngeal nerve also controls the majority of the intrinsic laryngeal muscles, which open and close the vocal folds to assist with airway protection. Finally, the hypoglossal nerve (XII) innervates all of the intrinsic lingual muscles as well as most of the extrinsic lingual muscles.

■ BRAINSTEM

The swallowing command center is contained bilaterally in the upper medulla and pontine areas of the brainstem and is part of the reticular formation. A complex network of neurons containing afferent portions, efferent portions, and interneurons are known as the central pattern generator for swallowing. The interneurons are separated into a dorsal group and a ventral group, with the dorsal neurons lying in the nucleus of the tractus solitarius and the ventral neurons lying in the nucleus ambiguus. The dorsal neurons of the nucleus tractus solitarius integrate information from the cortex as well as sensory information from cranial nerves V, IX, and X. The dorsal neurons of the nucleus tractus solitarius then activate the ventral neurons of the nucleus ambiguus, which activates the motor neuclei of cranial nerves V, VII, and X to trigger the swallow.

■ CORTEX

Research demonstrates that both cerebral hemispheres are responsible for swallowing. Esophageal and pharyngeal muscles have been found to have representation in the motor cortex. In addition, multiple studies agree to support the assertion that cortical control of swallowing is dominant in the left hemisphere in humans (Hamdy et al., 1996).

THE PHASES OF THE SWALLOW

In order to understand dysphagia, one must first have a clear understanding of normal swallow function. There are four commonly accepted phases of the swallow: The oral preparatory phase, the oral transit phase, the pharyngeal phase, and the esophageal phase. Typically, an SLP's scope of practice focuses on the first three phases of the swallow. While SLPs are knowledgeable about the esophageal phase of the swallow, they typically refer to a gastroenterologist for more formal evaluation, diagnosis, and treatment of esophageal conditions (eg, reflux). **Figure 70-1** provides an illustration of the oral preparatory, oral transit, and pharyngeal phases of the swallow.

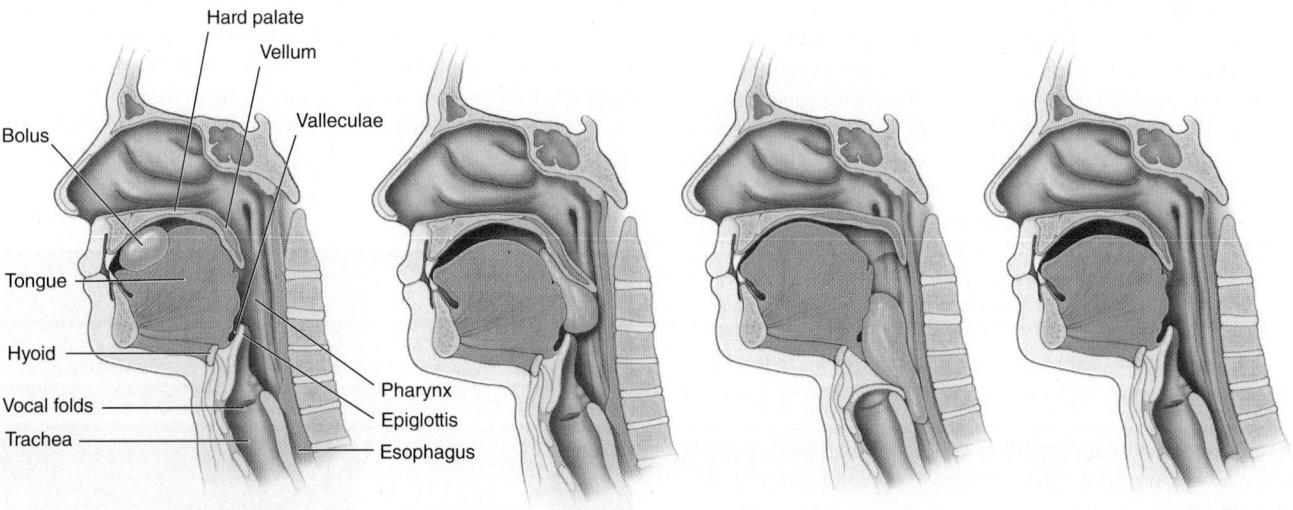

A Oral preparatory phase   **B** Oral transit phase   **C** Pharyngeal phase   **D** Esophageal phase

Figure 70-1 (A). *Oral preparatory phase:* The lips are sealed to prevent anterior bolus loss and velum makes contact with the tongue base to prevent posterior bolus loss. The tongue moves the bolus around the oral cavity to assist with mastication and to mix the bolus with saliva prior to forming the bolus into a cohesive ball. (*B*). *Oral transit phase:* The tongue elevates to make sequential contact with the palate in order to squeeze the bolus toward the posterior oral cavity and into the pharynx while the velum begins to elevate. (*C*). *Pharyngeal phase:* The velum is fully elevated to prevent bolus entry into the nasal cavity. The vocal folds adduct and the epiglottis deflects to protect the airway. The upper esophageal sphincter relaxes to allow the bolus to pass into the esophagus. (*D*). *Esophageal phase:* The epiglottis has returned to the home position, the vocal folds have reopened, the bolus has fully entered the esophagus, and the upper esophageal sphincter has closed.

ORAL PREPARATORY PHASE

Prior to any bolus manipulation, an individual must first open his or her mouth to accept the food or liquid. Once the food or liquid has entered the oral cavity, bilateral labial seal is necessary to prevent any portion of it from spilling back out of the oral cavity. With the food or liquid fully contained, bolus preparation can begin. The amount and type of manipulation necessary will depend on the texture of the material to be swallowed (eg, liquid vs solid). With liquids and most purees, the tongue will create a cohesive bolus in the center of the oral cavity. If mastication is required, the tongue will propel the bolus toward the dentition in order for mastication to occur. In adults, the mandible and tongue will move in a rotary fashion to mix solids with saliva, propel solids toward the teeth, and ultimately form a cohesive bolus of masticated food. During this process, tension is present in the buccal musculature, which prevents food from accumulating in the lateral sulcus that exists between the teeth and cheeks. With liquid and pureed boluses, the velum is in the descended position and making contact with the posterior portion of the tongue in order to keep the bolus in the oral cavity. With solids, particularly those requiring mastication, the velum is also in the descended position; however, it is normal for a portion of the bolus to exit the posterior oral cavity and begin to enter the pharynx during this phase.

ORAL TRANSIT PHASE

Once a bolus has been fully prepared and organized into a cohesive ball, the tongue will begin to propel it toward the posterior portion of the oral cavity. There is a sequential, anterior to posterior elevation of the tongue against the hard palate that causes the bolus to be squeezed toward the back of the oral cavity.

PHARYNGEAL PHASE

When the anterior aspect of the bolus passes any point between the anterior faucial arches and the area where the base of the tongue crosses the lower rim of the mandible, the pharyngeal phase of the swallow should be triggered. A number of events occur with the triggering of the pharyngeal swallow in which the bolus passes from the oral cavity, through the bilateral valleculae, along the aryepiglottic folds, and into the bilateral pyriform sinuses at the entrance of the upper esophagus. The velum elevates completely to prevent any portion of the bolus from entering the nasal cavity. The hyoid bone and larynx elevate and move in an anterior direction. The false vocal folds and true vocal folds adduct to protect the entrance of the larynx (respiration halts). The epiglottis deflects to offer further laryngeal closure and protection. The base of the tongue flattens and moves in a posterior direction to propel the bolus into the pharynx. The posterior pharyngeal wall moves in an anterior direction to make contact with the tongue base, and the pharyngeal constrictor muscles contract to squeeze the bolus through the pharynx into the esophagus. At the same time, the cricopharyngeus muscle (upper esophageal sphincter) relaxes to allow the bolus to pass into the esophagus. Respiration typically resumes with an exhale upon completion of the pharyngeal swallow response.

ESOPHAGEAL PHASE

Once the bolus has entered the esophagus through the upper esophageal sphincter, tension returns to the cricopharyngeus muscle to prevent the bolus from moving backward and reentering the pharynx. A series of peristaltic waves propel the bolus through the esophagus to the lower esophageal sphincter, which relaxes to allow for bolus passage into the stomach.

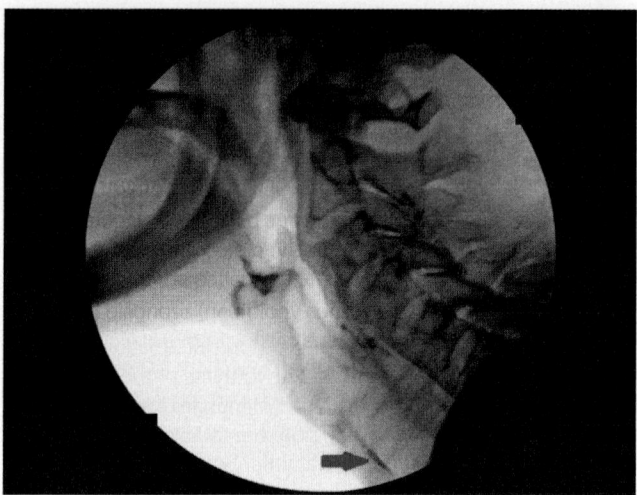

Figure 70-2 *Aspiration during videofluoroscopic swallow study.*

SIGNS AND SYMPTOMS OF DYSPHAGIA

Some people who experience difficulty swallowing will seek out the expertise of a health care professional. Others may develop clinical presentations that signal a possible swallowing problem (eg, recurrent pneumonia). When assessing a patient to determine if he or she has dysphagia, medical professionals are often observing the patient for signs and symptoms that suggest the presence of either aspiration or penetration on food, liquid, or secretions. Aspiration is commonly defined as the entrance of any food or liquid into the trachea below the level of the true vocal cords (**Figure 70-2**). Aspiration should trigger some type of visible and/or audible response such as throat clearing or coughing. However, some people with dysphagia present with silent aspiration in which there are no outward signs that aspiration has occurred. Penetration is commonly defined as the entrance of any bolus into the larynx or laryngeal vestibule up to but not below the level of the true vocal cords (**Figure 70-3**). Penetration may trigger a cough or throat clear; however, it may also be silent. It is important for clinicians to be able to identify the common signs and symptoms of dysphagia so that they can begin to differentially diagnose the problem as well as request appropriate consultative services as necessary (eg, Otolaryngology, Gastroenterology, Speech/Language Pathology). Some of

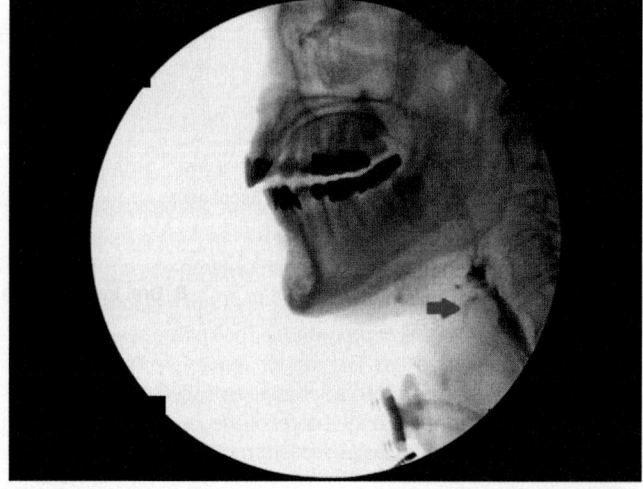

Figure 70-3 *Penetration during videofluoroscopic swallow study.*

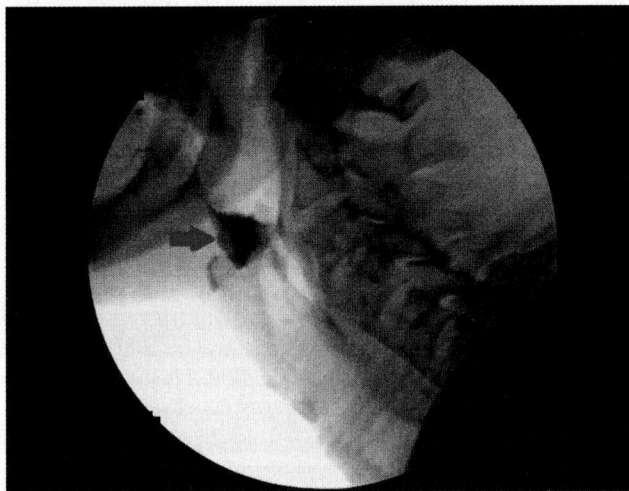

Figure 70-4 *Residue in the valleculae during videofluoroscopic swallow study.*

the most common signs and symptoms of dysphagia include the following:

- Residue, which is any portion of a bolus remaining in the oral cavity or throat after a swallow (**Figures 70-4 and 70-5**)
- Holding boluses in the oral cavity without triggering a swallow
- Food falling out of the oral cavity
- Additional time or effort needed to chew and swallow
- Wet or gurgly vocal quality
- Frequent coughing or throat clearing (particularly in the context of eating/drinking)
- Increased congestion including pneumonia
- Increased work of breathing or shortness of breath during eating/drinking
- Odynophagia, which is a complaint of pain with swallowing
- Globus, which is the sensation that food or liquid is stuck in the throat

DYSPHAGIA ASSESSMENTS

There are a variety of ways in which to assess for dysphagia. Choosing which assessment is most appropriate for your patient will depend both on your patient's presentation as well as on the

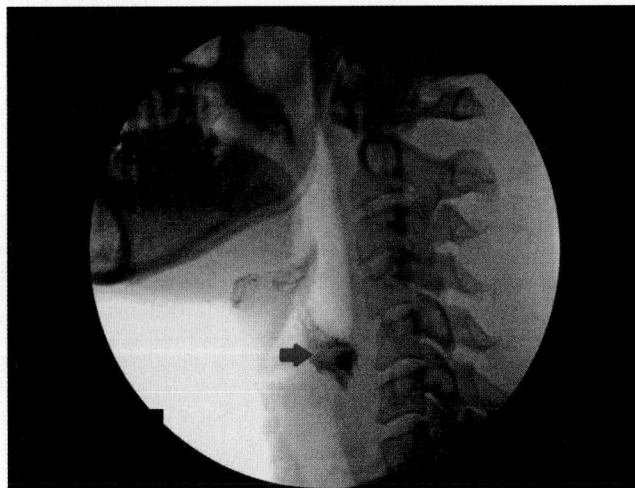

Figure 70-5 *Residue in the pyriform sinuses during videofluoroscopic swallow study.*

availability of various resources. The most common assessments include bedside swallow assessments, videoflouroscopic swallow studies, and fiberoptic endoscopic evaluations of the swallow.

■ BEDSIDE SWALLOW ASSESSMENT

Regardless of patient presentation, the majority of patients who present with signs or symptoms of dysphagia will first be seen for a bedside evaluation of the swallow. Ideally, due to their training in dysphagia diagnosis and treatment, an SLP would complete the bedside swallow assessment. However, other medical professionals including physicians, physician assistants, nurse practitioners, nurses, and occupational therapists can all be trained to administer a basic bedside swallow screening in the case that an SLP is not available. While a great deal of useful information can be obtained from the completion of a bedside swallow assessment, it is important to note that it is the most subjective type of swallow assessment discussed in this chapter.

The following is a description of a basic bedside swallow screening which can be used by physicians, particularly resident MDs who may find that they need to assess swallowing status in a hospitalized patient after hours or when an SLP is not immediately available for consultation, as may be the case in smaller facilities and/or more rural areas.

Cognitive/Linguistic Status: While it may seem obvious, it is important to ensure that the patient is awake and alert. If a patient has difficulty achieving or maintaining alertness, he/she may not be safe or appropriate for per os (PO) intake. It is also useful to determine if the patient is able to follow basic commands and express basic needs. However, keep in mind that while patients with communication disorders such as aphasia may not be able to express themselves or follow verbal commands, many of these patients retain the ability to interpret gestures and mimic behavior and can still participate in a bedside swallowing assessment.

Speech and Vocal Status: An informal, qualitative assessment of a patient's speech output and vocal quality can provide useful information related to strength and coordination of the oral musculature as well as respiratory drive and vocal fold mobility, which is important for airway protection during the swallow. Listen to the patient's speech quality. One who presents with imprecise articulation due to muscle weakness may demonstrate difficulty managing oral intake in the oral preparatory and/or oral transit phases of the swallow. If a patient has a wet or gurgly vocal quality, it may indicate that the patient is not managing his/her secretions appropriately due to a swallowing problem. If a patient has a vocal quality that is weak, breathy, hoarse, or harsh, it may indicate a problem with respiratory drive and/or a problem with vocal fold mobility. If the vocal folds are not functioning properly, they may fail to adduct and protect the airway during the swallow, which places the patient at a significantly greater risk of aspiration. It is also useful to determine if the patient can follow commands to clear his/her throat and cough, as these are protective mechanisms that can clear the airway of material if penetration or aspiration occurs.

Posture: Make note of the patient's habitual posture. Is the patient able to sit up straight in bed or in a chair? Upright posture typically allows for safer oral intake.

Respiratory Status: It is important to be aware of the patient's respiratory status, as those with a compromised respiratory system may experience an exacerbation of their respiratory symptoms when eating and drinking (eg, increased shortness of breath, increased need for supplemental oxygen, etc).

Oral Mechanism Exam: Prior to providing any food or drink, it is necessary to evaluate the strength, symmetry, and function of the muscles needed for eating and drinking. Observe the patient's face for signs of weakness and/or asymmetry. A useful set of basic commands to determine general strength and symmetry include:

1. Open your mouth and do not let me close it (apply upward pressure to the chin)
2. Close your jaw tightly and do not let me open it (apply downward pressure to the chin)
3. Close your lips tightly and do not let me open them (apply up/down pressure to the lips)
4. Smile
5. Pucker your lips
6. Fill your cheeks with air and do not let it out (apply pressure to the cheeks)
7. Stick out your tongue
8. Move your tongue to the left side and right side (use a tongue blade to provide resistance)
9. Open your mouth and say "ah" to assess for velar elevation

A patient who exhibits signs of labial weakness may experience difficulty sealing on a cup/straw, difficulty stripping food from utensils, or difficulty containing food/liquid in the oral cavity. If secretions are found pooled in a patient's oral cavity, it may indicate reduced oral sensation and/or difficulty swallowing. A patient who has inadequate dentition or who demonstrates difficulty opening/closing the jaw may have trouble with timely and/or efficient mastication. A patient who demonstrates signs of lingual weakness or reduced coordination may have trouble forming a cohesive bolus or moving food/liquid through the oral cavity. Lastly, a patient who exhibits reduced velar elevation may experience premature spillage of boluses out of the oral cavity prior to the onset of the pharyngeal swallow, which places them at greater risk for aspiration.

Oral Trials: In the next section of the bedside swallow evaluation, the patient should be provided with various liquids and solids to consume while the clinician assesses the patient's ability to manage these textures in the oral and pharyngeal phases of the swallow.

In the oral phases of the swallow, the clinician should assess the patient's ability to accept and contain food and drink in the oral cavity, chew, and propel the bolus from the oral cavity into the pharynx. After each swallow, the clinician should examine the oral cavity to determine if there is any residue left on the lingual surface, in the anterior sulcus, or in the lateral sulci. If residue is present, the patient should be cued to use a lingual sweep or finger sweep to clear the residue from the oral cavity. If the patient is unable to masticate food in a timely manner, or if he/she experiences consistent residue in the oral cavity, a softer solid or a pureed solid may be more appropriate.

In the pharyngeal phase of the swallow, the clinician should assess the patient's laryngeal elevation as it provides information about the timing, completion, and strength of the swallow. This is best done through a combination of visual and tactile assessment. Have the observer place the ring, middle, and index fingers on the anterior surface of the throat while keeping the index finger in the superior position with the thyroid notch between the middle and ring fingers. When the patient swallows, the thyroid notch should elevate above the middle finger at the height of the swallow if elevation is to be considered normal.

Throughout the assessment, the clinician should assess the patient for signs and symptoms of aspiration or penetration. It is useful to have the patient vocalize after every swallow in order to determine if his or her vocal quality sounds wet or gurgly. If an altered vocal quality is appreciated, cue the patient to cough or clear his/her throat and then perform a dry swallow. If other signs or symptoms of aspiration are observed (eg, more consistent coughing, throat clearing, vocal wetness), the patient may require an altered texture such as a softer solid or thickened liquid. If the signs/symptoms of aspiration persist, it may be necessary to recommend NPO status until an SLP can provide a more detailed assessment. Depending on the cause and severity of a patient's dysphagia, nonoral nutrition and hydration from a nasogastric tube or gastrostomy tube may be necessary.

■ VIDEOFLUOROSCOPIC SWALLOW STUDY (VFSS)

The videofluoroscopic swallow study or modified barium swallow (MBS) is a fluoroscopic procedure in which the patient is provided with various consistencies of barium to swallow under fluoroscopy. The resulting exam allows a trained SLP to watch a video of the liquids and solids passing from the oral cavity through the pharynx and into the upper esophagus. The VFSS is particularly useful as it allows the clinician to observe instances of penetration and aspiration that occur before, during, and/or after the swallow. In addition, this study affords the clinician the opportunity to observe the location and amount of residue in the pharynx (such as valleculae, pyriform sinuses), as well as the impact of trialing different viscosities and textures of liquids and solids. Finally, this study allows the clinician to see, in real time, the effectiveness of various safe swallow maneuvers and strategies (eg, chin tuck, head turn, etc.). Due to the fact that the VFSS allows the SLP to observe the entire swallow from the oral to the upper esophageal phase, it is often considered to be the gold standard of swallowing assessments.

■ FIBEROPTIC ENDOSCOPIC EVALUATION OF SWALLOWING (FEES)

The FEES is another objective evaluation of swallowing that can be completed by SLPs who have undergone specific training. During the FEES, a flexible endoscope is passed through the patient's nares, and held in place in the pharynx just above the tongue base in order to provide a view of the pharynx and larynx. Observations may be made regarding the presence and management of secretions, as well as informal observations of the integrity and mobility of the true vocal folds and other pharyngeal and laryngeal structures. Typically, patients are provided with various textures of food and liquid to swallow during this assessment, which allows the clinician to observe the passage of boluses through the pharynx to the upper esophageal sphincter. While the FEES is particularly useful for observation of secretions and residue in the pharynx as well as observation of vocal fold mobility, there are limitations to the FEES that are not present in the VFSS. The FEES does not allow visualization of the oral phases of the swallow. In addition, during the FEES, there is complete obliteration (known as "white out") of the image at the height of the swallow when the pharyngeal musculature contracts around the endoscope. Due to this period of white out, episodes of penetration and aspiration that occur during the swallow reflex are not observed, whereas episodes of penetration/aspiration that occur before and after the swallow are able to be visualized. It is often possible to see evidence of penetration/aspiration that occurred during the swallow if residue is left in the laryngeal vestibule or upper airway.

DYSPHAGIA MANAGEMENT

Once causes and characteristics of dysphagia are diagnosed, a variety of treatment approaches can be utilized. An SLP should be consulted to assist with diagnosing dysphagia and with creation of the treatment plan that will include a number of different strategies to maximize safe oral intake. Compensatory treatment approaches are often attempted first as they can quickly alter the flow of food/liquid to eliminate signs/symptoms of dysphagia, although they do not alter the physiology of the patient's swallow. Three types of compensatory treatment approaches include diet modifications, postural changes, and swallow maneuvers. Other approaches to dysphagia treatment can include exercises or surgery.

■ DIET MODIFICATIONS

Food and liquid may be presented in a variety of different textures. Solids may be modified so that they have increased moisture and/or require less mastication. In addition, liquids may be modified from a thinner consistency to a thicker consistency, which allows the swallowing mechanism more time to propel them safely through the pharynx to the esophagus.

■ POSTURAL ADJUSTMENTS

Some patients benefit from postural adjustments to alter the way food/liquid flows through the system, or to change the dimensions of the pharynx to improve safety. Two of the most common postural adjustments include a chin tuck (swallowing while looking down at one's chest) and a head turn (typically turning the head to look over the shoulder on the weaker side). However, it is critical to understand that there is no single postural adjustment that works for all patients, and some patients actually experience worsening symptoms of dysphagia if the wrong postural adjustment is utilized. Therefore, consultation with an SLP trained in dysphagia management is recommended prior to prescribing any postural adjustments.

■ SWALLOW MANEUVERS

Some patients benefit from performing additional maneuvers during the swallow, provided that their cognitive status is sufficient to allow for successful implementation of such maneuvers. Safety may be enhanced by placing different aspects of the pharyngeal swallow under voluntary control. One example of a swallow maneuver is called the supraglottic swallow. Here, the patient is instructed to hold his or her breath, then swallow, and then cough immediately after the swallow. This maneuver is intended to assist with volitional airway protection before, during, and after the swallow. A second swallow maneuver is the Mendelsohn maneuver. Here, the patient is instructed to try to prolong laryngeal elevation at the height of the swallow. This maneuver is intended to prolong the amount of time that the upper esophageal sphincter is relaxed, in order to allow a greater portion of the bolus to pass into the esophagus. A trained SLP is best suited for making recommendations regarding swallow maneuvers, and this is done only after thorough evaluation.

■ SWALLOW EXERCISES

The aforementioned compensatory techniques are not expected to alter swallow physiology. However, patients may be instructed to complete various swallow exercises to improve the strength or coordination of various muscles involved in swallowing. An SLP will be able to make appropriate exercise recommendations based on each patient's presentation. Some possible exercises include lingual resistance exercises, tongue base retraction exercises, and laryngeal elevation exercises.

■ SURGICAL INTERVENTIONS

Some swallowing disorders may benefit from surgical intervention to alter the feeding/swallowing anatomy. These include, but are not limited to, cervical osteophytes and dysfunction of the cricopharyngeal muscle. Bony prominences that grow on the cervical vertebrae may cause anterior bulging of the posterior pharyngeal wall and disrupt bolus flow. In severe cases, it may be necessary to surgically reduce the osteophyte in order to allow boluses to pass through the pharynx. In patients who have severe dysfunction of the cricopharyngeal muscle such that it does not relax properly to allow boluses to enter the esophagus, cricopharyngeal myotomy may be performed to allow for greater relaxation of this muscle during the swallow.

DIET LEVELS

While all medical facilities offer foods and liquids in a variety of different textures to accommodate the needs of those with dysphagia, there is a wide variety of terminology used to describe each of these diet levels. The American Speech/Language Hearing Association (ASHA), the governing body for SLPs, does not currently have an established diet level structure or recommended terminology to describe diet levels, nor does it provide guidelines for the types of food that should be included on a particular diet level.

In 2002, the American Dietetic Association established a set of guidelines known as the National Dysphagia Diet. While very few facilities specifically use this terminology to describe the diet levels available at their facility, the descriptions of each solid diet level are useful for illustrative purposes.

■ NATIONAL DYSPHAGIA DIET (NDD)

NDD 1 Dysphagia Pureed—all foods must be pureed and thickened (if necessary) to a pudding-like consistency. It must be lump free and little or no chewing is required.

NDD 2 Dysphagia Mechanically Altered—all foods are moist, soft-textured, and easily chewed. Meats are ground and served with gravy or sauce. Cooked cereals, soft breads, and well-cooked pastas are allowed. Some chewing is required.

NDD 3 Dysphagia Advanced—includes most regular consistency foods but excludes hard, dry, sticky, or crunchy foods. Food should be moist and in bite-size pieces. Dry breakfast cereals must be well moistened and meats must be tender.

NDD 4 Regular—No restrictions.

In general, medical facilities seem to have greater agreement among one another with the terminology used to describe different liquid viscosities. Typically, liquids may be described as thin (water consistency), nectar thick, honey thick, and pudding/spoon thick. A wide variety of products on the market offer prethickened liquids in various consistencies. In addition, there are numerous gels and powders available that can be added to thin liquid in order to create nectar thick, honey thick, or pudding thick liquids.

CONCLUSION

Dysphagia is a serious and sometimes life threatening condition, which affects millions of people each year. There are a wide range of causes for dysphagia, as well as a variety of management approaches. While SLPs working in the medical setting often specialize in the diagnosis and treatment of oropharyngeal dysphagia, it is critical that all members of the medical team recognize the signs and symptoms of dysphagia in order to expedite treatment with the ultimate goal of maximizing patient health and safety.

SUGGESTED READINGS

Bhattacharyya N. The prevalence of dysphagia among adults in the United States. *Otolaryn Head Neck Surg*. 2014;151(5):765-769.

Bosma J. Physiology of the mouth, pharynx and esophagus. In: Paparella M, Shumrick D, eds. *Otolaryngology, Volume 1: Basic Sciences and Related Disciplines*. Philadelphia, PA: Saunders; 1973:356-370.

Hamdy S, Aziz Q, Rothwell JC, et al. The Cortical topography of human swallowing musculature in health and disease. *Nat Med*. 1996;2(11):1217-1224.

Logemann JA. *Evaluation and Treatment of Swallowing Disorders*, 2nd ed. Austin, TX: Pro-Ed; 1998.

Mistry S, Hamdy S. Neural control of feeding and swallowing. *Phys Med Rehabil Clin N Am*. 2008;19(4):709-728.

Murray J. *Manual of Dysphagia Assessment in Adults*. San Diego, CA: Singular Publishing Group; 1999.

The National Dysphagia Diet Task Force. *The National Dysphagia Diet: Standardization for Optimal Care*. Chicago, IL: American Dietetic Association; 2002.

Palmer JB, Rudin NJ, Lara G, Crompton AW. Coordination of mastication and swallowing. *Dysphagia* 1992;7:187-200.

CHAPTER 71

Incontinence

Alayne D. Markland, DO, MSc
Catherine E. DuBeau, MD

Key Clinical Questions

1. How should you evaluate urinary and fecal incontinence in the hospital or rehabilitation setting?
2. How do you treat urinary and/or fecal incontinence?
3. What are the important elements of incontinence management in transitions of care?
4. What are the treatment options for urinary retention in hospitalized patients?
5. What are the guidelines for urinary catheter use and management in hospitalized patients?

INTRODUCTION

It has been estimated that 22% to 35% of patients on general medical wards have UI and 10% have FI. In the hospital setting, both UI and FI may coexist with urinary retention (UR). Incontinence may cause skin breakdown and pressure ulcers, and UI may cause increased use of indwelling catheters, and falls. Catheter-associated urinary tract infection (CAUTI) accounts for up to 70% to 80% of all hospital health care acquired infections (HAIs). Hospital-acquired CAUTI, a "never event," is both a marker of insufficient quality performance and negatively impacts reimbursement. The duration of catheter use is strong risk factor for CAUTI in hospital settings. Poor quality incontinence management also increases costs from absorbent and containment products and increased use of already limited resources (eg, nursing and aide time), and may lead to increased caregiver burden after discharge.

PRACTICE POINT

- Although continence care is often delegated to nursing staff, failure to recognize, evaluate, and treat incontinence and UR as significant "hazards of hospitalization," especially in older patients, may increase morbidity, length of stay, and functional impairment, even up to 30 days postdischarge.

NORMAL MICTURATION AND DEFECATION

Normal micturition and defecation involve similar neural control and muscular coordination. Continence results from effective storage during filling and efficient emptying during the voiding phase or defecation phase. Efferent nerves arising from the sacral micturition center at S2-S4 mediate bladder muscle (detrusor) contraction via muscarinic receptors. Sympathetic, adrenergic nerves arising from T11-L2 sustain contraction of smooth muscle in the proximal urethral and internal anal sphincters. The distal urethral sphincter and the external anal sphincter are voluntarily controlled via somatic cholinergic nicotinic nerves arising from the sacral micturition center. Urethral and anal closures are also maintained through contraction and support from striated muscle and fascial elements in the pelvic floor. A micturition center in the pons linked to subcortical and frontal centers that inhibit urgency and voiding controls coordination of bladder filling and emptying. Less is known about neurological control of defecation, although similar mechanisms have been proposed that coordinate relaxation of the external anal sphincter with the change of the ano-rectal angle with valsalva. Normal defecation also depends on stool consistency (affected by diet and colonic transit time), rectal compliance and sensation (ability to retain stool in the rectum and delay defecation until socially appropriate), and integrity of the internal and external anal sphincters and the puborectalis muscles.

INCONTINENCE

■ PATHOPHYSIOLOGY

Especially relevant in the hospital setting, urinary and fecal incontinence may result or be exacerbated by impaired function (eg, decreased mobility, altered manual dexterity from IVs) and cognition (eg, delirium), and the presence of comorbid conditions (**Table 71-1**) and medications (**Table 71-2**) that may directly or

TABLE 71-1 Comorbid Conditions Causing or Exacerbating Urinary and/or Fecal Incontinence

Comorbidity	Effect on Continence
Cardiovascular disease	
Acute coronary syndrome	Altered mental status
Congestive heart failure	Nocturnal polyuria; treatment with loop diuretics
Metabolic disease	
Diabetes mellitus	Osmotic diuresis from hyperglycemia, altered mental status from hyper- or hypoglycemia, urinary retention from constipation, gastroparesis, neuropathy
Hypercalemia	Diuresis, altered mental status
Vitamin-B12 deficiency	Impaired bladder sensation, peripheral neuropathy
Thyroid disease	Changes in cecal transit time from hypo- or hyperthyroidism
Neurologic disease	
Cerebrovascular disease, stroke	Upper motor neuron disease with impaired bladder sensation, acutely impaired physical function and cognition
Seizures	Acute loss of motor control/sphincter impairment
Delirium	Impaired cognitive function
Dementia	Impaired cognitive function
Parkinson's disease	Impaired CNS control impaired physical function, constipation
Spinal cord injury or impairment	Dependent on level: suprasacral—uninhibited contractions and dyssynergia between bladder and sphincter contraction; sacral—impaired detrusor contractility, sphincter incompetence
Psychiatric disease	
Affective disorders, psychosis	Decreased motivation; cognitive impairment
Alcoholism	Functional and cognitive impairments; acute intoxication: diuresis, diarrhea, urinary retention
Gastrointestinal disease	
Constipation	Urinary retention, impaired urgency sensation, impaction
Diarrhea (infectious causes)	Increase in rectal volume, impaired ability to voluntarily contract external anal sphincter
Malabsorptive syndromes	Loose stool, increase bowel frequency
Inflammatory bowel disease	Stool consistency changes, altered recto-anal anatomy, reduced rectal storage capacity
Others	
Musculoskeletal disease	Functional impairment, detrusor overactivity from cervical myelopathy in rheumatoid arthritis and osteoarthritis
Peripheral venous insufficiency	Nocturnal polyuria
Pulmonary disease	Exacerbation of stress incontinence and fecal leakage with chronic cough

Adapted from DuBeau CE. Incontinence. In: Durso SC, Sullivan GM, eds. *Geriatric Review Syllabus*, 8th ed. American Geriatric Society, 2013, pp. 244-253.

indirectly affect neural and muscular control of micturition and defecation. Recognition and management of these potentially remediable factors are essential for effective incontinence treatment and prevention. Procedures and monitoring in the acute care setting can also impact continence status (**Table 71-3**). Imposed bedrest makes toileting impossible, and predisposes to impaired bladder emptying, UR, and constipation that can lead to dual incontinence.

Iatrogenic changes in stool consistency are major causes of FI in the hospital setting. Constipation and impaction may cause UI by impairing bladder emptying by mechanical obstruction and/or a reflex sympathetic stimulation or when watery stool "leaks" around impacted stool. Impaction in the rectal canal also may impair afferent sensations of bladder and rectal fullness, leading to leakage without sensory awareness. Anal fissures, hemorrhoids, fistulas, and abscesses in close approximation to the anal sphincters may all lead to FI by impairing anal sphincter function. Large volume, watery diarrhea may cause FI by overwhelming the rectal capacity and voluntary anal sphincter contraction.

CLASSIFICATION

UI is typically classified into four main symptom types: urge, stress, mixed urge and stress, and impaired bladder emptying (formerly called "overflow") (**Table 71-4**). Hospitalized patients may have uncommon causes of UI, such as extra-urethral urine leakage from vesico-vaginal or vesico-rectal fistulas.

The main types of fecal leakage are urge (associated with urgent need to pass stool), passive (without sensation), mixed (urge and passive leakage), or seepage (low-volume staining in underwear).

EVALUATION

As noted above, hospitalized patients are at high risk for new or worsening UI and FI due to underlying and acute multiple medical conditions, pre-existing and new medications, immobilization, new functional impairment, IV fluid support, delirium, acute interventions and iatrogenic complications. The basic evaluation for UI should include a focused history, physical examination, laboratory evaluation, and, less frequently, radiology tests (**Table 71-5**)

TABLE 71-2 Medications Associated with Urinary and Fecal Incontinence

Medication	Effect on Continence
Alcohol	Frequency, urgency, sedation, delirium, immobility, change in stool consistency
α-Adrenergic agonists	Outlet obstruction (men)
α-Adrenergic blockers	Stress leakage (women)
Angiotensin-converting enzyme inhibitors	Associated cough worsens stress and urge leakage in persons with impaired sphincter function
Antibiotics/antifungals	Increase gastrointestinal side-effects, including diarrhea
Anticholinergics	Impaired emptying, retention, delirium, sedation, constipation, fecal impaction
Anticholinesterase inhibitors	Increased gastrointestinal side-effects, including diarrhea
Antipsychotics	Anticholinergic effects, rigidity, and immobility
Calcium channel blockers	Impaired detrusor contractility and retention, constipation, dihydropyridine agents increase pedal edema and may lead to nocturnal polyuria
Cholinesterase inhibitors	Urge incontinence
Colchicine	Increase in bowel frequency, diarrhea
GAGAnergic agents (gabapentin, pregablin)	Pedal edema leading to nocturia
Loop diuretics	Polyuria, frequency, urgency
Narcotic analgesics	Urinary retention, fecal impaction, sedation, delirium
Nonsteroidal anti-inflammatory drugs	Pedal edema leading to nocturnal polyuria, constipation
Nonsulfonurea glucose lowering drugs (metformin)	Alterations in stool consistency
Osmotic laxatives (lactulose, polyethylene glycol)	Diarrhea
Proton pump inhibitors	Diarrhea
Sedative hypnotics	Sedation, delirium, immobility
Thiazolidinediones	Pedal edema leading to nocturnal polyuria

Adapted from DuBeau CE. Incontinence. In: Durso SC, Sullivan GM, eds. *Geriatric Review Syllabus*, 8th ed. American Geriatric Society, 2013, pp. 244-253.

(**Figure 71-1**). Postvoiding residual volume should be checked in all hospitalized patients with acute UI.

If general measures do not immediately remediate incontinence, then the next step is to evaluate the possible role of multimorbidity (Tables 71-1 and 71-3) and medications (Table 71-2). Such acute or worsening UI and FI is frequently referred to as "transient," because the underlying precipitants may be reversible. However, some patients can leave the hospital with "transient" incontinence still in place if precipitants have not or cannot be resolved.

Urinalysis should be interpreted with caution to avoid over-treatment of asymptomatic bacteriuria which is found in at least 20% of older women (see Chapter 197 [Urinary Tract Infections]). Diagnosis of urinary tract infection (UTI) requires positive culture *and*

TABLE 71-3 Other Hospital-Acquired Causes of Urinary and Fecal Incontinence

Causes	Impact on Continence
Prolonged use of transurethral catheters	Stress UI from urethral damage; urge UI from bladder irritation
Prolonged use of rectal tubes	Fecal incontinence (urge and passive types) due to weakness in anal sphincters
Epidural or spinal anesthesia	Urinary retention, UI and FI from interruption of efferent and afferent pathways
Decreased mobility from physical or chemical restraints, Foley catheters, IV lines, casts, etc	Limit toilet access leading to UI and FI

relevant symptoms, including acute dysuria or fever *and* either new or worsening urgency, frequency, UI, suprapubic pain, hematuria, or costovertebral angle tenderness. Delirium with positive culture does not indicate UTI unless there are additional relevant symptoms or the patient has an indwelling urinary catheter. In catheterized patients, urine samples should be collected at the time of placement of a new catheter, and not from the side port or collection bag of a current catheter.

The basic FI evaluation is similar to that for UI, with particular focus on the perineal and anorectal exam (**Figure 71-2**). Further work-up

TABLE 71-4 Types of Urinary Incontinence

Type	Symptoms	Common Pathophysiology
Urge	Leakage associated with urgency, the relatively sudden and compelling need to void. Often coexists with urinary frequency and nocturia	Uninhibited bladder contractions due to: • Increased afferent signaling from the detrusor and urothelium • Impairment in CNS inhibitory control • Interruption/damage to suprasacral spinal pathways • Idiopathic
Stress	Leakage with increased abdominal pressure (coughing, laughing, change in position, straining)	• Impaired urethral support • Impaired urethral closure
Mixed	Combination urge and stress symptoms	Combination urge and stress causes
Incomplete emptying	Elevated postvoiding residual Other symptoms nonspecific; may include dribbling, urgency, stress, stranguria	• Urethral obstruction • Weak or absent detrusor contractility • Combination of both

TABLE 71-5 Evaluation of Incontinence in Acute Care

Focused history	• Acute vs chronic • Onset, duration, frequency, previous evaluation/treatment • Review of comorbid conditions, medications, mobility, access to toilet/commode • Review nursing assessment for bladder and bowel function • Fluid status—intravenous and oral

Physical examination	• General
	  • Volume status
	  • Abdomen (masses, suprapubic tenderness)
	  • Neurological (motor strength, sensation)
	  • Cognition (eg, MiniCog, Confusion Assessment Method, see Chapter 81 on delirium)
	  • Bedside pelvic (check for significant pelvic organ prolapse, pain on bimanual exam)
	  • Rectal (in all patients, check for impaction and masses; in patients with retention, check sacral nerve innervation by perineal sensation, sphincter tone, and anal wink and/or bulbocavernosus reflex*)
	  • Perineal skin (dermatitis, cellulitis, pressure ulcers)

Laboratory	• Urinalysis • If diarrhea, consider stool studies appropriate to patient's condition (eg, *Clostridium difficile* antigen, ova and parasites, culture, fecal leukocytes, fecal fat) • Other: if chronic UR, consider vitamin B12 level; with chronic diarrhea or constipation, thyroid studies
Radiology	• Postvoid residual volume (by bladder ultrasound, if available) • Abdominal KUB if constipation • Neurological and/or pelvic imaging if indicated by known or suspected comorbidity (eg, pelvic mass, new neurological deficits) • Indigo carmine or methylene blue testing if urinary tract fistula suspected

*To do anal wink, lightly scratch perineal skin lateral to anus and visually check for anal contraction; for bulbocavernosus reflex, lightly squeeze either the clitoris or glans and check for anal contraction (either visually or with finger inserted in rectum).

may include anoscopy, flexible sigmoidoscopy, or colonoscopy to exclude mucosal disease or to evaluate rectal bleeding.

■ PREVENTION

Prevention and Treatment of UI and FI in hospitalized patients begin with addressing contributing comorbidity, iatrogenic complications, and medications. General measures include removal of impediments that limit access to toilets or commode, regular toileting by staff (eg, every 2 hours while awake), bedside commodes, condom catheters, and handheld urinals.

■ TREATMENT OF URINARY INCONTINENCE

Indwelling (Foley) catheters should only be used for five specific indications (**Table 71-6**). Indwelling catheter should never be used for staff or patient convenience because of the high risk of catheter associated urinary tract infection (CAUTI). CAUTI increases the risk of a publicly reported marker of poor quality care and not reimbursed by Medicare. Clean intermittent catheterization has little role in the acute care setting.

PRACTICE POINT

Management of Urinary Incontinence
- Cognitive impairment: management starts with nonpharmacological approaches (prompted voiding, scheduled toileting); these patients are especially vulnerable to anticholinergic side effects.
- Heart failure: administer diuretics early in the morning and early afternoon to avoid nighttime fluid overload and nocturia.
- Actively dying: guidelines for catheter management may not apply; the goals of care focus on patient comfort and wishes.

Medications for urge UI include antimuscarinic agents oxybutynin, darifenacin, tolterodine, solifenacin, trospium, and fesoterodine, and the β-3 adrenergic agonist mirabegron. The antimuscarinic agents may cause dry mouth, constipation, and dyspepsia; hospitalized patients are at higher risk of an elevated PVR/partial retention with antimuscarinics because of their many other risk factors for UR. Antimuscarinics have also been associated with cognitive impairment. Antimuscarinics (with the exception of trospium and fesoterodine) are metabolized by CY34A and 2D6, with potential interactions with macrolide antibiotics, oral antifungals, and SSRIs. Antimuscarinics should not be combined with cholinesterase inhibitors used to treat dementia Mirabegron does not have anticholinergic side effects, but may elevate blood pressure and has significant drug interactions with metoprolol and digoxin. There are no medications to treat stress UI. Most patients with stress UI can be referred for appropriate gynecology or urology follow-up after discharge; however, in-hospital neurology consultation should be considered if neurogenic sphincter dysfunction is suspected because of other symptoms or signs for spinal cord injury. Treatment of UI with indwelling catheters should be reserved for only specific indications (Table 71-6). Clean intermittent catheterization has little role in the acute care setting.

■ MANAGEMENT OF FECAL INCONTINENCE

Management of FI with diarrhea may include medications (bulking agents and antidiarrheals); containment by absorbent products or external fecal collectors, bowel management systems, or diversion by rectal tube. Data on the efficacy and utility of most of these options in the acute care setting are limited. Diphenoxylate should be avoided because of potential drug interactions and cognitive changes. External fecal collectors are preferable to rectal tubes, which can damage anal sphincters continence and rectal mucosa, and block fecal passage as diarrhea resolves. They are contraindicated in patient with recent rectal or prostate surgery, recent myocardial infarction, rectal mucosal disease, clotting disorders, and impaired immune status. FI due to impaction is treated with oral laxatives and enemas; methylnaltrexone may be effective for opiod-induced constipation in palliative care settings. Evidence exists for the use of polyethylene glycol versus lactulose for chronic constipation.

■ MANAGEMENT OF INCONTINENCE IN SPECIAL POPULATIONS

Surgery: Catheters should not be used to manage incontinence or generalized bladder management in the perioperative period. Guidelines suggest that catheters may be used after specific urologic and pelvic surgery or surgery on structures contiguous to the

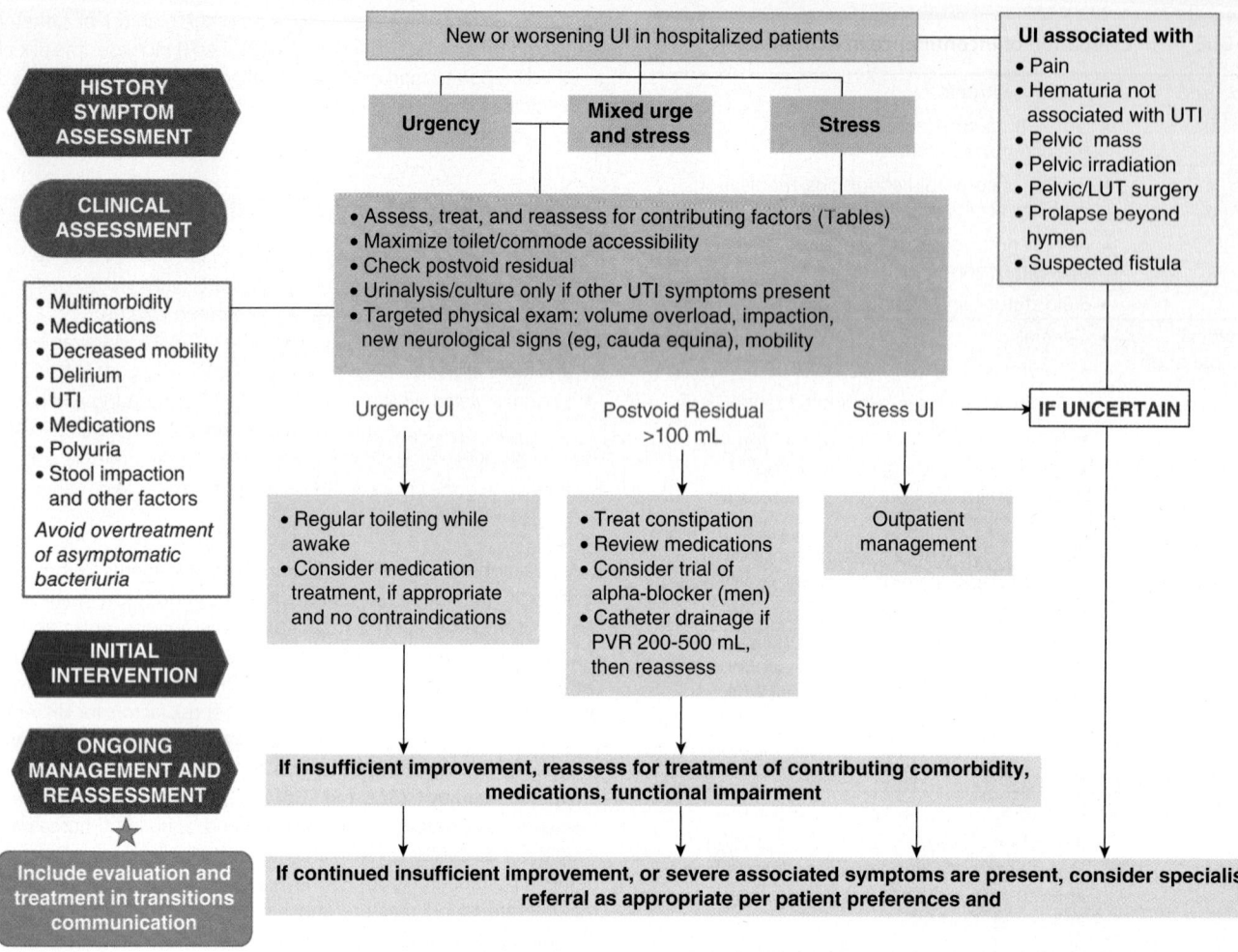

Figure 71-1 *Algorithm for treatment of new or worsening urinary incontinence in hospitalized patient.*

genito-urinary tract; anticipated long duration surgery (with catheter removal in postacute care unit); when there is a need for intraoperative urinary output measurement; and when large volume fluids or diuretics are required during surgery. In the postoperative period, catheters should be removed as soon as possible and appropriate toileting and use of bedside devices should be considered.

Dementia: Management of UI in patients with dementia in the hospital setting should focus on potentially reversible factors (see above) and nonpharmacological approaches (containment, prompted voiding, scheduled toileting). Antimuscarinic medications for urge UI should not be started in patients with dementia in the acute care setting because of the likelihood that new or worsening UI is due to "transient" causes, and because of the risk of worsening cognition. Antimuscarinics should not be given to patients taking cholinesterase inhibitors (eg, donepezil); mirabegron can be used instead, if there are no contraindications to its use.

Heart failure: Patients with diastolic and systolic heart failure may develop UI from new or higher doses of loop (but not thiazide) diuretics, and nocturia from remobilized lower-extremity edema. There is no specific evidence-based recommendation regarding timing of diuretics to prevent UI and nocturia in hospitalized patients. Data from a small, short term randomized trial in nonhospitalized patients showed that oral furosemide 40 mg given 6 hours before bedtime had no impact on nocturia episodes but did increase daytime frequency. Alteration in positioning and prolonged time supine also affect diuresis and natriuresis, and patients with CHF likely have other multimorbidity that contributes to incontinence and nocturia. Patients may benefit

from general HF management strategies, such as compression stockings and avoidance of medications causing edema and fluid retention, as well as repeated "n of 1" trials of optimal diuretic timing in individual patients. Catheter insertion to measure urine output should be avoided, especially outside of the critical care setting unless UI poses a significant barrier to accurate urine output measurement.

End of life: Urinary catheters are appropriate to use in dying patients for comfort, especially to avoid frequent changes of protective garments.

Neurologic diseases: Adults with complex neurologic diseases (eg, multiple sclerosis, spinal cord injury, Parkinson's disease, stroke) frequently have UI and FI because of direct effects on areas of the neuroaxis important for bladder and bowel function (especially prefrontal cortex, pontine and suprapontine areas, and thoracic and lower-lumbar spinal cord), as well as associated cognitive and functional impairments. These patients should always have PVR checked as part of the evaluation. Consideration of medications and other factors that may contribute to urinary retention is important prior to placing a urinary catheter (**Table 71-7**). Constipation can be common and contribute to urinary symptoms and FI.

Select patients (especially those with high PVR for UI and no external anal sphincter tone at rest or diarrhea with noninfectious etiology for FI) may need further evaluation by a specialist in urology, gynecology, gastroenterology, colorectal surgery, or neurology depending on the type of incontinence and potential etiologies. Nurses specializing in Wound, Ostomy, and Continence (WOC) care are also a valuable resource in the acute care setting.

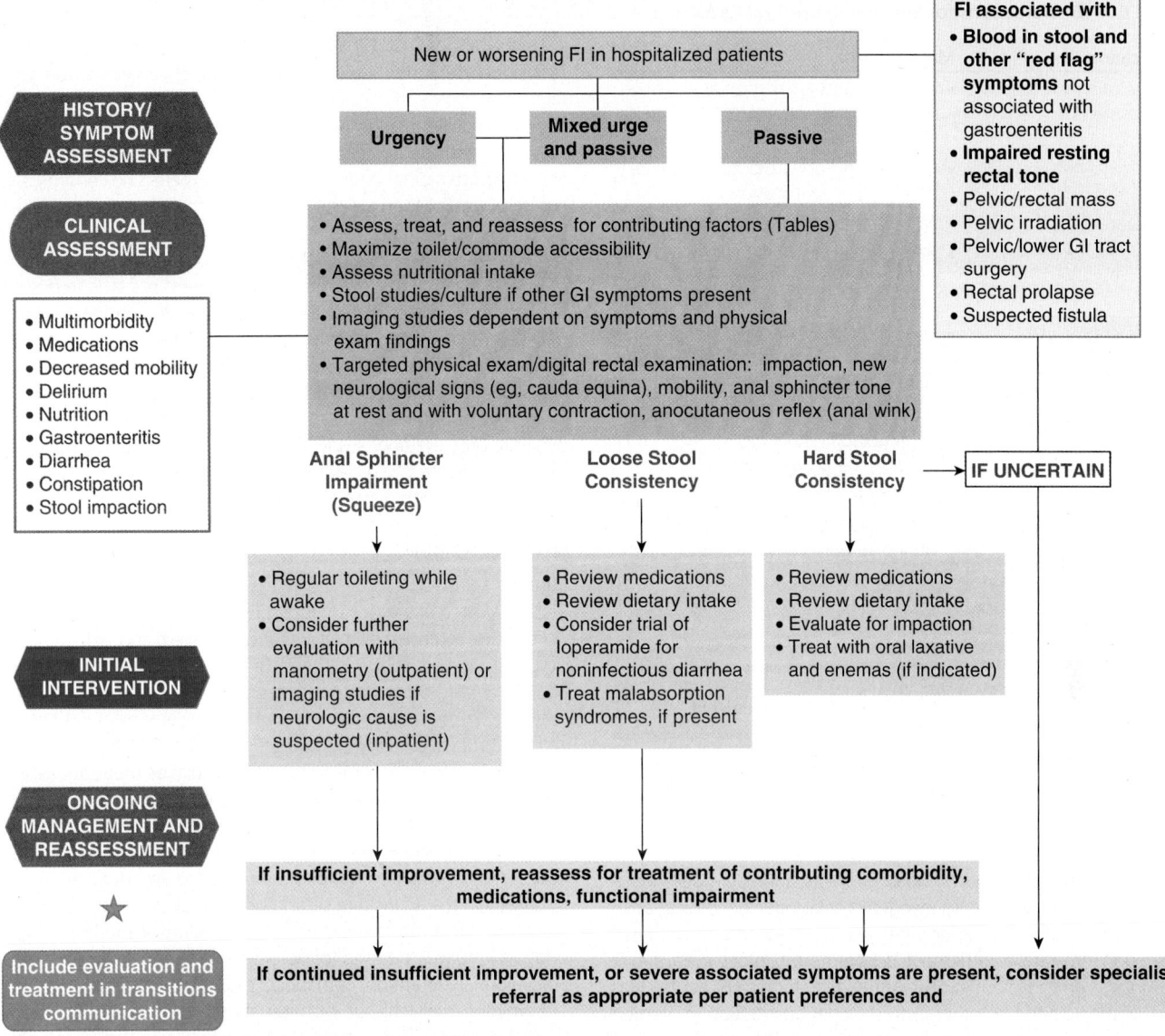

HISTORY/ SYMPTOM ASSESSMENT

CLINICAL ASSESSMENT

- Multimorbidity
- Medications
- Decreased mobility
- Delirium
- Nutrition
- Gastroenteritis
- Diarrhea
- Constipation
- Stool impaction

INITIAL INTERVENTION

ONGOING MANAGEMENT AND REASSESSMENT

★

Include evaluation and treatment in transitions communication

New or worsening FI in hospitalized patients

Urgency | **Mixed urge and passive** | **Passive**

FI associated with
- **Blood in stool and other "red flag" symptoms** not associated with gastroenteritis
- **Impaired resting rectal tone**
- Pelvic/rectal mass
- Pelvic irradiation
- Pelvic/lower GI tract surgery
- Rectal prolapse
- Suspected fistula

- Assess, treat, and reassess for contributing factors (Tables)
- Maximize toilet/commode accessibility
- Assess nutritional intake
- Stool studies/culture if other GI symptoms present
- Imaging studies dependent on symptoms and physical exam findings
- Targeted physical exam/digital rectal examination: impaction, new neurological signs (eg, cauda equina), mobility, anal sphincter tone at rest and with voluntary contraction, anocutaneous reflex (anal wink)

Anal Sphincter Impairment (Squeeze) | **Loose Stool Consistency** | **Hard Stool Consistency** → **IF UNCERTAIN**

- Regular toileting while awake
- Consider further evaluation with manometry (outpatient) or imaging studies if neurologic cause is suspected (inpatient)

- Review medications
- Review dietary intake
- Consider trial of loperamide for noninfectious diarrhea
- Treat malabsorption syndromes, if present

- Review medications
- Review dietary intake
- Evaluate for impaction
- Treat with oral laxative and enemas (if indicated)

If insufficient improvement, reassess for treatment of contributing comorbidity, medications, functional impairment

If continued insufficient improvement, or severe associated symptoms are present, consider specialist referral as appropriate per patient preferences and

Figure 71-2 *Algorithm for treatment of new or worsening fecal incontinence in hospitalized patients.*

PRACTICE POINT

Indications for referral for incontinence include (see also treatment algorithms):

- Urology: hematuria without UTI, pelvic mass, prior pelvic radiation, prior pelvic/lower urinary tract surgery, suspected bladder fistula
- Gynecology: pelvic pain not responding nonpharmacologic and pharmacologic treatments, pelvic mass, prior pelvic radiation, prior pelvic/lower urinary tract surgery, suspected fistula, prolapse beyond the hymen
- Gastroenterology: "Red flag" or alarm symptoms (chronic GI bleeding, progressive unintentional weight loss, progressive dysphagia, nocturnal symptoms, iron deficiency anemia, family history of colon cancer or inflammatory bowel disease), acute inflammatory bowel disease, pancreatitis, malabsorption syndromes, stool impaction not responding to pharmacologic treatment and enemas
- Colorectal surgery: rectal mass, colon cancer, congenital abnormalities, inability to reduce rectal prolapse

- Neurology: cauda equina or tumor, spinal cord injury, multiple sclerosis, stroke, prior back surgery with other neurologic findings
- Nurses specializing in Wound, Ostomy, and Continence (WOC): incontinence associated dermatitis, pressure wounds, management in spinal cord injury, special containment requests

URINARY RETENTION

PATHOPHYSIOLOGY

Urinary retention (UR) may be acute or chronic, and partial (patient may still void or leak urine) or complete (inability to void). Acute UR presents with a relatively sudden difficulty or inability to pass urine, usually with abdominal or suprapubic pain. Pain may be absent due to impaired sensory afferents (eg, with cauda equina syndrome), medication (eg, narcotics), or not recognized (eg, cognitive impairment). Chronic retention may be asymptomatic except for associated UI.

The causes of UR fall into three general categories: increased bladder outflow resistance (mechanical or dynamic); interruption of

TABLE 71-6 Indications for Indwelling Urethral Catheters

Indication	Management
Acute urinary retention or obstruction	• Remove catheter as soon as possible (eg, after reversible causes identified and removed) • Arrange appropriate outpatient care following hospitalization
Accurate measurement of urinary output in critically ill patients	• Minimize time with catheter inserted • Remove catheter when alternative means of urinary collection are available
Perioperative use	• Urologic surgery or other surgery on contiguous structures in the genitourinary tract • Anticipated long duration surgery (with catheter removal in PACU) • Need for intraoperative urinary output measurement • Large volume fluids or diuretics during surgery
Stage 2 or greater open sacral or perineal wounds in incontinent patients	• To improve healing and reduce exposure to moisture
Comfort care at the end of life	• When goal is to improve quality of life for patient and caregivers

Adapted from the Centers for Disease Control and Prevention: Guidelines for Prevention of Catheter-Associated Urinary Tract Infections 2009. http://www.cdc.gov/HAI/ca_uti/uti.html. Accessed April 1, 2015.

detrusor sensory afferents or motor efferents; and decreased detrusor contractility (neurogenic, myogenic, or iatrogenic [medications]) (Table 71-7). UR is common after spinal or epidural anesthesia. Although prostate enlargement is common in older men and if advanced can cause outlet obstruction and chronic UR, acute UR is usually precipitated by other factors. Outlet obstruction in women is uncommon; when present, it is usually due with prior anti-incontinence surgery or marked pelvic organ prolapse.

■ EVALUATION

The evaluation of urinary retention also is similar to that of UI and FI (Table 71-7). Risk factors for elevated PVR, in addition to medications (Table 71-2), include previous history of UR, new stroke, untreated

TABLE 71-7 Common Causes of Urinary Retention in Hospitalized Patients

Mechanical	Neurogenic	Medications
Stool impaction	Acute cauda equina syndrome	Anesthesia
Catheter obstruction (eg, blood clot, twisted catheter)	Sacral/subsacral spinal cord injury	Opiates
	Bedrest	Anticholinergics (eg, phenergan, metoclopramide, antispasmodics)
	Sacral herpes zoster	
	Urinary tract infection	
	Bladder overdistention from rapid dieresis	

UTI, hip fracture, fecal impaction, male gender, bedrest, and benign prostatic enlargement.

Neither abdominal palpation nor percussion is sensitive or specific for bladder distension. Only by bladder scan or catheterization accurately determines the presence or absence of UR accurately. If the patient can void, bladder volume should be determined only after they void, and the percentage emptying considered as well as the absolute postvoiding residual (PVR) volume. There is no consensus on cut-off values for "normal" PVR either from the perspective of definition or clinical relevance. Women may tolerate higher PVRs than men because they have less urethral resistance, and PVR up to 200 mL may not be clinically relevant unless the patient has UTIs, frequency, urgency, or UI. In men, PVR > 100 mL are generally considered abnormally elevated. In the absence of *new* renal impairment men and especially women have a low prior probability of hydronephrosis due to elevated PVR and upper-tract imaging is not necessary.

The gold standard for the diagnosis of outlet obstruction is urodynamic pressure-flow study; cystoscopy alone is nonspecific and insensitive. Acute UR, prostate infection, and urethral instrumentation/catheterization may elevate prostate specific antigen (PSA).

■ MANAGEMENT

Figure 71-3 presents a general management approach for patients with suspected acute urinary retention.

For acute retention, all patients should have bladder decompression with an indwelling catheter for several days. Antibiotic and antimicrobial catheters are not recommended for short-term hospital usage due to the relative lack of efficacy, as well as patient discomfort and cost. Following catheter insertion, patients should be treated for potentially remediable causes such as medications, and impaction. Medications may expedite catheter removal in selected patients. Alpha-adrenergic antagonists (eg, terazosin, doxazosin, tamsulosin, alfuzosin) can be used for UR due to prostatic obstruction. 5-Alpha reductase inhibitors (finasteride and dutasteride) are not useful in the acute care setting because of the delayed onset of treatment effect (up to 6 months). Methylnaltrexone (0.15 mg/kg of body weight) may be used for opioid-induced and possibly postoperative urinary retention. Bethanecol chloride is ineffective.

A voiding trial without catheter should follow decompression. With the patient adequately hydrated, the catheter is removed (*never* clamped), and a PVR checked after the first void (or bladder volume checked if there is no void after about 6 hours). If the PVR is <100 to 150 mL, the catheter can stay out but the patient should have close follow-up—both in the hospital and after discharge—to ensure that retention does not recur. If the PVR remains high, one can consider short-term intermittent catheterization or reinsertion of the catheter while further evaluation and treatment of the inability to void continues. Patients who must leave the hospital with catheter in place should have a follow-up appointment within 1 week and another voiding trial attempted at that time.

Select patients may need further evaluation by a specialist in urology, gynecology, gastroenterology, colorectal surgery, or neurology depending on the type of incontinence (UI with high PVR) and potential etiologies (cauda equina syndrome). Nurses specializing in Wound, Ostomy, and Continence (WOC) care are also a valuable resource in the acute care setting.

TRANSITIONS OF CARE

Medication reconciliation should consider possible drug interactions between previous or new bladder antimuscarinics and new medications at discharge. Hospital-acquired deconditioning may greatly impact continence; discussion with the patient, family, and other care providers must anticipate and help with new home needs such raised toilet seats, bedside commodes or urinals,

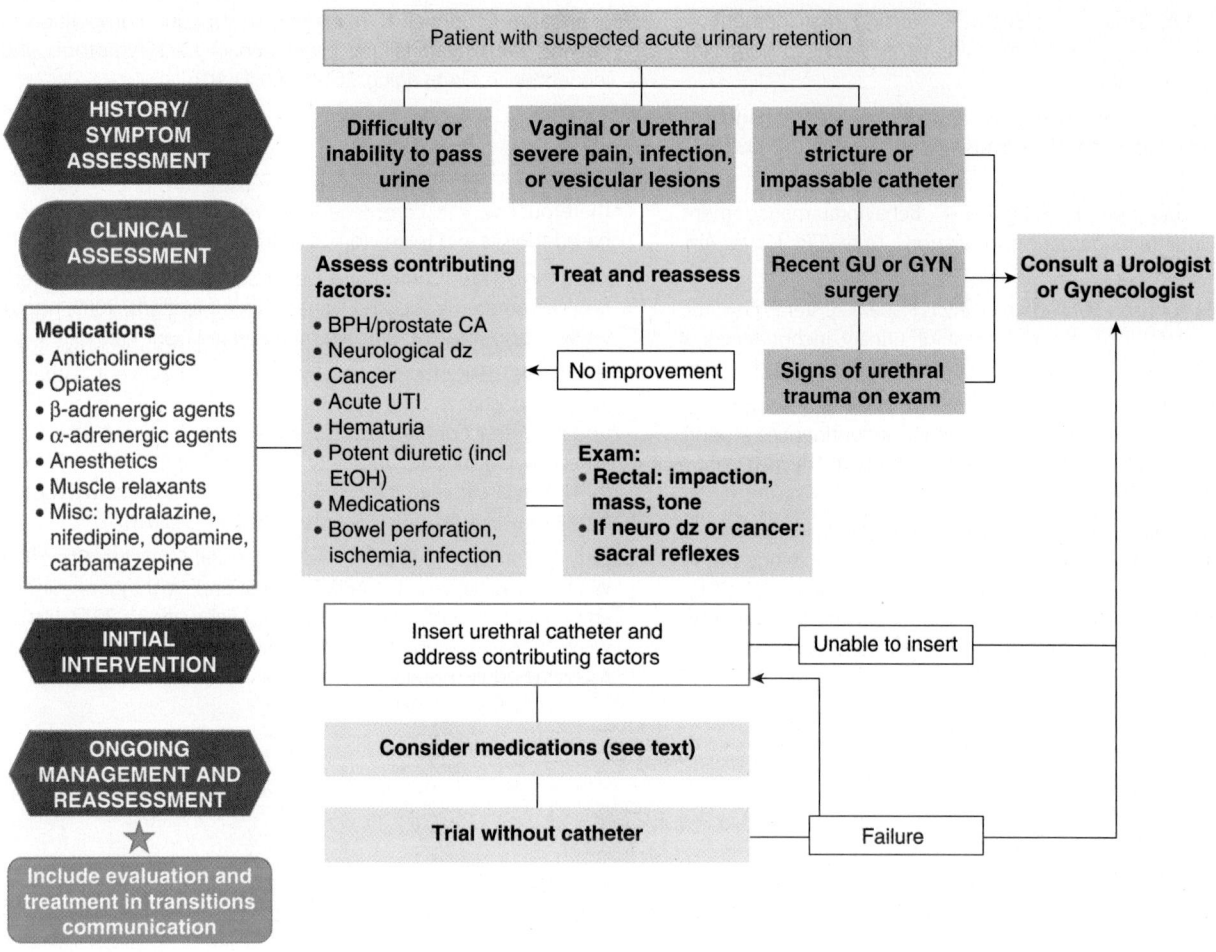

Figure 71-3 *Algorithm for treatment of patient with suspected acute urinary retention.*

protective garments, adsorbent products, and skin care. If long term catheter use is indicated, specific instructions for management and follow-up are needed for subacute care settings; nursing care should be arranged for patients returning home.

Management of UI in post acute care follows the same principles and management as in the acute care setting, with two differences. Prompted voiding and regular toileting may be more feasible. Two systematic reviews found prompted voiding was moderately effective in reducing daytime UI in post acute patients with cognitive impairment. At skilled nursing facilities institute prompted voiding was found to be somewhat effective at short-term follow-up in reducing daytime incontinence in two systematic reviews of randomized trials involving SNF patients with cognitive impairment and urinary incontinence. One study suggested a persistent benefit 4 months among long-stay patients after the intervention period. Most trials used research staff to provide the prompting intervention, and it is uncertain whether implementation with usual nursing staff would be similarly effective, given constraints of added cost and nursing time. An exercise program (graded strength and endurance training) may be considered as an adjunct to prompted voiding, although its effectiveness is uncertain, with benefit found in two trials and no benefit in one. Addition of medications for urge UI may be considered, especially if "transient" contributing factors have resolved or improved.

QUALITY IMPROVEMENT

Hospitals have implemented daily order renewal and review of indwelling catheter need to reduce the incidence of catheter-associated urinary tract infection. Screening and recognition of a prior UI, FI, and UR history upon hospital admission will identify hospitalized patients at risk for these conditions. Discussion of continence care and options for management may help reduce adverse effects of leakage on skin. Development of pharmacy reminders for medications that are associated with incontinence and UR among hospitalized patients may also help improve outcomes. Lastly, improvements in bowel regimens, especially for hospitalized patients on narcotics and at risk for constipation, are needed.

SUGGESTED READINGS

Candy B, Jones L, Goodman ML, Drake R, Tookman A. Laxatives or methylnaltrexone for the management of constipation in palliative care patients. *Cochrane Database Syst Rev.* 2011;(1):CD003448.

Centers for Disease Control and Prevention. Guidelines for Prevention of Catheter-Associated Urinary Tract Infections; 2009. http://www.cdc.gov/HAI/ca_uti/uti.html. Accessed April 1, 2015.

Gulur, DM, Mevcha AM, Drake MJ. Nocturia as a manifestation of systemic disease. *BJU Int.* 2011;107(5):702-713.

Lam TBL, Omar MI, Fisher E, Gillies K, MacLennan S. Types of indwelling urethral catheters for short-term catheterisation in hospitalised adults. *Cochrane Database Syst Rev.* 2014;(9):CD004013.

Lee-Robichaud H, Thomas K, Morgan J, Nelson RL. Lactulose versus polyethylene glycol for chronic constipation. *Cochrane Database Syst Rev.* 2010;(7):CD007570.

Lo E, Nicolle LE, Coffin SE, et al. Strategies to prevent catheter-associated urinary tract infections in acute care hospitals: 2014 update. *Infect Control Hosp Epidemiol.* 2014;35(5):464-479.

McCormick KA, Scheve AA, Leahy E. Nursing management of urinary incontinence in geriatric inpatients. *Nurs Clin North Am.* 1988;23(1):231-264.

Ostaszkiewicz J, O'Connell B, Millar L. Incontinence: managed or mismanaged in hospital settings? *Int J Nurs Pract.* 2008;14(6): 495-502.

Petrilli CO, Traughber B, Schnelle JF. Behavioral management in the inpatient geriatric population. *Nurs Clin North Am.* 1988;23(1):265-277.

Pfisterer MH, Johnson TM 2nd, Jenetzky E, Hauer K, Oster P. Geriatric patients' preferences for treatment of urinary incontinence: a study of hospitalized, cognitively competent adults aged 80 and older. *J Am Geriatr Soc.* 2007;55(12):2016-2022.

Sier H, Ouslander J, Orzeck S. Urinary incontinence among geriatric patients in an acute-care hospital. *J Am Med Assoc.* 1987;257(13):1767-1771.

Society for Hospital Medicine—Adult Hospital Medicine. Choosing Wisely®An Initiative of the ABIM Foundation. Five things physicians and patients should question. Released February 21, 2013. http://www.choosingwisely.org/doctor-patient-lists/society-of-hospital-medicine-adult-hospital-medicine/. Accessed April 1, 2015.

Tannenbaum C, Johnell K. Managing therapeutic competition in patients with heart failure, lower urinary tract symptoms and incontinence. *Drugs Aging.* 2014;31(2):93-101.

ONLINE RESOURCES

Catheterout.org. This comprehensive web site includes evidence-based toolkits and team work to reduce hospital-acquired CAUTI.

Centers for Disease Control and Prevention. Guidelines for Prevention of Catheter-Associated Urinary Tract Infections; 2009. http://www.cdc.gov/HAI/ca_uti/uti.html. Accessed April 1, 2015.

Lo E, Nicolle LE, Coffin SE, et al. Strategies to prevent catheter-associated urinary tract infections in acute care hospitals: 2014 update. *Infect Control Hosp Epidemiol.* 2014;35(5):464-479. Published by Cambridge University Press on behalf of The Society for Healthcare Epidemiology of America Stable. http://www.jstor.org/stable/10.1086/675718. Accessed June 17, 2016.

Society for Hospital Medicine – Adult Hospital Medicine. Choosing Wisely® An Initiative of the ABIM Foundation. Five things physicians and patients should question. Released February 21, 2013. http://www.choosingwisely.org/doctor-patient-lists/society-of-hospital-medicine-adult-hospital-medicine/. Accessed April 1, 2015.

CHAPTER 72

Pressure Ulcers

Courtney H. Lyder, ND, ScD(Hon), FAAN

Key Clinical Questions

1. What is a pressure ulcer? How are pressure ulcers staged?
2. Which patients are at risk for pressure ulcers?
3. What measures are effective in pressure ulcer prevention?
4. How should pressure ulcers be cleansed, debrided, and dressed?
5. What role do adjunctive therapies have in pressure ulcer treatment?

INTRODUCTION

Pressure ulcers, or bedsores, are a key clinical indicator of quality of care in hospitals. Their occurrence is widely seen as a marker for substandard care, triggering anger and sometimes litigation on the part of patients and families. However, they remain common in hospitalized patients. In 1993, pressure ulcers were diagnosed during 280,000 hospital stays in the United States, a number that rose to 503,300 in 2006. Up to 15% of elderly patients develop pressure ulcers within the first week of hospitalization. Mortality may be as high as 60% for older persons with pressure ulcers in the year after hospital discharge.

Pressure ulcers are also expensive, with an average charge per stay of $43,180. In 2007, the Centers for Medicare and Medicaid Services (CMS) made payouts of more than $11 billion for beneficiaries admitted to hospitals who developed Stage III and Stage IV pressure ulcers. The Centers for Medicare and Medicaid Services subsequently stopped reimbursement for hospital-acquired Stage III and Stage IV pressure ulcers in October 2008.

PATHOPHYSIOLOGY

Pressure ulcers are focal injuries of skin and subcutaneous tissue resulting from pressure, shear forces, friction, or some combination of these. They most often overlie bony prominences of the pelvis and lower extremities, such as the sacrum, greater trochanter of the hip, and heels, but they may appear in other locations, depending on patient positioning (**Figure 72-1**).

Tissue ischemia occurs when external pressures exceed perfusion pressures. Normal blood pressure within capillaries ranges from 20 to 40 mm Hg; 32 mm Hg is considered average. An external pressure 32 mm Hg usually suffices to prevent pressure ulcers. However, capillary blood pressure may be less than 32 mm Hg in critically ill patients due to hemodynamic instability and comorbid conditions.

Frictional forces, like those generated between the heels and bedsheets, can lead to blisters and skin breakdown, favoring the development of pressure ulcers. Bedbound patients are also prone to shear forces, which occur when bone and soft tissue move relative to the skin, which is held in place by friction.

Older patients are more susceptible to shear forces, as their soft tissues are atrophied and contain less elastin. Moisture, as in urine, stool, and sweat, acts synergistically with pressure, friction, and shear forces to facilitate skin breakdown.

PREVENTION

Pressure ulcer prevention requires a team effort, involving physicians, nurses (including wound, ostomy, and continence nurses), dietitians, and physical therapists. Studies have demonstrated that comprehensive pressure ulcer prevention programs can decrease incidence rates, although not to zero. For optimal effectiveness, pressure ulcer prevention must begin as soon as patients enter the hospital. There are five basic components to comprehensive pressure ulcer prevention: risk assessment, skin care, mechanical loading, support surfaces, and nutritional support.

■ RISK ASSESSMENT

The identification of patients at greatest risk of pressure ulcers involves the use of a risk assessment tool, skin assessment, and clinical judgment. More than 20 pressure ulcer prediction tools are used throughout the world, with the most popular being the Braden,

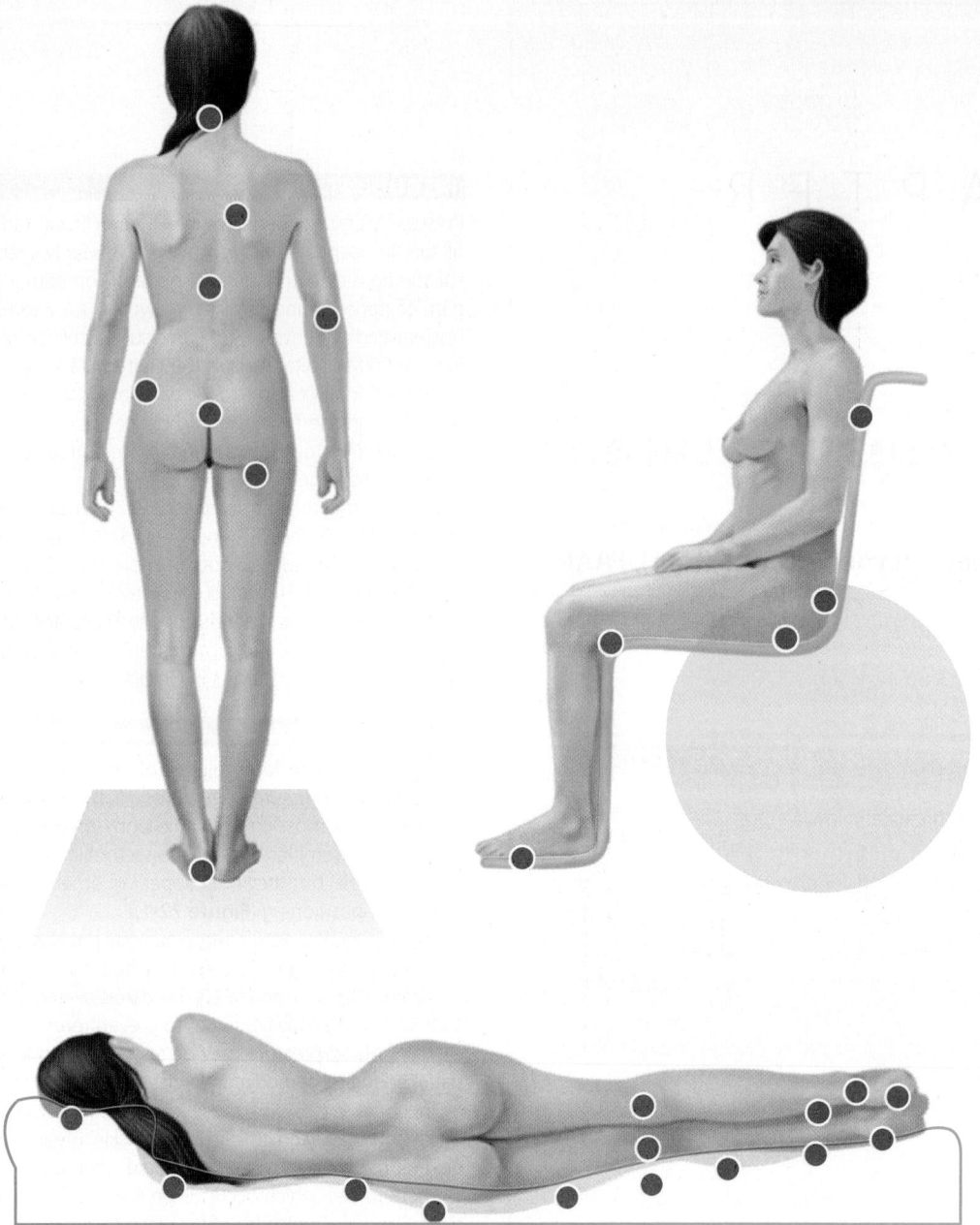

Figure 72-1 *Pressure ulcer locations. The most common sites of pressure ulceration are the sacrum and coccyx, heels, and greater trochanters of the hip.* (From *Preventing Pressure Ulcers: A Patient's Guide.* Washington, DC: U.S. Department of Health and Human Services; 1992, USGPO 617-025/68298.)

Norton, and Waterlow scales. The Braden Scale for Predicting Pressure Sore Risk is the most widely used in US hospitals. (The copyrighted tool is available at http://www.bradenscale.com/images/bradenscale.pdf.) The Braden Scale is designed for use with adults, and consists of six subscales: sensory perception, moisture, activity, mobility, nutrition, and friction and shear. Total scores on the Braden Scale range from 6 (high risk) to 23 (low risk); a score of 18 is the cut-off score for onset of pressure ulcer risk.

There is general consensus from most pressure ulcer clinical guidelines to do a risk assessment on admission, at discharge, and whenever the patient's clinical condition changes. Skin assessment should also be correlated with risk assessment. Close attention should be paid to greater trochanters, heels, sacrum, and coccyx, as >60% of all pressure ulcers occur at these locations.

■ SKIN CARE

The skin of patients at risk of pressure ulceration should be inspected regularly for erythema. This includes pressure points, as well as areas of contact with medical devices, such as catheters, oxygen tubing, ventilator tubing, and semirigid cervical collars, as these may also cause ulceration. Pain over an erythematous area may herald skin breakdown. It is not always possible to see redness on darkly pigmented skin. Depending on the degree of pigmentation, erythema may appear blue or purple, compared to adjacent skin. Erythema should be categorized as blanching or nonblanching. Localized heat, edema, and induration over pressure points are additional warning signs for pressure ulcer development. Patients may need more frequent inspection in response to any deterioration in condition.

Protecting skin from excessive moisture with barrier paste or other products is essential, as moisture and warmth impair the mechanical integrity of the stratum corneum. Massaging areas of reddened skin should be avoided, as these may contain damaged blood vessels or fragile skin. Skin emollients to hydrate dry skin should be considered.

MECHANICAL LOADING

Decreasing mechanical load and pressure exposure are crucial in preventing pressure ulcers. High pressures over bony prominences for short periods of time and low pressures over bony prominences for long periods of time are equally damaging. Repositioning frequency should be determined by the patient's skin condition and tissue tolerance, level of activity and mobility, general medical condition, overall treatment objectives, and support surfaces applied to the bed or chair. Turning and repositioning hospitalized patients every 2 hours while in bed, and every hour while seated, is reasonable for most hospitalized patients. Those who are critically ill may require hourly repositioning, while stable patients on specialty beds, such as low air loss or air fluidized, may only need repositioning every 4 hours.

The patient should be repositioned to relieve or redistribute pressure. Transfer aids that reduce friction and shear forces, such as the Hoyer lift or trapeze, should be used. Avoid positioning the patient directly on a bony prominence or directly onto medical devices, such as tubes or drains. The 30°-tilt position and the standard 90° side-lying position seem to be equivalent in protection against the development of pressure ulcers.

SUPPORT SURFACES

Pressure should be distributed as evenly as possible across the patient's body to reduce the incidence of pressure ulcers. The use of support surfaces may assist in pressure redistribution. The Centers for Medicare and Medicaid Services have divided support surfaces into three categories for reimbursement purposes. Group 1 devices are static and do not require electricity. Static devices include air, foam, gel, and water overlays or mattresses. These devices are ideal when a patient is at low risk for pressure ulcer development. The devices have some drawbacks: foam may degrade and lose its stiffness over time, and gel mattresses can increase skin heat and moisture. Group 2 devices are dynamic and powered by electricity or pump action. These devices include alternating and low-air-loss mattresses. These mattresses are better for patients at moderate to high risk for pressure ulcers, or who have full-thickness pressure ulcers (Stage III and Stage IV). Critically ill patients are excellent candidates for this group of support surfaces.

Group 3 devices, also dynamic, comprise only air-fluidized beds. These are electric, and contain silicone-coated beads that liquefy when air is pumped through the bed. These beds are used for patients at very high risk for pressure ulcers, patients with non-healing full-thickness pressure ulcers, and patients with numerous truncal full-thickness pressure ulcers. The National Pressure Ulcer Advisory Panel has suggested new definitions for support surfaces that move away from these categories and divide support surfaces into simply powered or nonpowered.

Approximately 20% of all pressure ulcers are found on the heels. Heel-protection devices should be considered for hospitalized patients at risk for pressure ulcers. The heels should be elevated and offloaded to distribute the weight of the leg along the calf without putting pressure on the Achilles tendon. The knee should also be in slight flexion to avoid hyperextension of the knee, which could lead to obstruction of the popliteal vein and deep vein thrombosis. Some hospitals may alternatively use a pillow to float the heels. If the use of a pillow is preferred, then the pillow should be placed under the calves to elevate the heels from the mattress.

NUTRITION

While nutritional status in patients with pressure ulcers is often poor, the evidence for a relationship between nutrition intake and pressure ulcer prevention is not always supported by randomized controlled trials. There is also a lack of empirical evidence to link the use of vitamin and mineral supplementation to the prevention of pressure ulcers. Therefore, while nutritional status should be optimized in patients at risk for pressure ulcers, overtreatment should also be avoided.

TREATMENT

When a pressure ulcer develops, the hospitalist must provide local care of the ulcer, but also assess the patient's overall physical health, nutritional status, pain level, and psychosocial health, considering the whole patient, not merely the ulcer. In addition to mechanical loading and support surfaces, as discussed above, pressure ulcer management includes the following.

ULCER ASSESSMENT

The ulcer bed should first be cleansed with a nontoxic solution. Cleaning removes necrotic debris and bacteria that may delay healing. Normal saline (0.9% sodium chloride) or water solutions are best, as neither is toxic to healthy tissue. Although the active ingredients in newer wound cleansers may be nontoxic surfactants, the inert carrier may be toxic to healthy granulation tissue.

The pressure ulcer should be assessed for location, stage, size (length, width, and depth), sinus tracts, undermining, tunneling, exudate (quality and quantity), necrotic tissue, and the presence or absence of granulation tissue and epithelialization. This comprehensive assessment establishes the baseline for measuring ulcer healing or deterioration. Ulcer assessment should be done at least weekly.

STAGING

Upon completing the pressure ulcer assessment, the ulcer should be staged. The most commonly used pressure ulcer staging system was developed by the National Pressure Ulcer Advisory Panel. Their system classifies skin changes into five levels of skin ulceration (**Table 72-1** and **Figure 72-2**).

This system rates the pressure ulcer from superficial tissue damage (Stage I) to full-thickness skin loss involving muscle or bone (Stage IV) and deep tissue injury. If the pressure ulcer is covered with necrotic tissue (eschar), it is noted as unstageable.

WOUND BED PREPARATION

A recent concept in the healing of chronic ulcers is wound bed preparation. The goal of wound bed preparation is to provide the ulcer with an optimal environment for healing: a wound bed that is highly vascularized, with minimal exudate. The three main principles are debridement, bacterial balance, and exudate control.

There is no optimal debridement method. The preferred method is determined by the goals of the patient, the presence or absence of infection, the amount of dead tissue present, and cost considerations. There are five common types of debridement: mechanical, autolytic, enzymatic, sharp, and biosurgery. *Mechanical debridement* uses wet-to-dry gauze to adhere to the necrotic tissue, which is then removed. Removal of the gauze dressing also removes necrotic tissue and wound debris. The challenge with mechanical debridement is the possibility that healthy granulation tissue may also be removed along with devitalized tissue, thus delaying wound healing. *Autolytic debridement* involves semiocclusive, transparent film dressings, and occlusive dressings, such as hydrocolloids and hydrogels, which create a favorable environment for the body's enzymes to break down the necrotic tissue. *Enzymatic*

TABLE 72-1 National Pressure Ulcer Staging System

Pressure Ulcer Stage	Definition	Description
Deep tissue injury	Purple or maroon localized area of discolored intact skin or blood-filled blister due to damage of underlying soft tissue from pressure and/or shear	• The area may be preceded by tissue that is painful, firm, mushy, boggy, warmer, or cooler, as compared to adjacent tissue • Deep tissue injury may be difficult to detect in individuals with dark skin tones • The area may rapidly evolve to expose additional layers of tissue, even with optimal treatment
Stage I	Intact skin with nonblanchable redness of a localized area, usually over a bony prominence	• The area may be painful, firm, soft, warmer, or cooler, as compared to adjacent tissue • Stage I may be difficult to detect in individuals with dark skin tones
Stage II	Partial thickness loss of dermis presenting as a shallow open ulcer with a red, pink wound bed without slough. May also present as an intact or open/ruptured serum-filled blister	Presents as a shiny or dry shallow ulcer without slough or bruising. This stage should not be used to describe skin tears, tape burns, perineal dermatitis, maceration, or excoriation
Stage III	Full-thickness tissue loss. Subcutaneous fat may be visible, but bone, tendon, or muscle are *not* exposed. Slough may be present but does not obscure the depth of tissue loss. *May* include undermining and tunneling	• The depth of a Stage III pressure ulcer varies by anatomical location. The bridge of the nose, ear, occiput, and malleolus do not have subcutaneous tissue, and Stage III ulcers can be shallow. In contrast, areas of significant adiposity can develop in extremely deep Stage III pressure ulcers • Bone/tendon is not visible or directly palpable
Stage IV	Full thickness tissue loss with exposed bone, tendon, or muscle. Slough or eschar may be present on some parts of the wound bed. *Often* includes undermining and tunneling	• The depth of a Stage IV pressure ulcer varies by anatomical location. The bridge of the nose, ear, occiput, and malleolus do not have subcutaneous tissue, and these ulcers can be shallow • Stage IV ulcers can extend into muscle and/or supporting structures (eg, fascia, tendon, or joint capsule), making osteomyelitis likely to occur • Exposed bone/tendon is visible or directly palpable
Unstageable	Full thickness tissue loss in which *actual* depth of the ulcer is *completely* obscured by slough (yellow, tan, gray, green, or brown) and/or eschar (tan, brown, or black) in the wound bed	• Until enough slough and/or eschar is removed to expose the base of the wound, the true depth, and therefore stage, cannot be determined. Stable (dry, or adherent, intact without erythema or fluctuance) eschar on the heels serves as the body's natural biological cover and should not be removed

debridement employs proteolytic enzymes, such as papain-urea, collagenase, and trypsin, to remove necrotic tissue. While enzymatic debridement is effective, it is slower than other types and often costly. *Sharp debridement* with scalpel or laser is probably the most rapid and effective type of debridement, and should be strongly considered when the patient is suspected of having cellulitis or sepsis. Finally, *biosurgery* (maggot therapy) is another effective and relatively quick method of debridement. Maggot therapy is very specific for devitalized tissue, although patient and provider unease have limited its acceptance.

Managing bacterial burden is an important consideration in wound bed preparation. All pressure ulcers contain a variety of bacteria. Bacteria are more likely to impede wound healing when their concentration exceeds 106 organisms per gram in the ulcer. Certain bacteria may impair ulcer healing at lower concentrations. Signs of ulcer infection include odor, purulent exudate, excessive draining, bleeding, and pain. If these are present, wound cultures should be obtained, and treatment with oral or intravenous antibiotics should be considered based on antimicrobial sensitivity testing. Other strategies to reduce bacterial bioburden include the use of silver impregnated dressings and topical sulfa silverdiazine.

Exudate management is the last component of wound bed preparation. Excessive exudate decreases ulcer healing, and may damage healthy surrounding tissue. Exudates are managed by

selecting an appropriate dressing. Dressings can be classified as gauze, petroleum-based nonadherent gauze, transparent films, hydrocolloids, foam islands, alginates, hydrogels, composites, and combinations (**Table 72-2**).

Whichever dressing is selected, the pressure ulcer should be kept moist to optimize healing. Since no studies exist that demonstrate that one dressing heals all pressure ulcers within an ulcer classification, a careful assessment of the pressure ulcer, patient needs, and environmental factors (frequency of dressing changes to increase adherence) must be considered.

Since wet-to-dry gauze dressings are a form of debridement, they should only be used in necrotic wounds. Once healthy granulation tissue is observed, wet-to-dry dressing should be stopped, and other dressings should be used. Negative pressure therapy, or vacuum-assisted closure (VAC) therapy, should also be considered for exudative ulcers. Negative pressure therapy removes excess exudate, increases local blood flow, and promotes granulation tissue. Negative pressure therapy should not be used in pressure ulcers with suspected osteomyelitis, eschar, or exposed blood vessels or viscera.

■ NUTRITION

Many patients with pressure ulcers are malnourished. High-protein diets in poorly nourished patients with pressure wounds are reasonable, although there is a paucity of evidence to support their use.

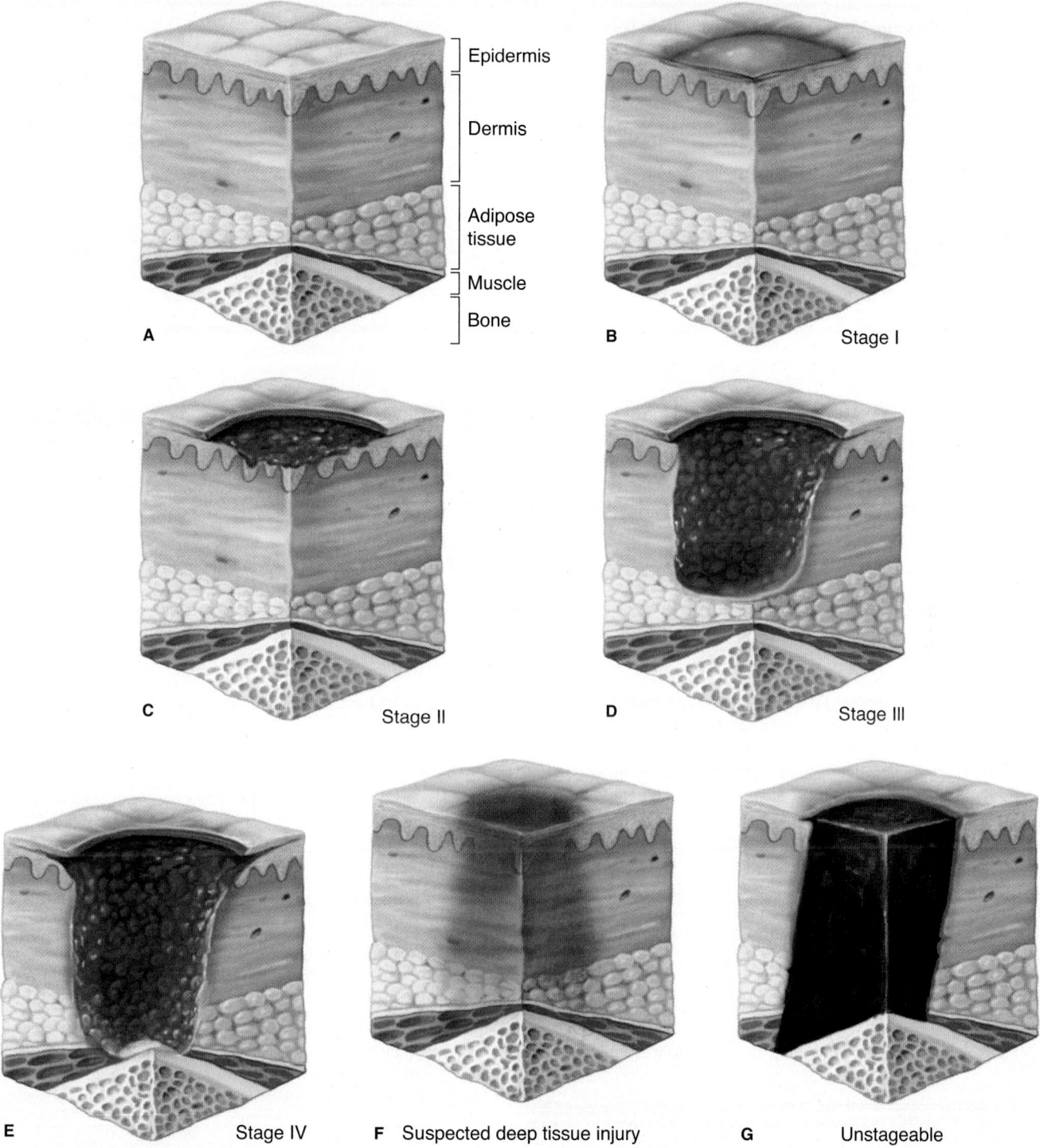

Figure 72-2 *National pressure ulcer staging system. (A) Normal skin. (B) Stage I pressure ulcer. (C) Stage II pressure ulcer. (D) Stage III pressure ulcer. (E) Stage IV pressure ulcer. (F) Deep tissue injury. (G) Unstageable pressure ulcer. (Reproduced with permission from the National Pressure Ulcer Advisory Panel, 2011.)*

■ PAIN MANAGEMENT

Pressure ulcers are often painful, especially Stage IV ulcers. Strategies to reduce pain include the use of dressings that may mitigate pain, such as those containing soft-silicone, and administering analgesic prior to dressing changes.

■ MONITORING HEALING

There is considerable debate regarding the use of reverse staging of pressure ulcers to monitor healing. Staging of pressure ulcers is only appropriate for defining the maximum anatomic depth of tissue damage. Since pressure ulcers heal to progressively more shallow depth, they do not replace lost muscle, subcutaneous fat, or dermis before they reepithelialize. Instead, pressure ulcers are filled with granulation (scar) tissue composed primarily of endothelial cells, fibroblasts, collagen, and extra cellular matrix. Thus, a Stage IV pressure ulcer cannot become a Stage III, Stage II, or subsequently Stage I. When a Stage IV pressure ulcer has healed, it should be classified as a healed Stage IV pressure ulcer, not a Stage 0. Therefore, reverse staging does not accurately characterize what is physiologically occurring in the pressure ulcer.

TABLE 72-2 Pressure Ulcer Dressing Classification Selection

Dressing Classification	Partial Thickness (Stages I and II)	Full Thickness (Stages III and IV)	Moderate Drainage	Heavy Drainage
Transparent films	X			
Hydrocolloids	X	X (As a secondary dressing)	X	X
Alginates	X (Stage II only)	X		X
Foams	X (Stage II only)	X	X	X
Composites	X (Stage II only)	X	X	X
Hydrogels	X (Stage II with dry wound bed only)	X (Dry wound beds only)		
Hydrofibers		X		X
Antirecalcitrant dressings		X	X	X

The Pressure Ulcer Scale for Healing (PUSH) and the Bates-Jensen Wound Assessment Tool (BWAT) are both valid and reliable for measuring pressure ulcer healing. The PUSH tool requires less time, having only three items, compared to the 13 items of the BWAT tool. For both tools, a lower score indicates a greater degree of healing. Both tools are usually used weekly.

■ **ADJUNCTIVE THERAPY**

When the pressure ulcer is not showing signs of healing within 2 to 4 weeks, adjunctive therapies should be considered. The most commonly adjunctive therapies include electrical stimulation, hyperbaric oxygen, growth factors, and autologous skin. Electrical stimulation is the use of electrical current to stimulate cellular processes important to pressure ulcer healing. These processes include increasing fibroblasts, neutrophils, and macrophages, collagen and DNA synthesis, and increasing the number of receptor sites for specific growth factors. Electrical stimulation is most effective in healing Stage III and IV pressure ulcers.

Hyperbaric oxygen is believed to promote wound healing by stimulating fibroblast, collagen synthesis, epithelialization, and control of infection. However, there remains a dearth of studies investigating the association of hyperbaric oxygen and healing pressure ulcers. The use of growth factors and skin equivalents in healing of pressure ulcers is relatively new. The use of cytokine growth factors, such as recombinant platelet-derived growth factor-BB (rhPDGF-BB) and fibroblast growth factors (bFGF), and skin equivalents are currently under study. Further research is needed to identify the appropriate ulcer environment for growth factors to be optimally effective.

PRACTICE POINT

- All wounds may be painful, and they may become more sensitive over time. Light touch or even air movement across a pressure ulcer may be exquisitely painful for some patients. Control of background pain and incident pain (pain with dressing changes) may require basal pain medication, as well as premedication for dressing changes. Nonpharmacologic measures that may reduce patient discomfort during dressing changes include measures that make the environment less stressful, such as noise reduction, engaging family members and ancillary personnel in hand holding when appropriate, frequent explanation and verbal engagement with the patient, and limiting wound manipulation and exposure to the minimum necessary.

DISCHARGE CHECKLIST

- ☐ Have the patient and outpatient caregivers been given clear instructions on wound care, turning, and positioning?
- ☐ Do outpatient caregivers have appropriate support surfaces, transfer devices, and wound dressings for the patient?
- ☐ Has the patient's nutritional status been optimized? Are additional measures necessary for nutritional support in the outpatient setting?
- ☐ Has outpatient follow-up been arranged with wound clinic, infectious diseases, and plastic surgery, as appropriate?

SUGGESTED READINGS

Ayello EA, Braden B. How and why to do pressure ulcer risk assessment. *Adv Skin Wound Care*. 2002;15:125-132.

Bolton LL, van Rijswijk L, Shaffer FA. Quality wound care equals cost-effective wound care: a clinical model. *Adv Skin Wound Care*. 1997;10(4):33-38.

Lyder C, Grady J, Mathur D, et al. Preventing pressure ulcers in Connecticut hospitals using the plan-do-study-act model for quality improvement. *Jt Comm J Qual Patient Saf*. 2004;30:205-214.

Lyder CH, Preston J, Grady J, et al. Quality of care for hospitalized Medicare patients at risk for pressure ulcers. *Arch Intern Med*. 2001;161:1549-1554.

National Institute for Health and Clinical Excellence. *The Prevention and Management of Pressure Ulcers in Primary and Secondary Care*. London: National Institute for Health and Care Excellence (UK); 2014. http://www.ncbi.nlm.nih.gov/pubmedhealth/PMH0068960/pdf/PubMedHealth_PMH0068960.pdf. Accessed September 12, 2016.

National Pressure Ulcer Advisory Panel, European Pressure Ulcer Advisory Panel and Pan Pacific Pressure Injury Alliance. In: Haesler E, ed. *Prevention and Treatment of Pressure Ulcers: Quick Reference Guide*. Perth, Australia: Cambridge Media; 2014. http://www.npuap.org/wp-content/uploads/2014/08/Updated-10-16-14-Quick-Reference-Guide-DIGITAL-NPUAP-EPUAP-PPPIA-16Oct2014.pdf. Accessed September 12, 2016.

Reddy M, Gill SS, Rochon PA. Preventing pressure ulcers: a systematic review. *JAMA*. 2006;296:974-984.

Patient Safety and Quality Improvement in Postacute Care

Mousumi Sircar, MD

Jatin K. Dave, MD

Matthew L. Russell, MD

Helen Chen, MD

Key Clinical Questions

1. Is each medication indicated for either an acute or chronic medical indication?

2. If the drug does not have an indication for either an acute or chronic condition, was it prescribed to treat an adverse effect of another medication?

3. Is the patient near the end of life?

4. If you plan to discontinue a medication, does the drug require tapering rather than abrupt discontinuation?

5. Are all underlying medical problems optimally treated with drug therapy according to established guidelines?

INTRODUCTION

Review of patient safety issues and opportunities for quality improvement in skilled nursing facilities (SNFs) begins with the index hospitalization and the necessary steps to guarantee a safe transition from the referring hospital to the receiving facility. The transition of care from hospitalization to postacute care presents a significant risk to the safety of the older adult patient. Two key areas that require the clinician's attention to ensure a safe transition of care are effective discharge communication including the discharge summary and the discharge medication reconciliation process. Safe and effective transitions reduce preventable readmissions and other adverse events.

PREVENTABLE READMISSIONS

The costs associated with the current transitions system illustrate the danger of care transitions and the need for a coordinated effort to ensure patient safety. Readmissions from skilled nursing facilities to the hospital increased by 29% from 2000 to 2006. Up to 24% of Medicare beneficiaries were readmitted to the hospital from a skilled nursing facility within 30 days at a cost of $4.34 billion in 2006. One-third of these occurred within just a week of initial discharge.

Older adults are at higher risk for readmission from skilled nursing facilities and more frequently experience care transitions. Patients who are frail or cognitively impaired often cannot actively participate in their transition processes and critical information (such as prehospital admission medications that were held) may be lost as a result.

Skilled nursing facilities are increasingly being held accountable for preventable readmissions. Similar to hospital metrics, Center for Medicare & Medicaid Services (CMS) is planning to use the 30-day readmission metric as a quality measure for skilled nursing facilities that provide postacute care (PAC). It is therefore important for individual clinicians to have a clear understanding of the PAC capabilities of their community SNFs. Clinicians and health care systems are creating preferred SNF networks based on readmission rate, length of stay, and other quality measures. Provider groups and hospitals are increasingly partnering with SNFs in quality improvement initiatives that help to ensure patient safety and reduce unnecessary utilization and readmissions.

PRETRANSFER CONSIDERATIONS IN THE SELECTION OF A SKILLED NURSING FACILITY

▪ STAFFING

Nurse and medical staffing ratios can be quite variable across facilities. Referring clinicians should be mindful that while the acuity level of PAC admissions has increased, nurse staffing ratios continue to remain far lower than those of acute care hospitals. Some nursing homes employ physicians and mid-level staff while others rely on as needed medical coverage from attending physicians in practice for whom "SNF rounding" is an additional responsibility, and who may not have special expertise in managing postacute care patients. Many postacute care transitions occur after hours or on weekends. Facilities with decreased after-hour staffing and coverage may not be ideal receiving facilities for highly medically complex patients. It is important for referring clinicians to understand and confirm what is reasonably available in these facilities to ensure that safer transitions can be supported (**Table 73-1**).

TABLE 73-1 Basic Considerations When Selecting a Skilled Nursing Facility

1. How many hours per day/week are physicians and mid-level clinicians on-site?
2. What is the after-hours staffing and coverage?
3. What is the facility's capacity to perform diagnostic testing?
4. Is there an on-site pharmacy or do medications need to be delivered from an off-site vendor?
5. What disciplines are available at the facility?
6. What quality data can be obtained from the facility? Do they have the capacity to respond to clinical quality of care concerns?
7. Are all readmissions to acute care hospitals regularly reviewed using a standardized tool such as INTERACT to identify root causes from preventable readmissions?

■ LOGISTICS OF PATIENT TRANSFER

Logistical aspects of patient transfer must be accounted for to ensure a safe transition. If the patient is transferred very late in the day or on the weekend, the clinician primarily responsible for the patient may not be available, and therefore an on-call physician may not receive critical information about the patient. This is particularly true for the high-risk patient who is cognitively impaired or delirious for whom a simple transfer to another site of care may cause decompensation. Nurse staffing also decreases at this time, which may slow the transfer from the receiving end. Late day transfers may occur near shift changes that create yet another transition of care for the patient as clinicians are changed. To minimize this, the patient should be transferred as early in the day as possible.

■ DIAGNOSTIC TESTING AND OTHER SERVICES

At baseline, postacute care skilled nursing facilities provide skilled nursing, rehabilitation therapies, and medical oversight. In some communities, some SNFs are differentiating themselves by offering advanced services such as in-house diagnostic testing, palliative care services, or specialty cardiac, pulmonary, or other condition specific medical care, as well as the ability to manage intravenous medications and other infusions.

THE DISCHARGE PROCESS

Inconsistencies with medications and follow-up care result in adverse health outcomes. Barriers to safe transitions include lack of standardization of the discharge process across institutions (often hindered by lack of financial incentive and fragmentation of communication). In addition, electronic medical records frequently cause data overload with multiple medication lists on admission and discharge. Transitions of care contribute to this problem through differences in medication lists that are not frequently explained in documentation.

■ MULTIDISCIPLINARY TEAMS

Daily interdisciplinary rounds at the hospital with careful planning of discharge with timely discharge summary and insurance authorization as well as warm handoff if necessary can minimize errors and last minute transfer issues. Interdisciplinary teamwork between social work, physicians, and nursing may accelerate the discharge to earlier in the day.

■ INTENSITY OF HANDOFF

Clinicians should pursue a more thorough handoff based on risks. (**Table 73-2**).

TABLE 73-2 Handoff Process

Identify high-risk patients

Complete discharge summary using joint commission requirements

Ensure safe medication reconciliation

Use step-wise approach (Project RED, Project BOOST) to provide safe transition for high-risk patients

Standardizing the handoff using evidence-based models such as RED (Re-Engineered Discharge) and Project BOOST (Better Outcomes for Older adults through Safe Transitions) is shown to reduce avoidable readmissions (**Tables 73-3, 73-4, and 73-5**).

■ THE DISCHARGE SUMMARY

The Joint Commission has recommended guidelines for discharge summaries including diagnosis (admission and discharge), key physical examination findings, key test results, discharge medications, follow-up appointments, patient and family education provided, and tasks to be completed. As anticoagulation is a specific high-risk intervention that can lead to adverse outcomes, it is particularly important to clearly communicate to community or PAC clinicians the goals for anticoagulation, current and recent INR levels (when appropriate), and current anticoagulants in use.

Clear language should be utilized on the summary, and any barriers in language or cognition should be elicited such that a translator in the former case and a caregiver in the latter may be made available. In addition, baseline and discharge mental status assessment should be clearly communicated so that receiving clinicians will be able to effectively assess for delirium or other changes in mental status. Red flags in terms of signs and symptoms should be elucidated such that the patient or clinician will know when rehospitalization may be required. Goals of care discussions should occur to ensure that the level of postacute care that has been chosen is consistent with the patient's self-defined quality of life. Should a Physician Order for Life-Sustaining Treatment form be available in the state, it should be utilized and transmitted to the PAC clinician to clarify resuscitation measures for the patient across all settings.

MEDICATIONS

■ MEDICATION RECONCILIATION FAILURES

The Joint Commission US Pharmacopeia Medmarx reporting program for medication reconciliation failures noted 2022 medication

TABLE 73-3 Re-engineered Discharge

1. Identify language barriers
2. Make follow-up appointments
3. Plan for follow-up of inpatient tests
4. Arrange outpatient services and equipment (eg, home oxygen)
5. Medication reconciliation with patient
6. Compare treatment plan with national guidelines
7. Teach patient using a written treatment plan
8. Educate patient regarding diagnosis and medications
9. Educate patient about what to do if a problem arises
10. Assess patient's understanding of plan
11. Send discharge summary to receiving physician
12. Provide telephone support for patient

TABLE 73-4 Start-to-Finish Guidelines for the Discharge Process That Have Been Published

Project BOOST (Better Outcomes for Older adults through Safe Transitions)	1. Identifies patients at high risk of rehospitalization 2. Targets specific interventions to mitigate potential adverse events 3. Improves flow of information between hospital and outpatient physicians and clinicians 4. Improves communication between clinicians and patients
CHAMP (Collaboration for Homecare Advances in Management and Practice)	Originally developed for home care of the geriatric patient, the CHAMP website now features a Care Transitions toolkit with 1. Validated tools to identify patients at risk for an unsafe transition 2. Intervention tools for patient safety 3. Tools for patients and caregivers 4. Tools to improve communication between clinician, patient, and caregivers
Community-Based Care Transition Program (CCTP)	In 2011, the Center for Medicare & Medicaid Services (CMS) began funding for acute-care hospitals with high readmission rates which partner with community-based organizations providing transition services to improve patient's transition from the acute to long-term settings. Application requirements for the Community-based Care Transition Program (CCTP) are described in detail on the CMS webpage

reconciliation errors, 66% occurring during change in level of care, 22% during admission to facility, and 12% discharge. Improper dose/quantity or omission of medications represented the majority of failures. In response, the Joint Commission in 2004 designated medication reconciliation as national patient safety goal, and in 2005, began requiring accredited organizations to develop and test a designated process for medication reconciliation. Despite these efforts, a 2012 article cited that medication discrepancies occur in up to 70% of patients at admission or discharge, and one-third of these have potential to harm the patient. Actual adverse drug events occur in up to 12% to 17% of patients postdischarge.

In 2006, Joint Commission advised the following as a process for medication reconciliation, which was defined as the process of comparing current medication orders to all medications the patient has been taking. This is expected to occur during any transition in setting, service, practitioner, or level of care. The requirement is represented by a five-step process.

1. Develop the current list by ensuring preadmission list is correct.
2. Develop updated list.
3. Compare the two lists.

TABLE 73-5 The Transition of Care from Hospital to Skilled Nursing Facility

Safe Transition	Unsafe Transition
• Education of patient and family	Complex, chronic conditions requiring multiple clinicians
• Coordination among health care professionals with timely exchange of information about complex care needs with a warm handoff for high-risk transitions	Absence of information specifying names of consultants, contact information, follow-up plans
• Goals of care/clinical status	Each clinician works alone lacking knowledge of:
• Logistical arrangements	- Problems addressed
	- Services provided
	- Information obtained
	- Medicines prescribed (discrepancies may result)

4. Make clinical decisions based on the comparison and adjust medications.
5. Communicate the new list to the patient and caregivers.

The current list, including immunization and allergies, should be shared with patients, nursing, and pharmacy. The reconciliation is required at all interfaces of care and patient should be guided in creating a personal/portable medication list with stop dates if appropriate. Prior to transition, it is essential to ensure that the facility, home care clinician or caregiver/patient is able to administer the planned medication in the new care setting. Orders such as IV diuretics may be essential in preventing rehospitalization but require staff/caregiver education and may not be available at all sites of care.

Improving transitions requires understanding common barriers to a safe reconciliation process and developing strategies to overcome them. Common barriers include:

- Cumbersome or difficult process of transferring or harmonizing information within the permanent medications record
- Lack of clinician reimbursement for completing the medication reconciliation
- Failure to assign responsibility for signing off on the reconciliation tool to one clinician
- Failure to assign responsibility to complete list and pass document from one clinician on to the next clinician
- Difficult process of transferring information from the medication reconciliation tool at the clinician's level to the patient's personal medication list

The reimbursement and implementation of Transitional Care Management Visits offers an opportunity to improve medication reconciliation after discharge.

■ PHARMACOKINETIC CHANGES WITH AGING

Pharmacokinetic changes with aging, which often increases half-life of many drugs (**Table 73-6**). Five classes of medications in which discrepancies can be particularly hazardous and common include anticoagulants, diuretics, ACE inhibitors, lipid-lowering agents, and proton-pump inhibitors.

■ POLYPHARMACY AND UNNECESSARY DRUGS

Few studies have measured the prevalence of unnecessary drug use in the elderly population and only one study has evaluated the prevalence of unnecessary drug use specifically in the inpatient setting. That study reported in a population of 384 frail hospitalized

TABLE 73-6 Pharmacokinetic Changes Leading to Adverse Effects

Body System	Changes Associated with Aging
Liver	↓ First-pass metabolism
Kidney	↓ Renal clearance of drugs
	• Serum creatinine unreliable
	• Cockcroft-Gault formula required for reliable prediction of renal function
Fat	↑ Distribution of lipophilic drugs due to ↑ fat
Total body water (TBW)	↓ Distribution of water-soluble drugs due to ↓ TBW

veterans aged 65 and older, 44% of patients had at least one unnecessary drug at time of discharge from the hospital. The reasons for a medication to be classified as unnecessary included lack of indication (33%), lack of efficacy (19%), and therapeutic duplication (8%). This study also noted that approximately 75% of those receiving an unnecessary drug were prescribed that medication prior to admission while the remaining 25% had an unnecessary drug started during hospitalization.

PRACTICE POINT

On admission, throughout hospitalization, and with any transition of care:

- Determine whether drug side effects are responsible for any new symptoms or exacerbating underlying medical conditions.
- Establish clear and practical therapeutic goals and monitoring plans.
- Review periodically medications and perform drug reconciliation with each transition, including screen for adverse drug reactions, therapeutic failures, and adverse drug withdrawal events.
- Taper or discontinue ineffective or redundant or possibly harmful medications.
- Minimize adverse effects by screening for drug-drug and drug-disease interactions before prescribing a medication to a patient.
- Develop expertise in prescribing a few select drugs—the medication's dosing, therapeutic and adverse effects—to manage common problems in the elderly.
- When in doubt, consult with a pharmacist.
- In older patients, if starting a new medication, start low and gradually titrate when possible.

Inappropriate polypharmacy is a particular danger that needs to be addressed both during hospitalization and during PAC. Half of the geriatric population is using more than five medications. Of these patients, 1 in 20 experiences an increase in morbidity and mortality. Not only does the patient suffer the adverse effects of the medication itself, but they also experience interactions between medications and incur additional cost. Therefore, prior to discharge, careful review and relevant de-prescribing should be done to the benefit of patients. Step to reduce polypharmacy include:

1. Identify potentially inappropriate medications (PIM) for the older adult using tools such as STOPP (Screening Tool of Older Persons' Potentially Inappropriate Medications) with the reasons for stopping each medication. Medications for which there is little evidence for beneficial effect should also

be discontinued. Down-titration is necessary prior to full discontinuation for β-blockers, opiates, sedatives, gabapentin, clonidine, and selective serotonin reuptake inhibitors. If a medication cannot be stopped, the dose should be lowered when possible.

2. Medications should be eliminated when not consistent with the patient's goals of care. Discontinuing some medications is appropriate if the patient is expected to pursue a palliative approach, or if estimated life expectancy is likely too limited to obtain benefit from a medication (such as a statin in the case of quickly progressive terminal cancer).

3. Medications that may pose higher risk for adverse effects in older adults according to the "Beers" list should be reassessed, including sedative hypnotics, antidepressants, anticoagulants/antiplatelet agents, hypoglycemic agents, opiates, and anticholinergic medications. There are often safer alternatives for many of these drugs that should be chosen. One algorithm for reducing polypharmacy is illustrated below in **Table 73-7A**, through stepwise evaluation of the patient's current medication risk and utility.

Another useful method, STRIP (Structured Tool to Reduce Inappropriate Prescribing) is a more concise, five-step process with a yearly review: obtain a drug history, perform an analysis of drugs, develop a treatment plan, review patient preferences, and provide follow-up and monitoring (**Table 73-7B**).

TABLE 73-7A Reducing Polypharmacy: Evaluation and Management*

Evaluation	Corresponding Management
1. Ensure medication list is correct	
2. Ascertain risk of adverse drug reaction - ≥8 Medications - Age >75 - High-risk medications	If 3 criterion met, reduce medication list to 5 or less medications
3. Prognosticate life expectancy	
4. Defines goals of care	If life expectancy <2 y, preserve function and quality of life instead of using medication to prolong life
5. Confirm indications for all drugs	Discontinue drugs that are ineffective or for which diagnosis no longer exists
6. Confirm need for preventative medications	Discontinue drugs that will not have benefit during limited lifespan
7. Determine benefit vs harm using a tool (www.mdcalc.com)	Discontinue drugs where harm exceeds benefit
8. Rank drugs from high to low utility	Remove low utility drugs
9. Obtain patient consent for discontinuing the above drugs	
10. Implement discontinuation or deprescribing plan (eg, tapering)	

*Adapted from Appropriate Prescribing and Important Drug Interactions in Older Adults.

TABLE 73-7B Stepwise Approach for Safe Prescribing

1. Develop the current list (ensure preadmission list is correct)
   - Identify high-risk drugs based upon the tables above
     A. Class of drug
     B. Pharmacokinetic changes
   - Identify drugs currently unnecessary/causing side effects
2. Develop updated list with the plan for deprescribing PIMs
3. Compare the two lists
4. Make clinical decisions based on the comparison
   - Adjust medications based upon table above for polypharmacy
5. Communicate the new list to the patient and caregivers

PREVENTING READMISSION

A fourth of Medicare beneficiaries discharged from hospitals to SNF are readmitted in 30 days. Reducing preventable readmissions require risk stratification and careful strategies for patients who are at higher risk for readmissions.

■ RISK STRATIFICATION TO PREVENT READMISSION

Discharge diagnoses with high risk of readmission include heart failure, chronic obstructive pulmonary disease, renal failure, urinary tract infections, and pneumonia. The immediate common cause of readmission is often delirium, polypharmacy, pressure ulcers, deconditioning, and iatrogenic illnesses.

Critical quality measures of care during hospitalization and SNF placement which predispose to readmissions

There are also practical measures that can be taken while the patient is hospitalized to reduce the risk of readmission back to the hospital. Some of these measures have been detailed by the American Medical Directors Association (now called the Society for Post-Acute and Long-Term Care Medicine).

Hospitalized patients should be mobilized from bed as soon as possible. Bedrest increases disability and delays rehabilitation. Lack of ambulation also increases risk for pressure ulcers, comorbid infections, and depression. The lack of rehabilitation then feeds forward to functional decline, which can increase the risk of rehospitalization.

Foley catheters without a specific medical indication should be discontinued as soon as possible to minimize the risk of catheter-related urinary tract infections that can occur upon receipt of the patient at the SNF. This increases the risk of delirium.

Patients may incur additional costs from transportation for diagnostic studies that are not available at the SNF. This should be taken into consideration before deferring inpatient studies to the outpatient setting. It is best practice to complete the diagnostic workup in the hospital to ensure that there is a clear, well-defined plan prior to a transfer to a SNF. Other factors of inpatient care that can subsequently affect outcome of care at the SNF and readmission are untreated pain and depression that can likely be identified prior to transfer with the assistance of the patient's bedside care team.

SNF Quality measures that impact readmission rates

The quality of care at the SNF may also affect readmissions. Quality SNF care begins with excellent communication between both nursing and medical clinicians. The Society for Post-Acute and Long-Term Care Medicine (formerly AMDA) has defined the following critical SNF quality measures.

- Timely removal of Foley catheters.
- Pressure ulcer prevention.
- Effective pain management.
- Timely response to delirium.
- Effective management of depression may also be relevant to preventing adverse outcomes.

Education of nursing staff including greater frequency of interdisciplinary meetings (weekly vs biweekly) may be helpful, as well as timely and effective discharge planning that includes communication with home care agencies and family or other caregivers.

The INTERACT (Intervention to Reduce Acute Care Transfers) is a useful tool for quality improvement to prevent avoidable hospitalization. INTERACT consists of the following:

1. Designating a team with leadership support that will be responsible for quality improvement
2. Early identification of changes in condition
3. Managing changes in condition early to prevent hospitalization
4. Increased utilization of advanced care planning, hospice, and palliative care
5. Improved communication between SNF, hospital, and family

■ THE CONTINUING NEED FOR QUALITY IMPROVEMENT IN THE DISCHARGE PROCESS

Despite the recommendations above, every health care system needs to reassess their own barriers to a safe and effective transition and then design interventions to account for these barriers as a continual process. The work of Eric Coleman illustrates three types of barriers: patient, clinician, and system.

Patient education: discharge planning checklist/personal health

Patient level barriers are lack of health literacy and self-efficacy. As mentioned above, patients may not be aware, able to understand or able to communicate their medical history or their medication list. Patients also are faced with new diagnoses while hospitalized requiring new medications, self-care, and monitoring of symptoms.

Clinician communication

Clinician level barriers are primarily in communication failures. Discharge summaries often do not arrive in a timely manner or fail to include key information including follow-up appointments and pending results. Phone call and e-mail communication between transitioning clinicians are infrequent. Clinicians often do not have a working knowledge of what can be done in the postacute care setting. This can include things such as frequency of vitals, staffing levels, and availability of timely diagnostics (x-rays, labs).

System level

Privacy measures limit sharing of clinician contact information. Differing formularies between institutions have led to multiple drug substitutions. Quality improvement projects can first identify and then target safety failures at each of these levels in order to ensure patient safety (**Table 73-8**).

SNF-level opportunities for quality improvement

Because health plans and other payers, including ACOs, are seeking ways to reduce readmissions, some nursing homes, particularly those with a substantial postacute patient population, are developing innovative strategies to better partner with their referring network hospitals. Some, such as the Community-based Care Transitions program, are highlighted above. In addition, because of health

TABLE 73-8 Best Practices for Continuous Quality Improvement to Improve Patient Safety

- IDENTIFY compromises in patient safety
  - Standardize medication reconciliation process
  - Identify barriers in medication reconciliation
  - Standardize discharge process
    - Identify patients at high risk for readmission
    - Increase handoff intensity
  - Identify patient, provider, and system barriers
- INITIATE continuing quality improvement projects based on safety failures identified using multiple interventions such as The Joint Commission recommendations, Project RED, or Project BOOST

care reform and the rapidly changing reimbursement environment, many SNF-level quality improvement initiatives are being driven by health plans, health systems, and newer payment models. A few models are highlighted below.

1. Bundled payment models: In 2013, expanded participation in the Bundled Payments for Care Improvement to include postacute care settings. As of 2015, there are 678 participants in BPCI Model 2 in which the postacute care clinician is held responsible for costs incurred within 30, 60, or 90 days of discharge for episodes of care related to specific conditions such as congestive heart failure or joint replacement. As a result, participating acute and PAC clinicians are developing the infrastructure to communicate effectively beyond the initial discharge period with skilled home care clinicians as well as patients and their families to ensure that the patients' needs are being appropriately met and so that readmissions can be prevented. It remains to be seen whether the BPCI models will result in significant and sustainable savings, however, on face, they are requiring a greater level of accountability and attention to transitional care improvement on the part of PAC clinicians. (https://innovation.cms.gov/initiatives/BPCI-Model-2/)

2. Direct partnerships with Accountable Care Organizations (ACOs): Understanding that many ACOs have a vested interest in managing total medical expenditure (TME) including costs incurred during stays in PAC facilities, some Pioneer ACOs have elected to directly manage the care of their attributed members while in PAC settings by deploying ACO clinicians to provide primary care in those settings. It is difficult to obtain published data regarding these interventions; however, anecdotal data from a Massachusetts ACO would support that the ACO physicians can reduce both average length of stay and readmission rates in their PAC patients. Additionally, patients have reported increased satisfaction with communication between the ACO PAC physician/midlevels and their primary care physicians because they are part of the same health system and share the same electronic health record. The use of ACO-medical staff in PAC settings is likely most successful in those PAC settings without an employed medical staff model.

3. Provision of palliative care within PAC settings: Patients transitioned to PAC settings often have serious and life-limiting illnesses such as stroke or congestive heart failure. They may or may not be able to actively participate in rehabilitation and some may fail to improve substantially. There is an increasing body of literature that as in other care settings, patients with serious and life-limiting illnesses in PAC settings benefit from palliative care. In addition to addressing symptomatic issues, palliative care teams can provide the needed education and support as well as assist families and patients in clarification of their goals of care. This can also prevent unnecessary or burdensome hospitalizations, particularly for conditions that are likely to worsen over time such as congestive heart failure.

4. Participation in waiver programs: Historically, fee for service Medicare beneficiaries have been required to have a qualifying 3-day hospital admission in order to receive Medicare coverage for postacute SNF care. With the rise of observation stays, many patients and their families have learned that they did not meet the criteria for a Medicare-covered SNF stay even though they assumed that they had officially been admitted. In 2014, CMS approved a 3-day SNF waiver program for beneficiaries attributed to a Pioneer ACO. These beneficiaries could be directly admitted to SNF from observation, ER or even from the physician's office or other sites of care. Each ACO has specific criteria for approving SNF participation in the 3-day waiver program. These criteria generally include quality of care metrics such as staffing, readmission rates, and average length of stay as well as the availability of physicians and other clinicians after hours. SNFs participating in the 3-day waiver program have been required to track and report their performance on quality metrics. It is too soon to deem the 3-day waiver program a success. However, in eastern Massachusetts, where there are 5 Pioneer ACOs, the 3-day waiver program has resulted in some improvements in average length of stay as well as acute care utilization rates.

5. Improvement of post-SNF discharge communication: Discharge from SNF to home or other care settings represents another transition of care that can be a risk to patient safety. Similar to hospital discharge, SNF clinicians need to ensure that there is complete and clear communication with the primary care physician or practitioner who will be caring for the patient in the community. The SNF clinician has the added responsibility of communicating any remaining issues that were identified as needing "primary care followup" during the acute care stay. Specific information that is important to include in SNF discharge communications are listed in the practice point box on discharge information. Increasingly, SNFs are employing templates and checklists to ensure that this information is being accurately documented and are also requiring that appropriate follow-up appointment scheduling occurs prior to SNF discharge. For some ACOs, particularly those who are participating in the CMS SNF 3-day waiver program, postdischarge communication, handoffs, and timely post-PAC follow-up are being monitored as quality metrics.

PRACTICE POINT

Discharge information from rehabilitation

- Detailed instructions for specific/high-risk drugs in addition to an updated, reconciled discharge medication list:

1. Anticoagulation

   Warfarin: start date, recent dosage changes, target INR, duration of treatment, date of next scheduled INR, responsible clinic or physician for monitoring.

   Low-molecular-weight heparin: duration of treatment, time of next scheduled dose, any insurance issues, as patients may not be able to afford medication after discharge from rehabilitation.

2. Antibiotics

Duration of treatment: Indications for an extended course of antibiotics and identification of who should be consulted in case problems arise, and monitor therapy if continued post rehabilitation. If patient is to be discharged on extended IV antibiotics, type and placement of line should be documented.

3. Narcotic/benzodiazepine dosing

Indication, therapeutic endpoint, recent changes, and reason.

4. Insulin therapy

Indicate exact doses, whether additional control was required by a sliding scale, and include amount of additional insulin in prior 24 hours as well as whether there were any issues relating to hypoglycemia.

- Nutrition

1. If discharged with tube feedings, discussion of who will administer and manage feedings. Special equipment and supplement supplies should be available at the patient's home or other site of care at the time of discharge.

2. Specify goals of therapy and who will follow-up if problems arise.

- Supplemental oxygen

1. Document O_2 saturation and requirement of O_2 to maintain O_2 saturation above 88%.

2. Ensure that O_2 delivery systems and transport O_2 are available at the time of discharge.

- Wound care

1. Documentation of specific wound care instructions.

2. If complex dressing/supplies are used that require special orders, this should be addressed prior to discharge.

Monitoring: particularly important if patients are being discharged to skilled home care or facility based long-term care.

1. Document monitoring, if required, for specific drugs or interventions.

2. Document discharge weight, especially if there will be need for ongoing diuresis.

- Summary information

1. Very brief description of reason for index rehabilitation admission, course, complications, how the patient is at time of discharge (cognitive, cardiopulmonary, and functional status).

2. Identify consultants by name and who to contact if a problem arises.

3. Brief summary of relevant and abnormal test results and identification of person responsible for follow-up of abnormal or pending test findings and unresolved issues as well as follow-up appointments with consultants and primary care physician.

4. Family spokesperson with numbers, code status, health care proxy.

Goals for continued rehabilitation (if needed) and contingency planning if patient does not respond to treatment.

CONCLUSION

The process of discharge from the hospital to a postacute facility is fraught with danger for the patient and can predispose to readmission. By standardizing safety into medication reconciliations and discharge summaries between facilities, adverse events to the patient may be prevented, thereby optimizing quality of patient care.

SUGGESTED READINGS

American Medical Directors Association. American Medical Directors Association Policy Resolution H 10. 2010. Accessed at https://www.nhqualitycampaign.org/files/Transition_of_Care_Reference.pdf.

American Medical Directors Association. Nursing Home Quality Improvement Initiative. Accessed at http://www.amda.com/consumers/initiative.cfm.

Berkowitz RE, Fang Z, Helfand BK, Jones RN, Schreiber R, Paasche-Orlow MK. Project ReEngineered Discharge (RED) lowers hospital readmissions of patients discharged from a skilled nursing facility. *J Am Med Dir Assoc*. 2013;14(10):736-740.

Butterfield S, Stegel C, Glock S, Tartaglia D. Understanding Care Transitions as a Patient Safety Issue. *Patient Safety & Quality Healthcare*. New York, Medicare Quality Improvement Organization, 2011.

Flint L. Transitions and Continuity of Care. In: Williams BA, et al, eds. *Current Diagnosis and Treatment Geriatrics*, 2nd ed. New York, NY: McGraw Hill; 2014:75-78.

Florida Atlantic University. Interventions to Reduce Acute Care Transfers. (2011). Accessed at https://interact2.net/.

Gnjidic D, Kouladjian L, Hilmer S. Deprescribing trials: methods to reduce polypharmacy and the impact on prescribing and clinical outcomes. *Clin Geriatr Med*. 2012;28:237-253.

Greenwald JL, Denham CR, Jack BW. The Hospital Discharge: A Review of a High Risk Care Transitions With Highlights of a Re-engineered Discharge Process. *J Patient Saf*. 2007;3(2):97-106.

Hajjar ER, Hanlon JT, Sloane RJ, et al. Unnecessary drug use in frail older people at hospital discharge. *J Am Geriatr Soc*. 2005;53:1518-1523.

Harris-Kojetin L, Sengupta M, Park-Lee E, Valverde R. Long-term care services in the United States: 2013 overview. National Center for Health Statistics. *Vital Health Stat*. 3. 2013;(37):1-107.

The Joint Commission. Sentinel Event Alert. 2006. Accessed at http://www.jointcommission.org/assets/1/18/sea_35.pdf.

Meulendijk MC, Spruit MR, Drenth-van Maanen AC, et al. Computerized Decision Support Improves Medication Review Effectiveness: An Experiment Evaluating the STRIP Assistant's Usability. *Drugs Aging*. 2015;32(6):495-503.

Mor V, Intrator O, Feng Z, Grabowski DC. The revolving door of rehospitalization from skilled nursing facilities. *Health Aff (Millwood)*. 2010;29:157-164.

Mueller SK, Sponsler KC, Kripalani S, Schnipper JL. Hospital-based medication reconciliation practices: a systematic review. *Arch Intern Med*. 2012;172(14):1057-1069.

National Transitions of Care Coalition. National Transitions of Care Coalition. 2016. Accessed at http://www.ntocc.org/WhoWeServe/HealthCareProfessionals.aspx. Accessed January 27, 2016.

Oakes SL, Gillespie SM, Ye Y, et al. Transitional care of the long-term care patient. *Clin Geriatr Med*. 2011;27:259-273.

Ouslander JG, Diaz S, Hain D, Tappen R. Frequency and diagnoses associated with 7- and 30-day readmission of skilled nursing facility patients to a nonteaching community hospital. *J Am Med Dir Assoc*. 2011;12(3):195-203.

Smith CM. Practice Brief. Documentation requirements for the acute care inpatient record. American Health Information Management Association. *J AHIMA*. 2001;72(3):56A-56G.

Society of Hospital Medicine. Project BOOST Mentored Implementation Program. 2015. Accessed at http://www.hospitalmedicine.org/boost/.

Wallace J, Paauw DS. Appropriate prescribing and important drug interactions in older adults. *Med Clin N Am*. 2015;99:295-310.

ONLINE RESOURCES

Champ transitions of care toolkit *http://www.champ-program.org/page/100/geriatric-care-transitions-toolkit*. Accessed January 27, 2016.

Project BOOST Toolkit *http://www.hospitalmedicine.org/Web/Quality_Innovation/Implementation_Toolkits/Project_BOOST/Web/Quality___Innovation/Implementation_Toolkit/Boost/Overview.aspx*. Accessed January 27, 2016.

Project RED website *http://www.ahrq.gov/professionals/systems/hospital/red/index.html*. Accessed January 27, 2016.

CHAPTER 74

Hospice

Julia M. Gallagher, MD

Hospice is a concept of care delivered by an interdisciplinary team that focuses on providing best supportive care to terminally ill patients and their families with the goal of maintaining the patient's comfort and quality of life. Hospitalists, caring for patients with chronic, progressive illness, many of whom are nearing the end of life, are uniquely positioned to improve the quality of care that these vulnerable patients receive and to more closely align their care with patient preferences. Hospitalization represents an opportunity to reassess patients' prognoses, their understanding of their illnesses and how available treatment options align with their care preferences. Hospice offers high-value end-of-life care and minimizes unwanted interventions and care transitions.

In the United States, "hospice" is an insurance benefit as well as a concept of care. More than 85% of patients enrolled in hospice in 2014 were covered under Medicare Hospice Benefit (MHB). Most commercial insurers, state Medicaid programs and other government insurance programs have eligibility requirements similar to those for Medicare. This chapter will review the hospice benefit and strategies to overcome common barriers to the timely transition of appropriate patients to hospice care.

VALUE BASED CARE

Out of 2.6 million total deaths annually in the United States, one in five occurs in the hospital setting. Many of those patients who died had multiple advanced chronic illnesses, suffered from progressive frailty and had a series of hospitalizations prior to their deaths. Many had a likely prognosis of less than 6 months during at least one of the hospitalizations preceding the terminal hospitalization. As payment reform shifts from an episodic, fee-for-service model to a longitudinal, shared risk model, an acute care hospitalization is no longer viewed as an isolated event along the patient's trajectory of illness. Hospitalists play an increasingly important role in this longitudinal model of care as each hospitalization represents an opportunity to reassess a patient's prognosis, his or her understanding of their illness and how goals of care may have changed in the face of disease progression. Hospitalists should consider referral for palliative care for those patients who require assistance with complex symptom management and advance care planning (**Figure 74-1**). For those patients without complex symptom management or advance care planning needs and who have a likely prognosis of less than 6 months and comfort as the primary goal, the hospitalist can manage the transition to best supportive care with hospice. The transition to hospice care may, at times, present a unique set of challenges from provider, patient and hospice standpoint.

STRATEGIES TO OVERCOME UNDERUSE OF HOSPICE

While the number of patients served by hospice has steadily risen over the years and the percent of patients who die while enrolled in the Medicare hospice benefit has increased, recent studies have raised concerns that hospice enrollment in and of itself is an incomplete marker of higher-quality end-of-life care. Many patients continue to experience multiple care transitions in the days to months before death including ICU admissions. The percentage of patients enrolled in hospice for 3 days or fewer has also increased and many of these patients are hospitalized just prior to enrolling in hospice.

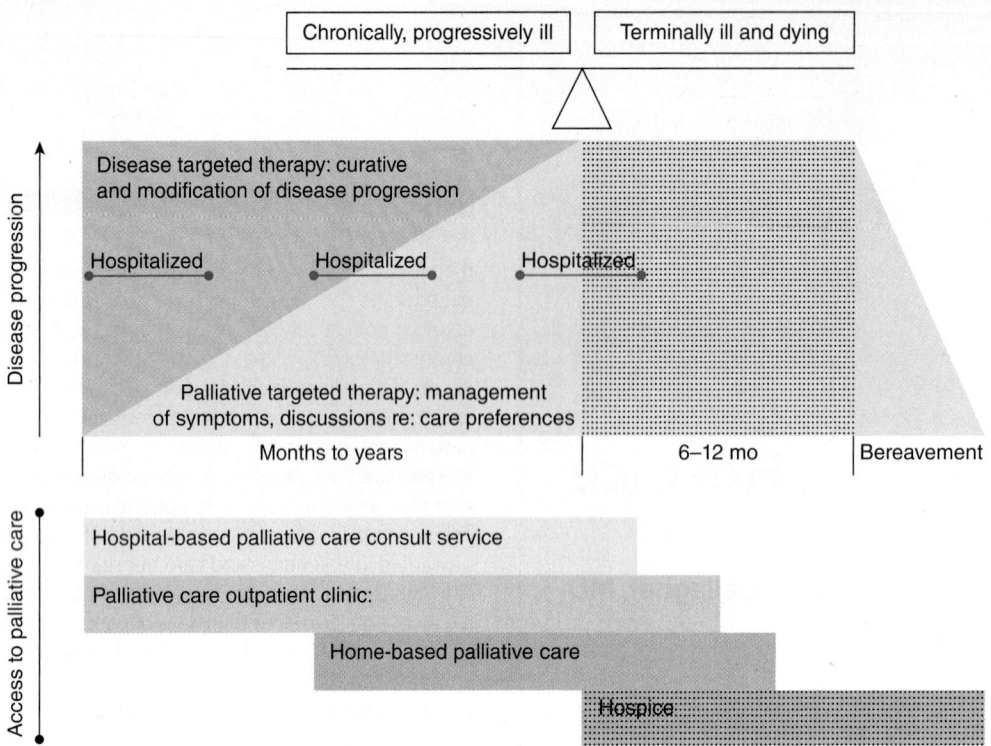

Figure 74-1 *Access to palliative care and hospice along the trajectory of disease.*

Timely transition to hospice requires an understanding of a patient's goals and values and how available treatment options based on a patient's prognosis align with those patient preferences. The patient and family meeting is a critical intervention during which the hospitalist gains an understanding of a patient's goals and values and then discusses his or her recommendations for treatment, including hospice when appropriate, based on those goals and values. Public policy efforts to increase awareness of the importance of advance care planning and medical school and residency educational programs to improve communication skills have likely led to improvements in these end-of-life care discussions over the last decade (**Table 74-1**).

However, despite improved end-of-life communication there are still multiple barriers and delays to appropriate and timely transitions to hospice including: discontinuities of care (replacement of primary specialist and/or primary care physician with multiple rotating hospitalists), frequent hospitalizations with transitions to other settings before these conversations take place, societal myths about hospice (especially for certain cultures) a lack of consensus among clinicians regarding prognosis as well as the appropriate timing of the hospice referral and insurance coverage that may involve financial disincentives to enrolling in the hospice insurance benefit. In addition, hospice providers' serving the same geographic area may have different enrollment policies, inconsistency in capability to handle advanced symptoms and variable availability of facilities such as hospice residences. **Table 74-2** reviews steps to hospice enrollment.

■ PROGNOSTICATION

Given the increasing attention to end-of-life care, many people, from health care administrators to health care researchers to patients and their families, are asking "*What if a patient dies* **without** *the support and management of a hospice team?*" rather than "*What if the doctor is wrong and the patient doesn't die within 6 months?*" Reframing the question in this way allows everyone involved in the

TABLE 74-1 Steps to Hospice Enrollment

Eligibility	Medicare Benefit Policy Manuel	To be eligible to elect hospice care under Medicare, an individual must be entitled to Part A of Medicare and be certified as being terminally ill with a projected life expectancy (<6 months)
Terminal status guidelines	Local coverage determinations (LCDs) as defined by Medicare and the applicable MAC*	While these guidelines are roughly similar, different MACs have developed slightly different LCD definitions of terminal status
Certification of terminal status	Hospice Medical Director and the Attending of Record** at enrollment; the Hospice Medical Director at each certification period thereafter	In addition to the LCD guidelines, the hospice medical director uses his or her clinical judgment to consider the terminal diagnosis, related conditions, the patient's likely clinical course

*LCDs are decisions by Medicare and their administrative contractors (MACs) that provide coverage information and determine whether services are reasonable and necessary. MACs are private organizations that carry out the administrative responsibilities of Medicare (Parts A and B); different MACs serve different geographic areas.

**The Attending of Record (AOR) is the physician whom the patient chooses to manage their care while on hospice; patients often chose the physician who has been most involved with their care and the management of their terminal illness.

TABLE 74-2 Levels of Care under the Medicare Hospice Benefit

	Routine Home Care	Continuous Home Care	General Inpatient Care
Approximate daily rate paid to the hospice agency	$150/d	$900/d	$700/d
Site of care	Home, skilled nursing facility, assisted living, rest home, hospice residence	Home	Hospital, skilled nursing facility, hospice residence
Services provided under the designated level of care	Routine nursing visits required approximately twice a week; participation of social worker, chaplain, home health aides, volunteers and therapists visits determined by the care plan; medical director dictated by clinical condition	Increased hospice team participation required during a period of crisis to support the patient and family at home: 8 h of support in a 24-h period, 4 h of which must be skilled nursing for ongoing pain and symptom management	Ongoing skilled nursing required to assess pain and symptom management, adjust medications and coordinate care with the attending physician and/or hospice medical director: daily visits by a hospice team member

care of the patient to consider the benefits forgone by the patient who dies without hospice care and helps to mitigate some of the internal biases regarding prognostication and the transition to hospice. Most patients and their families report high satisfaction with hospice care once they transition to their hospice insurance benefit. Furthermore, there is no penalty if a patient is referred to hospice and does not die within the current eligibility requirement of an expected prognosis of less than 6 months if the disease runs its natural course. The hospice eligibility requirement acknowledges the inherent uncertainty in prognostication and the role of best clinical judgment. Once enrolled in hospice, the hospice medical director assumes the responsibility for the ongoing assessment of the patient's prognosis and documenting that assessment in what is called a certification narrative. **Table 74-3** describes levels of care under the Medicare hospice benefit. See Chapter 105 (Using Prognosis to Guide Treatment).

■ COMMUNICATION WITH PATIENTS

When the Medicare hospice benefit was first enacted in 1982, the majority of patients cared for under the benefit had a cancer diagnosis and the transition between "treatment" and "best supportive care" was much starker. The regulation does not, in fact, use the words "cure" or "treatment" in defining hospice eligibility but this binary distinction has persisted. Today, only about a third of Medicare hospice beneficiaries have a diagnosis of cancer and the use of advanced palliative therapies has become commonplace blurring the distinction between cancer "treatment" and "best supportive care." Additionally, patients with a diagnosis of dementia, heart disease or lung disease are enrolling in hospice with increasing frequency and accounted for 14.8%, 14.7%, and 9.3%, respectively of Medicare beneficiaries enrolled in hospice in 2014. There is no cure for any of the above noncancer diagnoses: all are

TABLE 74-3 Poor Prognostic Factors

Recurrent hospitalization especially to intensive care unit

Activities of daily life (ADL) dependency

Weight loss

Recurrent falls, infections

Declining performance status and score on the palliative performance scale (PPS)

Laboratory findings: low albumin, low hemoglobin

chronic, progressive, life-limiting illnesses. All patients, regardless of their underlying chronic progressive illness, benefit from maximal medical management targeted toward disease modification *as well as* the involvement of palliative care whenever there is significant or complex symptom burden as is often encountered in the advanced stages of many illnesses. Therefore, in conversations regarding end-of-life care, it may be helpful to reframe the transition to hospice as the "standard of care" at that point along the disease trajectory when further disease modification is no longer possible and symptom burden becomes more prominent. When a patient transitions to hospice, clinicians should continue to provide maximal medical management in addition to palliation of symptoms in a way that is not unduly burdensome to the patient as many patients prefer to remain home and avoid burdensome care transitions if possible during the last weeks to months of life. Some patients and family members may continue to request that "everything be done" during this difficult transition from chronically, progressively ill to terminally ill and dying. This request is often made by the patient or family member looking for reassurance that they or their family member will not be "abandoned," that active medical management will continue and that long term care providers will remain involved supporting the patient and the family. When explored skillfully, the request may be less about seeking specific interventions and more about ensuring the ongoing involvement of the care providers. See Chapter 215 (Communication Skills for the End of Life Care).

■ HOSPICE ENROLLMENT POLICIES AND PATIENT CHOICE

Hospitalists often encounter barriers to hospice use at the level of the hospice provider due to restrictive and often variable enrollment policies and at the level of the patient and family due to the financial disincentives associated with some insurance coverage. While it is unclear how much hospice enrollment policies and patient choice due to financial concerns contribute to some of these observed hospices referral patterns, hospitalists may effectively navigate those barriers on behalf of their patients by working closely with case managers and hospice providers to clarify these barriers and identify alternative pathways to hospice enrollment.

■ CLARIFYING COMMON SOURCES OF CONFUSION

Palliative care versus hospice

Palliative care is delivered across the entire trajectory of illness and in parallel with curative therapy as well as with disease modifying

507

therapy. Hospice care is that small segment of palliative care that addresses the needs of patients and their families at the end of life, needs that are covered by the comprehensive hospice insurance benefit.

Hospice is "a place"

Hospice refers to a concept of care not a location. An interdisciplinary team provides hospice care to patients and their families and each member of the team visits a patient wherever the patient happens to live. The majority of patients who receive hospice care live in their own homes but hospice team members may also visit patients who live in nursing homes, rest homes, assisted living facilities or even the hospital. A "hospice house" generally refers to a freestanding hospice residence or house built by an individual hospice agency. Not all hospice agencies build or own a hospice residence. Patients may transition to a hospice residence for any number of reasons, including increasing care needs that the family can no longer manage or a desire not to die in their own home. All hospice residences must be licensed by the state in which they operate and are certified to provide either "routine level" of care or both "routine level" of care and "general in-patient" level of care. A hospice residence that provides "routine level" of care provides a supportive environment similar to that found in a patient's home with the addition of on-site home health aides, LPNs and often volunteers. Patients and their family are required to pay for room and board if they transition to a "routine level" of care residence. A hospice residence that provides "general in-patient" level of care provides an enhanced skilled nursing environment for patients who require more intensive skilled nursing assessment and medication administration, care that could not reasonably be provided in the home. Hospice agencies without a hospice residence certified for "general in-patient" level of care contract with either a local nursing home or acute care hospital in order provide this level of care. The "general in-patient" level of care is utilized during shorter, more intense periods of symptom management and the cost of room and board is included in the "general in-patient" level of care.

Role of hospice The interdisciplinary hospice team helps to support and guide the care of the patient while the patient is enrolled in hospice. For patients who chose to remain at home, the patient's family and/or caregivers manage the patient's physical care needs and administer all of the medications used to manage pain and symptoms. Patients and their families may call the hospice agency at any time and speak to a triage nurse who will respond to their questions and concerns over the phone. If the triage nurse is unable to adequately manage pain or symptoms over the phone, a responding nurse is sent to the home to further assess and manage the symptoms or to address patient and family concerns. Aside from these "as needed visits," the nurse care manager typically visits the patient once or twice a week for approximately an hour, depending on the care needs of the patient and the support and educational needs of the family. In complicated situations the nursing visit frequency may be increased to several times a week. The hospice social worker and chaplain assess patients and their families upon admission to hospice and determine their visit frequency based on identified needs. Likewise, the RN case manager arranges home health aides and volunteers based on the needs of the patient and family. The vast majority of patients cared for at home are cared for under this "routine level" of hospice care. If a patient experiences difficult to manage pain or symptoms and requires more frequent skilled nursing care, the hospice agency may provide for this more intense level of care under the "general in-patient" level of care discussed above.

Hospice coverage Chapter 9 of The Medicare Benefit Policy Manual details the hospice insurance benefit. Coverage of Hospice Services falls under Medicare Part A; Medicare Part B provides coverage for services such as laboratory tests and doctor visits. To be eligible to elect hospice care under the Medicare benefit, the patient must be entitled to Medicare Part A and be terminally ill which is defined as having a "life expectancy (of) 6 months or less if the illness runs its normal course" (**Table 74-1**). The language is straightforward and *does not* state that the patient must forego treatment related to the terminal illness. However, additional language in the regulation states that for care related to the terminal illness "only care provided by (or under arrangements made by) a Medicare certified hospice is covered under the Medicare hospice benefit." This subsequent language often shifts *the cost* of providing care related to the terminal illness to the individual hospice agency: the patient and his or her family are responsible for the cost of care not included in the hospice plan or care or arranged by the hospice agency. Stated another way, Medicare reimburses a hospice agency for care under a capitated payment system and the hospice assumes all of the financial risk for the cost of care related to the terminal illness. Please note that the services unrelated to hospice diagnosis continue to get reimbursed under traditional Medicare (ie, a patient admitted to hospice for end-stage COPD may be admitted to the hospital and have his or her care covered under Medicare Part B for an episode of GI bleeding related to diverticular disease).

In the 1980s, the financial implication of such language was not unduly burdensome: the majority of hospice patients had cancer, there were fewer disease modifying or palliative therapies and the trajectory toward death generally took place over a few short months and was predictable. Today, that language has led some hospice agencies to develop restrictive enrollment policies based on the cost of various treatments and medical management options. Hospice agencies receive a fixed "per diem" payment (**Table 74-2**). The hospice agency must cover all of their fixed operating costs (salaries and benefits, support staff, information technology, space) as well as the costs related to terminal illness (medication and palliative interventions, medical equipment, supplies) with daily reimbursement for routine hospice of about $150.00 per day per patient.

The number of palliative interventions and therapies we offer patients near the end-of-life has expanded tremendously since the 1980s and many of those interventions are often costly relative to the "per diem" the hospice agency receives. While the language of the Medicare hospice benefit does not *explicitly* exclude what a patient may or may not receive for care of their terminal illness, hospice agencies at times choose not to assume the cost for certain treatments based on their ability to absorb those costs and remain financially viable.

Impact of hospice on survival The goal of hospice is neither to hasten death nor to prolong suffering. The goal is to focus on quality of life for both the patient and his or her family through the support of a multidisciplinary team. Various studies have shown that hospice enrollment is not significantly associated with shorter survival. In fact, for a subset of patients with end-stage heart failure, colon cancer and lung cancer, hospice enrollment has been associated with longer survival times.

Barriers to hospice The following two cases review some of the barriers hospitalists frequently encounter when transitioning patients to best supportive care with hospice. These cases assume that the clinician has already determined that the patient has a likely prognosis of fewer than 6 months and has guided the patient and their family through the decision to transition to best supportive care with hospice.

CASE 74-1

An 82-year-old woman with moderate to advanced dementia developed mental status changes, hypotension, and pneumonia at home. She was initially admitted to the intensive care unit where she received peripheral partial nutrition (PPN) through a midline. Her past medical history included a similar presentation 6 months ago and a more recent hospitalization for a mechanical fall at home followed by several weeks of rehabilitation at a skilled nursing facility. Since returning home, the patient had become increasingly frail and wheelchair bound. She slept most of the day and had lost 15 pounds but still enjoyed eating small amounts of food, particularly ice cream. After several days without a change in her ability to swallow, the clinicians readdress goals of care with the family. Observing her decline, the family agrees with the recommendation to transition to best supportive care with hospice.

Hospice enrollment policies Overwhelmed by the rapidity of the patient's decline, the family asks that PPN be continued for a little while hoping that her swallowing improves. However, the hospice agency referred by the nursing facility does not accept patients on PPN likely due to cost.

Clinicians may take the following steps:

- They may call the hospice agency and ask to speak with the hospice medical director or the operations manager to review the case and request that they accept the patient in order to help support the family through the final steps of discontinuing PPN.
- They may call the nursing facility and ask the director to consider issuing a one-time contract with another hospice agency that might have less restrictive policies with regards to costly interventions such as PPN.

Barrier two—financial issues The patient is able to return to the nursing home on her Part A Medicare Skilled Nursing Care Facility benefit due to her "skilled needs" for PPN as well as speech and physical therapy. Medicare covers the full cost of the skilled services provided *as well as* the room and board at the facility for up to 100 days per a defined benefit period. If she elects to access her Part A Medicare Hospice Benefit, the patient forgoes her Skilled Nursing Care Facility benefit under the Part A Medicare while she is on hospice. While Medicare covers the cost of room and board under the skilled nursing benefit it *does not* cover the cost of room and board under the hospice benefit. This discrepancy is likely an unintended consequence of how the original benefit was structured given the expectation that most patients would be cared for at home. As a result, the patient and her family would have to pay the cost of room and board which is often costly and can average $400 a day.

While the patient cannot access her Medicare hospice benefit without significant financial implications for the family, the overall goal of care for the patient *does not change*. The goal remains to transition her back to her facility with best supportive care. Her advanced directives should reflect her goals of care and include orders for DNR and DNI. Additionally, an order for Do Not Hospitalize (DNH) should be discussed with the family as repeated hospitalizations for expected clinical complications related to her progressive dementia would be burdensome and not align with the goal of preserving the patient's comfort and dignity at the end of life. Clinicians should call the attending physician or the nurse practitioner caring for the patient at the facility to review and clarify the goals of care for the patient and to reassure the provider that the family understands and appreciates the order for DNH. The patient returns to the facility with the opportunity to improve with speech and physical and therapy interventions but with an overarching goal of best supportive care and avoidance of burdensome hospitalizations, even while she was not able to access her Medicare hospice benefit due to financial disincentives. The skilled nursing facility may also have access to certified palliative care physicians or nurse practitioners that it could consult for assistance with symptom control and ongoing decision support around goals of care. If the patient was experiencing difficulty to control symptoms that required ongoing skilled nursing assessment and medication titration, the patient could access their Medicare hospice "general in-patient" level of care and remain in the hospital until their symptoms stabilized: patients who are imminently dying but are otherwise comfortable and do not require ongoing skilled nursing interventions do not qualify for the "general in-patient" level of care benefit.

Patients with Medicaid and Medicare If this patient had both Medicaid and Medicare coverage (ie, dual eligibility), room and board at the facility may be covered. However, some skilled nursing facilities may discourage patients and their families from "disenrolling" from the Medicare skilled nursing care facility benefit because the facility is reimbursed under that benefit at a much higher rate than they are reimbursed by the hospice agency under the hospice benefit for dual eligible patients. Additionally, hospice agencies may suggest that some interventions such as speech and physical therapy are not necessarily part of "best supportive care" and may not actively offer those services as they add to the total cost of providing care for the patient. Such services *may be offered* under the Medicare hospice benefit and clinicians should advocate on the part of the patient and their family if this misunderstanding emerges as a barrier to transitioning a dual-eligible patient to the Medicare hospice benefit.

> ### PRACTICE POINT
>
> - Clinicians should become familiar with the enrollment policies of local hospice agencies, cultivate relationships with these hospices, and navigate potential gaps in insurance coverage that result in financial barriers to patients transitioning to end of life care.

CASE 74-2

A 58-year-old man receiving palliative chemotherapy for nonsmall cell lung cancer is hospitalized with new widespread metastasis to the bone and liver. He begins *radiotherapy* to his right femur. Based on his previous discussions with his oncologist, he understands that his prognosis is likely limited and he wants to go home as soon as possible.

Hospice enrollment policies None of the area hospices accept patients undergoing radiation therapy, likely due to the voluntary restrictive enrollment policies of individual hospice agencies. This patient is under 65-year old and likely has commercial insurance. Hospice agencies may contact a commercial insurer and request that they consider allowing what is called a "carve out" to their hospice coverage. Under a "carve out" agreement, the insurer allows the patient to access their hospice insurance benefit, and the insurer agrees to pay for the cost of a specific treatment such as radiation therapy separately: the hospice agency does not have to assume the cost of the palliative radiation. Peer to peer communication by the clinician to the hospice medical director may facilitate the necessary coverage by clarifying goals of care and asking the medical director to advocate on the patient's behalf.

The need for a primary caregiver None of the local hospice agencies will accept the patient if he lives alone and does not have a "primary caregiver." Hospice agencies prefer that patients have clearly identified family and/or caregivers who could support the patient as the patient declines and ensure that the patient is safe at home. However, a primary caregiver is not a requirement for care under the Medicare hospice benefit or under most other hospice insurance programs. It is the role of the hospice nurse care manager and social worker to work with the patient to establish a safe care plan when the patient is no longer able to care for himself at home.

Patient and family issues A limited number of hospice agencies have an "Open Access" policy and accept patients who are receiving a broad range of palliative and often costly interventions. These agencies hope that if they are responsive to the needs of their referral base (hospitalists, oncologists) that they will receive referrals for other patients who might not have such extensive care requirements. Hospice agencies also understand that when many patients transition to best supportive care with hospice, the team members can take the time to help support the patient and their family as they consider discontinuing what are often burdensome interventions.

Medicare has also recognized that many patients and their families benefit from the support and guidance of a hospice team during that difficult transition. Under new provisions enacted with the passage of the Affordable Care Act of 2010, Medicare will reimburse selected hospices under the Medicare Care Choices Model for routine and respite level care for patients who choose to continue to receive a range of interventions: phase one of the program is scheduled to begin January 2016 and a list of participating hospices is available on the Medicare Innovations website.

Patients with a military connection Patients with a military connection may be eligible to receive hospice care in an inpatient hospice unit at select Veterans Affairs facilities at little to no cost to the patient. However, the number of VA facilities with dedicated hospice units and care teams is limited, and families may not be able to shoulder the burden of the prolonged travel necessary to visit the patient at one of these facilities.

PRACTICE POINT

Clinicians and case managers should work together to:
- Identify opportunities for "carve out" options with commercial insurance carriers.
- Determine the availability of "Open Access" hospice agencies in their area and hospice agencies participating in the Medicare Care Choices Model.
- Identify patients who are eligible for VA benefits including transfer to an inpatient hospice unit at little to no cost to the patient.

CONCLUSION

Hospitalists encounter patients at their most vulnerable moments, and often at a time when they are transitioning from chronically, progressively ill to terminally ill and dying. In addition to the challenges associated with prognostication and communication at the end of life, clinicians are faced with deciphering the complexities of hospice insurance coverage. Addressing barriers to transitioning a patient to best supportive care with hospice, may both enhance the end-of-life care many patients receive and simultaneously facilitate the ability of clinicians and health care systems to meet quality metrics in an emerging value-based health care.

SUGGESTED READINGS

Aldridge Carlson MD, Barry CL, Cherlin EJ, McCorkle R, Bradley EH. Hospices' enrollment policies may contribute to underuse of hospice care in the United States. *Health Aff (Millwood)*. 2012;31(12):2690-2698.

Enguidanos S, Vesper E, Lorenz K. 30-day readmissions among seriously ill older adults. *J Palliat Med*. 2012:15(12):1356-1361.

Finucane TE. How gravely ill becomes dying: a key to end-of-life care. *JAMA*. 1999;282(17):1670-1672.

Holden TR, et al. Hospice enrollment, local hospice utilization patterns, and rehospitalization in Medicare patients. *J Palliat Med*. 2015:16(7):601-612.

Hooton TM, Roberts PL, Cox ME, Stapleton AE. Voided midstream urine culture and acute cystitis in premenopausal women. *N Engl J Med*. 2013;369:1883-1891.

Lin RJ, Adelman RD, Diamond RR, Evans AT. The sentinel hospitalization and the role of palliative care. *J Hosp Med*. 2014;9(5):320-323.

NHPCO Facts and Figures: Hospice Care in America. Alexandria, VA: National Hospice and Palliative Care Organization; October 2014.

Teno JM, et al. Change in end-of-life care for Medicare beneficiaries: site of death, place of care, and health care transitions in 2000, 2005, and 2009. *JAMA*. 2013;309(5):470-477.

Thomas JM, O'Leary JR, Fried TR. Understanding their options: determinants of hospice discussion for older persons with advanced illness. *J Gen Intern Med*. 2009;24(8):923-928.

PART IV
Approach to the Patient at the Bedside

CHAPTER 75

Acute Abdominal Pain

Norton J. Greenberger, MD, MACP

Key Clinical Questions

1 What are the important features in the history and physical examination that can help to determine the cause of acute abdominal pain?

2 What tests have the greatest impact in the diagnosis of patients with acute abdominal pain?

3 What are the important metabolic/endocrine disorders that cause acute abdominal pain simulating an acute abdomen?

4 What are the important hematologic/immunologic disorders that cause acute abdominal pain simulating an acute abdomen?

INTRODUCTION

Acute abdominal pain, particularly when severe, requires an expeditious evaluation because a missed or delayed diagnosis may lead to significant morbidity and mortality. The first step is to determine whether the patient has a life-threatening cause of acute abdominal pain. After the patient has been stabilized, the emergency physician or hospitalist must then determine whether the patient needs emergent surgery. The decision to obtain an emergency surgical consultation depends on the history and physical examination (with ancillary radiographic examinations of secondary importance), and when signs of an acute abdomen are present, a surgical consult should be requested, with concurrent diagnostic testing as appropriate. In other instances, a thorough history and physical examination is required with close observation and repeat examinations are often needed. Elderly patients and very young patients may present with atypical or nonspecific signs and symptoms that otherwise might be dismissed as insignificant.

Appendicitis, cholecystitis and choledocholithiasis, intestinal obstruction, pancreatitis, mesenteric ischemia, bowel perforation, and diverticulitis account for two-thirds of hospital admissions for acute abdominal pain and are associated with significant morbidity and mortality. In addition, physicians must be mindful of complications following procedures.

PATHOPHYSIOLOGY

Patients may experience visceral pain, parietal pain, and/or referred abdominal pain.

Visceral pain is typically dull or crampy in character. It is caused by stretching, torsion, distention, or contraction of organs. The visceral innervation of the gut and accessory organs comes via the anchoring mesentery, so pain does not always localize to the quadrant in which the pathology resides, and is often midline. Pain innervation corresponds to dermatomes that match the innervations of the injured organ. Epigastric visceral pain corresponds with organs proximal to the ligament of Treitz, including the hepatobiliary system and the spleen. Periumbilical visceral pain corresponds with injury to organs distal to the ligament of Treitz and the hepatic flexure of the colon. Lower abdominal visceral pain corresponds to injury to organs distal to the hepatic flexure.

Parietal pain is sharp in character and localized to the site of peritoneal inflammation or capsular. This pain is similar to skin and muscle pain and lateralization occurs due to unilateral parietal innervations.

Referred pain is typically well localized. It occurs because visceral afferent nerves carrying stimuli from an inflamed organ enter the spinal cord at the same level as somatic afferent nerves from remote locations.

PRACTICE POINT

Acute cholecystitis
- Initially there is visceral pain in the epigastric region due to stretch and distention of the gallbladder.
- Then parietal pain develops due to direct irritation of the peritoneal lining in the right upper quadrant (location).
- Ultimately, referred pain develops in the right shoulder.

Splenic hematoma

- Initially there is visceral pain in the epigastric region due to stretch and distention of the spleen.
- Then parietal pain develops due to direct irritation of the peritoneal lining in the left upper quadrant (location).
- Ultimately, referred pain develops in the left shoulder.

Acute appendicitis

- Initially there is visceral pain in the periumbilical region due to stretch and distention of the appendix.
- Then parietal pain develops due to direct irritation of the peritoneal lining in the right lower quadrant (location).
- Ultimately, referred pain develops in the flank, depending on the location of the appendix.

THE HISTORY

■ DID THIS PATIENT'S ABDOMINAL PAIN OCCUR ABRUPTLY?

Pain that occurs suddenly increases the likelihood of the following disorders:

- Obstruction (intestinal, ureteral, or biliary)
- An acute vascular problem (aortic dissection, rupture, or hemorrhage into the retroperitoneal space, or ischemia due to embolism)
- Perforation of a viscus
- Torsion of a visceral structure

Intermittent, colicky pain is more suggestive of obstruction of a viscus rather than the severe, persistent, or worsening pain of a perforation. The onset of pain associated with inflammation such as appendicitis is more gradual and in the early stages may not cause severe pain. Appendicitis should be considered in all patients with acute abdominal pain.

PRACTICE POINT

The alvarado clinical decision rule for appendicitis (LR+ = 3.1)

Variable score

Migration = 1
Anorexia-acetone = 1
Nausea-vomiting = 1
Tenderness in right lower quadrant = 2
Rebound pain = 1
Elevation of temperature = 1
Leukocytosis = 2
Shift to the left = 1
Maximum total score = 10
Positive ≥ 7

Data from does this patient have appendicitis? Wagner J, Simel DL, Rennie D, eds. *The Rational Clinical Examination*. New York, NY: McGraw-Hill; 2008:63.

Women should always be asked about the menstrual cycle, possible pregnancy, and birth control pills.

■ DID THIS PATIENT'S ABDOMINAL PAIN LOCALIZE?

Localization of pain may be useful in determining its cause.

Diffuse pain may result from gastroenteritis, peritonitis, perforation, gastrointestinal hemorrhage, abdominal abscess, acute pancreatitis, intestinal obstruction, early appendicitis, ileocolitis, sigmoid diverticulitis, strangulated hernia, inflammatory bowel

disease, mesenteric ischemia, aortic dissection or rupture, and traumatic injury. Angioedema of the bowel (hereditary, idiopathic or medication induced), familial Mediterranean fever, sickle cell crisis, acute porphyria, diabetic ketoacidosis, uremia, hypercalcemia, opiate withdrawal, and heavy metal intoxication may also cause diffuse pain.

Mid upper abdominal pain may be caused by peptic ulcer disease; pancreatic cancer, pancreatitis; biliary colic, cholecystitis, or ascending cholangits; esophagitis, gastroesophageal reflux disease, or pill-induced esophagitis, myocardial ischemia or pericarditis, mesenteric ischemia, rupture or dissection of the aorta, and traumatic injury.

Periumbilical pain may arise from early appendicitis, obstruction of the small bowel, gastroenteritis, mesenteric ischemia, aortic aneurysm rupture or dissection, and traumatic injury.

Right upper quadrant pain may result from acute cholecystitis, ascending cholangitis or biliary colic, acute hepatitis, hepatic abscess, hepatic congestion secondary to congestive heart failure, perforated duodenal ulcer, acute pancreatitis, retrocecal appendicitis, colitis, right-sided diverticulitis, myocardial ischemia, pericarditis, right lower lobe pneumonia, pulmonary embolism, subphrenic abscess, pyelonephritis, renal calculi, perinephric abscess, and traumatic injury.

Right lower quadrant pain suggests appendicitis, inflammatory bowel disease, right-sided diverticulitis, ileocolitis, ischemic colitis, gastroenteritis, hernia, Meckel diverticulosis, cecal diverticulosis, mesenteric adenitis, incarcerated strangulated groin hernia, leaking aneurysm, ruptured ectopic pregnancy, twisted ovarian cyst, pelvic inflammatory disease, salpingitis, Mittelschmerz, endometriosis, gynecologic cancer, pyelonephritis, renal calculi, prostatitis, seminal vesiculitis, psoas abscess, and traumatic injury.

Left upper quadrant pain may be caused by gastritis or peptic ulcer disease; acute pancreatitis or pancreatic cancer; splenic enlargement or infarction, rupture, infarction or aneurysm, myocardial ischemia, pulmonary embolism, subphrenic abscess, left lower lobe pneumonia, pyelonephritis, renal calculi, perinephric abscess, and traumatic injury.

Left lower quadrant pain may result from sigmoid diverticulitis, ischemic colitis, inflammatory bowel disease, ileocolitis, gastroenteritis, incarcerated or strangulated groin hernia, regional enteritis, leaking aneurysm, ruptured ectopic pregnancy, Mittelschmerz, twisted ovarian cyst or torsion, gynecologic cancer, salpingitis, pelvic inflammatory disease, endometriosis; pyelonephritis, perinephris abscess, ureteral calculi, seminal vesiculitis, prostatitis, psoas abscess, and traumatic injury.

With any lateralizing pain location (any of the four quadrants), particularly when there is a lack of clinical evidence for an intra-abdominal process, the physician should think about the possibility of herpes zoster (lateralizing sharp pain, classically band like along a dermatome, sometimes preceded by tingling), which may arise prior to development of the classic eruption. Abdominal wall processes and muscular processes (including hematoma, infection, and muscle strain) should also be considered in the appropriate setting.

■ DOES THIS PAIN RADIATE?

Gallbladder pain, liver disease, and referred pain from diaphragmatic irritation typically radiate to the back and/or shoulder. Liver disease and gallbladder disease may also radiate to the tip of the scapula. Pancreatitis, posterior perforation of an ulcer, kidney disease, and dissecting aneurysm can cause severe back pain due to inflammation in the retroperitoneum, occasionally with radiation to the shoulder. Other retroperitoneal structures such as kidney or ureter may also cause abdominal or flank pain that radiates to the back. Abdominal pain radiating to the groin/testicles may be due to an obstructing renal stone in the ureter.

■ WHAT IS THE SEVERITY OF THIS PATIENT'S PAIN NEAR THE TIME OF ONSET?

Although pain is experienced subjectively, there are certain types of pain that are classically intense within seconds or minutes of onset. Acute vascular insufficiency from torsion of a visceral structure or an acute embolic event (eg, in a patient with atrial fibrillation), perforation, hemorrhage, and dissection will often present with intense, acute pain. Renal colic also can present acutely, but waxes and wanes often with near-complete resolution between pain peaks.

■ HOW DOES THE PATIENT DESCRIBE THE QUALITY OF PAIN?

Abdominal pain in a patient with bowel obstruction is colicky in nature. Repeated episodes of colicky abdominal pain may suggest internal hernias as the cause of intermittent or acute intestinal obstruction. An intra-abdominal hernia occurs when an anomalous fold or outpocketing of the peritoneum traps an intestinal loop. Acute strangulation of the intestinal loop may result in compression of the vasculature or gangrene of the bowel (50% of patients) or volvulus (14% of patients).

Biliary colic is a misnomer, the pain does not wax and wane but builds over 15 to 60 minutes, then is steady for several hours and dissipates slowly (visceral pain).

Pain in cholecystitis usually lasts longer than 6 hours and is located in the right upper quadrant due to progressive inflammation (parietal pain).

Although peptic ulcer disease may be asymptomatic and occasionally a patient may report crampy abdominal pain, most patients characterize the pain as burning/gnawing pain.

Visceral pain in diverticulitis is initially crampy in character, followed by parietal pain as the inflammation progresses.

Pain in acute mesenteric ischemia is acute in onset and severe. The patient reports periumbilical visceral pain out of proportion to the physical examination. Parietal pain and localizing exam findings are ominous findings in mesenteric ischemia, suggesting that the bowel may have infarcted or perforated. A dissecting aneurysm usually manifests with sudden severe pain, sometimes described as tearing/ripping sensation that radiates to the back. The onset may be in the epigastric region but then may progress to involve the lower quadrants as the dissection proceeds. Often the intense pain occurs intermittently as new tearing episodes occur.

■ HOW HAS THE PAIN PROGRESSED?

Has the patient experienced similar episodes in the past? If so, have the patient describe them, and determine what prior evaluation has been performed and what presumptive diagnoses were obtained.

■ WHAT ARE THE ASSOCIATED SIGNS AND SYMPTOMS?

Is there a history of systemic symptoms, such as fever, anorexia, weight loss? Acute inflammatory symptoms such as fever, particularly when infectious diarrhea is not suspected, may suggest the need for urgent imaging. Fever may be due to a loss of bowel wall integrity (perforation or severe mucosal injury) or due to infection in other abdominal structures (eg, cholecystitis). Weight loss may suggest a chronic inflammatory condition, mesenteric ischemia, malignancy, a problem with absorption, or a stricture. Sometimes food avoidance due to fear of pain may be the cause of weight loss.

Vomiting preceding the pain suggests the diagnosis of gastroenteritis, intestinal obstruction, biliary colic, or ureteral colic. Gastroenteritis, however, is usually associated with diarrhea. In appendicitis, vomiting rarely precedes pain. Bilious vomiting suggests mechanical obstruction.

Obstruction caused by a tumor, diverticulitis, stricture, or less commonly by a colonic volvulus, may have nausea, vomiting, abdominal distention, and pain.

Dark urine and pale stools suggest biliary obstruction. Be cautious in interpreting these complaints, however, since loose stools in general are often paler than formed stools, and truly acholic stools are uncommon. Further, dehydration—common with poor oral intake—leads to concentrated urine, so the clinician should specifically seek a history of brown or tea colored urine rather than simply asking if the urine is "dark." Jaundice is often not present early on after a biliary obstruction since scleral icterus reflects bilirubin levels from days earlier.

■ WHAT FACTORS EXACERBATE THE PAIN?

The examiner should specifically inquire whether eating exacerbates the pain. If so, it is important to clarify the time course of the pain, the associated symptoms (such as nausea and vomiting), and the types of food or drink that cause the symptoms. If pain occurs during swallowing or immediately afterward, an esophageal problem such as stricture or achalasia is likely. Although dysphagia usually presents with chest discomfort and not abdominal pain, some patients will have epigastric pain. If the pain is exacerbated by acid-containing foods (eg, citrus fruits or tomato sauce), caffeine, or alcohol, mucosal pain (esophagitis, gastritis, duodenitis, and possibly ulceration) should be considered. These symptoms can occur shortly after ingestion, but sometimes will not start for up to 1 to 2 hours later. If fatty foods in particular seem to be a culprit, consider gallbladder or biliary disease, or perhaps pancreatitis if the pain is severe. Postprandial pain may also suggest chronic mesenteric ischemia (ie, "mesenteric angina") due to a fixed vascular obstruction.

A patient with esophagitis/gastroesophageal reflux disease will often have increased pain when lying down. Patients with pancreatitis report steady, boring pain that makes them uncomfortable when lying supine.

A patient with a perinephric abscess may experience more pain with bending toward the uninvolved side.

Pain associated with salpingitis or endometriosis is worse before and during menstruation.

■ IS THERE A HISTORY OF PRIOR ABDOMINAL SURGERY?

Adhesions are almost exclusively seen in patients with prior abdominal surgeries—regardless of when the surgery occurred—and are the main causes of partial and complete obstructions of the small bowel. If the surgery was recent, then acute infections (eg, abscess) must be considered.

Even seemingly minor procedures may be associated with serious complications. For example, upper endoscopy may be complicated by esophageal perforation, aspiration pneumonia, or bleeding. Colonoscopy may cause abdominal bloating, lower gastrointestinal bleeding, perforation, or (rarely) splenic rupture. Cardiac catheterization and closed renal biopsy may lead to retroperitoneal bleeding. Interventions involving the biliary or pancreatic ducts (ie, endoscopic retrograde cholangiopancreatography) are commonly complicated by pain and transient elevations of pancreatic enzymes, even in the absence of overt pancreatitis, but if the pain persists or worsens, true pancreatitis should be considered.

■ WHEN WAS THE PATIENT'S LAST BOWEL MOVEMENT?

A constipated patient with abdominal pain may be developing a serious complication, such as obstruction, ischemia, or perforation. Obstruction may precipitate new onset constipation or exacerbate chronic constipation. Volvulus should be considered in any patient experiencing a sudden onset of constipation associated with abdominal pain, distention, and nausea and vomiting. Patients with small bowel obstruction will often evacuate their bowels shortly after the obstruction occurs, sometimes in parallel with the onset of vomiting, due to accelerated peristalsis throughout the gut. With prolonged obstruction, a lack of bowel movements is the norm. See Chapter 80 for a detailed discussion of constipation.

Likewise, the presence of diarrhea may provide clues to the cause of the abdominal pain. See Chapter 82 for a detailed discussion of diarrhea.

■ WHAT ARE THE PATIENT'S RISK FACTORS FOR GASTROINTESTINAL DISORDERS?

Is there a history of excessive alcohol use?

Injury to the lumen of the upper gastrointestinal tract (esophagitis, gastritis, or duodenitis, with or without ulceration) is common in this setting, as are pancreatitis and acute alcoholic hepatitis.

Is there accompanying iron deficiency anemia, weight loss, or a personal or family history for colorectal cancer?

Does the patient have a prior history of gastrointestinal disease or surgery?

A stricture should be considered on the differential diagnosis in any individual who has had prior colonic resection, a history of diverticulitis, peritonitis, or inflammatory bowel disease.

Does the patient have a systemic disorder that predisposes him to the development of acute abdominal pain? (See **Table 75-1**.)

Known cardiovascular, cerebrovascular, or peripheral vascular disease increases the risk of bowel ischemia or aortoiliac disease. Regarding mesenteric ischemia, several historical features may suggest either an arterial or venous event as the cause of abdominal pain. Risk factors for either superior mesenteric arterial thrombosis due to atherosclerotic stenotic lesions or superior mesenteric arterial embolism of cardiac origin include the usual risk factors for cardiovascular disease and a history of vascular disease in several distributions (peripheral, cerebrovascular, cardiac). The examiner should specifically inquire about a history of intestinal angina suggested by postprandial pain and gut emptying, avoidance of food, and significant weight loss. Because collateral circulation will compensate for chronic occlusive disease of the superior, celiac, and inferior mesenteric arteries, mesenteric ischemia would not be expected to result unless one or two main vessels are thrombosed. When the third artery becomes occluded, the patient develops diffuse ischemia involving the liver, gallbladder, and much of the

TABLE 75-1 Nonsurgical Disorders Causing Acute Abdominal Pain

Category	Key Diagnostic Feature
Metabolic/Endocrine	
Diabetic ketoacidosis	High-serum glucose; ketoacidosis
Hyperthyroidism	High T4, low TSH
Hypercalcemia	High-serum calcium
Hypokalemia	Low-serum potassium
Hypophosphatemia	Low-serum phosphate
Addison disease	Low-serum cortisol, elevated ACTH
Porphyria	High prophobilinogen and delta ALA
Familial Mediterranean fever	Duration >1-2 d; pleuritis and peritonitis
Vascular/Cardiopulmonary	
Myocardial ischemia/infarction	Abnormal ECG, high troponin
Aortic dissection	Widened mediastinum and diagnostic CT angiography
Median arcuate ligament syndrome	MRA or CTA
Pneumonia/pleurisy	Chest x-ray
Pulmonary embolus	Well's score, high D-dimer, CT-PA
Drug/Toxin	
Salicylate	Tinnitus, confusion, mixed respiratory alkalosis and metabolic acidosis
Anticholinergics	Confusion, dilated pupils, tachycardia, ileus, urinary retention
Tricyclic anti-depressants	Delirium, anticholinergic symptoms, ECG changes, serum/urine TCA level
Cocaine	Tachycardia, HTN, systemic end-organ ischemia, positive toxic screen
Heavy metals	Renal, neurological toxicity, 24 urine assay
Vasculitis/Connective Tissue	
Systemic lupus erythematosus (SLE)	>4 of 11 SLE criteria are met
Systemic vasculitis	Multiorgan disease with + p-ANCA and ANA, low complement
Scleroderma	Skin changes, Raynaud's phenomenon and visceral disease
Hematologic/Immunologic	
Sickle cell crisis	History, periarticular pain, effusions
Henoch-Schoenlein purpura	Skin biopsy: leukocytoclastic vasculitis with IgA and C3 deposition
Hemolytic uremic syndrome	ARF with schistocytes on smear
Hereditary angioneurotic edema	Low C1 esterase inhibitor level
Systemic mast cell disease	High-serum tryptase and urinary histamine; increased tissue mast cells
Thrombotic thrombocytopenic purpura	Fever, confusion, thrombocytopenia, schistocytes

(Continued)

TABLE 75-1 Nonsurgical Disorders Causing Acute Abdominal Pain (*continued*)

Category	Key Diagnostic Feature
Infectious	
Staphylotoxin	Fever, hypotension, rash (CDC case definition)
Bornholm disease	Fever, rash, spasmodic pain, enterovirus (coxsackie/echo)
Yersinia enterocolitica	Diarrhea, fever, positive stool culture, ileal inflammation
Tuberculous mesenteritis	Fever, fatigue, diarrhea, right lower quadrant mass and ascites, positive biopsy
Dengue fever	Fever, HA, myalgias/arthralgias, low platelets, high LFTs, positive serology
Malaria	Fever, chill, diaphoresis, HA, myalgia, cough, multiorgan disease, red blood count smear
Musculoskeletal	
"Slipping rib" (lower rib margin) syndrome	Production of pain with rib compression only on affected side
Rectus sheath hematoma/neuroma	Carnett's sign
Chronic abdominal wall pain syndrome	Right upper quadrant (mainly) tenderness and positive Carnett sign
Neurologic/Psychiatric	
Herpes zoster	Unilateral, painful vesicular rash in dermatomal distribution, positive DFA of lesion or PCR of fluid
Abdominal migraine	Adolescents, cyclic occurrence
Temporal lobe seizures	Adolescents, aura, abnormal EEG
Radiculopathy	Mechanical pain in dermatomal distribution, positive MRI
Irritable bowel syndrome	Manning or Rome III criteria
Renal	
Nephro/ureterolithiasis	Hematuria and positive CT
Papillary necrosis	Hematuria, obstructive uropathy, diabetes, sickle cell disease

ACTH, adrenal corticotropin hormone; ALA, aminolevulinic acid; ANA, antinuclear antibody; ARF, acute renal failure; CDC, centers for disease control and prevention; CT, computed tomography; CT-PA, computed tomography-pulmonary angiography; CTA, computed tomography-angiography; DFA, direct fluorescent assay; ECG, electrocardiogram; EEG, electroencephalogram; HA, headache; HTN, hypertension; IgA, immunoglobulin A; LFT, liver function test; MRA, magnetic resonance angiography; MRI, magnetic resonance imaging; PCR, polymerase chain reaction; SLE, systemic lupus erythematosus; TCA, tricyclic antidepressants; TSH, thyroid stimulating hormone.
Data from Makrauer FL, Greenberger NJ. Acute abdominal pain: basic principles & current challenges. In: Greenberger NJ, Blumberg RS, Burakoff R, eds. *Current Diagnosis & Treatment: Gastroenterology, Hepatology, & Endoscopy.* New York, NY: McGraw-Hill; 2009:1-10.

colon and associated metabolic abnormalities. Embolism of the superior mesenteric artery may also cause acute abdominal pain because of the lack of preexisting arterial collaterals. Risk factors include cardiac arrhythmia, recent myocardial infarction, or proximal aortic disease. These patients typically do not have a history of intestinal angina. Cholesterol embolism may affect branches and terminal arteries leading to segmental bowel involvement and abdominal pain without focal findings until necrosis of the entire bowel wall occurs.

Mesenteric ischemia of venous origin is characterized by acute and chronic forms. The chronic form causes abdominal pain and diarrhea, but does not usually progress to acute abdominal findings. Risk factors include prior venous thromboembolism and primary hypercoagulable states, previous abdominal surgery, intra-abdominal cancer, inflammatory bowel disease, and portal hypertension. The acute form is more likely to involve a major venous vessel such as the portal or superior mesenteric vein. The chronic forms may develop in small peripheral veins and progress proximally.

Elderly vasculopathic patients are particularly prone to developing ischemic colitis—a clinically distinct entity from mesenteric ischemia—in which small vessel insufficiency results in sloughing of the metabolically active mucosal lining of the colon. This condition is often confused with inflammatory or infectious colitis since it often presents with crampy pain and diarrhea (often positive for occult blood, and sometimes grossly bloody), and often with fever. Since this condition results from small vessel insufficiency, there is rarely any role for evaluation of mesenteric vessels.

THE PHYSICAL EXAMINATION

■ DOES THE PATIENT LOOK SICK?

A patient who lies still, has his knees flexed, and has a rigid abdomen most likely has peritoneal inflammation. Patients who are restless, unable to get comfortable, and pace may have renal colic or an aortic dissection. Patients with a perinephric abscess may bend over toward the involved side.

■ WHAT ARE THE VITAL SIGNS?

Although lack of fever does not rule out an inflammatory process, especially in immunocompromised hosts, patients with renal failure, or the elderly, its presence requires further evaluation. Tachycardia may result from pain from any source, fever, and dehydration. Hypertension can arise from any severe pain but may also predispose to vascular events. It is initially present in more than 70% of patients with acute aortic dissection. Hypotension in association with acute abdominal pain raises the possibility of aortic rupture or dissection, sepsis, gastrointestinal bleeding, dehydration, and pump failure (acute myocardial infarction, pulmonary embolism). Patients may also develop nonocclusive mesenteric ischemia associated with a low-output state related to septic shock, myocardial infarction, and other causes of hypotension. Patients with chronic adrenal insufficiency may experience nonspecific abdominal pain and have relatively low blood pressures but otherwise appear well.

Tachypnea may be associated with anxiety, severe pain, sepsis, acute pulmonary embolism, pneumothorax, and other respiratory causes.

ARE THERE ANY SIGNS OF SYSTEMIC ILLNESS?

A general physical examination should be performed to determine the presence of systemic illness that may be associated with abdominal pain.

PRACTICE POINT

- The abdominal examination may confirm the clinician's pretest suspicion of an underlying disorder. However, most signs are useful if present but not if absent.
- For example, elderly patients may have acute cholecystitis without any signs or symptoms in the right upper quadrant. The clinician's gestalt has a reported LR+ 25 to 30 compared with a positive Murphy sign, LR 2.8 (0.8-8.6) and right upper quadrant tenderness, LR 1.6 (1.0-2.5).
- The presence of ecchymoses, signifying subcutaneous blood from intraperitoneal or retroperitoneal hemorrhage dissecting the skin overlying the flanks (Turner sign), a periumbilical bruise (Cullen sign) or a green or jaundiced discoloration at the umbilicus (Ransohoff sign of a ruptured bile duct) is helpful only if present. Prominent venous patterns may suggest portal hypertension or inferior vena caval syndrome but are also seen in normal elderly patients.
- Regarding ascites, the presence of a fluid wave has a reported LR+ 6.0 (3.3-11) and shifting dullness LR+ 2.7 (1.9-3.9). The absence of a fluid wave or shifting dullness does not rule out the presence of significant ascites in the patient with risk factors or symptoms of ankle swelling, weight gain, and abdominal distention.
- Palpating a liver edge below the right costal margin may increase the patient's pain and correlates poorly with the actual liver span (LR+ 2.0). For patients with risk factors for splenomegaly, the reported LR+ for percussion of Traube space is 2.3 (1.8-2.9) and palpation 8.2 (5.8-12).
- The sensitivity of abdominal palpation in patients with a ruptured abdominal aneurysm, especially in obese patients or those who cannot relax their abdomen, is sufficiently low that emergent surgical consultation and imaging is required if the index of suspicion is sufficiently high. The LRs vary with the size of the aneurysm; for aneurysms >4 cm the reported LR+ is 16 (8.6-29).

Data from Simel DL, Rennie D, eds. *The Rational Clinical Examination.* McGraw-Hill; 2008:27, 73, 147, 300, 613.

THE ABDOMINAL EXAMINATION

Inspection

The abdominal examination must be performed gently and carefully to elicit localized and generalized peritoneal signs. The examiner should first inspect the abdomen at the foot of the bed to detect visible peristalsis, asymmetry suggesting hernias or masses, and distention. Unless there are surgical scars or a prior term pregnancy, the umbilicus should be within 1 cm of the midpoint between the xiphoid and the pubis. Organomegaly, masses, or ascites may cause displacement of the umbilicus. Eversion or outward protrusion of an inverted umbilicus is not a reliable sign for chronic ascites. In generalized peritonitis, respiratory motion is not associated with movement of the abdominal wall. The clinician should also note any changes in skin color, the presence of ecchymoses, and the presence of scars. The presence of surgical scars increases the likelihood that abdominal adhesions may be causing acute pain. If the patient can attempt a modified sit-up that contracts his rectus abdominal muscles, a ventral hernia may be more visible than palpable.

Auscultation

In general, auscultation for abnormal bowel sounds should be performed prior to performing percussion or palpation of the abdomen. Of note, the absence of bowel sounds may be normally present between episodes of normal bowel motility and, hence, is not specific by itself for advanced intestinal obstruction or secondary ileus from inflammatory conditions such as pancreatitis, pyelonephritis, or peritonitis. In fact, some experts believe that the examiner must listen for at least 1 to 2 minutes before concluding that the bowel sounds are in fact absent. However, it is worthwhile to listen for the very high-pitched tinkles and rushes characteristic of small bowel obstruction. A succession splash suggests gastric outlet obstruction. An epigastric bruit with a diastolic component may suggest hemodynamically significant stenoses of branches of the aorta including the celiac axis and superior mesenteric artery as well as in disease of the aorta, or the renal arteries. Friction rubs may rarely be appreciated over an inflamed gallbladder, splenic infarct, and in cases of hepatoma, cholangiocarcinoma, and metastatic carcinoma. A murmur due to compression of the splenic artery may be appreciated in patients with pancreatic carcinoma.

Percussion

Light percussion to estimate the liver span (with >15 cm consistent with liver enlargement) is the most reliable method to check for the presence of hepatomegaly. If the patient's abdomen is distended, the examiner should look for signs of ascites (fluid wave, shifting dullness) or perhaps perform a bedside ultrasound. Likewise, the clinician should start with light percussion to determine whether splenomegaly is present. A full bladder is defined as at least 250 mL of urine. An enlarged bladder requires ultrasound confirmation due to the unreliability of the physical examination in detecting bladder distention.

Palpation

The examiner should always first explain to the patient what the examination will entail and examine the most painful area last. The patient should be asked to distinguish between pressure and pain during examination of all quadrants. During the abdominal examination the patient's hips and knees should be flexed to relax the abdominal musculature. Involuntary guarding and rebound tenderness may be an indication of parietal peritoneal (layer of the abdominal wall) involvement, a rough or cold examining hand, or due to patient apprehension. The examiner should ask the patient to point to the area of pain. A patient with appendicitis may be able to precisely localize the pain using one finger, especially after coughing or performing the Valsalva maneuver. A positive Murphy sign is elicited when the inflamed gallbladder descends to the examiner's thumb and causes pain sufficient to abruptly cease inspiration. The reported sensitivity of the Murphy sign is only 27% but increased with bedside ultrasound imaging the precise location of the gallbladder. Some experts do not recommend testing for rebound tenderness because the test is only useful if positive and it causes unnecessary pain. If the pain is significantly out of proportion to the physical findings, obstruction and ischemia should be suspected. To determine if abdominal pain is originating from an intraabdominal source or the anterior abdominal wall, check for the Carnett sign. Have patient lift their head off the pillow resulting in increased tension in the anterior abdominal wall muscles thus protecting the structures within the abdomen from the pressure of the examiner's hand. If the pain is lessened by this maneuver, it indicates that the pain is arising from an intraabdominal source. Conversely, if the pain is worsened, it indicates that the pain is arising from the anterior abdominal wall.

If the patient can relax, the abdomen should be deeply palpated a few centimeters above the umbilicus slightly left of midline to detect a widened aorta. A normal abdominal aorta is usually less than 3 cm wide. Obesity, voluntary guarding, firm musculature limit the sensitivity of the examination. Palpable kidneys are consistent with bilateral polycystic kidney disease or hydronephrosis. Pancreatic pseudocysts may also be palpable in approximately 50% of patients.

The abdominal examination should include a rectal and genital examination.

PRACTICE POINT

Findings	Systemic Disease That May be Associated with Abdominal Pain
Clubbing	Inflammatory bowel disease, pulmonary malignancy, cirrhosis, congenital heart disease, endocarditis (bacterial endocarditis), artrioventricular malformations, fistulas
Koilonychia	Iron deficiency anemia, systemic lupus erythematosus (SLE)
Onycholysis	Hyperthyroidism, amyloidosis, connective tissue disorders
Beau lines	Any severe systemic illness that disrupts nail growth
Yellow nail	Rheumatoid arthritis (RA), nephritic syndrome, tuberculosis, immunodeficiency
Terrys (white nails)	Hepatic failure, cirrhosis, diabetes, congestive heart failure (CHF), hyperthyroidism, malnutrition
Asure lunula	Wilson disease, silver poisoning
Half-and-half nails	Chronic renal failure, cirrhosis
Muehrckes lines	Hypoalbuminemia
Mees lines	Arsenic poisoning, Hodgkins disease, CHF, leprosy, malaria, carbon monoxide poisoning, other systemic insults
Splinter hemorrhage	Subacute bacterial endocarditis, SLE, RA, antiphospholipid syndrome, peptic ulcer disease, malignancies
Telangiectasis	RA, SLE, dermatomyositis, scleroderma
Skin lesions	Vasculitis, septic emboli
Gangrene, dependency rubor	Peripheral vascular disease
Pallor	Severe anemia (Hg < 7 g/dL)
Jaundice	Liver disease, biliary tract disease, biliary obstruction
Slate brown color	Addison disease
Rash and fever	Infection
Pyoderma gangrenosum	Inflammatory bowel disease
Bruits	Vascular disease
Heart murmurs, gallops	Significant heart disease
Pulmonary signs and symptoms	Pneumonia, pulmonary embolism, pneumothorax, empyema
Peripheral edema	CHF, ascites, deep venous thrombosis

CASE 75-1

A 57-year-old man developed acute right upper quadrant abdominal pain that radiated to his back. Similar to prior episodes, the pain was severe, abrupt onset, colicky in nature, lasting 45 to 60 minutes followed by an aching right upper quadrant discomfort lasting several hours. His laboratory tests, including CBC, comprehensive metabolic profile, serum amylase and lipase, urinalysis without the presence of bilirubin, and esophagogastroduodenoscopy, were all normal. Three ultrasound examinations obtained during three separate Emergency Department visits visualized the gallbladder but did not detect gallstones.

On physical examination the patient had normal vital signs and his blood pressure was equal in both arms. His heart and lung examination was normal. Examination of the abdomen revealed thump tenderness in the right upper quadrant but not the left upper quadrant, thump tenderness over the right lower anterior chest but not the left lower anterior chest, and a palpable liver that was tender to deep palpation. The gallbladder which is usually identified by the junction of the right lateral rectus muscle and the costal margin was not palpable.

Consistent with gallbladder disease but in the absence of stones, the clinical picture of this case is termed acalculous cholecystopathy. Delayed gastric emptying characterized by postprandial bloating and distention is less likely due to long intervals between acute attacks. A HIDA scan with injection of cholecystokinin would be the next test to perform. It should reproduce the patient's pain during his attacks and show a reduced gallbladder ejection fraction to <35%. If this test is positive it would obviate the need for further testing such as CT scan, MRI, CT angiogram, or MR angiogram.

The patient underwent a laparoscopic cholecystectomy from which pathologic specimens showed clear-cut evidence of chronic cholecystitis.

This case highlights that the finding of a normal ultrasound examination should not deter the clinician from seeking additional studies to help establish this diagnosis for patients who have symptoms clearly suggestive of gallbladder disease. Consultation with a radiologist about the bedside clinical information might have facilitated an earlier diagnosis.

ANCILLARY LABORATORY TESTS

Laboratory studies are often of limited value. A normal complete blood count (CBC) does not rule out appendicitis or other inflammatory processes. Complete blood count, liver enzymes, urinalysis, and pregnancy test are helpful when abnormal. A urinalysis may point to nephrolithiasis or urinary tract infection. Plain radiographs of the abdomen are not helpful in most cases of abdominal pain, but can be diagnostic in cases of small bowel obstruction or volvulus and when there is a perforated viscus. In patients with abdominal distention, pain and constipation, plain abdominal radiography can be helpful assessing the degree of constipation and ruling out obstruction. Abdominal radiographs may demonstrate a dilated colon or small bowel with air fluid levels indicative of obstruction. The presence of free air on plain abdominal radiograph would indicate perforated bowel. Calcifications in the pancreatic bed indicate the presence of chronic pancreatitis. (See Chapter 116.)

If abdominal radiography demonstrates colonic dilatation suggestive of an obstruction, additional imaging should be performed (**Table 75-2**). Computed tomography (CT) has led to the greatest improvement in the care of patients with acute abdominal pain, and is usually the next diagnostic test in a patient with unexplained pain

TABLE 75-2 Major Causes of Acute Abdominal Pain with Preferred Diagnostic Test for Each

Common Conditions	Key Diagnostic Test(s)
Acute appendicitis	CT scan
Acute cholecystitis, choledocholithiasis	Ultrasound
Acute diverticulitis	CT scan
Acute pancreatitis	Serum amylase/lipase, CT scan
Bowel perforation	CT scan
Acute mesenteric ischemia	CT angiogram, MRI
Ischemic colitis	Colonoscopy
Intestinal obstruction	Flat film, imaging study
Anterior abdominal wall pain (in rectus hematoma)	Carnett sign, Fothergill sign
Sigmoid volvulus	CT scan or Barium enema
Biliary duct or pancreatic duct rupture	MRCP, ERCP

CT, computed tomography; ERCP, endoscopic retrograde cholangiopan-creatography; MRCP, magnetic resonance cholangiopancreatography; MRI, magnetic resonance imaging.

Data from Makrauer FL, Greenberger NJ. Acute abdominal pain: basic principles & current challenges. In: Greenberger NJ, Blumberg RS, Burakoff R, eds. *Current Diagnosis & Treatment: Gastroenterology, Hepatology, & Endoscopy.* New York, NY: McGraw-Hill; 2009:1-10.

symptoms and clinical suspicion of significant abdominal pathology. Ultrasound is often the best modality to image a fluid filled body such as a cyst or gallbladder but CT is usually diagnostic in these conditions as well. Ultrasound is the modality of choice in any woman who may be pregnant.

CASE 75-2

An 86-year-old woman with a prior history of coronary artery disease, hypertension, cholecystectomy, and renal artery stenosis presented to an outside hospital with worsening postprandial abdominal pain for over 6 months. There was no history of diarrhea, hematochezia, or reflux symptoms. Studies performed within the prior 3 months included an unrevealing esophagogastroduodenoscopy and a colonoscopy. At the outside hospital laboratory testing reported an elevated serum amylase and lipase, and a noncontrast enhanced CT scan identified a 15 mm × 7 mm hypoechoic mass in the head of the pancreas. She was transferred to a tertiary hospital for further evaluation of superimposed acute-on-chronic abdominal pain and the pancreatic lesion.

Key questions to ask include:

- Has the patient ever had an episode of acute pancreatitis?
- Is the pain she is experiencing similar to the pain she experienced prior to her cholecystectomy?
- Does the size of the meal that she eats influence the severity of her postprandial pain?
- If she eats smaller quantities of food, does she experience less pain?
- Has she lost weight and if so, how much?

This patient's vital signs were notable for temperature 97.1°F, pulse 107 and regular, blood pressure 126/70 mm Hg, respirations 18, SaO$_2$ 98% on room air. Head/neck examination revealed no thyromegaly jugular venous distention or lymphadenopathy.

Lungs were clear to auscultation and cardiac examination revealed a regular rate and rhythm without murmurs. Abdominal examination revealed a soft, nondistended abdomen. However, she was tender to palpation in the right upper quadrant, left upper quadrant, and the periumbilical area. The abdominal pain seemed out of proportion to the fairly benign examination of the abdomen. There was no mention of an abdominal bruit, which would have been an important physical finding. There was no shake tenderness. A rectal examination revealed hemoccult negative stool.

Laboratory data included white blood cell count 15,500/mm³, hemoglobin 11.5 g/dL, hematocrit 33.6%, platelets 283,000. Metabolic profile sodium 140 mEq/L, potassium 3.8 mEq/L, chloride 105 mEq/L, and HCO$_3$ 25 mEq/L, BUN 44 mg/dL, creatinine 0.8 mg/dL, and blood glucose 188 mg/dL. Liver tests revealed serum ALT 11 U/L, serum AST 14 U/L, serum alkaline phosphatase 101 U/L, total bilirubin 0.4 mg/dL, serum amylase 140 U/L (normal < 120 U/L), and serum lipase 190 U/L (normal < 60U/L).

A magnetic resonance cholangiopancreatography revealed subcentimeter ill-defined irregular areas of decreased enhancement of the pancreas consistent with either sidebranch intraductal papillary mucinous neoplasm or pancreatic cancer. There were also findings consistent with chronic pancreatitis with irregularity of the main pancreatic duct. An endoscopic ultrasound examination to clarify the lesion in the pancreas revealed congestion and edema in the stomach, along with several small areas of erosion and shallow ulcerations also in the stomach. Endosonographic findings revealed an irregular mass-like lesion in the pancreatic head. Biopsy of the 15 mm by 7 mm hypoechoic lesion revealed only pancreatic tissue. Before a decision was made about whether she should undergo a laparotomy with biopsy of the pancreatic mass, she developed increasingly severe abdominal pain and continued tenderness in the abdomen.

A MR angiogram of the abdomen without contrast revealed the superior mesenteric artery arising with the celiac artery. There was moderate-to high-grade stenosis at the ostium of the celiac axis. The superior mesenteric artery was considerably narrowed but still retained some patency.

Shortly after the completion of these studies, the patient became increasingly confused, tachycardic, and hypotensive. Laboratory studies at that time revealed serum amylase 334 U/L (normal 20-70 U/L), serum lipase 276 U/L (normal 3-60 U/L), a low arterial blood gas pH 7.29, and elevated serum lactate level 5.0 mg/L.

At this juncture it seemed clear that she had severe mesenteric vascular ischemia and that she probably had developed gut infarction. She underwent exploratory laparotomy. There was marked ischemia and some transmural necrosis of the small bowel, from approximately 30 cm from the ligament of Treitz to the distal ileum, which was resected. She developed ST-segment elevation consistent with acute myocardial infarction. Thereafter, the patient's family requested comfort measures only and she died shortly thereafter.

The diagnosis of mesenteric vascular ischemia clearly explained virtually all the findings, and the lesions in the pancreas, while of some interest, were not the most important issue to address in this patient after she presented. Clues that this patient had significant mesenteric vascular ischemia included:

- Risk factors (hypertension, coronary artery disease)
- Postprandial pain, worse with larger meals, somewhat better with smaller meals or without eating
- Weight loss
- Abdominal pain out of proportion to any physical findings

The physical examination did not document whether she had an abdominal bruit, the presence of which would have increased the likelihood of mesenteric ischemia as the cause of her symptoms. Her clinicians also overlooked the possibility that the abnormal pancreatic enzymes resulted from gut ischemia.

The findings in the pancreas obfuscated the very real danger of mesenteric vascular ischemia. By the time any patient develops lactic acidosis and elevated liver enzymes, frank gut infarction has usually developed. A cardinal rule is that once the diagnosis of mesenteric vascular insufficiency is entertained, determining the status of the mesenteric vasculature becomes of prime importance and overrides virtually all other diagnostic considerations. It would have been more appropriate to do a MR angiogram early in the course of this patient's illness and upon the demonstration of severe mesenteric vascular ischemia a decision should then have been made as to how to address this diagnosis.

CONCLUSION

The possibility of an intrathoracic lesion must be considered in every patient with abdominal pain, especially if pain is in the upper abdomen. An orderly, painstakingly detailed history is vital, especially the chronologic sequence of events. Pelvic and rectal examinations are *mandatory* on every patient with acute abdominal pain. Laboratory studies may be of considerable value, but they infrequently establish the diagnosis. Sometimes, even under the best of circumstances, a definitive diagnosis cannot be established at the time of the initial examination.

SUGGESTED READINGS

American Gastroenterological Association Medical Position Statement. Guidelines on Intestinal Ischemia. *Gastroenterology* 2000;118:951-953.

Greenberger NJ. Sorting through the nonsurgical causes of acute abdominal pain. *J Crit Illn.* 1992;7:1602-1604, 1609.

Greenberger NJ. Techniques for physical assessment of acute abdominal pain: getting the most out of the history and physical exam. *J Crit Illn.* 1994;9:397-404.

Greenberger NJ, Hinthorn DR. The abdomen. In: *History Taking and Physical Examination: Essentials and Clinical Correlates.* St. Louis, MO: Mosby-Year Book, Inc.; 1993:199-261.

Greenberger NJ, Paumgartner G. Acalculous cholecystopathy. Diseases of the gallbladder and bile ducts. In: Fauci AS, Kasper DL, Longo DL, Braunwald E, Hauser SL, Jameson JL, Loscalzo J, eds. *Harrison's Principles of Internal Medicine*, 19th ed. New York, NY: McGraw-Hill; 2008:1996.

Grunkemeier DM, Cassara JE, Dalton CB, et al. The narcotic bowel syndrome: clinical features, pathophysiology, and management. *Clin Gastroenterol Hepatol.* 2007;5:1126-1139; quiz 1121-1122.

Lewis FR, Holcroft JW, Dunphy E. Appendicitis. A critical review of diagnosis and treatment in 1,000 cases. *Arch Surg.* 1975;110:677-684.

Makrauer FL, Greenberger NJ. Acute abdominal pain: basic principles & current challenges. In: Greenberger NJ, Blumberg RS, Burakoff R, eds. *Current Diagnosis & Treatment: Gastroenterology, Hepatology, & Endoscopy.* New York, NY: McGraw-Hill; 2009:1-10.

Rettenbacher T, Hollerweger A, Gritzmann N, et al. Appendicitis: should diagnostic imaging be performed if the clinical presentation is highly suggestive of the disease? *Gastroenterology.* 2002;123:992-998.

Saito YA, Locke GR, Talley NJ, et al. A comparison of the Rome and Manning criteria for case identification in epidemiological investigations of irritable bowel syndrome. *Am J Gastroenterol.* 2000;95:2816-2824.

CHAPTER 76

Acute Back Pain

John A. Flynn, MD, MBA

Key Clinical Questions

❶ What are the key questions that an examiner should ask when approaching a patient with acute back pain?

❷ What should the examiner look for on physical examination?

❸ What are "red flag" findings that should heighten your level of concern when approaching a patient with acute back pain?

❹ What are some nonspinal etiologies of back pain?

INTRODUCTION

Back pain has a major impact on patient well-being and health care budgets in developed nations. It is the fifth leading cause of hospital admissions and the third most common reason for surgical procedures. Back pain ranks second only to upper respiratory tract infections as a reason for primary care physician office visits. The annual prevalence of chronic low back pain ranges from 15% to 33%, and 7% of adult patients may have low back pain at any given time. In the United States, back pain, including chronic low back pain, is the leading cause of disability in subjects younger than 45 years of age. Individuals with spine pain in the United States account for nearly $90 billion yearly in direct health care expenditures with an additional $20 billion yearly in indirect costs related to lost productivity with approximately 2% of the US workforce compensated for back injuries each year.

Roughly 95% of visits for back pain stem from benign causes. However, in hospitalized patients, the percentage with serious pathology may be higher, so clinicians have to have a high index of suspicion. This chapter focuses on the initial evaluation of acute low back pain in patients admitted to the hospital as well as patients hospitalized for other reasons who develop back pain as a complication of hospitalization.

PATHOPHYSIOLOGY

The function of the anterior spine is to absorb the shock of body movements such as walking and running. The function of the posterior spine is to protect the spinal cord and nerves, and to stabilize the spine by providing sites for attachment of muscles and ligaments. The normal alignment of the spine is notable for the following:

- Lumbar and cervical lordosis and thoracic kyphosis on lateral view
- Straight column on anterior view

Movements of the cervical and lumbar regions are greater than the thoracic regions during activity. The elasticity of vertebral disks—largest in the cervical and lumbar regions—allows the bony vertebrae of the spine to move easily upon one another. Elasticity declines with age.

CASE 76-1

ACUTE ABDOMINAL AND BACK PAIN IN AN EMERGENT SETTING

An 81-year-old man with a history of myocardial infarction 10 years ago presented with new-onset low back pain and crampy abdominal pain that had begun 2 hours prior. He had never had this type of back pain before. His exam revealed a blood pressure of 110/70 mm Hg. His creatinine was 2.5 mg/dL with a glomerular filtration rate of < 35/mL/1.73 m² which is his baseline after his myocardial infarction 10 years ago. He had good pedal pulses, and his abdominal exam revealed a soft abdomen with diffuse tenderness without rebound or guarding and normal bowel sounds. The patient's back and abdominal pain improved after narcotic administration. A computed tomography (CT) scan without contrast showed an abdominal periaortic hematoma. A 2D echocardiogram did not identify a dissection in the ascending aorta or aortic arch. A stable descending abdominal dissection was diagnosed and a vascular surgery consultation obtained for further management.

Different types of pain suggest different etiologies.

■ VISCERAL OR REFERRED PAIN

Visceral pain is poorly localized pain that is usually bilateral. It may arise from distension of abdominal organs, torsion, or contraction. The pain radiates along the dermatomes that innervate the involved organ (**Figure 76-1**). For this reason, it is possible to have pain referred to the back (ie, the posterior portion of the spinal segment that innervates the diseased organ).

Because of visceral innervation, diseases involving the pelvic organs, kidneys, gastrointestinal (GI) tract, and thorax may initially cause isolated back pain.

In general, the referral patterns are as follows:

- Upper abdominal diseases: pain T8 to L1 or L2
- Lower abdominal diseases: L2 to L4
- Pelvic diseases to the sacral region

Usually, the patient has associated thoracic, abdominal, or pelvic pain depending on the location of the diseased organ. For example, sudden lumbar pain in a patient with a coagulopathy may indicate

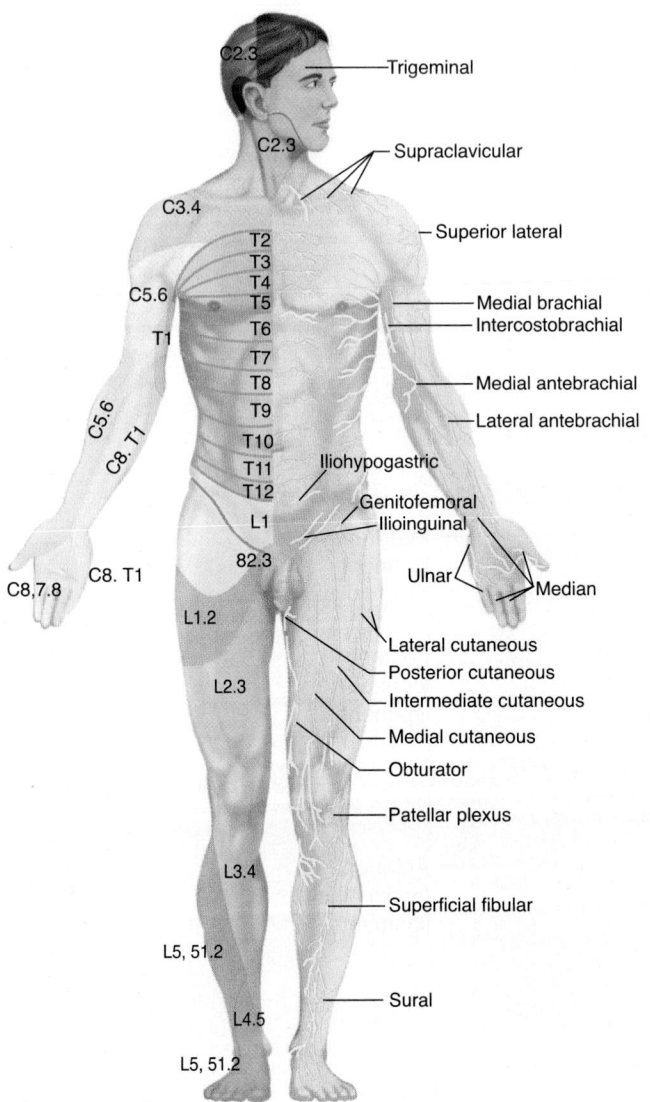

Figure 76-1 *Dermatomes.*

retroperitoneal hemorrhage. Changes in position do not usually affect visceral pain (**Table 76-1**).

■ LOCALIZED PAIN

Back pain may be produced by irritation or compression of local sensory nerve endings. Diseases of any of the pain-sensitive structures of the back—periosteum of the vertebrae, dura, facet joints, annulus fibrosus, epidural veins, and the posterior longitudinal ligament—may cause back pain without nerve root compression (**Figure 76-2**).

Back pain may result from direct injuries (usually musculoligamentous, but sometimes fractures with or without spinal cord trauma) and degenerative processes (spinal stenosis, disk herniation, changes in the intervertebral disks and other structural abnormalities). Ordinarily, the nucleus pulposus and inner annulus fibrosus do not have innervation. However, inflammatory cytokines, ingrowth of pain nerve fibers into the damaged disks, and nerve root injury due to disk herniation have been hypothesized as possible mechanisms of pain related to disk disease. Substantial genetic influences rather than age-related changes determine the incidence of disk disease which recurs in 40% of patients within 6 months. Pain from the lumbar spine may be felt in the coccyx, hips, or buttocks. The pain should not shoot down the posterior thighs without disk impingement on a nerve root.

Structural abnormalities specific to the spine include congenital and acquired anomalies. Spondylolysis is a defect in the pars interarticularis leading to vertebral body instability of the lumbar vertebral bodies that may lead to bilateral stress fractures. In such cases, the activity-related persistent back pain is the main feature of the disease.

Alterations of the microarchitecture of the vertebral body may lead to compression fractures and localized back pain (**Figure 76-3**). The pain may be exacerbated by movement, relieved by lying flat in bed, and may radiate to the extremities. Common underlying causes include immobilization, endocrine disorders (hyperparathyroidism, hyperthyroidism), malignancy (multiple myeloma, metastatic carcinoma), chronic glucocorticoid use, and osteoporosis and osteomalacia.

Bacteremia in the setting of endocarditis, pneumonia, or pyelonephritis may seed the vertebral bodies and disk, leading to osteomyelitis and discitis. Less commonly, vertebral osteomyelitis may arise from local infection, such as postoperative infection after surgery. Extension of infection can lead to meningeal involvement, with an epidural or subdural abscess. The thoracolumbar vertebral bodies are the usual sites of involvement, but any area of the spine may be affected. After spinal surgery, reverse extension of the infection from the disk space to the endplates may occur. *Mycobacterium tuberculosis* of the spine, also known as Pott disease, is common in patients from endemic regions and typically affects the lower thoracic spine.

Arthritic spine diseases include ankylosing spondylitis (AS), reactive arthritis, psoriatic arthritis, and inflammatory bowel disease associated with spondyloarthritis and undifferentiated spondyloarthritis. Patients may report insidious onset of low back pain and buttock pain. A suggestive feature is worsening pain with rest or back pain that awakens the patient at night. Patients with AS frequently report alternating upper buttock or lower lumbosacral pain, deep in nature, which worsens on long car rides or with prolonged sitting. The patient may improve on ambulation or exercise. Patients with psoriatic arthritis, as in reactive arthritis, have their spine involved much less frequently than in AS.

■ RADICULAR PAIN

Nerve roots exit from the vertebral bodies. They may be injured at any point along their intraspinal course to their exit at the intervertebral foramen. Facet joint hypertrophy can produce unilateral

TABLE 76-1 Referred Pain

Visceral Disease	Referred Pain	Pathology	Comments
Peptic ulcers, tumors of posterior wall of stomach or duodenum	Midline back or paraspinal pain	Retroperitoneal extension	
Pancreatitis, pancreatic tumors	Back pain to the right or left of the spine	Involvement of head of pancreas (right sided); body or tail (left sided)	See Chapter 157: Acute and Chronic Pancreatitis
Retroperitoneal structures	Paraspinal pain that radiates to the lower abdomen, groin, or testicles	Hemorrhage, tumors, pyelonephritis	
Abdominal aortic aneurysm	Isolated LBP (15%–20% of patients)	Contained rupture	Abdominal pain, shock, back pain <20% of patients; hypotension 50%; two of three features in 66%; typical patient elderly male smoker
Iliopsoas mass or abscess	Unilateral lumbar pain to groin, labia, or testicles		
Colitis, diverticulitis, or colon cancer	Midlumbar pain ± beltline distribution around body	Lesion in transverse or proximal descending colon (mid or left L2–3); sigmoid (upper sacral)	Lower abdominal pain or isolated back pain or both
Endometriosis, uterine cancers, uterine malposition, menstrual pain, remote radiation therapy to pelvis	Sacral pain	Lower back pain rare except in disorders involving uterosacral ligaments	
Pregnancy	Lower back pain radiating to one or both thighs	Last weeks of pregnancy	
Chronic prostatitis; prostate cancer metastatic to spine; ureteral obstruction from stones	Lumbosacral back pain		
Infectious, inflammatory, or neoplastic renal disease; renal vein thrombosis	Ipsilateral lumbar sacral pain		See Chapter 243: Kidney Stones; See Chapter 197: Urinary Tract Infections and Pyelonephritis
Hip pain	May mimic lumbar spine disease		Patrick sign or heel percussion sign may help distinguish from spine etiologies

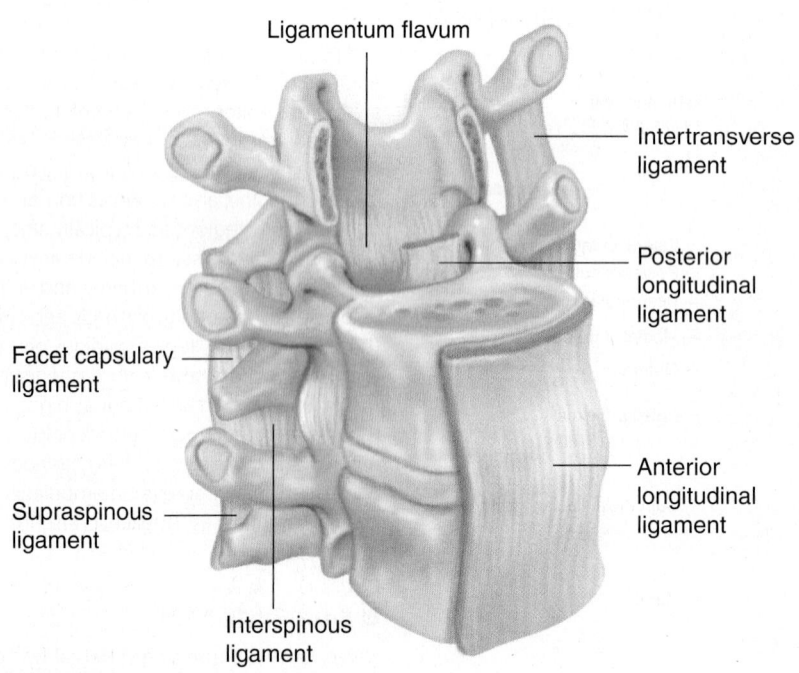

Figure 76-2 *Ligament structures in the lumbar spine.*

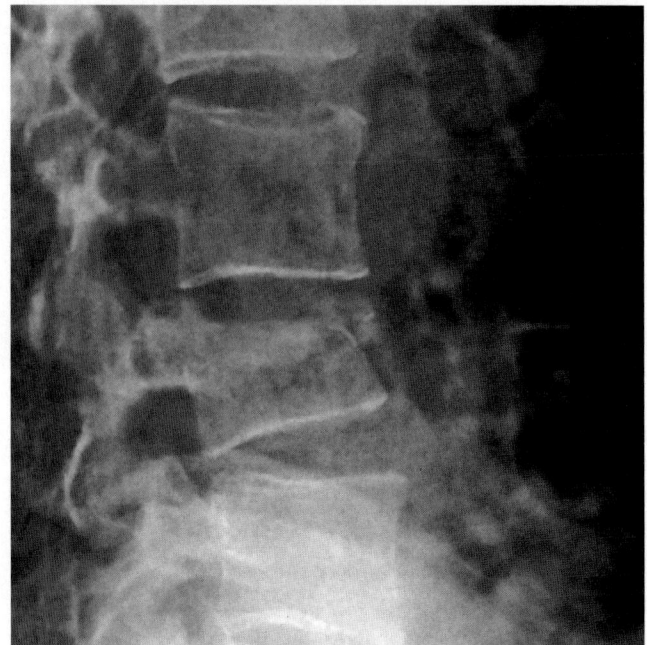

Figure 76-3 *Compression fracture on plain film.*

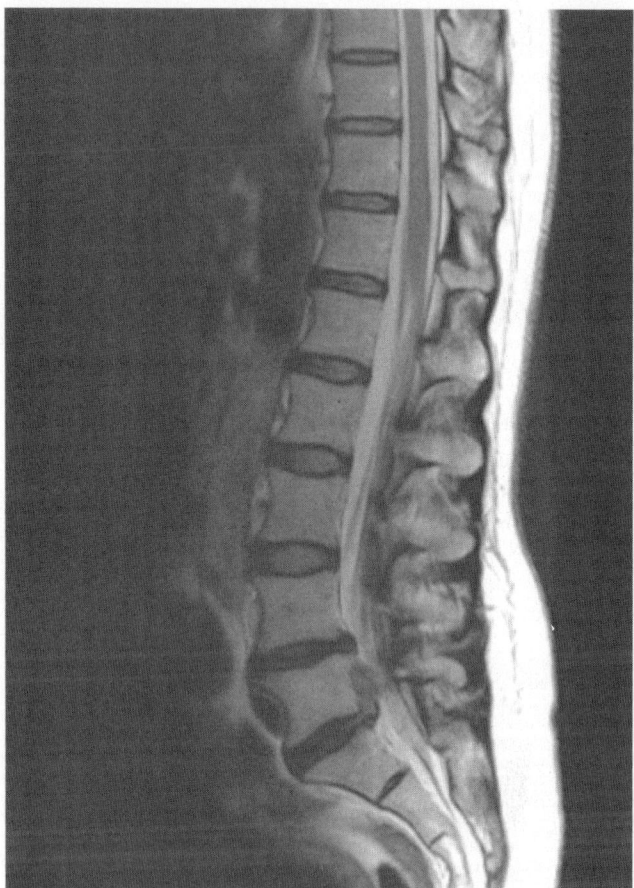

Figure 76-4 *MRI of L5–S1 disk herniation.*

radicular symptoms due to bony compression of the nerve roots. With worsening facet osteoarthritis, cysts may protrude and cause further narrowing of the spinal canal. Referred pain can be associated with radicular pain. For example, a retroperitoneal bleed can cause neuropathic pain along the femoral nerve.

Pain originating from spinal nerve roots may be referred to the extremities. For example, pain originating from the lumbar region may be referred to the buttocks or legs, or localized to the lumbar region. Diseases of the upper lumbar spine may cause pain localized to the lumbar region, groin or anterior thighs. Diseases of the lower lumbar region may cause pain referred to the buttocks, posterior thighs, or rarely, the calves or feet.

Radicular pain is often aggravated by postures that stretch nerves and nerve roots. Because the sciatic nerve (L5 and S1 roots) passes posterior to the hip, sitting increases pain arising from stretching of the sciatic nerve. Pain arising from the femoral nerve (L2, L3, and L4 roots), however, will not be stretched from the sitting position because the femoral nerve passes anterior to the hip.

Disc herniation may impinge upon a nerve root, thereby causing radicular pain. The L5 and S1 nerve roots are involved in close to 95% of lumbar-disk herniation (**Figure 76-4**). These patients will describe a subacute to chronic, deep, burning, aching lower back pain that involves the buttocks and radiates down the posterior thigh to the posterolateral aspect of the calf.

Radiating pain may be elicited by lifting heavy objects, straining to have a bowel movement, coughing, or sneezing.

Spondylolisthesis or anterior slippage of one vertebral body, pedicles, and superior articular facets over another may arise from congenital anomalies of the lumbosacral spine with one example being spondylolysis (**Figure 76-5**); other common causes include degeneration, osteoporosis, trauma, prior surgery, infection, and tumor. When symptomatic, it may cause low back pain, tightness of the hamstring muscles, and nerve root injury, most frequently of L5.

Lumbar adhesive arachnoiditis causes radicular pain due to injury of the subarachnoid space. Multiple lumbar operations, chronic spinal infections, spinal cord injury, intrathecal injection, demyelination polyneuropathies, or neoplastic infiltration can cause inflammation with subsequent fibrosis.

Lumbar spinal stenosis causes radicular pain due to a narrowed spinal canal that impinges on the spinal cord during certain postures. Spinal stenosis may develop secondary to congenital defects such as spondylolysis and acquired causes such as spondylolisthesis or adjacent to prior sites of fusion surgery. The discomfort, commonly referred to as neurogenic claudication, radiates from the lower back to the buttock, and even down to

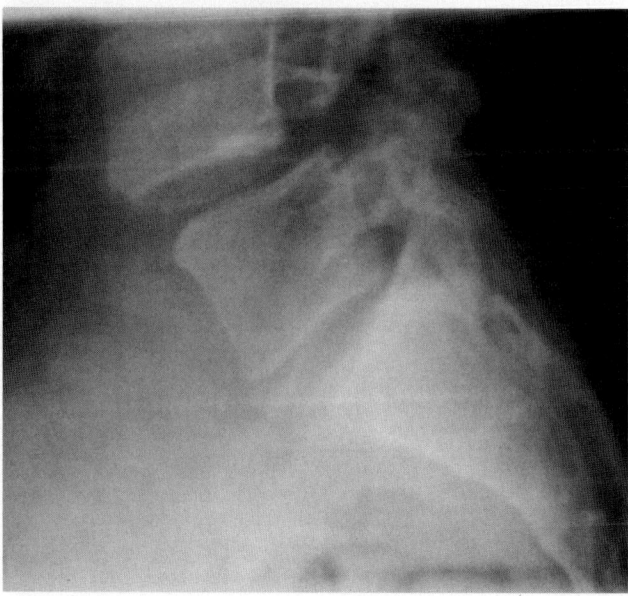

Figure 76-5 *Plain film showing spondylolisthesis.*

the proximal legs (**Figure 76-6**). The pain is worse with prolonged walking and standing and much better on sitting or change in posture—a clear distinction from the inflammatory back pain syndromes.

Cauda equina syndrome (CES) can cause acute or subacute back pain. By definition, it is associated with serious neurologic deficits, such as impairment of bladder, bowel, or sexual function and perianal "saddle" numbness. A centrally herniated disk is the most common cause of this syndrome. Less common causes of the CES include spinal injury, spinal stenosis, neoplasms, abscesses, tuberculosis, AS, spinal anesthesia, back manipulation, or postoperative complications such as hematoma. CES can present acutely as the first symptom of lumbar disk herniation, or insidiously with slow progression to numbness and urinary symptoms. CES need not present with complete urinary retention and reduced urinary sensation. The loss of desire to void and a poor stream are symptoms of an "incomplete" CES. This condition requires a high index of suspicion to make the diagnosis, especially if the patient has pre-existing urinary difficulties. In fact, patients have inappropriately undergone prostate surgery

with no improvement in their symptoms prior to reaching the correct diagnosis of CES.

■ MUSCLE SPASM PAIN

Spasms of taut paraspinal muscles will produce nonspecific localized dull pain aggravated by abnormal posture. Ninety percent of patients with the poorly defined muscle sprain or strain—the most common cause of nonemergent back pain—will recover within 2 weeks. Heavy lifting, pushing, pulling, prolonged walking and standing, and driving are associated with this type of back pain.

Systemic diseases such as primary or metastatic cancer, infection, or arthritic spine disease may cause back pain by multiple mechanisms, including stretching of the nerve fibers entering the spinal cord, disrupting bony structures, occupying space in the vertebral bodies, or referred pain from visceral structures. The most common malignancies that metastasize to the extradural space include breast, lung, prostate, thyroid, kidney, GI tract, multiple myeloma, and lymphomas. Primary tumors—chordomas, neurofibromas, osteoid osteomas, osteoblastomas, hemangiomas, and aneurysm bone cysts—rarely do this. Schwannomas, meningiomas, neurofibromas, and lipomas may grow in the intradural extramedullary space. Astrocytomas and ependymomas affect the intramedullary space. Leptomeningeal metastases, most commonly from leukemia, lymphoma, breast cancer, and lung cancer, may initially present with back pain or postural headache, and signs or symptoms at multiple sites in the spinal cord, brain, and cranial nerves. Pelvic cancer may cause a lumbosacral plexopathy.

PRACTICE POINT

● Thoracic pain suggests metastatic cancer or possibly Pott disease.

CASE 76-2

ACUTE AND SUBACUTE FOCAL LESIONS INVOLVING THE VERTEBRAL COLUMN

A 60-year-old diabetic farmer with a history of prostate cancer and normal prostate specific antigen (PSA) on lupron after radiation therapy 5 years ago reported 3 months of low back pain without numbness or tingling, urinary or bladder retention, or lower extremity weakness. He mentioned low-grade fevers between 100.5 and 102°F that had previously been treated with nonsteroidal anti-inflammatories. He reported a 5-lb weight loss in the past 3 months. He denied any recent trauma to his back but an episode of lower extremity cellulitis required oral antibiotics close to 4 months earlier. He was taking warfarin for stroke prophylaxis due to fibrillation and aspirin for cardiovascular protection given a strong family history of heart disease. His vital signs were normal and his examination significant for focal tenderness on palpating the spinous process of two vertebrae in the mid thoracic spine.

■ DIAGNOSIS

Acute back pain requires immediate assessment to avoid progressive morbidity and mortality that can arise from serious underlying causes. The challenge for the examiner at the bedside is to identify those patients who require emergent consultation and/or imaging due to evidence of:

1. Systemic underlying disease such as metastatic cancer or bacteremia
2. Neurologic compromise
3. Complications of hospitalization that require intervention

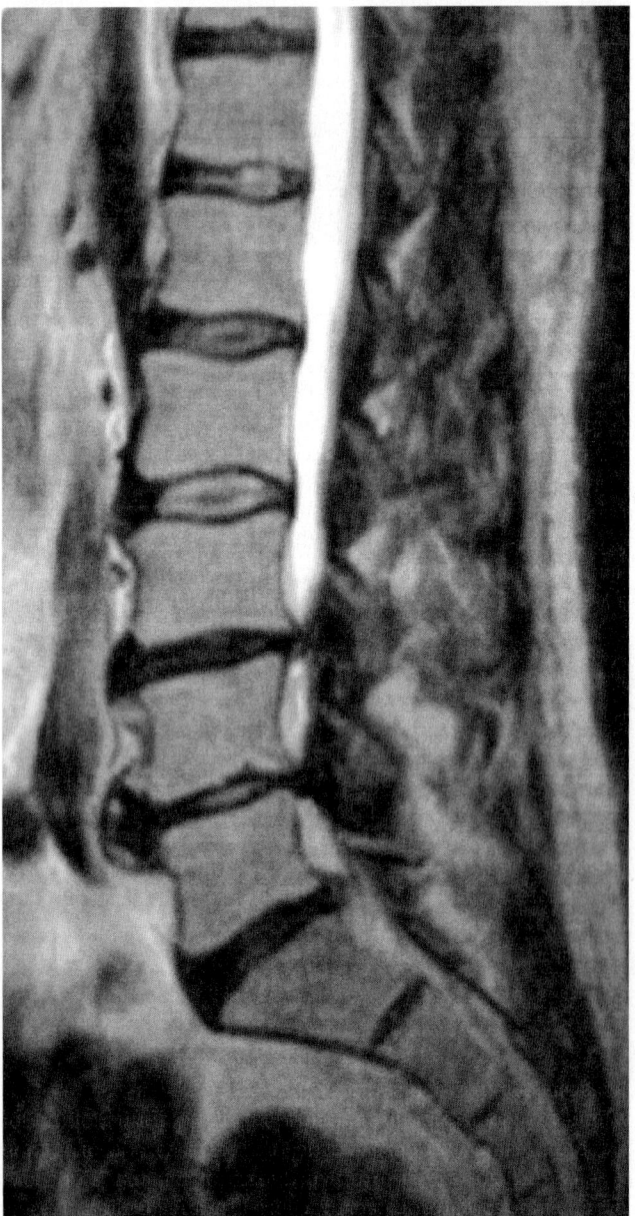

Figure 76-6 *MRI of a patient with lumbar spinal stenosis.*

TABLE 76-2 Chart Review Risk Factors for Serious Underlying Causes

History

- Age > 50 y
- Reason for admission: intractable pain, worse at rest, worse at night, failed conservative management, metastatic cancer, bacteremia (lung, urinary tract, skin), trauma, progressive neurologic problem (falling, weakness, urinary retention, or incontinence)
- Medication use: intravenous drug abuse, chronic steroids, immunosuppression
- Past medical history: cancer, chronic infections, immunosuppression, known coagulopathy or thrombocytopenia, known abdominal aortic aneurysm or significant vascular disease, unexplained weight loss, prior procedures

Medications

- Glucocorticoids
- Antibiotics that may not cover specific organisms likely to affect spine
- Warfarin, antiplatelet agents

Hospital course

- Procedures (epidural anesthesia, spine surgery, lumbar puncture, central lines)
- Unexplained fever

Physical examination

- Fever, hypotension
- Progressive focal neurologic deficits (signs of spinal cord injury, focal weakness or muscle atrophy, reflex changes, diminished sensation in the extremities)
- Percussion tenderness over spine
- Abdominal, rectal, pelvic mass

The hospitalist should expeditiously review the reason for admission to the hospital, past medical history, and hospital course, ask about the quality of pain, and seek neurologic symptoms and signs that suggest a worrisome diagnosis. Chart review, including any consultant notes and prior physical therapy evaluations, may reveal important historical and physical findings that may suggest structural causes (**Table 76-2**).

PRACTICE POINT

- Back pain following any procedure requires immediate communication with the surgeon or proceduralist.

The patient's primary nurse, who has spent time with the patient, should be consulted.

Although more recent systematic reviews on screening red flag questions have warned against their false-positive rates, they provide a framework for the overall clinical assessment and triage process usually in the primary care setting. Recommendations regarding the use of red flags in assessing patients with acute low back pain are summarized in **Table 76-3**.

PRACTICE POINT

- The mere fact that a patient is hospitalized is a "red flag" that the patient is at risk for a serious underlying cause of back pain.

THE PHYSICAL EXAMINATION

The physical examination is helpful if it confirms the examiner's provisional diagnosis. However, the absence of neurologic signs does not rule out catastrophic etiologies of acute back pain. Therefore, clinicians need to synthesize risk factors, past medical history, quality of pain, acuity, and severity of pain, as well as the physical examination, to determine whether emergent consultation and imaging are required.

Vital signs should be checked first. Hypotension, hypoxia, or fever point to systemic disease, such as ruptured aortic aneurysm or dissection, myocardial infarction, bacteremic seeding of the spine, retroperitoneal hemorrhage, perforated viscera, or injuries related to trauma. When there is hemodynamic instability, the focus should be on immediate stabilization and obtaining preliminary tests that do not require moving the patient, such as portable chest radiograph, electrocardiograph (ECG), blood work, and appropriate consultation and triage.

When vital signs are abnormal but stable, the examiner starts with a targeted examination for signs of systemic disease as well as performs a neurologic examination. For example, a widened pulse pressure may suggest aortic insufficiency, and the examiner should carefully perform cardiac auscultation to appreciate an aortic regurgitant murmur. Fever in any patient with back or buttock pain should prompt the clinician to examine the skin for evidence of an embolic process, vasculitis, or infection, listen for new murmurs that may suggest endocarditis, examine the lungs to assess for pneumonia, solicit spine percussion tenderness, which may suggest vertebral osteomyelitis, spondylodiscitis, or epidural abscess, check for costovertebral tenderness that would suggest acute pyelonephritis or renal abscess, examine the abdomen, and to order blood and urine cultures and appropriate imaging.

The back examination begins with observation. Clues to a systemic process include an assessment of whether the patient appears acutely ill, in severe pain, confused, or has evidence of skin abnormalities. The curvature of the spine should be examined for changes in the normal alignment, scoliosis, and other structural abnormalities. Forward bending or asymmetry of the paraspinal muscles is most consistent with muscle spasm. The presence of an indwelling Foley requires a consideration of progressive cord lesions, in addition to the usual causes of acquired urinary retention during hospitalization, such as deconditioning and administration of narcotics and sedatives.

PRACTICE POINT

- In patients with cord lesions, the blood pressure can be very labile. Avoid overtreatment of the blood pressure.

Examination should proceed with palpation of the paraspinal muscles. Palpation and percussion over the spine may reproduce bony pain originating from the spine. The examiner should note whether motion exacerbates the pain during changes in position. Motion exacerbates the pain from vertebral osteomyelitis and mechanical back pain, but rest only relieves mechanical etiologies. Referred pain from visceral structures is unaffected by positional changes. Vertebral tenderness, particularly when elicited by percussion with a fist over the affected area, is a sensitive sign of infection, but it lacks specificity, also being seen in metastatic disease to the spine, vertebral compression fractures, and other causes of localized pain. The bedside examination cannot exclude osteomyelitis. Fever is present in fewer than 50% of patients, and only 15% have motor and sensory deficits.

TABLE 76-3 Red Flags

Serious Considerations	Clinical Findings
Acute, severe back pain with associated chest, or abdominal pain in the majority of patients • Note: specificity of additional features such as ripping or tearing pain or migrating pain in the diagnosis of aortic dissection is unknown Aortic dissection not only causes pain but may be associated with neurologic compromise if the false lumen is supplying the spinal cord	Thoracic aortic dissection and myocardial infarction See Chapter 128: Acute Coronary Syndromes See Chapter 255: Diseases of the Aorta
Back pain that awakens the patient at night	Cancer, inflammatory back pain associated with ankylosing spondylitis (AS)
New-onset back pain in a patient age > 50 y, failure to improve with conservative therapy, pain > 1 mo, previous history of cancer, insidious onset, systemically unwell Pain from bony metastatic disease becomes constant, dull, unrelieved by rest, and worse at night unlike mechanical low back pain	Bony metastatic disease See Chapter 176: Hematologic Urgencies and Emergencies
Risk factors • Recent epidural anesthesia, spine surgery, procedure such as intrathecal devices • Anticoagulant use or coagulation disorder, thrombocytopenia **Symptoms** • Sudden, severe back or neck pain around the involved vertebrae with radiating pain • Within hours to days, ascending numbness, radicular paresthesia, and progressive paraparesis may develop **Treatment** • Early decompressive laminectomy with hematoma evacuation is essential	Spinal hematoma See Chapter 64: Common Complications in Neurosurgery
Risk factors • IV drug use or longer-term catheter placement, recent bacterial infection, immunosuppression from steroids, HIV, or organ transplantation **Symptoms** • Fever, neurologic symptoms	Osteomyelitis of the vertebral body or epidural abscess See Chapter 193: Osteomyelitis and Septic Arthritis
Risk factors • History of herniated disks **Symptoms** • Loss of bowel or bladder function, saddle anesthesia, widespread, or progressive motor weakness	Cauda equina syndrome
Risk factors • Age > 70 y, significant trauma, prolonged use of corticosteroids, altered sensation from trunk down, diagnosis of fracture **Symptoms** • When symptomatic, the pain with a compression fracture may be sharp or dull, localized and may arise acutely or insidiously. Sitting or moving may aggravate the pain while laying supine is usually the most comfortable position	Vertebral compression fracture Vertebral osteomyelitis (spondylodiskitis)
Risk factors • Family history of AS, personal history of psoriasis, uveitis, inflammatory bowel disease, or recent infection **Symptoms** • Gradual onset before the age of 40 y • Worse with rest and improved with exercise • Morning stiffness ≥ 0.5–1.0 h • Peripheral joint arthritis	Axial spondyloarthritis

---

PRACTICE POINT

• Most spine tumors compress rather than invade. In patients with a history of cancer and progressive spinal cord symptoms, especially involving bowel and bladder, assume that cord compression is the cause of their back pain until proven otherwise. Weakness usually affects the legs first, so be sure to check motor function of the lower extremities. Also check position and vibration sense, which are very sensitive for compression.

A straight leg-raising (SLR) test is performed with the patient supine, and the examiner's hand holding the leg straight and cupping the heel. This maneuver stretches the L5 and S1 nerve roots and the sciatic nerve. Passive dorsiflexion of the foot further increases the stretch. Reproducing the patient's back or extremity pain with leg elevation to less than 60° is considered a positive test. Tight hamstring muscles may limit the degree of elevation without pain but would not be expected to reproduce the patient's presenting pain. A positive crossed SLR test reproduces the patient's symptoms in the opposite leg from the

TABLE 76-4 Neurologic Examination

Lumbosacral Nerve Roots	Examination Findings			
	Reflex	Sensory	Motor	Pain Distribution
L2*	–	Upper anterior thigh	Psoas (hip flexion)	Anterior thigh
L3*	–	Lower anterior thigh Anterior knee	Psoas (hip flexion) Quadriceps (knee extension) Thigh adduction	Anterior thigh, knee
L4*	Quadriceps (knee)	Medial calf	Quadriceps (knee extension)[7] Thigh adduction Tibialis anterior (foot dorsiflexion)	Knee, medial calf Anterolateral thigh
L5§	–	Dorsal surface—foot Lateral calf	Peroneii (foot eversion)[7] Tibialis anterior (foot dorsiflexion) Gluteus medius (hip abduction) Toe dorsiflexors	Lateral calf, dorsal foot, posterolateral thigh, buttocks
S1§	Gastrocnemius/soleus (ankle)	Plantar surface—foot Lateral aspect—foot	Gastrocnemius/soleus (foot plantar flexion)[7] Abductor hallucis (toe flexors)[7] Gluteus maximus (hip extension)	Bottom foot, posterior calf, posterior thigh, buttocks

*Reverse straight leg–raising sign present—see "Examination of the Back."
[7]These muscles receive the majority of innervation from this root.
§Straight leg–raising sign present—see "Examination of the Back."
Reproduced, with permission, from Fauci AS, Braunwald E, Kasper DL, et al. *Harrison's Principles of Internal Medicine*, 17th ed. New York, NY: McGraw-Hill; 2008, Table 16-2.

flexed limb. This maneuver is less sensitive but more specific for lumbosacral radiculopathy. The examiner should also perform a hip examination because hip pain can be confused with low back pain and any patient with bacteremia can seed the hip as well as the spine.

The purpose of the neurologic assessment is to identify deficits that would require emergent neurosurgical consultation and to document a baseline examination in the event that the patient goes to surgery (**Table 76-4**). Ask the patient to walk. If a patient is unable to walk due to weakness, the examiner should look for focal weakness that may suggest a cord compression or spinal hematoma. In patients with spinal stenosis, walking in a forward-hunched position may relieve the pain with ambulation (anthropoid posture). These patients may have a positive Romberg maneuver, a wide-based gait, and claudication on forced lumbar extension, but are unlikely to have motor signs or weakness (**Table 76-5**).

Asymmetric reflexes may assist in localization of the defect:

- Hyporeflexia of the patellar reflex: disk herniation at L4; Achilles reflex: disk herniation at S1
- Hyperreflexia below the lesion: spinal cord compression, spinal hematoma, spinal stenosis. Note whether clonus is present
- Absent perirectal tone and perineal sensation: cauda equina syndrome

PRACTICE POINT

- The examiner should document the timing and nature of any bowel, bladder, motor, and sexual dysfunction once a diagnosis that may be associated with neurologic compromise is suspected. Be sure to record any deficits prior to surgical intervention.

USE OF IMAGING TO EVALUATE BACK PAIN IN HOSPITALIZED PATIENTS

Back pain is a common, often chronic, problem that may not require evaluation during hospitalization. Early magnetic resonance imaging (MRI) in outpatients without serious neurologic or systemic signs or symptoms does not alter treatment or overall quality of low back pain after 8 and 24 months. The presence of degenerative lumbar disk changes of herniation, degeneration, or an annular fissure do not correlate with symptoms, and are also seen in 14% to 50% of healthy volunteers. However, hospitalized patients are a different population. For patients with chronic pain in particular, it is important to determine whether the patient has had prior appropriate imaging, if the patient has had a procedure during or prior to hospitalization that might result in complications affecting the spine, and whether the patient's symptoms have changed or simply noted during review of symptoms.

The presence of additional signs, symptoms, and underlying chronic disease conditions determines the proper differential diagnosis and direct selection of imaging. New back pain demands careful consideration of causes for which prompt imaging will avoid catastrophic effects upon patient outcome. Aortic dissection is characterized by back pain and may be accompanied by chest pain or abdominal pain. Physical examination may reveal hypertension, differential blood pressures, pulsus paradoxus, and possibly a pulsatile aorta in addition to evidence of organ compromise, depending on the location and extent of dissection or it may be unrevealing. Recent angiography or other vascular intervention may also increase concern. The diagnosis of dissection and determination of extent must be undertaken emergently. In this case, the rapidity with which the examination can be performed outweighs the imaging modality selected. CT and MRI are both widely used for evaluation of the entire aorta. Dissection may also be diagnosed on angiography and ultrasonography although the extent of dissection

TABLE 76-5 Targeted History and Physical Examination of the Spine

Symptoms including reported neurologic deficits
Onset including precipitating factors: Examples: cord contusion following hyperextension of the spine due to severe trauma with underlying pathology causing stenosis or instability or rarely, spontaneous epidural hematoma following valsalva maneuvers with coughing and sneezing, cocaine use, back manipulation, and even exercise.
Pain (mild, moderate, severe; bilateral vs unilateral; radiating)
Bladder/bowel
Sensory
Motor
Vital signs
Lability of BP (very labile with cord lesions, especially during pain)
Specifically note presence of hypotension, fever in last 24 h
Cardiac examination
Murmurs (especially if fever present or known bacteremia)
Pulmonary
New signs suggestive of pneumonia (especially if fever or known bacteremia)
Abdomen
Bowel sounds
Check for tenderness, guarding, presence of pulsatile mass
Percussion of bladder if urinary retention suspected
Vascular
BP in both arms
Pulses, including examination of extremities for cyanosis
Bruits
Bowel/bladder
Presence of Foley catheter or diapers
Evidence of urinary retention
Spine
Alignment
Tenderness
Spasm
Deep tendon reflexes (biceps, triceps, brachioradialis, knee, ankle, Babinski)
If brisk, check clonus, spreading
If spine cord injury suspected, check abdominals, suprapubic, cremasteric, anal reflexes (place a gloved finger in the patient's anal canal to check the "anal wink" or contraction of external anal sphincter in response to noxious stimuli; place a finger on the perineum right behind the scrotum, pull on penis or bladder catheter to check the bulbocavernosus reflex or contraction of the cavernosus muscle)
Straight leg raise to reproduce patient's pain: L5, S1
Reverse straight leg raise: L3 or L4
Hip
FABER (put ankle on opposite knee; rotate knee toward examination table) positive for mechanical LBP or hip pathology but not for disk disease
Patrick sign (internal and external rotation at the hip with hip and knee in flexion)
Heel percussion sign (tapping heel when extremity extended)
Motor
Deficits (slow movements; fast but weak movements; arms compared to legs)
Atrophy
Fasciculations
Tone (rigidity, spasticity)
Gait
Sensory
Pin
Light touch
Temperature
Cranial nerves (if leptomeningeal metastases suspected)

may be outside the imaging that is being performed for other purposes. The careful evaluation of images by the radiologist makes a critical difference in patient care, particularly when dissection is the cause of back pain for which a spine MRI has been ordered.

Any condition leading to impending cord compression is a reason for emergent MRI examination. There is one exception—trauma. In the setting of trauma, since the most helpful identifications are of bone fragments, CT would be chosen over MRI for initial workup because calcium voids are a limitation of MRI. Regarding cancer and infection, it is the presence and degree of cord compression that is the real emergency issue, as opposed to whether the etiology is due to tumor or infection. Radiography, radionuclide bone scans, and CT scans are helpful for identifying musculoskeletal metastases from a wide variety of tumors but MRI allows identification of nerve roots and tumor extension into the thecal sac. If cancer is suspected, MRI imaging of the entire spine is indicated. Like cancer, epidural abscess usually requires rapid identification and treatment to prevent permanent neurologic deficit. CT may miss a significant epidural collection that could suddenly cause neurologic compromise; thus, MR is preferred. With concerns about the risks of IV contrast enhancement, higher field strengths may allow more alternatives to IV contrast enhancement of MR sequences.

PRACTICE POINT

- Consult with the radiologist at your institution to determine the best emergent imaging study and whether contrast is required to avoid unnecessary delays and to avoid imaging studies that do not rule out the condition you suspect.

In an elderly woman with known osteoporosis, back pain may arise from an acute compression fracture of a vertebra and be confirmed by chest radiographs or radiography of a single region of the spine. Osteoporosis is also associated with chronic disease and treatments, such as steroids making this an even more common possibility among hospitalized patients. Some conditions cause bone deformities that also increase potential for mild trauma to become devastating during a hospitalization. It is important to remember that endoscopic examinations and intubation can stress abnormal spines setting up catastrophic complications. In a patient with rheumatoid arthritis, new-onset neck pain may indicate a C1–C2 subluxation. In a patient with AS, new-onset neck pain may indicate an unstable fracture of the fused cervical spine. In either case neck immobilization should precede cervical spine imaging.

MANAGEMENT

CASE 76-3

NONEMERGENT HOSPITALIST ADMISSION FOR BACK PAIN

A 35-year-old construction worker was evaluated in the emergency department with severe low back pain that had been ongoing for 4 days and has culminated in limiting his ability to walk. He had never had back pain before and the pain was described as dull and constant but markedly worse on ambulation. The pain did not arouse the patient once he was able to fall asleep. Acetaminophen and ibuprofen taken intermittently had not relieved the pain. He denied any pain in his lower extremities, numbness, tingling, or any bowel or bladder symptoms, sexual dysfunction, chest pain, shortness of breath, nausea, vomiting, or abdominal pain. There had been no fever or weight loss. His review of systems was otherwise unremarkable. He drank six to ten beers on a daily basis

and had been smoking a pack a day for 7 years. He occasionally used intranasal cocaine on a recreational basis. He denied using intravenous illicit drugs and reported no HIV risk factors. He has recently started working in his current job, which involves heavy lifting. He reported that his mother has hypertension and his father has both hypertension and a prior history of a myocardial infarction. He also reported a younger brother who has psoriasis. On exam the patient was afebrile. His pulse was 88 beats per minute, and his blood pressure was 140/80 mm Hg. Respirations and pulse oximetry were normal while breathing ambient air. The examination was significant for a negative straight leg test. He had full range of motion of his cervical spine and tenderness to palpation of the paraspinal muscles at the lumbar and sacral spine. His upper extremity strength was 5/5 in all muscle groups but it was difficult to assess his lower extremity strength due to pain with any motion. His labs were significant for a white blood cell count of 9000/mm^3, a normal erythrocyte sedimentation rate, and normal PA and lateral films of the thoracic and lumbar spine. His pain was mildly improved with intravenous hydromorphone at 2 mg every 4 hours, but he was still not able to walk. The hospitalist on duty was contacted to assess this patient for a possible admission.

What emergent causes of back pain will need to be ruled out prior to discharge? What are the more common nonemergent causes of this type of back pain? What are the next steps in this patient's management? How can this patient be safely transitioned to the outpatient setting?

The above case represents a patient who did not appear to have "red flags" that would suggest an emergent cause that would warrant any further testing in an inpatient hospital setting. The history and physical examination in the ED were consistent with acute low back pain that did not portend serious underlying pathology. His presentation was not consistent with a cardiopulmonary pathology. He had no worrisome lab values consistent with an infection or an inflammatory state. His neurologic review of systems and exam did not suggest an acute lumbar disk protrusion leading to the cauda equina syndrome. He was not presenting a history or exam consistent with inflammatory back pain and a spondyloarthritis.

If the patient continued to have difficulty ambulating, an admission for IV ketorolac followed by a transition to oral ibuprofen (with or without a proton pump inhibitor given his alcohol consumption) might be warranted. Based on the patient's wishes and ability to ambulate within the next 12 hours, a social work consultation as well as an inpatient physical therapy consultation was recommended. The patient might be prescribed ibuprofen at 1800 to 2400 mg in three divided doses for 5 days, with consideration of a proton pump inhibitor upon discharge. He should see his primary care physician within 2 weeks of his hospitalization. The patient might also be prescribed cyclobenzaprine at a dose of 10 mg orally at night for the first 2 weeks. It is vital that person-to-person communication between the inpatient team and the primary care physician be established in all cases where compliance is in question or when other specific case peculiarities have arisen during the hospital stay.

Initial management requires a decision about consultation. For interhospital transfers and patients admitted through the emergency department, it is very important to consider a wide range of diagnostic possibilities, in addition to the provisional diagnosis. When a patient is transferred from an outside hospital for intractable back pain, conservative management generally has failed, and emergent consultation with specialists, including neurosurgery, should be considered. The outside films should be reviewed with a radiologist to guide the need for additional imaging. Emergent imaging may be required if there are red flags suggestive of infection or other serious pathology, or technical limitations of the outside films. See Chapter 99 (Pain).

PRACTICE POINT

- Indications for emergent neurosurgical consultation include decompression of the spine in the setting of epidural abscess, tumor, or hematoma; urgent need for a tissue diagnosis; spinal instability, with displaced bone or ligaments; and metastatic disease that has recurred despite radiation therapy.

CONCLUSION

Clinicians need to assimilate the history and physical examination within the context of a new patient—one whose personality, pain tolerance, and unique qualities may not be apparent during a single encounter. Clinically excluding life-threatening and neurologically serious possibilities may require taking advantage of all the resources in the hospital including careful review of the chart, communication with caregivers who know the patient best, framing appropriate questions about risk factors and antecedent events, and emergent consultation and imaging. Although in general, hospitalists should avoid the temptation to pursue unnecessary and expensive diagnostic imaging when chronic conditions do not require inpatient workups such as spinal stenosis, it is also critical to advocate for appropriate and emergent imaging studies in selected patients based on rational choices. The responsible attending should always ask the question: What are the kinds of things that cannot be missed such as acute cord compression that may require emergent surgery and radiation therapy? In these instances, MRI may be the only imaging modality that will give you the information that you need. Although there is a vast literature about back pain in the outpatient setting, it is always important to remember that hospitalized patients are a different population.

SUGGESTED READINGS

Caragee E. Persistent low back pain. Clinical practice. *N Engl J Med*. 2005;352:1891-1898.

Chou R, Hoyt Huffman L. Medications for acute and chronic low back pain: a review of the evidence for an American Pain Society/American College of Physicians Clinical Practice Guideline. *Ann Intern Med*. 2007;147:505-514.

Gilbert FJ, Grant AM, Gillan MG, et al. Low back pain: influence of early MR imaging or CT on treatment and outcome-multicenter randomized trial. *Radiology*. 2004;231:343-351.

Henschke M, Maher CG, Refshauge KM. A systematic review identifies five "red flags" to screen for vertebral fracture in patients with low back pain. *J Clin Epidemiol*. 2008;61(2):110-118.

Henschke N, Maher C, Refshauge K. Prevalence and screening for serious spinal pathology in patients presenting to primary care setting with acute low back pain. *Arthritis Rheum*. 2009;60:3072-3080.

Henschke N, Maher CG, Refshauge KM. Screening for malignancy in low back pain patients: a systematic review. *Eur Spine J*. 2007;16:1673-1679.

Katz JN, Harris MB. Lumbar spinal stenosis. *N Engl J Med*. 2008;358:818-825.

Klinberg E, Mazanec D, Orr D, et al. Masquerade: medical causes of back pain. *Cleve Clinic J Med*. 2007;74:905-913.

Lavy C, James A, Wilson-MacDonald J, et al. Cauda equina syndrome. *BMJ*. 2009;338:881-884.

Wilco C, Hans C, Wilbert B, et al. Surgery versus prolonged conservative treatment for sciatica. *N Engl J Med*. 2007;356:2245-2256.

CHAPTER 77

Evaluation of Anemia

Deborah M. Siegal, MD, MSc, FRCPC
Madeleine Verhovsek, MD, FRCPC

INTRODUCTION

According to the World Health Organization (WHO), anemia is defined as a hemoglobin concentration of less than 13 g/dL in men and less than 12 g/dL in women. Anemia is common among hospitalized patients. In this chapter, we focus on the evaluation of acute presentations of anemia in hospitalized patients, outlining a practical approach for assessment with emphasis on differentiating common disorders from rare potentially life-threatening conditions. We also provide case vignettes to illustrate typical presentations of anemia encountered in this setting.

CLASSIFICATION OF ANEMIA IN THE ACUTE CARE SETTING

Anemia can be classified broadly by the underlying pathophysiological mechanism of blood loss, increased RBC destruction, or reduced RBC production (**Table 77-1**).

■ BLOOD LOSS

Blood loss leading to anemia may be acute or chronic. With acute bleeding, the initial hemoglobin concentration and hematocrit do not accurately represent the actual volume of blood loss. Reductions in hemoglobin concentration may not become apparent for several hours after the onset of bleeding. Clinical presentation is often characterized by signs of hemodynamic compromise, including hypotension, tachycardia, and hypoperfusion. Acute blood loss may be overt (eg, hematochezia, melena, hematemesis, epistaxis) or occult (eg, retroperitoneal hemorrhage). A high index of suspicion for occult acute bleeding should be maintained in patients receiving antiplatelet or anticoagulant therapies, or those with known bleeding diatheses who present with acute anemia and no obvious source of bleeding. In the perioperative setting, worsening anemia should be investigated for occult bleeding at the operative site (eg, retroperitoneal, intra-abdominal, periprosthetic).

Chronic blood loss causes anemia through depletion of iron, which is required for erythropoiesis. Patients with chronic blood loss may present to hospital with progressive symptoms of anemia such as chest discomfort, palpitation, dyspnea, syncope, or severe fatigue requiring urgent assessment and management. Unexplained iron deficiency anemia requires endoscopic evaluation to exclude occult blood loss from gastrointestinal lesions including malignancy. For patients with prolonged hospital admissions, iatrogenic blood loss from frequent diagnostic testing may contribute significantly to blood loss leading to anemia.

PRACTICE POINT

- With acute blood loss, the initial hemoglobin concentration and hematocrit may not reflect the volume of blood loss. Reductions in hemoglobin concentration may not become apparent for several hours after the onset of bleeding.

■ REDUCED RBC PRODUCTION

Erythropoietin is a hormone produced predominantly by the kidneys, which stimulates RBC production in the bone marrow in the presence of adequate nutrients such as folate, vitamin B12, and iron. Impaired RBC production can result from an abnormality in erythropoietin production (eg, chronic kidney disease) or a disorder

TABLE 77-1 Classification of Anemia Based on Pathophysiology

Decreased RBC Production	Increased RBC Destruction (Hemolysis)	Blood Loss
Substrate deficiency (iron, folate, or vitamin B12 deficiency)	Immune mediated • Autoimmune • Alloimmune • Drug induced	Acute or chronic blood loss
Anemia of chronic inflammation	Nonimmune mediated • Microangiopathic (TTP/HUS, DIC, HELLP, SRC, malignant hypertension) • Mechanical (eg, cardiac valve hemolysis) • Thermal (eg, burn injury) • PNH	
Myelodysplastic syndrome		
Bone marrow infiltration (eg, lymphoma, myeloma, leukemia, myelofibrosis, metastatic malignancy)		
Bone marrow failure syndrome (congenital or acquired)	RBC membrane defect • Hereditary spherocytosis • Hereditary elliptocytosis	
Chronic kidney disease	Hemoglobin defect • Thalassemia • Sickle cell anemia	
Liver disease	RBC enzyme defect • G6PD deficiency • PK deficiency	

DIC, disseminated intravascular coagulopathy; G6PD, glucose-6-phosphate dehydrogenase; HELLP, hemolysis elevated liver enzymes low platelets; HUS, hemolytic uremic syndrome; PK, pyruvate kinase; PNH, paroxysmal nocturnal hemoglobinuria; RBC, red blood cell; SRC, scleroderma renal crisis.

affecting the ability of bone marrow precursors to respond to erythropoietin (eg, nutritional deficiency, bone marrow replacement, abnormal RBC maturation).

Iron deficiency is the most common cause of hypoproliferative anemia, especially among females of child-bearing age. Iron deficiency in males or postmenopausal females should prompt consideration of occult gastrointestinal blood loss or malabsorption.

Other disorders commonly associated with reduced RBC production include chronic inflammation, renal disease, liver disease, and hypothyroidism. Folate and vitamin B12 deficiency cause impaired DNA synthesis, and subsequent reduced erythropoiesis. Chemotherapeutic agents, immunosuppressive drugs, and ethanol commonly suppress RBC production. Infectious agents such as parvovirus B19, human immunodeficiency virus, may also be associated with hypoproliferative anemia.

RBC production can result from marrow infiltration by metastatic malignancy, hematologic malignancy (eg, lymphoma, myeloma, leukemia), or myelofibrosis. Myelodysplastic syndrome is a primary clonal bone marrow disorder resulting in abnormal maturation of bone marrow precursors leading to peripheral cytopenias, including anemia. Pure red cell aplasia and aplastic anemia are less common bone marrow failure syndromes.

Stable hospitalized patients frequently develop multifactorial anemia due to suppression of RBC production from infection, inflammation, malignancy, and/or renal impairment that can accompany acute medical illness.

■ INCREASED RBC DESTRUCTION

The normal RBC life span is approximately 120 days. Hemolysis is the premature breakdown of RBCs. The severity of anemia resulting from hemolysis depends on the rate of hemolysis and the ability of the bone marrow to compensate by increasing RBC production. Hemolysis may be congenital or acquired. Although some congenital hemolytic conditions present earlier in life (eg, thalassemia major, sickle cell disease), others associated with mild-to-moderate hemolysis may be clinically silent until later in life (eg, hereditary spherocytosis [HS], glucose-6-phosphate dehydrogenase [G6PD] deficiency, β-thalassemia intermedia, hemoglobin H disease).

Causes of hemolysis can be classified according to etiologies intrinsic or extrinsic to the RBC (see Figure 173-1). Intrinsic factors include abnormalities of the RBC membrane (eg, hereditary spherocytosis, hereditary elliptocytosis), hemoglobin (eg, thalassemias, sickle cell disease), or RBC enzymes (eg, G6PD deficiency, pyruvate kinase deficiency). Extrinsic causes include immune-mediated (allo- or autoantibodies) or nonimmune mediated (microvascular or macrovascular mechanical RBC damage).

Often extrinsic causes will present acutely in patients with no prior hemolytic issues. Patients with chronic hemolytic anemia may present to hospital with acute exacerbations of their underlying condition manifested generally as jaundice, fatigue, and exertional dyspnea.

In patients who have received RBC transfusion in the preceding 4 weeks, features of acute hemolysis may be due to a delayed hemolytic transfusion reaction (DHTR). DHTR occurs when patients develop an alloantibody to antigens on the transfused blood, which can be identified on antibody investigations by the transfusion medicine laboratory.

APPROACH TO DIAGNOSIS AND INITIAL MANAGEMENT

A systematic approach to diagnosis starts with a detailed history including medication review, physical examination, and laboratory testing.

In the acute setting, initial management should focus on assessment of hemodynamic stability in a monitored setting. For acute bleeding, resuscitative measures (eg, intravenous fluids, transfusion) and local hemostatic measures (eg, compression, packing, splinting) should be applied as necessary with early referral for procedural/surgical intervention. Laboratory tests evaluating possible etiologies of anemia including complete blood count (CBC), reticulocyte count, peripheral blood film, ferritin, transferrin saturation, vitamin B12, haptoglobin, lactate dehydrogenase (LDH), and direct antiglobulin test (DAT or Coombs test) should be considered as part of initial investigations prior to administration of RBC transfusion, which can interfere with the interpretation of these tests and the ability to correctly identify the underlying cause.

PRACTICE POINT

• Laboratory tests evaluating possible etiologies of anemia include complete blood count (CBC), reticulocyte count, peripheral blood film, ferritin, transferrin saturation, vitamin B12, haptoglobin, lactate dehydrogenase (LDH), and direct antiglobulin test (DAT or Coombs test). These tests should be considered as part of initial investigations prior to administration of RBC transfusion, which can interfere with the interpretation of these tests and the ability to correctly identify the underlying cause.

RBC transfusion is a scarce resource with associated health risks and should be reserved for patients with severe symptomatic anemia. In unstable bleeding patients, RBC transfusion should be provided to maintain hemoglobin over 7 g/dL, to replace the volume of blood lost and maintain oxygen carrying capacity. In stable critically ill patients, RBC transfusion should be provided when hemoglobin is less than 7 g/dL. Transfusion thresholds for patients with acute coronary syndromes are uncertain and RBC transfusion should be considered for such patients with low hemoglobin and signs of inadequate tissue oxygen delivery.

For patients with ongoing, brisk hemolysis, clinicians must take into account the patient's symptoms of anemia, rate of hemolysis, and reticulocyte response when determining whether to include RBC transfusion in initial management. Frequent serial monitoring of hemoglobin concentration is often required before deciding on necessity and volume of transfusion. For patients with sickle cell disease, we recommend against transfusion for uncomplicated sickle pain episodes, if hemoglobin concentration is near the patient's baseline, and there is appropriate reticulocytosis.

PRACTICE POINT

- In patients with acute bleeding, RBC transfusion should be provided to maintain hemoglobin above 7 g/dL. The threshold for RBC transfusion in stable critically ill patients is 7 g/dL. The transfusion threshold for patients with acute coronary syndrome is uncertain, but RBC transfusion should be considered if the hemoglobin is low and there are signs of poor tissue oxygen delivery.

■ HISTORY

A careful medical history can reveal important information regarding the time course and possible underlying etiologies. Fatigue is a nonspecific symptom but the onset and progression can be helpful to establish a timeline. The presence and progression of additional symptoms such as dyspnea, chest discomfort, palpitation, dizziness, syncope, jaundice, and dark urine can also be helpful. A history of overt bleeding (eg, hematochezia, melena, hematemesis, vaginal bleeding) should be sought. Fever, chills, drenching night sweats, unexplained weight loss, and mass lesions are concerning for underlying malignancy or infection. Excessive bruising and petechiae are suggestive of thrombocytopenia or coagulopathy that can accompany bone marrow failure/infiltration, disseminated intravascular coagulation (DIC), microangiopathic hemolytic anemia (MAHA), malignancy, or infection. Alcohol intake, illicit drug use, and history of sexually transmitted infections should also be evaluated. There may be a family history of anemia or other hematologic disorders.

Details regarding chronic medical conditions should be elicited with particular emphasis on hematologic/red blood cell disorders, renal disease, liver disease, chronic inflammatory conditions, disorders of malabsorption, and malignancy. Pharmacological agents can cause bone marrow suppression and hemolysis and a complete review of all prescription, over-the-counter, and naturopathic medications is essential (**Table 77-2**).

■ PHYSICAL EXAMINATION

A comprehensive physical examination should evaluate for the following:

- General appearance: pallor, jaundice, bruising, petechiae, cachexia, rash, koilonychia (spoon nails), angular cheilitis
- Vital signs: tachycardia, hypotension, tachypnea, hypoxemia, fever
- Cardiovascular system: jugular venous distension, systolic (flow) cardiac murmur
- Head and neck: lymphadenopathy, thyroid abnormalities
- Abdomen: masses, hepatomegaly, splenomegaly, digital rectal exam for blood or melena
- Central nervous system: level of consciousness, focal neurologic deficits

■ LABORATORY TESTING

Evaluation of the complete blood count (CBC), reticulocyte count, RBC mean corpuscular volume (MCV), and review of the peripheral blood film is essential for identifying potential etiologies (**Table 77-3**). **Table 77-4** shows suggested laboratory tests for investigation of anemia with low (microcytic), normal (normocytic), or high (macrocytic) MCV based on the suspected underlying cause.

In the setting of brisk hemolysis or blood loss, the peripheral blood film may show evidence of increased RBC production with the presence of less mature RBC forms including polychromasia (indicative of reticulocytosis) and nucleated RBCs (immature forms). Other findings suggestive of hemolytic conditions include spherocytes (autoimmune hemolytic anemia, hereditary spherocytosis), RBC agglutination (cold autoimmune hemolytic anemia), RBC fragments (DIC, microangiopathic hemolytic anemia, mechanical fragmentation), bite/blister cells (oxidative damage, G6PD), and copious target cells (thalassemias) (see Table 173-2).

The reticulocyte count is a marker of RBC production reported as an absolute count or as a percentage. The normal reticulocyte count is approximately 50,000/μL to 100,000/μL in the absence of anemia, although reference ranges vary between automated methods for measurement. Local reference ranges should be used. When expressed as a percentage, the reticulocyte count is corrected for hematocrit, age, and gender. In the setting of anemia, an absolute reticulocyte count <100,000/μL or corrected reticulocyte count less than 2% suggests a hypoproliferative state. An absolute reticulocyte

---

TABLE 77-2 Common Drugs Associated with Anemia and Their Mechanisms

Direct Bone Marrow Suppression	Aplastic Anemia	Immune Mediated	Hemolysis	
			Nonimmune Mediated (oxidative)	
Methotrexate	Chloramphenicol	Methyldopa	Dapsone	
Cyclophosphamide	Carbamazepine	Cephalosporins	Nitrofurantoin	
Etoposide	Penicillamine	Penicillin	Sulfa drugs	
Hydroxyurea	Acetazolamide	Diclofenac	Methylene blue	
		Procainamide		
		Quinine		
		Isoniazid		

TABLE 77-3 Classification Based on RBC Size

Microcytic Anemia (MCV < 80 fL)	Normocytic Anemia (MCV 80-100 fL)	Macrocytic Anemia (MCV > 100 fL)
Iron deficiency anemia	Acute blood loss	Megalobalstic anemia
Thalassemia	Hemolysis	Vitamin B12 deficiency
Anemia of chronic inflammation	Chronic kidney disease	Folate deficiency
Sideroblastic anemia	Anemia of chronic inflammation	Myelodysplastic syndrome
Lead poisoning	Hypothyroidism	Liver disease
Copper deficiency	Drugs (eg, chemotherapy, methotrexate, azathioprine)	Alcohol
		Hypothyroidism
	Bone marrow failure syndromes (aplastic anemia, pure red cell aplasia, congenital)	Reticulocytosis
		Drugs (eg, hydroxyurea)
	Bone marrow infiltration (metastatic malignancy)	
	Hematologic malignancy (eg, acute leukemia, myeloma, lymphoma, myelofibrosis)	

count ≥100,000/µL or corrected reticulocyte count greater than 2% suggests increased production of RBCs as a response to hemolysis or bleeding.

Coexisting thrombocytopenia may contribute to active bleeding or may be a sign of a process affecting both cell lines (eg, TTP, DIC, bone marrow failure, liver disease). Increased white blood cell count (WBC) should prompt review of the WBC differential, and consideration of relevant contributing processes (eg, infection, malignancy), while low WBC may be indicative of bone marrow underproduction or autoimmune conditions.

■ SUMMARY

Anemia is a common finding among hospitalized patients and is often multifactorial in nature. Infection, inflammation, malignancy, renal failure, and hepatic dysfunction contribute significantly to anemia in this setting. Preliminary investigations should be directed at excluding life-threatening and common causes of anemia. Subsequent specialized investigations should be directed by the results of preliminary testing or reserved for patients with persistent unexplained anemia following resolution of the acute illness.

Key questions to help guide investigations and emergent consultation:

- Is the anemia acute or chronic?
- Is there an identifiable reversible cause (eg, iron deficiency, vitamin B12 deficiency)?
- Is there overt bleeding?
- Has the patient had recent surgery?
- Are there abnormalities on the CBC or peripheral blood film suggesting a primary hematologic disorder (eg, schistocytes, spherocytes, target cells, thrombocytopenia, neutropenia, blasts)?
- Is the patient receiving medications known to cause anemia?
- Does the patient have underlying metabolic abnormalities (eg, renal or liver failure), infection, inflammation, or malignancy?

CASE VIGNETTES

CASE 77-1: ANEMIA IN THE INTENSIVE CARE UNIT

A 48-year-old previously healthy male was admitted to the intensive care unit 2 weeks ago with pneumonia, sepsis, and acute kidney injury requiring renal replacement therapy. He is being treated with antibiotics and remains on a mechanical ventilator

TABLE 77-4 Suggested Laboratory Tests Based on Initial RBC Size

Microcytic Anemia (MCV < 80 fL)	Normocytic Anemia (MCV 80-100 fL)	Macrocytic Anemia (MCV > 100 fL)
Initial tests	**Initial tests**	**Initial tests**
• CBC with reticulocyte count	• CBC with reticulocyte count	• CBC with reticulocyte count
• Peripheral blood film	• Peripheral blood film	• Peripheral blood film
• Ferritin	• Ferritin	• Vitamin B12 level
	• Hemolytic testing (eg, haptoglobin, free hemoglobin, bilirubin, LDH, DAT/Coombs)	• RBC folate
Supplementary tests	• Serum creatinine	• Liver enzymes and function (AST, ALT, ALP, GGT, albumin, bilirubin, INR)
• Iron studies (serum iron, iron saturation, iron binding capacity)	• Thyroid stimulating hormone	• Thyroid stimulating hormone
• Inflammatory markers (ESR, CRP)	**Supplementary tests**	**Supplementary tests**
• Hemoglobinopathy screen (hemoglobin electrophoresis)	• Iron studies (ferritin, serum iron, iron saturation, iron binding capacity)	• Bone marrow evaluation
• Lead level	• Inflammatory markers (ESR, CRP)	
• Copper level	• Serum protein electrophoresis ± urine protein electrophoresis	
	• Hemoglobinopathy screen	
	• Bone marrow evaluation	

ALP, alkaline phosphatase; ALT, alanine aminotransferase; AST, aspartate aminotransferase; CBC, complete blood count; CRP, C-reactive protein; DAT, direct antiglobulin test; ESR, erythrocyte sedimentation rate; GGT, gamma-glutamyl transpeptidase; INR, international normalized ratio; LDH, lactate dehydrogenase; RBC, red blood cell.

and hemodialysis. His hemoglobin decreased from 11 g/dL on admission to 8 g/dL. There is no bleeding. The MCV is 90 fL and reticulocyte count is 50,000/μL (normal range 30-90). The remainder of the CBC and peripheral blood film are normal. Nutritional and hemolytic investigations are negative.

This case illustrates multifactorial anemia commonly encountered in acutely ill-hospitalized patients. Infection and inflammation lead to the production of cytokines, which suppress RBC production through hepcidin-mediated suppression of iron utilization, and suppression of erythropoietin production and activity. Renal failure contributes to reduced erythropoietin production. Frequent laboratory testing leads to progressive iron losses also contributing to anemia. In stable critical care patients, RBC transfusion should be reserved for patients with hemoglobin concentration less than 7 g/dL.

CASE 77-2: ACUTE ANEMIA AND JAUNDICE

A 52-year-old previously healthy female presents to the emergency department (ED) with a 3-day history of fatigue, dyspnea, jaundice, and "blood" in her urine. Her vital signs are within normal limits. Examination is significant for jaundice and petechiae. Initial laboratory testing shows hemoglobin 6.5 g/dL, MCV 95 fL, reticulocyte count 200×10^9/L, platelet count 8×10^9/L, and white blood cell count 8.2×10^9/L. Peripheral blood film is significant for polychromasia and dense fragments/schistocytes. Creatinine is elevated at 1.64 mg/dL. Coagulation tests are within normal limits. Hemolytic indices show low haptoglobin, positive free hemoglobin, LDH 1200 U/L, and bilirubin 3.68 mg/dL. Urine shows "3+ blood" on dipstick testing, but no red blood cells on microscopy.

This case is an illustration of microangiopathic hemolytic anemia due to thrombotic thrombocytopenic purpura (TTP). Although the classic pentad of TTP includes MAHA, thrombocytopenia, renal failure, fever, and neurological findings, a provisional diagnosis of TTP can be made in the presence of MAHA and thrombocytopenia alone. This is to facilitate urgent treatment with plasma exchange due to the high mortality of TTP in the absence of appropriate therapy. Careful review of peripheral blood film is essential, with dense fragments or schistocytes, as the definitive RBC morphological finding in MAHA, alongside the presence of increased reticulocytes. As highlighted in this case, patients (and care providers) may mistakenly identify the red-colored urine as "hematuria"; while RBCs in the urine should be ruled out, this discoloration is typically due to hemoglobin released by RBC hemolysis/fragmentation.

CASE 77-3: G6PD DEFICIENCY

A 65-year-old man with chronic obstructive pulmonary disease (COPD) presents to the ED with acute jaundice 2 days after starting moxifloxacin and prednisone for pneumonia with COPD exacerbation. The patient is afebrile, with oxygen saturation on room air of 95%, blood pressure (BP) of 135/82, and heart rate of 98. He has jaundice and scleral icterus. Chest x-ray shows a consolidation in the right lower lobe. Hemoglobin is 6.2 g/dL, with normal WBC and platelet counts. Peripheral blood film shows polychromasia, bite cells, and blister cells. Blood film stained with brilliant cresyl blue is positive for Heinz bodies. Bilirubin is 4.1 mg/dL, reticulocyte count is 362, and haptoglobin level is undetectable. On further questioning, the patient recalls a prior similar episode in childhood, when he had eaten a large meal

of fava beans in his home country of Lebanon, and remembers being told that it was due to an inherited blood disorder.

The above case illustrates a classic presentation of acute hemolytic anemia due to a stressor in G6PD deficiency. Patients with less severe G6PD deficiency (WHO class II or III) may have only low-grade hemolysis at baseline, which is exacerbated by triggers including fava beans, oxidant drugs, certain chemicals (eg, naphthalene in moth balls), fever, and/or infection. Management of acute hemolytic episodes includes discontinuing the offending trigger and supportive care, which may include RBC transfusion. Prevention of acute hemolytic episodes requires patients and providers to be aware of the underlying G6PD deficiency diagnosis, and familiar with the list of exposures to avoid. Genetic counseling and testing of relevant family members is also important, as G6PD deficiency is an X-linked recessive disorder. Individuals with Hemoglobin H disease (alpha thalassemia) can also experience acute worsening of anemia with physiologic stress or exposure to oxidant drugs.

CASE 77-4: ANEMIA FOLLOWING TRANSFUSION

A 78-year-old male with transfusion-dependent myelodysplastic syndrome (MDS) is hospitalized for worsening fatigue and dyspnea over the previous week. His last RBC transfusion was 2 weeks ago. On examination his vital signs show BP 115/78, heart rate 105, and oxygen saturation 94% on room air. He appears pale and jaundiced. CBC shows hemoglobin of 5.7 g/dL (baseline maintained above 8 g/dL with RBC transfusion). His platelet count is 67 and WBC 2.3 consistent with his baseline values. Peripheral blood film shows spherocytes. Total bilirubin is 2.4 mg/dL which is predominantly unconjugated. Direct antiglobulin test is positive for IgG coating the RBCs. A new anti-E RBC alloantibody is identified.

Delayed hemolytic transfusion reactions (DHTR) result from the presence of recipient alloantibodies directed against donor RBC antigens. Alloantibodies develop during previous RBC transfusion or prior pregnancy. The antibodies are below the level of detection during the initial antibody screen. Re-exposure to donor antigens results in an anamnestic response and increased production of alloantibodies, which bind to donor RBCs and cause hemolysis. DHTRs typically occur within 2 weeks of transfusion and the majority of cases are self-limited. Patients present with evidence of hemolytic anemia including decreased hemoglobin, reticulocytosis, spherocytosis, elevated LDH, hyperbilirubinemia, positive DAT, and positive antibody screen. Patients with alloantibodies should receive compatible, antigen negative blood.

CASE 77-5: APLASTIC CRISIS IN PATIENT WITH SCD

A 25-year-old woman with sickle cell disease presents to her internist's office, complaining of increasing fatigue over the past week accompanied by headache, runny nose, and muscle aches. She works at a daycare and many of the children have recently been sick with "slapped cheek disease." Urgent blood tests drawn in the clinic show a hemoglobin of 5.6 g/dL (compared with her baseline hemoglobin of 8.0 g/dL), with normal WBC and platelet counts. Peripheral blood film shows moderate sickle cells. Reticulocyte count is 8, bilirubin 2.22 mg/dL, and haptoglobin level is undetectable. Blood group and screen is completed and she is sent directly to the Medical Daycare Area where she receives transfusion of three units of RBCs, with a plan to return the next day for follow-up.

Aplastic anemia due to parvovirus B19 can cause precipitous drop in hemoglobin for patients with chronic hemolytic anemia who rely on a steady, high rate of reticulocytosis to maintain hemoglobin levels. Awareness of this association is critical to rapid, accurate diagnosis. Management is supportive and typically includes RBC transfusion and close monitoring of hemoglobin and reticulocyte counts.

CASE 77-6: AUTOIMMUNE HEMOLYTIC ANEMIA–COLD AGGLUTININS DUE TO *MYCOPLASMA PNEUMONIAE*

A 32-year-old woman presents to the ED with fever, cough, fatigue, pallor, and jaundice increasing over the past 1 week. Initial evaluation shows BP 110/72, heart rate 118, and regular, oxygen saturation 97% on room air. Lung auscultation reveals rhonchi in the right base and left mid-zone, and scattered moist rales. Chest x-ray shows diffuse bilateral infiltrates, most prominent in the lower lobes. Hemoglobin is 101 g/dL, WBC 11.7 × 10⁹ with WBC differential showing absolute neutrophil count 8.0×10^9, and platelet count 443. Peripheral blood film shows RBC agglutination and polychromasia. Reticulocyte count is 189. DAT is strongly positive when tested with the monospecific reagent for C3 (complement). *Mycoplasma pneumoniae* ELISA test is positive for IgM. The patient is discharged home with a prescription for levofloxacin and instructed to follow up with his family physician in 1 to 2 weeks for clinical assessment and repeat CBC.

Cold agglutinins are IgM autoantibodies directed against RBC antigens, which bind at low body temperatures (eg, extremities, nose ears) and cause RBC agglutination on the peripheral blood film and complement-mediated hemolysis. Cold agglutinins are a common sequela of *M. pneumonia* infection, particularly in children and young adults. Infectious mononucleosis is also commonly associated with cold agglutinins. Hemolysis in this setting is mild and resolves within 2 to 4 weeks.

SUGGESTED READINGS

Bain B. Diagnosis from the blood smear. *N Engl J Med*. 2005;353:498.

George JN. Evaluation and management of patients with thrombotic thrombocytopenic purpura. *J Intensive Care Med*. 2007;22:82.

Hébert PC, Wells G, Blajchman MA, et al. A multicenter, randomized, controlled clinical trial of transfusion requirements in critical care. Transfusion Requirements in Critical Care Investigators, Canadian Critical Care Trials Group. *N Engl J Med*. 1999;340(6):409-417.

Koch CG, Li L, Sun Z, et al. Hospital-acquired anemia: prevalence, outcomes, and healthcare implications. *J Hosp Med*. 2013;8(9):506-512.

Otis S, Price EA. Hematology-oncology. Hemoglobinopathies and hemolytic anemias. In: Singh AK, ed. *Scientific American Medicine [online]*. Hamilton, ON: Decker Intellectual Properties; 2013. doi:10.2310/7900.1044. http://www.deckerip.com/products/scientific-american-medicine/. Accessed November 16, 2015.

Tefferi A. Anemia in adults: a contemporary approach to diagnosis. *Mayo Clin Proc*. 2003;78(10):1274-1280.

Weiss G, Goodnough LT. Anemia of chronic disease. *N Engl J Med*. 2005;10;352(10):1011-1023.

CHAPTER 78

Bleeding and Coagulopathy

Meridale V. Baggett, MD
Daniel P. Hunt, MD

Key Clinical Questions

1. What are the initial priorities for the patient with severe or life-threatening bleeding?

2. Is the bleeding medically remediable or does it require structural intervention (interventional radiology or surgery)?

3. Does the patient have a coagulopathy or a platelet disorder based on history and examination?

4. What explains an elevated international normalized ratio (INR), an elevated partial thromboplastin time (PTT), and a low platelet count?

5. How should coagulopathy be managed in the bleeding patient?

6. If a coagulopathy is present, what should be done to prepare a patient for an invasive procedure?

INITIAL BEDSIDE PRIORITIES

Initially, the goals for the hospitalist caring for a patient with bleeding should be resuscitation of the unstable patient, control of bleeding, and prevention of further bleeding. Bedside evaluation of patients with apparent brisk bleeding (gastrointestinal, pulmonary, and postpartum) includes vital sign measurement and assessment for adequate perfusion (mentation, capillary refill, urine output). Interpretation of vital sign measurements should take into account the patient's baseline blood pressure and any medications that may blunt the heart rate response to bleeding. Evidence of hemorrhagic shock mandates aggressive resuscitation using large bore intravenous access for intravenous fluids and blood products.

Life-threatening bleeding events may include intracranial hemorrhage (intracerebral, subdural, epidural, subarachnoid), gastrointestinal hemorrhage, massive hemoptysis, postpartum hemorrhage, and retroperitoneal hemorrhage. Spontaneous intracerebral hemorrhage portends a 25% to 30% in-hospital mortality. Upper gastrointestinal hemorrhage from varices predicts substantial in-hospital mortality.

Similar to management of severe traumatic hemorrhage, the bedside approach should minimize the time between recognition of severe or life-threatening bleeding and bleeding control. Each diagnostic intervention, including history, physical examination, laboratory testing, and radiographic testing, should have the potential to lead directly to therapeutic intervention. The adage of the trauma surgeon that "the only diagnostic test that is absolutely required before operating on the severely injured trauma patient is a type and cross for blood products" emphasizes the absolute focus on intervention that is required for acute, severe bleeding. In general, control of active bleeding requires a multidisciplinary approach that may involve surgery, interventional radiology, and/or endoscopy. **Table 78-1** provides guidance regarding the appropriate consultative services to engage urgently for each of the serious or life-threatening hemorrhagic problems along with the anticipated approach.

PRACTICE POINT

- Initial assessment: β-blockers or calcium channel blockers may blunt the usual heart rate response to severe bleeding.
- Among patients with chronic hypertension, a "normal" blood pressure may actually suggest relative hypotension.
- Bleeding from sites that cannot be directly visualized (gastrointestinal, intracerebral, bronchial tree) should prompt great wariness.

SECONDARY HISTORY AND PHYSICAL EXAMINATION FOR BLEEDING DISORDERS

Systematic assessment of bleeding disorders requires a working knowledge of normal hemostasis. The two major mechanisms that contribute to clotting in distinctive but interrelated fashion are (1) platelet adhesion, activation, and plugging ("primary hemostasis") and (2) the coagulation cascade that generates a fibrin clot ("secondary hemostasis") with resultant consolidation of the platelet plug. Endothelial injury that exposes the circulating blood to subendothelial tissue factor and collagen activates both clotting mechanisms. Platelets adhere to exposed collagen and to exposed

TABLE 78-1 Consultative Approach to Severe Bleeding

Bleeding Event	Urgent Consultation	Expected Intervention
Spontaneous intracerebral hemorrhage	Neurosurgery	*Assessment for surgical intervention.**

Traumatic brain injury associated hemorrhage
  -Extradural hematoma
  -Subdural hematoma
  -Intracerebral hemorrhage
	Neurosurgery
	Trauma surgery
		Assessment for surgical intervention.*

Upper gastrointestinal hemorrhage
  -Esophageal variceal bleeding
  -Nonvariceal bleeding
  -Bleeding peptic ulcer after endoscopic treatment
	Gastroenterology
	General Surgery
	Interventional radiology
		Upper gastrointestinal hemorrhage often amenable to endoscopic intervention.
		
		Surgery should be involved in most patients with substantial bleeding and should be consulted early.

Lower gastrointestinal hemorrhage	Gastroenterology General Surgery Interventional radiology	*Lower gastrointestinal hemorrhage may require angiography for localization and potential intervention.*
Retroperitoneal hemorrhage	General Surgery Interventional radiology (Urology)	*Although most patients are managed with conservative approaches and correction of coagulopathy/reversal of anticoagulation, surgical opinion should be obtained early.* *Ureteral compression may require urologic intervention.*
Postpartum hemorrhage	Obstetrics	*Assessment for surgical intervention.**
Massive hemoptysis	Thoracic Surgery Interventional radiology Pulmonary	*Bronchial artery embolization has a role in stabilizing patients and may be adequate primary treatment.*

*Surgical team may request assistance from Medicine in managing coexistent coagulopathy.

collagen-bound von Willebrand factor. Collagen exposure also activates the platelet, inducing a change in the shape of the platelet to a more irregular form that enhances adhesion and interaction with other platelets. Activated platelets discharge fibrinogen, fibronectin, von Willebrand factor, platelet factor IV, factor V, and factor VIII, promoting adhesion and aggregation of other platelets. In addition, activated platelets secrete adenosine diphosphate, adenosine triphosphate, and serotonin that also increase platelet activation. Thrombin generated by the coagulation cascade also aggressively activates platelets.

Exposure of blood to tissue factor in the subendothelium initiates the coagulation cascade, as depicted in **Figure 78-1**. This complex interaction of enzymes and cofactors generates fibrin clot that stabilizes the platelet plug. Deficiencies of components in the clotting cascade lead to bleeding disorders of varying severity depending on the qualitative and quantitative defect. Platelet adherence, activation, and aggregation in combination with the explosive production of a fibrin clot via the coagulation cascade have the potential to induce excessive thrombus formation. Antithrombin, tissue factor pathway inhibitor, and activated protein C limit the extent of clot propagation.

Clotting requires complex interaction of the injured endothelium with platelets and the coagulation cascade. Defects or deficiencies in any of these steps may lead to excessive bleeding or bleeding risk.

The history and physical examination are critical components in the evaluation of a patient with a suspected bleeding disorder. It is important to determine if the patient has had significant bleeding in response to past hemostatic challenges such as dental extractions, surgery, trauma, or childbirth. Ask about each previous surgery in detail, seeking surgical reports of bleeding, need for transfusion, repeated operations, or potential anatomic contributors to operative or perioperative bleeding. Immediate bleeding suggests primary hemostatic defects (ie, platelet abnormalities or vascular endothelial abnormalities, such as blood vessel fragility in senile purpura or scurvy), whereas secondary hemostatic defects (ie, clotting factor abnormalities) typically cause delayed bleeding.

Patients with defects in secondary hemostasis may report a history of hemarthrosis or other deep tissue bleeding. A history of mucosal bleeding usually indicates a defect in primary hemostasis. Examples of mucosal bleeding include epistaxis, oral bleeding, gastrointestinal or genitourinary bleeding (without a local cause such as malignancy), hemoptysis, and protracted menstrual bleeding. Inquiring specifically about transfusion requirements, interventions such as suturing or packing, and the need for hospitalization allows estimation of bleeding severity.

A history of bleeding since infancy or early childhood suggests an inherited disorder. Eliciting a family history of abnormal bleeding can be helpful when considering inherited bleeding disorders and coagulopathies. Lack of such a history, however, is not sufficiently sensitive to exclude a hereditary process. Genetic mutations can arise de novo. Variable penetrance may mask disease in relatives. Recessive genetic defects will not be clinically apparent in relatives with one functional copy of the gene. Further, sometimes congenital coagulopathy may be inapparent until a major hemostatic challenge.

Review of a patient's medication list should include assessment of prescribed, over-the-counter, and herbal remedies. Warfarin and heparin products cause iatrogenic defects in secondary hemostasis. New oral anticoagulants (NOACs) include the direct thrombin inhibitor dabigatran and the anti-Xa inhibitors rivaroxaban and apixaban. The NOACs are commonly used for patients with atrial fibrillation and venous thromboembolism and pose particular challenges in the management of bleeding. Platelet dysfunction induced by aspirin, clopidogrel, prasugrel, ticagrelor, or nonsteroidal anti-inflammatory drugs can contribute to bleeding in the setting of normal platelet counts and coagulation parameters. It is important

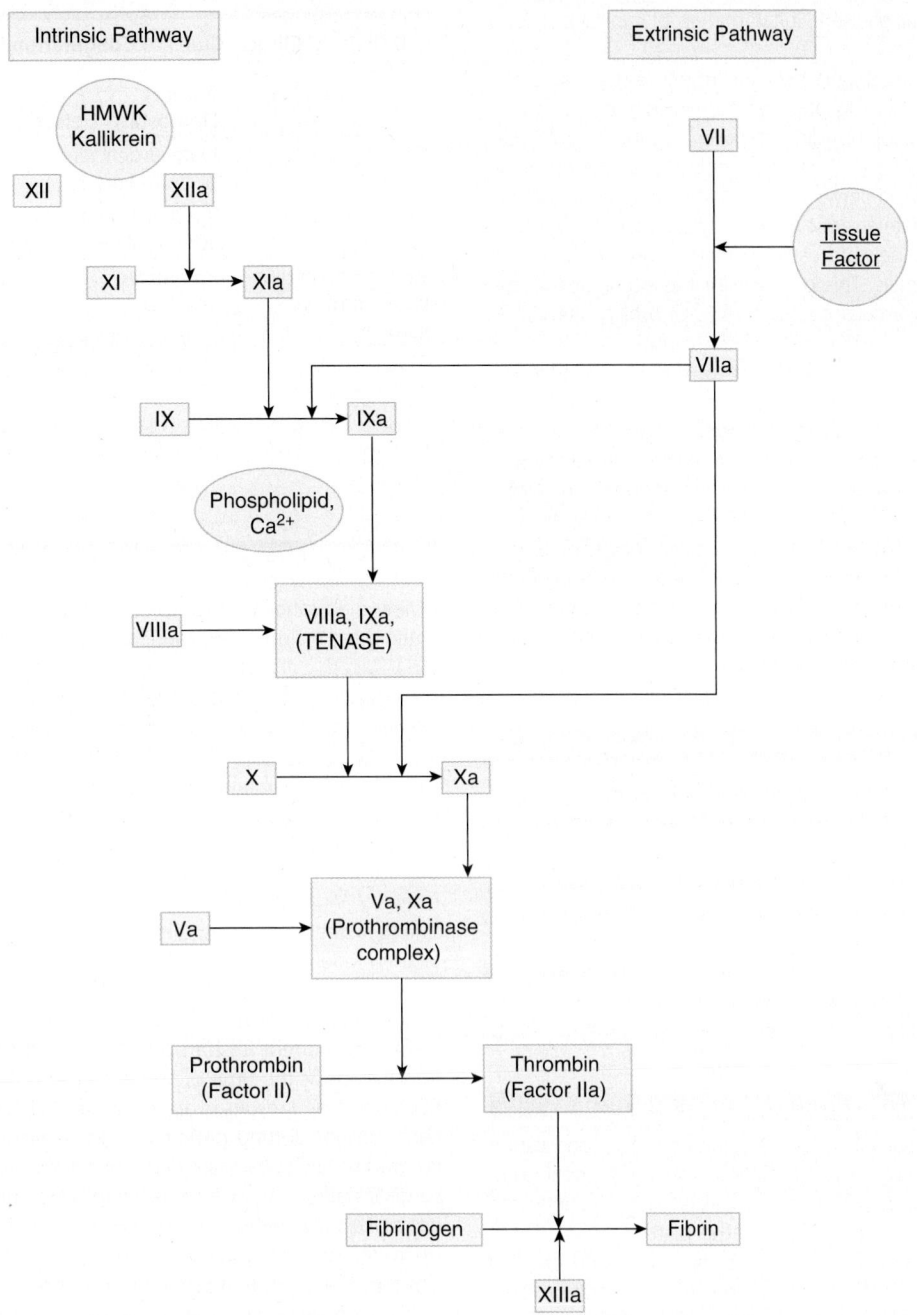

Figure 78-1 *Simplified coagulation cascade.*

for the hospitalist to determine the timing and dosage of any antithrombotic agents that the patient may have received as this information is key to management.

Other medications, such as sulfonamides and vancomycin, may contribute to bleeding through drug-induced thrombocytopenia. Quinine-containing beverages (such as tonic water) or medications can also cause thrombocytopenia. Herbal agents (particularly the "g" herbs such as ginseng, garlic, ginko) have been linked with bleeding.

Patients with irregular dietary habits, such as hospitalized patients, alcoholics, those with mental illness, and the elderly, are at higher risk for nutrition-related bleeding disorders. Vitamin K deficiency can lead to bleeding through coagulation factor deficiencies. Vitamin C deficiency may manifest as perifollicular hemorrhages due to impaired collagen synthesis leading to blood vessel fragility. Altered bowel flora due to recent antibiotic use is another cause of vitamin K deficiency in hospitalized patients.

Examination of the skin and mucous membranes are of central importance in the bedside approach to bleeding disorders. Purpura is caused by the extravasation of blood through the vessel walls into subcutaneous or intracutaneous tissues, resulting in nonblanching skin lesions. Over time, these lesions evolve in color from red (hemoglobin) to purple (deoxyhemoglobin) to green (biliverdin) to orange (bilirubin). Purpuric lesions are classified according to size, which along with location and the presence or absence of preceding trauma can be helpful in identifying platelet disorders and clotting disorders.

Petechiae are nonpalpable purpuric lesions less than 3 mm in diameter. Petechiae should be distinguished from telangiectasias, which are blanchable. Petechiae are most commonly found in gravitationally dependent areas, so attention should be directed to the lower legs, ankles, and feet. Petechiae typically result from platelet deficiency or dysfunction, but can also be the result of increased intravascular pressure, inflammation of capillary beds, or venous stasis.

Ecchymoses are nonpalpable purpuric lesions larger than 3 mm in diameter. The size and location of ecchymoses are helpful in determining the type of bleeding disorder causing them. Small, superficial ecchymoses are most commonly due to blood vessel fragility or multiple blood draws in the hospitalized patient, but may also be caused by platelet deficiency or dysfunction. Ecchymoses from fragile blood vessels are usually round or oval with smooth borders and no necrosis. This differs from the ecchymoses seen in disseminated intravascular coagulation (DIC), which often show central necrosis surrounded by stellate ecchymoses.

Lesions larger than 2 cm or evidence of deep tissue bleeding (eg, hematomas or hemarthroses) indicate a defect in secondary hemostasis. Large, spontaneous, and centrally located ecchymoses or hematomas are more concerning for underlying pathology than the peripheral bruising after trauma seen in patients with normal hemostasis.

Mucosal bleeding is generally due to platelet deficiency or dysfunction. Epistaxis, conjunctival bleeding, or gingival bleeding may be seen on exam. Hemorrhagic mucosal bullae ("wet purpura") typically indicate severe platelet deficiency or dysfunction, and a higher risk for spontaneous intracranial bleeding.

PRACTICE POINT

- Secondary history and examination: Aspirin or other antiplatelet agents are the most common cause of petechiae in hospitalized patients.
- Bleeding from a wound that begins several days after the initial procedure suggests nutritional deficiency or medication-induced coagulopathy.
- Hospitalized patients with limited nutrition or exposure to antibiotics are at risk for vitamin K deficiency.

LABORATORY TESTING FOR BLEEDING DISORDERS

The most useful initial laboratory assessments for coagulation defects include the prothrombin time (PT) that is now most commonly reported as the international normalized ratio, the activated partial thromboplastin time (aPTT), and the platelet count. These studies should be obtained in addition to the history and physical examination in an attempt to determine the presence of coagulopathy and to begin to define the specific cause of the defect.

■ CLOTTING ABNORMALITIES

Table 78-2 summarizes the common causes of elevated INR and/or prolonged aPTT. Prior to considering specific causes of abnormal INR or aPTT, the clinician should consider possible artifactual causes for these abnormalities. The aPTT and/or INR may be prolonged by incorrect collection of the blood specimen. Collection problems include an inadequate amount of blood in the specimen tube which results in elevated aPTT and INR. Additionally, obtaining the sample above or from a line that has been flushed with heparin can prolong not only the aPTT but also sometimes the INR. When artifactual elevation is suspected, the assays should be repeated on a specimen obtained by careful peripheral venipuncture. The measured aPTT may be artifactually prolonged in patients with polycythemia (hematocrit > 55), lipemia, icteric specimens, or hemolyzed specimens. In these situations, the clinical laboratory can be helpful in determining the appropriate approach.

To efficiently assess the etiology of an elevated INR or aPTT, the next step after exclusion of artifactual abnormality is to carefully

TABLE 78-2 Clinical Clues to Coagulation Defects

	Primary Hemostasis Defect	Secondary Hemostasis Defect
Etiology	Platelet deficiency or dysfunction	Coagulation factor abnormalities
	Vascular endothelial abnormalities	
Timing of bleeding post trauma or surgery	Immediate	Delayed
Characteristic bleeding sites	Mucosal	Deep tissue or hemarthrosis
Physical exam findings	Petechiae	Large, central, spontaneous ecchymosis
	Epistaxis	Hemarthrosis

review medications for the presence of anticoagulants (vitamin K antagonists including warfarin, heparins, or direct thrombin inhibitors). Systemic diseases that might prolong clotting time should be considered on the basis of the history and examination. For unexplained elevated INR or prolonged aPTT, a mixing study with normal plasma may help differentiate between a factor deficiency and the presence of an inhibitor. If the aPTT corrects in a mixing study, then specific assays for factors in the intrinsic pathway (Figure 78-1) are indicated. Correction of a prolonged prothrombin time in the mixing study implies deficiency of prothrombin, fibrinogen, or factors V, VII, or X. For a hospitalized patient with an elevated INR due to factor deficiencies, the most common causes are warfarin or vitamin K deficiency due to antibiotics and poor nutritional intake. Additionally, patients who receive large-volume RBC transfusions may develop low levels of remaining clotting proteins even if they receive concurrent fresh frozen plasma (FFP) along with their RBC transfusions at the time of surgery. Each unit (250 mL) of packed RBCs transfused results in approximately a 5% decrease in the concentration of clotting proteins, and the half-life of FFP is hours in contrast to RBCs which are in the order of weeks. For malnourished surgical patients who received significant transfusions, they may not make sufficient innate clotting factors quickly enough to make up for the recent blood loss.

If the mixing study shows a persistent prolongation of aPTT, this implies the presence of an inhibitor of the aPTT pathway. These inhibitors include unfractionated heparin, direct thrombin inhibitors (lepirudin, argatroban), lupus anticoagulant, or specific factor inhibitors including inhibitors of factor VIII or factor V. Additional studies that allow the laboratory to determine the presence of heparin or a direct thrombin inhibitor include the thrombin time (TT) and reptilase time. Either class of drugs will prolong the TT, but demonstrate a normal reptilase time.

Persistent prolongation of the prothrombin time despite mixing with normal serum implies an inhibitor of the PT pathway and generally is associated with prolongation and inhibition of the aPTT. These inhibitors include factor V inhibitors, direct thrombin inhibitors, excess heparin in the laboratory specimen, or, less commonly, a lupus anticoagulant.

If the examination demonstrates petechiae or there is significant mucosal bleeding, a quantitative or qualitative abnormality of platelets should be considered. There are many potential causes of thrombocytopenia in hospitalized patients. **Table 78-3** provides a framework for considering a low platelet count. Assessment of platelet function is more difficult, although the medication history is often revealing as the most common causes of petechiae or platelet

TABLE 78-3 Causes of Thrombocytopenia

Decreased Platelet Production		Increased Platelet Destruction	
Marrow Processes	Other Processes Affecting Production	Immune-Mediated Processes	Consumptive Processes
Myeloproliferative disorders	Drugs	Immune thrombocytopenia purpura (ITP)	Thrombotic thrombocytopenia purpura (TTP)
Aplastic anemia	B12 or folate deficiency	Drugs (eg, heparin)	Hemolytic uremic syndrome (HUS)
Radiation	Infections (such as HIV or parvovirus)	Infections	Sepsis
	Cirrhosis (decreased thrombopoietin)	Post-transfusion	Eclampsia/HELLP syndrome
			Disseminated intravascular coagulation
			Hypersplenism

dysfunction among hospitalized patients are antiplatelet medications. See Chapter 171 (Platelets).

Although the bleeding time was traditionally used as an initial screening test for primary hemostasis, recent guidelines argue against its use. The test requires a small incision of the skin followed be measurement of time to clot formation. Technical variables that make reproducibility of the test challenging include direction of the incision, exercise, cuff pressure on the tested arm, previous testing, patient anxiety, local edema, and excessive wiping of the incision make reproducibility of the test challenging. Numerous medications (including aspirin, nonsteroidal anti-inflammatories, antibiotics, calcium channel blockers) and clinical conditions (including von Willebrand disease, uremia, liver disorders, paraproteinemias, chronicmyeloproliferative disorders) may cause prolongation of the bleeding time (**Table 78-4**). A prolonged bleeding time, even assuming technical reliability, is a very nonspecific finding. Additionally, normal bleeding times do not assure hemostasis with invasive procedures, while prolonged bleeding times are not necessarily associated with excessive hemorrhage. A 1998 position statement from the College of American Pathologists and the American Society of Clinical Pathologists concluded that the bleeding time test failed as a screening test. Many hospital laboratories no longer offer the bleeding time test. Automated platelet function testing may provide better insight when patients are suspected to have defects

TABLE 78-4 Causes of Abnormal INR or aPTT

Test Result		Causes	
INR	aPTT	Inherited	Acquired
Elevated	Normal	Factor VII deficiency	Warfarin or other coumarins (such as rat poison)
			Neworal anticoagulants
			Liver disease
			Vitamin K deficiency
			Acquired factor VII deficiency
			Inhibitor of factor VII
Normal	Prolonged	Deficiency of factors VIII, IX, or XI	Heparin
		Deficiency of factor XII, prekallikrein, or high-molecular-weight kininogen (HMWK) (associated with abnormal labs but not bleeding)	Low molecular weight heparin (particularly when dosed excessively)
		von Willebrand disease	Neworal anticoagulants
			Inhibitor of factors VIII, IX, XI, or XII
			Acquired von Willebrand disease
			Lupus anticoagulant
Elevated	Prolonged	Deficiency of prothrombin, fibrinogen, or factors V or X	Liver disease
		Dysfibrinogenemia	Disseminated intravascular coagulation
		Combined factor deficiencies	Heparin
			Supratherapeutic warfarin, or other coumarins
			Vitamin K deficiency
			Combined warfarin and heparin
			Inhibitor of prothrombin, fibrinogen, or factor V or X
			Direct thrombin inhibitors (including dabigatran)
			Neworal anticoagulants (rivaroxaban, apixaban)
			Primary amyloidosis (factor X deficiency)

in primary hemostasis, but have normal PT, PTT, and platelet count. The Platelet Function Analyzer (PFA-100) has been adopted by many laboratories and has received considerable attention in the literature. This test stimulates platelets through interaction with a membrane coated with collagen and either adenosine diphosphate or epinephrine and then measures the time required for the platelets to close an aperture of the membrane. This is thought to simulate the adhesion and aggregation of platelets in vivo. A systematic review found that the sensitivity of the PFA-100 system is 82% to 89%, while the specificity is 67% to 86% for detection of a defect in primary hemostasis as determined by more comprehensive platelet function testing. For patients who are highly suspected of having a disorder of platelet function, a negative PFA-100 test would not absolutely exclude a functional problem. In these cases, consultation with a hematologist and with the clinical laboratory is advisable.

PRACTICE POINT

- Laboratory evaluation: If the INR and/or aPTT are unexpectedly elevated, the studies should be repeated to exclude artifact.
- Mixing studies are a key step in determining whether the apparent defect is a deficiency or an inhibitor of factor(s) in the coagulation pathway.
- Bleeding time is no longer used to assess platelet function.

TREATMENT OF COAGULOPATHY IN THE BLEEDING PATIENT

The bleeding patient should be assessed for concomitant acute or chronic defects in either primary or secondary hemostasis so that appropriate corrective treatment can be administered alongside hemodynamic support and transfusion of red blood cells in anticipation of any necessary structural interventions. **Table 78-5** summarizes treatment options to address hemostasis defects in bleeding patients.

It is useful to assess the degree of bleeding using the WHO bleeding grades when deciding interventions for coagulopathies. The grades are as follows: Grade 0 = no bleeding; Grade 1 = petechiae, ecchymosis, mucosal bleeding; Grade 2 = gross bleeding, including melena, hematemesis, hematuria, or hemoptysis; Grade 3 = bleeding that requires red blood cell transfusion; and Grade 4 = retinal bleeding with visual impairment, intracranial bleeds, and life-threatening bleeds (massive gastrointestinal hemorrhage, retroperitoneal hemorrhage, massive hemoptysis). For hemorrhage that is considered WHO Grade 2 or greater, platelet transfusions are indicated if thrombocytopenia is present although the specific threshold for transfusion should be individualized. In general, the target for the platelet count after transfusion should be greater than 50,000. Transfusion of platelets for patients with suspected platelet dysfunction is reasonable in the setting of substantial bleeding, although there are no readily available laboratory parameters to guide management.

Recent guidelines emphasize a preference for use of prothrombin complex concentrates (PCC) in the management of major bleeding in patients with vitamin K deficiency or warfarin therapy. PCC contains concentrated vitamin-K-dependent coagulation factors, does not require thawing, and is administered in a relatively small volume. Three-factor PCC that is available in the United States contains factors II, IX, and X (refer to Figure 78-1), while four-factor PCC contains factors II, VII, IX, and X. Emergent reversal of warfarin should be addressed with weight-based dosing of PCC along with IV vitamin K.

Fresh frozen plasma (FFP) contains plasma proteins including coagulation factors. It may be used for bleeding patients with vitamin K deficiency or warfarin therapy although it is considered suboptimal and should only be used if PCC is not available. FFP may also be used to manage bleeding and coagulopathies associated with liver disease, acute DIC with a treatable trigger, massive transfusion, and acquired deficiencies of single coagulation factors. Laboratory parameters that would prompt use of FFP to address bleeding in any of these conditions include significantly increased prothrombin time, INR, or aPTT, although massive red blood cell transfusion of greater than one blood volume should prompt consideration of FFP

TABLE 78-5 **Management of Coagulopathy in the Bleeding Patient**

Defect	Treatment	Suggested Initial Dose	Expected Response	Potential Complications
Primary Hemostasis				
Thrombocytopenia or platelet dysfunction (ie, NSAID use)	Platelet transfusion	6 pack (4-6 whole blood derived units pooled) or one apheresis unit	30-60,000/μL increase in platelet count	Infection Hemolytic transfusion reaction Transfusion-related acute lung injury (TRALI)
Secondary Hemostasis				
Elevated PTT with unknown factor deficiency	Fresh frozen plasma	10-15 mL/kg	Not well defined	Infection Hemolytic transfusion reaction TRALI Volume overload
Vitamin K deficiency (ie, nutritional deficiency or warfarin use)	Vitamin K* Prothrombin complex concentrate Fresh frozen plasma	10 mg IV Dosage varies dependent on manufacturer 10-15 mL/kg	INR improvement within 4-6 h Emergent reversal of vitamin K antagonists Not well defined	Anaphylaxis Overcorrection and warfarin resistance Potential risk of venous and arterial thrombosis See above

*For serious bleeding, administer prothrombin complex concentrate concurrently for immediate replacement of vitamin-K-dependent coagulation factors.

even if coagulation parameters are unknown. FFP carries a substantial risk of transfusion-related acute lung injury (TRALI) and a number of studies caution about its overuse, particularly for patients with minimally elevated INR (up to 1.7) or aPTT. Oral vitamin K is the preferred route of administration for most patients with mildly elevated INR in the absence of life-threatening hemorrhage.

PRACTICE POINT

- Correction of coagulopathy: Patients with severe bleeding and suspected platelet dysfunction (eg, from antiplatelet agents) should be considered for platelet transfusion despite normal platelet counts.
- FFP and platelet transfusions are associated with a higher risk of transfusion-related acute lung injury than red blood cell transfusions.

BLEEDING AND NOACs

The new oral anticoagulants (NOACs) present assessment and management challenges for practicing hospitalists. These agents have also been called novel oral anticoagulants or target specific oral anticoagulants (TSOACs).

Dabigatran is a direct thrombin inhibitor that is excreted by the kidneys. Although there are no readily available reliable laboratory tests for the anticoagulant effects of dabigatran, a normal aPTT and normal thrombin time suggest that high levels are not present in the bleeding patient. Hemodialysis would be expected to accelerate clearance of dabigatran, although this can be challenging to employ in an acutely ill, bleeding patient. For patients with ongoing life-threatening bleeding, options would include PCC, activated PCC (APCC), or recombinant Factor VIIa (rFVIIa), although these recommendations are based on case reports, animal studies, and expert opinion. A recent clinical trial of idarucizumab, a monoclonal antibody fragment with very high affinity for binding dabigatran, showed very rapid reversal of anticoagulant effect and may become standard of care for patients with life-threatening hemorrhage in the setting of dabigatran.

Rivaroxaban and apixaban are oral factor Xa inhibitors. Both agents are tightly protein bound and therefore are not removed by dialysis. There are no specific pharmacologic countermeasures for these agents, so for the majority of bleeding patients, the best approach is cessation of the drug and addressing the source of bleeding. For ongoing life-threatening bleeding, PCC, APCC, or rFVIIa could be considered. However, both APCC and rFVIIa incur an increased risk of thrombosis.

Hospitalists should strongly consider obtaining hematology consultation for patients receiving NOACs when faced with bleeding or when considering periprocedural or perioperative risks for these patients.

INVASIVE PROCEDURES IN THE COAGULOPATHIC PATIENT

Hospitalized patients are frequently subjected to invasive procedures for both diagnostic and therapeutic purposes, and hospitalists frequently consult on patients prior to surgical procedures. The potential for bleeding complications plays a central role in the discussion of risks and benefits of proposed procedures, and despite a lack of high-quality evidence to support indiscriminant preprocedural coagulation testing, it is common practice for patients to have coagulation testing in anticipation of most procedures. However, identifying patients at high risk for bleeding requires a clinical history and should not rely on laboratory testing alone. PT and PTT tests may be insensitive to rare but clinically important bleeding disorders. For example, patients with factor XIII deficiency (who usually have a positive

bleeding history) may have normal PT and PTT tests, but experience life-threatening surgical bleeding. Current recommendations from the British Committee for Standards in Hematology are to obtain a bleeding history in all patients undergoing invasive procedures or surgery, including bleeding following prior trauma or surgery, a family history of bleeding, and the use of prescription and nonprescription medications that predispose to bleeding.

Selected patients should undergo coagulation testing. Patients who may benefit from coagulation testing include those with a positive bleeding history, evidence of systemic disease that may affect coagulation (eg, liver disease), or risk factors for malabsorption or malnutrition. Patients planned for procedures associated with a higher risk of morbidity and mortality from bleeding complications (eg, intracranial, neurosurgical) typically have preoperative coagulation testing.

Patients with abnormal bleeding histories or other clinical indications warrant directed diagnostic testing guided by their clinical features and may require hematology consultation to help guide further workup and the plan for correction prior to undergoing procedures.

If diagnostic testing reveals prolongation of the PT, options for correction will be dictated by the underlying etiology. Those with nutritional deficiencies typically respond to administration of vitamin K. While oral administration of vitamin K is slower to take effect, there is less risk of anaphylaxis which has been associated with intravenous administration of vitamin K. Subcutaneous vitamin K works more slowly than oral vitamin K, and in one meta-analysis was similar to placebo in treating excessive anticoagulation.

Although widely practiced, the prophylactic use of FFP for patients with prolonged PT undergoing procedures lacks sufficient evidence to support or refute its efficacy and the potential hazards of transfusion are well documented. In patients with minimally prolonged PT, transfusion of FFP may have little effect on the PT, and the effects may be transient if the patient is not provided with substrate (vitamin K) to generate more clotting factors. Many inpatient procedures are performed by specialists and interventional radiologists, and the preference and comfort of the operator will largely drive the preprocedural testing and transfusion practice. See Chapter 43 (Hemostasis).

PRACTICE POINT

- Preprocedure evaluation for coagulopathy: Obtaining a bleeding history from a patient may help uncover coagulopathies not evident on routine testing.
- Oral vitamin K is the preferred treatment of nutrition-related coagulopathy in patients planned for nonemergent procedures.
- If possible, procedures should be delayed to allow clearance of the anticoagulant effect of NOACs.

CONCLUSION

The approach to a bleeding patient starts with emergent resuscitation if required, identification of the bleeding site, evaluation for the presence of a coagulopathy (initially PT, INR, aPTT, and platelet count), and management of bleeding which may require specialty consultation. A stepwise approach begins with a focused history and physical examination. The cause of a surgical patient's elevated INR and bleeding are most likely due to a number of factors: (1) poor nutrition causing relative vitamin K deficiency, (2) exposure to broad spectrum antibiotics, (3) exposure to anticoagulants, and/or (4) in cases of major trauma requiring recent large-volume RBC transfusion, low levels of remaining clotting proteins. Other considerations for an elevated INR in the absence of warfarin include: severe liver disease (history of alcohol use, abnormal liver function tests, clinical signs of cirrhosis, preoperative elevation of INR), acquired factor VIII inhibitors or factor VIII deficiency, von Willebrand disease causing some degree of factor VIII deficiency, DIC or significant renal or hepatic insufficiency resulting in supratherapeutic doses of low molecular weight heparin.

Evaluation of thrombocytopenia should include review of the peripheral smear. The timing of onset of thrombocytopenia is a valuable clue regarding its possible etiologies. In general, patients with low platelet counts or documented platelet function abnormalities who are bleeding are likely to benefit from platelet transfusions. However, unlike correction of anemia, not all causes of thrombocytopenia may be safely treated with the transfusion of platelet products. Conditions associated with immune destruction of platelets (such as immune thrombocytopenia or heparin induced thrombocytopenia) or microangiopathic hemolysis (thrombotic thrombocytopenic purpura) can be dangerously aggravated by platelet transfusions. See Chapter 77 (Anemia) and Chapter 172 (Bleeding Disorders).

SUGGESTED READINGS

Chee YL, Crawford JC, Watson HG, Greaves M. Guidelines on the assessment of bleeding risk prior to surgery or invasive procedures. British Committee for Standards in Haematology. *Br J Haematol.* 2008;140(5):496-504.

Crowther M, Crowther MA. Antidotes for novel oral anticoagulants: current status and future potential. *Arterioscler Thromb Vasc Biol.* 2015;35:1736-1745.

De Simone N, Sarode R. Diagnosis and management of common acquired bleeding disorders. *Semin Thromb Hemost.* 2013;39:172-181.

Hurwitz A, Massone R, Lopez BL. Acquired bleeding disorders. *Emerg Med Clin North Am.* 2014;32:691-713.

Kamal AH, Tefferi A, Pruthi RK. How to interpret and pursue an abnormal prothrombin time, activated partial thromboplastin time, and bleeding time in adults. *Mayo Clin Proc.* 2007;82(7):864-873.

Lippi G, Franchini M, Montagnana M, Favaloro EJ. Inherited disorders of blood coagulation. *Ann Med.* 2012;44:405-418.

Makris M, Van Veen JJ, Tait CR, Mumford AD, Laffan M. British Committee for Standards in H. Guideline on the management of bleeding in patients on antithrombotic agents. *Br J Haematol.* 2013;160:35-46.

Rossaint R, Duranteau J, Stahel PF, Spahn DR. Nonsurgical treatment of major bleeding. *Anesthesiol Clin.* 2007;25(1):35-48, viii.

Tanaka KA, Key NS, Levy JH. Blood coagulation: hemostasis and thrombin regulation. *Anesth Analg.* 2009;108(5):1433-1446.

CHAPTER 79

Chest Pain

Kittane S. Vishnupriya, MBBS
Arjun S. Chanmugam, MD, MBA

Key Clinical Questions

1. What signs and symptoms point to a serious cause of cardiogenic chest pain?

2. What key historical elements will help to narrow the differential diagnosis?

3. What studies should be ordered to evaluate a patient presenting with suspected cardiac ischemia?

INTRODUCTION

According to the 2006 National Hospital Ambulatory Medical Care Survey, 6,392,000 patients presented to emergency departments (ED) with a chief complaint of chest pain or related symptoms. Of those, 1,976,000 patients were admitted to the hospital, with a mean length of stay of 3.7 days. Chest pain was the principal admitting diagnosis in 5.4% of all admitted patients.

Because morbidity and mortality is high if clinicians "miss" a cardiac presentation of chest pain, a significant portion of these admissions are specifically for the purpose of ruling out myocardial ischemia or infarction. In one study of patients presenting to an emergency department with complaints consistent with cardiac ischemia, 17% ultimately had cardiac ischemia, while 27% had stable angina or other cardiac conditions. Fifty-five percent had noncardiac conditions diagnosed as the cause of their symptoms. The wide differential diagnosis for this heterogeneous group of patients includes nonischemic life-threatening etiologies as well as more benign causes. Despite the focus on cardiac causes, in this study, 2.1% of the patients with acute myocardial infarction were erroneously discharged; this figure and the concern it generates may play prominently in the low threshold to admit patients with chest pain.

Chest pain also occurs in patients already admitted to the hospital for other reasons. These patients have already suffered some degree of physical decompensation and an occurrence of chest pain may indicate illness, a complication of hospitalization, or a patient's response to a very stressful situation. The hospitalist must evaluate the possibility of an immediate life-threatening event, consider the entire differential of possible etiologies, and integrate this information with the patient's prior clinical diagnoses and course. The focus of this chapter will be on the initial evaluation of patients presenting with chest pain, specifically targeting the investigation of cardiac ischemia in those patients.

BEDSIDE APPROACH

■ INITIAL RAPID ASSESSMENT

The initial evaluation of a patient reporting chest pain requires the rapid identification and treatment of any life-threatening conditions. These include the five "do-not-miss" causes of chest pain: (1) aortic dissection, (2) acute myocardial infarction (MI), (3) pulmonary embolism (PE), (4) pneumothorax, and (5) esophageal rupture (**Table 79-1**). The electrocardiogram (ECG) is one of the most important screening tests for early risk stratification and is often performed at the point of triage as one of the "vital signs."

All potentially unstable patients with chest pain should have an intravenous line, supplemental oxygen, and a cardiac monitor placed as soon as possible. This can be accomplished even before the arrival of the physician at the patient's bedside. Empiric treatment with aspirin and sublingual nitroglycerin should be given if cardiac chest pain is suspected unless there are specific contraindications. An initial assessment should include a review of the ECG, analysis of current vital signs, and a targeted history and physical examination. A stat portable chest radiograph should be ordered. With this information, patients can be assigned to one of three classes which suggest high, intermediate, or low likelihood of acute coronary syndrome (ACS) which is described in detail below.

TABLE 79-1 Life-Threatening Causes of Chest Pain

Diagnosis	Risk Factors	Characteristic Findings	Diagnostic Testing
Aortic dissection	Hypertension, connective tissue disease, vasculitis, prior heart or valvular surgery, Turner syndrome, crack cocaine use, cardiac catheterization	New diastolic murmur, upper-extremity pulse deficit, neurologic complications of stroke	Computed tomography, magnetic resonance imaging, transesophageal echocardiography, angiography

Special considerations: Aortic dissection may be difficult to diagnose, but patients will most commonly present with chest pain; syncope may occur at the time of symptom onset. Dissections may be classified as Stanford type A (involving the ascending aorta) or type B (all others). In one study, 72.7% of patients reported chest pain, 90.6% reported severe or worst pain ever, and 84.8% had abrupt onset. Aortic insufficiency murmur was noted in 31.6% and pulse deficit was noted in 15.1%. Chest radiograph showed widened mediastinum in 61.6%, and ECGs were less helpful, being normal in 31.3%.* Medical treatment is initially indicated for type B dissections with strict blood pressure control (beta-blockade and nitroprusside). Given the high risk for life-threatening complications such as tamponade, aortic regurgitation, and myocardial infarction, type A dissections are treated as surgical emergencies.

Myocardial infarction	Age over 55, tobacco use, family history of coronary artery disease, diabetes, hypercholesterolemia, hypertension	S_4 or S_3 gallop, vomiting, diaphoresis, Levine sign (fist over center chest, low predictive value)	Electrocardiography, cardiac biomarkers

Special considerations: The diagnosis of ST-segment elevation myocardial infarction should be readily made from a 12-lead ECG and requires urgent intervention to improve survival. These patients will benefit from standard medical therapy as well as reperfusion. According to the 2007 ACC/AHA focused update on the management of patients with ST-elevation myocardial infarction, patients with acute STEMI will benefit from primary percutaneous intervention with a goal door-to-balloon time of <90 min. Fibrinolytic therapy within 30 min is preferred if transfer to a PCI-capable facility will make door-to-balloon time > 90 min. These guidelines are directed toward patients presenting to the hospital with STEMI, but may also help to decide when to transfer inpatients who develop STEMI during hospitalization.

Pulmonary embolism	Immobilization, recent surgery, stroke, paralysis, prior venous thromboembolism, malignancy, recent central venous instrumentation	Dyspnea, pleuritic pain, calf or leg pain or swelling, jugular venous distention	Computed tomography, ventilation-perfusion scan, pulmonary angiography

Special considerations: Thrombolytic therapy for submassive pulmonary embolism (PE) is a controversial treatment modality. It has been advocated for patients with evidence of right ventricular dilation or hypokinesis on echocardiography, but this indication for use is generally not widely accepted. Thrombolysis for cardiac arrest from PE has been successful in case reports, but does not seem to be helpful in cases of pulseless electrical activity.§ Thrombolytic regimens for PE range from 2 to 24 h infusions. For imminent or actual cardiac arrest, a bolus therapy is indicated. One such regimen is tPA, 0.6 mg/kg over 2 min.

Pneumothorax	*Pneumocystis jirovecii*, tuberculosis, chronic obstructive pulmonary disease, Marfans, familial, mechanical ventilation, smoking, cystic fibrosis	Decreased breath sounds, hyperresonant percussion, distended neck veins, tracheal deviation	Chest radiography, computed tomography

Special considerations: Of all emergency diagnoses, the only one that is immediately reversible is a tension pneumothorax. Needle decompression involves placing a 14-gauge angiocath in the second or third intercostal space in the midclavicular line. In a study of trauma patients with computed tomography scans of the chest, the mean chest wall thickness studied averaged 4.24 cm at this location, and almost a quarter of patients had chest walls thicker than 5 cm.¶ Therefore, one should use the longest catheter possible. Alternatives include using a spinal needle or rapid tube thoracostomy.

Esophageal rupture	Esophageal instrumentation, forceful emesis, ulcers or esophagitis	"Hammans sign" (mediastinal crunching sound), subcutaneous emphysema, odynophagia, hoarseness (cervical rupture)	Cervical and chest radiography, computed tomography, contrast esophagography

Special considerations: More than half of all cases of esophageal rupture occur as a complication of medical procedures that involve instrumentation of the esophagus, so knowledge of the inpatient course is paramount.** Spontaneous ruptures classically occur after forceful vomiting, but may also be associated with ingestion of caustic substances or pills, eosinophilic esophagitis, Barretts esophagitis, or ulcers.

*Hagan PG, Nienaber CA, Isselbacher EM, et al. The International Registry of Acute Aortic Dissection (IRAD): new insights into an old disease. *JAMA.* 2000;283:897.

†Antman EM, Hand M, Armstrong PW, et al. 2007 focused update of the ACC/AHA 2004 Guidelines for the Management of Patients With ST-Elevation Myocardial Infarction: a report of the American College of Cardiology/American Heart Association Task Force on Practice Guidelines (Writing Group to Review New Evidence and Update the ACC/AHA 2004 Guidelines for the Management of Patients With ST-Elevation Myocardial Infarction). *J Am Coll Cardiol.* 2008;51:210-247.

§Abu-Laban RB, Christenson JM, Innes GD, et al. Tissue plasminogen activator in cardiac arrest with pulseless electrical activity. *N Engl J Med.* 2002;346:1522.

¶Givens ML, Ayotte K, Manifold C. Needle thoracostomy: implications of computed tomography chest wall thickness. *Acad Emerg Med.* 2004;11(2):211-213.

**Pasricha P, Fleischer D, Kalloo A. Endoscopic perforation of the upper digestive tract: A review of their pathogenesis, prevention and management. *Gastroenterology.* 1994;106:787.

TABLE 79-2 Differential Diagnosis of Chest Pain

Cardiac	Pulmonary	Other
Aortic dissection	Pneumothorax	Esophageal rupture
Myocardial infarction	Pulmonary embolism	Mallory-Weiss tear
Angina	Pleuritis/serositis	Esophageal spasm
Coronary spasm	Pneumonia	Pancreatitis
Pericarditis	Cancer	Biliary tract disease
Myocarditis	Sarcoidosis	Costochondritis
Valvular disease		Musculoskeletal injury
Stress-induced cardiomyopathy		Peptic ulcer disease
		Gastritis/esophagitis/reflux
		Herpes zoster
		Mediastinitis
		Psychogenic/psychosomatic

PRACTICE POINT

- All patients with chest pain should be first evaluated for stability and possibility of any life-threatening conditions.

■ HISTORY

The history remains important in initial risk stratification because objective evidence including a diagnostic ECG is only present in a minority of patients. Once emergency conditions have been ruled out or stabilized, a targeted history can be used to identify and prioritize a list of differential possibilities (**Table 79-2**).

Classic symptoms of angina/cardiac ischemia include chest heaviness, pressure, tightness, or burning (sometimes with vigorous denial of pain), provocation by physical or emotional stress or cold, relief by rest, radiation to neck, jaw, or shoulder, duration >2 minutes and <20 minutes (>20 minutes could suggest myocardial infarction), dyspnea, nausea/vomiting, diaphoresis, presyncope, and palpitations. However, some recent studies have shown that a significant proportion of patients with STEMI (ST elevation myocardial infarction) and NSTEMI (non-ST elevation myocardial infarction) have either atypical chest pain (pleuritic, stabbing, or reproducible chest pain) or no chest pain at all. It should be noted that relief of chest pain with nitroglycerin does not predict ACS. While history alone is insufficient to rule out cardiac ischemia, it may be used in combination with exam and ECG testing, to identify patients who are at low risk for cardiac ischemia (**Table 79-3**).

RISK FACTORS

When it comes to initial diagnosis of ACS (acute coronary syndrome), risk factor evaluation does play a role and is helpful in stratifying patients for appropriate workup. Age over 55 years, family history of coronary artery disease (CAD), known CAD, vascular disease (cerebrovascular, peripheral vascular disease), diabetes mellitus, hypercholesterolemia, hypertension, and tobacco use are recognized as risk factors for CAD. Absence of risk factors does not rule out ACS. Given the high prevalence, morbidity, mortality, and liability issues surrounding the diagnosis of ACS, risk factors are always used in conjunction with clinical evaluation and diagnostic techniques in highly efficient pathways which are further detailed later in this chapter.

THE PHYSICAL EXAMINATION

The physical examination is often normal in patients with chest pain, even when serious pathology is present. However, certain signs may be helpful for risk stratification and for determining symptom etiology. Overall appearance of the patient combined with vital signs including pulse oximetry should be noted early in the assessment. Tachycardia and hypotension are ominous signs in the patient with chest pain and may require intervention to prevent cardiovascular collapse. Tachypnea may be subtle; the clinician should measure this vital sign independently if suspicion is high despite a normal documented respiratory rate, as it is one of the most common signs of pulmonary embolism (PE). New fever may direct the workup toward infectious etiologies but low-grade fever is a nonspecific finding and may also be associated with PE, myocardial infarction (MI), pneumonia, and pericarditis. New hypoxia is a clue to either cardiac (pump insufficiency with heart failure) or serious pulmonary pathology.

It is important to perform cardiac auscultation in a quiet room and ask the patient to lean forward. Using the diaphragm of the stethoscope, the examiner should listen for regurgitant murmurs and

---

TABLE 79-3 Likelihood that Signs and Symptoms Represent an ACS Secondary to CAD

	High Likelihood	Intermediate Likelihood	Low Likelihood
Feature	Any of the following	Absence of any high likelihood features and presence of any of the following	Absence of high or intermediate features but may have the following
History	Chest pain or left arm discomfort as chief complaint reproducing prior documented angina; known history of CAD, including MI	Chest or left arm pain or discomfort as chief symptom; age >70 y; male sex; diabetes mellitus	Probable ischemic symptoms in absence of any of the intermediate likelihood characteristics; recent cocaine use
Examination	Transient MR, hypotension, pulmonary edema or rales	Peripheral vascular disease	Chest discomfort reproduced by palpation
ECG	New ST deviation (≥0.05 mV) or T-wave inversion (≥0.2 mV) with symptoms	Fixed Q waves; abnormal ST segments not documented to be new	T-wave flattening or inversion with dominant R waves; normal ECG
Biochemical markers	Elevated troponin or CK-MB	Normal	Normal

ACS, acute coronary syndrome; CAD, coronary artery disease; CK-MB, MB fraction of creatine kinase; MI, myocardial infarction; MR, mitral regurgitation.
Reproduced, with permission, from Anderson JL, Adams CD, Antman EM, et al. ACC/AHA 2007 guidelines for management of patients with unstable angina/non-ST elevation myocardial infarction. *J Am Coll Cardiol*. 2007;50(7):e1-e157.

pericardial friction rubs. The finding of a new systolic mitral insufficiency murmur might indicate myocardial ischemia, a flail mitral leaflet, or decompensated heart failure and as such, puts the patient in a high likelihood category. A new murmur of tricuspid insufficiency might signal right ventricular overload from PE. A diastolic murmur may reflect acute aortic insufficiency and aortic dissection. Any new murmur, especially in the presence of fever, may signify endocarditis. See Chapter 255 (Diseases of the Aorta) and Chapter 189 (Infective Endocarditis).

Other examination findings of evidence of extracardiac vascular disease places the patient at intermediate risk of ACS. Chest pain reproduced by palpation is less likely to be from ACS but does not rule it out completely.

DIAGNOSTIC CONSIDERATIONS

■ ELECTROCARDIOGRAPHY

Myocardial ischemia

Patients reporting chest pain should have an ECG as soon as possible. ECGs that are obtained while the patient is having symptoms should be compared with any prior ECGs that may be available to assess for changes.

ST-segment elevation: The ESC/ACCF/AHA/WHF committee for the definition of myocardial infarction established specific ECG criteria for ST-segment elevation myocardial infarction including 2 mm of ST-segment elevation in ECG leads for men (1.5 mm for women) and greater than 1 mm in other leads. The elevations must be present in at least two contiguous leads, corresponding to a specific arterial territory. Although controversial, symptomatic patients with "new" or "presumed new" left bundle branch block (LBBB) should be considered as high risk similar to STEMI but need not be rushed to cardiac catheterization as was recommended previously. This is in light of recent studies which revealed that only a small number of these patients with LBBB had MI and two-thirds of these patients were discharged with alternative diagnoses.

Many patients will have alternate causes of ST-segment elevation (benign early repolarization, left ventricular hypertrophy or aneurysm, pericarditis, hyperkalemia), so experience interpreting ECGs, obtaining serial ECGs, and comparison with old ECGs is critical. In pericarditis, the lack of regional ischemic changes (ie, diffuse rather than localized ST elevations), PR depression, as well as a suggestive history and cardiac examination may help distinguish pericarditis from MI. See Chapter 130 (Myocarditis, Pericardial Disease, and Cardiac Tamponade).

Bundle branch block and paced rhythms make ECG interpretation challenging. The Sgarbossa criteria assign points to significant ECG findings in the presence of a left bundle branch block: concordant ST-segment elevation of 1 mm or more in any lead (five points), ST-segment depression of 1 mm or more in leads V1, V2, or V3 (three points), discordant ST-segment elevation of 5 mm or more (two points). A score of at least three is associated with high specificity for myocardial infarction but low sensitivity. In patients with LBBB or paced rhythms, the finding of ST-segment elevation ≥5 mm in leads with a negative QRS complex is highly specific for myocardial infarction.

Identification of inferior wall myocardial infarction should be followed by examination for evidence of posterior wall involvement (V_1 ST depression), conduction disturbance (Wenckebach, bradycardia, or complete heart block), and right ventricular infarction (right-sided ECG, lead rV_4).

ST-segment depression: ST-segment depression (0.5 mm or greater) predicts increased risk of myocardial ischemia. The greater the extent of depression, the higher the risk of MI and

death. In addition, ST depression in ≥2 mm in some precordial leads (V1–V4) may indicate transmural posterior injury; multilead ST depression with coexistent ST elevation in lead aVR has been described in patients with left main or proximal left anterior descending artery occlusion. Posterior leads may help differentiate the patient with anterior ST-segment depression who has ischemia from the patient who has an acute posterior wall MI.

T-wave inversion: These indicate lower risk than ST depressions. Likewise, the presence of Q-waves is less predictive of acute cardiac events.

Electrical alternans or low voltage: The findings of electrical alternans or low voltage in an ECG for a patient with chest pain should prompt consideration of pericardial effusion or hemorrhage. ECG abnormalities are common after stroke. Cerebral T waves (deep, symmetric T-wave inversions) can be seen with subarachnoid hemorrhage. ST-segment deviations may occur in stroke patients as well, sometimes making differentiation between stroke and myocardial infarction challenging in difficult-to-assess patients.

LABORATORY TESTING

Patients admitted to the hospital with chest pain or who develop chest pain while hospitalized should have basic laboratory tests performed, including a metabolic panel and complete blood count. Additional laboratory tests may be sent based upon clinical suspicion. Cardiac biomarkers are essential in the evaluation of patients suspected of having cardiac ischemia. Patients with possible intra-abdominal pathology should have liver enzymes and a lipase ordered as well as appropriate imaging. D-dimer testing may be appropriate in patients who present to the emergency department, but should not delay diagnostic imaging and treatment. D-dimer may not useful in hospitalized patients when PE is a consideration due to elevation in many disorders in addition to PE and will not exclude PE in patients with a high pretest probability of PE. See Chapter 253 (Diagnosis and Treatment of Venous Thromboembolism).

Cardiac biomarkers: A current definition of myocardial infarction involves typical rise and/or fall of cardiac biomarkers, along with ischemic symptoms, ischemic ECG findings (ST-segment deviation, Q waves), and/or coronary artery intervention.

Creatine kinase (CK) and the CK-MB isoform (unique to the myocardium) have similar temporal patterns in cases of myocardial injury, rising within 4 to 8 hours and peaking between 12 and 24 hours (slightly earlier for CK-MB). CK-MB is cleared within 36 to 48 hours, and CK is cleared within 3 to 4 days. Troponin levels rise within 6 hours, peak after 12 hours, and are cleared after 7 to 14 days.

Current cardiac troponin assays exhibit superior sensitivity and specificity when compared with CK and CK-MB for the diagnosis of myocardial infarction. The cardiac troponin assays are becoming the test of choice for many providers, replacing CK and CK-MB testing completely in these settings. Elevations in troponin identify patients who would benefit from aggressive treatment such as antithrombotic, antiplatelet, and coronary intervention. Hospitalists need to be aware of the reference range for the specific assay in use at their institution. The "normal range" of cardiac troponin is a troublesome concept, as any detectable troponin level has been shown to have prognostic significance and may be a marker of chronic as well as acute disease.

Troponins may be elevated in patients with renal failure who do not have evidence of myocardial damage. This is likely due to decreased clearance as well as increased incidence of comorbid pathology (including pathology seen at the cellular level). These patients also have a high rate of coronary disease. Therefore, an appropriate serial rise in troponin is more helpful than a single

TABLE 79-4 Differential Diagnosis of Elevated Troponin in the Absence of Acute Myocardial Infarction or Congestive Heart Failure

Cardiac and vascular disease	Aortic dissection, CVA
Respiratory disease	Acute PE, ARDS
Cardiac inflammation	Pericarditis, endocarditis, myocarditis
Muscular damage	Rhabdomyolysis
Infections	Sepsis, viral disease
Acute complications of inherited disorders	Neurofibromatosis, Duchenne muscular dystrophy, Klippel-Feil syndrome
Environmental exposure	Carbon monoxide, hydrogen sulfide, colchicine, evenomations (snake, jellyfish, spider, centipede, scorpion)
Chronic diseases	ESRD, cardiac infiltrative disorders (amyloidosis, sarcoidosis, hemochromatosis, scleroderma), HBP, diabetes, hypothyroidism
Iatrogenic disease	Invasive procedures (heart transplant, congenital defect repair, radiofrequency ablation, lung resection, ERCP), noninvasive procedures (cardioversion, lithotripsy), pharmacologic (chemotherapy)
Myocardial injury	Blunt chest trauma, endurance athletes
Miscellaneous	Kawasaki disease, stress cardiomyopathy, TTP, birth complications in infants, GI bleeding

ARDS, acute respiratory distress syndrome; CVA, cerebrovascular accident; ERCP, endoscopic retrograde cholangiopancreatogram; ESRD, end-stage renal disease; GI, gastrointestinal; HBP, high blood pressure; PE, pulmonary embolism; TTP, thrombotic thrombocytopenic purpura.
Data from Kelley WE, Januzzi JL, Christenson RH. Increases in cardiac troponin in conditions other than ACS and HF. *Clin Chem*. 2009;55(12):2098.

elevated, stable value for the diagnosis of myocardial infarction in these patients. Other conditions associated with increased troponin values include massive pulmonary embolism, myocarditis, cardiopulmonary resuscitation, cardioversion, heart failure, stroke, stress cardiomyopathy, and demand ischemia (**Table 79-4**).

NEW APPROACH TO PATIENTS PRESENTING TO EMERGENCY DEPARTMENTS WITH CHEST PAIN

Based on currently available technology, evidence, and resources, hospitals and emergency departments are now following a new approach based on clinical pathways. This typically involves the following steps:

1. Focused patient history and exam (see Table 79-3).
2. Stratification for risk of ACS
3. Use of observation unit or extended acute care unit
4. Appropriate testing based on initial risk stratification
5. Patient disposition and follow-up based on test results

RISK STRATIFICATION OF SUSPECTED CARDIAC CHEST PAIN PATIENTS

Recently, there have been several studies that focus on stratification of patients presenting to the emergency rooms with undifferentiated chest pain for risk of ACS. Several scores and algorithms

have been proposed. Some of these studies have used scores like TIMI (Thrombolysis in Myocardial Infarction) or GRACE (Global Registry of Acute Coronary Events) and more recently developed HEART score (history, ECG, age, risk factors, and troponin). These have also been prospectively studied and they all compare well and overall provide excellent prediction of 30-day MACE (major adverse cardiac events).

The TIMI score for NSTEMI continues to be an important tool due to its simplicity and also its usefulness in determining the patients disposition from the ED as outlined below. The TIMI risk score consists of the following elements: (1) age (>65 years), (2) three or more CAD risk factors (hypertension, current smoking, diabetes mellitus, hyperlipidemia, or strong family history of early CAD), (3) known previous CAD (coronary stenosis > 50%), (4) severe angina (>2 episodes in last 24 hours), (5) aspirin use in last 7 days, (6) ECG deviation >0.5 mm, and (7) troponin elevation. Each element that is present yields one point to the risk score with a maximum score of seven. In one useful algorithm, all the above elements except the troponin are used in the initial screening. (In other words, a modified TIMI or mTIMI score is used.) Then the troponin result is used to determine which type of hospital unit is best suited for the ED patient, which makes it consistent with using the whole TIMI score. See Chapter 128 (Acute Coronary Syndromes) (**Figure 79-1**).

USE OF OBSERVATION OR EXTENDED CARE ACUTE UNITS

Hospitalists are increasingly asked to manage the workup of chest pain patients who are at low, but not negligible, risk for coronary disease. The admission status of these patients will vary by institution. Chest pain "observation units" are becoming more popular and may be staffed by emergency physicians, hospitalists, cardiologists, or nonphysician providers. The general goal of these units is to expedite the workup of patients at low-to-intermediate risk for an acute coronary syndrome. The patients are placed on predetermined clinical pathways based on initial risk stratification. Patients that are identified as intermediate or high risk undergo additional testing and/or evaluation which may include noninvasive testing like exercise ECG, myocardial perfusion imaging (MPI), stress echocardiogram, or multislice CT coronary angiography.

Choosing which type of testing to use will depend on the characteristics of the patient, resources available, and the policies of the institution, as well as the information desired. Exercise testing with echocardiography or radionuclide myocardial perfusion imaging will allow localization of abnormalities. Patients who are unable to exercise can undergo pharmacologic stress testing with dipyridamole, adenosine, or dobutamine. Dobutamine echocardiography, however, should be avoided in patients who may be suffering from active or unstable ischemia.

There is now widespread availability of multislice CT (64 slice or higher) coronary angiography in many centers with good expertise at both generating high-quality images and their interpretation. This technique adds to our diagnostic testing kit and is best used for intermediate-risk patients with no known previous CAD as outlined in our algorithm (**Figure 79-2**). Several recent studies have shown its usefulness given its excellent negative predictive value (99%), reduced diagnostic time, and overall cost.

Coronary artery calcium (CAC) scoring is another marker of CAD. It is used as an estimate of coronary plaque burden and high CAC scores are associated with increased risk of coronary events. Additionally, in ED patients with undifferentiated chest pain a CAC of 0 is associated with a negative predictive value of almost 100% for up to 4 years of follow-up. While CAC score is available as an independent test, it is typically included as an option in current protocols of multislice CT coronary angiography which has the

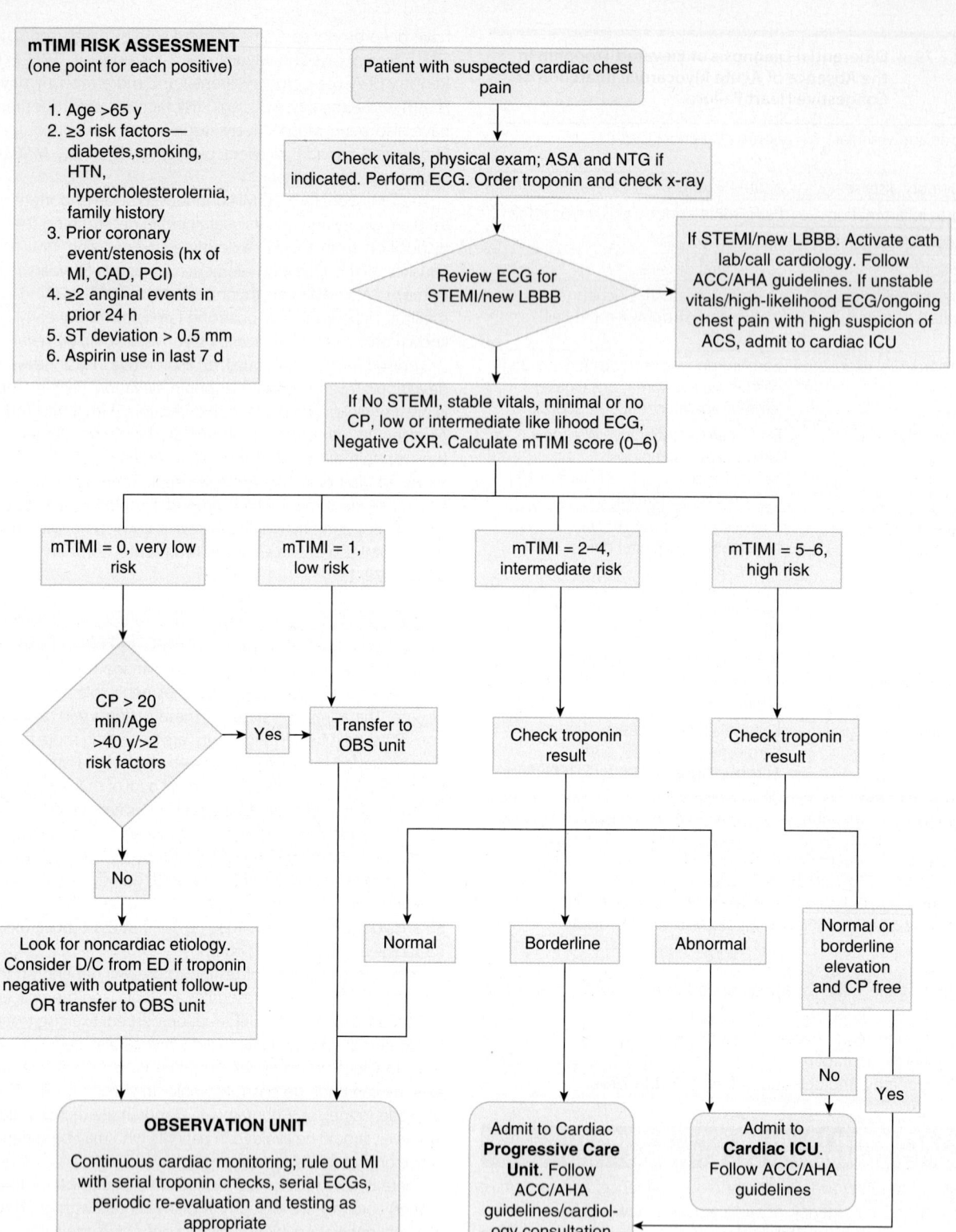

mTIMI RISK ASSESSMENT
(one point for each positive)

1. Age >65 y
2. ≥3 risk factors—diabetes, smoking, HTN, hypercholesterolemia, family history
3. Prior coronary event/stenosis (hx of MI, CAD, PCI)
4. ≥2 anginal events in prior 24 h
5. ST deviation > 0.5 mm
6. Aspirin use in last 7 d

Patient with suspected cardiac chest pain

Check vitals, physical exam; ASA and NTG if indicated. Perform ECG. Order troponin and check x-ray

Review ECG for STEMI/new LBBB

If STEMI/new LBBB. Activate cath lab/call cardiology. Follow ACC/AHA guidelines. If unstable vitals/high-likelihood ECG/ongoing chest pain with high suspicion of ACS, admit to cardiac ICU

If No STEMI, stable vitals, minimal or no CP, low or intermediate like lihood ECG, Negative CXR. Calculate mTIMI score (0–6)

mTIMI = 0, very low risk

mTIMI = 1, low risk

mTIMI = 2–4, intermediate risk

mTIMI = 5–6, high risk

CP > 20 min/Age >40 y/>2 risk factors — Yes → Transfer to OBS unit

No

Check troponin result

Check troponin result

Look for noncardiac etiology. Consider D/C from ED if troponin negative with outpatient follow-up OR transfer to OBS unit

Normal

Borderline

Abnormal

Normal or borderline elevation and CP free

No   Yes

OBSERVATION UNIT

Continuous cardiac monitoring; rule out MI with serial troponin checks, serial ECGs, periodic re-evaluation and testing as appropriate

Admit to Cardiac **Progressive Care Unit**. Follow ACC/AHA guidelines/cardiology consultation

Admit to **Cardiac ICU.** Follow ACC/AHA guidelines

Figure 79-1 *Algorithm for chest pain triage. (ACC, American College of Cardiology; AHA, American Heart Association; ASA, aspirin; D/C, discharge.)*

added advantage of direct visualization of the artery and coronary plaques.

Hospitalists should familiarize themselves with the availability, advantages, limitations, risks, and contraindications of the various modalities of stress testing and imaging. For example, stress echocardiography has the advantage of no radiation exposure but may be of limited use in case of obesity or pre-existing LBBB. Cardiac CT angiography has the advantages of not needing a full "rule out" by biomarkers prior to testing but is limited by ability of the patient to

hold their breath; in addition the concerns of radiation exposure and the impact on renal function especially if the patient has known kidney disease must be considered. A patient who is able to exercise should preferentially perform exercise stress testing. Patient selection via risk stratification is crucial. Applying these tests indiscriminately will adversely affect the positive predictive value and may lead to unnecessary downstream risk of additional testing and invasive coronary angiography. The indications for noninvasive testing for ACS in women are similar to men. However, the predictive

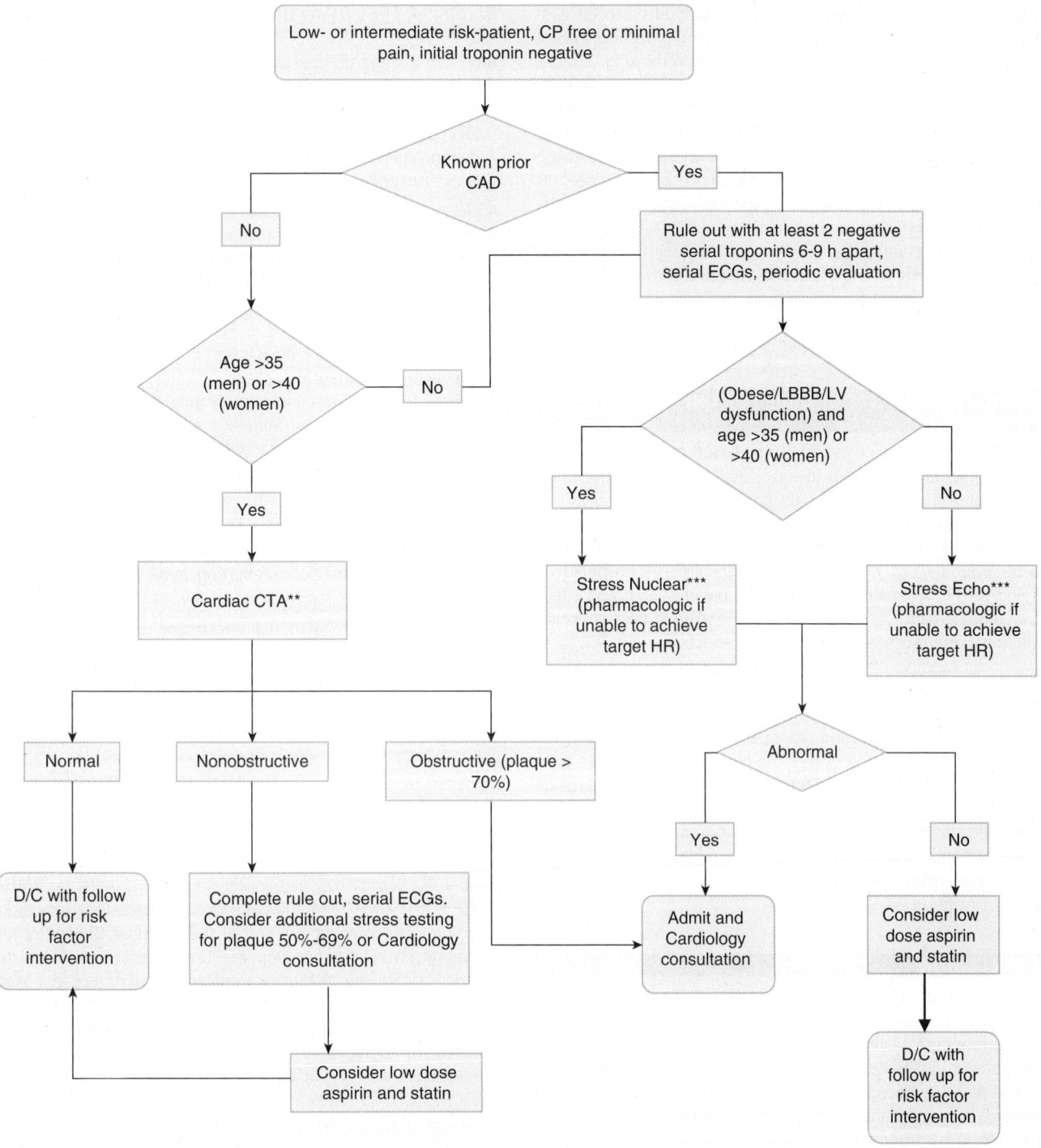

Figure 79-2 *Suggested work-up protocol for low-to-intermediate risk patients. (CTA, CT angiography; D/C, discharge.)*
**Relative contraindications include intolerance to betablocker, creatinine clearance <60 ml/min, unable to raise arm over shoulder, unable to breathe for 10s, very irregular heart beat or atrial fibrillation.
***One can consider non-imaging stress if baseline ECG is normal and TIMI score is 0 if additional resources are unavailable.

value of exercise ECG without imaging is less in women than in men primarily due to lower pretest probability of CAD and possibly from pre-existing ECG abnormalities.

Newer biomarkers such as high-sensitivity troponins are being used increasingly in emergency departments with turnaround times between 9 and 14 minutes. These biomarkers may help with earlier identification of low-risk patients. Small studies on use of stress cardiac magnetic resonance imaging have also been published recently, but this modality is still not widely available.

In a recent observational study, 1975 patients were placed on an accelerated diagnostic protocol (ADP) that included pretest probability scoring by TIMI score, ECG, and 0+2h troponin I as the sole biomarker. The primary end point was MACE (major adverse cardiac events) within 30 days. The study results revealed that the ADP successfully identified a group (392 patients—20%) who were at low short-term risk of MACE (0.25%) and thus were suitable for rapid discharge from the emergency department with early follow-up.

WORKUP ALGORITHM FOR OBSERVATION UNITS

The workup algorithm is depicted in Figure 79-2 and is based on current literature and guidelines.

We would like to emphasize that the described protocols cannot substitute sound clinical judgment. Ongoing or recurrent chest pain is always concerning and should prompt rethinking of initial stratification and protocol. Serial ECGs should be reviewed carefully even if troponins remain normal. Furthermore, not every patient can be easily classified into described categories and studies of accelerated diagnostic protocols are still fairly new and more studies are needed. A negative stress test while reassuring cannot be used as a "warranty" against the need for follow-up longitudinally in the outpatient setting. Some areas of uncertainty still exist and include testing of patients with known CAD who present with recurrent episodes of chest pain, testing of patients who present with chest pain in setting of cocaine use as these groups of patients are excluded from many trials.

IMPROVING QUALITY OF CARE FOR CHEST PAIN PATIENTS

As is true for many aspects of hospital-based medicine, hospitalists are uniquely positioned to enact quality improvement measures that will benefit chest pain patients. These measures will be institution specific, but several general considerations deserve attention. The health care cost of these patients is estimated to be around 10 to 13 billion dollars annually. The hospitalist is tasked with coordinating all aspects of a patient's care, and effective communication among health care workers is paramount. In addition, patient-centered care requires effective communication and understanding of the hospital experience from the patient perspective. Knowledge and respect for patients' needs and concerns can diminish the helplessness many feel during admission to the hospital. Standardizing chest pain algorithms, especially for acute coronary syndrome evaluation, can save considerable time and effort and if accepted institution-wide may allow discharge of low-risk emergency department patients who would have otherwise been admitted. Lastly, taking time to communicate and coordinate with primary care physicians will enable earlier discharges and improve overall patient care.

CONCLUSION

The symptom of chest pain suggests a wide differential diagnosis that can be narrowed by a careful history, physical examination, and appropriate testing to rule out life-threatening disorders. For patients suspected to have ACS, risk stratification and a clinical-pathway-based approach have proven to be safe and effective. Newer technologies such as multislice CT imaging and high-sensitivity troponins are additional tools that are becoming increasingly available and useful. Many chest pain patients will have evaluations that reveal non–life-threatening disorders. Although these patients likely do not require continued hospitalization, they should receive education about the most likely diagnosis, treatment, and the need for close follow-up. A key point is to review with the patient the symptoms that should prompt an urgent reassessment and where the patients should seek additional care. The importance of follow-up with their primary care physicians, cardiologist, or other longitudinal providers cannot be overstated.

ACKNOWLEDGMENT

With special thanks to Mary C. Westergaard, MD, who was an author of the previous edition of this chapter.

SUGGESTED READINGS

American College of Emergency Physicians, Society for Cardiovascular Angiography and Interventions, O'Gara PT, et al. 2013 ACCF/AHA guideline for the management of ST-elevation myocardial infarction: a report of the American College of Cardiology Foundation/American Heart Association Task Force on Practice Guidelines. *J Am Coll Cardiol*. 2013;61(4):e78-140.

Anderson JL, Adams CD, Antman EM, et al. ACC/AHA 2007 guidelines for the management of patients with unstable angina/non-ST-Elevation myocardial infarction: a report of the American College of Cardiology/American Heart Association Task Force on Practice Guidelines (Writing Committee to Revise the 2002 Guidelines for the Management of Patients With Unstable Angina/Non-ST-Elevation Myocardial Infarction) developed in collaboration with the American College of Emergency Physicians, the Society for Cardiovascular Angiography and Interventions, and the Society of Thoracic Surgeons endorsed by the American Association of Cardiovascular and Pulmonary Rehabilitation and the Society for Academic Emergency Medicine. *J Am Coll Cardiol*. 2007;50(7):e1-e157.

Antman EM, Cohen M, Bernink PJ, et al. The TIMI risk score for unstable angina/non-ST elevation MI: a method for prognostication and therapeutic decision making. *JAMA*. 2000;284(7):835-842.

Canto AJ, Kiefe CI, Goldberg RJ, et al. Differences in symptom presentation and hospital mortality according to type of acute myocardial infarction. *Am Heart J*. 2012;163(4):572-579.

Cullen L, Mueller C, Parsonage WA, et al. Validation of high-sensitivity troponin I in a 2-hour diagnostic strategy to assess 30-day outcomes in emergency department patients with possible acute coronary syndrome. *J Am Coll Cardiol*. 2013;62(14):1242-1249.

Goldstein JA, Gallagher MJ, O'Neill WW, Ross MA, O'Neil BJ, Raff GL. A randomized controlled trial of multi-slice coronary computed tomography for evaluation of acute chest pain. *J Am Coll Cardiol*. 2007;49(8):863-871.

Hendel RC, Berman DS, Di Carli MF, et al. ACCF/ASNC/ACR/AHA/ASE/SCCT/SCMR/SNM 2009 appropriate use criteria for cardiac radionuclide imaging: a report of the American College of Cardiology Foundation Appropriate Use Criteria Task Force, the American Society of Nuclear Cardiology, the American College of Radiology, the American Heart Association, the American Society of Echocardiography, the Society of Cardiovascular Computed Tomography, the Society for Cardiovascular Magnetic Resonance, and the Society of Nuclear Medicine. *J Am Coll Cardiol*. 2009;53(23):2201-2229.

Hoffmann U, Truong QA, Schoenfeld DA, et al. Coronary CT angiography versus standard evaluation in acute chest pain. *N Engl J Med*. 2012;367(4):299-308.

Jain S, Ting HT, Bell M, et al. Utility of left bundle branch block as a diagnostic criterion for acute myocardial infarction. *Am J Cardiol*. 2011;107(8):1111-1116.

Lee TH, Goldman L. Evaluation of the patient with acute chest pain. *N Engl J Med*. 2000;342(16):1187-1195.

Litt HI, Gatsonis C, Snyder B, et al. CT angiography for safe discharge of patients with possible acute coronary syndromes. *N Engl J Med*. 2012;366(15):1393-1403.

Lyon R, Morris AC, Caesar D, Gray S, Gray A. Chest pain presenting to the emergency department—to stratify risk with GRACE or TIMI? *Resuscitation*. 2007;74(1):90-93.

Pollack CV Jr, Sites FD, Shofer FS, Sease KL, Hollander JE. Application of the TIMI risk score for unstable angina and non-ST elevation acute coronary syndrome to an unselected emergency department chest pain population. *Acad Emerg Med*. 2006;13(1):13-18.

Six AJ, Cullen L, Backus BE, et al. The HEART score for the assessment of patients with chest pain in the emergency department: a multinational validation study. *Crit Pathw Cardiol*. 2013;12(3):121-126.

Than M, Cullen L, Aldous S, et al. 2-hour accelerated diagnostic protocol to assess patients with chest pain symptoms using contemporary troponins as the only biomarker: The ADAPT trial. *J Am Coll Cardiol*. 2012;59(23):2091-2098.

Wright RS, Anderson JL, Adams CD, et al. 2011 ACCF/AHA focused update incorporated into the ACC/AHA 2007 guidelines for the management of patients with unstable angina/non-ST-elevation myocardial infarction: a report of the American College of Cardiology Foundation/American Heart Association Task Force on Practice Guidelines developed in collaboration with the American Academy of Family Physicians, Society for Cardiovascular Angiography and Interventions, and the Society of Thoracic Surgeons. *J Am Coll Cardiol*. 2011;57(19): e215-367.

CHAPTER 80

Constipation

Linda A. Lee, MD
Eugenie Shieh, MD

Key Clinical Questions

1. What are the risk factor(s) for developing constipation in the hospital?

2. How do you prevent constipation in a hospitalized patient with a history of constipation?

3. What are the likely causes of new constipation in a hospitalized patient?

4. What is the treatment of common causes of new constipation?

CASE 80-1

An 82-year-old man with relapsed diffuse large cell lymphoma presents with severe abdominal pain, distention, and vomiting beginning 24 hours ago. The pain is intermittent, crampy, and diffuse. He has not had a bowel movement in 7 days. He has been receiving rituximab for his lymphoma. He has no history of abdominal surgery. He does have a history of thyroid disease, atrial fibrillation, gout, and diabetes.

The patient has a long-standing history of chronic constipation and has used polyethylene glycol (PEG) 3350 daily for 2 years. When he was hospitalized a week ago, he was given docusate sodium daily instead of his usual regimen. His other medications include warfarin, allopurinol, levothyroxine, glimepiride, and amlodipine.

His physical exam is remarkable for normal vital signs and a moderately protuberant abdomen. There are bowel sounds but no palpable masses. There is mild diffuse tenderness, but no rebound. The rectal exam reveals no stool in the vault. His laboratory tests are normal. An abdominal flat plate shows a large amount of stool in the right and transverse colon.

What are the causes of this man's constipation? What is the best way to manage his constipation acutely and chronically?

INTRODUCTION

Constipation has many meanings, but for the purposes of this chapter, the medical definition of constipation includes one or all of the following: fewer than three bowel movements per week; passing hard, lumpy stools; straining with defecation; or having a sense of incomplete evacuation. Constipation can newly arise in a patient hospitalized for other medical reasons, represent an exacerbation of a chronic problem, be the principal reason for hospitalization, or be a manifestation of an acute, possibly catastrophic, event.

Chronic constipation is a common complaint that compromises quality of life and frequently prompts use of health care services. Constipation results in 2.5 million physician visits and 92,000 hospitalizations per year in the United States. The prevalence of constipation in North America is estimated to range from 2% to 27%, with most studies citing a prevalence of 15%. This variation in prevalence reflects different diagnostic criteria for constipation and study design. The estimated prevalence of constipation in other developed countries is similar to that in North America at 17.1% in Europe, 14.3% in Hong Kong, and 16.5% in South Korea. Constipation is reported more often by females (2-3:1 predominance), non-whites, individuals of lower socioeconomic status, and the elderly (prevalence of 20%-24%). The cumulative incidence of constipation over more than one decade is about 1 in 6. This incidence increases dramatically in the setting of certain comorbidities.

Although most individuals with constipation do not specifically seek medical care, constipation contributes significantly to health care expenses. In the United States, the total health care cost of constipation diagnosis per patient exceeds $2500, and in 2001, $235 million dollars were spent for constipation, with more than half of the cost incurred from inpatient care. In the California Medicaid program, 0.6% of patients presenting to a physician with a medical complaint of constipation were admitted to a hospital, averaging almost $3000 per admission. This chapter will discuss how to distinguish, evaluate, and manage the conditions in which constipation occurs.

PATHOPHYSIOLOGY

The pathophysiology of constipation can be understood first by a very brief review of the elements required for normal colonic transit and defecation. Normal colonic transit requires segmental activity and propagated activity, which depends on both low-amplitude and high-amplitude propagated contractions. Normal defecation requires intact pelvic floor muscles and rectal compliance. The muscles of the pelvic floor include the internal anal sphincter, the external anal sphincter, and the puborectalis muscle. The internal sphincter muscle, which is tonically contracted, is innervated by the enteric nervous system. The external sphincter and puborectalis muscles are innervated by the pudendal nerves (S2, S3, and S4). During defecation, both must relax in order for normal defecation to occur. The puborectalis muscle forms a U-shaped sling around the rectum, and when contracted maintains the rectum at a 90° angle (ie, perpendicular) with respect to the anal canal. This muscle must relax with voluntary defecation so the angle can widen to 135° to allow unobstructed passage of stool from the rectum to the anal canal. Medications, medical illness, prior surgery, and other factors can diminish colonic contractions, contribute to pelvic floor weakness, alter rectal compliance, or cause obstruction.

NEW CONSTIPATION IN THE HOSPITALIZED PATIENT

New constipation commonly arises in hospitalized patients and has been attributed to multiple causes (**Table 80-1**). Lack of physical activity, change in diet, electrolyte disturbances, use of anesthetics and narcotics, medication side effects, and failure to continue the home laxative regimen may precipitate constipation. In the elderly, acute hospitalization further increases the prevalence of constipation in an already susceptible age group, with one-third of hospitalized geriatric patients requiring laxatives three times daily. The incidence of new-onset constipation at 4 weeks after a first stroke exceeds 50% and affects nearly 80% of post-stroke patients in a rehabilitation unit. Eighty percent of patients with spinal cord injuries will experience constipation. The incidence of constipation among cancer patients is 60%, but increases to 87% in those using opioids. Forty-four percent of patients who have had thoracolumbar surgery experience constipation despite being prescribed prophylactic laxatives. Constipation may also be part of a symptom complex representing a serious, acute event. If abdominal distention, high-pitched bowel sounds, and pain are present, then colonic obstruction must be considered. Accompanying fever and rebound tenderness should trigger an evaluation for perforation.

The patient's history is essential for identifying the cause of constipation and determining the best course of management. It is important to ask the patient to define the duration of constipation, the frequency of bowel movements, whether there is incomplete evacuation, straining, or passage of hard (scybalous) stool. Associated symptoms may suggest a cause for constipation. Blood or mucus in the stool may indicate an obstructive process, anal fissure, rectal prolapse, or hemorrhoids. Tenesmus suggests hard stool or possibly rectal obstruction. Overflow fecal incontinence or mental status changes can be presenting symptoms of fecal impaction in elderly patients.

Important elements of the past medical history include an obstetric and surgical history. A thorough review of all medications can reveal a drug-related cause of constipation. Common culprits of constipation-induced medications include prescription medications (opiates, anticholinergics, and calcium-channel blockers), over-the-counter drugs, and herbals (**Table 80-2**). In the elderly, home use of laxatives is the only identifiable risk factor for developing constipation in the hospital. A family history of bowel disorders should be sought. The social history should explore physical activity and dietary habits, including amount of fiber intake, fluid intake, number and timing of meals, and dehydration. Red flags for a serious underlying etiology of constipation include weight loss, abdominal pain, rectal bleeding, iron deficiency anemia, or a significant family history of colon cancer. Complaints of severe pain with abdominal distention could signal colonic obstruction or intestinal ischemia with potentially life-threatening complications.

A complete physical exam searching for signs of a systemic illness is essential, although it is often unrevealing. In particular, the abdominal exam should focus on palpating for stool in the left or right lower quadrant. Severe abdominal distention, high-pitched bowel sounds, and tenderness to palpation are suggestive of an obstructive etiology. Evaluation of the patient may sometimes reveal a fecolith palpable through the abdominal wall or on digital examination of the rectum. A complete neurologic examination may provide evidence of occult neurologic disease such as Parkinson's disease. The anorectum should be inspected for hemorrhoids,

---

TABLE 80-1 Causes of New Constipation in the Hospitalized Patient

Drugs and supplements

Reduced physical activity

Bedridden for length of time more than 2 wk

Postsurgical

Dietary change

Low-fiber diet

Dehydration

Electrolyte disturbances: hypercalcemia, hyponatremia, hypokalemia, uremia

Paraneoplastic syndrome

TABLE 80-2 Drugs by Class That Cause Constipation

Anticholinergics

Antidepressants

Antiparkinsonian drugs

Antipsychotics

Antispasmodics

Analgesics

Nonsteroidal anti-inflammatory drugs

Neurally acting agents

Adrenergics

Anticonvulsants

Antihistamines

Antihypertensives

Calcium channel blockers

Opiates

Vinca alkaloids

Cation-containing agents

Aluminum

Barium sulfate

Calcium

Iron supplements

anal fissures, skin tags, or rectal prolapse. If cauda equina syndrome is suspected, perineal sensation can be evaluated by using a Q-tip or sharp point of a pin to gently stroke all quadrants. An anocutaneous reflex ("anal wink") can be elicited by stroking the perineal skin; the absence of reflex contraction of the external anal sphincter would suggest a neuropathy. The digital rectal examination can evaluate sphincter tone, the contents of the rectal vault, and allow detection of blood in the stool. Fever, tachycardia, and other signs of hemodynamic instability are clues to complications of perforation or ischemia.

Pertinent laboratory tests in the evaluation of constipation include a complete blood count, electrolytes, including calcium, phosphorous, and magnesium, blood urea nitrogen, creatinine, glucose, and thyroid function tests. Other laboratory tests, such as serum protein electrophoresis, urine porphyrins, serum parathyroid hormone, and evaluation for adrenal hypofunction should be considered, if indicated by history or physical exam.

Diagnostic imaging is not a necessary component of every evaluation of constipation, but can provide critical information in the right clinical scenario. In patients with abdominal distention, pain, and constipation, plain abdominal radiography can be helpful in assessing the degree of constipation and ruling out obstruction. Abdominal radiographs may demonstrate a dilated colon or small bowel with air fluid levels indicative of obstruction. Plain abdominal radiographs can also help diagnose a sigmoid or cecal volvulus. The presence of free air on plain abdominal radiograph would indicate perforated bowel (see Chapter 116 [Basic Abdominal Imaging]).

If abdominal radiography demonstrates colonic dilatation suggestive of an obstruction, additional imaging should be performed. A flexible sigmoidoscopy or colonoscopy, barium enema, or CT scan can help define a colonic obstruction. Flexible sigmoidoscopy and colonoscopy can also identify a mucosal lesion, such as a malignancy or stricture. The timing of the latter studies would depend on the risk of perforation from performing the study. For example, acute diverticulitis causing obstruction would require treatment prior to performing a colonoscopy to rule out the possibility of an occult cancer underlying the inflammation.

DIFFERENTIAL DIAGNOSIS OF ACUTE CONSTIPATION

FECAL IMPACTION

Impaction of feces occurs in children, institutionalized individuals, and the elderly, and sometimes as a complication of opioid use. Large calcified fecoliths as well as seed bezoars have caused large bowel obstruction. Treatment of fecal impaction requires aggressive management since impaction may lead to urinary tract obstruction, perforation of the colon, dehydration, electrolyte imbalance, renal insufficiency, fecal incontinence, decubitus ulcers, stercoral ulcers, and rectal bleeding. Treatment of fecal impaction in part depends on where the impaction is located. Fecal impaction may require urgent manual disimpaction, especially in the elderly, a population in whom risk factors of immobility, dehydration, and multiple medications predispose it to complications of mental status changes, agitation, and worsening confusion.

In the left colon, manual disimpaction may be followed by enemas, which work primarily by stimulating rectal propulsion in this situation. Soapsuds enemas (composed of 6 g castile soap/L) are chemical irritants and promote intestinal fluid secretion. There are rare reports of colitis after administration of soapsuds enemas for more than 5 days in a row. Hypertonic solutions, like sodium phosphate, work by osmosis, drawing water into the lumen. Sodium phosphate enemas should be used with caution, because retention of the enema in the absence of defecation can lead to dehydration, hyperphosphatemia, and acute renal failure.

Large-volume oral laxative solutions are often effective for the treatment of fecal impaction, particularly if the impaction is proximal to the sigmoid colon. Polyethylene glycol (PEG) 3350 with electrolytes has been shown to be effective monotherapy for the treatment of fecal impaction in children and is superior to lactulose in preventing future episodes. Following disimpaction, all patients need preventative therapy, and maintenance with daily dosing with oral PEG 3350 (at least 17 g daily) is highly recommended. Occasionally, twice daily dosing with PEG 3350 is required to prevent recurrent constipation.

COLONIC OBSTRUCTION DUE TO TUMOR, STRICTURE, OR VOLVULUS

PRACTICE POINT

- In any patient experiencing a sudden onset of constipation associated with abdominal pain, distention, and nausea and vomiting, volvulus should be considered.
- Consulting a gastroenterologist and surgeon is advised when volvulus is suspected, even in the absence of frank perforation.

Obstruction may precipitate new-onset constipation or exacerbate chronic constipation. Obstruction may be caused by a tumor, stricture, or less commonly by a colonic volvulus, leading to nausea, vomiting, abdominal distention, and pain. Concern for a possible malignant growth would be heightened if there is accompanying iron deficiency anemia, weight loss, or a personal or family history raising the risk for colorectal cancer. A stricture should be considered in the differential diagnosis in any individual who has had prior colonic resection or history of diverticulitis.

Volvulus should be considered in the patient experiencing a sudden onset of constipation associated with abdominal pain, distention, and nausea and vomiting. A sigmoid volvulus caused by the twisting of the colon around the mesenteric axis accounts for up to 5% of colonic obstruction in the U.S. Cecal volvulus, which is rarer than sigmoid volvulus, occurs when there is a mobile cecum, and has been reported as a complication following left colectomy, cholecystectomy, and other laparoscopic procedures. It is thought that adhesions may serve as the fulcrum for torsion in some cases. Cecal volvulus has also been rarely reported following routine colonoscopy. Twenty-eight percent of patients with acute cecal volvulus occur in patients hospitalized for other medical reasons. Abdominal plain imaging may demonstrate marked distention of an ahaustral colon with an appearance of a large "coffee-bean" pointing toward the right upper quadrant (in the case of sigmoid colon) or left upper quadrant (in the case of cecal volvulus). However, this radiographic sign is not always present. If there is proximal bowel dilatation, the diagnosis of volvulus can be very difficult to make based on abdominal films alone. Computed tomography may demonstrate a "whirl sign," which represents a twisted loop of intestine and engorged mesenteric vessels. Another CT finding is a "bird's beak" appearance of dilated bowel tapering to a point at the site of torsion. CT signs of ischemia and/or perforation include circumferential wall thickening, pneumatosisintestinalis, increased density in the mesenteric fat, and pneumoperitoneum. If the diagnosis is suspected but remains uncertain, barium enema has been reported to be diagnostic in 88% of cases and even therapeutic. A barium enema should only be performed if there are no signs of ischemia or perforation. No colonic preparation is given for this test in this circumstance. Consulting a gastroenterologist and surgeon is advised when volvulus is suspected, even in the absence of frank perforation. Sigmoidoscopy may diagnose and treat a sigmoid volvulus, and is preferable to barium enema because of a lower risk of perforation.

OGILVIE SYNDROME/INTESTINAL PSEUDOOBSTRUCTION

PRACTICE POINT

- Laxatives, particularly those that can be fermented by colonic bacteria to produce gas, should not be given to patients with pseudoobstruction. Rare reports of colonic perforation exist when such patients are given lactulose. Endoscopic or pharmacologic decompression may be required if patients do not respond within 24 to 48 hours to supportive therapy or if the cecal diameter reaches 10 cm (thereby increasing the risk of perforation or ischemia).

Colonic dilatation without evidence of a mechanical obstruction may be due to intestinal pseudoobstruction or Ogilvie syndrome. First described in cancer patients with malignant infiltration of the celiac plexus, it is now known to arise in all types of patients, including those with trauma, cardiac disease, obstetrical or surgical conditions, or neurologic disease. The cause of Ogilvie syndrome has been attributed to imbalanced parasympathetic and sympathetic stimulation of the colon. Since the right colon receives its parasympathetic innervation by the vagus nerve and the left colon from S2 to S4, Ogilvie syndrome has been attributed to decreased colonic contractility of the left colon as a result of perturbed parasympathetic innervation. Other risk factors for Ogilvie syndrome include electrolyte disturbances and the use of opioids. Intestinal pseudoobstruction can be associated with collagen vascular disease, like scleroderma, or a paraneoplastic syndrome. Intestinal pneumatosis may be evident on abdominal films or CT. Serum antibodies (anti-Hu) directed against the myenteric plexus may be detectable in patients with some types of malignancies, especially small cell carcinoma.

In the absence of a definite obstructing lesion, the management of acute intestinal pseudoobstruction is supportive initially. Patients should be NPO and if vomiting, a nasogastric tube should be inserted and placed on low-intermittent suction. Laxatives should not be given, particularly those that can be fermented by colonic bacteria to produce gas. Rare reports of colonic perforation exist when such patients are given lactulose. Electrolyte abnormalities should be corrected and medications known to exacerbate constipation should be discontinued if possible.

Once the cecal diameter reaches 10 cm increasing the risk for ischemia or perforation, or when the patient continues to do poorly on supportive therapy for more than 24 to 48 hours, endoscopic or pharmacologic decompression may be required. The risk of colonic perforation is estimated to be at about 3% when the cecal diameter exceeds 12 cm and had been present for >6 days. Neostigmine 2.0 mg administered intravenously can be used to decompress patients with acute intestinal pseudoobstruction. The response usually occurs rapidly after intravenous administration. The dose may be safely repeated if colonic dilatation recurs. In a small placebo-controlled randomized study, 91% of those receiving neostigmine experienced a reduction in abdominal distention. However, patients must undergo cardiac monitoring while receiving IV neostigmine, and atropine must be on hand in the event that severe bradycardia is induced. Contraindications to neostigmine use include ischemia, active bronchospasm, serum creatinine >3 mg/dL, cardiac arrhythmias, pregnancy, or bowel obstruction.

Alternatively, colonic decompression can be achieved endoscopically, recognizing the risk of perforation as a result of the procedure. A bowel prep should not be administered prior to this procedure. If there are concerns about recurrence, a colonic decompression tube can be left in place temporarily. This is preferred to a rectal tube, which succeeds mostly in decompressing the left colon.

MANAGING NEW CONSTIPATION IN THE HOSPITALIZED PATIENT

The management of acute constipation in the hospitalized patient has two arms: relieving the current discomfort associated with the constipation and preventing the situation from arising again. The treatment of acute constipation should be dictated by these verities of the patient's symptoms and the cause for the constipation. For example, a patient who typically had daily bowel movements but while hospitalized has had no bowel movement for several days and complains of abdominal discomfort, bloating, or distention would probably achieve the most rapid relief by taking a stimulant laxative until a bowel movement is achieved. In patients with only mild symptoms of constipation, an osmotic laxative may achieve satisfactory results. Enemas may be helpful for eliminating stool from the left side of the colon, particularly if the patient complains of a sense of rectal fullness. An abdominal flat plate can sometimes be helpful in determining the location and extent of fecal retention. In those patients who are severely constipated, right colonic stimulation may be required, and an oral stimulant laxative is suggested. Alternatively, oral lavage using large-volume PEG 3350 solutions (as used for colonoscopy preparation) can be very effective, provided the patient is not experiencing nausea or vomiting. Reducing the amount of opioids and correcting electrolyte disturbances are paramount to the treatment and prevention of constipation.

In patients with symptoms of severe constipation, stool softeners are likely to be ineffective and add little to a preventative laxative regimen. Lactulose should also be avoided in this situation, since colonic fermentation of lactulose produces gas and increases distention and abdominal pain. Rare instances of colonic perforation have been reported when lactulose has been administered in this scenario. However, lactulose may be used later to prevent recurrent constipation.

PREVENTING RECURRENT CONSTIPATION IN THE HOSPITALIZED PATIENT

Once a satisfactory bowel movement has occurred, the patient should be placed on a laxative regimen to prevent constipation from occurring again. It is helpful to immediately start the patient on an osmotic laxative, such as lactulose or polyethylene glycol 3350, on a daily basis. Addition of a stimulant laxative may be required intermittently or daily, particularly in those individuals at high risk for recurrent constipation. This would include those who are immobile, have neurologic disease, or use opioids.

CHRONIC CONSTIPATION

Many patients who complain of constipation during their hospitalization have a history of chronic constipation prior to being hospitalized. It is important to recognize that the chronic constipation can be difficult to define due to differing patient and physician perceptions. Patients with chronic constipation often present with a variety of symptoms including hard or lumpy stools, infrequent stools, excessive straining, feeling of incomplete evacuation, and rectal fullness or discomfort. The Rome III classification accounts for this heterogeneity of symptoms by basing its criteria on symptoms. Using Rome III criteria, a diagnosis of functional constipation is made when two or more of the symptoms in **Table 80-3** are fulfilled, when loose stools are rarely present without laxative use, and when the criteria for irritable bowel syndrome with constipation (IBS-C) subtype in **Table 80-4** are not met. In addition, symptoms must have started ≥6 months ago and must have been present for the last 3 months.

TABLE 80-3 Rome III Criteria for Functional Constipation*

1. Must include *two or more* of the following:
   a. Straining during at least 25% of defecations
   b. Lumpy or hard stools in at least 25% of defecations
   c. Sensation of incomplete evacuation for at least 25% of defecations
   d. Sensation of anorectal obstruction/blockage for at least 25% of defecations
   e. Manual maneuvers to facilitate at least 25% of defecations (eg, digital evacuation, support of the pelvic floor)
   f. Fewer than three defecations per week
2. Loose stools are rarely present without the use of laxatives
3. There are insufficient criteria for IBS

Criteria fulfilled for the last 3 mo with symptom onset at least 6 mo prior to diagnosis.

TYPES OF CONSTIPATION

Constipation can be classified into three pathophysiologic subtypes: normal-transit, slow-transit, and pelvic outlet dysfunction. The three subtypes can overlap. *Normal-transit constipation*, the most common subtype, is characterized by normal colonic transit time and normal defecatory function. A subset of these individuals has reduced colonic tone or compliance. *Slow-transit constipation* is characterized by delayed transit of stool through the colon due to a myopathy or neuropathy. Slowed colonic transit arises from diminished motor activity, such as reduced high-amplitude contractions. This type of constipation is moderately predicted by stool form (scybalous or hard lumpy balls of stool). In contrast to slow-transit constipation, *pelvic floor dysfunction*, the most common subtype among women, is characterized by difficulty or inability to evacuate stool from the anorectum. Pelvic floor dysfunction can be caused by failure of the internal anal sphincter or pelvic floor muscles to relax or paradoxical contraction of the external anal sphincter or puborectalis muscle while straining during defecation. Pelvic floor dysfunction is also referred to as defecatory disorder, anismus, pelvic-floor dyssynergia, paradoxical pelvic-floor contraction, obstructed constipation, functional rectosigmoid obstruction, spastic pelvic-floor syndrome, and functional fecal retention in childhood.

EVALUATION

The initial evaluation of a patient presenting with chronic constipation should consist of a careful history, physical examination, laboratory testing, and imaging to exclude secondary causes, prior

TABLE 80-4 Rome III Diagnostic Criteria for Irritable Bowel Syndrome with Constipation (IBS-C)*

Recurrent abdominal pain or discomfort[?] at least 3 d per month in the last 3 mo associated with *two or more* of the following:
1. Improvement with defecation
2. Onset associated with a change in frequency of stool
3. Onset associated with a change in the form (appearance) of stool—hard or lumpy stools[§] ≥ 25% and loose (mushy) or watery stools[¶] < 25% of bowel movements**

*Criteria fulfilled for the last 3 mo with symptom onset at least 6 mo prior to diagnosis.
[?]Discomfort means an uncomfortable sensation not described as pain.
[§]Bristol Stool Form Scale 1–2 (separate hard lumps like nuts [difficult to pass] or sausage-shaped but lumpy).
[¶]Bristol Stool Form Scale 6–7 (fluffy pieces with ragged edges, a mushy stool or watery, no solid pieces, entirely liquid).
**In the absence of use of antidiarrheals or laxatives.

to pursuing a diagnosis of functional constipation. Symptoms alone cannot distinguish between the subtypes of functional constipation. Certain historical clues, however, should generate a high index of suspicion for pelvic outlet dysfunction as a cause of constipation, including a sense of obstruction in the anal region, and manual maneuvers to facilitate stool evacuation, including unusual postures on the toilet, support of the perineum, digital manipulation of the rectum, and posterior vaginal pressure.

While a thorough examination of the abdomen, perineum, and anorectum should be performed, the physical exam should pay particular attention to pelvic floor motion. The examiner should inspect for perineal abnormalities while the patient bears down, including pulling forward of the anus. While performing the digital rectal exam, the examiner should assess sphincter tone by having the patient bear down to elicit perineal descent and relaxation of the sphincter. Abnormal findings on palpation include high resting anal sphincter tone, descent of the perineum <1.0 cm or >3.5 cm while straining, posterior rectal wall tenderness, a palpable mucosal prolapse, or defect in the anterior rectum. Physiologic testing for functional constipation should be performed only after excluding secondary causes of constipation in cases refractory to a high-fiber diet and laxatives. Colonic transit studies with radiopaque markers (Sitzmarks) or scintigraphy are the initial tests of choice, allowing differentiation between normal transit, slow transit, and pelvic outlet obstruction. The patient ingests a capsule containing radiopaque markers and an abdominal flat plate is obtained 120 hours later. No markers will be retained in those with normal transit. However, markers retained throughout the colon are indicative of slow transit. Accumulation of markers in the left colon is suggestive of pelvic outlet obstruction, but could also be compounded by slow transit.

If the history and physical exam are suggestive of pelvic floor dysfunction, anorectal manometry, balloon expulsion testing, and defecography are useful tests. Anorectal manometry assesses rectal sensation and compliance, sphincter pressures, and anorectal reflexes. The test may suggest Hirschsprung disease. The balloon expulsion test can identify but cannot exclude dyssynergic defecation. As an adjunct to other testing, MRI or video defecography can be used to confirm or exclude pelvic floor dysfunction, and can identify a clinically significant rectocele, rectal intussusception, and rectal prolapse. Finally, electromyography of the anal sphincter muscles can evaluate for dysfunction of the striated pelvic floor muscles.

MANAGING CHRONIC CONSTIPATION

PRACTICE POINT

- No currently available stimulant laxatives have been associated with an increased risk for neoplasia. The evidence that chronic stimulant laxative use damages neurons and causes cathartic colon is very limited and remains controversial.

Understanding how each laxative type works is essential for proper management of acute and chronic constipation (**Table 80-5**). For those individuals with mild, intermittent constipation, use of an occasional stool softener or magnesium-based osmotic laxative can be effective. Nearly all patients can benefit somewhat from increasing daily fiber consumption to at least 30 g per day. Daily fiber, be it insoluble or soluble, can be consumed in the diet or by use of one of numerous fiber supplements available over the counter. Patients should be encouraged to use the equivalent of 5 to 10 g of fiber daily, be it in the form of a supplement or foods, such as a high-fiber cereal that gives 10 to 13 g per cup. When using fiber to manage constipation, patients must be informed before they become discouraged that they may not observe a change in their stool

TABLE 80-5 Pharmacologic Agents Used to Treat Constipation

Bulking agents containing psyllium

Osmotic laxatives: these draw water into the intestinal lumen and are useful in those who report hard or scybalous stool that is unresponsive to dietary fiber

    Polyethylene glycol

    Lactulose

    Magnesium and sulfate salts

Stimulant laxatives

    Anthraquinones: senna, aloe, cascara, frangula

    Polyphenolic (diphenylmethane) compounds: bisacodyl, sodium picosulfate

Detergents/stool softeners

    Docusate sodium

    Liquid paraffin

Prokinetic agents

    Colchicines

    Misoprostol

Chloride channel activator

    Lubiprostone

Opioid antagonists

    Methylnaltrexone

    Alvimopan

Enemas and suppositories

    Sodium lauryl sulphoacetate, osmotic agents, glycerol

    Saline and water enema

    Hypertonic sodium phosphate enemas

    Glycerin suppositories, bisacodyl suppositories or enema, oxyphenisatin

consistency for 7 to 14 days after initiating daily fiber supplementation. In addition, they may experience increased gassiness during this 2-week period as a result of increased bacterial fermentation. Patients with irritable bowel syndrome may be exquisitely sensitive to the gas produced by increased fiber intake and may be intolerant of it.

In patients who report passage of hard, scybalous, stool with either normalor slow-transit constipation, if fiber fails to alleviate the hard stool, addition of a daily osmotic laxative, such as lactulose or PEG 3350, is usually effective. Because osmotic laxatives are not the same as stimulant laxatives, patients must be told to assess the full impact of this regimen after 7 to 14 days have passed. After that, the dose and timing of the laxative can be adjusted to better suit the lifestyle and expectations of the patient. Lubiprostone, a calcium channel stimulator, draws water into the colon and can be used in patients with mild-to-moderate constipation. The advantage of lubiprostone is that it is available in pill form, but does cause nausea in a third of users, and therefore should be taken with food. In a clinical trial involving individuals with chronic constipation, the majority of individuals had a bowel movement within 24 to 48 hours of taking the medication. Lubiprostone has also been approved by the FDA for the treatment of IBS-constipation, but at a dose of 8 mcg bid as opposed to 24 mcg bid approved for functional constipation.

Linaclotide is also a secretory agent like lubiprostone, but linaclotide works through a different mechanism as a guanylate cyclase C agonist. It is taken orally, 30 minutes prior to the first meal. A fifth of users experience diarrhea. Patients who respond to linaclotide should expect improvement in bowel movement frequency and/or abdominal pain within 1 week. Linaclotide is FDA approved for the treatment of chronic idiopathic constipation at a dose of 145 mcg and is also approved for IBS-constipation at 290 mcg.

Prucalopride, a 5-hydroxytryptamine-4 (5-HT4) receptor agonist, stimulates intestinal motility, and is approved in Europe for the treatment of chronic constipation in women, but has been shown to increase the number of weekly bowel movements and improve symptoms in men.

In patients with pelvic floor dysfunction, use of a suppository can be helpful if rectal stimulation is required to initiate the bowel movement. These patients frequently benefit from using a stimulant laxative, such as a sennasoide, bisacodyl, or sodium picosulfate, every day or every other day. Occasional enema use can also help address the left-sided fullness and stimulate defecation. Patients with pelvic floor dysfunction may also report hard stool, so a regimen using both an osmotic and stimulant laxative is sometimes required.

Patients frequently express concern about long-term stimulant laxative use. They fear chronic use causes "dependency" or a "lazy colon." Many health care providers share this concern because of early reports of a possible relationship between chronic stimulant laxative use and cathartic colon. However, the evidence that chronic stimulant laxative use damages neurons and causes cathartic colon is very limited and remains controversial. While it is true that chronic use of an anthraquinone may cause the diffuse colonic pigmentation known as melanosis coli, this is of no clinical significance. An additional concern was that use of stimulant laxatives could increase cancer risk. Most phenolphthalein-containing laxatives were withdrawn from the market when they were shown to increase ovarian, adrenal, renal, and hematopoietic neoplasms in rodents. No other stimulant laxatives have been associated with an increased risk for neoplasia.

Special attention is given here to managing constipation in the patient who chronically uses opioids for pain management. Eighty-one percent of chronic users will report constipation. Opioids, which activate μ-receptors widely distributed among the neurons of the myenteric and submucosal plexus and immune cells in the lamina propria, inhibit excitatory neural pathways thereby delaying intestinal transit. They also inhibit water and electrolyte secretion into the gut lumen. Constipation is this patient population may be additionally managed by attempting to reduce the amount of opioids used. Another possibility is to consider substituting a central μ-opioid agonist and norepinephrine reuptake inhibitor, such as tapentadol, which appears to be less constipating compared to oxycodone. Finally, peripheral μ-receptor antagonists naloxone and methylnaltrexone can be used to treat opioid-induced constipation. Prolonged-release naloxone when given in combination with prolonged-release oxycodone does not reverse the analgesia but improves bowel function. Methylnaltrexone, which is FDA approved for the treatment of opioid-induced constipation in patients taking opioids for noncancer pain, is administered as a subcutaneous injection, and 50% to 60% will experience a bowel movement within 4 hours after injection. The injection may be repeated every other day. Another peripheral μ-receptor antagonist, alvimopan, is currently FDA approved only for the use in postoperative ileus.

TIMING OF CONSULTATION WITH A GASTROENTEROLOGIST OR A SURGEON

A GI and/or surgical consultation should be obtained for any constipated patient who has severe pain, pain out of proportion to exam, or who has signs suggesting development of a serious complication, such as ischemia, perforation, or obstruction.

A consultant may be particularly helpful in the management of suspected colonic obstruction. Treatment of sigmoid volvulus includes placement of a temporary rectal tube or endoscopic reduction as long as there are no clinical, radiological, or laboratory signs of ischemia or perforation. Barium enema may also be performed, but carries a higher risk of perforation than endoscopic decompression. Sigmoid volvulus is very amenable to initial endoscopic reduction, but recurrence rate may be as high as 70% so elective resection after decompression is recommended. Any sign of ischemia, such as bloody stool, during endoscopic reduction is an indication for urgent surgery. Endoscopic reduction of cecal volvulus is successful in only 30% of cases, so surgery is generally recommended as first-line treatment unless the patient is a poor surgical candidate. Benign or malignant colonic strictures can be diagnosed by colonoscopy and biopsy. Benign strictures can be dilated endoscopically using balloon dilators or colonic stents. Surgery may be necessary to resect benign or malignant colonic strictures.

PREVENTION

PRACTICE POINT

- Stool softeners are largely ineffective in patients who take opioids, have undergone surgery causing them to be bedridden, or have a history of chronic constipation. A major contributing factor to constipation emerging as an active issue in the hospitalized patient is the failure to (1) obtain an accurate history of chronic constipation and (2) continue the patient's home laxative regimen.

A major contributing factor to constipation emerging as an active issue in the hospitalized patient is the failure to obtain an accurate history of chronic constipation and not continuing the patient's home laxative regimen. In fact, it is very common for admitting orders on some services to ignore the patient's home laxatives and reflexively include an order for stool softeners. Stool softeners are largely ineffective in patients who take opioids, have undergone surgery causing them to be bedridden, or have a history of chronic constipation. In the acutely hospitalized older patient, the use of laxatives at home was a good predictor for constipation while in the hospital. There is also the mistaken impression that patients who are not eating will not have any bowel movements at all.

Identifying the risks for constipation, as well as a prior history of constipation, is essential for preventing constipation in the hospitalized patient. In those at high risk, starting a daily osmotic laxative can be highly effective, recognizing that their effectiveness may not be immediately apparent. In selecting an osmotic laxative, it is important to be aware that frequent administration of magnesium-based compounds raises serum magnesium levels in patients with chronic renal insufficiency. A daily stimulant laxative may be helpful in those at highest risk or in whom the history suggests pelvic floor dysfunction.

CONCLUSION

Constipation is a common problem in the hospitalized patient. New constipation may be precipitated by many factors associated with hospitalization. Recognizing the risks for constipation is the mainstay of managing and preventing constipation. The major risks are a prior history of chronic constipation, use of constipating medications, particularly opioids, and lack of physical activity due to medical illness or surgical recovery. Selecting the proper laxative for management or prevention of constipation requires familiarity with the different types of laxatives and educating patients about these differences to address their expectations about their efficacy. Finally, it is also essential for the hospitalist to recognize when constipation is actually a manifestation of an acute, possibly emergent event that requires immediate management by consultants.

SUGGESTED READINGS

American Gastroenterological Association, Bharucha AE, Dorn SD, Lembo A, Pressman A. American Gastroenterological Association medical position statement on constipation. *Gastroenterology.* 2013;144(1):211-217.

Bharucha AE, Pemberton JH, Locke GR 3rd. American Gastroenterological Association technical review on constipation. *Gastroenterology.* 2013;144(1):218-38.

Lal SK, Morgenstern R, Vinjirayer EP, Matin A. Sigmoid volvulus an update. *Gastrointest Endosc Clin N Am.* 2006;16:175-187.

Leppert W. Emerging therapies for patients with symptoms of opioid-induced bowel dysfunction. *Drug Des Devel Ther.* 2015; 9:2215-2231.

Rao SS. Constipation: evaluation and treatment of colonic and anorectal motility disorders. *Gastroenterol Clin North Am.* 2007;36: 687-711.

CHAPTER 81

Delirium

Karin J. Neufeld, MD, MPH
Laura K. Max, BA
Makeida B. Koyi, MD
Dale M. Needham, MD, PhD

Key Clinical Questions

1 What is the prevalence of delirium in hospitalized patients?

2 What are the most common causes of delirium?

3 Why is it important to detect delirium?

4 What are the symptoms of delirium?

5 How is delirium diagnosed?

6 How can delirium be prevented and treated?

INTRODUCTION

Delirium is common in hospitalized patients. The prevalence of delirium may be as high as 80% in mechanically ventilated patients in the intensive care unit (ICU), 50% in geriatric postoperative patients, and 10% to 40% in general medical patients. Patients who develop delirium frequently have multiple risk factors. These include nonmodifiable factors, such as increased age, pre-existing cognitive impairment, and a history of prior stroke or brain injury. Important modifiable risk factors include (1) exposure to deliriogenic medications, (2) infection, (3) metabolic derangement, (4) organ failure, (5) dehydration, (6) malnutrition, (7) surgery, (8) immobility, (9) use of physical restraints, (10) sensory impairment, (11) sleep deprivation, (12) pain, and (13) drug withdrawal or intoxication.

PRACTICE POINT

Delirium as a red flag
- Delirium is a nonspecific warning sign, like fever or hypotension, indicating that something serious may be wrong and requires further investigation. Thirty-nine percent of inpatients with delirium die within one year. *Do not ignore this red flag.*

Delirium is associated with increased mortality, morbidity, and length of stay. Estimates of annual US health care costs attributed to delirium range from $40 billion to $150 billion. Delirious patients require extra care following discharge from acute inpatient units and are at increased risk of being discharged to a skilled nursing facility rather than directly home. Patients often suffer from frightening memories of delirious episodes while hospitalized. Such experiences may result in appreciable anxiety and preoccupation long after delirium has cleared, impacting the patient's quality of life for months to years. Family members are often distressed by the changed demeanor and behavior of their loved one, making care and support more challenging.

PATHOPHYSIOLOGY

The central feature of delirium is an acute disturbance of consciousness accompanied by altered cognition or perception. Disruptions in brain function occur in the brainstem, thalamus, prefrontal cortex, fusiform cortex, and parietal lobes. This widespread cortical dysfunction is typically associated with diffuse and symmetric slowing of electrical activity on electroencephalography (EEG), although fast electrical activity occurs in some cases, especially in alcohol or sedative withdrawal.

PRACTICE POINT

- The diagnosis of delirium requires diminished attention and awareness, evolving over a short period of time (hours to days), waxing and waning in severity, and associated with other disturbances in cognition, such as memory deficits and disorientation. Delirium cannot be wholly explained by a pre-existing neurologic disorder. History, physical examination, laboratory testing, and imaging should reveal one or more inciting factors, such as electrolyte disturbances, infections, adverse effects of medications, or drug and alcohol withdrawal syndromes.

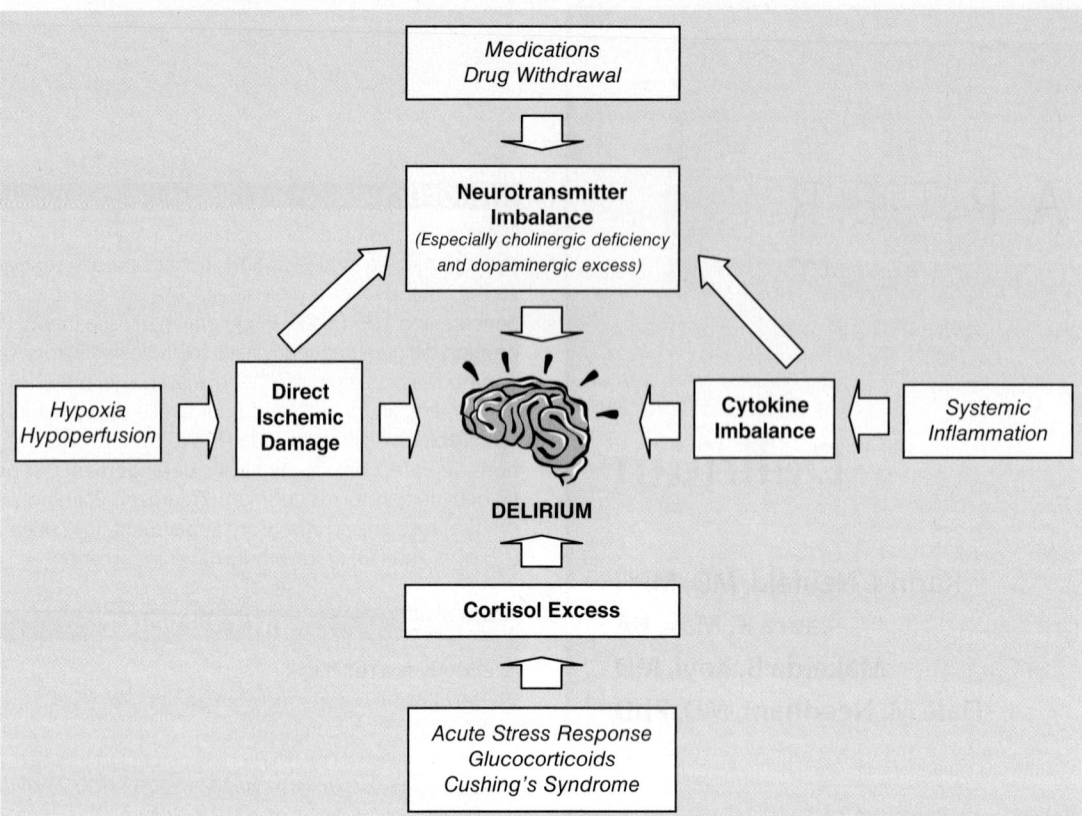

Figure 81-1 *Pathophysiology of delirium.*

Figure 81-1 depicts numerous potential pathways to delirium and underscores its complex pathogenesis. Neurotransmitter imbalances, especially cholinergic deficiency and dopaminergic excess, may play a key role in the development of delirium. This hypothesis is supported by the observation that anticholinergic and dopaminergic drugs frequently precipitate delirium, whereas antidopaminergic drugs, such as antipsychotics, have been used to treat the symptoms of agitation associated with delirium. Other neurotransmitters, such as glutamate, GABA, serotonin, norepinephrine, and histamine, have also been implicated in the pathogenesis of delirium. For example, norepinephrine and glutamate hyperactivity and GABA hypoactivity are associated with delirium tremens, while GABA hyperactivity is associated with hepatic encephalopathy.

Proinflammatory cytokines have a direct neurotoxic effect on the brain and affect the synthesis and release of neurotransmitters, thereby contributing to delirium. Finally, elevated cortisol levels and ischemic brain damage from hypoperfusion or hypoxia also have been linked to delirium.

DIAGNOSIS OF DELIRIUM

The diagnosis of delirium is based on a relatively abrupt alteration in the level of consciousness, which often waxes and wanes over the course of a day, with associated inattention and changes in cognition or perception. Due to inattention, patients may ask the same question repeatedly or perseverate on an issue. Cognitive deficits may affect short-term and intermediate recall, word finding, orientation, and the ability to learn new information. Perceptual disturbances, such as illusions or hallucinations, are also common. Illusions are misinterpretations of stimuli (eg, mistaking an intravenous line for a snake), while hallucinations are perceptions without stimuli. Hallucinations are most frequently visual (eg, seeing bugs crawling on the walls), but can be auditory (eg, hearing voices), or tactile (eg, feeling bugs crawling on the skin). These disturbances arise as physiologic

consequences of medical illness or from substance intoxication or withdrawal, rather than from an underlying psychiatric condition.

Other common features of delirium are not necessary for diagnosis but are noteworthy because they often mimic mental illness. Patients may develop fixed, false, idiosyncratic beliefs (delusions), often persecutory in nature. For example, delirious patients commonly believe that their nurses or doctors intend to harm them. Other frequent findings include speech that is difficult to follow or that frequently wanders off topic (disorganized speech). Patients may also experience significant and rapid shifts in emotional tone (affective lability), with bouts of tearfulness, anxiety, or increased irritability. Sleep-wake cycle disruption, with increased napping during the day and difficulty with sustained sleep at night, is present in most cases of delirium.

Subtypes of delirium are distinguished by the predominant level of psychomotor activity. The *hypoactive subtype* is characterized by decreased motor activity and increased somnolence. Patients appear quietly indifferent to their surroundings and have great difficulty arousing and sustaining attention. Treating physicians may misattribute this presentation to a depressive disorder. The *hyperactive subtype* is associated with increased motor activity and agitation. Patients are restless, talkative, and aroused. They may pull at intravenous lines and indwelling catheters or even strike out against caregivers. Although they appear fully alert, these patients have trouble sustaining attention. The *mixed subtype* includes features of both increased and decreased psychomotor activity. While hyperactive behavior is easy for nurses and doctors to identify, hypoactive delirium is often overlooked because these patients are not demanding, and their cognitive limitations must be elicited through direct cognitive examination. To avoid missing hypoactive delirium, physicians must maintain a high index of suspicion and should expect all patients to be easily arousable and able to perform basic cognitive tasks at their preadmission baseline.

There are many screening and delirium diagnostic tools available to rate the presence or absence and severity of delirium. Diagnostic algorithms such as the Confusion Assessment Method, or rating tools such as the DRS-98R or Memorial Delirium Rating Scale, are generally most valid when used by a clinical expert or trained evaluator. Because the rating of diagnostic tools and algorithms is based on a careful clinical examination that includes formal cognitive assessment, use of these tools takes much more time than delirium screening instruments.

Screening tools, designed for use by nonspecialist bedside personnel, can be performed in less than 2 minutes. For patients in the ICU setting, the CAM-ICU (a modified version of the CAM that can be administered to nonverbal, mechanically ventilated patients) has been demonstrated to be a valid and highly reliable screening tool (with pooled sensitivity and specificity of 76%-80% and 96%, respectively) that is easily administered by ICU nurses. Another validated instrument for the critical care setting is the Intensive Care Delirium Screening Checklist (ICDSC), a cumulative checklist that is completed during each nursing shift over a 24-hour period with sensitivity and specificity of 80% and 96%, respectively. Both the CAM-ICU and the ICDSC can be downloaded from the following website: http://www.icudelirium.org. The sensitivity of these particular instruments in a noncritically ill patient population is too limited for generalized use. Other tools for widespread use in noncritically hospitalized patients include the 4AT (available at http://www.the4at.com) which has been validated in a number of inpatient populations including older individuals with dementia and neurology inpatients. Other screening tests include the 3D-CAM, which has been validated in a geriatric population.

Finally, the EEG, which typically reveals diffuse slowing in the setting of delirium (except in delirium tremens, which is associated with fast activity), may help support a diagnosis of delirium or rule out nonconvulsive seizure activity. However, it should not be used as a primary diagnostic tool for delirium, as it is neither sufficiently sensitive nor specific.

DIFFERENTIAL DIAGNOSIS

Physicians frequently misattribute signs and symptoms of delirium to psychiatric illness. For example, distinguishing delirium from dementia can be challenging. Both diagnoses are associated with cognitive impairment. However, dementia without superimposed delirium does not result in fluctuating levels of consciousness. The patient's recent baseline physical and mental status, along with timing of onset, pattern of symptom fluctuation, and duration of symptoms will help to distinguish these two syndromes and should be carefully elicited from collateral informants such as the family and bedside nurse. Delirium has its onset over hours to days, while dementia involves a protracted decline over months to years. Sundowning refers to an increase in confusion and agitation during late afternoon and evening among a subset of patients with dementia. Some authors regard this as a delirium-related phenomenon. However, little systematic research has been conducted, and multiple other etiologies have been proposed. The phenomenon has been explained as a response to fatigue or to unmet physical or psychological needs, or as a consequence of underlying sleep disorders or inadequate daytime light exposure. It must be remembered that demented patients are at significant risk of developing delirium. Whenever there is a fluctuating level of consciousness, a workup for medical causes of delirium should be initiated.

Delirium, especially the hypoactive subtype, is also commonly confused with a depressive illness. Patients with either diagnosis may have significant psychomotor slowing, poor oral intake, and sleep disruption. They may appear withdrawn and sad, and they may even express a desire to die or end their lives. However, depressed patients do not experience alterations in level of consciousness. They may be inattentive and have problems with short-term recall, but they remain oriented. They also frequently have a personal or family history of depression and describe a gradual onset of symptoms, in contrast to the acute onset observed with delirium.

A number of other psychiatric disorders also may be misdiagnosed in the delirious patient. Hyperactive delirium may be confused with mania, and prominent hallucinations or delusions frequently raise concern for schizophrenia. Delirious patients who are anxious may be misdiagnosed with anxiety disorders. Moreover, those who are irritable (such that they refuse medical care) or inattentive (such that they fail to follow nursing instructions) may be considered "difficult" or "noncompliant," even when their behaviors result from delirium and are beyond their control. In all these cases, if there is a fluctuating level of consciousness or disorientation, delirium is more likely than any other psychiatric condition. The past psychiatric history and timing of symptom onset are also essential in making a diagnosis. Most psychiatric disorders present by early adulthood (although there are exceptions, such as depressive disorders). A geriatric patient suddenly seeing cats running across the hospital floor, or who is described by family members as usually "easy-going and slow-to-anger" but is now found to be "difficult," is more likely to have new-onset delirium, rather than a new-onset psychiatric disorder.

Because delirium can masquerade as almost any psychiatric disorder, it is imperative that physicians avoid basing any new psychiatric diagnoses on a patient's mental status while he or she is still delirious. Even if history obtained from collateral informants suggests that there is an underlying anxiety disorder or major depressive disorder, pharmacologic treatment of these disorders should not be initiated until the patient's delirium has cleared, since new medications may worsen the delirium, and response to a new medication cannot be properly assessed while a patient is still delirious. Physicians should also be wary of attributing psychiatric symptoms to a patient's known chronic psychiatric illness without thoroughly evaluating whether the symptoms are consistent with that illness. Just as demented patients can become delirious, so can patients with any other psychiatric disorder.

TREATMENT OF DELIRIUM

Delirium is an important medical indicator. It may be the first sign of a new life-threatening medical condition, such as organ failure, overdose, infection, or a central nervous system (CNS) event (see **Table 81-1** for a list of common causes). The most important goal in treating delirium is to discover and correct the underlying cause(s). The diagnostic workup of delirium is outlined in **Figure 81-2**. Clinicians should start by reviewing the history, doing a physical exam, including brief cognitive tests of mental status, and performing basic laboratory investigations.

■ WITHDRAWAL-RELATED DELIRIUM

As a first step, determine whether alcohol, benzodiazepine, or barbiturate withdrawal is a cause of the delirium. Obtain a history from the patient and collateral informants (including outpatient health care providers) to determine the duration, pattern, and quantity of alcohol intake; the extent of any prescription or illicit use of benzodiazepines or barbiturates; and whether there are any prior episodes of withdrawal symptoms. Review the street names for readily available prescription drugs in your area. For example, "pins" can refer to Klonopin (clonazepam) tablets, and "bars" can refer to 2-mg Xanax (alprazolam) tablets, which are commonly sold in illicit settings.

TABLE 81-1 Causes of Delirium: "DELIRIVM"

D Drugs/poisons
- *Medications* (see **Table 81-2**)
- *Drugs of abuse* (eg, alcohol, cocaine, PCP, inhalants)
- *Industrial poisons* (eg, organophosphates, heavy metals, organic solvents)
- *Animal, plant, and mushroom toxins*
- *Withdrawal* (from alcohol or sedatives/hypnotics)

E External insults
- *Closed-head injury*
- *Heat stroke*
- *Hypothermia*
- *Electrocution*

L Lesions from cancer
- *Primary brain cancer*
- *Meningeal carcinomatosis*
- *Metastatic lesions* (especially from melanoma and lung, breast, colon, and kidney cancers)

I Infections
- *Intracranial* (bacterial/viral/fungal encephalitis or meningitis, brain/epidural/subdural abscess, trichinosis, cerebral malaria, fungal infections, Creutzfeldt-Jakob disease, neurosyphilis; in HIV/AIDS: cytomegalovirus encephalitis, cryptococcal meningitis, progressive multifocal leukoencephalopathy, toxoplasmosis, tubercular meningitis)
- *Systemic* (sepsis, pneumonia, subacute bacterial endocarditis, influenza, mononucleosis, mumps, typhoid fever, Lyme disease, Behçet disease, brucellosis, psittacosis, Rocky Mountain spotted fever, typhus; in HIV/AIDS: disseminated herpes zoster, candidiasis)

R Remote effects of cancer (paraneoplastic syndromes)
- *Paraneoplastic limbic encephalitis* (especially with lung, breast, or testicular cancers; paraneoplastic syndromes may occur before there are any signs of cancer on imaging)

I Ictal/interictal/postictal (seizures)

V Vascular causes
- *Emboli from cardiac source*
- *Intracranial bleed or thrombosis*
- *Hypertensive encephalopathy*
- *Autoimmune* (lupus cerebritis, sarcoid, polyarteritis nodosa, thrombotic thrombocytopenic purpura)
- *Circulatory collapse* (shock)

M Metabolic causes
- *Hypoxia*
- *Hypoglycemia*
- *Electrolyte imbalance* (hyponatremia, hypernatremia, hypercalcemia, hypocalcemia, hypokalemia, hyperkalemia, hypomagnesemia, hypermagnesemia, hypophosphatemia)
- *Acidosis or alkalosis*
- *Errors of metabolism* (porphyria)
- *Vitamin deficiency* (vitamin B12, thiamine, nicotinic acid)
- *Vitamin intoxication* (vitamin A, vitamin D)
- *Organ failure* (kidney, liver, lungs, pancreas)
- *Endocrinopathies* (hyperthyroidism, hypothyroidism, hyperparathyroidism, hypopituitarism, Addison disease, Cushing syndrome, insulinoma, diabetic ketoacidosis, hyperosmolar nonketotic hyperglycemia)

If a patient is in withdrawal, physical examination will typically reveal autonomic arousal, with hypertension, fever, tachycardia, tongue and extremity tremor, pupillary dilation, sweating, and motor restlessness, or pronounced instability of vital signs. Peak autonomic withdrawal from alcohol occurs 72 to 96 hours from the last drink, while withdrawal from long-acting benzodiazepines such as diazepam may take up to 1 week to peak. Delirium may then extend several weeks beyond the presence of withdrawal signs. GABAergic agents such as chlordiazepoxide, diazepam, oxazepam, or lorazepam are the treatment of choice. Symptom-triggered dosing of a short-acting agent (eg, oxazepam 15-30 mg orally or lorazepam 1-2 mg IV every 2 hours as needed for symptoms of withdrawal, such as tremor, agitation, or insomnia) is associated with better outcomes than fixed titration schedules, but requires regular screening for symptoms of withdrawal by bedside staff. Another approach is to give a loading dose of a long-acting agent (eg, chlordiazepoxide 50-100 mg orally every 1-2 hours for mild-to-moderate withdrawal or diazepam 5-10 mg IV as frequently as every 5-10 minutes for severe withdrawal) until the patient is calm. The long half-life of these agents allows for a smooth self-taper after discontinuation. In the event of breakthrough withdrawal signs, additional medication (eg, chlordiazepoxide 25-50 mg orally or diazepam 5-10 mg IV) can be given every 2 hours as needed. Individuals with advanced liver disease should be treated with oxazepam or lorazepam preferentially, as these medications have shorter half-lives and no active metabolites. If the patient cannot be closely monitored for signs of withdrawal, then these short-acting agents should be given on a fixed schedule and tapered by 20% to 25% daily. Although symptom-triggered dosing has been associated with less total benzodiazepine administration and fewer days of delirium per patient than fixed schedule therapy, it is fully effective only when nurses have both the time and ability to monitor patients regularly and frequently.

If a patient's delirium worsens or fails to respond to treatment with benzodiazepines, the treating physician should consider alternative etiologies of the patient's continued delirium. For example, if a formerly agitated patient becomes sedated and confused, clinicians should consider both overuse of benzodiazepines and hepatic encephalopathy.

■ MEDICATION-RELATED DELIRIUM

Medication lists of delirious patients should always be reviewed to look for any new medication that coincided with the onset of delirium. In the setting of worsening kidney or liver function, a previously well-tolerated medication may cause delirium due to decreased drug clearance. The addition of new medications may render an old medication newly deliriogenic by inhibiting its metabolism, or old medications may cause delirium in the setting of new neurologic insults. Review the medication list for anticholinergic and other frequently implicated agents (**Table 81-2**) and discontinue or replace these medications.

If history and physical exam reveal little or no risk of withdrawal-related delirium, avoid using benzodiazepines (unless a patient was taking them prior to admission, in which case they should be continued at the preadmission dose). Avoid even the nonbenzodiazepine hypnotics, or "z" drugs used for sleep, such as zolpidem or zaleplon. These medications can also cause or contribute to delirium. Anxiety and agitation are common in delirious patients. Resist the urge to treat with benzodiazepines. If reassurance and redirection fail to calm a patient's severe agitation, try antipsychotics instead (**Table 81-3**), particularly if agitation is due to psychotic symptoms such as delusions or hallucinations.

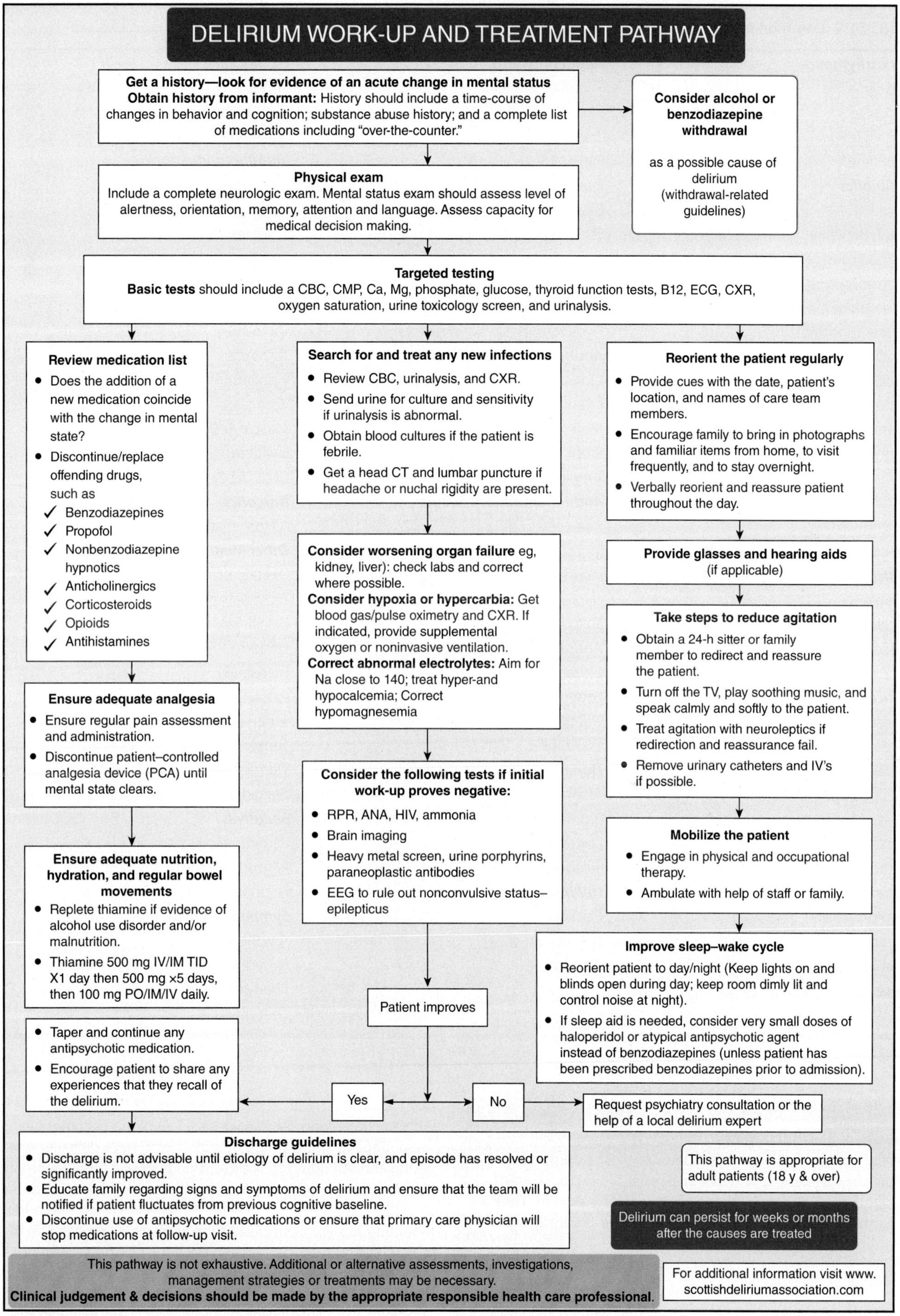

DELIRIUM WORK-UP AND TREATMENT PATHWAY

Get a history—look for evidence of an acute change in mental status
Obtain history from informant: History should include a time-course of changes in behavior and cognition; substance abuse history; and a complete list of medications including "over-the-counter."

Consider alcohol or benzodiazepine withdrawal

as a possible cause of delirium (withdrawal-related guidelines)

Physical exam
Include a complete neurologic exam. Mental status exam should assess level of alertness, orientation, memory, attention and language. Assess capacity for medical decision making.

Targeted testing
Basic tests should include a CBC, CMP, Ca, Mg, phosphate, glucose, thyroid function tests, B12, ECG, CXR, oxygen saturation, urine toxicology screen, and urinalysis.

Review medication list
- Does the addition of a new medication coincide with the change in mental state?
- Discontinue/replace offending drugs, such as
  ✓ Benzodiazepines
  ✓ Propofol
  ✓ Nonbenzodiazepine hypnotics
  ✓ Anticholinergics
  ✓ Corticosteroids
  ✓ Opioids
  ✓ Antihistamines

Ensure adequate analgesia
- Ensure regular pain assessment and administration.
- Discontinue patient–controlled analgesia device (PCA) until mental state clears.

Ensure adequate nutrition, hydration, and regular bowel movements
- Replete thiamine if evidence of alcohol use disorder and/or malnutrition.
- Thiamine 500 mg IV/IM TID X1 day then 500 mg ×5 days, then 100 mg PO/IM/IV daily.

- Taper and continue any antipsychotic medication.
- Encourage patient to share any experiences that they recall of the delirium.

Search for and treat any new infections
- Review CBC, urinalysis, and CXR.
- Send urine for culture and sensitivity if urinalysis is abnormal.
- Obtain blood cultures if the patient is febrile.
- Get a head CT and lumbar puncture if headache or nuchal rigidity are present.

Consider worsening organ failure eg, kidney, liver): check labs and correct where possible.
Consider hypoxia or hypercarbia: Get blood gas/pulse oximetry and CXR. If indicated, provide supplemental oxygen or noninvasive ventilation.
Correct abnormal electrolytes: Aim for Na close to 140; treat hyper-and hypocalcemia; Correct hypomagnesemia

Consider the following tests if initial work-up proves negative:
- RPR, ANA, HIV, ammonia
- Brain imaging
- Heavy metal screen, urine porphyrins, paraneoplastic antibodies
- EEG to rule out nonconvulsive status–epilepticus

Patient improves

Reorient the patient regularly
- Provide cues with the date, patient's location, and names of care team members.
- Encourage family to bring in photographs and familiar items from home, to visit frequently, and to stay overnight.
- Verbally reorient and reassure patient throughout the day.

Provide glasses and hearing aids (if applicable)

Take steps to reduce agitation
- Obtain a 24-h sitter or family member to redirect and reassure the patient.
- Turn off the TV, play soothing music, and speak calmly and softly to the patient.
- Treat agitation with neuroleptics if redirection and reassurance fail.
- Remove urinary catheters and IV's if possible.

Mobilize the patient
- Engage in physical and occupational therapy.
- Ambulate with help of staff or family.

Improve sleep–wake cycle
- Reorient patient to day/night (Keep lights on and blinds open during day; keep room dimly lit and control noise at night).
- If sleep aid is needed, consider very small doses of haloperidol or atypical antipsychotic agent instead of benzodiazepines (unless patient has been prescribed benzodiazepines prior to admission).

Yes | No

Request psychiatry consultation or the help of a local delirium expert

Discharge guidelines
- Discharge is not advisable until etiology of delirium is clear, and episode has resolved or significantly improved.
- Educate family regarding signs and symptoms of delirium and ensure that the team will be notified if patient fluctuates from previous cognitive baseline.
- Discontinue use of antipsychotic medications or ensure that primary care physician will stop medications at follow-up visit.

This pathway is appropriate for adult patients (18 y & over)

Delirium can persist for weeks or months after the causes are treated

This pathway is not exhaustive. Additional or alternative assessments, investigations, management strategies or treatments may be necessary.
Clinical judgement & decisions should be made by the appropriate responsible health care professional.

For additional information visit www.scottishdeliriumassociation.com

Figure 81-2 *Diagnosis and treatment of delirium.*

TABLE 81-2 Common Medications Linked to Delirium

Antiarrhythmics	**Antidepressants**	**H2 Blockers**
Disopyramide	Tricyclics	Cimetidine
Lidocaine	Phenelzine	Famotidine
Procainamide	Trazodone	Ranitidine
Quinidine	Paroxetine	**Immunomodulators**
Antibiotics	Fluoxetine	5-Fluorouracil
Acyclovir	Citalopram	Cyclosporine
Amphotericin B	Escitalopram	Chlorambucil
Aminogylcosides	Mirtazapine	Ifosfamide
Cephalosporins	**Antihistamines**	Interferon
Chloroquine	Diphenhydramine	Interleukin-2
Chloramphenicol	Hydroxyzine	Tacrolimus
Ganciclovir	**Antihypertensives**	Tamoxifen
Isoniazid	Clonidine	Vinblastine
Mefloquine	Nifedipine	Vincristine
Metronidazole	Methyldopa	**Muscle Relaxants**
Rifampin	Propranolol	Baclofen
Sulfonamides	Timolol	Cyclobenzaprine
Tetracyclines	**Anti-inflammatory Agents**	**Narcotics**
Vancomycin	Corticosteroids	All formulations
Voriconazole	Ibuprofen	**Other Medications**
Anticholinergics	Indomethacin	Digitalis preparations
Atropine	Naproxen	Dipyridamole
Benztropine	Sulindac	Disulfiram
Scopolamine	**Antipsychotics**	Lithium
Trihexyphenidyl	Clozaril	Pregabalin
Anticonvulsants	Low-potency typicals	Propylthiouracil
Ethosuximide	Quetiapine	Sildenafil
Carbamazapine	Olanzapine	Timolol ophthalmic
Gabapentin	**Dopamine Agonists**	Tramadol
Phenobarbital	Amantadine	Warfarin
Phenytoin	Bromocriptine	**Sedatives**
Primidone	Levodopa	Barbiturates
Valproic acid	Selegiline	Benzodiazepines
Antiemetics	**HIV Medications**	Nonbenzodiazepine hypnotics
Chlorpromazine	Efavirenz	**Sympathomimetics**
Metoclopramide	Nevirapine	Amphetamine
Promethazine	Zidovudine	Ephedrine
Prochlorperazine		Phenylephrine
		Theophylline

PRACTICE POINT

Beware of benzodiazepines
- Be wary of using benzodiazepines to treat agitation in a delirious patient who is not in alcohol or benzodiazepine withdrawal. Benzodiazepine use can be like **adding fuel to the fire, making agitation worse and prolonging delirium**.

Opioids can also contribute to delirium. Reduce the dose of opioids and consider nonopioid methods of pain management. Tramadol should be used with caution, as this medication has also been associated with the development of delirium. If a patient with a patient-controlled analgesia (PCA) pump becomes delirious, discontinue its use promptly. Patients who have difficulty remembering and attending to their surroundings will often unintentionally overuse the PCA, or alternatively, may not be organized and attentive enough to use the pump when indicated. In addition, mounting anxiety from delirium may result in frenetic use of the PCA, which, in turn, can worsen delirium. Use nurse-administered intravenous or oral agents instead. The management of pain in the delirious patient is a delicate balancing act. Just as the overuse of opioids can cause delirium, poorly controlled pain can precipitate or worsen delirium. Careful assessment and treatment of the patient's pain are vital.

TABLE 81-3 Considerations When Using Medications for Symptomatic Treatment in Delirious Patients[†]

- There is little evidence that any medication can **prevent** or **shorten** the duration of delirium.
- Benzodiazepines should be avoided unless specifically indicated (ie, alcohol withdrawal, serotonin syndrome) as they often worsen delirium.
- Antipsychotics are often used to treat the following symptoms associated with delirium:
  - Agitation or violence that places the patient or staff at risk of harm.
  - Hallucinations, delusions, fearfulness, or sleep cycle disruption.
- Before starting an antipsychotic:
  - Review/calculate QTc on ECG.
  - Check serum potassium (K^+), magnesium (Mg^{++}), and calcium (Ca^{++}).
- If QTc >450 msec in men or >470 msec in women, weigh the risks and benefits of starting a QTc-prolonging medication, such as an antipsychotic and do the following:
  - If possible, reduce dose or discontinue/substitute other prescribed medications that may be contributing to prolonged QTc.
  - Keep serum electrolytes K^+ >4 and Mg^{++} >2 mEq/L[††]. Normalize serum calcium.
- Antipsychotic use for the treatment of agitation in delirium is a temporary measure; ongoing use should be re-assessed daily.
  - Select an antipsychotic based on efficacy, available administration route (ie, by mouth [po], intravenous [IV], and intramuscular formulations [IM]) and cost.
  - Use the lowest effective dose to manage symptoms (eg, starting dose of haloperidol: 1–2 mg IV or 2–5 mg po in adults with severe agitation, with 50% dose reduction for frail or elderly patients). Repeat within 30 minutes if no effect is seen.
  - IM and IV administration of haloperidol results in double the peak drug levels compared to oral administration (ie, 1 mg of haloperidol IV = 2 mg po).
- Monitor for extrapyramidal side effects, such a sakathisia, dystonia, and Parkinsonian symptoms.
  - Akathisia—is a subjective sense of "inner restlessness" or "inability to stay still"; this side effect can be mistaken for worsening agitation because of the patient's motor restlessness.
  - Dystonia—includes oculogyric crisis (contraction of extraocular muscles resulting in sustained deviation of the eyes), or dystonia of neck or trunk muscles or of pharynx. Dystonia is very frightening, painful and can be life threatening (particularly pharyngeal dystonia). It should be treated immediately with diphenhydramine 25–50 mg IV or IM, or benztropine1–2 mg IV or IM.
  - Examinemuscular tone for cogwheel rigidity or tremor daily in elbow and wrist joints.
  - If side effects occur and the patient is on a high potency antipsychotic (such as, haloperidol or risperidone), lower the dose, or stop the medication, or consider switching to a lower potency medication (such as, olanzapine or quetiapine).
- Continue to search for and treat the underlying causes of delirium.
- Once the patient's agitation and sleep disruption have fully resolved, taper antipsychotic medication over a period of days with a goal, when feasible, to discontinue all antipsychotics **before hospital** discharge.

[†]No medication is approved by the U.S. Food and Drug Administration for the treatment of delirium.
[††]This recommendation comes from Huffman J, Stern T, Januzzi J. The Psychiatric Management of Patients with Cardiac Disease. In: Stern T, Fricchione G, Cassem N, et al (eds.). *Massachusetts General Hospital Handbook of General Hospital Psychiatry*, 5th ed. Philadelphia: Mosby, 2004, pp. 547–569. In our own experience, a magnesium level of > 2 mEq/L is hard to achieve. A more realistic goal may be to keep magnesium levels above the low end of normal (ie, > 1.3 mEq/L), aiming for the higher end of normal (ie, 2 mEq/L).

■ INFECTION, ELECTROLYTE IMBALANCE, AND ORGAN FAILURE

Look for new sources of infection and perform an appropriate workup. A relatively minor urinary tract or dental infection in a mildly demented elderly patient can trigger delirium. Electrolyte abnormalities such as hypo- and hypernatremia or hypo- and hypercalcemia are relatively common. Screen for these and correct any imbalances. Organ failure, including pulmonary compromise with hypoxia and hypercarbia, uremia, and hepatic failure are all potentially reversible causes of delirium. If history and physical examination are consistent with a neurologic condition (eg, history of headache, head trauma, anticoagulation, fever, stiff neck, or focal neurologic findings on physical exam), obtain brain imaging and lumbar puncture.

■ NONPHARMACOLOGIC MANAGEMENT OF DELIRIUM

1. **Orient patients by providing environmental cues.** Delirious patients have great difficulty acquiring and retaining new information. Because disorientation is common, staff and family should regularly remind patients of where they are and why they are in the hospital. Provide glasses and hearing aids if a patient has visual or auditory impairment. Familiarize patients with their surroundings by placing family photos, clocks, and calendars within their view. Encourage family members to visit or stay with patients, and make every effort to provide delirious patients with private rooms so that family members can stay overnight. Limit room and staff changes as much as possible.

2. **Reduce overstimulation.** Reduce noise, loud talk, and laughter. Delirious, disoriented individuals can easily assign sinister meanings to these random stimuli. Urge staff to use a quiet voice and to interact calmly with the delirious patient. Turn off the TV if the patient is not attending to it. Try music that may be soothing to the patient, based on their music preferences.

3. **Reduce restraint use.** Physical restraints can often worsen anxiety, make patients feel unsafe, and contribute to delusional beliefs about persecution. Round the clock observation of the patient by staff, family, or friends can minimize the need for restraints, especially when observers are skilled at redirecting

and reassuring the patient. Remember that a wide variety of medical equipment, including catheters and intravenous lines, function as restraints and may exacerbate agitation. Avoid their use as much as possible. If medical equipment is the focus of an illusion (eg, perceiving an IV line as a snake), try to disguise its presence by hiding or wrapping it in gauze.

4. **Improve sleep-wake cycle.** Strong circadian signals combat delirium-associated sleep disturbance. Thus, treatment of delirium should include opening window blinds during the day and shutting off or dimming lights at night. Instead of sedative medications, use back massage, warm milk or herbal tea, and relaxing music or white noise to help patients sleep at night. Minimize noise and patient care-related interruptions during night time.

5. **Mobilize early.** Get patients out of bed and involved in activity and mobilization as soon as possible. Studies have shown that decreased sedation and early mobilization dramatically reduce the prevalence of delirium with a commensurate drop in length of stay, even among critically ill individuals. If patients are bedbound, encourage exercise and activity that can be performed in bed, such as exercise bands and simple puzzles or games.

6. **Maintain nutrition, hydration, and oxygenation.** Monitor nutrition and hydration status, and maintain adequate oxygenation. Dehydration and hypoxia are common contributors to delirium. Ensure regular bowel movements and monitor urinary output, as constipation and urinary retention can both lead to agitation.

■ PHARMACOLOGIC MANAGEMENT OF DELIRIUM

The treatment of an agitated or combative delirious patient is particularly challenging. Treatment of agitation should begin with nonpharmacologic measures, such as reassurance and redirection of the patient. Medications should be considered only if nonpharmacologic management fails to control agitation and threatens the safety of the patient and staff, or if patients are experiencing distressing delusions or perceptual disturbances. The use of antipsychotics for the treatment of delirium has not been approved by the Food and Drug Administration and remains off-label. There are a limited number of randomized clinical trials examining the pharmacologic management of delirium. Meta-analysis of existing studies suggests that there is no evidence that antipsychotic medications decrease the duration or severity of delirium or the length of stay in the ICU or hospital. Current evidence suggests that there is no significant difference between low-dose haloperidol (≤3 mg/d) and atypical antipsychotics (such as olanzapine and risperidone) in decreasing the severity of delirium symptoms or in the incidence of extrapyramidal side effects (EPS). Higher daily doses of haloperidol are associated with an increased risk of EPS and may worsen delirium. Atypical antipsychotics may be associated with less EPS, but this has not been adequately evaluated in published randomized controlled trials of delirious patients. The main advantages of haloperidol are its availability in intravenous and intramuscular formulation, as well as its low cost.

Prolongation of the electrocardiographic QT interval leading to torsade de pointes is a rare, but recognized, complication of all antipsychotic agents, and can be made more severe by intravenous administration of these drugs, changes in liver or kidney function, and concomitant use with other QT-prolonged medications. Monitor the QTc regularly and titrate medications accordingly. Table 81-3 includes current guidelines for the use of antipsychotics in the delirious patient.

Benzodiazepines should be avoided as a treatment for agitated delirium, except in GABAergic-withdrawal-related delirious states, where benzodiazepines are a first-line treatment. Benzodiazepines

may make confusion and agitation much worse. The use of as-needed bolus, rather than continuous infusion, of sedation medications in the ICU has been associated with significantly fewer days of delirium. There is no convincing evidence to support any other pharmacologic approach to prevent the occurrence, or decrease the duration or severity of delirium once it has started.

■ THE ROLE OF PSYCHIATRIC CONSULTATION

The hospital physician will invariably encounter cases in which the diagnosis or management of delirium are not straightforward, even after following the guidelines presented in this chapter. In such cases, psychiatric consultation should be obtained. The psychiatric consultant can help clarify an ambiguous diagnosis, recommend further diagnostic studies, or suggest alternative management strategies when those suggested above prove insufficient.

> ### PRACTICE POINT
>
> **30% to 40% of delirium cases may be preventable through nonpharmacologic approaches**
> - It is easier to prevent than to treat delirium.
> - Address modifiable risk factors in patients at high risk for delirium.

■ PRIMARY PREVENTION

Delirium is often preventable. The most effective way to treat delirium is to prevent its occurrence. The nonpharmacologic interventions described above have been shown to decrease the incidence of delirium when used preventatively. In a landmark study of elderly patients admitted to a general medical service, a multicomponent intervention, including regular orientation and cognitive stimulation, use of nonpharmacologic methods to promote sleep, early mobilization, correction of dehydration, and proactive use of visual and auditory aids, significantly reduced the incidence of delirium to 9.9% in the intervention group ($n = 429$), compared to 15% in those who received usual care ($n = 429$). This striking reduction in the development of delirium suggests that these strategies should be considered a part of routine care for all high-risk hospitalized patients.

Other interventions have been studied in randomized controlled trials. A study of mechanically ventilated patients in the ICU showed that early introduction of routine, daily physical and occupational therapy reduced the median number of days of delirium per patient from 4 in control patients ($n = 55$) to 2 in study patients ($n = 49$). An Australian study demonstrated a decreased incidence of delirium when geriatric patients received rehabilitation services at home instead of in the hospital. The patients who received home rehabilitation were followed by a team that included physicians who proactively assessed and treated medical conditions such as infection in order to avoid readmission to the hospital.

Other preventative strategies include avoiding exposure to known deliriogenic medicines, especially anticholinergics and benzodiazepines, in patients at high risk for delirium. A detailed history of alcohol, benzodiazepine, and barbiturate use and prophylactic treatment with a benzodiazepine can also prevent withdrawal-related delirium in susceptible patients.

Early studies have suggested a role for a number of pharmacologic drugs including antipsychotics, cholinesterase inhibitors, and melatonergic agents for the prevention of delirium. However, convincing evidence is lacking for these drugs and routine use is not recommended. A number of small studies suggested that oral haloperidol and other antipsychotics might be useful in delirium prophylaxis; however, meta-analyses of studies regarding delirium prevention in perioperative or critically ill patients do not support this. A randomized controlled trial of the cholinesterase inhibitor rivastigmine, given as an adjunct to haloperidol treatment in critically ill delirious patients in the Netherlands, was stopped early due to increased mortality in the rivastigmine group. Although this difference in mortality did not reach statistical significance, the median delirium duration in the rivastigmine group was significantly longer than in the placebo group. Randomized controlled trials employing melatonin and other melatonergic agents have also resulted in mixed findings. A carefully conducted randomized controlled trial of melatonin in patients undergoing hip fracture repair in the Netherlands did not demonstrate any reduction in the incidence of postoperative delirium. Another trial of a melatonin agonist, ramelteon, in medically ill patients in Japan demonstrated a lower incidence of delirium, but this single study requires replication.

■ COMPLICATIONS

Delirium is associated with significantly increased morbidity and mortality. It can lead to a host of complications, including aspiration pneumonia, pressure ulcers, trauma from accidental falls or removal of medical devices, and decreased oral intake, all of which may contribute to an increased length of stay. The cumulative 1-year mortality rate for elderly patients with delirium has been reported to be 38%, compared to 21% for control subjects admitted to a community hospital. Studies have also found an association between delirium and subsequent long-term cognitive impairment. One study of nondemented patients aged 65 years and older reported that 18.1% of delirious patients were diagnosed with dementia by 3-year follow-up, compared to 5.6% of nondelirious patients. As discussed previously, the presence of mild cognitive impairment is a known risk factor for the future development of delirium. A prospective cohort of 821 critically ill patients demonstrated significant levels of cognitive impairment of survivors at 3 and 12 months of follow-up; longer duration of delirium was independently associated with worse global cognition at of these time points. Whether delirium actually causes long-term cognitive decline, or whether its association with cognitive decline can be attributed to pre-existing subclinical neurologic pathology, is currently being investigated.

Research does demonstrate that delirium is associated with psychological sequelae, including anxiety disorders, related to the frightening nature of perceptual experiences during delirium. A systematic review of the literature reported that the rate of clinically significant post-traumatic stress disorder (PTSD) symptoms up to 2 years after in-hospital delirium was 14%, with PTSD rates in ICU survivors even higher at 15% to 25% at 6 to 12 months after critical illness. Clinically significant depressive symptoms occurred in 31% of previously delirious patients.

CONCLUSION

Delirium is a medical emergency that can often be prevented if at-risk patients are identified and specific interventions are put in place. Although it is common in hospital settings, it may be missed on rounds, as delirious patients are often quiet and withdrawn. In order to identify hypoactive delirious patients, the treatment team must maintain a high index of suspicion and actively look for deficits in attention and cognition. Once a diagnosis of delirium has been made, triggers and sustaining factors must be identified and reversed, and specific nonpharmacologic treatments should be administered. Antipsychotic medications may be indicated if severe agitation fails to respond to nonpharmacologic measures or if delusions or perceptual disturbances are present. In ambiguous or difficult cases, psychiatric consultation should be obtained. The prevention and prompt identification and management of delirium may significantly reduce length of stay, morbidity, mortality, and health care costs. It can also save patients, family members, and caretakers considerable suffering and distress.

DISCHARGE CHECKLIST

- For patients with persisting delirium at the time of discharge, has 24-hour supervision been arranged?
- Have staff or family caretakers been educated in steps to prevent and manage delirium?
- Have deliriogenic medications, such as anticholinergics and benzodiazepines, been stopped?
- Have antipsychotic agents prescribed for the management of agitated delirium been stopped? Ideally, these medications should be stopped before discharge, as the risks of long-term antipsychotic use in older patients with dementia include increased risk of stroke and sudden death, extra pyramidal side effects, metabolic syndrome, and unnecessary expense. It is best to taper these medications slowly. If discharge occurs before this can be accomplished, it is important to communicate the plan for tapering and discontinuing antipsychotics after hospital discharge must be communicated to the patient's primary provider.

SUGGESTED READINGS

American Geriatrics Society Expert Panel on Postoperative Delirium in Older Adults. American Geriatrics Society abstracted clinical practice guideline for postoperative delirium in older adults. *J Am Geriatr Soc*. 2015;63:142-150.

Barr J, Fraser GL, Puntillo K, et al. Clinical practice guidelines for the management of pain, agitation, and delirium in adult patients in the intensive care unit. *Crit Care Med*. 2013;41:263-306.

Gusmao-Flores D, Martins JC, Amorin D, Quarantini LC. Tools for diagnosing delirium in the critically ill: is calibration needed for the less sedated patient? *Intensive Care Med*. 2014;40:137-138.

Hshieh TT, Yue J, Oh E, et al. Effectiveness of multicomponent nonpharmacological delirium interventions: a meta-analysis. *JAMA Intern Med*. 2015;175:512-520.

Inouye SK, Westendorp RG, Saczynski JS. Delirium in elderly people. *Lancet*. 2014;383:911-922.

Neto AS, Nassar AP Jr, Cardoso SO, et al. Delirium screening in critically ill patients: a systematic review and meta-analysis. *Crit Care Med*. 2012;40:1946-1951.

Pandharipande PP, Girard TD, Jackson JC, et al. Long-term cognitive impairment after critical illness. *N Engl J Med*. 2013;369:1306-1316.

Young J, Murthy L, Westby M, Akunne A, O'Mahony R, Guideline Development Group. Diagnosis, prevention, and management of delirium: summary of NICE guidance. *BMJ*. 2010;341:c3704.

CHAPTER 82

Diarrhea

Danielle B. Scheurer, MD, MSCR, SFHM
Talat H. Raja, MD

Key Clinical Questions

1. What questions in the diarrhea history will guide the need for diagnostic testing?
2. What is the yield of commonly ordered diagnostic stool tests?
3. What is a practical algorithm to guide rational diagnostic stool testing?
4. What are practical supportive therapies for hospitalized patients with diarrhea?
5. What are the key measures for preventing the spread of infectious diarrhea?

CASE 82-1

A previously healthy 45-year-old man sustained a motor vehicle accident resulting in multiple bone fractures and a traumatic brain injury. As such, he was admitted to the intensive care unit, intubated, sedated, and later taken to the operating room for repair of multiple fractures. On hospital day 3, the surgical team requested a medicine consultation for assessment and management of diarrhea. The patient had no history of diarrhea prior to admission, and his symptoms began on hospital day 2. The diarrhea was loose, semiformed, four to six times a day, without blood, mucus, or pus. The patient remained intubated and sedated. His vital signs were stable, he was afebrile, and his abdominal exam was benign. He received feedings via a nasogastric tube, reaching nutritional goals. His medications included subcutaneous heparin prophylaxis, a proton-pump inhibitor, docusate, senna, intravenous propofol, and intravenous morphine. He had normal laboratory tests, including a white cell count of 8000 per cubic millimeter.

INTRODUCTION

DEFINITION

The typical adult eating a Western diet excretes 100 to 200 g of fecal matter a day, consisting of water, electrolytes, indigestible matter, unabsorbed food, intestinal secretions, epithelial cells, and enteric bacteria. Diarrhea is defined as an abnormal increase in excretion of fecal matter to >200 g a day. Nosocomial diarrhea is an acute diarrheal episode not present during admission and occurring after >3 days of hospitalization.

The epidemiology of acute nosocomial and acute community-acquired diarrhea are quite disparate; this chapter will focus on the former. The usual bacterial, viral, and protozoal culprits in community-acquired diarrhea are rare in nosocomial diarrhea. They will be mentioned in this chapter as patients may acquire them prior to hospital admission, but they will be appropriately deemphasized as causes of diarrhea in hospitalized patients.

INCIDENCE

Diarrhea is a common affliction in the hospital, occurring in 33% to 50% of inpatients. Patients who acquire diarrhea while in the hospital have longer lengths of stay and higher mortality than those who do not. Diarrhea also is associated with more diagnostic testing (stool studies, imaging exams, electrolyte monitoring) and more interventions (intravenous fluids, electrolyte supplementation, and medication adjustments). It also creates cleanliness and quality-of-life issues, especially in patients that are not independent in mobility and self-care. The differential diagnosis for diarrhea in hospitalized patients is extensive, but is most conveniently dichotomized into infectious and noninfectious etiologies.

INFECTIOUS DIARRHEA

There are >200 million cases of infectious diarrhea in the United States each year, resulting in 1.8 million hospitalizations. Most are acquired from fecal-oral transmission, person-to-person contact, or food and liquids (although the latter is highly unusual in the hospital setting). Alteration of intestinal microbiome appears to play a role in most cases of infectious diarrhea. Contagious spread by person-to-person contact also includes transmission through fomites, such as stethoscopes, bedside commodes, or other medical equipment. The vast majority of infectious diarrhea in inpatients is caused by *Clostridium difficile*. Clinical studies have shown that 12% to 32% of hospitalized patients develop diarrhea and that <20% are due to *C. difficile*. A full discussion of *Clostridium difficile*-associated diarrhea (CDAD) diagnosis, management, and prevention can be found in Chapter 190 (*C. difficile* colitis).

■ BACTERIAL PATHOGENS

The bacterial pathogens that cause community-acquired diarrhea are rarely acquired in the hospital setting, although they may be already present in patients hospitalized with diarrhea acquired in the community. In the United States, there are 5.2 million cases of bacterial diarrhea, 46,000 hospitalizations, and 1500 deaths annually. The majority of these occur in outpatients as a result of food-borne transmission. Person-to-person transmission is less common and usually occurs with pathogens that only require a small inoculum to cause disease (**Table 82-1**). Bacterial etiologies make up 1.5% to 5.6% of cases of community-acquired diarrheal illness. The usual bacterial suspects include *Salmonella spp* (1.8%), *Shigella spp* (1.1%), *Campylobacter spp* (2.3%), and *Escherichia coli* 0157:H7 (0.4%).

Salmonella typhi is almost always acquired by person-to-person transmission, from an acutely infected or chronic carrier, but rarely can be transmitted through food or water. Such was the case of "Typhoid Mary" Mallon, a healthy Irish immigrant cook who, as an asymptomatic carrier, infected at least 22 people over 7 years before being identified. The rarity of *S. typhi* outbreaks in the United States is a reflection of exemplary hygiene and sewage standards. Transmissibility of the organism depends on the density of the organism in the infected person, and the infectivity of the strain. Generally, a high inoculum is required to result in clinical symptoms, based on voluntary experimental ingestions. Diarrhea is a variable finding in typhoid fever; some patients may have constipation.

Nontyphoidal *S. spp*, on the other hand, are rarely transmitted person-to-person, usually derive from an environmental animal reservoir (farm animals), and require a much lower inoculum to cause clinical infection. *Campylobacter spp*, similar to nontyphoidal *S. spp*, are rarely transmitted person-to-person, and are usually linked to contaminated food sources (meat, dairy, or water). Although a small inoculum is required for infection, widespread outbreaks rarely occur, because most patients remain asymptomatic.

E. coli 0157:H7 transmission also usually occurs through contaminated food (meats or fertilized fruits/vegetables), although secondary person-to-person transmission may subsequently occur. The infamous large outbreak in the early 1990s was linked to contaminated hamburger, and secondary infection was rampant, occurring in up to 20% of close contacts.

Shigella spp spreads from person to person or through contaminated food, but has no environmental reservoir (similar to *S. typhi*). It is highly contagious, with a low density of inoculum required to result in clinical infection. It therefore commonly causes outbreaks, usually within households and day care centers.

Occasional patients are seen with an antibiotic-associated hemorrhagic colitis that mimics *C. difficile* colitis. A small series of patients with this non-*Clostridium difficile* antibiotic-associated hemorrhagic colitis found that most cases were caused by *Klebsiella oxytoca*, which produces a cytotoxin leading to epithelial cell death. Patients have segmental mucosal ulceration and edema predominantly in the right and transverse colon. The diagnosis may be established by sending stool samples to the microbiology laboratory specifically to culture for *Klebsiella spp*. Rarely, non-*Clostridium difficile* antibiotic-associated hemorrhagic colitis may be due to enterotoxigenic strains of *Klebsiella pneumonia*, *Staphylococcus aureus*, and type A *Clostridium perfringens*.

Candida spp have also been implicated in nosocomial diarrhea. It is thought to cause a secretory diarrhea without evidence of colitis in critically ill or debilitated patients, but it is unclear how to treat or manage these patients.

■ VIRUSES/PROTOZOA

Viral outbreaks of diarrhea are much more common than bacterial outbreaks, both in the community and hospital setting. Viral causes of acute infectious diarrhea include caliciviruses (Norwalk and Sapporo viruses), rotavirus (primarily in children), adenovirus, and astrovirus.

The most common by far are the caliciviruses, which account for more than 90% of acute gastrointestinal outbreaks in the United States. They have high infectivity, with attack rates of up to 50% in close contacts, and an infectious inoculum as low as 10 viral particles. Cruise ships are notorious for these outbreaks, but they also occur in medical environments, including nursing homes and hospitals. Viruses are transmitted by infected food and water, as well as secondary person-to-person spread. Viral particles are present in both vomitus and feces (as opposed to bacterial enteritis, in which the bacteria are present only in stool), increasing the likelihood of person-to-person transmission. Unfortunately, these viruses also persist on environmental surfaces and are resistant to ordinary cleaning agents (although they are inactivated by household bleach).

Rotaviruses tend to cause symptomatic disease only in children. Similar to caliciviruses, they remain in the environment for prolonged periods of time and are difficult to eradicate with routine cleaning agents. Outbreaks of infection with astroviruses and enteric adenoviruses have occurred in the hospital setting. Although these pathogens are most common in pediatric populations, they also afflict the elderly, immunocompromised, and institutionalized.

Protozoal causes of acute diarrhea are most commonly caused by *Giardia lamblia*, *Cryptosporidium parvum*, and *Entamoeba histolytica*. These are usually connected with contaminated water sources, with secondary person-to-person transmission occurring via the fecal-oral route. They are transmitted via a very small inoculum and are therefore highly transmissible. These protozoa usually cause outbreaks in schools and day care settings, and outbreaks in the medical setting are highly unusual.

Immunocompromised patients (especially HIV with CD4 < 50) have a more extensive infectious differential diagnosis for nosocomial diarrhea. The additional organisms that should be considered include cytomegalovirus (CMV), norovirus, *Mycobacterium avium* complex (MAC), cryptosporidiosis, microsporidiosis, cyclosporiasis, isosporiasis, giardiasis, and strongyloidiasis.

TABLE 82-1 Transmissibility of Bacterial Diarrheal Diseases

Organism	Usual Transmission	Inoculum Required to Cause Disease
Salmonella typhi	Person-to-person food	High
Nontyphoidal Salmonella	Environmental animal reservoir	Low
Campylobacter	Food	Low
Escherichia coli 0157:H7	Food	Low
Shigella	Person-to-person food	Low

NONINFECTIOUS DIARRHEA

Most diarrhea in the hospital (>75%) is not caused by infection. Noninfectious nosocomial diarrhea can be due to a host of insults, including side effects of medical and nutritional therapy (drugs, foods, additives, enteral feedings, contrast agents, opiate withdrawal, radiation therapy), and new gastrointestinal pathology (fecal impaction, inflammatory bowel disease, transplant rejection, GI bleeding, fat malabsorption, and biliary obstruction).

■ SIDE EFFECTS OF MEDICAL AND NUTRITIONAL THERAPY

As medications are a major offender for nosocomial diarrhea, a careful review of medications is warranted (**Table 82-2**). The frequency of antibiotic-associated diarrhea (AAD) ranges from 2% to 25% (with no significant difference between intravenous and oral antibiotics). The spectrum of disease caused by antibiotic-associated diarrhea can range from uncomplicated loose stools to frank *C. difficile* colitis. Risk factors for AAD include advanced age, immune suppression, gastrointestinal disease or previous gastrointestinal surgery, and severe comorbidities. Antibiotics lead to diarrhea via many different mechanisms. Disruption of gut flora results in osmotic or secretory diarrhea by disrupting the metabolism of carbohydrates, short chain fatty acids, and bile acids, as well as impairing colonization resistance, resulting in a more favorable environment for diarrhea-genic organisms. Probiotics have been thought to possibly prevent AAD, but the recent PLACIDE trial involving nearly 3000 hospitalized patients found no evidence that probiotics prevented AAD or *C. difficile* colits.

New foods during the hospital stay can also result in diarrhea. Offending agents include sugar-free gum or candy, and new foods with dairy content in patients with previously unrecognized lactose intolerance. Medication elixirs often contain substances such as sorbitol, which causes osmotic diarrhea. Enteral feedings are also a common cause of osmotic diarrhea, which occurs in 15% of patients upon initiation of enteral feedings.

In patients taking narcotics before their hospital stay, a reduction or cessation of their usual amount can present with diarrhea as a symptom of opiate withdrawal. Since nausea and vomiting often accompany opiate withdrawal, vomiting up oral opiates may be an important exacerbating factor.

Oral contrast agents used in imaging present an osmotic load to the gut that can result in transient diarrhea. Radiation therapy in the abdominal and pelvic region can cause both acute and chronic diarrhea. The symptoms of acute radiation enteritis generally start during or shortly after radiation therapy, and usually improve within 2 to 6 weeks of cessation of the radiation, but may persist long-term.

■ NEW GASTROINTESTINAL PATHOLOGY

A number of new diagnoses during the hospital stay can result in diarrhea. Fecal impaction, especially in the elderly, psychiatric patients, and immobilized patients receiving high doses of opiates without an adequate bowel regimen, can develop diarrhea due to leakage around the impaction. New-onset inflammatory bowel disease should be entertained in cases of inflammatory diarrhea for which infectious causes have been ruled out. Bone marrow transplant patients can present with diarrhea as a symptom of graft versus host disease. GI bleeding can present with diarrhea, although the color of the stool should trigger an evaluation for bleeding. Fat malabsorption resulting from a new small bowel or pancreatic dysfunction can result in steatorrheic diarrhea. Biliary tract obstruction can result in bile-acid-associated diarrhea.

HISTORY

The onset, duration, frequency, color, consistency, and character of the diarrhea, as well as associated symptoms, provide clues to its etiology. The degree of volume depletion should be assessed (thirst, urine color and amount, lethargy). Patients should be queried about epidemiological risks for infectious diarrhea (health care or day care attendance or employment, pet or farm contacts, unpasteurized or raw foods, recent sick contacts). Medications should be reviewed to identify potential causes of drug-induced diarrhea. Infectious diarrhea is often accompanied by nausea, vomiting, fever, tenesmus, or abdominal pain, and the stool may be watery, malabsorptive, or dysenteric. Direct gross examination of the stool can be tremendously helpful in narrowing the differential diagnosis. Black tarry stools usually indicate digested blood, usually from the upper GI tract, and maroon, red, or pink stools indicate undigested blood, usually in the lower GI tract (or upper GI tract with rapid transit time). Greasy stools that float indicate fat malabsorption, and clay-colored stools point to biliary obstruction.

PHYSICAL EXAM

The physical exam should focus on the vital signs, general appearance, and the abdominal and rectal exams. The patient should be assessed for fever, signs of dehydration, and hemodynamic instability. The abdomen should be examined for pain, distention, and peritoneal signs. The rectal exam should include testing for gross or microscopic blood.

DIAGNOSTIC TESTING

An approach to rational diagnostic testing is presented in **Figure 82-1**. Several stool tests are available to help determine the etiology of diarrhea, most of which are discussed below. Physicians should adhere to the 3-day rule of diagnostic testing for bacterial or

---

TABLE 82-2 Medications Commonly Associated with Nosocomial Diarrhea

Antibiotics	Clindamycin
	Erythromycin
	Cephalosporins
	Ampicillin
Gastrointestinal agents	H$_2$ blockers
	Proton pump inhibitors
	Antacids (magnesium-containing)
	Misoprostol
Cardiovascular agents	Digitalis
	Quinidine
NSAIDs	All types (including aspirin)
Supplements	Magnesium
	Phosphorus
	Elixir additives (sorbitol/lactose)
Immunosuppressive agents	HIV medications (protease inhibitors)
	Chemotherapeutic agents
	Tacrolimus
	Cyclosporin
	Azathioprine
Other agents	Colchicine (dose limiting)
	Levothyroxine (dose related)
	Theophylline

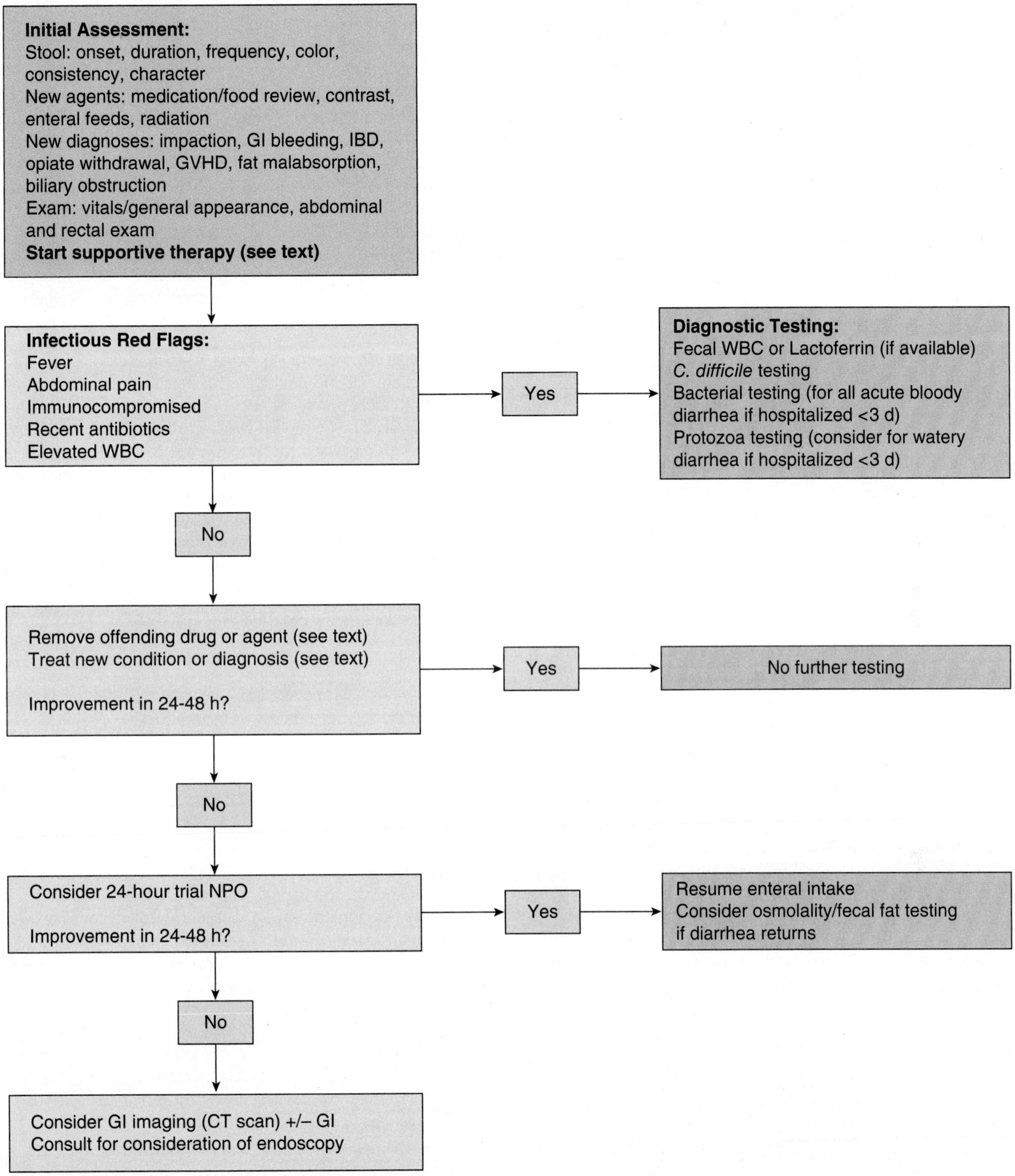

Initial Assessment:
Stool: onset, duration, frequency, color, consistency, character
New agents: medication/food review, contrast, enteral feeds, radiation
New diagnoses: impaction, GI bleeding, IBD, opiate withdrawal, GVHD, fat malabsorption, biliary obstruction
Exam: vitals/general appearance, abdominal and rectal exam
Start supportive therapy (see text)

Infectious Red Flags:
Fever
Abdominal pain
Immunocompromised
Recent antibiotics
Elevated WBC

Yes →

Diagnostic Testing:
Fecal WBC or Lactoferrin (if available)
C. difficile testing
Bacterial testing (for all acute bloody diarrhea if hospitalized <3 d)
Protozoa testing (consider for watery diarrhea if hospitalized <3 d)

No

Remove offending drug or agent (see text)
Treat new condition or diagnosis (see text)

Improvement in 24-48 h?

Yes → No further testing

No

Consider 24-hour trial NPO

Improvement in 24-48 h?

Yes → Resume enteral intake
Consider osmolality/fecal fat testing if diarrhea returns

No

Consider GI imaging (CT scan) +/– GI
Consult for consideration of endoscopy

Figure 82-1 *Diagnostic approach to nosocomial diarrhea.*

protozoal pathogens. That is, if the diarrhea developed after hospital day 3, it is unlikely to be due to these pathogens, and diagnostic testing for them is not cost effective.

A routine stool culture will usually yield *Shigella, Salmonella, Aeromonas,* and *Campylobacter.* Routine stool cultures will usually not identify *E. coli* 0157:H7, which requires sorbitol MacConkey agar and Shiga-toxin testing, *Vibrio cholera,* and *Yersinia enterocolitica,* which requires cold enrichment. Bacterial stool cultures remain the gold standard for detection, even though they have a generally low sensitivity >3 days after hospitalization or antibiotic treatment, are

laborious, and in <5% of cases yield a positive result. There are new nucleic acid amplification methods on the horizon that may have higher yield and quicker results. Generally, stool cultures should be ordered for patients with severe diarrhea (>6 stools/day), with fever or dysentery, or if there are clusters of patients with similar symptoms suggesting an outbreak. Stool cultures are not recommended in mild or watery diarrhea. A single specimen is sufficient in qualified laboratories. Stool cultures will usually not be able to distinguish colonization versus infection in toxin-mediated diarrhea secondary to *S. aureus, K. spp,* or *C. perfringens.*

A routine stool test for ova and parasites (O & P) consists of a gross and microscopic examination of the stool to look for parasites and their eggs. Direct antigen testing for *Giardia*, *Cryptosporidium*, and *Entamoeba* has a sensitivity of at least 95%. Acid-fast staining of the stool specimen can identify *Cyclospora* and *Isospora*, but this has a low sensitivity and low specificity (usually due to swallowing of sputum containing mycobacterial species which may or may not be pathogenic). In general, evaluation for parasites requires repeated testing, due to the periodic nature of their fecal excretion.

Viral testing of stool is rarely performed, outside of testing by local, state, or federal labs in the outbreak situation. Viral cultures can yield CMV, enteroviruses, and adenoviruses, but are rarely performed and take up to 14 days to yield an organism. Rotavirus antigen tests are available, but rarely performed in adults, as rotavirus rarely produces symptomatic illness in adults.

Testing stool for occult blood distinguishes blood from food and dyes in stool specimens that are grossly red or pink. The most common assays utilize the pseudoperoxidase activity of hemoglobin reacting with hydrogen peroxide to convert a colorless compound to one of a blue color. False-positive testing occurs between 1% and 10%. Causes of false-positive tests include dietary sources of peroxidase, such as turnips, horseradish, red meats, cauliflower, broccoli, cantaloupe, parsnips, mushrooms, apples, and bananas. Colchicine and contamination with iodine-containing antiseptics may also lead to false-positives. False-negatives are rare, but may be caused by foods and diets high in vitamin C.

Stool pH is rarely used as a diagnostic test for nosocomial diarrhea. Normal stool pH is about that of the body, with a normal range of 7.0 to 7.5. Stools with acidic pH may indicate a malabsorption syndrome that allow for fermentation of undigested food by gut bacteria. Conditions resulting in alkaline pH include antibiotic use, leading to impaired bacterial fermentation, and colonic inflammation.

PRACTICE POINT

Key historical points that might point to the need to perform an infectious workup include the presence of the following:
1. Immunosuppression
   - IgA deficiency, common variable hypogammaglobulinemia, chronic granulomatous disease
   - AIDS (common enteric and opportunistic pathogens)
   - Medication-related (chemotherapy, corticosteroids)
2. Malnutrition
3. Recent or current antibiotic use

Key historical points that might point to a specific cause of acute infectious diarrhea include the following:
1. Travel history
   - Latin America, Africa, Asia (enterotoxigenic *E. coli*, *Campylobacter*, *Shigella*, *Aeromonas*, *Salmonella*, norovirus)
   - Russia, wilderness areas (*Giardia*)
   - Cruise ships (Norwalk virus, other causes of infectious gastroenteritis)
2. Day care exposure
   - *Shigella*, *Giardia*, *Cryptosporidium*, rotavirus, norovirus
3. Recent food ingestion
   - Chicken (*Salmonella*, *Campylobacter*, *Shigella*)
   - Eggs (*Salmonella*)
   - Mayonnaise or creams (*S. aureus*, *Salmonella*)
   - Hamburger (hemorrhagic *E. coli* 0157:H7)
   - Raw seafood (*Vibrio spp*, *Salmonella*, acute hepatitis A)
   - Fried rice (*Bacillus cereus*)
4. Recent or current hospitalization or nursing home (*C. difficile*)
5. Recent or current antibiotic use (*C. difficile*)
6. Hemochromatosis (*Vibrio spp*, *Yersinia*)

Symptoms that suggest a particular etiology are as follows:
1. Prominent vomiting
   - Toxin-mediated syndromes (*B. cereus*, *S. aureus*), norovirus
2. Abdominal pain and fever
   - *C. difficile*, *Salmonella*, *Shigella*, *Campylobacter*, *E. coli* 0157:H7
3. Bloody diarrhea
   - *Salmonella*, *Shigella*, *Campylobacter*, *E. coli* 0157:H7, *Entamoeba histolytica*
   - *Aeromonas* species, *Vibrio parahaemolyticus*, *Yersinia*
4. Profuse watery diarrhea
   - *C. perfringens*, *V. cholerae*, enterotoxigenic *E. coli*, *K. pneumoniae*, *Aeromonas*, enteropathogenic and enteroadherent *E. coli*, *Giardia*, cryptosporidiosis, helminths

Leukocytes are not normally found in stool. Their presence indicates infection, with invasion of the intestinal wall, or inflammation, as in inflammatory bowel disease. For that reason, stool leukocytes are more likely to be present in invasive bacterial infections (*Salmonella*, *Shigella*, *Campylobacter*, *Yersinia*, invasive *E. coli*) than in viral infection, parasitic infection, or toxigenic bacterial infection. The sensitivity and specificity of stool leukocytes is relatively low, which limits its usefulness. However, a less readily available test, the immunoassay for the neutrophil marker lactoferrin, has higher sensitivity and specificity.

PRACTICE POINT

- Noninfectious etiologies of acute diarrhea in hospitalized patients include the following:
- Recent new medications or oral contrast
- Toxin or radiation exposure prior to admission
- Acute diverticulitis
- Inflammatory bowel disease
- Ischemic colitis
- Graft versus host disease

Fecal fat can be assessed by qualitative methods, which can be done on a random stool sample, with abnormal testing being >50 fat globules per high power field. Qualitative testing correlates well with quantitative testing, which is rarely required in inpatients.

Stool osmolality can be performed on a random stool sample. Normal values range from 275 to 295 mosm/L. The measured stool osmolality can be compared to calculated stool osmolality (2 × [Na + K]) to determine if there is an osmolar gap. A gap (>50) indicates an osmotic diarrhea, usually due to carbohydrates (sodium citrate, magnesium citrate, laxatives, lactulose, or sorbitol) or fat (mineral oil or castor oil). A stool osmolality >500 mg/dL is highly suspicious for factitious diarrhea (usually due to laxative abuse).

PRACTICE POINT

- Systemic manifestations associated with infectious diarrhea are as follows:
- Reactive arthritis (*Salmonella*, *campylobacter*, *Shigella*, *Yersinia*)
- Hemolytic-uremic syndrome (*E. coli* 0157:H7, *Shigella*)
- Thyroiditis, pericarditis, acute glomerulonephritis (*Yersinia*)

TREATMENT

■ STOP THE OFFENDING AGENT OR THERAPY

A careful review of new foods, additives, and medications may uncover an offending agent to be discontinued. Antibiotic-associated diarrhea usually responds to discontinuation of the agent.

There is little evidence that probiotics are effective in antibiotic-associated diarrhea, but their use is widespread, and there is little data to suggest harm, except in immunocompromised patients. Diarrhea related to new enteral feeds can be reduced by changing to a lower osmotic agent, reducing the rate, or adding antimotility agents, as discussed below. Contrast-associated diarrhea is self-limited; treatment is supportive care until resolution. Radiation-associated diarrhea is also treated supportively, unless intolerable symptoms dictate temporary cessation of the treatment.

■ TREAT NEW GASTROINTESTINAL DIAGNOSES

Treatment of bacterial causes of infectious diarrhea is summarized in **Table 82-3**. Empiric treatment for suspected bacterial pathogens with ciprofloxacin should be initiated in patients with acute febrile dysentery, but only after a fecal sample has been sent. In patients without fever or frank dysentery, empiric treatment is not warranted. For established diagnoses, patients should be treated according to Table 82-3. In patients with uncomplicated nontyphoidal *Salmonella* diarrhea, treatment with antibiotics does not reduce the duration of illness or fever, but does increase relapse rates and prolongs fecal shedding. However, patients with known or suspected bacteremia (toxic appearance or high fever) should be treated to prevent septicemia. *E. coli* 0157:H7 infection should not be treated with antibiotics, as this does not improve outcomes and increases the risk of hemolytic-uremic syndrome. *E. coli* 0157:H7 should be suspected in patients with bloody diarrhea, abdominal pain, and minimal fever.

Diarrhea related to fecal impaction usually requires a combination of mechanical and medical disimpaction. New symptomatic

TABLE 82-3 Treatment of Known or Suspected Bacterial Pathogens

Bacterial Pathogen	Antibiotic Options/Duration
Campylobacter jejuni	Azithromycin 500 mg 3 d
	Erythromycin 500 mg four times a day for 3 d
Vibrio cholera	Doxycycline 300 mg (single dose)
	Tetracycline 500 mg four times a day for 3 d
	Azithromycin 500 mg 3 d
	Erythromycin 250 mg three times a day for 3 d
Escherichia coli 0157:H7	Not recommended
Escherichia coli (enterotoxigenic, enteroaggregative, or traveler's diarrhea)	Ciprofloxacin 750 mg 1-3 d
	Azithromycin 1000 mg (single dose)
	Rifaximin 200 mg three times a day for 3 d
Salmonella (nontyphoid)*	Ciprofloxacin 500 mg 7 d
Salmonella (typhoid)	Azithromycin 500 mg 7 d
	Duration 14 d if immunocompromised
Shigellosis	Ciprofloxacin 750 mg 3 d
Aeromonas	Azithromycin 500 mg 3 d
Plesiomonas	
Escherichia coli (enteroinvasive)	
Noncholeraic vibrios*	

*Not recommended if uncomplicated.

IBD usually requires immunosuppressive agents and bowel rest to relieve symptoms. Treatment of opiate withdrawal symptoms and transplant rejection are beyond the scope of this chapter. Fat malabsorption warrants treatment of the underlying pancreatic or small bowel dysfunction, and usually requires enzymatic supplementation to correct. Biliary obstruction requires investigation and relief of the obstruction.

■ SUPPORTIVE THERAPIES

A trial of nothing by mouth for 24 hours is of reasonable diagnostic and therapeutic value. Osmotic diarrhea will improve with fasting, secretory diarrhea will not. Thereafter, diet can be resumed and advanced as tolerated. Use of a lactose-free diet, due to a transient lactase deficiency from mucosal injury, is usually recommended, although data to support its use are limited. Although probiotics have not been shown to prevent antibiotic-associated diarrhea, they may have a role in the treatment of infectious diarrhea, as a Cochrane review found that probiotics reduced the mean duration of diarrhea by 24 hours in this setting. There is not quality evidence supporting their role in noninfectious diarrheas. Patients who cannot tolerate oral hydration will need intravenous hydration. Isosmotic fluids are preferred, unless electrolyte abnormalities dictate otherwise. If warranted, repletion of potassium can usually be accomplished orally, but magnesium or phosphorus supplementation are generally preferred intravenously, as they can be caustic to the gut and exacerbate diarrhea.

PRACTICE POINT

- In patients with uncomplicated nontyphoidal *Salmonella* diarrhea, treatment with antibiotics does not reduce the duration of illness or fever, but does increase relapse rates and prolongs fecal shedding. However, patients with known or suspected bacteremia (toxic appearance or high fever) should be treated to prevent septicemia.
- Treatment of *E. coli* 0157:H7 increases the risk of hemolytic uremic syndrome and should be avoided.

■ ANTIDIARRHEAL AGENTS

Although hundreds of agents are claimed to relieve diarrhea, only three have Food and Drug Administration labeling to support their use. In general, antidiarrheal agents should be avoided in patients with suspected inflammatory diarrhea. These agents have been associated with prolonged fever with *S. spp*, hemolytic-uremic syndrome with *E. coli* 0157:H7, and toxic megacolon with *C. difficile*-associated diarrhea.

Loperamide (Imodium) inhibits peristalsis and has antisecretory effects. Bismuth subsalicylate reduces symptoms of nausea, diarrhea, and abdominal pain in patients with traveler's diarrhea, but its use in other types of diarrhea (especially nosocomial variants) is unstudied. Diphenoxylate (Lomotil) is an opiate agonist that is effective at reducing stool volume.

PREVENTION

Hospitalized patients experiencing diarrhea have longer lengths of stay and higher mortality than those who do not. They undergo more diagnostic testing, monitoring, and interventions. It is of paramount importance to prevent nosocomial diarrhea if possible. Prevention of infectious nosocomial diarrheas includes the usual hygiene provisions and universal precautions. Interventions to promote hand washing have been proven to reduce diarrheal episodes among children in institutions by 30% to 40%.

- It is of paramount importance to prevent nosocomial diarrhea if possible. Prevention of infectious nosocomial diarrheas includes the usual hygiene provisions and universal precautions. Alcohol-based solutions will not eliminate spores from *C. difficile*; practitioners should wash their hands with soap after contact with affected patients.

The patient's home diet and medications should be reviewed again on each care transition. Cessation or initiation of new foods, additives, or medications should be done with a careful review of the risks and benefits. Routine use of stool softeners in hospitalized patients is often unnecessary and may lead to diarrhea. If despite preventive interventions, a hospitalized patient does experience nosocomial diarrhea, a step-wise, rational approach to diagnostic testing should be initiated, as outlined in Figure 82-1. Therapeutic and supportive interventions should be initiated based on the diagnostic evaluation, in a timely and cost-efficient manner.

CASE 82-1 (CONTINUED)

Based on the algorithm outlined in Figure 82-1, the patient's diarrhea started in the hospital, had been present for 1 day, was occurring four to six times a day, and was brown and semiformed. His medication list included docusate, senna, and a proton-pump inhibitor, all of which can lead to diarrhea. He had recently received perioperative antibiotics for the prevention of surgical site infections, but was on no current antibiotic therapy and he was without any other infectious red flags. He had also recently been initiated on enteral feedings and had received oral contrast 2 days ago for abdominal imaging. The proton-pump inhibitor, colace, and senna were stopped, and the rate of his enteral feeds was reduced. His diarrhea resolved within 48 hours and no further diagnostic testing was performed.

SUGGESTED READINGS

Allen SJ, Martinez EG, Gregorio GV, Dans LF. Probiotics for treating acute infectious diarrhoea. *Cochrane Database Syst Rev.* 2010;(11):CD003048.

Allen SJ, Wareham K, Wang D, et al. Lactobacilli and bifidobacteria in the prevention of antibiotic-associated diarrhoea and *Clostridium difficile* diarrhoea in older inpatients (PLACIDE): a randomised, double-blind, placebo-controlled, multicentre trial. *Lancet.* 2013;382:1249-1257.

Bartlett JG. Antibiotic-associated diarrhea. *N Engl J Med.* 2002;346:334-339.

Dupont HL. Bacterial diarrhea. *N Engl J Med.* 2009;361:1560-1569.

Guerrant RL, Van Gilder T, Steiner TS, et al. Practice guidelines for the management of infectious diarrhea. *Clin Infect Dis.* 2001;32:331-350.

Pawlowski SW, Warren CA, Guerrant R. Diagnosis and treatment of acute or persistent diarrhea. *Gastroenterology.* 2009;136:1874-1886.

Polage CR, Solnick JV, Cohen SH. Nosocomial diarrhea: evaluation and treatment of causes other than *Clostridium difficile*. *Clin Infect Dis.* 2012;55:982-989.

Thielman NM, Guerrant RL. Acute infectious diarrhea. *N Engl J Med.* 2004;350:38-47.

CHAPTER 83

Disorders of the Eye

Ala Moshiri, MD, PhD
Prem S. Subramanian, MD, PhD

Key Clinical Questions

❶ Which conditions should prompt emergent ophthalmologic consultation?

❷ Which conditions require prompt imaging and/or consultation with neurologists or neurosurgeons?

❸ For hospital employees with viral conjunctivitis what are the recommendations to prevent nosocomial spread to hospitalized patients?

❹ What are the risks of topical corticosteroids in patients with allergic conjunctivitis?

INTRODUCTION

Ophthalmologic concerns in the hospitalized patient fall into two broad categories: signs and symptoms of the systemic condition for which the patient has been admitted, and unrelated but potentially urgent disorders of the eye that may threaten vision. While some of the conditions discussed in this chapter may relate to the former issue, our approach will be to describe common ophthalmologic disorders for which inpatient consultation is often considered, and to provide information on appropriate triage and workup prior to obtaining the consultant's opinion. In many cases, outpatient evaluation after the acute illness has passed may be more useful, since the patient's cooperation with subjective testing methods is much more reliable. Symptoms that may prompt urgent evaluation include red eyes (with or without pain), double vision, and subjective loss of vision. There are a number of bedside examination techniques that do not require specialized equipment but can yield important information to narrow the differential diagnosis and help determine the urgency of further testing.

The consulting physician should perform a focused but detailed eye history and physical examination prior to consulting an ophthalmologist. Time of onset, monocular or binocular nature, duration, and associated neurologic symptoms are especially important. Past medical and ocular history are relevant, as are recent interventions during the current hospitalization that might contribute to the visual complaints. The examination should ideally include best-corrected visual acuity (with glasses) measured for each eye, either with a near reading card, wall-mounted distance chart, or smartphone app. It should be noted whether the pupils are equal in size and reactive to illumination. Abnormal extraocular movements may be seen with new binocular double vision. Peripheral vision testing with a small red object (pinhead, marker cap) can detect up to 75% of clinically relevant deficits. Finally, a hand-light examination should be done at the bedside to look for eyelid swelling or redness, conjunctival hyperemia and discharge, corneal clarity or haze, and gross iris and anterior segment abnormalities. If a direct ophthalmoscope is available, examination of the fundus should be attempted. This is best done in dim lighting so that the pupil is somewhat large. If a normal appearance of the optic nerves, retinal vessels, and maculae can be confirmed, this can be very helpful. This requires some level of practice and proficiency, but is within the scope of physical examination techniques of every physician.

PRACTICE POINT

Ophthalmologic consultation is required for any condition that may cause severe and permanent vision loss, including
- Corneal ulcers
- Iritis
- Acute angle glaucoma
- Sudden visual loss
- Orbital mass, including orbital abscess
- Stevens Johnson Syndrome with mucosal involvement

TABLE 83-1 Differential Diagnosis of Common Red Eye Complaints

	Conjunctivitis	Iritis	Acute Glaucoma	Corneal Infection
Incidence	Very common	Common	Uncommon	Common
Discharge	Copious	None	None	Watery
Vision	Unaffected	Slightly blurred	Severely blurred	Usually blurred
Conjunctival injection	Diffuse	Circumcorneal	Circumcorneal	Circumcorneal
Pain	None	Moderate	Severe	Moderate to severe
Cornea	Clear	Usually clear	Steamy	Variable
Pupil size	Normal	Small	Mid-dilated	Normal
Pupillary light response	Normal	Sluggish	Fixed	Normal
IOP	Normal	Normal	Elevated	Normal

THE INFLAMED EYE

■ EMERGENT CONSIDERATIONS

In addition to the infections detailed below, loss of sympathetic innervation may give a mild red eye from vasodilation. When accompanied by ptosis (with or without miosis) as in Horner syndrome, this condition may be mistaken for ocular inflammation. Acute onset in a postpartum patient, with or without headache, may result from carotid artery dissection, and MR or CT angiography must be performed with consideration given to anticoagulation.

■ TEAR DYSFUNCTION SYNDROME (DRY EYE)

CASE 83-1

A 62-year-old woman is admitted for respiratory failure from a bacterial pneumonia. After 2 weeks of intubation in the intensive care unit on broad-spectrum antibiotics, her condition improves. She is extubated and transferred to the medicine ward, where she reports eye irritation. Both eyes appear slightly red, and she reports some tearing and sensitivity to bright lights. Her vision is mildly blurred, and measures 20/25 in each eye with her reading glasses using a pocket visual acuity card. The remainder of her eye exam is essentially normal.

This patient is likely suffering from exposure keratopathy or corneal abrasion (**Table 83-1**). Under normal conditions, the ocular surface and eyelid glands produce aqueous, oily, and proteinaceous tear secretions essential for normal eye health. Insufficient lubrication is common in the setting of an intubated and sedated patient and can lead to breakdown of the surface of the cornea with subsequent corneal infection and ulceration. For this reason, in such patients ICU protocols commonly include frequent lubrication of the eyes with ointments to prevent ocular surface disease. Despite this effort, mild damage to the cornea and conjunctiva, especially in a long hospitalization, may occur. Dry eye symptoms frequently include eye irritation, blurry vision, foreign body sensation, and mild eye redness. Other patients at risk include those with known facial nerve paresis, recent anesthesia with insufficient eyelid taping during the procedure, and dementia. Reassurance and further lubrication are warranted to relieve symptoms.

In contrast, a corneal ulcer presents as an opaque area in the cornea that may appear hazy or even white. The ulcer may have a significant mucopurulent exudate and will likely be very painful. The conjunctiva will frequently be bright red (**Figure 83-1**). At the bedside, the physician may use fluorescein dye to look for an epithelial defect. If corneal staining occurs, then the potential for corneal ulceration is high, even if an infiltrate is not yet seen and pain is minimal. Ophthalmologic consultation is required. Corneal ulcers may cause severe and permanent vision loss. The patient must be seen by an ophthalmologist that same day for culture of the corneal surface and broad-spectrum topical antibiotic therapy to prevent corneal perforation and endophthalmitis, which frequently will lead to loss of the eye. The ophthalmologist may prescribe fortified topical antibiotic drops to be applied every 30 to 60 minutes around the clock for the first 24 to 48 hours, and the nursing staff must be made aware of the importance of adherence to this very demanding but effective medical therapy.

■ CONJUNCTIVITIS

CASE 83-2

A 22-year-old man is admitted for respiratory distress attributed to an acute asthma attack. He is treated overnight with nebulized adrenergic agonists that are gradually weaned and prescribed systemic steroid therapy. It is also noted that he has mild eczematous changes on his hands that are not new. His roommate

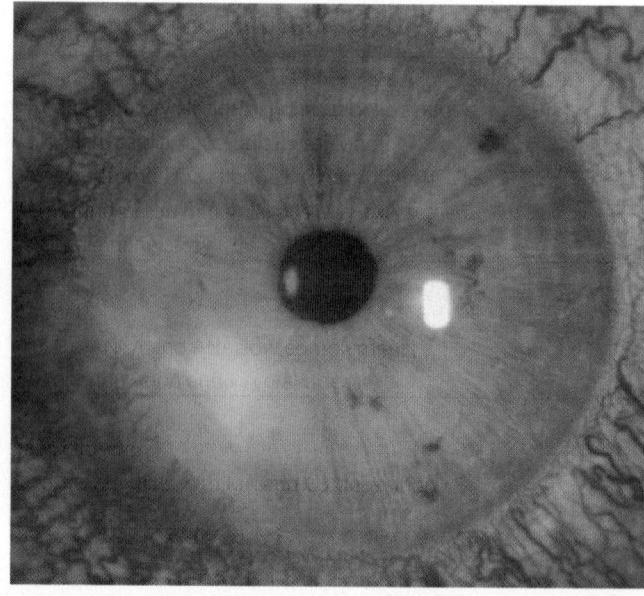

Figure 83-1 *Corneal ulcer with typical white exudate at the corneal limbus and severe conjunctival injection.*

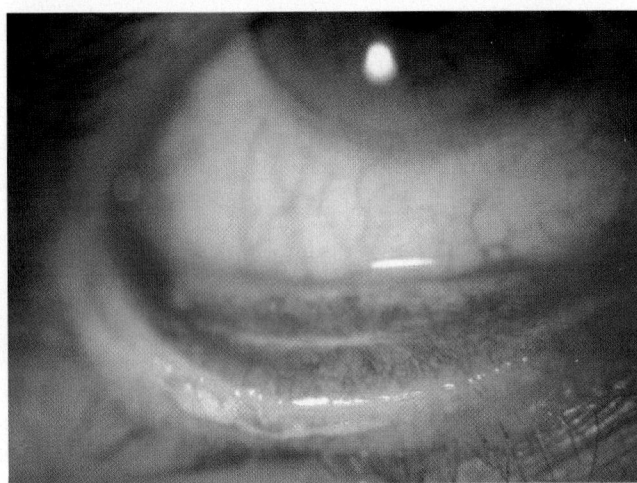

Figure 83-2 *Allergic conjunctivitis with formation of follicles in the inferior conjunctival fornix. Inspection alone does not allow differentiation from viral infection.*

notes that he has had red eyes for the past 2 days, which have been itching and tearing as well. There has been no crusting of the eyelashes upon waking up and there is no frank pain. The eyes are mildly irritated, but itching has been the prominent feature. The skin beneath his eyelids is also slightly hyperpigmented. He has had similar episodes of red eyes before, which had resolved without serious complication.

This case illustrates a classic example of allergic conjunctivitis. Severe itching is the most prominent symptom. Frequently, there will be generalized hyperemia (redness) of the conjunctiva and mild to moderate tearing (**Figure 83-2**). Visual blurring, if present, is mild and attributable to the tearing. Eye rubbing is typical, and the patient may have symptoms of allergic rhinitis as well, with associated rubbing of the nose. This rubbing can sometimes lead to mild eyelid edema and temporary hyperpigmentation (also known as allergic shiners, raccoon eyes) and a crease on the nose from manipulation as well. Common associations are with asthma, eczema, or history of other atopy. Symptoms can be managed with artificial tear lubricants and cool compresses if mild to moderate. If symptoms are severe or persistent, inpatient consultation with an ophthalmologist may be warranted, and treatment may require immune modulation with a topical antihistamine, mast cell stabilizer, or mild steroid. Topical corticosteroids should never be prescribed without active participation by the ophthalmologist, since untoward effects may include promoting viral infection (especially if there is a history of ocular herpes simplex) and intraocular pressure elevation.

■ VIRAL CONJUNCTIVITIS

Viral conjunctivitis also presents with bilateral red eyes. However, the symptoms will often have started in one eye 1 to 2 days prior to starting in the fellow eye. Often the eyes are very red with copious tearing, and the most prominent symptom is pain and burning. Mucous crusting of the eyelashes, especially in the morning, may be so copious as to preclude eyelid opening without manual assistance. A preauricular lymph node may also be palpated on exam and is relatively specific for viral etiology. Symptoms tend to worsen for the first few days of infection and generally resolve within 1 to 2 weeks. Household contacts may have had a recent URI or similar eye symptoms. Hand washing and contact precautions are crucial in preventing the spread of infection. If hospital workers become infected, they must be removed from patient contact for at least 7

days after symptoms start in the second eye to avoid nosocomial spread (spread to both eyes is very common even when infected persons are very cautious).

■ BACTERIAL CONJUNCTIVITIS

In contrast, bacterial conjunctivitis is often unilateral at presentation, which helps to distinguish it from allergic and viral etiologies, but it may spread to both eyes via the hands to become bilateral. Common organisms include Neisseria, pneumococcus, Staphylococcus, *Haemophilus influenzae*, Moraxella, and others. Copious mucopurulent discharge is the most prominent feature. Pain and irritation with severe hyperemia may occur, but there should not be frank vision loss. Bilateral cases can be challenging to distinguish from viral conjunctivitis, and an ophthalmologist should make this distinction. Debilitated patients are most prone to bacterial conjunctivitis, and suspicion for this diagnosis will be higher in such individuals. Treatment is usually with topical antibiotic ointments or drops, and may require cultures to determine the causative organism if the symptoms and signs are anything other than mild. Otherwise immunocompetent patients with unilateral disease may be treated empirically with topical fluoroquinolones such as moxifloxacin or gatifloxacin, both of which have broad-spectrum activity against the common organisms. If improvement is not seen within 48 hours, then cultures should be repeated and ophthalmologic consultation requested.

PRACTICE POINT

Conjunctivitis
- Allergic conjunctivitis: Topical corticosteroids should never be prescribed without active participation by the ophthalmologist, since untoward effects may include promoting viral infection and intraocular pressure elevation.
- Viral conjunctivitis: If hospital workers become infected, they must be removed from patient contact for at least 7 days after symptoms start in the second eye to avoid nosocomial spread.
- Bacterial conjunctivitis: Treatment is usually with topical antibiotic ointments or drops, and may require cultures to determine the causative organism if the symptoms and signs are anything other than mild. If improvement is not seen within 48 hours, then cultures should be repeated and ophthalmologic consultation requested.

■ IRITIS

CASE 83-3

A 32-year-old man is admitted for acute persistent diarrhea leading to electrolyte imbalances. Workup of his gastrointestinal distress reveals abnormal ulcerations on colonoscopy consistent with inflammatory bowel disease. During the first hospital day, the patient reports blurry vision and photophobia in the left eye only, which had started several days ago and has been gradually worsening. The eye is slightly red on examination and visual acuity is reduced to 20/40. The right eye is normal.

This patient has anterior uveitis associated with inflammatory bowel disease, but many autoimmune conditions can be associated with inflammation of the eye. The most prominent feature is photophobia. Often, patients are extremely sensitive to light; they may keep room lights off and blinds closed and even wear sunglasses indoors during an episode. Symptoms may be unilateral or bilateral, although the former is more common. Prior episodes also are common but vary in severity and laterality. Hyperemia is seen as a characteristic red ring of inflammation

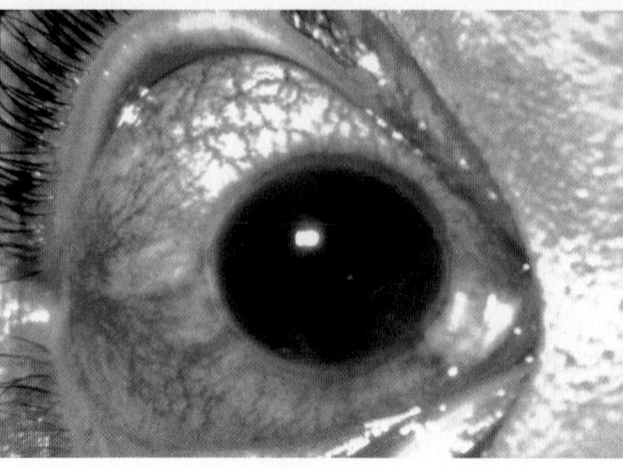

Figure 83-3 *Characteristic limbal flush (redness) seen in cases of acute iritis.*

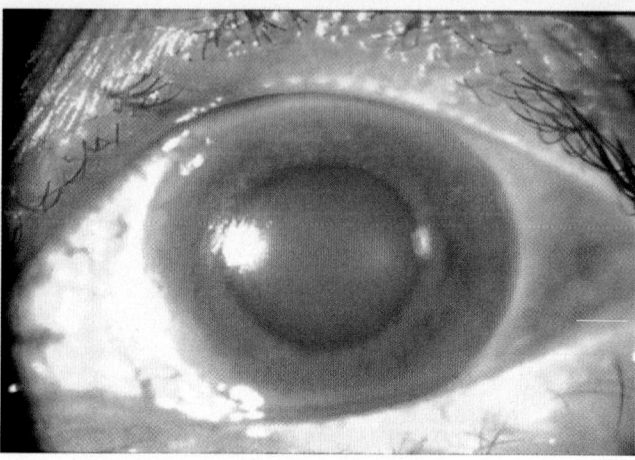

Figure 83-4 *Mid-dilated pupil and corneal clouding (seen as loss of typical corneal sheen and dulling of corneal light reflex) in a case of acute angle closure.*

around the edges of the cornea called limbal flush (**Figure 83-3**). Diagnosis requires a slit lamp, as inflammation cannot be diagnosed accurately without sufficient magnification of the anterior segment. Diagnosis, therefore, requires consultation with an ophthalmologist. While ocular inflammation may be related to autoimmune conditions as in the case above, it may also be the result of infection, and this must be ruled out in every case. The ophthalmologist will direct the appropriate investigations for possible infectious etiologies. Serum tests for syphilis, Lyme disease, toxoplasmosis, and serological (eg, QFT-GIT) and/or skin testing for tuberculosis exposure are commonly performed. In addition, the ophthalmologist may recommend chest imaging for sarcoidosis, and if the review of systems suggests a possible undiagnosed autoimmune disease, serum testing for HLA-B27 may be performed as well. Rheumatologic consultation also may be appropriate.

■ ANGLE CLOSURE GLAUCOMA

CASE 83-4

A 68-year-old Caucasian woman is hospitalized for workup of chest pain. Spending most of her day in a dimly lit hospital room watching TV, she suddenly develops a red, painful, blurry right eye. The pain and redness worsen over the next hour and do not remit. During this period of time, the vision is profoundly blurred. Visual acuity in the right eye is roughly 20/400, as is able to only make out the largest letters on the pocket vision chart. The vision does not improve even with the use of her glasses, which are bifocals that are somewhat thick. The patient reports she is far-sighted and has been for many years. The patient also reports that she has had similar episodes in the past several years on occasion, sometimes in the left eye, other times in the right eye, but never in both eyes simultaneously. She has attributed her symptoms to headache, and she has seen her primary care provider who diagnosed her with mild migraines and recommended Excedrin.

Acute angle closure attacks are virtually always unilateral. It is a rare but vision-threatening condition and should not be missed. Prompt ophthalmology referral is required to prevent permanent vision loss. It can be recognized by a very painful and red eye with profoundly decreased vision. Patients commonly present with a severe headache on the affected side, sometimes with associated nausea and vomiting; symptoms typically last for minutes to hours, not days or weeks. Similar episodes may

have occurred in the past in the same eye, or in the fellow eye, usually in dim lighting, such as a movie theatre, since pupillary dilatation bunches up the iris tissue in the angle. The pupil is usually slightly larger than the fellow eye and is unreactive. The cornea is often cloudy because the elevated pressure impairs corneal endothelial function, and this clouding makes it difficult to see the iris as clearly on the affected side in comparison to the fellow eye (**Figure 83-4**). There should be no discharge or exudate. This condition occurs more commonly in women and is associated with far-sightedness (hyperopia). The affected eye may feel much more hard (be difficult to indent) in comparison with the fellow eye when gently palpated through closed eyelids. This is indicative of a severely elevated intraocular pressure, which is the cause of the potential optic nerve damage in glaucoma. If this diagnosis is suspected, immediate ophthalmic consultation should be made for prompt reduction of the intraocular pressure, initially with topical agents. Ultimately this condition requires laser peripheral iridotomy in the affected eye as soon as possible, and in the fellow eye to prevent future episodes. Importantly, the vast majority of patients with glaucoma do not suffer from angle closure attacks, but rather primary open angle glaucoma, which is largely asymptomatic and has no commonality with an angle closure attack as described above. A patient with red eyes and a history of "glaucoma" for which they take eye drops on a regular basis is almost certainly not having an acute angle closure attack.

DIPLOPIA

■ EVALUATION

The evaluation of diplopia must begin with determination of whether or not the symptoms are binocular. Monocular diplopia, that is, double vision in one eye only, is virtually never an ophthalmic emergency. Many entities can cause double vision in one eye, such as cataract, corneal pathology, or incorrect spectacle prescription. Binocular diplopia, double vision due to misalignment of the eyes, virtually always requires ophthalmologic evaluation for proper diagnosis and treatment. Therefore, the first question to the patient who complains of diplopia should always be, "does the double vision go away when you cover either eye?" If the answer is yes, then the patient has binocular diplopia and an ophthalmologist should be called when the remainder of the evaluation is complete. The diplopia may be intermittent or constant and may change with position of gaze. Patients should be asked about associated neurologic symptoms such as headache, nausea or vomiting, vertigo, and weakness or tingling.

■ EMERGENT CONSIDERATIONS

A patient with new third nerve paresis (see below), especially if painful and/or incomplete, must be evaluated with urgent neuroimaging. Less commonly, a sixth nerve paresis may be accompanied by ipsilateral ptosis and miosis consistent with Horner syndrome, localizing the process to the cavernous sinus; acute onset can arise from cavernous sinus thrombosis or rapid tumor growth or hemorrhage.

■ SPECIFIC CAUSES OF DIPLOPIA

Cranial nerve paresis

CASE 83-5

A 73-year-old man is admitted with double vision that resolves upon covering either eye. He reports that his symptoms started that morning. He has also noticed the right eyelid drooping since this morning. He has not had any prior eye problems except for using reading glasses, and has had cataract surgery in both eyes 3 years ago. He has hypertension controlled with two oral antihypertensive medications, and no other chronic medical conditions. On examination, his visual acuity is 20/25 on the pocket visual acuity chart in each eye with his reading glasses on. The examination of the pupils reveals that the right pupil is larger than the left, and reacts more slowly than the left as well. He reports that no eye doctor has ever noted a pupillary abnormality before. His extraocular movements demonstrate limitation in elevation, depression, and adduction of the right eye. When he is looking straight, the right eye is misaligned downward and temporally. In addition, the right eyelid hangs lower than the left one (**Figure 83-5**). Visual fields tested by confrontation are grossly full. Hand-light examination reveals normal-appearing anterior segments without hyperemia or opacity of the cornea. Direct ophthalmoscopy reveals normal-appearing optic nerves, retinal vessels, and maculae in each eye, though the view was easier in the right eye due to the enlarged pupil.

This patient has an acute oculomotor (third cranial nerve) palsy. This may be due to ischemia of the nerve itself secondary to chronic microvasculopathy related to hypertension and/or diabetes, a cerebral aneurysm, a mass impinging on the nerve, viral infection, or trauma. The most concerning and potentially life-threatening cause is aneurysmal compression. Aneurysms often arise at the junction of the internal carotid and posterior communicating arteries. Because the pupillary fibers of the oculomotor nerve run peripherally within the nerve fascicle in the subarachnoid space, involvement of the pupil in an oculomotor

nerve palsy is indicative of a cerebral aneurysm impinging on the nerve until proven otherwise. Vascular insults to the third nerve generally spare the pupil and thus can be distinguished clinically from compressive lesions when the third nerve paresis is complete. An oculomotor nerve palsy affects the superior rectus, inferior rectus, medial rectus, and inferior oblique muscles, in addition to the iris and ciliary body. The lateral rectus and superior oblique muscles are intact, and hence the eye may rest in a "down and out" position. Limitations in elevation, depression, and adduction are typical but frequently are not complete, as some residual function may persist.

Trochlear (fourth cranial nerve) palsy results in double vision with images appearing tilted with respect to one another. Diplopia with a torsional component should make the examiner suspicious of this diagnosis. On examination, the affected eye appears higher than the fellow eye (hypertropia). This hypertropia increases when the affected eye looks down or in toward the nose. Congenital partial trochlear nerve palsy is relatively common and often well-controlled until adulthood, when it may decompensate and cause manifest diplopia. The patient in this scenario will have a history of tilting the head toward the affected side. This can be confirmed by looking at old photographs. Acquired trochlear paresis is also common and may be seen with even mild head trauma. It may also occur due to microvascular disease or cranial surgery.

Abducens (sixth cranial nerve) palsy results in horizontal diplopia with images appearing side by side due to limitation or absence of abduction of the eye. When the patient is looking straight ahead, the affected side may be misaligned with the eye pointing inward (esotropia). The remainder of the eye movements are normal. Frequently, the paresis is incomplete with some residual ability to abduct the affected eye. Most cases of abducens nerve palsy in older adults are related to microvascular disease from hypertension, diabetes, and hyperlipidemia, and these tend to resolve over weeks with no intervention. Careful ophthalmologic follow-up is required. If the abducens palsy does not resolve as expected, then tumor, arteriovenous fistulas, and other intracranial processes must be ruled out.

■ ORBITAL DISORDERS

Orbital masses may affect globe position and disturb normal extraocular muscle action with resulting binocular diplopia. Thyroid eye disease, most commonly associated with Graves disease but which can also be present in some hypothyroid and euthyroid states, is an infiltrative disease of the extraocular muscles and orbital fat that produces a congested orbit and proptosis. Unbalanced muscle involvement may lead to binocular diplopia. The diplopic patient must be asked about endocrine dysfunction. Orbital masses, in addition to causing double vision, frequently cause proptosis, which the astute observer will note even without exophthalmometry. If an orbital mass, including an orbital abscess, is suspected, prompt ophthalmic attention is required.

■ MYASTHENIA GRAVIS

Myasthenia gravis is a disease of the neuromuscular junction with antibodies against the nicotinic acetylcholine receptors on the motor end plate. It frequently presents (up to 75%) with ocular symptoms and may be limited to the eye. The most common presenting sign is ptosis, but any of the extraocular muscles may be involved. Therefore, ocular myasthenia gravis may mimic virtually any cranial neuropathy. The pupil is virtually never involved in myasthenia gravis. Thus, pupillary abnormalities are a helpful clinical sign that can distinguish this disease process from others. Diplopia in a patient with myasthenia typically waxes and wanes over the

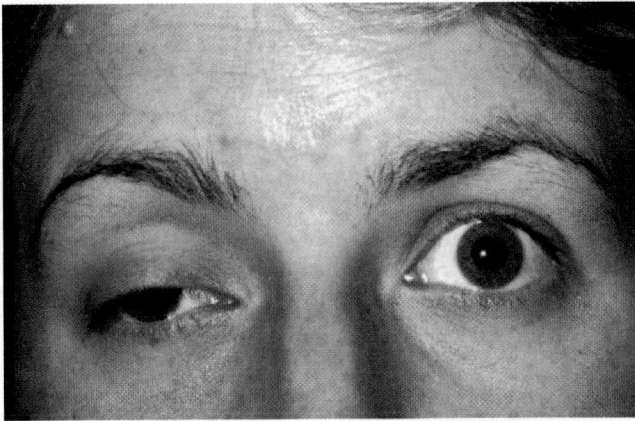

Figure 83-5 *Ptosis and ophthalmoparesis seen with third nerve palsy. Note dilation of the right pupil; this is not pharmacologic.*

course of a day, improves with rest, and often has symptoms that have been occurring for the previous months or years. Ocular myasthenia may be unilateral or bilateral. If this disease is suspected, the ophthalmologist may use tests of fatigability or the ice test to help in diagnosis, in conjunction with short-acting acetylcholinesterase inhibitors.

PRACTICE POINT

Cranial Nerve Palsies
- CN III: A patient with new third nerve paresis, especially if painful and/or incomplete, must be evaluated with urgent neuroimaging.
- CN IV: Trochlear palsy results in double vision with images appearing tilted with respect to one another; it arises from microvascular disease or neurosurgery.
- CN VI: The Horner syndrome (a sixth nerve paresis accompanied by ipsilateral ptosis and miosis) localizes the process to the cavernous sinus; acute onset can arise from cavernous sinus thrombosis or rapid tumor growth or hemorrhage.

Ocular myasthenia gravis may mimic virtually any cranial neuropathy but the pupil is virtually never involved.

SUDDEN VISION LOSS

Both visual acuity and confrontation visual field testing at the bedside must be performed and should help the clinician localize the vision loss to one eye or hemifield. If there is bilateral loss, then the degree of asymmetry is important to record. The presence of other ocular and orbital signs (redness, ocular motility disturbance, eyelid swelling, ptosis) should be noted, as they will assist in anatomic localization. Pupillary reactions provide objective evidence of afferent visual loss and may direct the workup even when other data are conflicting or unreliable.

If an obvious visual disturbance (severe unilateral vision loss with afferent pupillary defect, gross homonymous hemianopia) is not found, then further workup should be deferred and an ophthalmology consult obtained. Automated perimetric testing, dilated fundus examination, photography and advanced imaging of the retina and optic nerve, and even refraction performed by the ophthalmologist will allow for a much more directed investigation, and may reveal other benign causes of vision loss (**Table 83-2**).

CASE 83-6

A 76-year-old man with long-standing congestive heart failure is being treated with intravenous antibiotics for a community-acquired pneumonia. On hospital day 2, he complains of blurred vision in his left eye. He is unsure if it came on suddenly but notices it when he tries to read or watch television. There is no eye pain, and the eye and periorbital area are normal without erythema, warmth, or tenderness.

As in the assessment of diplopia, the first question to answer is whether the symptoms are monocular or binocular. Even very sophisticated patients may report vision loss in one eye when in fact they have a homonymous hemianopia on the side of reported monocular vision loss. Simple bedside testing with alternating eye occlusion is sufficient to get an answer. Most patients will have monocular symptoms. Painful vision loss often indicates a more acute process within the orbit, intracranial space, or systemically. Orbital or optic nerve infarction in giant cell arteritis is a rare but potentially life-threatening cause of severe, unilateral vision loss. Timing is the next crucial factor to determine. Vision loss may be discovered suddenly but be subacute in its true progression; the existence of an intercurrent acute illness may prompt attention to other organ systems as well. Finally, vision loss may be transient or fixed, and the differential diagnosis may be altered significantly (Table 83-2).

Bedside visual acuity is 20/20 OD, 20/70 OS. It does not improve with use of a pinhole. There is no relative afferent pupillary defect, and the fundi are difficult to see without dilation. Upon dilation, the consultant reports that the left retina has hemorrhages and lipid deposition superiorly, matching an inferior defect on perimetry (**Figure 83-6**). Fluorescein angiography confirms a branch retinal vein occlusion. CBC and coagulation panel are unremarkable, and a TTE/TEE are also found to be normal. Carotid duplex scans show no hemodynamic abnormalities. The patient is scheduled for outpatient ophthalmology follow-up in 30 days to screen for possible retinal neovascularization and resolution of macular edema. He is advised to maintain good glycemic and blood pressure control as an outpatient.

Acute vision loss from retinal or optic nerve disease can be precipitated by hemodynamic shifts in acutely ill patients or from adverse effects (hypotension, direct toxicity) of new medications. A thorough review of the patient's medical risk factors for vision loss

---

TABLE 83-2 Causes of Vision Loss in Hospitalized Patients

	Time of Onset	Severity	Unilateral vs Bilateral	Treatment
Cataract	Gradual	Usually mild or moderate	Bilateral >> unilateral	Observation, refraction, surgery
Glaucoma	Gradual	Severe when noticed by patient	Bilateral >> unilateral	Medication vs surgery
Macular degeneration	Gradual (dry) Rapid (wet)	Often severe	Bilateral >> unilateral	Intravitreal medication, laser therapy
Diabetic retinopathy	Gradual	Moderate to severe	Unilateral > bilateral	Laser therapy, intravitreal medication
Nonarteritic ischemic optic neuropathy	Sudden	Moderate to severe	Unilateral >> bilateral	Usually none
Arteritic ischemic optic neuropathy	Sudden	Severe	Unilateral >> bilateral	Immediate systemic corticosteroid therapy
Optic chiasm/ postchiasmal disease	Sudden > gradual	Moderate to severe	Bilateral	Varies by underlying cause

Table 83-2 is meant to be representative and is not exhaustive. A comprehensive ophthalmology text should be consulted if necessary.

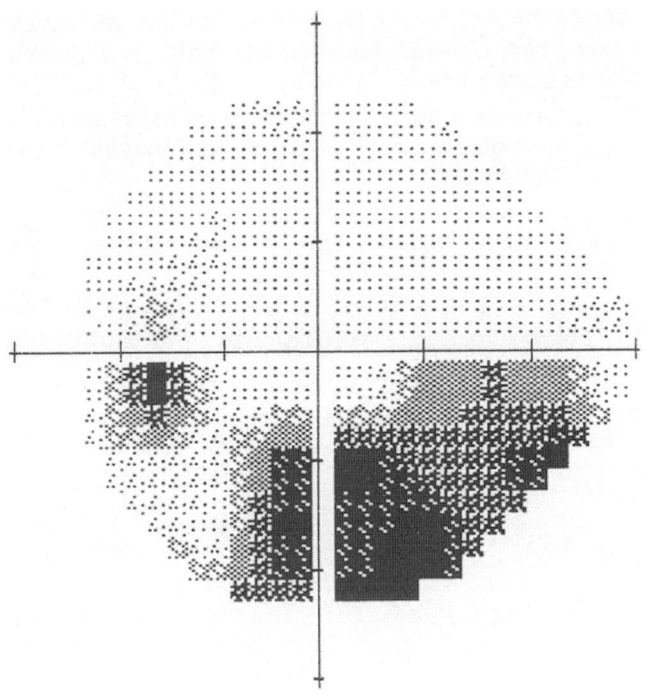

Figure 83-6 *Visual field testing showing loss of the inferior field of vision in a patient with superior branch retinal vein occlusion and retinal ischemia. The field defect respects the horizontal meridian, consistent with the distribution of the retinal vascular supply.*

is required so that no possibilities are overlooked. The acute treatment of these patients addresses the underlying hemodynamic or coagulation disorders that may be present and the systemic illness that may have precipitated the visual loss event. Careful ophthalmologic follow-up is essential, especially in cases of central retinal vein occlusion (CRVO), in which there is a high risk of later retinal neovascularization and development of severe glaucoma. If giant cell arteritis is suspected, then corticosteroids (preferably intravenous) should be started immediately. Waiting for an ophthalmology consultation and/or temporal artery biopsy is not necessary and may be harmful since it might delay treatment of a vision-threatening condition. While consultation and biopsy are necessary to confirm the diagnosis, they can be done after treatment begins and the patient is being protected from further events.

In the pregnant or immediate postpartum patient, hypertensive retinopathy with or without papilledema may occur at blood pressures below levels usually associated with malignant hypertension. Central vision loss is unusual except in severe or advanced disease; its presence should alert the clinician that urgent intervention is required to avoid permanent vision loss. Subtle optic disc swelling or hemorrhage may be difficult to appreciate with undilated fundoscopy, and ophthalmologic consultation should be obtained (inpatient if vision loss is present; otherwise, outpatient evaluation is indicated). The retinal changes should improve as better blood pressure control is obtained (**Figure 83-7**).

CONCLUSION

Hospitalized patients may develop a number of ocular disorders that will be brought to the attention of the treating physician. In many

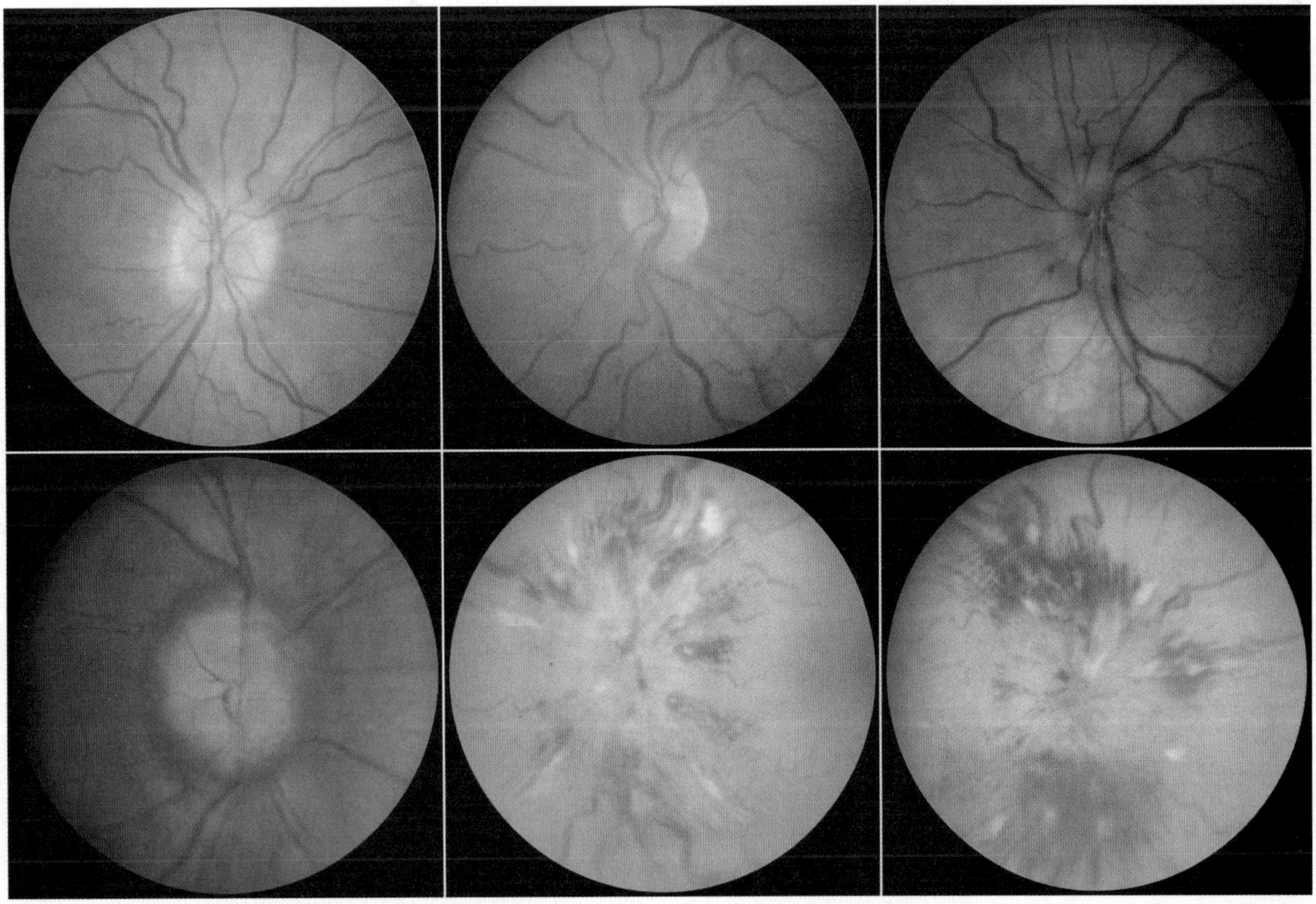

Figure 83-7 *Frisen Papilledema Scale, Grades 0-5.*

cases, the problems are simple and self-limited, especially when the patient's visual function is not impaired. Most of these issues are best managed in the outpatient setting, where the patient can see his/her general ophthalmologist. In more complex or concerning cases in which central or peripheral visual field loss is seen, or the patient reports severe pain, a basic bedside eye exam with attention to visual acuity ("the vital sign of the eye"), pupillary reaction, confrontational fields, and ocular motility will, along with basic inspection of the eye and adnexa, provide the ophthalmic consultant with invaluable information, allowing him or her to provide optimal care to the patient.

SUGGESTED READINGS

Dayan M, Turner B, McGhee C. Acute angle closure glaucoma masquerading as systemic illness. *BMJ*. 1996;313(7054):413-415.

Kerr NM, Chew SS, Danesh-Meyer HV. Non-arteritic anterior ischaemic optic neuropathy: a review and update. *J Clin Neurosci*. 2009;16(8):994-1000.

Prisco D, Marcucci R. Retinal vein thrombosis: risk factors, pathogenesis and therapeutic approach. *Pathophysiol Haemost Thromb*. 2002;32(5-6):308-311.

Sanders S, Kawasaki A, Purvin VA. Patterns of extraocular muscle weakness in vasculopathic pupil-sparing, incomplete third nerve palsy. *J Neuroophthalmol*. 2001;21(4):256-259.

Wilson LA. Acute bacterial infection of the eye: bacterial keratitis and endophthalmitis. *Trans Ophthalmol Soc UK*. 1986;105(1):43-60.

CHAPTER 84

Dizziness and Vertigo

Joseph M. Furman, MD, PhD

Key Clinical Questions

1 How do you determine whether a hospitalized patient has a benign cause of vertigo?

2 How might the physical examination confirm your suspicion of a benign cause of vertigo?

3 How do you treat vertigo?

INTRODUCTION

Dizziness and vertigo are common complaints and encompass a myriad of symptoms that may stem from many organ systems. A sensation of lightheadedness or faintness may relate to the presence of orthostatic hypotension, abnormalities of the cardiovascular system, altered ambulation as seen in patients with impaired vision and sensation of feet (multiple-sensory-defect dizziness), or imbalance experienced by older patients (benign disequilibrium of aging). Many patients describe dizziness in reference to impaired ambulation and fear of falling or when they have blurred vision or feel confused. Hyperventilation may also cause symptoms of dizziness. These symptoms may be associated with significant disability and possibly mortality.

PRACTICE POINT

- A sensation of lightheadedness or faintness may relate to the presence of orthostatic hypotension, abnormalities of the cardiovascular system, hyperventilation, altered ambulation as seen in patients with impaired vision and sensation of feet (multiple-sensory-defect dizziness), or imbalance commonly experienced by older patients (benign disequilibrium of aging).

A sensation of vertigo, which is defined as an illusion of movement of self or surroundings, is much more likely to be a reflection of an abnormality of the peripheral or central vestibular system. It may be physiologic, that is, occurring with seasickness or after spinning or pathologic of central or peripheral vestibular origin. The misuse of the term *vertigo* as a diagnostic term rather than as a symptom should be eschewed in favor of a recognized diagnostic entity. Simply assigning a diagnosis of *vertigo* could prematurely terminate the evaluation and thereby miss an opportunity for accurate diagnosis followed by appropriate treatment. In some cases, the term *vertigo* is used as shorthand for benign paroxysmal positional vertigo. Because of the high prevalence of this disorder in the outpatient setting, these patients may receive proper treatment despite sloppy documentation and failure to convey accurate information to colleagues.

This chapter primarily focuses on the symptom of vertigo in patients admitted to the hospital. Chapter 101 includes cardiac causes of presyncope. Other medical illnesses, drug toxicity, and substance abuse that may produce symptoms of dizziness and vertigo are covered elsewhere in this book. The published studies reviewing a systematic approach to the diagnosis and treatment of the symptom of vertigo relate to the outpatient or emergency room settings. Hospitalized patients are a different population. If symptoms of dizziness and vertigo are new experiences, the clinician should consider iatrogenic causes in addition to the usual suspects.

CASE 84-1

A 75-year-old woman with diabetes and hypertension underwent a total knee replacement. On the first postoperative day, she experienced vertigo when turning in her hospital bed. Each brief vertiginous episode was associated with mild nausea. The patient was essentially asymptomatic when sitting or lying still. She did not suffer any perioperative hypotension.

Physical and neurologic examinations revealed normal findings. What additional diagnostic testing should be considered?

THE VESTIBULAR SYSTEM

The vestibular system can be divided anatomically into the peripheral and central vestibular systems. The peripheral vestibular system consists of the left and right vestibular labyrinths and the eighth cranial nerve. The central vestibular system consists of the vestibular nuclei in the medulla and caudal pons and the pathways that subserve the vestibulo-ocular reflex, vestibulo-spinal reflexes, vestibular influences on spatial orientation, and the vestibulo-autonomic pathways that are important for the nausea and occasional vomiting that accompany vestibular system disease. Each vestibular labyrinth consists of three semicircular canals, which sense angular motion and two otolithic organs, the utricle and saccule, which sense linear acceleration and orientation with respect to gravity. The vestibular labyrinth senses motion of the head. This signal is conveyed to the vestibular nuclei via the eighth nerve. At that site, vestibular signals are combined with signals from the visual and somatosensory systems to provide the central nervous system with an accurate representation of head orientation. With this information, the central nervous system can accurately control eye position and postural stability. Note that eighth nerve afferents have a nonzero tonic resting activity, which is illustrated diagrammatically in **Figure 84-1**.

Tonic signals from the left labyrinth drive the eyes and the body to the right, whereas signals from the right vestibular labyrinth drive the eyes and body to the left. At rest, these influences are balanced. During movement, the afferent activity from one labyrinth increases while the afferent activity from the opposite labyrinth decreases. This imbalance leads to movement of the eyes or the body as appropriate to maintain stable vision and upright posture.

PATHOPHYSIOLOGY OF THE VESTIBULAR SYSTEM

Vestibular disorders can be either peripheral or central. Most peripheral vestibular disorders affect only a single labyrinth. Damage to a single labyrinth causes a left-right vestibular imbalance. This imbalance is interpreted as intense movement toward the intact labyrinth, which leads to excessive eye movement in the form of nystagmus, gait instability, spatial disorientation, and autonomic symptoms such as nausea, vomiting, and, in some patients, changes in heart rate and blood pressure (ie, either hypotension or hypertension). The effects of a unilateral vestibular loss are illustrated in **Figure 84-2**.

Over time, usually in a matter of days, central vestibular circuits rebalance despite the absence of a signal from one of the labyrinths. This process of rebalancing, known as *vestibular compensation*, leads to a gradual resolution of nystagmus and gait instability (see **Figure 84-3**).

Peripheral causes of vertigo include acoustic neuroma, aminoglycoside toxicity, benign positional vertigo, cholesteatoma, herpes zoster oticus, labyrinthine concussion related to head trauma, Ménière disease, perilymph fistula, otosclerosis, recurrent vestibulopathy, and vestibular neuronitis.

Central causes of vertigo include brain tumors, cerebellar or brainstem stroke, multiple sclerosis, vertebrobasilar transient ischemic attacks, and migraine-related dizziness.

HISTORY OF THE PATIENT WITH DIZZINESS OR VERTIGO

■ DOES THIS PATIENT HAVE VERTIGO?

The history is the most critical first step in distinguishing vertigo from other causes of dizziness and may pinpoint the etiology of the patient's symptoms in up to three-fourths of patients. The examiner should carefully ask the patient what is meant by these symptoms and what brings them on. Some patients may be unable to explain their symptoms at all and respond simply that "I'm just dizzy." Be sure to obtain an interpreter if English is not the primary language; do not make assumptions or characterize the symptoms for the patient in the interest of time. Most patients cannot adequately describe their symptoms because the sensation of dizziness and vertigo is not a normal sensation, and, unlike sensations such as vision and hearing, vestibular sensation does not have an associated vocabulary such as brightness, loudness, color, or pitch. Some patients complain

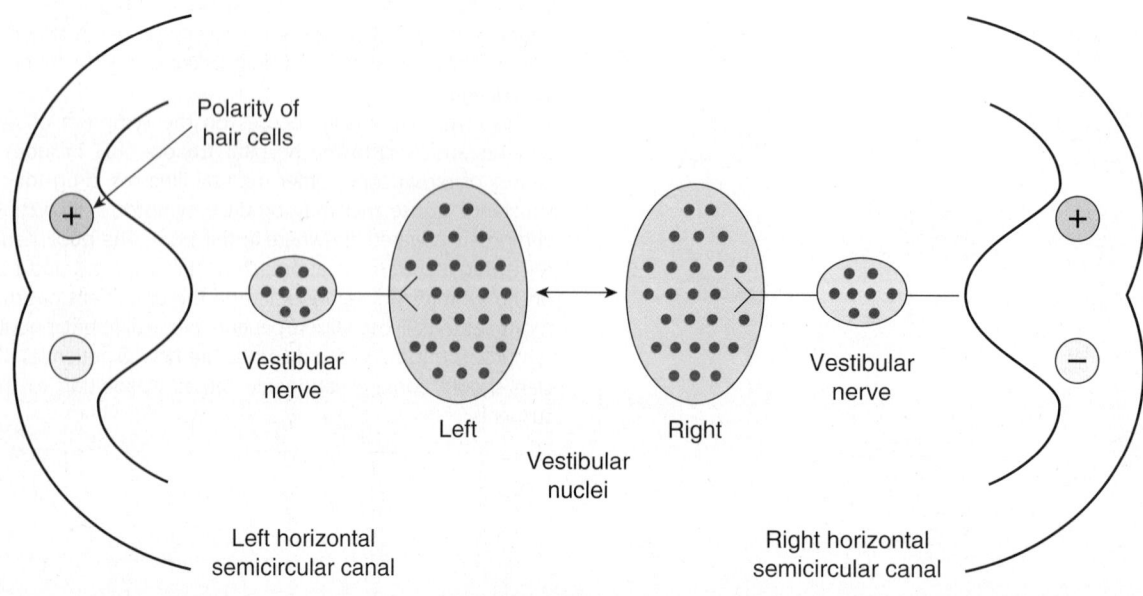

Figure 84-1 *Push-pull action of the horizontal vestibulo-ocular reflex, with no head movement, left and right vestibular influences are balanced.*

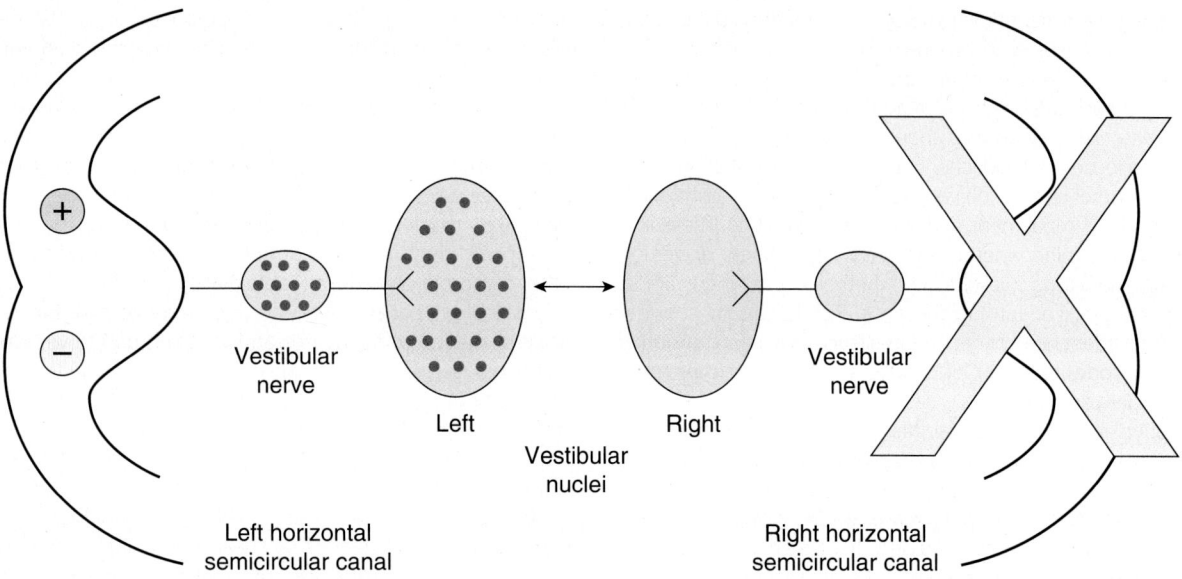

Figure 84-2 *The reciprocal push-pull interaction of the two labyrinths is disrupted after acute peripheral labyrinthine injury. For example, following the acute loss of right unilateral peripheral vestibular function, there is a loss of resting neural activity in the right vestibular nerve and right vestibular nuclei. Because the brain normally detects differences in activity between the two vestibular nuclear complexes, even when stationary the imbalance in neural activity is interpreted as a rapid head movement, in this case to the left.*

of a head sensation such as light-headedness, heavy-headedness, foggy-headedness, or presyncope. The three general types of dizziness symptoms, namely a sense of motion, imbalance, and head sensations, are not mutually exclusive. A nonspecific complaint of a head sensation, especially light-headedness, does not exclude the possibility of a vestibular disorder whether peripheral or central, and it may result from a metabolic derangement, drug effect, or other organ system disease. In fact, dysequilibrium, reduced cerebral perfusion, and vertigo can all be associated with the symptom of dizziness with standing. Ask whether or not the dizziness is characterized by a sense of motion such as spinning, rocking or tilting, imbalance when walking, veering to the right or left, or if the patient fears falling or has fallen.

PRACTICE POINT

- The history is the most critical first step in distinguishing vertigo from other causes of dizziness, and may pinpoint the etiology of the patient's symptoms in up to three-fourths of patients. The sensation of vertigo, defined as an illusion of movement of self or surroundings, is much more likely to be a reflection of an abnormality of the peripheral or central vestibular system. The misuse of the term *vertigo* as a diagnostic term rather than as a symptom should be eschewed in favor of a recognized diagnostic entity. If the physical examination confirms the presence of benign positional vertigo and the rest of the examination is unrevealing, then no further evaluation is necessary.

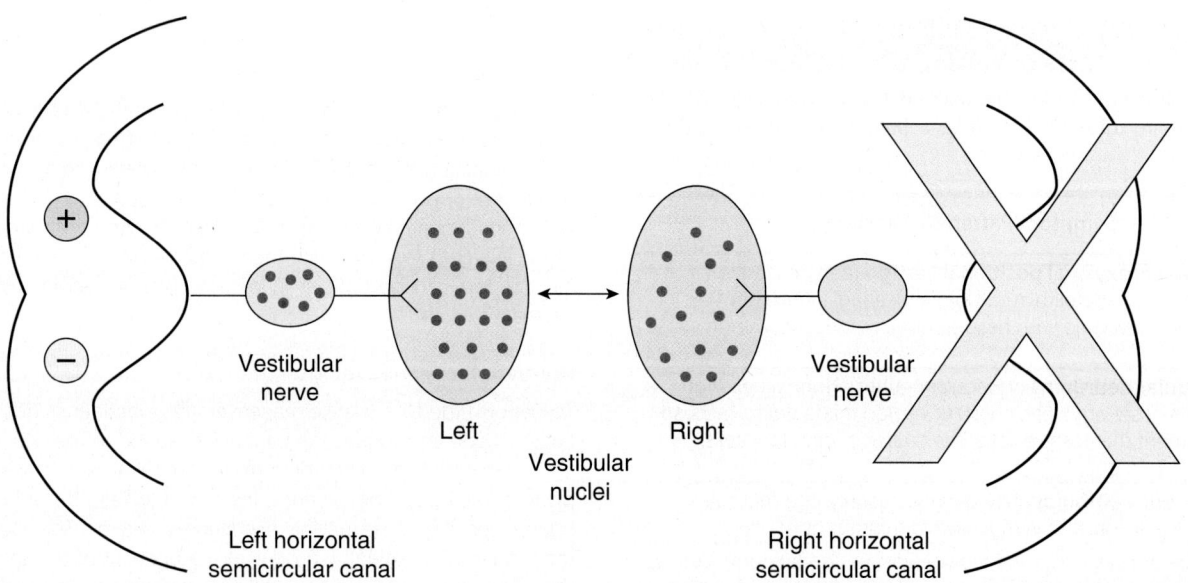

Figure 84-3 *When a peripheral vestibular injury is chronic, in this case on the right, the central nervous system is able, through vestibular compensation, to partially restore the lost resting activity within the deafferented vestibular nucleus, and thus reduce the asymmetry of neural activity between the vestibular nuclei at rest and partially restore the function of the vestibulo-ocular reflex.*

After giving the patient time to respond, sometimes asking about specific circumstances such as when the symptoms occur, other neurologic or otologic symptoms, and whether they are recurrent may help pinpoint the diagnosis more than the description of the dizziness. Associated symptoms should be specifically questioned: loss of consciousness, headache, tinnitus, decreased hearing, disturbance of other cranial nerves, trouble walking or controlling extremities, visual impairment, and nausea and vomiting. The examiner should determine whether the onset of dizziness or vertigo was sudden, how long it lasted, and whether worse when supine, standing, stooping, or turning the neck. Risk factors to consider include: antecedent head or neck trauma (such as hyperextension of the neck), episodes of low or high blood sugar, hypertension, prior stroke, and dehydration.

Medication review is essential. Many new medications and/or toxic levels of medications due to drug-drug interactions, changes in metabolism due to renal and/or liver derangements, or incorrect prescribing can cause dizziness. Typical examples include phenytoin toxicity and reactions to some antibiotics. Because nearly all medications can potentially cause "dizziness," clinicians should specifically inquire about new medications.

■ DOES THIS PATIENT HAVE A BENIGN CAUSE OF VERTIGO?

When formulating a differential diagnosis for a patient who presents with vertigo, consider whether the patient's abnormality is affecting the peripheral vestibular apparatus, the central vestibular system, or both and the nature of the disease process (eg, inflammatory, vascular, or neurochemical derangements). Note that peripheral vestibular disorders often are associated with otologic complaints such as hearing loss, tinnitus, or ear fullness. Central vestibular disorders are more likely to include associated neurologic symptoms such as numbness, weakness, and incoordination. A common misconception when obtaining a history from patients with dizziness is to insist that patients with vertigo indicate whether they or the world around them appear to be moving. Although it is helpful to elicit a history of self-motion and/or motion of the surroundings versus simply lightheadedness, making a distinction between motion of self and motion of surround has no diagnostic utility (**Table 84-1**).

THE PHYSICAL EXAMINATION OF PATIENTS WITH VERTIGO

The medical history identifies patients who have true vertigo. These patients are most likely to have a peripheral vestibular etiology.

TABLE 84-1 Symptom Patterns of Vertigo

Benign paroxysmal positional vertigo (benign positional nystagmus, cupulolithiasis): Normal hearing, intermittent episodes of vertigo with head turning, the most common cause of vertigo

Vestibular neuronitis (vestibular neuritis): Normal hearing, sudden onset of severe, constant vertigo made worse by head movement that resolves over the course of days to weeks, second in frequency

Recurrent vestibulopathy: Normal hearing, intermittent episodes of constant vertigo lasting minutes or hours

Toxins (drugs such as aminoglycosides or cis-platinum): Vertigo with or without hearing loss, bilateral labyrinthine dysfunction

Central causes of vertigo: Vertigo with symptoms of neurologic dysfunction including weakness, impaired speech, diplopia

Because true vertigo may be associated with other disorders, the evaluation of a patient complaining of vertigo should consist of a general physical examination, a neurologic examination, and, as appropriate, specialized bedside examination provocative tests. If the physical examination confirms the presence of benign positional vertigo and the rest of the examination is unrevealing, then no further evaluation is necessary. Hospitalized patients may be more likely to have multifactorial causes to their symptoms due to their medications, fluid and nutritional status, deconditioning, and other comorbid conditions (**Table 84-2**).

Hospitalized patients who are hypovolemic may have one or more of the following: nausea and vomiting due to vertigo, acute blood loss (surgical or medical), third spacing (severe liver disease), burns, or poor oral intake with limited fluid replacement. The first step is always to examine the patient's vital signs. The physical examination should include checking for orthostatic blood pressure changes, examining the tympanic membranes, and performing a cardiovascular examination along with listening for bruits. The criterion of a pulse increment of >30 beats per minute from the supine to standing position may have limited utility in patients taking nodal blockers or with conduction system disease. Deconditioning can lead to orthostatic blood pressure changes as can autonomic nervous system dysfunction and medications. Hence, clinical judgment is required to assess abnormal vital signs.

The bedside neurologic examination should include performing an eye examination, testing for hearing loss and checking other cranial nerves, assessing sensation of the feet, and an assessment of gait and station; see Chapter 104. An abnormal neurologic examination will likely localize the illness and determine the need for imaging.

■ SPONTANEOUS NYSTAGMUS

Vertical nystagmus is a central vestibular sign that usually warrants MRI specifically of the vestibular nuclei or of the cerebellar vermis. A unidirectional horizontal nystagmus that includes a slight torsional component is more likely caused by a peripheral abnormality. Upbeating nystagmus seen only on upward gaze is usually a benign finding akin to bidirectional horizontal gaze-evoked nystagmus.

If the patient does not have spontaneous nystagmus, the examiner should perform a provocative maneuver to test for positional nystagmus.

Head-impulse test

To perform the head-impulse test, the patient's head is abruptly rotated to the right or left while the patient attempts to fixate on a distant stationary object. The examiner looks for a small rapid eye movement opposite to the direction of head movement that signifies an inadequate vestibulo-ocular reflex resulting from a disorder of the labyrinth toward which the head has been moved. Performing this test can be difficult in patients with an acute vestibular imbalance.

Dix-Hallpike maneuver

To perform the Dix-Hallpike maneuver, the examiner stands at the patient's side and rotates the patient's head 45° to the nearside to align the ipsilateral posterior semicircular canal with the sagittal plane of the body. The patient is instructed to keep his or her eyes open, especially if he or she experiences vertigo. The examiner then moves the patient, whose eyes are open, from the seated to the supine ear-down position and then extends the patient's neck slightly so that the chin is pointed slightly upward. The latency, duration, and direction of nystagmus, if present, and the latency and duration of vertigo, if present, should be noted. A positive test

TABLE 84-2 The Clinical History and Physical Examination

Does this dizzy patient have vertigo?

- True vertigo accounts for roughly half of the causes of dizziness.
- Sometimes asking about specific circumstances such as when the symptoms occur, other neurologic or otologic symptoms, and whether symptoms are recurrent may help pinpoint the diagnosis more than the description of the dizziness.

Ask the following questions:

- Are the symptoms characterized by a sense of motion such as spinning, rocking, or tilting?
- Is there a sense of imbalance when walking, veering to the right or left, or concern about falling? If so, inquire whether the patient does not have symptoms of dizziness when sitting or lying down. Dysequilibrium accounts for roughly 3% of causes of dizziness.

Does this patient have a benign cause of vertigo?

- Forty percent of dizzy patients will have peripheral vestibular disorders affecting the inner ear and cranial nerve VIII.
- Benign paroxysmal positional vertigo and vestibular neuronitis are most frequent diagnoses.

Inquire about associated hearing loss.

- For patients without associated hearing loss, the likelihood of a cerebello-pontine mass as the cause of vertigo is low (probability 1×10^{-4}).

Inquire about whether the vertigo is episodic or persistent.

- No hearing loss and episodic, brief, intense vertigo is likely benign paroxysmal positional vertigo.
- No hearing loss and persistent vertigo lasting hours to days with nausea is likely vestibular neuronitis.

Inquire about associated otologic complaints.

- Peripheral vestibular disorders are often associated with otologic complaints such as hearing loss, tinnitus, or ear fullness.
- Hearing loss and episodic vertigo lasting hours with tinnitus and a sensation of ear fullness is most consistent with Ménière disease.
- Hearing loss and severe persistent vertigo lasting hours to days with nausea is most consistent with labyrinthitis.

Does this patient have a central cause of vertigo?

- Roughly 10% of all dizziness may be central in origin.

Inquire about associated neurologic complaints.

- Central vestibular disorders are more likely to be associated with numbness, weakness, and incoordination.

Inquire about antecedent trauma and other risk factors.

Review medication list.

Is this patient orthostatic?

Does this patient have an abnormal neurologic examination?

Does this patient have an abnormal ear examination?

- Ear drainage is seen as a complication of chronic otitis media along with hearing loss and vertigo (cholesteatoma).
- Ramsay Hunt syndrome may be identified by the presence of vesicles along with hearing loss and facial palsy.

Does this patient have spontaneous nystagmus?

- Spontaneous horizontal nystagmus with or without torsional nystagmus is usually seen in patients with vestibular neuronitis or in other peripheral disorders.
- Vertical nystagmus is a central vestibular sign.
- Upbeating nystagmus only on upward gaze and bidirectional horizontal gaze-evoked nystagmus are usually benign findings.
- Absence of nystagmus during vertigo may suggest psychogenic vertigo.

Does this patient have positional nystagmus that reproduces the patient's symptoms?

produces a paroxysmal upbeating-torsional nystagmus. The examiner observes the patient's eyes for the characteristic nystagmus that generally lasts for the duration of the patient's vertigo.

COMMON VESTIBULAR DISORDERS IN THE HOSPITAL

Common vestibular disorders that may lead to a hospital admission or that may present once a patient has been admitted for an unrelated ailment involve peripheral disorders, including vestibular neuritis, benign paroxysmal positional vertigo, and Ménière disease, and central disorders, including vestibular migraine, medication-induced dizziness and vertigo, and posterior fossa stroke. Note that patients admitted following trauma may experience dizziness or vertigo on either a peripheral or central basis and that some psychiatric illnesses, notably panic disorder, may include dizziness.

■ BENIGN PAROXYSMAL POSITIONAL VERTIGO

Benign paroxysmal positional vertigo (BPPV) represents a very common vestibular disorder in the outpatient and emergency room setting. BPPV may be encountered in the hospital setting, especially in patients who have undergone a surgical procedure or who require prolonged bed rest. BPPV is characterized by brief periods, generally 10 to 20 seconds, of intense rotational vertigo that may or may not be associated with nausea. Aside from attacks of positional vertigo, patients with BPPV are often asymptomatic. A definitive diagnosis of benign paroxysmal positional vertigo can be made at the bedside using the Dix-Hallpike maneuver. The nystagmus may be complex with a mixture of both upbeating and torsional (rotary) eye movement. Physical examination will be normal otherwise.

Treatment for benign paroxysmal positional vertigo consists of a particle repositioning maneuver to relocate otolithic debris from the posterior semicircular channel to the vestibule. Patients may be referred to a physical therapist for treatment or to the following website regarding the Epley maneuver for instruction in how to perform these exercises: www.charite.de/ch/neuro/vertigo.html.

Patients with chronic vertigo of vestibular origin may benefit from a vestibular rehabilitation program designed to facilitate central compensation.

■ VESTIBULAR NEURITIS

Vestibular neuritis generally presents with the acute or subacute onset of severe vertigo, nausea, vomiting, and disequilibrium sometimes as the sequelae of a flu-like illness or an afebrile viral illness. Symptoms are present at rest and are exacerbated by any head movement. Certain head positions may exacerbate or reduce symptoms. Severe symptoms usually last for 1 to 3 days during which acute management is required. Then, symptoms gradually resolve over a period of days or weeks.

Physical examination generally reveals a unidirectional horizontal nystagmus that increases when the patient gazes in the direction of the quick component of the vestibular nystagmus. Gait instability is the rule. Note, however, that patients with vestibular neuritis are able to ambulate although they may require assistance. The head-impulse test is generally abnormal in patients with vestibular neuritis. Imaging in patients with vestibular neuritis is normal and usually not indicated. If there was something clinically that did not quite fit with this diagnosis and generates some concern on the physician's part, a definitive diagnosis of vestibular neuritis can be established by caloric testing in the vestibular laboratory indicating a markedly reduced or absent caloric response unilaterally.

It is the standard of practice to treat with corticosteroids although their benefit has not been consistently shown. Antiviral agents have not been shown to be effective. Supportive measures may include vestibular suppressants such as meclizine, tranquilizers, and bedrest for a few days.

■ MÉNIÈRE DISEASE

Ménière disease is a term that should be reserved for patients who suffer from presumed endolymphatic hydrops, a pathophysiology that produces the triad of vertigo, unilateral hearing loss, and unilateral tinnitus. That is, the term Meniere disease should be reserved for the characteristic syndrome and should not be used to describe patients with presumed peripheral vestibular disease of uncertain etiology. These symptoms are frequently associated with unilateral ear fullness. Symptoms generally last from several minutes to several hours and occur in episodes; patients are usually asymptomatic between episodes. During episodes, patients may experience nausea, vomiting, and severe gait instability. They would be expected to exhibit a marked horizontal-torsional nystagmus independent of head position, worse with loss of visual fixation. Between episodes, patients may manifest unilateral low-frequency sensorineural hearing loss, which can be discovered using tuning forks and confirmed definitively with audiometry. Balance laboratory testing often reveals a reduced vestibular responsiveness on the same side as the patient's tinnitus and hearing loss. Treatment for Ménière disease consists of a reduction of dietary intake of sodium (<2 g/d) and pharmacotherapy with a combination of hydrochlorothiazide and triamterene.

■ MEDICATION-INDUCED DIZZINESS

Patients with medication-induced dizziness generally do not experience vertigo, and the mechanism by which medications produce dizziness is unknown. Patients may experience nonspecific head sensations and gait instability. Medications that are especially likely to cause dizziness include centrally acting agents such as benzodiazepines, anticonvulsants, antidepressants, and antirejection medications such as tacrolimus. These patients may never experience vertigo and may not experience dizziness or imbalance until their vestibular loss is severe because of the symmetric damage. A special circumstance relates to known ototoxic medications such as aminoglycosides and cis-platinum. These medications may produce bilateral peripheral vestibular loss via hair cell damage and lead to oscillopsia (jumbled vision) and gait ataxia. Patients with medication-induced dizziness may have postural hypotension and gait instability. Establishing a diagnosis of medication-induced dizziness may be challenging in that changing a patient's medication regimen may not be possible. Vestibular laboratory testing of such patients is generally unrevealing aside from nonspecific abnormalities of ocular motor function in patients receiving centrally acting drugs. Patients with ototoxicity will have decreased vestibular responses.

CEREBROVASCULAR DISEASES

Cerebrovascular accidents affecting the brainstem and cerebellum may present with dizziness and vertigo. The most commonly recognized conditions include Wallenberg syndrome, which is caused by ischemia in the territory supplied by the posterior inferior cerebellar artery, by ischemia in the territory supplied by the anterior inferior cerebellar artery, or by cerebellar hemorrhage. Symptoms and signs will of course depend upon the precise location of the central nervous system abnormality. In general, however, patients will present with definitive central nervous system symptoms and signs.

■ HEAD AND NECK TRAUMA

Patients admitted following traumatic injuries of the head and neck may experience dizziness. Diagnostic considerations include BPPV, which may be posttraumatic, and labyrinthine concussion. Some patients following trauma of the head and neck experience combined injury to the peripheral vestibular system and the central vestibular pathways. It is important to consider cervical injuries as exacerbating factors for dizziness because somatosensory neck muscles afferents that normally provide signals related to head position may be damaged. This damage can cause dizziness because of a mismatch between vestibular and somatosensory signals. Hyperextension of the neck as seen in motor vehicle accidents or during neck manipulation may result in injury of the vertebrobasilar system and subsequent dissection producing ischemic symptoms.

■ VESTIBULAR MIGRAINE

Vestibular migraine is an increasingly recognized disorder characterized by vestibular signs and symptoms in association with migrainous symptoms. Whereas patients with vestibular neuritis and benign paroxysmal positional vertigo experience clearly defined vestibular-related symptoms, patients with vestibular migraine often have more nonspecific symptoms, making diagnosis more challenging. Vestibular migraine should be considered especially in patients who have suffered from migraine headache over a span of many years and then begin to experience episodic attacks of vertigo and dizziness exacerbated by head movement. The duration of vestibular migraine episodes is highly variable; attacks can last for seconds, minutes, hours, or days. Examination is usually normal between attacks. During attacks, patients may manifest either peripheral vestibular signs, central vestibular signs, or both. Vestibular migraine remains a diagnosis of exclusion in that there are no pathognomonic signs or symptoms or laboratory test abnormalities to confirm this diagnosis. Approximately 25% of patients with migraine-related dizziness manifest a unilateral reduction of vestibular function when assessed in the vestibular laboratory. Treatment of vestibular migraine is similar to the treatment of migraine headache

TABLE 84-3 Medications Commonly Used to Reduce Dizziness, Vertigo, and Associated Nausea

Drug (Brand Name)	Pharmacologic Class	Dose	Primary Use	Adverse Reactions
Meclizine (Antivert, Bonine)	Anticholinergic Antihistamine	25 mg every 4-6 h orally	Dizziness	Drowsiness
Dimenhydrinate (Dramamine)	Anticholinergic Antihistamine	50 mg every 4-6 h orally	Dizziness	Drowsiness
Cyclizine (Marezine)	Anticholinergic Antihistamine	50 mg every 4-6 h orally or IM	Dizziness	Drowsiness
Diazepam (Valium)	Benzodiazepine	1-2 mg twice daily orally; 2-10 mg (1 dose) given acutely orally, IM or IV	Dizziness	Lethargy
Clonazepam (Klonopin)	Benzodiazepine	0.25-0.5 mg twice daily orally	Dizziness	Lethargy
Prochlorperazine (Compazine)	Phenothiazine	10 mg orally or IM every 6 h or 25 mg rectally every 12 h	Nausea	Extrapyramidal reactions, drowsiness, anticholinergic effects
Promethazine (Phenergan)	Phenothiazine	25 mg every 6-12 h orally or rectally	Nausea	Extrapyramidal reactions, drowsiness, restlessness
Trimethobenzamine (Tigan)	Substituted ethanolamine	250 mg every 6-8 h or 200 mg rectally or IM	Nausea	Extrapyramidal reaction (unusual)
Diphenhydramine (Benadryl)	Antihistamine	25-100 mg every 8 h orally	Nausea	Drowsiness
Ondansetron (Zofran)	Antiemetic	4-8 mg orally every 8 h	Nausea	Lethargy
Hydroxyzine (Vistaril, Atarax)	Piperazine derivative	25-50 mg every 8 h orally	Nausea	Drowsiness

as treatment may be preventative, abortive, or symptomatic. Preventive medication may consist of antidepressants, beta-blocking agents, anticonvulsants, and calcium channel-blocking agents. Symptomatic treatment may include vestibular suppressants. Abortive treatments with triptans may be efficacious.

PSYCHIATRIC DIZZINESS

Psychiatric dizziness represents a diagnosis of exclusion and should be used with caution in that many patients with vestibular system abnormalities develop psychiatric manifestations, notably anxiety, including panic attacks. However, some patients with primary anxiety disorders can present with dizziness, especially in association with panic attacks. Although some of these patients will suffer from an underlying vestibular disorder, many will not. Treatment of psychiatric dizziness consists of identifying the psychiatric disorder and treating it appropriately. For dizziness associated with panic attacks, treatment with antidepressants and benzodiazepines should be considered.

■ NONSPECIFIC DIZZINESS

Unfortunately, for many patients who experience dizziness and vertigo, no definitive diagnosis can be reached. If worrisome disorders are not a consideration, empiric treatment can be safely recommended. When considering treatment options, it is important to understand that the compensation process can be slowed by vestibular suppressant medications, such as meclizine and benzodiazepines.

The table provides a list of medications that should be considered for the symptomatic treatment of dizziness, vertigo, and associated nausea (**Table 84-3**).

Note that vestibular suppressant medications should not be continued indefinitely. Thus, if a patient is provided with a prescription for a vestibular suppressant upon discharge from the hospital, arrangements should be made for follow-up care.

CASE 84-1 (CONTINUED)

The patient was found to be suffering from BPPV based on a positive Dix-Hallpike maneuver. The patient underwent particle repositioning appropriate for posterior semicircular canal BPPV, which lead to complete relief from positional vertigo. The patient continued to experience some gait instability, which was thought to be related to her orthopedic problem primarily with a history of BPPV as a secondary component. Additional physical therapy for balance rehabilitation was ordered.

CONCLUSION

The history is the most critical first step in distinguishing vertigo from other causes of dizziness, paying attention to underlying systemic diseases and risk factors as well as possible medication related dizziness and vertigo. The examiner should check for orthostatic vital signs, perform a cardiovascular and neurologic examination and make an assessment of the patient's overall health. If the patient appears to have vertigo, the clinician should try to pinpoint a precise etiology, consistent with symptom pattern of vertigo the patient is describing. If a central cause of vertigo is suspected, the patient should proceed directly to imaging. If a peripheral cause of vertigo is suspected, a physical examination should confirm the absence of impaired speech, weakness, numbness, incoordination, or other neurologic signs suggesting a central etiology.

SUGGESTED READINGS

Baloh RW. Clinical practice. Vestibular neuritis. *N Engl J Med.* 2003;348(11):1027-1032.

Epley JM. The canalith repositioning procedure: for treatment of benign paroxysmal positional vertigo. *Otolaryngol Head Neck Surg.* 1992;107(3):399-404.

Furman JM, Cass SP. Benign paroxysmal positional vertigo. *N Engl J Med*. 1999;341(21):1590-1596.

Halmagyi GM, Curthoys IS. A clinical sign of canal paresis. *Arch Neurol*. 1988;45(7):737-739.

Shupak A, Issa A, Golz A, Margalit Kaminer, Braverman I. Prednisone treatment for vestibular neuritis. *Otol Neurotol*. 2008;29(3):368-374.

Strupp M, Zingler VC, Arbusow V, et al. Methylprednisolone, valacyclovir, or the combination for vestibular neuritis. *N Engl J Med*. 2004;351(4):354-361.

von Brevern M, Zeise D, Neuhauser H, Clarke AH, Lempert T. Acute migrainous vertigo: clinical and oculographic findings. *Brain*. 2005;128(Pt 2):365-374.

von Brevern M, Radtke A, Lezius F, et al. Epidemiology of benign paroxysmal positional vertigo: a population based study. *J Neurol Neurosurg Psychiatry*. 2007;78(7):710-715.

Wrisley DM, Sparto PJ, Whitney SL, Furman JM. Cervicogenic dizziness: a review of diagnosis and treatment. *J Orthop Sports Phys Ther*. 2000;30(12):755-766.

CHAPTER 85

Dyspnea

Jakob I. McSparron, MD
Tracy J. Doyle, MD
Richard M. Schwartzstein, MD

Key Clinical Questions

1. What are the underlying physiologic mechanisms that result in dyspnea?

2. How can a physician elicit a patient's personal description of shortness of breath in order to gain insight into the underlying diagnosis?

3. What physical exam findings are concerning for impending respiratory failure?

4. What are the key diagnostic studies a physician should order to further elucidate the cause of a patient's dyspnea?

5. How can the disease states associated with dyspnea be organized into a clinical framework?

CASE 85-1

■ INPATIENT ADMISSION

A 63-year-old woman describes shortness of breath on postoperative day 3 after a hip replacement. At 3 AM, the patient starts complaining that she "can't catch her breath" and feels as though she is suffocating. Sitting upright, she appears in acute distress with rapid, shallow breathing and expiratory grunting. Her blood pressure is 210/95 mm Hg with a heart rate of 120 beats per minute and an oxygen saturation of 92% while using supplemental oxygen at 6 L/min by nasal cannula. On physical examination, auscultation of the lungs reveals rales over the lower one-third of the lung fields with dullness at the bases, as well as significant peripheral pitting edema. A chest radiograph (CXR) demonstrates increased interstitial markings and blunting of the costophrenic angles bilaterally. Of note, the patient has been receiving intravenous normal saline at 100 cc/h since the surgery. The clinical picture is most consistent with acute pulmonary edema. Increased interstitial edema activates a variety of receptors that stimulate the respiratory controller and cause air hunger, while pleural effusions cause an increase in work of breathing by affecting the body's ventilatory pump. Note that while hypoxemia with low O_2 saturation can lead to dyspnea via stimulation of chemoreceptors, this patient was experiencing breathing discomfort despite an acceptable saturation with the use of supplemental oxygen.

The history, exam findings and CXR help to confirm the diagnosis of volume overload. Other potential causes of dyspnea in an older patient who has undergone major surgery include myocardial ischemia, aspiration, and pulmonary embolism. In addition to treating congestive heart failure (CHF), it is important to seek out any underlying error that may have caused the condition and effect a system change that can improve quality of care for future patients. In the above case, indiscriminant use of maintenance fluids was the culprit; focused provider education and adjustment of existing order sets may be needed.

PRACTICE POINT

- Indiscriminant use of maintenance fluids is a common and preventable cause of pulmonary edema in inpatients.

INTRODUCTION

Dyspnea, or "shortness of breath," is a common problem affecting up to half of patients in acute care hospitals and one quarter of ambulatory outpatients. This sensation of breathlessness can be associated with anxiety, fear, or depression and, thereby, cause substantial disability. The American Thoracic Society consensus statement on dyspnea describes it as "an uncomfortable sensation of breathing," which encompasses several qualitatively distinct sensations that reflect the subjective nature of the experience as well as the psychological, social, and environmental factors that contribute to the symptoms. A solid understanding of these distinct sensations and the pathophysiologic mechanisms underlying them can help physicians better understand, diagnose, and treat their patients.

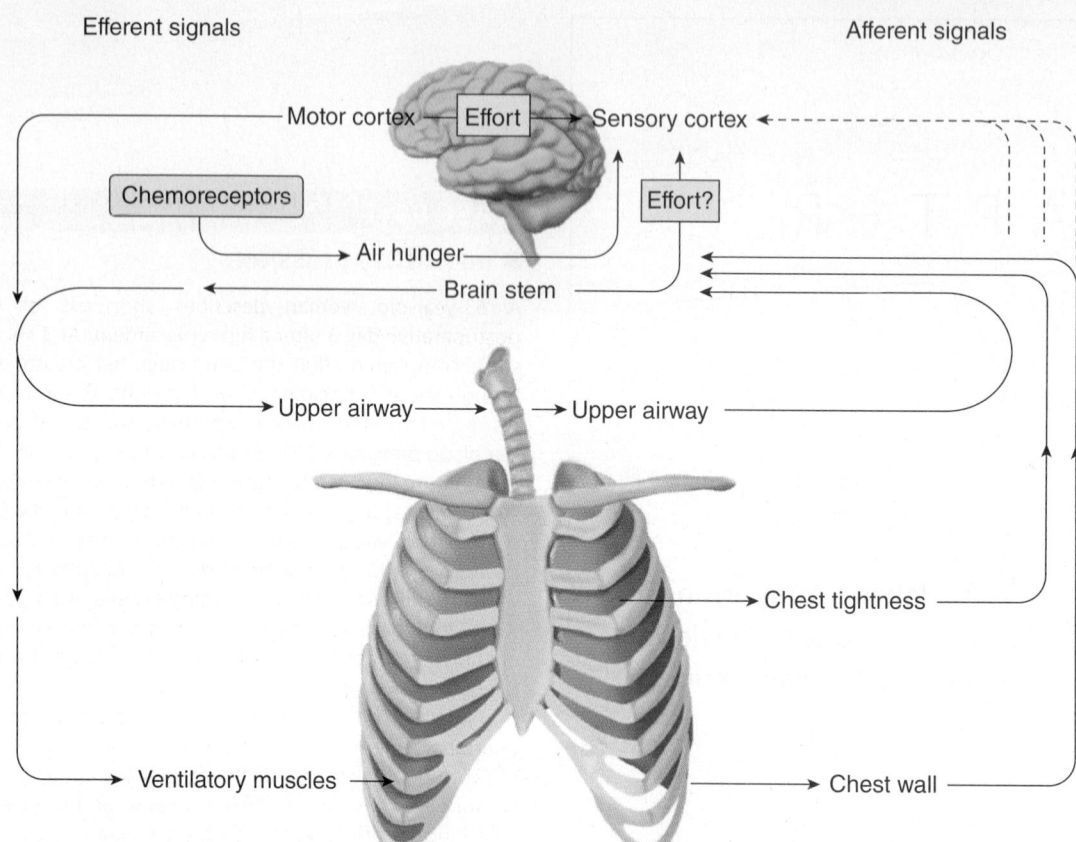

Efferent signals   Afferent signals

Motor cortex — Effort → Sensory cortex

Chemoreceptors   Effort?

→ Air hunger

Brain stem

→ Upper airway → → Upper airway

→ Chest tightness

→ Ventilatory muscles → → Chest wall

Figure 85-1 *The sense of respiratory effort is believed to arise from a signal transmitted from the motor cortex to the sensory cortex coincidently with the outgoing motor command to the ventilatory muscles. The arrow from the brain stem to the sensory cortex indicates that the motor output of the brain stem may also contribute to the sense of effort. The sense of air hunger is believed to arise, in part, from increased respiratory activity within the brain stem, and the sensation of chest tightness probably results from stimulation of vagal irritant receptors. Although afferent information from airway, lung, and chest-wall receptors most likely passes through the brain stem before reaching the sensory cortex, the dashed lines indicate uncertainty about whether some afferents bypass the brain stem and project directly to the sensory cortex. (Reproduced from Manning HL, Schwartzstein RM. Pathophysiology of dyspnea. N Engl J Med. 1995;333:1547-1533.)*

MECHANISMS OF DYSPNEA

Similar to the feelings of thirst or hunger, the complex sensation of dyspnea is a visceral experience that integrates information from a number of sensory receptors and, in the case of dyspnea, is the consequence of a variety of pathophysiologic mechanisms. Dyspnea begins with a physiological impairment or stimulus that activates a range of sensory receptors that transmit incoming or afferent information to the cerebral cortex and to respiratory centers in the brainstem. Central chemoreceptors located in the medulla respond to alterations in PCO_2 and pH, and peripheral chemoreceptors in the aortic arch and carotid bodies detect changes in the partial pressure of oxygen in the blood as well as alterations in pH and PCO_2. Mechanoreceptors in the airways, lungs, and chest wall detect alterations in the pressure, flow, and volume of the respiratory system, while stretch receptors in the pulmonary vasculature and right heart respond to change in pressure and intravascular volume. Activation of irritant receptors in the lungs may also stimulate breathing. Together, all of the elements of the system that alter rate and depth of breathing can be considered the "respiratory controller"—akin to a thermostat—whose function is to set the rate and depth of each breath. Additionally, the brain sends efferent or outgoing neural messages to the muscles of ventilation, activating the "ventilatory pump." Most often, a patient's dyspnea can be attributed to abnormalities in one or both of these components of the respiratory system, and any additional mismatch between this motor feed-forward message and sensory feedback (ie, unsatiated air-hunger) increases the intensity of dyspnea (**Figure 85-1**).

■ VENTILATORY PUMP

Patients with disorders that affect the ventilatory pump experience an increased sense of "effort to breathe" or "work of breathing." The ventilatory pump consists of peripheral nerves, muscles of ventilation, supporting skeleton, pleura, and airways—everything needed to move air from outside the body to the alveoli; any disorder that affects these components can lead to an increased sense of the work of breathing (see below section: Clinical Framework of Cardiopulmonary disease). Obstructive lung disease leads to dyspnea due to hyperinflation and increased airways resistance. Myopathies can produce muscular weakness, and kyphoscoliosis can lead to a stiff chest wall. Both of these conditions contribute to an increased sense of effort to breathe. Lastly, pleural effusions increase the work of breathing by expanding the chest wall and shortening inspiratory muscles, and may stimulate pulmonary receptors via associated atelectasis of regions of lung compressed by the fluid.

■ RESPIRATORY CONTROLLER

Patients with disorders that stimulate the respiratory controller experience the sensation of "air hunger." Activation of receptors throughout the respiratory system—for example, irritant and stretch receptors in the airways and lung parenchyma, flow receptors in the central airways, and chemoreceptors in the carotid bodies and medulla—lead to stimulation of the control centers in the brainstem. We observe this as an increase in ventilatory drive (increased rate and depth of breathing, use of accessory muscles of ventilation, etc), and patients perceive a sense of an increased urge to breathe or air

TABLE 85-1 Afferent Inputs Involved in Respiratory Control

Receptors	Disease States Causing Activation	Resulting Effect/Sensation
Chemoreceptors	Hypoxemia, acute hypercapnea, acidemia	Increase in ventilation; air hunger
J-receptors	Interstitial edema	Increase in ventilation; air hunger
C fibers	Inflammation	Increase in ventilation; air hunger
Pulmonary vascular receptors	Pulmonary embolism	Increase in ventilation; air hunger
Metaboreceptors	Exercise; increased metabolic rate	Increase in ventilation; air hunger
Mechanoreceptors lung	Bronchospasm	Increase in airway resistance and ventilation, hyperinflation; chest tightness
Mechanoreceptors muscles	COPD, asthma, chest wall abnormalities	Increase in airway resistance, hyperinflation; sensation of increased work of breathing, inability to get a deep breath

hunger. Interstitial edema activates J-receptors; inflammation activates C fibers; and acute changes in pulmonary artery pressure (eg, pulmonary emboli) activate C fibers in pulmonary vessels and pressure receptors in the pulmonary vasculature or right atrium. Changes in the metabolic rate during exercise affect metaboreceptors located in the skeletal muscle, which also contribute to uncomfortable breathing. Nondisease states, such as the hypoxemia associated with high altitude, pregnancy's high progesterone state, and drugs such as aspirin, can also stimulate the respiratory controller and cause dyspnea. Furthermore, some receptors provide afferent input that leads to other sensations that can be interpreted as dyspnea. For example, bronchospasm stimulates mechanoreceptors in the lungs, which we believe leads to a sensation of chest tightness, sensed through vagal afferents, and may act as another stimulus for dyspnea (**Table 85-1**).

Some disorders, such as pneumonia, pulmonary edema, aspiration, pulmonary embolism, asthma, and COPD, not only contribute to dyspnea by the mechanisms outlined above, but also result in abnormalities in gas exchange. The hypoxemia, acute hypercapnea, and subsequent acidemia associated with these conditions activate chemoreceptors in the carotid bodies and medulla and cause an increase in ventilation to compensate for the ventilation/perfusion abnormalities, thereby contributing to the sensation of dyspnea.

CASE 85-2

■ EMERGENCY ROOM

Recently diagnosed with asthma based on complaints of intermittent dyspnea and occasional wheezing, a 54-year-old man presents to the Emergency Department with progressive shortness of breath. He states that breathing is "a lot of work," he feels an increased urge to breathe, and sometimes he cannot get a full breath. His symptoms are worse with exertion. He denies problems when he goes out in cold air, but has a chronic cough productive of small amounts of gray sputum. He has a 30 pack-year history of cigarette smoking. His oxygen saturation is 88% while breathing ambient air. On physical exam, auscultation of the lungs reveals distant breath sounds and intermittent expiratory wheezing. A CXR demonstrates hyperinflation with no infiltrates or effusions; heart size is normal.

Physiologically, the patient is experiencing activation of his airway receptors and chemoreceptors, which stimulate the respiratory controller and increase his urge to breathe. Chronic hypoxemia and acute hypercapnia, may also be contributing to his sensation of dyspnea. Hyperinflation, which affects the efficiency of the ventilatory pump and leads to reduced inspiratory capacity,

contributes to the sensation of an unsatisfying breath (with increasing end-expiratory lung volume, the patient's inspiratory capacity may literally be constrained by the limits of his lungs and chest wall to expand, ie, total lung capacity). Lastly, this patient may have dynamic airway compression that is sensed through vagal afferents as another stimulus for dyspnea. These physiologic mechanisms, coupled with the physical exam and radiographic findings, are consistent with a diagnosis of COPD exacerbation. Other potential etiologies of dyspnea and wheezing in an obese smoker include CHF/pulmonary edema, pulmonary embolism, and myocardial ischemia; acute onset of asthma in a 50-year-old patient would be unusual without an antecedent respiratory infection. This case highlights the risk of anchoring bias, or the tendency to place too much importance on one piece of information, for example, a prior diagnosis of asthma. It is important to know what history is available before you see the patient, but you must then be disciplined to evaluate the patient with fresh eyes.

PRACTICE POINT

- Adult onset asthma is relatively unusual and generally does not result in resting hypoxemia unless the condition is severe.

APPROACH TO THE PATIENT WITH DYSPNEA

Dyspnea as a symptom must be differentiated from the physical signs associated with "respiratory distress," such as tachypnea, use of accessory muscles of respiration, or intercostal retractions. In describing a patient's dyspnea, one should be careful to elicit the patient's own qualitative descriptors of their dyspnea, rather than use general terms that reflect the physical signs observed, such as "labored breathing." Common to these individual descriptors is the concept of "discomfort in the act of breathing," but it is the subtle differences in a patient's descriptors that may help elucidate the underlying physiological mechanisms.

■ QUALITATIVE DESCRIPTORS OF DYSPNEA

The descriptor, "shortness of breath," reflects different sensations in patients with differing etiologies and mechanisms of their discomfort. The varied and overlapping vocabulary chosen by patients to describe their dyspnea relate to the different physiologic factors that produce each particular form of dyspnea (**Table 85-2**).

TABLE 85-2 Association of Qualitative Descriptors and Pathophysiologic Mechanism of Shortness of Breath

Qualitative Descriptor	Pathophysiologic Mechanism (Disease States)
Chest tightness or constriction	Bronchoconstriction (asthma), interstitial edema (myocardial infarction)
Increased work of breathing, effort to breathe	Airway obstruction (COPD, moderate to severe asthma), neuromuscular disease (myopathy), chest wall disease (kyphoscoliosis); dynamic hyperinflation
Air hunger, need to breathe, urge to breathe	Increased drive to breathe (CHF, PE), moderate to severe airway obstruction (COPD/asthma)
Cannot get a deep breath, unsatisfying breath	Hyperinflation (asthma, COPD), restricted tidal volume (pulmonary fibrosis, chest wall disorders), anxiety
Heavy breathing, rapid breathing, breathing more	Deconditioning

Data from Manning HL, Schwartzstein RM; Simon PM, et al; and Elliott MW, et al.

The sensitivity and specificity of these characteristic phrases, and of the use of a multidimensional dyspnea profile (MDP) to measure separate dimensions of dyspnea (eg, distinguishing the sensory quality from emotional content) are areas of active investigation. It may be helpful for the physician to think of dyspnea as an all-encompassing descriptor, such as pain. Pain arises from numerous mechanisms and is experienced differently depending on the origin and the patient's perception. In taking a medical history, we typically elicit common descriptive qualities of pain and link them to the underlying pathology, such as the "burning" pain from acid reflux or the "crushing" pain of a myocardial infarction. One reason our interviewing techniques for patients with dyspnea have not evolved along the same lines is the fact that healthy physicians rarely experience dyspnea other than with exercise, whereas many physicians (and their patients) have had varying types of pain throughout their lives; absent that shared experience, doctors are less likely to prompt patients about the quality of their breathing sensations.

■ HISTORY

A good place to start is asking the patient to describe the sensation of dyspnea in his or her own words. If the patient finds this difficult, suggest phrases such as chest tightness, increased effort to breathe, urge to breathe, cannot get a deep breath, or rapid breathing; or use a dyspnea questionnaire, which may help the patient describe the sensation he/she is experiencing (**Table 85-3**).

These phrases may give the physician clues to the underlying diagnosis as certain qualitative descriptors are associated with specific pathophysiologic mechanisms of dyspnea. Additionally, one must not overlook characteristic *forms of dyspnea*, such as the *orthopnea* or *paroxysmal nocturnal dyspnea* associated with CHF, or *platypnea* associated with left atrial myxoma and hepatopulmonary syndrome.

Once the quality of dyspnea has been explored, it is important to define the timing of and precipitating factors for the dyspnea. When did the dyspnea start? Was the onset sudden or gradual? Is it episodic or continuous? Does the dyspnea occur only with exertion, or at rest? Dyspnea on exertion can be a manifestation of underlying lung disease that becomes evident with the increased metabolic demands of activity, or it may reflect cardiovascular deconditioning. For example, patients with COPD or interstitial lung disease may experience an acute physiologic change while exerting themselves, such as hyperinflation, bronchospasm, or hypoxemia, or may be deconditioned due to the sedentary lifestyle that often accompanies chronic illness.

Precipitating factors associated with breathing discomfort are also important clues. For example, dyspnea that occurs following exposure to fumes or cigarette smoke may indicate a bronchospastic response typical of asthma or COPD. Worsening of symptoms when the patient is at home or at work followed by resolution of symptoms while on vacation suggests hypersensitivity pneumonitis, often due to an unrecognized exposure. Dyspnea that primarily occurs when lying down or bending over can be suggestive of diaphragm paralysis, usually idiopathic or as a result of phrenic nerve injury, or moderate to severe abdominal obesity.

Lastly, the patient needs to be questioned regarding other factors associated with his or her respiratory symptoms. For example, fevers, upper respiratory symptoms, and pleuritic chest pain indicate a possible pulmonary infection. Risk factors for venous thromboembolism (VTE), antecedent calf pain, and pleuritic chest pain may suggest pulmonary embolism. Chest pressure, nausea, and diaphoresis may indicate an acute coronary syndrome. Fatigue and muscle weakness could be symptoms of myasthenia gravis or amyotrophic lateral sclerosis. Rashes and joint symptoms may indicate a collagen-vascular disease and associated interstitial lung disease (ILD). It is important to remember that as the history is elicited, the physician must be aware of any concerning features that may indicate a life-threatening diagnosis requiring emergent intervention, such as

TABLE 85-3 Breathlessness Descriptor Questionnaire

Breathlessness Descriptor Statements

I feel that I am smothering.
I feel that I am suffocating.
I cannot get enough air.
I feel out of breath.
I feel hunger for air.
My breathing requires work.
My breathing requires effort.
My chest is constricted.
My chest feels tight.
My breathing is heavy.
I feel that my breathing is rapid.
I feel that I am breathing more.
My breathing is shallow.
My breath does not go out all the way.
My breath does not go in all the way.

Patients select statements that describe qualities of their breathlessness from the 15-item questionnaire above.
Data from Mahler DA, et al.

PRACTICE POINT

- Chronic dyspnea at rest is unusual in patients with cardiopulmonary disease due to the presence of physiological reserve, that is, at rest, patients are usually not operating at the limits of cardiopulmonary performance.

pulmonary embolism, tension pneumothorax, pericardial tamponade, acute myocardial ischemia, anaphylaxis, upper airway obstruction, or impending respiratory failure from pulmonary edema, pneumonia, or obstructive lung disease.

PHYSICAL EXAM

The physical exam starts as soon as you enter the patient's room. A quick assessment of the patient's overall respiratory status and a review of the vital signs may alert the clinician to impending respiratory failure. Concerning signs include use of accessory muscles of respiration, supraclavicular retractions, sitting in a tripod position (leaning forward with hands braced on the knees), pursed lip breathing, cyanosis, tachypnea, the inability to speak in full sentences without stopping to take a breath, audible stridor, or general distress with increased effort to breathe. An elevated heart rate, elevated blood pressure, rapid respiratory rate, and an exaggerated pulsus paradoxus (a fall in the systolic blood pressure greater than 10 mm Hg with inspiration) are all concerning findings. While pulsus paradoxus is seen in pericardial disease, this finding may also be present in obstructive lung disease due to large changes in intrathoracic pressure needed to overcome the forces associated with increased airways resistance and hyperinflation, which lead to changes in ventricular filling. In severe cases of pulsus paradoxus, a clinician may be able to manually palpate a diminished pulse during the inspiratory cycle, which allows a rapid assessment of the severity of the physiological insult. The oxygen saturation is another useful vital sign since the recognition of hypoxemia can be critical to a patient's evaluation (see Chapter 95 [Hypoxia]). However, normal oxygen saturation does not exclude a gas exchange problem. Hyperventilation may mask a large arterial-alveolar gradient, which defines the presence of a problem with the gas exchanger; oximetry merely tells you about oxygen saturation.

Physical exam findings can help elucidate the underlying physiologic mechanism of the patient's dyspnea. Increased work of breathing, as evidenced by the use of accessory muscles of respiration, supraclavicular retractions, and tripod positioning, is indicative of increased airway resistance, decreased compliance of the lungs and chest wall, or other disorders of the ventilatory pump. Pursed lip breathing helps reduce hyperinflation by slowing the respiratory rate and is commonly seen in patients with COPD. Rounding of the abdomen during expiration with an associated end-expiratory grunt can be a fairly specific sign of congestive heart failure (**Figure 85-2**). Inability of the patient to speak in full sentences without taking a breath indicates stimulation of the respiratory controller or reduced vital capacity. The clinician should also look for paradoxical movement of the

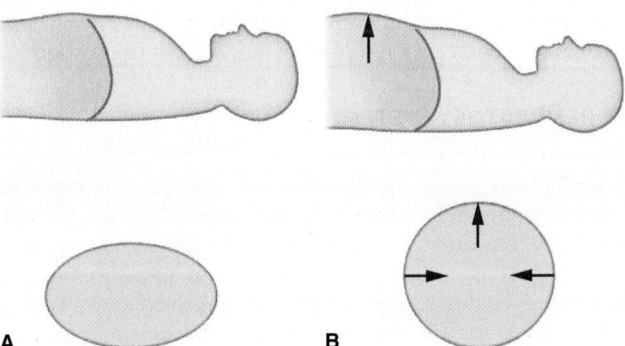

Figure 85-2 *Rounding of the abdominal cross-section during expiration.* (**A**) *Normal shape of the abdomen during expiration.* (**B**) *Rounding of the abdomen during expiration. This respiratory pattern is frequently observed in patients with congestive heart failure as a cause of dyspnea.*

abdomen with breathing. If the abdomen appears to be "sucked in" during inspiration, this suggests diaphragmatic weakness due to paralysis or fatigue. Conversely, in patients with high-thoracic or low-cervical spinal cord injuries, there may be retraction of the thoracic wall with inspiration resulting from paralyzed intercostal muscles.

If the patient appears clinically stable, then the physician should proceed with a full physical exam, focusing on the evaluation of the chest (respiratory and cardiovascular status) and extremities. Examination of the chest should include the elements of inspection (symmetry, kyphoscoliosis), auscultation (crackles/rales, wheezes, rhonchi, diminished breath sounds, prolonged expiratory phase), and percussion (dullness, hyperresonance). A cardiac examination should look for elevated jugular venous pressure, a prominent S_2, S_3/S_4 gallop, or a murmur suggesting cardiovascular dyspnea. A right ventricular heave, an accentuated P_2, a new soft systolic murmur of tricuspid regurgitation, or a pulsatile liver may indicate pulmonary hypertension. The extremities should be examined for clubbing (a possible sign of a thoracic tumor, congenital hypoxemia, or inflammatory or fibrotic lung disease) or cyanosis indicating severe hypoxemia, edema suggesting congestive heart failure or VTE, or rashes and/or joint deformities, which may indicate rheumatologic disease and associated ILD. If the patient is complaining of exertional dyspnea, you should consider walking with the patient while observing her performance and measuring her ambulatory oxygen saturation; both can provide very useful information. Normal oxygen saturation at rest with evidence of significant desaturation while walking is indicative of processes that destroy lung tissue (COPD, pulmonary fibrosis) or impair diffusion of oxygen from the alveolus into the pulmonary capillaries (eg, pulmonary vascular diseases, acute pulmonary edema, or interstitial pneumonia).

DIAGNOSTIC STUDIES

Further evaluation of the patient with unexplained dyspnea should begin with a CXR and an electrocardiogram (to rule out myocardial ischemia). Interpretation of the CXR should start with an evaluation of lung volumes. Decreased lung volumes can suggest pulmonary processes such as interstitial edema, fibrosis or atelectasis, or impaired chest wall or diaphragmatic motion, possibly from neuromuscular disease. Do not assume that low lung volumes are due to a "poor inspiration" by the patient! Unilateral elevation of the hemidiaphragm can point to diaphragmatic paralysis. Hyperinflation indicates obstructive lung disease.

Next, one can evaluate the pulmonary parenchyma for evidence of emphysematous changes, bullae, or interstitial changes. Pleural effusions can be bilateral (suggestive of CHF) or unilateral (concerning for carcinoma, liver failure, PE, or other such processes). An effusion associated with an infiltrate raises the concern for a parapneumonic process that will need urgent sampling and possible chest tube placement (see Chapter 236 [Pleural Diseases]). An enlarged cardiac silhouette and prominent pulmonary vasculature in the upper zones can point to mild CHF, while enlarged central pulmonary arteries suggest pulmonary arterial hypertension. When considering chest radiographic findings that support the diagnosis of a systemic disease, consultation with the radiologist is usually helpful.

An arterial blood gas (ABG) can be particularly useful in assessing the degree of hypoxemia or hypercarbia, as well as impending respiratory failure and acidemia. If possible, always perform an arterial blood gas with the patient breathing room air, that is, no supplemental oxygen, to enable you to assess the alveolar to arterial oxygen gradient (A-aDO$_2$). A gas exchange problem in the setting of either hyperventilation or hypoventilation is defined as an abnormal A-aDO$_2$. If the patient is receiving supplemental oxygen and it is removed, make sure the patient has been off oxygen long enough for the alveolar gas to reflect atmospheric gas (5-10 minutes in a healthy patient and up to 15-20 minutes in a patient with COPD) before the ABG is performed. Based on the CXR and suggestive elements of the history and physical, further testing modalities may include additional blood tests (CBC to assess for anemia, serum electrolytes to assess the acid-base status of the patient), a computed tomography angiogram (CTA), and/or transthoracic echocardiogram (TTE). Additional blood tests that may be useful include B-type natriuretic peptide (BNP or NT pro-BNP), to evaluate for volume overload (if not obvious on physical examination), and methemoglobin or carboxyhemoglobin levels if the patient has been on particular medications or has a history that suggests exposure to fumes from a fire or furnace. A D-dimer to assess for possible pulmonary embolus has low utility for acutely ill hospitalized patients (see Chapter 253). A CTA can diagnose (or exclude) acute pulmonary emboli while providing a more detailed look at the interstitium of the lung. A TTE is useful in patients with suspected cardiovascular dyspnea, as it can provide evidence of systolic or diastolic dysfunction, as well as occult valvular disease. The diagnostic accuracy of TTE for pulmonary hypertension is unfortunately not as reliable as many believe, but the presence of right-heart dysfunction with dilatation strongly suggests pulmonary hypertension. A right heart catheterization would be the diagnostic modality of choice to confirm the diagnosis of pulmonary hypertension.

PRACTICE POINT

- When possible, perform an arterial blood gas with the patient off supplemental oxygen in order to accurately determine the alveolar to arterial oxygen gradient.

In patients with persistent unexplained dyspnea, more specialized pulmonary testing may need to be performed, including pulmonary function testing (PFT), a sniff test, a methacholine challenge, and/or exhaled nitric oxide level. Standard PFTs consist of three parts: (a) spirometry, with pre- and postbronchodilator values to evaluate for obstructive lung disease and reactive airways disease, (b) lung volumes to assess for restrictive lung disease and hyperinflation, and (c) diffusing capacity to assess for interstitial lung disease, emphysema, or pulmonary vascular disease. In patients with respiratory muscle weakness who do not have an acute need for intubation, serial measurements of respiratory muscle capacity may assist with determining the need for mechanical ventilation. This can be accomplished at the bedside by measuring the negative inspiratory force (NIF) or the forced vital capacity (FVC), if a portable spirometer is available (small electronic hand-held devices are acceptable). If performed methodically, a low NIF may be more specific to muscle weakness, but the NIF does not add additional information if a FVC is available. While NIF is widely available, this test is less reproducible than FVC because it is difficult to control the lung volume from which the NIF maneuver is performed; starting at lower lung volumes yields a greater NIF. In addition, the FVC measurement provides information about both the inspiratory and expiratory muscles, as opposed to the NIF which only takes into account the inspiratory muscles. A NIF less than one-third of normal is highly concerning for impending respiratory failure. A forced vital capacity (FVC) less than 50% of predicted or a vital capacity (VC) less than one liter suggest impending respiratory failure and may indicate the need for mechanical ventilation; the patient should be observed in an intensive care setting if either of these findings are present.

PRACTICE POINT

- A NIF <1/3 of normal or forced vital capacity (FVC) less than 50% of predicted or a vital capacity (VC) less than 1 L suggest impending respiratory failure and may indicate the need for mechanical ventilation.

A 6-minute walk test is performed with continuous oxygen saturation monitoring and is useful to get a quick evaluation of a patient's exercise capacity and possible gas exchange problems. Maximal inspiratory and expiratory pressures are useful in assessing neuromuscular or diaphragmatic weakness. If unilateral hemidiaphragm paralysis is suspected, a fluoroscopic sniff test may confirm the suspicion by demonstrating paradoxical elevation of the paralyzed diaphragm with inspiration, although this test is increasingly being replaced by ultrasound evaluation of diaphragm movement during normal breathing. If a diagnosis of asthma is suspected, PFT laboratories can also perform bronchoprovocation testing with methacholine or measure exhaled nitric oxide levels, elevation of which is indicative of airway inflammation.

When the diagnosis is still unclear, a cardiopulmonary exercise test (CPET) can be helpful, especially in patients with an exertional component to their dyspnea or concurrent pulmonary and cardiovascular disease. This test includes a graded exercise protocol during which frequent measurements of respiratory and cardiovascular system mechanics and gas exchange are made. Arterial and right heart catheters may be included in the protocol when there are particular concerns about pulmonary vascular or cardiac disease. The resulting data can help determine what is physiologically limiting the patient's ability to exercise by differentiating between deconditioning, cardiovascular diseases (myocardial ischemia, heart failure, exercise-induced pulmonary arterial hypertension), and underlying lung disease.

PRACTICE POINT

- Many specialized tests to evaluate dyspnea can be deferred to the outpatient setting, and may yield better results when the patient is at her/his baseline clinical status.

CLINICAL FRAMEWORK OF CARDIOPULMONARY DISEASES

A reasonable clinical framework for approaching the common disease states associated with dyspnea is to divide them into those diseases associated with disorders of the respiratory system or those associated with problems of the cardiovascular system (**Figure 85-3**). Key elements of the history and physical exam, coupled with the diagnostic studies discussed above, can help determine into which broad pathophysiologic category a patient's dyspnea can be classified.

■ RESPIRATORY SYSTEM

As discussed above, respiratory system dyspnea can be divided into disorders of the ventilatory pump, respiratory controller, or gas exchanger. Acute bronchitis and pneumonia are common causes of respiratory system dyspnea. Pathophysiologically, acute bronchitis increases airway resistance due to sputum production and airway epithelial inflammation, and pneumonia may increase airway resistance due to airway edema. Pneumonia may also lead to decreased compliance of the respiratory system due to regions of lung consolidation. Both processes may impair gas exchange by disturbing ventilation-perfusion relationships, while some pneumonias are characterized by shunt physiology due to filling/collapse of

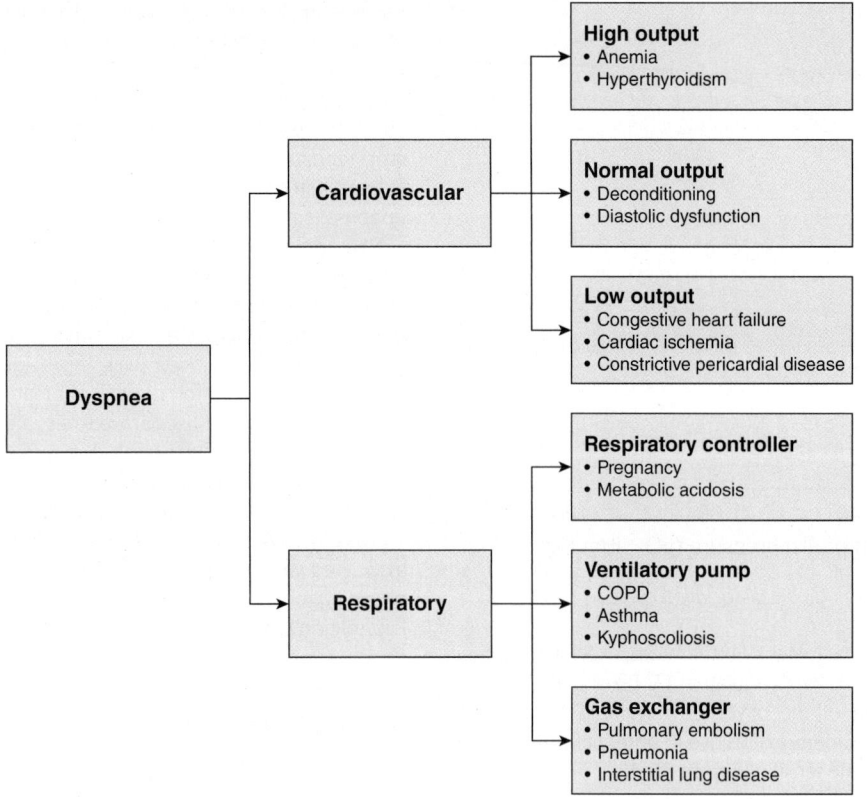

Figure 85-3 *Common causes of dyspnea due to disorders of the cardiovascular and respiratory systems.* (Adapted from Schwartzstein RM, Feller-Kopman D. Approach to the patient with dyspnea. In: Goldman L, Braunwald E eds. *Primary Cardiology.* 2nd ed. Philadelphia, PA: Saunders; 2003.)

alveoli with inflammatory material. Patients with acute bronchitis typically present with cough and sputum production and may have rhonchi on exam. In contrast, patients with pneumonia additionally will note fever, may complain of pleuritic chest pain, and have rales on exam. An infiltrate on CXR often confirms the diagnosis of pneumonia. Acute bronchitis is usually not treated with antibiotics unless the patient has preexisting lung disease such as COPD or bronchiectasis. The mainstays of treatment of pneumonia are antibiotics and supplemental oxygen. Aspiration pneumonitis has a very similar physiologic mechanism and clinical presentation to pneumonia, and should be suspected in patients who were obtunded or have swallowing difficulties due to a stroke or other neuromuscular problems. Although aspiration pneumonitis due to gastric acid does not need to be treated with antibiotics, most clinicians add antimicrobial coverage, particularly if there is an elevation in the patient's temperature or white blood cell count, as there may be an infectious component due to aspiration of oral or GI flora.

PRACTICE POINT

- It is important to protect patients against aspiration by elevating the head of the bed or by obtaining a formal swallowing evaluation if there is concern about the ability of the patient to protect her airway during oral intake.

Obstructive airway diseases, including asthma and COPD, are another common cause of dyspnea. These diseases affect the respiratory controller, ventilatory pump, and gas exchanger. Bronchoconstriction increases airway resistance, thereby overworking muscles of inspiration. The patient often develops hyperinflation (breathing at higher lung volumes than normal), which shortens the inspiratory

muscles (including the diaphragm) and makes them less effective. This is often accompanied by auto-PEEP (the persistence of positive pressure at the end of exhalation due to the prolonged exhalation time), which further increases the mechanical load on the inspiratory muscles, thereby augmenting the work of breathing. Severe airway obstruction can lead to hypoxemia and hypercarbia, which may have an additive effect on the respiratory controller. Patients with acute bronchoconstriction characteristically have hypocapnia (ie, hyperventilation) even in the absence of frank hypoxemia. This is evidence of increased respiratory drive that is believed to result from stimulation of airway receptors secondary to bronchospasm and airway inflammation. Patients with asthma often present with complaints of "chest tightness," a sensation attributed to stimulation of airway receptors, and a sensation of an "inability to take a deep breath" and "air hunger," which likely arises from the increased drive to breathe and limited inspiratory capacity resulting from hyperinflation.

On exam, these patients are found to be hyperinflated (low diaphragm on percussion, positive Hoover's sign [inward motion of the lower lateral rib cage on inspiration indicative of a "flat" diaphragm], increased antero-posterior diameter of the chest) with a prolonged expiratory phase and polyphonic expiratory wheezing on auscultation. CXR often confirms hyperinflation with flattened diaphragms and an increased antero-posterior chest diameter. Treatment for both asthma and COPD includes bronchodilators and steroids; anticholinergic inhalers may be more effective in COPD than in asthma. A COPD exacerbation can further be treated with antibiotics if there has been a change in the quality or color of their sputum or evidence of pneumonia; antibiotics are not indicated in most acute asthma attacks. Judicious use of oxygen in patients with COPD is important because high concentrations of supplemental oxygen may worsen hypercarbia (largely due to worsening

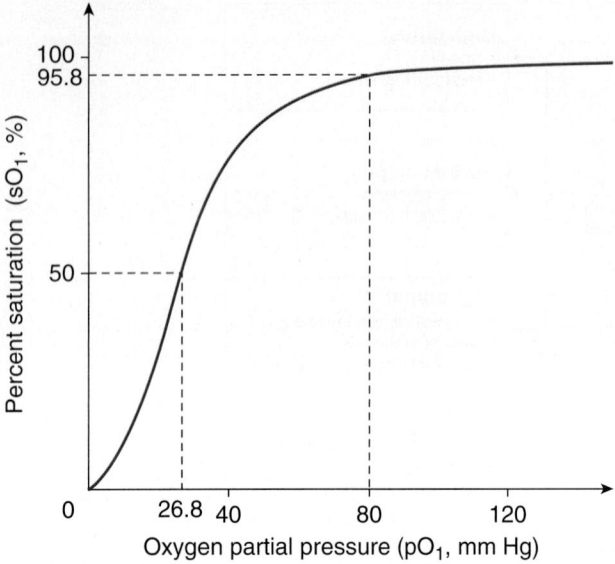

Figure 85-4 *Oxygen-hemoglobin dissociation curve.*

of ventilation/perfusion mismatch). Furthermore, excessive supplemental oxygen may mask hypoventilation by placing the patient far out on the plateau of the oxygen-hemoglobin dissociation curve, rendering pulse oximetry insensitive to potentially dangerous increases in carbon dioxide tension (**Figure 85-4**).

PRACTICE POINT

- In most clinical situations, patients with COPD who need supplemental oxygen should have a target oxygen saturation of 88% to 92%.

Stridor (wheezing on inspiration, typically localized to the neck), often due to anaphylaxis or foreign body obstruction, is a special form of upper airway obstruction that causes acute respiratory distress. In adults, the presence of stridor indicates significant airways narrowing with a diameter often less than 5mm. However, the absence of stridor does not rule out significant airway compromise. Acute airway obstruction is considered a medical emergency that may require emergent intubation or a surgical airway. Occasionally the patient can be temporized with administration of inhaled heliox (a mixture of helium and oxygen). Heliox has a lower density than nitrogen and oxygen, which lessens the work of breathing by reducing turbulent flow.

Pleural effusions can cause dyspnea by increasing the work of breathing due to alterations in the mechanics of the ventilatory pump and by activating pulmonary receptors if there is associated atelectasis. If the pleural effusions are associated with other conditions, such as pneumonia or pulmonary edema, the physiologic mechanisms of those disease states will also play a role in the sensation of dyspnea. Patients with pleural effusions usually present primarily with complaints of pleuritic chest pain or dyspnea as well as symptoms that relate to the underlying cause of the effusion, that is, cough and fever from pneumonia, abdominal pain and distension from ascites in liver disease, anuria in renal disease, or cachexia from metastatic malignancy. A CXR may demonstrate blunting of the costophrenic angle and associated atelectasis. The first step in the evaluation of a patient with a pleural effusion of unknown etiology is to sample the fluid and determine whether it is exudative or transudative. Pleural fluid should be analyzed for lactate dehydrogenase, protein, pH, glucose, cholesterol, microbiologic studies, and cytology. Any patient with an infiltrate and an effusion concerning for a

parapneumonic effusion needs a diagnostic thoracentesis urgently to assess for evidence of a complicated parapneumonic effusion or an empyema, which would require early surgical drainage or chest tube placement. For simple effusions, treating the underlying condition usually leads to resolution of the effusion, but if it is recurrent, repeated thoracenteses, chest tube placement, pleurodesis, video-assisted thoracoscopy (VATs), and decortication are available options. See also Chapter 236 [Pleural Diseases].

Neuromuscular diseases, such as myopathies, amyotrophic lateral sclerosis, or myasthenia gravis, can also lead to dyspnea. In these patients, the mechanics of the respiratory system are normal but the ventilatory muscles are weakened, so a greater neural drive is needed to move the chest wall. This heightened efferent output is sensed as increased effort or work of breathing. On exam, other findings consistent with muscular weakness are often seen. Patients with advanced neuromuscular disease may require noninvasive ventilation or chronic tracheostomies to facilitate intermittent invasive ventilation to assist the weakened respiratory muscles. Chest wall diseases, such as kyphoscoliosis, result in a stiffened chest wall and are also associated with an increased effort to breathe. As described above, obtaining measurements of NIF or vital capacity can provide valuable information regarding the development of respiratory failure.

■ CARDIOVASCULAR SYSTEM

Cardiovascular dyspnea can be subdivided into high cardiac output (anemia or shunt), normal cardiac output (diastolic dysfunction, myocardial ischemia, constrictive pericarditis, or deconditioning), or low cardiac output (congestive heart failure or pericardial effusions). Physiologically, high cardiac output dyspnea may result from reduced oxygen delivery to the tissues, as seen with severe anemia, or from the increased intracardiac pressures required to achieve the elevated cardiac output, as might occur with a large arteriovenous shunt. The exact mechanism by which anemia causes dyspnea, however, is unclear. These patients usually complain of dyspnea on exertion when an increased cardiac output is required to meet the demand of increased metabolic activity; remember, anemia does not cause hypoxemia although it does lead to reduced oxygen content of the blood. Patients with diastolic dysfunction have normal cardiac output at rest, but their stiffened left ventricle is unable to dilate with exercise to accommodate greater stroke volume without significant increases in left ventricular end diastolic pressure (LVEDP), which leads to interstitial edema and stimulation of pulmonary receptors as well as stiffening of the lung and increased work of breathing.

Patients with diastolic dysfunction present with dyspnea on exertion and signs or symptoms of pulmonary edema. They may also have a history and physical exam findings suggestive of the cause of their diastolic dysfunction, such as a history of hypertension, the systolic ejection murmur of aortic stenosis, or an episode of syncope, which may be associated with hypertrophic cardiomyopathy. These patients require a TTE to aid diagnosis. However, the presence of impaired diastolic filling or left ventricular hypertrophy alone may not be diagnostic since these findings are common among asymptomatic patients. Another cause of normal cardiac output dyspnea is myocardial ischemia. In any patient with risk factors for coronary artery disease, dyspnea should be considered as a potential anginal equivalent. The pathophysiology of dyspnea in ischemia is likely related to high left ventricular filling pressure secondary to the impaired contractility of the ischemic region of the heart, which causes pulmonary edema. These patients often describe sensations of chest tightness or heaviness and chest pain, in addition to dyspnea.

In patients with low cardiac output dyspnea, CHF is the predominant etiology. In this cardiovascular disease state, the respiratory controller is stimulated by elevated vascular pressures as well as the resultant interstitial edema. Pulmonary edema affects both the respiratory controller, through activation of J receptors in the lung, as well as the gas exchanger. Patients with CHF often complain of air hunger, an increased urge to breathe, or a sensation of not being able to get enough air. Additional complaints of nocturnal dyspnea, dyspnea on exertion, and orthopnea are also suggestive of cardiac dyspnea. On exam, patients usually have peripheral edema, an elevated jugular venous pressure, an S_3 gallop, and bibasilar crackles on auscultation. An "expiratory grunt," or rounding of the abdomen during expiration, has been found to be a fairly specific physical finding in CHF. The CXR typically shows an enlarged cardiac silhouette, vascular cephalization, perihilar or bibasilar alveolar infiltrates, and bilateral pleural effusions. A TTE is also exceptionally helpful in this population to assess myocardial contractility and acute valvular dysfunction. An optimal cardiac regimen includes diuretics, medications to reduce afterload and, in select cases, medications to enhance contractility (see Chapter 129 [Heart Failure]).

Pulmonary embolism is a unique cause of dyspnea. The mechanism leading to the symptom is complex and poorly understood and often the symptoms are out of proportion to the derangement in pulmonary mechanics or gas exchange. One possible mechanism contributing to the sensation of dyspnea is activation of C fibers in the pulmonary vasculature or stimulation of pressure receptors in the right atrium. Pulmonary emboli also cause hypoxemia due to ventilation perfusion mismatch and hypercarbia due to increased dead space. Although these derangements may contribute to the sensation of dyspnea, the dyspnea is largely independent of these gas transfer defects. The addition of supplemental oxygen to correct hypoxemia typically has little effect on the breathlessness associated with pulmonary embolism, and acute hypercarbia is unusual with small and medium size emboli. Clues to this diagnosis may include sudden onset of chest pain and dyspnea, possibly associated with unilateral lower extremity swelling (see Chapter 253 [Diagnosis and Treatment of Venous Thromboembolism]). Hospitalization is a major risk factor for VTE for all patients irrespective of VTE prophylaxis.

PRACTICE POINT

- A pulmonary embolus caused by inadequate DVT prophylaxis is a partially preventable cause of dyspnea. All inpatients should be considered for DVT prophylaxis.

On exam, these patients are tachycardic and tachypneic, but their chest exam and CXR are generally unremarkable. Pulse oximetry may remain normal despite the presence of a widened alveolar-arterial oxygen gradient because of the hyperventilation typical of acute pulmonary embolism. Usually the diagnosis is made with a PE-protocol CTA. Although a normal D-dimer has a high negative predictive value (in low-to-moderate-risk patients), its utility is limited for excluding clots in hospitalized patients who are usually high risk (see Chapter 253 for treatment options).

■ PERSISTENTLY UNEXPLAINED DYSPNEA

Occasionally neither the diagnosis nor the physiologic mechanisms of dyspnea are clear. These patients often have normal physical examinations and diagnostic workups. CPETs are particularly helpful in this population to assess the patient for evidence of deconditioning as well as to look for findings consistent with malingering or hyperventilation syndrome. Patients with hyperventilation syndrome typically complain of a sensation of inability to get a deep breath despite breathing with very large tidal volumes. They often have a concomitant anxiety disorder. Anxiety can also explain dyspnea out of proportion to the underlying cause, as it can alter the perception of sensory data and lead to breathing patterns that worsen physiologic abnormalities. Anxiety is particularly troublesome in patients

with hyperinflation since the behavioral issues lead to increased respiratory rate, which worsens hyperinflation and increases further the work of breathing in patients with expiratory airflow obstruction.

■ GOALS OF TREATMENT

Although not all dyspnea can be fully eliminated by efforts to correct the underlying disorder, there are ways to lessen the distress. For example, administration of oxygen can diminish the activation of chemoreceptors, pursed-lip breathing can lessen dynamic airway collapse, and inspiratory muscle training can strengthen the ventilatory pump. Many patients with chronic dyspnea, particularly those with COPD, can benefit from pulmonary rehabilitation to overcome the cardiovascular deconditioning that often accompanies chronic dyspnea.

CONCLUSION

Dyspnea is a complex symptom that encompasses many distinct sensations. Encouraging patients to choose their own qualitative descriptors can give the physician insight into the disease causing the dyspnea and its underlying physiologic mechanisms. This understanding, coupled with the physical exam and diagnostic data, can help the physician decide if the patient has dyspnea related to the respiratory or cardiovascular system and subsequently investigate the specific disease state responsible for the problem. The expectation is that this knowledge will help prevent common diagnostic errors, facilitate the correct management, and improve the quality of care of patients with dyspnea.

SUGGESTED READINGS

American Thoracic Society. Dyspnea: mechanisms, assessment, and management: a consensus statement. *Am J Respir Crit Care Med*. 1999;159:321-340.

Banzett RB, O'Donnell CR, Guilfoyle TE, et al. Multidimensional dyspnea profile: an instrument for clinical and laboratory research. *Eur Respir J*. 2015;45(6):1681-1691.

Berkman N, Avital A, Breuer R, et al. Exhaled nitric oxide in the diagnosis of asthma: comparison with bronchial provocation tests. *Thorax*. 2005;60(5):383-388.

Crapo RO, Casaburi R, Coates AL, et al. Guidelines for methacholine and exercise challenge testing-1999. This official statement of the American Thoracic Society was adopted by the ATS Board of Directors, July 1999. *Am J Respir Crit Care Med*. 2000;161:309.

Elliot MW, Adams L, Cockroft A, et al. The language of breathlessness: use by patients of verbal descriptors. *Am Rev Respir Dis*. 1991;144:826-832.

Mahler DA, Harver A, Lentine T, et al. Descriptors of breathlessness in cardiorespiratory disease. *Am J Resp Crit Care Med*. 1996;154:1357-1363.

Mahler DA, O'Donnell DE. Recent advances in dyspnea. *Chest*. 2015;147(1):232-241.

Manning HL, Schwartzstein RM. Pathophysiology of dyspnea. *N Engl J Med*. 1995;333:1547-1533.

Schwartzstein RM. Dyspnea. In: Fauci AS, ed. *Harrison's Principles of Internal Medicine*. 18th ed. New York, NY: McGraw-Hill; 2011.

Schwartzstein RM. The language of dyspnea. In: Mahler DA, O'Donnell DE, eds. *Dyspnea: Mechanisms, Measurement, and Management*. 2nd ed. Boca Raton, FL: Taylor & Francis; 2005.

Simon PM, Schwartzstein RM, Weiss JW, et al. Distinguishable types of dyspnea in patients with shortness of breath. *Am Rev Respir Dis*. 1990;142:1009-1014.

CHAPTER 86

Edema

Teresa L. Carman, MD

Key Clinical Questions

1. How may the history and physical examination findings direct the evaluation of lower-extremity edema?

2. What diagnostic or laboratory studies will help better delineate the differential diagnosis?

3. What therapeutic options may be beneficial in the management of edema?

CASE 86-1

A 42-year-old woman with a medical history of vascular disease presented to the emergency department with difficulty walking from painful leg and foot wounds present for 4 weeks. Her medical history includes traditional vascular risk factors, hypertension, diabetes, and hyperlipidemia, coronary artery disease (four myocardial infarctions, s/p percutaneous coronary intervention and stent placement, ischemic cardiomyopathy with ejection fraction of 25% and left apical thrombus, venous thromboembolism (deep venous thromboembolism, pulmonary embolism, s/p inferior vena caval filter placement), warfarin associated gastrointestinal bleeding, and partial amputation of her right foot due to osteomyelitis. She has not been taking her medications for 2 weeks. She complains of acute blisters of unknown etiology on her feet. The left is more involved than the right. She has been evaluated at an outside hospital for similar findings and a biopsy was done without defining an underlying etiology.

On examination vital signs include temperature 99.4°F; heart rate 116; blood pressure 133/93 mm Hg, respiratory rate 20, with a room air pulse oximetry at 100%. Her neck veins are distended and elevated to 14 cm. She is tachycardic with a regular rate with a 3/6 systolic murmur at the apex. No gallop is noted. Her lungs are clear without wheezes or crackles. Her abdomen is soft. No abdominal bruits are noted. She is tender to palpation in the right upper quadrant. Lower-extremity edema extends from the feet to the proximal hips and lower abdominal wall bilaterally. There are multiple punched-out fibrous-based wounds as well as intact fluid-filled blisters over the thighs and posterior knees. The left foot is completely involved with a partially hemorrhagic bulla. Pulses are not palpable.

Initial laboratory examination reveals hemoglobin of 7.7 g/dL, hematocrit 26.1%, albumin 1.8 g/dL, prealbumin 5.0 mg/dL, total protein 6.5 g/dL. BUN 21 mg/dL, creatinine 1.14 mg/dL, and glucose 401 mg/dL. Urinalysis demonstrates 3+ protein, 2+ blood, and 1000 mg/dL glucose. Further workup during the admission is directed at identifying the etiology of her volume overload, managing her edema, and local wound care.

INTRODUCTION

Edema or lower-extremity swelling is a common clinical complaint of both hospitalized and ambulatory patients. The differential diagnosis for lower-extremity swelling is quite extensive. Despite the clinical frequency of the complaint, few clinical series or studies address the etiology, evaluation, or diagnostic approach to lower-extremity swelling. Clinically, edema and lymphedema are often mistakenly used interchangeably to refer to soft tissue fluid accumulation. However, these conditions are very different with respect to their pathophysiology and clinical implications.

All swelling results from an increase in interstitial or tissue fluid, which is mostly water. The transcapillary tissue fluid may be predominantly water (edema), the result of abnormal intravascular hydrostatic pressure or oncotic pressure, or may be due to the inability or failure of the lymphatics to clear residual tissue fluid and proteinaceous material from the tissue space (lymphedema). All edema has some component of lymphatic failure—with the lymphatics being unable to clear the excess, residual, tissue fluid. This is not necessarily due to structural changes in the lymphatics but to overwhelming the normal carrying capacity. Venous return is responsible for approximately 80% of tissue fluid drainage and transportation from the interstitial space. The lymphatic system accommodates the return of protein, cellular debris, and the remaining 20% of interstitial fluid. Therefore, true lymphedema has a distinct pathophysiology resulting in regional increases in protein-rich fluid due to either decreased uptake or transport of tissue fluid. This will be discussed in more detail at the end of the chapter.

PATHOPHYSIOLOGY

Intravascular and extravascular fluid homeostasis requires stable capillary filtration supported by normal venous and lymphatic return to the systemic circulation. If the capillary fluid filtration rate exceeds the tissue drainage or transportation rate, fluid will accumulate within the extravascular or tissue space. Capillary filtration depends upon a normal, intact vascular endothelium and adequate serum oncotic pressure or protein/albumin content as well as equal ion distribution between the intravascular and extravascular compartments. In the most basic terms, if capillary filtration is adequately offset by vascular reabsorption, normal tissue fluid balance is maintained.

Maintaining endothelial integrity is the initial step in controlling edema. Vascular integrity is tightly regulated. As part of normal fluid homeostasis approximately 30% of postcapillary venule endothelial junctions are open and permeable. When regulation is disrupted, increased permeability may result in edema. This mechanism typically underlies the edema associated with inflammation, infection, trauma or burns, and medications. Most stimuli that affect vascular integrity are reversible and do not cause permanent endothelial impairment.

Even when there is no disruption in vascular permeability, edema may be caused by increased capillary filtration with a shift of intravascular fluid from the vessels into the extravascular space. This is usually due to physiological changes in oncotic pressure, changes in hydrostatic pressure, or changes in intravascular fluid volume (Table 86-1). In this case, normal homeostasis and fluid balance

between the intravascular and extravascular space is determined by hydrostatic pressure and oncotic gradients.

Intravascular oncotic pressure is influenced by protein and albumin content. If oncotic pressure within the vessels is decreased by nutritional depletion of albumin or protein, decreased synthesis as in liver disease, or by a loss of protein through the kidneys or the gastrointestinal tract, water will move from the vessels into the interstitium to maintain a constant oncotic pressure between the intravascular and extravascular compartments. Similarly, if the intravascular oncotic pressure is decreased due to increased intravascular fluid or volume accumulation this will also promote fluid shifts into the tissues and cause edema. Low serum albumin is a common hospital laboratory finding. Albumin is an acute phase reactant and decreases rapidly during illness. Patients with chronic inflammatory states or chronic medical conditions such as malignancy will frequently have low albumin levels. Protein malnutrition is underrecognized but is a frequent cause of edema especially in the elderly and institutionalized individuals. Nutrition screening should be considered for all patients with lower-extremity edema.

PRACTICE POINT

- The calf muscle pump is required to propel the column of venous blood back to the heart against a high pressure gradient along with competent venous valves to maintain normal venous return. Anything that disrupts or impairs the calf muscle pump may be associated with edema. Immobility, an impaired or shuffling gait frequently seen in the elderly or those with neurologic disorders, and paresis are common conditions that cause loss of the calf muscle pump.

A second important pressure gradient (hydrostatic pressure) occurs within the venous system. There is a static pressure within the veins that depends on the height of the column of blood. Any condition that raises the resting right heart pressures or intravenous pressure may cause edema (**Table 86-1**). Normal systemic venous return relies upon a normal cardiac pump, an intact calf muscle pump, intact venous valves to support antegrade venous return, and a pressure gradient between the ankle and the right heart. Chronic venous hypertension may result when any of these primary components are abnormal.

Venous valvular insufficiency due to loss of valve integrity or damage will frequently result in increased venous pressures, so-called venous hypertension. This may affect the deep veins as well as the superficial veins. The loss of valve integrity may be primary, related to varicose veins and valve degeneration, or secondary, from trauma or injury to the valves usually associated with venous thrombosis. This is termed post-thrombotic syndrome. Regardless of the etiology, loss of valve integrity may result in increased venous pressure due to the static column of blood within the vein and secondary increased capillary filtration along the pressure gradient.

The importance of the calf muscle pump, in conjunction with competent venous valves, must not be overlooked for normal venous return. Venous pressure at the ankle may be as high as 100 mm Hg in the standing position. The calf muscle pump is required to propel the column of venous blood back to the heart against this pressure gradient. Anything that disrupts or impairs the calf muscle pump may be associated with edema. Immobility, an impaired or shuffling gait frequently seen in the elderly or those with neurologic disorders, and paresis are common conditions that cause loss of the calf muscle pump. It is not uncommon to be able to trace the onset of the edema to the initial use of a cane, walker or other mobility aid.

A common cause of edema in hospitalized patients is an increase in plasma volume. Increased plasma volume caused by sodium and

---

TABLE 86-1 Etiology of Tissue Edema

Capillary filtration
  Inflammation or trauma
  Vasodilation or increased permeability
  Decreased intravascular oncotic forces
    Hepatic insufficiency with hypoalbuminemia
    Cirrhosis
    Hypoalbuminemia due to nutritional deficiency
    Low protein due to renal loss or protein-losing enteropathy
  Increased intravascular volume (plasma volume)
    Activation of the rennin-angiotensin-aldosterone system
    Heart failure and relative volume retention
    Decreased renal output/regulation of volume
    Hormonally related fluid retention
    Medications causing volume/sodium retention

Changes in venous pressure
  Elevated right heart pressures
    Decreased left ventricular ejection fraction
    Primary pulmonary hypertension or chronic thromboembolic disease
  Post-thrombotic changes with venous obstruction
  Valvular insufficiency with reflux
  Chronic limb dependency
  Gait abnormalities or immobilization with loss of the calf muscle pump

water retention results in secondary changes in both intravascular pressure as well as lowered oncotic forces. Plasma volume is maintained through intact renal excretion of ions followed by passive water excretion. Heart failure, renal disease, liver disease, medications, pregnancy, or any other condition that augments the neurohormonal reabsorption of sodium and water through activation of vasopressin or the renin-angiotensin-aldosterone system may result in secondary edema due to sodium and water retention.

In reality, most edema is multifactorial and many variables and pathophysiologic mechanisms may be contributing. Clinical clues and historical elements may help focus your evaluation of the patient. A thorough evaluation of edema should focus on evaluating for underlying cardiopulmonary, kidney disease, liver disease, contributing medications, and venous disorders.

PRACTICE POINT

- The approach to bilateral lower-extremity edema of an unclear etiology should focus on the most common clinical contributors. Testing should be used to evaluate the clinical conditions with the most significant impact. A thorough evaluation of edema should focus on evaluating for underlying cardiopulmonary disease, kidney disease, liver disease, contributing medications, and venous disorders.

The approach to lower-extremity edema of an unclear etiology should focus on the most common clinical contributors. Testing should be used to evaluate the clinical conditions with the most significant impact. Edema is frequently considered cosmetic, but the underlying clinical contributors may indeed be life threatening. The most important clinical questions that may help evaluate edema are the following:

1. Is the swelling unilateral or bilateral?
2. What is the age of the patient?
3. Are there associated clinical symptoms of pain, erythema, fever, or systemic illness?
4. What are the onset, duration, and progression of the symptoms?
5. Are there associated clinical examination findings?
6. What exacerbates or relieves the edema?
7. Is there coexisting medical illness, predisposing factors, or medications known to cause edema?

EVALUATION

■ UNILATERAL VERSUS BILATERAL EDEMA

The differential diagnosis of unilateral edema can be extensive (**Table 86-2**). Unilateral edema is typically due to a localized process affecting a single quadrant of the body as opposed to systemic factors. While it is common for patients with systemic illness, such as heart failure, to have a modest or moderate degree of asymmetry in their lower-extremity edema, complete sparing of one leg is not typical. In general, the initial evaluation of a patient with acute onset, unilateral edema should include testing to either diagnose or exclude deep venous thrombosis (DVT). The signs and symptoms of DVT are notoriously nonspecific and the consequences of venous thromboembolism may be severe. In addition, several clinical conditions have been associated with secondary DVT related to inflammation or venous compression, therefore evaluation to exclude the diagnosis of DVT should be pursued. This can be done using Well's criteria, D-dimer testing, and objective imaging. It is important to recognize that a patient with a high pretest probability on Well's criteria may require more than a simple venous duplex examination to exclude DVT. In particular, duplex ultrasound is often unable to diagnose or exclude common iliac or proximal external iliac vein

TABLE 86-2 Partial List of Differential Diagnoses Associated with Unilateral Limb Swelling. The Mnemonic VINDICATE may be Helpful to Expand Initial Considerations when Evaluating the Patient

Vascular: deep vein thrombosis, lymphedema, varicose veins, post-thrombotic syndrome, vascular compression (ie, May-Thurner syndrome)

Infectious/inflammatory: cellulitis, erysipelas, insect envenomation, inflammatory arthropathies

Neoplastic: soft tissue tumors may cause focal swelling or fullness, with compression of vascular structures, or lymphatics may also cause secondary edema, diffuse cutaneous tumor infiltration (while uncommon) may be perceived as edema

Drugs: unlikely to cause unilateral edema but a frequent case of bilateral swelling (Table 86-4)

Iatrogenic: disruption of lymphatics during surgery (ie, hernia or vein harvest), vascular intervention-related hemorrhage (ie, central line placement or cardiac catheterization)

Congenital/developmental/inherited: varicose veins, Klippel-Trenaunay syndrome, Parks-Weber syndrome, congenital or familial lymphedema

Anatomic: May-Thurner syndrome, popliteal vein entrapment

Trauma: sprain, strain, rupture of the medial gastrocnemius muscle, muscular hemorrhage, ruptured popliteal cyst, reflex sympathetic dystrophy/chronic regional pain syndrome

Environmental/endocrine: plant or insect exposure/hypersensitivity, myxedema

DVT, so computed tomography (CT) or magnetic resonance (MR) imaging may be needed if isolated proximal DVT is suspected (such as in a patient with recent pelvic or hip trauma). Once acute DVT has been excluded, other clinical or historical clues may lead one to suspect etiologies related to other clinical conditions (Table 86-2).

PRACTICE POINT

- The approach to unilateral edema should focus on a localized process—affecting a single body quadrant—as opposed to systemic factors. While it is common for patients with systemic illness, such as heart failure, to have a modest or moderate degree of asymmetry in their lower-extremity edema, complete sparing of one leg is not typical. In general, the initial evaluation of a patient with acute-onset, unilateral edema should include testing to either diagnose or exclude deep venous thrombosis (DVT).

Bilateral lower-extremity edema suggests a more central, that is, cardiac or central venous, or systemic etiology (**Table 86-3**). In patients with new onset bilateral edema, the clinician should conduct a thorough evaluation for underlying cardiac conditions, hepatic or renal insufficiency, and if these conditions are absent, bilateral or central venous thrombosis should be excluded. Evaluation for venous thromboembolism with venous duplex ultrasound is often still prudent, but may be lower yield. Many common medications are associated with edema (**Table 86-4**) and contribution from medications should not be overlooked. Symmetric bilateral lower-extremity swelling usually has a systemic predisposition (**Table 86-5**) whereas unilateral swelling will typically be related to a limb or localized body quadrant etiology. Bilateral swelling with an asymmetric characteristic may have an additional component of venous or lymphatic insufficiency in addition to the underlying systemic pathology.

TABLE 86-3 Systemic Contributors to Bilateral Edema

Elevated right-heart pressure
   Left or right ventricular failure
   Tricuspid regurgitation
   Pericardial constriction
   Cor pulmonale
   Pulmonary hypertension
   Obstructive sleep apnea
Endocrine disorders
   Myxedema (may be mistaken for edema)
   Cushing syndrome
Medications (see Table 86-4)
Metabolic dysfunction
   Protein imbalance
      Decreased hepatic production
      Excess protein losses
   Malnutrition
Vascular
   Varicose veins/venous insufficiency
   Caval occlusion

■ AGE-RELATED EVALUATION

Evaluation of edema should be directed primarily by ancillary clinical clues since the differential diagnosis, which is quite broad, may change considerably. Edema in children is uncommon and should raise immediate clinical concern. Protein-losing enteropathy, malnutrition, nephrotic syndrome, medication-induced, trauma, injury, infection, and cardiac conditions prevail. Venous thromboembolism is less common but increasingly recognized in pediatric populations and should not be overlooked especially in chronically ill or hospitalized patients.

TABLE 86-4 Pharmaceuticals Associated with Edema

Antidepressants
Antihypertensive agents
   Calcium channel blockers
   B-blockers
   Direct vasodilators
   Antisympathomimetics
Hormones
   Oral contraceptives
   Prednisone/Steroids
   Estrogen replacement
   Testosterone
Steroids
Nonsteroidal anti-inflammatory agents
Thiazolidinediones
   Pioglitazone
   Rosiglitazone
Antiepileptic drugs
   Gabapentin
   Pregabalin

TABLE 86-5 Partial List of Differential Diagnoses Associated with Bilateral Limb Swelling Using the Mnemonic VINDICATE

Vascular: bilateral deep vein thrombosis, acquired lymphedema, varicose veins, post-thrombotic syndrome, structural and hemodynamic cardiac conditions, obstructive sleep apnea

Infectious/inflammatory: cellulitis, erysipelas, inflammatory arthropathies, retroperitoneal fibrosis

Neoplastic: retroperitoneal tumors with compression of vascular structures or lymphatics, lymphoma, vascular invasion (ie, renal cell cancer)

Drugs: a frequent case of bilateral swelling (Table 86-4)

Iatrogenic: disruption of lymphatics during surgery (ie, hernia or vein harvest), vascular intervention-related thrombosis (ie, IVC* filters)

Congenital/developmental/inherited: congenital lymphedema

Anatomic: absent or atretic IVC

Trauma: IVC injury/ligation

Environmental/endocrine: myxedema, Cushing syndrome

*IVC, inferior vena cava.

The most common cause of edema in the second or third decade of life is idiopathic edema, also referred to as cyclic edema. Patients may report associated facial and hand swelling. Other systemic causes for swelling should be excluded. Diuretic abuse is common with this disorder. In middle-aged patients, chronic venous insufficiency is the most common diagnosis. However, patients with new onset edema after the age of 40 should be fully evaluated for underlying systemic causes.

Most chronic edema in the elderly is multifactorial. Gait and mobility assessment may be important since decreased ambulation is a frequent contributor to bilateral swelling. In addition, patients should be questioned regarding sleep habits. Due to physical disabilities, medical comorbidities, or sleep irregularities many patients sleep in a chair or recliner leaving their legs chronically dependent. This will only be discovered by direct questioning. All of the aforementioned differential diagnoses must be considered. In addition, obstructive sleep apnea is frequently overlooked as a cause of edema.

■ CLINICAL FINDINGS

Physical examination findings may help support diagnostic suspicion. All patients should be thoroughly evaluated for signs of systemic processes contributing to edema. Examination should include an assessment for jugular venous distension, extra heart sounds including gallops or murmurs, truncal telangiectasias, hepatojugular reflux, lung crackles, ascites, etc. Lower-extremity tenderness, increased warmth, and pitting are nonspecific findings frequently associated with edema. Inflammation is frequently associated with edema and contributes to these clinical findings. Dilated subcutaneous veins—"sentinel" veins—represent dilated collateral vessels that can be seen in the setting of venous obstruction. These are commonly visualized along the abdomen, anterior chest wall or extremities. Both acute and chronic conditions may present with this nonspecific constellation of symptoms. Soft doughy pitting in the absence of inflammation may be more consistent with hepatic dysfunction, renal protein losses or nephrotic syndrome, or acute/subacute cardiac etiologies; however, this can be quite variable. Chronic skin changes of hyperpigmentation or hemosiderin staining, eczema or dermatitis, and brawny skin thickening (called lipodermatosclerosis) are characteristic of chronic venous hypertension or chronic, persistent swelling. Chronic venous insufficiency is a nonspecific term used to identify edema associated with varicose veins and chronic venous hypertension. The term varicose veins collectively includes typical large ropey varicosities, small 1 to 3 mm subcutaneous reticular veins, and even dermal telangiectasias. The common clinical finding of clusters of small dilated veins at the ankles sometimes called corona phlebectatica is consistent with chronic venous stasis and chronic venous hypertension and frequently associated with edema.

Edema that terminates at the ankle and spares the foot may be consistent with lipoedema. Lipoedema is frequently mistaken for edema or lymphedema. This is typically identified in women. It may be considered a physiologic variant consisting of bilateral, symmetric deposition of adipose tissue.

ONSET, DURATION, EXACERBATING AND REMITTING FACTORS

Acute edema, especially when unilateral, is typically more concerning for a venous obstructive process and necessitates evaluation for DVT. Chronic, longstanding swelling is clinically relevant and certainly may impact the function and quality of life of the patient, thus evaluation and treatment is warranted. However, in most of these patients routine venous duplex is not indicated. In patients with long-standing swelling, a change in the characteristic or nature of the swelling, new onset pain or a change in pain quality, or other clinical findings may indeed provoke the need for imaging.

Edema related to venous disease will frequently improve overnight or with elevation due to the decrease in venous pressure. During the day patients with underlying venous disease typically experience an increase in swelling due to the dependent nature of the legs and increased pressure-drive venous filtration. Patients with underlying cardiac, hepatic, or renal issues predisposing to edema are less likely to notice dramatic daily changes in their edema but there is often a modest degree of diurnal variation.

DIAGNOSTIC TOOLS

Duplex ultrasound is both sensitive and specific for the diagnosis of venous thromboembolism as well as venous reflux in the visualized segments. The testing uses both compression imaging as well as Doppler insonation of the vessels (**Figures 86-1** and **86-2**). Vessels from the common femoral vein or even the distal external iliac vein through the popliteal vein and into the calf are easily imaged. If a segment cannot be imaged adequately due to bandaging, dressings, patient comfort, patient positioning, patient cooperation, obesity, or extensive edema adding significant tissue depth, then DVT cannot be fully excluded. It is important to recognize that duplex sonography is less sensitive for calf vein thrombosis than for proximal DVT. Therefore calf vein DVT may be missed by venous duplex examination. In a patient with high clinical suspicion for DVT and negative initial imaging it may be prudent to repeat testing in 5 to 7 days to exclude DVT. In addition, some vascular laboratories and radiology departments do not routinely visualize calf veins and therefore cannot exclude DVT involving these segments.

Subtle changes in the Doppler waveforms may suggest underlying conditions that require further evaluation. Normal venous flow is respirophasic—cessation of flow occurs with inspiration and flow resumes when the diaphragm is relaxed. Pulsatile venous flow—flow noted above and below the Doppler baseline—suggests elevated right-sided heart pressures, significant tricuspid regurgitation, or increased venous pressures (**Figure 86-3**). Monophasic flow, the absence of spontaneous respirophasic flow, or decreased return with distal augmentation suggests more proximal occlusion or obstruction and may require additional imaging of the pelvis or inferior vena cava (IVC) (**Figure 86-4**). In this setting, further imaging with abdominal/pelvic CT, CT venography, or magnetic resonance venography (MRV) may be helpful.

The ultrasound evaluation for venous insufficiency differs from venous duplex imaging for DVT. To evaluate for venous insufficiency, the patient is examined in a standing position with the index leg offloaded. The deep venous system is evaluated for evidence of

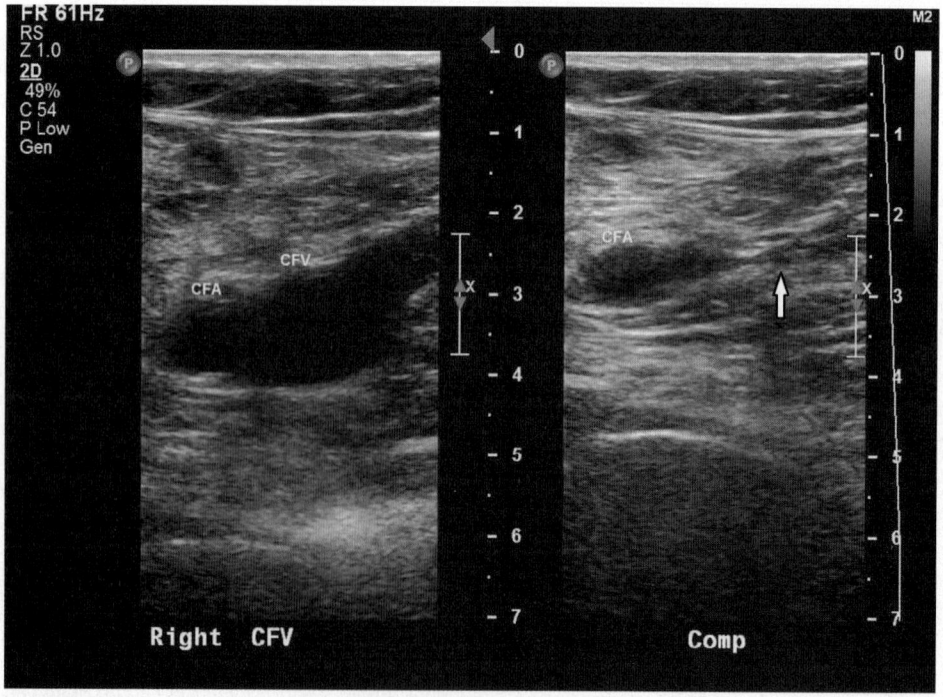

Figure 86-1 *Compression image of the artery and vein at the level of the groin demonstrating a normal common femoral artery (CFA) and vein (CFV). With compression over the vein, the walls of the vein coapt when the vein is free of thrombus.*

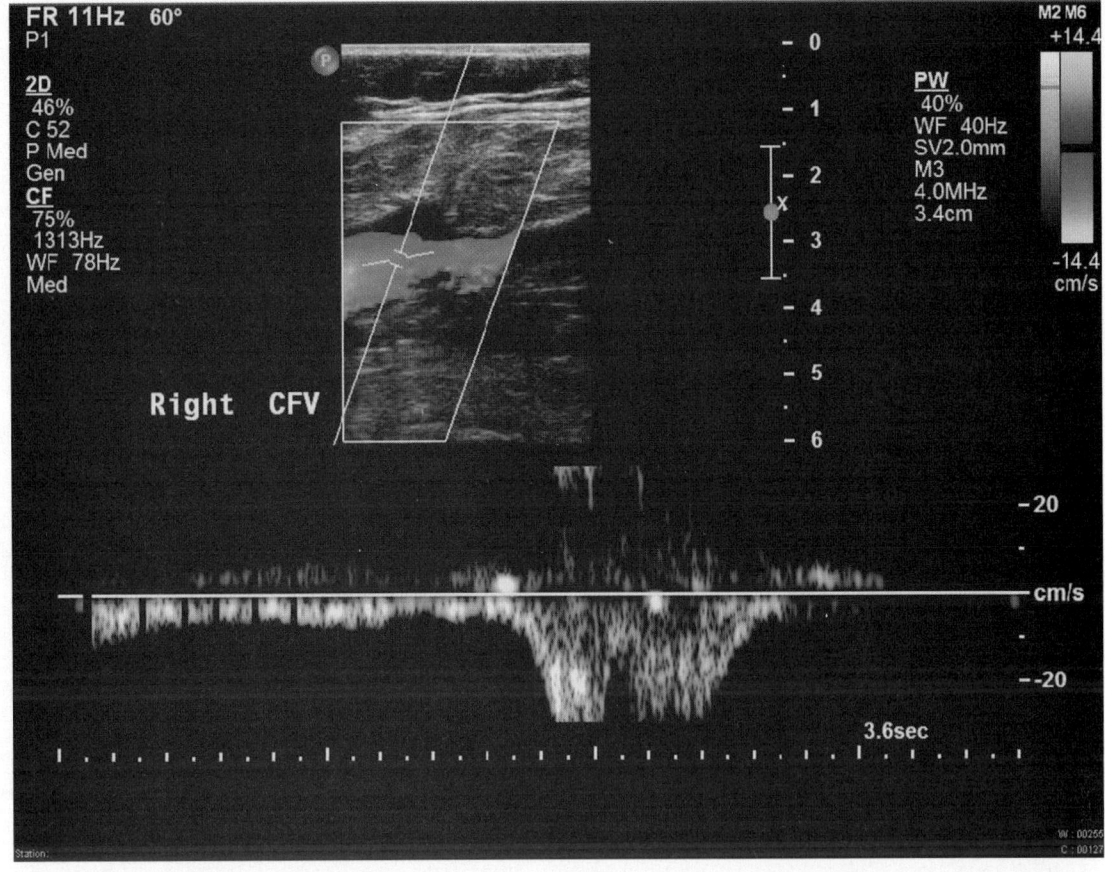

Figure 86-2 *A normal vein demonstrates spontaneous respirophasic flow and augmentation of venous return when the calf muscle is compressed.*

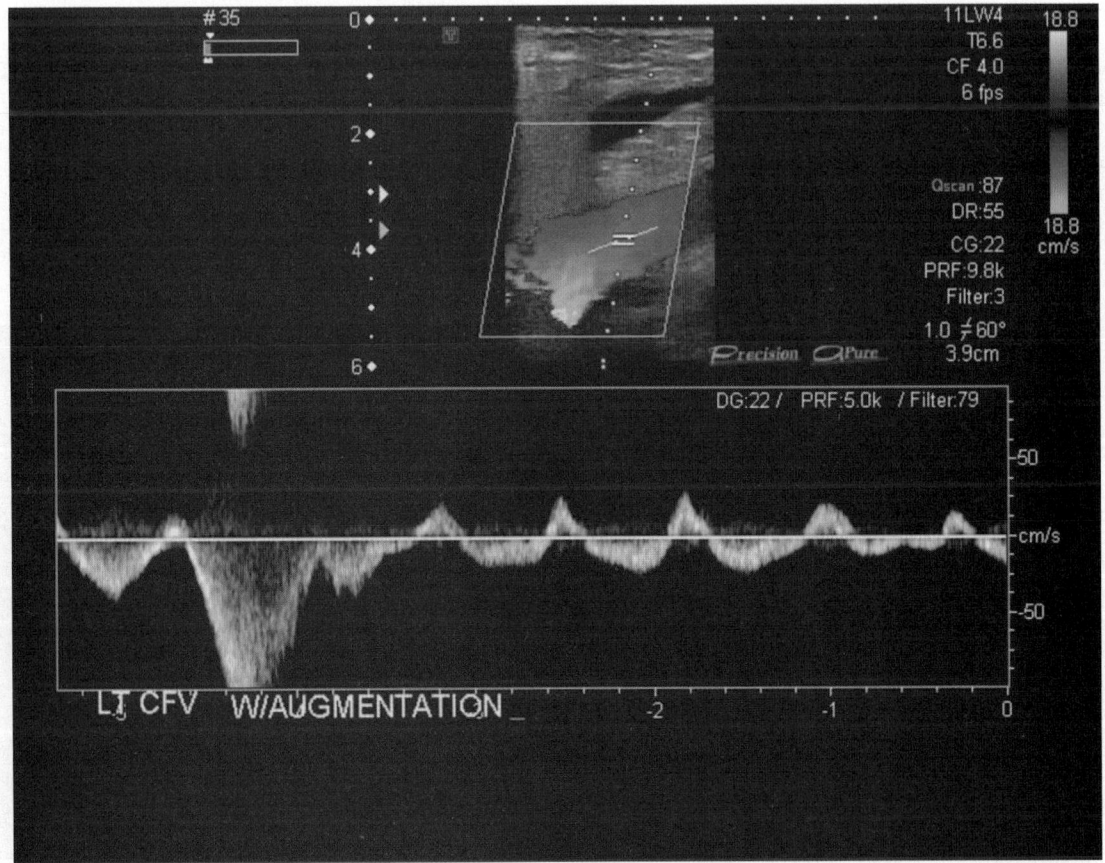

Figure 86-3 *Pulsatile venous waveforms are due to reflection of pressure down through the inferior vena cava. This is usually consistent with volume overload or elevated right heart pressures.*

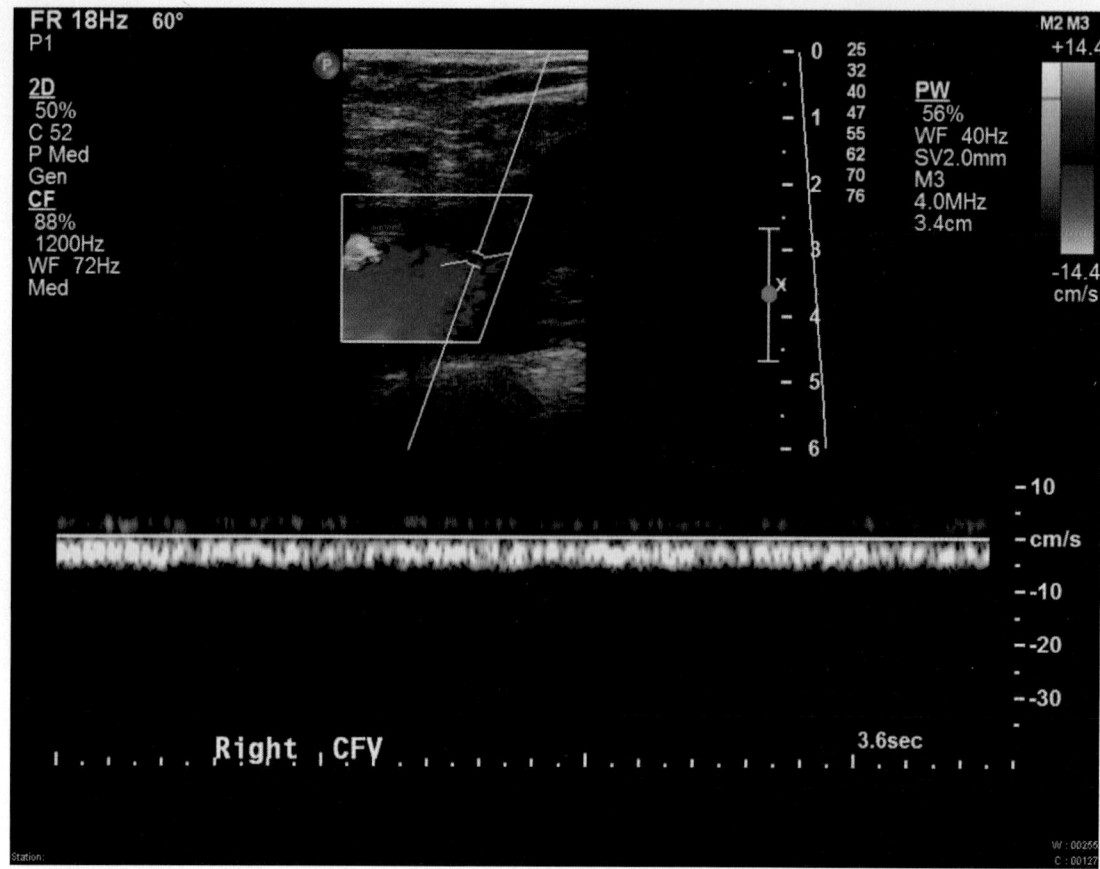

Figure 86-4 *Monophasic flow within the vein should raise concern for a more proximal obstruction within the venous system.*

DVT or venous reflux. In addition the technician spends considerable time evaluating all segments of the great and small saphenous veins for thrombosis as well as reflux with Valsalva or compression maneuvers. This test is time consuming, usually performed in the outpatient setting and is less likely warranted in a hospitalized patient.

Abdomen and pelvis CT with intravascular contrast may demonstrate obstruction or occlusion at the level of the inferior vena cava (IVC) or iliac veins as an etiology (**Figure 86-5**). The IVC may be visible on duplex ultrasound, but this is variable and not necessarily reliable. IVC and iliac imaging relies predominantly on Doppler insonation. CT venography, MRV, or conventional ascending contrast phlebography are the most reliable imaging for the IVC and iliac veins. They directly image veins for the presence of intraluminal thrombus or external compression as an etiology for edema. Intravascular pressure measurements or intravascular ultrasound combined with ascending phlebography may be required to evaluate subtle abnormalities to ensure that there is no hemodynamic significance to the changes. Typical limitations of CT and MR should be noted including the use of contrast, prolonged imaging times for MR, and the inability to image in the setting of some indwelling devices.

Patients with suspected cardiopulmonary etiology for their edema should have an ECG and chest x-ray as well as echocardiogram. Echocardiography can be used to assess hemodynamics including preload and afterload, ventricular function and contractility, pulmonary hypertension, or physiologic and anatomic valve abnormalities. Echocardiography should be included in the evaluation in patients with evidence of heart failure, unexplained volume overload, or murmurs on examination. In some cases central pressure monitoring and right heart catheterization may be useful. Sleep apnea and associated heart failure and pulmonary hypertension is

an under-recognized cause of lower-extremity edema. Edema that is worse upon awakening is sometimes reported, and is a major clue to the diagnosis. Polysomnography testing may be helpful.

■ LABORATORY EVALUATION

Further evaluation for a systemic etiology should include a basic laboratory evaluation. A complete metabolic panel will help exclude

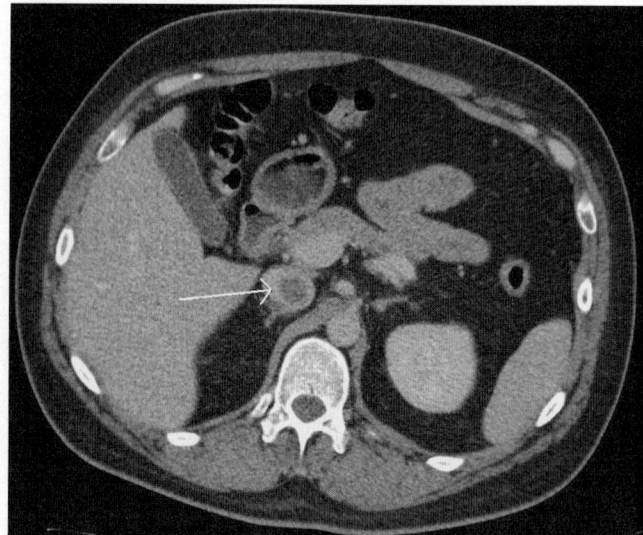

Figure 86-5 *Contrasted CT scan of the abdomen demonstrating partially occlusive thrombus within the inferior vena cava (arrow).*

low protein or albumin states and provide a basic assessment of liver integrity, renal function, and ion balance. Urinalysis is useful to identify renal protein loss. Prothrombin time (PT), albumin, and prealbumin provide an assessment of the synthetic function of the liver. Urinalysis should be performed to exclude significant proteinuria. Prealbumin should be ordered when there is suspicion for significant hypoalbuminemia or malnutrition. Calorie counts and evaluation by a dietician may be helpful. Brain natriuretic peptide (BNP) or NT-pro-BNP may be useful to exclude heart failure. Clinical clues suggestive of an underlying endocrinopathy such as Cushing syndrome or thyroid disease should prompt appropriate testing.

■ TREATMENT

Edema should be managed according to the underlying diagnosis. Venous thromboembolism should be treated with systemic anticoagulation. Consideration may be given to more aggressive management with pharmacomechanical thrombolysis in an effort to preserve venous valve function and minimize late effects of the post-thrombotic syndrome. Many practitioners treat edema with diuretics. However, in many cases edema is not due to excess intravascular volume and therefore diuretics are not indicated nor are they likely to be helpful. In cardiac conditions causing volume retention, and sometimes in liver disease or renally mediated volume retention, diuretics may be helpful. However, renal function and intravascular volume should be followed closely. Lifestyle modification and optimizing pharmacotherapy should be the primary focus.

Most patients benefit from an aggressive skin care regimen to prevent eczema and ulceration associated with increased tissue fluid. Decreasing edema through elevation and compression are mainstays of therapy. Elevating the foot of the bed by several inches will decrease the pressure gradient between the ankle and the right atrium and improve venous return. Combined elevation with active calf muscle exercise increases volume reduction when compared to elevation alone.

Patients with chronic venous insufficiency and lymphedema should wear compression stockings. Typically, 20 to 30 mm Hg or even 30 to 40 mm Hg compression is required. However, the most important factor when prescribing compression therapy is to tailor the therapy to the ability of the patient to don and doff the garment. In many cases, elderly patients are best served by a 15 to 20 mm Hg garment due to physical limitations of mobility, arthritis, and hand strength that may impede the use of a stronger compression. Thromboembolic deterrent (TED) hose may be helpful to decrease and control edema in hospitalized patients but these are typically not sufficient to control swelling in ambulatory patients. ACE wraps may also be used to control edema. However, the elastic nature of the compression typically causes variable constriction and relaxation which limits their use in ambulatory patients, and, if misapplied or bunched up such that the proximal pressures are higher than distal pressures, venous return may actually be impaired.

Compression may cause significant volume mobilization and therefore, should be used cautiously in patients with underlying left ventricular dysfunction or heart failure. Caution should also be used when applying compression to patients with underlying peripheral arterial disease (PAD). In general, compression stockings should be used with caution when the ankle-brachial index in <0.7 and compression is not be recommended for patients with PAD and an ankle-brachial index <0.5.

LYMPHEDEMA

Lymphedema is the accumulation of protein-rich interstitial fluid due to impaired lymphatic transport. This impairment may be due to either qualitative functional impairment or quantitative loss of function of the lymphatics. The lymphatics are responsible for

TABLE 86-6 Classification of Lymphedema

Primary	
Congenital	Onset <1 y of age
Preacox	Onset during adolescence or 20s
Tarde	Onset over age 40
Secondary	
Surgery	Lymph node dissection, hernia repair, vein harvest, groin exploration, any surgical disruption of lymphatic tissue
Malignancy	Tumor infiltration or related to treatment including radiation therapy
Infection/Inflammation	Most commonly cellulites or chronic stasis inflammation as seen in phlebolymphedema
Trauma/injury	Burns, crush injury, any significant soft tissue trauma

collecting and transporting cellular debris as well as interstitial fluid and protein not returned to the circulation by the venules. The lymphatic vessels are small blind-end vessels that begin in the dermis as lymphatic capillaries. These join to form precollector vessels and collecting vessels that through one-way transport move the lymphatic fluid into the lymph nodes and major lymphatic channels to the thoracic duct. Lymphedema may be primary (ie, no underlying etiology for the lymphatic failure can be identified) or it may be secondary to a myriad of acquired causes (**Table 86-6**). Lymphedema can be graded based on the clinical presentation (**Table 86-7**). Most patients present with painless swelling of the limb and dorsum of the foot. Clinically, squared, thickened, and edematous toes and a positive Stemmer sign—the inability to pinch a skin fold at the base of the second toe—are frequently present, especially with later presentations. When the clinical diagnosis is in doubt, lymphoscintigraphy can be used to evaluate lymphatic function and when abnormal it is diagnostic of lymphedema. It is important to note, however, lymphoscintigraphy cannot differentiate between primary and secondary causes of lymphedema. Patient education is paramount to successful management of lymphedema. This condition is not reversible and may indeed worsen if left untreated. Patients should be treated with an aggressive skin care regimen to prevent

TABLE 86-7 Lymphedema Grading Based on Clinical Presentation

Grade 1
Extremity swelling that typically pits and will decrease with elevation of the limb
Grade 2
Frequently is nonpitting. Little improvement is seen with overnight elevation. The skin becomes thickened and fibrotic. Skin may begin to develop changes with hyperpigmentation
Grade 3
Described as "elephantiasis." The edema is fixed and does not pit or change with elevation. The skin is brawny and thickened. The dermal elements may hypertrophy causing hyperkeratotic or verrucal changes to the skin

injury and secondary infection. Heavy emollients may help soften and even reverse the hyperkeratotic skin changes. Manual lymphatic drainage is therapist-directed lymphatic massage and limb wrapping designed to stimulate and drain the lymphatics. As a component of complex decongestive therapy, manual lymphatic drainage should be used to decrease limb volume and help restore function. Chronic compression therapy provides the maintenance phase for maintaining the gains of manual lymphatic drainage.

Phlebolymphedema is an under-recognized condition with characteristics of both venous insufficiency and lymphedema. The venous and lymphatic systems are intimately related both anatomically and physiologically. The diagnosis of phlebolymphedema is primarily based on clinical history and examination. The patient will typically have evidence of chronic venous hypertension with varicose veins but will also have significant swelling of the dorsum of the foot, squared toes, and skin changes mimicking lymphedema. The underlying pathophysiology is related to the chronic venous hypertension with accumulation of interstitial fluid. When the increased fluid exceeds the capacity of the lymphatics transport capacity a low-protein edema results. Treatment should focus on managing the underlying chronic venous hypertension. Compression therapy is a mainstay, while surgical or endovascular procedures to manage venous reflux or obstruction may be prudent.

CASE 86-1 (*continued*)

A limited study due to her edema, Duplex ultrasound demonstrated normal compressibility in the visualized segments and the proximal waveforms were pulsatile bilaterally (see Figure 86-3), consistent with intravascular volume overload and elevated right heart pressures. On echocardiogram her left ventricle ejection fraction was 20% to 25% with global hypokinesis and a restrictive diastolic filling pattern. The right ventricle was moderately dilated with decreased systolic function and a calculated systolic pressure of 85 mm Hg. A 24-hour urine collection demonstrated protein loss of 2071 mg/24 hours. Under the direction of the heart failure service she was managed with aggressive diuresis, sodium and fluid restriction, and control of her diabetes with the addition of an ACE inhibitor for renal protection. Nutrition consultation provided recommendations to optimize her nutrition while strictly limiting her salt and carbohydrate intake. Her underlying edematous state was felt to be related to her heart failure, malnutrition, and renal protein losses. This patient demonstrates the multifactorial nature of edema that may be encountered in some acutely ill patients who present for management of otherwise unrelated medical concerns.

CONCLUSION

Edema is not necessarily just a cosmetic issue. Diuretics are frequently recommended but may not be the optimal therapy. When confronted with a patient with lower-extremity swelling it is necessary to determine what pathophysiology is underlying the condition. Successful management should be directed at the pathophysiology and not at the physical finding of swelling. Edema is best managed by addressing the medical conditions related to the underlying volume retention, optimizing medical regimens; diuretic therapy may be helpful. In patients with chronic venous insufficiency and venous hypertension, diuretics have limited benefit. The mainstay of therapy should be directed toward managing the underlying venous hypertension using elevation and compression. Surgical management of venous reflux and incompetent perforators may be appropriate for some patients. Lymphedema is best managed by a combination of limb decongestion and maintenance with compression therapy. Attention to skin care and protection of the limb is also of paramount importance.

SUGGESTED READINGS

Blankfield RP, Finkelhor RS, Alexander JJ, et al. Etiology and diagnosis of bilateral leg edema in primary care. *Am J Med*. 1998;105:192-197.

Bunke N, Brown K, Bergan J. Phlebolymphedema: usually unrecognized, often poorly treated. *Perspect Vasc Surg Endovasc Ther*. 2009;21:65-68.

Ely JW, Osheroff JA, Chambliss ML, Ebell MH. Approach to leg edema of unclear etiology. *J Am Board Fam Med*. 2006;19:148-160.

Felty CL, Rooke TW. Compression therapy for chronic venous insufficiency. *Semin Vasc Surg*. 2005;18:36-40.

Kerchner K, Fleischer A, Yosipovitch G. Lower extremity lymphedema update: pathophysiology, diagnosis and treatment guidelines. *J Am Acad Dermatol*. 2008;59:324-331.

Meissner M, Moneta G, Burnand K, et al. The hemodynamics and diagnosis of venous disease. *J Vasc Surg*. 2007;46:4S-24S.

Murakami M, Simons M. Regulation of vascular integrity. *J Mol Med*. 2009;87:571-582.

Schrier RW. Water and sodium retention in edematous disorders: role of vasopression and aldosterone. *Am J Med*. 2006;119(Suppl 1):S47-S53.

Tan M, van Rooden CJ, Westerbeek RE, Huisman MV. Diagnostic management of clinically suspected acute deep vein thrombosis. *Br J Haematol*. 2009;146:347-360.

Yale SH, Mazza JJ. Approach to diagnosing lower extremity edema. *Comp Ther*. 2001;27:242-252.

CHAPTER 87

Falls

Rollin Wright, MD
Robert M. Palmer, MD

Key Clinical Questions

❶ Why is prevention of falls and management important in hospitalized adults?

❷ How can the hospitalist identify the patient at risk of falling with injury?

❸ What assessment can be performed at the bedside to identify patients at high risk for falling in hospital?

❹ What interventions reduce the incidence of falls and injuries?

❺ What is the bedside approach to the fallen patient?

CASE STUDY

An 85-year-old woman was admitted to the hospital 2 days ago after suffering a fall complicated by a left proximal humerus fracture. She subsequently fell in her hospital room after she stood from the bed and leaned forward to answer the phone located on the bedside table just out of her reach. She struck her forehead on the corner of the bedside table and twisted her right arm which she was using to grasp the bedrail and steady herself. Nurses report that she has been delirious, with episodes of restlessness and frequent attempts to get out of bed. Her past history includes macular degeneration in the left eye, osteoporosis, hypertension, mild cognitive impairment and recurrent falls at home. At the time of the fall in the hospital, her medications included: trimethoprim/sulfamethoxazole for a urinalysis suggestive of urinary tract infection; metoprolol for hypertension and irregular heart rhythm; calcium carbonate with vitamin D; subcutaneous enoxaparin for prophylaxis against thromboembolism; aspirin; hydrocodone for severe shoulder pain; and trazodone for sleep. The previous night she received 50 mg orally of quetiapine because of her restlessness and calling out for help.

At the bedside, this patient is awake, crying for help, lying prone on the floor by the bed and with her left arm in a sling under her. She has a bleeding laceration that will require suturing over the right zygomatic bone and a large hematoma forming over her right eye. She tells you her right hand and arm hurt.

This case illustrates risk factors for falls as well as common risk factors contributing to an in-hospital fall with injury (**Table 87-1**). Hospitalists have opportunities to improve the quality of patient care so as to reduce the risk for subsequent falls and fall-related injuries. This chapter provides a framework for efforts to prevent future falls and injuries and for the hospitalist's targeted evaluation of the fallen patient.

FALLS PREVENTION AND MANAGEMENT— THE HOSPITALIST'S OPPORTUNITY

Falls are the most common type of adverse event in acute care hospitals. Estimates suggest that 700,000 to 1 million falls occur in hospitals each year. Defined as an unplanned descent to the floor, the ground or any lower level, a fall may be further classified as *injurious* or *noninjurious*. A fall is considered injurious if it results in any injury (such as bruising or fracture) that leads to reduced physical function and an evaluation by a health care professional. An injurious fall is further characterized by the severity of injury or level of harm brought about by the fall (Table 87-1). Nearly one-third of falls that occur in the hospital result in an injury, making falls one of the most common causes of hospital-acquired injury reported.

Considered preventable and costly to the health care system, injurious falls remain a patient safety and quality improvement priority in hospitals. The Joint Commission estimates that a serious fall-related injury costs the hospital, on average, $13,000 in operational costs and increases length of stay by an average of 6.27 days. One-third of falls are thought to be preventable. The Center for Medicare and Medicaid Services (CMS) and regulatory organizations (eg, The Joint Commission's National Patient Safety Goals) and many insurance carriers have created incentives to hospitals to reduce the incidence of fall-related injuries of patients in hospital. The CMS no

TABLE 87-1 The National Quality Forum (NQF) Definitions of Harm and Examples of Common Injuries from Falls

Category	Action Required	Common Injuries
No harm	None	
Minor harm	Application of dressing, ice, topical medication	Minor limb contusions
		Lacerations
	Cleansing wound	Sprains
	Leg elevation	Minor head injury
Moderate harm	Suturing, steri-strips, splinting	Lacerations of arms, legs and head
		Sprained ankle, wrist
		Vertebral and rib fractures
		Minor traumatic brain injury and small subdural hematoma
Major harm	Surgery, casting, traction	Fractures of the hip, forearm, leg, ankle, pelvis, upper arm, hand, skull
	ICU monitoring	Traumatic brain injury such as a subdural hematoma epidural bleed
Death		Head and neck trauma
		Major internal organ damage and Hemorrhage

TABLE 87-2 Risk Factors for Falls

Intrinsic risk factors:
- lower-extremity weakness
- lower-extremity osteoarthritis or pain
- poor grip strength
- gait and balance deficits
- history of falls
- need for some help with daily activities
- requires 1:1 supervision or assistance with bed transfers and walking
- urinary incontinence
- sensory (visual, auditory) impairment
- cognitive impairment (delirium, dementia)
- depression
- orthostasis
- age

Extrinsic risk factors:
- use of four or more prescription drugs (polypharmacy)
- use of high-risk medications (benzodiazepines, antipsychotics)
- environmental challenges (poor lighting, slippery floors, bed height, and absence of grab bars or assistive devices)

longer pays for the added patient-care costs incurred as the result of an injurious fall in the hospital. In turn, this provides an opportunity for hospitalists to assume a medical leadership role with nursing and hospital administration to design processes of care that prevent injurious falls.

IDENTIFYING THE PATIENT AT RISK OF FALLING

A national database examined rates of falls among adult patients in 1263 hospitals on surgical, medical and medical-surgical nursing units, and found a rate of 3.56 falls/1000 patient days. Rates vary by hospital unit with fall rates of 4.03/1000 patient days and injurious fall rates of 1.08/1000 patient days on medical units; and fall rates on surgery units of 2.76/1000 patient days and injurious falls rate of 0.67/1000 patient days. The incidence of in-hospital falls is higher among the patients 65 years of age and older with estimates of 3 to 17 per 1000 patient days. Patients over the age of 85 who fall in the hospital are the most likely to incur injury because of the fall. These oldest patients fall at a rate of 3.3 to 11.5 falls and 0.9 injurious falls per 1000 patient days. Patient safety groups suggest a benchmark rate of 2.5 to 3.5 falls per 1000 patient days with an ambitious goal rate of no >0.1 injurious falls per 1000 patient days. Most falls in the hospital occur in patients' rooms and bathrooms during transfers between the bed and a chair or while using the toilet or shower. So how do hospitals and providers go about either lowering the rate of injurious falls through prevention efforts or of reducing the level of

harm incurred by an injurious fall? Falls prevention starts with recognition of risk factors that predispose a patient to falling.

Most falls occur because of a multifactorial etiology rather than a unifactorial (single) cause. A fall is a complex event that often results from an interaction between patient-related, *intrinsic*, characteristics and environmental, *extrinsic*, challenges imposed on the patient (**Table 87-2**). Some intrinsic risk factors, such as delirium or deconditioned state, may be preventable or modifiable. In the hospital setting, the presence of cognitive impairment due to dementia or delirium poses the highest risk of falling. Thus, predisposition to falling often exists in certain people, especially older patients, before they arrive at the hospital. The acuity and impact of illness in hospitalized adults over age 65 add to the risk of falling in the hospital.

Fall rates in hospitals vary by unit type, with falls on medicine units eclipsing the rate of falls on surgical and intensive care units. Once admitted to the hospital, patients rapidly decondition when kept immobile or confined to bed because of (1) medical reasons, (2) restraints or tethers (intravenous lines, urinary bladder catheters, oxygen tubing, feeding tubes), or (3) reservations of staff about transferring patients or allowing walking by patients with poor baseline physiologic reserve. Immobilizing patients within a day or two of admission leads to unintended consequences. Medically complex and seriously ill patients quickly become physically debilitated and unsteady to walk safely, placing them at risk of sustaining an injurious fall when they do attempt to get out of bed in the hospital and after transition to home or a postacute care facility.

Extrinsic factors include the added hazards imposed by the hospital's physical environment. Furthermore, unfamiliar obstacles or surroundings challenge the debilitated patient who tries to navigate a hospital room or hallway. Taking multiple medications, including anticholinergic medications and others that act on the central nervous system (CNS) adversely affects cognition, safety, and balance, adding to the environmental challenges implicated in falls. Examples of medications known to increase fall risk include those that cause orthostatic hypotension and cerebral hypoperfusion (specifically loop diuretics, antihypertensive medications such as α-blockers and vasodilators) and those that act directly on the CNS (antidepressants, antipsychotics, and sedative-hypnotics such as benzodiazepines).

Certain combinations of factors place some hospitalized patients at a particularly high risk of suffering a fall-related injury. The patient populations at highest risk of a serious injury caused by a fall in the hospital include patients over the age of 85, those with osteoporosis and other bone diseases, patients receiving anticoagulation treatment or have bleeding disorders, and patients with sutured wounds after a recent surgery (particularly amputation, abdominal, and thoracic surgeries). The presence of four or more intrinsic and extrinsic risk factors also seems to confer a higher risk of injury after a fall. In a common scenario where multiple risk factors for a fall coexist, a confused patient on intravenous fluids and anticoagulation therapy falls while getting out of bed at night to go to the bathroom in a poorly lit room without anyone to assist him. Where there are multiple risk factors predisposing patients to falling, there are multiple opportunities to implement interventions to prevent a fall.

■ BEFORE THE FALL: FALL PREVENTION

Fall prevention starts with (1) assessing the patient's likelihood or risk of falling and (2) identifying the presence of the risk factors most strongly associated with injurious falls. Many hospitals have formal systems in place for the nursing staff to conduct a routine fall risk assessment upon admission to the hospital. Some task physical therapists with assessing fall risk. Of note, communication between providers about the findings on these risk assessments is variable, and the documentation of the assessment can be challenging to find in the hospital record. Studies suggest that effective fall prevention requires an interdisciplinary (nursing, physician and/or advance practice provider, rehabilitation therapist, clinical pharmacist, care manager) team approach to the risk assessment, prevention, and treatment of someone potentially at risk of falling.

Fall risk assessment tools are divided into those that predict a probability of falling (risk screening tools) and those that assess factors that contribute to the patient's risk of falling (risk factor assessment tools). These tools are commonly used at health care systems level to stratify risk and target interventions to patients with the highest risk of falling. The most common validated tools used for risk screening are summarized in **Table 87-3**. But, none of them demonstrates both high predictive value and ease of administration. They have high false-positive rates (low specificity), low positive predictive value, and/or are cumbersome to perform. Ultimately, risk screening tools in clinical trials without multifactorial interventions have not proven effective at reducing the incidence of falls, and, in particular, injurious falls in the hospital.

Simple risk assessment, on the other hand, starts at the bedside, that is, at the patient level with team members identifying each patient's intrinsic and extrinsic risk factors for falling. But which risk factors are most strongly associated with falls that cause serious injury? One study found that use of certain medications, selective serotonin reuptake inhibitors, conferred the highest risk of sustaining a severe injury as a result of a fall. Other studies consistently suggest that use of CNS-active medications, including benzodiazepines, antidepressants and antipsychotic medications, places older patients in particular at increased risk of falling. Although falls risk factors are well established, empirical evidence suggests that risk

---

TABLE 87-3 Falls Risk Screening Tools

Tool	Items measured	Scoring	Comments
Morse Fall Scale	• History of falling • Secondary diagnosis of falls • Use of ambulatory aid • Intravenous therapy • Gait impaired • Mental status impaired	• Yes/No responses for each item • Each item is weighted • Total score = 0-125 • Low risk = 0-24 • Medium risk = 25-44 • High risk = 45-100	• Oldest of validated falls risk tools • Time consuming to complete • Low positive predictive value for incident falls • Low specificity
St. Thomas Risk Assessment Tool in Falling Elderly Inpatients (STRATIFY)	• Fall on or during admission to hospital • Agitation present • Vision impaired • Need frequent toileting • Transfer/mobility impaired	• Yes/No responses for each item • Total score = 0-5 • Fall risk ≥ 2	• Validated falls risk tool • Simple scoring • Low positive predictive value • The population and setting affect STRATIFY performance
Hendrich II	• Confusion/disorientation • Depression • Altered elimination • Dizziness/vertigo • Male gender • Administered antiepileptics • Administered benzodiazepines • Abnormal "Get up and Go" item #2 (rising from chair)	• Yes/No responses • Each item is weighted • Total score = 0-20 • High risk ≥ 5	• Validated falls risk tool • Brief tool • Only tool that includes at-risk medications • Slightly higher specificity than the Morse scale • Low positive predictive value

factors for injurious falls are not as easily identified by health care professionals. Perhaps that is due in part to the fact that injuries, notably serious injuries, from a fall in hospital occur at a relatively low rate of approximately 10%. Even so, a cognitively impaired patient (with delirium, dementia, or both) who is unable to transfer independently from bed to a chair or to stand up without assistance might be readily identifiable as a patient at high risk of falling and sustaining a serious injury. Furthermore, virtually any acutely ill older adult, previously not regarded as being at high risk, can become high risk due to incident functional and cognitive impairments, polypharmacy, prolonged bed rest and immobility, and an environment that is hostile to independent and safe patient activity.

WHAT WORKS TO REDUCE FALLS AND INJURIES?

Strategies to prevent falls and injuries can be divided into unifactorial or multifactorial interventions to reduce fall risk factors, changes to improve the safety of the patient environment, and education of patients/staff. In a leadership role, hospitalists have the opportunity to be engaged in each of these strategies. The first step requires fall-risk screening (Table 87-3) to identify patients considered at risk of falling and target them to receive universal and/or specific interventions. Universal falls prevention interventions are standard procedures applied to all patients admitted to the hospital, regardless of how many risk factors they may have. For example, nursing staff orient all

patients to the hospital environment. All patients' possessions and a call bell are placed within easy reach. Floor surfaces in all patients' rooms are clean and dry, and all patients receive nonskid socks to wear. The hospitalist's or physical therapist's initial assessment of the patient's baseline physical strength and mobility limitations should be noted during the medical history and physical exam. Common interventions in high-risk patients include 1:1 monitoring with a sitter or companion, use of bed and chair alarms, physical therapy, supervised and scheduled toileting, judicious review and modification of medication lists containing medications that increase risk of falls, or a combination of these in a multifactorial, patient-specific intervention.

Fall prevention interventions in hospitals are typically complex, involving multiple components that depend on leadership involvement and the cooperation of front-line staff from multiple disciplines (**Table 87-4**). The hospital leadership is responsible for making sure that hospital staff is adequately trained to assess each patient's risk of falling and that interventions are in place to prevent falls resulting in injury. But, which intervention or combination of interventions achieves meaningful risk reduction?

A recent systematic review of several aspects (implementation, components, adherence, and effectiveness) of hospital-based fall prevention programs demonstrates broad variability in both the interventions and the clinical outcomes. In the review of 59 studies, most interventions consisted of a multicomponent approach, including risk

TABLE 87-4 Interventions that May Potentially Prevent Falls and/or Fall-Related Injuries in Acute Care Hospitals

Intervention Domain	Intervention Type	Fall Prevention	Injury Prevention	Supportive Evidence Base
Exercises	Physical, occupational therapy	X		X
	General physical activity	X		
Medication Modification Targets	Antihypertensives	X	X	X
	Calcium	X	X	
Non pharmacologic Treatment	Vitamin D	X	X	
Substitution Targets	Reduce burden of medications active on the central nervous system (benzodiazepines, sleep aids, narcotics, antipsychotics, antidepressants)	X	X	
	Anticoagulation therapy		X	
	Parkinson's' disease medications	X	X	
	Reduce polypharmacy	X	X	
Toileting and Incontinence Management	Scheduled toileting assistance	X	X	
	Bladder catheter need assessment	X		
Education and Behavior Change	Video, reading material	X	X	X
	Teach back	X	X	
Environmental Modifications/Assistive Techniques	Nursing assistance with daily activities	X	X	
	1:1 supervision by family member or caregiver	X	X	
	Hip protectors		X	
	Bedside floor mats		X	
	Adjustable-height beds		X	
	Bed and chair alarms	X	X	
	Location close to nurses station	X		
	Helmets		X	
	Removal of physical restraints	X	X	
	Brightly-colored wrist bands, identifiers of risk	X		
	Sensory impairment aids (hearing aids, glasses)	X		
	Flooring modification	X	X	
Delirium prevention bundle/ Acute Care for Elders	Enhance mobility, physical functioning and cognition; multidisciplinary care; safe environment	X		X

assessments, visual risk alerts, patient education, care rounds, bed-exit alarms, and postfall evaluations. However, many of the clinical trials to decrease falls incidence took place in multiple institutional settings (such as subacute or rehabilitation units as well as the acute care hospital), limiting the ability to apply the study results to the acute care setting. Even when data from multiple randomized trials are analyzed together, the rate of falls is relatively low. The rate of falls with injuries is even lower, often too low to achieve significant point estimates.

While patients with multiple intrinsic risk factors seem to be at greater risk of falling, one study of 16 medical-surgical hospital units found that only a few independent variables, namely the use of certain classes of CNS-active medications, were associated with injury after a hospital fall. Only one randomized controlled trial designed specifically to prevent falls and restricted to acute care hospitals demonstrated a significant reduction in the incidence of falls. No studies showed benefits of a program on the incidence of injurious falls. However, there are numerous reports of quality improvement studies that show sometimes dramatic reductions in falls. Most quality improvement interventions combine multiple strategies and care processes to reduce falls. These may include risk assessment, visual alerts indicating risk, patient and family education, care rounds, bed-exit alarms, and post fall evaluations. Often, interventions are applied only to persons identified as being at high risk. In some quality improvement studies the benefits are not sustained over time, whereas sustained effects are seen in up to 5 years in others. In a quality improvement study a fall risk screening instrument linked to specific interventions administered by nurses, including strategies related to age >85 years, bleeding risk, increased risk of fracture such as osteoporosis, and recent surgery, reduced serious injury in two Veteran's Hospital medical-surgical units. Lean and rapid improvement event techniques, reflecting the commitment of hospital leadership, reduced total fall rates and falls with injury in a 16-month post-test. Reduction in falls related to injuries was observed in another hospital system that employed a rapid improvement event technique. A multidisciplinary team of health care professionals engaged in acute hospital care created effective screening techniques and interventions targeted at hospitalized patients at risk for falls with injury.

Most reported falls prevention interventions are multifactorial. Unifactorial interventions such as bed alarms have not been effective in reducing falls or injuries but are often included as part of a care-bundle in a multidisciplinary intervention.

> Best evidence: In older medical patients reducing risk factors for hospital-acquired delirium significantly reduces incident falls.

Risk factors identified as modifiable may be the most appropriate targets for unifactorial and/or multifactorial interventions (**Figure 87-1**). In a meta-analysis of 14 interventional studies designed to decrease the incidence of hospital-acquired delirium, the odds of falls decreased significantly among intervention patients in four studies by 62%; and in two randomized or matched trials the odds of falls decreased by 64%. The authors note that these results represent the equivalent of 4.26 falls prevented per 1000 patient days. A systematic review and meta-analysis of Acute Care for Elders shows that patients receiving the intervention have a significant 49% reduced risk of falls. Neither study reported the effect on the incidence of injurious falls.

Both acute care and delirium prevention models are multidisciplinary in focus and target reduction of risk factors for common geriatric conditions or syndromes such as hospital falls. Successful programs reduced the incidence of falls by enhancing the patient's performance of activities of daily living (ADL), mobility and cognition. Optimizing patient hearing and vision with aids and other devices, occupational therapy for enhancing physical functioning and assistive devices including adaptive equipment serve to enhance independent ADL functioning. Hospital providers enhance mobility by not writing orders that keep patients in bed, and avoid physically restrain patients "for safety," and minimizing use of various tethers. A mobility protocol targets therapies based on assessment of the patient's ability to move freely in bed, transfer from bed to chair, stand and initiate walking. Typically performed by bedside nurse or physical therapists, the mobility protocol includes guidance regarding transfers from bed to chair and for allowing patients to ambulate independently. Providers may help enhance cognition by avoiding

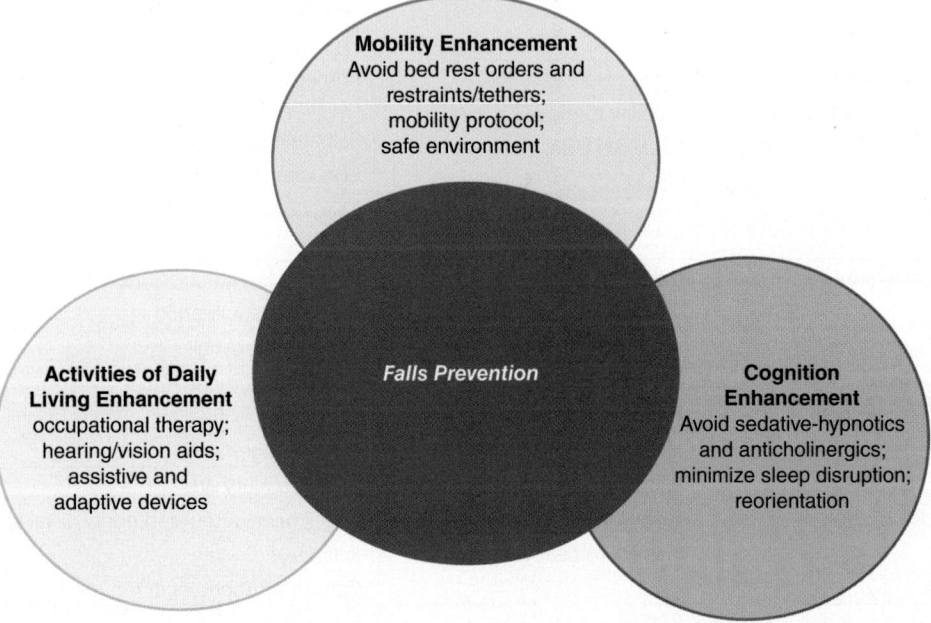

Figure 87-1 *Prevention of hospital falls by enhancement of patient performance of daily activities, mobility, and cognition.*

or reducing the use of medications that reduce brain perfusion and cause orthostasis (vasodilating medications, alpha adrenergic blockers) and by minimizing doses of CNS-active (antipsychotics, sedative hypnotics, and antidepressants) medications. Sleep protocols also enhance cognition by minimizing sleep disruption that occurs when vital signs or blood tests are obtained during sleeping hours. Reality reorientation by nursing staff, including reminders of the day, time, and upcoming events, and reintroduction of self to patients on rounds, all serve to enhance patient cognition and engagement in medical care. The hospitalist can identify other modifiable risk factors, such as generalized weakness (reducing mobility) or potential adverse medication effects, balancing benefits and harms of any treatment.

Another approach is to combine falls risk assessment with a "safe" physical environment that reduces the risk of falls for all patients irrespective of risk-factor screening scores or individual risk considerations. This systems approach is an extension of the concepts of continuous quality improvement where changes in the physical environment create congruence with patient needs and safety. Incongruence between the older patient's needs and a hospital environment may play an important role in this decline in functional capacity of hospitalized older patients, potentially leading to increased risk of injurious falls. Hence, adaptation of the physical environment to assure a patient's independent function and safety may be an effective way of reducing the rate of injurious falls. Previous experience has suggested that carpeted floors or highly resilient synthetic floor materials, hand rails in the hallways and in patient rooms to promote mobility, elevated toilet seats to enable safe toileting, adequate lighting to enable patients to exit rooms or toilet safely may enhance patient safety and reduce risk of falls. The Institute for Healthcare Improvement advocates a checklist approach to environmental fall risk assessment. In leadership roles, hospitalists may work with nurses, environmental engineers, physical and occupational therapists and patient safety teams to assure a safe physical environment that encourages patient mobility and reduces risk of serious injury in the event of an accidental fall. Environmental considerations include characteristics of patient rooms: adequate lighting, unobstructed path to the bathroom, safely arranged furnishings, furniture free of sharp edges, beds at the lowest setting whenever possible, patient's personal belongings within reach, handrails provided in patient bathroom are properly secured, and nonslip surfaces in patient showers. Other environmental considerations include: floor surfaces free of tripping hazards, hallways clear/clutter free to allow patient ambulation, and nonslippery floors.

Successful falls prevention programs are multifactorial. Unifactorial (isolated) interventions appear not to work. Hip protectors, movement (bed) alarms, and low beds do not appear to reduce falls or injury in the hospital setting. Modifiable intrinsic and extrinsic risk factors identified through risk assessment and strategies to create "safe" physical environments for patients may be the most appropriate targets for multicomponent fall prevention interventions.

APPROACH TO THE FALLEN PATIENT

Hospitalists are often called to the bedside to evaluate the fallen patient. Suggestions for the hospitalist's workup of a fallen patient are found in **Table 87-5**. A comprehensive approach to risk factor identification and possible injuries (Table 87-1) is advisable and often informs clinical decision-making. For example, patients with

---

TABLE 87-5 Suggested Workup of the Fallen Patient Based on Site-specific Injuries

Site of Injury	Type of Injury	Signs and Symptoms of Injury	Evaluation and Management Options
Head	Traumatic brain injury (concussion, subdural hematoma) Stroke	Altered consciousness, Acute/subacute confusion, Headache, Light-headedness, Visual changes, Focal neurologic deficit	Stop anticoagulation If anticoagulated and bleeding, consider administration of vitamin K Mental status assessment Neurology, Neurosurgery consult Perform neurologic assessments every 2 h for 24-48 h Imaging
Spinal Column	Cord injury Vertebral fracture	Absence of sensation. Inability to move Localized pain	Immediate stabilization of spine and immobilization with backboard, rigid cervical collar, lateral head supports Palpate entire spine Consult spine surgery for assessment Imaging with x-rays, CT scan Analgesia
Skin	Laceration	Bleeding Visible alteration of skin integrity	Hemostasis with pressure, ice Cleansing, sterilization Suturing, stapling Pain management
	Ecchymoses	Discoloration	Ice Pain management
Extremities	Fracture Dislocation	Pain Limb, joint deformity Inability to bear weight	Visualize injury site Check neurovascular integrity distal to injury site Splint site Consult orthopedics or reduce dislocation
Abdominal and Pelvic Injuries	Blunt trauma Pelvic fracture	Pain	Physical exam x-ray/CT

dementia, delirium, or altered mental status may not be able to provide accurate description of the fall and injury that occurred. They might not be able to verbalize or communicate important symptoms. Therefore, some detective work on the part of the hospitalist, along with a high index of suspicion for occult or serious injury, is required in order to avoid missing important injuries.

The assessment of a fallen patient begins with a documentation of the circumstances of the fall and the condition of the fallen patient. Assessment of the fallen patient includes a set of vital signs followed by a focused physical examination for the presence of injury to the brain, spine, or other musculoskeletal site. The hospitalist determines if the patient lost consciousness and whether to embark on a syncope evaluation. A thorough pain assessment is warranted along with prompt and appropriate analgesia (ice, splinting, analgesic medication) for the fallen patient in pain. The remaining workup concentrates on specific sites of injury (Table 87-5). Often, patients who have fallen are unaware of having hit their head on the floor. Any evidence of cervical or cranial injury should prompt the hospitalist to order frequent checks of mental status and vital signs and to order neuroimaging should there be any concern of intracranial hemorrhage, fracture or subdural hematoma. When clinical suspicion is high, multiple x-ray views are obtained for all injury sites. A computed tomography (CT) scan is recommended when clinical suspicion is high and x-rays are negative (especially for hip and vertebral compression fractures), as some fractures might not be evident on plain films. Lacerations and ecchymoses on face or scalp prompt further evaluation for concussion and traumatic brain injury.

In elderly or frail patients a pelvic fracture can be sustained from low energy trauma such as a fall from a standing position. Such pelvic fractures should not be overlooked as they are associated with significant bleeding and concomitant injuries including muscle contusions, and high mortality. Intra-abdominal organ injury is rare in falls, but is possible when the patient suffered blunt abdominal trauma.

Hospitalists are often asked to participate in a root-cause analysis with nursing staff after a patient falls with serious injury. Bundled interventions are often implemented after a fall with serious injury. The team analysis often identifies intrinsic and extrinsic factors predisposing to falls, which leads to interventions that are used to prevent incident falls. This experience helps the team calibrate its falls screening and prevention approaches, which are most effective in multidisciplinary settings. Hospitalists in a leadership role have the opportunity to improve patient safety and hospital-outcomes metrics while working with the multidisciplinary team.

CONCLUSION

Hospitals and their staff are now accountable for injuries that occur as a result of a fall in the hospital. The hospitalist plays both a role in efforts to prevent or reduce injurious falls and in the evaluation and management of patients who have fallen in the hospital. Key to both roles is the hospital physician's ability to recognize and modify, to the extent possible, each patient's intrinsic and extrinsic risk factors for falling and injurious falls.

SUGGESTED READINGS

Bouldin EL, Andresen EM, Dunton NE, et al. Falls among adult patients hospitalized in the United States: prevalence and trends. *J Patient Saf*. 2013;9:13.

Cameron ID, Gillespie LD, Robertson MC, et al. Interventions for preventing falls in older people in care facilities and hospitals. *Cochrane Database Syst Rev*. 2012;12:CD005465.

Hempel S, Newberry S, Wang Z, et al. Hospital fall prevention: a systematic review of implementation, components, adherence, and effectiveness. *J Am Geriatr Soc*. 2013;61:483.

Hshieh TT, Yue J, Oh E, et al. Effectiveness of multicomponent nonpharmacological delirium interventions. A meta-analysis. *JAMA Intern Med*. 2015;175:512.

Institute for Health Care Improvement (IHI). Transforming Care at the Bedside How-to Guide: Reducing Patient Injuries from Falls: http://www.ihi.org/resources/Pages/Tools/TCABHowToGuideReducingPatientInjuriesfromFalls.aspx. Accessed November 4, 2015.

Miake-Lye IM, Hempel S, Ganz DA, Shekelle PG. Inpatient fall prevention programs as a patient safety strategy. *Ann Intern Med*. 2013;158:390.

Mion LC, Chandler AM, Waters TM, et al. Is it possible to identify risks for injurious falls in hospitalized patients? *Jt Comm J Qual Patient Saf*. 2012;38;408.

National Quality Forum (NQF). A detailed guideline for the screening and detection of older patients at risk of falling. In: *Safe Practices for Better Healthcare–2010 Update: A Consensus Report*. Washington, DC: NQF; 2010.

Quigley PA, Hahm B, Powell-Cope G, Sarduy I, Tyndal K, White SV. Reducing serious injury from falls in two Veterans' Hospital medical-surgical units. *J Nurs Care Qual*. 2009;24:33.

CHAPTER 88

Fever and Rash

Shanta M. Zimmer, MD

Key Clinical Questions

1. What are the most common causes of fever and rash in the hospitalized patient?
2. What is the pathophysiology of fever and rash?
3. What other clinical symptoms and findings are associated with fever and rash?
4. How can laboratory tests help with diagnosis of the etiology of rash?

CASE 88-1

A 25-year-old graduate student who was living in student housing presented to the hospital complaining of a 4-day history of upper respiratory tract symptoms that have progressed to include fever and rash on his extremities. The rash began on his hands and feet as a pink, flat rash, but has progressed over the last several hours to be purplish in nature, and extends now to his trunk and face. He is admitted to your service for further evaluation and treatment.

The rapid progression of the patient's rash and the appearance of macular rash that progressed to petechiae and purpura raised immediate concern for meningococcemia. The patient was placed in droplet precautions, blood cultures were collected, and ceftriaxone therapy initiated. Vital signs revealed blood pressure of 110/60, pulse rate of 118, respiratory rate of 24, and temperature of 39.2°C. No nuchal rigidity was noted. The patient's respiratory status declined and he was admitted to the intensive care unit (ICU) and intubated. Blood cultures grew *Neisseria meningitidis* at 24 hours and laboratory findings were consistent with disseminated intravascular coagulation (DIC). A lumbar puncture was not performed due to severe thrombocytopenia. Multisystem organ failure developed rapidly.

INTRODUCTION

The clinical presentation of patients with rash and fever must first be divided into categories of those who are critically ill versus those who are not. Critically ill patients with rash often have the fulminant onset of both fever and rash, and must be diagnosed quickly to receive appropriate care. The timing of the rash is important for judging the severity of the disease, with rapid onset often portending a more rapidly progressive course. The most worrisome cause of fulminant onset of rash is septicemia, especially purpura fulminans of meningococcemia, which can progress over hours or even minutes. Gradual or waxing and waning rash and fever suggest a more chronic process, or one that may be noninfectious, such as rheumatological disease or malignancy.

PRACTICE POINT

- Patients presenting in the hospital with rash and fever must be divided into two categories: those who are critically ill and those who are not. Causes of critical illness include hemorrhagic fever, meningococcemia, Rocky Mountain spotted fever, toxic shock syndrome, Stevens-Johnson syndrome, toxic epidermal necrolysis, and acute vasculitis.

APPROACH TO FEVER AND RASH AT THE BEDSIDE

Some acute rash and fever syndromes are caused by infectious diseases that can be spread by airborne or respiratory droplets. Therefore, before beginning the history and physical, if such a transmissible disease is suggested, appropriate precautions should be instituted (**Figure 88-1**).

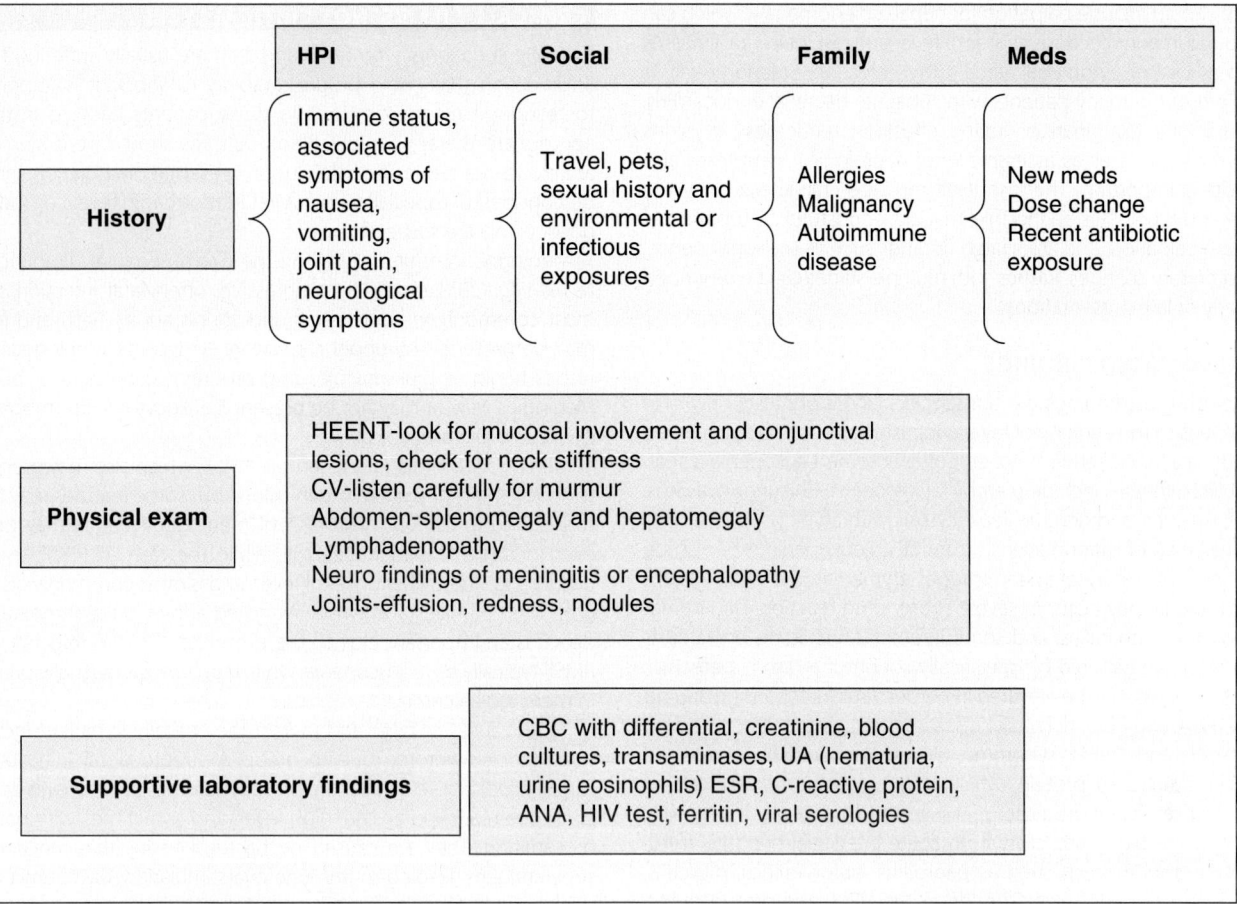

Figure 88-1 *History, physical, and laboratory tests in patients with fever and rash.*

HISTORY

The age of the patient and the season of the year provide important epidemiologic clues to the differential diagnosis. Patients should be asked about location of onset of rash and time sequence of progression of rash. Physicians should enquire about secondary changes to the rash possibly due to self-treatments, such as lotions and over-the-counter ointments, or from excoriation or picking. When multiple lesions are present, it may be helpful to ask the patient, "Can you show me an area that looks like how the rash started?" or "Are there any new lesions?" Associated symptoms of fever, sore throat, lymphadenopathy, and other systemic symptoms such as weight loss and joint pain should also be noted. Ask about new medications, recently discontinued medications, or dosing changes in old medications. While many allergic reactions occur within the first several days or weeks of an exposure to a new drug, some reactions do not occur until after more prolonged exposure; in particular, antiepileptic drugs such as phenytoin are notorious for presenting with fever and rash after a few weeks of exposure, and only rarely within the first few days. Family and personal history of fever syndromes or allergies can also be a clue to the risk of drug allergy. Although often

overlooked in adult patients, vaccination history and prior history of illnesses of childhood are important when evaluating fever and rash presentations. Family history of rheumatologic diseases should also be obtained, including history of lupus, vasculitis, or juvenile onset arthritis. Social, travel, and exposure histories are especially important when evaluating patients with fever and rash. Sexual history might suggest risk factors for acute human immunodeficiency virus (HIV) infection, syphilis, or gonococcal disease. Travel to endemic areas may suggest exposures to certain mosquito-borne illnesses such as dengue, Chikungunya fever, or malaria or tick-borne illnesses such as Rocky Mountain spotted fever (RMSF) or Lyme disease. Social history should include exposures to small children either through work (daycare, school teacher), or home.

PHYSICAL EXAM

As with all hospitalized patients, vital signs and general appearance contribute to the overall gestalt of the patient's condition. Pulse-temperature dissociation (elevated temperature without elevation pulse) may be a clue to infection with intracellular pathogens such as *Rickettsia*, and is often present with drug reactions. Localized, tender lymph nodes suggest a bacterial etiology, while diffuse lymphadenopathy suggests lymphoma or a disseminated viral infection such as Epstein-Barr virus (EBV) or HIV. There is growing recognition that drug reactions can be associated with lymphadenopathy. Drug rash with eosinophilia and systemic symptoms (DRESS) syndrome should be included in the differential of fever, rash and lymphadenopathy.

Careful attention to oral and genital membranes on physical exam can identify mucosal rashes or ulcers. Cardiac exam should include careful evaluation for a new murmur or evidence of congestive heart failure, which could point to endocarditis. Abdominal exam should include palpation for hepatosplenomegaly, which can be found in noninfectious causes of fever and rash or in viral illnesses such as EBV or cytomegalovirus (CMV) infection. Splenomegaly is also present in many patients with subacute bacterial endocarditis. Careful joint examination, noting effusions, tenderness, or signs of synovitis, as well as assessment for neurological symptoms and deficits is important. The rash itself must be characterized by the color and type of lesion (nodule, macule, or pustule), distribution of lesions, palpation, and associated findings such as scale, purulence, or secondary changes. Rashes with multiple stages can be described as early or late presentations.

■ ASSOCIATED FINDINGS

Although most findings are nonspecific, laboratory tests may provide clues to the etiology of fever and rash. Eosinophilia suggests an allergic reaction or cholesterol emboli syndrome. Leukopenia is seen with viral illnesses including arboviral infections, Chikungunya virus, CMV, measles, and dengue; leukocytosis with atypical lymphocytes is a hallmark of mononucleosis from EBV. Leukopenia may also be a prominent feature of systemic lupus erythematosus (SLE). Thrombocytopenia may occur in severe sepsis, drug reaction, DIC, hematological malignancies, and some infections, including ehrlichiosis and RMSF, and should be specifically sought if a rash is petechial. Transaminases may be elevated in herpes virus infections (including CMV, HSV, and EBV), rickettsial diseases, toxic shock, β-lactam drug reactions, and DRESS syndrome. Urinalysis should be performed for hematuria and protein, which may be a clue to vasculitis or endocarditis. When drug allergy is suspected, urinary sediment may reveal white blood cell casts from acute interstitial nephritis (AIN), associated with drugs such as penicillins, sulfonamides, diuretics, nonsteroidal anti-inflammatory drugs (NSAIDs), and proton pump inhibitors. However, the absence of urinary sediment changes does not exclude the diagnosis, and kidney biopsy may be needed if renal function is deteriorating.

THE RASH

Lesion appearance is critical to diagnosis and in communicating appropriately with consultants (**Table 88-1**). For a thorough description of all lesion types and associated differential diagnosis, a dermatology textbook should be consulted. Common lesions associated with fever and rash are limited, and for the most part include macules, vesicles and bullae, papules, nodules, and sometimes plaques.

PRACTICE POINT

- Appearance of the lesions is critical to determining the differential diagnosis and also in communicating appropriately with consultants.

CRITICALLY ILL VS. NOT CRITICALLY ILL

Critically ill patients with fever and rash are usually suffering from an infection that could progress rapidly to shock. It is important to recognize diagnostic signs in these patients early to institute appropriate therapy rapidly. Blood cultures should be drawn and antibiotics started immediately upon presentation. Isolation should be considered, especially when viral hemorrhagic fevers or meningococcemia are suspected.

Meningococcemia, caused by the Gram-negative diplococcus, *N. meningitidis*, is a rapidly progressive, often fatal infection seen most commonly in adolescents and young adults. Rash and fever may be preceded by upper respiratory symptoms. Meningococcal rashes begin as pink macules and progress to purpura or bullae. Meningitis may or may not be present. Leukocytosis, thrombocytopenia, and DIC are typical.

Meningococcemia may resemble RMSF, which also may progress to shock and multisystem organ failure, but some features may help to distinguish the two. The rash of meningococcemia may begin even before the patient feels ill, while the rash of RMSF usually occurs 3 to 5 days after onset of fever, and is most commonly distributed on the ankles and wrists. As noted above, pulse-temperature deficit is an important clue to the presence of RMSF. Patients with RMSF typically have leucopenia, while leukocytosis is usually present in meningococcemia.

Other causes of fever and rash in the critically ill patient include toxic shock syndrome due to group A streptococcal infection or *Staphylococcus aureus* infection. These syndromes present with diffuse erythroderma, hypotension, high fever, and sometimes with nausea or vomiting. They are caused by bacterial toxins that function as superantigens, leading to immune overstimulation; bacteremia may or may not be present. Treatment of the critically ill patient with fever and rash is directed at the underlying illness, and will often include empiric coverage for staphylococcal (both methicillin-sensitive and methicillin-resistant) and streptococcal infections. If toxic shock syndrome is suspected, an infectious disease specialist should be consulted for consideration of intravenous immunoglobulin infusion and appropriate antibiotic selection, including addition of clindamycin in streptococcal infections for its antitoxin effect. Early surgical consultation is mandated in patients with necrotizing fasciitis and myonecrosis, as rapid debridement of affected tissue can be life-saving.

CASE 88-2

A 57-year-old diabetic man with end-stage liver disease secondary to hepatitis C was admitted to the hospital for fevers and found to have methicillin-resistant *S. aureus* (MRSA) bacteremia. He was started on vancomycin on admission, but fevers persisted for the next 3 days. On hospital day 4, he developed a diffuse macular rash on his abdomen, chest, arms, and legs, as well as an increased temperature of 38.8°C.

TABLE 88-1 Description of Common Types of Skin Lesions and Examples of Pathologic Causes

Macule	Papule	Nodule	Vesicle/Bulla	Pustule	Plaque
Flat, in the plane of the skin, nonpalpable	Small, solid, raised, palpable	Larger papule, solid	Fluid-filled blister, usually clear or bloody fluid	Small, blister filled with pus	Flat, like a macule, but palpable and usually larger; may have secondary changes such as scale or crusting
Drug rash, viral exanthema, syphilis, HIV	Viral, allergic reaction, stigmata of endocarditis	Erythema nodosum, fungal or atypical mycobacterial infections	Varicella, HSV, bullous diseases, drug eruptions	Bacterial infection or superinfection	Psoriasis, MCTD, syphilis, atypical drug eruption, malignancy

The rash was most prominent on the trunk, and had a macular appearance with irregular borders and areas of confluence. The erythema was blanching and seemed to be spreading. The patient was otherwise well appearing, and complained of slight itchiness on his abdomen. Suspecting allergic drug eruption, his physicians checked carefully in the mouth and genital region for evidence of mucosal erythema, ulceration, or sloughing. Orders included repeat blood cultures, urinalysis with microscopy, urinary eosinophils, complete blood count (CBC) with differential, and a chemistry panel, including creatinine and transaminases. In the meantime, vancomycin was held.

Medication hypersensitivity is a common cause of fever and rash in hospitalized patients, and antibiotics are among the most often implicated agents in cutaneous adverse drug reactions (CADR). Several clinical clues suggest the medication as the cause of fever and rash. Timing of initiation of the drug is important, but not always helpful since patients may develop allergy to a medication at any time during its use. Allergic reactions to antibiotics commonly occur after 7 to 10 days of therapy, but may occur immediately or at a later time. Fever from drug rash is often very high (>38.8°C) and not associated with other symptoms of toxicity, such as tachycardia or hypotension. Skin findings usually include an erythematous macular rash that is sometimes papular and can involve any part of the body, including the palms and soles. Bullous lesions or mucosal ulceration are signs of severe disease and progression, so patients should be examined carefully for evidence of mucosal involvement, including oral, conjunctival, and genital areas. The presence of eosinophilia is supportive, but is not required for the diagnosis of drug reaction. Severe drug toxicity may also include hepatitis or renal involvement. In hospitalized patients, polypharmacy may make it difficult to determine which drug is responsible. Certain medications are more frequent causes of this presentation and should be eliminated first. Medication lists should be reviewed for new additions and unnecessary medications that can be eliminated or placed on hold.

Exanthematous (also known as morbilliform or maculopapular) drug eruption after administration of a new medication is the most common CADR in hospitalized patients, accounting for up to 90% of all drug rashes seen. Antibiotics (including sulfonamides, penicillins, and cephalosporins), antiepileptic medications, and NSAIDs are among the most commonly implicated agents.

Vancomycin is not among the most commonly cited causes of fever and rash, although this may change with the increased use of vancomycin for MRSA infections. Another cutaneous reaction associated with vancomycin, red person syndrome, consists of infusion-related flushing and erythema of the face, neck, and chest. This reaction abates with slowing the rate of infusion and antihistamine medications. Patients may have transient fever during the infusion, but prolonged fever with rash is more indicative of a true drug allergy.

The disease continuum of Stevens-Johnson syndrome (SJS)/toxic epidermal necrolysis (TEN) is life-threatening, albeit rare. SJS presents as an inflammatory reaction with erythroderma, mucosal involvement, and systemic symptoms. Mucosal involvement is a hallmark feature; another diagnosis should be considered if this is not present. Immune-mediated bullous diseases should be considered in the differential diagnosis. Although SJS/TEN may be idiopathic or occur in response to a viral infection, drugs are causative in approximately 70% of cases. Implicated drugs in one case-control study include sulfonamides, oxicam NSAIDs, anticonvulsants, and allopurinol. Surprisingly, corticosteroids were also associated with an increased risk of SJS. Coexisting conditions also increase the risk for SJS/TEN, especially HIV infection, SLE, and chronic EBV infection.

Treatment of SJS, which may be fatal in 5% to 15% of cases, includes immediate cessation of the offending drug. Multidisciplinary care is often required; dermatology and burn unit teams should be consulted promptly. Mucosal involvement may necessitate ophthalmology and urology involvement. Supportive care is the mainstay of therapy, including fluid and nutritional support. Corticosteroids are not recommended, but there is data to support a role for IVIG.

CASE 88-3

A 37-year-old woman with two small children presented to the hospital with fever, night sweats, and sore throat for several weeks. She also noted fatigue and knee pain. She denied travel, sick contacts, or exposure to pets or unclean water. She took no medications except ibuprofen, which alleviated some of her symptoms. Physical examination was notable for fever of 40°C and a macular rash over her chest, back, arms, and legs. The nonpalpable rash was lacy in appearance. Other notable findings include splenomegaly without other lymphadenopathy.

Her physicians are concerned about the possibility of lymphoma, mononucleosis-like illness, or a rheumatologic disease such as SLE or adult Still's disease. Blood cultures remained negative. Labs revealed elevated WBC, slight elevation in transaminases, evidence of prior infection with both EBV and CMV, elevated ESR, and ferritin of 15,000 ng/mL. ANA and RF were negative and complement levels were normal. CT scan of the chest, abdomen, and pelvis revealed splenomegaly and diffuse mediastinal and intraabdominal lymphadenopathy. Rheumatology was consulted for treatment of adult Still's disease.

The broad differential diagnosis of fever and rash includes bacterial syndromes such as bacteremia and endocarditis, viral illnesses such as EBV or CMV, SLE, adult Still's disease, familial Mediterranean fever and other periodic fever syndromes, vasculitis, or malignancy, especially lymphoma. Adult Still's disease is a diagnosis of exclusion because there is no gold standard and the overlap with rheumatologic and malignant diseases is great. In addition to exclusion of the above illnesses, the clinical criteria include arthralgias or arthritis, sore throat, and characteristic salmon-pink rash in an otherwise healthy patient with fever for greater than 2 weeks; additional laboratory features suggestive of this illness include a leukocytosis with a polymorphonuclear predominance and a markedly elevated ferritin level. Nonbulky adenopathy is common.

OTHER CLINICAL SYNDROMES

Viral illnesses in children cause many macular rashes with fever. Viral syndromes should also be considered in young adults or nonimmune adults with fever and rash. **EBV mononucleosis** presents with the familiar triad of fever, pharyngitis, and cervical lymphadenopathy. Liver involvement may be prominent in older patients with primary EBV infection. A rash is present in 10% of patients. Rash is more common in patients with EBV infection who receive amoxicillin and other antibiotics. The mechanism for this is unclear, but it does not seem to represent a true drug allergy.

Cytomegalovirus causes a mononucleosis-like syndrome in adults, with prolonged fever and malaise, mild hepatitis, and a rash in one-third of cases. Pharyngitis and cervical lymphadenopathy are less prominent in CMV mononucleosis, compared to EBV mononucleosis. **Parvovirus B19** in adults tends to present as a nonspecific flu-like illness. In children, parvovirus causes a maculopapular rash that clears centrally, leaving a lacy, reticular pattern. It may be prominent on the face, with a "slapped cheek" appearance. Although fever usually precedes the onset of rash in parvovirus by 2 to 5 days, in immunocompromised patients, the onset of fever can coincide with the rash. In adults, the rash is less pronounced. Adults with parvovirus often have a symmetric arthropathy of small joints that mimics rheumatoid arthritis; this is especially common in women.

Chikungunya virus, once an obscure tropical pathogen, has recently emerged from West Africa to become a scourge and nuisance in many parts of the world. In recent years, outbreaks have occurred in Italy, India, Indonesia, China, Malaysia, Thailand, the Caribbean, and much of Central and South America. Locally acquired cases have been reported in Florida and Puerto Rico. Chikungunya should be suspected in travelers to endemic regions returning with fever, rash, and distal arthritis and tenosynovitis which may be disabling.

Vesicular lesions should prompt concerns for **varicella**, as adults have more severe primary infection and are prone to pneumonia and respiratory failure, especially immunocompromised or pregnant patients. Varicella zoster (shingles) represents reactivation, rather than primary disease. It is usually limited to one or two dermatomes, but may disseminate in patients with immunodeficiency. **Primary HIV infection** is another important cause of fever and rash in adult patients. Although many different rashes have been described in the acute seroconversion syndrome associated with HIV infection, the rash is usually a diffuse, macular erythema typical of a viral exanthem. Patients suspected of having acute HIV infection should undergo testing with an HIV viral load rather than an HIV antibody, which is often negative in acute infection. HIV also increases the risk for drug reactions. Allergic reactions to sulfa antibiotics are especially common, even in patients who tolerated these drugs prior to HIV infection.

Syphilis, the great imitator, is another cause of fever and rash. The rash of secondary syphilis is variable, but is classically a papulosquamous eruption involving the palms and soles. A rash without a clear etiology should prompt an evaluation for syphilis with a treponemal antibody test. **Vasculitis** may cause fever and rash, with palpable purpura being typical. Dermatology and rheumatology consultation should be considered. Lesions often require biopsy for diagnosis. Multisystem involvement is the rule.

Finally, **malignancies** may present with fever and rash, especially lymphoma and some types of leukemia. Careful lymph node exam and examination of the peripheral blood smear are warranted when malignancy is considered. Skin and bone marrow biopsy may be required.

CONSULTATION

Critically ill patients with fever and rash should be treated empirically with appropriate antibiotics until infection has been excluded. Infectious disease consultation is prudent. Management of infection control questions and post-exposure prophylaxis for meningococcal infection can be facilitated by the hospital epidemiologist and infectious diseases service. For mild to moderate drug reactions due to antibiotics, infectious disease consultation can help choose alternative therapy. When toxic shock with necrotizing infection is suspected, timely surgical consultation should be done quickly as a life-saving and often limb-saving procedure may be needed. Dermatology should be consulted when the diagnosis of fever with rash is murky or when biopsy is indicated to diagnose suspected vasculitis or SJS/TEN. Rheumatology consultation may facilitate outpatient follow up for chronic conditions such as adult Still's disease, vasculitis, or SLE.

RISK MANAGEMENT

In drug-induced fever and rash, there may be questions of blame on the part of family members or patients. Although allergic drug reactions are often not avoidable if there is no known preexisting allergy, the severity and suddenness of the disease can be alarming. Communication with the patient and family members about the harm done by the medication is important in an ethical, professional, and open manner.

SUGGESTED READINGS

Coco A, Kleinhans E. Prevalence of primary HIV infection in symptomatic ambulatory patients. *Ann Fam Med*. 2005;3:400-404.

Fleming P, Marik PE. The DRESS syndrome: the great clinical mimicker. *Pharmacotherapy*. 2011;31(3):332.

Gruchalla RS, Pirmohamed M. Clinical practice. Antibiotic allergy. *N Engl J Med*. 2006;354:601-609.

Hazin R, Ibrahimi OA, Hazin MI, Kimyai-Asadi A. Stevens-Johnson syndrome: pathogenesis, diagnosis, and management. *Ann Med*. 2008;40:129-138.

Mahroum N, Mahagna H, Amital H. Diagnosis and classification of adult Still's disease. *J Autoimmun*. 2014;48-49:34-37.

Ramdial PK, Naidoo DK. Drug-induced cutaneous pathology. *J Clin Pathol*. 2009;62:493-504.

Ramos-e-Silva M, Pereira AL. Life-threatening eruptions due to infectious agents. *Clin Dermatol*. 2005;23:148-156.

Weaver SC, Lecuit M. Chikungunya virus and the global spread of a mosquito-borne disease. *N Engl J Med*. 2015;372:1231-1239.

CHAPTER 89

Headache

Rafael H. Llinas, MD

CASE 89-1

A 25-year-old, right-handed woman with a 3-year history of headaches is admitted to the hospital for "pain control." In the emergency department, she had a negative noncontrast head computed tomographic (CT) scan and was prescribed intravenous hydromorphone (Dilaudid).

Does the patient have any other medical problems or risk factors for intracranial pathology?

Her past medical history and review of systems is otherwise negative. Her family history is positive for migraine.

What factors worsen the headaches?

Tension and stress triggered her headaches, typically worse 2 or 3 days before her menstrual period begins. Alcohol, chocolates, and peanuts may aggravate her headache. She tried stopping the oral contraceptive and noticed no improvement in her headaches. Social history reveals that she is single and disabled from her headaches.

What medications has she tried?

She has tried many different medications, including analgesics, antidepressants, calcium channel blockers, and β-blockers. The only medications that help her are sumatriptan taken subcutaneously and narcotics, currently hydrocodone at least one tablet a day. She has been taking alprazolam 10 mg three times a day for a couple of years. She also uses promethazine for nausea. Recently she is beginning to have daily headaches and has to make trips to the emergency department to get shots of meperidine.

What has been her workup to date?

She has seen multiple neurologists. She has been treated with biofeedback and has seen psychologists. She had multiple CT scans and magnetic resonance imaging (MRI) of her head.

INTRODUCTION

Complaints of headache represent a major health problem due to their prevalence, chronicity, and the cost of ruling out life-threatening or serious underlying pathology that may cause significant morbidity and mortality.

The International Headache Society classifies headache as primary and secondary. Primary headaches account for at least 90% of all headaches and have benign outcomes. Primary headaches include migraine with or without aura, tension type headache, and less commonly, cluster headache. Some patients with a history of primary headaches have significant risk factors for developing secondary headaches. This chapter focuses on the diagnostic approach for the patient with headache in the hospital, and the reader is referred to subsequent chapters for specific management. Headache during hospitalization may occur due to:

- An initial presenting symptom of a systemic disease
- A complication of a diagnostic procedure or medical therapy acquired during hospitalization
- Coexisting benign headache syndromes (primary headaches)

For patients with preexisting headache syndromes, there may be significant drug interactions between medications used to treat chronic headache and those used to treat systemic disease, and there are also important contraindications to commonly used migraine medications that may limit the safety of these drugs in hospitalized patients.

PRIMARY HEADACHE

Elucidating the cause of a headache, particularly when severe, requires an understanding of the pathophysiology of the major headache types and recognizing the classic types of pain syndromes (and associated symptoms) they produce. Primary headaches should not cause focal neurologic signs and symptoms, except sometimes briefly during the aura phase of a complex migraine.

■ MIGRAINE

In general, migraine causes episodic severe headache pain associated with nausea, photophobia, and photophobia insensitivities to external stimuli. This disorder is typified as much by nausea and photophobia as it is by pain. Because of the severity of pain associated with migraines, it is the most common headache that leads patients to medical attention (even though it is not nearly as common as tension headaches). Environmental or physiologic stimuli trigger recurrent and stereotyped headache spells that may be associated with meningeal symptoms and signs. Many patients will describe an aura or warning beforehand. A history of recurrent headaches, similar in severity and character occurring with weather changes, the menstrual cycle, stress, sleep deprivation, excessive sleep, withdrawal from caffeine, or associated with ingestion of certain types of food are often migrainous headaches (**Table 89-1**). Migraine runs in families and can be associated with mitral valve prolapse. The precipitating etiology is probably electrical, much like seizures, rather than vasoconstriction followed by vasodilatation as previously thought.

In general, the most important question to answer when considering migraine is whether the patient has ever had a headache like this before. The classic question about the severity of headache—the worst headache ever—does not help distinguish between primary and secondary headache because every migraine sufferer will have the worst migraine of her life at some point, and the most severe headaches are more likely to trigger medical consultation. The evolution of symptoms may help distinguish migraine from other causes of neurologic deficit. Classically migraines begin mildly, following an aura, and worsen over minutes to hours to reach a pinnacle of pain. Patients can often predict when they are about to get a headache as they begin to feel ill or have mild photophobia as the symptoms begin to worsen over time. The pain is not maximal at onset.

PRACTICE POINT

Migraine

- Migraine sufferers usually experience positive phenomena (flashing lights) but complex migraine may be associated with speech or motor deficits.
- Migraine mimics such as stroke or transient ischemic attacks usually present with loss of function (weakness, lack of sensation, impaired vision, and language dysfunction).

At the bedside patients will often exhibit significant photophobia and complain of nausea, although not always with vomiting. They will often have some neck stiffness. Although migraines can occasionally present with focal neurological findings (termed complex migraines when such focal findings exist), it is best to assume that patients with severe headache and focal neurologic findings have something more ominous until proven otherwise.

TABLE 89-1 Diagnostic Criteria for Migraine

Migraine without aura

A. At least five attacks fulfilling criteria B-D below

B. Headache attacks lasting 4-72 h (untreated or unsuccessfully treated)

C. Headache has at least two of the following characteristics:
  1. Unilateral location
  2. Pulsating quality
  3. Moderate or severe intensity (inhibiting or prohibits daily activities)
  4. Aggravation by walking stairs or similar routine physical activity

D. During headache at least one of the following:
  1. Nausea and/or vomiting
  2. Photophobia and phonophobia

E. No evidence of contributing underlying disorder

Migraine with aura

A. At least two attacks fulfilling B

B. At least three of the following four characteristics:
  1. One or more fully reversible aura symptoms indicating focal cerebral cortical and/or brain stem dysfunction
  2. At least one aura symptom developing gradually over more than 4 min or two or more symptoms in succession
  3. No aura symptom lasting more than 60 min. If more than one aura symptom is present, accepted duration is proportionately increased
  4. Headache following aura with a free interval of less than 60 min. It may also begin before or simultaneously with the aura

C. No evidence of contributing underlying disorder

Headache Classification Committee of the International Headache Society. Classification and diagnostic criteria for headache disorders, cranial neuralgias and facial pain. *Cephalalgia*. 1988;8(Suppl 7):1-96.

■ TENSION OR MUSCLE CONTRACTION HEADACHES

Tension or muscle contraction headaches are a muscular pain syndrome similar to a strained muscle in any other portion of the body (**Table 89-2**). They commonly result from tension or spasm within the pain-sensitive muscles of the neck or temples in the setting of tight neck muscles, grinding of the jaw, and chronic stress. Patients do not describe disabling symptoms, photophobia, phonophobia, nausea, or vomiting.

PRACTICE POINT

Tension headache

- Muscular pain localizes poorly, and neck pain can present in many patients with referred pain to the cranial region.
- Giant cell arteritis can cause typical-sounding tension headaches. This diagnosis should be considered in patients over the age of 60, particularly when the headaches are new. Patients may give a history of transient visual loss or visual changes, or jaw claudication. The physical exam may reveal tenderness in the muscles of the shoulder as well the temples or scalp. There will almost always be an elevated erythrocyte sedimentation rate, commonly above 65 mm/h.

TABLE 89-2 Diagnostic Criteria for Tension Headache

A. At least 10 episodes fulfilling criteria B-D below (<180/y or <15/mo)

B. Headaches lasting from 30 min to 7 d

C. Headache has at least two of the following characteristics:

   1. Bilateral location

   2. Pressing/tightening (nonpulsatile) quality

   3. Mild or moderate intensity (may inhibit but does not prohibit activities)

   4. Not aggravated by routine physical activity such as walking or climbing stairs

D. Both of the following:

   1. No nausea or vomiting (anorexia may occur)

   2. Photophobia or phonophobia absent, or one but not the other present

E. No evidence of contributing underlying disorder

Data from Headache Classification Committee of the International Headache Society. Classification and diagnostic criteria for headache disorders, cranial neuralgias and facial pain. *Cephalalgia*. 1988;8(Suppl 7):1-96.

■ CLUSTER HEADACHES

Cluster headaches abruptly reach maximum intensity on one side of the head, last 1 to 2 hours, and have associated ipsilateral autonomic signs such as tearing, miosis, ptosis, or rhinorrhea. Patients should not have focal neurologic signs or symptoms (**Table 89-3**).

SECONDARY HEADACHE

■ HISTORY

"Do not miss headaches"

While the vast majority of headache pain may have benign causes, a small percentage result from underlying diseases that require further evaluation and treatment on an emergent basis (**Table 89-4**).

The presentation of intracranial hemorrhage depends on the location of the bleeding. Blood in the subarachoid space will cause

TABLE 89-3 Diagnostic Criteria for Cluster Headache

A. At least five attacks fulfilling B-D

B. Severe unilateral orbital, supraorbital, and/or temporal pain lasting 15-180 min untreated

C. Headache associated with at least one of the following signs, which must be present on the pain side:

   1. Conjunctival lacrimation

   2. Lacrimation

   3. Nasal congestion

   4. Rhinorrhea

   5. Forehead and facial sweating

   6. Miosis

   7. Ptosis

   8. Eyelid edema

D. Frequency of attacks from one every other day to eight per day

E. No evidence of contributing underlying disorder

Data from Headache Classification Committee of the International Headache Society. Classification and diagnostic criteria for headache disorders, cranial neuralgias and facial pain. *Cephalalgia*. 1988;8(Suppl 7):1-96.

meningeal irritation headache. Patients may have nausea and vomiting, photophobia, phonophobia, and unilateral or bilateral throbbing pain. Intracerebral hemorrhage will lead to increased intracranial pressure but more acute in onset than tumors.

Subarachnoid hemorrhage (SAH), carotid and vertebral artery dissections, venous sinus thrombosis, pituitary apoplexy, and hypertensive emergencies may present with the abrupt onset of excruciating pain. Cluster headaches may have a similar presentation, but tearing or rhinorrhea should be present, and the pain should remit within a couple of hours. Migraines gradually increase to a maximal level over 1 to 2 hours.

PRACTICE POINT

Intracranial hemorrhage

- Do not to assume that a headache is benign based on a known headache history. Many of the patients who present with acute and serious headache pathology will have had a prior history of primary headaches.
- Blood in the subarachnoid space can mimic the symptoms of migraine.
- Pain medications can reduce arousal and may reduce ventilation, thereby, worsening neurologic status as well as make the neurologic examination difficult. Nonsteroidal anti-inflammatory medications are not advisable due to their effect on platelets.
- Indications for neuroimaging include the presence of:
  - High risk historical features or risk factors for secondary headache
  - Altered mental status, depressed sensorium or neurologic signs
  - Antecedent head or neck trauma

Headache or migraine that coincides with stroke syndromes should raise the specter of hemorrhagic stroke. Twenty percent of strokes are associated with SAH (10%) and intracerebral hemorrhage (10%). Headache occurring at the onset of stroke should be assumed to signify SAH. In intracerebral hemorrhage, pain sometimes occurs acutely at the time of the hemorrhage but may be delayed until the hematoma expands and compresses pain-sensitive intracranial structures such as large arteries and meninges. In ischemic stroke involving large vessels, headache is usually not a feature but occasionally occurs prior to, during, or after the onset of stroke. Cerebrovascular dissection may cause both headache and stroke. Subcortical strokes (lacunar infarcts—pure motor, pure sensory, ataxic hemiparesis, clumsy hand dysarthria, sensorimotor where face, arm, leg more equally affected than in cortical infarcts) only rarely cause headache.

Space-occupying lesions in the brain tend not to cause pain unless they become large enough to compress pain-sensitive structures. The most common presenting symptom of brain tumors is seizure—not headache—although not infrequently patients with brain tumors will develop progressive headaches as the tumor becomes larger. They tend to be mild to moderate in intensity and unremitting. Patients often ignore these symptoms for some time since they tend not to interfere with activities of daily living and work. Increased intracranial pressure headaches can also occur from occlusion of the venous sinuses, which may present with severe headache, seizures, and bilateral papilledema. Most migraine headaches are relieved somewhat by rest. Patients with increased intracranial pressure will classically awaken from sleep with a severe, classically boring, bilateral headache. These patients may vomit due to slight hypoventilation during sleep, which leads to hypercarbic vasodilatation and increased intracranial pressure.

TABLE 89-4 "Do Not Miss Headaches"

Disorder	Risk Factors	Symptoms	Signs
Aneurysmal SAH	Polycystic kidney disease Coarctation of aorta Connective tissue disorders Neurofibromatosis Pituitary tumors AVM Sympathomimetic drugs Stroke	Prodrome: sentinel small bleed or aneurysmal dilation prior to rupture Rupture during activity Unusually severe or atypical H/A, especially if brief LOC, N/V, meningismus, or any focal findings	Cushing sign, fever Nuchal rigidity Ptosis of one eyelid with dilated nonreactive pupil, impaired adduction and vertical movement of affected eye Preretinal hemorrhages
Intracerebral hemorrhage	HBP Cerebral amyloid Stroke risk factors	AVM rupture commonly associated with seizure; fever	Typically hemorrhage into subcortical regions (putamen, thalamus, caudate) or if AVM, in that location
Rupture of bacterial abscess	Immunosuppression IV illicit drug use	Sudden severe pain, LOC	Fever, nuchal rigidity
Raised ICP of any etiology		Unilateral or bilateral Boring, aching pain typically without photophobia or phonophobia or environmental triggers Worse lying down; nocturnal awakening Seizures	Cushing sign Abducens paresis Bilateral papilledema, retinal hemorrhages Nuchal rigidity
Meningitis		Often a throbbing component of the headache, hypersensitivity to sound and light, nausea and sometimes vomiting	Fever, photophobia, nuchal rigidity, obtundation
Giant cell arteritis	>60 y of age	Severe throbbing but also dull, sharp or burning headaches, localized to the temples or diffuse, acute onset Systemic symptoms: painful stiff proximal extremities, myalgias, weight loss Jaw claudication Visual disturbances: sudden monocular blindness or stuttering, visual loss, amaurosis fugax, diplopia, or field cut	Asymmetric temporal arterial pulses, thickened or tender temporal arteries
Status post (s/p) neck injuries with muscle spasm **Dissection of great vessels** **Subdural hematoma** **Intracranial hemorrhage**	Seemingly minor trauma may however be associated with dissection and subdural hematoma	Tension-type or occipital headache Elderly patients receiving anticoagulants may suffer intracranial hemorrhage without severe headache Neck or upper shoulder pain LOC	Palpation of affected muscles will exacerbate the pain syndrome; reduced range of motion of the neck Focal signs
Carbon monoxide poisoning (or inhaled methyl chlorine)	Suspect when multiple family members have headache; seasonal and regional variation; workers who use methyl chloride or inhale paint remover	Diffuse headache Nonspecific symptoms (malaise, dizziness)	

AVM, arteriovenous malformation; BP, blood pressure; CN, cranial nerve; ECG, electrocardiogram; H/A, headache; HBP, high blood pressure; ICP, intracranial pressure; LOC, loss of consciousness; N/V, nausea and vomiting; SAH, subarachnoid hemorrhage, Cushing sign (↑ICP, ↑BP, bradycardia).

Increased intracranial pressure
- Intracranial pressure headaches typically occur as the meninges are stretched or the blood vessels are compressed.
- The most concerning symptom to suggest increased intracranial pressure is a history of worsening headache with lying down. Patients may describe a history of nausea and vomiting only when lying flat.
- Usually not acute in onset, they become slowly more severe over days to weeks to months.
- Focal neurologic signs are often present.

Patients with chronic headaches and new seizures should always be considered for the possibility of an intracranial mass. Patients, particularly those in middle age, with chronic headaches that do not appear to be analgesic withdrawal headaches and that lack migrainous components should generally undergo brain imaging.

Underlying systemic illness

A new or change in headache in a patient with risk factors for intracranial illness (such as cancer, hematologic disorders, infection) should also alert the clinician to the possibility of a serious headache etiology (**Table 89-5**). The neurologic presentations of systemic diseases should help the clinician order the appropriate studies. For example, patients with AIDS have increased risk for toxoplasmosis, abscess, lymphoma, and meningitis and should undergo neuroimaging prior to analysis of the spinal fluid. Patients with HIV may first present with aseptic meningitis. Similarly, a new, progressively worsening headache in any patient with malignancy should prompt MRI of the intracranial venous channels.

Head and neck trauma is a risk factor for subdural hematoma (SDH) as well as SAH and intracerebral hemorrhage. Injuries caused by abrupt flexion and extension of the neck (as in boxing, motor vehicle accidents), patients with connective tissue disorders, and severe straining (by pregnant women during delivery) may be associated with dissection of the extracranial vessels.

A decrease or loss of vision with headache may result from temporal arteritis, carotid dissection, and acute narrow-angle glaucoma.

Nausea and vomiting are seen with SAH, intracranial hemorrhage, acute angle glaucoma (as well as migraine). Narrow-angle glaucoma headaches are typically centered over the affected eye.

Headache precipitated by cough or Valsalva may be associated with cerebrovascular disease or underlying malignancy.

Toxins
- Toxins may cause headache. If multiple family members present with headache, consider carbon monoxide poisoning.

Medications that increase bleeding risk include anticoagulants, nonsteroidal anti-inflammatory drugs (NSAIDs), and antiplatelet agents.

Acute sinusitis, seizure, temporomandibular joint syndrome, hypercalcemia and/or hyperviscosity, and glaucoma sometimes present with headache in the hospital setting.

Drugs

Medications are an especially common cause of headache (**Table 89-6**).

Analgesic withdrawal headaches

Patients with analgesic withdrawal headaches are usually easy to diagnose but can be a challenge to treat. In general, the worst actors for analgesic withdrawal headaches are any medications that have significant amounts of caffeine, particularly short-acting medications. Even ibuprofen or acetaminophen taken frequently can cause analgesic withdrawal headaches. Anyone who takes medications on a daily basis for headaches more than 15 times a month probably has at least a component of analgesic withdrawal headaches. These headaches tend not to have associated meningeal signs. Historical aspects to make one suspicious of analgesic withdrawal headaches include the following:

1. Pain medications on chronic daily basis for at least 2 to 3 weeks
2. Occurrence of headaches in the morning as soon as the previous dose of medication wears off
3. Taking medications first thing the morning every day for at least 2 to 3 weeks
4. Resistance on the patient's behalf to change or discontinue the chronic daily medications

The physical examination, including the neurological examination, should be normal.

Analgesic withdrawal headache
- Headache is probably one of the only pain disorders that will often become worse with ongoing treatment.
- The classical analgesic withdrawal headache is the caffeine withdrawal headache. As long as patients take caffeine, they do not have pain. Once they acutely discontinue caffeine, they begin having throbbing and severe headaches that are only made better with caffeine.
- Withdrawal headaches can occur from almost any analgesic medication. Short-acting medications are more likely to cause analgesic withdrawal headaches once they are discontinued.

Low pressure headaches

Most common following lumbar puncture, low pressure within the cranial vault likely causes pain by traction or irritation of the meninges. Low pressure (LP) headaches can also be seen after neurosurgery or spontaneously after a particularly violent sneeze or cough, even with no significant trauma. The patient may experience positional bilateral throbbing, temporal, squeezing pain with photophobia and rarely phonophobia. However nausea and vomiting are generally absent for unknown reasons. The propensity for migraine headaches and younger age (due to less free space in the cranium) increases the likelihood of developing low pressure headache. There should be no cranial nerve deficits as long as the intracranial hypotension is not severe. Classically, when patients lie flat, the pain becomes much improved as the pressure equalizes between the low back and the cranium. As patients sit or stand, particularly if they move quickly, the headache will begin again. Although most migraine headaches will also worsen as patients stand up, complete or near-complete relief with recumbence is not typical for migraines. In general there are no physical exam findings that are particularly helpful, and the neurologic exam is nonfocal. See Chapter 104 (The Neurologic Examination).

Most post-LP headaches will resolve spontaneously over 1 to 5 days. Opiates are usually ineffective in the acute or chronic treatment of this disorder. Because there is some meningeal traction,

TABLE 89-5 Systemic Diseases and Headache

	Disorder	Symptoms and Signs	Pathophysiology
Cardiology	Atrial fibrillation	Sudden onset, severe headache	Cerebral embolism from cardiac surgery or associated heart disease
	Atrial myxoma	Focal symptoms and signs involving a vascular territory	
	Ventricular aneurysm		
	Severe dilated cardiomyopathies		
	Valvular heart disease		
	Myocardial infarction		
Endocrinology	Obesity	Chronic, recurring diffuse headaches with or without papilledema	Benign intracranial hypertension
	Menstrual disorders		
	Hypoparathyroidism		
	Adrenal insufficiency		
	Hypo- or hyperthyroidism Hyperparathyroidism Hyperaldosteronism		Intracranial vasodilatation
	Mineralocorticoid excess, Steroid withdrawal		
	Hypoglycemia		
	Pheochromocytoma	Diffuse, throbbing headache	Catecholamines
		Excessive perspiration, tachycardia, and labile hypertension	
	Tumors of the hypophyseal-pituitary axis	Visual field cuts with the presenting endocrinopathy	
Gastroenterology	Crohn disease and ulcerative colitis	Diffuse, sometimes hemicranial, recurrent headaches	Recurrence may be related to the severity of IBD
Hematology	Hypercoagulable states		Intracranial venous thrombosis
	Multiple myeloma, polycythemia vera, and other hematologic malignancies	Diffuse headache Blurring or loss of vision, diplopia Vertigo, nystagmus Tinnitus, sudden deafness Ataxia	Hyperviscosity (viscosity > 4 centipoise) due to paraproteinemias or Vascular congestion or venous occlusion from marked leukocytosis or thrombocytosis
	Cerebellar hemangioblastomas	Diffuse pain Posterior location of pain	Hyperviscosity due to tumor secretion of erythropoietin or hydrocephalus Location of tumor
	Leukemias, lymphomas	Diffuse, progressively severe headache Cranial nerve palsies, nuchal rigidity, papilledema, or hydrocephalus	Studding the cranial meninges
	Thrombocytopenia	Focal or diffuse headache or recurrent headaches similar to migraine	Brain hemorrhage or infarction
	Hemophilia	Sudden onset, severe headache	Cerebral hemorrhage from factor deficiency
	Anemia (usually <8 g/dL)	Diffuse, throbbing headache that is worse with exertion	Rarely, iron deficiency anemia has been associated with benign intracranial hypertension
	Sickle cell disease	Focal or diffuse headache Focal findings of stroke	Cerebral infarction

(Continued)

TABLE 89-5 Systemic Diseases and Headache (*Continued*)

	Disorder	Symptoms and Signs	Pathophysiology
Oncology	Brain tumors	Nondescript pain, not necessarily more likely in the early morning, with straining or bending over, or accompanied by vomiting	Lack of pain due to location in cerebral hemisphere
		Usually other neurologic symptoms predominate, such as weakness, confusion, seizures	
	Meningeal carcinomatosis	Diffuse, progressive, severe headache	Breast, bronchial, gastrointestinal, and melanoma most common cancers, sometimes present for months or years
		Often with vomiting, back pain, meningeal irritation, decreasing consciousness, cranial nerve palsies, papilledema, and diabetes insipidus	
	Lung cancer	Pain in the angle of the jaw or ear	Irritation of the pain fibers in the ipsilateral vagus nerve
	Mediastinal tumor	Worsening headache	Obstruction of the superior vena cava with death from increased intracranial pressure or cerebral hemorrhage
		Cough, dyspnea, hoarseness, airway obstruction	
Infectious disease	Bacterial endocarditis	Sudden severe headache	Septic cerebral embolism with resultant hemorrhage from a mycotic aneurysm
		Focal neurologic signs	
		Seizure	
	Brain abscess (bronchiectasis, empyema, TB)	Focal findings, seizure, altered mentation	Rupture of brain abscess may cause meningitis and sudden severe diffuse headache
			Mass effect symptoms analogous to brain tumor unless there is associated meningeal irritation
	Meningitis	Focal cranial nerve dysfunction seen with Listeria, TB, and fungal meningitis	Due to affecting basal meninges
	Many pneumonias, classically *Mycoplasma pneumoniae*	Diffuse headaches, which are worse with coughing	
	Infection in the paranasal or mastoid sinuses or lungs (such as *M. pneumoniae*) may serve as a nidus	Severe headache	Meningeal spread or development of brain abscess
		Meningeal signs, fever	
Pregnancy and postpartum period			
	Pre-eclampsia in the last trimester of pregnancy	May have headache as a presenting symptom in addition to hypertension, proteinuria, and edema	
	Arteriovenous malformations (AVMs) and subarachnoid hemorrhage (SAH)	Sudden severe headache	Bleeding more likely in the second trimester for AVMs and third trimester for SAH
	Carotid dissection during delivery	Horner's ± focal neurologic symptoms and signs	Straining during labor and delivery
Psychiatry	Intoxication	Severe diffuse headache	Cocaine due to hypertension or cocaine-induced migraine or SAH or intracranial hemorrhage
		Signs of sympathetic over activity	
	Withdrawal syndromes	Severe diffuse headache	Alcohol or opiate withdrawal
		Signs of sympathetic overactivity	
Pulmonary	Acute respiratory failure or chronic disorders (eg, OSA or severe COPD)	Morning headaches worse with coughing	pCO_2 retention and hypoxia $\rightarrow$ Cerebral vasodilation, may have associated polycythemia
		Low head position during sleep may increase cephalic congestion along with impaired respiratory efficiency	

(Continued)

TABLE 89-5 Systemic Diseases and Headache (*Continued*)

	Disorder	Symptoms and Signs	Pathophysiology
Renal	Rarely, uremia	Diffuse and throbbing headaches that abate following dialysis or renal transplantation	Cerebral edema and increased pressure
Rheumatology	Vasculitis	Migraine-like headaches	
	Cranial arteritis	Symptoms of meningitis	
	Aseptic meningitis	Focal neurologic defects (vasculitis)	
	Arthritis of cervical spine		
Surgery	Removal of acoustic neuroma	Dull headache in region of incision	Damage to regional nerves
	Carotid endarterectomy	Vascular headache	Removal of stenosis distends already dilated poststenotic vessels

AVM, arteriovenous malformation; COPD, chronic obstructive pulmonary disease; DIC, disseminated intravascular coagulation; IBD, Inflammatory Bowel Disease; ITP, idiopathic thrombocytopenic purpura; OSA, Obstructive Sleep Apnea; SAH, subarachnoid hemorrhage; TB, tuberculosis; TTP, thrombotic thrombocytopenic purpura.
Data from *Hospitalist Neurology*. Samuels M, Edmeads J, eds. *Headache*. Vol. 25. Waltham, MA: Butterworth Heinman; 1999. Chap. 1.

these headaches can be treated using an acute migraine protocol, which can include caffeine and migraine-specific medications. Maintaining a recumbent position will often help to keep the pain from becoming severe, and abdominal binders can be tried to increase pressure in the cerebrospinal fluid (CSF). When conservative measures fail and symptoms persist for more than 2 days, the leak can be sealed using an epidural blood patch. An anesthesiologist injects some of the patient's blood in the epidural space at the site of the prior LP and allows it to thrombose and seal the area. The patch will ultimately be absorbed, and there is minimal risk of infection.

Neuropathic pain syndromes

In general, neuropathic pain syndromes involving the face and skull present with focal areas of extreme, lancinating, shooting, or stabbing pain in the face within any of the distributions of the trigeminal nerve, or on the back of the skull within the distribution of the occipital nerve. Sometimes the stabbing, lancinating pain occurs within the eye or in the posterior pharynx. Neuropathic pain syndromes may have an area of anesthesia that when touched or irritated elicits the paroxysm of pain. Patients will often point to one area that is exquisitely tender, and as you move to examine this area there is a certain amount of guarding. These pain syndromes can be unremitting and severe. This syndrome can be precipitated by any etiology that leads to sensory nerve irritation such as viral infections, bony compression, demyelination, masses, or soft tissue compression. Herpes zoster can sometimes present with this type of pain before the vesicles appear.

PRACTICE POINT

Warning signs for serious pathologies include the following:
- New headache with meningeal symptoms and signs that is maximal at the time of onset
- Any headache associated with alteration of mental status or new cranial nerve findings
- Chronic or subacute headache in patients over the age of 50, particularly worse at night, awakening patients from sleep, especially with focal neurologic deficits
- New headaches in patients over the age of 60 that are associated with elevated markers of inflammation, and pain within the back of the neck, shoulders, and arms

---

CASE 89-1 *(CONTINUED)*

Does she appear acutely ill?

On examination she is a well-developed, well-nourished, young woman in no acute distress with normal vital signs. Her general physical examination is normal and noncontributory.

Is she confused?

Her mental status is normal and she does not appear intoxicated.

Does she have a "nonfocal" neurologic examination?

No bruits are heard over the orbits, cranial vessels, or temples. Cognitive function, language, and memory are all intact. Her cranial nerve examination is completely normal, including sharp optic discs and normal visual fields. She does not have meningeal signs. Her motor exam shows full and equal tone, power, and bulk in all four extremities. Her sensory exam is intact for all modalities, and the Romberg test is negative. Tests of coordination in the upper and lower extremities are all normal. There is no evidence of cerebellar dysfunction. Her gait and stance are normal, including tandem gait. Her reflexes are average in amplitude and equal bilaterally; both plantars are flexor. No pathological reflexes are elicited.

PHYSICAL EXAMINATION

■ DOES THE PATIENT APPEAR ACUTELY ILL?

If a patient appears toxic or hemodynamically unstable, the headache is more likely to have an underlying secondary cause. In severe meningitis, the patient may be sitting upright on the edge of the bed with knees and hips flexed, the neck extended with a lordotic curvature of the spine, and the arms brought back to support the thorax—the tripod position referred to as the Amoss or Hoyne sign.

■ WHAT ARE THE PATIENT'S VITAL SIGNS?

Does the patient have a fever? Fever may be associated with SAH, intracerebral hemorrhage, meningitis, encephalitis, rupture of brain abscess, septic cerebral emboli, or arterial dissection and may prompt the need for a spinal fluid examination, usually following neuroimaging to ensure the absence of serious mass effect. Of the classic clinical triad of fever, neck stiffness, and altered mental status, fever is the most sensitive sign of meningitis.

TABLE 89-6 Common Medical Interventions Associated with Headache

Cardiology
- Nitrates (diffuse throbbing headaches with initial use) and adrenergic inhibitors such as hydralazine, minoxidil, reserpine (vasodilators)
- Some calcium channel blockers (diltiazem and dihydropyridines)

Endocrinology
- Withdrawal of glucocorticoids (new headache or triggering preexisting migraine)

Gastroenterology
- Ranitidine and famotidine
- Sulfasalazine

Hematology
- Intravenous immune globulin (nondescript headache or trigger migraine in susceptible individuals)

Oncology
- Chemotherapy (nonspecific, sometimes change preexisting migraine pattern)
- Intrathecal methotrexate (acute aseptic meningitis)

Infectious disease
- Antibiotics especially trimethoprim-sulfamethoxazole (direct vascular effect or aseptic meningitis)
- Zidovudine (AZT) (unknown mechanism in first few weeks of treatment)
- Interferon-alpha
- Antimalarial drugs

Pregnancy
- Spinal headache (from epidural anesthesia that is actually a spinal tap)

Psychiatry
- Drug interactions (severe hypertension from sympathomimetic drugs such as meperidine or bronchodilators in patients already taking monoamine oxidase inhibitors)
- Benzodiazepines (dull nondescript headache during initiation)

Pulmonary
- Theophylline, albuterol, terbutaline

Renal
- Hemodialysis (recurrent nondescript headache associated with hemodialysis or part of the "dialysis disequilibrium syndrome" more commonly at the end of hemodialysis due to osmotic shifts)
- Central nervous system infections or lymphomas (from immunosuppression in renal transplant patients)

Rheumatology
- Nonsteroidal anti-inflammatory drugs (direct vascular effect, increased intracranial hypertension or aseptic meningitis)

Surgery
- Fasting prior to surgery especially in patients with preexisting migraines or unrecognized substance dependency

Does the patient have hypertension? Ordinarily, hypertension does not cause headache unless severe. However, hypertension and bradycardia may be a clue that the patient has increased intracranial pressure (Cushing sign).

■ DOES THE PATIENT HAVE SIGNS OF MENINGEAL IRRITATION?

For patients with meningeal irritation headaches, the examiner should note any historical information, symptoms and signs that would indicate a need for head imaging prior to consideration of a lumbar puncture. These include age >60, history of central nervous system (CNS) disease or recent seizure, immunocompromised state, decreased level of consciousness, inability to answer questions or follow commands, abnormal language or motor function, the presence of a gaze or facial palsy, or abnormal visual fields. The examiner should also note the presence of fever and nuchal rigidity.

Although fever occurs in the majority of patients with meningitis, followed by neck stiffness, immunocompromised patients and the elderly are less likely to have fever or nuchal rigidity. The classic signs of meningeal irritation include positive Kernig, Brudzinski, and contralateral signs and worsening of headache with the Jolt maneuver. A positive Kernig sign occurs when extension of the knee causes resistance or pain in the lower back or posterior thigh in a supine patient with hips flexed at 90 degrees. A positive Brudzinski sign occurs when passive neck flexion causes flexion of the knees and hips in a supine patient. The contralateral reflex occurs when passive flexion of the hip and knee results in flexion of the opposite leg. A positive Jolt test causes worsening of headache when the patient turns the head horizontally at a frequency of two to three rotations per second. The absence of all three signs of fever, neck stiffness, and altered mental status makes the diagnosis of meningitis much less likely, but no constellation of symptoms or signs are sufficiently sensitive with low negative likelihood ratios to rule out meningitis. Cryptococcal meningitis and localized inflammatory processes involving the meninges such as a neurosurgical wound are not associated with positive stretch signs. Positive stretch signs may be associated with noninfectious causes such as musculoskeletal problems, tumors, carcinomatous meningitis, Mollaret's meningitis, SAH, and other conditions. If meningitis is suspected, further diagnostic testing is required to confirm the diagnosis.

- Meningeal irritation syndromes often present with pain that is very similar in quality and associated symptoms to migraine headaches.
- Patients with meningeal irritation headaches in the setting of fever, alteration of mental status, or focal neurologic findings should never be diagnosed with migraine without a detailed evaluation for life-threatening pathology.

The most concerning cause of meningeal irritation headaches is blood within the meninges, particularly from an SAH. But meningitis, encephalitis, or any type of CNS infection/inflammation can present similarly. SAH tends to be a meningeal-type headache that can resemble by history a migraine headache. Since some patients with SAH happen to be migraine sufferers, it is crucial not to assume that all headaches in a patient with a history of migraines are due to migraines. In general, migraine sufferers who present with a new type of headache, particularly if maximal at onset, should have an evaluation for another cause of headache pain. Classically a very stiff neck is more common with the meningitis or SAH than with migraine, whereas photosensitivity and nausea tend to be more marked with migraine.

If SAH is strongly suspected and head imaging is negative, proceed with a lumbar puncture. The sensitivity of head computed tomography (CT) for identifying SAH depends on the size of the bleed (lower with minor bleeds) and timing relative to the rupture with the highest sensitivity in the first 12 hours after SAH (almost 100%).

PRACTICE POINT

Bloody spinal fluid

SAH	Traumatic tap
• ↑ RBC in both tubes 1 and 4 (although unreliable sign by itself) • ↑ WBC by 1 for ≈ every 500-700 RBC (if a normal WBC:RBC ratio in the peripheral blood) • Xanthochromia usually present (takes 2-4 hours to develop)	• Significant fall in RBC from tubes 1 to 4 • Mild increase in WBC explained by bloody contamination alone, with WBC:RBC ratio comparable to that observed in the patient's blood • Xanthochromia absent

---

If meningitis is suspected, but altered mental status, papilledema, or focal neurologic findings suggest the need for CT prior to lumbar puncture, antibiotics should not be delayed.

■ DOES THE PATIENT HAVE ALTERED MENTATION?

Acute meningitis, encephalitis, and SAH may cause confusion or obtundation. Alteration of the level of consciousness is extremely uncommon in migraine headaches unless the patient has been treated pharmacologically. Although assessing the patient's level of awareness involves determining whether the patient is oriented to person, place, and time, orientation is not sensitive enough to pick up confusion, and disorientation is nonspecific (and can be due to psychosis, aphasia, amnesia). Family members may be the first people to note altered mentation or a subtle personality change. It is essential to test attention before moving on to testing language, memory, calculation, construction, and abstraction, and looking for focal neurologic deficits by screening cranial nerve, reflex, motor,

and sensory exams. If a patient cannot sustain attention or if he has an altered level of arousal, proceed with a workup which includes neuroimaging and possibly an examination of the spinal fluid.

■ DOES THE PATIENT HAVE FOCAL NEUROLOGIC SIGNS?

Abnormalities on neurologic examination are often diagnostic for intracranial pathology. A neurologic evaluation should include a detailed cranial nerve exam to look for dilated or unreactive pupils, limitation in range of motion of the eyes, facial droop, lateralizing weakness, sensory loss, or asymmetric deep tendon reflexes. None of these findings should be seen in a migrainous disorder, except in the rare patient with complex migraines. Intra-axial (intraparenchymal) lesions cause conjugate eye deviation, visual field defects, asymmetrical motor tone, strength, reflexes, and Babinski signs. Focal neurologic findings are often, but not always, seen in SAH and meningitis.

If a dilated, nonreactive pupil is noted, consider the following diagnostic possibilities:

1. Eye drops containing anticholinergic medications, scopolamine patches, systemic atropine (patients are alert without focal neurologic symptoms or signs)
2. Holmes-Adie syndrome due to loss of parasympathetic neurons innervating the eye resulting in unopposed sympathetic dilation of the affected pupil (patients may have blurred vision, areflexia)
3. Aneurysmal cranial nerve compression leading to unilateral papillary dilation (patients may have associated oculomotor dysfunction and headache)
4. Uncal herniation due to large temporal lobe mass lesions (comatose patients)

If a Horner sign is appreciated in a patient with headache, carotid or vertebral dissection should be considered.

Focal findings along a vascular territory and headache should increase suspicion for extracranial large vessel disease (atherosclerosis, dissection, fibromuscular dysplasia, and aortic disease) and intracranial large vessel disease (inflammatory arteriopathies and atherosclerosis).

PRACTICE POINT

Vascular territory

Anterior circulation	Posterior circulation
• Motor dysfunction of contralateral extremity or face or both • Ipsilateral visual loss, homonymous hemianopia • Aphasia (dominant hemisphere) • Dysarthria • Sensory deficit of contralateral extremity or face or both • Aphasia, cortical sensory loss or weakness • MCA—predominantly face and arm > leg • ACA—leg > arm or face	• Motor dysfunction of ipsilateral face and/or contralateral extremity • Loss of vision of one or both eyes, homonymous visual fields • Sensory deficit of ipsilateral face and/or contralateral extremity • Typical associated symptoms (not diagnostic in isolation) • Ataxia • Vertigo • Diplopia • Dysphagia • Dysarthria

---

Cortical signs include aphasia, visual field defects, monoparesis (clumsy, weak, or flaccid), hemineglect, cortical sensory loss (numbness, paresthesias), and abulia.

If a patient has focal neurologic signs, proceed with neuroimaging and consider imaging of the large vessels at the same time, especially if the patient has signs and symptoms along a vascular territory. With CNS mass lesions, focal neurological deficits are usually present, although not invariably, and are often extremely subtle.

■ DOES THE PATIENT HAVE SIGNS OR SYMPTOMS OF INCREASED INTRACRANIAL PRESSURE?

Extra-axial processes (outside of brain tissue) commonly cause raised intracranial pressure and may cause the following signs to be present: evidence of raised intracranial pressure (Cushing reflex), ptosis of one eyelid (aneurysmal compression of the ipsilateral third cranial nerve), dilated nonreactive pupil (constriction controlled by ipsilateral third cranial nerve), impaired adduction and vertical movement of one eye (complete third cranial nerve compression), impaired lateral rectus muscle function (stretching of sixth cranial nerve from increased intracranial pressure), subhyaloid hemorrhage on retinal examination.

■ DOES THE PATIENT HAVE SIGNS OF AN UNDERLYING SYSTEMIC DISORDER?

A general physical examination should search for the source of any fever, with particular attention to the ears, sinuses, respiratory system, and skin due to the association with meningitis. Any infection may cause a toxic vascular headache characterized as bilateral throbbing headaches increased by exertion, bending, and straining or may trigger migrainous attacks. Like toxic vascular headache, bacterial, viral, fungal, or protozoal systemic infections may cause meningeal irritation.

A general physical examination may uncover a new diagnosis of cancer or evidence of metastatic disease. For example, approximately 50% of patients with meningeal carcinomatosis may have no history of systemic cancer. Patients with known cancer may develop headaches secondary to parenchymal or skull tumor metastases, carcinomatous meningitis, or intracranial venous thrombosis; however, they are more likely to have headaches from primary causes (migraine or tension headaches) or from fever and sepsis or from drug therapy. Because of the potentially subtle findings, new-onset headaches in older patients and headaches that fail to meet diagnostic criteria for primary functional headaches should prompt neuroimaging (see Tables 89-1, 89-2, and 89-3 for the diagnostic criteria by the International Headache Society).

Patients with rheumatologic disorders may have a number of different mechanisms for headaches, including recurrent headaches similar to migraine or chronic headaches due to vasculitis, pseudotumor cerebri, or aseptic meningitis. The signs and symptoms of cerebral vasculitis include multifocal neurologic deficits and headache, often associated with systemic inflammation and fever. Granulomata from Wegener disease, lymphomatoid granulomatosis, and sarcoidosis may infiltrate the meninges and produce headache and multiple cranial nerve deficits. Arthritis of the cervical spine may lead to neck stiffness and occipital headaches.

CASE 89-1 (continued)

NEUROLOGY CONSULTATION

Almost certainly too much medication has caused a syndrome of chronic daily headache superimposed on a history of migraine. The best course of action would be for her to consult a headache expert, to help her get on a program that would allow her to taper alprazolam and hydrocodone with the goal of discontinuation and start a more rational, abortive treatment program for her headaches. The general rule is that oral medications do not help much during migraine because of atony of the stomach. Subcutaneous sumatriptan has helped her but is very expensive. It may be better to use rectal indomethacin at the first sign of the headaches. Cyproheptadine, a mild antiserotonin drug, may cause some sedation, which in her case may be useful since sleep and rest make the headaches better.

FOLLOW-UP

Instead, the patient consulted a pain clinic, which continued her narcotics and added a number of new medications. She continues to periodically visit emergency departments for pain relief.

CONCLUSION

The history and physical examination are the most important parts of the evaluation of headache at the bedside. Headache symptoms of concern include sudden rapid onset, occipitonuchal radiation, or association with focal neurologic symptoms or altered mental status. Patient-specific risk factors include older age, coexistent malignancy, infectious disease, coagulopathy, or underlying immunosuppression. Precipitating factors of concern include onset during exertion or antecedent head or neck trauma. Physical examination findings of concern include toxic appearance, fever, meningismus, papilledema, altered mental status, and focal neurologic signs. Unfortunately, it can sometimes be difficult to differentiate each form of headache type from another, and the neurologic examination may be normal. This is why imaging is so often needed.

SUGGESTED READINGS

Attia J, Hatala R, Cook DJ, Wong JG. In: Simel DL, Rennie D, eds. *The Rational Clinical Examination.* Vol. 400. New York: McGraw-Hill; 2009;400:175-181.

Peter J. Goadsby, Richard B. Lipton, Michel D. Ferrari, et al. Migraine—the current understanding and treatment. *N Engl J Med.* 2002;346:257-270.

Rasmussen BK. Epidemiology of headache. *Cephalalgia.* 1995;15(1):45-68.

Samuels MA, ed. *Hospitalist Neurology.* Waltham, MA: Butterworth/Heinemann; 1999.

Sapira JD. *The Art and Science of Bedside Diagnosis.* Baltimore, MD: Urban & Schwarzenberg; 1990:469-470.

Stephen D. Silberstein, Richard B. Lipton, Martin Sliwinski, et al. Classification of daily and near-daily headaches. *Neurology.* 1996;47:871-875.

Sun-Edelstein C, Bigal ME, Rapoport AM, et al. Chronic migraine and medication overuse headache: clarifying the current International Headache Society classification criteria. *Cephalalgia.* 2009;29:445.

CHAPTER 90

Hemoptysis

Christopher Knudson, MD

Sukit Chaiyachati, MD

Alvaro Velasquez, MD

Key Clinical Questions

1. What is the initial approach in a evaluating a patient with suspected hemoptysis?
2. What are the causes of hemoptysis, and what clinical features can suggest the mechanism of hemoptysis?
3. What are the diagnostic tests that should be performed for a patient with hemoptysis?
4. What are treatment modalities for hemoptysis, and when is each appropriate?

DEFINITION

Hemoptysis is coughing or spitting up blood or blood mixed with phlegm as a result of bleeding in the lower respiratory tract. The lower respiratory tract is defined as any part of the respiratory system that is below the vocal cords or glottis. This includes the trachea, bronchi, and pulmonary parenchyma. This definition is important in that blood that is generated from other sources has a very different evaluation, triage and treatment.

ANATOMY OF HEMOPTYSIS

Hemoptysis may range from large amounts of frank blood to light streaks of blood in the sputum, which suggests that hemoptysis has diverse etiologies and pathology. Bleeding from the lower respiratory tract occurs from one of two sources: either the high-pressure systemic arterial blood supply or the lower pressure pulmonary arteries and their branches.

The lower respiratory tract blood supply starts proximally with the inferior thyroid arteries supplying the upper trachea. Next, the bronchial arteries, originating from the aorta at the level of T3 to T8, travel along the tracheobronchial tree with small penetrating arteries feeding the lower trachea and bronchi. The bronchial arteries end by anastomosing with branches of the pulmonary arteries, together forming the capillary bed around the alveoli. The pulmonary arteries travel alongside the bronchial arteries on the tracheobronchial tree, but only perform oxygen exchange once at the alveoli.

The significance of these anatomical considerations is that massive hemoptysis (defined below) is more likely coming from the systemic arteries, and the volume of blood may help elucidate the origin of the bleeding. Ninety percent of cases of massive hemoptysis are from bronchial arteries. The remaining 5% of cases are from the pulmonary arteries and 5% from other arteries.

It is also important to realize that bronchial, but not pulmonary arteries proliferate in the setting of inflammation. They can enlarge, become tortuous, and create pathologic high-pressure anastomosis with nearby pulmonary arteries. These abnormal vessels are highly prone to bleeding, and explain (in part) the hemoptysis encountered with chronic inflammatory disease (eg, cystic fibrosis, bronchiectasis), and facilitate our understanding of recurrent bleeding in these disorders.

ETIOLOGY OF SUSPECTED HEMOPTYSIS

There are many causes of hemoptysis, with some of the more common listed in **Table 90-1**. The differential diagnosis of hemoptysis depends primarily on the patient population. In the so-called developed world, the most common causes encountered are bronchitis, bronchogenic carcinoma, bronchiectasis, pneumonia, and tuberculosis. A recent review found that pulmonary embolism is also a common cause of hemoptysis. In contrast, developing countries encounter active infection or sequelae from infection as more common causes. Bronchitis, pneumonia, mycobacterial (eg, tuberculosis) and parasitic (eg, paragonimiasis) infections as well as mitral valve disorders from rheumatic fever, and bronchiectasis are generally seen most frequently.

INITIAL APPROACH TO A PATIENT WITH SUSPECTED HEMOPTYSIS

The first step during the evaluation of hemoptysis is to ensure that there is a patent airway, good gas exchange, and hemodynamic stability. Signs of respiratory or hemodynamic compromise such

TABLE 90-1 Causes of Hemoptysis

Cardiac and pulmonary vascular
Airway-vascular fistula
Aneurysm: Bronchial artery
      Pulmonary artery (Rasmussen aneurysm, mycotic, arteritis)
Arteriovenous malformations
Congenital cardiac or pulmonary vascular malformations
Heart failure
Mitral stenosis
Pulmonary embolism, infarct
Pulmonary hypertension

Hematological
Coagulopathy (congenital, acquired or iatrogenic)
Platelet disorders (platelet dysfunction, thrombocytopenia, von Willebrand Disease)

Infectious
Bacterial endocarditis with septic emboli
Mycetoma* and other fungal infections
Mycobacteria (tuberculosis* and nontuberculosis)
Necrotizing pneumonia* and lung abscess (*Klebsiella pneumoniae, Pseudomonas aeruginosa, Staphylococcus aureus, Streptococcus pneumoniae,* other *Streptococcus* spp. and *Actinomyces* spp.)
Parasitic (paragonimiasis, hydatid cyst)
Viral (Herpes simplex)

Neoplastic
Bronchogenic carcinoma*
Endobronchial tumors (carcinoid, adenoid cystic carcinoma)
Metastatic cancer to lungs
Sarcoma

Pulmonary
Bronchiectasis* (including cystic fibrosis)
Bronchitis
Alveolar hemorrhage and underlying causes

Rheumatologic disorders and vasculitis
Amyloid
Antiglomerular basement membrane disease (Goodpasture's syndrome)
Behçet's disease
Genetic defect of collagen (Ehlers-Danlos vascular type)
Granulomatosis with polyangiitis (Wegener's)
Systemic lupus erythematosus

Trauma and iatrogenic
Bronchoscopy with brushing, biopsy or needle aspiration
Interventional pulmonology procedures (dilation, metallic stent placement, high-dose brachytherapy)
Pulmonary artery catheter-induced vascular injury
Tracheal tube erosion into innominate artery
Transtracheal procedure
Blunt chest trauma
Penetrating chest trauma

Drugs and toxins
Anticoagulants, antiplatelet agents
Bevacizumab
Cocaine
Penicillamine
Solvents
Trimellitic anhydride

Miscellaneous
Endometriosis of lung
Lymphangioleiomatosis
Broncholithiasis
Cryptogenic
Foreign body aspiration
Lung transplantation

*The most common underlying causes of massive hemoptysis.

as dyspnea, hypoxemia or hypotension may require intubation, and at the very least monitoring in a setting where this could be performed quickly if deterioration occurs. If possible during intubation, bronchoscopy should be performed concurrently or soon after to attempt to localize and—if possible—suppress bleeding or clear areas of bleeding that may compromise oxygenation. Supplemental oxygen should be given as needed. Hemodynamics should be monitored at this time, with immediate intravenous (IV) access obtained and IV fluids or blood products administered as appropriate.

As early as possible in treating a patient with hemoptysis, positioning the patient is important. Laying the patient in the lateral decubitus position, keeping the suspected side of bleeding dependent, will theoretically prevent blood from spilling over to the unaffected lung and preventing aspiration. It may be difficult to determine on initial exam, but some clues may be discomfort on one side of the chest, focal crackles, or wheezes on exam. Initial radiologic studies are often necessary, and a rapid bedside chest radiograph may be helpful. With heavy bleeding patients sometimes cannot tolerate lying in the lateral decubitus position, and intubation and sedation may be necessary.

The next triage step is to determine the extent of bleeding. Traditionally, hemoptysis has been regarded as either massive or nonmassive, but there is no clear definition of massive hemoptysis. Different sources define anywhere from 100 to 1000 mL

of blood over 24 hours, with some definitions suggesting more than 100 mL/h. More important are the clinical implications of hemoptysis, and this so-called magnitude-of-effect definition includes features such as requiring transfusion, intubation, aspiration, airway obstruction or hypoxemia. We consider a significant magnitude of effect from hemoptysis as massive hemoptysis, particularly when employing the "Approach to the Patient with Hemoptysis" algorithm **Figure 90-1**.

Massive hemoptysis is a life-threatening event with a mortality rate ranging from 0% to 38%, and these patients should be monitored in an intensive care unit. Calling all consultants (pulmonary, interventional radiology, and cardiothoracic surgery services) immediately is important, as rapid intervention may be required. By doing so, if urgent intervention is needed, they will be aware of the case and can respond more quickly to an emergency.

BEDSIDE EVALUATION OF HEMOPTYSIS

The bedside evaluation is often performed concurrently with the initial triage and should be performed rapidly in the setting of severe bleeding. A common clinical difficulty is determining if the patient has hemoptysis or pseudohemoptysis. Pseudohemoptysis is bleeding that initially seems to be hemoptysis but is not from the lower respiratory tract. Hematemesis, or bleeding from the upper

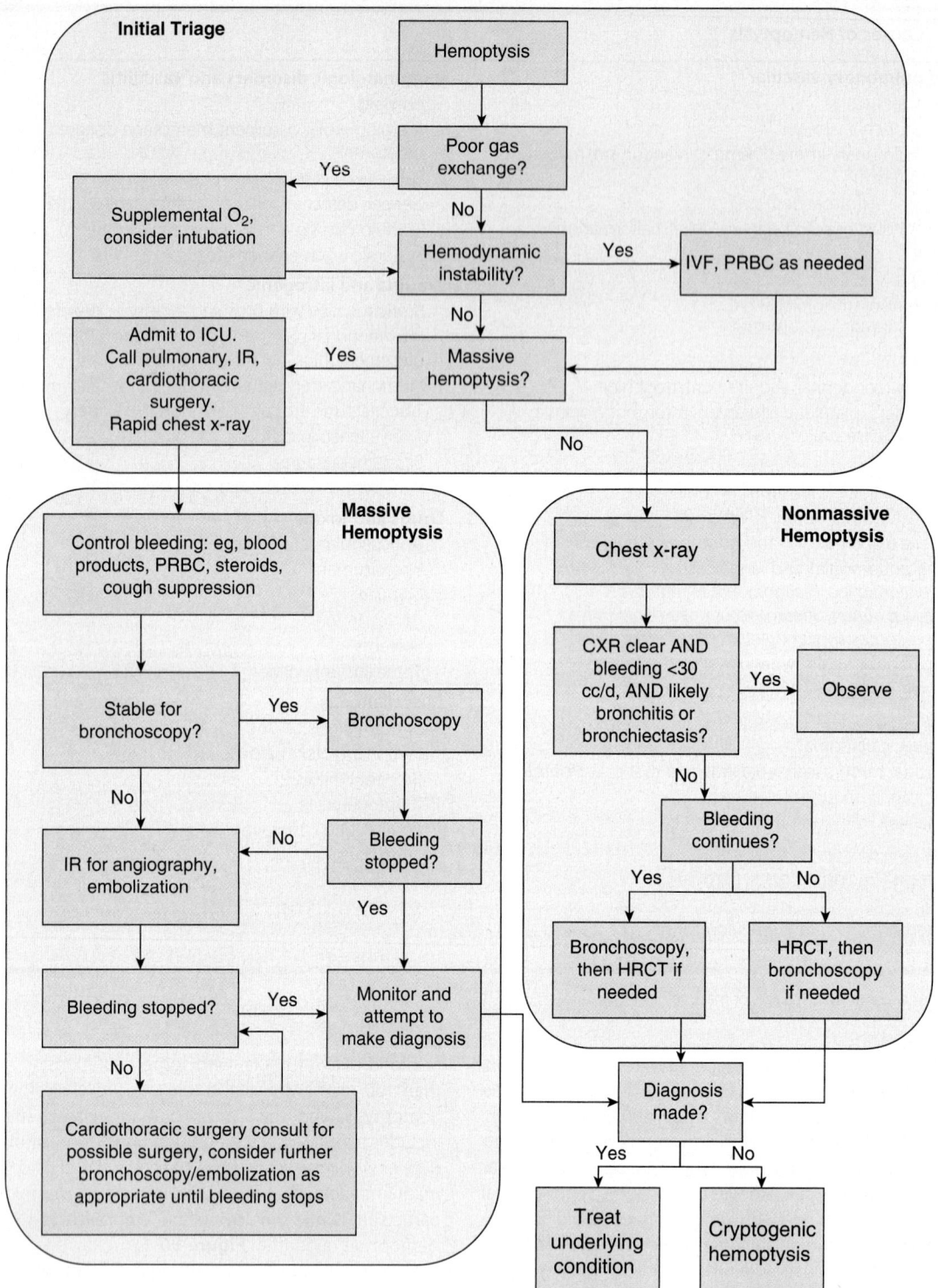

Figure 90-1 *Approach to the patient with hemoptysis.*

gastrointestinal tract, epistaxis, or bleeding from the nasal passages and oropharyngeal bleeding all fall within this definition.

It is often difficult to determine the exact mechanism of hemoptysis from the history, but it can often quickly differentiate true hemoptysis from pseudohemoptysis. Most patients with hemoptysis have significant symptoms involving their respiratory system (such as cough or shortness of breath) and this is often absent in pseudohemoptysis. Patients with epistaxis may have noticed bleeding from their nose prior to coughing up blood, and then noticed it in their saliva or aspirated the blood and coughed it back up.

Patients with hematemesis may have abdominal pain predominate over respiratory symptoms, nausea and vomiting, recent history of black stools, or an initial episode of bloody or blood-tinged vomitus followed by coughing up blood-tinged sputum. Pain in the mouth, tooth or gum disease, or recent surgeries within the oropharynx would suggest this source of bleeding.

There are several components of the history that may suggest the mechanism of hemoptysis, which should be asked so that more directed future testing (eg, laboratory tests) can be initiated quickly. Knowing the patient's risk factors for the most common causes of hemoptysis is important. Determining where the patient has lived is an important first step in establishing the epidemiologic likelihood of causes of disease. Many of the causes listed in Table 90-1 rely on a prior history of disease, and the physician should inquire about a past history of heart or valvular disease, cancer, rheumatologic conditions, HIV, cystic fibrosis, or other pulmonary disorders. Risk factors for tuberculosis should be elucidated, and respiratory isolation should be instituted if there is a likelihood of tuberculosis. Cancer risks (eg, smoking, age) and symptoms (eg, weight loss, night sweats) should be noted. The clinician should review if any recent procedures had been performed that could induce bleeding (eg, bronchoscopic biopsies, pulmonary artery catheterization). The review of systems should include inquiries that would catch the majority of causes as described in Table 90-1.

The physical exam may help define the location of the bleeding. Examine the nares for crusted blood, active sites of bleeding, or fissures. The oropharynx should be inspected, not only the mucosal tissue, but gums and teeth. Place a sputum cup at the bedside for the patient to generate sputum if not available to inspect during your exam. Frothy, light colored blood in sputum is characteristic of a respiratory source. Blood that is exposed to stomach contents is generally a darker red. Measurement of the pH is helpful; stomach acid makes the fluid more acidic, whereas respiratory sources are typically alkaline. Auscultation of the lung may reveal abnormalities consistent with local infection (focal finding), or diffuse bleeding (bilateral findings). Cardiac examination is important to evaluate for signs of valvular disease or heart failure. Some causes have coexisting dermatologic findings (eg, vasculitidies, infections, coagulopathic disorders) that may help diagnosis.

DIAGNOSTIC EVALUATION OF HEMOPTYSIS

Every patient with suspected hemoptysis should have a laboratory evaluation. If proper oxygenation is a concern, an arterial blood gas will be important in triaging a patient. Include a complete blood count, type and screen, and coagulation studies. In addition, the following studies may be appropriate in selected patients:

- Urinalysis and creatinine to screen for pulmonary-renal syndromes
- Sputum culture and microscopic examination for bacteria, acid fast, and fungal organisms in patients with a likely pulmonary infection although bronchoscopic lavage is generally more fruitful
- Antiglomerular basement membrane antibodies, antinuclear antibodies (ANA), antinuclear cytoplasmic antibodies (ANCA), and anticardiolipin antibodies if appropriate
- A brain natriuretic peptide (BNP) to diagnose heart failure

Chest radiography should always be performed (see Figure 90-1). The chest roentgenogram may show localizing bleeding, significant hemorrhage, bilateral findings of pulmonary edema or diffuse hemorrhage, radiopaque foreign bodies, or excluding pathology such as masses. Further workup is not necessary if the chest radiograph is normal, hemoptysis is mild (one study suggests <30 mL/d) and the clinical picture fits with simple infection (eg, bronchitis) or known chronic bronchiectasis. The diagnosis is most likely hematemesis when the chest radiograph is normal in patients with massive hemoptysis.

High resolution computed tomography (HRCT) should be performed in most patients, barring patient instability. HRCT is useful, particularly before bronchoscopy. HRCT often will either make the diagnosis (in roughly 60%-70% of cases), or greatly assist in narrowing the differential. It is complementary to bronchoscopy in diagnosis as it can visualize lung tissue that cannot be assessed visually or physically with bronchoscopy, and provides findings that may guide the bronchoscopic evaluation in terms of tissue sampling. However, if the patient is having continued hemoptysis, bronchoscopy should

be performed as soon as possible and not be delayed by performing HRCT.

Unless the diagnosis is clear from imaging and the clinical picture, bronchoscopy is often performed to evaluate hemoptysis. The airways are directly visualized, definitive diagnosis may be accomplished by biopsy and culture and active bleeding may be treated. If bronchoscopy takes place while the patient is experiencing bleeding, the diagnosis is made 93% of the time. If the bronchoscopy is performed after bleeding has stopped, the diagnostic yield decreases to 50%. Therefore, if the patient is having active hemoptysis and is stable for bronchoscopy, this diagnostic test should be performed as soon as possible, before other modalities (including HRCT).

Angiography may also help make the diagnosis and is often performed if massive hemoptysis persists after bronchoscopy is completed. Its role is mainly for treatment.

Roughly 30% of the time, no cause is discovered with the above testing, and the patient therefore has cryptogenic hemoptysis. This group of patients may be reassured that in most cases, outcomes are good and complete resolution of bleeding may be expected within 6 months. A minority (2%-6%) will eventually have carcinoma diagnosed.

TREATMENT OF HEMOPTYSIS

In many cases, once a diagnosis is made, the treatment for the underlying condition will resolve the hemoptysis. The first goal in treatment of hemoptysis is to administer therapy for any obvious contributor or cause of hemoptysis. Examples include treating a pulmonary embolism with anticoagulation, administering blood products to reverse a coagulopathy, and systemic steroids for vasculitis. In bleeding that persists despite interventions (or as a temporizing measure if interventions cannot be performed immediately), tranexamic acid can be administered orally or intravenously. Cough suppression with antitussive medications should be given to prevent worsening of bleeding.

Bronchoscopy should be performed immediately for continuous bleeding. If an area of bleeding is encountered, several treatment options are available based on clinical scenarios (eg, iced saline lavage, vasoconstrictors like epinephrine, ablative treatments including electric or cryoablation, application of fibrinogen or thrombin or balloon tamponade). Rigid bronchoscopy, as compared to fiber-optic bronchoscopy, has the benefit of improved clot clearance/suction, more interventional procedures possible, and more secure airway protection. The disadvantages are that anesthesia is required, it is not available at all facilities, and it cannot reach the upper lobes and more distal airways.

If the patient is not stable enough for bronchoscopy or significant bleeding continues despite bronchoscopy, the next step is arteriography with possible embolization. This may be performed instead of bronchoscopy if there is persistent bleeding and bronchoscopy would be too risky in unstable patients. This procedure does not look for active extravasation, but rather abnormal vasculature that may be the cause of the bleeding. The bronchial (higher pressure) arteries are evaluated first, as they are most likely the cause of a significant bleed (90% of the time). Embolization is attempted if an abnormal vessel is seen. Depending on the studies, embolization stops bleeding in 57% to 100% of cases. The long-term control of bleeding with embolization is roughly 70% to 90%, and recurrence is often due to a continuing disease process.

If the patient continues to have life threatening bleeding localized to one lung and the above treatments were unsuccessful, consideration of surgery is the next step. The morbidity and mortality are high from this final attempt to control bleeding, but may be the only option in severe cases. In cases from the 1960s to 1990s (mostly prior to the advent of bronchial artery embolization) patients with uncontrollable hemoptysis had a mortality rate ranging from 0% to

50% with surgery; however, the mortality rate was about 80% with medical management.

SUGGESTED READINGS

Kamangar N, et al. Hemoptysis. In: Monsenifar Z, Soo Hoo GW, eds. *Practical Pulmonary and Critical Care Medicine Disease Management*. New York, NY: Taylor & Francis Group; 2006:125-166.

Larici AR, Franchi P, Occhipinti M, et al. Diagnosis and management of hemoptysis. *Diag Interv Radiol*. 2014;20:299.

Sakr L, Dutau H. Massive hemoptysis: an update on the role of bronchoscopy in diagnosis and management. *Respiration*. 2010;80(1):38.

Uzun O, Atasoy Y, Findik S, Atici AG, Erkan L. A prospective evaluation of hemoptysis cases in a tertiary referral hospital. *Clin Respir J*. 2010;4(3):131.

CHAPTER 91

Hypertensive Urgencies and Emergencies

Joseph Varon, MD, FACP, FCCP, FCCM, FRSM

Key Clinical Questions

1. What is hypertension?
2. What is the prevalence of hypertensive crises?
3. What causes hypertensive crises?
4. What are key differences between a hypertensive urgency and emergency?
5. How can one diagnose a hypertensive crisis?
6. What is the treatment for a hypertensive crisis?

INTRODUCTION AND EPIDEMIOLOGY

Hypertension remains the most common reason for patients to seek medical attention in the United States. It affects over 75 million people in the United States, with global numbers approaching one billion. The annual costs of chronic hypertension, both direct and indirect, are estimated to be $50 billion in the United States alone.

The most popular classification of hypertension is that of the Seventh Report of The Joint National Committee on Prevention, Detection, Evaluation, and Treatment of High Blood Pressure (JNC VII). Blood pressure is classified as normal, prehypertension, stage 1 hypertension, and stage 2 hypertension (**Table 91-1**). The newer JNC VIII deals mostly with chronic hypertension, with less emphasis on the management of urgent and emergent situations.

Patients with untreated or inadequately treated hypertension are prone to sudden elevations in blood pressure and the development of **hypertensive crises**. Up to 1% of all hypertensive patients will have a hypertensive crisis in their lifetime. Hypertensive crises come in two forms. In a **hypertensive emergency**, a surge in blood pressure is accompanied by end-organ damage. **Hypertensive urgency** is an acute elevation in blood pressure without evidence of end-organ damage. There is no blood pressure threshold that defines a hypertensive crisis, although most patients with pressures exceeding 180/120 mm Hg can be considered to be in hypertensive crisis, with diastolic blood pressures over 120 mm Hg being most strongly associated with end-organ damage. Patients who develop a hypertensive crisis in settings other than chronic essential hypertension may develop end-organ damage at lesser degrees of blood pressure elevation, as they lack the vascular smooth muscle hypertrophy that provides some protection against uncontrolled hypertension.

PATHOPHYSIOLOGY

■ NORMAL BLOOD PRESSURE CONTROL

Many elements are involved in blood pressure regulation, such as the renin-angiotensin-aldosterone system (RAAS) of the kidney. Renin is released by the juxtaglomerular apparatus in response to low kidney perfusion, elevated sympathetic response, low dietary sodium, and other stimuli. Renin cleaves circulating angiotensinogen to form angiotensin I, which in turn is cleaved to angiotensin II by angiotensin-converting enzyme (ACE). Angiotensin II is a potent arteriolar constrictor that increases both systolic and diastolic blood pressure. It also signals the adrenal cortex to secrete aldosterone, which increases the reabsorption of sodium from urine, sweat, saliva, and bowel.

Catecholamines from the sympathetic nervous system greatly affect blood pressure, especially epinephrine. Binding of epinephrine to $\alpha 1$ receptors leads to vasoconstriction and increased peripheral vascular resistance, causing blood pressure to rise. Binding to β_1 receptors increases heart rate and cardiac output, which also raises blood pressure. The endothelium also locally produces vasoactive substances that affect blood pressure, such as the vasodilators nitric oxide, prostacyclin, and bradykinin, and the vasoconstrictor endothelin-1. Neutrophils are commonly attracted to the areas of vascular injury in acute hypertension.

Arterial baroreceptors are mechanoreceptors in the carotid sinuses and aortic arch. When blood pressure rises, the mechanoreceptors are stretched, decreasing their firing rate. This decreases central sympathetic outflow and increases parasympathetic tone, lowering blood pressure. Conversely, when blood pressure falls,

TABLE 91-1 Blood Pressure Classification Based on Guidelines from the Seventh Report of the Joint National Committee on Prevention, Detection, Evaluation, and Treatment of High Blood Pressure

	Normal	Prehypertension	Stage I	Stage II
Systolic blood pressure (in mm Hg)	<120	120-139	140-159	>160
Diastolic blood pressure (in mm Hg)	<80	80-89	90-99	>100

Data from Chobanian AV, Bakris GL, Black HR, et al. Seventh Report of the Joint National Committee on Prevention, Detection, Evaluation, and Treatment of High Blood Pressure. *JAMA.* 2003;289:2560-2572.

decreased stretching of mechanoreceptors increases their firing rate, stimulating sympathetic and inhibiting parasympathetic outflow. This feedback loop is sensitive to acute fluctuations in blood pressure, but in chronic essential hypertension, the set point rises and a higher basal blood pressure is tolerated.

■ PHYSIOLOGIC DERANGEMENTS IN HYPERTENSIVE CRISES

In general, hypertensive crises result from a breakdown in arterial adaptation to chronic hypertension, leading to a vicious cycle of vascular injury. The endothelium adapts to high blood pressure by smooth muscle hypertrophy and vasoconstriction. Prolonged smooth muscle contraction eventually leads to endothelial dysfunction, diminished nitric oxide production, and a failure of autoregulation. Focal vasodilation, endothelial damage, and increased vascular permeability result, with leakage and deposition of fibrinogen and plasma proteins in blood vessel walls. Monocyte chemoattractant protein-1 (MCP-1) recruits monocytes to the sites of vascular inflammation. The coagulation cascade is then activated, and fibrinous clot is formed, leading to ischemia, further endothelial injury, inflammation, and release of vasoconstrictive mediators, perpetuating the cycle of injury.

Under normal conditions, the brain autoregulates cerebral blood flow (CBF) to ensure that the high metabolic demands of neuronal cells are met, despite fluctuations in blood pressure. Normally, CBF is maintained at 50 mL blood per 100 g of brain tissue per minute (**Figures 91-1** and **91-2**). The upper limit of autoregulation is a mean arterial pressure (MAP) of >120 mm Hg for normotensive patients, and >180 mm Hg for hypertensive patients. (The higher threshold in hypertensive patients is due to vascular hypertrophy and other morphologic changes from chronic elevations in blood pressure.) If the upper limit of autoregulation is surpassed, endothelial dysfunction and damage may occur, the blood-brain barrier may break down, and cerebral edema and microhemorrhages may develop, giving rise to hypertensive encephalopathy.

The lower limit of CBF autoregulation also differs between hypertensive and normotensive patients. Hypertensive patients may show signs or symptoms of cerebral hypoxemia, including loss of consciousness, coma, or seizures, at MAP levels of 50 ± 5 mm Hg and below, whereas normotensive patients will show these symptoms at a MAP of 40 ± 5 mm Hg and below. This has important implications for the management of hypertensive emergencies: too rapid lowering of blood pressure in these patients poses a risk of significant cerebral hypoperfusion.

CAUSES

The most common causes of hypertensive crises are inadequate adherence to antihypertensive therapy and previously undiagnosed essential hypertension. Patients who stop taking some antihypertensive drugs may develop severe rebound hypertension, especially those who abruptly discontinue β-blockers or clonidine. Chronic renal insufficiency and sleep apnea are common medical causes of poorly controlled hypertension. Cocaine, amphetamines, phencyclidine, aminophylline, phenylephrine, diet pills, and other sympathomimetic drugs may cause hypertensive crises. Patients who take monoamine oxidase inhibitors (MAOIs), including the antibiotic linezolid and over-the-counter drugs with MAOI activity, such as St. John's wort, are at risk for developing hypertensive crisis with confusion if they also ingest selective serotonin reuptake inhibitors, tricyclic antidepressants, meperidine, tramadol, methadone, dextromethorphan, or tyramine-containing foods such as red wine, aged cheeses, smoked or pickled meats, and avocado. Bevacizumab, a monoclonal antibody against vascular endothelial growth factor that is approved for use in several advanced adenocarcinomas, may lead to hypertensive crisis.

Although most patients with a hypertensive crisis do not have a secondary cause of hypertension, such as renal artery stenosis, acute glomerulonephritis, preeclampsia, pheochromocytoma, scleroderma renal crisis, or Cushing syndrome, an evaluation for secondary hypertension should be considered, especially in the

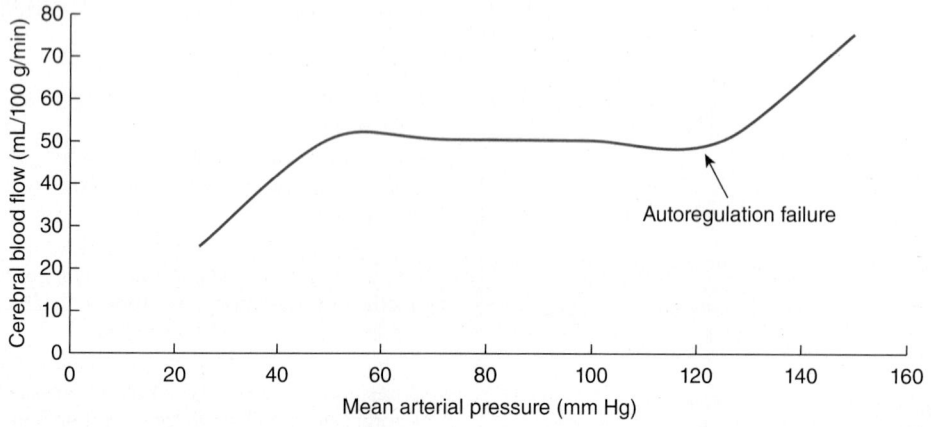

Figure 91-1 *Autoregulation of cerebral blood flow in response to changing mean arterial pressure in normotensive patient.* (Data from Strandgaard S, Olesen J, Skinhoj E, et al. *Br Med J.* 1973;1(5852):507-510.)

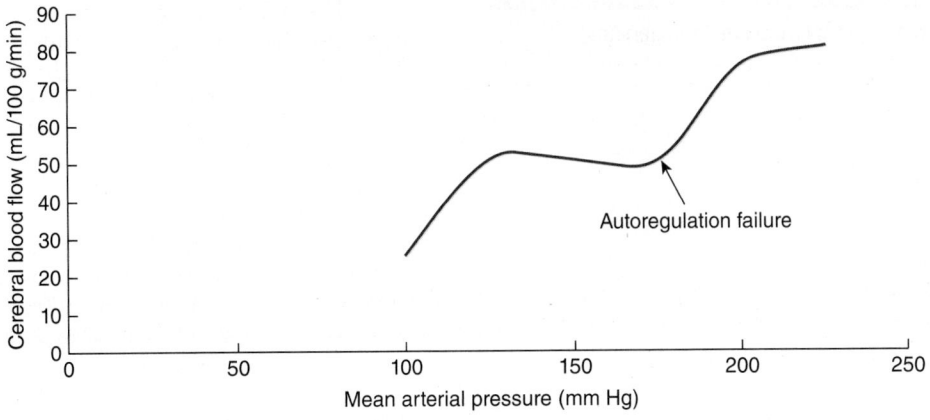

Figure 91-2 *Autoregulation of cerebral blood flow in response to changing mean arterial pressure in hypertensive patient.* (Data from Strandgaard S, Olesen J, Skinhoj E, et al. *Br Med J.* 1973;1(5852):507-510.)

presence of compatible signs and symptoms, as described in Chapter 244. Careful examination of the patient is required in all cases.

In the hospital, hypertensive crises may develop after surgeries. Postoperative hypertension is arbitrarily defined as a systolic blood pressure ≥190 mm Hg or a diastolic blood pressure ≥100 mm Hg on two consecutive readings following surgery. More than 50% of patients have a history of hypertension prior to surgery. Postoperative hypertension is most common after cardiac surgery, major vascular surgery (eg, carotid and aortic procedures), head and neck surgery, neurosurgery, trauma, and organ transplantation. Increases in sympathetic tone and vascular resistance are thought to underlie the condition.

CLINICAL MANIFESTATIONS

Clinical characteristics of the hypertensive crisis are summarized in **Table 91-2**. End-organ damage in hypertensive emergencies is summarized in **Table 91-3**, and discussed later in this chapter.

■ NEUROLOGIC

The central nervous system is the organ system most often involved in hypertensive emergency. Clinical events may include stroke, hypertensive encephalopathy, intracranial hemorrhage, and subarachnoid hemorrhage. Cerebral edema often develops, particularly in the white matter of the parietooccipital regions, leading to the posterior reversible encephalopathy syndrome (PRES) (**Figure 91-3**). Although patients with this syndrome may develop severe symptoms, including headache, nausea, delirium, visual disturbances, and focal neurologic findings, as the name suggests, many patients recover well as the cerebral edema resolves. The reason for the parietooccipital predominance is unknown, but may involve a relative paucity of sympathetic innervation in these regions.

■ CARDIAC

Myocardial ischemia is common, because of high myocardial oxygen demand, high-end diastolic pressures, endothelial damage, and previous myocardial hypertrophy, in patients with underlying essential hypertension. Congestive heart failure and pulmonary edema are common. Aortic dissection is a dreaded complication, and should be suspected in those with sudden tearing or ripping chest pain radiating into the back, discordant upper-extremity pulses, and new diastolic murmurs. It should be borne in mind that neurologic symptoms in hypertensive crises may also be caused by aortic dissection disrupting the cerebral circulation.

■ RETINOPATHY

Visual disturbances in hypertensive crisis may be due to hypertensive encephalopathy and the posterior PRES, but they may also be due to malignant hypertensive retinopathy, characterized by swelling of the optic disc, retinal hemorrhages, and soft exudates (cotton-wool spots).

■ RENAL

The kidney, like the brain, has a capacity to autoregulate its blood supply, but in the setting of a hypertensive crisis, this ability may be overwhelmed and a vicious cycle of kidney damage may ensue, characterized by vascular damage, endothelial dysfunction, fibrinoid necrosis, inflammation, and ischemic injury.

DIAGNOSIS OF HYPERTENSIVE URGENCIES AND EMERGENCIES

The initial assessment should include a thorough medical history, including the duration and severity of hypertension, comorbid cardiovascular and renal disease, all current prescription and

TABLE 91-2 Clinical Characteristics of the Hypertensive Emergency

Blood Pressure (mm Hg)	Neurologic Status	Cardiac Findings	Funduscopic Findings	Renal Symptoms	Gastrointestinal Symptoms
Not needed for diagnosis but usually ≥180/120 mm Hg	Headache, confusion, somnolence, stupor, visual loss, seizures, focal neurologic deficits, coma	Prominent apical pulsation, cardiac enlargement, congestive heart failure	Hemorrhages, exudates, papilledema	Azotemia, proteinuria, oliguria	Nausea, vomiting

Data from Vidt DG. Hypertensive crises: emergencies and urgencies. *J Clin Hypertens.* 2004;6:520-525; Chobanian AV, Bakris GL, Black HR, et al. Seventh Report of the Joint National Committee on Prevention, Detection, Evaluation, and Treatment of High Blood Pressure. *JAMA.* 2003;289:2560-2572.

TABLE 91-3 Examples of Hypertensive Emergencies

Acute aortic dissection

Acute ischemic or hemorrhagic stroke

Subarachnoid hemorrhage

Hypertensive encephalopathy

Acute myocardial ischemia/infarction

Acute heart failure

β-Blocker or clonidine withdrawal

Catecholamine excess states

Cocaine, phencyclidine hydrochloride use

Eclampsia

Head trauma

Hemorrhage

Pheochromocytoma crisis

Data from Hebert C, Vidt D. Hypertensive crises. *Primary Care: Clin. Office Pract.* 2008;35:475-487.

nonprescription medications, and recreational drugs, especially cocaine and other stimulants. Patients should be questioned in a nonjudgmental way about adherence to antihypertensive medications and possible obstacles to adherence.

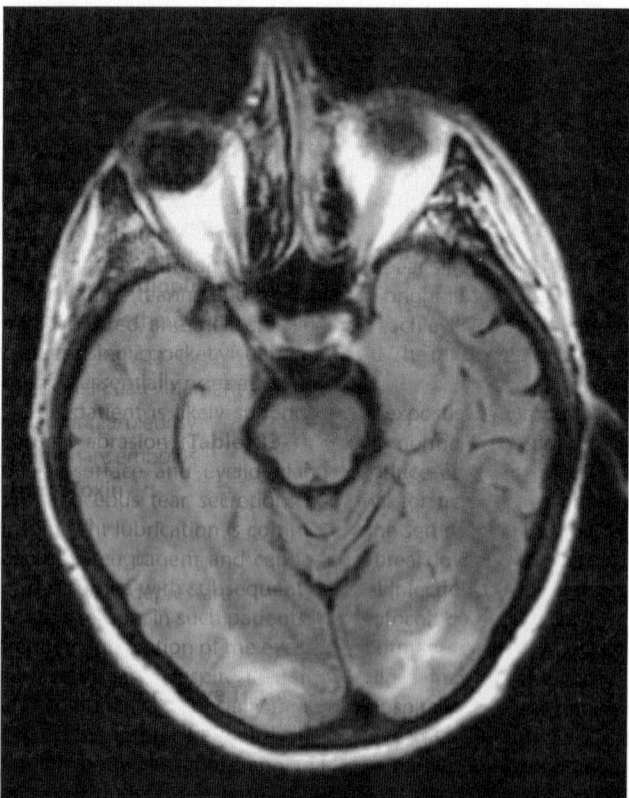

Figure 91-3 *Axial FLAIR MRI showing increased signal (white) in the occipital subcortical white matter and cortex bilaterally. These findings are typical of the reversible posterior leukoencephalopathy syndrome (RPLS) in the setting of hypertensive emergency, and probably represent reversible vasogenic edema. Other causes of RPLS include preeclampsia, cancer chemotherapy, and cyclosporine, tacrolimus, and other immunosuppressive drugs. (Reproduced, with permission, from Simon RP, Greenberg DA, Aminoff MJ. Clinical Neurology. 7th ed. New York, NY: McGraw-Hill, 2009. Fig. 1-10.)*

The review of systems should focus on symptoms that might indicate end-organ damage from hypertension, such as chest pain, shortness of breath, severe headache, changes in vision, dizziness, altered mental status or somnolence, oliguria, or anuria.

On examination, the first step in diagnosing a hypertensive crisis is accurate blood pressure measurement. This should be repeated at least twice, taking precautions to properly position the patient and use an adequately sized cuff. Blood pressure should be checked in both arms and in the lower limbs. A blood pressure difference of more than 20 mm Hg between arms suggests aortic dissection, but unfortunately is not a sensitive finding. The examiner should also focus on detecting new end-organ damage. On funduscopic examination, chronic hypertensive patients often have chronic findings, such as widening of the arterial stripe (copper-wire and silver-wire changes) and arteriovenous nicking. Greater significance is attached to acute changes, such as new hemorrhages, cotton-wool retinal exudates, and papilledema. Signs of heart failure, such as elevated jugular venous pressures, S3 heart sounds, and pulmonary rales, should be sought on cardiopulmonary examination. A new diastolic heart murmur suggests aortic insufficiency from aortic dissection.

TREATMENT

Excessive blood pressure lowering should be avoided in most patients with hypertensive crisis, as many of them have chronic hypertension with vascular changes and are at risk for cerebral ischemia if blood pressure falls too quickly. This is especially true of older patients. An approach to triage in patients with hypertensive crisis is summarized in **Table 91-4**. In patients with hypertensive urgency, blood pressure lowering may usually be accomplished with oral medications over a 24- to 48-hour period. These patients do not necessarily require hospital admission. They may be observed and treated with oral agents for several hours prior to discharge with close outpatient follow-up, assuming that their blood pressure falls into an acceptable range. However, if patients with hypertensive urgency are symptomatic or if there are concerns about adherence, it is reasonable to admit these patients.

Patients with hypertensive crisis often benefit from being in a quieter and less stressful environment, if such can be provided in the inpatient setting. There are very few randomized controlled trials of therapy in hypertensive crisis. In hypertensive urgency, a reasonable approach is to restart oral antihypertensives in patients who have been nonadherent, or to increase doses of current therapy in adherent patients. In patients not previously taking antihypertensive therapy, initial choices for drug therapy include an ACE inhibitor, β-blockers, or a calcium channel blocker. These patients are likely to require more than one agent for blood pressure control. Loop diuretics may be helpful in edematous patients. Sublingual nifedipine was once commonly used in the treatment of hypertensive crisis, but has fallen out of favor because of the risks of reflex tachycardia and hypotension. This agent must be avoided in all cases of hypertensive crises.

Patients with hypertensive emergencies ideally should be admitted to an intensive care unit for continuous monitoring of hemodynamics, neurologic status, urine output, and other manifestations of end-organ damage. Hypertensive emergencies are typically managed with short-acting titratable antihypertensive agents (**Table 91-5**). In the first hour of therapy, the goal is to lower mean arterial blood pressure by no more than 15% to 20%, with a diastolic blood pressure in the range of 100 to 110 mm Hg. Blood pressure is further reduced to 25% to 30% of the initial value within the next 4 to 8 hours. Oral antihypertensive agents should replace intravenous agents only when stable blood pressure control has been achieved, and there is no evidence of continuing end-organ damage.

Sodium nitroprusside used to be the preferred agent for hypertensive emergency, given its rapid onset of active, easy titration

TABLE 91-4 Algorithm for Triage Evaluation

| Parameter | Severe Hypertension (Urgency) | | Hypertensive Emergency |
	Asymptomatic	Symptomatic	
Blood pressure (mm Hg)	<180/120	<180/120	Usually >180/120
Symptoms	Headache, anxiety; often asymptomatic	Severe headache, shortness of breath	Shortness of breath, chest pain, nocturia, dysarthria, weakness, altered consciousness
Examination	No target organ damage, no clinical cardiovascular disease	Target organ damage; clinical cardiovascular disease present, stable	Encephalopathy, pulmonary edema, renal insufficiency, cerebrovascular accident, cardiac ischemia
Therapy	Observe at least 1-3 h; initiate, resume medication; increase dosage of inadequate agent	Observe at least 3-6 h; lower blood pressure with short-acting oral agent; adjust current therapy	Baseline laboratory tests; intravenous line; monitor BP; may initiate parenteral therapy in emergency room
Plan	Arrange follow-up within 3-7 d; if no prior evaluation, schedule appointment	Arrange follow-up evaluation in less than 72 h	Immediate admission to intensive care unit; treat to initial goal BP; additional diagnostic studies

Data from Vidt DG. Hypertensive crises: emergencies and urgencies. *J Clin Hypertens*. 2004;6:520-525.

and rapid cessation of action when infusions are halted. However, sodium nitroprusside is a powerful vasodilator, and most authors caution against its use in patients with increased intracranial pressure and other conditions. Thiocyanate toxicity, manifesting as confusion and lactic acidosis, is likely with nitroprusside infusions, especially when high doses are given in the setting of renal insufficiency. For this reason, nitroprusside infusions should not continue beyond 24 hours. The author strongly recommends against the use of this agent.

Other agents include labetalol (a β-1 and β-2 adrenergic blocking agent), which should be used with caution in the setting of bradycardia, atrioventricular block, heart failure, and bronchospasm, and the dihydropiridine calcium channel blocker nicardipine, which is associated with mild reflex tachycardia, headache, and flushing.

Fenoldopam is a selective dopamine-1 receptor antagonist and short-acting vasodilator. It seems as effective as sodium nitroprusside in hypertensive crisis, with the advantages of improved renal perfusion and promotion of diuresis, with less side effects. Tachyphylaxis usually develops after 48 hours. Nitroglycerin can be used in hypertensive emergencies, although high intravenous doses of this agent are required to lower blood pressure. This drug may be especially helpful in the management of hypertension with myocardial ischemia. Headache is common with both fenoldopam and nitroglycerin.

Clevidipine is a short-acting dihydropyridine calcium channel blocker that selectively inhibits the influx of extracellular calcium through the L-type channels. It has minimal effect on myocardial contractility. Side effects include headache, reflex tachycardia,

TABLE 91-5 Dose and Administration of Intravenous Agents Used in Hypertensive Emergencies

Drug	Dose and Administration
Clevidipine	Loading dose of 1-2 mg, followed by repeated incremental doubling of the dose at 90-s intervals until the desired blood pressure is achieved. As blood pressure approaches goal, increase the dose by less than double and lengthen the time between dose adjustments to every 5-10 min. An approximately 1-2 mg/h increase will generally produce an additional 2-4 mm Hg decrease in systolic pressure. The desired therapeutic response for most patients occurs at doses of 4-6 mg/h. Patients with severe hypertension may require doses up to 32 mg/h.
Enalaprilat	IV injection of 1.25 mg over 5 min every 6 h, titrated by increments of 1.25 mg at 12-24-h intervals to a maximum of 5 mg every 6 h.
Esmolol	IV loading dose of 500-1000 µg/kg over 1 min (1 mg/kg ideal body weight), followed by an infusion at 25-50 µg/kg/min, which may be increased by 25 µg/kg/min every 10-20 min until the desired response to a maximum of 300 µg/kg/min.
Fenoldopam	An initial IV dose of 0.1 µg/kg/min, titrated by increments of 0.05-0.1 µg/kg/min to a maximum of 1.6 µg/kg/min.
Hydralazine	5 mg bolus then 5-10 mg IV every 20-30 min as needed.
Labetalol	Initial bolus 20 mg, followed by boluses of 20-80 mg or an infusion starting at 1-2 mg/min and titrated up to until the desired hypotensive effect is achieved. Bolus injections of 1-2 mg/kg have been reported to produce precipitous falls in blood pressure and should therefore be avoided; maximum cumulative dose is 300 mg over 24 h.
Nicardipine	5 mg/h; titrate to effect by increasing 2.5 mg/h every 5 min to a maximum of 15 mg/h.
Nitroprusside	0.5 µg/kg/min; titrate as tolerated to maximum of 2 µg/kg/min.
Phentolamine	Sympathetic crisis: IV 5-20 mg. Treatment of pralidoxime-induced hypertension (unlabeled use): IV 5 mg. Surgery for pheochromocytoma/hypertension: IM, IV 5 mg given 1-2 h before procedure and repeated as needed every 2-4 h.

IM, intramuscular; IV, intravenous.
Data from Varon J. Treatment of acute severe hypertension: current and newer agents. *Drugs*. 2008;68:283-297.

nausea, and possibly atrial fibrillation. Another agent that is less commonly utilized is hydralazine. This drug has the concern of its prolonged and unpredictable antihypertensive effects. Hydralazine is still used in some cases of pregnancy-induced hypertension.

Hypertensive crisis from cocaine

- Acute and chronic effects of cocaine on the cardiovascular system include tachycardia, hypertensive crisis, myocardial infarction, stroke, aortic dissection, and cardiomyopathy. Hypertension in patients with cocaine intoxication relates to central stimulation of the sympathetic nervous system, as well as inhibition of neuronal catecholamine reuptake. β-blockers are *contraindicated* in cocaine intoxication, as they may lead to paradoxical worsening of hypertension via the unopposed α-adrenergic vasoconstrictive effects of cocaine. Although labetalol has both β- and α-blocking properties, it should also be avoided in this setting, as it is a more effective β-blocker than α-blocker. Therapeutic options for cocaine-induced hypertension include the α-blocker phentolamine, benzodiazepines such as diazepam or lorazepam, continuous infusions of calcium channel blockers, and occasionally oral clonidine.

DISCHARGE CHECKLIST

- Has the patient been transitioned to oral antihypertensives, with blood pressure consistently maintained ≤160/100 mm Hg?
- Has close outpatient follow-up been arranged to encourage adherence and to further titrate the patient's medications to achieve the target blood pressure? (Target blood pressure is generally < 140/90 mm Hg, but as low as <130/80 mm Hg in certain populations, including diabetics and patients with chronic renal disease).
- Have efforts been made to engage family members, friends, and outside resources, such as visiting nurses and pharmacists, to optimize medication adherence?

- Has the patient been advised about dietary sodium avoidance? Nutrition consult is often helpful in this setting.
- Have barriers to outpatient care been addressed, such as lack of health insurance, financial problems, poor home situation, knowledge gaps, comorbid psychiatric conditions, and untreated substance abuse? The involvement of social work providers may be very helpful in this regard.

SUGGESTED READINGS

Aggarwal M, Khan I. Hypertensive crisis: hypertensive emergencies and urgencies. *Cardiol Clin.* 2006;24:135-146.

Chobanian AV, Bakris GL, Black HR, et al. Seventh Report of the Joint National Committee on Prevention, Detection, Evaluation, and Treatment of High Blood Pressure. *Hypertension.* 2003;42:1206-1252.

Gore JM, Peterson E, Amin A, et al. Predictors of 90-day readmission among patients with acute severe hypertension. *Am Heart J.* 2010;160:521.e1-527.e1.

Karabacak M, Yiqit M, Turdogan KA, Sert M. The relationship between vascular inflammation and target organ damage in hypertensive crises. *Am J Emerg Med.* 2015;33:497-500.

Mayer S, Kurtz P, Wyman A, et al. Clinical practices, complications, and mortality in neurological patients with acute severe hypertension: The STAT Registry. *Crit Care Med.* 2011;39:2330-2336.

Varon J. Treatment of acute severe hypertension: current and newer agents. *Drugs.* 2008;68:283-297.

Varon J, Marik P. The diagnosis and management of hypertensive crises. *Chest.* 2000;118:214-227.

Varon J, Soto-Ruiz KM, Baumann BM, et al. The management of acute hypertension in patients with renal dysfunction: labetalol or nicardipine? *Postgrad Med.* 2014;126:124-130.

Vidt DG. Hypertensive crises: emergencies and urgencies. *J Clin Hypertens (Greenwich).* 2004;6:520-525.

CHAPTER 92

Hyperthermia and Fever

Chad S. Miller, MD, FACP, FHM
Jeffrey G. Wiese, MD, MHM, FACP

Key Clinical Questions

1. What is the difference between hyperthermia and fever?
2. What are the underlying mechanisms of hyperthermia and fever?
3. What are the implications of treatment for hyperthermia and fever?
4. Who is at greatest risk of developing hyperthermia?
5. What are the lasting effects of prolonged hyperthermia?

CASE 92-1

An 82-year-old man was brought to the emergency department with altered mental status. His neighbor found him unresponsive in his apartment on an extremely hot, humid summer day. He has a history of poorly controlled type 2 diabetes, hypertension, benign prostatic hypertrophy, and urinary urgency. He was currently taking glipizide, lisinopril, hydrochlorothiazide (HCTZ), doxazosin, oxybutynin, and diphenhydramine.

His temperature was 40°C, pulse rate was 120 beats/min, respiratory rate was 18 breaths/min, blood pressure was 90/60 mm Hg, and pulse oximetry was 98% on room air. He responds to sternal rub, but is otherwise nonresponsive and does not follow commands. His skin is flushed, warm, and dry. His pupils are 4 mm and minimally responsive to light. Bowel sounds are present.

What is the most likely cause of this patient's altered mental status and hyperthermia?

This man most likely has heat stroke, with multiple contributing factors. The ambient temperature is extremely hot, significantly increasing the risk of heat stroke. Older patients do not sense changes in temperature as well as young adults. He also takes oxybutynin and diphenhydramine, medications with anticholinergic properties that make him susceptible to anticholinergic poisoning and will lower his threshold for heat stroke. Although anticholinergic toxicity is possible, his lack of mydriasis and present bowel sounds suggest that this is not the primary contributing factor. Uncontrolled diabetes and HCTZ have also likely contributed to this man being chronically volume depleted, further lowering his threshold for heat stroke.

INTRODUCTION

The 99th percentile for healthy individuals defines the maximum oral temperature as 37.2°C (98.9°F) at 6 AM and 37.7°C (99.9°F) at 4 PM. Body temperature typically varies no more than 0.5°C (0.9°F) throughout the day. The hypothalamic thermoregulatory center maintains a normal temperature in the face of heat dissipation from the skin and lungs and heat generation from metabolic activity in muscle and liver. The postprandial state, pregnancy, and endocrine disorders may affect body temperature. The morning temperature tends to be lower in the 2 weeks prior to ovulation in menstruating women and then rises by 0.6°C (1.6°F) with ovulation until the next period (**Table 92-1**).

HYPERTHERMIA AND FEVER PRESENTATIONS

■ HYPERTHERMIA

Hyperthermia is defined as any elevation in the body's temperature beyond normal limits, with fever being considered a subset of hyperthermia. Hyperthermia is often used in a more specific fashion to denote elevated body temperature due to imbalances between metabolic heat production and heat loss, or exposure to extreme environmental heat. Fever results from inflammatory cytokine stimulation of the hypothalamus which changes the set point of the core body temperature. Fever should be considered when a morning temperature is greater than 37.2°C (98.9°F) or an evening temperature is greater than 37.7°C (99.9°F). However, in the hospital, a patient may not be considered to have a fever until the temperature

TABLE 92-1 Body Temperature Measurements

Type of reading	Normal 36.0-38.0°C	Core body temperature is tightly regulated between a normal diurnal range of 36.0 and 37.5°C
Rectal	0.4°C (0.7°F) higher than oral readings	May be 0.2-0.3°C higher than actual core body temperature
Oral	Lower readings due to mouth breathing	Influenced by eating, drinking, breathing devices, tachypnea, and mouth breathing
Tympanic membrane (TM)	Measures radiant heat from TM and nearby ear canal; more variable readings than oral or rectal modes	Preferred to oral measurements in patients with pulmonary disorders such as asthma or pneumonia
Axillary	Underestimates core body temperature	Not recommended

is greater than 38.0°C (100.4°F). The higher threshold increases the specificity of this vital sign. It is important to distinguish between fever and hyperthermia, as some causes of hyperthermia may be rapidly lethal, may respond poorly to antipyretics, and require additional means of decreasing the body temperature.

Body temperatures in hyperthermia may rise to levels greater than 41.1°C (106°F). This rise in temperature is not usually mediated by inflammatory cytokines and not usually caused by infection, except when the hypothalamic regulatory center has been affected by meningitis, encephalitis, or brain abscess. Brain or spinal trauma may also cause a marked rise in core body temperature, as experimental models have demonstrated that even a small amount of blood within the cerebrospinal fluid may induce hypothalamic dysregulation. However, most cases of classic hyperthermia are due to diseases causing imbalances in heat production and heat loss, such as malignant hyperthermia, neuroleptic malignant syndrome, serotonin syndrome, anticholinergic drugs, sympathomimetic drugs, thyrotoxicosis, and heat stroke (**Table 92-2**).

The most common presentation of hyperthermia is mental status changes or confusion. Altered mental status is an early finding in 80% of patients with severe hyperthermia. Heat stroke is often preceded by symptoms of heat exhaustion such as fatigue, malaise, nausea, muscle cramping, and headache. The progression to mental status changes such as confusion or coma is consistent with heat stroke and the inability to dissipate excessive heat. The core temperature usually exceeds 40.0°C. Hyperthermia can be difficult to distinguish from fever, but it should be considered in the presence of a high temperature and significant mental status changes, especially when infection has been excluded. Key historical clues include exposure to extremely high ambient temperatures or to certain medications, anesthetics, or recreational drugs. Common offending agents include halothane, isoflurane, succinylcholine, and the recreational drugs cocaine, ecstasy, and amphetamines.

Certain populations are at greater risk for hyperthermia. The very young, very old, bedridden, and those confined to poorly ventilated areas without air conditioning are at significant risk for nonexertional heat stroke. Young men tend to be at greatest risk for exertional heat stroke, but anyone engaging in strenuous activity, especially in high ambient temperatures, is at risk. Outdoor athletes, especially football players, and military recruits have a higher incidence. Dehydration,

medications with anticholinergic effects, and recreational drugs may accelerate the time to heat stroke in susceptible populations.

PRACTICE POINT

- Hyperthermia can be difficult to distinguish from fever, but should be considered in the presence of a high temperature and significant mental status changes, especially when infection has been excluded. Key historical clues include exposure to extremely high ambient temperatures or to certain medications, anesthetics, or recreational drugs.

Prolonged hyperthermia may result in irreversible neurologic damage. Severe morbidity and even death may result from disseminated intravascular coagulation, rhabdomyolysis, electrolyte disorders, and severe acid-base disturbances, often due to buildup of lactic acid.

PRACTICE POINT

- Prolonged hyperthermia may result in irreversible neurologic damage. Severe morbidity and even death may result from disseminated intravascular coagulation, rhabdomyolysis, electrolyte disorders, and severe acid-base disturbances, often due to build-up of lactic acid.

■ FEVER

Fever is the most common temperature disturbance in the hospital setting. Fever is the hypothalamic-mediated upregulation of the thermal set point in response to cytokine activation. These cytokines include interleukin (IL)-1, IL-6, and tumor necrosis factor (TNF-α). Fever is defined as a core body temperature greater than 38.0°C. Because most microbial organisms have a defined thermal range for survival, it is theorized that fever is an evolutionary adaptation for overcoming infection. However, there is no clinical evidence that fever hastens recovery from infection, or that the use of antipyretics delays recovery. While noninfectious causes of fever exist, the presumption should be that an infection is the cause of fever until excluded.

Many patients may be asymptomatic and have fever as the only sign of illness. In others, fever is one marker among a constellation of signs and symptoms. Symptoms that commonly accompany fever include diaphoresis, flushing, rigors, and chills. Rigors and chills are due to the rapid alteration in the body's thermal set point, causing the sensation that the body's current temperature under the new set point is too low, thus inducing a sensation of chills. Rigors, isometric contraction of muscles, are an effort to elevate the body's core temperature to meet the new thermal set point.

In the elderly and residents of long-term-care facilities, a decline in functional status, confusion, incontinence, falling, deteriorating mobility, reduced food intake, or failure to cooperate with staff should prompt a temperature measurement and evaluation for potential infectious causes. Fever is less common in hemodialysis patients, as the core body temperature is lost with each dialysis episode; over time, the baseline thermal set point is adjusted to a value lower than normal. Elevations in temperature between 0.5°C and 1.0°C in dialysis patients should prompt evaluation for infection.

Infections are the most common cause of fever, but many noninfectious inflammatory conditions cause the release of proinflammatory cytokines with a febrile response. Noninfectious disorders rarely cause a fever greater than 38.9°C, although notable exceptions

TABLE 92-2 Common Causes of Hyperthermia: Remember Them by Using the Mnemonic CHASE NMS

Central Nervous System Damage

Mechanism: damage of the hypothalamic regulatory center

Causes: subarachnoid hemorrhage, status epilepticus, hypothalamic injury

When to suspect: hyperthermia (>104°F) with associated head trauma, central nervous system infection, or history of seizures

Heat Stroke

Mechanism: inability to dissipate heat

Causes: exposure to high ambient temperatures, strenuous exercise

When to suspect: hyperthermia, dry skin, delirium in a patient exposed to high temperatures or having undergone severe exercise

Anticholinergic Poisoning/Exposure

Mechanism: central and peripheral muscarinic receptor blockade

Causes: antihistamines, atropine, belladonna alkaloids, carbamazepine, diphenhydramine, meclizine, phenothiazines

When to suspect: hyperthermia, altered mental status, dry mouth, lack of perspiration, flushing, and urinary retention

Serotonin Syndrome

Mechanism: overstimulation of 5-HT_{1A} receptors in the central grey nuclei and the medulla; 5-HT_2 receptors may also play a role

Causes and examples:

1. Excess precursors of serotonin or serotonin agonists—buspirone, L-dopa, lithium, LSD, L-tryptophan, trazodone
2. Increased release of serotonin—amphetamines, 3,4-methylenedioxymethamphetamine (MDMA), cocaine, reserpine, fenfluramine
3. Reduced uptake of serotonin—selective serotonin reuptake inhibitors (SSRIs), tricyclic antidepressants (TCAs), trazodone, venlafaxine, meperidine
4. Slowing of serotonin metabolism—monoamine oxidase inhibitors

When to suspect: hyperthermia, hyperhidrosis, confusion or agitation with significant autonomic and neurologic derangement

Endocrine

Mechanism: elevated endogenous metabolism

Causes: thyrotoxicosis, pheochromocytoma

When to suspect: hyperthermia, adrenergic symptoms, hypertension, and no associated drug exposures or heat exposures

Neuroleptic Malignant Syndrome (NMS)

Mechanism: unproven, but dopamine receptor blockade is thought to play a key role in precipitating NMS

Causes and examples:

1. Typical antipsychotic medications—haloperidol, chlorpromazine, loxapine
2. Atypical antipsychotic medications—aripiprazole, olanzapine, quetiapine, risperidone
3. Dopamine antagonists—metoclopramide, promethazine

When to suspect: hyperthermia, rigidity, altered mental status in a patient taking any of the classes of medications known to cause NMS

Malignant Hyperthermia

Mechanism: genetic disorder of calcium channels in skeletal muscle that allows an uncontrolled influx of calcium into the cell resulting in sustained muscle contraction and increased metabolism

Causes: inhalational anesthetics—halothane, enflurane, isoflurane; succinylcholine

When to suspect: hyperthermia in anyone receiving inhalational anesthetics or succinylcholine

Sympathomimetic Poisoning/Overdose

Mechanism: central and peripheral disturbances in thermoregulation

Causes: amphetamines, methamphetamines, cocaine, MDMA or ecstasy

When to suspect: recreational drug users and other high-risk populations with hyperthermia, mental status changes, and evidence of adrenergic stimulus

include adult Still's disease, lymphoma, transfusion reactions, biologic cytokine therapy, as well as agents implicated in hyperthermia. Any temperature above this threshold should prompt an evaluation for infection, as well as consideration of hyperthermia (hyperpyrexia) not mediated by inflammatory cytokines, but by disrupted thermoregulation.

THE FIREPLACE MODEL APPROACH

◼ HYPERTHERMIA

Hyperthermia is the result of a mismatch between heat production and heat loss, in the same way that overheating a home is due to a mismatch between heat production and heat loss from the home's fireplace. Overheating is caused by either too much firewood being burned (too much fuel), too much fire (metabolism), or too much insulation (heat retention).

The fuel (firewood) for basal metabolism must be adequate in order to generate heat. This includes normoglycemia, adequate nutrition, and adequate muscle mass. **Excess fuel** may sometimes be a contributing factor to hyperthermia. Increased muscle mass is a risk factor for malignant hyperthermia, due to increased metabolic demands. The body may reach higher temperatures more rapidly because the main means of increasing basal metabolism is through skeletal muscle.

Fuel excess is rarely the cause of hyperthermia; **excess body metabolism** (fire) is a much more common cause. Acute hyperthyroidism, malignant hyperthermia, neuroleptic malignant syndrome, and the serotonin syndrome are the common causes of acute elevations in metabolic rate. In these scenarios, the catalyst is endogenous (acute thyroid hormone elevations), or iatrogenic: anesthesia (in patients with a genetic predisposition), neuroleptics, or a combination of drugs that work on the serotonin receptors. The metabolism reaches levels too great for the normal compensatory mechanisms of heat loss to handle.

Once fuel supplies and metabolism have been excluded, **failure of heat elimination/excess heat conservation** (insulation) should be considered. The vasoconstriction associated with cocaine, sympathomimetics, and anticholinergic drugs may result in hyperthermia due to the inability to expel heat. Although mortality from cocaine overdose increases substantially in hot weather due to the inability to dissipate heat, cocaine has not been shown to affect core temperature in the absence of external heat stress. Anticholinergics competitively antagonize muscarinic receptors in sweat glands, decreasing the body's ability to sweat, a phenomenon dependent on cholinergic nerve fibers.

If the foregoing categories have been excluded, **altered thermal set point** (uncontrollable fire) should be considered. Core body temperature is maintained by balancing heat production and heat loss. This equilibrium is rigorously managed by the hypothalamus, brain stem, and cervical spinal cord. While damage to any of these components may result in hyperthermia or hypothermia, the most common etiology is the administration of antipsychotic drugs. Barbiturates, opioids, tricyclic antidepressants, and benzodiazepines can cause central thermoregulatory failure, resulting in either hypothermia or hyperthermia. Phenothiazines impair central thermoregulation and inhibit peripheral vasoconstriction.

Although this is usually obvious from the history, prolonged exposure to heat may cause hyperthermia. The history or manner in which the patient is brought into the hospital should provide the clinical clues.

FEVER

The approach to fever in the hospitalized patient should begin with the presumption that the fever is due to an infection, while simultaneously excluding noninfectious causes of fever and additional causes of hyperthermia.

Infectious causes

The approach to infectious causes of fever should begin with the usual suspects. The lungs, blood, urine, skin, and sinuses are the most common sites of infection. Evaluation of all five is suggested unless the source is clinically apparent. The presenting symptoms should guide the evaluation, but where symptoms are not present, the hidden sources of infection should be considered (see Table 92-1). Based upon the Centers for Disease Control and Prevention's (CDC's) "opt out" recommendations, all patients with a reasonable possibility of having HIV should be tested unless the patient opts out of testing. HIV status should be determined early, as this may broaden the search for opportunistic infections. The role of atelectasis as a cause of fever is unclear; however, atelectasis probably does not cause fever in the absence of pulmonary infection.

Noninfectious causes

The noninfectious causes fall into three categories: vascular, inflammatory, autoimmune and endocrine.

Vascular disruption may lead to fever. The decreased blood supply from vascular compromise leads to tissue necrosis, which releases inflammatory cytokines that may result in fever. Potential causes include cerebral infarction or hemorrhage, subarachnoid hemorrhage, myocardial infarction, ischemic bowel, fat emboli, deep venous thrombosis, pulmonary emboli, and gastrointestinal bleeding. It should be noted that hematomas may result in fever, not only from the underlying vascular injury, but due to the immune activation during resorption, especially for a large hematoma.

Inflammatory causes of fever may be due to a cytokine response to noninfectious antigens. The body responds as if infected, even though the inflammatory response is to a noninfectious antigen. Examples are posttransfusion fever, drug fever, organ transplant rejection, and intravenous contrast dye reactions. Other inflammatory causes may be due to tissue injury or immune dysfunction. These include aspiration pneumonitis, acute respiratory distress syndrome (ARDS), gout, pseudogout, and neoplastic fevers. Treatment with organ-specific cytokine therapy (eg, interferon-γ, interleukin-2) usually results in fever through the same mechanisms. After the age of 50, the incidence of fevers due to malignancy and autoimmune disease increases relative to infection.

Autoimmune disease overlaps the inflammatory and the vascular categories. By definition, autoimmune diseases have an inflammatory reaction to self antigens, and many autoimmune diseases have concomitant vasculitis.

PREVALENCE AND ADJUSTMENTS
BASELINE PREVALENCE

Death from extreme temperatures are relatively uncommon. Early diagnosis and treatment can often prevent mortality. In the United States, a total of 3442 deaths from exposure to extreme heat were reported between 1999 and 2003. Of these deaths, 2239 (65%) were recorded as exposure to excessive heat and 1203 (35%) were due to nonexposure hyperthermia. From 2003 to 2005, the number of cases of malignant hyperthermia related to anesthesia increased from 372 to 521 per year in the United States. The actual prevalence of serotonin syndrome is unknown, but it has been seen in approximately 14% of all patients who overdose with selective serotonin reuptake inhibitors (SSRIs). The prevalence of NMS is estimated to be anywhere from 0.02% to 2.44% of the population and appears to be decreasing with the increased reliance on atypical antipsychotic mediations.

FACTORS THAT IMPACT PREVALENCE

Age. There is a significant increased risk of dying from hyperthermia in adults over the age of 65. The ability to sense heat is reduced with age. The elderly have a higher threshold for sweating and cutaneous vasodilation. The use of medications, especially those with anticholinergic or diuretic effects, accentuate the risk of heat stroke in the elderly. Greater than 40% of all hypothermia- and hyperthermia-related deaths are in this age group. Diabetic patients 65 years or older have a slightly higher risk of dying on hot days than other subjects.

Gender. Men have a twofold increased risk of death due to hyperthermia as compared to women. The discrepancy is likely explained by exertional heat illness that occurs in previously healthy young men during exercise. Men, on average, have a higher skeletal muscle mass for a given surface area. Therefore, the ability to dissipate heat is decreased compared to women. Typical scenarios include military exercises undertaken by personnel recently arrived in a hot country, and long-distance races on excessively hot days. The one exception to the male predominance is malignant hyperthermia. There is a slightly greater mortality risk for female patients.

Race, ethnicity. While there is a hereditary risk for malignant hyperthermia in the setting of anesthetics, it is not tightly associated with any one race. The better approach is to inquire as to a family history of problems following the administration of anesthetics.

THE HISTORY

■ HYPERTHERMIA

The diagnostic approach to hyperthermia is summarized in **Figure 92-1**. The causes of hyperthermia are often apparent from events immediately preceding the temperature elevation, such as severe heat exposure, exertion, or ingestion of drugs that affect thermoregulation.

■ MALIGNANT HYPERTHERMIA

- *Has this patient recently been administered anesthetics or succinylcholine?* If yes, this increases the likelihood of malignant hyperthermia; a positive family history of adverse reactions to anesthetics increases this possibility.

Neuroleptic malignant syndrome

- *Is the patient taking neuroleptics?* If yes, this increases the possibility of neuroleptic malignant syndrome (NMS). High-potency neuroleptic drugs with strong D2 receptor antagonism, such as haloperidol and thiothixene, are more likely to cause NMS than lower-potency antipsychotics, such as chlorpromazine or thioridazine.
- *Is this patient taking antipsychotic medications?* If yes, this increases the likelihood of hypothalamic dysfunction resulting in extremes of temperature.

Serotonin syndrome

- *Is this patient taking selective serotonin receptor inhibitors (SSRIs), serotonin-norepinephrine reuptake inhibitors (SNRIs), monoamine oxidase inhibitors (MAOIs), meperidine, or linezolid, particularly in combination?* If yes, this increases the possibility of serotonin syndrome. Linezolid has weak, reversible, competitive and noncompetitive MAOI activity.

Sympathomimetic

- *Has this patient used cocaine or a sympathomimetic?* Drugs with sympathomimetic properties include amphetamines, as well as ephedrine and pseudoephedrine, which are present in over-the-counter decongestants and dietary agents (eg, Ma Huang). If yes, this increases the likelihood of heat illness due to inability to dissipate heat.

Anticholinergic

- *Is this patient taking anticholinergic medication?* Medications that have anticholinergic properties include antihistamines, parkinsonism medications, atropine, scopolamine, donnatal (belladonna alkaloids combined with phenobarbital), neuroleptics, antispasmodics, tricyclic antidepressants, and many plant species, the most common being jimsonweed.

Endocrine

- *Does this patient have a history of thyroid disease or is the patient currently taking thyroid medication?* Thyroid disease is the most common endocrine disease that may manifest with elevated core body temperature.

Heat stroke

- *Is the patient's temperature greater than 40°C?* If yes, this increases the likelihood that this is hyperthermia and not mediated by inflammatory cytokines.
- *Is it one of the hottest days of the year?* If yes, the patient's heat dissipation mechanisms may be altered even if the patient is otherwise healthy.

- *Has this patient recently undergone extreme exertion?* If yes, the patient's heat dissipation mechanisms may be altered even if the patient is otherwise healthy.

CNS injury

- *Does this patient have signs of CNS infection?* If yes, this may be the exception where both inflammatory mediators and hypothalamic derangement are contributing to the elevated temperature.
- *Has this patient sustained recent head trauma?* Intracranial hemorrhage may result in extremely high temperatures.
- *Is this patient taking anticoagulants?* This increases the potential for intracranial hemorrhage.

■ FEVER

Infectious causes

There are various risk factors for infection (**Table 92-3**).

- *Does this patient note any potential infectious symptoms?* If yes, the workup should proceed as appropriate for the differential diagnosis in question (eg, if sputum production and cough are present, further questioning and testing should address the diagnoses of pneumonia and bronchitis). If the patient has none of these symptoms, subsequent questions should be directed at risk factors for infection and hidden sources of infection.
- *Does this patient have any potential predisposing factors for infection?* If yes, the line of questioning should proceed as appropriate for the risk factor being considered (eg, if there is a recent sick-contact exposure, the nature of the exposure and the symptoms of the index case should be explored). For all affirmative answers, the physical examination, laboratory studies, and radiologic examinations should further evaluate the patient's risk.

Because noninfectious causes of fever are usually less life-threatening, the line of questioning for these diagnoses should proceed after the pretest probability for infection has been sufficiently reduced or excluded. Patients presenting to the hospital with fever on the day of admission are much more likely to have an infection than they are to have a noninfectious cause of their fever (90% vs 10%). As the hospitalization proceeds, however, the pretest probability for noninfectious causes increases (60% vs 40%), and this line of questioning should be routinely employed.

Vascular causes

- *Does this patient have signs of focal neurologic deficits or increased intracranial pressure?* If yes, evaluate for intracranial bleed.
- *Does this patient complain of chest pain and have risk factors for atherosclerosis?* If yes, consider myocardial infarction, especially if the fever is low grade.
- *Has this patient sustained a severe fracture?* If yes, the likelihood of fat emboli is increased.
- *Is this patient in a hypercoagulable state?* If yes, the likelihood of venous thromboembolism is increased.
- *Does this patient have signs or a history of vascular stasis?* If yes, the likelihood of venous thromboembolism is increased.
- *Has this patient recently been hospitalized or had surgery?* If yes, the likelihood of venous thromboembolism is increased.
- *Does this patient have risks for endothelial damage such as smoking or inflammatory diseases?* If yes, the likelihood of venous thromboembolism is increased.

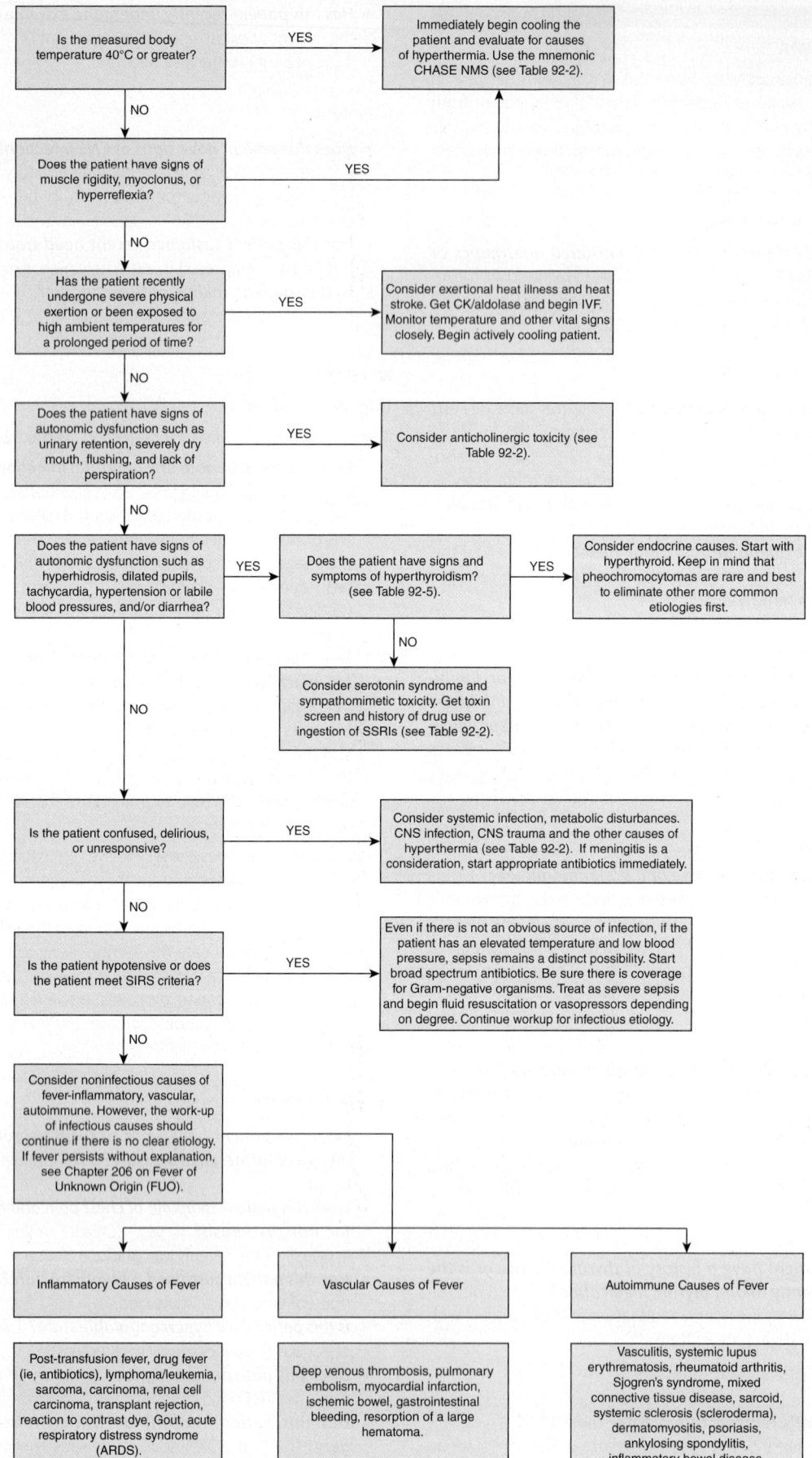

Figure 92-1 *Diagnostic approach to hyperthermia (for hospitalized patients with an elevated temperature >38.0°C and without an obvious source of infection).*

TABLE 92-3 Risk Factors for Infection

Exposure Risks

- Indwelling catheter (vascular or urinary)?
- Intravenous drug use?
- Open sores?
- Resides in long-term care facility?
- Sick contacts?
- Recent travel?
- Occupational exposures?
- Pets or animal contacts?
- Recent trauma or surgery?
- Recent hospitalization?

Innate Risks

- Is this patient HIV positive?
- Does this patient have diabetes?
- Is this patient on immunosuppressive medications?
- Is there a history of recurrent infections?

- **Does this patient have signs of bruising or bleeding?** If yes, these could be signs of vascular damage and tissue necrosis.
- **Does this patient have a large hematoma?** If yes, large hematomas may cause fever from both vascular injury and immune activation during resorption.
- **Has this patient recently had intravenous access or engaged in intravenous drug use?** This increases the likelihood for thromboembolism or infection.

Antigen stimulation and inflammatory causes

- **Has this patient received a transfusion of blood products in the last 24 hours?** If yes, this increases the likelihood of serum sickness or a reaction to blood products.
- **Is the patient receiving a medication, especially intravenous, known to cause drug fever (eg, antibiotics)?** If yes and infectious causes are unlikely, consider drug fever.
- **Are routine cultures negative for infection?** If yes, this decreases the pretest probability of common infections and must increase the likelihood of other causes, including noninfectious causes.
- **Is this patient at risk for aspiration?** If yes, consider aspiration pneumonitis.
- **Does this patient have a transplanted organ?** If yes, this increases the risk that the fever is from transplant rejection. However, unless there is a clear indication of transplant organ dysfunction, a thorough evaluation for infection must be completed before this etiology is pursued, because these individuals are at high risk of infection related to immunosuppressive medications.
- **Is this patient maintaining proper oxygen saturation?** If no, ARDS could be considered. Although many underlying causes of ARDS are infectious, a significant number are noninfectious (eg, pancreatitis).
- **Is this patient complaining of severe joint pain?** If yes, consider gout and pseudogout.
- **Has this patient received intravenous contrast in the previous 24 hours?** If yes, increase the risk for contrast dye reactions.
- **Has this patient had routine cancer screening?** If no, consider evaluating the patient for malignancy, based upon age and gender, among other factors.

- **Does this patient have additional risk factors for malignancy?** If yes, risk factors such as tobacco smoking, HIV, family history, should prompt additional evaluation if no other cause of fever is determined.

Inflammatory and vascular (autoimmune) causes

- **Does this patient or a family member have a history of autoimmune disease or vasculitis?** If yes, the likelihood of the patient having an autoimmune disease may be increased.
- **Does this patient have other complaints consistent with autoimmune disease such as arthralgias, arthritis, myalgias, rash, photosensitivity, Reynaud phenomenon, pulmonary/renal disease, or other signs of severe inflammation?** If yes, this should prompt a further workup for autoimmune disease.

Endocrine causes

- **Does this patient have a family history of thyroid disease, known thyroid disease, or symptoms suggesting hyperthyroidism?** Look for physical findings such as tachycardia, moist skin, thyroid enlargement, and eyelid retraction, and check serum thyroid-stimulating hormone.
- **Does this patient have a family history of pheochromocytoma, known pheochromocytoma, or symptoms suggesting pheochromocytoma?** If so, consider checking plasma free metanephrines.

THE EXAMINATION

■ HYPERTHERMIA

If the patient has a pontine hemorrhage, the temperature may have a significant role in prognosis (**Table 92-4**).

Thyrotoxicosis may cause elevated temperatures by increasing the basal metabolism, although it usually does not cause extremely high body temperatures. **Table 92-5** lists physical exam findings that may be helpful in making the diagnosis of hyperthyroidism.

The diagnosis of neuroleptic malignant syndrome (NMS) based upon Levenson and Sternbach requires meeting three major criteria, or two major and four minor criteria, plus a supportive history (**Table 92-6**). Infection, metabolic disturbances, and substance abuse must be excluded.

The Hunter Serotonin Toxicity Criteria have replaced Sternbach's criteria for serotonin syndrome (**Table 92-7**). The Hunter criteria are 84% sensitive and 97% specific for diagnosing serotonin toxicity, with a positive likelihood ratio of 28.0 and a negative likelihood ratio of 0.16. Key examinations features of serotonin syndrome include sweating, shivering, rigidity, hyperreflexia, myoclonus, and delirium, seizures, or coma in the setting of exposure to a serotonergic agent. There is a milder form of serotonin syndrome that may be misdiagnosed as it does not neatly fit the criteria described above. It presents with restlessness, insomnia, dilated pupils, akathisia, tachycardia, dyspnea, diarrhea, and autonomic instability. Unlike the full-blown serotonin syndrome, it may not be associated with hyperthermia or the same degree of delirium.

TABLE 92-4 Utility of Temperature Predicting Mortality in a Patient with a Pontine Hemorrhage

	+LR (95% CI)	−LR (95% CI)
Temperature >39°C predictive of mortality in a patient with a pontine hemorrhage	23.7 (1.5, 371)	0.4 (0.2, 0.6)

TABLE 92-5 Utility of Clinical Findings for Diagnosing Hyperthyroidism

	+LR (95% CI)	−LR (95% CI)
Pulse ≥90 beats/min	4.4 (3.8, 5.1)	0.2 (0.2, 0.3)
Skin moist and warm	6.7 (5.0, 9.1)	0.7 (0.7, 0.7)
Enlarged thyroid	2.3 (2.1, 2.5)	0.1 (0.1, 0.2)
Eyelid retraction	31.5 (16.6, 59.7)	0.7 (0.6, 0.7)
Eyelid lag	17.6 (9.2, 33.7)	0.8 (0.8, 0.8)
Fine finger tremor	11.4 (8.7, 14.8)	0.3 (0.3, 0.4)
Wayne index ≥20 points	18.2 (2.9, 113.5)	

PRACTICE POINT

- Hyperreflexia and ankle clonus are suggestive of serotonin syndrome in the appropriate clinical setting. Patients with neuroleptic malignant syndrome tend to have hyporeflexia and lead-pipe rigidity.

Distinguishing between serotonin syndrome and neuroleptic malignant syndrome is difficult. Typically, serotonin syndrome develops in minutes to hours after exposure to serotonergic agent, and NMS may occur at any time during treatment. Some have suggested that patients with NMS demonstrate higher fevers and more pronounced extrapyramidal effects, while patients with serotonin syndrome have lower fevers, myoclonus, and gastrointestinal symptoms.

■ FEVER

When pursuing infectious etiologies, the physical exam should be guided by the presenting complaints but still comprehensively evaluate all organs, including the skin. The possibility of pneumonia and bacteremia should be thoroughly evaluated, as these are two of the most common diagnoses in the inpatient setting.

The patient's perception of fever, or the examiner simply detecting an abnormally warm forehead, is associated with an increasing likelihood of fever before a fever has been objectively detected. The patient's perception carries a positive likelihood ratio of 2.9 (95% CI: 1.1-8.0) and the finding of a warm forehead carries a positive likelihood ratio of 2.9 (95% CI: 2.5-3.5).

Physical exam findings or maneuvers that may help in the diagnosis of bacteremia are listed in **Table 92-8**. The presence of hypotension is the most helpful for increasing the probability of bacteremia. Being below the age of 50 or having a temperature less than 38.5°C is the most helpful for ruling out bacteremia, assuming the patient is not HIV-positive.

TABLE 92-6 Criteria for the Diagnosis of Neuroleptic Malignant Syndrome

Major Criteria for NMS	Minor Criteria for NMS
Fever	Tachycardia
Muscular rigidity	Labile blood pressure
Elevated creatinine phosphokinase (or aldolase, creatine kinase)	Tachypnea
	Altered consciousness
	Sweating
	Leukocytosis

TABLE 92-7 Hunter Serotonin Toxicity Criteria

In the presence of a serotonergic agent, must meet one of the five criteria below

1. Spontaneous clonus
2. Inducible clonus and agitation or diaphoresis
3. Ocular clonus and agitation or diaphoresis
4. Tremor and hyperreflexia
5. Hypertonic and temperature >38°C and the presence of either ocular clonus or inducible clonus

---

Physical exam findings or maneuvers that may help with the diagnosis of pneumonia are listed in **Table 92-9**. The most helpful findings are diminished breath sounds, bronchial breath sounds, egophony, cachexia, percussion dullness, and a Heckerling score of 4 or 5. The absence of any of the findings above is not helpful for ruling out pneumonia.

For diagnosing meningitis, nuchal rigidity assessment can be helpful (**Table 92-10**).

For a few of the noninfectious causes of fever, there are significant physical exam findings that may aid in diagnosis. **Table 92-11** shows helpful findings in the diagnosis of pulmonary embolism, such as a high probability Wells score or unilateral calf pain. A temperature greater than 38°C suggests an alternative diagnosis. The findings helpful for detecting deep vein thrombosis are provided in **Table 92-12**. The most helpful findings are a history of active cancer, asymmetric calf swelling, and high pretest probability Wells score.

THE LABORATORY APPROACH

■ HYPERTHERMIA

A creatine phosphokinase or aldolase evaluation should be ordered. These tests are usually highly elevated in malignant hyperthermia, NMS, or serotonin syndrome, but they may also be elevated in sympathomimetic overdose, anticholinergic overdose, and heat stroke. However, there is no diagnostic test that distinguishes between these potential causes. If infection remains likely, an evaluation of the central nervous system (CNS) is warranted, and a diagnostic lumbar puncture should be performed if there are no signs of increased intracranial pressure or focal neurologic deficits.

Although not diagnostic, NMS typically presents with leukocytosis (10,000-40,000 white blood cells/μL), and low levels of serum magnesium, calcium, and iron. Often, patients initially have metabolic alkalosis, elevated liver enzymes, and elevated lactate dehydrogenase.

TABLE 92-8 Utility of Clinical Findings for Diagnosing Bacteremia

	+LR (95% CI)	−LR (95% CI)
Age 50 or greater	1.4 (1.2, 1.6)	0.3 (0.1, 0.8)
Temperature ≥38.5°C	1.2 (1.1, 1.3)	0.5 (0.2, 1.0)
Tachycardia	1.2 (1.1, 1.4)	0.7 (0.6, 0.9)
Respiratory rate >20	0.9 (0.8, 1.1)	1.2 (0.8, 1.7)
Hypotension	2.6 (1.6, 4.4)	0.9 (0.9, 1.0)
Confusion or depressed sensorium	1.5 (1.3, 1.8)	0.9 (0.8, 1.0)

TABLE 92-9 Utility of Clinical Findings for Diagnosing Pneumonia

	+LR (95% CI)	−LR (95% CI)
Diminished breath sounds	2.3 (1.9, 2.8)	0.8 (0.7, 0.9)
Bronchial breath sounds	3.3 (2.0, 5.6)	0.9 (0.8, 1.0)
Egophony	4.1 (2.1, 7.8)	0.9 (0.9, 1.0)
Crackles in patients with cough and fever	1.8 (1.2, 2.7)	0.8 (0.7, 0.9)
Absence of sore throat	1.8 (1.3, 2.5)	0.7 (0.6, 0.9)
Absence of rhinorrhea	2.2 (1.5, 3.2)	0.8 (0.7, 0.9)
Cachexia	4.0 (1.7, 9.6)	0.9 (0.8, 1.0)
Abnormal mental status	1.9 (1.2, 3.0)	0.9 (0.9, 1.0)
Temperature >37.8°C	2.0 (1.5, 2.6)	0.7 (0.6, 0.8)
Respiratory rate >28/min	2.0 (1.4, 2.8)	0.8 (0.7, 0.9)
Heart rate >100 beats/min	1.6 (1.4, 1.7)	0.8 (0.7, 0.9)
Percussion dullness	3.0 (1.7, 5.2)	0.9 (0.8, 1.0)
Heckerling score, 4 or 5 findings	8.2 (5.8, 11.5)	

FEVER

The history and physical exam should guide the laboratory approach based upon the pretest probability for serious infection or underlying malignancy. If serious infection remains likely, the laboratory approach should include a complete blood count, complete metabolic panel, blood cultures, urinalysis, and chest x-ray. A left shift in the white blood cell count with bandemia, toxic granulations, and Dohle bodies suggests bacteremia (**Figure 92-2**). A C-reactive protein level may be helpful to screen for the presence of disease in patients with low-grade or borderline fever.

If there is reversal of usual peak and trough temperatures, disseminated tuberculosis (TB) and typhoid fever could be considered. Temperature-pulse dissociation with relative bradycardia may be seen with typhoid fever, brucellosis, leptospirosis, babesiosis, malaria, legionella, viral hemorrhagic fevers, Gram-negative invasive rods (eg, *Escherichia coli*, *Salmonella*, *Shigella*), factitious fever, and some drug-induced fevers. Relative bradycardia in an obscure febrile illness in the hospital, in the absence of pneumonia, suggests a drug-fever-hypersensitivity reaction marked primarily by fever and a pulse-temperature deficit with no cutaneous manifestations. It is estimated that up to 10% of patients hospitalized in the United States have fevers due to drug hypersensitivity.

Fever patterns of hospitalized patients are usually of limited utility, but characteristic tertian (every third day) or quotidian (every fourth day) fevers should prompt consideration of *Plasmodium vivax* or *Plasmodium malaria*, respectively. If exposure is likely, this would guide test ordering to include thick and thin blood smears.

Fevers that last for 3 to 10 days followed by similar afebrile periods (Pel-Ebstein fevers) are seen with lymphomas, including Hodgkin lymphoma. Fevers every 21 days accompanying neutropenia are associated with a condition termed cyclic neutropenia. Additional information regarding the diagnostic approach to febrile patient is found in Chapter 206 (Undiagnosed Fever in Hospitalized Patients).

TABLE 92-10 Utility of Nuchal Rigidity for Diagnosing Meningitis

	+LR (95% CI)	−LR (95% CI)
Nuchal rigidity	3.0 (2.1, 4.2)	0.1 (0, 2.0)

TABLE 92-11 Utility of Clinical Findings for Diagnosing Pulmonary Embolus

	+LR (95% CI)	−LR (95% CI)
Temperature >38°C	0.4 (0.3, 0.7)	1.1 (1.0, 1.2)
Pulse >100/min	1.2 (0.9, 1.5)	0.9 (0.8, 1.1)
Respiratory rate >30/min	2.0 (1.5, 2.8)	0.9 (0.8, 0.9)
Systolic blood pressure <100 mm Hg	1.9 (1.1, 3.0)	1.0 (0.9, 1.0)
Wheezes	0.2 (0.1, 0.4)	1.1 (1.1, 1.1)
Unilateral calf pain or swelling	2.3 (1.8, 3.0)	0.9 (0.8, 1.0)
Wells score, moderate probability, 2-6 points	1.7 (1.5, 2.0)	
Wells score, high probability, 7 or more points	5.0 (2.5, 10)	

TREATMENT

HYPERTHERMIA

Once the diagnosis of hyperthermia is established, potential offending drugs should be discontinued. The central core temperature should be monitored continuously by rectal, esophageal, or tympanic probe. Vital signs should be closely monitored as well. Aggressive volume resuscitation is extremely important. If rhabdomyolysis is significant, intravenous fluids are essential to avoid the risks of myoglobinuria. Active measures should be taken to lower body temperature (**Table 92-13**). The best method is debated, but direct application of ice packs to the groin, axilla, and neck can be used. Evaporative cooling may be used, in which the naked patient is sprayed with alcohol and water and cooled with fans. Immersion in cool water is an option but may interfere with resuscitation and lead to complications from vasoconstriction. Other methods include extracorporeal bypass, cooling blankets, and iced peritoneal or gastric lavage. There has been much success with the rapid infusion of 30 mL/kg of iced (4°C) normal saline to induce hypothermia in comatose survivors of cardiac arrest, and this should be considered in patients with hyperthermia. To prevent excessive cooling, these methods should be halted when core body temperature reaches 38.5°C.

Dantrolene and bromocriptine are the main medications for the treatment of NMS. Intravenous clonidine, carbamazepine, amantadine, levodopa, and anticholinergic medications have been used in case reports. Treatment should continue for at least 10 days and then tapered slowly. If the insult is due to depot antipsychotics,

TABLE 92-12 Utility of Clinical Findings for Diagnosing Deep Venous Thrombosis

	+LR (95% CI)	−LR (95% CI)
Active cancer	2.9 (2.4, 3.6)	0.9 (0.8, 0.9)
Recent immobilization	1.6 (1.3, 2.1)	0.9, (0.8, 0.9)
Recent surgery	1.6 (1.3, 1.9)	0.9 (0.9, 1.0)
Any calf or ankle swelling	1.2 (1.1, 1.3)	0.7 (0.6, 0.8)
Asymmetric calf swelling, ≥2 cm	2.1 (1.8, 2.5)	0.5 (0.4, 0.7)
Swelling of entire leg	1.5 (1.2, 1.8)	0.8 (0.6, 0.9)
Superficial venous dilation	1.6 (1.4, 1.9)	0.9 (0.8, 0.9)
Wells score, high pretest probability	5.2 (3.2, 8.5)	

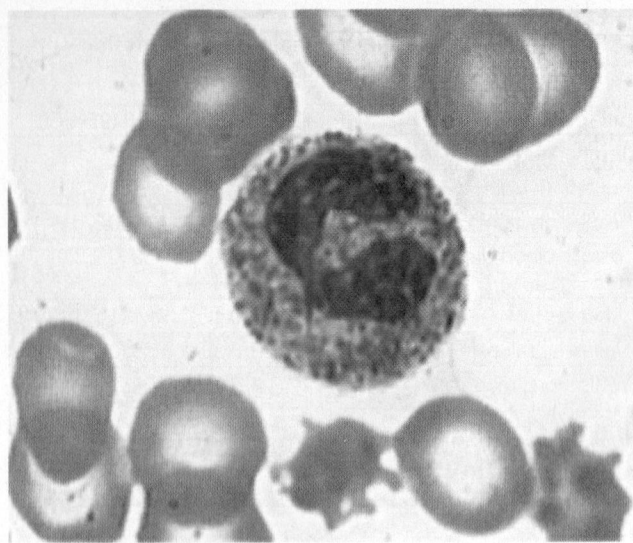

Figure 92-2 *Toxic granulations of a neutrophil.*

TABLE 92-13 Additional Treatments for Specific Causes of Hyperthermia

Cause of Hyperthermia	Specific Additional Treatments
1. Malignant hyperthermia	Dantrolene, hyperventilation with 100% oxygen
2. Neuroleptic malignant syndrome	Bromocriptine, dantrolene, muscle relaxants
3. Serotonin syndrome	Serotonin antagonists, propranolol, benzodiazepines, cyproheptadine
4. Sympathomimetic	Sympatholytics, benzodiazepines
5. Anticholinergics	Physostigmine (rarely needed), sedatives
6. Endocrine	Propranolol, methimazole
7. Heat stroke	Supportive care
8. CNS injury/infection	Antibiotics

treatment should extend for a total of 2 to 3 weeks. In cases refractory to medical treatment, electroconvulsive therapy may be used to improve fever, sweating, and delirium.

Most patients with serotonin syndrome will improve within 24 hours after stopping the causative agents and beginning supportive therapy. Besides rapid cooling, benzodiazepines can be used to induce muscle relaxation and decrease associated anxiety. Cyproheptadine and chlorpromazine may be used to combat many of the symptoms associated with serotonin syndrome. Cyproheptadine is considered to be the first line, as chlorpromazine can cause hypotension, which should be avoided in the setting of cardiovascular instability.

Antipyretics, such as nonsteroidal anti-inflammatory drugs (NSAIDs) or acetaminophen, have no role in hyperthermia because the actions of these medications are distinct from the underlying mechanisms of hyperthermia. Acetaminophen can hasten hepatic damage, and salicylates can worsen existing coagulopathy.

■ FEVER

NSAIDs and acetaminophen are useful for treating fever. NSAIDs decrease prostaglandin E2 through inhibition of cyclooxygenase (COX)-1 and COX-2. Acetaminophen is a poor inhibitor of COX in the periphery and is thought to work as an inhibitor of COX-3, which is located in the CNS. There is no convincing evidence that treating a fever changes time to recovery from infection. Preexisting cardiac, cerebrovascular, or pulmonary disease is aggravated by fever, and aggressive treatment should be considered. Aspirin should not be used for patients with thyrotoxic storm; it can displace thyroid hormone from thyroid binding globulin, and thereby increase free T4. Ultimately, the underlying cause of the fever should be targeted, whether it is infectious, inflammatory, vascular, or autoimmune in nature.

SUGGESTED READINGS

Gruber MP. Diagnosing neuroleptic malignant syndrome. *Chest.* 2004;125:1960-1961.

Marik PE. Fever in the ICU. *Chest.* 2000;117:855-869.

Martinez M, Devenport L, Saussy J, Martinez J. Drug-associated heat stroke. *South Med J.* 2002;95:799-802.

McAllen K, Schwartz D. Adverse drug reactions resulting in hyperthermia in the intensive care unit. *Crit Care Med.* 2010;38:S244-S252.

McGee SR. *Evidence-Based Physical Diagnosis.* 3rd ed. St. Louis, MO: Saunders Elsevier; 2012.

Musselman ME, Saely S. Diagnosis and treatment of drug-induced hyperthermia. *Am J Health Syst Pharm.* 2013;70:34-42.

Perry PJ, Wilborn CA. Serotonin syndrome vs neuroleptic malignant syndrome: a contrast of causes, diagnoses, and management. *Ann Clin Psychiatry.* 2012;24:155-162.

93

Hypotension

Danielle Jones, MD, FACP
Lorenzo Di Francesco, MD, FACP, FHM

Key Clinical Questions

1 What symptoms and signs should be assessed in the initial evaluation of a patient with reported hypotension?

2 What are the major categories of hypotension?

3 What are the common iatrogenic complications that produce hypotension in the hospital?

INTRODUCTION

Hypotension may be the presenting reason for hospital admission or it may develop during a patient's hospitalization, sometimes as an iatrogenic complication. Out of hospital nontraumatic hypotension is associated with increased in hospital mortality. Additionally, hypotension observed in the emergency room or that develops during management of acute decompensated heart failure, COPD and community acquired pneumonia or sepsis have all been associated with higher mortality. Because patients with hypotension may decompensate quickly, suffer irreversible end-organ damage, and ultimately die, clinicians must recognize the clinical presentation of patients with life-threatening or reversible causes of hypotension and appropriately intervene expediently.

Deviations from "normal" blood pressure must be considered in the context of the patient's baseline blood pressure. A patient's blood pressure normally varies depending on the time of day, even from minute to minute, and typically decreases during sleep by 10% to 20%. Arterial monitoring has shown that the systolic and diastolic blood pressure also varies with the respiratory cycle and with each heartbeat. Although hypotension typically refers to blood pressure lower than 90/60 mm Hg, some patients may be completely asymptomatic at such readings, whereas other patients may develop clinically important hypotensive symptoms at much higher readings. A patient with advanced cirrhosis, for example, may have a chronic stable systolic blood pressure of ~90 mm Hg that requires no intervention, whereas a severely hypertensive patient may experience a stroke, myocardial infarction, or renal insufficiency from relative hypotension with "normal" blood pressure readings. Acute decreases in mean arterial pressure (typically >25%), such as after receiving a parenteral antihypertensive medication, put patients at greatest risk for acute end-organ damage and potential morbidity and mortality.

CASE 93-1

The hospital's rapid response team (RRT) was summoned to the bedside of an 87-year-old man who had recently undergone a total hip replacement after sustaining a hip fracture from a mechanical fall. His vital signs were notable for no discernible blood pressure, a heart rate of 110, respiratory rate of 20, O_2 saturation of 95% (on 2 L via nasal cannula), and a temperature of 96° F. Telemetry review revealed sinus tachycardia. Postoperatively he had an agitated delirium, developed renal insufficiency, and became hypertensive. He had received 10 mg of intravenous (IV) hydralazine for a blood pressure of 180/100 mm Hg 30 minutes before the RRT call. His manual systolic blood pressure after placement in the Trendelenburg position was noted to be 70 mm Hg. Rapid infusion of normal saline was ordered. His usual antihypertensive medications were held, and he was transferred to the intensive care unit (ICU).

Of note, the effects of hydralazine, a potent vasodilator, may be unpredictable when used in acutely ill patients, especially the elderly. Renal insufficiency prolongs its half-life. Treatment of the underlying condition that caused this patient's hypertension (agitated delirium) is likely to be more effective and safer than using antihypertensive agents to treat the elevated blood pressure directly. Importantly parenteral antihypertensive agents should only be used for patients with true hypertensive emergencies (eg, hypertensive encephalopathy, acute cardiogenic pulmonary edema, malignant hypertension of the kidney, etc) or to control blood pressure in patients unable to receive enteral antihypertensive medications in particular in the postoperative period.

IS THE REPORTED BLOOD PRESSURE MEASUREMENT ACCURATE?

After quickly ensuring that the patient is alert and responsive and that advanced cardiac life support (ACLS) does not need to be initiated, the first step is to determine whether the reported blood pressure reading is a valid measure of intra-arterial blood pressure; this requires assessing the blood pressure *manually*. Many factors may affect the immediate accuracy of a blood pressure measurement, including the device used (cuff size, leaky bulb, faulty aneroid device), the technique or bias of the examiner (positioning of patient, placement of the cuff, inappropriately rapid deflation, excess bell pressure), and a noisy environment. Most errors overestimate the blood pressure, so a report of low blood pressure should alert the clinician to a possible impending emergency. In general, when assessing a hypotensive patient, the examiner should obtain a manual blood pressure reading.

DOES THE BLOOD PRESSURE READING REFLECT CENTRAL ARTERIAL PRESSURE?

After a low blood pressure is confirmed, the next step is to determine whether the blood pressure reading reflects an acute drop in central arterial pressure. In general during initial encounters with hypotensive patients, physicians should personally record blood pressure measurements in both arms and, depending on the reason for admission and comorbidities, obtain orthostatic blood pressure readings. In an asymptomatic patient who has a history of vascular disease, a targeted vascular examination should be performed. Any hemodynamically significant vascular stenosis in the arms could result in a systolic difference of at least 10 or 15 mm Hg. Uncommonly, patients may have bilateral stenosis in both subclavian arteries, resulting in falsely low blood pressure in both arms, but in this setting a low blood pressure reading would be unlikely to cause symptoms of decreased perfusion unless accompanied by vascular disease elsewhere. If upper extremity vascular disease is suspected as the etiology for inaccurate upper extremity blood pressure readings, large thigh cuffs can sometimes be used (with the patient reclined) to obtain accurate blood pressure measurements (**Table 93-1**).

PRACTICE POINT

Postural hypotension

- Normally the diastolic pressure remains the same or rises slightly and the systolic pressure stays the same or drops slightly when a patient stands.
    - The diastolic pressure almost never drops, and when it does, the drop is small and the systolic pressure will rise so that mean arterial pressure (MAP) = DBP + 1/3 [SBP – DBP] does not change
- Hypotension in the upright position compared with the recumbent position is caused by the following:
    - *Volume depletion* from hemorrhage, surgery, gastrointestinal losses, adrenal insufficiency, or diuretics
    - *Autonomic dysfunction*: Neurogenic factors from some antihypertensive medications, autonomic dysfunction due to diabetes mellitus, Shy-Drager syndrome, prolonged bedrest, severe heart failure due to inability to increase cardiac output with standing

- Failure of the heart rate to rise in response to an orthostatic drop in blood pressure suggests neurogenic factors rather than volume depletion.
    - Exceptions include patients receiving β-blockers or nondihydropyridine calcium channel blockers (eg, diltiazem, verapamil) and patients with predominant vagal insufficiency (diabetics, postcardiac transplant).
- Measure blood pressure and pulse after the patient has rested in the supine position for 5 minutes, then standing for at least 3 minutes.
    - Avoid measurement in the sitting position unless the patient is unable to stand due orthostatic symptoms prior to standing.
    - Orthostasis is defined as a fall in systolic blood pressure of ≥20 mm Hg or diastolic blood pressure of >10 mm Hg. Orthostatic hypotension is defined by systolic blood pressure <90 mm Hg upon standing.

TABLE 93-1 Etiologies and Classifications of Hypotension

Anaphylaxis/Anaphylactic Shock	**Neurologic**
Cardiogenic and obstructive	*Age-related*
Acute coronary syndrome	*Central nervous system*
Arrhythmias	Medullary stroke
Cardiomyopathy	Parkinsonism
Congestive heart failure	Shy-Drager syndrome
Valvulopathy	Wernicke syndrome
Pulmonary embolism	*Dysautonomia*
Pulmonary hypertension	Diabetes mellitus
Cardiac tumors	Postprandial
Cardiac tamponade	*Peripheral neuropathy*
Tension pneumothorax	Amyloidosis
Drug-induced	Diabetes mellitus
Alcohol	HIV
Anesthesia	*Sensory*
Antidepressants	Alcohol
Antihypertensives	Syphilis
Antipsychotics	*Vasomotor*
Anxiolytics	Emotional
General anesthesia	Micturition
Narcotics	**Orthostatic**
Endocrinologic	Anemia
Adrenal insufficiency	Endocrine-mediated
Diabetes mellitus (uncontrolled)	Medication-induced
Hypothyroidism	Neurally mediated
Hypovolemia	Pregnancy
Hemorrhage	Volume depletion
Volume Depletion	**Structural**
Dialysis	Pregnancy (pressure on the inferior vena cava)
Infectious	**Trauma**
Septic shock	**Vascular**
Measurement error	Aortic dissection or rupture
	Peripheral vascular disease
	Pulmonary embolism

DOES THE LOW BLOOD PRESSURE READING REFLECT THE PATIENT'S AVERAGE BLOOD PRESSURE?

The next step is to determine whether the patient is experiencing symptoms related to their hypotension. If the patient is asymptomatic, the clinician has more time to review the prior blood pressure measurements and hospital records with the goal to adjust any medications that may be contributing. Assuming a confirmed accurate low blood pressure reading, asymptomatic patients are more likely to be young and healthy, pregnant, or have systemic diseases such as severe hypothyroidism, chronic adrenal insufficiency, heart failure, cirrhosis, or vascular disease.

WHAT ARE THE SYMPTOMS AND SIGNS OF HYPOTENSION?

Symptoms and signs of hypotension depend on the etiology of the low blood pressure, the acuity of the drop, and the patient's overall health and age. Initially, patients may experience lightheadedness, dizziness, or a syncopal episode. The examiner should assess the patient's hemodynamic stability by assessing whether the patient appears acutely ill and obtaining a complete set of vital signs. An abnormal heart rate may affirm that the hypotension is uncompensated and, therefore, unstable. Either bradycardia or tachycardia should prompt the clinician to obtain an electrocardiogram (ECG). Pulsus paradoxus (>10 mm Hg) is by definition an exaggeration of the normal inspiratory respiratory fall in systolic blood pressure (normal ≤10 mm Hg). It is most commonly associated with cardiac tamponade (see Chapter 130 [Myocarditis, Pericardial Disease, and Cardiac Tamponade]) or severe obstructive lung disease, but it can also be seen in tension pneumothorax, massive pulmonary embolism, right ventricle infarction, hemorrhagic shock, large bilateral pleural effusions and in restrictive cardiomyopathy.

The initial examination should include an assessment of the patient's *volume status* (by estimating central venous pressure [CVP] and evaluating orthostatic blood pressures measurements), *cardiac output* (by examining heart and lungs), and *perfusion* of organs (by assessing the patient's mental status, urine output, and the warmth over the knee caps). Skin pallor and the degree of diaphoresis should be observed, and recent administration of vasoactive medications reviewed.

FRAMEWORK OF HYPOTENSION EVALUATION

The clinician must evaluate the hypotensive patient at the bedside and confirm the low blood pressure through a manual measurement (ie, with an analog sphygmomanometer, and not an electronic or automatic device). Then, if the patient appears unstable, lower the head of the bed, place the patient on a bedside monitor, and evaluate for the presence of a shockable tachyarrhythmia or evidence of severe bradyarrhythmia that might require administration of atropine or pacing. If the patient is in extremis, ACLS protocols should be followed (see Chapter 137 [Inpatient Cardiac Arrest and Cardiopulmonary Resuscitation]). **Figure 93-1** provides the initial assessment and stabilization algorithm for acute hypotension. The examiner should rapidly determine the likely mechanism of the patient's hypotension. Most causes of hypotension will respond to aggressive fluid resuscitation; however, excessive fluid expansion may worsen right and left ventricular failure. Treatment of cardiogenic shock, therefore, is directed at the underlying etiology and the pathophysiology.

While resuscitating a hypotensive patient, the clinician should communicate with the patient (when possible), family members (when available), the patient's bedside nurse and others familiar with the patient to help identify changes in mental status; and perform a focused chart review to assess recent vital signs, urine output, and risk factors for causes of hypotension. Always review the notes for the last 24 hours and the medications that have recently been administered (**Table 93-2**). Discontinue any medications that likely exacerbated or caused the hypotension. Order stat studies including 12-lead ECG, cardiac enzymes, complete blood count, comprehensive metabolic profile, coagulation profile, lactate, arterial blood gas, blood and urine cultures, and type and screen for possible blood transfusion if appropriate.

■ HYPOVOLEMIC SHOCK

The presentation of hypovolemic hypotension depends on the etiology, severity, and duration of the problem as well as the patient's age and underlying medical conditions. Patients typically have abnormal vital signs (tachycardia and tachypnea) and a narrow pulse pressure in addition to low blood pressure. Symptomatic patients appear pale with flattened neck veins and cool, clammy, or mottled extremities; poor capillary refill; diminished peripheral pulses; and altered mentation. Make note of any administrations of β-blockers and nondihydropyridine calcium channel blockers as they may mask some of the early symptoms and signs of acute blood loss and volume depletion, particularly the reflex increase in heart rate. β-blockers can also mask other signs of increased adrenergic tone, such as diaphoresis.

Hypovolemia is characterized by reduced blood volume or CVP and increased systemic vascular resistance in an effort to maintain perfusion. Acute blood loss triggers cardiovascular, respiratory, renal, hematologic, and neuroendocrine responses to increase heart rate and contractility, conserve sodium and water, control blood loss at the source of bleeding, and redistribute blood flow to preserve vital organ function. With progressive hemorrhage or continued volume depletion without resuscitation, cardiac output can no longer compensate, leading to arterial hypoperfusion.

If the examiner identifies symptoms and signs of hypovolemia, volume depletion and/or acute blood loss likely accounts for the hypotension. Volume depletion in the hospital setting may result from decreased fluid intake or from increased fluid losses, especially seen with vomiting, nasogastric suction, drains, diarrhea, and intentional diuresis. Increased rates of insensible losses can be dramatic when the skin is damaged (eg, burns, Stevens-Johnson syndrome) or when patients have a high fever and lose fluid via perspiration and a high respiratory rate. Hemorrhage may result from trauma, bleeding from the genitourinary or gastrointestinal tracts, and vascular etiologies. Hospital-acquired etiologies include trauma from surgery or procedures and drug interactions that lead to excessive anticoagulation and spontaneous bleeding.

PRACTICE POINT	
Hypovolemic shock	
Blood Loss (% circulating blood)	**Associated Signs**
<20%	Cool, clammy skin, cool knee caps, decreased capillary refill, ↓ pulse pressure
20%-40%	Tachycardia, tachypnea, postural blood pressure changes, confused or agitated; ongoing losses without resuscitation: hypotension, oliguria, deeper and faster respirations, mottling of skin
>40%	Tachycardia, profound hypotension, either tachypnea or irregular respirations, ↓↓ urine output, ↓ or absent pulses, pallor, lethargy, obtundation
Death from severe hemorrhage or severe Volume depletion	Respiratory arrest prior to circulatory arrest due to fatigue of respiratory muscles and bradycardic or asystolic rhythms or pulseless electrical activity (PEA)

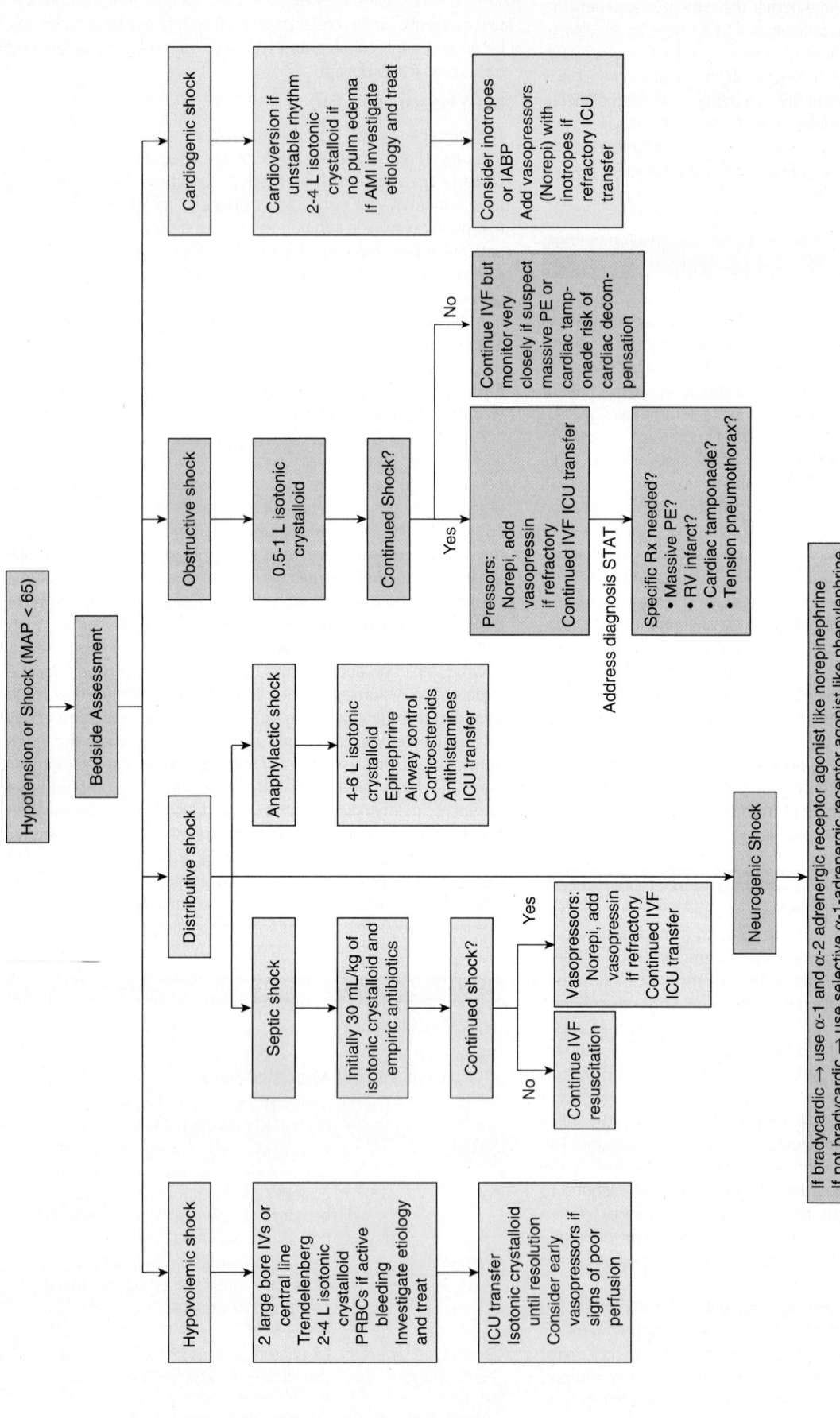

Figure 93-1 *Framework of Evaluation of Hypotension.* (AMI, acute myocardial infarction; CHF, congestive heart failure; ICU, intensive care unit; IVF, IV fluids; MAP, mean arterial pressure; NS, normal saline; PE, pulmonary embolism; RV, right ventricle.)

TABLE 93-2 Common Hypotension-Inducing Drugs

Drug	Mechanism of Hypotension
Alcohol	Potentiation of orthostatic hypotension via impairment of vasoconstrictor response
Alpha blockers	Loss of reflex vasoconstriction upon standing
Anesthesia (general and regional)	Vasodilatation and decreased cardiac contractility
Antihypertensives (including beta blockers and nondihydropyridine calcium channel blockers)	Decreased cardiac output via heart rate depression and negative inotropy
Antidepressants (including monoamine oxydase inhibitors and tricyclics)	Orthostatic hypotension
Antipsychotics	Alpha-adrenergic blockade, calcium blockade, inhibition of centrally mediated pressor reflexes, and a negative inotropic effect especially in older, typical antipsychotics
Anxiolytics (including benzodiazepines)	Central inhibition of sympathetic outflow
Diuretics	Orthostasis via hypovolemia
Nitrates	Vasodilatation
Opiates	Increase in histamine release, direct vasodilatation, depression of the medullary vasomotor center
Phenothiazines	Alpha-adrenergic blockade
Sildenafil	Vasodilation

■ CARDIOGENIC SHOCK

Decreased cardiac output and systemic hypoperfusion may result from a variety of insults affecting the heart itself or affecting the blood flow to the right or left ventricle. The presentation depends on the etiology, severity, and duration of the problem as well as the patient's age and underlying medical conditions. Signs of cardiogenic shock may include a narrowed pulse pressure, diaphoresis, elevated CVP, lung crackles, cool and clammy extremities and acute kidney injury.

If the patient's heart rate is sufficiently slow (generally <40 beats/min) or fast (>150 beats/min), bradyarrhythmias or tachyarrhythmias may contribute to the low cardiac output leading to hypotension. In emergency situations, review of the monitor strip lead V_1 may be sufficient to make a diagnosis and initiate appropriate treatment without wasting valuable time obtaining a 12-lead ECG and/or a right-sided 12-lead ECG. Arrhythmias may precipitate cardiogenic hypotension by a variety of mechanisms. Bradycardia reduces cardiac output directly but may also be associated with atrioventricular dyssynchrony, as in complete heart block. Ineffective ventricular contractions may occur in ventricular tachycardias. In patients with acute hypotension due to bradyarrhythmias or tachyarrhythmias, ACLS protocols should be initiated immediately. In atrial fibrillation and atrial flutter, some patients (particularly the elderly and other patients with stiff ventricles) may experience a modest degree of hypotension or heart failure symptoms due to a lack of left atrial "kick," but this can be confounded by the difficulty in accurately

determining blood pressure in the setting of an irregular rhythm with erratic stroke volumes.

■ OBSTRUCTIVE SHOCK

Obstructive hypotension occurs when left-sided cardiac output is impaired by a physiologic or anatomic limitation to flow, which may occur at any point in the circuit. In cardiac tamponade and tension pneumothorax and other causes of pericardial or superior vena cava compression, there is impaired filling of the right heart due to external compression. Pulmonary embolism, pulmonic stenosis, and decompensated severe pulmonary hypertension can lead to impaired flow of blood from the right heart to the left heart whereas in an acute right ventricular myocardial infarction, the acutely failing right ventricle is unable to provide enough cardiac output to the lung and the left hear. Importantly aggressive fluid resuscitation should complement standard acute myocardial infarction treatment to maximize the right ventricular contractility (by taking advantage of the Starling phenomenon) and increase blood through the pulmonary circulation to the left heart. A left atrial myxoma (and other cardiac tumors) can impair flow through the heart itself. Severe mitral stenosis, aortic stenosis or the presence of a dynamic left ventricular outflow obstruction due to hypertrophic cardiomyopathy impair flow through and out of the left heart.

PRACTICE POINT		
Cardiogenic and Obstructive Shock		
Clinical question	Pearls and signs	*The rational clinical exam reference*
Does this patient have abnormal central venous pressure?	• Use the abdominal pressure to identify the internal jugular vein. • Jugular venous pulsations (JVP) seen vertically greater than 3 cm above the sternal angle of Louis or a sustained JVP increase of at least 4 cm with abdominal compression: three- to fourfold increased likelihood of an elevated CVP.	Cook DJ, et al. *JAMA.* 1996;275(8): 630-634.
Does this patient have left-sided heart failure?	• A pulse >90-100/min and an SBP <90 mm Hg is associated with ↓ LVEF.	Badgett RG, et al. *JAMA.* 1997;277(21): 1712-1719.
	• The presence of an S3 (which may be easier to appreciate by palpation) likelihood ratio 11 for heart failure in patients with acute dyspnea.	Wong C, et al. *JAMA.* 2005;294(15): 1944-1956.
Does this patient have cardiac tamponade?	• Acute cardiac tamponade: hypotension, ↑ CVP, and quiet heart sounds (Beck's triad). • Medical patients with known pericardial effusion, occasionally a pericardial friction rub or the presence of pulsus paradoxus may support the diagnosis.	Roy CL, et al. *JAMA.* 2007;297(16): 1810-1818.

CHAPTER 93 Hypotension

661

DISTRIBUTIVE SHOCK

Sepsis, anaphylaxis, and neurogenic disorders may lead to distributive shock. The presentation of distributive shock depends on the etiology and severity of the underlying problem. Flushing, warm extremities, and a widened pulse pressure suggest distributive shock. However patients may also have signs of hyperthermia or hypothermia, tachycardia, tachypnea, and mental status changes depending on the underlying precipitating cause.

PRACTICE POINT	
Distributive shock	
Type of Shock	**Signs**
Septic	• Hypothermia, hyperthermia, flushing, warm extremities, purpura, petechial rash as well as obtundation
	• Important clue: acute hyperventilation with respiratory alkalosis ($PCO_2 < 30$ mm Hg)
Anaphylactic	• Urticaria; flushing or generalized erythema; tachypnea; angioedema most often involving head, neck, face, and upper airways; hoarseness; stridor; and wheezing
	• Vomiting and diarrhea
	• Cardiac dysrhythmias
Neurogenic	• Bradycardia and flaccid paralysis (spinal cord injury usually proximal to T4)

In the early stages of septic shock (see also Chapter 141 [Sepsis and Shock]) patients have warm extremities due to the predominance of vasodilatory mediators. There is an initial decrease in the right ventricular and left ventricular ejection fraction with an increase in both end-diastolic and end-systolic volume indices and normal stroke volume. Systemic vascular resistance and cardiac filling pressures decrease. When accompanied by the adult respiratory distress syndrome (ARDS), there is increased microvascular permeability in the lungs resulting in hypoxemia due to perfusion of underventilated alveoli and right-to-left shunting. Skin lesions associated with sepsis might include primary infection (cellulitis, erysipelas, fasciitis), disseminated intravascular coagulation (acrocyanosis and necrosis of peripheral tissues), and/or lesions related to infective endocarditis (microemboli, immune complex vasculitis). Retinal hemorrhages, cotton wool spots, conjunctival petechiae, endophthalmitis, and panophthalmitis are often found in patients with infective endocarditis as signs or complications of the bacteremia.

Anaphylaxis refers to the clinical syndrome of a severe hypersensitivity reaction characterized by cardiovascular collapse and respiratory compromise (see Chapter 230 [Allergy and Anaphylaxis]). Immediate hypersensitivity reactions occur within seconds or minutes after presentation of the antigen, most commonly antibiotics, aspirin, or nonsteroidal anti-inflammatory agents. Iodinated vascular contrast may elicit a similar reaction (sometimes referred to as *anaphylactoid* since it does not involve antibodies, but has similar clinical presentation to true anaphylaxis). Anaphylaxis usually has characteristic symptoms and signs that include urticaria, flushing, tachypnea, hoarseness or throat tightness. The skin and gastrointestinal tract are most commonly affected, but multi-organ involvement and failure may be rapid in onset. Although the diagnosis may be clear at the time of presentation due to the presence of urticaria and/or stridor, the severity of the reaction may not be appreciated initially.

Neurologic causes of hypotension are often accompanied by an abnormal heart rate. Although increases in intracerebral pressure lead to reflex hypertension, acutely subarachnoid hemorrhage may lead to hypotension with associated bradycardia (Cushing's reflex). Loss of consciousness, focal neurologic deficits, and severe headache are common. Spinal cord injury disrupts sympathetic stimulation to vessels, and loss of sympathetic tone causes arterial dilation and venodilatation, which may lead to reflex tachycardia. However, cardiac and thoracic vessel sympathetic innervation is from T1 to T8; spinal cord lesions or injury proximal to T4 may disrupt sympathetic, but spare vagal innervation, leading to bradycardia. Dysautonomia may also present as hypotension without the typical tachycardic response in patients with long-standing diabetes, amyloidosis, Parkinson disease and other forms of Parkinsonism (such as Shy-Drager syndrome), or other neurodegenerative diseases.

PHARMACOLOGIC SHOCK

Pharmacologic shock results from vasodilatation or myocardial depression. Medications are a leading cause of iatrogenic hypotension in hospitalized patients. Any medication that affects cardiac output, volume status, and/or systemic vascular resistance can potentially contribute to the development of pharmacologic shock (**Tables 93-3** and **93-4**).

INITIAL MANAGEMENT

With few exceptions an unstable, hypotensive patient should receive a bolus of IV fluid (IVF), usually a liter of normal saline or lactated ringers. In the absence of severe heart failure, many patients may in fact require very aggressive fluid resuscitation (5-7 L of isotonic crystalloid is not uncommon) prior to the initiation of vasopressors (or concomitantly with vasopressors) if hypotension persists.

PREVENTION

Patient safety considerations include daily review and adjustment of all medications whose metabolism may become altered due to drug-drug interactions or the development of liver or renal insufficiency. In elderly patients especially, clinicians should pay attention to initiate lower dosages of medications and eliminate unnecessary polypharmacy. Additionally, quality improvement initiatives may start with a review of all ICU transfers, and include information technology support to alert prescribers of drug-drug interactions and appropriate dosing.

CONCLUSION

This chapter provides a framework for the initial bedside assessment of the patient with hypotension. When a significant fall in mean arterial pressure occurs, the clinician must take steps to avoid acute end organ damage by directing immediate therapy, determining the need for emergent surgical and specialty consultation and ensuring an appropriate level of patient care. In general, IVF administration will raise the blood pressure until specific measures can be undertaken, but it must be prescribed with care for some causes of obstructive shock. Given the demonstrated mortality benefit, early initiation of empiric broad-spectrum antimicrobials (within 1 hour of severe sepsis or shock recognition) for suspected sepsis or septic shock should be implemented. For medication-induced hypotension, the offending agent should be discontinued and if necessary, reversed. Timely administration of epinephrine may be life saving in the treatment of anaphylaxis (see Chapter 230 [Allergy and Anaphylaxis]). The reader is referred to specific clinical conditions for a more detailed discussion of the management of specific causes of hypotension commonly encountered in the hospital setting.

TABLE 93-3 Initial Management of Common Types of Hypotension

Type of Hypotension or Shock	Initial Management	Pearls and Pitfalls
Hypovolemic	Aggressive IV fluid resuscitation	Caution in patients with CHF who are hypotensive due to overdiuresis
Obstructive or Cardiogenic Hypotension		
Fulminant dilated cardiomyopathy or necrosis of >40% of left ventricular mass	Inotropic and mechanical support with intra-aortic balloon	Avoid fluid resuscitation
Right ventricular infarct	IV fluid volume load and dobutamine	Obtain right-sided electrocardiogram to diagnose; avoid diuretics that decrease preload and worsen already poor cardiac output; avoid dopamine, which increases pulmonary vascular resistance
Rupture of papillary muscles or the ventricular wall	Cardiac surgery	
Acute, massive pulmonary embolism	Thrombolysis and IV fluids as needed	Paradoxical worsening of hypotension may develop if right ventricle is severely dilated and septal bowing compromises left ventricular filling
Tension pneumothorax	Needle aspiration, chest tube	Administer IV fluids carefully as excessive fluid expansion may worsen right ventricular failure
Cardiac tamponade (malignancy, autoimmune, infectious, hemorrhage)	Aggressive fluid resuscitation	Removal of even a small amount of fluid (eg, 10-20 mL) by pericardiocentesis can lead to dramatic improvement
Hypotension due to severe, decompensated pulmonary hypertension	Consider fluid retention if patient does not have neck vein distension; may need pressor support in an intensive care unit setting and urgent specialty consultation	Paradoxical worsening of hypotension may develop if right ventricle is severely dilated and septal bowing compromises left ventricular filling
Distributive Shock		
Septic shock	Aggressive fluid administration, pressors, antibiotics	
Anaphylaxis	Stop drug, aggressive fluid administration, epinephrine	
Neurogenic	Fluid administration	
Pharmacologic	Administer IV fluids and discontinue precipitants See **Table 93-4** for antidotes	Carefully review all medications, including as needed medications

TABLE 93-4 Agents Used to Reverse Medication-Induced Hypotension

Hypotension-Inducing Agent	Antidote	Antidote Dosing
Anticholinergics (eg, atropine)	Physostigmine	0.5-2 mg IV or IM (may repeat every 20 min until response occurs)
Benzodiazepines	Flumazenil	0.2 mg IV (may repeat)
Beta-blockers	Glucagon	5-10 mg IV
Calcium channel blockers	Atropine (if bradycardia present)	0.5-2 mg IV
	Calcium chloride (10%)	10 mL or 1-2 g IV (may repeat to max 10-12 g)
	Calcium gluconate (10%)	20 mL IV
	Glucagon	5-10 mg IV
Opiates	Nalmefene	Nonopioid-dependent: 0.5-1 mg/70 kg (may repeat)
	Naloxone	Opioid-dependent: 0.10.5 mg/70 kg (may repeat)
		0.4-2 mg IV (may repeat)
		IM and SQ available (longer onset to action)
Tricyclic antidepressants	Sodium bicarbonate	50-100 mEq IV bolus or norepinephrine 4-8 mcg/min IV infusion

Data from Olson K. Poisoning. In: McPhee SJ, Papdakis MA, eds. *Current Medical Diagnosis and Treatment* 2010. New York, NY: The McGraw-Hill Companies; 2009. Chap. 38.

SUGGESTED READINGS

Cook DJ, Simel DL. The rational clinical exam: does this patient have abnormal central venous pressure? *JAMA*. 1996;275(8):630-634.

Freeman MB. Neurogenic orthostatic hypotension. *N Engl J Med*. 2008;358:615-624.

Jones AE, Stiell IG, Nesbitt LP, et al. Nontraumatic out-of-hospital hypotension predicts inhospital mortality. *Ann Emerg Med*. 2004;43:106-113.

Levy JH. Treating shock—old drugs, new ideas. *N Engl J Med*. 2010;362:841-843.

Luciano GL, Brennan MJ, Rothberg MB. Postprandial hypotension. *Am J Med*. 2010;123(3):281.e1-281.e6.

Pickering TG, Hall JE, Appel LJ, et al. Recommendations for blood pressure measurement in humans and experimental animals. I. Blood pressure measurement in humans: a statement for professionals from the Subcommittee of Professional and Public Education of the American Heart Association Council on High Blood Pressure Research. *Circulation*. 2005;111:697-716.

CHAPTER 94

Hypothermia

Chad S. Miller, MD, FACP, FHM
Jeffrey G. Wiese, MD, MHM, FACP

Key Clinical Questions

1. What are the signs and symptoms of hypothermia?
2. What are the most common causes of hypothermia?
3. Does intoxication associated with hypothermia suggest a better or worse prognosis?
4. What are the dangers associated with hypothermia?
5. Who is most likely to die from hypothermia?

CASE 94-1

A 54-year-old man was brought to the hospital after being found unresponsive in his apartment. His family noted that he had been recently hospitalized for pneumonia and had been released from the hospital 3 days earlier. The ambient temperature of the apartment was normal per the EMS report.

His temperature was 32°C, his heart rate was 50 beats/min, his respiratory rate was 14 breaths/min, and his blood pressure was 90/60 mm Hg. His head and neck, cardiovascular, and abdominal examinations were normal. His skin was cool but warmer than expected given his core temperature; pulses were present in all extremities. There were decreased breath sounds and egophony in the right lower lobe; the signs of consolidation were confirmed by chest x-ray.

What is the cause of this man's mental status changes and what is his prognosis?

INTRODUCTION

Vital signs are routinely measured for all hospitalized patients on admission, during nursing shifts and when infusions are being administered. Clinicians should be able to recognize when abnormal temperatures require immediate action to avoid adverse consequences that may be potentially life-threatening.

HYPOTHERMIA PRESENTATIONS

Core body temperature is tightly regulated between a normal diurnal range of 36.0°C and 37.5°C. Temperatures below 36.0°C are considered abnormal. Patients admitted to the inpatient service frequently have temperature abnormalities on admission or may develop them during the hospital stay. Because of potential life-threatening causes, it is essential to obtain an accurate measurement of core body temperature. Temperature is most accurately measured by the gold standard methods of intravascular, esophageal, or bladder thermistors. Because these are logistically difficult, temperature is most commonly measured by rectal, oral, and tympanic membrane measurements. Axillary measurements routinely underestimate core body temperature and are not recommended. Interpretation of oral measurements requires consideration of influences that affect the results such as eating, drinking, breathing devices, tachypnea, and mouth breathing. Rectal temperatures may be two to three tenths of a degree Celsius higher than actual core body temperature. Infrared cutaneous, aural, and oral thermometers are not reliable in patients with hypothermia. The most accurate aural method is a thermistor probe in direct contact with the tympanic membrane, although the ear canal must be free of cerumen and debris for this to be precise.

◼ EXPOSURE HYPOTHERMIA

Exposure hypothermia is defined as an unintentional fall in core body temperature below 35.0°C from exposure to a cold environment. The most common cause is lack of shelter, warm clothing, or heat during the winter months. When environmental exposure to cold ambient temperatures is not obvious, making the diagnosis can be challenging because the presenting signs are often subtle and associated with numerous potential diagnoses. The initial phase

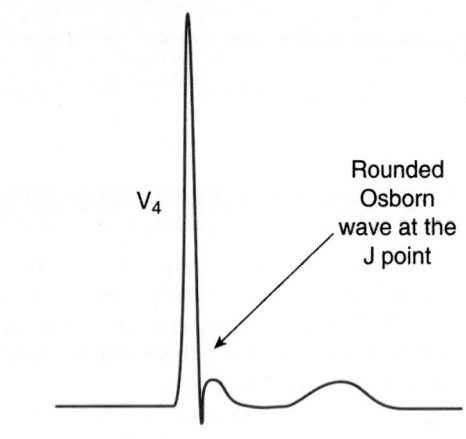

V_4

Rounded Osborn wave at the J point

Figure 94-1 *Osborn wave.*

of hypothermia usually consists of shivering, tachycardia, tachypnea, and peripheral vasoconstriction. Shivering may disappear if hypothermia is prolonged or progresses to severe levels. Other signs include confusion, drowsiness, dysarthria, decreased coordination, and arrhythmias. In moderate hypothermia (28.0-32.0°C), pupillary dilatation, hallucinations, and the phenomenon of paradoxical undressing—the removal of clothes as core temperature drops—may be present. Cardiac manifestations such as bradycardia and arrhythmias begin to develop. Electrocardiographic (ECG) findings, such as a prolonged QT interval as well as an Osborn wave, sometimes referred to as a J wave, may be present (**Figure 94-1**). The Osborn wave is also seen in severe hypercalcemia, but the QT interval is usually shorter and the patient is more likely to be tachycardic from volume depletion. Movement artifact from shivering may also be present on the ECG in patients with hypothermia, especially in the limb leads (with relative sparing of the precordial leads).

> **PRACTICE POINT**
>
> • Severe (<28.0°C) hypothermia may result in coma, hypotension, extreme oliguria, and peripheral areflexia.

At any stage of hypothermia, the precapillary vascular resistance may fail, with resultant vasodilation. The increased blood flow that follows may cause sufficient warming to restore vascular function and reinstate local vasoconstriction. The oscillation between dilatation and constriction is known as the Lewis-Hunting reaction and occurs primarily on the fingertips, toes, ears, and face resulting in paroxysms of flushing. Cold also directly inhibits the enzymatic reactions of both the intrinsic and extrinsic pathways of the clotting cascade, so hypothermic patients may have significant bleeding or hemorrhage.

■ NONEXPOSURE HYPOTHERMIA

Causes of nonexposure hypothermia include sepsis, metabolic disturbances that result in downregulation of the body's metabolic rate, such as euthyroid sick syndrome, hypothyroidism, and adrenal insufficiency.

■ THE FIREPLACE APPROACH TO DIAGNOSING HYPOTHERMIA

Hypothermia is ultimately the result of a mismatch between heat production and heat loss, in the same way that underheating a home is due to a mismatch between heat production from the home's fireplace and heat loss from the home's insulation. The resultant

problems stem from three components; not enough wood (fuel), not enough fire (metabolism), or not enough insulation (heat loss).

The *fuel* (wood) for basal metabolism must be adequate in order to generate heat. Hypoglycemia, malnourishment, and decreased muscle mass contribute to hypothermia as the patient has too little fuel to generate heat. Hypothermia from hypoglycemia is a result of glucopenia in the hypothalamus, resulting in a down-adjustment of the thermal set point that is presumptively to reduce metabolic rate in the setting of inadequate fuel supply. The chronic malnourishment of alcohol abuse places alcoholics at greater risk of hypothermia.

If fuel supplies are adequate, the *body's metabolism* (fire) should be evaluated as a potential cause of the hypothermia. Hypothermia from inadequate metabolism may be caused by hypothyroidism, adrenal insufficiency, and hypopituitarism. The body's metabolic rate simply cannot generate enough heat to keep up with the heat loss. Also included in this category is impaired central nervous system (CNS) thermoregulation, which may be seen with CNS injury from cerebrovascular accident, subarachnoid hemorrhage, trauma, or neoplasm. In these scenarios, the brain simply does not signal to the body to generate the appropriate amount of heat.

Once fuel supplies and metabolism have been excluded, *causes of heat liberation* (lack of insulation) should be considered. Hypothermia may result from induced vasodilation. This results in a greater amount of warm blood in the periphery, which allows a greater amount of heat to be lost to the environment. Acute alcohol consumption, vasodilatory medications, infections (ie, sepsis), and toxins are the common causes. Loss of the body's natural insulation due to burns or traumatic injury to the skin may result in hypothermia. Although usually obvious from history, prolonged exposure to cold (exposure hypothermia) results in too much heat lost to the environment.

> **PRACTICE POINT**
>
> • Nonexposure hypothermia should be considered sepsis until proven otherwise; the peripheral vasodilatation associated with progressive sepsis results in the inappropriate liberation of body heat, lowering the body's temperature.

■ PREVALENCE AND ADJUSTMENTS

Death from extreme temperatures remains relatively uncommon in the United States, and early diagnosis and treatment can often prevent mortality. Between 2003 and 2013, 13,419 deaths in the United States were due to hypothermia-related diagnoses, which is an annual rate ranging from 0.3 to 0.5 per 100,000 persons. Men accounted for 9050 (67%) of the deaths and rates were highest among those over the age of 65. A total of 1391 (10%) of hypothermia-related deaths were associated with alcohol or drug poisoning. A brief review of hypothermia related deaths in Wisconsin noted that nearly half of all deaths were individuals who lived alone, which likely led to delay in treatment. The overall rate of deaths related to hypothermia tends to be higher in the northern and western states, in particular, Montana, Wyoming, and Alaska.

Those at greatest risk for exposure hypothermia are the elderly, alcoholics, persons with psychiatric conditions, and the physically impaired. Aging results in a delayed vasoconstrictor response to cold as well as a decreased perception of cold. Although temperature homeostasis declines with age, of greater relevance to hypothermia are poor social circumstances, comorbidities, and the drugs used in treating these. Patients hospitalized for hypothermia and acute intoxication have a far better prognosis than patients found at home whose hypothermia was not linked to intoxication. Hypothermia portends a poor prognosis in sepsis as well as congestive heart failure. Patients over the age of 65 years admitted for congestive heart failure with a temperature below 35.2°C (<95.5°F) have an odds ratio of death of 4.46 (95% confidence interval [CI]: 1.38-14.3) compared to normothermic patients with congestive heart failure.

There is a significant increased risk of dying from hypothermia in adults over the age of 65. Greater than 40% of all hypothermia-related deaths are in this age group. The rate of death from hypothermia of individuals greater than 75 approaches six per 100,000 population, compared to less than three per 100,000 in individuals younger than 65 years. Men have a threefold increased mortality from hypothermia as compared to women. While mortality from hypothermia is lower in Caucasians, the discrepancy is likely due to social as opposed to physiologic reasons.

THE HISTORY

The following questions should be part of a thorough history; these can narrow down the most likely contributing causes of the hypothermia, and can help define the prognosis.

- **Was this patient brought in from home?** If yes, the prognosis is worse.
- **Was this patient found outside?** If yes, prognosis is better.
- **Does this patient drink excessive amounts of alcohol or engage in recreational drug use?** If yes, prognosis is better.
- **Is it winter, or one of the coldest days of the year?** If yes, the likelihood of cold ambient temperatures contributing to pathology increases.
- **Was this person submerged in cold water?** If yes, the likelihood of a good outcome is greater than submersion in warm water.
- **Is the patient greater than 65 years?** Increased age increases risk of hypothermia.
- **Has the patient recently had a fever? Is this patient at risk for infection? Does this patient have other signs or symptoms of infection or sepsis?** If yes, an infection is more likely and prognosis is worse.
- **Has the patient recently undergone extreme exertion under very cold conditions?** If yes, the patient may have exposure hypothermia.
- **Is the patient malnourished?** If yes, this decreases the patient's ability to increase basal metabolism.
- **Is the patient taking hypoglycemic medications?** If yes, the patient may have become unconscious and unable to avoid excessive cold.
- **Is the patient elderly or frail?** If yes, this decreases the patient's ability to increase basal metabolism.
- **Does this patient have a history of adrenal, thyroid, or pituitary disease?** If yes, this places the patient at greater risk because he or she cannot increase basal metabolism.
- **Is this patient taking medications that cause peripheral vasodilation?** If yes, this puts patient at risk for excessive heat loss.
- **Is this patient taking antipsychotics?** If yes, may cause significant temperature dysregulation.
- **Does this patient have a history of congestive heart failure?** If yes, portends a worse prognosis.
- **Did this patient just have surgery?** If yes, may be due to exposure hypothermia of the operating room or due to large amounts of cool fluids or blood products used during the surgery.

THE EXAMINATION

The hypothermic patient should immediately undergo a thorough evaluation for sepsis; intravenous lines or indwelling catheters should be considered potential sources and removed if indicated.

TABLE 94-1 Utility of Clinical Findings for Diagnosing Bacteremia

	+LR (95% CI)	−LR (95% CI)
Age 50 or greater	1.4 (1.2, 1.6)	0.3 (0.1, 0.8)
Tachycardia	1.2 (1.1, 1.4)	0.7 (0.6, 0.9)
Respiratory rate >20	0.9 (0.8, 1.1)	1.2 (0.8, 1.7)
Hypotension	2.6 (1.6, 4.4)	0.9 (0.9, 1.0)
Confusion or depressed sensorium	1.5 (1.3, 1.8)	0.9 (0.8, 1.0)

LR, likelihood ratio (higher number is better).

The physical exam should specifically note common sites of infection including the lungs, skin, genitourinary system, oropharynx, and sinuses. Physical exam findings or maneuvers that may help with the diagnosis of bacteremia are shown in **Table 94-1**.

Hypothyroidism is a common underlying cause of hypothermia. The findings in **Table 94-2** can help make the diagnosis.

If a hypothyroid patient becomes hypothermic and develops myxedema coma, the clinician should search for an underlying precipitant such as infection. It is critically important to diagnose this condition, because of the significant mortality, especially if the diagnosis is overlooked and because the treatment of hyperthermia differs from other causes.

The signs of adrenal insufficiency are often subtle and present insidiously, but usually include fatigue and hypotension. The physical exam should note the patient's general nutritional status as malnutrition is associated with hypothermia. Age and decreased muscle mass should be noted.

THE LABORATORY APPROACH

Patients should be evaluated for infection as well as endocrine disturbances. A complete blood count, blood cultures, chemistries, urinalysis, and chest x-ray are all potentially indicated. A thyroid-stimulating hormone (TSH) and a cosyntropin stimulation test should be considered. If there is a possibility of adrenal crisis, do not withhold corticosteroids for fear of interfering with the stimulation

TABLE 94-2 Utility of Clinical Findings for Diagnosing Hypothyroidism

	+LR (95% CI)	−LR (95% CI)
Cool and dry skin	4.7 (3.1, 7.1)	0.9 (0.8, 0.9)
Coarse skin	3.4 (1.4, 8.0)	0.7 (0.5, 0.9)
Dry palms	1.5 (1.0, 2.4)	0.8 (0.6, 1.1)
Hair loss of eyebrows	1.9 (1.1, 3.6)	0.8 (0.7, 1.0)
Slow pulse rate	4.1 (3.2, 5.3)	0.8 (0.7, 0.8)
Hypothyroid speech	5.4 (2.7, 10.7)	0.7 (0.5, 0.9)
Enlarged thyroid	2.8 (2.3, 3.4)	0.6 (0.6, 0.7)
Delayed ankle reflexes	3.4 (1.8, 6.4)	0.6 (0.4, 0.9)
Billewicz score 30+ points	18.8 (1.2, 300.5)	

LR, likelihood ratio (higher number is better).

test. An arterial blood gas (ABG) to determine pH and a lactate level are useful for prognosis and may influence choice of intravenous fluids (see below). An ECG should be performed. Supraventricular arrhythmias occur frequently in hypothermic individuals, and atrial fibrillation is the most common. Cardiac arrhythmias usually resolve spontaneously after rewarming.

DESIGNING MANAGEMENT WHILE THE DIAGNOSIS IS PENDING

An exposure hypothermia patient may recover neurologically intact after prolonged cardiac arrest. There have been reports of young adults with rectal or esophageal temperatures as low as 17.5°C. There are also reports of neurologically intact survival despite documented cardiac arrests of 4.5 hours at extremely low temperatures. Resuscitation efforts should continue unless arrest persists after a 35°C core temperature has been reached.

Most hypothermic patients should receive intravenous fluids, as a large amount of fluid is lost due to cold diuresis (the peripheral vasoconstriction due to hypothermia results in increased renal blood flow and renal fluid wasting, and the release of antidiuretic hormone is compromised in hypothermia). The intravenous fluids should be warmed to 38 to 42°C (100-108°F) before administration. Because large volumes of normal saline may exacerbate underlying acidosis, if the pH is low, other isotonic crystalloid solutions should be considered.

For mild hypothermia (32-35°C; hypothermia (HT) Stage I based upon the Swiss Staging System for the Management of Accidental Hypothermia) begin passive rewarming with warm environments, clothing, and active movement (as the patient allows).

For moderate hypothermia (28-32°C; HT Stage II), begin active external rewarming and minimally invasive rewarming techniques, such as warm intravenous fluids, forced-air heating packs or blankets, and a warm environment. If the patient is in cardiac arrest, begin cardiopulmonary resuscitation (CPR) and follow the Advanced Cardiovascular Life Support (ACLS) Protocol.

For severe hypothermia (<24-28°C; HT Stage III), begin active internal rewarming; follow ACLS protocol and consider extracorporeal membrane oxygenation (ECMO) for patients with cardiac instability that does not respond to medical management. Airway management may be required at this stage.

For very severe hypothermia (<24°C; HT Stage IV), follow management for HT II and HT III with the following exceptions: if the patient has cardiac arrest, begin CPR and up to three intravenous or intraosseous doses of 1 mg epinephrine. Strongly consider rewarming ECMO in these patients. Cardioactive medications may accumulate to toxic levels if given repeatedly and spacing out doses of epinephrine is prudent. Overall, ACLS management of cardiac arrest in hypothermia should focus more aggressively on core rewarming as the hypothermic heart may be unresponsive to cardiovascular drugs, pacemaker stimulation, and defibrillation.

Patients who are malnourished or alcoholic may develop Wernicke encephalopathy on rewarming due to thiamine deficiency.

Any patient that is malnourished or has a history of alcohol abuse should receive intravenous thiamine.

Congestive heart failure patients frequently have mild hypothermia, and isolated reports have shown that warming improves symptoms and hemodynamic variables.

If myxedema coma is being considered, immediate administration of intravenous tri-iodothyronine is recommended. Recognize that this may precipitate adrenal crisis if adrenal insufficiency coexists; it is prudent to also give intravenous corticosteroids. Although hypothermia in myxedema coma should be treated, active rewarming methods and direct heat should be avoided as this may lead to peripheral vasodilatation and worsen hypotension and shock. Passive rewarming with blankets and other methods is preferred. Because sepsis is common in patients with hypothermia but can be difficult to detect because classic features may not be present, broad-spectrum antibiotics may be indicated.

RARE CAUSES

There are only a handful of reports of recurrent episodic hypothermia associated with pathology of the hypothalamus. These include stroke, multiple sclerosis, brain tumors, and traumatic brain injury. Two specific syndromes of episodic hypothermia have been described. The first is Shapiro syndrome, with approximately 50 cases reported, comprising recurrent hypothermia and hyperhidrosis associated with agenesis of the corpus callosum. A second rare syndrome is called spontaneous periodic hypothermia. Patients present with cyclical hypothermia associated with hyperhidrosis, headache, vomiting, and abdominal pain. Neurological examination, endocrine studies, and imaging are all normal, and some speculate that it may be a migraine variant.

SUGGESTED READINGS

Brown DJ, Brugger H, Boyd J, Paal P. Accidental hypothermia. *NEJM* 2012;367:1930-1938.

Centers for Disease Control and Prevention. Hypothermia-related deaths—Wisconsin, 2014, and United States, 2003–2013. *MMWR Morb Mortal Wkly Rep.* 2015;64(06);141-143.

Epstein E, Anna K. Accidental hypothermia. *BMJ.* 2006;332:706-709.

Mallet ML. Pathophysiology of accidental hypothermia. *QJM.* 2002;95:775-785.

O'Grady NP, Barie PS, Bartlett JG, et al. Guidelines for evaluation of new fever in critically ill adult patients: 2008 update from the American College of Critical Care Medicine and the Infectious Diseases Society of America. *Crit Care Med.* 2008;36:1330-1349.

Vassal T, Benoit-Gonin B, Carrat F, Guidet B, Maury E, Offenstadt G. Severe accidental hypothermia treated in an ICU: prognosis and outcome. *Chest.* 2001;120:1998-2003.

CHAPTER 95

Hypoxia

Rebecca Dezube, MD, MHS
Noah Lechtzin, MD, MHS

Key Clinical Questions

1. What key clinical entities must be considered in the initial assessment of a hospitalized patient with hypoxia?
2. What are initial diagnostic tests and assessments that should be obtained in the hypoxic patient?
3. What are the potential pitfalls of reliance on pulse oximetry to define hypoxia, and how are these avoided?
4. How should supplemental oxygen be delivered in the hypoxic hospitalized patient?

CASE 95-1

A 63-year-old white female with a history of chronic obstructive pulmonary disease (COPD), requiring 2 L/min (LPM) home oxygen supplementation, coronary artery disease, hypertension, obesity, diabetes mellitus (DM), and lung cancer is admitted to the hospital from clinic with worsening shortness of breath. In the past few months, she has experienced worsening shortness of breath and dyspnea on exertion, and is now unable to walk to the bathroom without getting short of breath. She admits to orthopnea, lower-extremity edema, fatigue, and chest pain. She now requires 4 LPM of oxygen in order to maintain an oxygen saturation >89%.

Her lung cancer was diagnosed in 1996 and was treated with lobectomy and radiation therapy. She has a 50 pack-year tobacco history but quit smoking 12 years ago. Her physical exam is notable for an oxygen saturation of 94% on 4 L, but she desaturates to 81% when semirecumbent. Crackles are heard in the left lung base, and she becomes quite dyspneic and tachypneic upon minimal effort. A one-sixth systolic ejection murmur is heard, along with a loud P2 and paradoxical splitting of S2. Lower extremities have +1 pitting edema, and she has mild digital clubbing

What are the next steps needed to appropriately evaluate and treat this patient's hypoxia?

INTRODUCTION

Hypoxemia is defined as an abnormally low arterial oxygen tension (PaO_2). **Hypoxia** refers to insufficient oxygen in the tissues, and can be generalized or local. The two terms are often used interchangeably, but in actuality hypoxia can be caused by hypoxemia as well as other entities such as anemia or ischemia. This chapter discusses *hypoxemic* **hypoxia**.

A PaO_2 of 60 mm Hg approximately corresponds with the point on the oxygen-hemoglobin dissociation curve in which hemoglobin is 90% saturated. The curve is steep at this point, and further decreases in oxygen tension correspond with dramatic falls in hemoglobin saturation and resultant inadequate oxygen delivery to tissues (**Figure 95-1**). Oxygen affinity can be affected by pH, carbon dioxide (CO_2), 2,3-diphosphoglycerate (2,3-DPG), and temperature. As pH decreases and CO_2 increases, oxygen is more readily released, shifting the oxyhemoglobin curve to the right, increasing delivery of oxygen to the tissues. Red blood cells contain 2,3-DPG, which helps modulate oxygen affinity. Increasing levels of 2,3-DPG decrease the oxygen affinity, also shifting the dissociation curve to the right. Elevated body temperature shifts the dissociation curve to the right, helping to unload oxygen at a time when additional oxygen to tissues may be needed.

■ HYPOXIA IN THE INPATIENT SETTING

Hypoxia is a common and important cause of mortality and morbidity in the hospital. Therefore, rapid evaluation and treatment is critical to avoid serious complications resulting from hypoxia. History and physical exam alone is not sufficient to rapidly detect hypoxia, and other measurements should be used to accurately and efficiently detect hypoxia, including pulse oximetry and blood gas analysis. This chapter will cover the etiology and pathophysiology of hypoxia, considerations for the diagnosis of hypoxia, and treatment options to correct hypoxia.

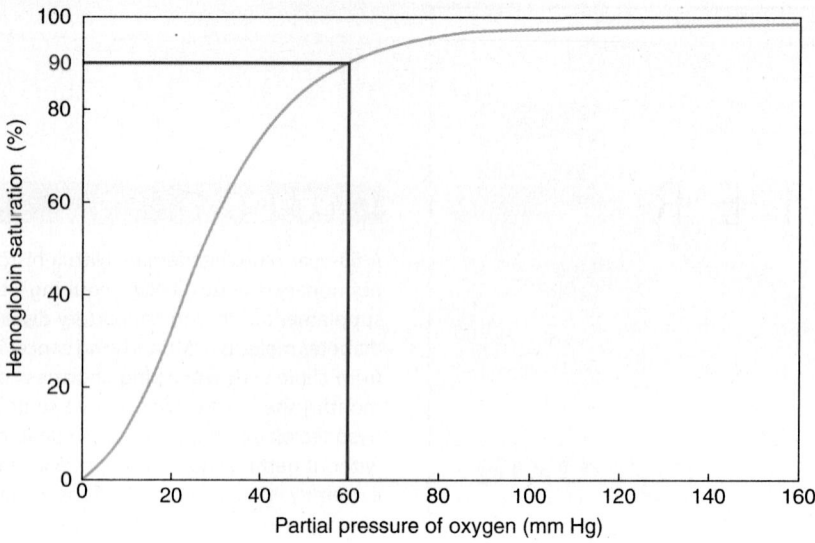

Figure 95-1 *The oxyhemoglobin dissociation curve.* (Levitzky MG. *Pulmonary Physiology.* 8th ed. New York: McGraw-Hill; 2013.)

PATHOPHYSIOLOGY AND MECHANISMS OF HYPOXIA

There are five general mechanisms that cause hypoxia: hypoventilation, ventilation/perfusion (V/Q) mismatch, right to left shunt, diffusion abnormalities, and reduced inspired oxygen tension (**Table 95-1**). Only the first four of these are clinically relevant in the inpatient setting, and only the first three generally cause hypoxia at rest. It is important for the clinician at the bedside to be familiar with these mechanisms and common disease states responsible for them, permitting more accurate diagnoses and facilitating appropriate therapy. The underlying cause of hypoxia can often be elucidated with simple tests such as arterial blood gas (ABG) assessment and chest radiographs. Additionally, assessing how much the PaO_2 increases with oxygen supplementation can help differentiate shunt from other causes of hypoxia.

In *hypoventilation*, alveolar CO_2 increases; as a result alveolar O_2 must decrease. Alveolar hypoventilation is a common occurrence in hospitalized patients. It can be caused by opioid analgesics and other central nervous system depressants or by central hypoventilation syndromes, such as obesity-hypoventilation syndrome. Conditions that cause weakness of the respiratory muscles such as

TABLE 95-1 Mechanisms of Hypoxia

Mechanism	Example	Diagnostic Clues
Hypoventilation	• Central nervous system depression • Narcotic analgesics • Obesity hypoventilation syndrome • Chest wall disorders (eg, kyphoscoliosis) • Respiratory muscle weakness (eg, myasthenia gravis, ALS, GBS)	• Normal A-a gradient • Elevated CO_2 • Readily corrected by oxygen supplementation
Ventilation/perfusion (V/Q) mismatch	• COPD • Asthma • Pulmonary embolism • Interstitial lung disease	• Increased A-a gradient • Hypoxia improved by relatively low levels of oxygen

Right to left shunt	• Anatomic shunts
	   • Intracardiac shunt
	   • Arteriovenous malformation
	 • Physiologic shunts
	   • Pneumonia
	   • Adult respiratory distress syndrome
	   • Atelectasis
		• Difficult to correct with oxygen supplementation

Diffusion impairment	• Pulmonary fibrosis • Pneumocystis pneumonia • Emphysema	• Hypoxia worsens with activity • Hypoxia corrects relatively easy with oxygen supplementation
Reduced inspired oxygen tension	• High altitude	• Hypoxia corrects relatively easy with oxygen supplementation

ALS, amyotrophic lateral sclerosis; COPD, chronic obstructive pulmonary disease; GBS, Guillain-Barré syndrome.

Guillain-Barré syndrome, amyotrophic lateral sclerosis, and myasthenia gravis may result in hypoventilation, as will disorders of the chest wall such as kyphoscoliosis. An ABG taken in the setting of hypoventilation will reveal an elevated CO_2 but will have a normal alveolar-arterial (A-a) gradient. The A-a gradient is the difference in PaO_2 between the alveoli and arterial blood (see later discussion for additional information). However, the A-a gradient may be increased if hypoventilation is coupled with atelectasis, as it frequently is. Furthermore, hypoxemia due to hypoventilation is readily corrected by an increase in fraction of inspired oxygen (FiO_2). However, one should use caution in patients with hypoxia due to hypoventilation. It is critical to treat the hypoxia, but patients with hypoventilation syndromes may have a blunted respiratory response to hypercarbia and may depend on their hypoxic respiratory drive. Their hypoventilation and CO_2 retention may worsen in response to supplemental oxygen, and CO_2 narcosis can ensue. Additionally, increasing PaO_2 without improving hypoventilation will mask the ability to detect ongoing hypoventilation with pulse oximetry. In other words, hypoventilation and hypercarbic respiratory failure may continue and worsen, but oxygen saturations will remain above 90%. Ventilatory assistance, frequently with noninvasive ventilation (see Chapter 138 [Respiratory Failure]), is often necessary to treat hypoxia due to hypoventilation.

The most common cause of hypoxia is V/Q *mismatch*. Areas of the lung with low ratios of ventilation to perfusion result in low alveolar oxygen (O_2) tension. In most situations of V/Q mismatch, there are areas with low V/Q ratios, areas with normal V/Q ratios, and areas with high V/Q ratios. While areas of high V/Q ratio will have a higher alveolar oxygen tension, this will not offset the low PaO_2 from low V/Q areas. This is because the hemoglobin saturation does not change very much from normal V/Q areas to high V/Q areas; therefore the increase in arterial oxygen content from these areas is small and does not offset the decrement in oxygen content from the low V/Q areas.

Common causes of V/Q mismatch include obstructive lung diseases such as asthma and COPD, but V/Q mismatch is seen in many other lung diseases including pulmonary embolism, pulmonary vascular diseases, and interstitial lung diseases. In a pulmonary embolism, gas exchange abnormalities occur from increased alveolar dead space, but hypoxia can also occur due to V/Q mismatch, right to left shunting, and a low mixed venous O_2 level, although hypoxia only occurs in approximately 25% of patients with pulmonary embolism. Low V/Q ratios develop because blood flow is redistributed away from the obstructed vessel, resulting in overperfusion of normal lung regions. Humoral mediators released by platelets stimulate bronchoconstriction, causing atelectasis, which complicates hypoxia. In addition, physiologic shunting occurs because of increased flow through some areas of low V/Q ratios. V/Q mismatch is characterized by an increased A-a gradient. Hypoxia caused by V/Q mismatch is improved by relatively low levels of supplemental oxygen.

Right to left shunt refers to conditions in which deoxygenated blood from the right side of the heart bypasses oxygenation in the lungs and goes to the left side of the heart. One way to consider shunt is in terms of V/Q ratios. The extreme case of V/Q ratio in which there is perfusion but no ventilation is synonymous with shunt. Shunt can occur due to anatomic abnormalities such as intracardiac shunts or arteriovenous malformations. Shunt also occurs due to alveolar filling processes such as pneumonia, acute respiratory distress syndrome, or alveolar collapse (ie, atelectasis). Shunt is less responsive to supplemental oxygen than other causes of hypoxia, which helps differentiate V/Q mismatch from hypoxia caused by a shunt, as a shunt is not readily corrected by increasing levels of FiO_2. Even with supplemental oxygen, shunted blood does not come into contact with alveoli with a higher PO_2. However, with supplemental

oxygen in V/Q mismatch, in the low V/Q regions, the PaO_2 increases with a higher FiO_2, and the blood flow to these regions will have a higher capillary oxygen content, therefore producing a higher PaO_2. Therefore, a response to supplemental oxygen can help distinguish V/Q mismatch and shunt.

Lung diseases that *impair diffusion* of oxygen across the alveolar capillaries and into the bloodstream can result in hypoxia. However, at rest, gas exchange is completed by the time blood has moved a third of the way through the alveolar capillaries. Therefore, even in the setting of severe decrements in diffusing capacity, there is usually enough time in the alveolar capillaries for gas exchange to be completed, and hypoxia does not occur. However, exercise and other conditions that decrease the transit time of blood in alveolar capillaries will lead to hypoxia in the setting of impaired diffusion. Common conditions that cause impaired diffusion by thickening the alveolar-capillary membrane are disorders of interstitial inflammation such as idiopathic pulmonary fibrosis or pneumocystis pneumonia. Diseases that result in loss of alveolar surface area, such as emphysema, will also lead to impaired diffusion. These diseases may also be associated with V/Q mismatch and have mixed etiologies for hypoxia. Hypoxia from impaired diffusion is often associated with desaturation with activity and corrects relatively easily with supplemental oxygen.

Hypoxia will occur if the *inspired oxygen tension is reduced*. Fortunately this does not occur in hospitals but is an important phenomenon in mountaineers. Compensatory mechanisms cause hyperventilation and the ABG value shows a low $PaCO_2$ and a low PaO_2. This condition also improves with supplemental oxygen.

CONFIRMING HYPOXEMIA AT THE BEDSIDE: MEASURES OF OXYGENATION

PULSE OXIMETRY

The use of pulse oximetry is ubiquitous in the hospital setting and provides valuable information quickly and noninvasively. Pulse oximetry is based on differences in the absorption of light by oxygenated hemoglobin and deoxygenated hemoglobin. Oxygenated hemoglobin reflects light more effectively than deoxygenated at 660 nm, whereas the reverse is true at 940 nm. Pulse oximeters calculate the relative amounts of oxygenated and deoxygenated hemoglobin based on the reflection of light at these two wavelengths. Pulse oximetry is very useful in that it can provide rapid and continuous information about arterial oxygen tension. Pulse oximetry results are inaccurate in the setting of methemoglobinemia and carbon monoxide poisoning. In carboxyhemoglobinemia, the pulse oximeter recognizes oxyhemoglobin and carboxyhemoglobin as identical because they reflect light at similar wavelengths, and therefore overestimates the oxyhemoglobin concentration (and therefore the oxygen saturation is incorrectly reported as high). Methemoglobinemia registers at both frequencies of the pulse oximeter and therefore at high concentrations (>35%) tends to result in a reading that is close to an 85% saturation, which fails to respond normally to changes in supplemental oxygen. (With lower concentrations of methemoglobin, pulse oximetry is falsely elevated.) Individuals with very dark skin pigmentation may have artificially low readings, and dark nail polish may also affect results (**Table 95-2**).

Co-oximetry can be performed to measure accurate levels of methemoglobin and carboxyhemoglobin. A co-oximeter measures absorption of different wavelengths, and the proportions of oxyhemoglobin, carboxyhemoglobin, and methemoglobin can be readily distinguished. When a patient presents with carbon monoxide poisoning, for instance, a co-oximeter can detect the carboxyhemoglobin and therefore report the oxyhemoglobin (and oxygen saturation) as markedly reduced.

TABLE 95-2 Pitfalls of Pulse Oximetry Interpretation

Source of Error	Result	Means of Accurate Diagnosis
• Methemoglobinemia • Drugs (anesthestics such as lidocaine, benzocaine, and prilocaine and dapsone) • Hereditary Methemoglobinemia	• Pulse oximetry shows a result ~85% • Oxygen supplementation does not raise O_2 saturation	• Place a co-oximeter (a device which measures absorption at different wavelengths and can accurately distinguish oxyhemoglobin from methemoglobin and carboxyhemoglobin) to confirm presence of methemoglobinemia
• Carboxyhemoglobinemia • Carbon monoxide poisoning	• Falsely high saturation (carboxyhemoglobin is measured as oxyhemoglobin)	• Place a co-oximeter to confirm presence of carboxyhemoglobinemia
• Dark skin pigmentation	• Artificially low readings	• Confirm hypoxemia with arterial blood gas (ABG)
• Dark nail polish	• Artificially low readings	• Confirm hypoxemia with ABG
• Bilirubin	• Falsely low saturation	• Use ABG to guide management
• Poor peripheral perfusion	• Low signal, unreliable results	• Use ABG to guide management

---

PRACTICE POINT

Oximetry pitfalls

• Pulse oximetry is a valuable tool but can occasionally be inaccurate. Clinicians must assure the pulse tracing is accurate and matches the cardiac monitor. Patients with poor peripheral circulation (eg, systemic sclerosis or severe hypotension and shock) frequently have inaccurate or unobtainable pulse oximetry. Patients with very dark skin pigmentation or dark nail polish may also have inaccurate pulse oximetry. Lastly, pulse oximetry is falsely elevated in patients with methemoglobinemia and carboxyhemoglobinemia.

PRACTICE POINT

• When an individual is on supplemental oxygen, the actual inspired FiO_2 depends on minute ventilation and respiratory patterns. Room air (PO_2 of ~21%) can be mixed in with delivered O_2, and it is difficult to determine the actual FiO_2 the patient is receiving. For example, four liters of oxygen deliver approximately 36% FiO_2. Yet, in a patient with COPD with a high minute ventilation and prolonged expiratory phase (who entrains more ambient air), the FiO_2 actually delivered may be 28%. Every 0.05 increase in the FiO_2 will decrease the calculated A-a gradient by 35 mm Hg. Therefore, in the COPD patient example, the calculated A-a gradient may be incorrectly high. We recommend always calculating the A-a gradient on room air.

■ ARTERIAL BLOOD GAS

Direct sampling of arterial blood provides the ability to measure arterial tensions of oxygen and CO_2 and arterial pH. The greatest advantage measuring ABGs has over pulse oximetry is that $PaCO_2$ can be accurately measured. This allows clinicians to determine whether hypoventilation is present and accurately calculate the A-a oxygen gradient. The A-a gradient is the difference in PaO_2 between the alveoli and arterial blood. To calculate the A-a gradient one must first use the alveolar gas equation to estimate the alveolar oxygen tension. The alveolar gas equation is: $P_AO_2 = FiO_2(P_B - PH_2O) - (PaCO_2/R)$, where FiO_2 is the fraction of inspired oxygen, P_B is the barometric pressure, PH_2O is the vapor pressure of water, and R is the respiratory quotient. If a patient is breathing room air and is near sea level FiO_2 equals 0.21, P_B equals 760 mm Hg and PH_2O equals 47 mm Hg and the equation simplifies to $PaO_2 = 150 - (PaCO_2/0.8)$.

To calculate the A-a gradient one simply subtracts the measured PaO_2 from the calculated P_AO_2. *A normal A-a gradient for a 20 year old ranges from 4 to 17 mm Hg and increases by 3 to 4 mm Hg per decade of age.* The A-a gradient will also normally increase with increasing levels of inspired oxygen. Therefore, it is best to calculate the A-a gradient on room air.

APPROACH TO HYPOXIA AT THE BEDSIDE

This section will focus on the presentation of hypoxia commonly seen in the hospital setting. It is important to recognize signs and symptoms of hypoxia, differentiate between a pulmonary etiology and other causes, and treat quickly and appropriately. The principles of management of acute hypoxia include identifying the correct clinical setting for the patient, airway management, correction of hypoxemia, and treatment of the underlying cause.

There are circumstances when acute hypoxia is considered a life-threatening condition, necessitating immediate action. Fulminant hypoxic respiratory failure and cardiopulmonary arrest are indications for emergent intubation and mechanical ventilation. In these situations, it is necessary to secure the airway first, attempt to correct the hypoxemia, and then work up the potential cause for the respiratory arrest.

Differential diagnosis

There are many different reasons an individual may become hypoxic. Abnormalities of the central nervous system can cause suppression of the neural drive to breathe, resulting in hypoventilation and hypercapnia. Examples include overdose of opioid or sedative drugs, meningoencephalitis, localized tumors of the medulla, strokes affecting the medulla, hepatic failure, and uremia. Drugs can particularly negatively affect individuals whose respiratory center is already desensitized by hypoventilation syndromes, such as obstructive sleep apnea or obesity hypoventilation. Disorders of the peripheral nervous system or muscles including Guillain-Barré, myasthenia gravis, muscular dystrophies, and disorders of the chest wall (kyphoscoliosis) can cause hypoventilation and hypoxemic respiratory failure. Obstruction of the upper airways is a common cause of acute hypoxemia, especially in pediatric populations. Upper airway examples include acute epiglottitis, foreign body aspiration, and tumors. Lower airway (bronchi or bronchiole) obstruction can be caused by COPD, asthma, or cystic fibrosis exacerbations (the latter often due to mucus plugging). Disorders of the alveoli themselves can result in hypoxemia, characterized by diffuse alveolar filling. This most commonly occurs in pulmonary edema, pneumonia, pulmonary hemorrhage, and aspiration.

Evaluation

After ensuring that the patient is not acutely decompensating, a comprehensive history should be obtained to help elucidate the possible cause of hypoxemia. Smoking status, possible occupational exposures, sick contacts, recent travel, and personal medical history may give diagnostic clues to the etiology of the hypoxemia. For instance, a history of COPD, coronary artery disease, cystic fibrosis, neuromuscular disorder, or stroke can give an indication of the cause of hypoxia.

A patient may display signs and symptoms of hypoxia including tachypnea, dyspnea, and cyanosis. Cardiac manifestations include tachycardia, palpitations, arrhythmias, hypotension, chest pain, diaphoresis, and shock. Hypoxia may be evident by the presence of altered mental status, delirium, headache, seizures, obtundation, or tremors. Clinicians must thoroughly assess for these signs and symptoms, and initiate the appropriate workup for the etiology of hypoxia.

Confirmation of the diagnosis of suspected hypoxia is based on arterial blood analysis. Evaluation must be initiated early, concurrent with the treatment of acute respiratory failure and/or hypoxia. The ABG value is used to assist in the diagnosis of hypoxia, differentiate between acute and chronic forms, and help guide treatment.

A chest x-ray (CXR) should be obtained to look for causes of hypoxia such as pneumonia, pneumothorax, pulmonary edema, or masses that can be further evaluated and treated. A noncontrast computed tomographic (CT) scan of the chest may also be warranted to follow up an abnormal CXR. A normal CXR in the setting of unexplained hypoxia should raise suspicion for possible pulmonary embolus (PE) as an etiology for acute hypoxia, and can be evaluated with contrast CT scan of the chest (PE protocol), lower-extremity Doppler ultrasound, or V/Q scan.

Treatment

The initial goal of treatment of hypoxemia is to provide adequate oxygen delivery to organs and tissues, keeping the $PaO_2 \geq 60$ mm Hg. Supplemental oxygen is supplied by low-flow or high-flow systems, based on the clinical circumstances. In more severe cases of hypoxemia, continuous positive airway pressure (CPAP) or bilevel positive airway pressure (BPAP) is necessary to provide sufficient oxygen delivery. However, if an acceptable PaO_2 cannot be obtained by these means, intubation is required.

■ HYPOXIA WITH A CLEAR CHEST X-RAY

One situation that is commonly faced in the hospital is a patient that presents with hypoxia but has a clear chest radiograph. Fortunately, the differential diagnosis is relatively limited, and the etiology can generally be discerned with a thorough history and readily available tests. Potential causes include pulmonary embolism, bronchospasm from obstructive lung disease such as asthma, early pneumonia (especially pneumocystic jiroveci/carinii pneumonia [PCP]), early interstitial lung disease, shunt due to intracardiac causes or arteriovenous malformations, hypoventilation, and lastly microatelectasis. It should be apparent that a history and physical exam can help narrow the etiology. Patients with asthma will often wheeze and have a history of asthma. Additionally they should respond to appropriate therapy such as bronchodilators and steroids. While the diagnosis of pulmonary embolism can be challenging (see Chapter 253 [Diagnosis and Treatment of Pulmonary Embolism]), there are items on the history that should make one suspicious. These include risk factors for deep venous thrombosis (DVT), and the acute onset of dyspnea and/or chest pain. Patients with early pneumonia will frequently have fever, cough, and sputum production.

Microatelectasis may be considered if no other causes are found. Even relatively small amounts of atelectasis can cause significant shunt physiology and hypoxia. Atelectasis should be identifiable on CT scan.

Hypoventilation will be detected with the correct clinical scenario and an ABG value showing an elevation in $PaCO_2$ without an increased A-a gradient.

TREATMENT CONSIDERATIONS

Oxygen supplementation can be given in a variety of ways, depending on the level of hypoxia and its underlying reason. Indications for acute oxygen therapy include hypoxemia ($PaO_2 < 60$ mm Hg or oxygen saturation [SaO_2] < 90%) or tachypnea with a respiratory rate >24 breaths/minute. Indications for long-term chronic oxygen therapy are $PaO_2 \leq 55$ or an $SaO_2 \leq 88\%$ at rest (or during sleep or during exertion). During oxygen supplementation, it is important to remember that a PaO_2 of 60 mm Hg is approximately equal to an SaO_2 of 90%. It is reasonable to aim for a goal of PaO_2 of 60 mm Hg in initial treatment of hypoxia, although in certain situations the acceptable threshold level may be adjusted up or down. For instance, in sickle cell anemia, hypoxia associated with cardiac disease, or chest pain, increases above a PaO_2 of 60 mm Hg may be important. Those with chronic CO_2 retention may need to have a lower goal (usually goal SaO_2 of 88%-92%) because of abnormal control of respiration.

There are two main oxygen delivery systems: low-flow and high-flow delivery systems. Low-flow systems include oxygen delivery by nasal cannula (NC), simple mask, and reservoir mask (partial rebreather and nonrebreather). Low-flow systems do not deliver a constant inspired oxygen concentration since there is room air entrained into the NC or mask. Changes in inspiratory flow rate and tidal volumes will entrain more or less room air, changing the actual FiO_2 received. High-flow oxygen delivery systems (eg, venturi masks) maintain the selected FiO_2 by using an oxygen flow rate that is higher than typical inspiratory flows or a reservoir bag.

Nasal cannulas can deliver up to 6 LPM of oxygen. Higher flow rates become uncomfortable for patients and often do not offer additional improvement in oxygen levels. One liter per minute of oxygen delivers approximately 24% oxygen (FiO_2 0.24), with each additional liter adding approximately 3% to 4% of oxygen (**Table 95-3**). However, these estimates are very crude and can vary greatly. Different respiratory patterns can affect how much room air is entrained into the mask, therefore mixing room air with delivered O_2, resulting in a lower or higher inspired FiO_2. Low minute ventilation and hypoventilation will increase the actual inspired FiO_2. Prolonged expiratory phase, increased metabolic rate associated with sepsis, and hyperventilation from exercise will decrease the actual FiO_2. Therefore, the percent of oxygen supplied by each liter is a rough estimate, and breathing patterns can alter the amount of oxygen actually delivered. *Simple masks* can deliver up to 50% to 60% oxygen, and require a 5 to 6 LPM flow rate to avoid buildup of carbon dioxide (CO_2) in the mask. A reservoir bag can be attached to a simple face mask to increase the delivered oxygen to 80% to 85%. A flow rate of at least 5 to 8 LPM is needed to ensure distention of the bag and to keep CO_2 out of the mask. A *nonrebreather mask* can deliver (in theory) nearly 100% FiO_2, by keeping inspiratory gases separate from expiratory gases by means of a one-way valve. Because these masks do not seal tightly on the patient's face, room air can leak in and the FiO_2 will be less than 100%.

Air entrapment masks, which are frequently called *venturi masks*, can deliver up to 50% FiO_2 and are able to supply a constant and predictable FiO_2. Oxygen (100%) flows through a one-way valve and passes by two open ports, incorporating room air. The amount of air entrained depends on the flow rate and size of the two open ports, and as the inflow rate increases, less entrained room air is included. Therefore, the resultant FiO_2 remains constant, which is the main advantage to the venturi mask over simple masks. The venturi mask is ideal in treatment of hypoxia caused by COPD or

TABLE 95-3 FiO$_2$ of Oxygen Delivery Devices

Oxygen Device	Approximate FiO$_2$ %
Nasal cannula	
1 L	24
2 L	28
3 L	32
4 L	36
5 L	40
6 L	44
Simple oxygen mask	
5-6 L	40
6-7 L	50
7-8 L	60
Simple mask with reservoir*	
6 L	60
7 L	70
8 L	80
9 L	90
10 L	>99
Nonrebreather	100
Venturi masks (manufacturer-dependent)	
2 or 3 L	24
4 L	28
6 L	31
8 L	35
10 or 12 L	40
15 L	50 or 60

Low minute ventilation and hypoventilation will increase the actual inspired FiO$_2$. Prolonged expiratory phase, increased metabolic rate associated with sepsis, and hyperventilation from exercise will decrease the actual inspired FiO$_2$. Therefore, the amount of oxygen delivered by each device is a rough estimate of the actual amount.

*In theory, reservoir masks can deliver near-100% FiO$_2$; however, the FiO$_2$ is often <100%.

chronic respiratory failure typified by hypercarbia because the FiO$_2$ can be accurately controlled, and a goal PaO$_2$ around 60 mm Hg (SaO$_2$ 88%-92%) can be obtained while decreasing the risk of worsening hypercarbia and acidosis. Nasal cannula or simple masks cannot accurately control the level of FiO$_2$ delivered, and providing too much oxygen can decrease respiratory drive and increase CO$_2$ retention.

An additional high-flow delivery system that has been recently developed is the *high-flow nasal cannula (HFNC)* system. Historically, it has been recommended to avoid flows greater than 6 LPM via nasal cannula due to patient discomfort, frontal sinus pain, and the risk of drying of the nasal mucosa. However, systems consisting of a heated, humidified high-flow nasal cannula that can deliver up to 100% oxygen at a maximum flow of 40 to 60 LPM were first developed in 2000 and continue to improve. The key components of HFNC include a patient interface, gas delivery system, and humidification mechanism. An air/oxygen blender (gas delivery system) is used to provide precise oxygen delivery, independent of the patient's work of breathing. HFNC has also been shown to provide low-level distending pressures to the airways (equivalent to positive

end-expiratory pressure [PEEP]). The advantages of HFNC include patient comfort/freeing of the mouth which allows speaking and eating, the ability to deliver high levels of FiO$_2$, and the ability to provide positive airway pressure. There has been recent evidence suggesting that HFNC can decrease rates of intubation when compared with noninvasive positive pressure ventilation (NPPV), described in the next section.

NPPV can be employed in certain types of respiratory failure (see Chapter 138 [Acute Respiratory Failure]) to avoid the complications of mechanical ventilation such as airway trauma and pneumonia. Oxygen delivery can be adjusted with NPPV by changing the FiO$_2$ or by changing the airway pressures. NPPV is beneficial in patients with COPD, congestive heart failure, chest wall disorders, obstructive sleep apnea, obesity hypoventilation and neuromuscular disorders. NPPV allows the patient to be awake and interactive and allows swallowing to take place. Treating appropriate patients with NPPV helps to avoid endotracheal intubation and the associated risk of ventilator-associated pneumonia. However, NPPV should be avoided in patients with significant altered mental status, respiratory or cardiac arrest, and aspiration risk. Mask options include nasal masks or full-face masks. Nasal masks tend to be more comfortable, cause less claustrophobia, and create less dead space. However, acutely dyspneic patients tend to breathe through their mouth; therefore full face masks are generally the better option in the acute setting.

More severe hypoxemia may require intubation and treatment with mechanical ventilation (see Chapter 138 [Acute Respiratory Failure]), ensuring delivery of required FiO$_2$. Some patients who require mechanical ventilation may have relatively normal ABG values but have signs of increased work of breathing with accessory muscle use, nasal flaring, paradoxical movement of the abdomen, and supraclavicular and intercostal retraction. These are all signs of respiratory fatigue and impending respiratory failure. In these cases early intubation and mechanical ventilation can relieve respiratory distress by improving gas exchange, decreasing the work of breathing, and reversing respiratory muscle fatigue, while allowing treatment of and recovery from the process that incited respiratory failure.

There are several different modes of mechanical ventilation (see Chapter 140 [Basic Ventilator Management]), but the mode that is used most frequently initially in medical intensive care units is assist volume control (A/C) ventilation. In A/C mode the ventilator delivers a preset tidal volume both at a set rate and when triggered by a patient's inspiratory effort. This mode allows patients to breathe above the ventilator's set rate but also gives them full support with each attempted breath, allowing respiratory muscles to rest. Initial parameters to set include respiratory rate, tidal volume (Vt), FiO$_2$, and PEEP. FiO$_2$ should initially be set at 100% and titrated down to keep PaO$_2$ > 60 mm Hg or SaO$_2$ > 90%. Pulmonary toxicity can occur at higher FiO$_2$ levels, and the goal should be to titrate down to 60% FiO$_2$ and below as tolerated. PEEP is normally set at 5 cm H$_2$O unless the patient has the acute respiratory distress syndrome, which may require higher levels of PEEP. Methods to increase oxygenation (improve PaO$_2$) include increasing FiO$_2$ and PEEP.

■ PULMONARY CONSULTATION

Frequently the cause of hypoxemia can be determined and treated without need for pulmonary consultation. However, in complicated cases, or cases in which a patient is unstable, or when considering invasive or expensive testing, a pulmonary consultation can be valuable. The pulmonary consultant should provide a reasonably complete but focused differential diagnosis for the patient's hypoxia, can assist in selecting the appropriate diagnostic tests to confirm the diagnosis, and should also assist in guiding appropriate therapy to correct the hypoxia and its underlying cause.

CASE 95-2

Our patient's initial workup included pulmonary function tests, chest CT, echocardiogram, and ABG. Pulmonary function tests showed a moderate obstructive defect, a moderate restrictive defect, and a severe gas transfer defect. A CT scan of the chest showed patchy interstitial thickening bilaterally, mild emphysematous changes, cardiomegaly, and a pericardial effusion.

ABG on four liters of oxygen revealed a pH of 7.49, $PaCO_2$ of 35 mm Hg, PaO_2 of 71 mm Hg, and bicarbonate of 26. B-natriuretic peptide (BNP) was 4347 (reference range 0-125 pg/mL). Echocardiogram showed a massively dilated right ventricle with evidence of pressure and volume overload. A bubble study was positive for a patent foramen ovale with right to left shunting. Severe pulmonary hypertension was also suggested on echocardiogram with a right ventricular systolic pressure of 78 mm Hg. Right heart catheterization confirmed pulmonary hypertension, showing a mean pulmonary artery pressure of 58 mm Hg.

The etiology of her hypoxemia was thought to be secondary to pulmonary hypertension, which was multifactorial in nature. Causes included COPD, interstitial disease from previous radiation therapy, and obstructive sleep apnea. She was aggressively diuresed, which resulted in improved oxygenation, and was able to be discharged on diuretic therapy with spironolactone and furosemide. She was then started on sildenafil, a phosphodiesterase-5 inhibitor, as an outpatient in a pulmonary hypertension specialty clinic. Her oxygenation and symptoms improved with this treatment, and she has improvement in her functional capacity. This patient is now able to leave the house to participate in daily activities, which she was unable to do previously. This case highlights multiple possible causes of hypoxia and the many diagnostic tools available to evaluate hypoxia.

CONCLUSION

In summary, hypoxia is common in the hospital setting and requires close monitoring and treatment. It is important to recognize signs and symptoms of hypoxia, differentiate between pulmonary etiologies and other possible causes, and treat quickly and appropriately.

SUGGESTED READINGS

Branson RD. The nuts and bolts of increasing arterial oxygenation: devices and techniques. *Respir Care.* 1993;38:672-686.

George RB. Ventilation, gas exchange, and oxygen delivery. In: George RB, Light RW, Matthay MA, Matthay RA, eds. *Chest Medicine: Essentials of Pulmonary and Critical Care Medicine.* 3rd ed. Baltimore: Williams and Wilkins; 1995:63-78.

Glenny RW. Teaching ventilation/perfusion relationships in the lung. *Adv Physiol Educ.* 2008;32:192-195.

Grippi MA. Respiratory failure: an overview. In: Fishman AP, Elias JA, Fishman JA, Grippi MA, Kaiser LR, Senior RM, eds. *Fishman's Pulmonary Diseases and Disorders*, 3rd ed. New York, NY: McGraw-Hill; 1998:2525-2535.

Hall JB, Schmidt GA, Wood LDH. Acute hypoxemic respiratory failure. In: Murray JF, Nadel JA, eds. *Textbook of Respiratory Medicine.* 2nd ed. Philadelphia, PA: WB Saunders; 1994:2589-2613.

The Acute Respiratory Distress Syndrome Network. Ventilation with lower tidal volumes as compared with traditional tidal volumes for acute lung injury and the acute respiratory distress syndrome. *N Engl J Med.* 2000;342:1301-1308.

Wahr JA, Tremper KK. Noninvasive oxygen monitoring techniques. *Crit Care Clin.* 1995;11:199-217.

Ward, JJ. High-flow oxygen administration by nasal cannula for adult and perinatal patients. *Respir Care.* 2013;58:98-122.

West JB. Ventilation-perfusion relationships. In: Coryell PA, ed. *Respiratory Physiology: The Essentials.* 5th ed. Baltimore, MD: Williams and Wilkins; 1995:51-69.

Williams AJ. ABC of oxygen: assessing and interpreting arterial blood gases and acid-base balance. *BMJ.* 1998;317:1213-1216.

Wood KE. Major pulmonary embolism: review of a pathophysiologic approach to the golden hour of hemodynamically significant pulmonary embolism. *Chest.* 2002;121:877-905.

CHAPTER 96

Sleep Disturbance in the Hospitalized Patient

Xi Chen, MD, PhD
Mihaela H. Bazalakova, MD, PhD

Key Clinical Questions

1. What are common causes of sleep disturbance in hospitalized patients?
2. How do you approach the patient complaining of sleep disturbance?
3. Which inpatient populations are at high risk of sleep disturbance, and what are the corresponding common primary or secondary sleep problems?
4. How do you choose a hypnotic agent based on etiology of insomnia and medical comorbidities?
5. What are the nonpharmacologic behavioral alternatives in cases of insomnia, hypersomnia, or sleep disturbance secondary to circadian mismatch?

EPIDEMIOLOGY

Sleep remains one of the least understood physiological processes, despite the significant percentage of our lives spent in the sleep state. As such, it is at the modern day frontier of not only scientific inquiry but also clinical knowledge and practice. Perhaps nowhere is this better illustrated than in the inpatient setting where, despite our increasing understanding of the wide-ranging role of sleep on a spectrum ranging from mood and attentiveness to metabolic physiology to molecular signaling in the healthy state, little effort is expanded to optimize sleep quantity and quality during acute illness and recovery. In fact, little is known about sleep architecture, duration, and disturbance in the inpatient setting, and correlates of sleep variables with clinical outcomes. However, it is estimated that approximately one-third of hospitalized patients have insomnia at the time of admission. Additionally, up to 69% of postsurgical patients continue to complain of prolonged sleep problems after hospital discharge. The high prevalence of sleep disturbance among this population warrants the evaluation and treatment of sleep problems as part of routine hospital care. Early recognition and treatment of sleep complaints may improve recovery among hospitalized patients.

Sleep disturbance in the outpatient population, primarily as investigated in the context of obstructive sleep apnea (OSA) associated both with recurrent hypoxemia but also recurrent arousals resulting in sleep fragmentation and sympathetic overactivation, has been implicated in increased morbidity and mortality in a variety of cardiovascular (refractory hypertension, congestive heart failure [CHF], atrial fibrillation, stroke), metabolic (insulin resistance, diabetes, obesity), and psychiatric (mood disorders, anxiety) phenotypes. Outside of OSA, self-reported, and therefore subjective, short (<6 hours) and long (>10 hours) overnight sleep duration have both been associated with increased cardiometabolic morbidity and mortality in large epidemiological studies. This, at first glance contradictory, proposed inverted U shape relationship of sleep duration and mortality may be due to two aspects of sleep. The first refers to the current leading hypothesis as to the primary purpose of sleep, namely a "restorative" anabolic function, perhaps especially of slow-wave or "deep" sleep, the latter necessary for growth hormone secretion. The hypothesis is that persistently shortened sleep duration, either due to overall shortened sleep zone or recurrent sleep interruption, may curtail the organism's chance of physiological restoration.

Indeed, studies of chronic partial sleep deprivation in humans demonstrate metabolic disturbance with decreased leptin (satiety hormone) and increased ghrelin (appetite stimulating hormone) secretion, hypothermia due to impaired temperature regulation, acute insulin resistance equivalent to a prediabetic state, and hypothalamic-pituitary-adrenal axis dysregulation with elevated levels of thyroid stimulating hormone (TSH) and increased evening cortisol secretion among others. Mice exposed to complete sleep deprivation die due to overwhelming sepsis, referencing another important physiological function of sleep, through incompletely understood mechanisms: immune system regulation and function.

The relationship between sleep and the immune system appears to be bidirectional, and objective hypersomnia or increased sleep duration is certainly observed in the context of increased proinflammatory cytokine secretion, including interleukins 6 (IL-6) and 1beta (IL-1β) and tumor necrosis factor-alpha (TNF-α), during acute illness. This has been hypothesized as a potential explanation for the association between subjectively reported long sleep and increased morbidity, with hypersomnia or at least subjective hypersomnolence the "readout" of underlying inflammation due to systemic illness.

As little as we know about sleep and hence our limited means to regulate not only sleep duration, but also sleep architecture or sleep stage cycling, given the relationships between sleep and physiology as described above, it is likely to serve acutely ill patients well to, at minimum, minimize sleep disruption in the inpatient and recovery setting.

A recent study examined risk factors for sleep disturbance during hospitalization and found that the severity of comorbid conditions and poor performance of activities of daily living (ADL) predicted sleep complaints during admission. Physician awareness of the impact of sleep disturbance in hospitalized patients is vital since about half of patients admitted on general medical wards will complain of sleep disruption. In this chapter, we will examine the major categories of sleep disturbance, common etiologies, and diagnostic and therapeutic approaches.

■ RISK STRATIFICATION—PATIENT POPULATIONS AT RISK FOR SLEEP DISTURBANCE

Multiple aspects of the inpatient experience lower the threshold for sleep disturbance, including environmental noise, pain, medication side effects, and psychophysiological stress. However certain patient populations may be at higher risk of notable sleep disruption, especially exacerbations of primary sleep disorders. Although by no means exhaustive, a list of patient populations predisposed to primary or secondary insomnia, circadian misalignment and hypersomnia, are summarized in **Table 96-1** and described below:

A. *Sleep maintenance or initiation insomnia and/or secondary daytime sleepiness/fatigue:*
1. **Obese** patients (body mass index (BMI) > 35 kg/m^2), especially with **truncal** pattern of obesity and/or large **neck** circumference (>17 in men, >14 in women), **crowded posterior**

oropharyngeal anatomy (Mallampati airway classification III-IV) due to relative macroglossia, narrowed anterior-posterior or lateral diameters and low-sloping soft palate, or craniofacial features including notable overbite or retrognathia, micrognathia, midface hypoplasia, or narrowed maxillary dental arch with high-arched palate; **postmenopausal women**, **African American**, and **Asian American** populations with above exam findings: these patients may be at high risk of **OSA** (which may present with nocturnal snoring, witnessed apneas, gasping arousals, sleep maintenance, and/or initiation *insomnia*) or daytime symptoms (excessive daytime sleepiness [EDS] or fatigue). While beyond the scope of this chapter, OSA evaluation with screening questionnaires such as the STOP-Bang, and typically outpatient, objective sleep testing once acute medical issues have stabilized, should be considered in all patients with **refractory hypertension** (resistant to three or more antihypertensive agents), early onset primary hypertension, **atrial fibrillation** (where central apnea or periodic obstructive breathing are also highly prevalent), **congestive heart failure**, and poorly controlled **diabetes** or **hypothyroidism**.

See Chapter 235 (Sleep Apnea and Obesity Hypoventilation Syndrome).

2. Diabetes and **hyperthyroidism** are associated with insomnia independently of OSA, due to a multitude of factors including painful neuropathy and diuresis, and anxiety and frequent awakenings respectively.
3. **Renal failure**, **pregnancy**, and **synucleopathies** (Parkinson disease [PD], multiple systems atrophy [MSA], Lewy Body Dementia [LBD]) are some of the conditions highly associated with **restless leg syndrome (RLS) and/or comorbid periodic limb movements of sleep (PLMS)**, at least partially due to a relative iron-deficiency state and/or dopaminergic dysregulation. Depletion of iron stores in the context of **frequent phlebotomy**, **bleeds** or **postoperatively**, is also likely to worsen RLS/PLMS acutely. Exacerbation of RLS/PLMS, which often

TABLE 96-1 Medical Comorbidities of Common Primary Sleep Disorders

Sleep Disorder	Clinical Features	Patient Populations at Risk
Sleep apnea, obstructive (OSA), central (CSA) or Cheyne Stokes respiration (CSR)	Nocturnal (snoring [less prominent in women], apneas, gasping arousals, sleep maintenance and initiation insomnia). Daytime (nonrefreshing sleep, fatigue (women), excessive daytime sleepiness (men), anxiety.	Obesity, early onset or refractory (three or more antihypertensive medications) hypertension, atrial fibrillation, heart failure, symptomatic postmenopausal women, DM, hypothyroid
Restless leg syndrome (RLS)	Sensory-motor leg, arm or torso disturbance described as "achy," "crawling," "pulling," "prickling," or "tingling," sensation, desire to move, sometimes involuntary hyperkinetic movements with triple flexion of the lower extremities, worsened by rest and circadian phase (worse at night), improvement by movement. May lead to sleep initiation and maintenance insomnia.	Iron deficiency anemia, hypoferritinemia (ferritin < 50), acute bleeds or phlebotomy, pregnancy, renal failure, synucleopathy (PD, MSA, LBD), rapid opiate taper (rebound RLS), prolonged immobilization, untreated OSA, TCAs, SSRIs, CCBs
Circadian misalignment	Mismatch between internal circadian sleep-wake cycles and the external environments. Insomnia resolves when patients are allowed to determine sleep timings and duration.	Elderly patients (advanced phase, irregular sleep-wake times); tauopathy (Alzheimer disease), TBI, hepatic cirrhosis, adolescents and young adults (delayed phase); congenital blindness (free-running non–24-h disorder)
Hypersomnia	Excessive sleepiness despite ample sleep opportunity.	TBI, hypoventilation (obesity, neuromuscular, scoliosis), hypothyroid
Insomnia	Difficulty initiating or maintaining sleep, early awakenings, nonrefreshing sleep, daytime dysfunction.	DM, hyperthyroid, mood disorders, anxiety, substance use disorder, withdrawal from hypnotics, sedatives, opiates

American Academy of Sleep Medicine. International *Classification of Sleep Disorders-3, Revised: Diagnostic and Coding Manual*. Chicago, IL: American Academy of Sleep Medicine; 2014.

present with sleep initiation and/or maintenance insomnia due to *sensory-motor disturbance (creepy-crawly or achy sensations and/or involuntary small amplitude nonsustained hyperkinetic movements)* involving the leg, arms, or torso, *worsened at rest, relieved by movement, and presenting in a circadian fashion typically worse in the evening*-night time hours, should also be considered in the context of **withdrawal or diminished dosing of long-standing opiates**, as opiates constitute one of the most effective RLS treatments, and taper or discontinuation can result in RLS-related insomnia, for example, in the postoperative setting where rapid opiate tapers are frequently used. **Tricyclic antidepressants, antiemetics** with antidopaminergic actions, such as metoclopramide or prochlorperazine, and **calcium channel blockers**, are among the known exacerbators of RLS/PLMD.

4. Patients with history of drug use disorders, notably **chronic alcohol use**, are likely to experience significant **sleep initiation and maintenance insomnia** upon **abrupt cessation of alcohol intake**. While acute alcohol ingestion results in shorter sleep latency and initial slow wave sleep increase, increased nocturnal awakenings and rapid eye movement (REM) sleep rebound are characteristic in the latter half of the sleep cycle, frequently resulting in *nonrefreshing sleep, nightmares, and lower arousal threshold with shortened overall sleep duration.* Abrupt abstinence due to hospitalization may not only cause short term sleep initiation difficulties, but may unmask underlying sleep initiation insomnia. High level of clinical suspicion should be maintained not only for primary insomnia but **comorbid anxiety or mood disturbance**, with alcohol use as self-medication for above.

B. **Circadian misalignment**, *or insomnia due to sleep-wake circadian mismatch.*

Frequently masquerading as sleep initiation insomnia, difficulty with sleep initiation is often due to mismatch between innate circadian sleep-wake timings and the environmental or social night-day cues. The key distinction is the *resolution of insomnia if the patient is allowed to sleep ad lib*, or whenever they feel sleepy and for as long as they require. Thus someone who requires >30 minutes and often-times on the order of hours in order to initiate sleep regardless of the time of day indeed should be considered as experiencing insomnia. In contrast, a patient who has difficulty initiating and/or sustaining sleep at 10 PM, but will easily fall asleep at 2 AM and subsequently sleep for an acceptable 7 to 8 hours, is displaying circadian mismatch with, in this example, delayed sleep phase. **Elderly patients** and patients with **neurodegenerative processes**, including but not limited to **Alzheimer disease**, are prime candidates for circadian disruption, as levels and circadian oscillation of melatonin, the endogenous hormone regulating circadian effects on sleep, appears to dampen with age and in neurodegeneration, including Parkinson disease. Medications, especially lipophilic β-blockers such as propranolol, have also been associated with melatonin suppression.

Patients may present with advanced (early sleep times and early awakenings) or delayed (late sleep onset and wake, to the point of **complete day-night inversion**) sleep phase respectively. Elderly patients with or without dementia are also more prone to **irregular sleep-wake cycles**, where sleep is poorly consolidated throughout the 24-hour cycle, and one or more daytime naps lower the sleep drive and contribute to sleep initiation and maintenance difficulties, and nocturnal awakenings with variable return latencies.

Patients with **hepatic cirrhosis, traumatic brain injury** (TBI) patients suffering from postconcussive syndrome, as well as **teenagers or young adolescents** are particularly prone to circadian mismatch with **delayed circadian sleep phase**, or the "night owl" sleep phenotype.

Congenitally blind patients, or patients with retinal pathology, including **retinitis pigmentosa**, are at risk of **non–24-hour or "free-running" circadian disorder** where the sleep zone drifts later or delays by minutes to hours on a daily basis, corresponding to our natural circadian period which is slightly longer than 24 hours, and which is not entrained to light/dark stimuli in blind patients, until the patient's sleep zone "marches around the clock."

C. **Hypersomnia**, *or excessive daytime sleepiness in the absence of sleep initiation or maintenance insomnia, or in the presence of adequate sleep opportunity.*

Certainly acute illness is frequently accompanied by hypersomnia or fatigue, likely in large part secondary to elevated cytokine secretion, including elevated levels of IL-6 and TNF-α. However, persistent sleepiness or fatigue in the postacute convalescence state can limit participation in physical and occupational therapy and opportunity for placement with higher level acute rehab due to lack of patient participation.

Patients with **primary hypersomnias such as narcolepsy or long (>10 hours/24 hours) sleep requirement at baseline** can experience *rebound hypersomnolence* in the context of inpatient **discontinuation of wake promoting agents** such as over the counter caffeine, frequently also self-prescribed for subjective fatigue or sleepiness; sympathomimetics (methylphenidate or amphetamine derivatives), modafinil/armodafinil, or amantadine, frequently used in attention deficit (ADD) or attention deficit and hyperactivity (ADHD) disorders or antidepression augmentation therapy, **or antidepressives with wake promoting properties** (including buproprion and venlafaxine). Prompt resumption in these medications should be considered as soon as the clinical circumstances allow it.

A likely underdiagnosed entity is **obesity hypoventilation syndrome** (OHS), which should be considered in patients with *hypersomnolence*, headaches upon awakening, morbid obesity or **BMI >35 to 40 kg/m², and serum HCO$_3$ >27 mEq/L** not explained by alternative causes, such as contraction alkalosis from diuretic use.

Both insomnia and hypersomnia have been described **posttraumatic brain injury (TBI)**, with hypersomnolence encountered more commonly. Rarely, significant TBI can result in **secondary narcolepsy**, with loss of hypocretin secreting hypothalamic neurons and resultant sleep attacks or **cataplexy** (emotionally induced weakness with preserved consciousness).

INSOMNIA

By far, insomnia is the most common sleep complaint among patients in both ambulatory and hospital settings. The prevalence of chronic insomnia is high, with approximately 20% to 30% of the general population reporting ongoing symptoms. Chronic insomnia is associated with decreased quality of life, daytime functional limitations, chronic pain, increased risk of medical and psychiatric illnesses, substance abuse, increased utilization of health services, and increased risk of death.

The *International Classification of Sleep Disorders* (ICSD-3), published by the American Academy of Sleep Medicine (AASM), defines insomnia as difficulty initiating or maintaining sleep, waking up too early, or sleep that is chronically nonrestorative or perceived to be poor in quality. To meet diagnostic criteria for insomnia, these symptoms *must* be associated with daytime mental or physical sequelae that impair the functional status of the individual. Insomnia may be a primary disorder or may be comorbid with another physical or mental illness.

EVALUATION

Assessment and evaluation of any sleep problem begins with an initial interview of the patient and family, as well as a review of the medical record for documentation of preexisting primary sleep disorders and any factor that could exacerbate or contribute to the current situation. Obtain a focused history by using questions listed in **Table 96-3** to characterize the onset, duration, frequency, and specific characteristics of the patient's current sleep patterns.

The first question in the evaluation of insomnia is whether sleep initiation and maintenance difficulty is dependent on timing of sleep. If a patient reports sleep initiation difficulties at a certain desired bedtime, but upon reflection they are not sleepy at this time (even though they may be fatigued), and they fall asleep readily and sleep well when naturally sleepy at an earlier or, more commonly, later time, then the problem is one of circadian mismatch, rather than insomnia.

Sleep regulation is a balance between a homeostatic "sleep drive" or "sleep debt" and the intrinsic body clock, or circadian pacemaker. The homeostatic sleep drive is directly proportional to wakefulness duration, that is, the longer one is continuously awake, the higher their sleep drive. The circadian variation of sleep and wake is regulated at least partially by melatonin, a hormone produced by the pineal gland under regulation from the master pacemaker, the suprachiasmatic nucleus. Melatonin levels begin rising 2 to 3 hours prior to the onset of the circadian night, remain elevated throughout the sleep zone, and decrease coincident to the end of the circadian night.

Next, establish whether the onset of the patient's sleep complaint began at the time of hospitalization. If the sleep disruption began with hospitalization, subsequent questions (**Table 96-4**) may then focus on hospital factors that may be impairing sleep, such as altered sleep hygiene or, more commonly, medication side effects **(Table 96-2)**. Inquire about the use or abuse of substances such as hypnotics (rebound insomnia and/or anxiety upon discontinuation), stimulants (including over-the-counter caffeine) (rebound hypersomnia and/or depression upon discontinuation), antidepressants and antiepileptic drugs (AEDs) (rebound insomnia or hypersomnia depending on the mechanism of action and individual agent), and opioids (rebound RLS exacerbation and/or pain resulting in insomnia). Ask questions about pain syndromes, nocturnal gastroesophageal reflux, and other symptoms that often impact sleep.

The next step is to assess for preexisting mood, anxiety, psychotic, and substance use disorders, all of which may be exacerbated during an acute hospitalization. Substance abuse disorders are also associated with sleep problems. Over half of patients undergoing alcohol rehabilitation exhibit symptoms of insomnia, such as increased sleep latency during the 6 months prior to entering treatment, and many report using alcohol for the purpose of initiating sleep. Indeed, untreated insomnia and other sleep problems may increase the risk of developing substance abuse problems due to "self-medicating" with alcohol and other substances to help with sleep. While alcohol and illicit substance intoxication and withdrawal are known to disrupt sleep directly, sleep disturbances may persist long after withdrawal symptoms have abated, sometimes years later.

Before prescribing a sleep agent, assess for the presence of suboptimally treated medical, neurologic, psychiatric conditions, or a primary sleep disorder (see **Tables 96-1** and **96-2**). Care should be taken to rely only on sound, documented evidence or a confirmatory medical history when formulating the diagnosis. For example, a patient may state that he has "apnea" because his wife speculates this, but he has never had a formal evaluation for OSA.

Lastly, evaluate the extent to which environmental factors such as noise level, various therapies, and hospital routines may be impairing sleep. Discuss the importance of maintaining a quieter environment with key staff members. When available, relaxation tapes, massage, and warm (noncaffeinated) beverages are preferable to pharmacologic strategies, as shown in **Table 96-6**.

In addition, limit potential iatrogenic causes of disrupted sleep by using alternative drugs or drug regimens, and consider altering

evaluation and treatment interventions to promote uninterrupted sleep at night. Carefully review the medication list and consider whether the drugs themselves, the dosing regimens, or the methods of administration are disrupting sleep (see Table 96-2). If possible consider changing drugs or altering the timing of administration.

An algorithm for diagnosing and treating sleep problems in hospitalized patients is outlined in **Figure 96-1**. By following these steps, the provider may develop a treatment plan that addresses primary sleep disorders, untreated comorbidities, and iatrogenic causes of poor sleep.

INPATIENT MANAGEMENT

1. Circadian mismatch

Light, especially blue-spectrum, but also high intensity (10,000 lux), physical activity, and food intake, are among the most potent "zeitgebers," or entrainers of the intrinsic circadian night to the external or environmental day/night light/dark cycle. Melatonin secretion is exquisitely sensitive to light but, and this is a crucial point for the clinical use of light therapy to modify sleep timings, in a time-dependent manner. Specifically, light exposure prior to the nadir or body temperature, delays the sleep zone or results in a "night-owl" phenotype. Conversely, light later than or following the body temperature nadir, advances the sleep zone, or results in a "morning lark" phenotype. The body temperature nadir is itself dependent on the circadian pattern, and in general occurs approximately 2 to 4 hours prior to the circadian wake time in a patient with a sleep zone of average duration (8 hours).

Thus, in a "normal" individual, with a sleep zone of 10 PM to 6 AM, the body temperature nadir may occur around 4 AM—light between 7 PM and 4 AM will delay the circadian phase and predispose to later bed and wake times, while light exposure between 4 AM and 8 AM will advance the circadian phase and predispose to earlier bed and wake times. Light in the middle of the day, that is, noon or early-afternoon has minimal effect on the circadian phase and sleep-wake timings. However, in a patient with a delayed sleep phase, and a sample sleep zone of 2 AM to 10 AM, light exposure at 6 AM will likely precede the body temperature nadir, and will in fact result in circadian delay, instead of the desired circadian advance to earlier bedtimes and wake time.

While the circadian phase may be determined with urinary or salivary melatonin measurements, this is a labor intensive procedure which ideally has to be performed in complete darkness, controlled physical activity and food intake levels, is not clinically validated in outpatients, and is likely to be affected by underlying pathophysiology in the hospitalized patient. Instead, to estimate the patient's underlying circadian "baseline" the question may be posed: "when healthy, and after a week of sleeping ad lib, for example during vacation, which would correct for sleep deprivation and resultant sleep rebound, what would you estimate as your ideal sleep zone timing and duration. In other words, when would you naturally prefer to go to sleep and wake up." Similarly, an estimation of the sleep pattern over the past 2 to 3 days by patient and/or family or nursing staff, either by recall or facilitated by sleep diaries, gives an idea of the current state of the patient's circadian phase.

Timed exposure to high intensity light (10,000 light boxes), as well as avoidance of light at crucial times, and low-dose melatonin (0.5-3 mg) may be used as chronotherapy to regulate the timing and consolidation of the sleep zone in the hospitalized patient. The general rules are as follows: avoid bright, high intensity and blue spectrum enriched light (which is emitted by screens including tablets, personal phones, laptops and TV screens) for 2 to 3 hours prior to desired bedtime; if screen use is necessary, use blue-light blockers or dim screen intensity. At that time also administer low-dose

TABLE 96-2 Selected Drugs, Common Clinical Uses and Side Effects

Drug Class	Examples of Drugs	Common Uses	Side Effects/Caution
CNS			
TCAs	Amitriptyline, imipramine, nortriptyline, desipramine, doxepin, clomipramine	Insomnia and comorbid migraine and mood disorders, concussive symptoms including tinnitus, headache, vertigo	*Very sedating.* Risk of daytime "hangover" sedation, urinary retention, constipation, orthostatic hypertension, weight gain. Can worsen RLS/PLMS, RBD, and suicidality in bipolar disorder
SSRIs	Fluoxetine, sertraline, citalopram, escitalopram, paroxetine	Insomnia and comorbid depression/anxiety. Suppress REM sleep and, therefore, reduce cataplexy	Some patients experience activation rather than sedation. Can worsen RLS/PLMD, unmask RBD, risk of suicidality with bipolar disorder
Buproprion		Hypersomnolence with comorbid depression/anxiety, RLS/PLMD (only antidepressant not associated with RLS/PLMD exacerbation). Smoking cessation	Can exacerbate headaches, insomnia. Known to increase REM sleep and thus exacerbate narcolepsy/cataplexy. May lower seizure threshold
SNRI	Venlafaxine, duloxetine	Insomnia and comorbid depression. Venlafaxine is effective for perimenopausal hot flashes and associated insomnia	*Activating* in some patients; *sedating* in 12%-31%. If keeps patient *awake*, switch to AM dosing. If *sedating*, switch to PM dosing. May cause vivid dreams or nightmares, and exacerbate underlying anxiety disorders such as posttraumatic stress disorder
Stimulants	Caffeine	Hypersomnia. Circadian mismatch	*Activating.* Avoid after 6 PM. Anxiety, GI upset, diuresis. However, appears safe to beneficial in dose-dependent fashion in CHF, cardiac arrhythmia patients
Sympatho-mimetics	Methylphenidate, amephatmine-derivatives	Hypersomnia, comorbid depression, ADD/ADHD, long sleepers, circadian mismatch	Relatively contraindicated in coronary artery disease (CAD), coronary vasospasm, hypertension, h/o susbstance use d/o. May worsen insomnia, anxiety, nausea, headaches, lower seizure threshold
Wake promoting	Modafinil, armodafinil	Same as sympathomimetics, but no cardiovascular side effects, preferred in comorbid HTN, CAD, h/o substance use d/o	Headaches, decrease OCP effectiveness, risk of SJS. May worsen insomnia, anxiety, nausea
Cardiovascular			
Lipophilic β blockers	Propranolol, pindolol, metoprolol, timolol		Fatigue, nightmares. Suppress melatonin secretion and can affect circadian phase. Atenolol is nonlipophilic and thus less associated with sleep disturbance
Ca²⁺ channel blockers	Amlodipine, verapamil, nifedipine		↓ Lower esophageal sphincter tone → nocturnal gastroesophageal reflux → sleep disturbance. Exacerbated RLS/PLMD
Diuretics	HCTZ, furosemide		Nighttime diuresis → frequent awakenings → ↓ sleep
Other			
Opioids	Codeine, morphine, oxycodone	Insomnia and comorbid RLS	Very effective for RLS/PLMD symptoms. Quick tapers or abrupt discontinuation can lead to rebound RLS and worsening of insomnia. Use with caution in hypoventilators
NSAIDs	Ibuprofen, indomethacin, celecoxib	Insomnia and comorbid pain	May increase nocturnal arousals and cause sleep fragmentation
Methylxanthine	Theophylline	Insomnia and comorbid nocturnal asthma	Causes less restful sleep. May increase arousal frequency
Antihistamines	Diphenhydramine, promethazine	Over the counter sleep aids	May have paradoxical effect on children. Can disrupt sleep if associated with delirium. Effective for sleep onset insomnia, but limited by quick tolerance and sedation "hangover." Can exacerbate RLS/PLMD
Corticosteroids	Dexamethasone, prednisone		Can disrupt sleep, ↑ anxiety, induce mania or psychosis
Quinolone	Ciprofloxacin, sparfloxacin, ofloxacin, grepafloxacin, levofloxacin		Activating. Consider sleep agent after maximizing sleep hygiene. Linezolid rarely causes sleep disturbances

(continued)

TABLE 96-2 Selected Drugs, Common Clinical Uses and Side Effects (*Continued*)

Drug Class	Examples of Drugs	Common Uses	Side Effects/Caution
Dopamine agonists	Ropinirole, pramipexole	Insomnia and RLS, synucleopathy (PD, MSA, LBD), comorbid depression	Can cause sedation or paradoxical insomnia. Watch out for augmentation or worsening of RLS (earlier onset, extension and worsening of symptoms), orthostasis, impulse control behavior dysregulation, including gambling, uncontrolled spending, sex, overeating
Dopa	Sinemet	Insomnia and RLS, synucleopathy (PD, MSA, LBD)	Insomnia with higher doses. Discontinuation may results in REM rebound with nightmares, increased awakenings, neuroleptic malignant syndrome. RLS augmentation

melatonin (0.3-3 mg). Melatonin at bedtime is rarely helpful as a hypnotic, although certain individuals are more sensitive to melatonin's effects than others. It is most effective as a chrono-agent administered 2 to 3 hours prior to bedtime, or 12 hours prior to wake times. Side effects of melatonin include headache, nightmares, and "hangover" in the morning.

Light should be minimized throughout the sleep zone, while bright light (preferably close to 10,000 lux, full spectrum or blue light-enriched), should be instituted as close to wake time as possible for a minimum of 15 to 30 minutes. Side effects of light therapy include mania and headaches. Direct retinal exposure should be avoided to minimize chance of photodamage.

It is essential to maintain the same wake time, rather than bed time, every day, as this resets the circadian cycle. Food and physical activity should be encouraged close to wake time. Daytime napping should be minimized. Initially, this may result in temporary sleep restriction, which in turn heightens the sleep drive and facilitates sleep initiation, maintenance and consolidation. In a patient with circadian mismatch, the same principles apply, with gradual change in wake times, bed times, time of melatonin intake and light exposure advanced or delayed by an hour every 1 to 3 days for delayed and advanced sleep phase phenotypes respectively.

2. Sleep disordered breathing

Treatment of OSA with positive airway pressure (PAP), continuous (CPAP) or more commonly auto (APAP), is shown to improve control of refractory hypertension, at least partially by restoring nocturnal blood pressure dipping by reducing arousals, sleep fragmentation, sympatho-activation and endothelial and oxidative damage due to recurrent hypoxemia; ejection fraction in CHF; recurrence of atrial fibrillation following cardioversion; and perioperative morbidity. AutoPAP should be avoided in congestive heart failure due to the high incidence of Cheyne Stokes respiration, periodic obstructive breathing, and PAP-exacerbated central apnea, all of which can be worsened by high pressures. Bilevel should be considered in the hypoventilating patient, where ventilation with CO_2 reduction is the goal, in addition to or instead of resolution of obstructive breathing and recurrent hypoxemia.

3. Pharmacological management of insomnia

Although nonpharmacologic therapies are ideal, it may be difficult to provide these in the hospital setting, or they may be only partially effective in resolving the sleep problem. In these instances, pharmacologic strategies may be needed. Care must be taken in choosing the appropriate drug due to increased risk of side effects and drug-drug interactions in sick patients. To choose an appropriate sleep agent, evaluate the drug's efficacy/pharmacokinetics, mechanism of action, and side-effect profile. Then match these characteristics with the patient's clinical condition(s). Some common scenarios include:

1. In patients with comorbid sleep and psychiatric problems, consider using a sedating psychotropic at bedtime to promote sleep.
2. Avoid TCAs or SSRIs in patients with RLS/PLMS. However, consider TCAs in patients with comorbid migraines or postconcussive syndrome.

TABLE 96-3 Summary of Questions in a Focused Sleep History of Hospitalized Patients

Focus	Examples of Questions
Sleep pattern	When did the sleep problem start? What time do you try go to sleep? How long does it take you to fall asleep? How often do you wake up during the night? What wakes you up at night? How long does it take you to fall back asleep? What time do you wake up? What wakes you up in the morning? How long are you sleeping during the day (naps)?
Behavioral factors	How does your sleep at home compare with your sleep in the hospital?
Environment	Does the lighting or noise level in the hospital disrupt your sleep? How so? Are you awakened from sleep for tests, monitoring, bathing, or other nursing/medical procedures?
Patient comfort	Is your pain adequately controlled at night? If not, are you on a scheduled analgesic regimen, or do you have to ask for pain medications? Do you have breathing problems, gastroesophageal reflux, or some other type of discomfort that keeps you from sleeping well?
Substances	Do you drink alcohol? How much, and how often? When was your last alcoholic beverage? Do you use cocaine, methamphetamine, marijuana, or other substances? When was your last use?
Psychosocial	How was your mood just prior to being hospitalized? How has your mood been since you were admitted? Have you experienced any emotionally or physically traumatic event just prior to your hospitalization? Have you had any treatments or procedures during this hospitalization that were particularly bothersome to you (eg, intubation, resuscitation, surgery, blood draws, magnetic resonance imaging scan)?

TABLE 96-4 Common Sleep Barriers in the Hospital and Potential Solutions

Barriers	Strategies to Optimize Sleep in the Hospital
Noise and lighting	Limit the volume level of audiovisual and other electronic equipment (eg, televisions, radios, handheld games).
	Promptly respond to alarm monitors; consider liberalizing the monitor alarm setting.
	Keep patients' doors closed, if appropriate.
	Post signs to remind staff to minimize conversations at or near the bedside.
	Switch beepers and other electronic devices to "vibrate" at night.
	Offer earplugs and eye masks.
	Encourage exposure to brighter light during the day (turn on the lights, open the curtains), and turn off the lights by 8 PM.
Visitors	In shared hospital rooms, have patients and their visitors meet in another location (eg, conference room, cafeteria).
	Request that patients and their visitors turn off the ringer on their cell phones.
	Adhere strictly to visiting hours.
	Encourage visitors to minimize discussing emotionally difficult topics with patients near bedtime.
	Encourage patients to limit contact with anxiety-provoking individuals, especially in the evening.
Substances	Minimize use of benzodiazepines for sleep. Try to wean patients off benzodiazepines prior to discharge.
	Avoid starting multiple medications at one time. Minimize use of sleep-disrupting medications.
	Change medication regimens to promote sleep (eg, avoid night-time diuretics if possible).
	No caffeine or cigarette smoking after 6 PM.
Routines	Encourage regular nocturnal sleep time, and discourage lengthy naps during the day.
	Minimize bathing, dressing changes, room switches, and other activities at night.
	Regularly review nighttime orders to see if you could decrease the frequency of overnight monitoring.
Delirium	Provide an updated calendar to facilitate cognitive orientation.
	Discontinue nonessential medications. Minimize use of benzodiazepines, barbiturates, opiates, antihistamines, and anticholinergic agents.
	Regularly provide verbal and other cues to orient patients to the date, time, location, and circumstances.
Nocturnal discomfort	Optimize nighttime glycemic control and maximize pain management.
	For patients with reflux: No oral intake after 8 PM, and keep head of bed elevated ≥30°.
	Provide nocturnal O_2, CPAP, and/or other medications, as appropriate. If patient is on CPAP, assess the mask's fit and comfort.

CPAP, continuous positive airway pressure.

3. Avoid benzodiazepines in patients with history of drug use disorders and hypoventilation, because of dependence/abuse potential and risk of respiratory depression, respectively.

The US Food and Drug Administration (FDA) has approved five classes of medications for the treatment of insomnia: benzodiazepine $GABA_A$ receptor agonists, nonbenzodiazepine $GABA_A$ receptor agonists (non-BzRAs), melatonin-receptor agonists, low-dose tricyclic antidepressants, and, most recently, orexin receptor antagonists (**Table 96-5**). Benzodiazepines include estazolam (ProSom), flurazepam (Dalmane), quazepam (Doral), temazepam (Restoril) (notable for intermediate half-life), and triazolam (Halcion) (notable for a short half-life). Flurazepam and quazepam have long half-lives, increasing the risks of side effects and drug interactions, and should generally be avoided in hospitalized patients. For similar reasons, it is prudent to avoid use of other long-acting benzodiazepines such as clonazepam (Klonopin) and diazepam (Valium), unless there is a specific indication such as RLS. All benzodiazepines except lorazepam, oxazepam, and temazepam have significant hepatic metabolism and should be used with caution in patients with liver disease.

Although non-BzRAs are structurally unrelated to benzodiazepines, they also act at the $GABA_A$ receptor, and have many similar characteristics and risks. These agents include eszopiclone (Lunesta), which is most effective in sleep maintenance insomnia due to having the longest half-life and has mild antianxiety properties due to affinity at the α 2 and 3 subunits of the $GABA_A$ receptor; zaleplon (Sonata) which can be used as needed for middle of the night awakenings due to its very short half-life, zolpidem (Ambien), and zolpidem extended-release (Ambien CR) which are useful for both sleep initiation and maintenance insomnia. Both benzodiazepines and non-BzRAs have a risk for abuse and dependence. Although there is much less risk of dependence with the nonbenzodiazepines, it appears prudent to avoid using all of these agents to treat insomnia in patients with a prior history of sedative-hypnotic or alcohol dependence.

Side effects of benzodiazepines include daytime sedation, anterograde amnesia, cognitive impairment, incoordination, dependence, tolerance, rebound insomnia, and, importantly, respiratory depression. The side-effect profile of non-BzRAs is generally similar but appears to be less severe. Additionally, zolpidem and eszopiclone have been associated with delirium-like episodes, hallucinations, and sleep behaviors, including sleep walking and sleep-related eating disorder, which can be exacerbated in the hospital setting. Long-acting agents should not be used in the elderly due to increased risk of falls, daytime sedation, and adverse cognitive effect. Ideally, the lowest possible dose and shortest acting formulations (ie, triazolam, temazepam, zaleplon, or zolpidem), should be used inpatient populations at risk of side effects, including the elderly.

Ramelteon (Rozerem) is a synthetic melatonin analogue. Ramelteon has demonstrated efficacy in decreasing sleep latency, as well as increasing total sleep time, but does not cause drowsiness the next

TABLE 96-5 Food and Drug Administration-Approved Drugs for Insomnia

Drugs	Adult Dose (mg)	Half-Life (h)	Onset (min)	Time to Peak Effect (h)	Major Effects/Clinical Comments
Benzodiazepine					**Caution** *in elderly patients*. **Tolerance develops to the sedative, hypnotic, anticonvulsant effects**
Estazolam (ProSom)	1-2	10-24	60	½-1½	Short-term (7-10 d) treatment for frequent arousals, early morning awakening. Not as useful for sleep onset. Avoid in patients with OSA. **Caution** *in elderly patients*, liver disease. High doses can cause respiratory depression
Flurazepam (Dalmane)	15-30	47-100	15-20	3-6	In general, avoid in hospitalized medical patients, especially elderly patients
Quazepam (Doral)	7.5-15	25-114		1½	In general, avoid in hospitalized medical patients, especially elderly patients
Temazepam (Restoril)	15-30	6-16		2-3	Short-term (7-10 d) treatment for sleep onset and maintenance. Doses ≥30 mg/d: morning grogginess, nausea, headache, and vivid dreaming
Triazolam (Halcion)	0.125-0.25	1.5-5.5	15-30	1.7-5	Maximum dose is 0.5 mg. Short-term (7-10 d) treatment. Rapid onset; should be in bed when taking medication. **Contraindicated** with atazanavir, ketoconazole, itraconazole, nefazodone, ritonavir
Non-BzRAs					
Eszopiclone (Lunesta)	1-3	6-9		1	In elderly: difficulty *falling* asleep: initially 1 mg; maximum 2 mg. Difficulty *staying* asleep: 2 mg. Rapid onset; should be in bed when taking medication. For faster sleep onset, do not ingest with high-fat foods. No tolerance after 6 mo
Zaleplon (Sonata)	10-20	1	Rapid	1	Short-term (7-10 d) treatment for falling asleep and/or next-day wakefulness is crucial (eg, shift workers)
Zopiclone (Imovane)	5-15	3.8-6.5 (5-10 in elderly)	30	<2	Transient and short-term (7-10 d) treatment. **Contraindicated** in severe respiratory impairment. **Caution** in liver disease and depression; elderly prone to side effects. Anticholinergic agents may ↓ plasma level
Zolpidem (Ambien)	5-10	1.4-4.5	30	2	Short-term (7-10 d) treatment for sleep onset and maintenance. Rapid onset; should be in bed when taking medication. For faster sleep onset, do not ingest with food. No tolerance after 50 wk
Melatonin agonist					
Ramelton (Rozerem)	8	1-2	30	1-1.5	For sleep *onset*. For faster sleep onset, do not ingest with high-fat foods. No tolerance. **Contraindicated** with fluvoxamine
Tricyclic antidepressant					
Doxepin (Silenor)	3-6 mg	8-24		2-3	For sleep onset and maintenance. Higher doses up to 75-100 mg qday for comorbid depression. Can worsen RLS, RBD, cause weight gain, constipation
Dual orexin receptor antagonist					
Suvorexant (Belsomra)	10-20	12 h	30-60	2	For sleep onset and maintenance insomnia. Relatively contraindicated in narcoleptics, possibility of cataplexy, sleep paralysis, sleep onset hallucinations. Hangover, suicidal ideation possible. Caution with hepatic impairment

A common algorithm would be: start with medium to long acting non-BzRA (zolpidem or eszopiclone). If not effective, switch to ramelteon (if sleep initiation insomnia) or sedative antidepressant (trazodone, doxepine, mirtazapine) or suvorexant. If monotherapy not effective consider dual therapy, starting with non-BzRA and low-dose sedative antidepressant.

day. Because ramelteon is not a general central nervous system (CNS) depressant, it would not be expected to decrease respiratory drive, and it appears safe in patients with COPD. Furthermore, ramelteon has been shown to lack abuse potential. Given its very short half-life, Ramelteon is most effective for sleep initiation insomnia, and is not expected to be helpful in sleep maintenance insomnia.

Doxepin (silenor), is a tricyclic antidepressant which has been approved by the FDA for treatment of sleep initiation and maintenance insomnia at doses (3-6 mg) much lower than doses typically used for treatment of depression. At these low doses, incidence of tolerance, withdrawal, sleep-related behaviors, amnesia or hangover appears to be very low.

TABLE 96-6 Alternatives to FDA-Approved Drugs for Insomnia

Drug	Pertinent Side Effects	Comments
Antidepressants		
Mirtazapine (Remeron)	Somnolence, ↑ appetite, ↑ weight, dry mouth	May be beneficial for comorbid depression and insomnia. Lower doses (≤15 mg) increase sedation, but not effective for antidepressant action. Avoid in RLS
Trazodone	Residual daytime sedation, headache, orthostatic hypotension, priapism, cardiac arrhythmias	May be beneficial for comorbid depression and insomnia. Not recommended as first-line agent for insomnia. May be an alternative if benzodiazepines are contraindicated (severe hypercapnea or hypoxemia or history of substance abuse). Tolerance usually develops within 2 wk. Lower doses (50-100 mg) than when used for depression (400 mg)
TCAs	Delirium, ↓ cognition, ↓ seizure threshold, orthostatic hypotension, tachycardia, acquired prolonged QT syndrome, heart block, acute hepatitis	**Avoid** in hospitalized patients due to their anticholinergic, antihistaminic, and cardiovascular side effects. May be beneficial for comorbid depression and insomnia. Avoid in RLS patients
Antihistamines		
Diphenhydramine (Benadryl)	Residual daytime sedation, delirium, orthostatic hypotension, ↓ psychomotor function, prolonged QT syndrome, blurred vision, urinary retention	Better than placebo to treat insomnia, but data are lacking to definitively endorse diphenhydramine for insomnia. Tolerance to antihistamines develops within a few days. **Avoid** in patients >60 y old
Hydroxyzine	Drowsiness, dry mouth, dizziness, agitation, ↓ cognitive function	Efficacy as anxiolytic for >4 mo use not established. Not FDA-approved for insomnia. **Avoid** in patients >60 y old, closed-angle glaucoma, prostatic hypertrophy, severe asthma, and COPD
Antipsychotics		
Quetiapine (Seroquel)	Sedation, orthostatic hypotension, hyperglycemia, ↑ appetite, ↑ weight, hyperlipidemia	The most sedating of the atypical antipsychotics, it is frequently used as a sleep aid. Not recommended for insomnia or other sleep problems unless there is a comorbid psychiatric disorder. Dosed lower (25-100 mg) when used for insomnia vs for FDA-approved indications (600-800 mg)
Olanzapine (Zyprexa)	Sedation, hyperglycemia, ↑ appetite, ↑ weight, hyperlipidemia, prolonged QTc.	Of atypical antipsychotics, olanzapine is the most likely to cause metabolic complications. **Should not** be used solely for insomnia
Haloperidol	Sedation, weight gain, prolonged QTc	Atypical antipsychotics should not be used in the elderly due to increased risk of death associated with atypicals. Haloperidol, a conventional antipsychotic can be given in low dose
Barbiturate		
Chloral hydrate	Over sedation, respiratory depression, nausea, vomiting, diarrhea, drowsiness, ↓ cognitive function, psychotic symptoms (paranoia, hallucinations), vertigo, dizziness, headache	Chloral hydrate has been used for the short-term (<2 wk) treatment of insomnia, but is currently not FDA-approved for that indication. Additive CNS depression may occur if given with other sedative-hypnotics. **Comes in liquid form and has high abuse potential.** Highly lethal in overdose and should be avoided in patients with risk of suicide

COPD, chronic obstructive pulmonary disease; FDA, U.S. Food and Drug Administration; TCAs, tri- and tetracyclic antidepressants (trimipramine, doxepin, amitriptyline, imipramine, nortriptyline, desipramine); ↑, increase; ↓, decrease.

Suvorexant (Belsomra), a hypnotic with a novel mechanism of action, namely dual orexin receptor antagonism, has only recently been approved by the FDA for insomnia. Similarly to ramelteon, suvorexant has a limited side effect profile, with no evidence for dependence, abuse potential, or respiratory disturbance due to CNS depression. The primary side effects are sedation and narcolepsy-like state including symptoms of cataplexy, or emotion (laughter, surprise, anger)-mediated weakness with loss of deep tendon reflexes. Because of the possibility of cataplexy, suvorexant is contraindicated in patients with narcolepsy. Suvorexant undergoes hepatic metabolism and is also contraindicated in severe hepatic impairment. Doses of 10-20 mg at baseline are suggested, and given the moderately long half-life, suvorexant is efficacious for both sleep initiation and maintenance insomnia.

Limited data exist on the efficacy of non-FDA-approved medications for insomnia, such as antihistamines, antidepressants other than doxepin, and conventional and atypical antipsychotics, examples of which are listed in Table 96-6.

The administration of antihistamines, barbiturates, chloral hydrate, and alternative/herbal therapies has been discouraged because the benefits rarely outweigh the risks associated with their use. Antihistamines are the most commonly used over-the-counter agents for chronic insomnia. Diphenhydramine (Benadryl) has been shown to be better than placebo to treat insomnia, but data are lacking to definitively endorse its use to promote sleep. Selecting a non-FDA-approved medication with a sedative effect can be appropriate when the patient has a concomitant illness that also requires treatment, such as a sedating antihistamine (diphenhydramine) in an individual with asthma who is also experiencing insomnia. The anticholinergic action of antihistamines may lead to orthostatic hypotension, urinary retention, or delirium in vulnerable patients. Therefore, diphenhydramine should probably be avoided in hospitalized patients.

Trazodone is the most commonly prescribed antidepressant for the treatment of insomnia. Trazodone is popular among prescribers because, unlike most benzodiazepines, trazodone does not

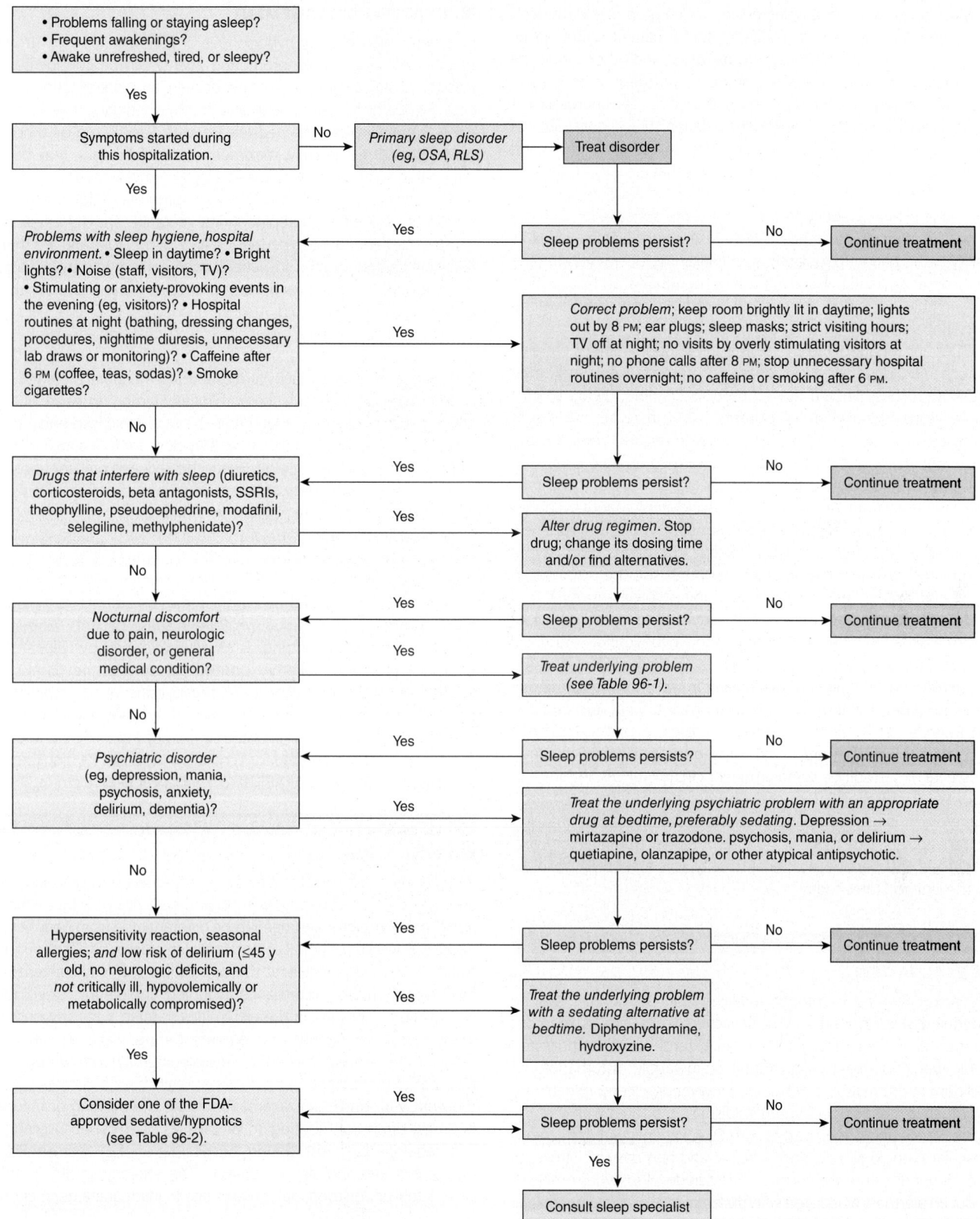

Figure 96-1 *A diagnostic and treatment algorithm for promoting sleep in hospitalized medical patients.* OSA, obstructive sleep apnea; RLS, restless leg syndrome; SSRIs, selective serotonin reuptake inhibitors; FDA, food and drug administration. (Data from Young JS, Bourgeois JM, Hilty DH, Hardin KA. Sleep in hospitalized medical patients. Part 2. Behavioral and pharmacological management of sleep disturbances. J Hosp Med. 2009;4(1):50-59.)

have a recommended limited duration of use and is perceived as being "safer." However, with long-term use, the hypnotic effects of trazodone diminish. In addition, trazodone has been associated with arrhythmias in patients with preexisting cardiac conduction system disease. For this reason, we recommend that trazodone be

used as a short-term alternative to benzodiazepines for patients with hypercapnia or hypoxemia, and in those with a history of drug abuse or dependence, but should not generally be prescribed for most patients with sleep disturbances who do not require treatment of depression.

Mirtazapine, a newer antidepressant, which promotes both sleep and appetite, may be particularly helpful for patients with cancer, acquired immunodeficiency syndrome (AIDS), and other conditions in which the triad of poor sleep, anorexia, and depression is common. Mirtazapine is a noradrenergic and specific serotonergic agent that causes inverse, dose-dependent sedation (15 mg doses are less sedating). To target sleeplessness, start with a dose between 7.5 and 15 mg. If this dose is ineffective, it is unlikely that increasing the dose will be of benefit for sleep. Interestingly, some patients with OSA appear to exhibit a reduction in the apnea-hypopnea index with this drug, but mirtazapine's tendency to cause weight gain may limit its utility in this patient population, and similar improvements are seen with other hypnotic classes, including non-BzRAs and trazodone, presumably by raising the arousal threshold and thus lowering transitional apnea.

TCAs are sedating and useful in a select population of patients who having underlying neuropathy or chronic pain syndromes. Otherwise, these should not be used as first-line agents to promote sleep in hospitalized patients. TCAs increase the risk of cardiac conduction abnormalities, decrease seizure threshold, and have significant anticholinergic and anti-α-adrenergic effects. In patients with dementia, the anticholinergic effect of TCAs may precipitate delirium. Also, conventional and atypical antipsychotics have a similar side-effect profile and should not be used routinely as first-line agents for insomnia, except in patients who have a psychiatric history where agitation may coexist or be precipitated by hospitalization, and in acute delirium. Atypical antipsychotics should be used cautiously in the elderly due to increased risk of death associated with them. Haloperidol, a conventional antipsychotic, may alternatively be given in a low dose. Electrocardiograms should be followed, particularly in patients with structural heart disease and those on medications that may prolong the QT interval. Lastly, chloral hydrate, the oldest hypnotic, has been displaced by barbiturates and subsequently benzodiazepines. However, it can still be useful in select circumstances. It comes in liquid or pill form and does not suppress epileptiform discharges; therefore, it is useful in patients where sedation may be masking seizure activity. Due to its high abuse potential, potential for lethal overdose, and hepatic and renal toxicity, it is essentially obsolete in the United States today.

HYPERSOMNOLENCE

■ EVALUATION

Hypersomnolence in the hospitalized patient, or EDS despite adequate sleep opportunity or, in other words, not as the consequence of sleep disturbance, is an extensive and complicated topic, with etiologies ranging from toxic-metabolic disturbance and delirium to prion disease. However, a few medical comorbidities are worthwhile mentioning. Hypothyroidism is associated with daytime somnolence and often coexists with OSA. Patients with intracranial vascular pathology including ischemic and hemorrhagic stroke, as well as venous sinus thrombosis (VST), can develop hypersomnia or reduced alertness associated with thalamic strokes, high intracranial pressures associated with intracranial bleeding or VST. Perhaps most relevant to the hospitalist, hypercapnic hypoventilation is a common contributor to hypersomnolence, and should be considered in obese patients (BMI > 40, with otherwise unexplained serum HCO_3 > 27), as well as patients at risk for hypoventilation due to myopathy (especially myotonic dystrophy which can have a narcolepsy-like presentation), neuromuscular junction dysfunction (myasthenia gravis), motor neuron disease, chest musculoskeletal deformity (kyphosis, scoliosis), primary lung pathology (restrictive or obstructive pulmonary disease), or hepato-pulmonary or intrapulmonary left to right shunts.

■ INPATIENT MANAGEMENT

In patients with primary hypersomnia or EDS secondary to stroke or other etiologies, wake-promoting agents can be considered if inability to stay awake hinders the recovery and rehabilitation process. Sympathomimetics, including methylphenidate or Adderall, either immediate or sustained release, with 5 to 20 mg q4-6 hour or bid dosing respectively, maximum 60 mg total daily, may be a reasonable starting point (see Table 96-2). However, sympathomimetics, which raise not only the wake-promoting dopaminergic tone, but also affect norepinephrine reuptake and release, can cause dose-dependent hypertension and tachycardia, and are thus relatively contraindicated in patients with coronary artery disease, hypertension, coronary vasospasm and seizures, as they can also lower the seizure threshold. Anxiety, headaches, insomnia, nausea and anorexia with weight loss include additional side effects.

Modafinil (Provigil) and armodafinil (Nuvigil) are not associated with hypertension and tachycardia, and are therefore preferred in patients with cardiovascular comorbidities. Starting doses are 50 to 100 mg qday to bid (but no later than 2-3 PM to avoid insomnia), and can be up- titrated to 400 mg max daily dose for modafinil, or 300 mg max daily dose for Provigil. Headache, reduced oral contraceptive efficacy and possibility of Stephens Johnson syndrome, as well as nausea and anxiety are possible side effects.

Noninvasive positive pressure ventilation (NPPV), starting with bilevel, improves sleep efficiency, total sleep time, and quality of life in patients with hypercapnic COPD without significantly improving gas exchange and should be considered as an adjunctive therapy for improving sleep and quality of life in these patients. A rough bedside calibration of settings is usually performed by respiratory technicians, where expiratory positive airway pressure (EPAP) is titrated to resolution of obstructive breathing (snoring, inspiratory or expiratory grunting, apneas) which is typically worst during supine and REM sleep, and pressure support of 4 to 6 cm H_2O above estimated EPAP can be used for ventilation purposes (ie, inspiratory positive airway pressure [IPAP] 10 to 12 cm over EPAP 6 cm.

SLEEP-RELATED MOVEMENT DISORDERS

■ EVALUATION

Patients with OSA, renal failure, synucleopathies, and pregnant or anemic patients frequently have concomitant RLS or PLMD, which are distinct problems and need to be differentiated from peripheral neuropathy and positional or nocturnal leg cramps. RLS is thought to affect as much as 40% of the population and is characterized by a sensory-motor disturbance including unpleasant "creeping" or "crawling" sensation in the extremities or torso, with or without involuntary hyperkinetic movements during wake. A cardinal feature is the desire to move the affected extremity, with symptoms relieved by movement. Symptoms classically have a circadian distribution, with onset or exacerbation in the late evening or before bedtime, often contributing to or causing sleep-onset insomnia. The requisite bed rest during hospitalization can worsen RLS, further exacerbating sleep problems. The etiology of RLS is not completely understood, but it may relate to inadequate generation or transport of dopamine due to iron deficiency or iron metabolism disturbance.

■ INPATIENT MANAGEMENT

Goal ferritin in RLS patients is >75 µg/L. Of note, ferritin is an acute phase reactant and is likely to be falsely elevated during acute illness. Therefore, not only serum ferritin, but percent transferrin saturation and total iron-binding capacity (TIBC) should be evaluated. High dose iron supplementation should be initiated if hypoferritinemia (ferritin < 50 µg/L) or iron deficiency with transferrin saturation < 20% or TIBC > 400 µg /L is present.

The equivalent of elemental iron 65 mg bid to tid dosing, with vitamin C or orange juice and avoidance of concurrent calcium supplements or alkaline dairy products for improved absorption is recommended. Various iron formulations (the most common being ferrous sulfate 325 mg) exist, which may be substituted in cases of nausea or constipation, the two most common side effects of iron supplementation.

Ferritin and iron studies should be repeated in the outpatient setting, 3 to 4 months after initiation of supplementation. Intravenous dextran infusions can be considered as alternatives to oral supplementation in cases of intolerable side effects or poor absorption.

Dopamine (DA) agonists, namely ropinirole (Requip) 0.25 to 2 mg 30 to 60 minutes prior to onset of RLS symptoms, or pramipexole (Mirapex) 0.125 to 0.75 mg 2 to 3 hours prior to onset of symptoms, used to be considered first line therapy (Table 96-2). However, high incidence of augmentation (or the earlier onset of more severe symptoms spreading to arms or torso), and side effects including nausea, sedation or paradoxical insomnia, orthostasis and impulse control dysregulation with behaviors such as compulsive gambling, spending, and hypersexuality have, in many cases, displaced the DA agonists as first line therapy.

Double-blind controlled studies have showed similar to higher efficacy and reduced or absent augmentation with $\alpha2\delta$ calcium channel agonists, including pregabalin (Lyrica) and gabapentin (Neurontin), which are increasingly becoming first line therapy for RLS, particularly in individuals with comorbid neuropathy, headaches or insomnia. Side effects of the $\alpha2\delta$ calcium channel agonists include sedation, weight gain, and orthostasis, as well as rebound anxiety.

Opiates, including methadone (typically in the 5-25 mg qhs range) and oxycodone (on average 25 mg total daily dose, tailored to timing of worst symptoms), are very effective in the treatment of RLS, and while it is a theoretical worry, incidence of dependence and abuse in RLS patients is low.

Clonidine and long acting benzodiazepines, such as clonazepam, can be considered as well in refractory cases. Selective serotonin uptake inhibitors (SSRIs), tricyclic antidepressants (TCAs), antihistamine agents, and alcohol may exacerbate RLS and should be avoided, if possible. Buproprion (Wellbutrin) is the one antidepressant which does not appear to exacerbate RLS.

SLEEP BEHAVIORS (PARASOMNIAS)
■ EVALUATION

Nonrapid eye movement (NREM) sleep parasomnias, including confusional arousals, sleepwalking, and night terrors, are disorders of partial/incomplete arousal from deep or slow wave (SWS, N3) sleep during the first third of the night when SWS tends to occur. They are characterized by complex, seemingly purposeful behavior without individual awareness and, in the case of night terrors, hyperarousal including diaphoresis, agitation, pupillary dilation, and fearful behaviors. Unusual manifestations reported in the inpatient setting including patients repeatedly pulling out intravenous or central lines in their sleep, with anterograde amnesia for the event. Sleep disruption and deprivation and psychophysiological stress are frequent risk factors. Overnight polysomnography may be required to rule out nocturnal seizures, but these are typically more stereotyped, of shorter duration, rarely result in leaving the bed, and are frequently accompanied by bizarre hypermotoric movements (in the case of frontal lobe epilepsy) or focal neurological signs and symptoms.

REM parasomnias: patients with neurodegenerative disorders, especially synucleopathies including PD, MSA, and LBD and, to a lesser extent, tauopathies such as Alzheimer disease, have an increased risk of REM sleep behavior disorder (RBD), which frequently precedes the motor manifestations of neurodegeneration by years to decades. RBD is characterized by dream enactment in the context of loss of typical muscle atonia during REM sleep. Upon awakening from an episode of dream enactment patients clearly recall vivid and, in the case of men especially, frequently violent dreams, with dream enactment such as punching, kicking, yelling, and sometimes launching themselves out of bed, corresponding to fighting, pursuit or fleeing in the corresponding dream. SSRIs commonly unmask RBD, but untreated OSA and RLS/PLMS can also precipitate RBD.

■ INPATIENT MANAGEMENT

Good sleep hygiene with regular sleep-wake times and adequate sleep duration are important because sleep deprivation may trigger arousals. Ensuring the safety of the environment is essential for these patients. Waking up patient or the use of restraint should be avoided in NREM parasomnias, as confronting patients could prolong the episode and may even worsen the behavior. Patient should be quietly guided back to bed. In the case of frequent occurrence or injury to patient, pharmacologic therapy could be considered.

Clonazepam 0.25 to 1 mg (commonly effective at 0.5 mg) is generally effective in both NREM and REM parasomnias, as it reduces both SWS and arousals. High dose melatonin (starting with 3 mg at bedtime, titrating up by 3 mg every 2-3 nights to max 12-15 mg at bedtime) is also an effective alternative for RBD, but not NREM parasomnias. Clonidine has also been trialed as treatment. Selective serotonin receptor inhibitors (SSRIs) frequently unmask RBD and if possible, use should be minimized. Sleep disturbance, for example from untreated OSA or RLS/PLMS, should be minimized as it may lead to lower arousals threshold and frequent sleep stage or sleep wake transitions also resulting in dream enactment.

SLEEP AND PSYCHIATRIC DISTURBANCE
■ EVALUATION

Sleep disturbance is a diagnostic criterion for mood, anxiety, substance abuse, and psychotic disorders. Thus, comorbid psychiatric disorders must be considered in hospitalized patients with sleep complaints, even if not previously diagnosed. Major depression is particularly common in hospitalized patients with early morning insomnia. Longitudinal studies have found that prior insomnia was associated with 2- to 5-fold increase in the odds of mood and anxiety disorders and suicide. Often, sleep disorders precede the onset of clinical depression, supporting the importance of assessing patient sleep quality during hospitalization.

■ INPATIENT MANAGEMENT

Traditionally, treatment of underlying mood disorder or anxiety has been prioritized temporally prior to treatment targeting comorbid insomnia specifically. However, it is increasingly recognized that pharmacological and nonpharmacological treatment of insomnia is synergistic to treatment of mood or anxiety disorders, and lower the likelihood of depressive episode recurrence. This growing recognition is paralleled by a body of research suggestive that insomnia is indeed a state of hyperarousal, with brain overactivation evident in functional brain imaging in insomniacs compared to "normals."

While comprehensive cognitive behavioral therapy for insomnia (CBT-I) can be pursued in the outpatient setting, pharmacological therapy should be considered in the inpatient setting, tailored to patient comorbidities and medication pharmacokinetics (see Table 96-6). Several hypnotics commonly used in comorbid anxiety/depression merit mention, including eszopiclone (lunesta), a long-acting hypnotic with action on the $\alpha2$ and 3 subunits of the GABA$_A$ receptor, thus mild antianxiety effects in addition to hypnotic effects; doxepin (silenor), a tricyclic antidepressant used for insomnia at 3 to 6 mg, doses much lower than doses used in management of depression; mirtazapine (Remeron), a norepineph-rine and serotonin specific antidepressant, has hypnotic effect at lower doses (7.5-15 mg at bedtime), which resolve at the higher doses used for depression (30 mg and higher); trazodone (desyrel), a tetracyclic antidepressant, had dual hypnotic and antianxiety properties; venlafaxine (Effexor), a serotonin-norepinephrine reuptake inhibitor (SNRI), has been validated for perimenopausal hot flashes and associated sleep disturbance despite its overall activating rather than sedating properties.

PRACTICE POINT: INSOMNIA IN THE HOSPITALIZED PATIENT

1. Poor performance of ADLs heralds a "red flag" for increased sleep disturbance during hospitalization.
2. There is an increasing recognition that primary insomnia represents a hypermetabolic, hyperactivated state, suggesting the value of at least short term pharmacological management when nonpharmacological interventions are insufficient. Avoid abrupt discontinuation of hypnotics, sedatives and pain medications if possible to avoid rebound insomnia.
3. Maintain high level of clinical suspicion for self-medication as the etiology of alcohol (for comorbid chronic insomnia, mood or anxiety disorders) or nicotine (for excessive daytime sleepiness/fatigue) use disorders.

PRACTICE POINT: CIRCADIAN MISMATCH IN THE HOSPITALIZED PATIENT

1. Clinicians should suspect circadian misalignment as a common etiology of sleep initiation insomnia in elderly patients with or without dementia, especially Alzheimer tauopathy, TBI/post-concussive syndrome, hepatic cirrhosis, congenital blindness, or adolescents. Recognize importance of behavioral measures, including restriction of time in bed, consistent wake times, avoidance or minimization of daytime naps, light/dark, and physical activity cues, and low-dose melatonin approximately 12 hours prior to daily wake time as chronoagent for sleep timing/circadian phase adjustment and sleep consolidation.
2. Low-dose (0.3-3 mg) melatonin administered 2 to 3 hours prior to desired bedtime, is typically more effective as a chronoagent, and typically minimally effective as a hypnotic, with doses as high as 5 mg or greater not currently indicated.
3. Recognize that timing of light exposure is critical in manipulation of the sleep zone—in patients with delayed circadian phase ("night owls") early morning light exposure may precede the body temperature nadir. and may thus further delay the sleep phase.

PRACTICE POINT: SLEEP DISORDERED BREATHING IN THE HOSPITALIZED PATIENT

1. It is a common error to assume that lack of desaturation below 90% on nocturnal oximetry "rules out" sleep apnea. In fact recurrent desaturations, even if above the 90% threshold, have long term adverse oxidative damage and sympatho-activation consequences. In fact, some patients with severe sleep apnea with frequency of obstructive respiratory events or apnea hypopnea index (AHI) >30 or as high as 100/hour, may never exhibit desaturation below the low 90s due to rapid cycling of respiratory events (desaturation "banding" rather than "umbrella desaturations" may be seen in those patients, but inpatient oximetry frequently does not have the resolution to allow for recognition of this pattern).
2. Have a high index of suspicion for obesity hypoventilation syndrome in hypersomnolent morbidly obese patients (BMI > 40)

and otherwise unexplained serum HCO_3 > 37, with or without associated sleep disordered breathing or hypoxemia.

PRACTICE POINT: SLEEP-RELATED MOTOR ACTIVATION

1. Have a high index of suspicion for RLS/PLMD contribution to sleep initiation, and maintenance insomnia should be sustained in patients with renal disease, pregnant patients, PD/MSA/LBD patients, patients with acute blood loss or anemia, and (post-op) patients on rapid opiate tapers (at risk of rebound RLS).

DISCHARGE CHECKLIST

1. Referral to sleep specialist has been considered for the patient with insomnia and at risk of OSA, hypoventilation, circadian mismatch, RLS/PLMD.
2. Referral to psychiatric specialist has been considered for the patient with insomnia and at risk for mood or anxiety disorder, including patients with substance use disorders.
3. Referral to neurology specialist has been considered for the patient with dream enactment behavior consistent with RBD and/or parkinsonian features (orthostasis, hyposmia, masked facies, psychomotor slowing or frank bradykinesia, tremor, rigidity).
4. A plan is in place for repeat check of ferritin and iron studies in RLS/PLMS patients following normalization of illness (and thus possibly falsely elevated ferritin levels given acute phase reactant properties) and/or 3 to 4 months following initiation of high dose oral iron supplementation.

SUGGESTED READINGS

Benca R. Clinical evaluation of sleep disorders. In: *Sleep Disorders: The Clinician's Guide to Diagnosis and Management*. New York, NY: Oxford University Press; 2012: 25-46.

Cundrle I, Calvin AD, Somers VK. Sleep deprivation and the cardio-vascular system. In: Bianchi MT, ed. *Sleep Deprivation and Disease*. New York, NY: Springer; 2014: 131-148.

Fava M, et al. Eszopiclone co-administered with fluoxetine in patients with insomnia coexisting with major depressive disorder. *Biol Psychiatry*. 2006;59(11):1052.

Gillis CM, et al. Inpatient pharmacological sleep aid utilization is common at a tertiary medical center. *J Hosp Med*. 2014;9(10):652.

Goldstein C. Management of Restless Legs Syndrome/Willis-Ekbom Disease in hospitalized and perioperative patients. *Sleep Med Clin*. 2015;10(3):303.

Mignot EJ. A practical guide to the therapy of narcolepsy and hyper-somnia syndromes. *Neurotherapeutics*. 2012;9(4):739.

Schutte-Rodin S, et al. Clinical guideline for the evaluation and management of chronic insomnia in adults. *J Clin Sleep Med*. 2008;4(5):487.

Unbehaun T, et al. Management of insomnia: update and new approaches. *Nat Sci Sleep*. 2010;2:127.

Young JS, et al. Sleep in hospitalized medical patients. Part 1. Factors affecting sleep. *J Hosp Med*. 2008;3(6):473.

ACKNOWLEDGMENT

Some of the material in this chapter was adapted from the previous edition chapter authored by Kimberly A. Hardin, MD, MS, FAASM, Kristina Antonson, MD, PhD, Anne B. McBride, MD, and Julie S. Young, MD, MS.

CHAPTER 97

Nausea and Vomiting

John O. Clarke, MD
Susan Y. Quan, MD

Key Clinical Questions

1. What key clinical entities must be considered in the initial assessment of a hospitalized patient with acute nausea and vomiting?

2. What is the clinical diagnostic approach to the inpatient with nausea and vomiting?

3. How should patients with nausea and vomiting in the hospital setting be treated?

CASE 97-1

A 28-year-old woman was admitted from clinic with refractory nausea and vomiting. She has a history of long standing type 1 diabetes mellitus, which has been complicated by retinopathy and neuropathy. From a gastrointestinal standpoint, symptoms began 3 years ago with the onset of early satiety, nausea, and vomiting. This has progressively worsened despite decent glycemic control and aggressive lifestyle modification. She reports constant nausea, which is worse with food, but present to some extent even if she has had nothing to eat. She also reports vomiting after most meals—this may be as soon as minutes after eating or as long as hours. Symptoms are present with both liquids and solids and may even be worse with liquid intake. She is taking ondansetron every 8 hours and promethazine as needed in between ondansetron doses. She has attempted therapy with metoclopramide in the past but did not feel any improvement and also developed a tremor (which reversed upon stopping metoclopramide). She had an attempted solid gastric emptying study but vomited the eggs shortly after ingestion. Her liquid emptying study was markedly abnormal. Prior endoscopy showed no evidence of gastritis, peptic ulcer disease, or gastric outlet obstruction. An upper gastrointestinal (GI) series with small bowel follow-through showed delayed gastric emptying, no abnormal distention, and apparently normal small bowel transit. She has now lost 70 pounds over the past year and was admitted for evaluation, rehydration, and further management.

INTRODUCTION

Nausea and vomiting are common and uncomfortable symptoms with a large number of underlying causes. Nausea is a subjective sensation, usually experienced in the epigastrium or throat when vomiting is imminent (although vomiting may or may not occur). Nausea may be followed by retching, which is repetitive active contraction of the abdominal musculature. Retching may occur in isolation without the forceful expulsion of gastric contents. In contrast, vomiting is a highly physical event that results in the evacuation of gastric contents. This should be distinguished from regurgitation, which is the effortless reflux of gastric or esophageal contents to the hypopharynx.

■ PATHOPHYSIOLOGY

Studies have suggested that the act of vomiting is controlled by a central neurologic center. Borison and colleagues have studied the mechanism of vomiting in cats and found that vomiting can be induced by electrical stimulation of a "vomiting center" located in the dorsal portion of the medulla. These studies, however, have not been repeated in human subjects. Experimental studies have also suggested that a chemoreceptor trigger zone (CTZ) activates the vomiting center when stimulated.

Emetic stimuli can cause vomiting by one of two mechanisms. One mechanism is by activation of afferent vagal and sympathetic neural pathways within the gastrointestinal tract that act directly on the vomiting center. Ablation of these pathways in experimental animals prevents vomiting induced by copper sulfate, which is known to cause vomiting. The second mechanism by which emetic stimuli can cause vomiting is via the CTZ. Unlike the vomiting center, the CTZ is not responsive to electrical stimuli, but only to chemical stimuli from the circulation that crosses the blood-brain barrier. These stimuli include drugs, uremia, diabetic ketoacidosis, and toxins derived from gram-positive bacteria. The exact neurotransmitters that are involved are not known, but there is strong evidence that both dopamine and serotonin may mediate vomiting—hence explaining their role in pharmacologic treatment of nausea and vomiting.

Regardless of the emetic stimulus or the mechanism by which the vomiting center is activated, the act of vomiting is initiated from the vomiting center. The efferent pathways are primarily somatic and involve the vagus, phrenic, and spinal nerves that supply the abdominal musculature.

■ APPROACH TO NAUSEA AND VOMITING

Three steps should be considered in approaching nausea and vomiting:

1. What is the etiology?
2. What are the consequences and/or complications that need to identified and corrected?
3. What therapy may be provided?

There are a vast number of causes of nausea and vomiting (**Tables 97-1** and **97-2**). The differential diagnosis can be approached with a careful history and physical examination. The acuity of symptoms should first be addressed. Acute nausea and vomiting are usually associated with acute infection (especially of the gastrointestinal tract), ingestion of toxins, gastrointestinal obstruction or ischemia, new medication, pregnancy, or head trauma/increased intracranial pressure. Chronic nausea and vomiting, which are usually defined as the persistence of symptoms for more than 1 month, suggest partial mechanical obstruction, intracranial pathology, dysmotility such as gastroparesis, metabolic or endocrine etiology, or a psychologic disturbance.

The timing of vomiting in relation to meals can also be important in elucidating the etiology of symptoms. Patients with a pyloric peptic ulcer or psychogenic vomiting may present with vomiting during or soon after a meal. Patients with gastric outlet obstruction as in diabetic or postvagotomy gastroparesis are more likely to experience delayed vomiting of more than 1 hour after eating. The content of the vomitus can further provide important information. Old food in the vomitus may suggest gastroparesis, gastric outlet obstruction, or a proximal small bowel obstruction, while presence of bile indicates patency between the stomach and proximal duodenum.

The physical examination may be helpful in determining the underlying etiology and is important in assessing the consequences of nausea and vomiting. The general examination can detect important findings such as tachycardia or orthostatic hypotension, which would suggest dehydration. Examination may also reveal jaundice, abdominal masses, or features suggestive of an endocrine process such as thyrotoxicosis or Addison disease. Abdominal examination should focus on presence or absence of bowel sounds, tenderness, distention, as well as evidence of masses, hernias, or prior surgical procedures.

The history and physical examination should direct which lab tests and radiologic studies to order. Basic laboratory testing includes a complete blood count and electrolyte panel. Sustained vomiting resulting in loss of water and electrolytes may lead to dehydration and a hypokalemic metabolic alkalosis. In women, a pregnancy test should be obtained not only to determine if pregnancy is the cause of vomiting, but also as a prerequisite for any radiologic studies. Further laboratory testing may include serum drug levels in patients who are taking certain medications, as well as thyroid function tests.

TABLE 97-1 Differential Diagnosis of Nausea and Vomiting

Abdominal Causes	Nervous System Causes
Mechanical obstruction	Autonomic system disorders
Gastric outlet obstruction	Demyelinating disorders
Small bowel obstruction	Hydrocephalus
Motility disorders	Congenital malformations
Chronic intestinal pseudo-obstruction	High intracranial pressure
Functional dyspepsia	Low-pressure hydrocephalus
Gastroparesis	Intracerebral lesions with edema
Irritable bowel syndrome	Labyrinthine disorders
Organic disorders	Labyrinthitis
Acute appendicitis	Meniere disease
Acute cholecystitis	Motion sickness
Acute hepatitis	Meningitis
Crohn's disease	Migraine headaches
Inflammatory intraperitoneal disease	Seizure disorders
Mesenteric ischemia	Visceral neuropathy
Mucosal metastases	**Other Causes**
Pancreatic cancer	Alcohol abuse
Pancreatitis	Anxiety and depression
Peptic ulcer disease	Cardiac disease
Retroperitoneal fibrosis	Congestive heart failure
Drugs (see Table 97-2)	Myocardial ischemia
Infectious Causes	Radiofrequency ablation
Acute gastroenteritis	Cyclic vomiting syndrome
Bacterial	Eating disorders
Viral	Functional disorders
Nongastrointestinal infectious	Hypervitaminosis A
Otitis media	Intense pain
Systemic	Paraneoplastic syndrome
Metabolic and Endocrine Causes	Postoperative state
Acute intermittent porphyria	Postvagotomy
Addison disease	Radiation therapy
Diabetes mellitus	Rheumatologic disorders
Hypercalcemia	Scleroderma
Hyperparathyroidism	Sjögren's syndrome
Hyperthyroidism	Systemic lupus erythematosis
Hyponatremia	Rumination syndrome
Hypoparathyroidism	Starvation
Pregnancy	
Uremia	

Flat radiographs of the abdomen or a computed tomographic (CT) scan may reveal mechanical obstruction. An upper gastrointestinal series or endoscopy is particularly helpful in making the diagnosis when the history and physical examination suggest that peptic ulcer disease or gastric outlet obstruction is likely. It is important to recognize that the serial imaging included with an upper GI series adds important diagnostic information that a single image obtained during a CT scan may not. The absence of obvious obstructive pathology on

TABLE 97-2 Common Medications Associated with Nausea and Vomiting

Antibiotics	Cardiovascular Drugs
Acyclovir	Antiarrhythmics
Antituberculosis drugs	Antihypertensives
Erythromycin	β-Blockers
Sulfonamides	Calcium channel antagonists
Tetracycline	Digoxin
Antidiabetic agents	Central nervous system drugs
Antigout agents	Antiparkinsonian drugs
Aspirin	Anticonvulsants
Cancer chemotherapy	Diuretics
Cis-platinum	Gastrointestinal medications
Cytarabine	Azathioprine
Dacarbazine	Lubiprostone
Etoposide	Sulfasalazine
5-Fluorouracil	Narcotics
Methotrexate	Nicotine
Nitrogen mustard	Nonsteroidal antiinflammatory drugs
Tamoxifen	Oral contraceptives
Vinblastine	Theophylline

a CT scan should not dissuade the clinician from obtaining an upper GI series or small bowel follow-through if appropriate. In patients with chronic nausea and vomiting who have a normal upper gastrointestinal series and endoscopy, further evaluation with a radionuclide gastric emptying study can be considered. Electrogastrography and antroduodenal manometry can also be considered if available; however, the clinical utility of these studies in most patients with chronic nausea is not well established, and these procedures are offered at only select tertiary facilities. In patients with normal gastric emptying and motility studies, evaluation with CT, ultrasonography or biliary scintigraphy may provide valuable information if a gallbladder, pancreatic, or hepatobiliary etiology is suspected. In addition, given that central nervous system processes can result in nausea, one should have a low threshold to perform neurologic imaging in the appropriate clinical context. Finally, a psychiatric consultation should also be considered if studies do not indicate any organic pathology.

When vomiting arises in the hospital, often it is medications that are to blame. Opiates, in particular, slow gastrointestinal transit and have additional direct emetogenic effects in some patients. Chemotherapeutic medications, antibiotics, and general anesthesia are also common precipitants of nausea in hospitalized patients. Abdominal procedures are also well known to result in nausea and delayed gut motility, independent of the anesthesia received. In many instances in which a clear precipitant is apparent, there is not a need to pursue aggressive diagnostic interventions; supportive care is adequate. However, if the symptoms are out of proportion to the clinical scenario or unusually prolonged (eg, persistent nausea and vomiting 4 days after general anesthesia for a nonabdominal procedure), diagnostic evaluation is wise. Additionally, other signs and symptoms such as fever or focal neurologic deficits should be sought out, and if present, should lead to prompt diagnostic evaluation. Finally, myocardial ischemia (particularly right-sided myocardial infarction) should be considered in hospitalized patients with cardiovascular risk factors. Diaphoresis, dyspnea, and changes in heart rate or blood pressure may suggest a cardiac etiology.

> **PRACTICE POINT**
>
> - In many instances in which a clear precipitant is apparent, there is no need to pursue aggressive diagnostic interventions; supportive care is adequate. However, if the symptoms are out of proportion to the clinical scenario or unusually prolonged (eg, persistent nausea and vomiting 4 days after general anesthesia for a nonabdominal procedure), diagnostic evaluation is wise.

■ TREATMENT

Treatment of nausea and vomiting involves correction of fluid and electrolyte imbalance if present, identification and treatment of the underlying cause if one exists, and relief of symptoms either by suppression or by elimination if the primary cause cannot be promptly identified and removed. Patients with long-standing chronic nausea and vomiting are at risk for developing malnutrition, and it is important to monitor for this in the hospital setting. If a patient is not able to tolerate adequate oral caloric intake after a 5-day period, consideration should be given for enteral or parenteral feeding. Enteral feeding is usually the first option; however, dislodgment of enteral feeds with acute vomiting is not uncommon and occasionally parenteral feeding may be required.

Pharmacologic treatment

There are many commonly employed antiemetic agents, and these medications can be divided into two main categories: central antiemetic agents and peripheral prokinetic agents. In practice, many drugs employ both mechanisms and many of the specific pathways by which these medications exert benefit are still being elucidated. The main antiemetics are detailed in the next sections.

Dopamine D2 receptor antagonists

Metoclopramide is the classic agent in this category and exerts a central antiemetic effect through antagonism of dopamine D2 receptors as well as a peripheral prokinetic effect through stimulation of peripheral 5-HT$_4$ receptors. Common indications include postoperative nausea and vomiting, chemotherapy and radiation therapy-induced nausea, and gastroparesis. The standard dose is 5 to 10 mg orally or intravenously three to four times daily. Metoclopramide is associated with significant side effects, including restlessness, anxiety, somnolence, extrapyramidal effects, QT interval prolongation, and, if used for a prolonged period of time, tardive dyskinesia in rare cases (which in some cases is irreversible). Metoclopramide is currently the only US Food and Drug Administration (FDA)-approved medication for diabetic gastroparesis; however, due to side effects it has a black box warning against use of greater than 12 weeks based on the risk of tardive dyskinesia.

Domperidone is a second agent in this category that crosses the blood-brain barrier poorly and is believed to act primarily through prokinetic function as a peripheral D2 receptor antagonist. Domperidone is a weaker antiemetic than metoclopramide, but as it is better tolerated, higher doses can be employed and the risk of anxiety and dystonia is significantly reduced. Domperidone is not approved for use in the United States; however, it can be obtained by filing an investigational new drug application with the FDA. Recent studies suggest QT prolongation and a potential increase in the risk of sudden cardiac death and if this is used clinically then close monitoring is essential.

Phenothiazines

Phenothiazines (chlorpromazine, promethazine) block D2 dopaminergic receptors in addition to muscarinic M1 receptors and histamine H1 receptors. These drugs induce relaxation and somnolence and are generally used parenterally or as suppositories in patients with acute intense vomiting of central origin (such as with migraine headaches and motion sickness). Although effective, side effects can be significant and often limit use. Of note, promethazine does have a black box warning from the FDA due to severe tissue injury; as a vesicant, if promethazine extravasates into subcutaneous tissues or is accidentally infused intra-arterially, severe local necrosis may occur.

Butyrophenones

Butyrophenones block D2 dopaminergic receptors and muscarinic M1 receptors and are believed to affect nausea through central antiemetic effects. Commonly used agents in this category include droperidol and haloperidol. As with the phenothiazines already mentioned, side effects and safety concerns have limited routine use of these agents, although they may be of benefit on an adjunct basis.

Antihistamines and antimuscarinic agents

These agents work primarily through blockage of histamine H1 receptors and muscarinic M1 receptors at a central level. Commonly used antihistamines are diphenhydramine, meclizine, and cyclizine. The most commonly used antimuscarinic agent is scopolamine. In addition, promethazine also has both antihistamine and antimuscarinic effects. Somnolence and drowsiness are the main limiting factors with these agents; however, anticholinergic effects can also be problematic—particularly for older patients. These agents are commonly used for treatment of motion sickness and nausea associated with vestibular disease.

Serotonin antagonists

Serotonin 5-HT$_3$ receptors seem to play a key role in nausea, and selective antagonists (such as ondansetron) are particularly effective through central nausea mediation. In addition, these agents may have a mild gastric prokinetic function. These agents are primarily used for postoperative nausea and after chemotherapy and radiation therapy; however, given their efficacy they are often used for refractory nausea related to other conditions. Of note, headache is a common side effect. For those patients that cannot tolerate oral agents, granisetron is available in transdermal form with a 7-day duration of action.

Serotonin agonists

Serotonin 5-HT$_4$ receptors seem to play a key role in gastric motility, and agonists of these receptors (such as metoclopramide, cisapride, and tegaserod) have significant prokinetic capabilities. Of these agents, cisapride has the most potent function and demonstrated efficacy for nausea associated with gastroparesis, pseudoobstruction, or other motility cause; however, cisapride was removed from the market due to QT-prolongation complicated by the risk of lethal ventricular arrhythmias. Tegaserod was also removed from the market due to increased associated cardiac events. At the moment, the only medication available in the United States that works through this mechanism is believed to be metoclopramide, and, as detailed earlier, this is but one mechanism by which metoclopramide is believed to exert benefit. Prucalopride has been approved in Europe and Canada, but is not yet available in the United States.

Motilin receptor agonists

The classic motilin receptor agonist is the antibiotic erythromycin, which acts as a motilin receptor ligand on smooth muscle cells and enteric nerves, increasing gastric and intestinal peristaltic motor activity. In clinical practice, erythromycin may be used to treat acute nausea and vomiting associated with delayed gastric emptying and is also used to clear the stomach of retained food and blood prior to endoscopy. Erythromycin is best used acutely and is, unfortunately, not a good agent for chronic use in most patients as it is associated with tachyphylaxis. Erythromycin also induces nausea in a significant subset of patients and is associated with QT interval prolongation. New synthetic motilin agonists devoid of antibacterial activity are in development; however, none are ready for clinical use at the present time.

Ghrelin is a peptic structurally similar to motilin that also accelerates gastric emptying. Ghrelin receptor agonists are under development and may play a role in the future; however, they are not available at present for clinical use.

Glucocorticoids

The antiemetic mechanism of glucocorticoids is not clear and numerous hypotheses have been raised, including inhibition of central prostaglandin synthesis, altered serotonin processing, and enhanced endorphin release. Regardless, glucocorticoids do appear to have an antiemetic effect and are often used for postoperative nausea or for treatment of nausea in the context of chemotherapy or radiation. In most cases, this use is as an adjunct therapy in combination with other agents rather than as a sole treatment modality.

Cannabinoids

Synthetic cannabinoids have entered the therapeutic armamentarium for treatment of nausea. Two oral formulations, dronabinol and nabilone, are approved by the FDA for chemotherapy-induced nausea and vomiting refractory to conventional antiemetic therapy. While attractive to many patients, use of these agents is often limited by hypotension and psychotropic reactions. Marijuana has also been used for treatment of chronic nausea; however, data and availability are limited and it is uncertain where this falls at present in the treatment algorithm.

Neurokinin-1 receptor antagonists

Neurokinin-1 (NK) receptor antagonists inhibit substance P/NK-1 and are potent antiemetics. These agents (aprepitant, fosaprepitant) appear to be particularly effective for treatment of postoperative vomiting and may be used as adjunct therapy for patients not responding to the foregoing measures. An ongoing large multicenter randomized trial is currently in progress evaluating the role of aprepitant in chronic nausea related to gastroparesis.

Benzodiazepines

Although not proven nor approved as therapy for nausea, anecdotal experience supports the use of benzodiazepines in patients with refractory nausea, particularly when there appears to be a psychological or anticipatory component (ie, the patient reports nausea at the smell or sight of food prior to ingestion).

Alternative and surgical treatment

For patients with refractory nausea despite the pharmacologic options already detailed, it is occasionally necessary to explore alternative and surgical options. Acupuncture has been studied for treatment of nausea in select clinical situations and has shown benefit. Gastric electrical stimulation has also been explored for chronic nausea associated with gastroparesis. The concept is that an implantable neurostimulator delivers brief, low-energy impulses to the stomach, which alters afferent sensation, particularly with regard to nausea. This is approved for humanitarian use by the FDA; however, the procedure is not without risk, and clinical improvement is not universal—with most studies suggesting approximately a 40% response rate. At the moment, this is only approved for chronic nausea in the context of gastroparesis; however, studies are ongoing that may broaden this indication. Other surgical options for chronic nausea do not appear to have sufficient data to pursue further at the present time, except for perhaps completion gastrectomy in patients with nausea in the context of postsurgical gastroparesis—and potentially pyloroplasty in patients with gastroparesis and pylorospasm.

CASE 97-1 (continued)

The patient was admitted for intravenous fluids and started on erythromycin, while being continued on the remainder of her regimen. She declined supplemental enteral or parenteral nutrition and after stabilization was discharged home. As an outpatient she was started on domperidone and seen in consultation by surgery for gastric stimulator placement, which she underwent later that year. Following gastric stimulator placement, she had a difficult postoperative recovery period and was discharged home on parenteral nutrition, which she was able to eventually taper off. She did well for a period of 3 months with marked improvement in nausea and significant weight gain, but unfortunately developed recurrent debilitating nausea and progressive weight loss, leading to a jejunal tube placement for enteral nutrition. At present, nausea remains a significant ongoing issue despite the efforts detailed here.

CONCLUSION

Nausea and vomiting are common in hospitalized patients and can occur due to a wide variety of causes. The initial step should be identifying whether the symptoms are acute or chronic. If acute, the differential diagnosis is somewhat more limited, and it is important to exclude life-threatening issues that require emergent action (shock, hypokalemia, perforation, cerebral edema, organ infarction, poisoning), and pregnancy. If chronic, the differential diagnosis is quite broad; however, by evaluating the patient's history, examination, and basic test results it is often possible to arrive at the etiology. The best treatment is removal of the causative factor. If this is not possible, then there is a wide array of treatment options available from a pharmacologic standpoint to at least ameliorate the symptoms. The choice of which pharmacologic agent to use is an individual decision based on the suspected etiology of nausea and concern for side effects.

SUGGESTED READINGS

Carlisle JB, Stevenson CA. Drugs for preventing postoperative nausea and vomiting. *Cochrane Database Syst Rev*. 2006;(3): CD004125.

Chepyala P, Olden KW. Nausea and vomiting. *Curr Treat Options Gastroenterol*. 2008;5:202-208.

Hasler WL, Chey WD. Nausea and vomiting. *Gastroenterology*. 2003;125:1860-1867.

Lacy BE. Neuroenteric stimulation for gastroparesis. *Curr Treat Options Gastroenterol*. 2015; 13:409-417.

Malagelada J, Malagelada C. *Nausea and Vomiting. Sleisenger and Fordtran's Gastrointestinal and Liver Disease*, 10th ed. Philadelphia, PA: Saunders Elsevier; 2015:207-220.

Matthews A, Haas DM, O'Mathuna DP, Dowswell T. Interventions for nausea and vomiting in early pregnancy. *Cochrane Database Syst Rev*. 2015;(9):CD007575.

Quigley EM, Hasler WL, Parkman HP. AGA technical review on nausea and vomiting. *Gastroenterology*. 2001;120:263-286.

CHAPTER 98

Numbness: A Localization-Based Approach

Aaron L. Berkowitz, MD, PhD

Patients may use the word numbness to describe an alteration in sensation (ie, paresthesia or sensory loss), strength (ie, weakness), or coordination (ie, clumsiness). Therefore, the approach to the patient presenting with numbness begins with clarifying what the patient means by the word. This chapter will focus on the evaluation of the patient with alteration in sensation.

Differential diagnosis in neurology requires determining the localization of the problem within the nervous system (brain, brainstem, spinal cord, nerve roots, peripheral nerves, neuromuscular junction, or muscle), the time course over which the problem has arisen (acute, subacute, or chronic), and any associated symptoms that accompany the chief complaint (eg, if the chief complaint is numbness, is there associated weakness or pain?).

OVERVIEW OF SENSORY PATHWAYS (FIGURE 98-1)

Sensory information from the body travels in peripheral nerves to dorsal root ganglia, then enters the spinal cord through the dorsal roots. After entering the spinal cord, different types of sensory information travel in different pathways en route to the brain. Pain and temperature sensation travel in the *spinothalamic (anterolateral) tracts*, whereas proprioception and vibration travel in the *dorsal (posterior) columns*. Light touch sensation travels to some extent in both pathways and is therefore of less precise localizing value.

The fibers destined for the spinothalamic tracts cross directly to the contralateral anterolateral spinal cord after entering the spinal cord, and ascend through the brainstem to the thalamus, and from the thalamus to the somatosensory cortex housed in the postcentral gyrus. A unilateral spinal cord lesion affecting the spinothalamic tract at any level therefore causes *contralateral* loss of pain and temperature below the level of the lesion. Since the entering fibers cross over several spinal levels, if this pathway is affected in the spinal cord, there may also be a small patch of ipsilateral sensory loss at and above the level of the lesion.

The dorsal column pathways remain ipsilateral in the spinal cord and cross at the level of the lower brainstem (the medulla), where it then ascends to the thalamus en route to the somatosensory cortex like the spinothalamic tract. Therefore, a unilateral spinal cord lesion affecting the dorsal column pathway causes *ipsilateral* loss of proprioception and vibration sensation below the level of the lesion, whereas a lesion superior to the medulla causes *contralateral* loss of proprioception and vibration sense.

Sensation on the face is subserved by the trigeminal nerves (cranial nerve V), which transmits information to the brainstem, where it ultimately crosses to join the corresponding somatosensory pathways from the body (ie, information from the left trigeminal nerve crosses to the right side of the brainstem to join the already-crossed ascending sensory pathways from the left side of the body).

All sensory information from the extremities and torso in both the spinothalamic and posterior column pathways is transmitted to the ventral posterior lateral (VPL) nucleus of the thalamus. Sensory information from the face is represented in the ventral posterior medial (VPM) nucleus of the thalamus. Somatosensory information from these thalamic somatosensory nuclei is transmitted to the somatosensory cortex in the postcentral gyrus of the parietal lobe, with the face represented on the lateral cortical surface, the lower-extremity superio-medially, and the upper extremity between these two regions.

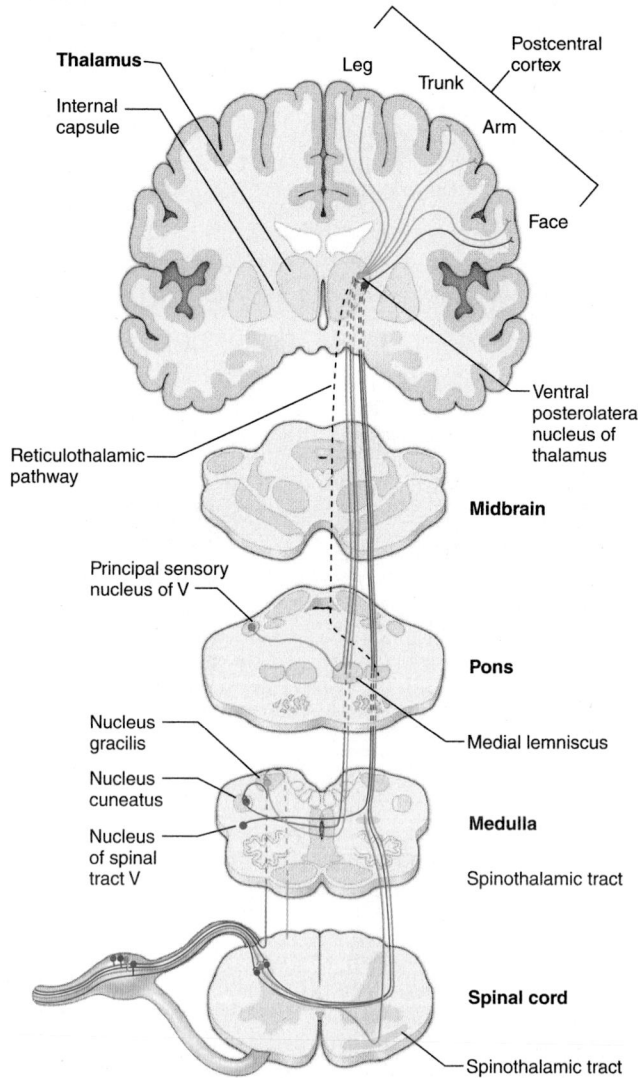

Figure 98-1 *Dorsal columns, spinothalamic tracts, and basic trigeminal pathway.*

LOCALIZATION OF SENSORY DISTURBANCES

Alterations in sensation may be localized to one or more peripheral nerves, dorsal root ganglia, one or more nerve roots, the spinal cord, the brainstem, or the brain (and within in the brain, in the thalamus, somatosensory cortex, or the subcortical white matter that connects them). Clinical localization may be determined from the pattern of sensory symptoms. Each level of the nervous system may be affected by distinct pathological processes, distinguished by the time course of onset and progression of symptoms, as well as any associated symptoms and signs. For example, sudden-onset hemi-body numbness is highly suggestive of an ischemic infarct or intracerebral hemorrhage, whereas insidious onset of the same symptoms may suggest an intracranial tumor. Rapid development of sensory disturbances affecting the distal bilateral lower extremities could signify early Guillain-Barré syndrome or transverse myelitis, whereas similar symptoms of chronic onset could suggest a polyneuropathy due to systemic illness or a spinal tumor.

■ PATTERNS OF SYMPTOMS (FIGURE 98-2)

Overview

Mononeuropathy and radiculopathy lead to sensory loss in a specific distribution, which may be accompanied by a pattern of weakness or reflex loss related to the nerve or root affected. Polyneuropathy leads to symmetric symptoms that often begin distally, leading to the 'stocking-glove' pattern. There are several patterns of sensory symptoms that can occur from spinal cord lesions, depending on whether the lesion is a complete transection, unilateral (Brown-Sequard syndrome), central (e.g., syrinx), anterior, or posterior (see below). Thalamic, subcortical, or cortical lesions cause contralateral sensory loss that may be complete (causing a hemisensory defect) or may affect only part of the contralateral body depending on the size and location of the lesion within these structures. A common pattern of sensory disturbance due to a unilateral brain lesion is a sensory disturbance affecting the contralateral face and hand, since these are the most highly represented regions of the body, and also since their representations are adjacent and both within the middle cerebral artery territory in the somatosensory cortex. Although it is possible to develop isolated sensory symptoms from a very small well-placed brainstem lesion, this is uncommon in practice. Given the large number of structures in a small anatomical region (eg, cranial nerve nuclei, descending motor pathways, connections between the brainstem and cerebellum), other neurologic features generally predominate over sensory symptoms and signs with brainstem lesions. A distribution of sensory symptoms that is unique to the lower brainstem is the presence of "crossed findings"—unilateral facial sensory disturbance with contralateral sensory disturbance in the rest of the body.

If the face is affected, this requires a lesion in the trigeminal nerve, the brainstem, or the cerebral hemispheres, whereas deficits in the arm(s) and/or leg(s) can localize anywhere along the neuraxis.

Peripheral nervous system

Neuropathy refers to pathology of one or more peripheral nerves. Symptoms depend on the fiber type affected and can therefore be sensory, motor, autonomic, or a combination of these. Sensory symptoms may include negative symptoms (ie, loss of sensation), positive symptoms (eg, paresthesias, pain), or both. Sensory loss can be multimodal or may be specific to pain/temperature or vibration/proprioception, depending on the fiber type(s) affected.

Mononeuropathy. When a single nerve is affected, symptoms occur in the distribution of that particular nerve. These symptoms may involve sensory disturbances and/or weakness depending on whether the affected nerve is sensory, motor, or mixed, and the degree to which the nerve is affected. Mononeuropathies are most commonly caused by trauma or compression, and patients with underlying polyneuropathy (eg, due to diabetes) can be predisposed to superimposed mononeuropathies. The most common mononeuropathy is carpal tunnel syndrome, in which the median nerve is compressed in the carpal tunnel, leading to sensory symptoms on the lateral palm sparing the medial and posterior surface, often with associated weakness of thumb abduction. Mononeuropathy can be difficult to distinguish clinically from radiculopathy, although radiating pain from the neck or back is more typical of radiculopathy.

Although numbness in the distribution of a single nerve (eg, carpal tunnel syndrome) is more commonly seen in the outpatient setting, the hospitalist should be aware of mononeuropathies that may arise in hospitalized patients. Focal numbness, weakness, and/or pain can develop postoperatively due to operative positioning leading to nerve compression or due to injury from retractors (eg, the femoral nerve in pelvic surgery). Unilateral or bilateral numbness in the medial (ulnar) portion of the hand(s) suggests ulnar neuropathy due to compression of the ulnar nerve at the medial elbow, which can occur in patients who are bedbound for prolonged periods. If severe, weakness of intrinsic hand muscles may be present. By a similar mechanism in bedbound patients, the peroneal nerve may be compressed at the fibular head, especially

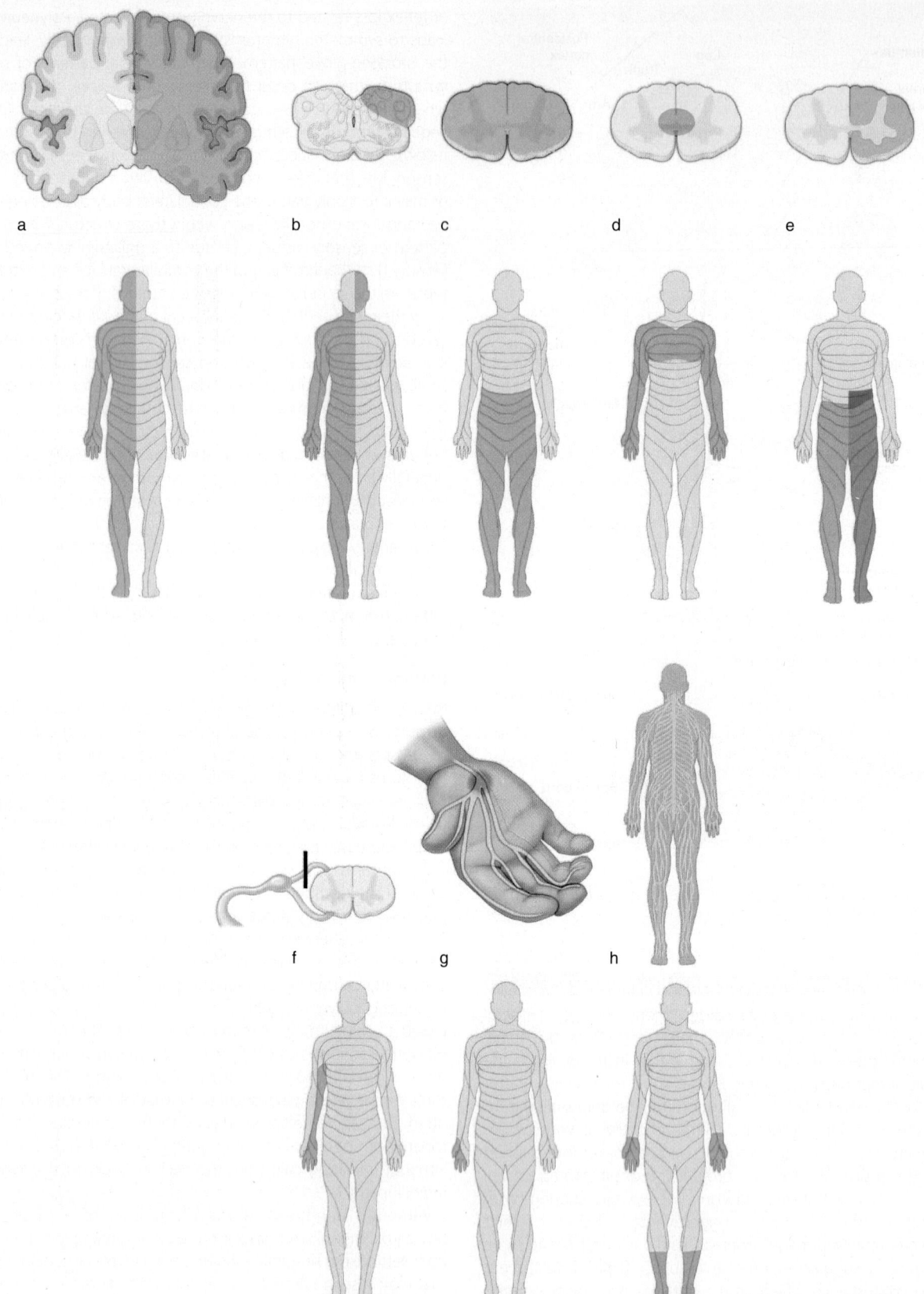

Figure 98-2 *Patterns of sensory disturbances.* **A.** *Brain hemisphere lesions cause contralateral sensory disturbances in the face and body.* **B.** *Brainstem lesions cause ipsilateral sensory disturbances in the face and contralateral sensory disturbances in the body.* **C.** *Transection of the spinal cord causes sensory disturbances bilaterally below the level of the lesion.* **D.** *Central cord lesions at the cervical level cause disturbances in pain and temperature sensation in a cape-like distribution.* **E.** *A lesion of one side of the spinal cord causes ipsilateral loss of vibration sense and proprioception and ipsilateral weakness below the level of the lesion and contralateral loss of pain and temperature sensation below the level of the lesion.* **F.** *A root lesion causes sensory disturbances in the region supplied by the affected root.* **G.** *A nerve lesion causes sensory disturbances in the region supplied by the affected nerve.* **H.** *Polyneuropathy causes sensory disturbances that begin in the distal extremities.*

if the legs are frequently crossed. The presence of foot drop in peroneal neuropathy is usually more salient than the sensory disturbance that affects the lateral calf and dorsum of the foot. Weakness of hip flexion and knee extension caused by femoral neuropathy requires evaluation for retroperitoneal hematoma in patients who are anticoagulated or who have undergone femoral artery catheterization; sensory disturbances (of the anterior thigh and medial leg) are typically less prominent than weakness.

Polyneuropathy. The clinical presentation and differential diagnosis of symmetric polyneuropathy is discussed in detail in Chapter 213. Most polyneuropathies are chronic, and although they may be present in hospitalized patients, are unlikely to be a cause for hospital admission.

Acute polyneuropathy is seen in Guillain-Barré syndrome. Although the classic presentation is one of ascending paralysis (legs before arms), the initial symptoms may be sensory in nature (classically paresthesias in the feet), and sensory-only variants do occur. Further details regarding the diagnosis and treatment of Guillan-Barré are discussed in Chapter 213 (Peripheral Neuropathy). The main differential diagnosis in a case of rapidly ascending weakness and/or sensory changes is Guillain-Barré syndrome versus a spinal cord lesion (eg, transverse myelitis or epidural abscess). Notably, upper motor neuron signs (hyperreflexia, clonus) may be absent in the acute phase of a myelopathy. The presence of early bowel and/or bladder dysfunction, back pain, and/or a spinal level are suggestive of spinal cord pathology. Other causes of acute polyneuropathy to be considered include heavy metal toxicity, porphyria, and HIV infection, particularly at the time of seroconversion.

Critical illness polyneuropathy is discussed in Chapter 213 (Peripheral Neuropathy). Weakness is generally the presenting feature rather than associated sensory loss. Sensory loss aids in the distinction between critical illness polyneuropathy and critical illness myopathy since the latter should have no associated sensory abnormalities, though the two commonly occur together.

Mononeuropathy multiplex refers to the sequential involvement of individual nerves. For example, a patient may develop a wrist drop (radial neuropathy) followed by a foot drop (peroneal neuropathy). This can be seen in systemic vasculitis due to nerve infarction, which is typically painful. Mononeuropathy multiplex can also be seen in leprosy, hepatitis C or HIV infection, and systemic autoimmune diseases (eg, sarcoidosis).

Radiculopathy typically causes radiating pain from the neck or back into the distribution of an individual nerve root, and may be accompanied by paresthesias, sensory loss, and/or weakness in the affected root distribution. Compression due to degenerative disc disease is a common etiology of radiculopathy. Polyradiculopathy can also be caused by local compression or invasion by malignancy or infectious radiculitis (eg, Lyme, HSV, CMV; CMV radiculitis is generally only seen when CD4 < 50). When polyradiculopathy is a cause of sensory or motor abnormalities, these tend to be painful and asymmetric, compared to polyneuropathy, which is more commonly symmetric.

Plexopathy. When unilateral sensorimotor symptoms do not fit into the distribution of a single nerve or root, the possibility of a lesion of the brachial or lumbosacral plexus should be considered. Motor features usually predominate over sensory disturbances in plexopathies, though the latter are commonly present. The brachial and lumbosacral plexuses can be affected by trauma (injuries that stretch the axilla or depress the shoulder for the brachial plexus; pelvic injuries for the lumbosacral plexus), malignancy (lung and breast for the brachial plexus; colorectal, gynecologic, urologic for the lumbosacral plexus), surgery (sternotomy for the brachial plexus; pelvic surgery for the lumbosacral plexus), radiation, and inflammatory conditions (eg, Parsonage-Turner syndrome for the brachial plexus; diabetic amyotrophy [also known as diabetic lumbosacral radiculoplexus neuropathy] for the lumbosacral plexus).

With the exception of trauma, it is rare for the entire plexus to be affected by the disease processes mentioned. When numbness occurs in an entire limb or an entire functional component of a limb that spans multiple nerves/roots (eg, the entire hand or the entire leg), a central nervous system etiology should be considered.

Ganglionopathy refers to disease processes affecting the dorsal root ganglia. Ganglionopathy causes sensory abnormalities including paresthesias and impaired proprioception. The proprioceptive deficit causes incoordination and gait unsteadiness due to sensory ataxia (ie, ataxia due to absence of proprioceptive input rather than due to cerebellar dysfunction). Reflexes are typically absent. Strength is generally spared since motor pathways are not involved. This is an important clinical syndrome to recognize as its differential diagnosis is somewhat circumscribed: autoimmune disease (most commonly Sjögren syndrome), infection (most commonly HIV), vitamin B6 toxicity, paraneoplastic syndrome (most commonly anti-Hu due to small cell lung cancer), and chemotherapy-induced (most commonly platin-based chemotherapies).

Central nervous system

Spinal cord

Lesions of the spinal cord cause deficits below the level of the lesion. The type (sensory, motor, or both) and extent of these deficits (arms, legs, unilateral, bilateral) depend on the location and size of the lesion. The spinal cord can be affected by trauma, vascular pathology (eg, epidural hematoma, dural arteriovenous fistula, infarction), infection (eg, viral myelitis, epidural abscess, tuberculosis, syphilis [tabes dorsalis], HIV-associated vacuolar myelopathy, HTLV-1, schistosomiasis, cysticercosis), inflammatory conditions (eg, multiple sclerosis, neuromyelitis optica, transverse myelitis, Sjögren's syndrome, systemic lupus erythematosis), neoplasm (eg, primary and metastatic tumors to the spinal column, cord, or dura mater), metabolic conditions (eg, vitamin B12 and copper deficiency), and degenerative conditions (eg, Friedreich's ataxia).

An initial differential diagnosis can be generated from the time course of symptom onset, associated symptoms presented in the history, and features of the physical examination, but MRI is often required to distinguish between underlying etiologies. It should be noted that an MRI of the entire spine can be useful to evaluate for spinal cord compression in the appropriate context, but often does not have the resolution of MRI of individual spinal levels (eg, MRI of the cervical spine). It is therefore ideal to attempt to localize the level of the lesion as precisely as possible on the physical examination. If the upper extremities are involved, the lesion must involve the cervical spine. It is important to note that the spinal cord ends at approximately L1, with only the roots of the cauda equina inferior to this level. Therefore, upper motor neuron findings on examination (brisk reflexes, Babinski sign, clonus, etc) in a patient with isolated bilateral lower-extremity symptoms suggest localization to the thoracic or cervical cord rather than the lumbar region.

A useful clinical sign of spinal cord pathology is the finding of a spinal level—a level on the back at which there appears to be a change in sensation with diminished sensation below the level and preserved sensation above it. This is not only quite specific for spinal cord pathology but can aid in localization so as to determine the level at which neuroimaging analysis should be focused.

The following are the main clinical patterns associated with different types of spinal cord lesions and their most common underlying etiologies.

Complete transection. A full-thickness lesion of the spinal cord will produce complete paralysis and sensory loss in all modalities below the level of the lesion. If the lesion is acute (eg, trauma, early transverse myelitis), the upper motor neuron signs that would be expected with a spinal cord lesion may not yet be present, leading to diagnostic uncertainty with respect to the possibility of

Guillain-Barré syndrome. Bowel and/or bladder dysfunction and a spinal level are suggestive of a spinal cord etiology of flaccid paralysis and/or sensory loss in the acute setting.

Hemicord/Brown-Séquard Syndrome affects one half of the spinal cord. In addition to ipsilateral paralysis below the level of the lesion, this syndrome is characterized by dissociated sensory loss: ipsilateral loss of proprioception and vibration and contralateral pain and temperature loss below the lesion (see above). This pattern of symptoms is generally caused by penetrating trauma, although a unilateral tumor or an eccentric demyelinating lesion may produce this syndrome.

Central cord syndrome. A syrinx is an enlargement of the central canal of the spinal cord, occurring most commonly at the cervical level. A syrinx can be caused by a spinal cord tumor, spine trauma, or can be associated with Chiari malformation type I. Enlargement of the central canal first affects the crossing anterolateral (spinothalamic) fibers leading to loss of pain and temperature in the upper extremities with sparing of vibration and proprioception. Due to the lamination of these pathways, the upper extremities are affected first, leading to the so-called "cape-like" distribution of sensory findings.

Subacute combined degeneration refers to combined degeneration of the corticospinal tracts and the dorsal columns. This is most commonly due to vitamin B12 deficiency, but can also be caused by copper deficiency. The combined pathology of the corticospinal tracts and dorsal columns leads to weakness with impaired proprioception and vibration sense. Impaired proprioception can lead to sensory ataxia, unsteady gait, and Romberg sign. Vibration sense is typically diminished distally. Since vitamin B12 deficiency and copper deficiency can also cause neuropathy, there may be both peripheral (lower motor neuron) and central (upper motor neuron) features on examination (eg, hyporeflexia with upgoing toes, or brisk knee reflexes with absent ankle reflexes), classified as *myeloneuropathy*. In addition to pernicious anemia and malabsorption, vegetarianism and gastric bypass can predispose to vitamin B12 deficiency. Excess zinc consumption (from denture cream or supplementation) and gastric bypass are common causes of copper deficiency.

Anterior cord syndrome. The anterior spinal cord is particularly vulnerable to ischemia due to lack of extensive collateralization. The anterior spinal artery territory comprises the anterior two thirds of the spinal cord, including the anterolateral and corticospinal tracts, but not the dorsal columns. Patients with anterior spinal artery infarction therefore present with bilateral paralysis and diminished or absent pain and temperature sensation below the level of the lesion, but preserved proprioception and vibration sensation. This is most commonly seen with abdominal aortic aneurysm (AAA) rupture or after surgical repair of AAA.

Tabes dorsalis. Tertiary neurosyphilis can affect the brain (causing dementia) and/or the spinal cord (causing tabes dorsalis). The posterior columns and dorsal roots are primarily affected in tabes dorsalis, and therefore the clinical features are predominantly due to impaired proprioception: gait unsteadiness, sensory ataxia, absent or diminished vibration sense and proprioception, and Romberg sign. Paresthesias, lancinating pain, bladder dysfunction, and Argyll Robertson pupils are common accompanying features.

Saddle anesthesia due to lesions of the cauda equina and/or conus medullaris. Sensory changes in the perineal region (saddle anesthesia), often accompanied by bowel and/or bladder dysfunction, should alert the clinician to the possibility of pathology affecting the conus medullaris (the most inferior portion of the spinal cord) or the cauda equina (the lumbar and sacral nerve roots). Classically, cauda equina syndrome is more likely to cause pain and asymmetric symptoms and signs compared to conus medullaris syndrome. However, the two can be difficult to distinguish clinically and both require MRI of the lumbosacral spine to evaluate for the underlying etiology. Potential pathology in this region includes compression by tumor or prolapsed disc, infection (eg, epidural abscess or viral polyradiculitis), and inflammatory diseases such ankylosing spondylitis and sarcoidosis.

Brainstem

As mentioned previously, the sensory pathways in the brainstem are rarely affected in isolation. When they are affected as part of the lateral medullary syndrome due to infarction in the territory of the posterior inferior cerebellar artery, the sensory loss is often 'crossed,' with facial sensory loss contralateral to sensory loss in the extremities and torso.

Trigeminal nerve

Isolated facial numbness can occur with lesions of the trigeminal nerve or with small lesions of the brain or brainstem. Patients also sometimes use the term numbness to describe the sensation of facial weakness that occurs in Bell's palsy, although true sensory deficits are not common in this condition. Facial numbness due to pathology of the trigeminal nerve can be caused by skull base lesions (eg, tumor, leptomeningeal metastases), inflammatory disease (eg, Sjögren's syndrome, sarcoidosis), perineural spread of head and neck cancers (particularly squamous cell cancer of the skin), and dental pathology. Numbness in the chin (*numb chin sign*) raises the specter of metastatic malignancy affecting the distal trigeminal branches in the mandible or the mandibular portion of the trigeminal nerve in the skull base, and may be the presenting feature of systemic malignancy.

Brain

A patient presenting with acute-onset numbness limited to one side of the body should be evaluated for stroke. Lacunar infarction of the thalamus can produce contralateral sensory loss in isolation. When cerebral infarction is the etiology of alteration in sensation, the patient generally describes sensory loss in the acute period rather than paresthesia or pain, although the latter may emerge later. Patients with isolated somatosensory cortex infarction may describe the affected limb to be functioning abnormally despite lack of clear deficits on routine motor and sensory examination. However, subtle signs such as agraphesthesia (inability distinguish numbers traced on the palm) or neglect to double simultaneous stimulation (inability to detect bilateral simultaneous sensory stimulation) may be clues to a cortical lesion.

In addition to vascular etiologies, the differential diagnosis for acute-onset unilateral neurologic deficits includes migraine and seizure. Sensory disturbances may accompany migraine and may precede the emergence of the headache, and sometimes occur in the absence of the headache in patients with a history of migraine (ie, migraine aura without headache, a.k.a. acephalgic migraine). In contrast to the loss of sensation commonly associated with acute stroke, migraine-associated sensory disturbances are typically positive phenomena such as paresthesias that tend to spread over minutes. Positive somatosensory phenomena may also be caused by seizures with origin in or spread to the somatosensory cortex, with paresthesias typically spreading over seconds.

The development of localized sensory loss over hours to days due to a lesion in the brain can suggest an inflammatory process (eg, a demyelinating lesion) or an infectious process (eg, cerebral abscess). A more indolent development of focal sensory disturbance of cerebral origin could be suggestive of neoplasm.

Nonneurologic causes of sensory disturbances

Electrolyte abnormalities (eg, hypocalcemia) and hyperventilation can cause paresthesias, classically perioral and in the distal extremities. Sensory disturbances can also accompany panic attacks.

APPROACH TO THE PATIENT WITH NUMBNESS

With the above patterns and their differential diagnoses in mind, the examiner seeks to elicit from the history the nature of the sensory complaint (ie, absence of sensation, paresthesia, or both), the location(s) of the symptoms (acknowledging that this can be challenging for patients to localize precisely), the timing of symptom onset (acute, subacute, chronic), associated symptoms (pain, weakness, incoordination), and any prior neurologic events or deficits.

The physical examination seeks to determine the distribution of the sensory abnormality, the modalities that are altered (ie, pain, temperature, vibration, and/or proprioception), and any associated features that provide clues to peripheral versus central nervous system etiology (eg, altered deep tendon reflexes, presence of pathologic reflexes such as a Babinski sign).

The sensory examination is considered by many practitioners to be the most subjective aspect of the neurologic examination, and can be challenging to interpret. One approach is to proceed from general comparisons to more specific ones. For example, one can begin by comparing pinprick sensation between the same points in the left and right hands in general for differences between the sides before seeking to circumscribe the extent of the deficit in the affected hand, or comparing the most distal point (the big toe) to a more proximal one (the thigh) before assessing for the precise location at which sensation changes when proceeding from distal to proximal.

Assessing for a spinal level (see above) is particularly useful when there are acute-onset deficits in sensation in the bilateral extremities such that the upper motor neuron features of myelopathy (if present) may have not yet emerged. With more subacute or chronic presentations of bilateral sensory disturbances, hyperreflexia, clonus, Babinski sign, and/or spasticity, if present, allow for localization in the spinal cord if the motor pathways are involved. Hyporeflexia or areflexia in this context suggest peripheral nervous system pathology.

A Romberg sign or sensory ataxia suggest a deficit in proprioception, which can localize to the peripheral nerves, dorsal root ganglia, or dorsal columns. Sensory ataxia due to impaired proprioception can be distinguished from cerebellar ataxia by several features on the finger-nose test. Sensory ataxia tends to lack the rapid oscillations perpendicular to the plane of movement seen in cerebellar ataxia, appearing as more of a searching movement that may circle toward the examiner's finger and the patient's nose. In sensory ataxia, finger-nose testing becomes highly inaccurate when the patient closes the eyes, whereas a patient with normal proprioception can maintain reasonable accuracy with the eyes closed.

The localization in conjunction with the time course yields an initial differential diagnosis. Sudden-onset sensory deficits localizable to the brain may be vascular, migrainous, or epileptic, but can also be due to acute electrolyte disturbances. Acute-onset sensory disturbances due to stroke, migraine, or seizure are typically unilateral, whereas systemic etiologies typically cause bilateral sensory symptoms. Sudden-onset symptoms localizing to the spine may be due to spinal cord infarction or spinal cord compression due to acute disc prolapse or spine fracture. Acute onset mononeuropathy suggests nerve infarction, especially when painful, as can be seen in vasculitis. Sensory disturbances of subacute onset can be seen in infectious or inflammatory/demyelinating conditions of the peripheral or central nervous system, but can also occur with metabolic abnormalities (eg, vitamin B12 deficiency). More chronic development of sensory alterations can occur with systemic disease (eg, peripheral neuropathy due to diabetes, cervical spinal cord compression due to rheumatoid arthritis); primary or metastatic malignancy of the brain, spine, or compressing the brachial or lumbar plexus; or degenerative conditions.

CT scan (of the brain or spine) is generally performed in the acute setting to evaluate patients with sudden-onset neurologic deficits, but MRI has higher resolution and sensitivity for the detection of nearly all types of pathology of the brain and spinal cord with the possible exception of acute hemorrhage. Contrast administration can aid in the detection and characterization of tumors, acute infectious or inflammatory lesions, and meningeal processes (infectious, inflammatory, or neoplastic). When the differential diagnosis includes neuropathy, radiculopathy, and/or plexopathy, electromyography (EMG)/nerve conduction studies can aid in localization, and can also provide an objective measurement of the extent of injury to a given nerve, which can be useful in prognosis for recovery.

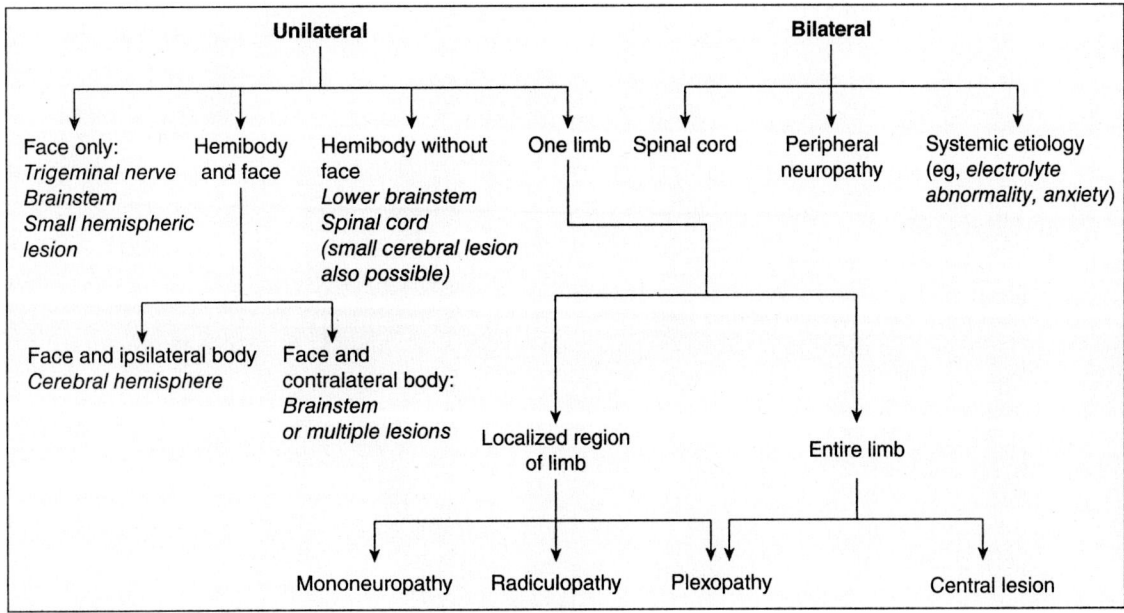

Figure 98-3 *Most common lesion localization for numbness by region of body.*

SUGGESTED READINGS

Biller J, Brazis PW, Masdeu JC. *Localization in Clinical Neurology.* 6th ed. Philadelphia, PA: Lippincott Williams and Wilkins; 2011.

Daroff RB, Fenichel GM, Jankovic J. *Bradley's Neurology in Clinical Practice.* 6th ed. Philadelphia: Elsevier; 2012.

Evans RW, Kirby S, Purdy RA. Numb Chin Syndrome. *Headache.* 2008;48:1520-1524.

Herskovitz S, Scelsa S, Schaumburg H. *Peripheral Neuropathies in Clinical Practice.* New York, NY: Oxford; 2010.

Mauermann ML, Burns TM, eds. Peripheral nervous system disorders. *Continuum.* 2014;20(5):1161-1525.

Ropper AH, Samuels MA, Klein JP. *Adams and Victor's Principles of Neurology.* 10th ed. New York, NY: McGraw-Hill; 2014.

Sheikh SI, Amato AA. The dorsal root ganglion under attack: the acquired sensory ganglionopathies. *Pract Neurol.* 2010;10:326-334.

CHAPTER 99

Pain

Samer Abdel-Aziz, MD
Meredith C.B. Adams, MD, MS

Key Clinical Questions

1. What are the goals of pain therapy?
2. How is the sensation of pain measured?
3. What are the types of pain?
4. How do patient comorbidities affect pain management?
5. What are the most appropriate and effective pain treatment options available?

CASE 99-1

A 76-year-old female with a history of dementia, hypertension, hypercholesterolemia, coronary artery disease, chronic obstructive pulmonary disease, and chronic low back pain suffered a right tibia fracture. The orthopedic surgery service surgically repaired her leg and transferred her to the primary service for management of multiple co-morbidities. On the second postoperative day, severe pain has limited her movement and ability to work with physical therapy or use the bathroom facilities. Home medications include atorvastatin, metoprolol, ramipril, hydrochlorothiazide, ipratropium, albuterol metered dose inhaler, and oxycodone controlled-release 20 mg twice a day. Her vital signs were: heart rate is 120 beats per minute, blood pressure 150/95 mm Hg, SpO$_2$ 95% on 2 L of oxygen, and temperature 37.2°C. Laboratory results were notable for a glucose level of 212 mg/dL. Her postoperative pain is managed by 2 mg of intravenous (IV) morphine every 3 hours. On this regimen she does continue to report severe right leg pain.

INTRODUCTION

DEFINITION AND CLASSIFICATION

Pain is the leading cause of both adult outpatient and emergency department visits, impacting both inpatient and outpatient care for over 100 million Americans annually. The International Association for the Study of Pain defines *pain* as an unpleasant sensory and emotional experience associated with actual or potential tissue damage, or described in terms of such damage.

Pain may be classified in multiple domains. Currently the majority of pain classifications rely on various parameters of pain experience such as anatomy, duration, etiology, body system, severity, functioning and mechanism. The first is the classification based on the underlying etiology of the pain. Nociceptive pain refers to the direct tissue injury from a noxious stimulus. Inflammatory pain refers to the release of inflammatory mediators that perpetuate and modulate nociceptive input. Direct injury to nerves results in a third type of pain, neuropathic pain, whereby the nature of sensory transmission is altered and accompanied by pain frequently described as a burning type of pain. Although these are described as discrete types of pain, they more often represent a continuum of the same injury. Surgical incision is a model of nociceptive injury that produces an inflammatory response. Incising the primary nociceptors in the skin with subsequent development of inflammatory neuritis can result in neuropathic pain.

The second domain of classification refers to the anatomic location of pain. In this category, pain can be described as either somatic or visceral. Somatic pain refers to a well-localized sensation related to skin, muscle, and bone, whereby visceral pain is poorly localized and is usually in response to distention of the internal organs such as the colon or small bowel, or compression or inflammatory injury, which occurs in pancreatic cancer or pancreatitis.

The third domain classifies pain based on the temporal nature of the pain. Acute pain usually refers to a neurophysiologic response to a noxious stimulus, a response expected to resolve with completion of wound healing. In contrast, chronic pain persists beyond the expected time course of an acute injury and its repair process. Chronic or persistent pain does not simply suggest that a given time interval has passed. Rather, such a diagnosis implies development of multiple neurophysiologic changes that alter the fundamental balance between noxious stimuli and their inhibitory mechanisms. Such changes occur from the peripheral nerve to the dorsal horn of the spinal column, interneurons throughout the spinal cord, to the thalamus and cortical circuits. These changes ultimately result in remodeling in the organization of the central nervous system.

> **PRACTICE POINT**
>
> - Although the clinician must be aware that the patient may manipulate the pain report, it is imperative to first validate the patient's understanding of his or her pain by receiving his or her report with an unbiased view.

■ EVALUATION OF PAIN

Pain is a subjective phenomenon and results from a patient's understanding of the physical and affective impact the sensation has had on them. There are multiple quantitative pain evaluation scales. Although these are subjective reports with no way to verify the answer's "truth," these scales have been used for decades and correlate well to experimental and clinical pain responsiveness. Numerous factors can influence perception of pain including cultural components, particularly when you define culture to include categorization such as Veterans, athletes, and other nonethnic cultures.

The patient's pain history has specific components to direct diagnostic and therapeutic options. Key pain specific information for the inpatient setting may involve the provocative and palliative components of pain. Many patients experience their pain primarily with activity, such as physical therapy. This may impact the design of therapeutic regimen to avoid oversedation at rest and sufficient pain control to facilitate participation in therapy. Another important aspect when assessing the inpatient with pain is to consider their baseline home pain scores. Patients may have baseline pain scores greater than 4 at home due to other co-morbid pain conditions. Normalization of pain scores to baseline home level that allows function may be a pragmatic goal in patients with higher scores at baseline.

The numerical rating scale (NRS) is the most commonly used tool for the evaluation of pain severity. Patients are asked to rate their pain on a scale of 0 to 10, with 0 translated as "no pain" and 10 the "worst pain imaginable." The visual analog scale (VAS) allows patients to mark a point on a 10-cm line that corresponds to the level of their pain. Using the 4-point verbal rating scale (VRS), patients categorize their pain as none, mild, moderate, or severe. The NRS and VAS demonstrate excellent agreement, and offer superior discriminating ability to the categorical VRS. All of these scales are subjective and can be useful only when comparing pain severity within the same patient at different times or during different activities, but are not useful in comparing pain severity in different patients since different patients have different perception of pain and its severity. Although the practitioner must be aware that the patient can manipulate the pain report, it is imperative to first receive the patient report with an unbiased opinion.

Patients with pain may have comorbidities that pose a challenge when it comes to pain evaluation. The above case study discusses a patient with dementia. Standard pain reporting scales are ineffective in demented patients, unconscious patients, or patients unable to communicate. Pain scales such as MOBID-2, Checklist of Nonverbal Pain Indicators, and Doloplus-2 have been designed for patients with dementia or in an assisted living facility. These scales have strong conceptual and psychometric support; however they are an indirect measure of the patient's pain and may be influenced by the intrinsic bias of the health care provider.

> **PRACTICE POINT**
>
> - Poorly controlled pain may present through multiple parameters including vital signs and laboratory values, reinforcing the impact of a patient under significant physiologic and psychological stress. Manifestations of this stress can include myocardial ischemia, immunosuppression, impaired wound healing, and thromboembolic events.

Timing and activity are relevant to the interpretation of pain scores. Reported pain scores may refer to the past hour, 24 hours, week, or month. Average, maximum, and minimum pain scores help ascertain the patient's range of pain. Twenty-hour pain scores may give the best information regarding overall trends of pain status. Pain scores may also be described as rest or static versus active or dynamic to correlate the given score with activity level. Pain scores reported by the patient when resting may not reflect pain-based limitations on activity. Because the goal of pain treatment usually includes improvement in mobility or function to decrease thromboembolic and pulmonary complications, addressing only rest/static pain may result in a failure to maximize the benefit of pain control.

The above scales are applied to all types of pain: acute, chronic/persistent, and cancer pain. The added complexity of chronic/persistent or cancer pain can require more multifaceted evaluation tools. Additional pain scales can be administered to these patients to better deliver more targeted pain care, but they will not be discussed as they are beyond the scope of this chapter. The history should be supplemented by a focused pain exam, incorporating knowledge of muscle innervation and dermatomes (**Table 99-1**) to define the patient's pain pattern and guide treatment approaches.

■ TREATMENT OF PAIN

Treatment of pain may utilize four primary modalities: medications, interventions, behavioral therapies and physical therapy/complementary treatments. This review will focus on the medical and interventional management of pain, although behavior and complementary treatments are essential components of improving the overall pain state in patients with persistent pain.

■ SYSTEMIC ANALGESIA

Opioids

Opioid analgesics remain the most common treatment for both acute and chronic pain. By activating the *mu* opioid receptor throughout the CNS, opioids modulate the perception and

TABLE 99-1 Sensorimotor Nerve Distribution

Movement	Nerve Root	Key Sensory Area
Shoulder abduction	C5	C5: lateral upper arm
Elbow flexion	C5-C6	C6: thumb
Elbow extension	C6-C7	C7: middle finger
Finger flexion	C8	C8: fifth finger
Finger abduction	T1	T1: ulnar forearm
Hip flexion	L2-L3	L2: medial midthigh
Knee Extension	L3-L4	L3: medial knee
Ankle dorsiflexion (heel walk)	L4-L5	L4: medial calf
Knee flexion	L5-S1	L5: lateral calf and dorsum foot
Ankle planterflexion (toe walk)	S1-S2	S1: posteriolateral foot and ankle

TABLE 99-2 Common Opioid Analgesics

Opioid	Dose	Dose Interval	Metabolism and Excretion	Conversion factor to PME
Morphine (IV)	2-5 mg	Every 4-6 h/as needed	H/R	1
Morphine (PO)	15-30 mg	2-3 times a day	H/R	0.33
Oxycodone- IR (PO)	5-10 mg	Every 4-6 h/as needed	H/R	0.5
Oxycodone-SR (PO)	15-20 mg	2-3 times a day	H/R	0.5
Hydromorphone (IV)	0.5- 2 mg	Every 3-4 h/as needed	R/H	6.7
Hydromorphone (PO)	2-4 mg	Every 3-4 h/as needed	R/H	1.3
Fentanyl (IV)	25-100 mcg	Every 3-4 h/as needed	H/R	100
Fentanyl transdermal	12 mcg/h	Every 72 h	H/R	25
Methadone (PO)	2.5-5 mg	3 times a day	H/R	1
Hydrocodone/ Acetaminophen (PO)	5/325 mg	Every 4-6 h/as needed	H	0.3
Codeine (PO)	15-60 mg	Every 4-6 h/as needed	H/R	0.05
Tramadol (PO)	50-100 mg	Every 4-6 h/as needed	H/R	0.07

H, hepatic; IR, immediate release; PME, parenteral morphine equivalent; R, renal; SR, sustained release.

transmission of painful stimuli. Opioid-based therapies are not limited by a ceiling effect; increasing doses will theoretically yield increasing analgesic effects even at extremely high doses. However, increasing doses of opioids are functionally limited by side effects such as nausea, vomiting, constipation, sedation, and respiratory depression.

When used for acute pain, the most common routes of systemic opioid administration include intravenous (IV), intramuscular (IM), and per os (by mouth) (PO). Parenteral routes may also include transdermal (TD), subcutaneous (SC), transmucosal (TM), or ionto-phoretic transdermal (ITD). Epidural and intrathecal administration is also used in a variety of settings.

Intravenous administration of opioids ensures a rapid, predictable onset and distribution of analgesic functioning, making this the favored route for the initial treatment of severe acute pain. Intra-muscular and enteral routes may result in delayed onset of effects, limiting their effectiveness in the acute pain setting. Similarly, TD (ITD excepted) and SC routes of administration have considerably delayed onset and are more often appropriate for long-term use such as in chronic pain or palliative care settings.

Table 99-2 lists several opioids commonly prescribed for acute and chronic pain medicine. Commonly, patients will experience excellent pain relief following administration of opioids. However, there may be a variable response to different formulations and pharmacologic compounds resulting from genetic polymorphisms involving *mu*-opioid receptor activation, receptor distribution, opioid metabolism, and the type of pain. Opioids are often best at treating static, nociceptive pain such as postsurgical pain; however they are less effective for dynamic or movement-related pain or neuropathic pain. Further, opioids are often ineffective in the treatment of bone fracture pain such as the pain experienced by the patient in the case study.

Opioid conversion: In the course of transitioning from severe acute pain to moderate, subacute pain, physicians will frequently transition the patient from parenteral to oral opioid administration.

1. Calculate the patient's 24-hour opioid use.
2. Convert this to "parenteral morphine equivalent" (PME).
3. The total oral dose prescribed to the patient is commonly less than 100% of the parenteral dose equivalent; this decision is guided by the clinical milieu of the patient including "the patient's recovery from his or her pain."

4. Consider the division of this requirement into short and/or long-acting opioids. This decision depends greatly upon the patient, the timing of his or her pain, and the nature of his or her pain.
5. Fifty percent of the 24-hour PME may be given as a sustained preparation, and 50% as shorter-acting, immediate-release medications ordered as needed.
6. Numerous conversion tables and calculators are available to assist the physician with opioid conversion. See www.hopweb.org.

Nonsteroidal anti-inflammatory agents (NSAIDs)

NSAIDs exert their analgesic effect via inhibition of the cyclo-oxygenase (COX) enzyme, thus interfering with prostaglandin (PG) production. Prostaglandins modify nociceptive thresholds at both peripheral and central sites. By limiting production of PG from COX-1 and COX-2, NSAIDs offer effective analgesia for mild to moderate pain. Further, this mechanism of action apart from the *mu*-opioid receptor provides a strong supplement to opioids during treatment of moderate to severe pain. Although opioid sparing, NSAIDs do have a ceiling effect, beyond which increasing doses will yield no increase in analgesia. Clinically, NSAIDs decrease pain associated with orthopedic injuries, and those with extensive prostaglandin involvement such as pain from uterine contraction and muscle inflammation. However, the risk of bleeding and mixed evidence regarding interference with union of fractures and spinal surgery necessitates involvement of the operative team in the decision to add NSAIDs.

Traditionally, NSAIDs were nonspecific for the isoforms of cyclooxy-genase, COX-1 and COX-2. COX-1 is constitutively expressed in nearly all human tissues, while COX-2 is focally expressed with inflammation. Blockade of COX-1 may promote development of gastrointestinal irritation and bleeding. NSAIDs as a class may also interfere with autoregulation of renal perfusion. To minimize the effects of gastrointestinal irritation and bleeding, drug development turned to selective COX-2 inhibitors. Although effective in minimizing gastrointestinal bleeding, selective COX-2 inhibitors may result in a prothrombotic milieu that may increase the risk of myocardial infarction.

Acetaminophen, a para-aminophenol derivative (not an NSAID), may represent a special class of NSAIDs. While its mechanism of action is not completely understood, there is evidence of antagonistic activity against COX-2, and a splice variant of COX-1 named COX-3. Notably, acetaminophen appears to not inhibit peripheral

TABLE 99-3 Neuropathic Pain Medication Guidelines

Drug	Start Dose	Maximum Dose	Documented Effect	Side Effects
Gabapentin	300 mg/d	3600 mg/d	PHN, PDN, mixed neuropathic pain	Sedation, dizziness, edema
Pregabalin	25 mg/d	600 mg/d	PHN, PDN, mixed neuropathic pain, central pain	Sedation, dizziness edema
Tricyclic antidepressants	25 mg/d (NB: plasma level)	75-150 mg/d (NB: plasma level)	PHN, PDN, central pain, mixed neuropathic pain	Cardiac, anticholinergic, sedation
Venlafaxine	37.5 mg/d	25-375 mg/d	Painful neuropathy	Sedation
Duloxetine	60 mg/d		Painful neuropathy	Sedation
Milnacipran	12 mg/d	100 mg/d	Painful neuropathy	Sedation
Carbamazepine (oxcarbazepine)	300 mg/d (NB: plasma level)	1200-1800 mg (1/3 higher dose for oxcarbazepine) (NB: plasma level)	Trigeminal neuralgia	Sedation, dizziness, ataxia
Tramadol	50 mg/d	400 mg/d	Painful neuropathies	Sedation, dizziness, obstipation
Lamotrigine	25 mg/d* (NB: plasma level)	400-600 mg/d (NB: plasma level)	Trigeminal neuralgia, poststroke central pain	Sedation, tremor, rash
Opioids	5–10 mg/d, titrate substitute with long-acting opioids	Variable	PHN, PDN, postamputation pain	Sedation, dizziness, tolerance, drug abuse
Lidocaine patch			PHN, traumatic nerve injury	Allergic reaction
Capsaicin cream	4×/d for 8 wk		PHN, PDN, HIV	

PDN, peripheral diabetic neuropathy; PHN, postherpetic neuralgia.

*To be titrated slowly.

Reproduced, with permission, from Jensen TS, et al. Pharmacology and treatment of neuropathic pains. *Curr Opin Neurol.* 2009;22:467-474.

COX-1, which may explain its favorable safety profile in regards to gastrointestinal, hematological, cardiovascular, and renal effects seen with other NSAIDs and selective COX-2 inhibitors.

In assessing comparative efficacy, the number of patients needed to treat (NNT) for at least a 50% reduction in pain after 4 to 6 hours for 1 g of acetaminophen is 4.4, which compares favorably to 650 mg of aspirin or 100 mg of ibuprofen. A more typical dose of ibuprofen, 400 mg, however, had an NNT of only 2.3. Celecoxib, a selective COX-2 inhibitor, has a NNT of 4.5 at 200 mg when compared with placebo for postoperative pain.

Anticonvulsants and antidepressants

Adjuvant medications can add value to a multimodal treatment plan (**Table 99-3**) depending on the pain indications. Selected anticonvulsants, like gabapentin and pregabalin are considered the first line therapy in the treatment of neuropathic pain. Gabapentin and pregabalin work by binding to voltage gated calcium channels on primary afferent neurons, reducing the release of neurotransmitters from their central terminals. The effective dose of gabapentin is 1800 to 3600 mg daily usually divided in three doses, while for pregabalin, the effective dose is 300 to 600 mg daily usually divided in two doses. Start at low doses and titrated up to the effective dose over several weeks to avoid or decrease the main side effects of these medications (somnolence and dizziness). The gabapentinoids have a clear role in the treatment of postoperative pain when given in the perioperative period (pre- and postoperatively) in a number of major orthopedic and gastrointestinal surgeries. In the acute and chronic pain setting, they have been shown to be opioid sparing and show promise as successful adjuvant analgesics.

Antidepressant medications, mainly tricyclic antidepressants (TCAs) and selective serotonin and norepinephrine reuptake inhibitors (SSNRIs) are commonly used in the treatment of neuropathic pain. TCAs, specifically amitriptyline and nortriptyline, are effective in treating neuropathic pain. The starting dose for TCAs is 25 mg at bedtime slowly titrated to decrease the side effect profile while achieving pain relief up to a maximum dose is 100 to 150 mg daily. Evening dosing takes advantage of one side effect, somnolence, and may facilitate sleep and decrease pain. The most common side effect of TCAs is dry mouth. TCAs are not recommended in patients with ischemic heart disease or in patients with dementia due to anticholinergic effects.

Selective serotonin and norepinephrine reuptake inhibitors (SSNRIs) like duloxetine and milnacipran effectively treat neuropathic pain. Their analgesic effect is separate from their antidepressant effects, and benefit chronic pain patients who have concomitant depression.

Duloxetine is effective at a dose of 60 mg once daily, while milnacipran is used at 100 mg daily divided in two doses. The most common side effects of these medications are nausea, somnolence and dizziness, they as well need to be started at low doses and titrated up to the effective dose.

Combining an anticonvulsant like gabapentin or pregabalin with an antidepressant like duloxetine or amitriptyline may be very effective in treating neuropathic pain allowing lower dosing and fewer side effects.

CASE 99-1 (*continued*)

In managing the postoperative patient with dementia the goal is to minimize her opioid requirement (and side effect burden) by using NSAIDs and gabapentinoids as adjuncts. The patient has no history of renal insufficiency or gastric ulceration, and scheduled

TABLE 99-4 Intravenous Patient-Controlled Analgesia Initial Settings

Opioid	Demand Dose	Lockout (Range)	Continuous Basal Infusion Rate*
Morphine	1-2 mg	10 min (6-10 min)	1-2 mg/h
Hydromorphone	0.2-0.4 mg	10 min (6-10 min)	0.2-0.4 mg/h
Fentanyl	20-50 mcg	5 min (5-10 min)	10-60 mcg/h
Sufentanil	4-6 mcg	5 min (5-10 min)	2-8 mcg/h

*Continuous infusion of opioids is not recommended in the opioid-naïve patient.

In patients already receiving opioid medications:

(a) If the patient is hospitalized, calculate the patient's 24-h opioid use and convert this into the IV opioid equivalent, and give 50%-75% of the total dose as the continuous infusion delivered over 24 h and the remaining 25%-50% as demand doses.

(b) If the patient is on home oral opioid or transdermal regimen, calculate the patient's 24-h baseline home regimen into the IV opioid equivalent and administer 75% of this as a continuous infusion and supplement with appropriate demand dose using the initial settings.

doses of ketorolac, ibuprofen, or celecoxib may be appropriate. However, this would require consultation with the operative surgeon due to associated bleeding risk and the possibility of impaired bone healing. In the absence of hepatic insufficiency, scheduled acetaminophen would also be appropriate. One may also consider starting low doses of pregabalin or gabapentin.

Patient-controlled analgesia

When compared to intermittent bolus dosing of opioids, IV patient-controlled analgesia (PCA) offers significantly greater analgesia and satisfaction. Both the strengths and risks of PCA systems depend upon a negative feedback loop: when in pain, the patient self-administers potent analgesics leading to pain relief, therefore limiting further opioid demands. An additional benefit of PCA dosing is that the patient is not dependent upon administration variables and has constant access to the prescribed dosing.

PCA systems allow for a continuous and demand dosing. Demand dosing is a preset amount that can be accessed at regulated intervals. This dosing also has an hourly maximum dose with lockout to prevent overmedication. **Table 99-4** lists common IV PCA programs for initial use with a variety of opioids.

As with any opioid-based therapy, PCA use may result in respiratory depression. If there is discordance between nociception (pain) and antinociception (opioid), a relative decrease in pain input or increase in opioid-based inhibition may each result in respiratory depression in the presence of opioids. Minimizing the use of background infusions in opioid-naïve patients mitigates this risk. Background infusions are best individualized to better control the overall pain state when incorporating a home opioid regimen. Home opioid dosing may be converted to background infusion dosing with the addition of patient controlled dosing to assess and treat in the acute pain phase. Once a stable regimen achieves adequate control of the patient's pain, the dosing requirement may be used to transition to an oral regimen that will reflect the patient's opioid requirements.

Some institutions use pulse oximetry monitoring to assess the respiratory depression associated with opioid administration. Unfortunately, this monitoring is not appropriately sensitive, nor is it in any way specific enough to capture the relationship between respiratory depression and opioid administration when it is used concomitantly with supplemental oxygen. Pulse oximetry then lends a false sense of security in addition to monitoring and administrative burden without the benefit of providing predictive value. Capnography, a much more specific correlate of respiratory depression, is best reserved for those patients who have substantial comorbidities that elevate the risks associated with opioid therapy.

■ INTERVENTIONAL TECHNIQUES

Peripheral nerve blocks

Peripheral nerve blocks, either as single injections or continuous infusions of local anesthetic, deliver analgesia and anesthesia around the target nerve. Peripheral nerve blocks may offer superior analgesia, decreased opioid consumption, improved pharmacokinetic titration, and increased patient satisfaction when compared with systemic analgesic techniques or placebo.

Using either land marks, nerve stimulators or ultra sound guided techniques, anesthesiologists may customize the regional anesthetic regimen to reflect each patient's surgical, perioperative, and rehabilitation requirements. Although single injections of local anesthetic may provide a block lasting up to 24 hours, placement of a perineural catheter through the needle allows the therapy to be extended for up to several weeks. Multiple injections and/or catheters may be needed to adequately anesthetize pertinent nerve distributions.

Neuraxial anesthesia

Neuraxial anesthesia refers to injections of local anesthetic and/or opioids into the epidural or intrathecal space, either through a needle as a single-injection or through an indwelling catheter.

Epidural anesthesia: Epidural anesthesia commonly refers to infusion of solutions containing local anesthetic and opioids through a catheter within the epidural space. As the solution infiltrates this potential space, it spreads superiorly and inferiorly within the spinal canal. This spread gives coverage along dermatomal distribution congruent with the level of the catheter or injectate. This spread is slightly affected by gravity and patient positioning; thus, patients may notice epidural effects predominating upon dependent locations when laterally positioned.

Epidural solutions commonly contain mixtures of local anesthetic and opioids. High local anesthetic concentrations will result in sympathectomy, sensory loss, and motor block depending upon the required dose for analgesia. In general, the low concentrations of local anesthetic used for analgesia offer a discriminatory block providing excellent analgesia, minimal sensory inhibition and nearly absent motor block. Opioid-only solutions avoid some side effects such as sympathectomy and motor block, but at the cost of nausea, pruritus, and less-potent analgesia. Solutions combining local anesthetic with opioids provide superior dynamic pain relief, decreased sensory block regression, and decreased local anesthetic dose requirement.

Epidural solutions are commonly delivered through continuous infusions rather than single shot administration. While effective, such infusions fail to account for the dynamic nature of painful conditions. The administration of epidural analgesia using patient-controlled epidural analgesia (PCEA) systems has become more common. The PCEA system allows the patient to self-administer an epidural bolus at a dose and schedule ordered by the physician, while providing continuous background infusion. Such systems allow for patient-controlled individualization of analgesic regimens. When compared with continual infusion-only regimens, PCEA systems offer lower drug use yet greater patient satisfaction.

Epidural side effects: As with all types of medications, epidural analgesia is not without side effects. Local anesthetics can result in anesthesia, motor blockade, and hypotension from sympathectomy. When placed in the lumbar and sacral epidural space, local anesthetics or opioids may result in urinary retention necessitating either bladder catheterization or frequent bladder scans. The lower-extremity weakness, and potential orthostatic hypotension associated with epidural analgesia, make appropriate fall precautions necessary.

Sympathectomies due to epidural analgesia may result in profound hypotension, although the incidence with postoperative epidural analgesia averages 0.7% to 3.0%. If the epidural is dosed to the upper thoracic dermatomes, blockade of the cardiac accelerator fibers may also lead to severe bradycardia. Frequent hemodynamic monitoring is therefore essential during initiation and modification of epidural analgesia involving local anesthetics.

Epidural opioid administration is generally devoid of the hemodynamic perturbations seen with epidural local anesthetics. Side effects are usually those also seen with systemic administration, such as nausea, vomiting, pruritus, and respiratory depression. Pruritus due to neuraxial opioids appears to be related to central activation of "pruritus pathways" that mediate nonhistamine itch. Intravenous naloxone, naltrexone, and nalbuphine each appear efficacious for treatment of opioid-induced pruritus without affecting analgesia when dosed appropriately.

The rate of respiratory depression from neuraxial opioids does not appear to differ from that of systemic opioid administration, ranging from 0.1% to 0.9%. The concern for respiratory depression stems from the cephalic spread and systemic distribution of neuraxial opioids. Respiratory depression appears early after bolus with lipophilic opioids such as fentanyl or sufentanil, and may be delayed up to 12 hours with hydrophilic opioids such as morphine. Risk factors include increasing dose, age, concomitant systemic opioid or sedative use, thoracic surgery, prolonged or extensive surgery, and the presence of applicable comorbidities.

Paravertebral anesthesia: Occasionally, situations arise in which a patient would benefit from epidural analgesia confined to a single side of the body, or in which an avoidance of large-segment sympatholysis becomes critical. This can be accomplished by delivering local anesthetics to the paravertebral compartment either through a single injection or via continuous infusion via catheter. Such techniques are finding increasing use for unilateral thoracic, breast, abdominal, and hip surgeries, and for pain from rib fractures.

Risks of regional anesthesia

As with all medical and surgical therapies, the risk-to-benefit ratios of regional anesthesia should be thoroughly discussed with patients prior to implementation. The American Society of Regional Anesthesia and Pain Medicine (ASRA) published guidelines on providing regional anesthesia for patients on anticoagulation medications. With regional anesthesia there is a rare but catastrophic risk of direct mechanical injury to the spinal cord or peripheral nerves. Bleeding and infection are likewise possible with any regional anesthetic, especially those related to the central nervous system. With regard

to neuraxial and paravertebral analgesia, development of an epidural hematoma may result in spinal cord hypoperfusion, injury, and subsequent permanent paralysis. Epidural hematoma formation may occur during needle or catheter placement, and during catheter removal. Concurrent use of neuraxial or paravertebral analgesia with systemic anticoagulation requires exceptional vigilance to prevent or minimize complications involving epidural hematomas. An epidural hematoma should be considered in a patient with severe back pain or neurologic deficit after an epidural placement or removal; this should warrant an immediate imaging and neurosurgical consultation.

Infection represents another major concern, especially with neuraxial analgesia. Serious infections resulting in epidural abscess or meningitis following epidural analgesia are quite rare (<1/1000 and <1/50,000, respectively), although catheter colonization rates may approach 35%.

CASE 99-1 (continued)

A peripheral nerve block using a femoral nerve catheter, a relatively low-risk intervention, may alleviate much, but not all of her pain. This would allow systemic anticoagulation with low-molecular-weight heparin without risk of an epidural hematoma. If a femoral nerve catheter does not sufficiently control her pain, an epidural placed in the low lumbar region may offer superior pain relief. This would require urinary catheterization, and appropriate precautions regarding anticoagulation. Either intervention may decrease or obviate the need for supplemental opioids. The ultimate goal with this patient is to improve functionality and have her out of bed and working with physical therapy. It is important to achieve a sensory blockade while maintaining motor function, decreasing her fall risk and improving her ability to work with physical therapy.

ALTERED DRUG METABOLISM

The older adult

Elderly patients have both multiple comorbidities and altered liver and kidney physiology, which impact their drug metabolism and clearance. Opioids, with the exception of buprenorphine, have increased active half-lives and metabolites. This requires decreased dosing and longer dosing intervals to minimize adverse events. Cognitive impairment is still a recognized sequelae and titration should be slow and gradual. Inappropriate medications in the older adult with dementia and/or delirium include flurazepam, pentazocine, and meperidine. Risky medications also include long-acting benzodiazepines such as diazepam. Ketorolac is a better alternative.

Hepatic disease

Hepatic disease may be associated with dysfunction in several pathways that impede pain control strategies. Coagulation issues may preclude interventional management techniques including regional anesthesia, nerve blocks, and other injections. Liver dysfunction may affect opioid metabolism and preclude the use of medications containing acetaminophen. Drugs with decreased hepatic clearance include meperidine, dextropropoxyphene, pentazocine, tramadol, and alfentanil. Morphine has decreased clearance and increased oral bioavailability. With the exception of meperidine, these drugs may be used but would require a decreased dose or increased dosing interval. An active metabolite of meperidine, normeperidine, may cause seizures. The metabolism of fentanyl, sufentanil, and remifentanil does not appear to be altered by hepatic disease.

Renal disease

The use of NSAIDs is associated with an increased rate and severity of side effects in patients with renal dysfunction. These effects may range from electrolyte abnormalities to chronic renal failure on a dose and exposure basis. This relationship is best correlated with the plasma concentration of the NSAIDs, which does not eliminate their usage entirely, but requires caution. Diclofenac is a topical nonsteroidal that has demonstrated benefit in the patch and gel format for osteoarthritis, but has only 2% renal clearance, decreasing that concern in patients with renal insufficiency/failure. Treatment modalities include oral and transdermal analgesics, topical NSAIDs (minimizing systemic absorption), interventional therapies (pain-state specific).

PRACTICE POINT

- A modified WHO ladder paradigm to treat nociceptive and neuropathic pain in end-stage renal disease (ESRD) patients (Barakzoy) includes:
  - Mild pain: acetaminophen and adjuvants
  - Moderate pain: tramadol, hydrocodone, oxycodone, nonopioid analgesics, and adjuvants
  - Severe pain: hydromorphone, fentanyl, and methadone in addition to the lower-tier recommendations

PRACTICE POINT

- Sedatives, anesthetics, and analgesics appear to selectively compromise patients with obstructive sleep apnea (OSA) compared to unaffected individuals. Optimize pain control while minimizing detrimental effects of treatment on respiratory mechanics. Use adjuvants, NSAIDs, tramadol, regional anesthetics, and the use of home CPAP. Avoid opioid and centrally acting agents that suppress respiratory drive as much as possible. Efficacy of CPAP has not been evaluated in the perioperative period or with concomitant use of analgesics or opioids.

PRACTICE POINT

- Patients with peripheral vascular disease and comorbidities that are not amenable to operable repair are left with medical analgesic therapy or spinal cord stimulation. Spinal cord stimulator treatment has been found to improve 12-month limb salvage and lower analgesic use in nonoperative patients compared with conservative therapy.

■ SPECIFIC PAIN CONDITIONS

Neuropathic pain

Diagnosis of the cause of the neuropathy (ie, diabetes mellitus, HIV, chemotherapy-induced peripheral neuropathy) should guide the management to prevent worsening of the neuropathy.

Oral and transdermal therapies are the primary modalities; spinal cord stimulation may benefit some patients who experience refractory pain. First-line medications include tricyclic antidepressants, selective serotonergic and noradrenergic reuptake inhibitors, calcium channel alpha 2-delta ligands (pregabalin and gabapentin), and topical lidocaine. Opioid analgesics and tramadol are considered second-line agents. Third-line agents include other anticonvulsants, antidepressants, mexiletine, N-methyl-D-aspartate (NMDA) receptors, and topical capsaicin (Table 99-3).

Stroke pain: central stroke pain

Central stroke pain is disabling sequelae of stroke in 8% to 14% of patients. First-line drugs include tricyclic antidepressants and neuropathic agents including pregabalin and gabapentin. Second-line drugs would include selective serotonin-norepinephrine reuptake inhibitors, lamotrigine, opioids, and drug combinations. Diagnosis is made by exclusion of other likely causes of pain in consultation with the neurology service.

Phantom limb pain

Phantom limb pain occurs in 50% to 80% of both traumatic and operative amputees. Pain and sensory alterations at the site of amputation predominate in the initial postoperative and posttraumatic period. Phantom limb sensations and pain generally develop within 1 month of the amputation with a second peak of development approximately 12 months postamputation. Preoperative analgesia has been evaluated as a possibility to improve outcomes, but neither regional anesthetic techniques nor oral regimens have been found to decrease incidence of the development of phantom limb pain.

Treatment of phantom limb pain may require a multimodal therapeutic regimen. First-line therapies include transcutaneous electrical nerve stimulation (TENS) and biofeedback. Medication options include anticonvulsants (gabapentin), opioids, and NSAIDs. Other treatment modalities that have not been investigated fully but have benefitted some patients include: acupuncture, mirror-box therapy, NMDA, and calcitonin receptor agonists. Patients should be evaluated for the need to adjust prosthesis, stump neuroma, referred pain, and care of the residual limb.

Chronic abdominal pain/distention

Treatment goals for patients with chronic abdominal pain include evaluating patients for a correctable cause in consultation with gastroenterology or gynecology, minimizing opioids, and maintaining motility. Exposing patients to opioids for nonmalignant pain puts them at higher risk for developing aberrant drug-related behaviors and illicit drug use. Opioid-induced constipation is a common side effect that limits the efficacy of this drug class for patients with abdominal pathology.

Narcotic bowel syndrome may cause an acute abdominal pain exacerbation. It is a diagnosis of exclusion in patients with greater than 2 weeks of moderate opioid usage with a compatible clinical presentation. Treatment of narcotic bowel syndrome includes recognition of the syndrome, developing a relationship with the patient to facilitate this process, graded withdrawal of the narcotic according to a specified withdrawal program, and

TABLE 99-5 WHO (Modified) Analgesic Ladder

Step 1	**Nonopioid analgesics** (eg, acetaminophen, NSAIDs [OTC and Rx], adjuvants, antidepressants, membrane stabilizers, local anesthetics [topical and enteral], bisphosphonates, and steroids)
	Pain procedural interventions
Step 2	**Nonopioid and "weak" opioid analgesics** (eg, codeine, hydrocodone, and tramadol)
	Pain procedural interventions
Step 3	**Nonopioid and "strong" opioid analgesics** (eg, morphine, hydromorphone, fentanyl, methadone, and oxycodone)
	Pain procedural interventions

the institution of medications to reduce withdrawal effects. Methylnaltrexone is a newer agent that can be used to counteract opioid-induced constipation with minimal central effects and lack of withdrawal potential. These patients should be screened for ileus or other obstructive causes of constipation prior to administration.

Chronic pancreatitis may develop as part of an increased neural density and hypertrophy resulting in a neuropathic pain state, similar to the state that develops in pancreatic adenocarcinoma. The neuropathic pain treatment paradigm may be used in its treatment. However, NMDA antagonists and tricyclic antidepressants may result in decreased gastrointestinal motility. Tramadol may be a useful alternative to stronger opioids with regard to pain control and GI motility side effects. Celiac plexus blocks/neurolysis are not permanent procedures with nerve regrowth within 3 to 6 months and have complication risks including paralysis. Spinal cord stimulation may prove to be a treatment strategy for refractory severe abdominal visceral pain.

Epidural analgesia may be used for treatment and management of chronic abdominal pain of multifactorial origin. The management is similar to that of postoperative abdominal pain as above.

CONCLUSION

Hospitalists have a primary role in managing pain by initiating the appropriate therapies and consulting the pain management service and other medical services when necessary. Treatment of pain begins with proper evaluation and identifying the causes of pain. This should be followed by an individualized treatment plan based on the type of pain and the patient's comorbidities. The treatment plan should be reassessed at appropriate intervals. A multimodal treatment approach gives the best results in patients with chronic pain. Managing pain properly improves the patient's health, functionality, and quality of life.

SUGGESTED READINGS

Breivik H, Borchgrevink PC, Allen SM, et al. Assessment of pain. *Br J Anaesth*. 2008;101:17.

Drossman D, Szigethy E. The narcotic bowel syndrome: a recent update. *Am J Gastroenterol*. 2014;2(1):22-30.

Gachaqo C, Draganov PV. Pain management in chronic pancreatitis. *World J Gastroenterol*. 2008;14:3137.

Hudcova J, McNicol E, Quah C, et al. Patient controlled opioid analgesia versus conventional opioid analgesia for postoperative pain. *Cochrane Database Syst Rev*. 2006;CD003348.

Hurley RW, Cohen SP, Williams KA, et al. The analgesic effects of perioperative gabapentin on postoperative pain: a meta-analysis. *Reg Anesth Pain Med*. 2006;31:237.

Kehlet H, Jensen TS, Woolf CJ. Persistent postsurgical pain: risk factors and prevention. *Lancet*. 2006;367.1618.

Nikolajsen L, Ilkjaer S, Christensen JH, et al. Randomised trial of epidural bupivacaine and morphine in prevention of stump and phantom pain in lower-limb amputation. *Lancet*. 1997;350:1353.

Ritter JM, Harding I, Warren JB. Precaution, cyclooxygenase inhibition, and cardiovascular risk. *Trends Pharmacol Sci*. 2009;30:503.

Thomas J, Karver S, Cooney GA, et al. Methylnaltrexone for opioid-induced constipation in advanced illness. *N Engl J Med*. 2008;358:2332.

Werawatganon T, Charuluxanun S. Patient controlled intravenous opioid analgesia versus continuous epidural analgesia for pain after intra-abdominal surgery. *Cochrane Database Syst Rev*. 2005;CD004088.

CHAPTER 100

Suspected Intoxication and Overdose

Nicholas J. Connors, MD
Edward C. Jauch, MD

Key Clinical Questions

1. What information should be obtained in a patient with an unknown exposure?
2. The physical examination should focus on what key areas?
3. What are the common toxidromes?
4. What are effective decontamination procedures?
5. How do you determine the disposition of the poisoned patient?
6. When should you consider delayed toxicity?
7. What are the roles of a poison center and poison information specialist?

CASE 100-1

A 27-year-old man was observed stumbling in a local park. The police brought him to the Emergency Department (ED) for evaluation of his altered mental status and possible drug intoxication. A history was difficult to obtain because he was mumbling incoherently, hallucinating, and extremely agitated. It was unknown whether the patient had an underlying psychiatric disorder.

Due to increasing agitation and combativeness, the patient was placed in physical restraints. Initial vital signs documented were blood pressure 158/94 mm Hg, heart rate 133 beats per minute (bpm), respiratory rate 20, temperature 101.5°F, and O_2 saturation 98%. Pupils were symmetric and approximately 6 mm and reacted poorly to light. A limited physical examination was notable for dry oropharynx, absence of cardiac murmurs, clear lungs, and a soft, nontender abdomen. Bowel sounds were present but very infrequent. Neurologically he was confused and combative but moving all extremities with good strength equal bilaterally. Occasional myoclonic jerks of the upper and lower extremities were noted. The skin was warm and dry, and flushing noted at the face and neck.

Laboratory studies revealed a fingerstick glucose of 100 mg/dL. Complete blood cell count, kidney function, and electrolytes were within normal limits. Serum ethanol concentration was <10 mg/dL. He received a 1 L normal saline fluid bolus and required a total of 4 mg of midazolam for sedation. The patient continued to be tachycardic and combative. He was admitted to the telemetry unit for monitoring and further treatment. How would you further manage this patient?

INTRODUCTION

The American Association of Poison Control Centers maintains a database, the National Poison Data System. Without the ability to verify the presence of a substance in blood or urine, all calls reported and suspicious for a particular substance are categorized as an exposure to that agent. Approximately 2.2 million human exposures were reported to US poison control centers in 2013, a slight decrease from 2012 and a continuation of the gradual decrease in reported cases since peaking at 2.5 million in 2008. Notably the number of cases with serious outcomes has increased, as has the number and proportion of cases reported by a health care facility compared to those reported from the general public. Children under 6 years old made up 48% of all calls, but only 2.4% of reported fatalities. The percent of total fatalities increased with each decade of life, peaking at 19% for cases between 50 and 59 years old, then declining steeply with further increased age; unintentional exposures represented 99% of exposures in children age <6, 60% in adults age <20, and only 33% in adults age >20. Analgesics, sedative/hypnotics/antipsychotics, and antidepressants were the top medication classes involved in exposures. Categories resulting in the largest numbers of adult fatalities were sedative/hypnotics/antipsychotics, cardiovascular drugs, opioids, stimulants, street drugs, and alcohols. Data from poison centers rely on voluntary reporting and the true incidences of exposure and serious outcome due to poisoning are likely underestimated.

Of cases reported to a poison center the vast majority (69%) are managed at the site of exposure (home, work, etc.), while 13% are treated and released from a health care facility and 7.6% are admitted for medical care. Many of these admitted patients will be managed and stabilized by hospitalists. A systematic approach to the poisoned patient is needed to provide effective, efficient, and timely care. In most cases, basic stabilizing measures involving protection of the airway and ensuring adequate breathing and circulation have already occurred in the ED, however, continued reassessment and care is required until each patient is medically stable and ready for discharge or transfer to psychiatry. This may involve continued decontamination of the gut, the administration of oxygen, intravenous fluids, antidotes, vasopressors, sedation, or the initiation of hemodialysis.

THE INITIAL EVALUATION

■ RECOGNIZE TOXIDROMES

Toxidromes are collections of signs and symptoms associated with toxicity from distinct drug classes that assist with diagnosis and guide appropriate therapy. Common toxidromes to consider include opioid, sympathomimetic, sedative/hypnotic, anticholinergic, cholinergic, serotonin toxicity, and neuroleptic malignant syndrome (NMS) (**Table 100-1**). Both opioid and sedative/hypnotic toxidromes are characterized by a range from somnolence to coma, but differ in the respiratory depression noted in opioid toxicity, whereas vital signs remain relatively normal with sedative/hypnotics. Cholinergic toxicity causes profuse secretions from sweat, tear, and salivary glands, and the gastrointestinal and urinary systems. The triad of hyperthermia, tachycardia, and hypertension can be seen with sympathomimetics, serotonin toxicity, and NMS; serotonin toxicity is more associated with clonus and tremor while NMS is more associated with increased tone and rigidity. Clinicians should also be aware of mixed ingestions causing features from multiple toxidromes, for example, unresponsiveness in the setting of tachycardia and hypertension that can be seen with concomitant cocaine and heroin use.

■ HISTORY

A common challenge in the assessment of poisoned patients is obtaining a complete history from the patient, acquaintances, bystanders, or first responders. The key elements in the toxicologic history include the medications or substances that were found at the scene, and what is suspected. The amount, formulation, concentration, route, and time of exposure are also critical. Additionally, clinicians should aim to obtain the patient's full medication list, whether they also use nonprescription medications and herbal supplements, drug and alcohol use, and the presence of other available substances, including medications or illicit drugs used by others in the same household. The intent of the patient is important, as unintentional exposures are usually much less severe than intentional overdoses. Symptoms experienced by the patient are crucial, but symptoms suffered by others in the household may suggest a common exposure (eg, carbon monoxide).

■ PHYSICAL EXAMINATION

The clinician may have to determine the type of exposure based solely on the physical examination findings. Frequent reassessment allows caregivers to modify treatment as toxicity develops and examination findings change. Vital signs may suggest a toxidrome. An abnormal respiratory rate or core temperature may help guide immediate treatment. A widened pulse pressure will suggest agents that enhance inotropy and peripheral vasodilation, namely beta-adrenergic agonists (such as albuterol, caffeine, and theophylline). The mental status may be "altered," though this term does little to adequately describe the patient, as "altered" can range from comatose to agitated delirium. The eye examination should note the size of the pupils and their relative reactivity to light. An abdominal examination with findings of an enlarged and palpable bladder and decreased bowel sounds suggest anticholinergic toxicity. The skin should be examined for tactile temperature, flushing, diaphoresis, abnormal dryness (best noted in the groin and axilla), cyanosis, and lesions such as needlestick wounds. Reflexes and muscle tone may suggest the exposure is related to a sympathomimetic or an agent with serotonergic or neuroleptic properties. In cases where no history is available, every clue should be utilized to identify a causative agent. Several toxicities are associated with characteristic odors including: garlic with organophosphates and thallium, mint with methylsalicylate, rotten eggs with hydrogen sulfide, and almonds with cyanide.

DIFFERENTIATING TOXIC VERSUS NONTOXIC CAUSES FOR ADMISSION

Patients with toxicity secondary to a medication or illicit drug appear very similar to those with infectious and metabolic illnesses. It is important to consider and adequately rule out these other causes. A patient with somnolence and confusion who is prescribed benzodiazepines and muscle relaxants and drinks alcohol nightly, may have toxicity due to of any of those, but depending on the history and physical examination, the patient should be evaluated for intracerebral hemorrhage, encephalitis, meningitis or other infectious or metabolic problems. It is reasonable to pursue multiple diagnostic avenues simultaneously to ensure that patients with emergent nontoxicologic pathology are not missed.

DIAGNOSTIC EVALUATIONS

Laboratory tests may yield data critical to the evaluation and treatment of poisoned patients. In any patient with altered mental status, from comatose to agitated, a point-of-care fingerstick glucose test should be performed and hypoglycemia addressed (if present). The pathophysiology of many toxins interferes with metabolic pathways. An evaluation of each patient's acid-base status with a venous blood gas with serum lactate and basic metabolic panel will guide the differential diagnosis. A complete blood count is infrequently helpful, other than cases where the serum white blood cells are expected to be abnormal (colchicine, levamisole, methotrexate, etc.) or when there is anemia from abnormal bleeding due to anticoagulants. Liver function tests should be reviewed in cases

---

TABLE 100-1 Common Toxidromes

	Mental Status	Heart Rate	Respiratory Rate	Pupils	Skin
Sympathomimetic	Agitated	Increased	Increased	Enlarged, briskly reactive	Wet
Anticholinergic	Confused	Increased	Normal	Enlarged, slowly reactive	Dry
Cholinergic	Normal	Decreased	Normal	Small	Wet
Opioid	Somnolent	Decreased	Decreased	Small	Normal
Sedative-hypnotic	Somnolent	Decreased	Normal	Normal	Normal

where acetaminophen and valproic acid ingestions are suspected. Coagulation studies may be helpful when the exposure is suspected to be an anticoagulant. Creatine kinase will show whether rhabdomyolysis is developing in the agitated patient with persistent motor activity or in the unresponsive patient found down (after a significant period without changing position).

Serum concentrations of several medications are commonly available. An acetaminophen concentration should be checked for every patient with a suspected intentional overdose. A patient with a significant acetaminophen ingestion may present without symptoms initially but will clinically worsen over the following 24 hours as the toxic metabolite (N-acetyl-p-benzoquinone imine [NAPQI]) is generated, resulting in liver toxicity. N-Acetylcysteine, the antidote, has excellent efficacy when administration begins within 8 hours of ingestion, but becomes less effective as the time from ingestion increases, with associated increases in the risk for hepatic failure and death.

Concentrations of salicylate, ethanol, digoxin, lithium, phenytoin, valproic acid, theophylline, and phenobarbital are commonly available, while concentrations of ethylene glycol, methanol, methotrexate, and others may only be available at certain centers or at certain times of the day. Other drug concentrations, like levetiracetam, lamotrigine, methanol, and ethylene glycol, may be available through an offsite laboratory. These results may be useful, but will not guide treatment during the first hours and days of an acute issue. Serum osmolarity may be used as a surrogate for toxic alcohols when direct measure of ethylene glycol and methanol are delayed, but should not be used to rule out methanol or ethylene glycol toxicity. Blood gas analysis for carbon monoxide and methemoglobin may be helpful depending on the clinical scenario.

An electrocardiogram in the poisoned patient can reveal much about the ingestion; abnormalities in the QRS and QT intervals may suggest agents with sodium and potassium channel blocking properties, respectively. The absence of an R wave in lead AVR effectively rules out a tricyclic antidepressant. In cases of tricyclic toxicity, a QRS interval of greater than 100 and 160 ms are predictive of seizures and arrhythmias, respectively. Digoxin use can be seen as repolarization abnormality in the QT segments and findings of regularized atrial fibrillation, premature ventricular contractions, and ventricular tachycardia suggest digoxin toxicity.

A source of controversy is the utility of toxicology screening tests or urine drug screens. Kellerman et al conducted a prospective study of 582 consecutive ED patients with suspected drug overdose and found that more than 95% of cases had no significant change in treatment or disposition in response to routine toxicologic screening. The urine drug screen provides information regarding what the patient has been exposed to over the last week to month, not necessarily what is causing the patient's current symptoms. Additionally, the drug screen is plagued by false positives and negatives, making interpretation difficult. See **Table 100-2** for tests to consider in ruling in or out other diagnoses that may be confused with ingestion.

TREATMENT OPTIONS

■ GASTROINTESTINAL DECONTAMINATION

The American Academy of Clinical Toxicology has developed expert consensus guidelines on each of the common techniques for GI decontamination. Syrup of ipecac is essentially inefficient and ineffective in decontaminating the gut, with unpredictable time of onset, and is no longer recommended for acute or chronic ingestions in the ED. Circumstances in which ipecac may be of benefit are rare, but may include an acute, serious ingestion with extended transport time to definitive care. It should not be used once the patient has arrived at the hospital. If considered, its use should be discussed with the local poison center or medical toxicologist.

TABLE 100-2 Tests to Consider in the Poisoned Patient

Tests for All Patients	Diagnoses to Consider
Rapid glucose test	Hypoglycemia, hyperglycemia
Electrocardiogram	Cardiotoxic effects of cardiovascular or psychotropic drugs (QRS widening and QTc prolongation)
Venous blood gas	Acidosis, hypercarbia
Electrolytes	Electrolyte abnormalities
BUN/Creatinine	Acute kidney injury
Acetaminophen	Acetaminophen overdose with potential hepatotoxicity
Tests to consider with specific clinical suspicion	
Complete blood cell count	Anemia, leukocytosis, leukopenia, blood dyscrasias
Serum osmolality	Toxic alcohol ingestion
Serum ethanol	Ethanol intoxication
Urinalysis	Ketones, crystaluria (may indicate ethylene glycol ingestion)
Computerized tomography	Intracranial process (mass, hemorrhage, other)
CSF studies	Meningitis, Encephalitis, Subarachnoid hemorrhage
Electroencephalogram	Seizure disorder

Activated charcoal may be beneficial in certain circumstances, but its routine use exposes patients to greater risk for adverse events (such as aspiration), without appreciable benefit, and routine administration for oral overdoses has little to no significant impact on hospital length of stay or patient outcomes; it should be reserved for those who:

- Present early following overdose as there is evidence for benefit within one hour of ingestion.
- Ingested a substance that is adsorbed by activated charcoal and for which there is no antidote, such as, aspirin.
- Have significant or life-threatening ingestions of carbamazepine, theophylline, phenobarbital, dapsone, and quinine.

Caustics, alcohols, and metals have little to no adsorption by activated charcoal, but charcoal does enhance the elimination of phenytoin and theophylline from the serum (likely by adsorbing medication from the enterohepatic circulation into the gastrointestinal system).

Gastric lavage is only indicated when a patient presents early after an ingestion with a high likelihood of mortality. Though performed routinely in the past, it is no longer commonly used in the management of overdoses. Although intuitively removing pills or fragments from the stomach should afford less medication to be absorbed into the circulation, clinical and experimental trials have failed to support a significant benefit. Lavage can be associated with significant morbidity, and should only be performed by those proficient in the technical aspects of the procedure. It is contraindicated in patients who are at risk of perforation (due to an underlying condition or the ingestion of caustics).

Whole bowel irrigation can be employed in patients who present greater than 2 hours postingestion, and who have ingested substances that should be cleared from the small and large intestine (sustained release or enteric coated preparations, especially lithium, iron, potassium, and packets of drugs). Irrigation can be accomplished by administering polyethylene glycol 1 to 2 L/h via nasogastric tube until the rectal output is clear.

■ RENAL REPLACEMENT THERAPY

Intermittent hemodialysis can enhance elimination of toxins such as salicylate, methanol, ethylene glycol, lithium, barbiturates, theophylline, and carbamazepine. Additionally, hemodialysis may correct metabolic derangements caused by toxins. Continuous renal replacement therapies provide far less clearance of toxin due to lower flow rates.

■ CONSULTING POISON CONTROL

The American Association of Poison Control Centers includes 57 centers that take calls from their regional catchment area. Both the public and staff at health care facilities can call 1-800-222-1222 and have access to guidance from Certified Specialists in Poison Information (CSPI). The specialists in poison information are trained in poisoning management and triage, and this group includes physicians, pharmacists, nurses, and other poison information providers. Poison control centers serve multiple functions for the medical community. They provide education and educational resources, collect epidemiological data enabling them to track emerging trends and epidemics, and provide clinical guidance. Through a combination of local management protocols, specific online and text resources, and quick access to medical toxicologists, the poison information specialists provide the necessary advice to guide the management of the patient at hand, and medical toxicologists are on call to provide support for the CPSI. When calling the poison center, specific information that is helpful includes the patient's age, weight, substance to which the patient was exposed, time of exposure, up-to-date clinical picture including vital signs, laboratory studies, and ECG results if applicable, treatments administered thus far, and specific questions regarding management. With that information CSPI can quickly provide advice about management, or if necessary, solicit the help of the medical toxicologist.

■ USE OF ANTIDOTES

Table 100-3 lists commonly recommended antidotes.

TRIAGE CONSIDERATIONS

The disposition of a patient with medication or drug toxicity depends on what was ingested, the treatments being administered, the expected course, and the level of care required. Hospitalists must pay close attention to mental status, hemodynamics, and any ancillary test results obtained in the ED.

A patient must have the ability to protect their airway and have adequate respiratory drive to be admitted to the general medical service. Indications for intensive care unit admission include:

- Hemodynamic instability
- Vasopressors support
- Intubation on a ventilator or concern that the airway may become compromised
- Likely worsening course, such as those recently post ingestion of a sustained release preparation or who have worsening vital signs or mental status
- Naloxone infusions due to the possibility of respiratory depression
- Hourly fingerstick glucose measurements
- Hemodialysis
- Chemical restraint required

Consultation with a medical toxicologist or the regional poison control center will help in making the decision on what level of care is anticipated (**Table 100-4**).

After admission, patients may develop delayed effects from their exposure. Like acetaminophen, other agents with delayed toxicity include hepatotoxic mushrooms, iron, colchicine, vitamin

TABLE 100-3 Common Antidotes

Toxin/Drug	Antidote
Acetaminophen	N-Acetylcysteine
Amphetamine, Methamphetamine	Benzodiazepines
Anticholinergic drugs	Physostigmine
Beta adrenergic antagonist	Glucagon, high-dose insulin euglycemia
Calcium channel antagonist	Calcium chloride, high-dose insulin euglycemia
Carbon monoxide	(Hyperbaric) oxygen
Cocaine	Benzodiazepines, phentolamine
Cyanide	Hydroxocobalamin, Cyanide antidote kit (sodium nitrite, sodium thiosulfate)
Cyclic antidepressant— sodium channel antagonists	Sodium bicarbonate
Digoxin, cardiac glycosides	Digoxin-specific Fab
Ethylene glycol, methanol	Ethanol, Fomepizole
Hydrofluoric acid (rust removers and glass etching)	Calcium gluconate
Insulin	Glucose/dextrose
Iron	Deferoxamine
Isoniazid, hydrazines	Pyridoxine
Lead, arsenic, mercury	Dimercapto-succinic acid (Succimer)
Methemoglobinemia	Methylene blue
Methotrexate	Glucarpidase
Opioids	Naloxone
Organophosphates	Atropine, pralidoxime
Sympathomimetics	Benzodiazepines
Valproic acid	L-Carnitine

K antagonist anticoagulants (eg, warfarin, brodifacoum), and thyroid hormone. Many medications, including long-acting insulin preparations, sulfonylureas, phenytoin, and amiodarone, may cause prolonged symptoms lasting at least 24 hours. In rare cases, patients may ingest packets of illicit drugs that may open or rupture to avoid arrest. In all cases, it is important to continue to reassess patients for changes in mental status and vital signs.

Another concern for the admitted patient is the development of withdrawal syndrome. Alcohol and benzodiazepine withdrawal cause a sympathomimetic toxidrome and may also cause seizures. Early recognition of increases in heart rate and blood pressure and the presence of mild tongue fasciculations and muscle tremor allow early treatment and prevention of severe sequelae.

WHEN TO CONSULT A MEDICAL TOXICOLOGIST

Often the toxicologist is involved in discussions of complicated or controversial management, or if the caller has questions that are beyond the scope of practice of the CSPI fielding the call. Since each poison center has toxicologists on call, callers may request to speak directly with that physician. This may be particularly useful in cases in which direct and immediate feedback is crucial. Some cases may require multiple conversations between the hospital provider and the toxicologist due to changes in management based on a dynamic clinical course and updated results. When patients are in extremis due to poisoning, early involvement of a medical toxicologist is recommended.

TABLE 100-4 Criteria for Triaging the Poisoned Patient to the ICU

Hemodynamic instability
- Hypotension
- Non sinus cardiac rhythm
- Hypothermia
- Hyperthermia
- Hypoxia
- Hypercarbia

End organ damage
- Unable to respond to verbal stimuli, GCS < 13, unable to protect airway
- Confusion requiring monitoring for respiratory depression, withdrawal states
- Renal failure or may require emergent dialysis for removal of toxin(s) or metabolites
- Hypertensive emergency
- Respiratory failure
- Heart block other than first degree AV block, QTc > 500 ms, Osborn wave
- Life-threatening electrolyte disturbances or hypoglycemia that requires ongoing frequent monitoring and treatment
- Rhabdomyolysis
- Disseminated intravascular coagulation (DIC)
- Seizures or other neurologic conditions requiring ICU care
- Impending multisystem failure

Nursing requirements
- 1:1 ICU nursing required to monitor and administer therapy
- Higher level of care due to limited resources on general medical floor

Clinical course expected to worsen

TABLE 100-5 Toxicology Resources for Hospitalists

Poison Center Hotline: 1-800-222-1222

Textbooks
- Goldfrank's Toxicologic Emergencies (Hoffman R, et al. [eds.] 10th ed.)
- Critical Care Toxicology: Diagnosis and Management of the Critically Poisoned Patient (Brent J, et al. [eds.])
- Poisonings and Drug Overdose (Olson K, et al. [eds.] 6th ed.)
- Handbook of Poisonous and Injurious Plants (Nelson LS, et al. [eds.])

Online Resources
- Erowid (www.erowid.org)
- A forum with reports from users and up to date names and categories of drugs of abuse and herbal products managed by biochemists
- American College of Medical Toxicology www.acmt.net
- American Academy of Clinical Toxicology www.clintox.org
- American Association of Poison Control Centers www.aapcc.org
- The Poison Review www.thepoisonreview.com

toxicology history, and when necessary, request timely consultation of experts in critical care, nephrology, and/or poison control/medical toxicology. There are many exposures where morbidity and mortality can be prevented with appropriate early management.

SUGGESTED READINGS

American Academy of Clinical Toxicology and European Association of Poison Centres and Clinical Toxicologists. Position statement and practice guidelines on the use of multi-dose activated charcoal in the treatment of acute poisoning. *J Toxicol Clin Toxicol.* 1999;37:731-751.

Ashbourne JF, Olson KR, Khayam-Bashi H. Value of rapid screening for acetaminophen in all patients with intentional drug overdose. *Ann Emerg Med.* 1989;18(10):1035-1038.

Benson BE, Hoppu K, Troutman WG, Bedry R, Erdman A, Hojer J, et al. Position paper update: gastric lavage for gastrointestinal decontamination. *Clin Toxicol (Phila).* 2013;51(3):140-146.

Bosse GM, Matyunas NJ. Delayed toxidromes. *J Emerg Med.* 1999;17(4):679-690.

Chyka PA, Seger D, Krenzelok EP, Vale JA. Position paper: Single-dose activated charcoal. *Clin Toxicol (Phila).* 2005;43(2):61-87.

Holubek WJ, Hoffman RS, Goldfarb DS, et al. Use of hemodialysis and hemoperfusion in poisoned patients. *Kidney Int.* 2008;74(10):1327-1334.

Kraut JA. Diagnosis of toxic alcohols: limitations of present methods. *Clin Toxicol (Phila).* 2015;26:1-7.

Mowry JB, Spyker DA, Cantilena LR Jr., McMillan N, Ford M. 2013 Annual Report of the American Association of Poison Control Centers' National Poison Data System (NPDS): 31st Annual Report. *Clin Toxicol (Phila).* 2014;52(10):1032-1283.

Skinner CG, Chang AS, Matthews AS, Reedy SJ, Morgan BW. Randomized controlled study on the use of multiple-dose activated charcoal in patients with supratherapeutic phenytoin levels. *Clin Toxicol (Phila).* 2012;50(8):764-769.

Thanacoody R, Caravati EM, Troutman B, Hojer J, Benson B, Hoppu K, et al. Position paper update: whole bowel irrigation for gastrointestinal decontamination of overdose patients. *Clin Toxicol (Phila).* 2015;53(1):5-12.

Another important role of the poison center, the poison center specialist, and the medical toxicologist is to help assess the need for the patient's transfer to another facility based on local and regional capabilities including adult and pediatric critical care, hyperbarics, and liver transplant. Using poison centers or hospital-based toxicologists may optimize management, thereby resulting in more efficient use of the health care system and reduced morbidity for poisoned or overdosed patients (**Table 100-5**).

CASE 100-1 *(continued)*

During the night, the patient received an additional 6 mg of midazolam for agitation and experienced intermittent visual hallucinations. Approximately 24 hours after being admitted, he was awake and oriented to person, place, and time. His pupils remained dilated and he remained amnestic to the previous day's events. He admitted to being homeless, having a history of depression and noncompliance with his antidepressant medications. Prior to being found in the park, he had ingested an unknown amount of over-the-counter sleeping pills. The pills contained an anticholinergic agent that caused the patient's toxidrome. He was subsequently evaluated by psychiatry and transferred to an inpatient mental health service.

CONCLUSION

This chapter has reviewed the approach to patients admitted for observation and management of intoxication and overdose. Hospitalists should be able to recognize the signs and symptoms associated with toxicity from different classes of drugs, obtain a focused

CHAPTER 101

Syncope

Frank E. Corrigan, III, MD

Kush Agrawal, MD

J. Richard Pittman Jr., MD, FACP

Daniel D. Dressler, MD, MSc, SFHM, FACP

Key Clinical Questions

1. How should the history, physical examination, and electrocardiogram be utilized to direct further testing or limit further testing in the evaluation of syncope?
2. What diagnostic testing should be considered for common causes of syncope?
3. When do patients require hospital admission for syncope?
4. What are the indications for advanced noninvasive or invasive tests in the evaluation of syncope?

INTRODUCTION

DEFINITION

Syncope is a sudden, transient *loss of consciousness and postural tone* with rapid onset and spontaneous recovery due to *reduced perfusion* to the brain's reticular activating system. Other causes of unconsciousness resulting from etiologies other than transient cerebral hypoperfusion should not be classified as syncope. Syncope can cause physical injuries, impact quality of life, and be a predictor of adverse cardiovascular outcomes.

EPIDEMIOLOGY

Syncope has a 3% incidence in the general population and 6% incidence in persons over age 75 years. It is responsible for 1% of emergency department (ED) visits, with more than 30% of ED syncope patients admitted, representing at least 2% of all hospital admissions. Older patients have higher rates of hospitalization and morbidity. The median cost of hospitalization of patients with syncope is approximately $8700, and up to 50% are discharged from the hospital without a specific diagnosis that caused the syncopal episode.

Syncope can present various diagnostic challenges, as many episodes of transient loss of consciousness may occur as unwitnessed events and with limited available history. Many testing modalities are also available in the evaluation of syncope, and judicious selection as well as timing and order of the most appropriate modalities can be challenging. However, following extended systematic evaluation (including outpatient evaluation when indicated), less than 20% of patients diagnosed with syncope will remain with a final diagnosis of unknown cause.

Estimates of syncope *recurrence* suggest that prior syncope, psychiatric illness, and age less than 45 years confer a higher risk of recurrent syncope. Surprisingly, severities of presentation, structural heart disease, and tilt table test response have no predictive value on syncope recurrence. Carotid sinus syndrome (CSS), the association of a syncopal event or events with carotid sinus hypersensitivity, has the highest prevalence (43%) in a population of patients presenting with recurrent syncope to the ED.

PATHOPHYSIOLOGY

Transient hypoperfusion of the brainstem or both cerebral hemispheres can result from either decreased cardiac output or significant decrease in peripheral vascular resistance. These two mechanisms form the basis of the pathophysiology behind all syncopal events (**Figure 101-1**). Specific diagnoses may then be derived based on symptoms, signs, and additional testing.

In patients with traumatic injury (eg, coup-contrecoup or concussion injury), transient loss of consciousness (T-LOC) is not associated with decreased blood flow. In nontraumatic transient LOC, clinicians should consider seizure and psychogenic etiologies. Rarer causes of transient LOC without syncope include tumor, metabolic etiologies, or intoxications. Several conditions may be incorrectly diagnosed as syncope (ie, "nonsyncope") (**Table 101-1**). Clinicians should consider anemia or pregnancy in the appropriate clinical setting.

DIFFERENTIAL DIAGNOSIS

Syncope etiologies are broadly divided into four major categories (reflex syncope, orthostatic, cardiac, and neurologic) in addition to unknown etiology (**Table 101-2**). Reflex syncope (most commonly

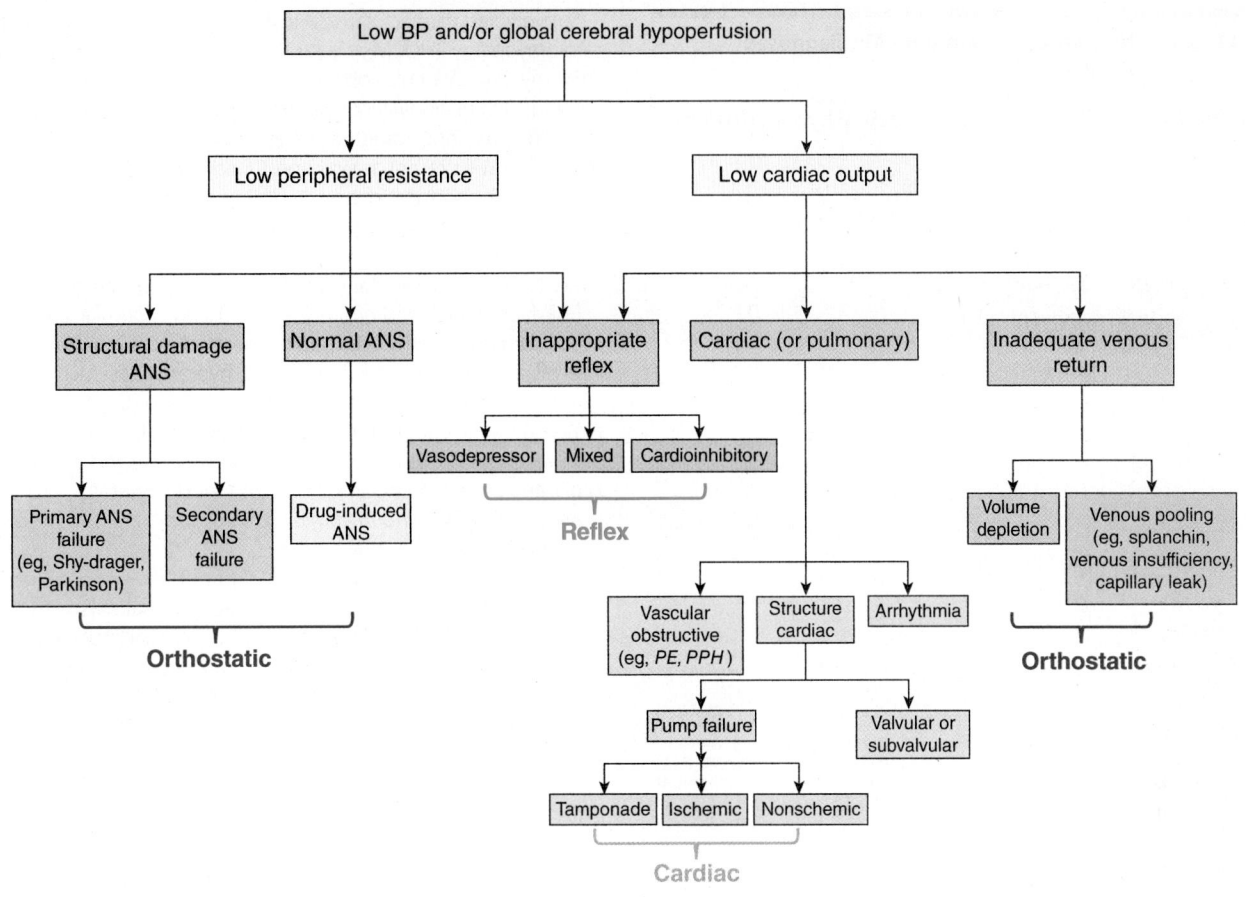

Figure 101-1 *Pathophysiologic basis of syncope.* ANS, autonomic nervous system; BP, blood pressure; PE, pulmonary embolus; PPH, primary pulmonary hypertension.

vasovagal) occurs most frequently, followed by cardiac etiologies. More than 70% of cardiac causes are due to arrhythmia, while the remainder is due to various types of structural heart disease.

Following identification of true syncope (ie, excluding nonsyncope based on history, physical exam, and initial testing), narrowing the differential diagnosis should be accomplished based on suggestive clinical features and appropriate diagnostic testing **(Table 101-3)**. The relative yield and contribution of advanced diagnostic modalities in syncope should be considered when selecting modalities in the diagnosis of syncope patients.

DIAGNOSIS

■ HISTORY

Determination if the event is truly syncope, rather than nonsyncope, can help include or exclude items within the differential diagnosis (Table 101-1). The relevant aspects of the history include the patient's symptoms experienced *prior to and following* loss of consciousness, the setting in which syncope occurred, past medical history, current medications, assessment of family history (including sudden death), and social history **(Table 101-4)**. Prior episodes and frequency of syncope episodes may also potentially help guide diagnosis and/or testing.

Did the patient actually experience a sudden, transient LOC? Was there spontaneous recovery without resuscitation?

Certain historical features may point toward a nonsyncopal event (Table 101-1). History should delineate if there was actual loss of consciousness. A mechanical fall or confusion (altered consciousness) would not be termed syncope or even LOC.

If the patient did actually lose consciousness, consideration of nonsyncopal etiologies of transient LOC including intoxications,

hypoglycemia, hypoxia, or severe anemia may be appropriate. These patients may have more gradual development of symptoms prior to a syncopal episode and/or delayed recovery (many minutes to hours) compared with true syncope.

When LOC is witnessed, description of tonic-clonic activity points toward seizure as a nonsyncopal etiology of transient LOC; however, lay person witnesses of seizure activity may not be reliable in description. When a seizure is not witnessed, historical features that may point toward seizure as an etiology include lateral tongue biting or laceration (reasonably specific for seizure, LR+ 8), pre-LOC aura, prolonged (more than 1 or a few minutes) confusion upon awakening. Bowel or bladder incontinence are nonspecific findings that may occur in syncope or seizure. Importantly, many patients with syncope are often misdiagnosed as seizure due to misinterpretation of body movements during the event. Any syncopal episode can lead to brief myoclonic activity (occurring in nearly 10% of patients with vasovagal syncope); and brief "full body stiffening" prior to awakening can occur in up to 1% of syncope patients. Many misinterpret this stiffening or myoclonic activity as seizure. Extended duration of actual LOC is referred to as coma rather than syncope (which is transient). Loss of consciousness that requires resuscitation or defibrillation to return a pulse and consciousness is referred to as sudden cardiac arrest and not syncope.

Cardiac syncope (inadequate cardiac output, arrhythmias)

Historical features suggesting cardiac etiologies of syncope include chest pain prior to syncope, syncope during exertion, and syncope while supine. In ventricular tachycardia, patients may present with syncope that has no prodrome. Often those patients recall no

TABLE 101-1 Nonsyncope: Conditions Misdiagnosed as Syncope

Conditions with LOC but no global cerebral hypoperfusion

1. Seizure
   a. Tonic-clonic seizure (not witnessed)
   b. Absence or partial complex seizure (LOC but no loss of postural tone)
2. Metabolic derangements
   a. Hypocapneic hyperventilation
   b. Hypoglycemia
   c. Hypoxemia
   d. Hyponatremia
   e. Severe anemia
3. Acute alcohol or other drug intoxication
4. TIA or stroke of *vertebrobasilar* origin
5. Increased intracranial pressure
   a. Tumor
   b. Edema
   c. Cough induced
6. Narcolepsy

Conditions without LOC

1. Cataplexy
2. TIA or stroke of *carotid* origin
3. Falls
4. Drop attacks
5. Psychogenic pseudosyncope
   a. Conversion or somatization disorders
   b. Panic disorder, major depressive disorder (MDD), or anxiety disorder
   c. Malingering, factitious disorder, or Munchausen syndrome

Conditions of cardiac arrest

1. Intervention, such as closed-chest compressions, medication, or defibrillation was required to regain a pulse and/or consciousness

LOC, loss of consciousness; TIA, transient ischemic attack.

specific symptoms prior to the syncopal episode, only recall awakening, and are often injured from a fall.

Pump failure

Is this patient having an acute MI?

Up to 7% of patients who present with syncope and no chest pain may have ischemia as the cause of their syncopal event (see Chapter 128 [Acute Coronary Syndromes]). In patients who have *syncope but no chest pain,* four factors are predictive of ACS as the etiology of the syncope: (1) arm, neck, shoulder, and throat pain, (2) history of stable angina (provoked by exercise), (3) the presence of rales on physical examination, and (4) electrocardiographic ischemic abnormalities.

Obstruction

Is there obstruction to flow resulting in inadequate cardiac output?

Patients may have valvular, subvalvular, or vascular obstruction leading to transiently reduced cardiac output and syncope. Valvular causes include aortic stenosis (AS), mitral stenosis, pulmonic stenosis (PS), or prosthetic valve malfunction. Historical features may include exertional syncope.

Subvalvular cardiac causes include hypertrophic obstructive cardiomyopathy (HOCM), classically with exertional syncope, and atrial myxoma. Vascular obstruction can occur due to pulmonary embolus (PE) or significant pulmonary hypertension. Although less than 1% of syncope admitted to the hospital is due to PE, up to 10% of PE cases will present as syncope. Clinicians should consider PE in patients with shortness of breath, elevated markers of cardiac injury without symptoms of acute coronary syndrome, or symptoms to suggest lower-extremity venous thromboembolism.

Are ventricular arrhythmias suspected as the cause of syncope?

Risk factors include coronary artery disease, valvular aortic stenosis, cardiomyopathy, congenital heart disease, prolonged QT interval, hypo- or hyperkalemia, and hypomagnesemia. Patients with ventricular arrhythmia causing syncope may present with no symptoms at all prior to the syncopal event, and injury occurs commonly. Various drugs prolong the QT interval (https://crediblemeds.org/), and place patients at risk for torsades de pointes.

Are supraventricular arrhythmias or bradyarrhythmias suspected as a cause of syncope?

Syncope occurs uncommonly in supraventricular tachyarrhythmias (SVTs), though it should be considered in patients with a history of atrial fibrillation, atrial flutter, or paroxysmal supraventricular tachycardia (eg, atrioventricular [AV] nodal reentrant tachycardia, atrial tachycardia). Bradyarrhythmias due to conduction system disease and/or the coadministration of AV nodal blocking agents may also lead to syncope.

Reflex syncope

Is the patient having a benign vasovagal episode?

Reflex syncope, also known as vasodepressor syncope, vasovagal syncope, neurocardiogenic syncope, or the "common faint," is the most common cause of syncope. Reflex syncope is mediated by inappropriate vasodepressor (ie, loss of vasoconstriction during standing) or cardioinhibitory (ie, reflex reaction characterized by bradycardia and/or asystole) responses to orthostatic challenge or emotional stress. It may also be precipitated by Valsalva (eg, micturition, defecation, swallowing) or mobilization after prolonged bed rest.

Diagnosis can often be made with a careful history. The *classic prodrome* exhibits by a *sympathetic response* (diaphoresis, palpitations/tachycardia, piloerection, anxiety, pallor) followed by a *parasympathetic* response (nausea and/or vomiting, warmth/venodilation, low heart rate). Individual patients may exhibit only a portion of the classic symptoms.

Reflex syncope related to carotid sinus hypersensitivity should be diagnosed by provocation through carotid sinus massage. Occasionally, these patients may describe syncope after rapid head or neck movements.

Orthostatic hypotension

Is orthostasis causing the patient's syncope?

Syncope due to orthostatic hypotension (OH) can occur with (1) inadequate venous return (low cardiac output), (2) structural damage to the autonomic nervous system (ANS), or (3) transient impairment of normal autonomic nervous system function (eg, medication induced). Inadequate venous return may be caused by volume depletion or venous pooling—in the peripheral venous system (eg, venous insufficiency) or in the splanchnic system (eg, following a meal). Low peripheral resistance can result from primary or secondary autonomic nervous system failure (Figure 101-1). With an intact ANS, drug-induced ANS failure or inappropriate vasodepression during a reflex response can cause syncope.

Postural orthostatic tachycardia syndrome is a poorly understood entity believed to occur due to autonomic dysfunction that can be

TABLE 101-2 Syncope Differential Diagnosis

Syncope Category	Approximate Frequency	Specific Etiologies
Reflex Syncope (ie, neurally mediated, neurogenic, or neurocardiogenic)	35%-40%	Vasovagal, Vasodepressor
		Situational (micturition, defecation, cough, valsalva, mobilization after prolonged bed rest, etc)
		Carotid sinus hypersensitivity
Cardiac	20%-25%	
Arrhythmia		• Tachyarrhythmias (eg, VT, SVT, torsades de pointe)
		• Bradyarrhythmias (third degree AVB, SSS, pacer malfunction)
Structural		• Valvular (aortic stenosis, mitral stenosis)
		• Obstructive (hypertrophic obstructive cardiomyopathy [HOCM], atrial myxoma)
		• Pump failure (large acute MI, cardiac tamponade)
		• Vascular (PE, PPH, subclavian steal, dissection)
Orthostatic	5%-15%	• Drug-induced ANS failure (eg, β-blocker, calcium channel blocker, digoxin)
		• Primary ANS failure (eg, Parkinson disease, Shy-Drager syndrome)
		• Secondary ANS failure (eg, diabetes mellitus, HIV, renal failure, collagen vascular disease)
Neurologic	10%-15%	• Vertebrobasilar TIA or stroke
		• Rare: SAH, migraine
Unknown	15%-25%	• (% after extended evaluation)

ANS, autonomic nervous system; AVB, atrioventricular block; HIV, human immunodeficiency virus; MI, myocardial infarction; PE, pulmonary embolus; PPH, primary pulmonary hypertension; SAH, subarachnoid hemorrhage; SSS, sick sinus syndrome (tachy-brady syndrome); SVT, supraventricular tachycardia; VT, ventricular tachycardia.

exacerbated by deconditioning. It is manifested by a pathologic excess of venous pooling, tachycardia (in which HR increases by 30 beats/min, or up to 120 beats/min with standing) and hemodynamic instability in response to the venous pooling. It may be associated with chronic fatigue syndrome.

In addition to drug-induced OH, two predominant forms of OH in the elderly include classical OH and delayed OH. In classical OH, chronic ANS failure impairs sympathetic vasoconstriction leading to low systemic vascular resistance in an orthostatic challenge. In delayed OH, a decline in venous return is coupled with inappropriately low cardiac output and impaired vasoconstriction, leading to syncope.

■ PHYSICAL EXAMINATION

Initial physical examination should focus on vital signs, including orthostatic assessment, and thorough cardiac and neurologic evaluations. Orthostatic vital signs are especially helpful in the evaluation of syncope though are infrequently documented (<40% of patients admitted with syncope), but can identify up to 20% of syncope etiology.

CLINICAL DIAGNOSIS AND RISK STRATIFICATION: ECG AND OTHER TESTING

Key historical features and physical examination should guide appropriate diagnostic direction (Table 101-4). The history and physical examination aid with rapid recognition of life-threatening etiologies and are critical for clinicians to make appropriate decisions regarding discharge versus further triage and management.

■ SIGNIFICANCE OF THE ECG

The electrocardiogram (ECG) contributes to the initial triage and risk stratification in syncope and should be obtained in all patients. Up to 50% of patients presenting with syncope have an abnormal ECG, though it is diagnostic in only about 5% of patients. An ECG can help diagnose ischemia, atrioventricular conduction abnormalities, pre-excitation (ie, Wolff-Parkinson-White), Brugada syndrome, long QT syndrome, and arrhythmogenic right ventricular cardiomyopathy. Findings considered *diagnostic* of syncope at the time of an event include high-grade AV block, symptomatic sinus bradycardia, sinoatrial exit block, alternating RBBB and LBBB, rapid paroxysmal supraventricular and ventricular tachycardia, sinus pause greater than 3 seconds, and pacemaker malfunction.

ECG is an important risk stratification tool. In the setting of syncope, an abnormal ECG, history of ventricular tachycardia, history of heart failure, and age greater than or equal to 65 years old are each clinical predictors of death within 1 year. Patients without any of these risk factors have less than 1% risk of death or ventricular arrhythmia at 1 year; compared to a more than 10% risk in those with two or more risk factors present. A history suggestive of a benign syncopal etiology and a normal ECG can help to identify low-risk patients who may be safe to discharge from an ED or hospital early in the evaluation process.

■ RISK STRATIFICATION

Several risk stratification algorithms or "rules" have undergone prospective validation and can be used to identify short-term or longer-term risk (**Table 101-5**). Two in particular, the San Francisco Syncope Rule (SFSR) and the Risk Stratification of Syncope in the Emergency Department (ROSE) study examined large cohorts prospectively. Both these scoring systems have high sensitivity though lack specificity and thus only have high negative predictive value within the syncope population. These tools can help clinicians stratify patients for possible early discharge from the ED or hospital versus continued evaluation based on estimated risk of adverse outcome.

TABLE 101-3 Major Causes of Syncope, Suggestive Clinical Features, and Relevant Further Testing

Pathophysiologic Mechanism	Subtypes/Specific Etiology	Examples	Suggestive Clinical/ Historical Features	Further Diagnostic Testing to Consider
1. Reflex Syncope (vasodepressor or cardio-inhibitory)	Vasovagal, from a stress on the orthostatic regulatory system	Emotional hyperactivity, pain, fear of blood	Precipitating event; nausea, diaphoresis, palpitation, bowel or bladder incontinence prior to attack; eyewitness account; abdominal discomfort; postprandial; recurrent nature	ECG Stress test or echocardiogram if history of cardiac disease. If negative, no further testing is needed
	Carotid sinus hypersensitivity/ syndrome		Neck movement; shoulder pain; age >40 y; neck tumor, syncope during shaving, due to tight shirt collars	Carotid sinus massage
	Situational	Valsalva due to cough, micturition, defacation, vomiting	See examples	None, if heart disease reasonably excluded
2. Orthostatic Hypotension	Primary ANF	Shy-Drager, Lewy body dementia, multisystem atrophy	History of neurologic disease	Orthostatic challenge
	Secondary ANF	Diabetes, uremia, spinal cord transection/injury, amyloidosis, HIV disease	History of diabetes, HIV, rheumatologic, oncologic or neurologic disease	Orthostatic challenge Neurologic testing to establish Dx, as needed
	Drug-induced OH	EtOH, diuretics, TCAs, SSRIs, vasodilators	Thorough medication review, including temporal relationship to fall	Orthostatic challenge
	Volume depletion	Hemorrhage, diarrhea, emesis, iatrogenic	Postural change; timing of standing to falling; prolonged standing; recent alpha-blocker or diuretic	Orthostatic challenge, volume challenge and retest
	Venous pooling	Postprandial, venous insufficiency	History of timing of syncope; varicosities or peripheral edema on examination	Orthostatic challenge
3. Cardiovascular Syncope A. Bradyarrhythmia B. Tachyarrhythmia	Arrhythmia	Bradyarrhythmia: SSS, AV conduction disease, pacer malfunction Tachyarrhythmia: Atrial: SVT, Afib, MAT, WPW Ventricular: VTach, torsades, ICD malfunction	Family history of SCD, congenital heart disease such as channelopathy; QT-prolonging agents; palpitations; antiarrhythmic; ECG findings such as bifascicular block, AV conduction abnormality, sinoatrial block or inappropriate bradycardia, VT, WPW, LQTS, Brugada pattern, ARVC pattern, Q waves suggestive of MI. VT classically will have no prodrome	ECG, telemetry, outpatient monitoring (Holter, ILR), EP study
	Structural cause A. Valvular B. Subvalvular C. Pump Failure	Valvular: AS, MR Subvalvular: HOCM, atrial myxoma Pump failure: ischemic CM (acute MI), DCM, restrictive CM, constrictive CM, tamponade	Exertional syncope; angina; palpitations; Q wave suggestive of MI	Echo, stress test
	Pulmonary vascular cause	Pulmonary HTN, PE, dissection	Exertional syncope; dyspnea; pleuritic CP, tearing CP	Echo, ECG, diagnostic cath if indicated, CT chest if indicated

Afib, atrial fibrillation; ANF, autonomic nervous system failure; ARVC, arrhythmogenic right ventricular cardiomyopathy; AS, aortic stenosis; AV, atrioventricular; CM, cardiomyopathy; CP, chest pain; CT, computed tomography; DCM, dilated cardiomyopathy; Dx, diagnosis; ECG, electrocardiogram; EP, electrophysiology; EtOH, alcohol; HIV, human immunodeficiency virus; HOCM, hypertrophic obstructive cardiomyopathy; HTN, hypertension; ICD, implantable cardioverter-defibrillator; ILR, implantable loop recorder; LQTS, long QT syndrome; MAT, multifocal atrial tachycardia; MI, myocardial infarction; MR, mitral regurgitation; PE, pulmonary embolus; SCD, sudden cardiac death; SSRIs, selective serotonin reuptake inhibitors; SSS, sick sinus syndrome; SVT, supraventricular tachycardia; TCAs, tricyclic antidepressants; VT, ventricular tachycardia; WPW, Wolff-Parkinson-White syndrome.

TABLE 101-4 Key Historical Points in the Evaluation of Syncope

Clinical Feature	Suggestive Syncope Etiology
History	
Sudden standing or sitting	Orthostatic hypotension
Prodrome: palpitations, lightheadedness, anxiety, sweating, piloerection, nausea, warmth	Vasovagal
Severe pain, fear, instrumentation	Vasovagal or (if structural heart disease present) Adrenergic-mediated Dysrhythmia
Situation: micturition, defecation, coughing	Vasomotor
During or immediately following exertion	Cardiogenic
Chest pain, shortness of breath	Cardiopulmonary
Focal neurologic symptoms: headache, diplopia, dysarthria, weakness	Neurologic (eg, ICH, vertebrobasilar ischemia)
Tonic-clonic activity, lateral tongue biting	Seizure
Prolonged postsyncope symptoms (eg, confusion) and prolonged duration of recovery (>few minutes)	Seizure
Poor oral intake, dehydration, GI bleed symptoms	Hypovolemia
Injury from fall	
Family history of sudden death or arrhythmia	Ventricular arrhythmia
Past Medical History	
Prior syncopal episodes: number, frequency, and surrounding history	
Coronary heart disease, heart failure, arrhythmias	
Psychiatric disease	
CVA, TIA	
Pulmonary hypertension	
Medications or Drugs	
Antihypertensives, antianginals, antidepressants, QT-prolonging drugs, CNS depressants (eg, opioids, sedatives), others (vincristine, digoxin, insulin, marijuana, alcohol, cocaine)	

CNS, central nervous system; CVA, cerebrovascular accident; GI, gastrointestinal; ICH, intracranial hemorrhage; TIA, transient ischemic attack.

■ FURTHER EVALUATION IN THE HOSPITALIZED PATIENT

Reasons for hospital admission include suspicion of a cardiac or neurologic cause of syncope, frequent or recurrent symptoms, and/or documented injury or high estimated risk for injury. Clinicians should strongly consider hospital admission and evaluation of syncope patients with structural heart disease, those with ECG or clinical findings suggestive of syncope due to arrhythmia or ischemia, and those with important comorbidities such as electrolyte alterations or significant/symptomatic anemia.

Syncope guidelines suggest clinical criteria for admission of patients presenting with syncope (**Table 101-6**).

■ INPATIENT ADMISSION VERSUS OBSERVATION ADMISSION

Patients with syncope often are admitted under observation status unless there is a clear etiology identified or significant risk of bodily injury, recurrent syncope, or high mortality risk. Average length of hospital stay is 3 days or less.

Figure 101-2 outlines a proposed algorithm for initial hospital evaluation of the patient and provides direction for further consultation and testing. In the patient without a clear cause of syncope, if historical features suggest a vasovagal cause or suspicion is low for cardiogenic syncope, the patient can be safely discharged with close follow-up.

■ OTHER INPATIENT TESTING

Additional testing considerations for inpatients and outpatients presenting with syncope are outlined in **Table 101-7**.

Telemetry monitoring

Although telemetry (inpatient continuous electrocardiographic monitoring) has been shown to have a poor diagnostic yield (1%-16%) in the setting of syncope, it should be employed for patients with a high pretest probability of arrhythmia. Telemetry monitoring during a hospitalization for syncope only occasionally identifies arrhythmia as syncope etiology, but may help document absence of arrhythmia during symptoms or a witnessed syncopal event.

Echocardiography and cardiac imaging

While seldom diagnostic of syncope in the absence of severe aortic stenosis, atrial myxoma, or cardiac tamponade, echocardiography is a valuable tool in assessing cardiac structure and function. The echocardiogram can rapidly identify structural abnormalities including left ventricular dysfunction, hypertrophic cardiomyopathy with or without outflow obstruction, right ventricular dysfunction in the setting of pulmonary embolism or pulmonary hypertension, and pericardial effusions or thickening in the setting of constrictive cardiomyopathy or cardiac tamponade.

In a patient with an unexplained syncope, an abnormal ECG, or a history of cardiac disease, an echocardiogram can help risk stratify patients by systolic function and can help identify a subset of patients who may benefit from implantable cardioverter-defibrillator (ICD) placement for the primary prevention of sudden cardiac death (SCD). However, one study showed that *patients with an unremarkable cardiac history and normal ECG* do not benefit from echocardiography in the evaluation of syncope.

The use of computed tomography, magnetic resonance imaging, and transesophageal echocardiography is limited to more

TABLE 101-5 Risk Stratification of Syncope Patients at Initial Evaluation Based on Prospective Cohort Studies

Study	Risk Factor	Score	End Points	Results
San Francisco Syncope Rule	• Abnormal ECG • CHF • SOB • Hematocrit < 30% • SBP < 90 mm Hg	No risk = 0 items Risk = ≥1 item	**7-d** serious events	Validation cohort: Sensitivity: 86%, Specificity 49% LR(+) 1.7, LR(−) 0.28
ROSE Score (BRACES)	• BNP level ≥ 300 pg/mL • Bradycardia ≤ 50 in Emergency Department or prehospital • Rectal examination showing fecal occult blood (if suspicion of gastrointestinal bleed) • Anemia—hemoglobin ≤90 g/L • Chest pain associated with syncope • ECG showing Q-wave (not in lead III) • Saturation ≤ 94% on room air	No risk = 0 items Risk = ≥1 item	**1-mo** serious outcome or all cause death	Sensitivity: 90% Specificity: 70% NPV: 98% LR (+): 3.0, LR (−) 0.15
Martin study	• Abnormal ECG • History of ventricular arrhythmia • History of CHF • Age >45 y	0-4 (1 point each item)	**1-y** severe arrhythmias or death	Score 0: 0% Score 1: 5% Score 2: 16% Score 3 or 4: 27%
OESIL Score	• Abnormal ECG • History of cardiovascular disease • Lack of prodrome • Age >65 y	0-4 (1 point each item)	**1-y** mortality	Score 0: 0% Score 1: 0.6% Score 2: 14% Score 3: 29% Score 4: 53%
EGYSIS Score	• Palpitations before syncope (+4) • Abnormal ECG and/or heart disease (+3) • Syncope while supine (+2) • Autonomic prodrome (−1) • Predisposing and/or precipitating factors (−1)	Sum of + and − points	**2-y** mortality	<3: 2% ≥3: 21%

BNP, beta natriuretic peptide; CHF, congestive heart failure; ECG, electrocardiogram; LR, likelihood ratio; NPV, negative predictive value; SBP, systolic blood pressure; SOB, shortness of breath.

TABLE 101-6 Indications for Hospital Admission in Syncope

Hospital Admission Indicated

- History, physical examination, or ECG suggestive of:
  a. Cardiac disease (eg, CAD/ischemia, CHF, arrhythmia, valvular disease, prolonged QT) or,
  b. Neurologic disease

Hospital Admission Possibly Indicated

- History suggesting:
  a. Sudden LOC with injury and no prodrome (may suggest ventricular tachycardia)
  b. Exertional syncope (may suggest HOCM or exertion induced high grade atrioventricular [AV] block)
  c. Medications likely to prolong QT (may increase risk for torsades de pointes)
  d. Frequent unexplained episodes
  e. Older age
- Physical Examination suggesting:
- Moderate to severe orthostatic hypotension

BBB, bundle branch block; CAD, coronary artery disease; CHF, chronic heart failure; CVA, cerebrovascular accident; ECG, electrocardiogram; HOCM, hypertrophic obstructive cardiomyopathy; LOC, loss of consciousness.

specific situations, such as in the evaluation of aortic dissection, cardiac masses seen on transthoracic echocardiography, pulmonary embolism, diseases of the pericardium/myocardium predisposing to restrictive/constrictive cardiomyopathy, and congenital coronary artery anomalies.

Cardiac enzymes

Cardiac enzymes have relatively low yield if ordered in unselected patients presenting with syncope, and can lead to additional significant health care costs with the average cost effectiveness of indiscriminate screening >$22,000 per diagnosis. However, at least one retrospective study suggested that up to 7% of patients with syncope and without chest pain had acute coronary syndrome as the etiology of the syncope. Given their relative low yield, it is important to reserve cardiac enzymes for those patients with intermediate to high pretest probability of coronary disease.

Exercise stress testing

While exercise testing for syncope evaluation has very low diagnostic yield, such testing can provide value when ordered for specific indications (**Table 101-8**). The 2006 ACC/AHA guidelines on syncope management recommend exercise testing in patients with history of coronary artery disease, after echocardiography has

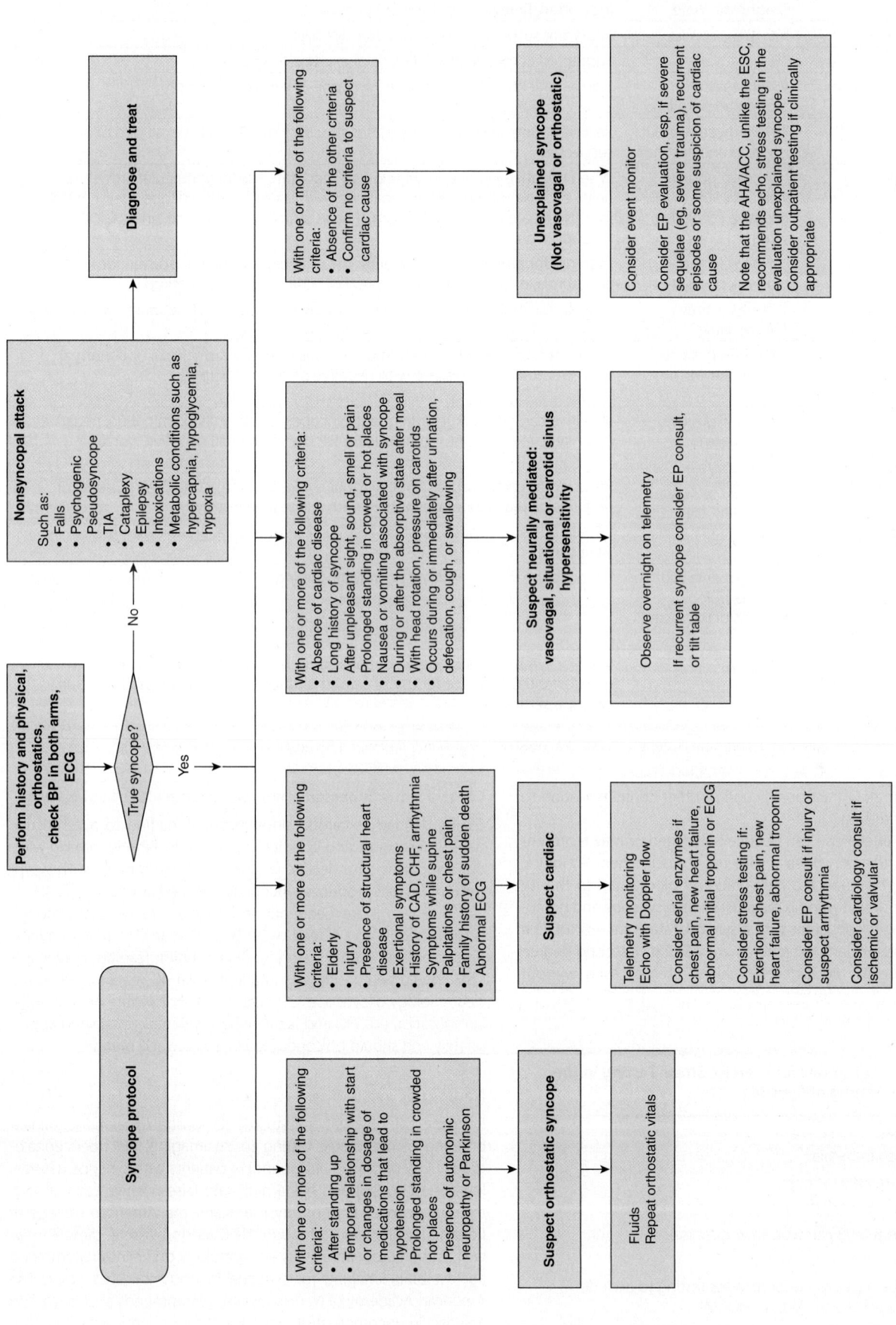

Figure 101-2 *Overview of syncope evaluation.* CAD, coronary artery disease; CHF, chronic heart failure; ECG, electrocardiogram; EP, electrophysiology; TIA, transient ischemic attack.

TABLE 101-7 Diagnostic Testing Modalities in Syncope and Estimated Yield

Test	Diagnostic Yield	Indication/Relevant Etiology of Syncope
Echocardiography	5%-10%	Known or suspected structural heart disease
Exercise stress test	1%	Suspected coronary artery disease or exertional syncope
Carotid sinus massage	45% in selected monitored population	Elderly patients with unexplained syncope or suggestive history
Tilt-table testing	49% in those without isoproterenol testing	Recurrent unexplained syncope after structural heart disease excluded or not suspected
Signal-averaged ECG	Unknown positive yield, but 90% negative predictive value	When negative in patients with low to moderate risk for ventricular arrhythmia, helps exclude this condition in patients with unexplained syncope. Ideal candidates for this test are patients with normal heart structurally, but who unexplained syncope without a prodrome
Electrophysiological study	60% in selected high-risk population	High risk for arrhythmia (frail, elderly, risk of injury/fall), high suspicion for arrhythmia, or structural heart disease with negative initial workup
Holter monitoring (test duration: 24-72 h)	19% (4% positive, 15% negative)	High suspicion for frequent arrhythmia, abnormal ECG, or structural heart disease
External loop recorder (test duration: 3-4 wk, or up to 2-3 mo)	34% (13% positive, 21% negative)	Frequent syncope (>1 episode/mo) with suspicion for arrhythmia or abnormal ECG/structural heart disease with negative cardiac workup
Implantable loop recorder (ILR, test duration: up to 36 mo)	59% (27% positive, 32% negative)	Negative cardiac workup, infrequent syncope, negative tilt examination, negative psychiatric examination. Some role for ILR use after initial negative workup
Psychiatric evaluation	21%	Recurrent unexplained syncope without evidence of structural heart disease or negative cardiac workup, especially with suggestive history
Electroencephalogram (EEG)	1%-2%	Witnessed seizure, postictal state, history of seizure, focal neurologic signs or symptoms
Head computed tomography (CT)	4% in patients with focal neurologic findings or witnessed seizure	History of head trauma, focal neurologic findings, or history consistent with seizure
Neurovascular imaging studies (eg, carotid ultrasound)	Unknown	Signs or symptoms suggestive of transient ischemic attack/stroke; at present no substantial evidence for use of carotid ultrasound or transcranial Doppler in syncope setting

Modified and reproduced, with permission, from Fuster V, O'Rourke RA, Walsh RA, et al. *Hurst's the Heart*. 12th ed. New York: McGraw-Hill; 2008. Table 48-5.

assessed for outflow tract obstruction or other contraindication to exercise stress testing.

Syncope after exercise can be reflex mediated or may represent underlying conduction disease with risk for permanent AV block, as tachycardia can induce a high-grade AV block distal to the AV node. Exercise stress testing is diagnostic when syncope and hemodynamic changes consistent with a syncopal state are reproduced and documented during exercise or when Mobitz II second degree or third degree AV block develop during exercise even without syncope.

TABLE 101-8 Indications for Exercise Stress Testing in the Setting of Syncope

- **Indications**
  1. Suspected ischemia
  2. Exertion-related syncope
  3. Exertion-induced tachyarrhythmias
  4. AVB w/BBB (AVB can worsen w/exercise)
- **Yield:** 1%
- Echo may be necessary prior to stress testing to exclude structural heart disease (eg, AS, HOCM)

AVB, atrioventricular block; AS, aortic stenosis; BBB, bundle branch block; HOCM, hypertrophic cardiomyopathy.

Carotid sinus hypersensitivity/syndrome (CSH/CSS) testing

CSH is defined as carotid sinus massage leading to a ventricular pause >3 seconds and/or a decline in systolic BP ≥50 mm Hg without symptoms (or a decline in systolic BP ≥30 mm Hg with symptoms). CSH that produces syncope is classified as CSS.

CSS occurs more frequently in patients >40 years old though is most frequent in elderly patients (>70 years). As many patients do not present with a history of neck rotation leading to syncope, CSM should be considered in patients over 40 years old without a clear etiology of syncope. CSM carries a very low rate of neurologic complication (<0.3%) and is safe when patients are selected appropriately and should be conducted in a structured manner.

Neurologic evaluation

Retrospective observational studies demonstrate that indiscriminate ordering of neurologic testing (brain imaging, electroencephalogram [EEG], or carotid ultrasound) in patients with syncope has very low yield (1%-2%) and has a high rate false-positive tests. In fact, the American College of Physicians and the American College of Emergency Physicians (through the Choosing Wisely® campaign) as well as the European Society of Cardiology guidelines recommend against brain imaging for syncope in uncomplicated cases. The American Academy of Neurology also recommends against carotid imaging in uncomplicated syncope without neurologic symptoms. Neurologic studies should be reserved for patients with neurologic symptoms and/or signs.

Neurologic causes of syncope are rare and a more thorough evaluation should be pursued if the initial assessment is suggestive of such an etiology. Dysautonomia can lead to autonomic nervous system failure in the elderly and should be evaluated as part of the orthostatic hypotension workup (Table 101-3).

Trauma and elevated intracranial pressure

While head trauma and conditions predisposing to increased intracranial pressure (eg, subarachnoid hemorrhage and intracranial neoplasm) can cause transient loss of consciousness, the patient's history and physical exam will generally identify neurologic findings.

Cerebrovascular event

Cerebrovascular disorders can rarely lead to syncope. Subclavian "steal" phenomenon is seen when there is retrograde blood flow in a vertebral artery in the setting of a proximally stenosed left subclavian artery and can lead to syncope or other symptoms of posterior cerebral ischemia during asymmetric arm exercise. A transient ischemia attack (TIA) or stroke of the carotid artery or anterior cerebral circulation does not cause transient loss of consciousness. However, cerebral ischemia of the vertebrobasilar circulation can lead to syncope.

Seizure

Up to 10% of all events described as syncope may be due to seizures. Some cases of syncope are misdiagnosed as seizure because cerebral hypoxia from any cause can lead to myoclonic jerking motions or involuntary movement. History is the most useful tool in distinguishing seizure from true syncope; seizure is more likely if an aura phenomenon is described preceding the event, classic automatisms are involved, postrecovery myalgia and fatigue are seen. Importantly, a postictal, prolonged (usually >1 minute) recovery state is suggestive of seizure rather than syncope. If seizure is suspected or if there is a provoked attack resulting in a suspected case of psychogenic pseudosyncope or pseudoseizure, an electroencephalogram is an important diagnostic tool. When syncope is the most likely cause, an EEG is usually inappropriate, because interictal EEGs are often normal and cannot rule out seizure.

■ ADDITIONAL OUTPATIENT TESTING FOR SYNCOPE

Syncope that is recurrent or which is not considered life threatening after 24 to 48 hours of inpatient monitoring can be evaluated safely in an outpatient setting.

Electrophysiology study

Electrophysiology (EP) studies evaluate cardiac conduction and can be helpful in assessing the function of the AV node and for ventricular or supraventricular arrhythmias. EP studies can identify intermittent significant AV nodal block in patients at risk (eg, bifascicular block on ECG). In patients with structurally abnormal hearts or those with other symptoms, signs, or testing to suggest ventricular arrhythmia risk, an EP study can help identify inducible ventricular arrhythmias. EP studies may also identify supraventricular tachyarrhythmias though this is most often only implored in the setting of invasive catheter-based therapy for supraventricular tachyarrhythmias.

Head-up tilt-table testing

Head-up tilt-table testing (HUTT) is most useful in patients with *recurrent* episodes in which reflex syncope is suspected. Unless there are occupational hazards or a high risk of injury associated with syncope, testing for a single or rare event is not indicated. HUTT may help distinguish syncope from epilepsy or to help identify the cause of syncope in the elderly with multiple falls. As reflex syncope can be

situational, the diagnostic utility can be limited. For reflex syncope, a positive study induces transient loss of consciousness in the setting of a vasodepressor and/or cardioinhibitory response. Additionally, the HUTT can be helpful in diagnosing dysautonomia and postural orthostatic tachycardia syndrome. Some protocols use provocative agents (eg, isoproterenol or nitroglycerin) to decrease vascular tone or increase heart rate. These agents increase sensitivity but reduce specificity and reproducibility.

Holter monitoring, external loop recorders and implantable loop recorders

Short-term or long-term electrocardiographic monitoring can help establish the diagnosis of arrhythmia as the cause of syncope or help in ruling out arrhythmia. In the patient whose syncope is not life threatening and in whom a definitive diagnosis has not been established, outpatient telemetry via Holter monitoring or loop recorders should be considered. In general, Holter recordings are most useful in patients with daily symptoms of lightheadedness or palpitations, whereas loop recorders are indicated for patients with less frequent symptoms.

Holter monitoring

Holter monitoring provides 24 to 72 hours of continuous ECG monitoring via surface electrodes at a cost of roughly $1000 per device and associated servicing costs. The yield for a diagnosis of syncope is from 1% to 4% and negative yield (ie, patients in whom an arrhythmia was not detected during a syncopal event, effectively ruling out arrhythmia) is near 15%. Holter monitoring carries a very high cost-per-diagnosis ratio due to the infrequency of arrhythmia in most patients with syncope of unknown etiology.

External loop recorder

An external loop recorder, also a portable system with cutaneous electrodes, can be used to retrieve data generated over 3 to 4 weeks and up to 2 to 3 months. External loop recorder continually store and delete ECG data. The patient is able to manually activate the recorder in the setting of symptoms and 5 to 15 minutes of preactivation ECG data is stored for analysis. From prospective studies, the positive yield to achieve diagnosis is approximately 15% to 25%, and the negative yield is approximately 20%, giving this modality also a high cost-per-diagnosis ratio. Patient compliance beyond 3 weeks is unusual and further limits the usefulness of this test.

Implantable loop recorders

Implantable loop recorders (ILRs) can provide ECG data up to 36 months and obtain higher diagnostic yield per device than other recording modalities such as the Holter monitor. Implantable loop recorders can have a diagnostic yield of 90% in patients with syncope of unknown etiology though they have a high initial cost more than $10,000. Newer implantable loop recorders are small and can be implanted subcutaneously as an office-based procedure with experienced providers.

Syncope in the patient with psychiatric illness

Antipsychotic medications and side effects from chronic use can lead to orthostatic hypotension and/or QT prolongation. Important medications to consider in syncope etiology include benzodiazepines, antidepressants (specifically SSRIs, tricyclics, and MAOIs), barbiturates, and neuroleptics, as well as drugs of abuse such as ethanol.

Pseudosyncope is believed to be a functional disorder which results in involuntary T-LOC. Patients often suffer T-LOC though show no signs of seizure during the attack, have a normal EEG, and have normal hemodynamics during a tilt table test. In pseudosyncope, history usually does not identify a trigger to the event. Attacks occur frequently and can last for several minutes—in contrast to only several seconds of T-LOC seen in true syncope. Psychiatric evaluation is indicated and can be valuable in patients with recurrent syncope without injury or when an exhaustive workup has not yielded a certain diagnosis.

■ SPECIAL CASE: RECURRENT SYNCOPE

Regardless of etiology, syncope recurs in 30% to 40% of patients followed for 3 years after the diagnosis. In patients with vasovagal syncope, prognosis is generally excellent. While age is not predictive of future risk of recurrence, shortened time to recurrence after diagnosis and number of previous syncopal episodes increase recurrence risk. Recurrent syncope does not confer a higher mortality risk than an isolated syncopal episode, but injury morbidity with recurrent episodes may impose restrictions on patient's quality of life.

■ SPECIAL CASE: ELDERLY PATIENTS WITH SYNCOPE

Elderly patients often have coexistence of many predisposing medical conditions that can lead to syncope. Common causes in the elderly population include orthostatic hypotension, reflex syncope, carotid sinus syndrome, and arrhythmias. Syncope of cardiac origin carries a similar mortality risk in both young and old.

As in all patients, a detailed but focused history and physical examination can yield a diagnosis in many initial evaluations. A comprehensive medication history focusing on temporal relationships between the falls/syncope and initiation of new medications or dosing changes is critical, as is consideration of changing drug levels due to dynamic renal or hepatic function. Any associated comorbidities such as deconditioning, dependence for activities of daily living, cognitive impairment, and performance status can also increase risk. A focused neurologic examination should be complemented by assessment of gait instability, orthostatic challenge, and balance. *Routine carotid sinus massage* (**Figure 101-3**) (when no contraindications) is recommended for elderly patients presenting with syncope in addition to the thorough initial assessment as used for younger patients.

PRACTICE POINT

- A high-yield approach at initial evaluation involves a thorough history; medication review; physical examination focused on postural blood pressure measurement, cardiac, and neurologic examinations; and electrocardiogram. Risk stratification should be carried out on initial evaluation in accordance with well-validated risk-scoring tools. In those with an unclear etiology, further testing should be done with a focus on efficiency and high-yield tools.

TREATMENT AND PRIMARY PREVENTION OF SYNCOPE

■ TREATMENT OVERVIEW

Treatment of syncope is directed at the underlying disorder causing the episode. Detailed discussion of those therapies is beyond the scope of this chapter; however, some generic principles are relevant to inpatient practice. Irrespective of establishing an etiology for syncope, the primary goals in the treatment of syncope are to reduce the risk of injury/trauma, improve survival, and evaluate and prevent recurrent syncopal events. Treatment is aimed at an underlying cause if one can be identified (**Figure 101-4**).

■ REFLEX SYNCOPE, AUTONOMIC DYSFUNCTION, AND ORTHOSTATIC HYPOTENSION/INTOLERANCE

In reflex/vasovagal syncope or autonomic dysfunction and consequent orthostatic hypotension, the aim is to prevent syncope recurrence and limit risk of bodily injury or harm to the patient. Treatment of reflex syncope includes patient education, reassurance, and avoidance of triggers. Recognition of triggers and recognition of a prodrome warning period, such as nausea, lightheadedness, and sense of impending fall or loss of balance can help abort a syncopal event.

Physical counter-pressure maneuvers (PCMS) to increase venous return can be instituted with success if done in a timely manner during prodrome or trigger recognition. These maneuvers involve causing a rapid increase in systolic and diastolic blood pressure through the timely initiation of either gluteal muscle tightening with concomitant leg crossing or arm tensing through interlocking handgrip and isometric contraction. In a multicenter, prospective trial, the burden of recurrent syncope enjoyed a relative risk reduction of near 40% when comparing patients who had received physical counterpressure maneuver training with those who did not.

Pharmacologic therapy for prevention and treatment of reflex syncope address peripheral vasoconstriction, volume expansion, prevention of paradoxical bradycardia and excess vagal activity, and treatment of anxiety (**Table 101-9**). No randomized controlled trial evidence establishes benefit of these therapies, and none of the medications commonly used for reflex syncope has Food and Drug Administration approval for this indication.

Treatment of orthostatic hypotension and intolerance should first seek to employ nonpharmacologic measures. Patients should change posture slowly, increase fluid and salt intake to 3 L and up to 10 g sodium per day if supine hypertension is not a comorbid illness, seek adjustment of antihypertensives with physician guidance, and avoid excessive durations of recumbency and sleep, while maintaining the head of the bed at 10° to 20°. Avoiding the rapid ingestion of cold water, limiting the size of meals and carbohydrate intake, and avoidance of alcohol help reduce postprandial hypotension. The use of tight lower-extremity elastic stockings and occasionally abdominal binders can help maintain venous return while standing. Finally, as in reflex syncope, all patients should be counseled on anticipatory physical counterpressure maneuvers. Pharmacologic measures for OH treatment are aimed at expanding central volume, improving vasoconstriction, and mitigating various factors such as anemia, nocturnal diuresis, and poor sympathetic tone (Table 101-9).

■ ARRHYTHMIAS

Specific to the nature of the arrhythmia, treatment of syncope due to arrhythmia varies from medication discontinuation to cardiac pacemaker or implanted cardioverter-defibrillator placement and even radiofrequency catheter ablation. See Chapter 132 (Supraventricular Tachyarrhythmias), Chapter 133 (Bradyarrhythmias), and Chapter 134 (Ventricular Arrhythmias) for more detailed information about treatment of related specific diagnoses that may lead to syncope. See Chapter 136 (Pacemakers, Defibrillators, and Cardiac Resynchronization Devices) for specific information regarding indications for those devices in relationship to syncope or arrhythmias.

Implanted pacemakers or ICDs can be associated with syncope. When suspected, device interrogation by a device specialist or trained cardiologist is helpful. In the setting of generator battery depletion or lead failure, device replacement is effective. ICDs may rarely be associated with syncope if the patient suffers an arrhythmia and loss of consciousness outside of the specific treatment thresholds set for the device. For example, a patient with ventricular tachycardia may suffer loss of consciousness before appropriate therapy if delivered. Reprogramming and/or the addition of antiarrhythmic medications may be necessary in this setting, in consultation with cardiology or electrophysiology specialists.

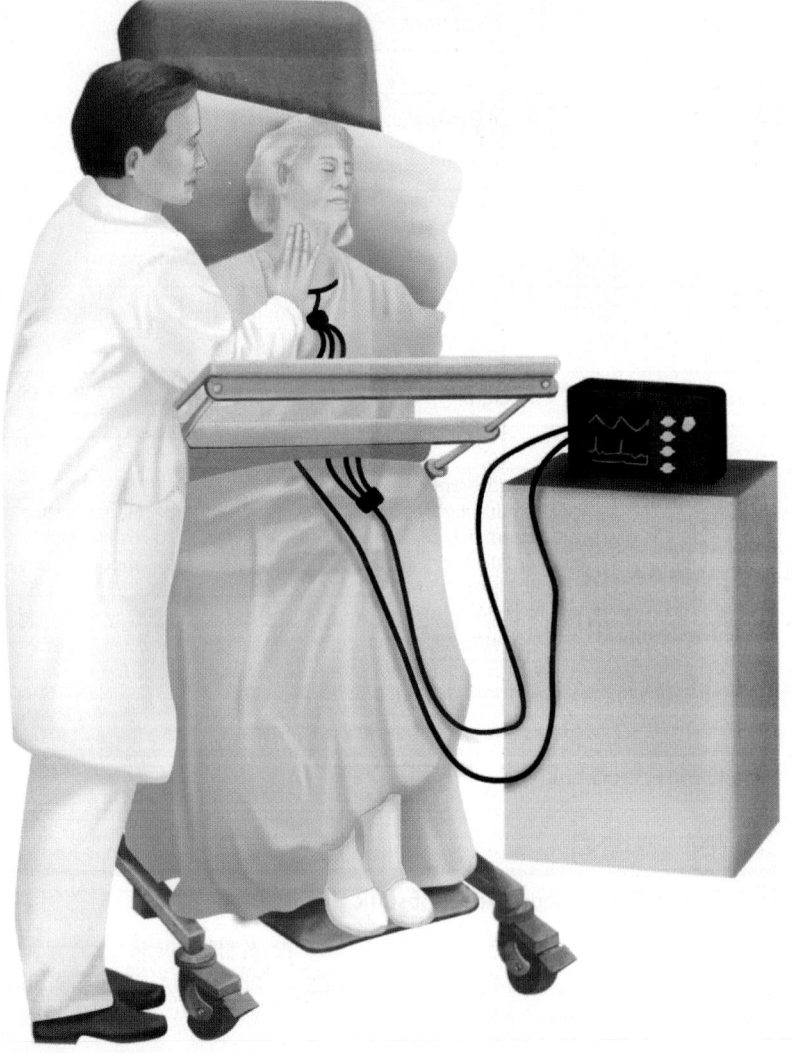

Figure 101-3 *Carotid sinus massage methodology.*

A. Contraindications: MI, TIA, or CVA in the past 3 months; history of VT or VF, or previous adverse reaction to carotid sinus massage (CSM).

B. Relative contraindications: carotid bruits require carotid ultrasound; if significant stenosis is present some recommend performing the CSM while the patient is supine. Others recommend against performing it.

C. With the patient supine (at least 5 minutes),

1. Record baseline ECG, SBP, DBP, HR.
2. Perform CSM on the right side while patient is supine. Another operator should record hemodynamic variable changes. Carotid sinus is located midway between the thyroid cartilage and angle of mandible; firm longitudinal massage on area of maximal carotid artery pulsation is carried out for at least 5 seconds.
3. During CSM for 5 seconds, the operator performing massage should indicate "CSM ON" and "CSM OFF" to indicate those time points on continuous ECG recording, done by the second operator.
4. Nadir SBP and DBP occur typically 15 seconds after stopping CSM. CSM should be discontinued if a sinus pause >3 seconds occurs. In the case of prolonged asystole, a precordial "thump" is advised.
5. Repeat the procedure in the left supine, right erect, and left erect, only after patient's HR has reached pre-CSM levels in each case. Upright position CSM has an additional 30% diagnostic yield.
6. If neurological complications arise, lay the patient supine, ensure BP is returned to baseline as soon as possible, give aspirin 325 mg if not contraindicated, and admit for observation.

CSM, carotid sinus massage; CVA, cerebrovascular accident; DBP, diastolic blood pressure; ECG, electrocardiogram; HR, heart rate; MI, myocardial infarction; SBP, systolic blood pressure; TIA, transient ischemic attach; VF, ventricular fibrillation; VT, ventricular tachycardia. (Reproduced, with permission, from Halter JB, Ouslander JG, Tinetti ME, et al. *Hazzard's Geriatric Medicine and Gerontology*, 6th ed. New York: McGraw-Hill; 2009. Fig. 57-4.)

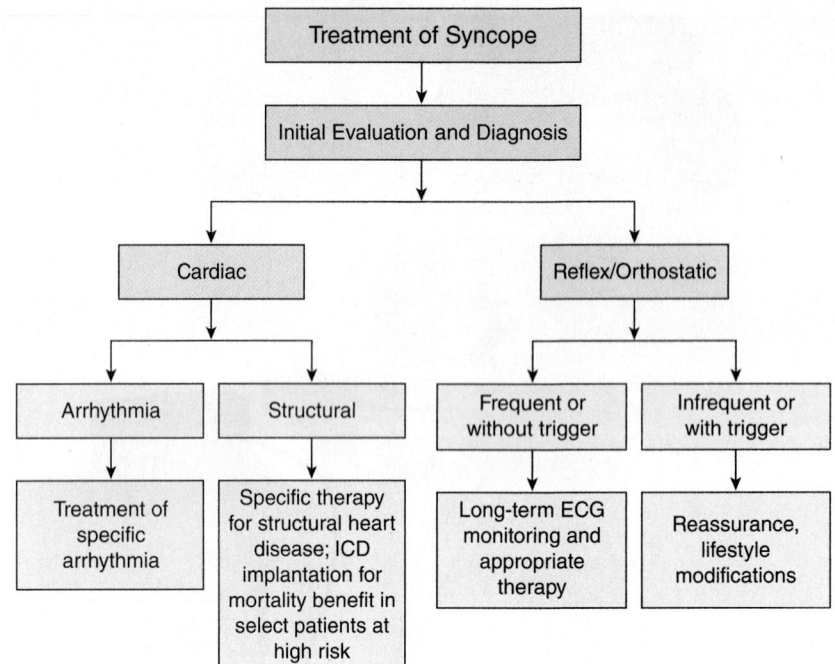

Figure 101-4 *Proposed inpatient algorithm for hospitalist management of syncope.*

TABLE 101-9 Selected Therapies for Reflex Syncope and Orthostatic Hypotension

Treatment	Application	Form Effective in				Problems
		NCS	PD	HA	OH	
Reconditioning	Aerobic exercise 20 min 3 times/wk	X	X	X	X	If done too vigorously may worsen symptoms
Physical maneuvers (tilt training, etc)	30 min 3 times per day	X				Noncompliance is common
Sleeping with head tilted upright	During sleep	X		X	X	
Hydration	2 L orally per day	X	X		X	Edema
Salt	2-4 g/d	X	X		X	Edema
Fludrocortisone	0.1-0.2 mg orally per day	X	X		X	Hypokalemia, hypomagnesemia, edema
Metoprolol	25-100 mg twice a day			X		Fatigue
Labetalol	100-200 mg orally twice a day			X		Fatigue
Midodrine	5-10 mg orally three times a day	X	X		X	Nausea, scalp itching, supine hypertension
Methylphenidate	5-10 mg orally three times a day	X	X	X		Anorexia, insomnia, dependency
Bupropion	150-300 mg XL every day		X	X	X	Tremor, agitation, insomnia
Clonidine	0.1-0.3 mg orally twice a day			X		Dry mouth, blurred vision
Pyridostigmine	30-60 mg orally per day		X		X	Nausea, diarrhea
SSRI-escitalopram	10 mg orally per day	X	X		X	Tremor, agitation, sexual problems
Erythropoietin	10,000-20,000 g subcutaneously every week	X	X		X	Pain at injection site, expensive
Octreotide	50-200 μgm SC three times a day		X	X	X	Nausea, diarrhea, gallstone
Permanent pacing		X				

HA, hyperadrenic postural orthostatic tachycardia syndrome; NCS, neurocardiogenic syncope; OH, orthostatic hypotension; PD, partial dysautonomia postural orthostatic tachycardia syndrome; SSRI, selective serotonin reuptake inhibitor.

STRUCTURAL HEART DISEASE MANAGEMENT

The primary aims in treating patients with structural heart disease are to identify the causative factor contributing to syncope and treat the primary process as well as to prevent sudden cardiac death. History is important as patients with underlying heart disease often have reflex and orthostatic syncope. Surgical therapy is indicated in the setting of syncope due to severe aortic stenosis or atrial myoxoma. Syncope in the setting of acute coronary syndrome, pulmonary embolism, or pericardial tamponade requires urgent condition-specific therapy. Patients with syncope due to underlying restrictive cardiomyopathy or severe pulmonary hypertension require symptomatic management which often cannot correct the underlying pathology. Syncope with hypertrophic cardiomyopathy requires arrhythmia specific therapy (often with medications) and consideration of an ICD for prevention of SCD. See Chapter 128 (Acute Coronary Syndromes), Chapter 130 (Myocarditis, Pericardial Disease, and Cardiac Tamponade), and Chapter 131 (Valvular Heart Disease) for management of specific related disorders that could lead to syncope.

Placement of an ICD has been established to prevent SCD in patients with (a) ischemic and nonischemic cardiomyopathy with severely reduced systolic function, (b) hypertrophic cardiomyopathy, (c) arrhythmogenic right ventricular cardiomyopathy, and (d) patients with primary electrical abnormalities (eg, long QT and Brugada syndromes).

CONSULTATION

Hospitalists should rely on their consultant colleagues when there is a therapeutic aim to address by the approached specialty. A particularly useful result of the frugal use of consultation is deciding with the consultant whether the patient needs further inpatient testing or treatment and whether outpatient follow-up is sufficient for an otherwise stable condition.

Inpatient cardiology consultation for diagnostic or therapeutic testing or interventions (eg, cardiac catheterization, tilt-table testing, carotid sinus massage, or electrophysiology study) may each be appropriate based on the clinical context of the syncope.

The routine use of neurologic testing in the initial evaluation of syncope in the absence of neurologic symptoms has poor diagnostic value and cost effectiveness. Presentation suggesting vertebrobasilar insufficiency may require neurology consultation, as would suspected seizure as etiology of unwitnessed syncope (especially if EEG or continuous EEG monitoring is believed indicated).

Consultation with a psychiatrist is indicated to identify psychosomatic conditions predisposing to syncope, such as conversion, somatoform, or factitious disorder. Establishing psychogenic pseudosyncope or another psychiatric diagnosis as syncope etiology may be useful in patients with recurrent symptomatic syncope who have undergone a thorough negative workup for cardiac, reflex, and orthostatic syncope as appropriate.

DISCHARGE PLANNING

Prior to discharge, patients should be educated on measures to prevent recurrent reflex syncope, recognition of prodromal symptoms, and warning signs that warrant emergency care. Of particular concern to patients is the fear of syncope recurrence while driving. Driving following a syncopal episode is regulated by individual states, and clinicians should refer to their specific state laws when making recommendations to patients, and clinicians should document clearly discussions with patients regarding driving following syncope. However, in general, private drivers usually have no restrictions on driving independent of those imposed by having an ICD according to current society guidelines. If, however, unexplained syncope occurs while driving and/or in the presence of structural heart disease, driving limitations may be necessary or legally required. For professional drivers, permanent restrictions may be recommended if an ICD has been implanted, occasional syncope occurs during high-risk activity, syncope is recurrent and severe and treatment has not been established, and in unexplained syncope if treatment has not been established. Long-term accident and insurance data indicate, reassuringly, that rates of vehicular accidents are no higher than in the general population without syncope. Timely follow-up with appropriate outpatient physicians (primary care physicians, cardiologists, neurologists, as indicated) should occur within 2 to 4 weeks of hospital discharge.

QUALITY IMPROVEMENT TO ADDRESS PERFORMANCE GAPS

One of the major areas of practice improvement related to syncope is resource utilization. Patients with syncope require a multidisciplinary approach in some cases and in other instances may be discharged safely from the emergency department or hospital with close follow-up.

In the United States, up to 1% of all ED patients present with syncope, with 32% admitted representing 2% of all ED admissions. This equates to >740,000 ED visits per year and >460,000 hospital admissions annually. With median cost of each US hospital admission for syncope of approximately $8700, it comes as no surprise that our annual expenditure for syncope is approximately $3.8 billion.

Hospitalists are keenly positioned to appreciate costs associated with syncope admissions and the benefits reaped by thoughtful resource utilization. Patients should be risk stratified using well-validated criteria, and further testing carried out to assess posthospital risk or injury and mortality. Early discharge from the ED or hospital should be considered in low-risk patients.

Testing should be limited to that necessary for immediate risk stratification and/or diagnosis confirmation or treatments of the syncopal event. In a retrospective analysis of costs associated with inpatient admission of syncope in elderly patients, researchers found that postural blood pressure recording (ie, orthostatics measurement) costs $17 per test affecting the diagnosis or management of a case of syncope. In contrast, the cost effectiveness of cardiac enzyme measurement was $22,397, head CT $24,881, ECG $1020, and telemetry $710 per clinically relevant finding affecting diagnosis or treatment (**Table 101-10**).

Three societies, The American College of Physicians (ACP), the American Academy of Neurology (AAN), and the American College of Emergency Physicians (ACEP) have identified overtesting in simple syncope as a key area of opportunity to reduce waste in health care, as part of the American Board of Internal Medicine (ABIM) Choosing Wisely® campaign. All three organizations suggest reduction of neurologic imaging in patients presenting with

TABLE 101-10 Test Value and Cost in Syncope Patients

Test	% Patients Receiving Test	% Patients Diagnosis Affected by Test	Cost per Diagnosis or Management
Postural BP	38%	26%	$17
EKG	99%	7%	$1020
Echo	39%	4%	$6272
Carotid U/S	13%	1%	$19,600
CV enzymes	95%	2%	$22,400
Head CT	63%	2%	$25,000
EEG	8%	1%	$33,000

"simple" syncope, where patients do not have focal or specific neurologic findings based on history or physical examination to suggest a neurologic etiology. The recommendations have a basis in clinical studies analyzing syncope testing patterns, diagnostic yields, and costs. Such studies consistently show low diagnostic impact at high cost if such tests are conducted indiscriminately in syncope patients. By following these recommendations, hospitalists can help reduce the unnecessary use of brain imaging and carotid imaging in patients presenting with syncope. Judicious use of testing will improve the diagnostic yield of tests ordered, without reducing the relevant diagnosis of neurologic etiologies of syncope. This practice is summarized in the UK's National Institute for Health and Clinical Excellence guidelines for transient loss of consciousness. Admission for the syncopal patient should not be unnecessarily prolonged. On the part of the hospitalist as coordinator of care, this may require earlier consultation with specialists to plan earlier testing, discharge, and follow-up. In prospective, randomized controlled trials incorporating strict adherence to syncope criteria for admission and utilization of Syncope Management Units (SMU) in the ED to triage syncope patients, there is a marked reduction of hospital length of stay, number of tests conducted per patient, and associated lower costs. SMUs involve staffing by ED physicians, cardiologists, and/or neurologists and ready access to echocardiogram, tilt testing, beat-to-beat blood pressure, and continuous telemetry monitoring for up to 6 hours with a decision reached to admit or discharge in that timeframe. Long-term follow-up to 2 years has shown no difference in morbidity and mortality in these patients. With careful selection, triage, and early discharge, hospitalists can make a lasting impact on the resources utilized in the management of syncope.

CONCLUSION

Syncope is characterized by sudden, transient, reversible loss of consciousness with prompt spontaneous recovery. Recurrent syncope can be distressing to the patient, carries a serious risk of bodily injury and harm, and can lead to significant lifestyle changes including loss of gainful employment. Diagnosis should occur in a timely, cost-efficient manner. At the time of discharge, the goal is to provide the patient with a reasonably confident estimate of prognosis, risk of recurrence, and goals and timing of further diagnostic studies and therapy.

A high-yield approach at initial evaluation involves a thorough history; medication review; physical examination focused on postural blood pressure measurement, cardiac, and neurologic examinations; and electrocardiogram. In those with an unclear etiology, further testing should focus on efficient and high-yield tools based on the thorough history and physical examination. Risk stratification should be carried out on initial evaluation in accordance with well-validated risk-scoring tools (Table 101-5).

Specific causes of syncope such as arrhythmias and structural cardiopulmonary disease should be quickly identified and treated in consultation with a specialist to expedite care as well as to establish adequate, timely follow-up after hospital discharge.

Finally, an area of active research in syncope is the use of SMUs, primarily in emergency departments. Success in Europe is the basis for ongoing investment of this concept in the United States. SMUs can help identify patients who would otherwise be deemed low risk by standardized triage protocols and discharged from the emergency department for rapid follow-up.

ACKNOWLEDGMENT

Special thanks to Robert Young, MD for his contributions to the first edition chapter.

SUGGESTED READINGS

Cooper PN, Westby M, Pitcher DW, Bullock I. Synopsis of the National Institute for Health and Clinical Excellence Guideline for management of transient loss of consciousness. *Ann Intern Med.* 2011;155:543-549.

Mendu ML, McAvay G, Lampert R, Stoehr J, Tinetti ME. Yield of diagnostic tests in evaluating syncopal episodes in older patients. *Arch Intern Med.* 2009;169(14):1299-1305.

Moya A, Sutton R, Ammirati F. Guidelines for the diagnosis and management of syncope (version 2009). The Task Force for the Diagnosis and Management of Syncope of the European Society of Cardiology (ESC). *European Heart Journal.* 2009;30:2631-2671.

Reed MJ, Newby DE, Coull AJ, Prescott RJ, Jacques KG, Gray AJ. The ROSE (Risk Stratification of Syncope in the Emergency Department) study. *J Am Coll Cardiol.* 2010;55:713-721.

Schnipper J, Kapoor W. Diagnostic evaluation and management of patients with syncope. *Med Clin N Amer.* 2001;85(2):423-456.

Serrano LA, Hess EP, Bellolio MF, et al. Accuracy and quality of clinical decision rules for syncope in the emergency department: a systematic review and meta-analysis. *Ann Emerg Med.* 2010;56:363-373.

Soteriades ES, Evans JC, Larson MG, et al. Incidence and prognosis of syncope. *N Engl J Med.* 2002;347:878-885.

Sun BC. Quality-of-life, health service use, and costs associated with syncope. *Prog Cardiovasc Dis.* 2013;55:370-375.

CHAPTER 102

Tachycardia

Geoffrey L. Southmayd, MD

Key Clinical Questions

1. How do you triage a patient with a new tachyarrhythmia?

2. What are the electrocardiographic features that suggest that a wide complex tachyarrhythmia is of ventricular origin?

3. What are the electrocardiographic features that suggest that a wide complex tachyarrhythmia is of supraventricular origin?

4. What is the differential diagnosis for short RP tachycardia? What is the differential diagnosis for long RP tachycardia?

5. How do you acutely manage a symptomatic tachyarrhythmia?

INTRODUCTION

This chapter will review the initial bedside approach to a hospitalized patient with a new, potentially life-threatening tachycardia, defined as a heart rate ≥100 beats per minute (bpm). The reader is then referred to subsequent cardiology chapters for definitive management of specific arrhythmias.

■ THE NORMAL CARDIAC CONDUCTION SYSTEM

The conduction pathway in the heart begins in the sinoatrial node, which spontaneously activates the right atrium, the interatrial septum, and then the left atrium. The initial portion of the P wave represents depolarization of the right atrium, and the terminal portion depolarization of the left atrium. Normally, the atrioventricular (AV) node, His bundle, and bundle branches transmit impulses in anterograde fashion from the atria to the ventricles. The QRS complex represents ventricular depolarization and the T wave represents ventricular repolarization (**Figure 102-1**).

■ TACHYARRHYTHMIAS AND CONDUCTION DISTURBANCES

Tachycardias are encountered frequently in inpatient practice. Symptoms from tachyarrhythmias are variable, and some patients are asymptomatic. When present, symptoms may include palpitations, shortness of breath, chest pain, anxiety, syncope, hypotension, or may manifest by hemodynamic collapse and sudden cardiac death.

In addition to the typical AV conducting pathway, anomalous bands of tissue—accessory pathways—may be able to conduct between the atria and ventricles in a retrograde or antegrade fashion that bypasses the normal conduction system. These pathways may or may not be visible on surface electrocardiogram (ECG).

Supraventricular tachycardias (SVTs) include all tachycardias that arise at or above the His bundle. Sinus tachycardia is easily the most common SVT, but does not represent a primary pathologic arrhythmia except in rare cases. Paroxysmal SVTs usually have narrow complexes with a normal QRS duration of <100 ms; however, some may have aberrant conduction notable for a different QRS configuration from the baseline ECG. Intraventricular conduction disturbances may manifest as incomplete (100-120 ms) or complete bundle branch blocks (QRS ≥ 120 ms in duration), and may be rate-dependent. A right bundle branch block (RBBB) configuration is more common than a left bundle branch block (LBBB) aberrant pattern. The altered depolarization causes secondary repolarization ST-T abnormalities and discordance of QRS-T wave vectors. Ischemia, electrolyte disturbances, and digitalis cause primary depolarization ST-T abnormalities independent of the QRS vector. Sudden death from SVT is rare.

Ventricular tachycardia (VT) arises from the ventricles and is more likely to cause cardiac compromise and sudden death.

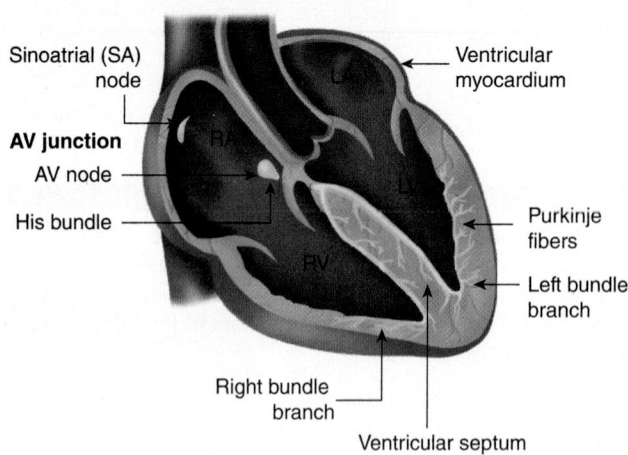

Figure 102-1 *Cardiac conduction system.*

INITIAL APPROACH

CASE 102-1

POSTOPERATIVE TACHYCARDIA

A 65-year-old female with past medical history of hypertension, osteoarthritis, and GERD underwent elective left total hip replacement.

After transfer to the floor, the patient had an asymptomatic 15-beat run of wide-complex tachycardia with a variable heart rate ranging from 60 to 120 bpm. Two hours later, the covering physician was notified about recurrence of the tachyarrhythmia identified on telemetry.

Initial data: Telemetry (**Figure 102-2**) showed a wide-complex tachycardia at a heart rate of 120.

Vital signs: Systolic blood pressure was 140 mm Hg, O$_2$ saturation 98% on nasal cannula, afebrile.

A systematic approach to the patient with tachyarrhythmia allows for rapid identification and triage of potentially life-threatening conduction abnormalities. Management of these patients often requires urgent or emergent treatment decisions by the clinician before a precise diagnosis can be made; by following an algorithmic approach, the physician at bedside can promptly differentiate various diagnostic groups and respond with timely and appropriate therapy.

■ IS THE PATIENT HEMODYNAMICALLY STABLE?

Critical assessment of a tachyarrhythmia requires a determination of whether the patient has a life-threatening arrhythmia. The

first step always begins with reviewing the patient's vital signs for hemodynamic stability, as well as identifying any artifacts that may have produced ECG findings mimicking cardiac arrhythmias. For example, motion artifact from muscle tremors or rigors may produce ECG changes that simulate cardiac tachyarrhythmias on a cardiac monitor tracing. If hemodynamic instability is present with tachyarrhythmia, clinicians should proceed promptly to direct-current cardioversion or defibrillation according to ACLS protocols. See Chapter 137 (Inpatient Cardiac Arrest and Cardiopulmonary Resuscitation). In the case of sinus tachycardia with hemodynamic instability, treatment should focus on the underlying cause of the rhythm (volume depletion, pain, anxiety, anemia, etc) rather than on the tachycardia itself.

PRACTICE POINT

- Critical assessment of a tachyarrhythmia requires a determination of whether the patient has a life-threatening arrhythmia. If hemodynamic instability is present, clinicians should proceed promptly to direct-current cardioversion or defibrillation according to ACLS protocols.

In hemodynamically stable patients, clinicians should try to determine the mechanism of tachycardia before initiating treatment.

ECG INTERPRETATION

The goal of ECG interpretation is to identify the location of the ectopic impulse formation causing the rhythm disturbance, baseline conduction abnormalities, and to look for evidence of myocardial ischemia. See Chapter 108 (The Resting Electrocardiogram).

■ ARE THE QRS COMPLEXES NARROW OR WIDE?

During the assessment of hemodynamic stability, the clinician should examine the monitor strip to determine whether the QRS complex is narrow (<120 ms) or wide (>120 ms). A regular wide complex tachycardia (WCT) suggests VT, SVT with aberrant conduction, or SVT with pre-excitation via an accessory pathway.

Distinguishing VT from SVT with aberrancy or SVT over an accessory pathway can be challenging, but has important management implications. Until proven otherwise, patients who have a WCT and a history of structural heart disease (coronary artery disease or cardiomyopathy) are presumed to have VT. The frequency of VT amongst these patients in the setting of WCT is greater than 90%.

PRACTICE POINT

- Until proven otherwise, patients who have a wide complex tachycardia and a history of structural heart disease (coronary artery disease or cardiomyopathy) are presumed to have VT.

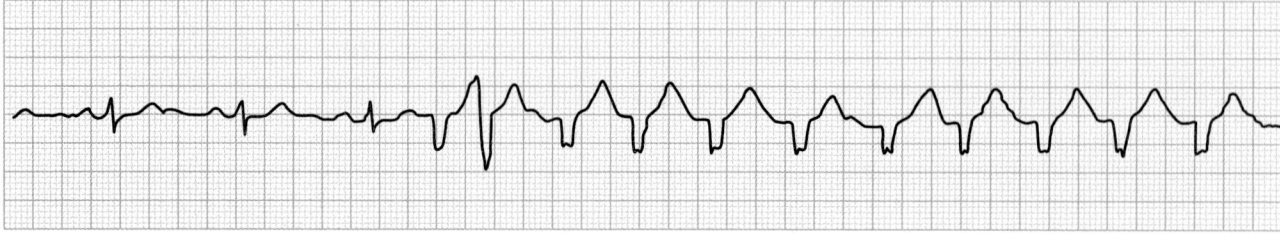

Figure 102-2 *Monitor tracing of the patient's heart rhythm showing wide complex tachycardia.*

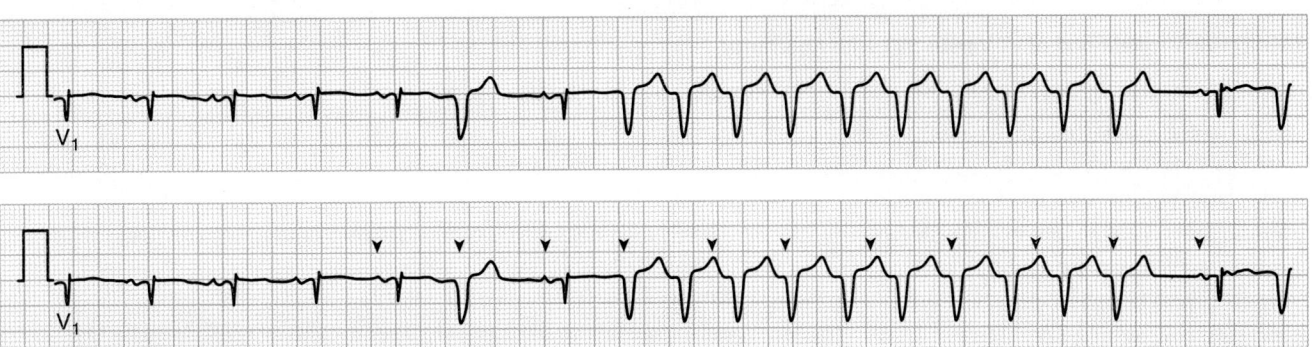

Figure 102-3 *Monitor strip showing AV dissociation. The arrows above the rhythm mark the location of the P waves as they "march" through the run of nonsustained ventricular tachycardia.*

Application of the Brugada criteria may help differentiate VT from SVT with aberrant conduction, but requires interpretation of a 12-lead ECG.

> ### PRACTICE POINT
>
> **Brugada criteria**
>
> - VT is diagnosed on the basis of (1) absence of RS complex in all leads V_1-V_6; (2) the interval from the beginning of the R wave to the nadir of the S wave >0.1 second in any precordial RS lead; (3) presence of AV dissociation, fusion, or capture beats; and (4) morphology criteria for VT present in both leads V_1 and V_6.
> - If none of these criteria are met, the diagnosis favors supraventricular tachycardia with aberration.

The presence of atrioventricular (AV) dissociation, fusion beats, and capture complexes generally favor the diagnosis of VT. AV dissociation is characterized by loss of dependence between atrial and ventricular depolarization, and is identified when the P waves "march" through the tachycardic sequence without any temporal relationship to QRS complexes. In these cases, the ventricular rate should be greater than or equal to the atrial rate. When present, AV dissociation is highly specific for VT, but recognition of P waves on the surface ECG during VT may be challenging. P waves are absent in up to 70% of VT cases, and so their absence should not reassure the examiner that the arrhythmia is supraventricular in origin (**Figure 102-3**).

Fusion beats, arising from simultaneous activation of the ventricle from two sources, have a QRS configuration that is intermediate between supraventricular and ventricular complexes. They form when the ventricle is depolarized simultaneously via the normal conduction system in addition to a ventricular focus. Similarly, capture beats are formed when a sinus nodal impulse successfully conducts down to the ventricles in the typical manner, resulting in a QRS complex that is identical to the baseline ECG (**Figure 102-4**).

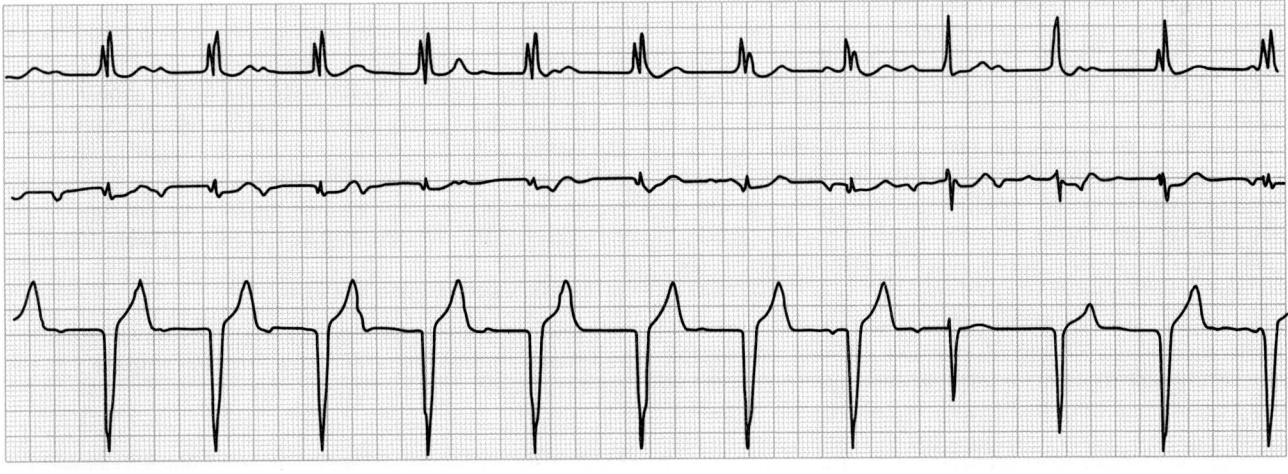

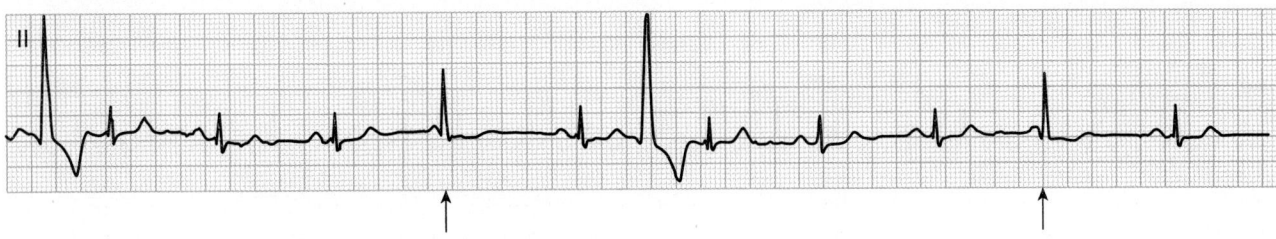

Figure 102-4 *Capture complex (above) and fusion beats (below, arrows).*

TABLE 102-1 Likelihood of VT Versus SVT with Aberrancy

Ventricular Tachycardia More Likely...	SVT with Aberrancy More Likely...
Hemodynamic instability or cardiac compromise	Hemodynamic stability
Structural heart disease	Patients with normal hearts
Wide complex tachycardia >0.14 s in duration	Narrow QRS
AV dissociation, capture, and/or fusion beats	Similar QRS morphology to QRS during normal sinus rhythm or during an aberrantly conducted PAC
Extreme axis deviation (northwest)	
Atypical bundle branch block	Presence of P waves
Ventricular concordance	Typical bundle branch block (<0.14 s if RBBB; <0.16 s if LBBB) if narrow QRS during sinus rhythm
Prolonged QT interval	
Tachyarrhythmia initiated by a PVC	Ventricular discordance (some QRS deflections in precordial leads positive, some negative)
	Tachyarrhythmia initiated by a PAC

A markedly widened QRS >140 ms supports the diagnosis of VT, especially if associated with northwest axis (−90° to +180°) of the QRS complex in the frontal plane. This is due to a shift in depolarization vector from cardiac apex toward the base. Similarly, the precordial leads V_4-V_6 would be expected to have negative QRS complexes. See Chapter 134 (Ventricular Arrhythmias). Activation of the ventricles by SVT over an accessory pathway generally results in less extreme frontal axis deviation, and predominantly positive QRS complexes in the lateral precordial leads (**Table 102-1**).

■ WHAT IS THE RATE?

In patients with SVT, atrial rates (measured using the P-P interval) and ventricular rates (measured using the R-R interval) may differ due to limitations of AV nodal conduction, and rate evaluation may provide useful clues to the etiology of the tachyarrhythmia. In cases of typical atrial flutter (AFL), atrial rates average near 300 bpm (range 240-340 bpm) due to a common macroreentrant circuit around the tricuspid valve. See Chapter 132 (Supraventricular Tachyarrhythmias). ECG typically shows classic "sawtooth" flutter waves that are predominantly negative (for *counterclockwise* type 1 AFL, most common) or positive (for *clockwise* type I AFL) in the inferior leads. With 2:1 AV nodal conduction, the ventricular rate falls to around 150 bpm (**Figure 102-5**).

Frequently, flutter waves are buried within the T waves, and can be difficult to distinguish from other SVTs. Recognition of a ventricular rate near 150 bpm should raise the clinician's pretest probability for AFL unless an alternate diagnosis is evident. In these cases, vagal maneuvers or adenosine may be useful to slow the ventricular rate and identify the underlying atrial rhythm. In cases of variable AV block, the ventricular rate will appear irregular. It is sometimes helpful to look for discrete R-R intervals that have a common divisor; for example, a rate of 150 bpm for some sequences and 100 bpm for others is consistent with AFL with variable block (2:1 and 3:1 with a stable atrial rate of 300 bpm) (**Figure 102-6**). Type II AFL has faster atrial rates in the range of 340 to 440 bpm, and may not demonstrate sawtooth pattern on ECG.

Sinus tachycardia classically has a maximum rate of 220 bpm minus the patient's age in years. Multifocal atrial tachycardia (MAT) more often occurs at rates between 100 and 150 bpm, and atrioventricular nodal reentry tachycardia (AVNRT) and atrioventricular reentrant tachycardia (AVRT) typically range from 150 to 250 bpm (**Figure 102-7**).

■ IS THE RHYTHM REGULAR OR IRREGULAR?

Regularity is defined by beat-to-beat variation in rate that does not exceed 10%, although most regular rhythms demonstrate even less variability. Sinus tachycardia, AFL with consistent AV conduction, AVNRT, AVRT, and atrial tachycardia cause regular tachyarrhythmias. In contrast, AF, MAT, and tachyarrhythmias due to multiple anterograde AV nodal pathways cause irregularly irregular rhythms (**Figures 102-8** and **102-9**). MAT may be distinguished from sinus tachycardia with frequent multifocal atrial premature complexes because it does not have any dominant atrial pacemaker. MAT is identified by ectopic P waves of at least three morphologies best seen in leads II, III, and V_1, a ventricular rate of >100 bpm, isoelectric baseline between P waves, and varying PP, PR, and RR intervals. Some P waves may be blocked due to their rapid rate. Atrial tachycardias with variable AV block may also appear irregular.

VT and SVT with aberrancy are typically regular forms of WCT. Monomorphic VT can occasionally produce slight irregularity, most commonly in the period immediately after onset (the so called "warm-up phenomenon"). An irregular WCT is more suggestive of polymorphic VT or AF with aberrant conduction (**Table 102-2**).

■ EXAMINATION OF P WAVES

Are P waves present during the tachyarrhythmia? What is the P wave morphology, and how do they compare with the baseline sinus ECG?

The next step is to identify the presence of atrial activity and to examine the relationship between the P wave and the QRS complex. P waves may be embedded at the end of the QRS complexes or

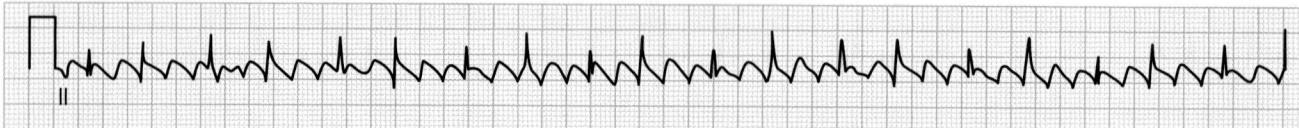

Figure 102-5 *A macroreentrant circuit in the right atrium causes atrial flutter "sawtooth" waveforms accompanied by an atrial rate that varies between 240 and 340 bpm.*

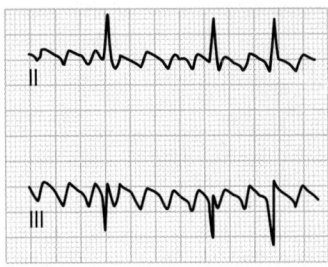

Figure 102-6 *Type 1 aflutter with variable block.*

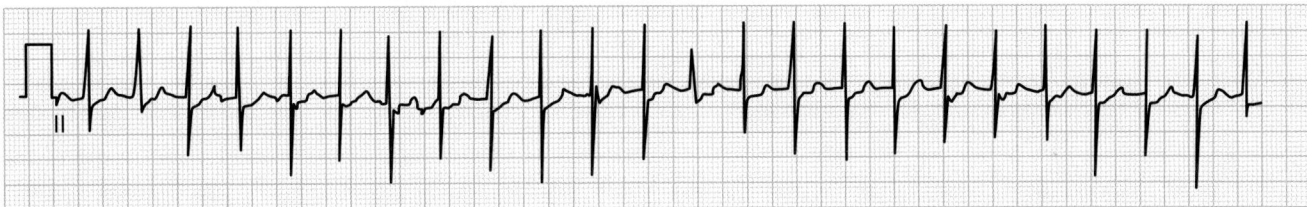

Figure 102-7 *A narrow QRS complex tachycardia in the range of 150 to 250 beats/min, often with P waves inscribed at the terminal portion of the QRS complex and reflecting retrograde atrial depolarization.*

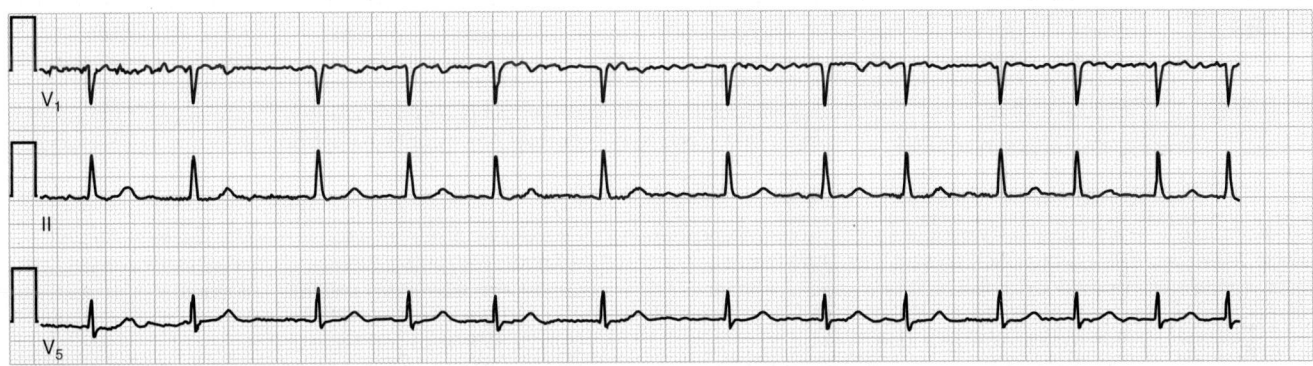

Figure 102-8 *An irregularly irregular narrow complex tachycardia consistent with atrial fibrillation.*

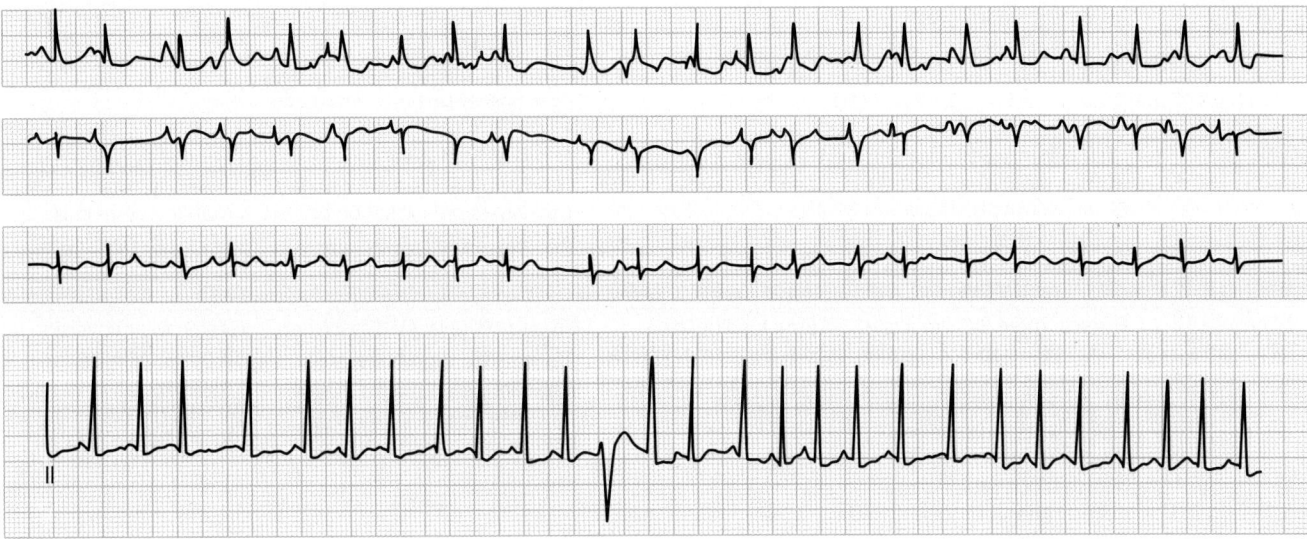

Figure 102-9 *MAT.*

TABLE 102-2 Tachyarrythmias

Rhythm	ECG Features	Predisposing Conditions	Electrical Physiology	Initial Management
Sinus Tachycardia	Regular narrow complex rhythm, normal P wave axis; Ventricular rate up to 220 minus the patient's age	Underlying disorder, hypermetabolic state or systemic stressor (anemia, fever, hypovolemia), drug effect	Sinus node the one dominant atrial pacemaker; Rapid narrow complexes usually similar to patient's baseline; PR interval may be short, normal, or prolonged	Treat underlying problem
Unifocal Atrial Tachycardia	Regular rhythm with atrial rate 150-250 bpm; Single nonsinus P wave morphology; Ventricular rate >100 bpm.	Uncommon; cardiopulmonary disease, drugs, status post AF ablation, digitalis intoxication	Ectopic atrial focus—either from enhanced automaticity or reentry; Paroxysmal if reentrant mechanism; incessant if enhanced automaticity	Adenosine terminates rhythm in 60%-80% of cases. Rate control with AV nodal blockade
Multifocal Atrial Tachycardia (MAT)	Rate 100-150 bpm, Irregularly irregular rhythm; P waves with at least three different morphologies; varying PR, RR, RP intervals	Acute illness, cardiopulmonary disease, sepsis, low K^+ and Mg^{++}	Enhanced automaticity; MAT does not require AV conduction and may persist during AV block	Treat underlying illness; replete K^+ and Mg^{++}; rate control; digoxin of no value; cardioversion ineffective
Atrial Flutter	Atrial rate of 240-340 bpm usually with 2:1 AV block; QRS may be normal or aberrant; rate and regularity depend on AV conduction	Usually underlying disease present (heart or lung); if no underlying cardiopulmonary disease, rule out thyroid disease or PE	Most cases due to reentry around tricuspid valve	Electrical cardioversion if hemodynamically unstable; vagal maneuvers slow rate and expose flutter waves
Atrial Fibrillation	Absent P waves; Atrial activity irregular with varying fibrillatory waves; Ventricular rate of 130-200 bpm, irregularly irregular rhythm

If rate >200 bpm and QRS >0.12 s varying in width, consider WPW | Atrial enlargement due to any cause including structural heart disease or CAD; lung disease, hyperthyroidism, low Mg^{++}, alcoholism, cocaine, physiologic stress | Increased automaticity and multiple reentrant wavelets predominantly in the left atrium around the pulmonary veins; ventricular rate may regularize in digitalis toxicity but atrial activity remains totally irregular | Rate control with AV nodal blockers; electrical cardioversion if unstable |
| AV-Nodal Reentrant Tachycardia (AVNRT) | Rate 150-250. P waves often hidden, but when present are retrograde near terminal portion of QRS. RP interval is short (*typical AVNRT*) or long (*atypical AVNRT*) | None. Most common SVT (>60%) | Reentry circuit confined to AV node, with antegrade conduction down slow pathway and retrograde via fast pathway (*typical*, 80%-90%) or antegrade via fast pathway and retrograde via slow (*atypical*, 10%-20%) | Usually terminates with vagal maneuvers or adenosine |
| AV Reentrant Tachycardia (AVRT) | Rate 150-250

Orthodromic: narrow complex, retrograde P waves with short RP interval

Antidromic: wide complex, retrograde P waves with long RP interval | None | Reentry circuit involving accessory pathway

Orthodromic: antegrade conduction via AV node, retrograde conduction via accessory pathway

Antidromic: antegrade conduction via accessory pathway, retrograde via AV node | *Orthodromic:* terminates with vagal maneuvers and adenosine

Antidromic: Caution with AV nodal blockade. Expert consultation. Electrical cardioversion for unstable patient |
| WPW | Most patients asymptomatic with no dysrhythmias; Short PR interval and delta wave present with widening of QRS. May be associated with AVRT, AFL, AF, and VT/VF | Congenital (Ebstein anomaly) and acquired | Accessory pathway (Kent bundle) bypasses the AV node and causes pre-excitation of ventricle (delta wave) | Electrical cardioversion if hemodynamic instability; ventricular rates >285 at greatest risk of degenerating to VF |
| Ventricular Tachycardia | Three or more PVCs at a rate >100/min in rapid succession; RR intervals usually regular; AV dissociation, capture and fusion beats, extreme axis deviation, atypical bundle branch block, prolonged QT interval; abrupt onset and end | Structural heart disease; hemodynamic instability or cardiac compromise | Brugada criteria: AV dissociation; RS complex absent in V_1-V_6; R to S interval >100 ms in any precordial lead; morphology criteria for VT in V_1-V_2 and V_6 | Electrical cardioversion for hemodynamic instability; Antiarrhythmic therapy for stable patients |

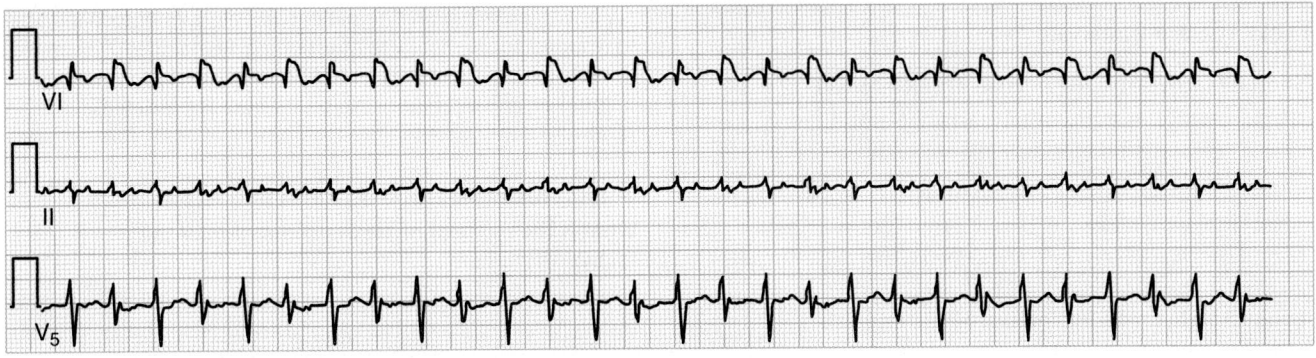

Figure 102-10 *Atrial tachycardia is characterized by a P-wave axis or morphology that is distinct from that of sinus rhythm, generally 150 to 250 beats/min, characteristically slower than that of atrial flutter.*

within the T wave; therefore, it is important to compare the tracing to prior ECGs to examine for changes in the QRS and T wave morphology. The normal sinus P wave is 0.08 to 0.11 seconds in duration and is always upright in leads I and II and negative in lead aVR. It is usually upright in lead aVF. Due to the location of the sinus node in the superior right atrium, the atrial depolarization vector first moves anteriorly to the right atrial tissue, and then posteriorly toward the left atrium. As a result, the P wave is usually biphasic in leads V_1 and V_2, positive in V_3-V_6, and may appear notched in the limb leads.

Leads II and V_1 are the most helpful places to assess P wave morphology. Ectopic atrial rhythms may have upright P waves arising from an atrial focus near the sinus node or inverted P waves arising from an ectopic focus in the lower atrium. The location of the ectopic focus relative to the AV conduction system and the presence or absence of delay in this system determines the duration of the PR interval (whether short, normal, or prolonged). The QT interval (representing the duration of ventricular depolarization and repolarization) is typically normal in ectopic rhythms. Ectopic P waves will have a different morphology from sinus P waves and may be easier to identify if there is an earlier ECG tracing of sinus rhythm used as a reference. P waves that are negative in aVL or terminally positive in V1 suggest a left atrial ectopic focus. Negative P waves in the inferior leads are seen in AVNRT and AVRT, as well as atrial tachycardias that originate in the lower atrium.

When ectopic P waves precede each QRS complex (even if the QRS complex is wide) then the tachycardia is supraventricular in origin. This is the case even when P waves are retrograde (inverted in lead II and upright in lead aVR), as would be seen in the setting of low atrial tachycardia. When ectopic P waves follow the QRS complexes, the origin of the tachyarrhythmia may be either supraventricular from the AV junction or ventricular. Tachycardia arising from the AV node more commonly has narrow QRS complexes, although AV junctional tachycardia may be associated with aberrant conduction causing a wide QRS complex tachycardia.

If P waves are present, what is the R-P interval?

Together with the P wave morphology, the R-P interval can assist distinguishing various causes of SVT. Long R-P tachycardia is defined by an R-P interval that is longer than half the R-R interval. Sinus tachycardia is a long R-P tachycardia. By definition, sinus tachycardia has sinus P waves, although these can be difficult to identify when the P wave fuses with the T wave of the preceding QRS complex. This situation usually occurs in critically ill patients with heart rates greater than 180 bpm, patients receiving vasopressors, or when there has been significant volume loss.

Besides sinus tachycardia, atrial tachycardia is the most common long R-P tachyarrhythmia. P waves in these instances will be abnormal. AV block may occur without interrupting the tachycardia because the AV node is not an integral part of the arrhythmia circuit. An ectopic atrial tachycardia with 2:1 block may be identified by finding a second P wave buried in the terminal portion of the QRS complex in the inferior leads. In this case, measurement of the timing of deflections will demonstrate that they occur exactly halfway between the more visible P waves (**Figure 102-10**). Suspect digitalis intoxication if paroxysmal tachycardia is associated with AV block.

Unlike sinus tachycardia, AFL and atrial tachycardias, the mechanisms of AVNRT and AVRT involve reentrant circuits within the AV node (for AVNRT) or via an accessory pathway (for AVRT). On ECG, AVNRT and orthodromic AVRT can be recognized by narrow complex, short R-P interval tachycardia. In many cases, these rhythms will appear without evident P waves, but if they are visible, P waves appear at the terminal portion of the QRS complex or superimposed on the ST segment or T wave, reflecting retrograde atrial depolarization. See Chapter 132 (Supraventricular Tachyarrhythmias). Differentiation between AVNRT and AVRT is often impossible by surface EKG alone, and may require electrophysiological evaluation. AVNRT is much more common than AVRT (**Figure 102-11** and **Table 102-3**).

CASE 102-1 (*continued*)

POSTOPERATIVE TACHYCARDIA

Per OR notes: In the operating room, the patient received 4 L of IV fluids with no intraoperative hypotension or tachycardia. Estimated blood loss was approximately 1 L. Subsequently, in the

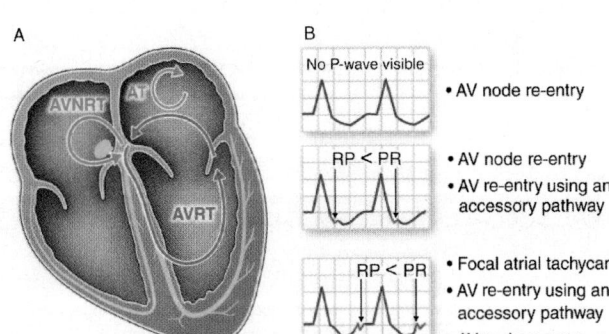

Figure 102-11 *RP interval in the assessment of SVT.* (From Michaud GF, Stevenson WG. Supraventricular tachyarrhythmias. In: Kasper DL, et al., eds. *Harrison's Principles of Internal Medicine,* 19th ed. New York: McGraw-Hill; 2015, Fig. 276-2.)

TABLE 102-3 R-P Intervals

Short RP tachycardia (RP interval <½ RR interval)

- Typical AVNRT (AV nodal reentry tachycardia)

- Orthodromic AVRT (AV reentrant tachycardia)

- Atrial tachycardia with first degree AV delay

- Junctional tachycardia

Note: If no P wave seen, likely embedded within QRS complex and therefore Short RP tachycardia

Long RP tachycardia (RP interval >½ RR interval)

- Sinus tachycardia

- Atrial tachycardia

- Atypical AVNRT

- PJRT (permanent junctional reciprocating tachycardia)

- Sinus node reentry tachycardia

recovery room she was noted to be hypoxic as O_2 sat declined to 70% while receiving 4 L of nasal oxygen while sleeping and was administered 100% NRB mask with improvement of her oxygenation level to ≥96%.

Back at the bedside: The covering team rapidly assessed the patient's airway, breathing and circulation, placed pads on the patient and brought a defibrillator to the bedside.

Her baseline ECG (**Figure 102-12**) was notable for sinus bradycardia, heart rate 54 bpm, normal intervals, normal axis, normal R wave progression, and no ST-T abnormalities. The baseline ECG was officially read by a cardiologist as normal.

History of present illness: No prior history of arrhythmia, coronary artery disease, or cardiomyopathy. She denied any chest pain, palpitations, shortness of breath, lightheadedness, dizziness, syncope, or diaphoresis. She had no history of substance abuse, including alcohol.

On review of systems, her only complaints related to her recent hip surgery.

Review of her home medications and her current medications were notable for her blood pressure medications (amlodipine, lisinopril, and hydrochlorothiazide), extended release bupropion, calcium, vitamin D, and omeprazole. New medications since hospitalization included enoxaparin, warfarin, and morphine via a patient-controlled analgesia (PCA).

Physical examination: The patient was alert, oriented, and able to respond appropriately to questioning. Remainder of exam was notable for a difficult to assess JVP, distant heart sounds, absence of murmur, and clear lungs. No bruits were appreciated.

■ PRE- AND POSTARRHYTHMIA ECG ASSESSMENT

What is the mode of onset or termination of the tachyarrhythmia?

Telemetry monitoring, Holter monitors, and pacemaker or defibrillator interrogation, if available, can provide useful information about the onset and termination of an abnormal rhythm. Premature atrial complexes (PAC) immediately prior to arrhythmia onset suggests paroxysmal SVT. Sudden onset or offset of SVT is typical for AVNRT, AVRT and atrial tachycardias, whereas sinus tachycardia and MAT typically have a gradual onset. In addition, response to vagal maneuvers or adenosine is indicative of AV nodal-dependent reentrant arrhythmias.

Is there a baseline ECG?

If the patient is stable, obtain a 12-lead ECG to look for any changes from the baseline ECG that might suggest cardiac ischemia and for the presence of pre-existing bundle block. The clinician should examine for evidence of a prolonged QT interval, AV dissociation, capture and fusion beats, extreme axis deviation, or atypical bundle branch block that might suggest pre-existing structural heart disease and increase the likelihood of ventricular arrhythmias. Although uncommon, ECG changes suggestive of Wolf-Parkinson-White (WPW), precordial ST abnormalities characteristic of the Brugada syndrome, and epsilon waves seen in arrhythmogenic RV dysplasia all have important management implications.

A baseline ECG may allow for comparison of the QRS complexes during the tachycardia with the configuration of isolated ectopic beats preceding the tachycardia. Pre-excitation apparent during normal sinus rhythm would indicate that the tachycardia is due to an accessory pathway. Isolated PACs may lead to atrial group beats, atrial tachycardia, AF or AFL. When the atrial tachyarrhythmias terminate, isolated PACs may follow. Likewise, when the QRS configuration during isolated PVCs before and after the tachycardia is identical to that present during the tachyarrhythmia event, the rhythm is confirmed ventricular. Of note, while frequent premature beats or runs of nonsustained VT could suggest the presence of structural heart disease, isolated premature beats on prior ECG are of little prognostic value. Amongst patients without known heart disease, 24-hour Holter monitoring reveals PACs in 99% of patients, and PVCs in 80%.

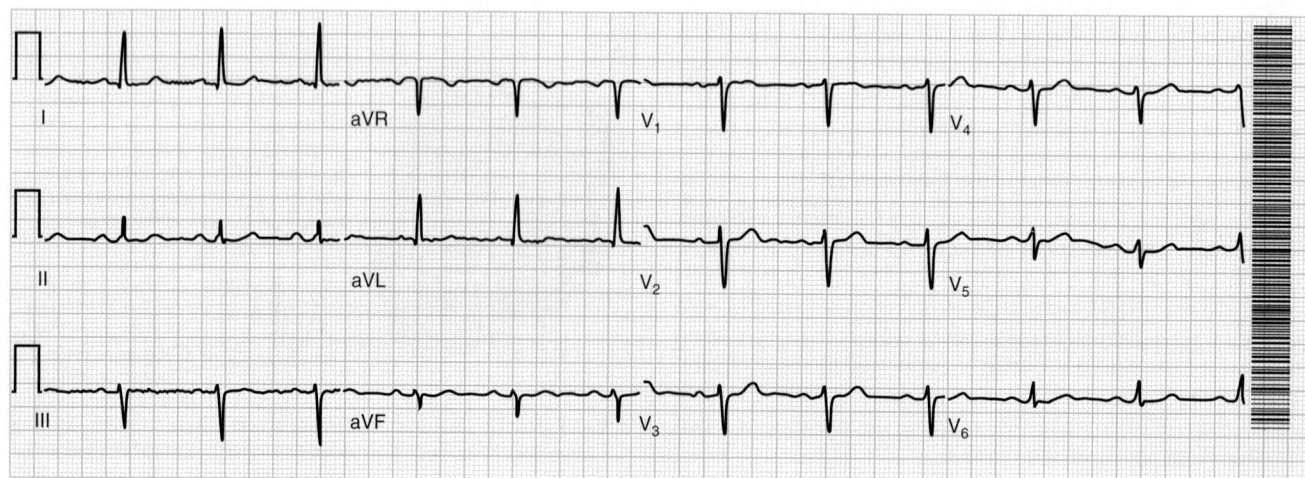

Figure 102-12 *Baseline ECG for Case 102-1.*

NEXT STEPS

◼ ADDITIONAL DATA

For hemodynamically stable patients, physicians should perform a targeted history and physical examination specifically looking for signs and symptoms of significant cardiopulmonary and vascular disease. The neck veins should be examined for the presence of cannon A-waves that match the rate of tachycardia due to atrial contraction during ventricular systole when the tricuspid valve is closed. Canon A-waves would not occur in sinus tachycardia, ectopic atrial tachycardia, or atrial flutter. Their presence does not differentiate the two principal types of AV reentrant tachycardia. Less commonly, cannon A-waves may occur in VT when retrograde AV conduction depolarizes the atria during ventricular systole.

For the postoperative patient, electrolytes, cardiac enzymes, and complete blood count should be obtained in addition to a resting ECG. Special attention should be made to repletion of potassium and magnesium. Oxygen should be administered as necessary and continuous ECG monitoring should be provided.

CASE 102-1 (continued)

POSTOPERATIVE TACHYCARDIA

Evaluation: 12-lead ECG (**Figure 102-13**) was notable for a regular heart rate of 118, a wide complex QRS with LBBB morphology, left axis deviation, and no visible P waves. There were no ST segment abnormalities, and T wave changes were appropriate in the setting of LBBB. Neither her baseline ECG nor this ECG demonstrated the hallmarks of WPW, and it did not meet Brugada criteria for the diagnosis of VT. Together with the absence of known structural heart disease, stable vital signs, and lack of ischemic symptoms, the clinician was most concerned for SVT with aberrant conduction.

◼ ATTEMPT TO SLOW OR TEMINATE THE TACHYCARDIA

The treatment options for tachycardia depend on identification of the underlying mechanism. Acutely ill patients often have difficulty performing the Valsalva maneuver, during which they maintain a forced expiratory effort against a closed glottis. The examiner may give the patient simple instructions to insert his index finger in his or her mouth, close the mouth around his or her finger, and exhale into a closed space. Auscultation for carotid bruits prior to performing

carotid massage is a reasonable but very imprecise way to determine whether cerebrovascular disease is present, but most experts would avoid carotid massage if they identified a cervical bruit.

Adenosine potently and transiently blocks AV nodal conduction, and would be expected to terminate AV-nodal dependent rhythms such as AVNRT or AVRT. In the setting of AFL or atrial tachycardia, transient AV block by adenosine may decrease ventricular rate and uncover atrial activity that was previously hidden and facilitate rhythm recognition. For WCTs not known to be ventricular in etiology, if the patient is hemodynamically stable and the rhythm is regular and monomorphic in pattern, then adenosine is a reasonable treatment option. Expected treatment or diagnostic response would be similar as for SVTs previously listed. VT does not typically respond to adenosine, although some forms of idiopathic VT (most commonly right ventricular outflow tract VT) may terminate with adenosine therapy. Before administering adenosine, physicians should specifically inquire about a history of asthma or reversible COPD and whether the patient is receiving dipyridamole. Adenosine can trigger acute bronchospasm in vulnerable patients and dipyridamole can potentiate AV block. At the time of administration, they should also warn the patient about transient sensations of chest tightness, nausea, and flushing.

CASE 102-1 (continued)

POSTOPERATIVE TACHYCARDIA

Management: Vagal maneuvers were attempted but had no effect on rhythm. Given the low suspicion for VT or pre-excitation, and ECG showing regular and monomorphic rhythm, adenosine was deemed appropriate for use. 6 mg Adenosine IV push was administered followed by rapid saline flush but had no effect. A 12 mg IV dose transiently decreased the heart rate without appreciable change in morphology. The clinician then administered 5 mg IV metoprolol for two doses, with resulting decrease in heart rate to less than 100 bpm, and P waves became clearly evident. After a few minutes at the lower heart rate, the QRS complexes transitioned to narrow complex morphology (**Figure 102-14**). The patient remained stable without change in vital signs.

Her repeat 12-lead ECG showed narrow QRS complexes, normal axis and intervals, and resolution of the previous LBBB morphology (**Figure 102-15**). Her laboratory tests including electrolytes and cardiac enzymes were unremarkable.

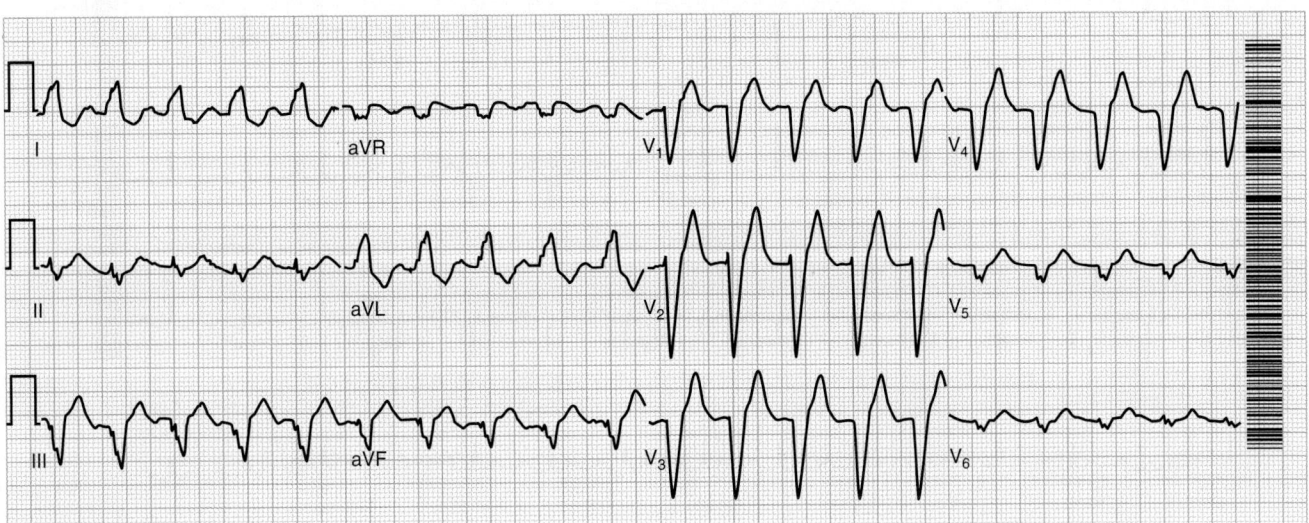

Figure 102-13 *Postoperative sinus tachycardia.*

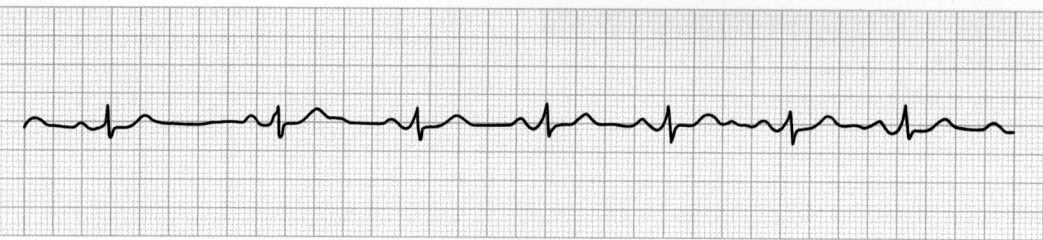

Figure 102-14 *Monitor tracing with slowing return to normal sinus rhythm with narrow complex QRS.*

Intravenous administration of AV nodal blockers may reduce the ventricular rate and alleviate distressing symptoms despite persistence of the rhythm disturbance. β-Blockers or nondihydropyridine calcium-channel blockers are preferable to adenosine in patients with atrial tachycardias. Importantly, AV nodal blockers are contraindicated in patients with pre-excitation AF, since slowing the native pathway may precipitate conduction down the accessory pathway, paradoxically increasing the ventricular rate. In these patients, antiarrhythmic therapy such as procainamide may be necessary for management, and expert consultation is recommended. For surgical patients already taking a β-blocker, the negative inotropic effects of calcium channel blockers may be accentuated. Calcium-channel blockers should not be used for rate control in the setting of severe heart failure (New York Heart Association Class III/IV) due to risk of cardiac decompensation. β-Blockers or digoxin are appropriate alternatives based on clinical status.

PRACTICE POINT

- Calcium-channel blockers should not be used for rate control in the setting of severe heart failure (New York Heart Association Class III/IV) due to risk of cardiac decompensation. β-Blockers or digoxin are appropriate alternatives based on clinical status.

CASE REVIEW—ASSESSMENT OF THE POSTOPERATIVE PATIENT WITH TACHYCARDIA

In this patient, the tachyarrhythmia proved secondary to sinus tachycardia with a rate-dependent LBBB morphology. Tachycardia-contingent bundle branch block may occur if either the right or left-sided bundle branch reaches its effective refractory period and cannot conduct impulses to match the rapid rate of the tachycardia. In a patient with paroxysmal SVT-related WCT and a structurally normal heart, the bundle branch pattern usually has a typical appearance, identical to conventional bundle branch morphology.

Sinus tachycardia is a common finding in the postoperative period due to the adrenergic drive that develops as a result of hypotension, volume shifts, acute blood loss, pain and/or anxiety. Further treatment of her tachycardia would focus on recognition and treatment of these primary causes.

During the patient's workup and treatment, the presence of P waves eliminated the possibility of atrial fibrillation, and no flutter waves were appreciated with slowing of the rhythm in response to vagal maneuvers. Pre-excitation or conduction over an accessory pathway may cause the QRS morphology to be wide during SVT, but without delta waves or shortened PR intervals on her baseline ECG, WPW with a reentrant circuit seemed unlikely. Other historical features to consider include the use of bupropion, which can cause tachycardia and arrhythmia.

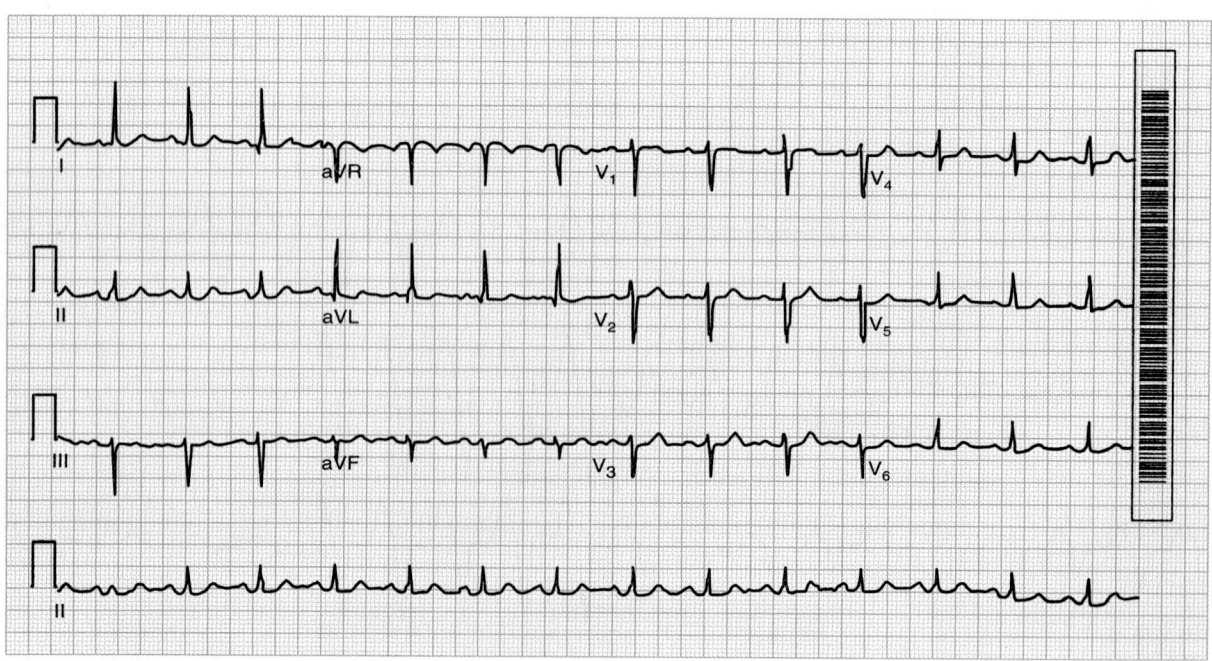

Figure 102-15 *ECG prior to discharge with resolution of rate-related LBBB pattern.*

CONCLUSION

A stepwise approach to a hospitalized patient with a tachyarrhythmia should begin with asking the following questions:

1. Is this patient hemodynamically stable?
2. Are the QRS complexes narrow or wide?
3. Is the rhythm more likely to be ventricular in origin?
4. If the origin of the rhythm is likely supraventricular, what is the rate of the tachycardia based on the R-R interval? Is the rhythm regular? Are P waves present, and if so, is their morphology the same as the baseline ECG in normal sinus rhythm? What is the R-P interval?

Management of tachyarrhythmia is influenced by hemodynamic status and presence of prior structural heart disease. For all patients, electrolytes, cardiac enzymes, and a complete blood count should be obtained in addition to a resting ECG. Oxygen should be administered as necessary and continuous ECG monitoring should be provided. Serum K^+ and Mg^{2+} should be repleted, hypoxia corrected, underlying precipitants such as failure to administer home medications, pain and withdrawal states identified and treated.

Clinicians should always anticipate the possibility of requiring emergent electrical cardioversion or defibrillation in the management of acute tachyarrhythmias. Persistent tachycardias unresponsive to the usual measures or clinical deterioration should prompt emergent specialty consultation.

SUGGESTED READINGS

Brugada P, Brugada J, Mont L, et al. A new approach to the differential diagnosis of a regular tachycardia with a wide QRS complex. *Circulation*. 1991;83:1649-1659.

Link MS. Clinical practice. Evaluation and initial treatment of supraventricular tachycardia. *N Engl J Med*. 2012;367(15):1438-1448.

Sauve JS, Laupacis A, Ostbye T, et al. Does this patient have a clinically important carotid bruit? In: Simel DL, Rennie D, eds. *The Rational Clinical Examination*. New York, NY: McGraw-Hill; 2009.

Whinnett ZI, Sohaib SMA, Davies DW. Diagnosis and management of supraventricular tachycardia. *BMJ*. 2012;345:e7769.

CHAPTER 103

The Geriatric History and Physical Examination

Arline D. Bohannon, MD

Peter A. Boling, MD

INTRODUCTION

The US population of adults aged 65 years and older will double within the next 20 years. This aging population includes many adults who use hospital care extensively. In 2005, an estimated 35 million nonfederal hospital discharges occurred in the United States excluding newborns, and while older adults (65+) comprise 12% of the population, they accounted for 35% of hospital stays and increasingly often enter through the emergency room. For example, for patients 80 years and older, 55% were admitted through the emergency room in 1997 compared with 64% in 2002.

Risk of intensive care unit (ICU) admission and ICU utilization also rise with age, peaking in the very old: in those aged 85 years or more there were 58.2 admissions per 1000 individuals and 195.8 days per 1000 individuals, compared with 3.8 admissions per 1000 individuals and 11.5 days per 1000 individuals in those 18 to 44 years old. Individuals 85 years old and older were 3.75 times more likely to be admitted to the ICU than those aged 18 to 44 years after controlling for comorbid illness. Risk of ICU admission rates increased with admission to surgical unit, and presence of multiple comorbid illnesses especially cardiovascular and renal disease. Risk of death is increased among elderly patient nearly 25% of all hospital deaths occurred in patients over 85 years old.

Normal aging reduces physiologic reserve and the ability to maintain homeostasis under physiologic stress even in the best of circumstances. Chronic disease, the stress of acute illness precipitating admission, and polypharmacy add to vulnerability in this heterogeneous population. Furthermore, the hospital experience disrupts normal life rhythms in a foreign environment away from familiar cues. Hospital procedures and policies enforce dependency and immobility that is often related to physical restraints; expose the patient to multiple unfamiliar people involved in direct patient care, further exacerbated by unit transfers. The hospital setting disrupts sleep and nutrition due to lighting, unit noise, and interruptions such as frequent blood drawing, performance of vital signs and tests. Use of sedatives or medications with anticholinergic side effects —sometimes unavoidable during general anesthesia — and inadequate pain management further exacerbate the risk of hospital acquired complications, including delirium, depression, infection, malnutrition, deconditioning, falls, and pressure ulcers. Adverse outcomes include death, a prolonged hospital stay, nursing home placement and increased long-term dependency.

The incidence of delirium during hospitalization ranges from 11% to 42% and functional deficits related to delirium may persist long after hospital discharge. Even in patients admitted for cardiovascular disease rather than infection or dehydration, delirium is associated with higher unexpected in-hospital death which is also an important quality measure. Studies have shown that 30% to 60% of older people develop new dependencies in activities of daily living (ADL) during their hospital stay. Pressure ulcers, considered a preventable complication of hospitalization, are also associated with increased length of stay and health care cost, to the point that they are being called "never" events for which Medicare will refuse to pay. The median incidence of pressure ulcers in hospitalized elderly persons varies from 5% to 16% and has not decreased in recent years. There is evidence that some pressure ulcers develop early during hospitalization, after only a few hours of immobility-induced pressure, yet the evidence of the tissue injury may not appear until days later, and may worsen even after the pressure is relieved. One large study found that 6% of patients developed one or more hospital-acquired pressure ulcers within 2 days of hospital admission. Risk factors for new pressure ulcers include increased age, male gender, African American ethnicity, immobility (requiring assistance with turning in bed), transfer from nursing home, nutritional compromise, body mass index (BMI) less than 18.5, the presence of a pressure ulcer at admission, and urinary and fecal incontinence. There are two things for hospitalists to consider: checking for evidence of skin injury on admission, a task shared with nurses, and looking for ways to prevent skin injury during the hospital stay. (See Chapter 149 [Pressure Ulcers] and Chapter 165 [Principles of Geriatric Care] for a discussion of evidence-based comprehensive models of care to prevent inpatient complications.)

Not only are the personal costs of acute illness and related complications high but also, in a rapidly growing older population, the impact on health care costs is also high. Examples include delirium and functional decline during hospital stays. The occurrence of delirium more than doubles the impact on health care costs, and with careful attention, some of this may be avoided. Annual estimated costs in the United States attributable to delirium range from $38 to $152 billon due to increased mortality and morbidity, prolonged hospital stay, functional decline and long-term institutional care. With 42% of the US national health care budget spent on inpatient care and readmissions accounting for one quarter of Medicare inpatient expenditures, reduction in readmissions is becoming a focal point in health care policy and hospitals may lose reimbursement when preventable readmissions occur. The elderly patient admitted to the hospital should be considered a "high-risk senior," defined as those at risk for developing health-related crises, simply by virtue of being hospitalized. The first hospitalization of an elderly patient, in particular, may offer a window of opportunity for identifying those at risk for further functional disability and clarifying targets for timely intervention to prevent or delay further decline and a cascade of readmissions. The hospitalist should provide an actionable assessment that will lead to an interprofessional, multidisciplinary patient-centered approach utilizing case management, therapies (OT and PT), appropriate consultation, disease management programs, and home care. Optimal practice involves targeting posthospital services and service design to be cost-effective and efficient: the right care in the right place at the right time, based on need.

The admission history and physical examination is a multistep process of acquiring partial data that will lead to a provisional diagnosis. Physicians are taught to seek a diagnosis that will explain all or most aspects of a patient's signs and symptoms at presentation. However, elderly patients commonly have multiple major comorbid conditions of varying severity that may affect the initial presentation of acute illness. Unlike younger patients, whose signs and symptoms usually refer to a diseased organ, ill elderly patients commonly present with nonspecific signs and symptoms such as lethargy, confusion, falls, and incontinence and decreased ability to perform ADLs. Painless myocardial infarction, pneumonia without cough, apathetic hyperthyroidism, and depression masquerading as dementia are examples of common yet atypical presentations. A change in mental status, gradual debilitation, and nonspecific symptoms is also characteristic of tuberculosis in the elderly which is fortunately uncommon but treatable and should not be overlooked. This patient population has changes in T-cell immune function leading to declining delayed hypersensitivity reactions so that only 5% to 10% of 90 year olds will have a positive PPD despite a 90% rate of prior TB exposure. In addition, in older patients there may not be one unifying diagnosis to explain all new symptoms, some of which may be drug-related. Therefore, clinicians need to maintain a high index of suspicion, incorporate risk factors into clinical decision making, carefully review all medications and treatments, obtain information from multiple sources, and perform a comprehensive examination.

Geriatric medicine focuses on four functional domains—physical, cognitive, psychological, and social—that may be used to assess quality of life and goals of care. In addition to treating the cause for admission, a multifaceted approach may improve outcomes by identifying disability, taking steps to improve functional performance, instituting preventative measures to limit iatrogenic complications and disability, and by promoting wellness and independence. This chapter will describe the essential history and physical exam components that should be routinely performed for hospitalized elderly patients in addition to the complete admission history and physical examination ordinarily performed for younger patients and explain how to factor this information into discharge planning.

GERIATRIC PATIENT HISTORY

A geriatric history must include an assessment of the cognitive, functional, psychological and social domains. In order to obtain a complete patient history, clinicians should communicate with family members and caregivers for information about baseline functioning and with the primary care provider on the day of admission. Inpatient providers need this information to define and then achieve goals of hospitalization, which include avoidance of complications that might exacerbate preexisting conditions that make the patient even more vulnerable to a prolonged hospital stay and need for permanent placement upon discharge. The team should encourage liberal visiting by family and friends especially during meals and evening hours, inform the family of the risks of hospitalization, and engage them in preventative measures such as orienting the patient, explaining the hospital routine, and assisting with ambulation. The family should bring in the patient's hearing aid, glasses, and any assistive devices that will facilitate optimal function.

Effective communication during the patient interview always begins with speaking in the patient's native language and at the level appropriate for the patient's educational background and cognitive function. The clinician should also take time to obtain a meaningful history from elderly patients by:

- Addressing the patient by his or her last name.
- Trying to minimize extraneous noise and interruptions.
- Sitting opposite the patient at eye level, smiling, and speaking slowly with a low voice.
- Inquiring about hearing deficits, confirming that the patient can hear the conversation, and asking him or her to repeat back what has been said.
- Raising the volume of his or her voice, if necessary, but not shouting (as shouting may be misinterpreted as anger).
- Writing the questions down in a large print, if the patient does not have his hearing aid or still cannot hear.
- Always allowing plenty of time for the patient to respond to questions.
- Trying to reassure the patient that he or she is in a safe environment.
- Engaging the patient to speak about his or her interests.
- Using visual aids in the room to identify caregivers and being readily available when family members visit.

THE COGNITIVE DOMAIN

The prevalence of cognitive impairment doubles every 5 years after the age of 65. Forty to fifty percent of 90 year olds will suffer from dementia. In the early stages of dementia, family members and friends often notice behavioral changes but may deny the symptoms or neglect to mention the symptoms to busy medical practitioners. Many patients do not complain or volunteer any information about memory loss unless specifically questioned. The interviewer should try to determine if the patient has an underlying dementia by inquiring whether the patient suffers from memory loss sufficient to interfere with social functioning in the months or years preceding the acute illness.

CASE 103-1

AN ELDERLY PATIENT WITH DEMENTIA

A 79-year-old female with hypertensive heart disease, mild chronic obstructive lung disease, and dementia is admitted to the hospitalist service after calling an ambulance for chest pain. On admission the plan of care was discussed by e-mail with her primary care physician who agreed with ruling her out for a myocardial infarction and then discharging her to home if her cardiologist agreed. She had not been seen in one year due to missed appointments. The cardiologist noted that she had had a recent negative pharmacologic stress test and did not recommend any further workup. The patient lives alone and denied any problems with ADLs or IDLs. Her son lived nearby but was unavailable. The team excluded a myocardial infarction and sent off some lab tests for causes of impaired cognition (thyroid function, B12, RPR) in addition to the admission blood work. She was dressed and eager to leave the hospital. She had normal fluent speech, attention, was well groomed, and able to walk without assistance.

Two days later, her attending hospitalist called her home to be sure that she would follow-up with her primary care physician. The patient answered the telephone, and then put the receiver on a table. For the rest of the afternoon the signal was busy. Concerned, the hospitalist discussed this with case management who contacted Elder Services. Apparently, this patient had not been functioning well at home, and, in fact, there had been multiple—too numerous to count—police visits to her apartment to check on her over the last year.

This case highlights the importance of a third party interview when questioning patients with dementia.

On admission, clinicians should interview caregivers about baseline cognition and recent changes in mental status. Delirium is an acute decline in attention and cognitive function characterized by waxing and waning mental status which likely started in the last few days or weeks. Delirium is subacute by nature and should not be confused with dementia which has an insidious onset, chronically present for years by the time of diagnosis, and usually does not progress abruptly. Recent changes in alertness, confusion, agitation, disruption of daily routines (sleeping more or less than normal, eating poorly) are common signs of delirium. These symptoms are sometimes subtle but noticeable to the people who live with the older adult and may sometimes precipitate a "social admission" for "placement" which may not be necessary when the delirium resolves. In such scenarios, caregiver burnout should be assessed and early involvement of social work help is vital to explore the social support situation.

Delirium itself is most often seen in patients with existing dementia, but it can occur in patients with no prior cognitive deficits if the new stress is severe enough. The examiner should probe for evidence of cognitive impairment pre-existing before the acute illness while also inquiring about other risk factors for developing delirium-poor baseline functional status, frailty, polypharmacy, CNS-active medications, chemical dependency, and number of medical comorbidities— particularly cerebrovascular and cardiovascular diseases, chronic liver or kidney disease, and visual or hearing impairment. See Chapter 81 (Delirium) and Chapter 166 (Agitation in Older Adults).

Each provider should spend extra time making sure that the "home medication list" is correct while obtaining the medical history. There is evidence that errors are frequently made on the admission medication list which leads to a high likelihood or errors

at the time of discharge. Someone on the inpatient team should verify home meds with patient, family and outpatient pharmacy, and question medications or doses that seem unusual or potentially ill-advised in an older patient. Hospital admission is a good time to re-evaluate the patient's regimen, working in concert with outpatient providers, who know the patient well.

■ THE PHYSICAL DOMAIN OF FUNCTION

The geriatric physical domain includes function, nutrition, vision, and hearing. Functional status should be assessed by determining the elder's ability to perform basic and instrumental ADL. Basic ADLs, essential to independent living, include seven items in a standardized, widely accepted scale: bathing, dressing, eating, toileting, transferring, ambulating, and maintaining continence. Bathing is the basic ADL with the highest prevalence of disability and often the reason why home health aids provide care of the elderly. As the patient perceives difficulty with bathing, he or she may change the task to sponge baths or neglect altogether. In patients without impaired cognition, self-report of daily function is reliable; in those with impaired cognition a third party interview should confirm this information. Mobility may be assessed by asking if the patient has difficulty walking outside, from room to room, or climbing a flight of stairs. Presence of new ADL deficits commonly acquired during hospitalization predicts both mortality and institutionalization.

Commonly the acute admitting illness is the result of progressive deteriorating chronic health status at home, which chronic conditions become apparent during the hospital stay, when underlying problems emerge such as malignancies, vascular disorders, and complications of longstanding metabolic illnesses like diabetes. The prevalence of sarcopenia which contributes to frailty in elderly hospitalized patients is high, reported in one study at around 22%[1]; this is another reason why functional assessment is particularly important when preparing for the consequences of immobility and catabolic states often seen during hospital care episodes and preparing patients for discharge.

Memory loss, medical illness, depression, inability to shop, and financial issues may impact nutritional status. Dysfunction and diseases of the oral cavity may affect overall health, social interactions, and increase the risk of malnutrition. Poor oral hygiene may be compromised due to alterations in vision, manual dexterity, upper extremity function, or alterations in salivary flow. The examiner should specifically inquire whether the patient has regular dental visits that may uncover untreated dental disease which is less likely to produce symptoms compared to younger patients. Dysphagia or the inability to initiate a swallow or the sensation that solids or liquids or both do not pass easily from the mouth to the stomach, odynophagia, and severe vascular disease that affects the celiac axis may cause fear of eating and result in malnutrition. Weakness of the soft palate or pharyngeal constrictor muscles can cause dysarthria and nasal regurgitation of food. In addition to direct observation of nutritional status, the interviewer should inquire about meals, whether the patient prepares them or has assistance, and whether the patient has changed the way he or she performs the IADLS such as using the telephone, shopping and cooking meals, managing finances, doing housework and laundry, and managing transportation. A weight loss of 10 pounds in the preceding 6 months or 5% in the past month indicates increased risk for malnutrition and predicts functional limitations. In this context, the examiner should consider all medications including over the counter medications such as antihistamines which can exacerbate cognitive impairment and may affect appetite and discover whether the

---

[1] Martinez BP, Menezes Santos Batista AK, Gomes IB, Olivieri FM, Camelier F, Camelie AA. Frequency of sarcopenia and associated factors among hospitalized elderly patients. BMC Musculoskelet Disord. 2015;16:108.

patient independently takes his or her medications. Anticholinergics, antihistamines, and certain antihypertensives can exacerbate poor dental hygiene by decreasing salivary flow. See Chapter 9 (Principles of Evidence-Based Prescribing) and Chapter 73 (Patient Safety and Quality Improvement).

Vision and hearing impairment increases the risk of falling and may be associated with depression, social isolation, and further decline. For hospitalized patients, vision and hearing impairment, referred to as sensory deprivation, not only interferes with communication but also increases the risk for delirium and hence morbidity. Visually impaired patients may not be aware of their deficits and may have no idea of who is examining them. There are many reasons for visual impairment, but the physician should inquire whether the patient is still driving, has difficulty seeing the television, reading or identifying people in the room. If a patient is visually impaired, there should be a sign in the room so that people identify themselves upon entering. Many elderly patients are also unaware of their hearing deficit due to the slowly progressive nature of usually symmetric sensorineural loss or deny it due to the stigma of wearing a hearing aid. Family members should be asked whether the patient hears them or plays the radio or television too loud. Clinicians may misinterpret hearing loss for cognitive impairment.

PSYCHOLOGICAL DOMAIN

Symptoms of depression have an adverse impact on quality of life, risk of physical disability, slower recovery from an acute illness, and a significant increase in the cost of medical services, even after adjusting for the severity of chronic diseases. Depression may be confused with dementia and may be chronic. However, orientation should be intact. The patient may be apathetic, express hopelessness, and make little effort to perform a task. For example, in the hospital a patient may refuse to work with physical therapy whereas demented patients with impaired cognition in multiple domains usually make an effort to perform an assigned task. Clinicians should ask the patient whether he or she often feels sad, more irritable or depressed, treat underlying depression, and address anxiety and worries that inevitably develop during hospitalization. Some patients may require help with the bereavement process if they have lost friends or family, as well as with loss of independence which can be equally damaging psychologically.

SOCIAL HISTORY DOMAIN

In addition to lifestyle habits such as tobacco and alcohol use that are commonly asked about, social history in geriatric patients should explore current living situation and any economic issues that interfere with patient wellbeing; plus support systems for daily activities that include meal preparation, mobility, bathing, dressing and toileting, transportation, and medication administration. In addition, the clinician should recognize symptoms that may suggest elder mistreatment or neglect. See Chapter 167 (Elder Mistreatment). The physician may then combine an awareness of functional limitations that is gained during the medical history with knowledge of social supports to enhance the posthospital care plan. The patient's caregiver support rather than the patient's primary diagnoses or functional disability often determines whether the patient can be discharged to his or her home. Often this information is best obtained from family and usual caregivers. The admission assessment should identify patient's primary support, health care proxy, and any potential barriers for return to the community.

GERIATRIC PHYSICAL EXAMINATION

The examiner should search for and document pre-existing conditions at the time of admission that predispose elderly patients to complications acquired during hospitalization such as malnutrition

and take steps to avoid further deterioration. The baseline neurologic examination should assess cognitive function (documenting the presence of delirium and depression), functional status (including evidence of deconditioning and the presence of pressure ulcers), and hearing and vision.

VITAL SIGNS

The first step is to review vital signs not only in the context of the complaint precipitating admission but also to assess prognosis and function. The pulse pressure (PP) and the systolic blood pressure (SBP) typically increase with age whereas the diastolic blood pressure (DBP) declines. According to Framingham data, age-related changes in blood pressure gradually shifts from the DBP as the strongest predictor of coronary artery disease in people less than 50 years of age to DBP, SBP, PP as approximately equal predictors in people aged 50 to 59 years, and SBP and PP as the strongest predictors in people over the age of 60 years. According to the Multiple Risk Factor Intervention Trial, isolated systolic hypertension (SBP > 140 mm Hg and DBP < 90 mm Hg) triples the risk of coronary heart disease and all-cause mortality in men over the age of 50. A higher PP >60 mg is an additional independent risk factor for myocardial infarction, carotid artery stenosis, end stage renal disease, renovascular hypertension, left ventricular hypertrophy, cardiovascular events, and mortality. A wide PP greater than 50% of the SBP is also seen in aortic regurgitation and may be a clue to high flow states such as hyperthyroidism, fever, symptomatic anemia, Paget's disease, or rarely severe exfoliative dermatitis.

A narrow pulse pressure PP less than 25% of the SBP coupled with cool extremities, altered mentation, Cheyne-Stokes respiration, and a resting tachycardia may portend severe ventricular dysfunction and impending cardiogenic shock. (Refer to Chapter 93 [Hypotension].) A narrow pulse pressure may also be seen in aortic stenosis, pericardial tamponade, constrictive pericarditis, and tachycardia.

Particularly if the patient or family have reported dizziness, syncope, or falling, the blood pressure and pulse should be recorded while the patient is supine and again after standing for 1 to 2 minutes to detect orthostatic changes. Postural hypotension is defined as a drop in mean blood pressure (MBP), namely, one-third SBP and two-thirds DBP, of 20% or more. Alterations of the conduction system by disease or medications such as β-blockers may prevent a change in pulse. Orthostatic or postural hypotension is common in older patients both on admission and later during the course of hospital care. This finding has been reported in 30% of hospital stays, is easily overlooked in a busy Emergency Department where patients are on stretchers, and also on the wards since vital signs are usually taken while the patient is in bed, and orthostasis may later contribute to falls, in the hospital or after discharge. Too often, hospitalized patients are only assessed when lying in bed.

The examiner should personally observe the patient's breathing and respiratory rate which is too often recorded incorrectly on the vital sign sheet. If tachypnea is noted at rest, the patient may have functional limitations due to respiratory insufficiency with hypoxia during exercise that may not be apparent at rest, or may have incipient heart failure from fluid administration during the acute illness or perioperatively, and increased work of breathing may be the only clue. An elderly patient with increased intracranial pressure following stroke or a patient with severe heart failure may have Cheyne-Stokes breathing. Kussmaul's breathing suggests metabolic acidosis. Biot's breathing with irregular periods of apnea often seen in the setting of multiple strokes carries a poor prognosis. During quiet breathing an examiner can check for pulsus paradoxus, an exaggeration of the normal decrease in SBP with inspiration. Normally during inspiration the SBP may drop 0 to 10 mm Hg. Many conditions may cause a pulsus paradoxus such as constrictive pericarditis, tamponade, pulmonary embolism, right ventricular failure, and asthma, and its presence is correlated with severity of illness.

The patient should be weighed on admission and periodically during the hospitalization. A measure of body size and indirect measure of body fat, a BMI of 18.5 kg/m³ or less is a practical measure of underweight.

■ OBSERVATION

Nothing tells the story like firsthand observation. If the patient is asleep, observe breathing before waking the patient up. Does the patient open his or her eyes when you enter the room? Does the patient fall asleep during your conversation? Does the patient appear well nourished? Are they eating during your visit? Does the patient have tethers that can be removed such as oxygen, Foley catheters, intravenous lines or other monitoring devices? Is the patient wearing a diaper? Can the patient sit up without assistance during the examination? The examiner should refrain from assisting the patient until the determination is made that the patient cannot do this on his or her own. If the patient can sit up without assistance, can the patient walk without risk of falling? Simply watching the hospitalized patient get out of bed and take a few steps or use the telephone provides valuable insight into the patient's ability to perform ADLs. There are formally validated measures such as timed walk or timed "Get Up and Go" which provide numeric data: 20 seconds on the Up and Go defines high risk of institutional care. (See Chapter 87 [Falls].) A physician who does not attempt to get the patient out of bed or pay attention to their ability to participate in self care will often miss the mark when it comes to making proactive plans for continuing care, resulting in last minute scrambling for alternative options and dissatisfaction.

■ PRESSURE ULCERS AND THE SKIN EXAM

There are both medical-legal and regulatory reasons for a thorough, documented skin assessment upon admission and at regular intervals during hospitalization, with special attention to high-risk areas. Much of this work can and should be done by nurses, but the physician should lead this initiative, "confirm nurses findings" when problems are found, and perform independent assessments based on clinical judgment and patient risk factors. In addition to the sacrum, ischial areas, and trochanters, physicians should pay attention to the heels, an area often overlooked, and be alert to erythema of intact skin in high pressure areas that does not resolve when pressure is removed (thus consistent with a Stage 1 pressure ulcer). Physicians should recognize immobility as a major risk factor for skin damage and when making rounds, ask the nurses about the skin, and examine the skin of immobilized patients. (See Chapter 72 [Pressure Ulcers].) Reducing the incidence of pressure ulcers requires a multi-disciplinary team approach, identifying patients at risk and intervening early. Preventive strategies shown to be effective include risk assessment on admission and 48 hours later.

Pressure ulcers observed early in the hospital stay may fall into two major groups: (i) superficial ulcers induced by friction or transient pressure and that are usually quickly resolved and (ii) deep ulcers reflecting a sustained, pressure-related ischemic injury to deep layers of the skin and subcutaneous tissues, occurring days earlier, sometimes before hospitalization, but delayed in clinical presentation and appearing days later. These wounds may take months to heal.

■ COGNITIVE DOMAIN

Although busy inpatient physicians cannot be expected to do an indepth mental status examination on every patient, the usual "alert and oriented" questions are inadequate to detect clinically significant cases of dementia and delirium. A more complete assessment is needed for every older inpatient. Memory loss is typically the first sign of dementia. The diagnosis of "dementia" is too often added to the patient's record when the real diagnosis is delirium or depression, or simply because the patient has been prescribed medications to enhance memory by another physician. If the patient cannot pay attention due to delirium, then screening for dementia will not reveal valid results. Dementia should be considered only when there is a history of chronic cognitive impairment dating back several months and sufficiently severe to affect social functioning. Several brief screening tools for delirium are available and should be familiar to inpatient care providers. The confusion assessment method (CAM) is the most studied. A positive CAM score requires evidence of an acute onset and fluctuating course plus a deficit in attention (the hallmark features), and at least one of two other features, which are disorganized thinking and change in level of alertness. The CAM-ICU version helps when patients cannot communicate verbally. The Delirium Rating Scale can be used to rate symptom severity.

Validated measures to screen for dementia in nondelirious patients are available, such as the Mini Mental State Exam (MMSE); these require 3 to 5 minutes and some components may be physically difficult for acutely ill patients to complete. One strategy is to use the most reliable single component within the MMSE as an initial screen. That component is three-item recall (learning a list of three words and repeating them after brief distraction) which is the most specific test of short-term memory, the common ground for all types of dementia. Three-item recall is a useful clue but is not sufficient by itself. Combining recall with clock drawing is the Mini-Cog and in testing for dementia, the Mini-Cog has comparable sensitivity and specificity to the full MMSE. Clock drawing may also be difficult in the inpatient setting. Nonetheless, whatever strategy is used by the hospital physician, it should go beyond simple orientation to person place and time. Baseline mental status testing should be a routine feature of all inpatient geriatric physical exams. And, when present, impaired cognition found in the hospital should be placed in context with the history.

■ DISCHARGE PLANNING

Despite recent advances in electronic records, patient pathways, and technology-assisted decision support, the following factors identified nearly 20 years ago still cause delayed discharge from hospital: inadequate assessment of the patient by health care professionals resulting in poor knowledge of the patient's social circumstances; and poor organization, for example, late booking of transport preventing timely discharge from hospital and poor communication between the hospital and providers of clinical services in the community after discharge.

Discharge planning should begin at the time of admission. When preparing for discharge, incorporating a solid understanding of the geriatric patient's functional status, clinical condition and social support needs and ensuring adequate provision of continuing care following discharge may reduce the likelihood of return to hospital with preventable problems such as falls. Discharge planning begun at the time of admission can have impressive results. One classic 1995 study found 50% fewer readmissions after applying focused care processes designed for selected older patients with recurrent admissions for heart failure related to uncontrolled hypertension or ischemia. Geriatric cardiologist medication review, intensive patient education, and specific home nursing follow-up were the main interventions.

The literature on discharge planning is extensive and offers both success stories and failures. The most successful studies select and concentrate on patients who are inherently vulnerable to poor transitions from hospital to home, and provide a focused, robust intervention. Between 2002 and 2006, comparing historical costs and postintervention costs incurred at our medical center, we saw a sharp reduction in readmissions and days in the hospital for selected patients when a Naylor model transitional care model helped complex patients posthospital and the same pattern continued through 2015.

Many discharge planning programs have reported increased quality of life and patient satisfaction. Neither optimal care nor health care utilization benefits occur when team members work in isolation. Multidisciplinary intervention: a combination that includes discharge planning, geriatric assessment with functional and cognitive evaluation, and medication review- is far more likely to be effective. In-person intervention (rather than telephonic care management) is found in the most successful models, and the experience and expertise of discharge planners also makes a difference. Of note, there are varied control group costs in the formal studies of transitional care interventions, and combined with the differences in magnitude of impact, one must conclude that each institution should consider targeted populations, usual care settings, and local resources when designing strategies. The Society of Hospital Medicine has identified transitions of care as a major quality issue and initiated BOOST (**B**etter **O**utcomes for **O**lder adults through **S**afer **T**ransitions) to improve transitions of care for the elderly in Pennsylvania and more recently in Michigan (**Table 103-1**).

TABLE 103-1 BOOST (Society of Hospital Medicine)

Project BOOST Facts

GOAL: The goal of Project BOOST (**B**etter **O**utcomes for **O**lder adults through **S**afe **T**ransitions) is to improve the care of patients as they transition from the hospital to home.

OUTCOMES:

By improving discharge processes, Project BOOST aims to:

- Reduce 30 d readmission rates for general medicine patients (with particular focus on older adults).
- Improve facility patient satisfaction scores.
- Improve the institution's H-CAHPS scores related to discharge.
- Improve flow of information between hospital and outpatient physicians.
- Ensure high-risk patients are identified and specific interventions are offered to mitigate their risk.
- Improve patient and family education practices to encourage use of the teach-back process around risk specific issues.

APPROACH:

1. **Create a national consensus for best practices.** Project BOOST's advisory board includes representatives from the Agency for Healthcare Research and Quality (AHRQ), The Joint Commission, Centers for Medicare and Medicaid Services, Blue Cross and Blue Shield Association, pharmacy, nursing, geriatricians, patient advocates, and others.
2. **Create resources to implement best practices.** Project BOOST created a resource room-BOOSTing Care Transitions Resource Room, for quality improvement teams including:
- Clinical toolkit (discharge planning tools, risk stratification tools).
- Data collection tools.
- Project Management Tools (guidance for gaining institutional support, creating and managing a team).
- Educational tools background information for professionals new to quality improvement.
- Review of key literature.
- Exchange Information and Share Success stories.
3. **Provide technical support.** Project BOOST offers several technical support options via the Project BOOST Mentoring Program. Participating sites will receive:
- Day long training sessions (fee-based).
- Year-long coaching/mentoring program (free, courtesy of grant from the John A. Hartford Foundation).

PARTICIPATING SITES

Any site can access the BOOST tool kit via the resource room free of charge at www.hospitalmedicine.org/BOOST. Over 265 sites have downloaded the complete Implementation Guide which serves as a portable version of the resource room and will walk you through the steps improve the discharge process. There are two cohorts participating in the Project BOOST Mentoring Program.

Cohort one, listed below started in September 2008.

Six hospitals were selected to participate in Project BOOST's pilot mentoring program:

- Piedmont Hospital, Atlanta, Georgia.
- Queens Medical Center, Honolulu, Hawaii.
- University of New Mexico Health Science Center School of Medicine, Albuquerque, NM.
- Hospital of the University of Pennsylvania, Philadelphia, PA.
- Southwestern Vermont Medical Center, Bennington, VT.
- ThedaCare: Appleton Medical Center, Appleton, WI; ThedaClark Medical Center, Neenah, WI.

(Continued)

TABLE 103-1 BOOST (Society of Hospital Medicine) (*Continued*)

Cohort two, listed below started in March 2009.

Twenty-four hospitals were selected to participate in Project BOOST's mentoring program:

- Banner Good Samaritan Medical Center, Phoenix, AZ.
- Kaiser Permanente Hospital West Los Angeles, Los Angeles, CA.
- California Pacific Medical Center, San Francisco, CA.
- University of California, San Francisco, San Francisco, CA.
- Greenwich Hospital, Greenwich, CT.
- Morton Plant Hospital, Clearwater, FL.
- Emory Crawford Long Hospital, Atlanta, GA.
- Emory University Hospital, Atlanta, GA.
- Rush University Medical Center, Chicago, IL.
- University of Kansas Hospital, Kansas City, KS.
- UMass Memorial Medical Center, Worcester, MA.
- University of Michigan, Ann Arbor, MI.
- SSM St. Mary's Health Center, St. Louis, MO.
- Billings Clinic, Billings, MT.
- Mission Hospital, Asheville, NC.
- Lakes Region General Hospital, Laconia, NH.
- Cooper Health, Camden, NJ.
- Huntington Hospital, Huntington, NY.
- Albert Einstein Healthcare Network, Philadelphia, PA.
- Medical University of South Carolina, Charleston, SC.
- Sanford USD Medical Center, Sioux Falls, SD.
- Baptist Hospital, Nashville, TN.
- Chesapeake Hospitalists, P.C., Chesapeake, VA.
- Aurora Medical Center, Summit, Milwaukee, WI.

■ AREAS FOR FUTURE RESEARCH

Care of the hospitalized elder is challenging and requires an interprofessional, multidisciplinary approach to prevent and manage complications like delirium and decline in functional status.

Geriatric focused history and physical exams are required to identify patient at increased risk. One method to improve documentation of risk factors is use of templates consultation notes or inpatient notes adapted to an electronic medical records. Templates provide cues to document physical function, mental status, social supports, advance directives and complete skin assessments. The electronic medical record can then trigger use of care sets or treatment protocols which restrict use of medications known to precipitate delirium, encourage early mobilization, and promote pressure relief. There remains a paucity of high quality published research on preventing complications in hospitalized elders, examining mortality, quality of life, caregiver issues, health care utilization and cost. As the aging population is growing exponentially, it is imperative that interventions are developed, tested and proven to be reproducible in order to systematically improve the care of hospitalized elders nationwide.

CONCLUSION

Limited physiologic reserves, high comorbidity and complex social issues make the needs of elderly inpatients relatively unique among adults. Circumstances vary across settings and studies, including such issues as financial assets, extent of managed care penetration in communities, availability of community assets, and strength of the local primary care workforce. Solid evidence shows that improved care processes including team-based assessments and rounds can materially reduce the incidence and consequences of delirium, pressure ulcers, and decrease length of stay, institutional care, hospital readmission, and avoidable health care costs. We have described the importance of the geriatric focused history and physical that can provide value information to target interventions to improve outcomes. Beyond what is known there is much research work yet to be done in further refining our clinical care of older patients. In particular, the roles of nonphysicians on the care team are an opportunity for sharing the work of structured and focused yet comprehensive assessment. In the near future, Medicare will require the team to document certain items, such as function and cognition, in all hospitalized patients.

CHAPTER 104

The Neurologic Examination

David J. Likosky, MD, SFHM, FAHA, FACP
S. Andrew Josephson, MD

Key Clinical Questions

① What elements of the history and examination are most useful in lesion localization?

② What elements of the neurologic examination can be assessed at the bedside without formal testing?

③ What tests can be performed on the unresponsive patient?

④ What scales and tools are used to document the findings of the neurologic exam?

INTRODUCTION

The neurologic examination is central to the evaluation of patients with neurologic complaints. It relies heavily on the history and on hypothesis-driven physical testing. The neurologic examination can provide a great deal of information quickly. Even when it is not diagnostic, it guides the appropriate choice of imaging and ancillary testing. However, if it is performed in a cursory fashion, one can easily miss clues to a diagnosis that may not be apparent on imaging. This chapter reviews the essential elements of the neurologic examination in evaluating patients in the hospital.

IMPORTANCE OF THE HISTORY

The history allows the hospitalist to narrow the range of diagnostic testing and perform a more focused and higher yield neurologic examination.

CASE 104-1

A 57-year-old right-handed man presents with an episode of syncope while typing a manuscript. He recalls no prior episodes but does have a history of well-controlled hypertension and hyperlipidemia. You are called by the emergency department physician to admit the patient to telemetry and rule out an arrhythmia. The patient recalls similar episodes that he has had for as long as he can remember. They were bothersome during school but are brief and infrequent now. He also notes that they were worse when he was tired.

When taking the neurologic history, the hospitalist should focus first on localizing the lesion, and then on developing a differential diagnosis. Missed diagnoses are common in neurology when one jumps to a conclusion before establishing where the problem lies. Tempo is helpful. Does the process wax and wane, as in delirium? Is it steadily progressive, as in dementia? Or does decline occur in a stepwise fashion, as with multiple strokes? In patients with muscle weakness, pay attention to the pattern of weakness. Difficulty rising from a chair, carrying heavy loads, or brushing or washing hair suggests proximal weakness. Problems with opening a jar, opening a car door, or turning a key in a lock suggest distal weakness. In patients with sensory symptoms, is there loss of sensation (negative phenomena), such as the numbness resulting from stroke, or inappropriate sensation (positive phenomena), such as tingling from nerve root compression?

CASE 104-1 (continued)

The patient's physical examination was unrevealing. A computed tomography (CT) scan of his brain was negative, but an electroencephalogram (EEG) showed occasional epileptiform discharges from the left hemisphere. The patient was begun on anticonvulsants at a very low dose and has had no further episodes.

Without a detailed history, this patient might have been admitted to telemetry and had extensive and inappropriate cardiac investigations. He might have been discharged with the diagnosis of unexplained syncope and gone on to have a seizure at an inopportune time. With a careful history, he leaves instead with a correct diagnosis and life-altering therapy.

LOCALIZING THE LESION

A major goal in neurology is to localize the lesion causing the patient's symptoms. Diagnosis in neurology, as in other domains of medicine, relies partly on pattern recognition. Important patterns include the hemiparesis and language deficit of a dominant middle cerebral artery stroke, the cranial nerve findings and crossed body involvement of a brainstem stroke, the distal neuropathy of diabetes, the ascending weakness of Guillain-Barré syndrome, and the diurnal variation of ptosis and diplopia in myasthenia gravis. However, many signs and symptoms in neurology are nonspecific, and may be produced by lesions in more than one anatomical site.

■ CENTRAL VERSUS PERIPHERAL

CASE 104-2

A 27-year-old man who has previously been healthy complains of strange sensations. You note that his mental status is normal, as are his cranial nerves, with the exception of an afferent papillary defect on the right. He has full strength, with increased muscle tone diffusely, and developed a mild right-sided foot drop about a year ago, for which he never sought treatment. Sensation is normal except for much of his left hemithorax. Reflexes are mildly hyperactive, and a Babinski sign is present.

A fundamental distinction in neurologic disease is deciding whether a central or peripheral lesion is responsible. Central lesions affect the brain and spinal cord, and peripheral lesions affect the anterior horn cells, peripheral nerves, neuromuscular junctions, or muscles. Localizing a lesion to the central or peripheral nervous system avoids excessive, shotgun imaging, in which may lead to inflated costs and overdiagnosis. In the case above, there are elements that are likely central (afferent pupillary defect, hyperactive reflexes, increased tone, and Babinski sign) and others that could be either (foot drop). It would be helpful to further define the abnormal sensation using dermatome and peripheral nerve maps (**Figures 104-1** and **104-2**). If the new abnormality does not conform to the distribution of a peripheral nerve or dermatome, a central lesion is probable, and neuroimaging is indicated. Ordering an electromyogram (EMG) in this setting would be inappropriate and of low yield.

In this case, the patient has lesions that are separated in space (different locations in the CNS) and time (old foot drop, new altered sensations). Magnetic resonance imaging (MRI) of the brain is ordered, which demonstrates multifocal T2 hyperintensities that particularly involve the periventricular white matter, consistent with demyelinating lesions of multiple sclerosis.

■ UPPER VERSUS LOWER MOTOR NEURON LESION

When patients have weakness, it is helpful to localize the lesion to either the upper or lower motor neuron (**Figure 104-3**). Severity of weakness does not distinguish between these anatomical sites, but examination of tone, reflexes, and other elements of the exam

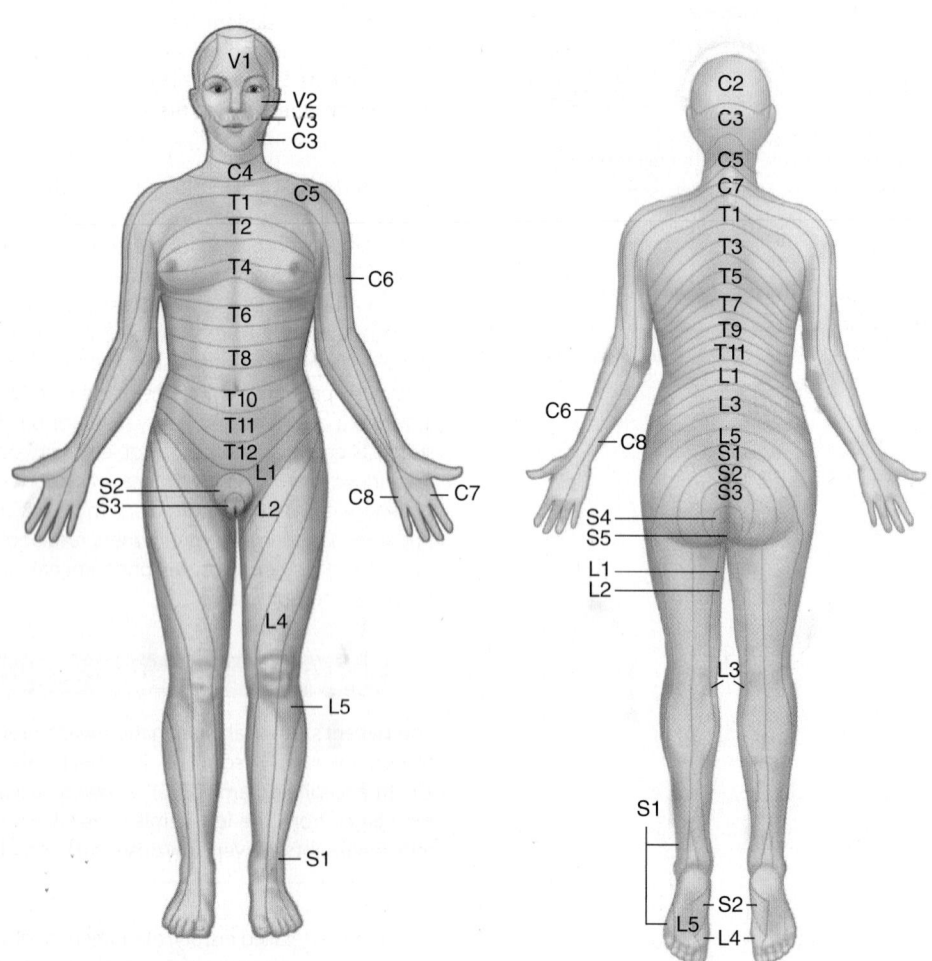

Figure 104-1 *Dermatome map.* (Reproduced, with permission, from Cunningham FG, Leveno KJ, Bloom SL, et al. *Williams Obstetrics,* 23rd ed. New York, NY: McGraw-Hill; 2010, Figure 19-3.)

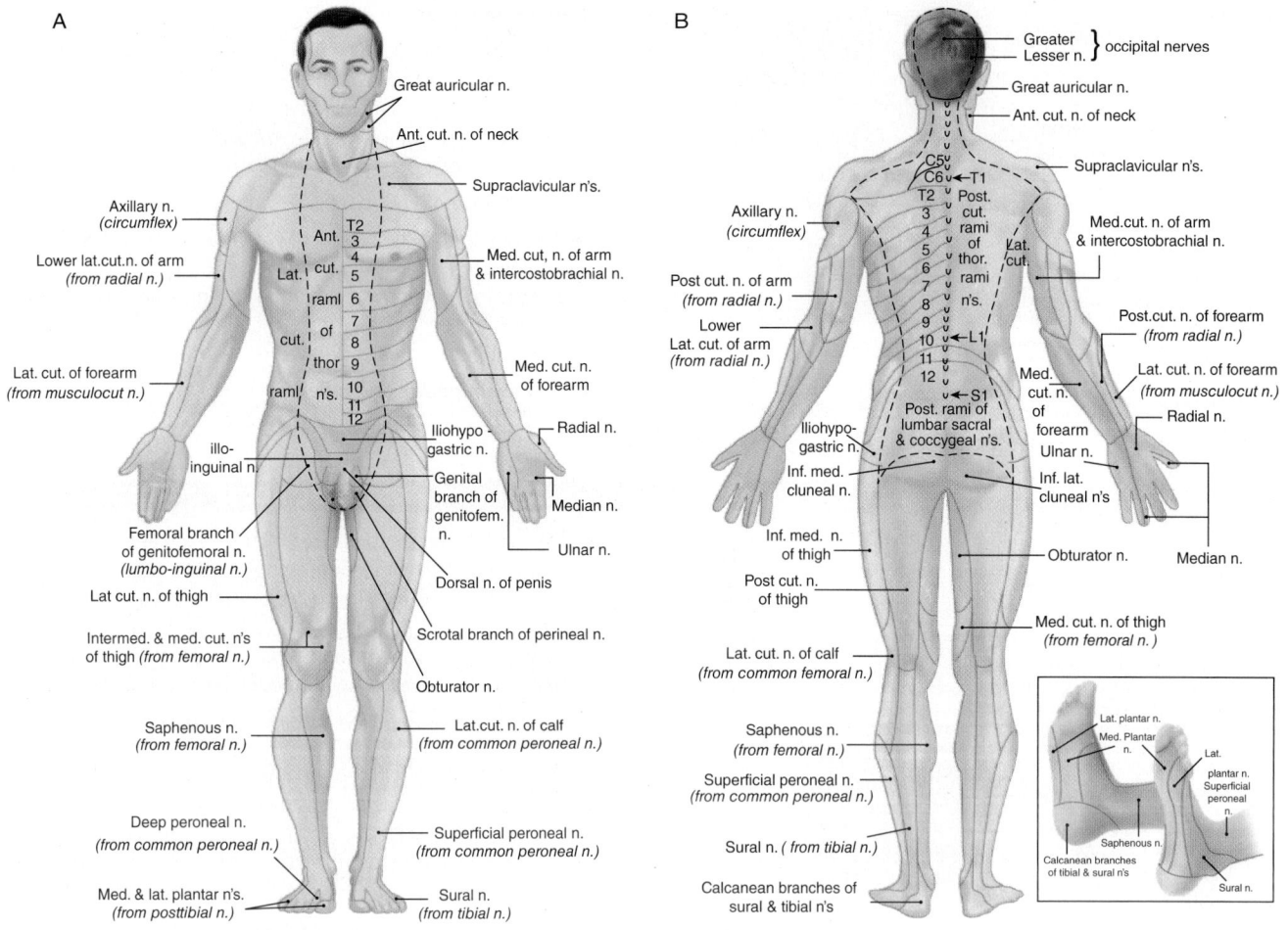

Figure 104-2 *Map of peripheral sensory nerves.* Front (A). Back (B). (Reproduced, with permission, from Haymaker W, Woodhall B. *Peripheral Nerve Injuries,* 2nd ed. Philadelphia, PA: Saunders; 1953.)

do (**Table 104-1**). When upper motor neuron weakness is present, the lesion must be in the brain or spinal cord. Lower motor neuron weakness may have multiple localizations (**Table 104-2**), none of which can be discerned through imaging studies of the brain and spinal cord; next steps may include EMG and nerve conduction studies (NCSs).

■ POSTERIOR FOSSA LESIONS

CASE 104-3

A 76-year-old woman is reportedly found "twitching" in the hallway of her apartment building, after having been seen to be well 1 hour prior. She is intubated for airway protection. In the emergency department, she has a recorded blood pressure of 240/130 mm Hg. On exam, her right eye is abducted in downgaze, and the right pupil is larger than the left. Cranial nerves are otherwise intact. She withdraws to painful stimulus with the right arm, which appears ataxic with movement. She is able to communicate intact sensation. She is hyporeflexic, and Babinski signs are present bilaterally.

The posterior fossa contains the brainstem and cerebellum. Due to their bony encasement, even minor swelling may obstruct the outflow of cerebrospinal fluid, leading to major morbidity and mortality. Brainstem signs include abnormal cranial nerve findings, such as unequal or misshapen pupils and facial asymmetry. In addition, crossed signs—contralateral findings in face and body—may

be present. Many of these are present in this case. Our patient had urgent neuroimaging that did not reveal a hemorrhage and recovered following thrombolysis for ischemic stroke.

ESSENTIAL ELEMENTS OF THE NEUROLOGIC EXAMINATION

An in-depth neurologic examination can take an exorbitant amount of time when not driven by a hypothesis. Many of the patients cared for by hospitalists warrant only a brief screening examination. It is particularly important to assess for underlying mental frailty due to underlying dementia, as neurologic illness often becomes more apparent due to the stresses of hospitalization. This may take the form of delirium unmasking dementia, or respiratory failure revealing underlying neuromuscular weakness.

Fortunately, much of the neurologic examination is observational. The attentive clinician may be able to document many essential elements of the exam without formal testing:

Mental status

- Established during history taking when asking specific questions
- Language fluency is apparent during the history

Cranial nerves

- Vision, eye movements, and sternocleidomastoid, as the patient watches the examiner walk between the sides of the bed
- Facial symmetry, lid strength, hearing, and tongue strength as the history is taken

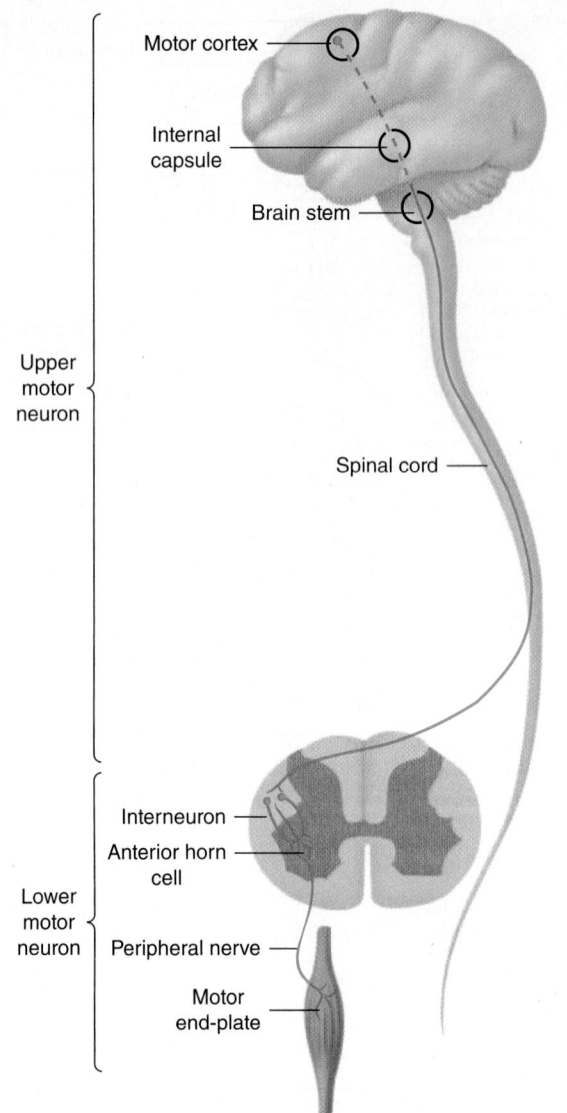

Figure 104-3 *Anatomical localization of upper and lower motor neuron lesions.* (Reproduced, with permission, from Waxman SG. *Clinical Neuroanatomy*, 26th ed. New York, NY: McGraw-Hill; 2010, Figure 5-22.)

TABLE 104-1 Upper Versus Lower Motor Neuron Weakness

	Upper Motor Neuron	Lower Motor Neuron
Pattern of weakness	Pyramidal	Variable
Function/dexterity	Rapid alternating movements slow and clumsy (indicates disease in cerebellar or corticospinal tracts)	Impairment of function is mostly due to weakness
Tone	Increased	Decreased
Tendon reflex	Increased	Decreased, absent, or normal
Other signs	Babinski sign, other central signs (eg, aphasia, visual field cut)	Atrophy (except with problems of the neuromuscular junction)

Motor examination

- Gross abnormalities can be seen as the patient moves in bed or between the bed and a chair
- Subtle signs, such as the external rotation of a foot, as evidence of upper motor neuron-type leg weakness
- Tremor may be noted at rest and with movement

Coordination

- Although getting the patient to walk may be difficult, it is often very revealing
- Observe the patient manipulating the nurse call button and moving the bedside tray, or ask the patient to retrieve a medication list from a purse or drawer

Sensory examination and reflexes

- Usually require formal testing for assessment

PRACTICE POINT

The ability to test higher cognitive functions such as memory and language is limited in patients who cannot sustain attention. Inattentiveness, or the inability to concentrate, often indicates delirium, particularly when accompanied by fluctuating mental status, alteration of consciousness, and disorganized thinking. Bedside tests useful in assessing attention and delirium include:

- Assessing the level of arousal (awake, drowsy, lethargic, or comatose); speak to nurses and family members to assess whether mental status is waxing and waning;
- Assessing the level of awareness (orientation to person, place, and time). Note that an oriented patient may still be confused, and a disoriented one may have psychosis, amnesia, or aphasia instead of delirium;
- Days of the week or months of the year, forward and backward (serial 7s and spelling words backward are not good tests, particularly for patients who are illiterate or uneducated).

Have the patient play a game that requires attention. For example, if the examiner taps once, the patient taps twice on the table; if the examiner taps twice, the patient does not tap on the table. Alternatively, have the patient tap the examiner's palm every time a certain letter of the alphabet is mentioned.

Many elements do require specific attention and testing, as one may miss significant findings or leave others poorly defined. These are typically symptom-driven, as in a patient presenting with suspicion of intracranial disease, spinal cord disease, peripheral weakness or numbness, or multifocal neurologic disease. If the patient cannot pay attention, as in the case of delirium, the examiner may erroneously assume that he or she has an underlying dementia. Therefore, formal neuropsychological testing is best delayed until the patient has recovered from acute illness and the delirium has resolved.

UNRESPONSIVENESS

CASE 104-4

A 62-year-old man is found unresponsive. His cranial nerves are tested individually and are intact, with the exception of unequal pupils, corneal reflexes, and abnormal eye movements. He does not respond to painful stimuli. Babinski sign is present on the left. MRI reveals a basilar artery thrombosis.

Frequently, the exam is erroneously thought to be of little use in patients who are unresponsive or comatose. At the very least,

TABLE 104-2 Patterns of Muscle Weakness

	Motor Neuron Disease	Neuropathy	Neuromuscular Junction	Myopathy
Weakness pattern	Variable	Distal	Diffuse	Proximal
Deep tendon reflexes	Increased, normal, or decreased	Decreased or absent	Normal or decreased	Normal or decreased
Atrophy	Yes	Yes	No	No
Fasciculations	Yes	Sometimes	No	No
Sensory symptoms and signs	No	Yes	No	No

pupillary, corneal, and gag or cough reflexes can be evaluated easily in the nonparalyzed patient. Facial strength, along with the motor and sensory systems, can be evaluated with response to painful stimuli.

Coma can result from two different localizations: bilateral cerebral hemispheric damage, as in head trauma or metabolic disturbances, such as hepatic encephalopathy or drug intoxication, and damage to the reticular activating system in the brainstem. Most cranial nerve nuclei (III to XII, except XI) are housed in the brainstem near the reticular activating system. If there are cranial nerve abnormalities, the lesion responsible for coma likely involves the reticular activating system, as in the patient vignette above. In the more common scenario where the cranial nerves are normal, bilateral hemispheric dysfunction is likely the culprit.

HEADACHE

CASE 104-5

A 45-year-old otherwise healthy woman presents with progressive headaches and left-sided weakness. She has had recent fevers. Her exam reveals bilateral papilledema, in addition to mild left-sided weakness.

Headache is a common element in patients with various underlying intracranial processes. These patients may have normal exams or relatively nonspecific exam findings. The character of the headache and nature of its onset are very important. A moderate headache of subacute onset is evaluated differently than a severe headache of acute onset. An exacerbation of a previously evaluated migraine syndrome may not warrant repeated imaging, but a sudden-onset "worst headache of my life" certainly does.

This patient has papilledema on exam, concerning for raised intracranial pressure, which may present solely with headache. Causes of high intracranial pressures include venous sinus thrombosis, cerebrovascular disease with edema, malignancy, meningoencephalitis, mass lesion, pseudotumor cerebri, and brain abscess. In these cases, historical elements such as blurred vision, diplopia, headache, and nausea will often be of more help in the differential diagnosis than the exam. Signs in patients with headaches due to focal lesions include a depressed level of consciousness, pupillary asymmetry, unilateral weakness, and pronator drift. However, even large subdural hematomas may be missed on a thorough examination, requiring a high index of suspicion from the history, and communication with family members who may report a subtle personality change.

CASE 104-5 (continued)

Further history reveals three spontaneous miscarriages. Over the next several hours, the patient develops bilateral weakness, increasing headache, and a left-sided seizure that generalizes.

Magnetic resonance venography (MRV) shows a venous clot and stroke with hemorrhagic conversion. She is subsequently found to have antiphospholipid antibody syndrome.

VERTIGO

CASE 104-6

A 54-year-old man with a history of myocardial infarction and stroke complains of vertigo. He is recovering from a recent upper respiratory infection. The emergency department physician calls you to admit the patient for a possible brainstem stroke.

Vertigo is a source of frequent consternation, as it may represent the common sequelae of an upper respiratory tract infection, or a harbinger of life-threatening posterior fossa disease. Key initial steps are to determine whether the patient has true vertigo, with the illusion of movement, or a different sensation, such as presyncope.

Elements of the history and exam that suggest a central cause of vertigo, such as brainstem stroke, intracranial mass lesions, or multiple sclerosis, include headache, persistent symptoms, neck pain, visual disturbances, speech difficulty, cranial nerve palsies, and ataxia. Horizontal nystagmus is common in both central and peripheral vertigo, but vertical nystagmus is more common with central rather than peripheral conditions. Hearing loss is uncommon with central disease.

CASE 104-6 (continued)

The patient's history is reassuring. The only finding on a detailed neurologic exam is two beats of horizontal nystagmus. He is sent home from the emergency department and does well.

COMPLAINTS REFERABLE TO THE SPINAL CORD

CASE 104-7

A 32-year-old woman with a distant history of tuberculosis and recent treatment with prednisone for an asthma exacerbation presents with midback pain and vague complaints of difficulty walking, along with a sensation of her legs giving way. On examination, her gait is tentative, and Babinski signs are present bilaterally.

TABLE 104-3 Tendon Reflexes and Their Associated Nerve Root Levels

Reflex	Peripheral Nerve	Nerve Root
Biceps	Musculocutaneous	C5, C6
Triceps	Radial	C7, C8
Brachioradialis	Radial	C5, C6
Abdominal	Segmental cutaneous nerves	T8-T9 (above umbilicus); T10-T11 (below umbilicus)
Patellar	Femoral	L3, L4
Achilles	Tibial	S1, S2

TABLE 104-5 Grading of Deep Tendon Reflexes

4	Very brisk, often with clonus (record the number of beats)
3	Brisk
2	Normal
1	Minimal
0	Absent

Few areas are more important in neurologic localization than the spinal cord. Because the spinal cord is tightly confined in a bony canal, irreversible damage with profound consequences can be millimeters or minutes away. Historical features that increase the risk of spinal cord compression include recent trauma, metastatic cancer, myeloma, and systemic infection, especially with bacteremia, which increases the risk of epidural abscess. Pain at the site of compression is usually the first symptom. Patients may have radicular pain at the level of compression, often exacerbated by coughing or straining. Leg weakness and sensory disturbances are also common. Cauda equina involvement may produce bowel and bladder disturbances.

Sensory testing must be performed to help define the level of involvement. This can be performed with a safety pin or tuning fork run quickly over the patient's back. This brief examination is of immense value in determining what level should be imaged. Reflex testing may also help to define the level, as well as the affected side if disease is unilateral (**Table 104-3**). Weakness, hyperreflexia, and Babinski signs may also be present.

CASE 104-7 (*continued*)

The patient's sensory exam reveals a clear change in sensation below T11. Subsequent evaluation confirms Pott's disease of the spine.

MULTIFOCAL DISEASE

Multifocal disease can be difficult to diagnose. Many neurologic diseases present with ill-defined symptoms, particularly in the early stages. There is a tendency to label a patient as a malingerer in the absence of an easily discernible pattern or localizable lesion. This risk

TABLE 104-4 Grading of Muscle Strength (Modified Medical Research Council Scale)

Grade 0	No movement whatsoever
Grade 1	Flicker or trace contraction
Grade 2	Moves only when gravity is eliminated (in the horizontal plane only)
Grade 3	Moves against gravity but not resistance
Grade 4-	Moves against gravity and light resistance
Grade 4	Moves against gravity and moderate resistance
Grade 4+	Submaximal movement against resistance
Grade 5	Full power

of misdiagnosis is increased in patients with vague complaints or barriers to communication.

Multifocal disease calls for an even more careful history and examination, as disease manifestations may be protean. Conditions such as polyarteritis nodosa, sarcoidosis, Sjögren syndrome, porphyria, and lead poisoning can be clinically confusing even when disparate sensory and motor symptoms are not part of the clinical picture. When these are the presenting symptoms, the difficulty in lesion localization may drive electrodiagnostic studies, as well as a wide-ranging laboratory evaluation.

DOCUMENTING THE EXAMINATION

When caring for patients with neurologic disease, documentation of the examination requires greater precision than "nonfocal" and general terms such as "weak." Whereas the sensory exam does not lend itself well to quantification, the motor strength and reflex testing do (**Tables 104-4** and **104-5**). It is important to record what areas are tested and the degree of weakness noted. This information is especially valuable when patients have fluctuating symptoms either in the hospital or after discharge.

Specialized instruments, such as the National Institutes of Health Stroke Scale (NIHSS), may be very helpful for the hospitalist (http://www.ninds.nih.gov/doctors/NIH_Stroke_Scale.pdf). In addition to quantifying the deficits in patients suffering acute stroke and determining eligibility for more aggressive intervention, the NIHSS is an excellent tool for documenting neurologic deficits. Many hospitals mandate recording of the NIHSS on admission and at intervals during a hospital stay. If the patient has a significant change, a covering physician or nurse will be able to quantify the degree of difference and determine whether additional interventions are needed. Free training courses are available online.

CONCLUSION

The neurologic examination is key in determining the cause of neurologic complaints. While the potential range of evaluation can be daunting, a focused examination that is informed by the history has a high yield. This is no less true for patients who are poorly responsive. By using standardized tools and scales, one can more easily communicate change and intervene with more certainty. With a core set of neurologic examination skills and knowledge, the practicing hospitalist plays a central role in the care of these patients.

SUGGESTED READINGS

Biller J, Gruener G, Brazis P. *DeMyer's The Neurologic Examination: A Programmed Text*, 6th ed. New York, NY: McGraw-Hill; 2011.

Booth CM, Boone RH, Thomlinson G, et al. Is this patient dead, vegetative, or severely neurologically impaired? In: Simel DL, Rennie D, eds. *The Rational Clinical Examination*. New York, NY: McGraw-Hill; 2009:215-226. Chap. 17.

Froehling DA, Silverstein MD, Mohr DN, Beatty CW. The Rational Clinical Examination. Does this dizzy patient have a serious form of vertigo? *JAMA*. 1994;271(5):385-388.

Goldstein LB, Simel DL. Is this patient having a stroke? In: Simel DL, Rennie D, eds. *The Rational Clinical Examination*. New York, NY: McGraw-Hill; 2009:627-641. Chap. 48.

Lance JW. The Babinski sign. *J Neurol Neurosurg Psychiatry*. 2002;73:360-362.

Lanska DJ, Goetz CG. Romberg's sign: development, adoption, and adaptation in the 19th century. *Neurology*. 2000;55:1201-1206.

Rao G, Fisch L, Srinivasan S, et al. Does this patient have Parkinson disease? In: Simel DL, Rennie D, eds. *The Rational Clinical Examination*. New York, NY: McGraw-Hill; 2009:505-514. Chap. 38.

Smetana GW and Shmerling RH. Does this patient have temporal arteritis. In: Simel DL, Rennie D, eds. *The Rational Clinical Examination*. New York, NY: McGraw-Hill; 2009:643-656. Chap. 49.

Tejus MN, Singh V, Ramesh A, Kumar VR, Maurya VP, Madhugiri VS. An evaluation of the finger flexion, Hoffman's and plantar reflexes as markers of cervical spinal cord compression. *Clin Neurol Neurosurg*. 2015;134:12-16.

CHAPTER 105

Using Prognosis to Guide Treatment

Rachelle E. Bernacki, MD, MS
Joshua R. Lakin, MD

Key Clinical Questions

1. How does the physician approach a patient with multiple comorbidities? How are they different than other patients?

2. How do multiple comorbidities and functional status affect a patient's prognosis?

3. How does the physician take prognosis into account when formulating treatment plans for patients?

CASE 105-1

A 79-year-old woman with moderately severe chronic diseases (obstructive pulmonary disease, osteoporosis, osteoarthritis, type 2 diabetes mellitus, and hypertension) was admitted to the hospital for a complicated urinary tract infection. She had recently moved to the area and needed to establish primary care following discharge. Her newly assigned primary care physician requested that "good maintenance medications" be prescribed for her chronic diseases prior to discharge. However, if the relevant clinical practice guidelines were followed, the patient would be prescribed 12 medications (her cost $406 per month) along with a complicated nonpharmacological regimen (see **Table 105-1**). The patient did not find these recommendations to be practical.

INTRODUCTION

The remarkable success of medicine combined with improved living conditions in the last century has led to an increase in life expectancy in the United States. In the 21st century, a 70-year-old woman in the top 25% percentile of health can expect to live an additional 21.3 years (see **Figure 105-1**). As more people are living into old age, the numbers of patients with multiple comorbitites are rising. In fact, very few patients have only hypertension or simply diabetes; many patients with chronic diseases have multiple comorbidities. In 2010, only 32% of Medicare beneficiaries had one or less chronic medical conditions and 37% had four or more. Health care costs for individuals with at least four chronic conditions accounted for 74% of Medicare's annual spending. Comorbidity is associated with higher health care use, physical disability, polypharmacy/adverse drug events, poor quality of life, and increased mortality. Improving care for this population is clearly important, but it is a challenge for physicians, including hospitalists, who need to balance and prioritize treatment of the acute conditions requiring hospitalization with the chronic morbidities that may complicate treatment.

Until recently there have been few guidelines on how to account for patients' comorbidities and formulate reasonable treatment plans. Care can be haphazard, scattered, and costly for the patient, provider and health care system. Some argue that the best way to approach the above patient is to consider her prognosis in making recommendations on how to treat her various conditions and take patient preferences into account.

To a large degree, how a medical team decides to treat a patient's particular condition or comorbidity depends on the patient's prognosis. *"How long do I have?"* is among the most common questions asked by patients. Prognosis is defined as "a prediction of the probable course and outcome of a disease" or alternatively, "the likelihood of recovery from a disease." More simply put, the question is: "What can I expect with the future of my illness?" which includes both the timeframe and the functional and experiential trajectory of the illness. Current textbooks of internal medicine present a diagnosis-based approach to disease and provide little information about the prognosis of diseases.

Prognosis guides individualized clinical decisions such as cancer screening or hospice, and identifies groups at high risk for poor outcomes in whom targeted interventions may be most useful. Importantly, prognosis can provide the foundation for discussing goals of care. Many patients want to discuss prognosis with physicians, and

TABLE 105-1 Treatment Regimen for Case 105-1

Treatment Regimen Based on Clinical Practice Guidelines for a Hypothetical 79-Year-Old Woman with Hypertension, Diabetes Mellitus, Osteoporosis, Osteoarthritis, and COPD*

Time	Medications[†]	Other
7:00 AM	Ipratropium metered dose inhaler 70 mg/wk of alendronate	Check feet Sit upright for 30 min on day when alendronate is taken Check blood sugar
8:00 AM	500 mg of calcium and 200 IU of vitamin D 12.5 mg of hydrochlorothiazide 40 mg of lisinopril 10 mg of glyburide 81 mg of aspirin 850 mg of metformin 250 mg of naproxen 20 mg of omeprazole	Eat breakfast 2.4 g/d of sodium 90 mmol/d of potassium Low intake of dietary saturated fat and cholesterol Adequate intake of magnesium and calcium Medical nutrition therapy for diabetes[§] DASH[§]
12:00 PM		Eat lunch 2.4 g/d of sodium 90 mmol/d of potassium Low intake of dietary saturated fat and cholesterol Adequate intake of magnesium and calcium Medical nutrition therapy for diabetes[§] DASH[§]
1:00 PM	Ipratropium metered dose inhaler 500 mg of calcium and 200 IU of vitamin D	
7:00 PM	Ipratropium metered dose inhaler 850 mg of metformin 500 mg of calcium and 200 IU of vitamin D 40 mg of lovastatin 250 mg of naproxen	Eat dinner 2.4 g/d of sodium 90 mmol/d of potassium Low intake of dietary saturated fat and cholesterol Adequate intake of magnesium and calcium Medical nutrition therapy for diabetes[§] DASH[§]
11:00 PM	Ipratropium metered dose inhaler	
As needed	Albuterol metered dose inhaler	

Abbreviations: ADA, American Diabetes Association; COPD, chronic obstructive pulmonary disease: DASH; Dietary Approaches to Stop Hypertension.

*Clinical practice guidelines used: (1) Joint National Committee on Prevention, Detection. Evaluation, and Treatment of High Blood Pressure VII. (2) ADA; glycemic control is recommended; however, specific medicines are not described. (3) American College of Rheumatology; recent evidence about the safety and appropriateness of cyclooxygenase inhibitors, particularly in individuals with comorbid cardiovascular disease, led us to omit them from the list of medication options, although they are discussed in the reviewed clinical practice guidelines. (4) National Osteoporosis Foundation; this regimen assumes dietary intake of 200 IU of vitamin D. (5) National Heart, Lung, and Blood Institute and World Health Organization.

[†]Taken orally unless otherwise indicated. The medication complexity score of the regimen for this hypothetical woman is 14 with 19 doses of medications per day, assuming two as needed doses of albuterol metered dose inhaler plus 70 mg/wk of alendronate.

[§]Dash and ADA dietary guidelines may be synthesized, but the help of a registered dietitian is specifically recommended. Eat foods containing carbohydrate from whole grains, fruits, vegetables, and low-fat milk. Avoid protein intake of more than 20% of total daily energy; lower protein intake to about 10% of daily calories if overt nephropathy is present. Limit intake of saturated fat (<10% of total daily energy) and dietary cholesterol (<200-300 mg). Limit intake of trans unsaturated fatty acids. Eat two to three servings of fish per week. Intake of polyunsaturated fat should be about 10% of total daily energy.

(Reproduced, with permission, from Boyd CM, Darer JD, Boult C, et al. Clinical practice guidelines and quality of care for older patients with multiple comorbid diseases: implications for pay for performance. *JAMA.* 2005;294(6):716-724. Copyright © 2005 American Medical Association. All rights reserved.)

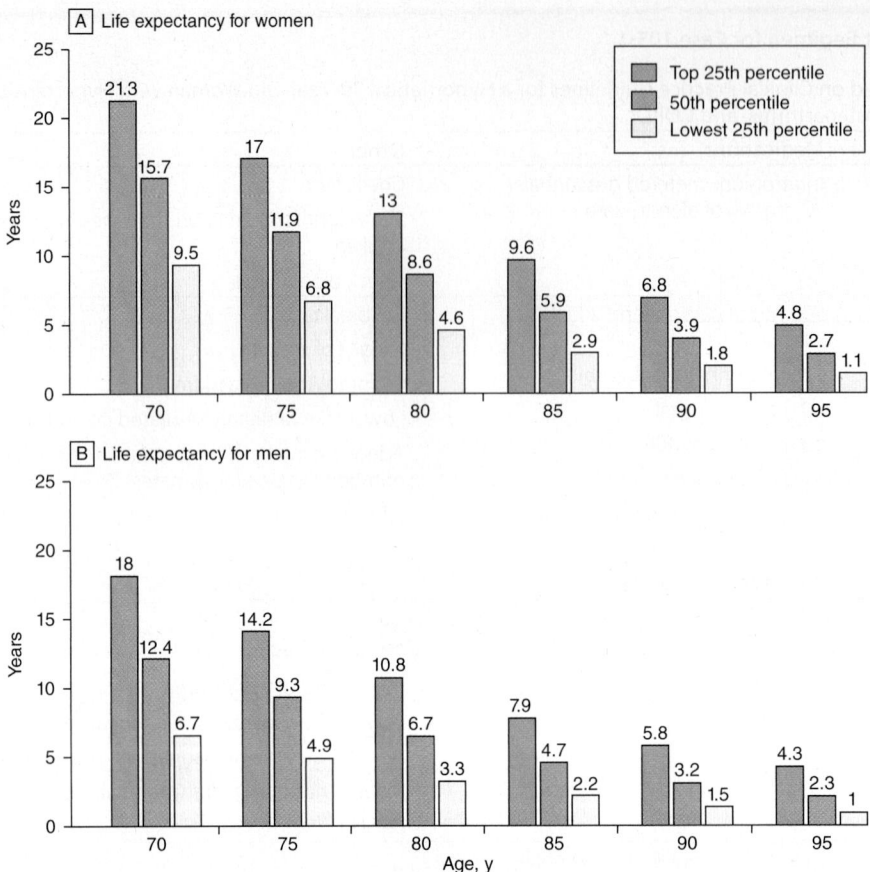

A | Life expectancy for women

B | Life expectancy for men

Age, y

Figure 105-1 *Upper, middle, and lower quartiles of life expectancy for women and men at selected ages.* (Reproduced, with permission, from Walter LC, Covinsky KE. Cancer screening in elderly patients: a framework for individualized decision making. *JAMA.* 2001;285:2750-2756. Copyright © 2001 American Medical Association. All rights reserved.)

inadequacy of prognostic information is often the greatest complaint patients/families have about end-of-life care.

PRACTICE POINT

- Patients expect their doctors to discuss the future of their illnesses with them.
- Hospitalists are obligated to provide patients with the information they need to make decisions in keeping with their core values.
- Hospitalists can initiate a conversation by stating: "I worry that this hospitalization means that you are getting sicker. Tell me what this means to you in the context of your discussions about your goals and fears that you have been having with your doctor?"

Despite the importance of prognosis, physicians are often reluctant to prognosticate. In a national survey of physicians, 90% felt they should avoid being specific about prognosis. Furthermore, 57% felt inadequately trained in prognostication. In another study looking at the accuracy of physician prognostic skill, physicians were asked to provide survival estimates of terminally ill patients at the time of hospice referral. Physicians were accurate 20% of the time and overestimated survival time by a factor of 5.3. In addition, if the duration of the physician-patient relationship increased, prognostic accuracy decreased, suggesting that physician feelings toward patients may alter their ability to prognosticate. In part for this reason, but also because hospitalists often see patients in the midst of a clinical deterioration, it is crucial that hospitalists do not defer prognostication and end-of-life decision making to the

outpatient provider. Clinicians sometimes struggle with how to initiate discussions about prognosis and providing structure can be helpful. Systematic means for doing so, such as that provided by the Serious Illness Conversation Guide (see **Figure 105-2**), provide a format for discussing prognosis and goals of care.

Furthermore, a recent small survey of physicians confirmed ongoing low rates of understanding and use of prognostic tools. One useful and quick clinical tool for prognostication is the Surprise Question, asking "Would you be surprised if this patient died in the next year?" The question is associated with hazard ratio of death of 3.5 (dialysis patients) to 8 (cancer patients) in the following year and has been validated in cancer and dialysis populations.

PRACTICE POINT

A core competency for hospitalists is the assistance in decision making for patients with serious and life threatening illness. This requires:

1. Knowledge about the patient's functional status and disease state
2. Communication with collaborating physicians
3. Shared and informed understanding of the patient's prognosis
4. Exploration of the patient's and family's understanding about their illness, goals, fears, and wishes

PROGNOSTIC MODELS

Prognostication can be difficult, as there are many different pathways to death (see **Figure 105-3**). Certain diagnoses, like metastatic cancer, may have a more predictable terminal period. However, only

Serious Illness Conversation Guide

CLINICIAN STEPS

☐ **Set up**

- Thinking in advance
- Is this okay?
- Hope for best, prepare for worst
- Benefit for patient/family
- No decisions necessary today

☐ **Guide** (right column)

☐ **Act**

- Affirm commitment
- Make recommendations about next steps
  - Acknowledge medical realities
  - Summarize key goals/priorities
  - Describe treatment options that reflect both
- Document conversation
- Provide patient with Family Communication Guide

CONVERSATION GUIDE

Understanding	What is your understanding now of where you are with your illness?
Information preferences	How much information about what is likely to be ahead with your illness would you like from me? For example: Some patients like to know about time, others like to know what to expect, others like to know both.
Prognosis	***Share prognosis as a range, tailored to information preferences***
Goals	If your health situation worsens, what are your most important goals?
Fears/worries	What are your biggest fears and worries about the future with your health?
Function	What abilities are so critical to your life that you cannot imagine living without them?
Tradeoffs	If you become sicker, how much are you willing to go through for the possibility of gaining more time?
Family	How much does your family know about your priorities and wishes? (Suggest bringing family and/or health care agent to next visit to discuss together)

Draft R4.3 4/14/15

Figure 105-2 *Serious illness conversation guide.* (Reproduced, with permission, from Bernacki R. *JAMA Intern Med.* 2014;174(12):1994-2003. Copyright Ariadne Labs.)

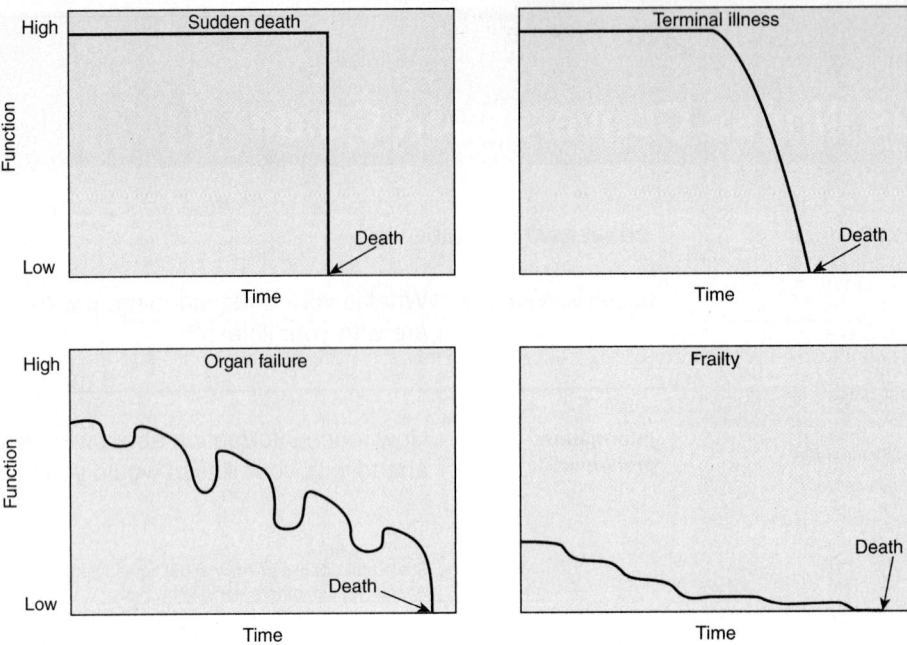

Figure 105-3 *Theoretical trajectories of disease.* (Reproduced, with permission, from Lunney JR, et al. Profiles of older Medicare decedents. *J Am Geriatrics Soc.* 2002;50:1108-1112.)

21% of Medicare beneficiaries die of cancer and less than 16% will die suddenly. Furthermore, even cancer can be difficult to predict, with up to a quarter of patients dying with no disability or chronic persistently severe disability, rather than the more traditional terminal disease trajectory. Many patients die of acute complications of a chronic condition in which the terminal period is much more uncertain, such as organ failure (20%). Patients who die from dementia or frailty (20%) may have long periods of debility with less predictable courses. A recent study followed actual patient pathways to death and found that only about a third of patients with a given disease follow a particular trajectory, mainly dementia and sudden death.

PRACTICE POINT

- There are four theoretical trajectories to death: sudden death, terminal disease, organ failure, and frailty.
- Determining which pathway your patient follows will help you prognosticate and communicate with patients and families.

Life expectancy tables can give rough estimates of prognosis (see Figure 105-1). Those at or above the top 25th percentile at each age are active patients with no significant comorbid illnesses; the 50th percentile is the median life expectancy at each age; and below the lowest 25th percentile at each age are patients with severe comorbid illnesses like dementia or congestive heart failure. Most hospitalized patients fall into the bottom 25th percentile and therefore, this portion of the life table can be used as an estimate for the "best" possible life expectancy for the typical hospitalized patient.

A prognostic index is a clinical tool that quantifies the contributions that various components of the history, physical exam, and laboratory findings make toward a diagnosis, prognosis, or likely response to treatment. Physicians can use prognostic indices to lend confidence to their judgments about prognosis and these indices provide an objective measure to support clinical intuition. Combining clinical estimates with prognostic indices results in more accurate estimates than either alone. Prognostic indices have many different names such as clinical prediction rules, decision rules,

and staging systems (eg, Goldman Index, Dukes staging system for colorectal cancer, and NYHA congestive heart failure class).

PRACTICE POINT

- Prognostic indices can be used to support clinical judgment and lend confidence to prognostic estimates.
- Prognostic The bottom 25th percentile of life expectancy at each age group can be used as an estimate for the "best" possible life expectancy for most hospitalized patients

CASE 105-2

An 81-year-old man with a history of mild congestive heart failure was admitted from home for nausea, vomiting, and abdominal pain. He improved with antibiotics prescribed for diverticulitis. During his hospitalization an echocardiogram reported an ejection fraction was 45%. An albumin of 2.9 g/dL prompted nutrition consultation which noted adequate caloric intake by the time he was ready for discharge. His physicians decided to transition him to a nursing home for assistance with activities of daily living (ADLs: bathing, dressing, and toileting). When asked by family members about his prognosis, how should his physicians respond?

Hospitalization is often a major health transition for elders and is often a time to reassess goals of care. Walter et al. developed an accurate and easy-to-use index to stratify older adults into groups by their risk for 1-year mortality after hospital discharge. The index was developed in a large heterogeneous group of patients aged 70+ admitted to a general medical service by identifying risk factors for mortality from multiple domains including demographics, comorbities, laboratory findings, and functional status. Kaplan Meier survival curves of the four risk groups demonstrate that the groups have markedly different survival trajectories (see Figure 105-3). Using only six accessible variables, (gender, congestive heart failure, cancer, creatinine, albumin, and ADL dependency at discharge), this prognostic index stratifies older adults according to 1-year mortality after hospitalization. For example, our patient in Case 105-2 would receive one point for being male, two points for a history of congestive heart failure, two points for being discharged to a skilled nursing facility, and two points for poor nutritional status (albumin 2.9) for a total of seven points (a patient with metastatic cancer receives eight points). His 1-year mortality is estimated at 68%. This study emphasizes the importance of considering multiple domains when assessing prognosis in older adults. Some hospices use the Walter criteria (>6 points) to enroll patients.

In 2012, a systematic review identified 16 prognostic indices, including the Walter Index described above, that predict mortality in a variety of clinical settings; however, only two indices have independent validation. The most clinically useful of these indices are available free for use at www.ePrognosis.org. This website categorizes patients depending on their location. For hospitalized patients, the website provides an online calculator using the Walter Index and provides both numerical and visual representation of 1-year mortality. A recent study evaluating the use of this tool found that 91% of users found the tool to be useful and 47% of health care professionals stated that the prognosis that they were presented affected their clinical decision making.

IMPORTANCE OF FUNCTIONAL STATUS

Functional status is of utmost importance when estimating prognosis in older adults. In the Walter index (see **Figure 105-4**), measures of functional status added important information about risk for 1-year mortality beyond that provided by medical diagnoses or physiologic or laboratory measures. Functional status reflects the severity and end result of many different illnesses and psychosocial factors. Hospitalists often do not routinely record functional status for their patients, but it is important for considering a patient's prognosis. A recent study confirmed the impact of functional status on critically ill hospitalized patients, showing a two to three fold increase in the risk of death for patients with prehospitalization disability.

PRACTICE POINT

- Functional status reflects the severity and end-result of many different illnesses and psychosocial factors and is the best prognostic tool available.

Estimating prognosis based on functional status began with oncology patients; the Karnofsky Index (100 = normal; 0 = dead)

and the ECOG scale (Eastern Cooperative Oncology Group) (0 = normal; 5 = dead) are the most commonly used scales. A median survival of 3 months roughly correlates with a Karnofsky score <40 or ECOG >3. Newer prognostic scales have also been developed. The simplest method to assess functional ability is to ask patients: *"How do you spend your time? How much time do you spend in bed or lying down?"* If the response is >50% of the time and this is increasing, estimate the cancer patients' prognosis at 3 months or less. An increasing number of physical symptoms, especially dyspnea, are also a good indication that time is short. The Palliative Performance Scale (PPS) uses five observer-rated domains correlated to the Karnofsky Performance Scale, commonly used to estimate prognosis in patients with cancer. The PPS is a reliable and valid tool and correlates well with actual survival and median survival time for patients (see **Tables 105-2** and **105-3**). It has been found useful for purposes of identifying and tracking potential care needs of palliative care patients, particularly as these needs change with disease progression.

CARDIOPULMONARY RESUSCITATION

Survival to discharge following cardiac arrest occurring in the hospital is infrequent. In a recent study examining 433,985 Medicare patients who underwent in-hospital CPR, 18.3% of patients survived to discharge. For some diseases such as cancer, the prognosis is poorer; a meta-analysis of survival rates for CPR revealed that 6.7% of cancer patients survived to discharge. Survival to discharge for ward cancer patients was better than ICU cancer patients: 10.1% versus 2.2%. CPR for hospitalized patients is associated with poor outcomes, as the cause of arrest is related to advanced life-threatening illness rather than a reversible acute cardiopulmonary event (eg, arrhythmia). Even if the patient survives, he or she may then have significant morbidity including permanent neurological and functional impairment, a fact that should be included when having discussions about preferences for CPR. The actual statistics about survival of CPR are in sharp contrast to what the general public sees. In a study of survival of CPR depicted on television, 75% of the patients survived the immediate arrest, and 67% appeared to have survived to hospital discharge. Thus, the portrayal of CPR on television may lead the public to have an unrealistic idea of CPR and its chances for success. Physicians should be aware of the images of CPR depicted on television and the confusion these images may create when discussing preferences about CPR with patients and families.

Not only is prognosis important for planning, but patients may change decisions based on perception of prognosis. In a study of older adults, subjects were asked about preferences for cardiopulmonary resuscitation (CPR). Before learning the true probability of

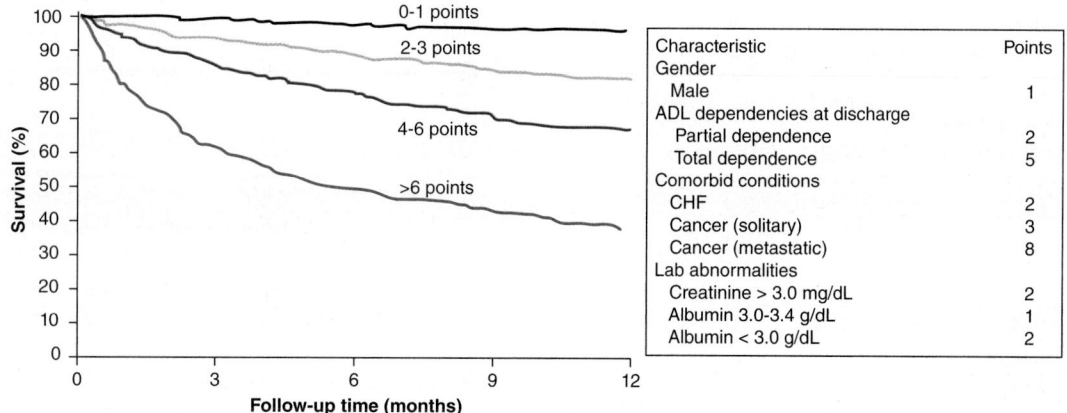

Figure 105-4 *Mortality at 1 year postdischarge.* (Reproduced, with permission, from Walter LC, et al. Development and validation of a prognostic index for 1-year mortality in older adults after hospitalization. *JAMA.* 2001;285:2987-2994. Copyright © 2001 American Medical Association. All rights reserved.)

TABLE 105-2 Palliative Performance Scale

PPS Level	Ambulation	Activity & Evidence of Disease	Self-Care	Intake	Conscious Level
100%	Full	Normal activity & work No evidence of disease	Full	Normal	Full
90%	Full	Normal activity & work Some evidence of disease	Full	Normal	Full
80%	Full	Normal activity *with* Effort Some evidence of disease	Full	Normal or reduced	Full
70%	Reduced	Unable Normal Job/Work Significant disease	Full	Normal or reduced	Full
60%	Reduced	Unable hobby/house work Significant disease	Occasional assistance necessary	Normal or reduced	Full or Confusion
50%	Mainly Sit/Lie	Unable to do any work Extensive disease	Considerable assistance required	Normal or reduced	Full or Confusion
40%	Mainly in Bed	Unable to do most activity Extensive disease	Mainly assistance	Normal or reduced	Full or Drowsy +/- Confusion
30%	Totally Bed Bound	Unable to do any activity Extensive disease	Total Care	Normal or reduced	Full or Drowsy +/- Confusion
20%	Totally Bed Bound	Unable to do any activity Extensive disease	Total Care	Minimal to sips	Full or Drowsy +/- Confusion
10%	Totally Bed Bound	Unable to do any activity Extensive disease	Total Care	Mouth care only	Drowsy or Coma +/- Confusion
0%	Death	-	-	-	-

Source: Ho F, et al. A reliability and validity study of the Palliative Performance Scale. *BMC Palliat Care.* 2008;4(7):10.

survival, 41% of subjects wanted CPR. After learning the true probability of CPR, 22% of subjects wanted CPR. If life expectancy was less than 1 year 5% of subjects wanted CPR.

PRACTICE POINT

- Survival of in-hospital CPR is low (18%) especially for those with diseases such as cancer (6.7% total, 2.2% for those with cancer in the ICU).

■ CANCER

Cancer follows the terminal disease model (see Figure 105-3), a more predictable disease trajectory. However, there is significant heterogeneity in disease courses between different types of cancers

TABLE 105-3 Palliative Performance Scale Survival Statistics

Initial PPS	Mean Survival Time in Days (95% CI)	Median Survival Time in Days (95% CI)	Range of Survival in Days
10%	5 (1, 9)	2 (1, 3)	<1-22
20%	14 (8, 21)	6 (4, 8)	<1-123
30%	32 (23, 41)	12 (9, 15)	1-249
40%	65 (36, 95)	31 (15, 47)	1-493
50%	58 (43, 72)	35 (29, 41)	2-320
60%	104 (61, 147)	50 (33, 67)	7-624
70%	168 (133, 203)	110 (77, 143)	3-607
80%	151 (92, 210)	71 (0, 196)	33-424

CI, confidence interval; *P* value < 0.001 for all data points.
From Lau F, et al. *J Pain Symptom Manage.* 2009;37(6):965-972.

and this holds true even within more narrowly defined areas such as "metastatic solid tumors."

The functional status based tools described above can prove very useful in this population. For example, for patients with metastatic cancers with longer survival times, such as prostate or breast cancer, a Karnofsky Performance Scale of less than 60, correlates with a median survival of less than 6 months. This is in contrast to cancers with shorter survival times, such as pancreatic or biliary cancers, which have a median survival of less than 6 months with a much higher KPS score (<90).

PRACTICE POINT

Prognosis estimates in older adults with cancer require:
- A functional status assessment
- Communication with patient's primary oncologist who can provide insight into the aggressiveness of cancer and treatment options

Certain cancer syndromes portend poorer prognosis (median survival):
- Less than 3 months: malignant hypercalcemia, malignant pericardial effusion, leptomeningeal disease, multiple brain metastases without radiation
- Less than 6 months: malignant ascites, malignant pleural effusion, malignant bowel obstruction, multiple brain metastases with radiation
---

■ CHRONIC OBSTRUCTIVE PULMONARY DISEASE (COPD)

COPD follows the organ failure model (see Figure 105-3), an unpredictable disease trajectory. The forced expiratory volume in 1 second (FEV1) is often used to grade severity of COPD, but a multidimensional grading system may better predict survival. The Bode index uses four factors to predict the risk of death: the body mass index (B), the degree of airflow obstruction (O), dyspnea (D), and exercise capacity (E), measured by the 6-minute-walk test. Comorbidity is also important in COPD; in one study of patients that required mechanical ventilation, the in-hospital mortality rate for the entire cohort was 28% but fell to 12% for patients with a COPD exacerbation but without a comorbid illness. In another study, patients ventilated more than 48 hours had a 50% 1-year survival. Severity of illness and functional status were associated with short-term mortality while comorbidity and age were associated with 1-year mortality. Last, hospitalization for exacerbation is an indicator of poorer prognosis in this patient population, with one study showing 1-year mortality of 28%.

CONGESTIVE HEART FAILURE (CHF)

CHF follows the organ failure model (see Figure 105-3), an unpredictable disease trajectory, and is modifiable by use of medications but is nevertheless subject to a high incidence of sudden death. Despite this unpredictable course, the need for hospitalization in this population is associated with a poorer prognosis, with up to 37% mortality at 1 year. Mortality increases with increasing hospitalization rates, with one study showing survival of approximately 7 months for older patients after four hospitalizations. In addition to hospitalization, other indicators associated with limited prognosis in CHF include severity of heart failure, cachexia, reduced functional capacity, kidney disease, hyponatremia, physical exam findings, and anemia.

Several models have been developed to help in determining mortality in heart failure patients. The Seattle Heart Failure model is a 24-variable risk model and estimates mean 1-, 2-, and 3-year survival and, importantly, incorporates clinical and laboratory variables, CHF medications, and device therapies. These prognostic indices require frequent updating for changing standards of CHF care and this makes accurate prognostication for patients with heart failure challenging.

DEMENTIA AND THE ELDERLY

Dementia is a syndrome of impaired cognition affecting memory, language, and problem solving. Depending on the cause, dementia can be irreversible, leading to progressive brain failure and death. Prognostication in dementia follows the frailty trajectory (see Figure 105-3) and progression is difficult to predict. The following factors have been associated with poorer prognosis: older age, male gender, comorbidity (including cancer, CHF, COPD, and diabetes mellitus), aspiration, bowel incontinence, recent weight loss, dehydration, fever, pressure ulcers, shortness of breath, dysphagia, poor oral intake, sleeping most of the day, and low body mass index (BMI). Hospitalized patients with end-stage dementia that reside in nursing homes have a particularly poor prognosis.

Functional assessment staging (FAST) identifies progressive steps of functional decline. Hospice guidelines state that a FAST stage 7A, ability to speak limited to six words, is appropriate for hospice enrollment if the patient also exhibits dementia-related comorbidities (aspiration, upper urinary tract infection, sepsis, multiple stage 3-4 ulcers, persistent fever, or weight loss >10% within 6 months). The reliability of the FAST scoring system in prognostication is limited. Also, many patients with dementia do not follow the stages sequentially, posing further challenges to accurate prognostication. Estimation of survival in terminal dementia may depend on the goals of care and decisions regarding the level of intervention that will be provided to treat acute medical problems such as urosepsis.

For the oldest old (>85 years), as highlighted by the prior discussion of life tables, hospitalized adults often fit into the lower quartile estimate for life expectancy, already placing a prognosis at hospitalization of 1 to 2 years. Based on this information alone, experts suggest discussing prognosis with this patient population. Furthermore, physicians frequently do not recognize this situation, even when complicated by comorbidity, as one where the expected life span should affect decision making, such as with cancer screening unlikely to yield clinical benefit. Furthermore, for elderly patients hospitalized for an illness requiring a first intensive care unit stay, 6-month mortality was recently demonstrated to be around 30%. Independent predictors of mortality in this group included, in descending order of contribution, presence of a do-not-resuscitate order, older age, burden of comorbidity, admission from or discharge to a skilled nursing facility, length of hospitalization, primary diagnosis of sepsis or hematologic malignancy, and male sex.

DISCHARGE CONSIDERATIONS

One in five patients enrolled in Medicare is readmitted within 30 days. Hospitalists' discharge plans for their patients need to be realistic. Improved prognostic skill allows physicians to discharge patients to appropriate settings, including home, skilled nursing facilities, and hospice. A frank and honest conversation about prognosis with the patient and family may save multiple frustrating readmissions in which little is accomplished. Hospitalists are in a unique position to spur these conversations, including prognostic disclosure, with patients and formulate discharge plans that are practical, sensible, and in line with prognosis and patients' goals of care.

CASE 105-1 (continued)

The patient with moderately severe chronic diseases expressed her wishes to keep her medications to a minimum. She did not want to spend the rest of her life eating bland food. She worried about a low blood sugar (HgA1c is 7.3%), particularly since she had been living alone since the death of her husband. Her physicians reduced her glyburide dose to 5 mg, a change likely to be associated with a slightly higher HgA1c. According to the life expectancy tables, she had 4.6 years of life left. A nutritionist educated her how to liberalize her diet to her satisfaction. Her wishes were communicated to her new primary physician who will periodically reevaluate the changes.

CASE 105-2 (continued)

A family meeting was arranged with the 81-year-old patient admitted with diverticulitis, his niece, and the medical team. After introductions, the patient and family were queried about their understanding of his hospitalization, his progress, and likely prognosis. His physicians reviewed his improvement in the hospital and recommended a discussion about the future. His niece asked them to explain this recommendation. The physicians explicitly responded that while they saw no immediate concerns, they would not be surprised if he became significantly more ill or died within the next year. This hospitalization identified congestive heart failure, poor nutritional status, and need for discharge to a skilled nursing facility for help with ADLs. The patient responded that while he was feeling better, he was not surprised and found the opportunity for a discussion a "relief." After determining that the patient had not specified advance directives, the discussion shifted to an explanation of why this was important. Subsequent family meetings gave the patient the opportunity to appoint his niece as his health care proxy and outline his wishes if he were to become more ill and unable to speak for himself.

CONCLUSION

Older adults with multiple comorbidities experience higher health care use, physical disability, adverse side effects related to polypharmacy, poor quality of life, and increased mortality. Functional status provides valuable information and prognostic indices are available and can aid in formulating prognoses. Evaluating comorbidity and estimating prognosis is a responsibility of clinicians, is important to patients, and is intimately linked to good individualized clinical decision making.

It takes courage to make a prognosis. Fullness of knowledge does not always bring confidence; the more one knows the more timidity may grow. The faculty which enables a man to look all around a question, to take a philosophical view of it, may be tempered with doubt, and an inability to reach a conclusion. A cocksure diagnosis and a positive prognosis may express the assurance of ignorance.

Sir William Osler. Lancet. 1910;1:973-977.

SUGGESTED READINGS

Bernacki R, Block R. Communication about serious illness care goals: a review and synthesis of best practices. *JAMA Intern Med.* 2014;174(12):1994-2003.

Boyd CM, Darer J, Boult C, et al. Clinical practice guidelines and quality of care for older patients with multiple comorbid diseases: implications for pay for performance. *JAMA.* 2005;294(6):716-724.

Ehlenbach WJ, Barnato AE, Curtis JR, et al. Epidemiologic study of in-hospital cardiopulmonary resuscitation in the elderly. *N Engl J Med.* 2009;361(1):22-31.

Ferrante LE, Pisani MA, Murphy TE, et al. Functional trajectories among older persons before and after critical illness. *JAMA Intern Med.* 2015;175(4):523-529.

Lamont EB, Christakis NA. Complexities in prognostication in advanced cancer: "to help them live their lives the way they want to." *JAMA.* 2003;290(1):98-104.

Lau F, Maida V, Downing M, Lesperance M, Karlson N, Kuziemsky C. Use of the Palliative Performance Scale (PPS) for end-of-life prognostication in a palliative medicine consultation service. *J Pain Symptom Manage.* 2009;37(6):965-972.

Levy WC, Mozafarrian D, Linker DT, et al. The Seattle Heart Failure Model: prediction of survival in heart failure. *Circulation.* 2006;113(11):1424-1433.

Mitchell SL, Teno JM, Kiely DK, et al. The clinical course of advanced dementia. *N Engl J Med.* 2009;361(16):1529-1538.

Yourman LC, Lee SJ, Schonberg MA, et al. Prognostic indices for older adults: a systematic review. *JAMA.* 2012;307:182-192.

ONLINE RESOURCES

Online Prognostication Tool. www.ePrognosis.org.

Seattle Heart Failure Model. https://depts.washington.edu/shfm/.

CHAPTER 106

Weakness: How to Localize the Problem

Joshua P. Klein, MD, PhD

Key Clinical Questions

1. Is the onset of weakness abrupt/acute, gradual/subacute, or insidious/chronic?
2. Is the weakness stable, progressively worsening, waxing and waning, or fatigable?
3. Is the weakness symmetric or lateralized?
4. Is the weakness length-dependent?
5. Are the involved muscles all weak to the same degree?
6. If a gradient of weakness exists, is it worse proximally or distally?
7. Are specific muscles or groups of muscles weak?
8. Do the involved muscles correspond to a myotome or a portion of the brachial or lumbar plexus?
9. Are there nonmotor deficits?

PRACTICE POINT

- The pace of onset of neurological symptoms, including weakness, is the best clue as to its etiology. Vascular events (ischemic and hemorrhage stroke) cause abrupt symptom onset, inflammatory and infectious symptoms tend to develop over hours to days, and symptoms resulting from neurodegeneration develop over weeks to years. There are, of course, exceptions.
- Defining the pattern of weakness as well as the presence or absence of other associated symptoms is the key to accurate neuroanatomic localization. In a given patient, one lesion causing all symptoms is more likely than several lesions each causing a single symptom.

PRACTICE POINT

- A major concern in a patient with progressive weakness is airway protection. Slurred speech, drooling, coughing, choking, a nasal or hoarse voice, weakness of neck flexion or extension, or gasping for air should alert the clinician to the possibility of neuromuscular airway compromise. The airway should be secured immediately.
- Bedside testing of pulmonary function including vital capacity and negative inspiratory force measurements are helpful but are dependent on patient cooperation and effort and should not replace or overly reassure one's clinical impression.
- Neurological conditions in which the airway may be particularly susceptible include acute ischemic and hemorrhagic stroke, acute inflammatory demyelinating polyneuropathy (Guillain-Barré syndrome), amyotrophic lateral sclerosis (ALS), and diseases affecting the basilar meninges and the lower cranial nerves.

INTRODUCTION

Weakness is a common neurological symptom that can result from dysfunction of many parts of the central and peripheral nervous system as well as from disorders of muscle itself. Familiarity with the anatomy of the motor system including the corticospinal tract and its peripheral projections, and the relationship of these pathways to nonmotor (sensory and autonomic) pathways, aids in the localization of neurological deficits.

The role of the clinician in the evaluation of a patient with weakness is to first establish the pace of onset and distribution of symptoms and then to formulate an anatomic localization of the lesion. Diagnostic testing including imaging and electrophysiologic examinations may follow, though these tests should always be hypothesis-driven so that the pretest probability of detecting a causative abnormality is increased, and the probability of detecting incidental and noncausative abnormalities is reduced.

The clinician should be mindful that patients may describe weakness as numbness, and vice versa. Furthermore, weakness is frequently reported as a symptom of fatigue, exhaustion, malaise, pain, or depression, all of which are not primary disorders of the motor pathways or muscles. Precision in history-taking reduces the mischaracterization of these and other symptoms and signs, and in turn reduces diagnostic ambiguity and error.

ANATOMIC CONSIDERATIONS

The neurological causes of weakness can be anatomically divided into (1) those resulting from dysfunction of central nervous system structures, (2) those resulting from dysfunction of peripheral nervous system structures, and (3) those resulting from diseases of the muscle itself. The principle motor pathway of the central nervous system is the *corticospinal tract* whose neurons (the "upper motor neuron") originate in the cortex and terminate in the spinal cord. The motor pathway of the peripheral nervous system (the "lower motor neuron") originates in the spinal cord and terminates at the neuromuscular junction.

CASE 106-1

A 70-year-old woman with hypertension and diabetes has abrupt onset of right sided weakness, numbness, and slurred speech. On physical examination she is alert and her speech is fluent although dysarthric. She is able to follow verbal commands. Her right lower face, right arm and right leg are weak. She feels that the sensation in her right face, arm, and leg is diminished as well.

The acute onset of symptoms suggests a vascular etiology of the patient's symptoms. The clinical syndrome is that of hemiparesis and hemianesthesia. The dysarthria is due to facial and oropharyngeal muscular weakness. The forehead muscles receive bilateral innervation from the cortex and are therefore spared in the setting of unilateral cerebral damage. The lack of dysphasia or altered mental state suggests that the lesion is small and deep rather than large and superficial.

Brain imaging revealed a small acute ischemic infarction affecting the posterior limb of the internal capsule (containing descending corticospinal fibers) and the adjacent posterior thalamus (containing ascending sensory fibers). Vascular imaging showed diffuse intracranial atherosclerosis. The etiology of the stroke was most likely due to microangiopathy related to chronic hypertension and diabetes, causing occlusion of a lenticulostriate artery and a lacunar infarction.

THE UPPER MOTOR NEURON

Weakness resulting from injury to the central nervous system implies damage to the upper motor neuron. This damage may affect the cell body of the neuron or its axon. The cell body of the upper motor neuron resides in layer V of the cortex in the precentral gyrus of the frontal lobe. The precentral gyrus, which runs in a transverse orientation from midline to lateral over the cerebral convexity, has a topography such that neurons near the midline subserve lower extremity motor function, neurons more lateral subserve upper extremity motor function, and neurons far lateral subserve facial motor function.

The axons of these upper motor neurons form the corticospinal tract, which projects inferomedially from the cortex via the corona radiata through the posterior limb of the internal capsule and into the cerebral peduncle of the ventral midbrain. As these axons course inferiorly, they condense into a compact band. After transiting the ventral pons, the axons decussate in the pyramids of the lower medulla and form the lateral corticospinal tracts of the spinal cord. Lesions above this decussation produce contralateral weakness and lesions below the decussation produce ipsilateral weakness. Axons destined to innervate specific muscles at each vertebral level exit the corticospinal tract and synapse in the anterior horn of the spinal cord at that level.

CASE 106-2

A 62-year-old man presents with 1 year of progressive weakness in his arms. He has no numbness and no pain other than occasional cramps in the weak muscles. On physical examination there is atrophy of the interosseous muscles of the right greater than the left hand. Occasional fasciculations are seen in the hand muscles as well. Sensation is normal to all modalities throughout. Deep tendon reflexes are abnormally brisk on the left and reduced on the right and a left extensor plantar response is elicited. MRI of the spine shows no spinal cord compression though subtle signal abnormality is reported in the anterior and lateral spinal cord with mild cord atrophy. Electromyography shows evidence of chronic denervation and reinnervation of arm and leg muscles with normal sensory and motor nerve conduction studies.

The insidious nature of symptom onset suggests an underlying degenerative process. In the absence of spinal cord compression, the patient's asymmetrical weakness, fasciculations, and abnormal deep tendon reflexes are concerning for a disorder of motor neurons, specifically ALS. In this disease, there is degeneration of corticospinal (upper motor) neurons and anterior horn (lower motor) neurons. This degeneration most often produces asymmetrical weakness, with hyperreflexia and spasticity where upper motor neurons are predominantly affected and hyporeflexia and muscle atrophy where lower motor neurons are predominately affected. Sensory neurons are spared. In some cases of ALS, atrophy of the corticospinal tracts and anterior horns is visible on MRI of the spinal cord.

THE LOWER MOTOR NEURON

The cell body of the lower motor neuron resides in the ventral horn of the spinal cord. The axons of these neurons exit the spinal cord via the *ventral root* and then exit the spinal canal adjacent to the dorsal root, through the neural foramen. All the muscles innervated by the lower motor neurons of one spinal vertebral level are termed a *myotome*. Depending on the extent and precise location of a nerve injury, some or all of the muscles of a myotome may be affected.

In the cervical and lumbosacral areas, the peripheral nerves containing lower motor axons form the brachial and lumbar plexi, respectively. Injury to these plexi will produce a pattern of muscular weakness that is different than the pattern associated with nerve root injury. Familiarity with myotome, plexus, and peripheral nerve innervation maps will aid in lesion localization.

When a single spinal nerve root is injured, as in neural foraminal stenosis, the resulting syndrome is designated a *radiculopathy*. When multiple spinal nerve roots are injured, the resulting syndrome is designated a *polyradiculopathy*. When a single peripheral nerve is injured, as in carpal tunnel syndrome, the syndrome is designated a *mononeuropathy*. When several nonadjacent peripheral nerves are injured, the syndrome is designated a *mononeuropathy multiplex*. When there is diffuse peripheral nerve injury, particularly when symmetric and length-dependent as in diabetic neuropathy, the syndrome is designated a *polyneuropathy*. In any of these cases, when inflammation is the cause of nerve injury, the radiculopathy or neuropathy is referred to as a *radiculitis* or *neuritis*.

CASE 106-3

A 40-year-old woman complains of progressively worsening weakness over 2 days which has not been relieved by rest. She also complains of patches of tingling and numbness in all of her limbs as well as pain in her lower back. She had a diarrheal illness 2 weeks prior to onset of symptoms. On physical examination she is alert with no neck pain and is diffusely weak in all four extremities with sensory loss in the legs. The muscular weakness in her extremities is worse distally than proximally and is fairly symmetric. Deep tendon reflexes are diminished in the arms and absent in the legs. There is no response to plantar stimulation.

The subacute progressive onset of symptoms suggests an inflammatory condition. The combination of sensory and motor deficits along with hyporeflexia implies a peripheral nerve injury that in this case is affecting many nerves. The symptoms are consistent with acute inflammatory demyelinating polyneuropathy, or Guillain-Barré syndrome (GBS). The recent diarrheal illness is notable in relation to the onset of GBS as several microorganisms, in particular *Campylobacter jejuni*, are known to induce an immune response that, through molecular mimicry, attacks the myelin of the peripheral nervous system. The length-dependent nature of the weakness (worse distally than proximally) reflects the probabilistic nature of demyelination, that is, that longer nerves have a greater probability of demyelination somewhere along their course than shorter nerves. A nerve conduction study showed temporal dispersion (slowing) of impulses in sensory and motor nerves, consistent with peripheral nerve demyelination. The patient underwent a lumbar puncture that showed albuminocytologic dissociation (elevated protein without pleocytosis), another characteristic feature of GBS. In its most severe form GBS can be fulminant with respiratory compromise from diaphragmatic weakness and end-organ complications from autonomic dysregulation.

THE NEUROMUSCULAR JUNCTION

Peripheral nerves subserving motor function terminate at the neuromuscular junction. When an action potential arrives at the presynaptic bouton of a peripheral motor nerve, membrane-bound voltage-gated ion channels are activated, facilitating the release of the excitatory neurotransmitter acetylcholine into the synaptic cleft. Acetylcholine binds to nicotinic receptors on the postsynaptic cell, the myocyte. Binding of the receptor activates voltage-gated ion channels that depolarize the muscle fiber and lead to muscle contraction. Disorders of the neuromuscular junction involve pathophysiologic processes that interfere with the transmission of information between the pre- and postsynaptic cells.

CASE 106-4

A 70-year-old man complains of fluctuating weakness throughout the day. The symptoms began subtly about 6 months earlier, but more recently the patient has experienced reduced exercise tolerance and endurance. He has no other constitutional symptoms. He presents to the emergency room after choking on food. On physical examination he is alert and speaks with a nasal voice. His language and cognition are normal and his speech is dysarthric. He is wearing a soft cervical collar which he explains is to support his head and to prevent it from dropping forward. Sensation and deep tendon reflexes are normal.

The fluctuating nature of the patient's slowly worsening weakness and the exacerbation of weakness with exercise are the key clinical features that suggest a myasthenic syndrome, in this case myasthenia gravis. In the most common form of this disease, antibodies elaborated against acetylcholine receptors at the postsynaptic neuromuscular junction inhibit the excitatory effects of acetylcholine and thereby inhibit muscle contraction. These antibodies are, in some cases, associated with tumors of the thymus gland as well as other systemic cancers. This patient has not only weakness of limb muscles, but also weakness of postural

(causing head drop) and pharyngeal (causing dysarthria and nasal voice) muscles. Weakness of pharyngeal and other proximal muscles places the patient at elevated risk of airway compromise (myasthenic crisis).

THE MUSCLE

Intrinsic disease of muscle can impair its function, leading to weakness. Both inherited diseases (ie, muscular dystrophy) and acquired conditions (ie, polymyositis) produce a disruption in normal muscle fiber contraction. Weakness can result from the presence of abnormal structural elements in the muscle fibers or from inflammation within the fibers themselves.

OTHER MOTOR PATHWAYS

Besides the corticospinal tract there are several other central nervous system pathways that influence motor function. The basal ganglia, comprised of the caudate nucleus, putamen, globus pallidus, subthalamic nucleus, and substantia nigra, influence the initiation and control of movement, while the cerebellum influences the rate, range, force, and direction of movement. Interestingly, diseases that affect the basal ganglia such as Parkinson and Huntington disease, as well as diseases that affect the cerebellum, do not generally produce frank muscle weakness though loss of motor control is apparent.

Additional central nervous system pathways such as the rubrospinal, reticulospinal, vestibulospinal, and tectospinal tracts mediate motor control over functions such as maintenance of posture, reflex movement of the head, and the automatic movements of locomotion. Like with damage to the basal ganglia and cerebellum, isolated damage to these pathways does not generally produce muscle weakness.

PATTERNS OF WEAKNESS

The clinical approach to weakness should focus on delineating the pace of symptom onset and the pattern of weakness. Is the distribution of weakness symmetric or lateralized? Are the involved muscles all weak to the same degree or is there a gradient? If a gradient exists, is the weakness worse proximally or distally? Are specific muscles or groups of muscles involved, and do the involved muscles correspond to a myotome?

Damage to an upper motor neuron causes spastic paresis and hyperreflexia whereas damage to a lower motor neuron causes flaccid paresis, muscle atrophy, and hyporeflexia. Hyperreflexia results from a loss of normal cortical inhibition of deep tendon reflexes. Hyporeflexia results either from muscle denervation, intrinsic muscle disease, or damage to the sensory portion of the deep tendon reflex arc. Spasticity and hyperreflexia following upper motor neuron injury develop over the course of days to weeks and are most often not present acutely (ie, immediately after an acute injury such as a cerebral infarction or spinal cord trauma).

Disorders of the neuromuscular junction produce fatigable weakness; deep tendon reflexes may be normal or reduced. Weakness may occur in muscles of the limbs or alternatively muscles under the control of cranial nerves such as the extraocular muscles (weakness causes diplopia), levator palpebrae superioris (weakness causes ptosis), or the oropharyngeal muscles (weakness causes dysphagia and dysarthria).

Myopathies result from a variety of acquired and inherited conditions and reflexes may be normal or reduced. Several patterns of weakness are characteristic of myopathies. Of these, the most common pattern is limb-girdle weakness, in which the proximal muscles near the origins of the limbs are affected out of proportion to the muscles of the distal extremities. Less common patterns include distal extremity predominant weakness (seen in myofibrillar myopathy and myotonic dystrophy), proximal arm and distal leg (scapuloperoneal) weakness (seen in humeroperoneal and facioscapulohumeral dystrophies, central core myopathy, and acid maltase deficiency), and distal arm and proximal leg weakness (seen in inclusion body myositis). As in the diseases of the neuromuscular junction, myopathies can affect muscles under the control of cranial nerves, producing ptosis, diplopia, dysarthria, and dysphagia.

LOCALIZATION AND NEIGHBORHOOD SIGNS

A key principle of neuroanatomic localization is that of diagnostic parsimony, which suggests that an aggregate of symptoms and signs is more likely to be due to a single lesion than many individual lesions. A lesion anywhere along the course of the upper motor neuron will produce a contralateral spastic paresis. The presence of other symptoms along with a lesion of the upper motor neuron can increase the precision of localization. For example, paresis of the right face along with expressive dysphasia suggests a left lateral frontal cortical lesion (affecting the face area of the motor cortex as well as Broca's area, which lies adjacent). A right-sided hemiparesis with a left oculomotor palsy suggests a lesion in the left midbrain (affecting the left cerebral peduncle and the left infranuclear oculomotor fibers exiting the ventral midbrain). In both of these cases a single lesion explains the combination of neurological deficits, and though exceptions exist, parsimony is most often the rule.

Unilateral lesions of the spinal cord affecting the descending corticospinal tract produce ipsilateral paresis below the level of the lesion, with or without sensory and autonomic disturbances depending on the extent of the lesion. Unilateral lesions of the spinal cord that damage the anterior horn cells produce weakness of the muscles of the myotome at that level.

Lesions of the proximal nerve roots produce weakness and numbness in the dermatome-myotome distribution of that nerve root. For example, a herniated intervertebral disk may cause external compression of a proximal nerve root. More distal nerve injuries affect only the specific muscles they innervate. For example, paresis of the tibialis anterior muscle limiting ankle dorsiflexion may result from injury to the L5 nerve root or from injury to the common peroneal (fibular) nerve. These may be differentiated by testing other muscles. The L5 nerve root also innervates the tibialis posterior muscle so with nerve root injury there will be weakness of ankle inversion in addition to weakness of dorsiflexion. With a common peroneal nerve injury, ankle inversion will be spared.

CONCLUSION

The clinical approach to weakness requires assessment of the pattern of deficits in the context of their pace of onset. Weakness often co-exists with other neurological deficits such as numbness, and the presence or absence of other deficits can help localize the cause of weakness.

SUGGESTED READINGS

Barohn RJ, Amato AA. Pattern recognition approach to neuropathy and neuronopathy. *Neurol Clin.* 2013;31(2):343-361.

Ivanhoe CB, Reistetter TA. Spasticity: the misunderstood part of the upper motor neuron syndrome. *Am J Phys Med Rehabil.* 2004;83(10 Suppl):S3-S9.

Jackson CE, Barohn RJ. A pattern recognition approach to myopathy. *Continuum (Minneap Minn).* 2013;19(6):1674-1697.

Klein JP. Imaging of progressive weakness or numbness of central or peripheral origin. *Handbook of Clinical Neurology.* 2016;136(47):927-941.

Liang CL, Han S. Neuromuscular junction disorders. *PM&R.* 2013;5:S81-S88.

Van Alfen N, Malessy MJ. Diagnosis of brachial and lumbosacral plexus lesions. *Handb Clin Neurol.* 2013;115:293-310.

PART V

Diagnostic Testing and Procedures

SECTION 1
Interpretation of Common Tests

CHAPTER 107

Basic Diagnostic Tests

Sylvia C. McKean, MD, SFHM, FACP
Francine L. Jacobson, MD, MPH

Key Clinical Questions

1. How do you quantify the diagnostic accuracy of a test?
2. Why is it important to address the problem of inappropriate test ordering?
3. With any test that entails more than negligible risk, the decision to perform the study must take into account what factors?

INTRODUCTION

Each field of medicine challenges clinicians to recommend a course of action for a specific patient at a particular time. To efficiently and safely obtain the right information through testing, physicians need to ask the right questions. Clinical expertise assumes that the physician has the ability to

- Comprehend the information that the test will provide relevant to the decision at hand.
- Appreciate the situation and consequences of each approach.
- Utilize the information rationally in the context of a coherent set of care goals and ethical values.
- Explicitly communicate choices regarding care to the patient or surrogate so that there is informed consent.

Prior to ordering any examination, clinicians should first question whether they require additional data collection to optimize medical decision making. Clinicians need to weigh (1) medical indications, (2) patient preferences, (3) quality of life, and (4) contextual features to reach a decision that is right for the patient. Deciding whether or not to perform a diagnostic study involves balancing its risks and costs versus the information it might provide and the benefits of having that information. As a general principle, clinicians should select the least invasive imaging examination that provides the needed information with the least amount of risk, including the smallest dose of ionizing radiation, and at the least cost.

PRACTICE POINT

- Diagnostic testing is rarely without risk or financial cost and almost never completely accurate. The pursuit of diagnostic tests may delay much needed treatment; thus physicians cannot pursue every diagnostic avenue, even if patients want all the information.

There are times when the physician's most important job is to know when to ask for assistance and where to go to get that assistance. Initial decisions regarding the care of an acutely ill hospitalized patient must be continually reassessed in light of both new data and the patient's ongoing course.

THE PROCESS OF CLINICAL REASONING

The process of clinical reasoning (data collection, problem formulation, and the generation of a hypothesis) ideally results in pursuing the most viable hypotheses. One of the most important first steps in approaching a patient is to frame the problem either in terms of a diagnosis or syndrome. The process of weighing the probability of one disease versus that of other diseases possibly accounting for a patient's illness leads to the creation of a differential diagnosis. This process requires both a pathophysiologic knowledge of the potential causes of a problem and an understanding of the effect of new data on the probability of each potential cause. It is important to consider all possible diagnoses but especially those that are either life-threatening or for which effective treatment exists.

Physicians generally develop a working hypothesis that is based on partial information. This is particularly true in the hospital when the patient is acutely ill and urgent decisions must be efficiently made, often without access to outside ambulatory records.

TABLE 107-1 Common Presentations in the older adult

Painless myocardial infarction
Apathetic hyperthyroidism
Pneumonia without cough
Tuberculosis as a change in mental status, gradual debilitation and nonspecific symptoms, and negative PPD due to declining delayed hypersensitivity reactions
Depression masquerading as dementia

Furthermore, the older adult commonly has multiple comorbidities, and decreased ability to perform activities of daily life (ADLs) or non-specific symptoms such as lethargy, confusion, incontinence, or falls may precipitate hospital admission (**Table 107-1**). Physicians must be willing to reassess initial decisions when there are new data and the patient's ongoing course runs counter to expectations.

INAPPROPRIATE TEST ORDERING

Inappropriate test ordering refers to both under and over utilization. Inappropriate testing results from not requesting the best test, underestimating the risk of testing, ordering tests "too soon" after the initial test, or ordering tests that are unlikely to affect patient management (**Table 107-2**). Physicians commonly repeat studies due to failure to properly review the medical record or because these tests are readily available and easier to obtain than outside information. How much imaging is too much? Does the average hospitalized patient receive CT imaging approximately every 4 days? To answer what may seem at first glance an appalling question, clinicians may need to review how much imaging their patients are actually receiving, including any films prior to CT scans. See Chapter 113 (Patient Safety Issues in Radiology).

Focused and deliberately considered ordering of medical tests may also benefit from the review of previous examinations. Newer imaging is not always better for hospitalized patients. The maxim, "The answer is in the jacket," provides power and rapid answer to a myriad of carefully framed specific questions. An old CT will frequently answer the question raised by subsequent health care teams. During the hospitalization, comparison of serial films, even bedside chest radiographs, may provide more information than can be derived over time by more sophisticated imaging. The rate of evolution of abnormalities, both regarding progression and resolution, may separate many abnormalities that have the same potential appearance at a particular moment in time.

Hospitalized dying patients frequently receive fully aggressive care up to and including life-sustaining treatment and resuscitation. Although distraught families sometimes drive this care, the core of the doctor-patient relationship is the need for guidance and direction from the clinician for these families. The patient's surrogate should not determine evaluation and/or treatment if it serves no meaningful purpose for the patient or may even contribute to distress. See Part I: The Value and Values of Hospital Medicine (Section VII: Principles of Medical Ethics and Medical-Legal Concepts) and Part VI: Clinical Conditions in the Hospital Setting (Section 11: Palliative Care).

It is important to reduce inappropriate test ordering due to limited resources, patient safety issues, and patient discomfort. To do this, clinicians need to take the time to do an appropriate targeted history and physical examination know what the symptoms and signs mean, and most importantly, make sure that each test is preceded by a conscious decision that the test is indicated based on best practices whenever possible. Will the test increase the pretest probability sufficiently to alter patient management? The whole

TABLE 107-2 Examples of Inappropriate Test Ordering in the Hospital

Common examples
- Under and over utilization
- Unlikely to affect patient management
- Repeat studies
- Not the best test
- Inadequate clinical information
- Underestimation of risk of testing
- Short interval of follow-up studies

Factors that lead to inappropriate testing include:
- Time constraints that limit the physician's willingness to contemplate data before ordering a test or to obtain "outside" information
- Diagnostic uncertainty, fear of missing a crucial diagnosis, concern about medical malpractice
- Availability of sophisticated technology and support services
- Pressure from patients and families
- Risk of treating without an established diagnosis
- Testing habits of the individual physician and the group practice

Over utilization
- Failure to examine the primary data when a patient has been hospitalized elsewhere and treatment may have impacted course of illness (fever of unknown illness): time constraints
- "Ruling out" unlikely diagnoses (inappropriate ordering of D-dimer tests leading to unnecessary PE-protocol CT): fear of missing a crucial diagnosis
- The availability of sophisticated technology and support services in the hospital
- Pressure from patients and families
- Risk of treating without an established diagnosis
- Testing habits
- Financial incentives

Under utilization
- Disparities of health care for minorities: see Chapter 3
- Financial incentives

Data from Putterman C, Ben-Chetrit E. Clinical problem solving. Testing, testing, testing… *N Engl J Med.* 1995;333(18):1208-1211.

point of a diagnostic test is to use it to make a diagnosis, so clinicians need to know the probability that the test will give the correct diagnosis. Will the test accurately distinguish between patients who do and do not have the disorder?

DIAGNOSTIC ACCURACY OF A TEST

The simplest diagnostic test is one in which the results of an investigation such as a physical finding, blood test, or radiographic study are used to classify patients into two groups according to the presence or absence of a symptom or sign. The terms positive and negative are used to refer to the presence or absence of the condition of interest.

Sensitivity and specificity is one approach for quantifying the diagnostic accuracy of a test. In clinical practice, however, the test result is all that is known. We want to know how good the test is at predicting an abnormality. How many patients with abnormal test results are truly abnormal? The sensitivity and specificity do not answer this question. Values of test sensitivity and specificity derived in one clinical population cannot be extrapolated to make predictions about a different population. Test sensitivity increases with increasing severity of disease. What this means is that there is a distribution of sensitivities and specificities across the spectrum of disease. The values of sensitivity and specificity are actually average values across the population. In addition to knowing the test's average sensitivity and specificity, the clinician must be aware of how the test performs in different segments of the population. As the prevalence falls, the positive predictive value falls and the negative predictive value rises. Clinicians will, on average, learn the most from a clinical sign, symptom, or laboratory test when the likelihood of disease is 40% to 60%. If the prevalence of disease is very low, the positive predictive value will not be close to one even if the sensitivity and specificity are high. Thus, in screening the general population, it is inevitable that many people with positive test results will not have the disease.

The likelihood ratio (LR) represents the likelihood that a test result would be expected in a patient with the target disorder compared with the likelihood that the same result would be expected in a patient without the target disorder. The LR indicates the value of the test for increasing certainty about a positive diagnosis. A high LR may show that the test is useful, but it does not necessarily follow that the test is a good indicator of the presence of disease. For LR > 1, the probability of disease goes up; for LR < 1, the probability of disease goes down. When the LR is close to 1, the probability of disease is unchanged because the finding is equally likely in patients with and without the disorder.

The LR is more stable than sensitivity and specificity when the prevalence of disease changes because the direction of change is the same for the numerator and denominator of the LR. Unlike sensitivity and specificity (which limit the number of test results to just two levels, "positive" and "negative"), a LR may be generated for multiple levels of the diagnostic test result. The LR may be used to calculate the increase in probability of disease from baseline prevalence with positive test (LR positive) and decrease in probability of disease from baseline prevalence with negative test (using alternative LR negative) for any level of disease prevalence. The likelihood ratio may be used to shorten a list of diagnostic hypotheses because the pretest "odds" (the ratio of the probabilities for and against a diagnosis) of the target disorder multiplied by the likelihood ratio for the diagnostic test result equals the posttest odds for the target disorder. The LR allows you to carry out sequences of diagnostic tests. The posttest probability for one test becomes the pretest probability for a second, independent test with a distinct pathophysiology. For example, a result whose likelihood ratio is 2 increases the probability about 15%, 5 about 30%, and 10 about 45%. Likelihood ratios of 0.5 decrease the probability about 15%, 0.2 about 30%, and 0.1 about 45%. For diagnostic tests to be meaningful, they should increase or decrease probability by at least 20% to 25% (corresponding to likelihood ratios with values >3 or <0.3). Although the posttest probability may be calculated by a series of equations, they are at most only approximations in clinical medicine.

Spectrum bias refers to disease factors that affect the sensitivity and specificity of a diagnostic test. The following factors may affect the sensitivity or specificity of a diagnostic test:

- Severity of disease
- Cyclic nature of disease activity
- Duration of disease
- Therapy
- Control group composition

Reporting bias refers to the tendency to report strongly positive (or negative) results and not report results that are not clinically relevant at that time. Availability heuristic is a bias that makes noteworthy outcomes more likely (eg, a radiologist overestimating the likelihood of cancer in abnormalities seen on Chest CT so as to not miss a malignant tumor).

Reproducibility refers to the consistency of test performance and result interpretation. Interobserver agreement is expressed using the kappa statistic. A κ-value =

- 0 is the same as that by chance
- 0.2 to 0.4, fair agreement
- 0.4 to 0.6, moderate agreement
- 0.6 to 0.8, substantial agreement
- 0.8 to 1.0, almost perfect agreement

For most diagnostic tests, interobserver agreement is less than perfect, with κ statistics over a wide range depending on the diagnostic study or physical sign. Interobserver disagreement commonly relates to interpretation of the test's significance but also to the specific study and the examiner's experience. Abdominal ultrasound examinations are more subjective and require more expertise than CT.

PRACTICE POINT

- Communication between the ordering clinician and radiologist interpreting imaging may change the pretest probability and diagnostic accuracy of a test. Consulting a radiologist with a discussion about the presentation of illness, including localization of symptoms, may compel another review of the imaging and clarification of next steps. In the absence of effective communication, the radiologist cannot be expected to be right more than 70% of the time.

ASSESSMENT OF THE PATIENT'S DATA

Hospitalists must ask the right questions to address those problems; gather pertinent data from many sources; efficiently, logically, and resourcefully sort through complex information; acknowledge personal biases that may hinder analysis; interpret data in the context of each patient before them; and expediently reach trustworthy conclusions that form (**Table 107-3**).

TABLE 107-3 Clinical Problem Solving

1. Frame a question to answer a problem.
2. Formulate a concise and coherent hypothesis devoid of irrelevant information.
   - Organize thoughts and articulate them concisely and coherently.
   - Strip a verbal argument of irrelevancies and phrase it in its essential terms.
3. Seek and gather critical data to test and evaluate hypothesis.
   - Use evidence skillfully and impartially.
   - Distinguish between logically valid and invalid inferences.
4. Draw reliable conclusions from the result.
   - Suspend judgment in the absence of sufficient evidence to support a decision.
5. Habitually question one's own views and attempt to understand both the assumptions that are critical to those views and the implications of the views.
6. Reassess a hypothesis when data does not support that approach.

ASKING THE RIGHT QUESTION

The hallmark of clinical problem-solving requires asking the right questions to obtain the right information. Without the right information, we cannot make the correct diagnosis or order the appropriate treatment. A thorough history and physical examination will in fact usually lead to the correct diagnosis, especially in complex or perplexing cases. During emergency medical conditions, clinicians, however, tend to order tests first and clinical problem solve after the results are known, especially with imaging studies. With this approach clinicians will not find out information if they skip the step of asking pertinent questions.

The evidence-based medicine (EBM) approach requires a series of steps, the first of which is to ask a clinical question that can be answered. Failure to follow the first step will result in an unproductive search that cannot be applied to the patient in front of you (**Table 107-4**).

For each test, the examiner should take a systematic approach in assessment, beginning with the history and physical examination. *What is the patient telling us? Does the physical examination confirm our suspicions? Do we need to ask additional questions and re-examine the patient?*

The admission data should then be reviewed in the context of the patient in front of us, including available information from outside records and the diagnostic quality of any imaging. The first step in making any diagnosis is to think of it. *Although one diagnosis is highly likely, does the diagnosis adequately explain this patient's symptoms? Or even if less frequent, what might cause this patient's death? Does the principal diagnosis explain all of the positive and negative findings? Are there no convincing alternative diagnoses?* A hypothesis generated by partial information requires diagnostic adequacy. At each step in the process as more data becomes available, certain hypotheses may be eliminated. A limited number of hypotheses should be tested at each step, not just ruling out one, to see whether the specific diagnoses fit the available information. This requires keeping an open mind until sufficient clinical data is obtained to favor one hypothesis over another, constantly reassessing the validity of the favored hypothesis in light of new data, and reexamining all data for any "minor" detail that might have been overlooked or in this case misinterpreted.

DISCORDANT DATA

An admitting diagnosis is not absolute and is still inferential. The sequential acquisition of partial data is a multistep process. Refinement of the hypothesis usually requires additional diagnostic testing to verify the diagnosis. Overlooking discordant data may result in failure to order appropriate studies to make the correct diagnosis. Hospitalization presents another opportunity to formulate an adequate and coherent diagnosis that may be verified with additional laboratory testing or appropriate imaging.

No test is infallible. For plain films, alignment of bones will provide information of whether the patient is properly positioned. Then the

---

TABLE 107-4 Evidence-Based Patient Care (the PICO Question)

1. Ask questions specific to your **P**atient that can be answered.
2. Search for evidence to support an **I**ntervention.
3. Assess the evidence for its validity and relevance and **C**ompare to other interventions.
4. Integrate the evidence with clinical expertise and the patient's values.
5. Evaluate **O**utcomes.

---

reviewer should have a mental checklist so that all aspects of the film are reviewed, not just the one area of concern. For chest radiography if the pathology is where you think it is, the localization of it should be correct on both frontal and lateral views. If not, the localization is incorrect, and a new hypothesis is needed. The fit between the data and the disease reveals itself over time and dialogue.

PRACTICE POINT

- Recent diagnostic technologies that have expanded our ability to define anatomic and physiological abnormalities have not reduced the frequency of misdiagnosis. Even the most recent CT scanners may be misleading due to technical limitations relating to body size or timing of contrast bolus, timing relative to onset of symptoms, the human factor in interpretation, and the significance of other findings.

Experience provides a context for anticipating diagnoses and interpreting clinical events. This process begins with reviewing imaging and consulting with radiologists interpreting the study. Specialists may provide the necessary expertise to improve diagnostic accuracy but specialty focus may limit the categories of illness considered. Therefore, it will always be the responsibility of generalists to know when to ask for help and where to go for that help.

THE DECISION TO PERFORM THE STUDY

Clinical problem solving relies upon inferential diagnosis to guide further action, whether in the selection of further testing or treatment. With any procedure that entails more than negligible risk, the decision to perform the study must take into account the following factors:

- The risk to the patient inherent in the procedure with the patient's comorbidity factored into the risk assessment
- The risk associated with missing a potentially dire diagnosis
- The likelihood that the procedure will result in a diagnosis relevant to the patient's care
- The cost of the procedure

Is additional testing in accordance with the patient's goals and values? Never leave the patient out of the equation.

GUIDELINES

With computerized order entry, data on individual ordering of imaging studies will become readily available and increasingly, imaging guidelines will be developed along with performance measures to define and measure quality. Built on consensus, guidelines are typically evolving documents developed to answer important questions. However, they may not reflect evolving technology or address conflicting recommendations from different societies in the ordering of imaging studies. They also may not be applicable to the acutely ill patient before you. Critical decision making will therefore remain central to the privilege of caring for sick persons.

COMMUNICATION

Optimal use of consultants, including radiologists, requires effective communication so that key questions are answered. The most crucial clinical information for radiologists is the location of symptoms. One example, CT, contains complex information about multiple organ systems and anatomy. Clinical information directs the radiologist's attention to a specific problem. Interpretation attributes the observed abnormalities to a disease process. Accuracy is improved by improving sensitivity (perception) without affecting specificity. Clinical information improves accuracy with respect to diagnostic imaging, including radiography, CT, MR, and mammography by refining the pretest probability for the radiologist. If the story changes as so often happens during the course of hospitalization, the study should be reread with the new defining information that would place the patient in a different population. A potentially different pretest probability might completely change the proper interpretation of a potentially ambiguous finding. This is true for pneumonia, heart disease, and a large variety of tumors. If the patient is presented as "normal" the potentially ambiguous radiographic finding is overwhelmingly "normal."

PRACTICE POINT

- Tests are often performed to "rule out" a particular problem. Beware of a signout or progress note communication that states "negative" without looking at the final report. Radiology does not negate or trump physical exam findings and the creation of the differential diagnosis.

Hospital care requires teamwork and effective communication, often through progress notes in the medical record. From hospital day one a patient should have an accurate problem list that reflects a formulation of the care plan and promotes clear decision making. Although the practice of "cutting and pasting" computer generated progress notes improves efficiency of documentation for billing and other purposes, failure to synthesize the information in a concise and up-to-date problem list may impede the transfer of necessary information and impact the recommendations of consultants who may not review the primary data.

CONCLUSION

Critical decision-making rests upon the foundation of common sense, informed and experienced clinical judgment, and one of the old medical virtues, humility. An unflinching self-awareness recognizes that subjective assessments of events are often affected by factors unrelated to true prevalence, errors in assessing diagnostic value of clinical evidence, and errors in revision of probability. Interpretation of Common Tests focuses on the "low-tech" tests that are routinely available on admission such as the ECG and urinalysis. Optimizing Utilization of Radiology Services addresses the selection of imaging tests, some of which carry significant risk and cost. The third section briefly summarizes common procedures performed by hospitalists for either diagnostic or therapeutic purposes and refers the reader to other on-line resources.

SUGGESTED READINGS

Berbaum KS, el-Khoury GY, Franken EA Jr, Kathol M, Montgomery WJ, Hesson W. Impact of clinical history on fracture detection with radiography. *Radiology.* 1988;168:507-511.

Berlin L. Accuracy of procedures: has it improved over the last five decades? http://www.ajronline.org/cgi/content/full/188/5/1173.

Halkin A, Reishman J, Scaber M, et al. Likelihood ratios: getting diagnostic testing into perspective. http://qjmed.oxfordjournals.org/content/91/4/247.short.

Houssami N, Irwig L, Simpson JM, et al. The influence of clinical information on the accuracy of diagnostic mammography. *Breast Cancer Res Treat.* 2004;85(3):223-228.

Kaplan DM. Clear writing, clear thinking, and the disappearing art of the problem list. *J Hosp Med.* 2007;2(4):201-202.

Leslie A, Jones AJ, Goddard PR. The influence of clinical information on the reporting of CT by radiologists. *Br J Radiol.* 2000;73:1052-1055.

Loy C, Irwig L. Accuracy of diagnostic tests read with and without clinical information. *JAMA.* 2004;292:1602-1609.

Peterson MC, Holbrook JH, Von Hales D, et al. Contributions of the history, physical examination, and laboratory investigation in making medical diagnoses. *West J Med.* 1992;156:163-165.

Richardson W, Wilson M, Nishikawa J, et al. The well-built clinical question: a key to evidence-based decisions (editorial). *ACP J Club.* 1995;123:A12-A13.

Sackett DL, Richardson WS, Rosenberg W, et al. *Evidence-Based Medicine: How to Practice and Teach EBM,* 2nd ed. Edinburg, Scotland: Churchill Livingstone; 1997.

Sackett DL, Rosenberg WMC, Gray JAM, et al. Evidence based medicine: what it is and what it isn't. *Br Med J.* 1996;312:71-72.

Wilczynski NL. Quality of reporting of diagnostic accuracy studies: no change since STARD statement publication—before-and-after study. http://radiology.rsna.org/content/248/3/817.

CHAPTER 108

The Resting Electrocardiogram

Timothy J. Poterucha, MD
Thomas P. Rocco, MD

Key Clinical Questions

① How does the resting electrocardiogram (ECG) assist in the diagnosis and management of acute coronary syndrome (ACS)?

② What is the differential for ST elevations, and what are the key differentiating electrocardiographic features of ACS versus acute pericarditis versus early repolarization?

③ How does the ECG assist in the diagnosis of acute pulmonary embolism?

④ How does the ECG assist in determining the cause of syncope?

⑤ What are the characteristic ECG findings of electrolyte disturbances?

⑥ What are the characteristic ECG findings of hypothyroidism, stroke, and drug effects?

INTRODUCTION

A graphic recording of electrical potentials generated by the heart, the electrocardiogram (ECG) is the most commonly performed cardiovascular laboratory procedure in the United States. As a noninvasive, versatile, reproducible, and inexpensive test, the ECG has utility in the evaluation of a range of signs and symptoms encountered by the hospitalist, including acute chest discomfort, breathlessness, syncope, and palpitations. While the ECG is useful in the detection of myocardial ischemia, structural changes of the myocardium, arrhythmias, and conduction system disease, clinicians should also be able to recognize normal variants that may mimic cardiac disease and electrocardiographic manifestations of noncardiac illness. Guidelines for the use of electrocardiograms in patients with and without pre-existing heart disease have been published by the American College of Cardiology and American Heart Association (ACC/AHA).

THE NORMAL RESTING ELECTROCARDIOGRAM

The electrocardiogram is a graphical recording of the difference in potential between electrodes placed on the body surface. The standard twelve lead ECG used commonly in clinical practice includes the six extremity (limb) and six chest (precordial) leads. The chest leads (V_1-V_6) record electrical activity in a horizontal plane, and the limb leads (bipolar leads I, II, and III; and unipolar leads aVR, aVL, and aVF) record potentials transmitted on the frontal plane. These standard twelve leads are categorized by their anatomic location into the following groups: inferior (II, III, aVF), septal (V_1-V_2), anterior (V_3-V_4), and lateral (V_5-V_6, I, aVL). In addition to the standard 12 leads, right-sided precordial leads (V_1R-V_6R) and the posterior leads (V_7-V_9) may be useful in the assessment of right ventricular and posterior infarctions, respectively. If a wave of depolarization spreads toward the positive pole of a lead, a positive deflection is recorded in that lead. Conversely, if a wave of depolarization spreads toward the negative pole of a lead, a negative deflection is recorded in that lead. The components of the normal resting electrocardiogram are the P-wave, generated by atrial contraction; the PR interval, representing conduction through the AV node; the QRS complex, generated by biventricular contraction; and the ST-T wave, reflecting biventricular recovery.

ACUTE CHEST DISCOMFORT

The initial diagnostic evaluation of the patient with acute chest discomfort centers on the recognition of life-threatening conditions, including ACS and pulmonary embolism.

■ ACUTE CORONARY SYNDROME

Electrocardiography is an indispensable tool in the diagnosis and management of ACS. The ECG changes in ACS include ST elevations, ST depressions, T-wave inversions, and Q-waves. ST segment elevations signify an acute transmural infarction and may be preceded by the appearance of tall, positive, hyperacute T-waves. These ST segment elevations are often accompanied by prominent reciprocal ST-segment depressions on leads overlying the contralateral surface of the heart. When ST-segment elevations are absent, ST-depressions and T-wave inversions represent active ischemia. Old infarctions frequently result in Q-waves. ST-segment elevations and Q-waves in ACS always localize to the affected area

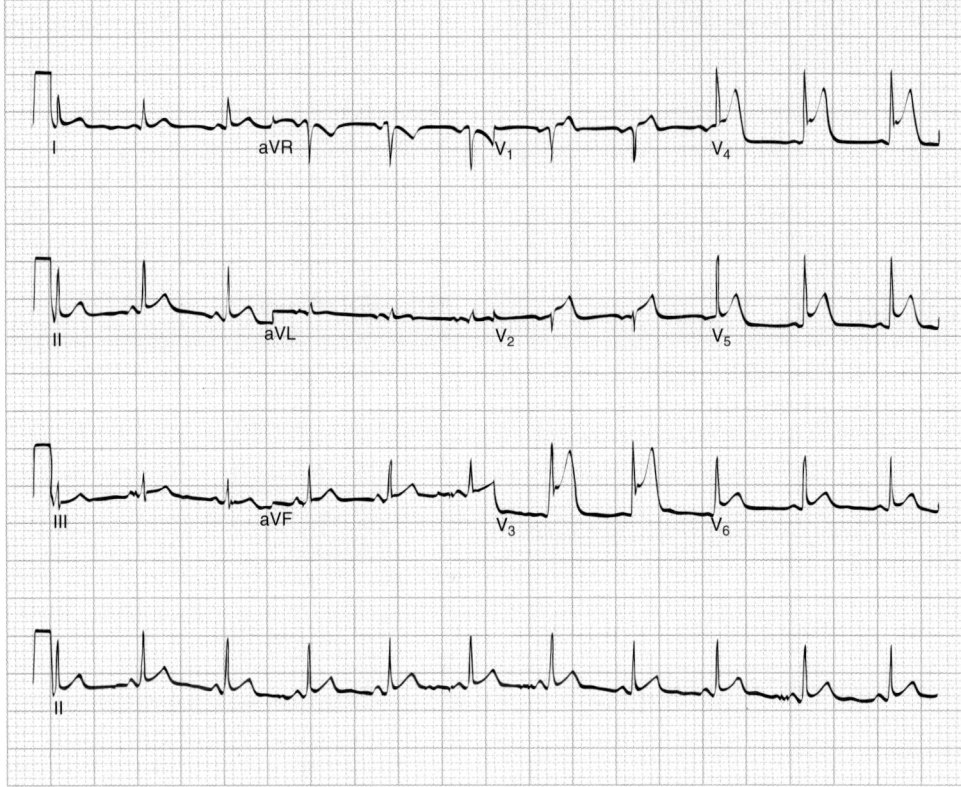

Figure 108-1 *Electrocardiogram reveals prominent anteroseptal and lateral ST-segment elevations, consistent with an acute anterolateral ST elevation MI. The patient was found to have an acute thrombosis within the proximal left anterior descending artery.*

of myocardium. For instance, ST-segment elevations in II, III, and aVF in the setting of an acute infarction will reliably indicate an infarction of the inferior wall. In contrast to ST-segment elevations, ST-segment depressions and T-wave inversions do not have this same dependable ability to localize ischemia. In the setting of an acute transmural infarction, the initial ST-segment elevations evolve with T-wave inversions and Q-wave formation (**Figures 108-1, 108-2, and 108-3**).

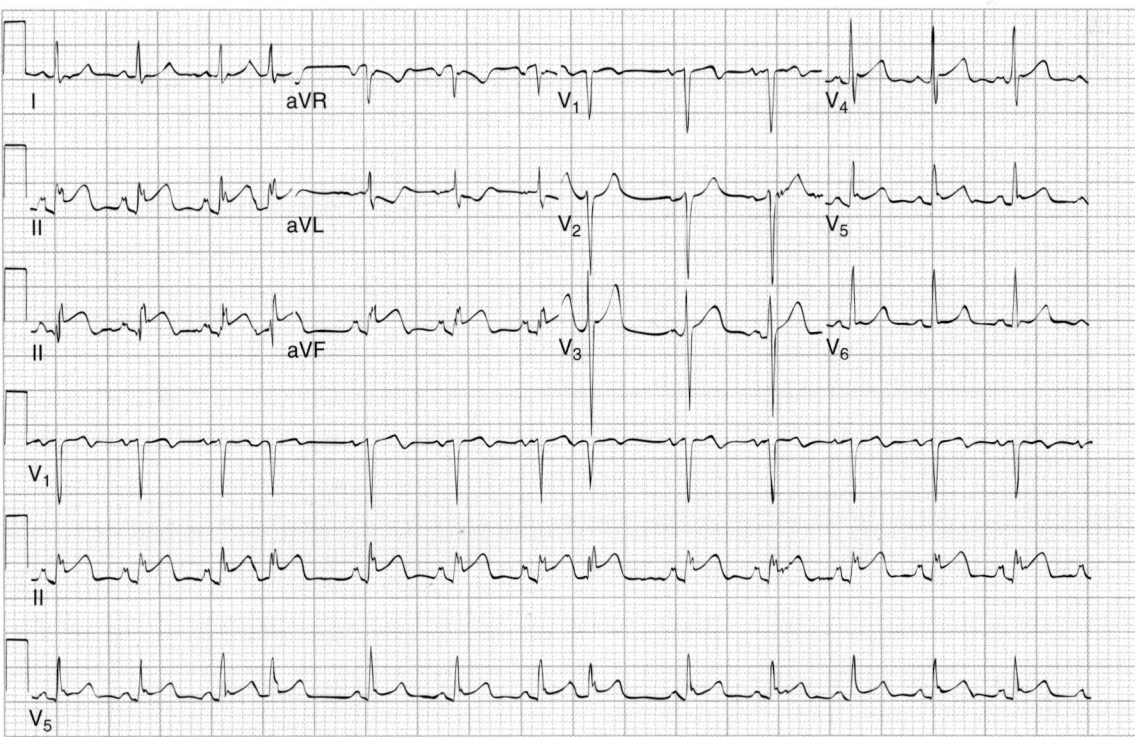

Figure 108-2 *59-year-old gentleman presenting with chest pain and prominent inferolateral ST-segment elevations. He was found to have acute thrombosis of the mid right coronary artery.*

PRACTICE POINT

Chest pain

Acute Myocardial infarction

- Epicardial injury or transmural ischemia is manifested by ST-segment deviation toward the ischemic zone, manifested by ST-segment depression or elevation.
- In the setting of ST-segment elevations, reciprocal ST-segment depressions in other leads support a diagnosis of ischemia rather than early repolarization.

Prior Myocardial infarction

- <1 mm ST-segment elevation in any lead and T-waves upright in the leads with pathological Q-waves (>1/3 of the R-wave amplitude with duration of >0.04 seconds).
- Suspect aneurysm or large akinetic region if wide deep Q-waves across the precordial leads in a stable pattern.

Early repolarization syndrome

- Most clinically urgent problem—distinguishes between early repolarization and ischemia.
- Diagnostic criteria:
  - Concave ST-segment elevation <5 mm and most prominent in the precordial leads.
  - Reciprocal ST depression usually seen in AVR.
  - T-waves usually asymmetric.
- Notching of the R-wave at its junction with ST-segment (≥50% of cases).
- During exercise the ST-segment elevation of early repolarization may return to baseline.

Acute pericarditis

- Depression of the PR segment, reflecting atrial injury, early in course.
- Commonly, ST-segment elevation in all leads, except aVR, which has ST-segment depression.

- Other leads, including V_1, aVL, and lead III, may not show ST-segment elevation.
- A relatively slow sinus rate is frequent with early repolarization and infrequent with acute pericarditis.
- Almost exclusively in pericarditis:
  - T-wave amplitude ≤3 mm in V_6.
  - Ratio of height of the onset of the ST-segment to the amplitude of the T-wave in V_6 ≥0.25 is more characteristic of pericarditis rather than early repolarization.

Pericardial effusion

- Low voltage, defined as limb leads <5 mm peak to peak and precordial leads <10 mm peak to peak, is seen in less than 1% of normal people.
  - Isolated low voltage in limb leads has no clinical significance.
- Low specificity of low voltage for pericardial effusion.
  - Any process that reduces the mass of electrically active myocardium (eg, MI, myocardial diseases, cardiac amyloidosis).
  - Interposition of air or tissue between the heart and surface electrodes such as in emphysema, pleural effusions, obesity, and myxedema.
- Abnormal position of heart within pericardial cavity may result in lack of normal R-wave progression in anterior leads.
- Beat-to-beat alternation of amplitude and direction of QRS (electrical alternans) seen in cardiac tamponade.
- Flattening of T-waves and sinus tachycardia (large pericardial effusions with tamponade physiology).
- The slow or normal heart rate seen in myxedema is not present with other etiologies. Myxedema may produce large pericardial effusions and tamponade with resulting electrical alternans on ECG. Inflammatory changes, such as those of acute pericarditis, depend on the etiology. Idiopathic and neoplastic effusions are often not associated with inflammation.

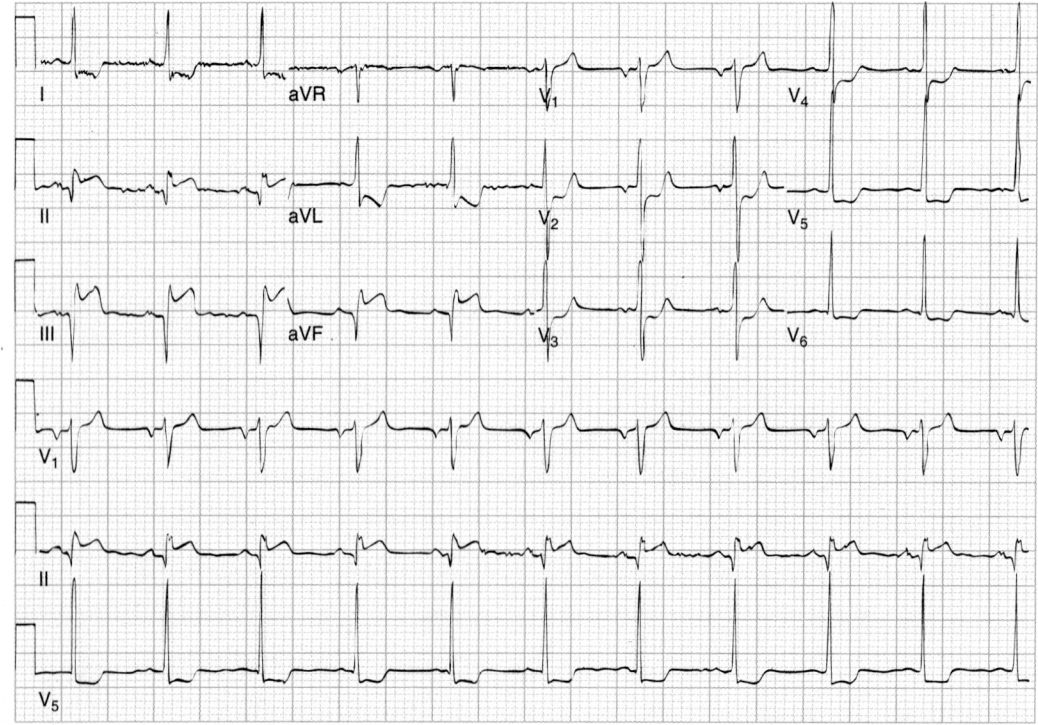

Figure 108-3 *Elevations of the ST-segment in the inferior leads is suggestive of a thrombotic lesion within the right coronary artery. Reciprocal changes are apparent in the lateral limb and precordial leads. A tall R-wave and ST-segment depression in lead V_2 suggest posterior involvement.*

TABLE 108-1 Electrocardiographic Changes and Localization of Lesions

Region(s) of Myocardium Affected	Location of Culprit Stenosis or Lesion(s)	Electrocardiographic Changes
Anterolateral wall and septum	Proximal left anterior descending artery	ST-segment elevations in leads V_1-V_6 and limb leads I and aVL with reciprocal ST-segment depressions in limb leads III and aVF
Anterior and inferior walls	"Wrap around" left anterior descending artery that extends onto the inferior wall or multivessel disease	ST-segment elevations in leads V_1-V_6, accompanied by ST elevations in limbs leads II, III, and aVF
Inferior	Right coronary or circumflex arteries	ST-segment elevations in limb leads II, III, and aVF (and greater in lead III than lead II), along with elevation in lead V_1 suggestive of occlusion of proximal or mid-right coronary artery
Posterior wall	Right coronary or circumflex arteries	ST-segment depressions in leads V_1 and V_2 with eventual appearance of prominent R-waves. Posterior leads V_7-V_9 (V_7, posterior axillary line; V_8, posterior scapular line; and V_9, left border of spine) may show ST-segment elevations
Right ventricle	Right coronary artery	ST-segment elevations in V_1R-V_6R (particularly V_4R) and limb leads II, III, and aVF, along with reciprocal ST-segment depressions in limb leads I and aVL

Patterns of ST-segment elevations may be useful in localizing the region of involved myocardium and may suggest the site of occlusion within the coronary arterial tree (**Table 108-1**).

Pathophysiologically, ST-segment elevations in ACS indicate complete or near-complete luminal obstruction. In clinical practice, this most commonly occurs due to atherosclerotic plaque rupture and occlusive intraluminal thrombus formation. However, spontaneous or drug-induced coronary vasospasm and can also lead to luminal obstruction (**Figure 108-4**).

When ischemia is primarily subendocardial, ST-segment depressions appear in the overlying leads (**Figure 108-5**).

Although hyperacute T-waves may precede or accompany ST-segment elevations, inversion of the T-wave or pseudonormalization of previously inverted T-waves may also indicate ischemia. Deep and symmetrically inverted T-waves in the anterior precordial leads, in particular, may indicate high-grade stenosis in the proximal left anterior descending artery, an exception to the rule that leads in which T-wave inversions are present do not correlate with the location of coronary stenoses (**Figure 108-6**).

Symmetric giant T-waves (amplitude > 10 mm in two or more leads) may be associated with pericarditis, pheochromocytoma, severe aortic insufficiency, myocarditis, and cerebrovascular disease. Commonly inverted in all precordial leads at birth, T-waves may remain inverted in the right precordial leads in normal persons in a persistent juvenile pattern. Inversion of the T-waves in leads III, aVR, and V_1 may also be a normal variant in adults.

While a normal ECG throughout the course of an acute infarct is uncommon, the ECG does not have perfect sensitivity or specificity in the diagnosis of ACS. Clinicians should recognize that ECG changes are not specific for myocardial ischemia and should be able to distinguish the changes associated with acute pericarditis and benign early repolarization from those seen with myocardial ischemia. In contrast to the regional ST-segment elevations and reciprocal ST-segment depressions created by myocardial infarction, acute pericarditis can cause diffuse ST-segment elevations with PR segment depression. Reciprocal PR segment elevation in aVR is another common finding in pericarditis. In contrast to the T-wave inversions that develop in an acute ST-segment

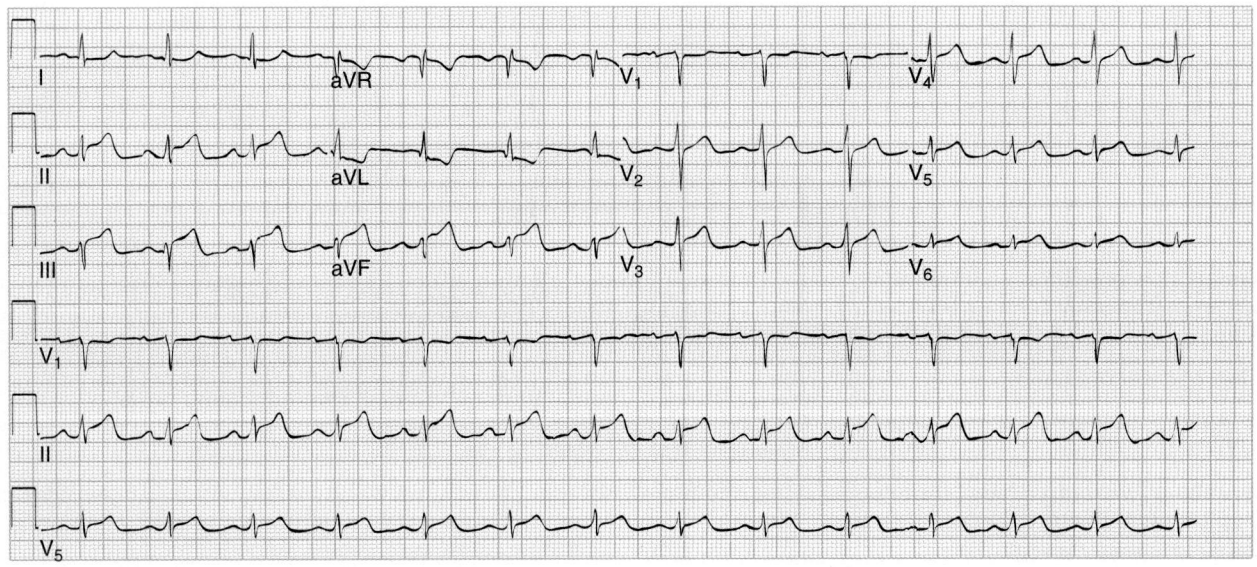

Figure 108-4 *55-year-old gentleman with nonobstructive coronary artery disease. Electrocardiogram reveals prominent inferolateral ST-segment elevations, attributed to coronary vasospasm and successfully treated with nitrates and calcium-channel blockade.*

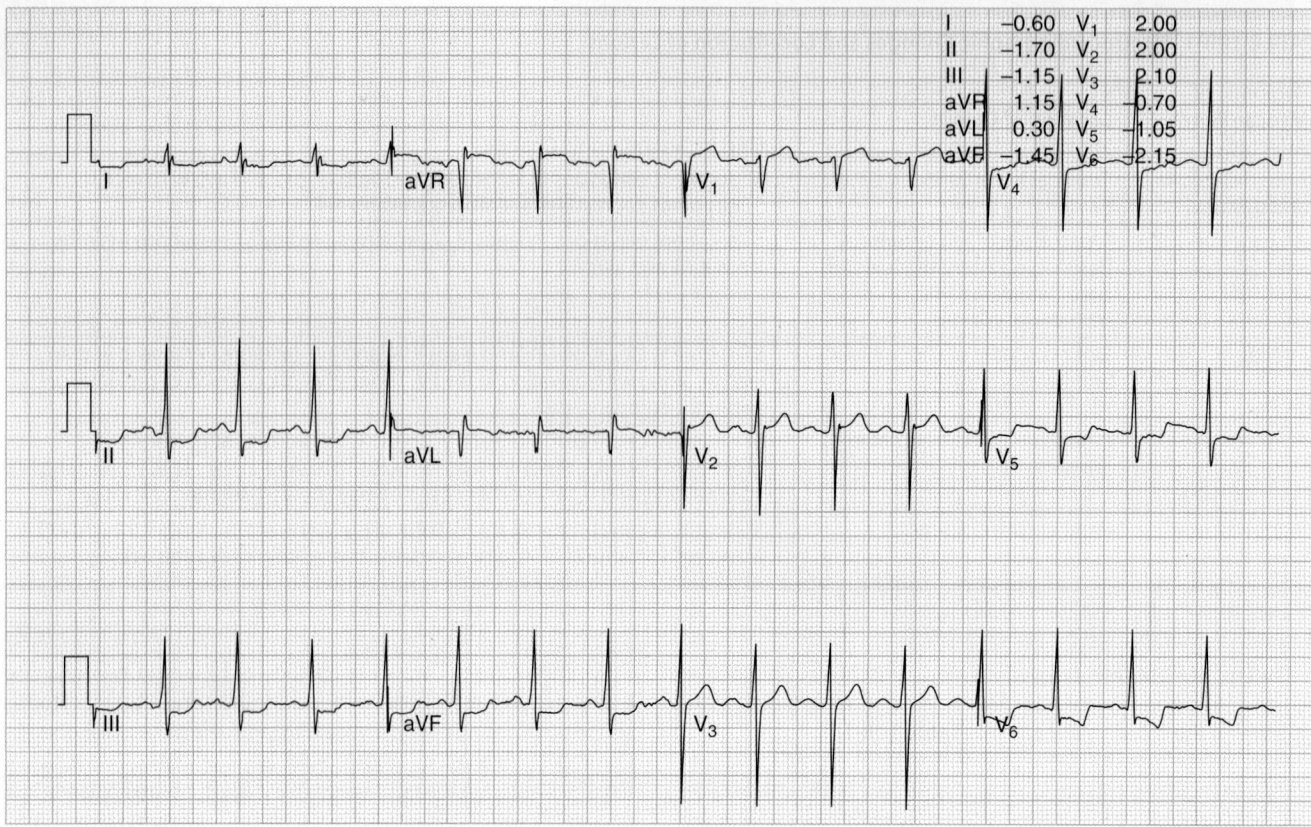

Figure 108-5 *When ischemia is subendocardial, ST-segment depressions with or without T-wave inversions may appear, as in this electrocardiogram of a 44-year-old gentleman with obstructive stenoses within the left anterior descending and left circumflex arteries on coronary angiography.*

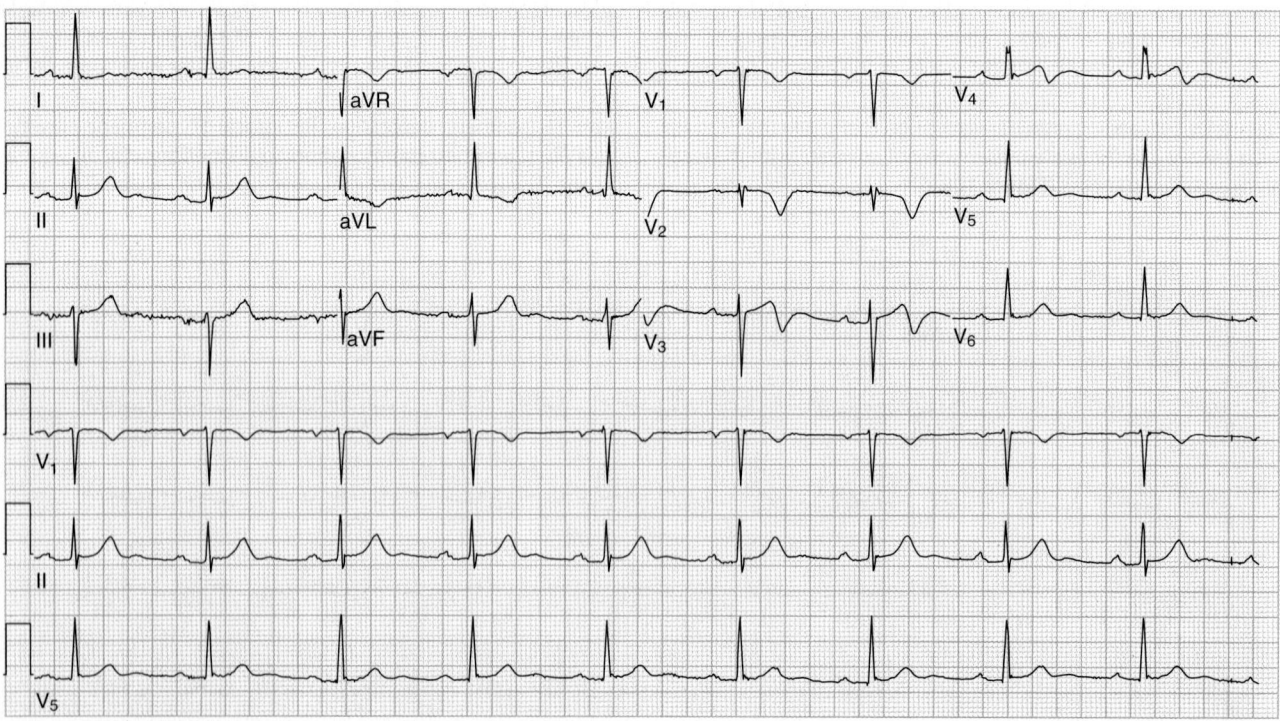

Figure 108-6 *Prominent and new T-wave inversions in the anterior precordial leads (also known as Wellen sign) may indicate a high-grade proximal stenosis within the left anterior descending artery. This 70-year-old gentleman had a 90% to 95% thrombotic and ulcerated obstructive lesion within the left anterior descending artery.*

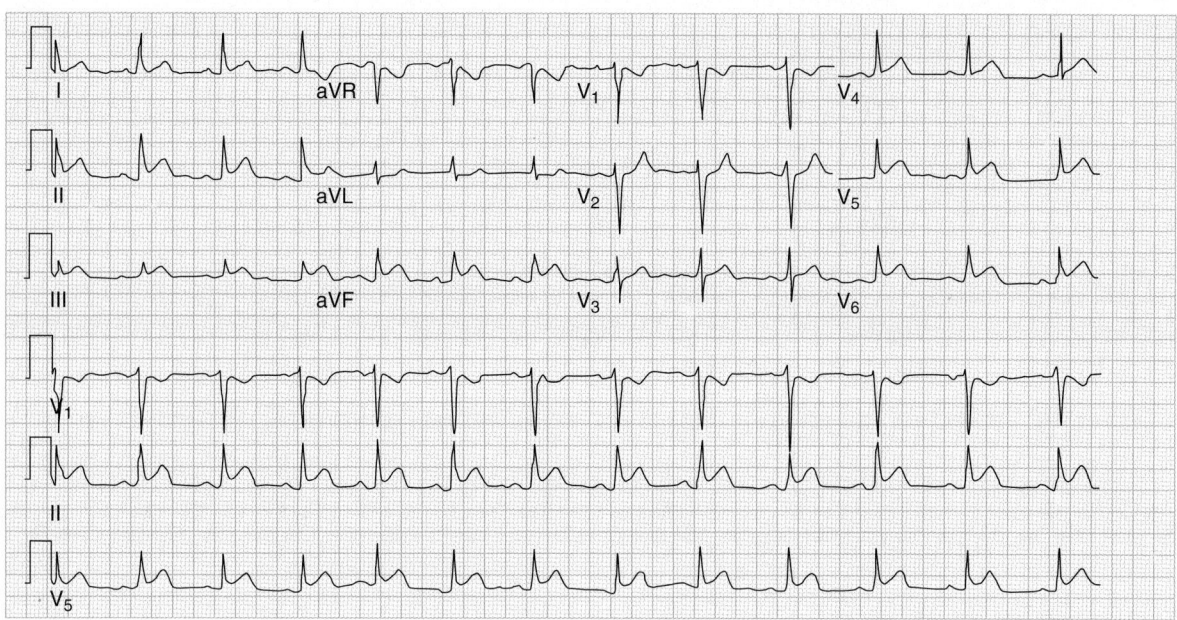

Figure 108-7 *Acute pericarditis creates diffuse ST-segment elevations, often in the presence of PR-segment elevation in aVR and reciprocal PR-segment depressions in the other leads.*

elevation MI, T-wave inversions in acute pericarditis generally do not develop until the ST-segments have returned to isoelectric baseline (**Figure 108-7**).

The electrocardiographic signature of early repolarization is ST-segment elevation, especially in the midprecordial leads and more commonly at slow heart rates and among young adult men (**Figure 108-8**).

In contrast to the convexity seen in ST-segment elevations associated with myocardial ischemia, those seen with early repolarization are generally concave in form and associated with notching of the

R-wave at its junction with the QRS complex. Biphasic T-wave inversions may also accompany the ST-segment elevations seen with early repolarization.

Among patients with ACS, the electrocardiogram also offers utility in the recognition of ischemia-related arrhythmias and postinfarct complications. The most common malignant rhythms observed in ACS include polymorphic ventricular tachycardia and ventricular fibrillation. Other more benign findings can include premature ventricular contractions and the accelerated idioventricular rhythm (AIVR). AIVR is a ventricular rhythm that can occur when the rate of

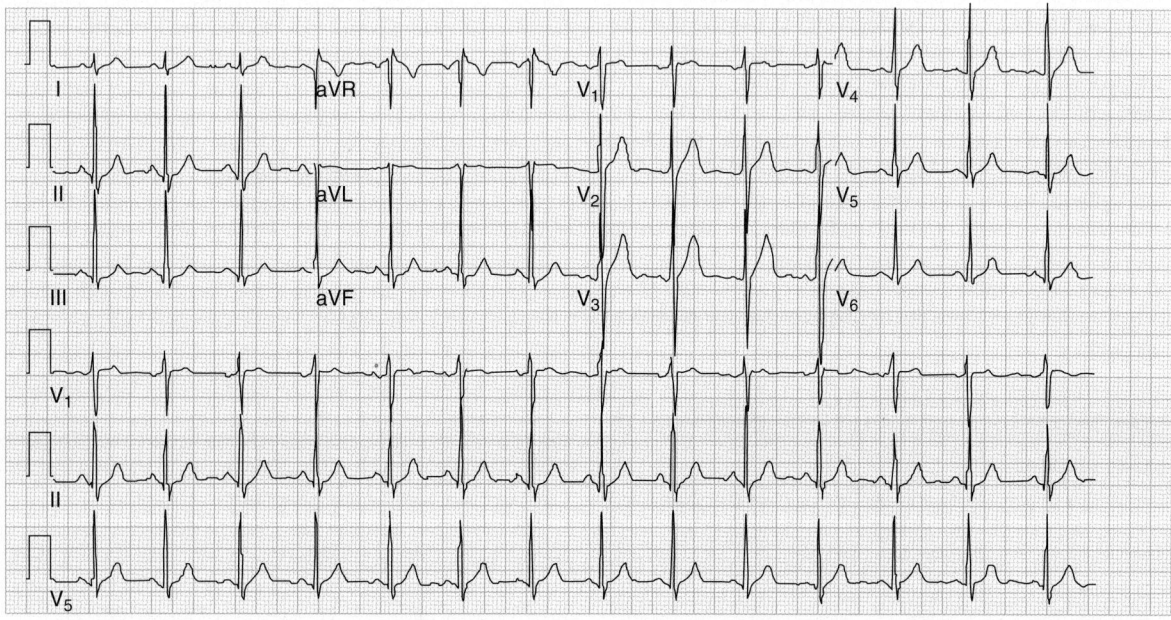

Figure 108-8 *The ST-segment elevation of early repolarization may mimic acute ischemia. In contrast to the convexity seen in ST-segment elevations associated with myocardial ischemia, ST-elevations seen with early repolarization are generally concave in form and associated with notching of the R-wave at its junction with the QRS complex, as in this tracing from a healthy 23-year-old gentleman. During exercise, the ST-segment elevations of early repolarization may return to baseline.*

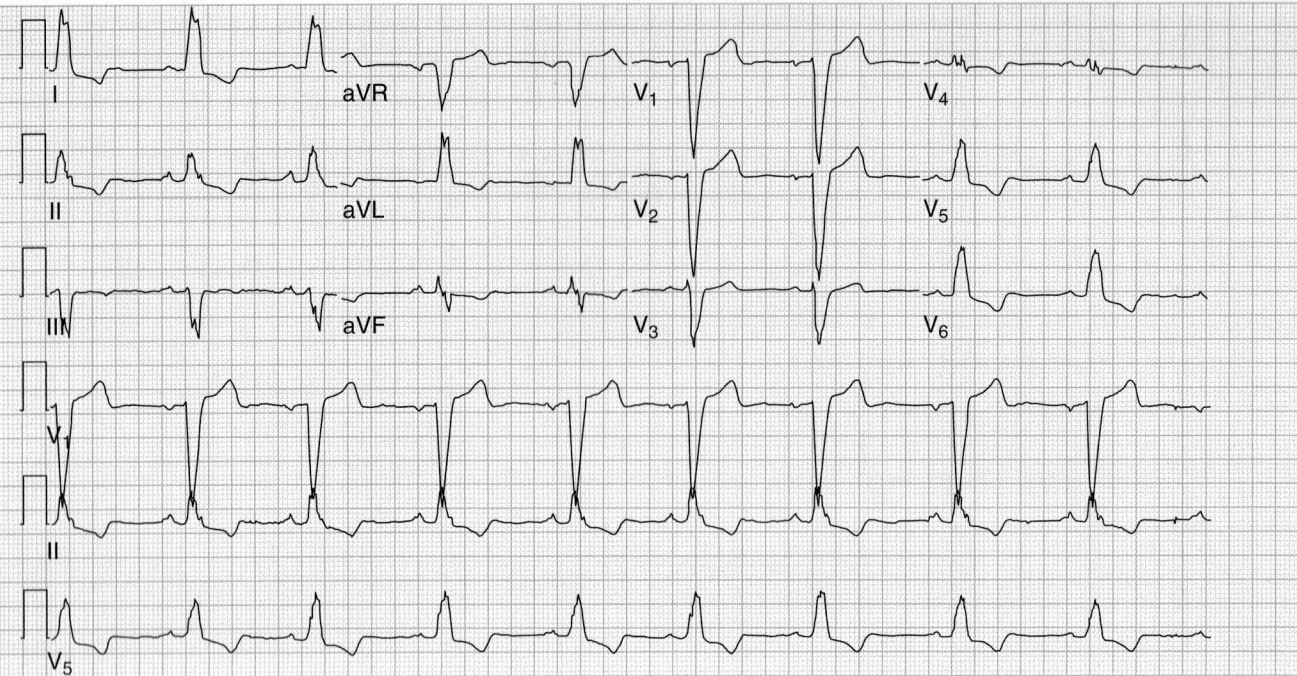

Figure 108-9 *New left bundle branch block, as shown in this electrocardiogram, may indicate a large, anterior wall acute MI in the appropriate clinical setting.*

an ectopic ventricular pacemaker exceeds that of the sinus node. It is typically benign and self-terminating.

Ventricular aneurysm may be suggested by ST-segment elevations that persist despite reperfusion.

A new left bundle branch block (LBBB) in the setting of symptoms consistent with acute MI may indicate a large, anterior wall acute MI (**Figure 108-9**).

Because the LBBB is spread over a large anatomic area, an infarct must be large in order to affect the entire bundle. At the same time, a LBBB impairs the ability of the clinician reading the ECG to assess for signs of ischemia. Therefore, a new LBBB in the setting of signs and symptoms of ACS is considered to be an ST-segment elevation equivalent. With a pre-existing LBBB, the diagnosis of acute STEMI may be obscured. However, the Sgarbossa criteria may be used to assess for signs of ischemia in the setting of a LBBB. These criteria include the following: ST-segment elevation ≥1 mm concordant with the QRS complex; ST-segment depression ≥1 mm in lead V_1, V_2, or V_3; or ST-segment elevation ≥5 mm discordant with the QRS.

Right bundle branch block (RBBB) may obscure the diagnosis of an acute anterior MI by interfering with the interpretation of ST-segment elevations in leads V_{1-3}, but the pseudonormalization of the normally discordant T-waves (ie, normally opposite the terminal deflection of the QRS complex) may suggest acute ischemia. The appearance of an RBBB can make the diagnosis of a posterior infarct more challenging.

PRACTICE POINT

Pulmonary embolism

ECG in pulmonary embolism is clinically helpful mainly in patients with no history of heart or lung disease. The following are the most common findings in pulmonary embolism:

- Sinus tachycardia
- $S_1Q_3T_3$ pattern
- Right atrial abnormality, right axis deviation, complete or incomplete RBBB
- T-wave inversions in V_1-V_3

■ PULMONARY EMBOLISM

While pulmonary embolism frequently may not generate electrocardiographic changes or only subtle nonspecific abnormalities, there are characteristic findings that may indicate right ventricular pressure overload. These electrocardiographic findings may include T-wave inversions in V_1-V_3 or a characteristic $S_1Q_3T_3$ with an S-wave in lead I and new Q-waves and T-wave inversions in lead III. Sinus tachycardia is most frequently observed rhythm in pulmonary embolism (**Figure 108-10**).

SYNCOPE, PALPITATIONS, AND SUDDEN CARDIAC DEATH

Syncope, the sudden transient loss of consciousness with associated loss of postural tone, may be arrhythmic in origin. Sinus node dysfunction, atrioventricular block, and ventricular tachycardia need to be considered in the evaluation of arrhythmic syncope. Sinus arrest, or sinus pause, is a form of sinus node dysfunction that occurs when the sinus node fails to depolarize on time and manifests as pauses that may last longer than 3 seconds. Pauses may also represent atrioventricular block (**Figure 108-11**).

Sick sinus syndrome is a disease predominantly of the elderly in which the sinus node fails to function normally. In most cases, this will cause an isolated bradycardia. This is an established indication for permanent pacing if it is associated with symptomatic chronotropic incompetence. In many cases of sick sinus syndrome, the sinus node dysfunction results in the tachycardia-bradycardia syndrome, which is defined as episodes of sinus or junctional bradycardia alternating with an atrial tachycardia. Management of this disorder often requires nodal blocking agents to control paroxysmal tachycardia. This intervention often results in therapy-related bradycardia, which necessitates pacemaker placement.

Atrioventricular disturbances are classified as first-, second-, or third-degree block. Often a consequence of AV-nodal slowing medications, first-degree atrioventricular block is characterized by prolongation of the PR interval beyond 200 milliseconds (**Figure 108-12**).

The hallmark of second-degree atrioventricular block is a failure of one or more, but not all, atrial impulses to conduct to the ventricles. Mobitz type I (or Wenckebach) block, characterized by a prolonging PR interval prior to a nonconducted atrial impulse, is often

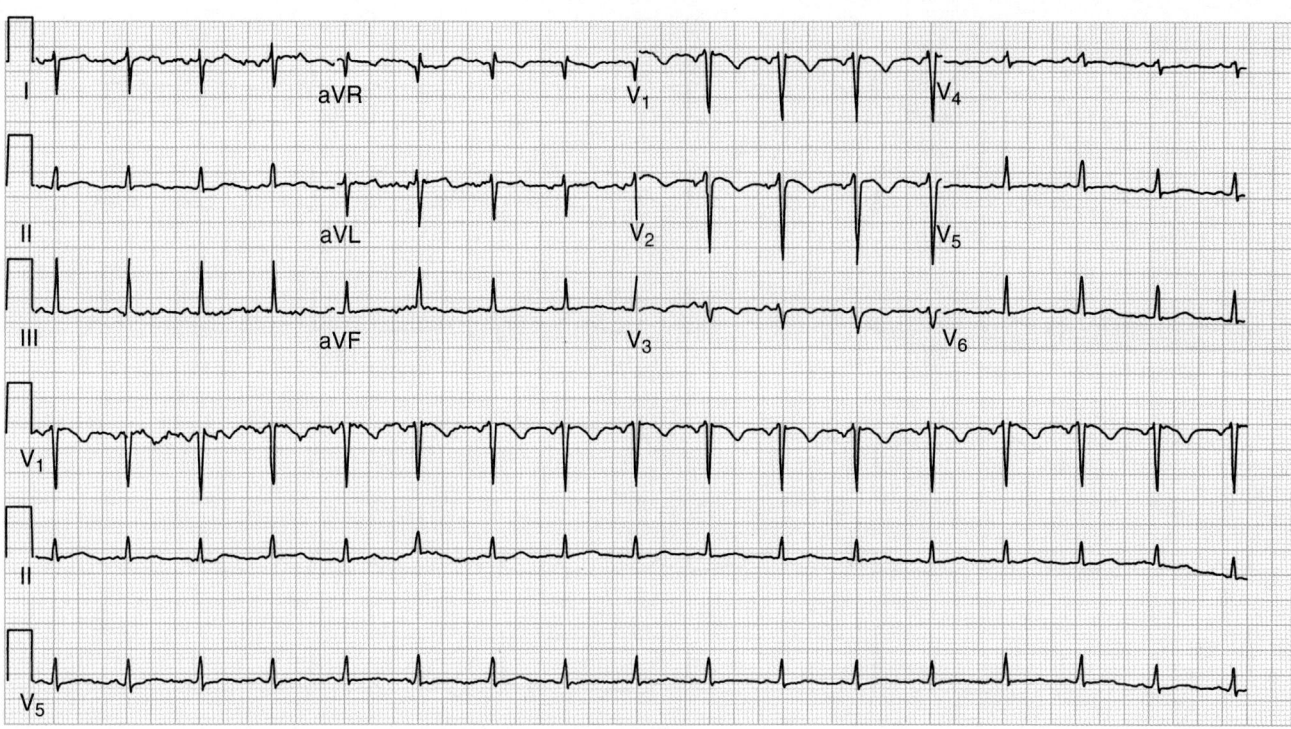

Figure 108-10 *This 35-year-old woman presented with an acute submassive pulmonary embolism 1 month after an ankle fracture. Her ECG shows right axis deviation, T-wave inversions in the anteroseptal leads, and poor R-wave progression all consistent with severe right heart strain.*

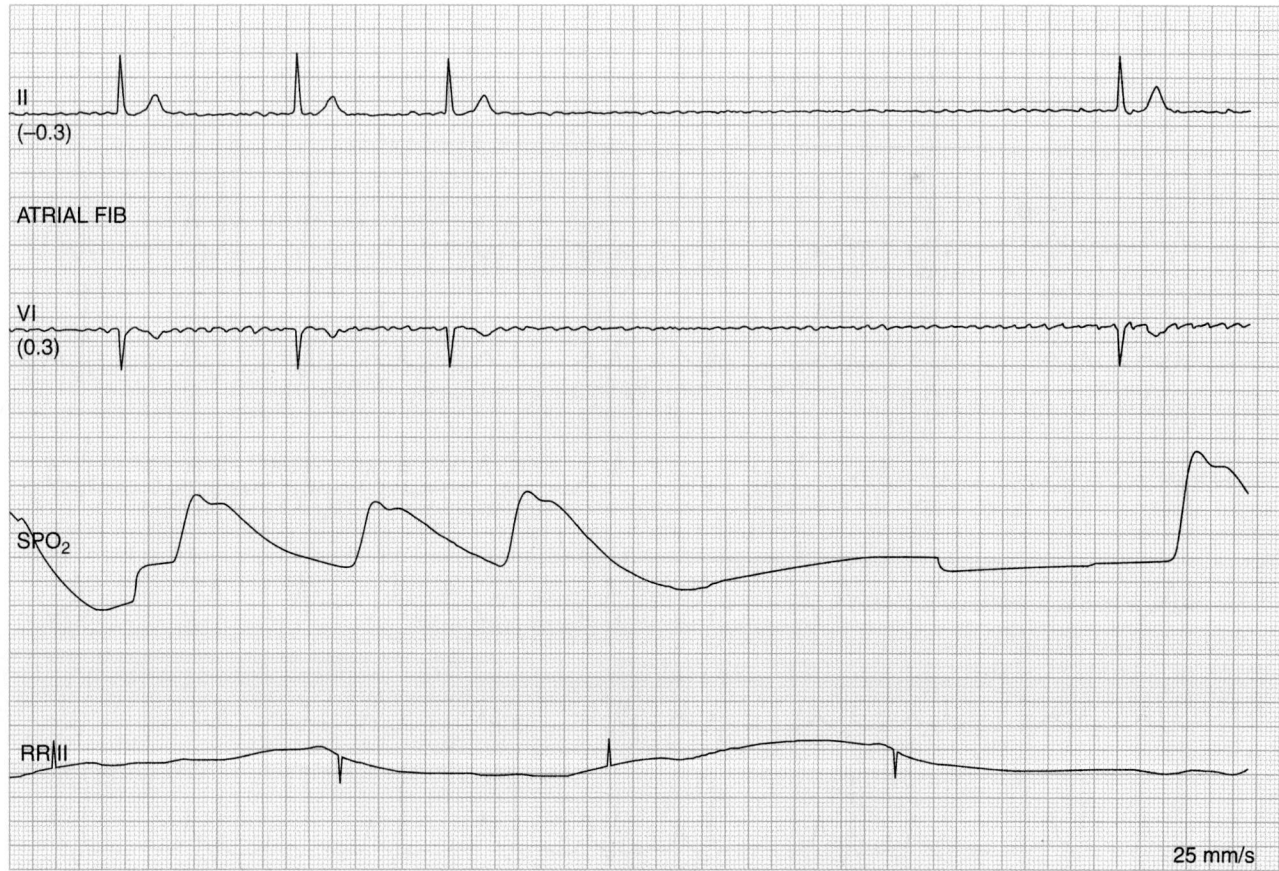

Figure 108-11 *A prolonged pause, as in this gentleman's electrocardiogram with underlying atrial fibrillation, signifies AV block and is generally an indication for permanent pacing.*

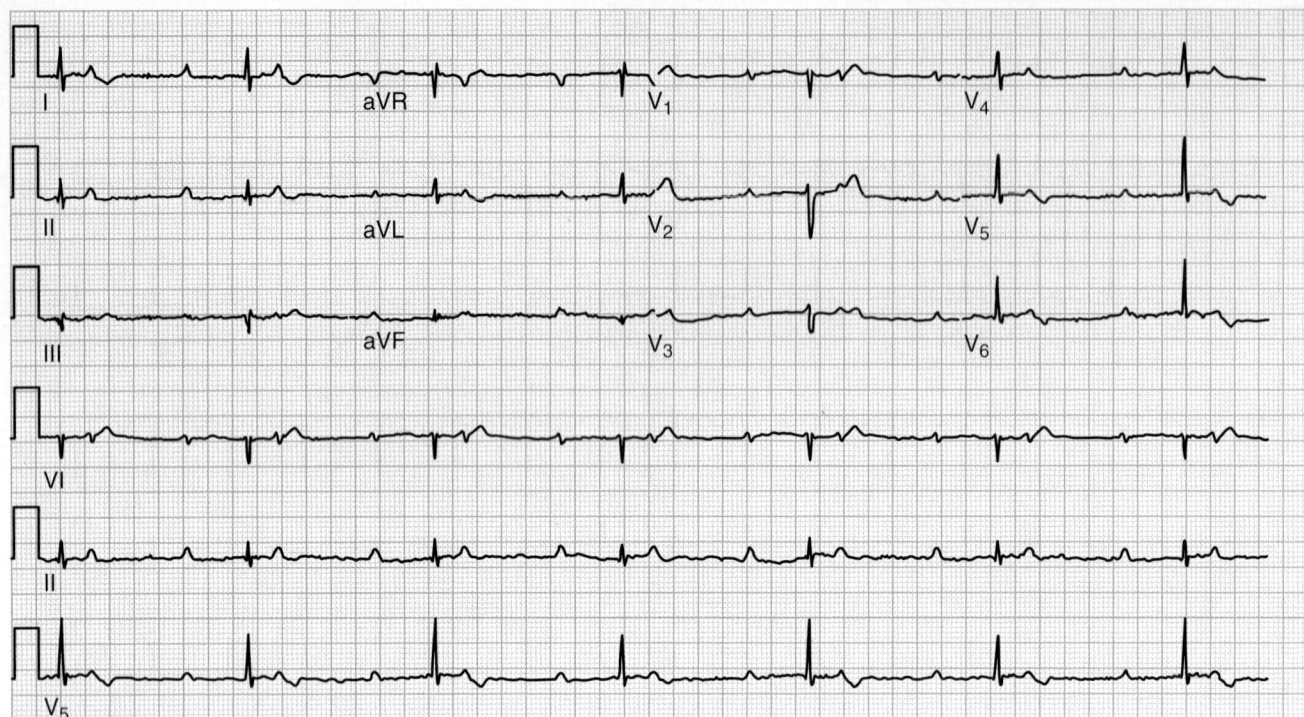

Figure 108-12 *First-degree atrioventricular block is characterized by prolongation of the PR interval beyond 200 milliseconds, as seen in this electrocardiogram from a 39-year-old man on AV nodal–slowing medication.*

secondary to a block at a level above the His bundle and generally does not require permanent pacing unless symptomatic bradycardia is observed (**Figure 108-13**).

Generally, more pathologic, high-grade atrioventricular block is described as Mobitz type II atrioventricular block and is electrocardiographically characterized by conducted impulses that are preceded by a constant PR interval (**Figure 108-14**).

The site of block is generally infrahisian and permanent pacing is often required. For 2:1 conduction patterns, it may be difficult to distinguish between Mobitz type I or type II atrioventricular block.

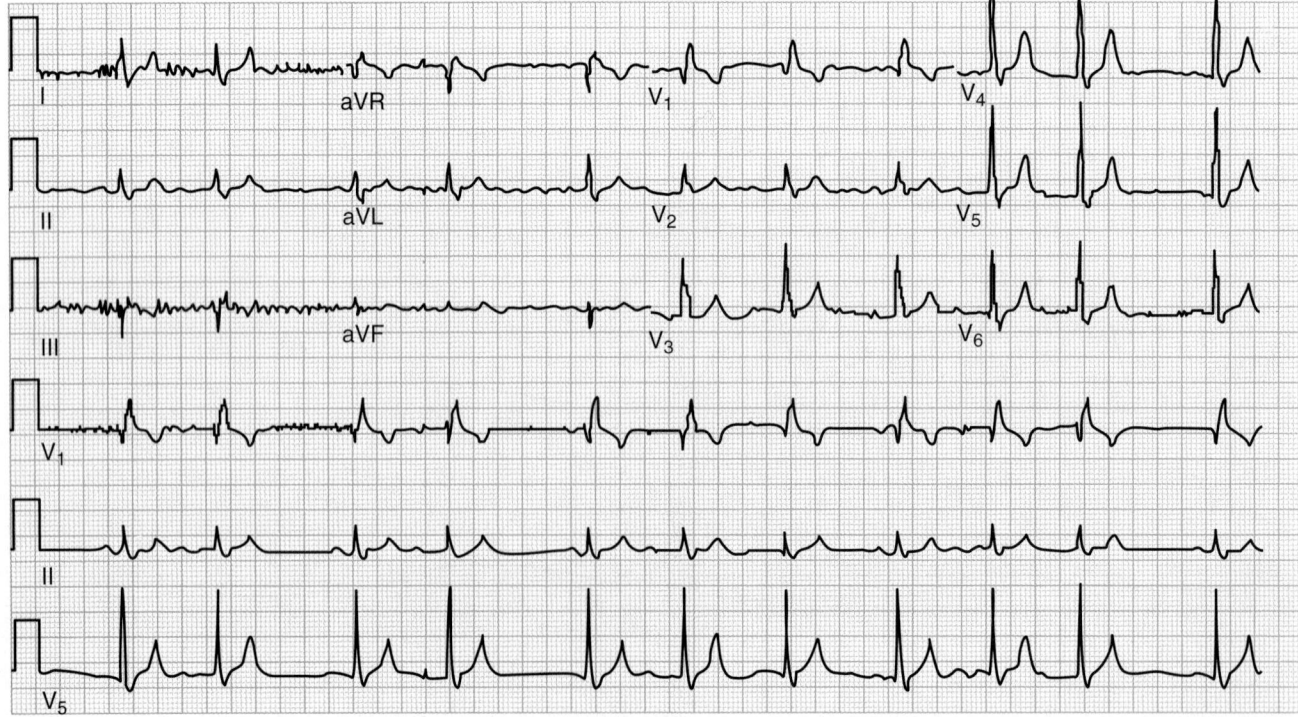

Figure 108-13 *Mobitz type I (or Wenckebach) block is characterized by a prolonging PR interval prior to a nonconducted atrial impulse, is often secondary to a block at a level above the His bundle. The tracing also shows a right bundle branch block, which, together with atrioventricular block, suggests significant underlying conduction system disease.*

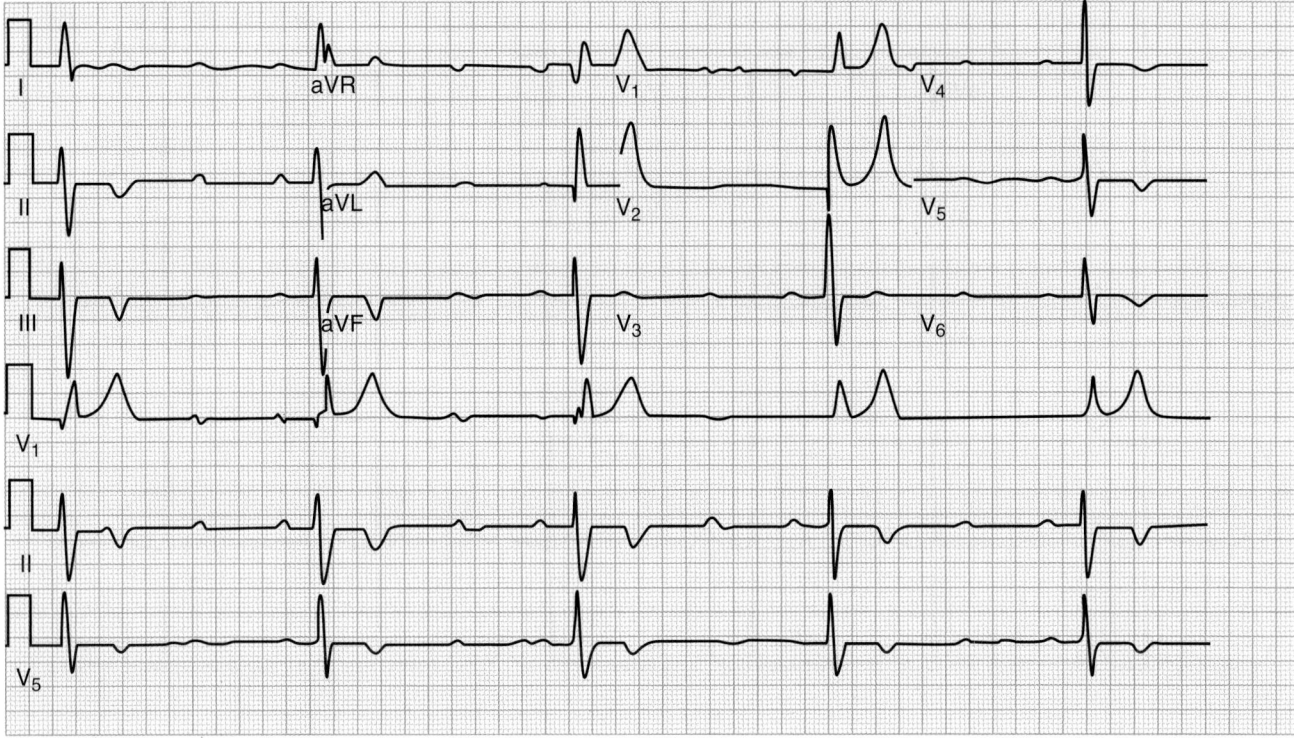

Figure 108-14 *Atrioventricular block with 3:1 conduction. The atrial rate is 90 with a ventricular rate of 30. An infra-Hisian origin of the conduction delay is suggested by the abnormal and prolonged QRS complex.*

Third-degree atrioventricular block is also known as complete heart block and is characterized by complete dissociation of the atrial and ventricular electrical activity (**Figure 108-15**).

Electrocardiographically, atrial activity is more rapid than ventricular activity in complete heart block.

PRACTICE POINT

Syncope, presyncope, sudden death secondary to cardiac arrhythmias

Cardiac syncope can be caused by both bradycardia and tachycardia and has a broad differential

- Bradycardia
  - Sick sinus syndrome
  - Second- and third-degree AV nodal blockade
    - ▶ Independence of atrial and ventricular depolarizations
    - ▶ The atrial rate is greater than the ventricular rate, unlike other forms of AV dissociation in which the ventricular rate is less than the atrial rate
- Tachycardia
  - Supraventricular tachycardia
  - Ventricular tachycardia and ventricular fibrillation
    - ▶ Monomorphic VT
    - ▶ Exercise-induced VT
    - ▶ Brugada syndrome: upwardly coved ST elevations associated with recurrent VT in patients with structurally normal hearts
    - ▶ Right ventricular outflow VT
    - ▶ Polymorphic VT
    - ▶ Torsades de pointes is a specific type of polymorphic VT which occurs as a result of QT prolongation and frequently degenerates into VF

The diagnosis of wide-complex tachycardia (WCT) is of particular concern to the hospital clinician. WCT is defined as having a rate greater than 100 beats/min with a QRS duration greater than 120 milliseconds. The differential diagnosis of WCT is ventricular tachycardia or supraventricular tachycardia (SVT) with aberrancy, and distinguishing between these two entities has important implications for management. Ventricular tachycardia (VT) is defined as three or more QRS complexes of ventricular origin at a rate exceeding 120 beats/min (**Figure 108-16**).

VT is first defined as either nonsustained (lasting <30 seconds) or sustained (lasting >30 seconds). Though frequently regular in rate and appearance, VT may be irregular and may be polymorphic. VT is more common than SVT with aberrancy, and clinical features that further increase the likelihood of VT are older age, known structural heart disease, coronary artery disease, and a history of heart failure. There are numerous algorithms for distinguishing VT from SVT, and the most commonly cited one is the Brugada criteria. The presence of atrioventricular dissociation, fusion beats, and capture complexes favors a diagnosis of VT over SVT with aberrancy.

PRACTICE POINT

Wide-complex tachycardia

The differential diagnosis of wide-complex tachycardia is either VT or SVT with aberrancy. The following criteria support a diagnosis of VT over SVT with aberrancy and make up the Brugada criteria.

- Absence of an RS complex in all precordial leads (V_1-V_6).
- R to S interval greater than 100 milliseconds on any one of the precordial leads.
- Signs of atrioventricular dissociation, such as lack of a clear relationship between P-waves and QRS complexes, fusion beats, and capture beats.
- Morphology criteria for VT.

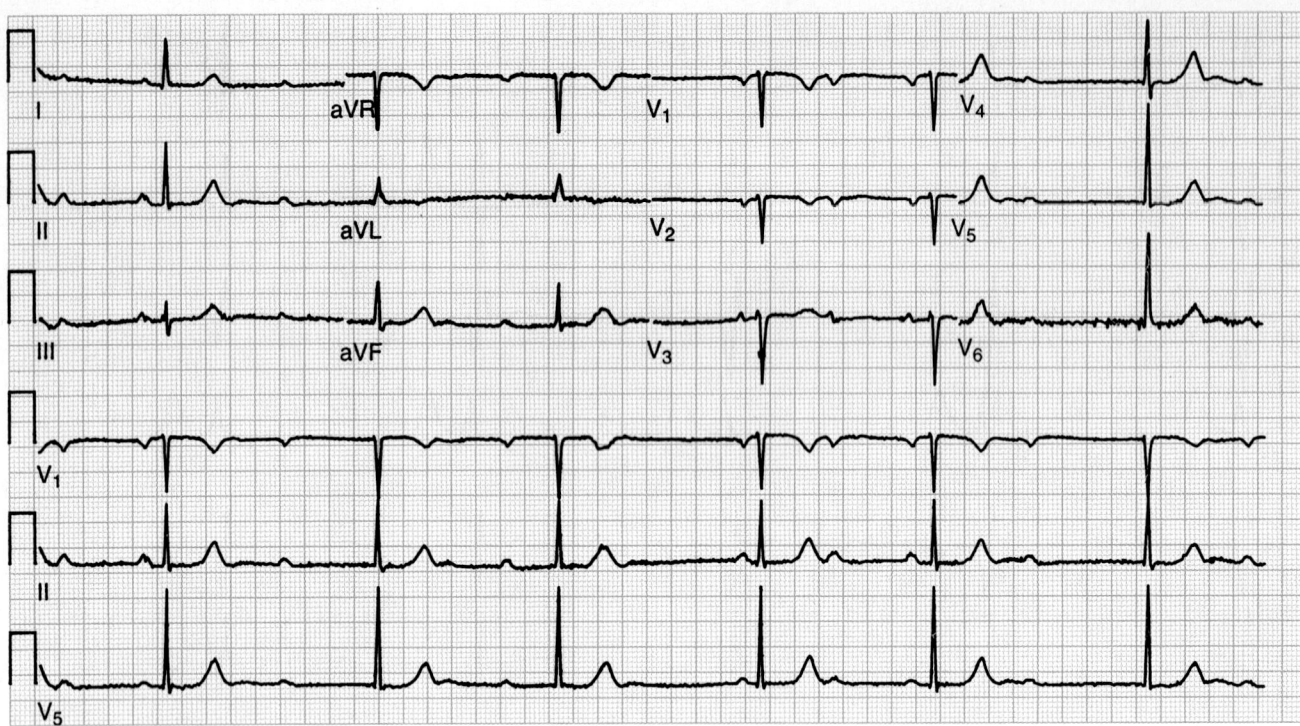

Figure 108-15 *Complete, or third-degree heart block, is characterized by atrioventricular dissociation, as seen in this electrocardiogram from a 78-year-old woman who presented with syncope. The ventricular rate is maintained by a junctional escape rhythm. Sinus arrhythmia is also seen.*

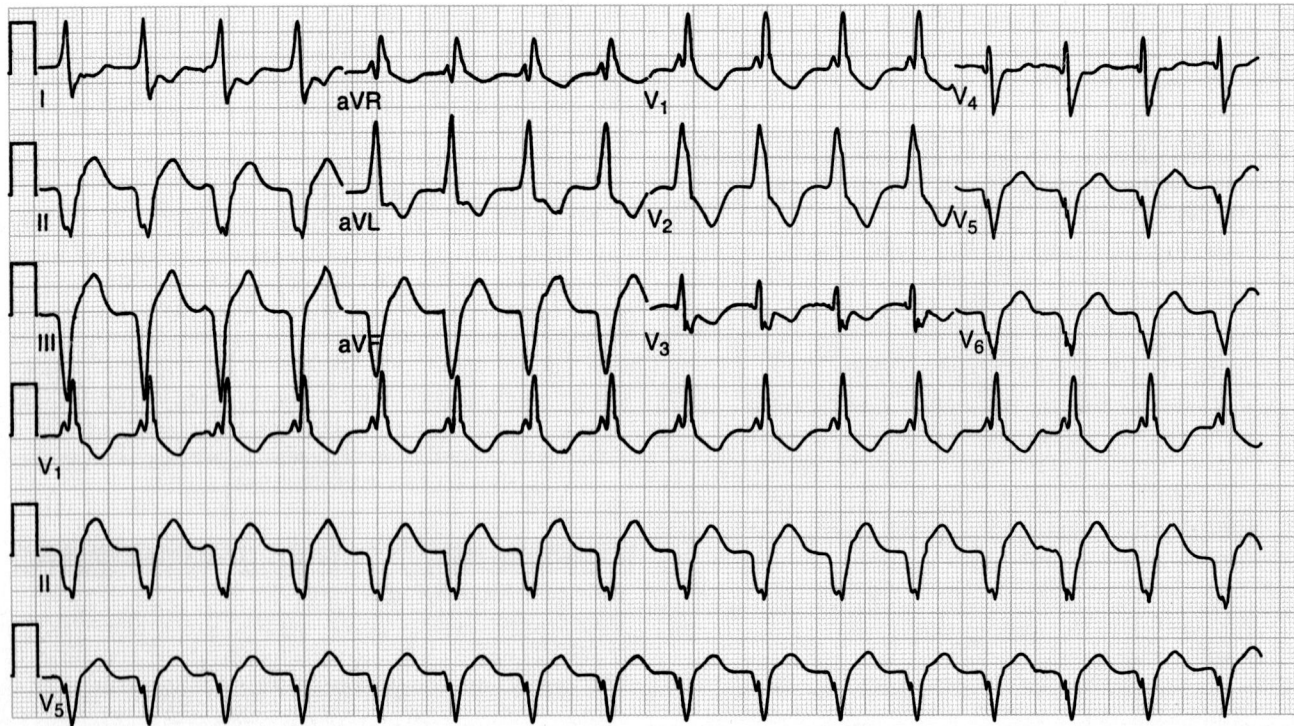

Figure 108-16 *Ventricular tachycardia is defined as three or more QRS complexes of ventricular origin at a rate exceeding 100 beats/min. This electrocardiogram is from a 61-year-old gentleman with extensive ischemic heart disease status post surgical and percutaneous revascularization. His ischemic substrate, as well as atrioventricular dissociation (with P-waves inscribed within the QRS complex), is suggestive of scar-related ventricular tachycardia. He continued to have ventricular tachycardia despite intravenous amiodarone and required ablation of his ventricular tachycardia.*

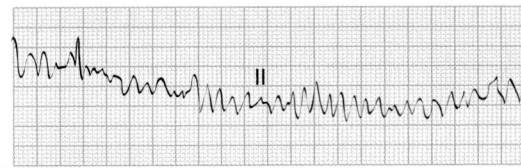

Figure 108-17 *Ventricular fibrillation, a chaotic nonperfusing ventricular rhythm that reflects no organized electrical activity, is uniformly fatal without advanced cardiac life support.*

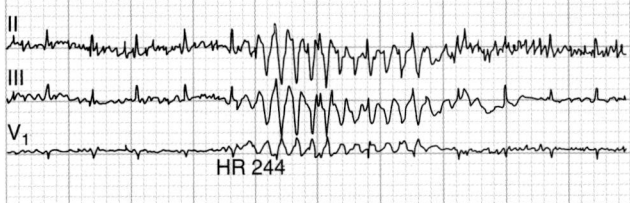

Figure 108-18 *Motion artifact should be distinguished from tachyarrhythmias. In this tracing, QRS deflections are visible at regular intervals throughout the region of artifact, making a ventricular arrhythmia much less likely.*

Ventricular fibrillation, a chaotic ventricular rhythm that reflects no organized electrical activity, is uniformly fatal without advanced cardiac life support (**Figure 108-17**).

The seasoned clinician should also be able to recognize motion artifacts simulating serious arrhythmias (**Figure 108-18**).

■ PALPITATIONS

Palpitations are defined as a subjective feeling of one's own heartbeat and can occur due to arrhythmias, ectopic ventricular or atrial contractions, hyperdynamic circulation, or sympathetic overdrive due to medical or psychiatric disease. Supraventricular tachyarrhythmias are a frequent etiology of palpitations. These tachycardias usually have the same QRS morphology as the patient's sinus rhythm and therefore are narrow-complex in the majority of patients. Such tachyarrhythmias, which may be regular or irregular in appearance, commonly occur in the hospital setting. When regular, the following need to be considered: sinus tachycardia, atrial flutter with consistent atrioventricular conduction, atrioventricular node reentrant tachycardia (AVNRT), atrioventricular reentrant tachycardia (AVRT), atrial tachycardia, and junctional tachycardia. Multifocal tachycardia, atrial flutter with variable conduction, sinus tachycardia with frequent premature atrial contractions, and atrial fibrillation account for irregular narrow-complex tachyarrhythmias.

Sinus tachycardia manifests as a sinus rhythm with a rate above 100 beats/min and generally reflects a highly active metabolic state, medication effect, or an underlying process such as fever, hypovolemia, or anemia (**Figure 108-19**).

Typical atrial flutter, characteristically the result of a macroreentrant circuit in the right atrium, is easily recognizable by the appearance of negatively directed "sawtooth" waveforms in the inferior leads accompanied by an atrial rate that varies between 280 and 340 beats/min (**Figure 108-20**).

The mechanism of AVNRT involves a reentrant circuit within the AV node that generates a narrow QRS complex tachycardia in the range of 150 to 250 beats/min, often with P-waves inscribed at the terminal portion of the QRS complex (reflecting retrograde atrial depolarization) (**Figure 108-21**).

Ventricular pre-excitation, any condition in which anterograde ventricular or retrograde atrial activation occurs partially or totally via an anomalous pathway, may lead to AVRT. Wolff-Parkinson-White (WPW) syndrome is a form of ventricular pre-excitation and electrocardiographically produces a short PR interval and

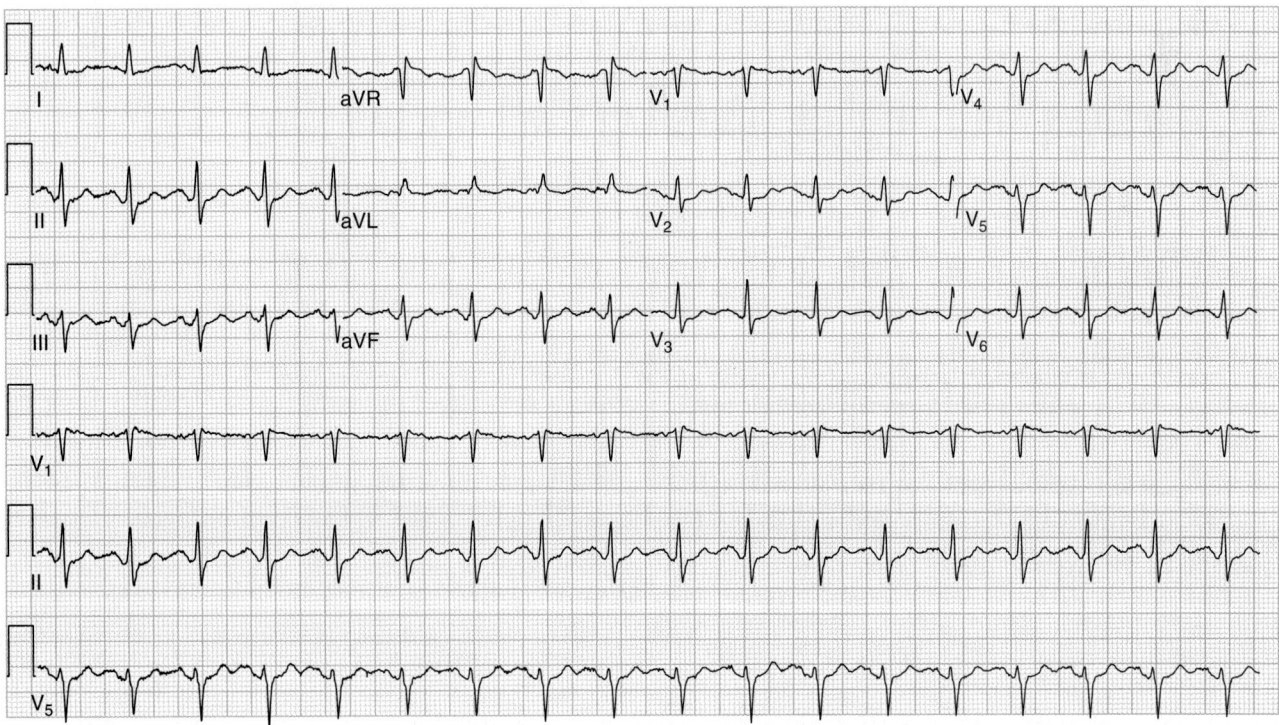

Figure 108-19 *Sinus tachycardia manifests as a sinus rhythm with a rate above 100 beats/min and generally reflects an underlying process (eg, fever, hypovolemia, or anemia), metabolic state, or medication effect. This electrocardiogram is from a 54-year-old woman affected by uncontrolled pain.*

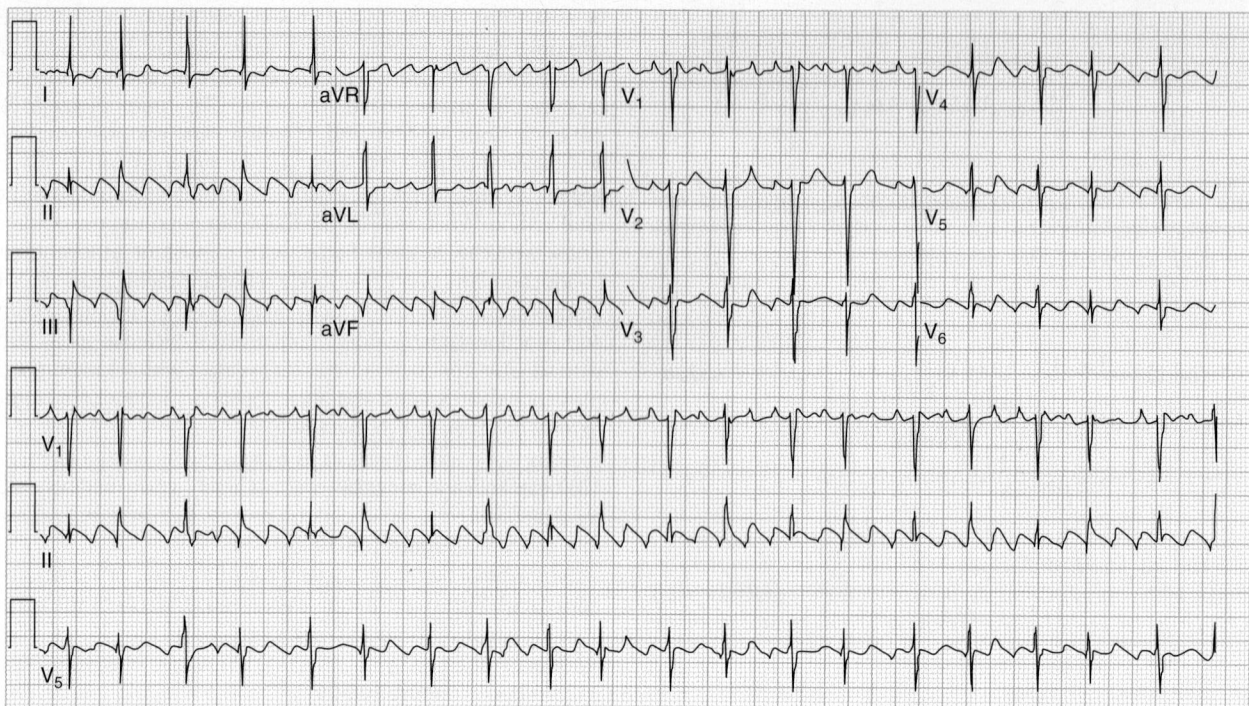

Figure 108-20 *Atrial flutter, characteristically the result of a macroreentrant circuit in the right atrium, is easily recognizable by the appearance of "sawtooth" waveforms accompanied by an atrial rate between 280 and 340 beats/min.*

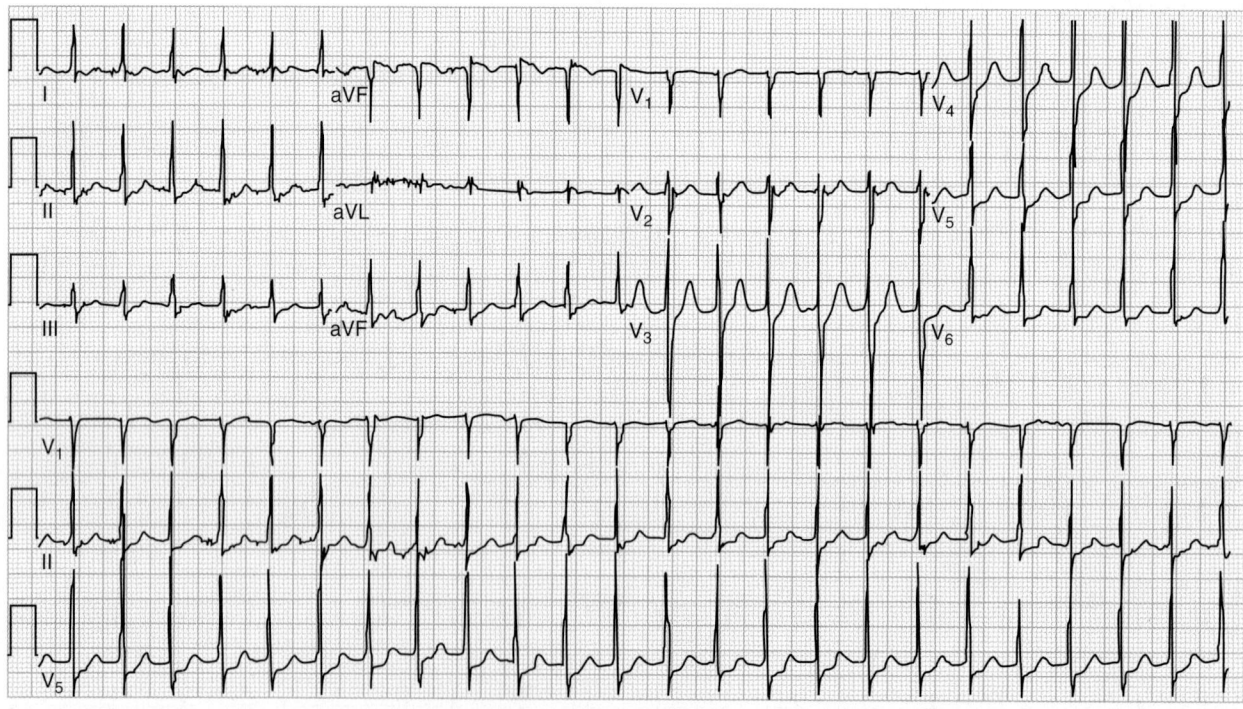

Figure 108-21 *The mechanism of AVNRT involves a reentrant circuit within the AV node that generates a narrow QRS-complex tachycardia in the range of 150 to 250 beats/min, often with P-waves inscribed at the terminal portion of the QRS complex and reflecting retrograde atrial depolarization, as in this electrocardiogram from a 66-year-old gentleman who presented with palpitations. Regional ST-segment depressions are also seen, suggestive of rate-related subendocardial injury. During electrophysiologic testing, dual AV node physiology was confirmed and radiofrequency ablation of the slow pathway was successfully performed.*

QRS prolongation with a delta wave, an initial slurring of the QRS complex signifying ventricular activation by the accessory pathway (**Figure 108-22**).

AVRT relies on a reentrant circuit composed of an accessory pathway and the AV node and can present with either orthodromic or antidromic conduction. In orthodromic AVRT, the ventricles are depolarized normally through the His-Purkinje system with the accessory pathway conducting the depolarization wave back into the atria. This will result in a narrow complex rhythm unless the patient has a baseline or rate-related bundle branch block. Antidromic AVRT occurs when the ventricles are depolarized by conduction through the accessory pathway and will always result in a wide QRS complex.

Characteristically, both AVNRT and AVRT may be terminated with adenosine, which suppresses AV-node conduction. Atrial

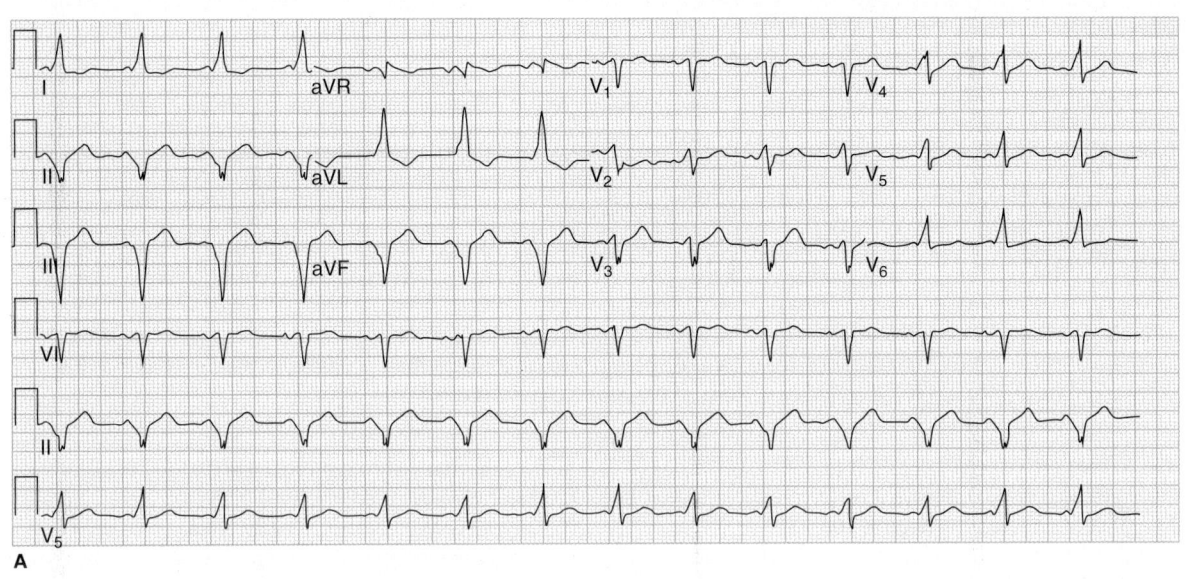

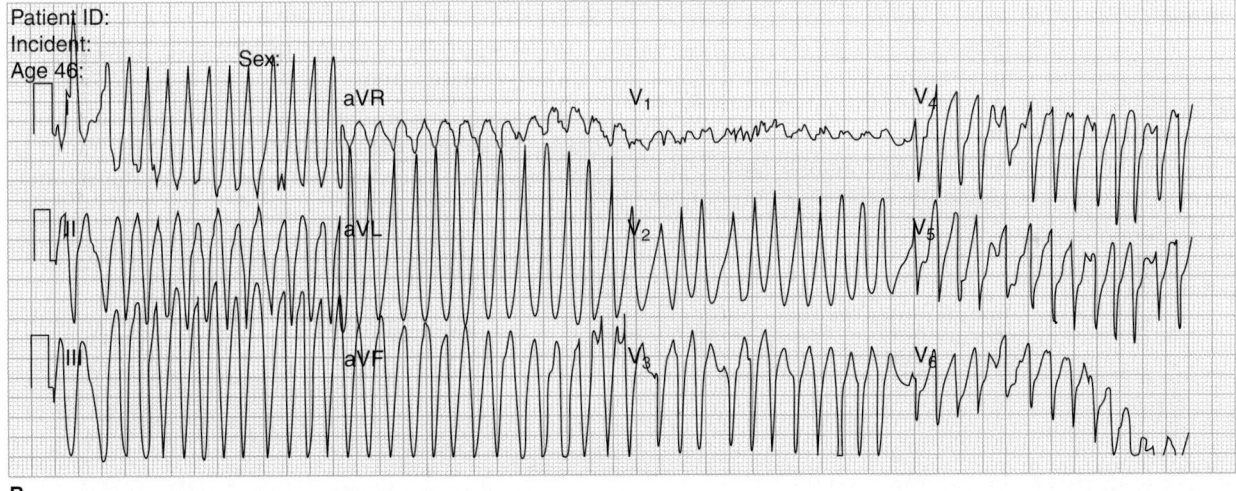

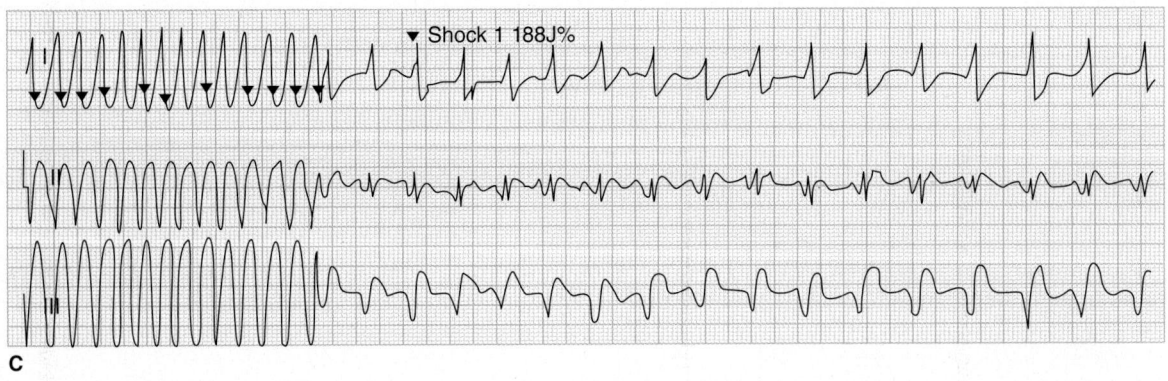

Figure 108-22 *Wolff-Parkinson-White (WPW) syndrome is a form of ventricular pre-excitation and electrocardiographically produces a short PR interval and QRS prolongation with a delta wave, an initial slurring of the QRS complex signifying ventricular activation by the accessory pathway, as seen in (A) from an initially asymptomatic 48-year-old woman. After a year of close follow-up, she developed near syncope with hemodynamic instability, presenting with the irregularly irregular wide complex tachycardia seen in (B) which represented atrial fibrillation with rapid conduction through the accessory pathway. She underwent direct current cardioversion (C), followed by successful ablation of a posteroseptal accessory pathway.*

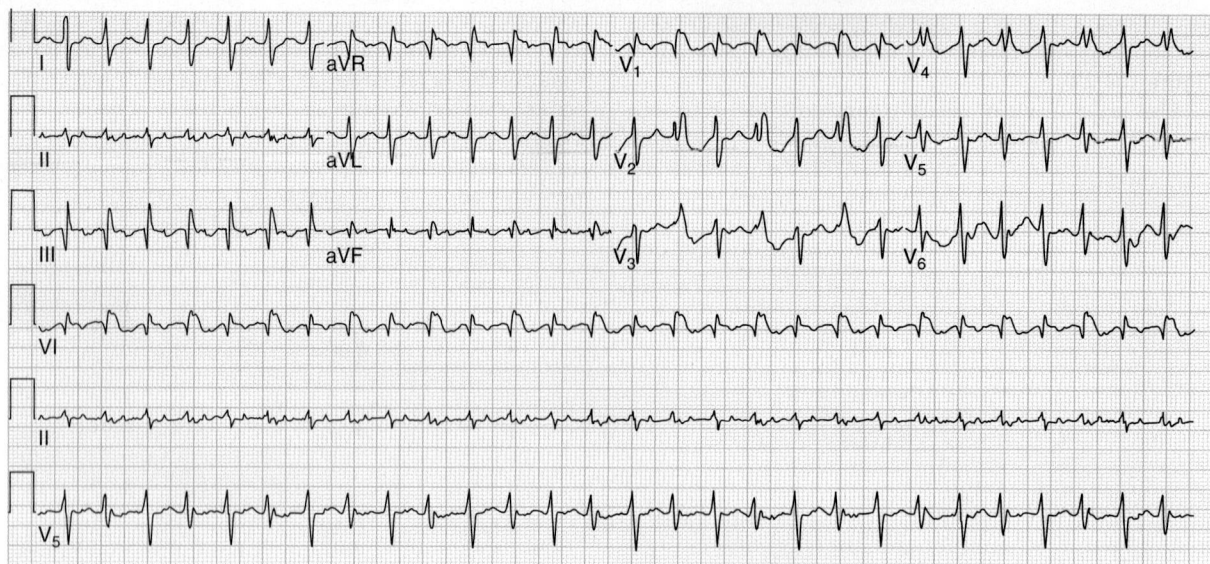

Figure 108-23 *Atrial tachycardia is characterized by a P-wave axis or morphology that is distinct from that of sinus rhythm, as in this electrocardiogram from a 64-year-old woman with palpitations. The atrial rate is generally 100 to 250 beats/min, characteristically slower than that of atrial flutter. Right axis deviation and an incomplete right bundle branch block are also seen in this tracing.*

tachycardia, in contrast, generally does not terminate with adenosine and is characterized by a P-wave axis or morphology that is distinct from that of sinus rhythm (**Figure 108-23**).

Atrial tachycardia with atrioventricular block is typically seen with digoxin toxicity. Multifocal atrial tachycardia, an irregular arrhythmia, is characterized by an atrial rate greater than 100 beats/min and P-waves with three or more different morphologies. It is frequently associated with concurrent pulmonary disease. A discussion of atrial fibrillation, the most common sustained tachyarrhythmia, is found elsewhere (**Figure 108-24**).

Often associated with physiologic stress, drugs, or chronic lung disease, atrial fibrillation may produce an irregularly narrow complex

tachycardia that likely represents increased automaticity and multiple reentrant wavelets predominantly in the left atrium around the pulmonary veins. Multifocal atrial tachycardia can be distinguished from atrial fibrillation by an isoelectric baseline between the P-waves.

■ ELECTROCARDIOGRAPHIC ASSOCIATIONS WITH SUDDEN CARDIAC DEATH AND GENETIC ARRHYTHMOLOGY

The seasoned clinician should be able to identify the electrocardiographic pattern associated with conditions associated with a high prevalence of sudden death such as the Brugada and long

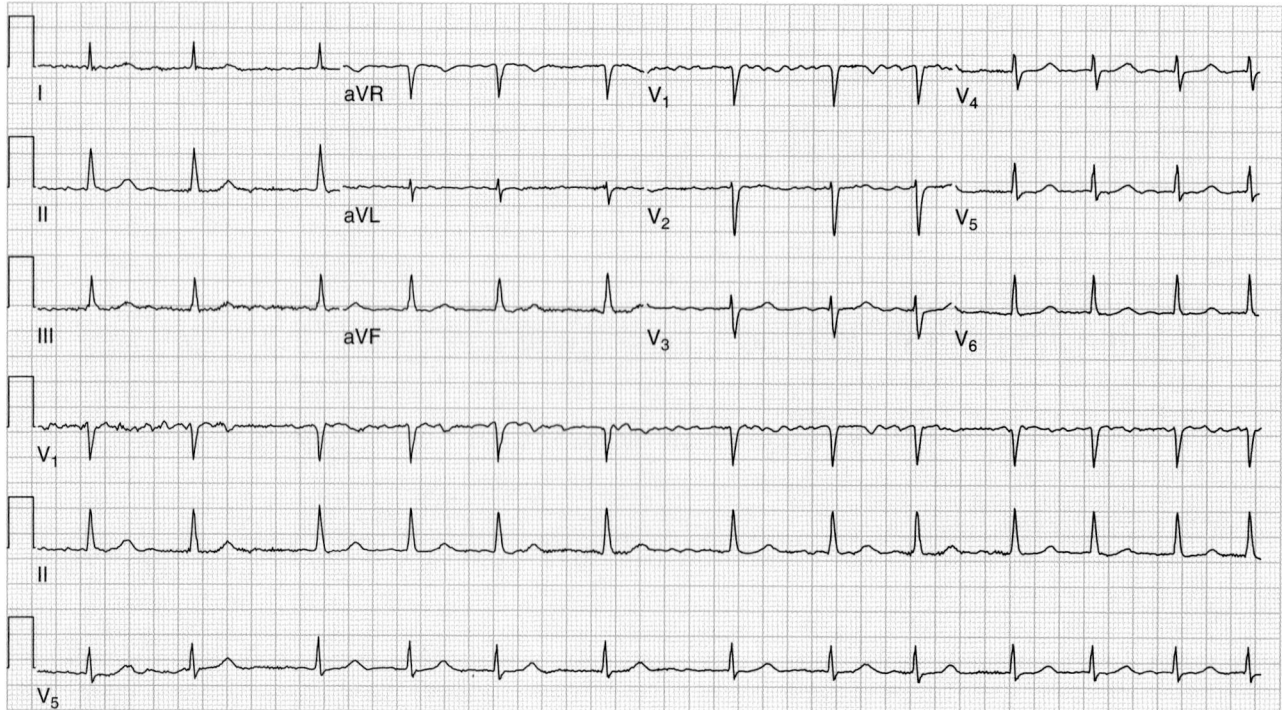

Figure 108-24 *Often associated with physiologic stress, sympathomimetic drugs, or chronic lung disease, atrial fibrillation may produce an irregularly narrow complex tachycardia. This electrocardiogram is from an 88-year-old gentleman with obesity-hypoventilation syndrome and sleep apnea.*

QT syndromes. Brugada syndrome is an inherited condition associated with sudden cardiac death and mutations linked to the *SCN5A* gene, encoding a cardiac sodium channel. Electrocardiographically, it is associated with RBBB with ST-segment elevation in leads V_1-V_3 (**Figure 108-25**).

Prolongation of the QT interval may be either congenital or acquired. Congenital prolonged QT syndrome is the result of genetic mutations, most commonly in genes expressing ion channels. Acquired QT prolongation occurs as a result of electrolyte derangements or ingestion of QT-prolonging medications such as macrolides, fluoroquinolones, and antipsychotics (**Figure 108-26**).

The QT interval, measured from the beginning of the QRS complex to the end of the T-wave in the lead with the longest interval, decreases as heart rate increases. The Bazett formula offers a mathematical means for relating the QT interval to heart rate as follows:

$$QT_{Corrected} = QT/(RR)^{1/2}$$

A prolonged QT interval may predispose to torsades de pointes, a type of polymorphic VT characterized by a typical "twisting of the points."

PRACTICE POINT

Medical illness
Hyperkalemia
- Sensitivity of the ECG for detecting hyperkalemia often depends on the chronicity of the derangement. Patients with chronic hyperkalemia may have relatively minor ECG changes such as peaked T-waves despite severe hyperkalemia whereas other patients may be at risk of unstable cardiac rhythms at lower serum potassium levels.
- Peaked T-waves usually at K^+ levels > 5.5 mEq/L.
- Atrial abnormalities such as P-wave flattening usually at K^+ levels > 6.5 mEq/L.
- QRS widening usually at K^+ levels > 7 mEq/L with higher levels causing wider complexes.
- Cardiac arrest due to ventricular fibrillation, asystole, or PEA arrest at K^+ levels > 9 mEq/L.
- QT intervals are normal or short unless there is concomitant hypocalcemia in which the QT can be prolonged.

Hypokalemia
- Marked QT prolongation with or without a prominent U-wave.
- Reduced amplitude of T-waves and ventricular arrhythmias in severe hypokalemia.

Hypothermia
- Osborn waves, deflections at the junction of the QRS and the ST-segments can be seen in leads V_2-V_6.
- Prolonged PR, QRS, and QT intervals.
- Sinus bradycardia, slow atrial fibrillation, and variable heart block.
- Shivering artifact can obscure ECG findings, especially in the limb leads.

Hypothyroidism
The ECG findings of hypothyroidism are varied and can occur due to reduced cardiac adrenergic activity, myocardial edema, and development of pericardial effusions.
- Bradycardia.
- Reduced amplitude of all ECG waveforms.

- Increase in PR interval (due to sympathetic withdrawal and slower AV nodal transmission).
- Prolonged QT with accompanying T-wave inversions.

Stroke
- ST-segment depression or elevation, T-wave inversions. U-waves, and/or prolongation of the QT interval in up to 75% of patients with subarachnoid hemorrhage and >90% of unselected patients with either ischemic stroke or intracerebral hemorrhage.
- Varied other ECG changes including heart block and SVT can be seen with insular cortex infarcts.

Drug therapy
- Digitalis Intoxication: atrial tachycardia with variable AV block, nonparoxysmal junctional tachycardias, second and third degree AV block, sinoatrial block, ventricular arrhythmias (including bidirectional VT), and near regularization of the ventricular rate in the presence of atrial fibrillation.
- Class IA agents (quinidine, procainamide, disopyramide): slight widening of the QRS at normal doses. In the setting of hypokalemia and bradycardia, quinidine can cause QT prolongation.
- Class IB agents (lidocaine, mexiletine, tocainide): no effect on ECG at therapeutic doses.
- Class IC agents (flecainide, propafenone): widening of the QRS and lengthening of the QTc interval due to QRS prolongation at normal doses.
- Class III agents (sotalol, ibutilide, and dofetilide): QT prolongation.
- SSRI's: QT prolongation, often in a dose-dependent manner.
- Lithium: prolonged QT and T-wave abnormalities.
- Tricyclic Antidepressants: sinus tachycardia, prolonged QRS complex, first degree AV block, prolonged QT interval, prominent R-wave in aVR.
  - A QRS duration <100 milliseconds favorable prognosis.
  - A QRS duration 100 to 160 milliseconds moderate risk.
  - A QRS duration >160 milliseconds high risk of seizures and ventricular arrhythmias.
- Carbamazepine: sinus tachycardia in massive overdose; bradyarrhythmias or AV conduction delay in elderly women with therapeutic or slightly elevated levels and abnormal renal function.

Chronic obstructive pulmonary disease pattern
- Pseudoinfarct pattern: right atrial abnormality, vertical P and QRS axes, dominant S-waves across precordium, low voltage of R-wave in V_6.
- Features that specifically suggest the presence of chronic obstructive pulmonary disease pattern disease if all present (>90% specificity and >50% sensitivity):
  1. P-waves with a rightward axis in the range of +70° to +90° (ie, negative P-wave in aVL). This reflects that atrial activation is directed more inferiorly than usual while the ventricular activation is more superiorly and posteriorly than normal due to the vertical suspension of the heart in the midline.
  2. The QRS complexes with low voltage in limb leads and precordial leads, reflecting increased lung volumes.
  3. The QRS axis is superior with negative complexes (QS or rS) in inferior leads.
  4. The precordial leads show predominant S-waves through V_6.
  5. The R-wave in V_6 is <5 mm in amplitude.
- P-pulmonale (tall peaked P-waves) from pulmonary hypertension is not required for the diagnosis.

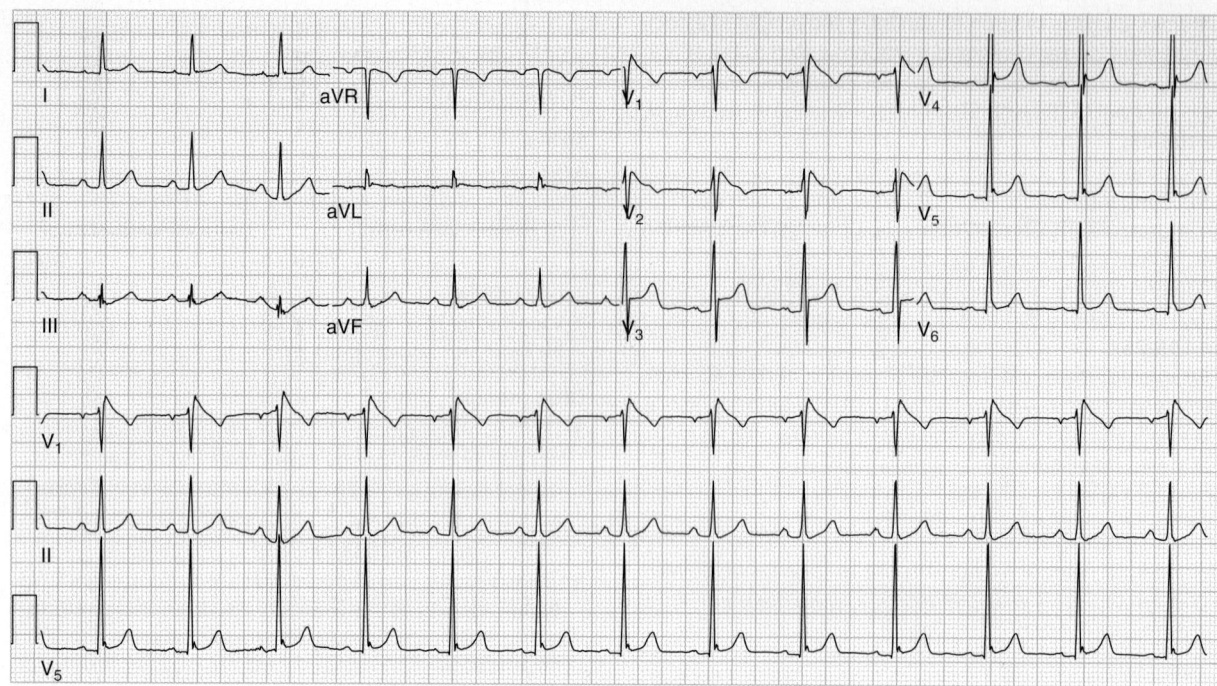

Figure 108-25 *Brugada syndrome is a condition associated with sudden cardiac death and mutations linked to the SCN5A gene, encoding a cardiac sodium channel. This electrocardiogram is from a 54-year-old gentleman with a syncopal episode. Coronary angiography revealed normal coronaries. The ST-segment elevations with biphasic T-wave inversions in V_1-V_3, along with his syncopal episode, implicated Brugada syndrome. He received a single-chamber implantable cardioverter-defibrillator (ICD) for secondary prevention.*

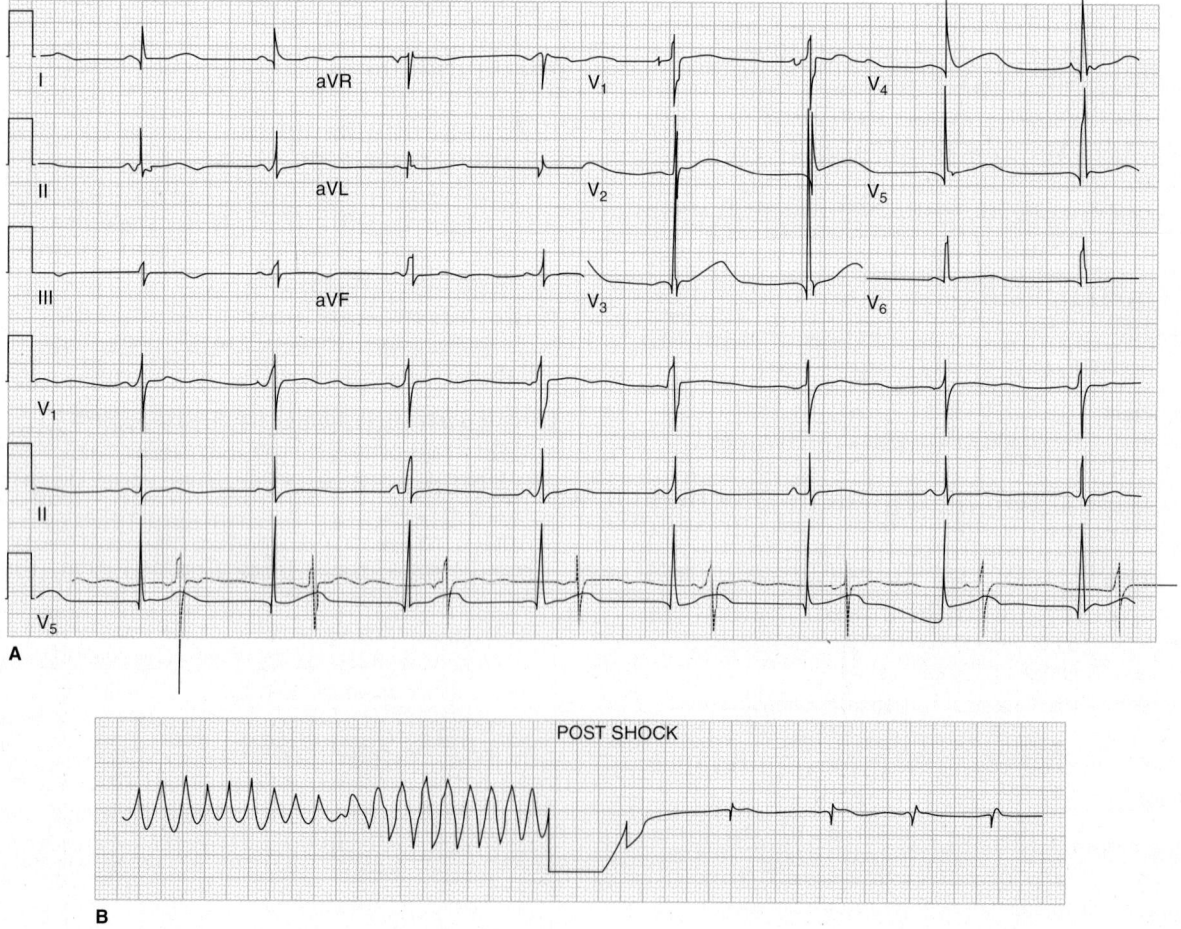

Figure 108-26 *Prolongation of the QT interval may be congenital or acquired due to electrolyte abnormalities or ingestion of QT prolonging medications. This electrocardiogram is from a gentleman with recent dose escalation of methadone. Prolongation of the QT interval is seen in (A). He developed torsades de pointes (B) requiring defibrillation.*

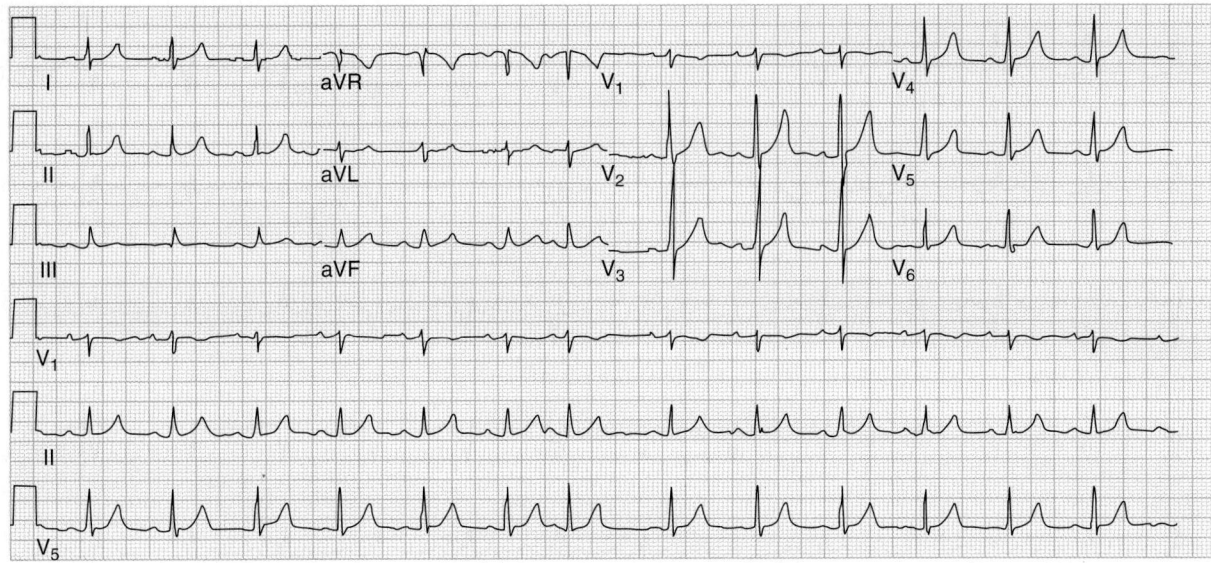

Figure 108-27 *Hyperkalemia may initially produce narrowing and peaking of the T-waves, followed by widening of the QRS complex and decrement in P-wave amplitude. This electrocardiogram is from a 68-year-old gentleman with end-stage renal disease on hemodialysis; his serum potassium was 6.8 mg/dL.*

ELECTROCARDIOGRAPHIC MANIFESTATIONS OF NONCARDIAC ILLNESS AND METABOLIC DISTURBANCES

Electrolyte abnormalities, acid-base disturbances, and systemic hypothermia may produce characteristic electrocardiographic changes. Changes in extracellular potassium balance, in particular, are associated with a distinctive sequence of electrocardiographic changes. Hyperkalemia may initially produce narrowing and peaking of the T-waves, followed by widening of the QRS complex and decrement in P-wave amplitude (**Figure 108-27**).

With increasing severity of hyperkalemia, there may be loss of P-waves, generating a sino-ventricular junctional escape rhythm. Hypokalemia, associated with myocardial hyperpolarization, leads to ST-segment depressions, T-wave flattening, increased U-wave prominence, and QT prolongation predisposing to torsades de pointes (**Figure 108-28**).

Changes in extracellular calcium content generally affect the action potential duration, with hypercalcemia and hypokalemia producing shortening and prolongation of the QT interval, respectively (**Figure 108-29**).

A late potential, the Osborn wave or convex elevation at the junction (J point of the ST-segment), may be associated with severe hypercalcemia and disappear with appropriate treatment. The Osborn wave is also seen in about one-third of hypothermic patients (**Figure 108-30**).

Hypothyroidism, related to decreased adrenergic activity, may produce bradycardia, prolongation of the PR interval, and reduced amplitude of all electrocardiographic waveforms (**Figure 108-31**).

This metabolic disturbance may also be associated with pericardial effusion, which, in addition to producing reduction of

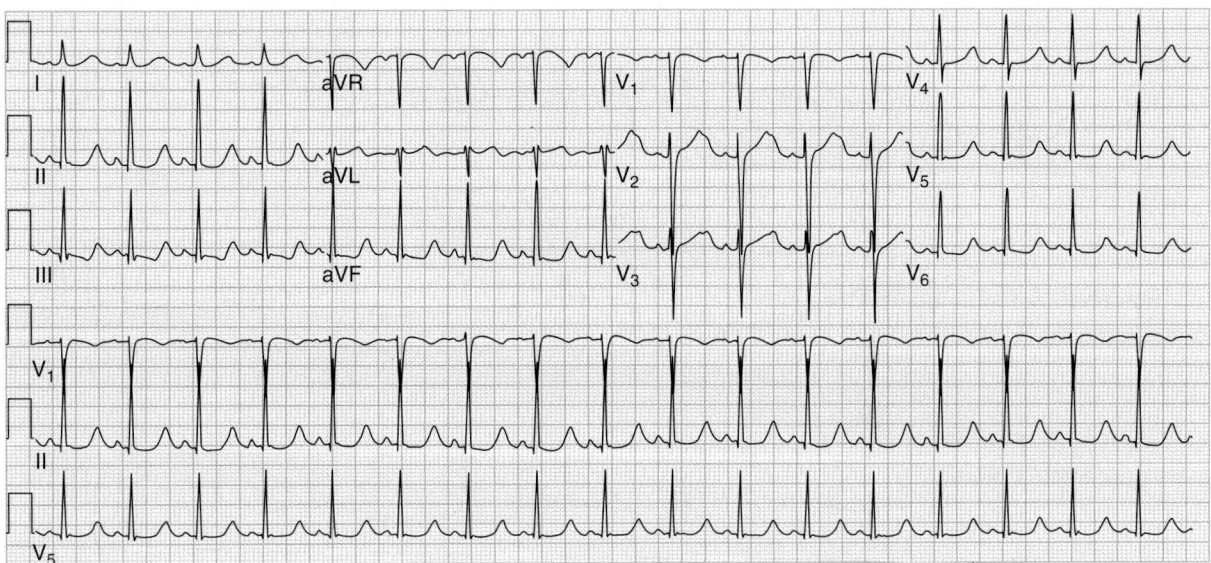

Figure 108-28 *Hypokalemia leads to ST-segment depressions, T-wave flattening, increased U-wave prominence, and QT prolongation. This electrocardiogram is from a 20-year-old woman with severe hypokalemia secondary to hyperemesis gravidarum. Resolution of QT prolongation was seen with electrolyte repletion.*

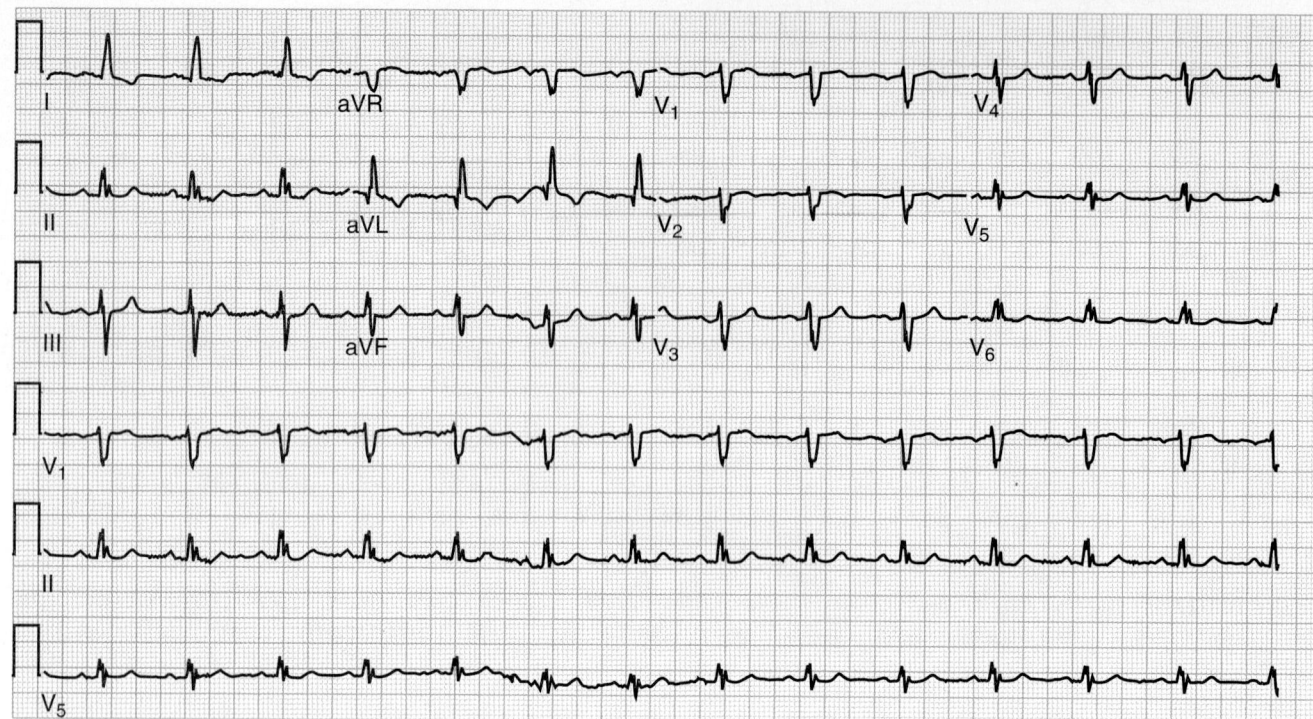

Figure 108-29 *Changes in extracellular calcium content generally affect the action potential duration, with hypercalcemia producing shortening of the QT interval, as in this electrocardiogram from a 58-year-old woman with excessive exogenous calcium intake.*

electrocardiographic waveforms, may produce electrical alternans (**Figure 108-32**).

Repolarization abnormalities in arrhythmias may occur in up to 70% of stroke patients. Prominent T-wave inversions, characteristically diffuse and often associated with changes in the ST-segment and QT prolongation, are often an electrocardiographic feature of a cerebrovascular accident, especially larger infarcts and hemorrhages.

Injuries to the insula in particular may be associated with characteristic cardiac findings. The right insula, as may be affected following a right middle cerebral artery infarct, may lead to tachyarrhythmias and hypertension. Bradycardia and vasodepression often occur in the setting of left insular injury. Among patients with cerebrovascular accidents, those presenting with electrocardiographic changes have a higher 6-month mortality.

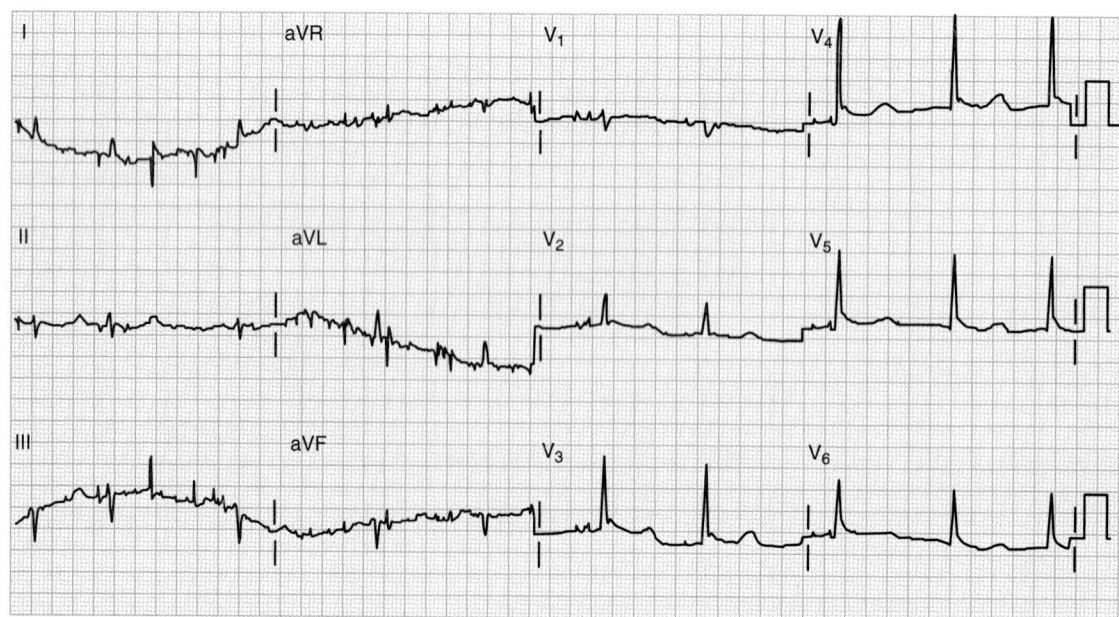

Figure 108-30 *Systemic hypothermia may generate a distinctive Osborn wave, a convex elevation at the junction (J point) of the ST-segment. This electrocardiogram is from a 90-year-old gentleman who was found unresponsive. Prominent artifact from his shivering is seen in the limb leads.*

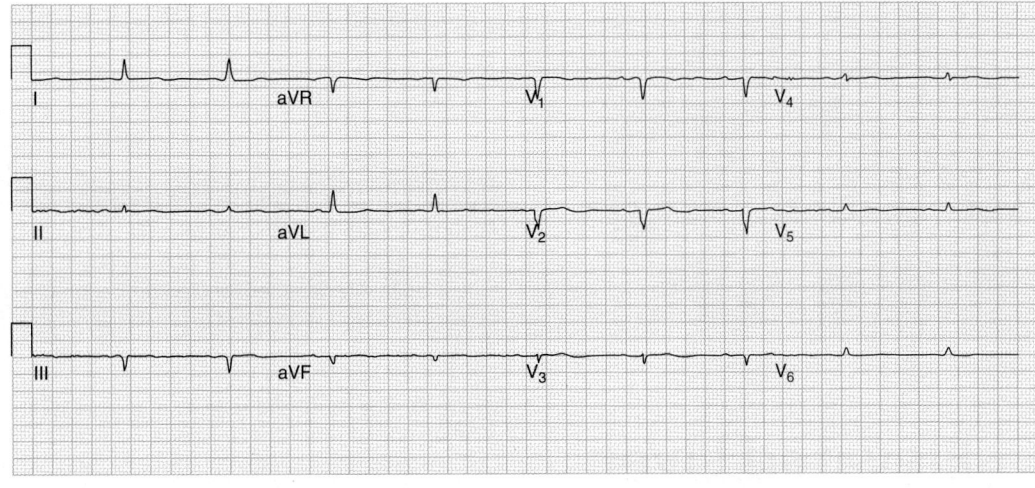

Figure 108-31 *Hypothyroidism, related to decreased adrenergic activity, may produce bradycardia, prolongation of the PR interval, and reduced amplitude of all electrocardiographic waveforms, as in this tracing from a woman with myxedema coma.*

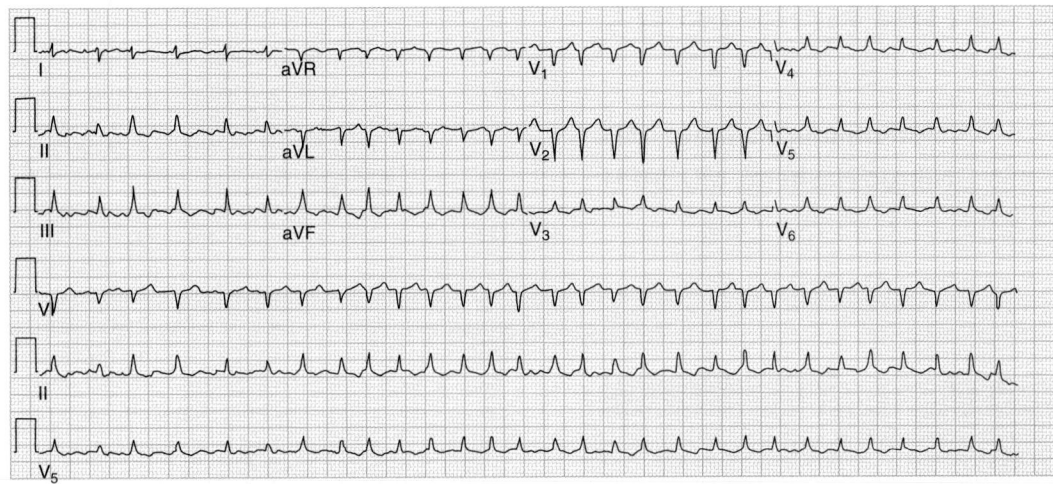

Figure 108-32 *Pericardial effusion may produce reduction in electrocardiographic waveforms, along with electrical alternans, as in this tracing from a 65-year-old woman with known lung cancer who presented with dyspnea and hemodynamic instability. Nearly 2 L of hemorrhagic pericardial fluid were withdrawn emergently; cytology revealed malignant cells consistent with lung adenocarcinoma. Atrial fibrillation with rapid ventricular response is also seen.*

CONCLUSION

The electrocardiogram quickly provides valuable information that may suggest acute life-threatening illness or underlying medical illness. It is a valuable bedside tool when properly interpreted in the clinical context of the patient's presentation.

SUGGESTED READINGS

Channer K, Morris F. ABC of clinical electrocardiography: myocardial ischemia. *BMJ.* 2002;324:1023-1026.

Goldberger AL. *Myocardial Infarction: Electrocardiographic Differential Diagnosis,* 4th ed. St. Louis, MO: Mosby-Year Book; 1991.

Klatsky AL, Oehm R, Cooper RA, et al. The early repolarization normal variant electrocardiogram: correlates and consequences. *Am J Med.* 2003;115:171.

Kligfield P, Gettes LS, Bailey JJ, et al. Recommendations for the standardization and interpretation of the electrocardiogram. Part I. The electrocardiogram and its technology: a scientific statement from the American Heart Association Electrocardiography and Arrhythmias Committee, Council on Clinical Cardiology; the American College of Cardiology Foundation; and the Heart Rhythm Society. *Circulation.* 2007;115:1306-1324.

Schlant RC, Adolph RJ, DiMarco JP, et al. Guidelines for electrocardiography. A report of the American College of Cardiology/American Heart Association Task Force on Assessment of Diagnostic and Therapeutic Cardiovascular Procedures (Committee on Electrocardiography). *J Am Coll Cardiol.* 1992;19:473.

Surawicz B, Parikh SR. Prevalence of male and female patterns of early repolarization in the normal ECG of males and females from childhood to old age. *J Am Coll Cardiol.* 2002;40:1870.

Wellens HJJ, Gorgels AP. The electrocardiogram 102 years after Einthoven. *Circulation.* 2004;109:562-564.

Zimetbaum PJ, Josephson ME. Use of the electrocardiogram in acute myocardial infarction. *N Engl J Med.* 2003;348:933-940.

CHAPTER 109

Elevated Liver Biochemical and Function Tests

Stephanie M. Cantu, MD

Nikroo Hashemi, MD, MPH

Key Clinical Questions

1. What is the approach to the hospitalized patient with abnormal liver function tests?

2. Explain the appropriate diagnostic and therapeutic algorithm for cholestatic liver injury?

3. What are the causes of acute hepatocellular injury?

4. What is the treatment algorithm for acetaminophen overdose?

5. Are there evidence-based interventions for alcoholic hepatitis?

6. What is the definition of acute liver failure?

7. When should a patient with acute liver failure be referred for liver transplantation?

INTRODUCTION

Abnormalities in liver function tests (LFTs) commonly occur in the inpatient setting, whether the primary cause for hospital admission, incidentally detected, or a complication of acute illness and its management. Diagnosis of hepatobiliary disorders may include laboratory tests, imaging studies, and liver biopsy. Individual tests, especially those of liver biochemistry, have limited sensitivity and specificity. The cause and severity of disease is often defined by a combination of tests. Certain scores such as Model of End-Stage Liver Disease (MELD), Child-Pugh score, and Maddrey Discriminant Function (mDF), have incorporated clinical and laboratory features to predict survival in patients with significant liver disease including those with decompensated cirrhosis and alcoholic hepatitis (AH).

It is important to discern between liver enzymes and LFTs. Serum aminotransferase levels and alkaline phosphatase (AP) levels are liver enzymes. Their elevation in the serum indicates hepatocyte and bile duct epithelial injury. Albumin, bilirubin, and prothrombin time are actual measures of hepatic function. However, they are affected by extrahepatic factors including nutrition, hemolysis and antibiotic use. For the purpose of this chapter, LFTs will be referred to liver enzymes. Here, we aim to provide a framework for the evaluation of abnormal LFTs in the hospitalized patient to distinguish acute-on-chronic liver injury from acute liver injury, to provide a framework for diagnosis of the many etiologies of liver injury, and to provide evidence-based management where it is available. Early recognition of acute liver failure (ALF), defined by encephalopathy and coagulopathy in a patient without preexisting liver disease, is an important aspect of inpatient care in order to facilitate prompt evaluation for liver transplantation or transfer to a liver transplantation center. Special consideration is given to acetaminophen overdose, the use of N-acetylcysteine (NAC), and the treatment of alcoholic hepatitis. The management of chronic liver disease and decompensated cirrhosis in the hospitalized patient is addressed elsewhere (see Chapter 160 [Cirrhosis and its Complications]).

EPIDEMIOLOGY

Abnormal LFTs are a frequent cause for hospitalization, the majority as a consequence of biliary pathology, including cholecystitis and cholangitis, or acute liver injury, in the form of hepatotoxins, such as alcohol and acetaminophen, and viral hepatitides. Approximately 2000 cases of ALF occur annually in the United States. Both ALF and cholangitis, in particular, can confer high mortality of 30% in ALF without transplantation and nearly 100% in untreated acute cholangitis. Acetaminophen overdose continues to be recognized as the most common cause of ALF, accounting for approximately one-third of cases, followed by idiosyncratic drug reactions and acute viral hepatitis. From 2006 to 2010, nearly one-half million emergency room visits were attributed to acetaminophen overdose, half resulting in hospitalization, and consequentially costing the health care system $1 billion annually (Altyar).

Latrogenic etiologies of abnormal LFTs encountered during hospitalization include liver injury as a result of a multitude of medications, and as a consequence of systemic illnesses including shock, congestive heart failure, and sepsis.

HISTORY

A comprehensive history may provide many important clues to the origin of abnormal LFTs. The initial step in evaluation is to determine whether the patient has known chronic liver disease or underlying cirrhosis, or a prior history of abnormal LFTs. If a history cannot be obtained from the patient or family, collateral history and prior laboratory testing should be requested from a primary care provider. It should be noted that nonalcoholic fatty liver disease is the most common cause of mild to moderate hypertransaminasemia, and if transaminase elevations are consistent with prior studies, further evaluation may be deferred to postdischarge follow-up.

Given the proportion of acute liver injury attributable to acetaminophen and other drugs, a detailed medication history should be obtained, including prescription, nonprescription, and herbal and dietary supplements. If the patient is not able to provide a history, this information should be sought through family members or others in close proximity to the patient. Both female gender and a history of self-harm have been associated with acetaminophen overdose. A history of alcohol ingestion or medications inducing cytochrome P450 may heighten the possibility of unintentional acetaminophen overdose (**Table 109-1**). A history of recent heavy alcohol use should also prompt consideration of alcoholic hepatitis. Intravenous drug use or recent travel to hepatitis endemic areas (Central and South America, Eastern Europe, parts of Asia and Africa), and a history of malaise or anorexia may suggest acute viral hepatitis. Additional history should include sexual history and possibility of pregnancy-related hepatic dysfunction, recent HIV status, and immunocompromised state including immunosuppressive medications, which predispose to viral hepatitides that are rare in immunocompetent patients. Heart failure is an important etiology of abnormal LFTs, and recent assessment of cardiac function should be reviewed if available. Further, critical illness and recent admission to an intensive care unit may suggest ischemic injury to the liver. A history of autoimmune disease may suggest autoimmune hepatitis. Hepatic vein thrombosis is most often identified in the presence of hypercoagulable state, such as inherited or acquired thrombophilias, malignancy, paroxysmal nocturnal hemoglobinuria, or inflammatory bowel disease. Signs of early emphysema or of neurologic dysfunction may suggest alpha 1 antitrypsin deficiency, or Wilson's disease, respectively.

With respect to evaluating cholestatic pattern of liver test abnormalities and identifying biliary pathology, pertinent history should include preceding postprandial or intermittent epigastric or right-upper quadrant (RUQ) discomfort, which may suggest cholelithiasis or choledocholithiasis. Charcot's triad—jaundice, fever, and RUQ pain—should prompt timely evaluation for cholangitis. Both jaundice, often first noted under the tongue or in the sclerae, and light colored stools may suggest biliary obstruction. Unexplained weight loss or anorexia may be the only clues to an occult pancreatic head tumor causing obstruction of the common bile duct. Sinusoidal obstruction syndrome, or veno-occlusive disease, is a distinctive and potentially fatal form of liver injury, which occurs after drug or toxin exposure, most commonly observed after conditioning chemotherapy for hematopoietic stem cell transplantation.

PHYSICAL EXAMINATION

There are two critical elements to be gathered by the physical examination: (1) signs of chronic liver disease or cirrhosis, and (2) signs of hepatic encephalopathy (HE). The latter should include an assessment of mental status, including changes in mood and orientation, presence of confusion, or lethargy noted by the patient or family members (**Table 109-2**). Asterixis (flapping tremor) is a motor disorder characterized by the inability to actively maintain a position and is demonstrated by jerking movements of the outstretched hands when extended at the wrists. It may be an early sign of HE, although it is not specific for hepatic dysfunction and may by present in other causes of metabolic encephalopathy such as uremia. Patients with evidence of HE may meet criteria for ALF if there is no history of chronic liver disease. Such patients require close monitoring and consideration of treatment in the intensive care setting and should be regarded as more ill than patients without HE given high mortality with delay in appropriate care. See Chapter 159 (Acute Liver Disease).

The physical examination may provide the only clue of underlying cirrhosis when the patient is unable to provide history and collateral information is not available. Examination may reveal scleral icterus or jaundice, muscle atrophy, signs of portal hypertension including ascites, splenomegaly, or caput medusa (visibly dilated abdominal veins), or signs of estrogen excess due to inadequate hepatic metabolism including spider angiomata distributed on the chest or trunk, palmar erythema, and in men, gynecomastia or testicular atrophy.

Fever may develop in viral or alcoholic hepatitis, as well as acute cholecystitis or cholangitis. Jaundice, occurring in both hepatocellular dysfunction and cholestatic disorders, is the most specific symptom of liver disorders. It is a yellowish discoloration of skin and mucous membranes caused by hyperbilirubinemia, which generally become visible when the bilirubin level is 2 to 3 mg/dL.

TABLE 109-1 Cytochrome P450-inducing Medications

Cytochrome P450 Inducers
Ethanol
Isoniazid
Rifampin or rifabutin
Phenobarbital
Glucocorticoids
Phenytoin
Pioglitazone
Omeprazole
Insulin
Carbamazepine
Nafcillin
HIV antiretrovirals (efavirenz, nevirapine)
St John's wort

TABLE 109-2 Grades of Encephalopathy

Grade	Clinical Picture
I	Mood instability
	Shortened attention span
	Insomnia
	Mild confusion
II	Lethargy
	Personality changes
	Moderate confusion/disorientation
III	Marked confusion
	Somnolence
	Incoherent
IV	Coma (unresponsive to verbal or noxious stimuli)

Examination of the abdomen is imperative. Right upper quadrant pain due to liver disorders usually results from inflammation of the liver capsule or distention (eg, by passive venous congestion or by mass effect from tumor). Marked hepatomegaly or ascites in the absence of chronic liver disease may suggest acute Budd-Chiari syndrome. Murphy's sign, pain on inspiration when the examiner's fingers are placed under the right costal margin next to the rectus abdominalis, is a finding associated with acute cholecystitis. Courvoisier sign, an enlarged, palpable and nontender gallbladder with painless jaundice, is associated with biliary obstruction from carcinoma of the pancreatic head. Splenomegaly may suggest a diagnosis of underlying malignancy, including lymphoma, or a hemolytic anemia.

On general examination, the internal jugular vein should be examined for evidence of fluid overload. Extremities should be evaluated for peripheral edema. Skin exam may reveal petechiae when thrombocytopenia or coagulopathy are present from chronic liver disease.

DIAGNOSIS

Aminotransferases (alanine and aspartate aminotransferase: ALT and AST) are not specific to the liver. ALT is produced in the liver, muscle, and kidney. AST is produced in the liver, muscle, heart, kidney, red cells, and brain. They may therefore be elevated from nonhepatic causes including hemolysis, myocardial infarction, acute renal injury, muscle injury, and infarcted bowel. Alkaline phosphatase is present in biliary epithelium, bone, placenta, intestine, and kidney. AP can be fractionated: bone fraction is heat labile and liver fraction is heat stable.

Characterization of elevated liver enzymes are based on chronicity (acute versus chronic) and pattern of injury (hepatocellular, cholestatic, or mixed). In general ALT/AP (both × upper limit of normal) >5 is hepatocellular and <2 is cholestatic. Whether the pattern of injury is hepatocellular or cholestatic may guide the diagnostic work-up and management.

As a general rule, attention should be given to three key steps when evaluating abnormal LFTs in the hospitalized patient:

1. Distinguish acute liver injury from acute-on-chronic liver disease.
2. Determine the etiology based on pattern of liver injury and exclude nonhepatic causes.
3. Determine the severity of liver injury; assess for complications such as coagulopathy, encephalopathy, or need for intervention.

Specific laboratory and imaging work-up based on pattern of injury and suspected etiology will be discussed further; however, all patients with liver injury should undergo a basic evaluation, including complete blood count with differential, basic metabolic panel to assess for electrolyte derangement, renal dysfunction, and acidosis, and coagulation profile. Albumin is synthesized solely in the liver and should be monitored in all patients with liver injury. Hypoalbuminemia may occur in chronic liver disease and if present may point toward underlying liver disease, malnutrition, or loss of albumin through nephrotic syndrome or enteropathy. In addition to albumin, synthesis of factor V and vitamin K dependent factors (II, VII, IX, X) also occurs in the liver. Prothrombin time and INR (international normalized ratio) should be obtained in all patients, because presence of coagulopathy signifies liver synthetic dysfunction and may be of prognostic significance. Characteristically, elevated INR in the setting of hepatocellular injury will not respond to parenteral vitamin K administration, while improvement in INR may be seen in cholestasis. With this framework in mind, the predominant pattern of liver injury allows the evaluation to be tailored to identify the most likely diagnoses.

TABLE 109-3 Causes of Isolated Elevated Alkaline Phosphatase

Thyroid dysfunction
Diabetes mellitus
Congestive heart failure
Hodgkin's lymphoma
Inflammatory bowel disease

ELEVATED ALKALINE PHOSPHATASE

Alkaline phosphatase is an enzyme found in liver, bone, intestine and, in late pregnancy, placenta. An elevation in AP may be an early indicator of cholestasis, biliary obstruction from intrahepatic or extrahepatic causes or both. Elevation in AP, up to 1.5 times the normal range is physiologic in those younger than 18 years of age, in those older than age 60, or in pregnant women. There may also be a small elevation from intestinal AP in patients with type O and B blood.

Because the AP enzyme is not specific to the liver, the first step in evaluation of elevated levels is to confirm that liver is the source. Both gamma glutamyl-transpeptidase (GGT) and 5'-nucleotidase can distinguish hepatic from nonhepatic sources of AL, given GGT is found in liver but not in the bone or other tissues. An elevation in GGT will confirm that AP is of liver origin, and should prompt further investigation. A number of medications may cause increased AP, and medication review should be the first step in the work-up of the hospitalized patient. A number of nonbiliary etiologies of elevated AP may also be considered (**Table 109-3**). In general, an elevation in AP greater than three to four times the upper limit of normal should prompt evaluation for intrahepatic or extrahepatic biliary obstruction with abdominal ultrasound, as well as serology for antimitochondrial antibody to assess for primary biliary cirrhosis. If no abnormality is found on ultrasound, and the level is unchanged or downtrending, outpatient evaluation soon after discharge may be appropriate.

CHOLESTATIC PATTERN OF INJURY: ELEVATION IN BILIRUBIN

Bilirubin is the pigment product released from senescent red blood cells via the degradation of heme proteins. Unconjugated (indirect) insoluble bilirubin is released from the red cell and transported to the liver, where it is conjugated to a water-soluble form (direct bilirubin) for excretion via bile into the intestine. In the intestine, bacteria convert bilirubin to urobilinogen which is either excreted as stercobilinogen via the stool, providing the dark color of stool, or as urobilinogen via the kidneys. Obstruction of the biliary system thereby leads to impaired bilirubin excretion in the bile, clinically evident as jaundice, pale stool or dark urine. Additionally, because unconjugated bilirubin is insoluble in water, and therefore not filtered by the kidneys, the presence of bilirubin in the urinalysis may support cholestasis.

Serum hyperbilirubinemia will be reported as elevation of either the direct or indirect component. An elevation in indirect bilirubin should prompt evaluation for hemolysis (elevated LDH, low haptoglobin, increased reticulocyte count). Gilbert's syndrome, impaired bilirubin uptake by hepatocytes due to decrease in the enzyme UDP glucuronyl transferase, may present as elevation in indirect bilirubin (most often below 4 mg/dL) in a patient with physiologic stress, for example, in the setting of acute illness, hospitalization, or surgery. Outpatient data may be helpful in identifying preceding episodes of asymptomatic elevations in indirect bilirubin elevation.

TABLE 109-4 Causes of Intrahepatic Cholestasis

Toxins:
- Medications
- Primary biliary cirrhosis
- Metastases
- Sepsis
- Cholestasis of Pregnancy
- Granulomas
- TPN
- Sickle Cell Crisis
- AIDS Cholangiopathy
- Chronic Hepatitis
- Infiltrative Disease: amyloidosis, sarcoidosis, tuberculosis, lymphoma

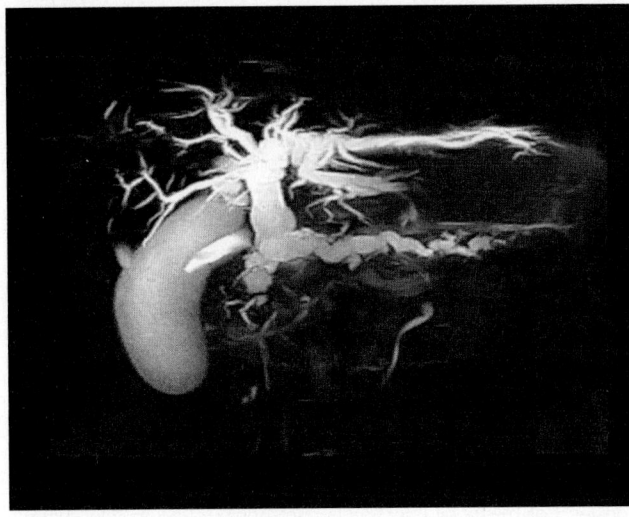

Figure 109-1 *Dilated gallbladder, bile ducts, and pancreatic duct in pancreatic head cancer.*

Elevations in direct bilirubin are indicative of cholestasis, which may be intrahepatic or extrahepatic. In cases of hepatocellular pattern of liver injury secondary to drug-induced liver injury or acute hepatitis, a higher degree of bilirubin elevation may portend worse prognosis. Intrahepatic cholestasis may be precipitated by a wide spectrum of disorders (**Table 109-4**). A number of medications may also cause cholestasis (**Table 109-5**).

Extrahepatic causes of cholestasis are primarily anatomic in nature, including tumor (cholangiocarcinoma, pancreatic head carcinoma, large nodal metastases), obstruction of the common bile duct (CBD) by choledocholithiasis, sphincter dysfunction, choledochal cysts, trauma, and less commonly obstruction by parasites (eg, ascaris). Primary sclerosing cholangitis, cholangiocarcinoma, and radiation may cause both intra and extrahepatic cholestatic liver disease.

The diagnostic evaluation of direct hyperbilirubinemia should begin with abdominal Doppler ultrasound to assess for dilatation of the CBD (normal <8 mm) with 90% to 95% sensitivity, which would be suggestive of obstruction. Ultrasound may also demonstrate cholelithiasis or evidence of cholecystitis. Doppler is imperative in determining patency of the hepatic and portal venous systems (**Figure 109-1**). When CBD dilatation is present, magnetic resonance cholangiopancreatography (MRCP) can provide high-resolution images of the biliary and pancreatic head anatomy to assess for the source of obstruction. If biliary obstruction is suspected, endoscopic retrograde cholangiopancreatography (ERCP), if available, can be used as a diagnostic and therapeutic modality, whereby choledocholithiasis, biliary strictures or masses may be visualized and stone or stricture treated endoscopically.

ACUTE CHOLANGITIS

Bacterial infection superimposed on an obstructed bile duct leads to acute cholangitis. Increased biliary pressure pushes the infection into the biliary canaliculi, hepatic veins, and perihepatic lymphatics, leading to bacteremia in 25% to 40% of cases. The most common organisms isolated in bile are *Enterococcus coli*, *Klebsiella* species, and *Enterococcus* species, in addition to polymicrobial infections. Historically, the mortality from untreated cholangitis was up to 100%. With the advent of ERCP, endoscopic sphincterotomy, stone extraction and biliary stenting, the mortality rate has significantly declined to 5% to 10%. For this reason, it is imperative to recognize the signs of cholangitis and expedite treatment. Charcot's triad of fever, RUQ pain, and jaundice was only present in 15% to 20% of patients with cholangitis in recent studies. Reynold's pentad adds altered mental status and sepsis to the triad. Cholangitis should be suspected in any patient who appears septic, especially in those who are elderly, jaundiced, or have abdominal pain. Fever is present in 90%, abdominal pain in 70%, jaundice in 60% and altered mental

TABLE 109-5 Medications Associated with Cholestasis

Cholestasis without hepatitis:	Cholestasis with hepatitis:	Characterized by ductopenia, or vanishing bile duct syndrome:
Oral contraceptives, estrogen	Macrolides	Amoxicillin-clavulanic acid
Anabolic steroids	Amoxicillin-clavulanic acid	Barbiturates
Tamoxifen	NSAIDs	Carbamazepine
Azathioprine	Isoniazid	Ciprofloxacin
Cyclosporine	Gabapentin	Diazepam
Infliximab	Carbamazepine	Clindamycin, erythromycin
	Tricyclic antidepressants	Trimethoprim-sulfamethoxazole
	Methyldopa	Tetracycline
	Halothane	Thiabendazole, phenytoin

status in 10% to 20%. Note that elderly patients may not have fever or may be too ill to localize their pain. Abnormal liver chemistries (elevated AP, alanine aminotransferase, aspartate aminotransferase) and inflammatory markers (white blood cell count, C-reactive protein) support the diagnosis. Imaging establishes the diagnosis if there is biliary dilation as well as a stricture, stone, or other etiologic abnormality.

Urgency of treatment depends on the severity of illness. Sepsis and shock from suspected acute cholangitis should be considered a medical emergency. Standard therapy of cholangitis consists of fluid resuscitation, parenteral empiric broad-spectrum antibiotics, ideally after blood cultures are drawn, and close observation to determine the need for emergency biliary decompression. The most common organisms isolated in bile are *E. coli*, *Klebsiella*, *Enterococcus* species, *Streptococcus* species, *Enterobacter* species, and *Pseudomonas aeruginosa*. The most common pathogens isolated in blood cultures are *E. coli*, *Klebsiella* species, *Pseudomonas aeruginosa*, and *Enterococcus* species. Polymicrobial infection is commonly found in bile cultures (30%-87%) and less frequently in blood cultures (6%-16%). See Chapter 158 (Biliary Disease: Jaundice, Obstruction and Acute Cholangitis).

Urgent biliary decompression via ERCP, or transfer to a center which can provide ERCP, is critical in the treatment of acute cholangitis. ERCP has a high success rate and is safer than surgical and percutaneous intervention. During ERCP, the gallbladder may be decompressed and stones may be removed, with sphincterotomy performed to prevent further episodes. Percutaneous cholecystostomy tube placement may be considered for decompression in the unstable patient with concomitant cholecystitis, or if ERCP is unavailable or unsuccessful. Resolution of the acute illness and complete decompression are required before hospital discharge. In the event of a percutanous cholecystostomy tube, home nursing may be requiring to assist with drain maintenance until outpatient follow-up.

HEPATOCELLULAR PATTERN OF INJURY: ELEVATION IN TRANSAMINASES

The release of AST and ALT into the serum signifies apoptosis and necrosis of hepatocytes. A rise in serum bilirubin may follow hypertransaminasemia and provide prognostic information; however if a hepatocellular pattern of injury predominates, the degree of elevation may be helpful in narrowing the differential diagnosis. Of the cases of ALF in the United States, acetaminophen overdose accounts for approximately one-third of cases, followed by medications and toxins comprising approximately one-tenth of cases. Medications known to cause drug-induced liver injury include outpatient or inpatient medications, and herbal or nutritional supplements. Drug-induced liver injury (DILI) may occur in a dose-dependent fashion; however most drug-induced liver injury is idiosyncratic, and may occur at any time in therapy. There is evidence that some patients with DILI may actually have hepatitis E and this diagnosis should be considered if there is a history of recent travel to a developing country where hepatitis E is endemic. In developed countries, sporadic infection may occur following consumption of uncooked/undercooked pork or deer meat. The National Institutes of Health provides an up-to-date online database of the diagnosis, causes frequency, patterns and management of liver injury attributable to prescription medications and nonprescription medications, herbals, and dietary supplements (www.livertox.nih.gov).

In the setting of acute illness in the hospitalized patient, elevations in AST and ALT less than 5 to 15 times are not uncommon and may result from nearly any cause of liver disease. Wilson's disease, autoimmune hepatitis, and reactivation of hepatitis B may lead to acute-on-chronic liver disease and high elevations in AST and ALT. Nonhepatic causes of moderate AST and ALT elevation include rhabdomyolysis, myopathy, hemolysis and tumor lysis, and thyroid

dysfunction. Transaminase elevations greater than 1000 U/L are most often caused by toxins, namely acetaminophen, acute viral hepatitides, or ischemia, such as in the setting of shock or post cardiac-arrest. The causes of hepatocellular liver injury and corresponding diagnostic tests that should be considered on initial evaluation, as well as those that should be considered based on clinical history and presentation are presented in **Table 109-6**.

PRACTICE POINT

- Drug-induced liver injury is most often idiosyncratic, and not dose-dependent. The offending agent should be stopped immediately. Transaminase elevation >1000 U/L is most often seen in acetaminophen or drug-induced liver injury, acute viral hepatitis, or ischemic hepatopathy.

LIVER BIOPSY

Liver biopsy has long been considered an important diagnostic adjunct in the evaluation of abnormal liver tests of unclear etiology, that is, when the diagnosis has not been elucidated after a thorough history, physical examination, laboratory and imaging studies. Several studies have shown that in a proportion of patients, liver histology will lead to change in management. It may also be helpful in the establishment of an unsuspected diagnosis, such as alcoholic liver disease. The risks and benefits of liver biopsy in the hospitalized patient should be carefully weighed and the decision to perform a liver biopsy should be individualized, when knowledge of a specific diagnosis is likely to alter the management plan.

ACETAMINOPHEN TOXICITY

From 2006 to 2010 nearly half a million Emergency Department visits were due to acetaminophen overdose, requiring hospital admission for near half of patients. Acetaminophen toxicity, whether intentional or unintentional, remains the leading cause of ALF. Up to one-quarter of patients will require liver transplantation to survive (Altyar). Toxicity can occur with as little as 3 to 4 g of acetaminophen ingestion in the setting of chronic alcohol abuse or with concurrent ingestion of medications that induce the cytochrome P450 system. In such therapeutic misadventures, the ability of the liver to detoxify acetaminophen metabolites via glutathione is overwhelmed, and hepatocyte necrosis occurs.

If acetaminophen ingestion is suspected, or severe elevation in transaminases is present with possible ingestion and without an alternate etiology, the patient should be considered for transfer to a liver transplant center early in the course for consideration of transplant, which may be the only life-saving option in up to a quarter of patients.

In the event of an acute ingestion, activated charcoal (1 g/kg) given within 4 hours of ingestion has been demonstrated to reduce liver injury and peak acetaminophen level and is recommended by American Association for the Study of Liver Diseases. N-acetyl cysteine (NAC) has been demonstrated to reduce hepatic injury regardless of acetaminophen level if given within 8 hours of ingestion and should be given to all patients with known overdose, or to those with known acetaminophen consumption within 24 hours presenting with transaminase elevation.

Use of the Rumack-Matthew nomogram may be helpful to determine efficacy of NAC based on time from ingestion and serum level (Dart). Serum acetaminophen level should be repeated after 4 hours to assess for peak concentration.

NAC may be given orally or intravenously if enteral access is unavailable (oral: 140 mg/kg loading dose, 70 mg/kg every 4 hours × 17 doses; intravenous: 150 mg/kg loading dose over 15 minutes,

TABLE 109-6 Causes of Hepatocellular Liver Injury

Cause	Diagnosis	Cause	Diagnosis
Acetaminophen	Serum acetaminophen level	Autoimmune Hepatitis	Antinuclear Ab
			Antismooth muscle Ab
			Anti liver-kidney microsomal Ab, IgG
Alcoholic Hepatitis	History of heavy or prolonged alcohol; serum alcohol level	Primary Sclerosing Cholangitis	Cholangiogram with beaded appearance
Amanita Phalloides	History of mushroom ingestion	Wilson Disease	AP/bilirubin < 2
			Ceruloplasmin, 24-h urine copper, Kayser Fleischer rings
Pregnancy-related - Acute Fatty Liver of Pregnancy - HELLP	Serum or urine HCG; CBC, LDH, haptoglobin, reticulocyte count	Alpha-1 Antitrypsin	Alpha-1 antitrypsin SPEP
Viral Hepatitis	Travel, health care worker, drug use, sexual history HAV IgM HCV Ab, consider RNA HBV sAb, sAg, c IgM HIV	Hemochromatosis	Iron, TIBC, Ferritin (% sat > 45, Ferritin > 300)
Viral Hepatitis (cont)	Immunocompromise CMV PCR, IgG EBV Panel HSV PCR	Nonhepatic - Rhabdomyolysis - Thyroid dysfunction - Celiac disease - Hemolysis - Babesiosis - Malaria	- - (AST) CK - TSH - Tissue transglutaminase Ab - Haptoglobin, LDH, peripheral blood smear - Peripheral smear; PCR - Thin smear
Vascular - VOD - Acute Budd-Chiari	- Portal flow by Doppler - RUQ ultrasound with Doppler		

50 mg/kg given over 4 hours, 100 mg/kg given over 16 hours). Administration may be limited by nausea, vomiting, or less commonly bronchospasm.

PRACTICE POINT

- N-acetylcysteine should be administered in acetaminophen overdose to reduce hepatic injury; it is most beneficial if given within 8 hours of acetaminophen ingestion. Activated charcoal should be administered within 4 hours of ingestion, prior to NAC.

ALCOHOLIC HEPATITIS

Alcoholic hepatitis should be considered in the patient with recent or prolonged heavy alcohol use, with or without fever, jaundice, and tender hepatomegaly, in patients with or without underlying alcoholic cirrhosis. The AST:ALT ratio is characteristically 2:1. Mortality in severe alcoholic hepatitis is high, with mortality of 34% at 28 days, and less than 25% survival at 6 months without treatment. The principles of management of alcoholic hepatitis are aimed at supportive care, diagnosing and treating concurrent infection, and on whether to initiate AH specific treatment. Patient with AH frequently have coexisting infection. Patients hospitalized with AH should undergo infectious work-up, including cultures of blood and

urine and if present, ascites, and chest x-ray if there is clinical suspicion for pneumonia. Appropriate antibiotics should be initiated if an infectious source is identified. There is no consensus on initiation of empiric antibiotics.

The most widely utilized prognostic score in AH is the mDF, which was originally described in 1978 to identify patients who may benefit from corticosteroid therapy.

$$MDF = 4.6 \times [\text{patient's prothrombin time (seconds)}$$
$$- \text{control prothrombin time (seconds)}] + \text{bilirubin (mg/dL)}$$

A score of equal or greater than 32 or presence of HE defines severe AH. The mDF should be calculated in all patients presenting with AH, and specific pharmacotherapy should be considered solely for patients with severe AH.

Corticosteroids (40 mg prednisolone daily for 28 days, with or without a 2-week taper) and pentoxifylline have been used to treat alcoholic hepatitis. Corticosteroids are contraindicated in significant infection, renal failure, or gastrointestinal bleeding. In the Steroids or Pentoxifylline for Alcoholic Hepatitis (STOPAH) trial, there was a nonsignificant trend toward improved 1-month survival of patients with severe AH and an increased risk of infection in the prednisolone treated arm. There was no short or long-term survival benefit seen in the pentoxyfylline arm. In one recent systematic meta-analysis of 22 randomized controlled trials, corticosteroids demonstrated decreased short-term mortality, with no effect on medium or long-term mortality. The addition of NAC has shown improved 1-month, but not 6-month, survival.

Given the risk of infection with corticosteroid treatment, the Lille score has been proposed to determine response to corticosteroid therapy. Calculated after 7 days, a score greater than 0.45 conveys a poor response to therapy and in these patients discontinuation of steroids should be considered. Six-month survival in steroid no-responders is extremely high (/0%) but may be improved with early liver transplantation in highly selected patients with AH. Resource allocation in patients with active alcohol use varies among liver transplant centers.

Lille score = 3.19 − 0.101 × age (years) + 0.147 × albumin on day 0 (g/L) + 0.0165 × the change in bilirubin between day 0 and day 7 of corticosteroid treatment (μmol/L) − 0.206 × renal insufficiency (rated as 0 if absent and 1 if present) − 0.0065 × bilirubin on day 0 (μmol/L) − 0.0096 × prothrombin time (seconds)

PRACTICE POINT

- Calculate the mDF in patients with suspected AH. In severe AH, mDF > 32 or presence of HE, consider treatment with corticosteroids (prednisolone 40 mg daily) if no contraindication, with or without NAC.
- Reassess response to corticosteroids after 1 week of treatment using the Lille score. If poor response (score > 0.45), discontinue therapy and consider evaluation by transplantation specialist, based on institutional practice.

ACUTE LIVER FAILURE

It is critical to recognize ALF—coagulopathy and encephalopathy in a patient with no known liver disease—due to high morbidity and mortality associated with complications of ALF. While acetaminophen overdose, toxin ingestion and viral hepatitis are the most common causes, any of the etiologies presented in this chapter may cause ALF, and up to one-fifth of cases are idiopathic.

Patients with ALF may present with hemodynamic instability and multiorgan failure. Transfer to a liver transplant center and management in an intensive care unit is most appropriate to allow for serial laboratory testing and examination, particularly to identify worsening encephalopathy and increased intracranial pressure, coagulopathy, bleeding, infection, and concomitant organ failure. Treatment is supportive and is aimed at addressing the complications of hepatic failure (**Table 109-7**).

In a prospective RCT by the National Institutes of Health, intravenous NAC administered to patients with nonacetaminophen induced ALF improved transplant free survival (52% vs 30%, $p = 0.010$) in early stage ALF (grade I/II encephalopathy alone), and was well tolerated (Lee Gastroenterology 2009). Additionally, there was a trend toward shorter hospital stay by 4 days in the NAC treated group of patients. Consequentially, NAC should be administered to patients with nonacetaminophen ALF given the potential benefit with limited adverse effects.

In the setting of ALF, the clinician pursue early transfer to a transplant center. Serial calculations of prognostic scores, such as the MELD score, are used to predict which patients will have a high mortality without liver transplant. A patient meeting all King's

---

TABLE 109-7 Organ-specific Management of Acute Liver Failure

Organ System	Complication(s)	Management
Neurologic	Cerebral edema and intracranial hypertension	1. Consider placing an intracranial monitor
		2. Maintain a cerebral perfusion pressure of 60-80 mm Hg
		3. Maintain an ICP < 25 mm Hg
		4. Maintain head of bed somewhat elevated (45°)
		5. Medical management of elevated ICP (see Figure 158-1)
		6. Avoid stimulation of patient
		7. Serial neurologic examinations
		8. Consider EEG
Pulmonary	Mechanical ventilation for either airway protection from altered mental status or due to respiratory failure from ALI/ARDS	1. Lidocaine IV or endotracheal during intubation
		2. Propofol for sedation
		3. Consider *cis*-atracurium paralysis
		4. Either volume or pressure controlled ventilation
		5. Low tidal volumes of 6 mL/kg of ideal body weight
		6. Maintain maximal plateau pressure < 30 cm H_2O
		7. Avoid bronchoscopy
Cardiovascular	Hypotension (hemodynamic collapse)	1. Arterial catheter for direct measurement
		2. Fluid resuscitation (often less volume than is required with sepsis)
		3. Vasopressor support with norepinephrine as first choice
		4. Avoid alpha-adrenergic agents
		5. Consider a pulmonary artery catheter
		6. Monitor mixed or central venous oxygen saturation
Renal	Acute kidney injury, volume overload, and metabolic disturbances	1. Early initiation of renal replacement therapy with CRRT preferred over HD
		2. Nephrology consultation
		3. Bicarbonate buffered hemofiltration
		4. Renal ultrasound

(Continued)

TABLE 109-7 Organ-specific Management of Acute Liver Failure (Continued)

Organ System	Complication(s)	Management
Hematology	Thrombocytopenia and coagulation abnormalities involving both a bleeding and thrombosis risk	1. Vitamin K 10 mg SQ × 3 d 2. Avoid FFP unless there is bleeding, and monitor serial INR/PT/PTT 3. Transfuse platelets based on Practice Point recommendations (p. 1293) 4. Subcutaneous heparin for DVT prophylaxis 5. Consider recombinant factor VII if placing an intracranial pressure monitor
Infectious Disease	Bacterial and fungal infections; acute viral causes of ALF	1. Maintain a low clinical threshold to culture and start empiric antimicrobials 2. Follow hospital protocols to reduce iatrogenic infections from central lines and catheters 3. Early antiviral therapy for acute hepatitis B, HSV, CMV, or VZV
Endocrine	Relative adrenal insufficiency	1. Maintain a low clinical suspicion if hypotension seems refractory 2. Consider stress dose steroid therapy
Electrolytes	Hypoglycemia, hypophosphatemia, hyponatremia, hypo- or hyperkalemia, low magnesium levels, metabolic acidosis	1. Frequent serum glucose checks; dextrose-containing fluids 2. Bicarbonate buffered solutions with CRRT 3. Replete phosphorous, potassium, and magnesium 4. Treat hyperkalemia 5. Early CRRT
GI/Nutrition	Stress ulcerations, severe catabolic state	1. Early enteral feedings should be considered 2. TPN if enteral feeds not possible (ileus, etc) 3. H2-blocker or PPI therapy

ALI/ARDS, acute lung injury/acute respiratory distress syndrome; CMV, cytomegalovirus; CRRT, continuous renal replacement therapy; DVT, deep vein thrombosis; EEG, electroencephalogram; HD, hemodialysis; HSV, herpes simplex virus; ICP, intracranial pressure; PPI, proton pump inhibitor; TPN, total parenteral nutrition; VZV, varicella zoster virus.

College Criteria (**Table 109-8**) has a likelihood ratio of 8.63 for a poor prognosis without liver transplant.

PRACTICE POINT

- All patients with ALF with stage I or II HE should receive NAC, regardless of etiology, to improve transplant free survival. Patient with ALF should be evaluated early at a transplant center. The King's College Criteria and MELD score may help in determining poor prognosis without liver transplant.

TABLE 109-8 King's College Criteria—Prognostic Model for Determining Poor Outcome without Liver Transplantation in Acute Liver Failure (ALF)

For acetaminophen-Induced ALF	For nonacetaminophen-Induced ALF
Arterial pH < 7.3	INR > 6.5
OR	OR
All three of the following:	Three out of five of the following criteria:
INR > 6.5	Age < 11 or > 40
Serum creatinine > 3.4 mg/dL	Serum bilirubin > 18 mg/dL
Grade III or IV encephalopathy	Time from jaundice to coma > 7 d
	INR > 3.5
	Etiology non-A or non-B viral hepatitis OR drug-induced liver injury

SUGGESTED READINGS

Altyar A, Kordi L, Skrepnek G. Clinical and economic characteristics of emergency department visits due to acetaminophen toxicity in the USA. *BMJ Open*. 2015;5(9):e007368.

Bhatia V, et al. Predictive value of arterial ammonia for complications and outcome in acute liver failure. *Gut*. 55;98:2006.

Chalasani N, Fontana RJ, Bonkovsky HL, et al. Causes, clinical features, and outcomes from a prospective study of drug-induced liver injury in the United States. *Gastroenterology*. 2008;135(6): 1924-1934, 1934.e1-4.

Dart RC, Rumack BH. Acetaminophen (Paracetamol). In: Dart RC, ed. *Medical Toxicology*, 3rd ed. Philadelphia: Lippincott Williams & Wilkins; 2004.

Dugum M, McCullough A. Diagnosis and management of alcoholic liver disease. *J Clin Transl Hepatol*. 2015;3(2):109-116.

Lee WM, et al. Acute Liver Failure Study Group. Intravenous N-acetylcysteine improves transplant-free survival in early stage non-acetaminophen acute liver failure. *Gastroenterology*. 2009;137(3):856-64, 864.

Leise MD, Poterucha JJ, Talwalkar JA. Drug-induced liver injury. *Mayo Clin Proc*. 2014;89(1):95-106.

Mathurin P, Moreno C, Samuel D, et al. Early liver transplantation for severe alcoholic hepatitis. *N Engl J Med*. 2011;365:1790-1800.

Mathurin P, O'Grady J, Carithers RL, et al. Corticosteroids improve short-term survival in patients with severe alcoholic hepatitis: meta-analysis of individual patient data. *Gut*. 2011;60:255-260.

Polson J, Lee WM. AASLD position paper: the management of acute liver failure. *Hepatology*. 2005;41:1179-1197.

Singh S, Murad MH, Chandar AK, et al. Comparative effectiveness of pharmacological interventions for severe alcoholic hepatitis: a systematic review and network meta-analysis. *Gastroenterology.* 2015;149(4):958-70.e12.

Smilkstein MJ, Knapp GL, Kulig KW, Rumack BH. Efficacy of oral N-acetylcysteine in the treatment of acetaminophen overdose. Analysis of the national multicenter study (1976 to 1985). *N Engl J Med.* 1988;319(24):1557.

Thursz MR, Richardson P, Allison M, et al. Prednisolone or pentoxifylline for alcoholic hepatitis. *N Engl J Med.* 2015;372:1619-1628.

ONLINE RESOURCES

LiverTox: *http://livertox.nih.gov*

CHAPTER 110

Pulmonary Function Testing

Joseph J. Miaskiewicz, Jr., MD, FHM

Key Clinical Questions

1. What information do pulmonary function tests provide in addition to the history and physical examination?
2. What specific tests might you order to evaluate the acutely ill hospitalized patient and how does each test influence diagnostic evaluation or management?
3. What operations require preoperative pulmonary function tests as part of the preoperative evaluation?
4. What are the predictors of increased postoperative risk?

INTRODUCTION

Pulmonary function tests (PFTs) objectively assess lung function. Along with measurement of arterial blood gases (ABGs), PFTs are used to evaluate how much a patient's symptoms or known lung disease impairs daily activities and the tests are helpful in management, such as when to treat a patient and in what setting. The purpose of PFTs is to evaluate dyspnea by assessing the mechanical function of the respiratory system, to quantitate the loss of lung function, and to monitor disease progression and response to treatment. PFTs also predict postoperative risk of pulmonary complications and which patients will likely have adequate pulmonary function after lung resection. Serial evaluations monitor respiratory muscular strength in progressive neuromuscular diseases such as Guillain-Barre, myasthesia gravis, and muscular dystrophy.

PFTs estimate the following:

1. Volumes or the ability of the lungs to fully expand (TLC, FRC, RV).
2. Flow rates or the rate of inflow and outflow of air (FEV1, forced expiratory flow [25%-75%]).
3. Maximum voluntary ventilation or airflow through major airways by rapid inspiration and expiration maneuvers (MVV).
4. Maximum inspiratory and expiratory pressure, a measure of respiratory muscle strength (Pi[max], Pe[max]).
5. Diffusing capacity (DLCO) or measurement of the ability of oxygen to get into the blood.

Interpretation will be (1) normal, (2) obstructive, (3) restrictive, or (4) combined obstructive and restrictive. For the majority of PFTs to be meaningful, patients must be able to physically perform the tests and to follow instructions. With the exception of oximetry, ABGs, and simple spirometry, PFTs are usually performed in the outpatient setting. Hospitalists should be able to (1) recognize patterns of pulmonary involvement when they review outside medical records, (2) know when to order specific tests to evaluate acutely ill patients, and (3) avoid unnecessary ordering of PFTs when they are of limited utility in hospitalized patients.

COMPONENTS OF TESTING

PFTs will detect significant increased resistance to airflow (airway obstruction) and increased resistance to expansion (parenchymal disease, weakness of respiratory muscles or abnormalities of the chest wall or diaphragm). ABGs supplement PFTs by measuring the effect of pulmonary and other illnesses on oxygenation and ventilation (**Figure 110-1**).

■ VOLUMES

TLC = Total lung capacity or the total volume of gas within the lungs after a maximal inspiration

RV = Residual volume or the volume of gas remaining in the lungs after a maximal expiration

VC = Vital capacity or the volume of gas expired after a maximal inspiration followed by a maximal expiration

FRC = Functional residual capacity or the volume of gas within the lungs at the end of expiration during normal tidal breathing at rest

To quantitate VC, ask the patient to breathe into a spirometer and obtain a spirometric tracing. To quantitate RV, FRC, and TLC, other methods such as dilution tests or body plethysmography are

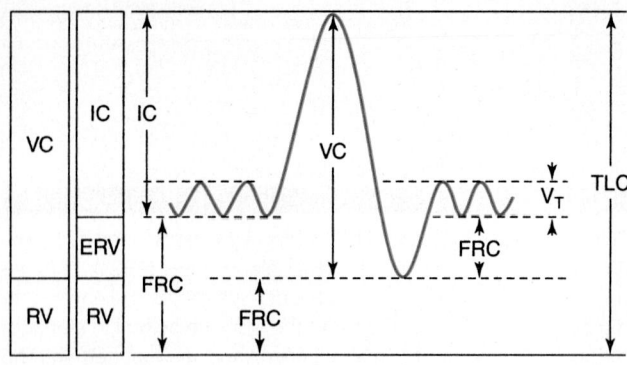

Figure 110-1 *Lung Volumes.* (Reproduced, with permission, from Weinberger SE. *Principles of Pulmonary Medicine,* 4th ed. Philadelphia: Saunders; 2004.)

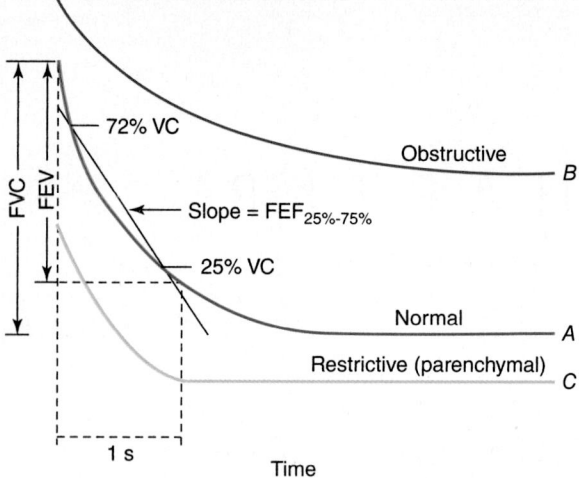

Figure 110-2 *Volume versus time.* (Reproduced, with permission, from Fauci AS, Braunwald E, Kasper DL, et al. *Harrison's Principles of Internal Medicine.* 17th ed. New York: McGraw-Hill; 2008. Figure 246-2, p. 1586.)

needed to measure the amount of air left in the lungs. These measurements require significant expertise on the part of the respiratory therapist in the PFT laboratory and maximal patient cooperation and ability to follow instructions. Inert gas dilution may underestimate lung volumes when there is airflow obstruction in patients who have air spaces such as bullae within the lung that do not communicate with the bronchial tree. Body plethysmography may overestimate lung volumes in airflow obstruction but may provide a more accurate measurement of intrathroacic gas volume in patients with noncommunicating airspaces within the lung.

Most diffuse lung disease is associated with decreased lung volumes. Restrictive PFTs means limitation to full expansion of the lungs. Volumes are decreased but flow rates are normal. Interstitial lung disease has reduced lung compliance and a restrictive defect. PFTs will reveal a decreased TLC, FRC, and RV. Although FEV1 and FVC may be decreased secondary to decreased volumes, the FEV1/FVC ratio is normal or increased. When the TLC and VC are decreased, the differential diagnosis includes restrictive lung disease (pulmonary fibrosis) or loss of lung volume (surgery, diaphragmatic paralysis, or skeletal problems). Decreases in the TLC, RV, and FRC can be interpreted as mild (60%-80% reduction), moderate (40%-60% reduction) or severe (<40% reduction). Marked decreases in the VC may also occur in certain neuromuscular diseases, and serial testing may be used to monitor disease progression in Guillain-Barre Syndrome, myasthenia gravis, and muscular dystrophy.

■ FLOW RATES

Measurement of flow rates requires that the patient breathe into a spirometer as hard and as fast as possible from TLC down to RV. The information can be displayed as a flow versus volume graph or a volume versus time graph. The volume expired during this test is the forced vital capacity or FVC. The amount expired during the first second is the forced expiratory volume in 1 second, or FEV1. This maneuver also reports the forced expiratory flow between 25% and 75% of VC (FEF 25%-75%), also referred to as the maximum mid-expiratory flow rate (MMEFE or MMFR), which is the rate of airflow during the middle one-half of the expiration capacity. It is not effort or technique dependent (**Figure 110-2**).

Obstructive lung disease such as chronic obstructive pulmonary disease (COPD) is a spectrum of disorders that have in common impairment in expiratory flow. Diagnosis is made by spirometry showing a permanent reduction in FEV1/FVC ratio below 75%. The slow vital capacity or SVC will be greater than the FVC when the FVC is decreased in the setting of obstruction. Decreases in both FEV1 and FVC and a normal FEV1/FVC would suggest restrictive disease. Spirometry can be used to determine the degree of reversibility of the airways to bronchodilators and adequacy of treatment

of obstructive airway disease. An increase in FEV1 of 200 cc or 12% is considered a significant response to bronchodilators and inadequately treated obstructive lung disease.

In addition to spirometry, flow rates may be measured using peak flow meters. Peak flow rates usually occur in the very early stages of the FVC maneuver and may be useful in measuring obstructive airway disease. Although a very simple test easily performed without too much training on the part of the operator or the patient, measuring the peak flow is very effort dependent and is not accurate enough to replace spirometry. The predicted values are rather nonspecific and the previously described prediction of severity of disease does not apply to these values. However, in the hospital it allows for a very simple, objective way of monitoring a patient's obstructive airway disease and response to therapy. Measuring the peak flow is a simple way for patients with asthma to objectively measure the degree of obstruction, starting in the hospital in preparation for discharge home when patients should monitor their peak flow and understand when they need to return for medical evaluation before they are so ill that they need to be rehospitalized. A peak expiratory flow calculator using age, sex, and height may be found at the link http://www.dynamicmt.com/PEFform.html.

■ THE FLOW VOLUME LOOP

The flow volume loop graphically records the maximal inspiratory and maximal expiratory maneuvers with flow on the *Y*-axis and volume on the *X*-axis. The patterns of the flow volume loops can be diagnostic of various types of obstruction including intra and extrathoracic obstruction, or fixed or variable obstruction. Although the beginning of a forced expiratory maneuver depends on effort, the latter part of forced expiration primarily reflects the mechanical properties of the lung and the resistance to airflow. The evaluation of the flow volume loop may be a qualitative visual analysis of the shape and concavity of the expiratory portion of the curve or a quantitative analysis comparing observed flow rates at specified volumes with predicted values.

In a fixed obstruction, changes in pleural pressure do not affect the degree of obstruction, and the inspiratory and expiratory portions of the curve reveal a plateau, reflecting a limitation in peak airflow of both inspiration and expiration.

In a variable obstruction, the location of the lesion and the effect of alterations in pleural and airway pressure with inspiration and expiration determine the amount of obstruction. If the lesion is intrathoracic, the flow volume loop will demonstrate airflow limitation during expiration. If the lesion is extrathoracic, the flow volume loop will demonstrate airflow limitation during inspiration (**Figure 110-3**).

In obstructive disease, the flow volume loop demonstrates a decrease in the expiratory loop, especially at the later part of the expiration (**Figure 110-4**).

■ MAXIMUM VOLUNTARY VENTILATION

This is the measurement of the maximum amount of air a patient can move in 12 to 15 seconds, using a spirometer. The results are expressed in liters/min. Because MVV tests airflow through major airways and muscle strength, consider weakness of respiratory muscles, especially the diaphragm, if MVV is low and flow rates are normal. Major airway lesions and neuromuscular disease result in a decreased MVV. Obstructive disease may also have a low MVV (MVV = FEV1 × 33). In theory, isolated restrictive disease should have a normal MVV; however, it is a nonspecific test and reductions are seen in pulmonary diseases (restrictive and airway obstruction) and in neuromuscular disease (loss of coordination, diminished cognitive function, and overall deconditioning).

Between 10% and 30% of patients with Guillian-Barre Syndrome will require ventilatory support. Patients most likely requiring mechanical ventilation present within 7 days of onset of symptoms, FVC <60% predicted, maximal inspiratory pressure (MIP) <30 cm H_2O, or an expiratory pressure <40 cm H_2O. These patients are at great risk of requiring mechanical ventilation and should be monitored carefully with serial FVC and inspiratory pressure measurements.

■ MAXIMUM INSPIRATORY AND EXPIRATORY PRESSURE

This is a good estimate of muscle strength, which would be presumed to be normal with a normal maximum inspiratory and expiratory pressure. Patients must be able to cooperate with the test.

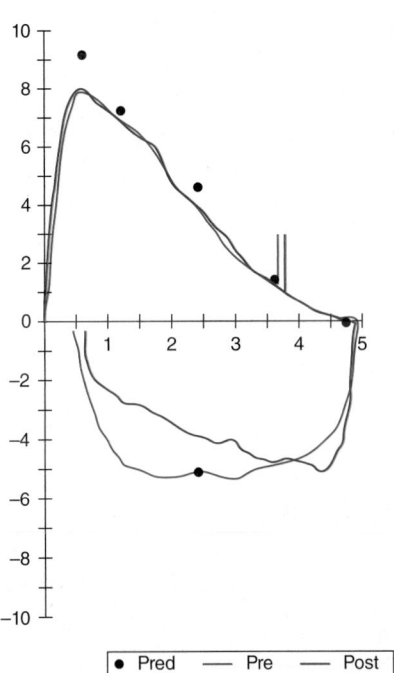

● Pred ── Pre ── Post

	Pre-Bronch			Post-Bronch		
	Actual	**Pred**	**%Pred**	**Actual**	**%Pred**	**%Chng**
---- SPIROMETRY ----						
FVC (L)	4.92	4.70	105	4.85	103	−1
FEV1 (L)	3.67	3.64	101	3.75	103	2
FEV1/FVC (%)	75	77	97	77	100	3
FEF 25% (L/s)	700	7.35	95	6.86	93	−2
FEF 75% (L/s)	1.08	1.56	69	1.14	73	6
FEF 25%-75% (L/s)	2.86	3.23	88	2.97	92	4
FEF Max (L/s)	8.01	9.32	86	8.32	89	4
FIVC (L)	4.42			4.20		−5
FIF Max (L/s)	5.30			5.03		−5
MVV (L/min)	152	145	105	164	113	8
---- LUNG VOLUMES ----						
SVC (L)	4.98	4.70	106			
IC (L)	3.89	3.24	120			
ERV (L)	1.09	1.46	75			
FRC–TGV (Pleth) (L)	3.18	3.32	96			
RV (Pleth) (L)	2.09	1.95	107			
TLC (Pleth) (L)	7.07	6.56	108			
RV/TLC (Pleth) (%)	30	30	99			

Figure 110-3 *Normal flow volume loop, spirometry, and DLCO.*

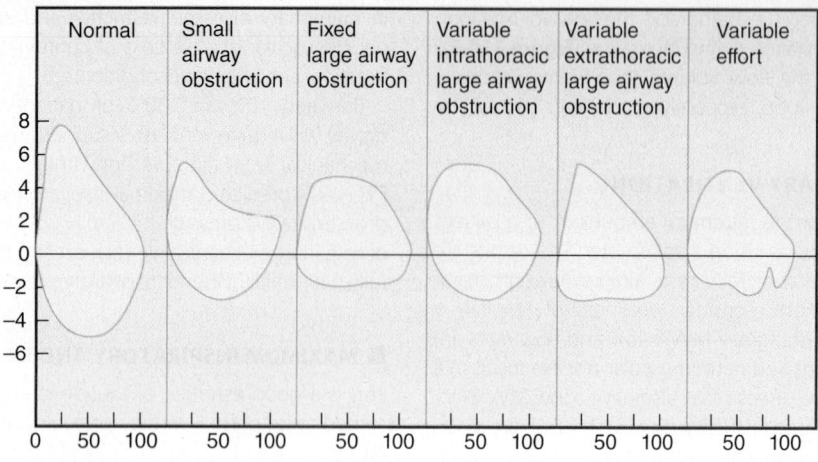

Figure 110-4 *Flow volume loop patterns.*

■ DIFFUSING CAPACITY (DLCO)

Usually measured as DLCO, diffusing capacity is the measurement of the rate of gas transfer from the alveolus to the capillary measured in relation to the driving pressure of CO across the alveolar-capillary membrane. It is reported as ml of CO/min/mm Hg. The CO behaves like O_2 and is usually measured in a single breath. The diffusing capacity is most dependent on the surface area available for gas exchange and the volume of blood or hemoglobin in the pulmonary capillaries available to bind to CO. The observed value of the diffusing capacity is corrected for the patient's hemoglobin level. The diffusing capacity should be normal in diseases that only affect the airway such as asthma and chronic bronchitis and not pulmonary parenchymal disease, such as interstitial lung disease or emphysema.

CASE 110-1

INTRATHORACIC OBSTRUCTION

This case demonstrates the PFT findings of a patient with a tracheal tumor. At the bedside the patient with a presumptive diagnosis of COPD exacerbation was found to have disproportionate upper airway wheezing.

The DLCO does not correlate with disease severity due to dependence on the Hgb level, pulmonary capillary volume, and thickness of the alveolocapillary membrane. Conditions that decrease the DLCO include:

1. Anemia, in which a decrease of 1 gm of Hg will decrease the DLCO by 7%.
2. Anatomical emphysema, pneumonectomy, pulmonary hypertension, and recurrent pulmonary emboli due to decreased pulmonary capillary volume.
3. Restrictive lung diseases such as interstitial lung disease due to increased thickness of the alveolar capillary membrane.

In the setting of obstructive disease, the DLCO helps distinguish between emphysema (decreased DLCO) and other causes of chronic airway obstruction such as asthma (normal DLCO). In the setting of restrictive disease, the diffusing capacity helps distinguish between intrinsic (or interstitial) lung diseases, in which DLCO is usually reduced, from other causes of restriction, in which DLCO is usually normal. Conditions that increase the DLCO include:

1. Alveolar hemorrhage, polycythemia, left to right shunt, and in some asthmatics due to increased pulmonary capillary volume.

2. The supine posture, after exercise, high cardiac output states.
3. Obesity.

The DLCO can be useful in the evaluation of diffuse pulmonary infiltrates when there is a large differential diagnosis.

■ HYPOXIA ALTITUDE SIMULATION TEST (HAST)

The purpose of the HAST is to simulate the oxygen tension while traveling by commercial airline flight. Aircraft pressure is maintained at an altitude of 8000 ft. The pO_2 at this level is approximately 55 mm Hg. If the pO_2 falls below 50 mm Hg, supplemental oxygen is supplied and the test repeated. Predictive of the risk of hypoxemia seen in flight, the HAST test identifies patients in need of supplemental oxygen when flying. Through a tight fitting mask the patient inspires air with 15.1% oxygen content. An ABG is obtained prior to the test and at 20 minutes. Continuous oxygen saturation and ECG monitoring is conducted. Symptoms are monitored.

■ INPATIENT PULMONARY COMPLIANCE STUDY

For intubated, mechanically ventilated patients, inpatient pulmonary compliance studies assess pulmonary mechanics by esophageal balloon. Esophageal balloon manometry provides an estimate of pleural pressure and lung compliance. Transpulmonary pressure can be recorded with PEEP and tidal volume titration. This information can be effectively used to improve oxygenation and respiratory system compliance in ventilated ARDS patients by identifying patients who derive benefit from higher levels of PEEP than would ordinarily be used.

■ PATTERNS OF PFT ABNORMALITIES

The obstructive pattern

Patients with asthma, chronic bronchitis, or emphysema typically have an obstructive pattern: decreased FEV1 with normal or decreased FVC.

The FEV1/FVC is normally decreased in obstructive lung disease, but may be near normal when the FVC is at very low volumes. The FEF 25% to 75% is usually quite low. The flow volume loop will be abnormal when flow rates measured by spirometry are reduced.

In addition to asthma syndromes and COPD, wheezing may be caused by tumors, laryngeal or vocal cord dysfunction due to GERD, postnasal drip or psychological states, allergic reactions, CHF, vasculitis, aspiration, and other pulmonary causes such as pulmonary embolism, bronchiectasis, sarcoidosis, and interstitial lung disease. Decreased FEV1 and FEV1/FVC are the hallmarks of obstructive

	Pre-Bronch			Post-Bronch		
	Actual	**Pred**	**%Pred**	**Actual**	**%Pred**	**%Chng**
---- SPIROMETRY ----						
FVC (L)	3.26	3.11	105	3.13	100	−4
FEV1 (L)	2.51	2.41	104	2.51	104	−0
FEV1/FVC (%)	77	78	99	80	103	4
FEF 25% (L/s)	2.84	4.81	59	3.45	72	21
FEF 75% (L/s)	1.72	1.25	137	0.92	74	−46
FEF 25%-75% (L/s)	2.41	2.30	105	2.30	100	−5
FEF Max (L/s)	2.98	6.07	49	3.56	59	19
FIVC (L)	2.63			2.94		12
FIF Max (L/s)	0.95			1.48		56
MVV (L/min)	53	88	60	43	49	−18
---- LUNG VOLUMES ----						
SVC (L)	3.04	3.11	98			
IC (L)	2.60	2.08	125			
ERV (L)	0.44	1.03	42			
FRC–TGV (Pleth) (L)	2.27	2.67	85			
RV (Pleth) (L)	1.83	1.86	98			
TLC (Pleth) (%)	4.87	4.75	102			
RV/TLC (Pleth) (%)	38	39	96			
Trapped Gas (L)						
---- DIFFUSION ----						
DLCOunc (mL/min/mm Hg)	23.68	21.56	110			
DLCOcor (mL/min/mm Hg)	23.26	21.56	108			
DL/VA (mL/min/mm Hg/L)	5.56	4.54	123			
VA (L)	4.18	4.75	88			
Hgb (g/dL)	14.0	12.18				

Figure 110-5 *No response to bronchodilators despite the presence of severe obstructive disease (FEV1, FEF25-75, and FEV1/FVC).*

disease. Flow volume loops can help identify if wheezing is originating from an intrathoracic or extrathoracic source and they can help identify if the obstructing lesion is fixed or variable. Measurement of the DLCO can be helpful in differentiating obstruction due to chronic bronchitis, emphysema, and asthma. The DLCO is lower in emphysema and is usually not affected in other forms of airway obstruction that cause wheezing. The presence of reversibility of airway obstruction suggests asthma or COPD requiring intensification of bronchodilator therapy. Measurements of ABGs can be obtained to evaluate severity of illness and need for home O_2 therapy (**Figures 110-5-110-8**).

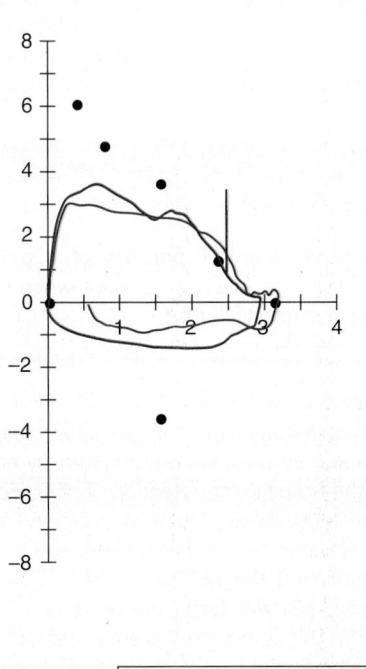

● Pred —— Pre —— Post

Figure 110-6 *An intrathoracic pattern by flow volume curve (a flattening of the expiratory portion of the curve with a preserved inspiratory portion of the curve).*

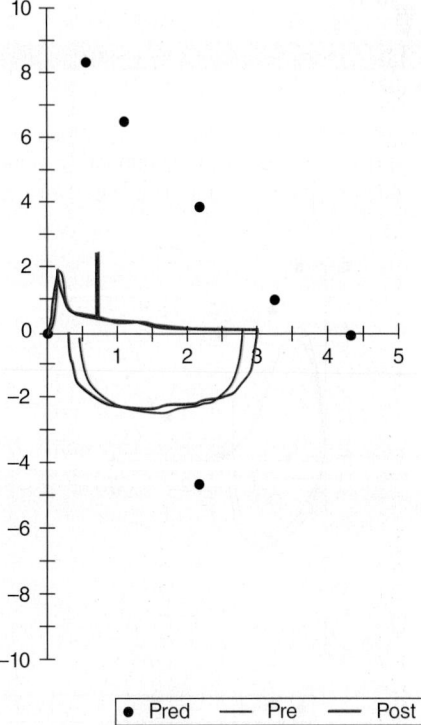

● Pred —— Pre —— Post

Figure 110-7 *A typical pattern of severe obstruction with a scooped terminal portion of the expiratory loop.*

	Predrug reported	Predrug predicted	% Predicted	Postdrug reported	% Predicted	% Change
FVC	2.69	5.42	50	3.30	61	23
FEV1	1.17	3.96	29	1.34	34	15
FEF 25%-75%	.50	3.87	13	.54	14	8
FEV1/FVC	43.55	73.45	59	40.63	55	−7
MVV	51.39	145.61	35			
TLC	7.72	776	99			
RV	5.31	2.34	227			
RV/TLC	68.80	30.17	228			
DLCO	2.97	3.87	77			

Figure 110-8 *A markedly decreased FEV1, FEF25-75, and FEV1/FVC with a significant response to bronchodilators consistent with severe COPD. The lung volumes suggest air trapping and the decreased DLCO the presence of emphysema.*

CASE 110-2

SEVERE OBSTRUCTIVE LUNG DISEASE

This case demonstrates the PFT findings of a patient with progressive and persistent obstructive symptoms; he would likely benefit from more intense therapy and pulmonary rehabilitation.

The restrictive pattern

Patients with severe skeletal deformities, diaphragmatic paralysis, s/p surgical repair, or pulmonary fibrosis typically have a restrictive pattern. A low TLC, a decrease in FEV1 and FVC with a normal FEV1/FVC, a normal or super-normal FEF 25% to 75%, and a low DLCO would suggest restrictive lung disease. The flow volume loop usually is normal in configuration but has low lung volumes (**Figures 110-9 and 110-10**).

The combined obstructive and restrictive pattern

Patients with cystic fibrosis, bronchiolitis obliterans, COPD and congestive heart failure, COPD and pneumonia, or COPD with obesity typically have a combined obstructive and restrictive pattern (**Table 110-1**).

ANCILLARY TESTS

■ OXIMETRY

Reflective of the percentage of hemoglobin molecules occupied by oxygen, oximetry can be used to continuously monitor oxygen saturation. Oximeters transmit light at different wavelengths. The light absorption of oxyhemoglobin is different from reduced hemoglobin. A photo detector usually placed on a finger or ear compares pulsatile and baseline light absorption at the different wavelengths of light to calculate the oxygen saturation. The results may be falsely low when there is poor blood flow and perfusion to the fingertips, vasoconstriction due to hypothermia or sepsis, anemia, dark skin pigmentation, obscuring nail polish, and vital dyes. In certain circumstances the concentration of carboxyhemoglobin, such as in smoke inhalation, can significantly affect the results, falsely elevating the values. Oximetry does not take into consideration the pCO_2 and therefore, does not reflect ventilation or acid-base status.

■ ARTERIAL BLOOD GASES (ABGS)

While PFTs objectively assess lung function, ABGs assess the effects of the cardiopulmonary system on oxygen delivery by measuring both oxygenation and ventilation. ABGs directly measure the pO_2, pCO_2, and pH. Below a pO_2 of 60 mm Hg corresponding to an O_2 saturation of 80%, the oxyhemoglobin saturation curve is steep, and large changes in oximetry can mean small changes in oxygenation. Below this level, oximetry may not correlate with oxygenation, and an ABG should be obtained (**Figure 110-11**).

The normal range for the pH is between 7.36 and 7.44 corresponding to a normal range of 36 to 44 torr for the pCO_2. Respiratory function and acid-base status determine the pCO_2 and pH. (See Chapter 238 [Acid-Base Disorders].) The normal range for the pO_2 is between 80 and 100 torr. Age and the pCO_2 determine alveolar O_2.

CASE 110-3

RESTRICTIVE LUNG DISEASE

This case demonstrates the PFT findings of a patient with restrictive lung disease who failed to improve when treated for presumptive congestive heart failure.

ABGs are primarily obtained to assess ventilation in hospitalized patients. A high-oxygen saturation may be falsely reassuring in patients whose respiratory drive is compromised by an increase of oxygenation in the hospital and retention of pCO_2. For patients with known severe lung disease, such as a history of oxygen-dependent O_2, an elevated serum bicarbonate may be a clue of chronic CO_2 retention and the ABG will confirm CO_2 retention. Neither oximetry nor ABGs will detect the presence of a reduced O_2 carrying capacity. This is because anemia, carbon monoxide poisoning, and methemoglobinemia do not affect the alveolar pO_2. An elevated carboxyhemoglobin will be required to make the diagnosis in carbon monoxide (CO) poisoning with levels above 20 diagnostic. Nonsmokers may have levels up to 3, smokers 10 to 15, and CO poisoning levels above 15. When there is CO poisoning, the

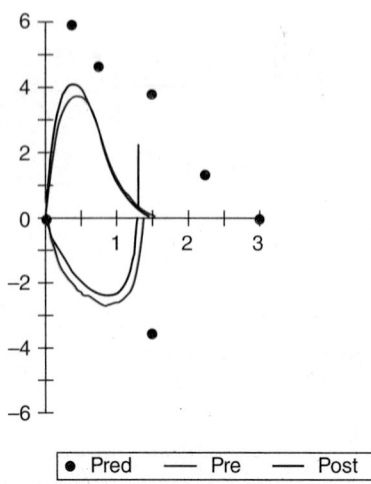

● Pred — Pre — Post

Figure 110-9 *The flow volume loop with a normal configuration but low lung volumes.*

	Predrug reported	Predrug predicted	% Predicted	Postdrug reported	% Predicted	% Change
FVC	1.59	2.84	56	1.67	59	5
FEV1	1.48	2.08	71	1.57	75	6
FEF 25%-75%	4.29	2.47	174	3.79	153	−12
FEV1/FVC	92.96	73.22	127	94.27	129	1
MVV	75.33	86.63	87			
TLC	2.26	4.52	50			
RV	.66	1.68	39			
RV/TLC	29.12	37.15	78			
DLCO	1.63	4.05	40			

Figure 110-10 *A decreased FEV1 and FVC, an increased FEV1/FVC and FEF25%-75%, and a decreased DLCO consistent with parenchymal disease.*

oximeter will report normal O_2 saturation. This is due to the inability to differentiate between hemoglobin molecules with CO attached and those with O_2 attached. ABGs will also report normal values because the PaO_2 is a measurement of the oxygen dissolved in the blood and not the number of O_2 molecules attached to hemoglobin molecules. Likewise, the presence of abnormal hemoglobins, such as sickle cell, fetal hemoglobin, and methemoglobin will not affect the ABG results.

■ A-A GRADIENT

The A-a gradient is the difference between the oxygen in the alveoli (PAO_2) and the oxygen dissolved in the blood (PaO_2).

A normal A-a gradient is around 10 to 15 torr. An increase in the A-a gradient represents increased difficulty in getting O_2 from the alveoli to the blood. The A-a gradient may normally increase in the absence of underlying lung diseases due

- Advancing age. A normal A-a gradient = 2.5 + 0.21 age in years
- Higher FiO_2 which disproportionately causes the PAO_2 to increase more than the PaO_2. When breathing 100% oxygen, older patients may normally have an A-a gradient as high as 80 torr and younger patients as high as 120 torr. It is best to calculate the A-a gradient on room air if possible

The A-a gradient will also abnormally increase in the presence of

- Diseases that affect the pulmonary interstitium, such as interstitial lung disease, pneumonia, and CHF
- Pulmonary vascular disease, such as pulmonary emboli, shunts, pulmonary hypertension
- Ventilation/perfusion mismatches of large vessels such as pulmonary or tumor emboli and of small vessels such as pulmonary hypertension, vasculitis, interstitial lung disease, and emphysema (**Table 110-2**). The following link may be useful for calculating the A-a gradient: http://www.mdcalc.com/a-a-o2-gradient

Calculating the A-a gradient is most useful for determining the severity of the underlying disorder and whether there is a component of hypoventilation. Especially for hospitalized patients who have been prescribed medications which may suppress respiration,

the A-a gradient is used to determine the relative contribution of hypoventilation to hypoxia due to underlying lung disease. If the A-a gradient is normal, the ABG abnormality is all due to hypoventilation.

■ CALCULATION OF THE A-a OXYGEN GRADIENT FROM ABG

The A-a oxygen gradient = $PAO_2 - PaO_2$

A-a O_2 Gradient = ([FiO_2] × [atmospheric pressure − H_2O pressure] − [$PaCO_2$/respiratory quotient] − PaO_2)

Inspired air at sea level, the FiO_2 of room air = 0.21
Atmospheric pressure = 760 mm Hg
PH_2O at 37°F = 47 mm Hg
Respiratory quotient = 0.8
Normal gradient estimate = (age/4) + 4

■ PREOPERATIVE PULMONARY FUNCTION TESTING

Pulmonary function testing is indicated for patients before undergoing lung resection, surgical coronary revascularization, and to evaluate optimization of medical management of respiratory obstruction or assessment of unclear respiratory symptoms. For patients scheduled for lung resection, combining the results of spirometry with radioisotope or CT lung scans predicts whether remaining lung function following lobectomy or pneumonectomy will be greater than 1 L. For patients scheduled for upper abdominal surgery, pulmonary function testing is important to evaluate respiratory obstruction to document optimization of medical management (**Figures 110-12** and **110-13**).

CONCLUSION

PFTs are usually deferred to the outpatient setting, when the acutely hospitalized patient has recovered sufficiently to be able to optimally perform the test. Review of outside records, including PFTs, may provide valuable information that cannot be obtained during acute illness, may point to an alternative diagnosis when a patient is not improving as expected, or provide important prognostic information. Interpretation of PFTs assumes "normal standards" based on

TABLE 110-1 Summary of Pulmonary Function Findings in Certain Diseases

Pattern	FVC	FEV1	FEV1/FVC	TLC	RV	DLCO
Normal	Normal	Normal	Normal	Normal	Normal	Normal
Obstructive	Normal ↑ or ↓	↓	Normal or ↓	Normal or ↑	Normal or ↑	Normal or ↓
Restrictive	↓	Normal or ↑	Normal or ↑	↓	Normal or ↓	↓
Neuromuscular	↓	↓	Normal or ↓	↓	Normal or ↑	Normal

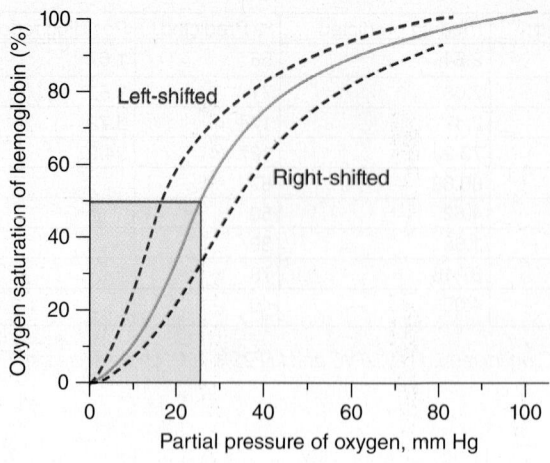

Figure 110-11 *Oxyhemoglobin dissociation curve.*

TABLE 110-2 **Causes of Hypoxemia**

	ABG	A-a gradient
Hypoventilation	Elevated pCO_2 and decreased PAO_2	A-a gradient is normal. The hypoxemia can be easily corrected with small amounts of O_2
V/Q mismatch	Occurs normally and as part of many disease processes. The PAO_2 is decreased. The pCO_2 can be normal, low, or elevated	The A-a gradient is increased and only a small to moderate amount of O_2 will correct the hypoxemia
Right to left shunt	Anatomic and physiologic The PAO_2 is decreased. The pCO_2 can be normal, low, or elevated	The A-a gradient is increased. The hypoxia can be difficult to correct with O_2
Diffusion limited	Interstitial disease. The PAO_2 is decreased. The pCO_2 can be normal, low, or elevated	The A-a gradient is increased

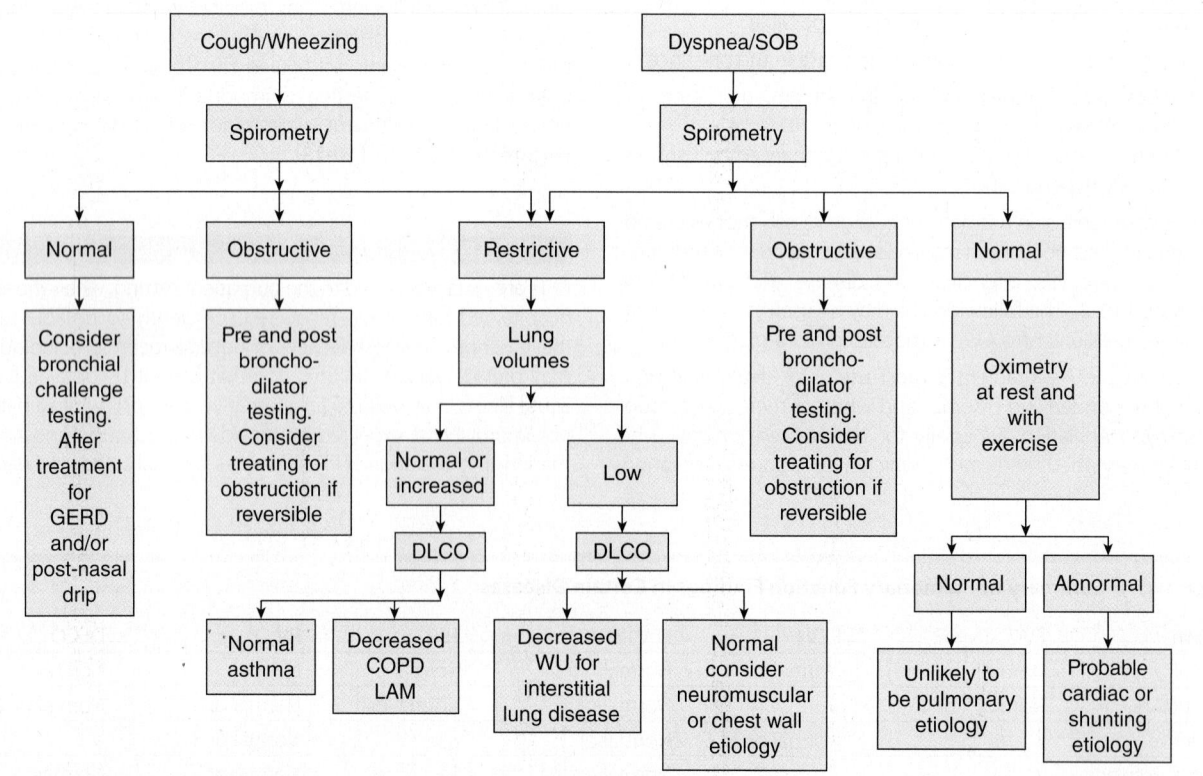

Figure 110-12 *Assessment of symptoms.*

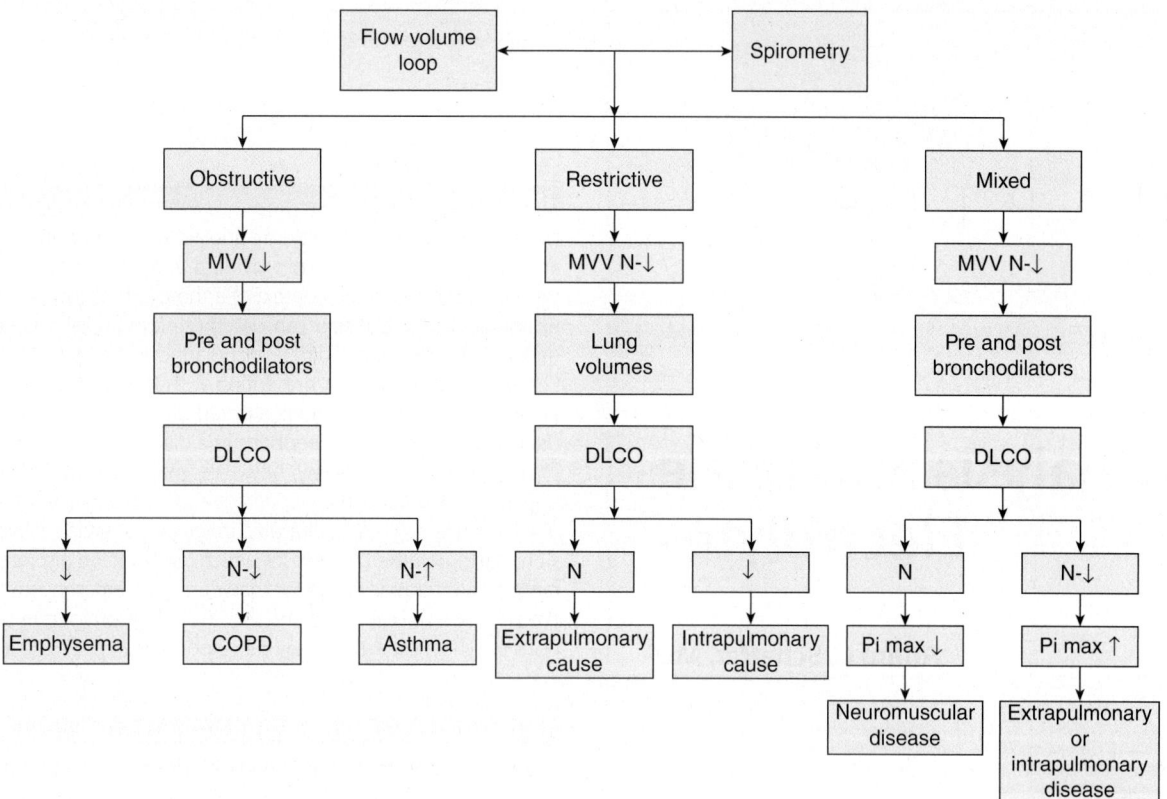

Figure 110-13 *Evaluation of abnormal PFTs.*

nonsmoking control subjects based on age, height, and gender. The standards may vary from laboratory to laboratory. Most "normal" values are greater than 80% with the exception of the FEV1/FVC ratio, which is normally predicted to be around 75% to 80%. There is no specific spirometric or lung volume pattern associated with pulmonary vascular disease; hence, in general, no matter what criteria are used to define normal lung function, it is important to take all of the data into account to determine if a pattern is consistently present.

SUGGESTED READINGS

Crapo RO, Morris AH, Gardner RM. Reference spirometric values using techniques and equipment that meet ATS recommendations. *Am Rev Respir Dis.* 1981;123:659.

Crapo RO. Pulmonary function testing. *N Engl J Med.* 1994;331:25.

Gass GD, Olsen GN. Preoperative pulmonary function testing to predict postoperative morbidity and mortality. *Chest.* 1986;89:127.

Guntupalli KK, Bandi V, Sirgi C, et al. Usefulness of flow volume loops in emergency center and ICU settings. *Chest.* 1997;111:481.

Hansen JE. Arterial blood gases. *Clin Chest Med.* 1989;10:227.

CHAPTER 111

Urinalysis and Urine Electrolytes

Adam C. Schaffer, MD

Key Clinical Questions

1 How does interpretation of the urinalysis and urine electrolytes guide clinical decision making?

2 What are the limitations of urinalysis and urine electrolytes?

3 When is it helpful to measure the urine osmolality, the fractional excretion of sodium and the fractional excretion of urea?

INTRODUCTION

Urine tests can be a valuable diagnostic tool, especially since they are easily obtained and can provide a wide range of information. When interpreted in the context of a thorough history and physical examination, the clinician can use the information obtained from urinalysis to narrow the differential diagnosis and guide treatment. For example, in a patient presenting with kidney disease, the presence of significant proteinuria and red blood cell (RBC) casts in the urine suggests glomerulonephritis as a diagnosis.

This chapter will review how the major components of the urinalysis—including the appearance of the urine, urine dipstick, urine microscopy, and urine electrolytes—can guide clinical decision making. Unlike blood tests, which usually have discrete normal ranges, the "normal" range for many urine parameters is a function the patient's clinical status and any metabolic or volume perturbations to which the kidney may be responding.

URINE COLOR AND APPEARANCE

The gross appearance of the urine may provide clues about volume status, source of bleeding, presence of infection, and medication use, as shown in **Table 111-1**.

Centrifugation of the urine can help distinguish hematuria from other causes. A red-colored pellet suggests intact RBCs, whereas a red supernatant may suggest myoglobinuria or hemoglobinuria. The gross appearance of the urine may suggest significant proteinuria (foamy urine) or lipiduria (greasy urine). Foul-smelling urine may suggest infection. Sweet-smelling urine raises the possibility of ketonuria.

URINE REAGENT STRIP (DIPSTICK) TESTING

■ SPECIFIC GRAVITY (AND URINE OSMOLALITY)

Specific gravity, which is measured using a urine dipstick, is the density of the urine relative to the density of water. This is a measure of the concentration of the urine. A related measure of urine concentration that is measured by the laboratory is urine osmolality, which the concentration of particles per kilogram of solution. Assessing the concentration of the urine is important when diagnosing primary polydipsia as the cause of hyponatremia and evaluating a patient with polyuria. The usual physiologic range of urine specific gravity is 1.005 to 1.030 and for urine osmolality is 50 to 1200 mOsmol/kg. Unlike osmolality, which measures the solute concentration and is not a function of the size of the particles in solution, specific gravity is affected by the mass of the particles in the urine. Therefore, large particles that are excreted in the urine, such as radiocontrast material, can cause an increase in the specific gravity. Nonetheless, under most conditions, urine specific gravity usually correlates fairly well with osmolality. Urine specific gravities of 1.001, 1.010, and 1.030 are approximately equal to a urine osmolality of 40, 320, and 1200 mOsmol/kg, respectively. In addition to the presence of radiocontrast in the urine, glucose and protein in the urine can also elevate the specific gravity.

TABLE 111-1 Urine Appearance and Associated Medications and Conditions

Appearance of Urine	Associated Medications	Associated Conditions
Pale yellow		Volume replete
Dark yellow		• Volume depleted • Jaundice
Orange	• Rifampin • Phenazopyridine (Pyridium)	
Red	• Senna • Doxorubicin Phenytoin	• Hematuria (sediment*) • Hemoglobinuria (supernatant*) • Myoglobinuria (supernatant*) • Porphyrins • Ingestion of beets • Ingestion of rhubarb • Ingestion of blackberries
Brown	• Metronidazole • Levodopa	Povidone-iodine contamination
Blue-green	• Indomethacin • Amitriptyline • Triamterene • Propofol (depending on pH)	*Pseudomonas aeruginosa* urinary tract infection
Milky	• Propofol (depending on pH)	Lipiduria Chyluria
Foamy		Proteinuria

*Upon centrifugation.

Data from Foot CL, Fraser JF. Uroscopic rainbow: modern matula medicine. *Postgrad Med J*. 2006;82:126-129; Fogazzi GB, Verdesca S, Garigali G. Urinalysis: core curriculum 2008. *Am J Kidney Dis*. 2008;51:1052-1067; and Raymond JR, Yarger WE. Abnormal urine color: differential diagnosis. *South Med J*. 1988;81:837-841.

PRACTICE POINT

• Clinically, urine osmolality—and so also urine specific gravity—will be elevated in cases in which antidiuretic hormone (ADH) is elevated.

• A urine osmolality > 100 mOsm/kg is inappropriate as in SIADH; the urine osmolality frequently will be higher than this and typically higher than the serum osmolality.

• A urine osmolality < 100 mOsm/kg in a hyponatremic patient suggests primary polydipsia.

• Patients with acute kidney injury (AKI) from acute tubular necrosis (ATN) will usually have a urine osmolality < 400 mOsm/kg due to compromise of the kidney's urinary concentrating ability.

• Patients with prerenal azotemia will usually have a urine osmolality that is >500 mOsm/kg.

ADH can be elevated appropriately in cases of hypovolemia, or inappropriately, as in cases of the syndrome of inappropriate antidiuretic hormone secretion (SIADH). In SIADH, the urine osmolality may not be absolutely high, but it is inappropriately high relatively speaking, given that the adaptive response to hyponatremia is to excrete free water.

In cases of polyuria, the urine osmolality can help distinguish a water diuresis from a solute diuresis. A urine osmolality >300 mOsm/kg is consistent with a solute diuresis, whereas a urine osmolality <150 mOsm/kg is suggestive of a water diuresis. In cases of a higher urine osmolality (>300 mOsm/kg) suggestive of a solute diuresis, possible causes include high salt intake, glucosuria, or mannitol. In cases of low urine osmolality (<150 mOsm/kg) suggesting a water diuresis, possible causes include diabetes insipidus or excessive water intake, as with primary polydipsia.

■ HEMATURIA

The initial test commonly used to evaluate for hematuria is the urine dipstick. The different cutoffs used for hematuria account, in part, for the different test characteristic numbers. Urine dipsticks have sensitivities of 91% to 100%, using 2 to >5 RBCs per high power field (HPF) on sediment microscopy as the reference standard. Urine dipsticks have specificities in the 65% to 99% range, using microscopy as the reference standard. There are a number of conditions that can cause positive results for hematuria in the absence of hematuria. Myoglobinuria and hemoglobinuria, from rhabdomyolysis and hemolysis, respectively, cause urine dipsticks to register positive for heme. The absence of RBCs on urine microscopy in the setting of a urine dipstick positive for heme suggests the possibility of rhabdomyolysis or hemolysis. In one series by Grover et al, examining patients with rhabdomyolysis, a urine dipstick showing moderate or large urine heme in the absence of hematuria had a sensitivity of 81% for detecting creatine kinase levels greater than 10,000 U/L. Another condition that can lead to false positives for heme on urine dipsticks includes some bacteria with pseudoperoxidase activity, such as certain species of staphylococci and streptococci. Ascorbic acid can result in false negative results for glucosuria due to its inhibition of the glucose oxidase reaction.

It is important to consider that urine dipsticks and microscopy signal hematuria, not necessarily disease. Epidemiological studies looking at the proportion of patients with hematuria who have serious disease have yielded inconsistent results, with rates of significant urologic disease among patients with microscopic hematuria varying from 17% to 56% in different studies. Mariani et al, evaluated 1000 consecutive adults with asymptomatic hematuria (microscopic or macroscopic). Of these patients, 9.1% had what was deemed a life-threatening condition, most commonly bladder transitional cell cancer or renal adenocarcinoma. Significant findings, such as nephrolithiasis or cystitis, occurred in 22.8% of patients. In 56.4% of patients, only insignificant findings resulted from the evaluation of their hematuria, and in the remaining 11.7% of patients, no diagnosis to explain the hematuria was obtained. The authors of this study assert that there is no lower limit to the number of RBCs in the urine that rules out serious underlying disease, given that 18.6% of patients with life-threatening conditions produced a urinalysis with fewer than three RBCs/HPF within 6 months of the cancer diagnosis.

Unexplained hematuria requires further evaluation. The most important goal of this further evaluation is to assess for the presence of cancer affecting the kidney or urinary tract. In general, patients with unexplained hematuria should undergo imaging, such as a CT scan, urine cytology testing, and also be referred to a urologist for cystoscopy and further evaluation.

Detection of hematuria should prompt the clinician to do the following:

- Review any prior abdominal imaging performed in the hospital to assess for the presence of cancer affecting the kidney or urinary tract.
- Consider whether the patient had any procedures including Foley catheter insertion that might account for hematuria.
- Include information about the presence of hematuria in the discharge summary, and communicate this information to the patient's PCP. In the majority of patient in whom hematuria is detected while in the hospital, further evaluation for this hematuria will occur as an outpatient, and so the need for this workup must conveyed to the patient's PCP.
- Inform the patient of the hematuria and further evaluation is required.

■ PROTEINURIA

Most urine dipsticks can detect albumin concentrations of 200 to 300 mg/L. There are semi-quantitative assays, usually reporting the amount of proteinuria as 1+ to 3+ or 4+. A limitation of urine dipstick testing for albuminuria is that it is affected by the concentration of the urine sample being used. Using the albumin-to-creatinine ratio as the reference standard, a study of 310 general hospitalized patients by Pugia et al, found that dipstick assessment for albuminuria had a positive predictive value of 82% and a negative predictive value of 99%. The authors concluded dipstick testing had good agreement with the quantitative albumin-to-creatinine ratio. Microalbuminuria refers to urinary albumin excretion of 30 to 300 mg/d. Microalbuminuria is commonly used to detect early renal disease in diabetic patients, and so is mainly used in the primary care setting rather than the inpatient setting.

Urine dipsticks are insensitive for nonalbumin proteinuria, such as the light chains that may occur in the setting of myeloma kidney (Bence Jones proteins).

- When there is a suspicion of nonalbumin proteinuria, other methods of assessing for proteinuria besides a dipstick should be used, such as a spot urine protein-to-creatinine ratio performed by the clinical laboratory.

Sulfosalicylic acid, when added to a urine sample, will cause turbidity in the presence of protein in the urine (both albumin and nonalbumin protein) and so can be used as a point-of-care test to detect nonalbumin proteinuria (with a reported sensitivity of 76.7% and specificity of 75.4%).

Measuring proteinuria is an important part of evaluating any patient with known or suspected renal disease, as heavy proteinuria can signal significant glomerular disease, or can be a consequence of renal involvement in a systemic disease, such as multiple myeloma. Proteinuria >150 mg/d is considered abnormal. When proteinuria exceeds 3.5 g/d, it is in the nephrotic range, and when accompanied by hypoalbuminemia, edema, and hyperlipidemia, full-blown nephrotic syndrome is present. Not only is the level of proteinuria diagnostically useful, but it is also a risk factor for progression of chronic kidney disease in both diabetic and nondiabetic patients. There are three different methods of assessing for proteinuria: (1) a 24-hour urine collection for protein excretion; (2) a spot (ie, untimed) urine protein-to-creatinine ratio; and (3) a urine dipstick.

The 24-hour urine collection, while often used as a reference standard, has a limited role in routine inpatient clinical practice. Under many circumstances, a spot urine can be obtained for a protein-to-creatinine ratio, which gives an estimate of the 24-hour protein excretion in the urine. Populations with a lower muscle mass—such as the elderly, underweight individuals, and women—are more likely to have a low urine creatinine. Consequently, a spot protein-to-creatinine ratio may overestimate the 24-hour urinary protein excretion in these populations.

One study by Lane, et al, which looked at 103 patients in a renal and hypertension clinic, concluded that as the level of proteinuria increased, the accuracy of the spot urine protein-to-creatinine ratio decreased, and that at levels of proteinuria above 1 g/24 h, the spot measurement was inadequately accurate, and a 24-hour collection should be used instead. The authors argue that the spot measurement is helpful in answering whether the patient has significant proteinuria, but if the exact amount of that significant proteinuria needs to be known (such as for following the effect of treatment), then a 24-hour urine collection should be used. Nonetheless, in the inpatient setting, a spot urine protein-to-creatinine ratio will in most cases provide the necessary information.

LEUKOCYTE ESTERASE, NITRITE, AND THE DETECTION OF INFECTION IN THE URINE

The urine dipstick features used to diagnose a urinary tract infection (UTI) include the presence of leukocyte esterase and nitrites. White blood cells (WBCs) on urine microscopy and an organism isolated on urine culture help confirm the diagnosis. Leukocyte esterase is an enzyme contained in WBCs, while nitrites are a product resulting from the metabolism of nitrates by certain bacteria. Bacteria that can convert nitrates to nitrites include *Escherichia coli* and other bacteria in the family *Enterobacteriaceae*. However, a number of important urinary pathogens do not produce nitrites, including *S. saprophyticus*, *Pseudomonas*, and enterococci. Certain factors can cause a misleading negative nitrite test on dipstick testing, including insufficient nitrates in the diet to be converted by the bacteria and a dipstick that has been exposed to the air for a prolonged period. It takes at least 4 hours for bacteria to convert nitrates to detectable levels of nitrite, and so this test may be negative in patients with UTIs whose urinary frequency does not provide adequate time for bacterial conversion of nitrates to nitrites. The presence of urine eosinophils or *Trichomonas* in the urine can lead to false positive results. Factors that can lead to false negative results include the presence of ascorbic acid, high levels of glucose or protein, and certain antibiotics, including cephalexin and tetracycline.

A systematic review by Hurlbut et al, of the test characteristics of dipstick leukocyte esterase and nitrite to detect UTI, which used >100,000 cfu/mL on the urine culture as the reference standard, found that considering either positive leukocyte esterase or positive nitrite to denote a positive test for UTI yielded the greatest area under the ROC curve. Considering either leukocyte esterase positive or nitrite positive to be a positive result for UTI yielded a sensitivity of 75% and a specificity of 82%. This review and other reviews concluded that in the setting of a high clinical suspicion, a dipstick negative for both leukocyte esterase and nitrite is not sufficient to exclude a UTI. A study of 408 women by Little et al, found similar results. Using either a dipstick positive for nitrite or positive for both leucocytes and blood to be a positive test yielded a sensitivity of 77% and a specificity of 70%, using culture data as the reference standard.

In assessing the relationship between the degree of pyuria and likelihood of bacteriuria, measuring the leukocyte excretion rate is the most diagnostically useful. However, this method is cumbersome, and so the method employed in most clinical laboratories to measure pyuria is counting the number of WBCs per HPF in the centrifuged urine sample. A common break point used by clinical laboratories is ≥10 WBCs/HPF as being abnormal pyuria, though the break points used by clinical laboratories vary. In general, the higher the number of WBCs, the more likely there is to be significant bacteriuria. One older study by Holm et al, found that among patients with 0 to 1 WBCs/HPF, 3% of patients had urine cultures with >10³ bacteria/mL, whereas among patients with >9 WBCs/HPF, 87% had >10³ bacteria/mL urine. A more recent study by Al-Daghistani et al, examining the diagnostic characteristics of pyruia, using >50,000 cfu/mL as representing a true UTI, found that of ≥10 WBCs/HPF has a sensitivity of 34% and a specificity of 86.5%. Pyuria on microscopy, as currently performed by most clinical laboratories, cannot by itself be used to make the diagnosis of a UTI, and must be used in conjunction with other diagnostic information. Pyuria with a negative urine culture ("sterile pyuria") can be seen in the setting of partially treated UTIs and UTIs due to *Chlamydia trachomatis*, *Ureaplasma urealyticum*, and *Mycobacterium tuberculosis*. Other settings in which sterile pyuria can be seen include polycystic kidney disease, urolithiasis, papillary necrosis, Kawasaki disease, and tubulointerstitial diseases.

The most commonly used break point for the diagnosis of bacteriuria is ≥10⁵ cfu/mL of urine. Some authors have suggested that it would be preferable to use a lower threshold, such as ≥10⁴ cfu/mL of urine to define significant bacteriuria, with other authors suggesting thresholds as low as ≥10² cfu/mL of urine. Three or more isolates each present in quantities of ≥10⁵ cfu/mL suggest contamination. A single isolate present in quantities of <10² cfu/mL is also a probable contaminant. Squamous epithelial cells seen on urine microscopy should raise suspicion of contamination.

PRACTICE POINT

- Assess for symptoms of a UTI in deciding whether antibiotic treatment is warranted.
- In pregnant women, in patients undergoing urologic procedures in which mucosal bleeding is expected, and in patients undergoing transurethral resection of the prostate, treatment of asymptomatic bacteriuria is indicated.
- Outside of these circumstances, treatment of asymptomatic bacteriuria is generally inappropriate.

The diagnosis of a UTI in patients with indwelling urinary catheters (Foley catheters) presents a challenge. In patients with indwelling urinary catheters, the association between pyruia and actual UTIs is weaker than in patients without such catheters. Therefore, in patients with indwelling urinary catheters, pyuria cannot be used to reliably diagnose a UTI. Moreover, many patients with indwelling urinary catheters who have UTIs may have minimal symptoms or be asymptomatic. According to a 2009 Infectious Diseases Society of America clinical practice guideline on catheter-associated UTIs by Hooton et al, a catheter-associated UTI is "defined by the presence of symptoms or signs compatible with UTI with no other identified source of infection along with ≥10³ colony forming units (cfu)/mL of ≥1 bacterial species in a single catheter urine specimen or in a midstream voided urine specimen from a patient whose urethral, suprapubic, or condom catheter has been removed within the previous 48 hours."

■ GLUCOSURIA

Once serum glucose levels increase above about 180 mg/dL, glucose will start to appear in the urine. The presence of ascorbic acid and bacteria may cause false negative glucosuria readings on dipsticks. Dipsticks that are left uncapped and so exposed to the air for extended periods may provide false positive glucosuria results. Glucosuria may occur in the absence of hyperglycemia (known as renal glucosuria) in certain inherited disorders and in patients with Fanconi syndrome, which is a syndrome of renal proximal tubular dysfunction. Causes of Fanconi syndrome include medications—such as antiretroviral drugs (especially tenofovir), aminoglycosides, ifosfamide, and cisplatin. As part of the syndrome of proximal tubular dysfunction, wasting of bicarbonate, phosphate, calcium, and amino acids also occurs. Elevated levels of these substances in the urine support the diagnosis of Fanconi syndrome.

Case 111-1 shows how urine dipstick and urine microscopy testing can be used together to help arrive at a diagnosis.

CASE 111-1

USING URINE DIPSTICK AND URINE MICROSCOPY RESULTS TO SUGGEST A DIAGNOSIS

A 68-year-old female with a history of coronary artery disease, hypertension, and hyperlipidemia presents with malaise, weakness, and diffuse muscle aches that have been present for the past 3 days. Medications the patient is taking include metoprolol, aspirin, atorvastatin, and gemfibrozil. She notes that her urine has seemed darker than usual, but she denies any dysuria, urinary hesitancy, or foul-smelling urine. She also denies any fevers. Her urinalysis shows a specific gravity of 1.014, and is negative for glucose, protein, leukocyte esterase, and nitrites. The urinalysis is positive for hematuria. Urine microscopy detects no RBCs or WBCs.

A urinalysis positive for hematuria with no RBCs found on urine microscopy raises the possibility of myoglobinuria from rhabdomyolysis or hemoglobinuria from hemolysis. In this patient with muscle aches who is on atorvastatin and gemfibrozil, a drug combination that is a known cause of rhabdomyolysis, this is the most likely diagnosis. It would be appropriate to start IV hydration with isotonic fluids while awaiting the results of serum tests, which can confirm the suspected diagnosis. This patient's serum tests showed a creatine kinase level of 15,125 U/L, confirming the diagnosis of rhabdomyolysis.

URINE MICROSCOPY

Urinary casts can provide important information corroborating a suspected diagnosis. In some cases, a careful examination of the urine sediment can point to a possible diagnosis that may not have initially been given prominent consideration. Urine that is to be examined for casts and other urinary elements should be fresh and should be examined as soon as possible after it is obtained. The procedure for preparing urine for examination is as follows. Ten milliliters of urine is centrifuged at 1500 to 2000 rpm for 5 to 10 minutes. Suction is used to remove 9.5 mL of the supernatant. The sediment at the bottom of the tube is resuspended in the remaining 0.5 mL of supernatant by tapping on the tube. Using a pipette, a single drop of the resuspended urine is placed on a slide and then a coverslip is placed on the urine drop. The sample should be examined under the low-power objective and the high-power objective of the microscope.

Not all casts are pathologic. For instance, hyaline casts can be a normal finding. The presence of most casts, however, suggests renal disease. The absence of casts cannot be used to exclude a diagnosis, as casts may be missed or may degrade due to specimen processing. In general, casts are composed of the diagnostic element within a matrix of Tamm-Horsfall glycoprotein. Hyaline casts, which are composed primarily of Tamm-Horsfall glycoprotein, are faint, nearly colorless casts that can be seen in patients without renal disease. Renal tubular epithelial cell casts, which are composed of renal tubular epithelial cells shed in the setting of tubular injury, are most commonly seen in patients with ATN. Granular casts represent a degradation product that can contain broken down renal tubular epithelial cells and also other cellular elements. Thus granular casts may be seen in ATN, but are nonspecific and may also be seen in other types of renal disease. A scoring system by Perazella et al, based on the number of renal tubular epithelial cells and granular casts was found to be useful in distinguishing prerenal AKI from ATN, as well as in predicting the worsening of either prerenal AKI or ATN. RBC casts are seen in pathologic states in which there is blood of glomerular origin, such as glomerulonephritis or vasculitis affecting the kidney. When reported, the morphology of any RBCs seen on microscopy can be helpful. Dysmorphic RBCs—particularly acanthocytes (ringform RBCs with blebs protruding off)—suggest the hematuria is glomerular in origin.

Leukocyte casts occur in pyelonephritis and acute interstitial nephritis, as well as in glomerulonephritis. Fatty casts, which contain lipid droplets and have a "Maltese cross" appearance under polarized light, may be seen in the setting of lipiduria, such as in patients with nephrotic syndrome. **Table 111-2** summarizes different casts and their clinical significance.

An important limitation in the use of casts as a diagnostic tool relates to the skill it takes to correctly identify urinary casts. One study by Tsai et al, comparing the performance of nephrologists with that of the clinical laboratory found that the nephrologists were more likely to identify renal tubular epithelial cells, granular casts, renal tubular epithelial cell casts, and dysmorphic RBCs, as compared to the clinical laboratory. The clinical laboratory identified more squamous epithelial cells than the nephrologists, raising the possibility that the clinical lab was incorrectly identifying other urinary elements, such as renal tubular epithelial cells, as squamous epithelial cells.

PRACTICE POINT

- Overall, nephrologists performed better than the clinical laboratory in deriving information from the urinalysis.
- Therefore, it is advisable to review a urine sediment with a nephrologist, rather than relying on the clinical laboratory, if the results of the sediment examination are crucial.

URINE EOSINOPHILS

Testing for urine eosinophils is frequently used to aid in the diagnosis of acute interstitial nephritis (AIN). Older data supporting the use of urine eosinophils in diagnosing AIN have not been borne out by more recent reports. A 1986 study by Nolan et al of 92 patients, focusing on the technical advantages of using Hansel stain rather than Wright stain to detect urine eosinophils, found that 10 of 11 patients with AIN were positive for urine eosinophils using Wright stain. Notably, however, eosinophiluria was also seen in cases of acute prostatitis, rapidly progressive glomerulonephritis, postinfectious glomerulonephritis, and acute cystitis. No eosinophiluria was detected among patients with ATN or acute pyelonephritis. Corwin et al, in 1989 reviewed 183 patients who had been tested for eosinophiluria, to evaluate the test characteristics of eosinophiluria in diagnosing AIN. The sensitivity (using Hansel stain) was 63% and the specificity was 93%. Eosinophiluria was also seen in two patients with UTIs, one patient with membranoproliferative glomerulonephritis, and in one patient with no diagnosis. The authors concluded that eosinophiluria was a good test for AIN.

Arriving at a different conclusion, a 1994 study by Ruffing et al, tested 148 patients with pyuria for eosinophiluria. Considering only those patients in whom testing for urine eosinophils had been recommended by a nephrologist because of a suspicion of AIN, the authors found eosinophiluria had a sensitivity of 40% and a specificity of 72%. Conditions beside AIN in which eosinophiluria was detected included glomerulonephritis and chronic renal failure. The conclusion from this study was that eosinophiluria alone was inadequate to make the diagnosis of AIN, and that both false positive and false negative test results are a problem. An influential 2008 study of the value of eosinophiluria in diagnosing AIN by Fletcher included 534 quantitative urinary eosinophil tests and reported a sensitivity of 25% and a positive predictive value of 3%. A common methodological problem in studies assessing the test characteristics of eosinophiluria for diagnosing AIN is that many of the cases of AIN were established based on clinical criteria, rather than the gold standard of renal biopsy.

The bottom line is that testing for eosinophiluria as a means of diagnosing AIN needs to be done with extreme caution, as its utility in diagnosing AIN is very limited. The presence or absence of eosinophiluria is not adequate to either establish or exclude the diagnosis of AIN. The results of testing for urine eosinophils must be viewed in the larger clinical context, and the presence of other clinical features typical of AIN, such as, in addition to kidney injury, fever, rash, eosinophilia, and arthralgias, need to be considered. Renal biopsy remains the gold standard for diagnosing AIN.

URINE CRYSTALS

Crystals, which are typically visualized in the urine using polarizing light microscopy, can precipitate in the kidney, resulting in AKI. For example, tumor lysis syndrome can occur with treatment of lymphoma or leukemia, in which cell death may lead to hyperuricemia and AKI as a result of the uric acid precipitating as crystals that obstruct the renal tubules.

Precipitation of crystals, due to limited medication solubility, is also an important mechanism of medication-induced AKI. The archetype is acyclovir, with one study finding nearly 50% of patients had an increase in their creatinine in the setting of receiving high-dose IV acyclovir. Principles of prevention of AKI as a result of medication precipitation include maintaining a high urine output, slowly infusing the medication, using caution in patients who have CKD, and adjusting the medication dose based on the patient's renal function. These same principles are generally applicable to other medications that may precipitate as crystals and cause AKI. Other culprit medications include indinavir, sulfonamides (such as sulfamethoxazole and sulfasalazine), and foscarnet. There have also been case reports of crystal nephropathy in association with ciprofloxacin.

URINE SODIUM AND OTHER URINE ELECTROLYTES

URINE SODIUM

The urine sodium and fractional excretion of sodium (FE_{Na}) are of particular value in helping to determine the etiology of oliguric AKI and in assessing a patient's volume status, such as in a patient with hyponatremia. However, as will be discussed below, these indices have a number of important limitations.

In oliguric patients, a urine sodium <20 mEq/L suggests renal hypoperfusion, as can occur with intravascular volume depletion. This condition is what is commonly referred to as a "prerenal" state. The low urine sodium results from the hypoperfused kidney responding by retaining sodium, so as to maximize intravascular volume. In the setting of ATN, the renal tubular cells are damaged, and so are unable to retain sodium, resulting in a higher urine sodium, usually >40 mEq/L. Urine sodium values between 20 and 40 mEq/L are indeterminate.

TABLE 111-2 Urinary Casts

Cast		Clinical Significance
Hyaline*		Nonspecific, may be seen in patients without renal disease.
Renal tubular epithelial cell†		Seen in cases of acute tubular necrosis.
Granular (fine)*		May represent degenerating renal tubular epithelial cell casts and so can be seen in cases of acute tubular necrosis. Also can represent other disintegrating cellular elements and proteins and so can be seen in a variety of renal diseases.
Granular (coarse)*		
Red blood cell*		Seen in cases of bleeding that are glomerular in origin, such as glomerulonephritis or vasculitis affecting the kidney.
Leukocyte*		Seen in pyelonephritis, acute interstitial nephritis, and glomerulonephritis.
Fatty*		Seen in cases of lipiduria, such as nephrotic syndrome. Has Maltese cross appearance under polarized light.

*Images courtesy of Agnes B. Fogo, Vanderbilt Collection.
†Image reprinted, with permission, from Fogazzi GB, Verdesca S, Garigali G. Urinalysis: core curriculum 2008. *Am J Kidney Dis.* 2008;51:1052-1067, copyright 2008, Elsevier.

A urine sodium >40 mEq/L may be seen in the following circumstances despite the presence of intravascular volume depletion:

- Diuretic therapy
- Renal salt wasting
- Metabolic alkalosis

In patients with metabolic alkalosis, the urine chloride can be checked instead of the urine sodium, as the chloride should be more reflective of the patients' volume status. A major limitation of the urine sodium is that it reflects free water handling in addition to sodium handling, which is why using the fractional excretion of sodium is generally preferred.

■ FRACTIONAL EXCRETION OF SODIUM

The fractional excretion of sodium (FE_{Na}) (%), calculated as [(urine sodium × plasma creatinine)/(plasma sodium × urine creatinine)] × 100, takes into account both filtration and reabsorption of sodium. In the setting of AKI, an FE_{Na} <1% suggests renal hypoperfusion (analogous to a urine sodium <20 mEq/L), whereas an FE_{Na} >2% suggests ATN (analogous to a urine sodium >40 mEq/L).

The FE_{Na} has a number of limitations. In patients with normal renal function with a moderate salt diet, an FE_{Na} <1% may be normal because, with a normal GFR, a large amount of sodium is filtered, and an FE_{Na} <1% may reflect the moderate sodium intake of the patient.

PRACTICE POINT

- The FE_{Na} should not be used in a patient with normal renal function, since it is unlikely to provide useful information about the patient's volume status in this setting.

Prolonged hypoperfusion itself may lead to ATN, and so a higher urine sodium. Thus an elevated FE_{Na} may represent a late consequence of renal hypoperfusion prolonged and severe enough to result in hypotension and ATN. There are certain clinical situations that are thought to be due to ATN, but when a low FE_{Na} often exists—including contrast induced nephropathy, AKI from myoglobinuria or hemoglobinuria, and glomerulonephritis. In patients with cirrhosis, congestive heart failure, and sepsis, the FE_{Na} may be low, due to decreased effective circulating volume.

Another major limitation in using the FE_{Na} is that its accuracy diminishes in patients receiving diuretics, a treatment commonly used in hospitalized patients. A study of 99 patients by Pepin et al, looked at the performance of the FE_{Na} in predicting which cases of AKI were transient (<7 days, and so likely the result of renal hypoperfusion), as opposed to prolonged AKI (which is more likely the result of ATN) in patients on diuretics and in patients not on diuretics. The sensitivity and specificity of the FE_{Na} in predicting transient AKI in patients not on diuretics was 78% and 75%, respectively. On diuretics, the sensitivity of the FE_{Na} goes down to 58%, but the specificity is not markedly changed at 81%. The area under the curve (AUC) for the FE_{Na} in patients without diuretics is 0.83, whereas in patients with diuretics, the AUC falls to 0.75. It is worth noting that in patients receiving diuretics, a low FE_{Na} can be helpful, because patients with a low FE_{Na} despite receiving diuretics clearly have kidneys that are sodium avid, and so likely have renal hypoperfusion. However, in patients receiving diuretics, an FE_{Na} that is high is unhelpful, because it is impossible to distinguish whether the high FE_{Na} reflects the effect of the diuretics or the actual lack of sodium avidity by the injured renal tubules (as would be expected in ATN).

■ FRACTIONAL EXCRETION OF UREA

In response to the limitations of the FE_{Na}, the fractional excretion of urea (FE_{urea}) has been proposed as an alternative. Using the FE_{urea}

is physiologically appealing in this setting, because urea is reabsorbed primarily in the proximal portion of the nephron, and so urea handling by the kidney would be expected to be less affected by diuretic administration than would salt handling. The FE_{urea} is calculated by the same method as the FE_{Na}, with the urine urea substituting for the urine sodium, and the plasma urea (blood urea nitrogen) substituting for the plasma sodium. The breakpoint used for the FE_{urea} is <35%, which, analogous to the <1% breakpoint used with the FE_{Na}, suggests an avid kidney responding to renal hypoperfusion. Pepin et al, also examined the performance of the FE_{urea} in distinguishing between transient and prolonged AKI. This study found that the FE_{urea} did not perform well, even in patients on diuretics. The sensitivity of the FE_{urea} for predicting transient AKI in patients on diuretics was 79% and the specificity was 33%. In patients not on diuretics, the FE_{urea} had a sensitivity of 48% and a specificity of 75%. Overall, the test characteristics were less favorable for FE_{urea}, which has an AUC of 0.56 for patients not on diuretics and 0.57 for patients on diuretics. This compares to an AUC for FE_{Na} of 0.83 in patients not on diuretics and 0.75 for patients on diuretics.

In contrast to the findings by Pepin et al, a study by Carvounis et al, supports the utility of the FE_{urea} in the setting of diuretic use. In this study, 102 episodes of AKI were categorized as being due to either prerenal azotemia in patients who were not treated with diuretics, prerenal azotemia in patients who were treated with diuretics, or due to ATN. FE_{urea} performed the best overall, with a sensitivity of 85% and a specificity of 92%. The AUC for FE_{urea} was 0.972, while the AUC for FE_{Na} was 0.889. Among prerenal patients on diuretics, 89% of them had an FE_{urea} <35%, whereas only 48% of them had an FE_{Na} <1%. FE_{urea} and FE_{Na} performed similarly in prerenal patients not on diuretics, with 90% of them having an FE_{urea} <35% and 92% having an FE_{Na} <1%.

Given these conflicting data, the FE_{urea} should be used as a diagnostic tool with caution. Outside of the setting of diuretic use, the FE_{Na} is preferred. In the setting of diuretic use, the available data do not clearly support using one over the other. One approach is to use both and to obtain urine electrolytes at multiple time points, and see if this larger pool of data is congruent so as to support a diagnosis of renal hypoperfusion or ATN.

■ URINE ELECTROLYTES IN ACID-BASE DISTURBANCES

Urine sodium and urine chloride should, in theory, correlate fairly closely with each other, though one report by Sherman et al, found that a dissociation between urine sodium and urine chloride >15 mEq/L occurred in 30% of patients. Urine sodium and urine chloride will diverge in acute acid-base disturbances. In the setting of an alkalosis, a normal kidney will excrete the excess bicarbonate. In order to maintain electroneutrality, the anionic bicarbonate excreted in the urine by the kidney will be accompanied by cations, such as sodium. Therefore, in the setting of an alkalosis, an elevated urine sodium may be a reflection of the renal compensation for the alkalosis, rather than the volume status. With an acidosis, a functioning kidney should respond by eliminating excess protons in the urine, which it does by excreting ammonium. For electroneutrality, the cationic ammonium is accompanied by anionic chloride. Thus in this setting, the urine chloride may be elevated primarily as a reflection of the kidney's effort to compensate for the acidosis, rather than the volume status. Case 111-2 shows the use of urine electrolytes in a patient having episodes of emesis.

CASE 111-2

URINE ELECTROLYTES IN A VOMITING PATIENT

A 45-year-old patient, with a history of alcoholic liver disease, presented with multiple episodes of vomiting. Initial vitals signs included a blood pressure of 100/80 mm Hg and a pulse of 90 beats/min. Serum electrolytes were notable for a blood urea nitrogen of 53 mg/dL and a creatinine of 7.0 mg/dL. Urine electrolytes showed an FE_{Na} of 2.4%.

Given the history of vomiting, intravascular volume depletion leading to AKI from a prerenal state would seem to be a leading diagnosis. However, the FE_{Na} of 2.4% suggests ATN as a cause of the AKI. This case illustrates a limitation of the FE_{Na} and how it can potentially be diagnostically misleading. In this patient, even if he does become intravascularly volume depleted because of vomiting, this vomiting will lead to a metabolic alkalosis due to the loss of gastric acid in the emesis. The resulting metabolic alkalosis will lead to a compensatory excretion of bicarbonate by the kidney, and with the excretion of bicarbonate in the urine, there will be the obligate excretion of sodium in order to maintain electroneutrality. Therefore, in this patient who is volume depleted due to vomiting, the FE_{Na} may be high because the increased urinary sodium loss as a result of compensation for the metabolic alkalosis may more than offset the sodium avidity that would be expected due to the intravascular volume depletion. In a case such as this, the urine chloride may be a more helpful guide. The urine chloride in this patient was low (<10 mmol/L), consistent with intravascular volume depletion. The patient's AKI improved with IV isotonic fluids.

■ THE URINE ANION GAP

These same principles described above underlie the urine anion gap, which is calculated as urine ($Na^+ + K^+ - Cl^-$). The urine anion gap is an indirect measure of urinary ammonium excretion, since urinary ammonium is an unmeasured cation, and increased ammonium excretion in the urine is accompanied by increased chloride excretion in the urine. Therefore, as urinary ammonium excretion is increased, urinary chloride is also increased, and so the urine anion gap decreases, and will often become negative. One of the main clinical situations in which the urine anion gap may be useful is in a nonanion gap (hyperchloremic) metabolic acidosis, in which one wants to help distinguish whether the nonanion gap metabolic acidosis is from diarrhea or either a type 1 (distal) or type 4 (hyperkalemic) renal tubular acidosis (RTA). In a nonanion gap metabolic acidosis in which the kidney is functioning normally, such as in a patient with diarrhea, the kidney will respond by increasing ammonium production, and so the urine anion gap will be negative. In one series of patients with diarrhea described by Batlle, et al, the average urine anion gap was –20. In a nonanion gap metabolic acidosis caused by either a type 1 or type 4 RTA, the defect is in the kidney, and so it will not be able to mount an appropriate increase

in ammonium excretion in response to the acidosis, and so the urine anion gap will be positive. Conditions that can render the urine anion gap less reliable include excretion of other unmeasured anions in the urine, such as ketoacids or lactic acid, and in certain types of dietary intake, such as cereals that provide chloride without Na^+ or K^+.

URINE TESTING IN THE DIFFERENTIAL DIAGNOSIS OF ACUTE KIDNEY INJURY

The results of the urinalysis and other urine testing can, in conjunction with the clinical picture, help elucidate the cause of AKI in hospitalized patients. Particularly in cases in which both prerenal and postrenal causes of AKI have been determined to be less likely, the results of urine tests can help distinguish among intrarenal causes of AKI—such as ATN, AIN, and glomerulonephritis. In ATN, the tubular cells are damaged and so are unable to reabsorb sodium, so an $FE_{Na} > 2\%$ (and an $FE_{urea} > 50\%$) would be expected, along with minimal proteinuria and muddy brown casts in the urine sediment. Most cases of AIN have only low-level proteinuria, except in cases of NSAID-induced AIN, which commonly involves nephrotic-range proteinuria. AKI from glomerulonephritis is characterized by elevated levels of proteinuria, RBC casts, and an FE_{Na} that is typically low. The use of urinary parameters in diagnosing AKI is summarized in **Table 111-3**.

URINARY BIOMARKERS

Multiple investigations have been undertaken with the goal of finding urinary biomarkers that could herald the onset of AKI prior to an increase in the serum creatinine, analogous to how serum troponins are used in cardiology for early identification of cardiac ischemia. Among the most studied urinary biomarkers for AKI are neutrophil gelatinase-associated lipocalin, and interleukin 18. Though these and other urinary biomarkers for AKI have performed well in some individual studies and in certain populations, none is expected to soon be widely used in clinical practice. Some of the reasons that these urinary biomarkers remain limited to investigational use are that they have performed well mainly in very specific situations (such as postcardiac bypass pediatric patients) and because many are confounded by the presence of pre-existing CKD.

CONCLUSION

All the urinary parameters discussed in this chapter have limitations. However, when taken together, these parameters can be very useful in arriving at a diagnosis. Beyond this use, rinary tests can assist in determining the cause of AKI, identifying the cause of hyponatremia, diagnosing rhabdomyolysis, and determining the etiology of an acid-base disturbance. Considering the relatively low cost and ease

TABLE 111-3 Urinalysis and Urine Electrolyte Findings in AKI

Etiology of ARF	Urine Na (mEq/L)	FE_{Na}	FE_{Urea}	Proteinuria	Urine Sediment
Prerenal	<20	<1%	<35%	Minimal	Bland
Intrarenal					
ATN	>40	>2%	>50%	Minimal	Granular casts
AIN	Variable	Variable	Variable	Variable	Eosinophils
GN	<20	<1%	<35%	>150 mg/d	RBC casts
Postrenal	Variable	Variable	Variable	Minimal	Bland or RBCs

AKI, acute kidney injury; ATN, acute tubular necrosis; AIN, acute interstitial nephritis; GN, glomerulonephritis.
Adapted from Albright RC Jr. Acute renal failure: a practical update. *Mayo Clin Proc.* 2001;76:67-74; Singri N, Ahya SN, Levin ML. Acute renal failure. *JAMA.* 2003;289:747-751; Weisbord SD, Palevsky PM. Acute renal failure in the intensive care unit. *Semin Resp Crit Care Med.* 2006;27:262-273; and Michel DM, Kelly CJ. Acute interstitial nephritis. *J Am Soc Nephrol.* 1998;9:506-515.

of obtaining most urinary tests, they are an important, and often overlooked, means to obtain important diagnostic information.

Evidence base and literature

Mariani AJ, Mariani MC, Macchioni C, Stams UK, Hariharan A, Moriera A. The significance of adult hematuria: 1,000 hematuria evaluations including a risk-benefit and cost-effectiveness analysis. *J Urol.* 1989;141(2):350-355.

Lane C, Brown M, Dunsmuir W, Kelly J, Mangos G. Can spot urine protein/creatinine ratio replace 24 h urine protein in usual clinical nephrology? *Nephrology.* 2006;11(3):245-249.

Pugia MJ, Wallace JF, Lott JA, et al. Albuminuria and proteinuria in hospitalized patients as measured by quantitative and dipstick methods. *J Clin Lab Anal.* 2001;15(5):295-300.

Hooton TM, Bradley SF, Cardenas DD, et al. Diagnosis, prevention, and treatment of catheter-associated urinary tract infection in adults: 2009. International Clinical Practice Guidelines from the Infectious Diseases Society of America. *Clin Infect Dis.* 2010;50(5):625-663.

Little P, Turner S, Rumsby K, et al. Dipsticks and diagnostic algorithms in urinary tract infection: development and validation, randomised trial, economic analysis, observational cohort and qualitative study. *Health Technol Assessment (Winchester, England).* 2009;13(19):iii-iv, ix-xi, 1-73.

Nicolle LE, Bradley S, Colgan R, Rice JC, Schaeffer A, Hooton TM. Infectious Diseases Society of America guidelines for the diagnosis and treatment of asymptomatic bacteriuria in adults. *Clin Infect Dis.* 2005;40(5):643-654.

Perazella MA, Coca SG, Hall IE, Iyanam U, Koraishy M, Parikh CR. Urine microscopy is associated with severity and worsening of acute kidney injury in hospitalized patients. *Clin J Amer Soc Nephrol.* 2010;5(3):402-408.

Perazella MA, Coca SG, Kanbay M, Brewster UC, Parikh CR. Diagnostic value of urine microscopy for differential diagnosis of acute kidney injury in hospitalized patients. *Clin J Amer Soc Nephrol.* 2008;3(6):1615-1619.

Tsai JJ, Yeun JY, Kumar VA, Don BR. Comparison and interpretation of urinalysis performed by a nephrologist versus a hospital-based clinical laboratory. *Amer J Kidney Dis.* 2005;46(5):820-829.

Corwin HL, Bray RA, Haber MH. The detection and interpretation of urinary eosinophils. *Arch Pathol Lab Med.* 1989;113(11):1256-1258.

Fletcher A. Eosinophiluria and acute interstitial nephritis. *N Engl J Med.* 2008;358(16):1760-1761.

Nolan CR, 3rd, Anger MS, Kelleher SP. Eosinophiluria—a new method of detection and definition of the clinical spectrum. *N Engl J Med.* 1986;315(24):1516-1519.

Raghavan R, Eknoyan G. Acute interstitial nephritis—a reappraisal and update. *Clin Nephrol.* 2014;82(3):149-162.

Ruffing KA, Hoppes P, Blend D, Cugino A, Jarjoura D, Whittier FC. Eosinophils in urine revisited. *Clin Nephrol.* 1994;41(3):163-166.

Carvounis CP, Nisar S, Guro-Razuman S. Significance of the fractional excretion of urea in the differential diagnosis of acute renal failure. *Kidney Int.* 2002;62(6):2223-2229.

Pepin MN, Bouchard J, Legault L, et al. Diagnostic performance of fractional excretion of urea and fractional excretion of sodium in the evaluations of patients with acute kidney injury with or without diuretic treatment. *Am J Kidney Dis.* 2007;50(4):566-573.

Batlle DC, Hizon M, Cohen E, Gutterman C, Gupta R. The use of the urinary anion gap in the diagnosis of hyperchloremic metabolic acidosis. *N Engl J Med.* 1988;318(10):594-599.

Nanji AJ. Increased fractional excretion of sodium in prerenal azotemia: need for careful interpretation. *Clin Chem.* 1981;27(7):1314-1315.

Sherman RA, Eisinger RP. The use (and misuse) of urinary sodium and chloride measurements. *JAMA.* 1982;247(22):3121-3124.

Vanmassenhove J, Vanholder R, Nagler E, Van Biesen W. Urinary and serum biomarkers for the diagnosis of acute kidney injury: an in-depth review of the literature. *Nephrol Dial Transplant.* 2013;28(2):254-273.

SUGGESTED READINGS

Espinel CH. The FE$_{Na}$ test. Use in the differential diagnosis of acute renal failure. *JAMA.* 1976;236:579-581.

Fletcher A. Eosinophiluria and acute interstitial nephritis. *N Engl J Med.* 2008;358:1760-1761.

Fogazzi GB, Verdesca S, Garigali G. Urinalysis: core curriculum 2008. *Am J Kidney Dis.* 2008;51:1052-1067.

Kamel KS, Ethier JH, Richardson RM, Bear RA, Halperin ML. Urine electrolytes and osmolality: when and how to use them. *Am J Nephrol.* 1990;10:89-102.

Mody L, Juthani-Mehta M. Urinary tract infections in older women: a clinical review. *JAMA.* 2014;311(8):844-854.

Perazella MA, Coca SG, Kanbay M, Brewster UC, Parikh CR. Diagnostic value of urine microscopy for differential diagnosis of acute kidney injury in hospitalized patients. *Clin J Am Soc Nephrol.* 2008;3:1615-1619.

Sherman RA, Eisinger RP. The use (and misuse) of urinary sodium and chloride measurements. *JAMA.* 1982;247:3121-3124.

Wilson ML, Gaido L. Laboratory diagnosis of urinary tract infections in adult patients. *Clin Infect Dis.* 2004;38:1150-1158.

SECTION 2
Radiology

CHAPTER 112

Introduction to Radiology

Francine L. Jacobson, MD, MPH
Sylvia C. McKean, MD, SFHM, FACP

Key Clinical Questions

1. What determines the ability of plain films to differentiate various substances and tissues? What are the limitations of a single radiographic view?
2. What are the limitations of ultrasound?
3. In addition to the five categories of density, computed tomography (CT) technology is able to detect what differences? What are Hounsfield units?
4. What are the limitations of magnetic resonance imaging (MRI)?
5. What are the advantages of nuclear imaging?

INTRODUCTION

The radiology examination that provides the required data with the least amount of radiation, expense, and need for extraneous follow-up supports the best practices of patient care. Although radiologic examinations have become vital adjuncts to clinical problem solving, they should not replace the process of developing a coherent problem list generated by the patient's concerns, medical history, and physical examination. The ordering physician critically contributes to the process of radiology interpretation not only by asking the right questions of individual patients, but by selecting the right examination and effectively communicating the questions that need to be answered by imaging to patients, technologists, and radiologists. The physician should request only those studies that will influence management, continually filter the results in the context of the patient, and ensure appropriate follow-up of abnormal and incidental findings. Practitioners must not only balance risks and benefits of a specific study for an individual patient but also be mindful of the impact of clinical decision-making on populations of patients even if the test is readily available.

Ever-expanding technologies will always require the expertise of radiologists in interpretation; however, physicians must have a basic understanding of various imaging modalities, their limitations, risks, and relative costs in order to select the right examination for a specific patient.

PRACTICE POINT

Framework for utilization of radiology

A golden rule for ordering imaging tests:

- Avoid ordering tests when the results will not impact patient care.
- Review tests previously performed to answer current questions.
- Order the best test to maximize quality, efficiency, and cost-effectiveness.
- Prepare your patient to minimize delays in getting studies done; in general, patients should be hemodynamically stable and able to cooperate as active participants in creating optimal images.
- Provide the necessary clinical information to radiology technicians to answer the question.
- Consult your radiologist when unsure about next imaging steps, the meaning of a radiology report, or the significance of a negative or incidental finding.
- Provide patient-centered care: inform, consent, educate.

This chapter will introduce general concepts for different imaging modalities, how to "interpret" the radiology report, and what to do about "incidental findings" in the context of care transitions and handoffs. Chapter 113 will review principles of patient safety—risks of contrast, radiation exposure, and gadolinium. Subsequent chapters will cover the application of specific imaging modalities.

CASE 112-1

ORDERING THE RIGHT IMAGING STUDY

A 64-year-old male with a past medical history of multiple myeloma, status post bone marrow transplant, and recent extraction of a molar heard a crack on the left side of his mandible accompanied by pain while eating. On physical examination, the patient had fever, moderate swelling, and tenderness of the left angle of the mandible.

A maxillofacial CT scan revealed a lytic lesion with a nondisplaced pathologic fracture at the site of the left posterior mandible in the area where the molar had been extracted. The differential diagnosis included osteomyelitis and multiple myeloma. A whole body bone scan did not show an area of metastasis or obvious involvement by multiple myeloma, nor was there evidence of osteomyelitis.

Would this second imaging study provide any new information that could guide management? Or how good is this second imaging study at identifying an abnormality?

To answer this question, the ordering clinicians need to select imaging studies in the context of the uncertainty that needs to be resolved in the patient in front of them and then integrate the clinical presentation with the reported new data. This process requires both a pathophysiologic knowledge of the potential causes of a problem and an understanding of the effect of new data on the probability of each potential cause. In this case, the clinicians should weigh the high likelihood of osteomyelitis (given the presentation and risk factors for infection) versus the much lower likelihood of recurrence of a previously treated multiple myeloma. Prior to ordering a specific imaging study, they should know the value of a positive test for increasing certainty about a diagnosis and likewise, the value of a negative test for decreasing probability of disease.

1. What is the likelihood that a whole body bone scan will diagnose the suspected diagnosis?

Even when lucencies within the bones are readily visualized by CT, a radionuclide bone scan may not identify multiple myeloma. A skeletal survey, which images most of the bones in the body while conserving radiation dose, is a better study to diagnose lytic lesions and other bone abnormalities. However, a bone scan can image metastases from solid tumors.

2. What is the likelihood that a whole body bone scan will diagnose an alternative explanation for the presentation?

In this patient the bone scan imaging was performed only 3 to 4 hours following injection of radiotracer. This approach is insensitive for the diagnosis of osteomyelitis.

The bottom line: for either diagnosis—multiple myeloma or osteomyelitis—a negative whole body scan would not change the likelihood of disease or put another way, resolve the uncertainty raised by the abnormal maxillofacial CT scan. Failure to understand this concept (which also applies to the use of blood cultures to diagnose osteomyelitis) resulted in overreliance on negative imaging and treatment delays.

On the sixth hospital day a positive WBC study in nuclear medicine led to surgical repair of the mandible. Pathologic examination of the resected pathologic fracture revealed osteomyelitis due to actinomycosis osteomyelitis, a soil organism that is radiographically possible to diagnose, due to the characteristic extension across bone, and through to the chest wall.

Given the high probability of osteomyelitis in this patient, what study should have been performed to confirm the diagnosis?

Three-phase bone scan augments the conventional radionuclide bone scan imaging at 3 to 4 hours with sequential images during and immediately following the injection to follow the tracer distribution in the soft tissues. It is possible to differentiate cellulitis from osteomyelitis by comparing radioisotope distribution in soft tissue and bone over time. The first "flow" phase provides a nuclear angiogram using two to five second images of a focal area of concern. The second phase "blood-pool" image is obtained approximately 5 minutes following injection. The third "bone image" phase is obtained after urinary excretion has decreased the amount of radionuclide in soft tissues.

Three-phase Radionuclide Bone Scan

Phase	Phase 1 Flow	Phase 2 Blood Pool	Phase 3 Bone Image
Cellulitis	Increased uptake	Increased uptake	Normal or diffusely increased
Osteomyelitis	Increased uptake	Increased uptake	Increased uptake

When clinical suspicion of osteomyelitis is high but three-phase bone scan is normal, a gallium scan may be considered. It is important to consult directly with the radiologist or nuclear medicine physician to correctly tailor the examination.

BASIC RADIOLOGY

Projection radiographs are viewed as the radiologist looks at the patient, placing the patient's right side at his own left side. Coronal cross-sectional images use the same orientation, generally presented, from anterior to posterior. Axial images are viewed from the perspective of standing at the supine patient's feet, again placing the patient's right side at the radiologist's own left side. Sagittal images are generally presented from the patient's left side to the right side, although this convention is not always applicable to all studies, particularly MRI. It is helpful to reconcile the position of the heart in determining whether sagittal images are on the right or left side of the patient's body. The Visible Human Project and the proliferation of web-based medical education materials now allow easy access to comparison images for anatomic identification in all three of these planes. Sophisticated image processing of volumetric CT data sets increasingly enables radiologists to provide data for surgery in the perspective of the surgeon. Surgeons have also learned to use conventional axial CT images to determine operability and plan specific surgeries.

The manner in which a standard radiological examination is performed may be modified to accommodate the inability of a hospitalized patient to have a more standard examination. Thus, a frontal chest radiograph may be made with the patient sitting up on a stretcher, sitting in a wheelchair, or lying in bed. In these instances, the radiograph will be made with projection from anterior to posterior rather than the standard erect imaging approach from posterior to anterior. The standing position facilitates obtaining radiographs in maximum inspiration. Gravitational effects are not as favorable in the supine position and other positions introduce a variety of variable complications. At minimum on an AP radiograph, the heart will appear larger due to magnification that varies with the inverse square law, whereby increasing the distance of the heart by a factor of 2 will increase the magnification by a factor of 4. This effect increases with increasing size of the patient, being particularly prominent when imaging an obese patient.

For a radiology examination to have maximal benefit in patient care, it should be performed at the right time. Sedation decreases cooperation and depth of respiration. Likewise, it may be better to presumptively treat an acutely tachypneic patient and obtain the diagnostic study after the patient is hemodynamically stable, able to lie flat, and breathe less rapidly for image acquisition.

PRACTICE POINT

- The acute hospitalization may not be the right time for obtaining many radiologic examinations. The patient participates in most imaging, whether by staying still, following breathing instructions, or moving through a series of positions. CT, MR, and fluoroscopic examinations that are not essential to address the immediate treatment of the acute process should not be performed when the images will most certainly be limited by uncontrolled respiration and superimposed acute processes. Clinicians rarely help patients by obtaining an inpatient CT or MR to either spare the patient the outpatient trip or to work up a nonacute incidental finding, such as an indeterminate subcentimeter pulmonary nodule.

■ PLAIN FILMS

The most fundamental undertaking of all radiology examinations is the largely noninvasive visualization of tissues that make up the body, with differentiation of normal structures from pathology. Projection radiographs detect five categories of density: air, fat, water (including soft tissue and muscle), calcium, and metal. The relative radiodensities of various substances and tissues will determine the ability of plain films to differentiate between them. For example, blood, muscle, and liver will have an almost identical medium gray appearance as will most solid or fluid filled organs and tissue masses, greater than air, but less than bone or metal. The muscular heart filled with blood will appear homogeneous relative to the air-filled lungs on both sides of it.

The radiologist is able to process two-dimensional data in three dimensions; focusing through various layers, perhaps starting with the posterior portions of the ribs and then the anterior, thinking about superimposed masses and the anatomic structures responsible for them. The lung is much thicker medially where it borders the mediastinum and inferiorly. There are more vessels superimposed on each other in the medial half of the lung field and in the lower half of the lung than the upper half. The radiologist notes an abnormal shadow by its proximity to a particular rib or interspace. "Fool's triangle" refers to the right cardiophrenic angle where many vascular trunks overlap due to the anteriorly placed middle lobe superimposed on the vessels of the posterior lower lobe. Novices in radiology interpretation may over read infiltrates in this area or note the most obvious abnormality, whereas radiologists systematically study each film looking at various structures in a deliberate order, concentrating on the anatomy of each, while excluding superimposed shadows of other structures. The integration of two orthogonal views provides the maximal localization of individual structures and abnormalities. A single radiograph will not be able to precisely locate a foreign body or support line. Bony fractures may not be apparent with a single film and a second film at right angles should be ordered to identify the lack of alignment and possible fragments.

Serial radiographs may be more helpful than more sophisticated imaging through the introduction of the fourth dimension, following the course of disease and physiology over time. Radiography can be performed at the bedside when the patient is unable to travel to the radiology department and can be made available very rapidly.

■ ULTRASOUND (US)

US imaging takes advantage of sonographic properties such as augmented transmission through fluid and textures that may be influenced by fat, blood vessels, and other structures. However, there are important limitations because ultrasound is stopped by air, limiting its utility in lungs and in the setting of gas collection throughout the body. Ultrasound cannot penetrate bone and many medical devices (such as joint replacement).

The Doppler shift refers to the change in frequency that occurs when a sound wave is reflected by moving blood. This change in frequency is proportional to the velocity of the blood flow in the vessel being sampled. Since World War II Doppler technology has evolved from crude, continuous-wave Doppler flow detectors blindly applied to the skin surface to color flow mapping systems. Duplex instruments combine pulsed Doppler techniques with real-time ultrasound imaging, made possible through the introduction of electronically steered, phased array transducer systems and the application of signal processing and display techniques for analyzing ultrasound echoes.

Duplex Doppler imaging with two-dimensional US provides anatomic information with pulsed-wave Doppler analysis to calculate a color overlay containing information about the direction and velocity of blood flow. Pulsed Doppler permits a smaller sample size, thereby permitting analysis of the arterial lumen without the associated vein. The spectral tracing is a quantitative depiction of red blood cell movement within a sample volume. A semiquantitative color encoding of the Doppler information is superimposed on the gray-scale, real-time image providing color Doppler imaging. The color depends on the mean velocity of flow and the direction of flow. Blue does not necessarily mean venous flow as seen in the reverse component of triphasic flow characteristic of normal arterial flow. Red does not necessarily mean arterial flow as seen in reflux of venous flow in incompetent veins. The hue reflects the relative blood velocity, so that fast flow just proximal to a critical stenosis may appear white whereas slow flow beyond the stenosis would have a deeper hue. Color duplex imaging increases the sensitivity of duplex imaging. Color Doppler imaging makes it easier to evaluate deep veins in obese or edematous individuals and to identify flow around a thrombus.

Doppler technology has largely replaced venography in the diagnosis of venous thrombosis involving the legs. Although noninvasive, safe, and less expensive, US may not always be able to image vessels for the following reasons using the 5 MHz probe: (1) the vessels too deep to be imaged due to overlying fat or edema, (2) iliac veins and the inferior vena cava obscured by overlying bowel gas and depth of vessels, (3) inability to visualize a segment of the distal superficial femoral vein in the adductor canal (isolated clot in this area unlikely), (4) the small caliber and multiple branches of the calf veins, (5) inability to definitively distinguish between acute and chronic thrombus, and (6) limited expertise of operator.

Duplex or color flow Doppler US may be used to confirm arterial perfusion of organ transplants and exclude venous thrombosis in portal, splenic, and renal veins. Doppler US indicates the direction of blood flow, which may be helpful in diagnosing subclavian steel or portal hypertension with altered hemodynamics or in the diagnosis of pseudoaneurysms or mesenteric ischemia. Doppler US may be used to characterize tumors, varices, or ectopic pregnancies that have characteristic flow patterns.

Pulse Doppler quantitates the degree of arterial stenosis. Real-time US may be able to characterize arterial plaque as calcified or soft. The reliability depends on whether the vessel can be imaged adequately, whether the vessel is straight or tortuous, whether there are tandem lesions, and on the skill of the sonographer. For vessels that can be imaged easily, the reliability of US is excellent. If the vessel is not well suited to imaging, the anatomic and hemodynamic information is unreliable, especially in inexperienced hands. The mere presence of a hemodynamically significant vascular lesion does not reliably prove that it is the cause of a particular symptom or that it is otherwise functionally significant.

Ultrasound guidance is being used with increasing frequency for central venous catheter placement, thoracentesis, and paracentesis. Owing to increased concerns about patient exposure to ionizing radiation, ultrasound is being used increasingly for novel applications including joint examination. It is actively being explored as an adjunct for bedside physical examination in ICU settings.

■ COMPUTED TOMOGRAPHY (CT) SCANS

In addition to the five categories of density, air, fat, water (includes soft tissue and muscle), calcium, and metal detected by plain films, CT scans are able to detect the differences between water and a variety of specific soft tissues including liver and kidneys and in the case of the brain, between white and gray matter. CT provides detailed anatomic images in which a variety of soft tissues can be recognized; the resulting basic transaxial images are the in vivo equivalent of transaxial anatomic pictures of a cadaver. State-of-the-art multidetector CT scanners are capable of acquiring ever-increasing numbers of individual slices of data at one time. Four-detector scanners image the chest in approximately 20 seconds, a practical time for patient breath holding. Readily available clinical models with the capability of producing 16 to 64 slices at one time can scan the chest in 10 seconds or less. Alternatively, very small structures may be studied using ever-smaller slice thickness. Along with cardiac gating, providing up to 320 slices at one time permits unprecedented in vivo evaluation of ultrastructure in lungs as well as the heart.

Specialized CT examinations are performed according to disease-specific algorithms. The reconstructed image thickness of the CT determines its sensitivity and specificity for identifying certain underlying conditions, based primarily on the size of the structure being assessed. For example, a PE-protocol CT requires thinner images than a venous-CT of the lower extremities.

Hounsfield units derive their name from the developer of the CT scanner, Nobel Laureate Sir Godfrey N. Hounsfield. The scale arbitrarily assigns water the attenuation value of zero, and air 1000, with the attenuation of other materials defined in relation to these set points. These numerical values of normalized x-ray attenuation define the gray scale of all CT images. The display windows highlight various structures based on the relationships between the underlying fundamental gray scale and the composition of various tissues in the body.

Intravenous iodinated contrast material commonly provides optimum delineation of vascular structures, particularly when they lie in close proximity to the pathologic entity. Thus, lung cancer staging is most often performed with IV contrast. Oral contrast is used to aid delineation of gastrointestinal (GI) tract structures. A routine abdomen/pelvis CT performed for nonspecific abdominal pain or cancer restaging typically employs both intravenous and oral contrast for optimal tissue characterization. Alternative routes of contrast material administration are also used for nonvascular examinations such as cystography and myelography. Nonionic contrast agents have replaced older ionic contrast agents as they produce fewer side effects. The use of well-functioning 20-gauge or larger peripheral IV is required for administration of iodinated contrast agents for optimal imaging, particularly for vascular CT applications that require high contrast flow rates. Whether in the GI fluoroscopy suite, CT fluoroscopy suite, or angiography suite, fluoroscopy provides physiologic information along with anatomic information but they are invasive tests, best preceded by appropriate subspecialty consultation.

Not all CT scans require IV or oral contrast material. For example, to diagnose the presence of a renal stone, a dedicated renal stone CT would not use intravenous or oral contrast as neither is needed to detect a high-density renal stone. High-resolution CT to assess interstitial lung disease is generally performed without contrast. Follow-up CT scans may be performed without contrast materials

depending upon the tissue contrast between the structures of continuing interest.

PRACTICE POINT

CT

- CT scans of contiguous body parts such as chest, abdomen, and pelvis are frequently performed together. The sequence of scanning and the volume of contrast material utilized will be selected to maximize scanning efficiency and answer the clinical questions posed.

- Separate doses of IV contrast material are generally not required. The same bolus of contrast material may be followed through the body with attention to circulation time and distribution of contrast material within organs to optimize imaging. Bolus tracking methods in modern scanners provide individualized selection of delay. The chest may easily be imaged during the delay required for liver enhancement on an abdomen CT scan.

- In many instances, the chest portion of the CT scan will be equally diagnostic with or without IV contrast enhancement. The chest portion of the CT scan should be performed prior to contrast administration to assess interstitial lung disease or detect calcification in very small lung nodules. Chest CT scanning may also be performed during the administration of IV contrast material for some contrast enhanced head CT scans.

To ensure that the CT scan is tailored to the clinical questions and patient-specific needs, speak directly to the radiologist before ordering the CT scan. The radiologist may suggest potentially valuable alternatives and prevent waiting for test results from the wrong test that cannot further clinical decision-making.

PET-CT is a lengthy examination that is often better suited to outpatient follow-up. Patients are asked to avoid strenuous activities the day before the examination and may be given special preparatory dietary instructions to consume a fatty meal the evening before the examination. The patient should be NPO for at least 4 to 6 hours. While PET-CT has become a central tool for the staging of malignancies, significant overlap in results between neoplastic and inflammatory processes limits the value of the study during hospitalization for acute illness.

■ MAGNETIC RESONANCE IMAGING (MRI)

MR uses very specific depolarizing pulse sequences to detect tiny differences in signal from soft tissues that may be otherwise indistinguishable. Gadolinium has paramagnetic properties that make it the most common contrast agent used for MR examinations. While inert, gadolinium does pose potential risk for nephrogenic systemic sclerosis (NSF), particularly in the setting of renal failure. MRI examinations are customized to the problem being evaluated. Coils used to perform the examination not only provide improved imaging but also control technical parameters such as field of view. The bore of the available MRI scanner, itself, may limit the size of patients who can have MRI. Larger bore and open scanners have decreased this limitation, but a patient may have to go to a special location to have such an examination.

Hospitalized patients are often unable to cooperate adequately to allow the full benefit of the MRI technology in their care. MRI examinations do not use ionizing radiation but may be quite lengthy, lasting 1 hour or more in duration. The request for wider coverage such as adjacent body parts is not easily accommodated in the same scanning session. It is therefore imperative to have a specific goal for the MRI from the outset. MRI and CT are equivalent for imaging lymphadenopathy. MRI imaging is by nature less than contiguous and should otherwise be viewed as complementary to CT imaging. In many instances, the patient will be better served by MRI as part of outpatient follow-up following recovery from the acute illness requiring hospitalization. The need for critical information determines the best study; MRI/MRA may more rapidly diagnose potentially surgical aortic disease such as aortic dissection compared with conventional angiography. Selected for the wrong reason, MRI will increase the stress on the acutely ill patient and delay institution of needed therapy.

Always inquire about patient claustrophobia before ordering the MRI examination. Patients often benefit from oral premedication; those with severe claustrophobia or difficulty remaining still in the confines of the scanner may require sedation with an anesthesiologist present during the scan. All patients should be screened for possible contraindications prior to scanning as routine practice. Contraindications to MRI include aneurysm clip, recent surgery (generally within 10 days) and incompatible cardiac pacing devices. Some patients who have metallic implants such as joint prostheses will experience unacceptable heating of the region that will prevent completion of the examination. This is sometimes quite specific to the location of scanning relative to the location of the implant. These effects vary with the field strength of the MRI unit. Relative contraindications also include cochlear implants and neurostimulators. In addition, patients who have potential to have a metallic foreign body in an eye, typically due to occupational or other machine shop exposure, may need to have radiographs or even CT scanning of the orbits prior to MRI. There is no known adverse effect of MRI on the fetus but the decision to scan during pregnancy should be made on an individual basis.

MRI exceeds CT for the multifactorial differentiation of fat and other tissue planes, properties that are particularly useful when studying the musculoskeletal system and in localizing boundaries of pathology, and fluids, including the differentiation of the various states of hemoglobin. In the brain, MRI images provide significantly more information than CT images, resulting in greater sensitivity for small and subtle lesions such as early brain metastases. The use of MRI for clinical problem solving is more apt to reflect the problem under consideration than a standardized approach. MR angiography (MRA) may provide high-quality images of many parts of the body often adequate to replace conventional angiography.

The use of MRI for direct acquisition of multiplanar, sagittal, coronal, and axial images has diminished with increasing availability of PET-CT as well as multidetector CT scanners that permit data to be acquired with voxels of equal dimension in all three planes, thus providing high-quality sagittal and coronal reformatted CT images. MRI imaging of calcium as a signal void is a particular pitfall in MRI imaging that highlights the complementary nature of CT for the study of bones and potentially calcified pathology.

NUCLEAR MEDICINE

Nuclear medicine images reflect the movement of tracer in the body as it travels and/or interacts with variably specific cells. Radiotracer may prove patency of central venous catheters, identify low-level bleeding otherwise difficult to localize, and evaluate function. For a patient with a normal chest x-ray, a normal perfusion scan alone still provides the finest exclusion of PE.

PRACTICE POINT

- Perfusion scan should be considered for exclusion of PE in a pregnant patient with a normal chest x-ray. With hydration and frequent voiding, the dose of ionizing radiation to the fetus can be lower level than from scattered radiation during a PE-CT of the chest.

Nuclear medicine is also used extensively for cardiac evaluation, even in the acutely ill. Tagged white blood cell scans may localize elusive infection in patients with unexplained fever. Likewise, three-phase bone scanning may pinpoint osteomyelitis. These are very worthwhile tests when chosen for the correct reason. Consultation with the nuclear medicine physician can result in performance of examination tailored to the specific pathophysiologic question, beyond the most exhaustive list of nuclear medicine studies. PET-CT has been adopted in many institutions as a nearly universal substitute despite availability of more specific physiologically-oriented nuclear medicine studies.

Radionuclide substances can increase the radiation dose received due to their persistence within the body following the imaging. Depending on the radioisotope, the clearance may range between hours and days with most eliminated via urine. Encouraging fluids and frequent emptying of the bladder are important ways to control the radiation dose. Allergic reactions have not been described and patients with renal insufficiency may safely undergo nuclear medicine examinations.

PATIENT PREPARATION

Fasting is required for safe performance of many imaging procedures. Overnight fasting is required for proper adhesion of fluoroscopically administered oral contrast agents for barium swallow and upper GI series examinations. Fasting is also required for interventional procedures. Common contrast agents require specific preparations. For iodinated intravenous contrast material, 4 hours of pretest fasting is preferred to minimize risk of aspiration because administration of contrast material on a full stomach significantly increases the probability that a patient will become nauseated and vomit while lying down in a scanner. In a true emergency, this requirement for fasting may be modified or waived.

Dietary changes and careful timing in the administration of oral contrast agents may significantly improve the value of radiology examinations, most particularly for patients who are ill enough to require hospitalization. Contrast agents are the drugs most frequently ordered by radiologists. These may be administered by mouth, feeding tube, intravascular catheter, or rectal tube. More than one may be used for the same examination. Oral contrast agents are selected for consistency and risk of leakage into lungs, mediastinum, and peritoneal cavity. Radiologists may also order or recommend hormones, beta-blockers, or steroids largely to support the use of contrast agents in specific radiology examinations. On occasion, particularly in ultrasound, water will be administered as an oral contrast agent to increase through transmission to the pancreas that is located behind the stomach.

COST

With limited resources and decreasing reimbursements of imaging, all physicians must consider not only the clinical value of tests they order in terms of efficacy and safety, but also cost. It may not be possible to determine the actual cost and charges for medical imaging due to differences in reimbursement based on separate contractual agreements, insurance policies limiting the number of reimbursable radiologic examinations to one each day, and bundling of inpatient costs under disease related groups (DRGs). Intensive labor by billing experts to capture reimbursement for the most expensive test performed each day and prolonged hospitalization due to test ordering or complications from imaging add to the costs of medical imaging. Although inpatient reimbursement will differ from patient to patient, nevertheless, clinicians should have a general awareness of relative costs of different radiologic tests. For example, automatic ordering of costly imaging studies such as MRI often fails to offer significant additional information that influences clinical management.

Cost-effectiveness analysis, which compares the clinical benefit a patient receives from an intervention compared to the cost of the intervention, is increasingly being applied to radiology testing.

RADIOLOGY REPORTS

Radiology reports provide the reason given for the examination, the technique with comments about limitations, findings, and an impression or conclusion. Increasingly, radiologists will communicate directly with the physician about significant findings and document this communication within the report. At the physician's request, a radiology report may be sent to the patient's primary care physician but this should not be relied upon as the primary documentation of communication with the primary care provider.

Maximizing the value of radiology examinations to acute patient care begins with consideration of prior radiology examinations. In an ideal world, the examinations would be reviewed directly within the new clinical context. Reading the reports, and even just recognizing what examinations have been performed, particularly the most recent prior radiology examinations can propel patient care forward without waste in time, resources, health care dollars, or patient radiation exposure. Many sophisticated and expensive radiology examinations have utility long after the original reason for performing the examination. This is especially true for cross-sectional imaging such as CT and MRI in which a single examination can serve as a permanent reference for anatomic variants that become confusing on projection radiographs in the course of acute care.

The review of a series of plain images over time with the radiologist may provide the most valuable pathophysiological data with the least amount of incidental findings for follow-up after hospitalization. The transfer of responsibility for follow-up of incidental findings unrelated to the admission is a crucial and often burdensome requirement for the physician who orders the radiology examination. It is important to document all such communication as directly as possible to avoid medico-legal disasters arising from lack of communication of findings such as potential lung cancer that could be treated successfully with prompt follow-up.

The busy clinician must always critically assess the data in the context of the patient. If the radiology report does not provide the best explanation for each constellation of symptoms and signs, the practitioner should consult the radiologist for a second look, perhaps to gain greater understanding for why a "false" diagnosis may be incorrect. In many instances this may require reviewing prior films whose interpretation may be altered by more recent events. In addition, without the proper clinical context, the practitioner may attach too much significance to incidental findings reported by radiologists who may not have received adequate clinical information to focus on a specific area or who do not want to overlook a potential malignancy.

A negative imaging examination in a patient with a compelling story and physical examination may not mean that a patient does not have the disease. The timing of the imaging study in the course of the disease and the limitations of the imaging study remind us that while positive x-ray findings may point to the diagnosis, incidental findings may mislead, and a negative study may prove less helpful. For example, the patient with miliary tuberculosis may not show the characteristic minute miliary densities in the lung parenchyma until several weeks after a presumptive clinical diagnosis has been made. An incidental pulmonary nodule may mislead the clinician into thinking that the underlying process for acute illness is lung cancer. Likewise, a PE-protocol CT may fail to reveal a pulmonary embolism if obtained weeks after the primary event or if there are technical limitations to the study. Yet concurrent illness may fail to explain the coexistence of pulmonary hypertension. At the same time, the clinician in consultation with the radiologist must be aware of the fallibilities of the imaging method for that same disease.

PRACTICE POINT

An important component of appropriate care in the 21st century

- Hospitalists play a central role in balancing the well-being of patients through their lifetimes (direct patient care) with prudent resource allocation. More judicious use of imaging studies that do not meaningfully contribute to patient management decisions is the responsibility of all physicians. The majority of interventions in patient care can be replaced by evidence-based strategies that are far more cost effective without diminishing quality of care. The ethical mandate is to ensure equally high-quality, affordable health services for all citizens.

CONCLUSION

The radiology chapters in this text are intended to provide the reader with a framework that may be applied over time, even as technology evolves, to clinical problem-solving relating to the diagnosis and treatment of the subpopulation of hospitalized ill patients. The results of any diagnostic imaging examination should always be germane to the patient's care during admission. Less expensive "low-tech" testing may provide valuable information regarding the next best imaging step to pursue. However, simple radiology films may falsely reassure the clinician that all is normal and may identify incidental findings that lead to more expensive testing. Ultrasound, MR, and nuclear medicine tests are more able to reveal physiologic function than CT and plain radiography. Optimal test ordering, therefore, requires asking the right question combined with an appreciation of the indications of a specific imaging test, the likelihood that a specific test will diagnose certain conditions depending on the patient population studied, the relative risks of different imaging modalities, absolute contraindications, and the inherent limitations of the testing, including impact of timing, body habitus, and observer variation among radiologists interpreting the same film. Clinicians should be able to inform patients about the indications, relative costs, preparation required, and risks. The input of radiologists will increase the value of the interpretation and often the rapidity with which the study will be interpreted.

SUGGESTED READINGS

Elgazzar, A. *Concise Guide to Nuclear Medicine.* New York, NY: Springer Publishing; 2011.

Hofer, M. *CT Teaching Manual: A Systematic Approach to CT Reading,* 4th ed. New York, NY: Thieme Medical Publishers; 2011.

Hofer, M. *Ultrasound Teaching Manual: The Basics of Performing and Interpreting Ultrasound Scans,* 2nd ed. New York, NY: Thieme Medical Publishers; 2005.

Westbrook, C. *MRI at a Glance,* 2nd ed. Hoboken, NJ: Wiley-Blackwell; 2010.

CHAPTER 113

Patient Safety Issues in Radiology

Srinivasan Mukundan, MD, PhD
Francine L. Jacobson, MD, MPH
Aaron Sodickson, MD, PhD

Key Clinical Questions

1. How do you estimate cumulative radiation dose and risk?
2. What is the latest theory about contrast-induced nephropathy?
3. What are the risk factors for contrast-related allergic reactions?
4. What are the risks associated with gadolinium-based contrast materials?

INTRODUCTION

One must not lose sight of the potential risks of short- and long-term adverse effects of modern imaging for an acutely ill patient whose hospitalization is one snapshot in time. There are risks associated with contrast administration, ionizing radiation, and the possibility of incidental findings generating additional studies.

CONTRAST MATERIALS

ORAL CONTRAST

Contrast materials may be administered intravenously, orally, rectally, and for problem solving, through a variety of support lines and tubes. The selection of a specific oral contrast agent is based on the risk for aspiration versus the risk for extravasation of the contrast material. Catastrophic aspiration requiring ICU admission may occur when oral contrast material is administered to a patient with achalasia or other significant risk factors for aspiration, especially while the patient is supine. Although inert, barium is permanent when aspirated into the lungs. Barium becomes concentrated as it passes through the GI tract and may contribute to constipation and obstipation, particularly at the concentrations administered for x-ray and fluoroscopic examinations. Gastrografin is more commonly used when there is concern for extravasation into mediastinum or peritoneal cavity. Although gastrografin will be reabsorbed, it may cause pulmonary edema due to its hypertonicity. Gastrografin contains iodine and should not be used in patients with a known iodine allergy, as a small amount is absorbed in the GI tract. Specialized contrast agents may also be used for purposes such as distending the bowel without obscuring mucosal enhancement.

IODINATED INTRAVENOUS CONTRAST

Low-osmolar nonionic contrast agents are almost universally used in current practice due to their reduced risk of fluid shifts and allergic reaction. In a labile patient, these risks may not be warranted for the increase in diagnostic information provided by the contrast enhancement. This is best determined in consultation with the radiologist, to explore how crucial the intravenous contrast is for the clinical question at hand (**Tables 113-1** and **113-2**).

RISK OF CONTRAST-INDUCED NEPHROPATHY (CIN)

Classic teaching is that it is best to avoid ordering multiple contrast studies in rapid succession and seek alternative imaging modalities whenever possible due to the perceived risk of contrast-induced nephropathy, defined as a rise in serum creatinine (usually between 25% and 50%) within 48 hours after administration of intravascular iodinated contrast. CIN was thought to be associated with higher morbidity and mortality as well as longer length of hospitalization. More recently, the very existence of CIN has been questioned. This is because the temporal association between contrast administration and decreased renal function is confounded by other treatments in sick hospital patients or even daily variations in creatinine levels in patients with chronic kidney disease. One large review of over 30,000 hospitalized patients, who did not even undergo contrast administration, demonstrated that over half demonstrated a 25% or greater increase in serum creatinine suggesting that this occurs at a high background level in hospitalized patients. Over the past 2 years, several large studies have attempted to account for this potential selection bias by using a propensity score adjustment and

TABLE 113-1 Conditions Associated with Adverse Reactions to Contrast Material

Risk factors for contrast-acquired renal failure

- Pre-existing renal insufficiency
- Diabetes with and without diabetic nephropathy
- Acutely rising Cr or other signs of AKI
- Hypertension, anemia, multiple comorbidities
- Urgent procedures
- Concurrent use of vasoconstrictive (nonsteroidal anti-inflammatory medications), nephrotoxic medications (aminoglycosides), and volume-depleting agents such as diuretics
- States of reduced perfusion such as hypotension, hypovolemia, cirrhosis, and congestive heart failure
- Large volume contrast load

Risk factors for contrast-related allergy reactions

- Previous anaphylaxis to contrast material
- Asthma
- Multiple medication allergies, including food or medication

propensity score matching; they demonstrated that CIN is much less common than previously believed. Four studies each with greater than 10,000 patients concurred that there was no evidence of CIN in patients with eGFR $\geq$ 45 mL/min/1.73 m^2, and that iodinated contrast was rarely implicated in patients with eGFR 30 to 44

TABLE 113-2 Patient Safety Measures for All Patients About to Receive Contrast

1. Is the study necessary? How important is the study? If contrast is not administered, will you obtain the information you need to make a clinical decision?
2. Does the patient have risk factors for contrast-induced nephropathy?
3. Does the patient have allergy to contrast and if so, which type?
4. Is there an alternative study that does not involve contrast?
5. Are there any modifiable risk factors?
   - Discontinue NSAIDs at least 24 h prior to the administration of contrast, particularly in patients at increased risk.
   - Discontinue metformin for 48 h prior to the administration of contrast if the creatinine is abnormal; if normal, discontinue and perform the study, if required, without delay. Metformin should be withheld for 48 h after contrast administration and not resumed until renal function is documented to be at least baseline.
   - Consider holding oral hypoglycemics on the day of the study as most patients will be npo, and prescribe replacement insulin as needed.
   - Hold diuretics on the day of the study.
   - Regarding ACE inhibitors, the data is mixed because there is increased risk as well as protective effects. Do not start ACE inhibitors on the day of the procedure.
   - Optimize volume status prior to the procedure.
6. Will the patient require another contrast study within 72 h?
7. If the patient is at increased risk for an ADE, has a discussion occurred with radiology to either reduce the risk or to consider an alternative study?

mL/min/1.73 m^2. In patients with eGFR < 30 mL/min/1.73 m^2, the studies were split while two studies implicated iodinated contrast as a risk factor for nephropathy while two did not.

Medical screening for factors associated with decreased renal function prior to contrast administration include: history of renal disease (including dialysis, renal transplant, single kidney, renal cancer, and renal surgery), hypertension, diabetes mellitus, and use of metformin or metformin containing drugs. If any of these are present, blood testing of serum creatinine should be performed. Recent data suggest that glomerular filtration rate (eGFR), calculated from the serum creatinine using the modified diet for renal disease (age, race, sex, SCr level, MDRD-4), more correctly identifies at-risk patients than serum creatinine values.

The risk of further renal injury may be decreased by volume expansion with isotonic fluids prior to and following contrast administration. Although sodium bicarbonate, N-acetylcysteine, diuretics (mannitol and fenoldopam) and other renal protective agents have been proposed, none have been demonstrated to be definitively helpful. Historically, radiologists have avoided administering iodine contrast agents to patients with multiple myeloma, systemic lupus erythematosus, urinary tract infections, or receiving medications such as NSAIDs, diuretics, amino-glycosides, and some cytotoxic agents. Routine screening for these in the general population has not been advocated as the risks posed by modern low-osmolar agents are considered to be low. However, many practices, especially in specialty hospitals such as cancer hospitals or university referral centers, do screen for these entities. Institutional guidelines may include renal function testing prior to contrast administration based on patient's age.

Administration of metformin (Glucophage) or metformin containing drugs, used to treat type II diabetes, may result in severe lactic acidosis in the setting of contrast-induced nephropathy. Metformin therapy is typically suspended for at least 48 hours following the administration of iodinated contrast material and resumed after the patient's renal function has confirmed to be at baseline. Adjustment of medications that are excreted by the kidneys may also be helpful.

Historically, patients with eGFR > 60 are considered by radiologists to have normal renal function for routine prescription of IV contrast. Both European and US guidelines now suggest that this level can be reduced to an eGFR $\geq$ 45 mL/min/1.73 m^2. Many practices reduce contrast dose for eGFR between 30 and 45, if the diagnostic quality of the scan may be preserved at lower contrast doses. If not, alternative diagnostic strategies should be pursued. When eGFR is less than 30, most practices avoid administration of IV iodinated contrast material, although this restriction is not absolute given a favorable risk-benefit analysis. Anuric patients with end stage renal failure on dialysis may receive IV contrast material when necessary if prior discussion with their nephrologists has taken place.

CASE 113-1

WEIGHING THE RISK OF CONTRAST

A 61-year-old female mentioned transient right-sided pleuritic chest pain to her nephrologist. When a CXR revealed a new moderate right-sided pleural effusion, he recommended a V/Q scan. Her glomerular filtration rate (eGFR) estimated at 32 mL/min might not preclude a contrast study according to hospital protocols but she had only one functioning kidney. Extensive changes of interstitial lung disease were also reported on CXR. Lower-extremity ultrasound did not reveal deep venous thrombosis.

Key question:

1. *Would a V/Q scan provide any meaningful information given her extensive interstitial lung disease, bronchiectasis, and bullous emphysema?*

This patient would most likely have an indeterminate or, perhaps, an intermediate probability scan. In a landmark PIOPED study, more than half of individuals with intermediate probability and indeterminate studies were found to actually have PE (pulmonary embolism).

2. *Would hydration and mucomist provide suitable protection for PE protocol imaging?*

Although hydration is definitely helpful, it may not provide adequate protection in patients with markedly compromised renal function. It is unlikely that mucomist would provide any additive benefit.

3. *Should such a patient receive hemodialysis following administration of IV contrast for CT if required for adequate diagnosis or selection of treatment?*

Hemodialysis will not adequately remove contrast material to conserve renal function.

4. *What are the risks of gadolinium in patients with compromised renal function?*

Gadolinium can no longer be recommended in patients with an eGFR below 30 mL/min/1.73 m^2 due to the risk of nephrogenic systemic fibrosis (NSF). If there is a high risk/benefit assessment, then class II agents only should be considered.

5. *Would there be any utility to performing MRI without gadolinium?*

MRI is infrequently used to address PE, and then almost always with gadolinium enhancement of vessels. MRI does not offer a practical solution for obtaining a diagnostic quality examination of pulmonary vessels in an acutely ill, dyspneic patient.

6. *What if this patient had pleuritic chest pain from active systemic lupus erythematosus (SLE)?*

If the patient has active SLE, it is possible that her renal insufficiency might become unstable, thereby further increasing her risk. This patient also had light chains in her urine consistent with multiple myeloma.

The bottom line: Standard hospital protocols would not have prevented this patient from undergoing a contrast study given her estimated GFR > 30 mL/min. Yet, the best balance of risk and benefit may preclude a valuable frequently performed imaging test. A search for diagnostic precision may subject the patient to risks that she would find unacceptable.

■ ADVERSE EVENTS DUE TO CONTRAST ADMINISTRATION

Acute events

Adverse events are best characterized as either "allergic-like" or "physiochemotoxic." Allergic-like reactions are similar to other "anaphylactoid" or "idiosyncratic" reactions in that they are not dose related and are of unclear etiology, although basophil and mast cell-mediated histamine release and IgE-mediated pathways have been implicated. These reactions run the spectrum from urticaria, edema, erythema, bronchospasm, to anaphylactic shock. Physiochemotoxic reactions are associated with dose- or concentration-related response that is related to chemo- or osmotoxicity of the agent. These reactions include nausea, vomiting, flushing, headache, dizziness, anxiety, hypertension, cardiac arrhythmias, cardiogenic pulmonary edema, vasovagal reactions, and rarely seizures. The distinction is important in that premedication is less helpful in avoiding physiochemotoxic reactions.

Mild physiochemotoxic reactions to contrast material include generalized warmth or flushing, a metallic taste in the mouth, and nausea and vomiting. These reactions are usually non–life-threatening, self-limited problems. The risk of vomiting in the supine position with a high probability of associated aspiration is the primary reason for fasting 4 hours prior to contrast administration. When this risk is less than the potential benefit, such as the finding of acute life-threatening injuries due to trauma, the examination will be performed without fasting.

Mild allergic-like reactions most frequently occur while the patient is having the examination. Acute bronchospasm, profound hypotension, and severe urticaria may occur during injection or within minutes of administration of contrast material and may occur in patients who have not been exposed to contrast material previously. Mild iodine contrast reactions present with signs and symptoms and are self-limited, without evidence of progression. Limited urticaria with mild pruritis and transient nausea with not more than one episode of emesis are most common. Rash, hives, nasal and facial swelling, and anxiety may be present. Treatment is limited to observation to confirm resolution or lack of progression. Patient reassurance is usually helpful. Hives may develop shortly following the examination and increase over the next 15 minutes. Observation or treatment with 25 to 50 mg of intravenous diphenhydramine may be indicated. Some centers include a dose of diphenhydramine 1 hour before CT scan in the pretreatment protocol for patients who have had contrast reactions.

Moderate signs and symptoms of contrast reaction are more pronounced and may include tachycardia or bradycardia, hypertension, generalized erythema, dyspnea, wheezing, bronchospasm, laryngeal edema, and hypotension. The clinical findings may require prompt treatment and careful observation for progression to a life-threatening event.

Severe signs and symptoms of contrast reaction are often life-threatening and may include severe or rapidly progressive laryngeal edema, convulsions, unresponsiveness, cardiopulmonary arrest, profound hypotention, and cardiac arhythmias. Prompt recognition and aggressive treatment are required. Patients who have had such reactions should not receive iodine contrast agents again even following pretreatment.

DELAYED REACTIONS

Delayed adverse reactions occurring 30 minutes to 1 week or more after the administration of contrast material are more likely following administration of an ionic contrast agent. The typical symptoms of delayed reactions involve urticaria or pruritis and are treated with antihistamines or topical steroids. Other manifestations resemble a flu-like syndrome and include fever, chills, nausea, vomiting, abdominal or joint pain, fatigue, and congestion. Recognizing these symptoms as a delayed reaction to contrast administration for CT or angiography may help limit the workup of the new symptoms in the hospitalized patient. Typically treatment consists of expectant management, and referral to an allergist may be helpful.

EXTRAVASATION OF CONTRAST

Extravasated contrast material may lead to a compartment syndrome if enough contrast material leaks into surrounding tissue. The use of well-functioning 20-gauge or larger peripheral IV catheters in the antecubital fossa for administration of iodinated contrast agents decreases the potential for extravasation of contrast material at the high injection rates required for optimum imaging, ranging up to 4 to 6 cc/s for vascular examinations. Immediate treatment includes elevation of the extremity and cold compresses. Initial assessment should include outlining the extravasation, evaluation of distal pulses and capillary refill, and performing a neurological exam of the extremity. Plastic surgery consultation should be sought and may be initiated by the radiologist.

■ PRETREATMENT FOR CONTRAST ALLERGY

Consulting with the radiologist prior to ordering examinations that may require iodine contrast agents is most imperative when the patient

TABLE 113-3 Pretreatment Steroid Comparisons

Corticosteroid	Route of Administration	Equivalent Strength Dosage	Premedication for Iodine Contrast
Prednisone	PO	5 mg	40-50 mg
Methylprednisolone		4 mg	32-40 mg
Medrol	PO		
Solu-Medrol	IV		
Hydrocortisone		20 mg	200 mg
Cortef	PO		
Solu-Cortef	IV		
Dexamethasone	IV, IM, PO	0.75 mg	7.5 mg

has previously had an adverse reaction to iodine contrast material. Anaphylactic reactions are the most serious and potentially life-threatening allergic reactions associated with the administration of contrast material. Patients with a history of anaphylactic reactions to contrast material are more likely to have a similar reaction on repeat exposure. Patients with a history of multiple food and medication allergies or asthma have double the risk of developing adverse reactions compared to the general population. No substantive data support the myth that patients with seafood allergy are at higher risk of developing allergic reactions to contrast media.

Patients who have previously had mild contrast reactions may be pretreated with steroids in order to perform necessary iodine contrast enhanced CT scan. Pretreatment regimens vary; therefore specific guidance should be sought from the radiologist in your institution. Enough time should be allowed for two doses of steroids such as prednisone beginning 12 or more hours before the examination. It is important to provide the doses in addition to steroids being given for any other reason; 25 to 50 mg of diphenhydramine may be administered 1 to 2 hours prior to the scan. A new alternative is 10 mg of ceterizine which has similar antihistaminic effect to diphenhydramine but is nonsedating. Coordination with the CT technologists should be started at the time of CT ordering in order to perform the scan at the prescribed interval after pretreatment (**Table 113-3**). Pretreatment with steroids is not typically indicated in patients with delayed reaction to contrast agents, although consultation with an allergist may be helpful.

■ USE OF IODINE CONTRAST MATERIAL DURING PREGNANCY

The extent of potential mutagenesis of fetal tissue due to iodine contrast material is not known. It is paramount when balancing the risks and benefits of any imaging procedure performed during pregnancy to weigh the value of the procedure and need for contrast materials to safeguard the health care of the mother.

PRACTICE POINT

A general rule for pregnant patients:
- The clinical needs of the mother should take precedence in determining the diagnostic approach.
- X-ray exposure to less than 5 rads has not been associated with fetal anomalies or pregnancy loss, but is thought to increase risk of childhood leukemia.
- Contrast material and radiation should be avoided when possible in pregnant women.
- There are no known associations of MRI with fetal abnormalities. Gadolinium administration is typically avoided in pregnancy.
- Ultrasound is the best imaging modality to use, when possible, for pregnant patients.

■ GADOLINIUM-BASED CONTRAST MATERIALS

Magnetic Resonance Imaging uses gadolinium-based contrast materials (GBCM) as contrast agents. Unlike iodinated agents used in x-ray-based imaging, GBCMs are not associated with contrast-induced nephropathy, and the occurrence of anaphylactic reactions is very rare. Over the last decade, an entity known as nephrogenic systemic fibrosis (NFS) has been linked to administration of gadolinium contrast agents as a rare late complication in patients with impaired renal function. Increasing concern for NSF led to a black box warning for patients with impaired renal function. With proper selection criteria, the incidence of NSF has fallen essentially to zero. Criteria vary slightly from institution to institution based upon the availability of specific contrast agents, as different GBCMs vary in the degree with which they are associated with NSF. In general, GBCMs are best avoided in patients with an eGFR less than 30 mL/min 1.73 m². It is best to consult the radiologist beforehand to maximize the value of the MRI examination as special scanning sequences may sometimes be used to provide the needed information without any contrast agent.

At the time of writing, the FDA has also announced that it is reviewing a new issue that has been identified regarding some GBCMs, gadolinium retention in the brain. At this time, the FDA does not have enough evidence to suggest a change in clinical practice, but it has suggested that physicians remain judicious in the use of GBCMs.

RADIATION EXPOSURE

Much of what we know about radiation biology comes from long-term follow-up of atomic bomb survivors, and relatively small studies of medical or occupational exposure. These studies have demonstrated increases in cancer incidence for exposures on the order of 50 to 100 mSv, but controversy persists about the shape of the dose-response curve from smaller exposures or from fractionated or prolonged exposures. Until more data become available that directly explores risk models in these lower-dose regimes, radiation risk estimation will typically be performed using a linear-no-threshold (LNT) model in which cancer risk is assumed to rise linearly as a function of exposure. Recently, several large epidemiologic studies have demonstrated increases in cancer risks from low-dose exposures that do appear to support the LNT assumption.

Figure 113-1 shows results from the widely used BEIR-VII (Biological Effects of Ionizing Radiation) report that uses an LNT model. For a given exposure, female patients are at higher risk than male patients, and risk per dose increases at younger ages, due to both the increased radiation sensitivity of younger tissues and the longer timeline remaining in which a radiation-induced cancer may develop. The lifetime attributable risk (LAR) represents an additive risk above baseline cancer rates (42% in the US population).

These curves may be used for rough estimates of risk levels, based on the patient's age, gender, and level of exposure. However, it is

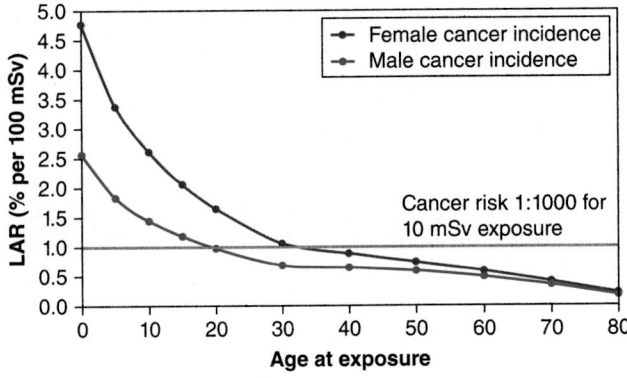

BEIR-VII Lifetime Attributable Risk (LAR) of radiation-induced cancer above baseline

- Female cancer incidence
- Male cancer incidence

Cancer risk 1:1000 for 10 mSv exposure

Figure 113-1 *Expected lifetime attributable risk of radiation-induced cancer (data extracted from Table 12D of BEIR-VII). For a 10 mSv exposure (solid horizontal line), approximate cancer risk is 1 in 1000 for a 33-year-old woman or a 19-year-old man.*

important to realize that these models assume standardized US life expectancies. Radiation-induced cancers typically have a 10 to 20 year latency (depending on the organ), so patients with short remaining life expectancy have very little associated risk from radiation exposure.

Radiation risks have been alternately downplayed and exaggerated in the literature and lay media, resulting in great confusion about the magnitude of these risks. While conventional x-ray, fluoroscopy, and nuclear medicine studies also expose patients to ionizing radiation, CT has appropriately received the greatest scrutiny because of the relatively high radiation dose per exam. Although it comprises about 15% of all medical imaging procedures, it produces approximately half of the population's medical radiation exposure. It is therefore most valuable to consider the approximate levels of risk imparted by CT, and the factors influencing these risks, to encourage a more rational decision-making process by enabling risk estimates to be weighed against the perceived benefits of imaging. It is important to note that while the "typical" radiation dose values of **Table 113-4** are reasonable estimates, there are many strategies to

TABLE 113-4 Approximate Effective Doses from Common Imaging Procedures

Imaging Study	Approximate Effective Dose per CT (mSv)
X-ray: PA and lat chest	0.1
X-ray: abdomen	0.7
X-ray: lumbar spine	1.5
X-ray: hip	0.7
Mammography	0.4
CT: head, face	2
CT: C-spine, neck	2
CT: chest, PE, T-Spine	8
CT: abdomen/pelvis, L-Spine	15
CT: abdomen or pelvis alone	7.5
Nucs: cardiac rest-stress MIBI	12
Nucs: cardiac stress-rest thallium	40
Nucs: V/Q	2.5
Nucs: FDG PET	14

reduce dose to patient, including continued rapid improvements in the dose reduction technologies available on modern scanners. Patient size is an important determinant of radiation dose, with smaller patients typically receiving substantially lower dose than is required for diagnostic quality scans in larger patients.

■ CUMULATIVE RISK

The risk from most individual CT scans is small, but many patients undergo large numbers of imaging studies over time. As radiation risks are generally believed to accumulate additively, recurrent imaging may lead to large cumulative risks over time. One may make a rough estimate of a patient's cumulative risk (**Table 113-5**). Regardless of the estimation of cumulative risk, clinicians may take steps to reduce the cumulative risk (**Table 113-6**).

> **PRACTICE POINT**
>
> **The most important guiding principles:**
> - Focus imaging on the acute problem and limit the gathering of data that is outside the scope of the current illness.
> - Use prior imaging in clinical context to provide additional/new information.
> - Minimize radiation and contrast exposure when diagnostic quality of the exam can be preserved.
> - Separate examinations that require administration of intravenous contrast material by at least 24 h, even in patients with normal renal function.

TABLE 113-5 Estimation of Cumulative Risk

Approach for rough estimation of cumulative risk:

1. Count all prior chest and abdomen/pelvis CT scans.
2. Divide by 10 (this assumes approximately 10 mSv per scan). The result is the approximate LAR in percent above baseline.

To incrementally improve these estimates:

3. Adjust for scan type. The simplified approach above assumes that each CT scan imparted a 10 mSv effective dose. If all the scans were abdomen/pelvis, increase by 50% (see Table 113-1). If there are many head CTs, these can be included by adding 1/5 of them to the "scan count" of step 1.
4. Adjust for patient size. Assuming appropriate dose modulation techniques, increase by a factor of 2 for extremely obese patients, decrease by a factor of 2 for small patients.
5. Adjust for age and gender. Multiply by the appropriate y-axis value from Figure 113-1.
6. Understand that these estimates are high for patients with life expectancy substantially shorter than age- and sex-matched peers.

Example:

1. A moderately obese 60-year-old man has had 40 CT scans of the abdomen/pelvis.
2. The crude LAR estimate is 4% above baseline.
3. As all of these scans are relatively higher dose abdomen/pelvis scans, adjust to 6%.
4. Then adjust to 9% for moderate obesity.
5. Finally, multiply by 0.5 from Figure 113-1 to adjust for his gender and age.

The result is an LAR estimate of 4.5% above baseline, potentially increasing his expected lifetime cancer risk from 42% to 46.5%.

6. If the patient is unlikely to survive this hospital admission, radiation risk estimation is irrelevant (step 6).

TABLE 113-6 Patient Safety: Reduce Radiation Exposure

Methods to reduce radiation risk:

- Only order scans that will impact management.
- Review the patient's prior imaging history as thoroughly as possible, not just the last one or two studies.
- Move beyond the incremental risks of the single scan being considered at present, and balance the benefits of recurrent imaging against cumulative radiation risks.
- Take a longitudinal view of the patient. If numerous prior scans for the same complaint have been unrevealing, a new approach may well be warranted.
- Consider other imaging or diagnostic alternatives for focused questions, if the desired information is available by other means.
- Increase spacing between scans when possible.

- Consult radiology personnel prior to ordering invasive radiologic procedures.
- Address incidental and nonemergent findings responsibly.

CONCLUSION

This chapter provides a framework for assessing the risk of radiographic imaging so that the clinician can take steps to minimize risk. Radiology studies may provide more extensive and valuable information than plain films; however, it is important to follow the guiding principle to order only the tests necessary for management of the acute illness. Direct consultation with the radiologist in choosing and scheduling the optimal imaging test may prompt review of prior studies and avoid unnecessary testing. If imaging with contrast is required, the temporary discontinuance or delay in starting of a particular medication that will adversely affect patient hydration at the time of iodinated intravenous iodine contrast administration may attenuate risk for a specific patient. An eGFR based on MDRD-4 is suggested as a better screening laboratory test with new cutoffs (ie, an eGFR value of 45 mL/min/1.73 m^2 and 30 mL/min/1.73 m^2) in patients receiving IV contrast. Allergic reactions to IV contrast are now subdivided into "allergic-like" and "physiochemotoxic" with different pretreatment implications.

SUGGESTED READINGS

Contrast

American College of Radiology Manual on Contrast Media (v10.1 2015). http://www.acr.org/quality-safety/resources/contrast-manual.

Choyke PL, Cady J, DePollar SL, Austin H. Determination of serum creatinine prior to iodinated contrast media: is it necessary in all patients? *Tech Urol.* 1998;4(2):65-69.

Davenport MS, Khalatbari S, Cohan RH, Dillman JR, Myles JD, Ellis JH. Contrast material-induced nephrotoxicity and intravenous low-osmolality iodinated contrast material: risk stratification by using estimated glomerular filtration rate. *Radiology.* 2013;268(3):719-728.

Davenport MS, Khalatbari S, Cohan RH, Ellis JH. Contrast medium-induced nephrotoxicity risk assessment in adult inpatients: a comparison of serum creatinine level and estimated glomerular filtration rate-based screening methods. *Radiology.* 2013;269(1):92-100.

Davenport MS, Khalatbari S, Dillman JR, Cohan RH, Caoili EM, Ellis JH. Contrast material-induced nephrotoxicity and intravenous low-osmolality iodinated contrast material. *Radiology.* 2013;267(1):94-105.

European Society of Urogenital Radiology Guidelines on Contrast Media (version 8.1 2015). http://www.esur.org/guidelines/.

McDonald JS, McDonald RJ, Carter RE, Katzberg RW, Kallmes DF, Williamson EE. Risk of intravenous contrast material mediated acute kidney injury: a propensity score-matched study stratified by baseline-estimated glomerular filtration rate. *Radiology.* 2014;271(1):65-73.

McDonald RJ, McDonald JS, Bida JP, et al. Intravenous contrast material-induced nephropathy: causal or coincident phenomenon? *Radiology.* 2013;267(1):106-118.

Newhouse JH, Kho D, Rao QA, Starren J. Frequency of serum creatinine changes in the absence of iodinated contrast material: implications for studies of contrast nephrotoxicity. *AJR Am J Roentgenol.* 2008;191(2):376-382.

Tippins RB, Torres WE, Baumgartner BR, Baumgarten DA. Are screening serum creatinine levels necessary prior to outpatient CT examinations? *Radiology.* 2000;216(2):481-484.

Allergy

Beaty AD, Lieberman PL, Slavin RG. Seafood allergy and radiocontrast media: are physicians propagating a myth? *Am J Med.* 2008;121(2):158.e1-e158.

Bettman MA. Frequently asked questions: iodinated contrast agents. *Radiographics.* 2004;24:S3-S10.

Davenport MS, Cohan RH, Caoili EM, Ellis JH. Repeat contrast medium reactions in premedicated patients: frequency and severity. *Radiology.* 2009;253:372-379.

Greenberger PA, Halwig JM, Patterson R, Wallemark CB. Emergency administration of radiocontrast media in high-risk patients. *J Allergy Clin Immunol.* 1986;77(4):630-634.

Greenberger PA, Patterson R, Radin RC. Two pretreatment regimens for high-risk patients receiving radiographic contrast media. *J Allergy Clin Immunol.* 1984;74(4 pt 1):540-543.

Harjai KJ, Raizada A, Shenoy C, et al. A comparison of contemporary definitions of contrast nephropathy in patients undergoing percutaneous coronary intervention and a proposal for a novel nephropathy grading system. *Am J Cardiol.* 2008;101(6):812.

Pannu N, Wiebe N, Tonelli M. Prophylaxis strategies for contrast induced nephropathy. *JAMA.* 2006;295(23):2765-2779.

Scanlon PJ, Faxon DP, Audet AM, et al. ACC/AHA guidelines for coronary angiography. A report of the American College of Cardiology/American Heart Association Task Force on practice guidelines (Committee on Coronary Angiography). Developed in collaboration with the Society for Cardiac Angiography and Interventions. *J Am Coll Cardiol.* 1999;33(6):1756-1824.

Sinert R, Doty CI. Evidence-based emergency medicine review. Prevention of contrast-induced nephropathy in the emergency department. *Ann Emerg Med.* 2007;50(3):335-345, 345.e1-e2.

Tramèr MR, von Elm E, Loubeyre P, Hauser C. Pharmacological prevention of serious anaphylactic reactions due to iodinated contrast media: systematic review. *BMJ.* 2006;333(7570):675.

Radiation

Amis ES Jr, Butler PF, Applegate KE, et al. American College of Radiology white paper on radiation dose in medicine. *J Am Coll Radiol.* 2007;4(5):272-284.

Leuraud K, Richardson DB, Cardis E, et al. Ionising radiation and risk of death from leukaemia and lymphoma in radiation-monitored workers (INWORKS): an international cohort study. *Lancet Haematol.* 2015;2(7):e276-e281.

Mathews JD, Forsythe AV, Brady Z, et al. Cancer risk in 680 000 people exposed to computed tomography scans in childhood or adolescence: data linkage study of 11 million Australians. *BMJ.* 2013;346:f2360.

Mettler FA Jr, Bhargavan M, Faulkner K, et al. Radiologic and nuclear medicine studies in the United States and worldwide: frequency, radiation dose, and comparison with other radiation sources—1950–2007. *Radiology.* 2009;253(2):520-531.

Mettler FA Jr, Huda W, Yoshizumi TT, Mahesh M. Effective doses in radiology and diagnostic nuclear medicine: a catalog. *Radiology.* 2008;248(1):254-263.

National Research Council (U.S.). Committee to Assess Health Risks from Exposure to Low Level of Ionizing Radiation. Health risks from exposure to low levels of ionizing radiation: BEIR VII, Phase 2. Washington, DC: National Academies Press; 2006.

Pearce MS, Salotti JA, Little MP, et al. Radiation exposure from CT scans in childhood and subsequent risk of leukaemia and brain tumours: a retrospective cohort study. *Lancet.* 2012;380(9840):499-505.

Sodickson A. Strategies for reducing radiation exposure in multi-detector row CT. *Radiol Clin North Am.* 2012;50(1):1-14.

Sodickson A, Baeyens PF, Andriole KP, et al. Recurrent CT, cumulative radiation exposure, and associated radiation-induced cancer risks from CT of adults. *Radiology.* 2009;251(1):175-184.

114

Basic Chest Radiography (CXR)

Maria F. Barile, MD
Francine L. Jacobson, MD, MPH

Key Clinical Questions

1 What are the different types of plain chest radiographs and when would you order them?

2 What are the limitations of the anteroposterior (AP) film?

3 How does the chest radiography differentiate between different types of pneumonia from atelectasis?

4 What are the radiographic changes you should look for when considering acute, potentially life-threatening causes of chest pain?

5 What radiographic abnormalities require follow-up?

INTRODUCTION

The majority of hospitalized patients routinely have chest radiographs on admission or prior to surgery. Chest radiographs provide a snapshot of the patient's physiologic health and insights into a wide variety of systemic diseases. Chest radiographs have the highest yield when obtained to evaluate acute cardiopulmonary signs or symptoms, or to assess the possibility of a complication following a procedure. Chest x-rays are also used to monitor critical illness in the intensive care unit (ICU), response to therapy as in congestive heart failure or pneumonia, and stability of pulmonary nodules.

The clinician can minimize unnecessary test ordering and delays in diagnosis by recognizing the indications for different types of radiographs and their limitations. **Table 114-1** summarizes the different types of chest projections, indications, and technical considerations. A posteroanterior (PA) radiograph provides more information than an anteroposterior (AP) projection. Due to magnification based on distance from the image data collector or film, the heart will appear larger on bedside AP chest radiographs and also in obese individuals. Hence, an AP image may suggest heart failure (upper lobe diversion, cardiomegaly, wide mediastinum, and high hemidiaphragms) in patients without fluid overload and significant pulmonary pathology may not be obscured. An AP film is also more likely to miss a small pneumothorax due to anterior collection of air, and diffuse shadowing may signify either poor inspiration or a posterior pleural effusion. Therefore, a PA radiograph may be required for more definitive diagnosis and is the preferred initial study. However, the patient must be able to cooperate and be clinically stable in order to be transported to another area in the hospital for acquisition of a posteroanterior radiograph. Although the standard chest radiograph may provide information about the overall health of the bones, special views should be obtained to properly assess the thoracic spine and shoulder joints in cases of trauma or infection. Rib fractures in particular may indicate more severe pulmonary injury than what is readily apparent from the plain film.

The interpretation of any radiographic test begins with assessing the adequacy and technical quality of the film(s) in view. Normal chest radiograph anatomic structures contribute to the radiographic appearance of the chest (**Figures 114-1** and **114-2**). The right hemidiaphragm should reach the anterior end of the right sixth or seventh rib or the posterior end of the ninth rib on full inspiration. The degree of inspiration affects the appearance of the lower zone vessels that seem more prominent with poor inspiration. The clinician may mistakenly diagnose basilar pneumonia or cardiomegaly if the radiograph has the domes of the diaphragms at the posterior end of seventh ribs or higher. Comparison with prior radiographs that look like the current examination can be most helpful when viewing radiographs without a radiologist. This is analogous to comparing a current electrocardiogram to a baseline electrocardiogram in a patient with possible cardiac ischemia. Then the examiner should carefully inspect the heart, lungs, mediastinum, and chest wall. The bones should be examined for fracture and metastatic disease. The examiner should also routinely check for the presence and position of any invasive medical equipment such as central lines, feeding tubes, or endotracheal tubes (**Table 114-2** and **Figure 114-3**).

TABLE 114-1 Types of Chest Radiographs

Type of Film	Indications	Technical Considerations
Posteroanterior radiograph	Preferred image unless patient unstable to evaluate acute signs and symptoms of the chest	Patient stands with anterior chest against film cassette; exposure is full inspiration
Anteroposterior radiograph	Alternative to PA chest for unstable patients	Film cassette placed behind patient, portable x-ray machine used Rotation is more likely than with a PA film
Lateral view	To localize an abnormality seen in another view; to identify abnormalities obscured by the heart or costophrenic recess	
Lateral decubitus view	To identify a small pleural effusion or to distinguish from pleural thickening; to determine if raised hemidiaphragm due to subpulmonary hemothorax; to confirm clinical impression that pectus excavatum with depressed sternum is cause of unusual cardiac contour or cardiomegaly	Patient lying with his abnormal side down
PA inspiration-expiration views	To identify pneumothorax; expiration to identify inhaled foreign body when gas trapping is evident	
Apical lordotic views	To examine the lung apex usually obscured by clavicle and upper ribs	

PRACTICE POINT

- Clinicians should always provide radiologists with sufficient information to interpret a radiograph in the clinical context of the patient. Otherwise, the radiologist may generate a wide differential diagnosis that may lead to unnecessary additional imaging or overlook subtle signs of infection in an immune-compromised host.
- Consideration of chest radiographic findings that support a new diagnosis of a systemic disease almost always benefits from direct consultation with the radiologist; a study requisition does not allow an interchange of specific clinical information that can alert the radiologist to findings that might otherwise be ignored.

CHEST RADIOGRAPHIC TERMINOLOGY

The Fleischner Society Lexicon (Tuddenham 1984) is the standard reference resource for chest radiographic terminology (Table 114-3). The term opacity is used to describe the addition of substances to lungs that results in lighter gray to white appearance of normally dark-gray lungs. The term density is not used because density is a photographic term for increasing blackness in the image.

THE HEART

The simplest measurement of the cardiac silhouette, the transverse diameter of the heart, compares the measurements of the widest width of the heart with the widest width of the thorax on standard PA chest radiographs. Cardiomegaly is a nonspecific finding in fluid overload states. The heart may enlarge from baseline without

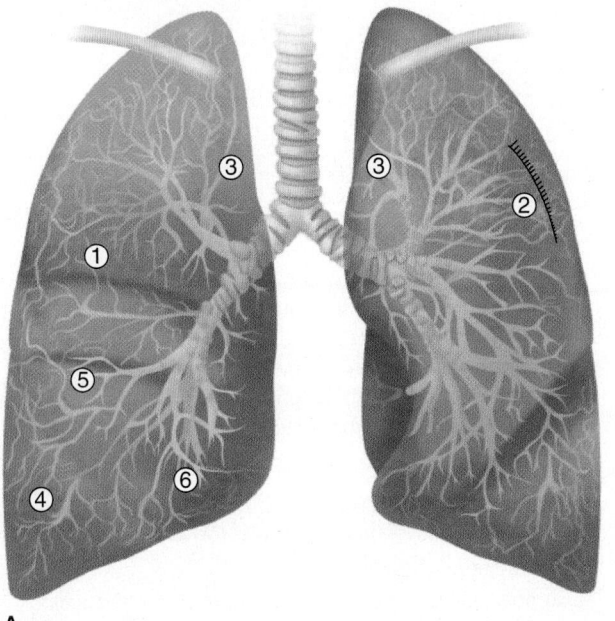
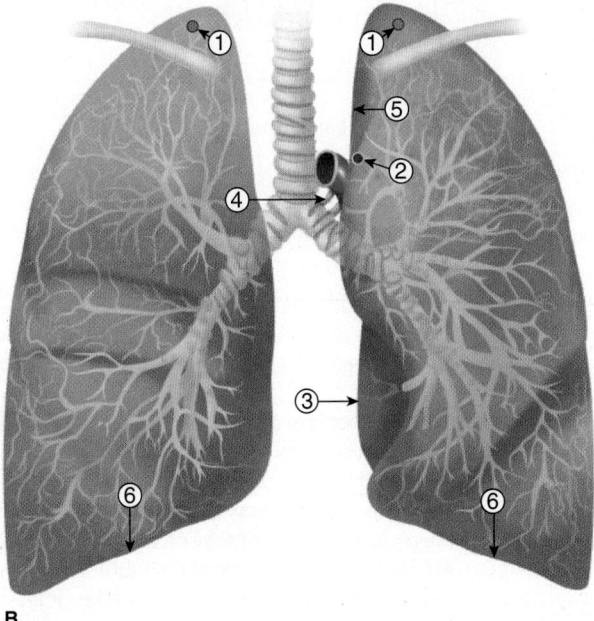

A   B

Figure 114-1 (A) Normal chest radiograph anatomic schematic drawing of fissures on PA radiograph. 1, minor fissure; 2 to 4, major fissure; 5, superior accessory fissure; 6, inferior accessory fissure. (B) Normal chest radiograph anatomy schematic drawing of structures on PA radiograph 1, normal apical opacity; 2, aortic nipple; 3, descending aortic interface; 4, air in esophagus; 5, aortic pulmonary stripe; 6, diaphragm.

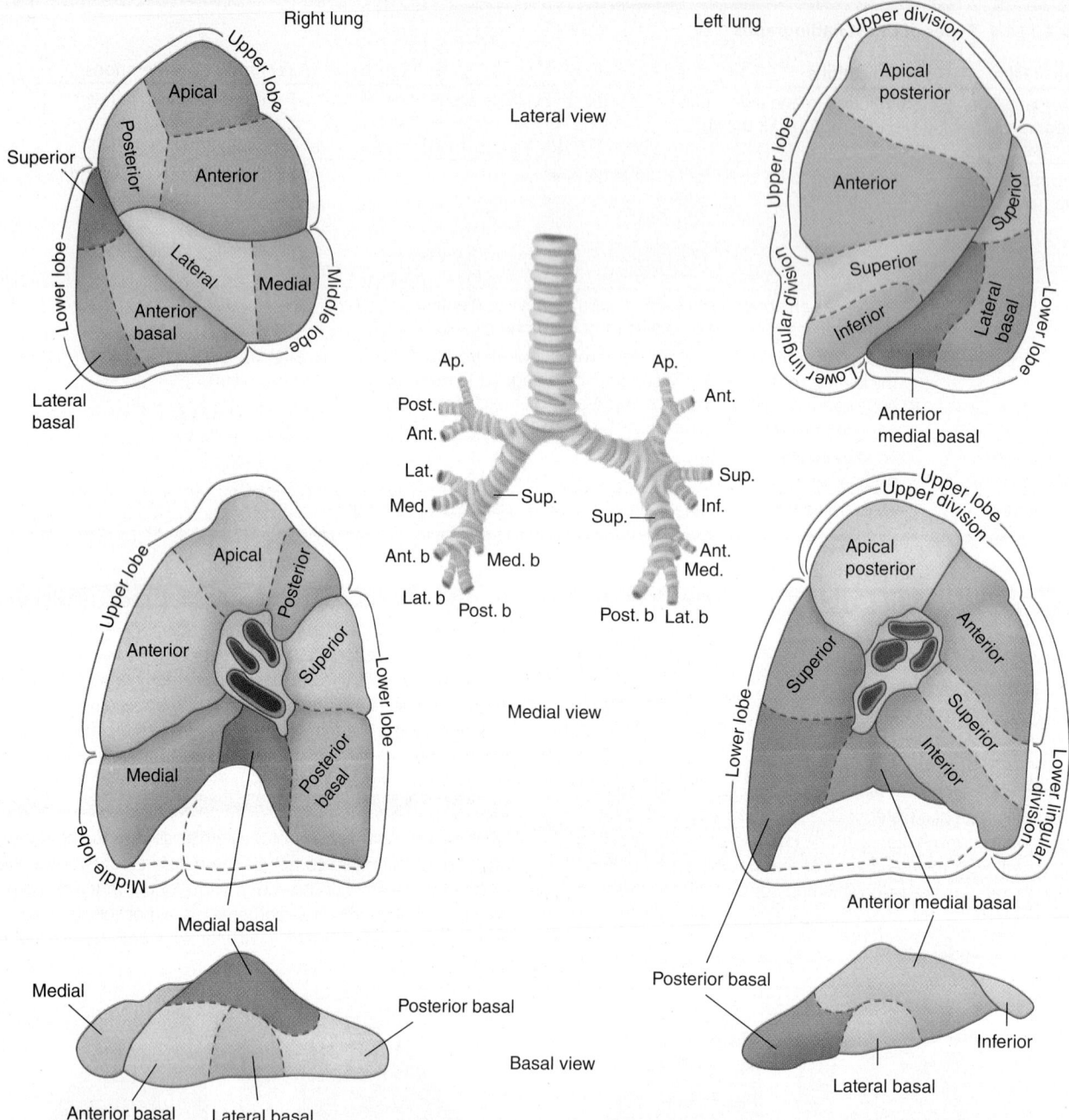

Figure 114-2 *Lobar and segmental anatomy of lungs.* (Reproduced, with permission, from Doherty GM. *Current Diagnosis & Treatment: Surgery.* 13th ed. New York: McGraw-Hill; 2010. Fig. 18-7.)

meeting criteria for cardiomegaly, be normal in the setting of acute lung injury, or enlarged for other reasons. Viewing images with prior plain films provides a more reliable assessment of the presence of cardiomegaly due to a wide range of normal and abnormal heart sizes. An important sign of a possible pericardial effusion, separation of epicardial and pericardial fat, should prompt comparison with prior films to determine if there has been rapid enlargement and development of a globular configuration. A characteristic cardiac contour may suggest left ventricular enlargement, but right ventricular enlargement will, for the most part, be indistinguishable from right ventricular displacement in an enlarged heart. It takes at least 2 years of untreated hypertension to result in a hypertensive cardiovascular silhouette with ectasia of the aorta and more horizontal axis of the heart on PA chest radiograph. For patients with "labile" hypertension, the presence of target end organ damage would be an

indication for treatment. Calcification and a change in contour may suggest left ventricular aneurysm, and bulging of the lower third of the left cardiac border may signify aortic valve disease. Prominence of left heart border or posterior enlargement of the left atrium may suggest the possibility of mitral stenosis.

PRACTICE POINT

- Pericarditis
- Compare current chest radiograph with prior chest radiographs to determine if there is
- A new separation of epicardial and pericardial fat
- Oligemic appearance of lungs

TABLE 114-2 Support Lines

Support Device	Optimum Placement	Proximal Limit	Distal Limit	Common Malposition
Endotracheal tube	Middle of intrathoracic trachea	Tip even with top of clavicle	Tip 2 cm from carina	Tip in right mainstem bronchus
Central venous catheter	Superior vena cava	Brachiocephalic vein	Cavoatrial junction	Right atrium; inferior vena cava; azygous vein following arch posteriorly; internal mammary vein with slight lateral direction; persistent left superior vena cava can be acceptable depending on vessel size
Peripherally inserted central catheter	Depends on use; localization will change with arm position	Arm for long-term peripheral access	Cavoatrial junction	Visiting Nurse Association (VNA) service may require superior vena cava
Swan-Ganz catheter	Right or left main pulmonary artery	Right ventricle	Interlobar descending pulmonary artery	Distal placement only when wedged
Nasogastric tube	Stomach			Side vent marker needs to be distal to gastroesophageal junction

Anatomic landmarks within the heart are only identified if they are calcified or associated with radiopaque markers, such as coronary stents, prosthetic valves, and closure devices for patent foramen ovale.

THE LUNGS

Forty percent of the lung area and 25% of the lung volume may be obscured by the heart and mediastinum on a PA or AP chest radiograph. Both lungs should be equal in size. Fissures should not be wider than hairline. The outline of the hemidiaphragms is usually smooth, arcuate, with the highest point medial to the midline of the hemithorax. Normally, airways are invisible unless they are abnormally thickened or pass through an area of consolidation. Consolidation is the hallmark of airspace disease. Air bronchograms are seen on projection radiographs as lucent tubular branching structures within a larger opacity produced by confluent filling of airspaces by fluid and other substances (Figure 114-3). Volume loss in the region may also contribute to the opacity.

Some terms suggest a broad differential diagnosis that may be considerably narrowed by the clinical context. Large irregular opacities may result from consolidation, lobar collapse, carcinoma, pleural abnormalities, or chest wall lesions. Single or multiple nodular opacities may reflect malignant causes (primary bronchogenic carcinoma, solitary or multiple metastasis) and benign causes (granulomas, arteriovenous malformations [AVMs], intrapulmonary bronchogenic cysts, bronchial atresia, and traumatic hematomas). Collapse is often reserved for lobar collapse but by definition, atelectasis is correct at all levels whether a subsegment, segment, lobe, or complete atelectasis of the entire lung. The differential diagnosis for collapse is most importantly an obstructing lesion; an endobronchial tumor may be primary lung cancer (including carcinoid that has recently been reclassified as a flavor of lung cancer); endobronchial metastasis (particularly breast, gastrointestinal tract, and renal cell carcinoma); foreign bodies (such as a peanut or bullet); and secretions as mucoid impaction (particularly important in an intubated patient). Pneumonia may occur with collapse related to secretions and in particular aspiration pneumonias may be more likely to be associated with atelectasis. Atelectasis commonly occurs in the postoperative setting due to low lung volumes. In babies, atelectasis may also reflect decreased surfactant—unusual in adults. Radiographic clues to the presence of atelectasis include: crowding of airways and vessels within the lobe, crowding of ribs, shift of mediastinum and other

structures, raised hemidiaphragm, compensatory hyperexpansion of ipsilateral lobe and contralateral lung. Additional terms are presented in **Table 114-3**.

> ### PRACTICE POINT
>
> **Acute airspace disease = water, pus, blood.**
> - Bilateral symmetric disease favors water.
> - Focal air space disease favors pneumonia.
> - Bilateral asymmetric and sparing of periphery are associated with hemorrhage.

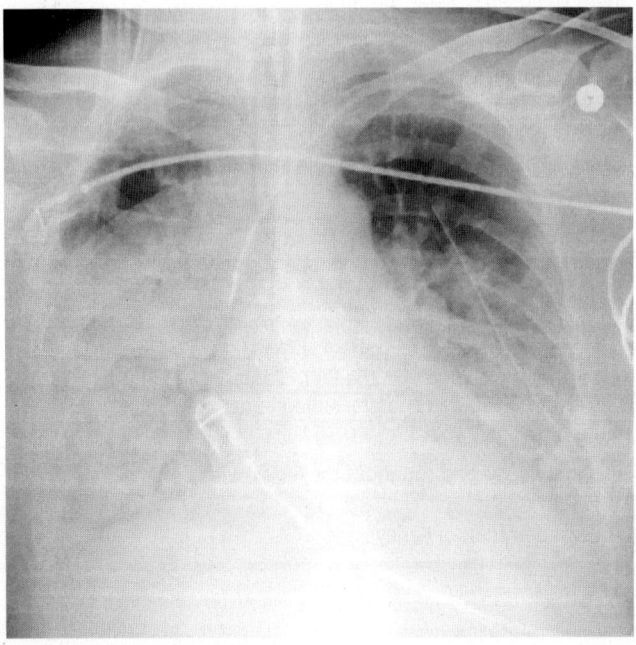

Figure 114-3 *ICU patient with dense consolidation and air bronchograms well seen in right lung base corresponding with pneumonia. Support lines include endotracheal tube, left subclavian central venous catheter and left chest tube placed for pneumothorax that may be due to line placement or barotrauma in setting of multiorgan system failure with injury pulmonary edema present.*

TABLE 114-3 Glossary of Terms

Descriptive Term	Differential Diagnosis
Infiltrate • Pathologic term often used clinically (but not radiographically)	A relatively acute development of a diffuse process that includes little if any consolidation, corresponds with acute interstitial pneumonia (AIP), injury pulmonary edema, corresponding to clinical diagnosis of adult respiratory distress syndrome (ARDS)

Solitary pulmonary nodule
• Typically homogeneous parenchymal lesion with sharply defined margins, ≤3 cm
• Usually standard chest radiograph will not detect nodules <1 cm
• Nodules between 1 and 2 cm in size may be missed due to overlapping bones or vascular structures
	Malignant nodules
	• Primary bronchogenic carcinoma
	• Solitary metastasis
	• Clues to origin:
	  • Smoker, past medical history (PMH) of head & neck cancer (lung)
	  • PMH extrathoracic cancer (metastasis from original site)
	Benign Diseases
	• Benign tumors
	  • Hamartomas, bronchial adenomas
	• Non-neoplastic processes
	  • Granulomas, intrapulmonary bronchogenic cysts, bronchial atresia, traumatic hematomas, AVMs
	• Clues to benign (as opposed to malignant)
	  • Calcification in a typical benign pattern
	  • No growth on serial chest radiograph over 2-y period
	  • Nonsmoker <35 y old

Atelectasis • Decreased lung volume, at any level of lung organization • May be associated with other signs of volume loss in the hemithorax (ipsilateral shift of the mediastinum, decreased spacing of ribs and elevation of the diaphragm) • Collapse refers to complete lung atelectasis • Subsegmental and segmental atelectasis refer to discoid or plate-like atelectasis based on projection	Pneumonia, pulmonary embolism, and abdominal fluid or pain that causes splinting Mucoid impaction at the level of any bronchus, leading to collapse patterns that are specific for each lobe In the case of the bronchus intermedius, atelectasis may involve both the right middle and right lower lobes • Atelectasis of both right middle and lower lobes (bronchus intermedius) • Irregular bands of atelectasis (adhesion of airways possibly related to mucus) Low lung volumes and expiration (focal atelectasis)
Kerley A lines • Longer (at least 2 cm) unbranching lines coursing diagonally from the periphery toward the hila in the inner half of the lungs • Never seen without Kerley B or C lines also present	Distention of anastomotic channels between peripheral and central lymphatics of the lungs
Kerley B lines • Short (<2 cm long), straight, horizontal parallel lines (<1 mm thick) at the lung periphery that end at right angles against the pleura • Generally absent along fissural surfaces in any zone but most frequently observed at the lung bases at the costophrenic angles on the PA radiograph, and in the substernal region on lateral radiographs	Fluid in interlobular septa, or dilated lymphatic channels visible with elevation of the pulmonary capillary wedge pressure (usually 25 mm Hg or higher) Associated with congestive heart failure (CHF) and interstitial lung diseases (ILD)
Kerley C lines • Short, fine lines throughout the lungs, with a reticular appearance • Least common of Kerley lines	Thickening of anastomotic lymphatics or superimposition of many Kerley B lines

Normally, blood vessels should be much more apparent in the lower lung zones than in the upper lung zones. Lines seen within 2 cm of the chest wall probably represent interstitial abnormalities such as edema, fibrosis, or metastatic disease.

THE MEDIASTINUM

PRACTICE POINT

Mediastinal contour abnormalities

- Lymphoma: Typically, a lobulated anterior mediastinal mass that most likely represents matted lymph nodes with associated mediastinal lymph nodes. Lymphadenopathy can also occur in sarcoidosis and infection.
- Thymoma: More focal and unilateral than lymphoma, not associated with paratracheal lymphadenopathy, seen in older patients.
- Germ cell tumor: Characteristic fat and calcification particularly in young patient.
- Metastatic disease: Middle mediastinum more likely to be involved by metastatic disease from testicular germ cell tumors, renal cell carcinoma, or melanoma.
- Vascular congenital anomaly or in a patient who has had cardiac surgery pseudoaneurysm at bypass pump cannulation site.

■ ANATOMY

The mediastinum is divided into radiographic compartments that differ somewhat from the anatomic divisions of the mediastinum.

1. The anterior mediastinum includes the retrosternal clear space seen on lateral chest radiograph. Radiologists may use either the anterior surface of the aorta or the anterior wall of the trachea as the posterior boundary of this compartment.
2. The middle mediastinum extends from this boundary to 1 cm behind the anterior surface of the vertebral bodies on the lateral view.
3. The posterior mediastinum extends posteriorly from the middle mediastinum to the posterior chest wall. The structures in this region all lie posterior to the mediastinum.

It is sometimes useful to apply the term superior mediastinum to the region above the aortic arch although not a compartment. The vascular pedicle is assessed on the frontal view with greater magnification expected on bedside anteroposterior radiographs than standard posteroanterior radiographs. Distention of the azygous vein to greater than 11 mm in diameter along right side of trachea just above bifurcation signifies pulmonary vascular engorgement.

The hila are often considered with the mediastinal structures. The border-forming structures are the pulmonary arteries. The left pulmonary artery is approximately 2 cm higher than the right pulmonary artery. This slope, sometimes referred to as the hilar angle, may be altered as in the case of right upper lobe volume loss elevating the right hilum. The direction of the right and left central pulmonary artery differs resulting in expected mild asymmetry. The upper limit of normal currently used on CT scans for the main pulmonary artery is 24 mm with borderline to 29 mm. The upper limit of the normal range in size of the right interlobar descending pulmonary artery most easily measured on chest radiographs is 16 mm for a man and 14 mm for a woman. Increased intravascular pressure may be temporary as in the case of pulmonary edema or long standing as in the case of pulmonary artery hypertension.

■ MEDIASTINAL MASSES

The differential diagnosis of a mass in the anterior mediastinum includes thyroid enlargement (continuous with the thyroid gland causing deviation of the trachea), a thymoma or thymic cyst (typically marginated and sometimes lobulated), lymphoma and small-cell lung cancer (which may involve multiple lymph node groups), or a germ cell tumor (sometimes evidenced by fat, hair, and teeth). The differential diagnosis of middle mediastinal masses includes tumors involving the esophagus, thyroid, and lymph nodes, duplication cysts including bronchogenic cysts (most frequently at the bifurcation of trachea and central airways, sometimes para-esophageal or intraparenchymal), lymphadenopathy, pericardial cysts (characteristically adjacent to the heart, especially in the cardiophrenic sulcus and smoothly marginated), intrathoracic goiter (with heterogeneous tissue), tracheal tumors, and vascular variants. Posterior mediastinal masses may represent neurogenic tumors, extramedullary hematopoiesis, and esophageal abnormalities.

■ HILAR ADENOPATHY

In an otherwise healthy adult, bilateral, noncalcified hilar adenopathy suggests sarcoid. In a patient with a prior history of malignancy, the presumption has to be malignancy. Most common malignancies that cause hilar adenopathy include bronchogenic carcinoma, lymphoma, bronchial carcinoid, and extrathoracic primary tumors metastasizing to the chest. Nonmalignant causes include pulmonary arterial or venous dilation or tortuosity, cysts, granulomatous adenopathy, and benign tumors. Reactive and malignant adenopathy may be radiographically indistinguishable unless there is obvious calcification. Vascular abnormalities are often asymmetric and can simulate adenopathy. The first step is to compare with prior films. Consultation with a radiologist and serial review of images will facilitate differentiation of hilar lymphadenopathy from pulmonary artery enlargement.

■ MEDIASTINAL SHIFT

Both whole lung atelectasis and pleural effusion may cause complete whiteout of a hemithorax. The direction of mediastinal shift may suggest the likely possibility. The shift will be toward the opaque hemithorax when the lung collapses. Pleural effusion on the other hand occupies space and can cause contralateral shift of the mediastinum. Since both can be present at the same time, it is possible for the mediastinum to be midline with balanced volume loss due to atelectasis and pleural effusion. A low diaphragm will cause a right shift of the mediastinum, and a high diaphragm will cause a left shift.

Fluid overload

Fluid overload typically has characteristic radiographic signs that may be correlated with the severity of the process. Early changes include minimal cardiomegaly and equalization of flow to upper and lower zones corresponding to pulmonary capillary wedge pressure of 15 to 25 mm Hg. The diameter of the upper lobe vessels is less than or equal to the lower lobe vessels at the same distance from the hilum, and pulmonary vessels in the first intercostal space are greater than 3 cm. Kerley B lines are present at the basal aspects of the lung with progressive worsening of heart failure. These markings cannot represent blood vessels because vessels are not normally seen as lung markings in the peripheral quarter of the lungs. Frank pulmonary edema (fluid accumulation in the alveolar spaces) becomes evident radiographically when bilateral, predominantly basilar and perihilar alveolar infiltrates are seen, and vessels near the hila become indistinct due to interstitial fluid accumulation.

Pulmonary edema may occur under special circumstances. Up to one-third of opiate overdoses develop pulmonary edema. Pulmonary edema due to inhaled or intravenous opiate abuse or inhalation of solvents or "crack" cocaine may have permeability edema with normal cardiomediastinal silhouette. Rapid clearing of edema is typical and pneumomediastinum or pneumothorax is occasionally associated.

Pulmonary hemorrhage may produce similar acute radiographic signs to pulmonary edema but the patient should have risk factors for pulmonary hemorrhage, should not have signs of fluid overload on examination, and the changes would resolve over a few days into a coarse interstitial pattern. Iatrogenic acute fluid overload would be expected to resolve very quickly with appropriate treatment (**Figure 114-4**).

PRACTICE POINT

Radiographic criteria of pulmonary edema
- Any fissure wider than hairline
  Pulmonary vascular redistribution
- Cephalization in upright patient
- Lateralization in dependent lung of patient lying primarily on one side
- Equalization when neither upper or lower lobe vessels predominate
- Perihilar "bat-wing" pulmonary edema
- Kerley B lines in lower zones
Enlargement of hilar pulmonary vessels
- Cardiomegaly is nonspecific and not invariably present radiographic finding.
Limitations of the chest plain film in the diagnosis of fluid overload
- Poor inspiration (less than the seventh rib) makes the lower zone vessels appear more prominent.
- Patients with severe parenchymal lung disease may have atypical radiographic changes for edema.
- The AP chest film may be misleading regarding cephalization and heart size.

PNEUMONIA

The chest radiograph is mandatory for patients suspected of pneumonia, for acutely ill patients with new respiratory complaints or hypoxia, for patients with an exacerbation of chronic obstructive pulmonary disease, for immunocompromised patients with fever, and for elderly patients with confusion. The diagnosis of pneumonia can only be made through radiographic imaging, but a chest film cannot definitively identify the causative pathogen or rule out noninfectious causes (**Table 114-4**). Clinical pneumonia in the immune-compromised host can present with a normal chest radiograph, as classically seen with *Pneumocystis jiroveci* (formerly PCP). Unlike a normal host, patients with neutropenic fever may have only subsegmental atelectasis or focal peribronchial thickening in the presence of a bacterial infection. Hence, with the knowledge of the patient's immune status and exposure history, the radiologist will lower the threshold for detection of subtle abnormalities and compare with a baseline study whenever possible.

A patient who is dehydrated will have decreased pulmonary vessel sizes with resulting overall decrease in vascularity on chest radiography. After rehydration signs of pneumonia may "bloom."

■ ASPIRATION PNEUMONIA

Inhaled food is usually translucent, but if the inhalation has occurred some time previously, there may be segmental or lobar collapse. It is also possible for as little as 25 mm of sterile gastric contents to be aspirated more widely, resulting in Mendelson syndrome with visual appearance on chest radiograph that may be indistinguishable from

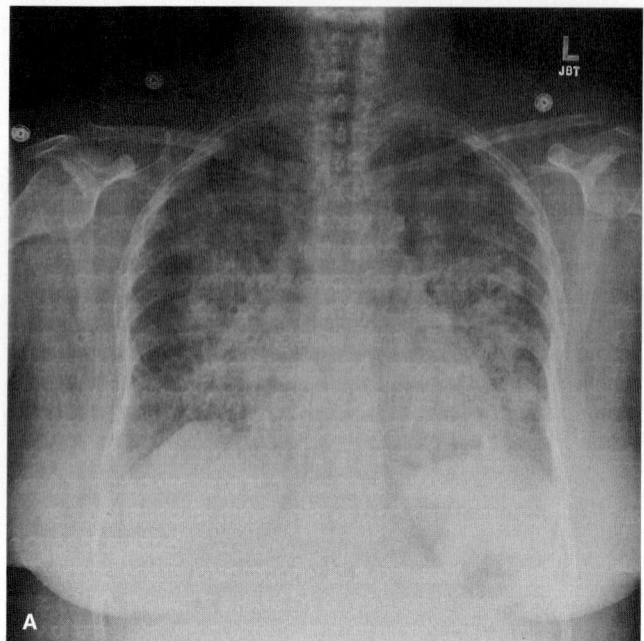

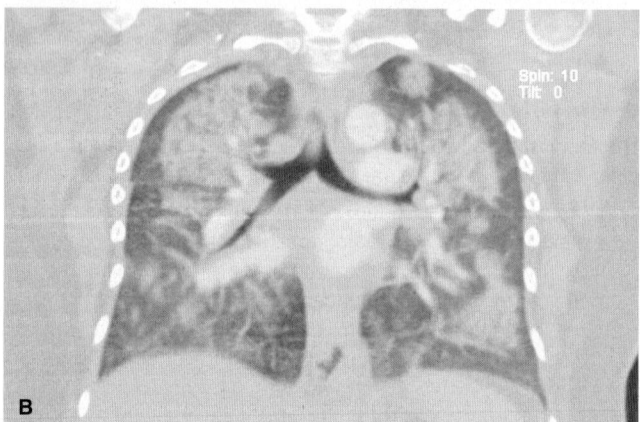

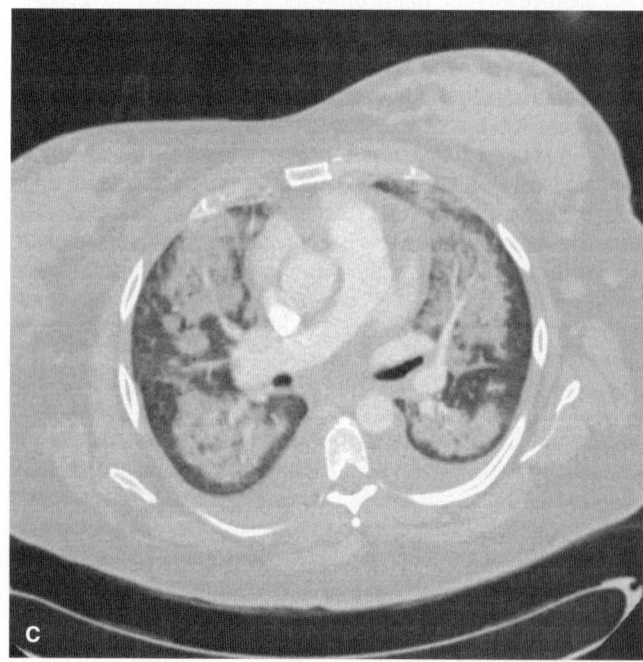

Figure 114-4 *(A) Perihilar airspace opacities are consistent with non-cardiogenic pulmonary edema. Note sparing of lung bases and normal size of heart. (B) Coronal chest CT in the same patient with pulmonary edema. (C) Axial chest CT.*

TABLE 114-4 Typical Pneumonia Patterns

Multilobar Pneumonia	S. pneumoniae and L. pneumophilia More Common
Bilateral diffuse pulmonary infiltrates in an immunocompetent patient	More likely due to congestive heart failure or inhalation of a toxin or allergen than to a pneumonia caused by an atypical pneumonia
Community-acquired pneumonia due to methicillin-resistant *Staphylococcus aureus*	Often bilateral cavitary lesions
Aspiration pneumonia	In a supine patient: left lower lobe (LLL) due to more posteriorly directed left mainstem bronchus
	Time course: More homogeneous consolidation within 2 days of aspiration
	• Necrotizing pneumonia (Gram-negative and anaerobic organisms)
	• Cavities sometimes becoming thick walled over a period of a few weeks, thereby mimicking tuberculosis (TB). Unlike TB, lymphadenopathy is uncommonly associated
Cavitary lesions	*S. aureus, Pseudomonas*; TB; *Aspergillus* infections (pulmonary infarct picture)
	Mixed flora including anaerobes, aspiration (along with empyema)
	Klebsiella (may have a bulging fissure sign), *E. coli*
	Thin-walled cavities: *Coccidioides immitis*
Mass-like lesions	Acute histoplasmosis: Hilar adenopathy and focal alveolar infiltrates
	Disseminating form: Multiple nodules and hilar adenopathy
	Blastomycosis: Mass-like opacities

pulmonary edema, although pulmonary vasculature is unlikely to be engorged by this process. Gravity directs the location, and underlying bronchiectasis may increase the likelihood of developing active infection. Patient position at the time of aspiration may lead to logical patterns besides the classically described pattern, involving the superior segments of the lower lobes and posterior basilar segments of the lower lobes.

■ FUNGAL PNEUMONIA

Fungal infections in healthy individuals are most frequently due to endemic species in particular locations. Travel history can be vital to the radiologist in identifying the likely organism and decreasing the number of serologic tests required to confirm the specific diagnosis. The size, number of nodules, and associated findings, including more chronic calcification from reactivation of prior infection, may help distinguish histoplasmosis from coccidiomycosis. Small, numerous nodules associated with mediastinitis (evidenced by linear calcifications), large calcified lymph nodes, and tiny calcifications in the spleen suggest an infection with histoplasmosis. The largest calcified lymph nodes, often referred to as histoplasmomas, may, for technical radiologic reasons, not appear calcified on standard chest radiographs with the high kilovolt techniques that decrease conspicuity of bones. Fewer large nodules with associated adjacent pleural thickening suggest coccidiomycosis.

PRACTICE POINT

Radiographic signs of pneumonia

- Consolidation from pneumonia may maintain, increase, or decrease the volume of the affected lung with air bronchograms present.
- Atelectasis, irregular aeration, peribronchial thickening and interstitial prominence may characterize more subtle pulmonary infections.
- Reactive lymphadenopathy is most common in ipsilateral hilum.
- Infection and infarction can have identical appearances on imaging studies.

Actinomycosis is the most frequent pneumonia to extend through the chest wall, characterized by suppurative and granulomatous inflammation that can lead to abscess formation and even sinus tracts through the skin that may be found on physical examination.

■ VARICELLA PNEUMONIA

Varicella pneumonia occurs most frequently in pregnant women. Varicella pneumonia presents as diffuse, 5 to 10 mm nodular opacities that are poorly defined and may coalesce as the nodules increase in size. Although hilar lymph nodes may enlarge, they do not usually calcify. Healing can result in small calcific opacities throughout the lungs that are smaller in size and less uniform than that observed with prior histoplasmosis (**Table 114-5**).

TUBERCULOSIS (TB)

The hematogenous spread of primary TB infection is radiographically inapparent in normal hosts. Miliary TB can be associated with primary progressive and reactivation of TB, particularly in immune-compromised patients. The visualization of micronodules on radiographs represents superimposition of multiple such shadows most likely seen at lung bases. Late presentation of miliary TB may result in greater visibility of nodules in lung apices due to the oxygen-rich environment favored by TB. Postprimary TB initially images as heterogeneous, poorly marginated opacities in the apical or posterior segments of the upper lobes or in the superior segments of the lower lobes, and later forms reticular and nodular opacities. Cavitation typically occurs within an area of consolidation and may result in endobronchial spread. Scarring, atelectasis, traction bronchiectasis, nodules, and calcification characterize healing. The presence of back or neck pain should be communicated to the radiologist to insure maximal study of the spine for osteomyelitis. The most frequently visible sign of Pott's Disease is vertebra plana representing complete collapse of the affected vertebral body.

PULMONARY DISEASES

■ SCATTERED OPACITIES

Usual interstitial pneumonia (UIP), rheumatoid lung, scleroderma lung, chronic hypersensitivity pneumonitis, asbestosis, and

TABLE 114-5 Classic Presentations of Pneumonia

Organism	Primary Finding	Secondary Findings	Evolution
Streptococcus pneumoniae	Consolidation with air bronchograms that begins at the periphery and spreads to involve the entire segment or lobe; less likely with early appropriate treatment	Small pleural effusion (50%) Possible hilar adenopathy; air bronchograms Cavitation unusual for most serotypes but lymphadenopathy rare	Transient round pneumonia 24-48 h, progresses to lobar consolidation, resolves by fading slowly
Mycoplasma pneumoniae	Bronchial wall thickening	May have focal opacities Nonspecific findings	Subtle persistent symptoms more prominent than radiographic findings
Legionella pneumophila	A focal homogeneous opacity that may mimic a tumor followed by rapid progression to bilateral parenchymal involvement with associated pleural effusions without evidence of lympadenopathy	Sharply demarcated peribronchovascular opacity Cavity formation may occur in immunocompromised patients but is uncommon in normal hosts	Bilateral asymmetric opacities may range from ground-glass to dense consolidation
Staphylococcus aureus *Klebsiella pneumoniae* *Pseudomonas aeruginosa*	Consolidation with cavitation	Reactive lymphadenopathy May have sympathetic effusion	*Staphylococcus* may develop thin-walled cyst called a pneumatocele *Klebsiella* may appear as enlarged, consolidated lobe
Pneumocystis (carinii) jiroveci	Diffuse bilateral, fine to medium reticulonodular subtle opacities that could easily be overlooked Chest radiograph may be normal (10%)	Pneumatoceles (10%) Pneumothoraces (5%-6%) No pleural effusion	Insidious can lead to consolidation
Aspergillus	Nodular opacities with ground-glass halo	May be solitary or multiple May also have consolidation	Solid opacity that cavitates
Mucormycosis (Zygomycetes)	Nodular opacity with ground-glass center	May be solitary or multiple	Evolves as infarction
Mycobacterium avium-intracellulare (MAI) and mycobacterium avium-complex (MAC)	Bronchiectasis with tree-in-bud opacities	Lymphadenopathy may be present	Chronic colonization may not progress without treatment
M. tuberculosis			
Primary Infection	Unilateral hilar lymphadenopathy and ipsilateral pleural effusion	Ipsilateral mediastinal lymphadenopathy Consolidation may be radiographically absent	Develop Ghon complex with granulomas that calcify within 2 y
	Miliary opacities of hematogenous TB become visible	Lymphadenopathy and pleural effusion may be present or absent	Primary progressive TB
Reactivation TB	Bronchiectasis and cavity particularly in upper lobe	Upper lobe volume loss	Development of new opacities

pulmonary drug toxicity may all produce similar radiographic abnormalities. Typically, UIP shows a pattern of bibasilar irregular linear opacities, which on high-resolution CT appear as ground-glass opacities, traction bronchiectasis, and honeycomb cysts in the periphery without associated adenopathy or pleural effusions. The presence of rheumatoid nodules and pleural effusion may help to radiographically distinguish rheumatoid lung from UIP. Small nodules or an upper lobe predominance may suggest chronic hypersensitivity pneumonitis. Pleural effusion or pleural plaques are a clue to the diagnosis of asbestosis. Pulmonary drug toxicity (amiodarone, bleomycin, methotrexate, nitrofurantoin) may also produce fibrosis (honeycomb cysts, architectural distortion, traction bronchiectasis).

Bronchiolitis obliterans typically appears as scattered air space consolidations (or as ground-glass opacities and consolidations without evidence of fibrosis on CT) in a peripheral and subpleural distribution with slightly reduced lung volumes. Bronchial wall thickening or bronchiectasis is commonly present. Bronchiolitis

obliterans may have associated pleural effusions, nodules, or irregular linear opacities in a smaller number of patients. When parenchymal opacities are present, it is considered part of cryptogenic organizing pneumonia (COP, formerly BOOP). Pulmonary lymphoma and multifocal adenocarcinoma may have a similar radiologic appearance to COP on plain film imaging. Subtle ground-glass opacities seen on CT are often inapparent on chest radiographs.

Eosinophilic pneumonia from alveolar and interstitial infiltration by eosinophils and other inflammatory cells classically has peripheral and upper lobe opacities. The classic "reverse pulmonary edema" occurs in less than 50% of cases. Etiologies include pulmonary vasculitis (Churg-Strauss syndrome), allergic bronchopulmonary aspergillosis, and drug reactions.

■ EMPHYSEMA

Panlobular emphysema typically has regional or generalized decreased lung attenuation preferentially affecting the lung bases.

Initially, centrilobular emphysema preferentially affects the apices as 2 to 10 mm lucencies without walls that later form large regions of decreased lung attenuation.

■ BRONCHIECTASIS

Parallel lines (tram tracks), ring shadows, and mucus plugs are characteristic images of bronchiectasis. Basilar bronchiectasis may result from viral pneumonia (such as adenovirus or measles in childhood), repeated aspiration, or prior bronchiectasis. Cystic fibrosis typically involves the upper lobes more than the lower lobes. Allergic bronchopulmonary aspergillosis may show cylindrical or saccular central, but not peripheral, bronchiectasis and preferentially involves the upper lobes.

■ SARCOID

Up to 90% of patients will have abnormality on chest radiographs at some time over the course of their illness. Tissue diagnosis showing microscopic noncaseating granulomas present in lungs, even when the radiographic appearance of the chest is normal, establishes the diagnosis. The most classic radiographic presentation includes bilateral symmetric hilar and mediastinal lymphadenopathy, particularly in subcarinal and right paratracheal regions. Differential diagnosis includes lymphoma. Less common, asymmetric hilar lymphadenopathy may result from sarcoid. Metastatic disease, TB, and other infections are unlikely to produce symmetric hilar lymphadenopathy. Irreversible end-stage lung disease seen in stage IV sarcoid has the greatest correlation between imaging findings and symptoms (**Table 114-6**).

■ INTERSTITIAL LUNG DISEASE OR DIFFUSE PARENCHYMAL LUNG DISEASE

The interstitium is the potential space between the alveoli and capillaries. Collagen deposition in the interstitium produces a radiographic appearance of diffuse interstitial opacification.

It is difficult and usually unnecessary to work up chronic interstitial lung disease during hospitalization for an unrelated acute illness. Fluid overload states cause pulmonary vascular engorgement from

TABLE 114-7 Interstitial Lung Disease

Cause	Radiographic Finding
Asbestosis (prolonged exposure to asbestos)	Lower-lung field predominance of infiltrates, pleural calcification, plaques
Silicosis	Hilar egg-shell calcifications
Sarcoidosis	Bilateral symmetrical hilar and paratracheal lymphadenopathy
Lymphangioleiomyomatosis (LAM)	Pneumothorax in a premenopausal woman, chylous effusions

interstitial pulmonary edema producing thickening of interlobular septae on plain imaging. Repeated episodes of interstitial edema may lead to hemosiderin deposition, creating permanent visualization of interlobular septae even without pulmonary vascular engorgement or intrinsic interstitial lung disease. A nodular form of interstitial pulmonary edema may be reported as tiny nodular opacities or micronodules due to superimposed shadows. The clinical context is critical because micronodules may also represent hematogenous dissemination of infection (miliary TB or other fungal infections) or tumor. Visualization over time may help to avoid unnecessary evaluations for potential cancer. Unless directly related to the reason for admission, postdischarge follow-up after recovery of the acute illness would be advisable. See **Table 114-7** for examples of common radiographic findings that may suggest an underlying chronic disease process or exposure.

■ PULMONARY NODULES

Admission chest radiographs frequently identify incidental pulmonary nodules. By definition, a lung nodule measures up to 3 cm in diameter while a lung mass measures more than 3 cm in diameter. In clinical practice, these terms are not always used correctly. Doubling in less than 30 days generally indicates benign disease even when a lesion is large. Features of a nodular lesion and accompanying findings help to create a patient-specific differential diagnosis. Miliary TB, for example, may show diffuse 1 to 3 mm nodules that represent superimposition of micronodules not individually resolved by radiography. The larger volume of lung in the lung bases usually makes it more apparent in the bases than the apices, although a patient with a late presentation of miliary TB can have larger, and therefore more easily seen, tiny nodules in the lung apices due to the affinity of TB for the oxygen-enriched apical regions of the lungs.

When one solid pulmonary nodule is noted, the answer may be "in the jacket" (ie, 2 years of radiographic stability ensures that a solid nodule is benign). When multiple pulmonary nodules are present, necessary workup may be limited to explaining a prior infection. Nodules measuring less than 5 mm in diameter that are very well seen on chest radiographs, are likely calcified, and represent sequela of prior infection and require no further workup. Serial radiographs 6 months apart establish baseline when the patient has a positive PPD associated with scarring.

New nodules, nodules that increase in size, or nodules that have worrisome features should be evaluated by CT but not necessarily during the current hospitalization. Acute findings, such as atelectasis, pneumonia, pulmonary edema, and pleural effusions, often obscure important parenchymal findings. It may take 2 months or more for the appearance of the lung parenchyma following acute pneumonia to reach a new baseline. A plain film at that time may be sufficient to document complete clearing and the absence of

TABLE 114-6 Staging of Sarcoidosis

Stage	Findings	Location
0	Normal chest radiograph	
I	Lymphadenopathy	Bilateral hilar, subcarinal, right paratracheal regions
II	Lymphadenopathy and pulmonary parenchymal opacities	Opacities along bronchovascular bundles, particularly in upper lobes Small nodules that may also be seen peripherally
III	Pulmonary parenchymal opacities *without* lymphadenopathy	Peribronchial thickening, small nodules
IV	Honeycombing and traction bronchiectasis	Subpleural fibrosis accompanied by bronchiectasis Lung opacities seen in stages II and III may also be present
	Alveolar sarcoid (stages II to IV)	Consolidation due to interstitial granulomas filling alveoli

an underlying nodule or central lesion causing a postobstructive pneumonia. The probability of cancer increases with the size of the nodule, although the size required for detection on chest radiographs varies with location. The best-quality chest CT scan requires the patient to be able to perform the breath-hold maneuvers. **Figure 114-5** provides an algorithm for further evaluation of solitary pulmonary nodules. CT-based evaluation strategy is presented in Chapter 115.

■ BENIGN TUMORS

Arteriovenous malformation

Typically, arteriovenous malformations appear as round, lobulated, well-defined masses ranging in size from less than one to several centimeters in diameter in the medial third of the lung. A chest radiograph may identify the enlarged feeding artery and draining vein, and a change in size may be apparent when erect versus supine radiographs are compared. Feeding vessels leading to the pulmonary nodule are prominent, enlarging rather than tapering along their often tortuous course. Small AVMs may require echocardiographic bubble study for detection. Radiographs may underdiagnose the number of AVMs present. It is therefore important to look

for telangiectasias. Osler-Weber-Rendu syndrome is also known as hereditary hemorrhagic telangiectasia.

Hamartoma

Hamartomas are solitary nodules usually less than 4 cm in diameter located peripherally in 90% of cases and may have a "popcorn-like" appearance due to calcification.

Granuloma

Granulomas form in response to inflammatory processes including TB and sarcoidosis. Radiographic confirmation of calcification, often possible for nodules measuring less than 5 mm in diameter, confirms the benign nature of the nodule.

■ MALIGNANT TUMORS

Carcinoid

Bronchial carcinoid tumors occur 85% of the time within the central bronchi as hilar masses with or without associated atelectasis or obstructive pneumonia. The other 15% of tumors arise peripherally as solitary, well-circumscribed pulmonary nodules.

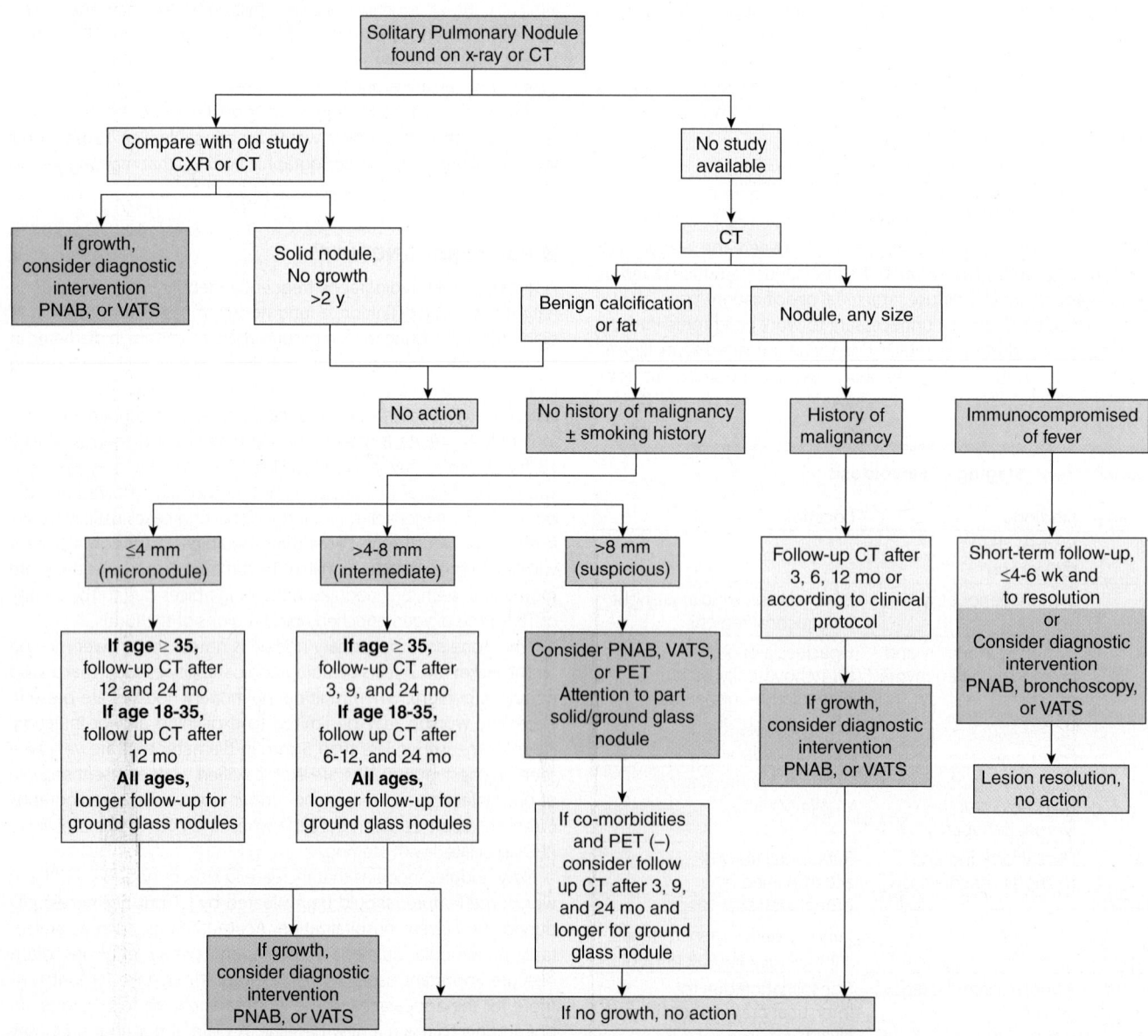

Figure 114-5 *Workup of solitary pulmonary nodule.*

Bronchogenic carcinoma

Bronchogenic carcinoma may present as a smoothly marginated or spiculated nodule or mass. Adenocarcinoma has become the most frequent type of lung cancer. Early adenocarcinoma of lung can mimic an inflammatory process that might only be seen on CT scan. Even a very well-defined ground-glass opacity may be too subtle to see on chest radiographs because it does not obscure vessels.

Pleural tumors

Malignant pleural mesothelioma may image as a unilateral pleural mass, either focal or diffuse, is often associated with pleural effusion, and may locally invade the chest wall, mediastinum, or diaphragm. Pleural plaques from asbestos may be seen on the contralateral side, and are usually larger and more numerous in the mid to lower lung. More commonly encountered pleural tumors include solitary fibrous tumor and metastases.

■ PULMONARY INFARCT

Septic or bland infarcts, typically wedge-shaped and peripheral, are more numerous in the lung bases. Septic infarcts, usually 1 to 2 cm in diameter, cavitate in about 50% of nodules with moderately thick and irregular walls that decrease in size and eventually resolve, leaving in some cases a peripheral linear scar. Pleural effusions may be associated with septic or bland infarcts.

■ PULMONARY CAVITIES

When the lesion has a central cavity, the description of the wall is most valuable. The course over time is also helpful. One-third to one-half of Wegener granulomatosis lesions progress from solid nodules to thick-walled cavities, to thin-walled cavities, and finally resolve without necessarily leaving a scar. Ten percent of patients may also develop diffuse pulmonary hemorrhage. An individual patient may have a mixture of these findings at the same time or over time. The presence of a fluid level in a cavity indicates communication with the tracheobronchial tree. It does not necessarily mean the cavity is infected. Cavitation is not always obvious on chest radiographs and superimposition of small and coalescing opacities may simulate a cavity without one being present. CT scanning is most reliable for identification and description of a cavitary lesion. Large cavitary lesions will also be apparent on magnetic resonance imaging (**Table 114-8** and **Figure 114-6**).

■ PNEUMOTHORAX

To identify a pneumothorax, first look at the boundary of a pneumothorax, which remains a thin white line parallel to the chest wall, in locations where it will be oblique to the ribs. Extensive lung opacities may obscure the thin white line, thereby creating a smooth boundary. Large bullae may be distinguished radiographically from a pneumothorax by their ring shadow or capsule. The sizing of a pneumothorax is often more reliable on chest radiographs than CT scans. Although symptoms dictate treatment of a pneumothorax rather than size, a reference for size ranges predicts the likelihood that intervention will not be required in an asymptomatic patient. In the absence of a continuing air leak, a small pneumothorax that is only visible above the lung apex will resolve in 5 days or less, at the rate of 1% of total volume of the hemithorax per day. In the erect patient, gas collection will only be seen above the lung apex, and pleural apposition will be maintained down the lateral chest wall. The apposition of lateral pleura is lost in a moderate pleural effusion, resulting in decreased resorption of pleural fluid and greater chance of requiring intervention. Large pneumothoraces allow separate visualization of lobes of the lung and may be associated with tension physiology including hypotension due to a potentially catastrophic decrease in venous return to the heart (**Figure 114-7**).

PRACTICE POINT

Pneumothorax

- On the supine AP chest radiograph in the adult, one of the most reliable signs of pneumothorax is the deep sulcus sign. If air is in the pleural space, it can easily track down making the costophrenic angle deeper and more acute.
- Quantitative measurements, whether percentage pneumothorax or centimeters of displacement from the chest wall, are less useful than expert radiologic consultation, particularly when chest radiographs are obtained at the bedside.
- The sizing of pneumothoraces and pleural effusions is often more reliable on chest radiographs than CT scans.
- When a patient also has significant pleural effusion providing opacity outside the lung, it may become nearly impossible to detect the pneumothorax on a supine bedside chest radiograph.

■ PLEURAL EFFUSION

Normally, a thin white line represents the apposition of the parietal and visceral surfaces. Pleural disease, however, may cause expansion of the pleural space along with lobar collapse. Plain chest radiographs, rather than chest CT scans, may provide more reliable sizing of pleural effusions. An average of 300 cc of fluid is required to completely blunt a posterior costophrenic sulcus on a lateral chest radiograph. A *small pleural effusion* may not be visible on PA chest radiograph. A *moderate pleural effusion* is well seen on both PA and lateral views, and the distance between the stomach bubble and lung base may be increased. Subpulmonic collections may laterally displace the hemidiaphragmatic peak on the PA view. This does not in itself mean that the collection is trapped or loculated. Loculation may be associated with empyema, especially when it occurs in a patient who becomes increasingly ill despite improvement in treated pneumonia. A *large pleural effusion* severely restricts lung expansion, but retains visible lung on chest radiographs. A *very large*

TABLE 114-8 Cavitary Lesions

Wall Thickness	Inner Surface	Outer Surface	Significance
Thin wall	Smooth	Smooth	Cyst, bulla, pneumatocele
Thick wall	Smooth	Irregular	Abscess with or without adjacent pneumonia
Thick wall	Irregular	Smooth, may be lobulated	Malignant lesion particularly squamous cell carcinoma
Air-crescent	Smooth	Well-defined, may have ground-glass halo	Invasive aspergillosis (occurs in immune-compromised host)

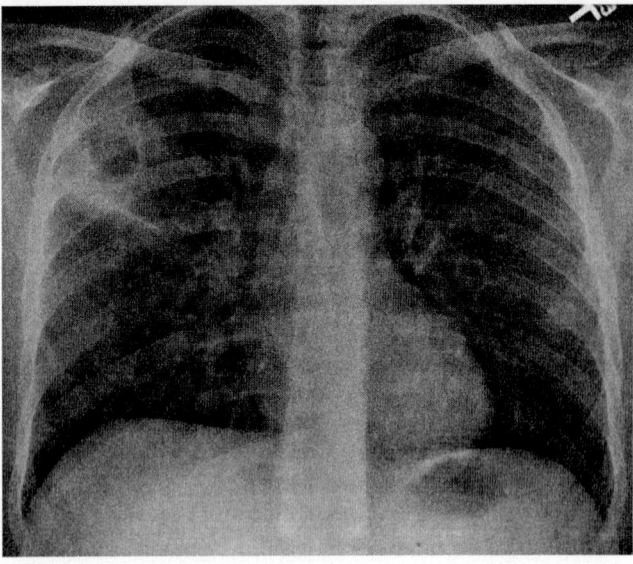

Figure 114-6 *Right upper lobe opacity with volume loss elevating the lateral aspect of the minor fissure contains a large central cavity due to necrosis. Gram-negative bacteria, such as Pseudomonas aeruginosa or anaerobic bacteria from oral flora is likely cause of this necrotizing pneumonia that has resulted from aspiration.*

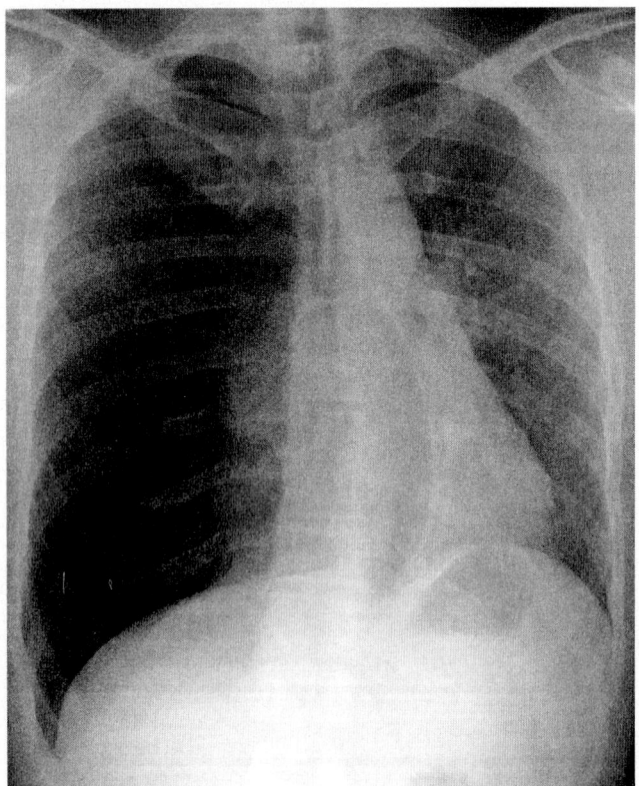

Figure 114-7 *Tension pneumothorax. Expiratory radiograph of right tension pneumothorax increases the apparent shift of midline structures including the azygoesophageal line, seen here behind the heart, to the left of the spine. The three lobes of the right lung are seen separating from each other centrally with complete absence of lung markings peripherally. Increased space between ribs and depression of the right hemidiaphragm also indicate expansion of the space occupied by the pneumothorax.*

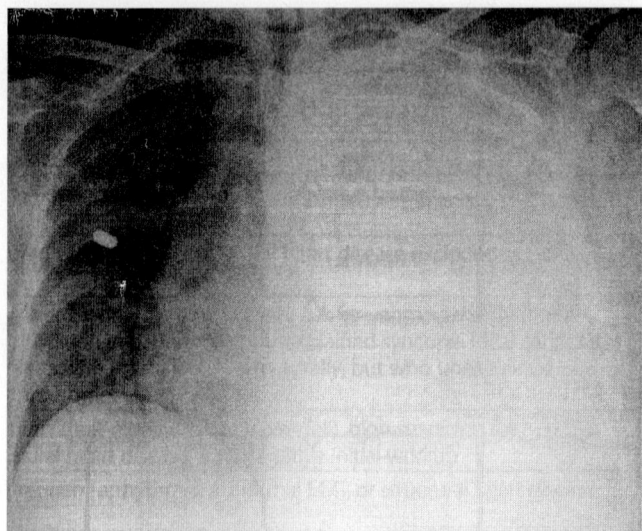

Figure 114-8 *A very large pleural effusion can also cause tension physiology. Note contralateral shift of the mediastinum.*

pleural effusion may result in complete whiteout of the hemithorax (**Figure 114-8**).

When a patient has a significant pleural effusion providing opacity outside the lung, it may become nearly impossible to detect the pneumothorax on a supine bedside chest radiograph. In this case, usually from barotraumas or line placement, the abnormal gas collection may take up to 5 days to become apparent, at which time the patient will have developed a pneumoperitoneum from a pneumomediastinum that communicated through the tight retroperitoneal cavity and dissected through the mesentery. Pneumoperitoneum has to be attributed to rupture of a hollow viscus until proven otherwise. For intubated patients who cannot be examined for an acute abdomen, this requires consultation with radiologists and other specialists and correlating with instrumentation.

EVALUATION OF CHEST PAIN AND/OR DYSPNEA

Commonly, chest radiographs are urgently ordered to evaluate causes of chest pain and to look for complications such as asymptomatic pulmonary edema in the setting of myocardial ischemia. Although the chest radiograph may be normal despite a life-threatening condition, such as an aortic dissection or pulmonary embolism (PE), plain chest radiographs may facilitate immediate identification if abnormal signs are present in addition to expediting management and further investigation.

PRACTICE POINT

Thoracic dissection: radiographic clues that should prompt advanced imaging

- Widening of superior mediastinum >8 cm
- Blurring of the aortic contour
- Opacification of the angle between the aorta and the left pulmonary artery
- Tracheal shift to the right
- Depression of the left main bronchus to an angle <40° with the trachea

Note: Aneurysms of the aorta are defined by the following measurements:

- >3.5 cm aortic arch
- >5 cm ascending thoracic arch
- >3 cm abdominal aorta

Typical life-threatening disorders that can alter the contour of the cardiomediastinal silhouette are acute vascular emergencies (ie, leaking thoracic aortic aneurysm or aortic dissection). If prior films are available for comparison, changes in aortic vessel diameter between two films are likely to be significant. For a stable patient, differentiating great vessel pathology from mediastinal disease requires advanced imaging unless there are prior images for comparison. If the plain chest imaging shows an abnormality of the mediastinum (eg, widening or distorted contour) or a displacement or narrowing of the trachea, the following potentially life-threatening diagnoses should be considered: primary and metastatic malignancy (bronchogenic and esophageal carcinoma, germ cell tumors, lymphoma, and thymoma), aortic disease (aneurysm, coarctation, dissection), congenital cysts, and vascular abnormalities. Benign diagnoses include asymmetric fat deposition, intrathoracic goiter, esophageal hernia, and vascular tortuosity.

Although a chest radiograph lacks specificity in the diagnosis of PE, it provides valuable data to use in the selection of further imaging to evaluate for PE, especially when pretest probability of PE is low. A chest film may identify abnormalities that explain the patient's symptoms or make interpretation of a ventilation scan indeterminate. If the chest radiograph is normal, a normal nuclear medicine perfusion study provides the best possible exclusion of PE. The patient with normal radiography will have an unambiguous ventilation/perfusion scan, and the normal CT will only add radiation and contrast without benefit as well as potentially lead to additional CT scans to prove stability of incidentally identified small lung nodules.

THE EVOLUTION OF RADIOGRAPHIC FINDINGS

The evolution of radiographic findings over time can correctly single out the likely diagnosis to explain a chief complaint. While acute consolidation of lung can be due to hemorrhage, pneumonia, or pulmonary edema, each of these processes undergoes a different evolution over time. The clinical presentation provides supporting data, including suggestive symptoms in the setting of known risk factors such as anticoagulation or heart disease, abnormal vital signs, or confirmatory physical signs. Hemorrhage occurs suddenly and resolves over several days with a coarse interstitial pattern as it resolves. The radiographic features of pulmonary edema depend upon the rapidity of onset; an interstitial pattern that may be accompanied by small pleural effusions may be seen when symptoms have a gradual onset, whereas perihilar consolidation is more commonly seen with symptoms that arise suddenly. Both forms can clear quite quickly, often within 24 hours, especially in patients on dialysis who can have wide fluctuations in fluid status. Pneumonia will cause increasing opacity; as it resolves, it will fade slowly, often over a prolonged period of time, well beyond the hospitalization.

The evolution of these processes suggests the optimum time for follow-up imaging. For example, an elderly patient with pneumonia would not be expected to have radiographic resolution of a significant pneumonia at the time of his first follow-up appointment with his primary care physician in a week's time. The timing of follow-up films should depend on the need to confirm a diagnosis or to assess response to treatment. One film obtained after the acute illness has likely resolved may be all that is necessary as a new baseline for future patient care. The timing of a chest radiograph to check for resolution of pneumonia depends on the age of the patient, the severity of the pulmonic process, and whether there is a high likelihood of postobstructive pneumonia (lobar collapse).

FINDINGS THAT REQUIRE FURTHER FOLLOW-UP IMAGING

It may be useful to divide such findings into two broad categories: (1) follow-up is needed to ensure the chest has returned to normal and (2) follow-up is needed to evaluate a previously unknown finding of potential significance, such as a lung nodule. The further workup of incidental nodules that require CT scanning is best deferred until the patient has recovered and the appearance of the chest has otherwise returned to normal. This is also true of investigations for interstitial lung disease. The central question regarding pulmonary nodules is whether the nodule is likely to be benign or malignant. Solitary pulmonary nodules may be an early manifestation of lung cancer. In one study, 40% of lung cancers were originally detected as a solitary pulmonary nodule. Opacification and consolidation with radiodense bone lesions in multiple ribs would suggest that disease has already become metastatic. It is also important to examine the hilum and mediastinum, especially in patients with a prior history of cancer. Variations of appearance based on visual features about margins, calcification, cavitation, and wall thickness may evolve over time. The presence of a mixture of solid, thick-walled cavities, thin-walled cavities, and resolution of prior nodules without scarring is far more specific for Wegener granulomatosis when these features are all seen in the same patient over time (Figure 114-8).

CONCLUSION

Chest radiographs are the most frequently obtained medical imaging during acute illness. The radiographs can provide physiologic as well as anatomic data. A baseline follow-up examination following resolution of the acute abnormality is mandatory for the care of patients with pneumonia and extremely helpful for the care of patients who have episodes of congestive heart failure, exacerbations of chronic obstructive pulmonary disease, or a tendency to develop acute abnormalities superimposed on chronic changes. As more data are accumulated during the workup of the acute illness, reconsideration of prior chest radiographs may rapidly provide additional information without additional radiography or more advanced imaging. Increasing the clinical information provided to the interpreting radiologist will result in more specific answers to clinical questions. The radiologic differential diagnosis will also be reduced through consideration of the evolution of the radiographic findings over time.

SUGGESTED READINGS

Austin J, Simon M, Trapnell D, Fraser RG. The Fleischner Society glossary: critique and revisions. *AJR.* 1985;145:1096-1098.

de Lacey G, Morley S, Berman L. *The Chest X-Ray: A Survival Guide.* Philadelphia, PA: Saunders; 2008.

Hall FM. Language of the radiology report: primer for residents and wayward radiologists. *AJR.* 2000;175:1239-1242.

Ketai L, Meholic A, Fofgren R. *Fundamentals of Chest Radiology*, 2nd ed. Philadelphia, PA: Elsevier Saunders; 2006, p. 304.

Khan AN, Al-Jahdali H, AL-Ghanem S, Gouda A. Reading chest radiographs in the critically ill (Part I): normal chest radiographic appearance, instrumentation, and complications from instrumentation. *Ann Thorac Med.* 2009;4(2):75-87.

Khan AN, Al-Jahdali H, AL-Ghanem S, Gouda A. Reading chest radiographs in the critically ill (part II): radiography of lung pathologies common in the ICU patient. *Ann Thorac Med.* 2009;4(3):149-157.

MacMahon H, Austin JHM, Gamsu G, et al. Guidelines for management of small pulmonary nodules detected on CT scans: a statement from the Fleischner Society. *Radiology.* 2005;237:395-400.

Martin GS, Ely EW, Carroll FE, Bernard GR. Findings on the portable chest radiograph correlate with fluid balance in critically ill patients. *Chest.* 2002;122:2087-2095.

Miller JC. Evaluating pulmonary nodules. MGH Radiology Rounds. 4(8). 2006. http://www.mghradrounds.org/index.php?src=gendocs&link=2006_august.

Mittl RL Jr, Scwab RJ, Duchin JS, Goin JE, Albeida SM, Miller WT. Radiographic resolution of community-acquired pneumonia. *Am J Respir Crit Care Med.* 1994;149:630-635.

Tuddenham WJ. Glossary of terms for thoracic radiology: recommendations of the Nomenclature Committee of the Fleischner Society. *AJR.* 1984;143:509-517.

Advanced Cardiothoracic Imaging

Maria F. Barile, MD
Francine L. Jacobson, MD, MPH

Key Clinical Questions

1. What are the advantages of noncontrast computed tomography (CT) compared with other CT studies?

2. What are the indications for noncontrast CT with thin-section reconstruction?

3. When is the use of IV contrast with CT imaging mandatory?

4. What are the limitations of positron-emission tomography (PET)-CT?

5. What are the Fleischner Society Guidelines recommendations concerning follow-up of incidental solid and subsolid pulmonary nodules?

6. What are the main indications for cardiac-CT?

7. What are the disadvantages of cardiac magnetic resonance with late gadolinium enhancement?

8. Complementary to two-dimensional echocardiography, transesophageal echocardiography (TEE) is able to provide superior visualization of what cardiac structures?

9. What calcium score would preclude contrast computed tomography angiography (CTA)?

INTRODUCTION

The overwhelming majority of advanced chest imaging for hospitalized patients is performed by computed tomography (CT), with ultrasound, magnetic resonance imaging (MRI), and nuclear medicine reserved for specific indications. The evolution of disease processes in the chest is central to the diagnostic process, necessitating integration between modalities in choosing comparison studies over time. An experienced radiologist may provide interpretation of serial bedside chest radiographs with physiologic and pathologic information that may not be available from more advanced imaging that reflects only a single snapshot in time.

The chief complaint and clinical differential diagnosis should guide decisions about the extent of medical imaging necessary for the proper diagnosis and treatment of the acute illness. The systematic way in which a clinician completes a history and physical examination is similar to the way in which a radiologist systematically analyzes and interprets an image. Both use a checklist that will identify the truly incidental and unrelated findings as well as separate seemingly unrelated findings that complete the picture of acute illness.

Many patients who require hospitalization for successful care of their acute illness have underlying medical conditions and chronic disease processes. Pre-existing heart disease, lung disease, and systemic disease findings help to develop the personalized differential diagnosis for the reporting of the imaging studies whether obtained as radiographs, CT, MRI or any other modality. Diabetes, collagen vascular diseases, chronic obstructive pulmonary disease, atherosclerosis, and suppression of the immune system may lead the radiologist to different conclusions about the significance of particular findings in an individual patient.

This chapter will focus on the abnormalities that most frequently require advanced imaging for diagnosis and the common incidental findings that require mandatory follow-up postdischarge.

NORMAL VERSUS ABNORMAL FUNCTION OF LUNGS

Blood flow is greater to the lower lobes than the upper lobes, and greatest in the right lower lobe. Hematogenous spread of tumor likely begins in the lung bases due to greater blood flow to this area, particularly the right lower lobe. Pulmonary emboli and septic emboli also occur more often in lower lobes. Oxygenation is greater in the upper lobes. Oxygen-loving mycobacterium organisms prefer the lung apices. Warm cigarette smoke rises most directly to the apical segment of the right upper lobe, not surprisingly causing the right upper lobe to be the most frequent site of primary lung cancer. The diametrically opposed oxygenation of the apices and perfusion of the bases creates a pH gradient from 7.52 in the lung apices to 7.39 in the lung bases. In the setting of hypercalcemia, as in renal failure, serum calcium will be precipitated in the lung apices. "Metastatic" deposition of calcium into normal tissues, reversible with correction of the hypercalcemia, only occurs in a base environment.

CT SCANNING

■ NONCONTRAST CHEST CT

The most basic enhanced chest CT scan without oral or intravenous (IV) contrast requires no special patient preparation other than breath-holding in inspiration. Multidetector CT scanners rapidly provide many images without respiratory motion artifacts despite continuous patient breathing; their use is preferred in the acutely ill hospitalized patient and the scanning room can generally accommodate ventilators and extensive support devices. Visualization of great vessels is generally adequate due to the presence of fat in the mediastinum in the absence of IV contrast material. The aerated lung parenchyma provides exquisite contrast for branches of the pulmonary arteries and pulmonary veins without requiring the addition of oral contrast agents.

Common indications for a noncontrast chest CT include:

- Further characterization of abnormalities identified on chest x-ray (CXR), including parenchymal consolidation, pulmonary nodules and masses, and pleural abnormalities
- Monitoring response to therapy of a known parenchymal disease
- Evaluation for interstitial lung disease

The noncontrast chest CT should not be used to assess hilar lymph nodes, particularly when small to borderline in size, pulmonary emboli (PE), and acute cardiovascular disease.

◼ NONCONTRAST ENHANCED CHEST CT WITH THIN-SECTION RECONSTRUCTION

Noncontrast enhanced chest CT with thin-section reconstruction is the standard imaging study of intrinsic, interstitial lung disease. Expiratory scans may be used to evaluate air trapping. A second scan during forcible expiration will best demonstrate central airway narrowing and thereby identify tracheomalacia, one of the causes of difficulty weaning a patient from ventilatory support. At end-expiration, thin-section reconstruction will clearly image lung parenchyma and air trapping in small airways. Prone images to more

completely evaluate the extent of interstitial lung disease are more easily performed following resolution of the acute illness.

High-resolution computed tomography (HRCT) uses slice thickness ≤ 2 mm with high spatial frequency reconstruction to image lung structure distal to all but the most peripheral vasculature (the secondary pulmonary lobule). HRCT images do not require contrast enhancement, which may confound the findings (see **Table 115-1**).

◼ CONTRAST-ENHANCED CHEST CT

Contrast-enhanced chest CT examinations differ by rate of injection and delay before imaging (slightly longer for the evaluation of aortic dissection). Cardiac gating may be used in some institutions to provide a triple-rule-out scan for the coronary arteries, the aorta and pulmonary arteries.

The use of IV contrast material is mandatory for CT pulmonary angiography (CT-PA). Patients who have had prior mild to moderate contrast allergy reactions may receive prophylaxis over approximately 12 hours prior to CT-PA. If the history of allergic reaction is severe, such as anaphylaxis, an alternative test should be chosen. See Chapter 113 (Patient Safety Issues in Radiology).

Ideally, the patient should be fasting for 4 hours prior to the administration of IV contrast material but a nonfasting patient may have CT-PA without delay when necessary. A large bore, minimum 20-gauge catheter is required in order to inject contrast material at a high velocity of approximately 4 cc/second. Using a tenuous or smaller IV for the study will almost certainly result in an inadequate opacification of pulmonary arteries and a nondiagnostic study. Pulmonary emboli may be seen on standard contrast-enhanced chest CT scans, so clinicians should review any recent prior CT scans with

---

TABLE 115-1 Radiologic Features and Differential Diagnosis of Idiopathic Interstitial Pneumonias

Histologic Pattern	Radiographic Features	Distribution on CT	HRCT Features	Differential Diagnosis
AIP (DAD)	Progressive diffuse ground-glass opacity leading to consolidation ARDS	Diffuse	Early: lobular sparing Late: traction bronchiectasis	Hydrostatic edema Pneumonia Acute eosinophilic pneumonia
COP (BOOP)	Patchy bilateral consolidation	Subpleural	Consolidation Nodules (small or large)	Infection, vasculitis, sarcoidosis, BAC, lymphoma, pneumonia, NSIP
RB-ILD	Bronchial wall thickening Ground-glass opacity Normal in 14%	Diffuse	Bronchial wall thickening Centrilobular nodules Patchy ground-glass opacity Emphysema	DIP NSIP Hypersensitivity pneumonitis
NSIP	Nonspecific Normal in 7%	Peripheral, subpleural, bases, symmetric	Centrilobular opacities Irregular lines Microcystic honeycombing	UIP DIP OP Hypersensitivity pneumonitis
DIP	Ground-glass opacity Normal in 3-22%	Peripheral bases Diffuse in 18%	Ground-glass attenuation Reticular lines Honeycombing	RB-ILD Hypersensitivity pneumonitis Sarcoidosis PCP
IPF (UIP)	Basal predominant reticular abnormality with volume loss Normal in 10-15%	Peripheral bases Subpleural	Reticular Honeycombing Traction bronchiectasis Bronchiectasis Architectural distortion Focal ground-glass	Asbestosis Collagen vascular disease Hypersensitivity pneumonitis Sarcoidosis

the radiologist in light of new suspicion for PE prior to subjecting the patient to the risks of additional radiation and contrast.

THORACIC PET-CT

Thoracic PET-CT uses a radionuclide that binds to a D-glucose analogue to produce FDG. Because glycolysis is upregulated in tumor cells as well as in normal cells during anaerobic conditions, PET-CT can identify tumors when other imaging is indeterminate. PET-CT recognizes tumor through inflammatory characteristics; hence, high uptake of fludeoxyglucose (FDG) may falsely suggest malignancy in metabolically active infections and inflammatory conditions. Originally, PET-CT was used to evaluate solitary pulmonary lesions that may be cancerous. However, infectious granulomas (eg, tuberculosis or fungal), hyperplastic thymic tissue in the anterior mediastinum, and brown adipose tissue at the base of the neck, supraclavicular area, or superior mediastinum in adults may avidly take up FDG. Decreased FDG uptake may occur when there is acute hyperglycemia because FDG and glucose compete for the same receptor.

Positron-emission tomography CT (PET-CT) is usually used for staging *known* cancer. PET-CT may reliably evaluate 8 mm pulmonary nodules of unclear etiology, but some well-differentiated adenocarcinomas of the lung can be very slow growing and, therefore, reveal little or no FDG-glucose avidity.

Although PET-CT does not require contrast, the dose of ionizing radiation that the patient receives from the CT scan for attenuation correction is not negligible. The CT scan performed for attenuation correction of the PET scan is not a diagnostic quality CT scan. The uncertain and incidental findings will also lead to significant additional imaging. This long and very expensive examination should not be undertaken when the patient cannot adequately cooperate or has acute processes that may interfere with interpretation and are expected to resolve in a short interval of time.

CARDIAC COMPUTED TOMOGRAPHY (CCT)

Cardiac-computed tomography (CCT) visualizes nonstenotic calcified and noncalcified coronary plaques with a very high negative predictive value (91%-100%) to rule out the presence of coronary artery disease (CAD). Excellent images may be obtained within 5 minutes, thereby facilitating rapid triage from the emergency department in some institutions. Its primary use in acute chest pain should be reserved for patients with an intermediate pretest probability of coronary artery disease or for those patients at increased risk for aortic dissection and segmental pulmonary embolism that may be visualized at the same time. Patients with a low pretest probability should not be subjected to the risk of radiation; patients with a high pretest probability of CAD and suspected non-ST elevation myocardial infarction (NSTEMI) or unstable angina (UA) would not benefit because a negative CCT would not alter the pretest probability. Cardiac CTA requires the administration of contrast.

LUNG CANCER SCREENING CT

The United States Preventative Services Task Force (USPSTF) recommends annual lung cancer screening with low-dose CT (LDCT). Screening begins at age 55 in adults who have a 30 pack-year history, either currently smoke or have quit within the past 15 years, and are in their usual state of health. Annual screening ends once a person has not smoked for 15 years or develops a health problem that substantially limits life expectancy or the ability or willingness to have curative lung surgery. Exclusion criteria also include treatment for nonskin cancer within the preceding 5 years. This screening is performed in the outpatient setting along with counseling for smoking cessation. Entry into a screening program begins with a "shared decision making" visit, ordinarily with the patient's primary care physician. The guidelines for this test will undoubtedly evolve.

The American College of Radiology maintains very complete and up-to-date resources.

DIAGNOSIS-DRIVEN IMAGING

PULMONARY EMBOLISM

The diagnosis of pulmonary embolism (PE) has remained difficult despite successive improvements and refinements in imaging modalities. Patients who require hospitalization for acute care, particularly with advancing age, have comorbidities that increase the pretest probability of PE. Evaluation of ventilation-perfusion scanning by PIOPED investigators suggests that more than 50% of patients likely to be seen by hospitalists will fall into the category most at risk for actually having PE when the result is intermediate or indeterminate. As a result, CT-PA has been widely adopted as the primary diagnostic test for PE *although a normal perfusion scan still provides greater exclusion of PE* (**Table 115-2**).

Pulmonary emboli may be hard to detect even in lobar arteries and the detection of the smallest peripheral emboli may be difficult to put in clinical perspective. The number of vessels present in each lung and each segment within each lung is daunting for complete assessment by conventional angiography. Pulmonary emboli are easier to identify in the larger vessels in the lower lobes that are also more readily examined in the axial plane. With increasing use of coronal and sagittal reformatted images and advanced image processing, the detection of upper lobe pulmonary emboli and smaller vessels will continue to improve. The lungs normally trap and make harmless the much more frequently occurring subclinical microemboli; as a result these microemboli fail to pass through the capillaries in the lungs, thereby do not reach other organs. At what point should this normal function be deemed clinically significant pathology requiring treatment? The existence of significant sources of additional clot may inform the decision-making process more than the current miniscule burden of clot.

TABLE 115-2 Acute Chest Pain, Suspected Pulmonary Embolism

Radiologic Procedure	Appropriateness	Radiation Level
X-ray chest—do not expect to be definitive	9	1
CTA chest with contrast	9	3
Tc-99m V/Q scan lung	8	3
US lower extremity with Doppler	7	3
Ateriography pulmonary with right heart catheterization	5	4
MRA pulmonary arteries with and without contrast	4	0
MRA pulmonary arteries without contrast	3	0

The evaluation of potential PE by CT initially included pelvic and lower extremity imaging to assess for DVT. This portion of the CT-PA examination is now largely historical as it required significant additional radiation and was rarely helpful. When the value of identifying DVT as a source for future PE is important, lower extremity noninvasive imaging (LENI) with ultrasound is preferred and may also obviate the need for CT-PA in the pregnant patient. The absence of clot is less helpful in the diagnosis of acute PE because one-third or more patients will have no evidence of clot in their lower extremities despite acute PE. The normal perfusion scan remains the single best test to exclude PE when the CXR is normal.

PRACTICE POINT

Pulmonary embolism (PE)

If the result of a "negative" PE-protocol CT does not support the clinical pretest probability and the lungs are not normal for a perfusion strategy, the options in order of descending preference are as follows:

1. Consult with your chest radiologist to obtain a "second opinion" about the original CT.
2. Consider an MRA versus a conventional pulmonary angiogram to address the areas in question on CT. The choice will vary depending on institutional resources.
3. Consider repeating the CT-PA; however, the yield is likely to be low unless there was a quality issue with the first scan (such as timing or velocity of administration of contrast bolus, respiratory motion).

As always, the result must be interpreted in the context of the patient sitting in front of you, including weighing the risk of empiric anticoagulation for a defined period of time. For example, if a patient had severe acute airspace disease or severe end-stage lung disease, a significant PE would likely lead to intubation. Of course the patient may have a real but tiny left lower lobe PE (LLL PE). In the setting of all the rest, it is not the problem.

The radiographic evolution between acute PE and infarction occurs over several days. It is not infrequent for pulmonary emboli to no longer be visible, particularly when peripheral, so that multiple subsegmental defects may elude detection several days after the acute symptoms such as pleuritic chest pain occur. It then becomes more important to consider whether any secondary signs of PE or right heart strain are present on the scan already obtained. Chronic changes that may result from prior PE include pulmonary artery wall thickening and segmental bronchiolitis obliterans with marked diminution of pulmonary vessels.

The detection of pulmonary emboli also varies due to patient factors, including respiratory factors and artifacts that can be minimized by relocating foreign bodies such ECG leads for the test. A shallower inspiratory breath-hold will maximize vessel opacification particularly in young and relatively healthy patients. Clinicians should prepare patients to expect to raise their arms and to hold their breath for the study. Respiratory motion and bolus quality often conspire to limit the exclusion of PE to central PA branches in the acutely ill patient. The interpreting radiologist should report the bolus quality and use variable display window and level settings to better visualize emboli.

■ CHEST PAIN OF UNCLEAR ETIOLOGY

In some institutions, patients with chest pain of less clear etiology may receive CT scans even while still in the emergency department. IV contrast material will be used to provide greatest opacification of the primary region suspected to be the cause of a particular

patient's chest pain. Thus, a longer delay will be needed for contrast enhancement of the aorta than the pulmonary arteries. In fact, by the time the aorta is well opacified, the standard bolus of contrast material may no longer be visible in the pulmonary arteries. In a patient who may suffer from an aortic dissection that may decrease perfusion of the kidneys, it is not advisable to increase the dose of IV contrast material to maintain contrast enhancement through pulmonary and systemic circulation simultaneously (**Figure 115-1** and **Table 115-3**).

PRACTICE POINT

Aortic dissection

- Dissection is imaged by CT angiogram of the chest and abdomen which is usually the most rapidly available modality in the institution.

PRACTICE POINT

The triple CT scan

- The best quality CT scan will be achieved through pretest consideration of probability as well as a more complete description of the patient's chest pain, whether pleuritic, radiating to the neck, radiating to the back, or crushing. Accompanying signs and symptoms, such as elevated blood pressure and shortness of breath also contribute to the decision-making process and, of course, CT should not be used as a substitute for complete history and physical examination.

■ PERICARDIAL DISEASE

Visibility on chest radiographs of the separation of epicardial and pericardial fat depends upon a fortuitous relationship to the diverging x-ray beam. A change in the shape or sudden increase in size of the cardiac silhouette suggests a pericardial effusion and requires confirmation with echocardiography. It is quite common to have discrepancy in reporting of pericardial effusion between CT scans and echocardiography, particularly when the anterior pericardial recess is used as an acoustical window in the course of transthoracic echocardiography. The recess itself may give the impression of being part of a more generalized effusion. Measured in millimeters on CT scans, a 1 cm pericardial effusion is comparatively large.

Calcification associated with constrictive pericarditis will be seen on plain radiographs and CT scans. On MRI it will appear as a signal void. Additionally, cardiac MR can demonstrate the altered function quite elegantly.

■ LUNG CANCER

Nonsolid and part solid adenocarcinoma of lung

Adenocarcinoma commonly begins with noninvasive, lepidic growth along alveolar walls that results in very well-defined, though subtle, nonsolid or ground-glass opacities on CT images. Over time, the ground-glass nodules continue to grow in size and increase in density, developing solid components (**Figure 115-2A**).

The solid components indicating focal invasion on histology are visible on CT scans along with small cystic spaces in the tumor that may resemble airways and other parenchymal features. The progressive evolution of solid components leads to the type of nodule that is most worrisome for cancer, the part-solid nodule. Additional features may raise suspicion even higher, particularly when focal linear extensions are seen to cross the lung to pleural surfaces that may be remote from the lesion and focal pleural thickening when

Stanford A:
Involves the ascending aorta, may also involve descending aorta
Typically treated surgically

Stanford B:
Involves the descending aorta
Typically treated medically

DeBakey I:
Dissection involves ascending aorta, arch, and descending aorta

DeBakey II:
Dissection involves ascending aorta only

DeBakey III:
Dissection involves descending aorta only

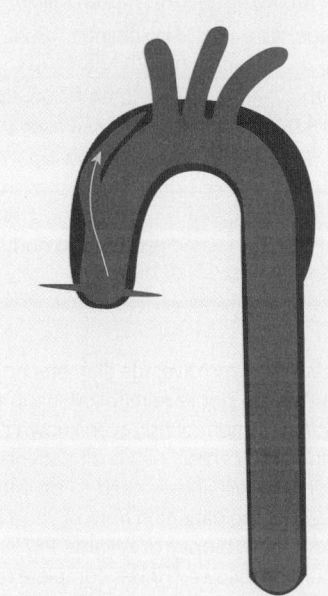 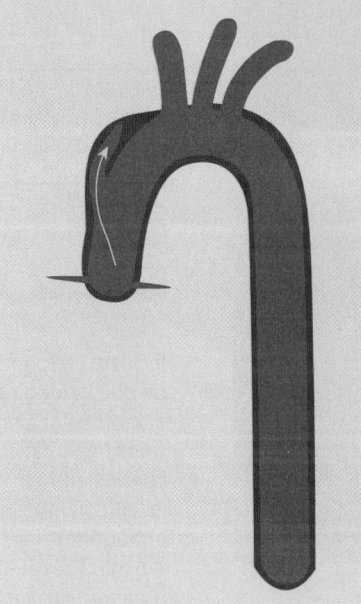 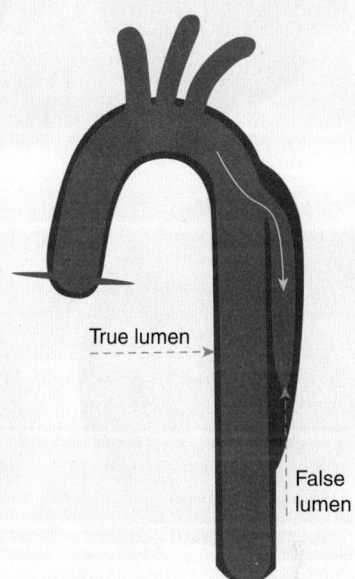

True lumen

False lumen

Debakey I / Stanford A

Debakey II / Stanford A

Debakey III / Stanford B

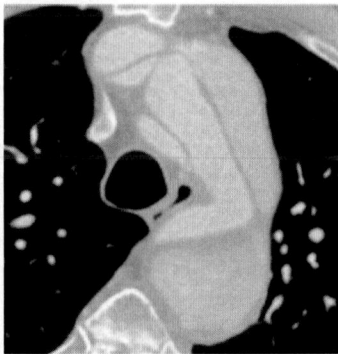 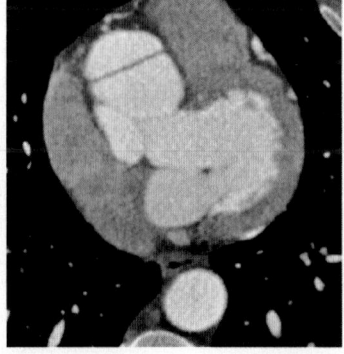 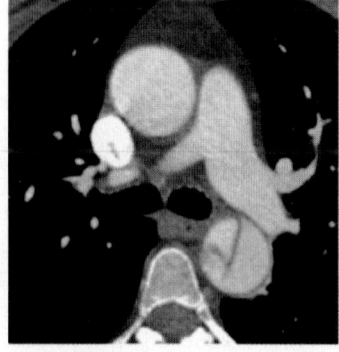

Dissection of the ascending and descending aorta

Dissection of the ascending aorta only

Dissection of the descending aorta only

Figure 115-1 *Aortic images dissection.* (Reproduced, with permission, from Jacob C. Mandell, MD, Brigham and Women's Radiology.)

TABLE 115-3 Acute Chest Pain, Suspected Aortic Dissection

Radiologic Procedure	Appropriateness	Radiation Level
X-ray chest—do not expect to be definitive	9	1
CTA chest and abdomen	9	4
MRA chest and abdomen	8	0
US echocardiography transesophageal	8	0
Aortography chest and abdomen	5	4
US echocardiography transthoracic	4	0

the lesion is adjacent to the pleura. The presence of multiple lesions does not exclude cancer although acute infection and hemorrhage associated with nodules may be more common (**Figure 115-2B**).

Further evaluation and treatment for early lung cancer should be deferred during an acute illness. Needed coronary artery revascularization and valve replacement are generally performed prior to lobectomy or other treatment for lung cancer.

Lymphangitis carcinomatosis

Lymphangitis carcinomatosis most commonly represents the end process of hematogenous dissemination of a tumor with tumor cells in the lymphatics that course along with the pulmonary venous structures in the septae of the secondary pulmonary lobule. To differentiate from interstitial edema, it is helpful to look for pulmonary

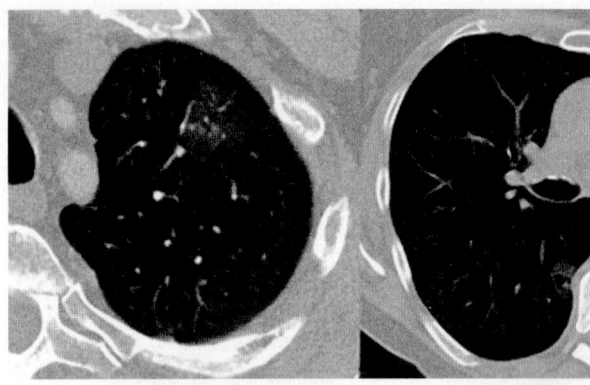

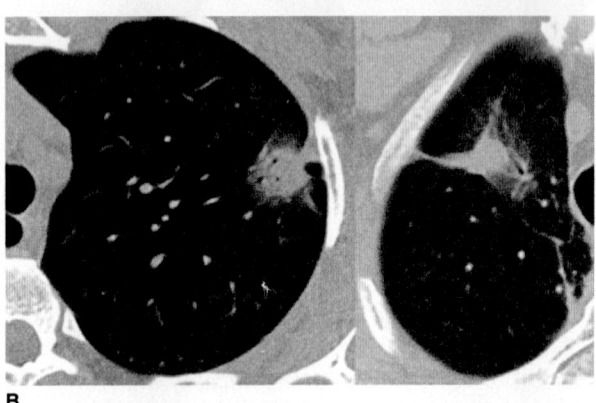

Figure 115-2 *(A) Images of early adenocarcinoma of lung demonstrating well-defined ground-glass opacity without additional distinguishing features (left), and areas of increased density and small cystic spaces, with more specific features (right). Long-term follow-up (>2 years) often required for confident diagnosis, as PET-CT will demonstrate little, if any, FDG-glucose avidity. (B) Images of progressive adenocarcinoma of the lung with thin extensions to distant pleura, focal pleural thickening, and sharp demarcation between the ground-glass opacity and the adjacent normal lung, unlike inflammatory lesions such as pneumonia.*

nodules, even micronodules, and nodular thickening of the fissures. The findings will not abate with diuresis. The finding no longer signifies imminent death within 6 months as patients often live 3 or more years with treatment. Twenty percent of lymphangitis is due to obstruction of central lymphatics rather than actual tumor. This is particularly likely when a central hilar mass such as a lung cancer obstructs the lymphatics. In this case, lymphangitis will generally be unilateral instead of bilateral when due to hematogenous dissemination of tumor. Breast cancer may also be associated with unilateral lymphangitis carcinomatosis.

■ INCIDENTAL PULMONARY NODULES

Purely solid pulmonary nodules

The most reliable sign of benign disease is solid or central calcification in a pulmonary nodule. The presence of contrast material, regardless of timing, may limit the detection of calcium in a nodule. Contrast enhancement of nodules to identify malignancy is infrequently performed in most centers that have PET-CT scanning readily available. The Fleischner Society 2005 Recommendations and other guidelines address indeterminate incidental pulmonary nodules found on chest CT scans (**Table 115-4**).

The Fleischner Society Guidelines recommend follow-up of incidental solid pulmonary nodules based on size and features of the nodule but do not apply to patients less than 35 years of age or to patients who have a known malignancy. It is extremely unusual for

TABLE 115-4 **Fleischner Society Small Nodule Follow-up Recommendations**

Nodule Size	Low Risk Patient	High Risk Patient
≤4 mm	None	12 month If no change, stop
4-6 mm	12 month follow-up If no change, stop	6-12 month follow-up If no change, 18-24 month follow-up
6-8 mm	6-12 month follow-up If no change, 18-24 month follow-up	3-6 month follow-up If no change, 18-24 month follow-up
>8 mm	CT scan at 3, 9, 24 months Consider PET-CT (in some centers also nodule enhancement chest CT) or biopsy	

incidentally found, tiny, less than 4 mm average diameter nodules to be due to lung cancer so they do not require follow-up in patients at low risk for lung cancer. Assessment of risk, even known cigarette smoking, is difficult and in some centers nearly all patients will be considered high risk. Guidelines will always need to be interpreted in light of the clinical context of the patient in front of you. Not large enough for transthoracic needle biopsy or reliable PET scan, the 4-6 mm size category should be followed unless complete resection is performed. It is appropriate to refer the recommended follow-up to either a pulmonologist or thoracic surgeon who is accustomed to following these lesions and promptly acting upon the results when necessary.

Subsolid nodules

Management strategies for incidentally found subsolid nodules, including pure ground glass nodules and part solid, part ground glass nodules, differ from the management of purely solid nodules. In 2013 The Fleischner Society published recommendations for the management of subsolid pulmonary nodules detected on CT (**Table 115-5**). These recommendations reflect the indolent nature of peripheral adenocarcinomas (formerly referred to as bronchoalveolar carcinomas [BAC]) which often initially present as subsolid nodules. Subsolid nodules should be followed for greater than 2 years to ensure stability, given their slow rate of growth.

PRACTICE POINT

Pulmonary nodules

● It is not appropriate to follow-up previously identified nodules during acute pulmonary processes just because the patient is in the hospital. Pulmonary nodules require direct communication with the patient and the patient's primary care physician (PCP) to make certain the findings are not overlooked after the acute illness resolves.

Transthoracic CT-guided biopsy may be performed for actionable lesions in the 1 cm range.

Tiny, indeterminate pulmonary nodules

Multidetector CT scans are exquisitely sensitive for detection of solid nodules measuring 2 to 3 mm in diameter. These are seen in more than 50% of patients and will be overwhelmingly benign. In populations with high rates of endemic granulomatous infections, 90% or more of patients cared for by hospitalist physicians will have

TABLE 115-5 Fleischner Society Pulmonary Nodule Recommendations

Nodule Type	Initial Management Recommendations	Additional Follow-up Considerations
Solitary ground-glass >5mm	Initial Follow-up in 3 mo	CT follow-up yearly for minimum of 3 y
		Solid-component ≥5 mm requires diagnostic evaluation that may include PET-CT, biopsy, or resection
Multiple ground-glass nodules ≤5 mm	Follow-up CT at 2 and 4 y	Consider alternative causes
Multiple ground-glass nodules >5 mm	Initial follow-up in 3 mo	CT follow-up yearly for minimum of 3 y
Part-solid nodules >5 mm solid	Follow-up CT in 3 mo	Persistent lesion has high risk of lung cancer-consider surgical resection

tiny indeterminate nodules. Through studies in Japan and the Early Lung Cancer Action Project, follow-up of thousands of such nodules reveals an extremely low rate of cancer in these tiny nodules that most often represent granulomas and intrapulmonary lymph nodes. In the lung cancer screening CT trials, the rare cancer identified at a site of indeterminate tiny nodule on a prior CT was so low that such nodules receive at most one follow-up CT scan. The rare nodule of this type that becomes a lung cancer generally grows in a short amount of time. A solitary pulmonary nodule identified on chest radiographs may prove to be one of multiple pulmonary nodules by CT. The primary purpose for CT scanning of a dominant pulmonary nodule with significant probability of malignancy is to stage lung cancer (see **Table 115-6**).

The most conservative approach to an incidental pulmonary nodule seen on abdominal CT is to obtain a chest CT to identify all lung nodules that might be present. This follow-up CT scan may be deferred when the incidental finding will not affect immediate treatment decisions.

■ INCIDENTAL FINDINGS OUTSIDE THE LUNG PARENCHYMA

Incidental findings of the aorta, kidneys, liver, and gallbladder will be frequently encountered on chest CT scans. When the finding is in the upper abdomen or lower neck, the follow-up will be with the more appropriate focal examination. Follow-up of findings with potential for imminent catastrophe, such as aortic rupture, and findings that might completely change the immediate decisions about the course of therapy should be worked up promptly during the hospitalization. Otherwise, it is appropriate to defer the workup until the patient is well and transient acute findings such as pleural effusion have resolved. For example, an aberrant right coronary artery arising from the left aortic leaflet is at risk for obstruction by adjacent structures; it is unlikely to suddenly become symptomatic while the patient is acutely ill, although it makes the radiologist reporting the study uncomfortable. Incidental findings in the abdomen can be managed by following the recommendations of the American College of Radiology (ACR). Hospitalists should communicate incidental findings and the radiologist's recommendations so that the patient does not undergo unnecessary repetition of imaging (**Figure 115-3**).

MAGNETIC RESONANCE IMAGING (MRI)

Organizing an MRI for a hospitalized patient is not a simple undertaking and examinations are frequently suboptimal when patients are acutely ill. All support lines and tubes must be specifically approved for imaging by MRI. In rare cases, the examination will require general anesthesia. In centers that can perform the examination under anesthesia, a radiologist and an anesthesiologist will generally both be required continually throughout the procedure, lasting on average 1 hour. See Chapter 112 (Introduction to Radiology) regarding contraindications to MRI.

TABLE 115-6 Differential Diagnosis of Solitary Pulmonary Nodule

Primary considerations:

Lung cancer, including all neuroendocrine lung tumors (carcinoid-small cell)

Hamartoma

Granuloma

AVM

Solitary pulmonary metastasis

Specialized considerations:

Hematoma following trauma with laceration to lung parenchyma

Infection due to fungus, parasite, or atypical organism

Infarction, particularly from Swan-Ganz catheter

Noninfectious inflammatory process such as Wegeners granulomatosis

Vasculitis

Primary pulmonary lymphoma

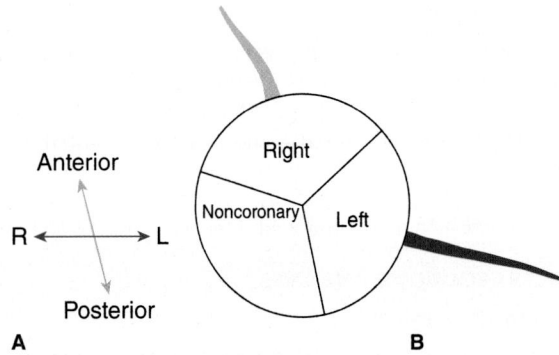

Figure 115-3 *There are most commonly two coronary artery origins from the proximal aorta, at the junction between the sinuses of valsalva and the aorta. The right coronary artery arises from the anterior right coronary cusp and the left coronary artery arises from the posterior left coronary cusp. Drawing (A) and CT scan image (B) provide axial image orientation. (Reproduced, with permission, from Jacob C. Mandell, MD, Brigham and Women's Radiology.)*

Magnetic resonance imaging examinations in the chest are most frequently performed with a gadolinium-based contrast agent. Gadolinium is no longer considered inert and without risk. The dose of gadolinium will be adjusted based on the patient's weight to minimize the risk of nephrogenic systemic fibrosis (NSF). If a patient has had a severe allergic reaction to iodinated contrast material used for CT, consultation with a radiologist will facilitate a decision between choosing noncontrast enhanced chest CT and MRI. MRI and CT provide equivalent information regarding the mediastinum and the presence of lymphadenopathy. MRI may be superior to CT in examination of pleural fluid and pleural masses and can confirm the presence of blood despite a mass-like appearance. The degradation of red blood cells provides changes in appearance of extravascular blood over time that can be used to estimate the duration of the abnormality. MRI provides greater definition of fat planes and chest wall masses. MR angiography (MRA), coupled with cardiac gating, can provide high quality images in place of conventional angiography. Computed tomography may complement MRI for the study of bones due to the signal void on an MRI examination caused by calcification. Without correlative imaging, whether chest radiographs or CT scan, such signal voids may cause confusion. Any outside imaging that might bear on this issue should be brought to the attention of the interpreting radiologist.

Cardiac magnetic resonance (CMR) with late gadolinium enhancement may provide information about proximal coronary anatomy, myocardial perfusion, myocardial viability, acute versus chronic changes, and global and regional cardiac function. It may identify specific myocardial regions at risk and thereby provide additive information not only pertinent to risk stratification but also help target revascularization in patients with UA/NSTEMI. Cardiac magnetic resonance is a rapidly evolving technology and the reported specificity, positive predictive value, and overall accuracy is likely to reflect expanded protocols. The disadvantages of CMR include cost, length of time required for scanning, the use of gadolinium in patients with reduced renal function, and contraindications (implanted pacemakers and defibrillators).

ULTRASOUND (US)

◼ ADVANTAGES

Ultrasound can be brought to the patient at the bedside or performed in the radiology department. Ultrasound of the chest requires no special preparation, can be done in a variety of positions, and does not expose the patient to ionizing radiation.

◼ LIMITATIONS

Patient body habitus and comorbidities may become limiting for ultrasound examinations, including echocardiography. Adipose tissue attenuates ultrasound and decreases the penetration, limiting the depth that can be examined. Air stops the transmission of ultrasound. Ultrasound is not routinely used to image lung parenchyma and the presence of an overlying lung can limit visualization even in normal individuals. Destructive lung disease such as emphysema causes greater obscuration due to increased anterior extension of lung.

◼ ULTRASOUND OF THE CHEST

Noncardiac ultrasound

The most frequent use of noncardiac ultrasound of the chest is for planning and performance of thoracentesis. Ultrasound can differentiate complex fluid and pus from free fluid, detect septal structures that become dilated due to interstitial pulmonary edema. Ultrasound lung comets (ULC), an echographic sign of extravascular lung water, originate from water-thickened interlobular septa. Ultrasound may occasionally image extrathoracic soft tissues and accessible vascular structures.

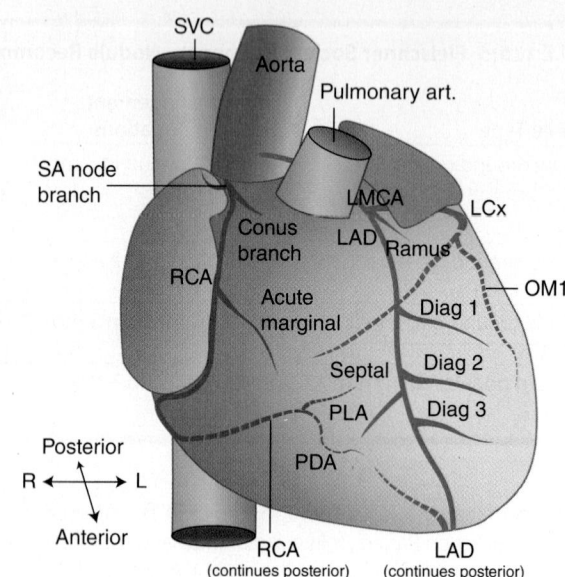

Figure 115-4 *Normal coronary anatomy.*

Cardiac ultrasound

Cardiac ultrasound two-dimensional (2D) echocardiography with color Doppler is frequently the first imaging acquired for the internal structure and functional evaluation of the heart, including ejection fraction. It may be ordered without prior chest radiographs for a young patient with a heart murmur. Coupling anatomic detail with physiologic function, it can assess a wide range of abnormalities from mitral valve prolapse to pulmonary artery hypertension and critical aortic stenosis. A bedside two-dimensional echocardiography will detect abnormalities of wall motion in all cases of STEMI and hence, may be indicated when there is uncertainty about the diagnosis (pericardial effusion, RV infarction, ventricular aneurysm, or LV thrombus), the need for emergent reperfusion therapy, or prognosis (reduced left ventricular function) (**Figure 115-4**).

Complementary to 2D echocardiography, transesophageal echocardiography (TEE) is able to provide superior visualization of the posterior cardiac structures. The acoustical window provided by the esophagus allows excellent evaluation of the ascending aorta and a significant portion of the heart and descending thoracic aorta without intervening lung and bone. In institutions where transesophageal echocardiography is readily available with high level of skill at the bedside, it may be used as the first, and potentially only, diagnostic test for aortic dissection that requires emergent surgical intervention. Since air stops sound waves, the region of the aortic arch is not completely imaged with this modality. Extension into great vessels is better assessed by CT or MRI.

In addition to suspected aortic dissection, TEE may be used as an initial test to guide percutaneous interventions for structural heart disease, assess the cause of fever in patients with intracardiac devices, and to evaluate the possibility of left atrial thrombus prior to cardioversion or radiofrequency ablation. Contraindications include esophageal problems and poor cooperation due to altered mental status. Patients with coagulopathy may have increased risk of bleeding. Complications are usually minor such as transient bronchospasm, hypoxia, nonsustained ventricular tachycardia, atrial fibrillation, hemoptysis, vomiting, or hematoma. Patients should fast for 4 to 6 hours prior to the procedure.

NUCLEAR MEDICINE

Nuclear medicine can provide powerful problem-solving information in tailored examinations. Radiotracer can prove patency of central venous catheters, identify spleen when present in the pleural

TABLE 115-7 Radioactive Tracer Material

MIBI

- Technetium-99m (99mTc) labeled methoxy-isobutyl-isonitrile, aka 99mTc-sestamibi
- T1/2 = 6 h
- Lipophilic molecule that passively diffuses through myocyte membrane
- Higher photon energy
- Minimal redistribution, stays fixed in myocyte, giving a snapshot at time of injection

Thallium (Tl-201)

- T1/2 = 73 h
- Low photon energy
- Potassium analogue that enters normal myocytes
- Peak myocardial activity occurs 5-15 min after injection
- Intracellular concentration of thallium depends on vascular supply and membrane function
- Does not remain fixed in myocyte, redistributes

space, identify low level bleeding that is difficult to localize and evaluate function. For a patient with a normal chest x-ray, a normal perfusion scan alone still provides the finest exclusion of PE.

Nuclear medicine is also used extensively for cardiac evaluation, even in the acutely ill where pharmacologic stress can safely evaluate the heart muscle (**Table 115-7**).

PRACTICE POINT

Cardiac testing options

Exercise stress test: sensitivity 68%, specificity 77%

- No need to be fasting
- Still the best test for women with low pretest clinical probability even if more false positives
- Low risk (<1% annual cardiac mortality) clinical patients without ETT abnormalities do not benefit from further imaging
- Intermediate risk (2%-3% annual cardiac mortality)
- High risk (4% annual cardiac mortality) clinical patients should proceed directly to the cardiac catheterization laboratory without further imaging

Pharmacologic agents

- Dobutamine (broad adrenergic receptor agonist, titrated to heart rate response)
  - Contraindicated if ACS, VT, afibrillation with RVR
  - Fasting at least 4 hours
  - May use with atropine
- Vasodilators (stimulate adenosine A2a receptors): adenosine, persantine (dipyramidole), regadenoson (Lexiscan)
  - Contraindicated if bronchospasm, AV block
  - Fasting at least 4 hours, no caffeine for 24 hours
  - No aggrenox

SPECT reported: sensitivity 88%, specificity 77%

- May be exercise or pharmacologic
- Total time 2 to 4 hours

ECHO reported: sensitivity 76%, specificity 77%

- May be exercise or pharmacologic
- Requires good US windows and can be enhanced by contrast

CT

- Requires contrast
- Must be pharmacologic
- Patient must be supine
- Total time 30 minutes

In general, exercise is preferred if patients can walk as long as they do not have contraindications. Absolute contraindications include acute coronary syndrome (ACS), myocardial infarction within the previous 48 hours, unstable arrhythmias, decompensated congestive heart failure, symptomatic severe aortic stenosis, acute pulmonary embolism, acute myocarditis or pericarditis, aortic dissection, and acute pulmonary embolism. Relative contraindications include left main stenosis, uncontrolled hypertension, tachy- or bradyarrhythmia, left ventricular outflow obstruction, inability to exercise adequately, ventricular pacing, and left bundle branch block (LBBB). Perfusion imaging is preferred for patients whose baseline ECG has ST-segment abnormalities, digitalis therapy, LBBB, or pacing, and for those who have a significant pretest likelihood for coronary artery disease (CAD) or a history of previous revascularization to determine extent of ischemia. If patients can exercise safely, they should have an exercise imaging study. Pharmacologic stress imaging is indicated for those patients who cannot exercise and do not have contraindications to the agent such as severe hypertension (dobutamine) or acute bronchospasm or hypotension (adenosine).

The selection of imaging modality for the heart will vary with expertise and availability of services in each institution. Stress echocardiography can be performed with exercise or pharmacologic agents. In nuclear medicine, myocardial perfusion imaging is commonly performed with thallium (Tl-201) or sestamibi, creating planar or SPECT images. The nuclear medicine physician or radiologist who performs nuclear medicine studies can provide guidance in selection of pharmacologic stress testing. Both agents are highly sensitive in detecting ischemia and scarred myocardium. Thallium is better for detecting viable myocardium, particularly "hibernating myocardium" because of its redistribution. Since sestamibi is used in larger doses, image quality will be higher and there will be more flexibility in the imaging protocol because the radioisotope does not redistribute in tissue over time. Preparation for these examinations includes abstaining from caffeine for 12 hours prior to the test and abstaining from food and tobacco for 2 hours prior to the test. The test itself may take 2 or more hours. SPECT images are obtained in the cardiac axes, short, long, and vertical. Normal myocardial perfusion imaging is associated with less than 1% annual mortality while abnormal high risk findings predict 3% annual mortality and should be evaluated for coronary revascularization.

In some centers, cardiac PET-CT may be performed with rubidium-82, nitrogen-13 ammonia, or F-18 fluorodeoxyglucose. It can be performed with or without stress, particularly if the SPECT study is inconclusive or there is discordance between prior cardiac imaging tests. It may help determine the significance of an anatomic abnormality or coronary stenosis.

■ SCREENING FOR CORONARY ARTERY CALCIUM

At the initiation and progression of an atherosclerotic plaque, active processes cause calcium deposition in the coronary arteries. Best seen on cardiac-gated noncontrast CT, coronary calcification independently predicts cardiovascular events in intermediate risk patients and therefore provides additional prognostic data beyond traditional risk factors of age, diabetes, smoking, hyperlipidemia, and family history (**Table 115-8**). Calcium screening may be more beneficial in women than in men because traditional risk factors less accurately predict the presence of coronary artery disease in

TABLE 115-8 Coronary Calcium (CAC) Scores, a Surrogate of Total Atheroma Burden Independent of Pretest Relative Risk of MI or Cardiac Death

CAC Score: Lifetime Impact of All Atherosclerotic Risk Factors, Known & Unknown	Relative CAD Risk Proportional to Score based on Population Studies	Comments: Not a Functional Test, Does Not Signify Location or Severity of Blockage	Next Steps
0	Excludes most clinically relevant CAD	Even in high-risk asymptomatic or symptomatic populations	Healthy lifestyle and guideline-based treatment of individual risk factors; consider other diagnoses if symptomatic
≤10	Very low likelihood of CAD (<1%)	Considered a negative test	Healthy lifestyle and guideline-based treatment of individual risk factors; consider other diagnoses if symptomatic
11-100	2:1	Score 11-400 high risk >2% risk of future cardiac events; future risk of score higher if younger	Consider functional study along with intensive risk factor modification
100-400	3-6:1	Test + for atherosclerosis & ↑ risk	Intensive risk factor modification; further cardiac testing
400-1000	5-10:1 Majority of coronary events in people with high calcium scores & scores >75th percentile relative to age- & sex-matched controls	>400 indicate extensive coronary artery disease with 90% probability of >70% stenosis of a coronary artery; ≈ 5% per year risk of developing symptomatic heart disease	Intensive risk factor modification; further cardiac testing
>1000	10-30:1	Very high risk	Intensive risk factor modification

this population. Although there is no data supporting imaging for coronary calcification in low risk patients, it may be useful in asymptomatic intermediate risk patients to identify those patients who might benefit from the most aggressive risk factor modification or for imaging stable patients with chest discomfort to exclude

obstructive coronary artery disease. The total (Agatson) score is based on the deposition of calcium in the left main, left anterior descending, left circumflex, and right coronary artery. A calcium score of more than 400 would preclude a contrast CTA given the significant decrease in positive predictive value (**Figure 115-5**).

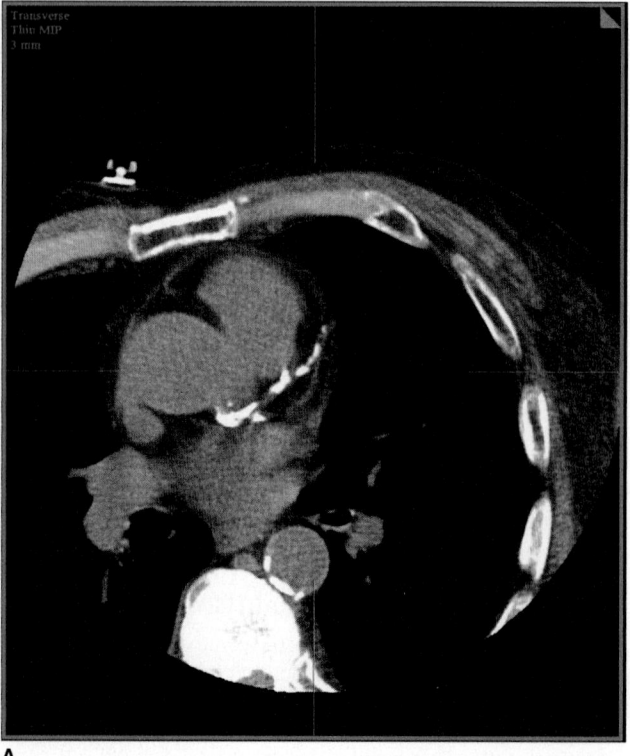
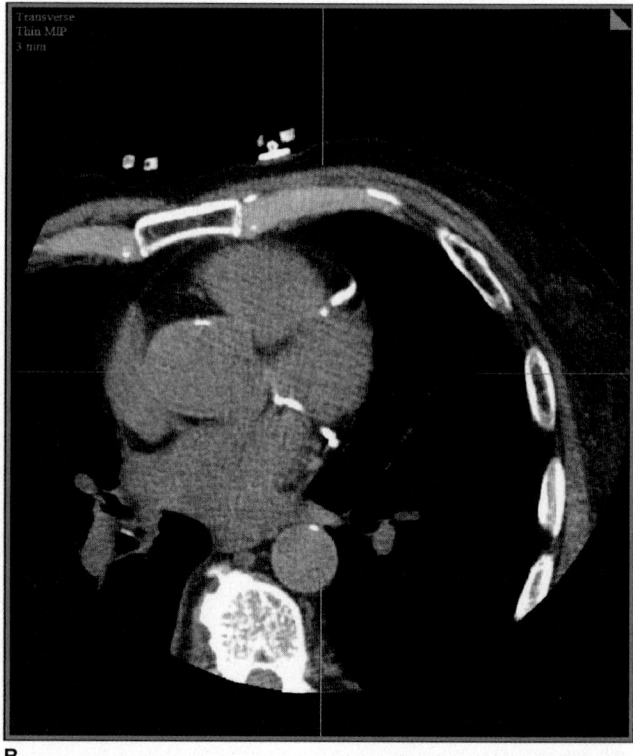

A   B

Figure 115-5 *Calcium score high, >3000; normal Rubidium-82 PET scan. (A and B) Calcification in left main coronary artery (left) continues in branches (right) seen on axial images from noncontrast enhanced cardiac-gated coronary CT scan. (C) Coronary artery calcifications not always indicative of obstructive CAD as in the same patient with no demonstrated functional impairment. Calcium scoring in a young patient more predictive of future risk.*

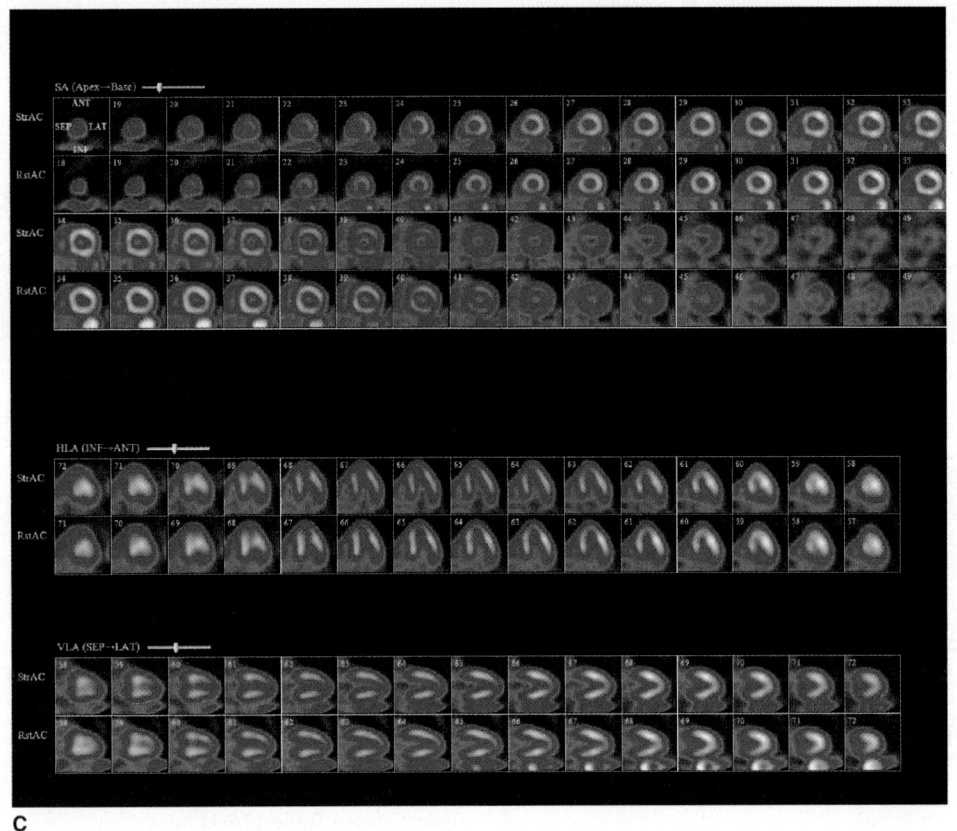

C

Figure 115-5 *(Continued)*

CONCLUSION

Computed tomography scanning is the primary advanced imaging for the chest in hospitalized patients. Through augmentation of chest radiographic data, the CT scan may answer questions that arise long after it is obtained. Accepting a negative result for definitive patient management is not appropriate when it is at odds with the pretest probability of the abnormality being present, particularly when the abnormality is one that cannot be missed, such as PE. In that situation, reviewing the images together with the radiologist may bring the report into agreement with the clinical impression that the likely abnormality is actually present. Consultation with radiology will also clarify the next steps, whether to treat the patient without further workup or order a different specific test. In the case of potential PE and other life-threatening possibilities, it is usually better to select a different modality. It is also important to consider the probability that the test will be adequate in relation to the interval since an acute event, particularly in the case of PE.

SUGGESTED READINGS

American Thoracic Society/European Respiratory Society International Multidisciplinary Consensus Classification of the Idiopathic Interstitial Pneumonias. *Am J Respir Crit Care Med.* 2002;165(2):227-304.

Berland LL, Silverman SG, Gore RM, et al. Managing incidental findings on Abdominal CT: White paper of the ACR incidental findings committee. *J Am Coll Radiol.* 2010;7(10):754-773.

MacMahon H, Austin JH, Gamsu G, et al. Guidelines for management of small pulmonary nodules detected on CT scans: a statement from the Fleischner Society. *Radiology.* 2005;237:395-400.

McClelland RL, Chung H, Detrano R, Post W, Kronmal RA. Distribution of coronary artery calcium by race, gender, and age: results from the Multi-Ethnic Study of Atherosclerosis (MESA). *Circulation.* 2006;113(1):30-37.

Mueller-Mang C, Grosse C, Schmid K, Stebellehener L, Bankier AA. What every radiologist should know about idiopathic interstitial pneumonias. *Radiographics.* 2007;27(3):595-615.

Naidich DP, Bankier AA, MacMahon H, et al. Recommendations for the management of subsolid pulmonary nodules detected at CT: a statement from the Fleischner Society. *Radiology.* 2013;266:304-317.

ONLINE RESOURCES

http://www.acr.org/SecondaryMainMenuCategories/quality_safety/app_criteria.aspx.

http://jakemandell.com/iip/.

interactive medical education

PE algorithm

http://www.guideline.gov/algorithm/5885/NGC-5885_2.pdf.

Cardiac imaging

http://info.med.yale.edu/intmed/cardio/imaging/.

http://www.ccsnm.org/pdfs/2010/radiologist-help-info/CardiacPracticeGuidelinesSummary.pdf.

http://www.acr.org/Quality-Safety/Resources/Lung-Imaging-Resources.

CHAPTER 116

Basic Abdominal Imaging

Francine L. Jacobson, MD, MPH

John M. Braver, MD

Sylvia C. McKean, MD, SFHM, FACP

Key Clinical Questions

1. What views are standard to evaluate the acute abdomen?

2. Which radiograph view is the most sensitive for detecting a small pneumoperitoneum?

3. What are the conditions simulating air under the diaphragm?

4. What are the causes of air-fluid levels on an erect abdominal image?

5. How do you quantify the amount of gas normally seen in the bowel?

6. What are the radiologic signs of bowel ischemia?

7. What are the most common abnormalities associated with acute pancreatitis?

Despite the availability of newer imaging modalities to look for intestinal obstruction or perforation, the supine abdominal radiograph (KUB) remains indispensable for evaluating a patient with abdominal pain due to the ease and ready availability for rapidly screening patients with abdominal pain. The standard field of view extends from the lung bases to the pubic symphysis, thereby framing the genitourinary system, imaging kidneys, ureters, and bladder. Additional views include an erect chest radiograph, erect abdominal view, and left lateral decubitus.

Figure 116-1 is a line diagram pointing out the twelfth ribs, lumbar transverse process, kidneys, psoas line, inferior liver edge, terminal ileum, sacroiliac spine, gas in the ileum and jejunum, gas and feces in the transverse colon, haustral folds, and descending colon. A thin layer of adipose tissue should be visible as a lucent line between the transverse abdominal muscle and the peritoneum extending from above the lateral margin of the liver to below the iliac crest and between the dome of the bladder and the pelvic peritoneum.

The abdominal radiograph is not symmetric and in fact there is significant variation in a "normal" KUB as seen in **Figure 116-2**. Systematic review of examinations may be facilitated by use of a checklist (see **Table 116-1**).

In order to better perceive structures on abdominal radiographs and to better correlate physical exam and imaging findings, it can be helpful to study coronal anatomy images of computed tomography (CT) or magnetic resonance imaging (MRI) (see Chapter 117, **Table 116-2**).

Air helps to identify hollow viscous structures on radiographs. The anatomic rendering reveals the colon coursing from the right side of the pelvis, up to the liver, across to the spleen, and then down to the rectum. The presence of adipose tissue may assist interpretation. For example, a thin layer of fat is often seen between the dome of the bladder and the pelvic peritoneum as a lucent line. Location of this layer may be an important clue signifying an enlarged bladder (or urinary retention) as the cause of the patient's abdominal pain. Tissue-fat interfaces with the adjacent bowel facilitate assessment of organ size.

The erect chest radiograph is used to detect pneumoperitoneum, but it may also provide important clues to other causes from the chest that mimic an acute abdomen, including congestive heart failure from acute myocardial infarction, widened aorta seen in aortic dissection, pneumothorax, pneumomediastinum, pneumonia, and pleural fluid collections. The erect abdominal radiograph does not provide additional information to the standard KUB and erect chest film.

Working films may also be obtained for the management of support lines and tubes. The placement of tubes into the stomach and small bowel may be confirmed using a somewhat hybridized view of lower chest and upper abdomen.

RADIATION EXPOSURE

The KUB delivers a higher dose of ionizing radiation than a posteroanterior (PA) chest radiograph because the abdomen is almost always a thicker body part. The greater penetration provides enhanced visualization of lung bases and may identify lower lobe lung processes or pleural effusions associated with abdominal pain. It is particularly important to communicate with the radiologic technologist regarding the priority areas for imaging when the patient is

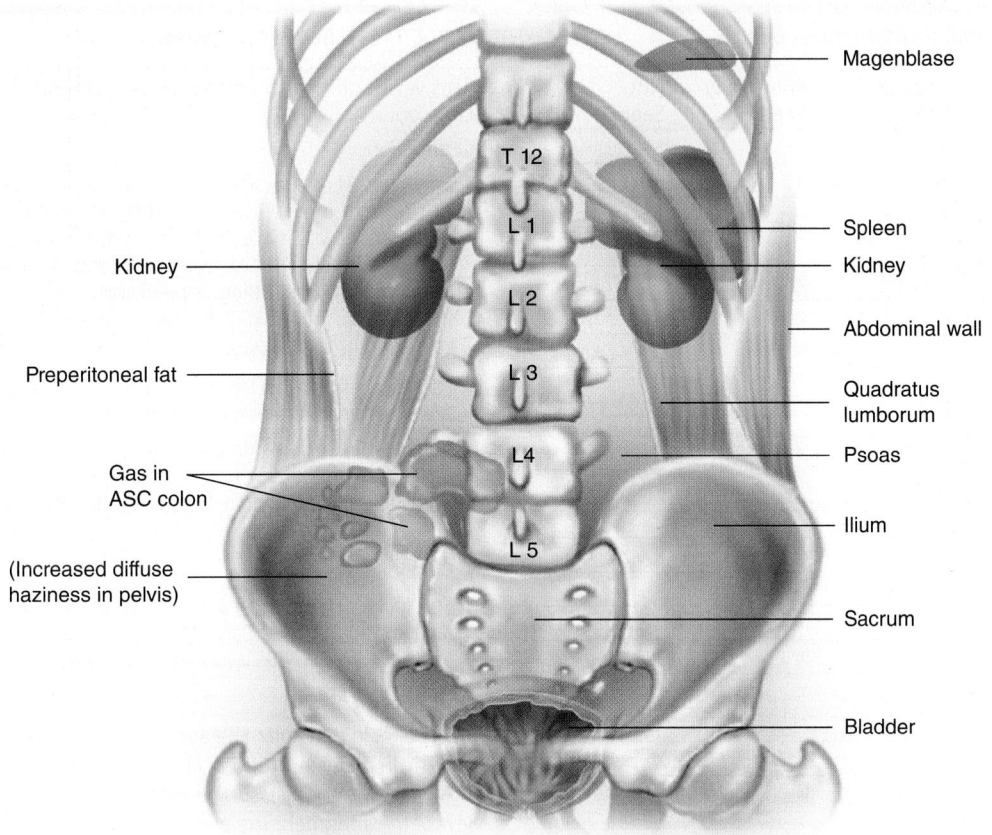

Magenblase

T 12

L 1

Spleen

Kidney

Kidney

L 2

Abdominal wall

Preperitoneal fat

L 3

Quadratus
lumborum

L4

Psoas

Gas in
ASC colon

Ilium

L 5

(Increased diffuse
haziness in pelvis)

Sacrum

Bladder

Figure 116-1 *Anatomic line drawing (including right kidney, psoas line, properitoneal fat line, inferior liver edge, terminal ileum, sacroiliac joint; twelfth rib, left psoas, haustral folds, lumbar transfer process, gas and feces in transverse colon, gas in jejunum, descending colon, gas in ileum).*

too large for a single 14 × 17 in image. This can decrease duplication of exposure for completion of examination and repeated examinations that delay patient care.

PRACTICE POINT

Communication
● Provide specific localizing clinical information. This facilitates radiograph interpretation and limits radiation exposure when the patient is too large for a single 14 × 17 in image.

TABLE 116-1 Checklist for Interpretation

- Diagnostic quality: Does the radiograph include the area from the diaphragm to the hernia orifices? Is the properitoneal lucency (flank stripe) separating the transverse abdominal muscle and parietal peritoneum visible?

- Alignment and integrity of bones, bone margins, joints: Are there any fractures of the lower ribs? Lumbar transverse processes? If so, worry about soft tissue injury to liver, spleen, and kidney. Is the acetabulum intact bilaterally?

- Soft tissues, fat-tissue interfaces.

- Air patterns: Look for pneumoperitoneum, abnormal bowel gas patterns, and air in biliary tree or portal vein.

- Size of organs.

- Calcification: Check for abnormal calcification (kidney stones, gall stones, pancreatic or splenic calcifications).

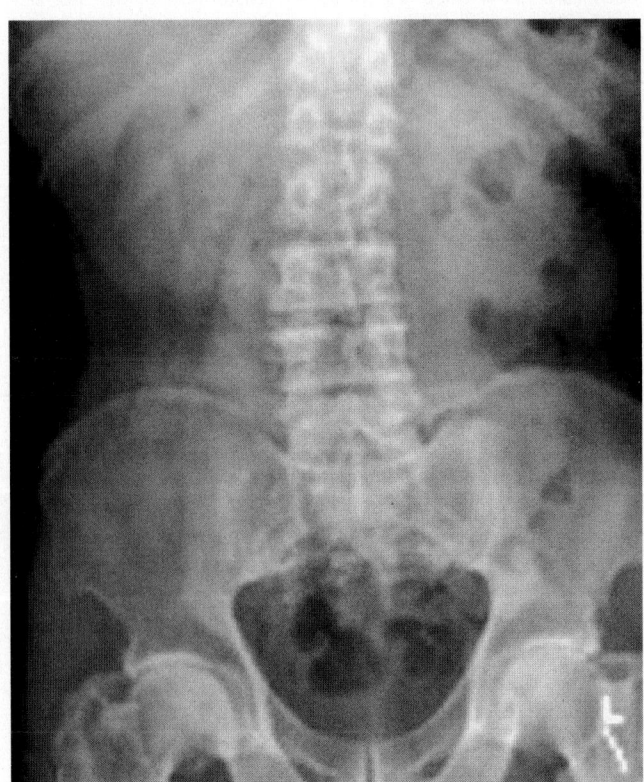

Figure 116-2 *Normal supine abdominal radiograph.*

TABLE 116-2 Visibility of Structures on KUB

Organ	Usually Seen	Potentially Seen	Not Seen
Liver	X		
Spleen	X		
Kidneys	X		
Stomach	X		
Duodenum		X	
Small intestine	X		
Cecum		X	
Colon	X		
Bladder	X		
Prostate		X	
Retroperitoneal fat	X		
Gallbladder			X
Pancreas			X
Adrenal glands			X
Ovaries			X
Uterus		X	
Ureters		X	
Lymph nodes			X
Mesentery			X
Vasculature			X

Calcification may localize otherwise inapparent organs.

SCREENING PLAIN FILMS

■ BONES

Plain films readily image ribs; lumbar vertebrae and appendages, especially transverse processes; sacrum; pelvis (iliac crests, acetabula, pubis); femoral head; and neck and may provide important clues to the patient's overall health. Patients with end-stage renal disease or endocrine disorders have characteristic bony changes and a screening plain film may uncover an underlying malignancy that has a prediction to bony metastasis.

Ribs, spine, and pelvic fractures can suggest location of soft tissue injury. If fractures are identified in the lower ribs and lumbar transverse processes, consider soft tissue injury to the liver, spleen, or kidney. Spine and sacroiliac (SI) joints may indicate chronic arthritic changes.

■ GAS PATTERNS

Normal

Air and fluid are both normally present in the gastrointestinal (GI) tract. Fluid is secreted into the GI tract even when a patient has no oral intake. The movement of gas through the system over time is valuable data for functional evaluation even from a single radiograph. The stomach and small and large bowels will normally distend to accommodate gas. The amount of gas normally seen in the small bowel is <2.5 cm in diameter and <5.5 cm in diameter for the colon. The cecum can normally be somewhat larger, up to 8 cm (**Table 116-3**).

■ PNEUMOPERITONEUM

The acute abdomen is assessed by two types of radiographs, the abdominal flat plate "KUB" with the patient in the supine position, and at least one more radiograph of either the chest or abdomen in the erect or decubitus position in order to look for gravitational

TABLE 116-3 Bowel Gas Patterns

Ileus versus obstruction: air-fluid levels, distention of small and large bowels

Obstruction

- Small bowel obstruction: 3-5 h after onset of complete obstruction, progression marked by collapse of distal bowel and absence of air in colon; central distribution, absence of feces, close valvulae conniventes extending across entire diameter of bowel, string of pearl sign.
- Large bowel obstruction: Peripheral distribution, haustral sacculations, presence of feces.
- Pseudoobstruction: Diffuse dilation of small and large bowel, often with prominent gastric distension.
- Volvulus: Closed obstruction of loops, leading to proximal and distal occlusion of portions of bowel, most commonly cecum (haustral sacculations present) and sigmoid colon.

Ileus

- Postoperative ileus.
- Sentinel loop sign focal adynamic ileus as in duodenum adjacent to inflamed pancreas.

effects and, in particular, the abnormal gas pattern of pneumoperitoneum. In many institutions, an acute abdomen series will include a PA view of the chest, supine view of the abdomen, and an erect view of the abdomen. The erect chest radiograph is the most sensitive for detecting a small pneumoperitoneum; however, the best gravity view is the left lateral decubitus view for patients unable to stand. The patient should be placed in position for a minimum of 10 minutes prior to obtaining this view to allow air to rise above the liver where it will become radiographically apparent.

Although the 2 to 3 mm thick diaphragm provides a useful silhouette for free intraperitoneal air, both benign and pathologic conditions can mimic pneumoperitoneum. Distention of the stomach thin walls may cause concern for pneumoperitoneum actually due to air in a distended or overdistended stomach. Interposition of the colon between the right hemidiaphragm and liver, called Chilaiditi's syndrome, may raise concern for free air when the air is actually contained within the colon. Basilar pneumothorax causes thickening of the pleura or subsegmental atelectasis when parallel to the hemidiaphragm. The presence of gas within the bowel wall itself, pneumatosis coli, can also raise concern for pneumoperitoneum even when it is a benign finding.

■ AIR-FLUID LEVELS AND DILATATION

Pain anywhere in the body can cause increased gas due to swallowed air. Abnormal gas patterns may suggest acute perforation, gastroparesis, adynamic ileus, small bowel obstruction, large bowel obstruction, and toxic megacolon. However, fluid levels are not pathognomic of obstruction. In addition to ileus and obstruction, air-fluid levels on erect abdominal plain film may normally be seen (if <2.5 cm in length) or related to gastroenteritis, electrolyte disturbances (hypokalemia), uremia, and ischemia. If on plain film of the abdomen the diameter of the small bowel exceeds 3 cm, it suggests either an obstruction or an ileus. If the small bowel dilatation is > 4 cm, an obstruction is more likely. The key to the differentiation of colonic obstruction and paralytic ileus on plain film is whether there is dilation of the cecum. If the transverse colon is more dilated than the cecum, a diagnosis of ileus is most likely. The cecum is the most dilated segment of the colon in obstruction. Megacolon refers to a dilation of the transverse colon >5.0 to 6 cm. The cutoff is not precise because it depends on the clinical context. For example, as

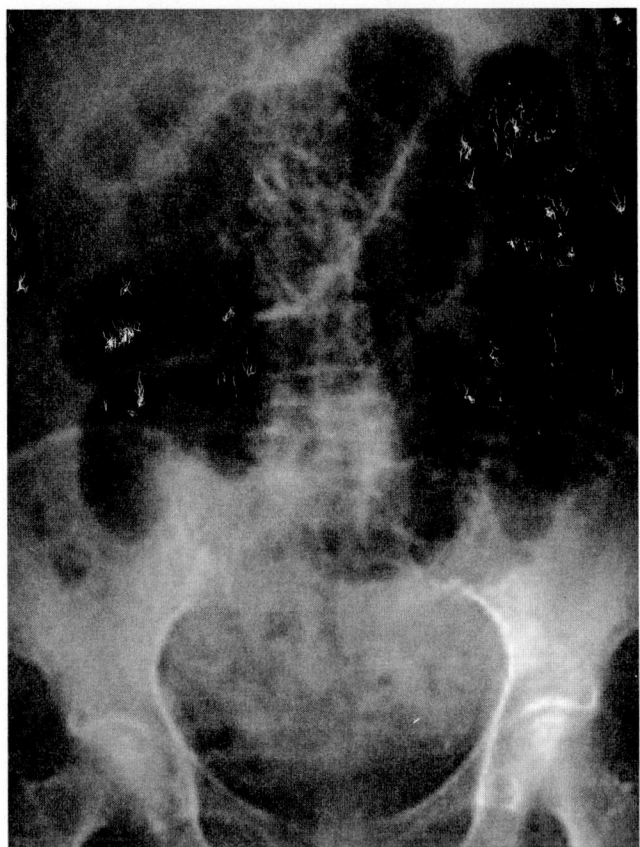

Figure 116-3 *Small bowel dilatation.*

patient size increases, magnification increases so that a normal look-ing large colon that still has haustration may be read as normal in an asymptomatic obese individual. When there is acute colonic disten-tion with the cecum >9 cm, there is an emergent risk of perforation (**Figure 116-3**).

The distribution of distention may localize the obstruction, which may be partial or complete. Small bowel dilated loops (central loca-tion and close valvulae across entire diameter) are usually evident within 3 to 5 hours after complete obstruction. Proximal to an obstruction, peristalsis increases as an attempt to move the bowel contents beyond a site of mechanical obstruction. The hyperperi-stalsis continues beyond the obstruction resulting in the clearing of the GI tract distal to the point of obstruction. These correlate with tinkles and rushes heard through the stethoscope. If dilated small bowel extends to the lower portion of the abdomen, it indicates that the obstruction is at least in the distal small bowel or perhaps in the proximal colon. Small bowel obstruction (SBO) will result in an emptied colon and central stair-step configuration of fluid levels in the small bowel. If air is seen distally in the colon or rectum, either a partial small bowel obstruction or an acute complete small bowel obstruction may be present (as some of the air distal to the obstruc-tion site has not yet been expelled). Gallstone ileus from the passage of a gallstone into the GI tract infrequently produces signs of small bowel obstruction or gas in the biliary tree.

PRACTICE POINT

Guiding principles
Ensure that a patient receives the least radiation during imaging.
- Make sure that the study is necessary.
  - Do you need an initial KUB if you are planning to order an abdominal CT anyway?
  - Do you need an erect abdominal radiograph? The erect abdominal radiograph does not provide additional information to the standard supine abdominal radiograph and erect chest radiographs.
- You can save repeated examinations with consequent expense, added radiation, and attendant delay of clinical care by communicating your clinical concerns that the examination will address.
  - The size of a patient's abdomen is frequently larger than what can be captured by a single view.
  - The technologist performing the examination will need to cut off the anatomy depending on the clinical information provided.
  - To ensure that a patient receives the least radiation in the course of abdominal imaging, the order must include the clinical concern that the examination is supposed to address.
- When in doubt about the utility of an additional test, consult your radiology team.

Radiographic features of large bowel obstruction include periph-eral location of dilatation, thick haustral sacculations that do not extend across the entire diameter, and the presence of feces. If the ileocecal valve is competent, there is a greater risk of cecal perfora-tion. Pseudoobstruction may involve diffuse dilatation of both the small and large bowel as well as the stomach.

PRACTICE POINT

Obstruction
- If the small bowel dilatation is >4 cm an obstruction is more likely. The key to the differentiation of colonic obstruction and paralytic ileus on plain film is whether there is dilation of the cecum. If the transverse colon is more dilated than the cecum, a diagnosis of ileus, is most likely. The cecum is the most dilated segment of the colon in obstruction. Megacolon refers to a dilation of the transverse colon >6 cm.

Adynamic ileus, most often seen in postoperative patients on large doses of pain medications, differs from the appearance of SBO because the small bowel and colon dilate to accommodate the large amounts of swallowed gas that is able to move freely within the bowel, even without the patient being able to pass gas.

Other abnormal gas patterns include "a string of pearls" sign, sentinel loop sign, and omega loop. As the lumen of an obstructed small bowel fills with fluid, small bubbles of air are trapped in most of the superior aspect of the lumen between the valvulae conni-ventes, looking like "a string of pearls." The sentinel loop sign refers to an ileus localized to a segment of bowel from a focal inflamma-tory process such as appendicitis, cholecystitis, or pancreatitis. The omega loop sign, referring to a massively dilated loop of colon that looks like an inverted U projecting out of the pelvis toward the right upper quadrant, suggests sigmoid volvulus (which is three times more common than cecal volvulus). Here there is a closed obstruc-tion of loops resulting in complete occlusion of both the proximal and distal portions of the involved bowel.

An abdominal radiograph may also reveal emphysematous collections (typically in diabetics) referring to air outlining the gall bladder or urinary bladder. Pneumatosis coli is a benign condition presenting radiographically as intramural gas limited to the colon.

ABDOMINAL ORGANS

Differentiation between various soft tissue structures on radiographs is largely based on relationships between organs, adjacent gas-containing bowel, and fat planes. The soft tissue densities of the liver, spleen, and kidneys can be measured to determine their size. The liver typically measures 21 to 22.5 cm across the widest point, 15 to 17.5 cm in cranial-caudal extent, and 10 to 12.5 cm from front to back. The size and shape of the liver, however, varies. Riedel lobe refers to its posterior edge, extending downward to the iliac crest. The spleen measures approximately 11 cm; autosplenectomy is common in sickle cell disease. The kidneys normally measure 12 to 14 cm. Asymmetry in kidney size may be an important clue to the presence of significant underlying kidney disease. In some instances the kidney size may be increased as in polycystic renal disease. The aorta normally measures 3 cm in diameter. Unless calcified, the pancreas will not be visualized on plain film.

CALCIFICATIONS

Pelvic phleboliths due to pelvic vein thrombosis and lymph nodes are the most common calcifications seen on KUB. Approximately 15% of gallstones and 85% of kidney stones appear radio-opaque and radiographs can reveal a staghorn calculus filling the intrarenal collecting system or the tiniest calcification at the ureteropelvic junction responsible for producing renal colic.

DO NOT MISS DIAGNOSES

With the exception of free peritoneal air, the diagnosis of most life-threatening disorders relies upon nonspecific radiographic signs in the clinical context of the patient. Concern about any of these possibilities should prompt further imaging or life-saving surgical exploration.

PNEUMOPERITONEUM

A supine radiograph may reveal intraperitoneal air under the inferior aspect of the liver or hepatorenal recess (Morrison pouch). Air may be evident between adjacent loops of bowel such that air is seen on both sides of the bowel wall (Rigler sign). The Cupula sign refers to larger air collections under the central tendon of the diaphragm creating a central crescentic lucency. Following abdominal surgery, a pneumoperitoneum may be visible for up to a week or more, depending on the amount of gas and the body habitus of the patient. Pneumoperitoneum may be continually seen in the presence of a percutaneous gastrostomy.

SPLENIC INJURY

Risk factors for splenic injury include trauma, domestic violence, and complications from procedures. Splenic injury cannot be excluded by a normal abdominal or chest radiograph. Possible nonspecific clues to splenic injury may be found in the erect chest radiograph, such as raised left hemidiaphragm, pleural effusion, basal atelectasis, and lower rib fracture. The KUB may reveal a left upper quadrant mass and medial displacement of gastric air bubble, inferomedial displacement of splenic flexure, splenic enlargement due to subcapsular hemorrhage, or signs of hemoperitoneum.

RETROPERITONEAL HEMORRHAGE

Risk factors for retroperitoneal hemorrhage include spontaneous bleeding due to a coagulopathy and procedure-related complications. Absence of a right psoas shadow may be normal in one-fifth of the population due to superimposed bowel contents or may be a clue to retroperitoneal hemorrhage due to free blood, psoas hematoma, or fractures of the vertebral spinous process. Other clues to retroperitoneal hemorrhage include bulging of the lateral margin of psoas shadow due to bleeding into the muscle fascia, loss of definition of the ipsilateral kidney, and ipsilateral fractures of the lower ribs or lumbar transverse processes.

AORTIC DISSECTION

Calcifications associated with an abdominal aortic aneurysm may increase suspicion for a leaking aneurysm and prompt scrutiny of surrounding soft tissues, which may be more prominent due to associated inflammation from blood. An increased soft tissue density between the descending colon and properitoneal line may signify blood in the left paracolic gutter (which may result from procedures, dissection, and splenic rupture).

HEPATIC INJURY

Fracture of the right lower rib and a subphrenic fluid collection are nonspecific signs that may prompt additional imaging.

SEVERE ABDOMINAL PAIN

The more severe the abdominal pain, the greater the likelihood that the initial plain film will be abnormal. By screening for abnormal gas patterns, distention of bowel loops, organomegaly, calcification, and masses, the KUB and upright may indicate the need for additional imaging of a specific location.

ACUTE PANCREATITIS

Acute pancreatitis usually is associated with normal plain films, and less commonly with dilated duodenal sentinel loop surrounding the inflamed pancreas, loss of left psoas sign, signs of gastric outlet obstruction, and left-sided pleural effusion. The colon may appear distended by gas through the transverse segment with a "colon cutoff sign" with absence of gas in colon distal to the splenic flexure. Additional clues include sympathetic pleural effusion and the presence of radio-opaque gallstones (gallstone pancreatitis). Evidence of prior episodes of acute pancreatitis include loss of fat planes and masses that might represent pseudocysts and punctuate pancreatic calcifications.

BOWEL ISCHEMIA

Bowel ischemia does not necessarily produce radiographic abnormality until late in the clinical course and it can also be intermittent. Nonspecific signs include bowel wall thickening and bowel wall dilatation. Pneumatosis intestinalis may be present. Bowel ischemia initially mimics mechanical obstruction, but with progression the bowel wall becomes severely thickened due to edema and necrosis. Ischemic colitis usually affects splenic flexure and descending colon imaged as thumb printing due to submucosal hemorrhage, with progressive linear gas in the bowel wall due to necrosis, and free air from perforation. Gas in the portal vein is a poor prognostic sign.

ACUTE INFLAMMATORY COLITIS

Initially, in ulcerative colitis the distribution of feces may indicate the extent of inflammation, where there is usually an abrupt cutoff from normal bowel. With progression, there may be pseudopolyps, which represent extensive mucosal ulceration leaving small mucosal islands, a gasless colon, and finally, toxic megacolon when the transfer colonic diameter exceeds 5.5 cm.

SELECTION OF MORE SPECIFIC ABDOMINAL IMAGING

Specific diagnoses may require advanced imaging without a prior screening KUB (**Table 116-4**).

The KUB may be used to select more specific abdominal imaging. Ultrasound examination may be directed to the kidneys or the

TABLE 116-4 Suspected Diagnoses Not Requiring the KUB Before Going Directly to Advanced Imaging

- Appendicitis: Skip KUB and go directly to CT (specifying appendix).
- Biliary colic, acute cholecystitis, cholangitis: Skip KUB and go directly to right upper quadrant ultrasound.
- Diverticulitis: Skip KUB and go directly to CT abdomen.
- Gastric or duodenal ulcer: Esophagogastroduodenoscopy; the erect chest radiograph is the most sensitive X-ray for detecting a small pneumoperitoneum.
- Intestinal obstruction if abdominal CT planned anyway.
- Pancreatitis: Skip KUB and go directly to right upper quadrant ultrasound to rule out gallstone pancreatitis.
- Abdominal CT in selected circumstances (see Chapter 117).

gallbladder based on history and physical examination as well as KUB. CT scanning is commonly used to image a larger area, typically including the pelvis with the abdomen, although the radiation dose required is relatively large (approximately 25 mSv). MRI is not commonly chosen based on KUB but can be valuable for assessment of specific organs and for patients who are allergic to the iodinated intravenous contrast material required for CT examination of vascular structures in the abdomen. Nuclear medicine is useful for investigation of gastric emptying and gastrointestinal bleeding.

Even a completely normal KUB may be helpful in patients with severe abdominal pain by directing additional testing. Ischemic bowel may have a grave prognosis, in part due to the discordance between signs and symptoms if the diagnosis is not suspected. These patients may not be further evaluated until the bowel is gangrenous and has perforated. (See Chapter 117.)

ALTERNATIVE ABDOMINAL SCREENING

Depending upon presentation of the current illness, initial imaging of the abdomen may be directed to a more specific organ system leading to appropriate selection of an alternative screening examination. The ability of ultrasound (US) to study physiologic effects and localize symptoms is also valuable when screening the abdomen. Even without signs and symptoms specific to the GU or GI tract, screening of the abdomen can be performed with abdominal ultrasound examination. Although US does not image gas patterns well due to US properties, it provides superior information regarding solid organs and can assist the performance of paracentesis. Readily available, it can be performed at the patient's bedside, it costs less than CT and MRI examinations, and it limits patient exposure to ionizing radiation, particularly during pregnancy.

SERIAL FILMS

Although a change in patient condition is the best indication of when to order a follow-up KUB, serial abdominal films will demonstrate worsening GI tract dysmotility that might require emergent surgical consultation to avoid acute perforation. When doubt exists, follow-up studies will demonstrate the resolution of GI tract dysmotility from gastroparesis, small bowel obstruction, and adynamic ileus or the passage of kidney stones. Serial films over time monitor the evolution of such processes without more direct abdominal or GI tract imaging. This approach minimizes radiation both by decreasing the number of images and also because of the lower radiation dose.

Serial abdominal films can be very useful during hospitalization. The resolution of GI tract dysmotility and restoration of normal bowel gas pattern are reassuringly demonstrated on follow-up studies. Progress of renal calculi through the ureter may be evaluated on follow-up studies as well. Change in patient condition is the best indicator of when to order a follow-up KUB. Bleeding with mass-like hematoma formation, bowel perforation due to stress, and return of abdominal pain related to adhesions from prior surgery are examples of situations in which working abdominal radiographs can quickly and inexpensively provide the information to optimize health care and minimize length of stay.

Serial working chest radiographs over time may monitor abdominal gastrointestinal disease processes such as gastroparesis, small bowel obstruction, and adynamic ileus without more direct abdominal or GI tract imaging. This is helpful for minimizing radiation both by decreasing the number of images and also because the radiation dose for the chest radiograph is less than for the KUB.

CONCLUSION

This chapter presents a framework for ordering plain abdominal imaging and stresses the importance of providing key clinical information and asking the right questions to get the most out of a radiologist's interpretation. The KUB most frequently identifies the presence of obstruction, calculi, gallstones, or ileus for patients with acute abdominal pain. Working with abdominal radiographs can quickly and inexpensively provide actionable information in acute abdominal pain related to surgical adhesions, bleeding with mass-like hematoma formation, and bowel perforation. The KUB may be used to select more specific abdominal imaging. Modalities used to image the abdomen include ultrasound, CT, nuclear medicine, and MRI.

SUGGESTED READING

Begg JD. *Abdominal X-Rays Made Easy*, 2nd ed. London, England: Churchill Livingstone Elsevier; 2006.

CHAPTER 117

Advanced Abdominal Imaging

Cheryl A. Sadow, MD
Francine L. Jacobson, MD, MPH
John M. Braver, MD

Key Clinical Questions

1. What are the advantages and limitations of abdominal ultrasound?
2. What are the indications for gastrointestinal (GI) fluoroscopy?
3. What are the advantages of computed tomography (CT) when compared with magnetic resonance imaging (MRI) for imaging abdominal structures?
4. What are the indications for nuclear medicine imaging studies?

INTRODUCTION

Radiologists expect to provide guidance in the use of advanced medical imaging tests in the care of acutely ill patients requiring hospitalization. This chapter is intended to present the thought processes that radiologists commonly use rather than dictate a particular test for a particular patient or situation.

Before ordering advanced imaging, it is always important to consider whether the information may be provided by prior studies. The kidneys, ureter, and bladder (KUB), a generic term for a frontal radiograph of the abdomen, is often not only ordered as a screening examination but also serves as the initial default imaging examination when selection of a more specific test cannot be made, as when a patient has diffuse abdominal pain without any localizing signs. No preparation is required. The radiation exposure is slightly higher than a chest radiograph. Although originally IV and oral contrast material was administered in conjunction with plain film radiography, this is no longer common practice. However, in the acutely ill patient who has received one or more contrast agents for a prior study, the KUB can provide additional information without readministration of contrast material, especially for patients with abdominal pain occurring during or shortly after imaging of a different region of the body. A rudimentary intravenous pyelogram (IVP) can be obtained following contrast-enhanced head or chest CT or even cardiac catheterization. The period of time over which the visualization persists will be inversely proportional to the patient's estimated glomerular filtration rate (eGFR) over several hours. The oral contrast material administered for an abdominal CT scan will be concentrated within the colon and often remain visible for several days.

ULTRASOUND OF THE ABDOMEN

Ultrasound can be the best possible examination for the acutely-ill hospitalized patient. It is relatively inexpensive, uses no ionizing radiation, and tailored examinations can be performed at the patient's bedside if necessary. Ultrasound is enhanced by passage through water and stopped by air and bone. It is therefore able to detect a pleural effusion and guide thoracentesis of small to moderate pleural effusions. The information provided depends very much on the operator even with complete video recording. Ultrasound is a very useful tool for the interventional radiologist and may be chosen by the radiologist for a variety of biopsies including liver and prostate.

▪ ABDOMINAL US

In the abdomen, renal and gallbladder ultrasounds are standard examinations. A screening abdominal ultrasound will also include images of the liver, spleen, and pancreas. The confirmation of a simple cyst can exclude more significant pathology in many organs, including ovaries, kidneys, and liver. In order to visualize the pancreas, the ultrasonographer will either compress the air out of the stomach or have the patient drink water to allow the stomach to act as an acoustic window, enhancing the through transmission of the sound waves to the pancreas behind the stomach. The tail of the pancreas may be inadequately examined due to air in the adjacent small bowel.

▪ PELVIC US

Pelvic ultrasound may be performed transabdominally through a full urinary bladder to provide an acoustic window or transvaginally for imaging ovaries and uterus. Ultrasound routinely evaluates pregnancies for diagnosis, prognosis, and on occasion, treatment of fetal disease.

■ VASCULAR US

Vascular ultrasound can identify DVT that prevents veins from collapsing when compressed. This is most helpful in the lower extremities and cannot be performed in regions, such as the pelvis, in which the veins cannot be directly compressed.

GASTROINTESTINAL (GI) FLUOROSCOPY

Limited GI fluoroscopy involves contrast administration followed by obtaining a KUB. A full fluoroscopic examination includes a physical examination by the radiologist to localize the patient's pain with palpation of the opacified structures of the gastrointestinal tract. During fluoroscopy, x-rays strike a fluorescent screen on which an image can be simultaneously formed and viewed. In early fluoroscopy units, the image was inferior, especially with larger patients, and the examination had to be performed in the dark (always literally, sometimes figuratively!) after the radiologist had first adapted his eyes to the dark by wearing red goggles. With modern equipment, which incorporates an image intensification system, the images can be viewed on a television monitor in comfortably subdued light.

The nature of the fluoroscopic examination provides physiologic as well as anatomic and pathologic information. The patient's position or physiologic state may be changed to provoke the chief complaint. The study begins with a supine view of the abdomen and continues with the radiologist at the bedside during the administration of contrast. With fluoroscopy, the radiologist can view the image directly on a television screen in real time without exposing an image and waiting for it to be processed. This "real-time" evaluation is especially useful for studying a dynamic process, such as gastroesophageal reflux. Attached to the image intensification tower is a device for making and transferring digital images to a picture archiving and communication system (PACS). During the examination, the radiologist will "spot image" areas of interest that he or she discovers fluoroscopically, and areas not optimally demonstrated on the overhead images, such as the convolutions of the sigmoid colon and the duodenal bulb. The spot images are not meant to replace or necessarily duplicate the overhead images the technologist takes. Many areas need to be "unfolded" and will be seen well only on adequately positioned spot images. The advantage of this system is that a permanent record can be made when the patient is perfectly positioned; otherwise one runs the risk of missing the abnormality on the overheads, which are exposed according to a set routine. Movie cameras (cine) and magnetic tape or computer-based recorders can be adapted to the basic system; the advance allows a dynamic recording of the constantly-in-motion GI tract for later review, and permanent storage, if desired. This advance is particularly useful for interpreting and storing a videofluoroscopic study of the swallowing mechanism.

■ PATIENT PREPARATION

Patient preparation varies from no preparation, to nothing orally and full bowel preparation, depending on the examination. Patient preparation should also include planning for the excretion of contrast material that will be concentrated in the colon and potentially cause severe constipation. Fluid and physical movement, such as walking, are most helpful. Should follow-up working images of the abdomen or chest be obtained, one should pay attention to whether retained barium is present.

It is useful to watch several of these studies being performed in order to realize the best studies require active participation by the patient, moving through a series of positions that may include prone and every angle between prone and supine. Gastrointestinal fluoroscopy examinations that require fasting are generally scheduled in the morning. In the afternoon, the same fluoroscopy suite may be used to study swallowing function in patients who are at risk for aspiration. Non-GI fluoroscopic examinations including retrograde cystography, joint arthroscopy, and chest fluoroscopy will also generally be scheduled after the completion of the GI fluoroscopy schedule.

■ ADVANCE COMMUNICATION WITH RADIOLOGIST TO TAILOR STUDY TO THE PATIENT

Examinations can be tailored to the specific needs and issues of the patient. Discussion in advance with the radiologist allows for more input than generally conveyed when ordering the examination. The examination types are used as starting points. A video swallow examination of the oropharynx is performed with a variety of liquid and solid contrast materials to determine risk for aspiration and identify protective positions in which a patient may swallow particular types of food safely. A barium swallow examination will briefly study the oropharynx and then focus on the esophagus itself in the erect position followed by the supine position. The stomach may be incompletely studied although the term "barium swallow" is also sometimes used as a synonym for the upper GI examination that includes the barium swallow with detailed examination of the stomach and duodenum. Delayed images to follow oral contrast material through the small bowel add the element of a small bowel follow-through to the upper GI examination.

The small bowel can be difficult to completely image and specialized small bowel enema, or enteroclysis, can be performed to identify rare small bowel lesions. For this examination, a feeding tube is placed through the nose to allow the contrast material to be delivered directly into the duodenum. The preparation may involve laxatives as well as a liquid diet for 24 hours or more prior to the enteroclysis. Medications that slow transit through the GI tract may need to be discontinued prior to the examination. Barium enema examinations may be performed with single or double contrast material. A limited study may be adequate to localize colonic obstruction such as seen with apple core colon cancer lesions in the sigmoid colon. Retained fecal material can interfere with the detection of polyps. Barium enema may be performed following incomplete colonoscopy to supplement the examination without repeating the preparation. The appendix and terminal ileum may be filled by the retrograde flow of contrast material.

CT SCAN OF THE ABDOMEN

Abdominal CT scanning may be performed as a screening examination or with a very specific protocol focusing on a single region or physiologic process. Thus it is very important to convey the reason for the examination to the radiologist in order for the examination to provide the needed diagnostic information. The information provided to the radiologist will determine the suitability of the examination performed to answer clinical questions at the time of examination and later on during the course of patient hospitalization. In many institutions, the pelvis will be included in a complete abdomen CT, while in some institutions a specific order may be required to include the pelvis. Pelvic CT can generally be ordered without an abdominal CT although this is most commonly done for pelvic fractures.

■ ABDOMINAL PAIN

Scanning is generally performed at least 70 seconds following the initial administration of IV contrast material. Such a scan will provide contrast enhancement of the liver, spleen, adrenal glands, kidneys, and GI tract including stomach, small bowel, and colon, the latter structures best appreciated if the scan is preceded by enteric contrast administration. This type of study is performed for the evaluation of abdominal pain and will allow detection of a wide variety of pathology, including abscesses, organ-specific masses, selected functional abnormalities and metastases, especially to liver and bones. It should be noted that on occasion, iodinated contrast material will decrease the visibility of liver metastases. This is particularly true of breast cancer metastases. In oncology centers, the liver may be imaged before and after the administration of IV contrast material to evaluate for potential breast cancer metastases.

Flank pain is most often addressed with CT performed without oral or intravenous contrast material. Intravenous contrast material is unnecessary for the detection of commonly calcified stones. In this setting, following of the ureter is generally facilitated by ureteral obstruction causing the renal colic.

Obstruction of biliary ducts and pancreatic ducts also makes these structures more apparent and more easily measured. In the liver, the basic examination is generally adequate. The smaller pancreas benefits from a thin-section examination with optimal parenchymal enhancement at 45 seconds after contrast material administration, earlier than that of the liver.

The gastrointestinal tract is increasingly imaged with CT, particularly for abnormalities that can also involve lymph nodes, such as lymphoma, and for abnormalities that lead to fistulae as a complication, such as Crohn disease. Intermittent symptoms may be due to intussusception or internal hernia. The identification of these abnormalities may be less straightforward and benefit from direct consultation with the radiologist. Appendicitis can be diagnosed on CT although the increasing concern to limit patient exposure to ionizing radiation may increase the use of ultrasound in the future.

■ HEMANGIOMAS

Sometimes focused CT scanning is performed to differentiate hemangiomas from metastases or from simple cysts. Hemangiomas in the liver are most often an incidental finding because they do not cause symptoms until very large. They have a greater tendency to lobulation and can overlap in appearance to metastases. In order to diagnose a benign hepatic hemangioma , a dedicated liver protocol is used which includes dynamic contrast phases through the liver in the late arterial and portal venous phases which should show a peripheral discontinuous nodular enhancement pattern in the lesion in the late arterial phase which typically fill in at least partially by the portal venous phase. When the differentiation appropriately can be delayed until the patient is an outpatient, MRI or CT may be used for this purpose.

PRACTICE POINT

- When an "incidental" finding suggests the possibility of a malignancy or the need for follow-up studies, always review prior imaging. Imaging studies obtained for other reasons sometimes years earlier are often helpful and may reveal pre-existing "stable" abnormalities. Any prior noted abnormalities should be clearly documented, added to the patient's current problem list, and include an assessment and follow-up plan based on radiologic consultation and communication with the patient's primary care physician.

■ ADRENAL GLANDS

The adrenal glands are seen in the upper abdomen on CT. The most common lesion, often an incidental finding, is an adrenal adenoma. These are characterized by low attenuation on scans without intravenous contrast enhancement. Contrast can interfere with this determination, although the distinct smooth margin can make this the most likely lesion present. Adrenal metastases, most associated with lung cancer, generally have poorly defined margins and may infiltrate surrounding fat. The adrenal glands are generally included and reported specifically on chest CT scans. Functional tumors such as a pheochromocytoma may not be identified by CT when their physiologic effect is far greater than their size. Pheochromocytoma can also occur in the mediastinum, increasing the region of concern.

■ CT ANGIOGRAPHY

Computed tomography angiography is used increasingly to spare patients the invasiveness and radiation exposure of conventional angiography. It is particularly useful when vascular disease is part of a larger differential diagnosis. Pain out of proportion to findings on examination is a classic presentation of mesenteric ischemia. This can be difficult to assess in the acutely-ill patient and may need to be considered in the planning of an abdominal CT scan.

■ PATIENT PREPARATION

Patient preparation most frequently involves fasting followed by oral administration of contrast material prior to the scan. Iodinated intravenous contrast material is frequently used, although different timing is selected for different purposes. Renal function testing is generally required prior to contrast administration in order to safeguard renal function that may be diminished, particularly in acutely-ill patients.

MRI OF THE ABDOMEN

Most alternatives are preferable for hospitalized patients. Magnetic resonance imaging can be a very difficult examination for the acutely-ill patient due to the length of the procedure, confinement, and noise. When the patient is unable to lie still, follow commands, and perform repeated breath-holds, the sought-after benefit will be elusive. For a patient who has had anaphylaxis in response to iodinated contrast material, MRI can be used in lieu of CT, particularly when lesion characterization is needed. Magnetic resonance imaging provides a high level of tissue characterization and is useful for diagnosing specific lesions in the liver, kidneys, spleen, pancreas, adrenal glands, ovaries, and prostate. When pathology is identified on female pelvic ultrasound, the next examination may be MRI rather than CT. Magnetic resonance imaging is inferior to CT for characterization of calcification, which appears on MRI only as a signal void. The data from CT and MR are often complementary, with MRI providing greater soft tissue characterization and fascial plane discrimination while CT provides higher spatial resolution and better definition of calcifications.

Magnetic resonance imaging cannot be performed for patients who have just had surgery. Most MRI facilities are unable to offer MRI to a patient who has a pacemaker. Cerebral aneurysm clips placed many years ago are not safe in MRI. Patients who have worked with metals or could, for any other reason, have metal foreign bodies in their eyes must have screening radiographs of the orbits. Most patients with indwelling orthopedic hardware can have MR examination as long as the heating of the metal during the MRI is not excessive. Magnetic resonance imaging technologists will screen patients to ensure patient safety. In cases in which the patient is unable to communicate adequately with the technologist, it is important to enlist the aid of a family member or advocate. This person can safely remain in the imaging suite if that increases the ability of the patient to undergo the MRI examination.

Magnetic resonance imaging examinations are performed using surface coils that have finite sizes. The imaging range may need to be adapted to make sure the area of greatest interest is imaged. The use of Vitamin E capsules can be helpful when a palpable mass is present or the patient can point to a specific painful location. Unlike CT, in which extending the examination of the abdomen to include the pelvis is easily done, each type of MRI examination will require a separate setup and imaging sequence. The abdomen and pelvis are separate examinations, as is the lumbar spine, which would each constitute a separate MRI examination with each requiring the full time for a MRI. Above all else, MRI is not a screening examination but rather an examination to solve a very specific problem.

Gadolinium contrast material is used for most but not all MRI examinations. Dosing is based on patient weight and may be completely avoided in patients with severe renal compromise (generally eGFR < 30) to prevent the rare complication of nephrogenic systemic fibrosis (NSF). Allergic reactions to gadolinium-based contrast agents are less common than to iodinated contrast agents but are not rare as previously thought based upon the inert nature of gadolinium.

NUCLEAR MEDICINE

The three most basic abdominal examinations for hospitalized patients are HIDA, GI bleeding, and gastric emptying studies. Specialized functional studies can be performed to identify endocrine tumors.

The radiotracer, most commonly technetium 99-m, is attached to an appropriate ligand to demonstrate the physiology of interest and is administered intravenously. While the radiation dose is small, the duration of exposure is most significant. The half-life of technetium 99-m is 6 hours. Other radiotracers used in nuclear medicine studies imaged with gamma camera have generally longer half-lives. New ultra-short half-life radiotracers are emerging for PET-CT scanning and will be used more extensively over time as molecular imaging agents. Patients should be instructed to drink freely and void often following the examination.

SELECTION OF ADVANCED IMAGING STUDIES

■ FIRST, REVIEW PRIOR IMAGING

Adequate diagnostic information is often available from multiple modalities when imaging the abdomen and pelvis. Reviewing any pre-existing imaging with the radiologist does not add expense or risk of radiation or contrast and may save time. Review of imaging studies obtained for other reasons may identify pre-existing calcifications and small caliber of vessels that would put an elderly patient at greater risk for developing mesenteric ischemia as the cause of pain. In general, a tailored study to address specific questions will provide the best study possible (see **Tables 117-1** and **117-2**).

PRACTICE POINT

- While modern CT scanners make it easy to perform CT scan of the complete abdomen and pelvis, it should not be used as a replacement for the bedside physical examination. The localization of abdominal pain is crucial to the correct selection of imaging and optimal interpretation of images.

■ SECOND, TRY TO LOCALIZE THE ABDOMINAL PAIN

While modern CT scanners make it easy to perform CT scan of the complete abdomen and pelvis, it should not be used as a replacement for the bedside physical examination. The localization of abdominal pain is crucial to the correct selection of imaging. While true throughout the abdomen, it is particularly helpful in localizing disease affecting the GI tract that might not otherwise be apparent on CT scans. As the patient's experience of pain guides the examiner's hand to the location of pain, critical communication of this

TABLE 117-1 Specific Abdomen Imaging Examinations

Organ System	Preferred Initial Examination	Alternate Examination
Gallbladder	US	HIDA, MR, ERCP
Liver	US	CT or MR
Pancreas	CT	US, MR, ERCP
Kidneys	US	CT, MR
GYN	US, transvaginal	MR or CT
Small bowel	UGI-Small bowel follow through	CT enterography, MR enterography
Colon	Colonoscopy, BE	CT colonography
Vascular	US or CT	MR or angiography

information guides the radiologist's eye to specific sites of active clinical disease (see **Figure 117-1A** and **B**).

■ THIRD, CONSIDER THE CHARACTER OF THE PAIN AND HOW IT IS EVOLVING OVER TIME

The characterization is also very important, as different causes of abdominal pain will evolve differently over time. Serial examinations of the abdomen at the bedside are most helpful in this regard. Radiology tests are not continually needed to document the evolution whether from periumbilical pain to pain over McBurney point or intermittent symptoms from ureteral stone that will cause different descriptions of pain by the patient over time, perhaps moving from flank pain and nausea early in the course of the acute episode followed by groin pain and diarrhea when the stone approaches the ureteral vesicular junction (UVJ) (see **Table 117-3**).

CASE 117-1

■ FLANK PAIN IN A YOUNG WOMAN

An adolescent female with a negative past medical history developed sharp, severe pain in her lower back over a 2-week period.

Associated symptoms included a couple of days of abdominal pain and nausea, most recently with two episodes of vomiting. She also described premenstrual cramps (LMP 4 weeks ago), perhaps with some urgency but without dysuria, fever or chills.

Acetaminophen may have provided minimal relief. Her mother reported no family history of kidney stones and the patient was not sexually active. The patient was alert and able to cooperate with her examiners. On examination, she had normal vital signs.

Pertinent findings included a soft, nontender abdomen with normal bowel sounds and significant midlumbar spine tenderness, somewhat worse over the right flank.

Negative laboratory tests included a complete blood count, metabolic profile, and pregnancy test. The only positive findings were on urinalysis (5019 WBC and 50-100 RBC/hpf)

Plain abdominal radiographs revealed a calcified structure in the right lower quadrant just caudal to the right side of the sacrum measuring approximately 5 mm × 10 mm. A nondiagnostic abdominal ultrasound reported the presence of mild hydronephrosis of her right kidney. An intravenous urography (IVP) revealed prompt excretion of contrast from the left kidney with delayed excretion of contrast from the right kidney.

Oblique radiograph with contrast in right ureter, however, did not coincide with the calcification. The medical team consulted a urologist regarding the ureteral obstruction and a general surgeon regarding the possibility of appendicitis. An abdominal CT scan was ordered but not performed due to the radiologist's reticence

TABLE 117-2 Patient Preparation

Radiologic Procedure	Purpose	Preparation	What to Expect
Abdominal radiographs: KUB Acute Abdomen	Screen abdomen	None	Breathing instructions, expiration may need to stand or lie on left side
US examinations: tailored to region physiology anatomy	Examine: gallbladder kidneys pelvis vascular structures	NPO for gallbladder Full bladder for pelvis	Patient may be asked to drink water to facilitate imaging of organ such as pancreas through an acoustic window
CT abdomen: oral contrast IV contrast	Examine abdomen, multiple organ systems; pelvis may be included	NPO prior to oral contrast material steadily consumed for 1-2 h	IV contrast material causes warmth
MRI: liver vascular pelvic	Problem solving: liver vasculature pelvis	Exclusions: foreign body metal in eyes pacemaker aneurysm clip; remove watch and metal jewelry; fasting may be required	Long examination, confined space, and loud noises; can be provided with earplugs
Nuclear medicine: HIDA bleeding infection gastric emptying	Specific physiologic tests	Dependent upon examination	Scanning may be performed over an extended period of time; most imaging agents are excreted by kidney—helpful to increase fluids and void frequently after the exam

IV contrast administration: NPO for 2-4 hours prior to examination decreases risk of aspiration.

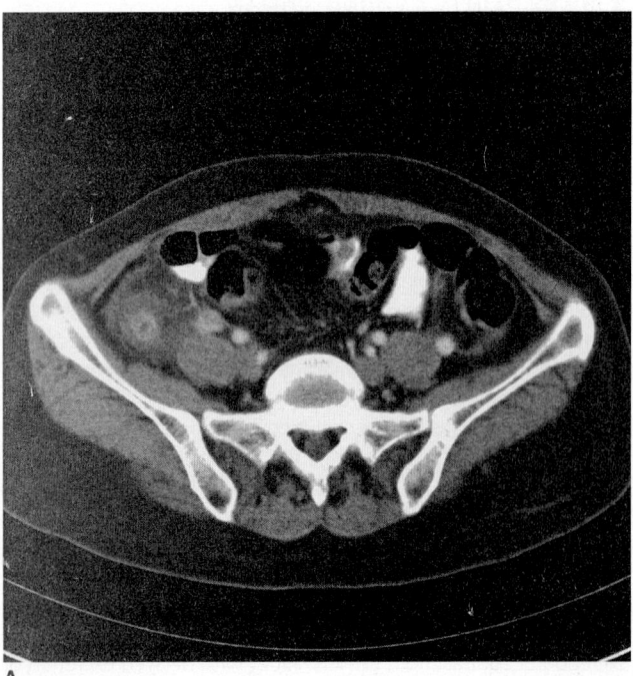

A

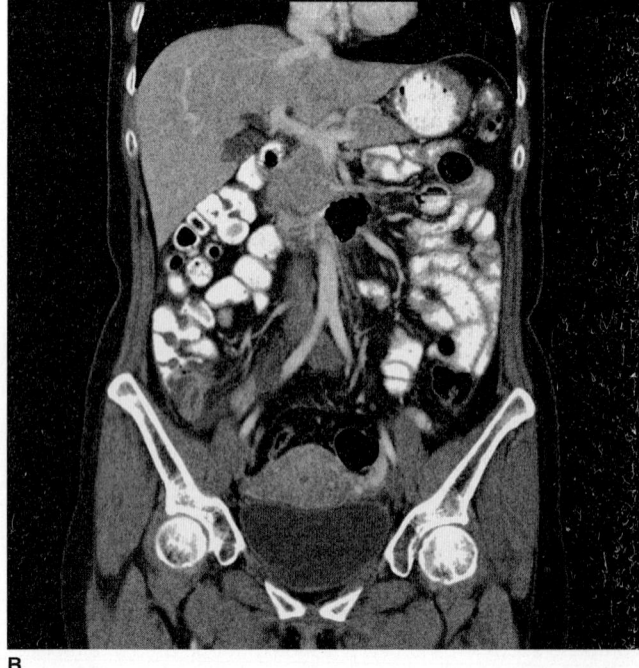

B

Figure 117-1 *(A) Appendicitis on axial CT image. Compare the dark gray, nearly black fat in left side of pelvis with irregular and lighter gray fat surrounding appendix, identified by its caliber and often also by its relationship to the ileocecal valve that may contain well-seen fat. (B) Appendicitis on coronal CT image. The infiltration of fat may seem less apparent on this image from the same CT scan, but it is useful also for orientation and correlation with physical examination. This scan has been performed with oral and IV contrast material maximizing the identification of GI tract and vascular structures.*

TABLE 117-3 Localization of Acute Abdominal Pain

Site of Pain	Imaging Modality					
	KUB	US	GI fluoro	CT	Nucs	MRI
Diffuse	X			X		
RUQ		X			X	
LUQ				X		
Flank	X			X		
Epigastrium		X		X	X	
RLQ		X		X		
Pelvis		X	X	X		X

to administer a second dose of IV contrast material. Passage of a small amount of tissue containing a tiny stone in her urine did not relieve her worsening abdominal pain. The patient underwent surgical exploration which identified the cause of her symptoms—early appendicitis caused by an appendicolith.

■ SYNTHESIS

The stone was rather large for a ureteral stone raising the possibility of other causes of obstruction and calcifications in the right lower quadrant such as an appendicolith. Types of calcifications that can be present in the pelvis include very common vascular calcifications in veins and arteries and reproductive system calcifications frequently seen in middle-aged and older individuals.

■ RADIOLOGY PRACTICE POINT

Initial imaging with CT scanning both before and after administration of contrast material has largely replaced IVP in most institutions so that more information is acquired with the single dose of contrast material. The CT dose is relatively high so it is appropriate to also consider ultrasound, particularly in patients of child-bearing age, as long as the patient can cooperate adequately for complete examination.

Source: Yamamoto LG. A Large Calcified Kidney Stone. Radiology Cases in Pediatric Emergency Medicine. Vol. 7, Case 6. From the Kapiolani Medical Center for Women and Children, University of Hawaii John A Burns School of Medicine.

Available at http://www.hawaii.edu/medicine/pediatrics/pemxray/v7c06.html.

■ IS THE PAIN OUT OF PROPORTION TO PHYSICAL EXAMINATION?

Strong discordance between the patient's complaint of pain and findings on physical examination that are not due to medication raise concern for potentially catastrophic mesenteric ischemia in the right setting. (See Chapter 75, second case.)

CONCLUSION

The selection of modality will vary with availability of testing and other local factors, especially where multiple modalities can provide the needed diagnostic evaluation. Sometimes patients can be spared the risk of contrast and radiation simply by reviewing past images or employing ultrasound to dynamically augment the physical examination. For example, depending on the physician's gestalt and skill at performing ultrasound, bedside ultrasonographic evidence of gallstones and a positive sonographic Murphy sign increase the likelihood of acute cholecystitis as the cause of pain. In addition, when the results are not as expected, nuclear medicine employs a small amount of radiation to provide functional information and allows imaging over time without added radiation exposure. (See Chapter 75, first case.)

Imaging complements but must never replace the history and physical examination. Despite technologic advances the localization of abdominal pain at the bedside will remain crucial to the correct selection of imaging and optimal interpretation of images and should always be communicated to the radiologist.

SUGGESTED READING

Berland LL, Silverman SG, Gore RM, et al. Managing incidental findings on Abdominal CT: White paper of the ACR incidental findings committee. *J Am Coll Radiol*. 2010;7(10):754-773.

CHAPTER 118

Neurologic Imaging

Francine L. Jacobson, MD, MPH

Liangge Hsu, MD

Key Clinical Questions

1. What are the indications for a noncontrast head computed tomography (CT)?
2. What are the indications for a contrast head CT?
3. What are the limitations of CT neuroimaging?
4. What are the indications for magnetic resonance imaging (MRI) neuroimaging?
5. What are the limitations for MRI imaging in the hospital setting?

INTRODUCTION

This chapter will present the thought processes behind general guiding principles for neurologic imaging. This chapter does not provide an exhaustive array of images because the goal is not to train hospitalists to interpret medical images but rather to provide a framework so that they can more effectively communicate with radiologists and order the most appropriate imaging modality to optimize timely evaluation and treatment. It will always be the responsibility of practitioners to provide radiologists with relevant clinical information so that recommendations regarding specific imaging and the actual interpretation are made in the context of the patient. A number of cases will be presented that highlight the limitations of imaging when this process does not occur.

Any patient with new neurologic symptoms and signs requires prompt imaging and appropriate specialty consultation to avoid catastrophic effects upon patient outcome. This is particularly true for processes that profoundly affect the homeostasis of anatomy and physiology with or without preexisting abnormality. Therefore, this chapter will review the characteristic findings to be expected for key "do-not-miss" diagnoses that would require the practitioner to contact the appropriate specialty services for emergent consultation and/or initiate steps for transfer to a tertiary care facility.

CORRELATION OF NEUROLOGICAL EXAMINATION WITH IMAGING

Correlation of the neurological examination with any imaging study obtained is of paramount importance. Anatomic references may help clinicians localize abnormalities. When subtle, as at the onset of a stroke syndrome, the conviction that a potential finding is in the precise location indicated by the focal neurological deficit can make the difference between the radiologist overlooking the possibility and confidently confirming the abnormality. In turn, this approach leads to decreased imaging during the acute illness. The workup of incidental findings can also then be deferred for outpatient workup when the imaging study will often be of higher quality due to the greater ability of the recuperated patient to understand and cooperate for the imaging study.

Several drawings accompany this text to refresh memory of neuroanatomy. It can be invaluable to consult an interactive Internet atlas, especially when immediate radiologic consultation is not available, and particularly in situations in which the patient condition evolves during the hospitalization. The clarity of anatomy is greater on MRI than CT so it may prove most helpful to use an MRI reference atlas, even for looking at the more commonly obtained in the acute care setting CT scan (**Figure 118-1**).

SELECTION OF IMAGING MODALITY

Neurologic imaging requires considerations of anatomy and function and an appreciation for the limitations of each imaging modality. Computed tomography has the highest spatial resolution; however, the superior tissue characterization of MRI allows the most exquisite demonstration of neuroanatomy in a physiologically relevant manner. Computed tomography images lesions by the degree of hyperdensity in the following decreasing order of density: bone (the highest density); clotted blood; liquid blood; subacute or approximately 2 weeks of blood similar to brain tissue; CSF equal to the density of water (0-10 HU), and fat the least dense (a negative HU value). This means that a resolving phase of

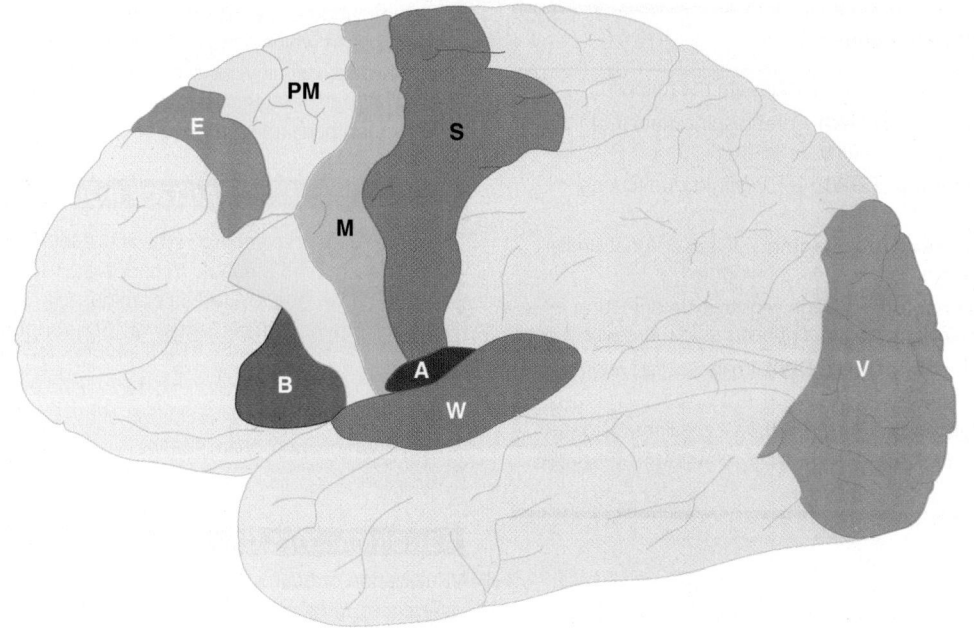

Figure 118-1 *Brain areas commonly resulting in stroke syndrome deficits: E is frontal eye field, PM is premotor, M is primary motor, S is primary sensory, V is visual, B is Broca's, W is Wernicke's, and A is primary auditory.*

hemorrhage may have a density equal to brain tissue, making it inapparent. Hyperdense lesions suggest recent blood hemorrhagic lesions such as metastases, hypercellular lesions like lymphoma, and meningioma, calcification, and bone. Hypodense abnormalities include infarcts greater than 12 hours, brain tumors, inflammation, old blood, edema, traumatic changes, fat, cysts, and air. Enlargement of the ventricles suggests atrophy, obstruction, or NPH. Magnetic resonance imaging can identify enhancing lesions (abscess, partially thrombosed aneurysm, resolving stroke or infection, metastatic lesions, active demyelination, and radiation necrosis), amyloid angiography, arteriovenous malformations, brainstem lesions (especially if thin cuts obtained), dissection of cranial vessels, edema, hemorrhage (although in general not as well as CT in the acute setting), and tumor (with characteristic T1 and T2 densities for each type, location, presence, or absence of hemorrhage, edema, calcification) (**Tables 118-1** to **118-3**).

TABLE 118-1   CT Images of Common Abnormalities

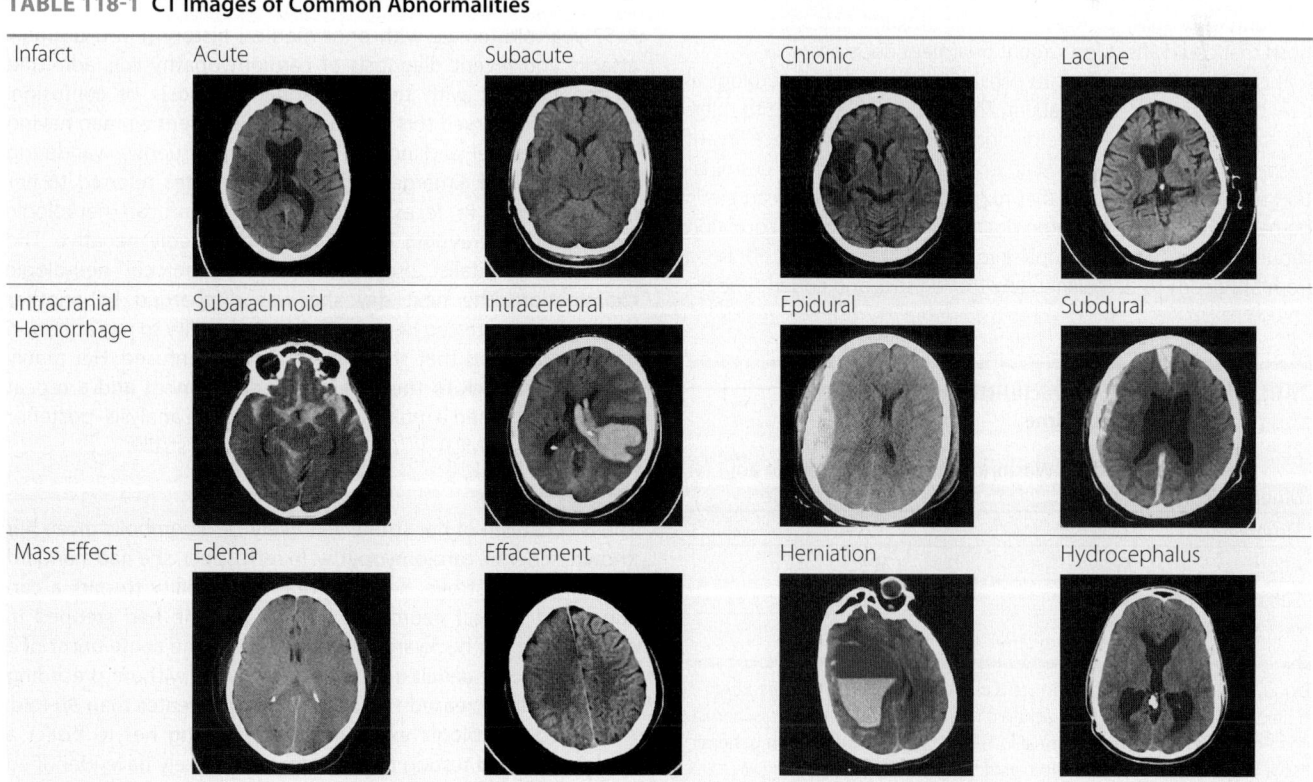

Infarct	Acute	Subacute	Chronic	Lacune
Intracranial Hemorrhage	Subarachnoid	Intracerebral	Epidural	Subdural
Mass Effect	Edema	Effacement	Herniation	Hydrocephalus

TABLE 118-2 MRI Techniques

Commonly used MR imaging techniques are the following:

- **T1-weighted imaging (T1-WI)**: Cerebrospinal fluid (CSF) is dark due to *long relaxation time*.
- **T2-weighted imaging (T2-WI)**: CSF is bright due to *long relaxation time*.
- **Proton density–weighted imaging**: CSF has a signal similar to brain tissue *as it is neither T1 nor T2 weighted*.
- **Gradient echo imaging**: Has high sensitivity in detecting *hemorrhage or mineralization that appears as low intensity*.
- **Diffusion-weighted imaging (DWI)**: Images *reflect relative flow of water molecules*.
- **Perfusion-weighted imaging (PWI)**: Fast gradient weighted MR sequences are based on passage of MR contrast through brain tissue.

Nuclear medicine tests such as SPECT brain scan can provide functional information regarding Alzheimer's and other neurodegenerative diseases, stroke, and seizure. Positron emission tomography–computed tomography (PET-CT) scans, increasingly being used to provide global assessment for metastases in patients with known cancer, have important limitations. The total body PET-CT does not provide adequate screening for brain metastases. In many centers, the application of this to the head is regarded as a separate examination. Centers that include the head on total body PET-CT scans may be doing so primarily to compare foci of increased activity with brain activity as a standardization procedure.

Computed tomography and MRI are both utilized for a wide variety of increasingly specific examinations, although the choice of CT or MRI may not be based upon the small differences in the value of the data obtained. One primary issue is the rapidity with which the examination can be obtained and interpreted. In acute neurological disease changes, time is of the essence, negating any benefit of more sophisticated imaging even if it would result in less ionizing radiation or possibly provide further information or a specific diagnosis that could affect less urgent treatment decisions.

It is extremely important to consider the effect the neurological event is having upon the patient. The ability of the patient to tolerate the examination may be diminished by the neurological event even as it is evolving. A CT scan is a significantly shorter examination than a MRI. The value that might be added by MRI can easily be negated by patient motion during the lengthy data acquisition sequences; thus the additional information that is often obtained from MR needs to be balanced by the logistics and added time for

TABLE 118-3 Signal Characteristics of Blood on MRI with Time

Mnemonic	George Washington Bridge	The layers of an Oreo® cookie
Time	T1WI	T2WI
Acute	**G**ray	**B**lack
Subacute	**W**hite	**W**hite
Chronic	**B**lack	**B**lack

Blood, hemosiderin, and calcium are dark on gradient echo images. FLAIR is helpful for detection of subarachnoid hemorrhage. DWI detects ischemia immediately and may be abnormal in TIA. ADC is decreased when ischemic tissue may still be viable. Diffusion restriction considers DWI and ADC together—bright on DWI and dark on ADC map.

MR examination on a case by case basis. The one exception is in acute stroke in which a fast diffusion sequence (a minute and half) can provide a definitive answer, especially when the CT is negative. Neurologic imaging for chronic neurological findings may be deferred and performed on an elective basis following discharge.

PRACTICE POINT

- Neuroimaging screening in the acute setting may be helpful in a patient who is unable to cooperate for a neurologic examination due to altered consciousness, agitation, or other factors. However, the images may be suboptimal and a high index of suspicion of an underlying disorder or identification of an acute focal neurologic defect based on a thorough history and physical examination of the patient is critical to the selection of appropriate studies.

ABNORMALITIES ON NEUROIMAGING

Visualization of brain structure on imaging is generally based upon differences in gray and white matter and upon alterations of CSF spaces. Some disease processes are diffuse and others are focal. Focal abnormalities may be accompanied by changes in surrounding tissue. The importance of the identification of blood cannot be overstated, whether in an extra-axial collection, subarachnoid hemorrhage, or hemorrhage into brain tissue itself. Blood degradation over time leads to different MRI signal characteristics that identify blood and provide a timeline (**Tables 118-4** and **118-5**).

STROKE SYNDROMES

In the setting of stroke, the exclusion of blood can be the most valuable outcome of the noncontrast enhanced screening head CT, allowing prompt thrombolytic therapy.

CASE 118-1

CONFUSION

A 57-year-old female with prior medical history (PMH) of panic attacks and recent diagnosis of cardiomyopathy was admitted to the hospital with the provisional diagnosis of confusion. Neighbors observed this previously independent woman having difficulty parallel parking her car and subsequently wandering in her backyard. Emergency department notes referred to her being covered in feces and having a "nonfocal" neurologic examination. Screening head CT was reportedly negative. The admitting hospitalist also documented a "nonfocal" neurologic examination. The next day she was discharged by another hospitalist who tested her orientation and ability to pay attention and documented that she was no longer confused. Her family brought her back to the emergency department and a repeat head CT confirmed a multiple correspondence analysis–posterior cerebral artery (MCA–PCA) watershed parietal stroke.

Synthesis

The mechanism of her stroke was likely cardioembolic given her known ischemic cardiomyopathy. In retrospect, she had standard risk factors for stroke, her presentation (inability to park a car) suggested a focal neurologic deficit, and she had stepped in dog feces in her backyard (due to neglect). The acute onset of a focal neurologic deficit during the prior week without preceding head trauma increased the odds of stroke greater than 90-fold. A focused neurologic examination (eg, asking her to bisect a straight line and testing for neglect) would likely have identified her parietal deficit at the time of her first hospitalization.

TABLE 118-4 Neuroimaging Abnormalities

Disease Process	Findings on CT and MR	Clinical Information
Acute ischemic stroke	Diffusion MR + in 30 min-h CT normal for up to 6 h	
Early evolution of ischemic stroke	Decreased gray-white differentiation, effacement of sulci, increasing *swelling* of gray matter	Cytotoxic edema
Continued evolution of stroke 24 to 48 h	Edema results in hypodense region may have mass effect	Mass effect on midline structures can lead to herniation
Extra-axial bleed	Crescentic collection that crosses	Subdural hematoma
Extra-axial bleed	Lentiform between sutures	Epidural hematoma requires emergency evacuation
Toxoplasmosis	Ring enhancing lesions better seen on MRI CT dDX abscess or tumor	MRI is more sensitive CT dDX abscess or tumor
Lymphoma	Periventricular enhancing lesions for primary lymphoma	Higher glucose utilization on PET-CT than toxoplasmosis
Astrocytoma/Glioma	Variable depending on grade, location and size	Variable presentation
Metastases	Can be solitary or multiple with no or extensive edema	Lung, breast, kidney, GI tract, melanoma
Leukoencephalopathy	Subcortical involvement Atrophy and white matter changes	AIDS dementia complex Impaired memory and slowing of motor skills, ataxia, hyperreflexia
Central pontine myelinolysis	Abnormal symmetric signal in central pons on MRI Widespread destruction of myelin pattern reverse of infarction	Coma, facial diplegia, spastic quadriparesis after rapid correction of hyponatremia

Radiology practice point

It is important to remember that CT imaging is often normal in patients with acute ischemic symptoms and may not become abnormal for 6 to 48 hours, even in those with persistent symptoms (Table 118-1, evolving stroke). New clinical information—focal abnormalities rather than confusion—should be brought to the attention of the radiologist who would then take another look at the right parietal region. Retrospective review of the first CT did in fact identify subtle abnormalities in this region.

The head CT must be obtained to rule out the presence of bleeding prior to consideration of reperfusion therapy. The evolution of a clinical stroke syndrome may begin with the most severe deficit at the time of a completely normal head CT scan. Even without reperfusion therapy, patients may often improve over the first several days. This may be due to the salvaging of neurons through the luxury perfusion that is seen in the periphery of the affected brain territory, limiting the ultimate extent of abnormality and corresponding defect. Over time, the transfer of function to other neurons will also augment the improvement, although much of this occurs over a longer period of time with rehabilitation in the nonacute care setting. Hence, the CT complements the neurologic examination rather than replaces it. A "normal" CT report should not mislead clinicians into assuming that a patient does not have a focal neurologic deficit. Correlation of clinical findings from an

TABLE 118-5 Incidental Findings

Virchow-Robin space: Enlarged perivascular spaces (EPVS) surround blood vessels and serve as pathways for drainage of interstitial fluid; may be incidental in older patients but are likely to be abnormal in young adults.

Empty Sella Syndrome (ESS): Primary ESS is caused by CSF pressure flattening the pituitary and it is associated with obesity and high blood pressure in women. Secondary ESS is due to regression of the pituitary gland after trauma, surgery, or radiation therapy with destruction of the pituitary gland affecting fertility and menstrual periods.

Lacunes: Evidence of prior strokes usually due to atherosclerosis of deep penetrating arteries. These minute holes can be caused by a succession of transient ischemic attacks and over the years can lead also to dementia.

Subcortical Arteriosclerotic Encephalopathy (SAE): Disease process in deep white matter that causes periventricular lucency and dementia.

PCOM and ACOM Aneurysms: Small aneurysms of the anterior and posterior communicating arteries can be incidental findings during acute hospitalization.

Meningioma: Small meningiomas that are asymptomatic may be incidental findings in acute clinical context, particularly in elderly patients.

Calcifications: Basal ganglia calcifications are frequent incidental findings. They are easier to detect on CT, although characteristic signal voids are seen on MRI.

Normal Pressure Hydrocephalus (NPH): Chronic communicating hydrocephalus in which intracranial pressure is stable with mild elevation due to equilibration between formation of CSF and absorption. Triad: gait difficulty, urinary incontinence, and mental decline. NPH is a cause of potentially reversible dementia.

in-depth neurological examination and study of CT scans may also identify evidence of chronic as well as acute stroke. The pattern of strokes can often point to more central vascular abnormalities, both in the brain, the great vessels and heart that require intervention to prevent additional strokes in the future.

CASE 118-2

STEREOTYPED "SPELLS"

A 65-year-old man with a PMH of hypertension and hyperlipidemia developed a 5-minute spell of heaviness of the right side of his face and right arm. One hour later he experienced another spell, this time with word finding difficulty, lasting 5 minutes with complete resolution. He then experienced a third stereotyped episode during his examination in the emergency department. Electrocardiogram (ECG) and initial laboratory tests were normal.

Synthesis

This patient had experienced sudden symptoms in a vascular territory involving the anterior circulation of the left hemisphere. Three stereotyped spells in one vascular territory suggested an increased likelihood of a stenosis of the MCA or extracranial ICA. The pretest probability of extracranial internal carotid stenosis is 15% to 20%. For secondary stroke prevention this patient might benefit from a carotid endarterectomy if he had, for example, a stenosis >70%.

Radiology practice point

Screening CT radiography would not routinely image the carotid circulation unless specified by the examiner. Therefore, a CT angiogram would be appropriate as the initial test.

Any patient with symptoms of anterior circulation transient ischemic attacks (TIAs) as suggested in this patient who had motor dysfunction of the contralateral extremity and face, followed by difficulty word finding, would require an evaluation of his carotid circulation as the first step.

CASE 118-3

MOTOR VEHICLE ACCIDENT (MVA)

A 45-year-old female with a PMH notable for three successful pregnancies and one miscarriage sustained a MVA. She was hit from behind, leaving her with a stiff, sore neck. Three days later she suddenly developed unsteady walking, numbness on the right side of her face, and in her left hand and leg. Her voice became hoarse and she choked while drinking water. Initial laboratory tests were normal including initial head CT, CBC, INR, ESR, electrolytes, antiphospholipid antibodies, and ECG.

Synthesis

This patient had experienced sudden symptoms in a vascular territory involving the posterior circulation of the right hemisphere: motor dysfunction of ipsilateral face and contralateral extremity with associated symptoms of ataxia and dysphagia. Her neurologic examination would be expected to show sensory loss on the right side of her face, left hand and leg, reduced palatal elevation on the right, smaller pupil on the right with mild right ptosis, and hemitaxia on the right. Given a likely flexion-extension injury during a recent MVA, a posterior circulation dissection was the most likely cause of her deficits. Other less likely possibilities in a younger patient include PFO and antiphospholipid antibody syndrome.

Radiology practice point

Suspicion of localization to the posterior circulation is valuable information to share with the radiologist. Screening CT would not ordinarily include imaging of the right vertebral artery. In some institutions, a separate request for a neck CT or CT angiogram would be required. Tailoring the imaging to the specific patient avoids diagnostic delays, increased risk, and costs from performing multiple examinations.

The clinical information of a flexion-extension injury should be conveyed to the radiologist who would recommend imaging of the extracranial vessels in addition to the brain, and then specifically look at areas of the brain likely to be affected.

These cases highlight the importance of answering the following questions when a patient presents with neurologic symptoms and signs.

1. Are the symptoms consistent with stroke or TIA?
2. Where does the ischemic event localize (anterior circulation, posterior circulation, cortical vs subcortical)?
3. What is the mechanism of the ischemic event, cardioembolism, extracranial carotid stenosis, dissection (anterior or posterior circulation), septic emboli, hypercoagulable states, giant cell arteritis, among other possibilities?

Only by asking the right questions can the practitioner determine what tests are needed and how urgently.

Serial CT scans may be obtained as working films, much as serial chest radiographs are obtained in acutely ill patients. A patient who has an acute nonhemorrhagic infarction of the brain will acutely have a normal or nearly normal head CT. Several days later, the evolving infarction may be identified by "luxury perfusion" resulting in greater enhancement of the affected area on a contrast-enhanced head CT. In patients who are known to have a subacute stroke by history, contrast may not be required to document the extent of the infarction because it will become more apparent even on noncontrast enhanced CT. Remote infarctions may be recognized by the prominence of CSF spaces and changes of encephalomalacia. This may be seen as dilatation of the lateral ventricles or cortical sulci or as one or more small lucencies within the brain parenchyma, particularly in putamen, caudate, thalamus, pons, internal capsule, and corona radiate. Hypertensive lipohyalinosis may be the underlying cause of such lacunar infarcts that are best managed medically with optimization of blood pressure.

Cerebellar strokes may present with vertigo, nausea and vomiting, ataxia, and frequently with brainstem signs. Patients often complain of headache. Large cerebellar strokes (>3 cm) are a neurosurgical emergency due to the risk of herniation, which may occur within hours of presentation.

CASE 118-4

VERTIGO

A 51-year-old right-handed man with a PMH of high blood pressure was conducting a business meeting when he suddenly developed severe vertigo, a feeling of imbalance while standing, and nausea. He vomited while calling 911. He did not have a PMH of other traditional vascular risk factors (diabetes mellitus, smoking, known occlusive vascular disease, structural heart disease, or atrial fibrillation). He did not have a history of neurologic disease (multiple sclerosis), or migraine headache. He denied recent head trauma, flexion-extension injury or headache. He also denied symptoms of diplopia, reduced vision, dysarthria, dysphagia, or focal sensory or motor deficits that might be expected with acute vertigo and brainstem stroke. He did not have antecedent hearing loss, a pressure sensation in either ear, or a history of Meniere syndrome. He experienced no antecedent viral symptoms to suggest acute labyrinthitis. He did have a history of bilateral tinnitus with normal audiograms in the past. His physical examination in the emergency department was notable for a middle-aged man who appeared extremely uncomfortable and reluctant to move. Horizontal nystagmus remained in the same direction when his gaze changed and was suppressed with visual fixation. He was able to walk without falling although he veered to his left. His neurologic examination was normal, including motor strength, the absence of dysmetria or sensory changes, and he had normal reflexes. Head CT imaging did not reveal any abnormalities of the cerebellum and fourth ventricle or the presence of multiple white matter lesions. The patient was admitted to the hospital for observation. The next morning he denied any symptoms of vertigo to the medical and neurology teams. His neurologic examination was completely normal and nystagmus was no longer present. At the recommendation of the neurology attending he underwent CT angiography which was negative. He was discharged home.

Synthesis

His history and normal neurologic examination did not suggest the possibility of dissection and he underwent an unnecessary CT angiography with its attendant risks of contrast and radiation exposure. If his first head CT had revealed a cerebellar infarction, emergent neurosurgical consultation and triage to an intensive care unit or to a stroke center would have been necessary.

Radiology practice point

CT scans of the cerebellum are usually normal in the first few hours following a cerebellar infarction; hence, the importance of a focused neurologic history and examination looking for cerebellar symptoms and signs, none of which were identified by multiple examiners over a 24-hour period of observation. If there were concern about cerebellar infarction or hemorrhage despite a "negative" CT, the clinician should consult with the radiologist. Routine MR imaging will likely detect an inferior cerebellar infarction but it is less sensitive for identifying a hemorrhage. The radiologist can arrange for MR sequences that would maximize identification of infarction and hemorrhage in the posterior fossa.

The mechanism of the stroke depends on the artery involved: superior cerebellar artery strokes are usually embolic but rarely cause hydrocephalus, posterior cerebellar artery strokes are equally likely to arise from stenosis or embolism, and anterior inferior cerebellar artery strokes are rare, and usually thrombotic with associated brainstem infarct.

ACUTE IMAGING OF BRAIN

Neuroimaging in the acute care setting relies on noncontrast enhanced head CT scanning both as the screening and, often, the definitive examination. For acute neurologic symptoms and signs and following trauma, timely initiation of the appropriate treatment requires identification of the presence and location of blood and/or mass effect. In many cases, this may be the only imaging required for the care of the patient.

Noncontrast enhanced CT scan is also the most important imaging to obtain when a patient presents with sudden onset of severe headache without any focal signs (assuming a complete neurologic examination) or symptoms suggesting focality. Most scans performed for this presentation will be negative.

Blood identified on noncontrast enhanced head CT scan must be localized to direct further workup and treatment of primary and secondary neurological disease. Subarachnoid hemorrhage indicates bleeding from within the brain parenchyma or bleeding into the CSF space not related to parenchyma. Subarachnoid hemorrhage is most commonly associated with bleeding intracranial aneurysms (75% of cases) or arteriovenous malformation (AVM) (10% of cases). The finding of edema in addition to blood may reflect metastasis of tumor from another organ, such as lung or breast. The specialized team providing care for the individual patient may involve interventional radiology or surgery to select further imaging and plan for treatment.

On occasion, a patient with or without a previously known tumor may present with new onset seizure due to a brain lesion (mass effect or bleeding) or with new cranial nerve findings due to involvement of the leptomeninges. When no more specific reason for seizure is known, a screening head CT potentially followed by contrast enhanced CT or MRI examination should be considered.

CASE 118-5

SEIZURE

A 42-year-old female with a history of hypertension suddenly developed a severe headache and suffered a seizure. She had no history of substance abuse or known vascular disease. In the emergency department her blood pressure was initially 260/140 mm Hg. Screening head CT was negative for blood. Fundoscopic examination was not documented. Her neurologic examination was notable for altered mental status attributed to her seizure. The covering neurologist was concerned about subtle occipital changes appreciated on subsequent MRI and worried about the possibility of the basilar scrape syndrome. Anticoagulation was recommended, initially with heparin as a bridge to therapeutic warfarin. Her blood pressure normalized with treatment consisting of lisinopril and hydrochlorothiazide and her clinicians attributed the initial high blood pressure elevation to her having suffered a seizure and possible noncompliance with her outpatient regimen. After her discharge to home, she collapsed, and reimaging revealed a large hemorrhage with evidence of transtentorial uncal herniation.

Synthesis

In retrospect, her diagnosis was hypertensive crisis complicated by seizure. A fundoscopic examination might have revealed exudates, hemorrhages, and papilledema.

Radiology practice point

Subtle occipital changes appreciated on MRI likely reflected hypertensive changes. Diffusion-weighted MR imaging may reveal vasogenic edema in hypertensive encephalopathy without ischemia or infarction. This finding may have therapeutic implications.

Head trauma can occur in the elderly from a fall with or without direct impact upon the skull. Extra-axial collection of blood forming a lentiform-shaped epidural hematoma that is confined between adjacent sutures can accumulate quickly and cause life-threatening mass effect requiring prompt surgical drainage. The longer more crescentic collection that crosses the adjacent suture is usually a more slowly accumulating subdural collection adjacent to torn bridging vessels that may be watched if small. Such a collection will sometimes go undiagnosed until other indications require a head CT scan. In the chronic phase, it will appear as a subdural hygroma filled with CSF fluid. The head CT scan may thus also provide additional history, such as prior strokes and prior falls and other trauma, particularly when a patient is unable to speak. In the elderly, these processes can be interrelated as the patient with a preexisting motor or balance–affecting deficit will also be at greater risk of falling. A patient who has had a stroke that affects his or her ability to communicate may also be less able to describe the present illness. Complete bedside examination for coincidental trauma can be helpful in reconstructing the series of events leading to the hospitalization. A patient fall while in the hospital requires much the same attention to neurological and total body surface examination for correct treatment.

NEUROIMAGING OF THE SPINE

Radiographs of the chest, abdomen, and pelvis may provide the initial screening examination of the spine. The appearance of the spine can remain normal until loss of 40% of the bone mineralization. The spine may not be studied in depth or specifically reported by the radiologist when the patient has imaging for other indications. It is very helpful to inquire specifically about the possibility of lesions when signs and symptoms suggest their presence. A comparison with prior studies that image the region of abnormality are very helpful for the assessment of acuity and potential significance that may range from a benign osteoporotic fracture to osseous metastasis. The spinal cord itself will not be imaged. Spine MRI is the imaging modality of choice when looking for impending cord compression and it is a widely recognized reason for emergent MRI examination. Computed tomography is an alternative choice if MRI is contraindicated. Radiography, radionuclide bone scans, and CT scans are helpful for identifying musculoskeletal metastases from a wide variety of tumors. Magnetic resonace imaging allows identification of nerve roots and tumor extension into the thecal sac. Radiographs, even when not specifically obtained for the bones, can be particularly helpful adjuncts in the evaluation of MRI and radionuclide bone scans. In patients who have had previous back surgery, intrathecal contrast material may be required for adequate CT examination. In cases in which hardware has been placed, artifacts can limit both CT and MR imaging. Such patients may not benefit from MRI due to artifacts, even if they tolerate the adjacent tissue heating that is likely to occur during the examination.

Oncologic patients often require specialized neurological imaging. The need may be less quickly recognized as part of the initial diagnosis. This is particularly true for back pain due to osseous metastases. If a patient has a known or suspected tumor, suspicion for cord compression requires prompt imaging to diagnose and intervene in order to preserve neurological function. Subtle presentation of impending cord compression is best addressed with outpatient MRI. While MRI is a standard examination for this indication, the hospitalized patient may not be able to adequately cooperate with the lengthy, complete spine MRI usually performed. A more limited examination may be considered based upon clinical examination. Very extensive bone destruction may be adequately studied for urgent treatment planning with CT scanning.

CASE 118-6

SEPSIS

A 51-year-old female with a PMH of a remote gastric bypass and a recent outside hospitalization for pneumonia was referred from an outside hospital (OSH) for MRI imaging of her spine. For the last couple of days she had been bedridden in her apartment and her family reported confusion. At the OSH her vital signs were notable for a BP of 90/55 mm Hg, pulse 110, regular, RR 24, T 100. She

appeared acutely uncomfortable and described severe myalgias. A black eschar was noted on her fifth digit, which was attributed to trauma. At the tertiary hospital she was admitted for pain control after having a reportedly negative MRI of her spine in the ED. She had an aortic murmur, which had not been described previously. She was unable to externally rotate her right hip secondary to severe pain. Her multiple blood cultures revealed *Staphylococcus aureus*. Interventional radiology drained 5 cc of pus from her right hip, which required debridement in the operating room. She subsequently underwent an aortic valve replacement.

Synthesis

This case highlights the importance of performing a physical examination to direct imaging. Magnetic resonance imaging of her back was negative because she did not have an epidural abscess. In this case relying on the provisional diagnosis from the emergency department and performing a limited history and physical examination led to performing the wrong test and delays in diagnosis and treatment. In retrospect, she was septic; the black eschar was due to a septic embolism.

Radiology practice point

Hospitalized patients are often unable to cooperate adequately to allow the full benefit of the MRI technology in their care. Magnetic resonance imaging examinations do not use ionizing radiation but can be quite lengthy, lasting an hour or more in duration. The request for wider coverage, such as adjacent body parts, is not easily accommodated in the same scanning session. It is therefore imperative to have a specific goal for the MRI from the outset.

CASE 118-7

READMISSION FROM REHABILITATION FACILITY

A 68-year-old female with PMH notable most recently for hiatal hernia repair with multiple postoperative complications, hypertension, and right breast carcinoma was transferred from acute rehabilitation to the medical service. She has been either at rehabilitation or in the hospital for most of the past year and returned from rehabilitation with a cough, bilateral sacral and sciatic pain, decreased ability to ambulate, and complaints of bilateral leg weakness. Pain was present only with movement, especially with attempts to ambulate; she described this pain as a "cramping" or "tightness" in the back of her thighs that ached increasingly with movement. She denied saddle anesthesia, change in bowel or bladder function or sensation, or leg numbness or tingling. The patient has been on multiple antibiotics for hospital-acquired infections. She currently had chest tube, J tube, and G tube in place. Examination was notable for a fully alert and appropriately interactive female. Her vital signs were normal. Her neurologic examination was diffusely abnormal including tongue fasciculation, motor weakness with fasciculations in her lower extremities, hypertonic reflexes with spasticity, clonus and bilateral Babinski signs. Rectal tone was normal. A STAT MRI of the L-spine was obtained and was reportedly negative. Patient was given 1 mg of lorazepam prior to MRI of her cervical and thoracic spine but her coughing in the supine position precluded the examination. She was subsequently transferred to the intensive care unit after elective intubation.

Synthesis

The differential diagnosis for a causative lesion in the spine is quite broad and spans infection, structural, neoplastic, and vascular.

Her examination suggested a myelopathic process involving the upper motor neurons of both legs. The lack of bowel, bladder, or saddle anesthesia symptoms made a full cauda equina syndrome less likely. As the patient has been NPO for some time, and has had many interruptions in her nutrition, a metabolic cause of her myelopathic picture should also be considered.

Radiology practice point

Selected for the wrong reason, MRI will increase the stress on the acutely ill patient and delay institution of needed therapy. In this case, the already debilitated patient likely required intubation due to respiratory suppression from lorazepam administration, deconditioning, and aspiration.

CONCLUSION

The scope of neuroradiology varies between institutions. In some centers, spine services are separately organized within neuroradiology or musculoskeletal radiology. Consulting the radiologists in your institution is important for understanding the availability and expertise in a variety of specialized examinations that might be available. The evolution of neurological findings over time can be very dynamic and inadequately conveyed on an imaging requisition. Continuing consultation during admission will provide the most clinical relevant data for patient treatment using the smallest number of scans and the least amount of contrast material possible.

SUGGESTED READINGS

Arslan A, Karaarslan E. Diffusion weighted MR imaging in non-infarct lesions of the brain. *EJR*. 2008;65:402-416.

Orrison WW Jr. *Atlas of Brain Function*, 2nd ed. New York, NY: Thieme; 2008.

Scarabino T, Salvolini U, Jinkins JR, eds. *Emergency Neuroradiology*. Heidelberg: Springer Science+Business Media; 2006.

ONLINE RESOURCES

1. http://headneckbrainspine.com/.
2. http://jakemandell.com http://www.lesionlocalizer.comhttp://jakemandell.com/headct/.
3. The Whole Brain Atlas MRI views of the normal and diseased human brain. Collaboration of MIT and Harvard University. www.med.harvard.edu/aanlib/.
4. http://www.neuroanatomy.ca/stroke_model/cross_section_anatomy.html.

CHAPTER 119

Interventional Radiology

Randall Czjakowski, MS, RRA, RT(R)(CT)
Francine L. Jacobson, MD, MPH

The purpose of this chapter is to provide a basic guide for the approach to interventional procedures and the patient issues that are common to all interventional procedures. Available procedures and the organization within the radiology department in a particular hospital will reflect the patient population being treated and professional collaborations through which specialized procedures are performed. The American College of Radiology website provides evidence-based guidance for a wide variety of procedures through Interventional Radiology Practice Parameters developed in collaboration with medical specialty societies. Practice parameters are continually reviewed and updated to respond to new issues and health care developments.

INTERVENTIONAL RADIOLOGY PROCEDURES DURING HOSPITALIZATION

The performance of minimally invasive diagnostic and therapeutic procedures has increased dramatically in the 21st century. Such procedures contribute significantly to decrease in length of stay and successful shift of care to the outpatient setting. Central venous catheter placement, thoracentesis, and paracentesis are straightforward procedures that may be organized through one or more divisions within the department of radiology. In some institutions, these will be performed by thoracic radiologists, abdominal radiologists, and angio-interventional radiologists while in other institutions all three will be performed by radiologists in a single interventional radiology division. Many procedures that have previously required open surgery may now be performed in angiography and other specialized radiology suites. The organization of service lines varies among hospitals as will the frequency with which individual procedures are performed. Learn how the service or services are organized in your institution and what procedures are offered. In this introduction, we will present issues that are common to the widest variety of procedures and also examples of how the service may be organized. Minimally invasive procedures are performed in radiology suites using very similar guidelines and procedures to those used for surgery. Inpatient acuity will generally prioritize patients for care although hospitalized patients often require more preparation and coordination for the safe performance of procedures.

ORGANIZATION OF SERVICES

Interventional services may be provided by one group of radiologists who are prepared to perform procedures in a variety of locations, including angiographic suite, ultrasound, and specialized CT and MR suites. In a hospital with strong modality-based organization of services, the radiologists may specialize in performance of procedures within a particular modality such as US, CT, or angiography. If your hospital has subspecialty groups of radiologists who are dedicated to specific organ systems, the interventional services may be performed by the radiologists who also perform and interpret diagnostic procedures in the same organ system regardless of the modality chosen for the procedure.

RADIOLOGY CONSULTATION

Consultation with radiology is as fundamental as consultation with surgery prior to selection and performance of any procedure. The radiologist with whom you normally consult can advise you regarding the organization of services within your hospital. The radiologist who will perform the procedure is best able to guide you in selection of biopsy site and modality as well as necessary preparation of the patient. The radiologist will also explain the procedure, including risks and benefits with your patient in order to obtain informed consent. Critically ill patients may also require anesthesia consultation for safe performance of minimally invasive procedures.

The purpose of the initial consultation is to consider the risks and benefits of performing a particular procedure. In an ideal world, every procedure performed would provide the correct diagnosis or complete treatment without any morbidity or mortality. In the real world the interactions between these factors are of primary importance. Can the target be reached safely using a closed or minimally invasive technique? Will the location, appearance or size of the target require an approach that increases the risk of complications? The patient's ability or inability to follow directions and actively participate in the procedure will also affect safety and success. When a patient cannot remain still and follow commands, general anesthesia may be necessary for patient safety. Interventional radiology procedures can provide valuable data for clinical decision making and, in some situations, rapid treatment.

▓ BEFORE THE PROCEDURE

The diagnostic process that leads to the decision to ask for an interventional procedure generally includes relevant diagnostic imaging from which the radiologist can discuss the potential benefits and risks of the interventional procedure, including how a particular structure can be safely approached and what types of specimens would realistically be obtained. Planning the procedure is poorly served by performance of diagnostic imaging in the same visit to radiology as an interventional procedure. The imaging guidance during the procedure will be initiated based upon prior available imaging. How recent the imaging will need to be varies with the pace of the patient's disease process.

When consulting the radiologist about the possibility of performing an interventional radiology procedure, it is important to disclose comorbidities, medications, and lab abnormalities that may adversely affect the safe performance of the procedure. Patient hearing, preferred language, and ability to give informed consent are also important considerations.

Informed consent

It is helpful to give the patient and family members a preliminary introduction to what will be done for a procedure to set the stage for the discussion with the radiologist and allow time for the patient and family members to think about the procedure and identify the questions they want answered.

Procedures are akin to surgery and will be performed with similar sterile techniques. Needles, wires, and catheters are very small but methods for stopping bleeding are more limited than in the OR where electrocautery and surgical clips can rapidly stop bleeding. It can be very helpful to observe the performance of a procedure you will be ordering frequently. This experience improves communication with the radiologist and with the patient. The radiologist performing the procedure will secure and document informed consent for invasive diagnostic or therapeutic procedure as well as moderate conscious sedation.

Preprocedure laboratory testing is intended to minimize bleeding risks and confirm adequate hemoglobin and platelets to deal with expected bleeding. If an intravenous contrast agent will be administered as part of the procedure, adequate renal function will also require confirmation. Patients with pancytopenia and anticoagulation will require additional testing to document adequate platelets and correction of coagulopathy.

Most procedures will require a minimum of 6 hours of preprocedure fasting. When procedures are added on to a schedule and

will occur late in the day, the patient may be allowed to have clears through the morning rather than being made NPO from midnight as might be done for a procedure being performed in the morning. Medications may need to be withdrawn for variable lengths of time to ensure adequate hemostasis during the interventional procedure. Cardiology consultation is recommended regarding management of Clopidogrel (Plavix). An invasive procedure may need to be deferred when this type of drug cannot be stopped for 5 days. This may also enter into a decision to pursue an open biopsy during which electrocautery can be employed to control bleeding.

▓ SPECIFIC PROCEDURES

Simple procedures

Procedures that can alternatively be performed at the bedside without preprocedure testing such as *thoracentesis and PICC line placement* are often performed with limited preinterventional procedure testing. The risk of bleeding is extremely small and preprocedure imaging is not required for basic procedure planning. This principle also applies to procedures such as lumbar puncture that is also frequently performed for diagnostic myelography imaging. Procedures in this category are brief and often performed without prolonged fasting or conscious sedation.

Drainage procedures

A wide variety of fluid collections can be drained using percutaneous approach with imaging such as ultrasound and CT. Abscess, pleural effusion, empyema, ascites, and obstructed kidneys can be drained with drainage tubes that are meant to be left in place or removed at the conclusion of the procedure. It is extremely important to have a clear understanding of how long the tube is expected to remain, how the decision will be made to remove it, and who will manage the tube during and, if necessary, after the patient is discharged.

Biopsy procedures

Lung biopsy is often viewed differently from other biopsies because of the potential complication of pneumothorax. The need for genomic testing of tumors has led to increased use of core biopsy needles to deliver larger specimens for pathologic examination. This and performance of multiple passes are undertaken to increase the yield and decrease the need for repeating the biopsy.

Embolization and specialized procedures

Transjugular intrahepatic portosystemic shunts (TIPS), vascular embolization, and thoracic duct embolization are not performed in every hospital. The TIPS procedure is performed to treat complication of portal hypertension. The creation of the channel through the liver shunts blood from the portal vein to a hepatic vein, reducing the portosystemic pressure gradient, effectively treating uncontrolled variceal hemorrhage and refractory ascites. Embolization of a feeding vessel may be requested by the surgeon prior to surgery in order to limit bleeding during the procedure. Thoracic duct embolization is more often performed following thoracic surgery to treat chylothorax. The role of the hospitalist may vary between institutions and even surgical services within a single institution. It is very important to have participation by the surgical services even if the hospitalist is providing the routine perioperative care for the surgical patient.

Range of sedation and analgesia

The range of sedation is very broad from minimal anxiolysis to general anesthesia. Minimal sedation is defined by the Joint Commission and the American Society of Anesthesiologists as "a drug-induced state during which the patient responds normally to verbal commands." The ability of the patient to do so contributes to the

TABLE 119-1 American Society of Anesthesiologists (ASA) Score

I	Completely healthy and fit patient
II	Mild systemic disease
III	Severe systemic disease, not incapacitating
IV	Incapacitating disease, ie, a constant threat to life
V	Moribund patient not expected to live 24 h

safety of many interventional radiology procedures. Cognitive function and coordination may be diminished but normal ventilator and cardiovascular functions will remain normal.

Patient-related risks for conscious sedation

Moderate sedation minimally depresses the level of consciousness without impairing the patient's ability to maintain protective reflexes and patent airway. The patient can be aroused by physical or verbal stimulation. The provision of moderate sedation and analgesia requires preprocedure evaluation, monitoring of patient during and after the procedure, specialized medications and availability of reversal agents. Patients who are American Society of Anesthesiologists (ASA) class I or II qualify for sedation and analgesia outside of the operating room by personnel other than anesthesiologists. Patients who are ASA III or IV require consideration of comorbidities, current condition, and expectation for goals of sedation (see **Table 119-1**). Consultation with an anesthesiologist may be required for the safe performance of procedures for critically ill patients.

■ AFTER THE INTERVENTIONAL RADIOLOGY PROCEDURE

The interventional radiologist will prepare orders and communicate with the service or services managing the patient's care regarding patient activity, resumption of diet, and follow-up imaging requirements such as chest radiographs to rule out or monitor pneumothorax following thoracentesis or lung biopsy. These orders may require clinical cosignature for activation. Verbal communication and confirmation of clock time (rather than elapsed time following procedure or prior radiograph) is most helpful for ensuring timely follow-up. The dialog between services immediately following the procedure should also include complete recap of participating services and the specific functions each will perform. This will avoid the unfortunate confusion that can easily surround a drain or chest tube with no one designated to manage the tube. Feedback between the

services does not end with the transfer of care back to the clinical service. The continuing sharing of data and feedback regarding the outcome of individual procedures is a cornerstone in the evolution of patient care through minimally invasive procedures. The radiologist can provide further guidance when the pathology report does not answer the clinical question. He or she can help to select the next course of action when pathology is "nondiagnostic." This may occur because the pathologic absence of tumor supports the imaging findings that are consistent with inflammation. In this case, the "nondiagnostic" for tumor may itself confirm a benign etiology. The next step or plan could be follow-up imaging, an open surgical biopsy, or a repeated biopsy. Follow-up imaging is often chosen when a lesion is very small and might be more adequately biopsied if it increases in size. An open surgical biopsy can provide more tissue for pathologic evaluation. In the case of a large lesion, an additional test such as PET/CT may be performed to improve the selection of biopsy site within a large lesion. A repeat biopsy may also be performed with the same modality if the patient was unable to adequately follow commands or a complication, such as bleeding or pneumothorax required premature termination of the procedure. Deferring biopsy until after discharge often serves the patient better than performing a biopsy during a hospitalization to address comorbid disease.

PROCEDURE RISK CATEGORY

Category 0: Procedures with Very Low Risk of Bleeding
LP, myelogram, spine or joint (including pubic symphysis, SI joint, iliopsoas bursa, trochanteric bursa) injections for pain

Category I: Procedures with Low Risk of Bleeding
Paracentesis, thoracentesis, superficial biopsy (eg, superficial inguinal node or subcutaneous mass), superficial needle aspiration or catheter drainage of fluid (eg, subcutaneous fluid collections and Baker's cysts), drainage catheter exchange (excluding catheters within solid organs, eg, liver, kidney), biopsy of intramuscular masses, bone biopsies including bony pelvis but excluding spine

Category II: Procedures with Moderate Risk of Bleeding
Fine needle biopsy of visceral solid organs or lung, drainage catheter exchange (within solid organ), retroperitoneal nonsolid organ catheter drainage, alcohol ablations; all neck or spine biopsy procedures

Category III: Procedures with Significant Bleeding Risk, Difficult to Detect or Control
Large needle (core) biopsies of solid organs (parenchymal or focal masses) or lung, thermal ablations (RF, Cryo, Microwave), intraperitoneal catheter drainage, solid organ catheter drainage

■ PREPROCEDURE LABS

Lab	Procedure Risk	Acceptable	Reason(s) to Measure
PTT	Category 0 or I	PTT < 2×	Unfractionated heparin, uncharacterized bleeding history/risk factor
	Category II or III	PTT < 1.5×	Routine, unless previous normal documented value and no risk factors
PT	Category 0 or I	INR ≤ 2	Warfarin, known/suspected liver disease, uncharacterized bleeding history/risk factor
	Category II or III	INR ≤ 1.5	Routine, unless previous normal documented value within 30 d and no risk factors
CBC	Category 0 or I	PLT ≥ 50K	Suspected thrombocytopenia, DIC, sepsis, malignancy and/or chemotherapy, medications including chloramphenicol, colchicine, H_2 blockers, hydralazine, indomethacin, isoniazid, quinidine, streptomycin, sulfonamide, thiazide diuretics, tolbutamide
	Category II	PLT ≥ 50K	Routine (also provides baseline Hct) within 30 d
	Category III	HCT ≥ 25	Routine (also provides baseline Hct) within 30 d
		PLT ≥ 50K*	

*Consider PLT ≥ 90K prior to liver cryoablation.

■ MEDICATION MANAGEMENT

Aspirin

Do not stop if used for secondary prophylaxis (eg, prior CV event such as CVA, MI, or coronary stent placement) without cardiovascular or PATC consult. Benefits versus risks must be carefully considered. Many procedures can be performed while on ASA with minimal increased risk of bleeding complications.

Primary prophylaxis, 81 mg:
  Category 0, or I: continue ASA
  Category II or III: stop 5 days before, restart >24 hours after

Primary prophylaxis, >81 mg:
  Category 0: continue ASA
  Category I: stopping prior to procedure is optional, timing is at the discretion of the radiologist, restart >12 hours
  Category II or III: stop 5 days before, restart >24 hours
  Nonelective/emergency: ignore

Clopidogrel (plavix) or prasugrel (effient)

Do not stop if used for secondary prophylaxis (eg, prior CV event such as CVA, MI, or coronary stent placement) without cardiovascular or PATC consult. Benefits versus risks must be carefully considered.

Consider deferring elective procedures or employing bridging strategy if procedure is critical to care.

Primary prophylaxis:
  Category 0: optional to stop ≥5 days, restart >12 hours
  Category I: stop >5 days, restart >12 hours
  Category II or III: stop >5 days, restart >24 hours

Nonelective/emergency procedures: Consider PLT transfusion if stopped <5 days; transfuse at least 6 hours after last dose

Heparin (unfractionated, IV or SQ)

SQ, Prophylactic dose:
  Category 0: ignore
  Category I-III: stop 4-6 hours, do not need to recheck PTT; restart >12 hours

Therapeutic dose:
  Category 0 or I: stop for 4 to 6 hours; restart >12 hours
  Category II or III: stop for 4 to 6 hours; optional recheck PTT, restart >24 hours
  Nonelective/emergency: consider protamine reversal (by referring medical/surgical team)

LMW heparin (low-molecular weight, eg, Lovenox, Dalteparin/Fragmin)

Prophylactic dose, 5000 IU once per day:
  Category 0: ignore
  Category I: stop 12 hours before, restart >12 hours
  Category II or III: stop 12 hours before, restart >24 hours

Therapeutic dose, ≥5000 IU once per day:
  Category 0: optional stop 24 hours before, restart >12 hours
  Category I: stop 24 hours before, restart >12 hours
  Category II or III: stop 24 hours before, restart >24 hours

Urgent procedure: ignore prophylactic LMWH, can perform 8 to 10 hours after last therapeutic dose

NSAIDs (other than ASA)

  Category 0 & I: ignore
  Category II or III: consider stopping 48 hours (optional)
  Nonelective/emergency: ignore

Warfarin (Coumadin)

Consider LMW heparin bridge if high risk for VTE, for example, heart valve surgery, recent PE, DVT.
  Category 0: optional to stop ≥5 days, restart >12 hours
  Category I: stop >5 days, restart >12 hours
  Category II or III: stop >5 days, restart >24 hours
  Nonelective/emergency: consider FFP/Vit K

■ OTHER ANTICOAGULANTS

Category I, II, or III:
  Direct thrombin inhibitor (nonreversible): dabigatran (Pradaxa), Factor Xa inhibitors: Fondaparinux (Arixtra), rivaroxaban (Xarelto), apixaban (Eliquis)—stop for 48 hours
  Antiplatelet: Tirofiban (Aggrastat) or eptifibatide (Integrilin): stop for at least 6 hours
  Reversible direct thrombin inhibitors (do not cause HIT): Argatroban -stop for 4 hours, consider checking PTT; also Bivalirudin (Angiomax) infusion: stop for ≥2 hours
  Phosphodiesterase inhibitor (inhibits PLT aggregation)—cilostazol (Pletal); stop 4 days

■ REVERSAL AGENTS

Kcentra is FDA approved only to urgently reverse warfarin (Coumadin) anticoagulation in adult patients with acute major bleeding. Any other use is "off-label" and should be considered only in emergency situations and in consultation with the referring physician or hematologist. Serious adverse events may include stroke, pulmonary embolism, or deep vein thrombosis.

SUGGESTED READINGS

O'Connor SD, Taylor AJ, Williams EC, Winter TC. Coagulation concepts update. *AJR Am J Roentgenol* 2009;192:1656-1664.

Patel IJ, Davidson JC, Nikolic B, et al. Consensus guidelines for periprocedural management of coagulation status and hemostasis risk in percutaneous image-guided interventions. *J Vasc Interv Radiol* 2012;23:727-736.

Patel IJ, Davidson JC, Nikolic B, et al. Addendum of newer anticoagulants to the SIR consensus guideline. *J Vasc Interv Radiol* 2013;24:641-645.

ONLINE RESOURCES

http://www.sirweb.org/patients/minimally-invasive-treatments/.
http://www.radiologyinfo.org/en/info.cfm?pg=tips.
http://www.acr.org/Quality-Safety/Standards-Guidelines/Practice-Guidelines-by-Modality/Interventional. Accessed November 15, 2015.

SECTION 3
Procedures

CHAPTER 120

Vascular Access

Karl D. Wittnebel, MD, MPH
Bradley T. Rosen, MD, MBA, FHM

A central venous catheter (CVC) is any vascular access device whose tip terminates in a large vessel in the body, most commonly the superior vena cava or inferior vena cava. Because indwelling lines pose definite risks to patients, steps should be taken whenever possible to minimize the risk of complications. Always seek operators with skill and experience, employ ultrasound for guidance, take the time to properly position patients, and employ meticulous sterile technique. The indications and necessity for central venous access must be critically reviewed prior to proceeding with a CVC insertion and each CV must be regularly reassessed for ongoing necessity and promptly removed as soon as the risks exceed the benefits.

There are no absolute contraindications to CVC placement provided that the likelihood and severity of potential complications are outweighed by the benefits of immediate venous access. Given the severity of illness generally associated with the requirement of a CVC, establishing adequate venous access is frequently a matter of ensuring survival. Although it is common practice to check coagulation parameters and to correct abnormalities, many CVCs may be safely placed in patients with coagulopathies; an actively hemorrhaging patient may require immediate placement of a large bore catheter regardless of INR or platelet levels. Bacteremic patients without peripheral access may require CVC in order to receive proper intravenous antibiotic treatment and/or monitoring. These patients are at high risk for developing secondary catheter related-bacterial superinfection (CR-BSI) due to the seeding of the CVC from circulating bacteria. In these patients, waiting 48 hours or longer until the bacteremia has cleared prior to placing a CVC may not be feasible. For these patients antibiotic-impregnated catheters are highly recommended along with prompt removal of the CVC as soon as it is no longer required. See **Table 120-1** for details on CVC indications and relative contraindications, site selection considerations, types of CVCs, and potential complications, and **Table 120-2** for practical CVC placement tips and recommendations.

For patients requiring peripheral venous access with poor vascular options, portable real time 2D ultrasound may identify deep veins in the forearm, brachial, and shoulder, thereby avoiding, at least temporarily, the need for central venous catheterization. Veins should be compressible and nonpulsatile. Bedside ultrasound can also be used to visualize the superficial external jugular vein and facilitate placement of midline catheters. The tip of midline catheters is inserted into an upper arm vein, (usually brachial or cephalic), and does not extend beyond the axillary line. Although short 3 cm peripheral intravenous (IV) lines require replacement every 3 days, 20 cm long midline catheters may remain in place for a longer period of time and they are appropriate for all intravenous fluids that would normally be administered through a short peripheral IV. Although they cost the same as peripherally inserted central catheters (PICC) lines, they do not require a chest film postinsertion and may facilitate early discharge to another setting. There are limitations as to the type of solution that can be used and the rate at which that infusate can be delivered through a peripheral midline.

Percutaneous translumbar placement of an inferior vena cava catheter by an interventional radiologist is a viable option in patients who have few or no other access sites and is not intended as a primary means of central venous access. Such catheters have been used for TPN, long-term antibiotic therapy, systemic chemotherapy, hemodialysis, and stem cell harvesting for bone marrow transplantation. Complications associated with this procedure include catheter thrombosis, fibrin sheath formation, infection, and migration of the

TABLE 120-1 Basic Considerations for Central Venous Catheters (CVC)

Indications	Prior to Insertion of CVC	Comments
• CPR (rapid infusion) • Transvenous pacing • Monitoring (central pressures) • Administration of phlebitic or vasoactive medications (chemotherapy, calcium chloride, pressors) • Hemodialysis, ultrafiltration, plasmapheresis, other blood filtering processes • TPN • Prolonged IV therapy • Recurrent and/or difficult phlebotomy	• Is this necessary? • Is insertion time critical as a matter of life and death? • What type of catheter is required? • Which site is preferred?	Because length and diameter of catheter determine flow rates, type of catheter selected depends on indication • 3 cc/min CT contrast • 70 cc/min pheresis • >300 cc/min HD Long-term IV therapy • PICC lines • Ports • Tunneled catheters Hemodynamic monitoring of LVEDP and cardiac output • Pulmonary artery (Swan-Ganz) catheters

Contraindications to CVC	Options	Comments
No absolute contraindication when need for immediate access outweighs other risks • Infection at insertion site • Venous clot • Coagulopathy • Bacteremia	Pick another site if local infection or venous clot Weigh risks and benefits for individual patients depending on the presence of coagulopathy, need for future HD, and other factors	Ideally, INR <1.5, platelets >50K • Patients kept "line free" for at least 48 h and/or until bacteremia clears prior to placing a new central line with reliance on peripheral lines for administration of antibiotics

Types of Catheters	Advantages	Disadvantages
Subclavian Vein Tip termination in superior vena cava (ideally at the cavoatrial junction corresponding to the right mainstem bronchus on CXR)	Lowest risk infection, clot Bony landmarks (obese patients) Most comfortable	↑ risk of pneumothorax relative to other sites; may have in ↑ risk in patients with COPD, asthma, high PEEP, upper thoracic trauma Unable to compress if bleeding; might consider other sites in patients with coagulopathy Not recommended for chronic HD (risk of thrombosis)
Internal Jugular Vein Tip termination in superior vena cava (ideally at the cavoatrial junction)	**Internal Jugular Vein** ~complication risk to subclavian but lower risk of pneumothorax Easier to control bleeding	**Internal Jugular Vein** ↑ risk of carotid puncture Technically difficult if intubation, tracheostomy, excessive pulmonary secretions, obese necks; avoid if postoperative cervical spine
Femoral Vein Tip termination in inferior vena cava (ideally at the cavoatrial junction)	**Femoral Vein** Easiest during code, no risk of pneumothorax	**Femoral Vein** Medication delays during code Highest risk of infection, clot Requires immobilization after insertion Avoid if vena cava clot, extrinsic compression or if IVC
PICC Peripherally inserted central catheters via mid arm through basilic or cephalic vein	**PICC** Lower risk of infection than nontunneled central lines and can be used for extended periods of time postdischarge	**PICC** A PICC line catheter tip should be located at the inferior aspect of the SVC (the arch of the azygous vein)
Tunneled Central Lines Typically indicated for long term (>2 wk) use Subcutaneous tunnel ~8-10 cm long on chest wall Outpatient HD most common indication (Hickman, Quinton, Permacath)	**Tunneled Central Lines** Lower risk of infection because all elements buried beneath skin, no dressing when not in use	**Tunneled Central Lines** More frequent vascular access →↑ risk of infection as skin over PORT limited in its ability to tolerate repeated use while retaining its ability to function as a barrier to infection
Port Cannisters implanted in SQ pocket (chest—Port-a-cath, arm—PAS-port)	**Port** Indicated for patients who require intermittent, repeated, >3-mo vascular access for infusion and/or phlebotomy	

(Continued)

TABLE 120-1 Basic Considerations for Central Venous Catheters (CVC) (Continued)

Line Complications	Types of Complications	Comments
>15% of patients will have a complication	**Mechanical**	**Mechanical**
	Subcutaneous emphysema or fluid infiltration, retained foreign object (guidewire or catheter), failed cannulation or line malposition, central vein perforation, nerve injury, bladder injury	Likelihood of mechanical complication depends more upon skill and experience of operator; have help readily available, avoid pulling on catheter
	Vascular	**Vascular**
	Arterial puncture or laceration	Withdraw needle, apply pressure for 5 min. If arterial puncture with dilator or catheter vascular surgical emergency
	Hematoma	
	AV fistula creation	If hematoma IJ, possible airway, carotid complications
	Central venous clot	
	Cardiac	A new pleural effusion following line placement, consider extravasation of fluid from line or pleural hematoma
	Arrhythmias due to stimulation of myocardium by catheter or guidewire myocardial	
	pericardial tamponade	**Cardiac**
	Pulmonary	Typically resolves with withdrawal of catheter or guidewire
	Pneumothorax, may require Chest Tube or emergency treatment if hemodynamic instability (tension pneumothorax)	**Pulmonary**
		↑ risk: COPD, bleb, bullous disease
	Air embolism	Prevention: select optimal site for insertion, use **US guidance**
	Infection	Air embolism ↑ risk: hypovolemia, low CVP, large negative intrathoracic pressure
	Local infection, bacteremia usually >72-h postinsertion	Prevention: keep hub occluded and catheter flushed with saline during insertion, patient in Trendelenburg until procedure done
	Decision to remove line suspected to be infected based	
	on available evidence, how difficult and necessary future vascular access will be to obtain	Treatment: place patient in left lateral decubitus postion and Trendelenburg to trap air in right ventricle
		Infection
		Antibiotic-coated catheters may have a RRR of 21% compared to traditional catheters
		Femoral lines higher incidence of late infectious complications
		Promptly remove CVC when no longer needed

Line Removal Complications	Prevention	Comments
• Bleeding	All preventable with proper positioning and removal technique. Trendelenburg	To minimize bleeding: reverse coagulopathy prior to removal and immediate manual pressure for 5-10 min or longer depending on site and bleeding
• Air embolism	(reverse Trendelenburg for femoral lines)	
As little as 100 mL of air can cause circulatory collapse at ambient pressure in a matter of seconds	If tunneled line, must be removed by IR or by dialysis service	To minimize risk of air embolism from thoracic sites, ↑ intrathoracic venous pressure prior to removal from upper body. To do this:
• Catheter fracture with or without embolism of retained fragment		• Position patient in Trendelenburg
		• Instruct patient to continuously hum or Valsalva or fully exhale during line removal
		• Apply an occlusive dressing over thoracic site following removal
		To avoid catheter fracture: do not forcefully tug at catheter if met with resistance during removal process

TABLE 120-2 Technical Tips

Type of Catheters	Positioning	Prevention
Determine the safest and most appropriate insertion site for each patient	Properly position patient, taking the time to ensure all comfortable before proceeding	If time not an issue, obtain help from experienced operator
	To prepare skin, use chlorhexidine scrub for at least 30 s of continuous scrubbing	Estimate insertion distance to SVC prior to catheterization
	Proper sterile draping to cover majority of patient	Meticulous sterile technique
		Use of **US guidance** to directly visualize target vein and to confirm anatomy (ideal)
Subclavian Vein Insert needle 2 cm below clavicle at the junction of the lateral $1/3$ and medial $2/3$ of the clavicle; use the deltopectoral groove to guide angle of approach and first aim for 2 cm above suprasternal notch	Trendelenburg position; remove pillow, place towel between scapulae, externally rotate arm to ↑ deltopectoral groove	Approximate length of line: Right subclavian 15 cm Left subclavian 18 cm
Internal Jugular Vein	Trendelenburg position; remove the pillow from underneath patient's head; **real-time US** ↓ complication rate during insertion	Approximate length of line: Right IJ 15 cm Left IJ 20 cm
Femoral Vein Vein always medial to artery The point of insertion one finger breath medial to artery and two finger breaths inferior to inguinal ligament	Patient should lie flat on back Use silk tape to assist with pannus retraction in the obese patient Always have one hand on femoral artery, the other to guide the insertion	Approximate length of line 20 cm or longer

catheter tip. Outward migration of the catheter into the retroperitoneal soft tissues may result in clinically insignificant hematoma, and loss of access. The catheter may also migrate into the iliac veins but, in most instances, endovascular retrieval techniques can reposition the catheter thereby avoiding catheter removal. Translumbar access is not straightforward in patients with indwelling IVC filters and/or in patients with a history of multiple thrombosis due to hypercoagulability because of the increased risk of caval thrombosis with multiple devices in situ. For most patients, translumbar catheter should be considered an access of last resort.

When intravascular access is not quickly available during emergency resuscitation, intraosseous (IO) access provides immediate access to the vascular system and has roughly the same absorption rate as CVC access. Any medication that can be introduced via IV can be introduced via IO. Intraosseous is also preferred over endotracheal (ET) drug administration. The latter allows only specific drugs that have relatively low toxicity to lung tissue and must be limited to low volumes to avoid drowning the patient. Using a mechanical or powered adjunct to place the catheter, the needle is injected through the bone's hard cortex and into the soft marrow interior. Intraosseous access has now become the preferred method of quickly establishing vascular access for patients experiencing cardiac arrest, major trauma, airway compromise, severe dehydration, and/or hypoperfusion (shock). Intraosseous is also an alternative route for patients who typically have poor peripheral vasculature or challenging vascular access. Intraosseous can be maintained for 24 to 48 hours, after which another route of access should be obtained.

Central venous access may also be required for monitoring purposes if the benefits outweigh the risks (higher rate of complications and availability of other safer options). Pulmonary artery (PA) catheters are no longer routinely used to obtain hemodynamic data to guide fluid management and therapeutic decision making. Pulmonary artery catheters are still indicated for some patients to distinguish cardiogenic versus noncardiogenic pulmonary edema and to determine the physiologic basis of shock (sepsis versus cardiac). Pulmonary artery catheters may also be used to titrate vasodilator therapy for patients with severe pulmonary hypertension. Other indications might include monitoring for selected patients with pretransplant decompensated heart failure or right ventricular infarction, or confirming the diagnosis of tamponade if echocardiology not available.

SUGGESTED READINGS

Chopra V, Flanders SA, Saint S, et al. The Michigan Appropriateness Guide for Intravenous Catheters (MAGIC): results From a multispecialty panel using the RAND/UCLA Appropriateness Method. *AnnIntern Med*. 2015;163(6 Suppl):S1-S40.

McGee DC, Gould MK. Preventing complications of central venous catheterization. *N Engl J Med*. 2003;348:1123-1133.

National Institute for Clinical Excellence (NICE) Report: Guidance on the Use of Ultrasound Locating Devises for Placing Central Venous Catheters; 2002.

Schoenfeld E, Boniface K, Shokoohl H. ED Technicians can successfully place ultrasound-guided intravenous catheters in patients with poor vascular access. *Am J Emerg Med*. 2011;29(5):496-501.

ONLINE RESOURCES

Graham AS, Ozment C, Tegtmeyer K, et al. Videos in Clinical Medicine. Central Venous Catheterization. Vol. 356; 2007:321. http://content.nejm.org/cgi/content/short/356/21/e21.

PACEP.org (PA catheters)

CHAPTER 121

Intubation and Airway Support

Bisan A. Salhi, MD
Todd A. Taylor, MD
Douglas S. Ander, MD

Airway management can significantly affect outcomes for hospitalized critically ill patients. Failure to deliver adequate oxygen may cause irreversible brain damage or preclude successful resuscitation. Options for management may range from assisted ventilation with a bag-valve-mask (BVM) to noninvasive ventilation (NIV) support to endotracheal intubation (**Table 121-1**). A successful outcome in any intubation demands proficiency in patient assessment, knowledge of the equipment (basic and advanced), requisite technical skills, appreciation of individual limitations, and an alternative plan to deal with the difficult or failed airway.

A small survey published in 2010 noted that individual hospitalists ($n = 175$) performed, on average, only 10 endotracheal intubations in the previous year with a range of 3 to 20. For those performing endotracheal intubation, it is important to maintain this essential skill, and to be aware of their own practices and skill limitations. Depending on their clinical environment and work setting, the expectations for different hospitalists in advanced airway management will vary. However, all hospitalists should be versed in initial airway management and stabilization, including effective use of oral and nasal airway and BVM devices.

Successful intubation requires not only knowledge of the basic procedural steps, but also knowledge of airway anatomy, landmarks, and locations of various airway structures relative to each other.

INDICATION FOR INTUBATION

All indications for endotracheal intubation can be classified as (1) failure to maintain a patent airway, (2) failure of oxygenation and/or ventilation, and (3) anticipation of a rapidly deteriorating clinical course (**Table 121-2**).

PREDICTORS OF A DIFFICULT AIRWAY

A *difficult airway* refers to complex or challenging BVM or endotracheal intubation. Difficult oxygenation is the inability to maintain the oxygen saturation >90% despite using a BVM and 100% oxygen. A *failed airway* refers to the inability to either ventilate or intubate a patient after three intubation attempts by the same operator. A higher rate of poor clinical outcomes occurs when the airway is managed as an emergent (rather than elective) procedure. In addition, an increased number of airway attempts predicts poorer outcomes; thus, a backup plan is necessary if initial intubation attempts are not successfully executed. The LEMON rule is one popular rule for assessment for difficult intubation (**Table 121-3**).

BAG-VALVE-MASK (BVM) VENTILATION

The most important skill required for inpatient clinicians in airway management is use of a BVM and airway adjuncts to ventilate and oxygenate the patient. BVM ventilation can effectively maintain airway patency while an alternative plan is developed and implemented. However, patients with a high risk of failing BVM ventilation may require more rapid and definitive airway evaluation and management. Predictors of difficult BVM are summarized in **Table 121-4**.

PROCEDURAL STEPS

Rapid sequence intubation (RSI) is now the predominant and preferred method in managing the emergent airway, precluding the apneic patient requiring a crash airway (ie, cardiac or respiratory

TABLE 121-1 Overview of Emergency Airway Management

Technique	Description	Notes
Rapid Sequence Intubation (RSI)	Defined by the simultaneous administration of a sedative and paralytic agent to assist in endotracheal intubation, usually via direct laryngoscopy	Avoids insufflation of the stomach Minimizes risk of aspiration with assisted BVM ventilation
Bag-Valve-Mask (BVM) Ventilation	The ability to ventilate a patient can be an effective bridge prior to intubation and is a requirement prior to use of any paralytic agents	Prior to ventilating with a BVM, place an airway adjunct to maintain patent airway and to optimize ventilation: • Nasopharyngeal airway if patient's airway (gag) reflexes intact • Oropharyngeal airway if absent airway reflexes If patient has dentures, they should be left in place during BVM ventilation and removed just prior to insertion of laryngoscope If the operator is having problems maintaining a seal or ventilating, two-hand BVM should be attempted
Endotracheal Intubation	Airway control established usually through direct laryngoscopy and orotracheal intubation	Any operator attempting intubation, particularly if using paralytic agents, should be very comfortable with the technique, equipment, rescue devices, and with other resources for assistance, have a plan to address any contingency

TABLE 121-2 Indications for Intubation

Indication	Suggestive Signs	Comments
Failure to maintain a patent airway	• Inability to phonate • Inability to swallow or handle secretions • High risk of aspiration	• The presence/absence of a gag reflex does NOT effectively assess airway patency • The gag reflex is physiologically absent in 20% of normal adults • Stimulation of the gag reflex increases risk of vomiting/aspiration
Failure to oxygenate or ventilate	• Unresponsiveness to noninvasive oxygenation or ventilation methods	• Assess patient's clinical appearance including vital signs, mentation • Monitor oxygenation with continuous pulse oximetry and/or ABG analysis • Monitor ventilation with capnography, ABG, or VBG analysis.
Anticipate deterioration in clinical condition	• Patient must be unaccompanied for testing • Patient unable to maintain current work of breathing • Likely further studies or surgery etc	• Consider clinical factors such as severe metabolic acidosis with inadequate respiratory compensation; neuromuscular weakness (impaired maximal inspiratory pressure); etc

TABLE 121-3 Assessment for Difficult Intubation (Mnemonic: LEMON)

Look	Injury, large incisors, large tongue, beard, receding mandible, obesity, abnormal face or neck pathology or shape
Evaluate the 3-3-2 rule	Mouth opening < 3 fingers, mandible length < 3 fingers, or larynx to floor of the mandible < 2 fingers
Mallampati	Class III (see base of uvula) and class IV (soft palate is not visible)
Obstruction	Any upper airway pathology that causes an obstruction (abscess, edema, masses, epiglottitis)
Neck mobility	Limited mobility of neck (eg, trauma with cervical spine immobilization, arthritis, congenital defect)

TABLE 121-4 Assessment for Difficulty with Bag-Valve-Mask (BVM) Ventilation (Mnemonic: MOANS)

Mask seal	Inadequate mask seal (beard, blood/emesis, facial trauma, operator small hands)
Obesity	BMI > 26 kg/m^2
Age	>55 y
No teeth	No teeth (impairs BVM effectiveness)
Stiff ventilation	Asthma, COPD, ARDS, term pregnancy

ARDS, acute respiratory distress syndrome; BMI, body mass index; BVM, Bag-valve-mask; COPD, chronic obstructive pulmonary disease.

TABLE 121-5 Equipment for Endotracheal Intubation

Endotracheal tubes (assortment of sizes) with stylet

Intubation blade (direct or video)

Oxygen

Bag-valve-mask

Suction with Yankuer tip

Airway adjuncts (oral and nasal)

Confirmation device (end-tidal CO_2 detector)

Stethoscope

Lubricant

arrest). Rapid sequence intubation is defined as the simultaneous administration of a sedative and paralytic agent to assist in endotracheal intubation, usually via direct laryngoscopy (**Table 121-5**). **Central to the concept of RSI is the avoidance of assisted BVM ventilation to avoid insufflation of the stomach and minimize the risk of aspiration.** Outcomes evidence supports RSI as a safe and effective technique for emergency airway management that maximizes the patient and physician likelihood of timely, successful airway management (**Table 121-6**).

In general, RSI is safer and more successful than awake intubation. However, *RSI is not advised if difficulty with BVM is predicted* or the ability to intubate via direct laryngoscopy is in question (eg, upper airway obstruction, stridor, angioedema, head and neck cancers). In select patients in which awake intubation is indicated, it should be approached with caution, and may require backup rescue airway methods and/or the involvement of consultants (eg, anesthesiology or otolaryngology).

COMPLICATIONS OF RSI (TABLE 121-7)

Various complications can occur during the course of accessing an advanced airway in a patient.

CONTRAINDICATIONS (TABLE 121-8)

Contraindications to endotracheal intubation can be divided into either absolute or relative but these need to be tailored to the specific clinical situation.

NONINVASIVE VENTILATION (TABLE 121-9)

In select patients, NIPPV may result in decreased need for intubation, serious complications, decreased hospital length of stay, and/or improved likelihood of survival to hospital discharge.

TABLE 121-6 Procedural Steps of Rapid Sequence Intubation (RSI)

Preparation	Equipment	Medical Team
Assessment of the airway, adequate IV access, continuous oxygenation monitoring, RSI medications (sedative and paralytic)	Laryngoscope with functioning light & blades of multiple sizes, working suction, oxygen, Medications (code cart nearby), Backup airway devices, BVM, Monitors (telemetry, pulse oximetry, BP)	Engage team of appropriately trained staff; backup nearby, Utilize the assistance of respiratory therapists early, Call for help early
Preparation	**Risk Factors**	**Assessment**
Anticipate a difficult airway (a complex or challenging intubation) with a backup plan such as fiberoptic intubation	*Congenital* Pierre Robin syndrome, Down syndrome, anterior epiglottis *Acquired* Ludwig angina, abscess, epiglottis; RA, AS, scleroderma, temporomandibular joint dysfunction; Adenomas, goiter, lipoma, hygroma, carcinoma tongue, larynx, thyroid; Facial injury, cervical spine injury; Obesity, acromegaly; Active burns, inhalation injury; Subglottic stenosis	**Look** for injury, large incisors, large tongue, receding mandible, obesity, abnormal face or neck pathology or shape **Evaluate the 3-3-2 rule (LEMON rule)** Mouth opening <3 fingers Mandible length <3 fingers Larynx to floor of mandible <2 fingers **Mallampati** Class III (see base of uvula) Class IV (soft palate not visible) **Obstruction** Any upper airway pathology that causes an obstruction **Neck Mobility** Limited neck mobility
Preparation	**Five Independent Risk Factors (MOANS):**	
Assess difficulty with bag-valve-mask (BVM) ventilation	1. Inadequate mask seal (beard, blood, emesis, facial trauma, operator small hands) 2. Obesity (BMI > 26 kg/mm³) 3. Age > 55 y 4. Absence of teeth 5. Stiff ventilation (asthma, COPD, ARDS, term pregnancy)	Difficult oxygenation—the inability to maintain oxygen saturation >90% despite BVM and 100% oxygen RSI by trained operators preferred, but other techniques and backup methods should be considered if difficulty with BVM is predicted

(Continued)

TABLE 121-6 Procedural Steps of Rapid Sequence Intubation (RSI) *(Continued)*

Preoxygenation	100% supplemental oxygen to induce nitrogen washout and maximize time for intubation without oxygen desaturation	Patients will have 7-9 min prior to desaturation in normal, healthy adult; less time in ill patient with comorbidity or critically ill
Premedication (Optional)	Administration of drugs 3-5 min before induction and paralysis	To blunt effects of direct laryngoscopy, including bronchospasm and a strong sympathetic response. This step is often omitted
Paralysis Sedatives for induction; paralytics for intubation Sedative regimen should provide reliable amnesia; paralytics ↓ metabolic demands, ↓CO_2 production, ↑chest compliance Unless contraindicated, commonly etomidate for sedation and succinylcholine for paralysis	**Sedatives** Etomidate …Onset 45-60 s for 5-10 min Propofol …Onset 45-60 s for 5-10 min …Short-acting, allows frequent monitoring of neurologic status Midazolam (Versed) …Often used in combination with fentanyl bolus …Anticonvulsant properties Fentanyl …Used to reduce pain from laryngoscopy, not always required …Higher potency, faster onset, shorter duration than morphine **Paralytics** Succinylcholine …First-line for RSI outside of ICU …Rapid onset, short acting Rocuronium …Alternative to succinylcholine …Rapid onset, minimal CV effects	**Side Effects** Etomidate Minimal hypotension, possible adrenal insufficiency Propofol Hypotension, depresses myocardial contractility; ↑triglycerides, pancreatitis Midazolam (Versed) Less hypotension than propofol, delirium, slower onset, respiratory depression, long half-life; contraindications: narrow-angle glaucoma Fentanyl Respiratory depression, constipation; contraindications: end-stage liver disease, severe respiratory disease if not intubated Succinylcholine Bradycardia, ↑ICP, histamine release; contraindications: …Hyperkalemia (ESRD, rhabdomyolysis, burns >10% BSA, crush injury) …Neurologic (stroke, spinal cord injury, ALS, MS,↑ICP, history of malignant hyperthermia, eye injury) …Prolonged immobility >48-72 h Rocuronium Caution with difficult airway: longer acting than succinylcholine
Proper Positioning to Optimize Visualization of Vocal Cords	Place a folded towel under the occiput to raise head by ~ 3-7 cm This "sniffing" position lines up the oral, pharyngeal, and laryngeal axes, thereby optimizing the view of the cords during laryngoscopy	Visualize the arytenoids and the vocal cords prior to insertion of endotracheal tube (ETT) by elevating epiglottis which lies just above larynx and vocal cords
Placement of ETT Typically advanced to 23 cm marker at the lip of adult male, 21 cm adult female	Multiple methods to confirm correct placement: …Condensation of ETT …Bilateral breath sounds …Absence of breath sounds over epigastrium …End-tidal CO_2 detection …CXR (ETT tube 2-3 cm above carina)	Gold standard for confirming appropriate tube placement: use of end-tidal carbon dioxide detection
Postintubation Care	Proper stabilization of ETT to prevent movement or accidental dislodgment. Patients who are medically paralyzed require sedation and pain control	Placement of a nasogastric or orogastric tube can help decompress any insufflated air that occurred during BVM use and will help ↓risk of emesis and aspiration

TABLE 121-7 Endotracheal Intubation Complications

Directly Related to Laryngoscopy	Notes
Hemodynamic changes including hypertension, hypotension, tachycardia, and bradycardia	A pneumothorax needs to be considered in a patient with hypoxia and hypotension and should be evaluated for all patients with postprocedure chest radiography
Hypoxemia	Routine preoxygenation with high flow oxygen via non-rebreather mask is standard in healthy, nonobese adults. Consider using noninvasive ventilation in critically ill patients with ill patient with compromised lungs or abnormal body habitus. Consider apneic oxygenation
Airway trauma/perforation	Proper technique is essential to avoid any local trauma to oral anatomy and airway structures
Laryngospasm and bronchospasm	
Trauma to teeth, lips, and tongue	
Right mainstem bronchus intubation	Evaluate with postprocedure chest radiography
Raised intracranial and intraocular pressure	Unclear clinical significance
Esophageal intubation	Prompt recognition of an esophageal intubation will allow immediate removal of the ETT and reventilation and oxygenation with a BVM prior to reattempting intubation
Failed intubation	Clinicians should assess patients for a difficult airway in an effort to prevent a failed intubation attempt. When a difficult intubation is predicted, consultation should be initiated early and backup equipment should be readily available
Related to Endotracheal Intubation	
Tension pneumothorax	A pneumothorax needs to be considered in a patient with hypoxia and hypotension and should be evaluated for all patients with postprocedure chest radiography
Aspiration	Placement of a nasogastric (NG) or orogastric (OG) tube following endotracheal intubation can help decompress any insufflated air that occurred during BVM use and will help reduce the risk of emesis and aspiration
Obstruction of endotracheal tube	Suction the endotracheal tube
Accidental extubation	Accidental dislodgment of the ETT should be avoided by proper stabilization of the tube with appropriate sedation of the patient

TABLE 121-8 Contraindications to Endotracheal Intubation

		Notes
Absolute	Total airway obstruction (eg, angioedema)	During cardiac or respiratory arrest, oxygenation and ventilation are of paramount importance, and therefore the use of BVM, intubation, or both should be attempted despite any contraindications. In these patients it is advised to perform an early cricothyrotomy as endotracheal intubation will be extremely difficult
	Total loss of facial or oropharyngeal landmarks (eg, blunt or penetrating trauma to the face)	
Relative	Anticipated difficult airway	If a difficult airway is anticipated early consultation is strongly advised. Other options include awake intubation, video laryngoscopy or use of the difficult airway adjuncts

TABLE 121-9 Noninvasive Positive Pressure Ventilation (NIPPV)

Indications	Contraindications	Notes
COPD (moderate to severe exacerbation)	Impending circulatory or pulmonary arrest	BIPAP preferred to intubation: ↓need for intubation, ↓LOS, ↓mortality
Acute CHF exacerbation, Asthma, Pneumonia in some selected cases	Altered mental status	BIPAP, CPAP ↓wall stress, ↓afterload, ↑oxygenation
	Inability to handle secretions	↓mortality (likely due of ↓VAP)
	Recent facial trauma or surgery	NIPPV not shown to be helpful and may be harmful in following situations:
	Recent upper airway or GI surgery (gastric distention)	ALI, ARDS
	Inability to properly fit mask	Postextubation respiratory failure (↑mortality by delaying intubation)
	Inability to adequately monitor patient for decompensation	Failure of ABG to improve after 1 h of therapy also highly predictive of subsequent impending respiratory failure

SUGGESTED READINGS

Bair AE, Filbin MR, Kulkarni RG. The failed intubation attempt in the emergency department: analysis of prevalence, rescue techniques, and personnel. *J Emerg Med.* 2002;23:131-140.

Caplan RA, Benumof JL. Practice guidelines for management of the difficult airway: an updated report by the American Society of Anesthesiologists Task Force on management of the difficult airway. *Anesth.* 2004;101:565.

Cattano D, Paniucci E, Paolicchi A, Forfori F, Giunta F, Hagberg C. Risk factors assessment of the difficult airway: an Italian survey of 1956 patients. *Anesth Analg.* 2004;99:1774-1779.

Kheterpal S, Han R, Tremper KK, et al. Incidence and predictors of difficult and impossible mask ventilation. *Anesthesiology.* 2006;105:885-891.

Masip J, Roque M, Sanchez B, Fernandez R, Subirana M, Exposito JA. Noninvasive ventilation in acute cardiogenic pulmonary edema: systematic review and meta-analysis. *JAMA.* 2005;294:3124-3130.

Pistoria M, Amin A, Dressler D, McKean S, Budnitz T. Core competencies in hospital medicine. *J Hosp Med.* 2006;1(S1):87.

Ram FSF, Picot J, Lightowler J, Wedzicha JA. Non-invasive positive pressure ventilation for treatment of respiratory failure due to exacerbations of chronic obstructive pulmonary disease. *Cochrane Database of Systematic Reviews* 2004, Issue 3. Art. No.: CD004104.

Ram FSF, Wellington SR, Rowe BH, Wedzicha JA. Non-invasive positive pressure ventilation for treatment of respiratory failure due to severe acute exacerbations of asthma. *Cochrane Database of Systematic Reviews* 2005, Issue 3. Art. No.: CD004360.

Thakkar R, Wright SM, Alguire P, Wigton RS, Boonyasai RT. Procedures performed by hospitalists and non-hospitalist. *J Gen Intern Med.* 2010;25(5):448-452.

Vital FMR, Saconato H, Ladeira MT, et al. Non-invasive positive pressure ventilation (CPAP or bilevel NPPV) for cardiogenic pulmonary edema. *Cochrane Database of Systematic Reviews* 2008, Issue 3. Art. No.: CD005351.

Weingart SD, Levitan RM. Preoxygenation and prevention of desaturation during emergency airway management. *Ann Emerg Med.* 2012;59(3):165-175.

CHAPTER 122

Arterial Blood Gas and Placement of A-line

Joseph J. Miaskiewicz, Jr., MD

Critically ill patients require arterial blood gas (ABG) analysis to assess oxygenation and ventilation due to limitations of noninvasive oximetry measurements. Below a pO_2 of 60 mm Hg corresponding to an O_2 saturation of 80%, the oxyhemoglobin saturation curve is steep and large changes in oximetry may mean small changes in oxygenation. Below this level oximetry may not correlate with oxygenation, and an arterial blood gas (ABG) should be obtained (**Table 122-1**).

By measuring both oxygenation and ventilation ABG analysis assesses the effects of the cardiopulmonary system in oxygen delivery. ABG analysis directly measures the pH, pCO_2, and pO_2. The normal range for the pH is between 7.36 and 7.44 corresponding to a normal range of 36 to 44 torr for the pCO_2. The normal range for the pO_2 is between 80 and 100 torr. However, age and the pCO_2 also determine alveolar O_2.

Oximetry does not measure pCO_2 and does not reflect ventilation or acid-base status. Ventilation may be defined in terms of movement of a volume of air into and out of the lungs, removing carbon dioxide from the blood and providing oxygen. Alveolar ventilation is defined in terms of ventilation of CO_2. High oxygen saturation may be falsely reassuring in patients whose respiratory drive is compromised by an increase of oxygenation due to supplemental O_2. Assessment of alveolar ventilation is the key to determining whether a patient is receiving enough oxygen. A raised $PaCO_2$ reflects reduced alveolar ventilation. See Chapter 238 (Acid Base Disorders). An approach to interpreting arterial blood gases is essential when caring for hospitalized patients (**Table 122-3**).

Respiratory failure is classified as hypoxemic respiratory failure (hypoxemia without carbon dioxide retention [$SaO_2 < 95\%$, $PaO_2 < 80$ on room air]) or hypercarbic respiratory failure ($pCO_2 > 45$ mm Hg). Calculation of the gradient between the alveolar and arterial oxygen tensions (the A-a gradient) in respiratory failure will help to determine whether the patient has associated lung disease or just reduced alveolar ventilation (**Table 122-2**). See Chapter 138 (Acute Respiratory Failure).

Neither oximetry nor ABGs will detect the presence of a reduced O_2-carrying capacity because anemia, and carbon monoxide (CO) poisoning, and methemoglobinemia do not affect the alveolar pO_2. When there is CO poisoning, the oximeter cannot differentiate between hemoglobin molecules with CO attached and those with O_2 attached and will report normal O_2 saturation. ABGs will also report normal values because the PaO_2 is a measurement of the oxygen dissolved in the blood and not the number of O_2 molecules attached to hemoglobin molecules. In CO poisoning an elevated carboxyhemoglobin will be required to make the diagnosis. Nonsmokers may have levels up to 3, smokers 10 to 15, and CO poisoning levels above 15. Likewise, the presence of abnormal hemoglobins, such as sickle cell, fetal hemoglobin, and methemoglobin, will not affect the ABG results.

Oximetry may also not correlate with oxygenation with falsely low results when there is poor blood flow and perfusion to the fingertips, vasoconstriction due to hypothermia or sepsis, anemia, dark skin pigmentation, obscuring nail polish, and vital dyes. In certain circumstances, the concentration of carboxyhemoglobin, such as in smoke inhalation, may significantly affect the results, falsely elevating the values.

TABLE 122-1 Obtaining an Arterial Sample and Placement of an Arterial Line

	ABG	A-Line
Indications	In hospitalized medical patients, an ABG is primarily obtained to confirm the severity and likely cause of the disturbance • Level of oxygenation, especially in settings when the oximeter measurements are thought to be unreliable or difficult to obtain • Need for intubation: refractory hypoxemia (pO_2 < 55 on 100% O_2 NRB mask) or hypercapnic respiratory failure (pCO_2 > 55 with acidemia pH < 7.25) • Severity metabolic acidosis and adequacy of respiratory compensation when ↑ work of breathing • Contribution of ↑pCO_2 versus other causes in somnolent patient	Usually in the ICU setting for • Frequent ABG sampling • Continuous blood pressure monitoring in use of inotropic or vasopressor agents
Contraindications	Impaired collateral circulation • Raynaud • Thromboangiitis obliterans • Cyanosis	Impaired collateral circulation
Preparation	Allen test: occlusion of the radial and ulnar arteries by firm pressure while the fist is clenched followed by opening of the hand and release of the arteries one at a time to assess adequacy of returning blood flow to the hand	Assess collateral circulation with Allen test Avoid brachial and femoral arteries (inadequate collateral supplies)
Technical Tips The radial artery at the wrist best site (near the surface, relatively easy to palpate, and stabilize with good ulnar collateral supply)	Apply local anesthetic with 1% lidocaine in the conscious patient Immobilize hand on a wrist board or towel and dorsiflex wrist	Same as for ABG If lose ability to palpate pulse, likely arterial spasm precluding successful cannulation. Wait until subsides or choose another site If unsuccessful, apply pressure for several minutes to avoid hematoma formation (which will make subsequent attempts more difficult) and consider use of ultrasound to visualize vessel Reassess perfusion of hand after placement
Complications	Transient obstruction of blood flow may ↓ arterial flow in distal tissues unless adequate collateral arterial vessels available in the setting of • Spasm • Intraluminal clotting • Bleeding and hematoma formation	Remove catheter immediately if any sign of vascular compromise Use nondominant hand preferred

TABLE 122-2 Calculation of the A-a Oxygen Gradient from the ABG

The Alveolar-Arterial Oxygen Gradient

The A-a oxygen gradient = $PAO_2 - PaO_2$

Estimated normal gradient ~ (Age/4) + 4

The Alveolar Gas Equation

$PAO_2 = (FiO_2 \times [Patm - PH_2O]) - (PaCO_2/R)$

• Inspired air at sea level, the FiO_2 of room air = 0.21
• Atmospheric pressure, Patm = 760 mm Hg
• PH_2O at 37 F = 47 mm Hg
• Respiratory quotient, R = 0.8

Hypoxemic Respiratory Failure with Normal A-a Oxygen Gradient

• Alveolar hypoventilation (oversedation, obesity hypoventilation syndrome, muscular weakness, neurologic disease)
• High altitude (low inspired FiO_2)

Hypoxemic Respiratory Failure with ↑ A-a Gradient

• Ventilation-perfusion mismatch (pulmonary embolism, COPD, ARDS, pulmonary artery vasospasm)
• Right-to-left shunt (anatomic: cardiac, pulmonary AVM, hepatopulmonary syndrome; physiologic due to fluid preventing ventilation of perfused alveoli: pneumonia, atelectasis)

Disorders of the lung structure reduce the efficiency of oxygen transfer and widen the A-a gradient. The prolonged respiratory depression may lead to collapse of some areas of lung and an increase in the A-a gradient.

Hypercarbic Respiratory Failure, Hypoxemia from Impaired Ventilation with Normal A-a Oxygen Gradient

• Inadequate alveolar ventilation (without shunting from fluid or collapse of alveoli)
• Ventilatory pump failure (respiratory muscle weakness, neurolgic disease, thoracic cage issues)

TABLE 122-3 Blood Gas Interpretation

Step 1: Acid-base (ventilation)

pH	PaCO$_2$	Interpretation
↓	↑	In acute respiratory failure the change in pH will be accounted for by the high carbon dioxide concentration.
↓	↓	A severe metabolic acidosis or some limitation on the ability of the respiratory system to compensate.
Normal	↑	Alveolar hypoventilation (raised PaCO$_2$) with a normal pH most likely a primary ventilatory change present long enough for renal mechanisms to compensate. Increased serum bicarbonate may also be a clue of chronic CO$_2$ retention.
		A similar picture may result from carbon dioxide retention due to reduced ventilation compensating for a metabolic alkalosis, although such compensation is usually only partial.
Normal	↓	A primary metabolic acidosis in which the respiratory system has normalized the pH. Calculate the anion gap.
↑	↓	Acute alveolar hyperventilation if the pH is appropriately raised for the reduction in PaCO$_2$.
		Chronic alveolar hyperventilation if the pH is between 7.46 and 7.50 as the renal system seldom compensates completely for an alkalosis.

Step 2: Oxygenation (pO$_2$, %saturation)

pO$_2$	PaCO$_2$	pH	
Normal	Normal	↑	A primary metabolic alkalosis to which the ventilatory system has not responded.
↓	Normal	↓	Hypoxemia: when patients with chronic CO$_2$ retention increase usual level of ventilation (acute pulmonary embolism in chronic lung disease).

Step 3: Calculate the A-a gradient to determine whether carbon dioxide retention is related to an intrapulmonary cause

A-a	Explanation	Etiology
Gradient	Calculating the A-a gradient is most useful for determining the severity of the underlying disorder and whether there is a component of hypoventilation.	Especially for hospitalized patients who are prescribed medications that may suppress respiration, the A-a gradient is used to determine the relative contribution of hypoventilation to hypoxia due to underlying lung disease.
Normal	A normal A-a gradient is ~10-15 torr. Advancing age results in increases of the normal A-a gradient. A-a gradient = 2.5 + 0.21 × age in years.	The ABG abnormality is all due to hypoventilation.
Elevated	An elevated A-a gradient represents ↑ difficulty in getting O$_2$ from the alveoli to the blood. A higher FiO$_2$ disproportionately increases the PAO$_2$ more than the PaO$_2$.	• Diseases that affect the pulmonary interstitium including interstitial lung disease, pneumonia, and CHF. • Pulmonary vascular disease: pulmonary emboli, shunts, pulmonary hypertension. • Ventilation/perfusion mismatches of large vessels (pulmonary or tumor emboli) and small vessels (pulmonary hypertension, vasculitis, interstitial lung disease and emphysema). • When breathing 100% oxygen, older patients may normally have an A-a gradient as high as 80 torr and younger patients as high as 120 torr.

Step 4: Does the result correlate with the clinical setting?

Possible Source of Error	Prevention
Presence of heparin in syringe	Express any heparin out of syringe prior to sampling
Air bubbles (resulting in equilibrium between air and arterial blood: ↓PaCO$_2$, ↑PaO$_2$)	Inspect sample and remove air bubbles
Inadequate sample	Obtain at least 3 mL aterial blood
Metabolically active cellular constituents of blood (resulting in changing arterial gas tensions over time)	Cool sample on ice Analyze sample within 1 h
Sampling of venous blood	Pay attention to technique

SUGGESTED READING

Williams AJ. ABC of oxygen: assessing and interpreting arterial blood gases and acid-base balance. *BMJ*. 1998;317(7167):1213-1216.

ONLINE RESOURCES

http://www.nejm.org/doi/full/10.1056/NEJMvcm1213181. radial A line insertion. Accessed July 28, 2016.

http://www.nejm.org/doi/full/10.1056/NEJMvcm0803851. arterial puncture for ABG. Accessed July 28, 2016.

http://www.mdcalc.com/a-a-o2-gradient. A-a gradient calculator. Accessed July 28, 2016.

http://accessmedicine.mhmedical.com/SearchResults.aspx?q=arterial+blood+gas#q=arterial+blood+gas&fl_TopLevelContentDisplayName=Multimedia&fl_ChildLevelContentDisplayName=Videos&instanceName=SearchResults&controller=Solr&action=SearchResultsWithHighlights&updateTargetSelector=#divSearchResults. Access Medicine video series. Accessed July 28, 2016.

CHAPTER 123

Feeding Tube Placement

Sylvia C. McKean, MD, SFHM, FACP

Nasogastric tube insertion is performed in the hospital setting for a variety of indications, including enteral feeding. The actual process of nutrients passing through the gastrointestinal (GI) tract appears to stimulate a complex series of responses that affect immunologic integrity. There is a lower incidence of infection, multiorgan failure, and mortality associated with enteral feeding than with total parenteral nutrition (TPN). Feeding tubes will not prevent microaspiration from oropharyngeal contents in cognitively impaired patients (see **Table 123-1**).

Although relatively simple to perform, it is probably one of the most uncomfortable procedures for the hospitalized patient and carries with it a risk of potentially life-threatening complications. It is crucial to take the necessary steps to ensure patient comfort, obtain a CXR for confirmation of correct placement of the tube, and to take a few simple measures to reduce aspiration risk during enteral feeding (see **Table 123-2**).

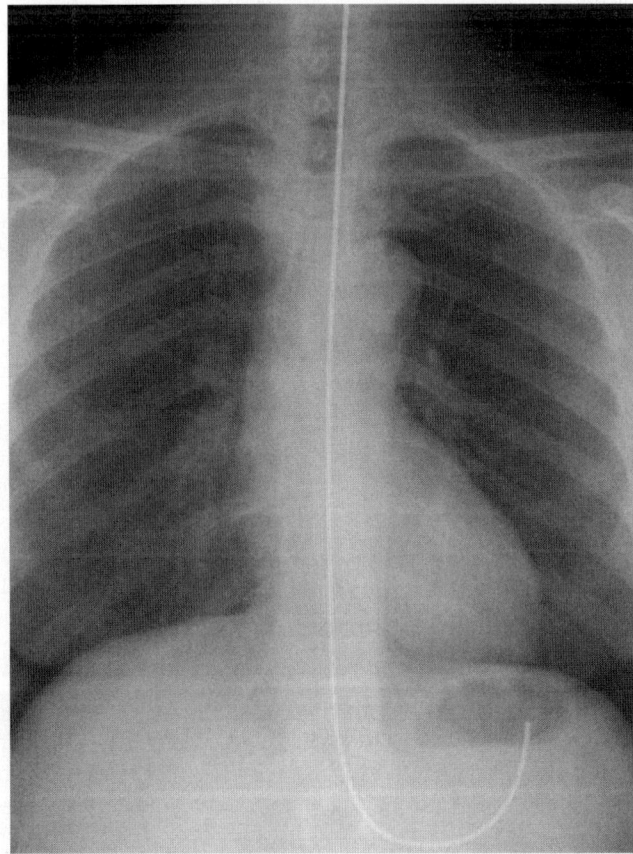

Figure 123-1 *Chest radiograph showing properly placed nasogastric feeding tube with tip visible below the diaphragm.*

TABLE 123-1 Basic Considerations

Indications	Prior to Insertion	Comments
Drain gastric contents	Is this indicated?	Nutritional support cannot be provided in complete obstruction
Prevent aspiration of stomach contents	Will the patient be able to cooperate?	Comatose patients require prior intubation because the procedure may precipitate vomiting and aspiration
Decompress GI tract proximal to obstruction	Does the patient have risk factors for misplacement of NG tubes?	Risk factors for misplacement (especially tracheobronchial tree):
Administer medications in patients who are NPO	What type of feeding tube is required?	Altered mental status, sedation
Provide enteral feeding	Who will perform the procedure?	Advanced age
		Recent prolonged endotracheal intubation (due to ↓airway reflexes)
		Patient s/p radiation therapy for head and neck cancer may not be able to swallow due to edema, mucositis, abnormal anatomy, and sensation
CONTRAINDICATIONS	Absolute	RELATIVE
NG Tubes	Severe maxillofacial trauma	↑risk of perforation due to esophageal abnormalities (recent ingestion of caustic substances, strictures, diverticula)
	Repair of choanal atresia and transnasal transphenoidal surgery	Lung transplant
		Prior pulmonary complication from NG tube placement
		Altered mental status and/or sedation
Types of Feeding Tubes	Advantages	Disadvantages
NG Tubes	*NG Tubes*	*NG Tubes*
A large tube inserted blindly through patient's nose until its tip lies ~10 cm below the GE junction	Can be rapidly inserted at the bedside in the following settings: drug overdose, poisoning; trauma; acute stroke, other neurologic states; severe UGI bleeding in preparation for endoscopic visualization; gastric motor failure, partial small bowel obstruction, postoperative ileus, palliation in metastatic cancer	Acutely agitated patients may pull out tube or be unable to cooperate with placement
Postpyloric Dobhoff Tubes		For enteral feeding, patients should generally have normal gastric emptying; enteral feeding limited to <1 mo
Nasoduodenal/nasojejunal small-bore feeding tubes may require endoscopic placement for tube to go beyond pylorus by GI or IR; flexible transnasal endoscopes can pass small-diameter (5-6 mm) feeding tubes over a guide wire with simultaneous gastric decompression via double-lumen	*Postpyloric Dobhoff Tubes*	Tube may become clogged due to medication administration; skilled nursing facilities may require alternative type of tube
	Allow for nutritional support beyond the ampulla of Vater in setting of poor gastric emptying due to critical illness or from gastric motor failure	*Postpyloric Dobhoff Tubes*
Gastrostomy (G-Tube)	In severe acute pancreatitis feeding can be given without pancreatic stimulation if placed more than 40 cm into jejunum, past ligament of Treitz	Reduced risk of aspiration of enteral feeding compared with NG tube
Percutaneous or surgical placement		*Gastrostomy (G-Tube)*
Jejunostomy (J-Tube)	*Gastrostomy (G-Tube)*	Stoma care necessary
Endoscopic or surgical placement	Long-term (>4 wk) feeding in patients with normal gastric emptying	Potential for fistula after tube removal
	Jejunostomy (J-Tube)	*Gastrostomy (G-Tube) and Jejunostomy (J-Tube)*
	Long-term (>4 wk) feeding in patients with high risk of aspiration with impaired gastric emptying; severe acute pancreatitis	For patients who do not recover sufficient swallowing function to allow for oral feedings, there are guidelines to assist in the decision-making process
NGT Placement Complications	Prevention	Comments
Intracranial injury	For patients with cribriform plate disruption (trauma, surgery), orogastric tube insertion instead	Since misplacement can have such dire consequences, confirmation of placement is critical to NGT insertion procedure
Epistaxis, sore throat	Be prepared to perform emergent suctioning during insertion	No medications or feeding via NGT until correct placement confirmed by CXR
Bleeding, perforation (esophageal, gastric, intestinal)		

(Continued)

TABLE 123-1 Basic Considerations (*Continued*)

Tube knotting and impaction	If NGT misplacement, remove as quickly as possible
Tube double backing and kinking	
Tube breakage	Placement of NGT can induce gagging or vomiting
Intravascular penetration (erosion into a retroesophageal aberrant right subclavian artery, right internal jugular vein to right atrium)	~50% of pneumothoraces require chest tube, rarely thoracotomy to remove tube
Pneumothoraces (~60% of complications)	
Aspiration pneumonitis	
Tracheobronchopleural complications (2% incidence, 0.3% mortality)	

Late Complications	Prevention	Comments
Sinusitis	Remove as soon as feasible Consultation with speech and swallow to assess dysphagia	Prolonged NGT use → damage of nasal mucosa, thereby ↑risk of sinusitis; insert G-tube if >4 wk
↑risk of GI reflux gastritis, GI bleeding, aspiration	Head of bed should always be elevated by 30°-40°;	First 48 h of use check gastric residual volume every 4 h to ensure <400 mL. If gastric residual high, a prokinetic drug like metoclopramide or a PPI to reduce gastric acid secretion
NGT syndrome due to postcricoid ulceration affecting the posterior cricoarytenoid muscles (rare)	Feeds should be started slowly (eg, 25 mL/h) and ↑ according to patient tolerance; continuous feeding without bolus	Can cause life-threatening laryngeal obstruction, due to vocal cord abduction paralysis and upper airway obstruction

TABLE 123-2 Technical Tips

Estimate the length of the tube that needs to be inserted	Measure the distance from the xiphoid process to the angle of the mandible and then to the nostril
Cool tube in an ice bath	Especially in case of small bore tubes, eases placement, less uncomfortable for patient
Provide local anesthesia because NG placement one of the most uncomfortable procedures for hospitalized patients	4% lidocaine delivered by nebulizer provides excellent anesthesia of both nasal and oral mucosa; lubricate 2-4 in of end of NGT with viscous lidocaine
Properly position patient	Flexion of patient's head to chest (chin-tuck) to narrow trachea and open esophagus
	Rotate patient's head toward right or left shoulder to deviate tube tip away from midline laryngeal opening
If resistance during passage, do not advance tube as this may mean you are in the wrong location or that the tube has coiled	If the patient starts to gag (indicating possible resistance to passage of the tube through the posterior pharynx), stop advancing the tube and ask the patient to sip ice-water through a straw. As the patient swallows, the epiglottis will cover the trachea and you may advance the tube further.
If changes occur in patient's respiratory status, or if unable to talk or if respirations can be heard through NGT, withdraw tube immediately	Never assume that cuffed endotracheal tube will always prevent inadvertent passage into trachea
Always use a CXR *read by a radiologist* to confirm placement of tube in all patients, including intubated patients prior to use	Inadvertent placement of a feeding tube into an airway may not be clinically apparent, yet life-threatening
An abdominal plain film will miss most of the important complications of NGT placement (penetration of the esophagus, passage of tube into trachea, bronchus)	…Signs suggestive of correct tube placement—absence of coughing, facile placement to 60 cm, inspection of NGT aspirate, epigastric auscultation—may be misleading
	…Bubbling of tube under water (pulmonary misplacement) can be falsely negative if portholes of NGT plugged
	…Phonation may be unaffected if a small fine bore tube in the bronchus has not interfered with the vocal cords
	A single view portable CXR may be difficult to interpret
	…Do not assume correct placement merely by identifying the tube tip over the gastric bubble
	…Make sure that the tube does not follow the path of a bronchus by examining the entire outline of the feeding tube
	…Make sure that the tube is inserted far enough into the stomach with at least 10 cm of the tip should be in the stomach

ACKNOWLEDGMENT

This chapter was adapted and updated from first edition version by Ruma Rajbhandari, MD, MPH, and Stephen C. Wright, MD.

SUGGESTED READINGS

Bankhead R, Boullata J, Brantley S, et al. Enteral nutrition practice recommendations. *J Parenter Enteral Nutr.* 2009;33(2):122-167.

O'Keefe SJD. A guide to enteral access procedures and enteral nutrition. *Nat Rev Gastroenterol Hepatol.* 2009;6:207-215.

Pillai JB. Thoracic complications of nasogastric tube: review of safe practice. *Interact Cardiovasc Thorac Surg.* 2005;4:429-433.

Shiamovitz GX, Shah NR. Nasogastric tube treatment & medication. eMedicine Specialties from WebMD. http://emedicine.medscape.com/article/80925-treatment. Accessed August 2, 2016.

Thomsen TW, Shaffer RW, Setnick G. Nasogastric intubation. *N Engl J Med.* 2006;354:e16.

CHAPTER 124

Thoracentesis

Sylvia C. McKean, MD, SFHM, FACP

Physicians or other clinicians perform an estimated 173,000 thoracenteses in the United States every year. The strict indications for thoracentesis are the presence of pleural fluid of unknown etiology where the physician cannot initiate care prior to diagnosis and severe dyspnea (**Table 124-1**).

Pleural effusions develop secondarily to systemic changes (transudates) or to local causes (exudates). Systemic causes that lead to the formation and absorption of pleural fluid most commonly include left ventricular heart failure, pulmonary embolism, cirrhosis, and renal disease. Acute pancreatitis may cause a left-sided pleural effusion. Pleural effusions commonly occur after abdominal surgery due to the porous diaphragm and are usually benign. Renal diseases that can cause pleural effusion include the nephrotic syndrome and urinothorax from hydronephrosis. Myxedema and cerebrospinal fluid leak to the pleura are other causes of transudates.

Local causes (exudates) are most commonly bacterial pneumonia, viral infection, malignancy, and pulmonary embolism. Parapneumonic effusions start out as sterile, reactive effusions and can rapidly progress to loculated empyema in immunocompromised patients or when there is a delay in administration of appropriate antibiotics. Failure to identify those patients with empyema or significant inflammation necessitating pleural drainage can result in trapped lung. Other infectious causes include tuberculosis, fungal infection and intra-abdominal abscess. Pancreatic pseudocyst, postcoronary artery bypass grafting or cardiac contusion, pericardial disease, drug-induced pleuritis, rheumatologic disease, uremia, and gynecologic disorders may also cause exudates. The most common causes of malignant pleural effusions in descending order of frequency are lung cancer, breast cancer, and lymphoma. In a patient with a prior history of asbestos exposure, mesothelioma should be suspected, especially if the pleural effusion is grossly hemorrhagic. (See Chapter 236 [Pleural Diseases].)

While dullness to percussion and reduced tactile fremitus are valuable findings to help identify a pleural effusion (positive likelihood ratio [LR+], 8.7 and 5.7, respectively), the physical examination is usually not helpful in diagnosing the cause of the pleural effusion or in ascertaining the best location to perform the thoracentesis.

The first step is to determine whether there is fluid by radiographic imaging. On chest x-ray (CXR), a pleural effusion will characteristically push the heart to the opposite side. If, however, the opacified space does not shift the heart, it is possible that the patient has significant atelectasis as the cause. A lateral decubitus film should reveal whether there is free-flowing fluid, and should be ordered to document free flow in most patients prior to thoracentesis. If there is doubt, ultrasonography can identify solid from liquid pleural effusions with 98% accuracy when combined with CXR. Computed tomography (CT) imaging may be indicated prior to definitive drainage in some instances, and CT-PE protocol imaging should be performed if pulmonary embolism is suspected. (See Chapter 114 [Basic Chest Radiography] and Chapter 115 [Advanced Cardiothoracic Imaging].)

In general, the procedure is usually safe and well tolerated (**Table 124-2**). However, when iatrogenic pneumothorax does occur, chest tube insertion may be required for up to 50% of the patients with an increased average length of stay of approximately 4 days. This complication not only incurs substantial increase in cost, but also increases morbidity and mortality. Ultrasound guidance has become the standard of care for the evaluation of free-flowing effusions. Real-time ultrasonography is helpful in delineating the

TABLE 124-1 Basic Considerations

Indications	Diagnostic Thoracentesis	Comments
	Perform if presence of pleural effusion of unknown origin or fails to respond to treatment (CHF, kidney disease, cirrhosis)	In general, not required in patients with a clear etiology such as pulmonary edema in heart failure, bilateral pleural effusions in patients with anasarca or the nephrotic syndrome, left-sided effusion in patients with acute pancreatitis, or effusions arising in patients having undergone certain surgical procedures
	Indications for parapneumonic effusions:	
	• 1 cm in depth on lateral decubitus film	Not all parapneumonic effusions require thoracentesis. See algorithm for evaluation of parapneumonic effusions
	• ↑ effusions despite appropriate antibiotics	Large volume thoracentesis will ↓ intrathoracic volume and ↓ diaphragmatic distention
	• Persistent unilateral effusion with fever, tachycardia despite appropriate antibiotics	
	• Possibility of loculated effusion or empyema by imaging (CXR, chest CT)	
	Therapeutic thoracentesis	
	Perform for symptomatic relief of dyspnea, hypoxia, pain	
Contraindications	Infection over entry site	Pick another site
	Coagulopathy	Weigh risks vs benefits for each patient:
	Mechanical ventilation	• No cutoff for diagnostic taps
	Hemodynamic or respiratory instability	• Consider reversal if INR>2, and/or platelets <50,000 mm^3 for therapeutic taps
		Some studies suggest thoracentesis can be safely performed in fully anticoagulated patients
		Use caution (positive-pressure ↑ risk of tension pneumothorax) stabilize first
Procedural Preparation	**Imaging**	**Comments**
Imaging to determine whether there is free-flowing fluid	CXR: a pleural effusion will push heart to opposite site; if no shift, opacification may represent atelectasis	Lateral decubitus film to document free-flowing fluid
		US to distinguish solid from liquid pleural effusions when in doubt
Determine who is the best person to perform the procedure	**Consultation**	Technically difficult taps include:
	Consider IR consultation for likely technically difficult taps	• Small effusions (<1 cm on lateral decubitus film)
Arrange for US guidance during the procedure	Consider thoracic surgery consultation for chest tube insertion and/or possible thoracic surgery in selected situations	• Effusions not free flowing
		• Complex, loculated effusions
		Indications for surgical consultation include:
		• Patients with a very high likelihood of hemothorax
		• Pleural effusions >50% of thorax
		• Trapped lung, lung abscess, empyema
Complications during Procedure	Pneumothorax (3%-30%)	Risk factors: multiple taps, blind taps, inexperience, draining more than 1.8 L of fluid
	Hemorrhage	Risk factors: coagulopathy, multiple taps, inexperience, blind taps
	Vasovagal syncope	Obtain CXR to rule out more serious conditions such as pneumothorax, hemorrhage
	Laceration of liver or spleen	Suspect if bloody, dry tap
		Obtain abdominal CT
Complications after Procedure	Re-expansion pulmonary edema	Risk factors: >2 L fluid removal
	Infection with local pain at site, redness, fever, purulent drainage	Risk factors: multiple taps, immunosuppression
		Consider chest CT

TABLE 124-2 Technical Tips

Properly position patient under locally sterile conditions, taking the time to ensure all comfortable before proceeding	Patient sitting up, leaning forward slightly on bedside table, monitored on a pulse oximeter.
Ensure an almost painless procedure	Reduce burning sensation of cutaneous injection of xylocaine by warming vial between palms.
Select the easiest location	Usually the posterolateral back 6-8 cm lateral to spine (to avoid neurovascular bundle), above the diaphragm but below the fluid level just above the rib (to avoid hitting any neurovascular structures).
Avoid blind taps	Use bedside ultrasound guidance. If unavailable, US marking by radiology with patient placed in same position in which thoracentesis will be performed.
Avoid negative pleural pressure to reduce risk of re-expansion pulmonary edema	Decrease flow rate into vacutainer by crimping tubing if rapid; limit amount of fluid drained to 1-1.5 L.
Address problems during the procedure	*Dry tap*: reimage. *Slowing of fluid removal*: check tubing, catheter; have patient Valsalva to increase intrathoracic pressure. *Air bubbles in syringe* (high negative pressure applied to pleural fluid), hypotension, desaturation, tachypnea: immediately halt procedure, obtain CXR, perform immediate needle-decompression if tension pneumothorax suspected prior to imaging. *Coughing* (a sign of re-expanding lung): stop procedure if excessive. *Bloody fluid* (cancer, pulmonary infarct, postcardiotomy syndrome, trauma, injury from thoracentesis): depending on clinical setting may require further evaluation (monitoring of vital signs, serial hematocrits, CT imaging).
During catheter removal avoid the possibility of air entering into the pleural space	Having the patient hum during catheter removal will prevent him from taking a breath in and creating negative intrathoracic pressure.
Consider postprocedure CXR in selected patients	Although not routine in uncomplicated thoracentesis, obtain if any procedural complication (air, blood in removed fluid, dry taps), patient symptoms (chest pain, dyspnea, or change in vital signs). Consider for patients for whom pneumothorax is more likely (small effusions, multiple needle sticks, blind taps, therapeutic taps).

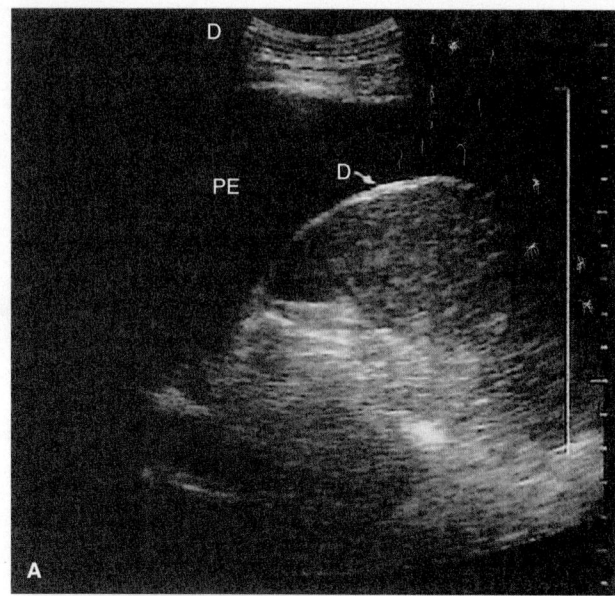
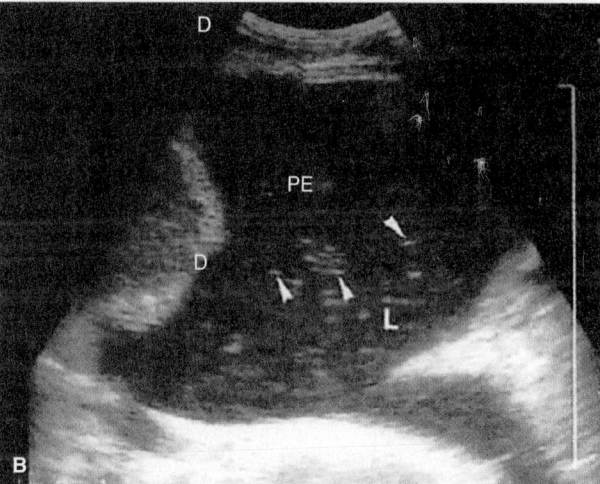
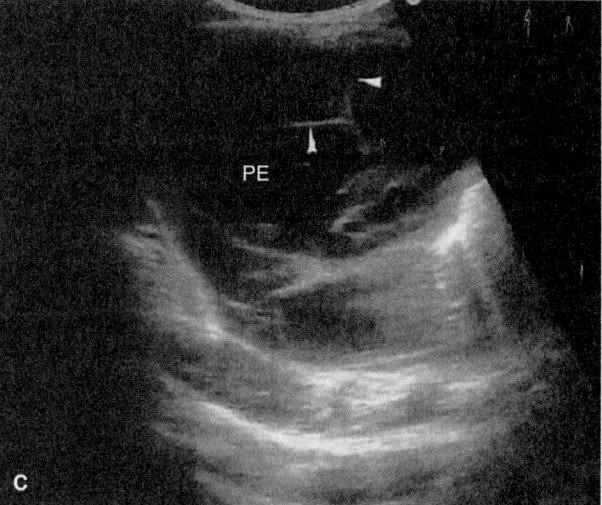

Figure 124-1 *(A) Pleural effusion is represented by an echo-free space (D, diaphragm; PE, pleural effusion). (B) Complex nonseptated effusion suggesting a transudate (arrows show echogenic foci in the pleural effusion). (C) Complex septated effusion (arrows indicate septations and potential need for surgical approach).*

TABLE 124-3 Normal Test Results

Test	Normal Value
Appearance	Clear, colorless
Amount	6-12 cc in the space between the visceral pleura lining the lung and the parietal pleura lining the chest wall and diaphragm
Transudate signifying the absence of pleural pathology	See Table 124-4
Imaging	No visible pleural effusion

TABLE 124-4 Characteristic Disease States

Tests	Transudate	Exudate
Always check cell count and differential, LDH and total protein, Gram stain and culture; send simultaneous serum total protein and LDH, glucose; hematocrit if fluid grossly bloody only check other tests if clinically indicated	CHF (most common) Cirrhosis Nephrotic syndrome Hypoalbuminemia Peritoneal dialysis Early acute atelectasis Pulmonary embolism (PE) Superior vena cava obstruction Early mediastinal malignancy Misplaced subclavian catheter, Myxedema	*Infection* (parapneumonic effusion, empyema; TB empyema; parasitic including amoeba, hydatid cyst, filarial; fungal; PCP, Nocardia, Cryptococcus, toxoplasmosis, histoplasma, mycobacteria) *Vascular* (PE, dissection) *Malignancy* (Kaposi sarcoma, lymphoma, Castleman disease, lung cancer in HIV; adenocarcinoma of lung, breast, ovary, lymphoma, mesothelioma) *Trauma* (abdominal surgery, hemothorax, pneumothorax) *Immunologic* (RA, SLE, hepatitis, Wegener, Sjogren, post-MI, postcardiac surgery, vasculitis) *Drug* (dantrolene, bromocriptine, nitrofurantoin, methysergide, hypersensitivity, asbestos exposure) *Chemical* (uremic, pancreatic, esophageal rupture, subphrenic abscess) *Lymphatic* (irradiation, Chylothorax) *Miscellaneous* (Meigs syndrome)
Gross appearance	Clear, pale yellow Bloody fluid from traumatic tap should clot within several minutes; nonuniform color during aspiration	Usually cloudy Blood present for more than several hours defibrinated, will not form good clot; uniform color, hemosiderin-laden macrophages, crenated RBCs Milky (chylous): trauma, obstruction of duct; check triglycerides, cytology, cultures including TB Greenish yellow, turbid: RA Green: biliopleural fistula Dark, red-brown: amebiasis Black: Aspergillus niger Foul odor: anaerobic empyema
Specific gravity	≤1.012	>1.012
Protein content	≤3 g/dL	>3 g/dL
Serum—pleural albumin	≥1.2 g/dL	<1.2 g/dL
Pleural protein/serum protein	≤0.5	>0.5
Pleural LDH/serum LDH	≤0.6 or <2/3 upper limit normal	>0.6 or >2/3 upper limit normal
Pleural glucose/serum glucose	≤0.8	>0.8
Glucose	≥60 mg/dL	<60 mg/dL empyema, sometimes low in TB, malignancy, SLE effusion, <30 mg/dL in >95% RA effusion
pH	>7.4 CHF, cirrhosis >7.3 PE	Low in empyema, esophageal rupture, urinothorax, malignancy, SLE, TB
Lymphocyte predominant		TB, chylothorax, lymphoma, rheumatoid pleurisy, sarcoidosis, lung transplant rejection, >2 months CABG
Polymorphonuclear predominant		PE, pneumonia, empyema; acute RA, SLE effusion; rupture of esophagus, pancreatitis

(Continued)

TABLE 124-4 Characteristic Disease States (*continued*)

Mononuclear predominant	<1000 CHF, cirrhosis, PE, atelectasis	TB, malignancy, chronic RA, SLE effusion
Eosinophilic		Pneumothorax, hemothorax, benign asbestosis, PE, parasitic, fungal, drug, lymphoma, carcinoma, Churg-Strauss syndrome, TB, sarcoidosis
RBC count (cells/μL)	<1000	Parapneumonic effusion, empyema <5000
		TB < 10,000
		Pulmonary infarction 100 to >100,000
		Pancreatitis, esophageal rupture 1000-10,000
		Malignant effusion 100 to several hundred thousand

See Figure 236-3, management of parapneumonic effusions.

potential characteristics of the pleural effusion, the potential of a complicated effusion, and the presence of adhesions and septations (**Figure 124-1**). These findings may be crucial in the management of pleural effusions and the potential need for a more invasive approach than a simple thoracentesis. The bottom line: only attempt blind taps when ultrasound guidance is not available. In this case consider the next best alternative of ultrasound marking in the radiology department. During radiology ultrasound marking, the patient must be placed in the same position that the thoracentesis will be performed. **Table 124-3** lists normal results. **Table 124-4** lists differential diagnosis depending on whether the fluid is a transudate or exudate.

ACKNOWLEDGMENT

This chapter was adapted and updated from Chapter 117 in the first edition by Christopher Parks, MD, and Rabih Bechara, MD.

SUGGESTED READINGS

Feller-Kopman D. Ultrasound-guided thoracentesis. *Chest*. 2006;129(6):1709-1714.

Schoonover GA. Risk of bleeding during thoracentesis in anticoagulated patients. *Chest*. 2006;130(4 Suppl):141S-1142S.

Soubani AO, Valdivieso M. Complications of thoracentesis. *Intern Med J*. 2009;39(9):628.

Wong CL, Holroyd-Leduc J, Straus SE. Does this patient have a pleural effusion? *JAMA*. 2009;301(3):309-317.

ONLINE RESOURCES

Videos in Clinical Medicine: Thoracentesis. http://www.nejm.org/video. Accessed March 22, 2016.

Harrison's video (Access Medicine): http://accessmedicine.mhmedical.com/content.aspx?sectionid=79758112&bookid=1130&Resultclick=2&q=thoracentesis. Accessed March 22, 2016.

CHAPTER 125

Lumbar Puncture

Claude Killu, MD
Mark J. Ault, MD

Lumbar puncture (LP) is performed to sample the cerebrospinal fluid (CSF) surrounding the brain and spinal cord. The majority of the CSF is in the subarachnoid space, where the arachnoid membranes bridge the sulci of the brain, in the basal cisterns and around the spinal cord. Cerebrospinal fluid moves within the ventricles and subarachnoid spaces under the influence of hydrostatic pressure generated by the production of CSF by the choroid plexus of the lateral third and fourth ventricles. The volume of CSF in humans is 140 to 150 mL of which only 30 to 40 mL is actually in the ventricular system, with a production rate of 21 mL/h. The turnover rate of total CSF is about 5 hours for an average sized human. Cerebrospinal fluid cushions the brain, regulates brain extracellular fluid, allows for distribution of neuroactive substances, and collects the waste products produced by the brain.

Computed tomography (CT) scan performance before an LP in cases of suspected meningitis is not warranted or recommended unless the patient has grossly altered mental status, active and recent seizures, focal neurologic signs, or papilledema. Patients with these findings or clinical risk factors should have a CT scan to identify mass lesions and other causes of increased intracranial pressure (ICP).

The authors routinely use bedside ultrasound to map the anatomic landmarks prior to virtually all LP attempts. Fluoroscopy-guided LP may be considered for the extremely challenging patient in which bedside LP has failed or in patients with spinal hardware. Fluoroscopy-guided LP shows the bony structures of the lumbar spine and provides real-time information about the position of the needle as it is being inserted. Fluoroscopy-guided LP is usually performed by an interventional radiologist in the radiology suite. Use of fluoroscopy requires the patient to lie in the prone position which makes the measurement of opening pressures more challenging.

TABLE 125-1 Basic Considerations

Indications	Diagnostic	Comments
	Infections, SAH, inflammatory conditions, multiple sclerosis, carcinomatosis	CSF sample for examination
		Pressure measurements (NPH)
	Therapeutic	Reduction of CSF pressure
	Cryptococcal meningitis, SAH, hydrocephalus with communication between all the ventricles, pseudotumorcerebri	Spinal anesthetics, antitumor agents, antibiotics
		Radio-opaque substance Radioactive agent
	Drug administration	
	Imaging	
	Myelography	
	Radionuclide cisternography	
Contraindications	Increased risk of fatal cerebellar or transtentorial herniation	When papilledema is the result of a CNS lesion, especially asymmetric lesions near the tentorium or foramen magnum
	Coagulopathy	
	Infection over puncture site	Consider reversal; hold enoxaparin for 12 h (prophylactic dosing)/24 h (therapeutic dosing)
	Spinal block requiring a sample of cisternal fluid or myelography above the lesion	
Procedural Preparation	Imaging	CT or MRI whenever increased CSF pressure suspected
		Ultrasound to directly visualize location of needle insertion
Complications during Procedure	Sciatic pain during needle insertion	Needle placement too laterally
	Slowing of fluid removal	Slowly elevate patient's head
	Herniation with high opening pressure (>400 mm H$_2$O)	Abort procedure or obtain smallest amount of necessary sample, then administer hyperosmolar agent such as mannitol, ideally observing fall in pressure; corticosteroids for vasogenic cerebral edema from tumors
Complications after Procedure	Headache (~1/3rd of patients)	Risk factors: history of migraine
	Likely due to reduction of CSF pressure from leakage of fluid at puncture site, tugging on cerebral and dural vessels when erect	Prevention: use of atraumatic needle (reduction by 50%), use of smaller needle, less CSF fluid removed the better, stylet re-inserted when removing needle
	Bleeding into spinal meningeal or epidural spaces	Risk factors: INR > 1.4, platelet counts <50,000/mm^3, impaired platelet function (alcoholism, uremia)
	Purulent meningitis, disc space infections (rare)	Prevention: reversal of coagulopathy prior to tap
		Prevention: meticulous local sterile technique, positioning

TABLE 125-2 Technical Tips

Properly position patient under locally sterile conditions, taking the time to ensure all comfortable before proceeding	Patient on left side for right handed physicians, hips and knees flexed, head as close to knees as comfort allows, hips vertical, back near edge of bed, pillow under patient's ear
Ensure an almost painless procedure	Reduce burning sensation of cutaneous injection of xylocaine by warming vial between palms
Select the easiest location	L3-L4 interspace, corresponding to the axial plane of iliac crests or at interspace above or below
Use atraumatic spinal needle	Smallest size practical (ie, 22g). If cutting needle needed insert with bevel oriented in longitudinal plane of the dural fibers. Slow advancement with slight cephalad angle, aiming toward umbilicus
If an unsuccessful tap despite 2-3 trials, sit patient up and then help him lie on one side for pressure measurements	The "dry tap" despite 2-3 trials usually result of malposition of needle rather than proteinaceous or viscous CSF, or obliteration of subarachnoid space from tumor or adhesive arachnoiditis
Consider fluoroscopy for likely technically difficult taps	For any obese patient in whom palpation of spinal landmarks not possible, any patient s/p several unsuccessful attempts, patients with spinal hardware or unclear anatomy
Obtain opening pressure measurements in all patients, looking for a few mL fluid oscillation in response to respiration, promptly rising with coughing, straining, abdominal compression	Attachment of manometer to needle in subarachnoid space with a relaxed patient in lateral decubitus position, legs straightened; lack of oscillations and low pressure likely result of needle aperture not fully in subarachnoid space
Drain the amount of fluid you need by checking in advance what is required	Only ~2 cc necessary for each of tubes 1-4, additional specialized tests require more fluid

TABLE 125-3 Normal Test Results

Test	Normal Value
Opening Pressure	6-14 mm Hg
Normal Appearance	Clear, colorless
Traumatic tap due to blood from epidural venous plexus	Decreasing number of RBCs in subsequent tubes and normal CSF opening pressure; occasionally clots; colorless supernatant with prompt centrifugation; 1-2 WBCs per 1000 RBCs assuming normal hematocrit but wide variation
Appearance in SAH	No clots due to dilution by CSF; erythrochromia within a few hours (pink-red color) due to hemolysis of RBCs; xanthochromia (yellow-brown) if >1 d following SAH; % WBCs to RBCs increase as RBC hemolyze but wide variation
Appearance in other conditions	Xanthochromia (severe jaundice, elevation of CSF protein >150 mg/100 mL from any cause in proportion of albumin-bound fraction of bilirubin); Yellow tint (hypercarotenemia, hemoglobinemia due to oxyhemoglobin, blood clots in subdural or epidural space)
WBCs	<5/μL, mainly lymphocytes. Elevated WBC = a reactive process to infection, blood, chemicals, inflammation, neoplasm, vasculitis
Protein	45-50 mg/dL with the cause of modest elevations 75 mg/dL often obscure. If serum protein normal, CSF protein should increase by ~1 mg/1000 RBCs (from same tube). In traumatic tap but higher ratio in SAH due to irritation of hemolyzed RBCs on leptomeninges
Glucose	45-80 mg/dL (about two-thirds of that in blood). Low CSF glucose <35 mg/dL: bacterial, TB, fungal meningitis, some patients with widespread neoplastic infiltration of meninges, or occasionally, sarcoid, SAH (first week), chemical induced inflammation
Osmolality	295 mOsm/L identical to plasma; rise in osmolality after administration of hypertonic solutions delayed up to several hours

TABLE 125-4 Characteristic Disease States

Condition	Cells	Protein	Glucose	Other Features
Bacterial infection	WBC < 50/mm³, often greatly increased	100-250 mg%	20-50 mg%; usually lower than half of blood glucose level	Gram stain shows organisms; pressure increased
Viral, fungal, spirochetal infection	WBC 10-100/mm³	50-200 mg%	Normal or slightly reduced	Special culture techniques required; pressure normal or slightly increased
Tuberculous infection	WBC > 25/mm³	100-1000 mg%	>50, often markedly reduced	Special culture techniques and PCR may be needed to detect organisms
Subarachnoid hemorrhage	RBC > 500/mm³; slight increase in WBC	60-150 mg%	Normal; slightly reduced later	Must be distinguished from traumatic lumbar puncture by presence of xanthochromia of spun sample; greatly increased pressure
Cerebral hemorrhage, trauma	RBC 50-200/mm³; higher if ventricular rupture of blood	50-150 mg%	Normal	Pressure may be elevated
Ischemic stroke	Normal or few WBC	Normal	Normal	Normal pressure unless brain swelling
Multiple sclerosis	Normal or few WBC	Normal or slightly increased	Normal	Increased IgG fraction and oligoclonal bands
Meningeal cancer	WBC 10-100/mm³	Usually elevated	Normal or depressed	Neoplastic cells in CSF; elevation of certain protein markers (eg, β_2-microglobulin)

IgG, immunoglobulin G; PCR, polymerase chain reaction; RBC, red blood cells; WBC, white blood cells.
From Ropper AH, Samuels MA, Klein JP. *Adams and Victor's Principles of Neurology*, 10th ed. New York, NY: McGraw-Hill; 2014, Table 2-1.

Is the information crucial to the diagnosis of neurologic disease and to guide management? Do you suspect conditions that require CSF analysis—infection, inflammatory diseases, SAH, and/or processes that alter intracranial pressure?

↓ Yes

Is there a contraindication to performing the procedure?
- Increased intracranial pressure
- Infection at or near puncture site
- Coagulopathy

↓ No

Is it necessary to obtain a CT before the LP?
For patients with suspected meningitis, if negative to all of the following risk factors, 97% negative predictive value for brainstem herniation:
- Age > 60 y
- Immunocompromised state
- CNS disease (mass, stroke, and/or focal CNS infection)
- Seizure in past week prior to presentation
- Neurologic findings (altered mental status, inability to answer questions or follow two commands correctly, and/or any focal neurologic findings such as gaze palsy, arm drift)

↓ Patient does not require CT (or CT negative)

Is the patient able to give informed consent?

↓ Informed consent provided

Is there a coagulopathy that requires reversal prior to the procedure? INR > 1.4, platelets < 50,000 mm^3, platelet dysfunction (uremia). Has enoxaparin, if previously administered, been withheld? 12 hours prophylactic dosing, 24 h therapeutic dosing.

↓ Absence of coagulopathy

Are there technical factors that will require specialty consultation to perform the procedure? Anatomical (spinal hardware in place, spinal block, inability to locate the intervertebral space between the posterior iliac crests), inability of the patient to cooperate with the procedure.

↓ No

Do you know which additional studies need to be performed? Always check cell count with differential, Gram stain, glucose, total protein, and culture. Specialized tests require different amounts of fluid and different tubes for processing.

Figure 125-1 *Practice algorithm: diagnostic lp.*

SUGGESTED READINGS

Armon C, Evans RW. Therapeutic and Technology Assessment Subcommittee of the American Academy of Neurology. Addendum to assessment: prevention of post-LP headaches: report of the Therapeutic and Technology Assessment Subcommittee of the American Academy of Neurology. *Neurology.* 2005;65:510-512.

Hasbun R, Abrahams J, Jekel J, Quagliarello VJ. CT of the head before LP in adults with suspected meningitis. *N Engl J Med.* 2001;345(24):1727-1733.

Straus SE, Thorpe KE, Holroyd-Leduc J. How do I perform a LP and analyze the results to diagnose bacterial meningitis? *JAMA.* 2006;296(16):2012-2022.

Strupp M, Schueler O, Straube A, Von Stuckrad-Barre S, Brandt T. "Atraumatic" Sprotte needle reduces the incidence of post-lumbar puncture headache. *Neurology.* 2001;57(12):2310-2312.

Williams J, Ley DC, Umapathi T. Diagnostic LP: minimizing complications. *Intern Med J.* 2008;38(7):587-591.

ONLINE RESOURCES

Lumbar Puncture Video. http://www.nejm.org/video.

McGraw Hill Access Medicine. http://accessmedicine.mhmedical.com/content.aspx?sectionid=79758128&bookid=1130&Resultclick=2&q=lumbar%20puncture.

CHAPTER 126

Paracentesis

Sally Wang, MD

Paracentesis is a procedure that removes ascitic fluid from the abdominal cavity with a needle or a catheter. A diagnostic paracentesis may determine the cause of ascites and rule out spontaneous bacterial peritonitis. A therapeutic paracentesis will remove excess fluid.

The mechanism for the development of ascites (excess fluid accumulation in the peritoneal space) is not well understood. Cirrhosis is the leading cause of ascites due to portal hypertension. Capillary pressure increases with obstruction of venous blood flow through the damaged liver. Reduced hepatic metabolism of aldosterone increases renal sodium and water retention. Reduced hepatic synthesis of albumin contributes to fluid moving from the vascular space into the peritoneal space. In addition to cirrhosis, other causes of portal hypertension include right heart failure, portal vein thrombosis, Budd-Chiari syndrome, and liver metastases. Pancreatitis, chylous fluid accumulation, nephritic syndrome, serositis, colitis, peritoneal carcinomatosis, tuberculous peritonitis, and peritonitis may cause ascites through a different mechanism.

Any amount of peritoneal fluid withdrawn during paracentesis is abnormal. A diagnostic test (60 cc of fluid) includes:

- Cell count and differential (few mL)
- Gram stain and culture (ideally, 5 mL in an anaerobic and aerobic blood culture bottle)
- Simultaneous serum albumin to calculate a serum albumin ascites gradient (few mL)
- Cytology (the more fluid, the greater yield)

Other studies such as amylase, triglycerides, and AFB are performed only if clinically indicated.

TABLE 126-1 Basic Considerations

Indications	Diagnostic Paracentesis	Comments
	New onset ascites of unclear etiology	Etiology: • Portal hypertension: liver disease, heart failure • Nonportal hypertensive causes: malignancy, pancreatitis, malnutrition, protein wasting
	Any change in the clinical status of the patient with known ascites, including hospital admission	To rule out spontaneous bacterial peritonitis, even in the absence of signs of infection
	Suspected peritonitis relating to peritoneal dialysis	
	Therapeutic paracentesis	
	To relieve abdominal discomfort and dyspnea	
Contraindications	Acute abdomen DIC Coagulopathy	There is no recommendation of INR or platelet cutoffs for patients with liver disease; it is generally accepted to reverse INR to <1.5 for patients on warfarin. There are inadequate data relating to antiplatelet agents
Site specific	Infected abdominal wall at entry site	Choose another site
	Distended bowel or bladder	
	Pregnancy	
	Abdominal adhesions	
	Caput medusa or superficial veins	
	Hernia at chosen site	
	Scar tissue (vascularity)	
Procedural preparation	Confirm location, amount of fluid, nearby vessels	US best modality
	Visualize structures (history of adhesions, presence of scars)	Consider abdominal CT
	Visualize suspectedwidespread malignancy	Have patient urinate prior to tap
	Empty bladder	
Complications during procedure	Hypotension	Risk factors: hypovolemia
	Bowel perforation	Risk factors: blind tap, inexperience
	Sheared-off catheter fragments hemoperitoneum, hematoma	Risk factors: coagulopathy
Complications after procedure	Persistent leak of ascitic fluid	Place a temporary ostomy bag, repeat therapeutic thoracentesis, or suture the opening
	Infection (peritonitis)	
	Renal failure	Risk factors: poor technique Risk factors: hypovolemia, large volume paracentesis, pre-existing renal disease

TABLE 126-2 Technical Tips

Make sure that patient does have enough ascites that can be tapped	US to confirm fluid location and amount, especially if very small amount of fluid or fluid primarily localized to structures such as liver
Properly position patient under locally sterile conditions, taking the time to ensure all comfortable before proceeding	Patient supine with head of bed elevated 30°-40°
Ensure an almost painless procedure	Reduce burning sensation of cutaneous injection of xylocaine by warming vial between palms; give the rest of the lidocaine once you get into the peritoneal space, the most sensitive part.
Select best location several cm below level of percussed dullness	US usage at bedside becoming standard of care Avoid inferior epigastric vessels, tap lateral to rectus abdominus muscle; go where the fluid is located
Location of tap (tense ascites)	Consider tapping LLQ, followed by midline, then RLQ • Lateral 2-4 cm medial, cephalad to anterior superior iliac spine • LLQ preferred for obese patients (thinner abdominal wall, deeper depth of ascitic fluid) and for cirrhotics (who may have recanalized umbilical vein) • Midline 2 cm below umbilicus, preferred in patients without cirrhosis (linea alba normally devoid of blood vessels)
Large-volume paracentesis	For each liter removed over 5 L, 6-8 g albumin (~25 cc of 25% IV albumin/L of ascites) AASLD Class IIA recommendation (studies controversial, no survival benefit, albumin expensive)

TABLE 126-3 Characteristic Disease States

Test Result	Condition	Additional Testing
Bloody fluid	Hemorrhagic ascites (RBC >50,000) likely due to trauma, malignancy, or TB	To correct for a traumatic tap, subtract 1 polymorphonuclear cell (not WBC) per 250 RBCs. SBP >250 PMNs/hpf
Ascitic PMN ≥250 cells/mm³ or + ascitic culture of typical organisms	Spontaneous bacterial peritonitis	
SAAG (serum albumin ascites gradient) <1.1 g/dL	Nonportal hypertension • Peritoneal carcinomatosis • Peritoneal tuberculosis • Pancreatic ascites • Nephrotic syndrome • Serositis	Total protein >2.5 g/dL Cytology AFB, adenosine deaminase Amylase: may be > serum Urine protein
SAAG (serum albumin ascites gradient) >1.1 g/dL	Portal hypertension • Total protein <1 g/dL: cirrhosis • Total protein >2.5 g/dL: CHF, Budd-Chiari syndrome • Liver metastasis	Additional imaging

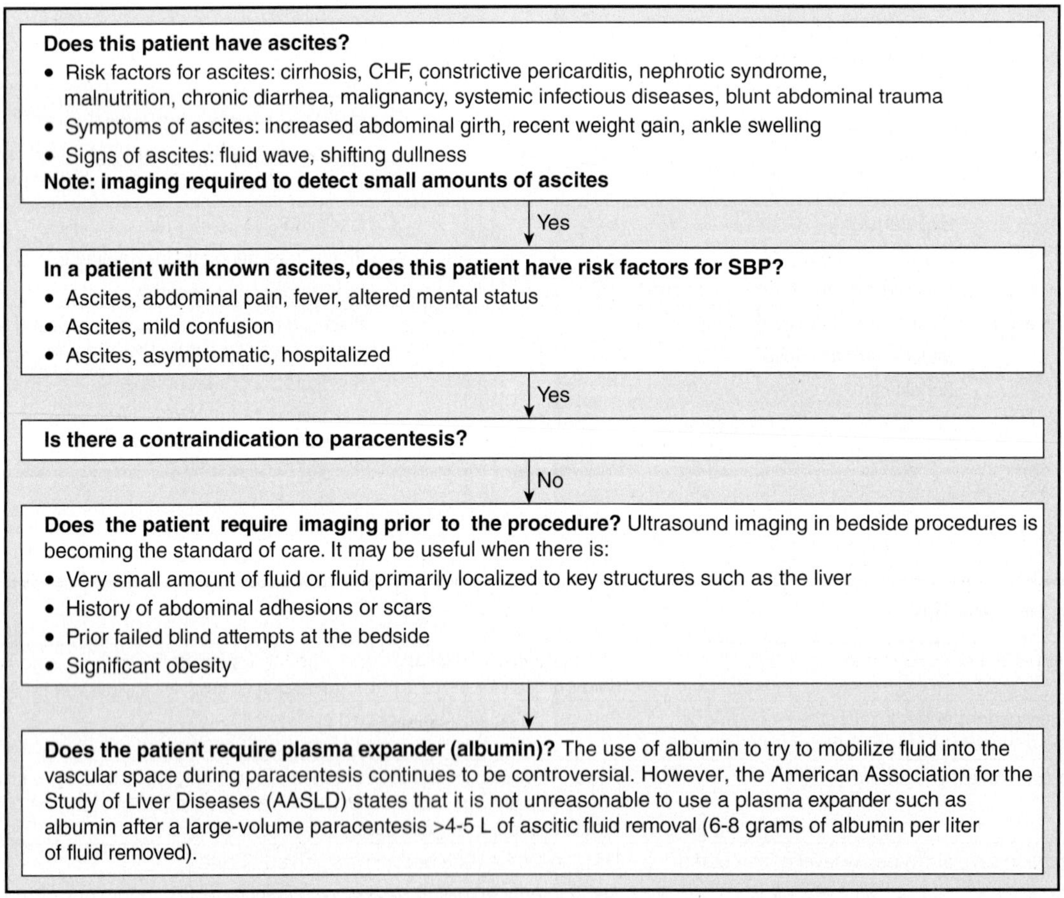

Does this patient have ascites?
- Risk factors for ascites: cirrhosis, CHF, constrictive pericarditis, nephrotic syndrome, malnutrition, chronic diarrhea, malignancy, systemic infectious diseases, blunt abdominal trauma
- Symptoms of ascites: increased abdominal girth, recent weight gain, ankle swelling
- Signs of ascites: fluid wave, shifting dullness
Note: imaging required to detect small amounts of ascites

↓ Yes

In a patient with known ascites, does this patient have risk factors for SBP?
- Ascites, abdominal pain, fever, altered mental status
- Ascites, mild confusion
- Ascites, asymptomatic, hospitalized

↓ Yes

Is there a contraindication to paracentesis?

↓ No

Does the patient require imaging prior to the procedure? Ultrasound imaging in bedside procedures is becoming the standard of care. It may be useful when there is:
- Very small amount of fluid or fluid primarily localized to key structures such as the liver
- History of abdominal adhesions or scars
- Prior failed blind attempts at the bedside
- Significant obesity

↓

Does the patient require plasma expander (albumin)? The use of albumin to try to mobilize fluid into the vascular space during paracentesis continues to be controversial. However, the American Association for the Study of Liver Diseases (AASLD) states that it is not unreasonable to use a plasma expander such as albumin after a large-volume paracentesis >4-5 L of ascitic fluid removal (6-8 grams of albumin per liter of fluid removed).

Figure 126-1 *Practice algorithm: preprocedure preparation.*

SUGGESTED READINGS

Moore KP, Aithal GP. Guidelines on the management of ascites in cirrhosis. *Gut*. 2006;55(Suppl 6):vi1-vi12.

Runyon BA. AASLD Practice Guideline Management of Adult Patients with Ascites Due to Cirrhosis: Update 2012. *Hepatology*. 2013;57(4):1-27. https://www.aasld.org/sites/default/files/guideline_documents/adultascitesenhanced.pdf. Accessed September 15, 2016.

ONLINE RESOURCES

Harrison's medical video

http://www.nejm.org/video Paracentesis video

CHAPTER 127

Arthrocentesis

Elinor Mody, MD

Excluding cases of trauma, pain with passive motion of a joint or palpation of the joint capsule suggests synovitis and requires further investigation. In the hospital setting, arthrocentesis is usually performed to diagnose whether a patient has a septic joint and to narrow antibiotic therapy once the cultures are known (**Figure 127-1**). Although radiography is essential in the diagnosis of trauma, it has no role in the early diagnosis of a joint infection. Neither CT or MRI or radionuclide scanning can distinguish between septic and noninfectious causes of inflammatory synovitis. Imaging is indicated, however, in patients with suspected:

- Sternoclavicular joint infection: to look for mediastinal extension.
- Sacroiliac joint infection: to look for pelvic involvement.
- Osteomyelitis.

See Figure 193-4, approach to the patient with suspected septic arthritis.

In the vast majority of cases, septic joints are a result of hematogenous seeding. Inflamed and artificial joints have an increased risk of being seeded by bacteria. The vasculature of the synovium does not have a basement membrane, thereby allowing bacteria to enter the joint space. Direct trauma to the joint such as an animal bite is a much rarer cause of joint infection. Polyarticular involvement is uncommon, but is sometimes seen in patients with rheumatoid arthritis. Although bacterial infections may affect less than 20% of all cases of acute arthritis, failure to diagnose bacterial infection may lead to permanent cartilage damage, destruction of bone, loss of joint function, and, in extreme cases, loss of limb and death. Aspiration almost always yields a diagnosis, and in the case of the septic joint, is akin to draining an abscess (see Chapter 193 [Osteomyelitis and Septic Arthritis] and Chapter 194 [Prosthetic Joint Infections]).

Arthrocentesis or aspiration of tophi is needed to establish the diagnosis of crystal deposition disease and to distinguish between pseudogout and gout. Classic radiographic findings of gout occur only very late in the disease. Likewise, radiographic findings of chondrocalcinosis and cystic erosions without marked joint space narrowing may suggest pseudogout but cannot confirm that the patient's sudden increase in pain is caused by this disease and not by coexisting bacterial infection. Arthrocentesis should be performed before initiating chronic hypouricemic therapy indicated for gout but not for pseudogout. Luckily, in the vast majority of cases, aspirating a joint is a simple and safe procedure rarely complicated by infection (see Chapter 247 [Gout, Pseudogout, and Osteoarthritis]). See **Tables 127-1** to **127-4**.

Is this patient at higher risk for septic arthritis?
- Preexisting joint disease (history of joint inflammation or injury, recent joint surgery)
- Rheumatoid arthritis (combination of joint damage, immunosuppressive medications, poor skin quality)
- Unprotected sexual activity (GC)
- Systemic illness and other conditions (immunosuppression, diabetes, renal disease, liver insufficiency, IV drug abuse)
- Skin lesions as a portal for occult bacteremia
- Involvement of small joints of the hand (usually direct inoculation or bite)
- Involvement of joints of the feet (usually progression of contiguous soft tissue infection or osteomyelitis, common in diabetics or patients with vascular insufficiency)
- Age > 80 y

Does this patient physical examination suggest the possibility of septic arthritis?
- Joint warmth, pain, swelling, restricted motion
- Monoarthritis
- Trauma with joint effusion
- Monoarthritis in a patient with chronic arthritis
- Polyarthritis, especially in patients with impaired immunity
- Sacroiliac and sternoclavicular involvement, especially in IV drug users
- Skin lesions (portal of entry, clinical syndrome of disseminated GC), signs of systemic illness

Does this patient require imaging prior to arthrocentesis?
- Trauma
- Sternoclavicular joint infections to look for mediastinal extension
- Osteomyelitis
- Sacroiliac joint infection to look for pelvic involvement

Does this patient require emergent specialty consultation?
- Suspected prosthetic joint infection (orthopedics)
- Joints ordinarily not aspirated by internists (hip, sacroiliac, small joints of hand, foot, etc)
- Small effusions, uncertainly about best diagnostic approach

What other studies should be performed at the same time as arthrocentesis in patients suspected of having septic arthritis?
- Blood cultures, possibly echocardiography (endocarditis)
- Peripheral CBC and differential, inflammatory markers (not specific but elevated WBC with left shift or elevated ESR, CRP at the beginning of treatment may help track response to treatment)
- For patients suspected of GC arthritis samples of GU, rectum, oropharynx (as synovial fluid cultures positive in <50% of patients)

Figure 127-1 *Practice algorithm: Diagnostic arthocentesis.*

TABLE 127-1 Basic Consideration

Indications	Diagnostic Arthrocentesis	Comments
	Monoarthritis	Patients with a sudden ↑ pain in a previously damaged joint and may not have prodromal symptoms or fever (>40% cases); fever may be associated with other conditions that cause joint pain, including gout
	Trauma with joint effusion	
	Monoarthritis in a patient with chronic polyarthritis	
	Suspected septic arthritis, gout, pseudogout, hemarthrosis	Always contact orthopedic service if concern about a septic prosthetic joint
	Therapeutic Arthrocentesis	**Comments**
	To administer steroids or anesthetics	Steroid injection of a joint, tendon sheath, or bursa may provide pain relief without significant side effects and shorten LOS
	To drain large effusions, hemarthroses	
Contraindications	Injecting a septic joint with cortisone	Even a small dose of cortisone can be disastrous; steroids can also exacerbate glaucoma and ↑ blood sugars in diabetics
	Risks of seeding infection by aspirating through cellulitis	No literature to support this theory; risk of not aspirating a septic joint outweighs risk
	Fracture	Possibility of making a closed fracture an open one
	Clotting diathesis	Severe thrombocytopenia is most worrisome; most joints can be safely aspirated but if INR excessive or if hemophilia, partial correction may be appropriate

(continued)

TABLE 127-1 Basic Consideration (*Continued*)

Indications	Diagnostic Arthrocentesis	Comments
Procedural Preparation	**Plain Radiographs**	**Comments**
	Plain films are not essential in uncomplicated septic arthritis but may identify complicating factors. Plain radiographs may identify foreign bodies, osteomyelitis, periarticular soft tissue swelling seen in early septic arthritis, joint space loss, periosteal reaction, marginal and central erosions, destruction of subchondral bone	Plain films, CT, MRI, or radionuclide scanning cannot distinguish between septic and noninfectious causes of synovitis. Only arthrocentesis will guide management
	Advanced Imaging	
	CT and MRI nonspecific joint inflammation, effusion, subchondral cysts, articular cartilage destruction	
Complications during Procedure	Trauma, pain, bleeding, infection	
Complications after Procedure	Reaccumulation of effusion, skin atrophy after steroid injections	Affected joint should be closely followed during treatment for recurrent signs and symptoms of infection
		Septic joints may require repeated irrigation and drainage even after appropriate antibiotic therapy and initial drainage

TABLE 127-2 Technical Tips

Properly position patient under locally sterile conditions, taking the time to ensure all comfortable before proceeding	Patient lying on his back, with the affected knee in a very slight passive flexion, obtained by placing a rolled towel under knee (see **Figure 127-2**)
Ensure an almost painless procedure	Reduce burning sensation of cutaneous injection of xylocaine by warming vial between palms; may also use ethyl chloride spray
Select easiest location	Approach knee either medially or laterally. Aim needle parallel to and just inferior to the patella so that it slips in, just underneath, into the joint itself
Dry tap	Perform with CT or US guidance, consider specialty assistance

TABLE 127-3 Normal Test Results

Test	Normal Value
Obtain cell count, differential, Gram stain, culture of synovial fluid and crystals	Insufficient fluid to tap
	Synovial fluid normally clear, colorless <200 WBCs/mm^3, <25% of polymorphonuclear cells

TABLE 127-4 Characteristic Disease States

	Color	Turbidity	Crystals
Septic	Yellow	Very	–
Inflammatory	Yellow	Very	–
Crystal	Yellow	Very	+
Osteoarthritis	Yellow	No	–

Note: A synovial fluid WBC count of more than 50,000 cells/mm^3 and neutrophil predominance is neither specific nor sensitive for septic arthritis. Crystalline arthropathy commonly causes synovial WBC counts in this range while immunosuppressed patients may not be able to mount synovial leukocytosis. A typical joint pathogen such as Mycobacterium tuberculosis or fungi may be associated with synovial WBC of lower magnitude. Synovial protein and glucose studies are neither sensitive nor specific and should not be checked.

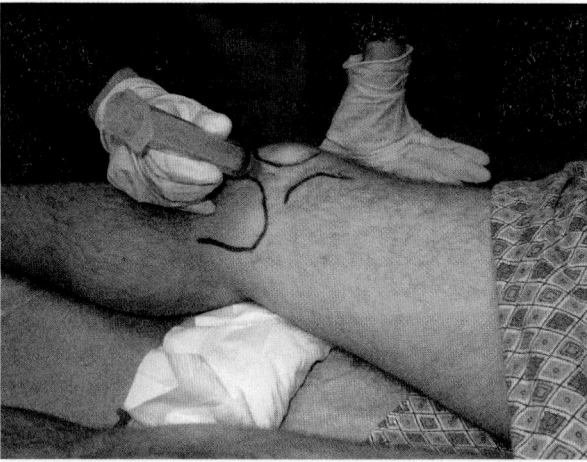

Figure 127-2 *Knee aspiration: Position the patient lying down on his/her back, with the affected knee in very slight passive flexion; this can be obtained by putting a rolled towel or sheet under the knee. The joint can be approached medially or laterally. In either case, aim the needle parallel to and just inferior to the patella, so that it slips in just underneath, into the joint itself.*

SUGGESTED READINGS

Bettencourt RB, Linder MM. Arthrocentesis and therapeutic joint injection: an overview for the primary care physician. *Prim Care.* 2010;37(4):691-702.

Coakley, G, Matthews C, Field M, et al. BSR & BHPR, BOA, RCGP and BSAC guidelines for the management of the hot swollen joint in adults. *Rheumatology.* 2006;45:1039-1041.

Goldenberg DL. Bacterial arthritis. *Curr Opin Rheumatol.* 1995;8(4):310-313.

Margaretten ME, Kohlwes J, More D, et al. Does this adult patient have septic arthritis. In: Simel DL, Rennie D, eds. *The Rational Clinical Examination.* New York, NY: McGraw-Hill; 2009.

ONLINE RESOURCES

arthrocentesis. http://www.nejm.org/video. Accessed September 13, 2016.

Harrison's video series. http://accessmedicine.mhmedical.com/content.aspx?sectionid=79758153&bookid=1130&Resultclick=2&q=arthrocentesis. Accessed March 13, 2016.

PART VI

Clinical Conditions in the Inpatient Setting

925

SECTION 1
Cardiovascular Medicine

CHAPTER 128

Acute Coronary Syndromes

Michael McDaniel, MD, FSCAI

Key Clinical Questions

❶ What is the optimal care and management of patients with ST-segment elevation myocardial infarction?

❷ What is the optimal care and management of patients with non-ST segment elevation acute coronary syndrome?

INTRODUCTION

The term acute coronary syndrome (ACS) refers to the spectrum clinical presentations related to acute myocardial ischemia or infarction due to the abrupt reduction in coronary blood flow. ACS is divided into ST-segment elevation myocardial infarctions (STEMIs) and non-ST segment elevation acute coronary syndromes (NSTE-ACSs). The NSTE-ACS is further subdivided on the basis of elevated cardiac biomarkers of myocardial necrosis. Patients with elevated cardiac biomarkers are defined as non-ST segment elevation myocardial infarction (NSTEMI) and those without elevated biomarkers are termed unstable angina (UA).

This chapter will focus on the diagnosis, risk stratification, and treatment of patients with ACS based on the American College of Cardiology Foundation and American Heart Association (ACCF/AHA) practice guidelines for STEMI and NSTE-ACS. All guideline recommendations will be cited in this chapter and referenced according the American College of Cardiology Foundation/American Heart Association classification scheme (**Table 128-1**).

■ EPIDEMIOLOGY & PATHOPHYSIOLOGY

ACS is common, with over 780,000 patients experiencing an ACS event every year in the United States. Of these events, approximately 70% are classified as NSTE-ACS. ACS is related to an acute imbalance of myocardial oxygen consumption and demand, usually related to a sudden coronary artery obstruction. Autopsy studies suggest that most ACS events are related to acute coronary thrombosis, with acute plaque rupture being the most common etiology. The atherosclerosis at sites of plaque rupture is characterized by large lipid-laden necrotic cores overlying a disrupted thin fibrous cap. The second most common cause of acute coronary thrombosis is plaque erosion, characterized by thrombus formation at an area of denuded endothelium. These plaques are characterized by smaller plaques with less lipid necrotic core and thicker fibrous caps compared to plaque rupture sites. Plaque erosion is actually the most common etiology of acute coronary thrombosis in younger female patients, especially those who smoke tobacco. More rare causes of coronary thrombosis are due to the calcified nodule which is not well characterized and is mostly seen in the elderly, and cardioembolic etiologies which are usually noted in distal coronary locations. Nonthrombotic sudden progressions in coronary arteries may be related to acute intraplaque hemorrhage without thrombosis. Rarely, acute coronary insufficiency may be caused by vasospasm, coronary arteritis, or spontaneous dissection.

■ HISTORY AND PHYSICAL

The most common clinical presentation of ACS is new onset pressure-like chest pain that occurs at rest (>10-20 minutes in duration) or with minimal activity. The pain is often retrosternal and can radiate to the arm (likelihood ratio [LR] 2.7), neck, or jaw and may be associated with diaphoresis (LR 2.0), dyspnea, or nausea (LR 1.9). However, chest pain can be absent in one-third of patients. Less common presentations of ACS include syncope, abdominal pain, hypotension, pulmonary edema, or unexplained fatigue. While older women and patients with diabetes most commonly present with typical symptoms of ACS, atypical ACS presentations are most common in these patients. Symptoms that are not characteristic of myocardial ischemia included pleuritic pain (LR 0.2), sharp or stabbing pain localized to a single location (LR 0.3), pain reproduced by

TABLE 128-1 ACCF/AHA Classification of Recommendations and Level of Evidence

Class I	Class IIa	Class IIb	Class III
Benefit >>>	*Benefit >> Risk*	*Benefit ≥ Risk*	*Risk ≥ Benefit*
Risk Procedure/ Treatment SHOULD be performed/ administered	*Additional studies with focused objectives needed*	*Additional studies with broad objectives needed; Additional registry data would be helpful*	*No additional studies needed*
	IT IS REASONABLE		Procedure/Treatment should NOT be performed/administered
	to perform procedure/administer treatment	Procedure/Treatment	SINCE IT IS NOT HELPFUL AND MAY BE HARMFUL
		MAY BE CONSIDERED	

Level A: Recommendation based on evidence from multiple randomized trials or meta-analyses
Level B: Recommendation based on evidence from a single randomized trial or non-randomized studies
Level C: Recommendation based on expert opinion, case studies, or standard of care

From O'Gara PT, et al. 2013 ACCF/AHA guideline for the management of ST-elevation myocardial infarction: executive summary: a report of the American College of Cardiology Foundation/American Heart Association Task Force on Practice Guidelines. *J Am Coll Cardiol.*2013;61(4):485-510.

palpitation (LR 0.2-0.4), or brief episodes lasting only seconds. Risk factors for ACS include older age, male sex, family history of coronary artery disease (CAD), peripheral arterial disease, diabetes mellitus, renal insufficiency, and prior CAD. The differential diagnosis for ACS is listed in **Table 128-2**.

The physical examination may be completely normal in many patients with ACS. Signs and symptoms of new congestive heart failure, mitral regurgitation, and/or shock suggest higher risk and usually require more emergent triage, treatment, and often invasive therapies. Signs of low cardiac output may be suggested by tachycardia, cool extremities, diaphoresis, confusion, and/or reduced urine output. Signs of congestive heart failure include elevated jugular venous distension, pulmonary edema, audible S3, and/or lower extremity edema.

■ ELECTROCARDIOGRAM

To rapidly identify STEMI, an electrocardiogram (ECG) should be performed within 10 minutes of arrival to the emergency department (ED) in all patients with signs and symptoms of ACS (Class I, Level of Evidence [LOE] C). In addition, Emergency Medical Service (EMS) personnel should perform a 12-lead ECG on site in all patients with suspected ACS and transport patients with STEMI to percutaneous coronary intervention (PCI)-capable facilities, where available.

STEMI is defined on ECG by new ST-elevation in at least two contiguous leads ≥2 mm in leads V_2-V_3 or ≥1 mm in the other chest leads or limb leads. Abnormalities alone on the EKG are insufficient to make a diagnosis of STEMI and the ECG must be interpreted in the appropriate clinical context. While new left bundle branch block (LBBB) was once considered as an STEMI equivalent, guidelines now recommend the LBBB in isolation should not be considered diagnostic of acute myocardial infarction (AMI) and specific ECG criteria have been proposed to diagnose STEMI in LBBB (**Table 128-3**). In addition, ST depressions in V_1-V_4 may indicate posterior injury (**Figure 128-1**) and isolated ST-elevation in aVR and/or V_1 with diffuse ST depression may suggest acute left main or proximal left anterior descending artery occlusion (**Figure 128-2**). Rarely, hyperacute T-waves can be seen early in patients with STEMI. When the initial ECG is nondiagnostic and the patient remains symptomatic, serial ECGs should be performed at 15 to 30 minute intervals during the first hour or if symptoms recur (Class I, LOE C).

The 12-lead ECG may suggest a diagnosis of NSTE-ACS, but is not required to make the diagnosis. Horizontal or downsloping dynamic ST-segment depression is highly suggestive of NSTE-ACS. In addition, significant deep precordial T-wave inversion (Wellen's sign) may suggest critical left anterior descending stenosis (**Figure 128-3**).

TABLE 128-2 Differential Diagnosis for NSTE-ACS

Nonischemic Cardiovascular
- Aortic dissection
- Expanding aortic aneurysm
- Myocarditis
- Pericarditis
- Hypertrophic cardiomyopathy
- Pulmonary embolism

Pulmonary
- Pneumonia
- Pleuritis
- Pulmonary hypertension
- COPD
- Pneumothorax

Gastrointestinal
- Gastroesophageal reflux
- Esophageal spasm
- Esophagitis
- Esophageal hypersensitivity
- Peptic ulcer
- Pancreatitis
- Biliary obstruction

Musculoskeletal
- Cervical disk radiculopathy
- Costochondritis
- Rheumatic disease
- Trauma

Other etiologies
- Sickle cell crisis
- Herpes zoster
- Depression and anxiety
- Drug intoxication
- Pheochromocytoma

Reprinted from Amsterdam EA, Wenger NK, Brindis RG, et al. 2014 AHA/ACC Guideline for the Management of Patients with Non-ST-Elevation Acute Coronary Syndromes: a report of the American College of Cardiology/ American Heart Association Task Force on Practice Guidelines. *J Am Coll Cardiol.* 2014;64(24):e139-228 with permission from Elsevier, Inc.

TABLE 128-3 ECG Criteria for Diagnosis of STEMI in the Setting of Left Bundle Branch Block (Sgarbossa Criteria)

Criterion	Odds Ratio (95% CI)	Score
ST-elevation ≥1 mm and concordant with QRS complex	25.2 (11.6-54.7)	5
ST-segment depression >1 mm in leads V_1, V_2, or V_3	6.0 (1.9-19.3)	3
ST-elevation >5 mm and discordant with QRS complex	4.3 (1.8-10.6)	2
A score >3 had a 98% specificity for acute myocardial infarction, but a score of 0 does not rule out STEMI.		

From O'Gara PT, Kushner FG, Ascheim DD, et al. 2013 ACCF/AHA guideline for the management of ST-elevation myocardial infarction: a report of the American College of Cardiology Foundation/American Heart Association Task Force on Practice Guidelines. *J Am Coll Cardiol.* 2013 29;61(4):e78-140. Reprinted with permission from Elsevier, Inc.

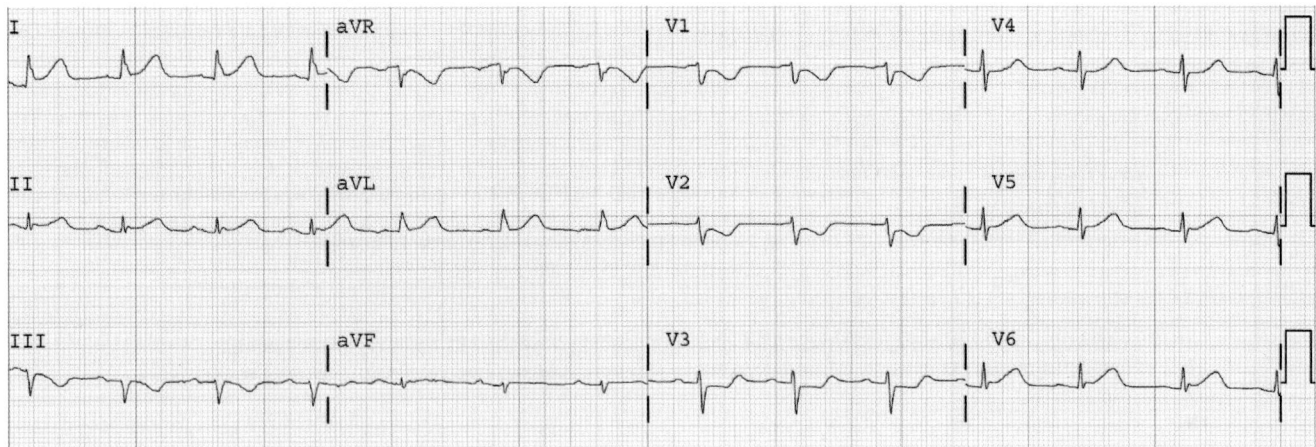

Figure 128-1 *EKG with and ST-depression in V_1-V_3 suggestive of acute posterior injury.* (Reproduced, by permission, from Knoop KE, et al eds. *The Atlas of Emergency Medicine,* 3rd ed. New York, NY: McGraw-Hill; 2010. ECG contributor: Ian D. Jones, MD.)

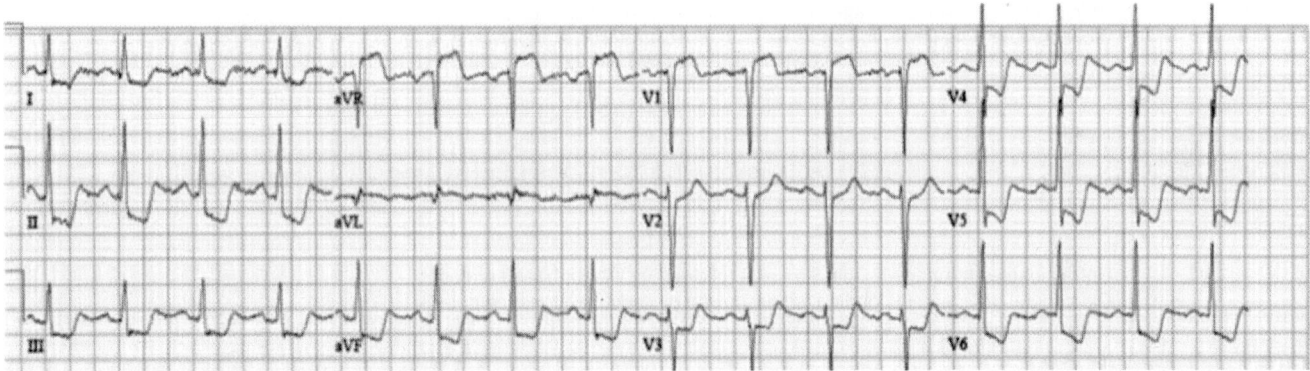

Figure 128-2 *ST-elevation in aVR with diffuse ST depression consistent with acute left main or very proximal left anterior descending artery occlusion.*

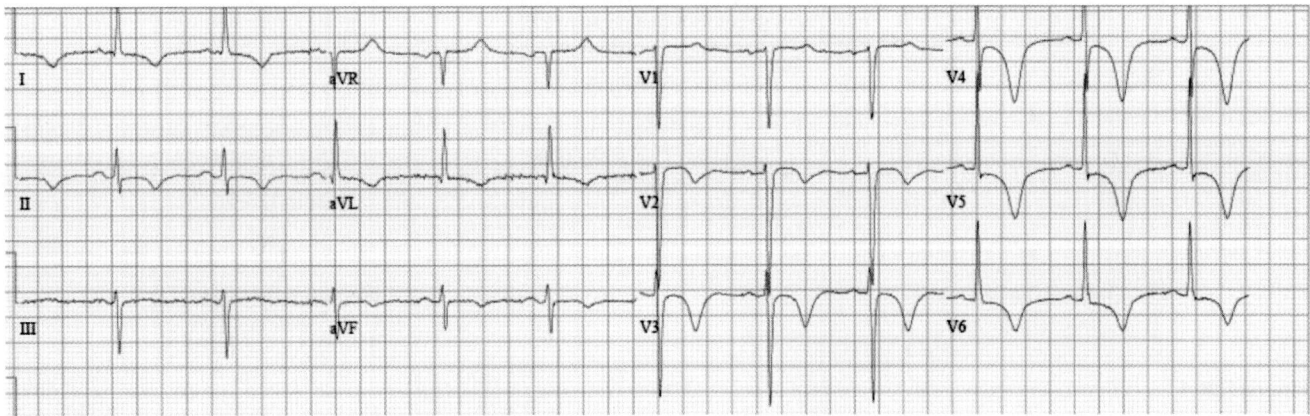

Figure 128-3 *Deep T-wave inversion in the precordial leads suggestive of ischemia in the left anterior descending coronary artery (Wellen's sign).*

More nonspecific ST-T changes are less diagnostic. Significant Q-waves can suggest a prior myocardial infarction (MI), but do not suggest ACS.

ST-SEGMENT ELEVATION MYOCARDIAL INFARCTION (STEMI)

■ MANAGEMENT OF STEMI AT PCI-CAPABLE HOSPITALS

All hospitals should develop coordinated regional approaches to STEMI care and participation in programs such as Mission:Lifeline (American Heart Association's Mission: Lifeline: http://www.heart.org) and the D2B Alliance is recommended (Class I, LOE B). These initiatives promote prehospital ECG to diagnose STEMI, EMS and ED activation of cardiac catheterization labs ("cath labs"), single calls to central paging operator to activate the cath team, cath lab staff arrival within 20 to 30 minutes of notification, and timely data feedback to all members of the STEMI team.

Once the diagnosis of STEMI is made, the most important therapy for patients is emergent revascularization within 90 minutes of first medical contact (FMC) (Class I, LOE A). As such, it is preferred for patients to bypass the ED and present directly via EMS to the cath lab when possible to optimize reperfusion times (**Figure 128-4**). Most patients arriving by EMS with ACS will receive aspirin 325 mg by EMS personnel (Class I, LOE A). Patients should also receive an unfractionated heparin (UFH) bolus (50-70 units/kg, max 5000 units) as soon as possible upon hospital arrival (Class I, LOE C). In addition, all patients presenting with STEMI should receive a *loading dose* of an oral antiplatelet P2Y12 antagonist as early as possible (Class I, LOE B). Presently, there are three options of the oral antiplatelet P2Y12 antagonists: clopidogrel 600 mg, prasugrel 60 mg, and ticagrelor 180 mg. Choosing between these agents will be discussed later in the *Dual Antiplatelet Therapy Section of Late Hospital & Hospital Discharge* part of the chapter.

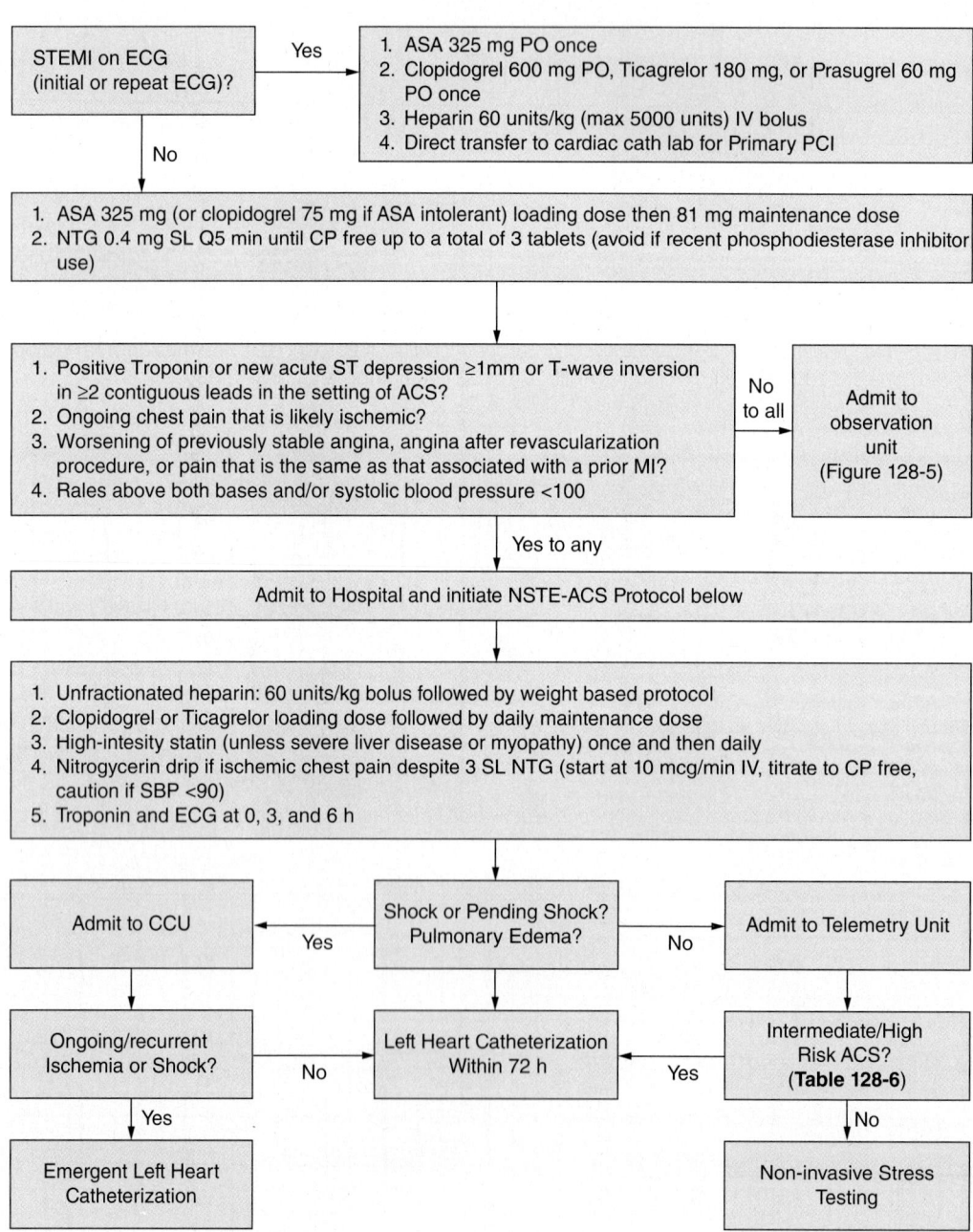

Figure 128-4 *Algorithm for evaluation and management of acute coronary syndrome for PCI-capable hospitals.* ACS, acute coronary syndromes; ASA, aspirin; CCU, coronary care unit; CP, chest pain; ECG, electrocardiogram; Non-STE ACS, Non-ST segment elevation acute coronary syndrome; NTG, nitroglycerin; PCI, percutaneous coronary intervention; PO, Per Os; SL, sublingual; STEMI, ST-segment elevation myocardial infarction.

There is little benefit to intravenous (IV) glycoprotein IIb/IIIa inhibitors (GPIs) prior to angiography in STEMI (Class IIb, B). However, GPIs are indicated in many patients during and *after PCI for STEMI* as it blocks the final common pathway of platelet activation. While a comprehensive review of the GPI trials is beyond the scope of this chapter, a few general principals regarding GPIs deserve mention. GPIs provide very rapid inhibition of platelets, much greater and faster than oral P2Y12 inhibitors. In addition, pooled studies suggest that GPIs reduce recurrent 30-day unplanned revascularization and mortality in STEMI. In a meta-analysis of 7414 patients from multiple randomized trials, patients undergoing PCI for STEMI receiving GPIs have about a 25% relative decrease in mortality compared to no GPI. However, GPIs are clearly associated with about a 50% relative increase in bleeding complications, especially with femoral access. This bleeding is attenuated but not eliminated by radial access. Currently, there are three GPI agents available for clinical use. There are two small molecule agents, eptifibatide and tirofiban, and one large molecule agent abciximab. Randomized trials, registries, and meta-analyses suggest that the large and small molecule GPI agents have similar efficacy and safety in patients undergoing primary PCI. As such, the choice of GPI may be driven more by cost considerations.

Bivalirudin is a direct thrombin inhibitor that has been studied extensively in primary PCI in STEMI, but its use is controversial given conflicting recent studies. In both the 3602 patient Harmonizing Outcomes with Revascularization and Stents in Acute Myocardial Infarction (HORIZONS AMI) and the 2218 patient European Ambulance Acute Coronary Syndrome angiography study (EUROMAX) trials, there were significantly less bleeding complications in patients randomized to bivalirudin compared to the combination of UFH and planned or provisional GPI. However, there was also significant more acute stent thrombosis, and the bleeding reduction was attenuated in patients with radial access. More recently, the benefits of bivalirudin compared to UFH alone have been questioned. In the How Effective Are Antithrombotic Therapies in Primary PCI (HEAT PPCI) trial, 1812 patients with STEMI were randomized to bivalirudin or UFH, both with provisional use of GPI. In this trial, there was no reduction of bleeding with the use of bivalirudin and actually higher major cardiac events with bivalirudin. It should be noted however that the use of provisional GPI was low and similar in both groups and most patients underwent PCI using the radial approach. Given the significantly higher cost compared to UFH, it is controversial if bivalirudin provides value compared to UFH, and further studies are warranted to best define the optimal role of bivalirudin in STEMI.

The radial access is increasingly utilized in STEMI as this strategy decreases access-site complications compared to PCI via femoral access (Class IIa, LOE A). In the 1001 patient Radial versus Femoral Randomized Investigation in ST Elevation Acute Coronary Syndrome trial, patients randomized to radial access had lower bleeding at 30 days (7.8% vs 12.2%, number needed to treat [NNT]23, P = 0.026) and cardiac mortality (5.2% vs 9.2%, NNT25, *P* = 0.02) compared with patients randomized to femoral access. Similar findings were noted in a meta-analysis of 5055 patients from 11 randomized trials in STEMI.

■ MANAGEMENT OF STEMI AT NON-PCI-CAPABLE HOSPITALS

Not all patients with STEMI present to hospitals that can perform primary PCI. These patients should be transferred to a PCI-capable hospital for primary PCI if this transport can occur rapidly and achieve revascularization at the receiving hospital with FMC-to-device time less than120 minutes (Class I, LOE B). If this time goal cannot be met, fibrinolytic therapy is recommended in the absence of contraindications within 30 minutes of hospital arrival (Class I, LOE B). Fibrin-specific agents (Tenecteplase, Reteplase, and Alteplase) are

TABLE 128-4 Contraindications to Fibrinolysis in STEMI

Absolute Contraindications
- Prior intracranial hemorrhage
- Structural cerebral vascular lesions
- Malignant intracranial neoplasm
- Ischemic stroke within 3 mo
- Suspected aortic dissection
- Active bleeding
- Significant closed-head or facial trauma within 3 mo
- Intracranial or intraspinal surgery within 2 mo
- Severe uncontrolled hypertensions unresponsive to therapy

Relative Contraindications
- Significant hypertension (SBP >180 mm Hg or DBP >110 mm Hg)
- History of ischemic stroke >3 mo
- Dementia
- Prolonged CPR >10 min
- Major surgery within 3 wk
- Recent internal bleeding within 2-4 wk
- Noncompressible vascular punctures
- Pregnancy
- Active peptic ulcer
- Oral anticoagulant therapy

preferred over non-fibrin-specific agents (Streptokinase). Absolute and relative contraindications to fibrinolytic therapy are listed in **Table 128-4**. In addition, patients presenting with cardiogenic shock, high bleeding risk, or presentations >3 to 4 hours after symptom onset should usually be transported to a PCI-capable hospital regardless of transport times.

All patients who receive fibrinolysis should also receive aspirin 325 mg PO loading dose, clopidogrel 300 mg PO loading dose, and unfractionated heparin bolus and infusion. In addition, all patients should be transferred emergently to a PCI-capable hospital for urgent/emergent angiography as part of either a rescue PCI strategy (for failed lysis) or a pharmocoinvasive strategy as both strategies have been shown to improve outcomes compared to conservative management strategies.

■ COMATOSE PATIENTS WITH OUT-OF-HOSPITAL CARDIAC ARREST

Comatose patients with out-of-hospital cardiac arrest (OHCA) due to ventricular fibrillation (VF) or pulseless ventricular tachycardia (VT) with return of spontaneous circulation (ROSC) deserve special mention. These patients have about a 10-fold increase in mortality compared to STEMI patients without cardiac arrest. Survival is optimized when CPR and defibrillation are initiated early. Importantly, the neurologic exam should not be used in the acute setting to predict future neurologic recovery or survival. While patients with longer pulseless times, unwitnessed arrests, and longer CPR durations have worse neurologic outcomes, there are no absolute predictors in the acute setting of neurologic recovery with intervention. As such, the neurologic status should not solely be used to guide decisions about invasive procedures in the acute setting.

Immediate angiography and PCI should be strongly considered for all comatose patients with OHCA and ROSC with STEMI on initial ECG (Class I, LOE B). In addition, targeted temperature management (TTM) should be started as soon as possible to target 32°C to 34°C for

12 to 24 hours (Class I, LOE B). Two randomized trials have reported improved neurologic survival when TTM was initiated before or at the time of PCI, and the combination of early angiography/intervention and TTM is associated with the highest survival and neurologic recovery. More recently, other randomized clinical trials of TTM in postresuscitated patients have found equally impressive survival rates, whether cooled to 33°C versus 36°C or whether initiated in the field or after arrival at the hospital. Several methods for hypothermia are available, but there are insufficient data to recommend one technique over another and local expertise should guide decisions between external cooling pads, intravascular cooling, cooling blankets, and ice packs. Of note, iced saline should rarely be used as the volume may precipitate pulmonary edema in patients at risk for heart failure and this can lead to more rapid fluctuations in body temperature.

While there is not a consensus to the optimal management of patients with OHCA due to VF/VT with ROSC without ST-elevations on ECG, most of the studies also support early angiography, PCI, and TTM for these patients as up to 25% to 30% of these patients will have culprit lesions at angiography despite a normal ECG. However, given the greater heterogeneity of these patients, consultation should be undertaken with interventional cardiology prior to cath lab activation for these patients.

PRACTICE POINT

STEMI

- Rapid ECG with interpretation is recommended *prehospital by EMS* or *within 10 minutes of arrival* to the hospital to rapidly identify patients with STEMI and optimize reperfusion times.
- When the initial ECG is nondiagnostic and the patient remains symptomatic, serial ECGs should be performed at 15- to 30-minute intervals during the first hour or if symptoms recur.
- Left Bundle Branch Block in isolation should not be considered diagnostic of acute myocardial infarction and specific ECG criteria have been proposed to diagnose STEMI in LBBB (Table 128-3).
- All patients with STEMI should receive an aspirin loading dose (325 mg), unfractionated heparin bolus (50-70 units/kg, max 5000 units), and a P2Y12 inhibitor loading dose prior to or at the time of angiography.
- Primary PCI is recommended within 90 minutes of first medical contact for PCI-capable hospitals.
- Transfer for primary PCI from a non-PCI-capable hospital is recommended when the first medical contract to device time (balloon or aspiration catheter) can be accomplished within 120 minutes. When this is not possible, fibrinolysis is preferred within 30 minutes of hospital arrival.
- The optimal use of glycoprotein IIb/IIIa inhibitors and Bivalirudin in STEMI remains controversial. When GPIs are used, they should usually be deferred until angiography is performed.
- Most comatose patients with out-of-hospital cardiac arrest due to VT/VF and return of spontaneous circulation should undergo emergent angiography and targeted temperature management.

NON-ST SEGMENT ELEVATION ACUTE CORONARY SYNDROMES (NSTE-ACS)

■ MORPHINE, OXYGEN, NITROGLYCERIN, AND ASPIRIN

"MONA" (Morphine, Oxygen, Nitroglycerin, and Aspirin) has been part of the classic teaching for patients with ACS for decades. However, aside from aspirin, there are now reasons to caution the routine use of these other agents in ACS.

Morphine should probably be avoided in most patients with active angina as it can mask ongoing ischemia or infarction in patients who may benefit from emergent revascularization, and its use has been downgraded in recent guidelines (Class IIb, LOE B) based on observational studies suggesting an association with adverse events and morphine use in ACS. While this may be related to the fact that sicker patients get morphine, morphine may mask the pain of ongoing infarction resulting in delays in revascularization and larger infarctions. Furthermore, morphine may impair the absorption of the oral antiplatelet agents. For most patients with active angina despite IV nitroglycerin, urgent coronary angiography should be considered instead of morphine.

Supplemental oxygen therapy is recommended only in patients with ACS and arterial oxygen saturation less than 90% or in respiratory distress (Class I, LOE C). The benefits of routine oxygen use without hypoxia have never been demonstrated, and some studies suggest that oxygen therapy may actually increase vascular resistance, reduce coronary flow, and result in larger infarctions. Furthermore, in a pooled Cochrane analysis of 430 patients from four randomized trials demonstrated a twofold higher risk of death in patients with AMI treated with oxygen. Taken together, routine oxygen therapy is probably not necessary in most patients with ACS unless hypoxia is present.

Nitrates are endothelium-independent vasodilators that relieve angina by decreasing cardiac preload and reducing ventricular wall tension. Sublingual (SL) nitroglycerin is recommended for patients with active angina (Class I, LOE C). If the angina continues despite 3 SL nitroglycerin, IV nitroglycerin should be given and titrated until chest pain free or limited by side effects such as hypotension or headache (Class I, LOE B). While nitroglycerin is effective at reducing the symptoms of angina, randomized trials have never demonstrated improved morbidity or mortality outcomes with nitrates. In addition, nitroglycerin should be avoided in patients with hypotension, right ventricular infarctions, and recent phosphodiesterase inhibitor-5 (sildenafil, vardenafil, or tadalafil) use due to risk of significant hypotension (Class III, LOE B).

All patients with ACS should receive nonenteric-coated ASA of 325 mg as soon as possible followed by 81 mg daily maintenance dose (Class I, LOE A). Aspirin is a mainstay of ACS therapy, results in thromboxane A2 inhibition via irreversible COX-inhibition, and results in approximately 30% to 45% relative reductions in death and recurrent myocardial infarction across a large spectrum of ACS. *Enteric-coated* aspirin should be avoided in the early setting of ACS due to delayed absorption.

■ SERIAL TROPONIN ANALYSIS

Increasingly, a troponin-only biomarker strategy (without ordering creatine kinase [CK] and creatine kinase myocardial enzyme [CK-MB] fraction) is used for the evaluation of AMI in NSTE-ACS. Although damaged cardiac myocytes release several biomarkers, troponins are preferred based on their superior sensitivity and specificity. Cardiac troponin will rise within 2 to 4 hours of symptom onset and will remain elevated for several days. *Shorter intervals of serial troponin measurements (such as 0, 3, and 6 hours) more rapidly diagnose and/or rule out AMI (Class I, LOE A).* Contemporary sensitive troponin assays now permit earlier serial sampling (in 3 hours vs previous 8 hours) for earlier detection and treatment of AMI. Furthermore, **a negative troponin value 6 hours from presentation essentially excludes the diagnosis of AMI** (unless recurrent symptoms), leading to earlier diagnostic testing or hospital discharge. It is important for physicians to be aware of the troponin assay used in their local hospital, as troponin measures >6 hours from onset may be required with less sensitive older assays. In addition, testing at longer intervals is required (up to 24 hours) if information about infarct size is required.

TABLE 128-5 Causes of Elevated Cardiac Troponin Values Due to Myocardial Injury

Injury related to primary myocardial ischemia

Plaque rupture

Intraluminal coronary artery thrombus formation

Injury related to supply/demand imbalance

Tachy-/bradyarrhythmias

Aortic dissection or severe aortic valve disease

Hypertrophic cardiomyopathy

Cardiogenic, hypovolemic, or septic shock

Severe respiratory failure

Severe anemia

Hypertension

Coronary spasm

Coronary embolism or vasculitis

Coronary endothelial dysfunction

Injury not related to myocardial ischemia

Cardiac contusion, surgery, ablation, pacing, or defibrillator shocks

Rhabdomyolysis with cardiac involvement

Myocarditis

Cardiotoxic agents, like anthracyclines

Multifactorial or indeterminate myocardial injury

Heart failure stress (Takotsubo)

Pulmonary embolism or pulmonary hypertension

Sepsis

Renal failure

Severe acute neurological diseases, such as stroke or subarachnoid hemorrhage

Infiltrative diseases, like amyloidosis or sarcoidosis

Strenuous exercise

Modified by permission from Thygesen K. Third Universal Definition of Myocardial Infarction. *JACC.* 2012;60(16):1586 (table 1). Elsevier Inc.

There is very little value to using other cardiac biomarkers in addition to troponin, as they are both less sensitive and less specific. Furthermore, moderate-sized registries suggest that the addition of CK-MB adds no additional diagnostic information compared to troponin alone. With contemporary troponin assays, CK-MB and myoglobin are not useful in the diagnosis of ACS and the current guidelines recommend against their use (Class III, LOE A). Importantly, elevated troponin values alone are insufficient to make a diagnosis of NSTEMI and should be evaluated in the appropriate clinical context. There are many reasons other than ACS for elevated troponin values (**Table 128-5**).

■ EARLY HOSPITAL TRIAGE IN NSTE-ACS

Patients with possible or definite NSTE-ACS represent a broad population with various levels of risk. Of patients presenting to the ED with possible ACS, less than 25% will be diagnosed with UA or AMI. However, on the opposite end, up to 5% of patients with ACS are inappropriately discharged from the hospital without appropriate diagnostic workup. To address these conflicting issues, *observation units* have been developed in many hospitals and are recommended for low-risk patients with possible ACS. These units have been associated with lower rates of missed acute MI, lower costs, improved patient satisfaction, and decreased admissions for

chest pain. While there are several tools used to risk stratify patients for observation units, many hospitals use modifications of the Goldman's prediction rule as these criteria predict MACE within 72 hours of presentation (Figure 128-4). The modified rule uses four criteria: (1) positive troponin or new acute ST depression ≥1 mm or T-wave inversion in ≥2 contiguous leads in the setting of ACS; (2) ongoing chest pain that is likely ischemic; (3) worsening of previously stable angina, angina after revascularization procedure, or pain that is the same as that associated with a prior MI; (4) rales above both bases or systolic blood pressure <100 (Figure 128-4). The absence of these four factor identifies patients at very low risk of subsequent cardiac events and appropriate for the observation unit (**Figure 128-5**). In observation units, dual antiplatelet therapy and anticoagulation is usually avoided. Patients undergo serial troponin evaluation, cardiac monitoring, and repeated ECGs. For patients with normal serial troponins and ECGs, stress testing before discharge or within 72 hours of discharge should be considered (Class IIa, LOE B). If patients have recurrent chest pain suggestive of ischemia, increased cardiac biomarkers, or dynamic ECG changes, they are then admitted to the hospital and managed according to inpatient pathways described below.

■ ANTIPLATELET THERAPY AT ADMISSION

Patients who are not low risk and/or patients with recurrent symptoms, ECG changes, or positive troponin values are admitted to the hospital for inpatient management (Figure 128-4). In addition to aspirin, dual antiplatelet therapy is recommended as soon as possible after admission to the hospital. There are two oral P2Y12 inhibitor options for upstream management in NSTE-ACS: clopidogrel (600 mg loading dose followed by 75 mg a day) and ticagrelor (180 mg loading dose followed by 90 mg twice a day). Both of these agents are options for both the invasive (Class I, LOE B) and ischemia-guided (Class I, LOE A) strategies. Choice between these agents will be discussed later in the *Dual Antiplatelet Therapy Section of Late Hospital & Hospital Discharge* part of the chapter.

The early benefit of clopidogrel was first noted in the Clopidogrel in Unstable Angina to Prevent Recurrent Events (CURE) trial, where there was a 34% relative reduction in major cardiac events in first 24 hours in patients randomized to clopidogrel and aspirin compared to aspirin alone. Furthermore, in a large meta-analysis of 37,814 patients undergoing PCI from six randomized control trials and nine observational studies showed a significant reduction in major adverse cardiac events (9.8% vs 12.3%, NNT = 40, $p < 0.001$) and trends toward improve mortality (1.5% vs 2.0%, $p = 0.17$) with dual antiplatelet therapy pretreatment compared to aspirin alone. The downside to routine upstream clopidogrel is increased bleeding in patients who require coronary artery bypass graft (CABG) surgery. However, CABG is only required in approximately 11% of patients with ACS, and if not emergent, surgery can be delayed 5 days until the antiplatelet effects have reversed.

The oral P2Y12 inhibitor prasugrel is not recommended prior to cardiac catheterization in patients with NSTE-ACS, based on the results of the ACCOST (A Comparison of Prasugrel at the Time of Percutaneous Coronary Intervention or as Pretreatment at the Time of Diagnosis in Patients With Non–ST-Elevation Myocardial Infarction) trial where 4033 patients with non-STE ACS were randomized to upstream or intraprocedural prasugrel. In this trial, there was no reduction in major adverse events but only increased bleeding complications in patients pretreated with prasugrel. It has been suggested that the lack of efficacy in this trial may relate to short time interval from pretreatment to catheterization and the rapid onset of action of the drug in the cardiac cath lab.

Upstream (prior to the cath lab) GPIs are usually not necessary for most patients with ACS in the setting of upstream oral dual antiplatelet therapy. Two randomized studies in NSTE-ACS have

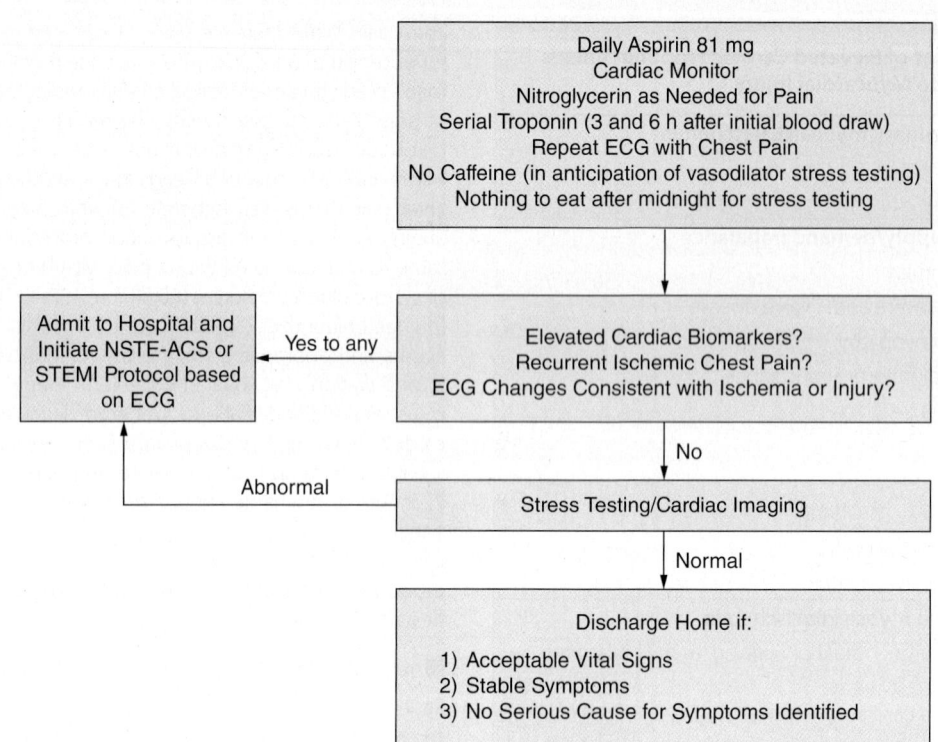

Figure 128-5 *Observation unit low-risk acute coronary syndrome (ACS) protocol.*

noted similar efficacy with a deferred GPI strategy (given at the time of PCI) compared with a routine upstream strategy. In the 10,500 patient Early Glycoprotein IIb/IIIa Inhibition in Patients With Non-ST-Segment Elevation Acute Coronary Syndrome trial, there were similar major adverse events (9.3% vs 10%, *p* = 0.23) with more bleeding in the routine upstream GPI use. Similar findings were noted in the Acute Catheterization and Urgent Intervention Triage strategY Timing Trial.

■ ANTICOAGULANT THERAPY AT ADMISSION

All patients admitted to the hospital with NSTE-ACS should receive IV anticoagulation prior to cardiac catheterization as well as during PCI. While the optimal anticoagulation strategy in patients with NSTE-ACS is unknown, the most widely used agent is UFH 60 units/kg bolus (maximum 4000 units) followed by an initial infusion of 12 units/kg/h (maximum 1000 units/h) adjusted per activated partial thromboplastin time to maintain therapeutic anticoagulation (Class I, LOE B). UFH does not break down existing thrombus, but does prevent further thrombus formation. While large studies investigating UFH in ACS are lacking, meta-analysis suggest about a 33% reduction (relative risk 0.67 [0.44-1.02], NNT = 40) in recurrent ischemia and infarction with the addition of UFH to aspirin. While low molecular weight heparins (LMWHs) offer an alternate option (to UFH) in NSTE-ACS (Class I, LOE A), large randomized trials and meta-analyses suggest essentially similar clinical efficacy and safety compared to unfractionated heparin. However, LMWH must be dose adjusted in patients with low glomerular filtration rates and can significantly delay the sheath removal in the cath lab due to longer durations of action. For these reasons, many interventional cardiologists prefer UFH to LMWH in the cardiac cath lab for patients with NSTE-ACS.

The factor X inhibitor fondaparinux is a synthetic pentasaccharide that indirectly inhibits factor Xa. While lower bleeding complications were noted with fondaprinux compared to LMWH in the OASIS (Organization to Assess Strategies in Ischemic Syndromes)-5 trial, its use should only be considered in a ischemia-guided strategy where

invasive procedures are unlikely due to increased rates of catheter thrombosis in patients undergoing PCI. Additional anticoagulation with either unfractionated heparin or bivalirudin is recommended when PCI is warranted with fondaparinux (Class I, LOE B). Furthermore, fondaparinux is contraindicated in patients with GFR < 30 mL/min and the long half-life (17 hours) can delay sheath removal in the cath lab when manual closure is performed. For these reasons, this drug is not ideal for patient with NSTE-ACS in patients with an invasive strategy.

Bivalirudin is an intravenous direct thrombin inhibitor that has been widely studied in patients with NSTE-ACS undergoing an invasive management strategy (Class I, LOE B). Several studies have demonstrated similar efficacy and reduced bleeding complications with bivalirudin compared to routine heparin and GPI use in NSTE-ACS. In the 13,819 patient ACUITY trial, there was a similar composite ischemic endpoint (7.8% vs 7.3%, *p* = 0.32) but significantly lower major bleeding complications (3.0% vs 5.7%, *p* < 0.001) with bivalirudin compared to UFH and GPI. Similar findings were noted in ISAR-REACT 4 trial. However, the benefits of bivalirudin over UFH in patients with NSTE-ACS undergoing PCI using the radial access are unknown.

■ EARLY INVASIVE STRATEGY VERSUS ISCHEMIA-GUIDED STRATEGY

All NSTE-ACS patients with refractory angina, electrical instability (eg, ventricular fibrillation or ventricular tachycardia), and/or cardiogenic shock should undergo immediate angiography within 2 hours of hospital presentation no matter the ECG findings (Class I, LOE A). However, for patients that are hemodynamically and electrically stable without ongoing angina, clinicians must select between an early invasive strategy or an ischemia-guided strategy.

An early invasive strategy is defined as angiography within 72 hours of admission to risk stratify patients based on coronary anatomy. The advantages to an early invasive strategy include rapid evaluation, early revascularizaton, and earlier discharge. An early

TABLE 128-6 Intermediate or High Risk Non–ST-Elevation Acute Coronary Syndrome (NSTE-ACS) Criteria

Intermediate or High risk NSTE-ACS is defined by *one or more* of the following:

1. Recurrent angina/ischemia at rest with low-level activities despite intensive medical therapy
2. Elevated troponin
3. New/dynamic ST-segment depression
4. Signs/symptoms of heart failure or new/worsening mitral regurgitation
5. High-risk findings from noninvasive testing
6. Hemodynamic instability
7. Sustained ventricular tachycardia (>30 s and/or hemodynamic instability)
8. PCI within 6 mo
9. TIMI risk score ≥3
10. Newly reduced left ventricular function (LVEF < 40%)

invasive strategy is indicated for initially stabilized patients with NSTE-ACS without contraindications to angiography and elevated risk of recurrent events (**Table 128-6**). Multiple studies and meta-analyses suggests that an early invasive strategy is preferred to an ischemia-guided strategy in higher-risk patients with NSTE-ACS as it is associated with lower rates of repeat hospitalization, myocardial infarction, and mortality. In a combined analysis of multiple randomized trials, there was an 11.1% absolute reduction (NNT9) in death and myocardial infarction in the highest risk NSTE-ACS by 5-year follow-up. An early invasive strategy is also associated with less angina and improved quality of life. It should be remembered that these are strategy trials, and not a comparisons of revascularization and medical therapy. Patients undergo revascularization with CABG or PCI revascularization in about 70% of patients randomized to an early invasive strategy and in 40% to 50% of patients randomized to an ischemia-guided strategy.

In contrast, an ischemia-guided strategy aims to avoid routine angiography unless patients experience refractory or recurrent angina, hemodynamic instability, or objective evidence of severe ischemia. An ischemia-guided strategy is preferred in patients at low risk for recurrent events, especially in troponin negative NSTE-ACS with low TIMI risk scores (≤2) (**Table 128-7**). Patients undergoing an ischemia-guided strategy should undergo noninvasive testing

TABLE 128-7 Thrombolysis in Myocardial Infarction (TIMI) Risk Score for Non–ST-Elevation Acute Coronary Syndrome (NSTE-ACS)

TIMI Risk Score	14-day Risk of Mortality, Recurrent MI, or Severe Ischemia Requiring Revascularization
0-1	4.7%
2	8.3%
3	13.2%
4	19.9%
5	26.2%
6-7	40.9%

TIMI risk score is determined by presence of seven variables on admission and one point given to each of the following: age ≥ 65 y, ≥3 cardiac risk factors, prior CAD defined as stenosis ≥50%, ST deviation on ECG, ≥2 anginal events in 24 h, use of aspirin in prior 7 d, and elevated cardiac troponin.

prior to discharge (Class I, LOE B). The optimal test depends on the patient's baseline ECG, available technologies, and local expertise. Due to low costs and simplicity, the exercise treadmill testing is preferred in patients when the baseline ECG is free of ST changes or LBBB (Class I, LOE C). If there are abnormal ST changes on the baseline ECG, then imaging (Single Photon Emission Computed Tomography or Echocardiogram) can be added to the exercise test (Class I, LOE B). Pharmacologic stress testing with imaging is recommended for patients unable to exercise due to physical limitations (Class I, LOE C).

PRACTICE POINT

NSTE-ACS

- Low-risk patients with possible ACS do not need admission to the hospital and can be safely monitored in an observation unit.
- All patients admitted to the hospital should receive the following on admission: aspirin 325 mg followed by 81 mg a day, an oral P2Y12 antagonist (clopidogrel or ticagrelor) loading dose followed by maintenance therapy, and anticoagulation (unfractionated heparin preferred if invasive management possible).
- Morphine and oxygen should be avoided in most patients.
- Nitroglycerin should be avoided in patients with right ventricular infarctions, hypotension, and/or recent phosphodiesterase-5 inhibitor use.
- Upstream glycoprotein IIb/IIIa inhibitors are not indicated in patients with NSTE-ACS when upstream dual antiplatelet therapy (aspirin + oral P2Y12 antagonist) is used.
- Serial troponin-only testing at *0, 3, and 6 hours* can be used to diagnose or rule out myocardial infarction. There is little role for other cardiac biomarkers (CK, CKMB, or myoglobin).
- Patients with refractory angina or cardiogenic shock should undergo emergent angiography within 2 hours of admission, even if there is no evidence of ST-elevations on ECG.
- Initially stabilized patients at intermediate or high risk should undergo an angiography with intent to perform intervention within 72 hours of admission. Patients at low risk should undergo an ischemia-guided strategy with noninvasive stress testing.

LATE HOSPITAL CARE & HOSPITAL DISCHARGE

DUAL ANTIPLATELET THERAPY

All patients with ACS should receive aspirin therapy indefinitely. Regardless if medically managed or revascularized with PCI or surgery, patients should receive low dose 81 mg daily as it appears to be equally efficacious as higher doses but with lower bleeding complications. In addition to aspirin, all patients with ACS should receive a P2Y12 antagonist for *1 year* regardless if treated with a bare metal stent or a drug eluting stent or without PCI. There are three options for patients who undergo PCI for ACS: clopidogrel, prasugrel, or ticagrelor. There are two options for patients who are medically managed without PCI: clopidogrel or ticagrelor. There is no consensus to the optimal P2Y12 antagonist in ACS at present.

The benefits of 1 year of dual antiplatelet therapy was established from the CURE trial, where dual antiplatelet therapy (clopidogrel and aspirin) resulted in a 20% reduction (NNT = 48) in cardiovascular death, myocardial infarction, or cerebrovascular accident compared with aspirin alone in 12,562 patients with ACS. This benefit was noted in patients who were managed both conservatively and invasively with PCI. Now that clopidogrel is generic, the low cost makes it an attractive option in ACS.

Prasugrel is a P2Y12 antagonist that is more efficiently metabolized to its active metabolite with greater potency and more rapid onset of action than clopidogrel. In 13,608 patients with ACS in the TRITON TIMI 38 trial, there were lower composite of death, myocardial infarction, and stroke in patients randomized to prasugrel compared to clopidogrel (9.9% vs 12.1%, NNT45, $p < 0.001$). However, there was significantly more major bleeding with prasugrel (2.4% vs 1.8%, NNH167, $p = 0.03$). Furthermore, patients over 75 years of age, body weight less than 60 pounds, and a history of stroke or transient ischemic attack had worse outcomes with prasugrel and there is a *black box warning* to avoid prasugrel in these patients. Despite the warning, up to 18% of patients in real word practice receive received prasugrel with these contraindications. In addition, there is little benefit to prasugrel in patients medically managed for ACS without PCI. In the TRILOGY ACS (Targeted Platelet Inhibition to Clarify the Optimal Strategy to Medically Manage Acute Coronary Syndromes) trial, prasugrel failed to reduce cardiac event rates compared to clopidogrel in patients with ACS undergoing medical therapy.

Ticagrelor is a direct acting P2Y12 antagonist that does not require metabolic activation. In 18,624 patients with ACS in the PLATO trial, ticagrelor reduced the composite of death, myocardial infarction, and stroke compared to clopidogrel (9.8% vs 11.7%, NNT53, $p = 0.003$). This benefit was noted in patients undergoing PCI and those medically managed without PCI. Using the same bleeding definition used in TRITON TIMI 38 (non-CABG TIMI major bleeding), there was again more major bleeding with tiacagrelor compared to clopidogrel (2.8% vs 2.2%, NNH167, $p = 0.03$). Interestingly, patients randomized in the United States and Canada did not derive a benefit with ticagrelor and trended toward harm. While this finding may be due to chance, interactions with the higher aspirin dose may also explain this finding. Therefore, in the United States ticagrelor is approved for use only with the lower aspirin dose (81 mg) with a warning against the use with the higher aspirin dose.

How is one to choose between these three P2Y12 antagonist agents: clopidogrel, prasugrel, and ticagrelor? All three agents have a similar recommendation in the ACCF/AHA guidelines (Class I, LOE B). However, these medications have very different costs, efficacy, and safety considerations. While both ticagrelor and prasugrel were shown to be superior to clopidogrel in large randomized trials, the benefits of these medications over clopidogrel seem to be most pronounced in patients with abnormalities in clopidogrel metabolism. Clopidogrel is a prodrug that requires two-step metabolism into an active metabolite. Patients with abnormalities in the CYP2C19 allele have impaired metabolism, higher on-treatment platelet reactivity, and worse outcomes with clopidogrel. Up to 30% of the US population has abnormalities in this CYP2C19 allele, and clopidogrel carries a warning of reduced efficacy in these patients. In the genetic subgroup analysis of the TRITON TIMI 38 trial, prasugrel and clopidogrel had similar outcomes in patients with normal CYP2C19 alleles. In contrast, the benefit of prasugrel was much greater in patients with abnormal CYP2C19 alleles (NNT16) compared to overall trial (NNT50). A similar trend was noted for ticagrelor in the genetic subgroup analysis of the PLATO trial. Taken together, these trials suggest that the benefits of prasugrel and ticagrelor are most pronounced in patients with abnormal CYP2C19 alleles with clopidogrel. However, for the remaining 65% to 75% of the ACS population, clopidogrel may be as effective, safer, easier to use, and more cost effective. Whether a tailored strategy based on genotype or platelet function testing is safe and effective with improved value is unknown and randomized trials are warranted.

BETA BLOCKERS

Oral β-blockers are recommended *within 24 hours* of presentation for patients with STEMI (Class I, LOE B) and NSTE-ACS (Class I, LOE A) and should be continued at discharge. β-Blockers decrease heart rate, contractility, blood pressure, and myocardial oxygen consumption. While *early* β-blockers do not reduce short-term mortality in patients with ACS, they decrease ischemia, reinfarction, and ventricular arrhythmia. Furthermore, β-blockers improve long-term survival in patients with MI complicated by heart failure and ventricular arrhythmia. The long-term duration of routine β-blocker therapy after myocardial infarction without heart failure or hypertension has not been prospectively addressed, but guidelines recommend a 3-year treatment course then reassess the clinical need for the medication. Meta-analysis from the reperfusion era suggests β-blockers can reduce MI (RR 0.72 [95% CI, 0.62-0.83], NNT = 209) and angina (RR 0.80 [95% CI, 0.65-0.98], NNT = 26) at the expense of increased heart failure (RR 1.1 [95% CI, 1.05-1.16], NNH = 79) and increased cardiogenic shock (RR 1.29 [95% CI, 1.18-1.41], NNH = 90) with no significant impact on mortality. While oral β-blockers are an important part of ACS management, IV β-blockers should usually be avoided as they increase the risk for shock (Class III, LOE B). In addition, oral β-blockers are contraindicated in patients with signs of acute heart failure, evidence of low-output state, increased risk for cardiogenic shock, second- or third-degree heart block, and active asthma. When β-blockers are contraindicated due to asthma exacerbation, then nondihyophyidine calcium channel blockers could be considered as long there are no contraindications (Class I, LOE B).

RENIN-ANGIOTENSIN-ALDOSTERONE SYSTEM INHIBITORS

Angiotensin Converting Enzyme (ACE) inhibitors have been shown to lower mortality in patients with recent myocardial infarction and reduced left ventricular ejection fractions (LVEF) less than 40% (Class I, LOE A). Furthermore, ACE inhibitors should be strongly considered in patients with diabetes mellitus and stable chronic kidney disease (Class I, LOE A). In patients who are intolerant to ACE inhibitors, angiotensin receptor blockers (ARBs) should be considered. While meta-analyses suggest a small (0.48% absolute, NNT = 208) reduction in 30-day mortality with ACE inhibitors in ACS, the clinical significance of this finding is unclear and ACE inhibitor should be used with caution without the above indications given the risk for renal dysfunction and hypotension.

Aldosterone antagonists (eg, eplerenone, spironolactone) are recommended for patients with AMI and LVEF less than or equal to 40% (Class I, LOE B). In the EPHESUS (Eplerenone Post-Acute Myocardial Infarction Heart Failure Efficacy and Survival) study, demonstrated significantly reduced rates of death from cardiovascular causes or hospitalization for cardiovascular events (relative risk, 0.87; 95% CI, 0.79-0.95; $P = 0.002$, NNT = 30) in patients with eplerenone initiated within days of admission.

HIGH-INTENSITY STATIN THERAPY

High-intensity statin therapy should be given to all patients with ACS without contraindications (Class I, LOE A). Statins should be started at moderate to high doses as soon as possible on admission and continued indefinitely. The benefits of statin therapy are well known in the primary prevention for high-risk patients and in secondary prevention for patients with CAD. There may also be an early acute benefit in patients with NSTE-ACS. Several studies have demonstrated reduced rates of periprocedural MI with high-dose statin loading before PCI; therefore, a statin is recommended before PCI when possible (Class IIa, LOE A for statin naive).

ANTICOAGULATION USE WITH ANTIPLATELET THERAPY IN ACS

The choice of stent, P2Y12 antagonist, duration of dual antiplatelet therapy, and anticoagulant is important for patients that require anticoagulation after ACS. This includes patients with atrial fibrillation, venous thromboembolism, mechanical heart valves, and left ventricular thrombus. When anticoagulation is warranted, warfarin is the most common anticoagulant agent and clopidogrel and aspirin the most common antiplatelet agents used. Very little data support the safety of the novel anticoagulants and P2Y12 inhibitors in this setting. In addition, patients with a history of gastrointestinal bleeding who require anticoagulation and antiplatelet therapy should also receive proton pump inhibitors (PPIs) (Class I, LOE C). A PPI can also be considered in patients without history of gastrointestinal bleeding when anticoagulation and antiplatelet therapy are warranted (Class IIa, LOE C). While there were early concerns over potential interactions with certain PPIs and clopidogrel metabolism, more recent registry and randomized trials suggest reductions in bleeding complications without increased cardiac events with the combination of PPIs and clopidogrel.

Triple therapy (aspirin, clopidogrel, and warfarin) after PCI is associated with two- to fivefold greater risk of major bleeding compared to dual antiplatelet therapy. Recent studies suggest that aspirin can often be omitted when anticoagulation is warranted after PCI. In the 573 patient randomized WOEST trial, omission of aspirin decreased major bleeding complications (44.4% vs 19.4%, NNH [by adding aspirin] 4, $p < 0.0001$) without any increase in ischemic events. Similar findings were noted in a meta-analysis of 1263 patients from six randomized trials as well as a larger real world registry of 12,165 patients undergoing PCI requiring anticoagulation.

Left ventricular (LV) mural thrombus is found in 3% to 15% of anterior MIs treated with percutaneous coronary revascularization. Pooled studies have noted a fivefold increased risk for systemic embolism with LV thrombus after anterior MI, and anticoagulation therapy decreases this embolic risk. Thus, anticoagulation is recommended for patients with acute MI and asymptomatic LV mural thrombus (Class IIa, LOE C). Anticoagulation after anterior MI without mural thrombus formation is controversial. Currently, the guidelines suggest that anticoagulation therapy may be considered for patients with STEMI and anterior apical akinesis or dyskinesis (IIb, LOE C). However, in a recent retrospective analysis of 460 undergoing PCI for anterior MI without LV thrombus, anticoagulation was actually associated with an increased incidence of stroke (3.1% vs 0.3%, $p = 0.02$), major bleeding (8.5% vs 1.8%, $p < 0.0001$), mortality (5.4% vs 1.5%, $p = 0.04$), length of stay, and readmissions. Furthermore, after propensity matching, anticoagulation was still associated with a fourfold greater incidence of net adverse cardiac events. These findings certainly question the routine use of triple therapy in this population without LV thrombus. Until larger randomized trials are conducted, if anticoagulation is used in this setting, clinicians should probably omit aspirin, add proton pump inhibitors, target lower INR ranges, shorten the anticoagulation course (3 months), and use radial access when possible.

■ SECONDARY PREVENTION

All patients with ACS should be referred to a comprehensive cardiovascular rehabilitation program (Class I, LOE B). These programs provide patient education, regular exercise, monitor risk factors, and address lifestyle modification. The pneuomococcal vaccine is recommended for patients 65 years and older and high-risk patients with cardiovascular disease (Class I, LOE B). In addition, annual influenza vaccination is recommended for all patients with ACS (Class I, LOE C), and based on randomized controlled trial data has been shown to reduce MACE (NNT = 17) and hospitalization for ACS (NNT = 31). NSAIDs have been associated with increased cardiovascular risk and should largely be avoided in patients with ACS (Class III, LOE B). For patients with chronic musculoskeletal pain, acetaminophen, nonacetylated salicylates, tramadol, or low dose narcotics should be used as required (Class I, LOE C). If NSAIDs are required when these therapies are insufficient, then the nonselective naproxen is preferred over other NSAIDS (Class IIa, LOE C).

PRACTICE POINT

Late Hospital ACS Care and Hospital Discharge

- All patients with ACS should be discharged with dual antiplatelet therapy.
  - Options for P2Y12 antagonists include clopidogrel, prasugrel, and ticagrelor after PCI.
  - Options for P2Y12 antagonists include clopidogrel and ticagrelor with medical management without PCI.
- All patients with ACS should receive high-intensity statin therapy.
- All patients with MI should receive oral β-blocker therapy for at least 3 years after myocardial infarction and indefinitely for patients with congestive heart failure and/or hypertension.
- All patients with reduced LVEF ≤ 40% should receive an ACEI or ARB and aldosterone antagonist unless contraindications.
- When anticoagulation is warranted in patients with PCI for ACS, warfarin is preferred and aspirin can usually be omitted.
- All patients should be counseled about smoking cessation, diet, and exercise.
- All patients should be referred to cardiac rehabilitation programs at discharge.

Discharge checklist

- Dual antiplatelet therapy
- High-intensity statin
- Referral to cardiac rehabilitation
- Smoking cessation education
- β-Blocker if myocardial infarction and no contraindications
- ACE inhibitor (or ARB) if diabetic, chronic renal failure, or LVEF≤40% and no contraindications
- Aldosterone inhibitor if LVEF≤40% and no contraindications

SUGGESTED READINGS

American Heart Association's Mission: Lifeline: http://www.heart.org/HEARTORG/HealthcareResearch/MissionLifelineHomePage/Mission-Lifeline-Home-Page_UCM_305495_SubHomePage.jsp

Amsterdam EA, Wenger NK, Brindis RG, et al. AHA/ACC Guideline for the Management of Patients with Non-ST-Elevation Acute Coronary Syndromes: a report of the American College of Cardiology/American Heart Association Task Force on Practice Guidelines. *J Am Coll Cardiol*. 2014;64(24):e139-e228.

Bangalore S, Makani H, Radford M. Clinical outcomes with β-blockers for myocardial infarction: a meta-analysis of randomized trials. *Am J Med*. 2014;127(10):939-953.

Dewilde WJ, Oirbans T, Verheugh FW, et al. Use of clopidogrel with or without aspirin in patients taking oral anticoagulant therapy and undergoing percutaneous coronary intervention: an open-label, randomized, controlled trial. *Lancet*. 2013;381:1107-1115.

Jolly SS, Yusuf S, Cairns J, et al. Radial versus femoral access for coronary angiography and intervention in patients with acute coronary syndromes (RIVAL): a randomized, parallel group, multicenter trial. *Lancet*. 2011;377:1409-1420.

Keller T, Zeller T, Peetz D, et al. Sensitive troponin I assay in early diagnosis of acute myocardial infarction. *N Engl J Med*. 2009;361(9):868-877.

McDaniel M, Ross M, Rab ST, et al. A comprehensive acute coronary syndrome algorithm for centers with percutaneous coronary intervention capability. *Crit Pathw Cardiol*. 2013;12(3):141-149.

Naghavi M, Libby P, Falk E, et al. From vulnerable plaque to vulnerable patient: a call for new definitions and risk assessment strategies: Part I. *Circulation*. 2003;108(14):1664-1672.

O'Gara PT, Kushner FG, Ascheim DD, et al. ACCF/AHA guideline for the management of ST-elevation myocardial infarction: a report of the American College of Cardiology Foundation/American Heart Association Task Force on Practice Guidelines. *J Am Coll Cardiol*. 2013;61(4):e78-e140.

Osborne AD, Ali K, Lowery-North D, et al. Ability of triage decision rules for rapid electrocardiogram to identify patients with suspected ST-elevation myocardial infarction. *Crit Pathw Cardiology*. 2012;11:211-213.

Panju AA, Hemmelgarn BR, Guyatt GH. The rational clinical examination. Is this patient having a myocardial infarction? *JAMA*. 1998;280(14):1256-1263.

Rab T, Kern KB, Tamis-Holland JE. Interventional Council, American College of Cardiology. Cardiac arrest: atreatment algorithm for emergent invasive cardiac procedures in the resuscitated comatose patient. *J Am Coll Cardiol*. 2015;66(1):62-73.

CHAPTER 129

Heart Failure

Omar Wever-Pinzon, MD
James C. Fang, MD, FACC

Key Clinical Questions

Heart Failure With Reduced Ejection Fraction (HFrEF)

1. What is the definition and classification of HF?
2. What is the mortality and morbidity of HF?
3. What is the recommended testing for a patient with newly diagnosed HF?
4. What are the standard therapies for HF?
5. How can we remove congestion in HF?

HF With Preserved Ejection Fraction (HFpEF)

1. How do you diagnose HF?
2. What are the predisposing risk factors for HFpEF?
3. What is the recommended evaluation for patients newly diagnosed with HF?
4. How do you treat HF?

HEART FAILURE WITH REDUCED EJECTION FRACTION (HFrEF)

■ EPIDEMIOLOGY/OVERVIEW

Heart failure (HF) is a condition that affects nearly 6 million people in the United States and 870,000 people are newly diagnosed each year. Its incidence increases with age, with rates approaching 10 per 1000 people after 65 years of age. Heart failure is a leading cause of hospital admissions in the United States and is responsible for over half a million emergency room visits, 1 million admissions and nearly 2 million office visits annually. Over the past decade, the rate of hospital admissions with a primary diagnosis of HF has remained elevated. After a hospital admission for HF, 25% of patients will be readmitted within a month, 50% within 6 months. Those at highest risk have an inpatient mortality as high as 20% to 25%.

The incidence and absolute number of HF deaths has continued to increase steadily (despite advances in HF therapy), in part due to aging of the population and improved survival after acute myocardial infarction (MI). Despite improvements in HF survival, mortality remains high; 50% of patients with HF will die within 5 years of the diagnosis. Approximately, 300,000 patients die of HF in the United States each year. The estimated direct and indirect cost of HF is $30.7 billion per year, and this total cost is expected to increase to 70 billion in the next 15 years.

The socioeconomic impact and significant burden that HF imposes on health care systems have led to the development of initiatives to reduce health care costs and improve patient outcomes. For example, the *American Heart Association (AHA) Get With The Guidelines–Heart Failure* Program is a collaborative quality improvement registry designed to improve adherence to evidence-based HF care of hospitalized patients, which has resulted in improved outcomes (eg, a reduction in 30-day readmission rates). The HF achievement measures of this program include:

- Angiotensin-converting enzyme (ACE) inhibitor or angiotensin receptor blocker (ARB) at discharge
- Evidence-based use of specific β-blockers
- Measurement of left ventricular (LV) function
- Postdischarge appointment for HF patients

In addition, The Joint Commission on Accreditation of Health care Organizations has developed core measures for advanced certification in the management of HF (**Table 129-1**).

■ PATHOPHYSIOLOGY

Heart failure is a complex clinical syndrome that can result from any structural or functional cardiac disorder that impairs the ability of the ventricle to fill or eject blood and maintain metabolic demands of the body. The signs and symptoms of HF include dyspnea, fatigue, exercise intolerance, abdominal bloating, early satiety, and peripheral edema. The nonspecific nature of these findings can make diagnosis challenging.

Heart failure may result from disorders of the pericardium, heart valves, myocardium, or coronary circulation as well as rhythm disturbances. The majority of patients have symptoms due to an impairment of LV myocardial function, with or without a reduced ejection fraction. The etiologies for LV dysfunction are broad, with coronary artery disease being the leading cause in developed countries (**Table 129-2**).

TABLE 129-1 Performance Measures for Advanced Certification in HF

Inpatient

1. Beta-blocker therapy (ie, Bisoprolol, Carvedilol, or sustained release Metoprolol Succinate prescribed for LVSD) at discharge
2. Postdischarge appointment for HF patients
3. Care transition record transmitted
4. Discussion of advance directives/advance care planning
5. Advance directive executed
6. Postdischarge evaluation for HF patients

Outpatient*

1. Hospital Outpatient Beta-blocker therapy (ie, Bisoprolol, Carvedilol, or sustained release Metoprolol Succinate prescribed for LVSD)
2. Hospital outpatient ACEI or ARB prescribed for LVSD
3. Hospital outpatient aldosterone receptor antagonist prescribed for LVSD
4. Hospital outpatient NYHA classification assessment
5. Hospital outpatient activity recommendations
6. Hospital outpatient discussion of advance directives/advance care planning
7. Hospital outpatient advance directive executed

*Reporting of outpatient core measures is optional, but highly encouraged. ACEI: Angiotensin-converting enzyme inhibitor; ARB: Angiotensin receptor blocker; LVSD: Left ventricular systolic dysfunction; NYHA: New York Heart Association.

Heart failure is generally a progressive disorder following an insult or stress to the myocardium, resulting in impaired diastolic and systolic ventricular performance and abnormal hemodynamics (eg, volume and pressure overload). Over time, the acute physiologic compensatory responses to myocardial dysfunction remain unchecked and lead to myocyte hypertrophy and apoptosis, myocardial fibrosis, and changes in calcium cycling. These cellular

TABLE 129-2 Etiologies of Left Ventricular Systolic Dysfunction

Coronary artery disease

Idiopathic dilated cardiomyopathy

Familial cardiomyopathy

Neuromuscular disorders (eg, muscular dystrophies)

Chagas cardiomyopathy

Toxins (eg, alcohol, cocaine)

Medications (eg, adriamycin)

Diabetes mellitus

Myocarditis (lymphocytic, hypersensitivity, giant cell)

Infiltrative (amyloidosis, sarcoidosis, hemochromatosis)

Metabolic disorders (hypothyroidism)

Peripartum

Untreated valvular heart disease (aortic stenosis or regurgitation, mitral regurgitation)

Tachyarrhythmias (atrial and/or ventricular arrhythmias)

Autoimmune disorders (lupus, rheumatoid arthritis)

Hypertension

and molecular changes result in increases in LV mass and size as well as changes in LV geometry and shape, collectively referred to as cardiac remodeling. These processes further increase hemodynamic wall stress causing a progressive decline in myocardial mechanical performance and ventricular enlargement in a vicious cycle. In some cases, the remodeling process produces functional incompetence of the mitral valve and valvular regurgitation. Mitral regurgitation leads to decreased forward stroke volume, elevated pulmonary venous pressure, increased wall stress, and ultimately more remodeling.

The acute response to a decline in LV performance is mediated through activation of numerous neurohormonal systems (in particular, the renin-angiotensin-aldosterone and adrenergic systems) to provide short-term hemodynamic stabilization. Elegant studies in HF have demonstrated elevated circulating or tissue levels of norepinephrine, angiotensin II, aldosterone, endothelin, vasopressin, and cytokines. However, when chronically stimulated, these systems act to adversely affect cardiac structure and function as described above. Neurohormonal activation also exacerbates the hemodynamic stress on the myocardium through sodium and fluid retention and peripheral vasoconstriction. This vicious cycle leads to the progression of HF and subsequent worsening of symptoms, development of arrhythmias, and ultimate death.

The ACCF/AHA task force developed a classification scheme outlining four stages in the evolution of the HF syndrome (**Figure 129-1**), resembling the cancer paradigm. This scheme recognizes cardiovascular risk factors, structural cardiac abnormalities, asymptomatic and symptomatic phases, and appropriate therapeutic interventions at each stage.

Acute decompensated HF (formerly "congestive HF" or ADHF) is often used to describe the HF state when there is an exacerbation of HF symptoms in the setting of clinically evident volume overload with or without a decrease in perfusion. This condition usually leads to an encounter with health care providers in the form of unplanned visits to the clinic or emergency room, resulting in hospitalization. In this setting, the volume overload leads to an elevation in left ventricular end-diastolic pressure as well as pulmonary venous and arterial hypertension. If the process occurs rapidly and/or associated with massive volume overload, the net result may be transudation of excess fluid into the alveolar spaces, leading to decreased diffusing capacity, hypoxemia, and shortness of breath. Inadequate cardiac output and poor end organ perfusion may also complicate ADHF and is a poor prognostic feature.

■ DIAGNOSIS

Clinical manifestations vary among individuals but the HF diagnosis can usually be established at the bedside. The chronicity, severity, and degree of hemodynamic decompensation as well as patient specific factors such as age, gender, and other comorbidities influence both signs and symptoms. However, clinical signs and symptoms of HF lack sensitivity and specificity. It should be noted that surprisingly, exercise intolerance does not correlate with LV dysfunction as assessed by ejection fraction. The New York Heart Association (NYHA) functional classification is often used to assess exercise tolerance and should be determined in the ambulatory and compensated state. By definition, the patient hospitalized for ADHF is NYHA class IV.

I = No symptoms
II = Symptoms with moderate or marked levels of activity
III = Symptoms with mild activity
IV = Symptoms at rest

Elevated left ventricular end-diastolic pressures are responsible for "congestive" symptoms such as shortness of breath, cough,

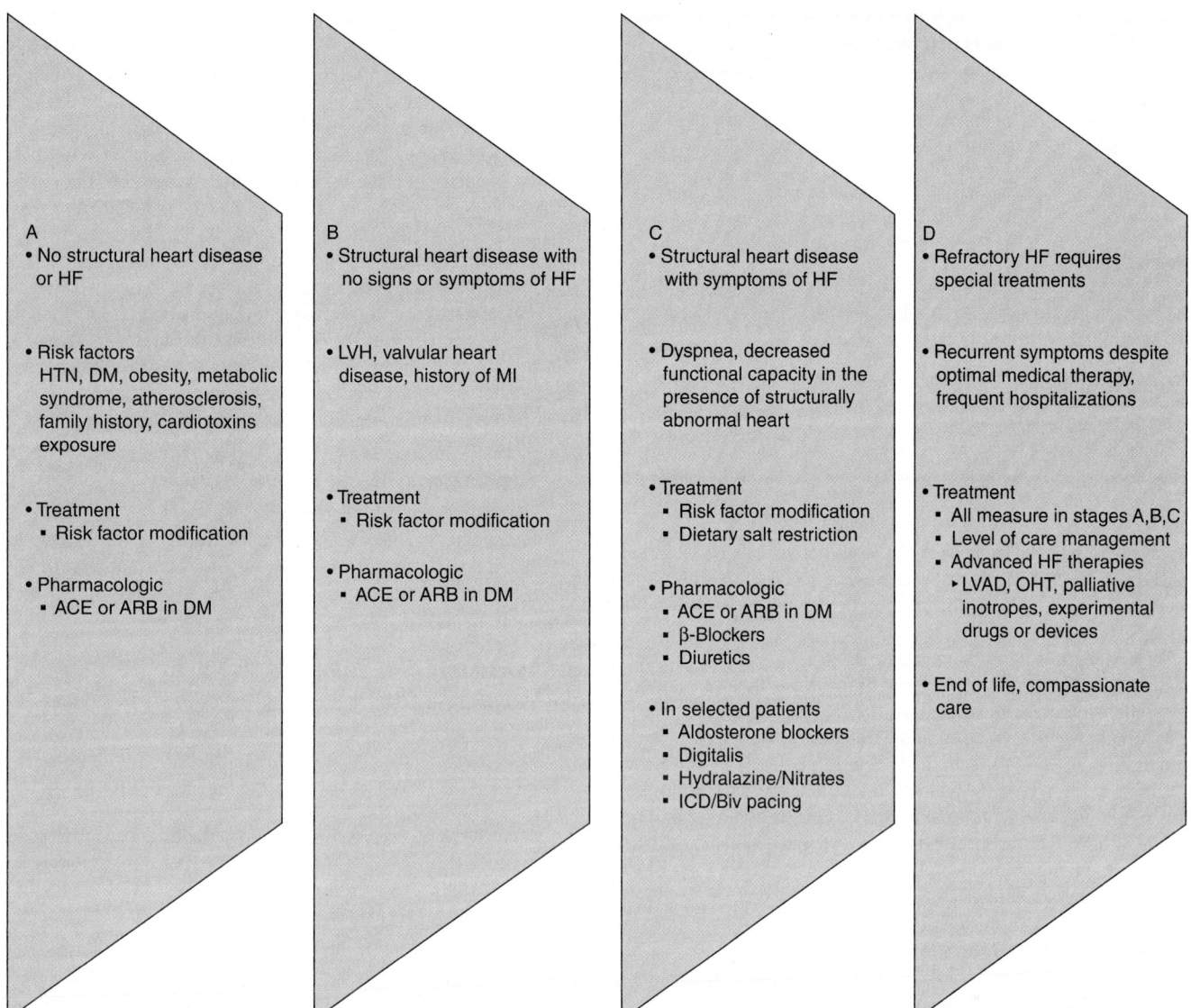

Figure 129-1 *Stages in the development of heart failure/recommended therapy by stage. ACEI, angiotensin-converting enzyme inhibitor; ARB, angiotensin II receptor blocker; EF, ejection fraction; FHx CM, family history of cardiomyopathy; HF, heart failure; LV, left ventricular; LVH, left ventricular hypertrophy; and MI, myocardial infarction.*

orthopnea, paroxysmal nocturnal dyspnea, and peripheral edema. Early satiety, right upper quadrant tenderness, and anorexia may be subtle signs of volume overload. A reduced cardiac output may be manifest as easy fatigability, mental status changes, nausea, and/or a decrease in exercise tolerance. Bendopnea, or dyspnea with bending forward, may be present when there is significant volume overload in the presence of decreased cardiac output. Angina may be present in both ischemic and nonischemic cardiomyopathies. A search for potential precipitating causes (eg, arrhythmias, use of nonsteroidal medications, variable medication, and dietary compliance) should also be explored upon presentation.

A detailed physical examination is the cornerstone of the evaluation of patients with HF. The examination should focus on determining the hemodynamic status along two axes: degree of volume overload ("wet" or "dry") and adequacy of perfusion ("warm" or "cold"). Almost all patients with ADHF should have evidence of volume overload. Findings consistent with fluid overload include elevated jugular venous pressure, hepatojugular reflux, gallops (S_3 and S_4), murmurs of tricuspid or mitral regurgitation, pulmonary rales, hepatomegaly, ascites, and edema. The presence of peripheral edema and pulmonary rales, although relatively specific, is not

sensitive and may be absent. A narrow pulse pressure, cool extremities, altered mentation, Cheyne-Stokes respiration, and resting tachycardia may suggest a reduction in cardiac output. Hypotension may indicate severe ventricular dysfunction and impending cardiogenic shock. The etiology of cardiac dysfunction may also be apparent on exam (eg, peripheral stigmata of atherosclerosis) although one should entertain a broad differential diagnosis (**Table 129-3**).

Electrocardiogram, full laboratory assessment, and a chest x-ray should be performed in all patients presenting with HF. Echocardiography is also critical in the initial evaluation of patients with new onset HF to obtain information on left ventricular wall thickness, end-diastolic and end-systolic dimensions, right ventricular function, ejection fraction, valvular and pericardial disease. Serial assessments may be useful after optimizing medical and device therapy or a change in clinical status. Echocardiography can also be used to complement the bedside assessment of the hemodynamic profile.

Brain natriuretic peptide (BNP) or N-terminal pro-BNP (NT-proBNP) (secreted by the ventricles in response to wall stress) can be useful when the diagnosis in patients presenting with dyspnea is uncertain. Natriuretic peptides have good negative predictive values to exclude HF and can also provide prognostic information if HF is

TABLE 129-3 Mimickers of Heart Failure

Myocardial ischemia

Pulmonary disease (pneumonia, asthma, chronic obstructive pulmonary disease, pulmonary embolus, pulmonary arterial hypertension)

Sleep disordered breathing

Obesity

Malnutrition

Hepatic failure

Renal failure

Hypoalbuminemia

Venous insufficiency

Depression and deconditioning

Pericardial disease

confirmed. Their use to guide therapy has not yet been established and is under active investigation. Screening for sleep disorders, HIV, rheumatologic disorders, and pheochromocytoma are reasonable in select situations.

Coronary angiography should be performed in patients presenting with new onset HF, especially if they have angina or evidence for ischemia (eg, EKG changes, positive troponins), unless they are not candidates for revascularization. Coronary angiography is rarely indicated in ADHF in the setting of known chronic HF. Endomyocardial biopsy is reserved for patients in whom a specific diagnosis is suspected (eg, hemochromatosis, amyloidosis, sarcoidosis); routine biopsy is not recommended. Right heart catheterization may also be useful if the hemodynamic profile is not apparent from the history and physical examination.

■ TRIAGE AND INITIAL MANAGEMENT

At initial triage, the cause for decompensation (**Table 129-4**) should be explored and the hemodynamic profile should be defined by using the physical examination and history. As noted above, the hemodynamic profile can be described as one of four states on the basis of a 2 × 2 matrix: volume status (overload ["wet"] or euvolemic ["dry"]) and perfusion or cardiac output (well perfused ["warm"] or low output ["cold"]) (**Figure 129-2**). The hemodynamic profile provides both prognostic information and a basis for an initial treatment plan. Compensated patients (eg, warm and dry) have a good short-term prognosis and rarely require admission; decompensated patients with signs and symptoms of congestion and hypoperfusion (eg, wet and cold) have an extremely poor prognosis.

TABLE 129-4 Precipitating Factors in Acute Decompensated Heart Failure

Acute coronary syndrome

Uncontrolled hypertension

Acute arrhythmia (ventricular or supraventricular)

Valvular heart disease

Acute severe myocarditis

Medical or dietary noncompliance

Infections

Perioperative volume resuscitation

Drug or alcohol abuse

Initial laboratory evaluation of patients with ADHF should include complete blood count, urinalysis, serum electrolytes (including calcium and magnesium), blood urea nitrogen, serum creatinine, fasting blood glucose, liver function tests, thyroid function tests, and cardiac biomarkers. As described above, measurement of natriuretic peptides should be considered. Elevations of troponin are common and are generally not due to acute coronary syndromes but rather to chronic myocardial injury seen in chronic heart failure. A twelve-lead electrocardiogram should be obtained to assess for rhythm, conduction system abnormalities, and acute ischemic changes. A chest x-ray is useful and should be examined for cardiomegaly, pulmonary congestion, and concomitant pulmonary disorders such as pneumonia or chronic obstructive pulmonary disease.

A risk stratification tool developed from the Acute Decompensated National Registry identified the following variables as predicting increased risk for in-hospital mortality from ADHF:

- Blood urea nitrogen >43 mg/dL
- Admission systolic blood pressure <115 mm Hg
- Serum creatinine >2.75 mg/dL

Other parameters associated with poor clinical outcomes include age, HF etiology (eg, ischemic cardiomyopathy has poorer prognosis), anemia, hyponatremia, B-type natriuretic peptide levels, and inability to tolerate ACE inhibitors and/or β-blockers.

■ TREATMENT AND COMPLICATIONS

The management of ADHF can be divided into two temporal periods: (1) the acute period when identifying precipitating factors, improving symptoms and addressing the role of comorbidities in the acute decompensation are the priorities and (2) the transition time to the outpatient setting which is directed at preserving functional capacity, preventing rehospitalizations, and improving long-term survival.

■ ACUTE MANAGEMENT OF ADHF

Most patients presenting with ADHF will be volume overloaded yet adequately perfused (so-called wet and warm). The relief of congestion is therefore a predominant goal of acute therapy.

Intravenous **loop diuretics** (eg, furosemide) will produce a diuresis and are accompanied by a decrease in filling pressures with subsequent relief of dyspnea (**Table 129-5**). Intravenous loop diuretics may also exert a vasodilatory effect. The dose of diuretic should generally be doubled from the outpatient setting to achieve a sufficient timely improvement in symptoms.

The peak diuretic effect occurs 30 minutes after administration and should be titrated to response. The administration of a thiazide diuretic, such as metolazone, 30 minutes prior to a dose of furosemide can potentiate its effect. Continuous infusions may be considered but are comparable in effect to properly dosed bolus treatment. Overly rapid diuresis with an excessive rapid reduction in intravascular volume may result in symptomatic hypotension and/or worsening renal function.

Morphine may be useful because it induces vasodilatation and relieves breathlessness as well as anxiety. **Supplemental oxygen** should be initiated and pulse oximetry monitored. Noninvasive positive pressure ventilation, if necessary for acute respiratory failure, has been associated with a reduction in the need for tracheal intubation and mechanical ventilation.

Vasodilator therapy should be initiated in the absence of symptomatic hypotension. Short-acting angiotensin-converting enzyme inhibitors, angiotensin receptor blockers, or hydralazine are the drugs of choice in most situations. Intravenous vasodilator therapy may be considered if rapid improvement of congestive symptoms is needed but requires close hemodynamic monitoring, ideally in an ICU setting. **Nitrates** decrease systemic and pulmonary

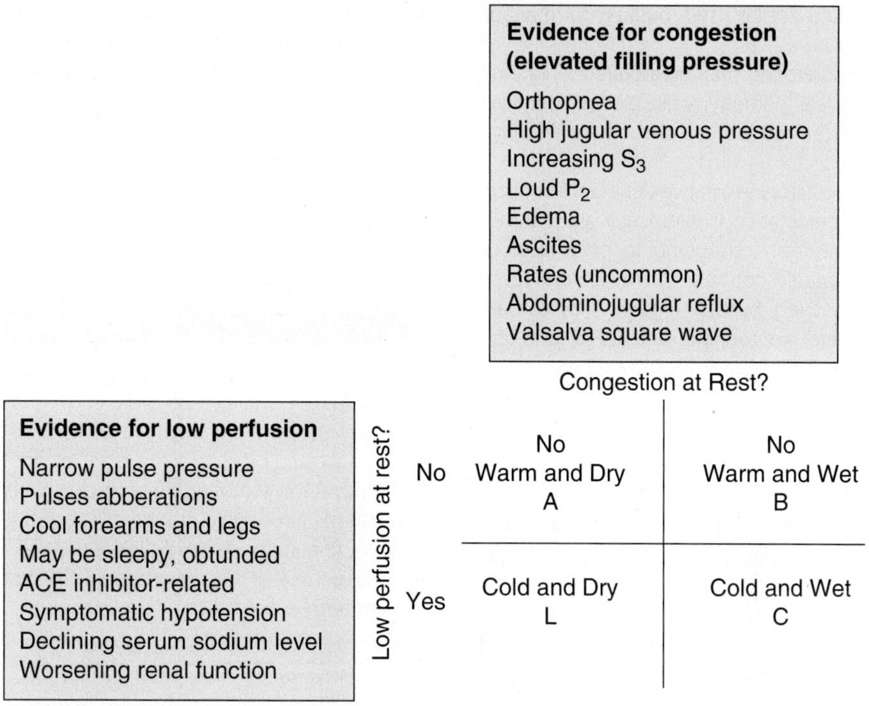

**Evidence for congestion
(elevated filling pressure)**

Orthopnea
High jugular venous pressure
Increasing S_3
Loud P_2
Edema
Ascites
Rates (uncommon)
Abdominojugular reflux
Valsalva square wave

Congestion at Rest?

Evidence for low perfusion

Narrow pulse pressure
Pulses abberations
Cool forearms and legs
May be sleepy, obtunded
ACE inhibitor-related
Symptomatic hypotension
Declining serum sodium level
Worsening renal function

Low perfusion at rest?	Congestion at Rest? No	Congestion at Rest? Yes
No	Warm and Dry A	Warm and Wet B
Yes	Cold and Dry L	Cold and Wet C

Diagram indicating 2 x 2 table of hemodynamic profiles for patients presenting with heart failure. Most patients can be classified in a 2-min bedside assessment according to the signs and symptoms shown although in practice some patients may be on the border between the warm-and-wet and cold-and-wet profiles. This classification helps guide initial therapy and prognosis for patients presenting with advanced heart failure. Although most patients presenting with hypoperfusion also have elevated filling pressure (cold and wet profile), many patients present with elevated filling pressures without major reduction in perfusion (warm and wet profile). Patients presenting with symptoms of heart failure at rest or minimal exertion without clinical evidence of elevated filling pressures or hypoperfusion (warm and dry profile) should be carefully evaluated to determine whether their symptoms result from heart failure.

Figure 129-2 *Hemodynamic profiles in heart failure. (Reprinted, with permission, from Nohria A, Lewis E, Stevenson WL. Medical management of advanced heart failure. JAMA. 2002;287(5):628-640. Copyright 2002 American Medical Association. All rights reserved.)*

TABLE 129-5 Suggested Diuretic Dosing in Heart Failure

Drug	Initial Dose	Maximum Daily Doses
Loop diuretics		
Bumetanide	1 mg	5-10 mg
Torsemide	20 mg	100-200 mg
Furosemide	40 mg	160-320 mg
Thiazide diuretics*		
Hydrochlorothiazide	25 mg	100 mg
Chlorothiazide	250-500 mg IV once or twice daily plus loop diuretic	
Metolazone	2.5-10 mg orally once or twice daily with loop diuretic	
IV continuous infusion		
Bumetanide	1 mg IV load then 0.5-1 mg/h	
Torsemide	20 mg IV load then 5-10 mg/h	
Furosemide	20-80 mg IV load then 5-20 mg/h	

*Given 30 min before loop diuretic to augment diuresis.

vascular pressures and are also coronary vasodilators. **Nitroprusside** is indicated when there is a need for acute combined afterload and preload reduction (hypertensive emergency, acute aortic regurgitation, acute mitral regurgitation). **Nesiritide** has venous, arterial, and modest coronary vasodilatory properties that reduce preload and afterload and has no direct inotropic effects. It is currently approved for the acute relief of dyspnea in the patient with ADHF. Because of its hypotensive effects, it should be used only at recommended doses and with caution.

Tolvaptan is a vasopressin V2 receptor antagonist that was evaluated in a large randomized controlled trial (EVEREST) program of patients hospitalized with HF. It failed to show a reduction in the dual endpoints of all-cause mortality and cardiovascular death or HF hospitalization. However, it significantly reduced dyspnea, body weight, edema and improved hyponatremia compared with placebo at a dose of 30 mg per day. Tolvaptan is approved by the Food and Drug Administration for the management of severe and/or symptomatic hyponatremia in patients with HF. Careful monitoring of liver function is required.

Intravenous inotropic agents (dobutamine, milrinone, dopamine) can be considered where there is evidence for systemic hypoperfusion (eg, hypotension, impaired renal function) with or without pulmonary edema refractory to the above treatment modalities. The benefit of hemodynamic improvement may outweigh the risk of arrhythmias and increase in oxygen demand caused by these agents. The use of these agents may require surveillance in intensive units. However, these agents should only be used for short-term circulatory support and should not be used routinely for management of ADHF.

Invasive hemodynamic monitoring may be required in carefully selected situations (eg, unclear hemodynamic picture, medically refractory hypotension) but the routine use of such monitoring is not recommended.

Temporary mechanical circulatory assistance (intra-aortic balloon counterpulsation pump or percutaneous ventricular assist device) may be indicated in patients not responding to pharmacologic therapy when there is reasonable potential for myocardial recovery with specific interventions (eg, bypass surgery). They can also be considered to help "bridge" appropriate patients to long-term mechanical circulatory support or cardiac transplantation.

Continuous electrocardiographic monitoring is recommended during ADHF.

■ SUPRAVENTRICULAR ARRHYTHMIAS (SVTs)

Supraventricular arrhythmias often complicate the course of patients with HF. In particular, atrial fibrillation and flutter are common and affect 10% to 30% of HF patients. It may occur as a primary disorder or secondary to the heart failure syndrome. Atrial arrhythmias are associated with a decrease in exercise capacity and worse long-term prognosis. Atrial fibrillation/flutter is poorly tolerated in HF due to the following:

1. The loss of atrial-ventricular synchrony and the atrial "kick," which may account for 15% to 20% of the cardiac output.
2. Rapid ventricular rates increase myocardial oxygen demand and decrease coronary perfusion.
3. Rapid ventricular rates impair ventricular relaxation and diastolic filling.
4. Blood stasis in fibrillating atria predisposes to systemic and pulmonary embolism.

The primary management strategy for atrial arrhythmias complicating ADHF is to control the ventricular rate and to provide anticoagulation to reduce thromboembolic complications. A target heart rate <110 beats/min is a reasonable goal. Rate control with β-blockers and digoxin should be considered, but overly aggressive β-blocker therapy may be poorly tolerated. Intravenous diltiazem is commonly used but may also be poorly tolerated, particularly when there is poor perfusion and/or presenting hypotension. Improvements in volume status alone or the use of vasodilators may decrease the rate of the ventricular response. Early involvement of a cardiovascular medicine specialist should be considered, since restoration of sinus rhythm (eg, cardioversion, antiarrhythmics, catheter ablation) may be of benefit in carefully selected patients.

■ RENAL INSUFFICIENCY

Renal insufficiency complicating HF management is known as the cardiorenal syndrome. Patients with HF often have baseline impaired renal function as a result of decreased renal perfusion, intrinsic renal disease, elevated central and renal vein pressure, neurohormonal activation, and/or drugs used to treat HF. Renal function may also acutely decline during treatment with diuretics and ACE inhibitors. Although these changes may be short-lived, asymptomatic and reversible, such declines in renal function often result in a prolonged hospitalization and portend a poor prognosis. As HF worsens, an accompanying decline in renal perfusion limits the ability of the kidneys to respond to diuretic therapy. In this situation, higher doses of diuretics and/or the addition of other diuretics with synergistic effects (eg, sequential nephron blockade) may be effective. Current studies suggest no significant advantage to the use of continuous intravenous diuretic regimens over intravenous bolus dosing, if appropriate dosing is used (eg, double the outpatient

dose). If diuretic management is ineffective or complicated by progressive renal insufficiency, mechanical fluid removal (ultrafiltration) may be considered in well-selected patients. Its routine use, however, is not supported by a limited number of randomized trials. Cardiovascular and renal consultation should be sought when cardiorenal syndrome is present. Right heart catheterization may be required to document poor cardiac output as the cause of the cardiorenal syndrome; in this setting, cardiovascular consultation is essential.

PRACTICE POINT

● Current studies suggest no significant advantage to the use of continuous intravenous diuretic regimens over intravenous bolus dosing. If diuretic management is ineffective or complicated by progressive renal insufficiency, mechanical fluid removal (ultrafiltration) may be considered in well-selected patients, although current data suggest that there is no benefit in terms of weight loss and renal function preservation in patients that are responsive to diuretics. Cardiovascular and renal consultation should be sought when cardiorenal syndrome is present.

■ CHRONIC MANAGEMENT

A crucial goal in the management of HF is optimizing the pharmacologic regimen in the chronic ambulatory state when the patient stabilizes. Goals shift to enhancing survival, minimizing symptoms and disability, improving functional capacity, and delaying disease progression. All patients should receive dietary instructions, including a daily sodium restriction of less than 2 to 3 g. Fluid restriction (eg, < 2 L per day) is generally recommended and is especially important in patients with hyponatremia (eg, serum sodium <135 mEq/L). Patients should record their weight on a daily basis and be given instructions for diuretic management when there is weight gain. See Figure 129-1 and below for recommended pharmacologic therapy by HF stage.

■ THERAPIES FOR HF WITH LEFT VENTRICULAR SYSTOLIC DYSFUNCTION

Diuretics treat the sodium and fluid retention of HF. Once a decompensated HF patient achieves a compensated volume status, an oral regimen using the lowest diuretic doses to maintain euvolemia should be determined. Possible and frequent complications of poorly monitored diuretic management include hypotension and worsening renal function.

ACE inhibitors are vasodilators and potent neurohormonal antagonists that have been shown to alleviate symptoms, improve clinical status, and reduce the risk of death and hospitalization and should be prescribed to all patients with HFrEF unless contraindicated (angioedema, pregnancy, significant renal artery stenosis, or hyperkalemia) (**Table 129-6**). Renal insufficiency (eg, serum creatinine >2.0-2.5 mg/dL) and cough are relative contraindications. Treatment with an ACE inhibitor should be initiated at low doses and gradually increased as tolerated to the target doses used in clinical trials (eg, captopril 50 mg three times a day, enalapril 10 mg twice a day, lisinopril 20 -40 mg daily). When excessive hypotension is a concern, short-acting ACE inhibitors should be considered with a transition to long-acting agents. Adverse effects of ACE inhibitors include hypotension, worsening renal function, hyperkalemia, cough, rash, leukopenia, dysgeusia, and angioedema. In patients who are hemodynamically or clinically unstable, it is recommended to interrupt treatment with the ACE inhibitors temporarily until the

TABLE 129-6 Selected Angiotensin-converting Enzyme Inhibitor Trials in Heart Failure

Clinical Trial	No. Patients	Inclusion	Study Drug	Initial Dosing	Target Dose	Relative Risk, Mortality
Save	2231	3 d post MI survivors with LVEF <40% without HF	Captopril	6.25 mg three times a day	50 mg three times a day	0.81 (0.68-0.97); $P = 0.019$
Consensus	253	NYHA IV Symptoms with heart size >600 mL/m²	Enalapril maleate	2.5 mg twice a day	10 mg twice a day	0.60; $P = 0.002$; power 90%
Solvd	2569	HF with LVEF <35%	Enalapril maleate	2.5 mg twice a day	10 mg twice a day	0.82 (0.74-0.95); $P < 0.0036$

patient stabilizes. **Angiotensin receptor blockers** should be used in patients who are ACE inhibitor intolerant (**Table 129-7**).

Neprilysin is a neutral endopeptidase that degrades endogenous vasoactive peptides, including natriuretic peptides, bradykinin, and adrenomudullin. Its inhibition counteracts the neurohormonal stimulation seen in HF that leads to vasoconstriction, sodium retention, and cardiac remodeling. The combination of the ARB, valsartan, and the neprilysin inhibitor, sacubitril (LCZ696), at 200 mg twice a day has recently been shown to be superior to enalapril 10 mg twice a day in reducing death from cardiovascular causes or hospitalization for HF (Table 129-7). It has not yet been established that a change to LCZ696 from either an ARB or an ACE inhibitor after an episode of ADHF is warranted.

β-blockers decrease the symptoms of HF as well as reduce the risk of death and hospitalization. β-blockers antagonize the sympathetic nervous system and thereby block the adverse consequences of adrenergic stimulation in HF. Three β-blockers have been shown to be effective in reducing the risk of death in patients with chronic HF: bisoprolol, sustained-release metoprolol succinate, and carvedilol. β-Blockers should be prescribed to all patients with stable compensated HFrEF unless they have a contraindication to their use (**Table 129-8**). β-Blocker therapy should be initiated once there is no or minimal evidence of fluid overload or volume depletion and no recent treatment with an intravenous positive inotropic agent.

Treatment with a β-blocker should be initiated at very low doses followed by gradual increments to target doses used in the clinical trials (eg, carvedilol 25-50 mg twice a day, metoprolol succinate 200 mg daily, bisoprolol 10 mg daily). Initiation of β-blockers can cause fluid retention, fatigue, bradycardia, heart block, and hypotension; therefore close monitoring and follow-up is necessary. If patients develop fluid retention with or without symptoms on β-blockers, the β-blocker can be continued while the dose of diuretic is increased. If a patient deteriorates to the point of hypoperfusion or the need for intravenous inotropic drugs, it is recommended to stop or reduce treatment with β-blockers temporarily until the patient stabilizes (Table 129-8).

Aldosterone receptor antagonists (spironolactone and eplerenone) have been shown to reduce mortality and hospitalizations and improve functional class in patients with advanced HF (spironolactone) as well as patients with HF after an acute MI (eplerenone). Addition of an aldosterone receptor antagonist is recommended in patients with NYHA class II to IV symptoms and HFrEF who can comply with laboratory monitoring to assess renal function and potassium concentration. Creatinine should be less than or equal to 2.5 mg/dL in men or less than or equal to 2.0 mg/dL in women (or estimated glomerular filtration rate >30 mL/min/1.73 m²) and the serum potassium should be less than 5.0 mEq/L in order to reduce the risk of hyperkalemia (**Table 129-9**).

TABLE 129-7 Selected Angiotensin-receptor Blocker Heart Failure Trials

Clinical Trial	No. Patients	Inclusion	Study Drug	Initial Dose	Target Dose	Relative Risk, Mortality
Val-Heft	5010	NYHA II-IV LVEF <40% EDD 2.9 cm.m²	Valsartan	40 mg twice a day	160 mg twice a day	1.02 (0.88-1.18); $P = 0.8$
CHARM-Added	2548	NYHA II-IV LVEF <40%	Candesartan	4-8 mg daily	32 mg daily	0.85 (0.75-0.96); $P = 0.011$
VALIANT	14,703	0.5-10 d post-MI with clinical or radiologic signs of HF and LVEF <35% by echo or <40 by LV gram	Valsartan	40 mg twice a day	160 mg twice a day	1.00 (0.90-1.11); $P = 0.98$
Paradigm-HF	8442	NYHA II-IV LVEF ≤40%	Valsartan + Sacubitril (LCZ696)	100 mg BID	200 mg BID	0.80 (0.73-0.87) $P < 0.001$ Combined endpoint of CV death or HF hospitalization

TABLE 129-8 β-Blocker Use in Heart Failure

Clinical Trial	No. Patients	Inclusion	Study Drug	Initial Dose	Target Dose	Relative Risk, Mortality
CIBIS II	2647	NYHA III-IV Symptomatic HF with EF <35%	Bisoprolol	1.25 mg daily	10 mg daily	RR 0.66 (0.54-0.81); $P < 0.0001$
Copernicus	2289	NYHA III-IV HF with EF <25%	Carvedilol	3.125 mg twice a day	25-50 mg twice a day	RR 0.65 (0.52-0.81); $P = 0.000013$
Comet	3029	NYHA II-IV Symptomatic EF <35%	Carvedilol	3.125 mg twice a day	25-50 mg twice a day	RR 0.83 (0.74-0.93); $P = 0.002$
US Carvedilol HF study	1094	NYHA II-III Mostly ischemic etiology	Carvedilol	3.125 mg twice a day	25-50 mg twice a day	RR 0.35 (0.20-0.61); $P < 0.001$
Merit HF	3991	NYHA II-IV Symptomatic HF with LEF <40%	Metoprolol succinate	12.5-25 mg/d	200 mg daily	RR 0.6 (0.53-0.81); $P < 0.001$

Ivabradine, a selective sinus node inhibitor, has been shown to reduce cardiovascular death or rehospitalization for HF in patients with symptomatic HF with an LVEF ≤35%, in normal sinus rhythm, who have a heart rate equal or greater than 70 beats/min despite guideline-derived medical therapy including a β-blocker (Table 129-9). Its use has been limited to its initiation in the outpatient setting.

Digitalis can improve symptoms, quality of life, exercise tolerance, and reduce hospitalization rates in patients with mild-to-moderate HF, but has no effect on mortality. Because of its narrow therapeutic window, it is currently considered second-line therapy for chronic HF (eg, Class IIa recommendation in ACC/AHA HF guidelines).

TABLE 129-9 Other Drugs Used in Heart Failure

Clinical Trial	No. Patients	Inclusion	Study Drug	Initial Dose	Target Dose	Relative Risk, Mortality
Rales	1663	NYHA III-IV LVEF <35%	Spironolactone	25 mg daily	25 mg daily	0.7 (0.60-0.82); $P < 0.0001$
Ephesus	6642	3-14 d post MI with LVEF <40% and HF symptoms	Eplerenone	25 mg daily	50 mg daily	0.85 (0.75-0.96); $P = 0.008$
Emphasis-HF	2737	NYHA II LVEF ≤35%	Eplerenone	25 mg daily	50 mg daily	0.63 (0.54-0.74) $P < 0.001$ Combined endpoint of CV death or HF hospitalization
V-Heft	642	Chronic CHF with LVEF <45% peak O_2 consumption <25 mL/kg/min	Hydralazine Isosorbide dinitrate	25 mg four times a day 10 mg four times a day	75 mg four times a day 40 mg four times a day	0.66 (0.46-0.96); $P < 0.082$
A-Heft	1050	NYHA III-IV LVEF <35% or <45% with EDD >6.5 cm by echo self ID Black	Hydralazine Isosorbide dinitrate	37.5 mg three times a day 20 mg three times a day	75 mg three times a day 40 mg three times a day	0.57 (0.1-1.9); $P = 0.01$
DIG	6800	HF and LVEF <45% and sinus rhythm	Digoxin	0.125 mg daily	0.25 mg daily	1.01
Shift trial	6558	NYHA II-IV LVEF ≤35% Sinus rhythm with heart rate ≥70 beats/min	Ivabradine	5 mg BID	7.5 mg BID	0.82 (0.75-0.90) $P < 0.0001$ Combined endpoint of CV death or HF hospitalization

The ACC/AHA HF guidelines suggest that the addition of **hydralazine**, an arterial vasodilator, and **nitrates** is reasonable in patients with HFrEF who have persistent symptoms despite target doses of ACE inhibitors and β-blockers for symptomatic HF. The combination can also be considered in symptomatic patients who cannot tolerate an ACE inhibitor or ARB. A prospective, double-blind randomized trial conducted in African American patients with NYHA class III/IV HF demonstrated a mortality/morbidity benefit of isosorbide dinitrate plus hydralazine when added to a standard HF regimen. Time to first hospitalization and quality of life were also improved. The target doses used in this trial were hydralazine 75 mg three times a day and isosorbide dinitrate 40 mg three times a day.

Anticoagulation with **warfarin** is indicated in patients with HF who have experienced a previous thromboembolic event or who have paroxysmal or persistent atrial fibrillation. Anticoagulation should also be considered in patients with underlying disorders that may be associated with an increased thromboembolic risk (eg, amyloidosis, myocarditis). The evidence for benefit of chronic warfarin anticoagulation in patients with systolic HF in the absence of these previous indications is limited and is considered a Class II indication.

Certain drugs should be avoided or used with caution in HF patients. Nonsteroidal anti-inflammatory drugs can cause sodium retention, peripheral vasoconstriction, and precipitate renal insufficiency. If analgesia is required, acetaminophen and judicious use of narcotics should be considered. Thiazolidinediones have been associated with increased peripheral edema and symptomatic HF, particularly in those with NYHA III/IV symptoms. Most calcium channel blockers should generally be avoided because of their cardiodepressant effects. Routine combined use of an ACE inhibitor, ARB, and aldosterone antagonist is not recommended given the risk for hyperkalemia, particularly in diabetic patients.

■ DEVICE THERAPY: INTRACARDIAC DEFIBRILLATORS (ICD) AND CARDIAC RESYNCHRONIZATION THERAPY (CRT)

Patients with HF and reduced ejection fraction are at risk for sudden cardiac death due to ventricular arrhythmias. Intracardiac defibrillators have been shown to decrease sudden death and all-cause mortality in several randomized prospective clinical trials of patients with left ventricular systolic dysfunction. The impact of ICD therapy is limited to a reduction in death from lethal arrhythmias; they do not improve quality of life or symptoms due to HF. The use of ICD therapy in primary prevention of sudden death must always be weighed against other factors that may affect long-term survival and individualized quality of life. Current Class I guideline recommendations for ICD therapy include:

1. Secondary prevention to prolong survival in patients with current or prior symptoms of HF and reduced LVEF who have a history of cardiac arrest, ventricular fibrillation, or hemodynamically destabilizing ventricular tachycardia.
2. Primary prevention to reduce total mortality by a reduction in sudden cardiac death in patients with either ischemic heart disease (at least 40 days post-MI) or nonischemic cardiomyopathy (at least 9 months) who have an LVEF less than or equal to 35%, with NYHA functional class II or III symptoms while on chronic guideline-directed medical therapy, and have reasonable expectation of survival of more than 1 year.

Intracardiac defibrillators are not recommended in patients with refractory symptoms of HF (stage D) and poor candidates for advanced therapies or in patients with concomitant diseases that would shorten their life expectancy independent of HF.

Electromechanical dyssynchrony (as evidenced by a prolonged QRS duration) has been associated with increased myocardial oxygen consumption, mitral regurgitation, ventricular remodeling, and neurohormonal activation in patients with HFrEF. Dyssynchronous contraction can be alleviated by electrically activating the right and left ventricles in a synchronized manner with a biventricular pacemaker device (known as cardiac resynchronization therapy). Cardiac resynchronization therapy improves symptoms and quality of life as well as improving ventricular size and function and decreasing mitral regurgitation. These benefits result in improved survival and decreased hospitalizations in patients with symptomatic HF despite optimal medical therapy who have prolonged QRS duration. The ACC/AHA/HRS Class I recommendation for cardiac resynchronization therapy is for patients with LVEF less than or equal to 35%, sinus rhythm, and NYHA functional class II, III or ambulatory class IV symptoms despite recommended, guideline-directed medical therapy and who have cardiac dyssynchrony, which is currently defined as a QRS duration equal or greater than 150 ms.

■ REVASCULARIZATION

The 2013 ACC/AHA guidelines on HF suggest coronary artery revascularization with coronary artery bypass graft (CABG) surgery or percutaneous intervention in the following situations unless the patient is not eligible for revascularization of any kind:

1. Heart failure patients on guideline-derived medical therapy who have angina and suitable coronary anatomy, especially for a left main stenosis or equivalent disease (Class I). In patients with both HF and angina, coronary revascularization can relieve symptoms of myocardial ischemia.
2. Coronary artery bypass graft to improve survival is reasonable in patients with mild-to-moderate LV systolic dysfunction (LVEF of 35%-50%) and significant multivessel coronary artery disease (Class IIa).
3. Coronary artery bypass graft or medical therapy is reasonable to improve morbidity and cardiovascular mortality for patients with severe LV dysfunction (LVEF <35%), HF and significant CAD (Class IIa).

Observational data have suggested that patients who have ischemic cardiomyopathy and reduced LVEF (≤35%) and no symptoms of angina, but have viable myocardium (by noninvasive imaging) have improvement in LV function and survival with revascularization compared with medical therapy. However, in the randomized STICH trial, all-cause mortality was similar between patients initially randomized to CABG in addition to optimal medical therapy versus patients initially randomized to optimal medical therapy alone and was surprisingly independent of the presence of viability as assessed by stress echocardiography and SPECT. Of note, there was a greater crossover from medical therapy to CABG than CABG to medical therapy and an as-treated analysis suggested a benefit to CABG. Moreover, more sophisticated viability assessments using either positron emission tomography or cardiac MRI were not used in the trial and the STICH conclusions may not be extended to these techniques. An extended follow-up through 10 years of this trial (STICHES) showed a reduction in all-cause mortality, death from cardiovascular causes, and death from any cause or hospitalization for cardiovascular causes among patients who underwent CABG compared with those in the the medical therapy group.

■ CARE TRANSITIONS (DISCHARGE CONSIDERATIONS)

Rehospitalization occurs in 30% to 50% of patients within 6 months following HF hospitalization and prevention remains an operational challenge for most health care systems. Failure to meet a set of discharge criteria may increase the likelihood for readmission. Such criteria for discharge have included:

1. Achieving optimal volume status, resolution of HF symptoms, and use of appropriate medications that are tolerated without hypotension or renal insufficiency.

2. An understanding of the discharge instructions by patients and their families regarding medications, diet, activity, daily weights, identification of symptoms, and scheduled follow-up.

3. Precipitating factors and comorbidities have been addressed.

Follow-up with a health care provider within a week of discharge has been associated with decreased rehospitalization and is strongly encouraged to assess the patient's clinical status, tolerance of medications, and to repeat laboratory evaluation. Closer follow-up after discharge may be necessary by telephone to assure stable weights or continuing weight loss if needed and to adjust diuretic dosing. Direct communication with the outpatient provider or disease management team should be standard practice. Hospital or practice-based disease management programs are of great benefit if available and have been shown to improve patient quality of life and reduce HF hospitalizations. Cardiology consultation should be strongly considered during inpatient care and is critical for follow-up to address the multiple issues relevant to the management of chronic HF. This consideration is particularly relevant since HF admissions are markers for subsequent mortality.

Patients with advanced HF, or stage D HF, have marked symptoms at rest despite maximal medical therapy and are best cared for by a multidisciplinary HF team. These patients are at high risk for readmission and mortality (see Table AA). Select patients may be eligible for specialized advanced treatments, such as mechanical circulatory support, procedures to facilitate fluid removal (ultrafiltration or dialysis), invasive hemodynamic guided therapy, or cardiac transplantation. End-of-life and palliative care should also be reviewed and offered when appropriate (**Figure 129-3**).

■ DISEASE MANAGEMENT STRATEGIES AND QUALITY IMPROVEMENT

The prevention of HF hospitalization is a primary benefit of multidisciplinary disease management programs. Such programs can also improve functional status and quality of life for these patients. Heart failure patients with a history of multiple readmissions, moderate to severe HF, multiple comorbidities, and/or those at high risk due to cognitive impairment or persistent nonadherence should be referred to HF management programs whenever possible. A multidisciplinary team made up of physicians, HF nurses, dietitians, and pharmacists can provide support to the patient as well as family members and other care providers in the form of:

- Individualized education and counseling that emphasizes self-care
- Assistance with medication and dietary compliance
- Optimization of drug therapy
- Medicine reconciliation
- Low-cost scales to measure daily weights
- Increased access to health care
- Early attention to signs and symptoms of fluid overload
- Close telephone follow-up after hospital discharge

Hospitalists play a critical role in leading the transition of the patient from inpatient to outpatient care. They can also initiate quality improvement efforts to facilitate patient education and discharge planning, ensure adherence to evidence-based guidelines, and implement national quality measures. Initiatives include the use of HF clinical pathways and preprinted HF discharge

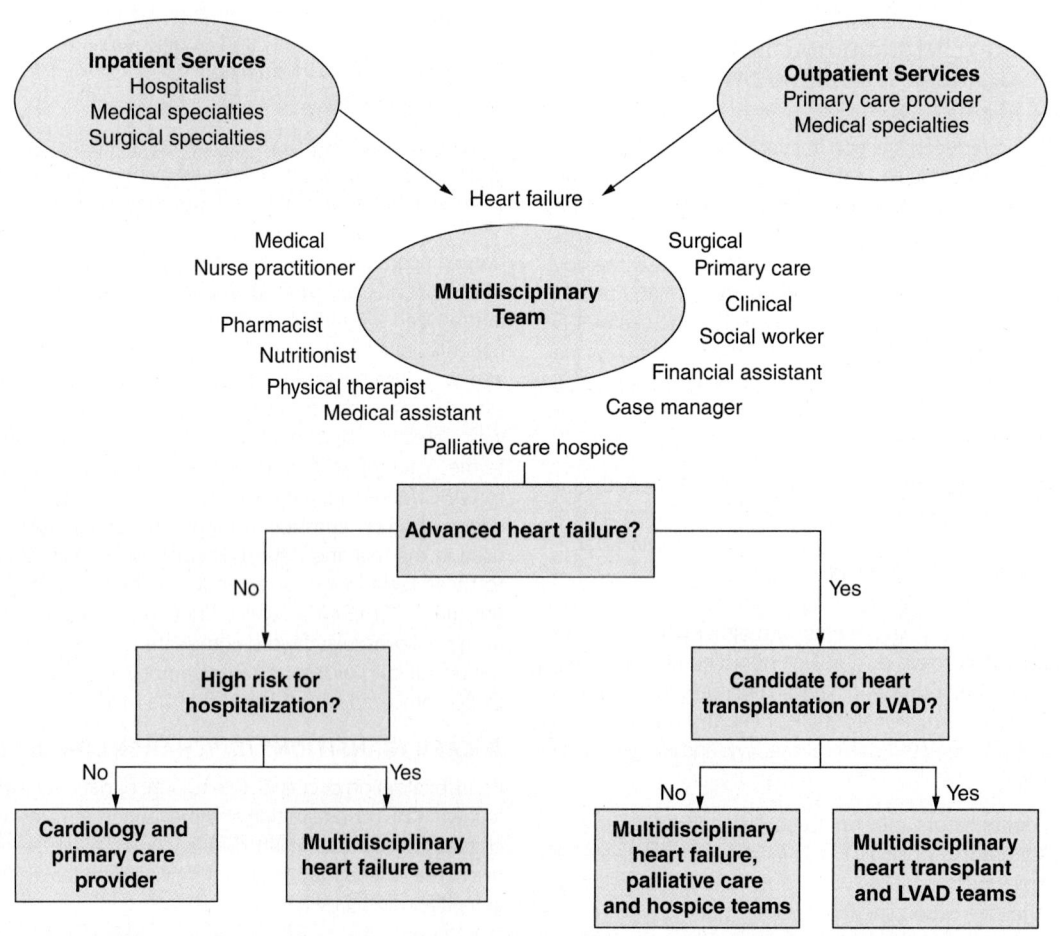

Figure 129-3 *Structure of multidisciplinary team and goal based algorithm management of patients with advanced heart failure.*

instructions as well as educational material. The hospitalist should participate in discharge planning to ensure a visiting nurse or telephone follow-up soon after discharge and a clinic visit within 1 week of discharge.

Educating patients with HF and their families is critical and should start early in the hospitalization. This can be achieved through discussions, videotapes, and reading materials at the appropriate educational level in the patient's native language. The aim of education should be to empower patients and their families to embrace the patient's self-care so they may recognize symptoms, implement therapy, and self-evaluate the effect of treatments. Patient noncompliance with medications and diet is a common cause of clinical deterioration and readmission and should be addressed prior to discharge.

Discharge instructions should address the following:

- Medications (prescribed and what to avoid)
- Dietary restrictions (low-salt diet and fluid restriction)
- Activity recommendations
- Signs and symptoms of HF and a subsequent action plan
- Plans for follow-up
- Weight monitoring (and a treatment algorithm for weight gain)

Other issues that should be addressed include:

- Smoking cessation counseling
- Exercise training or referral to cardiac rehabilitation program (now covered by CMS)
- Influenza and pneumococcal vaccination

■ EXERCISE TRAINING AND CARDIAC REHABILITATION

Exercise training in patients with HF has been shown to be safe and effective in improving functional capacity, exercise tolerance, quality of life, reducing hospitalization and improving survival. These data are derived from numerous prospective non-randomized and randomized controlled trials. HF-ACTION is the largest randomized controlled trial that showed a 15% reduction in cardiovascular mortality or HF hospitalization on adjusted analysis. Current recommendations include:

- Exercise training and HF disease-related self-care counseling is useful and effective in HF to improve functional status (AHA/ACC Class I).
- Cardiac rehabilitation can be useful in stable patients with HF to improve functional capacity, exercise duration, HRQOL, and mortality (AHA/ACC Class IIa).

Ambulatory patients with AHA/ACC stage C stable HF with stable NYHA II-III despite guideline-directed medical therapy should be considered for supervised cardiac rehabilitation. Contraindications for cardiac rehabilitation include uncontrolled diabetes or hypertension, moderate-severe aortic stenosis, significant ischemia at <2 METs of workload, any comorbidity preventing exercise participation, or acute myocarditis (or other acute cardiomyopathy) until stabilized. As in any other therapy, compliance with the exercise regimen is essential for the success of the exercise-training program.

HF WITH PRESERVED EJECTION FRACTION (HFpEF)
■ EPIDEMIOLOGY/OVERVIEW

HFpEF, previously known as diastolic HF, is as common as HFrEF as a cause for HF admissions. It is estimated that half of patients with HF have preserved LVEF. The prevalence of this condition is increasing due to the aging population, the increasing incidence of hypertension and diabetes mellitus, and a growing awareness and ability to make the diagnosis. The rate of HF hospitalizations and death rates are similar in patients with HFpEF and HFrEF.

Patients with HFpEF are more likely to be older, female, and have a history of hypertension and atrial fibrillation when compared with patients with HFrEF. Obesity, anemia, and diabetes are also commonly present. In contrast to HFrEF, HFpEF has been studied in fewer clinical trials and no therapy to date has been shown to improve survival in this type of HF.

■ PATHOPHYSIOLOGY

HFpEF is a poorly understood, heterogeneous disorder. HFpEF is the preferred designation, since it remains unclear if the primary abnormality in this syndrome is diastolic dysfunction. What constitutes a "preserved" LVEF is variable in both clinical trials and in practice and can range from >40% to 60%. HFpEF has traditionally been attributed to reduced diastolic ventricular compliance and abnormal relaxation. Abnormal renal sodium and water handling, reduced vascular compliance, and anemia also appear to play roles in HFpEF. Diastolic function is often abnormal in patients with HFrEF as well as those with preserved LVEF. The nature and extent of diastolic dysfunction is variable in HFpEF. Cardiac output, especially during exercise, may be limited by abnormal filling characteristics of the left ventricle as well as chronotropic incompetence and lack of vasodilator reserve. In restrictive cardiomyopathies, the "purest" form of HFpEF, ventricular chamber dimensions are reduced, intraventricular pressures are elevated, and cardiac output is essentially heart rate dependent. Chronic hypertension with resultant left ventricular hypertrophy is commonly present in HFpEF. Elevations in systemic blood pressure increase left ventricular wall stress and systolic load, which can impair myocardial relaxation in patients with HFpEF. Both macrovascular and microvascular coronary artery disease may also play important roles in this syndrome as well.

Several myocardial disorders may present as HFpEF and should be considered in the differential diagnosis, including restrictive (eg, infiltrative) and hypertrophic cardiomyopathies. Patients with HFpEF may have difficulty tolerating atrial fibrillation since the loss of atrioventricular synchrony can greatly reduce left atrial emptying, left ventricular filling, and LV stroke volume. Patients with HFpEF may not tolerate tachycardia since increases in heart rate shorten the duration of diastole and truncate the late phase of diastolic filling. Paradoxically, tachycardia may be important to preserve exercise tolerance when stroke volume is limited. Ischemia can worsen diastolic dysfunction and symptoms of HF. Ischemia can result from coronary heart disease and/or LV hypertrophy with subendocardial ischemia.

■ CLINICAL PRESENTATION AND MAKING THE DIAGNOSIS

Diastolic dysfunction alone is insufficient to make the diagnosis of HFpEF. Signs and symptoms of HF must be present. The signs and symptoms of HFpEF are similar to those in HFrEF and cannot be used to distinguish one from the other. Echocardiography remains the cornerstone of distinguishing HFpEF from HFrEF. (See **Table 129-10** for differential diagnosis in a patient presenting with HFpEF.)

Heart failure, whatever the etiology, is a clinical diagnosis. The diagnosis is generally based on the presence of typical signs or symptoms of HF in a patient who has preserved systolic function, currently defined by an EF >50%. There may or may not be evidence of abnormal left ventricular relaxation, filling, or stiffness. Evidence for diastolic dysfunction is often made by Doppler echocardiography but is load dependent. Echocardiographic signs of diastolic

TABLE 129-10 Diagnostic Considerations in Heart Failure with Preserved Ejection Fraction Syndrome

Valvular pathologies

Infiltrative heart disease

    Amyloidosis

    Sarcoidosis

    Hemochromatosis

Constrictive pericarditis

Systemic hypertension

Ischemic heart disease

High output states

    Anemia

    Thyrotoxicosis

    AV communications

Obesity

Pulmonary hypertension associated with pulmonary vascular disorders

Right-sided heart failure resulting from chronic lung disease

TABLE 129-11 Therapeutic Recommendations for Heart Failure with Preserved Ejection Fraction Syndrome

Class I (Level of evidence: B)
Systemic blood pressure control according to current guidelines
Class I (Level of evidence: C)
Diuretic use to control pulmonary congestion and peripheral edema
Rate control in patients with atrial fibrillation
Class IIa (Level of evidence: C)
Coronary revascularization is reasonable in patients with coronary artery disease in whom symptomatic or demonstrable myocardial ischemia is judged to be having an adverse effect on cardiac function
Class IIa (Level of evidence: C)
Management of atrial fibrillation in order to improve HF symptoms
Class IIa (Level of evidence: C)
Use of β-blocking agents, ACE inhibitors, and ARBs for hypertension in HFpEF
Class IIb (Level of evidence: B)
Use of ARBs might be considered to decrease hospitalizations in HFpEF

dysfunction include abnormalities in mitral inflow, tissue Doppler, and pulmonary venous inflow. Plasma concentrations of BNP and N-terminal pro-BNP may be increased in patients with HFpEF and can improve diagnostic accuracy. A documented abnormal elevation in left ventricular end-diastolic or pulmonary capillary wedge pressure (eg, >15-18 mm Hg) at either rest or provokable is also diagnostic of HFpEF if the ejection fraction is preserved.

■ TRIAGE AND INITIAL MANAGEMENT

Regardless of the cause of acute HF, initial treatment should focus on improving symptoms, hemodynamics, and oxygenation (if hypoxemia present) and searching for precipitating causes. No proven therapy for HFpEF currently exists. Treatment should be directed toward symptoms, comorbid conditions, and physiologic factors known to contribute to impaired ventricular relaxation, such as control of systolic and diastolic hypertension, the ventricular rate in atrial fibrillation, volume overload, and coronary heart disease. See **Table 129-11** for a summary of treatment recommendations.

Occult coronary heart disease is a potentially reversible cause of diastolic HF and should be excluded in patients with angina or demonstrable ischemia despite guideline-directed medical therapy (AHA/ACC Class IIa recommendation). Identification and treatment of obesity, anemia, and sleep disordered breathing are also important.

Angiotensin receptor blockers may decrease HF hospitalization in HFpEF; in the randomized CHARM study, candesartan reduced HF hospitalizations in patients with NYHA class II-IV and LVEF >40%, although there was no difference in cardiovascular mortality. Some authorities believe that aldosterone antagonism may play an important therapeutic role in HFpEF. In the landmark TOPCAT trial, the aldosterone antagonist, spironolactone, decreased HF hospitalizations; but the trial failed to meet the primary combined endpoint of cardiovascolar death and HF hospitalization.

However, other trials have failed to demonstrate a significant benefit for other ARBs or β-blockers. (See **Table 129-12** for a summary of randomized clinical trials in HFpEF.) Other agents have also been tried without success. Sildenafil failed to improve oxygen consumption as measured by cardiopulmonary exercise testing in the RELAX-HF trial. Isosorbide mononitrate did not improve (and

actually worsened) daily activity as measured by an accelerometer in the NEAT-HF trial. The combination of the ARB valsartan and the neprilysin inhibitor sacubitril, LCZ696, is currently under investigation in HFpEF (PARAGON-HF).

■ DISEASE MANAGEMENT STRATEGIES

Similar to HFrEF, high-risk patients (multiple readmissions, high risk due to cognitive impairment or multiple comorbidities, persistent nonadherence) should be referred to HF management programs if available. As discussed previously, a multidisciplinary team made up of physicians, HF nurses, dietitians, and pharmacists can provide individualized education and counseling to the patient, family members, and caregivers that emphasize self-care, optimization of drug therapy, increased access to health care, early attention to signs and symptoms of fluid overload, and close telephone follow-up after hospital discharge to assess symptoms and daily weights, adjust diuretic dosing, and answer questions regarding diet and medications.

■ CARE TRANSITIONS

Heart failure patients can be discharged once optimal volume status is obtained, symptoms have resolved, and appropriate medications have controlled heart rate and blood pressure without hypotension or renal insufficiency. Patient and family should demonstrate an understanding of the discharge instructions regarding medications, diet, activity, daily weights, worsening symptoms, and follow-up. Close follow-up with a primary care physician or cardiologist within a week is mandatory to assess the patient's clinical status, tolerance of medications, and to check for electrolyte abnormalities. Closer follow-up by telephone may be necessary to monitor weights and symptoms. Direct communication with the outpatient provider should be standard practice.

ACKNOWLEDGMENT

The authors would like to thank Dr Julio Barcena for his important contributions to the previous edition's version of this chapter.

TABLE 129-12 Outcomes of Randomized Clinical Trials in Heart Failure with Preserved Ejection Fraction

	CHARM-Preserved	I-Preserve	PEP-CHF	Seniors (s)	Relax	Topcat
Therapy	Candesartan	Irbesartan	Perindopril	Nebivolol	Sildenafil	Spironolactone
Age (y)	>18 (67)	≥60 (72)	≥70 (75)	≥70 (76)	≥18 (69)	≥18 (68.7)
EF (%)	≥40 (mean 54)	≥45 (mean 60)	≥40 (mean 65)	≥35 (mean 49)	≥50 (mean 60)	≥45 (median 56)
Patients (N)	3023	4128	850	752	216	3445
Female (%)	40%	60%	55%	38%	48%	52%
Primary endpoint	CV death or HF hospitalization	Death or CV hospitalization	Death or HF hospitalization	Death or CV hospitalization	Change in peak oxygen consumption after 24 weeks of therapy	Cardiovascular death or HF hospitalization
Relative risk	0.89 (0.77-1.03); $P = 0.051$	0.95 (0.86-1.05); $P = 0.35$	0.92 (0.70-1.21); $P = 0.545$	0.88 (0.73-1.05); $P = 0.21$	-0.20 vs -0.20 mL/kg/min ($P = 0.90$)	0.89 (0.77-1.04) $P = 0.14$

SUGGESTED READINGS

Bhatia RS, Tu JV, Lee DS, et al. Outcome of heart failure with preserved ejection fraction in a population-based study. N Engl J Med. 2006;355:260-269.

Borlaug BA, Redfield MM. Diastolic and systolic heart failure are distinct phenotypes within the heart failure spectrum. Circulation. 2011;123:2006-2014.

Cleland JGF, Daubert JC, Erdmann E, et al. The effect of cardiac resynchronization on morbidity and mortality in heart failure. N Engl J Med. 2005;352:1539-1549.

Fang JC, et al. Advanced (Stage D) heart failure: a statement from the heart failure Society of America Guidelines Committee. J Cardiac Fail. 2015;21:e519-e534.

Fonarow GC, Adams KF, Abraham WT, et al. Risk stratification for in-hospital mortality in acutely decompensated heart failure. JAMA. 2005;293:572-580.

Gheorghiade M, Filippatos GS, Felker GM. Diagnosis and management of acute heart failure syndromes. In: Bonow RO, Mann DL, Zipes DP, Libby P, eds. Braunwald's Heart Disease. A Textbook of Cardiovascular Medicine, 9th ed. Philadelphia, PA: Elsevier Saunders; 2012:517-542.

Heart Failure Society of America. 2010 Comprehensive heart failure practice guideline. J Card Fail. 2010;16(6):e1-e194.

McMurray JJ. Systolic heart failure. N Engl J Med. 2010;362:228-238.

McMurray JJ, et al. ESC Guidelines for the diagnosis and treatment of acute and chronic heart failure 2012. Eur Heart J. 2012;33:1787-1847.

McMurray JJ, Packer M, Desai AS, et al. Angiotensin-neprilysin inhibition versus enalapril in heart failure. N Engl J Med. 2014;371: 993-1004.

Mueller C, Scholer A, Laule-Kilian K, et al. Use of B-type natriuretic peptide in the evaluation and management of acute dyspnea. N Engl J Med. 2004;350:647-654.

Nohria A, Lewis E, Stevenson W L. Medical management of advanced heart failure. JAMA. 2002;287(5):628-640.

Owan TE, Hodge DO, Herges RM, et al. Trends in prevalence and outcome of heart failure with preserved ejection fraction. N Engl J Med. 2006;355:251-259.

Pitt B, Pfeffer MA, Assmann SF, et al. Spironolactone for heart failure with preserved ejection fraction. N Engl J Med. 2014;370: 1383-1392.

Pitt B, Zannad F, Remme WJ, et al. The effect of spironolactone on morbidity and mortality in patients with severe heart failure. N Engl J Med. 1999;341:709-717.

Rees K, Taylor RS, Singh S, et al. Exercise-based rehabilitation for heart failure. Cochrane Database Syst Rev. 2004;(3):CD003331.

Swedberg K, Komajda M, Böhm M, et al. Ivabradine and outcomes in chronic heart failure (SHIFT): a randomized placebo-controlled study. Lancet. 2010;376:875-885.

Taylor AL, Ziesche S, Yancy C, et al. Combination of isosorbide dinitrate and hydralazine in blacks with heart failure. N Engl J Med. 2004;351:2049-2057.

Velazquez EJ, Lee KL, Deja MA, et al. Coronary-artery bypass surgery in patients with left ventricular dysfunction. N Engl J Med. 2011;364:1607-16.

Velazquez EJ, Lee KL, Jone RH et al. Coronary-artery bypass surgery in patients with ischemic cardiomyopathy. N Engl J Med. 2016;374:1511-1520.

Wever-Pinzon O, Drakos SD, Fang JC. Team-based care for advanced heart failure. Heart Fail Clin. 2015.

Yancy CW, et al. 2013. ACCF/AHA Guideline for the Management of Heart Failure. Circulation. 2013;128:e240-e327.

Yusuf S, Pfeffer MA, Swedberg K, et al. Effects of candesartan in patients with chronic heart failure and preserved left-ventricular ejection fraction: the CHARM-preserved trial. Lancet. 2003;362:777-781.

Myocarditis, Pericardial Disease, and Cardiac Tamponade

Daniel L. Molloy, Jr., MD

Matthew E. Certain, MD

Stephen D. Clements, Jr., MD

Key Clinical Questions

1. How do you diagnose pericarditis and myocarditis?
2. Which imaging modality is most accurate in diagnosing myocarditis?
3. How do you diagnose and manage cardiac tamponade?
4. How does the treatment of constrictive pericarditis differ from cardiac tamponade?

MYOCARDITIS

■ INTRODUCTION

Acute myocarditis is an inflammatory infiltration of the myocardium characterized by areas of myocardial necrosis with lymphocytic infiltration. The clinical sequelae range from subclinical disease to fulminant cardiogenic shock.

■ PATHOPHYSIOLOGY

The most common cause of myocarditis is a viral pathogen. However, other infectious, autoimmune, and toxic causes occur as well. Initial studies in the latter half of the 20th century indicated Coxsackie B virus as the frequent causative agent in endomyocardial biopsies. However, since the 1990s adenovirus has emerged as the more frequent viral agent. Additionally, parvovirus, HIV, HCV, EBV, and CMV have been seen in the biopsy results of patients with myocarditis. The model for the development of acute myocarditis from these viral agents involves viral entry into the cells via specific membrane receptors with subsequent viral replication and myocyte necrosis. Cellular necrosis leads to exposure of the intracellular contents including proteins such as myosin and thus an autoimmune activation, which may last 3 to 5 days. Subsequent autoimmunity and activation of the lymphocytes may last weeks to months and is the driving force behind the time course of myocarditis.

Infectious etiologies other than viruses have been implicated as a cause of myocarditis, including mycoplasma, *Corynebacterium diphtheriae* and *Borrelia burgdorferi* (Lyme disease). In developing countries, *Trypanosoma cruzi* has been known to infect the myocardium causing Chagas disease.

■ PRESENTATION

The clinical presentation of patients with myocarditis ranges from mild dyspnea and chest discomfort to fulminant cardiogenic shock. Patients may report a viral prodrome in the weeks preceding presentation, including fevers, respiratory, or gastrointestinal symptoms. According to the European Study of Epidemiology and Treatment of Inflammatory Heart Disease, patients with myocarditis present with dyspnea (72%), chest pain (32%), and arrhythmias (18%). Patients may also present with symptoms related to congestive heart failure, including fatigue, orthopnea, paroxysmal nocturnal dyspnea, palpitations, and syncope.

As an infiltrative process, the amount of affected myocardium can be highly variable in myocarditis. Some patients may present with ventricular arrhythmias if the conducting system is involved while other patients may present with a dilated cardiomyopathy.

The physical examination of patients with acute myocarditis may correlate with the patients' symptoms. Signs of myocarditis are nonspecific, correlating with the severity of heart failure.

■ DIAGNOSIS

The electrocardiogram (ECG) in myocarditis is neither sensitive nor specific, but may show the following:

- Sinus tachycardia, nonspecific ST-segment changes and T-wave inversion.
- ST-segment elevation and Q-waves that suggest acute myocardial ischemia.

- Bundle-branch blocks, atrioventricular block, or ventricular tachyarrhythmias.
- Diffuse ST-segment elevation in addition to PR-segment depression (myopericarditis).

The ECG may add prognostic value, as it has been shown that QTc greater than 440 or an abnormal QRS are both predictors of poor clinical outcomes, and QRS duration of greater than 120 is an independent predictor of cardiac death.

PRACTICE POINT

ECG findings in acute pericarditis include:
- Diffuse ST-segment elevation
  - Hexaxial and precordial leads with the exception of AVR and V_1 which may have ST-segment depression
  - Concave shape and not accompanied by reciprocal changes
  - No T-wave inversion and no associated Q-waves
- PR depression, all leads except AVR and V_1 which may show PR elevation
- ECG changes lasting up to 2 weeks
- QTc of greater than 440 and abnormal QRS portend poor clinical outcome

---

Patients with myocarditis may have elevated biomarkers, such as troponin-I, CK-MB, and CPK. Troponin-I levels are more commonly elevated than other cardiac biomarkers. However, troponin-I elevation has a low sensitivity (34%) for myocarditis. Likewise, nonspecific markers of inflammation such as the C-reactive protein may be elevated in the setting of myocarditis, but normal values do not exclude the diagnosis.

The white blood cell count may range from completely normal to a mild leukocytosis. Viral myocarditis may cause a nonspecific lymphocytic predominance. Eosinophilia may be associated with drug-induced myocarditis or an infiltrative disease such as Churg-Strauss. Thrombocytopenia may be present due to the acute viral illness, or from splenic sequestration due to splenomegaly, accompanying congestive heart failure.

Severely affected individuals may have chemistries that correlate with congestive heart failure, including hyponatremia due to sodium dysregulation and reduced kidney function due to poor cardiac output. Elevated liver transaminases (AST and ALT) along with markers of synthetic function (PT/INR, PTT) may be elevated due to hepatic congestion.

Serologies for the most common viral etiologies offer little clinical benefit. Only 5% of the serologies were positive for the same entity noted on endomyocardial biopsy.

Chest radiography may reveal pulmonary vascular congestion and cardiomegaly due to a dilated cardiomyopathy or pneumonia if caused by mycoplasma.

Echocardiography has been the traditional imaging modality of choice; however, it can be normal in less severe cases of myocarditis. Even in severe cases of myocarditis, echocardiography may only identify a dilated cardiomyopathy or, less commonly, hypertrophic or restrictive cardiomyopathies. Regional wall motion abnormalities may mimic changes commonly seen with ischemia. The role of echocardiography in the diagnosis of myocarditis is used to exclude other causes of chest pain and acute decompensation.

Computed tomography (CT) or magnetic resonance imaging (MRI) may be useful in the diagnosis of myocarditis when echocardiography is nondiagnostic. Magnetic resonance imaging identifies myocarditis in 30% of patients with chest pain, elevated troponins, and normal coronary arteries. In cases where edema, capillary leak,

and necrosis can be assessed, cardiac MRI has a sensitivity of 67%, a specificity of 91%, and a diagnostic accuracy of 78%. The shortfall of cardiac MRI lies in its inability to differentiate myocarditis from the infiltrative diseases such as giant cell myocarditis or sarcoidosis, which have different management strategies.

Endomyocardial biopsy remains the gold standard for diagnosing myocarditis. However, the procedure carries risks, varies by interpreter, lacks prognostic value, and has a low sensitivity due to sampling error. For these reasons, endomyocardial biopsy should be reserved for cases when other infiltrative disorders are in the differential diagnosis, such as cardiac sarcoidosis or giant cell myocarditis. Histologically, an inflammatory cellular infiltrate may be seen with or without myocyte necrosis.

■ MANAGEMENT

The low incidence of myocarditis precludes performing randomized controlled trials with sufficient power to assess therapeutic regimens. The basis of therapy for patients with myocarditis remains largely supportive. The majority of patients with myocarditis will recover fully. For the patients with a stable clinical course, the basis of therapy resides in angiotensin-converting enzyme inhibitors, β-blockers, and diuretic therapy. Patients with severe left ventricular (LV) dysfunction may rapidly progress to cardiogenic shock. These patients may require a left ventricular assist device or extracorporeal membrane oxygenation as a bridge to cardiac transplantation.

Patients with myocarditis may have an increased risk of arrhythmias, requiring temporary pacemakers for bradycardia or complete heart block, or antiarrhythmic agents such as amiodarone for ventricular tachyarrhythmias. For patients with ventricular arrhythmias after the diagnosis of myocarditis, implantable cardiac defibrillators (ICDs) may be considered once the acute phase of the illness has resolved. In addition to patients with ventricular tachycardia or fibrillation, those patients with an ejection fraction less than 35% following resolution of the acute phase of myocarditis, should be considered for ICD implantation. It should be noted that patients under consideration for ICD placement should have a life expectancy longer than 1 year and be on optimal medical therapy.

While myocarditis is a lymphocytic infiltrative disease, immunosuppressive agents show only marginal beneficial effects. One small trial suggests that patients with human leukocyte antigen expression on biopsy have modest benefit (ejection fraction improvement and New York Heart Association [NYHA] class) from prednisone and azathioprine.

PERICARDITIS

■ INTRODUCTION

Acute pericarditis is defined as signs and/or symptoms consistent with pericardial inflammation of less than 3 weeks' duration. The true incidence of pericarditis is difficult to quantify since many cases go undiagnosed. Pericarditis may account for up to 1% of cases of ST elevations on ECG, and account for 5% of emergency room visits. Eighty to ninety percent of cases of pericarditis are idiopathic. A significant portion of patients with acute pericarditis present with recurrent pericarditis, which has been shown to plague 15% to 30% of patients after the first episode. Recurrent pericarditis presents similarly to acute pericarditis, but can be difficult to manage due to further recurrence.

■ PATHOPHYSIOLOGY

Pericarditis may be an acute, subacute, or chronic process. The etiology of acute pericarditis is often idiopathic or viral, although the pericardium may be affected by numerous other disease processes including infectious, neoplastic, autoimmune, and traumatic causes (**Table 130-1**).

TABLE 130-1 Causes of Pericardial Heart Disease

Idiopathic

Infectious

Bacterial (*Pneumococcus, Streptococcus, Staphylococcus, Haemophilus influenzae, gram-negative rods, Brucella melitensis, Francisella tularensis, Legionella pneumophila, Neisseria gonorrhoeae, Neisseria meningitidis, Borrelia burgdorferi* [Lyme disease], *Mycoplasma*)

Viral (Coxsackievirus, echovirus, adenovirus, varicella, influenza, cytomegalovirus, HIV, hepatitis B, mumps, infectious mononucleosis)

Mycobacterial (*Mycobacterium tuberculosis, Mycobacterium avium-intracellulare*)

Fungal (*Histoplasma, Coccidioidomycosis, Blastomyces, Candida albicans, Nocardia, Actinomyces*)

Protozoal (*Toxoplasma, Echinococcus, amebae*)

AIDS associated

Neoplastic

Primary (mesothelioma, fibrosarcoma)

Secondary (breast, lung, melanoma, lymphoma, leukemia)

Immune/Inflammatory

Connective tissue diseases (rheumatoid arthritis, systemic lupus erythematosus, scleroderma, acute rheumatic fever, dermatomyositis, mixed connective tissue disease, Wegener granulomatosis)

Arteritis (temporal arteritis, polyarteritis nodosa, Takayasu's arteritis)

Acute myocardial infarction and post myocardial infarction (Dressler syndrome)

Postcardiotomy, posttraumatic

Metabolic

Nephrogenic, myxedema, amyloidosis, aortic dissection

Drugs

Hydralazine, procainamide, daunorubicin, isoniazid, anticoagulants, cyclosporine, methysergide, phenytoin, dantrolene, mesalazine

Traumatic

Blunt trauma, surgical trauma, penetrating trauma, instrument/device trauma (implantable defibrillators, pacemakers, catheters)

Congenital

Pericardial cysts, congenital absence of pericardium, Mulibrey nanism

The pericardium serves many functions within the thorax although it is not required to support life. The pericardium is composed of two layers. An inner layer, the visceral pericardium, adheres to the epicardial surface of the heart and consists of a layer of mesothelial cells. The outer layer, an avascular, fibrous parietal pericardium, consists of elastin fibers embedded within compact layers of collagen. The visceral pericardium reflects back near the great vessels and forms the inner layer of the parietal pericardium. The pericardial space is formed from these two layers and normally contains up to 50 mL of an ultrafiltrate of plasma. In the pericardium, villi and cilia enhance the resorption of fluid. The capacity of the pericardium to accept increased fluid volume depends on the rate of accumulation. A rapid addition of 50 to 200 mL will dramatically increase pressure and affect cardiac function, whereas a very slow accumulation of large amounts of fluid as in myxedema will have little effect on pressure or hemodynamics.

The collagen matrix of the parietal pericardium gives the pericardium its unique mechanical properties. Functionally, the pericardium facilitates contraction and relaxation of the ventricles and atria, allowing pressure changes on one side of the heart to be transmitted to the other side. Additionally, the pericardium's mechanical properties may determine cardiac output during exercise via the pericardium's direct limitation of the cardiac filling volumes.

■ **PRESENTATION**

Acute pericarditis presents with chest pain of abrupt onset as the most common complaint. The pain may be quite severe, sharp in character, and nearly always pleuritic in nature. The sharp pain of acute pericarditis differs from the pressure-like discomfort of myocardial ischemia. The pain may be located substernally or located in the anterior chest, and radiation to the neck, arms, and shoulders may also occur (**Figure 130-1**).

The phrenic nerve, which innervates the trapezius muscles, traverses the pericardium; therefore, radiation to the trapezius ridge of the left shoulder is very specific for pericardial pain. Classically, the pain associated with pericarditis will improve with sitting up and leaning forward and worse by lying flat or with slight changes in position. Common symptoms include dyspnea from splinting due to pain, cough, myalgia, arthralgias; occasionally, patients report hiccoughs.

Vital signs in patients with pericarditis may be normal or show low-grade fever, tachycardia, and tachypnea. High fever may indicate a bacterial cause, and these patients should undergo echocardiographic evaluation. The most specific, and pathognomonic, sign associated with pericarditis is the pericardial friction rub, likely the result of inflamed visceral and parietal pericardium rubbing against each other. Classically, there are three components correlating with ventricular systole, ventricular diastole, and atrial systole. All components, two components, one component, or none may be present, as the finding is not sensitive. Two components would be expected in atrial fibrillation due to loss of the atrial component; rapid heart rates may only produce two components due to summation of the early diastolic rub and presystolic rub. The rub may be composed solely of the ventricular component, which is the last to leave over the course of illness. These rubs, described as triphasic, biphasic, or monophasic, may be confused with other cardiac abnormalities, especially in patients with a monophasic rub, which may be mistaken for a murmur.

The pericardial friction rub is best heard at the left sternal border, often in a well-localized spot but may be heard only at the apex. Therefore, the examiner needs to take a systematic approach to auscultation; position the patient forward or even on his hands and knees with the chest down or lying on his abdomen propped up on his elbows; use the diaphragm of the stethoscope against the chest wall with forced expiration; and listen over the entire left precordium. Frequent examinations may be required to hear the friction rub given its fleeting nature. The sound has been described as the sound produced when walking through snow, or pulling apart two pieces of Velcro. The rub of pericarditis may sound very similar to the harsh sound of Hamman crunch (heard in some patients with pneumomediastinum); care should be taken to differentiate these two auscultatory findings. In uncomplicated pericarditis, the jugular venous waveforms remain unchanged.

■ **DIAGNOSIS**

The initial testing includes ECG, cardiac enzymes, basic chemistry, complete blood count, erythrocyte sedimentation rate or C-reactive protein, and chest radiograph. Electrocardiogram abnormalities

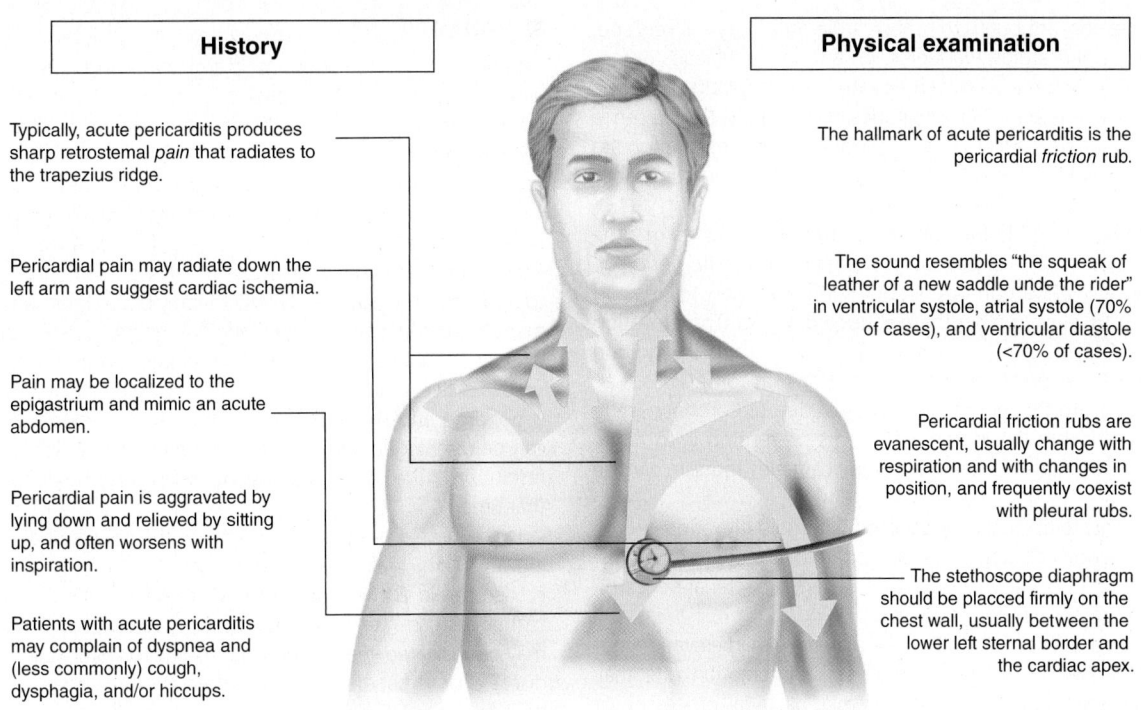

History

Typically, acute pericarditis produces sharp retrostemal *pain* that radiates to the trapezius ridge.

Pericardial pain may radiate down the left arm and suggest cardiac ischemia.

Pain may be localized to the epigastrium and mimic an acute abdomen.

Pericardial pain is aggravated by lying down and relieved by sitting up, and often worsens with inspiration.

Patients with acute pericarditis may complain of dyspnea and (less commonly) cough, dysphagia, and/or hiccups.

Physical examination

The hallmark of acute pericarditis is the pericardial *friction* rub.

The sound resembles "the squeak of leather of a new saddle unde the rider" in ventricular systole, atrial systole (70% of cases), and ventricular diastole (<70% of cases).

Pericardial friction rubs are evanescent, usually change with respiration and with changes in position, and frequently coexist with pleural rubs.

The stethoscope diaphragm should be placed firmly on the chest wall, usually between the lower left sternal border and the cardiac apex.

Clinical note: The quality, severity, and location of pain vary greatly. Repeat examinations often prove necessary to detect friction rubs, which may be confused with cardiac murmurs, with sounds due to pneumomediastinum, and most commonly, with artifacts produced by skin rubbing against a loosely placed stethoscope head.

Figure 130-1 *Clinical features of acute pericarditis. A prodrome of fever, malaise, and myalgia may herald the chief complaint of chest pain.* (Modified, with permission, from Fuster V, O'Rourke RA, Walsh RA, et al. *Hurst's the Heart*, 12th ed. New York: McGraw-Hill; 2008. Fig. 84-3.)

are found in approximately 90% of the patients (**Figure 130-2**). The most sensitive ECG change of acute pericarditis is ST-segment elevation due to abnormal repolarization secondary to pericardial inflammation. Classically, ST elevation develops in the hexaxial and precordial leads with the exception of AVR and V_1 which may demonstrate ST-segment depression. Differences in the shape of the ST-segment elevations and time course help to distinguish acute pericarditis from ischemia:

- The ST elevations have concave shape and are not accompanied by reciprocal changes in acute pericarditis; the slope of ST elevation is more often convex in shape and accompanied by reciprocal changes in ischemia.
- ST-segment elevation typically occurs during the first few days of pericardial inflammation and may last up to 2 weeks. T-wave inversion does not occur at the time of ST-segment elevation nor are there associated Q-waves.

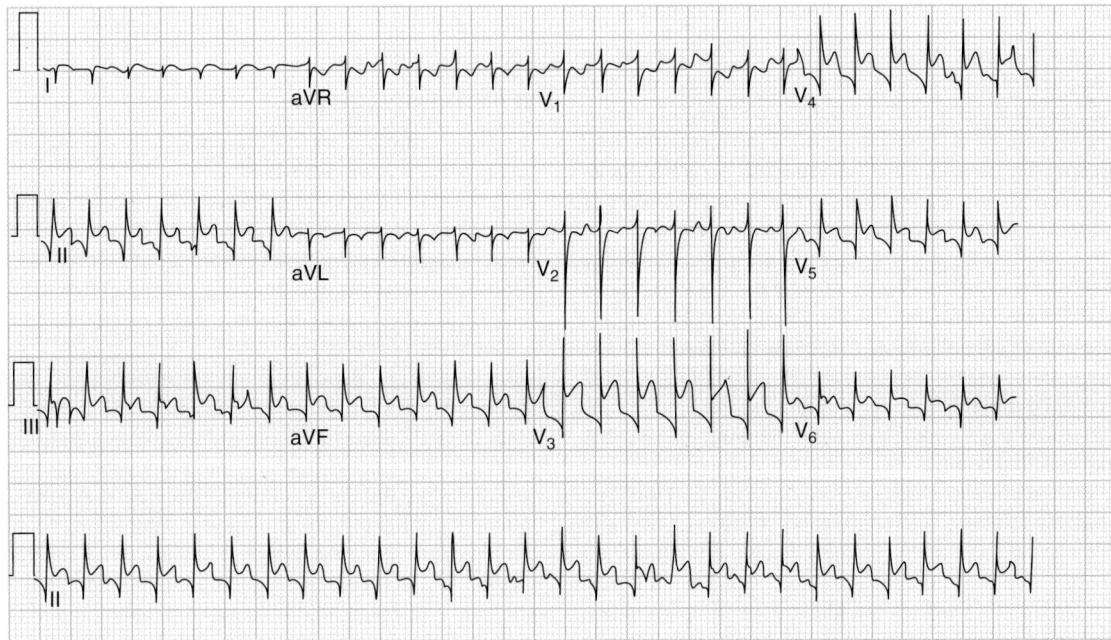

Figure 130-2 *Twelve-lead electrocardiogram of patient with acute pericarditis.* (Modified, with permission, from Fuster V, O'Rourke RA, Walsh RA, et al. *Hurst's the Heart*, 12th ed. New York: McGraw-Hill; 2008. Fig. 84-4.)

PR depression, attributed to subepicardial atrial injury, is very specific of acute pericarditis. PR depression is found in all leads except AVR and V_1, which may show PR elevation. Electrical alternans, the presence of alternating QRS amplitudes, may suggest the presence of a significant pericardial effusion. Serial ECGs at presentation are especially useful because of how the changes evolve in contrast to acute myocardial ischemia or J-point elevation.

Creatinine kinase MB fraction and/or troponin-I values may be elevated in 8% to 22% of patients presenting with acute pericarditis. Evidence of elevated troponin or CK-MB laboratory values correlate with ST elevation on the electrocardiogram. The elevation of cardiac enzymes may represent silent myocarditis in addition to pericarditis, or the epicardial inflammation that sometimes seen in acute pericarditis. Endocardial ischemia due to coronary artery disease should be considered in patients presenting with acute pericarditis who have concomitant significant elevations in cardiac biomarkers.

Acute pericarditis may be associated with mild elevations in the total white blood cell count. Viral or idiopathic pericarditis may present with a lymphocytic predominance, whereas bacterial pericarditis may have a neutrophilic predominance.

The erythrocyte sedimentation rate may have mild elevation, but significant elevations in the erythrocyte sedimentation rate may suggest an autoimmune etiology, uremia, bacterial processes, or tuberculosis.

The chest radiograph may be completely normal in viral or idiopathic acute pericarditis. Pericardial effusion should be suspected in the setting of an abnormal cardiac silhouette. An accumulation of more than 200 mL of pericardial effusion will enlarge the cardiac silhouette, indistinguishable from other causes of cardiomegaly. As more fluid accumulates, however, a "water-bottle" configuration may develop. In the absence of pulmonary venous congestion, considerable cardiomegaly may be a clue that a pericardial effusion is present. Fluid between the two pericardial layers may show separation of the epicardial fat pad from the outer border of the cardiac silhouette. An abnormal chest radiograph may suggest the etiology for the pericarditis, or a different diagnosis. An infiltrate on chest x-ray may suggest bacterial pericarditis as the etiology. An upper lobe infiltrate, or a completely normal chest x-ray may accompany tuberculosis pericarditis. Pulmonary congestion may suggest ischemia or myocarditis.

Echocardiography is the imaging modality of choice in acute pericarditis because of its availability, lack of radiation exposure, and ability to rule out potentially fatal complications such as tamponade. An echocardiogram is recommended for most patients with pericarditis, especially patients with fever, currently on anticoagulation therapy, in an immunocompromised state, a recent history of trauma, or if there is suspected myocardial involvement. Echocardiography in patients with uncomplicated acute pericarditis may be completely normal. A small effusion may be present which does not necessitate intervention. Large pericardial effusions are uncommon in acute pericarditis and should trigger the clinician to pursue other diagnoses. Focal wall motion abnormalities may suggest that myocarditis may be present.

Computed tomography and MRI are emerging as valuable methods for detecting complicated pericarditis. The inflamed pericardium in both acute and chronic pericarditis can be visualized by MRI. The ability to assess fluid attenuation on both CT and MRI allows a noninvasive assessment of the etiology. The thickened pericardial layers and any pericardial effusion can be effectively visualized on cardiac MRI. Furthermore, MRI may be the noninvasive imaging modality of choice for the diagnosis of myocarditis, which can accompany pericarditis.

MANAGEMENT

Patients with a history, physical examination, and testing consistent with pericarditis should receive nonsteroidal anti-inflammatory drugs (NSAIDs) as the initial treatment. Aspirin is preferred over NSAIDs if acute myocardial infarction is the cause of acute pericarditis, as NSAIDs may promote ventricular rupture. Therapeutic options include: aspirin (2-4 g daily), ibuprofen (1600-3200 mg daily), or other NSAIDs at high therapeutic dosing for 2 to 4 weeks' duration. Recent meta-analyses have shown that the addition of colchicine to traditional therapy with NSAID therapy has a significant improvement in outcomes (lower incidence of recurrent pericarditis) when directly compared to lone NSAID therapy. Colchicine has minimal serious side effects, limited to mostly gastrointestinal upset. If there is no large effusion and cardiac enzymes are normal, the patient can be discharged and followed up within 2 to 4 weeks to ensure resolution. If the pain has resolved, therapy may be discontinued at that time.

In the past, a prednisone taper over the course of a week, starting at 60 mg orally was used; however, caution is warranted for corticosteroid administration for acute pericarditis due to a much higher relapse rate than with other medications. Corticosteroids may be indicated in acute pericarditis due to systemic inflammatory diseases or in patients who are refractory to or have contraindications to aspirin, NSAIDs, and colchicine. However, *corticosteroids may promote the development of recurrent pericarditis*. Additionally, corticosteroids should not be used in patients with acute pericarditis due to bacterial infection or tuberculosis or in patients with postinfarction pericarditis due to the risk of ventricular aneurysm formation.

PERICARDIAL EFFUSIONS AND CARDIAC TAMPONADE

INTRODUCTION

Many inflammatory and noninflammatory conditions lead to excess fluid in the pericardial space, thereby, overwhelming the villi and cilia that physiologically reabsorb fluid and optimize the movement of the pericardial layers over one another (Table 130-1). Often, pericardial effusions accompany episodes of pericarditis and share the same etiology. Sometimes, pericardial effusions are incidentally noted during imaging for other indications. Therefore, clinicians need to quickly determine if a pericardial effusion is a factor in the patient's clinical syndrome, identify any hemodynamic consequences of the effusion, and then appropriately manage with the help of consultants.

PATHOPHYSIOLOGY

Pericardial effusions most commonly form due to an inflammatory process involving the pericardium and less commonly due to accumulation of lymphatic drainage or blood (hemopericardium). Ascending aortic dissection, perforation of the atrial or ventricular walls, or direct injury to the pericardium itself may result in hemopericardium. Patients with anasarca, uremia, or myxedema may also develop significant pericardial effusions.

Cardiac tamponade may develop irrespective of the underlying pathophysiology responsible for the effusion. The hemodynamic consequences of a pericardial effusion are determined by the amount of increased pressure within the pericardial sac and the heart's ability to compensate or accommodate this increased pressure. Rapid accumulation of pericardial fluid may lead to very high intrapericardial pressures within a very short amount of time causing hemodynamic collapse despite a small volume effusion. The pericardium is a compliant collagen-based structure with the intrinsic ability to stretch and accommodate a large amount of fluid without causing hemodynamic consequences when effusions accumulate subacutely or chronically. However, even large chronic effusions will

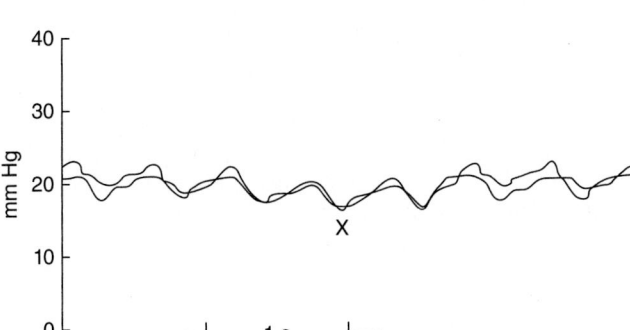

Figure 130-3 *Simultaneous right atrial and pericardial pressures from a patient with severe cardiac tamponade. The pressures are elevated and equal to one another, and only the x descent on the right atrial tracing is present; the y descent is absent. The pressures fall normally during inspiration. (Reproduced, with permission, from Fuster V, O'Rourke RA, Walsh RA, et al. Hurst's the Heart, 12th ed. New York: McGraw-Hill; 2008. Fig. 84-10.)*

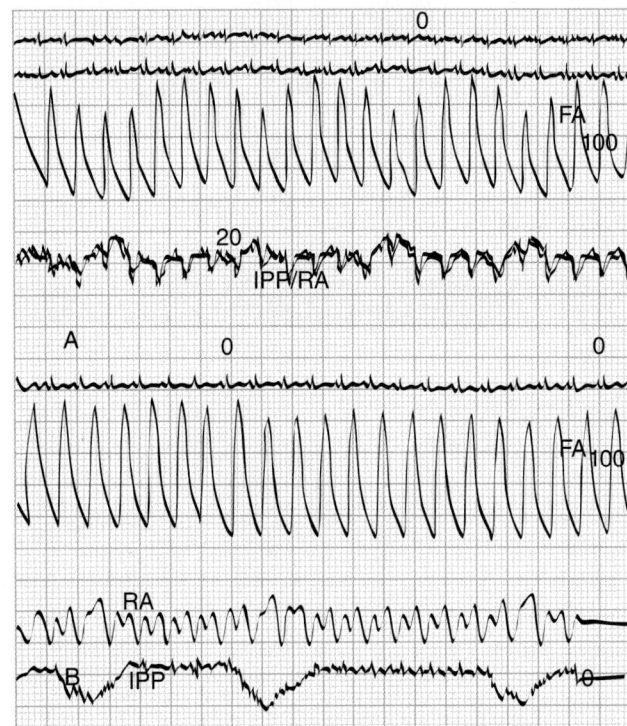

Figure 130-4 *Hemodynamic record from a patient with cardiac tamponade before (A) and after (B) pericardiocentesis. (A) Pulsus paradoxus is evident from the femoral artery (FA) pressure tracing. Note the absent y descent on the right atrial (RA) tracing and the equal and elevated RA and pericardial (IPP) pressures. (B) After removal of pericardial fluid, pericardial and right atrial pressures decrease and the pulsus paradoxus disappears. (Modified, with permission, from Fuster V, O'Rourke RA, Walsh RA, et al. Hurst's the Heart, 12th ed. New York: McGraw-Hill; 2008. Fig. 84-15.)*

eventually reach a critical volume at which intrapericardial pressures will lead to hemodynamic collapse.

Right atrial and ventricular diastolic pressures rise as intrapericardial pressure increases. Eventually, these pressures equalize at which time the hemodynamic consequences of cardiac tamponade become clinically evident. These hemodynamic effects are best appreciated as loss of the y descent in the RA venous waveform (**Figure 130-3**) and the presence of a paradoxical arterial pulse. Total heart volume is fixed while the inspiratory augmentation of venous return to right-sided circulation is retained in cardiac tamponade. Intrathoracic pressure changes are transmitted through the pericardium in contrast to the hemodynamics of constrictive physiology.

The y descent represents the decrease in RA pressure during passive filling of the right ventricle (RV) immediately after the tricuspid valve opens signifying the beginning of ventricular diastole. In cardiac tamponade, the normal pressure gradient between the right atrium (RA) and right ventricle is lost since diastolic pressures in all four cardiac chambers are equalized causing an abbreviated and minimized decrease in RA pressure represented by a "blunted" y descent (**Figure 130-4**).

The paradoxical pulse or "pulsus paradoxus" is defined as a greater than 10 mm Hg decrease in systolic blood pressure during inspiration. The decreased intrathoracic pressure accompanying inspiration leads to increased filling of the right heart. Since total cardiac volume is fixed, this increase in right-sided filling comes at the expense of decreased left heart volumes mediated through interventricular dependence or exaggerated leftward shift of the interventricular septum. Consequently, there is decreased LV filling and therefore stroke volume. The increased right-sided filling does lead to increased RV stroke volume. However, several cardiac cycles are required before this causes increased LV filling. As intrapericardial pressure increases, total intracardiac volume is further diminished, and the above hemodynamic effects are accentuated, potentially leading to hemodynamic collapse.

■ PRESENTATION

Pericardial effusions do not usually cause symptoms beyond those associated with any concomitant pericardial inflammation. However, cardiac tamponade commonly causes chest pain, dyspnea, or chest fullness. Additionally, symptoms of hepatic and visceral

congestion, fever, fatigue, and lethargy have been reported. Importantly, these symptoms may be absent or unobtainable in patients with acute cardiac tamponade if they are in shock or critically ill. Of these symptoms dyspnea has the highest sensitivity reported in observational studies of 87% to 88%.

The presence of a pulsus paradoxus is the most helpful bedside test for cardiac tamponade. Pulsus paradoxus may be initially appreciated by the disappearance of the radial pulse on inspiration. Smaller degrees of pulsus paradoxus may be noted while gradually reducing finger pressure on the radial or femoral artery similar to the gradual lowering of blood pressure from the point of obliterating the pulse to the point when only expiratory pulses are felt to the point of feeling all pulses. The accurate measurement of the paradoxical pulse is quantified using cuff sphygmomanometry, represented by the differences in recorded pressures between that recorded when the first Korotkoff sound is auscultated and that at which Korotkoff sounds are heard with every heart beat. Importantly, a paradoxical pulse may be absent when preexisting conditions exist that elevate LV diastolic pressures such as aortic regurgitation, LV hypertrophy, or LV failure, and conditions that limit right heart filling such as pulmonary hypertension. When cardiogenic shock develops, pulsus paradoxus may be difficult to detect. A paradoxical pulse may be present in the absence of tamponade in patients with a multitude of disorders including COPD, asthma, pulmonary embolism, or shock. The presence of a paradoxical pulse has a reported sensitivity of 98%, specificity of 83%, a positive likelihood ratio (LR+) of 5.9, and a negative likelihood ratio (LR-) of 0.03. Elevated jugular venous pressure and tachycardia have good sensitivity (76% and 77%,

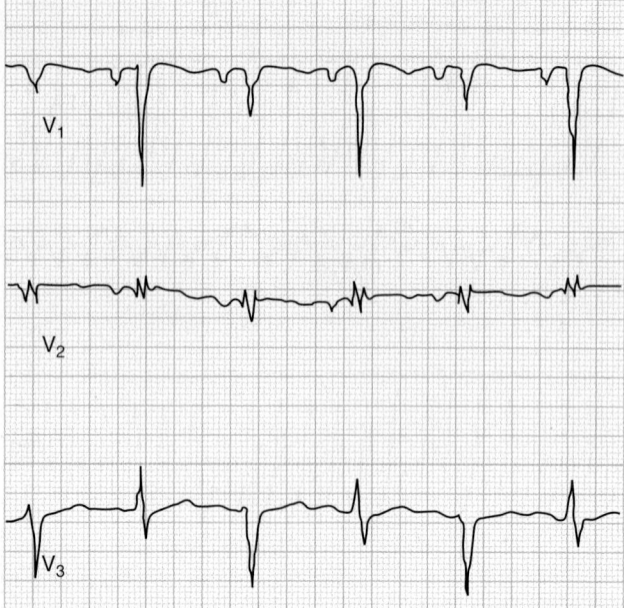

Figure 130-5 *Electrocardiogram (leads V$_1$-V$_3$) of a patient with cardiac tamponade demonstrates marked electrical alternans, with varying or alternating amplitude of the QRS complex with each cardiac contraction.*

respectively) that, when absent, decreases the likelihood of cardiac tamponade. Hypotension and distant heart sounds are insensitive physical findings in the assessment of cardiac tamponade (see Suggested Readings, Roy, C et al).

■ DIAGNOSIS

Electrocardiographic findings of low voltage, electrical alternans, and PR depression have specificities ranging from 89% to 100%, but are very insensitive findings for the diagnosis of pericardial effusions. Electrical alternans is caused by "swing" of the heart within the fluid-filled pericardium (**Figure 130-5**). Similarly, the finding of an enlarged cardiac silhouette on chest radiography has a high sensitivity (~89%) and low specificity (~50%) for pericardial effusions. The cardiac silhouette may appear flask like with "tenting" that often obscures the left heart border at the level of the left atrial appendage (**Figure 130-6**).

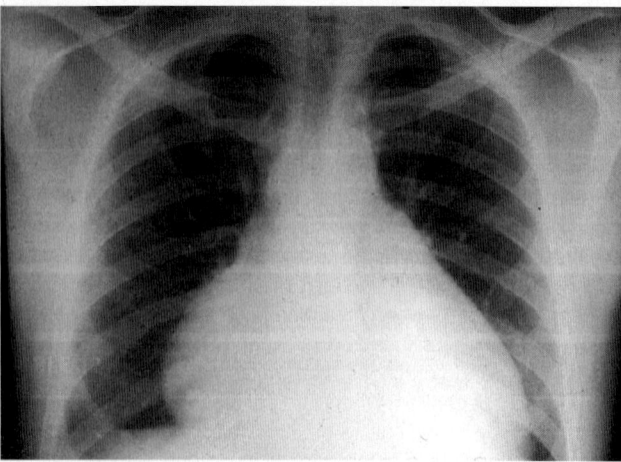

Figure 130-6 *Chest x-ray (anterior) of a patient with rapidly increasing pericardial effusion and hemodynamic evidence of cardiac tamponade. Note how the cardiac silhouette is rounded in its lower portion and tapers at the base of the heart, resembling a plastic bag filled with water sitting on a table ("water-bottle" heart).*

The primary diagnostic imaging modality for cardiac tamponade is transthoracic Doppler echocardiography, a noninvasive study that provides accurate information regarding the hemodynamic effects of a pericardial effusion. Echocardiography can accurately detect and quantify effusions of any size and serve as a useful tool to evaluate effusions on a serial basis. Collapse of the right atrium and right ventricle during early ventricular diastole signify that an effusion is severe enough to cause some degree of hemodynamic compromise. RA collapse is the most sensitive finding, while RV collapse is the most specific finding for cardiac tamponade (**Figure 130-7**). Large pleural effusions may also cause these findings to be present. Exaggerated respiratory variation of right- and left-sided venous and valvular flow patterns is highly specific for tamponade as well.

Both CT and MRI are useful adjuncts to echocardiography, providing accurate quantification of pericardial effusions and real-time imaging to quantify septal shift and chamber collapse with accuracy similar to that of echocardiography as well as identifying other pathology occurring within the chest.

■ MANAGEMENT

Management of pericardial effusions begins with echocardiography assessment of the effusion. The presence of cardiac tamponade should be considered a medical emergency, warranting admission to an intensive care unit with prompt consultation of a cardiovascular diseases specialist to determine the need for urgent pericardiocentesis. Invasive hemodynamic monitoring with pulmonary artery catheter can be useful in patients whom the decision to perform pericardiocentesis has been deferred. Volume resuscitation may benefit some patients with hypovolemia. However, in the absence of hypovolemia, excessive fluid resuscitation may cause increased intracardiac and pericardial pressures, thus decreasing the transmural myocardial pressures and cardiac filling eventually leading to circulatory collapse. It may be reasonable to give a fluid challenge and monitor closely for clinical improvement or deterioration if the patient's volume status is difficult to determine. The use of inotropes, specifically dobutamine, has some temporizing benefit in animal studies; however, in most patients with tamponade physiology compensatory mechanisms are already maximized.

PRACTICE POINT

- The presence of cardiac tamponade should be considered a medical emergency, warranting admission to an intensive care unit with prompt consultation of a cardiovascular diseases specialist to perform an urgent pericardiocentesis. If the patient becomes pulseless, pericardiocentesis should be performed immediately, even by inexperienced practitioners.
- Volume resuscitation is beneficial in patients with hypovolemia, but can be detrimental in the euvolemic or hypervolemic patient.

Removal of the pericardial fluid with pericardiocentesis is the definitive treatment for cardiac tamponade. When available, pericardiocentesis is performed in the cardiac catheterization laboratory using echocardiographic guidance. In the emergent situation, this may be performed blindly at the bedside. If the procedure is performed by a cardiovascular disease specialist, a pigtail catheter can be placed over a wire to facilitate further drainage of the effusion; however, this may not be possible in the emergent setting. Repeated echocardiography should be performed immediately postprocedurally to evaluate for hemodynamic improvement.

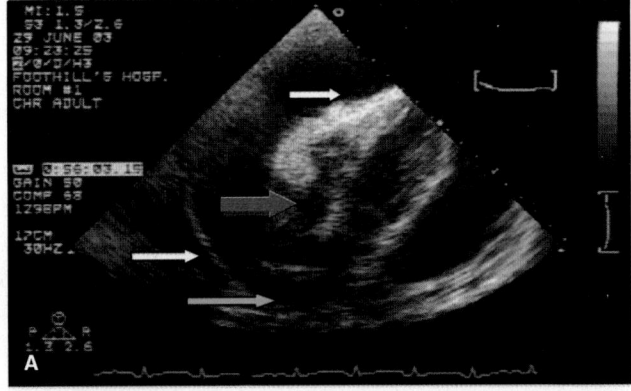

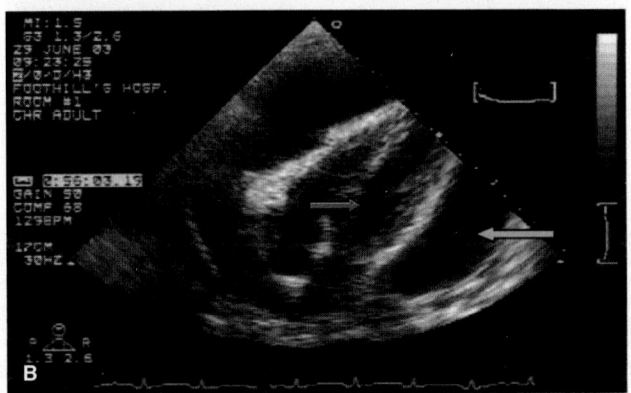

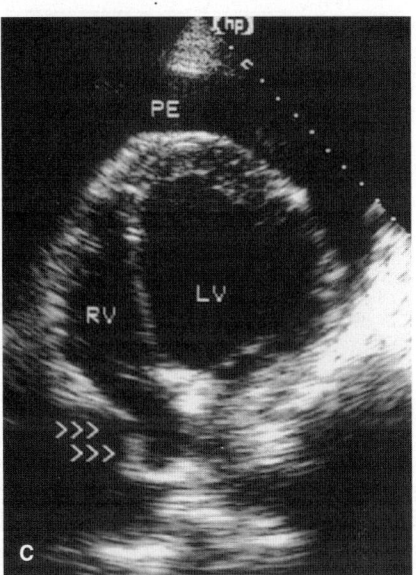

Figure 130-7 *(A) An early diastolic frame of a two-dimensional echocardiogram in a patient with cardiac tamponade. There is a very large pericardial effusion (white arrows) and right atrial (blue arrow) and right ventricular (red arrow) collapse. (B) A late diastolic frame from the same cardiac cycle; both ventricles are underfilled. Right and left ventricles labeled with red and blue arrows, respectively. (Reproduced, with permission, from Hall JB, Schmidt GA, Wood LDH. Principles of Critical Care. 3rd ed. New York: McGraw-Hill; 2005. Fig. 28-7.) (C) Two-dimensional echocardiogram in the apical four-chamber view. During late diastole, there is inversion of the lateral wall of the right atrium. (Reproduced, with permission, from Fuster V, O'Rourke RA, Walsh RA, et al. Hurst's the Heart, 12th ed. New York: McGraw-Hill; 2008. Fig. 16-138.)*

PRACTICE POINT

- Pericardiocentesis procedure: Patient is positioned at a 30° head-up angle to allow pericardial fluid to pool at the apex. A long 16- or 18-gauge pericardiocentesis needle attached to a stopcock and a large syringe filled with 10 to 15 cc of 1% lidocaine is inserted in the subxiphoid area one fingerbreadth below the left medial costal margin. Anesthetize along the anticipated needle path. The needle is slowly advanced at a 15° to 30° angle directed at the left shoulder with the injection of lidocaine as needed to minimize discomfort to the patient. Intermittent aspiration should occur during advancement of the needle. Once fluid is aspirated, the operator should immediately turn the stopcock to pressure to verify the location of the needle. In cardiac tamponade the pressure waveform will resemble that of the right atrium. A RV waveform is abnormal and the needle should be promptly withdrawn. Usually only 50 to 100 cc of fluid needs to be removed before hemodynamic improvement is observed.

Pericardial fluid should be sent to the laboratory for analysis, including cell count with differential, hematocrit, total protein, LDH, Gram and acid fast bacilli stains, as well as bacterial, fungal, and acid fast bacilli cultures when appropriate. Additionally, cytology may be helpful if there is a suspicion of a malignant etiology. Lights criteria, commonly used to evaluate pleural effusions, may be applied to determine if pericardial fluid is exudative or transudative. In the setting of pericarditis, a pericardial biopsy is often required to make a diagnosis.

Long-term management involves treating the underlying pathology causing the effusion and serial echocardiography to monitor for recurrence of effusion. We recommend a repeat transthoracic echocardiogram 48 to 72 hours following initial drainage of a pericardial effusion:

- No evidence of recurrence: then further transthoracic echocardiography performed as clinically indicated.
- Evidence of recurrence within the first 72 hours: repeat pericardiocentesis, or moredefinitively, a pericardial window performed by a cardiothoracic or thoracic surgeon.

Transudative pericardial effusions are more likely to recur and to require a pericardial window procedure. Follow-up for 2 weeks following hospital discharge is indicated for patients diagnosed with a pericardial effusion with a cardiovascular disease specialist.

CONSTRICTIVE PERICARDITIS

■ INTRODUCTION

Constrictive pericarditis is the late stage manifestation of any inflammatory process resulting in constriction and loss of elasticity of the pericardium. In the developed world, the three most common etiologies are postviral (idiopathic), postsurgical, and radiation induced. In less developed parts of the world, tuberculosis is still a major infectious etiology of constrictive pericarditis.

■ PATHOPHYSIOLOGY

Once scarring of the pericardium takes place, its intrinsic elasticity is lost. An inelastic pericardium results in restricted filling of both

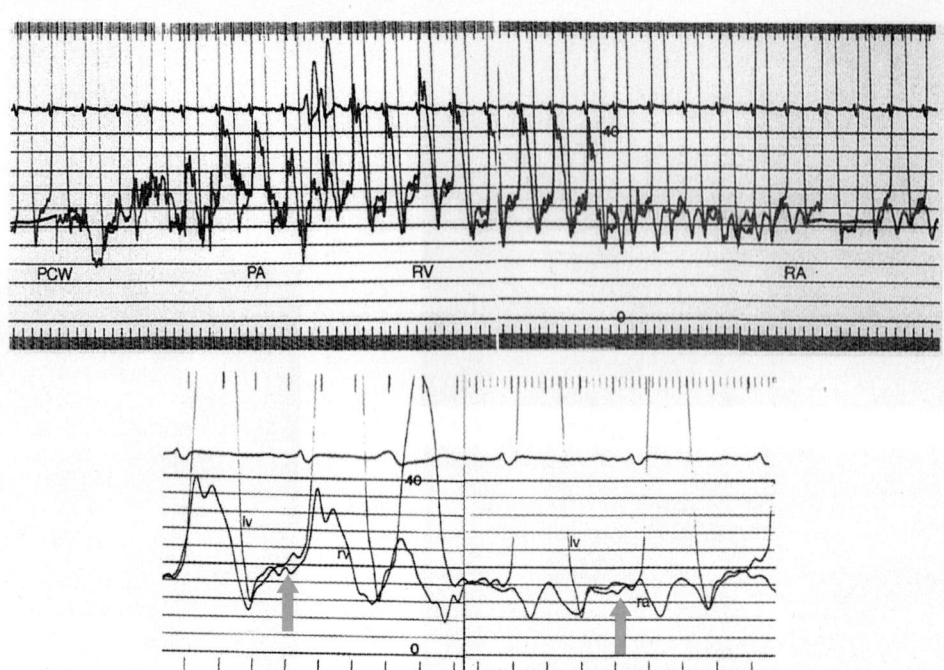

Figure 130-8 *Hemodynamic record of a patient with surgically proven constrictive pericarditis. Top: Slow-paper-speed recording of high-gain left ventricular (LV) pressure and simultaneous right heart pullback from pulmonary capillary wedge (PCW) to pulmonary artery (PA), right ventricle (RV), and right atrium (RA). Bottom: Fast-paper-speed recording of LV and simultaneous RV and RA pressure tracings. Note the increased and equal atrial and diastolic pressures (blue arrows), the prominent x and y descents on the RA tracing, and the dip and plateau on the RV and LV tracings during longer diastoles. (Reproduced, with permission, from Fuster V, O'Rourke RA, Walsh RA, et al. Hurst's the Heart, 12th ed. New York: McGraw-Hill; 2008. Fig. 84-22.)*

atria and ventricles. The stiffened pericardium effectively limits total cardiac volume causing equilibration of filling pressures in all four chambers of the heart. As a result elevated atrial pressures drive accentuated ventricular filling during early diastole. This rapid early filling continues until mid-diastole when the ventricles reach their filling limit set by the stiffened pericardium. At this point, ventricular filling ceases and filling pressures equalize throughout the heart. The rapid early ventricular filling is represented by an accentuated y descent in both right and left atrial pressure tracings. This presents as a dominant negative wave in the already distended neck veins. The equalization of ventricular filling pressures is represented by the "square root" sign seen on diastolic ventricular pressure tracings (**Figure 130-8**), both of which are distinguishing features of constrictive physiology. Overall, cardiac output is decreased as a result of under filling of the ventricles and systemic venous pressure is increased. Decreased cardiac output leads to increased sympathetic activity and up regulation of the renin-angiotensin, aldosterone system, enhancing sodium and water retention leading to volume overload. Significantly increased systemic venous pressures lead to congestive hepatopathy and cachexia in advanced stages of disease. Ventricular contraction is usually preserved; however, it may be slightly diminished because of a decreased preload effect.

The decrease in intrathoracic pressure seen with inspiration is not transmitted to any of the intracardiac chambers, but is transmitted to the pulmonary vasculature. This results in the following during inspiration:

- A diminished filling gradient between the pulmonary veins and the left atrium.
- A decrease in mitral inflow velocities and decreased filling of the left ventricle.
- Enhanced RV filling via right to left septal shift.

These events are reversed during expiration. This physiology differs from the hemodynamics seen in restrictive cardiomyopathy and cardiac tamponade.

Effusive-constrictive pericarditis develops when tamponade physiology results from a pericardial effusion in the setting of a fibrotic pericardium. Once the pericardial fluid is removed, constrictive physiology remains. The most common etiologies are malignancy, radiation therapy, connective tissue disease, and idiopathic pericarditis.

■ PRESENTATION

Patients with constrictive physiology usually present with complaints of volume overload, dyspnea on exertion, and fatigue. Additionally symptoms of hepatic congestion may also be prominent, sometimes leading to the misdiagnosis of chronic hepatic disease.

A Kussmal sign (lack of decline in jugular venous pressure with inspiration) may be seen in 20% of cases but may also be present in cases of severe right-sided heart failure and tricuspid valve disease. Other signs include a paradoxical pulse, appreciated in 20% of cases, and uncommonly, a pericardial friction rub and pericardial knock.

■ DIAGNOSIS

There are no specific features on electrocardiogram to aid in the diagnosis of constrictive pericarditis. Atrial fibrillation, low voltage, and nonspecific ST-T wave changes can be seen in up to 33% of cases, however these findings are nonspecific. Chest radiography may reveal ringed calcification of the cardiac silhouette, especially on the lateral view (**Figure 130-9**).

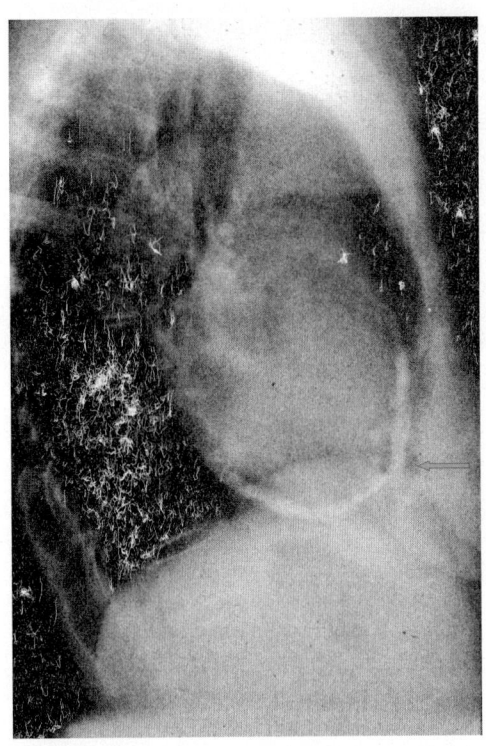

Figure 130-9 *Standard lateral view of a chest x-ray of a patient with constrictive pericarditis. Note the calcification appreciated in the apical region denoted by the blue arrow.*

Transthoracic Doppler echocardiography, a class I recommendation by the American College of Cardiology, remains a useful imaging modality in the evaluation of constrictive pericarditis to obtain hemodynamic and anatomic information. Both cardiac CT and MRI provide direct visualization of the pericardium and allow for precise measurement of pericardial thickness. Cardiac MRI may also provide useful information regarding hemodynamics, and is considered by some to be the imaging modality of choice for pericardial diseases. In some cases, the diagnosis of constrictive pericarditis cannot be made based solely on noninvasive imaging modalities. In these cases, a right and left heart catheterization is required to determine the diagnosis.

■ MANAGEMENT

Pericardiectomy is the treatment of choice for chronic symptomatic constrictive pericarditis (**Table 130-2**). Complete pericardiectomy (which has been likened to peeling an orange) is preferred to partial resection as recurrence rates decrease with complete resection. Additionally, patients surgically treated with complete pericardiectomy achieve more rapid normalization of hemodynamics and have lower long-term mortality rates when compared with those treated with partial pericardial resection, 83.8% versus 73.9%, respectively. Patients with very early or very advanced disease are not optimal surgical candidates because a small percentage of patients with acute pericarditis will also have some constrictive symptoms that will spontaneously resolve. The mortality associated with pericardiectomy can reach 30% to 40% in patients with advanced disease

TABLE 130-2 Evidence-Based Medicine: Key References for Pericardial Diseases

Reference	Methodology	Results	Limitations	Bottom Line
Imazio M, et al. Colchicine as first-line therapy for recurrent pericarditis. *Arch Intern Med.* 2005;165:1987-1989	A prospective, randomized, open-label design comparing the addition of colchicine to standard therapy with aspirin vs standard therapy alone	Treatment with colchicine significantly decreased the recurrence rate (actuarial rates at 18 mo were 24.0% vs 50.6%; $P = .02$)	Open-label trial design	Colchicine therapy led to a clinically important and statistically significant benefit over conventional treatment, decreasing the recurrence rate in patients with a first episode of recurrent pericarditis
Roy CL, et al. Does this patient with a pericardial effusion have cardiac tamponade? *JAMA.* 2007;297(16):1810-1818	Meta-analysis of 787 sources from 1966 to 2006. Systematically reviews the accuracy of the history, physical examination, and basic diagnostic tests for the diagnosis of cardiac tamponade	Five features occur in the majority of patients with tamponade with statistically significant sensitivities: dyspnea, tachycardia, pulsus paradoxus, elevated jugular venous pressure, and cardiomegaly on chest radiograph	Significant heterogeneity in study population, design, and reference standard for the diagnosis of cardiac tamponade	A pulsus paradoxus >10 mm Hg among patients with a pericardial effusion helps distinguish those with cardiac tamponade from those without. Diagnostic certainty of presence of tamponade requires additional testing
Bertog SC, et al. Constrictive pericarditis: etiology and cause-specific survival after pericardiectomy. *J Am Coll Cardiol.* 2004;43:1445-1452	A retrospective case review of 163 patients who underwent pericardiectomy for CP over a 24-y period at a single surgical center	Perioperative mortality was 6%. Idiopathic CP had the best prognosis followed by postsurgical and postradiation CP	Retrospective review with results from a single surgery center, significant heterogeneity of patient population, present cardiac physiology, and severity of disease at time of surgery	Long-term survival after pericardiectomy for CP is related to underlying etiology, LV systolic function, renal function, serum sodium, and PAP

CP, constrictive pericarditis; LV, left ventricular; PAP, pulmonary artery systolic pressure.

and NYHA class IV symptoms. Medical therapy with diuretics and digoxin may provide some minor clinical improvement as well. In selected patients, cardiac transplantation may be an option. In patients with tuberculous involvement, rapid treatment with appropriate antimicrobial therapy should be initiated.

SUGGESTED READINGS

Cooper LT Jr. Myocarditis. *N Engl J Med.* 2009;360:1526-1538.

Curtiss E, Reddy, Uretsky B, Cecchetti A. Pulsus paradoxus: definition and relation to the severity of cardiac tamponade. *Am Heart J.* 1988;115:391-398.

Lange RA, Hillis LD. Clinical practice. Acute pericarditis. *N Engl J Med.* 2004;351:2195-2202.

Little WC, Freeman GL. Pericardial disease. *Circulation.* 2006;113: 1622-1632.

Raval J, Nagaraja V, Eslick G, Denniss R. The role of colchicine in pericarditis—a systematic review and meta-analysis of randomized trials. *Heart Lung Circu.* 2015;23:1-7.

Reddy P, Curtiss E, O'Toole J, Shaver J. Cardiac tamponade: hemodynamic observations in man. *Circulation.* 1978;58:265-272.

Roy CL, Minor MA, Brookhart MA, Choudhry NK. Does this patient with cardiac pericardial effusion have cardiac tamponade? *JAMA.* 2007;297(16):1810-1818.

Spodick D. Acute cardiac tamponade. *N Engl J Med.* 2003;349:684-690.

Spodick DH. Acute pericarditis. *JAMA.* 2003;289:1150-1153.

Troughton RW, Asher CR, Klein AL. Pericarditis. *Lancet.* 2004;363: 717-727.

CHAPTER 131

Valvular Heart Disease

Jose F. Condado, MD, MS

Brian W. Kaebnick, MD

Vasilis C. Babaliaros, MD

Key Clinical Questions

1. What are the key factors that determine when to proceed to aortic valve replacement for patients with aortic stenosis? What guides decision making relating to aortic surgery for acute and chronic aortic regurgitation?

2. Which patients with aortic stenosis should be considered for transcatheter therapies such as valvuloplasty or transcatheter aortic valve replacement?

3. What are the indications for surgery in patients with mitral stenosis? What are the goals of medical therapy for mitral regurgitation and when should patients be considered for mitral valve repair or replacement?

4. When should patients with mitral regurgitations be considered for transcatheter mitral valve procedures?

5. What are the objectives of treatment of pulmonic valve disease? When should a patient be referred for surgery or transcatheter valve replacement?

6. What are the factors that determine medical versus surgical treatment of tricuspid stenosis or tricuspid regurgitation?

INTRODUCTION

Valvular heart disease is a common disorder seen by hospitalists. Often a cardiologist and/or cardiac surgeon is consulted to comanage these patients; however, a comprehensive understanding and appropriate screening by an internist is important for both an inpatient and outpatient practice. This chapter provides practical information regarding the pathophysiology, diagnosis, and therapy of the valvular abnormalities that commonly affect each of the four valves.

AORTIC VALVE DISORDERS

■ AORTIC STENOSIS

Pathophysiology

Aortic stenosis (AS) is the obstruction of blood flow through the aortic valve due to thickened or immobile leaflets. Aortic stenosis may be categorized into three disease processes: rheumatic, congenital, and degenerative. Rheumatic is the most common type of AS worldwide, but is rarely seen in industrialized countries due to improvements in therapy and diagnosis. Since it remains prevalent in developing nations, rheumatic disease should still be considered in immigrant populations. Congenital AS is caused by malformed aortic leaflets resulting in bicuspid or unicuspid aortic valve and is typically seen in symptomatic patients that are in their fourth or fifth decade of life. Degenerative AS (also known as calcific or senile AS) is the leading cause of valvular cardiac surgery in US adults, with an estimated prevalence of 2% to 7% in populations over the age of 65 years. Other less common causes of AS include connective tissue diseases, radiation therapy, and hyperlipoproteinemia syndromes.

Degenerative aortic disease represents a spectrum ranging from aortic sclerosis, defined as leaflet thickening without significant obstruction, to severe AS that significantly obstructs blood flow and requires replacement. Several risk factors have been associated with aortic sclerosis including smoking, hypertension, diabetes mellitus, and elevated low-density lipoprotein cholesterol and C-reactive protein. Recent data support the hypothesis that aortic valve calcification is an active process that may not completely reflect patient age or "wear and tear" of the valve. Abnormalities of blood flow across the valve can lead to damage of the valvular endothelium. Endothelial injury initiates an inflammatory process similar to atherosclerosis and ultimately leads to deposition of calcium on the valve and eventual stenosis. Patients with congenitally abnormal valves are exposed to more profound abnormalities in blood flow and develop AS earlier than trileaflet valves, usually in their fifth to sixth decade, but it can occur as early as their fourth decade. In rheumatic disease, an autoimmune inflammatory reaction is triggered by prior *Streptococcus* infection that targets the valvular endothelium leading to inflammation, leaflet thickening, and commissural fusion. Eventual calcification is also seen in rheumatic AS but often less than other disease processes.

Stenosis of the aortic valve occurs slowly and is subclinical until the disease is fairly advanced. Progressive calcium deposition and inflammation limit aortic leaflet mobility and impose a pressure burden on the left ventricle. This increased afterload causes the ventricle to concentrically hypertrophy in order to maintain normal wall stress. As the stenosis worsens, the adaptive mechanism fails and left ventricular wall stress increases leading to a decline in ventricular function and heart failure symptoms.

Three symptoms are commonly associated with severe AS: dyspnea, angina, and syncope. The compensatory concentric left ventricular hypertrophy (LVH) results in a decrease of chamber compliance and size, which consequently contributes to an increase of left ventricular end-diastolic pressure during periods of increased cardiac output leading to the patient's sensation of dyspnea. In addition to elevated filling pressures, the hypertrophied heart muscle requires more blood flow than a normal heart muscle during exercise due to the increase oxygen required to supply the hypertrophied ventricle. This can result in oxygen supply-demand mismatch leading to demand ischemia manifesting as chest pain even in the absence of coronary atherosclerotic disease. These areas of relatively ischemic heart muscle are potential sources of arrhythmia that can result in ventricular tachycardia with syncope and sudden cardiac death.

Diagnosis: does the patient have AS?

Aortic stenosis may exhibit a variety of possible clinical presentations and symptoms (**Table 131-1**). An electrocardiography (ECG) is indicated in the initial workup of all patients with valvular disease and is abnormal in more than 90% of patients with AS (**Figure 131-1**). The most common abnormality seen on the ECG is LVH due to pressure overload. Evidence of LVH and absent Q-waves helps distinguish AS from other conditions such as aortic sclerosis with ischemic heart disease. Patients with AS often have conduction disease manifesting as atrioventricular block, hemiblock, or bundle branch block.

Transthoracic echocardiography (TTE) is the ideal test for the initial evaluation of suspected valvular heart disease, such as AS, and should be performed in patients with pathologic murmurs detected on physical examination (**Figure 131-2**). Transthoracic echocardiography can visualize the leaflet mobility and anatomy to help determine the etiology of AS. Doppler assessments can accurately measure the pressure gradient across the aortic valve and estimate aortic valve area. Transthoracic echocardiography is also a comprehensive assessment of the heart anatomy and can assess left ventricular function and the presence of LVH. Information obtained from a TTE is usually enough to grade the severity of the AS from mild, moderate, or severe based on the calculated aortic valve area, maximal velocity (V_{max}), and aortoventricular mean gradient (**Table 131-2**). Clinicians need to recognize that TTE measurements may underestimate the severity of AS in patients with severely depressed left ventricular function. In these cases (low flow/low gradient AS), a dobutamine stress echocardiogram is critical for diagnosing a true severe symptomatic AS.

Cardiac catheterization is no longer the first test of choice used for the diagnosis of AS, but can be used in patients with inconclusive findings on TTE or with discrepancies between noninvasive findings and the physical examination.

Treatment

The need for aortic valve replacement in patients with severe AS is determined by the onset of symptoms or new reduction of left ventricular function. The onset of symptoms portends a poor prognosis with an average survival of only 2 to 3 years unless replacement is performed. Symptomatic patients are also at risk of sudden death (8%-34%), and thus, a strategy of "watchful waiting" should never take the place of prompt referral. Patients with failing left ventricular function and severe AS should be referred for treatment regardless of symptoms. Some patients may not report significant symptoms due to sedentary lifestyle or modifying their behaviors to accommodate their severe AS. In these patients, an exercise stress test may be considered to accurately delineate symptomatic from asymptomatic patients. Patients that have a drop in blood pressure, develop angina, or poor exercise tolerance should be considered symptomatic.

Balloon aortic valvuloplasty (BAV) can temporarily improve the symptoms caused by severe AS. This percutaneous procedure is performed in the cardiac catheterization laboratory by dilating a balloon in the aortic valve and thus, relieving the stenosis and symptoms. However, most patients will experience restenosis of their valve at 6 to 12 months, and there is no survival benefit to BAV when used in isolation. However, BAV can be useful as a palliative therapy in patients with a life expectancy shorter than 2 years or as a bridge for either surgical or transcatheter aortic valve replacement.

Surgical aortic valve replacement (SAVR) is a therapy for AS with proven survival benefit (**Figure 131-3**), and is the standard of care for patients with severe AS with low surgical risk. A thorough discussion between the surgeon and patient exploring the risks and benefits of valve replacement should take place before proceeding with surgery. Physicians should also discuss the merits and drawbacks of the different types of valves (bioprosthetic vs mechanical) before the operation. Current bioprosthetic valves are made of porcine or bovine pericardial tissue and require reoperation 10 to 20 years after implantation due to valve degeneration; these valves do not require long-term anticoagulation. Mechanical valves are not

TABLE 131-1 Symptoms and Physical Examination Findings in Aortic Stenosis

Aortic Stenosis Symptoms	Aortic Stenosis Physical Examination Findings
Decreased exercise tolerance	Late peaking systolic ejection murmur best auscultated at the right second intercostal space, which can obscure S_2 when severe
Dyspnea on exertion	
Chest pain	Gallavardin phenomena (A dissociation between the harsh and musical components of the systolic murmur, often heard loudest at the right upper sterna border but can also be heard along the left upper sternal border and apex of the heart)
Syncope/near syncope	
Heart failure	
	Murmurs radiating to the carotid arteries
	Delayed and diminished carotid upstroke (parvus et tardus)
	Jugular venous distension (in patients with pulmonary hypertension secondary to AS)

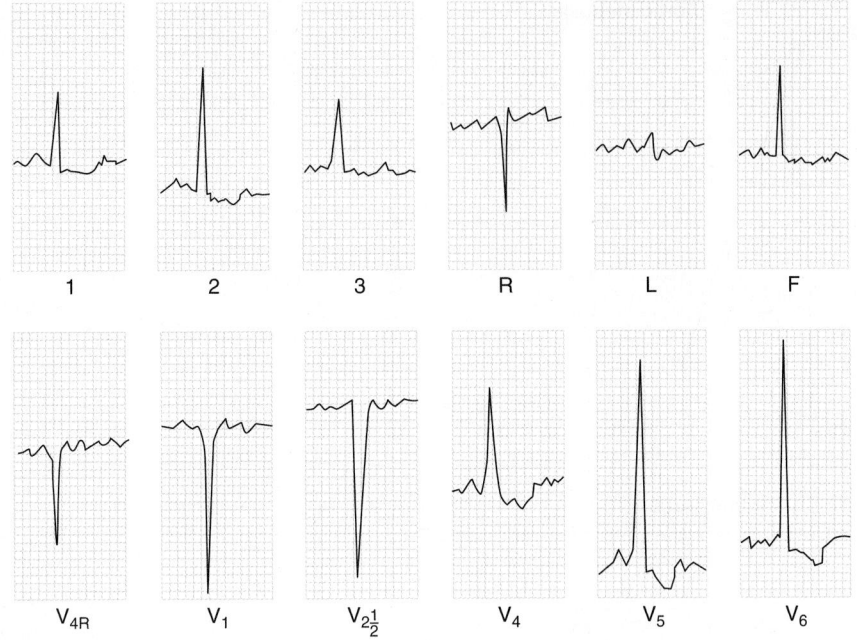

Figure 131-1 *ECG of a patient with aortic stenosis is consistent with severe left ventricular hypertrophy.* (Reproduced, with permission, from Fuster V, O'Rourke RA, Walsh RA, et al. *Hurst's the Heart*, 12th ed. New York, NY: McGraw-Hill; 2008. Fig. 82-23.)

prone to degeneration but patients are exposed to the risks of life-long anticoagulation. Therefore, the patient's bleeding risks are very important when selecting the type of valve to implant.

Transcatheter aortic valve replacement (TAVR): Transcatheter aortic valve replacement (placement of a stent-mounted bioprosthetic aortic valve using a catheter delivery system) has now become the treatment of choice of nonoperable patients, and is a comparable, or even superior, alternative to surgical aortic valve replacement in high-risk patients with severe symptomatic AS. This procedure initially performed more than a decade ago, allows the replacement of the diseased aortic valve by expanding a bioprosthesis using a percutaneous approach. The most common and preferred approach is the transfemoral access (insertion from the femoral artery), which may not be feasible in patients with

small femoral/iliac arteries or in patients with advanced peripheral arterial disease. Alternative approaches have been developed to include: transapical (by performing a small incision underneath the breast and between the ribs), transaortic (by performing a small sternotomy for catheter insertion), transcarotid (by using the carotid artery), or transcaval (by percutaneously creating a communication between the inferior vena cava and aorta). The results of the PARTNER and Corevalve US pivotal trial have proven the safety and feasibility of this technology in patients with severe AS who are at high surgical risk, and have led to The Food and Drug Administration (FDA) approval of two valves in the US: the Sapien valve (Edwards Lifescience, Irvine, CA) and Corevalve (Medtronic inc, Dublin, Ireland). Clinical trials are underway to further compare this technology in lower surgical risk patients and to further compare new valves or new generations of the exiting valves.

◼ AORTIC REGURGITATION

Pathophysiology

Aortic regurgitation (AR) is the diastolic reversal of blood flow from the aorta back into the left ventricle. It occurs as result of inadequate coaptation of valve leaflets due to either valve abnormalities or dilation of the aortic root. Aortic regurgitation is a serious cardiac abnormality and may occur as part of systemic or congenital disease. While rheumatic heart disease is the most common cause of AR in developing countries, bicuspid aortic valve and aortic root dilatation account for most of the cases in developed countries. Other causes of aortic root dilatation include connective tissue disorders such as Marfan syndrome, and aortitis related to syphilis,

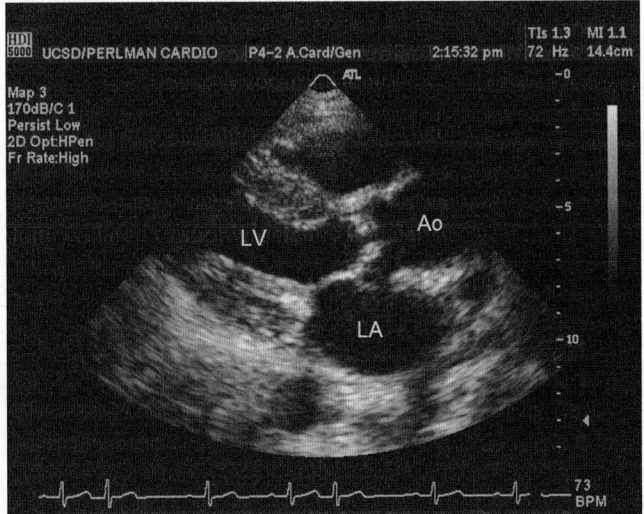

Figure 131-2 *Cardiac echocardiography in the parasternal long axis view shows thickened, stenotic aortic valve and left ventricular hypertrophy. Ao, aorta; LA, left atrium; LV, left ventricle.* (Reproduced, with permission, from Fuster V, O'Rourke RA, Walsh RA, et al. *Hurst's the Heart*, 12th ed. New York: McGraw-Hill; 2008. Fig. 16-59.)

TABLE 131-2 Severity of Aortic Stenosis Based on Echocardiogram Parameters

	Mild	Moderate	Severe
Valve area (cm²)	≥1.5	1.0-1.5	≤1.0
Maximal velocity (ms)	≤3	3-3.9	≥4
Mean gradient (mm Hg)	≤25	25-40	≥40

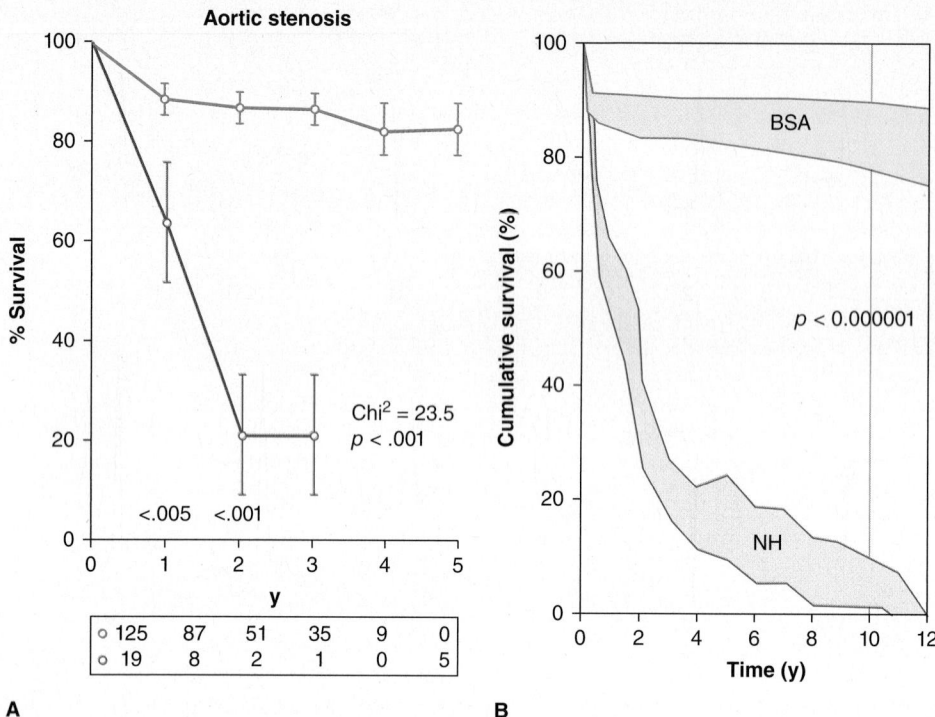

A

B

Figure 131-3 *Plot of survival versus time in patients with severe, symptomatic aortic stenosis that underwent surgical valve replacement (blue lines, BSA) versus best medical therapy (red lines, NH, natural history of aortic stenosis).* (Reproduced, with permission, from Fuster V, O'Rourke RA, Walsh RA, et al. *Hurst's the Heart,* 12th ed. New York: McGraw-Hill; 2008. Fig. 75-6.)

Behcet, Takayasu, reactive arthritis, or ankylosing spondylitis. Endocarditis can lead to the valve degeneration, rupture of leaflets, and vegetations on the valvular cusps that may cause inadequate closure of leaflets. Aortic root dissection can also affect leaflet function and lead to AR.

The overall prevalence of at least mild AR is approximately 13% in men and 8.5% in women, and increases with age. Of asymptomatic people over the age of 55, 29% have AR of which a minority (13%) have moderate to severe AR. In younger patients (23-35 years), the prevalence of AR is 1.3%.

Understanding the chronicity of the AR is also important as patients with acute AR have different clinical findings and management from those patients with chronic AR. Acute AR is often caused by acute aortic dissection, endocarditis, or direct trauma (motor vehicle accident), which results in a sudden increase in left ventricle end-diastolic volume and pressure. This increase in volume and pressure leads to a compensatory increase of heart rate and left ventricular contractility to augment cardiac output. However, in the setting of moderate or severe AR, these compensatory mechanisms may be insufficient to maintain the normal stroke volume and heart failure ensues. In chronic AR, the slow increase in preload allows for a compensatory left ventricular eccentric hypertrophy and dilation, which delays the occurrence of symptoms for months to years. However, as the AR progresses, left ventricle systolic dysfunction develops from continued cardiac remodeling and left ventricle end-diastolic pressure rises, resulting in symptomatic congestive heart failure. Timing aortic valve repair/replacement before irreversible myocardial dysfunction develops is of critical importance.

Diagnosis: does the patient have aortic regurgitation?

The signs and symptoms of AR depend on the acuity of disease. In acute AR, patients present with sign and symptoms of pulmonary edema, hypotension, cardiogenic shock, myocardial ischemia, or aortic root dissection. Physical examination may reveal a short

and soft diastolic murmur due to equalization of diastolic pressure between aorta and ventricle and/or an apical diastolic rumble (Austin Flint murmur, see below) (**Figure 131-4**). Pulse pressure may not be increased if systolic pressure is also reduced but patient will often have low diastolic pressures <50 mm Hg. In chronic AR, patients present with worsening signs of congestive heart failure and palpitations, and the typical physical examination findings of a high-pitched diastolic murmur, heard loudest in the left sternal border. Other commonly described findings of chronic AR include the: Becker sign (visible pulsation of retinal arteries), wide pulse pressure (palpable as a "water hammer" pulse and auscultated as "pistol shot" pulse), de Musset sign (pulsatile motion of patients head), Quincke sign (visible pulsation of fingernail beds after compression of the fingernails).

In addition to history and physical examination findings (**Table 131-3**), TTE is needed to confirm the diagnosis and further evaluate the severity and etiology of AR (**Figure 131-5**). Echocardiography evaluates the valvular anatomy, aortic root, and impact of AR on ventricular size and function.

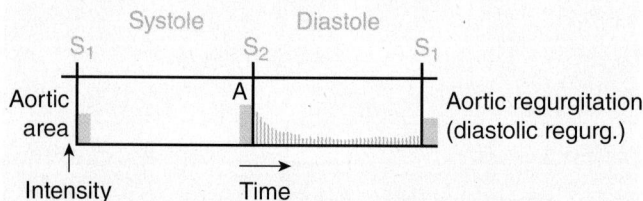

Figure 131-4 *Diagram representation of the heart murmur of aortic regurgitation. The murmur is a decrescendo murmur in early diastole that can also continue into late diastole when listening at the apex (Austin Flint murmur).* (Reproduced, with permission, from LeBlond RF, DeGowin RL, Brown DD. *DeGowin's Diagnostic Examination,* 9th ed. New York, NY: McGraw-Hill; 2009. Fig. 8-39.)

TABLE 131-3 Symptoms and Physical Examination Findings in Aortic Regurgitation

Aortic Regurgitation Symptoms	Physical Examination Findings
Decreased exercise tolerance	Arterial pulse shows rapid rise and a quick collapse (Corrigan pulse or water hammer pulse) resulting in widened pulse pressure >50 mm Hg
Shortness of breath on exertion	
Chest pain	High-pitched early-peaking diastolic, decrescendo blowing murmur, which is heard best with the diaphragm of the stethoscope just after A$_2$
Syncope/near syncope	
Heart failure	The murmur is usually soft and can be accentuated with the patient sitting up, leaning forward, and breath holding at the end of expiration
	Maneuvers that increase arterial pressure, such as squatting, accentuate the murmur; inhalation of amyl nitrate or Valsalva maneuver, which lower arterial pressure, decrease the intensity of the murmur

---

PRACTICE POINT

- In aortic regurgitation, timely aortic valve replacement can lead to reversal of left ventricular dilatation and improvement in ejection fraction (EF). Aortic valve replacement should be performed before the EF is ≤50% and/or before the left ventricular end systolic dimension is ≥55 mm to preserve the left ventricle even in asymptomatic patients.
- Medical therapy with vasodilators (hydralazine, nifedipine, and angiotensin-converting enzyme inhibitors) may temporarily improve symptoms but does not improve mortality.

In addition to TTE, other assessment tools are available if the results of echocardiogram (transthoracic and transesophageal) are of insufficient to determine the severity of AR or if the impact of the AR on the patient is unclear. Patients with chronic AR may undergo treadmill exercise testing to assess the functional status and symptomatic response in sedentary patients. Multigated Acquisition Scan (MUGA) or magnetic resonance imaging (MRI) can be used to assess left ventricular function. Fluoroscopic angiography evaluates AR and concomitant coronary disease preoperatively, which is particularly useful in patients undergoing valvular surgery that have risk factors for coronary disease (men > 35 years, premenopausal women > 35 years, and postmenopausal women).

Treatment

Acute severe AR is a surgical emergency. Surgery should be performed as soon as possible in patients with hemodynamic instability or congestive heart failure. Recommended initial management for patients with acute AR awaiting surgery includes airway management (intubation), positive inotropic agents (dobutamine), and a vasodilator therapy (nitroprusside).

Chronic AR has a protracted course and patients may remain asymptomatic for decades. Many patients with mild or moderate AR remain stable and may never require corrective surgery. Treatment of chronic AR depends on the following factors: severity, symptoms, left ventricular function, degree of left ventricular dilatation, and operative risk. Medical therapy with vasodilators (hydralazine,

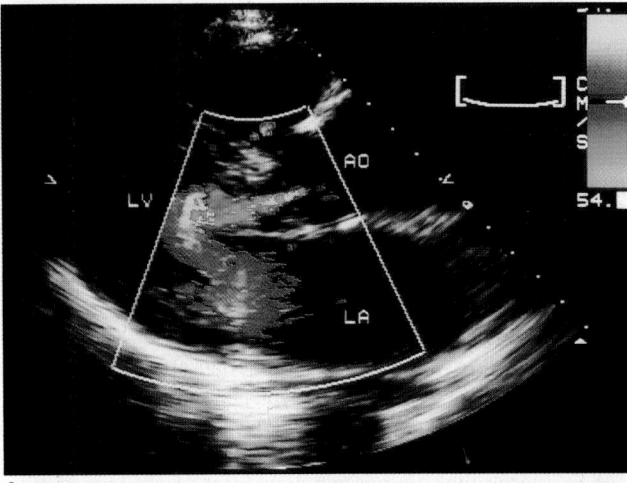

A

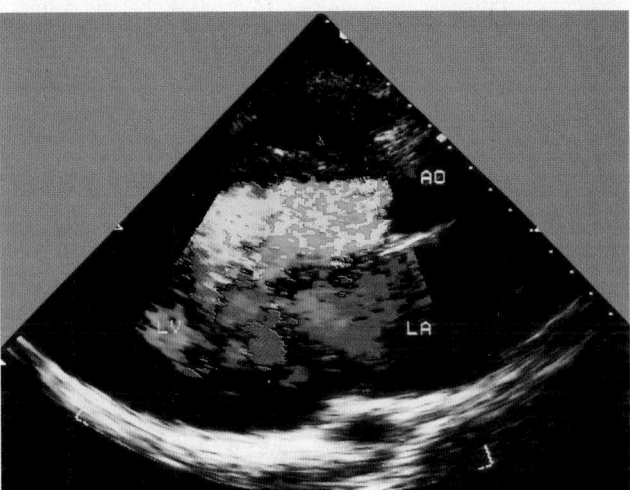

B

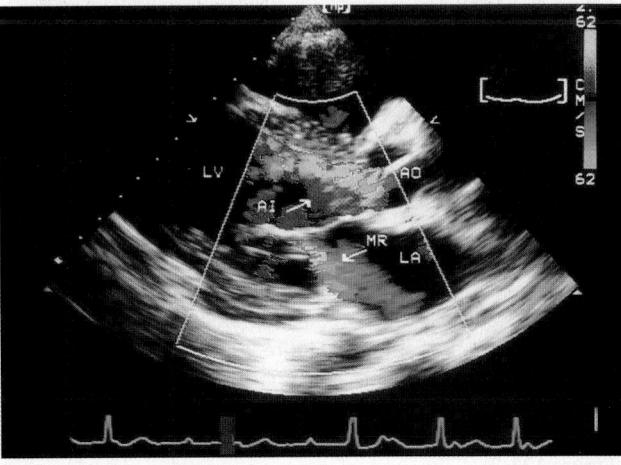

C

Figure 131-5 *Cardiac echocardiography in the parasternal long axis view shows mild (A) and severe (B and C) aortic regurgitation by color Doppler (seen as turbulent color flow originating from aortic valve). Ao, aorta; AI, aortic insufficiency; LV, left ventricle; LA, left atrium; MR, mitral regurgitation. (Reproduced, with permission, from Fuster V, O'Rourke RA, Walsh RA, et al. Hurst's the Heart, 12th ed. New York, NY: McGraw-Hill; 2008. Fig. 16-64.)*

nifedipine, and angiotensin-converting enzyme inhibitors) does not improve mortality but can help to manage symptoms. Aortic valve replacement is performed in the majority of patients requiring surgery, though aortic valve repair may be possible in selected patients at specialized centers. After valve replacement, the majority of the patients show reversal of left ventricular dilatation and improvement in ventricular function. Preoperative left ventricular function is the best predictor of long-term prognosis in patients undergoing surgery. Patients with normal preoperative EF or a brief duration of left ventricular dysfunction (<14 months) have greater improvement in left ventricular dimensions and early and late postoperative improvement in left ventricular function. Patients with impaired preoperative ventricular function have a greater risk of developing congestive heart failure postoperatively. In general, surgery should be performed before the EF is ≤ 50% and/or before the left ventricular end systolic dimension is ≤55 mm to preserve the left ventricle even in asymptomatic patients. Transcatheter aortic valve replacement has been used in selected patients with high or inoperable surgical risk with good success. However, current commercially available TAVR valves have only been studied in patients with AS, and as a result they are not approved for the treatment of AR at this time. Fortunately, there are new TAVR valves that are currently being evaluated in clinical trials specifically for the treatment of AR (ie, Jenavalve, Munich, Germany) and may be an option in the future for the treatment of this condition.

MITRAL VALVE DISORDERS

■ MITRAL STENOSIS

Pathophysiology

Mitral stenosis (MS) impedes the blood flow from the left atrium into the left ventricle, and is most commonly caused by a prior history of rheumatic fever (RF). Rheumatic heart disease accounts more than 95% of diagnosed cases of MS in the United States, presenting as isolated mitral valve (25%) or multivalve disease (35%, aortic and mitral), the tricuspid or pulmonic valves are rarely involved. In the United States, the decreased prevalence of streptococcal strains that cause RF and early detection and treatment of streptococcal pharyngitis has played a large role in the marked decreased incidence of rheumatic heart disease (1 in 150,000). However, rheumatic MS is still commonly seen in young patients coming from developing nations, where RF is highly prevalent (50 per 100,000).

Rheumatic MS results from an autoimmune process between the streptococcal protein and the valvular tissue causing inflammation and edema of the leaflets during bouts of RF, which leads to thickening of leaflet edges, commissural fusion, chordal shortening, and calcification of the mitral apparatus. These changes, which can occur over the course of years, culminate in valve stenosis and/or regurgitation. Aschoff bodies (another pathological finding of RF) are more consistently found in the myocardium and rarely seen on the valvular tissue at autopsy (**Figure 131-6**). The valvular pathological changes of RF mainly affect the anterior leaflet and result in a "doming" motion during ventricular diastole and the characteristic "fish-mouth" appearance seen by transthoracic echocardiogram (**Figure 131-7**).

As MS progresses, the normal mitral valve opening area (>4 cm²) can be restricted to a mild (1.5-2.0 cm²), moderate (1.0-1.5 cm²), or severe (<1.0 cm²) degree. The reduction in valve orifice leads to an elevated transmitral gradient, elevation in left atrial and pulmonary pressures, enlargement of the left atrium, and atrial fibrillation with high risk of thromboembolic disease. Patients with mitral stenosis usually are not symptomatic until the mitral valve area is <1.0 cm² or the valve stenosis is moderate with associated tachycardia. Tachycardia for any reason decreases the time for diastolic emptying of the left atrium, and therefore increases left atrial and pulmonic pressures, elevates transmitral gradient, and reduces cardiac output (underfilling of the left ventricle). Dyspnea and acute pulmonary edema can occur suddenly in an asymptomatic MS patient that develops tachycardia, such as atrial fibrillation with rapid ventricular response.

PRACTICE POINT

- Patients with mitral stenosis usually are not symptomatic until the mitral valve area is <1.0 cm² or the valve stenosis is moderate with associated tachycardia.

Diagnosis: does the patient have mitral stenosis?

Mitral stenosis is a slowly progressive disease and thus patients can remain asymptomatic for many years. Dyspnea is the most common presenting complaint along with fatigue during minimal exertion; other signs and symptoms of more advanced disease includes orthopnea, paroxysmal nocturnal dyspnea, and pulmonary edema. Symptoms in MS can be precipitated by changes in heart rate or volume status, such as atrial fibrillation, emotional stress, pregnancy, fever, or exercise. Other symptoms include hemoptysis (due to rupture of bronchial vessels in patients with pulmonary hypertension), chest pain, palpitations, and hoarseness because of compression of the left recurrent laryngeal nerve from the dilated left atrium and pulmonary artery (Ortner syndrome).

An irregular pulse is the most common but nonspecific finding on physical examination due to the high prevalence of atrial fibrillation with MS. Increased jugular venous pressure and posterior displacement of the left ventricular apex can be seen in patients with pulmonary hypertension and right ventricular failure. Classically, the auscultatory findings of MS are more evident when listening at the apex with the patient in the left lateral decubitus position. There is an accentuated first heart sound and an opening snap (snapping open of the domed leaflets into the left ventricle) though calcification and valvular thickening can reduce leaflet excursion and both sounds may be absent with severe MS. The diastolic murmur is low pitched and best heard with the bell of the stethoscope; the intensity of the murmur does not correlate with the severity of the MS as it can be altered by numerous factors, especially exercise. Repeat auscultation after exercise makes the murmur of MS more audible.

PRACTICE POINT

- Symptoms in MS include hemoptysis, chest pain, palpitations, and hoarseness and can be precipitated by changes in heart rate or volume status, such as atrial fibrillation, emotional stress, pregnancy, fever, or exercise. An irregular pulse due to atrial fibrillation is the most common finding on physical examination.

Echocardiography is the most accurate tool for assessment of the valve anatomy, valve area, transvalvular gradient, and the presence of multivalvular disease. Due to the posterior location of the left atrium, TTE images are often suboptimal, and thus a transesophageal echocardiogram (TEE) may be needed to delineate the valvular apparatus and evaluate for clots in the left atrium or left atrial appendage. Using TTE and TEE parameters, the severity of valve stenosis can be categorized as mild, moderate, or severe. Electrocardiography is nonspecific for the diagnosis of MS, though left atrial and right atrial abnormalities with right-axis deviation of the QRS complex should alert the clinician of the possibility of MS (**Figure 131-8**). Chest x-ray may show left atrial enlargement (splaying of the main stem bronchi), left atrial appendage enlargement (straightening of the left cardiac silhouette), enlargement of the pulmonary arteries and pulmonary edema.

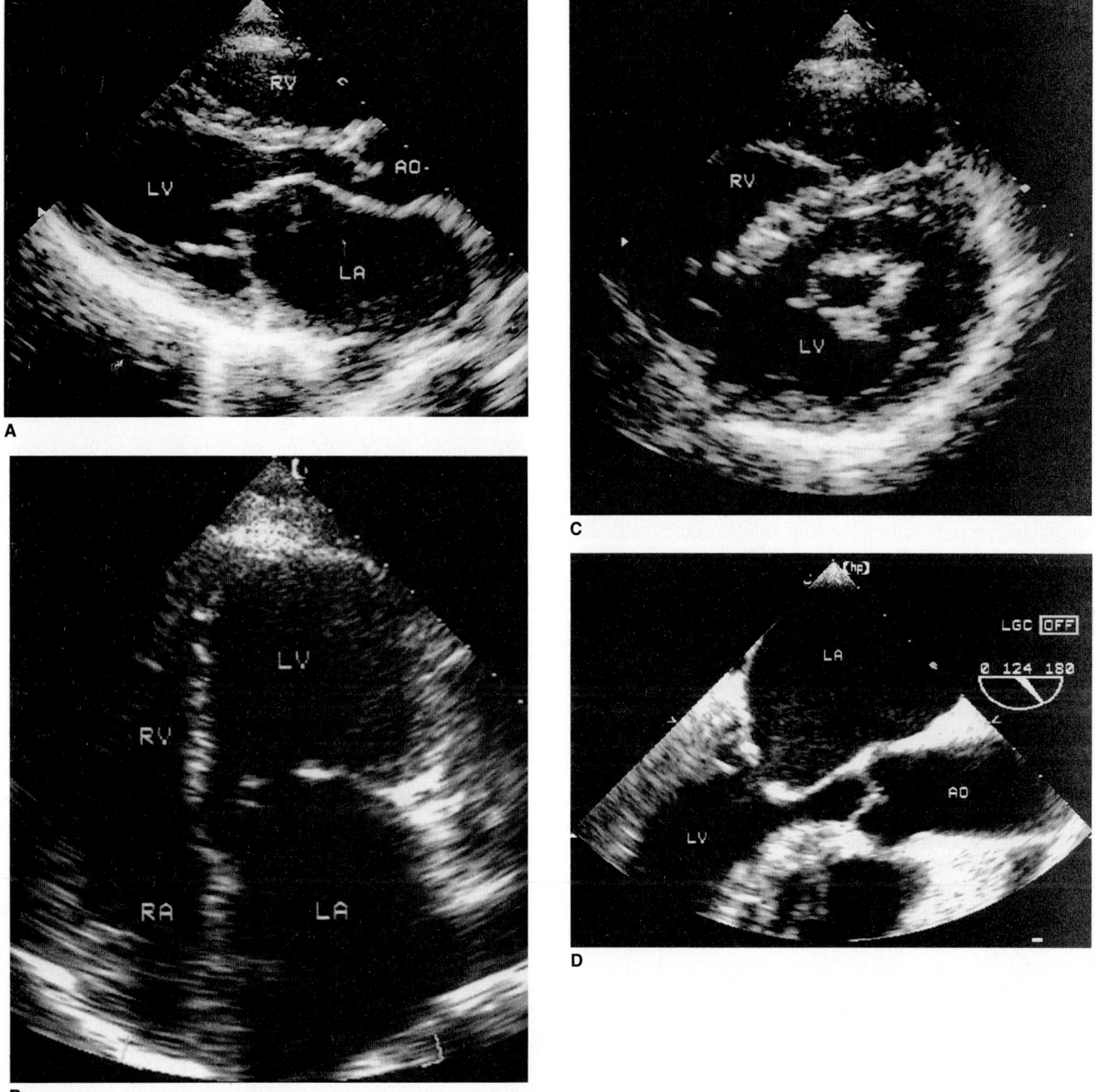

Figure 131-6 *Cardiac echocardiography in the parasternal long axis view (A), apical four-chamber view (B), short axis view (C), and three-chamber TEE (transesophageal) view (D) shows thickened and stenotic mitral valve. Ao, aorta; LA, left atrium; LV, left ventricle; RV, right ventricle. (Reproduced, with permission, from Fuster V, O'Rourke RA, Walsh RA, et al. Hurst's the Heart, 12th ed. New York: McGraw-Hill; 2008. Fig. 16-73.)*

Diagnostic catheterization can be helpful for quantifying trans-valvular gradient and valve area, if the echocardiographic data is inconsistent with clinical findings.

Treatment

Patients with mild-to-moderate MS can remain asymptomatic for years; therefore, medical management of MS is focused on preventing further complications and recurrences of RF, optimizing hemodynamics, treatment of atrial fibrillation with anticoagulation, and appropriate monitoring of disease progression to allow referral for surgical or nonsurgical intervention (**Table 131-4**).

Asymptomatic patients with moderate MS can be evaluated with an echocardiogram every 3 to 5 years while those with severe

AS without coexisting pathologies (pulmonary hypertension, atrial fibrillation, or left atrial enlargement) should be sent for yearly echocardiogram. Symptomatic or asymptomatic patients with coexisting pathologies listed above with moderate-to-severe MS, however, should be referred for percutaneous or surgical therapy, as the 5-year survival rate without intervention is approximately 40%. The therapy recommended for the patient is usually made after consultation with a cardiologist or cardiothoracic surgeon who has experience in percutaneous balloon mitral valvuloplasty (BMV) or surgical mitral repair or replacement. BMV, if feasible, is the first-line therapy recommended for patients need relief of their MS. Balloon mitral valvuloplasty is also a treatment option for patients that develop symptoms from MS during pregnancy, however, great

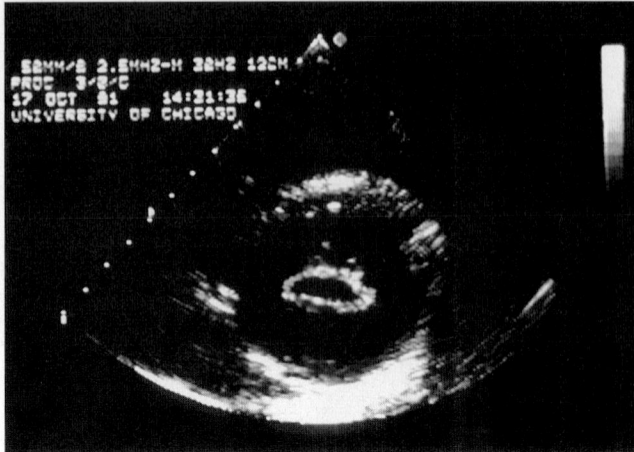

Figure 131-7 *Characteristic "fish-mouth" appearance of mitral stenosis seen by transthoracic echocardiogram.* (Reproduced, with permission, from Hall JB, Schmidt GA, Wood LDH. *Principles of Critical Care*, 3rd ed. New York: McGraw-Hill; 2005. Fig. 29-7.)

care should we used to limit the fetus radiation exposure during the procedure.

PRACTICE POINT

- Symptomatic patients with severe MS or asymptomatic patients with new atrial fibrillation, pulmonary hypertension, or atrial enlargement should be referred for percutaneous or surgical therapy as the 5-year survival rate without intervention is approximately 40%.

In appropriately selective patients, complications associated with BMV are uncommon and include embolism with stroke, severe mitral regurgitation, pulmonary edema, and complications during

TABLE 131-4 Treatment of Mitral Stenosis

Rhythm Maintenance: Maintain sinus rhythm if patients develop atrial fibrillation/flutter with antiarrhythmics such as class III and 1C agents and cardioversion.

Rate Control: Rate controlling agents, such as beta-blockers, calcium antagonists, and digoxin, will help in controlling heart rate moderating transvalvular gradients.

Optimize Volume Status: Maintain a low sodium intake, and patients often benefit from scheduled diuretics to optimize fluid status.

Anticoagulate Atrial Fibrillation: Anticoagulation in MS patients is recommended for atrial fibrillation (paroxysmal or permanent) regardless of CHADS2 score, as this is a high-risk population even in sinus rhythm.

the transseptal puncture (perforation of the left atrium or the aorta requiring surgical repair). Patients who are not favorable candidates for BMV, usually because of extensive leaflet calcification or significant mitral regurgitation, are considered for surgical valve repair or replacement with either a mechanical or bioprosthetic valve, depending on variables, such as patient age and ability to take anticoagulation.

■ MITRAL REGURGITATION

Pathophysiology

Mitral regurgitation (MR) occurs when the coaptation between the mitral leaflets is inadequate to prevent blood from returning back to the left atrium from the left ventricle during systole. A thorough understanding of MR requires knowledge of the mitral valve anatomy and function (**Figure 131-9**). The mitral valve apparatus consists of the anterior and posterior leaflets, which are attached at their base to the fibrous skeleton of the heart at the anterior annulus and to the left ventricle at the posterior annulus respectively. The leaflet

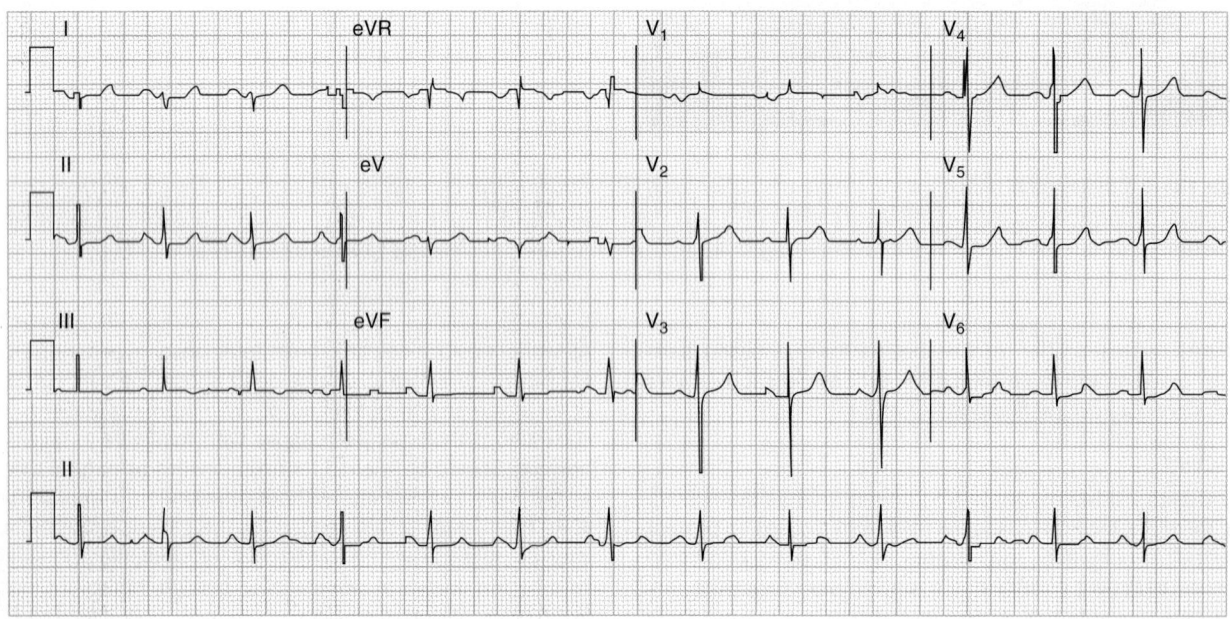

Figure 131-8 *ECG of a patient with mitral stenosis shows left and right atrial abnormality and right-axis deviation of the QRS.* (Reproduced, with permission, from Fauci AS, Braunwald E, Kasper DL, et al. *Harrison's Principles of Internal Medicine*, 17th ed. New York, NY: McGraw-Hill; 2008. Fig. 19-15.)

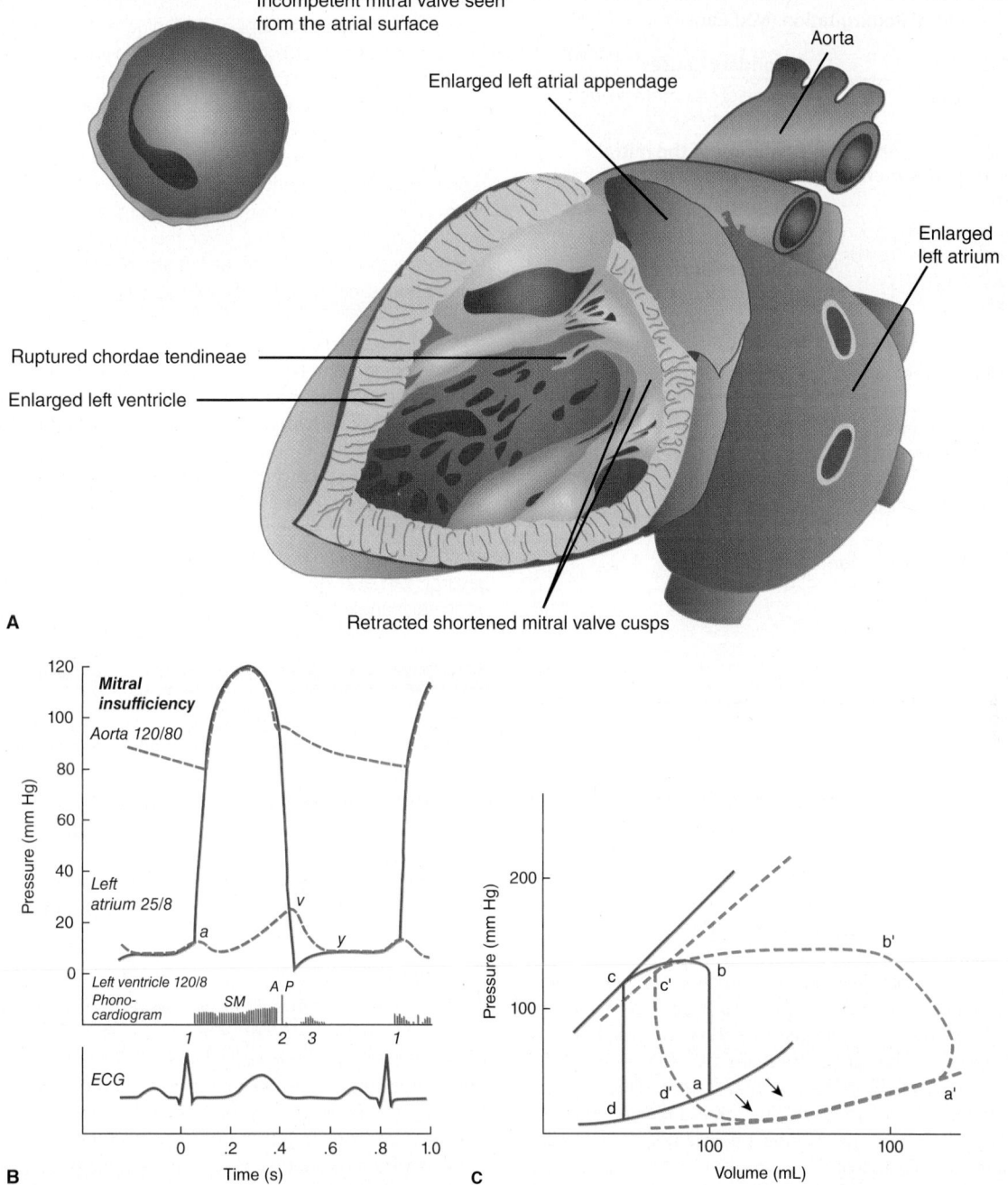

Incompetent mitral valve seen
from the atrial surface

Aorta

Enlarged left atrial appendage

Enlarged
left atrium

Ruptured chordae tendineae

Enlarged left ventricle

A

Retracted shortened mitral valve cusps

B

C

Figure 131-9 *Anatomical drawing (A), pressure tracings (B), and pressure-volume flow loop (C) in a patient with mitral regurgitation.* (Reproduced, with permission, from McPhee SJ, Hammer GD. *Pathophysiology of Disease: An Introduction to Clinical Medicine*, 6th ed. New York: McGraw-Hill; 2010. Fig. 10-26.)

tips are connected by the chordae tendineae to the papillary muscles, which originate from the left ventricle. During systole, contraction of the left ventricle and papillary muscles constricts the mitral annulus and steadies the position of the leaflets via the chordae tendineae, allowing adequate coaptation of the anterior and posterior leaflets. The pathophysiology of MR can involve derangements in one or all components of the mitral apparatus (**Table 131-5**).

During the acute phase of MR, left ventricle experiences enhanced emptying and decreased afterload because a portion of the stroke volume regurgitates into the low pressure left atrium. This decreased afterload allows for a normal left ventricle to have an exaggerated ejection fraction (eg, EF 75% or 85%). As regurgitation becomes more chronic and severe, the left ventricle hypertrophies and dilates to maintain cardiac output. As the heart continues to

remodel the cardiac output and left ventricle ejection fraction will eventually decrease, which will lead to left atrial dilation, pulmonary hypertension, and congestive heart failure symptoms.

Diagnosis: does the patient have mitral regurgitation?

Differentiating between primary (degenerative) and secondary (functional) MR is important as the prognosis and management is different. In primary MR, the regurgitation is caused by a derangement of the valvular apparatus, such as myxomatous leaflet, valve damage from endocarditis, or chordae tendinae rupture. Patients with mild MR usually remain asymptomatic for several years unless an acute event occurs such further chordae rupture result in increased leaflet fail and worsening regurgitation. Symptoms develop as left atrial pressure and pulmonary hypertension

TABLE 131-5 Mitral Regurgitation (MR) Causes

Primary Causes	Secondary Causes
Disease of the leaflets	Disease of the ventricle with normal leaflets
Redundancy, retraction, deformity, or perforations of the leaflets: • Myxomatous degeneration (ie, mitral valve prolapse or fibroelastic deficiency) • Rheumatic fever (RF) • Endocarditis **Abnormalities of the chordae** • Shortening (inflammation secondary to RF or endocarditis) • Lengthening (mitral valve prolapse) **Papillary muscle dysfunction** • Coronary ischemia/infarct • Can cause severe MR because of leaflet tethering or flail leaflet	**Dilatation of the mitral annulus** • Left ventricular dilation • Mitral annular calcification **Ischemia causing regional myocardial dysfunction at the papillary muscle insertion** • May result in papillary dysfunction with resultant MR

increases. Fatigue and exhaustion can be subtle clues to significant MR with progressively decreasing cardiac output and elevating pulmonary pressure with preserved ejection fraction. At times, significant and sometimes irreversible ventricular dysfunction has occurred by the time symptoms develop. Secondary or functional MR develops as a consequence of left ventricular dilation and remolding in patients with an underlying cardiomyopathy. This remodeling pulls the papillary muscles and chordae apart leading to failure coaptation of the otherwise normal mitral leaflets. Patients who have had an isolated myocardial infarction and scaring of the inferior wall involving the papillary muscles may also develop focal dilation and functional MR. In these setting, is often difficult to differentiate the MR role in symptoms. Physical examination findings of MR (regardless of the cause) include a holosystolic murmur and diastolic rumble (**Table 131-6**).

TABLE 131-6 Mitral Regurgitation Physical Examination Findings

Severe MR Physical Examination

Diminished S_1 due to defective leaflet closure and loud P_2 component of S_2 heralding significant pulmonary hypertension

Audible diastolic rumble and an S_3 due to the increased volume across the valve into the ventricle

Holosystolic murmur, high pitched, at the apex, sternum or back depending on the direction of the regurgitant jet

When the murmur is not holosystolic it is likely not severe and one should consider mitral valve prolapse, which exhibits a late peaking murmur and is preceded by a midsystolic click

Evaluation and management of MR requires echocardiography to evaluate for complications and candidacy for medical or surgical interventions. Echocardiography aids the diagnosis, quantification, etiology, and potential for surgical repair of MR. Transthoracic echocardiography can assess left atrial size, pulmonary pressures, and LV dimensions, which can be followed serially for subtle progression of disease prior to symptom onset. Transesophageal echocardiography provides better visualization of the mitral valve for assessing etiology and repair options. Mitral regurgitation severity is often qualified by the size of the color regurgitant jet and whether it reaches the posterior wall of the left atrium. Other echocardiogram parameters used to quantify MR severity include the effective regurgitant orifice, the regurgitant volume, the regurgitant fraction and the reversal of the pulmonary vein flow during systole. Electrocardiography typically shows left atrial abnormality and/or atrial fibrillation and may show signs of right ventricular enlargement if pulmonary hypertension is significant (**Figure 131-10**). On chest radiography, LV enlargement, left atrial enlargement, and pulmonary edema may be seen (**Figure 131-11**). Cardiac magnetic resonance imaging can also be used to accurately quantitate regurgitant volume and assess details of the valve apparatus, particularly when the echocardiogram is difficult to interpret. Regurgitant severity can also be assessed in the catheterization lab with left ventricular angiography.

PRACTICE POINT

- Symptoms in mitral regurgitation correlate with progression of left atrial pressure and pulmonary hypertension rather than left ventricular function. Therefore, fatigue and exhaustion can be subtle clues to significant MR.
- Echocardiographic findings of left atrial size, pulmonary pressures, and LV dimensions can be followed serially for progression of disease prior to symptom onset.

Treatment

Medical therapy is targeted at decreasing the amount of MR and treating the underlying left ventricular dysfunction. The amount of MR depends on the size of the regurgitant orifice and the pressure difference between the left ventricle and left atrium. Decreasing left ventricular preload and afterload will decrease the pressure (and size) of the ventricle and thus, medical therapy consists of preload reducing agents (eg, diuretics) and afterload reducing agents (eg, angiotensin-converting enzyme inhibitors). These therapies are effective for acute MR. In chronic MR however, the systemic vascular resistance is usually decreased and debate regarding benefit of afterload reduction in affecting forward volumes and preserving systolic function leads to some practice variation. In patients with primary LV dysfunction and secondary MR, medical therapy consists of optimal medical therapy for heart failure including beta-blockers and angiotensin-converting enzyme inhibitors.

Asymptomatic patients with significant MR and normal ejection fraction and dimensions should be followed with serial transthoracic echocardiograms every 6 to 12 months along with regular physical examinations. Ultimately, surgical or percutaneous intervention should be considered for patients with primary MR associated with significant symptoms and/or deteriorating ventricular function. Outcomes of surgical valve repair or replacement are significantly improved if the ejection fraction is >60% and/or left ventricular end systolic dimensions are <40 mm at time of surgery. Indications for valve repair or replacement in secondary MR are more controversial, particularly for ischemic MR, and should be discussed in detail with

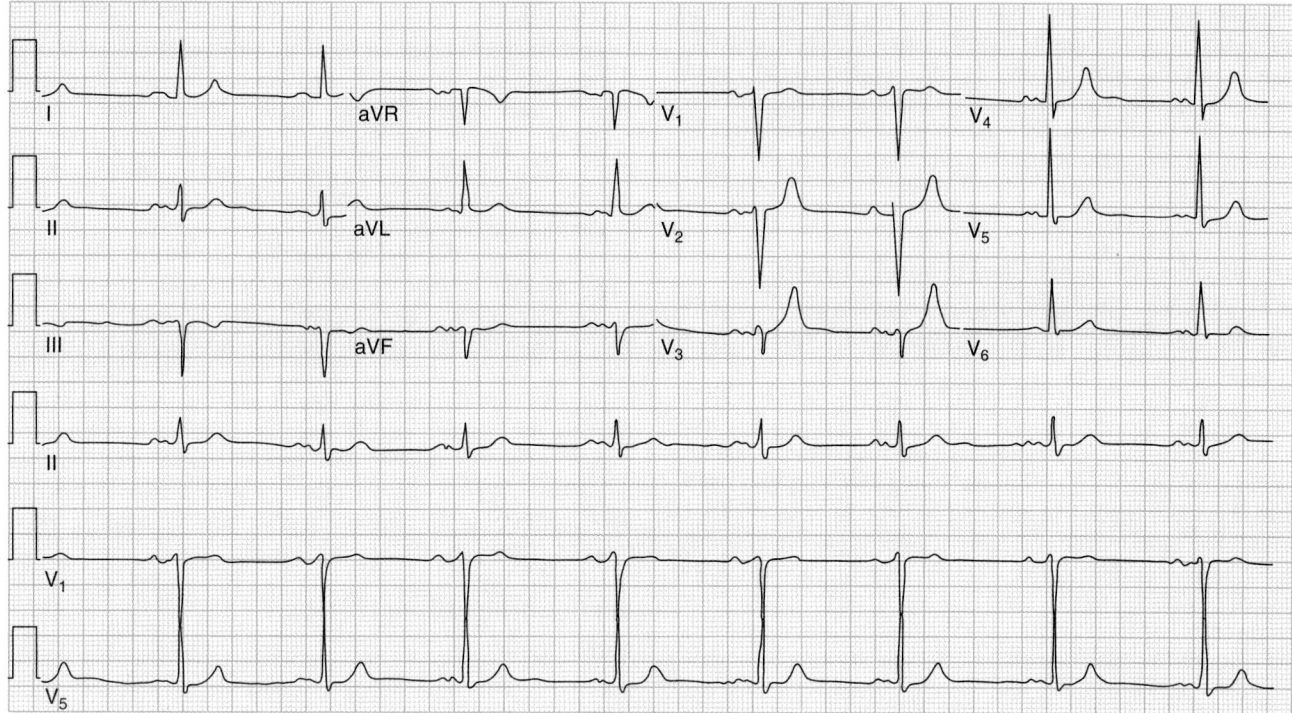

Figure 131-10 *ECG in a patient with mitral regurgitation demonstrating left atrial abnormality, based on p-wave with a "double-hump" in leads II, V4, V5, and V6.* (Reproduced, with permission, from Fuster V, O'Rourke RA, Walsh RA, et al. *Hurst's the Heart*, 12th ed. New York: McGraw-Hill; 2008. Fig. 76-9.)

a cardiac surgeon and cardiologist who have extensive experience in valvular heart disease.

Surgical treatment consists of mitral repair or replacement. Mitral valve repair is preferred over replacement at experienced centers if possible and consists of leaflet reconstruction and annuloplasty ring. Repair also offers greater chance for preservation of the subvalvular apparatus and a lower risk of thromboembolism, structural deterioration, or endocarditis compared with valve replacement. Patients with deformed leaflets secondary to rheumatic heart disease, rigid calcified leaflets second to end stage renal disease, and

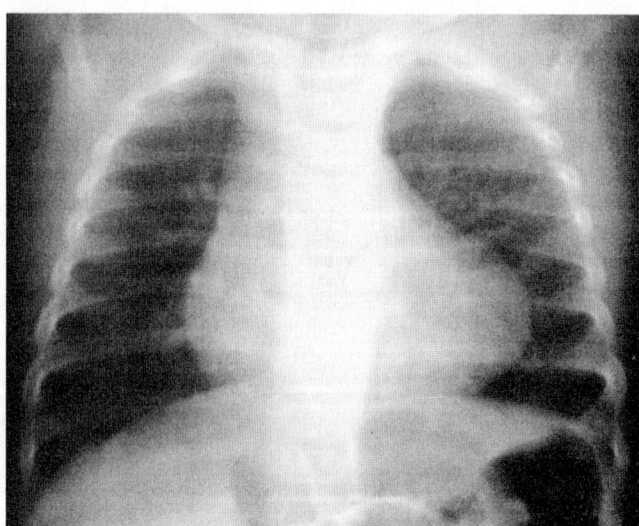

Figure 131-11 *Chest radiograph from a patient with mitral regurgitation shows enlarged left atrium, left ventricle and mild pulmonary edema.* (Reproduced, with permission, from Chen MYM, Pope TL, Ott TJ. *Basic Radiology.* New York: McGraw-Hill. Fig. 3-36.)

older patients may have better outcomes with valve replacement. Regardless of whether repair or replacement is selected, preservation of the chordae and papillary muscles helps preserve left ventricular function. Mitral valve repair or replacement has the potential to significantly improve ventricular function when the valve has primary dysfunction, whereas functional or secondary MR has less potential for ventricular recovery, as the primary problem is the cardiomyopathy.

Transcatheter mitral interventions are now emerging as feasible treatment for patients with degenerative or primary MR, especially in those patients with very high surgical risk. The MitraClip (Abbot vascular, Menlo Park, CA) is a transcatheter therapy, which is commercially available for the treatment of primary MR that decreases the regurgitant orifice by performing an edge-to-edge anastomosis of the central portions of the anterior and posterior leaflets. Access is gained with catheters inserted through the femoral vein and crossed into the left atrium with a transseptal puncture. MitraClip has been shown to cause sustained improvement of MR severity, symptoms and mortality in properly selected patients based on etiology and amenable anatomy for the procedure. New devices for transcatheter mitral valve replacement are currently enrolling patients in early-phase clinical trials.

PULMONARY VALVE DISORDERS

■ PULMONIC STENOSIS

Pathophysiology

Pulmonic stenosis (PS) is a valvular abnormality that obstructs blood flow between the right ventricle and the pulmonary arteries. Pulmonic stenosis is uncommon and when present is usually secondary to congenital PS, prevalent in 8% to 10% of pediatric and up to 15% of adult congenital cases. A congenitally malformed valve can range from a trileaflet valve with fusion at the commissures, a thickened dysplastic valve, an imperforate membrane, or atresia. PS can occur in isolation or as part of a multiorgan congenital disease such as Noonan syndrome. Acquired etiologies such as rheumatic heart disease are rare and rheumatic disease usually involves other valves if present on the pulmonic valve. Malignant carcinoid can involve the pulmonic valve in addition to the tricuspid valve. Obstruction of the valve can also be extrinsic to the valve as a consequence of cardiac tumors or sinus of valsalva aneurysm. The right ventricle usually tolerates mild-to-moderate obstruction well, with minimal dilatation or reduction in function.

Diagnosis: does the patient have pulmonic stenosis?

Adults with mild-to-moderate obstruction usually remain asymptomatic and infrequently progress to significant PS. In 15% to 20% of the patients, the obstruction can worsen with outflow tract obstruction leading to symptoms of fatigue, dyspnea, and chest pain. On physical examination, the murmur of PS depends on the pliability of the valve. The murmur is best auscultated in the left upper sternal border and may be associated with an ejection click. Often, a singular second heart sound without an ejection click is heard if the valve motion is significantly restricted. The ECG may be normal in mild-to-moderate cases. As severity progresses, right ventricular hypertrophy and strain may appear on the ECG as a tall R-wave or an "rSR" in lead V_1 with predominant S-waves in the lateral leads (**Figure 131-12**). Chest radiography reveals normal heart borders and vasculature in mild-to-moderate disease but with severe obstruction there can be right atrial and ventricular enlargement. Echocardiography is the definitive tool to assess for severity, cause, and characterization of the valve to determine appropriate therapy. A peak gradient >50 mm Hg across the pulmonic valve is consistent with significant disease.

Treatment

The options for therapy for PS focus on relief of the obstruction but depend on the status of the valve and cause of obstruction. A membrane or atresia usually requires creation of a tract and dilatation surgically. If stenosis is secondary to a valve with commissural fusion, balloon valvuloplasty can be performed with excellent long-term results. Even in the setting of a dysplastic valve, the results with valvuloplasty are usually favorable, though not as long lasting as with commissural fusion. For patients who are not candidates for valvuloplasty, surgical replacement of the valve is indicated usually in conjunction with patch repair of any supravalvular obstruction. Transcather pulmonary valve replacement with a Melody valve (Medtronic) has now emerged as a feasible treatment of patients with symptomatic PS and/or severe pulmonary regurgitation, and can be used as an alternative to surgery in these congenital patients (that often have had multiple cardiac surgeries). Regardless of the therapy, the prognosis of PS is excellent if there is adequate relief of the obstruction and preserved right ventricular function and size.

■ PULMONIC REGURGITATION

Pathophysiology

The most common etiology of pulmonic regurgitation (PR) is dilatation of the annular ring secondary to pulmonary hypertension (eg, pulmonary hypertension with MS), or connective tissue disorder (eg, dilation of the pulmonary artery with Marfan syndrome). Less commonly, diseases that cause deformation in the architecture of the leaflets can lead to regurgitation. These include rheumatic heart

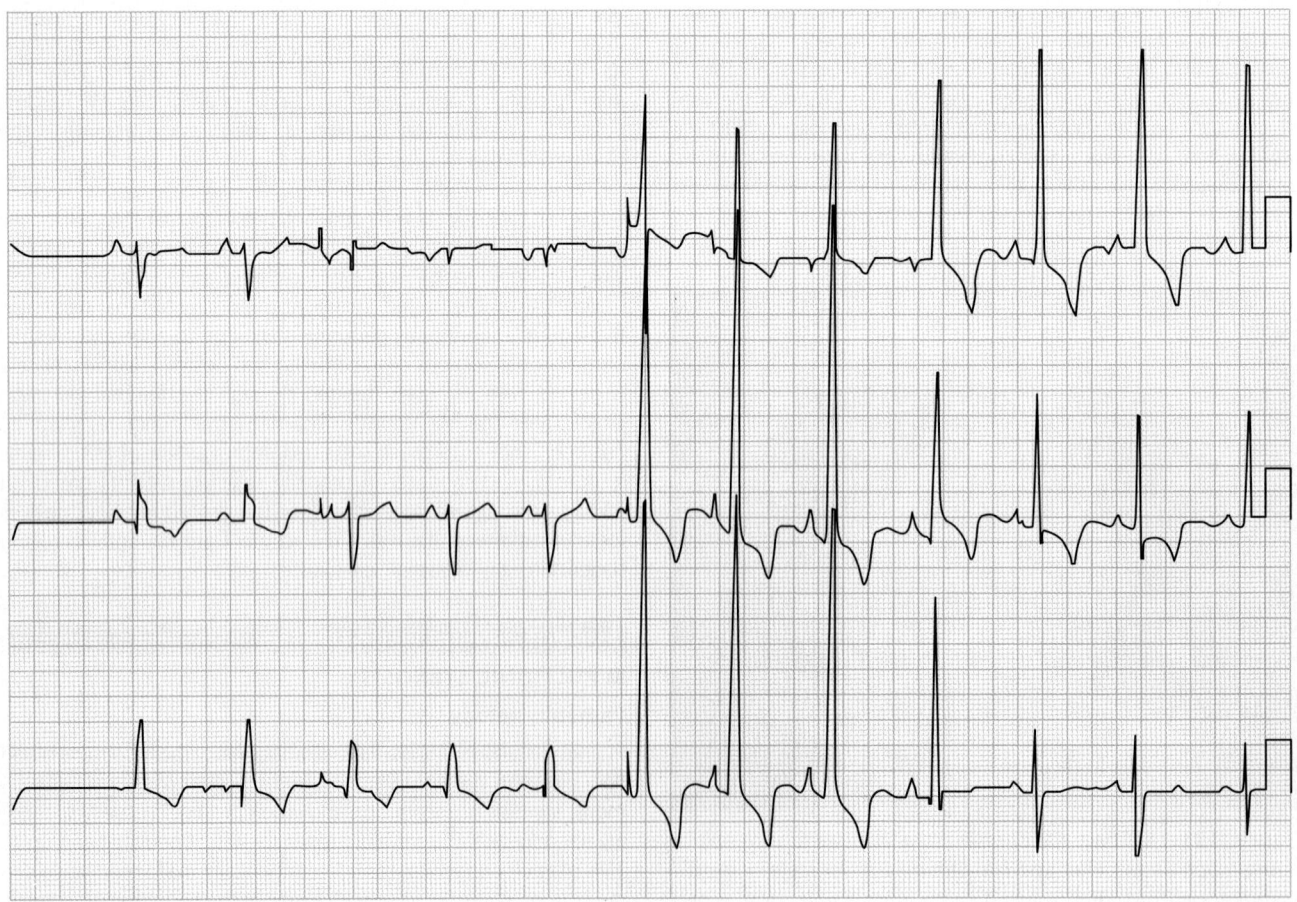

Figure 131-12 *Electrocardiograph in congenital pulmonic stenosis with severe right ventricular hypertrophy and marked right-axis deviation.* (Reproduced, with permission, from Crawford MH. *Current Diagnosis & Treatment: Cardiology,* 3rd ed. New York, NY: McGraw-Hill; 2009. Fig. 28-3.)

TABLE 131-7 Pulmonic Regurgitation Physical Examination Findings

Diastolic murmur best auscultated at the left parasternal third to fourth intercostal spaces, usually low pitched, occurring immediately after P_2

The murmur can be high pitched in the presence of significant pulmonary hypertension (Graham Steell murmur)

P_2 accentuated in the presence of pulmonary hypertension

Palpable tap in the second intercostal space, reflecting pulmonic valve closure at elevated pressures

disease, endocarditis, malignant carcinoid, and congenital malformation of the valve (also associated with other cardiac anomalies such as Tetralogy of Fallot and pulmonic stenosis). Direct trauma from right heart catheterization or surgical misadventure has been documented.

Diagnosis: does the patient have pulmonic regurgitation?

Pulmonic regurgitation can lead to right ventricular volume overload and is usually tolerated well over years without symptoms unless right ventricular failure or pulmonary hypertension ensues. Patients with PR from endocarditis can have septic pulmonary emboli, which can lead to pulmonary hypertension. If pulmonary hypertension develops, PR can progress and worsen right-sided failure. Most patients complain of dyspnea and fatigue. In addition to classic cardiac examination findings (**Table 131-7**), physical examination findings can include peripheral edema and ascites with liver dysfunction with severe right heart failure.

The electrocardiogram often is normal in mild-to-moderate cases but will begin to reflect right ventricular overload and hypertrophy as failure worsens and pulmonary hypertension ensues. The chest radiograph is usually nonspecific but may show pulmonary artery and right ventricular enlargement at the borders. Cardiac magnetic resonance is especially usefully in quantifying the regurgitant volume and assessing the valve structure, geometry, and function of the right ventricle. Echocardiography remains the gold standard for assessing regurgitant severity, valve anatomy, and pulmonary hypertension. Criteria for severity of PR by echocardiography are similar to that of AR.

Treatment

Though PR is usually tolerated, severe PR should be treated at early sign of right ventricle or right atrium dilation, increasing tricuspid regurgitation (TR) and/or symptoms. Often therapy directed at the causal event (eg, MS) will relieve PR by decreasing pulmonary hypertension. Surgical therapy for primary PR is indicated for progressive right heart failure and volume overload. As a rule, a pulmonic allograft or porcine bioprosthesis is typically chosen. Catheter-based valve implantation is currently available for high surgical risk patients with PR and/or PS.

TRICUSPID VALVE DISORDERS

■ TRICUSPID STENOSIS

Pathophyisology

Tricuspid stenosis is an uncommon condition that obstructs the flow of blood from the right atrium to the right ventricle during diastole. Distortion of the tricuspid valve apparatus with commissural fusion, shortened chordae, and decrease in valve orifice are the findings of TS regardless of etiology. Because the pressures in the right side of the heart are normally low, a pressure gradient ≥5 mm Hg across the tricuspid valve can result in elevated right atrial pressures.

Chronically elevated right atrial pressures lead to signs and symptoms of systemic venous congestion, including prominent jugular venous pulsations with an exaggerated a-wave, lower-extremity edema, ascites, and liver congestion/dysfunction. In more severe forms of TS, pulmonary blood flow is significantly decreased and cardiac output can become limited, especially with exercise. Right atrial enlargement and hypertrophy can contribute to the development of atrial fibrillation, which significantly exaggerates the symptoms of venous congestion.

The most common etiologies of TS include rheumatic heart disease (most common cause), carcinoid disease, congenital heart disease, and infective endocarditis. The overall incidence of TS in patients with rheumatic heart disease has been estimated at 9% to 15%, with clinically significant and more severe forms occurring in only 5%. Isolated tricuspid valve involvement is rare, and clinical TS is usually discovered concomitantly with mitral and aortic valve disease. Carcinoid heart disease occurs in patients who have primary intestinal tumors with metastasis to the liver. The incidence of carcinoid heart disease is approximately 1 in 300,000 of the population. The metastatic carcinoid tumors produce paraneoplastic substances (serotonin), which lead to the characteristic endocardial fibrous white plaque formation within the valve leaflets and tricuspid valve chordal apparatus. These fibrous depositions lead to valve distortion with foreshortened leaflets that are unable to open or close (frozen valve), resulting in TS and often tricuspid valve regurgitation. Infective endocarditis affecting the tricuspid valve can also lead to TS and is most common among those who are intravenous illicit drug users or those who have anatomically abnormal tricuspid valves at baseline. Congenital TS is extremely rare with an incidence occurring in less than 0.1% of the population.

Diagnosis: does the patient have tricuspid stenosis?

Patients with symptomatic TS usually present in their third or fourth decade of life, complaining of fatigue, lower-extremity swelling, abdominal discomfort, or dyspnea that is slowly progressive over a period of months to years. Antecedent history of rheumatic fever or heart murmur should be elicited on evaluation, but the absence of RF history should not exclude the diagnosis. Many adult patients with rheumatic heart disease may have not been diagnosed during childhood or may only remember an illness with a prolonged fever, rash, or severe joint pain requiring prolonged bed rest and absence from school. A history of persistent heart murmur beginning in late childhood that has been passed off as benign or innocent may also be the only historical clue to antecedent episode of RF.

Features of flushing, diarrhea, and bronchospasm should raise the possibility of carcinoid syndrome, and these patients have a 50% chance of cardiac involvement. The vast majority of patients with cardiac involvement present with signs of right heart failure secondary to severe dysfunction of the tricuspid and pulmonary valves. Tricuspid stenosis patients may also present with symptoms and signs of endocarditis, including unremitting or recurrent fever with generalized malaise and other physical stigmata. The patient may have an antecedent history of tricuspid valve replacement or intravenous drug use.

Cardiac findings on physical examination can be subtle or misinterpreted (**Table 131-8**). The presystolic murmur of TS is often missed or attributed to mitral valve stenosis. Although characteristics of the two murmurs can help differentiate one from the other, a high index of suspicion must be maintained for tricuspid valve involvement in a patient with multivalvular rheumatic heart disease. Patients with endocarditis-associated TS may present with the physical stigmata of bacterial endocarditis (eg, splinter hemorrhages, Osler nodes, and Janeway lesions).

A comprehensive metabolic profile helps evaluate for significant hepatic congestion associated with systemic venous hypertension and serves as a surrogate for end-organ dysfunction (eg, renal insufficiency). Twenty-four hour urinary excretion of 5-hydroxy-indole

TABLE 131-8 Signs of Tricuspid Stenosis

Physical Examination

Jugular venous pulsations elevated and a prominent presystolic a-wave during atrial contraction

Hepatomegaly, ascites, and peripheral edema with moderate-to-severe TS

Low-frequency presystolic murmur usually auscultated at the lower left sternal border in the fourth intercostal space, intensified with maneuvers that increase blood flow across the valve (eg, inspiration, squatting, and isotonic exercise)

An opening snap sometimes heard, but diminishes as severity worsens

acetic acid (5-HIAA) may be used to determine whether carcinoid heart disease is present. Blood cultures can help evaluate the possibility of bacterial endocarditis.

Ancillary tests should include chest x-ray, ECG, echocardiogram, and possibly cardiac catheterization. Although there are no clearly defined criteria for tricuspid stenosis severity, severe TS is often defined by the onset of overt symptoms accompanied by a mean gradient by echocardiogram or cardiac catheterization of >3 mm Hg, though a gradient >8 to 10 mm Hg is often observed. Mild-to-moderate TS is usually asymptomatic, and has no clearly defined gradient range beyond the definition of TS diagnosed with a gradient of ≤3 mm Hg.

Treatment

The main goal of treatment is to relieve the symptoms that result from restricted diastolic filling of the right ventricle and diminished pulmonary blood flow. Medical care consists of (1) assessment and treatment of the underlying etiology for the valvular pathology (eg, antibiotics for bacterial endocarditis or somatostatin analogs for carcinoid syndrome); (2) fluid and sodium restriction; (3) medications to treat cardiac arrhythmias secondary to right atrial distension (usually atrial fibrillation and/or flutter); and (4) pharmacotherapy with diuretics to reduce morbidity associated with systemic venous congestion.

Surgical valve replacement or commissurotomy is indicated if right heart failure persists or if low cardiac output develops. Successful percutaneous balloon valvotomy has been performed when the subvalvar structures are normal.

■ TRICUSPID REGURGITATION

Pathophyisology

Tricuspid regurgitation occurs commonly and depending on the severity usually not pathologic. Often it is asymptomatic and discovered initially by echocardiography. Tricuspid regurgitation is characterized by backflow of blood into the right atrium from the right ventricle during systole. Since the right atrium is compliant, no major hemodynamic consequences manifest in mild or moderate TR. However, with severe TR the right atrial and venous pressures rises and patients present with signs and symptoms of right-sided heart failure (**Table 131-9**).

An association between TR and the combined use of the anorectic drugs fenfluramine and phentermine has been described. The dopamine agonist pergolide may induce TR by a mechanism similar to that of anorectic drugs and carcinoid syndrome.

Does the patient have triscupid regurgitation?

The findings of mild-to-moderate TR are not striking other than an audible murmur. With severe TR, patients may exhibit right-sided

TABLE 131-9 Causes of Tricuspid Regurgitation

Functional causes

Dilatation of the right ventricle/tricuspid annulus from any cause

Secondary causes

Primary leaflet such as

- Ebstein anomaly
- Infective endocarditis
- Trauma
- Rheumatic Fever
- Carcinoid syndrome
- Papillary muscle dysfunction or rupture
- Marantic endocarditis
- Myxomatous degeneration

Tricuspid valve injury from

- Permanent pacemakers
- Implantable cardioverter-defibrillators
- Endomyocardial biopsies

Anorectic drug (eg, fenfluramine and phentermine, "Fen-Phen")

Carcinoid syndrome

congestive heart failure including painful hepatosplenomegaly, ascites, and peripheral edema as well as a sensation of pulsation in the neck (from distended and pulsatile jugular veins). In some patients however, no symptoms manifest for many years despite severe regurgitation. Tricuspid regurgitation is most commonly seen in association with left heart failure and/or left side valvular disease, and thus, the significance, prognosis, and treatment are difficult to determine.

PRACTICE POINT

- In severe tricuspid regurgitation, symptoms of right-sided congestive heart failure (painful hepatosplenomegaly, ascites, and peripheral edema) and a sensation of pulsation in the neck (from distended and pulsatile jugular veins) may occur. Jugular venous distension may be more prominent with inspiration. However, patients may have no symptoms for many years despite severe regurgitation.

Physical examination findings can suggest the presence of TR even in the absence of significant symptoms (**Table 131-10**). The jugular veins of patients with severe TR are distended and prominent, which reflects elevation in right atrial pressure. A prominent "c-v" wave due to systolic regurgitation into the right atrium is seen. Jugular venous distension may be more prominent with inspiration; this finding may not be obvious with marked venous distension. A systolic thrill may be palpated over the jugular vein in patients with severe TR.

The abdominal examination may reveal an enlarged, tender, and pulsatile liver. The murmur associated with severe TR can be auscultated over the liver coupled with a palpable thrill. The abdominal examination can also reveal ascites, peripheral edema, and in very severe cases anasarca. Unilateral or bilateral pleural effusions may occur in the presence of pulmonary hypertension or left-sided cardiac disease.

The ECG often reveals no characteristic changes unless other concomitant disorders are present such as right ventricular infarction, pulmonary hypertension, and pulmonary embolism. Chest

TABLE 131-10 Signs of Tricuspid Regurgitation

Physical Examination

Holosystolic murmur best heard at right or left mid-sternal border or at the subxiphoid area

Physical maneuvers that result in an increase in venous return (leg raising, exercise, hepatic compression) intensify the murmur of TR

Deep inspiration increases venous return to the right ventricle and the murmur of TR becomes louder and longer (Rivero-Carvallo sign)

Right ventricular heave on precordial palpation of the chest due to a dilated right ventricle

Abdominal examination with an enlarged, tender, and pulsatile liver; ascites, peripheral edema, and/or anascara

Unilateral or bilateral pleural effusions when pulmonary hypertension is present

radiographs of patients with TR reveal cardiomegaly due to right ventricular enlargement. A prominent cardiac silhouette is observed on the right in the PA view, and the enlarged right ventricle fills the retrosternal space in the lateral view. Additional findings may include right atrial enlargement, a prominent azygos vein, pleural effusion, and upward displacement of the diaphragm due to ascites. When the etiology of the TR is pulmonary hypertension secondary to a left-sided cardiac abnormality, other radiographic findings may be seen, particularly prominent right and left pulmonary artery hilar segments.

Echocardiography is the mainstay of testing in the evaluation of the TR. Tricuspid valve motion may be normal or abnormal. Characteristic primary valvular abnormalities that can be seen by echocardiography include Ebstein anomaly, carcinoid heart disease, RF, prolapse, flail leaflet, and endocarditis. The right ventricle and right atrium are usually dilated in the presence of moderate to severe TR, unless the TR is acute. Doppler color flow establishes the severity of TR. The major Doppler criteria for severe TR are a color jet (vena contracta) width >0.7 cm and systolic flow reversal in the hepatic veins. Systolic flow reversal may not be accurate when atrial fibrillation is present. Other findings include a dilated tricuspid annulus and paradoxical, interventricular septal motion, which reflect increased volume within the right ventricle (diastolic overload).

Cardiac catheterization and contrast right ventriculography are often not helpful for the diagnosis or evaluation of TR. However, in some patients, invasive evaluation may be performed to determine pulmonary vascular resistance or to evaluate the left heart pressures for causes of functional TR.

Treatment

The treatment of TR depends on the etiology. In functional TR, correction of high pulmonary artery pressures can result in improvement in TR. This has been demonstrated in patients with reversible causes of pulmonary hypertension such as mitral stenosis and chronic thromboembolic pulmonary hypertension. Among patients who undergo surgery for correction of left-sided heart disease, concurrent tricuspid valve annuloplasty is often performed (eg, mitral valve repair with concurrent tricuspid valve repair). Tricuspid annuloplasty for functional TR is rarely ever performed as an isolated procedure as the recurrence rate is high. Treatment of primary TR (often replacement with a tissue or mechanical valve) should be done by a cardiac surgeon that has experience in congenital heart or valvular heart disease.

CONCLUSION

Valvular heart disease is rapidly emerging as a separate subspecialty within cardiology and cardiac surgery. It encompasses multiple pathophysiologic processes due to a myriad of systemic and congenital diseases. Therapies for valvular heart disease continue to evolve as minimally invasive surgical and catheter-based approaches gain experience. The internist and hospitalist remain the gatekeepers of these patients and should maintain a working understanding of diagnoses and therapies to optimize patient care. Collaboration with a cardiologist or cardiac surgeon that has expertise in this area is essential.

SUGGESTED READINGS

Asgar AW, Mack MJ, Stone GW. Secondary mitral regurgitation in heart failure: pathophysiology, prognosis, and therapeutic considerations. *J Am Coll Cardiol.* 2015;65(12):1231-1248.

Carabello BA. Is it ever too late to operate on the patient with valvular heart disease? *J Am Coll Cardiol.* 2004;44:376-383.

Carabello BA, Crawford FA Jr, Valvular heart disease. *N Engl J Med.* 1997;337:32-41.

Gössl M, Holmes DR Jr. An update on transcatheter aortic valve replacement. *Curr Probl Cardiol.* 2013;38(7):245-283.

Lancellotti P, Tribouilloy C, Hagendorff A, et al. Recommendations for the echocardiographic assessment of native valvular regurgitation: an executive summary from the European Association of Cardiovascular Imaging. *Eur Heart J Cardiovasc Imaging.* 2013;14(7):611-644.

Nishimura RA, Otto CM, Bonow RO, et al. 2014 AHA/ACC guideline for the management of patients with valvular heart disease. A report of the American college of cardiology/american heart association task force on practice guidelines. *J Am Coll Cardiol.* 2014;63(22):2438-2488.

Saikrishnan N, Kumar G, Sawaya FJ, Lerakis S, Yoganathan AP. Accurate assessment of aortic stenosis: a review of diagnostic modalities and hemodynamics. *Circulation.* 2014;129(2):244-253.

132

Supraventricular Tachyarrhythmias

Elbert B. Chun, MD
Gerard M. McGorisk, MD, FACC, MRCPI

Key Clinical Questions

1. What electrocardiographic findings help differentiate between the common supraventricular tachyarrhythmias (SVTs)?

2. What acute and chronic management strategies are indicated for various SVTs?

3. What comorbid conditions increase the risk of thromboembolic complications in patients with atrial fibrillation?

4. Which patients with atrial fibrillation deserve anticoagulation, and which of these patients need bridging anticoagulation until oral warfarin attains therapeutic international normalized ratio (INR)?

5. Which SVTs deserve electrophysiologic intervention over medical management?

EPIDEMIOLOGY

Supraventricular tachyarrhythmias (SVTs) comprise an array of narrow-complex arrhythmias that originate above the ventricles and include both the most commonly encountered arrhythmia, atrial fibrillation (AF), and the uncommon ones, such as Wolfe-Parkinson-White (WPW) syndrome. Based on Medicare and a sampling of national community hospital discharge database, AF occurs 10-fold more frequently than paroxysmal SVTs such as AVnRT. This chapter describes in detail the common atrial arrhythmias encountered by hospitalists, and explains the uncommon arrhythmias that hospitalists should recognize and manage with cardiologist or electrophysiologist consultation or referral. The chapter will briefly describe arrhythmia mechanisms while focusing on arrhythmia diagnosis, management options in the acute setting, and long-term management strategies—all essential for a seamless transition beyond the inpatient setting.

PRESENTATION

Common presenting symptoms of SVTs include rapid palpitations, chest discomfort, dyspnea, presyncope, and syncope. Additionally, atrial fibrillation and atrial flutter may present with new stroke symptoms. Particularly in the elderly with atrial fibrillation, palpitations and chest discomfort are often absent and excessive fatigue is the predominant symptom.

■ RISK STRATIFICATION

As SVT is a heterogenous disorder describing different arrhythmias with vastly different clinical prognosis. As such, the crucial initial step is the proper recognition of the rhythm disorder to individualize treatment strategy and prevention of adverse events.

RHYTHM IDENTIFICATION

When evaluating patients with a narrow-complex arrhythmia, the QRS complex is by definition less than 120 ms. The regularity of the RR intervals then helps reduce the numerous possibilities, as indicated in the SVT recognition algorithm (**Figure 132-1**). Only four possibilities exist if the RR intervals are *irregular*: (1) atrial fibrillation, (2) atrial flutter with variable atrioventricular (AV) node blockade, (3) atrial tachycardia with variable AV node blockade, and (4) multifocal atrial tachycardia (MAT).

More challenging to diagnose is the SVT with a regular RR interval. If, however, no P-wave can be identified, this indicates the most common form of *paroxysmal* SVT: atrioventricular nodal reentrant tachycardia (AVnRT). The P-wave in typical AVnRT is buried within the QRS complex. If the P-wave is identified then determine if there is more than one P-wave for each conducted QRS. If so, then only atrial flutter or atrial tachycardia remains as possible diagnoses.

Finally, if only a one-to-one relationship between the P-waves and QRS complexes exists, measuring the RP interval will further narrow the likely rhythms (**Figure 132-2**). The response of the rhythm to bedside vagal maneuvers or intravenous adenosine can be used to better differentiate the regular narrow-complex arrhythmias by transiently slowing the AV conduction and revealing the P-waves,

SVT recognition algorithm

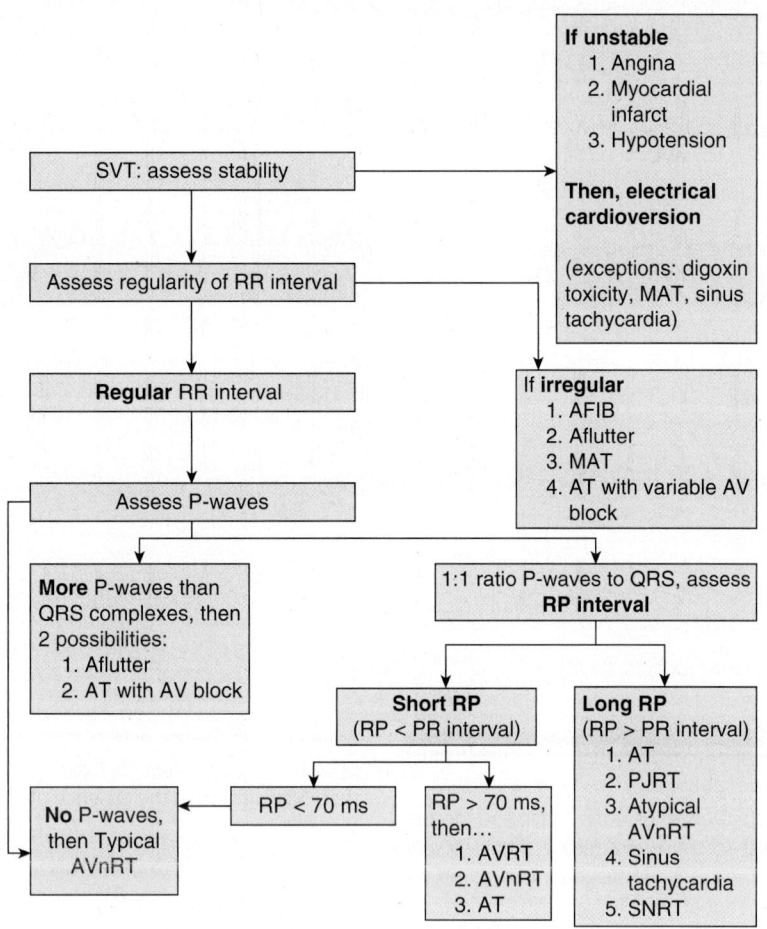

Figure 132-1 *Supraventricular tachyarrhythmia recognition algorithm. AF, atrial fibrillation; Aflutter, atrial flutter; AT, atrial tachycardia; AV block, atrioventricular block; AVnRT, atrioventricular nodal reentrant tachycardia; AVRT, atrioventricular reentry tachycardia; MAT, multifocal atrial tachycardia; PJRT, paroxysmal junctional reentrant tachycardia; SNRT, sinus node reentry tachycardia.*

converting the rhythm to sinus, or gradually slowing and reaccelerating the tachycardia (**Table 132-1**).

Proceeding through the SVT recognition algorithm (see Figure 132-1) using a sample ECG (**Figure 132-3**), the clinician first recognizes that the rate is greater than 100 beats per minute (bpm). The QRS complexes are narrow, thus leading to a generic diagnosis of SVT. Following the SVT recognition algorithm, the regularity of the RR intervals is assessed, and the absence of P-waves leads to the conclusion that the SVT is attributable to typical AVnRT (see Figure 132-3).

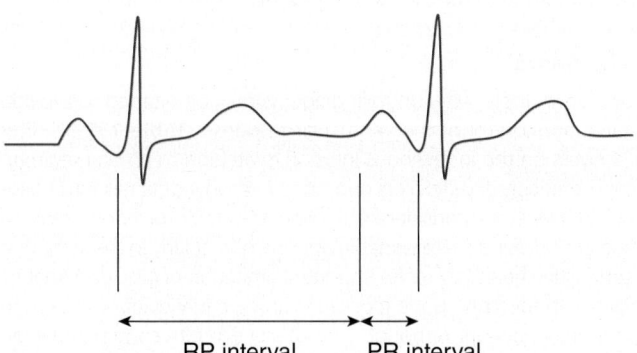

Figure 132-2 *ECG rhythm intervals demonstrating how to measure the PR and RP intervals.*

TABLE 132-1 Effect of Transient Atrioventricular Node Blockade on Supraventricular Tachyarrhythmia Diagnosis

Rhythm	Response to Transient AV Node Blockade (Vagal Maneuvers or IV Adenosine)
AVnRT	Sudden termination
AVRT	Sudden termination
Sinus reentry tachycardia	Sudden termination
Focal atrial tachycardia	Sudden termination, or gradual slowing and reacceleration
Ventricular tachycardia (high septal or fascicular origin)	No response
Sinus tachycardia	Gradual slowing, then reacceleration
Nonparoxysmal junctional tachycardia	Gradual slowing, then reacceleration
Atrial flutter	Persistent atrial tachycardia and transient high-grade AV blockade
Macro reentrant atrial tachycardia	Persistent atrial tachycardia and transient high-grade AV blockade

AVnRT, atrioventricular nodal reentrant tachycardia; AVRT, atrioventricular reentry tachycardia; VTACH, ventricular tachycardia.

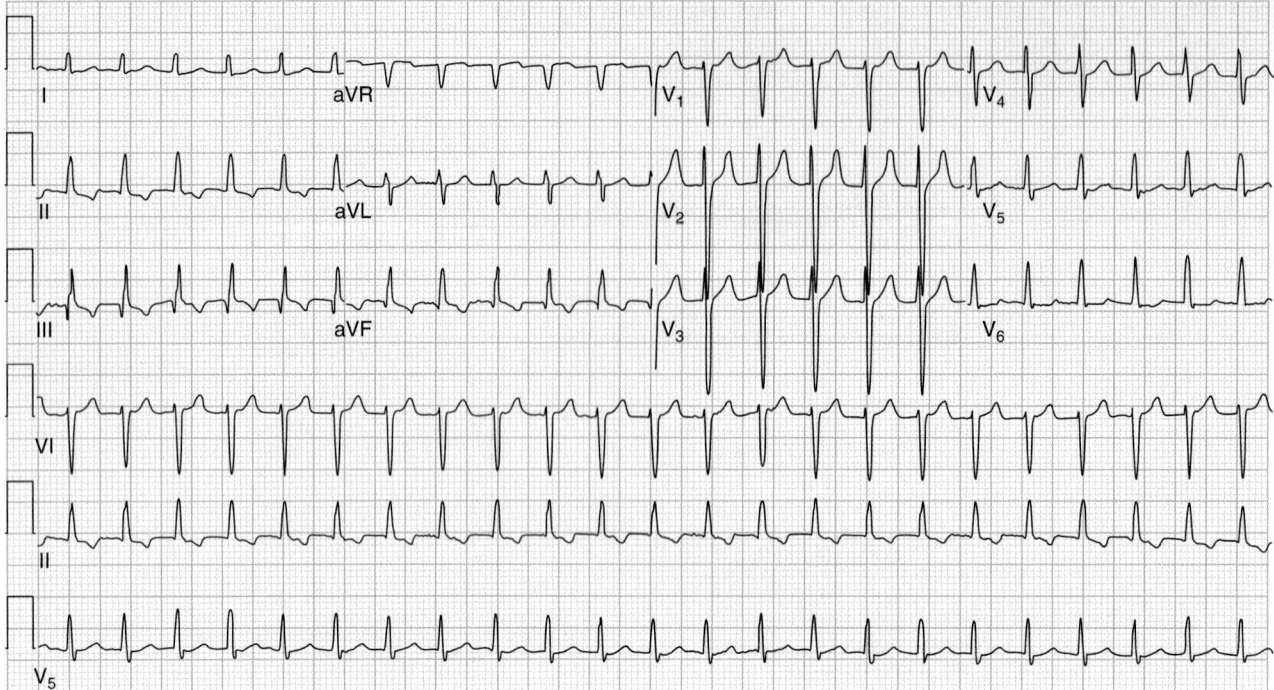

Figure 132-3 *Atrioventricular nodal tachycardia (AVnRT).*

ATRIAL FIBRILLATION

■ EVALUATION

Before the age of 60, the prevalence of atrial fibrillation occurs uncommonly, in stark contrast to the prevalence estimate of 8% among those older than 80 years. As AF is the most common arrhythmia encountered by the inpatient clinician, this section will address the questions pertaining to the valvular and nonvalvular etiology of this arrhythmia, judicious utilization of cardioversion, thromboembolic and other complications, methods for estimating risk of stroke, and management strategies in the acute and chronic settings.

Patients with atrial fibrillation are classified in one of three categories: (1) paroxysmal AF, (2) persistent AF, or (3) permanent AF (**Table 132-2**).

The atrium in patients with AF shows evidence of fibrosis and increased extracellular mass changes that are seen both in the myocardium of the elderly and in ischemia-induced hibernating myocardium. Within this scarred milieu, a focal-enhanced automaticity and variance in atrial tissue refractory and conduction times (known collectively as the *multiple wavelet hypothesis*) leads to this common arrhythmia. The enhanced automaticity often can be isolated to atrial tissue near the pulmonary veins. In addition to the aging process, any medical condition that leads to elevated left atrial pressure and dilated atrium—hypertension, mitral stenosis or regurgitation, and any cardiomyopathy—will predispose the patient to atrial fibrillation. Hyperadrenergic states—sepsis, alcohol ingestion or withdrawal, postoperative state, and thyrotoxicosis—also predispose to AF. *Lone atrial fibrillation* describes AF in patients younger than 60 years old in the absence of any predisposing factor.

■ INPATIENT MANAGEMENT

Hemodynamic compromise versus stable tachycardia

Common clinical scenarios for hospitalized patients with AF include those with stable tachycardia and those with hemodynamic compromise. For those with hypotension, a trial of *short-acting* rate-controlling agents (eg, esmolol) could be attempted to determine if slowing the tachycardia may improve the hemodynamics, keeping in mind that these very agents may exacerbate hypotension. Intravenous digoxin and amiodarone are options if hypotension prevents the use of β-blockers and calcium channel blockers. Synchronized direct cardioversion should be performed if the hypotension does not resolve (see Chapter 125). Currently there are two types of defibrillators: monophasic and biphasic. Biphasic defibrillators are now significantly more common and require less energy and reduced number of shocks delivered to achieve successful cardioversion. Biphasic defibrillators also have reduced skin injury. The monophasic device should be set at a minimum of 200 J and a maximum of 400 J. The biphasic device demonstrates effective cardioversion at 200 J and often times at just 100 J for AF.

Rate control

One or multiple rate-controlling agents may be needed to provide adequate control of the ventricular response (**Table 132-3**). After 24 hours on the intravenous infusion, switching to an oral regimen can be initiated. β-Blockers and nondihydropyridine calcium channel blockers are considered first-line agents. Intravenous digoxin and amiodarone are reasonable options, particularly in the setting of congestive heart failure. An important limitation of digoxin is that its vagally induced AV node blockade can be easily overcome in non-sedentary patients. Although very effective in rate control and even rhythm conversion, amiodarone has a long-term side effects profile which relegates its use as a distant second option. Clinicians should target a heart rate under 110 bpm at rest but consider patient symptoms in modification of rate control.

TABLE 132-2 Atrial Fibrillation Nomenclature

Paroxysmal AF	Episodes lasting <7 days and spontaneously converting to sinus rhythm
Persistent AF	Episodes lasting >7 days unless chemical or electrically cardioverted to sinus rhythm
Permanent AF	AF resistant to multiple attempts at cardioversion
Lone AF	AF in patients younger than 60 years old in the absence of any predisposing factor

AF, atrial fibrillation.

TABLE 132-3 Intravenous Medications for Rate-Control in Atrial Fibrillation or Atrial Flutter

Medication	Loading Dose	Maintenance Dose	Side Effects
Esmolol	500 mcg/kg over 1 min	60-200 mcg/kg/min IV	Hypotension
Metoprolol	2.5-5 mg IV over 2 min Up to 3 doses	NA	Hypotension
Diltiazem	0.25 mg/kg IV over 2 min	5-15 mg/h	Hypotension
Verapamil	0.075-0.15 mg/kg IV over 2 min	NA	Hypotension
Digoxin	0.25 mg IV every 2 h up to total dose 1.5 mg	0.125-0.375 mg/day IV or orally	Digoxin toxicity, heart block
Amiodarone	150 mg IV over 10 min	0.5-1 mg/min IV	Pulmonary toxcity, hepatitis, skin discoloration, thyroid dysfunction, corneal deposits, optic neuropathy

The presence of an accessory pathway would be an absolute contraindication in the use of AV node-blocking agents. As electrical impulses are conducted nondecrementally via the accessory pathway, the ventricular response in AF will actually increase and may degenerate into ventricular fibrillation (VFIB).

Rhythm control and consultation

After assessing clinical stability and adequately controlling the rapid ventricular response, the clinician should determine if the rhythm event is new, recurrent, or an exacerbation of a permanent form of the arrhythmia. If the condition is a new event or a paroxysmal one with infrequent yet very symptomatic recurrences and has been present for *less than 48 hours*, cardioversion—chemical or electrical—followed by an attempt to maintain a sinus rhythm may offer symptom benefit and is recommended by the ACC-AHA AF guidelines from 2006 (**Table 132-4**). If the AF duration is longer than 48 hours, cardioversion remains an option after transesophageal echo (TEE) is negative for left atrial thrombus. Cardioverting those with new-onset AF provides the theoretical benefit of curtailing the risk of developing permanent AF.

Cardioversion can be achieved not only with electrical means, but also chemical means (**Table 132-5**). The antiarrhythmics used for cardioversion should be considered after consultation with cardiology service. A class III agent, ibutilide, can be used in select patients that have no evidence of systolic dysfunction, normal magnesium and potassium levels, and a normal corrected QT interval (QTc). Due to the risk of torsades de pointes, this should be performed in a setting equipped to handle this potential complication. Ibutilide has the advantage of increasing the success of electrical cardioversion following a failed chemical cardioversion. An oral class III agent, tikosyn, can be used to both convert to a sinus rhythm and also maintain a sinus rhythm. This medication should be reserved for cardiology consultants due to the need for close monitoring of the QT interval, renal dose adjustments, and limitations of use in patients with liver

dysfunction. If the QT interval is greater than 500 ms, this medication should not be initiated or should be discontinued. The use of medications to maintain a sinus rhythm should remain under the care of a cardiologist due to the frequency of treatment failure and significant risk of malignant ventricular arrhythmias.

Anticoagulation

The unorganized atrial contractions during AF will lead to the formation of thrombus or spontaneous echo contrast (SEC) within the left atrium or the left atrial appendage posing a substantial risk of thromboembolic phenomena to the arterial circulation, which usually manifests as stroke and, less commonly, mesenteric ischemia or an acutely ischemic limb. The transthoracic echocardiogram is considered the diagnostic test of choice for initial evaluation. It is useful in assessing left atrial size and left ventricular function, but cannot exclude atrial thrombus. The transesophageal echocardiogram provides high resolution of the left atrium and left atrial appendage and to exclude thrombus and permit *early cardioversion*. Thrombus or dense SEC would preclude the option for early cardioversion and necessitate the need for full anticoagulation for 4 weeks prior to cardioversion. In the absence of thrombus or SEC on TEE, the patient may receive early cardioversion in the setting of anticoagulation. For AF recognized greater than 48 hours after onset in patients who do not undergo TEE, full anticoagulation for 4 weeks is recommended followed by cardioversion, if indicated.

In either strategy, anticoagulation for a minimum of 4 weeks postcardioversion is necessary to reduce the risk of thromboembolic complications. The risk of embolic stroke is approximately 1% with either approach. Stroke risk postcardioversion is due to a "stunning" effect on the left atrium after any form of cardioversion (electrical, chemical, or even spontaneous). This stunning refers to a delay in the resumption of mechanical contraction of the left atrium, providing an environment ripe for stasis and thrombus formation. Benefits from an early cardioversion approach include quicker conversion to a sinus rhythm, accelerated care for the patient, and potentially less bleeding complications associated without the preceding 4 weeks of anticoagulation.

TABLE 132-4 Indication for R-Wave Synchronized Cardioversion in Atrial Fibrillation

Rapid ventricular response not responding to pharmacologic measures in setting of ongoing angina, heart failure, myocardial ischemia, or symptomatic hypotension
Pre-excitation with rapid ventricular response or hemodynamic instability
Stable hemodynamics, but poorly tolerated symptoms
Early relapse of atrial fibrillation after attempted cardioversion, proceed with administration of antiarrhythmic medications first, then repeat cardioversion
Consider patient preferences in the setting of infrequent relapses

> **PRACTICE POINT**
>
> - Transesophageal echocardiogram is a highly sensitive test to rule out thrombus within the left atrium and left atrial appendage to permit an early cardioversion strategy, if indicated.

Ablation strategies

Invasive management options for atrial fibrillation should be considered secondary options following failure of medical therapies and recurrent admissions due to symptomatic palpitations or heart

TABLE 132-5 **Medications for Pharmacologic Cardioversion of Atrial Fibrillation**

Medication	Antiarrhythmic Class	Dosing	Route	Comments
Amiodarone (codarone, pacerone)	III	400 mg orally twice a day for 2 wks (10 g load), then 200 mg orally every day	Orally	Outpatient option: oral load (gastrointestinal side effects common)
		150 mg IV over 10 mins, then 1 mg/min for 6 h, then 0.5 mg/min for 18 h (1 g load)		Other side effects common and severe: pulmonary fibrosis, corneal deposits, thyroid dysfunction, hepatitis, skin deposition
Ibutilide (corvert)	III	If weight >60 kg, 1 mg IV once; may repeat dose if no response in 10 mins	IV	Inpatient only usually cardioverts within 1 h monitor for QT prolongation
		If weight <60 kg, then 0.01 mg/kg IV; may repeat if no response after 10 mins		Torsades 4% (more common in women)
				Must monitor K^+ and Mg^{+2}
Dofetilide (tikosyn)	III	500 mcg orally twice a day (restricted distribution in the US to trained prescribers and facilities)	Orally	Inpatient initiation only; adjust for renal function, age, body size
				QT prolongation
				Many drug interactions (CYP3A4)
				Contraindicated with Bactrim, HCTZ, verapamil
Flecainide	Ic	Start 50 mg orally twice a day, may increase 100 mg/d every 4 days; max dose 300 mg every day	Orally or IV	Contraindicated in structural heart disease
				Adjust dose for renal dysfunction
Propafenone	Ia	Start 150 mg orally three times a day, then may increase to 225 mg orally three times a day after 4 days, then, up to 300 mg orally three times a day	Orally or IV	Contraindicated in structural heart disease including significant LVH, CHF, severe obstructive lung disease

failure exacerbations. The palpitations associated with atrial fibrillation can be distressing to some individuals, particularly younger patients, and have significant negative impacts on quality of life. If the use of antiarrhythmic regimens has failed, options for catheter-based interventions or even intraoperative left atrial ablation, also known as the Maze procedure can be offered. One catheter-based approach called *ablate-and-pace*, entails ablating the AV node and then pacing the ventricle. Another catheter-based approach involves isolating the focus of automaticity, usually near the pulmonary veins of the cavoatrial isthmus, ablating the foci, and initiating anticoagulation therapy thereafter. The latter approach is relatively new and long-term outcome research is still pending. The short-term safety of the procedure in centers with established experience has been proven with death rates or stroke rates under 1% and overall major complications about 6% based on international survey data. However, the mean age of the patients enrolled in these trials was 55 years old with intact systolic function and relatively nondilated atrial diameters. More long-term outcome data will be needed before catheter-based interventions can be considered a parallel option to medical treatment. A final option usually reserved for those who are undergoing open heart bypass or valve replacement is the Maze procedure, and even left atrial appendage resection, both of which may prevent the occurrence of postoperative atrial fibrillation.

Death or significant neurologic deficits occur in 71% of patients with their first episode of embolic complications associated with AF. Reducing this risk is a crucial component in the management of AF. The annual risk of strokes for AF is approximately 4.5% per year, which is reduced by two-thirds (to 1.5% per year) if patients are fully anticoagulated. However, not all patients with this condition carry the same risk of embolic events and, therefore, should be managed based on risk. Clinicians must diagnose the etiology of AF, as that will help determine risk and direct management. The vast majority of AF is *nonvalvular*, but *valvular* etiologies such as significant mitral stenosis must be considered. A severalfold increase in thromboembolic risk occurs with mitral valve stenosis-associated atrial fibrillation, and mandates full anticoagulation regardless of other

stroke risk factors present. Patients with other risk factors leading to atrial fibrillation have variable levels of evidence supporting full anticoagulation, and some patients with few stroke or embolism risk factors may not attain benefit from anticoagulation that outweighs its risks (**Table 132-6**).

TABLE 132-6 **Antithrombotic Recommendations for Atrial Fibrillation by Etiology**

AF Risk Factor	Therapy Recommendation	Level of Evidence
Thyrotoxicosis	Full anticoagulation (eg, warfarin)	Level C: Expert opinion (ACC/AHA guidelines)
Mitral stenosis	Full anticoagulation (eg, warfarin)	Level C: Expert opinion (ACC/AHA guidelines)
Mechanical valve	Full anticoagulation (eg, warfarin)	Level 1A (ACCP guidelines 2008)
$CHADS_2$ score ≥ 2	Full anticoagulation (eg, warfarin)	Level 1A (ACCP guidelines 2008)
$CHADS_2$ score = 1	Full anticoagulation (eg, warfarin) or aspirin (75-325 mg daily)	Level 1A (anticoagulation) Level 1B (asprin) (ACCP guidelines 2008)
$CHADS_2$ score = 0	Aspirin therapy (75-325 mg daily)	Level 1B (ACCP guidelines 2008)

ACC/AHA, American College of Cardiology/American Heart Association; ACCP, American College of Chest Physicians.
Level 1A (ACCP): Consistent evidence from randomized controlled trials without important limitations or exceptionally strong evidence from observational studies.
Level 1B (ACCP): Evidence from randomized controlled trials with important limitations (inconsistent results, methodologic flaws, indirect or imprecise), or very strong evidence from observational studies.
Level C (ACC/AHA): Recommendation based on expert opinion, case studies, or standards of care.

TABLE 132-7 CHADS₂ Score and Stroke Risk

Number of Factors	Risk of Stroke (%/y)
0 (lower risk)	1.9 (1.2-3.0)
1 (intermediate risk)	2.8 (2.0-3.8)
2 (high risk)	4.0 (3.1-5.1)
3	5.9 (4.6-7.3)
4	8.5 (6.3-11.1)
5	12.5 (8.2 -17.5)
6	18.2 (10.5-27.4)

CHADS₂ score is calculated by adding 1 point for each of the following: Recent **C**ongestive heart failure, **H**ypertension, **A**ge ≥75 years, **D**iabetes mellitus; and 2 points for prior **S**troke/transient ischemic attack.

When considering the more common scenario of nonvalvular atrial fibrillation, multiple risk stratification strategies have been published over the decades to estimate the risk of thromboembolic complications, and to date the one most widely used and derived from large cohort data is known as the CHADS₂ score. **C**ongestive heart failure, **H**ypertension, **A**ge ≥ 75, and **D**iabetes each contributes one point in this risk stratification tool whereas **S**troke contributes two points. The total number of points corresponds to a level of risk (incidence) of embolic stroke each year (**Table 132-7**).

By using this risk stratification tool clinicians can balance the benefits of therapeutic anticoagulation against the well-known complication, bleeding. With no risk factors for thromboembolic phenomena, as in the scenario of *lone atrial fibrillation*, the risk of bleeding complications with coumadin outweighs the benefit of stroke prevention. An acceptable alternative stroke risk-reduction strategy for patients who have low baseline risk (CHADS₂ = 0) or who have contraindications to anticoagulation is antiplatelet therapy with aspirin (81-325 mg daily).

For patients with intermediate risk (CHADS₂ score = 1), one should implement an additional risk stratification tool known as the CHA₂DS₂-VASc (**Table 132-8**) to better define the risk of thromboembolic stroke. As recommended by national cardiology organizations, anticoagulation should be strongly considered if the score is 2 or greater. If the score 1 point, then either aspirin or anticoagulation are viable options. Major bleeding complication risk with anticoagulation can be estimated using a risk stratification scheme with the acronym HAS-BLED (**Table 132-9**).

The HAS-BLED score contains the variables hypertension, abnormal renal function, abnormal liver function, stroke, previous

TABLE 132-8 CHA₂DS₂-VASc

Number of Factors	Risk of stroke (%/y)
0	0
1	1.3
2	2.2
3	3.2
4	4.0
5	6.7
6	9.8
7	9.6
8	6.7
9	15.2

CHA₂DS₂-VASc score is calculated by adding 1 point for each of the following: Recent CHF, hypertension, Age 65-74, DM, female gender, Vascular disease (PVD, CAD, aortic plaque); and 2 points for Age ≥75 and prior Stroke/TIA.

TABLE 132-9 HAS-BLED Score

Letter	Clinical Characteristic	Points
H	Hypertension	1
A	Abnormal renal or liver disease	1 for each
S	Stroke	1
B	Previous major bleeding	1
L	Labile INR	1
E	Elderly (age >65)	1
D	Drugs or alcohol	1

Hypertension – SBP >160 mm Hg
Abnormal renal function: dialysis or serum creatinine >2.26 mg/dL (200 umol/L)
Abnormal liver function: cirrhosis, or elevated AST or ALT >3 X upper limit of normal
Labile INR: unstable INR or TTR (time in therapeutic range) <60%
Drugs: aspirin, other antiplatelet medications, NSAIDS, or alcohol abuse

bleeding, labile INR's, age >65 years old, concomitant use of aspirin or antiplatelet agent, and excessive alcohol consumption with each counting as a point. The final score then correlates with the risk of major bleeding per 100 patients per year (ie, % major bleeds per year with anticoagulation therapy).

These risk estimation tools can be used to counsel patients regarding treatment choices, including benefits and risks, and help identify patients who might gain more overall benefit from antiplatelet aspirin therapy rather than anticoagulation. The HAS-BLED tool might also be used to help determine which patients deserve more intensive outpatient monitoring of their anticoagulation (eg, in an anticoagulation clinic). National organizations recommend using caution when the HAS-BLED score ≥ 3 and a detailed discussion of risk and benefits with the patient.

More data over the past several years have demonstrated a larger role of AF in patients with cryptogenic strokes. Insertable cardiac monitors in a study published in 2015 have been utilized in this cohort of patients and have detected up to 8.9% patients with AF at 6 months compared to just over 1% in the cohort following standard of care monitoring. The most recent national medical organizations do not provide strong guidance in the intensity and duration of monitoring for potential AF detection in cryptogenic, but this data suggests a 24-hour Holter monitor is vastly insufficient.

■ ATRIAL FIBRILLATION AND OLDER PEOPLE: WARFARIN CONTROVERSY

Often a difficult clinical management decision, the use of anticoagulation in older patients is controversial. Atrial fibrillation is the etiologic factor for 36% of strokes in individuals over the age of 80. The morbidity and mortality of a first stroke due to this disease is 71%. Meta-analysis data estimate the overall risk reduction with vitamin-K antagonists at 66% and with aspirin at 21%. Recent data have also demonstrated that patients over the age of 85 benefit more from anticoagulation than younger cohorts. Thus, the argument for anticoagulation with warfarin in this group is compelling. However, the risk of major bleeding complications is still relevant. The rate of intracranial hemorrhage (ICH) while taking warfarin is approximately 0.3% to 0.6% per year (RR ~ 2, compared to control). Aspirin also carries an increased risk of ICH (RR ~ 1.4 compared to control). Although the risk of ICH seems low, this estimate may be underestimated as older patients were underrepresented in the early randomized trials performed almost 20 years ago. More recent observational studies have estimated the risk of a major bleeding complication in individuals over the age of 80 to be 13% per year including a 2.4% per year risk of ICH.

Additional concerns for anticoagulation in older people are the increased risk for falls, likely drug interactions due to polypharmacy, complexity of coumadin regimens, need for close monitoring, and the large representation of nursing home patients. Even in research trials studying the efficacy of coumadin to prevent strokes, only two-thirds of the INRs were in the therapeutic range. Some of these concerns can be addressed with the novel oral anticoagulants that reduce the need for frequent laboratory monitoring and reduce the concerns for drug interactions associated with polypharmacy. The data comparing coumadin with the direct thrombin inhibitor, dabigatran, demonstrate better stroke prevention with the higher dose of dabigatran at 150 mg orally twice a day and even a trend toward an overall mortality benefit after a median follow-up period of 2 years. The downside is the increased propensity of gastrointestinal bleeding compared to warfarin. The lower dose, 110 mg orally twice a day, was found to have an equivalent reduction of stroke risk and a lower risk of major bleeding complications but is not available in the United States. There are also three factor Xa inhibitors that Food and Drug Administration (FDA) approved to prevent strokes in the setting of nonvalvular AFIB, rivaroxaban, apixaban, and edoxaban. Rivaroxaban has been shown to be noninferior in stroke prevention, major bleeding complications, and mortality with warfarin. Apixaban however has been shown to prevent slightly more strokes, reduce risk of major bleeding outcomes, and reduce risk for mortality compared to warfarin. The most recent FDA approval of edoxaban in January 2015 was based on randomized trial data demonstrating superior stroke prevention compared to warfarin, less major bleeding complications, but slightly higher gastrointestinal bleeding complications. All of the novel anticoagulants compared to Coumadin have half as many intracranial bleeds. As no head-to-head studies have been conducted among the novel agents, all are considered viable options for stroke prevention for nonvaluvular AFIB.

PRACTICE POINT

- Novel anticoagulants reduce the need for frequent laboratory monitoring and reduce the concerns for drug interactions associated with warfarin and polypharmacy. These medications (dabigatran, rivaroxaban, apixiban, edoxaban) are approved for use in atrial fibrillation for stroke prevention. However, the cost may be prohibitive if not insured.

- Apixiban received FDA approval in 2015 for use in patients with ESRD on hemodialysis despite the absence of randomized control data but supported by pharmacokinetic data.

- Risk scores such as CHADS2, CHA_2DS_2-VASc apply only to nonvalvular AFIB. AFIB related to mechanical valves, *mitral stenosis* or rarely *hyperthyroidism* are at much higher risk for thromboembolic phenomena and require anticoagulation.

- The novel anticoagulants have not been FDA approved in patients with mechanical heart valves. In fact, dabigatran has been shown to have been inferior to coumadin in preventing embolic stokes with mechanical heart valves.

- The ACCP 2012 guideline on antithrombotics recommends the use of bridging anticoagulation in AF in high risk patients with a $CHADS_2$ score of 5 and 6. This has been supported by 2015 randomized trial BRIDGE which demonstrated more bleeding complications and no change in stroke prevention in those undergoing a bridging strategy.

- Bridging anticoagulation for those with low or moderate risk AFIB increases the risk of major bleeding complications and has not been proven to prevent more thromboembolic events via recent observational data and large randomized control trial in 2015.

TABLE 132-10 Risk of Postoperative Atrial Fibrillation (POAF) Based on Type of Surgery

Surgery Type	POAF/SVT %
Thoracic (noncardiac)	9-29%
Cardiothoracic	20-40%
Orthopedics	4%

Randomized trial data for the use of other antiplatelet agents (clopidogrel) in addition to aspirin for stroke prevention has been equivocal with respect to outcomes, with modest risk reduction of stroke but similar risk increase for major bleeding complications. Dual antiplatelet agents for stroke prevention are, therefore, not currently recommended.

■ POSTOPERATIVE ATRIAL FIBRILLATION

Postoperative atrial fibrillation (POAF) is the most common arrhythmia after surgery and observational data suggest an increased risk of short- and long-term mortality, increased length of stay, hospital costs, ICU length of stay, and stroke risk with this arrhythmia. Recent observational data in 2014 strongly suggest a twofold increase in stroke risk in patients with POAF compared to those with who didn't develop AF after noncardiac surgery at 1 year. This was also true in those who underwent cardiac surgery but to a lesser degree (hazard ratio 1.3, CI 1.1, 1.6). POAF is also the most common reason for hospital readmission after open heart surgery. The risk of developing this arrhythmia varies based on the type of surgical intervention, with open heart procedures bearing the highest risk (**Table 132-10**). Some of the risk factors associated with POAF include age, atrial enlargement, procedures related to the heart such as valvular repair, and β-blocker discontinuation.

The peak incidence of POAF occurs on the second postoperative day, and the majority occurs within 5 days postoperative. The majority of recurrent episodes of POAF occurred within several days of the first episode. The majority of POAF rhythms will spontaneously revert to sinus rhythm by the sixth postoperative week. However, if POAF is poorly tolerated due to hemodynamic compromise, anticoagulation and cardioversion would be recommended. Preoperative β-blockade leads to significant reduction in POAF incidence, but conflicting data mire the actual effect on hospital length of stay, postoperative strokes, and mortality. The ACC/AHA 2006 guidelines for AF offer a class I recommendation of perioperative β-blockers for prevention of POAF in patients undergoing coronary revascularization surgery (CABG).

■ POSTACUTE CARE: ATRIAL FIBRILLATION

If a patient is discharged on warfarin, rapid follow-up within 3 to 5 days is warranted as the risk of major bleeding complications is known to occur with initiation of anticoagulation. If an anticoagulation clinic is available, it would be strongly recommended to be monitored there. Within a week or two, the heart rate response can be reassessed as most patients will require AV nodal blocking agents to prevent a rapid ventricular response. The patient's symptoms can be periodically reassessed to determine whether the treatment strategy, either rate-control or rhythm control, needs to be changed. It should be noted that the latter approach has not been proven to reduce mortality, but only to improve symptoms and quality of life for a select group a patients with intolerable palpations and fatigue associated with AFIB.

■ DISCHARGE CHECKLIST: AFIB

- Transthoracic echocardiogram should have been performed recently to differentiate between valvular and nonvalvular AFIB and assess ventricular function and left atrial size.

- Thyroid function tests should have been completed to evaluate for hyperthyroidism.
- For new onset AFIB, early consultation with cardiology should be considered to evaluate the potential benefits of a rhythm control strategy.
- Ensure stroke risk stratification with $CHADS_2$ or CHA_2DS_2-VASc has been discussed with the *nonvalvular* AFIB patient and documented.
- Ensure risk stratification for major bleeding complications via HAS-BLED has been discussed with patients on anticoagulation.
  - For those on vitamin-K antagonists, rapid follow-up within 3 to 5 days should occur to avoid the perils of major bleeding complications.
  - For those on novel anticoagulants, ensure dosing has been based on level of renal function as FDA-approved antidotes are not available for the factor Xa inhibitors.
  - For those with cryptogenic stroke, strongly consider longer-term monitoring via an event monitor or insertable cardiac monitor to sufficiently evaluate for potential unrecognized AF.

ATRIAL FLUTTER

■ EPIDEMIOLOGY

Atrial flutter is the next most common form of SVT after atrial fibrillation and can manifest into the typical and atypical pattern. The typical pattern, also known as *counterclockwise flutter* due to the pattern of the macro reentry electrophysiologic mechanism, manifests as a sawtooth pattern, typical for the P-wave negative deflections (**Figure 132-4**). The second form of atrial flutter has the opposite pattern with positive deflections in the P-wave sawtooth pattern (**Figure 132-5**). Even though the atrial rate ranges from 240 to 300 beats/min, the AV nodal block will prevent all the atrial impulses from reaching the ventricle. The block at the AV node is frequently 2:1 but can also manifest as 3:1 and 4:1 or even variable block. The individuals that develop atrial flutter usually have a disorder that directly or indirectly involves the right atrium. Tricuspid

valvular disease, various pulmonary disorders, postsurgical repair of congenital heart disease, or any process leading to the enlargement of the right atrium increase the risk for atrial flutter.

> ### PRACTICE POINT
>
> - Any disease process leading to the enlargement of the right atrium increases the risk for atrial flutter.

■ EVALUATION

Practice guidelines from national and international organizations recommend to approach atrial flutter in the same manner as atrial fibrillation. A priority should be to ensure hemodynamic stability in the setting of a rapid ventricular rate and use of early anticoagulation barring contraindications. An echocardiogram will evaluate for any potential structural heart disease and clinical evaluation for any medical condition leading to increased right-sided heart disease.

■ MANAGEMENT

The management of atrial flutter is similar to the management of atrial fibrillation. Ventricular rate control is achieved by increasing the block at the level of the AV node to reduce ventricular response to the rapid atrial rate. Certainly if the patient is hemodynamically compromised, direct cardioversion should be performed (biphasic 100 J, monophasic 200 J). In contrast to AF, using calcium channel blockers or β-blockers alone are frequently insufficient in rate controlling the rhythm. It is often necessary to consider the addition of a class Ic antiarrhythmic, such as flecanide, to achieve satisfactory results. The class I agents are able to suppress the frequency of premature atrial beats, which trigger the development of this arrhythmia. Other agents to consider would be class III agents such as ibutilide for chemical cardioversion. Sotalol and amiodarone may also be used, but side effects need to be considered in chronic management.

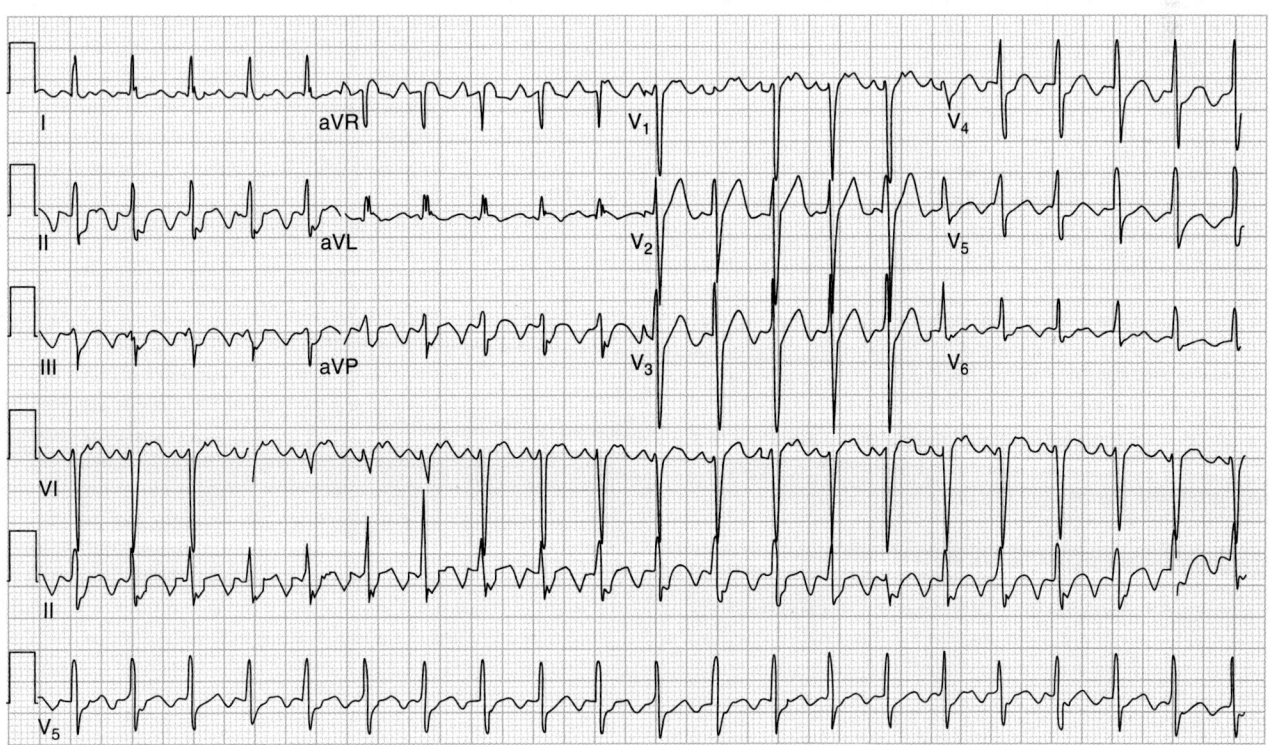

Figure 132-4 *Atrial flutter (2:1 block) with typical negative deflection P-waves revealing the classic "sawtooth" pattern.*

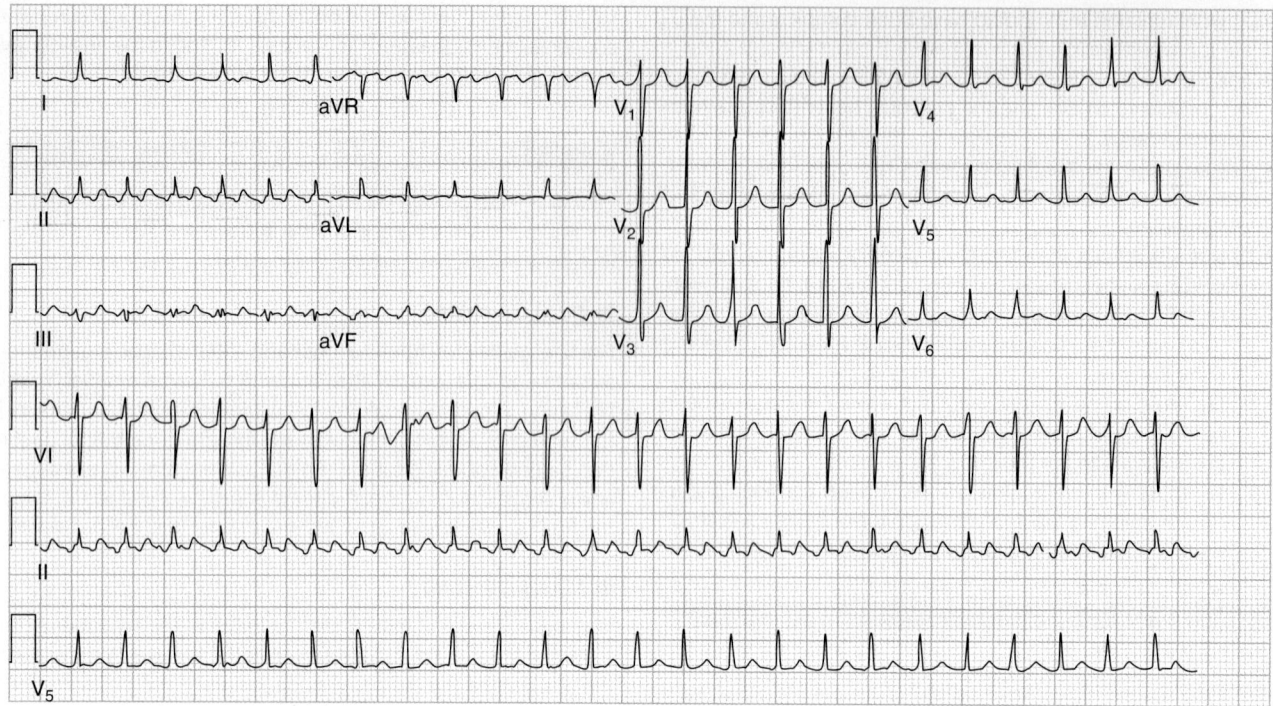

Figure 132-5 *Atrial flutter (2:1 block) with positive deflection P-waves revealing an upward "sawtooth" pattern.*

PRACTICE POINT

- In atrial flutter, avoid using flecainide as the sole treatment due to its ability to decrease the reentry circuit cycle length and potentially induce a fast, unstable 1:1 ventricular response and subsequent degeneration into ventricular fibrillation.

The risk of thromboembolic complications in atrial flutter is thought to be similar to that of atrial fibrillation, although there is a relative paucity of data compared with AF. For these patients, full anticoagulation should be strongly considered. Additionally, approximately 75% patients with atrial flutter also develop atrial fibrillation.

In contrast to atrial fibrillation, catheter-based intervention should be considered early in atrial flutter with rapid ventricular rate as medical therapy is frequently suboptimal. Success rates approaching 90% are reported with radiofrequency ablation (RFA) of the cavotricuspid isthmus, leading to a bidirectional block inhibiting the macro reentry mechanism of flutter. Due to the remaining anatomic or electrophysiologic conditions that remain after the RFA, the procedure is not considered curative. The recurrence rate is 10% to 20% over a period of 2 years but compares very favorably to the 60% recurrence rate of medical treatment alone. Less-frequent hospitalizations, lack of concern for medication side effects, and improved sense of quality of life are other factors weighing favorably toward a catheter-based ablative approach to atrial flutter management.

PRACTICE POINT

- A strong consideration of catheter-ablation strategy should be considered in patients with atrial flutter and rapid ventricular rate as medical management of rapid ventricular rate is frequently suboptimal.

ATRIOVENTRICULAR NODAL REENTRANT TACHYCARDIA

◼ EPIDEMIOLOGY

Atrioventricular nodal reentrant tachycardia (AVnRT) is the most common form of paroxysmal SVT, responsible for almost two-thirds of episodes; it is estimated that 10% of the general population has AVnRT. The palpitations characteristically start abruptly and may last for just a few minutes to as long as a few hours. They terminate as abruptly as they start. Additional symptoms include chest discomfort, dyspnea, lightheadedness, neck pulsations, and associated anxiety. These symptoms are often misdiagnosed as panic attacks if the arrhythmia is not caught while on a monitor. Signs of the arrhythmia include regular tachycardia with a heart rate between 120 and 200 bpm. Vagal maneuvers such as carotid sinus massage or the Valsalva maneuver can break the reentry circuit. This arrhythmia is usually not associated with structural heart disease and carries very little risk of death.

The mechanism of this tachyarrhythmia is a reentry circuit composed of the atrium, AV node or perinodal tissue, and the ventricle. The perinodal tissue or AV node exhibits a dual conduction physiology that reveals a slow pathway with an inherently short refractory period and a fast pathway with a relatively long refractory period.

There are three variants of AVnRT that depend on the routes of conduction. Approximately 90% of AVnRT is called typical AVnRT based on its antegrade conduction via the slow pathway and retrograde conduction via the fast pathway. With this typical conduction the surface ECG has the characteristic P-waves either buried within the QRS complex or just after the QRS. As expected with fast retrograde conduction, the RP interval is shorter than the PR interval. Recognizing the relative length of the RP and PR intervals can further differentiate between the other SVTs. The ECG for the typical AVnRT often demonstrates a pseudo-R'- wave in V_1 and pseudo-S'-waves in inferior limb leads. The less common variants include fast/slow and slow/slow, which will demonstrate clear P-waves, inverted in the inferior limb leads with an RP interval longer than the PR interval.

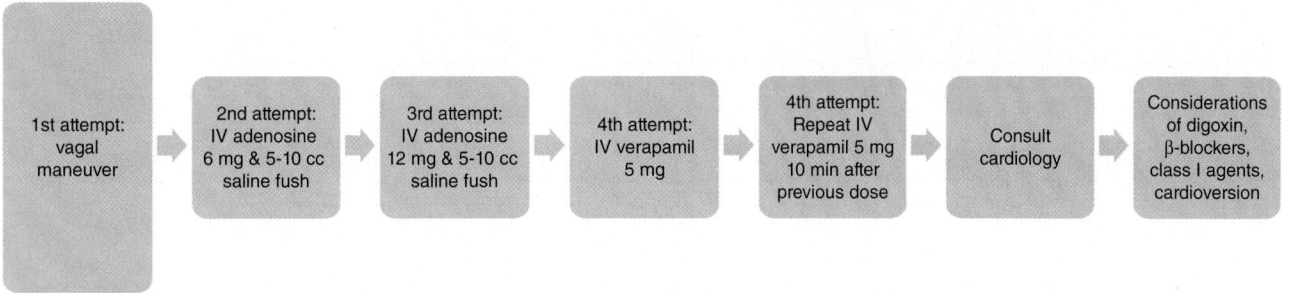

Figure 132-6 *Treatment sequence for atrioventricular nodal reentrant tachycardia (AVnRT).*

■ MANAGEMENT

Initial hospital management

Management of AVnRT can follow a straightforward treatment sequence (**Figure 132-6**). Vagal maneuvers such as the carotid sinus massage and Valsalva maneuver can break the reentry circuit 25% of the time. If the tachycardia is refractory to these maneuvers, adenosine will convert the rhythm to sinus in approximately 90% of patients. Due to its very short half-life of less than 10 seconds, it is crucial that adenosine be given as a rapid bolus and immediately followed by 5 to 10 mL of saline. Adenosine is typically dosed in 6 mg increments, but patients usually respond to a 12-mg dose. The expected symptoms with the infusion are dyspnea, facial flushing, and chest discomfort that last under a minute. When using adenosine, the patient's rhythm should be monitored by telemetry via a continuously running 12-lead ECG to observe the response that occurs within 30 seconds.

PRACTICE POINT

- AVnRT can be converted to sinus rhythm with vagal maneuvers in 25% of cases and with adenosine in 90% of cases. Adenosine must be given as a rapid IV bolus and immediately followed by 5-10 mL of saline. The expected symptoms with the infusion are dyspnea, facial flushing, and chest discomfort that last under a minute. When using adenosine, the patient's rhythm should be monitored continuously with rhythm strip or 12-lead ECG to monitor the response, which occurs within 30 seconds.

- Recent randomized data demonstrated in 2015 that a "modified Valsalva maneuver" converted 40% of patients with SVT compared to just 17% of those who underwent the standard Valsalva maneuver. The steps to this modified maneuver is as follows:
  a. semirecumbent position—head of bed at 45° angle
  b. have patient blow into a 10-cc syringe for ~15 seconds with enough pressure to just move the plunger
  c. then, immediately lay patient in the supine position and raise the legs up to ~45°

Typically, adenosine will convert the AVnRT to a sinus rhythm, but other possible rhythms include ventricular ectopy, transient sinus pause, transient bradyarrhythmias, atrial fibrillation or atrial flutter uncommonly, and, very rarely, polymorphic ventricular tachycardia. The risk of torsades de pointes is increased in patients with a baseline prolonged QTc. Factors that could decrease the efficacy of intravenous adenosine push include the use of methylxanthine products such as theophylline and caffeine, which block the A1 receptors. The use of dipyridamole (persantine, aggrenox) can augment the efficacy of adenosine by slowing its clearance. Due to the potential for exacerbating bronchospams, asthma is a relative contraindication for adenosine use. The transplanted heart is hypersensitive to adenosine, therefore a reduced dose or abandoning this approach altogether is appropriate in such patients.

Other options beside adenosine for the acute management of AVnRT include verapamil, β-blockers, and direct cardioversion. Verapamil, a nondihydropyridine calcium channel blocker, will block both fast and slow pathways. Dosing for acute management is 5 mg IV every 10 minutes and has been reportedly 90% effective. The downside to verapamil is the potential for hypotension that could be severe and long lasting. Another option includes digoxin, although this approach is not optimal due to its delayed effect. Direct cardioversion with 10 to 50 J is a final option if the previous interventions prove ineffective.

Outpatient longitudinal therapeutics

If the patient has frequent episodes that negatively impact quality of life, the use of invasive catheter ablation may be considered. The consensus approach by the ACC/AHA guidelines recommends ablation of the slow pathway due to its high efficacy (97%) and low risk of high-grade AV block (1%). The patient does need to consider the possibility of pacemaker placement if high-degree block develops as a complication. Long-term medical management is another option and includes medications such as verapamil, propanolol or class I antiarrhythmic agents such as flecanide and propafenone. The medications can be used on a daily basis to reduce the frequency of occurrences and the length of episodes. Additionally, the "pill-in-the-pocket" method obviates the daily use and could be used just during the episode. Cardiology consultation is indicated when using class I antiarrhythmics due to the risk of malignant ventricular arrhythmias.

ATRIOVENTRICULAR REENTRY TACHYCARDIA

■ EVALUATION

The next most common form of a paroxysmal SVT is atrioventricular reentry tachycardia (AVRT), which is characterized by an accessory conduction pathway between the atrium and ventricle that serves as a conduit for macro reentry. This pathway is a muscular bundle with variable properties of conduction, sometimes with bidirectional properties and in others just unidirectional capabilities. A commonly cited example of AVRT is Wolf-Parkinson-White syndrome, a narrow-complex tachyarrhythmia that manifests symptomatically with palpitations, chest discomfort, dyspnea, presyncope or syncope, and, very rarely, sudden cardiac death.

A baseline ECG when in sinus rhythm may ("revealed") or may not ("concealed") demonstrate the *delta wave* (**Figure 132-7**). The accessory pathway depolarizes the ventricular myocardium before the normal conduction system and is thus considered "pre-excitation." On the ECG, this will appear as the short PR interval. Due

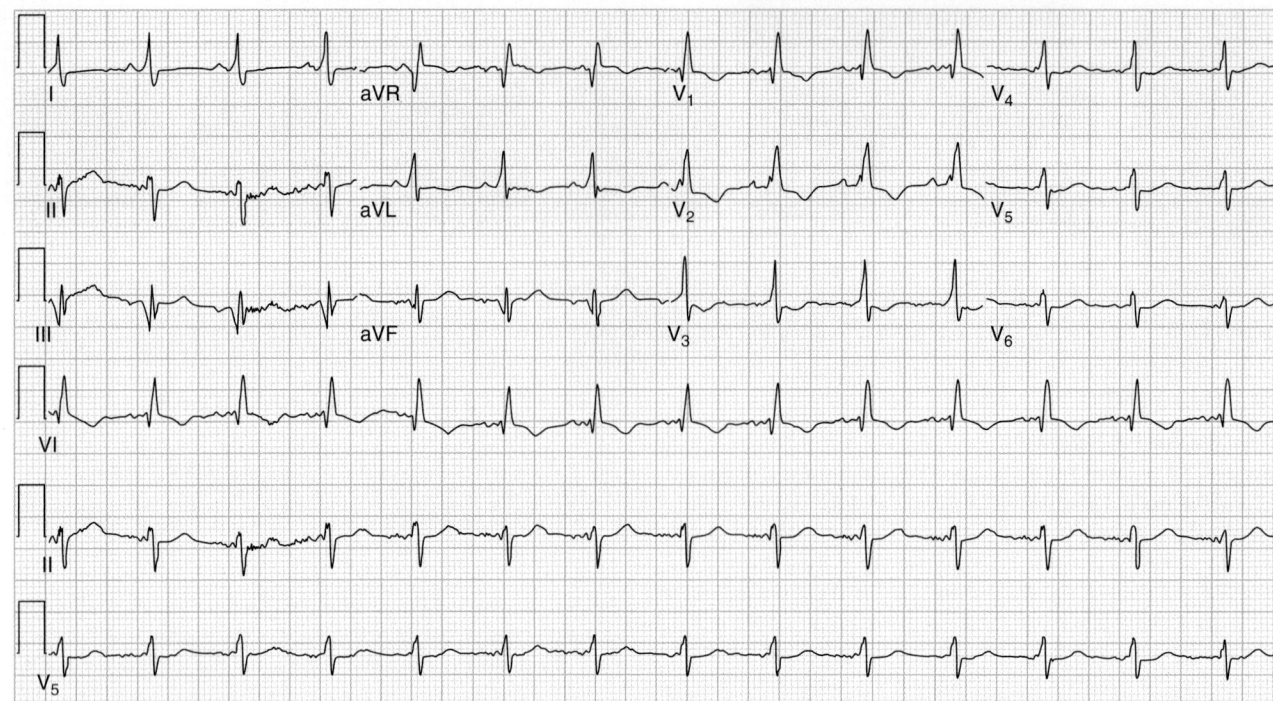

Figure 132-7 *Atrioventricular reentry tachycardia (AVRT). Wolf-Parkinson-White (WPW) syndrome with characteristic short PR interval and delta wave best seen in I, aVL, V3, and V4.*

to the relatively inefficient conduction from myocardial to myocardial cell (in contrast to the efficient His-Purkinje system), the initial portion of the QRS is slurred (delta wave) and gives the QRS a widened appearance (Figure 132-7). This accessory pathway, known as the bundle of Kent in WPW syndrome, provides the electrical wave front a conduit to move from the ventricle to the atrium, completing the macro reentry circuit.

■ INPATIENT MANAGEMENT

Management of this macro reentry arrhythmia is identical to the management for nodal reentry tachycardia with vagal maneuvers as a first option and intravenous adenosine push if unsuccessful. As discussed previously, adenosine administration usually converts the rhythm to sinus; however, less frequently atrial fibrillation or atrial flutter can develop. In very rare situations, the electrical impulse could conduct antegrade via the accessory pathway, leading to a very rapid ventricular rate, ventricular instability, and polymorphic ventricular tachycardia. This very rare complication of adenosine in AVRT requires having a crash-cart available during adenosine administration.

In some types of AVRT, the accessory pathway may not be recognizable on the ECG (considered concealed). When the accessory pathway conducts unidirectionally only from the ventricle to the atrium, the characteristic delta wave, short PR interval, and widened QRS are absent. The management remains the same as in the revealed WPW syndrome with very little concern for polymorphic ventricular tachycardia, as the accessory pathway will only conduct unidirectionally in a retrograde fashion from the ventricle to the atrium.

Beyond the acute management of AVRT, the frequency and severity of the palpitations will guide long-term treatments. Infrequent episodes that are short in duration and hemodynamically tolerable require only rest and time to resolve. A pill-in-the-pocket regimen could be considered with class Ia, Ic, or III antiarrhythmics or AV nodal-blocking agents as an option in this scenario in the absence of pre-excitation. However, if the episodes are frequent and prolonged, daily use of these medications can be considered.

These antiarrhythmics will prolong the refractory period for both the accessory pathway and the AV node, effectively preventing the arrhythmia or breaking the circuit during the episodes. Radiofrequency ablation of the accessory pathway provides another option (with a very high success rate and low complication rate) for permanent rhythm control that obviates the need for chronic medication in AVRT.

PRACTICE POINT

Wolf-Parkinson-White with atrial fibrillation:

- Atrial fibrillation (AF) in a very young patient should lower clinicians' threshold to consider WPW syndrome. AF occurs in up to one-third of patients with WPW and is the root cause for sudden death in these patients.
- The patient with a "revealed" WPW and atrial fibrillation will demonstrate a wide QRS complex on ECG due to the delta wave (often misinterpreted as atrial fibrillation with bundle branch block, BBB).
- WPW with AF should *not* be rate controlled with AV node-blocking agents, as atrial impulses would be forced to the incrementally conducting accessory pathway. The ventricular response would become 1:1, leading to unstable ventricular tachycardia (see **Figures 132-8** and **132-9**).
- Treatment: IV procainamide or IV amiodarone or electrical cardioversion.

The presence of a delta wave on a resting ECG does not require a cardiology consultation. However, a delta wave with a history of palpitations, syncope, or presyncope, or with a history of atrial fibrillation does require cardiology consultation. The electrophysiologist can perform invasive procedures to stratify some patients with the WPW syndrome for risk of sudden cardiac death, especially when the refractory period for the accessory pathway is short (RR interval of < 250 ms).

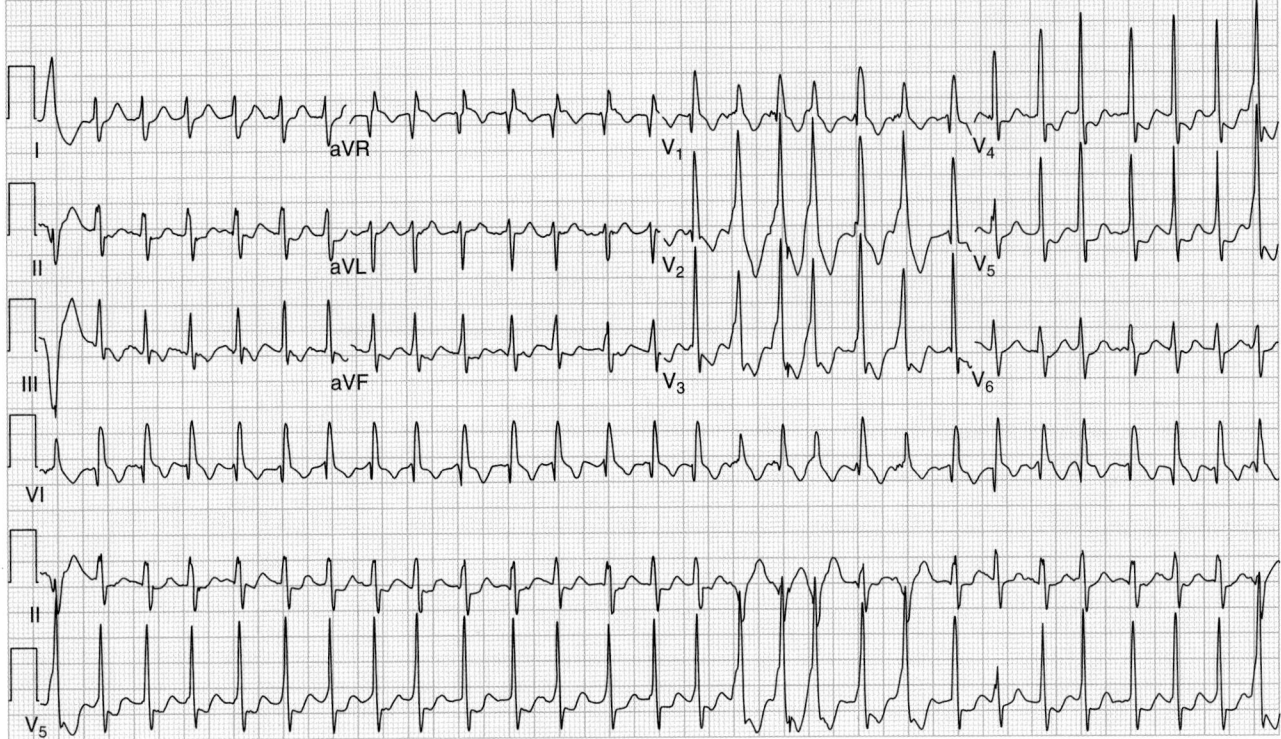

Figure 132-8 *Atrial fibrillation with brief run of aberrant conduction and noticeably wider conduction in the latter half of the ECG strip.*

MULTIFOCAL ATRIAL TACHYCARDIA

■ EVALUATION

Multifocal atrial tachycardia (MAT) is recognized on the surface ECG by the presence of tachycardia, at least three distinct P-waves, and at least three distinct PR intervals (**Figure 132-10**). Correct identification of this arrhythmia helps avoid improperly treating it as another arrhythmia.

Inpatient management

Multifocal atrial tachycardia usually results from another primary problem that leads to right heart strain or dysfunction (eg, severe COPD with exacerbation or pulmonary embolism). By treating the underlying condition, the arrhythmia usually resolves. However, if the tachycardia needs to be slowed based on clinical effects of the rate, β-blockers represent the first-line treatment. A short-acting

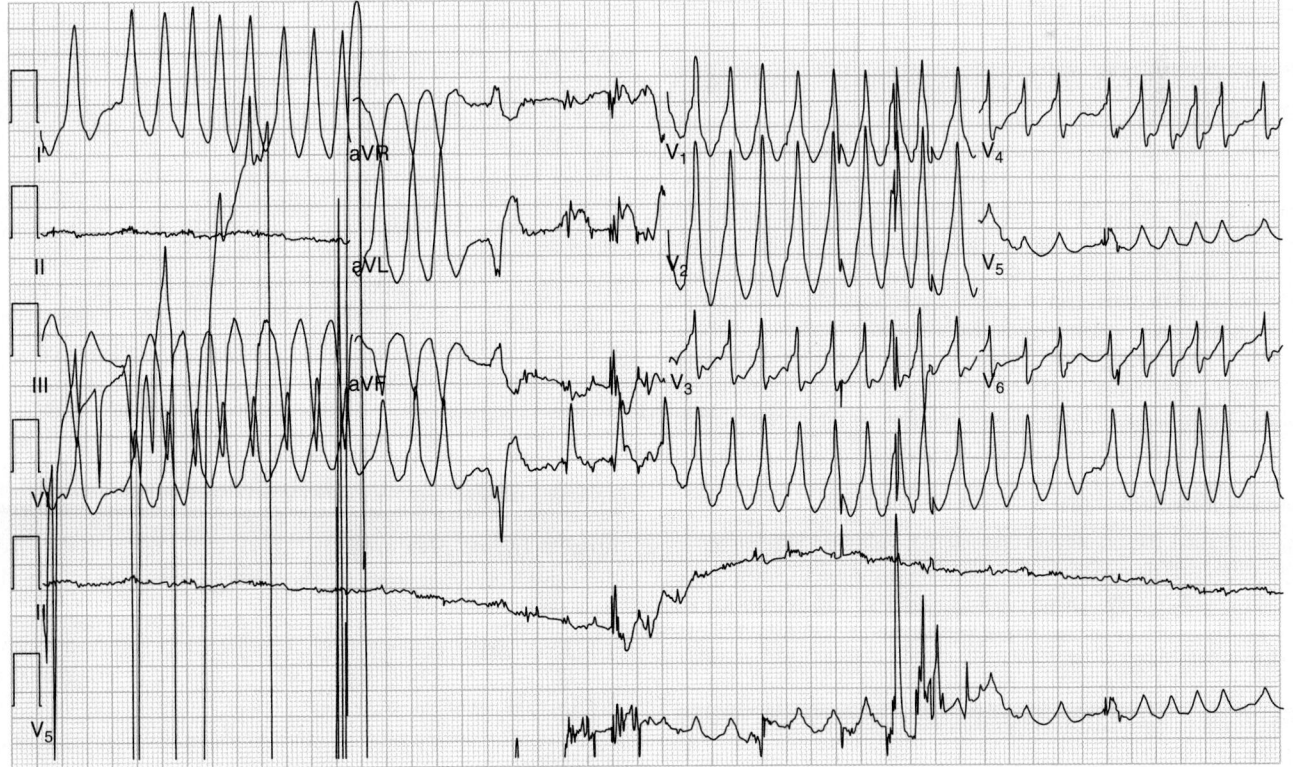

Figure 132-9 *Unstable ventricular tachycardia after patient was given IV adenosine. This AV nodal-blocking agent effectively shunted the atrial electrical impulses to the accessory pathway, which is characterized by nondecremental conduction.*

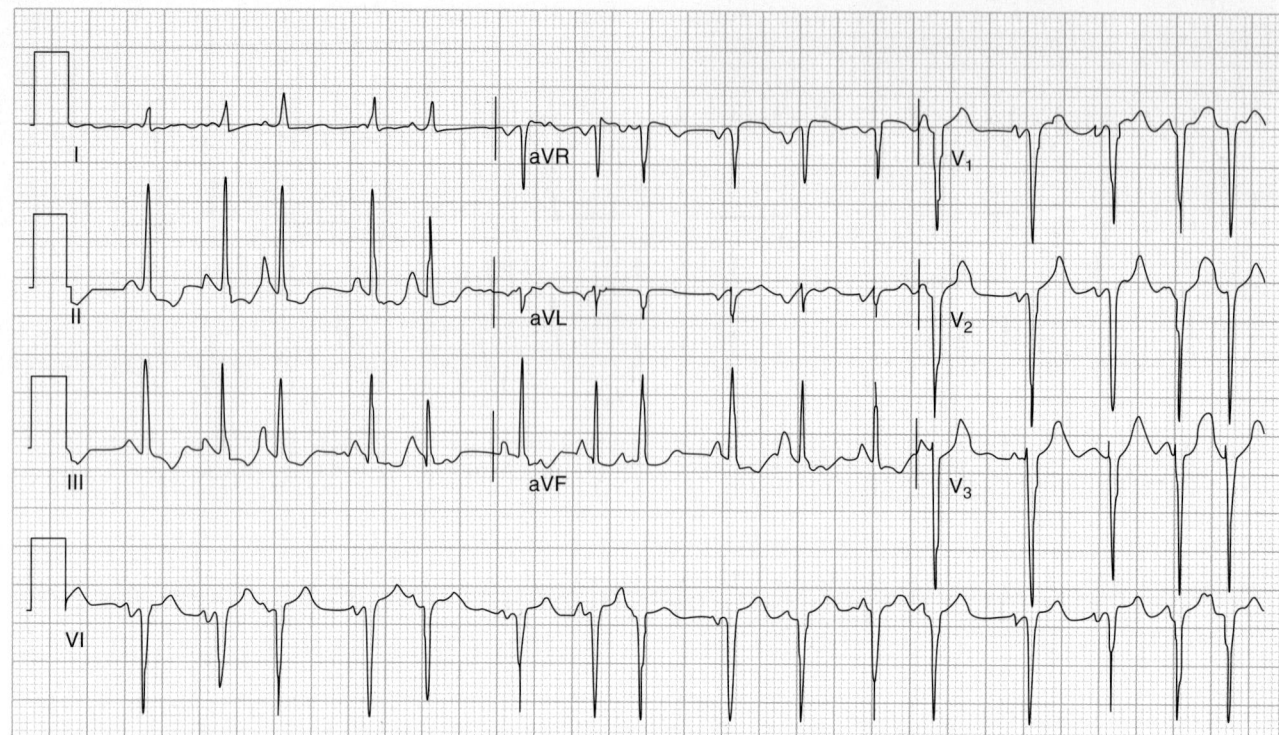

Figure 132-10 *Multifocal atrial tachycardia (MAT). Three or more distinct P-wave morphologies with an irregular rhythm.* (Reproduced, with permission, from Knoop KJ, Stack LB, Storrow AB, et al. *Atlas of Emergency Medicine*, 3rd ed. New York, NY: McGraw-Hill; 2009, Fig. 23-29A. Photo contributor: James V. Ritchie, MD.)

β-blocker, IV esmolol, may be considered if concern for bronchospasm or hypotension exists. Some trials support administration of IV magnesium to slow or convert the arrhythmia; however, this has not been well studied. Finally verapamil is another therapeutic option, but may be limited by hypotension. *Electrical cardioversion is not effective and thus not recommended.* Exacerbating factors for MAT may include commonly used medications for COPD such as β-agonists and theophylline.

JUNCTIONAL TACHYCARDIA
■ EVALUATION

Junctional tachycardia originates from the AV node or the bundle of His. The paroxysmal form is considered a rare occurrence in the adult population, but the nonparoxysmal form occurs most notoriously in the setting of digoxin toxicity. Particularly with digoxin toxicity, a Wenckebach conduction block in conjunction with junctional tachycardia can manifest. Other settings in which this arrhythmia may manifest include hypokalemia, postcardiac surgery, chronic lung disease, myocardial ischemia, myocarditis, and rarely, underlying sinus node dysfunction. Presentation of the arrhythmia under these circumstances allows the clinician to differentiate it from AVnRT, AVRT, and atrial tachycardia (AT).

Inpatient management

By addressing the underlying condition, the rhythm will correct. In the setting of digoxin toxicity, withholding the medication is the treatment of choice. Digoxin binding agents should be considered for judicious use in the setting of ventricular arrhythmias or high-grade AV block.

ATRIAL TACHYCARDIA
■ EVALUATION

An uncommon arrhythmia that falls under the category of SVT is atrial tachycardia. The incidence of this arrhythmia in young persons is less than 1%, however this arrhythmia is comprised of approximately 5% to 15% of patients undergoing electrophysiology studies. The arrhythmia can be seen on 24-hour Holter monitoring, but the asymptomatic patient should not be treated. If symptomatic, the patient may have typical symptoms accompanied with the SVT, including palpitations, lightheadedness, dyspnea, and perhaps syncope or presyncope.

The surface ECG can usually help differentiate AT from the more common rhythm sinus tachycardia by the following three features. Compare the EKG's in **Figures 132-11** and **132-12** which were obtained in the same patient. The former captures an episode of AT with a different P-wave axis and different PR interval. The second EKG, the patient is in a sinus rhythm with a normalized P-wave axis. Review of EKG's while not in an arrhythmia can be helpful in identifying the SVT. The P-wave axis is usually different from the sinus P-wave, which is upright in leads I and II. The onset and termination of atrial tachycardia is usually very rapid, occurring over a few beats, in contrast to the 30 seconds or minutes it takes sinus tachycardia to develop or terminate. Finally, the PR interval can be variable, which is also known as *unhooking*.

PRACTICE POINT

Atrial tachycardia features:
- P-wave axis is usually different from the sinus P-wave
- Onset and termination are very rapid
  - Occurring over a few beats (contrast to the 30 seconds or minutes it takes sinus tachycardia to develop or terminate)
- PR interval variable
- Potential for developing tachycardia-induced cardiomyopathy (>70% of untreated patients) if the incessant variety
  - Reversible with correction of the tachycardia

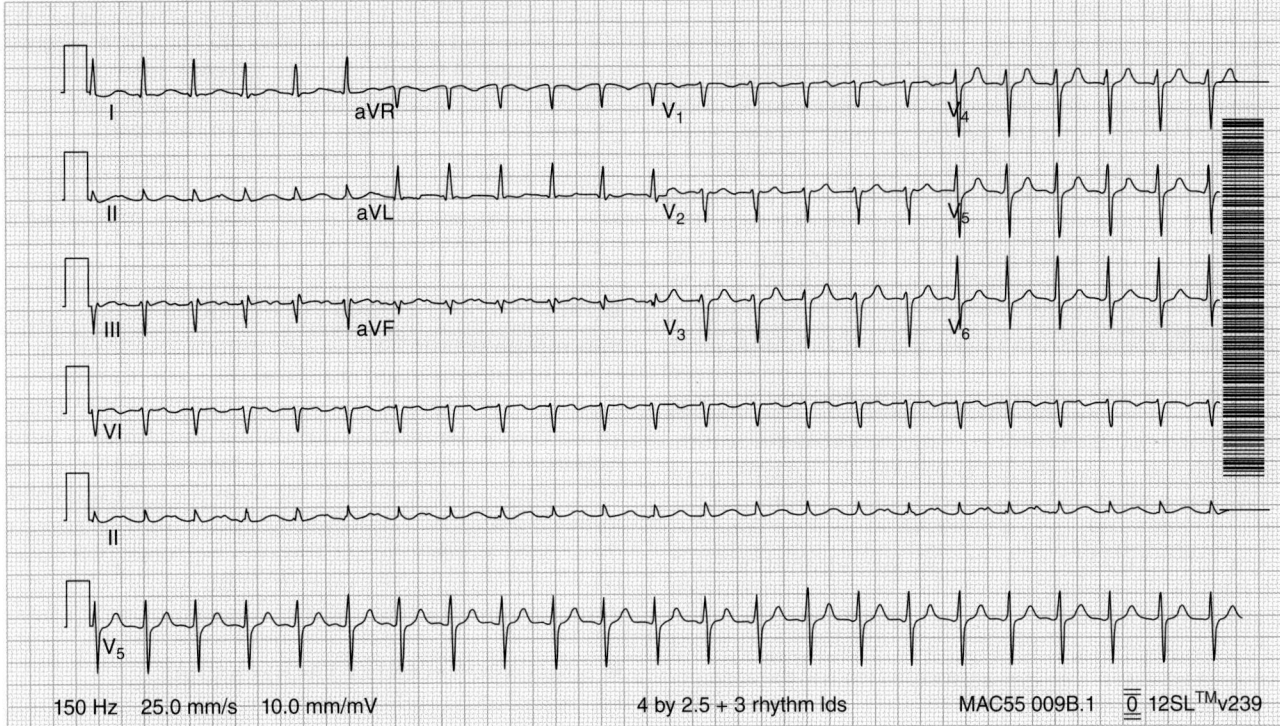

Figure 132-11 *Atrial tachycardia. Discernible P-waves best seen in III and aVF. Notice the RP interval is greater than the PR interval. The tachycardia started abruptly and spontaneously and abruptly terminated after 20 minutes.*

Difficulty differentiating this rhythm from a sinus tachycardia occurs when the focus of the arrhythmia is close to the superior portion of the cristas terminalis thereby mirroring the normal P-wave axis (positive in I, II). The importance of rhythm recognition lies in the potential for developing a tachycardia-induced cardiomyopathy if left untreated. Some studies have demonstrated that with an incessant form of atrial tachycardia, over 70% patients demonstrate decreased left ventricular function. Fortunately, this complication is reversible with correction of the tachycardia. Studies have demonstrated that patients with early-onset atrial tachycardia (before the age of 25) frequently spontaneously develop a normal sinus rhythm (Figure 132-12). AT could also be difficult to distinguish from AVRT and AVnRT, but clues such as variable RP intervals make AT more likely. If in doubt, the electrophysiologist should be consulted.

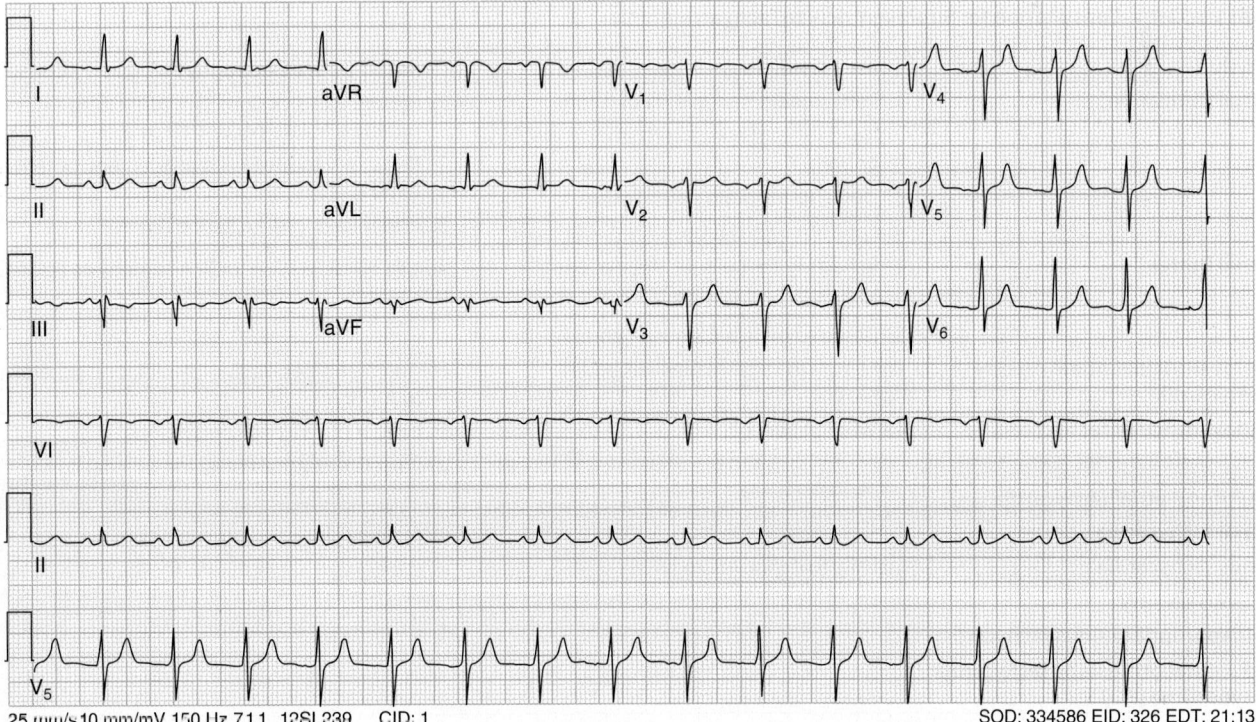

Figure 132-12 *Normal sinus rhythm of the patient after spontaneous resolution of atrial tachycardia. Notice the distinctly different P-wave morphology between the two ECGs.*

Inpatient management

In the acute setting, AV node-blocking calcium channel blockers (diltiazem, verapamil) or β-blockers can at times terminate the arrhythmia, or simply slow the ventricular rate via increased blockade at the AV node. Adenosine can also terminate the arrhythmia. The alternatives that are considered efficacious are sotalol and amiodarone; however, the side effects do need to be considered, especially if amiodarone is used for chronic management. The vagal maneuvers usually do not work, but electrical cardioversion may work, especially if the underlying reason for the AT is micro reentry or triggered activity. Long-term management may include the medications discussed previously or electrophysiologic ablation.

SINUS TACHYCARDIAS

The sinus tachycardias represent a heterogeneous group of arrhythmias comprised of normal sinus tachycardia, inappropriate sinus tachycardia, postural orthostasis tachycardia syndrome (POTS), and sinus node reentry tachycardia (SNRT). All have the same ECG findings, which include a pulse rate >100 bpm, upright P-waves in limb leads I and II (normal P-wave vector). The clinical presentation varies from the asymptomatic to regular palpitations accompanied by syncope or presycope. Normal sinus tachycardia, as one would expect, is a result of physiologic demand and requires the appropriate workup.

■ POSTURAL ORTHOSTASIS TACHYCARDIA SYNDROME

Postural orthostasis tachycardia syndrome (POTS) is usually found in a young population between the ages of 18 and 50 with a female predominance of 5:1. The postulated mechanisms include partial dysautonomia and the less common central β-hypersensitivity form. POTS also has pronounced sympathetic characteristics such as tremors, anxiety, and palpitations. The evaluation of this condition includes the head-up tilt-table (HUTT) test documenting the

patient's symptoms and tachycardic response greater than 30 bpm over baseline and usually greater than 120 bpm. Other diagnostic studies include 24-hour urine sodium collection, serum norepinephrine measurement (>600 pg/dL), and postganglionic antibody testing. The use of physical maneuvers to increase muscle tone in the lower extremities, compression garments, volume expanders (ie, mineralocorticoids, increased salt diet, increase fluid intake), peripheral vasoconstrictors, and centrally acting β-blockers (ie, pindolol) are the therapeutic options, however they have limited efficacy.

■ INAPPROPRIATE SINUS TACHYCARDIA

Inappropriate sinus tachycardia (IST) characteristically has daytime tachycardia at rest or with minimal exertion and normalization of the pulse during sleep. The sinus node regulation is dysfunctional with enhanced sensitivity to sympathetic stimulus or decreased regulation by the parasympathetic system. In contrast to sinus node reentry tachycardia (SNRT), the onset and termination of this rhythm is gradual, and atrial overdrive pacing has no influence on the arrhythmia. Treatment of IST requires high doses of β-blockers or calcium channel blockers. Other treatment options include antiarrhythmics or even catheter ablation in the event of medical failure.

■ SINUS NODE REENTRY TACHYCARDIA

Sinus node reentry tachycardia (SNRT) originates within or very close to the sinus node. It usually starts and ends abruptly. Bedside interventions such as vagal maneuvers or intravenous adenosine or verapamil can terminate this arrhythmia. Following the SVT recognition algorithm (see Figure 132-1), this rhythm is categorized within the arrhythmias with an RP interval greater than the PR interval.

CONSULTATION AND REFERRAL

A variety of instances of SVTs meet indications to consult general cardiology or electrophysiology cardiology (**Table 132-11**).

TABLE 132-11 Consultation for Supraventricular Tachyarrhythmias

Rhythm	Consult Cardiology	Consider Direct Electrophysiology (EP) Consult
Atrial fibrillation	1. Refractory to multiple medications 2. Need for cardioversion (chemical, electrical, or both) 3. Desire to maintain sinus rhythm 4. Lone atrial fibrillation	1. Presence of sick sinus syndrome (SSS)—potential ablate-pace strategy 2. Refractory to medical management: potential for RFA 3. Presence of pre-excitation (WPW)
Atrial flutter	1. Refractory to multiple medications 2. Need for cardioversion 3. Desire to maintain sinus rhythm	Strong consideration for RFA strategy as first-line treatment
Atrioventricular nodal reentry tachycardia	Refractory to vagal maneuvers and IV adenosine	Frequent and debilitating palpitations: potential need for RFA
Atrioventricular tachycardia	All WPW patients	1. History of syncope/ presyncope 2. Presence of atrial fibrillation or atrial flutter
Multifocal atrial tachycardia		
Atrial tachycardia		Incessant: risk of cardiomyopathy
Sinus tachycardia • **Sinus reentry** • **Inappropriate sinus tachycardia** • **Postural orthostatic tachycardia syndrome (POTS)**	Inability to define etiology	
Junctional tachycardia	Concern for digitalis toxicity	

RFA, radiofrequency ablation; SSS, sick sinus syndrome; WPW, Wolff-Parkinson-White syndome.

TABLE 132-12 Evidence-based Medicine: Key References for Supraventricular Tachyarrhythmias

Reference	Methodology	Results	Bottom Line
AFFIRM Wyse DG, et al. *N Engl J Med.* 2002;347(23):1825-1833.	Randomized trial (rate control vs rhythm control for atrial fibrillation) • N = 4,060 • Patients age >65 or risk factors for stroke	No difference in overall mortality after 5 years of follow-up 23.8% vs 21.3% P = 0.08	Rhythm control not better than rate control
AF CHF Roy D, et al. *N Engl J Med.* 2008;358(25):2667-2676.	Randomized trial (rate control vs rhythm control for atrial fibrillation in systolic CHF) • N = 1376 • Ejection fraction ≤35%	No difference in time to death from cardiovascular causes (25% vs 27%) after 37 months	Rhythm control not better than rate control in systolic CHF
Validation of Clinical Classification Schemes for predicting stroke. Gage BF, et al. *JAMA.* 2001;285(22):2854-2870.	Comparison of $CHADS_2$ to AFI and SPAF risk classification schemes	$CHADS_2$ c statistic of 0.82 compared to 0.68 and 0.74 for AFI and SPAF respectively	$CHADS_2$ performs better at predicting strokes than prior classification schemes
RE-LY: Randomized evaluation of long-term anticoagulation therapy study group. Connolly SJ, et al. *New Engl J Med.* 2009;361:1139-1151.	Randomized trial in atrial fibrillation warfarin versu dabigatran • N = 18113 patients • Dabigatran 2 doses: 110 mg twice a day, 150 mg twice a day • primary outcome • stroke or systemic embolism • follow-up 2 years	Coumadin event rate= 1.69%/ year Dabigatran 110 mg = 1.53%/y RR 0.91 P < 0.001 for noninferiority Dabigatran 150 mg = 1.11%/y RR 0.66 P < 0.001 for superiority	Higher-dose dabigatran prevents more strokes, but has equal major bleeding complications as coumadin

CHF, congestive heart failure.

CONCLUSION

A systematic algorithmic approach to SVTs will aid in differentiating the common from the uncommon (see Figure 132-1). In the setting of hemodynamic instability, other concerns fall to the wayside, and direct cardioversion should be performed without delay (except with sinus tachycardia, where the underlying cause should be identified and treated) (**Table 132-12**).

SUGGESTED READINGS

Blomström-Lundqvist C, Scheinman M, Aliot E, et al. ACC/AHA/ESC guidelines for the management of patients with supraventricular arrhythmias: a report of the American College of Cardiology/ American Heart Association Task Force and the European Society of Cardiology Committee for Practice Guidelines (writing committee to develop guidelines for the management of patients with supraventricular arrhythmias). *J Am Coll Cardiol.* 2003;42:1493

Fuster V, Ryden, L, Cannom M, et al. ACC/AHA/ESC 2006 guidelines for the management of patients with atrial fibrillation: a report of the American College of Cardiology/American Heart developed in collaboration with the European Heart Rhythm Association and the 2001 guidelines for the management of patients With atrial fibrillation) Cardiology Committee for Practice Guidelines (writing committee to revise association task force on practice guidelines) and the European Society of Fibrillation: a report of the American College of Cardiology/American Heart. *J Am Coll Cardiol.* 2006;48:e149.

Hylek E, Evans-Molina C, Shea C, et al. Major hemorrhage and tolerability of warfarin in the first year of therapy among elderly patients with atrial fibrillation. *Circulation.* 2007;115;2689-2696.

January C, Wann LS, Alpert JS, et al: 2014 AHA/ACC/HRS Guideline for the management of patients with atrial fibrillation: executive summary. *J Am Coll Cardiol.* 2014;64;2246.

Kay G, Plumb V, Jayam V, et al. Atrial fibrillation, atrial flutter, and atrial tachycardia. Supraventricular tachycardia: AV node reentry and Wolff-Parkinson-White syndrome. *Hurst's The Heart*, 11th ed. New York, NY: McGraw-Hill; 2004:825-874.

Olgin J, Zipes D, Miller J. Specific arrhythmias: diagnosis and treatment. *Braunwald's Heart Disease: A Textbook of Cardiovascular Medicine*, 8th ed. Philadelphia, PA: Elsevier Saunders; 2008: 863-923.

Pisters R, Oostenbrugge R, Knottberus I, et al. The likelihood of decreasing strokes in atrial fibrillation patients by strict application of guidelines. *Europace.* 12:779-784.

Singer D, Albers G, Dalen J, et al. Antithrombotic therapy in atrial fibrillation: American College of Chest Physicians evidence-based clinical practice guidelines, 8th ed. *Chest.* 2008;133;546S.

Wyse D, Waldo A, DiMarco J, et al. A comparison of rate-control and rhythm control in patients with atrial fibrillation. *N Engl J Med.* 2002;347:1825.

CHAPTER 133

Bradycardia

Stacy Westerman, MD

Michael Manogue, MD

Michael H. Hoskins, MD

Key Clinical Questions

1. What is the epidemiology of bradycardia?
2. What are the conduction abnormalities that lead to bradycardia?
3. What external factors can cause bradycardia?
4. When is treatment necessary for bradycardia?
5. When is pharmacologic versus pacemaker therapy indicated?

INTRODUCTION AND EPIDEMIOLOGY

Bradycardia is commonly encountered in clinical practice. It is usually defined as a heart rate of less than 60 beats/min, and its clinical significance varies depending upon the underlying etiology and the population being studied. For example, a low heart rate is an accepted signal of superior health in trained athletes and, in this population, has been associated with better long-term cardiovascular outcomes. In contrast, a resting heart rate below 62 beats/min in certain elderly populations is an independent risk marker of mortality when compared to age matched controls with higher resting heart rates. The appropriate approach to bradycardia requires an understanding not only of the underlying conduction system of the heart, but also of the patient in whom it is observed and the associated symptoms in order to determine its prognostic significance and the appropriate treatment.

Bradycardia can result from intrinsic disease of the conducting tissues of the heart or as a result of extrinsic and often reversible influences that may be metabolic, autonomic, iatrogenic, or toxic. Sinus node dysfunction, or sick sinus syndrome (SSS), is generally a disease of the elderly, occurring in 1 out of 600 cardiac patients older than 65, and accounts for approximately 50% of all pacemaker implantations in the United States. While it is associated with a high risk of syncope, the presence of SSS is not associated with an increased risk of mortality in population-based studies, independent of pacemaker therapy. Bradycardia resulting from high grade AV block (Mobitz type II or complete AV block) is rare in healthy population and generally associated with significant underlying heart disease and increased morbidity and mortality. Prognosis for bradycardia resulting from extrinsic influences on the heart largely depends upon the underlying diagnosis. For example, transient, asymptomatic asystole associated with obstructive sleep apnea is not associated with adverse outcomes compared to sleep apnea patients without bradycardia, and has been shown to resolve with effective CPAP treatment.

NORMAL ELECTRICAL ACTIVATION OF THE HEART

The electrical activation of the heart originates in the sinoatrial (SA or sinus) node, which is located in the right atrium and functions as the normal pacemaker of the heart. The sinus node is located in the subepicardial tissue on the lateral wall of the right atrium near the junction of the SVC and the right atrium. It is on average 10 to 20 mm in length. Its vascular supply is from the SA nodal artery, a branch of the right coronary artery (~60% of people) or the left circumflex artery (~40% of people). It contains the principal pacemaker cells that spontaneously depolarize, causing atrial depolarization. It has extensive input from both the parasympathetic and sympathetic nervous systems via the vagus nerve and the sympathetic chain, respectively. The parasympathetic effects on the sinus node, via acetylcholine, are negative chronotropy, prolongation of intranodal conduction time, and increased refractoriness. The concentration of acetylcholine in the atria, and the SA node in particular, is significantly greater than that in the ventricles, and there is tonic parasympathetic stimulation of the SA node. Sympathetic effects include positive chronotropy via an increase in the rate of sinus node discharge and decreased refractoriness.

After the sinus node discharges, the electrical impulse travels across the atria to the atrioventricular (AV) node, the electrical communication between the atria and ventricles. The AV node is a multiregional structure that includes the compact portion and His

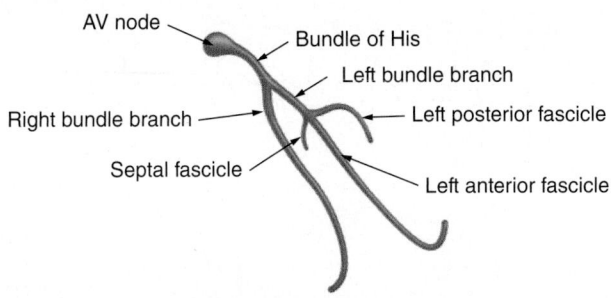

Figure 133-1 *Cardiac conduction system anatomy.*

bundle. The compact portion of the AV node is located anterior to the coronary sinus ostium and just superior to the septal insert of the tricuspid valve. The vascular supply of the AV node is from a branch of the right coronary artery in 85% to 90% of people, and from the left circumflex artery in 5% to 10% of people. The AV node's primary function is to delay electrical conduction from the atria to the ventricles, allowing for sequential and coordinated atrial and ventricular mechanical contraction.

Conduction continues from the compact AV node to the bundle of His, located in the membranous septum (**Figure 133-1**). The bundle of His gives way to the right and left bundle branches, which form at the top of the muscular interventricular septum. The right bundle travels intramyocardially to the apex and the anterior papillary muscle of the right ventricle. The left bundle branch can have variable anatomy, but is traditionally thought of having an anterior and a posterior fascicle, coursing to the anterolateral and posteromedial papillary muscles of the left ventricle. The blood supply to the upper muscular interventricular septum is via the left anterior descending and posterior descending arteries. This dual vascular supply can protect the conduction system at this level from ischemic events.

The AV node is under direct influence of the parasympathetic and sympathetic nervous system; parasympathetic input decreases conduction speed in the AV node and increases refractoriness, and sympathetic input increases conduction speed and shortens refractoriness. In contrast, normal conduction in the His bundle is not significantly influenced by the autonomic nervous system.

The ends of the bundle branches connect with specialized terminal Purkinje fibers, forming networks on the endocardium of the right and left ventricles. The Purkinje fibers penetrate the inner one-third of the endocardium, and the electrical impulse spreads through myocardial muscle to the epicardium, providing for simultaneous depolarization of both ventricles.

BRADYCARDIA

Bradyarrhythmias may be caused by abnormal function at any point in the conduction system of the heart. Mechanistically, the two broad categories of pathology include disorders of impulse formation and disorders of impulse conduction. Anatomically, bradyarrhythmias may be divided into either sinus node dysfunction or disorders of AV nodal conduction. Abnormal conduction may be due to disease states that are intrinsic to the conduction system, affecting structure, or extrinsic to the system. Not all bradycardia is pathologic, especially when originating at higher levels in the conduction system. In general, a heart rate <40 beats/min in the absence of sleep or highly trained athletes is considered abnormal, though symptom correlation is still critical to determine proper management.

SINUS NODE DYSFUNCTION

Sinus node dysfunction is a common clinical syndrome and includes both failure of impulse formation and impulse transmission to the atrial tissue. Etiologies include anatomic changes to the sinus node

TABLE 133-1 Causes of Sinus Node Dysfunction

Intrinsic	Extrinsic
Senile degeneration of the sinus node and atrial tissue	Medications (β-blocker, calcium channel blocker, antiarrhythmic drugs, digoxin, centrally active antihypertensive agents)
Myocardial ischemia or infarction	
Infiltrative disease	Endocrine abnormalities (hypothyroidism)
Collagen vascular disease	
Surgical injury or trauma	Hypothermia
Inflammatory diseases	Electrolyte disturbances (Hyperkalemia)
Neuromuscular diseases	
Pericardial disease	Autonomic dysfunction (vasovagal syncope, carotid sinus hypersensitivity)
Hypertensive heart disease	
	Increased intracranial pressure
	Sepsis
	Hypoxia

(including idiopathic degeneration, as seen with advanced age), ischemia, medication effects, increased vagal tone (as in sleep) or decreased sympathetic stimulation, iatrogenic injury during cardiac surgery, infection, electrolyte imbalances, hypothermia, and hypoxemia/hypercapnia (**Table 133-1**). Sinus node dysfunction is often asymptomatic, even in cases that are not physiologic.

■ SUBTYPES OF SINUS NODE DYSFUNCTION

Sinus bradycardia

Sinus bradycardia is defined by a sinus node discharge rateless than 60 beats/min. It is commonly observed in well-trained athletes or young adults during sleep due to an increase in vagal tone. Symptom correlation is essential, as bradycardia is often a benign arrhythmia; even significant sinus bradycardia may be asymptomatic and thus not require treatment. However, symptomatic patients may require treatment.

Chronotropic incompetence

Chronotropic incompetence is the inability of the sinus node to appropriately increase its rate with exercise. General definitions include the inability to achieve a heart rate of 100 to 120 beats/min or 70% of age-expected maximal heart rate with exercise. While often clinically silent, chronotropic incompetence may cause symptoms of exertional fatigue or dyspnea. Since the patient's resting heart rate may be normal in this scenario, detailed questioning and ambulation of the patient is required to make this diagnosis.

Sinus arrhythmia

Sinus arrhythmia is defined by a variation in the sinus rate of greater than 10% or 120 ms (**Figure 133-2**). It is manifest on ECG as varying P-P intervals. The P-wave morphology and PR interval is usually stable, though subtle variations may be present due to slight alterations in pacemaker focus within the sinus node. Sinus arrhythmia is considered a normal event, commonly seen in the young, and can occur with the respiratory cycle. (The P-P interval shortens with inspiration and lengthens with expiration.) It tends to occur less frequently with older age. Symptoms are rare, and generally occur only when pauses between sinus beats are significant.

Sinus arrest/sinus pause

Sinus arrest occurs when there is a loss of impulse formation from the sinus node. Asystole can occur as a consequence, though

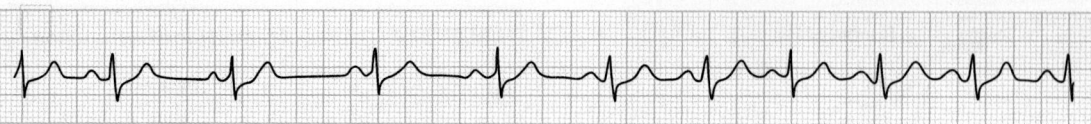

Figure 133-2 *Sinus arrhythmia.*

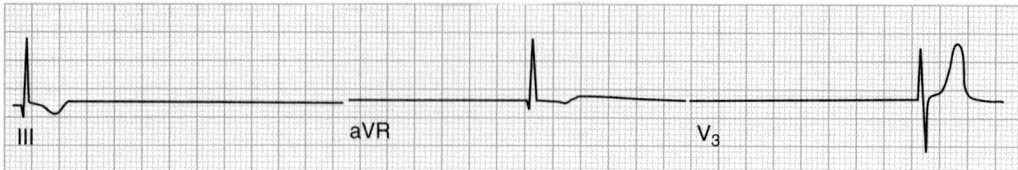

Figure 133-3 *Sinus arrest.*

frequently secondary pacemaker cells found in the atria, AV junction, or ventricles may provide an escape rhythm that prevents prolonged pauses (**Figure 133-3**). Causes of sinus arrest include high vagal tone (sleep apnea, vasovagal syncope), acute myocardial infarction, and degenerative changes to the sinus node.

PRACTICE POINT

- In general, pauses less than 3 seconds, asymptomatic patients, and patients with a transient cause for sinus arrest with a robust escape rhythm do not require pacing.

Persistent atrial standstill

Atrial standstill is a rare phenomenon of complete atrial inactivity with an inability to electrically stimulate the atria. Causes include infiltrating diseases such as amyloidosis, familial cases, inflammatory myocarditis, and certain myotonic dystrophies.

Sinoatrial exit block

SA exit block is a disorder of impulse transmission from the SA node to the atrial tissue. Like other etiologies of sinus node dysfunction, SA exit block may be due to medication effects, increased vagal tone, myocardial infarction, or degenerative changes of the sinus node and atrial tissue. Similar to AV block, SA exit block is characterized as first, second, or third degree. First-degree SA exit block is clinically silent and cannot be discerned on ECG; it is a prolongation of the time necessary for the sinus impulse to transmit to the atrial tissue. Second-degree SA exit block can be type I, in which there is

progressive lengthening of the SA node conduction time before the complete block of a sinus impulse, or type II, in which SA node conduction time remains constant before the complete block of a sinus impulse. Surface ECG is best able to diagnose second-degree SA exit block. This block will manifest as a pause due to the absence of a P-wave. In type I second-degree SA exit block the P-P intervals will shorten prior to the loss of a P-wave, and the pause will be less than two P-P cycles (**Figure 133-4**). In type II second-degree SA exit block the P-P intervals will remain constant prior to the loss of a P-wave, and the pause will be an exact multiple of the preceding P-P interval (**Figure 133-5**). Third-degree SA exit block has complete loss of impulse transmission from the sinus node, despite normal sinus node implies formation. Because the sinus node impulses do not conduct to the surrounding atrial tissue, cardiac activation relies on a lower pacemaker escape rhythm. Third-degree SA exit block requires an electrophysiologic study to diagnose. SA exit block is often transient, and symptoms depend on duration of pauses.

Tachycardia-bradycardia syndrome

Tachycardia-bradycardia syndrome, or tachy-brady syndrome, describes intermittent and alternating paroxysms of atrial tachyarrhythmias (most commonly atrial fibrillation) with sinus bradycardia or sinus pauses. Sinus node suppression that occurs during an atrial tachyarrhythmia may result in prolonged pauses after spontaneous or electrical cardioversion. These pauses are often highly symptomatic and may result in syncope. Tachy-brady syndrome is due to abnormal function of the sinus node, and should be distinguished from atrial fibrillation with intermittent fast and slow ventricular rates, which is a problem with AV node function.

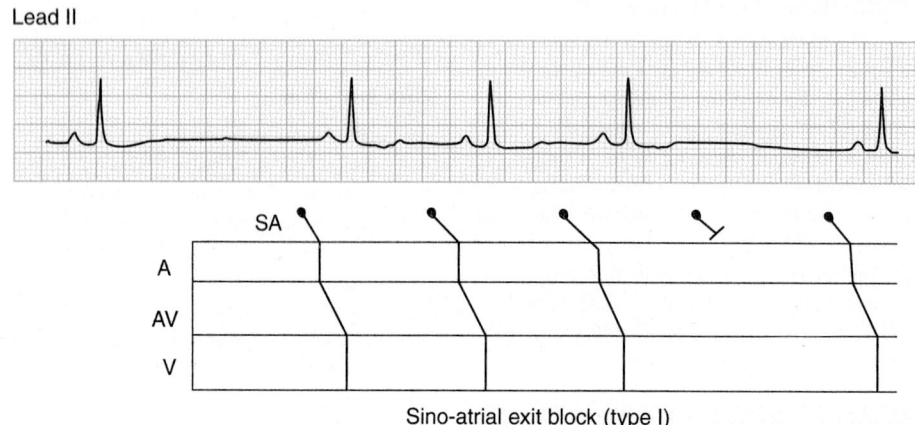

Figure 133-4 *SA exit block, type 1 second degree. Note the P-P intervals shorten prior to the loss of a P-wave, and the pause is less than two P-P cycles. As depicted in the accompanying ladder diagram, the SA discharge rate remains the same but the time it takes for impulse transmission to the atrium lengthens until there is complete block of a sinus impulse.*

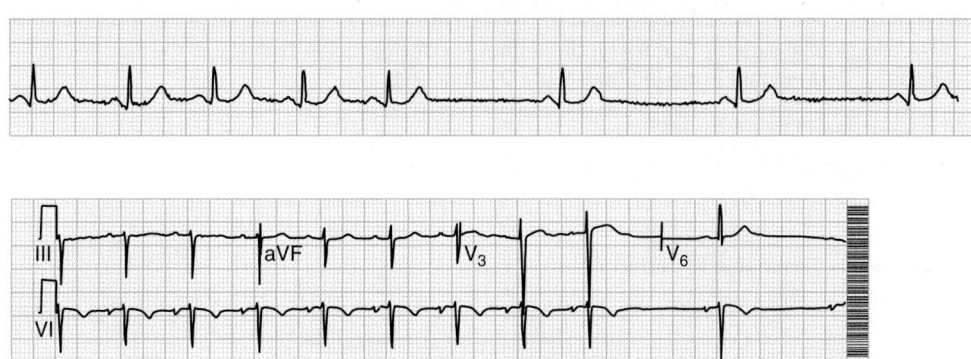

Figure 133-5 *SA exit block, type 2 second degree. Note the prolonged P-P interval is twice the length of the preceding P-P intervals.*

▉ DIAGNOSIS OF SINUS NODE DYSFUNCTION

Symptoms of sinus node dysfunction may be nonspecific and include fatigue, dizziness, dyspnea, angina, presyncope, and syncope. Symptoms result from decreased cardiac output as a result of bradycardia. It is critical to correlate symptoms to documented occurrences of bradycardia. The diagnosis of sinus node dysfunction can routinely be accomplished with noninvasive methods that include surface 12-lead ECGs, inpatient telemetry, ambulatory holter monitors, or longer-term event monitors. Ambulatory monitors typically have accompanying diaries to correlate symptoms with bradycardia. Exercise testing can be useful if chronotropic incompetence is suspected. Implantable loop recorders are an option for longer-term monitoring of more infrequent arrhythmias. Invasive electrophysiology studies can assess sinus node function and sinoatrial conduction time, but are generally required only when noninvasive methods of investigation prove nondiagnostic.

▉ MANAGEMENT OF SINUS NODE DYSFUNCTION

The management of sinus node dysfunction depends on the presence of symptoms, symptom severity, and identification of reversible causes. If bradycardia due to sinus node dysfunction is symptomatic, offending causes should be removed if possible. In the setting of acute symptomatic sinus node dysfunction in which reversible causes cannot be eliminated, such as with acute myocardial infarction, pharmacologic treatment or temporary pacing may be needed (**Table 133-2**). Pharmacologic options include atropine (0.5 mg IV boluses), dopamine (2-10 µg/kg/min IV drip), epinephrine (2-10 µg/min IV drip) or isoproterenol (1 µg/min IV drip), which may be effective in the short term. Temporary pacing options typically include a temporary transvenous pacing wire. In general, temporary transcutaneous pacing is not required for bradycardia due to sinus node dysfunction. If reversible causes are not present

TABLE 133-2 Acute Management for Persistent Symptomatic Bradycardia in a Patient with Signs of Hemodynamic Compromise. An Algorithmic Approach Adapted from ACLS 2010 Guidelines for Management of Bradycardia

1. Removal and/or reversal of offending agent if medication-associated

2. Administration of atropine 0.5 mg IV boluses, every 3-5 min. Maximum dose of 3.0 mg

3. If atropine not effective:

   Transcutaneous pacing, or

   Dobutamine infusion (2-10 µg/kg/min IV drip) or

   Epinephrine infusion (2-10 µg/min IV drip)

and symptomatic bradycardia persists, a permanent pacemaker may be indicated. Of note, there is no mortality benefit with pacing in circumstances of bradycardia due to sinus node dysfunction. See **Table 133-3** for indications for permanent pacemaker placement in sinus node dysfunction. In general, pacing is only indicated for overt symptoms due to bradycardia or equivocal symptoms with a sinus rate <40 beats/min. Cases of syncope of unidentified etiology but with an EPS revealing sinus node dysfunction are also an indication for pacemaker.

ATRIOVENTRICULAR BLOCK

Block of an electrical impulse as it travels through the AV node may be a physiologic or pathologic finding, depending upon the circumstances. Underlying autonomic tone and decremental conduction delay in the AV node are the primary factors mediating physiologic AV block. Parasympathetic tone slows conduction velocity in the AV node, which typically manifests as lengthening of the PR interval. In cases of intense vagal tone or well-trained athletes, more advanced degrees of block may occur. Decremental conduction is a physiologic property of the AV node in which conduction delay in the node increases in direct proportion to prematurity of the arriving impulse, such as a premature atrial contraction.

AV conduction abnormalities are divided into first-, second-, and third-degree AV block which in most cases can be distinguished by the surface electrocardiogram. First-degree AV block (or AV delay) is characterized by a prolonged, but stable, PR interval of >200 ms. Second-degree AV block may be further subdivided into type I and type II patterns. Type I second-degree AV block (Mobitz I or Wenckebach) is characterized by progressive prolongation of the PR interval until AV conduction fails. Type II second-degree AV block (Mobitz II) is characterized by a stable PR interval with intermittent P-waves that fail to conduct to the ventricle (**Figures 133-6** to **133-11**).

The ECG pattern of AV block provides insight as to the anatomic location of the failure of conduction. First-degree AV delay and Mobitz I patterns typically indicate that the location of conduction abnormality is within the compact AV node, proximal to the bundle of His. This is often physiologic and may be due to medications or enhanced parasympathetic tone. Conversely, Mobitz II and third-degree AV block typically occur at the level of or distal to the bundle of His. These more distal conduction abnormalities are associated with disease of the specialized His-Purkinje conduction system and are more likely to result in sudden loss of conduction and asystole. Occasionally, AV conduction will occur in a 2:1 pattern. This may represent Mobitz I or Mobitz II physiology. Further investigation may be required to determine the exact degree of conduction abnormality in this situation. Features suggesting Mobitz I are a narrow QRS and improvement in AV block with exercise or increased adrenergic tone, and features suggesting Mobitz II include a broad QRS and worsening of AV block with exercise or increased sympathetic tone.

TABLE 133-3 ACC/AHA/HRS 2008 Guideline Summary: Guidelines for Device Based Therapy of Cardiac Rhythm Abnormalities: Indications for Permanent Pacing in Sinus Node Dysfunction

Class I—Permanent pacing should be performed

1. Documented symptomatic bradycardia, including frequent symptomatic sinus pauses

2. Symptomatic chronotropic incompetence

3. Symptomatic sinus bradycardia due to drug therapy required for medical conditions

Class IIa—Permanent pacing is reasonable to perform

1. Heart rate < 40 beats/min, but without documentation of a clear association between significant symptoms and actual presence of bradycardia

2. Syncope of unexplained origin and sinus node dysfunction provoked or discovered with electrophysiologic testing

Class IIb—Permanent pacing may be considered

1. Heart rate chronically <40 beats/min while awake in minimally symptomatic patient

Class III—Permanent pacing should NOT be performed and may be harmful

1. Sinus node dysfunction in an asymptomatic patient

2. Symptoms suggestive of bradycardia have been documented to occur in the absence of bradycardia

3. Symptomatic bradycardia due to nonessential drug therapy that can be stopped

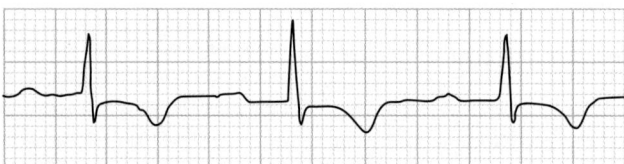

Figure 133-6 *First-degree AV block.*

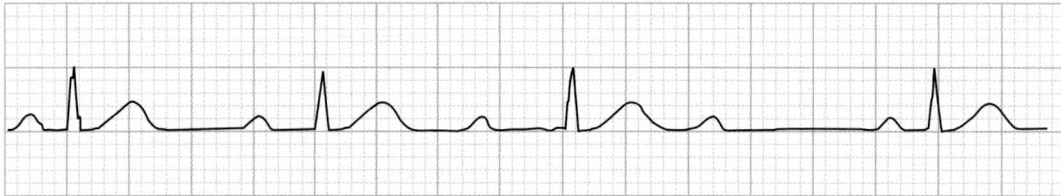

Figure 133-7 *Second-degree AV block, Mobitz type I.*

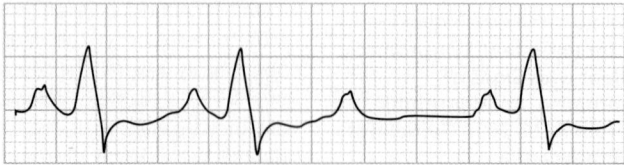

Figure 133-8 *Second-degree AV block, Mobitz type II.*

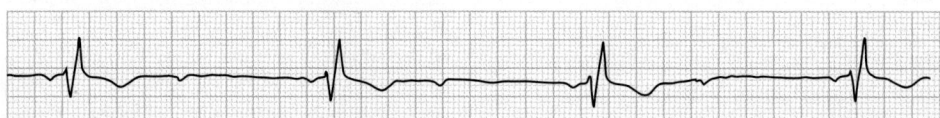

Figure 133-9 *2:1 AV block.*

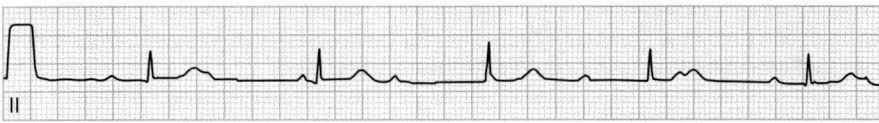

Figure 133-10 *Complete or third-degree AV block.*

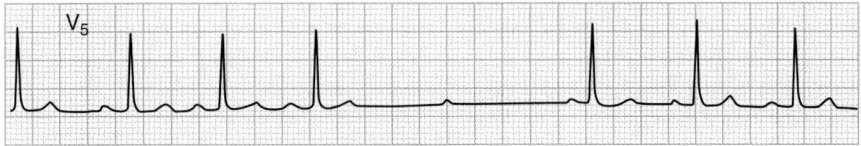

Figure 133-11 *Enhanced vagal tone resulting in nonconducted P-wave. Note the transient lengthening of P-P interval concurrent with dropped QRS complex.*

■ DIAGNOSIS OF AV NODAL CONDUCTION ABNORMALITIES

AV nodal conduction abnormalities are typically diagnosed by surface ECG tracings. While the ECG patterns described above are useful in the majority of cases, occasionally more subtle ECG clues are required. When evaluating the level of AV block, the primary focus should be to determine the anatomic location of conduction failure as this determines the risk of asystole. Clues that suggest that conduction delay occurs within the compact AV node include a prolonged PR interval and narrow QRS. Conversely, consistently short PR intervals and wide QRS complexes suggest that failure of conduction occurs within a diseased His-Purkinje system. The observed response of AV block to exercise or atropine administration is another useful adjunctive technique to localize the level of conduction block. An increase in adrenergic tone characterizes both interventions, which generally enhances conduction in the AV node with little effect on conduction in the His-Purkinje system. Thus, improvement in AV block with exercise suggests block within the compact AV node, while no change or worsening in AV block suggests block in the His-Purkinje system. When noninvasive maneuvers and surface tracings are not sufficient to determine the severity of conduction abnormality, an electrophysiologic study can often provide a definitive diagnosis.

Recognition of pathologic AV block should prompt a diligent search for underlying causes with initiation of appropriate treatment. Etiologies of pathologic AV block are diverse, with various underlying disorders listed **Table 133-4**. Once AV block is identified, attention must be devoted to determining the expected disease course of the underlying etiology. The importance of this is reflected in the fact that even high grade AV block in certain scenarios may not necessarily require a permanent pacemaker, such as in heart block due to digitalis toxicity in which the conduction system generally makes a full recovery with drug cessation. On the other hand, AV block in other contexts entails poor prognosis and should be treated without delay, such as development of Mobitz II with bundle branch block in the setting of myocardial infarction.

■ MANAGEMENT OF AV NODAL CONDUCTION ABNORMALITIES

Management of AV nodal conduction abnormalities depends on the degree of AV block and the presence of symptoms. Asymptomatic patients with first-degree or Mobitz I AV block generally do not require specific therapy. Conversely, patients with Mobitz II or complete AV block generally require pacing regardless of symptoms.

The primary treatment for AV block is a pacemaker. Pacing therapy can be delivered in a variety of forms, ranging from temporary transcutaneous or transvenous administration in the emergency setting to treat acute hemodynamic collapse to permanent pacemaker implantation for AV block with more insidious symptom onset. The decision of how to administer pacing therapy relies upon the acuity, symptoms, and hemodynamic effect of AV block. For instance, patients with asymptomatic first-degree AV block do not benefit from pacemaker implant. The decision to implant pacemaker for the patient with second-degree AV block rests upon two primary factors: the presence of correlating symptoms and determination of the site of block. Symptomatic patients with both forms of second-degree AV block benefit from pacemaker implantation. Because Mobitz Type II second-degree AV block may suddenly progress to more advanced AV block, it is reasonable to implant pacemakers in asymptomatic patients. In rare cases, even patients with Mobitz I may require pacing if they are sufficiently symptomatic.

TABLE 133-4 Causes of Atrioventricular Block

Ischemic heart disease
 Acute coronary syndrome, chronic ischemic CAD

Congestive heart failure
 Ischemic or nonischemic

Medication-induced
 β-Blocker, calcium channel blocker, digitalis, adenosine

Iatrogenic
 Surgical, radiofrequency ablation, alcohol septal ablation, transcatheter aortic valve replacement (TAVR)

Infiltrative cardiomyopathies
 Amyloidosis, sarcoidosis

Infectious cardiomyopathies
 Bacterial/fungal endocarditis, Lyme disease, Chagas disease

Metabolic derangements
 Hyperkalemia, myxedema

Structural congenital heart disease
 Congenitally corrected transposition of the great arteries (L-TGA), endocardial cushion defect, primum ASD, etc

Inherited disorders of conduction system
 Lenegre's disease, neuromuscular disease (myotonic muscular dystrophy, Erb's dystrophy, Kearns-Sayre syndrome, maternal systemic lupus erythmatosis)

Hypoxia

Hypothermia

Excessive parasympathetic tone

TABLE 133-5 ACC/AHA/HRS2008 Guideline Summary: Guidelines for Device Based Therapy of Cardiac Rhythm Abnormalities: Indications for Permanent Pacing in Acquired Atrioventricular Block

Class I—Permanent pacing should be performed

1. Third-degree block and advanced second-degree block at any anatomic level and any one of the following conditions:
   - Bradycardia with symptoms or ventricular arrhythmias due to AV block
   - Arrhythmias or other conditions that require medications that lead to symptomatic bradycardia
   - Asymptomatic awake patients in sinus rhythm with documented periods of asystole ≥3 s, an escape rate <40 beats/min, or an escape rhythm originating below the AV node
   - Asymptomatic awake patients in atrial fibrillation and bradycardia with pauses ≥5 s
   - After catheter ablation of the AV junction
   - Postoperative AV block after cardiac surgery, ie, not expected to resolve
   - Associated with neuromuscular diseases with AV block (eg, myotonic muscular dystrophy)
2. Second-degree AV block of any type with symptomatic bradycardia
3. Asymptomatic persistent third-degree AV block if average waking heart rate is <40 beats/min, or if >40 beats/min in cases of cardiomegaly or LV dysfunction, or if the block is below the AV node
4. Second- or third-degree AV block during exercise in the absence of ischemia

Class IIa—Permanent pacing is reasonable to perform

1. Persistent third-degree heart block with escape rate >40 beats/min, in absence of symptoms and cardiomegaly
2. Asymptomatic second-degree AV block at intra- or infra-His levels discovered with EP study
3. First or second-degree AV block with hemodynamic compromise or symptoms like those of pacemaker syndrome
4. Asymptomatic type II second-degree AV block with a narrow QRS

Class IIb—Permanent pacing may be considered

1. AV block in presence of drug use or toxicity when block is expected to recur even after drug is discontinued
2. Neuromuscular diseases associated with AV block with any degree of AV block even in absence of symptoms, due to unpredictable course of AV conduction disease

Class III—Permanent pacing should NOT be performed and may be harmful

1. Asymptomatic first-degree AV block
2. Asymptomatic type I second-degree AV block at the supra-His level
3. AV block, ie, expected to resolve and unlikely to recur (drug toxicity, Lyme disease, transient high vagal states)

Third-degree AV block, unless due to a reversible condition and expected to resolve, should be treated with pacemaker therapy. This is especially true of third-degree AV block associated with syncope, where pacemaker therapy reduces mortality (see **Table 133-5**).

SUGGESTED READINGS

Epstein AE, DiMarco JP, Ellenbogen KA, et al. ACC/AHA/HRS 2008 Guidelines for Device-Based Therapy of Cardiac Rhythm Abnormalities: a report of the American College of Cardiology/American Heart Association Task Force on Practice Guidelines (Writing Committee to Revise the ACC/AHA/NASPE 2002 Guideline Update for Implantation of Cardiac Pacemakers and Antiarrhythmia Devices): developed in collaboration with the American Association for Thoracic Surgery and Society of Thoracic Surgeons. *Circulation.* 2008;117(21):e350-408.

Mangrum JM, DiMarco JP. The evaluation and management of bradycardia. *N Engl J Med.* 2000;342(10):703-709.

Moulopoulos SD, Darsinos J, Sideris DA. Atrioventricular block response to exercise and intraventricular conduction at rest. *Br Heart J.* 1972;34:998-1004.

Olgin JE, Zipes DP. Specific arrhythmias. In: Mann DL, Zipes DP, Libby P, et al., eds. *Braunwald's Heart Disease: A Textbook of Cardiovascular Medicine*, 10th ed. Philadelphia, PA: Elsevier/Saunders; 2015: chap 37

Rubart M, Zipes DP. Genesis of cardiac arrhythmias. In: Mann DL, Zipes DP, Libby P, et al., eds. *Braunwald's Heart Disease: A Textbook of Cardiovascular Medicine*, 10th ed. Philadelphia, PA: Elsevier/Saunders; 2015.

Talwar KK, Dev V, Chopra P, et al. Persistent atrial standstill—clinical, electrophysiological, and morphological study. *Pacing ClinElectrophysiol.* 1991;14(8):1274-1280.

Vijayaraman P, Ellenbogen KA. Bradyarrhythmias and pacemakers. In: Fuster V, Walsh RA, Harrington RA, et al., eds. *Hurst's the Heart*, 13th ed. New York, NY: McGraw-Hill; 2011: chap 43.

Yen Ho S, Becker AE. Anatomy of electrophysiology. In: Fuster V, Walsh RA, Harrington RA, et al., eds. *Hurst's the Heart*, 13th ed. New York, NY: McGraw-Hill; 2011.

CHAPTER 134

Ventricular Arrhythmias

Mikhael F. El-Chami, MD, FACC, FHRS
Luis Fernando Mora, MD

Key Clinical Questions

1. What is the clinical and prognostic significance of frequent premature ventricular complexes (PVCs) and nonsustained ventricular tachycardia (NSVT), and how should they be managed?

2. In the setting of a wide-complex tachycardia (WCT), what features favor a diagnosis of ventricular tachycardia (VT)?

3. What types of ventricular tachycardia or ventricular fibrillation (VF) can occur in the absence of structural heart disease and what types can be precipitated by exercise?

4. How should a clinician distinguish between stable VT, unstable VT, and pulseless VT diagnostically and therapeutically?

5. Which patients deserve implantable cardiodefibrillators (ICDs) for primary or secondary prevention of sudden cardiac death (SCD), and what is the role of antiarrhythmic drug therapy in primary and secondary prevention of SCD?

INTRODUCTION

Ventricular arrhythmias are a heterogeneous group of cardiac rhythm disturbances that range from benign, asymptomatic premature ventricular complexes (PVCs) to malignant and often fatal arrhythmias, such as ventricular fibrillation (VF). They can occur both in the absence and presence of overt heart disease and have a wide spectrum of clinical significance and prognostic implications. The risk of sudden cardiac death (SCD) with some of these arrhythmias has led the medical community to identify patients susceptible to such events, and thus justify potentially dangerous and expensive treatments. Evidence gathered from clinical trials in the last three decades has helped establish clear epidemiological patterns for most types of ventricular rhythm abnormalities. These patterns have proven to be vital in the development of widely accepted, evidence-based guidelines for therapy and prevention.

The purpose of this chapter is to describe the epidemiology, pathophysiology, clinical presentation, diagnosis, treatment, and prevention of the most commonly encountered ventricular arrhythmias in current hospital practice. Care has been taken to include and cite evidence when appropriate. References to guidelines from the American College of Cardiology (ACC), American Heart Association (AHA), European Society of Cardiology (ESC), and the Heart Rhythm Society (HRS) are also found throughout the text.

PREMATURE VENTRICULAR COMPLEXES

■ INTRODUCTION AND EPIDEMIOLOGY

Premature ventricular complexes, also known as ventricular premature beats, ventricular extrasystoles, or ventricular premature depolarizations, are a frequent form of ventricular arrhythmia that occur both in the presence or absence of heart disease. Their prevalence depends on various demographic factors such as age, the presence or absence of heart disease, and the method used to detect them. In the Atherosclerosis Risk in the Community study, a review of over 15,000 healthy patients, the overall prevalence of any PVC on a 2-minute electrocardiogram (ECG) was 6% with a 34% rise for every 5-year increment in age. Conversely, published studies of healthy individuals evaluated with 24-hour ambulatory monitoring have found the prevalence of PVCs to be as high as 80%. In the background of acute myocardial infarction (AMI), the prevalence of PVCs may rise up to 93%.

Despite theoretical concerns of PVCs as a risk factor for heart disease, the occurrence of PVCs in healthy subjects has not been shown conclusively to have an impact on morbidity or mortality. A subanalysis of the Multiple Risk Factor Intervention Trial found a significant threefold increase in sudden cardiac death among healthy white males with any PVC on a 2-minute rhythm strip. An analysis of the Framingham Heart Study data also found significant increases in mortality when frequent or complex PVCs were identified in 1-hour ambulatory monitoring or when PVCs were identified during exercise testing. Nevertheless, several other studies do not support an association between PVCs and cardiovascular events or mortality and currently no consensus exists regarding the relevance of finding them in an otherwise healthy population. Interestingly, with the exception of frequent (>10/hour) and complex (primarily nonsustained VT) in post-MI patients, PVCs alone do not seem to be an independent predictor of outcomes in patients with known heart disease such as left ventricular hypertrophy and dilated or hypertrophic cardiomyopathy (HCM).

PRESENTATION

Symptoms related to PVCs are infrequent but important to recognize. The association of specific symptoms with PVCs, along with the perceived intensity of the symptoms, has important implications for treatment. Patients may complain of palpitations, which are usually due to postextrasystolic hypercontractility or the feeling of a "missed beat" secondary to the postextrasystolic pause. Patients may also describe neck pulsations or lightheadedness. Rarely, frequent PVCs can decrease cardiac output and cause exacerbation of underlying heart disease, particularly coronary disease and congestive heart failure. Physical exam findings vary according to the hemodynamic and electrophysiological consequences of the premature beat. Jugular venous pulsation may reveal cannon A waves (larger than normal, sporadic, jugular venous a-waves) if there is atrial activation (normal sinus beat) simultaneous with ventricular activation by the PVC. If there is functional atrioventricular (AV) block, a variable intensity first heart sound may be heard. A PVC that has a right bundle branch block morphology (ie, originating in the left ventricle) will generate a widely split P2. Finally, murmurs vary predictably in relation with PVCs and careful auscultation following the extrasystolic beat may provide important clues (decreased intensity in mitral valve prolapse murmur, increased dynamic obstruction in hypertrophic cardiomyopathy).

PATHOPHYSIOLOGY

The mechanisms responsible for the generation of PVCs are similar to those causing most tachyarrhythmias. Although increased automaticity, reentry, and triggered activity can all be causes of PVCs, each mechanism may have some distinguishing features on the surface ECG. PVCs often occur with a predictable and constant relationship to the preceding sinus beat (ie, fixed coupling). When this is the case, the mechanism of PVC generation is usually reentry. Examples of this type of PVC include bigeminy (a PVC after every sinus beat), trigeminy (a PVC after every two sinus beats), and quadrigeminy (a PVC after every three sinus beats). When fixed coupling is not present, the mechanism responsible for the generation of the PVC is generally increased automaticity or triggered activity from one or more ectopic ventricular foci.

MANAGEMENT

Currently no data support suppressive treatment of PVCs in asymptomatic healthy individuals except in the presence of high PVC burden (ie, 20% burden on a Holter monitor) and left ventricular (LV) dysfunction. In this particular group, PVC suppression with antiarrhythmic drugs or elimination with a successful ablation is associated with reverse remodeling and improvement in LV function. The evidence describing long-term mortality risk in healthy patients with PVCs is conflicting. These patients should be reassured and offered standard cardiac risk factor evaluation and modification. The clinician should also thoroughly investigate possible exacerbating factors such as current medications (eg, stimulants), possible comorbidities (eg, hyperthyroidism), and electrolyte abnormalities.

When PVCs are clearly *symptomatic*, intervention should also be aimed at reducing anxiety and identifying precipitating factors but consideration can be given to suppression of the PVCs with antiarrhythmic agents. The decision to treat with antiarrhythmics, however, must be carefully balanced. While most antiarrhythmic agents are effective at decreasing PVCs, many of these agents have known proarrhythmic properties that may render the net outcome as harm rather than benefit. As an example, in the Cardiac Arrhythmia Suppression Trials (CAST I and II), patients with a prior myocardial infarction and frequent PVCs were randomized to receive placebo versus one of three antiarrhythmic agents (flecainide, encainide, or moricizine). Although antiarrhythmic therapy proved efficacious in suppressing PVCs, the study was discontinued after 2-year follow-up because of an increase in overall mortality in the group that was randomized to antiarrythmic agents. Similarly, more recent trials using amiodarone for suppression of PVCs in the setting of post-MI patients and heart failure patients have shown antiarrhythmic therapy to be effective at reducing ventricular ectopy and arrhythmic mortality but have failed to demonstrate an effect on overall mortality. Based on the available evidence, even if PVCs may have some prognostic value in the setting of certain specific cardiac conditions, there is no indication to treat PVCs in the presence or absence of heart disease to reduce mortality risk. Nonetheless, the presence of structural heart disease may warrant therapy with PVC-suppressing agents, such as β-blockers, even when the primary aim is not to treat the PVCs (ie, β-blockers in heart failure and post-MI).

If PVCs do warrant therapy based on clinically significant symptoms, β-blockers are first-line therapy. This class of drug is particularly useful for daytime PVCs or PVCs that are related to stress, thyrotoxicosis, and mitral valve prolapse. The lowest possible dose that alleviates symptoms should be used. Other pharmacological alternatives include amiodarone and sotalol but referral to a cardiologist is generally warranted before initiation of these latter medications. The 2006 ACC/AHA/ESC guidelines for management of patients with ventricular arrhythmias, radiofrequency ablation (RFA) for PVCs may be offered (class IIa indication) if PVCs are frequent, symptomatic and have proven refractory to medical therapy if the patient is otherwise at low risk for sudden cardiac death (ie, does not meet criteria for device therapy).

VENTRICULAR TACHYCARDIA

INTRODUCTION AND EPIDEMIOLOGY

Ventricular tachycardia (VT) is another common form of ventricular arrhythmia that has a variety of different presentations. In the most severe of cases, VT may precipitate cardiac collapse and cause sudden cardiac death. Sudden cardiac death, commonly defined as death from an arrhythmic cause occurring within 1 hour of the onset of symptoms, accounts for up to 460,000 deaths annually in the United States. Ventricular tachycardia and ventricular fibrillation lead to more than 80% of monitored cases of SCD. Although VT may occur in the setting of structurally and genetically normal hearts, most patients with potentially malignant ventricular arrhythmias will have some form of underlying heart disease. Approximately 70% of patients with SCD will have severe coronary disease. Furthermore, over 50% of patients treated for recurrent VT will have ischemic heart disease and most others will have some form of cardiomyopathy. The prognosis of VT largely depends on the presence of underlying heart disease. Ventricular tachycardia in the presence of structural heart disease usually confers a high risk of SCD whereas VT in the absence of structural heart disease or inherited sudden cardiac death syndromes generally has a good prognosis.

■ PRESENTATION

In VT, symptoms are nonspecific and depend largely on the *degree of hemodynamic compromise* that occurs—*determined by the duration of the arrhythmia, the ventricular rate, and the presence of underlying heart disease.* Palpitations, heart failure, symptomatic hypotension or hemodynamic collapse and sudden cardiac death may all be presenting features of VT. Ventricular tachycardia may occur with minimal hemodynamic consequences and the absence of symptoms, and hemodynamic instability does not necessarily favor the diagnosis of another type of arrhythmia (ie, supraventricular tachycardia with aberrancy). Specific physical exam findings, as occurs with PVCs, include cannon A waves (secondary to AV dissociation), first heart sound variability, and split second heart sounds.

■ PATHOPHYSIOLOGY

The mechanisms responsible for the generation of VT are identical to those discussed for tachyarrhythmias and PVCs (ie, reentry, increased automaticity, or triggered activity) and vary according to the clinical context in which they are encountered (ie, normal heart, long QT interval, ischemic heart disease).

■ DIAGNOSIS

Ventricular tachycardia is defined as the occurrence of three or more consecutive ventricular beats at a rate of more than 100 beats per minute (bpm). Although ventricular beats typically originate in

ventricular muscle, they can also be initiated anywhere in the specialized conduction tissue distal to the bifurcation of the His bundle. *Because of its ventricular origin, the QRS in VT is usually wide (>120 ms), bizarre, and has a T-wave vector opposite the main QRS deflection* (**Figure 134-1**). Rarely however, ventricular beats originating in the basal septum or high in the fascicular system may produce a narrow complex QRS (< 5% of all VTs). Ventricular tachycardia is usually regular but slight R-R variability may exist. The rate varies anywhere from 60 to 250 bpm depending on the specific type of VT.

To classify VT, the morphology of consecutive beats and the duration of the VT episode are considered. The morphology of consecutive ventricular beats may be close to identical (ie, monomorphic VT) or may vary from beat to beat (polymorphic VT). Occasionally, the QRS axis will alternate predictably from beat to beat, a VT that is known as bidirectional VT (**Figure 134-2**), usually seen in the setting of digitalis toxicity, cardiomyopathy, or catecholaminergic polymorphic VT. The duration of VT also helps classify the tachycardia as nonsustained (arbitrarily defined as lasting < 30 seconds), or sustained (lasting more than 30 seconds or requiring termination due to hemodynamic collapse).

■ DIFFERENTIAL DIAGNOSIS

The differential diagnosis of wide-complex tachycardias (WCTs) includes three major categories: VT, supraventricular tachycardia (SVT) with aberrant conduction, and SVT with antegrade conduction through an accessory pathway (ie, pre-excitation). Though a clear distinction is often difficult to make, several clues support a diagnosis of VT in the setting of a WCT (**Table 134-1**). The most important clinical predictor of VT is the presence of structural heart disease. As such, a patient with a reduced ejection fraction or previous myocardial infarction and a wide-complex tachycardia should always be presumed to have VT (over SVT with aberrancy or pre-excitation) unless there is very compelling evidence otherwise.

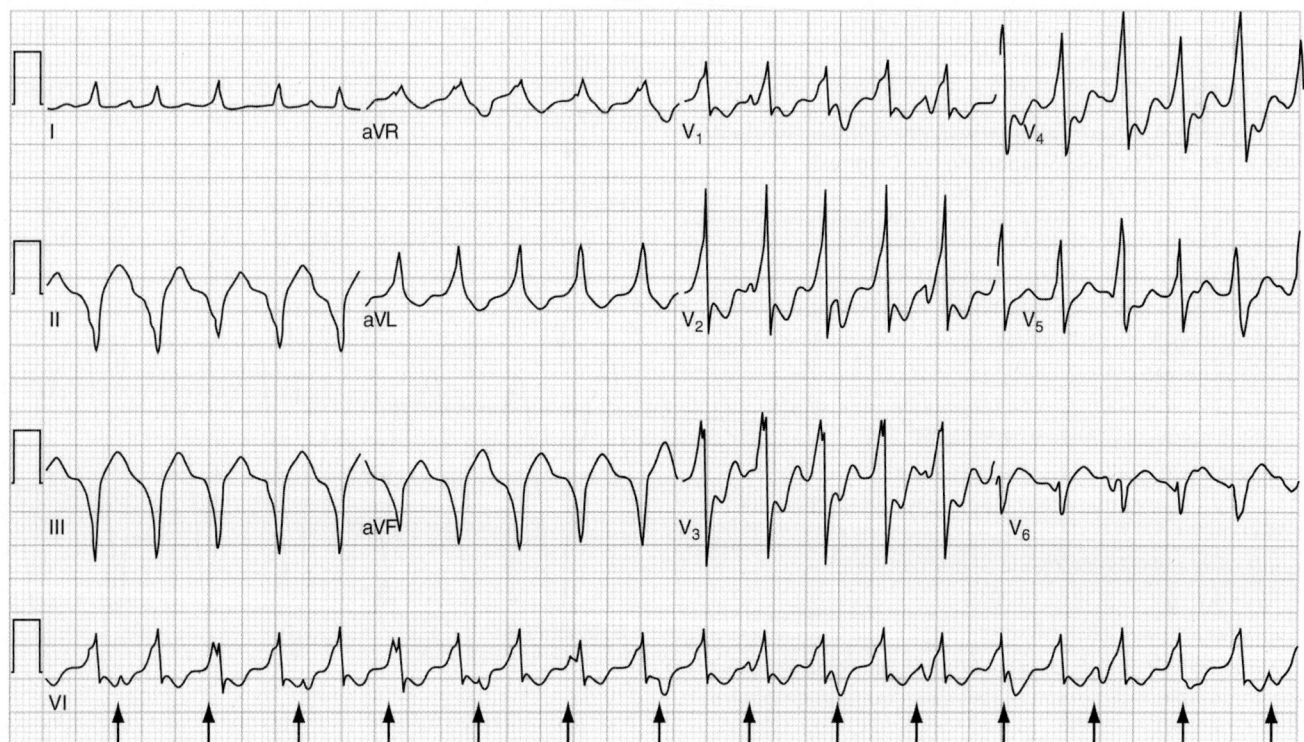

Figure 134-1 *Ventricular tachycardia. EKG showing a wide-complex tachycardia with independent atrial activity (arrows). AV dissociation (seen here), although not always present, is very specific for a tachycardia of ventricular origin.* (From Marchlinski F. The tachyarrhythmias. In: Fauci AS, et al, eds. *Harrison's Principles of Internal Medicine*, 17th ed. New York, NY: McGraw-Hill; 2008. Fig. 226-10.)

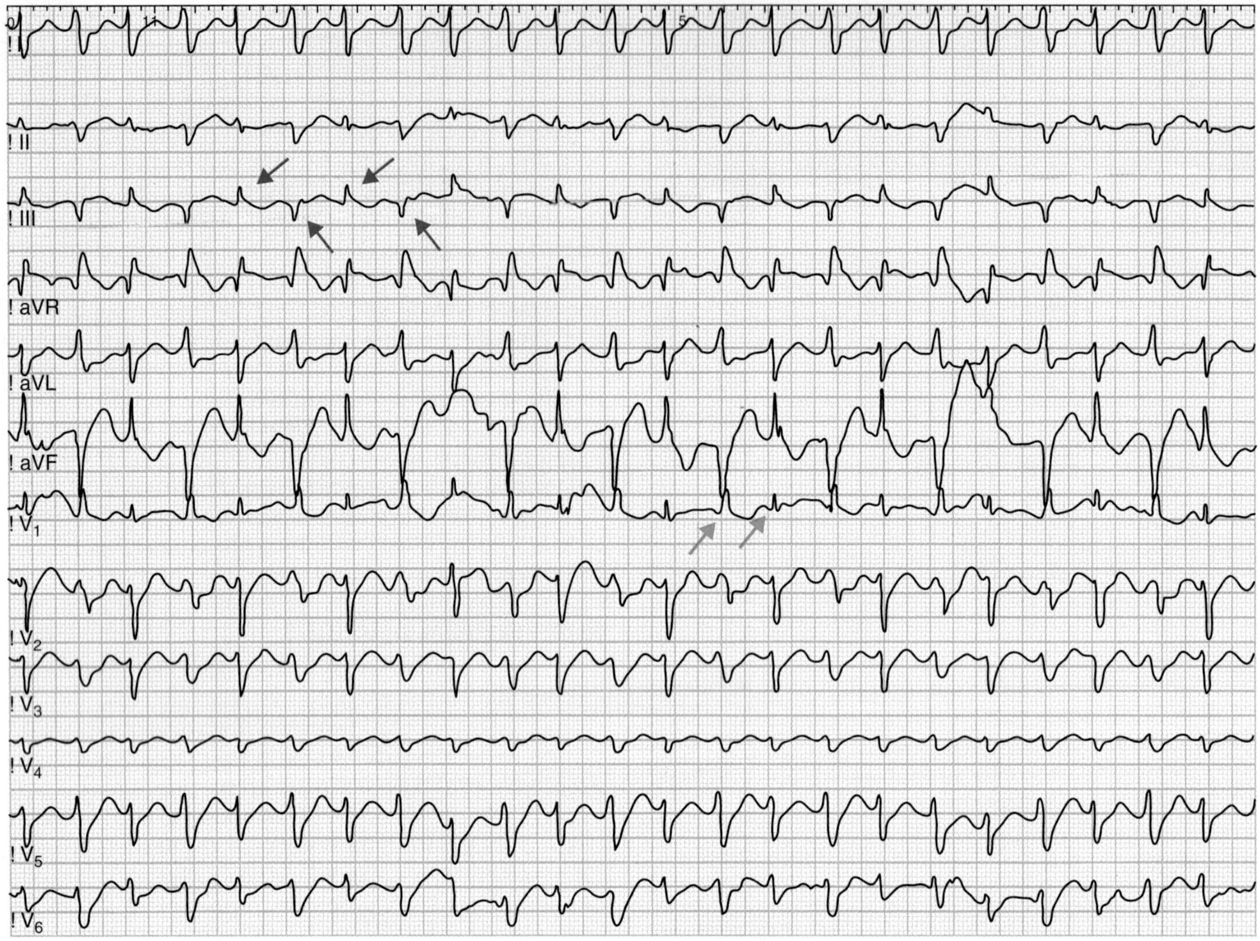

Figure 134-2 *Bidirectional ventricular tachycardia. Wide QRS tachycardia with relatively narrow QRS complex with right bundle branch block (RBBB) (green arrows) morphology and alternating inferior (red arrows) and superior (blue arrows) axes.*

In addition, careful observation of the ECG tracing for evidence of fusion beats, capture beats, or AV dissociation will provide important clues for the diagnosis. Fusion and capture beats (**Figures 134-3** and **134-4**) imply activation of the ventricle from two different electrical sites during the tachycardia. Because both fusion and capture beats result in a QRS that is narrower than the QRS seen during the rest of the tachycardia, they imply intermittent partial (fusion) or complete (capture) conduction to the ventricles from a supraventricular focus and thus rule out a supraventricular origin for the tachycardia. Although evidence of AV dissociation during a WCT has long been considered a forceful argument in favor of VT, retrograde activation of the atria (ie, ventricular to atrial conduction) is seen in up to 25% of VT. Thus, identification of independent atrial activity

---

TABLE 134-1 ECG Clues Supporting the Diagnosis of Ventricular Tachycardia

Known ischemic heart disease or cardiomyopathy
AV dissociation (atrial capture, fusion beats)
QRS duration > 140 ms for RBBB type V_1 morphology; V_1 > 160 ms for LBBB type V1 morphology
Frontal plane axis −90° to 180°
Delayed activation during initial phase of the QRS complex
LBBB pattern—R-wave in V_1, V_2 > 40 ms
RBBB pattern—onset of R-wave to nadir of S > 100 ms
Bizarre QRS pattern that does not mimic typical RBBB or LBBB QRS complex
Concordance of QRS complex in all precordial leads
RS or dominant S in V_6 for RBBB VT
Q-wave in V_6 with LBBB QRS pattern
Monophasic R or biphasic qR or R/S in V_1 with RBBB pattern

Note: AV, atrioventricular; RBBB/LBBB, right/left bundle branch block.

From Marchlinski F. The tachyarrhythmias. In: Longo DL, et al, eds. *Harrison's Principles of Internal Medicine*, 18th ed. New York, NY: McGraw-Hill; 2012, 1878-1900, Table 233-6.

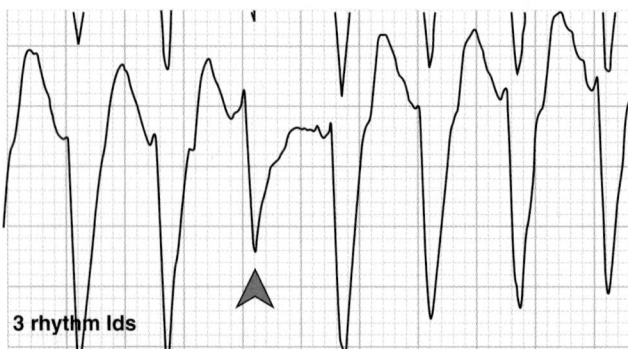

Figure 134-3 *Fusion beat. The QRS that is highlighted by the arrowhead represents fusion of a QRS originated from both a supraventricular focus and the ventricles.* (From Ritchie JV, et al. ECG abnormalities. In: Knoop KJ, et al, eds. *The Atlas of Emergency Medicine*, 3rd ed. New York, NY: McGraw-Hill; 2010. Fig. 23.32C. ECG contributor: Marc Mickiewicz, MD.)

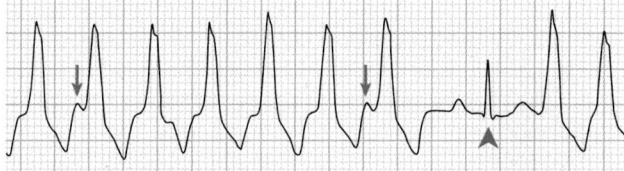

Figure 134-4 *Capture beat. Ventricular tachycardia with AV dissociation (arrows show P-waves). A capture beat occurs following a lapse in the VT (arrowhead).* (From Ritchie JV, et al. ECG abnormalities. In: Knoop KJ, et al, eds. *The Atlas of Emergency Medicine*, 3rd ed. New York, NY: McGraw-Hill; 2010. Fig. 23.32B.)

and AV dissociation during a WCT is helpful in identifying VT but is not always present (Figures 134-1 and 134-4); and if present may represent retrograde conduction. If the patient is stable and there is any doubt that the rhythm is VT versus SVT, immediate expert consultation should be sought.

■ MANAGEMENT

Initial hospital treatment

Stable and unstable VT with a pulse

The initial management of suspected ventricular rhythm disturbances requires careful assessment of stability. Stable patients bear no significant hemodynamic consequences related to the arrhythmia. Treatment of significant hemodynamic consequences (eg, extreme hypotension) or other symptoms related to hypoperfusion (ie, angina, heart failure, altered mental status) in the setting of a suspected ventricular arrhythmia should occur emergently (ie, within seconds to minutes), precluding any further diagnostic maneuvers. The diagnostic exercise of distinguishing VT from SVT with aberrancy or pre-excitation by using historical, clinical, and EKG data should only be undertaken in stable patients. Synchronized cardioversion with 100 to 200 J (monophasic) or 50 to 100 J (biphasic) is the treatment of choice in patients who are unstable as a result of VT. Required knowledge and practice of both basic life support process and algorithms and advanced cardiac life support process and algorithms aid successful resuscitative measures in unstable ventricular arrhythmias.

PRACTICE POINT

- Treatment of significant hemodynamic instability in the setting of a suspected ventricular arrhythmia should occur emergently, within seconds to minutes. The diagnostic exercise of distinguishing VT from SVT with aberrancy or pre-excitation by using historical, clinical and EKG data should only be undertaken in stable patients.

Clinically stable VT allows more time to identify the diagnosis and plan specific therapy. The yearly incidence of SCD in patients who present with stable VT is only 2%. Nonetheless, patients should be hospitalized and a judicious search for underlying, reversible conditions (ischemia, heart failure, and electrolyte abnormalities) should be performed, as correction of an underlying disorder may decrease or abolish the arrhythmic phenomena without any other antiarrhythmic therapy. If the diagnosis of VT is certain, nonemergent synchronized cardioversion, starting at monophasic doses of 100 to 200 J, remains a first-line option for treatment. If antiarrhythmic agents are used, amiodarone, procainamide, and lidocaine are all options. The medication choice depends on patient-specific information (eg, avoidance of procainamide in heart failure or renal

failure). Amiodarone is most often used in current hospital practice. Other therapeutic strategies are effective in specific circumstances. Magnesium sulfate, for example, has a specific role in *torsade de points*. Adenosine and verapamil can be used in certain types of idiopathic VT (see below). Digitalis-induced VT must be treated with digoxin specific Fab fragments (Digibind). In selected cases (eg, VT associated with a scar from a previous MI), the tachycardia can be acutely suppressed by overdrive pacing (also known as anti tachycardia pacing). In the absence of a previously implanted device (ie, implantable cardiodefibrillators [ICDs]), overdrive pacing requires placement of a pacemaker lead in the right ventricle (RV) to pace at a rate higher than that of the arrhythmia, reserved for specialized EP cardiology teams.

PRACTICE POINT

- Synchronized cardioversion serves as treatment of choice in unstable (but not pulseless) VT and in stable VT, when the diagnosis of VT is certain, cardioversion energy dosing is 50 to 100 J (biphasic) or 100 to 200 J (monophasic). Narcotic sedative and/or analgesic agents should be administered intravenously prior to cardioversion when possible.

Pulseless VT

VT with no discernible pulse is defined as pulseless arrest and not unstable VT. This has important implications for treatment. Pulseless VT and ventricular fibrillation are both nonperfusing rhythms that require immediate defibrillation to restore effective circulation. Early identification of the rhythm with earliest possible defibrillation is the most critical aspect of care. In VF, survival decreases by approximately 7% to 10% with every minute of VF that goes unattended. The selection of energy for defibrillation depends on the mechanism of delivery.

PRACTICE POINT

- Pulseless VT and VF are both nonperfusing rhythms that require immediate defibrillation (starting dose 120 J biphasic, 360 J monophasic) to restore effective circulation.

Though defibrillation is essential in pulseless VT or VF, adequate chest compressions also affect outcomes. *Pulse checks are no longer recommended after defibrillation and other interruptions in chest compressions.*

Following initial stabilization from any serious ventricular arrhythmia, efforts should continue in identifying and correcting the underlying cause. Most patients will need monitoring in an intensive care unit (ICU) setting for further stabilization and quick recognition of recurrences and complications. Antiarrhythmic medications (eg, amiodarone or lidocaine) that successfully aborted the arrest should be continued as an IV drip after successful resuscitation. Nearly all patients should be treated with a β-blocker agent following arrest due to a ventricular arrhythmia if the patient's blood pressure and heart rate will tolerate it. Induced hypothermia to mitigate postarrest anoxic brain injury should be employed in postresuscitative care, based on randomized controlled trial data and guideline recommendations. Cooling to 36°C (or preventing hyperthermia) is noninferior to cooling 32°C to 34°C for 12 to 24 hours in survivors of VF arrest, and health care facilities should have ICU processes in place for cooling or preventing hyperthermia in patients postarrest.

- Induced hypothermia to mitigate postarrest anoxic brain injury should be employed in postresuscitative care. Preventing hyperthermia and cooling to less than 36 C for 12 to 24 hours in survivors of VF arrest improve mortality outcomes.

■ LONGITUDINAL/OUTPATIENT THERAPEUTICS: PRIMARY AND SECONDARY PREVENTION

Long-term therapy for secondary prevention ventricular arrhythmias is aimed at preventing symptomatic recurrences and SCD. Consequently, not all patients with VT or VF will require long-term treatment. For example, episodes of asymptomatic nonsustained ventricular tachycardia (NSVT) in patients without structural heart disease will usually not be treated with chronic antiarrhythmic therapy or device implantation. Primary prevention may be indicated in selected patient populations based on their risk factor profile.

Primary prevention: Considerable evidence supports primary prevention for patients at high risk of SCD. Reduced left ventricular ejection fraction has consistently proven to be an independent risk factor for SCD. The Candesartan in Heart Failure Assessment of Reduction in Mortality and Morbidity study showed a 39% relative risk increase of SCD for every 10% reduction in EF below 45%. Though anti-arrhythmic drugs still may have a role in some patients for *symptom* control, the implantable cardioverter-defibrillator provides the most significant impact on primary prevention strategies.

The European and Canadian Myocardial Infarct Amiodarone Trials demonstrated reduced arrhythmic mortality with pharmacological therapy (amiodarone) but failed to show an impact on total mortality. Other large antiarrhythmic trials such as CAST and SWORD (Survival With d-Oral Sotalol) actually reported increased mortality in the treatment arms. These and other trials have provided a strong foundation for endorsing avoidance of antiarrhythmic drugs for purposes of primary prevention of SCD. The experience with ICD therapy has been quite the opposite. Initial trials like the Multicenter Automatic Defibrillator Implantation Trial (MADIT) and the Multicenter Unsustained Tachycardia Trial focused on patients with known coronary disease and low EF who had inducible VT; mortality was significantly reduced in both these trials. MADIT-II later showed improved mortality in the ICD arm with patients selected only based on EF and not presence/absence of inducible VT. Subsequent trials that included patients with both nonischemic and ischemic CM and low EF also demonstrated improved mortality in the ICD treatment arms. Based on these results, the AHA/ACC/ESC have provided clear recommendations for the use of ICD for prevention of sudden cardiac death (**Table 134-2**). Patients post-MI with low EF have a class I recommendation for ICD implantation only *after 40 days following the initial event*. One trial that specifically examined early implantation (5-32 days post-MI) of an ICD in patients with low EF following MI failed to show a significant effect on overall mortality.

Secondary prevention: Patients who have survived an episode of SCD are at very high risk for recurrent, life-threatening arrhythmic events. Secondary prevention trials have shown significant mortality benefit associated with ICD implantation. The Cardiac Arrest Study Hamburg, Antiarrhythmics versus Implantable Defibrillators, and Canadian Implantable Defibrillator Study trials all demonstrated reduced mortality in cardiac arrest survivors randomized to ICD. Although drugs like amiodarone have also been shown to be superior to placebo, comparisons favor ICD therapy. A meta-analysis of secondary prevention ICD trials showed a mortality benefit in the ICD population when compared to amiodarone. The benefit however was restricted to patients with EF lower than 35%. AHA/ACC/HRS guidelines provide class I recommendation for ICD implantation in patients who present with SCD from VF or sustained VT,

irrespective of EF. Additionally, patients who have near-normal hearts and sustained VT that does not result in cardiac arrest have a class IIa recommendation for ICD implantation.

The role of antiarrhythmic therapy currently is relegated to patients who refuse, or are poor candidates for, ICD therapy and for patients who have recurrent arrhythmias and ICD shocks. Poor candidates include patients who do not have a reasonable expectation of survival (>1 year) with an acceptable functional status, patients with incessant VT/VF or VT/VF that is amenable to catheter ablation, and patients with no structural heart disease and ventricular dysrhythmias due to a completely reversible disorder (eg, electrolyte imbalance, drugs, or trauma). Amiodarone effectively reduces the frequency of ventricular arrhythmias that result in symptoms or shocks and may also reduce the ventricular rate enough to allow for pace-termination of the arrhythmia. When amiodarone fails, other drugs such as sotalol, procainamide, or flecainide may be used. Radiofrequency ablation may also be effective in selected patients (ie, VT/VF precipitated by pre-excitation, RV or LV outflow tract VT, idiopathic VT or fascicular VT in the absence of structural heart disease).

VENTRICULAR FLUTTER AND FIBRILLATION

■ INTRODUCTION AND EPIDEMIOLOGY

Ventricular flutter (VFl) and fibrillation (VF) are extreme derangements of the electrical activity in the heart that usually terminate fatally within minutes if no intervention is made. As with VT, the incidence of VF can be inferred from the epidemiology of sudden cardiac death; *VF is the implicated arrhythmia in approximately 70% of reported cases of monitored SCD (including those preceded by VT)*. VF likely is responsible for the majority of unmonitored, out-of-hospital cardiac arrests. Though most cases of VF happen in the setting of underlying ischemic heart disease, VF may also be a manifestation of myocardial viral infection, valvular disease, hypertrophic cardiomyopathy, long and short QT syndromes, dilated cardiomyopathy, drugs (eg, class I and III antiarrythmics, digoxin, tricyclic antidepressants, cocaine), hypoxia, ion channel disorders, and electrolyte and acid base disorders. VF can also happen in the setting of atrial fibrillation (AF) with rapid antegrade conduction over an accessory pathway (eg, AF in Wolf-Parkinson-White syndrome [WPW]).

■ PRESENTATION

Patients with VF always present in complete hemodynamic collapse. Blood pressure is unobtainable, heart sounds are absent, and agonal breathing or apnea is typical. Asystole and death are the inevitable result if prompt resuscitation efforts are not initiated.

■ PATHOPHYSIOLOGY

Ventricular fibrillation happens as a consequence of multiple localized areas of microreentry, usually seen in structurally or genetically abnormal hearts that harbor an environment of heterogeneous ventricular depolarization and dispersion of ventricular repolarization. Electrical impulses traveling through myocardium with these derangements get fragmented and multiple areas of functional reentry are produced. This results in multiple, dynamic, reentry spiral waves of myocardial activation that manifest on the surface ECG as VF.

■ DIAGNOSIS

Ventricular flutter is a very fast (usually 150-300/min), sine wave appearing rhythm that is almost invariably associated with hemodynamic collapse (**Figure 134-5**). Under normal circumstances it cannot be differentiated from rapid VT or atrial flutter with

TABLE 134-2 2012 ACC/AHA/ESC Guidelines Focused Update

CLASS I

1. ICD therapy is indicated in patients who are surviors of cardiac arrest due to VF after evaluation to define the cause of the event and to exclude any completely reversible causes. (*Level of Evidence: A*)(16,319-324)

2. ICD therapy is indicate in patients with structural heart disease and spontaneous sustained VT, whether hemodynamically stable of unstable. (*Level of Evidence: B*)(16,319-324)

3. ICD therapy is indicated in patients with syncope of undetermined origin with clinically relevant, hemodynamically significant sustained VT of VF induced at electrophysiological study. (*Level of Evidence: B*)(16,322)

4. ICD therapy is indicated in patients with LVEF ≤35% due to prior MI who are at least 40 days post-MI and are in NYHA functional Class II or III. (*Level of Evidence: A*)(16,333)

5. ICD therapy is indicated in patients with nonischemic DCM who have functional Class II or III. (*Level of Evidence: B*)(16,333,369,379)

6. ICD therapy is indicated in patients with LV dysfunction due to prior MI who are at least 40 days post-MI, have an LVEF ≤30% and are in NYHA functional Class I. (*Level of Evidence: A*)(16,332)

7. ICD therapy is indicated in patients with nonsutained VT due to prior MI, LVEF ≤40%, and inducible VF or sustained VT at electrophysiogical study. (*Level of Evidence: B*)(16,327,329)

CLASS IIa

1. ICD implantation is reasonable for patients with unexplained syncope, significant LV dysfunction, and nonischemic DCM. (*Level of Evidence; C*)

2. ICD implantation is reasonable for patients with sustained VT and normal of near-normal Ventricular function. (*level of Evidence: C*)

3. ICD implantation is reasonable for patients with patients with HCM who have 1 or more major[†] risk factors for SCD. (*Level of Evidence: C*)

4. ICD implantation is reasonable for the prevention of SCD in patients with ARVD/C who have 1 or more risk factors for SCD. (*Level of Evidence: C*)

5. ICD implantation is reasonable to reduce SCD in patients with long-QT syndrome who are experiencing syncope and/ or VT while reciving beta blockers. (*Level of Evidence: B*)(349-354)

6. ICD implantation is reasonable for nonhospitalized patients awaiting transplantation. (*Level of Evidence: C*)

7. ICD implantation is reasonable for patients with Brugada syndrome who have had syncope. (*Level of Evidence: C*)

8. ICD implantation is reasonable for patients with Brugada syndrome who have documented VT that has not resulted in cardiac arrest. (*Level of Evidence: C*)

9. ICD implantation is reasonable for patients with catecholaminergic polymorphic VT who have syncope and/or documented sustained VT whlle receivingbeta blockers. (*Level of Evidence: C*)

10. ICD implantation is reasonable for patients with cardiac sarcoidosis, giant cell myocarditis, or chagas disease. (*Level of Evidence: C*)

CLASS IIb

1. ICD therapy may be considered in patients with nonischemic heart disease who have an LVEF of ≤35% and who are in NYHA functional Class I. (*Level of Evidence: C*)

2. ICD therapy may be considered for patients with long-QT syndrome and risk factors for SCD. (*Level of Evidence: B*)(16,349-354)

3. ICD therapy may be considered in patients with syncope and advanced structural heart disease in whom thorough invasive and noninvasive investigations have falled to define a cause. (*Level of Evidenve: C*)

4. ICD therapy may be considered in patients with a famllial cardiomyopathy associated with sudden death. (*Level of Evidence: C*)

5. ICD therapy may be condiderd in patients with LV noncompaction. (*Level of Evidence: C*)

CLASS III

1. ICD therapy is not indicated for patients who do not have a reasonable expectation of survival with an acceptable functional status for at least 1 year, even if they meet ICD implantation criteria specified in the Class I, IIa, and IIb recommendations above. (*Level of Evidence: C*)

(From *J Am Coll Cardiol*. 2013;61(3):e6-e75.)

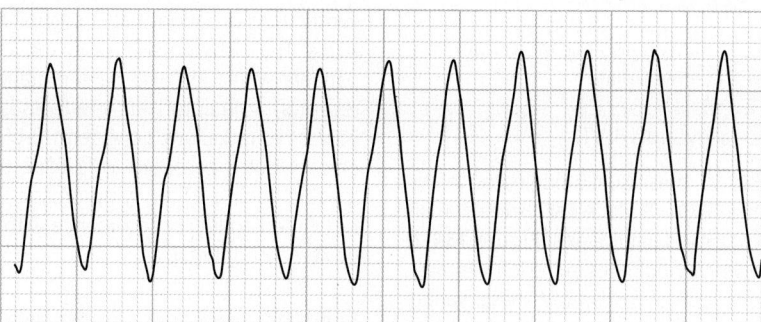

Figure 134-5 *Ventricular flutter. Very rapid, regular, wide-complex tachycardia with sine-wave appearance. The rate in this example is 330 bpm. Differential diagnosis includes WPW with atrial flutter. (From Ritchie JV, et al. ECG abnormalities. In: Knoop KJ, et al, eds.* The Atlas of Emergency Medicine, *3rd ed. New York, NY: McGraw-Hill; 2010. Fig. 23.33B.)*

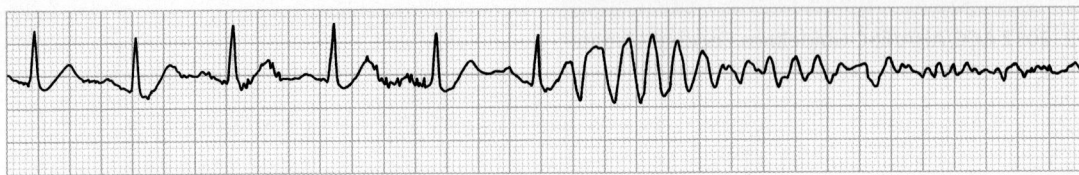

Figure 134-6 *Ventricular fibrillation. After six beats, sinus rhythm degenerates into ventricular fibrillation.* (From Stone CK, Humphries RL. *Current Diagnosis & Treatment: Emergency Medicine,* 7th ed. New York, NY: McGraw-Hill; 2011. Fig. 35-19.)

underlying pre-excitation. Ventricular fibrillation is characterized by a very rapid, irregular and polymorphic ventricular rhythm with no clearly defined QRS or T-wave (**Figure 134-6**). The absence of organized electrical activity precludes the generation normal myocardial contraction and cardiac output becomes negligible leading to hemodynamic collapse. Most cases of VF are preceded by an increase in ventricular ectopy (ie, PVCs) and repetitive nonsustained arrhythmias that include both monomorphic and polymorphic VT.

■ MANAGEMENT

Ventricular flutter and ventricular fibrillation are medical emergencies. Acute treatment has already been detailed in the management section of pulseless VT within this chapter. Long-term primary and secondary prevention of malignant ventricular arrhythmias has also been discussed previously.

SPECIFIC SUBTYPES OF VENTRICULAR TACHYCARDIA AND VENTRICULAR FIBRILLATION

Ventricular flutter and ventricular fibrillation occur most commonly in the setting of identifiable heart disease. One autopsy report found that 95% of patients who presented with SCD had evidence of structural abnormalities. Moreover, many patients with SCD and seemingly normal hearts have nonstructural cardiac pathology in the form of conduction disease, inherited ion channel abnormalities, or structural protein derangements. Nonetheless, a small subset of patients with VT/VF will have no detectable cardiac abnormality.

The fact that VT and VF can occur in either the absence or presence of structural heart disease leads to considerable heterogeneity in clinical features and implications. Specific examples are detailed in the following sections.

■ VT/VF IN THE ABSENCE OF STRUCTURAL HEART DISEASE

Idiopathic VT

Idiopathic monomorphic VT (10% of all VT referrals) occurs in structurally normal hearts and has a relatively benign prognosis. These tachycardias represent the nonmalignant end of the spectrum for VT and are considered specific syndromes rather than compensated forms of malignant VT. Although terminology varies, there are at least three well established forms of idiopathic VT:

(1) Repetitive monomorphic VT (RMVT, also known as right ventricular outflow tract [RVOT] tachycardia),
(2) Paroxysmal sustained VT, and
(3) Idiopathic left ventricular tachycardia (ILVT).

RMVT is a type of idiopathic VT that usually originates in the septal or anterior aspect of the RVOT. Surface EKG reveals a left bundle branch (LBBB) morphology and inferior axis (**Figure 134-7**) because of the origination site. RMVT originates in the left ventricular outflow tract in about 10% to 15% of cases. RMVT has a variety of synonymous descriptions in the literature, most relevant of which are catecholamine-sensitive VT, verapamil-sensitive VT, and exercise-induced VT. Typically, RMVT presents as nonsustained VT in young to middle-aged patients during periods of high levels of circulating catecholamines (such as stress or exercise). The pathophysiology of the arrhythmia involves abnormalities in cardiac sympathetic function and triggered activity. Prognosis for patients with RMVT is usually good but malignant variants have been described. These are, however, the exception and most cases of RMVT will not be treated as malignant unless certain high-risk features such as syncope, fast VT (>230 bpm) or frequent ectopy are present. The treatment of RMVT is relatively unique because the arrhythmia is sensitive to adenosine, verapamil, and β-blockers. Any of these drugs may be used to terminate the acute episode and verapamil and β-blockers are usually prescribed for prevention of recurrence. Class III antiarrythmics such as amiodarone and sotalol can also be used. Radiofrequency ablation is an alternative for refractory symptomatic patients that is being used with increased frequency and that has a success rate that ranges from 80% to 100% (for typical RVOT RMVT).

Paroxysmal sustained VT is another type of right ventricular idiopathic VT that also typically arises from the RVOT and that may respond to drugs like adenosine. Because of its obvious similarities with RMVT, it is considered by some not to be a distinct syndrome. Treatment for paroxysmal sustained VT is similar to that of RMVT.

ILVT usually originates in the inferoapical or midseptal region of the left ventricle. Because of its location, the QRS on the surface ECG will usually be relatively (0.12-0.14 seconds) narrow with a right bundle branch block (RBBB) morphology and a left superior axis. It typically presents as palpitations in young adults, and usually not often precipitated by exercise; sudden cardiac death is rare. Reentry has been proposed as the underlying electrophysiological mechanism. ILVT is especially sensitive to verapamil in the acute setting and is often used for long-term treatment. As with RMVT, RFA is an option for patients who are drug refractory or drug intolerant.

Catecholaminergic polymorphic VT

Polymorphic VT is less common than monomorphic VT in the absence of structural heart disease and inherited ion channel disorders. When clearly associated with a family history of SCD or stress-induced syncope, it is known as catecholaminergic polymorphic VT (CPVT). There is also a sporadic version in which no family history is identified. The disorder typically presents in childhood or adolescence as life-threatening VT (that is often bidirectional VT) or ventricular fibrillation that is precipitated by physical or emotional stress. The arrhythmia is easily inducible during EP testing. Many patients with CPVT will have mutations in the cardiac ryanodine receptor, a receptor that mediates calcium release from the sarcoplasmic reticulum. Long-term β-blockade has variable reported efficacy but is accepted as first-line treatment. Most patients with life-threatening VT or symptomatic VT despite β-blockers should be offered an ICD in accordance with ACC/AHA/HRS guidelines for device-based therapy.

Long QT syndrome (congenital, acquired) and *torsade de pointes*

The QT interval on a surface ECG represents the time it takes for myocardial cells to depolarize and repolarize. Although the

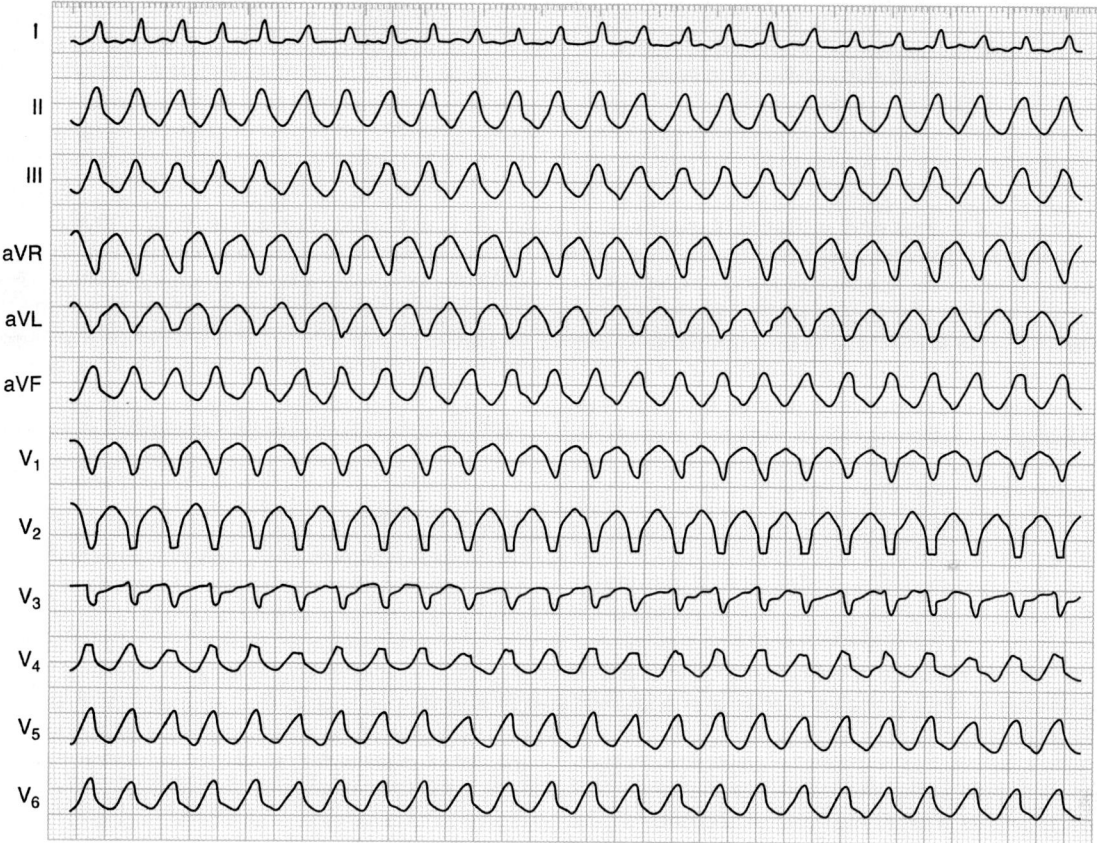

Figure 134-7 *Repetitive monomorphic ventricular tachycardia. Twelve-lead electrocardiogram that is typical of ventricular tachycardia (VT) in the absence of structural heart disease, originating in the right ventricular outflow tract. There is left bundle branch block morphology with late transition (V₄) in the precordial leads and an inferior axis in the limb leads. Negative QRS complex in lead avL suggests a septal origin.* (Reproduced, with permission, from Badhwar N et al. *Curr Probl Cardiol.* 2007;32:7.)

normal value for a corrected QT (QTc, adjusted for heart rate) is usually quoted as <440 ms, normal QT length also depends on other variables such as age and gender. Measurements are usually made in the lead with the longest clearly identifiable QT. Though expert opinion varies, U-waves, when present, should probably only be included as part of the QT when they are clearly merged with the T-wave. The long QT syndromes (LQTSs) are a heterogeneous group of disorders that are due to defects in the ion currents that are responsible for repolarization. These defects may be acquired or congenital and are especially important because they can lead to a very serious form of polymorphic ventricular tachycardia that is termed *torsade de pointes* (TdP). TdP is a polymorphic VT that is characterized by QRS complexes that vary in amplitude and cycle length in a pattern that seems to "twist" around the baseline (**Figure 134-8**). It is by definition associated with a long QT, usually in excess of 600 ms. The pathophysiology, clinical presentation, and management of the acquired and congenital forms of LQTS have several distinctive features.

> ### PRACTICE POINT
>
> - *Torsade de pointes* (TdP) is a polymorphic VT that is characterized by QRS complexes that vary in amplitude and cycle length in a pattern that seems to "twist" around the baseline (Figure 134-8). It is by definition associated with a long QT, usually in excess of 600 ms.

Acquired: Acquired LQTS is by far more common than congenital LQTS and is usually secondary to medications or electrolyte imbalances such as hypomagnesemia, hypokalemia, and hypocalcemia. The TdP that is seen in acquired LQTS tends to start after a PVC with a compensatory pause or during bradycardia. Although not a clearly a cause in itself, bradycardia aggravates potential that certain drugs have to prolong the QT interval and precipitate TdP.

Many drugs have been implicated in acquired LQTS. A more detailed list, that is updated frequently, is available on the Internet

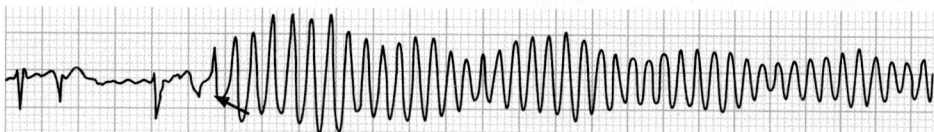

Figure 134-8 *Torsade de pointes. A polymorphic, "twisting," tachycardia is preceded by a short R-R interval followed by a long R-R interval with a PVC falling during repolarization; the R on T phenomenon (arrow).* (From Fuster O, O'Rourke RA, Walsh RA, et al, eds. *Hurst's The Heart*, 12th ed. New York, NY: McGraw-Hill; 2008. Fig. 94-4.)

(https://crediblemeds.org/). The medications most frequently responsible for QT prolongation and TdP are antiarrhythmics, macrolides, azole antifungal agents (eg, fluconazole, voriconazole), some antipsychotics and antihistamines. However, in recent years other commonly used medications (other antimicrobials [eg, quinolones], antinausea medications [eg, ondansetron], the narcotic analgesic methadone) have been implicated in prolonging QT interval and increasing risk of SCD. The overall incidence of drug-induced LQTS varies according to the drug and population studied. Two commonly cited drugs, sotalol and cisapride, have reported TdP incidences of 2% to 4% and 5.7%, respectively. Though drug-related LQTS is thought to be an idiosyncratic event, most patients who develop the syndrome will have one or more risk factors. These risk factors include female sex, concomitant electrolyte disturbances or bradycardia, baseline QT prolongation or silent congenital LQTS mutations, underlying heart disease, high drug concentrations, and concurrent use of medications that prolong the QT interval (eg, erythromycin and cimetidine).

Hypomagnesemia, hypokalemia, and hypocalcemia can also cause acquired LQTS and predispose to TdP. The QT prolonging effects of these electrolyte imbalances are likely a consequence of decreased activity in normal outward repolarizing currents and enhanced drug-related blockade of these currents. Other causes of acquired LQTS include stroke (both ischemic and hemorrhagic) and nutritional disorders.

Treatment for acquired LQTS is focused on rapid identification and correction of reversible causes and acute management of TdP when present (as detailed in the VT management section).

Congenital: The incidence of the congenital long QT syndromes in the general population is estimated to be 1 in 2500 to 1 in 10,000 and account for approximately 3000 to 4000 cases of SCD in the US annually. Two clinical phenotypes have been described. They are differentiated based on their inheritance pattern and presence of sensorineural hearing loss. The *Romano Ward syndrome* is the autosomal dominant variant of the LQTS and is not associated with hearing loss. The *Jervell and Lange-Nielsen syndrome* is the autosomal recessive variant of the LQTS that is associated with sensorineural hearing loss. In addition to the clinical phenotypes, the LQTS may be classified based on their underlying genetic mutation. Over ten different types of genetic mutations (LQT1-LQT8) have been described. However, mutations within LQT1, LQT2, and LQT3 represent over 90% of cases.

Symptoms related to congenital LQTS are nonspecific and are mostly a consequence of the development of arrhythmias. In the International QT registry, an ongoing study of patients with LQTS and their families started in 1979, 76% of proband patients (ie, index subjects with LQTS) had a cardiac event defined as cardiac arrest, SCD or syncope.

The pathophysiology of LQTS is incompletely understood but congenital LQTS is generally accepted a disease of ion channels. The common denominator of all these mutations is abnormal repolarization and prolongation of the QT interval. In the setting of a long QT, triggered activity (ie, early afterdepolarizations [EADs] that reach threshold potential) are thought to be the most common initiating factor for VT. The development of EADs and malignant arrhythmias is facilitated by bradycardia, electrolyte disturbances, and increased sympathetic activity.

The diagnosis of congenital LQTS is clinical and based on historical data (eg, family history, syncope), ECG findings (long QT interval, especially QTc >480 ms), and exercise testing (abnormal shortening of the QT interval is insensitive but may help in the diagnosis). Genetic testing is not used routinely for diagnosis but may be useful to identify family members of patients with a known diagnosis of congenital LQTS, to confirm the diagnosis in cases where clinical criteria are not conclusive, and to identify patients with LQT1, where strenuous exercise is particularly dangerous and β-blockers are especially useful.

The treatment of congenital LQTS is focused on the prevention of malignant arrhythmias and SCD. Avoidance of drugs that prolong the QT and close monitoring of electrolyte abnormalities is paramount. Restriction of activity to low-intensity exercise is also recommended, especially in confirmed LQT1 cases. Beta-blockers should be prescribed in all patients with congenital LQTS, as they reduce cardiac events and overall mortality in this population. Mexilitine may be used as add-on therapy in patients with LQT3. Based on ACC/AHA/HRS guidelines for cardiac device therapy, primary prevention of SCD with ICD implantation is recommended (class IIa) only for patients with LQTS who have VT or syncope while on β-blocker therapy. Other therapeutic strategies considered by electrophysiologists may include left cardiac sympathetic denervation, cardiac pacing, and RFA.

Brugada syndrome

The Brugada syndrome (BS) is a distinct form of inherited ion-channel disorder that can lead to VF and SCD in hearts with no evident structural abnormalities. The prevalence of ECG findings compatible with BS ranges from 0.4% in a report from the US to 1.0% in a report from Japan. BS has an autosomal dominant genetic pattern of inheritance, and occurs more commonly in men. Up to one-third of families with BS have mutations in the SCN5A gene that encodes the alpha subunit of the cardiac sodium channel. Collectively, mutations in the SCN5A gene may lead to a wide range of different phenotypes including sudden unexpected nocturnal death syndrome (SUNDS), atrial standstill, LQT3 and isolated progressive cardiac conduction defect. The mutations seen in BS are "loss of function" mutations that result in defective sodium channels with impaired activation or accelerated inactivation. These alterations ultimately reduce the duration of normal cardiac action potentials.

The characteristic ECG changes in the BS are thought to arise from differential expression of these defective channels within the layers of the right ventricle. It has been proposed that epicardial cells in the RV, which are preferentially affected, lose their action potential dome and thus promote a current directed towards them from the unaffected RV endocardial cells. This results in the typical ST segment changes seen in the three types of BS. The heterogeneity of electrophysiological properties within the RV also provides the substrate for reentry arrhythmias (phase 2 reentry). The typical ECG in BS has a pseudo-RBBB pattern with permanent ST segment elevation in the anterior precordial leads. Specific alterations in the appearance of the ST segment differentiate the syndrome into three "types" (**Figure 134-9**).

Diagnosis of BS, as with LQTS, is based on a combination of electrocardiographic, historical and clinical findings. Genetic testing, while available, is not routinely recommended due to its lack of sensitivity and specificity. EP testing is also not routinely performed but may have a role in risk stratifying asymptomatic patients with characteristic ECG findings.

The ACC/AHA/ESC currently recommends ICD therapy for patients with BS and previous cardiac arrest (class Ia), BS and previous VT without arrest (class IIa) and patients with BS and syncope (class IIa). Some groups also advocate ICD use in asymptomatic patients with inducible VT or VF during EP testing. Antiarrhythmic therapy is reserved for patients with frequent, recurrent episodes of VT and VF to reduce the amount of ICD discharges.

VT/VF and ischemic heart disease

The incidence of VT/VF in ischemic heart disease depends on the underlying pathology. In the GUSTO-1 trial, which included over 40,000 patients with ST-elevation MI (STEMI) treated with

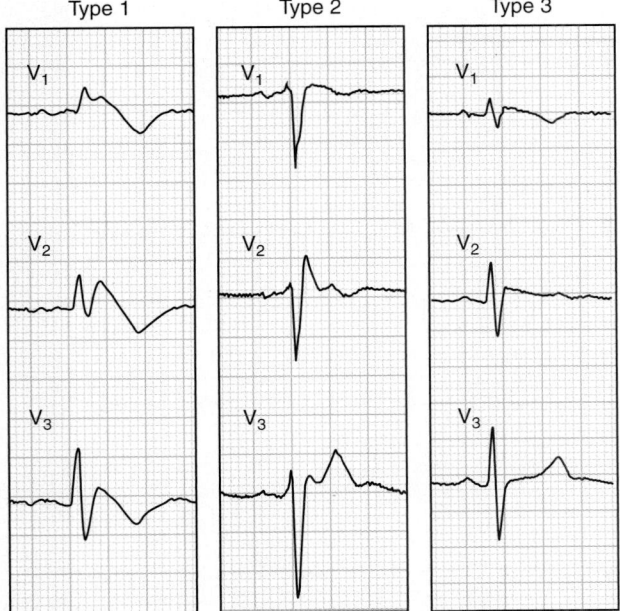

Type 1	Type 2	Type 3
V₁	V₁	V₁
V₂	V₂	V₂
V₃	V₃	V₃

Figure 134-9 *ECG patterns in Brugada syndrome (BS). Only type 1 ST-segment elevation is considered diagnostic for BS when associated with clinical features such as syncope and spontaneous/inducible ventricular arrhythmias. Types 2 and 3 may lead to suspect the presence of BS but drug challenge is required for diagnosis. The ECGs in the right and left panels are from the same patient before (right panel, type III) and after (left panel, type I) intravenous administration of 1 mg/kg of ajmaline in 10 minutes.* (From Fuster O, O'Rourke RA, Walsh RA, et al, eds. *Hurst's The Heart*, 12th ed. New York, NY: McGraw-Hill; 2008. Fig. 33-7.)

thrombolysis, the incidence of VT and VF was 3.5% and 4.1%, respectively. In a pooled analysis of over 25,000 patients with non-STEMI or unstable angina, the incidence of VT and VF was only 0.8% and 1%, respectively.

Patients with ischemic heart disease are at risk for developing ventricular arrhythmias from a variety of different mechanisms. As an example, acute ischemia leading to VT or VF is likely a consequence of local electrophysiological alterations in ischemic myocardium. Other rhythm disturbances, such as accelerated idioventricular rhythm (AIVR), are usually seen in the setting of reperfusion. Ventricular tachycardia in the patient with a remote history of an MI is usually due to reentry circuits around/in scarred myocardium tissue.

The pathogenesis of abnormal ventricular rhythms in ischemic heart disease varies according to the timing of the ischemic insult. The various time-dependent changes in ischemic myocardial cells provide a substrate for all the possible electrophysiological mechanisms of arrhythmia induction (ie, reentry, triggered activity, increased automaticity). Specifically, acute ischemia causes resting cardiomyocyte membrane potential to become less negative. In addition, acute ischemia significantly reduces the duration, amplitude, and velocity of the cardiac myocyte action potential. These alterations in resting membrane potential and conduction may lead to reentry, triggered activity, and increased automaticity. Chronic consequences (ie, scar) of an acute ischemic insult incite reentry as the predominant mechanism for ventricular arrhythmia. Although some ventricular rhythms may occur in the setting of reperfusion ("reperfusion arrhythmias"), these appear not to be life threatening and do not seem to carry any prognostic significance. Moreover, while the appearance of a typical reperfusion rhythm (AIVR) has long been considered a marker of relieved coronary occlusion, it is neither sensitive nor specific for successful reperfusion. AIVR, also

known as "slow VT," is identified on the EKG as a wide-complex ventricular rhythm with a rate of 40 to 100 bpm (usually 60-100 bpm).

VT/VF in hypertrophic cardiomyopathy

Patients with hypertrophic cardiomyopathy are at increased risk for malignant ventricular arrhythmias and SCD. In one community-based study of patients with HCM, the incidence of SCD was 1.1% at 5.5-year follow-up. Despite this, the use of routine electrophysiological testing as a screening tool is controversial. Instead, major society guidelines have advocated prevention and treatment decisions based on clinical data. High-risk clinical features for the development of VT include family history of SCD, syncope (especially exercise induced or repetitive), NSVT, failure to increase BP during exercise testing, and massive (≥30 mm LV thickness) left ventricular hypertrophy.

Current evidence for treatment of HCM is limited. As randomized controlled trial data are lacking, the ACC/AHA/HRS guidelines recommend ICD implantation, based on observational data, for patients with HCM who: (1) are survivors of an episode of sustained VT or SCD, (2) have one of the five high-risk features (see sidebar), or (3) have end stage HCM with LV dysfunction and dilation.

VT/VF in arrhythmogenic right ventricular cardiomyopathy (ARVC)

Arrhythmogenic right ventricular dysplasia (ARVC), a specific type of cardiomyopathy that is characterized by fibrofatty replacement of ventricular myocardium, initially affects the right ventricle producing typical wall motion abnormalities and RV dysfunction. Though predominantly described as a disease of the RV, the left ventricle (LV) is eventually involved in up to 60% of cases. *The mean age at diagnosis is 30 years and exercise is often a precipitating factor.*

Approximately 50% of patients with ARVC present with symptomatic ventricular arrhythmias. The patchy nature of the fibrofatty infiltration presumably provides a substrate for re-entry. Monomorphic VT is the most common form of arrhythmia in this population and is characterized by an LBBB pattern with an inferior axis, similar to RV outflow VT. Though rare, polymorphic VT associated with sympathetic stimulation may also be present in some forms of ARVC. *The resting ECG in sinus rhythm is normal in up to 50% of cases.* When abnormal, EKG findings include incomplete or complete RBBB, inverted T-waves in the right precordial leads and increased QT dispersion (variability in the QT between leads). A terminal notch following the QRS, commonly known as an *epsilon wave*, is seen only in 30% of patients (**Figure 134-10**).

The diagnosis of ARVC is based on clinical criteria that include the presence of ventricular arrhythmias, ECG findings, echocardiographic and historical information. Myocardial biopsy is insensitive owing to the segmental nature of the disease.

Treatment, as with HCM, focuses on the prevention of SCD. Patients with ARVC are instructed to avoid high demand physical activities, including competitive sports. Implantable cardiodefibrillators are recommended as secondary prevention for patients with sustained VT or VF and as primary prevention in patients with high-risk features (eg, extensive RV involvement, LV involvement, family with SCD, unexplained syncope). Antiarrhythmics are used in cases where ICDs are contraindicated or when ventricular arrhythmias and ICD discharges are frequent. Radiofrequency ablation is an option for patients who have failed antiarrhythmic therapy.

■ ELECTRICAL STORM

Electrical storm (ES) is commonly used to describe the occurrence of multiple episodes of unstable VT or VF in a short amount of time. Definitions vary but most authors agree that at least more than two episodes in a 24-hour period constitute ES. Electrical storm is a

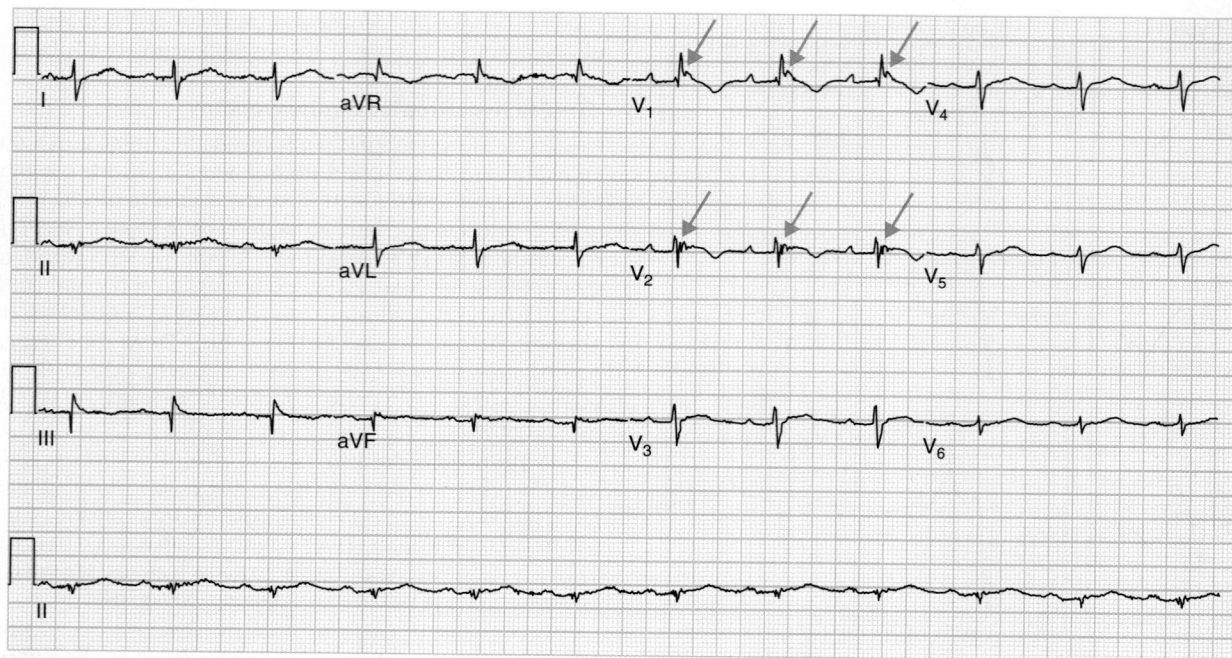

Figure 134-10 *Epsilon waves (arrows) in a patient with arrhythmogenic right ventricular cardiomyopathy. This is an important diagnostic feature for this condition.* (From Fuster O, O'Rourke RA, Walsh RA, et al, eds. *Hurst's The Heart*, 12th ed. New York, NY: McGraw-Hill; 2008. Fig. 39-3.)

relatively rare phenomenon in the absence of a known predisposition to ventricular arrhythmias but prevalence as high as 23% per year has been reported in secondary prevention ICD trials. Secondary prevention trials also have found ES to be an independent predictor for mortality, including cardiac nonsudden death. The most common identifiable precipitating factor for ES is ischemia.

The cornerstone of ES management is identifying and correcting any possible reversible cause. Ischemia, decompensated heart failure, and electrolyte disturbances must all be considered and treated accordingly. Patients who present with ES and have not had an ICD implanted previously should be resuscitated according to current advanced cardiac life support guidelines. Reperfusion, β-blockade, and IV antiarryhmics are essential in ES secondary to ischemia. Once stabilized, most patients who survive an episode of ES should undergo implantation of an ICD. Although antiarryhmics may be used, ICD therapy has proven to significantly improve mortality for survivors of cardiac arrest from ventricular arrhythmias when compared to drugs alone. For patients who already have an ICD, antiarryhmics, especially amiodarone, are often used for suppression of frequent symptomatic arrhythmic episodes and ICD discharges. Overdrive pacing, RFA, and spinal cord modulation are also alternatives in selected cases.

SUGGESTED READINGS

Antzelevitch C, Brugada P, Borggrefe M, et al. Brugada syndrome: report of the second consensus conference: endorsed by the Heart Rhythm Society and the European Heart Rhythm Association. *Circulation.* 2005;111:659.

Epstein AE, DiMarco JP, Ellenbogen KA, et al. ACC/AHA/HRS 2008 Guidelines for Device-Based Therapy of Cardiac Rhythm Abnormalities: a report of the American College of Cardiology/American Heart Association Task Force on Practice Guidelines (Writing Committee to Revise the ACC/AHA/NASPE 2002 Guideline Update for Implantation of Cardiac Pacemakers and Antiarrhythmia Devices): developed in collaboration with the American Association for Thoracic Surgery and Society of Thoracic Surgeons. *Circulation.* 2008;117:e350.

Hohnloser SH, Al-Khalidi HR, Pratt CM, et al. Electrical storm in patients with an implantable defibrillator: incidence, features, and preventive therapy: insights from a randomized trial. *Eur Heart J.* 2006;27:3027.

Huikuri HV, Castellanos A, Myerburg RJ. Sudden death due to cardiac arrhythmias. *N Engl J Med.* 2001;345(20):1473-1482.

Neumar RW, Shuster M, Callaway CW, et al. Part 1: Executive Summary: 2015 American Heart Association Guidelines Update for Cardiopulmonary Resuscitation and Emergency Cardiovascular Care. *Circulation.* 2015;132(18 Suppl 2):S315-S367.

Priori SG, Blomström-Lundqvist C, Mazzanti A, et al. 2015 ESC Guidelines for the management of patients with ventricular arrhythmias and the prevention of sudden cardiac death. *Europace.* 2015;17(11):1601-1687.

Rho RW, Page RL. Ventricular arrhythmias. In: Fuster V, Walsh RA, Harrington RA, et al, eds. *Hurst's The Heart*, 13th ed. New York, NY: McGraw-Hill; 2011, 1006-1024.

Sanders GD, Hlatky MA, Owens DK. Cost-effectiveness of implantable cardioverter-defibrillators. *N Engl J Med.* 2005;353:1471.

Zipes DP, Camm AJ, Borggrefe M, et al. ACC/AHA/ESC 2006 Guidelines for Management of Patients With Ventricular Arrhythmias and the Prevention of Sudden Cardiac Death-Executive Summary. A Report of the American College of Cardiology/American Heart Association Task Force and the European Society of Cardiology Committee for Practice Guidelines (Writing Committee to Develop Guidelines for Management of Patients With Ventricular Arrhythmias and the Prevention of Sudden Cardiac Death). *J Am Coll Cardiol.* 2006;48:1064.

CHAPTER 135

Cardioversion

J. Ryan Jordan, MD
Michael Manogue, MD
B. Robinson Williams III, MD

INTRODUCTION

Electrical cardioversion is an effective, rapid, and safe technique that has become a routine procedure in the management of patients with cardiac arrhythmias. Cardioversion disrupts the abnormal electrical circuit(s) in the heart and restores a normal heartbeat. The shock causes a critical mass of cardiac myocytes to depolarize simultaneously, thereby interrupting and terminating the abnormal electrical rhythm. This split second interruption of the abnormal beat allows the heart's electrical system to regain control and restore a normal rhythm. The delivery of energy during the shock is synchronized to the QRS complex, which represents cardiac depolarization, in order to terminate the arrhythmia safely and allow sinus rhythm to resume.

Defibrillation, on the other hand, delivers nonsynchronized energy to treat life-threatening arrhythmias such as pulseless VT or VF. Defibrillation is the treatment of choice for the arrhythmias most commonly associated with sudden cardiac arrest. The electrical shock delivered during cardioversion or defibrillation can be delivered externally to the heart using electrodes (external pads or paddles) placed on the chest (most common); directly to the heart using internal paddles during an open chest surgery; or through the electrodes of a permanently implanted cardioverter defibrillator (ICD).

Pharmacologic or chemical cardioversion uses antiarrhythmic medication instead of an electrical shock to restore the heart's normal rhythm.

MECHANISM OF CARDIOVERSION

Electrical cardioversion appears most effective in terminating arrhythmias that arise from a single reentrant circuit such as AFL, atrioventricular nodal reentrant tachycardia (AVNRT), atrioventricular reentrant tachycardia (AVRT), and monomorphic VT. The high-energy shock depolarizes the myocardium and the conduction tissue involved in the reentry circuit of the arrhythmia simultaneously. The depolarization of the myocardium is followed by a period of refractoriness that has the effect of interrupting the reentrant circuit, thereby breaking the repeating cycle and terminating the arrhythmia. When the reentrant circuit is broken and the arrhythmia stops, the sinus node begins to fire again and a normal heart rhythm is restored. This mechanism of action does not explain how electrical cardioversion terminates AF, which typically arises from multiple reentrant circuits. As a result of the multiple circuits, successful cardioversion of AF often requires higher energy (eg, 120 J) for termination. Other arrhythmias, such as junctional tachycardia and multifocal atrial tachycardia, originate from ectopic sites (ie, nonpacemaker) in the heart. Cardioversion is not effective for these types of arrhythmias.

TYPES OF DEFIBRILLATORS

Cardioverter defibrillators deliver energy in a variety of waveforms, broadly characterized as monophasic or biphasic. Monophasic devices provide a unidirectional pulse of energy, meaning that electrons flow in a single direction through the heart. Monophasic energy is highly effective, and monophasic cardioverter defibrillators remain widely used. Alternatively, biphasic devices deliver a sinusoidal biphasic waveform whereby the initial phase of energy is positive followed by a phase of opposite polarity, which means that during the shock the polarity and electron flow reverse. Biphasic cardioverter defibrillators deliver a more consistent magnitude of current, which terminates arrhythmias more effectively and at lower energies compared to monophasic devices. Biphasic cardioverter defibrillators have now become the standard for transchest defibrillation. Clinicians must distinguish which type of cardioverter defibrillator is available for use, as this will dictate how much energy is required for successful cardioversion.

■ INDICATIONS AND CONTRAINDICATIONS

Indications for electrical cardioversion include patients in whom the rate of the arrhythmia (eg, AF) cannot be adequately controlled medically or patients who poorly tolerate the arrhythmia (**Tables 135-1** and **135-2**). The most common reason for the elective cardioversion of atrial arrhythmias is to enhance cardiac performance by restoring sinus rhythm, particularly in patients with mitral stenosis, left ventricular hypertrophy (aortic stenosis, hypertrophic cardiomyopathy), and diminished myocardial reserve (heart failure, myocardial ischemia, and infarction). Urgent cardioversion may be required for patients with atrial or ventricular arrhythmias who have myocardial ischemia, acute heart failure (pulmonary edema) or hypotension.

TABLE 135-1 Indications and Contraindications of Cardioversion

Indications	Contraindications
AF/AFL	Known atrial thrombus
1. Patient with AF/AFL >48-h duration and anticoagulation for >3-4 wk (INR 2-3)	Sinus rhythm or tachycardia
	Multifocal atrial tachycardia
	Junctional tachycardia
2. Acute onset AF/AFL with associated hemodynamic instability including the following:	Accelerated idioventricular rhythm
	Digitalis toxicity (digitalis-induced tachyarrhythmias)
Angina pectoris	Severe electrolyte imbalance
Myocardial ischemia/infarction	Hypokalemia
Hypotension/shock	Unknown duration of AF/AFL in a stable patient not receiving therapeutic antecedent anticoagulation in the absence of a TEE
Heart failure	
Pulmonary edema	
Mitral stenosis	Patient that cannot be safely sedated
Preexcitation (WPW syndrome)	
Left ventricular hypertrophy	
AS	
HTN	
HOCM	
3. AF/AFL of unknown duration and absence of thrombus in left atrium or atrial appendage by TEE	
4. AF/AFL <48-h duration	
Atrioventricular nodal reentry tachycardia	
Atrioventricular reentry tachycardia	
Ventricular tachycardia with a pulse	

AF, atrial fibrillation; AFL, atrial flutter; AS, aortic stenosis; HOCM, hypertrophic obstructive cardiomyopathy; HTN, hypertension; TEE, transesophageal echocardiogram; WPW, Wolff-Parkinson-White.

TABLE 135-2 Indications and Contraindications of Defibrillation

Indications	Contraindications
Pulseless ventricular tachycardia	Expressed wishes by patient or patient's surrogate not to be resuscitated
Ventricular fibrillation	

Because electrical cardioversion is a low-risk procedure if properly performed, some authorities believe that every patient deserves one chance to achieve sinus rhythm by cardioversion, even if the short- or long-term prognosis of maintaining sinus rhythm is generally unfavorable. Other experts suggest that not all patients with newly discovered AF warrant an attempt at restoring sinus rhythm since several large, randomized trials have shown that the maintenance of sinus rhythm confers no survival (or other outcome) advantage over rate control. Treatment must be determined based on clinical parameters, clinician judgement and patient preferences.

Contraindications to electrical cardioversion include rhythms that do not respond to electrical cardioversion (eg, sinus rhythms, multifocal atrial tachycardia), digitalis toxicity, severe electrolyte imbalance (eg, hypokalemia), and known or suspected atrial thrombus. In AF or AFL, suspicion of atrial thrombus should be high if the rhythm onset is unknown or not clearly within the prior 48 hours. Transesophageal echocardiography (TEE) evidence that the left atrium is free of thrombus may permit cardioversion for AF or AFL with unknown or >48-hour onset.

■ TRIAGE/HOSPITAL ADMISSION

Cardioversion is routinely performed in most hospitals in a closely monitored setting, such as an intensive care unit, an emergency department, or a specially equipped procedure room. Although patients with atrial arrhythmias are often admitted to the hospital electively for cardioversion, outpatient cardioversion is a low-risk, effective, and economical procedure. Overnight hospitalization is seldom required.

TREATMENT

■ PREPROCEDURE CHECKLIST

Prior to performing electrical cardioversion, structured measures should be integrated for all patients (**Figure 135-1**) as follows:

1. Informed consent (patient or decision maker)
2. Fasting for 6 to 8 hours prior to cardioversion (if elective)
3. History and physical examination
   a. History should include current medications, allergies, previous adverse drug reactions or contraindications to sedation, diseases/disorders, prior hospitalizations, pregnancy status, oral intake status, and anticoagulation status (if presenting arrhythmia is AF/AFL).
   b. Use history to estimate duration of AF/AFL duration and determine need for anticoagulation and/or TEE evaluation.
   c. Physical examination should include vital signs, oxygen saturation, pulmonary and cardiovascular examination, and oral cavity and airway examination. Patients who have an abnormal airway exam should be considered to be at increased risk for airway obstruction during sedation and may potentially have a difficult airway to manage if mask ventilation or intubation becomes necessary. Patients who present with any high-risk features (**Table 135-3**) should be considered for anesthesiology consultation prior to the initiation of the procedure.

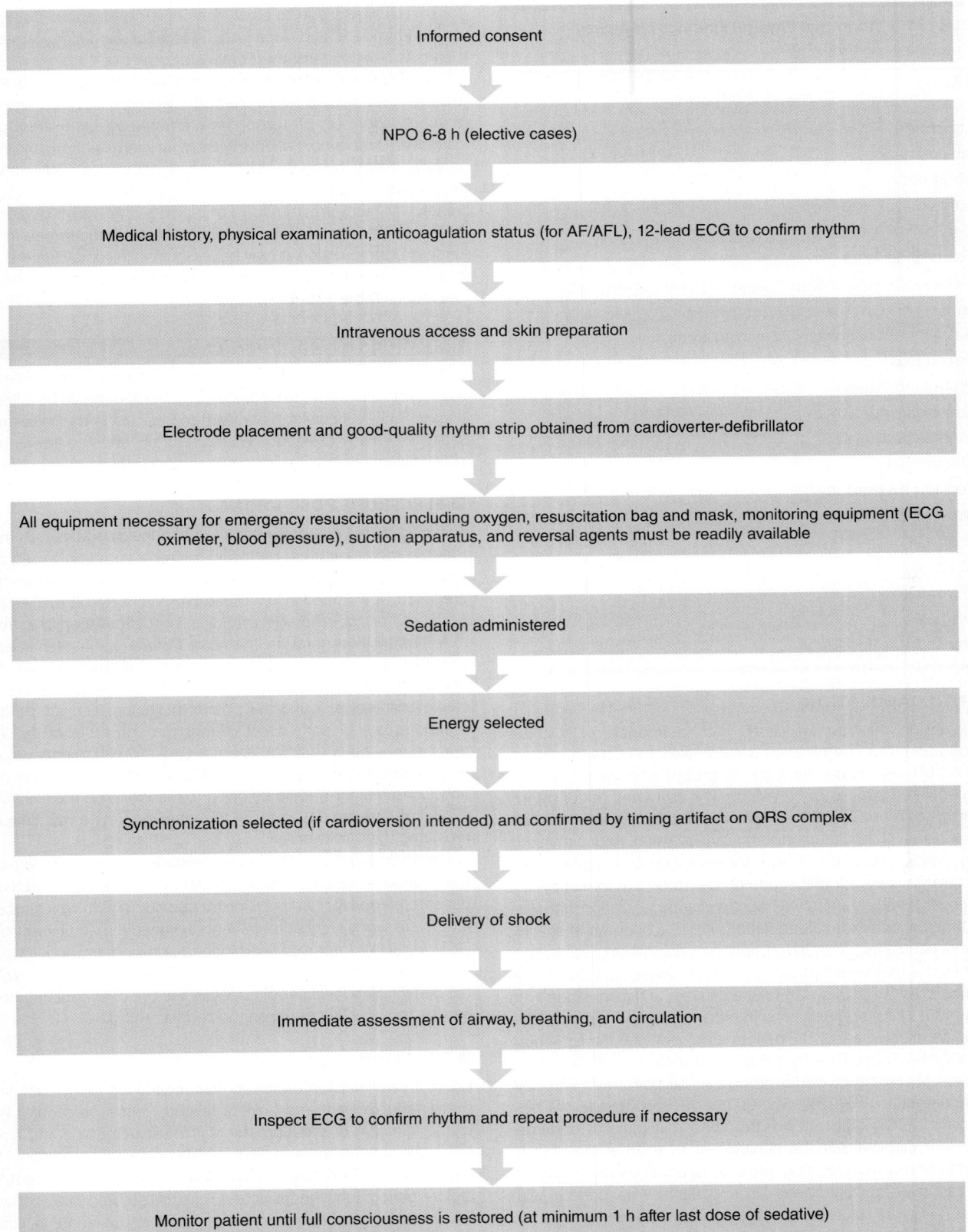

Informed consent

NPO 6-8 h (elective cases)

Medical history, physical examination, anticoagulation status (for AF/AFL), 12-lead ECG to confirm rhythm

Intravenous access and skin preparation

Electrode placement and good-quality rhythm strip obtained from cardioverter-defibrillator

All equipment necessary for emergency resuscitation including oxygen, resuscitation bag and mask, monitoring equipment (ECG oximeter, blood pressure), suction apparatus, and reversal agents must be readily available

Sedation administered

Energy selected

Synchronization selected (if cardioversion intended) and confirmed by timing artifact on QRS complex

Delivery of shock

Immediate assessment of airway, breathing, and circulation

Inspect ECG to confirm rhythm and repeat procedure if necessary

Monitor patient until full consciousness is restored (at minimum 1 h after last dose of sedative)

Figure 135-1 *Algorithm for external electrical cardioversion (preprocedure preparation and procedure).*

4. A 12-lead electrocardiogram (ECG) is used to confirm rhythm.
5. If any electrolyte abnormality (hypokalemia, hyperkalemia) or drug toxicity (digitalis) is suspected, appropriate blood levels should be checked.
6. Peripheral venous access (for preprocedure sedation and post-procedure medications or fluids if needed) is obtained.

7. Skin preparation includes shaving of the chest hair, if present (with electric clippers rather than a blade) to ensure good contact of the skin and electrode pads. High-quality continuous ECG from the cardioverter defibrillator will confirm proper contact of electrode pads to the skin.
8. Emergency resuscitation equipment available (Figure 135-1).

TABLE 135-3 Abnormal Physical Findings on Airway Examination

Habitus
  Significant obesity (especially involving the neck and facial structures)
Head and neck
  Short neck
  Limited neck extension
  Cervical spine trauma
  Tracheal deviation
  Decreased hyoid–mentum distance (<3 cm in an adult)
Mouth
  Small mouth opening (<3 cm in an adult)
  Edentulous
  Protruding incisors
  Loose or capped teeth
  High-arched palate
  Macroglossia
  Tonsillar hypertrophy
  Nonvisible uvula
Jaw
  Micrognathia
  Retrognathia
  Trismus
  Significant malocclusion

■ ANTICOAGULATION

Cardioversion may be associated with pulmonary or systemic embolization. This complication is more likely to occur in patients with AF/AFL >48 hours (ie, high-risk group) who have not been anticoagulated prior to cardioversion. The estimated risk of thromboembolism is between 1% and 5% in nonanticoagulated patients with AF/AFL >48 hours undergoing cardioversion. Anticoagulation before cardioversion allows time for resolution of any preexisting atrial thrombus and for prevention of new thrombus formation.

In patients with AF/AFL >48 hours, oral anticoagulation with warfarin (International Normalized Ratio [INR] 2.0-3.0) or target specific oral anticoagulants (TSOACs) (eg, apixaban, dabigatran, rivaroxaban) for at least 3 to 4 weeks prior to cardioversion reduces the thromboembolic risk to 0.5% to 0.8%. Alternatively, anticoagulation with intravenous unfractionated heparin or low molecular weight heparin can be initiated and a TEE performed to evaluate the left atrium and left atrial appendage for evidence of thrombus. If there is no evidence of thrombus, cardioversion can be performed with low thromboembolic risk (0.8%). The 2008 American College of Chest Physicians (ACCP) guidelines recommend that patients undergoing urgent cardioversion be heparinized as soon as possible to prevent thrombi from forming due to atrial appendage dysfunction after cardioversion. Cardioversion in patients who present with acute AF/AFL <48 hours (ie, low-risk group) is associated with a low clinical rate of thrombembolism (0.8%).

Late thromboembolic events after cardioversion are probably due to both the development of thrombus as a consequence of atrial stunning and the delayed recovery of atrial contraction after cardioversion. Pooled data from 32 studies of cardioversion of AF/AFL suggest that 98% of clinical thromboembolic events occur within 10 days of cardioversion. Anticoagulation after the procedure prevents thrombus formation from occurring before normal atrial mechanical activity has resumed, a process that may be delayed for several weeks due to atrial stunning. The American College of Chest Physicians and American College of Cardiology/American Heart Association, and the European Society of Cardiology (ACC/AHA/ESC) guidelines therefore recommend continuation of warfarin therapy for at least 4 weeks after cardioversion. This recommendation only addresses protection from embolic events related to the cardioversion period. Patients with AF at high risk from thromboembolic events based on risk scoring algorithms (ie, CHADS2-Vasc) may require long-term anticoagulation (refer to Chapter 132 [Supraventricular Tachyarrhythmias]). For patients with known duration of AF/AFL of less than 48 hours and low risk of thromboembolism who undergo cardioversion, it may be reasonable in some circumstance to omit pre- and postcardioversion anticoagulation at the clinician's discretion (**Table 135-4**).

PROCEDURE TECHNIQUE

Following preprocedure preparation, a standardized procedure algorithm for performing electrical cardioversion should be followed (Figure 135-1), including ECG lead and electrode pad placement, sedation, energy selection, synchronization, shock delivery, postshock patient and ECG assessment and postprocedure monitoring.

■ ELECTRODE POSITIONING

Two electrodes (self-adhesive pads or handheld paddles) determine the transthoracic current pathway. The most commonly used electrodes for external cardioversion are self-adhesive (ie, hands-free), pregelled, low-impedance, disposable-pad electrodes. Electrode positions for transthoracic cardioversion/defibrillation that maximize current flow through the heart include apex-anterior, apexposterior, and anterior-posterior positions (**Figure 135-2**). Less energy may be required to accomplish a higher rate of successful cardioversion of AF using the anterior-posterior electrode position. Anterior-posterior pads direct current through more of the atrial mass compared with apical anterior pads. Some patients who do not respond to one method occasionally respond to another position. Consideration should be given to repositioning the electrodes if initial shocks are unsuccessful in terminating the arrhythmia and repeating the cardioversion.

Handheld paddles with manual pressure may be more effective than self-adhesive pads. This was illustrated in a randomized trial of patients referred for cardioversion for persistent AF, in which success rates were slightly higher for patients assigned to paddle electrodes (96% vs 88%). Improved electrode-to-skin contact and reduced transthoracic impedance with handheld electrodes may explain the benefit. Handheld paddles require the use of conducting gel to ensure good contact between the paddles and skin.

■ SEDATION

External cardioversion under conscious sedation or general anesthesia reduces pain and anxiety related to the procedure. Prior to the initiation of sedation, the staff must determine and document the availability of a responsible adult to accompany the patient home if discharge is planned in the immediate postprocedure period. Intravenous access must be secured in all patients. All equipment necessary for emergency resuscitation including oxygen, oxygen equipment/supplies, resuscitation bag and mask, monitoring equipment (ECG, pulse oximeter, blood pressure), functioning suction apparatus/catheters and agents to reverse the effects of drugs administered to produce the moderate sedation (eg, naloxone, flumazenil) must be readily available. Crash cart/defibrillator and emergency airway equipment should be immediately accessible. A physician skilled in airway management (eg, anesthesiologist) should be present or immediately available. Short-acting intravenous sedatives and short-acting analgesic agents that

TABLE 135-4 2014 ACC/AHA/ESC Guideline Summary: Prevention of Thromboembolism in Patients with Atrial Fibrillation Undergoing Cardioversion

Class I—There is evidence and/or general agreement that the following approaches are effective for the prevention of thromboembolism in patients with AF undergoing cardioversion

1. For patients with AF or atrial flutter of 48-h' duration or longer, or when the duration of AF is unknown, anticoagulation with warfarin (INR 2.0-3.0) is recommended for at least 3 wk before and 4 wk after cardioversion, regardless of the CHA2DS2-VASc score and the method (electrical or pharmacological) used to restore sinus rhythm. (Level of evidence: B.)

2. For patients with AF or atrial flutter of more than 48-h duration or unknown duration that requires immediate cardioversion for hemodynamic instability, anticoagulation should be initiated as soon as possible and continued for at least 4 wk after cardioversion unless contraindicated. (Level of evidence: C.)

3. For patients with AF or atrial flutter of <48-h duration and with high risk of stroke, intravenous heparin or LMWH, or administration of a factor Xa or direct thrombin inhibitor, is recommended as soon as possible before or immediately after cardioversion, followed by long-term anticoagulation therapy. (Level of evidence: C.)

4. Following cardioversion for AF of any duration, the decision about long-term anticoagulation therapy should be based on the thromboembolic risk profile. (Level of evidence: C.)

Class IIa—The weight of evidence or opinion is in favor of the usefulness of the following approaches for the prevention of thrombembolism in patients with AF undergoing cardioversion

1. For patients with AF or atrial flutter of 48-h duration or longer or of unknown duration who have not been anticoagulated for the preceding 3 wk, it is reasonable to perform transesophageal echocardiography before cardioversion and proceed with cardioversion if no left atrial thrombus is identified, including in the left atrial appendage, provided that anticoagulation is achieved before transesophageal echocardiography and maintained after cardioversion for at least 4 wk. (Level of evidence: B.)

2. For patients with AF or atrial flutter of 48-h duration or longer or when duration of AF is unknown, anticoagulation with dabigatran, rivaroxaban, or apixaban is reasonable for at least 3 wk before and 4 wk after cardioversion. (Level of evidence: C.)

Class IIb—The weight of evidence or opinion is less well established in the usefulness of the following approaches for the prevention of thrombembolism in patients with AF undergoing cardioversion

1. For patients with AF or atrial flutter of <48-h duration who are at low thromboembolic risk, anticoagulation (intravenous heparin, LMWH, or a new oral anticoagulant) or no antithrombotic therapy may be considered for cardioversion, without the need for postcardioversion oral anticoagulation. (Level of evidence: C.)

produce conscious sedation enable rapid recovery after the procedure (**Table 135-5**). A typical medication combination for conscious sedation would include intravenous midazolam plus fentanyl.

Conscious sedation is assessed by lack of response to tactile and verbal stimuli. The patient's ability to communicate should be preserved. Heart rate and rhythm, blood pressure, oxygen saturation, respiratory rate, and response to verbal stimuli (level of consciousness) should be continuously monitored until the patient regains consciousness and makes a full recovery. The patient usually awakens 5 to 10 minutes after the cardioversion. The patient should be monitored until full consciousness is restored and at least 1 hour (preferably several hours) after the last dosing of a sedative or an analgesic.

ENERGY SELECTION AND TRANSTHORACIC IMPEDANCE

Successful cardioversion depends on the adequate delivery of energy to the heart, determined by the amount of energy provided by the cardioverter defibrillator and the patient's transthoracic impedance. The minimum effective energy dose for shocks should be administered initially, and energy dose can be titrated up for additional shocks when the clinical situation permits (**Table 135-6**). For cardioversion, lower energies effectively convert to sinus rhythm in most hemodynamically stable patients. More organized arrhythmias, such as AFL and VT, terminate with lower energy compared to AF and VF. In urgent settings, such as hemodynamic collapse

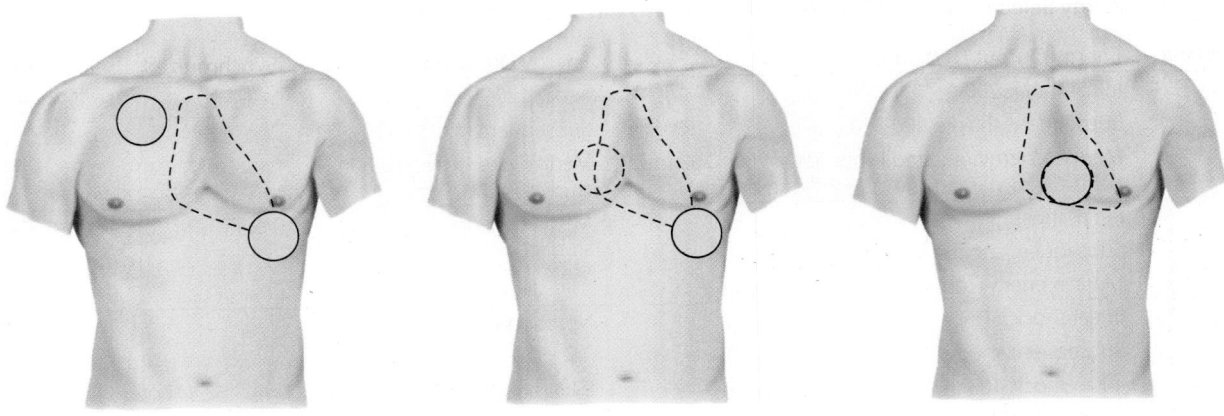

Apex-Anterior   Apex-Posterior   Anterior-Posterior

Figure 135-2 *Electrode positions commonly used for transthoracic defibrillation and cardioversion.* (From, with permission, Kerber RE. Transchest cardioversion: optimal techniques. In: Tacker WA, ed. *Defibrillation of the Heart: ICDs, AEDs and Manual.* St. Louis, MO: Mosby-Year Book; 1994:163.)

TABLE 135-5 Dosage and Dose Adjustments of Commonly Used Sedative/Analgesic Drugs

Drug	Class and Mechanism of Action	Dosing Guidelines (IV Administration)	Onset, Peak Effect, and Duration of Action	Adverse Drug Reactions	Reversal
Midazolam (Versed)	Benzodiazepine (Binds to GABA receptor resulting in CNS depression)	Adults 18-64 y of age: 0.05 mg/kg repeated every 2-3 min to adequate sedation up to a max dose of 0.2 mg/kg. Elderly (>65) and those with COPD, CHF, or chronic debilitation: 0.02 mg/kg repeated every 2-3 min to adequate sedation up to a max dose of 0.2 mg/kg	Onset: 1-3 min. Peak effect: 5-7 min. Duration of action: 20-30 min	Respiratory and cardiovascular depression may occur. May also cause ataxia, dizziness, hypotension, bradycardia, blurred vision, and paradoxical agitation	Flumazenil (Romazicon): 0.2 mg over 15 s, may repeat at 1 min as needed
Lorazepam (Ativan)	Benzodiazepine (Binds to GABA receptor resulting in CNS depression)	Adults 18-64 y of age: 0.02-0.05 mg/kg repeated every 3-4 min up to a max dose of 4 mg. Elderly (>65) and those with COPD, CHF, or chronic debilitation: 0.02 mg/kg repeated every 3-4 min up to a max of 4 mg	Onset: 3-7 min. Peak effect: 10-20 min. Duration of action: 6-8 h	Respiratory and cardiovascular depression may occur. May also cause ataxia, dizziness, hypotension, bradycardia, blurred vision, and paradoxical agitation	Flumazenil (Romazicon): 0.2 mg over 15 s, may repeat at 1 min as needed
Fentanyl (Sublimaze)	Opioid narcotic (Binds to opioid receptor in the CNS)	Adults 18-64 y of age: 0.5-1 µg/kg given in small incremental doses of 25-50 mcg up to a max dose of 250 µg. Elderly (>65): 0.5-1 µg/kg given in small incremental doses of 25 µg up to a max dose of 100 µg. The elderly are more susceptible to CNS depression	Onset 1-2 min. Peak effect: 10-15 min. Duration of action: 30-60 min	Hypotension, bradycardia, respiratory depression, nausea, vomiting, constipation, biliary spasm, and skin rash	Naloxone (Narcan): 0.4 mg initially followed by 0.1-0.2 mg every 2-3 min as needed. Caution: Naloxone can result in a surge in sympathetic tone, hypertension, and ultimately pulmonary edema, in some cases

CHF, congestive heart failure; CNS, central nervous system; COPD, chronic obstructive pulmonary disease; GABA, gamma-aminobutyric acid.

associated with VT or VF, high-energy defibrillation (ie, 200 J max with a biphasic defibrillator; 360 J max with a monophasic defibrillator) should be used. There is no benefit and the potential to cause harm in using greater than 360 J.

Transthoracic cardioversion must deliver an adequate current to compensate for transthoracic impedance. High transthoracic impedance, defined as the resistance of the chest to the flow of electrical current, degrades current flow through the heart. Obesity

TABLE 135-6 Energy Selection for Cardioversion of Commonly Encountered Arrhythmias

Arrhythmia	Energy Output (J) Monophasic	Energy Output (J) Biphasic	Synchronized	Success Rate
AF	Initial shock: 200. Subsequent shocks: 200-360. Median energy required in studies = 200 >200 may be required, particularly of AF of long duration	Initial: 120. Subsequent shocks: 120-200. Median energy required in studies = 100	Yes	75%-94%
AFL	Initial shock: 50. Subsequent shocks: 50-200. Median energy required in studies = 200	Median energy required in studies = 50	Yes	90%-100%
AVNRT, AVRT	Initial shock: 50. Subsequent shocks: 50-200	Not reported	Yes	Not reported
Stable VT	Initial shock: 100. Subsequent shocks: 100-200	Initial shock: 50. Subsequent shocks: 50-100	Yes	>90%

AF, atrial fibrillation; AFL, atrial flutter; AT, atrial tachycardia; AVNRT, atrioventricular nodal reciprocating tachycardia; AVRT, atrioventricular reciprocating tachycardia; VT, ventricular tachycardia.

and severe obstructive lung disease increase impedance. Measures to reduce impedance include applying pressure to the pads, shocking during end-expiration, improving skin-electrode interface and the use of conducting gels. Care should be taken to ensure that a nonconducting barrier (eg, a double gloved hand or dry towel) exists between the clinician applying pressure to the electrode pads to avoid injury from inadvertent return current pathway. The repeat administration of shocks also lowers impedance and improves efficacy of cardioversion. Conversely, increasing the distance between electrodes or increasing the amount of tissue or lung parenchyma between the electrodes increases impedance.

■ SYNCHRONIZATION

A rhythm strip should confirm the rhythm and synchronization with the QRS complex. If the QRS is low amplitude or synchronization occurs with the T-wave, the lead used for monitoring and synchronization on the cardioverter defibrillator should be switched until appropriate synchronization with each QRS complex is confirmed. The accidental delivery of an electrical shock to the T-wave may result in life-threatening ventricular arrhythmias (ie, torsades de Pointes). For this reason, synchronized cardioversion, rather than nonsynchronized defibrillation, should be used to treat hemodynamically stable arrhythmias (**Figure 135-3**). The mode must be switched to asynchronous if defibrillation is intended, as the lack of an identifiable QRS complex will prevent the cardioverter defibrillator from discharging in the synchronous mode.

■ SHOCK DELIVERY

Shock delivery involves the following sequential steps: positioning electrode pads, selecting the appropriate energy and mode (synchronized or nonsynchronized), confirming adequacy of patient sedation, charging the cardioverter defibrillator capacitors, reminding all staff to stand clear of the patient, and finally, charging and delivering the shock. The patient is examined for adequacy of airway, breathing, and circulation, and a 12-lead ECG confirms the rhythm. The procedure can be repeated as necessary with higher-energy shocks and/or changing the electrode pad position if the first attempt is unsuccessful until the arrhythmia terminates or a decision is made to abandon electrical cardioversion.

EFFICACY OF CARDIOVERSION

The overall immediate success rate of electrical cardioversion with AF is 75% to 94% and is inversely proportional to the duration of AF and size of the left atrium (Table 135-6). After electrical cardioversion only 20% to 40% of patients maintain sinus rhythm for the first year compared to 29% to 53% in patients treated with antiarrhythmic drugs before electrical cardioversion and throughout

follow-up. Most recurrences of AF occur within the first month after electrical cardioversion. Pretreatment with antiarrhythmic drugs (eg, amiodarone, flecanide, ibutilide, propafenone or sotalol), may enhance the success of electrical cardioversion and prevent recurrent AF. Pretreatment with pharmacological agents may have the greatest efficacy in patients who fail to respond to cardioversion and in those who develop acute or subacute recurrence of AF. In addition, prophylactic antiarrhythmic drug therapy may obviate the need for electrical cardioversion or reduce the energy required for the procedure by lowering the cardioversion threshold. In randomized trials of electrical cardioversion, patients pretreated with intravenous ibutilide were more often converted to sinus rhythm compared to untreated controls. In addition, patients in whom cardioversion initially failed could more often be converted when the procedure was repeated after treatment with ibutilide.

PHARMACOLOGIC CARDIOVERSION

Although pharmacologic and electrical cardioversion have not been directly compared, pharmacologic approaches appear simpler but are less effective. The major risk is related to the toxicity of antiarrhythmic drugs such as drug-induced torsades de pointes. Medications indicated for the pharmacologic cardioversion of AF less than or equal to 7 days' duration include flecanide, dofetilide, propafenone, ibutilide, or amiodarone. Pharmacologic cardioversion of AF present for more than 7 days includes dofetilide, amiodarone, or ibutilide.

Ibutilide, a class III antiarrhythmic drug (potassium-channel blocker), prolongs the time for repolarization in atrial and ventricular myocardium. Approved for the acute termination of AF/AFL of recent onset, it is more effective for conversion of AFL. The 2014 practice guidelines from ACC/AHA/ESC recommend intravenous ibutilide for the pharmacologic cardioversion of AF/AFL provided there are no contraindications to the medication (class I recommendation). In most patients who respond to ibutilide, arrhythmia terminates within 40 to 60 minutes after initiating the infusion. Ibutilide has a conversion rate of up to 75% to 80% in recent-onset AF and AFL; the conversion rate is higher for atrial flutter than for atrial fibrillation. Ibutilide has a 4% risk of torsades de pointes and should be avoided in patients with heart failure, uncorrected hypokalemia or hypomagnesemia, or prolonged QT interval.

Ibutilide should be administered with continuous ECG monitoring at a dose of 0.01 mg/kg infused over 10 minutes for patients weighing less than 60 kg and at a dose of 1 mg over 10 minutes for patients weighing more than 60 kg. If the arrhythmia does not terminate 10 minutes after the end of the infusion, a second bolus (same dose over 10 minutes) can be given. The infusion should be stopped when the presenting arrhythmia is terminated or the

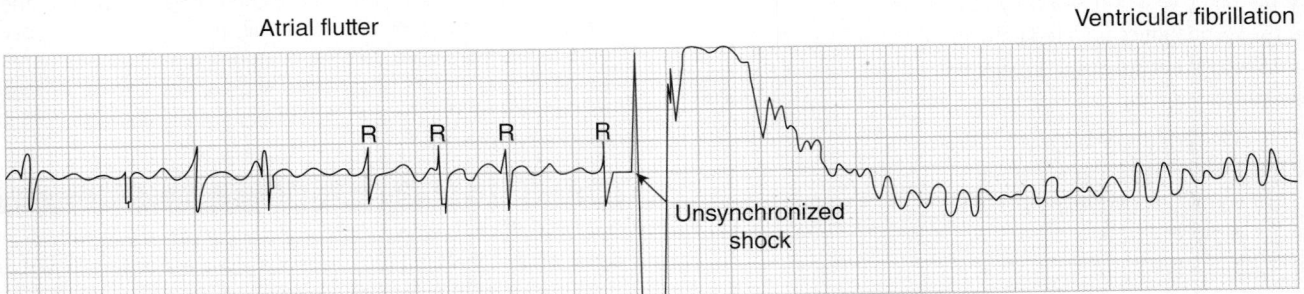

Figure 135-3 *A complication of cardioversion: induction of ventricular fibrillation. The ventricular arrhythmia occurred because the operator failed to enable the synchronizer, resulting in an inadvertent delivery of the shock on the vulnerable T-wave instead of the intended delivery on the R-wave. This complication is preventable by enabling the synchronizer and checking that it is properly functioning before shock delivery.* (From, with permission, Kerber RE. Transchest cardioversion: optimal techniques. In: Tacker WA, ed. *Defibrillation of the Heart: ICDs, AEDs and Manual*. St. Louis, MO: Mosby-Year Book, 1994:164.)

patient develops sustained or nonsustained VT or marked prolongation of the QT interval. Because of the risk of QT prolongation and arrhythmias, patients treated with ibutilide should be observed with continuous ECG monitoring for at least 4 hours after the infusion or until the QT_c interval has returned to baseline. There is no evidence that the risk of thromboembolism with pharmacologic cardioversion differs from electrical cardioversion. Recommendations for anticoagulation are therefore the same for both methods.

COMPLICATIONS

Complications after electrical cardioversion are uncommon but can be serious and are mainly related to thromboembolism and arrhythmias (**Table 135-7**).

■ THROMBOEMBOLISM

Pulmonary and systemic embolization may occur after cardioversion (spontaneous, pharmacologic, or electrical) if an embolus becomes dislodged from the atria as the heart begins to contract normally. Age, female gender, CHF, and diabetes mellitus are independent predictors of embolism. If patients with AF/AFL are appropriately anticoagulated for 3 to 4 weeks before cardioversion, the incidence of thromboembolism is 0.5% to 0.8%, with similar incidence in TEE-guided cardioversion. The risk of thromboembolism is highest in patients with rheumatic (or other) mitral stenosis,

TABLE 135-7 Complications (and Incidence When Known) of Electrical Cardioversion

Electrocardiographic changes
   ST segment depression (35%)
   ST segment elevation (15%-19%)
   T wave changes
Arrhythmia and conduction abnormalities
   Premature atrial contractions
   Premature ventricular contractions
   SVT (primarily sinus tachycardia) (30%)
   Bradycardia (25%)
   Left bundle branch block
   Sinus arrest
   High-degree atrioventricular heart block (15%)
   NSVT (5%)
   VT
   VF (usually the result of an asynchronous shock)
Embolization (pulmonary and systemic)
   1%-5% nonanticoagulated patients
   0.5%-0.8% anticoagulated patients
Myocardial necrosis
Myocardial dysfunction
   Atrial stunning
   Left ventricular dysfunction
Transient hypotension
Pulmonary edema rare
Airway compromise
Painful skin burns (20%-25%)
Physical trauma rare

NSVT, nonsustained ventricular tachycardia; SVT, supraventricular tachycardia; VF, ventricular fibrillation; VT, ventricular tachycardia.

large left atrium, chronic AF, diabetes, hypertension and prior cardiac embolic stroke.

■ ARRHYTHMIAS

Premature atrial or ventricular beats are not uncommon after cardioversion, and atrial arrhythmias, primarily sinus tachycardia, are seen in up to 30% of patients. Bradycardia occurs in up to 25% of patients immediately after cardioversion since cardioversion increases vagal tone. In one study of 75 patients undergoing cardioversion, sinus bradycardia occurred in 18 patients (24%), high-degree atrioventricular block occurred in 11 (15%), and temporary pacing was required in 10 (13%). Nonsustained VT occurs in up to 5% of patients, including those without structural heart disease. Patients receiving antiarrhythmic drugs are more prone to develop bradycardia and asystole post cardioversion. Temporary transthoracic pacing should be readily available at the time of cardioversion. The occurrence of ventricular arrhythmias does not appear to be related to the number of shocks and cannot be prevented by antiarrhythmic therapy. Electrolyte imbalances, such as hypokalemia, and digitalis toxicity increase the risk of ventricular tachyarrhythmias.

AIRWAY COMPROMISE

Oversedation occurs most frequently in the elderly and in patients with renal and hepatic impairment and can cause respiratory depression. Dose adjustment should be considered in those populations. The patient's airway and oxygenation should be monitored carefully until complete recovery. Reversal agents for opiates and benzodiazepines should be readily available during the procedure.

CHEST WALL INJURY AND SKIN BURNS

First-degree skin burns of the chest wall have been described with electrical cardioversion. In order to reduce the frequency and severity of burns, good skin-electrode interface should be confirmed, liberal conductive gel utilized (when using handheld paddles), and the lowest effective amount of energy should be used. Skin burns are more likely with improper technique and placement of electrodes. The incidence of skin burns has been substantially reduced with the use of pregelled pads and biphasic defibrillators.

ELECTROCARDIOGRAPHIC CHANGES AND MYOCARDIAL INJURY

Electrocardiographic changes, including ST segment and T-wave changes, can occur immediately after cardioversion. The frequency and extent of ST segment changes are lower with biphasic defibrillators. Electrocardiogram findings are nonspecific, typically resolve within 5 minutes, and should not be used as the sole criteria for identifying an acute ischemic event. The pathogenesis of ST elevation is uncertain since elevations in creatine kinase MB isoenzyme or troponin are uncommon and are usually minimal when they occur. Some myocardial tissue damage or stunning may occur as a result of high-energy shocks or repeated shocks. Any decline in cardiac function after cardioversion is typically temporary and does not produce symptoms.

INJURIES TO THE OPERATOR

Operator injuries during cardioversion occur very rarely, with an incidence of less than 1 in 1700. Cases of major electrocution have been described in extremely rare instances and have all been associated with equipment failure.

PHYSICAL TRAUMA TO THE PATIENT

Physical trauma to the patient is a rare complication and results from vigorous body movements during the delivery of the electric shock.

TROUBLESHOOTING

Failure of the monitor to work properly typically reflects a mechanical problem. The power source, lead connections, ECG leads and electrode pads should be checked and confirmed. If the timing artifact during synchronization mode falls on the T-wave, the monitoring lead should be changed until the correct position of the timing artifact is confirmed on the QRS complex. If the capacitor fails to discharge, this probably represents a failure to identify a QRS complex while in synchronized mode. The monitoring lead should be switched, synchronization on the QRS complex confirmed, and cardioversion reattempted.

CARDIOVERSION UNSUCCESSFUL

Important factors that determine the immediate and long-term success of cardioversion of atrial arrhythmias include the duration of the arrhythmia, the extent of atrial fibrosis, the size of the left atrium, and underlying structural heart disease (**Table 135-8**). If cardioversion is unsuccessful, a repeat ECG should be obtained to confirm the underlying rhythm. Next, the cardioversion telemetry strips should be carefully examined to distinguish between true failure to cardiovert and successful cardioversion that is followed by recurrence of arrhythmia. Patients with recurrence of arrhythmia might benefit from antiarrhythmic therapy before repeat attempts at cardioversion. For patients who truly fail to cardiovert, a higher level of energy, an alternate electrode pad configuration, or a biphasic device can be used on repeat attempts. In patients in whom AF recurs acutely or cardioversion fails, the combination of AV nodal blocker plus intravenous loading with amiodarone, procainamide, or ibutilide may pharmacologically restore sinus rhythm. If the AF persists, repeat cardioversion can be performed, and if successful the patient may be placed on long-term antiarrhythmic therapy. Electrolyte disturbances, digitalis toxicity, and thyrotoxicosis may result in failure to cardiovert and should be corrected prior to cardioversion.

PREGNANCY

Successful cardioversion has been performed in all three trimesters of pregnancy without adverse consequences to the mother or fetus. Cardioversion does not affect the rhythm of the fetus though it is recommended that the fetal heart rhythm be monitored during the procedure.

IMPLANTABLE PACEMAKERS AND CARDIOVERTER DEFIBRILLATORS

Several precautions are necessary when performing cardioversion in a patient with a permanent implanted device (pacemaker or ICD). Electrical cardioversion may change the settings of the device and may damage the pulse generator, the lead system, or myocardial tissue resulting in device dysfunction. To prevent this, the electrode pads should be placed at least 15 cm from the implanted device, preferably in the anterior-posterior position. Elective cardioversion should be initiated at low energies to reduce the risk of damage. The implantable device should be interrogated before and after cardioversion to ensure normal device function. When these precautions are employed, cardioversion with either monophasic or biphasic shocks is safe and effective in patients with implantable devices. In patients who are pacemaker-dependent, cardiology consultation is recommended prior to attempt at cardioversion given the potentially dire consequences of pacemaker malfunction in this context.

CONSULTATION

In 2000, an ACC/AHA task force on clinical competency published recommendations for technical and cognitive skills needed to perform external electrical cardioversion. The ACC/AHA also recommends that the minimum training necessary for competence to perform external electrical cardioversion should include competence in the interpretation of 12-lead ECGs. Previous ACC/AHA task forces recommended a minimum of eight supervised electrical cardioversions as a minimum requirement. The competence in electrical cardioversion may be achievable without formal training in cardiovascular disease. Cardiac consultation is advised for physicians without adequate experience with electrical cardioversion. Cardiology referral for initiation of an antiarrhythmic drug, if required, may also be indicated unless the physician is experienced with and knowledgeable of administration of these drugs. Because most antiarrhythmic agents can also be proarrhythmic and because many have dangerous side effects to monitor, their initiation and maintenance should be performed by a clinician experienced in their use.

QUALITY IMPROVEMENT TO ADDRESS PERFORMANCE GAPS

SECONDARY PREVENTION

Maintenance therapy with antiarrhythmic drugs is not typically recommended after electrical cardioverson in patients with a first episode of AF, particularly those at low risk for recurrence (eg, short duration and normal left atrial size) or those with a reversible cause (eg, cardiac surgery, pulmonary embolus, or hyperthyroidism). In other patients with recurrent paroxysmal or persistent AF, maintenance antiarrhythmic drug therapy may be administered to reduce the risk of recurrence if a rhythm control strategy is chosen. Because of the adverse effects associated with antiarrhythmic drugs and apparent lack of mortality benefit from a rhythm control strategy, many authorities reserve the use of long-term antiarrhythmic drug therapy to patients that remain symptomatic with rate control.

TRANSITIONS OF CARE

After cardioversion, all patients should receive oral anticoagulation with warfarin or TSOAC therapy for at least 4 weeks. A plan for anticoagulation and follow-up with INR monitoring with a primary physician, cardiologist or specialized anticoagulation clinic should be established. Patients with AF deemed to be at high risk for thromboembolic events may require longer-term anticoagulation. Patients with new-onset AF should undergo thyroid function testing and receive an echocardiogram. Patients with no recurrence follow up with their primary care physicians as outpatients and do not require any additional testing. Patients with either recurrent, symptomatic AF (despite attempts at rate control) or patients who prefer a rhythm control strategy should be referred to a cardiologist.

TABLE 135-8 Factors Associated with Failed Cardioversion of Atrial Fibrillation

- Structural heart disease (eg, congestive heart failure, valvular disease)
- Underlying illness (eg, thyrotoxicosis)
- Dilated left atrium
- Extent of atrial fibrosis
- Longer duration of atrial fibrillation
- Too low energy
- Technique

SUGGESTED READINGS

Botto GL, Politi A, Bonini W, et al. External cardioversion of atrial fibrillation: role of paddle position on technical efficacy and energy requirements. *Heart*. 1999;82:726-730.

January CT, Wann LS, Alpert JS, et al. 2014 AHA/ACC/HRS Guideline for the management of patients with atrial fibrillation: executive summary: a report of the American College of Cardiology/American Heart Association Task Force on Practice Guidelines and the Heart Rhythm Society. *J Am Coll Cardiol*. 2014;64:2246-2280.

Kerber RE. Indications and techniques of electrical defibrillation and cardioversion. In: Fuster V, O'Rourke RA, Walsh RA, Poole-Wilson P, eds. *Hurst's the Heart*, 12th ed. New York, NY: McGraw-Hill; 2008:1102-1108.

Klein AL, Grimm RA, Murray RD, et al. Assessment of cardioversion using transesophageal echocardiography investigators. Use of transesophageal echocardiography to guide cardioversion in patients with atrial fibrillation. *N Engl J Med*. 2001;344:1411-1420.

Manegold JC, Israel CW, Ehrlich JR, et al. External cardioversion of atrial fibrillation in patients with implanted pacemaker or cardioverter-defibrillator systems: a randomized comparison of monophasic and biphasic shock energy application. *Eur Heart J*. 2007;28:1731-1738.

Niebauer MJ, Brewer JE, Chung MK, et al. Comparison of the rectilinear biphasic waveform with the monophasic damped sine waveform for external cardioversion of atrial fibrillation and flutter. *Am J Cardiol*. 2004;93:1495-1499.

Oral H, Souza JJ, Michaud GF, et al. Facilitating transthoracic cardioversion of atrial fibrillation with ibutilide pretreatment. *N Engl J Med*. 1999;340:1849-1854.

Stambler BS, Wood MA, Ellenbogen KA, et al. Efficacy and safety of repeated intravenous doses of ibutilide for rapid conversion of atrial flutter or fibrillation. Ibutilide Repeat Dose Study Investigators. *Circulation*. 1996;94:1613-1621.

Tracy CM, Akhtar M, DiMarco JP, et al. American College of Cardiology/American Heart Association clinical competence statement on invasive electrophysiology studies, catheter ablation, and cardioversion: a report of the American College of Cardiology/American Heart Association/American College of Physicians–American Society of Internal Medicine task force on clinical competence. *Circulation*. 2000;102:2309-2320.

CHAPTER 136

Pacemakers, Defibrillators, and Cardiac Resynchronization Devices in Hospital Medicine

Michael H. Hoskins, MD
David B. De Lurgio, MD

Key Clinical Questions

1. What are the components of an implantable pacing or defibrillation system?
2. How do pacemakers interact with the heart's natural rhythm to know when to and when not to pace?
3. What do the common pacing codes (ie, VVI, DDD) mean, and how do they affect the electrocardiogram (ECG)?
4. When should patients be referred for cardiac resynchronization therapy (CRT)?
5. How should clinicians evaluate the patient who has received an implantable cardiac defibrillator (ICD) shock?
6. When should a pacemaker or ICD be interrogated in the inpatient setting?

INTRODUCTION

Advances in technology and the expansion of indications have greatly increased the numbers of patients receiving pacemakers and implantable cardiac defibrillators (ICDs). Approximately 200,000 pacemakers and 100,000 defibrillators are implanted annually for the management of cardiac arrhythmias, treatment of congestive heart failure, and the prevention of sudden cardiac death. These devices have progressed from relatively simple components with basic pacing and defibrillation features, to more advanced systems with a significant impact on patient morbidity and mortality. The increasing number and complexity of devices encountered in hospitalized patients frequently presents a clinical management challenge. The purpose of this chapter is to introduce basic concepts of pacing and defibrillation, review standard indications for cardiac rhythm devices, and highlight pertinent clinical considerations for hospitalist care of patients with these devices.

EQUIPMENT AND HARDWARE

Cardiac pacing and defibrillating systems consist of pulse generators and leads. The pulse generator is the "device" that contains the battery, circuitry, and capacitors. It is typically encased in a titanium housing that ranges in size and shape depending on the manufacturer. Defibrillator pulse generators are about 2 to 3 times larger than pacemakers (**Figure 136-1**).

The leads are connected to the pulse generator at the time of implant and are attached distally to the myocardium. They are secured to the myocardium either "actively" by means of a small screw or "passively" by means of small tines near the lead tip. Pacemaker leads consist of conducting wires, a silicone or polyurethane insulation coating, and platinum electrodes used for pacing. Defibrillation leads have one or two additional wire coils capable of delivering high-voltage impulses for defibrillation (**Figure 136-2**).

Many of the long-term complications related to cardiac rhythm devices are specific to transvenous leads. These complications include infection, malfunction, or venous stenosis. Lead extraction required as a result of these complications is associated with potentially serious adverse outcomes. Consequently, important recent advancements in cardiac rhythm device technology include the development of leadless pacemakers and subcutaneous defibrillators.

Leadless pacemakers are currently in clinical trial use, but may be encountered in the inpatient setting. These devices are similar in shape and size to a large vitamin and are inserted directly into the right ventricular apex. They are attached to the myocardium either actively or passively, similar to standard leads. These small devices contain the entire pacemaker system, including the battery, circuitry, and electrodes. Recently published data has demonstrated that they are a safe and effective alternative to standard devices. Currently, only ventricular pacing can be obtained with these devices (**Figure 136-3**).

Subcutaneous defibrillators are an alternative to standard defibrillators that offer the advantage of eliminating the need for transvenous leads. These devices are implanted in the subcutaneous tissue in the left thorax in the midaxillary region. The lead for this device is then tunneled in the subcutaneous space anteriorly toward the xiphoid process, then superiorly toward the sternal notch. These devices are safe and effective in the detection and treatment of ventricular tachyarrhythmias. However, they have limited pacing capabilities (**Figure 136-4**).

1025

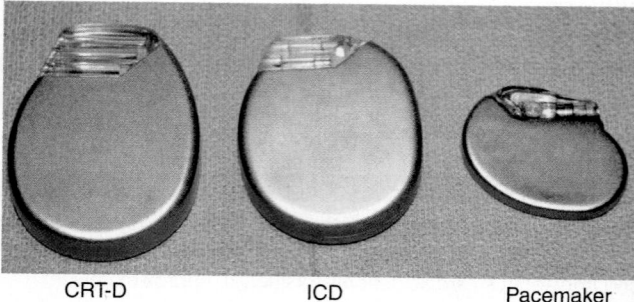

CRT-D   ICD   Pacemaker

Figure 136-1 *Examples of cardiac resynchronization therapy with defibrillator (CRT-D), implantable cardiac defibrillator (ICD), and pacemaker devices. Note the size difference between the defibrillator and pacemaker devices.*

Another important advancement in cardiac rhythm device technology is the development of "MRI-conditional" pacemakers. These devices have unique construction characteristics that potentially make them safer for patients to undergo MRIs. Currently, only MRI-conditional pacemakers have been approved by the FDA. MRI-conditional defibrillators are currently being evaluated in clinical trials. Standard cardiac rhythm devices may be able to safely pass through an MRI scanner, but this practice should be limited to specific circumstances and done under the guidance of an electrophysiologist.

Technologic advancements in the field of cardiac rhythm devices have resulted in smaller batteries with increased lifespans. Most batteries used in modern devices are lithium-based and are non-rechargeable with a finite lifespan. Typically, a pacemaker battery will last approximately 10 years, while an ICD battery will last approximately 8 years. Once exhausted, these batteries must be exchanged.

PRACTICE POINT

- Pacemaker batteries will last approximately 10 years, while an ICD battery will last approximately 8 years. Once exhausted, these batteries must be exchanged.

Battery longevity depends on several factors, the most important of which include pacing output, the relative amount of time pacing is required, and the number of programmable features that are activated on the device. Furthermore, frequent ICD therapies represent a common cause for battery drain. The cardiologist managing the patient will tailor device programming to maximize battery life without sacrificing the clinical function of the device.

The remaining life of a battery is displayed each time the device is interrogated. As battery life declines, the device will enter a period

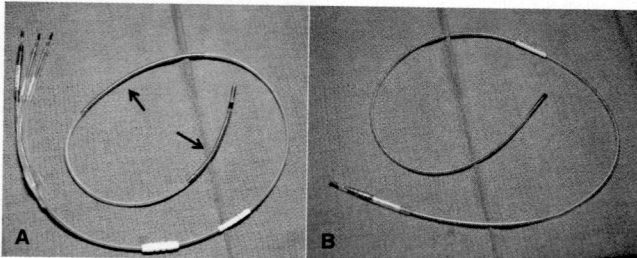

Figure 136-2 *Examples of (A) an implantable cardiac defibrillator (ICD) lead and (B) a pacemaker lead. Note the high-voltage defibrillation coils on the ICD lead (indicated by arrows).*

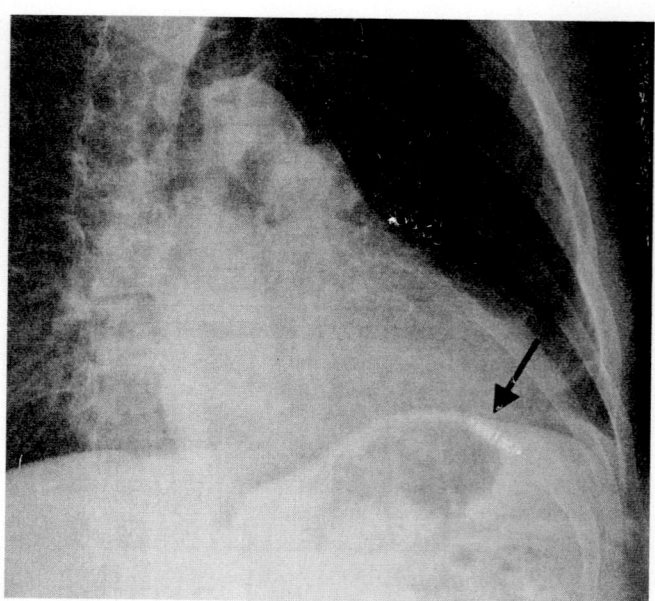

Figure 136-3 *Chest x-ray showing a leadless pacemaker inserted in the right ventricular apex (arrow).*

called *elective replacement interval* (ERI). This alerts the physician that there are approximately 2 to 3 months of remaining battery life and the patient should be scheduled for elective replacement of the device. Further depletion of the battery will lead to the *end-of-life* (EOL) period, an indication that the battery should be replaced as soon as possible. Importantly, as batteries enter the ERI and EOL periods, certain features of the device will automatically turn off to preserve as much battery life as possible. This may result in a reduction in the clinical benefit a patient receives from the device.

BASIC PACING CONCEPTS

■ SENSING AND PACING

The two primary functions of pacemakers are *sensing* and *pacing*. Sensing refers to the ability of the device to detect native impulses originating from the heart. These sensed events are used to time subsequent events based on programmable settings. The ability of the device to sense a native impulse depends on the amplitude of the electrical signal generated by the heart, as seen by the device. *Undersensing* occurs when the amplitude of the signal is insufficient for detection by the pacemaker and results in inappropriate pacing by the device (**Figure 136-5**). *Oversensing* occurs when the device inappropriately interprets signals as native impulses. Oversensing leads to inappropriate inhibition of pacing and may occur as a result of internal or external "noise" detected by the device (**Figure 136-6**). When oversensing occurs in an ICD, the device can misinterpret the signals as a ventricular arrhythmia and inappropriately shock the patient.

PRACTICE POINT

- *Undersensing* occurs when the amplitude of the signal is insufficient for detection by the pacemaker and results in inappropriate pacing by the device (Figure 3). *Oversensing* occurs when the device inappropriately interprets signals as native impulses. Oversensing leads to inappropriate inhibition of pacing and may occur as a result of internal or external "noise" detected by the device (Figure 4).

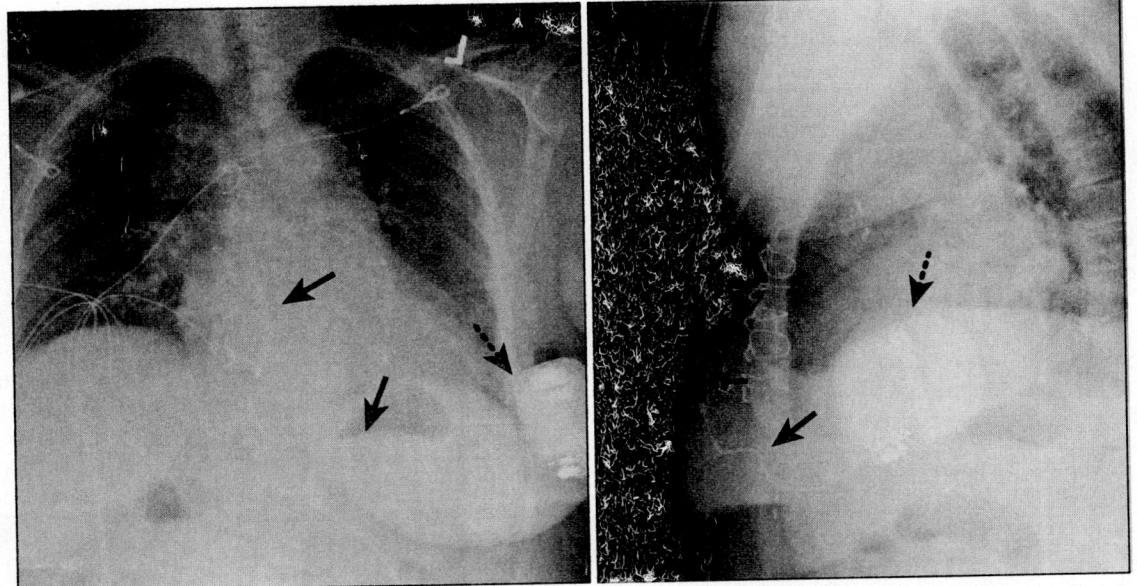

Figure 136-4 *PA and lateral chest x-rays showing position of a subcutaneous defibrillator device (dashed arrow) and lead (bold arrows).*

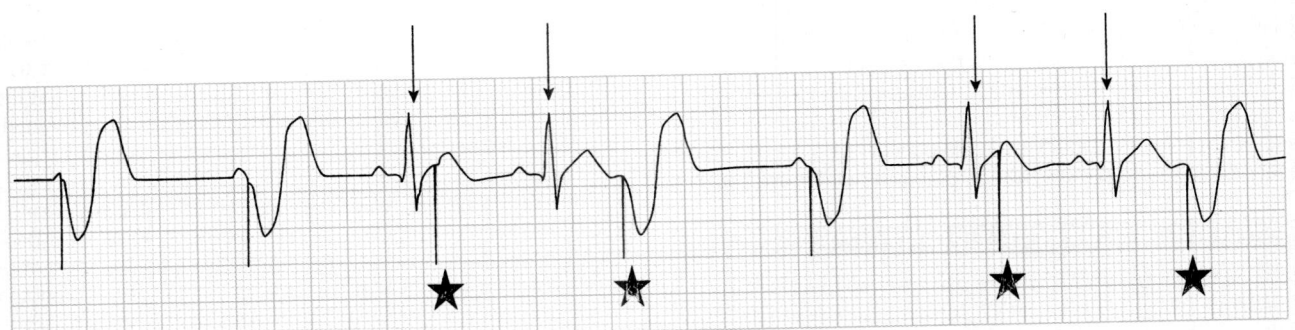

Figure 136-5 *Ventricular undersensing. The QRS complexes marked with arrows are not sensed by the pacemaker. As a result, the device continues to deliver pacing stimuli inappropriately (stars).*

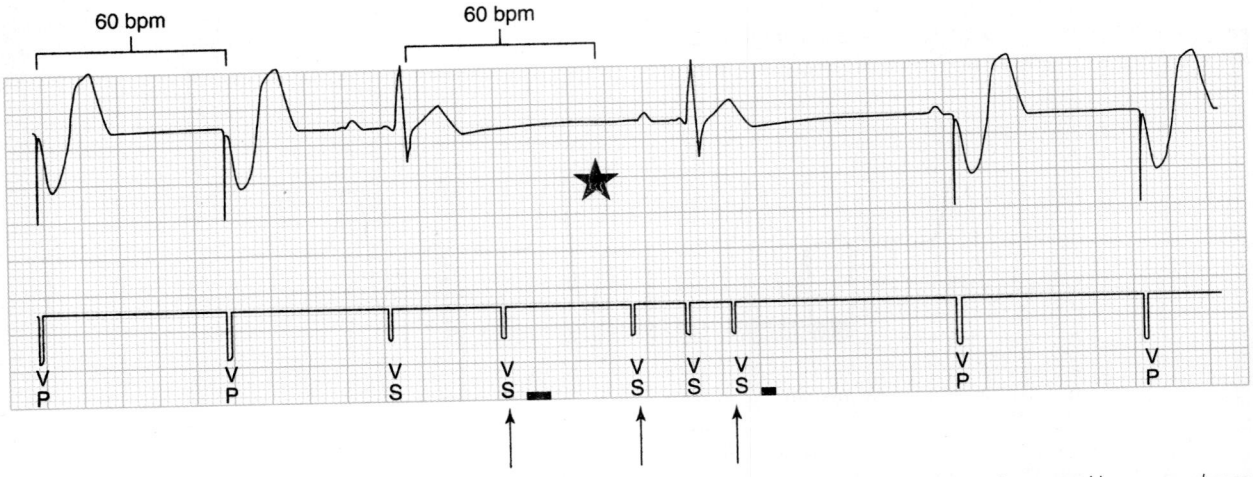

Figure 136-6 *Ventricular oversensing. This device is programmed VVI with a lower rate limit of 60 bpm. The markers noted by arrows show where ventricular oversensing occurs (VS). This causes an inhibition of pacing. Had oversensing not occurred, pacing would have occurred at the point marked by the star.*

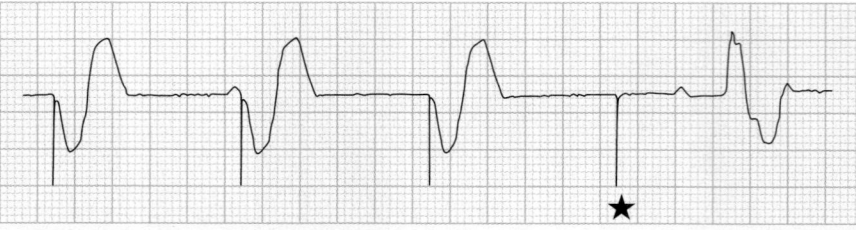

Figure 136-7 *Failure to capture. Ventricular pacing spikes precede the first three QRS complexes. The fourth pacing spike (star) fails to capture the ventricle and is not followed by a QRS complex.*

Pacing output is the electrical stimulation that results in myocardial depolarization and contraction of the heart. The minimal amount of electrical energy required to cause depolarization is termed the *capture threshold* and is a function of the electrode-tissue interface. Pacing output is programmed sufficiently above the capture threshold to provide an adequate safety margin. This output is seen on surface electrocardiograms as a discrete "spike," called a pacing stimulus artifact. Importantly, modern devices with bipolar pacing and low energy outputs can generate a relatively small stimulus artifact that may be difficult to see on surface tracings. Careful attention to the tracing will usually reveal these small artifacts.

When insufficient energy is delivered by the device, the electrical stimulus may fail to depolarize the myocardium. This is called *failure to capture*. It is recognized when a pacing stimulus artifact is not followed by a P-wave or QRS complex (depending on which chamber is being paced), and occurs as a result of either inappropriately low output or poor electrode-tissue interface from lead dislodgement. Failure to capture is relatively uncommon in chronic devices with stable leads. When failure to capture occurs in patients who are pacemaker dependent, dangerously low heart rates may result (**Figure 136-7**).

> **PRACTICE POINT**
>
> - Failure to capture occurs when a pacing stimulus artifact is not followed by a P-wave or QRS complex (depending on which chamber is being paced) and occurs as a result of either inappropriately low output or poor electrode-tissue interface from lead dislodgement.

■ TIMING INTERVALS

There are multiple programmable intervals pacemakers use to determine when to deliver pacing output. The most important of these include *lower rate limit*, *AV interval*, and *upper rate limit* (**Figure 136-8**). The *lower rate limit* is the slowest rate that a pacemaker will allow the

heart to reach. When the heart rate drops below this rate, the pacemaker will begin pacing. However, as long as the heart rate exceeds this rate, pacing will not occur. Therefore, lack of pacing on a surface ECG in this instance does not indicate device malfunction.

> **PRACTICE POINT**
>
> - Pacemaker *lower rate limit* is the slowest rate that a pacemaker will allow the heart to reach. When the heart rate drops below this rate, the pacemaker will begin pacing. However, as long as the heart rate exceeds this rate, pacing will not occur.

The *AV (atrioventricular) interval* is the time allowed after an atrial event before ventricular pacing will occur. This is analogous to the PR interval. As long as native AV conduction occurs within this interval, ventricular pacing will be inhibited. However, if the AV interval expires before native AV conduction occurs, then ventricular pacing will occur.

The AV interval is typically programmed sufficiently long to promote native conduction, as chronic right ventricular pacing increases morbidity in certain patient populations. The most important exception to this is in the case of cardiac resynchronization in patients with biventricular pacemakers. In this situation, the AV interval is programmed relatively short, to provide the physiologic benefits of biventricular resynchronization.

The *upper rate limit* is a programmed rate above which the pacemaker will not pace. In patients with sinus or atrial tachycardia that exceeds the upper rate limit, the pacemaker will pace the ventricle only as fast as the upper rate limit. This may result in atrial events that are not followed by ventricular pacing and may lead to misinterpreting pacemaker function from the surface electrogram.

Most surface electrograms in patients with pacemakers can be explained by these basic pacing functions. However, there are an increasing number of programmable features in modern devices

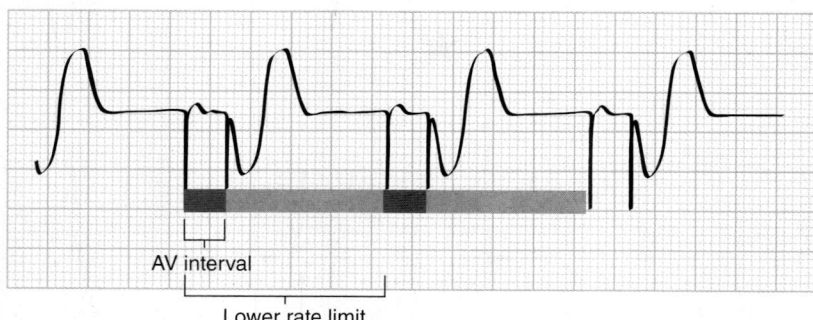

Figure 136-8 *Schematic demonstrating the concepts of lower rate limit and AV interval. This device is programmed DDD. An atrial event is not sensed before the lower rate limit expires, so atrial pacing occurs at the programmed rate. Native AV conduction does not occur within the programmed AV interval, so ventricular pacing occurs. See the text for details.*

designed to enhance overall pacing function. These features may mimic device malfunction in the form of oversensing, undersensing, or other strange phenomena, and may require the assistance of a cardiologist to interpret. While true device malfunction does occur, it is relatively uncommon. Apparent malfunction based on surface electrograms can usually be explained by normal device function.

■ NOMENCLATURE (NASPE CODES)

One common source of confusion is interpretation of the nomenclature used to describe pacemaker function. The current system in use was revised in 2002 by the North American Society of Pacing and Electrophysiology (NASPE) and uses a letter system to describe pacemaker function (**Table 136-1**). The first and second letters are used to identify the chamber(s) in which there is pacing and sensing, respectively. The third letter indicates the effect of sensing on subsequent pacing stimuli. Sensed events can induce (trigger) pacing, inhibit pacing, or both.

Modern pacemakers also have mechanisms to detect patient activity and increase the pacing rate accordingly to compensate for increased physiologic demands. This is particularly useful in patients with chronotropic incompetence who cannot increase their heart rate on their own. Depending on the manufacturer, patient activity may be sensed either by physical motion or changes in minute ventilation. When this feature is activated, a fourth letter, R (for Rate response), is used in the pacing code.

Most modern devices have the ability to pace in all modes, as long as they are connected to both the atrium and ventricle. The most commonly used modes are described below:

AAI/VVI

AAI and VVI modes function to pace and sense only in the atrium or ventricle respectively. The "I" in the third letter position refers to the fact that sensed events in a given chamber will inhibit pacing in that chamber. For instance, in AAI mode, if the atrial lead senses a native atrial depolarization, the pacemaker will inhibit pacing until the lower rate limit is exceeded. If a subsequent atrial event has not been sensed within that time, pacing will occur.

AAI mode is typically used for patients with isolated sinus node dysfunction to prevent sinus bradycardia or sinus pauses. The device will pace the atrium at a programmed lower rate unless the sinus node rate exceeds the lower rate limit. This mode has the benefit of limiting ventricular pacing but requires intact AV conduction. Similarly, VVI mode is used to pace and sense only in the ventricle. This mode is usually used as a "back-up" mode to prevent the heart rate from dropping below a programmed lower rate. It is commonly used in patients with permanent atrial fibrillation and high-grade or complete AV block.

DDD

Pacemakers in DDD mode offer the ability to pace and sense in both chambers. This mode provides the benefit of maintaining AV synchrony. DDD mode is programmed with lower and upper rate limits. A native atrial (sinus) impulse that occurs before the lower rate limit has "timed-out" is sensed by the device. If a native impulse does not occur in this time, an atrial pacing stimulus is delivered. The device then waits for native AV conduction, with a subsequent ventricular sensed event, to occur within a programmed AV interval. If a ventricular sensed event does not occur within this period, a ventricular pacing stimulus is delivered. **Figure 136-9** illustrates the various ways DDD pacing can manifest on the EKG.

VOO

VOO mode is often referred to as "asynchronous" pacing. This mode will pace the ventricle at a programmed rate, whether or not a native ventricular impulse occurs. Sensing (and thus inhibition) does not occur. This mode is typically used to prevent inappropriate inhibition (ie, from electromagnetic interference) in the pacemaker-dependent patient. It is commonly used during surgery in pacemaker-dependent patients to avoid inhibition of pacing caused by noise from electrocautery devices.

DEVICE INDICATIONS

■ PACEMAKERS

Multiple common cardiac conditions serve as indications for permanent pacemaker implantation for patients with sinus and/or AV node dysfunction (**Table 136-2**).

The indications for permanent pacemaker implantation relate primarily to bradycardia caused by sinus and/or AV node dysfunction. In general, permanent pacemakers should be considered in patients with sinus node dysfunction only when the patient is symptomatic as a result of bradycardia. Sinus node dysfunction that manifests as symptomatic sinus bradycardia, sinus pauses, or chronotropic incompetence (inability of the sinus node to adequately accelerate in response to physical activity) are Class I indications for pacing. Additionally, when drugs (ie, β-blockers) that may result in symptomatic sinus bradycardia are required for other indications, pacing should be considered.

The indications for cardiac pacing in patients with AV node disease are more varied. Similar to sinus node dysfunction, pacing is generally used in symptomatic patients. However, in the case of AV node disease, permanent pacemakers are required in certain conditions even in asymptomatic patients. For instance, patients with third-degree AV block or type 2 second-degree AV block (Mobitz 2) should be considered for pacing regardless of symptoms. Even in patients with type 1 second-degree AV block (Mobitz 1 or Wenkebach) pacing should be used if the patient is symptomatic. Occasionally, evaluation of the AV conduction system during electrophysiologic study is required to identify patients with advanced AV node disease. In this situation, certain criteria exist to suggest the need for pacing.

Slow AV conduction during atrial fibrillation is a common indication for permanent pacing. This may occur as a result of native

TABLE 136-1 Coding System for Pacemakers

I	II	III	IV	V
Chambers paced	Chambers sensed	Response to sensing	Rate modulation	Multisite pacing
O = None	O = None	O = None	O = None	O = None
A = Atrium	A = Atrium	T = Triggered	R = Rate modulation	A = Atrium
V = Ventricle	V = Ventricle	I = Inhibited		V = Ventricle
D = Dual (A+V)	D = Dual (A+V)	D = Dual (T = I)		D = Dual (A+V)

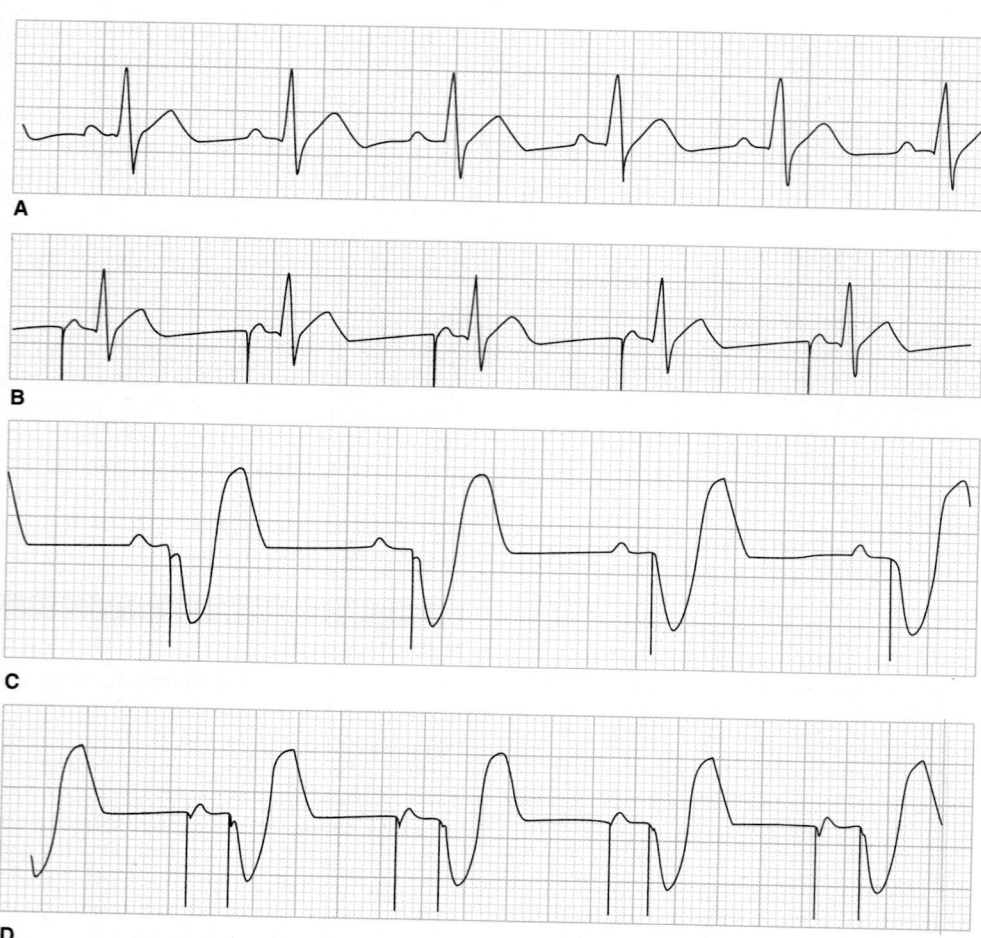

Figure 136-9 *Four appearances of DDD pacing. In each panel, the device is programmed DDD with a lower rate of 60 bpm and an AV interval of 200 ms. (A) The underlying sinus rate exceeds the lower rate limit, so atrial pacing does not occur. Native AV conduction is faster than 200 ms, so ventricular pacing does not occur. (B) The atrial rate has slowed to a rate below the lower rate limit, so atrial pacing occurs at 60 bpm. However, native AV conduction is still faster than 200 ms, so ventricular pacing does not occur. (C) The atrial rate exceeds the lower rate limit, so atrial pacing does not occur. However, native AV conduction is slower than the AV interval. Therefore, ventricular pacing occurs 200 ms after the atrial event is sensed. (D) Both the atrial rate and AV conduction are slower than the programmed intervals. Therefore, atrial pacing occurs at a rate of 60 bpm and ventricular pacing occurs 200 ms later.*

TABLE 136-2 Common Indications for Permanent Cardiac Pacemakers

Sinus node dysfunction

—Symptomatic sinus bradycardia

—Symptomatic sinus pauses

—Symptomatic chronotropic incompetence

—Required use of a medication that causes symptomatic sinus node dysfunction

Atrioventricular nodal dysfunction

—Symptomatic type I second-degree AV block (Mobitz I or Wenkebach)

—Type II second-degree AV block (Mobitz II)

—High-grade or complete AV block

—Atrial fibrillation with symptomatic slow ventricular response

—AV block caused by ablation of the AV node

—Required use of a medication that causes symptomatic AV nodal dysfunction

---

AV nodal disease, medications that slow AV conduction but are required for other indications, or iatrogenic ablation of the AV node for rapid ventricular rates. With the exception of patients who have undergone AV nodal ablation, pacing should be used only in patients who have symptoms from slow ventricular rates. However, in patients with atrial fibrillation and pauses of 5 seconds or longer, pacing is indicated even in the absence of symptoms.

■ DEFIBRILLATORS

Multiple cardiac conditions serve as common indications for ICD implantation (**Table 136-3**). ICDs were initially designed for patients who survived cardiac arrest from sustained ventricular tachycardia (VT) or ventricular fibrillation (VF). However, in the past two decades, indications for ICDs have expanded significantly. Multiple trials have established their superior mortality benefit when compared to antiarrhythmic medications for primary prevention of sudden cardiac arrest. Their current use can be divided into primary prevention of sudden cardiac arrest or secondary prevention for patients who have survived cardiac arrest from VT or VF.

The use of ICDs for primary prevention of sudden death is indicated in patients with ischemic or nonischemic cardiomyopathy,

TABLE 136-3 Common Indications for Implantable Cardiac Defibrillators

Primary prevention of sudden cardiac arrest

—Ischemic cardiomyopathy, EF <35%, NYHA class II-III, at least 40 d after myocardial infarction

—Ischemic cardiomyopathy, EF <30%, NYHA class I

—Nonischemic cardiomyopathy, EF <35%, NYHA class II-III

Secondary prevention of sudden cardiac arrest

—Survivors of sudden cardiac arrest from VF or sustained VT without reversible causes

—Structural heart disease and sustained VT

—Syncope with inducible hemodynamically significant VT of VF during EP study

Special patient populations

—Long QT syndrome with VT or syncope

—Brugada syndrome with VT or syncope

—Hypertrophic cardiomyopathy with risk factors for sudden cardiac arrest*

—Arrhythmogenic right ventricular dysplasia with risk factors for sudden cardiac arrest

*Risk factors include nonsustained VT, syncope, severe LVH, and hypotension with exercise.

ejection fraction less than or equal to 35%, and New York Heart Association (NYHA) class II-III heart failure symptoms. Patients with ejection fraction less than or equal to 30% and class I symptoms may also be candidates for ICD implantation. When properly selected, these patients experience a 25% to 30% relative reduction in mortality when implanted with an ICD. Primary prevention is the largest indication for ICDs and remains an important way for hospitalists to intervene on long-term patient outcome. When hospitalists encounter these patients, inpatient cardiology or electrophysiology consult can help determine if an ICD is appropriate.

Patients who have survived cardiac arrest from VT or VF should undergo ICD implantation regardless of the presence or absence of structural heart disease, unless a clearly reversible cause of the arrest can be identified and corrected. In patients with moderately reduced ejection fraction (≤40%), nonsustained VT, and inducible VT or VF during electrophysiologic study, ICD implantation is appropriate.

There are several considerations when timing ICD implantation. For patients with newly diagnosed nonischemic cardiomyopathy, the exact timing of ICD implantation varies. An ICD is indicated when the cardiomyopathy is nonreversible and patients are receiving appropriate heart failure medications. In patients with ischemic cardiomyopathy from myocardial infarction, ICDs should not be implanted within the first 40 days after the infarct. This recommendation is based on data that suggests no overall mortality benefit from ICDs implanted within this periinfarct period.

Other patient populations who may benefit from ICD therapy in certain situations include those with hypertrophic cardiomyopathy, long QT syndrome, Brugada syndrome, and cardiac sarcoid.

■ CARDIAC RESYNCHRONIZATION THERAPY

Patients with advanced heart failure and a severely reduced ejection fraction often have intraventricular conduction disturbances that result in mechanical "dyssynchrony" of the left ventricle. This dyssynchrony leads to inefficient ventricular contraction and increased maladaptive ventricular remodeling. Prolongation of the QRS duration (in particular, left bundle-branch block) is often used as an electrical surrogate for mechanical dyssynchrony. Many of these patients benefit from biventricular pacing (otherwise known as *cardiac resynchronization therapy* or CRT). Cardiac resynchronization is obtained by positioning a lead in the coronary sinus to pace the lateral wall of the left ventricle, in addition to the standard right ventricular lead. A CRT device can be programmed to pace the right and left ventricles at specific times to maximize cardiac output.

The ideal candidates for cardiac resynchronization include patients in sinus rhythm with ejection fractions <35%, NYHA class III symptoms, and left bundle-branch block with a QRS >120 ms. When patients are properly selected for this therapy, they experience approximately a 30% reduction in heart failure hospitalizations and mortality. Roughly two-thirds of patients who undergo CRT implantation will receive clinical benefit from this therapy.

PRACTICE POINT

- Candidates for cardiac resynchronization therapy (CRT) include patients in sinus rhythm with ejection fractions <35%, NYHA class III symptoms, *and* left bundle-branch block with a QRS >120 ms. When patients are properly selected for this therapy, they experience approximately a 30% reduction in heart failure hospitalizations and mortality.

Chronic right ventricular apical pacing may worsen heart failure symptoms and ejection fraction. Thus, another patient population that may benefit from CRT is patients with decreased ejection fraction and a need for chronic ventricular pacing. Cardiac resynchronization in these patients may reduce maladaptive left ventricular remodeling and preserve ejection fraction. One common example of CRT used in this setting is a patient with decreased ejection fraction and atrial arrhythmias who undergoes ablation of the AV node for control of rapid ventricular rates.

IMPLANTABLE CARDIAC DEFIBRILLATOR (ICD) THERAPY

ICDs are used to treat ventricular tachyarrhythmias. To do this, the device must recognize the arrhythmia, and then treat it appropriately. Ventricular arrhythmias are initially recognized by the device when the ventricular rate exceeds a programmed rate cutoff. If this ventricular rate is maintained for a given number of beats, the device will recognize the fast rhythm as VT or VF and begin to treat the arrhythmia. Nonsustained VT typically does not last long enough to meet criteria for the device.

Because the initial detection of the arrhythmia is based entirely on rate, it may be difficult for the device to discern whether a fast rhythm is ventricular or supraventricular in origin. Therefore, once VT or VF has been identified by the rate cutoff, ICDs use a series of programmable algorithms to discriminate true ventricular arrhythmias from other tachyarrhythmias such as sinus tachycardia, supraventricular tachycardia, or atrial fibrillation with rapid ventricular rates. These algorithms are designed to limit ICD therapy to only true VT or VF. These algorithms are very effective but not perfect. When optimally programmed, inappropriate shocks due to nonventricular rhythms can be minimized. Nonetheless, inappropriate ICD shocks remain one of the most common adverse events associated with ICD use.

The goal of ICD therapy is to terminate potentially lifethreatening ventricular arrhythmias. Modern devices perform this function with a combination of high-voltage defibrillation shocks and less painful bursts of rapid pacing. Typical programming

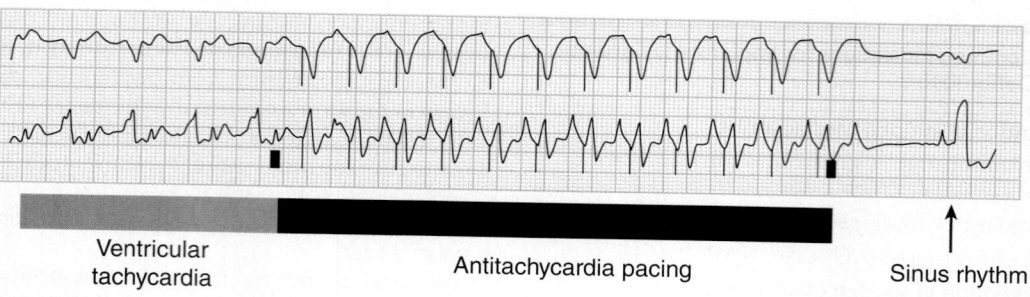

Figure 136-10 *Telemetry strip showing antitachycardia pacing (ATP) for ventricular tachycardia (VT). The patient is initially in a slow VT (approximately 130 bpm). A 12 beat burst of ATP is administered by the implantable cardiac defibrillator (ICD), which terminates the VT. A sinus beat is seen at the end of the strip.*

includes several initial attempts to pace the ventricle at a rate slightly faster than the ventricular tachycardia (termed "antitachycardia pacing"). In some patients, this will terminate the arrhythmia, and a shock can be avoided. However, if antitachycardia pacing is not successful, then the device will deliver a series of high-voltage shocks until the arrhythmia terminates (**Figures 136-10 and 136-11**).

> ### PRACTICE POINT
>
> - The goal of ICD therapy is to terminate potentially life-threatening ventricular arrhythmias. Often, initial attempts to overpace the ventricle at a rate slightly faster than the ventricular tachycardia (termed "antitachycardia pacing") will terminate the arrhythmia, and a shock can be avoided.

■ EVALUATING THE PATIENT WITH ICD SHOCKS

Approximately 15% to 30% of patients will experience an appropriate ICD shock within 3 years of implant. When a patient receives an ICD shock, the goal of the physician is to determine whether the therapy was appropriate. An important consideration is the number of shocks a patient receives. Most often, a single shock represents appropriate therapy for VT or VF. If the patient is otherwise stable, hospitalization is usually not warranted. A common practice is to have the patient call his or her physician's office to arrange follow-up within 24 hours. In this situation, if it is determined that the ICD shock was appropriate, the focus should be on addressing any exacerbating factors, most often congestive heart failure.

When a patient receives more than two shocks within 24 hours they should be evaluated immediately, as this may indicate inappropriate shocks, failed device therapy, or recurrent ventricular

arrhythmias. Whereas shocks preceded by syncope or presyncope are usually appropriate, shocks without such a prodrome may be inappropriate. Inappropriate shocks may result from sinus tachycardia, SVT or atrial fibrillation with rapid ventricular response, external electromagnetic interference (electrical "noise"), or true device or lead malfunction. The precise management of inappropriate ICD shocks will depend on the underlying cause.

> ### PRACTICE POINT
>
> - When a patient receives a single ICD shock, it often represents appropriate therapy for VT or VF. If the patient is otherwise stable, hospitalization is usually not warranted. When a patient receives two or more shocks within 24 hours they should be evaluated immediately, as this may indicate inappropriate shocks, failed device therapy, or recurrent ventricular arrhythmias.
> - Inappropriate shocks may result from sinus tachycardia, SVT or atrial fibrillation with rapid ventricular response, external electromagnetic interference (electrical "noise"), or true device or lead malfunction.

The term *electrical storm* describes multiple appropriate shocks within 24 hours and indicates recurrent VT or VF. This is a potentially life-threatening condition, and these patients should be hospitalized with a focus on correcting any underlying causes such as ischemia, electrolyte abnormalities, or worsening heart failure. Often, these patients will require short- or long-term antiarrhythmic medications to suppress recurrent ventricular arrhythmias.

Even single ICD shocks can result in considerable distress and anxiety for the patient and can reduce their quality of life. Attention should be paid to the patient's psychological status after any ICD shock, and when needed, anxiolytic medications should be offered. Less commonly, professional psychological treatment may be required.

IMPLANTATION AND PERIOPERATIVE CONSIDERATIONS

Implantation of pacemakers and defibrillators should be performed by experienced physicians with appropriate training, and in a sterile environment with trained ancillary staff. Usually this is done in an electrophysiology (EP) laboratory or in an operating room with fluoroscopic capabilities. Most often, conscious sedation is used in combination with local anesthesia. An incision is made in the upper anterior chest or in the delto-pectoral groove.

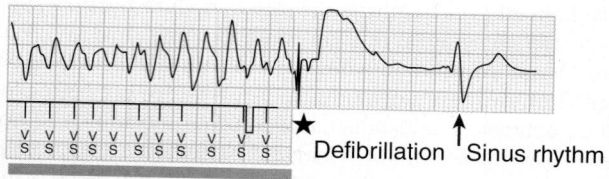

Figure 136-11 *Intracardiac electrograms during an implantable cardiac defibrillator (ICD) interrogation shows ventricular fibrillation that is successfully treated with a shock, indicated by the star. The resultant rhythm is sinus.*

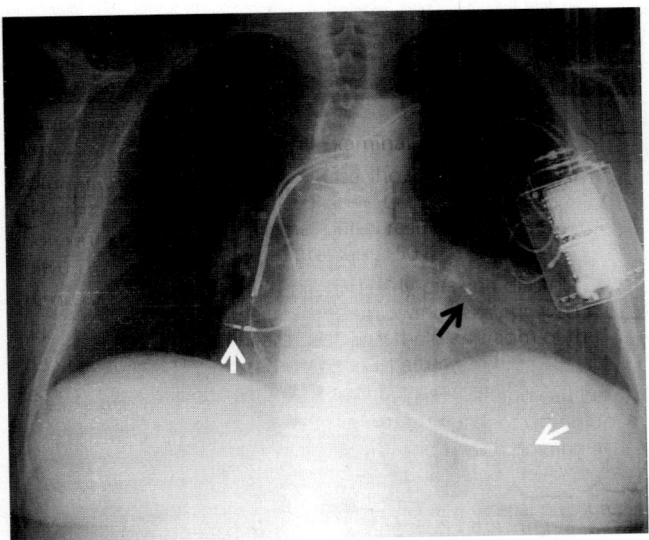

Figure 136-12 *Chest x-ray showing proper placement of a cardiac resynchronization therapy with defibrillator (CRT-D) device. Note the positions of the right atrial and right ventricular leads (white arrows). The left ventricular lead is positioned in the coronary sinus (black arrow).*

A pocket is then made in the subcutaneous or subpectoral space to house the pulse generator. Venous access is obtained either by needle puncture of the subclavian or axillary vein, or by direct cut-down of the cephalic vein. The leads are then advanced transvenously into the heart and positioned in their appropriate locations (**Figure 136-12**). The proximal ends of the leads are connected to the pulse generator which is then inserted into the pocket. The incision is sutured closed and dressed with a sterile dressing.

While implantation of cardiac rhythm devices is a relatively safe procedure, complications may develop. Complications that occur at the time of implant may include bleeding, air embolism, pneumothorax, cardiac perforation, and tamponade. Postoperative complications (occurring within approximately 30 days) include infection, pocket hematoma, wound dehiscence, or lead dislodgement.

Patients receiving cardiac rhythm devices often concomitantly receive anticoagulation therapy with aspirin, clopidogrel, warfarin, novel anticoagulants (dabigatran, rivaroxaban, apixaban, and edoxaban), and/or heparin products for other medical conditions. Each of these agents increases the risk of postoperative bleeding complications, albeit to varying degrees. In general, anticoagulation should be continued around the time of device implantation as medically indicated. However, as heparin and enoxaparin place the patient at particularly high risk of developing a hematoma, avoiding these agents whenever possible for 12 hours prior to the procedure and 1 to 2 days after the procedure may reduce the risk of hematoma formation. The use of novel anticoagulants may also increase the risk of bleeding. Our practice is to hold novel anticoagulants for 48 hours before and after device implantation whenever possible. Therapeutic treatment with warfarin usually does not cause significant bleeding complications if the INR is kept below 2.5. When withholding anticoagulation is not possible (ie, mechanical heart valves), the timing of the procedure is considered on a case-by-case basis.

Guidelines for antibiotic therapy in the perioperative period for cardiac rhythm devices are not well defined. While the risk is of infection is relatively low (<1%), patient morbidity and associated health care costs with cardiac device infection can be high.

Therefore, intravenous antibiotics to cover Gram-positive skin flora are given at the time of implantation. In general, postoperative antibiotics are not required.

DISCHARGE PLANNIG: OUTPATIENT DEVICE FOLLOW-UP

When patients are discharged from the hospital after device implantation, they should have explicit follow-up instructions. They should be seen by a physician or nurse approximately 1 week after implantation to have their wound examined and any stitches removed. Thereafter, regular follow-up with a cardiologist or a specialized device clinic should be arranged every 3 to 6 months. Newer devices have accompanying home monitoring systems that are capable of transmitting device data telephonically. These systems allow the physician to monitor the status of the device and communicate with the patient by phone, thereby reducing the frequency of office visits for the patient.

INDICATIONS FOR DEVICE INTERROGATION AND CONSULTATION

Interrogation of cardiac rhythm devices should be scheduled as an outpatient on a regular basis (every 6 months). Routine inpatient interrogation of a device is usually not warranted unless there if specific concern for a device-related issue. Examples of such issues include recent ICD shocks, failure of proper capture or sensing, decompensated heart failure, and specific patient complaints such as palpitations or syncope.

Occasionally patients will describe a vibration or beeping that originates from the device. These are programmed alerts designed to notify the patient to have their device interrogated. The majority of the times, these alerts are used to indicate battery depletion or lead malfunction.

> ### PRACTICE POINT
>
> - Routine *inpatient* interrogation of a device is usually not warranted unless there if specific concern for a device-related problem. Examples include recent ICD shocks, failure of proper capture or sensing, decompensated heart failure, syncope, or palpitations.
> - Occasionally patients will describe a vibration or beeping that originates from the device. These programmed alerts notify the patient to have their device interrogated (often indicate battery depletion or lead malfunction).

Cardiac rhythm devices are typically interrogated by a trained nurse or device company representative. The information collected is then routinely reviewed by an electrophysiologist or cardiologist. If abnormal device function is identified, simple programming changes can often correct the problem. However, an electrophysiologist should be consulted if a hospitalist has any concerns about device function that cannot be managed with programming changes. The most common examples of such concerns include frequent ICD shocks, lead malfunction/fracture, or device infection.

While most device evaluations can be done with the help of surface tracings (ECGs), when necessary consultation with a cardiologist or electrophysiologist can assist with diagnostic and management strategies.

QUALITY IMPROVEMENT TO ADDRESS PERFORMANCE GAPS

■ COST UTILIZATION

Implantable defibrillators are associated with increased cost to the health care system. The estimated cost per life-year added is between $30,000 and $50,000, which compares with the standard

TABLE 136-4 Evidence-Based Medicine Key References

Study	Methodology	Results	Limitations	Bottom Line
AVID Investigators, *N Engl J Med*. 1997;337:1576	Multicenter, randomized trial comparing antiarrhythmics vs ICDs in patients with decreased EF (<40%) and surviving sustained ventricular arrhythmias	1016 patients enrolled; patients receiving ICDs had 31% RRR in mortality at 3-y follow-up	No control group; amiodarone dosing was empiric and not determined by electrophysiologic testing	For secondary prevention, ICDs reduce mortality in survivors of life-threatening ventricular arrhythmias with reduced EF
Moss AJ, Zareba W, Hall WJ, et al. Prophylactic implantation of a defibrillator in patients with myocardial infarction and reduced ejection fraction. *N Engl J Med*. 2002;346:877	Multicenter, randomized trial comparing ICDs vs standard medical therapy in patients with prior myocardial infarction and reduced EF (<30%)	1232 patients randomized; patients receiving ICDs had HR for risk of death of 0.69 at 4-y follow-up	No control group; patients receiving ICDs had higher rates of heart failure exacerbations	For primary prevention, ICDs reduce mortality in patients with coronary disease and reduced EF
Abraham WT, Fisher WG, Smith AL, et al. Cardiac resynchronization in chronic heart failure. *N Engl J Med*. 2002;346:1845	Multicenter, randomized trial comparing cardiac resynchronization vs standard medical therapy in patients with moderate to severe CHF, EF ≤ 35%, and QRS ≥130 ms	453 patients enrolled; patients receiving CRT had improvement in quality of life, 6 min walk distance, and functional class. CRT patients had a 7% ARR in CHF hospitalizations	Investigators only blinded for initial 6 mo after randomization	In patients with moderate to severe CHF, reduced EF, and interventricular conduction delay, CRT improves clinical parameters and reduces CHF hospitalizations

benchmark of $50,000 for renal dialysis. The exact cost-effectiveness depends on a patient's individual risk for sudden death and his or her other comorbidities. Proper patient selection is necessary for this therapy to remain cost-effective. However, when restricted to appropriate patients, the cost-effectiveness of ICD implantation is comparable to other long-term cardiovascular therapies.

■ DISPARITIES IN CARE

Gender and ethnic disparities persist in patients who receive cardiac rhythm devices. Female gender and nonwhite race are both associated with decreased rates of device implantation (odds ratio of 0.86 [95% CI 0.791-0.927] and 0.70 [95% CI 0.66-0.76], respectively), even after accounting for multiple clinical and demographic variables. The causes behind these disparities are likely multifactorial, but may include differences in access to health care and physician-patient relationships among patients of varying race and gender.

SUGGESTED READINGS

Abraham WT, Fisher WG, Smith AL, et al. Cardiac resynchronization in chronic heart failure. *N Engl J Med*. 2002;346:1845.

Bardy GH, Lee KL, Mark DB, et al. Amiodarone or an implantable cardioverter-defibrillator for congestive heart failure. *N Engl J Med*. 2005;352:225.

Bernstein AD, Daubert J-C, Fletcher RD, et al. The revised NASPE/BPEG generic code for antibradycardia, adaptive-rate, and multi-site pacing. *Pacing Clin Electrophysiol*. 2000;25:260.

Buxton AE, Lee KL, Fisher JD, et al. A randomized study of the prevention of sudden death in patients with coronary artery disease. *N Engl J Med*. 1999;341:1882.

El-Chami MF, Hanna IR, Bush H, et al. Impact of race and gender on cardiac device implantations. *Heart Rhythm*. 2007;4:1420.

Epstein AE, DiMarco JP, Ellenbogan KA, et al. ACC/AHA/HRS 2008 Guidelines for Device-Based Therapy of Cardiac Rhythm Abnormalities: A Report of the American College of Cardiology/American Heart Association Task Force on Practice Guidelines (Writing Committee to Revise the ACC/AHA/NASPE 2002 Guideline Update for Implantation of Cardiac Pacemakers and Antiarrhythmia Devices) Developed in Collaboration with the American Association for Thoracic Surgery and Society of Thoracic Surgeons. *J Am Coll Cardiol*. 2008;51:e1.

Germano JJ, Reynolds M, Essebag V, et al. Frequency and causes of implantable cardiovertor-defibrillator therapies: Is device therapy proarrhythmic? *Am J Cardiol*. 2006;97:1255.

Hohnloser SH, Kuck KH, Dorian P, et al. Prophylactic use of an implantable cardioverter-defibrillator after acute myocardial infarction. *N Engl J Med*. 2004;351:2481.

Moss AJ, Zareba W, Hall WJ, et al. Prophylactic implantation of a defibrillator in patients with myocardial infarction and reduced ejection fraction. *N Engl J Med*. 2002;346:877.

The Antiarrhythmic Versus Implantable Defibrillators (AVID) Investigators. A comparison of antiarrhythmic-drug therapy with implantable defibrillators in patients resuscitated from near-fatal ventricular arrhythmias. *N Engl J Med*. 1997;337:1576.

SECTION 2

Critical Care

CHAPTER 137

Inpatient Cardiac Arrest and Cardiopulmonary Resuscitation

John E. Moss, MD
Jason Persoff, MD, SFHM

Key Clinical Questions

1 What are the fundamental goals of cardiopulmonary resuscitation?

2 Which components of resuscitation are considered vital to success?

3 How can the common pitfalls of resuscitation be surmounted?

4 What treatments should be instituted immediately upon successful resuscitation?

5 How should outcomes in resuscitation shape the discussion of advanced directives?

INTRODUCTION

Cardiopulmonary resuscitation is a time-dependent, team-based effort to reverse physiologic events that may culminate in a patient's imminent death. Biblical and ancient Egyptian hieroglyphic texts allude to mouth-to-mouth ventilation in divine contexts, but other texts indicate Jewish midwives used mouth-to-mouth resuscitation as early as 3300 years ago to revive stillborn children.

In the United States an estimated 375,000 to 750,000 hospitalized patients suffer in-hospital cardiac arrest (IHCA) requiring advanced cardiac life support (ACLS) annually. The incidence of IHCA is estimated to be as high as 1% to2% of all patients admitted to academic hospitals with a prevalence of approximately 65 people per 100,000 nationally.

In-hospital cardiac arrest encompasses a spectrum of disorders from insufficient cardiac output to generate appreciable cerebral perfusion such as arrhythmia or shock to complete cessation of cardiac activity. Vital sign anomalies may often herald impending inpatient cardiac arrest by minutes to hours, but many cardiac arrests occur suddenly and without warning. Acute pulmonary arrest (very common in pediatric populations, often due to airway obstruction; but much less common in adults) may precede IHCA and may occur from sedative or opiate analgesic overdose.

This chapter focuses on (1) the techniques that are essential to successful cardiopulmonary resuscitation especially with attention to good neurologic recovery (as defined by the cerebral performance category of zero or one), and (2) decision making based on patient resuscitation status.

TRIAGE

Since standardization of closed chest cardiac massage (CCCM)—that is, chest compressions—was first described systematically in the medical literature in 1960, CCCM has remained the only reliable means of reviving a patient in cardiopulmonary collapse. It is an effective and powerful intervention that, when unnecessarily delayed, may lead to poor patient outcomes. In one study, survival dropped from 34% to 14% if CCCM was delayed even as little as 60 to120 seconds from the time the patient collapsed. Therefore, clinicians must recognize and respond to cardiac arrest immediately for resuscitation measures to be effective.

Advanced cardiac life support combines basic life support (BLS) measures with specific interventions, such as medication, defibrillation, transthoracic pacing, and advanced airway management.

While often considered adequate for institution credentialing purposes, completion of American Heart Association (AHA) courses fails to result in long-term meaningful skill performance. Health care providers' capabilities to demonstrate appropriate technique for CCCM and capabilities to successfully navigate the steps of cardiopulmonary resuscitation begin to degrade just weeks following course completion. Therefore, for the whole medical team to respond concisely and in a coordinated fashion, clinicians must have extensive medical knowledge, training, drilling practice, continued education, and feedback.

Many providers are reluctant to initiate CCCM without complete assurance that the patient is truly in cardiopulmonary arrest (confirmed by vital signs or electrocardiographic rhythm), often leading to unnecessary delays in initiation of potentially lifesaving treatment. Furthermore, fundamental pulse assessment, even in nonemergency situations, cannot reliably and accurately predict the presence or absence of a pulse. One study tasked providers to determine whether or not patients had palpable pulses during elective cardiopulmonary bypass surgery. Ultimately providers took around 20 seconds to assess the pulse and were less than 70% accurate.

Time spent gathering cardiac monitoring, attaching leads, and setting up equipment can further delay promptly needed interventions to prevent death. In fact, clinicians may need to initiate CCCM prior to confirming cardiopulmonary arrest. Prompt initiation of CCCM for any patient who appears to be in extremis (ie, unarousable or clinically unstable with suspicion of cardiopulmonary arrest) should occur until confirmatory evaluation, often by a multispecialty resuscitation team, offers a high degree of confidence that CCCM can be discontinued. Providers should share a culture of support that accentuates that the greater harm to patients is in failing to initiate CCCM in contrast to the potential harms of CCCM (rib fracture, pneumothorax, organ perforation).

PRACTICE POINT

- Providers should initiate closed chest cardiac massage to any patient who appears in extremis without awaiting 100% confirmation that the patient is in cardiopulmonary arrest. Even delaying CCCM by as little as 30 seconds confers worse survival outcomes for patients in cardiopulmonary arrest.

PATHOPHYSIOLOGY

Cardiopulmonary arrest heralds death and may be an expected outcome in many hospitalized patients. However, rarely is cardiopulmonary arrest the first manifestation of physiologic events that ultimately culminate in collapse: patients frequently have alteration in mental status or significant vital sign changes (pyrexia, hypotension, bradycardia, decrease in oxygen saturation, change in respiratory rate), often hours before developing cardiac arrest. Intervention during this prearrest period may prevent cardiac arrest altogether. Alternatively, health care personnel may identify patients who are at the end of life and may thus benefit from a meaningful discussion about limiting resuscitative measures, including offering "Do Not Resuscitate" or "Allow Natural Death" orders. Many patients are not well informed about the resuscitative process and may have inflated images of routine successful resuscitation shaped from popular culture embodied by television and film. Clinicians often perform cardiopulmonary resuscitation on patients without informed consent—a discussion of the relevant risks, benefits, and alternatives to therapy along with the clinicians' recommendations. Thus the prearrest period may offer an unparalleled opportunity to give patients an active role in deciding whether resuscitation is desired (see Chapter 215 [Communication Skills for End of Life Care]).

While no one specific condition results in cardiopulmonary collapse, many health-care-associated interventions predispose patients to arrest and often require minimal intervention early on to alter the course of catastrophe (**Table 137-1**). Intervention during impending cardiac arrest requires a detailed history of recent interventions ranging from invasive procedures to recent sedation or anesthesia.

Responses to inpatient emergencies require multiple individuals who take on specific roles and integrate as a team. For care to function effectively and seamlessly during health care emergencies, each clinician must assume a narrowly focused essential function or task (such as assessing a patient's airway, recording data in a flowsheet, or ensuring chest compressions are adequate) and perform the task with high quality to facilitate the best possible patient outcome engendered by the team as a whole.

TABLE 137-1 Interventions to Specific Conditions that may Prevent Evolution to Cardiopulmonary Arrest in Hospitalized Patients

Cause	Intervention
Hypoxia due to medication or anesthesia	Supportive oxygen, reversal agents (naloxone for opiates, flumazenil for benzodiazepines)
Acidemia due to hypercapnic respiratory failure from medication or obstructive sleep apnea	Ventilation support (noninvasive or mechanical ventilation)
Pulmonary embolism	Appropriate VTE prophylaxis (pharmacologic unless significant contraindication); high index of suspicion and timely treatment
Cardiac arrhythmia due to acute coronary syndrome	Appropriate early intervention including antiplatelet therapy, beta-blockers, anticoagulation and early percutaneous coronary intervention (PCI)
Hyperkalemia	Calcium, sodium bicarbonate, insulin with dextrose, consideration of early hemodialysis; check for acid-base derangements
Hypokalemia	Correction of magnesium (first) followed by potassium; check for acid-base derangements
QT prolongation	Attention to medications known to prolong the QT interval (such as fluoroquinolones) and consideration of cardiac monitoring
Hypotension from severe sepsis	Early massive volume resuscitation with consideration of inotropes
Anticipated end-of-life care	Discussion of appropriate "Do Not Resuscitate" or "Allow Natural Death" orders and palliative care in appropriate patients

RAPID RESPONSE TEAMS AND THE PREARREST PERIOD

Recognizing that early intervention in impending cardiopulmonary arrest may prevent the arrest altogether, many hospitals have implemented rapid response teams (RRTs), consisting of any combination of critical care nurses, respiratory therapists, pharmacists, and/or physicians to attend to patients who exhibit one or more parameters of clinical instability but are not yet in extremis. Rapid response teams facilitate earlier communication with and transfer of care to intensive care units under the care of critical care teams and (when available) intensivists, which appear to reduce mortality in some centers, and need for crisis activation of cardiopulmonary arrest teams (ie, code teams). Additionally, RRTs have seen a marked expansion and elaboration in many disease states, such as improved identification of patients with sepsis and rapid implementation of early goal-directed therapy in patients with sepsis; and stroke teams in patients with neurological crises. Consistently, RRTs prompt discussion with patients and families about advanced directives (do not resuscitate orders or limitations of care), and reduce escalation of care in patients who do not desire such aggressive interventions and when the medical condition is expected to be immediately terminal.

Hospitalists must foster a culture of safety where any provider (or patient or family member) may initiate an RRT for any reason without fear of reprisal or judgment. Hospitalists should always thank other clinicians for calling RRTs and keeping the patients' safety of the utmost concern.

RESPIRATORY ARREST

Respiratory arrest from medications (anesthesia, benzodiazepines, or opiates) may lead to cardiac arrest through hypoxia and changes in the pH due to combined metabolic and respiratory acidosis. Respiratory arrest is often masked for some time due to the ubiquity of oxygen administration in hospitalized patients, which may lead to a prolonged period of hemoglobin oxygenation while ventilation may have already decreased or stopped. Overreliance on pulse oximetry as a sole source of interpreting ventilation effort may delay response to respiratory arrest until the patient is hypoxic and has developed profound acidemia. Systemic hypoxia causes pulmonary artery constriction, right ventricular failure, and systemic hypotension from poor right heart output coupled with loss of vascular tone from hypoxia (circulatory shock).

CARDIAC ARREST

Cardiac arrest may occur from multiple distinct mechanisms. True cardiac arrest (cardiac standstill) occurs either as a primary mechanism (from arrhythmias like ventricular fibrillation that prevent normal cardiac function) or as a secondary mechanism (from asystole or from an extended period of failed resuscitation and cardiac myocyte death). Most cardiopulmonary arrest episodes do not occur due to true cardiac standstill but rather from marked impairment in cardiac output resulting in systemic arterial hypotension, tissue hypoxia, and organ failure. Precardiac, intracardiac, or postcardiac mechanisms may independently or in combination result in cardiopulmonary arrest (**Table 137-2**).

TABLE 137-2 Cardiac Arrest Etiology by Anatomic Location

Precardiac	Intracardiac/ intrapulmonary	Postcardiac
Hypovolemia	Pulmonary embolism	Aortic dissection
Shock (septic, distributive)	Myocardial infarction	Hemorrhage
Pericardial Tamponade	Shock (cardiac)	Postcardiac
Pneumothorax	Cardiac arrhythmia (ventricular or atrial)	
Hypoxia	Left ventricular rupture	
	Hypertrophic cardiomyopathy	

SUBTYPES OF CARDIAC ARREST

Once appropriate resuscitation equipment has arrived, clinicians should immediately begin to differentiate whether the cardiac arrest is due to a "shockable" or "nonshockable" cardiac rhythm.

Shockable rhythms

Transthoracic electrical shocks can terminate some pathological cardiac rhythms that inhibit normal cardiac function. These can include ventricular fibrillation, ventricular tachycardia, AV nodal reentrant tachycardia, atrial fibrillation, and atrial flutter. While ventricular fibrillation has a very characteristic pattern, the other rhythms may be difficult to differentiate during an emergency and in the absence of 12-lead electrocardiography. In the setting of an unconscious patient in severe distress, who is obtunded or clinically severely unstable, all of these rhythms are considered pathologic and warrant immediate electrical shock.

Despite recommendations by the International Liaison Committee of Resuscitation (ILCOR) (the subsection of the American Heart Association responsible for publication of the ACLS guidelines) that differentiation of the exact cardiac arrhythmia may dictate very different types of cardiac intervention, ranging from dose (in joules) of electrical therapy to medication selection, confirming an exact rhythm diagnosis may not be practical. Thus, it is reasonable to treat all of these rhythms similarly in a cardiopulmonary arrest in the event of clinical uncertainty. Fundamentally similar to administration of CCCM, delays in electrical therapy may significantly negatively impact patient outcomes with even minimal delays. If a patient is not critically ill, then time allows for conscientious assessment of cardiac rhythm via 12-lead electrocardiogram (ECG) with appropriately targeted therapies for the underlying arrhythmia. (see Chapter 132 [Supraventricular Tachyarrhythmias] and Chapter 124 [Ventricular Arrythmias]).

Ventricular fibrillation results from disorganized myocardial electrical activity, and the heart is unable to generate a contraction to produce cardiac output. Hospitalists should be able to identify ventricular fibrillation confidently on rhythm strip (**Figure 137-1**).

The characteristic physiologic phases of ventricular fibrillation arrest underscore the importance of rapid electrical therapy. During the first few minutes of ventricular fibrillation (reflecting the combination of the "acute" and "electrical" phases of arrest, lasting up to 5-6 minutes), the myocardium is highly responsive to counter shock. This explains in part why successful defibrillation is so common on commercial airlines and in casinos where employees are trained to rapidly attach and initiate automated external defibrillators (AEDs). The acute and electrical phases can be extended when CCCM is initiated promptly, thus underscoring how critical CCCM is as an immediate therapy while definitive defibrillation equipment is located, attached, and initiated.

In the absence of CCCM, patients will degenerate into the "circulatory" phase where electrical therapies are less effective due to progressive tissue hypoxia and myocyte death. During this phase, CCCM may need to be performed for several minutes antecedent

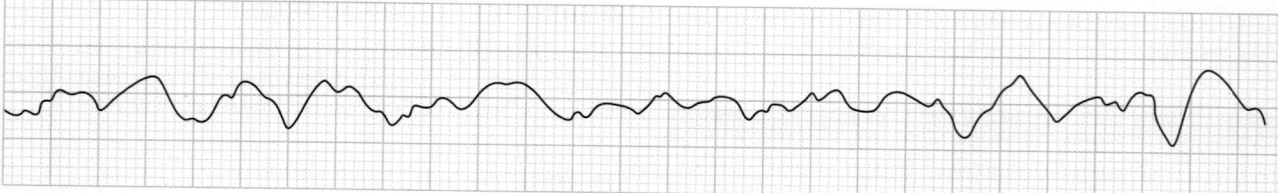

Figure 137-1 *Rhythm strip of a patient with ventricular fibrillation.*

to successful defibrillation. However, during the initial moments of a pulseless arrest, immediate rhythm identification and defibrillation of shockable rhythm takes precedence over CCCM.

Unchecked, patients will eventually enter the "metabolic" phase of ventricular fibrillation starting around the tenth minute of cardiac arrest. In the absence of effective CCCM, irreversible brain damage occurs. While there remains a slim hope of successful cardiac resuscitation at this point, survival to hospital discharge rapidly becomes improbable.

Ventricular tachycardia resulting in cardiopulmonary arrest fundamentally is identical to ventricular fibrillation in treatment: CCCM and early electrical shock are indicated.

Perhaps the most overwhelming change to resuscitation in recent years is the acknowledgment of severe ventricular stunning following electrical shock. For several minutes following defibrillation—and extending for a variable duration thereafter—the heart is mechanically dysfunctional and unable to generate an adequate cardiac output for organ perfusion or brain function. Consequently, it is absolutely critical to reinitiate CCCM for 1 to 2 minutes after defibrillation whether or not the shock is successful at aborting the ventricular arrhythmia.

PRACTICE POINT

- Even when defibrillation is successful, patients require at least 1 to 2 minutes of CCCM immediately following the shock due to stunning of the left ventricle. Resumption of a sinus rhythm does *not* equate to resumption of normal mechanical heart function.

Nonshockable rhythms

Nonshockable unstable or pulseless rhythms (characterized by bradycardia, asystole, and pulseless electrical activity [PEA]) constitute the majority of inpatient cardiac arrests. Deterioration in clinical status signified by deviations in mental status or marked changes in vital signs often foreshadows these types of cardiopulmonary arrests, and they may be preventable.

Bradycardia may be due to a primary arrhythmia (such as sick sinus syndrome or arterioventricular [AV] block), or may be due to a secondary cause such as medications (particular AV nodal blocking agents) or excessive vagal tone (due pain or nausea). Bradycardia severe enough to cause hemodynamic instability warrants immediate correction and treatment of the underlying cause. Atropine is a vagolytic that can potently reverse excessive vagally mediated bradycardia. However, with unpredictable effects and a narrow therapeutic window (too high or too low a dose of atropine can potentially paradoxically worsen bradycardia), its use is confined to select patients and only for short-term use. Chronotropic agents such as dopamine can be administered if time allows setup of an intravenous drip.

Bradycardia may respond to transcutaneous pacing, but this must be instituted rapidly. In conscious bradycardic patients transcutaneous pacing may prove to be exceptionally uncomfortable but should be used to bridge to transvenous pacing. Patients may require analgesia or sedation during transcutaneous pacing while awake.

Asystole as a primary cause of cardiac arrest is uncommon. Asystole typically is the end result of another pathophysiologic process, such as sustained hypoxia or coronary thrombosis. As such, asystole is a fairly late finding. Fine ventricular fibrillation may appear electrocardiographically similar to asystole. Clinicians should always confirm suspected asystole by checking multiple defibrillator leads and increasing the electrical gain. Doing such should clarify if the rhythm is actually asystole (vs masked fine ventricular fibrillation). Whereas defibrillation is likely to benefit a patient in ventricular fibrillation (and is necessary to terminate the rhythm), shocking a patient in asystole may result in depleting the heart of any remaining adenosine triphosphate (ATP) and with it any chance of successful resuscitation. In general, if clinicians are not certain whether asystole or ventricular fibrillation is the underlying rhythm, defibrillation is favored due to the overwhelming benefit patients with ventricular fibrillation receive from defibrillation compared to the minimal excess risk posed to those already in asystole.

Pulseless electrical activity represents a complex spectrum of disorders where patients appear to have an electrocardiographic rhythm that would be anticipated sufficient to generate a cardiac output, but clinical examination reveals no evidence of a palpable pulse. By definition, PEA is not a rhythm derangement, and therefore will not respond to any form of electrical shock. Pulseless electrical activity is a problem with either too little cardiac preload (vasodilation, pulmonary embolism, or profound volume depletion), ineffective cardiac output (due to cardiac failure or stunning), or extrinsic compression of the heart muscle (tension pneumothorax, severe airway obstruction, or pericardial tamponade). While seeking a cause, clinicians must pursue concomitant treatment with CCCM in spite of the apparently normal-appearing cardiac rhythm. Clinicians should use epinephrine and intravenous fluids along with the goal to furnish targeted treatment of the apparent cause of PEA (intubation for hypoxia or respiratory distress, needle decompression or chest tube insertion for tension pneumothorax, pericardiocentesis for tamponade, intravenous calcium for hyperkalemia, etc).

MANAGEMENT

While the approach to cardiac arrest has changed considerably over the past 5 decades, survival has improved little since initial reports on CCCM in 1960. ILCOR has published basic and advanced cardiac life support guidelines every 5 years, becoming the de facto standard of care in the United States and internationally. Despite their evidence base, criticism exists that many find the guidelines to be too complex and difficult to remember even just weeks following life support course completion. Also discordantly, the single most effective stratagem in resuscitation—effective chest compressions—frequently is not taught well or performed well during or following courses, with a time-dependent loss of skill following course completion.

While many clinicians learned that resuscitation begins with the "A-B-Cs," evidence now suggests that establishing an airway and initiating rescue breathing (accomplished in most hospitals via bag-valve-mask [BVM] ventilations) are not nearly as important as CCCM during the early phases of most adult inpatient cardiac arrests (**Figure 137-2**). Guidelines therefore now recommend focusing on "C-A-Bs," emphasizing that restoring circulation with compressions

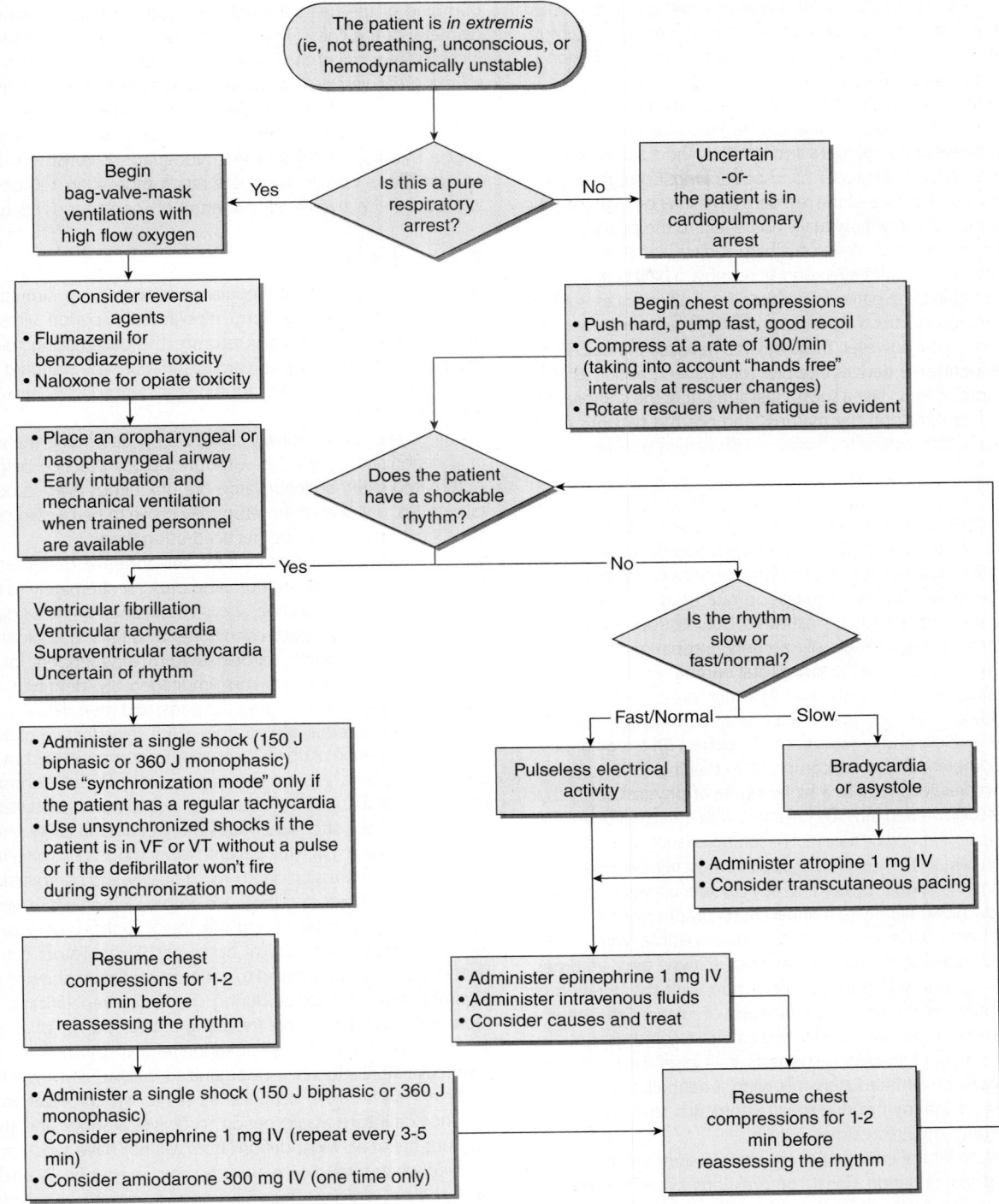

Figure 137-2 *Flow diagram of assessment and treatment during cardiac or pulmonary arrest.*

and early defibrillation are of critical importance. Certainly, in primary respiratory arrest (such as from medications) and in children (in whom respiratory arrest is much more common than cardiac arrest), management of airway and respiration must occur rapidly (Figure 137-2).

■ CHEST COMPRESSIONS (CLOSED CHEST CARDIAC MASSAGE)

When an apparently unconscious patient cannot be aroused, clinicians should assume that the patient might be in cardiopulmonary arrest and should institute chest compressions without delay. The mantra for quality chest compressions is to push hard, pump fast, and allow good chest recoil.

PRACTICE POINT

● Good chest compression technique requires pushing hard, pumping fast, and allowing adequate chest recoil.

Push hard

Many providers are concerned with pushing down on the sternum too hard; however, evidence does not support the assertion that pushing too hard occurs. Current recommendations suggest a compression depth of at least 2 inches, but that measurement is very difficult to extrapolate in clinical terms during resuscitation. The best advice is for rescuers to push as deeply as possible with arms locked and with the rescuer's shoulders directly over the patient's sternum with the rescuer using his or her body weight and waist flexion to deliver the compression.

Because most patients go into cardiopulmonary arrest in hospital beds, achieving proper positioning may be difficult, particularly when a patient is obese or the rescuer's arm length is short; a stool or other lift may prove critical for proper hand positioning. Compressing the chest solely with the force of the rescuer's arms may be highly kinetic in appearance but will offer virtually no benefit to the patient.

Compressions must be done on a hard surface, something a hospital mattress does not offer. As soon as possible, a backboard should be inserted behind the patient. Real-time feedback devices, such as accelerometers, may offer the best opportunity for ensuring adequate compression depth; however, these devices have technological limitations. Frequently the devices interpret total patient motion as compression depth when in fact a substantial amount of the compression is expended compressing the mattress and not the patient's chest. Compression depth indirectly correlates with patient survival.

Pump fast

Since ideal chest compressions result in only one-third normal cardiac output, about 10% of normal cerebral blood flow, and <5% of normal cardiac blood flow, compression rate has a substantial effect on tissue perfusion. Target compression rate of at least 100 compressions per minute should be instituted, but interruptions in chest compressions during change of rescuers, intubation, or rhythm analysis all result in a markedly lower total number of compressions over time. Studies consistently show that compressions are almost uniformly lower than 100 per minute, underscoring the need for practice, simulation, and feedback for all rescuers on a regular basis following completion of chest compression training.

Good compressions require a high degree of physical ability, but frequent rescuer rotation must be balanced with the need for uninterrupted compressions. While automated solutions (such as mechanical compression devices) may eventually replace most rescuer-performed compressions in inpatients, current devices are unwieldy or have failed to show noninferiority to manual chest compressions.

Some aspects of resuscitation are incompatible with ongoing chest compressions (such as rhythm analysis and, at times, intubation). In these situations, rescuers must limit the duration of the interruption as return of spontaneous circulation and neurologically intact survival are directly tied to chest compression rate. Furthermore, current evidence suggests it is essential to resume chest compressions immediately following a defibrillation attempt independent of the rhythm due to left ventricular stunning associated with highly impaired cardiac output.

Lastly, the beneficial effects of chest compressions are lost within seconds of discontinuation. Chest compressions' benefits appear to be additive to one another over time with subsequent compressions improving circulation and perfusion pressures; if compressions are widely spaced or stopped for any length of time, the benefits of the previous compressions' vascular effects are lost. Defibrillation success also depends on short "hands off" intervals (time when no compressions occur) as the chances of successful defibrillation diminish within seconds. This latter finding suggests that there is very little latitude for prolonged rhythm analysis during a cardiac arrest.

Good chest recoil

At the completion of a chest compression, rescuers must extend at the waist allowing the patient's chest to rise back to its rest position. The mechanisms by which compressions exert their physiologic effect appear to be a combination of increased intrathoracic pressure leading to compression of the great vessels and direct

pumping of the heart through reduction of the anterior-posterior diameter of the chest. The recoil phase is effectively "diastole," and incomplete recoil of the chest thus results in impaired blood return to the great vessels and heart resulting in further impairment in circulation in an already desperate perfusion environment. If recoil is consistently poor, rescuers will be incapable of surmounting this critical phase of circulation with adequate or consistent depth of compressions. Compression rate much more than 140 per minute will reduce effective recoil and return of spontaneous circulation.

■ ELECTRICAL THERAPY

Defibrillation is used to depolarize all myocytes simultaneously in order to achieve a uniform repolarization period whereby the sinoatrial node theoretically resumes the pacemaking role of the heart, thus restoring normal cardiac function. The standard dose for defibrillation is 120 to 200 J for biphasic defibrillators (and 360 J for monophasic defibrillators).

Caregivers will be unlikely to accurately determine the workings of a defibrillator in a crisis without copious practice beforehand. Automated external defibrillators are ubiquitous even in nonhospital settings, but even their setup may prove to be puzzling during a crisis if providers have not practiced using them.

Most manual defibrillators have self-adhesive defibrillator pads that are applied to the sternum and back (or alternately to the sternum and left midaxillary line, about the location of the cardiac apex) to deliver shocks. The pads concomitantly offer a "quick look" mode, displaying the patient's cardiac rhythm independent of cardiac leads. This means rescuers can simultaneously identify a patient's cardiac rhythm while charging the pads, and then deliver a shock.

Automated external defibrillators utilize self-adhesive pads as well but require a period of up to 20 seconds for computer rhythm analysis, during which time rescuers are not performing CCCM. All hospitalized patients in cardiac arrest should have self-adhesive defibrillator pads attached as these offer continuous monitoring and allow rescuers to deliver shocks or to pace the patient. Newer models also offer real-time feedback to compression depth, recoil quality, and compression rate.

Most defibrillators in clinical use employ a biphasic waveform, in which polarity reverses during the shock. Biphasic devices appear to confer better neurological outcomes. Defibrillators can deliver shocks that are synchronized to patients' cardiac rhythms to prevent administration of a shock during the critical repolarization phase represented by the T-wave (resulting in the "R on T" phenomenon and concomitant risk for precipitation refractory arrhythmias). Since ventricular fibrillation is a disorganized cardiac rhythm where no discrete T-waves exist, defibrillators set to "synchronization mode" may not delineate a safe period to deliver a shock and therefore may not fire at all. Most defibrillators will not have synchronization enabled when turned on without a clinician specifically enabling it. Nevertheless, clinicians must have good familiarity with the location of the synchronization button along with all functions on their hospitals' defibrillators so that when a defibrillator fails to fire, clinicians know where and how to deactivate synchronization prior to another attempt at defibrillation.

Rescuers should attempt to defibrillate a patient as soon as the code cart arrives and the defibrillator is fully set up and ready to deliver a shock. Compressions should continue unabated until the defibrillator is fully prepared, otherwise unnecessary hands-off intervals will result in poorer patient outcomes. Early defibrillation is critical as soon as a shockable rhythm is diagnosed or suspected clinically since the window for successful defibrillation decreases as patients progress from the electrical phase of ventricular fibrillation into the circulatory and metabolic phases. Chest compressions extend this window for a limited period of time, maintaining patients' responses to defibrillation.

RESPIRATORY THERAPY

Positive pressure ventilation via BVM provides oxygenation and ventilation. The design of the BVM is such that a one-handed squeeze provides the appropriate tidal volume for most adults in cardiopulmonary collapse: roughly 750 mL. Often, however, rescuers will use two hands to squeeze the bag, resulting in larger tidal volumes that may exceed 1000 mL. Data suggest that rescuers often deliver BVM ventilations at rates well beyond the recommended 1 ventilation every 5 seconds, with at least one report where ventilation rate exceeded the chest compression rate.

PRACTICE POINT

- The ideal technique for bag-valve-mask use involves three hands: two to properly seal the mask over the patient's mouth and nose while tilting the head back, and one hand (from a second rescuer) to squeeze the bag. The BVM is designed for a one-handed squeeze, which provides the appropriate tidal volume (750 mL) for most adults in cardiopulmonary collapse. Two-hand BVM squeeze may lead to hyperventilation and auto-positive end-expiratory pressure. The rate of BVM ventilations should be 1 ventilation every 5 seconds.

Well-intentioned rescuers often believe that hyperventilation will result in improved oxygenation, improved carbon dioxide levels, and improved acid-base balance, but in fact hyperventilation sets off a cascade of pathophysiologic changes that culminate in very high intrathoracic pressures, decreased cerebral and coronary circulation, and decreased survival. Since tissue perfusion (and by convention intact circulation) is a prerequisite to oxygenation, hyperventilating a patient without attending to proper chest compressions fails to bolster tissue oxygen levels. While carbon dioxide levels rise rapidly in circulatory collapse, carbon dioxide can only be off-gassed via ventilation if venous blood flow is able to enter the thorax and thereby the lungs. The single most effective treatment for the combined respiratory and metabolic acidosis uniform in cardiopulmonary arrest is resumption of physiologically normal circulation. Therefore, the proper route to achieve rescuers' intents is via high-quality chest compressions with supplemental oxygen administered via BVM ventilations (if rescuers are competent in its use) or via passive "blow-by" oxygen administered from a nonrebreather mask (if rescuers' skills are in doubt).

During cardiopulmonary arrest, the upper airway musculature may become lax, resulting in the tongue and jaw occluding the airway. Proper head positioning during ventilations will help decrease the risk of airway obstruction, but frequently other measures are required. Placement of either an oropharyngeal airway (in unconscious patients) or nasopharyngeal airway (in conscious patients) requires little training and may help stabilize the upper airway sufficiently to provide effective BVM ventilations. Nevertheless, rescuers may need to obtain an advanced airway (via laryngeal mask, endotracheal tube, or tracheostomy) in order to properly ventilate the patient. Only medical personnel with considerable training and experience in advanced airways should attempt to place an invasive airway. Experience is necessary in part to limit the duration of time needed to achieve the airway (during which CCCM frequently is halted) and to minimize the risk of complications (laryngeal spasm, esophageal intubation, induction of vomiting).

Almost all patients who suffer cardiopulmonary arrest will require an invasive airway to allow for ventilation in the postresuscitation period, but controversy exists as to the ideal timing to attempt airway stabilization. The airway is the key focus in patients in pure respiratory arrest, but increasingly it appears that CCCM and initial

defibrillation attempts should supersede airway priority in patients in cardiac arrest. In fact, recently ILCOR removed ventilation as a component of layperson adult resuscitation (out-of-hospital cardiac arrest) to further emphasize the importance of chest compressions as the single most important intervention during cardiopulmonary collapse. Further data suggest that a delayed approach to intubation (waiting >5 minutes into a cardiac arrest) results in equivalent survival to hospital discharge as earlier intubation.

MEDICATIONS

Vasoactive medications have traditionally played a large role in treatment of cardiac arrest care. Two vasoactive medications, epinephrine and vasopressin, are guideline recommended for use during cardiac arrest. Epinephrine is a sympathomimetic agent with beta-1, beta-2, and alpha-1 agonist properties. Beta-1 stimulation increases heart rate (chronotropy) and also increases contractility (inotropy), allowing for increased cardiac output secondary to higher heart rate and stroke volume. Beta-2 stimulation causes arterial vasodilation, yet its effect is mostly countered by the alpha-1 stimulation, which causes arterial vasoconstriction. Epinephrine continues to be the primary adrenergic agent used during resuscitation care. The alpha-adrenergic stimulating properties of epinephrine have been found to increase coronary perfusion pressure, but its beta-adrenergic effects are potentially detrimental, having been found to increase postresuscitation myocardial dysfunction and possibly worsen reperfusion injury. High-dose epinephrine (1 mg followed by 3 mg and then 5 mg of epinephrine depending on response) is definitely injurious, resulting in higher rates of successful cardiac resuscitation but disproportionately higher rates of poor neurologic outcomes.

One milligram of epinephrine should be administered intravenously after the rescuers deliver the first defibrillation and then every 3 to 5 minutes thereafter. Interruption of chest compressions to place a central line is not acceptable, especially if intraosseous (IO) access is available or the femoral vein is accessible. If no intraosseous or intravenous access is available, double-dose epinephrine may be administered down an endotracheal tube. Other medications that may be administered via endotracheal tube if indicated include naloxone, atropine, vasopressin, epinephrine, and lidocaine (NAVEL mneumonic).

Forty units of intravenous vasopressin may be used instead of epinephrine initially as a one-time dose. Clinical studies on vasopressin generally fail to demonstrate significantly improved outcomes over epinephrine, however. Neither vasopressin nor epinephrine have demonstrated improved neurological outcomes or survival to hospital discharge.

Atropine is an anticholinergic medication that increases heart rate via blockade of acetylcholine-mediated bradycardia. Atropine use should be confined to symptomatic bradycardia, as this medication has no role in other forms of cardiopulmonary arrest. Atropine has a narrow therapeutic window requiring at least 0.5 mg per dose, and not exceeding 3 mg cumulative dose, and may paradoxically worsen bradycardia. The 2010 ACLS guidelines recommend use of antiarrhythmic therapy for patients suffering cardiac arrest due to ventricular fibrillation or pulseless ventricular tachycardia. Amiodarone (300 mg delivered as an intravenous bolus) has proven to be superior to lidocaine based largely on out-of-hospital data showing improved rates of return of spontaneous circulation. No studies demonstrate that neurologic outcomes or survival to hospital discharge are better in patients receiving antiarrhythmic therapy, however.

Other medications, including sodium bicarbonate, calcium, and magnesium, have very specific roles in resuscitation, but their use is beyond the scope of this chapter. None of these medications is indicated routinely, and all have been associated with worse overall outcomes in nonselected patients in cardiopulmonary arrest.

Recent data suggest that a structured combination of intravenous **v**asopressin plus **s**teroid (methylprednisolone) plus **e**pinephrine (VSE therapy) improves good neurologic outcomes (Cerebral Performance Category 0-1) and is particularly effective at reducing postresuscitation shock. Wide scale adoption of VSE therapy awaits further clinical trials or guideline recommendation, but potentially improves the possibility of robust neurological survival postarrest (number needed to treat for good neurological outcome = 11).

■ RECOMMENDED APPROACH TO THE PATIENT IN CARDIOPULMONARY ARREST

The patient in apparent cardiopulmonary arrest requires prompt initiation of CCCM with very close attention to proper rate, depth, and recoil of compressions. Concomitantly the patient should be placed on a nonrebreather at >15 L/min of oxygen until adequate personnel are available to initiate stabilization of the airway.

Electrical shock serves as the penultimate goal in patients suffering from a shockable arrhythmia and in those in whom certainty of the underlying rhythm is not possible. While initial studies looking at further reducing the hands-off period of compressions by continuing CCCM during defibrillation appeared to suggest the potential safety of this approach, some data suggests possible risk to providers touching patients during defibrillation. Thus, the optimal strategy to minimize the hands-off interval is to charge the defibrillator while compressions are in progress, and then perform rhythm analysis with a countershock if indicated, prior to promptly resuming compressions.

Rescuers should attempt an initial "quick look" using manual defibrillator pads after charging the pads (120-150 J with a biphasic defibrillator or 360 J with a monophasic defibrillator). If indicated, personnel should deliver the shock and then resume resuscitation efforts.

Closed chest cardiac massage should continue with minimal interruption (5-15 seconds) for rhythm analysis and shock delivery.

Following the shock, CCCM should resume immediately without further rhythm analysis until at least an additional 150 compressions are delivered over the next 60 to 90 seconds due to the possibility of postshock ventricular stunning. After the first shock is delivered, rescuers need to embark on securing intravenous access and managing the patient's airway and breathing.

Initial airway maneuvers should focus solely on oxygen delivery and alleviating any upper airway flow resistance with temporary placement of an oropharyngeal or nasopharyngeal airway. If personnel with adequate airway training, practice, and experience respond to the cardiopulmonary arrest, BVM ventilations can be initiated at a rate of 5 ventilations per minute. An invasive airway should not be placed until the patient has received adequate chest compressions and an initial shock.

Once the rhythm is reassessed following 2 minutes of CCCM, if the patient remains in a shockable rhythm, a second shock is administered (at higher dose if appropriate) and epinephrine 1 mg or vasopressin 40 IU should be administered intravenously followed by another 2 minutes of compressions to allow for adequate circulation of the medication. The rhythm is then reassessed and another shock (at higher dose if appropriate) delivered if the arrhythmia is still present once again with a focus on resumption of chest compressions as soon as the shock is completed.

Clinicians should administer amiodarone 300 mg as an intravenous bolus if the arrhythmia continues followed by an additional shock 1 minute later. By this point in the cardiopulmonary collapse, clinicians with specialty training in hospital medicine, intensive care medicine, or emergency medicine should determine the next steps, if any, at ongoing resuscitation attempts.

In the case of a nonshockable rhythm, the defibrillation attempts and antiarrhythmic therapy would not be warranted, but otherwise the resuscitation should proceed in a similar manner.

In all cases of resuscitation, clinicians should attempt to determine the underlying cause while avoiding the pitfall of inaction (**Table 137-3**).

TABLE 137-3 Pitfalls in Cardiopulmonary Resuscitation and High-Impact Countermeasures to Abrogate Them

Pitfall	Cause	Countermeasure
• Failure to initiate closed chest cardiac massage (CCCM)	• Concern about potentially causing harm (rib fractures, organ perforation, pain, etc) • Uncertainty about whether the patient is truly in cardiopulmonary arrest	• Initiate CCCM immediately as the greater harm is in delaying treatment
• Focusing on airway and bag-valve ventilation preferentially to CCCM	• Possibility of improving oxygenation and ventilation	• Place the patient on a nonrebreather with oxygen delivery >15 L/min • Consider placing an oropharyngeal or nasopharyngeal airway
• Incorrect CCCM technique	• Providers pushing too shallowly, too slowly, or failing to release compression adequately	• Remember the adage: "Push Hard, Pump Fast, Good Recoil"
• Delay in transthoracic shock due to uncertainty in cardiac rhythm	• Concern about causing torsades-de-pointes or ventricular fibrillation • Concern about misidentification of a benign rhythm for a malignant one • Lack of familiarity with equipment and its use	• Transthoracic shocks are the only intervention, other than CCCM, that have meaningfully valuable impacts on patient survival, but survival begins to decrease every second a patient remains in a shockable rhythm. Early shocks lead to improved outcomes • Torsades-de-pointes and ventricular fibrillation are themselves shockable rhythms • Recognize that correct rhythm diagnosis may not be possible early on in a resuscitation • Recurrent training, practice, simulation, and feedback are essential to educate those who are expected to use resuscitation equipment in an emergency

POSTRESUSCITATION CARE AND TERMINATING THE RESUSCITATION

No criteria exist to guide clinicians when resuscitation is futile except in cases of obvious rigor mortis, evidence of decapitation, or evidence of decomposition. Complicating matters further, most resuscitation research is confined to the first minutes of resuscitation, leaving clinicians to use their best judgment as to whether resuscitative measures should continue. In general, clinicians should factor in the length of time the brain has been exposed to hypoxia and inadequate perfusion in deciding whether or not the hallmark of successful resuscitation—neurologically intact survival—is likely.

> ### PRACTICE POINT
>
> - The decision to forgo further resuscitation efforts should be made by the entire resuscitative team in a manner that considers premorbid level of function, duration of the resuscitative effort, and all team members' opinions and suggestions.

Literature supports allowing family members the decision to view the resuscitation prior to termination of efforts (with evidence suggesting that family members who witness the resuscitation have lower incidences of pathological mourning, anxiety and post-traumatic stress). Including family members in viewing resuscitation efforts requires a structured approach and an experienced team member assigned to family members to answer questions or address concerns.

Postresuscitation hypothermia

In those in whom resuscitation appears successful, clinicians should consider initiation of therapeutic hypothermia. Extensive research has demonstrated that inducing hypothermia following cardiac arrest improves neurologic outcomes (as defined by cerebral performance category) when patients develop cardiopulmonary arrest due to a shockable rhythm. The data for improved neurologic recovery are not as strong in PEA or asystole.

Therapeutic hypothermia requires continuous central temperature monitoring via specialized equipment such as bladder thermography. The goal of therapeutic hypothermia is rapid coolingcore temperature via external cooling devices (ice packs or specialized cooling pads), internal cooling (utilizing chilled saline), or a combination of both. Since human physiology will attempt to usurp hypothermia through shivering, patients may require paralysis to prevent shivers. After 24 hours, paralytics and cooling devices may be discontinued with the patient being allowed to passively rewarm.

The majority of the literature concerning therapeutic hypothermia has concentrated on a goal temperature of 33°C for 12 to 24 hours postcardiac arrest. However, current data suggests that avoidance of hyperthermia (maintaining temperature less than 36°C) and fever—which may be damaging to neurons—provides similar benefit to maintaining lower temperatures. Since therapeutic hypothermia requires specialized equipment, its use is often confined to centers with experience and established institutional protocols for hypothermia. In the absence of these, clinicians should strive to maintain patient normothermia and avoid even minuscule elevation of body temperature above normal.

Patients in whom an acute coronary syndrome is posited to be the cause of cardiac arrest should undergo cardiac revascularization as soon as possible to prevent recurrent arrhythmias.

INTRAVASCULAR VERSUS INTRAOSSEOUS ACCESS

Access to the circulation is needed in patients during cardiac arrest. Traditionally this has been in the form of peripheral venous access or central venous access. Peripheral IVs are fairly straightforward and simple to obtain, even in patients in cardiac arrest. However, in patients with little available immediate IV access, including patients who are IV drug users or dialysis patients, another route may be needed. Central venous lines (internal jugular, subclavian vein, or femoral vein) are one option, but require a clinician skilled in their placement. They also carry risk of pneumothorax (internal jugular and subclavian), arterial puncture and thrombosis.

Intraosseeous needle insertion is a rapid (usually <1 minute placement time) and effective method of obtaining access in adult populations. Gazin et al showed the success rate of establishing intraosseous access to be 97% after training, including a 60 minute lecture and 1 hour practical session. The IO access proved to be effective for fluid resuscitation, ACLS drug delivery, and sedative/paralytic drug delivery. Therefore, when IV access is unobtainable or difficult, IO access provides a safe and effective method to obtain access to the circulation for fluid and drug delivery. Some hospital systems are even utilizing IO as the primary access when patients in cardiac arrest do not have adequate vascular access.

PROGNOSIS

Only approximately one in seven patients survive in-hospital resuscitation to discharge, and of those who initially survive, only 19% are still living 6 months after IHCA. Fifty-one percent of survivors initially present in a shockable rhythm (ventricular fibrillation or ventricular tachycardia), but shockable rhythms are outnumbered in incidence to nonshockable rhythms (asystole or pulseless electrical activity) by nearly three to one in the inpatient setting.

Successful resuscitation preserves patients' neurologic function that the AHA defines using the Cerebral Performance Category score (**Table 137-4**).

Between 14% and 23% of survivors—whose prearrest neurological function was normal—develop moderate to severe cognitive deficits after resuscitation (Cerebral Performance Category 2-3). Fewer than 2% of survivors of IHCA will suffer prolonged coma or persistent vegetative state. While gender does not appear to predict outcomes in cardiopulmonary arrest, increased age may predict worse outcomes and lower survival probably less on the basis of age itself but rather through the accumulation of myriad comorbidities (particularly chronic kidney disease, coronary disease, and malignancy). Further multivariate data from the national registry of cardiopulmonary resuscitation (NRCPR) ultimately may help settle whether age is an independent predictor of short and long-term survival.

TABLE 137-4 Cerebral Performance Category Score and Related Neurologic Outcome

Cerebral Performance Category	Level of functioning
CPC 1	A return to normal cerebral function and normal living
CPC 2	Cerebral disability but sufficient function for independent activities of daily living
CPC 3	Severe disability, limited cognition, inability to carry out independent existence
CPC 4	Coma
CPC 5	Brain death

QUALITY IMPROVEMENT

Debriefing with clinicians after every resuscitation event allows team members to contribute their intellectual and emotional concerns. Debriefing, even just a few minutes, should occur after every resuscitation event. All resuscitations require careful post hoc analysis for team compliance with established resuscitation protocols. One very valuable source of feedback is participation in NRCPR. This international collective of nearly 15% of all U.S. hospitals, and all of the Canadian Health Care System plus several other international sites, was created by the American Heart Association to collect standardized data on all inpatient cardiac arrests. Participating institutions receive quarterly reports on their resuscitations that may be compared to local, regional, national, and international norms established by all other participating institutions. These data may offer areas where improvement is needed (such as time to initial defibrillation from onset of cardiopulmonary arrest) and may serve as valuable reinforcement to team members of areas in which mastery has been accomplished. Furthermore, NRCPR data continue to help refine the cutting edge in resuscitation research and therefore meaningfully impact future patients' outcomes from cardiopulmonary arrest.

Post hoc resuscitation analysis offers a partial intervention to impact future care, but continual retraining of providers offers the most proactive means to deliver high-quality care. Simulation labs offer an opportunity to objectively quantify team members' capabilities at performing chest compressions, BVM ventilations, and other logistics of team flow that may elude analysis during real-life resuscitations. Since studies show rapid degradation in resuscitation skills (both manual and intellectual) within days of biannual resuscitation training, clinicians require continual feedback over the intervening months to ensure an adequate skill set. Whether this feedback occurs in a formal simulation environment or one on one with a manikin is probably less important than ensuring that skills are adequate and reinforced over time.

SUGGESTED READINGS

Abella BS, Alvarado JP, Myklebust H, et al. Quality of cardiopulmonary resuscitation in adult inpatients. *JAMA*. 2005;293:305-310.

Arrich J, Holzer M, Herkner H, et al. Hypothermia for neuroprotection in adults after cardiopulmonary resuscitation. *Cochrane Database*. 2009;4:CD004128.

Ehlenach WJ, Barnato AE, Curtis JR, et al. Epidemiologic study of in-hospital cardiopulmonary resuscitation in the elderly. *N Engl J Med*. 2009;361:22-31.

Field JM, Hazinski MF, Sayre MR, et al. Part 1: Executive Summary: 2010 American Heart Association Guidelines for Caridiopulmonary Resuscitation and Emergency Cardiovascular Care Science. *Circulation*. 2010;122:S640-S656.

Hazinski MF, Nolan JP, Billi JE, et al. Part 1: Executive summary: 2010 International Consensus on Cardiopulmonary Resuscitation and Emergency Cardiovascular Care Science with Treatment Recommendations. *Circulation*. 2010;122(16 Suppl 2):S250-S275.

Mentzelopoulis SD, Malachias S, Chamos C, et al. Vasopressin, steroids, and epinephrine and neurologically favorable survival after in-hospital cardiac arrest. *JAMA*. 2013;310:270-279.

Nielsen N, Wetterslev J, Cronberg T, et al. Targeted temperature management at 33°C versus 36°C after Cardiac Arrest. *N Engl J Med*. 2013;369:2197-2206.

Olasveengen TM, Sunde K, Brunborg C, et al. Intravenous drug administration during out-of-hospital cardiac arrest. *JAMA*. 2009;302:2222-2229.

Reades R, Studnek JR, Vandeventer S, Garrett J. Intraosseous versus intravenous vascular access during out-of-hospital cardiac arrest: a randomized controlled trial. *Ann Emerg Med*. December 2011;58:509-516.

Salvatierra G, Bindler RC, Corbett C, et al. Rapid response team implementation and in-hospital mortality. *Crit Care Med*. 2014;42(9):2001-2006.

CHAPTER 138

Acute Respiratory Failure

Eric M. Siegal, MD, SFHM, FCCM

Key Clinical Questions

1 How should a clinician rapidly assess the severity and stability of a patient with acute respiratory distress?

2 How can principles of respiratory physiology be effectively applied to guide diagnosis and therapy?

3 What are the indications and contraindications for noninvasive positive pressure ventilation (NIPPV) and what outcomes does this intervention affect?

4 When does a patient require advanced airway management?

CASE 138-1

You are called to emergently assess a 53 years old with COPD who is hospitalized with acute pancreatitis. He has received substantial fluid resuscitation and parenteral morphine for severe epigastric pain. He has become increasingly confused and somnolent and his oxygen saturation has acutely decreased to 82% on 2 L per nasal cannula. On a nonrebreather face mask, his SpO_2 is now 98%. He appears uncomfortable, is tachycardic, tachypneic and moderately confused. His expiratory phase is prolonged, and breath sounds are nearly absent at the lung bases. He has moderate peripheral edema and his epigastrium is moderately tender.

INTRODUCTION

Acute respiratory failure is a common inpatient medical emergency that mandates rapid patient assessment and initiation of potentially lifesaving therapy, often with a paucity of diagnostic information. The clinician must enter this time-pressured, high-risk scenario with a preestablished diagnostic and therapeutic schema that facilitates an efficient and comprehensive approach, which can be broken into four key steps:

1. Rapidly assess the severity and instability of the presentation
2. Determine the likely cause or causes
3. Initiate treatment
4. Assess efficacy of treatment

PATHOPHYSIOLOGY AND DIFFERENTIAL DIAGNOSIS

Oxygen binds hemoglobin after it diffuses across a pressure and concentration gradient from the alveoli to the pulmonary capillaries, which is generated by the mean airway pressure (primarily positive end-expiratory pressure, or PEEP) and the fraction of inspired oxygen (FiO_2). Carbon dioxide exits the pulmonary circulation across a reverse gradient, but needs to be continually expired from the mouth for that gradient to be maintained. Thus, CO_2 elimination depends upon minute ventilation (expiratory tidal volume × respiratory rate). The key implication of this physiology is that oxygenation is entirely driven by the fraction of inspired oxygen (FiO_2) and the pressure under which oxygen is delivered. Hyperventilation has no impact upon hypoxemia, but it does increase CO_2 elimination.

PRACTICE POINT

Oxygenation is entirely driven by the fraction of inspired oxygen (FiO_2) and the pressure under which oxygen is delivered. Hyperventilation has no impact upon hypoxemia, but it does increase CO_2 elimination.

Understanding the pathophysiologic underpinnings of acute respiratory failure simplifies the diagnostic approach and informs therapeutic interventions that are physiologically sound. Respiratory failure can be broken into five major categories:

- Shunt [Perfusion (Q) > Ventilation (V)]
- Dead space(V > Q)
- Impaired diffusion
- Decreased mixed venous oxygen saturation
- Alveolar hypoventilation

■ SHUNT

Shunt occurs when pulmonary blood flow does not participate in gas exchange, causing deoxygenated blood to enter the systemic circulation. *Physiologic shunts*, the most common cause of acute hypoxemia in the hospitalized patient, develop when pulmonary perfusion is inappropriately maintained to injured, atelectatic or collapsed alveolar units. A relatively small area of infiltrate or atelectasis, especially in a dependent lung segment, may cause profound hypoxemia if perfusion is maintained to that area. *Anatomic shunts* are physical conduits that divert deoxygenated blood into the systemic circulation, such as right to left intracardiac or intrapulmonary shunts. As the degree of shunt (shunt fraction) increases, the partial pressure of arterial oxygen (PaO_2) becomes increasingly independent of the FiO_2. Once the shunt fraction exceeds 50%, the PaO_2 becomes decoupled from the FiO_2. Stated differently, when the shunt fraction is high, increasing the FiO_2 does little to increase the PaO_2.

■ DEAD SPACE

Physiologic dead space is the opposite of shunt, that is, inadequate perfusion of ventilated lung areas. Any process that reduces alveolar surface area (eg, emphysema), or impairs pulmonary perfusion (eg, alveolar overdistension, decreased venous return, impaired cardiac output, pulmonary arterial obstruction) will increase dead space. Worsening dead space is characterized primarily by hypercarbia rather than hypoxemia. As a case in point, marked hypoxemia is uncommon in otherwise healthy patients with acute pulmonary embolism (PE). Patients who become markedly hypoxemic after acute PE generally have other lung pathology (eg, chronic lung disease or pneumonia) or acute right to left intracardiac shunting due to acute right ventricular (RV) pressure overload.

PRACTICE POINT

- A relatively small area of infiltrate or atelectasis, especially in a dependent lung segment, may cause profound hypoxemia if perfusion is maintained to that area.

■ IMPAIRED DIFFUSION

Processes that damage or thicken the alveolar-capillary membrane, such as pulmonary edema, inflammation, fibrosis or hemorrhage increase gas transit time across alveolar-capillary membrane. At rest, gas exchange occurs early as hemoglobin transits the pulmonary microcirculation. As cardiac output increases to meet metabolic demand (eg, during sepsis or exercise), the rate of blood flow also increases, commensurately decreasing the amount of time for gas exchange in the pulmonary microcirculation. Impaired diffusion capacity becomes clinically evident when the time required for gas exchange exceeds the amount of time that hemoglobin spends in the pulmonary capillary. This explains why measuring exercise capacity in disorders characterized by progressive impairment of diffusion capacity, such as pulmonary fibrosis, remains the most sensitive and predictive indicator of disease progression.

■ DECREASED MIXED VENOUS OXYGEN SATURATION

Mixed venous oxygen saturation (SvO_2) is the saturation of hemoglobin returning to the pulmonary artery. As metabolic demand exceeds oxygen delivery (DO_2), tissue oxygen extraction (VO_2) increases, and hemoglobin progressively desaturates. If returning hemoglobin is sufficiently desaturated, there may be inadequate time for hemoglobin to fully reoxygenate before re-entering the systemic circulation, especially when cardiac output is elevated. Consequently, as metabolic demand increases and gas exchange worsens, the SvO_2 plays an increasingly important role in dictating the PaO_2.

■ ALVEOLAR HYPOVENTILATION

Alveolar hypoventilation is characterized by decreased minute ventilation due to impaired control or efficacy of the mechanics of breathing such that gas exchange does not meet metabolic demand.

DIAGNOSIS

Acute respiratory failure is often multifactorial and physiologic derangements can be synergistic. The patient with an opiate overdose may initially present with alveolar hypoventilation, but subsequent atelectasis or aspiration may lead to physiologic shunting, while hypotension may worsen dead space.

Dead space, shunt and diffusion abnormalities all reflect derangements in pulmonary gas exchange, while hypoventilation results from impaired mechanics or control of ventilation. The alveolar-arterial (A-a) gradient, calculated from an arterial blood gas differentiates abnormal gas exchange from abnormal ventilatory control.

$$\text{A-a gradient} = FiO_2 \times (P_{barometric} - P_{H_2O}) - PaO_2 + PaCO_2/0.8$$

At *sea level* breathing room air:

$$\text{A-a gradient} = 0.21 \times (760 - 50) - PaO_2 - (PaCO_2 \times 1.25)$$
$$\text{A-a gradient} = 150 - PaO_2 - (PaCO_2 \times 1.25)$$
$$\text{Normal A-a gradient} = (Age/4) + 4$$

For every 10% increase in the FiO_2, the A-a gradient increases by approximately 6 mm Hg, possibly due to blunting of normal pulmonary hypoxic vasoconstriction. A healthy patient with an A-a gradient of 10 mm Hg at room air will have an A-a gradient of 60 mm Hg when breathing 100% oxygen. Thus, the A-a gradient becomes increasingly difficult to interpret as the FiO_2 increases. In patients with high FiO_2 requirements, the ratio of oxygenation to supplementation (PaO_2/FiO_2 ratio) more reliably reflects gas exchange impairment.

PRACTICE POINT

- In patients with high FiO_2 requirements, PaO_2/FiO_2 ratio is a more sensitive and reliable gauge of impairment than the A-a gradient.

Despite its limitations in severely hypoxemic states, using the A-a gradient is a useful first step in a physiologic approach to acute respiratory failure (**Figure 138-1**). However, while it is vital to understand respiratory failure based on physiologic principles, it is equally instructive to categorize respiratory failure based upon the *systems* required for respiration; specifically central control of respiration, respiratory mechanics, the airway, the lung parenchyma, and vascular perfusion (**Table 138-1**). Using a system-based approach to acute respiratory failure in conjunction with a pathophysiologic approach facilitates rapid and comprehensive diagnosis and treatment.

Once a provisional diagnosis has been established, clinicians must rapidly initiate therapy that is specifically targeted to addressing the pathophysiology.

TRIAGE

■ RAPID ASSESSMENT OF SEVERITY AND STABILITY

Assessing the severity and stability of acute respiratory failure at the extremes of illness is generally straightforward. The awake patient who can speak in full sentences and appears relatively comfortable is unlikely to acutely decompensate or require emergent intervention. At the other extreme, the patient who is obtunded,

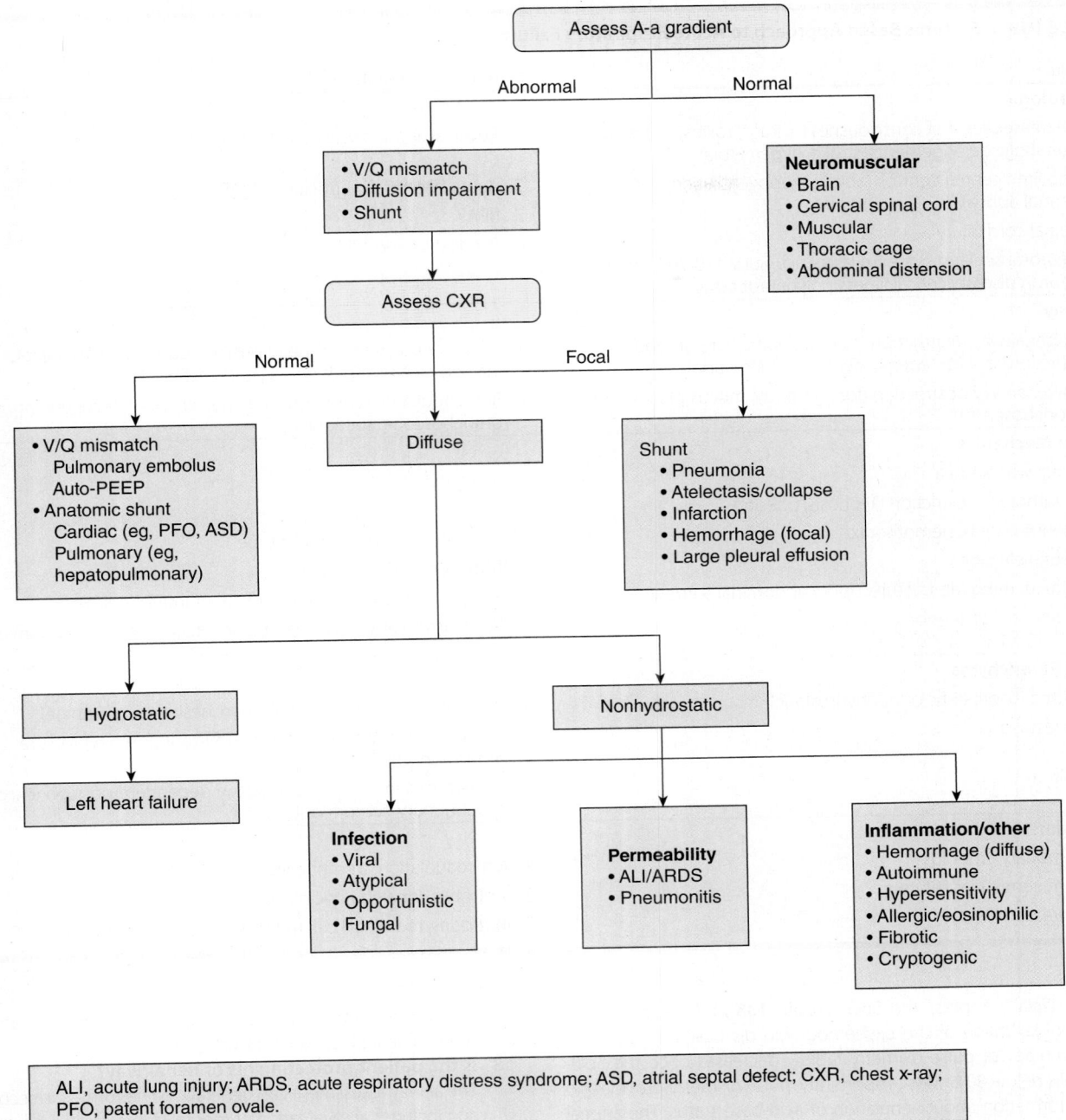

Figure 138-1 *A physiology-based algorithm for acute hypoxemic respiratory failure. (Adapted with permission from Kenneth E Wood, DO.)*

profoundly hypoxemic, hemodynamically unstable, or exhausted due to respiratory effort should almost always be immediately intubated and mechanically ventilated. The challenge lies in responding to presentations that fall between these two extremes. The initial survey must occur quickly and systematically to determine the degree of respiratory distress, the patient's stability and the likelihood of further deterioration. This assessment can be distilled to four key questions.

1. How severe is the patient's respiratory distress?

The degree of respiratory distress is quickly and accurately assessed with a physical examination that focuses upon level of consciousness (LOC), degree of respiratory effort and underlying physiological reserve. Decreased LOC, use of accessory muscles of respiration (sternocleidomastoid, scalene, intercostals, and abdominal musculature), degree

tachypnea and adrenergic stimulation (tachycardia, diaphoresis, hypertension, and agitation) suggest severe respiratory distress and impending respiratory failure. These findings should be taken in context of the patient's estimated physiologic reserve. Intuitively, a fit 25 year old will tolerate sustained respiratory distress far better than a chronically ill 75 year old.

2. Is gas exchange adequate?

Clinical signs of hypoxemia or hypercarbia are nonspecific and include headache, altered mental status, cyanosis, or acute end organ failure. Pulse oximetry is generally the first measurement available at the bedside and provides rapid, real-time quantification of peripheral oxygenation. Carboxy- or met-hemoglobinemia may falsely elevate SpO_2, while motion artifact, hypoperfusion due to occlusive arterial disease, hypotension, or vasoconstriction may degrade signal quality and

TABLE 138-1 Systems Based Approach to Acute Respiratory Failure

Cause	Potential Intervention
Neurologic	
1. Decreased level of consciousness: (drugs, toxins, infection, metabolic derangements, stroke, hypercarbia)	1. Reversal agents (naloxone, flumazenil)
2. Impaired central control: (obesity-hypoventilation, central apnea)	2. Acute bag-mask ventilation, BPAP
3. Spinal cord injury	3. BPAP
4. Neuromuscular disease (myasthenia, Guillain-Barre', motor neuron disease, critical illness polyneuropathy)	4. Pyridostigmine, BPAP
Airway	
1. Upper airway obstruction (tumor, trauma, foreign body, infection/abscess, edema, dynamic obstruction)	1. Foreign body removal, head positioning, oral airway, heliox, inhaled racemic epinephrine, corticosteroids
2. Lower airway obstruction (foreign body, mucus plug, tumor, bronchospasm)	2. Bronchodilators, corticosteroids, heliox, catheter suctioning, bronchoscopic suctioning
Chest Mechanics	
1. Chest wall trauma	1. Analgesia
2. Extrathoracic restriction (kyphosis, obesity)	2. BPAP
3. Pneumothorax, hemothorax	3. Tube thoracostomy ("chest tube")
4. Pleural effusion	4. Thoracentesis
5. Pain/splinting (rib fracture, upper abdominal surgery)	5. Analgesia: oral, parenteral, epidural or intercostal block
6. Abdominal distension	6. Nasogastric decompression, paracentesis, release of abdominal binder
Lung Parenchyma	
1. Edema (hydrostatic or nonhydrostatic)	1. Diuresis, vasodilators (nitroglycerin, nesiritide, morphine)
2. Atelectasis	2. Cough, incentive spirometry, intermittent positive pressure ventilation, chest percussion
3. Infiltrate	3. Position patient with "good" side in dependent position (except in pulmonary hemorrhage)
Vascular	
1. Pulmonary embolus	1. Anticoagulation, thrombolysis
2. Right ventricular failure	2. Inotropes, inhaled nitric oxide
3. Decreased MvO_2	3. Inotropes, red blood cell transfusion

artificially depress the SpO_2 (**Table 138-2**). Due to the sigmoidal shape of the oxyhemoglobin dissociation curve, the accuracy of pulse oximetry rapidly decreases once the SpO_2 falls below 80%. Most importantly, pulse oximetry provides no information about ventilation or acid-base status. The arterial blood gas, while mildly invasive and more difficult to obtain than pulse oximetry, remains the gold standard in the assessment of acute respiratory failure.

3. Is the patient protecting his or her airway?

The airway assessment can generally be performed in seconds, and includes an evaluation of mental status, ability to manage secretions, risk for aspiration, and airway patency. The patient who is awake, responsive, managing secretions, and phonating clearly is protecting his/her airway. Contrary to popular teaching, the gag reflex is not a reliable gauge of airway protection. Twenty five percent of healthy adults do not have an inducible gag reflex, while comatose patients may gag (and potentially vomit) if a foreign body is inserted into their posterior pharynx. Coma, defined as a Glasgow Coma Scale score of eight or less, is a much more reliable predictor of airway compromise (**Table 138-3**), and if not rapidly reversible (eg, naloxone for opiate overdose) mandates immediate endotracheal intubation.

TABLE 138-2 Factors Affecting the Accuracy of Pulse Oximetry

Falsely lowered SpO_2

- Probe malposition
- Impaired perfusion (peripheral vasoconstriction, peripheral arterial disease)
- Dark skin pigmentation
- Nail polish
- Methylene blue
- Motion artifact

Falsely elevated SpO_2

- Carboxyhemoglobin
- Methemoglobin
- Hypothermia

PRACTICE POINT

- A patient who is awake, responsive, managing secretions and phonating audibly is protecting his airway. The gag reflex does not reliably indicate whether the patient is protecting the airway.

TABLE 138-3 The Glasgow Coma Scale

		Score
Best eye opening	Spontaneous	4
	To voice	3
	To pain	2
	None	1
Best verbal response	Oriented	5
	Confused	4
	Inappropriate words	3
	Incomprehensible	2
	None	1
Best motor response	Obeys commands	6
	Localizes to pain	5
	Withdraws from pain	4
	Flexion to pain	3
	Extension to pain	2
	None	1
Total		**15**

The ability to manage secretions depends upon LOC, competency of the swallow mechanism, and volume of secretions or other fluids (saliva, sputum, blood, or gastric contents). As respiratory effort and confusion worsen, patients become increasingly unable to manage secretions and this too should be factored into the assessment.

The airway assessment must also include a projection of the expected clinical course. The comatose patient with acute hypercarbia may awaken quickly with noninvasive positive pressure ventilation (NPPV), while the patient with mild airway compromise due to acute epiglottitis may rapidly progress to complete airway obstruction. Unless rapid and sustained improvement is expected, patients with potentially threatened airways should be intubated quickly. Extreme caution should be exercised if the airway is compromised due to anatomic compression or obstruction, as these intubations are often extremely challenging. It may be safer to delay intubation until an expert in difficult airway management is available rather than risk a catastrophic procedural complication.

4. What is the likely progression of the acute presentation?

Predicting the natural history of acute respiratory distress is as important as assessing its severity. Patients with diabetic ketoacidosis with severe metabolic acidemia and tachypnea are rarely intubated because they are generally young and because the acidemia rapidly resolves with insulin. In contrast, patients with a similar degree of acidemia due to septic shock and lactic acidosis rarely improve quickly, and in all likelihood will continue to deteriorate. These patients are almost always intubated.

Using these four screening questions, a clinician can rapidly and efficiently obtain a snapshot of the severity of the presentation, the patient's "reserve" and the expected natural course of the condition. Any patient who "fails" one or more of these screening questions should be at minimum closely monitored if not immediately intubated.

MANAGEMENT

■ OXYGEN SUPPLEMENTATION AND OXYGEN FLOW DEVICES

Supplemental oxygen therapy improves arterial oxygenation by increasing the oxygen diffusion gradient across the alveolar-capillary membrane (see Chapter 95 [Hypoxia]). Each liter per minute of supplemental oxygen increases the FiO_2 by approximately 3%. Basic oxygen delivery devices such as the nasal cannula and simple face mask deliver *low flow* oxygen to supplement inspired room air. They are widely available, comfortable and generally well tolerated, but they cannot be set to deliver a precise FiO_2. Furthermore, each breath admixes room air with supplemental oxygen, limiting the maximum effective FiO_2 to approximately 40%. As respiratory distress worsen and minute ventilation increases, low flow devices lose efficacy because patients entrain an increasing proportion of room air relative to supplemental oxygen, thus diluting the inspired FiO_2.

Venturi masks rely upon the Venturi principle, whereby a jet of high flow oxygen entrains room air through a side port, mixing supplemental oxygen with room air. As in low flow systems, the effective FiO_2 is limited to about 40%, but they can be set to deliver a relatively precise FiO_2. The high flow of a venturi mask may better match the respiratory demand of a patient with high minute ventilation.

Closed systems such as the nonrebreather or reservoir face mask deliver oxygen into a reservoir bag from which the patient breathes. A tight face seal and a one-way exhalation valve on the side of the mask minimize entrainment of room air and rebreathing of exhaled gas. *In theory, reservoir masks can deliver near 100% FiO_2, but in real-world application, the FiO_2 rarely exceeds 70%.* Closed oxygenation systems may exacerbate acute hypercarbia and should be used cautiously (if at all) for this indication.

High flow nasal cannulas are a relatively recent innovation in supplemental oxygen therapy, delivering very high flow (generally humidified) oxygen at up to 60 L/min. This exceptionally high flow markedly exceeds minute ventilation in even the most distressed patient, thus eliminating inspiratory admixture of room air. These devices also provide a small amount of PEEP, which may recruit collapsed alveoli and reduce atelectasis. High flow nasal cannulas are generally more comfortable than face masks, allowing patients to eat, speak, and expectorate much more freely.

■ VENTILATORY SUPPORT

The physiology of positive pressure ventilation

The effects of positive pressure ventilation (PPV) on cardiopulmonary performance are complex and vary depending upon intravascular filling pressures, autonomic tone, lung compliance, and cardiac performance.

Positive pressure ventilation decreases work of breathing for patients with acute respiratory distress by reducing the metabolic load imposed upon respiratory muscles. At rest, respiration consumes roughly 3% of the resting cardiac output, increasing to up 40% during acute respiratory distress. PEEP (synonymous with continuous positive airway pressure [CPAP]) increases the mean airway pressure, which prevents end-expiratory collapse of damaged lung units and increases the oxygen gradient from alveoli to the pulmonary capillary bed. However, positive pressure ventilation can also be deleterious. The distribution of acute lung injury is heterogeneous, with areas of injured and noncompliant lung juxtaposed with uninjured areas with normal compliance. Positive pressure will preferentially distend compliant lung, potentially overdistending healthy lung segments and impairing their perfusion. This may increase dead space ventilation, worsen hypercarbia, increase work of breathing, and provoke barotrauma.

PEEP also has important hemodynamic effects, including reducing right ventricular preload and stroke volume as well as left ventricular afterload. The net effect is to unload the left ventricle (LV) by decreasing both LV preload and afterload, making PEEP a physiologically attractive treatment for acute cardiogenic pulmonary edema. High levels of PEEP (generally >10 cm H_2O) may impair venous return to the RV, leading to hypotension during hypovolemia, impaired RV function, pericardial tamponade, or severe pulmonary hypertension.

Noninvasive positive pressure ventilation (NPPV)

In appropriately selected patients, NPPV offers the benefits of mechanical ventilation without the morbidity and discomfort of an endotracheal tube (**Figure 138-2**). The two most commonly used NPPV modalities are continuous positive airway pressure CPAP and bi-level positive airway pressure (BPAP). (Note: "Bi-PAP" is a registered trademark). BPAP is CPAP with cyclic inspiratory positive pressure added to augment ventilation. The three main BPAP settings are the inspiratory positive airway pressure (IPAP), the expiratory positive airway pressure *(EPAP: synonymous with CPAP)* and the FiO_2. Generally, the initial EPAP is set between 5 and 10 cm H_2O and the IPAP is set at 5 to 15 cm H_2O *above* the EPAP. IPAP and EPAP are additive; thus a setting of EPAP: 5 and IPAP: 10 means that the patient is receiving 15 cm H_2O of pressure during inspiration. Higher EPAP settings may be required to compensate for extra thoracic pressure exerted by obesity, kyphoscoliosis, or abdominal distension. Increased IPAP may be necessary to meet the high inspiratory flow needs of patients who are young and fit, or in diseases characterized by inspiratory air hunger, such as COPD or asthma.

NPPV may be delivered through a face mask, nasal mask, or nasal prongs. As patients in respiratory distress almost invariably mouth-breathe, the face mask is the preferred initial choice in acute respiratory failure. However, the face mask is generally less comfortable than the nasal mask and restricts access for suctioning secretions or administering oral medications. Face masks should be used with extreme caution when there is potential for vomiting or aspiration. NPPV rarely induces barotrauma or adversely impacts hemodynamics because overly pressurized air usually leaks from the mask seal at the face, effectively serving as a pop-off valve. The primary side effects of NPPV include discomfort or claustrophobia due to dyssynchrony with positive pressure breaths, sinus pressure or discomfort, mild gastric distension, and pressure injury to the bridge of the nose or face after extended use.

Patient selection for NPPV

Patient selection is the most important predictor of successful response to NPPV, as the modality is most effective in patients who are young, have low critical illness severity scores, and who can calmly interface with the device. A good face mask seal is mandatory to maintain positive pressure, so NPPV is less effective in patients who have abnormal facial anatomy, are edentulous or who have copious facial hair. The best indicators of NPPV efficacy are visible reduction in respiratory effort and decreased respiratory acidosis (as measured with an arterial or venous blood gas). Patients who fail to respond to NPPV within 1-2 hours of therapy initiation are unlikely to improve and should be promptly intubated and mechanically ventilated.

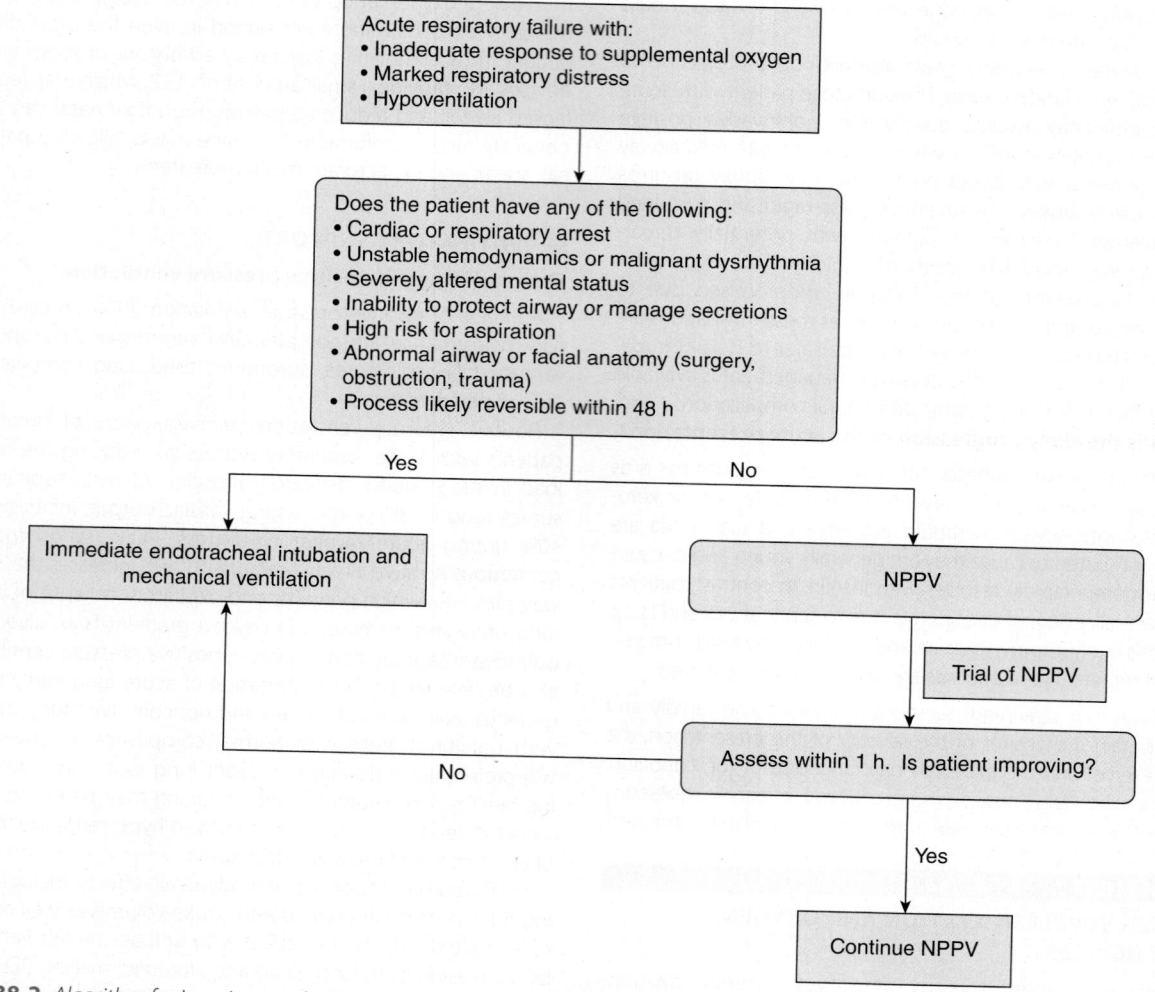

Figure 138-2 *Algorithm for invasive ventilation versus noninvasive ventilation decision making in patients with acute respiratory failure.*

An unprotected airway and high aspiration risk are near-absolute contraindications to NPPV (Figure 138-2). Cautious exceptions may be made for patients who are transiently obtunded due to hypercarbia and who are expected to rapidly improve after initiation of NPPV. Patients with acute cardiac or respiratory arrest, nonrespiratory acute organ failure, multiorgan failure, or significant hemodynamic instability should be intubated. NPPV is a short-term bridge rather than a durable treatment for acute respiratory failure, and it should generally be restricted to patients who are expected to improve within 48 to 72 hours after initiation of therapy.

NPPV may be considered as salvage therapy for "do-not-resuscitate" patients, but it should be implemented with a clear understanding of the goals to be achieved. NPPV is unlikely to "save" the patient with a diagnosis that typically requires endotracheal intubation. It may, however, reduce dyspnea or prolong life sufficiently for a patient to meaningfully interact with friends and family. These benefits should be weighed carefully against the potential adverse consequences of NPPV (discomfort, difficulty speaking, aspiration). NPPV is not a substitute for effective symptom palliation at the end of life.

NPPV for chronic respiratory failure should be conceptualized very differently than NPPV initiated for acute respiratory failure. Patients who chronically require NPPV for indications such as obesity-hypoventilation or neuromuscular disease generally wear these devices at home, and can be safely managed in most inpatient hospital units. In contrast, NPPV implemented as a treatment for *acute respiratory failure* implies instability and high risk for rapid progression to endotracheal intubation. Hospital units that accept NPPV for acute respiratory failure must offer close patient monitoring and have the resources necessary for emergent endotracheal intubation and mechanical ventilation.

The two primary indications for NPPV in acute respiratory failure are hypercarbic COPD exacerbations and acute cardiogenic pulmonary edema.

COPD exacerbation

NPPV is the treatment of choice for patients with moderate to severe acute hypercarbic COPD exacerbation (pH 7.10-7.35). A meta-analysis of 14 randomized trials comparing NPPV versus conventional therapy demonstrated that NPPV decreased *mortality* and *intubation* rates by approximately 50% (Number-Needed-to-Treat 10 and 4, respectively) and substantially reduced hospital lengths of stay. NPPV offers no advantages over supplemental oxygen therapy for patients with nonhypercarbic COPD exacerbations (pH > 7.35) and is often poorly tolerated in this population.

Acute cardiogenic pulmonary edema

Due to its salutary effects on left ventricular function, NPPV is an attractive nonpharmacologic therapy for acute cardiogenic pulmonary edema. The physiologic benefit of NPPV in decompensated heart failure primarily derives from CPAP or PEEP, which recruits or maintains inflation of alveoli. The use of inspiratory positive pressure (IPAP) in the absence of acute hypercarbia appears to offer no additional benefit and may increase patient discomfort. Meta-analyses agree that NPPV in acute cardiogenic pulmonary edema reduces the likelihood of endotracheal intubation and improves respiratory distress. The impact on mortality is unclear, as randomized controlled trials and meta-analyses have demonstrated conflicting results. Nonetheless, there is broad consensus that NPPV is a reasonable emergency therapy for acute cardiogenic pulmonary edema.

Other indications for NPPV

NPPV may reduce complications and mortality rates in patients with acute hypoxemic respiratory failure due to pneumonia. This benefit is most prominent in immunocompromised patients, primarily due to elimination of the infection risks associated with endotracheal intubation. However, as ventilator-associated pneumonia rates have declined with improved prophylaxis, the benefits of NPPV may have diminished over time. NPPV is also frequently used for treatment of status asthmaticus, but this remains controversial, as it is based on limited studies performed primarily in emergency departments. NPPV is reasonable first-line therapy for status asthmaticus when no contraindications exist with the clear recognition that these patients can decompensate very rapidly. It is imperative to monitor them closely and maintain a very low threshold for emergent intubation.

NPPV has also been studied for preintubation and postextubation management. A single trial demonstrated that NPPV is more effective than bag-valve-mask ventilation for preoxygenation prior to emergent intubation. Patients who received preintubation BPAP rather than standard bag-valve-mask ventilation had fewer desaturations and fewer severe hypoxemic episodes during intubation. NPPV may also expedite patient liberation from mechanical ventilation by providing a "step down" mode between mechanical ventilation and supplemental oxygen therapy. *Postextubation NPPV* is indicated as a weaning strategy for most or all COPD exacerbation patients being liberated from invasive mechanical ventilation. Meta-analyses from randomized controlled trials of patients with COPD exacerbation who had been intubated had significantly reduced mortality, ventilator-associated pneumonia, tracheostomy, and hospital length of stay when treated with NPPV postextubation. Postextubation NPPV is beneficial *only* if it is initiated prospectively, *before* a patient redevelops respiratory failure after extubation. A well-designed randomized trial demonstrated that NPPV for postextubation respiratory failure delayed inevitable reintubation and almost doubled mortality (25% vs 14%). Thus, most patients who develop postextubation respiratory failure should be promptly reintubated rather than attempting salvage treatment with NPPV.

Finally, NPPV may be a lifesaving temporizing intervention for patients with airway compromise from anatomic obstruction or compression. Clinicians with advanced airway management skills and equipment should manage difficult airways. In situations where difficult airway support is not immediately available, NPPV can occasionally be used to physiologically stent a compromised airway, buying crucial time to marshal the resources necessary to facilitate a safe intubation or a surgical airway.

The decision to intubate

The decision to intubate rests upon the four key questions posed at the beginning of this chapter (Figure 138-2):

1. How severe is the patient's respiratory distress?
2. Is the patient protecting his or her airway?
3. Is gas exchange adequate?
4. What is the likely progression of this acute presentation?

The most important question in acute respiratory failure is whether the preponderance of evidence supports safe management without an endotracheal tube. A prudent approach is to assume that every patient with acute respiratory failure will require endotracheal intubation until proven otherwise (Figure 138-2) (see also Chapter 140 [Basic Ventilator Management]).

SUGGESTED READINGS

Burns KE, et al. Noninvasive ventilation as a weaning strategy for mechanical ventilation in adults with respiratory failure: a meta-analysis. *CMAJ.* 2014;186:E112-E122.

Esteban A, Frutos-Vivar F, Ferguson ND, et al. Noninvasive positive-pressure ventilation for respiratory failure after extubation. *N Engl J Med.* 2004;350:2452-2460.

Masip J, Roque M, Sanchez B, Fernandez R, Subirana M, Exposito JA. Noninvasive ventilation in acute cardiogenic pulmonary edema: systematic review and meta-analysis. *JAMA.* 2005;294(24): 3124-3130.

Ram FS, Picot J, Lightowler J, Wedzicha JA. Non-invasive positive pressure ventilation for treatment of respiratory failure due to exacerbations of chronic obstructive pulmonary disease. *Cochrane Database Syst Rev.* 2009;(3):CD004104.

West JB. *Respiratory Physiology: The Essentials,* 9th ed. Baltimore, MD: Lippincott Williams & Wilkins, Wolters Kluwer Publishing Co; 2012.

Winck JC, Azevedo LF, Costa-Pereira A, Antonelli M, Wyatt JC. Efficacy and safety of noninvasive ventilation in the treatment of acute cardiogenic pulmonary edema—a systematic review and meta-analysis. *Crit Care.* 2006;10(2):R69.

OTHER RESOURCES

An excellent and entertaining review of critical care and respiratory pathophysiology. http://www.derangedphysiology.com/php/Respiratory-failure-and-mechanical-ventilation/index.php. Accessed March 05, 2016.

Exhaustive coverage of many topics in critical care medicine, all formatted as brief, bullet-pointed synopses. Excellent for quick review when time is limited. www.lifeinthefastlane.com. Accessed March 05, 2016.

CHAPTER 139

Pain, Agitation, and Delirium in the Critical Care Setting

Gary Margolias, MD
Michael Sterling, MD

Key Clinical Questions

1. What are the clinical and pharmacologic effects of single agent versus multiple agent sedative and analgesic administration?

2. What is the best way to dose sedative, analgesic, and paralytic agents in the intensive care unit (ICU)?

3. How do the pharmacokinetics and dosing of sedative, analgesic, and paralytic agents change with duration of infusion?

4. What is the proper sequence to initiate sedatives, analgesics, and/or paralytics, and how does dosing refinement affect time to weaning and other predictors of favorable outcome?

5. How do you select individual sedative, analgesic, or paralytic agents in critically ill patients?

6. When do you decide to paralyze a ventilated patient?

INTRODUCTION

Our understanding of pain, agitation, and delirium (PAD) has been a journey of discovery. In 1995, the Society of Critical Care Medicine (SCCM) published the relatively modest Practice Parameters for Intravenous Analgesia and sedation for Adult Patients in the Intensive Care Unit, six recommendations based mostly on expert opinion. The American College of Critical Care Medicine subsequently developed evidence-based guidelines in 2002 and most recently in 2013.

ICU patients experience significant nonprocedural as well as procedural pain. The development of reproducible and validated tools for assessing pain, sedation, agitation, and delirium have been essential in allowing clinicians to know not only when to treat, but how effective a given treatment is. Furthermore, the recognition that pain agitation and delirium may be a risk factor for the post ICU syndrome characterized by weakness, cognitive dysfunction, and post-traumatic stress disorder (PTSD), has further underscored the importance of their early recognition and effective treatment. In the following chapter, we will review the current concepts in the assessment, treatment, and monitoring of PAD in the ICU population.

■ DOSING PRINCIPLES

Sedative, analgesic, and paralytic therapies are administered by intravenous (IV) *bolus* or by IV *infusion*, as intramuscular and enteral titration are unreliable.

Principles of dose initiation and maintenance

Bolus dosing has the advantage of a rapid onset of action, but has the associated risk of either overshooting or undershooting the therapeutic goal. As such, nursing vigilance with frequent assessment and bolus titration to defined therapeutic outcomes is necessary. On the other hand, infusion drug dosing reflects a more gradual and refined titration to clinical effect, but does carry a greater risk of drug accumulation with protracted infusion. As such, an unwanted prolongation of time to awakening may occur when clinical circumstances allow for drug discontinuation. For this reason, infusions should only be undertaken in the ICU when bolus dosing has failed to produce the desired sedative effect.

Clinicians should follow a structured algorithm for ICU sedation, pain control, and paralysis and become familiar with the ACCM PAD guidelines (**Figure 139-1**). While sedative and analgesic agents help to maintain mechanical ventilation, their prolonged use can become an obstacle to liberation from life support. Because planning for weaning should occur as soon as ventilatory support is begun, the sedative and analgesic goals should be defined and dosing plan structured for each individual agent such that their sum individual dosing requirements are minimized.

Analgesic goals should be addressed first. Once adequate analgesia is achieved, sedation may be targeted to the patient's clinical need. For instance, a patient with acute respiratory distress syndrome (ARDS) ventilated with a high-frequency oscillator may require deep sedation and analgesia (and possibly neuromuscular blockade), whereas a patient requiring minimal volume ventilation or pressure support may need only mild analgesia and no sedation. An initial targeted focus on the patient's analgesic need will help curtail sedative requirements, as adequate pain control decreases anxiety and sedative need.

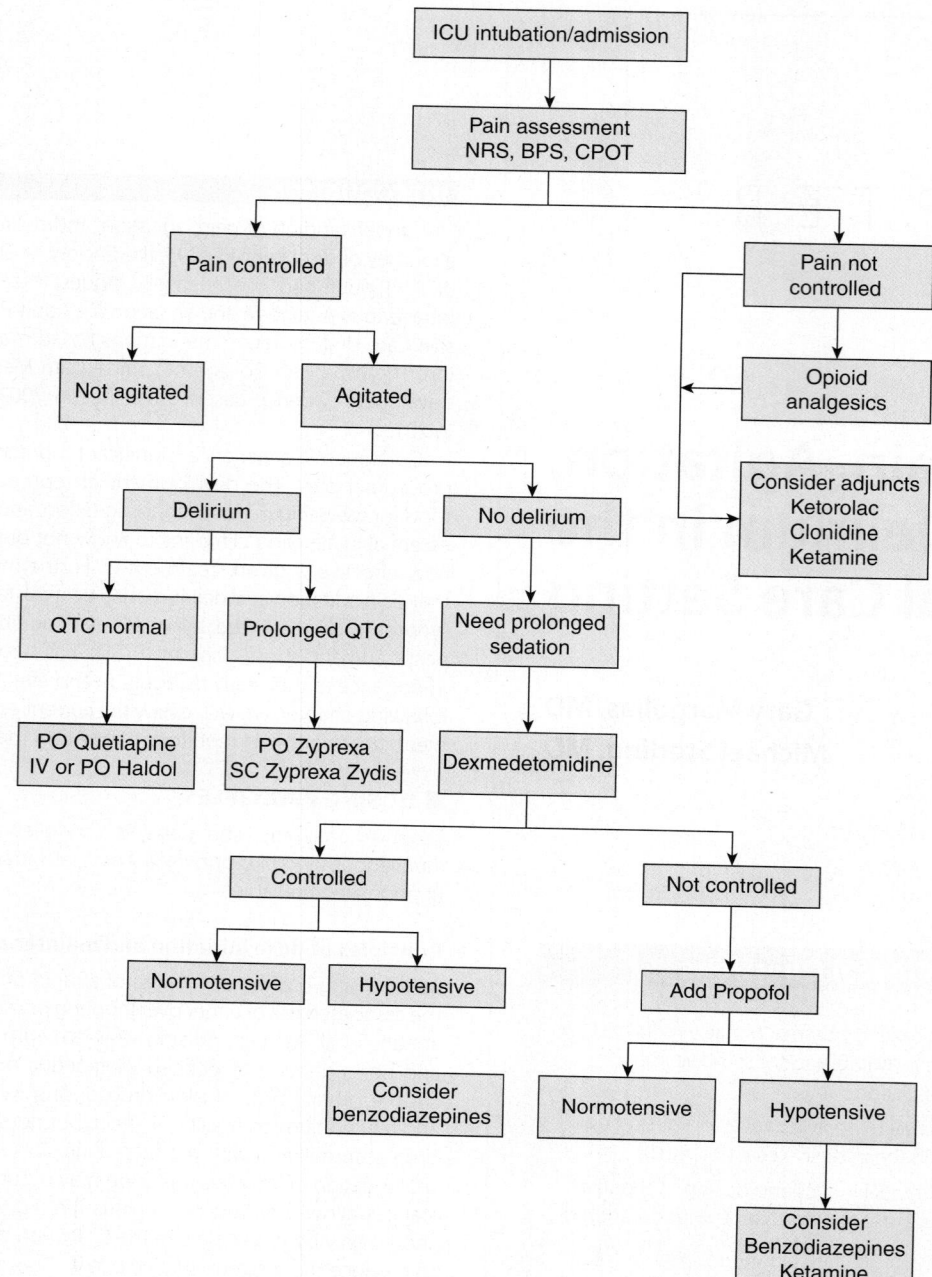

Figure 139-1 *Algorithm for ICU sedation, pain control, and paralysis.*

Recent clinical evidence supports that sedation need not be applied as a routine aspect of ICU care even in the most severely ill intubated patients provided that adequate bolus analgesia (opioids) is carefully administered. Patients treated in this manner demonstrated shorter ICU stays and fewer ventilator days without suffering any untoward clinical outcomes. It may be reasonable to consider only analgesia in some patients and utilize sedation only for patients who remain anxious or agitated after achieving adequate analgesia.

During the initiation phase of sedation and analgesia, the patient's chronic comorbid conditions must be considered in guiding analgesic requirement. For instance, the patient may have a source of chronic pain such as musculoskeletal pain or neuropathy. This could be an overlooked source of discomfort if not factored in the appraisal of a patient's analgesic need. Similarly, preexisting psychiatric disorders such as psychosis should be taken into account in targeting sedation and anxiolysis.

Medication maintenance

Active management of analgesia and sedation should continue throughout the ICU stay. If the patient's dissynchrony with the ventilator is primarily a manifestation of untreated pain, but sedative medications are escalated instead of analgesics, unnecessary hemodynamic compromises and drug accumulation may occur. This underscores the need for employing valid and reliable tools for scoring pain and agitation.

Medication weaning and discontinuation

Rapid withdrawal of sedative and analgesic medications can result in the development of delirium that may impede liberation from mechanical ventilation and trigger an unnecessary diagnostic workup. This type of delirium is common, having been reported in upward of one-third of patients who have been sedated in the ICU for greater than a week.

A sensitivity to the signs of withdrawal from opioids (diaphoresis, tachycardia, papillary dilatation, lacrimation, piloerection, hypertension, vomiting, abdominal cramping, restlessness, anxiety, fever, yawning) and benzodiazepines (tremor, diaphoresis, anxiety, tachycardia, nausea) should be maintained. Some advocate a 10% decrement in narcotic use every day, but a tailored approach may be appropriate for some patients.

■ PHARMACOKINETIC PRINCIPLES

Caring for critically ill patients represents an extremely dynamic practice in which drug regimens with rapid clinical effects and short durations of action are frequently best suited. In general, drugs without active metabolites and with few pharmacologic interactions offer the greatest efficacy with the fewest side effects. Furthermore, medications with smaller volumes of distribution are more easily titrated. Drugs that do not manifest significant tachyphylaxis also lend themselves to titration in ICU practice. Sedatives and analgesics with increased risk of hemodynamic side effects are avoided when possible, as are medications with higher risk of withdrawal symptoms upon their discontinuation.

Table 139-1 contains a list of the pharmacologic characteristics of the ideal drug. While no single drug possesses every one of these ideal properties, sedative and analgesic medications are selected on the basis of these parameters and the individual patient's clinical condition. ICU patients can have depressed or changing hepatic and renal clearance profiles, as well as dynamic hepatic synthetic function and nutritional flux. Drug concentrations and protein binding can change as well. Similarly, alterations in gut absorption affect serum levels of enterally administered agents. Each patient's predominant physiology as well as the response to sedative and analgesic therapy should impact the titration of sedative, analgesic, and paralytic medications in the ICU.

Drugs do not attain an immediate steady state, as they are influenced by the volume of distribution (V_d) within the patient and the variable redistribution into different anatomic compartments. Upon administration, drugs are preferentially distributed to vessel-rich organ systems. Drugs with lipophilic biochemical properties (eg, fentanyl, midazolam) are more rapidly distributed to the lipid-rich regions of the body, which includes the central nervous system (CNS) (**Figure 139-2**). Hydrophilic drugs (eg, morphine) on the other hand penetrate fatty tissue relatively poorly and are confined more to the lower V_d that is the plasma, with slower CNS penetration and clinical effect.

An administered drug will undergo renal and hepatic metabolism, but certain highly lipophilic drugs with relatively long elimination half-times by kidney and liver distribute rapidly at first into the vessel-rich group (including CNS), and then redistribute into a second "compartment" (plasma), thereby rapidly terminating

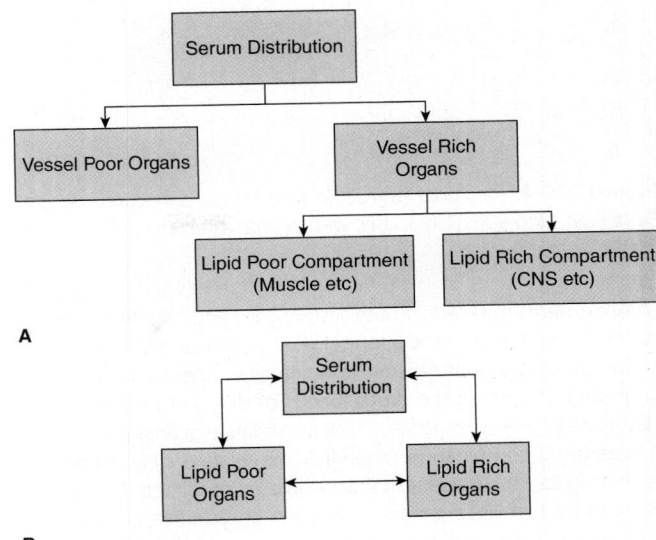

A

B

Figure 139-2 *(A) Distribution of lipophilic drug with initial bolus dosing. (B) Redistribution of lipid-rich organs over time.*

their clinical (sedative) effect. With time and ongoing infusion, this termination of clinical effect by redistribution becomes attenuated as a new steady state is established between compartments (**Figure 139-3**). Broadly, these phenomena of variable pharmacokinetics contribute to the context-sensitive half-time of an agent. This principle represents a clinically useful way to understand how greater length of infusion prolongs clinical effect. Classical ways of thinking about drug elimination half-lives after bolus dosing by renal and hepatic metabolism have little clinical utility with ongoing infusion and changing distribution between compartments. The concept of *context-sensitive half-time* describes changing time to elimination of half of the current plasma concentration with discontinuation of a drug at that point in time. These dynamic pharmacokinetics have important implications in the ICU setting. Suitable arousal for ventilator weaning is very much dependent on CNS concentration of sedative agents at that particular point in time, which in turn is reliant on the context-sensitive half-time of the drug. With passing time, and with continued administration, lipophilic drugs that have come to a steady state within lipid-rich

TABLE 139-1 Characteristics of the Pharmacologically Ideal Drug

Clinical onset	Rapid
Clinical effect	Short
Active metabolites	None
Pharmacologic interactions	None
Volume of distribution	Small
Tachyphylaxis	None
Hemodynamic side effects	None
Withdrawal symptoms	None

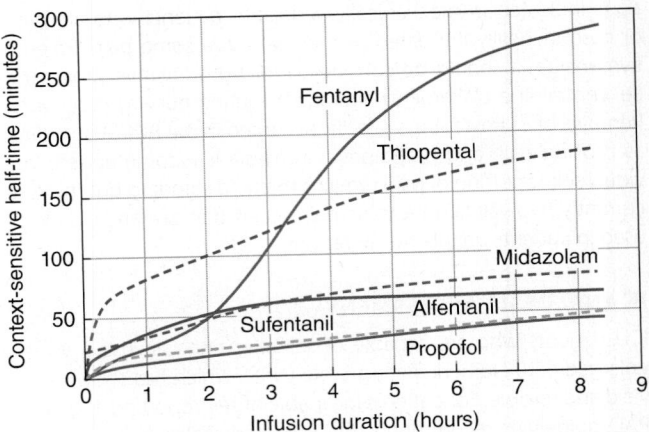

Figure 139-3 *Context-sensitive half-time of various sedative and analgesic drugs. (Reproduced, with permission, from Longnecker DE, Brown DL, Newman MF, et al. Anesthesiology. New York, NY: McGraw-Hill; 2008. Fig. 68-5.)*

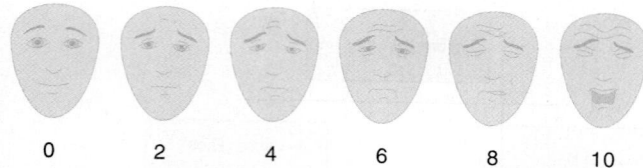

Figure 139-4 *The Faces Pain Scale. (The Faces Pain Scale—Revised. From Pain. 2001;93:173-183. Used with permission from IASP.)*

compartments may redistribute systemically and manifest a declining dose requirement and a longer time to clinical awakening.

Concomitant use of sedative and analgesic agents will affect the properties of each of the drugs. Drugs of different pharmacologic classes may have synergistic or additive sedative or analgesic effects. A synergistic combination magnifies the relative clinical effect of each drug to a greater extent than would be predicted on the basis of its individual dose potency, whereas an additive combination finds a clinical effect that approximates each drug's individual relative potency. Benzodiazepine sedatives and opiate analgesic agents display synergism in analgesia, sedation, and respiratory depression. Therefore, more pronounced clinical effects occur when these two classes of drugs are used in combination than when each is used individually at higher doses. Because of this, unpredictable clinical effects can occur when drugs are coadministered, and combining these classes of medications should be done with extreme caution in the nonventilated or weaning patient.

Similarly, changing individual doses of drugs in a combination regimen should be done with the same care as the administration of a new drug because an entirely new pharmacodynamic state is established with differing combination drug concentrations. Drugs that are not primarily considered sedative agents, but nonetheless have sedating properties (eg, anticholinergic agents or neuroleptics), should also be used with cognizance of their potential additive or synergistic sedative capability. Finally, many commonly used sedative medications, such as propofol, have no individual analgesic properties or potentiation when used in combination with opioids while other medications such as dexmedetomidine (dex) clearly have opioid sparing effects.

PAIN IN THE ICU

The awareness and recognition that ICU patients experience significant procedural as well as nonprocedural pain should help guide the assessment and treatment of ICU patients. For example, analgesia is indicated in mechanically ventilated patients who are orally or nasotracheally intubated as they will have some pain. Preemptive analgesia should be considered for both invasive procedures (ie, central line placement) and some routine nursing procedures. Removal of a chest tube is specifically noted in the ACCM guidelines as causing pain and preemptive analgesia is recommended. Individual self-reporting of pain remains the gold standard but there are currently two validated reliable pain scales that can and should be used in patients unable to self-report.

■ ANALGESIA ASSESSMENT

ICU patients who are capable of self-reporting can use a visually enlarged 0-10 Numeric Rating Scale (NRS), which has shown to be valid and reliable. For patients incapable of self-reporting, the ACCM PAD guidelines recommend two validated scales: Behavioral Pain Scale (BPS) (**Table 139-2**) and the Critical Care Pain Observation Tool (CPOT) (**Table 139-3**). Both of these scales have been validated in adult ICUs with medical, postoperative, and trauma patients (excluding brain-injured patients).

TABLE 139-2 Behavioral Pain Scale[a]

Item	Description	Score[b]
Facial expression	Relaxed	1
	Partially tightened (eg, brow lowering)	2
	Fully tightened (eg, eyelid closing)	3
	Grimacing	4
Upper limb movements	No movement	1
	Partially bent	2
	Fully bent with finger flexion	3
	Permanently retracted	4
Compliance with mechanical ventilation	Tolerating movement	1
	Coughing but tolerating ventilation for most of the time	2
	Fighting ventilator	3
	Unable to control ventilation	4

[a]Source: Aissaoui Y, et al. *Anesth Analg.* 2005;101(5):1470-1476.
[b]Score ranges from 3 (no pain) to 12 (maximum pain).

■ ANALGESIC MEDICATION SELECTION AND PRECAUTIONS

Intravenous (IV) opioids should be considered the first line of treatment of nonneuropathic pain in ICU patients. Nonopioid analgesics, such as acetaminophen and nonsteroidal anti-inflammatory medications, are suggested adjuncts for analgesic treatment in the ICU. Ketamine and α-agonist drugs (eg, dexmedetomidine) also have analgesic properties, but they are utilized primarily for their sedative properties rather than their analgesic sparing properties.

Opioid pharmacology

Opioid analgesics provide the clinically desirable effects of pain control and a blunting of the sensation of dyspnea. Various opioid agents exhibit slightly different time to onset and varying durations of effect (Table 139-3). Dosing and cost of different agents also vary widely. The analgesic action of these drugs occurs primarily due to interaction with the mu (μ) receptors in both the CNS and periphery. More lipid-soluble drugs (eg, fentanyl) have more rapid onset of action, as they are quickly distributed to the lipid-rich CNS tissue. Conversely, these same agents will have a protracted redistribution phase after they have been discontinued, as they will continue a slow release into circulation from these same lipid-rich compartments. Drugs with greater hepatic or renal metabolism may have extended activity in patients in whom comorbid disease or age impacts the function of these organ systems. Agents that are metabolized to active compounds usually have longer clinical effect, and the pharmacologic properties of metabolites may be clinically important.

Equianalgesic assessment is made using morphine as the standard-bearer to which other agents are compared (**Table 139-4**). These comparisons are extrapolated from studies with intramuscular dosing in healthy volunteers, and entirely different pharmacokinetics might exist with infusion dosing, opioid switching, and especially in critically ill patients with attendant renal and hepatic compromise as well as altered volume of distribution (V_d) and protein-drug binding.

Opioid selection

Fentanyl, hydromorphone, morphine, and methadone are the agents most often used in the ICU. Intravenous fentanyl, often the

TABLE 139-3 Critical-Care Pain Observation Tool[a]

Indicator	Description	Score	
Facial expression	No muscular tension observed	Relaxed, neutral	0
	Presence of frowning, brow lowering, orbit tightening, and levator contraction	Tense	1
	All of the above facial movements plus eyelid tightly closed	Grimacing	2
Body movements	Does not move at all (does not necessarily mean absence of pain)	Absence of movements	0
	Slow, cautious movements, touching or rubbing the pain site, seeking attention through movements	Protection	1
	Pulling tube, attempting to sit up, moving limbs/thrashing, not following commands, striking at staff, trying to climb out of bed	Restlessness	2
Muscle tension	No resistance to passive movements	Relaxed	0
Evaluation by passive flexion and extension of upper extremities	Resistance to passive movements	Tense, rigid	1
	Strong resistance to passive movements, inability to complete them	Very tense or rigid	2
Compliance with the ventilator (intubated patients)	Alarms not activated, easy ventilation	Tolerating ventilator or movement	0
	Alarms stop spontaneously		
OR	Asynchrony: blocking ventilation, alarms frequently activated	Coughing but tolerating	1
		Fighting ventilator	2
Vocalization (extubated patients)	Talking in normal tone or no sound	Talking in normal tone or no sound	0
	Sighing, moaning		
	Crying out, sobbing	Sighing, moaning	1
		Crying out, sobbing	2
Total, range			0-8

[a]Source: Gélinas C, Fillion L, Puntillo KA, et al. Validation of the critical-care pain observation tool in adult patients. *Am J Crit Care*. 2006;15(4):420-427. Table 1. Available at http://ajcc.aacnjournals.org/content/15/4/420.short. © 2006 American Association of Critical-Care Nurses. Used with permission.

first choice for IV opiate use, is a highly lipophilic agent with no active metabolites, attains almost immediate CNS effect, but may accumulate after prolonged infusion and in patients with renal dysfunction. Fentanyl patches are avoided in the ICU due to delayed and unpredictable onset and offset.

Hydromorphone can be used IV or PO and compared to morphine induces less histamine release and has fewer accumulating metabolites in renal failure patients.

Morphine, on the other hand, has an active metabolite (morphine-6-gluconoride) that can also accumulate in patients with renal dysfunction and may result in prolonged respiratory depression. Additionally, this agent has more histamine-releasing effects than other opioid agents.

Methadone, an opioid with associated N-Methyl-D-aspartic acid (NMDA) receptor antagonist properties, may be utilized for the treatment of chronic neuropathic pain. Its long duration of action also makes it useful for weaning from shorter-acting agents.

Meperidine has a neurotoxic metabolite (normeperidine) that may accumulate, especially in patients with renal dysfunction, and therefore its use in ICU patients should be avoided.

Once an opioid agent is selected, medications may be bolus dosed—utilizing careful assessment of analgesic effect (eg, pain scales)—as bolus dosing is less likely to result in drug accumulation, and steady states and analgesic effect will be more rapidly apparent than with titration of narcotic infusions. Narcotic dosing should be guided by clinical effect and not by defined "upper dose limits," as determined in pharmacologic manuals. When dose escalation fails to demonstrate analgesia, a different opioid medication should be tried because opioid receptor affinity may change with continued exposure to a single agent.

Opioid precautions

Clinically undesirable effects of opioids include the ablation of the hypoxic respiratory drive and the displacement of the carbon dioxide

TABLE 139-4 Pharmacologic Properties of Commonly Used Intravenous Opioids

Opioid Medications	Equianalgesic IV Dose	Intermittent Dosing	Infusion Dose	Onset (min)	Half-Life (h)	Lipophilicity	Active Metabolites
Fentanyl	100-200 mcg	0.35-0.5 mcg/kg every 0.5-1 h	0.7-10.0 mcg/kg/h	Immediate	1.5-6	+++	Yes
Morphine	10 mg	0.01-0.15 mg/kg every 1-2 h	0.07-0.5 mg/kg/h	<5	3-7	+	Yes
Hydromorphone	1.5 mg	10-30 mcg/kg every 1-2 h	7-15 mcg/kg/h	<5	2-3	++	No
Meperidine	70-100 mg	Not recommended	Not recommended	<5	3-4	+++	Yes
Methadone	10 mg	10 mg every 6 h	Not recommended	10-20	15-30	+++	No

response curve rightward. These effects increase the likelihood of respiratory acidosis and respiratory failure. Worsening hypotension may also occur in hemodynamically compromised patients due either to an indirect blunting of intrinsic catecholamine-mediated vasomotor tone during a stress response, or, rarely, from the direct vasodilating effect of histamine release with bolus doses of certain opioids (eg, morphine, meperidine). Opioid analgesics may also cause or potentiate reduced gut transit or ileus as well as urinary retention in critically ill patients. Rarely opioid use (especially with morphine) may cause release of histamine associated with hypotension, bronchospasm, flushing, and urticaria. For those with compromised hemodynamics or reactive airways disease, the concern for histamine release may factor into the choice of analgesic agent.

Rapid tapering of opioids may lead to withdrawal in patients exposed to high doses of narcotics for more than 1 week. Opioid infusions should not be decreased more than 25% per day.

Analgesia reversal

Naloxone is the most widely used competitive inhibitor of opioid medications. It is primarily used in the ICU setting to reverse the acute respiratory depressant effects of narcotic drugs. Its use in this manner is likely safe in most instances; however, clinically important nuances to using this drug include the following:

- Use of the drug in a patient in the early postoperative setting may result in acute analgesic reversal and an associated hyperadrenergic surge that can be devastating (eg, ventricular arrhythmias, acute congestive heart failure, hypertension), and incremental naloxone dosing is usually curtailed tenfold in these patients.
- Administration of the drug to those chronically dependent on opioids (eg, cancer patients, opioid abusers) might precipitate severe withdrawal.

If naloxone is used, it can be administered intravenously, subcutaneously, or intramuscularly. Intravenous dosing (in patients who are not postoperative) is 0.4 mg intravenously, repeated as needed. Intravenous infusion (eg, 0.4 mg/h) might be necessary to prevent recurrent narcotic sedation, as the drug half-life is fairly short (1-4 hours).

SEDATION IN THE ICU

■ SEDATIVE MEDICATION SELECTION AND PRECAUTIONS

There is a growing body of literature associating agitation and anxiety with poorer clinical outcomes. The priority with these patients should be early identification of agitation and anxiety using the available, validated assessment tools, identifying reversible causes such as pain, hypoxemia, hypotension, disruption of the sleep/wake cycle, and substance withdrawal syndromes. Attempts at mitigating agitation and anxiety should be made without sedatives if possible by addressing reversible causes first.

There is now a large body of literature demonstrating that maintaining light sedation (arousable and purposeful patient) is preferable to deep sedation (unresponsive to painful stimuli) and associated with improved outcomes, shorter lengths of stay (both hospital and ICU) and fewer days on a mechanical ventilator. The use of sedation should be protocolized and the use of sedation scales routine.

The use of nonbenzodiazepine sedation such as propofol and dexmedetomidine has markedly changed the way patients are sedated in the ICU and their use has been associated with less delirium and less post ICU cognitive dysfunction. Dexmedetomidine (dex) is a selective α-2 receptor antagonist that exhibits sedative, and opioid sparing properties. It major side effects include hypotension and bradycardia. Pts sedated on dex are easily arousable and

follow commands. It causes minimum respiratory depression and is approved for sedation in nonintubated patients. However, it can cause loss of airway and therefore nonintubated patients on dex need to have their respiratory status monitored closely.

Despite the availability of these relatively new agents, benzodiazepines are still used widely for sedating critically ill patients. Both benzodiazepines and propofol, despite being different classes of drugs, potentiate GABA inhibition within the CNS with anxiolytic, sedative, and hypnotic effects. Both have similar amnestic potential, which may be desirable within the ICU setting, and both have similar respiratory depressant effects due to shifting of the carbon dioxide (CO_2) response curve rightward (decreased respiratory drive at physiologic CO_2 levels) and blunting of hypoxic drive. Both benzodiazepines and propofol are lipid soluble. However, propofol is carried in a lipid emulsion that renders it much more lipophilic, which in turn accounts for the very rapid uptake into the lipid-rich and highly vascular CNS with subsequent quick redistribution out of the CNS after bolus dosing or brief infusions. This redistribution rapidly terminates propofol's clinical sedative effect. Like all lipophilic agents, propofol and benzodiazepines will demonstrate a prolongation of clinical effect once they have been discontinued if their protracted use has resulted in saturation of the body's "lipid compartment."

The choice of which agents to use depends on pharmacokinetic considerations and the matching of the time needed for sedation in a particular clinical circumstance to the pharmacokinetic properties of the drug. Propofol has been the agent of choice for sedation for brief procedural interventions or short-term mechanical ventilation (<1-3 days), whereas in the past, benzodiazepines have been used as a more cost-effective approach for sedation that is expected to last more than a few days. An alternative to benzodiazepines, dexmedetomidine may have considerable benefits. Benzodiazepines may still have a preferred role in the treatment of alcohol and other drug withdrawal syndromes or in patients who are unable to tolerate dexmedetomidine or propofol either due to drug intolerance or hemodynamic instability.

Benzodiazepines

Pharmacologic properties of commonly used benzodiazepine agents vary (Table 139-4) as do dosing regimens and costs of both benzodiazepine and opioid drugs (**Table 139-5**). The pharmacokinetic properties and dosing of sedative and analgesic agents were derived from studies of healthy volunteers who have received single bolus drug doses. These data may not accurately reflect dynamic context-sensitive half-times with continuous infusion, especially in critically ill patients with shifting volumes of distribution, serum drug-protein binding, severely compromised hepatic perfusion, and metabolism changes.

Midazolam and lorazepam are the most commonly used benzodiazepines in the ICU. Although midazolam is thought of as a rapid-onset, short-acting agent, when used in the short term, its high lipid solubility results in accumulation and prolonged action with extended infusions. This characteristic, along with the fact that its

TABLE 139-5 Equianalgesic Comparison of Commonly Utilized Opioids

Opioid Agent	Equianalgesic Potency (mg)
Morphine	1
Fentanyl	75-125 (mcg)
Hydromorphone	0.15
Meperidine	0.1

primary metabolite (1-hydroxymidazolam glucuronide) is clinically active for up to 36 hours after drug cessation, makes lorazepam a preferred sedative especially in the obese and in patients requiring greater than 48 hours of sedation.

Benzodiazepine precautions

Benzodiazepine withdrawal can occur with weaning from these drugs. Longer-acting agents such as diazepam, lorazepam, or even clonazepam may be used as a bridge to complete discontinuation of sedation. Patients receiving greater than 50 mg total dose or greater than 1 mg/kg of IV lorazepam per day are at risk for toxicity from *propylene glycol*, a solvent in which the drug is dissolved. Propylene glycol toxicity can cause renal injury and acute tubular necrosis (ATN), tissue necrosis, and significant anion-gap acidosis. Patients receiving greater than the recommended daily dose of this drug should be monitored for toxicity with daily osmolar gap measurements and serum lactates.

Propofol

Propofol, a hydrophobic drug, demonstrates rapid onset and offset due to its ability to rapidly penetrate the CNS with initiation and then redistribute to other tissues with discontinuation. The drug is metabolized to inactive products by the liver and then excreted by the kidneys. In general, *hepatic and renal diseases do not alter clinical effect in any appreciable manner*. Prolonged infusion times and deeper depths of sedation result in drug accumulation and sedation. Propofol use is associated with fewer ventilator days compared to patients treated with bolus dosing of lorazepam. Propofol has no individual analgesic properties or potentiation when used in combination with opioids.

Propofol precautions

The lipid emulsion of the drug has a significant caloric load (1.1 kcal/cc) that should be factored as part of the daily intake. Propofol is also associated with the development of hypertriglyceridemia, especially in those predisposed to this condition or in those receiving concurrent total parenteral nutrition.

In patients receiving high-dose propofol infusions (>83 mcg/kg/min for >48 hours), a rare (39 published cases) but serious condition—propofol-related infusion syndrome (PRIS)—associated with rhabdomyolysis, myocardial failure, acute renal failure, severe metabolic acidosis, Brady arrhythmias, cardiac arrest, and hypotension has been described. PRIS occurs more often in patients receiving vasopressors or glucocorticoids or those with mitochondrial metabolic deficiencies.

Dexmedetomidine

Dexmedetomidine is a water soluble primarily α-2 receptor agonist. While chemically related to clonidine it is approximately eight times more specific for the α-2 receptor making it more effective than clonidine for sedation and its analgesic sparing effect. Its onset of action is about 15 minutes and peak concentrations are usually achieved within an hour of starting the IV infusion. It is primarily metabolized by the liver and clearances can be decreased by more than 50% in patients with severe liver disease. There are no known active metabolites. IV loading of dexmedetomidine is no longer recommended because of the increased incidence of hemodynamic instability noted in critically ill patients.

Dexmedetomidine is especially useful for short-term sedation, has very little respiratory depressant effect, and has some analgesic properties. These characteristics frequently permit—unlike the other sedative agents—ventilator weaning without full discontinuation of the drug, a property advantageous in patients whose weaning is hindered by primarily nonpulmonary considerations such as pain and agitation.

Other sedative drugs

Other drugs used less frequently as alternatives for sedation in the ICU include neuroleptic drugs such as haloperidol and ketamine. Haloperidol can be given 2 mg IV/IM (doubled as needed every 15 minutes) for acute severe agitation, but its use should be avoided in the setting of a prolonged QTc interval (≥500 ms), and monitored with intermittent ECGs secondary to the increased incidence of torsade de pointes. Other medications that might prolong the QT interval (azole antifungal drugs, amiodarone, macrolides, etc) should be used with caution in combination with these medications and electrolyte balance (especially magnesium) should be maintained. Cumulative haloperidol dose (>35 mg) has been shown to increase the risk of torsade as has higher-dose IV administration (>20 mg) and prior cardiac disease. Extrapyramidal symptoms and neuroleptic malignant syndrome are other clinical entities associated with neuroleptic medication use and close monitoring of these patients is recommended.

Ketamine offers similar pharmacologic advantages to dexmedetomidine, as well as bronchodilator properties, but its use is limited by undesirable, dose-dependent, psychotropic effects. While Ketamine may be considered in patients who are intolerant of dex and propofol and have a bronchospastic component to their disease process, there is currently no outcomes data regarding its use as an ICU sedative.

■ MONITORING AND MANAGEMENT OF SEDATION

Evidence now demonstrates improved clinical outcomes with light as opposed to deep sedation in the ICU. A strategy that emphasizes nonbenzodiazepine sedation along with daily awakening for mechanically ventilated patients should be employed. Daily awakening of intubated patients permits reassessment of sedative and analgesic requirements on a routine basis, and once the patient has demonstrated lucidity and is examined by the provider, sedative protocols can be reinitiated at half their previous dose, which allows a stepwise decrement in sedative requirements. This sedation strategy has been shown to reduce the number of ventilator days and ICU LOS.

PRACTICE POINT

- Light sedation and daily awakening of intubated patients is an evidence-based practice and part of routine ICU care. Daily awakening protocols reduce ICU length of stay and decrease tracheostomy procedures, diagnostic studies ordered, and the amount of sedating drugs required. Daily awakening may also reduce the incidence of PTSD. Light sedation and daily awakening should not be employed in patients requiring neuromuscular blockade.

Sedation assessment

Several tools have been developed to assess the level of sedation and aid in the titration of sedating medications. The therapeutic goal of sedative-analgesic medications in intubated patients is to achieve comfort that includes a calm and cooperative disposition and ability to follow commands. However, for patients with a need for higher levels of mechanical ventilator support, deeper sedation goals may be necessary.

The Richmond Agitation-Sedation Scale (RASS) and the Sedation-Agitation Scale (SAS) are the two sedation assessment tools noted by ACCM PAD guidelines to be the most valid and reliable.

In the intubated comatose ICU patient or the patient who requires neuromuscular blockade, objective tools for measuring brain function should be employed as subjective assessments are unobtainable. Examples include EEG monitoring, Bispectral Index (BIS) monitoring and auditory evoked potentials (AEPs). BIS monitoring uses an algorithmic processing of the electroencephalogram to produce a number from 0 to 100 where 100 is a fully awake and 0 is absence of brain activity. AEPs use an auditory stimulus to evoke an electrophysiological response which is recorded. EEG monitoring should be used when nonconvulsive seizures are suspected or when a patient with neuromuscular blockade has known or suspected seizures.

Sedation reversal

Flumazenil is a benzodiazepine derivative with high affinity for the benzodiazepine receptor and acts as a competitive inhibitor for benzodiazepine drugs. Although this intrinsic effective inhibition has found indications for use in clinical practice, especially for reversal of benzodiazepine anesthetic use, the drug has little benefit in the ICU setting. Use of flumazenil after prolonged benzodiazepine use in the ICU might provoke withdrawal symptoms or seizures. The drug has no indication in those with any clinical predisposition toward seizure (eg, epilepsy, intracranial pathology, electrolyte disturbances, benzodiazepine, or alcohol dependence) or in the setting of cyclic antidepressant overdose. Use of the drug is also complicated by the relatively short elimination half-life (1 hour) that might result in benzodiazepine resedation after flumazenil metabolism. A better approach for a patient thought to be suffering respiratory compromise due to benzodiazepine overdose might be supportive.

PARALYSIS IN THE ICU

Neuromuscular blocking (NMB) use has been declining in ICUs over the last two and a half decades. Associated with increased mortality, LOS, ventilator days and an increase incidence of Critically Ill Polyneuropathy (CIP), their use has been critically reevaluated. Suggested uses may still include severe ARDS (a recent study showed improved outcomes when cis-atracurium was used early and for a limited period of time), and rapid sequence intubation (RSI). Additionally, a recent review article suggested the following uses for NMBs in the ICU setting:

(1) Status asthmaticus to mitigate patient ventilator dyssynchrony and limit barotraumas.
(2) Abdominal hypertension syndromes including abdominal compartment syndrome where prolonged abdominal pressures exceeding 20 mm Hg can lead to organ dysfunction and failure. NMBs may decrease intra-abdominal pressure by decreasing abdominal muscle tone and thereby give the clinicians time to treat the underlying cause.
(3) Therapeutic Hypothermia after out of hospital cardiac arrest. NMBs have been primarily use to treat shivering as part of a Therapeutic Hypothermia protocol.

Certainly there are other instances where NMBs may be considered, but NMB should only be used by clinicians experienced in their use and as part of protocolized care plan.

■ PARALYTIC MEDICATION SELECTION AND PRECAUTIONS

Neuromuscular blocking agents are broadly divided between the depolarizing agent succinylcholine and the myriad of other nondepolarizing agents (eg, vecuronium, rocuronium, cis-atracurium). Succinylcholine results in depolarization of the motor endplate with the onset of paralysis, whereas the nondepolarizing agents do not. Succinylcholine is used primarily for intubation because of its short onset and short duration of action. However, the use of succinylcholine in disease states where chronically denervated muscle groups exist (eg, stroke, metabolic acidosis, renal failure, burns, trauma) is not recommended. In these cases, an upregulation of Ach receptors at the motor endplate has occurred, and the use of succinylcholine could result in massive exaggerated muscle depolarization with attendant dangerous hyperkalemia.

Nondepolarizing NMBs are often used for intubation (rocuronium) and for the maintenance of paralysis (cis-atracurium).

In critically ill patients, density of the nicotinic acetylcholine (Ach) receptor (nAChR) at the nerve terminal increases over time. The result of this increase in receptor density in clinical practice is tachyphylaxis to the nondepolarizing NMB agents. With time, a greater concentration of NMB is needed to achieve sufficient receptor saturation and paralysis (**Table 139-6**).

PRACTICE POINT

● Tachyphylaxis is defined as rapid decrease in the response to a drug due to previous (long-term) exposure to that drug. Increasing the dose of the drug will not increase the pharmacologic response. Tachyphylaxis may develop with an initial dose. This can sometimes be caused by depletion or marked reduction of the amount of neurotransmitter responsible for creating the drug's effect.

Neuromuscular blocking agents

Multiple NMB agents are available for use in the ICU setting. Pharmacology and dosing varies based on the agent selected (**Table 139-7**). Vecuronium and rocuronium are commonly used paralytics in the ICU setting, serving as a cost-effective options and they only impacted to a minor degree by moderate renal and hepatic disease. Cis-atracurium has the benefit of *Hoffman degradation*, a pH-dependent serum elimination that is not influenced at all by kidney or liver function. Cis-atracurium has been shown in one recent trial to improve

TABLE 139-6 Pharmacologic Properties of Commonly Used Intravenous Sedatives

Drug	IV Dose	Intermittent Dosing	Infusion Dosing	Time to Onset	Half-Life	Lipophilicity	Active Metabolites
Midazolam	0.5-4.0 mg	0.02-0.08 mg/kg every 0.5-2 h	0.04-0.2 mg/kg/h	2-5 min	3-12 h	+++	Yes
Lorazepam	0.04 mg/kg	0.02-0.06 mg/kg every 2-6 h	0.01-0.1 mg/kg/h	5-20 min	10-20 h	++	No
Diazepam	2-10 mg	0.03-0.1 mg/kg every 0.5-6 h	NA	2-5 min	20-50 h	+++	Yes
Propofol	Infusion dosing	NA	5-80 mcg/kg/min	1-2 min	1.5-12.4 h	+++	No

TABLE 139-7 Pharmacology of Commonly Used Neuromuscular Blocking Agents

Drug	Intubating Dose (mg/kg)	Infusion Rate (µg/kg/min)	Onset to Intubating Conditions (seconds)	Duration of Action	Clinical Niche
Rocuronium	0.9-1.2	9-12	60-90	Intermediate	Rapid-onset nondepolarizing NMB
Vecuronium	0.08-0.12	1-2	90-150	Intermediate	Cost effective
Atacurium	0.5	3-12	90-150	Intermediate	ESRD/cirrhotic patients (nonrenal/hepatic metabolism)
Cisatacurium	0.15-0.2	1-3	90-120	Intermediate	Similar to atracurium but without risk of histamine release
Succinylcholine	1.5	NA	30-90	Very short	Emergent airway (most rapid onset)

outcomes in ARDS when used early and for a limited time. Elimination is not influenced by kidney or liver function and may be used in patients with severe renal or hepatic impairment. Bolus or continuous infusion is appropriate dosing for paralysis. Switching or combining NMB agents is generally not recommended as this might result in unanticipated synergistic potentiation and prolonged neuromuscular blockade.

Various medical conditions, medications, and clinical circumstances affect the duration of action and degree of neuromuscular weakness (**Table 139-8**). If sedation and analgesia fail to allow adequate ventilatory support and neuromuscular agents are thought to be clinically indicated, they should be utilized in patients who are normothermic, free of electrolyte or acid-base disturbances, lack concomitant neuromuscular disease, and are not receiving steroids or specific antibiotics that are known to potentiate neuromuscular blockade.

TABLE 139-8 Clinical Effect of Drug and Metabolic States on Neuromuscular Blockers

Agent or Clinical Condition	Effect on Neuromuscular Blockers
Phenytoin	Decrease sensitivity
Carbemazepine	
Ranitidine	
Azathioprine	
Aminoglycosides	Potentiate action
Polymyxin	
Tetracycline	
Clindamycin	
Lidocaine	
Quinidine	
Hypermagnesemia	Enhance weakness
Hyperthermia	Decrease sensitivity
Respiratory alkalosis	
Hypercalcemia	
Hypokalemia	Increased sensitivity
Hyponatremia	
Hypocalcemia	
Respiratory acidosis	
Metabolic alkalosis	
Hypophosphotemia	
Hypothermia	Prolonged action

Paralysis assessment

The paralytic effect of NMB agents is usually evaluated with neuromuscular monitors (with train-of-four [TOF] appraisal) rather than by clinical assessment of neuromuscular strength. Whenever a paralytic agent is used, the TOF test measures the degree of neuromuscular blockade using a peripheral nerve stimulator. A baseline measurement is performed prior to starting the paralytic agent to determine the current necessary to obtain twitch. The clinician should complete the TOF test and document until a TOF ratio of either 1/4 or 2/4 is achieved. TOF assessments should occur every 4 hours while a patient is receiving an NMB agent (intermittent bolus or infusion) for continued paralysis.

PRACTICE POINT

Instructions for train-of-four (TOF) assessment prior to and during paralysis

1. Attach two electrodes along the course of the ulnar nerve (temporal nerve may be used).
2. Connect the lead to the peripheral nerve stimulator by inserting the jacks into the proximal (red) and distal (black) output jacks. Connect the other end to the patient electrodes.
3. Turn the stimulator on. Select the current necessary (usually 20 mA) for that patient to twitch when the stimuli are applied.
4. Press the TOF once. It will deliver a train of four pulses where each is 0.5 seconds apart. Do not use the other buttons on the stimulator.
5. Count the number of twitches the patient had out of four (0/4, 1/4, 2/4, 3/4, 4/4). Adjust the medication as ordered. The goal ratio is between 1/4 to 2/4 twitches.

Paralytic precautions

The decision to use NMB agents should be made with care as their use is not without potential harm or clinical compromises. For example, their use can alter a clinician's ability to detect patient distress or potentially lethal medical conditions such as stroke, peritonitis, myocardial infarction, or hypoglycemia. A paralyzed patient shows no obvious outward signs of distress, and inadvertent ventilator disconnection could be lethal. Inadequate sedation in an otherwise paralyzed patients can occur and may result in significant psychological trauma. Additionally, with ongoing NMB use, up to 10% of patients may develop critical ill polyneuropathy (CIP) or myopathy, especially with concomitant steroid use. Secondary nerve or soft tissue injury may also arise (eg, decubitus ulcer) from the pressure of limbs and dependent body segments against hard surfaces in pharmacologically immobilized patients. For all of these reasons, paralytic use should, when not contraindicated, be punctuated by "drug holidays" during which a clinical appraisal of ongoing need and a survey for occult complications is undertaken.

CONSULTATION

Consulting critical care, anesthesia, or other specialties to assist with the use of sedative, analgesic, or paralytic medications in the ICU should be left to the individual clinician's experience and comfort level in utilizing these agents. As part of a planned and measured strategy for use of these agents (Figure 139-3), a hospitalist should solicit assistance early in the ICU course with management of comorbid psychiatric, rheumatologic, or other chronic uncontrolled painful disease as well as for management of long-standing opioid or drug dependence. Consultation by a critical care specialist is recommended for patients with complex multiorgan dysfunction or failure who may require advanced hemodynamic support, unconventional mechanical ventilation modes and the use of NMBs. Anesthesia consultation in particular should be considered in patients when a complex or very difficult intubation is anticipated, when preexisting neurologic or metabolic disease preclude the use of succinylcholine, or when hemodynamic compromise may complicate anesthetic induction at the time of intubation.

Prolonged ICU stays that require longer-term use of sedative, analgesic, or paralytic agents may benefit from consultation with various health care professionals. Clinical pharmacists guide dosing as pharmacokinetics shift with the clinical picture and the length of drug utilization. Nutritionists guide assessment of caloric need in the setting of ongoing propofol infusion. Wound care specialists may help prevent and treat soft-tissue breakdown when prolonged sedation or neuromuscular blockade is used.

While weaning off sedation and IV analgesia, consultation with psychiatry or a pain specialist may be indicated if a patient suffers delirium or drug withdrawal symptoms that preclude successful liberation from the ventilator. Such consultation should be done on a case-by-case basis.

QUALITY IMPROVEMENT

While the use of sedative, hypnotic, and neuromuscular blocking regimens represent an integral part of ICU care, they should be carefully monitored with validated scales and adjusted to specific patient needs. Nursing and both physician and nonphysician providers should work in concert to assess and implement an appropriate level of sedation that allows for ongoing ventilator needs without representing an impediment to efficient weaning, as increased ventilator-dependent days are associated a greater complication rate, and increased costs associated with longer length of stays and resource utilization. Protocolization of both the weaning process and the management of PAD in the ICU will optimize patient care and result in the minimum number of ventilator days, and ICU days for the individual patient.

SUGGESTED READINGS

Aissaoui Y, Zeggwagh AA, Zekraoui Abidi K, Abouqal R. Validation of a behavioral pain scale in critically ill, sedated and mechanically ventilated patients. *Anesth Analg*. 2005;101(5):1470-1476.

Barr J, Fraser GL, Puntillo, K, et al. Clinical Practice Guidelines for the management of pain, agitation and delirium in adult patients in the Intensive Care Unit. *Crit Care Med*. 2013;41:263-306.

Devlin J, Roberts R. Pharmacology of commonly used analgesics and sedatives in the ICU: benzodiazepines, propofol, and opioids. *Crit Care Clin*. 2009;25:431-449.

Gelinas C, Fillion L, Puntillo K, Veins C, Fortier M. Validation of the critical care pain observation tool in adult patients. *Am J Crit Care*. 2006;15(4):420-427.

Greenberg SB, Vender J. The use of neuromuscular blocking agents in the ICU: where are we now? *Crit Care Med*. 2013;41:1332-1344.

Kress JP, Gehlbach B, Lacy M, et al. The long-term psychological effects of daily sedative interruption on critically ill patients. *Am J Respir Crit Care Med*. 2003;168:1457-1461.

Kress JP, Pohlman AS, O'Connor MF, et al. Daily interruption of sedative infusions in critically ill patients undergoing mechanical ventilation. *N Engl J Med*. 2000;343:814-815.

Ostermann ME, Keenan SP, Seiferling RA, et al. Sedation in the intensive care unit: a systematic review. *JAMA*. 2000;283:1451-1459.

Sessler C, Varney K. Patient-focused sedation and analgesia in the ICU. *Chest*. 2008;133:552-556.

Strom T, Martinussen T, Toft P. A protocol of no sedation for critically ill patients receiving mechanical ventilation: a randomised trial. *Lancet*. 2010;375:475-480.

CHAPTER 140

Mechanical Ventilation

Bishoy Zakhary, MD
Amit Uppal, MD

Key Clinical Questions

1. How should I select an initial mode of mechanical ventilation? What are the distinguishing features of the various modes of mechanical ventilation?

2. How can patient ventilator dyssynchrony be rapidly identified and managed?

3. When and how should a patient on mechanical ventilation be assessed for liberation from mechanical ventilation?

INTRODUCTION

■ HISTORY OF MECHANICAL VENTILATION

One of the earliest descriptions of artificial ventilation is credited to the Belgian physician Andrea Vesalius, who, in his 1653 work, *De Humani Corporis Fabricia*, stated that "an opening must be attempted in the trunk of the trachea, in which a tube of reed or cane should be put; you will then blow into this so that the lung may rise again and the animal take in air." Over the ensuing decades, with the development of a bellows drive mechanism, the successful use of ventilators to treat victims of drowning and patients with neuromuscular weakness was reported.

Widespread use of mechanical ventilators, however, did not occur until the polio epidemic of the 1940s and 1950s. Thousands of patients were supported with negative pressure ventilators, which create a negative pressure outside the thorax so as to expand the lungs. With the development of the cuffed endotracheal tube (ETT), positive pressure ventilation became possible and increased in popularity.

Ventilator technology continued to improve, including a reduction in the size of the machines and the development of microchips able to respond to changes in patient characteristics. With these advancements, mechanical ventilation helped form the specialty of critical care medicine.

■ PHYSIOLOGIC CONSIDERATIONS

During quiet spontaneous breathing, inspiration is an active process, dependent on the contraction of the diaphragm and other respiratory muscles to expand the thoracic cage and draw air in. Exhalation is a passive process, during which relaxation of the same muscles returns the thoracic cage to its prior state to expel air out. During positive pressure ventilation, inspiration is an active process whereby the ventilator exerts a pressure at the tip of the endotracheal tube higher than the alveolar pressure such that air flows from the ventilator into the lungs and exhalation is a passive process whereby the pressure at the tip of the endotracheal tube is reduced and air passively flows back from the lungs into the ventilator.

To understand ventilatory air flow and the relation of pressure, flow, and volume, it is necessary to discuss two important physiologic variables—resistance and compliance.

Resistance

In mechanical ventilation, resistance refers to the degree to which the flow of air is obstructed.

Poiseuille's law defines the variables which affect resistance to airflow through a hollow tube:

$$R = 8\eta l/\pi r^4$$

where R is resistance, η is the viscosity of air, l is the length of the tube, and r is the radius of the tube. Because resistance (R) is inversely proportional to the fourth power of the tube radius (r), small reductions in r can have dramatic increases in R.

In a mechanically ventilated patient, we generally refer to the resistancesof the circuit tubing of the ventilator, the ETT, and the patient's tracheobronchial tree. We can deduce that factors which increase resistance to airflow include excessively long circuit tubing (increase in circuit l), patient biting on the ETT (decrease in ETT r),

TABLE 140-1 Factors which Can Increase Airway Resistance

Circuit Tubing	Excessive length (increases *l*)
	Fluid buildup (decreases *r*)
	Kink or Compression (decreases *r*)
Endotracheal Tube	Narrow tube selected (decreases *r*)
	Secretion buildup (decreases *r*)
	Patient biting (decreases *r*)
Airways	Secretion buildup (decreases *r*)
	Bronchospasm (decreases *r*)

and bronchoconstriction (decrease in tracheobronchial *r*). Important factors that can increase airway resistance are listed in **Table 140-1**.

Compliance

In mechanical ventilation, compliance refers to the degree of dispensability of the respiratory system.

The following equation defines compliance:

$$C = \Delta V / \Delta P$$

where *C* is compliance, ΔV is the change in volume, and ΔP is the change in pressure. Note that objects which require a high pressure to deliver a specific volume are said to have low compliance.

In a mechanically ventilated patient, we generally refer to the compliances of the lungs and of the chest wall. We can deduce that diseases which stiffen the lung (those that require a higher pressure to deliver a specific tidal volume) will reduce compliance. The majority of lung pathologies, such as pulmonary edema, the acute respiratory distress syndrome (ARDS), and pneumonia, reduce lung compliance. Similarly, diseases which limit chest wall expansion, such as kyphosis or obesity, reduce chest wall compliance. Important factors that can decrease respiratory system compliance are listed in **Table 140-2**.

MODES OF MECHANICAL VENTILATION

Over the years, a number of different modes of mechanical ventilation have been developed with purported benefits in specific patient populations. In general, no mode has proven superior to others, and choice is typically based on provider preference and patient tolerance. Here, we will review the most common modes encountered in a typical intensive care unit (ICU).

■ THE MECHANICAL VENTILATION BREATH PHASES

The mechanical ventilation breath is typically divided into four phases (**Figure 140-1**): initiation, delivery, termination, and exhalation. Initiation is defined by opening of the inspiratory valve; delivery is the period during which air flows from the ventilator into the

TABLE 140-2 Factors which Can Reduce Respiratory System Compliance

Lung	Alveolar collapse—atelectasis, pneumothorax
	Alveolar filling—edema, pneumonia, hemorrhage
	Intrinsic positive end expiratory pressure (PEEP)
Chest Wall	Chest wall deformity—kyphosis, burns, chest wall binder
	Abdominal distention

patient; termination is defined by closure of the inspiratory valve with cessation of inspiratory air flow; and exhalation occurs when the expiratory valve opens and air flows out of the patient back to the ventilator. Note that inspiration is comprised of three phases and exhalation one phase.

■ THE MECHANICAL VENTILATION BREATH VARIABLES

In discussing the different modes of mechanical ventilation, it helps to understand control variables and phase variables. The different modes of ventilation can then be defined as permutations of these variables.

Control variables are the independent variables set by the ventilator operator (ie, the physician and respiratory therapist). The most common ones used are: inspiratory pressure (*P*), tidal volume (V_t), flow ($\dot{V}$), and inspiratory time (I_t). Other variables that can be set are respiratory rate (RR), fractional inspiration of oxygen (F_iO_2), and positive end-expiratory pressure (PEEP).

Phase variables are those that control the different phases of the mechanical ventilation breath. They are trigger, limit, and cycle. The trigger variable initiates the breath. This can be done by the ventilator (time-triggered based on a set respiratory rate) or by the patient (pressure-triggered as sensed by the ventilator when the patient breathes in and decreases the pressure in the circuit). The limit variable defines how the breath is delivered, typically according to a set pressure or flow. The cycle variable terminates the breath. This can occur when a set volume is delivered, a set inspiratory time has elapsed, or inspiratory flow falls below a predefined amount.

■ THE MECHANICAL VENTILATION BREATH TYPES

The mechanical ventilation breath can be one of three types: controlled, assisted, or spontaneous. Controlled breaths are triggered by the ventilator and have limit and cycle variables set by the ventilator operator. Assisted breaths are similar to controlled breaths, in that limit and cycle variables are set by the operator, but in contrast to controlled breaths are triggered by the patient. Spontaneous breaths are triggered and cycled by the patient.

■ MODE: VOLUME CONTROL

In volume control (VC) ventilation, a set tidal volume is delivered with each breath. Control variables that are set are tidal volume and flow (V_t and $\dot{V}$, respectively)—these make up the independent variables. We can thus deduce that inspiratory pressure, *P*, is a dependent variable.

In VC, breaths can be triggered by the ventilator (controlled breaths) or by the patient (assisted breaths). The limit variable is flow such that the breath can be delivered at a constant flow rate (square waveform) or a declining flow rate (descending ramp waveform). The cycle variable is V_T—once the set tidal volume is delivered, the ventilator cycles off.

Tracing through an assisted VC breath (**Figure 140-2**)—with $V_T = 500$ ml, $\dot{V} = 60$ L/min and square waveform, and PEEP = 5 cm H_2O—we can map out the different parts of the waveform. The breath is initiated when a certain time has passed or when the patient breathes in (seen as a negative deflection in pressure) triggering the ventilator to deliver a mechanical breath. The flow quickly rises to 60 L/min causing a concomitant rise in pressure. As the breath is delivered, flow is held constant while inspired volume gradually rises causing a continued rise in pressure. Once the inspired volume reaches 500 ml, the ventilator cycles off and the breath ends. The expiratory valve opens and the patient exhales, reflected in a negative flow waveform. Pressure decreases back to 5 cm H_2O, while flow and volume gradually return to zero.

One important note is that during VC, pressure is a dependent variable and varies with changes in respiratory mechanics. For example, if

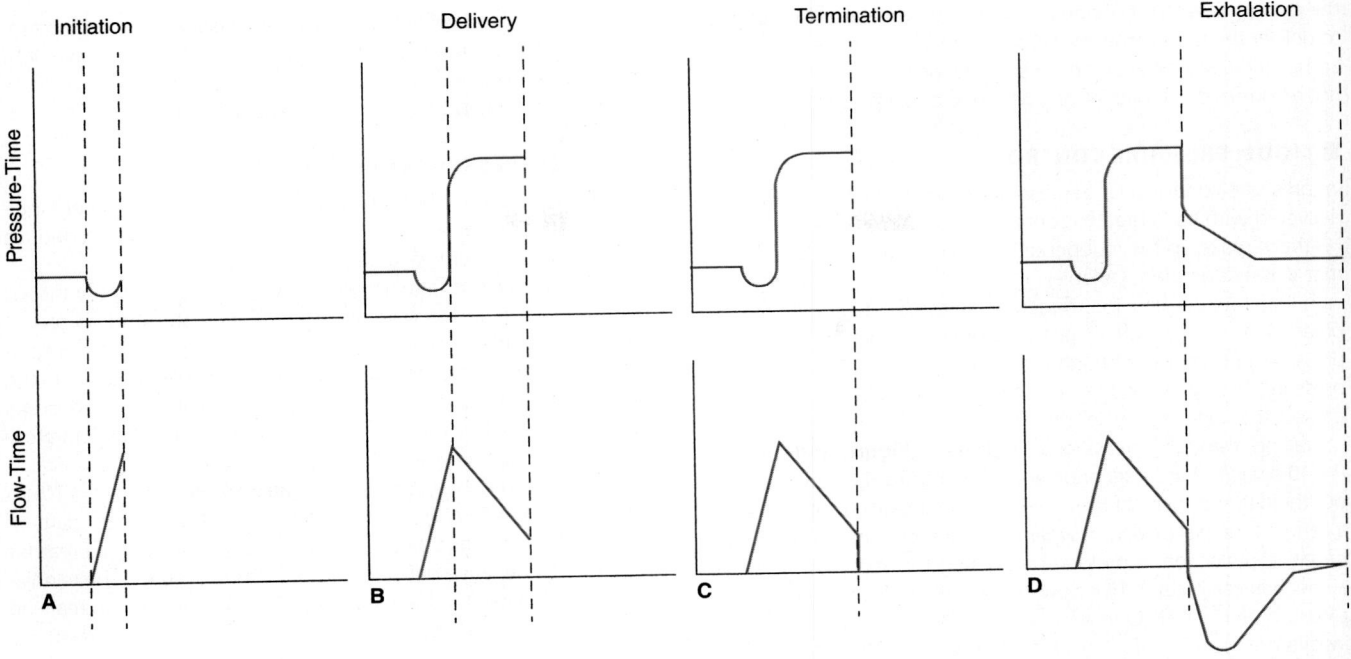

Figure 140-1 *Phases of the mechanical ventilator breath, shown in pressure versus time curves and flow versus time curves. Initiation (A), delivery (B), termination (C), and make-up inspiration. The final phase is exhalation (D). The represented breath in this figure is a patient-triggered pressure-control breath (see text).*

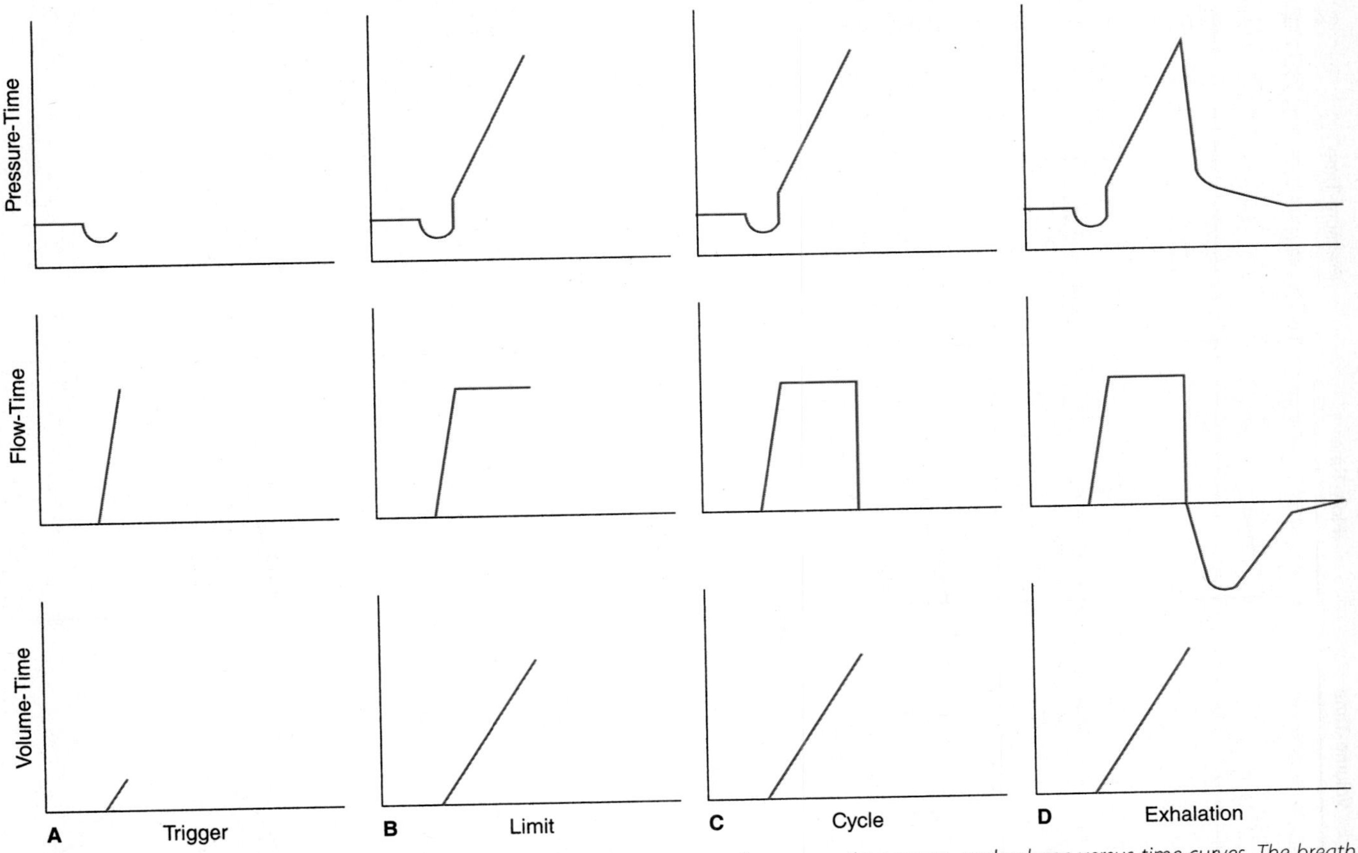

Pressure-Time

Flow-Time

Volume-Time

| A | Trigger | B | Limit | C | Cycle | D | Exhalation |

Figure 140-2 *Volume control breath, shown in pressure versus time curves, flow versus time curves, and volume versus time curves. The breath is patient- or time-triggered, flow-limited, and volume-cycled. The patient (A) initiates the breath as sensed by a drop in pressure. The breath is (B) delivered at a constant flow. The breath (C) terminates once the set tidal volume is delivered. The last stage is (D) exhalation.*

the patient develops pulmonary edema, the ventilator will continue to deliver the preset V_T at the preset $\dot{V}$, but, due to the reduced lung compliance, will require higher inspiratory pressures to do so. If this is not recognized, the patient can be at risk for barotrauma.

■ MODE: PRESSURE CONTROL

In pressure control (PC) ventilation, a set inspiratory pressure is delivered with each breath. Control variables that are set are P and I_t—these make up the independent variables. We can thus deduce that V_T is a dependent variable.

In PC, breaths can be triggered by the ventilator (controlled breaths) or by the patient (assisted breaths). The limit variable is pressure such that the breath is delivered at a constant inspiratory pressure. The cycle variable is I_t—once the set inspiratory time has passed, the ventilator cycles off.

Tracing through an assisted PC breath (**Figure 140-3**)—with $P = 10$ cm H_2O, $I_t = 0.9$ seconds, and PEEP = 5 cm H_2O—we can map out the different parts of the waveform. The breath is initiated when a certain time has passed or when the patient breathes in (seen as a negative deflection in pressure) triggering the ventilator to deliver a mechanical breath. The flow quickly rises to create an airway pressure of 15 cm H_2O (comprised of a PEEP of 5 cm H_2O plus an inspiratory pressure of 10 cm H_2O). As the breath is delivered, pressure is held constant while inspired volume gradually rises and flow gradually falls. Once 0.9 seconds has passed, the ventilator cycles off and the breath ends. The expiratory valve opens and the patient exhales, reflected in a negative flow waveform. Pressure decreases back to 5 cm H_2O, while flow and volume gradually return to zero.

One important note is that, during PC, volume is a dependent variable and varies with changes in respiratory mechanics. For example, if the patient develops bronchoconstriction, the ventilator will continue to deliver the breaths at the preset P and for the preset I_t, but, due to the elevated airway resistance, will result in lower V_T. If this is not recognized, the patient can develop respiratory distress or, if the patient is heavily sedated or paralyzed, hypercapnea.

■ MODE: PRESSURE SUPPORT

In pressure support (PS) ventilation, the ventilator aids patient initiated breaths. The only control variable set is P. We can thus deduce that V_T is a dependent variable.

In PS, all breaths are triggered by the patient (spontaneous breaths)—there are no ventilator triggered breaths and no set RR. The limit variable is pressure such that the breath is delivered at a constant inspiratory pressure. The cycle variable is flow—as the patient's inspiratory flow declines through the breath, and drops below a prespecified value (usually 20%-30% of the initial inspiratory flow), the ventilator cycles off.

Tracing through two PS breaths (**Figure 140-4**)—with PS = 10 cm H_2O and PEEP = 5 cm H_2O—we can map out the different parts of the waveform. The first breath is initiated when the patient breathes in (seen as a negative deflection in pressure) triggering the ventilator to deliver a mechanical breath. The flow quickly rises to create an airway pressure of 15 cm H_2O. As the breath is delivered, pressure is held constant—inspired volume gradually rises while flow gradually falls. Once the inspiratory flow drops below 25% of the initial flow rate, the ventilator cycles off and the breath ends. The expiratory valve opens and the patient exhales, reflected in a negative flow waveform. Pressure decreases back to 5 cm H_2O, while flow and volume gradually return to zero. The next breath is similar except the patient has a higher initial flow and a longer I_t.

One important note is that during PS, I_t can vary from breath-to-breath dependent on the patient's inspiratory demands. As such,

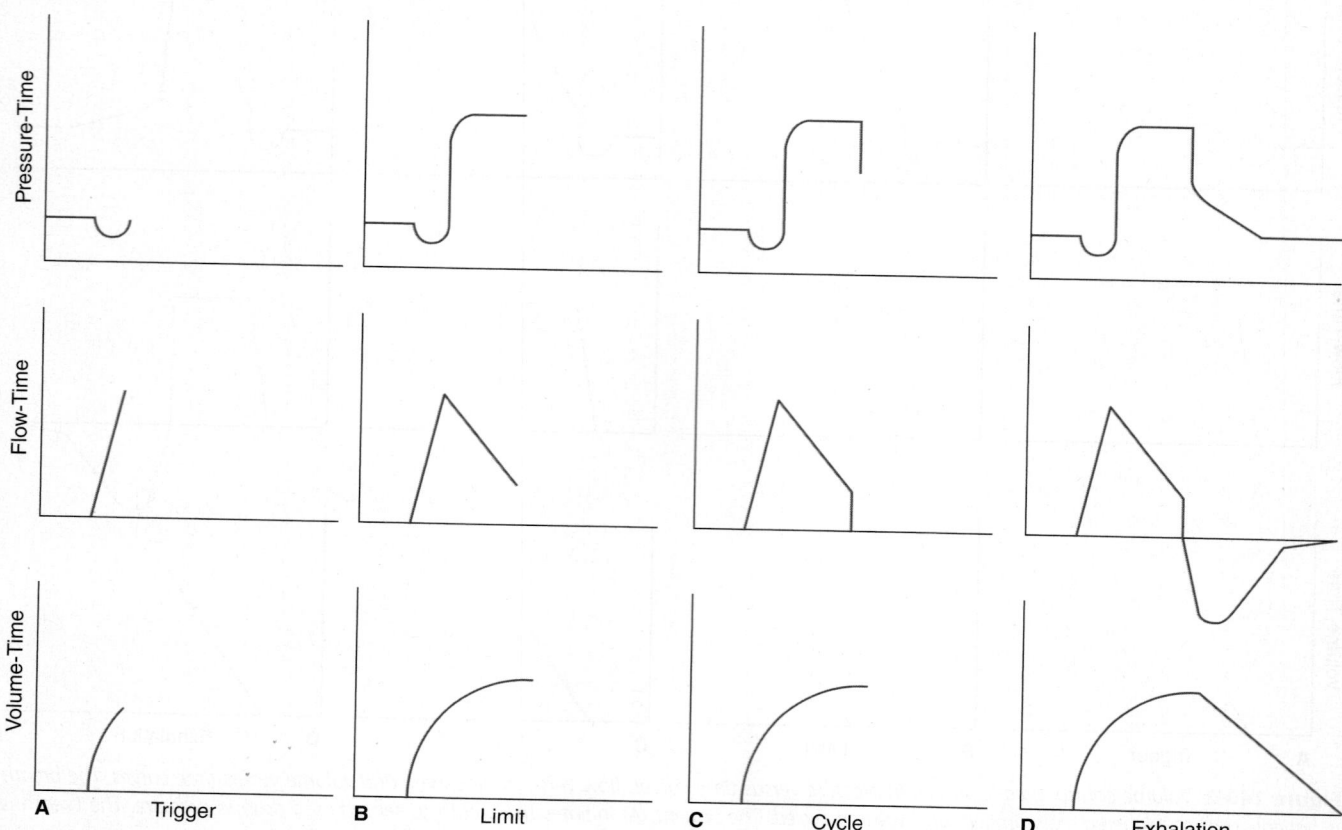

Figure 140-3 *Pressure control breath, shown in pressure versus time curves, flow versus time curves, and volume versus time curves. The breath is patient- or time-triggered, pressure-limited, and time-cycled. The patient (A) initiates the breath as sensed by a drop in pressure. The breath is (B) delivered at a constant pressure. The breath (C) terminates once the set inspiratory time has elapsed. The last stage is (D) exhalation.*

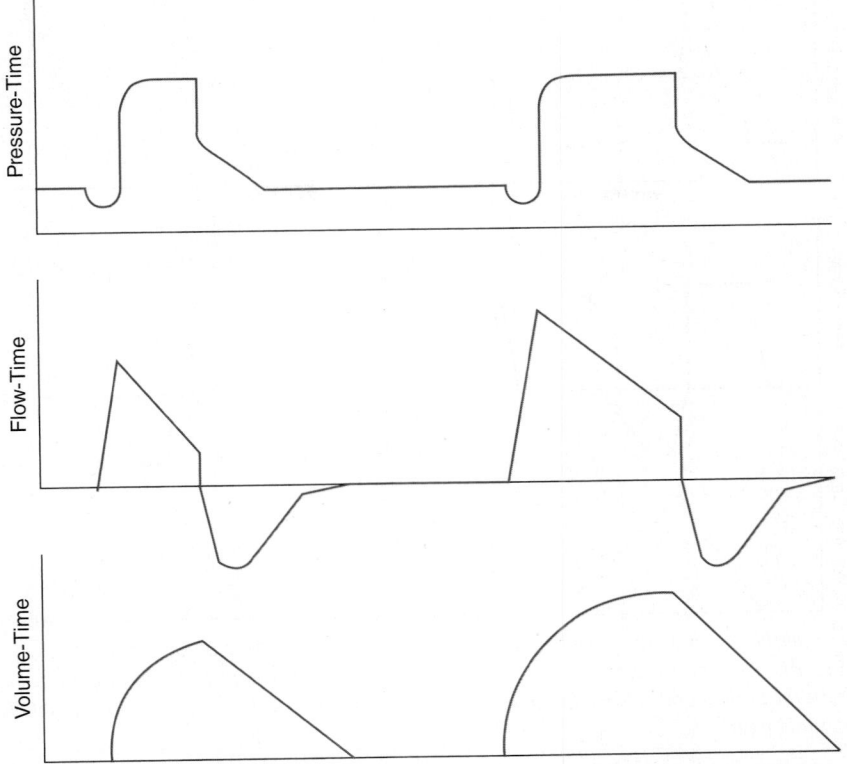

Figure 140-4 *Pressure support breaths, shown in pressure versus time curves, flow versus time curves, and volume versus time curves. The patient must initiate all breaths. Note that the inspiratory time and tidal volume can differ from breath to breath.*

V_T ($= \dot{V_I}$) will also vary from breath to breath. While PS is frequently more comfortable for patients, allowing for more autonomy over inspiratory variables, it is not suited for a patient with a depressed respiratory drive (such as in opiate overdose) since both RR and V_T are dependent on patient effort.

■ MODE: SYNCHRONIZED INTERMITTENT MANDATORY VENTILATION

Synchronized intermittent mandatory ventilation (SIMV) is a mode of ventilation thatcan be considered a hybrid of ventilatory breaths (either VC or PC) and spontaneous breaths. Mechanical breaths are synchronized to the patient's spontaneous breathing pattern while spontaneous breaths can be interspersed between.

In SIMV, breaths can be triggered by the ventilator (controlled breaths) or by the patient (assisted and spontaneous breaths). One unique aspect of SIMV is that, if the patient initiates a breath close to (usually within 0.5 s) of a scheduled mandatory breath, the ventilator provides a fully supported assisted breath. On the other hand, if the patient initiates a breath separate from a scheduled mandatory breath, the breath is a spontaneous one.

Tracing through several SIMV breaths (**Figure 140-5**)—with $V_T = 500$ mL, $\dot{V} = 60$ L/min and square waveform, PEEP = 5 cm H_2O, RR = 10 breaths/min, and PS = 10 cm H_2O—we can map out the different parts of the waveform. The first breath is initiated by the machine as a controlled VC breath. The patient takes a breath in 2 seconds after, but, since this is far from the next scheduled breath (delivered approximately every 6 seconds given the RR of 10 breaths/min), it is a spontaneous PS breath. The patient takes another breath soon after that one, and given that it does fall close to the next scheduled breath, the machine delivers an assisted VC breath.

The purported benefit of SIMV is that this mode allows for gradual weaning of the ventilator (by steady decrements of the RR such

that a greater proportion of breaths are spontaneous). It should be noted, however, that comparison of this mode to other modes of weaning has not demonstrated superiority.

VENTILATOR DYSSYNCHRONY

While a patient is on mechanical ventilation, it is necessary to ensure patient comfort. However, in 40% to 90% of mechanically ventilated patients, there is patient-ventilator dyssynchrony, defined broadly as a mismatch between ventilator gas delivery and patient demand. This can result in patient distress, increased energy expenditure, and hemodynamic instability. Although this can often be alleviated with heavy sedation and paralysis, simple recognition of dyssynchrony and adjustment of ventilator parameters can often result in improvement.

Ventilator dyssynchronies can be classified according to the phase of the breath during which they occur. As such, they are termed trigger, flow, and cycle dyssynchronies.

■ TRIGGER DYSSYNCHRONY

Trigger dyssynchronies occur during the initiation of the breath. The most common type is ineffective trigger. As discussed previously, a patient can trigger a breath by breathing in and causing a drop in circuit pressure. The ventilator senses either the pressure drop (pressure triggered) or the flow created by the pressure gradient (flow triggered), recognizes it as patient effort, and delivers a breath.

The amount of negative pressure (or inspiratory flow) required to trigger a breath is set manually. If the threshold for triggering a breath is set inappropriately high, the patient can make inspiratory efforts and not receive mechanical breaths. Consider a patient with neuromuscular weakness—he or she may not be able to generate enough negative pressure to trigger a desired breath.

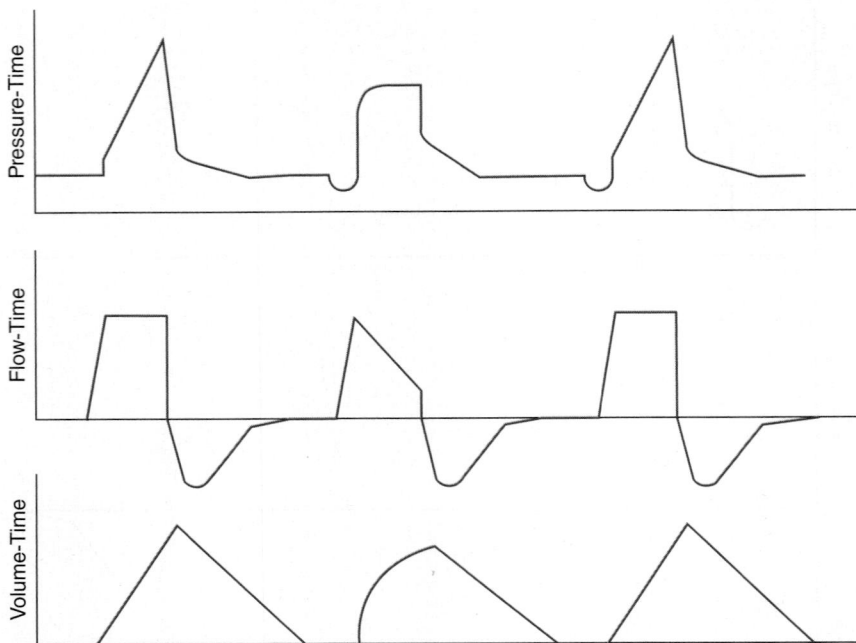

Figure 140-5 *Synchronized intermittent mandatory ventilation breaths, shown in pressure versus time curves, flow versus time curves, and volume versus time curves. The first breath is a controlled breath initiated by the ventilator and delivered as a volume control breath. The second breath is a spontaneous breath initiated by the patient and delivered as a pressure support breath. The third breath is an assisted breath initiated by the patient and delivered as a volume control breath.*

Ineffective triggers can be recognized clinically by seeing the patient make inspiratory efforts that are not followed by a mechanical breath. In the case of neuromuscular weakness, in which the patient may not have the strength to make efforts that are visibly apparent, the pressure-time tracing may display small negative deflections not followed by a positive pressure breath. These are termed ineffective triggers (**Figure 140-6**).

When ineffective triggers are recognized, the cause must be sought. In the case of neuromuscular weakness, the solution may be to lower the threshold for triggering. However, this comes with the risk of inadvertent triggering, where breaths are triggered even though the patient did not make a respiratory effort.

Of special note, in a patient with obstructive lung disease with air trapping and elevated intrinsic PEEP, the prevalence of ineffective triggers can be very high. This is because the patient starts at a higher end expiratory pressure than normal and must create additional negative inspiratory pressure to compensate for the intrinsic PEEP before reaching the pressure trigger (**Figure 140-7a**). In this case, the best way to reduce ineffective triggering is by increasing the applied PEEP (**Figure 140-7b**), so as to reduce the gradient the patient needs to overcome before triggering a breath. However,

reducing the respiratory rate is a key component in the ventilator strategy for such patients. Thus, the management of ineffective triggers in this case may be to suppress the patient's respiratory drive until their acute illness has improved.

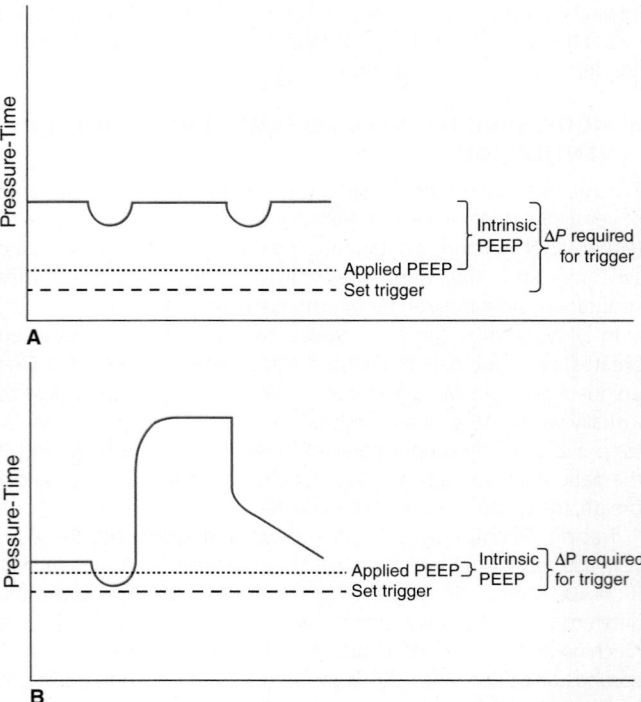

Figure 140-7 *Ineffective trigger in the setting of intrinsic PEEP. (A) Due to the presence of significant intrinsic PEEP, patient attempts to trigger a breath are inadequate to reach the threshold. (B) When the applied PEEP is increased, the drop in pressure required to reach the threshold is reduced, and the same patient effort is sufficient to trigger a breath.*

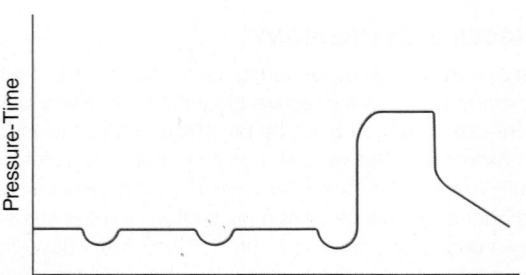

Figure 140-6 *Trigger dyssynchrony—ineffective trigger. Several attempts to initiate a breath, seen as negative deflections in pressure, fail to trigger the ventilator. The last attempt, with a larger negative deflection reaches the trigger threshold and a breath is delivered.*

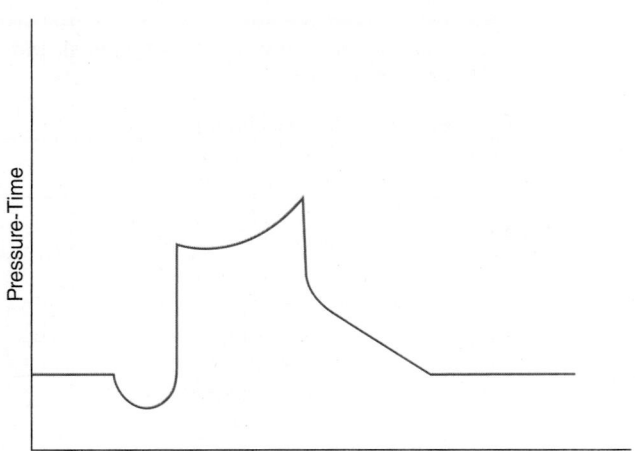

Figure 140-8 *Flow dyssynchrony—inadequate flow. Downward scooping of the pressure curve suggests insufficient inspiratory flow.*

■ FLOW DYSSYNCHRONY

Flow dyssynchronies occur during the delivery of the breath. The most common type is inadequate flow to meet the patient's needs. It is important to keep in mind that the state of the critical care patient is in continuous flux such that conditions which increase respiratory drive (such as infection or reduction in sedation) are common and that the ventilator, a static device, should be adjusted to meet these demands.

Inadequate flow can be recognized by seeing downward scooping of the pressure-time tracing (**Figure 140-8**). This occurs because the patient is creating a large negative airway pressure while the ventilator is attempting to deliver a positive pressure breath. If there is significant discrepancy, the preset flow (in VC) or pressure (in PC) is not maintained and scooping is seen.

If inadequate flow is recognized, various measures can be taken to address it. If in VC mode, increasing the set flow rate or switching to a descending ramp flow mode can help. Switching to a PC mode (which typically have high initial flow rates) can be attempted. If it is felt that the excessively high inspiratory demands are detrimental to the patient (such as in a patient with the acute respiratory distress syndrome), a trial of increased sedation may be considered.

■ CYCLE DYSSYNCHRONY

Cycle dyssynchronies occur during the termination of the breath. The most common types are premature and delayed cycling. While we can set a ventilator I_t, patients have a neural I_t which can vary significantly.

Cycle dyssynchrony can be recognized by analyzing the flow-time or pressure-time tracings. Premature cycling (**Figure 140-9a**), where neural I_t is longer than ventilator I_t, is seen as a positive deflection in flow (indicating continued patient inhalation) after the breath has terminated and flow has become negative. Delayed cycling (**Figure 140-9b**), where neural I_t is shorter than ventilator I_t, is seen as a positive deflection in pressure (indicating active patient exhalation) prior to the breath terminating and flow becoming negative.

If cycle dyssynchrony is recognized, ventilator I_t should be adjusted to match neural I_t. In VC, this is accomplished by reducing V_T or increasing $\dot{V}$. In PC, I_t can be directly altered.

TROUBLESHOOTING VENTILATOR EVENTS:HYPOXIA

While intubation and mechanical ventilation are utilized to treat patients with respiratory failure, patients can have clinical events while on the ventilator which lead to hypoxia. In such scenarios, familiarity with the peak inspiratory pressure (PIP) equation can be helpful.

■ VENTILATOR PRESSURES

There are three ventilator pressures of importance—PEEP, plateau pressure (P_{Plat}), and PIP.

Positive end-expiratory pressure is a positive pressure applied at the end of expiration in an attempt to maintain distal airways open and prevent at electasis. Although PEEP is set by the operator, in patients with obstructive lung disease, intrinsic PEEP may be higher than applied PEEP. In such cases, PEEP can be measured by applying an expiratory hold maneuver on the ventilator. When this is done, at the end of exhalation, the inspiratory valve does not open and the pressure in the circuit is measured directly (**Figure 140-10**). If the measured PEEP is higher than the applied PEEP, intrinsic PEEP is present. Note that to obtain an accurate PEEP measurement, the patient should not be actively breathing during the maneuver.

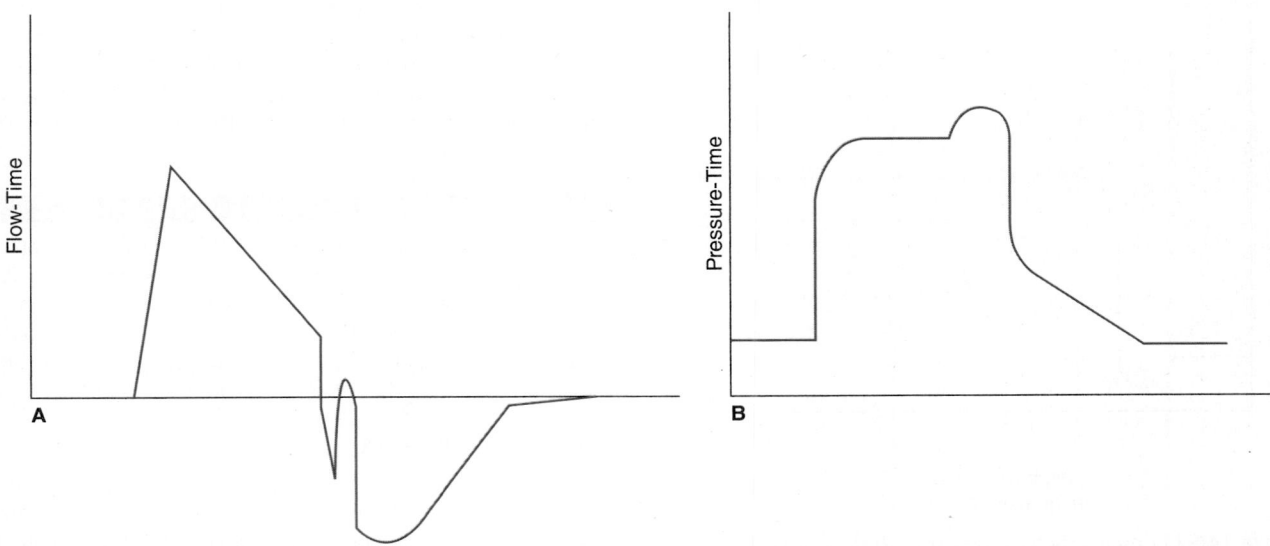

Figure 140-9 *Trigger dyssynchrony. (A) Premature cycling is seen as a positive deflection in flow after the mechanical breath has terminated indicating continued patient inhalation. (B) Delayed cycling is seen as a positive deflection in pressure prior to the breath terminating indicating active patient exhalation.*

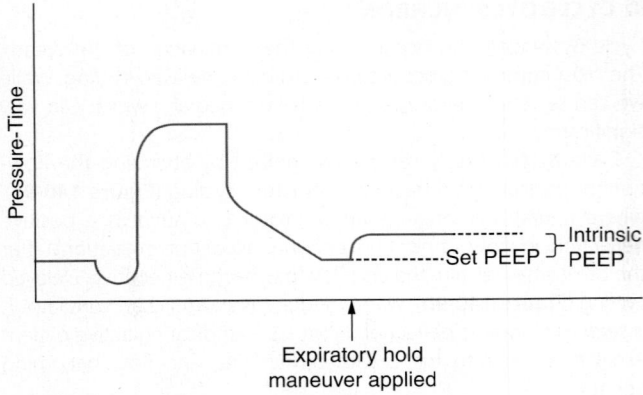

Figure 140-10 *Expiratory hold maneuver. At the end of exhalation, the inspiratory valve does not open and the pressure in the circuit is measured. A rise in pressure from the applied PEEP value is consistent with intrinsic PEEP.*

P_{Plat} is the airway pressure at the end of inspiration when flow has ceased. Since there is no flow, there is also no resistance, and so P_{Plat} is a reflection of the elastic (inverse of compliance) pressures. Plateau pressure can be measured by applying an inspiratory hold maneuver on the ventilator. When this is done, at the end of inspiration, the expiratory valve does not open and the pressure in this no flow circuit is measured directly (**Figure 140-11**). Note that to obtain an accurate P_{Plat} measurement, the patient should not be actively breathing during the maneuver.

Peak inspiratory pressure is the highest pressure obtained during the inspiratory cycle. Peak inspiratory pressure, in contrast to P_{Plat}, is measured during flow and thus reflects both resistive and elastic pressures. Peak inspiratory pressure measurement requires no special respiratory movements and is measured and displayed directly on the ventilator monitor (Figure 140-11).

■ THE PIP EQUATION

The *PIP* equation is as follows:

$$PIP = \dot{V} \cdot R + V_T/C + PEEP$$

where $\dot{V} \cdot R$ represents the resistive component, V_T/C represents the elastic component, and PEEP is the total PEEP.

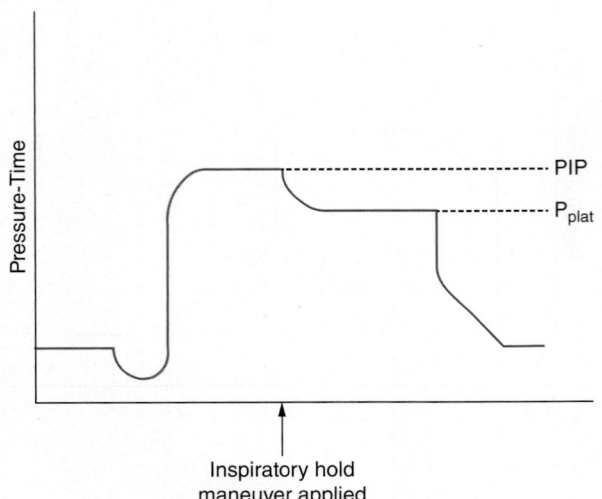

Figure 140-11 *Inspiratory hold maneuver. At the end of inspiration, the expiratory valve does not open and the pressure is measured. This pressure is the plateau pressure. The highest pressure during a breath is the peak inspiratory pressure.*

TABLE 140-3 Differential Considerations Based on Peak and Plateau Pressures

PIP	P_{Plat}	Interpretation	Possible Etiologies
↓		Air leak	Air leak (tube disconnection, cuff leak)
NC	NC		Vascular compromise (pulmonary embolus)
↑	NC	↑ resistance	Tube obstruction—biting, secretions
			Airway obstruction—mucous plug, bronchospasm
↑	↑	↓ compliance	Alveolar collapse—atelectasis, pneumothorax
			Alveolar filling—edema, pneumonia, hemorrhage
			Intrinsic PEEP
			Chest wall deformity/abdominal distention

ARDS, acute respiratory distress syndrome; NC, no change; PIP, peak inspiratory pressure; P_{Plat}, plateau pressure.

The majority of conditions that lead to hypoxemia on the ventilator lead to an elevation of PIP. If this is seen, note that the elevation can come from any of the three components of the equation, and it is necessary to determine which.

The first step is to obtain a P_{Plat} by performing an inspiratory hold maneuver. When this is done, note that $\dot{V} = 0$, and so the equation reduces to

$$P_{Plat} = V_T/C + PEEP$$

If P_{Plat} is also elevated, perform an expiratory hold maneuver to determine PEEP. If intrinsic PEEP is significantly higher than set PEEP, air trapping is likely to be contributing to the decompensation and should be addressed. If intrinsic PEEP is similar to set PEEP, then either V_T has been increased or C has decreased. Diseases which can decrease compliance include the development of pulmonary edema, ARDS, or pneumothorax.

If P_{Plat} is not elevated, then the elastic load has increased—either $\dot{V}$ has been increased or R has increased. Diseases which can increase R include secretions in the tubing or bronchoconstriction.

The benefit of the PIP equation depends on intermittent assessment of peak and plateau pressures in order to detect changes. **Table 140-3** lists some common problems that can be identified using the PIP equation.

LIBERATION FROM MECHANICAL VENTILATION

The overarching goal of intubation and mechanical ventilation is to support the patient while treating or awaiting the underlying cause of respiratory failure to sufficiently improve such that the patient can resume independent breathing. To this end, it is important to identify patients who may be candidates for liberation from mechanical ventilation and assess their ability to breathe unsupported.

■ WEANING CRITERIA

Several studies have now demonstrated that, for the majority of patients on mechanical ventilation, scheduled daily sedation breaks and consideration for spontaneous breathing trials (SBT) shorten the duration of mechanical ventilation. In general, evaluation of four broad categories is helpful to determine whether a patient is a good candidate for a SBT (**Table 140-4**).

TABLE 140-4 General Criteria to Evaluate an Intubated Patient for a Spontaneous Breathing Trial

Disease	Primary etiology sufficiently improved
Neuro	Pt alert, following commands, initiating breaths
	Able to hold head up
Pulm	$PaO_2 \geq 60$ with $FiO_2 \leq 40\%$ and PEEP ≤ 8
	Able to cough
	Suctioning $\leq$ every 4 h
CV	Hemodynamically stable with minimal vasoactive support

First, the reason that the patient required intubation and mechanical ventilation should have sufficiently improved such that the patient can support his or her own respiratory function. For example, if a patient was originally intubated for opiate overdose, there should be sufficient improvement in mental status such that the patient can maintain adequate minute ventilation. Similarly, if a patient was originally intubated for pneumonia, there should be sufficient improvement in gas exchange such that the patient can be adequately supported with supplemental oxygen (such as by face mask or nasal cannula). Note that complete resolution of the disease process is not required but sufficient improvement such that the patient is no longer dependent on ventilatory support.

Neurologically, it is desirable that the patient be alert, following commands, and able to initiate a breath. The ability to lift and hold the head off the pillow has been correlated with respiratory muscle strength. While an awake and cooperative patient is ideal, there are cases where patients with a depressed or inadequate mental status (such as patients with head trauma or delirium) can, after careful evaluation, be successfully extubated.

From a respiratory standpoint, patients should have an oxygen requirement of $FiO_2 \leq 40\%$ and a PEEP ≤ 8 cm H_2O. These numbers are chosen as they can be safely provided non-invasively. Additionally, the patient should have a strong cough and require secretion clearance at a frequency no more than every 4 hours.

Finally, the patient should be hemodynamically stable and on minimal inotropic or vasopressor support. This is of particular relevance in the heart failure population where the hemodynamic changes associated with removal of positive pressure ventilation can add significant strain on cardiac function.

During daily sedation interruption, if a patient is felt to meet the above criteria, he or she should undergo an SBT.

■ SPONTANEOUS BREATHING TRIALS

A SBT is a reduction or cessation of mechanical ventilatory support (with the ETT in place) to identify patients who could likely be liberated from mechanical ventilation and extubated successfully. The two most common forms of SBT are the pressure support (PS) trial and the T-piece trial.

The PS trial is the most commonly used SBT. During a PS trial, the patient is placed on PS mode with a reduced inspiratory pressure, typically 5 to10 cm H_2O. A PEEP of 5 cm H_2O is also commonly applied. Note that this still involves some small degree of mechanical ventilatory support. However, the patient is required to initiate all breaths and control V_T by varying I_t.

The T-piece trial involves disconnecting the mechanical ventilator from the patient's ETT and connecting flow-by oxygen across the external tip of the ETT (forming the shape of a "T"). Note that this, as opposed to a PS trial, involves cessation of positive pressure ventilation and artificial PEEP. As such, the patient is "liberated from the ventilator" and required to perform all the work of breathing.

In both cases, once an SBT is initiated, it is important to clinically evaluate the patient for signs of success or failure. A successful SBT is one where the patient continues to breathe comfortably with stable vital signs and a stable arterial or end-tidal CO_2 tension. An unsuccessful SBT is one where the patient develops respiratory distress, progressive hemodynamic instability or hypoxemia, or a significantly rising arterial or end-tidal CO_2 tension.

It may seem intuitive that a slow and deep pattern of breathing is preferred to a rapid and shallow one in order to maintain adequate minute ventilation. This has been found to be the case and has been quantified by the rapid shallow breathing index (RSBI) equation:

$$RSBI = RR/V_T$$

where RR is respiratory rate (in breaths/min) and V_T is tidal volume (in liters).

Note that a typical RSBI for a normal person breathing a tidal volume of 0.5 L at a rate or 10 breaths/min is 20. For intubated patients, an RSBI < 105 has been found to have sensitivity of up to 96% and specificity of up to 76% for predicting which patients could tolerate extubation without subsequent reintubation. It is important to keep in mind that, although this equation is commonly used for patients during either T-piece or PS trials, it has only been validated with the T-piece trial.

The optimal duration of spontaneous breathing trials typically lasts 15 to 30 minutes, which is sufficient to evaluate a patient. For T-piece trials, however, it is important to visually monitor the patient throughout the trial since, if respiratory distress or hypoxemia ensue, there is no ventilator to alarm or initiate a backup mode of ventilation.

■ EXTUBATION

Once a patient has a successful SBT, it is time to extubate the patient. This is best performed in a multidisciplinary fashion with a nurse, respiratory therapist, and physician at bedside. The patient should be sitting up and informed of the process. Secretions in the mouth and pharynx as well as in the ETT are cleared. The ETT holder is subsequently disconnected from the ETT, the balloon deflated, and the ETT removed in a swift motion. Secretions are then suctioned again and the patient encouraged to cough.

Neck and lung auscultation to rule out stridor should be performed. Supplemental O_2 can be administered as needed and the patient should be closely monitored for a period to ensure that he or she does not require reintubation.

SUGGESTED READINGS

Chang D. Operating modes of mechanical ventilation. In: *Clinical Application of Mechanical Ventilation*, 4th ed. New York, NY: Delmar Cengage Learning; 2013:81-123.

Gilstrap D, MacIntyre N. Patient-ventilator interactions: implications for clinical management. *Am J Respir Crit Care Med*. 2013;188: 1058-1068.

Girard T, Kress JP, Fuchs BD, et al. Efficacy and safety of a paired sedation and ventilator weaning protocol for mechanically ventilated patients in intensive care (awakening and breathing controlled trial): a randomised controlled trial. *Lancet*. 2008;371:126-34.

McConville J, Kress JP. Weaning patients from the ventilator. *N Engl J Med*. 2012;367:2233-2239.

Slutsky A. History of mechanical ventilation: from vesalius to ventilator-induced lung injury. *Am J Respir Crit Care Med*. 2015 (ahead of print).

CHAPTER 141

Sepsis and Shock

Kevin Felner, MD
Robert L. Smith, MD

Key Clinical Questions

1. What is the definition of systemic inflammatory response syndrome (SIRS) and how do you differentiate SIRS from sepsis, severe sepsis, and septic shock?

2. Which patients presenting with sepsis need admission to the intensive care unit (ICU)?

3. Which septic patients require invasive monitoring (arterial catheter, central venous catheter)?

4. What interventions in the treatment of sepsis improve mortality?

5. Which septic patients deserve empiric steroids as part of the therapeutic regimen?

INTRODUCTION

Sepsis is a clinical syndrome that complicates severe infection and is characterized by systemic inflammation and widespread tissue injury. The incidence and number of sepsis-related deaths has increased yearly from 1979 to 2009 with a combined peak of both primary and secondary sepsis in 2009 greater than 1 million patients in the United States; and sepsis is the ninth most common cause of death in the United States. Despite the rising number of cases, earlier identification of sepsis and improved intensive medical care has been shown to reduce the overall mortality rate to approximately 17.9%. Severity is correlated with mortality (**Table 141-1**).

Initially successful shock resuscitation may still be associated with considerable morbidity and mortality. Multiple organ dysfunction syndrome (MODS) refers to severe acquired dysfunction of at least two organ systems lasting at least 24 to 48 hours in the setting of sepsis, trauma, burns, or severe inflammatory conditions so that homeostasis cannot be maintained without intervention. Mortality is directly correlated with the number of dysfunctional organs and the duration of dysfunction (**Table 141-2**). An uncontrolled hyperinflammatory response is believed to be the cause of multiple organ dysfunction.

The American College of Chest Physicians (ACCP) and the Society of Critical Care Medicine (SCCM) defined the following terms to describe the spectrum of systemic inflammation and sepsis (the International Sepsis Definitions Conference, 2001):

- *Systemic inflammatory response syndrome* (SIRS) is a clinical syndrome that results from activation of the immune system whether due to infection, trauma, burns, or a noninfectious inflammatory process. This syndrome includes at least two of the following:
  (1) Temperature >38°C or <36°C
  (2) Heart rate >90 beats/min
  (3) Respiratory rate >20 breaths/min or $PaCO_2$ < 32 mm Hg
  (4) White blood cell count >12,000 cells/mm³, or <4000 cells/mm³, or >10% immature (band) forms
- *Sepsis* is a clinical syndrome that results from activation of the immune system with a documented infection. The definition of sepsis includes the above SIRS criteria plus a culture-proven infection or presumed presence of an infection.

A recent study has brought into the question the sensitivity of the current definition, suggesting that many patients, usually older, do not actually even have two out of four SIRS criteria when they are septic. These caveats have not been adopted into any formal guidelines at this time. Clinicians should have a lower threshold for considering sepsis, especially in older patients with a suggestive presentation despite not fulfilling the above criteria.

The severity of sepsis is graded according to the associated organ dysfunction and hemodynamic compromise. *Severe sepsis* refers to the presence of sepsis and one or more organ dysfunctions. *Organ dysfunction* may be defined as hypotension, acute lung injury including acute respiratory distress syndrome (ARDS), disseminated intravascular coagulation (DIC), thrombocytopenia, altered mental status, mottled skin, capillary refill greater than 3 seconds, renal dysfunction, hepatic dysfunction, cardiac dysfunction based on echocardiography or measurement of cardiac index, or lactic acidosis indicating hypoperfusion. The phenomenon of sepsis-induced myocardial dysfunction occurs when patients have normal cardiac function prior to their infection and the sepsis induces a global cardiac dysfunction, seen on echocardiography as global hypokinesis, which may impair the expected high cardiac output usually associated with a vasodilated circulation.

TABLE 141-1 Sepsis Syndromes, Definitions, and Mortality Risk

Syndrome	Definition	Approximate Mortality
Systemic inflammatory response syndrome (SIRS)	At least two of the following four clinical features: 1. Temperature >38°C or <36°C 2. Heart rate >90 beats/min 3. Respiratory rate >20 breaths/min **or** $PaCO_2$ <32 mm Hg 4. White blood cell (WBC) count >12,000 cells/mm³, **or** <4000 cells/mm³, **or** >10% immature (band) forms	10%
Sepsis	SIRS criteria plus a culture-proven infection *or presumed presence of an infection*	20%
Severe sepsis	Sepsis plus presence of one or more organ dysfunctions including: • Pulmonary dysfunction (eg, acute respiratory distress syndrome) • Cardiac dysfunction • Renal dysfunction • Hepatic dysfunction • Neurologic dysfunction (altered sensorium) • Hematologic dysfunction (eg, disseminated intravascular coagulation [DIC], thrombocytopenia) • Lactic acidosis (indicating end-organ hypoperfusion)	20%-40%
Septic shock	Sepsis and refractory hypotension with mean systemic blood pressure lower than 65 mm Hg unresponsive to crystalloid fluid challenge of 20-40 cc/kg	40%-60%

Septic shock refers to the presence of sepsis and refractory hypotension with mean systemic blood pressure lower than 65 mm Hg that is *unresponsive to crystalloid fluid challenge of 20 to 40 cc/kg.* Septic shock leads to acute circulatory collapse.

PATHOPHYSIOLOGY

Sepsis is as an uncontrolled inflammatory response to an infection in which a dysregulated host immune response leads to multiorgan involvement not limited to the source infected organ. Microbial antigens such as lipopolysaccharides (LPS) from Gram-negative bacteria bind to Toll-like receptors on inflammatory cells, thereby causing a complex immune reaction involving T-cells, macrophages, neutrophil, endothelial cells, and dendritic cells. Cytokines (such as IL-1, IL-6, IL-8), growth factors (such as TNFa), high-mobility group box-1 (HMGB-1), arachidonic acid metabolites, and nitric oxide and host genetics likely determine the nature of the response. The complement cascade, coagulation cascades, platelets, and leukocytes interact at the vascular endothelium level resulting in microvascular injury, thrombosis, and loss of endothelial integrity, which altogether results in tissue ischemia. This diffuse endothelial disruption is responsible for the various organ dysfunctions and global tissue hypoxia that accompany severe sepsis and septic shock. Multiple mechanisms including decreased preload, vasoregulatory dysfunction, myocardial depression, and impaired tissue extraction due to microcirculatory dysfunction or mitochondrial dysfunction (cytopathic hypoxia) cause global tissue hypoxia. Some noninfectious processes (eg, pancreatitis) may also lead to a dysregulated host immune response and multiorgan dysfunction, and these conditions are categorized using the term SIRS. These patients appear septic without a clear infectious source.

DIFFERENTIAL DIAGNOSIS

The differential diagnosis for conditions that cause sepsis includes conditions that present with high-output nonshock states. Common disorders that meet SIRS criteria include nonmassive pulmonary embolus, alcohol withdrawal, even COPD exacerbations. Thyrotoxicosis, aortic regurgitation, arteriosclerosis, and cirrhosis may mimic sepsis with high cardiac output state and wide pulse pressure without shock.

Conditions that belong to the category of vasodilatory or high cardiac output shock include anaphylaxis, adrenal insufficiency, and neurogenic shock in addition to septic shock. The other causes of shock all fall into a category of low-output states, including cardiogenic shock, hypovolemic shock, and obstructive shock (**Table 141-3**).

TABLE 141-2 Correlation between Organ Failure and Mortality in Sepsis

Organ Failure	Mortality
One organ lasting more than 1 d	20%
Two organs lasting more than 1 d	40%
Three organs lasting more than 3 d	80%

TABLE 141-3 Differential Diagnosis of Shock

Vasodilatory shock	Sepsis
	Anaphylaxis
	Adrenal insufficiency
	Neurogenic
Low-output shock states	Cardiogenic (eg, massive myocardial infarction, myocarditis, valvular disease)
	Hypovolemic (eg, hemorrhagic, gastrointestinal losses, burns, pancreatitis)
	Obstructive (eg, massive PE, tension pneumothorax, auto-PEEP, tamponade, abdominal compartment syndrome)

PE, pulmonary embolus; PEEP, positive end expiratory pressure.

DIAGNOSIS

Presentation of sepsis often varies according to infection source, patient age, underlying comorbidities (including immune system function and cardiac status), and timing of presentation relative to onset of sepsis. Early manifestations of sepsis (tachycardia, oliguria, and hyperglycemia) may be subtle and easily overlooked in the hospitalized patient. In addition, a patient with underlying poor cardiac function who becomes septic may not be able to generate the high cardiac outputs expected in sepsis and may not have the typical findings on physical examination of a septic patient. Signs of established sepsis include altered mental status, metabolic acidosis and respiratory alkalosis, hypotension with decreased systemic vascular resistance (SVR) and elevated cardiac output, and coagulopathy. Late manifestations include acute lung injury (ALI), ARDS, acute renal failure, hepatic dysfunction, and refractory shock.

Sepsis may be related to a systemic inflammatory response to any infectious source. Less than 50% of septic patients will have positive blood cultures, and 20% to 30% of patients will have no microbial cause identified from any source. Aggressive clinical evaluation includes a detailed history and review of systems. A complete physical examination can assess for sometimes inconspicuous and missed infection sources, including skin and soft tissue, central nervous system, gastrointestinal tract, and indwelling devices.

It is critical to stabilize the patient and identify the cause of the ongoing immunologic response. Obtaining cultures for blood, urine, and other fluids early, prior to administration of antibiotics, should be a high priority and helps preserve the integrity of results, but the evaluation should not be at the expense of administering antibiotics expediently. Identification of the underlying source remains paramount, and lack of source identification and control may render choice of antibiotics meaningless. The most common sites of infection in sepsis are the urinary and respiratory tracts, but any organ system may be involved. Urinary sources include cystitis, pyelonephritis, and perinephric abscess. Patients with kidney stones may develop Gram-negative septicemia. Sinusitis, mastoiditis, pneumonia, lung abscess, and empyema may be associated with sepsis. Gastrointestinal sources of sepsis may include esophageal rupture or perforation following a procedure or after vomiting, cholangitis, cholecystitis, intestinal infarction or perforation, acute pancreatitis, *Clostridium difficile* colitis, diverticulitis, and intra-abdominal abscess. Postoperative mediastinitis and acute bacterial endocarditis may lead to sepsis. Skin and soft tissue sources of sepsis include infected decubitus ulcer, postoperative wound infection, soft tissue abscess, or necrotizing fasciitis. Vascular causes of infection include central and peripheral lines, arterial catheters, dialysis catheters, ventriculoperitoneal shunts and septic thrombophlebitis. Infected articular prosthetic devices have also been associated with sepsis. Meningitis and intracranial abscess, sometimes associated with neurosurgery, are also considerations.

Relevant diagnostic studies based on symptoms, signs, and clinical suspicion in patients may include chest or abdominal radiography and culture of blood, urine, sputum, or other relevant body fluids that may be infected such as cerebrospinal fluid (CSF) analysis, paracentesis in patients with ascites, or thoracentesis in patients with pleural effusions. When plain films, blood cultures, and fluid cultures do not yield a likely infectious culprit, advanced imaging with chest and abdominal computed tomography may identify pulmonary infiltrates, intra-abdominal abscesses, and obstructing renal stones. Biliary pathology may be better imaged with ultrasound. In hemodynamically stable patients, magnetic resonance imaging (MRI), or endoscopic retrograde pancreatography (ERCP) may be indicated. Many patients undergo echocardiography to assess cardiac function and to identify the presence of vegetations.

TRIAGE AND HOSPITAL ADMISSION

All patients with a presentation of *severe sepsis* or *septic shock* should be admitted to or transferred to a monitored setting that is capable of continuous vital sign monitoring with the ability to measure central venous pressure (CVP) and central venous oxygen saturations (ScvO$_2$).

PRACTICE POINT

- Recent data suggest that most septic shock patients may be managed without the use of CVP or ScvO$_2$ monitoring; however the values may still be used to assess response to therapy in selected patients with undifferentiated or mixed shock and in patients with underlying organ dysfunction such as chronic kidney disease and cognitive impairment.

Those patients with SIRS and sepsis should be monitored closely if not placed in an intensive care unit setting so that they can be treated promptly if they start to show signs of deterioration. Vital signs should be monitored frequently in addition to telemetry and continuous pulse oximetry. Intermediate care units (sometimes called *step-down units* or *transitional care units*) vary from facility to facility in their capabilities for invasive monitoring and use of vasoactive agents. The protocols and policies at individual institutions will help determine placement of these patients, based on monitoring requirements and response to initial resuscitation in the emergency department or on a medical floor.

PRACTICE POINT

- Early aggressive resuscitation, early antibiotics (within 1 hour of severe sepsis or septic shock identification), and early source identification and control improve outcomes in patients with severe sepsis and septic shock. These patients require timely evaluation to determine admission location, and patients with marginally stable clinical parameters should be admitted to an intensive care unit setting to expeditiously meet early care goals to improve outcomes.

MANAGEMENT

Management of severe sepsis and septic shock requires a structured approach that ensures proper diagnostic evaluation and implementation of evidence-based interventions in an expedient manner to improve outcomes (**Figure 141-1**). This approach requires (1) empiric antibiotic coverage of an infectious source while cultures are pending, (2) optimal fluid resuscitation, (3) pressor and/or inotrope therapy for selected patients, and (4) consideration of additional therapies such as drainage of abscesses, removal of lines, moderate (but not intensive) control of hyperglycemia, and (5) consideration of steroids in selected patient subsets when indicated.

ANTIBIOTIC THERAPY

Initial emergency department management of patients with sepsis begins with a heightened awareness of the condition by assessing all patients for the presence of SIRS criteria. Numerous studies have shown that early and appropriate antibiotics are associated with markedly improved outcomes. Antibiotics should be directed against the likely organisms based upon the presumptive infection source. In many situations, especially when the presumptive source of infection is not obvious, multiple antibiotic agents should be

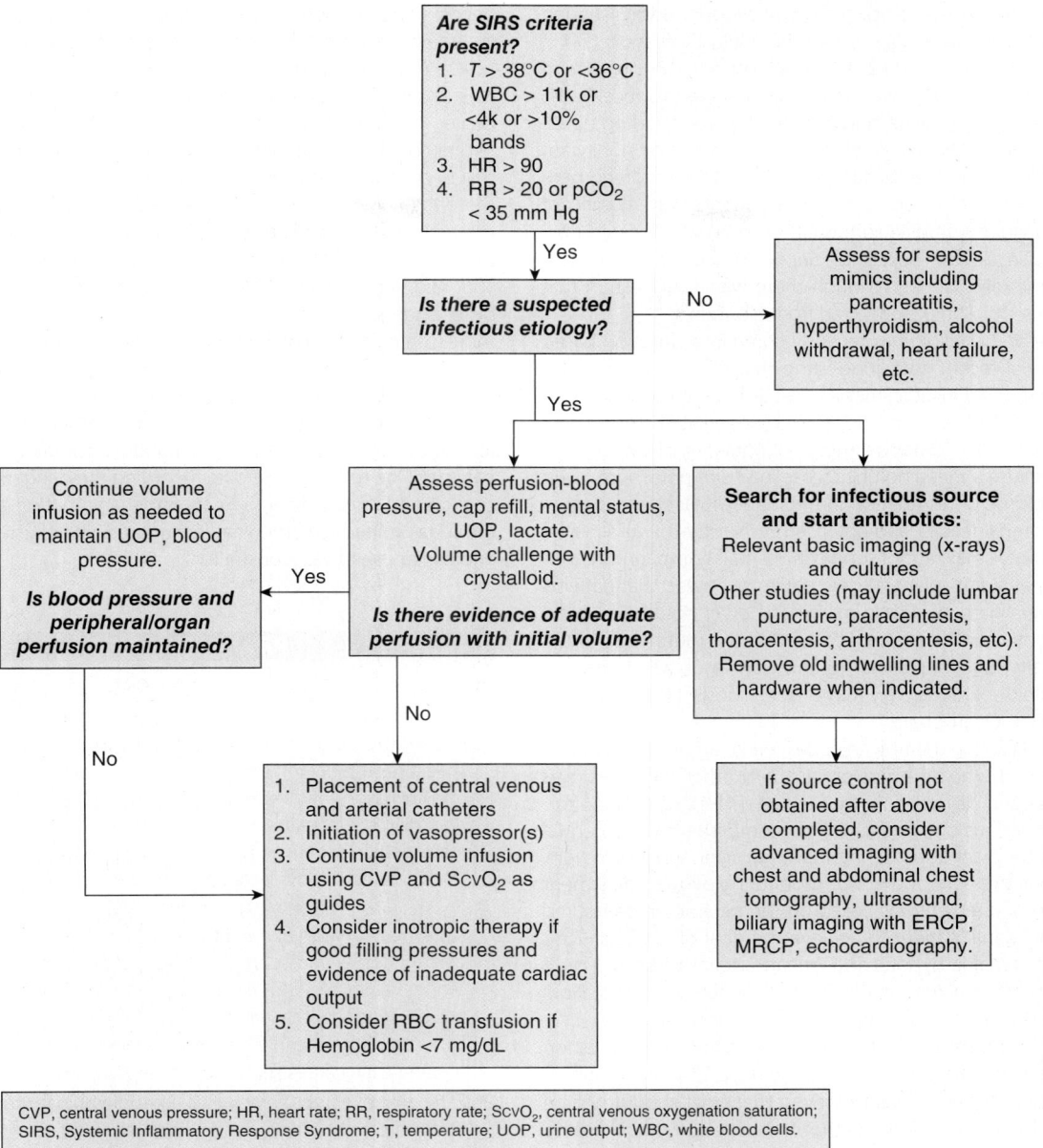

Figure 141-1 *Sepsis algorithm.*

CVP, central venous pressure; HR, heart rate; RR, respiratory rate; ScvO₂, central venous oxygenation saturation; SIRS, Systemic Inflammatory Response Syndrome; T, temperature; UOP, urine output; WBC, white blood cells.

initiated to offer broad antimicrobial coverage. Such broad coverage should then be re-evaluated daily to optimize dosing and minimize drug interactions and the development of resistance. Choice of antibiotic depends upon penetration into the suspected infection site, local resistance patterns, efficacy against the most likely organisms, prior exposure to specific antibiotics, and risks of side effects. Therapeutic drainage of an infected space is critical to diagnose the source of infection, guide the choice of antibiotic therapy, and facilitate recovery. In patients with devices, clinicians may need to evaluate and consider early and rapid removal of potentially or known infected invasive devices including central venous catheters (CVCs), peripherally inserted central venous catheters (PICCs), urinary catheters, and other implanted hardware.

Recent evidence suggests that mortality increases with delay of antibiotics more than 1 hour after identification and management of severe sepsis or septic shock. Patients at risk of fungal infections (ie, recent abdominal surgery, total parenteral nutrition (TPN) administration, chronic steroid use) may benefit from empiric antifungal agents in addition to the antimicrobial regimen.

More data is needed before recommending use of procalcitonin levels in septic patients. While there is reasonable evidence that procalcitonin may be useful in the management of community acquired pneumonia and COPD exacerbations, the evidence for its use in decisions to discontinue antibiotics in septic patients is less robust. Studies comparing a calcitonin-guided algorithm with standard management show no difference in the amount of time spent on antibiotics.

INTRAVENOUS FLUIDS

Volume resuscitation should begin simultaneously with empiric antibiotic therapy in patients suspected of having sepsis. In the vasodilatory state low blood pressures with decreased venous return lead to an underfilled, but hyperdynamic heart. Rivers and colleagues showed that early goal-directed therapy (EGDT), initiated in the emergency department, improved mortality in patients with severe sepsis and septic shock.

For routine use in sepsis, crystalloid fluid should be used first due to evidence of benefit, markedly lower expense, and demonstrated safety (lacking the inherent risks of blood product administration with albumin). The Saline Versus Albumin Fluid Evaluation (SAFE) study evaluated nearly 7,000 critically ill patients, 18% of whom had severe sepsis. Patients were randomly assigned to receive 4% albumin versus normal saline, and investigators reported no differences in mortality at 28 days. Additionally, there were no significant differences seen in the sepsis subgroup. Despite a theoretic benefit to using albumin in highly selected patients with significant volume overload, no studies support this approach. The Albumin Replacement in Severe Sepsis or Septic Shock (ALBIOS) study showed no mortality benefit, though there was a suggestion that patients with septic shock benefitted from albumin.

The choice of crystalloid has recently come into question based on the results of recent data suggesting that normal saline (NS) is associated with renal insufficiency as well as hyperchloremic metabolic acidosis. Alternatives include lactated ringers (LR) and plasmalyte and Normosol. LR contains 4 mEq/L of potassium; however, this is unlikely to cause a meaningful increase in serum potassium levels due to the volume of distribution in the intracellular space, even in patients with renal failure, and any rise is offset by the alkalinizing effect of LR. Three small randomized control trials comparing NS versus LR in perirenal transplant surgery patients showed that patients receiving several liters of LR had marginally lower potassium levels. There is currently insufficient data to support the routine use of the more costly alternatives, plasmalyte and Normosol, which are balanced crystalloid solutions; they may offset acidosis with anions that are converted to bicarbonate.

Early goal-directed therapy includes early aggressive volume resuscitation in the first 6 hours of care, and other measures over the first hours and days of care (see Figure 141-1). Close monitoring of central venous pressure (CVP) is accomplished with a central venous catheter placed in the internal jugular or subclavian vein. Central venous pressure and $ScvO_2$ monitoring allows adjustment of or addition of interventions based on the parameters measured within the individual patient to achieve the goal of $ScvO_2$ at 70%, if the patient remains hypotensive (mean arterial pressure [MAP] < 65 mm Hg) after a reasonable fluid challenge with crystalloid (approximately 20-40 cc/kg) to optimize filling pressures.

The EGDT algorithm, whose utility has come into question with three recent trials, uses a CVP goal of 8 to 12 cm H_2O, which is a reasonable estimate goal. However, that goal should not be applied blindly to all patients without knowledge of coexisting conditions including pulmonary arterial hypertension, dilated cardiomyopathy, and old right ventricular infarction. Clinicians may follow the trend of the CVP and correlate it with the $ScvO_2$, patient hemodynamics, and evidence of organ perfusion including mental status and urine output. Ample data suggest that the CVP serves as a poor predictor of volume responsiveness, and multiple factors are necessary to determine the need for continued volume resuscitation including passive leg raising and pulse pressure variation. Passive leg raise is a technique in which a spontaneously breathing patient is placed with the legs elevated, essentially transferring approximately 300 cc of intravascular fluid into the thorax, followed by measurement of cardiac output. This technique avoids the administration of exogenous fluid. The measurement of $ScvO_2$ carries valuable information and weight, offering the clinician an assessment of cardiac function and oxygen delivery balanced against oxygen consumption.

Despite strong evidence from the original Rivers et al. EGDT trial more than a decade ago, recent publications of the PROCESS (Protocolized Care for Early Septic Shock) trial, the ARISE (Australasian Resuscitation in Early Septic Shock) trial, and the PRoMISe (Protocolized Management in Septic Shock) trial have challenged the utility of the Rivers EGDT algorithm. The three trials showed that with early recognition of septic shock in the emergency department, management according to the Rivers' EGDT algorithm, including placement of central lines and measurement of CVP and $ScvO_2$, did not improve any outcome measures when compared to standard management. The results of these three large, multi-center, randomized control trials have seriously challenged what had become axiomatic since the publication of Rivers original EGDT trial. A change in management, however, may not be immediate as more than 50% of the patients in the EGDT and non-EGDT arms of the trials had central lines placed, and use of vasopressors without placement of a central line has not gained mainstream acceptance. That said, some patients with early positive response to IV fluids and other aggressive measures may not require a central line. Furthermore, use of lactate levels (rather than $ScvO_2$ ± CVP measurements) should provide adequate evaluation of response to therapy, supported by recent studies.

In addition, there has been a change in the paradigm that calls for the use of large volume resuscitation in the treatment of septic patients. Due to the ample data regarding the dangers of over resuscitation and its deleterious effects on organ function, fluid management has shifted to somewhat less aggressive volume resuscitation and earlier use of vasoconstrictors.

PRACTICE POINT

- Central venous saturation ($ScvO_2$) is a measure of oxygen saturation taken from the distal tip of a central venous line inserted just proximal to the right atrium. The $ScvO_2$ measures the balance between oxygen delivery and oxygen consumption, with normal $ScvO_2$ ranging between 65% and 75%. Lower values reflect a high oxygen extraction state, usually seen in states of shock with low cardiac output (cardiogenic, hypovolemic, obstructive).

- In sepsis, as in other vasodilatory or high cardiac output states, low oxygen extraction—possibly due to mitochondrial dysfunction—leads to higher values of $ScvO_2$. Often, these higher values of $ScvO_2$ are not apparent until the patient has been adequately resuscitated with intravascular volume expansion. The mean $ScvO_2$ in the Rivers study was 55%, which is lower than values seen in other sepsis trials.

- Early goal-directed therapy (EGDT) studies initially suggested that clinicians should augment therapeutic interventions when $ScvO_2$ is less than 70% in patients with severe sepsis or septic shock. Three recent studies have shown that outcomes are no worse when $ScvO_2$ is not used to guide management. More recent studies suggest that lactate clearance of at least 10% at a minimum of 2 hours after beginning volume resuscitation is a valid way to assess the efficacy of intravenous fluid administration.

- For EGDT the order of therapy augmentation included: volume expansion (to achieve CVP 8-12 mm Hg) → pressor agents (to achieve MAP ≥ 65 mm Hg) → transfusion of packed RBCs (to achieve an $ScvO_2$ ≥ 70%) → inotropic agents (to achieve an $ScvO_2$ ≥ 70%). This sequence has been challenged by the same three studies comparing EGDT versus standard treatment. A less codified algorithm might include 20-30 cc/kg fluid administration, pressor administration for patients who remain hypotensive with signs of hypoperfusion, further evaluation of the need for additional fluid, along with lactate clearance after the first 2 hours of therapy. Placement of a CVL and measurement of $ScvO_2$ should be individualized, and not routinely used in the care of many patients with sepsis. Of highest importance is early antibiotic administration and intravenous fluids via a secure peripheral or central venous line.

BLOOD TRANSFUSION

Patients with severe sepsis or septic shock who have been resuscitated adequately will usually demonstrate the physiology of a low oxygen extraction state with high ScvO$_2$ values, but importantly, preresuscitation values may make patients appear as high oxygen extractors, with low ScvO$_2$ values more consistent with a low cardiac output state. Early goal-directed therapy protocol includes transfusing red blood cells if the hematocrit is less than 30% and the ScvO$_2$ remains less than 70% after meeting CVP and blood pressure goals. While a subgroup analysis in the original EGDT trial favored transfusions to improve outcomes, potential deleterious effects from red blood cell transfusions, including questionable efficacy of older stored blood, the immuno-modulating effects of red blood cell transfusions, and the risk of transfusion reactions, make this part of the EGDT protocol more difficult to recommend broadly for every patient meeting EGDT criteria. The 2013 Surviving Sepsis Guidelines were revised for red cell transfusions due to the controversy and conflicting data regarding the benefits and risks of red blood cell transfusions. Current recommendations employ a transfusion threshold of 7 gm/dL once tissue hypoperfusion has resolved, except in the setting of active cardiac ischemia, blood loss, severe hypoxemia, and ischemic heart disease. The target goal recommendation is 7 gm/dl to 9 mg/dL, and transfusion for hemoglobin threshold less than 7 g/dL has been shown to have equivalent outcomes for mortality and other relevant outcomes as transfusion for a hemoglobin threshold less than 9 g/dL in patients with septic shock based on the 2014 TRISS trial.

VASOACTIVE MEDICATIONS

An important aspect of sepsis management includes vasoactive medications. Vasopressors are often required to maintain mean arterial blood pressures (MAP) above a target value and the choice of agent depends on the physiologic need (**Table 141-4**). The EGDT protocol recommends vasopressor agents to maintain MAP ≥ 65 mm Hg. There is no firm evidence favoring one vasopressor agent over another, but norepinephrine likely has the greatest vasoconstrictor potency along with some inotropic effect. The most recent Surviving Sepsis Guidelines recommend epinephrine as the second line vasopressor of choice after norepinephrine based on several randomized studies suggesting worse outcomes with use of dopamine (compared to norepinephrine). Epinephrine's most concerning side effects include arrhythmias and elevated lactate levels, which are due to beta receptor agonism rather than ongoing organ ischemia. Dopamine may be used if a more inotropic and chronotropic effect is desired and should be avoided if cardiogenic shock is suspected due to demonstrated increased mortality and arrhythmias in that patient population. Low-dose dopamine does *not* provide renal protection, and should not be used solely for that purpose. Phenylephrine may be the preferred agent for blood pressure elevation in patients with prohibitive tachycardia or arrhythmias. Vasopressin, a pure vasoconstrictor, has been used to lessen the doses of adrenergic vasopressor agents; however, current available data does not support its routine use in severe sepsis or septic shock.

The reversible global myocardial dysfunction that often occurs during sepsis may manifest as poor organ perfusion or as persistently low ScvO$_2$ values despite seemingly adequate filling pressures. Echocardiography or a pulmonary artery (PA) catheter may aid in this diagnosis; however, a PA catheter is rarely necessary in the management of septic shock. The identification of impaired cardiac function may be quite valuable in the management of septic patients. Recognizing cardiac dysfunction may help to avoid the administration of excess volume resuscitation, with consequent pulmonary edema, both cardiogenic and noncardiogenic, and earlier initiation of a vasopressor and/or inotrope to maintain organ perfusion. There has been a rising trend of focused echocardiographic training of noncardiologists which will allow the intensivist and inpatient caregivers to make real-time, noninvasive assessments of their patients at any hour of the day and avoid delays in recognition of this important and increasingly common phenomenon. The addition of an inotropic agent such as dobutamine or milrinone may be temporarily required until the myocardial dysfunction improves.

NUTRITION

Septic patients typically have increased catabolic physiology (breakdown of protein in order to generate amino acids for gluconeogenesis) due to inflammatory response. Supplying calories early in the clinical course of sepsis limit catabolic activity; gut integrity and immune function may be better maintained, leading to decreased infections in critically ill patients. In general, gastrointestinal (GI) tract (enteral) feeding should begin when patients are unable to feed themselves or meet nutritional goals on their own. Several studies have shown a decrease in infectious complications and stress ulcer complications in patients who are started on early (<48 hours) enteral nutrition. Multiple factors, including existing nutritional status as well as the potential for harm from temporarily withholding enteral nutrition or starting parenteral nutrition, play into the decision of initiating enteral nutrition. Patients who are hemodynamically unstable or on high-dose vasopressors may bear risk of bowel ischemia if fed enterally. Total parenteral nutrition (TPN) should be reserved for a minority of patients, typically patients post gastrointestinal surgery. TPN leads to more infectious complications (including fungemia) than enteral feeding, though there is no data showing that enteral feeding improves mortality versus TPN.

GLYCEMIC CONTROL

Guidelines recommend moderate glycemic control (blood glucose [BG] 140-180 mg/dL) in medical ICU patients, including septic patients. Tight glycemic control (keeping BG 80-110 mg/dL) in critically ill medical patients leads to worse mortality outcomes. No significant mortality benefit is achieved with tight glycemic control in critically ill patients except for those undergoing cardiothoracic surgery.

CORTICOSTEROIDS

Relative or functional adrenal insufficiency refers to suboptimal adrenal response to severe sepsis. While some debate has focused around when to prescribe corticosteroids to septic patients and how to make that decision, recent guidelines offer some assistance to clinicians making this decision (**Table 141-5**). In patients with septic shock, defined by systolic blood pressure less than 90 mm Hg despite volume resuscitation and vasopressor medications, corticosteroids offer benefit. The duration of the corticosteroids should be less than 7 days, and mineralocorticoids should not be prescribed. A 2009 meta-analysis summary of randomized controlled trial data suggests that low-dose (<300 mg hydrocortisone per day) short-course (<5 days) therapy offers significant mortality benefit (relative risk reduction 16%, number needed to treat 14) and length-of-stay reduction (average reduction 4.5 days) for patients with severe sepsis or septic shock.

TABLE 141-4 Vasoactive Medications in Sepsis

Medication (Dose)	Inotropy	Chronotropy	Arterial Vasoconstriction	Practical Uses
Norepinephrine 0.01-3.00 mcg/kg/min; 8-30 mcg/min typical dosing	Yes	Yes (but less than dopamine)	Yes	• First line for many patients with severe sepsis or septic shock • Significant vasoconstriction with inotropy which is helpful for patients with poor left ventricular reserve or sepsis-related cardiomyopathy
Dopamine 1-5 mcg/ kg/min, increased renal blood flow; 5-10 mcg/ kg/min, increased chronotropy/inotropy; >10 mcg/kg/min, predominant vasoconstriction, increased blood pressure	Yes	Yes	Yes	• *Not* a first line vasopressor for severe sepsis or septic shock. May be useful for severe bradycardia and mild hypotension • Randomized comparison to norepinephrine showed no significant differences in mortality, but *increased arrhythmias with dopamine and increased mortality in cardiogenic shock* • More tachycardia than with norepinephrine • More potent inotrope than norepinephrine • Differing effects at escalating doses with vasoconstriction at highest dose • Available in premixed or preprepared bags and therefore can be initiated quickly during emergent need
Epinephrine	Yes	Yes	Yes	• Second line vasopressor after norepinephrine in severe sepsis, septic shock. Similar to dopamine with differing effects with escalating doses • Increased production of lactate and significant tachycardia has kept this as a *second-line* medication. Lactate often related to beta receptor agonism rather than hypoperfusion
Phenylephrine 0.4-9.1 mcg/kg/min	No	No	Yes	• Pure vasoconstrictor • Used primarily in sepsis in patients with excessive tachycardia or arrhythmias to avoid medications with chronotropic effect • Used in severe aortic stenosis with hypotension to raise mean arterial pressure and preserve coronary perfusion • Decrease outflow tract gradient in patients with hypertrophic cardiomyopathy
Vasopressin 0.01-0.04 units/min	No	No	Yes	• Used due to relative depletion of vasopressin in sepsis • Nonadrenergic vasoconstrictor • Data not clear on role and effect, but does spare adrenergic receptors • Concern over decrease in splanchnic perfusion • *Should not be used as the sole vasopressor agent in sepsis, and should* not *be titrated for effect*
Dobutamine 2.5-20.0 mcg/kg/min	Yes	Yes	Vasodilator	• Used for patients exhibiting evidence of low-output state with sepsis due to underlying poor cardiac reserve or sepsis-induced cardiomyopathy • May lead to *hypotension*, and should be used with a vasoconstrictor initially if hypotension occurs due to vasodilatory effects
Milrinone 0.375-0.75 mcg/kg/min	Yes	Yes	Vasodilator	• Similar to dobutamine, though works through nonadrenergic receptors. May be useful in patients on long-acting beta blockers who need inotropy/chronotropy • Dose adjustment needed in renal failure

TABLE 141-5 Recommendations for Use of Steroids in Septic Shock

- Intravenous hydrocortisone (300 mg/d, split into every 6 h or every 8-h dosing) for adult patients in septic shock when hypotension responds poorly to fluid resuscitation and vasopressors. Avoid steroids in absence of shock (unless patient's underlying endocrine history requires it).
- ACTH (Corsyntropin) stimulation test is not recommended.
- Hydrocortisone is preferred to dexamethasone.
- Steroid therapy may be weaned once vasopressors are no longer required.

ACTH, adrenocrticotropic hormone.

CONSULTATION

The multidisciplinary environment of the ICU often requires many different consultants to aid in the care of critically ill patients with sepsis, severe sepsis, and septic shock. Critical care nursing, intensivists, infectious disease specialists, nephrologists, endocrinologists, surgeons, palliative care experts, nutritionists, social workers, and many others may be necessary to optimize the care of patients with sepsis. Clinicians caring for patients in the critical care setting should have a low threshold to involve necessary services in the care of their critically ill patients to optimize care quality and efficiency.

Many patients with sepsis will not require the care of an intensivist. Indications for consultation include:

- Persistent hemodynamic instability
- Incipient progression to multiorgan failure
- Advanced airway and/or ventilator management
- Uncertainty regarding diagnosis or management
- Invasive management, including placement of central venous and arterial catheters, and if placement of pulmonary artery catheters is contemplated
- Consideration of corticosteroid administration in the setting of septic shock

COMPLICATIONS AND PROGNOSIS

Uncomplicated sepsis that is treated appropriately and aggressively will often have very few untoward outcomes and patients may return to baseline within a very short time frame. Sepsis that progresses to severe sepsis or septic shock more frequently leads to a complicated course for the patient (Table 141-1). Patients will often require invasive procedures including central venous catheter and arterial catheter placement, as well as possible endotracheal intubation and mechanical ventilation to manage airway, refractory hypoxemia, and/or increased work of breathing. Patients with acute lung injury, also known as noncardiogenic pulmonary edema or acute respiratory distress syndrome (ARDS), may require a prolonged course of mechanical ventilation; their lung function typically improves over time, though not back to baseline. Other patients may suffer kidney injury requiring dialysis therapy. The typically reversible acute tubular necrosis may take days, weeks, or months to resolve, and some patients may require chronic hemodialysis permanently. A relatively common neurologic disorder encountered in sepsis is the development of critical illness polyneuropathy, which will typically manifest as difficulty liberating a patient from mechanical ventilation due to profound weakness. This condition usually resolves, but may often take several months. Psychological stress, often described as posttraumatic stress disorder, is related to the common complication of ICU delirium. Daily awakening in the ICU may minimize delirium.

DISCHARGE PLANNING

Patients may transition from a closely monitored setting—either intensive care unit or intermediate care unit—to a medical floor when they are hemodynamically stable (ie, off vasoactive medications) and not in need of frequent CVP and $ScvO_2$ measurement. Any septic patient requiring mechanical ventilation, or even noninvasive mechanical ventilation intermittently, should remain in an ICU setting until their gas exchange or work of breathing problems have resolved and they no longer require supportive devices. Discharge from the hospital may occur quickly if a patient has mild sepsis that is treated and resolves quickly. For a more prolonged hospitalization including mechanical ventilation, a patient may require significant physical rehabilitation within an acute or subacute rehabilitation facility before returning to the home environment (see Section III [Rehabilitation and Skilled Nursing Care]).

QUALITY IMPROVEMENT TO ADDRESS PERFORMANCE GAPS

Institutional sepsis protocols likely will standardize and improve overall care for septic patients admitted to hospitals and ICUs. Since outcomes in severe sepsis and septic shock highly depend on expeditious administration of evidence-based interventions, institutions and individual clinicians should consider measuring process outcomes (eg, time to antibiotics in sepsis) as well as patient outcomes to help best delineate areas of heterogeneous care and help drive consistent evidence-based or guideline-based practice to improve overall outcomes.

Sepsis prevention requires early recognition of disease and prompt treatment to prevent progression to severe sepsis and septic shock. The importance of early recognition has led to the development of "sepsis" teams which are often comprised of an intensivist, and ICU nurse, and in some places a pharmacist and can be activated similarly to rapid response and code teams. Small single center studies have shown decreased mortality, shorter length of ICU stay and lower costs when sepsis teams are employed.

A lower threshold for sepsis evaluation and aggressive therapy needs to be applied to immunosuppressed patients, including patients with HIV, asplenia, neutropenia, and patients receiving immunosuppressive agents. Early removal of urinary catheters, central venous catheters, and liberation from mechanical ventilation to prevent ventilator-associated pneumonia will lower the incidence of sepsis. The cost of caring for septic patients exceeds $22,000 per hospitalization, and much opportunity exists to improve outcomes and reduce hospital lengths of stay and costs for a medical condition that bears high morbidity and mortality (**Table 141-6**).

TABLE 141-6 Evidence-Based Medicine: Key References for Sepsis

Reference	Methodology	Results	Limitations	Bottom Line
The ProCESS Investigators. *N Engl J Med.* 2014;370:1683-1693	Multicentered randomized controlled trial of 1341 patients assigned to protocol-based early goal directed therapy (EGDT), protocol-based standard therapy, or to usual care.	Hospital mortality at 60 d was 21% for EGDT group, 18.2% for protocol-based standard therapy, and 18.9% for usual care. No statistical differences in 90-d or 1-y mortality or need for organ support.	No blinding. Possible incorporation of EGDT protocol into the protocol based standard therapy or usual care groups. Single-center study and bundled elements included transfusion of reblood cells in a way that has been proven to be unnecessary and possibly harmful. The utility of the central venous pressure to guide fluid responsiveness has been proven unreliable.	EGDT did not decrease mortality among patients presenting to the emergency department with early septic shock when compared to protocol-based standard therapy or usual care. Raises doubts regarding the value of incorporating EGDT into international guidelines as a standard of care is questionable.
Rivers, et al. *NEJM.* 2001;345(19): 1368-1377	Single center randomized controlled trial of 263 patients with sepsis or severe sepsis assigned to receive 6 h of early goal-directed therapy (EGDT) vs standard of care in the emergency room prior to admission to the intensive care unit. In-hospital mortality was the primary outcome.	Hospital mortality was 30.5% for the EGDT group vs 46.5% for the control group ($p = 0.009$).		The importance of early and aggressive volume resuscitation in septic patients is emphasized. The difference in the two groups is essentially related to the amount of volume they each received in the first 6 h. It is not clear that using the CVP and the hematocrit are ideal ways to manage sepsis resuscitation as there is strong independent evidence against both of them.
Ibrahim, et al. *CHEST.* 2000;118:146-155	Prospective cohort study of 142 patients with blood stream infections admitted to intensive care units comparing hospital survival and adequacy of antimicrobial therapy.	Hospital mortality rate of patients on inadequate antimicrobial treatment (61.9%) was greater than the hospital mortality (28.4%; CI 1.77-2.69; $p < 0.0001$) of the patients on adequate antimicrobial treatment.	Single-center study. Mixed group of medical and surgical patients may not be applicable to other types of intensive care unit patients. Antibiotic decisions based on physician judgment, which may differ from places where guidelines/protocols are in place and mandatory.	Appropriate antibiotics are crucial in caring for patients with bloodstream infections. Suggests using broad coverage initially and allowing culture data to narrow later to limit inappropriate use, which can breed resistance and not be cost effective.
Gaieski, et al. *Crit Care Med.* 2010;38:1045-1053	Prospective cohort study of 261 patients with severe sepsis or septic shock undergoing EGDT to study the association between time to antibiotic administration and survival.	Mortality was markedly better for patients who received appropriate antibiotics both <1 h from triage (mortality 19.5% vs 33.2%) and <1 h from qualification for EGDT to appropriate antibiotics (25.0% vs 38.5%).	Single-center study. May not be applicable to other institutions not using an ER-initiated EGDT algorithm.	Early appropriate antibiotics are essential for patients with severe sepsis or septic shock. This cohort was treated with EGDT, which controls for volume resuscitation, and the vasoactive medication aspects of sepsis. The results support this important intervention.

(Continued)

TABLE 141-6 Evidence-Based Medicine: Key References for Sepsis (*Continued*)

Reference	Methodology	Results	Limitations	Bottom Line
The NICE-SUGAR Study Investigators. *N Engl J Med.* 2009;360:1283-1297	Multicenter randomized controlled trial of 6104 medical and surgical intensive care unit (ICU) patients expected to require ICU care for three or more consecutive days. Patients were assigned to intensive glucose control with target of 81-108 mg/dL or a conventional-control target of <180 mg. Primary outcome was death at 90 d.	Significant mortality day 90 seen in patients in the intensive-control group vs the conventional-control group (27.5% vs 24.9%, $p = 0.02$). Severe hypoglycemia found in 6.8% of the intensive-control group vs 0.5% in the conventional-control group ($p < 0.0001$).	Open-label design, imbalance between the study groups with respect to number of patients on glucocorticoid therapy.	No additional benefit in lowering blood glucose levels below the range of approximately 140-180 mg/dL in critically ill patients.
Sprung, et al. *N Engl J Med.* 2008;358:111-124	Multicenter, randomized, double-blind, placebo-controlled trial of 499 patients with septic shock with study patients assigned to 50 mg intravenous hydrocortisone every 6 h for 5 d and tapered over 6 d vs placebo. Primary outcome was death at 28 d.	At 28 d there was no significant difference in mortality between the two groups with mortality 34.3% in the steroid group vs 31.5% in the placebo group ($p = 0.51$). There was no significant difference in mortality between the patients in the two study groups who did not have a response to cosintropin or between those who had a response to cosintropin.	The use of etomidate in 26% of the patients, which can inhibit corticosteroid production. Study lacked power due to early stop in patient enrollment due to slow recruitment, termination of funding, and time expiration of the study drug.	Based on this study, general use of corticosteroids for septic shock is not recommended. As well, corticotropin testing cannot be recommended to determine which patients should receive corticosteroid therapy. Steroids did lead to more rapid reversal of shock, but no change in mortality. Subgroup with refractory septic shock showed a mortality benefit from steroids, similar to Annane study. Patients on hydrocortisone also had more cases of superinfection and hyperglycemia.
Annane, et al. *JAMA.* 2002;288:862-871	Multicenter, randomized, double-blind, placebo-controlled trial of 300 patients with septic shock with study patients receiving hydrocortisone 50 mg every 6 h intravenously and once daily administration of 50 mcg of fludocortisone via nasogastric tube vs indiscernible placebos for total 7 d. Primary outcome was 28-d survival in nonresponders to the short corticotropin test.	There were 229 nonresponders to the corticotropin test and 70 responders to the corticotropin test with equal numbers of study and placebo in each group. In nonresponders, there was a significant ($p = .02$) decrease in death in the corticosteroid group and withdrawal of vasopressor therapy within 28 d in the corticosteroid group ($p = .001$) compared to placebo. No significant differences seen between responders.	The patients studied were in refractory shock, defined as systolic blood pressure <90 mm Hg after 1 h despite fluid resuscitation and vasopressor therapy. Significant number of patients received etomidate (24%) prior to enrollment, which is known to cause transient adrenal insufficiency.	Significant reduction in risk of death in patients with refractory septic shock given 7-d treatment with low-dose hydrocortisone and fludrocortisone with relative adrenal insufficiency (nonresponders to corticotropin stimulation).

This is one of three similar multicenter trials which arrived to similar conclusion. The trials, ARISE and ProMise are referenced in bibliography.

SUGGESTED READINGS

Annane D, Bellissant E, Bollaert PE, et al. Corticosteroids in the treatment of severe sepsis and septic shock in adults: a systematic review. *JAMA.* 2009;301(22):2362-2375.

Dellinger RP, Levy MM, Carlet JM, et al. Surviving sepsis campaign: international guideline for management of severe sepsis and septic shock. *Intensive Care Med.* 2013;39(2):165-228. *Crit Care Med.* 2013;41(2):580-637.

Ferrer R, Martin-Loeches I, Phillips G, et al. Empiric antibiotic treatment reduces mortality in severe sepsis and septic shock from the first hour: results from a guideline-based performance improvement program. *Crit Care Med.* 2014;42:1749-1755.

Finfer S, Chittock DR, Su SY, et al. Intensive versus conventional glucose control in critically ill patients. *N Engl J Med.* 2009;360(13):1283-1297.

Heffner AC, Horton JM, Marchick MR, et al. Etiology of illness in patients with severe sepsis admitted to the hospital form the emergency department. *Clin Infec Dis.* 2010;50(6):814-820.

Mouncey PR, Osborn TM, Power GS, et al. Trial of early, goal-directed resuscitation for septic shock. *N Engl J Med.* 2015;372(14):1301-1311.

Peake SL, Delaney A, Bailey M, et al. Goal-directed resuscitation for early septic shock. *N Engl J Med.* 2014;371(16):1496.

Rivers E, Nguyen B, Havstad S. Early goal-directed therapy in the treatment of severe sepsis and septic shock. *N Engl J Med.* 2001;345(19):1368-1377.

Yealy DM, Kellum JA, Huang DT, et al. A randomized trial of protocol-based care for early septic shock. *N Engl J Med.* 2014; 370(18):1683.

Yunos NM, Bellomo R, Hegarty C, Story D, Ho L, Bailey M. Association between a chloride-liberal vs chloride-restrictive intravenous fluid administration strategy and kidney injury in critically ill adults. *JAMA.* 2012;308(15):1566-1572.

CHAPTER 142

Acute Respiratory Distress Syndrome

Corey D. Kershaw, MD

Greg S. Martin, MD, MSc

Key Clinical Questions

1. What are the predisposing diseases/conditions that lead to acute respiratory distress syndrome (ARDS)?

2. How do you differentiate ARDS from other causes of hypoxemic respiratory failure?

3. How do you manage mechanical ventilation in ARDS?

4. What adjunctive therapies may benefit patients diagnosed with ARDS?

INTRODUCTION

The acute respiratory distress syndrome (ARDS) describes a common disorder encountered in the critical care unit that remains a significant cause of morbidity and mortality. In the last decade standardization of ventilator strategies and overall improvement in critical care management has resulted in significant improvements in outcomes. Early vigilance in patient triage to a higher level of care (eg, transferring to the ICU), efficient identification of predisposing syndromes, and initiation of appropriate ICU interventions may prevent progression to ARDS and can minimize morbidity and mortality.

DEFINITION

◼ ACUTE LUNG INJURY (ALI)

American-European Consensus Conference (AECC) defined ALI by the following three criteria:

(1) $PaO_2:FiO_2 \leq 300$.
(2) Bilateral infiltrates on chest x-ray (see **Figure 142-1**).
(3) Absence of left atrial hypertension or a pulmonary artery occlusion pressure ≤18 mm Hg. The third criterion excluded pulmonary edema of hydrostatic or cardiogenic origin.

◼ ARDS

ARDS was defined by the same criteria but with worse oxygenation ($PaO_2:FiO_2 \leq 200$), representing the subset of ALI patients with more severe hypoxemia. The AECC established a basis for years of publications on ARDS epidemiology, management, and outcomes research that could be easily applied to all patients by establishing a standard set of parameters to define ARDS.

◼ BERLIN DEFINITION OF ARDS

The European Society of Intensive Care Medicine updated the diagnostic criteria to reflect more recent research and to address the limitations of the AECC criteria. Published in 2012, the Berlin definition eliminated the term *acute lung injury* that was frequently misused and created three separate and exclusive categories to reflect severity (**Table 142-1**).

The European Society of Intensive Care Medicine used a combination of expert opinion and data validation to assess the performance of the new definition. This led to the exclusion of some other parameters in the AECC definition, such as static compliance or a high PEEP requirement. In the current era of more standardized ventilation strategies, the degree of hypoxemia is the best predictor of outcome, and stratifying ARDS into mild, moderate, and severe categories seems to better inform future clinic trials and direct more aggressive therapies to the patients at highest risk of poor outcome.

As a general rule, a precipitating cause of ARDS should be identified, and the onset of symptoms or signs of respiratory failure will occur within 7 days of that identified cause. In the presence of an inciting factor, the presence or absence of heart failure or even hypervolemia does not exclude the diagnosis of ARDS in this definition whereas previously these were largely considered mutually exclusive conditions. However, in the absence of a precipitating cause of ARDS, hydrostatic edema must be excluded. The committee suggested echocardiography for volume and cardiac assessment compared to the prior recommendation for pulmonary artery catheterization with a pulmonary capillary wedge pressure (PCWP) of <18 cm H_2O. This reflects the evolving ICU practice in which routine pulmonary artery catheters are now placed infrequently for these patients.

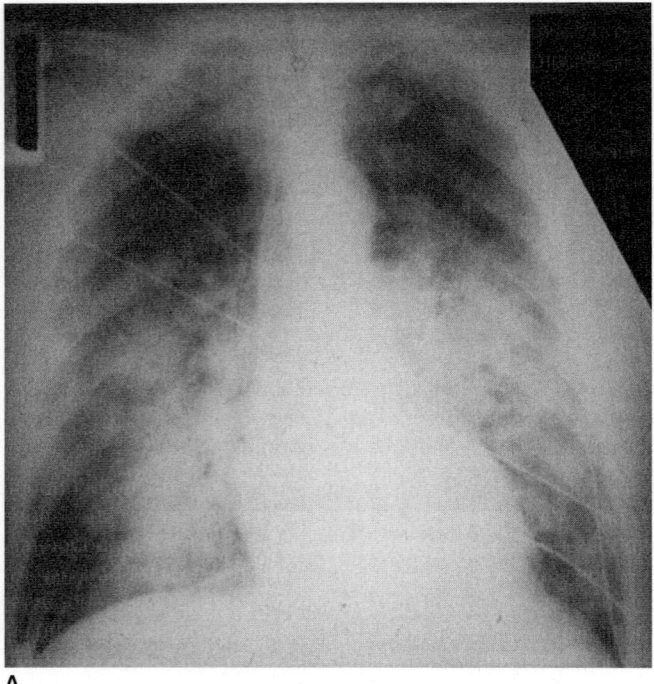

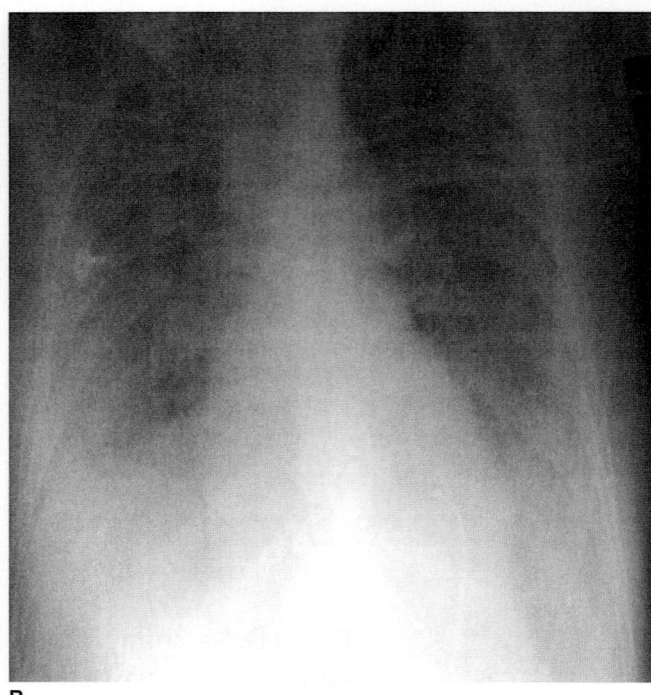

A

B

Figure 142-1 *Chest radiographs depicting ARDS with a patchy airspace pattern (A). ARDS can progress to a more confluent airspace pattern over time (B).*

EPIDEMIOLOGY

The reported incidence ranges widely from 1.3 to 34 cases per 100,000 person-years. When rigorous screening for ALI and ARDS was applied in King County, Washington in 2000, investigators reported an incidence of 86.2 cases/100,000 person-years and 64.0 cases/100,000 person-years, respectively. Inaccuracies in true incidence are magnified by a nonspecific case definition—mostly the AECC ARDS criteria that have been recently changed—and the relative lack of validation studies of the previous criteria.

PRESENTATION

Patients presenting with ALI or impending ARDS may be difficult to differentiate initially from other causes of hypoxemic respiratory failure. Identification of an underlying cause or inciting event is important in differentiating ARDS from other lung diseases or syndromes

TABLE 142-1 The Berlin Definition of the Acute Respiratory Distress Syndrome

Timing	Within 7 d of precipitating cause or onset of new/worsening respiratory symptoms
Chest imaging	Bilateral airspace opacities that cannot be explained otherwise (eg, by effusions, nodules, or atelectasis)
Origin of chest imaging abnormality	Not fully explained by cardiac failure or volume overload; Hydrostatic edema must be excluded if predisposing cause not present (eg, echocardiogram)
Oxygenation	
Mild	$200 < PaO_2/FiO_2 \leq 300$ with PEEP or CPAP ≥ 5 cm H_2O
Moderate	$100 < PaO_2/FiO_2 \leq 200$ with PEEP ≥ 5 cm H_2O
Severe	$PaO_2/FiO_2 \leq 100$ with PEEP ≥ 5 cm H_2O

that may be misidentified as ARDS. Pulmonary and nonpulmonary sepsis most commonly causes ARDS (**Table 142-2**).

PRACTICE POINT

- The evolution from inciting cause to ARDS typically occurs within 3 to 5 days. Severe hypoxemia is part of the diagnostic criteria of ARDS. Concomitant hypercapnia in the face of tachypnea indicates failure of compensatory ventilation, is especially worrisome, and warrants immediate attention.

The presenting complaint (shortness of breath, dyspnea, and cough) may be nonspecific. Fever and sputum production may indicate a pulmonary infection. Hypoxemia requiring high fractions of inspired supplemental oxygen suggests evolving ALI with worsening ventilation-perfusion (V/Q) mismatching and worsening shunt physiology. Patients may experience a declining level of consciousness secondary to severe hypoxemia or concomitant hypercapnia. Concerning findings such as altered mentation and hypercapnia usually warrant immediate endotracheal intubation. Tachypnea and auscultation of rales on physical examination is typical of ARDS but may also present in other causes of acute respiratory failure such as heart failure, pneumonia, or occult interstitial lung disease. Laboratory studies such as leukocytosis are not specific for ARDS but may suggest the predisposing cause as in severe pneumonia or sepsis.

TABLE 142-2 Common Predisposing Causes of ARDS

Direct Lung Injury	Indirect Lung Injury
Pneumonia	Nonpulmonary sepsis
Gastric aspiration	Acute pancreatitis
Chest trauma/lung contusion	Severe nonchest trauma
Inhalation injury	Blood transfusions
Near-drowning	Surface burns

Chest radiography reveals bilateral, diffuse airspace infiltrates. Patchy infiltrates may become more confluent as the syndrome evolves (Figure 142-1). Cardiomegaly suggests preexisting cardiac disease and thus left ventricular dysfunction as an etiology for the patient's hypoxemia and chest radiograph abnormality. In cases where there is concern about coexistent or predominant heart failure, additional testing with echocardiography, CT imaging, or pulmonary artery catheterization may be required to confirm the diagnosis of ARDS or rule out other conditions.

PATHOPHYSIOLOGY

■ EXUDATIVE STAGE

The predisposing injury leading to ARDS occurs at every level of the alveolar-capillary compartment (**Figure 142-2**). Integrity of the alveolar-capillary membrane is required to maintain a dry alveolar space and to ensure adequate gas exchange between the alveolar epithelium across the interstitial space to the pulmonary capillaries.

The alveolar epithelium is composed primarily of two types of cells. Type I pneumocytes function primarily in architectural support as well as fluid and solute transport through its aquaporin-5 surface proteins. Capable of differentiating into type I cells, type II pneumocytes primarily produce and recycle surfactant. Injury of the type I cell leads to a disruption of barrier integrity during the early phases of ARDS (the *acute, exudative phase*). Impaired surfactant function contributes to atelectasis and worsening pulmonary compliance.

In ARDS, the alveolar-capillary barrier loses its ability to limit egress of fluids, proteins, and debris from the vascular space on the capillary endothelial side. The combination of vascular hydrostatic and protein osmotic pressures, together with vascular integrity, sets the stage for accumulation of proteinaceous pulmonary edema according to Starling's equation:

$$J_v = K_{f,c}[(P_c - P_i) - \sigma(\pi_{pp} - \pi_{ip})].$$

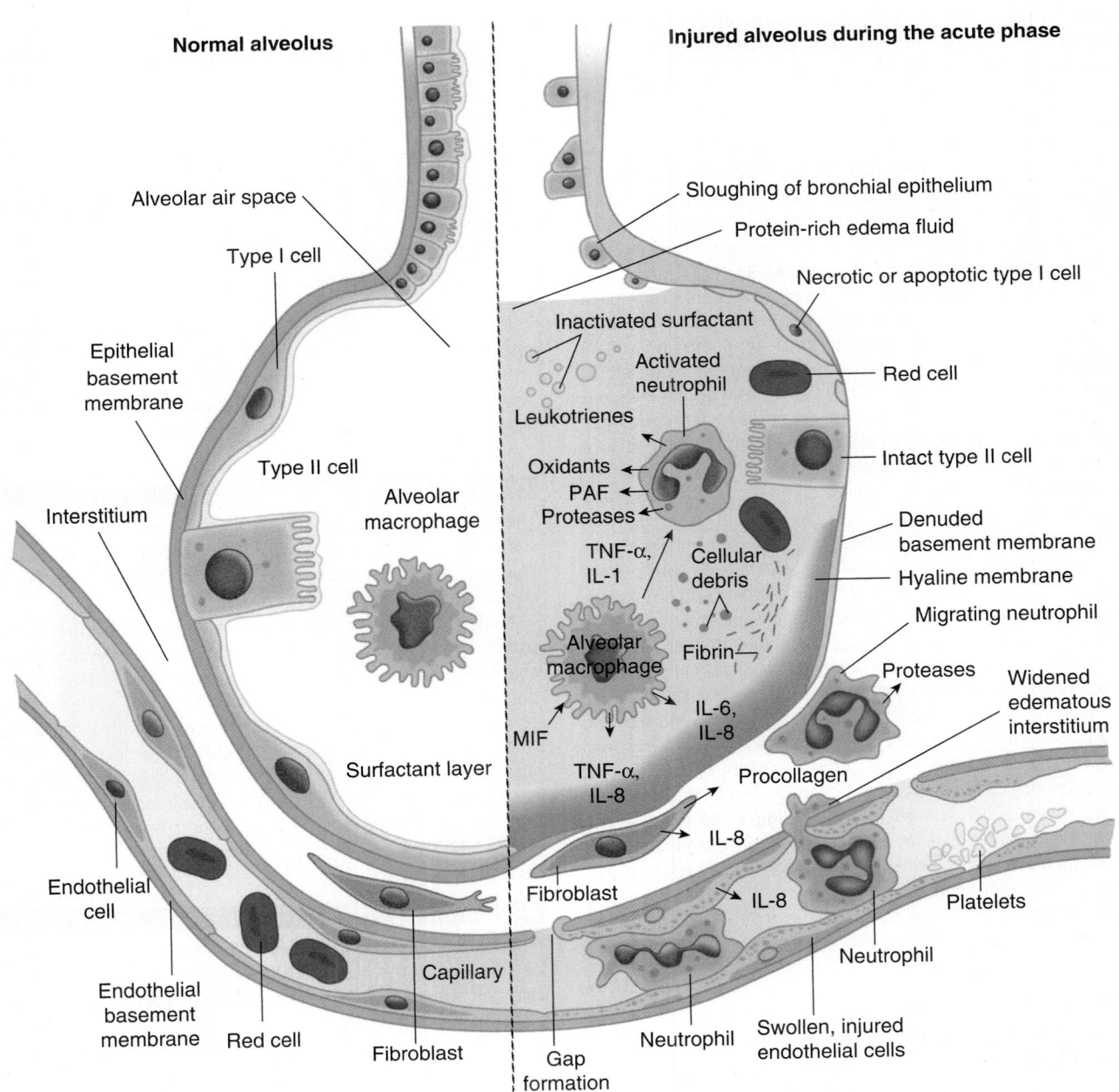

Figure 142-2 *Normal alveolus on the left and injured alveolus during the acute phase of the acute respiratory distress syndrome on the right.* (Reproduced, with permission, from Ware LB, Matthay MA. The acute respiratory distress syndrome. *N Engl J Med.* 2000;342:1334.)

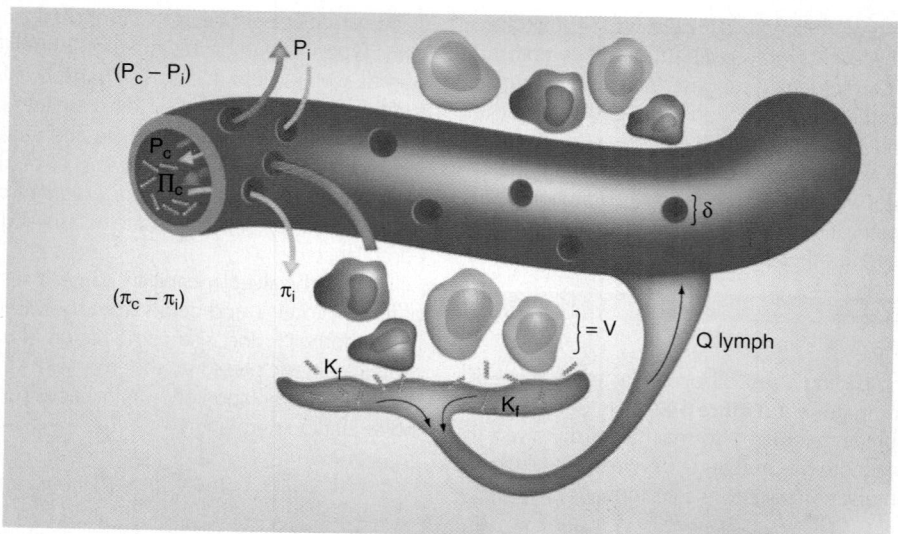

Figure 142-3 *Illustration of the relationships between hydrostatic and oncotic pressures, as described by the Starling Equation.* (Cribbs, SK, Martin GS. Fluid balance and colloid osmotic pressure in acute respiratory failure: optimizing therapy. *Expert Rev Resp Med.* 2009;3(6):651-662. http://www.informaworld.com.)

The Starling equation states that movement of fluid across a capillary barrier into an interstitial space is governed by balances in the hydrostatic pressure in the capillary and interstitium (P_c and P_i, respectively) and the plasma and interstitial oncotic pressures (π_{pp} and π_{ip}, respectively). The relationship between hydrostatic and oncotic pressures is illustrated in **Figure 142-3**.

Increases in capillary hydrostatic pressure or decreases in capillary oncotic pressure will result in net movement of fluid out of the plasma space and in to the interstitial sub-compartment. The capillary reflection coefficient (σ) and the bulk transfer coefficient (K_f) describe the integrity of the capillary barrier: as σ approaches zero the barrier loses its ability to segregate oncotically active substances, while increases in K_f linearly increase movement of fluid across the membrane. The injury seen early in acute lung injury facilitates movement of fluid out of the capillary compartment by a combination of these changes.

In this early stage of ARDS, shunting and hypoxemia dominate the clinical picture. The flooding of the alveolar unit with *proteinaceous edema* leads to worsening V/Q mismatching and physiologic shunt that is increasingly refractory to oxygen supplementation. The *atelectasis* caused by surfactant defects requires higher pressures to maintain alveolar patency for ventilation. *Increases in pulmonary artery pressures* secondary to hypoxemic pulmonary vasoconstriction, decreases in pulmonary circulation due to *microthrombi* and direct damage to the vascular endothelium lead to worsening dead space ventilation. Together, each of these contributes to increased work of breathing. The histological change seen in the exudative phase is known as *diffuse alveolar damage* (**Figure 142-4A**). Nonspecific for ARDS, diffuse alveolar damage is not considered diagnostic and a lung biopsy is not necessary unless other alternative diagnoses are seriously considered.

These changes in the exudative phase of ARDS are heterogeneous and of variable duration, typically lasting 7 to 10 days.

■ PROLIFERATIVE STAGE

The second stage of disease is known as the *proliferative phase* (**Figure 142-4B**). Type II pneumocytes begin to regenerate in order to reconstitute the surfactant layer, and type I cells rebuild the damaged alveolar epithelium. Depending on the effectiveness of this reparative process, recovery from ARDS in days 7 through 21 may

be rapid. Some patients, however, have a prolonged course as procollagen III is deposited in the interstitial space with subsequent fibrosis. A dominant or exaggerated fibrotic phase increases the risk for prolonged morbidity or mortality and may require prolonged mechanical ventilation. As the vascular changes that occur in the exudative phase become more irreversible, pulmonary hypertension may result.

In summary, the acute respiratory failure secondary to ARDS results from both permeability damage—from either direct injury to the alveolar-capillary membrane or an overzealous inflammatory response to the injury—and decreased lung compliance that deranges the normal gas exchange mechanisms.

DIFFERENTIAL DIAGNOSIS

The diagnosis of ARDS is based on clinical criteria and requires exclusion of other diseases presenting in a similar manner. This challenge illustrates the limitation of using clinical parameters to diagnose a complicated syndrome such as ARDS.

Acute infectious pneumonias that cause either an interstitial pattern or diffuse airspace disease may be clinically indistinguishable from ARDS. *Pneumocystis jiroveci* pneumonia (previously PCP), pneumonitis secondary to viral infection, or a severe bacterial community-acquired pneumonia may present with a similar chest x-ray and refractory hypoxemia without the same cellular toxicity seen in ARDS. Furthermore, these pulmonary infections may lead to the development of ARDS. Multiple noninfectious diseases may mimic the refractory hypoxemia and chest x-ray pattern in ARDS (**Table 142-3**).

TRIAGE

A patient presenting with new-onset or worsening hypoxemia must be admitted to the hospital. Admission to the ICU or progressive care unit should be pursued for patients requiring closer monitoring or higher levels of nursing care than can be provided in a typical medical or surgical floor setting. Indications for ICU admission include patients with respiratory distress or hypoxemia refractory to supplemental oxygen and those requiring initiation of mechanical ventilation. In some facilities, noninvasive ventilation also requires a higher level of monitored care.

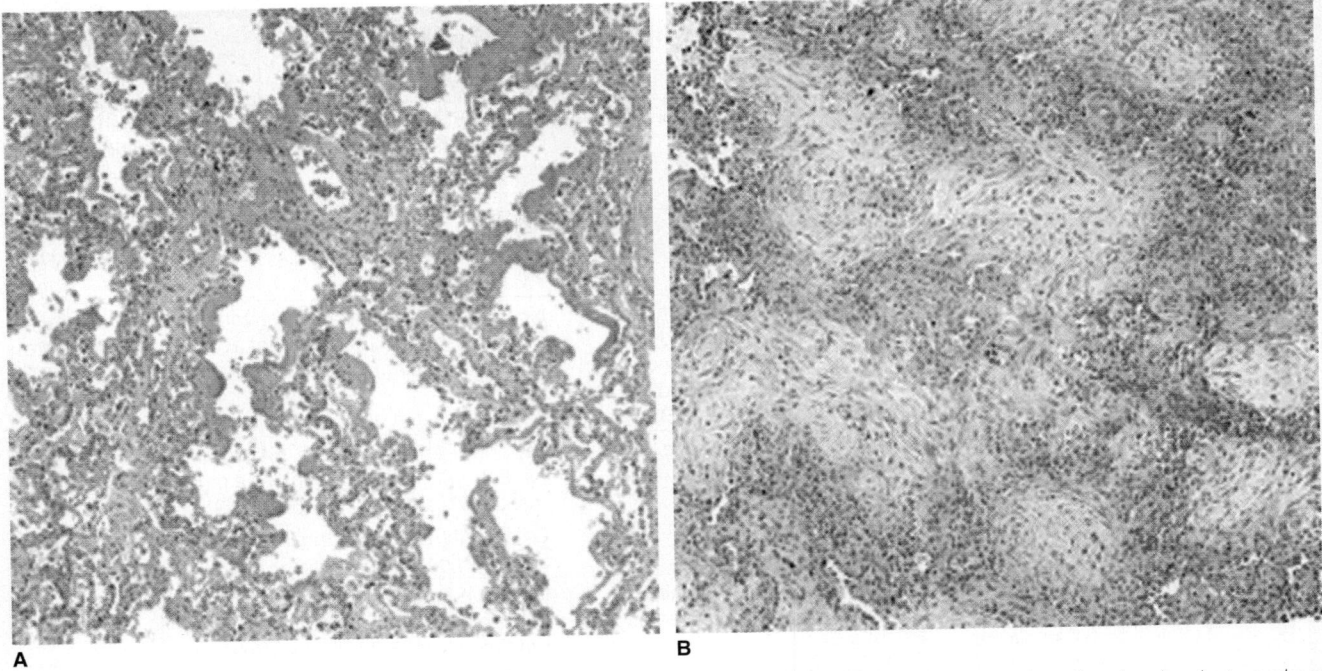

Figure 142-4 *(A) Exudative phase, diffuse alveolar damage: Prominent eosinophilic hyaline membranes line the alveolar ducts and sacs. (B) Proliferative phase, organizing diffuse alveolar damage: Extensive young fibroblastic proliferation fills the alveolar spaces and interstitium. (Courtesy of Anthony A. Gal, MD.)*

MANAGEMENT

Mechanical abnormalities in the lung parenchyma caused by ALI require increased work of breathing in order to adequately ventilate. While noninvasive methods of oxygen delivery may temporarily eliminate hypoxemia, definitive management often requires invasive mechanical ventilation to correct hypoxemia. **Table 142-4** summarizes the management strategies that have been studied in ARDS.

TABLE 142-3 Differential Diagnosis of Diseases Causing Diffuse Airspace Pattern on Chest Radiography and Severe Hypoxemia

Infectious

Pneumocystis jiroveci pneumonia

Viral pneumonitis

Severe community-acquired or nosocomial pneumonia

Noninfectious

Hydrostatic pulmonary edema: heart failure or other volume overload state

Aspiration pneumonitis

Acute interstitial pneumonia (Hamman-Rich syndrome)

Diffuse alveolar hemorrhage

Acute eosinophilic pneumonia

Lymphangitic spread of cancer or leukemic infiltration

Acute onset of cryptogenic organizing pneumonia

Drug toxicity (eg, amiodarone, methotrexate, bleomycin)

Immunologic (eg, lupus pneumonitis, Goodpasture disease, granulomatosis with polyangiitis)

Hypersensitivity pneumonitis

■ MECHANICAL VENTILATION STRATEGIES

Application of mechanical ventilation allows decreased work of breathing by off-loading respiratory muscles and improving effective minute ventilation. As the work of breathing decreases, CO_2 production is decreased and overall acid-base status is improved. The poor lung compliance and heterogeneity of ARDS, however, places the lung in a position of vulnerability from the positive pressure generated by the ventilator. Atelectatic segments, especially those in an area of transition near normal lung, are especially susceptible to overstretching during the inspiratory phase of respiration. The abnormalities in surfactant physiology characterizing ARDS lead to excessive closure of some alveoli during expiration. Repeated closure and over distention leads to additional alveolar damage, a phenomenon known as ventilator-induced lung injury.

Strides in improving overall survival from ARDS were realized by using low tidal volume ventilation in a lung-protective strategy. In 2000 the ARDS Network, a consortium of academic centers in the United States funded by the National Institutes of Health (NIH), reported an 8.8% absolute reduction in mortality when using 6 cc/kg target tidal volume compared with the standard target tidal volume (12 cc/kg). The investigation employed aggressive management of acid-base derangements and used a standardized protocol for the application of positive end-expiratory pressure (PEEP) for a given FiO_2. A follow-up study published in 2004 examined a higher PEEP/FiO_2 strategy in comparison to the use of low tidal volume ventilation that was used in the ARDS Network study of 2000. While there was no mortality difference between the two treatment arms, the mortality was similar to the earlier trial.

A hypothesis-generating paper from early 2015 challenges the concept that low tidal volume ventilation may be the best strategy for all patients with ARDS. The authors reviewed 3562 patients with ARDS from nine previous randomized trials. By employing a statistical method known as multilevel mediation analysis, they were able to isolate the effect of "driving pressure" on survival compared to tidal volume and PEEP. Driving pressure (ΔP) is the ratio of tidal

TABLE 142-4 Summary of Management Strategies for Acute Respiratory Distress Syndrome

Management Strategy	Effect	Reference
Low-tidal volume ventilation	Reduced mortality, shortened duration of mechanical ventilation	NHLBI ARDS Clinical Trials Network. Ventilation with lower tidal volumes as compared with traditional tidal volumes for acute lung injury and the acute respiratory distress syndrome. *N Engl J Med.* 2000;342:1301-1308.
Fluid restriction and/or diuretics	Reduced duration of mechanical ventilation	NHLBI ARDS Clinical Trials Network. Comparison of two fluid-management strategies in acute lung injury. *N Engl J Med.* 2006;354:2564-2575.
Corticosteroids	Reduced duration of mechanical ventilation and shock, improved oxygenation and respiratory-system compliance. Higher rates of neuromuscular weakness and increased mortality at 60 and 180 days if treated >14 days after ARDS onset of ARDS	NHLBI ARDS Clinical Trials Network. Efficacy and safety of corticosteroids for persistent acute respiratory distress syndrome. *N Engl J Med.* 2006;354:1671-1684.
Inhaled nitric oxide	Improved oxygenation; no impact on the duration of mechanical ventilation or survival	Taylor RW, et al. Low-dose inhaled nitric oxide in patients with acute lung injury: a randomized controlled trial. *JAMA.* 2004;291(13):1603-1609. Griffiths MJ, Evans TW. Inhaled nitric oxide therapy in adults. *N Engl J Med.* 2005;353:2683-2695.
Albumin and diuretics	Improved oxygenation and hemodynamics; no impact on the duration of mechanical ventilation or survival	Martin GS, et al. Albumin and furosemide therapy in hypoproteinemic patients with acute lung injury. *Crit Care Med.* 2002;30:2175-2182. Martin GS, et al. A randomized, controlled trial of furosemide with or without albumin in hypoproteinemic patients with acute lung injury. *Crit Care Med.* 2005;33:1681-1687.
Surfactant	No impact on duration of mechanical ventilation or survival	Spragg RG, et al. Effect of recombinant surfactant protein C-based surfactant on the acute respiratory distress syndrome. *N Engl J Med.* 2004;351:884-892.
Beta-agonists	Smaller trials suggested improvement in extravascular lung water; subsequent large clinical trials stopped early due to possible harmful effect in treatment group	Gao Smith F, et al. Effect of intravenous β-2 agonist treatment on clinical outcomes in acute respiratory distress syndrome (BALTI-2): a multicenter, randomized controlled trial. *Lancet.* 2012;379:229-235. NHLBI ARDS Clinical Trials Network. Randomized, placebo-controlled clinical trial of an aerosolized b2-agonist for treatment of acute lung injury. *Am J Respir Crit Care Med.* 2011;184:561-568.
Prone positioning	Early application in an experienced ICU for at least 16 h per day may improve mortality	Guérin C, et al. Prone positioning in severe acute respiratory distress syndrome. *N Engl J Med.* 2013;368:2159-2168.
Recruitment maneuvers	Potential improvements in oxygenation; possibly reduced duration of mechanical ventilation and other organ dysfunction	Meade MO, et al. Ventilation strategy using low tidal volumes, recruitment maneuvers, and high positive end-expiratory pressure for acute lung injury and acute respiratory distress syndrome: A randomized controlled trial. *JAMA.* 2008;299:637-645. Mercat A, et al. Positive end-expiratory pressure setting in adults with acute lung injury and acute respiratory distress syndrome: A randomized controlled trial. *JAMA.* 2008;299:646-655.
High-frequency oscillatory ventilation	Survival not improved in two randomized clinical trials	Ferguson ND, et al. High-frequency oscillation in early acute respiratory distress syndrome. *N Engl J Med.* 2013;368:795-805. Young D, et al. High-frequency oscillation for acute respiratory distress syndrome. *N Engl J Med.* 2013;368:806-813.
Extracorporeal membrane oxygenation	An experienced center with ECMO capabilities may improve 6-m survival; 24% of patients in ECMO group did not need ECMO	Peek GJ, et al. Efficacy and economic assessment of conventional ventilator support versus extracorporeal membrane oxygenation for severe adult respiratory failure (CESAR): a multicentre randomised controlled trial. *Lancet.* 2009;374:1351-1363.
Neuromuscular blocking agents	Early neuromuscular blockade for 48 h may improve mortality at 90 d, perhaps via improved patient-ventilator synchrony. ICU-acquired paresis was not increased	Papazian L, et al. Neuromuscular blockers in early acute respiratory distress syndrome. *N Engl J Med.* 2010;363:1107-1116.

volume (V_T) to respiratory-system compliance (C_{RS}), which uses the functional V_T as opposed to the predicted tidal volume for the patient's size ($\Delta P = V_T/C_{RS}$). By examining this variable, the study authors were able to take into account the severity of the patient's lung disease and its effect on the respiratory system as a predictor of survival. They reported that ΔP was most strongly associated with survival, more so than V_T or PEEP, even in patients receiving low tidal volume ventilation. This suggests that simply limiting tidal volumes or optimizing PEEP, without considering the pressure changes (as opposed to the associated static plateau pressure), may not provide optimal care for every ARDS patient. Airway pressure, measured as driving pressure (ΔP), is more important than tidal volume itself, and delivery of low tidal volume ventilation is most likely to improve outcomes when it results in small changes in ΔP. The standard of care remains the delivery of lung protective/low tidal volume ventilation for patients with ARDS, and this study helps us to individualize and prioritize ventilator settings.

Beyond low tidal volume strategies, novel or alternative methods of mechanical ventilation have long been an area of interest as to how and when to integrate them in patient management. New publications in the last 5 years have added important knowledge to this field, but applicability remains uncertain.

Administering mechanical ventilatory support in the prone position is known to confer improvement in respiratory mechanics that should be advantageous to ARDS patients. Clinical trials, however, have been inconsistent in improving outcomes. Most recently, a multicenter study from France and Spain enrolled 474 patients with ARDS, randomized to usual care versus prone ventilation for at least 16 hours per day. Mortality at 28 days was significantly better in the prone group without an increase in complications such as unplanned extubations. Comfort with this methodology is important, as all centers involved were very experienced in prone ventilation prior to the trial. Applicability of this study should take into account the competency level of the ICU staff with this technique. Whether prone ventilation becomes a true first-line therapy for ARDS management is not yet clear.

High-frequency oscillatory ventilation (HFOV) is a more advanced ventilator mode that employs very high respiratory rates with very small tidal volumes. The technology allows for maximal alveolar recruitment but with a lower risk of over distention because of the smaller tidal volumes delivered. Because of the high frequency, gas exchange is adequate despite the small volumes. Prior to 2013 small clinical trials suggested that HFOV may be helpful if applied early, but wide variability in ventilator management and patient population warranted larger, randomized clinical trials. Enthusiasm for this mode of ventilation for *routine* treatment of ARDS has waned following two publications in 2013. In two independent studies, over 1300 patients were randomized with ARDS to receive early HFOV or conventional ventilation management. Hypoxemia at enrollment in both trials was significant, $PaO_2/FiO_2 < 150$ on average. Each study varied in the ventilator protocols and in the severity of illness in their subjects. But, neither trial demonstrated an improvement in mortality, and one trial was stopped early due to worse survival in the HFOV group. At least for now, HFOV would seem to have a role only as a possible rescue therapy from conventional ventilation in a patient with refractory hypoxemia.

Other advanced modes of ventilation, such as adaptive support ventilation (ASV) or airway pressure-release ventilation (APRV), are becoming more prominent as ventilator technology advances. In ASV a target percentage minute ventilation is set. Using a closed loop algorithm, the ventilator delivers an appropriate frequency and tidal volume combination based on its determination of the lung's mechanics. Spontaneous breaths are delivered with either pressure support or in a pressure-controlled manner, the amount of which is determined by the ventilator. APRV, like HFOV, employs a stable distending pressure, but with a periodic decrease in pressure—the "release"—for CO_2 removal. The patient can breathe spontaneously above the distended pressure. Neither of the modes has been extensively studied in well-designed clinical trials of ARDS.

NONVENTILATORY STRATEGIES

The management of ARDS entails more than attention to proper ventilatory support, particularly as it relates to fluid status. In a trial published by the ARDS Network investigators in 2006, a conservative fluid management strategy reduced the number of days of ventilator support and ICU stay without causing nonpulmonary organ dysfunction. The same study found that use of a pulmonary artery catheter to direct fluid management was not superior to central venous catheter use, and resulted in more cardiac arrhythmias.

Based on the pathophysiological mechanisms in ARDS, multiple targets for pharmacotherapy have been identified. Despite numerous trials of various therapies, no definitive agent has shown a benefit in clinically important outcomes. These include surfactant therapy, inhaled nitric oxide, lisofylline, ketoconazole, phosphodiesterase inhibitors, activated protein C, and many others.

Corticosteroids have been studied extensively in differing doses and timing, yet no trial has yet defined a clear benefit in patients with ARDS. The best trial to date reported improvements in lung and cardiovascular physiology and a shortened duration of mechanical ventilation; however, mortality did not improve and steroid administration was associated with neuromyopathy.

Extracorporeal membrane oxygenation (ECMO) has the advantage of supporting hypoxemia without the potentially injurious ventilator settings sometimes needed in severe ARDS. In the CESAR trial, 180 patients were randomized to conventional ventilation versus referral to an ECMO center for management. Mortality was better in the ECMO group at 6 months, and at least in the UK, appeared to be cost effective in terms of quality-adjusted life-years. Much like prone ventilation and HFOV, center experience must be taken into account in interpreting this study. If ECMO is considered, transfer to a skilled facility should be initiated. Not every patient transferred to the ECMO site underwent ECMO (22 of 90 patients randomized to ECMO did not receive ECMO). Thus, some of the positive results may reflect that centers comfortable with ECMO may also be expert in general ARDS management. As with prone ventilation, ECMO's place in the ARDS treatment algorithm is not certain.

The underlying source of the patient's ARDS must always be addressed. Preventive measures should be employed to prevent ICU-related complications. This includes appropriate prophylaxis against stress ulcers bleeding and deep venous thrombosis, raising the head of the bed at least 30° to guard against ventilator-associated pneumonia, and daily screening for readiness-to-liberate from the ventilator in conjunction with daily interruption of all sedative and analgesic infusions. Clinicians should minimize procedures to those deemed absolutely necessary.

CONSULTATIONS

Clinicians with special expertise in critical care medicine and/or management of mechanical ventilation should be involved in the care of patients with ARDS. Transfer to a tertiary or quaternary medical center with expertise in advanced ARDS management (ECMO experience, for example) may be necessary. Most patients die of multisystem organ failure and nosocomial infection. Appropriate consultation of multiple services may be required to optimize care. Studies of physical and occupational therapy suggest that starting these therapies in the ICU, even in patients still requiring mechanical ventilatory support, leads to quicker and better functional recovery months after discharge.

PROGNOSIS AND COMPLICATIONS

■ PREDICTORS

The Berlin definition of ARDS stratifies severity based on degree of hypoxemia, because as stated above, it is the best predictor of outcome in the era of more standardization of ventilator techniques. Another important prognostic predictor regarding oxygen requirements is the time to recovery. Patients not demonstrating lower oxygen requirements by day 7 of presentation have a more protracted ICU course, are at increased risk for long-term ventilator dependency, and face a longer recovery to regain strength and conditioning should they survive to hospital discharge. Additional factors, such as increasing age, length-of-stay, net positive volume status, and sepsis as the predisposition to ARDS are also predictors of higher morbidity and mortality.

PRACTICE POINT

Management strategies:

- Low tidal volumes: 8.8% absolute reduction in mortality (NNT = 11) when using 6 cc/kg target tidal volume in ARDS compared with the common standard of 12 cc/kg.
- Prone ventilation: Early application of prone ventilation for at least 16 hours per day may decrease 28- and 90-day mortality, based on a trial performed in experienced centers.
- Fluid management: Conservative fluid management strategy, compared to aggressive fluid resuscitation, reduces ventilator days and ICU length of stay.
- Cardiopulmonary monitoring: Pulmonary artery catheter-directed fluid management does not improve outcomes compared to central venous catheter directed management, and results in more arrhythmias.
- Corticosteroids: After extensive study, no trial data has delineated a clear benefit of steroids in ARDS patients.

■ SURVIVAL

Studies differ in regard to the current trend in ARDS mortality. Disparity exists in trends between academic and community medical centers, as mortality has improved in the last 10 to 15 years in the former but perhaps not the latter. Analyzing pooled mortality over time in retrospective literature reviews demonstrates a *mortality rate of 35% to 50%*. Consensus is lacking on whether this number is truly static or decreasing on an annual basis, and it further depends on the patient population investigated and the site in which the investigation occurred. As an example, there has been an improvement in mortality from 35% to 26% in the last 15 years in patients enrolled in studies as part of the ARDS Network. This trend may not be widely generalizable.

Any reduction in mortality may be due to overall improvement in ICU care over time in addition to the administration of low tidal volume ventilation. In the ARDS Network mortality analysis, the mortality improvement trend persisted after adjusting the statistical

model for low tidal volume ventilation and other clinical covariates. Simple interventions such as daily ventilator liberation screening, proper oral care, venous thromboembolic disease prophylaxis, and other routine applications have likely made a significant impact on ARDS survival.

■ COMPLICATIONS

Patients who survive ARDS have surprisingly few respiratory system sequelae at 1 and 2 years after hospital discharge. A review of 1-year ARDS survivors found that none of the patients were requiring oxygen supplementation and their lung function testing, with the exception of low diffusion capacity, had returned to normal (see **Table 142-5**). Most frequently patients experienced functional limitation caused primarily by muscle weakness and fatigue. Corticosteroid administration and prolonged duration of respiratory failure are associated with more functional sequelae in these ARDS survivors.

Inability to perform functionally at premorbid levels adversely impacts patients' overall sense of well-being after going home. Their health-related quality of life is self-rated as lower than normal, a finding that is still present at 2 years from discharge. Half of survivors at 2 years report significant anxiety and depression not present prior to their critical illness. They also perform poorly on standardized neurocognitive tests, especially those assessing memory, attentiveness, and executive function (such as planning or abstract thinking).

DISCHARGE PLANNING

Patients who survive to ICU and hospital discharge have functionally limiting deficits. Early planning for referral to a physical rehabilitation facility is often indicated.

PRACTICE POINT

- The degree of hypoxemia is a good predictor of outcome, worsening with the degree of ARDS (mild, moderate, and severe oxygenation categories in the Berlin definition).
- Physical and occupational therapy initiation in the ICU—even in patients still requiring mechanical ventilatory support—leads to quicker and better functional recovery months after discharge.

For patients who do not recover quickly from ARDS or who require prolonged mechanical ventilation, the rehabilitation phase will likely involve some time in a long-term acute care (LTAC) facility. LTACs—health care facilities that provide lower intensity acute inpatient care—permit a smoother transition to physical rehabilitation while still providing a higher level of care in patients who are near ventilator liberation or have a tracheostomy in place. The ultimate goal of complete liberation from the ventilator and decannulation of the tracheostomy tube may be accomplished in parallel with physical, occupational, and speech/swallowing therapies. The transfer to a long-term acute care facility can be difficult on families as they adjust to a less intensive level of care as their loved ones recover. Hospitals make use of liaisons between the two facilities to make this transition easier (see Chapter 68 [Rehabilitation Options]).

TABLE 142-5 Evidence-based Medicine: Key References for Acute Respiratory Distress Syndrome

Study Title/Reference	Methodology	Results	Limitations	Bottom Line
NHLBI ARDS Clinical Trials Network. *N Engl J Med.* 2000;342:1301-1308.	Randomized, double-blind trial of 6 vs 12 cc/kg predicted body weight tidal volume for ventilation in ARDS	861 patients enrolled; 8.8% absolute reduction in mortality and 2 additional days free of mechanical ventilation in low tidal volume ventilation group	High tidal volume in control group may not represent standard practice	Low-tidal volume ventilation with increased PEEP at higher inspired oxygen levels and aggressive pH management improves mortality
Rubenfeld GD, et al. *N Engl J Med.* 2005;353:1685-1693.	Prospective, population-based, cohort study to identify incidence and outcomes of acute lung injury	Incidence of ALI was 79.8 per 100,000 person-years, with a mortality of 38.5%, estimated US deaths 74,500 per year	Single-region cohort (Pacific Northwest); demographics may differ in other regions; relied on medical and public health records for data—some cases may have been misclassified	Incidence of ALI in the US may be higher than expected and carries a substantial burden on public health
Herridge MS, et al. *N Engl J Med.* 2003;348:683-693.	Longitudinal, prospective cohort study; 109 survivors of ARDS followed to assess pulmonary and nonpulmonary function at 1 y after ICU discharge	Except DLCO, lung function normal at 6 mo no oxygen requirements; patients reported functional limitation, primarily due to muscle weakness and fatigue	Small number of patients followed; no control group (non-ARDS ICU survivors)	ARDS survivors have persistent functional disability, more due to weakness than pulmonary dysfunction 1 y after ICU discharge
NHLBI ARDS Clinical Trials Network. *N Engl J Med.* 2006;354:2564-2575.	Prospective, randomized study of conservative vs liberal fluid management in patients with early acute lung injury	1000 patients; no difference in 60-d mortality; conservative-strategy cohort had 2.5 more days alive and free of mechanical ventilation and shorter ICU length of stay; organ failures not increased	Strategy to guide fluid management may be challenging to apply in clinical practice	In hemodynamically stable patients with acute lung injury, targeting a central venous pressure of <4 mm Hg improves time off the ventilator and in the ICU without an increase in organ failure
Amato MPB, et al. *N Engl J Med.* 2015;372:747-755.	Multilevel mediation analysis of ARDS patients enrolled in prior randomized trials; assess the importance of respiratory system variables (V_t, PEEP, driving pressure) in ARDS survival	3562 patients analyzed; driving pressure (V_t/C_{RS}) independently associated with survival when isolated from tidal volume or PEEP settings. Low tidal volume specifically did not improve survival if not also associated with reduction in driving pressure	Study was retrospective analysis. Whether prospectively controlling driving pressure as an intervention is unknown	Driving pressure, even in the face of low tidal volume for predicted body weight, may be more important in ventilator-induced lung injury. May lead to future prospective studies to determine whether controlling driving pressure or tidal volume is most important

SUGGESTED READINGS

The ARDS Definition Task Force. Acute respiratory distress syndrome: the Berlin definition. *JAMA.* 2012;307:2526-2533.

Briel M, Meade M, Mercat A, et al. Higher vs lower positive end-expiratory pressure in patients with acute lung injury and acute respiratory distress syndrome: systematic review and meta-analysis. *JAMA.* 2010;303:865-873.

Marcelo BP, Amato MD, Meade MO. Driving pressure and survival in the acute respiratory distress syndrome. *N Engl J Med.* 2015;372:747-755.

Martin GS. The role of invasive monitoring in acute lung injury. *Semin Respir Crit Care Med.* 2013;34:508-515.

Neamu RF, Martin GS. Fluid management in acute respiratory distress syndrome. *Curr Opin Crit Care.* 2013;19(1):24-30.

NHLBI ARDS Clinical Trials Network. Comparison of two fluid-management strategies in acute lung injury. *N Engl J Med.* 2006;354:2564-2575.

NHLBI ARDS Clinical Trials Network. Efficacy and safety of corticosteroids for persistent acute respiratory distress syndrome. *N Engl J Med.* 2006;354:1671-1684.

NHLBI ARDS Clinical Trials Network. Ventilation with lower tidal volumes as compared with traditional tidal volumes for acute lung injury and the acute respiratory distress syndrome. *N Engl J Med.* 2000;342:1301-1308.

Putensen C, Theuerkauf N, Zinserling J, et al. Meta-analysis: ventilation strategies and outcomes of the acute respiratory distress syndrome and acute lung injury. *Ann Intern Med.* 2009;151:566-576.

CHAPTER 143

Prevention in the Intensive Care Unit Setting

Nishay Chitkara, MD

INTRODUCTION

Critical illness places patients at high risk for iatrogenic complications during hospitalization. Invasive monitoring devices, mechanical ventilatory support, immobility, and debility increase susceptibility to these complications. Previously considered unavoidable consequences of critical illness, many ICU-related complications may be prevented.

The Institute for Health Care Improvement (IHI) and other national organizations have advocated the adoption of a series of "bundles" with the goal of reducing the rate of complications in the ICU. Bundles aggregate evidence-based practices relevant to a diagnosis or procedure into a single intervention. The rationale for the use of bundles is that, when their elements are reliably applied together, they allow more uniform application of best practices and, thus, improve patient outcomes. Bundles represent one of many tools needed to prevent ICU-related complications (**Table 143-1**).

For each preventable ICU complication, this chapter will address epidemiology, strategies for prevention, and goals of care. Members of the critical care team should incorporate a worksheet for daily goals of care to ensure that the essential elements of preventive care are implemented in the ICU.

COMMON COMPLICATIONS

■ CENTRAL LINE-ASSOCIATED BLOOD STREAM INFECTIONS

Central line-associated blood stream infections (CLABSIs) cause significant morbidity and mortality in the ICU, increased length of stay and cost. Primary blood stream infections are most often related to infected intravascular devices, mostly central venous catheters. At least 80,000 new cases of CLABSIs occur in the ICU each year in the United States. Extra costs due to bloodstream infections among survivors averaged greater than $40,000 per patient.

Hospital-acquired infection rates now serve as a publicly reported quality indicator. Many states in the United States currently require mandatory reporting of CLABSIs to the centers for disease control and prevention (CDC), and some states have made hospital-specific data publicly available. These publicly reported infection rates are based on the National Health Care Safety Network (NHSN) surveillance definition (**Table 143-2**). As of October 1, 2008, the Centers for Medicare and Medicaid Services (CMS) no longer reimburse hospitals for costs associated with some hospital-acquired conditions, including CLABSIs.

The organisms most commonly causing BSIs include coagulase-negative *staphylococci* (31%), *Staphylococcus aureus* (20%), *Enterococcus* species (9%), *Candida* species (9%), and *Escherichia coli* (6%) (**Table 143-3**). Increased usage of intravascular catheters and the selection pressure created by broad spectrum antibiotic use has caused the emergence of coagulase-negative staphylococcal infections and *Candida* species as virulent organisms.

A number of intrinsic host factors including malnutrition, burns, loss of skin integrity, neutropenia, extremes of age, severity of underlying illness, and immunosuppression have increased susceptibility to CLABSIs. The single most important extrinsic factor related to development of primary BSIs is the catheter itself. Peripheral intravenous catheters have the lowest associated rate of infection (0.5 per 1000 catheter days), while pulmonary artery catheters have the highest rates of CLABSIs (3.7 per 1000 catheter days), followed by

TABLE 143-1 Components of the Institute for Health Care Improvement Central Line and Ventilator Bundles

IHI Central Line Bundle*	IHI Ventilator Bundle†
1. Hand hygiene	1. Elevation of the head of bed (to between 30° and 45°)
2. Maximal barrier precautions	2. Daily interruption of sedation and assessment of readiness to extubate
3. Chlorhexidine skin antisepsis	
4. Optimal catheter site selection, with avoidance of the femoral vein for central venous access in adult patients	3. Prophylaxis for peptic ulcer disease
5. Daily review of line necessity, with prompt removal of unnecessary lines	4. Prophylaxis for deep venous thrombosis
	5. Daily oral care with chlorhexidine

*5 Million Lives Campaign. *Getting Started Kit: Prevent Central Line Infections How-to Guide.* Cambridge, MA: Institute for Healthcare Improvement; 2008 (available at www.ihi.org).
†5 Million Lives Campaign. *Getting Started Kit: Prevent Ventilator-Associated Pneumonia How-to Guide.* Cambridge, MA: Institute for Healthcare Improvement; 2010 (available at http://www.ihi.org).

TABLE 143-2 National Health Care Safety Network Surveillance Definition of Central-Line-Associated Bloodstream Infection

Laboratory-confirmed bloodstream infection requires one of the following criteria:

1. A recognized pathogen cultured from one or more blood cultures; the organism is not related to an infection at another site

2. The patient has at least one of the following signs or symptoms: fever (>38°C), chills, or hypotension and signs and symptoms and positive laboratory results are not related to infection at another site

3. Organisms considered to be usual skin contaminants require that the patient have fever, chills, or hypotension, as well as one of the following: (1) the common skin contaminant is isolated from two blood cultures drawn on separate occasions, and the organism is not related to infection at another site, or (2) the common skin contaminant is isolated from a single blood culture in a patient with an intravascular access device and appropriate antibiotic therapy is instituted

4. A patient <12 mo of age has one of the following: fever (>38°C), hypothermia (<37°C), apnea, bradycardia, as well as one of the above organism criteria

Clinical sepsis is defined by either of the following criteria:

1. One of the following clinical signs or symptoms with no other recognized cause: fever (>38°C), hypotension (systolic pressure <90 mm Hg), oliguria (<20 mL/h). ALSO, blood culture is not done or no organism or antigen is detected in blood, and there is no apparent infection at another site.

2. The patient is <12 mo of age with one of the following signs or symptoms and no other recognized cause: fever (>38°C); hypothermia (<37°C); apnea; bradycardia and the following conditions all apply: blood culture is not done or no organism or antigen is detected in blood; there is no apparent infection at another site.

TABLE 143-3 Most Common Pathogens Isolated from Nosocomial Bloodstream Infections

	Percentage of BSIs	
Pathogen	Total	ICU
Coagulase-negative staphylococci	31.3	35.9
Staphyloccocus aureus	20.2	16.8
Enterococcus species	9.4	9.8
Candida species	9.0	10.1
Escherichia coli	5.6	3.7
Klebsiella species	4.8	4.0
Enterobacter species	4.3	4.7
Pseudomonas aeruginosa	3.9	4.7
Acinetobacter baumanii	1.7	2.1
Serratia species	1.3	1.6

central venous catheters (2.7 per 1000 catheter days for nonmedicated, nontunneled central venous catheters).

Some of the most effective measures to reduce CLABSIs include (1) appropriate site selection for the catheter (subclavian venous site or if not available, internal jugular site), (2) use of proper skin antiseptic agents (chlorhexidine rather than iodine-based antiseptic solutions), (3) use of maximal sterile barrier precautions during the procedure (**Table 143-4**), (4) early central catheter removal when no longer needed, and (5) use of antimicrobial-impregnated catheters. Table 143-1 summarizes the elements of the IHI's central line bundle for reduction of CLABSIs. The insertion of catheters into the subclavian vein has been associated with a significantly lower rate of infection compared to the femoral vein in a randomized controlled trial. Observational data suggest that the subclavian site is also associated with a lower risk of infection than the internal jugular site. However, a recent meta-analysis of two randomized controlled trials and eight cohort studies found no difference in the rate of CLABSIs among the three sites. The subclavian site may be associated with higher rates of mechanical complications, such as bleeding and pneumothorax, or subclavian stenosis in patients with advanced kidney disease. The femoral site has been associated with an increased risk of thrombotic complications. Decisions regarding site selection for CVC insertion should take into account the clinical circumstances of the individual patient.

Skin antisepsis at the catheter insertion site should be performed with 2% aqueous *chlorhexidine* gluconate. Tincture of iodine, an iodophor, or 70% alcohol may be used as alternatives if chlorhexidine is contraindicated, but is less effective than chlorhexidine in infection prevention. Maximal sterile-barrier precautions should always be used during catheter insertion (Table 143-4).

TABLE 143-4 Maximal Sterile Barrier Precautions during Central Venous Catheter Insertion

1. Persons placing the central venous catheter should wear a cap, mask, sterile gown, and sterile gloves

2. A large sterile drape should cover the patient from head to toe, with an opening at the site of insertion

3. A sterile sleeve should be used to protect pulmonary artery catheters during insertion

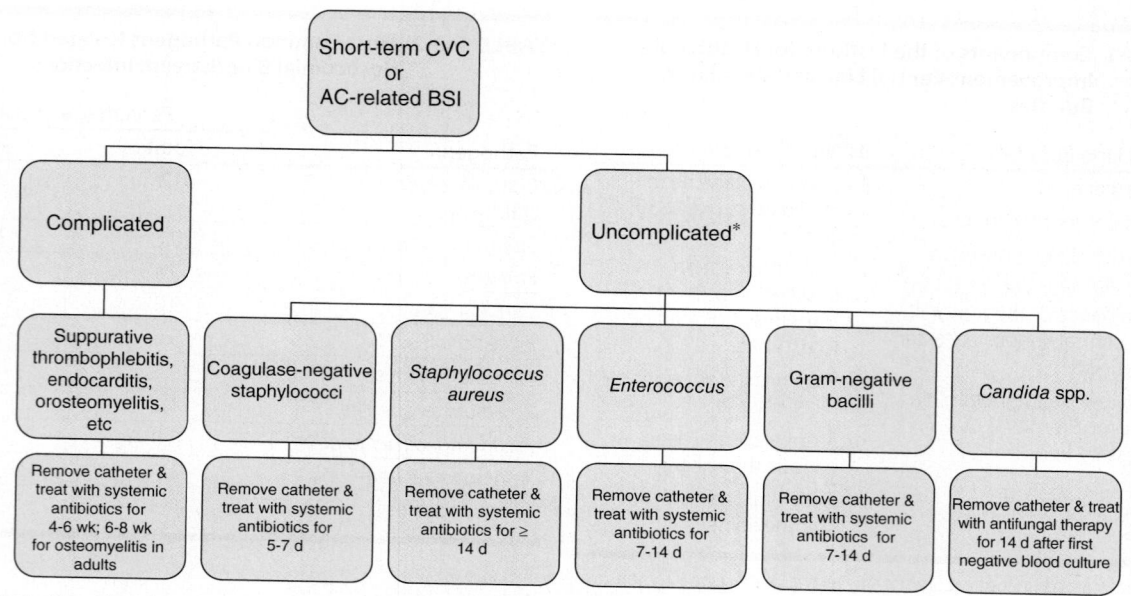

Figure 143-1 *Algorithm for management of patients with short-term CVC-related or arterial-catheter-related blood stream infection. AC, arterial catheter; BSI, blood stream infection; CVC, central venous catheter. *Uncomplicated BSI: resolution of BSI within 72 hours; no intravascular hardware; no evidence of endocarditis, suppurative thrombophlebitis, or S. aureus infection; no active malignancy; and no immunosuppression.*

The use of antimicrobial-impregnated catheters significantly reduced the rate of CLABSIs and reduced overall medical costs in randomized clinical trials. Three such types of catheters are currently available: chlorhexidine and silver sulfadiazine impregnated, platinum and silver impregnated, and minocycline and rifampin impregnated. Centers for disease control and prevention guidelines recommend the following; (1) use of an antimicrobial- or antiseptic-impregnated central venous catheter (CVC) in adults whose catheter is expected to remain in place more than five days if an institution's rate of CLABSI remains high, or above the institutional goal, despite education of staff who insert and maintain catheters; (2) use of maximal sterile barrier precautions; (3) and use of 2% chlorhexidine preparation for skin antisepsis during CVC insertion.

Central venous catheters should be removed promptly when they are no longer needed or when a peripheral IV can be reasonably inserted and serve the same function as the CVC. Maintaining a CVC when it is not absolutely necessary increases the risk of bacterial colonization and subsequent CLABSIs over time. Routine catheter changes do not reduce the risk of CLABSIs, and routine guidewire catheter exchanges may actually increase the rate of infections. Therefore, routine or scheduled CVC changes should not be performed. Rather, catheters should be changed only when concern arises for infection or catheter malfunction. If a catheter infection is suspected and a CVC is still needed, a new catheter should be placed at a different insertion site. Antibiotic ointments promote emergence of antibiotic-resistant bacteria when applied to catheter-insertion sites and therefore should be avoided.

Clinical manifestations of CLABSIs are often limited to fever, but more specifically can include inflammation or purulence at the site of catheter insertion and bacteremia with no apparent source. The diagnosis of CLABSIs requires microbiological data to fulfill the CDC criteria for a laboratory-confirmed bloodstream infection (LCBI).

When a CLABSI is suspected in a patient with fever and a CVC in place, the possibility of bacteremia should be evaluated with two cultures of blood from peripheral sites. A positive blood culture from the central venous catheter does not differentiate catheter colonization or hub contamination from a true CLABSI. A negative blood

culture from the catheter makes a CLABSI unlikely. When diagnosis of a CLABSI is highly suspected or confirmed—either clinically or microbiologically—the catheter should be removed immediately and antibiotics should be rapidly initiated. When the organism is identified antibiotics should be tailored to the sensitivity of the organisms grown in culture (**Figure 143-1**).

■ VENTILATOR-ASSOCIATED PNEUMONIA

Ventilator-associated pneumonia (VAP) is commonly considered a subtype of hospital-acquired pneumonia, which develops in mechanically ventilated patients more than 48 to 72 hours after endotracheal intubation. It is an important nosocomial infection, which has more recently become a subset of the broader category of ventilator-associated events (VAE). Incidence estimates range from 9% to 27% of mechanically ventilated patients, and the development of VAP is associated with increased mortality, increased ICU and hospital length of stay, and increased cost. Common pathogens include *Staphylococcus aureus, Klebsiella pneumoniae, Pseudomonas aeruginosa, Escherichia coli, Enterobacter species*, and *Acinetobacter* species. The diagnosis of VAP should be considered in mechanically ventilated patients with fever, change in respiratory secretions, leukocytosis, or change in oxygen requirements; and with a new or persistent infiltrate on chest radiography. A lower respiratory tract sample should be obtained for culture when VAP is suspected, prior to the initiation of antibiotics. Samples may be obtained bronchoscopically or nonbronchoscopically. Bronchoscopically obtained cultures may lead to narrower-spectrum antibiotic coverage and more frequent deescalation of therapy, but have not been convincingly shown to decrease mortality. As bronchoscopy may not always be available at all hospitals, initiation of antibiotics should not be delayed and a sample from an endotracheal aspirate or mini-bronchoalveolar lavage should be sent.

Multiple interventions can reduce the incidence of VAP, as demonstrated in well-designed trials. The IHI recommends the routine use of the IHI ventilator bundle (see Table 143-1) for the care of all mechanically ventilated patients. Elements of the IHI ventilator

TABLE 143-5 Strategies for the Prevention of Ventilator-Associated Pneumonia

Head-of-bed elevation	Elevation of the head of the bed to at least 30°-45° decreases the risk of aspiration of gastric contents compared to the supine position. A single RCT demonstrated a decrease in VAP incidence in patients managed in the semirecumbent position.
Subglottic suction	Continuous aspiration of subglottic secretions may decrease aspiration and risk of VAP. Studies have suggested that endotracheal tubes designed to permit continuous subglotttic suction are most effective in patients who are intubated for greater than 72 h.
Silver-coated endotracheal tubes	Silver-coated endotracheal tubes may reduce bacterial colonization and biofilm formation. A large RCT published in 2008 demonstrated an absolute risk reduction of 2.7% (NNT = 37) and a relative risk reduction of VAP of 35.9% for patients intubated longer than 24 h. There was also a delayed time to occurrence of VAP with silver-coated endotracheal tubes.
Oral care	Decontamination of the oropharynx may decrease the burden of microbes that are aspirated. Use of chlorhexidine for oral decontamination has been demonstrated to decrease the risk of VAP in patients after cardiac surgery and in patients intubated greater than 24 h, but does not impact mortality. A single large RCT using a combination of tobramycin, colistin, and amphotericin B for oral decontamination found a decrease in the risk of VAP and a reduction in the odds ratio of death (0.86 (95% CI 0.74-0.99), NNT = 35).
Selective digestive tract decontamination	Selective digestive tract decontamination typically refers to topical (oropharyngeal or through a nasogastric tube) administration of a combination of nonabsorbable antibiotics and antifungals, sometimes in combination with intravenous therapy to reduce oropharyngeal and gastric colonization. A large RCT of SDD (topical application of tobramycin, colistin, and amphotericin B in the oropharynx and stomach every 6 h until ICU discharge, and intravenous cefotaxime for four days) demonstrated a modest decrease in mortality without any short-term increase in bacterial resistance. Some clinicians remain concerned about longer-term effects on bacterial resistance patterns.
Stress ulcer prophylaxis	Modification of gastric pH may decrease the risk of stress ulcer bleeding, but may increase the risk of VAP. One RCT demonstrated a lower incidence of VAP with less change in gastric pH in patients receiving sucralfate for stress ulcer prophylaxis compared to antacids or H2 receptor blockers. More recent data has suggested that use of PPI increases the risk of hospital-acquired pneumonia. H2 blockers and PPIs may be more effective at reducing the risk of stress ulcer bleeding than sucralfate, but may confer an increased risk of VAP. Selection of stress ulcer prophylaxis should consider all these factors as well as local cost.
Ventilator circuit changes	Currently the Center for Disease Control recommends changing ventilator circuits no more frequently than every 48 h while the American Association of Respiratory Care recommends against routine changes. More frequent changes are associated with increased risk of VAP.

H2, Histamine-2; NNT, number needed to treat; PPI, proton pump inhibitors; RCT, randomized controlled trial; SDD, Selective digestive tract decontamination; VAP, ventilator-associated pneumonia.

bundle include: head-of-bed elevation of 30 to 45 degrees, daily interruption of sedation, daily assessment of readiness to extubate, stress ulcer prophylaxis, and deep venous thrombosis prophylaxis. While the ventilator bundle does not specifically address VAP prevention and observational studies have reported mixed results as to the bundle's effect on VAP prevention, use of the ventilator bundle is recommended in the care of all mechanically ventilated patients. Strategies for the prevention of VAP may include subglottic suction, silver-coated endotracheal tubes, oral care, and limiting ventilator circuit changes (**Table 143-5**).

■ HOSPITAL-ACQUIRED VENOUS THROMBOEMBOLISM

Venous thromboembolism (VTE) is a significant cause of morbidity, preventable illness, and mortality in the ICU. Hospitalization is associated with approximately 25% of all cases of VTE, with a majority of cases occurring on medical services. In high-risk patients not receiving any prophylaxis, prospective studies have detected deep vein thrombosis in 10.5% to 14.9% of patients by venography, and in 5.0% of patients by ultrasonography. Pulmonary embolism occurred in 0.3% to 5.0% of these patients. One county-based study from 1980 to 1990 detected the age- and sex-adjusted incidence of VTE to be 130 times greater among hospitalized patients compared with community residents. Thrombosis may be asymptomatic in over 70% of cases. Pulmonary embolism is still the leading cause of preventable hospital death.

Admitting medical conditions associated with a high rate of VTE include acute infectious diseases, congestive heart failure, acute myocardial infarction, acute respiratory disease, stroke, acute renal injury, malignancy, and rheumatic disease. Sepsis and the systemic inflammatory response syndrome are associated with hypercoagulopathy. Clinical characteristics or past history increasing the risk for VTE include previous VTE, older age, recent surgery or trauma, immobility or paresis, obesity (body mass index [BMI] > 30), central venous catheterization, inherited thrombophilic states, varicose veins, estrogen therapy (oral contraceptives and hormone replacement), pregnancy, and active tobacco use (**Table 143-6**).

No formal, prospectively validated risk assessment models exist for determining the need for pharmacologic prophylaxis for medical patients. However, patients who will benefit from pharmacologic prophylaxis for VTE include those over 40 years of age, those having limited mobility for three days or more, and those possessing at least one thrombotic risk factor (see Table 143-6). Presence of multiple risk factors increases the risk (see Chapter 252 [Prevention of Venous Thromboembolism in Medical Patients]).

Pharmacologic prophylaxis, as provided with unfractionated heparins (UFH), low-molecular-weight heparins (LMWHs), or fondaparinux, is the preferred preventive therapy for VTE (**Table 143-7**). In various studies of hospitalized patients at high risk for VTE, LMWHs, low-dose unfractionated heparin, and fondaparinux

TABLE 143-6 Risk Factors for Venous Thromboembolism in Hospitalized Patients

Admitting Conditions	Clinical Characteristics
Acute infectious disease	Previous venous thromboembolism
Congestive heart failure (New York Heart Association Class III or IV disease)	Advanced age (particularly >75 y)
Acute myocardial infarction	Recent surgery (especially orthopedic) or trauma
Acute respiratory disease	
Stroke	Immobility or paresis
Rheumatic disease (ie, acute arthritis)	Obesity (body mass index >30)
Inflammatory bowel disease	Central venous catheterization
Malignancy	
Spinal cord injury	Inherited or acquired thrombophilic states
Pregnancy/peripartum	Varicose veins
Nephrotic syndrome	Estrogen therapy
Sepsis or septic shock	Mechanical ventilation

have each significantly reduced the rate of VTE. No mortality benefit has been shown, and data on rates of major bleeding with pharmacologic prophylaxis are inconsistent.

Nonpharmacologic prophylaxis should be implemented in patients with contraindications to pharmacologic prophylaxis, including those at high risk for bleeding, such as patients with active or recent gastrointestinal bleeding, those with hemorrhagic stroke, or those with defects of hemostasis (ie, severe thrombocytopenia). Currently, no data on the use of graduated compression stockings are available from large studies of hospitalized medical patients, but a Cochrane Systematic Review has shown them to be effective in reducing VTE in postoperative hospitalized patients by 50%. Intermittent pneumatic compression devices offer another option for nonpharmacologic prophylaxis, preventing venous stasis by enhancing blood flow in

TABLE 143-7 Prophylaxis for Venous Thromboembolism

Drug	Subcutaneous Dose
Pharmacologic options	
Unfractionated heparin	5000 U every 8 h
Low-molecular-weight heparins	
Dalteparin	5000 units once daily
Enoxaparin	40 mg once daily
Fondiparinux	2.5 mg once daily
Nonpharmacologic options*	
Ambulation	
Exercises involving foot extension	
Graduated compression stockings	
Pneumatic compression devices	

*Nonpharmacologic prophylaxis is recommended for patients at high risk for bleeding, including those with recent or active gastrointestinal bleeding, patients with hemorrhagic stroke, and patients with severe thrombocytopenia or other coagulopathic conditions.

the deep veins and reducing plasminogen activator inhibitor-1 (thus increasing endogenous fibrinolytic activity). A Cochrane Systematic Review has shown them to be effective in reducing the incidence of VTE, and even more so when used in combination with pharmacologic prophylaxis. Pneumatic compression devices should not be used in the setting of peripheral vascular disease.

Protocols that promote increased use of pharmacologic VTE prophylaxis in hospitalized patients, and particularly in ICU patients, may improve prophylaxis rates and reduce VTE events and complications. Educational programs, computer prompts reminding physicians to consider VTE prophylaxis, and computer programs identifying high-risk patients have all increased the use of prophylaxis by clinicians.

■ STRESS ULCER BLEEDING

Stress ulcer bleeding may lead to significant morbidity in at-risk hospitalized patients. In one large North American study, 1.5% of ICU patients developed clinically relevant overt bleeding due to stress ulceration. Postulated mechanisms include excessive acid secretion, mucosal ischemia, and impaired mucus production. Risk factors identified in the large Canadian cohort study included respiratory failure (mechanical ventilation >48 hours) and coagulopathy (INR > 1.5, PTT > 2 times the upper limit of normal, or platelet count < 50,000/μL). Patients with one or both of these risk factors had a 3.7% rate of clinically important bleeding, compared to 0.1% in patients without either risk factor. Other likely risk factors for stress ulcer bleeding include

- Burns, major trauma, head injury
- Sepsis, hypotension
- Mechanical ventilation, coagulopathy, acute renal failure

Histamine receptor-2 antagonists (H2 blockers) and proton pump inhibitors (PPI) increase gastric pH and have been shown to be equally effective at reducing the risk of overt gastrointestinal bleeding (**Table 143-8**). Some data suggest that these drugs,

TABLE 143-8 Pharmacologic Therapies for Stress Ulcer Prophylaxis*

Sucralfate suspension, 1 gram via nasogastric tube every 6 h

H2-receptor blockade†

   Cimetidine, continuous infusion (up to 50 mg/h IV) or bolus dose (up to 300 mg IV every 6 h)

   Ranitidine, bolus dose (50 mg IV every 8 h)

   Famotidine, bolus dose (20 mg IV twice daily)

Proton pump inhibitors†

   Omeprazole, bolus dose (40 mg orally or via nasogastric tube daily)

   Pantoprazole, bolus dose (40 mg orally, via nasogastric tube, or IV daily)

   Esomeprazole, bolus dose (40 mg orally, via nasogastric tube, or IV daily)

   Lansoprazole, bolus dose (30 mg orally or via nasogastric tube daily)

   Rabeprazole, bolus dose (20 mg orally daily)

*This table includes the most commonly used medications for stress ulcer prophylaxis. Due to numerous side effects, antacids are rarely used to prevent stress ulcers. Prostaglandin analogs (such as misoprostol) are not effective in preventing stress ulcer formation.

†IV preparations are unnecessary and costly unless patient is unable to tolerate enteral-route medication.

particularly PPIs, may increase the risk of hospital- or ventilator-associated pneumonia. Sucralfate, a drug that does not alter the gastric pH, is associated with a lower rate of nosocomial pneumonia, but does not appear to be as effective as H2 blockers in the prevention of stress-ulcer-related bleeding. A trial of 1200 mechanically ventilated patients compared the H2 blocker ranitidine with sucralfate and found a significant reduction in clinically important GI bleeding with ranitidine (1.7% of patients) compared to sucralfate (3.8% of patients). A meta-analysis has shown stress ulcer prophylaxis with a PPI to confer a 4% absolute risk reduction in GI bleeding compared with prophylaxis with an H2 blocker (NNT = 25). Enteral nutrition may also reduce risk of stress ulcer bleeding, by promoting the integrity of the gastrointestinal mucosal barrier.

Recent studies have highlighted the emerging dangers of acid suppressive therapy, particularly as care for critically ill patients continues to advance. An increased incidence of hospital-acquired pneumonia and *Clostridium difficile* enteritis are possible consequences of stress ulcer prophylaxis. The quality of data supporting the use of stress ulcer prophylaxis has recently come into question, and additional evidence is necessary to better define the benefit of acid-suppressive therapy in critically ill patients.

Currently, guidelines from the American Society of Health System Pharmacists suggest that stress ulcer prophylaxis should be limited to patients at high risk of overt gastrointestinal bleeding, including patients with respiratory failure (mechanical ventilation > 48 hours) or coagulopathy (INR > 1.5 or platelet count < 50,000/μL), or two or more of the following risk factors: sepsis, ICU admission lasting more than one week, occult GI bleeding lasting 6 or more days, and glucocorticoid therapy (more than 250 mg of hydrocortisone or the equivalent daily). Local cost considerations should guide the selection of either an H2 blocker or PPI.

Stress ulcer pharmacologic prophylaxis should be discontinued when risk factors resolve or when patients transfer out of the ICU to the medical floor.

■ PRESSURE ULCER RISKS AND PREVENTION

The European Pressure Ulcer Advisory Panel (EPUAP) defines a pressure ulcer as "an area of localized damage to the skin and underlying tissue caused by pressure, shear, friction, or a combination of these." Pressure ulcers occur when the balance of compressive or shearing forces overwhelms the tissue tolerance for pressure or the tissue tolerance for changes in oxygen concentration. Additionally, external pressure exceeding capillary pressure results in occlusion and thrombosis of the capillary, leading to tissue anoxia, release of toxic metabolites, cell death, and formation of ulcers. Classification of pressure ulcers:

- Grade I: Nonblanchable erythema of intact skin; indicators may also include discoloration, warmth, edema, induration
- Grade II: Partial thickness skin loss involving epidermis, dermis or both; a superficial ulcer
- Grade III: Full-thickness skin loss, with damage or necrosis of subcutaneous tissue
- Grade IV: Destruction, tissue necrosis, or damage to muscle, bone, or supporting structures; full-thickness skin may or may not be present

Sedated, ventilated, and confined to bed for long periods, critically ill patients are invariably at risk for the development of skin breakdown. No risk assessment scales have been developed and validated for ICU patients. The four most significant external factors for development of pressure ulcers are: pressure (in excess of arteriolar pressure), shearing forces, friction (which can cause abrasion), and moisture. Host risk factors include immobility, incontinence, nutritional compromise, tissue perfusion (which may be

compromised by hypotension, dehydration, vasoconstriction in shock states, and heart failure), and neurologic diseases (leading to immobility).

Prevention of pressure ulcers requires relief of high degrees and extended durations of pressure. Frequent patient repositioning is the cornerstone of prevention and should be employed every 2 to 3 hours. Regular turning reduces interface pressure and maintains microcirculatory perfusion. Pressure-reducing support surfaces for bedbound patients come in numerous types. Nonpowered support surfaces are made of gel, foam or water, and distribute local pressure over a wider body surface area. Powered (dynamic) surfaces use electricity to alternate air currents in order to redistribute pressure on the body.

Supportive interventions are equally important for reducing the rate of pressure ulcers. Immobility may be prevented through physical therapy and the interruption of sedative medications. Incontinence should be managed since excess moisture contributes to skin breakdown. However, urinary catheters should not be used to prevent stress ulcers, but may be considered for patients to prevent the progression of otherwise severe or evolving pressure ulceration. Adequate nutrition prevents ulcer formation, and promotes healing of ulcers. Skin assessment should recognize changes in integrity, color, turgor, and moisture status. The skin should be kept clean and dry, with the use of mild cleansing agents that minimize irritation.

Regulatory organizations, such as the Joint Commission, now consider significant pressure ulcers that develop during a hospital stay as a "never event" and a marker of poorer-quality care. Additionally, the CMS may no longer reimburse facilities for pressure ulcers that develop during a hospital stay. Health care organizations should work to systematically implement interventions that help ensure prevention of pressure ulcers in hospitalized patients who are at risk for developing this condition (see Chapter 72 [Pressure Ulcers]).

ESSENTIAL ELEMENTS OF CARE IN THE ICU

High-quality ICU care requires:

1. **Hand hygiene and infection control:** In this era of increasing microbial resistance to antibiotics, adherence to hand hygiene and appropriate infection control precautions is a central tenet in safe ICU (and hospital) care. Scrupulous adherence to hand hygiene has been demonstrated to help terminate infectious outbreaks in health care facilities, reduce transmission of multidrug-resistant organisms, and reduce overall hospital-acquired infection rates. The CDC guidelines highlight the importance of handwashing with soap and water when hands are visibly soiled or contaminated, and before and after direct patient contact. Alcohol-based solutions may be used when hands are not visibly soiled. In the presence of *Clostridium difficile* infection, handwashing with soap and water is essential to preventing the transmission of infectious spores.

2. **Interdisciplinary communication:** The ICU is an extremely complex environment and patient safety research has identified the common association of poor communication between ICU nurses and doctors with critical incidents in the ICU. All members of the interdisciplinary Intensive care unit team must be committed to promoting teamwork and open communication across disciplines. Use of daily goals checklists in the ICU has been shown to improve interdisciplinary communication, improve team members' understanding of patient care plans in the ICU, and decrease ICU length of stay (**Table 143-9**).

3. **Communication with patients and families:** Good quality, early communication with patients and families in the ICU

TABLE 143-9 Sample Daily Goals Checklist for ICU Care

Date				
Problems to be addressed today				
What is the patient's greatest safety risk?				
Discharge plan or needs				
Pain management/sedation				
Cardiac/volume status				
Pulmonary/ventilation				
Mobilization (Risk for falls?)				
Medication changes (Can any be discontinued?)				
Diet/nutrition				
Consultations today				
Tests/procedures				
Nursing bedside treatments				
Can catheters or invasive devices be removed?				
Is this patient receiving venous thromboembolic and stress ulcer bleeding prophylaxis?				
Patient/family safety concerns; patient/family education and communication				
Print name/title				
Signature				
Print name/title				
Signature				

should be a priority for all members of the interdisciplinary ICU team. Communication with physicians consistently receives low marks in family satisfaction surveys of ICU care. One study found that half of the families of ICU patients surveyed failed to comprehend the patient's diagnoses, prognosis, or treatment plan. Among patients that died in the hospital, one in four had concerns about communication with their physician and half wanted more contact with their physicians. In addition, family members of critically ill patients have a high prevalence of symptoms of anxiety, depression, and posttraumatic stress disorder (PTSD) associated with having a loved one in the ICU. In 2007, an important study from France showed that implementing a program of a pro-active ICU family conference in combination with a bereavement pamphlet decreased anxiety, depression, and PTSD among family members 3 months after a death in the ICU. In a separate study, family meetings within the first three ICU days for patients at highest risk for poor outcomes achieved significant reductions in ICU length of stay and conflict over the goals of care (see Chapter 215 [Communication Skills for End of Life Care]).

4. **Daily interruption of sedation and daily assessment of readiness to extubate:** Both excessive and insufficient sedation and analgesia in mechanically ventilated patients may increase the risk of iatrogenic complications and potentially impede recovery. Kress and colleagues randomized 128 adult patients on mechanical ventilation to daily interruption of sedation or interruption at the clinician's discretion. Daily interruption of sedation resulted in a significant reduction duration of mechanical ventilation from 7.3 to 4.9 days ($p = 0.004$). Paired spontaneous awakening trials (daily interruption of sedation) and spontaneous breathing trials were assessed in the awakening and breathing controlled (ABC) trial. This approach to interruption of sedation and spontaneous breathing resulted in an increased number of days free from mechanical ventilation, decreased ICU and hospital length of stay, and decreased 1-year mortality. A recent single-center study demonstrating the feasibility and safety of mechanical ventilation without sedation will likely prompt further research.

5. **Assessment of delirium:** Delirium, a fluctuating disturbance of consciousness with reduced ability to focus, sustain, or shift attention, develops rapidly in the ICU setting. Delirium is a significant contributor to ICU and hospital length of stay, morbidity, and mortality in the ICU, and patients with delirium have lower 6-month survival rates. Intensive care unit patients, therefore, require frequent monitoring to assess for delirium. The Confusion Assessment Method in the ICU (CAM-ICU) allows physicians, nurses, and other clinicians to rapidly perform a bedside delirium assessment. This tool (available at http://www.icudelirium.org/docs/CAM_ICU.pdf) permits evaluation of changes in mental status, attention level, thought organization, and level of consciousness. The assessment of ICU delirium should be performed every shift. Patients' delirium risk may be reduced by modification of some factors, including sedative and analgesic medications. Strategies for prevention and treatment are currently being investigated in multiple studies (**Table 143-10**).

6. **Early mobilization:** Survivors of critical illness are subject to severe functional impairment due to ICU-acquired weakness, a syndrome of profound neuromuscular weakness resulting from prolonged immobility in the setting of systemic inflammatory conditions. Sedating medications contribute significantly to ICU-acquired weakness. Care of critically ill patients now favors wakefulness over sedation. Additional benefits of early mobilization include reduction in ICU delirium, reduction in duration of mechanical ventilation, reduction in ICU and hospital length of stay, and improvements in functional independence as well as physical strength. A team of consisting of physical and occupational therapists, a nurse, a respiratory therapist, and a physician should work together to mobilize patients in a progressive manner. The physical and mental benefits of early mobilization will have great consequence for patients following discharge from the ICU.

TABLE 143-10 Evidence-Based Medicine Key References: Prevention in the ICU

Study	Methodology	Results	Limitations	Bottom Line
Catheter-related blood stream infections				
Pronovost P, Needham D, Berenholtz S, et al. An intervention to decrease catheter-related infections in the ICU. *N Engl J Med*. 2006;355(26):2725-2732.	Prospective, observational	• 103 intensive care units in Michigan instituted a central line bundle consisting of (1) handwashing, (2) using full barrier precautions, (3) skin prep with chlorhexidine, (4) avoiding the femoral site, and (5) discontinuing unnecessary catheters. • Median infection rates decreased from 2.7 per 1000 catheter days to 0 per 1000 catheter days after 3 mo.	Before and after study design	Catheter-related blood stream infections are largely preventable with use of a central line bundle.
Ventilator-associated pneumonia				
Drakulovic MB, Torres A, Bauer TT, et al. Supine body position as a risk factor for nosocomial pneumonia in mechanically ventilated patients: a randomised trial. *Lancet*. 1999;354:1851-1858.	Randomized trial of the effect of supine vs semi-recumbent positioning of mechanically ventilated patients on incidence of ventilator associated pneumonia	• 90 patients randomized, 86 patients included for analysis. • Frequency of clinically suspected VAP was lower in the semirecumbent group vs the supine group—8% vs 34%; ($p = 0.003$). • Frequency of microbiologically confirmed pneumonia was lower in the semirecumbent group vs supine group—5% vs 23%; ($p = 0.018$).	• Single center • Analysis not intention to treat	Semirecumbent body position may decrease the incidence of VAP.
Kollef MH, Afessa B, Anzueto A, et al. Silver-coated endotracheal tubes and incidence of ventilator-associated pneumonia: the NASCENT randomized trial. *JAMA*. 2008;300(7):805-813.	Multicenter randomized, controlled, single-blind trial of silver-coated vs standard low-pressure, high-volume endotracheal tubes and incidence of VAP	• Among patients intubated for ≥24 h, rates of microbiologically confirmed VAP were 4.8% (95% CI, 3.4%-6.6%) in the group receiving the silver-coated tube and 7.5% (95% CI, 5.7%-9.7%) ($p = .03$) in the group receiving the uncoated tube (NNT = 37).	• Single-blind study • VAP rates low in both groups	Patients receiving a silver-coated endotracheal tube had a statistically significant reduction in the incidence of VAP.
Hospital-acquired venous thromboembolism				
Geerts WH, Bergqvist D, Pineo GF, et al. Prevention of venous thromboembolism: American College of Chest Physicians evidence-based clinical practice guideline (8th edition). *Chest*. 2008;133:381S-453S.	Evidence-based clinical practice guideline for prevention of venous thromboembolism	• Evidence-based recommendations for prevention pf venous thromboembolism in various patient populations.	Clinical practice guideline	Synthesis of many clinical trials with evidence-based recommendations.
Stress ulcer bleeding				
Cook DJ, Fuller HD, Guyatt GH, et al. Risk factors for gastrointestinal bleeding in critically ill patients. *N Engl J Med*. 1994;330(6):377-381.	Prospective observational study of intensive care unit patients	• 4.4% of patients had overt bleeding and 1.5% of patients had clinically important bleeding. • Respiratory failure (odds ratio 15.6) and coagulopathy (odds ratio 4.3) were strong independent risk factors for clinically important bleeding.	Observational study	Respiratory failure (mechanical ventilation for >48 h) and coagulopathy are risk factors from clinically important stress ulcer bleeding in ICU patients.
Pressure ulcers				
Reddy M, Gill SS, Rochon PA. Preventing pressure ulcers: a systematic review. *JAMA*. 2006;296(8):974-984.	Systematic review of randomized controlled trials of pressure ulcer prevention	• Use of support surfaces, repositioning the patient, optimizing nutritional status, and moisturizing sacral skin are appropriate strategies to prevent pressure ulcers.	Systematic review	Multiple strategies may help prevent pressure ulcers.

CI, confidence interval; NNT, number needed to treat; VAP, ventilator-associated pneumonia.

SUGGESTED READINGS

American Society of Health-System Pharmacists therapeutic guidelines on stress ulcer prophylaxis. *Am J Health Syst Pharm*. 1999;56(8):729.

Cook DJ, Fuller HD, Guyatt GH, et al. Risk factors for gastrointestinal bleeding in critically ill patients. Canadian Critical Care Trials Group. *N Engl J Med*. 1994;330(6):377.

Geerts WH, Bergqvist D, Pineo GF, et al. Prevention of venous thromboembolism: American College of Chest Physicians evidence-based clinical practice guidelines (8th edition). *Chest*. 2008;133:381S-453S.

Girard TD, Kress JP, Fuchs BD, et al. Efficacy and safety of a paired sedation and ventilator weaning protocol for mechanically ventilated patients in intensive care (awakening and breathing controlled trial): a randomised controlled trial. *Lancet*. 2008;371(9607):126-134.

Guidelines for prevention of intravascular catheter-related infections, 2002. Center for Disease Control and Prevention. http://www.cdc.gov/ncidod/dhqp/gl_intrvascular.html. Accessed May, 2015.

Lautrette A, Darmon M, Megarbane B, et al. A communication strategy and brochure for relatives of patients dying in the ICU. *N Engl J Med*. 2007;356(5):469.

Niederman MS, Craven DE. Guidelines for the management of adults with hospital-acquired, ventilator-associated, and healthcare-associated pneumonia. *Am J Respir Crit Care Med*. 2005;171:388.

Pronovost P, Needham D, Berenholtz S, et al. An intervention to decrease catheter-related infections in the ICU. *N Engl J Med*. 2006;355(26):2725.

SECTION 3
Dermatology

CHAPTER 144

Flushing and Urticaria

Joseph C. English, III, MD
Timothy J. Patton, DO

Key Clinical Questions

1. What mechanisms cause cutaneous flushing?
2. How does one differentiate benign and malignant etiologies of flushing?
3. What tests and studies are useful to evaluate each potential diagnosis?
4. What treatments are available for each etiology?
5. What is the difference between acute and chronic urticaria?
6. What are the common causes of acute urticaria and chronic urticaria?
7. What is the appropriate workup for patients with acute or chronic urticaria?
8. In what clinical scenario is a skin biopsy indicated?
9. What is the appropriate workup when vasculitis is present on skin histology?
10. What therapies are available for acute and chronic urticaria?

FLUSHING

Flushing results from vasodilation in the skin, produced by the release of vasoactive mediators or activity of the vasomotor nerves. It is characterized by sudden warmth and visible erythema, affecting the head (**Figure 144-1**), neck, and upper chest, regions of abundant superficial cutaneous vasculature. Flushing may be episodic or constant. When persistent, it may produce fixed facial erythema with a cyanotic tinge, secondary to the development of telangiectasias and large cutaneous blood vessels, containing slow-moving, deoxygenated blood (**Figure 144-2**).

The overwhelming majority of patients with flushing have common and relatively innocuous causes, with only a small proportion of cases being associated with tumors and other significant underlying medical problems (**Table 144-1**).

■ RISK STRATIFICATION

While the majority of patients with cutaneous flushing will be diagnosed as having a benign entity such as emotionally-induced flushing or rosacea, patients must be appropriately evaluated as to not miss a rare, but more life-threatening condition such as carcinoid syndrome or pheochromocytoma. While episodic flushing can be a normal physiologic response to external factors such as heat or alcohol, persistent flushing (>1 hour) is uncommon and should raise a red flag to the clinician that further investigation is warranted. Flushing is seldom the primary indication for hospital admission. However, the hospitalist should be familiar with the causes of flushing, as they may be seen in patients hospitalized for other reasons. Associated signs and symptoms may help to guide decision making and workup (**Figures 144-3** and **144-4**). Flushing can be seen in patients with fever, patients having reactions to medications or IV contrast, and patients with intoxications. Flushing in patients with hypertension suggests pheochromocytoma; flushing with wheezing and dyspnea suggests carcinoid syndrome or anaphylaxis, flushing with profuse diarrhea suggests carcinoid or pancreatic VIPoma.

PRACTICE POINT

- The majority of flushing patients have benign causes. However, flushing patients with concomitant diarrhea, hypertension, tachycardia, bronchoconstriction or hypotension may have potentially life-threatening conditions.

■ BENIGN CUTANEOUS FLUSHING

Evaluation

Flushing is most often physiologic (benign cutaneous flushing). It is more common in women than men. Common precipitants include fever, exercise, warm temperatures, spicy foods, and alcohol. In fair-skinned persons, flushing (or blushing) often occurs in response to strong emotion, stress, or anxiety. Although blushing historically was thought attractive, it may produce distress in some contemporary patients.

Inpatient management

Whether the patient tends to flush with emotion or stress can be determined from the patient or family. Inpatient admissions for other causes may induce anxiety and distress, with prominent

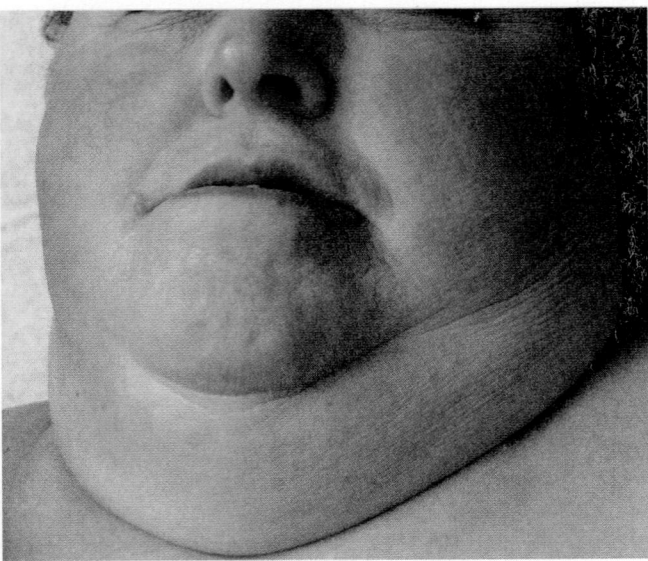

Figure 144-1 *Acute flushing.*

flushing. This is transient and should fade quickly. Emotional flushing has been treated anecdotally with nonselective β-blockers, such as nadolol, with mixed results. Topical ibuprofen has been shown to inhibit flushing during embarrassment and aerobic exercise in flushing-prone patients.

■ ROSACEA

Evaluation

Rosacea is categorized as being one or combination of the following: erythematotelangiectatic, papulopustular, phymatous, and ocular. It is characterized by acneiform inflammation of the central face, with erythema, flushing episodes, telangiectasias, and often papules and pustules. Eye lesions, such as blepharitis, conjunctivitis, episcleritis, and keratitis with corneal ulcers also occur. It is common in fair-skinned patients of middle age, with around 13 million adults in the United States being affected; the prevalence among Caucasian women in the United States is approximately 16%. The exact etiology is unknown; there seems to be a genetic predisposition. *Helicobacter pylori* and the face mite *Demodex folliculorum* have been invoked as possible causes, with equivocal data. Antimicrobial peptides (AMPs) have also been suggested to play a role. These

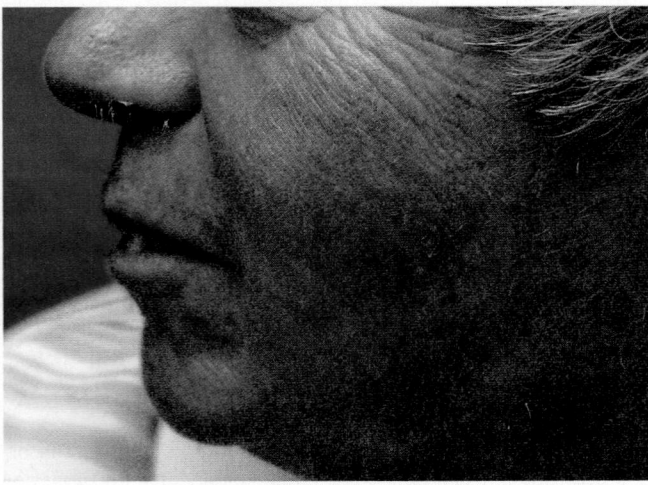

Figure 144-2 *Chronic persistent flushing.*

TABLE 144-1 Differential Diagnosis of Flushing

Common Causes of Benign Flushing
Physiologic
Emotional/stress/anxiety
Fever
Exercise
Hyperthermia
Rosacea
Climacterium (menospausal)
Drug-induced (partial list)
Niacin, calcium channel blockers, β-blockers, ACE inhibitors, nitroglycerin, sildenafil, vancomycin, NSAIDs, chemotherapy, morphine and other opiates
Alcohol
Food
Uncommon to Rare Potentially Life-Threatening Flushing
Neoplasms
Carcinoid syndrome
Pheochromocytomas
Medullary carcinomas of the thyroid
Systemic mastocytosis
VIPomas
Renal cell carcinoma
Anaphylaxis
Neurologic disorders
Parkinson disease, multiple sclerosis, migraines, brain tumors, epilepsy,
dysautonomia and orthostatic hypotension, autonomic hyperreflexia, Horner syndrome, Frey syndrome
Scombroid poisoning

peptides, such as cathelicidins and β-defensins, are components of the innate immune system, with broad antimicrobial activity. They are released with any injury to the skin. LL-37 canthelicidin is expressed in abnormally high amounts in the skin of rosacea patients, compared to controls. When LL-37 has been injected into the skin of mice, the mice demonstrate a phenotype similar to rosacea patients, with erythema, inflammation and telangiectasias. LL-37 also increases UVB-triggered inflammasome activation in rosacea patients with sun sensitivity.

Inpatient management

Rosacea with flushing is usually an incidental finding in the hospitalized patient. However, the differential diagnosis of the red face is at times difficult to parse clinically. Rosacea must be distinguished from acute cutaneous lupus erythematosus (ACLE), photosensitivity eruptions, seborrheic dermatitis, and other inflammatory dermatoses. The diagnosis of rosacea is made on clinical grounds, as there is no confirmatory laboratory test. Rosacea is usually confined to the face, and is not associated with systemic symptoms; lesions elsewhere on the body or systemic symptoms strongly suggest another etiology, such as lupus. Patient with ACLE in the midst of a systemic lupus erythematosus flare are usually significant ill with generalized malaise. The classic malar rash of SLE differs from rosacea, lacking papules or pustules.

When rosacea flushing has predictable triggers, such as spicy foods, hot drinks, alcohol, caffeine, and extremes in temperature,

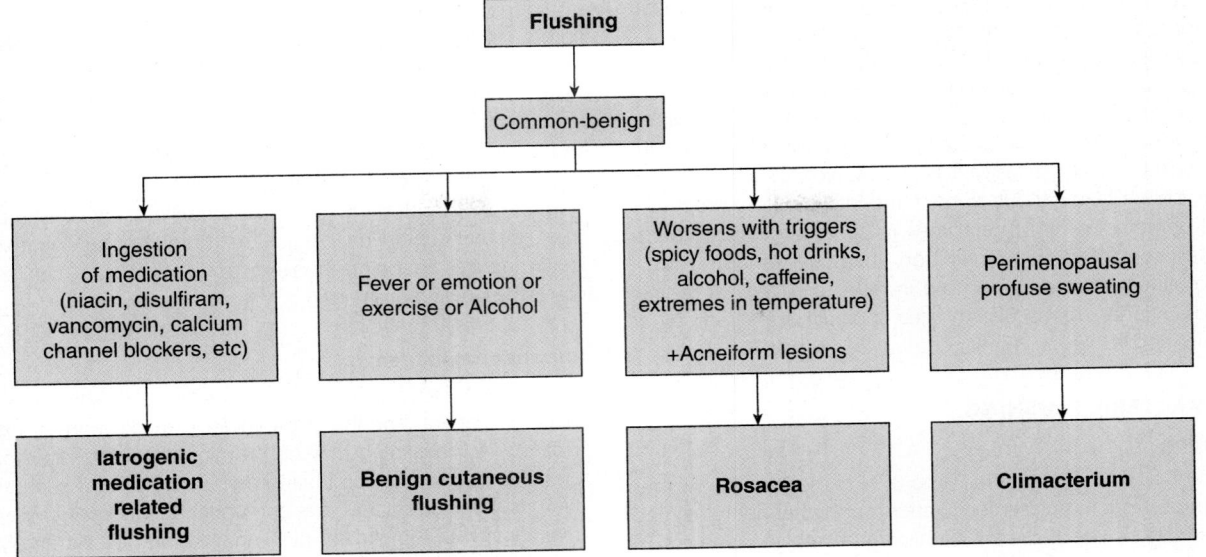

Figure 144-3 *Diagnostic approach to common causes of flushing.*

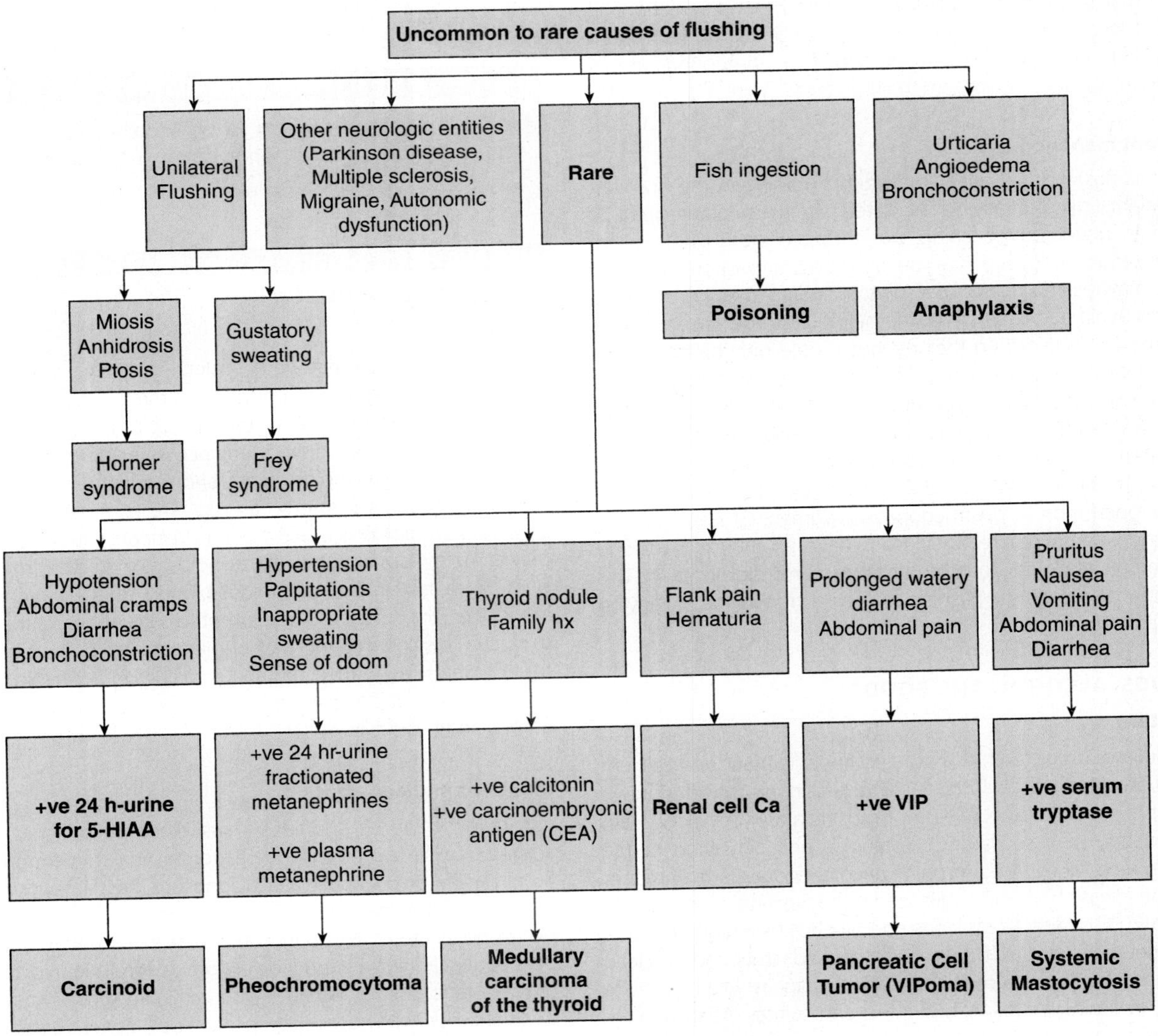

Figure 144-4 *Diagnostic approach to uncommon causes of flushing.*

avoidance is the best treatment. Rosacea of at least moderate severity is treated with combination therapy, including a topical wash, such as sulfacetamide 10%/sulfur 5%; topical antibiotics, such as metronidazole gel, clindamycin gel, dapsone gel, or ivermectin cream; and oral antibiotics, such as doxycycline or minocycline. Flushing in rosacea may be treated with pulsed dye laser to eliminate facial telangiectasias, as well as oral antibiotics such as doxycycline that blunt flushing due to their anti-inflammatory properties. Topical brimonidine, which activates α-2 adrenergic receptors to cause vasoconstriction, and inhibition of vascular smooth muscle with botulinum toxin may be used in refractory cases of rosacea flushing. Patients with ocular rosacea should be assessed by an ophthalmologist.

◼ CLIMACTERIC FLUSHING

Evaluation

Climacteric flushing occurs in 50% to 85% of menopausal women not taking estrogen replacement. Patients at higher risk for climacteric flushing include those with a history of smoking, depression, and oral contraceptive use. The hot flush is experienced as a wave of heat radiating outward from the upper body, typically lasting 3 to 4 minutes, with concomitant facial flushing. Skin temperature is elevated about 1°C during hot flashes, and heart rate also rises. The physiology is poorly understood, but may relate to changes in hypothalamic thermoregulation associated with fluctuations in estrogen levels. Levels of neurokinin B, a hypothalamic neuropeptide, are high in menopause, and infusion of this compound induces flushing in women.

Inpatient management

Climateric flushing is usually an incidental finding in the hospitalized patient. Episodes may be associated with the same precipitants as benign physiologic flushing, but they are often unprovoked. Concentration and sleep may be disturbed, and depression and fatigue may result. Lifestyle measures, including keeping the body cool and avoiding triggers, may be helpful. Estrogen replacement is the most effective drug therapy, but should only be prescribed after a detailed discussion of risks and benefits. The diagnosis of climacteric-related flushing is supported by laboratory testing of hormone levels, including follicle-stimulating hormone (FSH), which is elevated, and estradiol, which is diminished. Venlafaxine may decrease flushing frequency and severity by decreasing cutaneous microperfusion in postmenopausal women. Of note, women with moderate to severe hot flushes have an increased carotid intima-media thickness compared to those who did not flush. This suggests that climacteric flushing may be a marker for underlying cardiovascular disease.

◼ DRUGS, ALCOHOL, AND FOODS

Evaluation

All vasodilator drugs, such as nitroglycerine, sildenafil, and calcium channel blockers, may lead to flushing. Niacin-induced flushing is due to the subcutaneous release of prostaglandin D2, along with the formation of vasodilatory prostanoids and activation of the capsaicin receptor TRPV1. Morphine and other opiates may trigger histamine release from mast cells, leading to flushing.

Up to 70% of Americans consume alcohol beverages. Alcohol and its metabolite acetaldehyde are both vasodilators, and may lead to flushing. Wines may contain several substances which provoke flushing, including tyramine, histamine, and sulfites. Asian populations have a prevalence of alcohol-related facial flushing of up to 36%, often related to an inherited deficiency of aldehyde dehydrogenase 2 (ALDH2*2 allele), which leads to a buildup of acetaldehyde.

Foods containing tyramine, such as aged cheeses and soy products, foods containing sulfites, such as wines and dried fruits, nitrite-containing foods, such as cured meats, and spicy foods may lead to flushing. Scombroid poisoning results from fish left at room temperature too long, leading to conversion of histidine to histamine by surface bacteria. Histamine is not broken down by cooking, leading to flushing when ingested. Scombroid is not a true allergy. Ciguatera fish poisoning is a foodborne illness by consumption of reef fish that contain microalgae that produces the ciguatoxin. This toxin induces gastrointestinal distress, neurologic manifestations paresthesias, and flushing.

Inpatient management

Medication reactions are a common cause of flushing in the hospitalized patient. The list of provocative medications is extensive (Table 144-1). Flushing may be prominent in intoxicated patients. However, alcohol in combination with medications such as disulfiram, sulfonylureas, and oral antifungal agents may cause severe reactions with significant flushing. Flushing is extremely common with niacin, which is available over the counter as well as by prescription.

Flushing due to niacin, usually taken to lower lipids, occurs within 20 minutes to 1 hour after niacin dosing, generally lasts less than 1 hour. Coadministration with aspirin and apple pectin with niacin may reduce the incidence of flushing.

PRACTICE POINT

- Alcohol may cause flushing on its own, or it may play a supporting role in food- or medication-induced flushing.

NEOPLASMS

◼ CARCINOID SYNDROME

Evaluation

Carcinoid tumors are rare neuroendocrine tumors which originate most often in the gut, less commonly in the lungs, and rarely in the reproductive tract. The 5-year survival rate is up to 75%, regardless of stage or site. Carcinoid syndrome occurs in approximately 10% of all patients with carcinoid tumors, and results from tumor-derived mediators, such as serotonin and kallikreins, entering circulation. Carcinoid syndrome is usually seen in patients with lung primaries or liver metastases from bowel carcinoids, as mediators from the gut primary released into portal venous blood are usually broken down in the liver. The most common symptoms are abdominal pain, diarrhea, and flushing. Patients may also experience palpitations, shortness of breath, rhinorrhea, pruritus, and a pellagra-like skin rash (due to tryptophan depletion). Cardiac manifestations include valvular fibrosis and heart failure.

Inpatient management

Carcinoid syndrome should be suspected in selected patients admitted with symptoms of gastrointestinal hypermotility and flushing. The gold standard for diagnosis is the 24-hour urine level of 5-hydroxyindoleacetic acid (5-HIAA). Levels greater than 25 mg per 24 hours are usually diagnostic. CT scan, CT enterography, and octreotide scanning are used for anatomical localization of the tumor or metastatic disease. Patients with carcinoid tumors may have a carcinoid crisis, with flushing, bronchospasm, tachycardia and hemodynamic instability, during anesthesia or tumor manipulation during procedures. Early disease is treated with surgery; advanced disease is treated with chemotherapy and biologics therapy. Symptomatic flushing related to carcinoid syndrome can be treated with soma-tostatin, octreotide, or lantreotide, which decrease the secretion of vasoactive mediators.

PHEOCHROMOCYTOMA

Evaluation

Pheochromocytomas are rare catecholamine-producing tumors of the adrenal medulla that lead to hypertension and palpitations. They are said to follow the rule of tens: 10% are extra-adrenal, 10% are malignant, 10% are bilateral, and 10% are not associated with hypertension. Approximately 10% are familial, associated with genetic syndromes such as type 2 multiple endocrine neoplasia, von Hippel-Lindau disease, and neurofibromatosis. Both pallor and flushing are described in pheochromocytoma; to confuse matters, patients may associate episodes of pallor with a subjective sensation of flushing, perhaps due to rebound vasodilation after a paroxysm of catecholamine release. Whether pallor or flushing occurs may depend on whether α-adrenergic effects (leading to vasoconstriction) or β-adrenergic effects (leading to vasodilation) predominate.

Inpatient Management

Pheochromocytoma should be considered when flushing is associated with paroxysmal hypertension, headaches, palpitations, tachycardia, inappropriate sweating, anxiety, tremulousness, nausea, and vomiting. Measurement of plasma free metanephrines is the preferred screening test with 24-hour urine fractionated metanephrines testing for confirmation. False positive results are associated with the use of monoamine oxidase inhibitors, tricyclic antidepressants, serotonin-norepinephrine reuptake inhibitors, cocaine, and caffeine, as well as alcohol and benzodiazepine withdrawal syndromes. Contrast CT scan of the abdomen is the preferred initial test for tumor localization. Magnetic resonance imaging is useful to define the extent of metastatic disease. Successful treatment of pheochromocytoma requires surgical consultation for possible laparoscopic adrenalectomy, with the perioperative use of α-receptor blockers such as phenoxybenzamine or doxazosin, in conjunction with endocrinology. Patients are at significant risk for postoperative hypotension and hypoglycemia.

MEDULLARY CARCINOMA OF THE THYROID

Evaluation

Medullary carcinoma of the thyroid gland (MCT) is a tumor of the parafollicular cells (C cells) of the thyroid gland. It is an uncommon neuroendocrine malignancy associated, accounting for 1% to 2% of thyroid tumors in the United States. A minority of cases of MCT with advanced disease may present with flushing and diarrhea. A mutation in the RET codon M918T is associated with aggressive sporadic MCT. This malignancy is also seen in type 2 multiple endocrine neoplasia; evaluation of these patients to rule out pheochromocytoma and hyperparathyroidism is warranted. The flushing and diarrhea occasionally seen in MCT is believed to be due to overproduction of calcitonin and carcinoembryonic antigen (CEA).

Inpatient management

The initial assessment for suspected MCT includes blood testing for calcitonin and CEA and thyroid ultrasound. Fine needle aspiration of thyroid nodules >1.0 cm, with immunohistochemical staining for calcitonin, chromogranin, and CEA, is needed to confirm the diagnosis. Once the diagnosis of MCT is confirmed, patients may require total thyroidectomy and lymph node dissection, with or without radiation therapy. Computerized tomography or MRI is performed to assess for metastatic disease.

SYSTEMIC MASTOCYTOSIS

Evaluation

Systemic mastocytosis is caused by mast cell accumulation in skin, bones, and viscera. It is due to the D816V mutation of the KIT gene, a receptor tyrosine kinase. This mutation leads to persistent activation of the tyrosine kinase, and uncontrolled proliferation of mast cells. The symptoms of systemic mastocytosis result from the release of mast cell mediators, especially histamine, with flushing, pruritus, nausea, vomiting, abdominal pain, peptic ulcers, diarrhea, headache, osteopenia, and anaphylaxis.

Inpatient management

Serum total tryptase is used to screen for systemic mastocytosis. Levels in excess of 20 ng/mL warrant hematology consultation for possible bone marrow biopsy. Treatment of mastocytosis varies by subtype. Cutaneous mastocytosis without visceral involvement usually has a favorable prognosis. Treatment is aimed at symptom relief, with antihistamines, cromolyn sodium, phototherapy, and avoidance of triggers. Patients with systemic mastocytosis may also require therapy with interferon-α, cladribine, or tyrosine kinase inhibitors such as imatinib mesylate, in addition to symptomatic treatment. Patients with systemic mastocytosis are at higher risk for allergic reactions to IV contrast dye and various medications.

VIPOMA

Evaluation

Pancreatic neuroendocrine neoplasms of the gut include insulinoma, gastrinoma, glucagonoma, growth hormone-releasing factor secreting tumors (GRFomas), and vasoactive intestinal peptide secreting tumors (VIPomas). Vasoactive intestinal peptide secreting tumors are vanishingly rare tumors of the delta cells of the pancreas. They are associated with watery diarrhea, abdominal pain, and flushing. Due to voluminous diarrhea, patients develop hypokalemia and achlorhydria (Verner-Morrison syndrome). Vasoactive intestinal peptide relaxes cutaneous vascular smooth muscle, leading to cutaneous flushing.

Inpatient management

Serum VIP levels should be obtained in patients admitted with flushing associated with high-volume watery diarrhea which persists with fasting. Patients with elevated VIP levels in the presence of secretory diarrhea should have abdominal imaging with contrast CT, MRI, somatostatin receptor scintigraphy, or functional PET imaging. Initial treatment is geared toward rehydration and correction of electrolyte disturbances. Octreotide treatment reduces VIP levels and usually leads to improvement in diarrhea. In disease localized to the pancreas, surgical resection with regional lymph node dissection and splenectomy is definitive therapy. Liver metastases are traditionally treated with streptozocin-based chemotherapy and hepatic artery embolization. Sunitinib, bevacizumab, and everolimus have emerged as promising new agents.

> ### PRACTICE POINT
>
> - Neuroendocrine tumors, although rare, need to be considered in the differential diagnosis of all patients presenting with symptomatic flushing.

ANAPHYLAXIS

Evaluation

Anaphylaxis is a severe type 1 hypersensitivity immune reaction caused by mast cell and basophil degranulation, with the release of mediators such as histamine and PGD2. These produce symptoms which may include diffuse erythema, pruritus, flushing, urticaria, angioedema, bronchospasm, laryngeal edema, hyperperistalsis, hypotension, and life-threatening cardiac arrhythmias. Common causes of anaphylaxis include foods such shellfish, peanuts, and tree nuts, medications such as aspirin and IV contrast, and envenomation from stinging insects. Although the incidence of anaphylaxis is increasing in the United States, case fatality rates of have fallen to 0.3%, which likely reflects earlier recognition and management.

Inpatient management

Anaphylaxis is a medical emergency. Initial management includes ensuring airway patency, providing ventilatory support if necessary, and supporting blood pressure with IV fluids. Epinephrine and H1-antihistamines should be given as quickly as possible. Epinephrine is better absorbed with intramuscular injection than subcutaneous injections; intravenous epinephrine is used in unresponsive patients. Corticosteroids are also useful, but they are slower-acting and are a lower priority medication in anaphylaxis than epinephrine and H1-antihistamines. Due to the unpredictable natural history of anaphylaxis, observation up to 72 hours after onset is recommended. Education of the patient about trigger avoidance and the use of self-injectable epinephrine may be life-saving outside the hospital environment.

■ NEUROLOGIC DISEASE

Evaluation

Neurologic disorders that affect the autonomic nervous system, such as Parkinson disease, multiple sclerosis, and migraine, may occasionally lead to flushing. Cluster headache and paroxysmal hemicrania may cause ipsilateral facial pain and autonomic disturbances, including flushing. Patients with Horner syndrome may have ipsilateral ptosis, miosis, anhidrosis, and loss of flushing. Flushing is preserved on the contralateral side, leading to asymmetric physiologic flushing (harlequin syndrome). The patient may erroneously perceive the contralateral flushing as the abnormality. Causes of Horner syndrome include Pancoast tumors of the lung, carotid aneurysm, brainstem stroke, and multiple sclerosis. Aberrant nerve regeneration after parotid gland injury or surgery may result in ipsilateral flushing and sweating with eating and salivation (Frey syndrome). Additional associations include epilepsy, dysautonomia, and autonomic hyperreflexia.

Inpatient management

Flushing associated with new neurologic symptoms sometimes portends a serious condition, such as Horner syndrome due to a Pancoast tumor or internal carotid artery dissection, or autonomic hyperreflexia from a spinal cord lesion. In these patients, appropriate imaging studies should be performed. Alternatively, the patient may have a known neurologic diagnosis which is sometimes associated with flushing, such as multiple sclerosis, migraines, or Parkinson disease. In these patients, the patient's neurologist should be consulted regarding symptom alleviation.

DISCHARGE CHECKLIST FOR BENIGN FLUSHING

■ ROSACEA

- Is the patient going home with appropriate topical and oral antibiotics?
- Does the patient have a follow-up appointment with dermatology (and ophthalmalology, if there is ocular involvement)?

■ CLIMATERIC FLUSHING

- Has the use of estrogen or venlafaxine therapy been considered?
- Does the patient have a follow-up appointment with gynecology or endocrinology?

■ FLUSHING ASSOCIATED WITH FOODS, DRUGS, AND ALCOHOL

- Has the patient been counseled regarding trigger avoidance?
- If patient is an alcoholic, is there an outpatient plan for maintenance of sobriety?

DISCHARGE CHECKLIST FOR LIFE-THREATENING FLUSHING

■ NEOPLASMS

- Does the patient have appropriate follow-up with medical oncology and surgical oncology?

■ ANAPHYLAXIS

- Has the patient been educated about signs and symptoms of anaphylaxis?
- Does the patient have prescriptions for epinephrine auto-injectors? Have they been counseled about auto-injector storage? Epinephrine auto-injectors should be protected from light and not exposed to extremes of heat or cold, as in a parked car.
- Has the patient been instructed to return to the hospital if they self-administer epinephrine outside the hospital?
- Does the patient have scheduled follow-up with allergy?

■ NEUROLOGIC

- Does the patient have a follow-up appointment with a neurologist?

URTICARIA

Urticaria is a cutaneous disorder characterized by the presence of transient, pruritic, erythematous, slightly edematous plaques. Urticaria, or hives, is not a specific disease. Rather, it is a descriptive term for a cutaneous reaction with a number of potential etiologies. The lesions of urticaria tend to be pruritic, last for a few minutes to several hours, and are irregularly shaped with an adjacent zone of pallor (**Figure 144-5**). Individual lesions commonly last less than 24 hours. Crops of lesions recur for a period of less than 6 weeks in acute urticaria, and over a period of more than 6 weeks in chronic urticaria. Urticaria is occasionally accompanied by edema of deeper tissues, known as angioedema. In highly sensitive individuals, the inflammatory processes that lead to urticaria and angioedema can

Figure 144-5 *Urticarial wheals with circumferential pallor.*

progress to anaphylaxis, with symptoms of airway compromise and hypotension.

In one study, the cumulative incidence of acute urticaria was 18.7% among individuals 18 and older, in agreement with prior studies that measured the lifetime incidence of acute urticaria. The prevalence of chronic urticaria in the same population was estimated as 0.6%.

The primary effector in the pathogenesis of urticaria is the mast cell. In response to various stimuli, the mast cell releases multiple mediators of the urticarial response, including histamine, interleukins, prostaglandins, and leukotrienes. The stimuli leading to the release of these mediators may be immunologic or nonimmunologic. Some medications, such as opioids, directly stimulate mast cell degranulation. Neuropeptides and complement may also act directly on the mast cell. Immunologic causes of mast cell degranulation usually work through the high-affinity IgE receptor (FcεRI) on the surface of the mast cell. The allergen-IgE-FcεRI complex that forms on mast cells leads to mediator release. Antibodies directed against the FcεRI receptor or the IgE molecule itself can also stimulate mast cell degranulation.

■ RISK STRATIFICATION

The vast majority of patients with urticaria do not require hospital admission. While pruritus may affect quality of life, the condition is not life-threatening. Occasionally urticaria can be associated with serious underlying disease, such as a malignancy or a connective tissue disease, but without suggestive findings on the history and physical exam, a workup for these conditions is not warranted. Hospital admission may be warranted when urticaria occur in the setting of angioedema, anaphylaxis, or vasculitis.

PRACTICE POINT

- Causes of urticaria include physical stimuli, medications, infections, and autoimmune disease. In many cases, the etiology is unknown. The vast majority of patients with urticaria do not have non-life threatening conditions.

■ ACUTE URTICARIA

Evaluation

Acute urticaria is defined as hives present for less than 6 weeks. Patients should be asked about changes in medications or diet, as well as recent illnesses, such as viral or streptococcal infection. In many instances, there may be no clear cause of urticaria from the patient's history.

Urticarial lesions which remain in a fixed position for more than 24 hours, are associated with a burning sensation rather than itching, and heal with purpura formation are suggestive of urticarial vasculitis. Urticarial vasculitis is most often idiopathic. However, if urticarial vasculitis is diagnosed or suspected, patients should be assessed for systemic lupus erythematosus, Sjögren syndrome, granulomatosis with polyangiitis, viral hepatitis, and Epstein-Barr virus infection.

Inpatient management

NSAIDs and opioids may make urticaria more recalcitrant to therapy, and should be minimized if possible. Any medications which were initiated at around the same time as the onset of urticaria should be discontinued. Most patients with urticaria are prescribed H1-antihistamines as first-line therapy. Some patients are prescribed a combination of a first-generation antihistamine in the evening, due to a potential side effect of drowsiness, and a second-generation antihistamine during the day. More recent consensus groups recommend only using the second-generation nonsedating antihistamines only, using up to four times the recommended maximum dose if needed. While some studies suggest that the addition of a H2-antihistamine may be helpful, these are not routinely prescribed. Systemic corticosteroids are effective, but are not first-line therapy in acute urticaria because of their litany of possible adverse side effects, and the self-limited nature of the condition.

In patients with urticaria which burn, rather than itch, which last greater than 24 hours, and which resolve with purpura, a 4 mm punch biopsy is indicated to exclude urticarial vasculitis. Additional laboratory workup may include complete blood count, liver function tests, serum creatinine, urinalysis, antinuclear antibody, complement levels, antinuclear cytoplasmic antibody, antibodies to SS-A and SS-B, C3/4, serology for hepatitis B and C, cryoglobulins, and heterophile antibody. Treatment for urticarial vasculitis often requires the initial use of oral corticosteroids, with a transition to steroid-sparing agents such as hydroxychloroquine or mycophenolate mofetil. Underlying associated conditions should also be treated.

■ PHYSICAL URTICARIAS

In some patients with urticaria, specific physical stimuli can be identified as the cause of the lesions. Physical urticarias may be suspected based on patient history, and confirmed with either office or home testing. Some examples of physical provocation tests include ice cube application to the skin to provoke cold urticaria, or exposing the skin to ultraviolet or visible light to provoke solar urticaria. Urticaria usually have a similar appearance, no matter what the etiology may be. One exception is cholinergic urticaria, in which the lesions appear as small urticarial papules on an erythematous base (**Figure 144-6A, B**). These lesions can be duplicated in the clinic by having the patient run in place in the examination room. The most common form of physical urticaria is dermatographism, which occurs when the release of histamine from mast cells is stimulated by scratching or rubbing the skin (**Figure 144-7**). Testing for dermatographism can be easily performed in the office setting by stroking the skin with a fingernail or the wooden end of a cotton tip applicator. Other types include vibratory urticaria, delayed pressure urticaria, aquagenic urticaria, and galvanic urticaria.

Inpatient management

Diagnosis and management of physical urticarias would not likely be a significant part of inpatient management. Avoidance of the inciting trigger should be instituted when possible. If certain triggers are unable to be avoided as part of the hospital stay, the medical management would be similar to the management of acute urticarias (see above).

■ CHRONIC SPONTANEOUS URTICARIA

Urticaria lasting longer than 6 weeks without an identifiable external trigger is designated as chronic spontaneous urticaria. Many triggers have been implicated in chronic spontaneous urticaria, including infections, autoimmune diseases, and parasitic infestations. In some of these conditions (eg, *H. pylori* infection), the association between the condition and the urticaria, and whether or not the treatment of the underling condition leads to resolution of urticaria, is controversial. Performing an exhaustive workup to rule out other conditions is not likely to benefit the vast majority of patients with chronic spontaneous urticaria. An autologous serum skin test, while frequently

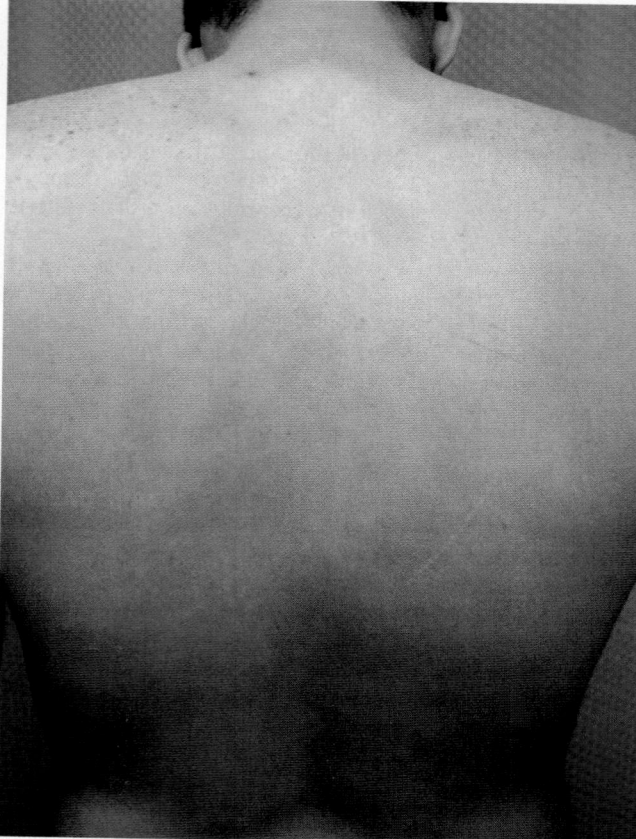

A

B

Figure 144-6 *Cholinergic urticaria. (A) Multiple erythematous flares, typically provoked by sweating and changes in body temperature. (B) Close-up view reveals pruritic papules on a red base.*

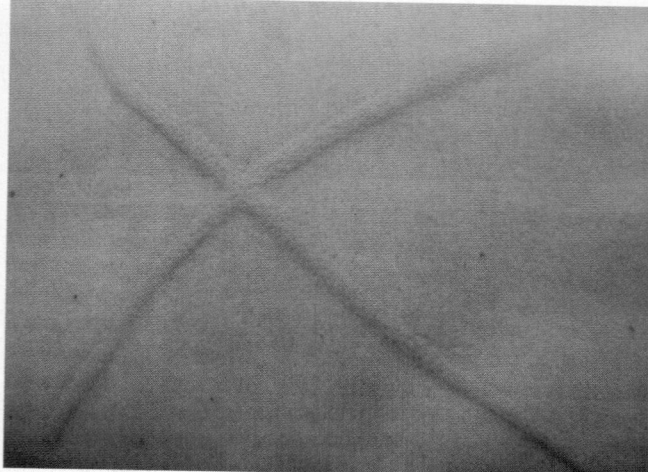

Figure 144-7 *Dermatographism.*

Inpatient management

The treatment algorithm for chronic spontaneous urticaria is similar to that of acute urticaria (**Figure 144-8**). Second-generation nonsedating antihistamines are recommended as first-line therapy, either as single daily doses or in doses up to four times the recommended maximum dose. Addition of an H2-blocker, montelukast, or a first-generation antihistamine is the next step in management. Systemic corticosteroids can be given for acute relief of severe flares, but should not be prescribed as long-term therapy. Options for third-therapy include montelukast, cyclosporine, azathioprine, mycophonlate mofetil, or omalizumab. Cyclosporine is not FDA-approved for the treatment of chronic spontaneous urticaria, but two randomized placebo-controlled trials have confirmed its effectiveness. Doses of 300 to 400 mg a day are recommended. Patients must be monitored for kidney function and hypertension while on therapy. Mycophenolate mofetil also is not FDA-approved, but has been reported as successful treatment at doses of 1000 to 3000 mg divided twice daily. Omalizumab, an anti-IgE antibody, has received FDA approval for the treatment of chronic spontaneous urticaria for patients refractory to H1-antihistamine therapy and montelukast. The recommended dose is either 150 mg or 300 mg subcutaneously every 4 weeks. Dosing is not based on serum IgE level, as it is in patients with asthma. The majority of patients with urticaria eventually achieve remission and are able to discontinue systemic therapy, with the exception of patients with physical urticarias, who tend to have persistent symptoms.

DISCHARGE CHECKLIST FOR URTICARIA

- Was the patient been instructed to avoid food and medication triggers, if these were identified?
- Was the patient instructed on the use of over the counter second-generation antihistamines as first-line therapy?
- Does the patient have a follow-up appointment with dermatology?
- Does the patient have a prescription for a short course of prednisone if needed for a severe flare?

ACKNOWLEDGMENT

In memory of Lisa Grandinetti, MD (August 12, 1976 to February 27, 2015). Her contributions to the first edition (Chapter 141) are with us in the second edition.

mentioned as a tool to diagnose chronic spontaneous urticaria, is rarely performed. More recently, laboratory tests which allow for the detection of antibodies to the high-affinity FcεRI or antibodies to IgE have become available. While this may serve to elucidate the cause of urticaria in some instances, the treatment plan is not significantly altered by the presence of these antibodies. Some also advocate testing for thyroid autoantibodies, but without overt thyroid disease, it is not always clear what the presence of these antibodies indicates in terms of the management of the patient.

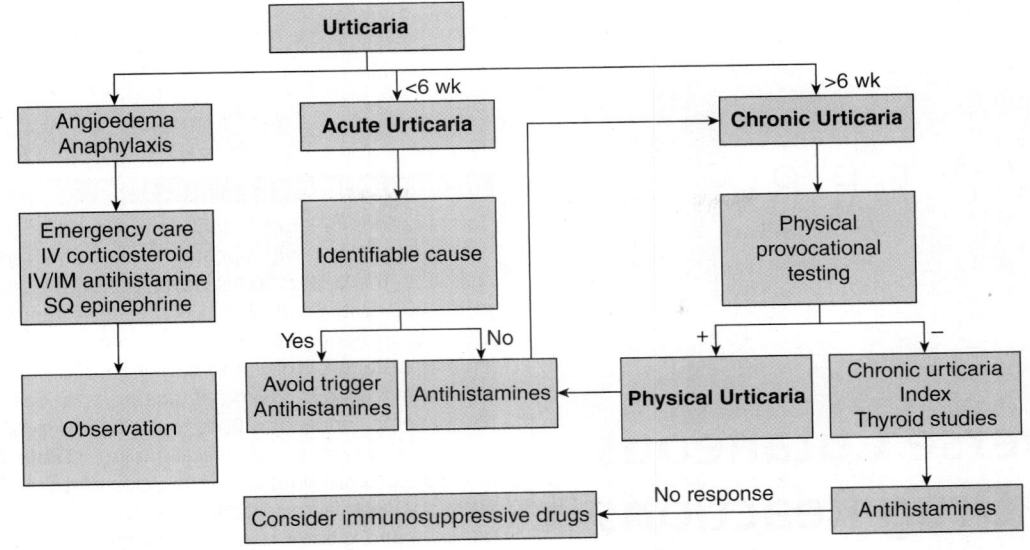

Figure 144-8 *Diagnostic approach to urticaria.*

SUGGESTED READINGS

FLUSHING

Bonadonna P, Lombardo C, Zanotti R. Mastocytosis and allergic disease. *J Investig Allergol Clin Immunol.* 2014;24:288-297.

Ikizoglu G. Red face revisited: Flushing. *Clin Dermatol.* 2014;32:800-808.

Lenders JW, Duh QY, Eisenhofer G, et al. Pheochromocytoma and paraganglionoma: an Endocrine Society clinical practice guideline. *J Clin Endocrinol Metab.* 2014;99:1915-1942.

Ma L, Danoff TM, Borish L. Case fatality and population mortality associated with anaphylaxis in the United States. *J Allergy Clin Immunol.* 2014;133:1075-1083.

Moore LE, Kemp AM, Kemp SF. Recognition, treatment and prevention of anaphylaxis. *Immunol Allergy Clin N Am.* 2015;363-374.

Nandy N, Dasanu CA. Management of advanced and/or metastatic carcinoid tumors: historical prespectives and emerging therapies. *Expert Opin Pharmacother.* 2013;14:1649-1658.

URICARIA

Kaplan AP, Greaves M. Pathogenesis of chronic urticaria. *Clin Exp Allergy.* 2009;39:777-787.

Kibsgaard L, Lefevre AC, Deleuran M, Vestergaard C. A case series study of eighty-five chronic spontaneous urticaria patients referred to a tertiary care center. *Ann Dermatol.* 2014;26: 73-78.

Marzano AV, Tavecchio S, Venturini M, et al. Urticarial vasculitis and urticarial autoinflammatory syndromes. *G Ital Dermatol Venereol.* 2015;150:41-50.

Zimmerman AB, Berger EM, Elmariah SB, Soter NA. The use of mycophenolate mofetil for the treatment of autoimmune and chronic idiopathic urticaria: experience in 19 patients. *J Am Acad Dermatol* 2012;66:767-770.

Zuberbier T, Maurer M. Omalizumab for the treatment of chronic urticaria. *Expert Rev Clin Immunol.* 2015;11:171-180.

CHAPTER 145

Adverse Cutaneous Drug Reactions

Steven T. Chen, MD, MPH

Nicole F. Velez, MD

Arturo P. Saavedra, MD, PhD

Key Clinical Questions

1. What are the red flags that should alert the hospitalist to an adverse cutaneous reaction?
2. When must the offending drug be discontinued?
3. How do you treat through a cutaneous reaction?
4. What is the recommended treatment for Stevens-Johnson syndrome/toxic epidermal necrolysis?
5. When should you call a dermatology consult?
6. How do you counsel the patient at the time of discharge?

INTRODUCTION

Complications of drug therapy are the most common adverse events associated with inpatient admissions and hospital discharge. In the United States, adverse drug events account for up to 140,000 deaths and $136 billion in costs annually. Skin involvement occurs frequently in drug reactions and may be the presenting manifestation. While most cutaneous reactions are benign and self-limiting, serious adverse cutaneous reactions affect 2% to 3% of inpatients and lead to 0.1% to 0.3% of hospital fatalities. However, early recognition of clinical findings (**Table 145-1**) is critical to ensure prompt drug discontinuation and prevent further complications. Risk factors include female gender, age, immunosuppression, and greater number of medications. Common culprits are penicillins, sulfonamides, and nonsteroidal anti-inflammatory agents (NSAIDs).

PATHOPHYSIOLOGY

Cutaneous drug reactions occur by both immunologic and non-immunologic mechanisms. Genetic predisposition, host characteristics, and probably other poorly understood factors also play important roles.

Nonimmunologic mechanisms are predictable drug reactions, related to overdose, cumulative toxicity, and delayed toxicity. Immunologic mechanisms are often unpredictable. They are classified into four categories. Type I reactions are IgE-mediated responses that activate mast cells, and produce urticaria, angio-edema, and hemodynamic instability. Type II reactions involve cytotoxic IgG responses, and often cause blood cell dyscrasias, such as hemolytic anemia, thrombocytopenia, and leukopenia. In type III reactions, immune complex deposition and complement activation lead to a vasculitis or serum sickness-like presentation. Finally, type IV reactions are T-cell mediated and account for most drug exanthems. The character of the skin rash may depend on the type of T-cell response elicited. For example, T-helper 2 responses produce interleukin-4 and interleukin-5 secretion, and the classic morbilliform rash with both erythematous macules and papules (**Figure 145-1**). A predominantly cytotoxic T-cell response may lead to keratinocyte necrosis and vesicular and pustular eruptions. The T-cell response elicited is determined by the antigenic epitopes of the drug, which depend upon the drug's chemical reactivity, prior metabolism, and protein binding. In Stevens-Johnson syndrome (SJS) and toxic epidermal necrolysis (TEN), keratinocyte death is also influenced by activation of fatty acid synthetase (Fas) receptors, leading to caspase activation and keratinocyte apoptosis.

Host characteristics that influence drug reactions include alterations in drug metabolism pathways, concurrent medications, immunosuppression, and underlying disease. Patients with low levels of the enzyme epoxide hydrolase who are taking aromatic anticonvulsants, such as phenytoin, carbamazepine, and phenobarbital, accumulate toxic metabolites (arene oxides). This predisposes to the development of drug reaction with eosinophilia and systemic symptoms (DRESS). Reactivation of latent viral infections, such as human herpesvirus 6 and 7, also predispose patients to more severe cutaneous drug reactions.

TABLE 145-1 The "Red Flags" of Adverse Cutaneous Drug Reactions

Cutaneous signs
  Blisters
  Palpable purpura
  Confluent erythema
  Epidermal necrosis
  Ulcers
  Mucosal involvement
  Facial edema

Systemic signs
  Fever (>40°C)
  Skin tenderness
  Lymphadenopathy
  Arthralgias
  Shortness of breath, wheezing
  Hypotension

Laboratory findings
  Liver function tests >3× normal
  Eosinophilia (>1500/mm³)
  Neutropenia

DOES THIS PATIENT HAVE AN ADVERSE CUTANEOUS DRUG REACTION?

■ EXANTHEMATOUS DRUG REACTION (THE "COMMON DRUG RASH")

Exanthematous or morbilliform eruptions account for more than 90% of drug reactions. Skin lesions may appear within 4 to 14 days of drug initiation, and typically consist of pink to red macules

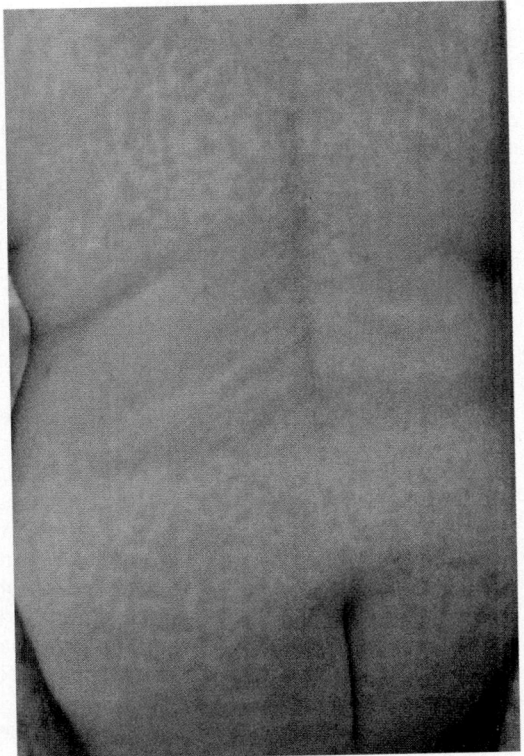

Figure 145-1 *Morbilliform drug rash. Erythematous macules and papules coalescing in dependent areas.*

and papules that begin symmetrically on the trunk and upper extremities. The eruption is polymorphic, spreads distally, and often becomes confluent on the trunk. Pruritus is a common complaint. The benign drug rash lacks mucosal involvement, skin tenderness, and signs of end organ damage. Symptomatic management consists of both sedating (eg, diphenhydramine or hydroxyzine 25 mg po every 6 hours) and nonsedating (eg, cetirizine 5-10 mg po daily or fexofenadine 180 mg po daily) antihistamines. Potent (class I) topical steroids, such as clobetasol 0.05% ointment, can be applied up to twice daily to the trunk and extremities. Sensitive areas, including the face, axilla, inframammary skin, and genitals, should be treated with a mild (class 5-7) topical steroid, such as hydrocortisone 2.5% cream. Topical steroid use should be limited to 2-week intervals to avoid side effects such as skin atrophy, striae, pigmentary change, contact dermatitis, and infection. Hypothalamus-pituitary-adrenal axis suppression is rare, unless the steroid is applied to large areas of denuded skin or mucosal surfaces where absorption levels are higher.

■ FIXED-DRUG ERUPTION/GENERALIZED BULLOUS FIXED-DRUG ERUPTION

Fixed-drug eruptions are characterized by well-demarcated pink to violaceous plaques, with or without blisters. Lesions favor the face, extremities, and genitalia, and typically occur at the same sites upon re-exposure. Affected areas resolve with postinflammatory hyperpigmentation. Onset is usually within 1 to 2 weeks of first exposure to the culprit medication, and then within 24 hours of subsequent exposures. In generalized bullous fixed-drug eruption (GBFDE), there are multiple cutaneous lesions, often with central blisters and areas of detached epidermis. Histopathology may reveal necrotic keratinocytes and resemble Stevens-Johnson syndrome or toxic epidermal necrolysis. However, unlike more severe drug reactions, GBFDE has limited mucosal involvement, mild systemic symptoms, no visceral involvement, and good prognosis. The history of similar lesions at the same sites upon prior medication exposure is most helpful in distinguishing this entity. These patients usually do not require transfer to a burn unit.

■ THE FEBRILE PATIENT WITH MUCOSAL SYMPTOMS

Stevens-Johnson syndrome and toxic epidermal necrolysis

Mucosal symptoms should always prompt the clinician to consider an early cutaneous drug reaction. Although the incidence of SJS and TEN are low (1.2-6 per million and 0.4-1.2 per million, respectively), they are associated with a combined mortality of 20% to 25%. SJS and TEN represent a clinical spectrum of disease which should not be confused with erythema multiforme. Whereas erythema multiforme is typically a postinfectious process with limited skin findings (**Figure 145-2**) and low morbidity, SJS/TEN represents a drug-induced systemic spectrum of disease characterized by epidermal necrosis, mucosal membrane involvement, rapid course, and poor prognosis (**Table 145-2**).

Diagnosis should be suspected in the patient with fever, mucosal symptoms, and progressive skin findings. There may be a prodrome of fever, malaise, and upper respiratory tract symptoms. Conjunctival lesions are seen in 85% of cases and range from asymptomatic hyperemia to keratitis, corneal erosions, and pseudomembrane formation. Erosions of the trachea, bronchi, gastrointestinal tract, and urethra may also occur, leading to respiratory compromise, impaired alimentation, and painful micturition. Ill-defined erythematous and violaceous macules with two zones of colors (atypical target lesions) begin on the upper trunk and spread to the extremities over 1 to 4 days. Keratinocyte necrosis produces flaccid blisters that spread with pressure (positive Nikolsky sign) and lead to epidermal sloughing (**Figure 145-3**). Although controversial, the distinction

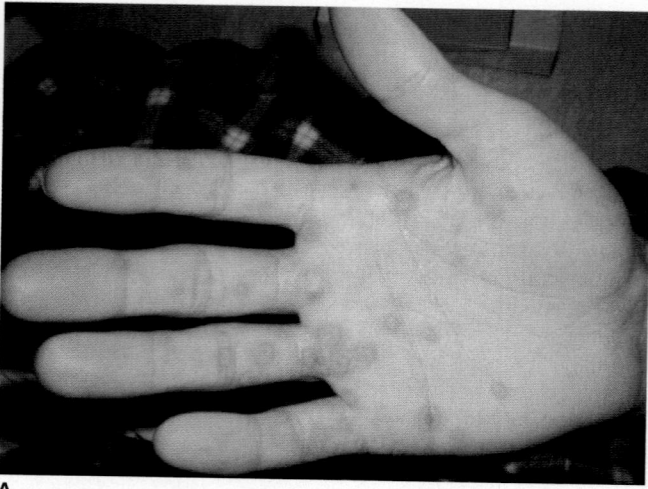

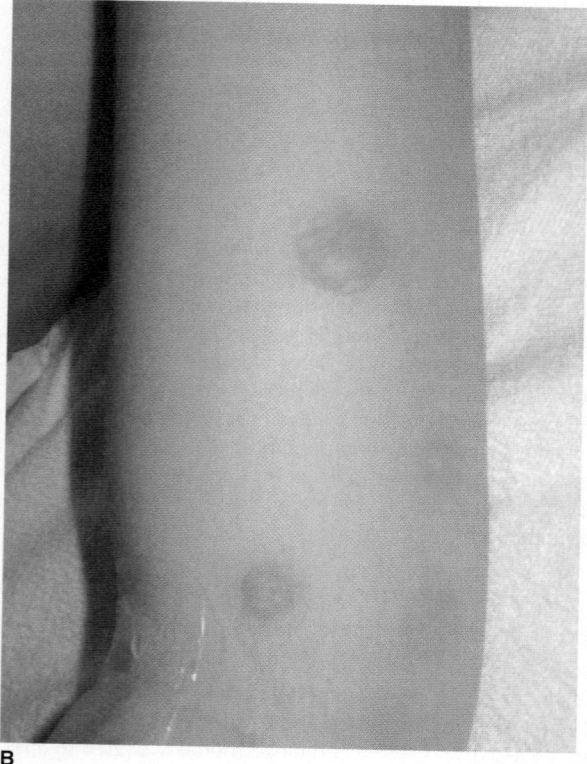

Figure 145-2 *Erythema multiforme. (A) Typical target lesions with three zones of color on the palm. (B) Similar target lesions with three zones of color (dusky and bullous center surrounded by an erythematous ring and an outer, light pink halo) with limited skin involvement.*

■ THE PATIENT WITH CUTANEOUS FINDINGS AND SIGNS OF END ORGAN DAMAGE

Drug reaction with eosinophilia and systemic symptoms (DRESS)

Previously associated with the aromatic anticonvulsant agents, DRESS is now known to be associated with other medications, including sulfonamides, antibiotics, calcium channel blockers, antivirals, and allopurinol. Symptoms usually begin 2 to 6 weeks after drug initiation (Table 145-2). Diagnosis should be suspected in the febrile patient with an evolving morbilliform rash (**Figure 145-4**), lymphadenopathy, eosinophilia (>1500/mm³), atypical lymphocytes, and transaminitis. Macules and papules evolve to form edematous and confluent plaques with perifollicular accentuation. Facial edema may be prominent. The cutaneous findings may resemble SJS if vesicles form secondary to dermal edema. Rarely, small pustules are observed, and the diagnosis may be confused with acute generalized exanthematous pustulosis. Dermatologic consultation and a skin biopsy can help distinguish these entities (**Table 145-3**). Evidence of visceral involvement may also be a distinguishing feature of DRESS. Up to 50% of patients develop a potentially life-threatening hepatitis (compared with 10% of patients with SJS/TEN). Other visceral complications include arthralgias, pericarditis, pulmonary infiltrates, and interstitial nephritis. Reactivation of human herpesvirus 6 (HHV-6) is frequently found in these patients and may predispose them to immunosuppression and subsequent bacterial infections. No prognostic factors have been identified. Mortality is 10%. DRESS can also induce an autoimmune thyroiditis; thyroid function tests should be checked 6 weeks after diagnosis, as prolonged hypothyroidism has been reported.

Drug-induced pseudolymphoma (**Table 145-4**) may also present with infiltrated plaques, lymphadenopathy, and similar histologic findings on lymph node biopsy. However, unlike DRESS, pseudolymphoma presents insidiously, lacks systemic involvement, and has a much better prognosis.

Urticaria, angioedema, and anaphylaxis

In a patient with urticaria, facial edema, or stridor and wheezing, drug-induced angioedema and anaphylaxis must be considered. IgE-mediated hypersensitivity reactions can occur within minutes to hours of drug exposure. The presence of urticaria, defined as itchy, edematous papules, and plaques of varying size with central pallor, may signal an IgE-mediated reaction. Pale, pink swellings of the face and mucosal surfaces that are painful rather than itchy, often persisting for >24 hours, are suggestive of angioedema, and must be evaluated more closely. Anaphylaxis, or cardiopulmonary compromise in the setting of systemic vasodilatation, is rare (80-100 cases/million/year). Drug allergies account for 18% of cases of anaphylaxis. The most common drug culprits are penicillins, anesthetic agents, and radiocontrast.

Non–IgE-mediated mechanisms also produce angioedema. Angiotensin-converting enzyme inhibitors (ACEI)-induced angioedema affects up to 0.1% to 0.7% of patients taking this class of medications. It presents as acute-onset nonpitting edema that may occur weeks to years after the medication was started. African-Americans, hemodialysis patients, and those with a history of idiopathic angioedema are at higher risk. While swelling of the lips and anterior tongue are the most common presentations and often the most visibly concerning, clinicians should carefully evaluate the palate and oropharynx, as swelling of these sites is more predictive of need for intubation.

Other causes of urticaria and angioedema that must be considered include infections and exposures, such as insect bites and food. Urticaria without angioedema can also be seen in common drug rashes, vasculitis, neutrophilic dermatoses, and early bullous

between SJS and TEN is based on the percentage of body surface area (BSA) with epidermal detachment (<10% SJS, >30% TEN, 10%-30% overlap SJS/TEN). This is important for prognosis and treatment. Laboratory findings may include anemia and lymphopenia. Neutropenia is rare and associated with worse prognosis.

Diagnosis is clinical, but skin biopsy and immunofluorescence studies may be of value in excluding other bullous and mucosal disorders, such as staphylococcal scalded skin syndrome, bullous pemphigoid, linear IgA, pemphigus vulgaris, and paraneoplastic pemphigus. The hospitalist should also ask about risk factors for other blistering disorders, such as thermal burns, phototoxic burns, and pressure blisters.

TABLE 145-2 Characteristics of Major Severe Cutaneous Drug Reactions

Drug Reaction	Cutaneous Findings	Mucosal Involvement	Percentage That Are Drug Induced (%)	Time Interval from Start of Drug and Onset of Reaction	Mortality (%)	Selected Responsible Drugs
Stevens-Johnson syndrome	Dusky, atypical target lesions, <10% of BSA	Yes	50	1-3 wk	5	Sulfonamides
						Anticonvulsants
Toxic epidermal necrolysis	Confluent erythema, large sheets of necrotic epidermis, >30% BSA	Yes	>80	1-3 wk	30	NSAIDs
						Allopurinol
DRESS	Facial edema, edematous plaques with perifollicular accentuation	No	70-90	2-6 wk	5-10	Anticonvulsants
						Sulfonamides
						Allopurinol
						Minocycline
						Lamotrigine
AGEP	Widespread erythema with nonfollicular sterile pustules	Rare (20%)	70-90	<4 d	1-2	Beta-lactam antibiotics
						Macrolides
						Calcium channel blockers

AGEP, acute generalized exanthematous pustulosis; BSA, body surface area; DRESS, drug reaction with eosinophilia and systemic symptoms.

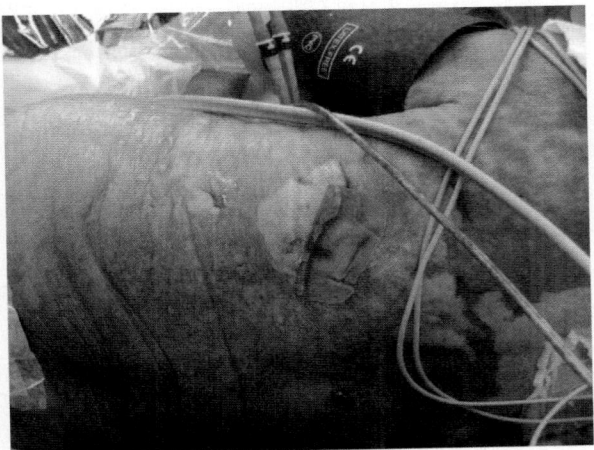

Figure 145-3 *Toxic epidermal necrolysis. Large dusky patches with flaccid blisters and areas of desquamation.*

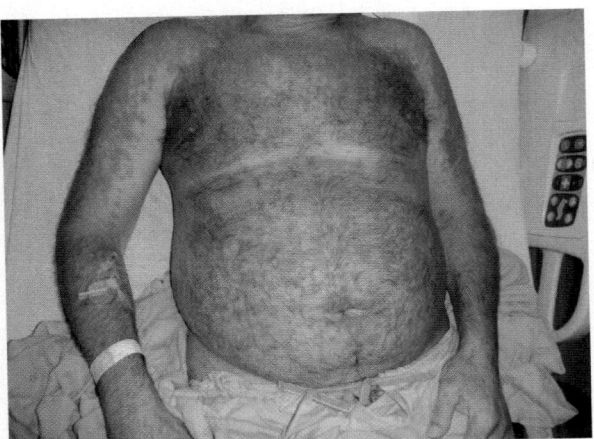

Figure 145-4 *Drug reaction with eosinophilia and systemic symptoms. Erythematous to violaceous macules and papules coalescing into patches on the chest and abdomen of a patient with early drug reaction with eosinophilia and systemic symptoms.*

pemphigoid. When angioedema occurs without urticaria and drug reactions have been excluded, the clinician should consider C1 esterase deficiency.

Drug-induced vasculitis

Adverse drug reactions account for approximately 10% of cases of leukocytoclastic vasculitis, or cutaneous small vessel vasculitis. Blood vessel inflammation and even necrosis may occur from drug-induced immune complex deposition, complement activation, and granulocyte recruitment. Common medication culprits are NSAIDs, penicillins, cephalosporins, sulfonamides, allopurinol, and propyl-thiouracil. Signs and symptoms begin within 1 to 2 weeks of first exposure and less than 3 days after re-exposure. Palpable purpura on the lower extremities is the classic cutaneous finding, but hemorrhagic blisters, ulcers, nodules, and urticaria may also be observed. While systemic involvement is rare, blood vessel inflammation can become widespread and affect the kidney, liver, gastrointestinal tract, or nervous system. Patients should be screened for systemic symptoms including fever, headache, abdominal pain, hematuria, and peripheral neuropathy. Urinary sediment and fecal occult blood should be checked in addition to a complete blood count and basic metabolic panel. Histopathology shows fibrinoid necrosis and direct immunofluorescence may reveal IgM and C3 deposits in the capillary wall. Patients who develop drug-induced vasculitis to propylthiouracil, hydralazine, or minocycline may have a positive antimyeloperoxidase antibody.

TABLE 145-3 Indications for Considering Dermatologic Consultation in Adverse Cutaneous Drug Reaction

Uncertainty regarding indication for skin biopsy

Uncertainty regarding indication for systemic steroids or intravenous immunoglobulin in patient with Stevens-Johnson syndrome and toxic epidermal necrolysis

Clinicopathologic correlation

TABLE 145-4 Drug Reactions That Mimic Systemic Disease

Presentation	Clinical Findings	Time Between Start of Drug and Onset of Symptoms	Resolution with Drug Discontinuation	Common Drug Culprits
Erythema nodosum	Bilateral, tender, erythematous nodules (mainly on shins)	Weeks	Yes	Oral contraceptive pills Estrogens Sulfonamides Penicillin Bromides Iodides Azathioprine
Subacute cutaneous lupus-like reaction	Psoriasiform or annular lesions on trunk, arms, and extensor surfaces	At least 1 y	Sometimes	Hydrochlorothiazide Calcium channel blockers Terbinafine NSAIDs Griseofulvin Docetaxel PUVA Interferon
Systemic lupus-like reaction	Fever, weight loss, serositis; cutaneous findings are uncommon	Variable	Yes	Procainamide Hydralazine Chlorpromazine Isoniazid Methyldopa Propylthiouracil Quinidine Practolol D-penicillamine PUVA Minocycline
Neutrophilic eccrine hidradenitis	Erythematous papules and plaques surrounding eccrine glands	7-14 d	Yes	Cytarabine Mitoxantrone Bleomycin Anthracyclines Methotrexate Cyclophosphamide Acetaminophen
Sweet syndrome (acute febrile neutrophilic dermatoses)	Painful, erythematous plaques (mainly on face and upper extremities)	Days	Yes	G-CSF All-*trans*-retinoic acid
Pseudoporphyria	Skin fragility, erosions, blisters, and scarring (mainly on dorsal hands, face and extensor surfaces of legs)	Variable	Yes	NSAIDs Furosemide Tetracycline Retinoids UVA exposure (including tanning beds) Hemodialysis
Pseudolymphoma	Solitary or widespread erythematous to violaceous papules, plaques, and nodules; lymphadenopathy and erythroderma may occur	Months to years	Yes	Phenobarbital Carbamazepine Chlorpromazine Promethazine Imatinib mesylate Angiotensin-2–receptor antagonists

(Continued)

TABLE 145-4 Drug Reactions That Mimic Systemic Disease (*Continued*)

Presentation	Clinical Findings	Time Between Start of Drug and Onset of Symptoms	Resolution with Drug Discontinuation	Common Drug Culprits
Pemphigus	Flaccid blisters, erosions of skin, and mucous membranes	Weeks to months	Sometimes	Penicillamine ACE inhibitors Gold sodium thiomalate Pyritinol
Linear-IgA bullous dermatosis	Tense vesicles in an annular configuration	1-15 d	Yes	Vancomycin Beta-lactam antibiotics Captopril NSAIDs
Granulomas	Firm, mobile cutaneous nodules; may be tender and ulcerate	Years	No	Injection of talc or starch products
Skin necrosis	Painful plaques and hemorrhagic blisters evolve into necrotic ulcers and ischemic infarcts; most common sites: breasts, thighs, and buttocks	2-5 d	No	Warfarin Heparin

ACE, angiotensin-converting enzyme; G-CSF, granulocyte colony-stimulating factor; NSAID, nonsteroidal anti-inflammatory drug; PUVA, psoralen ultraviolet-A radiation.

In the evaluation of a suspected drug-induced vasculitis, the possibility of an underlying infection must be excluded first. Other diagnostic considerations include Henoch-Schönlein purpura, polyarteritis nodosa, and granulomatosis with polyangiitis (Wegener granulomatosis). These entities may all present as small vessel vasculitis of the skin; features of leukocytoclastic vasculitis, in isolation, would not discriminate among these entities. Skin biopsies in certain conditions are only high-yield when taken within the first 2 days of cutaneous eruption, so a dermatology consult should be called early if it is deemed necessary. If the vasculitis is thought to be drug-related, symptoms should resolve with discontinuation. Systemic steroids are only indicated in visceral involvement.

■ THE PATIENT WITH CONFLUENT ERYTHEMA

Acute generalized exanthematous pustulosis

Acute generalized exanthematous pustulosis (AGEP) is a rare drug reaction with low mortality that may present with widespread erythema, and mimic other more life-threatening entities. AGEP presents within the first few days of drug exposure. Initial signs include high fevers (38°C), and widespread erythema that begins on the face and spreads centrifugally, favoring the intertriginous areas. Numerous, small, nonfollicular, sterile pustules appear on top of the erythema (**Figure 145-5**). Pustules may persist for up to 10 days. A characteristic pinpoint pattern of desquamation follows. Edema of the hands and face may be observed. Patients frequently report skin pain and burning. Mucosal involvement occurs in only 20% of patients, and usually presents as a localized oral erosion. Leukocytosis (>10,000/mL) and a mild eosinophilia may be present in a third of patients. Systemic involvement is rare. Estimated incidence is 1 to 5 cases/million. The most common culprits are beta-lactam antibiotics, macrolides, calcium channel blockers, and antimalarials.

Distinguishing AGEP from pustular psoriasis and Sneddon-Wilkinson disease (a recurrent, superficial pustular dermatosis with a polycyclic pattern and flexural accentuation) may be challenging. Features that distinguish AGEP include its short course, association

with new drug exposure, and histopathologic characteristics (superficial dermal edema, leukocytoclastic vasculitis, eosinophils, and focal keratinocyte necrosis). If the pustules are not appreciated on exam, the disease may resemble drug-induced erythroderma, toxic epidermal necrolysis, or staphylococcal scalded skin syndrome. Skin biopsy and dermatologic consultation may be of value if the diagnosis is unclear (Table 145-3).

Erythroderma

Erythroderma, or exfoliative dermatitis, is defined as a generalized erythema and scaling that involves more than 90% of the skin surface. Common associated signs and symptoms include fever, lymphadenopathy, edema, and pruritus. Medications are the second most common cause of erythroderma (20%). Other causes include

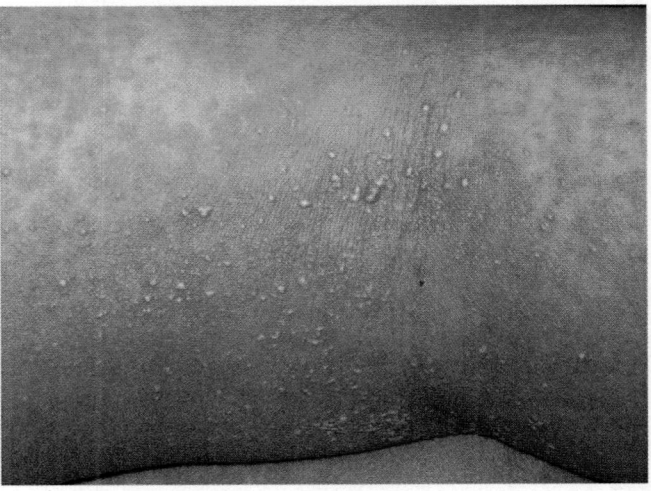

Figure 145-5 *Acute generalized exanthematous pustulosis. Widespread erythema with numerous, pinpoint, nonfollicular, sterile pustules.*

TABLE 145-5 Differential Diagnosis of Erythroderma

1. Primary dermatoses
   - Atopic dermatitis
   - Seborrheic dermatitis
   - Psoriasis
   - Pityriasis rubra pilaris
   - Pemphigus foliaceous
2. Infections
   - Human immunodeficiency virus
   - Staphylococcal scalded skin syndrome
   - Hepatitis
3. Neoplasm
   - Cutaneous T-cell lymphoma
   - Sezary syndrome
   - Malignant histiocytosis
   - Acute and chronic leukemias
   - Solid tumors (colon, lung, prostate, thyroid, fallopian tubes, larynx, and esophagus)
   - Reticular cell sarcoma
4. Medications (common examples)
   - Allopurinol
   - Beta-lactam antibiotics
   - Aromatic anticonvulsants
   - Sulfonamides
5. Idiopathic

generalization of an underlying dermatosis (50%) such as psoriasis, atopic dermatitis, seborrheic dermatitis, or contact dermatitis, neoplasms (10%), and infections (**Table 145-5**). No etiology is identified in up to 25% of cases. Drug-induced erythroderma is characterized by its acute onset, initial morbilliform appearance, and relatively short course, resolving within 2 to 6 weeks of drug discontinuation. Increased peripheral blood flow can produce facial edema, hepatomegaly, and systemic complications including tachycardia, high output heart failure, and thermoregulatory disturbances. A high prevalence of erythroderma has been reported among patients with human immunodeficiency virus (HIV), and an HIV test should be checked in all patients with risk factors. Of the many medications implicated, the most common culprits include allopurinol, beta-lactam antibiotics, and aromatic anticonvulsants. Histopathology is often helpful in ruling out other potential causes, and multiple skin biopsies may be required if the initial pathology is inconclusive.

■ THE PATIENT WITH A BULLOUS ERUPTION

While some patients develop bullae secondary to necrosis of the epidermis or dermal and epidermal edema, others will develop a primary bullous eruption that is autoimmune in nature. When evaluating a bullous eruption, the clinician can gather important information from the morphology of the blister and its characteristics. Testing for the Nikolsky sign is performed by rubbing skin adjacent to a blister and observing whether the blister spreads laterally. If the blister spreads easily, it is a positive Nikolsky sign, as may be seen in pemphigus vulgaris. If bullae are tense and fail to spread with adjacent pressure (negative Nikolsky sign), one should consider an autoimmune blistering disease affecting the hemidesmosome at the basement membrane zone, such as bullous pemphigoid. Flaccid

bullae, with a positive Nikolsky sign, are usually indicative of autoimmune processes that occur from defects in proteins located more superficially in the epidermis.

Drug-induced bullous pemphigoid

Bullous pemphigoid (BP) is an autoimmune blistering process due to circulating autoantibodies that target bullous pemphigoid antigens 1 and 2 (BPAG-1 and BPAG-2). These antigens are found in the hemidesmosome at the junction of the epidermis and dermis. Histopathologically, one sees an inflammatory infiltrate of eosinophils with marked epidermal and dermal edema. Patients may complain of pruritus. On clinical exam, tense bullae filled with serous fluid are seen (**Figure 145-6**). The oropharynx is involved in roughly 20% of the afflicted. A pruritic, urticarial, "prebullous phase" will often precede the development of frank bullae. BP is usually an acquired autoimmune condition not linked with medication usage, but occasional cases of drug-induced BP are seen in patients who have recently started a new medication. The most common culprits are furosemide, captopril, enalapril, penicillins, sulfonamides, and penicillamine. If this diagnosis is suspected, dermatology consultation may help to distinguish this entity from other blistering disorders. Biopsy with direct immunofluorescence (DIF) is performed when the dermatologist deems it necessary; it requires the use of an appropriate preservative when collecting the skin tissue sample. In DIF, the patient's skin is used as a substrate, and fluorescent-labeled anti-IgG, IgA, IgM, or C3 antibodies are mixed with the sample so that preexisting antibody complexes on the patient's skin can be further tagged by the new fluorescent-labeled antibody. In doing so, one is able to identify not only the subtype of immune complex on the patient's skin but also the location at which the concentration of immune complexes is highest. In this way, one can differentiate superficial and deep blistering processes. Furthermore, the pattern of fluorescence can give clues as to the underlying diagnosis. DIF in BP shows a linear band of IgG and C3 along the basement membrane.

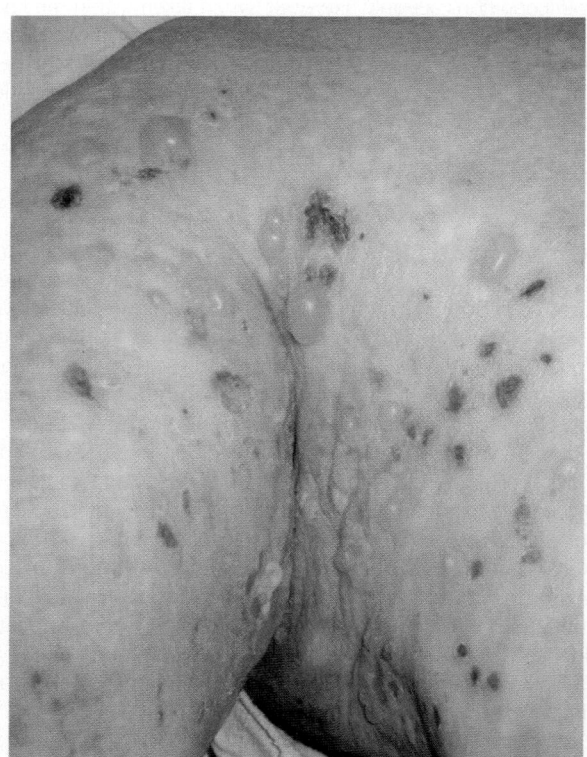

Figure 145-6 *Drug-induced bullous pemphigoid. Tense bullae on urticarial and pink plaques, with areas of hemorrhagic crusting.*

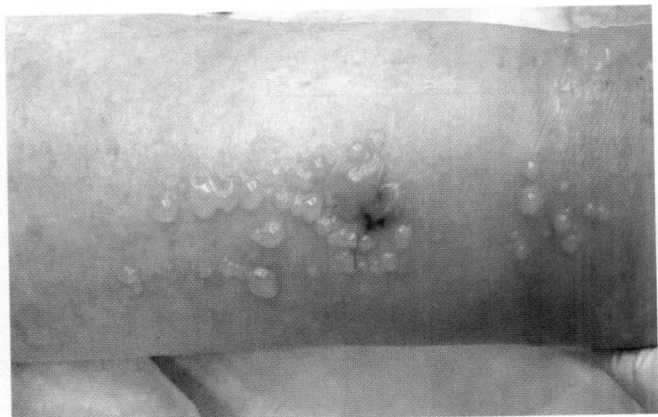

Figure 145-7 *Linear IgA. Tense bullae in an annular and serpiginous configuration.*

Linear IgA bullous dermatosis

Linear IgA bullous dermatosis is characterized by tense bullae filled with serous fluid, similar to BP. However, most patients develop these lesions in an annular configuration (**Figure 145-7**). Half of these patients also have mucosal involvement, which can lead to scarring. Much like BP, this entity is from autoantibodies, targeting BPAG2 more often than BPAG1. As opposed to BP, direct immunofluorescence demonstrates a linear band of IgA at the basement membrane zone (hence the name). Vancomycin is the drug most commonly linked to this type of eruption. Lithium, amiodarone, carbamazepine, penicillins, moxifloxacin, furosemide, phenytoin, diclofenac, statins, ACE inhibitors, and angiotensin-receptor blockers have also been implicated. A different form of this disease occurs in the pediatric population, which is usually not drug-induced.

Drug-induced pemphigus vulgaris

Drug-induced pemphigus vulgaris (PV) presents as flaccid bullae with serous fluid. While BP is typically associated with pruritus, PV usually induces a burning pain. In many cases, bullae may not be present on exam, and the clinician may only observe erosions and collarettes of scale at sites of previous blisters. PV is an autoimmune process from autoantibodies targeting desmoglein 3, with or without involvement of desmoglein 1. These proteins are in the desmosome, a structure that joins keratinocytes. Patients usually have mucosal sloughing characterized by desquamative gingivitis, with erosions also occurring elsewhere in the oropharynx. When PV presents in a patient who has recently started a new medication, a drug-induced eruption should be considered. Common culprit drugs include angiotensive converting enzyme (ACE) inhibitors, penicillins, calcium channel blockers, and rifampin. A dermatology consultation should be considered, as flaccid bullae with mucosal involvement should trigger the practitioner to exclude SJS/TEN as a potential entity. Unlike SJS/TEN, PV patients are less systemically ill, and rarely have fever or other systemic symptoms and signs unless superinfection is present.

■ THE PATIENT WITH AN ACNEIFORM ERUPTION

Steroid-induced acneiform eruption

Patients on systemic steroids can develop an acneiform and pustular eruption. This is typically acute and widespread in nature, involving the face, trunk, and upper arms. As opposed to acne vulgaris, steroid-induced acne is composed of clusters of monomorphic, often follicular, papules and pustules with an inflammatory base. Comedonal lesions are rare. Patients can develop this eruption even with courses of steroid as short as 3 to 5 days. Treatment includes

topical antibiotics, such as clindamycin, and topical retinoids, such as tretinoin, a vitamin A analog. If particularly bothersome or severe, systemic antibiotics can be used for their anti-inflammatory properties as well. Of note, topical steroids, especially the fluorinated types, can also induce an acneiform eruption.

Acneiform eruption related to EGFR inhibitors

Ninety percent of patients on epidermal-growth factor receptor (EGFR) inhibitors report cutaneous side effects, with acneiform eruptions being most common. This papulopustular eruption is dose-dependent and usually occurs 7 to 10 days after initiation of the therapy. Patients often complain of pruritus. The head, neck, and upper back are the most commonly affected sites. Clinical exam demonstrates follicular papules and pustules without comedones. The severity of the eruption is correlated with response to therapy, so some oncologists titrate the dosage to the eruption. Treatment can include topical antibiotics, topical steroids, or tretinoin. Oral antibiotics may be used. In severe cases, oral retinoids, such as isotretinoin or acitretin, have been helpful.

■ THE PATIENT WITH ACRAL ERYTHEMA

Palmoplantar erythrodysesthesia/hand-foot syndrome (HFS)

Usually seen in the oncologic population, this reaction occurs in a dose-dependent manner with certain chemotherapeutic agents and may be related to the high concentration of sweat glands in the hands and feet. Patients usually experience tingling in the palms and soles first, followed by painful, symmetric erythema, and edema (**Figure 145-8**). Flexural areas may also be affected. Erythema may spread to involve the rest of the body. Over time, the erythematous skin may blister and desquamate, eventually re-epithelializing. The most common chemotherapeutic agents that cause this reaction include 5-fluorouracil, doxorubicine, and cytosine arabinoside. Graft-versus-host disease (GVHD) should be considered, as this also occurs in oncology patients and has a predilection for the acral surfaces. Treatment is supportive, including ice packs and elevation. Oral pyrodoxine may be preventative.

Hand-foot skin reaction (HFSR)

HFSR is usually associated with multityrosine kinase inhibitors, such as sorafenib and sunitib. Like HFS, HFSR also has a predilection for the acral surfaces and is a dose-dependent reaction. However, HFSR is accompanied by hyperkeratosis of the weight-bearing areas of the feet, as well as the friction-prone areas of the hands. There is usually

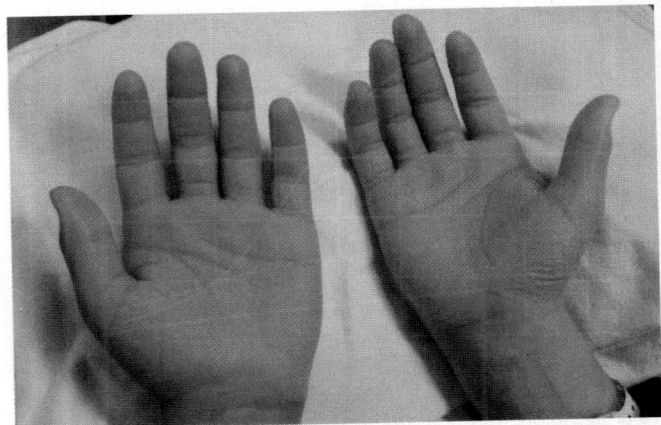

Figure 145-8 *Acral erythema, hand-foot syndrome. Severe erythema on the palms. Note the abrupt end to the eruption at the base of the hand.*

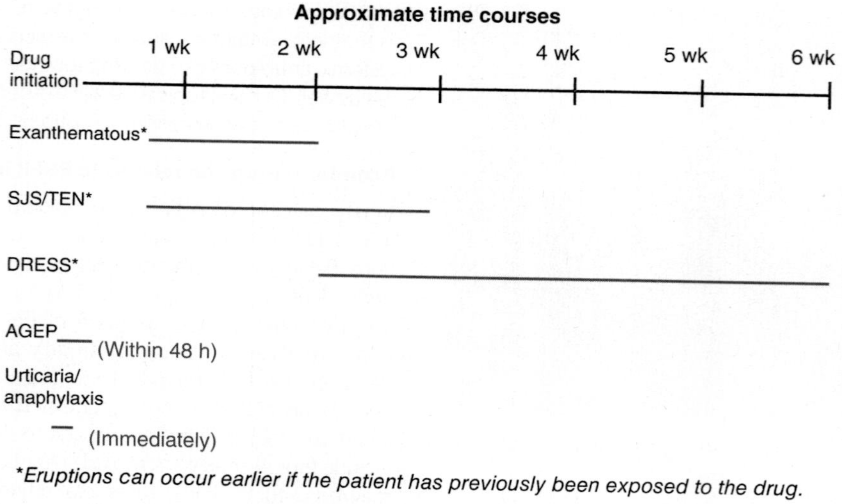

Approximate time courses

Figure 145-9 *Relative time courses. Describes when each particular type of drug eruption occurs in relation to stopping the drug.*

less erythema and pain than in HFS. Treatment targets areas of hyperkeratosis with urea cream, topical retinoids, and topical steroids.

■ USING THE TIMELINE TO IDENTIFY THE CULPRIT

The morphology and timeline of drug-induced eruptions can assist the clinician in deciding which drug is the likeliest offender. This is critical, as most drug eruptions can be terminated by discontinuation of the responsible agent. By knowing the time course associated with each type of adverse cutaneous eruption, one can usually identify the likely culprit drug (**Figure 145-9**). For certain eruptions, such as urticaria, anaphylaxis, and AGEP, only a single exposure to the drug is necessary. However, in exanthematous drug eruptions, SJS/TEN, and DRESS, the drug has usually been administered for multiple days.

■ SPECIAL CONSIDERATIONS IN THE IMMUNOCOMPROMISED POPULATION

Studies of adverse cutaneous drug reactions consistently demonstrate that patients with underlying immunosuppression, including malignancy, connective tissue disease, liver failure, renal failure and HIV, are at increased risk for drug rashes. Diagnosis is more challenging in these populations, because they are also at risk for other clinical syndromes with skin findings that may mimic a drug eruption.

Among HIV-positive patients, drug-related eruptions are 100 times more common than in the general population. Contributing factors include multiple medications, altered drug metabolism, increased oxidative stress, and immune dysregulation. Higher risk of rash is associated with decreasing CD4+ cell count, age, underlying skin disease, and viral reactivation. If the medication is necessary and the reaction is limited to the skin, the medication may be continued. However, the clinician should be aware that HIV patients are more liable to progress to SJS/TEN. Other serious conditions that may masquerade as a morbilliform exanthem in the HIV patient include Kawasaki disease, recalcitrant erythematous desquamating disorder (a chronic staphylococcal infection), and exacerbations of underlying dermatoses.

Morbilliform rash in the transplant population is most often due to an antibiotic or chemotherapeutic agent. As these patients are frequently thrombocytopenic, the eruption may appear more purpuric. Other diagnoses that must be considered include eruption of lymphocyte recovery, acute cutaneous graft-versus-host disease

(GVHD), engraftment syndrome, and viral infection. Acute GVHD may be difficult to distinguish from a drug reaction, and skin biopsy may not be diagnostic. Features that suggest acute GVHD include a rash that favors the scalp, ears, hands and feet, associated diarrhea, and elevated liver function tests. Once acute GVHD is suspected, systemic steroids should be initiated.

Some immunocompromised patients develop cutaneous drug reactions as expected side effects of their potent medications. An example is the papulopustular eruption associated with epidermal growth factor receptor inhibitors. This reaction is rarely life-threatening, and most patients are able to continue the medication with symptomatic treatment for the rash.

■ PATIENTS WITH SIGNS OF NEW SYSTEMIC DISEASE

Medications may provoke a wide spectrum of systemic diseases, including lupus, erythema nodosum, and neutrophilic dermatoses. In a patient on multiple medications who presents with signs or symptoms of a new systemic disease, a drug reaction should always be excluded prior to initiating treatment. Drug-induced syndromes usually resolve once the medication is discontinued. Table 145-4 provides a brief overview of the major classes of systemic disease which may be drug-induced, the most common culprits, and the effect of medication discontinuation.

DIFFERENTIAL DIAGNOSIS

■ BACTERIAL INFECTIONS

Bacterial infections should always be excluded before diagnosing an adverse cutaneous drug reaction. Staphylococcal scalded skin syndrome (SSSS) presents with fever, skin tenderness, and confluent erythema with overlying superficial blisters, which may initially resemble TEN. Although generally a disease of infants, SSSS can occur in adults with renal failure, immunosuppression, malignancy, chronic alcohol abuse, or HIV. The disease is mediated by an exfoliative toxin of *Staphylococcal aureus* that targets desmoglein 1, causing interdesmosomal splitting and blistering in the superficial epidermis. Features that distinguish SSSS from TEN include the superficial nature of the blister and its fragility (TEN forms subepidermal blisters), a negative Nikolsky sign, although this test is imperfect, and the absence of significant mucosal findings. Cultures of bullae are negative, but *S. aureus* may be isolated from the nasopharynx or blood. Early diagnosis is critical, as mortality among adults can be greater than 50%.

Staphylococcal and streptococcal toxic shock syndromes are characterized by fever, macular erythema, and multiorgan system failure, and may also resemble SJS/TEN. Recent surgery, upper respiratory tract infection, or tampon use are classically associated with staphylococcal toxic shock syndrome, whereas a history of recent trauma or soft tissue infection may be more suggestive of streptococcal toxic shock. In patients with this constellation of signs and no recent medication exposure, these diagnoses should be strongly considered. Blood cultures are positive in 15% of staphylococcal toxic shock cases and 50% of streptococcal toxic shock cases.

■ VIRAL INFECTIONS

Many viral infections present with prodromal symptoms, a morbilliform eruption, and systemic features that may mimic an adverse cutaneous drug eruption. Measles and rubella are still reported among communities with poor vaccination rates, and are rarely complicated by secondary bacterial infections, encephalitis, or thrombocytopenic purpura. In adults, parvovirus B19 presents with a diffuse, web-like (reticulate) rash, fever, and arthralgias. Epstein-Barr virus (EBV) usually follows a self-limited course with fever, pharyngitis, and lymphadenopathy. A macular rash is seen in 10% of patients, but the incidence may be as high as 90% in patients who have received ampicillin or amoxicillin. Severe complications of EBV include hepatitis and airway compromise. In bone marrow transplant patients, the most common viral infection is cytomegalovirus, which typically presents 30 to 100 days after transplant, and may lead to fatal pneumonitis. Patients may develop a morbilliform eruption and perianal erosions. Some centers perform weekly antigen tests in post-transplant patients. Finally, primary HIV infection must always be considered. A nonpruritic, photodistributed, macular rash is seen in 40% to 50% of patients during acute HIV infection (2-6 weeks postexposure).

■ ANGIOIMMUNOBLASTIC T-CELL LYMPHOMA

Angioimmunoblastic T-cell lymphoma (AITL), the second most common peripheral T-cell lymphoma, may present acutely with a diffuse, pruritic morbilliform rash, fever, and lymphadenopathy. The constellation of symptoms and the frequent accompanying eosinophilia may closely resemble drug reaction with eosinophilia and systemic symptoms. Distinguishing features of AITL include a polyclonal hypergammaglobulinemia (seen in 80% of patients), hemolytic anemia, and specific findings on lymph node biopsy. Treatment involves corticosteroids or cytotoxic agents. Prognosis is poor, with mortality of 50% to 72%, and a median survival of 11 to 30 months.

■ PRIMARY DERMATOLOGIC DISEASE

Exacerbation of an underlying dermatologic disease may have an acute and impressive presentation. Patients with psoriasis who are treated with systemic steroids for another condition may experience a severe generalized pustular version of psoriasis when the steroids are discontinued. A review of the patient's past dermatologic history should be performed when evaluating a potential drug reaction.

TRIAGE/HOSPITAL ADMISSION

Hospital admission is not required for reliable patients with classic morbilliform eruptions related to a known culprit, in the absence of mucosal or systemic involvement. These patients may be observed in the outpatient setting and managed symptomatically, as long as they are aware of possible complications (the "red flags" of Table 145-1) and have access to an emergency department. In these patients, the culprit drug should be discontinued. In extraordinary circumstances where the culprit drug is required, no alternative exists, and the cutaneous eruption is benign, the drug may be continued with frequent monitoring for systemic involvement. Symptomatic treatment of associated pruritus includes oral antihistamines and topical steroids.

Hospital admission is indicated for any patient with a progressive cutaneous eruption of unclear etiology or the patient with a known cutaneous drug reaction who has mucosal involvement, immunocompromise, blisters, or signs of a systemic inflammatory response, including two or more of the following: fever, tachycardia, tachypnea, and leukocytosis or leukopenia.

COMPLICATIONS
■ MUCOSAL DAMAGE

Ocular sequelae may affect up to 35% of patients who survive SJS/TEN. The most common complication is a dry eye syndrome. More serious sequelae include corneal scarring and ocular vascularization, which may lead to permanent visual loss. Ocular sequelae cannot be predicted by percentage of body surface area involved, currently used SJS/TEN severity scores, or ocular symptoms during the acute stage. No preventive treatment regimens have been identified, but early studies suggest that amniotic membrane transplantation may be of use in some cases as an anti-inflammatory mediator. All patients with SJS/TEN should be evaluated routinely by ophthalmology during hospitalization and after discharge.

■ HEPATITIS

Fulminant hepatitis is the most common cause of death associated with DRESS. Liver biopsies show an eosinophilic infiltrate, granulomas and hepatocyte necrosis. Early recognition of DRESS and discontinuation of the culprit drug are critical to prevent hepatic damage. High-dose steroids can be considered. Of note, hepatitis may persist for several weeks after drug withdrawal, and patients should be monitored closely.

■ SEPSIS

In patients with toxic epidermal necrolysis, sepsis is the most common cause of death. Early transfer to an intensive care unit, daily wound care, and periodic blood cultures can help prevent the morbidity and mortality associated with sepsis.

TREATMENT
■ SJS/TEN

Early discontinuation of the culprit drug reduces mortality and should be the primary intervention. All medications, especially those introduced within 1 month of the reaction, should be considered as a possible culprit, and discontinued. If widespread skin involvement is present (>30% BSA), the patient should be transferred to an intensive care unit or burn unit. A severity scoring system has been developed to predict prognosis (**Table 145-6**). Important complications to consider are fluid loss (approximately 3-4 L daily in adults with 50% BSA involved), renal insufficiency, diffuse interstitial pneumonitis, and sepsis. Treatment includes supportive measures such as daily wound care, eye lubrication, pain control, nutritional support, and fluid replacement. All patients should have a routine ophthalmologic evaluation, and gynecologic evaluation should be considered when appropriate. Patients may require mechanical ventilation.

There is no clear consensus on systemic treatment. As SJS/TEN is rare, randomized placebo-controlled trials are challenging. Thalidomide, cyclosporine, and cyclophosphamide have been studied to date, with mixed results. Several studies support the use of systemic corticosteroids in SJS, advocating that if administered within the first 2 days, mortality may be decreased. An ongoing controversy exists on the role of human intravenous immunoglobulin (IVIg). A proposed mechanism argues that IVIg may provide FAS-blocking antibodies which interfere with FAS ligand-induced keratinocyte apoptosis. Of the eight clinical studies of IVIg use in adults with SJS/TEN to date (with >10 patients), five showed reduction in

TABLE 145-6 SCORTEN: Severity-of-Illness Score for Toxic Epidermal Necrolysis

Variables	Points
Age (≥40 y)	1
Heart rate (≥120/min)	1
BSA involved at day 1 > 10%	1
Serum urea level (>10 mmol/L)	1
Serum bicarbonate level (>14 mmol/L)	1
Score	**Mortality**
0-1	3
2	12
3	35
4	58
≥5	90

BSA, body surface area.
Data from Bastuji-Garin S, et al. *J Invest Dermatol.* 2000;115:149-153.

mortality associated with a total dose of > 2 g/kg of IVIg over 3 to 4 days. Effect of IVIG likely depends on timing of treatment in disease course, variability in the IVIG batch, dosing, and the patient's comorbidities (particularly renal insufficiency). More recently, the use of cyclosporine has been promising in some small studies, however, practice patterns vary widely depending on the institution and clinician. Importantly, immunosuppressants should be avoided in cases where infection has been proven or is highly suspected.

■ DRESS

In addition to withdrawal of the offending medication, systemic corticosteroids are often advocated for treatment of DRESS, especially when there is associated inflammation of the heart and lungs. The typical starting dose is prednisone 1 mg/kg/d. Steroid dose should be tapered slowly over several weeks, to reduce the risk of relapse.

■ ANGIOEDEMA

All patients with progressive angioedema or possible anaphylaxis should be hospitalized and closely monitored. Severe angioedema must be treated with epinephrine. Otolaryngology should be consulted for airway management. Oral antihistamines, systemic steroids, or both, along with discontinuation of the culprit drug, are the treatment of choice in other cases.

■ AGEP

Treatment of AGEP consists of withdrawal of the culprit medication, topical corticosteroids, and antipyretics. Once the culprit medication is discontinued, resolution of symptoms occurs in a few days.

■ ERYTHRODERMA

Patients with erythroderma and signs of systemic inflammatory response or a history of immunosupression should be hospitalized to avoid complications related to high output heart failure, thermoregulatory disturbances, and the hypercatabolic state. Systemic therapies must be carefully guided by the underlying cause of the erythroderma. While steroids may be beneficial in drug-induced erythroderma, they exacerbate psoriasis, and are contraindicated in staphylococcal scalded skin syndrome (Figure 145-7).

DISCHARGE CONSIDERATIONS

- Has the adverse cutaneous drug reaction been recorded as an allergy in the patient's medical record? Documentation should include the date the culprit drug was initiated and discontinued,

the time of onset of the reaction, associated symptoms, systemic complications (if any), and the treatment provided. Patients who develop symptoms that are known side effects of a medication (eg, nausea while on doxycycline) should not be listed as allergic to the medication.

- Has the patient been clearly educated on what classes of medications to avoid? Patients with a history of DRESS associated with an aromatic anticonvulsant should avoid all other aromatic anticonvulsants (phenytoin, phenobarbital, and carbamazepine), as cross-reactivity approaches 70% to 80%. However, patients with adverse cutaneous drug reactions to sulfonamide antibiotics may not need to avoid other nonantibiotic sulfonamide agents. Research shows that while these patients are at a higher risk of future adverse drug reactions, there may not be cross-reactivity between the antibiotic and nonantibiotic sulfonamide agents.
- If a culprit agent has not been clearly identified, consider outpatient allergy referral.
- Is the patient aware of signs and symptoms that require emergency department evaluation?
- Is the patient aware that certain reactions may rebound with tapering of steroids?

PRACTICE POINT

- Benign morbilliform drug reactions can be impressive in appearance. They will frequently generalize and develop a violaceous hue in dependent areas. Outpatient management of a cutaneous drug reaction is appropriate if the patient is reliable, immunocompetent, well appearing, without mucosal membrane involvement or systemic symptoms, and if the culprit medication is identified. Patients who are not hospitalized should understand what signs and symptoms require further evaluation. Patients should also be aware that their skin findings and the associated pruritus may persist for up to 2 weeks after drug discontinuation.

SUGGESTED READINGS

Barron SJ, Del Vecchio MT, Aronoff SC. Intravenous immunoglobulin in the treatment of Stevens-Johnson syndrome and toxic epidermal necrolysis: a meta-analysis with meta-regression of observational studies. *Int J Dermatol.* 2015;54:108-115.

Frigas E, Park MA. Acute urticaria and angioedema: diagnostic and treatment considerations. *Am J Clin Dermatol.* 2009;10: 239-250.

Gruchalla RS, Pirmohamed M. Antibiotic allergy. *N Engl J Med.* 2006;354:601-609.

Kardaun SH, Jonkman MF. Dexamethasone pulse therapy for Stevens-Johnson syndrome/toxic epidermal necrolysis. *Acta Derm Venereol.* 2007;87:144-148.

Pavlos R, Mallal S, Ostrov D, et al. T cell-mediated hypersensitivity reactions to drugs. *Annu Rev Med.* 2015;66:439-454.

Schneck J, Fagot JP, Sekula P. Effects of treatments on the mortality of Stevens Johnson syndrome and toxic epidermal necrolysis: a retrospective study on patients included in the prospective EuroSCAR Study. *J Am Acad Dermatol.* 2008;58:33-40.

Strom BL, Shinnar R, Apter AJ, Margolis DJ. Absence of cross-reactivity between sulfonamide antibiotics and sulfonamide nonantibiotics. *N Engl J Med.* 2003;349:1628-1635.

Yawalkar N. Drug-induced exanthems. *Toxicology.* 2005;209: 131-134.

CHAPTER 146

Psoriasis and Other Papulosquamous Disorders

Anne E. Allan, MD
Timothy R. Quinn, MD, CM

Key Clinical Questions

1. When should a patient with an erythematous scaly eruption be evaluated for an underlying infectious process?
2. How should the patient with diffuse erythroderma be evaluated?
3. What are the best topical treatments for psoriasis?
4. Are oral steroids useful in the treatment of psoriasis?
5. Are there physical findings that help differentiate between contact and irritant dermatitis?

INTRODUCTION

Papulosquamous disorders are a group of unrelated dermatologic conditions in which patients present with red, raised lesions with scale. While psoriasis is the prototypical papulosquamous disorder, similar skin lesions may be seen in infections, lymphomas, and allergic conditions. The conditions described in this chapter are ubiquitous, and primarily inflammatory in nature. From a clinical point of view, the history, the distribution of the lesions, and careful evaluation of the primary lesion are most helpful in helping establish the diagnosis. Ancillary tests include a KOH preparation, a skin biopsy and, if necessary, dermatologic consultation. It should be remembered that treating a condition without a definitive diagnosis can lead to unnecessary patient aggravation and added expense.

PSORIASIS

Psoriasis, a chronic relapsing condition with genetic and environmental triggers, can be readily diagnosed on skin examination. It is very common. Approximately 2% of the population is affected by psoriasis. In the United States, the prevalence may be as high as 4.6%.

PATHOGENESIS

Psoriasis was formerly likened to "wound healing gone wrong." It was blamed on abnormally rapid keratinocyte growth and maturation, with a reduction of the epidermal turnover time from the normal 4 weeks to only 3 to 4 days. However, psoriasis is now recognized to be a T-cell–mediated disease. Several T helper lymphocyte-associated cytokines drive epidermal proliferation, such as interferon-α, tumor necrosis factor, and certain interleukins, particularly IL-17. Circulating levels of IL-22 are especially correlated with disease activity. Biopsy reveals epidermal hyperplasia with tortuous papillary dermal blood vessels, and a loss of the granular layer with abundant parakeratotic scale. In pustular lesions, neutrophils form collections in the epidermis.

CLINICAL FEATURES

The lesions are well demarcated and associated with a characteristic silvery white, plate-like adherent scale (**Figure 146-1**).

When the thick scale is forcibly removed, small punctate bleeding points develop (the Auspitz sign) (**Figure 146-2**).

Psoriasis may affect the entire body surface, including the nails. As injury can trigger psoriasis, lesions are typically seen on the elbows, knees, and buttocks (**Figure 146-3**).

While some patients are only troubled by pruritus, most are ashamed of their appearance and the unsightly scaling. Variants include the chronic plaque type, guttate psoriasis, and pustular psoriasis, all of which can evolve into the erythrodermic variant.

In plaque-type psoriasis, the most common presentation, patients develop well-demarcated erythematous scaly plaques distributed symmetrically over the extremities, often involving both elbows and knees. Psoriasis of the gluteal cleft is also common (**Figure 146-4**).

The lesions are chronic and persistent. In the guttate variant, which usually involves a younger age group, the lesions develop acutely, are smaller, have less scale, and are distributed widely over the trunk and buttocks (**Figure 146-5**).

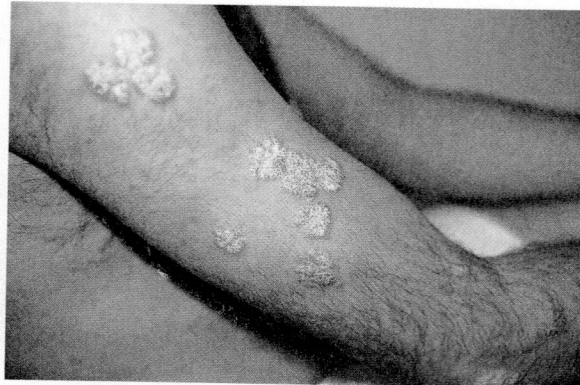

Figure 146-1 *Chronic plaque psoriasis with classic scale.*

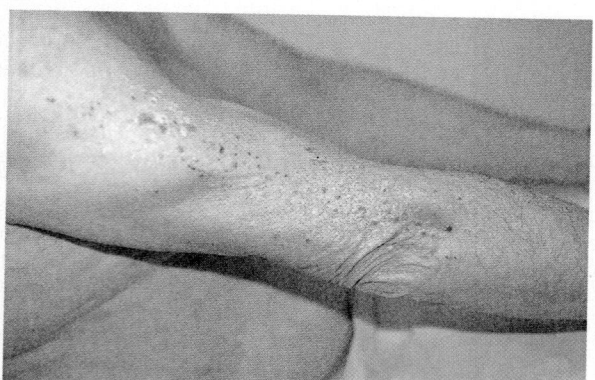

Figure 146-2 *Chronic plaque psoriasis with Auspitz sign.*

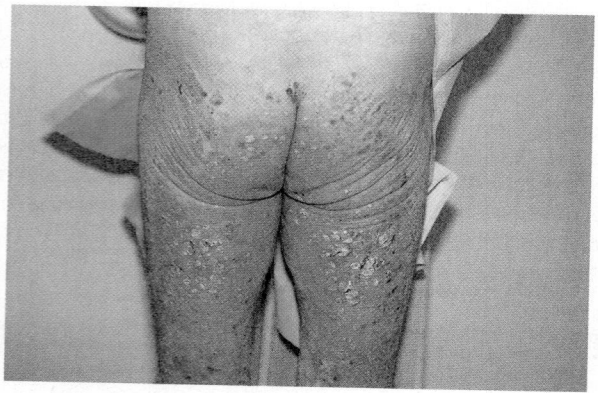

Figure 146-3 *Jockey with worsening psoriasis in areas of trauma.*

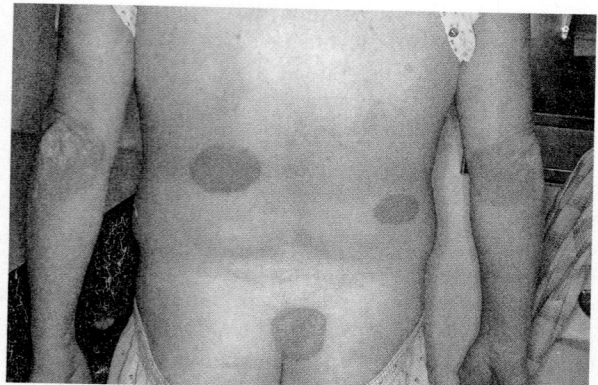

Figure 146-4 *Symmetrical involvement of psoriasis.*

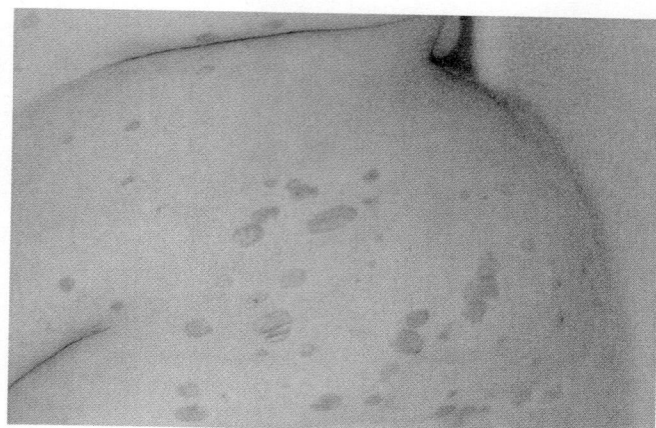

Figure 146-5 *Guttate psoriasis in the typical distribution.*

This variant is often triggered by an antecedent upper respiratory infection. In the rarer pustular variant, numerous pustules can be seen in a limited distribution involving acral sites (pustulosis of the palms and soles) or in a more generalized distribution associated with diffuse erythema (von Zumbusch variant). Common nail changes in psoriasis include nail pitting (**Figure 146-6**), onycholysis (separation of the nail plate from the nail bed), and subungual hyperkeratosis.

Occasionally, a yellow shiny lesion (oil spot) develops in the nail bed. About 10% of patients have concomitant arthritis, which may be severe.

DIFFERENTIAL DIAGNOSIS

In a patient with a few isolated, red, raised lesions, tinea corporis, atopic dermatitis, contact and irritant dermatitis, seborrheic dermatitis, and cutaneous T-cell lymphoma should be considered. In tinea corporis the lesions are more annular with central clearing and have a raised border, often with only fine peripheral scale. A KOH preparation of the scale demonstrating fungal hyphae is diagnostic. In atopic, contact, and irritant dermatitides, the lesions are not so well demarcated and the distribution is different. Cutaneous T-cell lymphoma often presents on the buttocks and posterior thighs, but the plaques are thin and somewhat less red. A skin biopsy revealing atypical T lymphocytes within the epidermis is helpful in confirming this diagnosis. The differential diagnosis of the guttate variant includes drug eruption, viral exanthem, secondary syphilis, and pityriasis rosea. In the pustular variant involving the palms and soles,

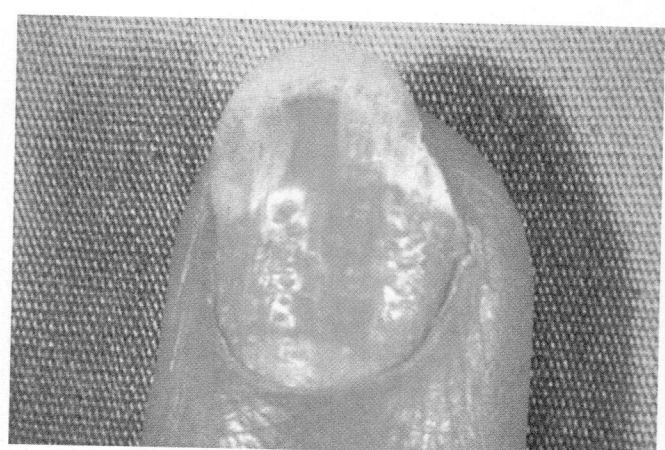

Figure 146-6 *Nail pitting in psoriasis.*

infections and impetiginized dyshidrotic eczema are in the differential diagnosis. In the more generalized pustular variant of psoriasis, pustular drug eruption and acute generalized exanthematous pustulosis (AGEP) should be excluded.

TREATMENT

In the hospitalized patient with chronic plaque-type psoriasis, it is reasonable to continue the patient's outpatient regimen. Topical steroid creams and ointments containing the vitamin D derivative calcipotriol or the retinoid tazarotene are mainstays of treatment. Both modify epidermal proliferation. Anthralins and tars are also effective, but not as widely used. Patients with a few lesions of the guttate variant may be treated with topical steroids alone. However, underlying streptococcal pharyngitis should be excluded and treated if present. Systemic high-dose corticosteroids should be used with great caution in patients with psoriasis, as a severe flare of psoriasis with total body erythroderma may occur as glucocorticoids are tapered.

In patients with more generalized lesions of the chronic type and the guttate variant, which often involve 20% of the body or more, therapeutic options include ultraviolet (UV) therapy with narrow or broadband UVB, or psolaren UVA therapy, combining oral methoxypsoralen with UVA radiation. The guttate variant usually resolves spontaneously over 3 months, but phototherapy hastens resolution. Additional therapies for diffuse recalcitrant psoriasis include acitretin, cyclosporine, methotrexate, and apremilast. Biologic agents, including the anti-TNF agents adalimumab, etanercept, and infliximab, the IL-17A inhibitor secukinumab, and the anti-IL-12/23 antibody ustekinumab, may be considered for use in moderate to severe psoriasis under the supervision of a dermatologist and after careful consideration of the risk of infection.

ERYTHRODERMA

Erythroderma, or exfoliative dermatitis, refers to extensive body redness often associated with scale. Diffuse erythroderma may be produced by several different underlying skin conditions. In 25% of cases, no clear cause is found. Erythroderma is rare, with a reported incidence of 1 to 2 per 100,000 of the population. Men are more often affected. The mean age of onset is 60 years.

PATHOPHYSIOLOGY

In erythroderma, inflammation leads to diffuse cutaneous vasodilation, with thermoregulation problems due to rapid heat loss through the skin. Patients may become hypothermic. Shunting of blood to the periphery may increase cardiac output and aggravate underlying heart disease. High-output cardiac failure has been reported. Inflammation also leads to epidermal hyperplasia and shortened transit time of keratinocytes through the epidermis. The new stratum corneum is poorly formed, compromising the normal barrier function of the epidermis, and leading to increased transepidermal water and protein loss. The risk of skin infection is also increased. As careful fluid, electrolyte, and cardiac monitoring are needed, patients with erythroderma are best managed in the hospital setting with dermatology consultation.

CLINICAL FEATURES

Over 90% of the patient's body surface area is diffusely erythematous (**Figure 146-7**). There is minimal scale early on, with more developing a week after the onset of the erythema. The skin is warm. The patient complains of pruritus and feels cold. On physical examination, 50% of patients have diffuse lymphadenopathy. When the exfoliative dermatitis is chronic, there may be associated hair loss and nail thickening. Hyperkeratosis of palms and soles also

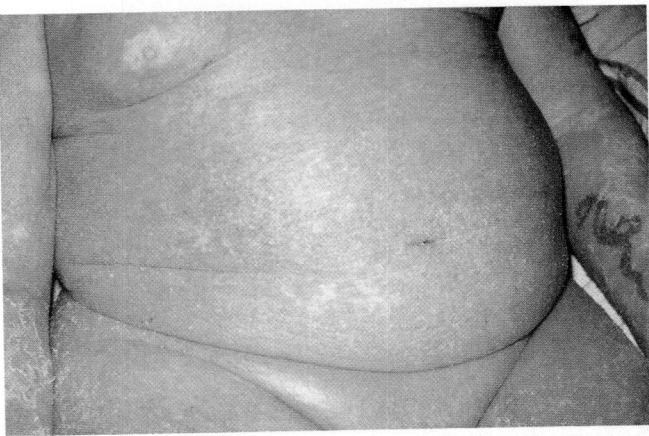

Figure 146-7 *Erythroderma.*

develops over time. Chronic periorbital edema and scale may lead to bilateral ectropion.

DIFFERENTIAL DIAGNOSIS

In evaluating the patient with diffuse erythema, it is important to seek a history of a prior skin condition (**Table 146-1**). In more than 50% of patients, erythroderma results when a preexisting skin condition such as atopic dermatitis, psoriasis, or cutaneous T-cell lymphoma becomes generalized. A complete drug history should also be obtained; over 60 different drugs have been implicated in erythroderma. Skin biopsy determines the cause of erythroderma in over 60% cases, revealing subtle changes of the underlying chronic condition on microscopy. Patients with apparently idiopathic erythroderma (red person syndrome) must be monitored and reevaluated over time.

Erythroderma usually develops gradually in those with a preexisting dermatosis, but may evolve rapidly and explosively when caused by lymphoma or a drug hypersensitivity reaction. Over 90% of patients present with pruritus. This is particularly severe in those with Sézary syndrome, and the erythrodermic variant of cutaneous T-cell lymphoma. Generalized lymphadenopathy is seen in half of those affected. It is usually dermatopathic in nature, driven by T cell expansion in response to antigen presentation by dendritic cells in the setting of skin inflammation. However, if lymphadenopathy is prominent, a Sézary count on peripheral blood and biopsies of skin or lymph node may be needed to rule out lymphoma.

TABLE 146-1 Underlying Causes of Erythroderma

Preexisting conditions: psoriasis, atopic dermatitis, seborrheic dermatitis, contact dermatitis, pityriasis rubra pilaris, ichthyoses, cutaneous T-cell lymphoma, stasis dermatitis, scabies, sarcoid, bullous pemphigoid, pemphigus foliaceus, lichen planus, graft-vs-host disease, reactive arthritis, connective tissue disease, human immunodeficiency virus

Drugs: allopurinol, amiodarone, antimalarials, aspirin, anticonvulsants, angiotensin-converting enzyme inhibitors, cimetidine, ranitidine, furosemide, thiazides, isoniazid, lithium, nonsteroidal anti-inflammatory drugs, quinidine, sulfonamides

Lymphoma: cutaneous T-cell lymphoma, Sézary syndrome, extracutaneous lymphoma

Idiopathic: unclear cause at time of presentation, follow-up over time required; some will be reclassified into the lymphoma group at a later date

TREATMENT

Definitive therapy of erythroderma depends on the underlying condition. Emollients and topical mild to mid-potency corticosteroid ointments under occlusion (to enhance absorption of the steroids) are helpful in most cases. Antihistamines can be given for pruritus. Cessation of all unnecessary drugs, including over-the-counter supplements, is advisable while the patient is being evaluated. Oral corticosteroids may be used in erythroderma due to drugs, but they are generally avoided in erythroderma secondary to underlying psoriasis. General care includes attention to the underlying metabolic and hemodynamic changes, and correction of fluid and electrolyte abnormalities.

SEBORRHEIC DERMATITIS

Seborrheic dermatitis is an erythematous, scaly eruption that develops in skin that is rich in sebaceous glands. Affected locations vary depending on the patient's age. In babies, the scalp and diaper regions are the major areas affected. In adults, the face, scalp, and chest are commonly involved. The prevalence is approximately 3% to 5%.

■ PATHOPHYSIOLOGY

The pathogenesis of seborrheic dermatitis has not been clearly established. Factors that may play a role include infection with the lipophilic yeast *Malassezia globosa*, increased sebaceous secretions, and genetic susceptibility. Patients with alcoholism and neurologic disorders such as Parkinson disease have an increased incidence of this condition, perhaps because of a reduced ability to perform skin care and hygiene. It is also common in HIV, presumably because of immune perturbations.

■ CLINICAL FEATURES

In adults, flaky, erythematous, thin, poorly demarcated patches and plaques are identified over the scalp, eyebrows, nasolabial folds, and ears. The chest can also be involved. The scale is yellower and greasier than that seen in psoriasis.

■ DIFFERENTIAL DIAGNOSIS

The presence of yellow scale and the absence of well-demarcated lesions help to distinguish seborrheic dermatitis from psoriasis. Actinic keratoses occur on sun-damaged areas, especially in fair-skinned persons; the scale is drier and crustier than that of seborrheic dermatitis. Additional entities that may be confused with seborrheic dermatitis include both contact and irritant dermatitis.

■ TREATMENT

Seborrheic dermatitis is generally a chronic relapsing condition. Topical therapies include a mild to mid-potency topical steroid cream combined with an antifungal cream, usually ketoconazole (2% cream applied daily). Attention to scalp involvement is also important, with frequent shampooing with 2% ketoconazole and antidandruff (zinc pyrithione) shampoos. In hospitalized patients with new onset or worsening seborrheic dermatitis, HIV testing should be considered. Seborrheic dermatitis is one of the most common cutaneous manifestations of AIDS, affecting between 20% and 80% of patients. Rarely, underlying zinc deficiency in those receiving parenteral nutrition has been also associated with this condition.

PITYRIASIS ROSEA

Pityriasis rosea is a self-limited skin eruption with a striking appearance, usually lasting 6 weeks, and most common in those between the ages of 10 and 35 years. The prevalence is 0.13% in women and 0.14% in men.

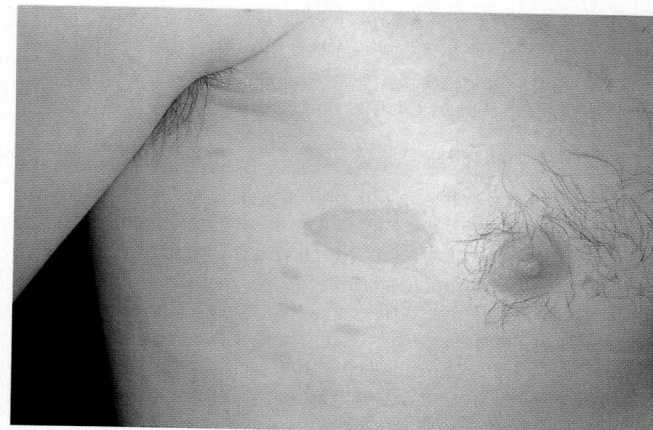

Figure 146-8 *The classic oval herald patch of pityriasis rosea with associated smaller lesions.*

■ PATHOPHYSIOLOGY

A viral etiology for pityriasis rosea has long been suspected, as it is more prevalent in cooler months in the temperate zones, and outbreaks occur in confined populations. In addition, many patients report low-grade fever and upper respiratory symptoms prior to the eruption. Recent studies have implicated human herpesvirus 6 and 7 (HHV-6 and 7), but these are not conclusive.

■ CLINICAL FEATURES

The typical patient develops a single red scaly lesion, 2 to 10 cm in diameter, usually on the trunk or extremity (**Figure 146-8**). This lesion, termed the herald patch, is usually slightly raised and salmon-red. This plaque or patch is ringed by a fine, wrinkled scale that forms a collar (collarette scale). After a few days to 2 weeks, additional smaller oval lesions with the same collarette scale develop over the trunk, distributed over the back along skin tension lines, a pattern likened to the drooping limbs of a Christmas tree. Most patients report some pruritus. The palms and soles are spared.

■ DIFFERENTIAL DIAGNOSIS

Classic pityriasis rosea is unlikely to be mistaken for other conditions by experienced clinicians. Unfortunately, atypical presentations occur. Patients may lack a typical herald patch. When only a few lesions are present, tinea corporis should be excluded, and a KOH examination performed. In those with more diffuse involvement, a drug eruption, a viral exanthem, guttate psoriasis, and secondary syphilis should be considered. Serologic testing for syphilis should be performed if the clinical diagnosis of pityriasis rosea is not definitive. Rarely, drugs such as captopril, hydrochlorothiazide, and imatinib have been reported to cause pityriasis rosea-like drug eruptions.

■ TREATMENT

Most patients only require reassurance that the eruption will dissipate and does not cause additional problems. Patients must be informed that the eruption can last for as long as 12 to 14 weeks. Oral antihistamines and topical steroids may mollify the pruritus. Broadband UVB with daily erythemogenic dosages of UVB may also relieve pruritus and hasten the resolution of the eruption. There is also some data to suggest that acyclovir may speed the resolution of rash. All therapies work best when begun within 2 weeks of the onset.

ATOPIC (ECZEMATOUS) DERMATITIS

Atopic dermatitis (AD) is the prototype of the group of eczematous dermatitides. It is a chronic pruritic eruption commonly found in individuals with a personal or family history of an atopic diathesis (atopic dermatitis, asthma, allergic rhinitis). The prevalence in children in northern Europe, America, and Australia ranges from 10% to 20%, with a slight female preponderance. While it usually arises before the age of 5 years, the disorder may persist into childhood and adulthood. Clinical findings include an erythematous exudative papulovesicular rash involving the flexural and extensor surfaces of the upper and lower extremity. Over time, scaly lichenified patches and plaques appear, and tend to localize to the flexural regions. AD is associated with xerosis, and an increased susceptibility to exogenous irritants.

■ PATHOGENESIS

Immunologic factors contributing to atopic dermatitis include respiratory and food allergies, and possibly autoallergy. The impaired barrier function of the skin in AD makes it susceptible to environmental factors such as microbial pathogens, irritants, and allergens which exacerbate the inflammatory process. Genetic factors also play a role in AD. Up to 73% of patients have a family history of atopy. Chromosomal regions 3q21 and 5q31 have been linked to elevated serum IgE levels and AD. Genes mapping to loci that are involved in T-cell activation, Th-2 cytokines, the high-affinity IgE receptor, and mast cell chymase have also been linked to AD.

■ CLINICAL FEATURES

While acute dermatitis predominates in childhood, and chronic changes are characteristic of adulthood, lesions may show acute, subacute, or chronic epidermal patterns at any age. Acute lesions are characterized by erythematous and edematous papules and plaques. In severe cases, these progress to vesicles with extensive crust. Superimposed excoriations are frequently present. Subacute and chronic lesions are characterized by increased epidermal thickening and hyperkeratosis with lichenification. Papular eczema with perifollicular accentuation is a variant commonly observed in patients with Asian and African heritage. In adults, AD is localized predominantly in a flexural distribution involving the antecubital and popliteal fossae and posterior neck. Wrists, hands, and feet are also commonly involved. Characteristic secondary findings include pruritus, xerosis, keratosis pilaris, ichthyosis vulgaris, and if lichenification is severe, prurigo nodularis. Erythroderma may develop at any stage of AD.

■ DIFFERENTIAL DIAGNOSIS

In adults, diagnostic considerations include allergic or irritant contact dermatitis, cutaneous T-cell lymphoma (CTCL), psoriasis, asteatotic eczema, lichen simplex chronicus, scabies, fungal infection, and drug reactions. The history and pattern of distribution should allow separation of AD from contact dermatitis and drug eruption. Biopsy will distinguish AD from most cases of psoriasis, CTCL, infection, and lichen simplex chronicus.

■ TREATMENT

Prevention and supportive care includes reducing triggers such as soaps and chemicals. Liberal use of emollients to avoid xerosis helps maintain the barrier function of the skin. Drug therapy includes topical corticosteroids and topical calcineurin inhibitors, such as tacrolimus and pimecrolimus. Adjunctive therapies include antihistamines for pruritus and antimicrobials for superinfection. Phototherapy, systemic steroids, and immunosuppressant therapies such as cyclosporine, methotrexate, and azathioprine are used in patients with severe and recalcitrant disease.

ALLERGIC CONTACT DERMATITIS

Allergic contact dermatitis (ACD) is a delayed-type hypersensitivity reaction from exposure to an allergen to which an individual has been previously sensitized. Common triggers include nickel-containing jewelry, cosmetics, topical medications, plants, and chemicals at home and in workplace. ACD is common, representing approximately 4% to 7% of all dermatologic consultations. No specific age, race, or sex difference can be observed when controlled for exposure patterns.

■ PATHOGENESIS

Re-exposure to an allergen after sensitization results in antigen presentation to primed T-cells, ultimately producing an eczematous epidermal reaction pattern. On biopsy, ACD is characterized by spongiotic microvesicles in the epidermis, imparting a Swiss cheese appearance. Subacute and chronic lesions are indistinguishable from other forms of chronic eczematous dermatitis.

■ CLINICAL FEATURES

ACD presents as a pruritic papulovesicular eruption, often exhibiting discrete or bizarre-appearing patterns, depending on the extent of contact with the allergen. Classic examples include linear streaks on the legs after contact with poison ivy, and lesions under earrings, necklaces, or watches in individuals with nickel allergy.

■ DIFFERENTIAL DIAGNOSIS

The differential diagnosis includes other forms of eczematous dermatitis, such as irritant contact dermatitis, atopic dermatitis, stasis dermatitis, and seborrheic dermatitis. Hand and foot contact dermatitis should be distinguished from psoriasis and tinea. The history and the pattern of distribution are generally most helpful in making a diagnosis. Patch testing and biopsy evaluation may be useful when the history and physical exam is not diagnostic.

■ TREATMENT

If the allergen is identified, removal of the offending agent and patient education are paramount for avoiding future contact reactions. Topical and systemic corticosteroids in the case of severe reactions are useful to reduce inflammation. Generous use of emollients will allow the reestablishment of the barrier function of the skin.

IRRITANT CONTACT DERMATITIS

Irritant contact dermatitis (ICD) is a localized nonimmune-mediated reaction secondary to the direct cytotoxic effect of an irritant compound. Offending agents include soaps, detergents, feces, urine, solvents, and wool. ICD is a leading cause of occupational morbidity in the hospital setting.

■ EPIDEMIOLOGY

ICD represents approximately 80% of all cases of contact dermatitis. High at-risk occupations with frequent irritant exposure include hospital workers; kitchen and catering staff; hair stylists; chemical, metal, and textile workers; and dry cleaner workers. Epidermal barrier function has a direct bearing on susceptibility to ICD, with infants and the elderly being more often affected. Any substance that reduces the barrier function of the skin, such as water or detergents, commonly increases the incidence of ICD.

■ PATHOGENESIS

Offending agents commonly associated with ICD may either act acutely, by provoking cytotoxic damage to keratinocytes, or chronically, gradual damaging cell membranes by disrupting the barrier function of keratinocytes and surface lipids. After keratinocyte injury, T-cells are activated, with cytokine production resulting in epidermal proliferation and an eczematous irritant epidermal reaction. On biopsy, epidermal necrosis with mild spongiosis is characteristic.

■ CLINICAL FEATURES

Skin findings include erythema, eczematous changes, vesiculobullous lesions, and frank epidermal necrosis. The lesions have sharply demarcated borders and are limited to the area of irritant exposure.

■ DIFFERENTIAL DIAGNOSIS

In most cases, ICD is a diagnosis of exclusion, with ACD being the most important differential consideration. Clinically, patients frequently report a sensation of burning or stinging, rather than the pruritus of ACD.

■ TREATMENT

Avoidance of and protection from causative agents is the principal treatment for ICD. Preventive measures include protective equipment, barrier ointments, and emollients. Topical steroids and immune modulators are generally not helpful in the treatment of ICD.

SUGGESTED READINGS

Boehncke WH, Schön MP. Psoriasis. *Lancet*. 2015;386:983-994.

Chang C, Keen CL, Gershwin ME. Treatment of eczema. *Clin Rev Allergy Immunol*. 2007;33:204-225.

Drago F, Broccolo F, Rebora A. Pityriasis rosea: an update with a critical appraisal of its possible herpesviral etiology. *J Am Acad Dermatol*. 2009;61:303-318.

Levine D, Gottlieb A. Evaluation and management of psoriasis: an internist's guide. *Med Clin North Am*. 2009;93:1291-1303.

Mansouri Y, Goldenberg G. New systemic therapies for psoriasis. *Cutis*. 2015;95:155-160.

Naldi L, Rebora A. Clinical practice: seborrheic dermatitis. *N Engl J Med*. 2009;360:387-396.

Nosbaum A, Vocanson M, Rozieres A, Hennino A, Nicolas JF. Allergic and irritant contact dermatitis. *Eur J Dermatol*. 2009;19:325-332.

CHAPTER 147

Diabetic Foot Infections

John M. Embil, MD, FRCPC

Elly Trepman, MD

Key Clinical Questions

1 What clinical screening methods may detect the risk of potential foot problems in a diabetic patient?

2 What treatment options are available for a foot ulcer?

3 How are skin and soft tissue infections of the lower extremities classified and treated in diabetic patients?

4 How is osteomyelitis diagnosed and treated in diabetic patients?

5 How is the Charcot foot diagnosed and treated?

6 What preventive measures may be taken to protect the diabetic foot?

EPIDEMIOLOGY

During the past decade, the number of patients in the United States with known diabetes mellitus has increased by 38%, from 15.2 million people (2004) to 21 million people (2014). This rising prevalence is associated with soaring numbers of the overweight and elderly in the population. Patients with diabetes mellitus are susceptible to peripheral neuropathy, peripheral vascular disease, and foot and ankle ulcers. Approximately 15% diabetics develop a foot ulcer during their lifetime. Ulcers may heal or may be complicated by cellulitis, abscess formation, osteomyelitis, gangrene, and amputation. The financial burden of a foot ulcer is approximately $28,000 within 2 years of diagnosis, and the lifetime cost of an amputation is approximately $50,000. Diabetic patients with foot ulcers are susceptible to amputation and death. Nonhealing ulcers precede 84% lower-extremity amputations in diabetic patients. The mortality rate of diabetic patients after lower-extremity amputation ranges from 11% to 41% within 1 year and 39% to 68% by 5 years.

PATHOPHYSIOLOGY

Diabetic foot infections usually are caused by direct bacterial invasion from a skin ulcer or break in the skin barrier, such as from tinea pedis. Other contributing factors include oxidative stress, poor nutrition, impaired neutrophil function associated with hyperglycemia, and tissue ischemia from vascular insufficiency and inflammation.

Peripheral neuropathy in diabetic patients may cause sensory, motor, and autonomic disturbances that increase the risk of developing foot ulcers. In individuals with normal sensation in their feet, minor injuries cause pain, leading to rest and treatment that promote healing. However, diabetic sensory neuropathy leads to loss of protective sensation. Injuries, including repetitive minor trauma or persistent pressure from poorly fitting footwear, may go unnoticed and evolve into necrotic lesions. Motor neuropathy causes contracture of intrinsic muscles and secondary claw toe deformities, with the development of pressure points on the toes or metatarsal heads. Autonomic neuropathy may cause skin dryness and cracking, allowing bacteria to invade and destroy the subcutaneous tissues.

Charcot neuroarthropathy may also contribute to ulcer development in diabetics. Charcot neuroarthropathy arises from repetitive microtrauma in the absence of protective sensation, leading to macroscopic fracture and joint injury. Furthermore, arteriovenous shunting associated with autonomic neuropathy may contribute to abnormal bone vascularity and osteopenia, resulting in increased susceptibility to fracture and joint injury. Damage to the bones and joints may collapse the longitudinal arch of the foot, leading to bony prominences, pressure points, and instability that may result in ulcer.

When an ulcer occurs, there may be initial bacterial colonization of the wound base. Subsequent bacterial invasion may occur with the development of overt infection, such as cellulitis, osteomyelitis, septic tenosynovitis, septic arthritis, or abscess. Rapid spread of infection along tissue planes may be facilitated by impaired immune function and poor vascularity. Therefore, a minor abrasion caused by a poorly fitting shoe may rapidly evolve to a limb-threatening septic tenosynovitis, sometimes within 1 or 2 days.

EVALUATION AND DIAGNOSIS

Evaluation of the diabetic patient, with or without a foot lesion, includes the history and physical examination, with attention to the foot and ankle (**Table 147-1**). Guidelines for frequency of screening

TABLE 147-1 Evaluation of the Diabetic Foot

History

Duration of diabetes

Previous foot ulcer

Previous Charcot neuroarthropathy

Trauma, injury

Erythema

Swelling

Increased warmth

Dependent rubor

Pain or paresthesias

Exertional pain

Nail problems

Shoes

Changes in blood sugar control

Fever, rigors, chills

Physical examination

Inspection: erythema, swelling, increased warmth, dryness, dependent rubor

Joint stiffness

Tendon contractures

Ulcers: probe to bone

Deformity

Corns, calluses

Neuropathy: Semmes-Weinstein monofilament (10 g)

Vascular: pulses, capillary refill

Laboratory investigations

Blood sugar, especially changes in glucose control

Hemoglobin A_{1c}

Complete blood count and differential

Erythrocyte sedimentation rate

C-reactive protein

Albumin

Blood cultures

Wound cultures

Biopsy and culture of infected tissue

Vascular studies

Ankle-brachial index (ABI)

Doppler waveforms

Toe pressures

Imaging studies

AP, lateral, and oblique foot radiographs

AP, lateral, and mortise ankle radiographs

Nuclear medicine (technetium bone scan, indium-labeled white blood cell scan, gallium scan)

Ultrasonography

Computed tomography

Magnetic resonance imaging (with or without gadolinium enhancement)

AP, anteroposterior.

TABLE 147-2 Risk Categories and Preventive Management of Diabetic Patients with Peripheral Neuropathy[*]

Risk Category[†]	Classification[†]	Preventive Management
0	Protective sensation intact	Patient education and daily self-examination
	Foot morphology normal	Foot examination at each visit or at least four times per year
		Appropriately fitted footwear
1	Protective sensation absent	Patient education and daily self-examination
	Foot morphology normal	Foot examination at each visit or at least four times per year
	No history of ulcers	Appropriately fitted footwear with soft insoles
2	Protective sensation absent	Patient education and daily self-examination
	Foot deformity present	Foot examination at each visit or at least four times per year
	No history of ulcers	Appropriately fitted footwear with a suitable insole
3	Protective sensation absent	Patient education and daily self-examination
	Foot deformity	Foot examination at each visit or at least four times per year
	History of plantar ulcer or amputation	Appropriately fitted footwear with a suitable insole (may need custom-made footwear)

[*]Modified from Foot screening: care of the foot in diabetes. The Carville approach. Department of Health and Human Services, USA. US Government Printing Office, 1994.

[†]The Semmes-Weinstein 10-g monofilament assessment for the presence of peripheral neuropathy is used in conjunction with a history of ulcers to establish the risk category. Higher risk category is associated with a greater risk of ulceration.

evaluations and use of protective footwear are based on the presence of neuropathy, history of ulcer, and foot deformity (**Table 147-2**).

HISTORY

Relevant history includes diabetes control and associated complications such as neuropathy and vascular disease. Prior foot ulcers are associated with a high risk of a new foot ulcer or infection. Trauma, even if minor, may cause tissue necrosis leading to an ulcer or initiate Charcot neuroarthropathy. The earliest indication of a diabetic foot infection may be a worsening of blood glucose control, which may precede fever, rigors, and local signs of sepsis.

PHYSICAL EXAMINATION

Physical examination includes inspection for ulcer, skin cracks, drainage, erythema, nail problems, and deformities (**Table 147-3**). Sensory neuropathy is confirmed by the absence of sensation upon contact with a 10-gram (Semmes-Weinstein) monofilament. Inspection between the toes may reveal maceration, ulcer, or purulent drainage,

TABLE 147-3 Common Foot Complications in Diabetic Patients

Clinical Manifestations	Explanation	Treatment Suggestions
Nonblanching erythema over pressure points	Indicates unrelieved pressure; skin can break down, leading to ulcer; appropriate footwear and orthoses may reduce pressure	Custom-made, pressure-relieving insole If deformity present, custom-made orthopedic footwear and/or corrective surgery
Calluses and corns	Ongoing unrelieved mechanical pressure or friction causing the keratin layer of skin to thicken May act as abnormal points of high plantar foot pressure and lead to skin ulcers and undermining of the underlying soft tissues Subkeratotic hematoma or hemorrhage in or under the callus is a sign of unrelieved pressure and underlying soft tissue injury A corn is a callus with a hard central core	Paring (debridement) to relieve pressure Care to avoid trauma to underlying intact skin Patient, family member, or caregiver may use a pumice stone to minimize buildup If visual impairment is present or the area to be treated with the pumice stone cannot be adequately visualized, then a care provider must be designated to perform this foot care Callus around the rim of a neuropathic ulcer is debrided to visualize ulcer and promote healing Appropriate footwear to minimize callus formation
Tinea pedis	Fungal infection, often related to increased moisture in the web spaces between toes Complications include fissuring of skin, which may act as a portal of entry for bacteria	The web spaces in between the toes must be kept dry; foot powder, lamb's wool, and footwear with a wide toe box may be helpful Topical antifungal therapy
Onychomycosis	Fungal infection of the toenails White/yellow discoloration of the nail, with nail hypertrophy and irregularity Most frequently due to *Trichophytin rubrum* and *T. mentagrophytes* Yeasts such as *Candida albicans* and other nondermatophyte molds have been associated with onychomycosis Topical creams and ointments are ineffective because microorganisms have invaded the nail bed and plate With conventional oral therapy, disease-free nail can be achieved in approximately 25%-50% patients	Nail clippings may be submitted to the microbiology laboratory for culture and identification of the dermatophyte Systemic therapy may be necessary to eradicate the infection in the nail bed and plate Oral therapy may include itraconazole, terbinafine, or fluconazole, but the risks and benefits of these agents must be carefully considered before embarking upon lengthy treatment courses For most people, treatment of onychomycosis is not necessary, as the clinical and cosmetic effects are minor Treatment may be indicated for recurring paronychia or psychological complications
Onychogryphosis	Hypertrophic nails that are thickened and horn-like These nails may disintegrate, get caught in socks, traumatize adjacent toes, or get torn off inside footwear	Regular nail care every 3-6 wk may minimize complications Nails are cut straight across and the edges smoothed down Nail care provided by caregiver knowledgeable about diabetic foot complications, with avoidance of injury to surrounding tissues
Onychocryptosis	Ingrown toenail Results from altered fit of the nail plate in the lateral nail groove as a result of improper footwear and poor nail-trimming technique Classification: Stage I—mild complications with local inflammation and slight infection Stage II—worsening of the process with infection and marked discomfort Stage III—most advanced process with lateral wall hypertrophy and infection; infection may be severe and lead to amputation	Regular nail care and properly fitted footwear may minimize occurrence Stage I disease may be treated by proper nail trimming and elevation of the nail edges Stage II disease may require systemic antimicrobial therapy and more aggressive surgical debridement of the nail Stage III disease may require partial nail avulsion and destruction of the nail matrix
Paronychia	Infection of the lateral nail fold May be a consequence of an ingrown toenail	Best treated by partial nail excision, twice-daily saline solution soaks, antimicrobial therapy, and adequate nail care Systemic antibiotics and local surgical debridement may be indicated Assess appropriateness of footwear

especially between the fourth and fifth toes. Erythema, swelling, and warmth may be seen in Charcot neuroarthropathy, but when associated with an ulcer or history of a prior ulcer should increase suspicion for an associated infection. Erythema associated with infection persists during foot elevation, but erythema associated with Charcot neuroarthropathy may decrease when the foot is elevated. Palpable pulses do not exclude serious microvascular disease.

When an ulcer is present (**Figure 147-1**), hospitalists should document the size (diameter), depth, location, odor, drainage, associated deformity, and the presence of visible bone, joint, or tendon tissue. The ulcer base may consist of moist red granulation tissue or dry gray necrotic debris. Drainage may be serous, serosanguinous, or purulent. When the ulcer base is explored with a sterile metal probe, palpation of exposed bone suggests the presence of osteomyelitis unless proven otherwise. Ulcers are classified based on depth, the presence or absence of exposed deep structures and infection, and the status of distal perfusion (gangrene). The Wagner classification system is the most commonly used (**Table 147-4**).

VASCULAR ASSESSMENT

Vascular assessment may include determination of toe blood pressures, oxygenation, and Doppler arterial waveforms. The normal ratio of arm to ankle blood pressure, or ankle-brachial index (ABI), is 0.8 to 1.0. Ratios of less than 0.8 are often associated with delayed wound healing. A ratio of less than 0.5 indicates inadequate arterial inflow and a very poor chance of wound healing. Normal ABI results may be misleading because heavily calcified blood vessels can lead to spuriously elevated occlusion pressures at the ankle. Toe pressures less than 40 mm Hg may indicate inadequate arterial inflow for wound healing, and vascular surgical consultation should be considered. Radiographs may reveal calcified small blood vessels in the forefoot or toes, bony changes consistent with osteomyelitis, or fractures and dislocations indicative of Charcot neuroarthropathy.

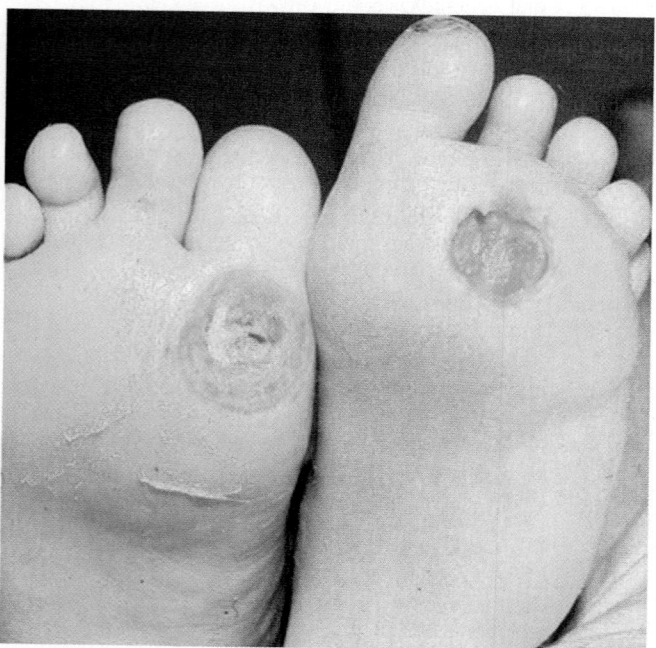

Figure 147-1 *This patient has an ulcer under the right first metatarsal head and sesamoids with central eschar and necrosis, and a clean granulating ulcer under the left second metatarsal head. Neuropathic deformities are also present.* (Reproduced, with permission, from Wolff K, Johnson RA, Suurmond D. *Fitzpatrick's Color Atlas & Synopsis of Clinical Dermatology*, 5th ed. New York, NY: McGraw-Hill; 2005. Fig. 15-3.)

Osteomyelitis and Charcot neuroarthropathy may be present concurrently, especially when ulcers are present.

IMAGING STUDIES

Plain radiographs should be obtained in all patients presenting with diabetic foot infections to assess for bony destruction and deformity, and also to assess for soft tissue gas and foreign bodies. Magnetic resonance imaging (MRI) is the study of choice for patients who require further imaging. Unfortunately, MRI is sensitive but less specific for infection, and the specificity of gadolinium enhancement for infection is unproven. Nuclear medicine studies may be obtained when MRI is contraindicated or unavailable, but specificity is lower than MRI. Technetium bone scintigraphy may be abnormal in osteomyelitis, fracture, or Charcot neuroarthropathy, and false negative results occur in patients with vascular disease or abscess. Indium-labeled white blood cell scans and gallium scintigraphy may be positive in either infection or Charcot neuroarthropathy, and may fail to distinguish these conditions.

WOUND CULTURES

Wound cultures by means of a swab from the ulcer base may be misleading, because the results frequently do not correlate with those of a deep wound or bone culture. Specimens for culture are best obtained from infected tissue that does not communicate with the skin surface. The ideal specimen for culture assessment of infection is a curettage specimen from the base of the ulcer or bone biopsy specimens when osteomyelitis is suspected. If such specimens are not available, cultures of purulent exudate from within the ulcer base or sinuses may be an acceptable alternative. However, in the absence of a current or previous foot ulcer, a swollen, warm, erythematous foot may indicate presence of early Charcot neuroarthropathy, and open biopsy has the risk of potentially causing a deep, limb-threatening infection.

TREATMENT

Diabetic foot infections require antibiotics, wound care, and attention to complications and patient factors (**Table 147-5**).

Some early localized diabetic foot infections may be treated in outpatients. However, many foot infections present with associated systemic sepsis and may be both limb- and life-threatening. If the patient has signs of systemic sepsis or a foot-at-risk because of abscess or septic tenosynovitis, then hospital admission, surgical and infectious diseases consultation, extensive operative debridement, and parenteral antimicrobial therapy usually are required. Timing of surgical debridement is based on clinical judgment and patient factors. In some instances, delay of surgical debridement may be prudent to allow reduction of swelling and abscess localization with parenteral antimicrobial therapy and bedrest, and to improve hemodynamic stability of the septic patient prior to anesthesia. However, in other cases, emergency debridement may be limb or life saving. Radical debridement includes excision of all purulent and necrotic tissue, including bone, joint, and tendon, and may include amputation of gangrenous portions of the foot. Emergency amputation is uncommon, but may be indicated for life-threatening, rapidly spreading infection such as gas gangrene or necrotizing fasciitis.

Antimicrobial treatment for diabetic foot infection may include parenteral, oral, and combination (parenteral and oral) antimicrobial therapy. Many diabetic foot infections are polymicrobial, and initial treatment may include empiric broad spectrum antimicrobials for coverage of gram-positive cocci, gram-negative rods, and anaerobic organisms. After culture results are available and clinical improvement is noted, culture-directed antimicrobial agents are chosen. Suggested empiric regimens for the treatment of infection in the diabetic foot are listed in Table 147-5.

TABLE 147-4 Diabetic Foot Ulcers: Wagner Classification and Treatment Options

Grade	Wagner Classification (Wagner, 1981)	Treatment Options
Grade 0	Skin intact, no open lesions Callus may be present at sites of localized pressure Nonblanching erythema may be present at sites of unrelieved pressure	Pare calluses Footwear and orthoses fitted for weight displacement
Grade 1	Superficial skin ulcer, often at high pressure areas (metatarsal heads, toes)	Pare calluses to expose ulcer base Deep swabs or curettage specimen from ulcer base for bacterial culture if clinical evidence of infection present Radiographs to exclude unsuspected bone infection (if this is detected, the ulcer is classified as a Grade 3 lesion) Moist dressings such as moist-to-dry saline gauze or hydroactive gel Infected ulcers (cellulitis) treated with systemic antimicrobials Pressure relief with appropriate footwear, crutches, wheelchairs, specialized casting (casts are applied by an experienced individual and monitored on a regular basis) Surgical debridement may be indicated
Grade 2	Deeper ulcer that may involve ligament, tendon, joint, bone, or fascia, usually associated with infection such as cellulitis	Treatment similar to Grade 1 lesions
Grade 3	Ulcer extends to deeper tissue layers such as bone If bone can be probed at the base of an ulcer, osteomyelitis is present unless proven otherwise Tendinitis, tenosynovitis, and deep space abscesses may also be present	Noninvasive assessment of the adequacy of peripheral circulation (ankle-brachial index) Radiographs to screen for foreign bodies, gas, and magnitude of bony involvement Aggressive surgical debridement of infected bone, especially when abscess or systemic sepsis is present Appropriate antimicrobial therapy. Antimicrobials may be administered orally in most patients, but parenteral therapy may be of benefit, depending on the extent of involvement Vascular surgical opinion may be necessary when vascular insufficiency is present
Grade 4	Localized gangrene (toes, forefoot, heel) Gangrene may be dry or wet Infection may or may not be present	Treatment as for a Grade 3 lesion Urgent noninvasive assessment of peripheral circulation and vascular surgical opinion, possibly including angiography Angioplasty or bypass surgery may be indicated when a suitable stenotic lesion is demonstrated on angiography Local surgery to remove gangrenous tissue may be attempted, but single ischemic toes may be kept dry and allowed to mummify and autoamputate Painting gangrenous toes with povidone-iodine may prevent or minimize the risk of progression to wet gangrene
Grade 5	Gangrene of entire foot	Urgent assessment as outlined for Grade 4 lesions Control of diabetes and infection Amputation guided by the level and adequacy of circulation

The duration and route of administration of antibiotics may vary, depending on clinical response, infection severity, availability of outpatient intravenous therapy, cost, and patient adherence issues. Infections confined to the skin and soft tissue infections usually are treated with oral antibiotics alone, or a brief course of parenteral antibiotics followed by oral therapy. Osteomyelitis may require surgical debridement and a prolonged course of parenteral or oral antimicrobial therapy. Recommendations about route and duration of antimicrobial therapy frequently are not evidence-based; therefore, clinical course and response to therapy are the best guides to the treatment approach. Foot infections restricted to soft tissue are commonly treated for 1 to 4 weeks, depending on severity. When bone is infected and complete debridement of nonviable bone and tissue has been performed, treatment duration typically is 4 to 6 weeks. When diabetic foot infections involve bone and debridement has not been performed or there is residual dead bone after debridement, failure rates of antibiotic treatment are high. Some clinicians treat for 3 months or longer in this scenario.

Antibiotic response is assessed by frequent clinical examination and monitoring of the white blood cell count, differential, and C-reactive protein. The erythrocyte sedimentation rate may remain elevated, despite adequate initial control of infection. Radiographs or CT scanning may demonstrate bony consolidation and maturation of healed bone, or regions of ongoing bone destruction or sequestrum that may require further surgical debridement. The role of routine follow-up cultures is controversial and is considered on a case-by-case basis; repeating specimens for cultures may be

TABLE 147-5 Empiric Therapy for Infection in the Diabetic Foot*

Infection Severity	Antimicrobial Agent†
Mild infections Neither limb nor life threatening Usually associated with cellulitis surrounding an ulcer Purulent debris may be present at the base of the ulcer Usual organisms: aerobic Gram-positive cocci Frequently treated with outpatient oral antimicrobial therapy	• Cephalexin • Cloxacillin • Trimethoprim-sulfamethoxazole (TMP-SMX) • Clindamycin • Amoxicillin-clavulanic acid • Linezolid • Doxycycline
Moderate infections More extensive cellulitis, plantar abscess Initial antimicrobial therapy directed against staphylococci, streptococci, anaerobes, and common *Enterobacteriaceae* species Patients who are not toxic may be treated with debridement and oral antimicrobial therapy Patients who are ill or toxic despite moderate local signs are treated as having a severe infection (see below)	• TMP-SMX and metronidazole • TMP-SMX and clindamycin • Ciprofloxacin (or levofloxacin) and clindamycin • Ciprofloxacin, linezolid, and metronidazole • Amoxicillin-clavulanic acid • Moxifloxacin • Linezolid
Severe infections Limb or life threatening Patients may be critically ill or toxic and usually are treated with initial parenteral therapy until stable, then oral therapy Frequently polymicrobial Immediate hospitalization, early surgical debridement, and parenteral antimicrobial therapy If MRSA is present or suspected, addition of an agent effective against MRSA should be considered	• Cefoxitin • Third generation cephalosporin (ceftriaxone or cefotaxime) and metronidazole • Combination of β-lactam antibiotic and β-lactamase inhibitor (eg, piperacillin and tazobactam) • Clindamycin and third generation cephalosporin (ie, cefotaxime, ceftriaxone, or ceftazidime) • Carbapenem (ie, imipenem/cilastatin, meropenem, or ertapenem) • Tigecycline
Osteomyelitis Treated with intravenous therapy or long-term oral antimicrobial therapy with agents that are well absorbed from the gastrointestinal tract and have good distribution to bone and tissue Surgical debridement indicated to remove necrotic debris, abscess, or sequestrum If MRSA is present or suspected, addition of an agent effective against MRSA should be considered	Parenteral options • Combination of β-lactam antibiotic and β-lactamase inhibitor (eg, piperacillin and tazobactam) • Clindamycin and third generation cephalosporin (ie, cefotaxime, ceftriaxone, or ceftazidime) • Carbapenem (ie, imipenem/cilastatin, meropenem, or ertapenem) Oral options (when supported by culture data) • Cloxacillin • Cephalexin • TMP-SMX • Clindamycin • Amoxicillin-clavulanic acid • Linezolid • Doxycycline • TMP-SMX and (metronidazole or clindamycin) • (Levofloxacin or ciprofloxacin) and (metronidazole or clindamycin)

*Antibacterial therapy should be guided by available culture results. When in doubt about the most appropriate antimicrobial regimen, discussion with an infectious diseases consultant may be prudent.

†Dosage may depend on renal function and drug levels. Prior to initiating antimicrobial therapy, verify creatinine clearance and modify dose and interval accordingly.

The agents suggested in this section are for empiric therapy prior to the availability of final culture and susceptibility results. Knowledge of local epidemiology also must guide therapeutic choices. Some agents (β-lactams) are ineffective against methicillin-resistant *Staphylococcus aureus* (MRSA). Parenteral agents effective against MRSA include vancomycin, linezolid, daptomycin, oritavancin, telavancin, and ceftobiprole.

Many of the agents identified in this table do not have a specific Food and Drug Administration (FDA) indication for the treatment of diabetic foot infections including osteomyelitis, but may have an indication for the treatment of skin and soft tissue infections or may have antimicrobial activity effective against the typical pathogens encountered in osteomyelitis of the diabetic foot. Therapy must be refined based on the final culture and susceptibility profiles for the pathogens recovered.

Duration of therapy is based on clinical response. However, typical treatment courses for skin and soft tissue infections range from 7 (mild) to 21 (severe) d, and the treatment of osteomyelitis may require 4 to 6 wk of parenteral or several months of oral antimicrobial therapy. When possible, it is desirable to switch to oral antimicrobial therapy to avoid complications from parenteral administration.

indicated when clinical response to therapy is incomplete or recurrent infection is suspected.

Wound care may include offloading, wound dressings, and surgical reconstruction. Offloading—removal of mechanical factors that impede wound healing—may include crutches and non–weight-bearing gait, removable walker boots, bivalved or other casts, wheelchairs, and periodic bedrest. The risks of immobilization, including thromboembolic disease and deconditioning, must be weighed against the risks of ambulation, such as spread of infection and delayed wound healing.

Despite the development of diverse (and sometimes costly) wound dressings, effective and cost-efficient basic wound care is based on maintaining a moist wound environment to expedite healing. The mainstay of wound treatment consists of basic gauze dressings moistened with saline and allowed to dry. This helps the debridement process and provides a moist environment for granulation tissue. Excess moisture in the applied gauze is avoided because of the potential for maceration of the wound margins (hence, the term "moist-to-dry" instead of "wet-to-dry" dressing). After necrotic debris has been removed from the wound base, gauze dressings may be continued until the wound is healed. Other commercially available (and more costly) dressing products, such as hydroactive gels or paraffin-impregnated gauzes, may be used to maintain a moist environment. Topical antimicrobial dressings are not recommended. There are limited data to support any added benefit to their use, and complications include hypersensitivity reactions and the development of antimicrobial-resistant pathogens. The development of suction sponge wound systems, such as the Vacuum Assisted Closure™ device, that decrease edema and wound size to facilitate wound healing after debridement, have shown some benefit in the treatment of acute surgical wounds in the diabetic foot.

Treatment of associated complications, such as peripheral vascular disease and Charcot deformity, may help control infection and prevent recurrence. If an infection does not respond to antimicrobial and wound treatment because of ischemia, peripheral vascular reconstruction may be indicated if the patient has an occlusion amenable to angioplasty or surgical correction. Charcot deformity may cause ongoing wound pressure and breakdown, and surgical reconstruction may be indicated to remove areas of bony pressure or to control instability. The healed foot is often provided with custom-molded orthoses and orthopedic footwear to decrease the risk of recurrent ulceration and infection.

PREVENTION OF RECURRENCE

Preventive programs have the potential to reduce the enormous personal morbidity and societal costs of diabetic foot ulcers (**Table 147-6**). Patient education may improve awareness of the importance of daily self-examination of the foot and shoes, and early evaluation of seemingly minor symptoms. For the patient with established neuropathy,

TABLE 147-6 Prevention of Diabetic Foot Ulcer and Infection

Patient education (classes, handouts)
Self-examination
Footwear and orthoses
Lotion and lamb's wool
Nutrition and glycemic control
Foot screening examinations
Aggressive early evaluation and treatment of foot lesions
Multidisciplinary clinic setting
Antimicrobial prophylaxis for elective surgery

specialized footwear and orthoses may protect the limb from external pressure and shear stresses that may result in ulcers or abrasions. Lotions may prevent cracking of dry exposed skin, and lamb's wool may prevent maceration and skin breakdown between the toes. Attention to nutrition with a low-glycemic program may reverse the early signs of metabolic syndrome and type 2 diabetes mellitus.

PRACTICE POINT

- Poor footwear may lead to foot injury in diabetics. The shoes of diabetics should be evaluated to ensure that they fit properly, provide support, and are in good repair. Inspection of the shoes may reveal blood stains, foul odor, rough seams, or an embedded foreign body, such as a thumb tack or nail. Diabetics should wear shoes with a wide, high toe box to prevent chafing and injury of the toes and metatarsal heads, and removable insoles to accommodate molded orthotics, if necessary.

DISCHARGE CHECKLIST

- Have systemic symptoms subsided, and has control of infection been established?
- Has long-term vascular access been obtained and arrangements made for home administration for patients being discharged on intravenous antibiotics?
- Have outpatient providers been informed about diagnosis, antibiotic duration, and required laboratory monitoring? C-reactive protein is followed to assess for residual infection, and complete blood counts, creatinine, and liver function tests are typically followed periodically in patients discharged on long-term antibiotics to monitor for toxicity.
- Has infectious diseases follow-up been arranged for patients with osteomyelitis?
- Has the patient's diabetic regimen been modified if glycemic control is inadequate?
- Has the patient been educated about diabetic foot care, and have foot care specialists been involved to assess for orthotics and footwear in the inpatient or outpatient setting?

SUGGESTED READINGS

Apelqvist J, Bakker K, van Houtum WH, Schaper NC. International Working Group on the Diabetic Foot (IWGDF) Editorial Board. Practical guidelines on the management and prevention of the diabetic foot. *Diabetes Metab Res Rev*. 2008;24(Suppl 1):S181-S187.

Embil JM, Rose G, Trepman E, et al. Oral antimicrobial therapy for diabetic foot osteomyelitis. *Foot Ankle Int*. 2006;27:771-779.

Embil JM, Trepman E. Microbiological evaluation of diabetic foot osteomyelitis. *Clin Infect Dis*. 2006;42:63-65.

Lipsky BA, Berendt AR, Cornia PB, et al. 2012 infectious Diseases Society of America clinical practice guidelines for the diagnosis and treatment of diabetic foot infection. *Clin Infect Dis*. 2012;54:e132-173.

Pinzur MS, Slovenkai MP, Trepman E, Shields NN. Guidelines for diabetic foot care: recommendations endorsed by the Diabetes Committee of the American Orthopaedic Foot and Ankle Society. *Foot Ankle Int*. 2005;26:113-119.

Sella EJ. Diagnostic imaging of the diabetic foot. *Foot Ankle Int*. 2009;30:568-576.

Trepman E, Bracilovic A, Lamborn KK, et al. Diabetic foot care: multilingual translation of a patient education leaflet. *Foot Ankle Int*. 2005;26:64-107.

Trepman E, Nihal A, Pinzur MS. Current topics review: Charcot neuroarthropathy of the foot and ankle. *Foot Ankle Int*. 2005;26:46-63.

CHAPTER 148

Venous Ulcers

Afsaneh Alavi, MD, FRCPC
Katherine L. Brown, MD, MPH
Tania J. Phillips, MD, FRCPC

Key Clinical Questions

1. Does this patient have a venous ulcer?
2. What is the diagnostic approach to a patient with a suspected venous ulcer?
3. What are appropriate treatments for venous ulcers?
4. How might patients prevent venous ulcers?

INTRODUCTION/EPIDEMIOLOGY

The prevalence of leg ulcers is rising. Up to 1% of adults in developed countries have leg ulcers, with venous disease as the cause in up to 80% of cases. Because of their often chronic course, venous ulcers impose a significant economic burden, accounting for 1% to 3% of the total health care budgets in developed countries. Venous ulcers also result in substantial indirect costs, including an estimated loss of 2 million working days per year in the United States, as well as decreased work productivity, premature disability, and diminished quality of life.

Risk factors associated with venous leg ulcers are listed in **Table 148-1**. Up to 60% of patients with venous ulcers have a prior history of deep venous thrombosis. Annual recurrence rates of venous ulcers are high, ranging from 6% to 27%, perhaps reflecting the high prevalence of underlying venous insufficiency.

PATHOPHYSIOLOGY

The lower-extremity venous system is made up of superficial, communicating, perforating, and deep veins. The deep system lies beneath the muscle fascia. The superficial system is located between the muscle fascia and skin, and includes the saphenous veins. The perforating system connects the superficial system to the deep system, and communicating veins connect veins within the same system. Veins have one-way valves that prevent reflux, and promote cephalad blood flow with leg muscle contraction.

Venous ulcers typically occur in the setting of chronic venous insufficiency, due to reflux through incompetent valves, venous outflow obstruction (as in venous thrombosis), or failure of the calf-muscle pump. Valvular incompetence may occur in the superficial or deep venous systems, or both. Obesity, leg immobility, inflammatory conditions of muscles or joints, fibrosis, and neuropathies can result in calf-muscle pump failure.

Several mechanisms contribute to the development of venous ulcers. Gravity plays a key role, as most venous ulcers are located on the lower extremities. Venous hypertension increases shear stress on vessel walls, leading to endothelial dysfunction and cytokine release. Inflammation stimulates the release of matrix metalloproteinases and other enzymes, with further damage to veins and soft tissue. Wound healing is handicapped by decreased oxygen diffusion to tissues in the setting of venous congestion, setting up a vicious cycle of endothelial activation, unchecked inflammation, soft tissue damage, inadequate repair, and ongoing venous injury.

The CEAP (clinical, etiologic, anatomical, and pathophysiological) system is used to stage the severity of venous insufficiency and venous ulcers (**Table 148-2**).

DIFFERENTIAL DIAGNOSIS

Most leg ulcers are due to venous or arterial disease. However, when pain is severe, the ulcer is of long duration, exhibits unusual morphology or location, or fails to improve with treatment, one should consider the possibility of concomitant infection, allergic contact dermatitis to topical wound treatments, malignancy, or other causes.

■ INFECTION

All nonhealing ulcers should be evaluated with *tissue* cultures (not surface cultures) for bacterial, fungal, viral, mycobacterial, and atypical mycobacterial infection.

TABLE 148-1 Risk Factors

Heredity

Age (peak prevalence between 60 and 80 y)

Female sex (1.6 female: 1 male)

Obesity

History of

   Leg injury

   Varicose vein surgery

   Phlebitis

   Deep vein thrombosis

   Congenital absence of valves

   Venous valve or wall degeneration

   Arteriovenous shunts

Pregnancy

Prolonged standing

Taller height

Inadequate treatment of chronic venous insufficiency or edema

■ MALIGNANCY

Patients with chronic nonhealing ulcers should have a skin biopsy to evaluate for malignancy. As the population ages, the prevalence of malignant leg ulcers is increasing. A low threshold for biopsy of atypical ulcers helps early detection of malignant wounds.

■ ARTERIAL LEG ULCERS

Arterial ulcers can present with claudication or rest pain, and are often exquisitely painful. They are usually sharply demarcated, punched-out ulcers with a fibrinous yellow base or black necrotic eschar, sometimes with exposure of deep tissues, such as tendons. Arterial ulcers often occur distally, especially on the foot, typically at the dorsum or lateral margin of the foot or over bony prominences.

■ INFLAMMATORY CONDITIONS

Inflammatory conditions associated with ulceration include pyoderma gangrenosum and vasculitis. Pyoderma gangrenosum often begins as a small pustule that rapidly enlarges. It develops violaceous, undermined borders with a cribriform (perforated, sieve-like) base, and tends to worsen with trauma, including debridement.

TABLE 148-2 CEAP (Clinical, Etiologic, Anatomical, and Pathophysiological) Classification of Chronic Venous Disease

Class	Definition
C_0	No visible or palpable signs of venous disease
C_1	Telangiectasias (dilated venules, <1 mm diameter), reticular veins (dilated nonpalpable veins, ≤3 mm diameter), malleolar venous flare (arrays of small veins about the ankles)
C_2	Varicose veins (dilated, palpable veins, >3 mm diameter)
C_3	Edema without skin changes
C_4	Skin changes*
C_5	Skin changes* with healed ulceration
C_6	Skin changes* with active ulceration

*As described in Table 148-3.

Two-thirds are associated with inflammatory bowel disease, rheumatoid arthritis, or hematologic malignancies. Vasculitis can be associated with palpable purpura (nonblanching red to blue papules), livedo reticularis (netlike, red-purple erythema, especially on the legs), and necrosis. Rheumatoid arthritis, systemic lupus erythematosus, scleroderma, and other connective tissue diseases may also be associated with lower-extremity ulcers in the absence of overt vasculitis.

■ PROCOAGULANT DISORDERS

Sickle cell anemia, anticardiolipin antibodies, and other procoagulant disorders can result in chronic wounds similar to venous ulcers.

APPROACH TO PATIENTS WITH SUSPECTED VENOUS ULCERS

■ EVALUATION

Clinical signs of venous disease are listed in **Table 148-3**, and **Table 148-4** outlines key components of ulcer evaluation. Patients should be assessed for risk factors for venous ulcers, associated symptoms and modifying factors, ulcer course, and response to prior treatments. Patients with venous ulcers have variable symptoms that tend to be worse at the end of the day, are aggravated when the legs are dependent, and improve with leg elevation. These include aching, cramping, swelling, heaviness, tingling, itching, burning, restless legs, and copious, sometimes malodorous drainage. It is not unusual for venous ulcers to persist for years or to recur at the same site. Claudication (calf pain or cramping with ambulation) is more consistent with arterial disease. Pyoderma gangrenosum ulcers typically enlarge after trauma, such as mechanical debridement. Ulcers may also be multifactorial and have secondary complications, such as bacterial superinfection.

Patients with venous ulcers may struggle with impaired mobility, depression, and social isolation.

TABLE 148-3 Clinical Signs of Chronic Venous Disease

Sign	Description
Pitting edema	Swelling of lower legs that retain an indentation after applying firm pressure
Venous eczema/stasis dermatitis	Redness, scaling, itch, ± exudates
Dyspigmentation	Reddish-brown discoloration, especially around the ankle
Purpura	Nonblanching red to purple spots
Hemosiderosis	Cayenne pepper-appearing specks on shins
Varicosities	
Malleolar venous flares	Arrays of small veins around the ankles
Varicose veins	Large tortuous superficial veins
Atrophie blanche	Stellate white scars
Induration/dermatosclerosis	Hardening of the skin
Lipodermatosclerosis	
Early changes	Acute noninfectious cellulitis with redness and swelling
Late changes	Sharply demarcated hardening associated with skin discoloration of the distal third of the lower leg, giving the lower leg the silhouette of an inverted champagne bottle

TABLE 148-4 Diagnostic Workup of Lower Extremity Ulcers

History	Screen for risk factors (Table 148-1)
	Are symptoms worse in the dependent position and alleviated with elevation?
	Does the patient have other systemic diseases?
	Does the patient experience calf pain or cramping with walking (claudication)?
	Does he or she complain of numbness or altered sensation?
	Does the ulcer historically worsen with invasive procedures (eg, following debridement)?
Physical examination	Ulcer location
	Surrounding skin changes (Table 148-3)
	Palpate pulses
	Measure ankle-brachial index (ABI)
	Test sensation with 10 g Semmes-Weinstein monofilament
Studies	Duplex ultrasonography (gold standard) for confirming venous reflux, and excluding thromboses
	Segmental arterial pulse waveform analysis, magnetic resonance angiography, arteriography if arterial disease suspected
	If osteomyelitis is suspected, consider bone scans, magnetic resonance imaging (MRI), computed tomographic scans (CT), and bone biopsy
Laboratory testing for possible underlying systemic disease	Antinuclear antibody (ANA)
	Glucose, HbA1c
	Anticardiolipin antibody
	Lupus anticoagulant antibody
	ANCA
	Protein C, protein S, antithrombin III
	Cryoglobulins
	Cryofibrinogens
	Rheumatoid factor (RF)
	Factor V Leiden, prothrombin gene mutation
Biopsy (for any nonhealing ulcer)	For histopathologic examination
	For tissue cultures (bacterial, viral, fungal, mycobacterial, atypical mycobacterial)

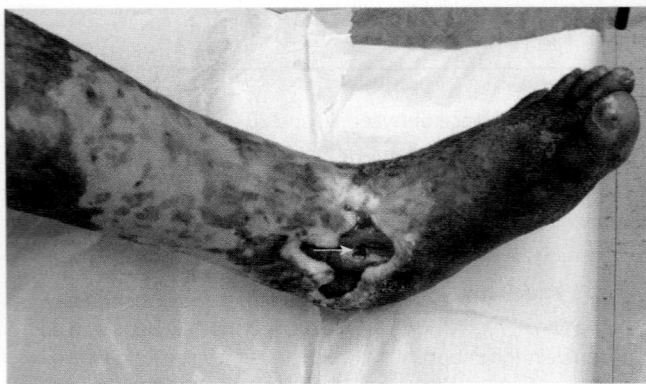

Figure 148-1 *Venous ulcer overlying the medial malleolus. Note the irregular shape of the ulcer, the fibrinous yellow exudate in the wound bed (yellow arrow), and the skin changes involving the gaiter region (the area between the mid-calf and ankle). In addition, this patient has pitting edema, hyperpigmentation related to hemosiderin deposition, skin hardening, and decreased ankle range of motion.*

medial malleolus or within the gaiter area (the distal third of the leg, from the mid-calf to the ankle). Ulcers outside this area should raise the possibility of another cause.

Venous insufficiency may be complicated by lipodermatosclerosis. This is a form of panniculitis, or inflammation of subcutaneous tissues, characterized by fat necrosis, septal fibrosis, and moth-eaten-appearing elastic fibers. The skin is tender and indurated. As fat lobules are obliterated and replaced by fibrosis, the calves take on the appearance of an upside-down champagne bottle (**Figure 148-3**).

Distal pulses should be palpated to assess for arterial disease. An ankle-brachial index < 0.8 supports an arterial component to the ulcer. The exclusion of concomitant significant arterial disease is mandatory before application of compression therapy.

The duplex ultrasound scan is preferred for evaluating venous anatomy and diagnosing venous insufficiency, due to its accuracy, noninvasiveness, and reproducibility. When ordering duplex ultrasonography, ask for evaluation of venous insufficiency (reflux). Failure to do so may result in testing for only the presence or absence of deep vein thromboses (DVT). Other less common studies include continuous-wave Doppler studies for superficial vein anatomic information, and air plethysmography or photoplethysmography for evaluating calf-muscle pump function. Invasive phlebography is reserved for evaluation before vascular surgery.

Most venous ulcers are diagnosed by clinical evaluation. Venous ulcers typically have ragged, ill-defined, irregular borders, and a shallow wound bed with a yellowish fibrinous exudate or pink granulation tissue (**Figure 148-1**). Around the ulcer, there can be skin dyspigmentation (darkening or lightening), purpura, and thickening of the skin. Although venous ulcers are usually less painful than other ulcer types, up to 75% of venous ulcer patients complain of pain. Deep ulcers around the ankles and ulcers with surrounding *atrophie blanche* (stellate white scars) are particularly painful (**Figure 148-2**). While the edema of cardiac, renal, and hepatic disease is typically soft and painless, venous disease is associated with hard, indurated edema. Venous ulcers tend to be located over the

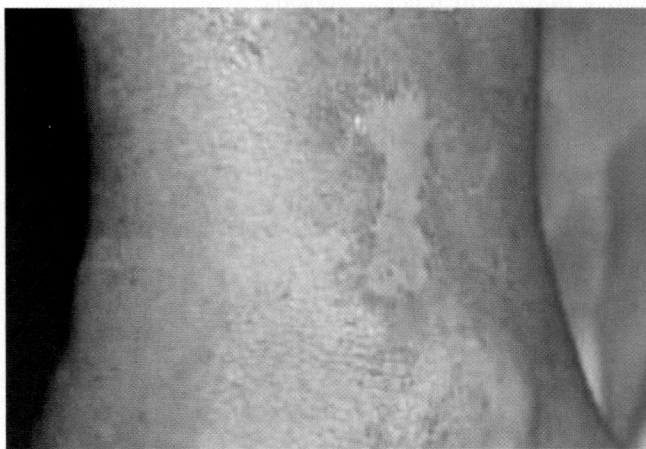

Figure 148-2 *Atrophie blanche, appearing as a whitish scar with stellate borders near the medial malleolus.*

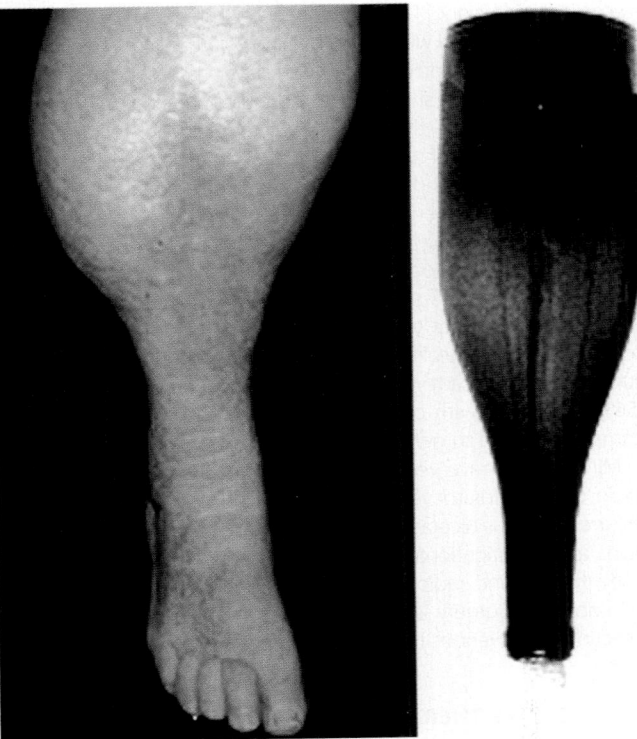

Figure 148-3 *Lipodermatosclerosis presents as redness, swelling, and skin hardening that gives the lower leg the silhouette of an inverted champagne bottle.*

PRACTICE POINT

- When ordering duplex ultrasonography as part of the workup for a suspected venous ulcer, specify that assessment for venous insufficiency and reflux is desired. Otherwise, the technician may only look for the presence or absence of deep venous thrombosis.

State-of-the-art ulcer care will fail unless underlying related diseases are first addressed. Laboratory testing may be performed to exclude concurrent inflammatory, infectious, and coagulopathic diseases, depending on the degree of clinical suspicion. Any nonhealing ulcer should be biopsied for histological examination and tissue cultures. This can be accomplished with either two small punch biopsies or one large wedge biopsy that is bisected with a scalpel, providing a sample for each study. Tissue should be cultured for bacteria, fungi, viruses, and mycobacteria, including atypical mycobacteria.

INPATIENT MANAGEMENT

◼ COMPRESSION

By raising local hydrostatic pressure and lowering superficial venous pressure, compression therapy (typically 35-40 mm Hg at the ankle) reduces edema and vascular leakage, increases cutaneous blood flow and lymph transport, approximates valve leaflets, and increases ulcer healing rates compared to controls. Contraindications to compression therapy include arterial insufficiency and decompensated congestive heart failure. Adequate blood supply, reflected by ankle-brachial index of 0.8 to 1.2, is required for safe application of compression of 40 mm Hg or higher. Walking and exercise involving the calf-muscle pump enhance the effectiveness of compression therapy. Unfortunately, patients with severe lipodermatosclerosis may have difficulties with the ankle dorsiflexion required in these exercises.

Compression choices include multicomponent compression wraps, graduated compression elastic stockings, orthotic compression devices, and compression pumps. Compression bandages are classified as either long stretch (elastic, with extensibility 100% 200%) or short stretch (inelastic, with extensibility limited to 40%-90%). An example of an inelastic bandage is the zinc oxide paste bandage or Unna boot.

The Unna boot is a zinc-impregnated, semirigid paste bandage applied with the foot at a 90° angle. It has a soothing effect on the skin, and improved patient adherence compared to compression stockings. The inelasticity of the Unna boot provides low resting pressures when the leg is inactive or supine, but high pressures during ambulation and activity. Thus, the Unna boot works with the action of the calf-muscle pump to promote venous return. However, it does not provide effective compression for immobile patients. Other disadvantages of the Unna boot include the need to keep it dry when bathing, unpleasant odor from wound exudate, inability to accommodate large leg volume fluctuations, need for frequent clinic visits, and potential for contact dermatitis.

Alternatively, there are a number of elastic compression therapies. Compression bandages are commonly applied spirally, with a 50% overlap from right above the toes to just below the knees, producing a double layer of wrapping with each component. As a result, even single-component bandages are not a single layer. Different application techniques, such as the figure of eight bandages, increase the compression.

Compression bandages may be adjusted for changes in leg volume, provide increased rest and working pressures, conform to the leg better than more rigid bandages, and allow for more frequent dressing changes. Disadvantages include complications related to improper application, unraveling, and patient adherence. Single-component compression bandages range from light compression (class I) to the moderate-high pressure (class III) bandages (eg, Tensopress, Setopress, and Surepress) used for severe edema, post-thrombotic venous insufficiency, and severe varicosities. Multicomponent bandage systems, like Dynaflex and Profore, provide 40 to 45 mm Hg of support, can adapt to changing leg sizes, and are more cost-effective despite higher upfront costs. They are effective in immobile patients, but have high resting pressures and should not be used for patients with concomitant arterial disease. Multicomponent bandages work better than single-component bandages, and multicomponent systems including an elastic bandage appear more effective than those composed mainly of inelastic components.

Orthotic compression devices consist of multiple Velcro straps. They are adjustable for changes in leg circumference, and easily removed for frequent dressing changes. Intermittent pneumatic compression (IPC) devices, originally designed for deep venous thrombosis prophylaxis, work by inflating and deflating an airtight bag around the leg. They require immobility for several hours per day. Studies of IPC have demonstrated increased healing relative to no compression. It is unclear whether IPC is equivalent to other forms of compression, or whether it may be used as an adjunct to other compression therapies.

◼ DEBRIDEMENT

Frequent venous ulcer debridement may facilitate healing by removing impediments to wound bed granulation and epithelialization. There are four types of wound debridement. **Autolytic** debridement uses occlusive dressings to maintain contact between the wound and enzyme-rich bodily fluids to selectively liquefy necrotic tissue. **Enzymatic** debridement employs commercially available topical agents, like collagenase (Santyl). **Mechanical** debridement includes wet-to-dry dressings, hydrotherapy, and irrigation for nonselectively removing viable and necrotic wound tissue. As this may be painful, many clinicians apply topical anesthetic agents, such as lidocaine/prilocaine combinations (marketed as Eutectic Mixture of Local Anesthetics or EMLA) during mechanical debridement. **Surgical** debridement is typically performed under anesthesia for wounds with a large amount of necrotic tissue.

■ WOUND PREPARATION AND TOPICAL TREATMENTS

Chronic wounds including venous ulcers should be kept moist and cleansed with physiologic saline. Topical antiseptics such as hydrogen peroxide, povidone iodine, acetic acid, and sodium hypochlorite should be avoided, as they are toxic to healthy granulation tissue as well as bacteria. Topical antibiotics are potent allergens and should be avoided. Uncomplicated venous eczema without ulceration that is wet and oozing usually improves with topical corticosteroid creams. Ointments may be used for venous eczema that is dry, thickened, and pruritic.

■ DRESSINGS

Dressings differ in many characteristics, including absorptiveness (**Table 148-5**). The wound should be covered with a moisture-retentive dressing, such as hydrocolloid or hydrogel, to promote autolysis of necrotic material and soothe pain. Highly absorptive dressings, such as foams and alginates, should be reserved for profusely exudative wounds. Dressings should be applied with adequate margins around the wound, and the frequency of dressing changes should be adjusted to avoid leakage. Compressive therapy should be applied over dressings.

■ SKIN GRAFTING AND VENOUS SURGERY

Skin grafts may be considered for refractory venous ulcers. Grafts may be harvested or grown from the patient's own intact skin (autografts) or bioengineered from donor cells (allografts). Treatment with skin grafts plus compression results in a greater number of healed ulcers at 6 months and a shorter time to wound closure, compared to compression alone. The combination of skin grafts and compression is also associated with better healing of large ulcers, deep ulcers, and ulcers of >6-month duration. Two-layer tissue-engineered skin grafts have also been shown to increase ulcer healing.

Adjunctive surgical therapies aim to reduce ulcer recurrence by stopping flow through incompetent superficial veins, thus decreasing venous reflux and hypertension. Surgical therapies include venous stripping, superficial vein ligation, and deep perforator vein ligation. Sclerotherapy is a nonsurgical means of accomplishing the same goal by injection of incompetent veins with an irritant solution. The ESCHAR study, a randomized controlled trial of 500 patients, showed that venous ulcer surgery with compression did not hasten ulcer healing compared to compression alone, but surgery did significantly reduce rates of ulcer recurrence at 3 years (56% recurrence with compression alone vs 31% recurrence with compression and surgery).

Minimally invasive venous surgical techniques include subfascial endoscopic perforator vein ligation (SEPS) for patients with chronic or recurrent venous ulceration associated with incompetent perforator veins, and investigational percutaneous techniques (eg, endovenous laser therapy and radiofrequency ablation) for greater saphenous vein ablation. Surgery is contraindicated in patients at high risk of infection, deep venous thrombosis, or anesthetic complications.

■ ADJUNCTIVE THERAPIES

Adjunctive therapies may be considered in patients whose wounds fail to heal despite appropriate dressings and compression therapy. These include systemic medications, growth factors, alternative medicine, and hyperbaric oxygen therapy. Evidence to support these therapies is limited.

Diuretics have a limited role in chronic venous insufficiency. They may help reduce edema that is difficult to mobilize, but may also lead to volume depletion. Though most venous ulcers are heavily colonized with bacteria, routine administration of topical

TABLE 148-5 Dressings

Type	Indications	Pros	Cons
Simple, nonadherent Telfa, Vaseline Adaptic	Minimal to mild exudate Superficial wound	Less expensive	Require second dressing
Films Tegaderm, Omiderm, Opsite, Bioclusive, Blisterfilm, Transeal	Minimal exudate	Clear Adhesive Bacterial barrier	Wound adherence Fluid collection
Hydrocolloids Duoderm, NuDerm, Comfeel, Cutinova, Replicare, Granulex, Tegasorb, Biofilm	Mild to moderate exudate Deep wounds	Autolytic debridement Absorbent Bacterial barrier	Opaque Odor
Hydrogels Vigilon, Tegagel, Curagel, Clearsite, Curafil, Elasto-Gel, Solosite wound gel, 2nd Skin	Painful wounds Dry or mild exudate Crusted exudate	Semitransparent Soothing Hydrating No wound adherence	Require second dressing Frequent dressing changes
Foams Allevyn, Flexzan, Hydrasorb, Lyofoam, Vigifoam	Moderate to heavy exudate Pressure relief Protection of bony prominences	Absorbent Conforms to contours	Opaque Require second dressing
Alginates Algiderm, Algisite, Algisorb, Kaltostat, Curasorb, Polymen, SeaSorb, Sorbsan, Cutinova	Heavy exudate Deep wounds	Highly absorbent Hemostatic No wound adherence Fewer dressing changes	Require second dressing

or systemic **antibiotics** does not improve healing rates, and may be complicated by emergence of resistant organisms and contact dermatitis. Antibiotics should be reserved for ulcers with signs of infection, such as increasing erythema, pain, and ulcer size. Tissue cultures should be obtained prior to starting antibiotics. Empiric treatment should cover both Gram-positive and Gram-negative bacteria, including *Pseudomonas*, and should be tailored according to culture results.

Although one small trial found a benefit of **aspirin** in speeding healing of venous ulcers, there is currently insufficient evidence to recommend it as routine therapy. No growth factors are currently approved by the FDA for venous ulcer treatment. **Pentoxifylline** is a methylxanthine derivative with antiplatelet and anti-inflammatory effects, which also reduces blood viscosity. It appears effective as an adjunct to compression bandaging and is possibly effective in the absence of compression for enhancing venous ulcer healing.

There is limited evidence to support the use of **herbal remedies**, such as horse chestnut extract, rutoside extracts, and pycnogenol (French maritime pine bark extract). It is unclear whether these substances provide additional benefit to patients on standard therapy, as most patients in these studies were not treated with compression therapy.

In **hyperbaric oxygen therapy** (HBOT), very high arterial oxygen tensions are achieved by placing patients in an airtight chamber filled with pure oxygen at pressures greater than one atmosphere. It may improve short-term wound healing, but no improvement in long-term outcomes has been shown.

PRACTICE POINT

- Caregivers should encourage patients with venous disease to elevate their legs above the level of the heart whenever possible. Lesser degrees of elevation, such as placing the feet on a footstool or ottoman while seated in an armchair, are ineffective in increasing venous return.

PROGNOSIS

The strongest predictors of failure of venous ulcers to heal are ulcer size and duration (**Table 148-6**). Healing occurs in 64% of venous ulcers present for less than 1 year, 48% of ulcers present for 1 to 3 years, and 24% of ulcers present more than 3 years. With regard to size, 72% of venous ulcers with baseline areas < 5 cm² heal, while only 40% of ulcers with a baseline area > 5 cm² heal.

PREVENTION

Compression stockings are effective in improving venous hemodynamics and edema and preventing primary and recurrent ulcers in patients with venous disease. Since recurrence rates are as high as 72%, patients with healed venous ulcers should wear lifelong compressive elastic stockings. There are four classes of compression stockings: class I (20-30 mm Hg, for varicose veins and mild edema), class II (30-40 mm Hg, for moderate venous insufficiency, moderate edema, and severe varicosities), class III (40-50 mm Hg, for severe edema), and class IV (≥60 mm Hg, for elephantiasis and severe venous insufficiency with post-thrombotic edema).

Elderly patients and those with arthritis find it difficult to put on compression stockings. Helpful tips include washing new compression stockings prior to wear to reduce stiffness, and applying stockings early in the morning when edema is least. Some stockings have modifications like silk liners or zippers for easier application and removal. There are also various aids (eg, Stocking Donner, Easy Slide, and Circaid) to assist with application of traditional compression stockings.

TABLE 148-6 Prognostic Indicators of Venous Ulcer Healing

Favorable	Unfavorable
Baseline ulcer surface area <5 cm²	Baseline ulcer surface area >5 cm²
Ulcer duration <1 y	Previous operations (eg, knee or hip surgery)
Ankle-brachial index (ABI) > 0.8	ABI < 0.8
Reduction in calf circumference ≥3 cm during the first 50 d of treatment	History of venous ligation or venous stripping
	Body mass index (BMI) > 33 kg/m²
	Daily walking distance <200 m
Emergence of new skin islets on >10% of wound in 50 d	History of surgical wound debridement
	>50% of wound covered with fibrin
	Wound depth >2 cm
	Fixed ankle joint
	Reduced ankle range of motion
	Calf:ankle circumference ratio <1.3

DISCHARGE CHECKLIST

- Has a provider been identified who will primarily manage the venous ulcer in the outpatient setting, such as a dermatologist, vascular surgeon, or both?
- Has the patient been assessed for compressive therapy and appropriate dressings for wounds? Does the patient have adequate financial resources and health care insurance to cover the costs of these? Are patients and caregivers able to handle the logistics of dressing application and compression therapy?
- Has arterial disease been excluded by measurement of the ankle-brachial index in patients who are candidates for compression therapy?
- Has the patient been educated about the role of leg elevation? (Ideally this should be 30 minutes, four times daily.)
- If wound cultures and biopsies were obtained, has follow-up been arranged for these?
- Has adjunctive pentoxifylline therapy been considered?

SUGGESTED READINGS

Briggs M, Nelson EA, Martyn-St James M. Topical agents or dressings for pain in venous leg ulcers. *Cochrane Database Syst Rev.* 2012;11:CD001177.

Fonder MA, Lazarus GS, Cowan DA, et al. Treating the chronic wound: a practical approach to the care of nonhealing wounds and wound care dressings. *J Am Acad Dermatol.* 2008;58:185-206.

Gohel MS, Barwell JR, Taylor M, et al. Long term results of compression therapy alone versus compression plus surgery in chronic venous ulceration (ESCHAR): randomised controlled trial. *BMJ.* 2007;335(7610):83.

Green J, Jester R, McKinley R, Pooler A. The impact of chronic venous leg ulcers: a systematic review. *J Wound Care.* 2014;23:601-612.

Jones JE, Nelson EA, Al-Hity A. Skin grafting for venous leg ulcers. *Cochrane Database Syst Rev.* 2013;1:CD001737.

Jull AB, Arroll B, Parag V, Waters J. Pentoxifylline for treating venous leg ulcers. *Cochrane Database Syst Rev.* 2012;12:CD001733.

Kranke P, Bennett MH, Martyn-St James M, Schnabel A, Debus SE, Weibel S. Hyperbaric oxygen therapy for chronic wounds. *Cochrane Database Syst Rev.* 2015;6:CD004123.

Liu YC, Margolis DJ, Isseroff RR. Does inflammation have a role in the pathogenesis of venous ulcers? A critical review of the evidence. *J Invest Dermatol.* 2011;131:818-827.

Milic DJ, Zivic SS, Bogdanovic DC, Karanovic ND, Golubovic ZV. Risk factors related to the failure of venous leg ulcers to heal with compression treatment. *J Vasc Surg.* 2009;49:1242-1247.

Nelson EA, Mani R, Thomas K, Vowden K. Intermittent pneumatic compression for treating venous leg ulcers. *Cochrane Database Syst Rev.* 2011;2:CD001899.

O'Donnell TF Jr, Passman MA, Marston WA, et al. Management of venous leg ulcers: clinical practice guidelines of the Society for Vascular Surgery and the American Venous Forum. *J Vasc Surg.* 2014;60(2 Suppl):3S-59S.

O'Meara S, Cullum N, Nelson EA, Dumville JC. Compression for venous leg ulcers. *Cochrane Database Syst Rev.* 2012;11:CD000265.

Phillips TJ, Machado R, Trout R, et al. Prognostic indicators in venous ulcers. *J Am Acad Dermatol.* 2000;43:627-630.

CHAPTER 149

Dermatologic Findings in Systemic Disease

Jennifer K. Tan, MD

Ruth Ann Vleugels, MD

Key Clinical Questions

1. What are the most common cutaneous manifestations of gastrointestinal, renal, rheumatologic, and endocrinologic disease? What are rare but important cutaneous findings which should not be missed?
2. How does systemic amyloidosis manifest in the skin?
3. What key features are necessary to recognize nutritional deficiencies?
4. What is the systemic approach to purpura?
5. When should an inpatient dermatology consultation be obtained?

INTRODUCTION

This chapter will focus on the integument and its unique ability to exhibit disease that lies beneath. A lesion may represent *skin involvement* from an internal condition, such as amyloidosis or cutaneous metastases, or a *reactive process* to underlying disease, such as neutrophilic dermatoses related to inflammatory bowel disease, or cutaneous vasculitis due to drug hypersensitivity. Cutaneous lesions can also be characterized as *specific* to an underlying systemic process, or as *nonspecific* manifestations that may occur in many disorders. Skin findings may represent the sole clinical manifestation of a systemic disorder. A basic knowledge of these conditions is essential not only for recognizing an underlying association, and for determining when an inpatient dermatology consult may be useful in the diagnosis and management of an otherwise puzzling patient.

CUTANEOUS MANIFESTATIONS OF GASTROINTESTINAL DISEASE

■ GASTROINTESTINAL HEMORRHAGE

Disorders in which vascular lesions are found in both skin and viscera may present with gastrointestinal (GI) hemorrhage. Though rare, these disorders should be considered in patients with gastrointestinal bleeds, particularly in the setting of recurrent bleeds, family history of hemorrhage, or multiple vascular lesions on the skin.

Telangiectasia in the setting of GI or pulmonary vascular lesions raises suspicion for **hereditary hemorrhagic telangiectasia** (HHT, also known as Osler-Weber-Rendu syndrome). This is a familial autosomal dominant or spontaneous disorder, characterized by cutaneous telangiectasias and visceral arteriovenous anomalies. Epistaxis in childhood is often the presenting sign, followed by the development of well-defined 2 to 3 mm macular or papular telangiectasias on the face, lips, tongue, ears, and chest during late childhood to young adulthood (**Figure 149-1**). Telangiectasias represent dilations of the superficial capillary network, which typically blanch upon pressure. Gastrointestinal bleeding from mucosal telangiectasias occurs in about 20% to 40% of cases, with onset typically after the fourth decade. The stomach and duodenum are often sources of this potentially life-threatening bleeding. Additional visceral manifestations of HHT include hepatic or pulmonary arteriovenous fistulae, which may lead to shunting, dyspnea, hemoptysis, or systemic embolism and infection, and cerebral arteriovenous malformations, which may lead to intracranial hemorrhage.

Blue rubber bleb nevus syndrome (BRBNS) is a spontaneous or autosomal dominant inherited disorder characterized by venous malformations of the skin, GI tract, and other viscera. Cutaneous findings include multiple dark blue to violaceous compressible, rubbery skin lesions known as blebs, most commonly located on the trunk and upper extremities. Initially characterized in the literature as hemangiomas, the lesions associated with BRBNS are actually venous malformations that may appear macular, papular, or nodular. The classic "blue rubber nipple" demonstrates delicate crumpling when compressed with slow refill upon release. Notably, cutaneous lesions tend not to bleed but are characteristically tender due to the high content of vascular smooth muscle. Most blebs are present at birth or by 2 years of age, but may enlarge and become more prominent with age. It is important for hospitalists to be familiar with BRBNS, as potentially life-threatening GI bleeding is generally the most serious complication of BRBNS. Patients thought

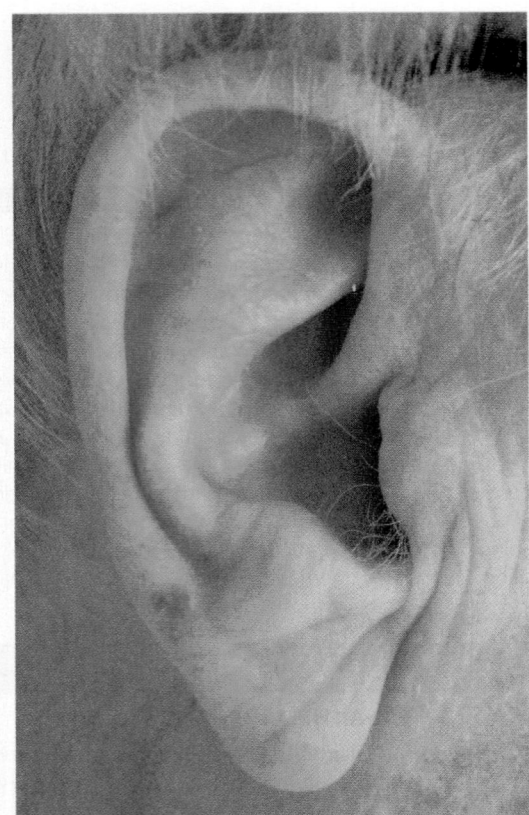

Figure 149-1 *Telangiectasia on the ear of a patient with hereditary hemorrhagic telangiectasia.*

to have BRBNS should be screened with colonoscopy to evaluate for potential GI involvement.

Henoch-Schönlein purpura (HSP) is a systemic vasculitis characterized by involvement of the skin, gastrointestinal tract, kidneys, and joints. Often considered a disease of childhood, HSP also occurs in adults. The major cutaneous manifestation of HSP is palpable purpura, the hallmark of small vessel vasculitis, which present as 2 to 5 mm erythematous to violaceous papules that do not blanch with pressure (**Figure 149-2**). These lesions typically

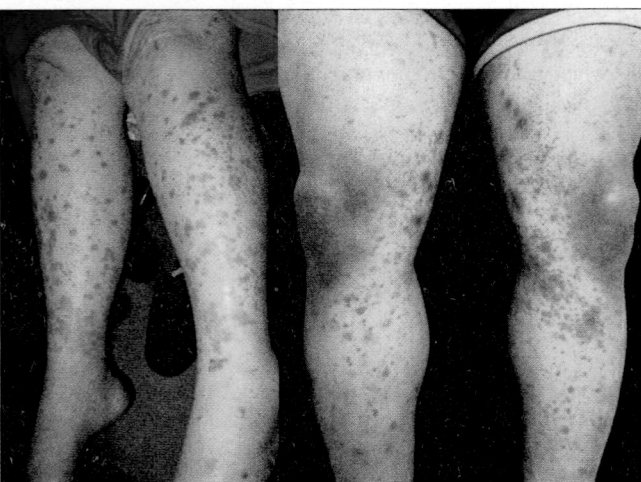

Figure 149-2 *Palpable purpura on the legs of two patients with Henoch-Schönlein purpura. This small vessel vasculitis results in non-blanchable papules that appear red to violaceous, depending on skin type and lesion duration.*

appear on the buttocks and lower extremities in HSP; lesions above the waist are anecdotally associated with an increased risk of renal involvement. Periumbilical purpura have also been noted to occur. Gastrointestinal signs and symptoms include abdominal pain, bleeding, and intussusception; these symptoms may precede the cutaneous findings. Gastrointestinal bleeding is often occult, and is thought to occur in 40% to 60% of cases. If findings are limited solely to the skin, no treatment is necessary. If renal or GI involvement is present, more aggressive systemic immunosuppressive therapy may be necessary. Other systemic vasculitides, such as microscopic polyangiitis and polyarteritis nodosa, can also result in GI hemorrhage.

Kaposi sarcoma (KS) may occasionally present with gastrointestinal bleeding, though KS in general is much less common since the advent of highly active antiretroviral therapy for HIV. Cutaneous KS is a vascular neoplasm associated with human herpesvirus-8. The epidemic form of KS, which occurs in association with HIV, presents with violaceous patches, plaques, or nodules, most commonly on the chest, face, and oral cavity (**Figure 149-3**). Among patients with epidemic KS, gastrointestinal tract involvement occurs in 50% to 80% of patients with cutaneous disease, and more than 90% of patients with oral disease.

Pseudoxanthoma elasticum (PXE), a rare genetic disorder resulting in degeneration of elastic tissue, may affect the elastic media of blood vessels and lead to hemorrhage. Upper GI bleeding is more common than lower GI bleeding, and often presents in the third to fourth decade. Unlike the other disorders discussed in this section, the dermatologic manifestations of PXE do not typically include cutaneous vascular lesions. Instead, PXE manifests as yellow, cobblestoned papules that resemble chicken skin on the neck, axillae, antecubital fossae, and groin. Similar lesions or diffuse superficial erosions may be observed on mucosal surfaces during endoscopy. Ophthalmic signs of PXE include retinal neovascularization, producing angioid streaks. Systemic manifestations include hypertension, premature vascular disease, cardiac disease, and cerebral hemorrhage. Gastrointestinal hemorrhage can be devastating in patients with PXE, and hemorrhage may precede the classic dermatologic and ophthalmologic signs.

MALABSORPTION SYNDROMES

Malabsorption syndromes often produce nutritional deficiencies due to vitamin and mineral loss. An associated cutaneous eruption may suggest the correct diagnosis. Zinc deficiency may result from autosomal recessive genetic abnormalities in zinc absorption, or be acquired from poor diet, geophagia (clay eating), chronic diarrhea, cystic fibrosis, total parenteral nutrition, renal disease, liver disease, alcoholism, or medications such as diuretics and sodium valproate. Zinc deficiency leads to a characteristic skin eruption known as **acrodermatitis enteropathica**. Eczematous, vesicular, or pustular skin lesions typically appear in an acral, perirectal, or perioral distribution. The diaper area is frequently involved. Alopecia, glossitis, and nail dystrophy may also be observed. Diagnosis is made via plasma zinc level, though alkaline phosphatase, a zinc-dependent enzyme, is also often low in this deficiency.

Dermatitis herpetiformis (DH) is characterized by a pruritic papulovesicular eruption on the extensor surfaces of the limbs, especially the forearms, elbows, and knees (**Figure 149-4**). The buttocks and posterior scalp are also often affected. As DH is intensely pruritic, patients often present only with excoriations, rather than well-defined vesicles, in the classic areas of involvement. Dermatitis herpetiformis is a cutaneous manifestation of gluten-sensitive enteropathy (celiac disease). Though more than 85% of DH patients demonstrate small bowel inflammation on biopsy, less than 10% have severe malabsorption. Patients may demonstrate an associated

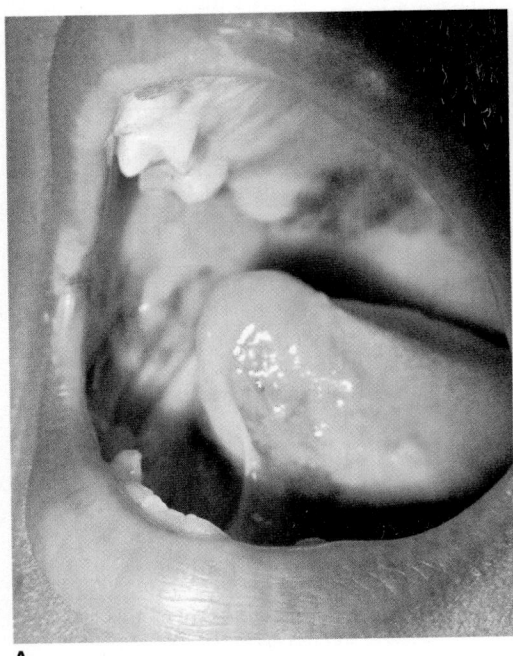
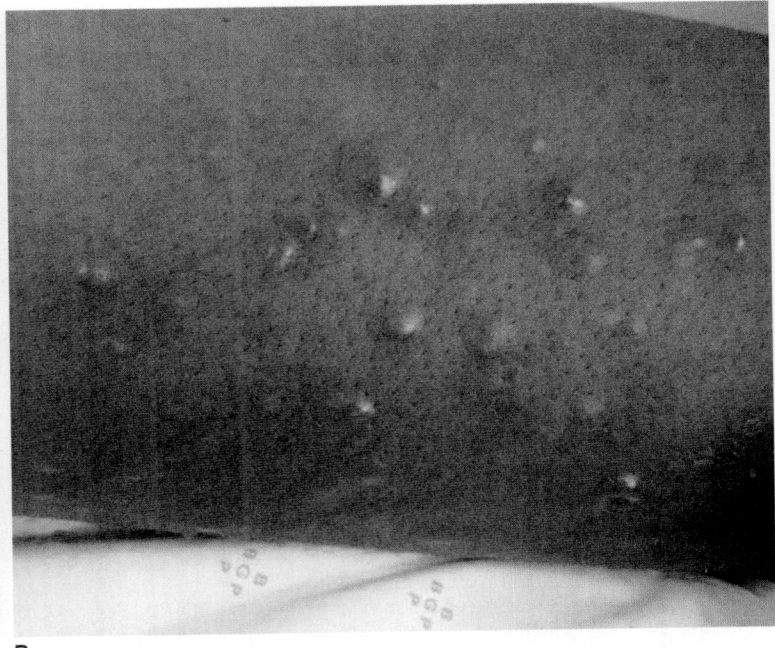

A **B**

Figure 149-3 *Kaposi sarcoma of the oral cavity (A) and thigh (B) in patients with AIDS. Lesions may appear as brown to violaceous patches, plaques, nodules, or tumors.*

autoimmune disease or endocrinopathy, including thyroid disease, diabetes mellitus, or Addison disease. Treatment of DH includes gluten avoidance and antineutrophilic agents such as dapsone.

INFLAMMATORY BOWEL DISEASE

Ulcerative colitis (UC) and Crohn disease (CD) produce skin findings in up to one-third of affected patients. Clinical manifestations range from specific lesions, such as fistulae formation and metastatic disease, to nonspecific reactive conditions. Many of

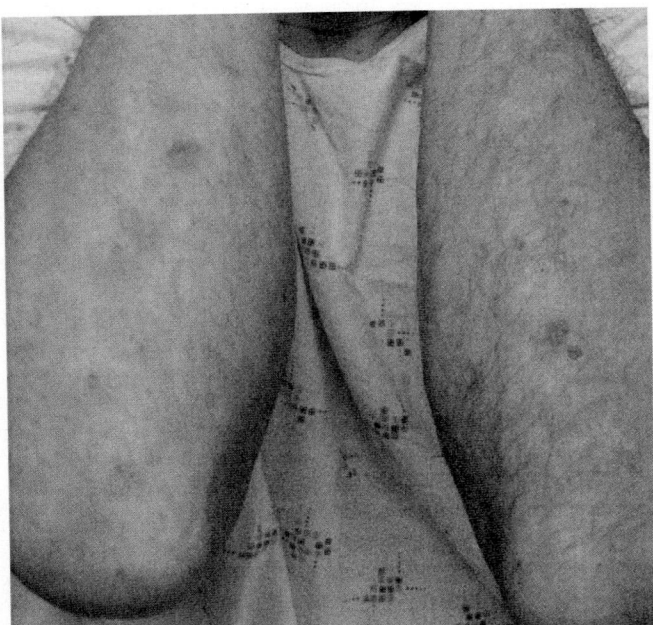

Figure 149-4 *Grouped erosions and bullae on the elbows and forearms in a patient with dermatitis herpetiformis. Small crusted papules and vesicles may also occur.*

these skin lesions may be seen in either UC or CD, though some findings are more often associated with a specific entity. Erythema nodosum and pyoderma gangrenosum will be discussed in detail. Other cutaneous manifestations of inflammatory bowel disease are listed in **Table 149-1**.

Erythema nodosum is the most common panniculitis, or inflammatory disorder of fat. It presents with erythematous, tender nodules, characteristically on the shins (**Figure 149-5**). It is not specific for inflammatory bowel disease (IBD). Erythema nodosum is often a hypersensitivity reaction to systemic disease or an antigenic trigger, although 30% to 50% of cases are idiopathic. Fever, malaise, and arthralgias may occur, and females are affected more commonly than males. It is typically self-limited and resolves within several weeks, with lesions appearing bruise-like later in the disease course. Ulceration usually does not occur. Erythema nodosum may herald the onset of IBD or occur concomitantly with a disease flare. It occurs in 1% to 10% of patients with UC and in less than 2% of patients with CD. Common associations, evaluation, and treatment are provided in **Table 149-2**. The differential diagnosis includes other forms of panniculitis, such as connective tissue panniculitis, infectious panniculitis, pancreatic panniculitis, and erythema induratum or nodular vasculitis, which is often associated with tuberculosis.

In 1930, Brunsting and colleagues characterized painful ulcers in several patients with underlying bowel disease. These skin lesions, which they called ***pyoderma gangrenosum*** (PG), were pustules that evolved into undermined ulcers with overhanging, gray borders and peripheral erythema (**Figure 149-6**). Although they were correct in identifying an association with bowel disease, the condition is not due to bacterial infection, as they had originally postulated. Pyoderma gangrenosum is now recognized as an inflammatory disorder sometimes associated with systemic diseases, including IBD, paraprotenemia, malignancy, and rheumatoid arthritis, although many cases are idiopathic. Though IBD is the single most common cause of PG, only 1% to 5% of patients with inflammatory bowel disease develop PG. In the setting of IBD, PG is usually associated with active colitis and may be an indication for surgery. Pyoderma gangrenosum typically presents on the leg, but lesions can present

TABLE 149-1 Cutaneous Manifestations of Inflammatory Bowel Disease

Disease	Cutaneous Exam Findings	Association	Treatment
	Nonspecific associations		
Urticaria	Transient, edematous, pruritic wheals	UC, Crohn	Antihistamines
Aphthous ulcers	Painful oral erosions	UC, Crohn	Topical steroids
Small vessel vasculitis	Multiple, small (~3-5 mm), nonblanchable red to purple macules and papules, known as "palpable purpura"	UC, Crohn	Systemic steroids if there is systemic involvement, otherwise supportive care
Erythema nodosum	Tender erythematous nodules on anterior shins, representing inflammation of the fat (panniculitis)	UC > Crohn	NSAIDs, bedrest, potassium iodide, systemic steroids, dapsone, colchicine
Neutrophilic dermatoses 1. Pyoderma gangrenosum 2. Sweet syndrome 3. Behçet disease 4. Bowel bypass syndrome	1. Pustules and boggy ulcerations with gray borders, typically on legs; can be peristomal 2. Very edematous, tender red to purple plaques and nodules, typically on face/neck/upper extremities and trunk 3. Recurrent oral and genital ulcerations, acne-like and erythema noduosum-like lesions 4. Red or purple papulovesicles on proximal extremities and trunk	UC >> Crohn	Treat underlying IBD (if present), systemic steroids, dapsone, colchicine, cyclosporine, mycophenolate mofetil, infliximab *AVOID debriding these lesions; the cutaneous eruption may worsen due to pathergy*
Cutaneous polyarteritis nodosa	Purple lacelike eruption on legs (livedo), with nodules or ulcerations	Crohn	Systemic steroids, cytotoxic agents such as cyclophosphamide if systemic involvement
	Specific associations		
Fissures and fistula	Painful erosions and draining sinus tracts, most commonly in the perineum	Crohn > UC	Treat underlying Crohn; sinus tracts may require surgery
Cutaneous or metastatic Crohn	Cutaneous granulomas manifesting as erythematous plaques, nodules, and linear ulcerations, typically in inguinal crease	Crohn	Treat underlying Crohn
Mucosal Crohn	Cobblestoning and ulceration of oral mucosa appearing identical to bowel lesions	Crohn	Treat underlying Crohn
	Rare associations		
Erythema multiforme	Target lesions on extremities and trunk ± ocular inflammation, hemorrhagic crusting on lips, oral/genital mucosal erosions	UC and Crohn (as well as infections and medications)	Supportive care, possible systemic steroids
Vitiligo	Depigmented macules on extremities, face, trunk	UC and Crohn (also thyroid disease)	Topical steroids, phototherapy
Epidermolysis bullosa acquisita (EBA)	Bullae and ulcerations with scarring over elbows and knees; may be peristomal (with differential diagnosis often including PG)	UC and Crohn	Treat underlying IBD, supportive care to bullae

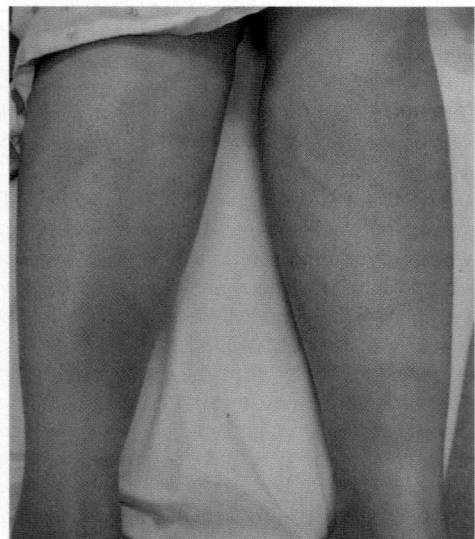

Figure 149-5 *Erythema nodosum: typical erythematous, tender nodules involving the pretibial region.*

anywhere. Peristomal PG is also common in IBD patients. Disease associations and treatment are summarized in **Table 149-3**.

Pyoderma gangrenosum is a neutrophilic dermatosis, with diffuse skin infiltration by mature neutrophils. Other neutrophilic dermatoses include Behçet disease, neutrophilic eccrine hidradenitis, bowel bypass syndrome, rheumatoid neutrophilic dermatitis, and Sweet syndrome (acute febrile neutrophilic dermatosis). An important characteristic of each of these entities is the phenomenon of **pathergy**, meaning that pustular, neutrophil-rich skin lesions develop or worsen following intradermal trauma. The pathergy test used in the diagnosis of Behçet disease is based on this phenomenon. Evidence of pathergy may be found within sites of vaccinations, venipuncture, indwelling catheters, or recently performed procedures (**Figure 149-7**).

It is useful to differentiate pathergy from another term commonly used in dermatology known as the **Koebner phenomenon**. First described in patients with psoriasis by Heinrich Koebner in the late 19th century, the Koebner phenomenon more generally refers to the development of lesions after minor trauma. It occurs in up to 25% of patients with psoriasis, often resulting from a sunburn or scratch (**Figure 149-8**). In addition to psoriasis, skin conditions that may demonstrate the Koebner phenomenon include lichen

TABLE 149-2 Causes, Diagnostic Considerations, and Treatment for Erythema Nodosum

Select Causes	Diagnostic Considerations	Select Treatment
Idiopathic (30%-50%)	(as appropriate)	**General**
Infections	CBC	Identify and treat underlying cause
Bacterial: streptococcal (most common), GI (*Yersinia, Salmonella, Campylobacter*)	HCG	Bed rest and leg elevation
	ESR or C-reactive protein	**Recommended based on large case series**
	CXR	
Viral: respiratory, HBV	Antistreptolysin O or anti-DNAse B titers	Potassium iodide
Fungal: coccidioidomycosis, histoplasmosis	Throat swab (for streptococcal infection)	**Recommended based on small series or case reports**
Mycobacterial: tuberculosis	Tuberculin test	Nonsteroidal anti-inflammatory drugs
Medications: OCPs, estrogens, sulfonamides, penicillin, others	Stool ova and parasite	Systemic corticosteroids
	Hemetest stool	Dapsone
Sarcoidosis	Biopsy	Colchicine
Inflammatory bowel disease		Mycophenolate mofetil
Pregnancy		Hydroxychloroquine, Tetracycline, Prophylactic penicillin
Neutrophilic dermatoses: Behçet disease, Sweet syndrome		

TABLE 149-3 Systemic Associations and Treatment Options for Pyoderma Gangrenosum

Select Systemic Associations	Select Treatment
Gastrointestinal	**General**
Inflammatory bowel disease	Rule out infection (biopsy, tissue culture for bacteria, mycobacteria, fungi)
Diverticulosis	
Primary biliary cirrhosis	
Chronic hepatitis	Avoid trauma/debridement/excision (given pathergy response)
Rheumatologic	
Rheumatoid arthritis	
Ankylosing spondylitis	Careful local wound care in conjunction with specialist
Polychondritis	
Systemic lupus erythematosus	**Recommended based on prospective controlled trial**
Wegener granulomatosis	Infliximab
Hematologic	**Recommended based on retrospective trial or large case series**
Leukemia	
Myeloproliferative disease	Prednisone
Myelodysplasia	Intralesional corticosteroids
Monoclonal gammopathy	Cyclosporine
Myeloma	Thalidomide
Solid organ malignancy	Oral antibiotics (eg, minocycline)
Colon	
Breast	Clofazamine
Prostate	Dapsone
Lung	Topical tacrolimus
Endocrinologic	Intravenous immunoglobulin
Diabetes mellitus	**Recommended based on small series or case reports**
Thyroid disease	
Idiopathic	High-potency topical corticosteroids
	Colchicine
	Tacrolimus
	Methotrexate
	Mycophenolate mofetil
	Azathioprine
	Cyclophosphamide
	Potassium iodide
	Topical cromolyn sodium
	Hyperbaric oxygen
	Etanercept

planus, vitiligo, and leukocytoclastic vasculitis. Unlike pathergy, koebnerization involves the development of lesions characteristic to an underlying disorder, and it is not a phenomenon limited to the neutrophilic dermatoses.

LIVER DISEASE

Cholestasis and cirrhosis have several cutaneous findings that are not specific to any particular etiology of liver disease. Diffuse **pruritus** and **xerosis** of the skin are common. **Jaundice** results from the binding of bilirubin to elastin, and may be observed initially in the conjunctivae, lingual frenulum, and on the soft palate, where elastic fibers are highly concentrated. **Spider angiomata**, with

punctate central arterioles and branches toward the periphery (**Figure 149-9A**), are common in chronic liver disease, but may also be seen with oral contraceptive use, increasing age, alcohol use, and in chronic inflammatory conditions. **Palmar erythema**, affecting the thenar and hypothenar eminences, is another clinical sign of liver disease (**Figure 149-9B**). It is also seen in pregnancy, rheumatoid arthritis, lupus, thyrotoxicosis, diabetes, and neoplasms, where it is thought to result from systemic release of angiogenic factors. It may also be an idiopathic condition. In liver disease, the pathogenesis of spider angiomata and palmar erythema is thought to involve increased levels of circulating estrogens.

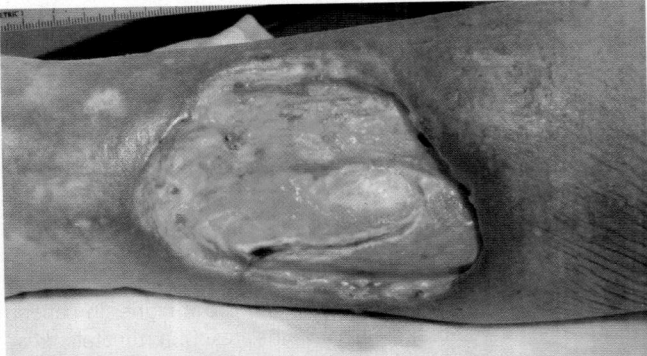

Figure 149-6 *Pyoderma gangrenosum in a patient with ulcerative colitis. Note the large, deep ulceration with overhanging, gray-colored borders.*

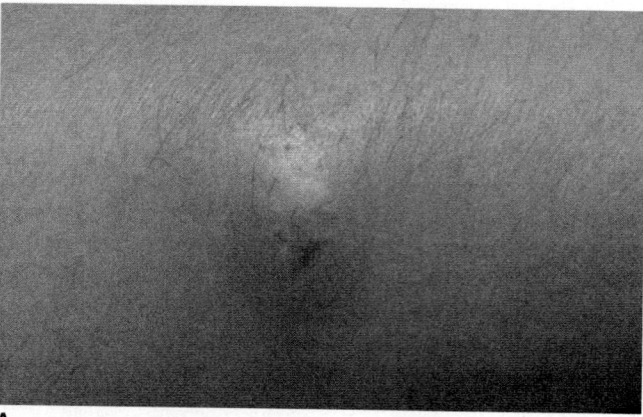

A

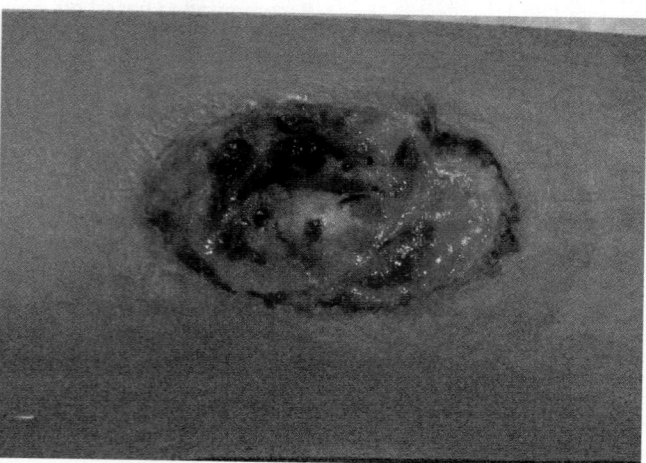

B

Figure 149-7 *Demonstration of pathergy in a patient with pyoderma gangrenosum. A large pustule developed in this patient with ulcerative colitis (A), which was initially suspected to represent an infectious process; all cultures were negative. Following debridement of the lesion, an ulcer characteristic of pyoderma gangrenosum developed (B). This patient's condition improved with systemic corticosteroids.*

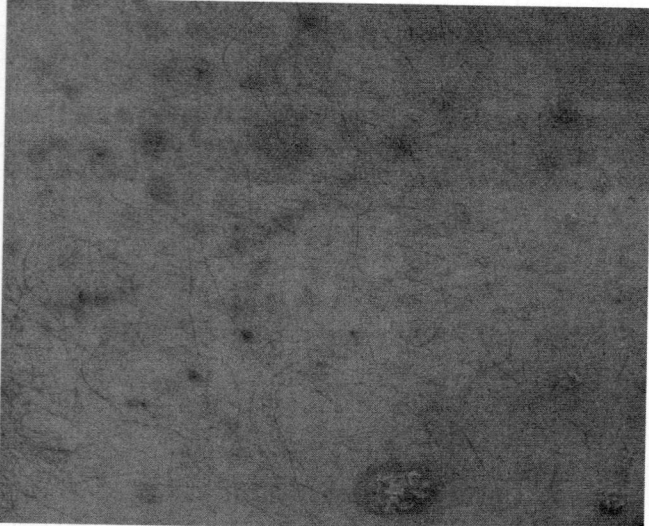

Figure 149-8 *Koebner phenomenon in a patient with psoriasis. Erythematous, scaly papules developed in a linear array after scratching. Typical psoriasiform papules and plaques are also seen in this patient.*

Dupuytren contracture, a thickening of the palmar aponeurosis that may lead to fixed flexion of the fourth and fifth digit, is seen in some cirrhotic patients. It has also been associated with diabetes, anticonvulsant use, a positive family history, and possibly repetitive trauma. The nails are also commonly affected in liver disease. **Terry nails**, the classic nail finding in liver failure, demonstrate whitening of the majority of the nail plate, with retention of only a small band of pink nail plate along the distal portion of the nail (**Figure 149-9C**). Terry nails are also seen in renal disease and malnutrition. Chronic infection with **hepatitis B virus** (HBV) or **hepatitis C virus** (HCV) may be associated with these nonspecific findings of liver disease. Several skin disorders are also specifically associated with either HBV or HCV (**Table 149-4**).

CUTANEOUS MANIFESTATIONS OF CHRONIC RENAL DISEASE

■ COMMON AND BENIGN CUTANEOUS DISEASE

The most common cutaneous complication of chronic renal failure is **pruritus**, which occurs in more than 50% of hemodialysis (HD) patients. Renal pruritus may be generalized, localized, sporadic, or continuous. It is exacerbated by HD. Though the precise etiology is unknown, it is suspected to involve an interplay between xerosis, neuropathy, mast cells, and possibly the HD membrane. Treatment strategies include emollients, narrowband phototherapy, which should be used with caution in transplant patients or transplant candidates due to an increased risk of non-melanoma skin cancer, particularly squamous cell carcinoma, antihistamines, gabapentin, serotonin reuptake inhibitors, and opiate receptor antagonists.

Chronic renal failure is also associated with nail changes. Approximately 10% of patients with chronic renal failure demonstrate **Lindsay nails**, also known as half-and-half nails, in which the proximal portion of the nail appears white, while the distal half appears normal. In nephrotic syndrome, multiple white bands may appear parallel to the lunula of the nail; these bands are known as **Muehrcke lines**, and may also be seen with hypoalbuminemia due to liver disease or malnutrition.

Acquired perforating dermatosis is an uncommon, nonspecific manifestation of chronic renal disease (**Figure 149-10A**). These lesions, characterized by relatively small, dome-shaped papules with a hyperkeratotic central core or plug, occur in up to 10% of dialysis patients. Most patients have end-stage renal disease due to diabetic nephropathy and are undergoing HD. However, lesions may develop prior to dialysis, as well as in patients without renal disease who have diabetes, liver disease, or malignancy. The arms and trunk are predominantly affected, particularly on the extensor aspects. No intervention is necessary for these benign lesions, although associated pruritus may be challenging to manage.

■ RARE AND SERIOUS DISEASE

Nephrogenic systemic fibrosis (NSF), previously known as nephrogenic fibrosing dermopathy, is a progressive, fibrotic thickening of the skin, beginning on the lower extremities. As the disease progresses, joint contractures may occur, limiting mobility and ultimately disabling the patient. The pathogenesis of NSF seems to relate to oxidative tissue damage from free gadolinium ions in patients, typically those with renal failure, who undergo magnetic resonance imaging (MRI) contrast imaging studies. The risk is increased with progressive degrees of renal insufficiency, which lead to a longer tissue half-life of gadolinium, and is higher in patients who receive less-stable gadolinium chelates. Unfortunately, treatment options for NSF are limited. Patients should undergo physical therapy to limit loss of movement and avoid additional exposure to gadolinium. Immunosuppressive medications, thalidomide, and

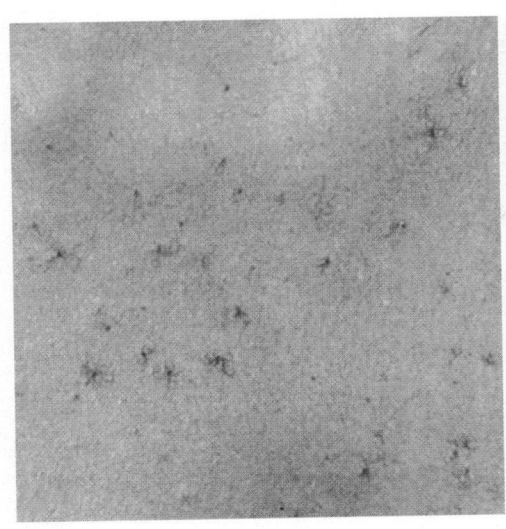

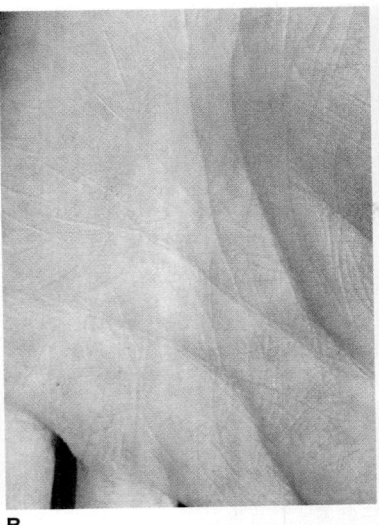

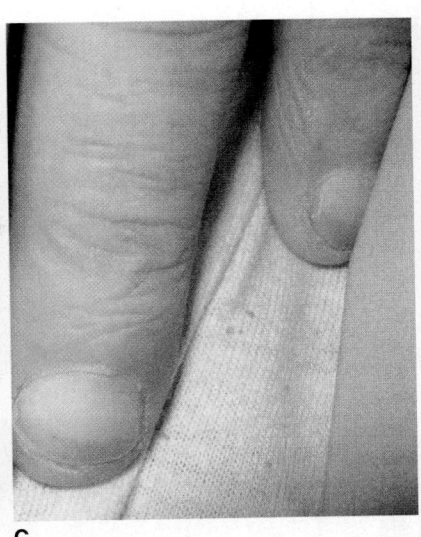

A   **B**   **C**

Figure 149-9 *Cutaneous manifestations of liver disease. (A) Multiple spider angiomata.* (Reproduced, with permission, from Wolff K, Johnson RA, Suurmond D. *Fitzpatrick's Color Atlas & Synopsis of Clinical Dermatology*, 5th ed. New York, NY: McGraw-Hill; 2005, Fig. 151-9.) *(B) Palmar erythema.* (Reproduced, with permission, from Wolff K, Johnson RA, Suurmond D. *Fitzpatrick's Color Atlas & Synopsis of Clinical Dermatology*, 5th ed. New York, NY: McGraw-Hill; 2005, Fig. 151-8.) *(C) Terry nails.* (Courtesy of Dr. Adam Lipworth.)

phototherapy have only a modest effect. Imatinib has shown some promising results in small uncontrolled series. Three gadolinium-based contrast agents are now contraindicated in patients with either chronic severe kidney disease or acute kidney injury.

Calciphylaxis is a serious, potentially lethal condition that affects 1% to 4% of patients with end-stage renal disease on dialysis. Calciphylaxis can also occur in other settings, including coumadin use

and primary hyperparathyroidism. It is a cutaneous vasculopathy characterized by arterial wall calcification and proliferation with subsequent fibrosis and thrombosis. The overlying skin develops progressive ischemia, with resultant severe pain and necrosis (**Figure 149-10B**). The pathophysiology is likely multifactorial, but may be related to prolonged hyperphosphatemia from secondary or tertiary hyperparathyroidism.

TABLE 149-4 Cutaneous Manifestations of HBV and HCV

Hepatitis	Disease	Cutaneous Manifestations	Systemic Manifestations
HBV	Serum sickness reaction	Urticarial or morbilliform eruption	Proteinuria, hematuria, arthritis, hypocomplementemia
	Polyarteritis nodosa	Purple lacelike eruption on legs (livedo), with nodules or ulcerations	Fever, abdominal pain, arthralgias, myalgias, mononeuritis multiplex, congestive heart failure, renal hypertension
	Papular acrodermatitis of childhood (Gianotti-Crosti Syndrome)	Skin-colored to red raised papules on extremities, buttocks and face, with sparing of the trunk	None
HCV	Urticaria/urticarial vasculitis	Edematous wheals	Arthralgias, abdominal pain, nausea, vomiting, diarrhea, proteinuria, hematuria
	Cryoglobulinemia	Red to violaceous raised papules on legs (palpable purpura), purple lacelike eruption on legs (livedo), ulceration of skin	Arthralgias, neuropathy, membranoproliferative glomerulonephritis; rheumatoid factor (RF) positive in cases associated with HCV
	Lichen planus	Violaceous, pruritic, polygonal papules, often on extremities. Can demonstrate Koebner phenomenon. Oral involvement is most closely associated with HCV	None
	Porphyria cutanea tarda (PCT)	Vesicles and bullae, predominantly on dorsal hands. Hyperpigmentation and fragility of skin, milia formation, hypertrichosis	Porphyrins are typically detectable in the urine. Bright coral red fluorescence of patient's urine with a Wood lamp allows for bedside diagnosis
	Necrolytic acral erythema	Papulosquamous or vesicobullous eruption on hands and feet	May be associated with zinc deficiency
	Sarcoidosis (associated with interferon and ribavirin therapy for HCV)	Red to brown papules, plaques, rarely subcutaneous nodules	Hilar lymphadenopathy, respiratory or cardiac involvement, hepatomegaly, arthralgias/arthritis, nervous system involvement, ocular involvement (including lacrimal gland enlargement, uveitis)

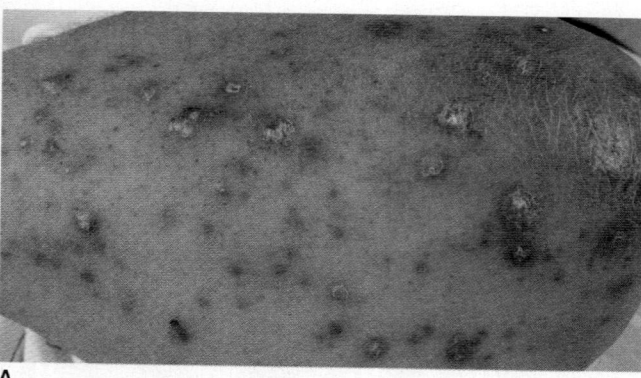

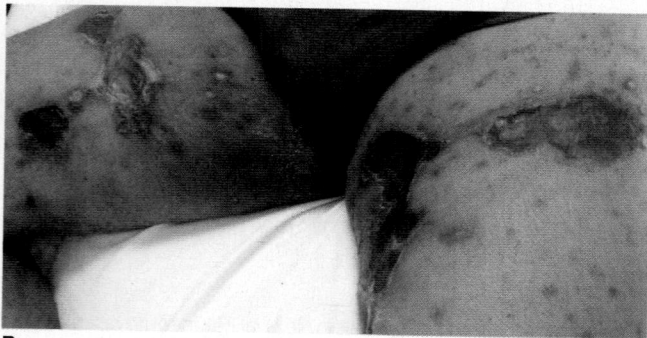

Figure 149-10 *Cutaneous manifestations of renal disease. (A) Acquired perforating dermatosis: dome-shaped papules with hyperkeratotic central cores. Lesions are often pruritic. (B) Calciphylaxis: painful necrotic ulcers on the thighs.*

Clinically, calciphylaxis manifests as red to violaceous plaques that progress to nodules and deep, necrotic ulcers. Lesions may have an overlying eschar and appear stellate, or star-shaped, outlining the area of vascular compromise. There may be associated livedo racemosa or retiform purpura, a patchy, net-like pattern of violaceous erythema on the skin. There is a predilection for the thighs, abdomen, breasts, and other areas with a thick layer of adipose tissue. Women who are obese or who have type 2 diabetes are at increased risk.

Calciphylaxis can be rapidly progressive and potentially fatal, requiring prompt recognition and treatment. A skin biopsy should be performed for confirmation of diagnosis. Treatment options are limited (**Table 149-5**). Therapies aim to mitigate hyperparathyroidism and the attendant hypercalcemia and hyperphosphatemia. There is low-quality evidence to support the use of sodium thiosulfate, which sequesters calcium ions in the form of highly soluble calcium thiosulfate complexes. The severe pain associated with tissue ischemia must be addressed. Complications are common, including infection and poor wound healing due to chronic ischemia. Overall, the prognosis is poor, with a mortality rate of up to 85% following diagnosis. Proximal lesions have a higher mortality. The major cause of mortality in patients with calciphylaxis is sepsis from wound infections, indicating a crucial need for meticulous wound care.

RENAL-CUTANEOUS SYNDORMES

Several rare but important syndromes are associated with cutaneous lesions and renal disease, including renal cell carcinoma. In many, the cutaneous findings may precede the development of malignancy. Thus, recognition of these syndromes may lead to earlier diagnosis of renal cancer. The cutaneous manifestations, gene defects, and renal manifestations of these rare entities are listed in **Table 149-6**.

TABLE 149-5 Calciphylaxis: Diagnostic and Therapeutic Considerations

Clinical Associations	Suggested Workup	Treatment Options
ESRD	BUN/Creatinine	Sodium thiosulfate
Alcoholic liver disease	Calcium	Parathyroidectomy
Coumadin use	Phosphorus	Cinacalcet
Protein C and S deficiency	Serum PTH	Etidronate
Primary hyperparathyroidism		Thrombolytics
Malignancy		Surgical debridement (controversial)
Diabetes		Pain management
Crohn disease		Meticulous wound care
		Discontinuation of calcium and vitamin D supplementation
		Lowering of serum phosphorus

RHEUMATOLOGIC DISEASE AND THE SKIN

■ LUPUS ERYTHEMATOUS

Cutaneous lupus erythematosus has three main subtypes: acute (ACLE), subacute (SCLE), and chronic (CCLE), as summarized in **Table 149-7**. Localized acute cutaneous lupus erythematosus manifests as the characteristic malar or butterfly rash (**Figure 149-11**). Subacute cutaneous disease commonly presents as scaly, red psoriasiform plaques or annular lesions (**Figure 149-12**). Chronic cutaneous lupus is further subdivided into discoid lupus, tumid lupus, and lupus panniculitis. These cutaneous lupus variants have different risks of systemic involvement, autoantibody profiles, and cutaneous findings, depending on the location and depth of the inflammatory infiltrate. Acute cutaneous lupus has the strongest association with systemic disease, and is always considered a manifestation of active SLE, followed by subacute and chronic cutaneous lupus, which may or may not be associated with SLE. Additional variants of cutaneous lupus include tumid lupus, lupus panniculitis, and neonatal lupus erythematosus.

Drug-induced SLE presents with arthralgias, serositis, and other systemic findings, with less frequent cutaneous involvement, whereas drug-induced SCLE presents with cutaneous findings similar to SCLE, without systemic findings. Drug-induced SLE has been associated with hydralazine, isoniazid, procainamide, quinidine, propylthiouracil, minocycline, statins, and tumor necrosis factor-α inhibitors, among others. Drug-induced SCLE has been associated with hydrochlorothiazide, calcium channel blockers, angiotensin converting-enzyme inhibitors, interferons, griseofulvin, and terbinafine. Minocycline, a commonly prescribed tetracycline antibiotic, has been associated with more than 75 cases of drug-induced SLE, sometimes with positive serology for C-ANCA.

In addition to photoprotection and topical corticosteroids, antimalarials such as hydroxychloroquine are a mainstay of therapy for cutaneous lupus. If systemic disease is present or if cutaneous disease is refractory to antimalarial therapy, oral steroids or steroid-sparing immunosuppressive agents is necessary.

■ SYSTEMIC SCLEROSIS/CREST

Systemic sclerosis is an autoimmune connective tissue disease characterized by fibrosis of skin and internal organs and extensive damage to the microvasculature. Cutaneous fibrosis without internal organ involvement can occur, and is known as localized scleroderma or morphea. This discussion will focus only on systemic sclerosis.

TABLE 149-6 Renal-Cutaneous Syndromes

Disease	Gene Defect, Inheritance Pattern	Cutaneous Findings	Renal Manifestations
Birt-Hogg-Dube	Folliculin, AD	Achrochordon, fibrofolliculomas, trichodiscomas (may be a variant of fibrofolliculoma)	Renal cell carcinoma, especially the chromophobe and oncocytic types
Fabry disease	α-Galactosidase A, X-linked recessive	Angiokeratoma corporis diffusum	Glomerulonephritis and "Maltese crosses" in the urine
Familial leiomyomatosis (Reed syndrome)	Fumarate hydratase, AD	Multiple skin colored leiomyomas (patients may also have uterine leiomyomas)	Renal cell carcinoma, papillary type
POEMS Syndrome (Polyneuropathy, organomegaly, endocrinopathy, monoclonal gammopathy, and skin changes)	No known genetic defect, cases are sporadic	Scleroderma like thickening of the skin, hyperpigmentation, glomeruloid hemangiomas (of the skin), hypertrichosis	Proteinuria, hematuria, and renal failure
Tuberous sclerosis	Hamartin, AD Tuberin, AD	Ash-leaf macules, facial angiofibromas, connective tissue nevi (shagreen patch), periungual fibromas	Angiomyolipomas, multicystic kidneys

Systemic sclerosis can be divided into localized and diffuse systemic sclerosis, depending on the extent of cutaneous involvement. In both localized and diffuse cases, Raynaud phenomenon is often the first manifestation of disease. Severe Raynaud may lead to pitted scars and ulcerations of the fingertips. Gangrenous digital lesions and fingertip amputation may ensue. Patients often go through a phase of hand swelling and edema, followed by progressive sclerosis. Both localized and diffuse systemic sclerosis initially demonstrate symmetric induration and fibrosis of the skin on the hands (**Figure 149-13A**), fingers, and face. Diffuse disease may then progress to involve the proximal extremities, trunk, and pelvis. Facial involvement characteristically affects the mouth, leading to decreased oral aperture, and occasionally the nose, giving it a beaked appearance. Patients may initially note a loss of wrinkles, and they may appear younger than their stated age. Loss of facial movement and microstomia develop as the disease progresses. Diffuse hyperpigmentation of the skin, or patchy follicular hypopigmentation along with hyperpigmentation (salt-and-pepper appearance), may also be observed (**Figure 149-13B**).

CREST syndrome refers to a subset of patients with localized systemic sclerosis, characterized by calcinosis cutis, Raynaud phenomenon, esophageal dysmotility, sclerodactyly, and telangiectasias (**Figure 149-13C**). Not all patients with localized systemic sclerosis have all of the diagnostic criteria for CREST, and some patients with diffuse disease have multiple features of CREST. Patients with limited disease and exaggerated CREST features have a higher frequency of anticentromere autoantibodies, and a higher incidence of pulmonary hypertension and gastrointestinal complications.

Organ involvement may develop before or after the characteristic cutaneous eruption in both localized and diffuse systemic sclerosis. Common extracutaneous manifestations include interstitial lung disease and pulmonary hypertension, esophageal dysmotility and reflux, right- or left-sided heart failure, and renal hypertension. Pulmonary hypertension is now the most common cause of death. Scleroderma renal crisis was formerly the leading cause of death, but outcomes have improved with aggressive angiotensin-converting-enzyme (ACE) inhibitor treatment. Patients with diffuse systemic sclerosis and antitopoisomerase I autoantibodies generally have a worse prognosis, and are more likely to develop early, severe internal organ involvement. Localized systemic sclerosis has a better prognosis, with patients tending to develop internal organ involvement years later in the course of their disease.

The pathogenesis of fibrosis in systemic sclerosis is unknown, though autoimmunity is thought to be involved. Most patients have a positive antinuclear antibodies (ANA). Patients with localized systemic sclerosis also may have anticentromere antibodies, while patients with diffuse systemic sclerosis may have anti-Scl-70 (antitopoisomerase) antibodies. However, the sensitivity of each of these autoantibodies is relatively low. Cytokines and growth factors, particularly TGF-β and connective tissue growth factor (CTGF), may contribute to the pathogenesis by increasing collagen synthesis. Current treatment is directed toward the manifestations of systemic sclerosis, rather than the underlying pathogenesis. Raynaud phenomenon responds well to calcium channel blockers. Phosphodiesterase inhibitors such as sildenafil citrate and endothelial receptor antagonists such as bosentan have been used for both refractory Raynaud phenomenon with ulcerations and pulmonary hypertension. Angiotensin-converting-enzyme inhibitors have substantially reduced the mortality associated with renal hypertension, and immunosuppressive therapies have shown effectiveness in pulmonary fibrosis. Cutaneous disease has been treated with agents including D-penicillamine, methotrexate, mycophenolate mofetil, imatinib mesylate, and cyclophosphamide, amongst others, although prospective studies are essentially lacking. Most recently, antibodies to TGF-β and CTGF have been studied in clinical trials, but the results have been limited.

■ DERMATOMYOSITIS

Dermatomyositis (DM) is an autoimmune connective tissue disease involving skin and proximal muscles. However, the characteristic rash may occur without notable muscle involvement, as in amyopathic or hypomyopathic dermatomyositis. Muscle involvement without a skin eruption (polymyositis) is now thought to occur through a different mechanism.

The cutaneous eruption of dermatomyositis typically begins on the face, with noticeable eyelid edema and violaceous-colored erythema (heliotrope rash). Erythema and poikiloderma (atrophy, telangiectasia, hyperpigmentation, and hypopigmentation) may develop on the mid-face or on the upper back and shoulders, called the shawl sign (**Figure 149-14A**). Dilated blood vessels or telangiectasias at the nailfold, with overgrowth of the cuticle, may be present (**Figure 149-14B**). Nail bed telangiectasias may also be seen in other connective tissue diseases. Pruritus, particularly of the scalp, can be a frustrating symptom for patients. Erythematous to violaceous papules and plaques, with or without scale, may develop on the dorsal hands with prominent involvement over the joints,

TABLE 149-7 Overview of Cutaneous Lupus, and Strength of Association with Systemic Lupus

Lupus Type	Cutaneous Findings	Systemic Findings	Autoantibody Profile	Treatment Options
Acute cutaneous lupus (ACLE)	Bilateral malar erythema (butterfly rash) Erythematous eruption on dorsal fingers, with sparing over the joints Periungal erythema Photosensitivity	*Strongest association with SLE* Oral ulcers Arthritis Renal involvement CNS involvement Pleuritis/pericarditis Blood abnormalities (leukopenia, anemia, thrombocytopenia)	ANA+ Anti-ds DNA+ (correlates with renal involvement) Anti-Ro, La, Sm+ Anti-phospholipid antibodies	Sun protection Topical corticosteroids Antimalarials (hydroxychloroquine) Oral steroids Steroid-sparing immunosuppressants (including methotrexate, azathioprine, mycophenolate mofetil)
Subacute cutaneous lupus (SCLE)	Lesions are often strikingly photodistributed (V of chest, back, arms) with sparing of mid-face. Types: 1. Annular (ring shaped) or polycyclic, erythematous plaques with clear center 2. Erythematous, psoriasiform scaly plaques	50% of patients meet criteria for SLE; however, a much lower percentage have renal or CNS involvement 40%-50% with arthritis/arthralgias 20% with leukopenia	80% with ANA+ Anti-Ro+ (correlates with photosensitivity)	Sun protection Topical corticosteroids Antimalarials (hydroxychloroquine) Immunosuppressants for refractory cases Topical tacrolimus or pimecrolimus
		Chronic cutaneous lupus (CCLE)		
Discoid lupus (DLE)	Hyperpigmented plaques with central atrophy and scarring; lesions favor the scalp, nose, malar areas, and ears	5%-10% of patients develop systemic involvement (increased if lesions on body in addition to face/scalp)	20% ANA+	Sun protection Topical or intralesional steroids Antimalarials (hydroxychloroquine) Immunosuppressants for refractory cases
Tumid lupus	Erythematous, edematous plaques on mid-chest, back, and face	5%-10% of patients develop systemic involvement	40% ANA+	Sun protection Topical corticosteroids Antimalarials (hydroxychloroquine)
Lupus panniculitis	Firm, tender subcutaneous nodules with normal overlying skin or with discoid lupus changes on overlying skin; typically on proximal upper extremities, thighs, buttocks, or face. Chronic lesions become depressed plaques	5%-10% of patients develop systemic involvement	30% ANA+	Antimalarials (hydroxychloroquine) Immunosuppressants
Neonatal lupus	Annular (ring-shaped), polycyclic, or scaly erythematous plaques with clear center, similar to SCLE. Typical involvement on face, particularly around eyes. Mother often has anti-Ro+ SCLE, and must be evaluated.	50% of children will have permanent third degree heart block (must therefore check ECG); hepatobiliary disease; thrombocytopenia	Anti-Ro, La, or U1RNP antibodies passively acquired from mother	If no heart block or systemic disease, supportive care only, as once the antibodies are degraded by the child, cutaneous eruption resolves If there is heart block, must involve cardiology Mother should be evaluated and treated for SCLE/autoimmune disease

known as Gottron's papules (**Figure 149-14C**). By contrast, patients with lupus can have an erythematous eruption, which typically involves the interphalangeal components of the dorsal fingers, with joint sparing.

Symmetric proximal muscle weakness is common in dermatomyositis, with particular involvement of the shoulders and hips. Myopathy can be diagnosed by measuring creatine kinase and aldolase levels or by obtaining an electromyogram. Muscle biopsies and MRI studies are also used. In addition, patients may develop arthritis and

arthralgias, as well as pulmonary fibrosis or even cardiac involvement. Esophageal involvement can present as either reflux or dysphagia. Baseline esophageal studies, pulmonary function tests with diffusion studies, and electrocardiogram are recommended. Similar to other autoimmune connective tissue diseases, specific autoantibodies can be associated with systemic involvement in DM (**Table 149-8**).

Between 10% to 50% of cases of DM in adults are associated with underlying cancer. The diagnosis of malignancy may precede or follow the diagnosis of DM. Underlying malignancies include

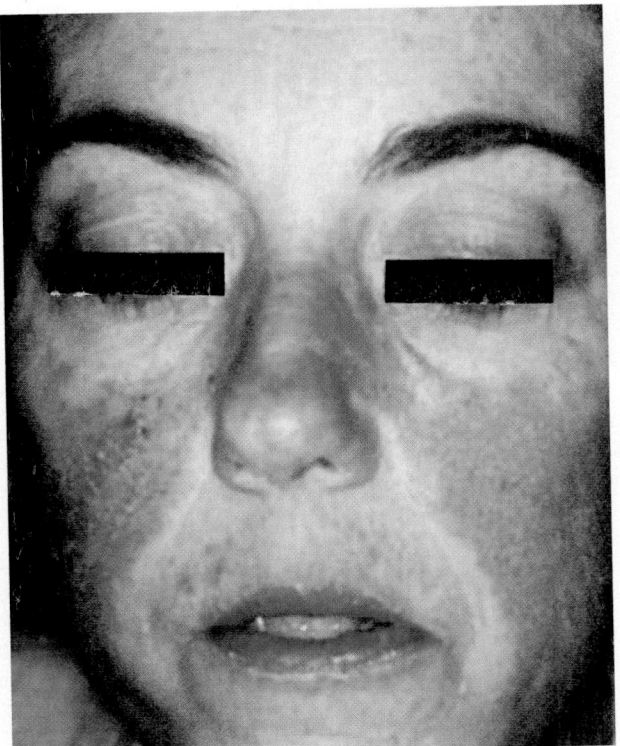

Figure 149-11 *Acute cutaneous lupus erythematosus (ACLE) typically manifests as the characteristic malar "butterfly" rash.* (Reproduced, with permission, from Wolff K, Johnson RA, Suurmond D. *Fitzpatrick's Color Atlas & Synopsis of Clinical Dermatology*, 5th ed. New York, NY: McGraw-Hill; 2005, Fig. 156-3.)

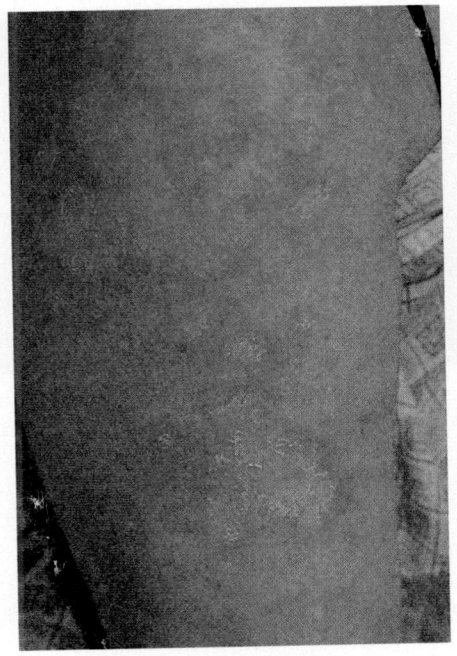

A

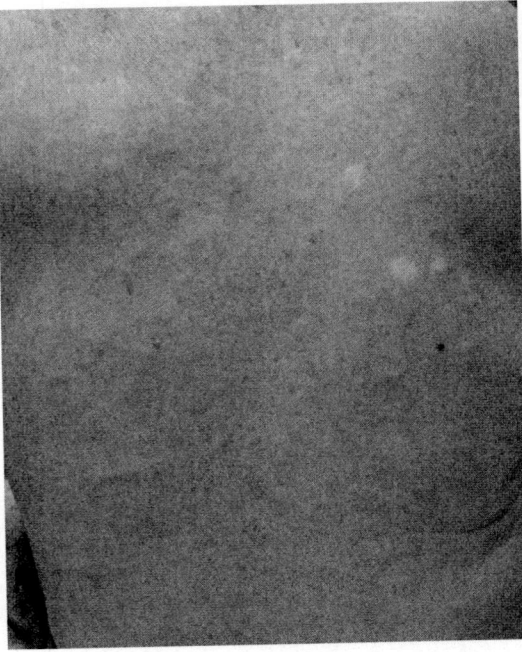

B

Figure 149-12 *Subacute cutaneous lupus (SCLE). There are two main clinical variants: psoriasiform, scaly erythematous plaques (A) and erythematous, annular plaques (B).*

adenocarcinoma of the ovary, lung, pancreas, colon, and stomach, as well as lymphoma. In female patients, there is a strong association with ovarian cancer, and in Southeast Asian patients, there is an association with nasopharyngeal carcinoma. Routine malignancy screening is not considered sufficient to detect potentially associated malignancies, and more advanced laboratory and imaging studies, such as computed tomography (CT) of chest, abdomen, and pelvis, along with a transvaginal pelvic ultrasound in women, are warranted. Screening tests should be performed at the time of diagnosis and annually for the next 3 to 5 years to detect possible malignancies (**Table 149-9**). Juvenile dermatomyositis is usually not associated with underlying malignancy, but may instead be associated with an increased risk of calcinosis cutis and vasculitis, particularly of the GI tract.

Oral steroids remain the initial treatment of choice for myositis. Steroid-sparing agents, such as methotrexate, azathioprine, or mycophenolate mofetil, may also be beneficial. For patients who have failed these treatments, intravenous immunoglobulin (IVIG) or rituximab may help. Cutaneous disease is treated with strict photoprotection, topical corticosteroids, antimalarials including hydroxychloroquine, and immunosuppressive medications in more refractory cases.

CUTANEOUS MANIFESTATIONS OF ENDOCRINE DISORDERS

■ THYROID DISEASE

Similar to its role elsewhere in the body, thyroid hormone is instrumental in regulating the development and homeostasis of the skin and hair. Specifically, thyroid hormone regulates skin thickness, protein synthesis, cell division, and temperature. As a result, hypo

and hyperthyroidism result in characteristic cutaneous findings, in addition to systemic manifestations.

Hypothyroidism results in a decreased metabolic state with reduced core temperature, vasoconstriction, and xerosis (dry skin). As a result, acquired ichthyosis or keratoderma may develop, in addition to brittle nails. The skin may be slightly yellow from carotenemia, as hypothyroidism diminishes the transformation of carotene to vitamin A. The patient may have ***myxedema***, swollen, pale, and waxy skin, with diffuse deposits of mucopolysaccharides. There is often associated swelling of the eyelids, lips, and tongue. Finally, loss of the lateral aspects of the eyebrows (madarosis) and scalp hair can also occur in hypothyroidism.

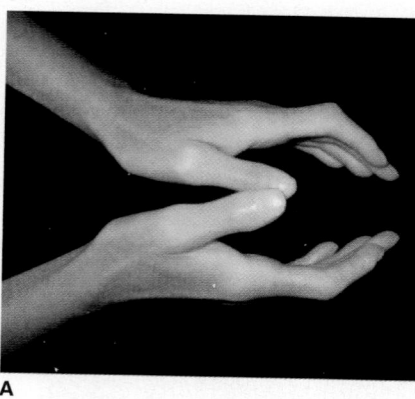
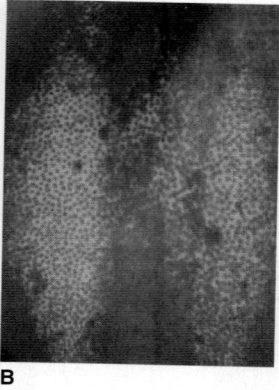
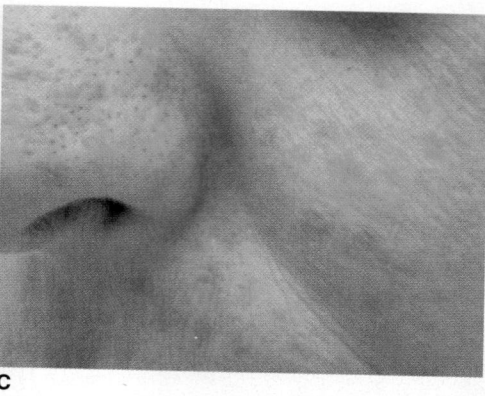

Figure 149-13 *Cutaneous findings in systemic sclerosis. (A) Sclerodactyly, or thickening of the skin of the digits of the hands and feet. Digital ulceration, calcinosis, and joint contractures may also develop. (B) Salt-and-pepper appearance of the skin, produced by a combination of patchy hyperpigmentation and follicular hypopigmentation. (C) In the CREST variant of systemic sclerosis, mat telangiectasias are common on the face, upper trunk, and extremities.*

Hyperthyroidism can also produce diffuse alopecia. However, in contrast to hypothyroidism, hyperthyroidism results in cutaneous thinning and warm, moist skin. Hyperhidrosis may also occur due to increased vasodilation. Finally, hyperpigmentation similar to that observed in Addison disease may be associated with hyperthyroidism.

The most common cause of hyperthyroidism is **Graves disease**, caused by autoantibodies to the thyroid-stimulating hormone (TSH) receptor. Up to 25% of patients with Graves disease develop ophthalmopathy (or orbitopathy), with exophthalmos and proptosis caused by orbital fat accumulation and edema of the ocular muscles. Hyperthyroid patients may have lid retraction and widening of the palpebral fissures without necessarily having Graves ophthalmopathy.

About 4% of patients with Graves disease have **pretibial myxedema** or dermopathy, manifesting as symmetric, indurated, firm plaques and nodules with a peau d'orange texture on the anterior shins. Rarely, patients with Graves disease have **thyroid acropachy**, consisting of the triad of digital clubbing, soft tissue swelling of the hands and feet, and periosteal bone formation.

■ DIABETES MELLITUS

Type 1 and type 2 diabetes mellitus are complicated by a variety of cutaneous manifestations (**Figure 149-15**). Contributing factors include vascular insufficiency, microangiopathy, metabolic derangement, neutrophil dysfunction from hyperglycemia, poor wound healing, and neuropathic complications.

Skin infections occur in 20% to 50% of diabetic patients. These include candidal intertrigo, tinea, diabetic foot infections, malignant otitis externa due to *Pseudomonas*, and mucormycosis in the setting of ketoacidosis. It is particularly important to recognize and treat tinea pedis in this population, as skin breakdown from tinea often serves as a portal of entry for diabetic foot infections.

Irregular, red-brown papules or plaques on the pretibial areas should raise suspicion for **diabetic dermopathy**. Once the inflammatory stage has subsided, these lesions heal over months to years, leaving atrophic, hyperpigmented scars. Diabetic dermopathy may precede the onset of abnormal glucose metabolism, and has been associated with a greater susceptibility for microvascular complications such as retinitis, nephropathy, and neuropathy. There is no specific therapy. Glycemic control should be optimized. Insulin resistance is associated with the development of **acrochordons** (skin tags), fleshy, soft papules on the eyelids, neck, axillae, and inguinal folds, and **acanthosis nigricans**, velvety, hyperpigmented, asymptomatic plaques in the neck, axilla, and groin.

Patients with diabetes often develop **nail changes**. In type 2 disease, 40% to 50% of patients demonstrate yellow nails, often most prominent along the distal portion. This may be confused with onychomycosis. In addition to yellow nails, patients may develop periungual telangiectasia, with ragged cuticles and nailfold erythema.

Necrobiosis lipoidica (NL) manifests as yellow to red-brown plaques with atrophy and telangiectasia on the lower legs. Central atrophy may develop, sometimes with painful ulceration. Though NL is seen in less than 2% of patients with diabetes, a third of patients with NL have frank diabetes, and another third have impaired glucose tolerance. Topical or intralesional corticosteroids may arrest the progression of plaques. Ulceration usually responds to topical wound care. **Diabetic bullae** (bullosis diabeticorum) also occur on the lower legs. These are noninflamed, asymptomatic blisters on the dorsal and lateral legs, which heal with supportive care in 2 to 6 weeks. Wound care is necessary to prevent bacterial secondary infection.

Patients with both types of diabetes may demonstrate skin thickening, ranging from nonspecific thickening of the dorsal hands (observed in 20%-30% of diabetics), to marked thickening of the upper back, known as **scleredema diabeticorum** (2.5%-14% of diabetics). Diabetes is responsible for only about a third of scleredema cases; scleredema may also be seen in paraproteinemia, hyperparathyroidism, and as a postinfectious streptococcal complication.

Similar to patients with chronic renal failure, diabetes has been associated with **acquired perforating dermatoses** and **calciphylaxis**, though less frequently. It is unknown whether these conditions tend to affect patients with diabetes alone, or patients who have concomitant diabetes and renal failure. **Vitiligo**, which presents with depigmented patches of skin, is observed in 1% to 7% of patients with type 1 diabetes. The coexistence of these two conditions suggests the polyglandular autoimmune syndrome.

Disseminated granuloma annulare is weakly associated with type 2 diabetes. This condition consists of hundreds of small, oval to ring-shaped thin pink papules that appear over the trunk and limbs. It tends to resolve spontaneously over time. Treatment options include topical or intralesional corticosteroids, amongst other anti-inflammatory therapeutic regimens.

AMYLOIDOSIS

Amyloid is a homogenous, eosinophilic, waxy material that can be deposited in any of the body's organ systems. Amyloidosis may be either acquired or hereditary, and may be further subdivided into

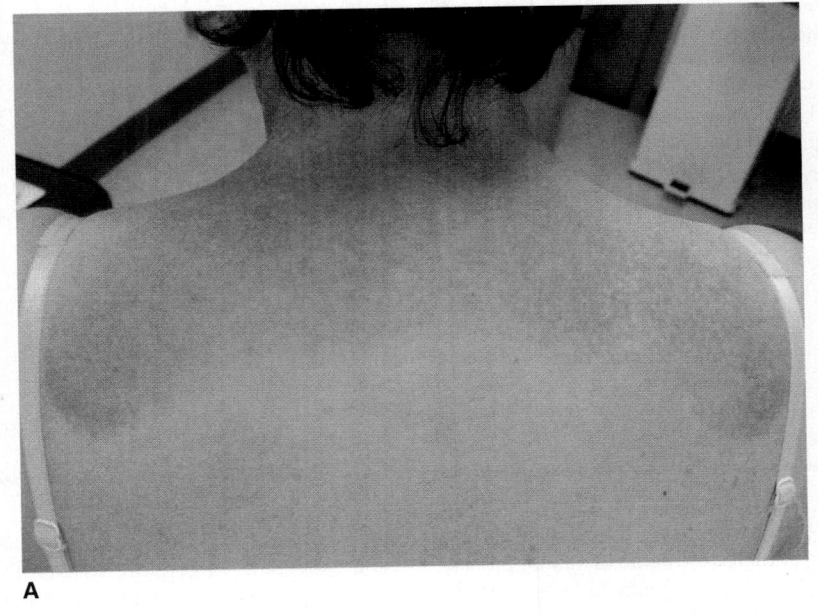

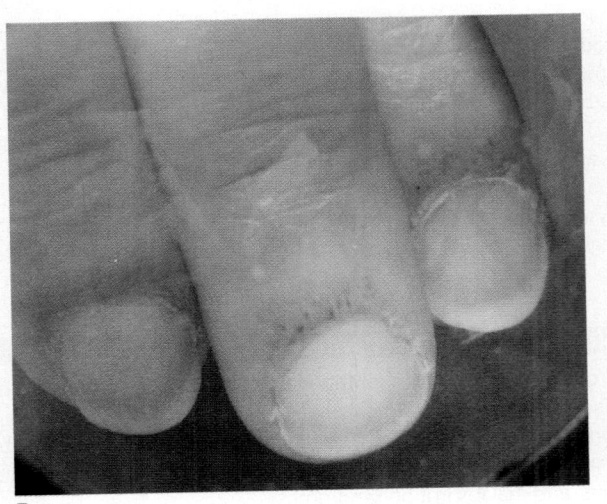

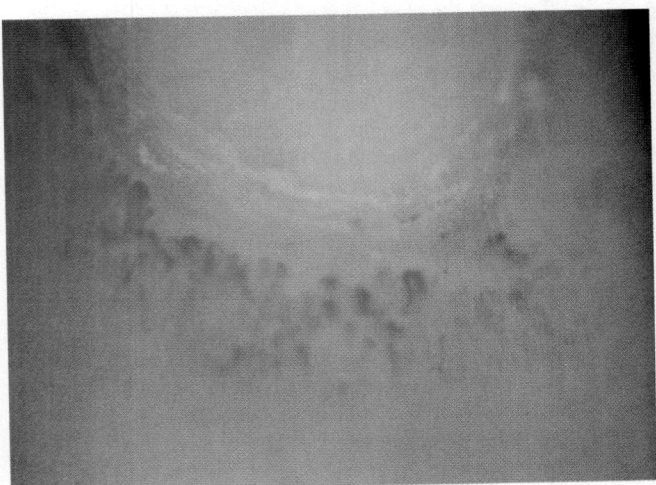

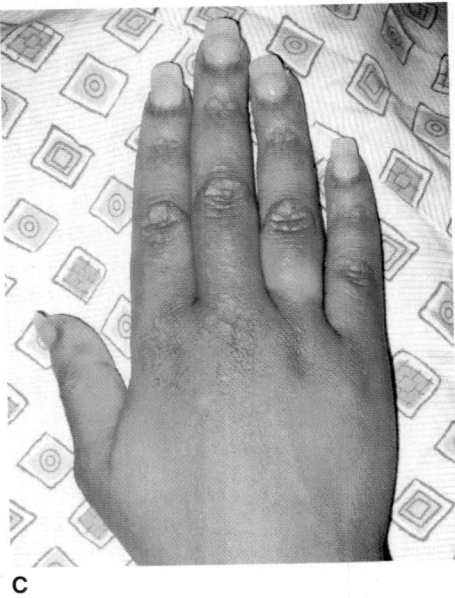

Figure 149-14 *Cutaneous findings in dermatomyositis. (A) Typical shawl sign demonstrating poikiloderma (atrophy, telangiectasia, hyperpigmentation, and hypopigmentation). (B) Dilated capillary loops within the nailfold, along with hypertrophic cuticles. (C) Gottron papules: violaceous papules overlying the joints. (Courtesy of Dr. Peter Lio.)*

TABLE 149-8 Autoantibodies Associated with Dermatomyositis, Systemic Sclerosis, and Mixed Connective Tissue Disease

Autoantibody	Cutaneous Findings	Systemic Findings
Anti-Mi2	Classic cutaneous dermatomyositis, particularly shawl sign and cuticular overgrowth	Better prognosis, better response to treatment, less risk of pulmonary fibrosis
Anti-tRNA synthetases (including Jo-1)	Erythema and nonpruritic, scaly patches on the hands, particularly lateral and volar fingers, so-called mechanic's hands	Increased risk of interstitial lung disease; fever, arthritis, myositis, Raynaud (so-called antisynthetase syndrome)
	Raynaud phenomenon	
Anti-PM-Scl	Sclerodermoid skin changes (thickening and induration of the skin)	Increased risk of systemic sclerosis
	Sclerodactyly	
Anti-U1RNP	Mixed connective tissue disease, with overlapping cutaneous features of lupus, systemic sclerosis, and dermatomyositis	Myositis, arthritis, increased risk of pulmonary fibrosis, decreased risk of nephritis compared to lupus

systemic and localized forms. Acquired amyloidosis may be primary, due to deposition of monoclonal immunoglobulin light chains, or secondary, due to accumulation of serum amyloid A in patients with longstanding systemic inflammatory conditions, as in untreated tuberculosis or rheumatoid arthritis.

The clinical presentation depends on the organ of deposition. Cutaneous lesions range from hyperpigmented patches, seen in macular amyloid, to macroglossia and pinch purpura, seen in primary systemic disease. **Table 149-10** summarizes the different subtypes of amyloidosis, as well as their cutaneous manifestations and treatment options.

Primary systemic amyloid is a clonal disorder of plasma cells. While myeloma is sometimes complicated by amyloidosis, most patients with primary systemic amyloid do not meet diagnostic criteria for myeloma. Organ involvement in primary amyloidosis includes the skin, gastrointestinal tract, kidneys, and especially the cardiovascular system; the most common causes of death are refractory heart failure and ventricular arrhythmia. Cutaneous involvement is observed in 40% of patients with primary systemic amyloidosis. Skin findings include macroglossia, often manifesting with indentations on the side of the tongue from the teeth, waxy or shiny nodules, and purpuric papules and nodules, particularly around the eyes, oral cavity,

and extremities. In contrast, visceral disease predominates in secondary systemic amyloid from inflammatory states or infection, and skin lesions are usually absent. Despite the ostensible lack of skin involvement in secondary systemic amyloidosis, biopsy of clinically normal skin may demonstrate perivascular amyloid deposition in 50% of cases; sensitivity may be increased by use of rectal biopsies, rather than abdominal fat pad biopsies.

Treatment is directed at the underlying causative disease. Primary systemic amyloid requires hematology-oncology consultation for evaluation and treatment of a potentially associated plasma cell dyscrasia. Secondary systemic amyloidosis, on the other hand, requires evaluation to determine the chronic inflammatory or infectious etiology.

NUTRITIONAL DEFICIENCIES

In developing countries, nutritional deficiencies arise from malnutrition or starvation, particularly in infants and young children. In contrast, nutritional deficiencies in developed countries are often manifestations of alcoholism, total parenteral nutrition, restricted diets, and malabsorption syndromes.

As many essential nutrients are involved in interrelated steps in metabolic pathways of fatty acids, vitamin deficiencies may have similar cutaneous eruptions (**Table 149-11**). These include: acral or intertriginous desquamative eruptions, which may initially be confused with atopic dermatitis or fungal infections; seborrheic eruptions, consisting of scaly erythematous plaques on the mid-chest, back, perioral areas, and central face; glossitis; diffuse alopecia; and peripheral edema. Unfortunately, these lesions are nonspecific and may be subtle. The histopathologic findings of the different nutritional deficiencies are also nonspecific, consisting of pallor of the epidermis with edema and bulla (blister) formation.

Patients with nutritional and vitamin deficiencies are often initially misdiagnosed. Frequently, children are diagnosed with atopic dermatitis, but do not respond to traditional eczema treatments. Adults are often misdiagnosed as having seborrheic dermatitis or psoriasis, but similarly fail to improve.

Diagnosing a possible nutritional deficiency requires a detailed dietary history, including total food intake, use of dietary supplements or suppressants, and a prior history of GI disease, including inflammatory bowel disease and previous gastrointestinal surgery. Physicians should consider coexisting psychiatric issues, such as alcoholism, substance abuse, anorexia, or bulimia. Laboratory values can be beneficial, including complete blood count, zinc levels, alkaline phosphatase levels (a zinc-dependent enzyme), vitamin A, vitamin B and subtypes, vitamin C, and vitamin D. In

TABLE 149-9 Malignancies Associated with Dermatomyositis and Suggested Evaluation

Malignancies associated with dermatomyositis (reported frequency 10%-50%)	Suggested malignancy workup (consider annually for 3-5 y following diagnosis)
Genitourinary, especially ovarian cancer	Full physical examination
Colon	CBC, complete metabolic panel, TSH, U/A
Breast	Stool occult blood testing
Lung	Breast and gynecologic in women; Pap smear and mammography
Gastric	
Pancreatic	
Lymphoma	CT of the chest, abdomen, and pelvis
Nasopharyngeal carcinoma (overrepresented in Southeast Asians)	Transvaginal pelvic ultrasound in women
	CA-125, CA 19-9
	Gastrointestinal endoscopy (age-appropriate)

infants, metabolic nutritional panels can be checked for possible inborn errors of metabolism causing dietary deficiency. Once the deficiency is determined, appropriate supplementation can be initiated (**Figure 149-16**).

CUTANEOUS SARCOIDOSIS

Sarcodoisis is a disease of unknown etiology that most commonly affects the lungs, eyes, lymphoid organs, liver, and skin. Approximately 70% of patients with cutaneous involvement actually have systemic sarcoidosis. Diagnosis is made on clinical exam and confirmed by the presence of noncaseating granulomas on histology. Nonspecific cutaneous conditions are also associated with sarcoid, including erythema nodosum, pruritus, erythema multiforme, and erythroderma.

Sarcoidosis mimics many types of cutaneous disease. The most common presentation is **papular sarcoid**, presenting as small, 3 to 5 mm red-brown to violaceous papules typically on the face (**Figure 149-17A**). Papules may coalesce into larger, annular plaques that appear serpiginious (**Figure 149-17B**). Lesions may be hypopigmented on darker skin. When the scalp is involved, there may be scarring alopecia. Sarcoidosis sometimes produces red, indurated plaques with telangiectasias on the central face or neck, a condition known as ***lupus pernio***; involvement of the nasal rim indicates increased risk for upper airway involvement. Sarcoidosis may develop within scars (**Figure 149-17C**) or areas previously affected by infection, trauma, or radiation. Less common manifestations of cutaneous sarcoidosis include ichthyosis-like lesions, pustular lesions, verrucous lesions, and subcutaneous sarcoid.

MALIGNANCY AND THE SKIN

Malignancy may manifest in the skin as direct metastatic spread, or by inducing an inflammatory dermatosis or other paraneoplastic skin changes. These paraneoplastic phenomena may resolve following treatment of the underlying malignancy.

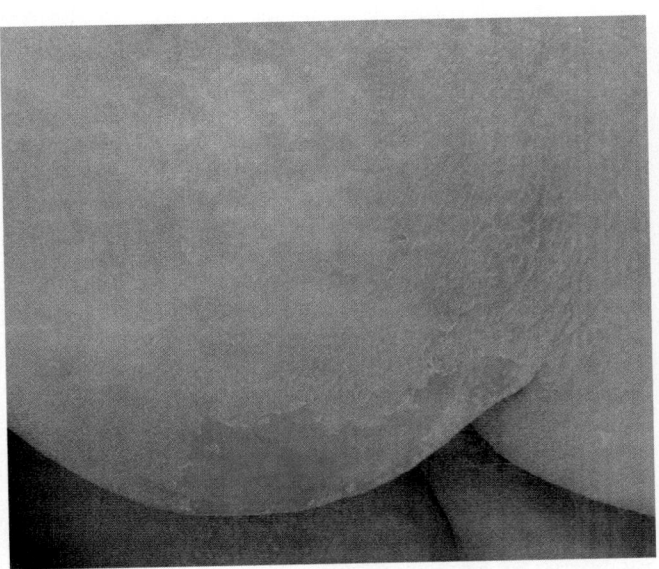
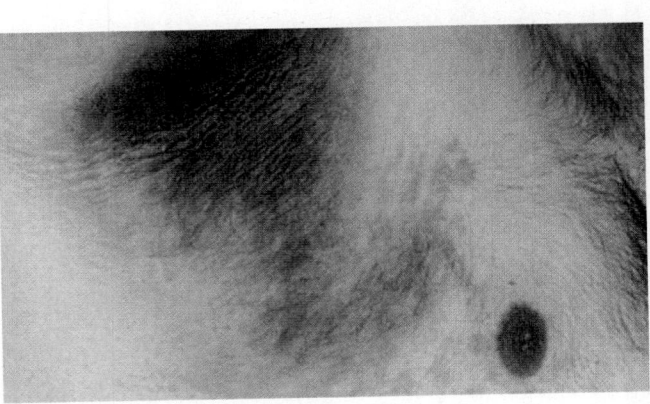
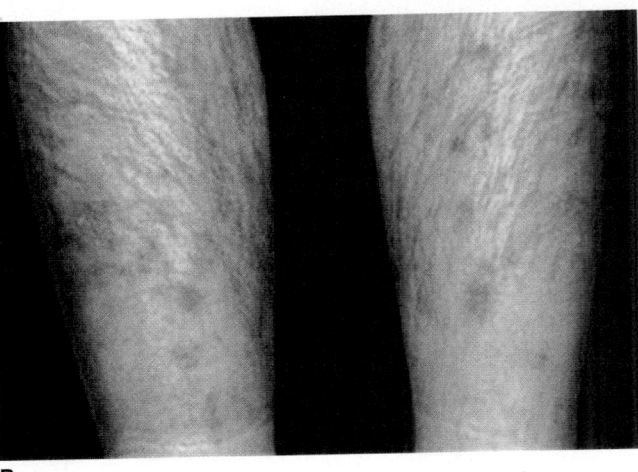
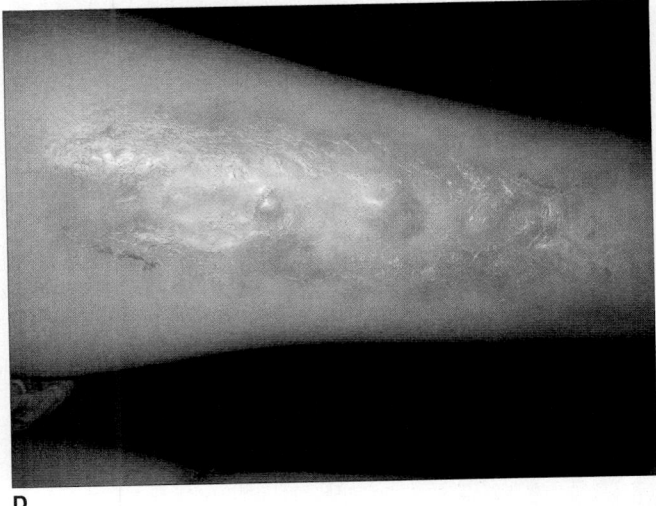

Figure 149-15 *Cutaneous manifestations of diabetes. (A) Eroded plaques with satellite papules and pustules, characteristic of cutaneous candidiasis. (B) Diabetic dermopathy: brown papules and plaques on the pretibial region. (Reproduced, with permission, from Wolff K, Johnson RA, Suurmond D. Fitzpatrick's Color Atlas & Synopsis of Clinical Dermatology, 5th ed. New York, NY: McGraw-Hill; 2005, Fig. 152-8.) (C) Acanthosis nigricans: typical hyperpigmented, velvety, verrucous axillary plaques. (Reproduced, with permission, from Wolff K, Johnson RA, Suurmond D. Fitzpatrick's Color Atlas & Synopsis of Clinical Dermatology, 6th ed. New York, NY: McGraw-Hill; 2005, Fig. 5-1.) (D) Yellow to red-brown plaques of necrobiosis lipoidica, with atrophy of the overlying epidermis and telangiectasias. (E) Disseminated granuloma annulare, many small, oval to ring-shaped pink papules over the trunk and limbs. (F) Depigmented patches on the lips in vitiligo. (G) Yellow nail changes.*

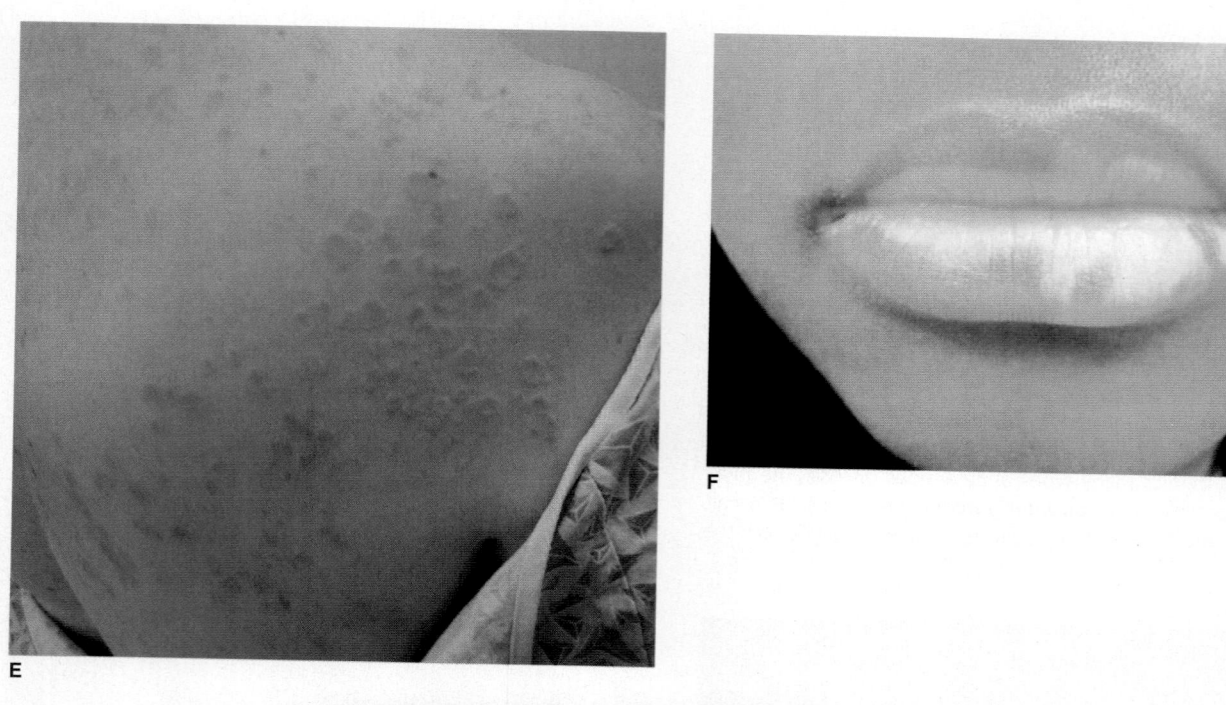

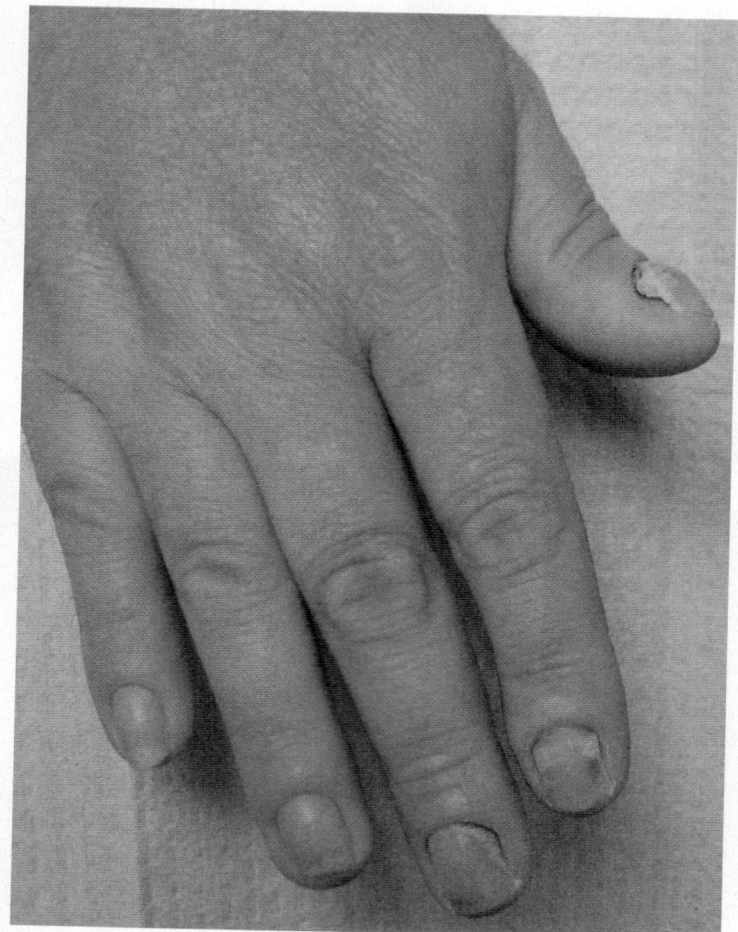

Figure 149-15 *(continued)*

TABLE 149-10 Summary of Amyloidosis

Disease	Underlying Disease	Type of Amyloid Deposited	Clinical Manifestations	Treatment
Systemic amyloidosis: involvement of multiple organ systems				
Primary systemic amyloid	Multiple myeloma or other plasma cell dyscrasias	AL amyloid	Cutaneous: macroglossia, pinch purpura (petechial and purpuric papules/nodules around eyelids, neck, axilla), and waxy or purpuric papules/plaques on body Systemic: Carpal tunnel syndrome, arthritis, CHF, hepatomegaly, neuropathy	Treat underlying myeloma/plasma cell dyscrasia, typically with chemotherapy
Secondary systemic amyloid	Chronic inflammatory conditions (such as RA) or chronic infections (such as TB)	AA amyloid	Cutaneous: usually none Systemic: amyloid deposited around parenchymal organs (kidneys, liver, spleen)	Treat underlying causative inflammatory or infectious condition
Localized amyloidosis: involvement of a single organ system				
Primary cutaneous amyloid	Deposition of amyloid likely due to chronic rubbing and irritation of the skin	Keratin-derived amyloid	Cutaneous lesions: 1. Macular amyloid: rippled, hyperpigmented patches, typically located on upper back between scapula 2. Lichen amyloid: hyperpigmented, scaly, pruritic papules, typically located on anterior shins or extensor surfaces Systemic: none	Avoid scratching and rubbing the area, as this worsens the hyperpigmentation Topical steroids Phototherapy
Primary cutaneous amyloid (AL-derived)	Cause unknown, but amyloid likely from localized plasma cells	AL amyloid	Nodular amyloid: single or multiple nodules on trunk, extremities or face	No treatment necessary Surgical excision or destruction may be useful
Secondary cutaneous amyloid	Amyloid deposited in pre-existing skin tumors, such as basal cell carcinomas, dermatofibromas, seborrheic keratoses	Keratin-derived amyloid	Cutaneous lesions: amyloid not appreciated clinically, but seen only on microscopic examination. Systemic: none	No treatment necessary for the amyloid
Cerebral amyloidosis	Alzheimer disease		Cutaneous lesions: none Systemic: CNS amyloid deposits	No effective treatment
Hereditary amyloid syndromes: may involve multiple organ systems				
Familial Mediterranean fever (FMF)	Mutations in pyrin gene, leading to increased secretion of interleukin-1β	AA amyloid	Cutaneous: erysipelas-like eruption on lower extremities Systemic: fever, pleuritis, peritonitis, synovitis, amyloid deposition in kidneys	Colchicine (anti-neutrophil agent)
Muckle-Wells syndrome	Proinflammatory mutation in cryopyrin gene	AA amyloid	Cutaneous: urticaria Systemic: fever, limb pains, deafness, amyloid deposition around kidneys	Anakinra (IL-1 receptor antagonist)

■ PARANEOPLASTIC CUTANEOUS SIGNS

Sweet syndrome, or acute febrile neutrophilic dermatosis; presents with fever, neutrophilia, and painful red-purple papules, nodules, and plaques that often appear indurated or vesiculated (**Figure 149-18**). It has three main types: classical, malignancy-associated, and drug-induced (**Table 149-12**). Malignancy-associated Sweet syndrome may precede, appear concurrently with, or arise after the patient's cancer diagnosis; it is often associated with hematologic malignancies, especially acute myelogenous leukemia. Sweet syndrome occurs relatively frequently, in comparison with other paraneoplastic phenomenon. Not surprisingly, it is often confused with an infectious process due to the presence of fever, leukocytosis, and tender skin lesions. Pustular lesions may develop in sites of trauma (pathergy). Systemic complications include pulmonary infiltrates, oral ulcers, hepatosplenomegaly, aortitis, glomerulonephritis, sterile osteomyelitis, blepharitis, and conjunctivitis.

Seborrheic keratoses are waxy, wart-like lesions with a stuck-on appearance, sometimes confused for melanoma when they are dark colored. **The sign of Leser-Trélat**, or the sudden appearance or growth of extensive seborrheic keratoses, has been associated with underlying adenocarcinoma, including colon, breast, stomach, lung, kidney, liver, and pancreas. High levels of epidermal growth factor

TABLE 149-11 Cutaneous and Other Manifestations of Vitamin Deficiencies

Vitamin/Nutrient Deficiency	Clinical Manifestations
Vitamin A	Night blindness; some patients demonstrate a follicular hyperkeratotic eruption that resembles toad skin (phrynoderma)
Vitamin B (and subtypes)	Cutaneous manifestations vary based on subtype. Pellagra (B3 deficiency) consists of photodistributed (forearms, face, neck, and V of chest) eczematous eruption. Other vitamin B deficiencies cause seborrheic dermatitis-like eruption, glossitis, and cheilitis
Vitamin C (scurvy)	Easy bruising, bleeding gums, corkscrew hairs with perifollicular hemorrhage
Zinc (acrodermatitis enteropathica)	Eczematous dermatitis, with crusting, in seborrheic distribution (perioral, inguinal regions) as well as acral sites (hands/feet)
Marasmus (caloric deficiency)	Shrunken, wasted appearance with height and weight >2 standard deviations below normal
Kwashiorkor (protein deficiency)	Edema, ascites, xerosis (dry skin)

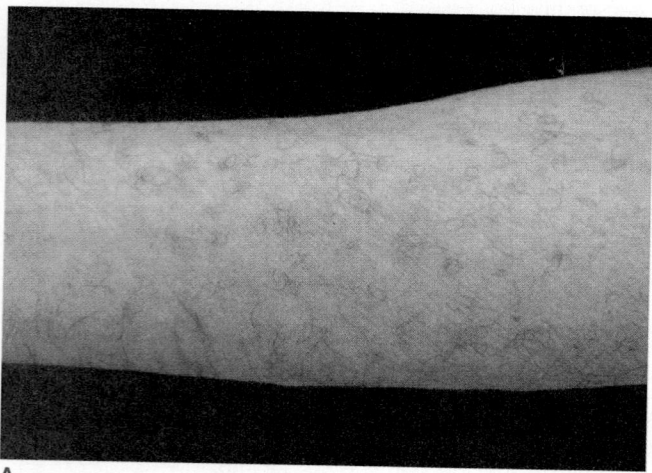

A

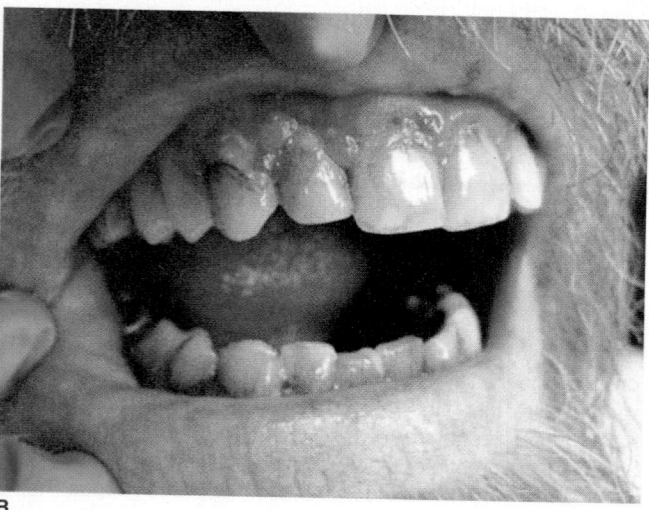

B

Figure 149-16 *Clinical features of vitamin C deficiency (scurvy): corkscrew hairs (A) and gingival friability and bleeding (B).*

and other cytokines have been suggested as a possible mechanism. The presence of many such lesions is extremely common in the adult population, and is most often a normal variant. The validity of this association has also been questioned in recent years.

Acanthosis nigricans, focal, symmetric, thickened, velvety plaques in the intertriginous folds of the axillae, groin, posterior neck, and oral mucosa, may occur in conjunction with underlying malignancy. It may be associated with adenocarcinoma of the GI or GU tract, particularly with gastric cancer, though associations with ovarian, endometrial, and lung cancers have also been reported. However, most cases of acanthosis nigricans are associated with obesity and insulin resistance, and it may also be seen in patients taking nicotinic acid, corticosteroids, growth hormone, and oral contraceptives. Familial forms also exist.

Tripe palms, a thickened, moss-like covering of the palms resembling the coarse folds of gastric rugae, are often a paraneoplastic phenomenon. When tripe palms and acanthosis nigricans are observed together, they are associated with gastric cancer; tripe palms occurring in isolation are most often related to underlying lung cancer.

Thickening of pressure-point areas on the soles can be seen in **Howel-Evans syndrome**. This autosomal dominant condition results in an acquired, focal keratoderma (thickening of the skin on the palms and soles), and is associated with esophageal cancer. Diffuse thickening of the skin on the palms and soles (acquired palmoplantar keratoderma) has also been observed with lung, breast, renal, and colon carcinoma.

Bazex syndrome, also known as acrokeratosis paraneoplastica, is an acquired keratoderma associated with malignancy, most commonly squamous cell cancer of the head and neck, as well as lung and esophageal cancer. Bazex syndrome has three progressive phases that parallel the course of the tumor. The initial eruption consists of violaceous, ill-defined, thin, slightly scaly papules on acral regions, including the fingers, toes, ears, and nose. Palmoplantar keratoderma appears in the second stage, along with spread of the initial lesions. In the third stage, the eruption generalizes, though the acral predominance, violaceous-color, and thickened palms and soles predominate.

Paraneoplastic pemphigus (PNP) is characterized by severe mucosal erosions and ulcers as well as variable skin lesions, ranging from lichenoid papules to erythema multiforme-like target lesions and frank blisters. In fact, PNP is often mistaken for severe erythema multiforme or Stevens-Johnson syndrome. Common associated malignancies include lymphoma, thymoma, and other lymphoproliferative disorders, such as Castleman disease. Patients with PNP must be followed carefully for involvement of the respiratory tract epithelium, manifesting as a rapidly progressive and potentially fatal form of brochiolitis obliterans with organizing pneumonia.

Generalized redness, swelling, and scaling of the skin is known as **erythroderma** (**Figure 149-19**). Though most cases are caused by an underlying skin disease such as psoriasis, seborrheic dermatitis, or ichthyosis, amongst others, 10% to 15% of cases may be paraneoplastic. Leukemia and lymphoma are common associations, including cutaneous T cell lymphomas. Viral infections such as HIV can also result in erythroderma. Erythema in a serpiginous, figurate pattern may represent a rare entity called **erythema gyratum repens**. Lesions demonstrate a polycyclic appearance resembling wood grain. This condition is nearly always associated with a malignancy, particularly underlying lung carcinoma.

Recurrent and migratory thrombophlebitis is known as **Trosseau syndrome**. Veins on the neck, chest, abdomen, and legs are typically involved, possibly by an underlying coagulopathy. This syndrome is associated with adenocarcinomas with abundant mucin production, such as pancreatic or prostate cancer.

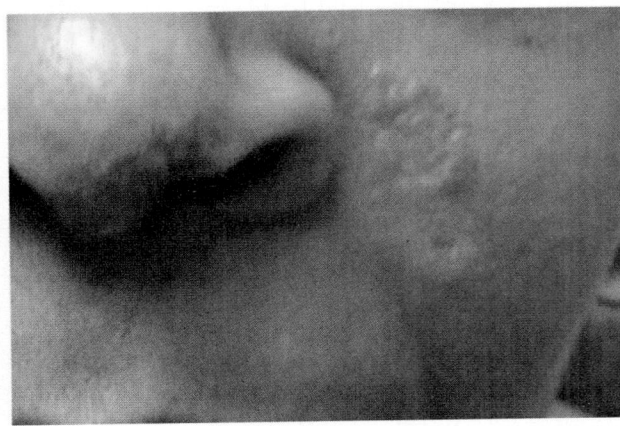

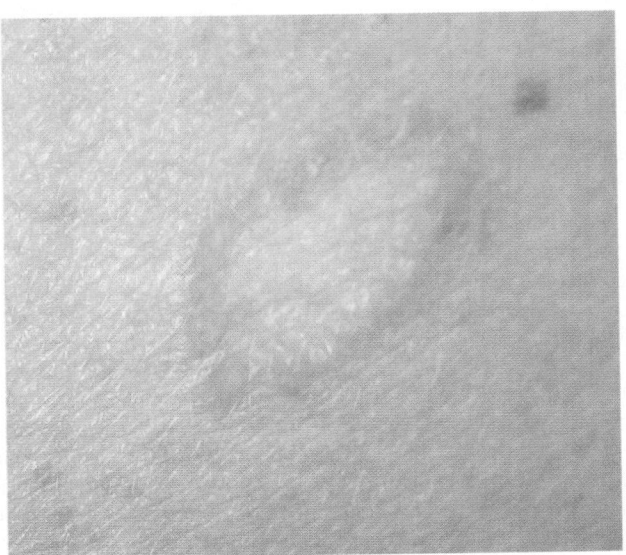

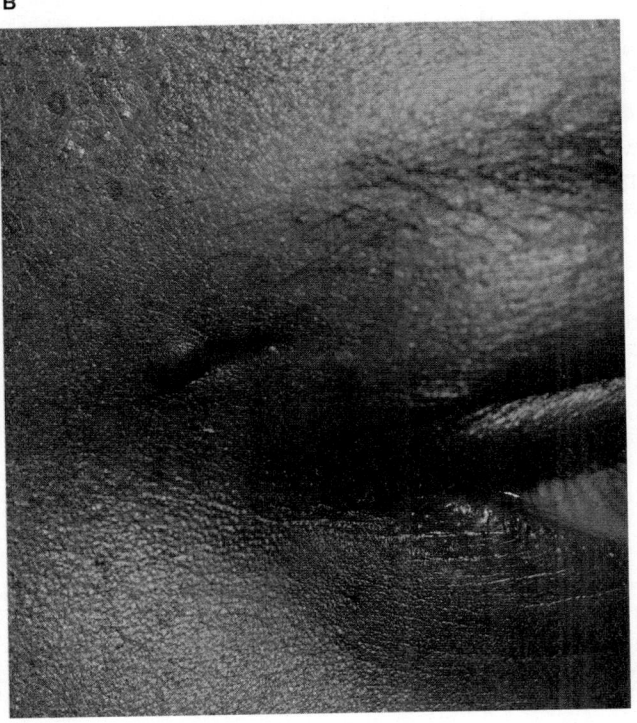

Figure 149-17 *The variable presentations of sarcoidosis: (A) papular sarcoid on the face; (B) orange-brown, annular plaque on the trunk; (C) in a scar. (Courtesy of Dr. Richard A. Johnson.)*

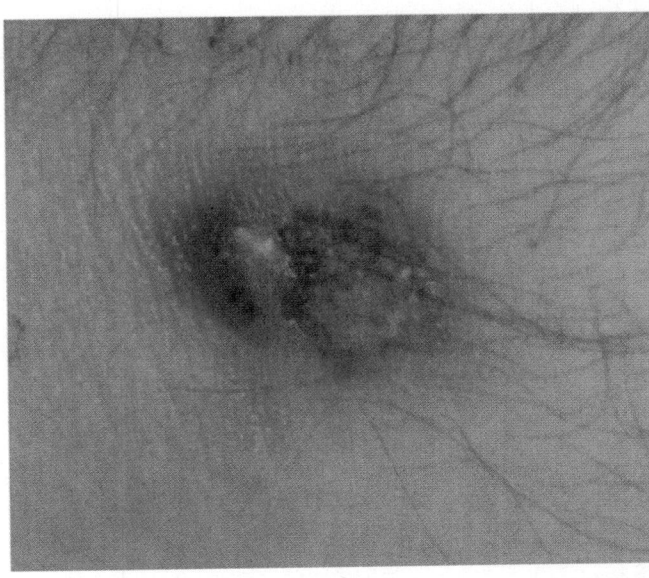

Figure 149-18 *Acute febrile neutrophilic dermatosis (Sweet syndrome). Edematous, violaceous, vesiculated plaques and papulonodules.*

METASTATIC DISEASE

Though uncommon, metastases to the skin can be the first sign of malignancy, affording a relatively straightforward opportunity for diagnosis. It may be difficult to discern the origin of a metastatic tumor on physical examination alone. Patient gender may be helpful in suggesting likely sources (**Table 149-13**). Skin lesions are often firm papules, plaques, or nodules. There may be secondary ulceration. Lesions are often violaceous in color, and individual lesions tend to vary in size and shape (**Figure 149-20**). The distribution is usually irregular, but lesions are sometimes found close to the primary tumor. Biopsy and histologic analysis are required for definitive diagnosis.

CUTANEOUS FINDINGS IN LEUKEMIA AND LYMPHOMA

The skin lesions associated with leukemia and lymphoma may also be reactive, or less often, the result of direct skin infiltration with malignant cells. Reactive skin conditions in hematopoietic malignancies include acquired ichthyosis, pruritus, erythroderma, and purpuric lesions. Direct infiltration of the skin with leukemic or lymphomatous cells often presents with skin colored to red or violaceous papules, plaques, nodules, or ulcers (**Figure 149-21A**). Size and distribution is variable, and the lesions often demonstrate a firm or rubbery texture. Rarely, patients may present with friable gingiva, exuberant responses to insect bites, or leukemic cells within cutaneous sites of inflammation such as a recent outbreak of herpes zoster (**Figure 149-21B**). The pathophysiology underlying these clinical presentations is poorly understood.

In acute myelomonocytic or monocytic leukemia, lesions may actually present several months before systemic disease is apparent. This phenomenon, known as aleukemic leukemia cutis, occurs when atypical blast cells appear in the skin prior to evidence of disease within the blood and bone marrow.

PURPURA

Purpura results from the extravasation of blood into the skin. Clinical manifestations range from nonpalpable purple macules to red-purple papules to large net-like plaques with hemorrhage and blister formation. Older lesions may have a greenish-yellow tinge from hemoglobin breakdown. Purely purpuric lesions are nonblanching,

TABLE 149-12 Sweet Syndrome: Associations, Diagnostic Criteria, and Treatment

Associations	Diagnostic Criteria*	Treatment
Classical	Major criteria	Prednisone (1 mg/kg/d, tapered over wks-mos)
• Infection (URI, GI)	• Abrupt onset of typical skin lesions	Potassium iodine (900 mg/d)
• Inflammatory bowel disease	• Pathology consistent with Sweet syndrome	Colchicine (0.6 mg three times in a d)
• Pregnancy		Dapsone (100-200 mg/d)
• Idiopathic	Minor criteria	Indomethacin (150 mg/d for 1 wk, then 100 mg/d)
Malignancy-associated	• Preceded by associated infection, vaccination; accompanied by associated malignancy, disorder, or drug	Cyclosporine (2-3 mg/kg/d, tapered over weeks)
• AML and other hematologic malignancies		
• GU, GI, breast	• Fever, constitutional signs, and symptoms	
Drug-induced	• Leukocytosis	
• G-CSF or GM-CSF	• Response to corticosteroids	
• All-trans retinoic acid		
• Antibiotics: trimethoprim-sulfamethoxazole, tetracyclines		
• OCPs		

*Proposed by Su and Liu in 1986. Diagnosis requires two major and two minor criteria.

although some purpura may partly blanch due to an associated inflammatory component.

Purpura may arise from intravascular, vascular, or extravascular pathology. Intravascular etiologies include platelet or coagulation hemostatic abnormalities. Vascular causes include inflammatory disorders, such as vasculitis, and noninflammatory conditions such as microvascular occlusion syndromes and thrombosis. Scurvy, corticosteroids, tissue swelling, and trauma are examples of extravascular causes of purpura.

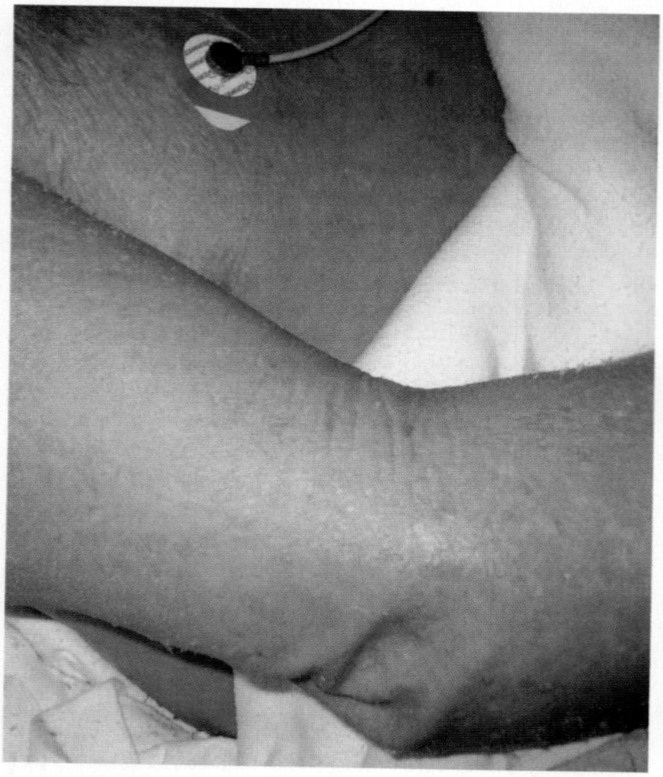

Purpura commonly develops in hospitalized patients, especially with the use of anticoagulation for prevention of deep vein thrombosis. Although purpura may result from incidental trauma, it can also represent the sole manifestation of overwhelming sepsis and thrombosis. The history should ascertain purpura duration, how the lesions began and progressed, distribution, and associated systemic symptoms. The patient's reason for hospital admission, comorbidities, and recent medication history should be reviewed. Physical examination should include a complete cutaneous examination, as well as cardiovascular, pulmonary, abdominal, and neurologic examinations, to determine whether the patient has a systemic illness or disease limited to the skin.

■ **MACULAR PURPURA**

Macular purpura (**Figure 149-22**) are the most common type of purpura. They present as flat, red-purple lesions. Petechiae are the smallest type, presenting as 2 to 3 mm round purpuric macules. Larger lesions are known as ecchymoses (bruises). The largest and deepest of these lesions are known as hematomas.

Macular purpura in the community is frequently caused by minor trauma and skin fragility related to aging (actinic or senile purpura). Macular purpura in the hospital setting is often related to a bleeding diathesis, as from therapeutic anticoagulation with heparin or warfarin, disseminated intravascular coagulation, platelet dysfunction from uremia, or drug-induced thrombocytopenia.

Small macular purpuric lesions are not concerning. However, as the macular purpuric lesions become larger or more confluent,

Figure 149-19 *Subacute erythroderma, presenting as full-body redness and scaling. Psoriasis, seborrheic dermatitis, ichthyosis, and other underlying skin diseases, along with medications, HIV, and malignancy can all result in erythroderma.*

TABLE 149-13 Most Common Malignancies Producing Cutaneous Metastases

Women	Men
• Breast	• Lung
• Colon	• Colon
• Melanoma	• Melanoma

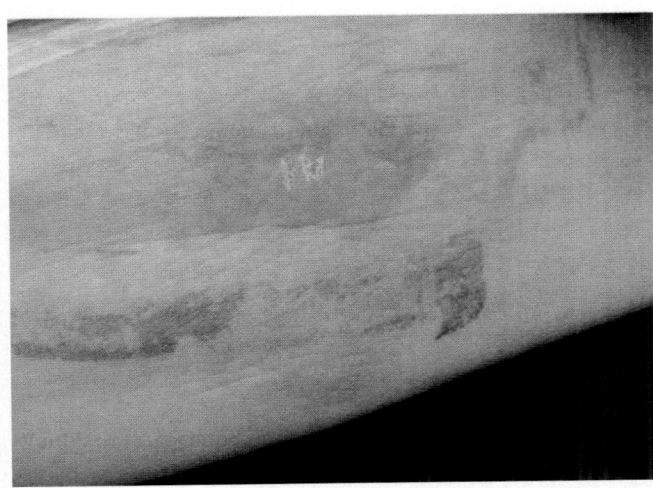

Figure 149-20 *Metastatic breast cancer to the skin. A firm, indurated, violaceous to erythematous plaque on the chest wall. The lesion was asymptomatic.*

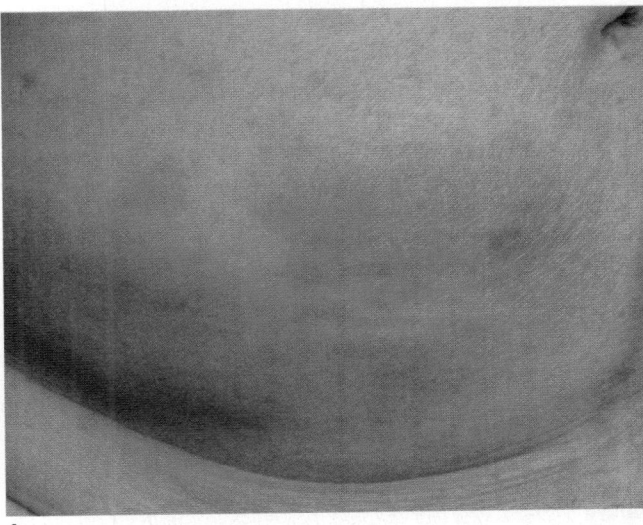

A

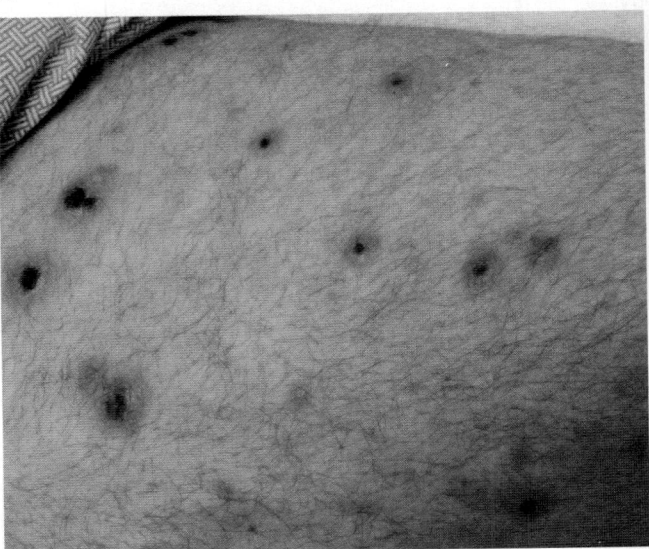

B

Figure 149-21 *Cutaneous findings in leukemia and lymphoma. (A) Several infiltrated, erythematous papules and plaques in a patient with lymphoma. Skin biopsy confirmed cutaneous involvement of lymphoma and lesions resolved with chemotherapy. (B) Seeding of recently active lesions of herpes zoster (shingles) with leukemic cells in a patient with CLL, producing chronic, violaceous nodules.*

the level of concern should increase. **Purpura fulminans** is the most aggressive and dangerous form of macular purpuric lesions. Purpura fulminans may begin as small petechial lesions, but rapidly progresses to large ecchymoses, particularly over the extremities and pressure points. The eruption subsequently generalizes with hemorrhagic skin necrosis on the hands, feet, and other acral areas. When this occurs, patients are typically hypotensive, septic, and unstable. Infectious causes of purpura fulminans include meningococcal meningitis, streptococcal or pneumococcal sepsis, or bacteremia of any organism. Noninfectious causes include antiphospholipid antibody syndrome, deficiencies of protein C or protein S, or factor V Leiden.

Purpura fulminans can be rapidly fatal. Patients who do survive may require amputation of several digits. Thus, it is imperative to recognize these patients and begin treatment as soon as possible. As soon as the diagnosis is suspected, blood cultures should be performed, and patients should be started on broad spectrum antibiotics and receive aggressive supportive care, including intubation, hemodynamic support, and replacement blood products, if necessary.

■ PALPABLE PURPURA

These lesions are typically small 0.5 to 1 cm purpuric papules and plaques that are slightly elevated and firm to the touch (**Figure 149-23**). There is often mild surrounding inflammation. Palpable purpura most commonly results from inflammation of the small vessels of the skin, known as leukocytoclastic vasculitis. In the hospitalized patient, palpable purpura are most often due to a drug hypersensitivity reaction. Common offenders include antibiotics, NSAIDs, thiazides, and allopurinol. Infections are another common cause of palpable purpura, typically bacterial infections or hepatitis B and C. Less common causes of palpable purpura and leukocytoclastic vasculitis include Churg-Strauss syndrome, microscopic polyangiitis, Henoch-Schönlein purpura, and cryoglobulinemia.

Palpable purpura alone requires only symptomatic treatment with topical corticosteroids. However, as palpable purpura implies cutaneous vasculitis, it is important to evaluate for potential systemic vasculitis. Systemic small vessel vasculitis may affect the cardiovascular, renal, gastrointestinal, pulmonary, neurologic, and musculoskeletal systems. Typical systemic manifestations include fever, arthralgias, weakness, shortness of breath, chest pain, abdominal pain, hemoptysis, hematuria, and hematochezia. Patients with

systemic vasculitis may require more aggressive treatment with systemic corticosteroids or steroid-sparing immunosuppressive agents. Thus, all patients with palpable purpura should be evaluated closely for signs of systemic vasculitis; a careful review of systems, blood pressure evaluation, blood urea nitrogen, creatinine, urinalysis and urine microscopy, and testing for fecal occult blood are warranted.

■ RETIFORM PURPURA

Retiform purpura form a net-like pattern of interconnecting blue or purple lines (**Figure 149-24**). Livedo reticularis, a physiologic manifestation of cool skin, appears clinically similar, but is nonpurpuric; the pattern is blanching, and resolves with warming of the skin. Retiform purpura are due to slow blood flow or occlusion of the cutaneous vessels, resulting in localized areas of decreased blood supply to the skin. Frank necrosis of the skin, manifested as a dusky

Figure 149-22 *Macular purpura: petechiae in a patient on anticoagulant therapy.*

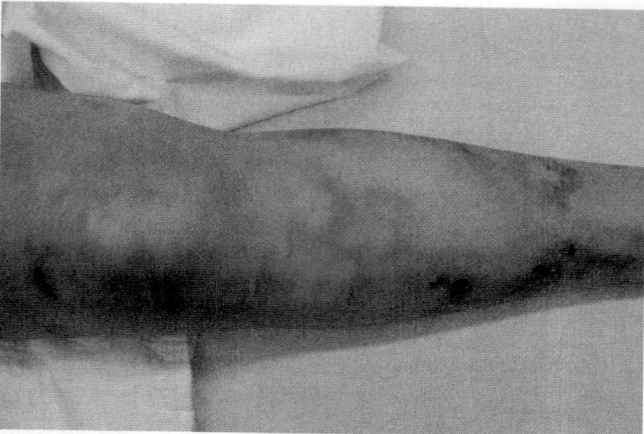

Figure 149-24 *Retiform purpura manifesting as net-like, nonblanchable erythema with minimal surrounding inflammation. This patient presented with Gram-negative sepsis with superficial cutaneous thrombosis.*

violaceous to gray color, may also be present. Ulcerations often develop in extensive cases, with acral hemorrhage or gangrene being relatively common.

Potential pathophysiologic causes include microvascular platelet plugs, such in thrombocytosis or thrombotic thrombocytopenic purpura, cold-related agglutination, as with cryoglobulins, and angioinvasive organisms, such as mucormycosis or *Aspergillus*. Other causes include altered coagulation, as in heparin-induced thrombocytopenia, sepsis and coumadin skin necrosis, crystal deposition, such as cholesterol emboli or calciphylaxis, red blood cell occlusion, as in sickle cell anemia, and inflammatory vasculitis, particularly medium vessel vasculitides such as rheumatoid vasculitis or polyarteritis nodosa, which can also present with nodules and ulcers.

Patients with retiform purpura should be considered extremely ill. Since retiform purpura is a cutaneous manifestation of vascular occlusion, vascular occlusion of internal organs may also be present. These patients may rapidly decompensate and require aggressive

supportive measures, including intubation and hemodynamic support. The underlying cause should be identified as quickly as possible to initiate specific therapy (**Figure 149-25**).

WHEN SHOULD AN INPATIENT DERMATOLOGY CONSULTATION BE OBTAINED?

As a general rule, if a patient is admitted for a complex skin condition, such as a diffuse blistering disorder, generalized erythroderma, or a severe cutaneous drug reaction, a dermatology consult should be obtained to facilitate diagnosis and management. Consultation should also be considered in cases that appear to be atypical presentations of an otherwise routine skin condition, such as a refractory or exuberant cellulitis or drug hypersensitivity reaction. Finally, consultation should be obtained early in the course of patients with dermatologic emergencies, such as Stevens-Johnson syndrome/toxic epidermal necrolysis, bullous graft-versus-host disease, staphylococcal scalded skin syndrome, meningococcemia, and retiform purpura.

Dermatology involvement may help to make an accurate diagnosis earlier and decrease the patient's length of stay. Dermatologists may also maximize the patient's topical and systemic therapy, helping the patient to improve more rapidly. Although inpatient dermatology consults are not readily available at all hospitals, there has been a move to increase access to prompt, high-quality dermatologic care through the establishment of dermatology hospitalist programs at some institutions. Indications for dermatology consultation are summarized in **Table 149-14**.

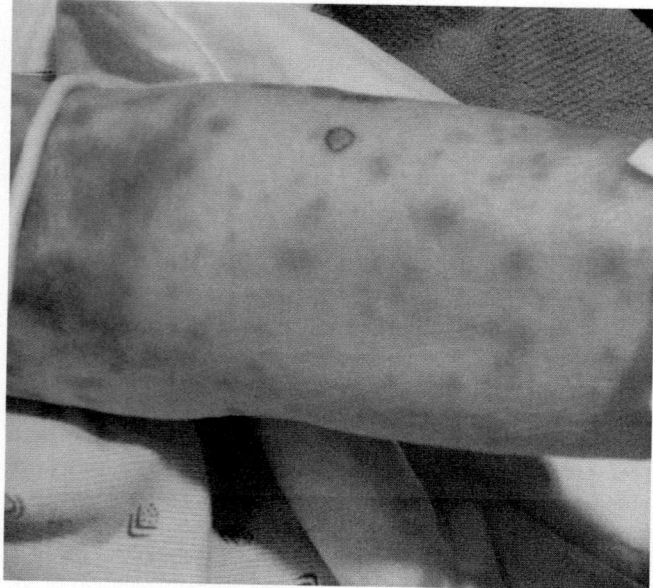

Figure 149-23 *Palpable purpura in a patient with small vessel vasculitis.*

TABLE 149-14 When Should an Inpatient Dermatology Consult be Obtained?

- Patient is admitted for a skin disorder
- Atypical presentation of common condition
- Common condition not responding to appropriate therapy
- Diagnostic challenge with cutaneous manifestation
- Suspected dermatologic emergencies (including Stevens Johnson Syndrome/Toxic Epidermal Necrolysis, bullous graft vs host disease, staphylococcal scalded skin syndrome, meningococcemia, and retiform purpura)
- Prompt diagnosis may result in early discharge

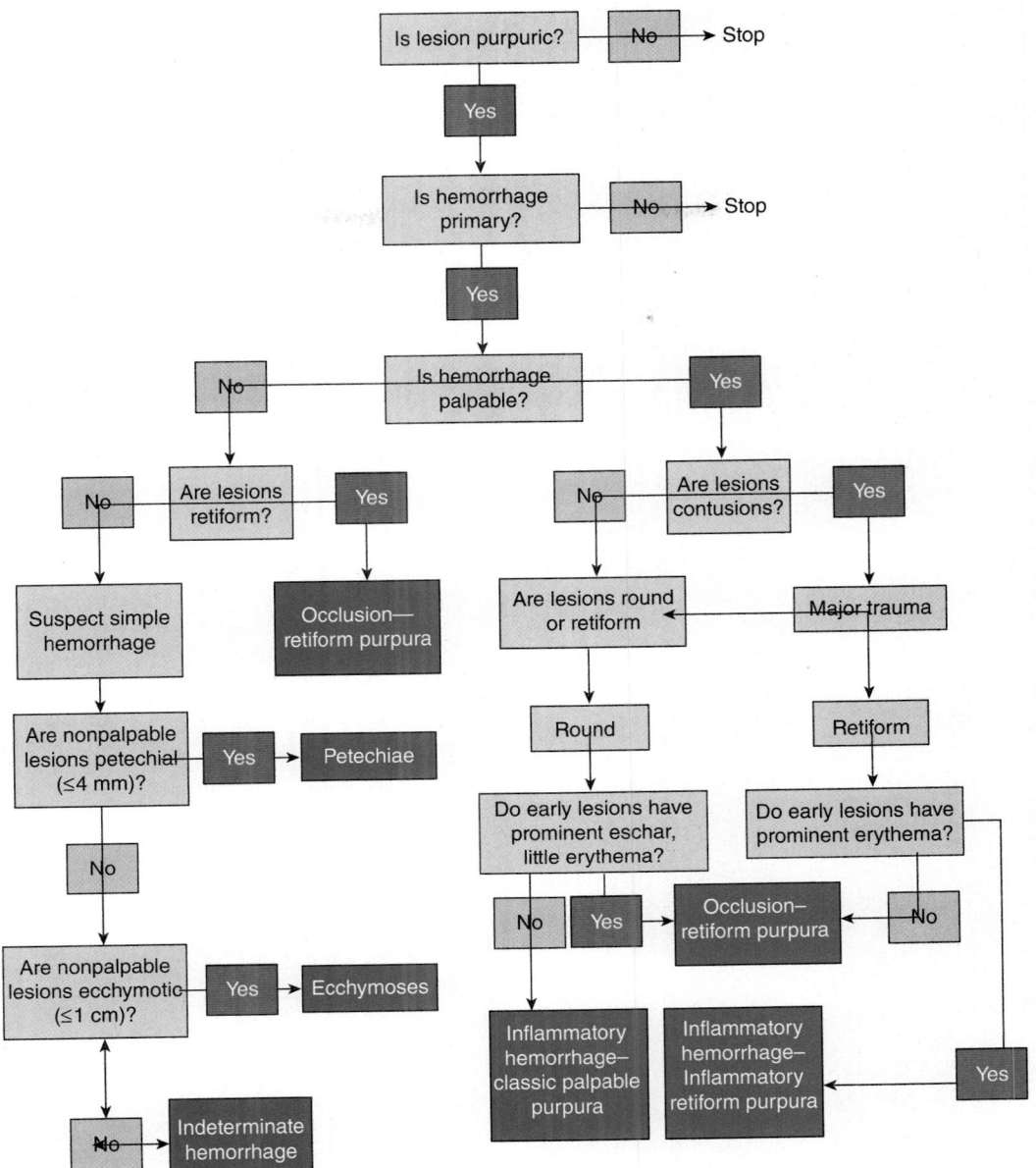

Figure 149-25 *Diagnostic algorithm for purpura.* (Reproduced, with permission, from Fauci AS, Braunwald E, Kasper DL, et al. *Harrison's Principles of Internal Medicine*, 17th ed. New York, NY: McGraw-Hill; 2008, Fig. 145-1.)

SUGGESTED READINGS

Anzalone CL, Cohen PR. Acute febrile neutrophilic dermatosis (Sweet's syndrome). *Curr Opin Hematol.* 2013;20:26-35.

Callen JP, Jorizzo JL, Bolognia JL, Piette W, Zone JJ, eds. *Dermatological Signs of Internal Disease*, 4th ed. London, UK: Elsevier; 2009.

Chen KR, Carlson JA. Clinical approach to cutaneous vasculitis. *Am J Clin Dermatol.* 2008;9:71-92.

Costner MI, Grau RH. Update on connective tissue diseases in dermatology. *Semin Cutan Med Surg.* 2006;25:207-220.

Dyachenko P, Shustak A, Rozenman D. Hemodialysis-related pruritus and associated cutaneous manifestations. *Int J Dermatol.* 2006;45:664-667.

Robinson-Bostom L, DiGiovanna JJ. Cutaneous manifestations of end-stage renal disease. *J Am Acad Dermatol.* 2000;43:975-986.

Ruocco E, Sangiuliano S, Gravina AG, Miranda A, Nicoletti G. Pyoderma gangrenosum: an updated review. *J Eur Acad Dermatol Venereol.* 2009;23:1008-1017.

Sontheimer RD. Skin manifestations of systemic autoimmune connective tissue disease: diagnostics and therapeutics. *Best Pract Res Clin Rheumatol.* 2004;18:429-462.

Van Hattem S, Bootsma AH, Thio HB. Skin manifestations of diabetes. *Cleve Clin J Med.* 2008;75:772, 774, 776-777.

Wanat KA, Rosenbach M. A practical approach to cutaneous sarcoidosis. *Am J Clin Dermatol.* 2014;15:283-297.

SECTION 4
Endocrinology

CHAPTER 150

Glycemic Emergencies

Margo S. Hudson, MD
Graham T. McMahon, MD, MMSc

Key Clinical Questions

1. How are diabetic ketoacidosis (DKA) and hyperosmolar hyperglycemic syndrome (HHS) diagnosed and treated?
2. How is hypoglycemia treated?
3. What are the causes of hypoglycemia in nondiabetic patients?
4. How is hypoglycemia avoided in the hospital?

INTRODUCTION

Admissions with diabetic ketoacidosis as the primary diagnosis have increased over the past 30 years, with 140,000 recorded in the United States in 2009. However, mortality has been reduced to less than 5%. Hyperosmolar hyperglycemic syndrome is less common, but it is associated with a mortality of up to 11%, because of the greater age and comorbid conditions of the at-risk patient population.

DIABETIC KETOACIDOSIS

■ PATHOPHYSIOLOGY

Diabetic ketoacidosis arises in patients with absolute or severe insulin deficiency. The resulting hyperglycemia combined with an increase in counter-regulatory hormones, including glucagon, catecholamines, cortisol, and growth hormone, precipitate proteolysis and lipolysis. Lipolysis causes the accumulation of acidic ketones, and hyperglycemia leads to osmotic diuresis and electrolyte loss, precipitating the characteristic metabolic acidosis and severe dehydration.

■ SYMPTOMS AND SIGNS

Symptoms of DKA generally develop over a short period of time and include polyuria, polydipsia, and weight loss. Abdominal pain and vomiting are common with acidosis, and must be distinguished from an acute abdomen. Decreased mentation and deep labored Kussmaul respirations are advanced findings. Additional features of an intercurrent illness should be sought. Leukocytosis and hyperamylasemia are often detectable at presentation and normalize with treatment.

■ DIAGNOSIS

The diagnostic criteria for DKA include five laboratory conditions: plasma glucose greater than 250 mg/dL (13.9 mmol/L), anion gap of greater than 10 mEq/L, the presence of ketonuria or ketonemia, serum bicarbonate below 18 mEq/L, and arterial pH less than 7.30. Diabetic ketoacidosis is graded as mild, moderate, or severe, with increasing severity associated with lower pH and deterioration in mental status. Arterial blood gas measurement should be obtained at the outset; measurements of venous blood pH can be used to track the resolution of the acidosis thereafter. Typical laboratory findings at presentation of DKA are shown in **Table 150-1**.

As 3-β-hydroxybutyrate is the most abundant ketone in the early stages of DKA, but is not measured in the nitroprusside assay for ketones, assessment should also include direct measurement of 3-β-hydroxybutyrate when available; a level over 3 mmol/L is considered clinically significant. Although a glucose of at least 250 mg/dL is included among the diagnostic criteria, patients who are pregnant or who have a high glomerular filtration rate can be in DKA at glucose levels under this threshold.

■ PRECIPITANTS

Precipitating factors fall into three categories: lack of insulin, initiation of a diabetogenic medicine, or development of another illness. Approximately one-quarter of DKA admissions occur at the onset of diabetes. Although type 1 diabetes accounts for the majority of these initial presentations, as many as half of adult African Americans and Hispanics with new-onset diabetes

TABLE 150-1 Laboratory Values in Diabetic Ketoacidosis (DKA) and Hyperglycemic Hyperosmolar State (HHS) (Representative Ranges at Presentation)

	DKA	HHS
Glucose,[a] mmol/L (mg/dL)	13.9-33.3 (250-600)	33.3-66.6 (600-1200)
Sodium, meq/L	125-135	135-145
Potassium[a,b]	Normal to ↑	Normal
Magnesium[a]	Normal	Normal
Chloride[a]	Normal	Normal
Phosphate[a,b]	Normal	Normal
Creatinine	Slightly ↑	Moderately ↑
Osmolality (mOsm/mL)	300-320	330-380
Plasma ketones[a]	++++	+/-
Serum bicarbonate,[a] meq/L	<15	Normal to slightly ↓
Arterial pH	6.8-7.3	>7.3
Arterial P_{CO_2},[a] mm Hg	20-30	Normal
Anion gap[a] (Na − [Cl + HCO₃])	↑	Normal to slightly ↑

[a]Large changes occur during treatment of DKA.
[b]Although plasma levels may be normal or high at presentation, total-body stores are usually depleted.
From Powers AC. Diabetes mellitus: management and therapies. In: Kasper DL, et al (eds). *Harrison's Principles of Internal Medicine*, 19th ed. New York: McGraw-Hill Education; 2015, Table 418-6.

presenting in DKA may actually have type 2 diabetes, and ultimately may be able to discontinue insulin therapy. In patients with a prior history of diabetes, poor adherence to insulin is the most common precipitating factor, particularly in adolescence and substance abuse. Technical problems with pumps, improper storage of insulin, or psychological or cognitive disorders should also be considered. Diabetogenic medicines such as atypical antipsychotics, glucocorticoids, and tacrolimus have been reported to precipitate DKA.

Infections, such as pneumonia or urinary tract infection (UTI), are a particularly common precipitating factor and must be assiduously excluded. Other intercurrent illnesses that may provoke DKA include myocardial infarction, stroke, pancreatitis, and surgery.

■ DIFFERENTIAL DIAGNOSIS

Diabetic ketoacidosis is not the only cause of an anion gap acidosis. Differential diagnoses include alcoholic ketoacidosis, starvation ketosis, severe chronic renal failure, lactic acidosis, and toxic ingestions such as salicylates, methanol, ethylene glycol, and paraldehyde. These conditions, especially toxic ingestions, should be considered when the clinical picture is not straightforward.

■ TREATMENT

Treatment of diabetic ketoacidosis should simultaneously address each of the components that contribute to the syndrome: dehydration, hyperglycemia, electrolyte loss, and acidosis. A stepwise approach can facilitate management of these patients (**Table 150-2**). Most patients with DKA are managed initially in critical care units, but local experience may facilitate management in a monitored general unit.

TABLE 150-2 Management of Diabetic Ketoacidosis

1. Confirm diagnosis (↑ plasma glucose, positive serum ketones, metabolic acidosis).
2. Admit to hospital; intensive care setting may be necessary for frequent monitoring or if pH < 7.00 or unconscious.
3. Assess:
    Serum electrolytes (K⁺, Na⁺, Mg²⁺, Cl⁻, bicarbonate, phosphate)
    Acid-base status—pH, HCO³⁻, PCO₂, β-hydroxybutyrate
    Renal function (creatinine, urine output)
4. Replace fluids: 2-3 L of 0.9% saline over first 1-3 h (10-20 mL/kg per hour); subsequently, 0.45% saline at 250-500 mL/h; change to 5% glucose and 0.45% saline at 150-250 mL/h when plasma glucose reaches 250 mg/dL (13.9 mmol/L).
5. Administer short-acting insulin: IV (0.1 units/kg), then 0.1 units/kg per hour by continuous IV infusion; increase two- to threefold if no response by 2-4 h. If the initial serum potassium is <3.3 mmol/L (3.3 meq/L), do not administer insulin until the potassium is corrected.
6. Assess patient: What precipitated the episode (noncompliance, infection, trauma, pregnancy, infarction, cocaine)? Initiate appropriate workup for precipitating event (cultures, CXR, ECG).
7. Measure capillary glucose every 1-2 h; measure electrolytes (especially K⁺, bicarbonate, phosphate) and anion gap every 4 h for first 24 h.
8. Monitor blood pressure, pulse, respirations, mental status, fluid intake and output every 1-4 h.
9. Replace K⁺: 10 meq/h when plasma K⁺ <5.0-5.2 meq/L (or 20-30 meq/L of infusion fluid), ECG normal, urine flow and normal creatinine documented; administer 40-80 meq/h when plasma K⁺ <3.5 meq/L or if bicarbonate is given. If initial serum potassium is >5.2 mmol/L (5.2 meq/L), do not supplement K⁺ until the potassium is corrected.
10. See text about bicarbonate or phosphate supplementation.
11. Continue above until patient is stable, glucose goal is 8.3-13.9 mmol/L (150-250 mg/dL), and acidosis is resolved. Insulin infusion may be decreased to 0.05-0.1 units/kg per hour.
12. Administer long-acting insulin as soon as patient is eating. Allow for a 2-4 hour overlap in insulin infusion and SC insulin injection.

Abbreviations: CXR, chest x-ray; ECG, electrocardiogram.
Source: Adapted from M Sperling, in Therapy for Diabetes Mellitus and Related Disorders, American Diabetes Association, Alexandria, VA, 1998; and AE Kitabchi et al: Diabetes Care 32:1335, 2009.

Fluid replacement

Patients with diabetic ketoacidosis are invariably dehydrated. Initial fluid resuscitation in the average adult without cardiac dysfunction should be 1 L of 0.9% sodium chloride, infused over 1 hour. Subsequent fluid replacement will depend on the degree of dehydration and corrected sodium level. Equations that are helpful in guiding therapy are presented in **Table 150-3**.

Normal saline should be infused until euvolemia is achieved.

After that, hypotonic fluids are appropriate if either corrected sodium level or serum osmolarity remain elevated. Typical total body water deficit in DKA in adults is 6 L, which should be replaced in the first 24 to 36 hours. Once serum glucose falls to between 200 and 250 mg/dL (11.1-13.9 mmol/L), dextrose should be added to the intravenous fluids to maintain glucose between 150 and 200 mg/dL (8.3-11.1 mmol/L).

TABLE 150-3 Estimating Water and Electrolyte Deficits in DKA and HHS

Calculation	Equation	Normal Range
Corrected Na (CNa)	Na (in mEq/L) + .016 (glucose [in mg/dL] – 100)	135-145 mEq/L
Effective osmolarity	$2\ Na(mEq/L)+\dfrac{glucose\ (mg/dL)}{18}$	280-290 mOsm/L
Water deficit	0.6 (wt in kg) ([CNa – 140]/140)	<0.5 L

Insulin

Intravenous insulin therapy is the standard of care for the management of hyperglycemia in DKA, although subcutaneous insulin algorithms have been used successfully in some patients with mild and uncomplicated DKA. The goal of intravenous insulin therapy is to lower serum glucose by approximately 50 to 70 mg/dL (2.8-4.2 mmol/L) per hour. This is usually accomplished with a 0.1 U/kg intravenous bolus of regular insulin, followed by a 0.1 U/kg/h insulin infusion, with the drip rate adjusted as needed to achieve the desired decrease in glucose. A bolus dose of insulin may not be necessary with an infusion rate of 0.14 U/kg/h.

Intravenous insulin should be continued until ketoacidosis has resolved. The current American Diabetes Association consensus criteria suggest that the patient can be transitioned to subcutaneous insulin when the glucose is below 200 mg/dL (11.1 mmol/L), the serum bicarbonate is greater than 18 mEq/L, and the venous pH is greater than 7.30. In addition, intravenous insulin should not be stopped prior to normalization of the anion gap. Urinary ketosis may remain detectable after clearance of serum ketones, and therefore is an unreliable indicator for resolution of the acidosis.

Once DKA has resolved, intravenous insulin should be continued for 2 to 4 hours after the first subcutaneous dose of basal and rapid-acting insulin; premature discontinuation of the insulin infusion is the most common reason for recurrence of DKA in the hospitalized patient. Subcutaneous insulin must be dosed to ensure that both basal needs and prandial needs are met when the patient resumes eating. A well-established outpatient insulin dose can be used to determine the insulin replacement strategy in patients with known diabetes. Patients new to insulin can be started on a weight-based dose of 0.5 to 0.6 U/kg/d, divided into 0.25 U/kg/d of long-acting insulin for basal requirements and 0.1 U/kg of a rapid-acting insulin before meals.

Potassium

Acidosis tends to raise serum potassium, even when total body potassium stores are depleted. Intravenous insulin, fluid replacement, and correction of acidosis lower serum potassium and can precipitate serious hypokalemia. In the absence of hyperkalemia, between 20 and 30 mEq of potassium should be added to each liter of intravenous fluids during treatment of DKA. Intravenous insulin treatment in a patient who is hypokalemic can be dangerous. If serum potassium is less than 3.3 mEq/L at the initial evaluation, potassium should be administered through a central line, and the patient should be monitored in the intensive care unit. Adequate renal function should be established prior to starting potassium replacement.

Bicarbonate

Bicarbonate is not recommended for the management of acidosis in patients with DKA as long as the initial pH is greater than 7.0, as it may provoke hypokalemia in adults and cerebral edema in children.

Judicious use of bicarbonate may be helpful for patients whose pH is less than 7.0.

Phosphate

Serum phosphate may be normal or high at the time of presentation of DKA, despite total body phosphate deficits. Serum phosphate falls rapidly with treatment. Aggressive phosphate replacement in DKA is generally not recommended, because of concerns of precipitating hypocalcemia and an absence of proven efficacy. If phosphate is below 1 mg/dL, it can be replaced in intravenous fluids as potassium or sodium phosphate at a dose of 20 to 30 mEq infused over 6 to 12 hours. When the patient is eating and drinking again, milk is an excellent source of phosphate.

■ COMPLICATIONS

Cerebral edema is the most feared complication of DKA treatment. It is extremely rare in adults, but occurs in up to 1% of episodes in children and is associated with a high mortality in this group. A high rate of initial fluid resuscitation or bicarbonate therapy has been associated with cerebral edema, but its etiology has not been clearly determined. Treatment with intravenous mannitol is recommended if cerebral edema develops, but outcomes are often poor.

■ PREVENTION

Patients should be educated about the dangers of insulin omission and guidelines for insulin adjustment during illness. In the hospitalized patient, diabetic ketoacidosis is preventable with adequate monitoring and should never occur de novo. Diabetic ketoacidosis can develop in hospitalized patients with diabetes if glucose levels are not monitored, or when only correctional (sliding scale) insulin is prescribed, omitting basal insulin from the patient's regimen.

HYPEROSMOLAR HYPERGLYCEMIC STATE

■ PATHOPHYSIOLOGY

Though DKA and hyperosmolar hyperglycemia (HHS) exist on a hyperglycemic continuum, HHS is associated with more severe hyperosmolarity and is not associated with acidosis or ketosis. Diagnostic criteria are listed in Table 150-1. Hyperosmolar hyperglycemic syndrome tends to occur in older patients, and is not seen in patients with type 1 diabetes. This may be because patients who develop HHS retain some insulin production and can suppress ketogenesis, and are therefore less prone to acidosis.

■ CLINICAL PRESENTATION

Most patients present with several days to weeks of increasing polyuria and polydipsia, with the gradual onset of mental status changes. Patients often have additional factors that contribute to the inability to maintain hydration, such as diuretic therapy or poor functional status. Patients with severe metabolic changes can present with obtundation, seizures, and hemiparesis or other focal neurological findings. On presentation, patients are severely dehydrated, frequently hypotensive, and may have hyperthermia or hypothermia.

■ PRECIPITANTS

Intercurrent illness, especially infection, is the most common precipitating event of HHS. Other causes can include myocardial ischemia, stroke, pancreatitis, corticosteroid use, and initiation of diuretics.

■ TREATMENT

A stepwise approach to the treatment of HHS is outlined in Table 150-2. Rehydration is the mainstay of management.

Fluids

Fluid resuscitation is the most important and urgent treatment modality, but must be managed with care. The effective osmolarity and the total body water deficit should be calculated using the corrected sodium (Table 150-3). In the absence of cardiac decompensation, the initial therapy will generally be 1 L of normal sodium chloride over 1 hour. Normal saline is used since it is hypotonic to the patient's serum when profound dehydration is present. The remaining calculated fluid deficit should be replaced over 24 to 36 hours. Typical fluid deficits are as high as 9 L. The serum osmolarity should be corrected gradually, as rapid correction has been associated with slower neurologic recovery.

Insulin

Subcutaneous insulin is not appropriate for patients with HHS because poor tissue perfusion limits the absorption of insulin from the skin. Intravenous insulin is recommended, using a similar protocol to that used in DKA. Once the serum glucose falls to below 300 mg/dL (16.7 mmol/L), dextrose infusion should be initiated, with a target glucose of between 250 and 300 mg/dL (13.9-16.7 mmol/L), until mental status and serum osmolarity have normalized.

Potassium

Potassium should be replaced carefully in HHS, since these patients have more significant renal insufficiency than in DKA, and potassium may accumulate.

HYPOGLYCEMIA IN HOSPITALIZED PATIENTS

Hypoglycemia is relatively common among hospitalized patients, and is almost always a complication of the treatment of diabetes mellitus. However, hypoglycemia can also be the presenting feature of an underlying disease. True spontaneous hypoglycemia is likely only when Whipple triad is present. This triad is comprised of: (1) typical hypoglycemic symptoms, (2) low measured plasma glucose, and (3) reversal of symptoms with restoration of normal glucose levels. A plasma value for glucose lower than 55 mg/dL (3.1 mmol/L) is generally needed for diagnosis. However, because some people normally have glucose levels below this cut-off and laboratory errors are possible, it is important that the other components of Whipple triad be present before initiating an evaluation.

Hypoglycemia symptoms are due to either autonomic activation or neuroglycopenia. Autonomic symptoms due to sympathetic and parasympathetic activation, including palpitations, tremors, sweating, and hunger, appear as the plasma glucose falls below 65 mg/dL (3.6 mmol/L). Neuroglycopenic symptoms such as behavioral changes, obtundation, focal neurologic deficits, seizures, and ultimately coma emerge as the glucose falls below 40 mg/dL (2.2 mmol/L). Patients with frequent hypoglycemia, with or without underlying diabetes, may develop hypoglycemia unawareness, and have attenuated or absent autonomic symptoms, leaving them more prone to develop severe neuroglycopenia. Many hospitalized patients have significant baseline neurologic or autonomic impairment, and may be unable to manifest the typical symptoms other than seizure or coma. Consequently, caregivers must be vigilant to recognize hypoglycemia in the hospitalized patient, particularly if consciousness is blunted. Diabetic patients with longstanding poor glycemic control may also develop symptoms of hypoglycemia at higher glucose levels than normal persons, because of alterations in cerebral glucose transport.

Glucose values are usually measured in the hospital using point-of-care testing devices that are not as precise as laboratory measures. Although 95% of values obtained on a glucometer are within 20% of the laboratory measured value, only 69% are within 10% at values below 70 mg/dL. Therefore, when unexpected hypoglycemia is noted at the bedside, the findings should be confirmed in the laboratory. When accurate measurement is critical, the blood glucose should be sent to the laboratory in a tube with an inhibitor of glycolysis, and the plasma separated from formed blood elements as quickly as possible.

EVALUATION AND TREATMENT OF HYPOGLYCEMIA IN PATIENTS WITHOUT DIABETES

■ CLINICAL PRESENTATION

Hypoglycemia should be evaluated in patients who fulfill Whipple triad. If hypoglycemia is recurrent, expeditious evaluation is imperative. To avoid misinterpretation, diagnostic testing must be performed during a hypoglycemic episode, which may need to be provoked by fasting. Precipitants of hypoglycemia, timing of the hypoglycemia in relation to fasting or food intake, and the patient's overall condition can be helpful clues to establishing the diagnosis, as discussed below.

■ CAUSES OF HYPOGLYCEMIA

The causes of hypoglycemia can be divided into two categories: those associated with high insulin levels and those associated with suppressed insulin levels (**Table 150-4**). An excess of endogenous insulin can cause hypoglycemia even in the presence of a robust counter-regulatory hormone response. Insulinomas are rare, with an incidence of 4 cases per 1 million patient-years. These islet cell tumors usually occur sporadically, but can be associated with multiple endocrine neoplasia syndromes. Fasting hypoglycemia is the most common presentation, but some patients present exclusively with postprandial hypoglycemia. Postprandial hypoglycemia is the most common presentation of two recently described conditions featuring diffuse islet cell hypertrophy (nesidioblastosis):postgastric

---

TABLE 150-4 Causes of Hypoglycemia

I. Insulinmediated
   A. Insulinoma
   B. Noninsulinoma pancreatogenous hypoglycemia
   C. Postgastric bypass hypoglycemia
   D. Oral diabetes secretagogue medications
      1. Glyburide
      2. Glipizide
      3. Gimepiride
      4. Gliclazide
      5. Repaglinide
   E. Genetic mutations
   F. Antibody-mediated
   G. Exogenous insulin (factitious or malicious)
II. Noninsulin mediated
   A. Critical illness
      1. Hepatic, renal, cardiac failure
      2. Sepsis
      3. Inanition/malnutrition
   B. Adrenal insufficiency
   C. Nonislet cell tumor
   D. Toxins
      1. Alcohol
      2. Salicylate excess
      3. Hypoglycin

bypass hypoglycemia (which usually occurs 1-2 years following the surgery) and the less well characterized condition called noninsulinoma pancreatogenous hypoglycemia.

Glyburide, glipizide, and other sulfonylurea medications, as well as meglitinides, boost endogenous insulin secretion. Repaglinide appears to be the only available member of the meglitinide class that causes significant hypoglycemia. Surreptitious use of any of these drugs can present with typical manifestations of insulinoma. Some genetic defects can cause hyperinsulinemic hypoglycemia, but these are rare and usually present early in life. Even rarer, antibodies to insulin or the insulin receptor may lead to fluctuations in serum insulin levels and hypoglycemia in nondiabetic patients who typically have other autoimmune diseases. Surreptitious insulin injection must always be considered as a cause of cryptic hypoglycemia with elevated insulin levels.

Noninsulin-mediated hypoglycemia may develop during critical or chronic illness. Severe protein and calorie malnutrition in the hospital setting impairs the ability to maintain normal glycogen stores, increasing susceptibility to hypoglycemia. Hepatic and renal insufficiency decrease gluconeogenesis and glycogenolysis. Patients with sepsis are particularly prone to hypoglycemia, and its presence in infection is associated with increased mortality. Hypoglycemia in heart failure is usually related to secondary hepatic dysfunction. Adrenal insufficiency, either primary or secondary to hypopituitarism, is only rarely a cause of hypoglycemia, but it should be considered in the appropriate clinical context.

Nonislet tumors producing insulin-like growth factor 2 (IGF-2) may cause hypoglycemia. Although IGF-2 has its own receptor, it can bind to the insulin receptor and have insulin-like effects. Tumors producing IGF-2 tend to be bulky and intra-abdominal or retroperitoneal, and include sarcomas, hepatomas, lymphomas, and teratomas. They produce a precursor form of IGF-2 ("big" IGF-2). This form is not measured by conventional assays, but is implied by suppressed levels of insulin, growth hormone, and IGF-1. Insulin-like growth factor 1 (IGF-1) secreting tumors leading to hypoglycemia have also been described.

Toxins should be considered in the evaluation of the hypoglycemic patient. Ethanol inhibits hepatic gluconeogenesis and suppresses the release of counter-regulatory hormones. Hypoglycemia is especially common in poorly nourished alcoholics. Salicylates in high doses also suppress hepatic glucose output. Excess consumption of Jamaican ackee fruit can cause hypoglycemia; the fruit contains the compound hypoglycin, which interferes with hepatic gluconeogenesis. A variety of medications (**Table 150-5**) have been reported to cause hypoglycemia, with variable levels of evidence. Pentamidine, quinine, fluoroquinolones, glucagon, and rarely sulfonamides may lead to hypoglycemia by enhancing endogenous insulin release. Mechanisms of hypoglycemia for other listed drugs are diverse, if known, or uncertain.

■ DIAGNOSTIC TESTING

Initial investigation of the patient with confirmed hypoglycemia should include tests of hepatic and renal function and a complete blood count. Biochemical testing comprising levels of insulin, C-peptide level, β-hydroxybutyrate, and cortisol should be obtained when the patient is symptomatic and the serum glucose is less than 55 mg/dL (3.1 mmol/L). Screening for sulfonylureas, meglitinides, alcohol, and salicylates should be considered. While "big" IGF-2 cannot be measured, growth hormone, IGF-1, and native IGF-2 can be obtained if a nonislet cell malignancy is suspected. Insulin antibodies can be measured if an autoimmune disease is suspected and the patient has not been previously treated with insulin. If surreptitious insulin use is suspected, hospital evaluation may need to include send out testing for newer analog insulins. Insulin assays may vary widely in ability to measure analog insulins.

β-Hydroxybutyrate levels are generally low (<2.7 mmol/L) when hypoglycemia is insulin-mediated, as insulin suppresses lipolysis. This test is rapidly available, and can incriminate insulin before other laboratory results return. Because high levels of insulin generally suppress glycogenolysis, an increase in the glucose level of more than 25 mg/dL (1.4 mmol/L) after administration of 1 mg of glucagon intravenously while hypoglycemic can also be used as an indicator of hyperinsulinemia. If hypoglycemia does not occur spontaneously, a monitored fast of up to 72 hours until hypoglycemia develops or a mixed meal challenge can be used to induce hypoglycemia and obtain necessary samples. **Table 150-6** outlines expected test results in various hypoglycemic disorders.

■ TREATMENT

Normoglycemia should be maintained until definitive treatment for the underlying diagnosis can be initiated. Normoglycemia can usually be accomplished with an initial dose of 25 g of glucose given intravenously, followed by a constant infusion of 5% or 10% dextrose in water. Symptoms generally resolve within 15 to 20 minutes after the glucose level normalizes. The time to recovery can be prolonged if the patient has had a recent seizure or is comatose. If endogenous insulin is felt to be the cause of hypoglycemia and intravenous dextrose is not sufficient for maintaining normoglycemia, octreotide, or diazoxide therapy can be initiated.

HYPOGLYCEMIA IN DIABETIC PATIENTS IN THE AMBULATORY SETTING

■ EPIDEMIOLOGY

Improved glucose control has been associated with reductions in diabetes-related morbidity and mortality. However, tight glucose control is generally associated with an increased incidence of hypoglycemia, which can sometimes be severe and dangerous. Severe hypoglycemia is variably defined, but any episode requiring assistance of another person generally qualifies. The rate of severe hypoglycemic episodes is approximately 115 and 35 events per 1000 outpatients per year with type 1 and type 2 diabetes, respectively. Among inpatients, hypoglycemia is generally defined as any glucose level below 70 mg/dL (3.9 mmol/L) and severe hypoglycemia as any confirmed glucose level below 40 mg/dL (2.2 mmol/L). Patients with either type 1 or type 2 diabetes, particularly those with autonomic insufficiency, can develop hypoglycemia unawareness and may be especially susceptible to severe hypoglycemia.

TABLE 150-5 Drugs Associated with Hypoglycemia with Moderate Confidence

Cibenzoline

Fluoroquinolones

IGF-1

Indomethacin

Lithium

Pentamidine

Propoxyphene/dextropropoxyphene

Quinine

Data from Murad MH, Coto-Yglesias F, Wang AT, et al. Drug-induced hypoglycemia: a systematic review. *J Clin Endocrinol Metab.* 2009;94:741-745.

TABLE 150-6 Differential Diagnosis of Hypoglycemic Disorders

	Insulinoma	Oral Hypoglycemics	Exogenous Insulin	NIPH/Gastric Bypass	IGF-2	Insulin Ab or Insulin-receptor Ab	Cortisol Deficiency
Insulin (high when >3 µU/mL)		↑	↑	↑	↓	↑	↓
C-peptide (high when >0.2 nmol/L)	↑	↑	↓	↑	↓	*	↓
β-Hydroxy-butyrate (high when >2.7 mmol/L)	↓	↓	↓	↓	↓	↓	↑
Cortisol (suggestive if <15 µg/dL when hypoglycemic)	↑	↑	↑	↑	↑	↑	↓
Sulfonylurea/meglitinide screen	–	++	–	–	–	–	–
IGF-2 associated findings†	–	–	–	–	++	–	–
Insulin antibody	–	–	+/–	–	–	++	–

*Free-C-peptide reported to be low.
†See text.
Data from Cryer PE, Axelrod L, Grossman AB, et al. Evaluation and management of adult hypoglycemic disorders: an Endocrine Society Clinical Practice Guideline. *J Clin Endocrinol Metab.* 2009;94:709-728.

CONSEQUENCES

Acute effects of hypoglycemia are primarily neurologic and have been previously discussed. However, acute hypoglycemia may also predispose to a prolonged QTc interval and precipitate major cardiovascular events. Long-term effects on cognitive function of recurrent hypoglycemia are unclear at this time, with some studies showing no significant effects and others demonstrating neurologic sequelae.

SIGNS AND SYMPTOMS

When hypoglycemic symptoms and signs are typical, the diagnosis is generally straightforward, given the wide availability of point-of-care testing. Nevertheless, diabetic patients with any change in neurologic status should have their glucose measurement checked, given the broad spectrum of neuroglycopenic symptoms.

CAUSES

Hypoglycemia develops in diabetic patients because of a mismatch between insulin (either injected or endogenously produced with the aid of a secretagogue) and carbohydrate availability. Accidental or intentional overdose of medications, deterioration in renal function, exercise, and a missed or delayed meal are common precipitants of hypoglycemia in the community. Alcohol ingestion suppresses hepatic glucose output such that oral hypoglycemic drugs in conjunction with alcohol can cause severe and prolonged hypoglycemia. This is particularly the case with metformin, which usually will not cause hypoglycemia independently.

TREATMENT

Initial treatment is 15 to 20 g of carbohydrate orally, such as 4 oz (120 mL) of juice or full-calorie soda, or 8 oz (240 mL) of nonfat milk. If the patient cannot take oral glucose, it should be given as an intravenous bolus of 25 g of dextrose 50% in water. In the absence of a functioning intravenous line, 1 mg of glucagon can be administered intramuscularly, although this may induce emesis. Glucose should be rechecked in 15 to 20 minutes and the treatment repeated if necessary.

PRACTICE POINT

- Factitious, or self-induced, hypoglycemia should be considered in all patients with unexplained hypoglycemia. Patients are more likely to be female, have a health care background, and have psychiatric comorbidities. In patients without diabetes, clinicians should attempt to determine if the patient has access to hypoglycemic drugs through work, friends, or family members. Patients with factitious hypoglycemia due to insulin injection will have a suppressed C-peptide, indicative of the exogenous origin of circulating insulin, sometimes with very high serum insulin levels, in contrast to the slightly high or inappropriately normal insulin levels typical of patients with hypoglycemia from insulinoma. Patients should be screened for sulfonylurea and meglitinide use as well. It should be born in mind that medication-induced hypoglycemia may be accidental, as in the older patient who mistakenly uses a spouse's pill bottle that resembles his or her own. Outbreaks of hypoglycemia due to the use of counterfeit medications have also occurred, such as sexual enhancement products contaminated with sulfonylureas.

Medication-induced hypoglycemia can result in prolonged and recurrent hypoglycemic episodes. The duration of action of the responsible medication can be used to determine the required duration of monitoring. Many sulfonylureas have a duration of action close to 24 hours. The duration of action of insulin varies by formulation, but is prolonged with higher doses, intentional overdose, and renal failure. Since many types of insulin are transparent, patients may not correctly recall which insulin was administered in error, so clinicians should be cautious in prematurely discharging patients with insulin-induced hypoglycemia.

Prevention of future episodes necessitates an understanding of the underlying cause of the precipitating episode. Medication adjustment, adequate glucose monitoring, and patient education are all important. A glucagon emergency kit should be prescribed to patients at risk for recurrence.

HYPOGLYCEMIA IN THE HOSPITALIZED PATIENT WITH DIABETES

■ HYPOGLYCEMIA IN THE INTENSIVE CARE UNIT

The association of hyperglycemia with poor inpatient outcomes has prompted more aggressive management of glucose in patients with known diabetes and those with new-onset hyperglycemia. Maintaining glucose in the normal range during critical illness has been associated with reductions in morbidity and mortality in some studies, and has resulted in widespread use of intravenous insulin administered using titration protocols. However, tighter control of glucose in critically ill patients results in an increased incidence of hypoglycemia, with 6% to 17% of patients experiencing at least one glucose value below 40 mg/dL (2.2 mmol/L). Concerns about the effect of hypoglycemia on patient outcomes have led to recommendations to change the glucose range for critically ill patients to between 140 to180 mg/dL (7.8-10 mmol/L). Increasing the familiarity of staff with the chosen intravenous insulin protocol and frequent monitoring appear to offer protection from hypoglycemia.

■ HYPOGLYCEMIA IN THE NON-ICU PATIENT

Oral agents are cumbersome to adjust and potentially dangerous in the hospital setting and generally should be stopped on admission. Subcutaneously administered insulin is the preferred medication for management of hyperglycemia in the noncritically ill hospitalized patient. Insulin is among the top 10 drugs causing preventable adverse drug events during hospitalization; some 69% of inpatient hypoglycemia events are preventable. Many situations that lead to insulin-induced hypoglycemia can be anticipated. Careful attention to glucose testing, timing of insulin delivery, and synchrony with meals can play an important role in the prevention of hypoglycemia. Hypoglycemia in non-ICU patients with diabetes has recently been associated with higher inpatient mortality, as well as mortality at 1 year post discharge, highlighting the need for prevention.

■ TREATMENT OF HYPOGLYCEMIA IN THE HOSPITAL

Both ambulatory and inpatient areas of the hospital should have protocols in place to deal with hypoglycemia. Caregivers must be able to act quickly and independently to restore normoglycemia. Initial response is as outlined above. To avoid repeat episodes, patients should be assessed regarding the need for an intravenous glucose infusion after initial stabilization.

■ PREVENTION OF HYPOGLYCEMIA IN HOSPITALIZED PATIENTS

To avoid unnecessary hypoglycemia, insulin is optimally dosed in three components, including basal insulin, prandial insulin (for the patient taking meals), and correctional (often called sliding scale) insulin. A combination of these three elements can achieve more stable glucose levels during hospitalization than sliding scale insulin alone. Initial dosing of insulin in the hospitalized patient can be difficult because of many changing factors that contribute both to hyperglycemia, such as infection and corticosteroids, and hypoglycemia, such as poor oral intake. In the well-controlled patient on established insulin as an outpatient, a 20% decrease from the usual outpatient dose is recommended.

■ DISCHARGE CHECKLIST

Hyperglycemia

- Has a precipitant of hyperglycemia been identified?
- Have volume deficits and electrolyte disturbances been corrected?
- Does the patient have access to diabetic medications? Does the patient have a functioning glucometer and glucose test sticks?
- Are obstacles to care present, such as substance abuse, language barriers, psychiatric illness, or visual or cognitive impairment? If so, is there a plan to deal with them?
- Does the patient or caregiver understand any changes to the outpatient medication regimen? Would the involvement of a visiting nurse be helpful?
- Does the patient have scheduled outpatient follow-up with his or her diabetes physician?

Hypoglycemia

- Does the patient or caregiver understand any changes to the outpatient medication regimen? Would the involvement of a visiting nurse be helpful?
- Does the patient have a functioning glucometer and glucose test sticks?
- Are obstacles to care present, such as substance abuse, language barriers, psychiatric illness, or visual or cognitive impairment? If so, is there a plan to deal with them?
- Do the patient and caregivers understand what to do in the event of symptoms suggestive of hypoglycemia?
- Does the patient have a medical alert bracelet?
- Does the patient have glucagon emergency kit?
- Does the patient have scheduled outpatient follow-up with his or her diabetes physician?

SUGGESTED READINGS

Arya VB, Mohammed Z, Blankenstein O, De Lonlay P, Hussain K. Hyperinsulinaemic hypoglycaemia. *Horm Metab Res*. 2014;46:157-170.

Cryer PE, Axelrod L, Grossman AB, et al. Evaluation and management of adult hypoglycemic disorders: an Endocrine Society Clinical Practice Guideline. *J Clin Endocrinol Metab*. 2009;94:709-728.

Kitabchi AE, Umpierrez GE, Murphy MB, et al. Hyperglycemic crises in adult patients with diabetes: a consensus statement from the American Diabetes Association. *Diabetes Care*. 2009;32:1335-1343.

Moghissi ES, Korytkowski MT, DiNardo M, et al. American Association of Clinical Endocrinologists and American Diabetes Association consensus statement on inpatient glycemic control. *Diabetes Care*. 2009;32:1119-1131.

Murad MH, Coto-Yglesias F, Wang AT, et al. Clinical review: drug-induced hypoglycemia: a systematic review. *J Clin Endocrinol Metab*. 2009;94:741-745.

Turchin A, Matheny ME, Shubina M, et al. Hypoglycemia and clinical outcomes in patients with diabetes hospitalized in the general ward. *Diabetes Care*. 2009;32:1153-1157.

Zapatero A, Gómez-Huelgas R, González N, et al. Frequency of hypoglycemia and its impact on length of stay, mortality, and short-term readmission in patients with diabetes hospitalized in internal medicine wards. *Endocr Pract*. 2014;20:870-875.

CHAPTER 151

Inpatient Management of Diabetes and Hyperglycemia

Jeffrey L. Schnipper, MD, MPH, FHM

Key Clinical Questions

1. Why control diabetes and hyperglycemia in the hospital?

2. What are the goals of glycemic management in critical care and noncritical care settings?

3. When should patients be treated with oral agents, with subcutaneous insulin, and with continuous insulin infusions?

4. Is it safe to prescribe subcutaneous insulin for the first time in a hospitalized patient?

5. How should insulin orders be adjusted in response to poor inpatient glucose control?

6. What should be considered when discharging a patient with diabetes or inpatient hyperglycemia?

7. How may the quality of glucose management be improved in hospital settings?

INTRODUCTION

Diabetes mellitus is common in hospitalized patients. In 2013, diabetes was listed as a diagnosis in approximately 23% of all hospital discharges in the United States. Because discharge diagnoses may not capture undiagnosed diabetes or hospital-related hyperglycemia, the true prevalence of diabetes or hyperglycemia in hospitalized patients is likely much higher. For example, in one study of general medicine and surgery admissions, hyperglycemia (defined as a fasting plasma glucose of ≥126 mg/dL or a random plasma glucose of ≥200 mg/dL) was found in 38% of patients. Of these, 68% had known diabetes, but the other 32% had no previous diagnosis and consisted of patients with undiagnosed diabetes, prediabetes unmasked by the stress of illness, and pure stress hyperglycemia.

Hyperglycemia is associated with worse outcomes among hospitalized patients, including infections, increased length of stay, decreased independent living after discharge, and increased mortality. Hyperglycemia among known diabetics in the hospital carries a 2.7 relative risk of in-hospital death; even more dramatic is the 18-fold increased risk of death associated with hyperglycemia among those without a previous diagnosis of diabetes. Similar results have been seen in patients with pneumonia, myocardial infarction, chronic obstructive pulmonary disease, stroke, and those receiving total parenteral nutrition. Some of this excess mortality reflects the role of hyperglycemia as a marker for physiologic stress and severity of underlying disease. However, even when rigorous adjustment for severity of illness is conducted, excess mortality remains.

RATIONALE FOR INPATIENT GLUCOSE CONTROL

Does correcting inpatient hyperglycemia improve outcomes? In the noncritical care setting, this question has remained unanswered until recently.

RABBIT Surgery was a dual-site randomized controlled trial of 211 patients with type 2 DM admitted to general surgery services. The intervention group received a basal-bolus regimen with glargine once daily and glulisine before meals with a goal premeal glucose of 100 to 140 mg/dL. The control group received sliding scale regular insulin four times daily for glucose >140 mg/dL. Mean glucose for the hospitalization was 157 versus 176 mg/dL in favor of the intervention. Proportion of patients with any glucose <40 mg/dL was 3.8% in the intervention group and 0% in the control group. Most importantly, the primary outcome, a composite of hospital complications including postoperative wound infection, pneumonia, respiratory failure, acute renal failure, and bacteremia, occurred in 24% in the control group and only 9% in the intervention group (p = .003; number needed to treat of 7 to prevent one complication).

In the critical care setting, several studies of tight glycemic control have been performed, with mixed results. Early studies, such as the Leuven study conducted by van den Berghe, et al, in surgical intensive care unit (ICU) patients, were clearly positive. In Leuven I, patients were randomized to an insulin infusion protocol triggered when the blood glucose was >100 mg/dL or a protocol that was triggered when glucose was >215 mg/dL. The mean achieved glucose was 103 versus 153 mg/dL. Outcomes in the intervention arm included a 46% reduction in sepsis, 41% reduction in the need for dialysis, 50% reduction in blood transfusions, 44% reduction in polyneuropathy, and a 34% reduction in inpatient mortality. However, subsequent studies have not been so favorable. A follow-up study on medical ICU patients conducted by the same group was equivocal: mortality did not improve except in a post hoc analysis of patients with an ICU length of stay of 3 days or more, although patients in the intervention group did have faster weaning from mechanical ventilation, earlier discharge from the ICU, and earlier discharge from the hospital. Rates of severe hypoglycemia were much higher in the intervention arm (19% vs 3% of patients with at least one glucose <40 mg/dL). More recently, the NICE-SUGAR study was even less favorable to tight glucose control. In this open-label study of 6104 critically ill patients (medical and surgical), the intervention arm had a slightly increased 90-day mortality rate (27.5% vs 24.9%), and a much higher rate of severe hypoglycemia (6.8% vs 0.5%).

Some providers have interpreted NICE-SUGAR as justifying lax glucose control in critically ill patients. There are many reasons to avoid this approach:

1. In the NICE-SUGAR study, control patients actually had reasonably good glucose control: 69% were on an insulin infusion, and the median glucose was 141 mg/dL.
2. The high rates of hypoglycemia observed may be a specific problem with the Leuven insulin infusion protocol. Lower rates of hypoglycemia are seen with the use of other insulin infusion protocols, such as Yale and Glucommander, which are easier to administer and take better account of trends in glucose control over time (**Table 151-1**).
3. Septic patients may be particularly prone to hypoglycemia (medical ICU patients in these studies always have higher rates of hypoglycemia than surgical ICU patients). The rational clinical response should be higher glucose targets in these patients, not lack of any target at all.
4. Insulin is one of the highest risk medications used in the hospital, and yet its inpatient use has been historically haphazard and irrational. A standardized approach to insulin use can prevent both severe hyperglycemia and hypoglycemia, which are both hazardous to patients.
5. Several quality improvement studies, including several conducted by hospitalists, have shown the ability to institute processes that reduce hyperglycemia, while maintaining or even reducing the rate of hypoglycemia.

In response to recent studies, the American Association of Clinical Endocrinologists (AACE) and the American Diabetes Association (ADA) have updated their guidelines. In critically ill patients, extrapolating from NICE-SUGAR's control group, they recommend starting insulin infusions at a threshold no higher than 180 mg/dL, and aiming for a target range of 140 to 180 mg/dL. Recommendations for noncritically ill patients remain essentially unchanged: goals of premeal glucose readings <140 mg/dL and random glucose readings <180 mg/dL, with more or less stringent goals depending on previously achieved control and medical comorbidities.

The Endocrine Society's 2012 Guideline for the noncritical care setting is similar, with a few additional recommendations based on studies such as RABBIT Surgery: treat insulin-requiring patients with scheduled subcutaneous insulin in the hospital, avoid use of sliding scale insulin alone, use basal, rapid acting, and correctional insulin in patients who are eating, and reassess therapy when blood glucose levels are less than 100 mg/dL. These are explained in more detail below. It should also be noted that the National Quality Forum now has two measures for inpatient glycemic control, with the Center for Medicare/Medicaid Services as the steward: average proportion of hyperglycemic hospital days, and rate of hypoglycemia events following administration of an antidiabetic agent.

PATHOPHYSIOLOGY

Even short-term hyperglycemia may be hazardous in medically ill patients. Hyperglycemia is associated with immune dysfunction, specifically neutrophil impairment and complement inhibition. Hyperglycemia leads to protein glycation and overproduction of free fatty acids, reactive oxygen species, ketones, and lactic acid, all of which may lead to cellular injury (including mitochondrial injury and endothelial dysfunction), inflammation, and defective wound repair. These adverse effects are likely to be most evident in patients with infections (eg, pneumonia), wounds (eg, sternotomy), and infarction or ischemia (eg, myocardial infarction, stroke), exactly the populations in which observational data linking hyperglycemia to increased mortality are the strongest. Hyperglycemia may also lead to fluid and electrolyte imbalances once thresholds for glucosuria are reached (generally around 200 mg/dL). These can be potentially catastrophic in patients already suffering from acute renal failure, hypernatremia, and lactic acidosis. Good inpatient glucose management may also lead to better glucose control after discharge, for example, triggering a change to insulin use in a patient poorly controlled on maximal doses of oral agents. Measures to improve outpatient glucose control can have sustained effects on long-term diabetic complications such as neuropathy, nephropathy, retinopathy, and cardiovascular disease.

DIAGNOSIS

Hyperglycemia is not usually the primary reason for hospitalization in diabetic patients. When it is, it is usually clinically obvious, as in diabetic ketoacidosis (DKA) in patients with type 1 diabetes, and hyperglycemic hyperosmolar state (HHS) in patients with type 2 diabetes. Diagnostic errors in the management of patients with diabetes and hyperglycemia may include the following:

1. Failure to recognize hyperglycemia in a patient without a previous diagnosis of diabetes (eg, failure to notice a routine laboratory glucose of 200 mg/dL as abnormal). Any routine glucose reading over 180 mg/dL should trigger further evaluation and

TABLE 151-1 Rates of Severe Hypoglycemia in Trials using Different Insulin Infusion Protocols

Study	Patient Population	Hypoglycemia Rate*
Leuven protocol		
Leuven 1 (*N Engl J Med*. 2001;345: 1359-1367)	Surgical	5.1%
Leuven 2 (*N Engl J Med*. 2006;354:449-461)	Medical	19%
Glucontrol (*Intensive Care Med*. 2009;35: 738-748)	Medical/ Surgical	8.6%
VISEP (*N Engl J Med*. 2008;358:125-139)	Medical	17%
NICE-SUGAR (*N Engl J Med*. 2009;360: 1283-1297)	Medical/ Surgical	6.8%
Yale protocol		
Yale 1 (*J Cardiothorac Vasc Anesth*. 2004;18:690-697)	Surgical	0%
Yale 2 (*Diabetes Care*. 2004;27:461-467)	Medical	4.3%
Glucommander protocol		
Glucommander 1 (*Diabetes Care*. 2005;28: 2418-2423)	Surgical	2.6%

*Proportion of patients with any glucose <40 mg/dL.

monitoring, including at least 24 hours of point-of-care (POC) glucose testing before meals and a hemoglobin A1c test. The hemoglobin A1c may be useful in the diagnosis of type 2 diabetes and helps assess the prior 90 days of glucose control, enabling the provider to distinguish diabetes from stress hyperglycemia. It is also extremely useful for discharge planning.

2. Failure to recognize type 1 diabetes, as opposed to type 2 diabetes. While the diagnosis may be obvious in a young, thin patient who presents for the first time in DKA, it should also be considered in the patient with chronic pancreatitis and pancreatic insufficiency, the patient who has had complete or partial pancreatectomy for malignancy, and other situations in which beta cell failure may be the predominant problem. These patients must receive insulin at all times, are more insulin sensitive, and typically have more labile glucose control due to the lack of pancreatic reserve. Many of these patients would benefit from endocrinology input for both diagnosis and management.

Glucose monitoring should be obtained in any patient with a history of diabetes, inpatient hyperglycemia, or receiving treatment that might cause hyperglycemia (such as systemic corticosteroids). In the setting of corticosteroids, monitoring can be stopped after 24 hours if hyperglycemia is not observed and increases in glucocorticoid doses are not planned. Patients eating discrete meals should generally be tested before each meal and before bedtime, while patients who are receiving nothing by mouth (NPO), receiving continuous enteral nutrition (tube feeds), or total parenteral nutrition (TPN) should be tested every 6 hours. Additional testing is optional depending on the circumstance. For example, testing at 3 AM can be used to rule out nocturnal hypoglycemia, while testing 1 to 2 hours after meals can be used to test the adequacy of nutritional insulin dosing. Recent studies indicate that there is no benefit to correcting bedtime hyperglycemia, so if it is checked, it should only be used to adjust scheduled insulin orders (see below).

TRIAGE

Patients with severe DKA may be best admitted to an ICU. Insulin infusions are usually required for these patients, as well as frequent (every 1-2 hours) monitoring and repletion of fluids and electrolytes. These considerations alone may mandate ICU-level care. However, some hospitals may be able to safely manage patients with less severe DKA (eg, venous pH > 7.25) in intermediate care areas. Beyond DKA, if the clinical situation otherwise requires intravenous (IV) insulin infusions, and such infusions can only be delivered in an ICU, then that would also mandate triage to an ICU.

TREATMENT

The management of inpatients with diabetes or hyperglycemia is inherently unstable. Patients suffer from nutritional and clinical instability, from acute illness and stress-related hyperglycemia that is dynamic and difficult to measure and predict, and from the use of diagnostic and therapeutic interventions that impact glycemic control and the actions of antihyperglycemic therapies. Most patients will require changes from their home regimen to an inpatient regimen that takes these factors into account.

■ USE OF ORAL ANTIDIABETIC AGENTS

Broadly speaking, there are three options for controlling inpatient hyperglycemia: oral agents, IV insulin infusions, and subcutaneous insulin injections. Most experts recommend against the routine use of oral agents in the hospital for a variety of reasons.

1. They are slow acting and difficult to titrate.
2. Insulin secretagogues such as glipizide, glyburide, and repaglinide inhibit pancreatic autoregulation and can easily cause hypoglycemia, especially in the setting of reduced oral intake. Many are also long acting.

3. Metformin can cause nausea, vomiting, and diarrhea, and is contraindicated in conditions that can predispose to lactic acidosis, including renal failure, use of intravenous iodinated contrast, heart failure, and liver failure.
4. Thiazolidinediones such as pioglitazone and rosiglitazone are very slow acting and can cause fluid retention and pulmonary and peripheral edema.
5. Newer oral agents (eg, dipeptidyl peptidase 4 inhibitors) do not have a well understood safety profile in hospitalized patients and are often not on formulary.

Oral agents should only be continued in patients with good glucose control before and at the time of admission, who are not very ill, have a short projected length of stay, will not be NPO for any procedure, and will not be undergoing studies that use IV contrast. Oral agents should also be avoided in hospitalized patients who either have or are at risk for developing renal failure, heart failure, liver failure, or peripheral edema during the hospitalization. In the small population of patients who are eligible to continue oral agents, glycemia should be closely monitored. If glucose control is poor, oral agents should be stopped and insulin begun.

■ USE OF INTRAVENOUS INSULIN INFUSIONS

Intravenous insulin infusions are rapidly effective and generally safe with frequent glucose monitoring. The benefit of IV insulin infusion is most proven in the settings of critical illness, before major surgical procedures, after organ transplantation, acute myocardial infarction, DKA, prolonged fasting in a patient with type 1 diabetes, and labor and delivery. Insulin infusions should be used in critically ill patients with hyperglycemia in accordance with updated AACE/ADA guidelines. Insulin infusions are generally underutilized in noncritically ill patients, especially in patients with infections, wounds, or organ damage with several days of poor glucose control on subcutaneous regimens. In these patients, an insulin infusion can usually restore good glucose control within hours. Policies can usually be adopted to protect patients and staff from unsafe situations, such as restricting their use in noncritical areas to daytime hours and only for 1 day, and guaranteeing availability of clinical personnel to adjust the drip rate every hour.

■ SUBCUTANEOUS INSULIN

The best treatment for most inpatients with diabetes and hyperglycemia is subcutaneous insulin injections, prescribed in an anticipatory and physiologic fashion. Three types of insulin orders should be provided: basal, nutritional (bolus), and correctional. **Basal insulin** is required in all patients with type 1 diabetes, and most patients with type 2 diabetes, to maintain euglycemia by preventing gluconeogenesis. It mimics the continuous, low-level endogenous insulin produced by the body at all times (**Figure 151-1**). Long-acting insulins such as glargine, detemir, and NPH are most appropriate for use as basal insulin (**Figure 151-2**). **Nutritional insulin** provides for the spike in blood glucose with meals, mimicking the rapid rise in blood insulin levels in response to eating. It should not be given to patients who are NPO. In patients eating discrete meals, rapid-acting insulins such as insulin lispro, aspart, and glulisine are most appropriate. For patients on continuous tube feeds, a short- to intermediate-acting insulin, such as regular insulin every 6 hours, is appropriate. In nondiabetics, the amount of basal insulin produced is approximately equal to the amount of nutritional insulin produced in any 24-hour period. This 50/50 ratio of basal-to-nutritional insulin is therefore generally recommended for the treatment of inpatient hyperglycemia.

Correctional insulin is extra insulin given to correct hyperglycemia that occurs despite basal and nutritional insulin. Correctional insulin has replaced the use of the term "sliding scale," to emphasize that correctional insulin should not be used alone and is ineffective in maintaining euglycemia without scheduled basal and nutritional insulin. It is often written in a stepped format, so that more severe

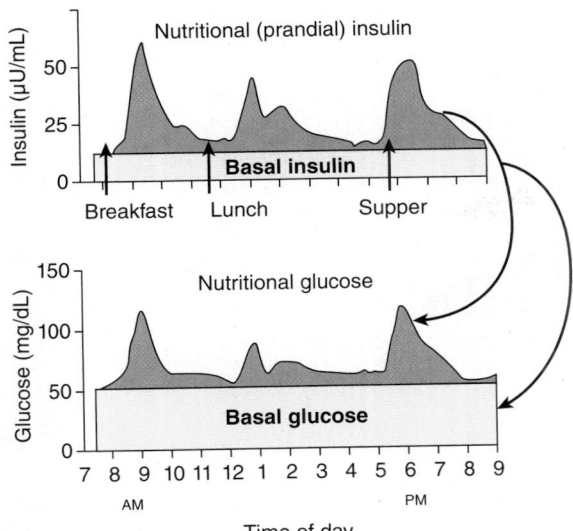

Figure 151-1 *Physiologic relationship between basal and nutritional glucose levels and basal and nutritional insulin levels in nondiabetic individuals.*

hyperglycemia is treated with higher doses. The steps should be customized to the patient, based on the patient's estimated insulin sensitivity (so that a patient receiving 100 units of scheduled insulin a day is not receiving a 1-5 unit scale). Correctional insulin that is required consistently (eg, two or more times a day) suggests a need to modify the scheduled basal or nutritional insulin doses.

Physiologic subcutaneous insulin regimens should be used in

- All patients with type 1 diabetes, unless they require an insulin infusion.
- Patients with type 2 diabetes that are already insulin requiring, are poorly controlled despite oral agents, or known to require high doses of oral agents that will be held in the hospital.
- Any patient with blood glucose levels during hospitalization consistently above the target range (eg, >180 mg/dL in non-critical care patients).

■ HOW TO ORDER PHYSIOLOGIC SUBCUTANEOUS INSULIN IN THE HOSPITAL

Most experts recommend a stepwise approach to physiologic insulin dosing in the hospital:

1. Decide if a patient is appropriate for subcutaneous insulin, and discontinue all oral antidiabetic agents.
2. Calculate the estimated total daily dose (TDD) of insulin.

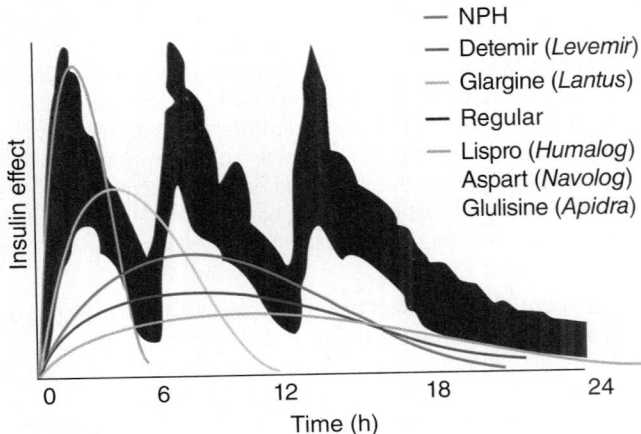

— NPH
— Detemir (*Levemir*)
— Glargine (*Lantus*)
— Regular
— Lispro (*Humalog*)
Aspart (*Navolog*)
Glulisine (*Apidra*)

Figure 151-2 *Pharmacokinetics of various types of insulin.*

3. Determine the distribution of the TDD, based on the patient's nutritional regimen.
4. Re-evaluate and adjust the TDD daily, based on the glycemic control of the previous 24 hours.

■ CALCULATING THE TOTAL DAILY DOSE

The TDD can be estimated in several ways. For patients well controlled on a preadmission insulin regimen, we recommend adding up all the scheduled insulin doses to derive the TDD. For patients not on insulin prior to admission, a weight-based calculation is most appropriate. A typical starting dose is 0.4 to 0.6 units/kg/d. Patients with recent hypoglycemia, who are older, thin, or insulin sensitive (eg, type 1), should start at the lower end of this range (or even 0.3 units/kg/d if multiple risk factors for hypoglycemia apply). Recent studies show that patients with renal failure (GFR < 45, not on renal replacement therapy) should start at a TDD of 0.25 units/kg/d. In contrast, patients who are obese, on corticosteroids, or have a history of hyperglycemia should start at the higher end of this range, and may in fact eventually need much higher doses. For patients transferred out of an ICU whose glucose level has been well controlled on an insulin drip at a stable dose for at least 6 hours, the TDD can be estimated by multiplying the hourly drip rate by 20. This is likely to slightly underestimate the TDD, but is done to avoid hypoglycemia. This also assumes that the patient was receiving nutrition in the ICU (eg, tube feeds); if the patient was not being fed, the above calculation estimates the basal insulin requirement only, and the TDD would be double this amount.

■ DIVIDING THE TOTAL DAILY DOSE INTO BASAL AND NUTRITIONAL COMPONENTS

Once the TDD has been estimated, the daily basal dose can be calculated as approximately half of the TDD, while the daily nutritional dose can be estimated as the other half of the TDD. Basal insulin can be given as one daily dose (eg, insulin glargine at night), or split (eg, NPH at morning and at night). The type, dose, and frequency of nutritional insulin will depend on the patient's nutritional status (**Figure 151-3**). For example, for patients receiving discrete meals, it can be written as rapid-acting insulin before meals (ie, split in three doses; **Figure 151-3A**). For a patient receiving continuous tube feeds or total parenteral nutrition, it can be written as regular insulin every 6 hours (ie, split in four doses; **Figure 151-3B**). Even in patients on continuous tube feeds, this approach is recommended over giving the entire TDD as insulin glargine, for example, in case tube feeds have to be discontinued (eg, for testing, or because of gastric tube malfunction or GI transit issues). In this case, the basal dose can remain unchanged, nutritional insulin can be discontinued, and the risk of hypoglycemia should persist for no more than 6 hours, rather than 24 hours. Nutritional insulin is not ordered in patients who are NPO.

In patients with unpredictable oral intake (eg, resuming PO intake after pancreatitis, nausea and vomiting, or recent GI surgery), it may be appropriate to wait until the meal has been eaten before giving nutritional insulin. If a patient eats all the food provided to him/her, the entire dose of rapid-acting insulin can be given immediately after the meal. If half the food is eaten, the dose can be halved, and so on. Assuming a patient has been written for a consistent carbohydrate meal (which is recommended), this approach resembles "carb-counting" (multiplying the carbohydrate intake by a factor to determine the insulin dose) but is easier to implement.

■ ORDERING CORRECTIONAL INSULIN

Correctional insulin is usually given in the same form as the patient's nutritional insulin. It may be given at the same time as nutritional insulin (eg, 6 units standing nutritional insulin, plus 4 units for a glucose of 260 mg/dL, for a total of 10 units rapid-acting insulin given before the meal). In patients who are NPO, it can be written as

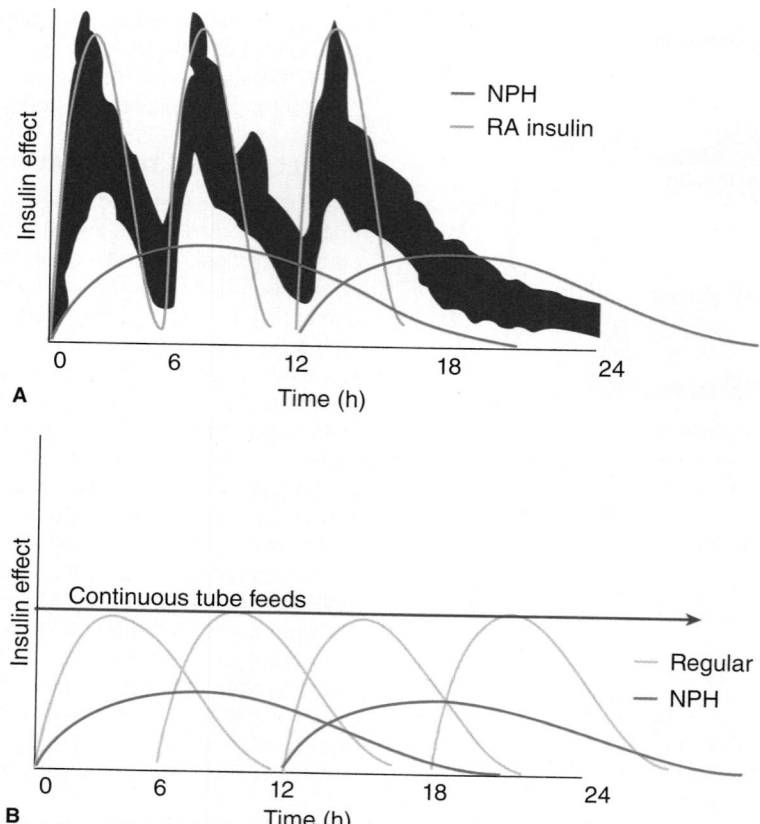

Figure 151-3 *Examples of insulin regimens for patients with different kinds of nutritional intake. (A) Patients eating discrete meals. (B) Patients receiving continuous enteral nutrition (tube feeds).*

regular insulin every 6 hours or rapid-acting insulin every 4 hours. As noted above, stepped dosing orders should take insulin sensitivity into account. One way to do this is to have three different strengths of sliding scales using the TDD as the estimate of insulin sensitivity (see **Table 151-2** as an example).

■ DANGERS OF SLIDING SCALE INSULIN USED ALONE

In patients well controlled on oral agents at home, or in nondiabetics started on corticosteroids, it may be appropriate to write for routine point-of-care glucose testing and a correctional insulin protocol alone. But if this approach results in hyperglycemia, it should be abandoned in favor of the approach described above. Correctional insulin by itself does not work: by definition, it is reactive and predictably causes hyperglycemia, it leads to a roller-coaster pattern of glycemia (which in itself may be dangerous), it increases the risk for stacking of insulin doses and hypoglycemia, and it promotes an illusion of control and clinical inertia. Several studies have shown that

sliding scale insulin alone leads to higher rates of hyperglycemia, compared with any other approach to glucose management. Moreover, even in the patients described above, starting physiological insulin on the first hospital day is completely safe. In anyone with a functioning pancreas (ie, anyone except patients with type 1 diabetes), endogenous insulin production will automatically adjust as exogenous insulin is given. Patients will not become hypoglycemic, as long as the TDD given is less than or equal to the patient's true insulin requirements, the dosing principles above are followed, and the patient is not receiving an insulin secretagogue. In our experience, patients with mild or no diabetes do well on physiologic insulin regimens because of the degree of pancreatic reserve.

■ INSULIN ADJUSTMENT

As a rule, insulin orders require daily adjustment in response to changes in patient status and glucose control. Unfortunately, there is currently no consensus on the best method of daily insulin adjustment. Some experts recommend adjusting the basal dose separately from the nutritional dose (eg, using the morning fasting glucose to guide basal dose adjustment, and glucose levels later in the day to guide nutritional dose adjustment). Others recommend using global glucose control to guide adjustments to the TDD and then distributing it into basal and nutritional components. We recommend the following approach based on the RABBIT Surgery trial given its benefits on hard patient outcomes in a randomized controlled trial:

1. If fasting and predinner blood glucose (BG) 100 to 140 mg/dL in absence of hypoglycemia previous day: no change.
2. If fasting and predinner BG 140 to 180 mg/dL in absence of hypoglycemia previous day: increase TDD by 10%.
3. If fasting and predinner BG >180 mg/dL in absence of hypoglycemia previous day: increase TDD by 20%.

TABLE 151-2 Examples of Correctional Insulin Scales Based on Total Daily Insulin Dose

	Low Scale	Medium Scale	High Scale
Premeal blood glucose	<40 units insulin/d	40-80 units insulin/d	>80 units insulin/d
150-199 mg/dL	1 unit	1 unit	2 units
200-249 mg/dL	2 units	3 units	4 units
250-299 mg/dL	3 units	5 units	7 units
300-349 mg/dL	4 units	7 units	10 units
>349 mg/dL	5 units	8 units	12 units

4. If fasting and predinner BG 70 to 99 mg/dL in absence of hypo-glycemia previous day: decrease TDD by 10%.
5. If hypoglycemia (<70 mg/dL), decrease TDD by 20%.

Then redistribute the TDD 50% basal, 50% nutritional.

Practically speaking, while not used in the RABBIT Surgery trial, we will often then adjust the basal and nutritional components of the TDD separately, keeping in mind that the morning fasting glucose is the best indicator of the adequacy of the basal insulin dose, while glucose readings 1 to 2 hours after eating are the best indicators of nutritional plus correctional insulin.

COMPLICATIONS

Common inpatient complications include hypoglycemia and iat-rogenic DKA. Hypoglycemia often occurs because of unexpected reductions in nutritional intake, such as vomiting or tube feeds that have to be held. This can be prevented with the following measures.

1. Proactively identifying patients at risk for hypoglycemia, includ-ing patients with type 1 diabetes, patients who are older, have renal dysfunction, or have unpredictable nutritional intake, and reduce insulin doses and monitor glucose levels more frequently in these patients.
2. Writing balanced basal and nutritional insulin doses. Many patients have preadmission regimens that are predominantly basal insulin because they are easier to administer. But when these patients have reduced oral intake in the hospital, hypo-glycemia may result. This is why we recommend splitting the patient's home TDD in half as the basal insulin dose, even if this results in a basal dose lower than that prescribed at home. The nutritional insulin can then be written based on the patient's degree of nutritional intake.
3. Giving nutritional insulin after meals in patients with unpredict-able oral intake, as described above.
4. Being aware of patients with inpatient insulin requirements that are much higher than preadmission requirements because of physiologic stress, and that these high requirements may resolve quickly as a patient's illness improves.

Iatrogenic DKA is best prevented by ensuring that all patients with type 1 diabetes (including patients with pancreatic disease) are receiving basal insulin at all times.

DISCHARGE CHECKLIST

- Has a hemoglobin A1c been obtained to assess the adequacy of preadmission glycemic control, if one is not available from the previous month? The hemoglobin A1c may be misleading if patients have recently undergone rapid red cell turnover, as in bleeding, transfusion, and hemolytic anemia. If the hemoglobin A1c is close to 7, then most patients can be discharged on their preadmission regimen, with the possible exception of patients being discharged on a long course of high-dose corticosteroids. If the A1c is significantly greater than 7, then the home regi-men probably needs to be adjusted once dietary or medication nonadherence has first been explored as the possible cause. This adjustment might include higher doses of preadmission oral agents, or minor (10%-20%) increases in preadmission insulin doses. Some patients may require more injections per day than previously; this requires full buy-in from patients, caregivers, and outpatient providers before attempting. Regimens that worked well in the hospital may not work for patients after discharge. In particular, inpatient regimens may be more complex than some patients can manage. Patients on maximum doses of two oral agents prior to admission with an elevated hemoglobin A1c pose a particular challenge. If possible, these patients should be discharged on insulin, using the simplest regimen possible (eg, insulin glargine once a day plus metformin twice a day).

- Have patients being started on insulin at discharge received inpatient insulin teaching? It should be determined as early as possible if the patient will require home fingerstick glucose monitoring and insulin, and if so, what type(s) of insulin and what means of injection (needle and syringe or insulin pen). Once these decisions are made, education can be tailored accordingly for patients or their caregivers. Education should focus first on survival skills, such as recognizing symptoms of hypoglycemia and how to manage it, and when and who to call for problems.
- Does the patient have insurance coverage for insulin, needles, and syringes, as well as a glucometer and test strips?
- Does the patient have adequate cognitive function and eyesight to self-administer insulin? Are there family members or other care-givers who can assist the patient in these tasks?
- For patients being discharged on insulin, has follow-up monitoring by a visiting nurse been arranged immediately following discharge, as well as follow-up with a diabetes educator and endocrinologist? Patients require ongoing diabetic education and reinforcement, even if they received diabetic teaching as an inpatient.

SUGGESTED READINGS

Davidson PC, Steed RD, Bode BW. Glucommander: a computer-directed intravenous insulin system shown to be safe, sim-ple, and effective in 120,618 h of operation. *Diabetes Care*. 2005;28:2418-2423.

Finfer S, Chittock DR, Su SY, et al. Intensive versus conven-tional glucose control in critically ill patients. *N Engl J Med*. 2009;360:1283-1297.

Moghissi ES, Korytkowski MT, DiNardo M, et al. American Association of Clinical Endocrinologists and American Diabetes Association consensus statement on inpatient glycemic control. *Endocr Pract*. 2009;15:353-369.

Preiser JC, Devos P, Ruiz-Santana S, et al. A prospective randomised multi-centre controlled trial on tight glucose control by intensive insulin therapy in adult intensive care units: the Glucontrol study. *Intensive Care Med*. 2009;35:1738-1748.

Schnipper JL, Liang CL, Ndumele CD, et al. Effects of a computer-ized order set on the inpatient management of hyperglycemia: a cluster-randomized controlled trial. *Endocr Pract*. 2010;16:209-218.

Society of Hospital Medicine. Glycemic Control Implementation Toolkit. 2015. http://www.hospitalmedicine.org/Web/Quality_Innovation/Implementation_Toolkits/Glycemic_Control/Web/Quality___Innovation/Implementation_Toolkit/Glycemic/Overview.aspx?hkey=ef88fb8f-7b6b-46bc-b9bd-ad02985ebe86. Accessed November 2, 2015.

Umpierrez GE, Isaacs SD, Bazargan N, You X, Thaler LM, Kitabchi AE. Hyperglycemia: an independent marker of in-hospital mortality in patients with undiagnosed diabetes. *J Clin Endocrinol Metab*. 2002;87:978-982.

Umpierrez GE, Hellman R, Korytkowski MT, et al. Management of hyperglycemia in hospitalized patients in non-critical care setting: an endocrine society clinical practice guideline. *J Clin Endocrinol Metab*. 2012;97:16-38.

Umpierrez GE, Smiley D, Jacobs S, et al. Randomized study of basal-bolus insulin therapy in the inpatient management of patients with type 2 diabetes undergoing general surgery (RABBIT 2 Surgery). *Diabetes Care*. 2011;34:256-261.

Van den Berghe G, Wilmer A, Hermans G, et al. Intensive insulin therapy in the medical ICU. *N Engl J Med*. 2006;354:449-461.

Van den Berghe G, Wouters P, Weekers F, et al. Intensive insulin ther-apy in the critically ill patients. *N Engl J Med*. 2001;345:1359-1367.

CHAPTER 152

Thyroid Emergencies

Jill M. Paulson, MD
Anthony N. Hollenberg, MD

Key Clinical Questions

1. How does one interpret thyroid function tests in the inpatient setting?

2. How can one distinguish nonthyroidal illness from other thyroid conditions?

3. How does myxedema coma differ from a normal hypothyroid state and how is it treated?

4. What characterizes thyroid storm and how is it distinct from thyrotoxicosis?

5. How is thyroid storm treated?

INTRODUCTION

Thyroid disease is important to hospitalists for two reasons. Rarely, patients are admitted to the hospital with myxedema coma or thyrotoxicosis, conditions that must be recognized early, as prompt diagnosis and treatment reduce patient morbidity and mortality. More often, patients have thyroid function tests performed in the hospital because of nonspecific symptoms such as fatigue, weight loss, and palpitations, and the hospitalist has to distinguish between true thyroid disease and nonthyroidal illness syndrome (euthyroid sick syndrome). To understand the diagnosis and treatment of thyroid disease, it is necessary to review the normal physiology of thyroid hormone.

THYROID HORMONE PHYSIOLOGY AND TESTING

Thyroid hormone usually refers to both thyroxine (T_4) and triiodothyronine (T_3). The thyroid synthesizes primarily T_4, but also synthesizes T_3. T_3 is thought to be the biologically active form of the hormone; T_4, which has a longer half-life, functions as a prohormone. Eighty percent of T_3 is produced by deiodination of the tyrosine rings of T_4 by tissue deiodinases. Both type 1 and 2 deiodinases convert T_4 to T_3. In contrast, type 3 deiodinase converts T_4 to inactive reverse T_3 (rT_3), and also inactivates T_3.

T_4 and T_3 gain access to cells by transporters which are still being elucidated. T_3 acts mainly in the nucleus, binding to thyroid hormone receptors to regulate gene expression. This genomic action accounts for many physiologic effects of T_3, including thermogenesis, decreased systemic vascular resistance, and increased cardiac chronotropy and inotropy.

T_3 feeds back at the level of the hypothalamus and pituitary to regulate thyrotropin-releasing hormone and thyroid-stimulating hormone (TSH) synthesis and secretion, respectively. Thyroid-stimulating hormone governs the amount of thyroid hormone synthesized by the thyroid gland. Thyroid-stimulating hormone is a heterodimeric glycoprotein hormone that can be measured by rapid, sensitive, and reliable immunoassays in the laboratory. A suppressed TSH demonstrates excessive thyroid hormone and hyperthyroidism, while an elevated TSH indicates inadequate thyroid hormone and hypothyroidism (**Figure 152-1**).

In certain clinical scenarios, including patients with central hypothyroidism (secondary hypothyroidism) due to hypothalamic-pituitary dysfunction, patients treated with medications such as dopamine and glucocorticoids, and patients who are critically ill, TSH does not reliably indicate thyroid status and should not be used as a screening test (**Table 152-1**).

Thyroid status can also be assessed by measuring circulating T_4 and T_3 levels. Because thyroid hormones are protein bound, the most common test used to measure peripheral thyroid hormone is an analogue free T_4 (fT_4) assay. While this assay is usually reliable, the indirect methodology used may make it difficult to interpret in severe illness or pregnancy. In these circumstances, measurement of total T_4 (TT_4) and total T_3 (TT_3), together with an index of protein binding such as thyroxine binding globulin (TBG) or resin uptake, is the preferred method. Also available, but rarely used due to high cost and lack of availability, is direct measurement of fT_4 by equilibrium dialysis. Free T_3 levels can also be measured, but have lesser clinical utility. When thyroid disease is clinically suspected, it is usual to screen with a TSH, and if abnormal proceed to determine circulating thyroid hormone levels by measuring fT_4 and potentially TT_3.

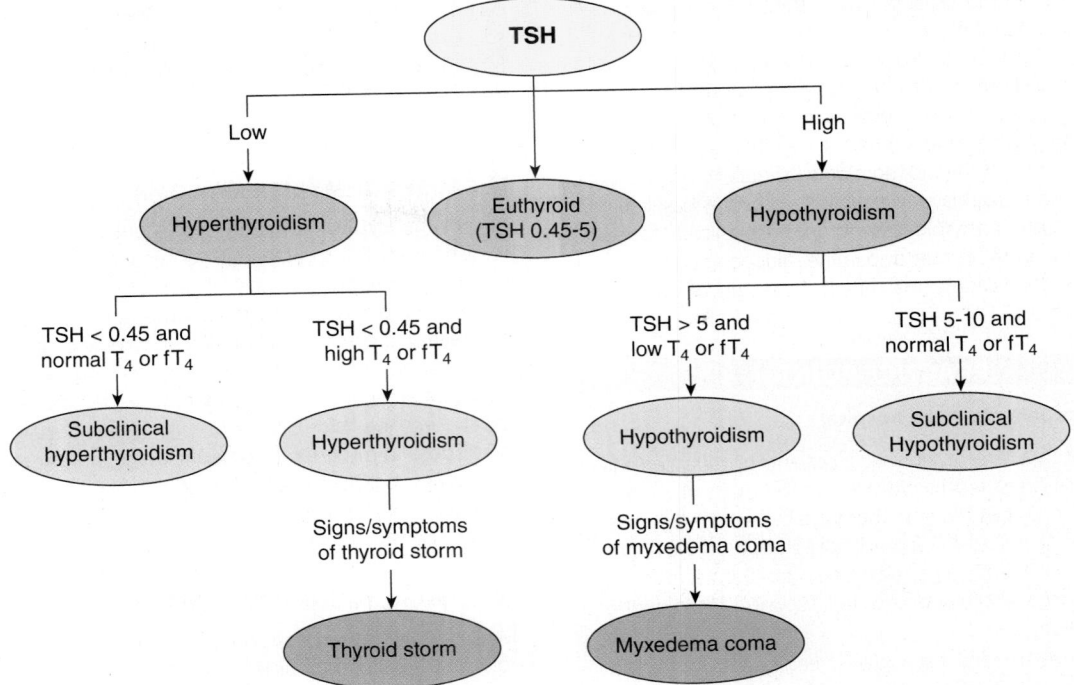

Figure 152-1 *Algorithm for thyroid function tests. This algorithm does not apply in patients with hypothalamic-pituitary disease, serious illness, or those who are taking certain medications such as amiodarone, glucocorticoids, and dopamine.*

However, in the critically ill patient with suspected thyroid dysfunction, it is reasonable to obtain a full panel of thyroid tests, including TSH, fT_4, TT_4, and TT_3.

NONTHYROIDAL ILLNESS SYNDROME (EUTHYROID SICK SYNDROME)

ALTERATED THYROID FUNCTION IN NONTHYROIDAL ILLNESS SYNDROME

Routine laboratory testing of thyroid function is best done outside the hospital. In severe illness, changes in thyroid function make it difficult to determine whether thyroid disease is present. Thyroid function tests are abnormal in 40% to 70% of intensive care unit (ICU) patients. Nonthyroidal illness syndrome, known as the euthyroid sick syndrome or low T_3 syndrome, is characterized by low serum T_3, high rT_3, normal-low T_4, and normal-low TSH. As these changes somewhat resemble central hypothyroidism, the clinical scenario must be taken into consideration when interpreting thyroid testing. The nonthyroidal illness syndrome is due to a complex interplay of changes in the hypothalamic-pituitary-thyroid axis and the

peripheral metabolism of thyroid hormone. There is controversy over whether these changes are maladaptive or adaptive, but it is likely that they are an effort to decrease energy utilization during extreme stress and illness.

LOW T_3 AND HIGH rT_3 IN NONTHYROIDAL ILLNESS

Nonthyroidal illness syndrome is sometimes termed low T_3 syndrome, as this is the earliest and most persistent abnormality. Uniformly, T_3 is low and rT_3 is high, with the T_3 level bearing an inverse relationship to the severity of disease. In acute illness, these changes may occur within hours. Alterations in deiodinase activity appear to be responsible. Type 1 deiodinase is inhibited, leading to diminished conversion of T_4 to T_3. There is an increased activity of type 3 deiodinase, which metabolizes T_4 to inactive rT_3, and also lowers T_3 by increasing its degradation. Thus, T_3 levels are rapidly lowered and rT_3 levels are elevated.

T_4 AND TSH IN NONTHYROIDAL ILLNESS

TSH and T_4 levels may be normal in nonthyroidal illness. However, a normal TSH in nonthyroidal illness may be inappropriate in the face of an already low T_3 level. In a healthy individual with an intact hypothalamic-pituitary-thyroid axis, this would lead to an increase in TSH. As the patient's underlying illness worsens, changes in hypothalamic and pituitary action also occur, leading to low TSH levels. TSH is usually detectable in this setting (>0.05 μU/mL), whereas in clinical thyrotoxicosis it is completely suppressed. Once TSH falls, serum T_4 usually follows suit. However, severe illness can also cause decreased binding of T_4 to its serum binding proteins. As a result, fT_4 concentrations can be low, normal, or high in nonthyroidal illness depending on the assay used. When TSH is low, the possibility of secondary hypothyroidism should also be considered. Production of other pituitary hormones is usually also affected, and it is important to remember that both gonadotropins and growth hormone can be suppressed in acute illness.

In recovery from nonthyroidal illness, the axis tends to reset from the top down. Thyroid-stimulating hormone rises, sometimes above

TABLE 152-1 Commonly Used Medications that Affect Thyroid Function Tests

Drug	Effect on Thyroid Function Tests
Amiodarone	Acute effects (up to 3 mo after initiation): Transient increase in TSH (<10 μU/mL) Increase in T_4 and fT_4 Decrease T_3 Long-term can lead to hypo- or hyperthyroidism
Dopamine	Decreases TSH (not undetectable)
Glucocorticoids	Decreases TSH (not undetectable)
Interferon-alpha	Hypothyroidism and hyperthyroidism can occur (transient in many cases)

the normal range in the initial period of the recovery, though typically not above 20 μU/mL, in order to allow for the recovery of T$_4$. However, T$_3$ may still remain low in this setting. Thyroid-stimulating hormone eventually returns to its physiologic normal level as the recovery continues. If TSH concentrations rise above 20 μU/mL in presumed nonthyroidal illness, primary hypothyroidism should be considered. Outpatient thyroid function tests prior to hospitalization may be very helpful, as this may establish a previous baseline.

When interpreting thyroid testing in hospitalized patients, it should be borne in mind that dopamine, glucocorticoids, amiodarone, and other medications may affect the results of thyroid function testing (Table 152-1).

PRACTICE POINT

Thyroid function tests in the hospital

- Thyroid tests are often abnormal in patients hospitalized with nonthyroidal illness (euthyroid sick syndrome). For this reason, thyroid testing is best done in the outpatient setting, unless thyroid disease is suspected on clinical grounds. If the patient has had a TSH recently checked in the outpatient setting, this is likely to be more helpful than a TSH performed during hospitalization.
- TSH is generally the most sensitive screening test for thyroid function. However, it may not accurately reflect thyroid status in patients with central hypothyroidism or those taking medications that alter thyroid function (Table 152-1).
- Typical laboratory findings of euthyroid sick syndrome include normal-low TSH, normal-low T$_4$, and low TT$_3$. Reverse T$_3$ (rT$_3$) is usually high. Thyroid-stimulating hormone may be elevated in the recovery phase.
- In euthyroid sick syndrome, TSH is usually detectable (>0.05 μU/mL), while in thyroxicosis, TSH may be suppressed to undetectable levels.
- Thyroid hormone treatment in euthyroid sick syndrome does not improve patient outcomes.

■ SHOULD NONTHYROIDAL ILLNESS SYNDROME BE TREATED?

In patients with a persistently low T$_3$ from nonthyroidal illness, the T$_3$ level is an independent predictor of morbidity and mortality. Does replacement of thyroid hormone to normal levels in such patients lead to lower morbidity and mortality? Treatment of nonthyroidal illness with T$_4$ therapy has not shown to be of clinical benefit. In one study of ICU patients with nonthyroidal illness, those treated with T$_4$ to normalize serum T$_4$ values did not have a significant rise in their T$_3$ levels. Furthermore, the T$_4$-treated group had the same mortality rate as the untreated control group.

Thyroid hormone replacement with T$_3$ has been tried in patients with low T$_3$ in a variety of clinical settings, including renal failure, congestive heart failure, and coronary artery bypass graft (CABG). T$_3$ replacement has not been found to be beneficial in the majority of studies. Although T$_3$ supplementation appears to temporarily improve hemodynamics in critically ill patients with cardiac disease, there is no evidence of a mortality benefit. Because of the potential for morbidity and harm with both T$_4$ and T$_3$ replacement, we do not believe that there is adequate evidence to treat patients who have nonthyroidal illness with thyroid hormone.

MYXEDEMA COMA

Myxedema coma is a rare and life-threatening manifestation of decompensated or previously undiagnosed hypothyroidism. Hallmarks include hypothermia, altered mental status, and a precipitating cause, such as concomitant severe illness, cold exposure, or drugs such as lithium or sedatives. As mortality rates are greater than 50% in many case series, clinical suspicion must be high, as survival depends on early recognition, treatment of the underlying illness, and thyroid hormone replacement.

■ CAUSES OF MYXEDEMA COMA

Approximately 90% to 95% of cases are due to primary hypothyroidism, with 5% to 10% due to secondary hypothyroidism. Precipitating factors are almost always present in myxedema coma. Underlying infection must be assumed until ruled out, and should be treated promptly and empirically. Leukocytosis and fever will often be absent in infection in the setting of myxedema. Cold exposure increases susceptibility to myxedema coma, although the exact mechanism for this is not fully understood. Many drugs may predispose to myxedema coma, including lithium, narcotics, benzodiazepines, barbiturates, and amiodarone. Surgery, trauma, burns, hypoxia, hypercapnia, acidosis, gastrointestinal bleed, and infections are also commonly implicated.

■ CLINICAL MANIFESTATIONS OF MYXEDEMA COMA

Most cases of myxedema coma occur in older women, as hypothyroidism is five to eight times more common in women. About 80% to 90% of cases of myxedema coma occur in winter. The patient interview should assess for symptoms of hypothyroidism, such as cold intolerance, decreased appetite, and fatigue. The patient should be asked about a history of thyroid disease, adherence to thyroid medications, a history of head and neck irradiation, and radioactive iodine treatment.

On examination, defective thermoregulation is always present, usually with marked hypothermia resulting in rectal temperatures less than 35.6°C (96.0°F). In patients with an underlying infection, body temperature may be close to normal, when fever would usually be expected. Other signs of severe hypothyroidism are common, but not all classic findings are present in all patients. The skin may be dry, with a thickened and doughy feel. The face may be swollen, with periorbital edema and macroglossia. The hair may be coarse, dry, and brittle, with the eyebrows missing the outer one-third of the hair (**Figure 152-2**). Deep tendon reflexes will have a delayed relaxation phase. Goiter or a thyroidectomy scar may be found.

Neurological manifestations are invariably present. The patient may display somnolence, lethargy, depression, and rarely coma (myxedema coma is a misnomer, as coma is not necessary for diagnosis). Seizures are present in up to 25% of cases. Sensory and motor peripheral neuropathies may be present. Neurogenic dysphagia may lead to aspiration events.

Cardiovascular involvement includes bradycardia, dilated cardiomyopathy, pericardial effusion, and QT prolongation. In long-standing compensated hypothyroidism, the pulse pressure may be narrowed, with an elevated diastolic blood pressure from increased systemic vascular resistance. However, in myxedema coma, cardiac contractility, stroke volume, and cardiac output may all be reduced, and hypotension and shock may occur. Hypotension in myxedema cannot be reversed without thyroid hormone therapy.

Other organ systems are also involved in myxedema. Pneumonia may be a complication of myxedema or a precipitant of it. Decreased respiratory drive, diaphragmatic weakness, pleural effusions, and airway obstruction from macroglossia may all lead to hypercapnic respiratory failure. Constipation is frequent in hypothyroidism. In myxedema coma, this may progress to paralytic ileus and megacolon. Ascites may also be found. The glomerular filtration rate is often reduced from decreased cardiac output and vasoconstriction, and most patients have hyponatremia from decreased

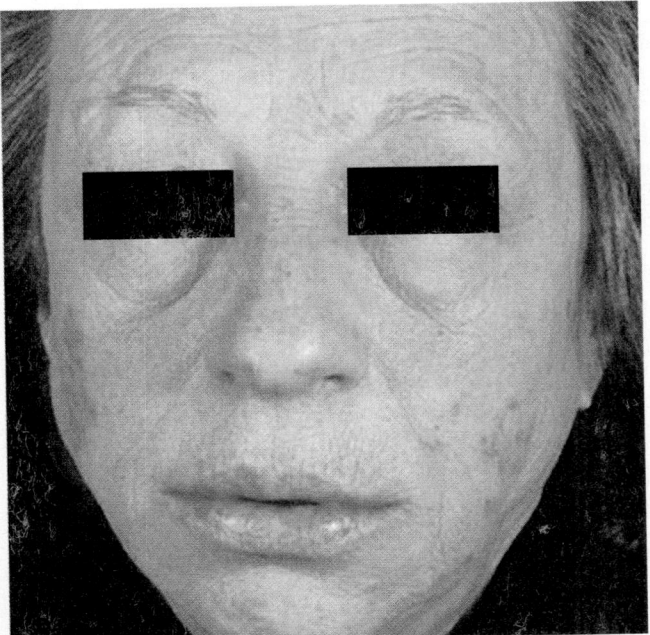

Figure 152-2 *Typical features of severe hypothyroidism, including dry doughy skin, coarse hair, periorbital puffiness, lateral thinning of the eyebrows, and a dull and apathetic facial expression.* (Reproduced with permission from Wolff K, Goldsmith LA, Katz SI, et al. *Fitzpatrick's Dermatology in General Medicine*, 7th ed. New York, NY: McGraw-Hill; 2008. Fig. 152-12.)

free water excretion. Features of myxedema coma are summarized in **Table 152-2**.

■ LABORATORY FINDINGS IN MYXEDEMA COMA

Individuals with myxedema coma have profoundly elevated TSH, with low T_4 and T_3, in addition to neurological aberrations, hypothermia, and usually a precipitating illness. In myxedema due to secondary hypothyroidism, TSH may be low or normal, and there may be other evidence of pituitary dysfunction. Routine blood testing may reveal hyponatremia and renal insufficiency. Hypoglycemia may result from hypothyroidism, concurrent adrenal insufficiency in secondary hypothyroidism, or impaired gluconeogenesis in critical illness and starvation. Hypercarbia and hypoxia may be present. There may be a mild normocytic anemia. Creatinine kinase and serum total cholesterol are often elevated.

■ THYROID REPLACEMENT IN MYXEDEMA COMA

Thyroid hormone replacement in myxedema must be adequate to reverse symptoms, but not be excessive, as atrial arrhythmias and cardiac ischemia may result. Unfortunately, there are no randomized prospective trials of treatment. Various thyroid replacement protocols have been proposed, including T_3 alone, T_3 and T_4 together, and T_4 alone.

It is also unclear whether such patients should be treated with intravenous or oral T_4 replacement. We favor intravenous thyroid replacement initially, as patients may be prone to aspiration because of altered mental status, and ileus may compromise absorption. Many experts prefer to use T_3 in myxedema coma due to its rapid onset, shorter half-life, and the decreased conversion to T_4 to T_3 in myxedema. Our preference is to use T_4 alone, particularly if the diagnosis is questionable and the patient appears stable. For patients in true myxedema coma, administration of both T_4 and T_3 is reasonable to restore thyroid levels quickly. Dosing of T_4 depends on the patient's age, comorbidities, cardiovascular function, and

TABLE 152-2 Potential Features of Myxedema Coma

Defective thermoregulation (can be normal temperature)
Thyroid
Goiter
Neurological
Somnolence, lethargy, depression, coma
Seizures in 25%
Sensory and peripheral neuropathies
Reflexes with delayed relaxation phase
Skin
Dry, coarse, myxedematous skin
Periorbital edema
Macroglossia
Cardiovascular
Bradycardia
Dilated cardiomyopathy
ECG abnormalities (prolonged QT)
Pericardial effusion
Elevated diastolic blood pressure
Hypotension and shock
Respiratory
Pneumonia
Aspiration events
Pleural effusions
Diaphragmatic weakness
Hypoventilation and hypoxemia
Edema of tongue and pharynx
Gastrointestinal
Paralytic ileus
Megacolon
Ascites

severity of illness. It is estimated that the total body pool of T_4 is 500 μg; many give high doses of T_4, up to 500 μg as a loading dose. We often give 200 to 250 μg of IV T_4 as an initial loading dose; in older patients and those with comorbid medical conditions, we withhold a loading dose. If a loading dose was given, we start replacement therapy with T_4 24 hours later based on body weight. We change to oral T_4 replacement when the patient is swallowing safely, and adequate absorption can be ensured. In selected patients, therapy with T_3, at a dose of 5 to 10 μg every 8 to 12 hours, may be given until clinical improvement is observed, usually for 1 to 3 days.

PRACTICE POINT

Treatment of myxedema coma

- It is generally safer to give thyroid replacement in myxedema coma as the prohormone T_4 (levothyroxine), rather than the biologically active form T_3 (liothyronine). This is especially true if the diagnosis of myxedema coma is unsettled.
- We give 200 to 250 μg of IV T_4 as an initial loading dose, followed by a weight-based daily maintenance dose of T_4 starting 24 hours later. In older patients and those with comorbid medical conditions, we forgo a loading dose. Intravenous levothyroxine may be switched to oral therapy

when the patient is clinically improved and able to swallow. Intravenous T$_4$ is twice as potent as oral therapy.

- If the diagnosis of myxedema coma is certain, therapy with T$_3$, 5 to 10 µg every 8 to 12 hours, may be given until clinical improvement is observed, usually for 1 to 3 days.
- Patients with hypothermia are best treated with passive rewarming, rather than active rewarming, which is more likely to lead to vasodilation and decreased blood pressure.
- Corticosteroids should be given until adrenal insufficiency is excluded. A random cortisol should be checked prior to starting glucocorticoids, unless a cosyntropin stimulation test has already been performed.

■ GENERAL CARE IN MYXEDEMA COMA

Thyroid hormone replacement alone will not reverse myxedema coma. Patients need vigorous supportive care and treatment of precipitating conditions. All patients should be considered for ICU admission. An infectious workup should be performed, including chest radiograph, blood cultures, urinalysis, and urine culture. Vasopressor support and hydration may be required for hypotension and shock. Due to the potential for arrhythmia and heart failure, cardiovascular status should be closely watched. Hypothermia should be treated, preferably with passive rewarming with blankets and other methods. Active rewarming methods and direct heat should be avoided, as this may lead to peripheral vasodilatation and worsen hypotension and shock. Noninvasive ventilation or mechanical ventilation may be necessary for patients with hypercapnia and hypoxia. Parenteral nutrition may be required until swallowing is found to be safe.

Though most cases of myxedema coma are due to primary hypothyroidism (90%-95%), failing to diagnose secondary hypothyroidism greatly increases the risk of death. Most cases of secondary hypothyroidism are due to pituitary dysfunction, and both thyroid and adrenal dysfunction may be present. If adrenal insufficiency cannot be excluded, glucocorticoids should be administered intravenously at stress dose levels. If possible, a random cortisol should be checked prior to administration, as there may not be time to perform a cosyntropin stimulation test. These patients usually will require formal testing of the adrenal axis at a later date, after glucocorticoids doses are tapered.

THYROID STORM

Thyroid storm, also called thyrotoxic crisis, decompensated thyrotoxicosis, and accelerated thyrotoxicosis, is a life-threatening form of severe hyperthyroidism. The distinction of thyroid storm from compensated thyrotoxicosis is clinical, as thyroid function test abnormalities are similar in the two conditions. In addition to typical features of hyperthyroidism, such as tachycardia and tremulousness, thyroid storm is accompanied by other features, such as fever, mental status changes, diarrhea, vomiting, hepatitis, arrhythmia, myocardial ischemia, and congestive heart failure. Mortality may be as high as 20% to 30%.

■ CAUSES OF THYROID STORM

Graves' disease is the most common cause of hyperthyroidism and thyroid storm. It is caused by autoantibodies to the TSH receptor, leading to enhanced production and release of thyroid hormone. Toxic adenoma (hot nodule) and toxic multinodular goiter may also cause hyperthyroidism and thyroid storm. Subacute thyroiditis is a common cause of thyrotoxicosis but rarely leads to thyroid storm. Other rare causes of thyrotoxicosis include TSH-producing pituitary adenomas, trophoblastic tumors producing hCG, which is able to bind to the TSH receptor, and struma ovarii, a rare ovarian tumor that produces ectopic thyroid hormone.

As with myxedema coma, infection is the most common precipitant of thyroid storm in patients with underlying thyrotoxicosis. Other precipitants include trauma, myocardial infarction, diabetic ketoacidosis, pulmonary embolism, surgery, pregnancy, stroke, emotional distress, poor adherence to antithyroid medications, sympathomimetic drugs such as pseudoephedrine, and salicylates, which displace thyroid hormone from binding proteins. Iodine loads from radiocontrast agents or amiodarone also predispose to thyroid storm. In the past, hyperthyroid patients undergoing thyroidectomy were at risk of thyroid storm due to release of thyroid hormones after thyroidal manipulation, in addition to the acute stress of surgery. This is currently rare because of pretreatment with antithyroidal medications. Uncommonly, patients go into thyroid storm after receiving radioactive iodine to treat underlying hyperthyroidism, probably from excessive thyroid hormone release from radiation thyroiditis.

■ CLINICAL MANIFESTATIONS OF THYROID STORM

Features of thyroid storm are summarized in **Table 152-3**. Patients should be questioned about common symptoms of thyrotoxicosis, including weight loss despite ample appetite, poor energy, difficulty sleeping, heat intolerance, hyperdefecation, palpitations, chest pain, anxiety, emotional labilitiy, and diplopia from ophthalmopathy. Additionally, a history of past thyrotoxicosis, recent radioactive iodine treatment, and recent surgery should be sought.

On physical examination, a goiter with possible bruit, ophthalmopathy, and rarely pretibial myxedema will help make the clinical diagnosis of Graves' disease. Thyroid exam may reveal nodules or diffuse enlargement. Skin may be moist. On cardiovascular exam, the patient may have sinus tachycardia and a hyperdynamic precordium. Atrial fibrillation is present in 10% to 35% of thyrotoxic individuals. Congestive heart failure, persistent arrhythmias, and

TABLE 152-3 Potential Features of Thyroid Storm

Fever (can have hyperpyrexia, temperatures >105°F)
Thyroid
Nodule
Diffuse enlargement
Ophthalmologic
Ophthalmopathy
Neurological
Anxiety, psychosis, or coma
Seizure
Hyperreflexia
Skin
Moist
Pretibial myxedema
Cardiovascular
Sinus tachycardia
Hyperdynamic precordium
Atrial fibrillation
Other arrhythmias
Congestive heart failure
Gastrointestinal
Nausea/vomiting
Diarrhea
Severe abdominal pain
Jaundice
Hepatosplenomegaly/vascular congestion

cardiovascular collapse may be present. The patient may have neurologic and psychiatric pathology, including anxiety, mania, psychosis, seizure, or coma. Muscles may be weak and wasted, and reflexes are brisk. Fever is present, often with hyperpyrexia in excess of 40.5°C (105°F). There may be severe nausea, vomiting, and abdominal pain. Jaundice, hepatosplenomegaly from vascular congestion, and hepatic necrosis are seen in severe cases.

Elderly patients with thyroid storm may have a clinical picture dominated by apathetic thyrotoxicosis, with blunting of hyperadrenergic symptoms. The major clinical features are apathy, depression, somnolence, and coma, in addition to typical symptoms of hyperthyroidism such as weight loss, weakness, and arrhythmias. Apathetic thyrotoxicosis and thyroid storm should be in the differential diagnosis of altered mental status and coma of unclear cause.

Burch and Wartofsky have developed a point system to help distinguish severe thyrotoxicosis from thyroid storm (**Table 152-4**). Diagnostic criteria include fever, central nervous system effects, gastrointestinal and hepatic dysfunction, tachycardia and atrial fibrillation, congestive heart failure, and the presence of a precipitating factor. A score of 45 or greater is highly suggestive of thyroid storm. However, the Burch-Wartofsky score has not been validated prospectively.

TABLE 152-4 Diagnostic Criteria for Thyroid Storm (Burch-Wartofsky Score)

Thermoregulatory Dysfunction		Cardiovascular Dysfunction	
Temperature		Tachycardia	
99-99.9	5	90-109	5
100-100.9	10	101-119	10
101-101.9	15	120-129	15
102-102.9	20	130-139	20
103-103.9	25	≥140	25
≥104	30		
Central nervous system effects		**Congestive heart failure**	
		Absent	0
Absent	0	Mild	5
Mild	10	Pedal edema	
Agitation		Moderate	10
Moderate	20	Bibasilar rales	
Delirium		Severe	15
Psychosis		Pulmonary edema	
Extreme lethargy			
Severe	30		
Seizure			
Coma			
Gastrointestinal-hepatic dysfunction		**Atrial fibrillation**	
		Absent	0
Absent	0	Present	10
Moderate	10	**Precipitating event**	
Diarrhea		Absent	0
Nausea/vomiting		Present	10
Abdominal pain			
Severe	20		
Unexplained jaundice			

A score of 45 or greater is highly suggestive of thyroid storm; a score of 25-44 is suggestive of impending storm, and a score below 25 is unlikely to represent thyroid storm. (Adapted, with permission, from Burch HB and Wartofsky L. *Endocrinol Metab Clin North Am.* 1993;22:263-277.)

■ LABORATORY FINDINGS IN THYROID STORM

As above, thyroid function tests are similar in patients with compensated thyrotoxicosis and thyroid storm; only the clinical manifestations distinguish the two. Thyroid-stimulating hormone is suppressed, except in the extremely rare case of a thyrotropin-secreting pituitary adenoma. Both T_4 and T_3 are markedly elevated. T_3 may be lower than expected due to concurrent nonthyroidal illness syndrome. Because TBG may be low in the patient with thyroid storm, and other inhibitors of protein binding may be present, the response to therapy is best followed by checking total T_4 with either TBG or resin uptake, yielding a free thyroxine index. The TSH may remain suppressed for months, so this is not followed acutely. Other laboratory findings may include hyperglycemia, due to increased glycogenolysis and catecholamine-mediated inhibition of insulin release. Mild hypercalcemia and elevated alkaline phosphatase occur, perhaps due to bone resorption provoked by thyroid hormone. Elevation of liver transaminases and total bilirubin occurs. There may be a slight leukocytosis and left shift, even in the absence of infection. While hepatic metabolism of cortisol is accelerated, and conversion of biologically inactive cortisone to active cortisol is decreased, there is also increased synthesis of cortisol, and adrenal function is usually normal. In long-standing thyrotoxicosis, adrenal cortical reserve is impaired. Diagnostic nuclear scanning of the thyroid should be delayed until the patient is stable.

■ TREATMENT OF HYPERTHYROIDISM IN THYROID STORM

In thyroid storm, one must treat the underlying precipitant, treat multiorgan and systemic complications, and decrease circulating levels of thyroid hormone. Patients need intensive monitoring and likely should be in the ICU.

Treatment of hyperthyroidism in thyroid storm or accelerated thyrotoxicosis involves four steps (**Figure 152-3**): suppression of thyroid hormone synthesis; preventing T_4 and T_3 release from the thyroid; inhibition of peripheral conversion of T_4 to T_3; and blocking the action of thyroid hormone on target organs.

Thionamides, such as propylthiouracil (PTU) and methimazole, inhibit thyroid hormone synthesis, and they may also have immunomodulatory effects. Because PTU inhibits peripheral conversion of T_4 to T_3 and methimazole does not, PTU has been favored for treatment of thyroid storm in the past. However, due to the longer half-life of methimazole and the use of other agents in thyroid storm that prevent peripheral conversion of T_4 to T_3, many clinicians now prefer methimazole, especially as PTU has more side effects, particularly hepatic. Our practice is to use either high doses of methimazole, typically 20 to 30 mg every 6 hours, or PTU 200 to 400 mg every 4 to 6 hours orally or through the nasogastric tube, until the patient's thyroid function and clinical condition is improving. We then decrease the antithyroidal medication dosage accordingly. Patients who cannot take oral medications, or who do not have a nasogastric

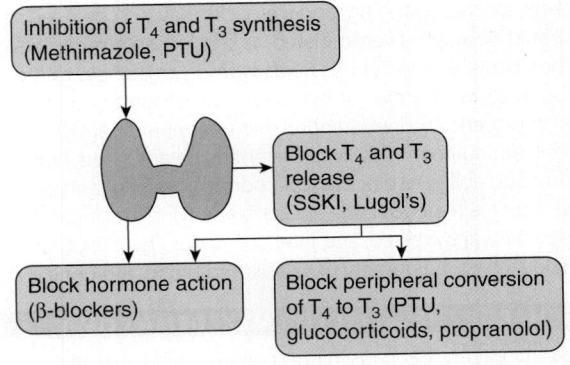

Figure 152-3 *Treatment of thyroid storm.*

tube, may be treated with methimazole or PTU in enema or suppository form. Major side effects of thionamides include rash or urticarial reactions in 5%, agranulocytosis in 0.2% to 0.4%, and liver function abnormalities in approximately 0.2%.

Iodine is given to prevent stored T_4 and T_3 release from the thyroid. In high doses, iodine inhibits iodine organification in the thyroid (Wolff-Chaikoff effect). Iodine may be given as a saturated solution of potassium iodide (SSKI), up to five drops every 6 hours, or Lugol's solution, up to eight drops every 8 hours. Radiocontrast iodine agents can also be used orally but because of the paucity of data we prefer SSKI or Lugol's. Iodine should be given only after antithyroidal medication has been started, waiting at least 1 hour, because of the potential for patient deterioration from increased iodination of thyroid hormone. In patients allergic to iodine, lithium may be given at a dose of 300 mg every 8 hours. This is rarely done, as lithium levels require close monitoring, and alternative agents are usually available. In patients who require an antiarrhythmic, amiodarone may be desirable. Amiodarone is 37.3% iodine by weight, inhibits thyroid hormone release, and also blocks conversion of T_4 to T_3.

Peripheral conversion of T_4 to T_3 should also be inhibited in thyroid storm. This may be accomplished with PTU, as noted above. Glucocorticoids are also effective. We prefer hydrocortisone 100 mg every 8 hours, with dexamethasone 4 mg every 12 hours as an alternative. As steroid breakdown is accelerated in thyrotoxicosis, high doses of hydrocortisone may need to be given for several days prior to tapering. This has the added benefit of treating the relative adrenal insufficiency that may be present. Iopanoic acid, which is no longer available in the United States, is another potent inhibitor of peripheral conversion of T_4 to T_3.

β-Blockade is useful to antagonize the effects of T_3 on the heart and sympathetic nervous system. Propranolol is most often used, as it also inhibits T_4 to T_3 conversion. An intravenous loading dose up to 1 mg can be given, followed by oral doses of 60 to 80 mg every 4 to 6 hours, with appropriate titration. Some authorities prefer intravenous esmolol, due to its short half-life and ability to be rapidly titrated. Cardioselective β-blockers can also be used, such as atenolol and metoprolol.

Rarely used therapies include potassium perchlorate, which is a competitive inhibitor of iodine transport. It has fallen out of favor because of its side effect profile, which includes aplastic anemia and nephrotic syndrome. Cholestyramine reduces enterohepatic thyroid hormone absorption, but may also interfere with absorption of a number of other medications. Treatments of last resort include plasmapheresis or emergency thyroidectomy, which is avoided if at all possible because of substantial perioperative mortality.

TREATMENT OF SYSTEMIC DECOMPENSATION

Besides lowering thyroid hormone levels, the multiorgan and systemic complications need to be treated. Hyperpyrexia and fever should be treated with acetaminophen, as aspirin at high dosages can displace thyroid hormone from TBG, increasing fT_4. Cooling blankets, alcohol sponging, and ice packs may also be needed. Fluids should be aggressively repleted, as sensible and insensible losses can be extensive. Intravenous fluids with dextrose help to replenish glycogen stores. Cardiac arrhythmias and congestive heart failure may be present and need aggressive treatment. If arrhythmias are present, amiodarone may be a preferred therapy, as its high iodine content and ability to block thyroid hormone release and peripheral conversion are beneficial side effects. Underlying precipitants should be identified and treated, and infection should be excluded by performing a chest radiograph, urinalysis, and blood and urine cultures.

DISCHARGE CHECKLIST FOR MYXEDEMA COMA

- Has the patient been discharged on levothyroxine, and told how to take it according to usual precautions? The medication should be taken fasting, 30 to 60 minutes before eating or 2 hours after eating, without other medications. It should be taken at least 4 hours away from calcium, iron, and multivitamins.
- Was the patient previously on levothyroxine? If the patient was on stable on a previously known levothyroxine dose, which they were not adherent with, they should resume that dose, adjusted as necessary based on new data.
- Has the levothyroxine dose on discharge been adjusted based on age? Elderly patients typically need lower levothyroxine replacement dosages.
- Has outpatient follow-up been arranged? Thyroid function tests should be done 6 weeks after discharge.
- Have interventions to improve medication adherence been considered, such as the use of pillboxes and support from visiting nurses and family members?

DISCHARGE CHECKLIST FOR THYROID STORM

- Has the patient been switched to methimazole, if not already on it? Methimazole is preferred to PTU due to its lower frequency of dosing, higher compliance rate, and better side effect profile. PTU now has a black box warning for severe liver injury and acute liver failure.
- Has outpatient follow-up with endocrinology been arranged?
- If the cause of hyperthyroidism is unclear, have arrangements been made for a radioactive iodine uptake scan? This is usually coordinated through endocrinology.
- Have once-daily β-blockers been prescribed for better adherence?
- Have barriers to care been identified during discharge, and have steps to ameliorate them been taken? Patients hospitalized for complicated thyrotoxicosis are more likely to be of lower socioeconomic class, uninsured, or covered by Medicaid.

SUGGESTED READINGS

Adler SM, Wartofsky L. The nonthyroidal illness syndrome. *Endocrinol Metab Clin North Am*. 2007;36:657-672.

Angell TE, Lechner MG, Nguyen CT, Salvato VL, Nicoloff JT, LoPresti JS. Clinical features and hospital outcomes in thyroid storm: a retrospective cohort study. *J Clin Endocrinol Metab*. 2015;100:451-459.

De Groot LJ. Dangerous dogmas in medicine: the nonthyroidal illness syndrome. *J Clin Endocrinol Metab*. 1999;84:151-164.

Hodak SP, Huang C, Clarke D, Burman KD, Jonklaas J, Janicic-Kharic N. Intravenous methimazole in the treatment of refractory hyperthyroidism. *Thyroid*. 2006;16:691-695.

Jonklaas J, Bianco AC, Bauer AJ, et al. Guidelines for the treatment of hypothyroidism. Prepared by the American Thyroid Association Task Force on Thyroid Hormone Replacement. *Thyroid*. 2014;24:1670-1751.

Klubo-Gwiezdzinka JK, Wartofsky LW. Thyroid Emergencies. *Med Clin N Am*. 2012;96:385-403.

Nayak B, Burman K. Thyrotoxicosis and thyroid storm. *Endocrinol Metab Clin North Am*. 2006;35:663-686.

Pingitore A, Galli E, Barison A, et al. Acute effects of triiodothyronine (T_3) replacement therapy in patients with chronic heart failure and low-T_3 syndrome: a randomized, placebo-controlled study. *J Clin Endocrinol Metab*. 2008;93:1351-1358.

Tsatsoulis A, Johnson EO, Kalogera CH, Seferiadis K, Tsolas O. The effect of thyrotoxicosis on adrenocortical reserve. *Eur J Endocrinol*. 2000;142:231-235.

Walter RM Jr, Bartle WR. Rectal administration of propylthiouracil in the treatment of Graves disease. *Am J Med*. 1990;88:69-70.

Wartofsky L. Myxedema coma. *Endocrinol Metab Clin North Am*. 2006;35:687-698.

CHAPTER 153

Adrenal Insufficiency

Jennifer C. Passini, MD
Elaine Chiewlin Liew, MD, FRCA
Ann M. Sheehy, MD, MS
Kenneth E. Wood, DO, FCCP
Douglas B. Coursin, MD, FCCP

Key Clinical Questions

1. What are the types of adrenal insufficiency?

2. What are normal and stress production levels of endogenous corticocosteroids?

3. Which patients are at high risk for development of adrenal insufficiency or critical illness-related corticosteroid insufficiency and therefore may benefit from physiologic or pharmacologic steroid treatment of their illnesses?

4. For those patients who need corticosteroid supplementation, which agents should be used, at what dose and for how long?

INTRODUCTION

Adrenal insufficiency (AI) was described by Thomas Addison in 1855 as a fatal disease caused by tuberculous adrenalitis and adrenal gland failure. In 1949, the synthesis of cortisone resulted in lifesaving therapy for Addison disease. However, this was shortly followed by reports of patient deaths from presumed adrenal crisis due to abrupt cortisone withdrawal in the perioperative period. These reports resulted in a new standard of administration of high doses of supplemental corticosteroids during periods of physical stress, although this practice may not be universally warranted.

Primary AI (Addison disease) refers to primary adrenal gland dysfunction. It has a prevalence of 40 to 110 cases per million people and an incidence of six cases per million people per year. Secondary AI denotes pituitary disease with adrenocorticotropic hormone (ACTH) hormone deficiency. The prevalence of secondary AI is approximately 150 to 280 per million. Hypothalamic dysfunction is responsible for tertiary AI. It usually arises after abrupt withdrawal or reduction in corticocosteroid dose, in the setting of chronic exogenous corticosteroids, and is reasonably common in the hospital setting, although the exact prevalence is unknown (**Table 153-1**).

PRACTICE POINT

- Common scenarios for AI in the hospital include patients on long-term glucocorticoid therapy not receiving adequate replacement or supplemental glucocorticoids during major illness, and critically ill patients with sepsis. Other patients at risk include those with a history of brain injury or intracranial aneurysm.

PATHOPHYSIOLOGY

The adrenal gland consists of a cortex that produces steroid hormones, and a medulla that produces catecholamines. The adrenal cortex is divided into three layers. The outermost layer, the zona glomerulosa, produces mineralocorticoids, primarily aldosterone. The middle layer, the zona fasciculata, produces glucocorticoids, primarily cortisol, and to a lesser extent, cortisone. The zona reticularis, the innermost layer, produces adrenal androgens.

The release of glucocorticoids is controlled by the hypothalamic-pituitary-adrenal (HPA) axis. The hypothalamus secretes corticotropin-releasing hormone (CRH), which acts on the pituitary to produce adrenocorticotropic hormone. Adrenocorticotropic hormone stimulates the adrenal glands to produce cortisol, which inhibits further production of CRH. Cortisol secretion is diurnal, with the highest levels in the morning, and the lowest around midnight. Daily endogenous secretion of glucocorticoid is equivalent to 5 to 7 mg/d of oral prednisone or 20 to 30 mg/d of hydrocortisone. During stress, cortisol synthesis can increase 10-fold.

All cells in the human body have glucocorticoid receptors, reflecting the integral role of glucocorticoids in physiologic homeostasis. Glucocorticoids regulate carbohydrate, lipid, and amino acid metabolism, facilitate catecholamine production and action, and maintain cardiovascular integrity, with additional effects on wound healing, the immune system and the nervous system.

TABLE 153-1 Primary, Secondary, and Tertiary Adrenal Insufficiency

Type	Incidence	Features	Etiologies

Primary	Prevalence: 40-110 cases/ million
	
	Incidence: 6 cases/million/y
		ACTH-independent
		
		>90% of destruction of adrenal cortex
		
		Loss of mineralocorticoid and glucocorticoid production
		
		Patients may be hyperpigmented
		
		Requires lifetime therapy
			Autoimmune
			  ~80% of cases in the United States
			  Isolated autoimmune adrenalitis
			  APS-1—associated with hypoparathyroidism, chronic mucocutaneous candidiasis
			  APS-2—associated with thyroid disease, type 1 diabetes mellitus
			Infection
			  Tuberculous
			  AIDS—CMV, MAC, Kaposi sarcoma
			30% of patients with AIDS develop AI
			  Fungal infections (histoplasmosis, coccidiomycosis, blastomycosis)
			Inflammation
			Cancer
			  Metastases from breast, lung, and melanoma may infiltrate and replace normal adrenal tissue
			Acute Addisonian crisis
			  Infectious—meningococcemia with purpura fulminans (Waterhouse-Friederichsen syndrome); sepsis with other bacteria
			  Stress
			  Hemorrhage
			  Shock
			Drug-induced adrenal insufficiency
			  Mitotane, ketoconazole, suramin, etomidate, aminoglutethimide

Secondary	Prevalence: 150-280 per million	Pituitary disease that interferes with ACTH secretion
		
		Clinical features due to loss of glucocorticoid function
		
		Intact mineralocorticoid function
		
		Rarely hypovolemic, more commonly hypoglycemic
			Panhypopituitarism
			  Pituitary tumors, craniopharyngomas
			  Infection
			  Infiltrative diseases
			  Head trauma
			  Intracranial artery aneurysms
			  Sheehan syndrome
			Isolated ACTH deficiency
			  Rare, likely autoimmune process

Tertiary	Most common form	Processes that interfere with hypothalamic CRH secretion	Abrupt cessation of glucocorticoid therapy Correction of Cushing syndrome

APS, autoimmune polyglandular syndrome 1 (APS-1); MAC, mycobacterium avium complex.

CAUSES OF ADRENAL INSUFFICIENCY

■ PRIMARY ADRENAL INSUFFICIENCY

Primary AI arises when greater than 90% of adrenal tissue is destroyed, resulting in loss of glucocorticoid and mineralocorticoid function. Absence of glucocorticoids result in an increase in ACTH and melanocyte-stimulating hormone levels, while the absence of aldosterone results in increased renin levels.

Autoimmune adrenalitis

In developed nations, 80% of primary AI is due to autoimmune disease, which may occur in isolation or as a manifestation of a polyglandular autoimmune syndrome. Autoimmune polyendocrine syndrome type I (APS-1) underlies up to 15% of autoimmune adrenalitis. It usually presents with hypoparathyroidism or chronic mucocutaneous candidiasis during childhood, with adrenal insufficiency developing by 10 to 15 years of age. It is also frequently associated with primary hypogonadism, childhood alopecia, and malabsorption. It

is caused by mutations in the autoimmune regulator (AIRE) gene, inherited in an autosomal recessive fashion. Mutations in AIRE interfere with the normal culling of autoreactive T-cells, leading to the eventual autoimmune destruction of endocrine glands.

Autoimmune polyglandular syndrome type II (APS-2) is more prevalent than APS-1, and has autosomal dominant transmission with incomplete penetrance. In half the cases, AI is the first manifestation, often associated with the later development of autoimmune thyroid disease and type 1 diabetes mellitus. The clinical spectrum may also include hypogonadism, vitiligo (seen in up to 15% of primary AI), myasthenia gravis, rheumatoid arthritis, antiphosholipid antibody syndrome, and celiac disease.

Infectious adrenalitis

Tuberculosis is the most common cause of primary AI worldwide, and was the cause of adrenal failure in most of Addison's original patients. Adrenal involvement in tuberculosis is not common except in disseminated disease, in which it is found in up to 50% of cases.

Although recovery of adrenal function is possible after appropriate antituberculous treatment, it often does not occur. AIDS is currently the principal infectious cause of AI in the United States. Causes of AI in AIDS patients include cytomegalovirus, *Mycobacterium avium-intracellulare*, cryptococcosis, and metastatic Kaposi sarcoma. Other factors may contribute to AI in HIV patients, such as peripheral resistance to glucocorticoid action from chronic inflammation, or use of the appetite stimulant megestrol acetate, which has intrinsic glucocorticoid activity and suppresses the hypothalamic-pituitary-adrenal axis. The endemic mycoses, such as histoplasmosis, coccidoidomycosis, and blastomycosis, may rarely cause granulomatous disease of the adrenals severe enough to cause AI.

The adrenal glands may be infiltrated by metastatic disease, most commonly from lung, breast, stomach, or colon cancer, melanoma, or lymphoma. However, metastases rarely destroy enough adrenal tissue for AI to manifest.

Hemorrhagic infarction

The adrenal gland is vascular and somewhat prone to hemorrhage. Bilateral adrenal hemorrhage may cause AI. It may result from meningococcal septic shock with disseminated intravascular coagulation (Waterhouse-Friderichsen syndrome), as well as overwhelming sepsis with other organisms, including *Staphylococcus aureus*, *Streptococcus pyogenes*, *Streptococcus pneumoniae*, *Pseudomonas aeruginosa*, and *Escherichia coli*. Other risk factors for adrenal hemorrhage include anticoagulants, coagulopathy, trauma, carcinoma, adrenal vein thrombosis, pregnancy, and any acute medical or surgical illness. Patients often present with back pain and hypotension; computed tomography imaging reveals enlarged adrenal glands with high attenuation.

Drugs

Drugs cause AI by various mechanisms. Etomidate, ketoconazole, metyrapone, and suramin inhibit cortisol synthesis. However, AI only becomes evident in patients with limited pituitary or adrenal reserve, and those previously on glucocorticoid therapy. Phenytoin, rifampin, and barbiturates accelerate the metabolism of cortisol, as well as the metabolism of synthetic steroids, such as dexamethasone and fludrocortisone.

Miscellaneous

Rare causes of primary AI include adrenoleukodystrophy, congenital adrenal hypoplasia, glucocorticoid insensitivity, and defective cholesterol metabolism.

■ SECONDARY ADRENAL INSUFFICIENCY

Any process that interferes with pituitary ACTH secretion may lead to secondary AI. Unlike primary AI, mineralocorticoid secretion is preserved because it is under the control of the renin-angiotensin system. Another distinguishing characteristic of secondary AI is decreased or absent plasma ACTH levels, compared to normal or elevated ACTH levels in primary AI. The most frequent cause of secondary AI is panhypopituitarism, and less commonly isolated ACTH deficiency.

Panhypopituitarism

Panhypopituitarism may result from pituitary tumors, traumatic brain injury, intracranial aneurysm, and pituitary surgery or radiotherapy. Up to 30% of patients with head trauma experience pituitary dysfunction months or years after the initial insult. Less often, panhypopituitarism can be caused by infection (tuberculosis, histoplasmosis), infiltrative diseases, and autoimmune lymphocytic hypophysitis. Although pituitary metastases are frequently found in patients with disseminated cancer, these metastases rarely impede hormone secretion. Sheehan syndrome is massive peripartum blood loss precipitating hypovolemic shock and anterior pituitary infarction. Pituitary apoplexy from hemorrhage into an enlarging

pituitary adenoma may also lead to panhypopituitarism during or after pregnancy.

Isolated ACTH deficiency

Isolated ACTH deficiency is a rare cause of secondary AI and may have an autoimmune origin. It is frequently associated with autoantibodies to pituitary cells and with other autoimmune endocrine disorders, most commonly thyroid disease.

■ TERTIARY ADRENAL INSUFFICIENCY

Tertiary AI occurs due to any process that involves the hypothalamus and interferes with the secretion of CRH and subsequent ACTH release. The most common cause of tertiary AI is abrupt cessation of glucocorticoid therapy. While patients on daily oral glucocorticoids are most likely to develop tertiary AI, patients on intermittent corticosteroids and those receiving frequent musculoskeletal corticosteroid injections are also at risk for tertiary AI. Patients on chronic inhaled corticosteroids or potent topical corticosteroids can very uncommonly develop tertiary AI.

Chronic glucocorticoid therapy

Prolonged corticosteroid therapy in excess of 5 mg/d of prednisone or its equivalent suppresses CRH and ACTH secretion, resulting in adrenal atrophy. Tertiary iatrogenic AI may then become apparent with abrupt cessation of exogenous glucocorticoid therapy, or when inadequate supplementation is provided in times of physiologic stress. There are inconsistent data to accurately predict the degree of adrenal suppression that occurs with exogenous glucocorticoid therapy. However, a reduced response to exogenous ACTH has been reported after discontinuation of oral prednisone 25 mg twice a day for as brief a period as 5 days. Patients who receive 5 mg/d or less of prednisone appear to have an intact HPA axis. It may require more than a year for the HPA axis to recover after cessation of exogenous glucocorticoids.

CLINICAL PRESENTATION

The diagnosis of AI may be delayed because signs and symptoms are nonspecific, and frequently misleading (**Table 153-2**). Most patients encounter several physicians prior to diagnosis, and many are only diagnosed after presenting with adrenal crisis. Recognition of patients at risk facilitates diagnosis. Common scenarios for AI in the hospital include patients on long-term glucocorticoid therapy not receiving adequate replacement or supplemental

TABLE 153-2 Clinical Features of Adrenal Insufficiency

Glucocorticoid Deficiency	Mineralocortocoid Deficiency	Adrenal Androgen Deficiency
Fatigue	Salt craving (primary AI)	Dry and itchy skin
Anorexia, weight loss	Dizziness	Loss of libido
Abdominal pain		Loss of pubic hair
Nausea, vomiting	Hypotension, orthostatic symptoms	
Myalgia		
Hypotension	Hyponatremia	
Anemia, lymphocytosis, eosinophilia	Hyperkalemia (primary AI)	
Hypercalcemia		
Hypoglycemia		
Increased TSH (primary AI)		

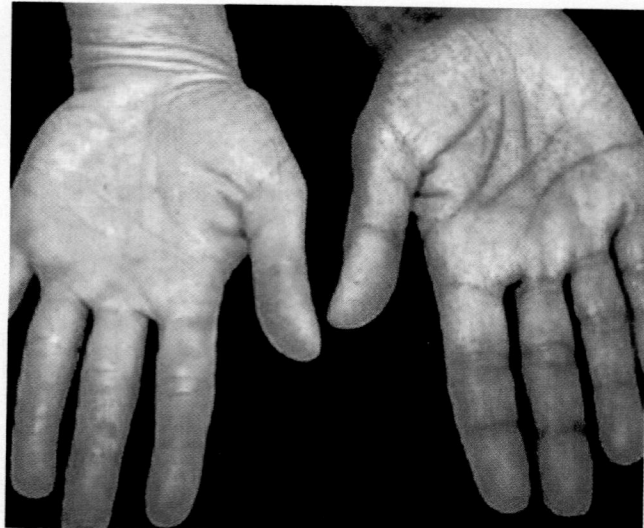

Figure 153-1 *Hyperpigmentation of the palmar creases in primary adrenal insufficiency is seen in the hand at the right, with the hand of an unaffected individual at left. Hyperpigmentation and freckling in primary adrenal insufficiency is more marked in sun-exposed areas, gums, buccal mucosae, axillae, pressure points, genitals, nail beds, nipples, areolae, and recent scars.* (Reproduced, with permission, from Wolff K, Goldsmith LA, Katz SI, et al. *Fitzpatrick's Dermatology in General Medicine*, 7th ed. New York, NY: McGraw-Hill, 2008. Fig. 152-16.)

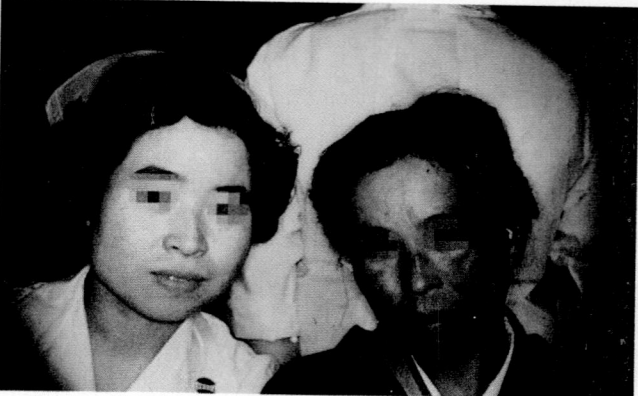

Figure 153-2 *Addison disease. Japanese patient in whom tuberculosis was the etiology of the adrenal insufficiency. Note the striking contrast in the skin color of a normal Japanese female nurse compared to the diffuse brown hyperpigmentation in the patient with Addison disease.* (Reproduced, with permission, from Fitzpatrick TB, Johnson RA, Polano MK, et al. *Fitzpatrick's Color Atlas and Synopsis of Clinical Dermatology: Common and Serious Diseases*, 2nd ed. New York, NY: McGraw-Hill, 1992. Fig. 647.)

glucocorticoids during major illness, and critically ill patients with sepsis. Other patients at risk include those with a history of brain injury or intracranial aneurysm.

Clinical features of AI include weakness, fatigue, anorexia, nausea, diarrhea, abdominal pain, weight loss, and hypotension. Hypotension occurs as a result of depressed myocardial contractility, reduced responsiveness to catecholamines, and hypovolemia with hyponatremia. Patients with Addison disease or primary adrenal failure also exhibit salt craving and a characteristic diffuse hyperpigmentation, with accentuation in the palmar folds, scars, and oral mucosa (**Figures 153-1** and **153-2**). Vitiligo may be present in up to 15% of patients, particularly in those with autoimmune-related adrenal failure. Low sodium and increased potassium are associated with mineralocorticoid deficiency. Adrenal crisis is life-threatening, and typically presents with severe, refractory hypotension. In addition to other signs of AI, hypoglycemia, fever, confusion, or coma may also be present.

DIAGNOSIS

PRIMARY AI

Hospitalized patients with suspected AI should have a morning cortisol drawn between 6 AM and 8 AM. Cortisol values less than 3 µg/dL or greater than 18 to 19 µg/dL essentially rule in or out the disease, respectively. Patients with cortisol between 3 and 18 µg/dL should receive a 250 µg cosyntropin (ACTH) stimulation test. A cortisol level drawn 30 to 60 minutes following injection of cosyntropin should be greater than 18 µg/dL, with lower values indicating adrenal insufficiency. (Of note, the cortisol rise of less than 9 µg/dl sometimes used to diagnose AI in the critical care literature is not used in noncritically ill patients.)

Adrenocorticotropic hormone levels should be drawn to differentiate primary AI from secondary and tertiary AI, with high values suggesting primary AI. Abdominal CT may be performed in patients with primary AI of unclear etiology; adrenal glands affected by autoimmune disease are usually small and atrophic. Brain MRI may be considered for those with suspected secondary AI (**Figure 153-3**).

SECONDARY AND TERTIARY AI

In secondary (pituitary origin) or tertiary (hypothalamic origin) adrenal insufficiency, serum cortisol and ACTH are both low when these are measured simultaneously in the absence of exogenous glucocorticoids. This may be confirmed with the 48-hour ACTH-stimulation test. Patients with secondary or tertiary adrenal insufficiency should boost cortisol production with prolonged ACTH dosing, whereas no effect on cortisol production will be seen in those with primary AI. Secondary and tertiary adrenal insufficiency can be distinguished by the corticotropin-releasing hormone test. Administration of CRH to patients with tertiary AI will result in a surge in ACTH levels, but will not boost ACTH levels in patients with secondary AI. (This distinction usually does not affect patient management.)

MANAGEMENT

ACUTE ADRENAL INSUFFICIENCY

Acute AI should be treated immediately. Diagnostic testing must not delay treatment of the patient in adrenal crisis. Management should proceed as follows:

1. Draw blood for serum cortisol, renin, ACTH, and chemistries.
2. Fluid resuscitation: 1 to 3 L 0.9% saline (or 5% dextrose in 0.9% saline, if hypoglycemic), titrated to volume status and urine output. Avoid hypotonic saline, which will worsen hyponatremia.
3. 100 mg IV hydrocortisone or 4 mg IV dexamethasone (if performing cosyntropin stimulation). If dexamethasone is given rather than hydrocortisone, also give fludrocortisone 0.1 mg po daily.
4. 250 µg cosyntropin-stimulation test, with 30-minute cortisol level if dexamethasone administered.
5. Intravenous hydrocortisone 200 mg continuous infusion over 24 hours, or 50 mg every 6 hours. In uncomplicated cases, an oral maintenance dose should commence after taper of IV therapy over 1 to 3 days.
6. Diagnostic evaluation to determine the cause of AI (Figure 153-3).

CHRONIC ADRENAL INSUFFICIENCY

In chronic AI, glucocorticoid replacement is usually given in morning and evening doses to mimic diurnal cortisol secretion. Oral administration of a total daily dose of 15 to 25 mg hydrocortisone is equivalent to the daily cortisol production of 5 to 10 mg/m². The optimal

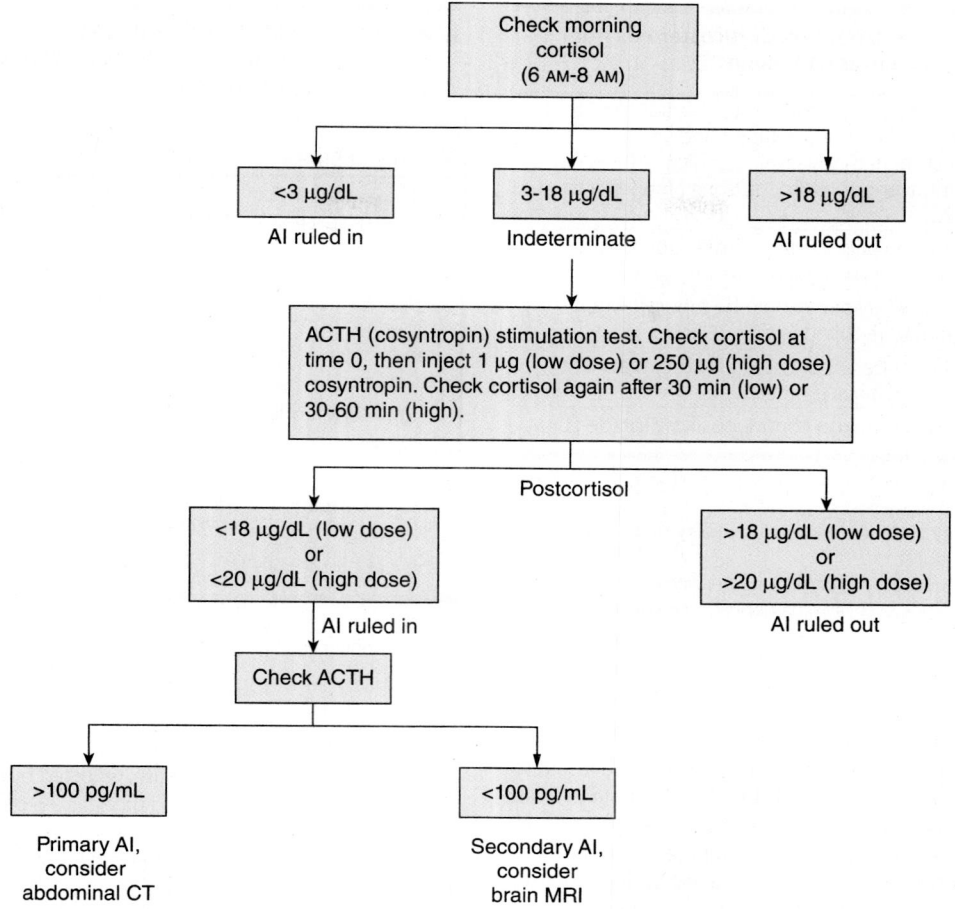

Figure 153-3 *Diagnostic evaluation of adrenal insufficiency.*

dose is that which avoids signs and symptoms of glucocorticoid excess, while relieving symptoms of glucocorticoid deficiency.

The short half-life of hydrocortisone enables dosing to mimic the normal physiologic diurnal variation. The morning dose (about one-half to two-thirds of total) should be given as soon as possible after waking, with the evening dose administered about 6 to 8 hours later. Long-acting glucocorticoids, such as prednisolone and dexamethasone, may be preferred for patients with afternoon fatigue or who are poorly adherent. Monitoring of the adequacy of glucocorticoid replacement is clinical, because reliable, objective measurements are lacking. Undertreatment with glucocorticoid manifests as an impaired sense of well-being, while overtreatment causes osteoporosis, excessive weight gain, and features of Cushing syndrome.

Patients with primary AI require replacement with both glucocorticoids and mineralocorticoids. Fludrocortisone, a potent synthetic mineralocorticoid, is typically started at 0.1 mg/d, with a dose range of 0.05 to 0.2 mg/d. Signs of excess mineralocorticoid replacement include hypertension, edema, and hypokalemia. Monitoring of mineralocorticoid replacement includes measurement of orthostatic blood pressure, serum sodium, potassium, and plasma renin. If hypertension develops, the dose of fludrocortisone should be reduced, with close monitoring of serum sodium and potassium. As the sodium-retaining effects of fludrocortisone require several days to develop, sodium deficits in acute AI should be replaced with intravenous normal saline. Mineralocorticoid doses do not need to be increased during stress or minor illness, as stress doses of hydrocortisone have mineralocorticoid properties. However, mineralocorticoid dosing may need to be increased during periods of increased salt loss, such as hot weather, and liberal salt intake should be encouraged in these circumstances.

Dehydroepiandrosterone (DHEA) levels, which are diminished in patients with primary AI, may be initially replaced with a 25- to 50-mg daily dose, with subsequent doses titrated to clinical response. Dehydroepiandrosterone replacement may have modest effects on sense of well-being and quality of life, although evidence to support claims of improved sexual function and satisfaction in women is not robust.

USE OF CORTICOSTEROIDS IN PATIENTS WITH CRITICAL ILLNESS

CRITICAL ILLNESS-RELATED CORTICOSTEROID INSUFFICIENCY (CIRCI)

The stress response in critical illness is a well-recognized physiologic phenomenon that parallels the adaptive "fight-or-flight" response seen in animals. This phenomenon involves activation of the HPA axis and the sympathetic nervous system, with resultant increases in cortisol, epinephrine, norepinephrine, and cytokines and other inflammatory mediators. However, in some critically ill patients, there may be inadequate production of corticosteroids and decreased peripheral responsiveness to corticosteroids, resulting in what has been called critical illness-related corticosteroid insufficiency (CIRCI). The prevalence of CIRCI may be as high as 60% in septic shock patients.

The definition and treatment of CIRCI remain controversial. Universal use of glucocorticoids in septic shock patients has not been shown to be beneficial. Two criteria that have been used for diagnosis are a random cortisol of less than 10 µg/dL in the presence of critical illness and a cortisol rise of less than 9 µg/dL on ACTH-stimulation testing. However, ACTH-stimulation testing does not identify patients who benefit from glucocorticoids. At present, the American College

TABLE 153-3 Recommendations on Corticosteroids from Surviving Sepsis Campaign

Do not use intravenous hydrocortisone to treat adult septic shock patients if adequate fluid resuscitation and vasopressor therapy are able to restore hemodynamic stability. If this is not achievable, suggest intravenous hydrocortisone alone at a dose of 200 mg/d (grade 2C).
Do not use the ACTH-stimulation test to identify adults with septic shock who should receive hydrocortisone (grade 2B).
In treated patients, hydrocortisone should be tapered when vasopressors are no longer required (grade 2D).
Corticosteroids should not be administered for the treatment of sepsis in the absence of shock (grade 1D).
When hydrocortisone is given, use continuous flow (grade 2D).

Grade A: High quality of evidence (several high-quality studies with consistent results)
Grade B: Moderate quality of evidence (one high-quality study or several studies with some limitations)
Grade C: Low quality of evidence (one or more studies with severe limitations)
Grade D: Very low quality of evidence (expert opinion; no direct research evidence)
Strength of recommendations: 1 = strong; 2 = weak

TABLE 153-4 Guidelines for Adrenal Supplementation Therapy for Patients on Chronic Corticosteroids*

Severity of Stress	Corticosteroid Dose	Frequency and Duration of Therapy
Mild Mild febrile illness Endoscopy	25 mg intravenous hydrocortisone	Day of procedure only
Moderate Routine abdominal surgery Significant febrile illness	50-75 mg intravenous hydrocortisone	Day of procedure, with 1-2 d taper back to usual dose
Severe Major surgery (cardiac) Severe pancreatitis	100-150 mg intravenous hydrocortisone	Day of procedure, with 1-2 d taper back to usual dose

*Patients using less than 5 mg/prednisone equivalent a day typically do not require supplementation in the setting of medical or surgical stress.

of Critical Care Medicine recommends consideration of corticosteroids in patients remaining in shock despite adequate fluid resuscitation and vasopressor administration (**Table 153-3**). If steroids are administered, intravenous hydrocortisone 50 mg every 6 hours for 7 days should be used, and subsequently tapered off. Fludrocortisone use merits further study, but is considered optional per the recent Society of Critical Care Medicine consensus statement.

As the current literature has mostly focused on intensive care unit patients with septic shock, these recommendations cannot be applied to other critically ill patients without sepsis, or to noncritically ill patient populations. Additionally, side effects of steroid use in the critically ill are substantial, and include hypertension, electrolyte abnormalities, volume overload, immunosuppression, delayed wound healing, neuromuscular weakness, and hyperglycemia. These side effects, the narrow scope of existing literature, and the lack of robust proven benefit make glucocorticoids a treatment modality that should be used in critically ill septic patients on a case-by-case basis only.

■ PRE-EXISTING ADRENAL INSUFFICIENCY AND NEED FOR CORTICOSTEROID AUGMENTATION

Patients with primary and secondary adrenal insufficiency, as well as the many patients on oral glucocorticoid therapy at risk of tertiary AI, may require supplemental steroids in the setting of acute illness. Patients on potent topical corticosteroids may also be at slight risk for tertiary AI. While dose augmentation in the setting of surgical procedures or severe illness should be considered for patients receiving more than 5 mg/d of prednisone or its equivalent, there is a debate over optimal duration and dose recommended. Suggested glucocorticoid dosing is found in **Table 153-4**, based on existing evidence and expert opinion. Mineralocorticoid use is a topic of ongoing investigation. Currently, supplementation is not routinely recommended except in patients with primary AI and selected patients with refractory septic shock.

■ GLUCOCORTICOID USE IN SELECT POPULATIONS

There are many other hospitalized patients for whom corticosteroid use should be considered. However, aside from studies in septic shock patients, large randomized controlled trials are lacking for most other patient populations. Several recent trials in patients with the

acute respiratory distress syndrome (ARDS) have shown improved outcomes with glucocorticoid use, reflected by decreased mechanical ventilation time and reduced mortality. In patients with severe or critical, relatively early ARDS (<2 weeks), methylprednisolone doses of 1 mg/kg/d continuous infusion is currently recommended for at least 14 days, followed by slow taper over 1 month.

Despite more limited data, such as small randomized trials, observational data, and expert opinion, recommendations supporting routine corticosteroid use can still be made for several other patient populations. These guidelines can be found in **Table 153-5**, and with comparative data on different corticosteroid medications in **Table 153-6**. Because data are limited for many patient groups, suggested doses, duration of therapy, and the choice of a particular corticosteroid are largely empiric, or based upon expert opinion. Risks need to be considered in any decision about corticosteroid use, particularly in situations in which benefits are not well defined.

PRACTICE POINT

- If adrenal crisis is suspected and a cosyntropin (ACTH) stimulation test has not yet been performed, dexamethasone 4 mg IV every 6 hours is preferred to hydrocortisone, as it is less likely to interfere with test interpretation.

DISCHARGE CHECKLIST FOR ADRENAL INSUFFICIENCY

- Have patients and their families been educated on the importance of taking corticosteroid replacement therapy as directed, and the potentially fatal consequences of failing to do so?
- Has the patient been instructed to take glucocorticoids until antibiotic therapy is completed, if the patient was discharged on antibiotics?
- Has the patient been instructed to check blood sugars and reduce insulin as glucocorticoids are weaned (if the patient was started on insulin for steroid-induced hyperglycemia)?
- Has the patient been instructed on stress-related glucocorticoid adjustment, and advised to double their hydrocortisone dose during infections requiring antibiotics or associated with fever?

TABLE 153-5 Recommended Uses of Supplemental Corticosteroids

Clinical Condition*	Recommended Dose†	Notes
Critical illness-related corticosteroid insufficiency (CIRCI)	50 mg IV hydrocortisone every 6 h for 7 d	Recommended for patients with shock refractory to volume and vasopressor administration, ACTH stimulation should not be used to determine who may benefit
Acute respiratory distress syndrome (ARDS)	1 mg/kg/d IV methylprednisolone for 14 d	Start within 14 d, taper slowly over 1 mo
Pneumocystis pneumonia (PCP)	40 mg oral prednisone twice daily for 5 d, then 40 mg daily for 5 d, then 20 mg daily for 11 d	Steroids indicated only for hypoxic patients (partial pressure of oxygen <70 mm Hg or alveolar-arterial gradient >35); doses recommended are for HIV patients, non-HIV patients with PCP pneumonia may require higher doses than listed
Chronic obstructive pulmonary disease (COPD) exacerbation	30-60 mg of oral prednisone for 7-10 d	
Asthma exacerbation	40-80 mg of oral prednisone in divided doses daily for 10-14 d	
Solid organ transplant	Doses vary	
Bacterial meningitis	Dexamethasone 10 mg IV every 6 h for 4 d	First does given before or with first dose antibiotics
Alcoholic hepatitis	40 mg oral prednisolone for 4 wk followed by taper	When discriminant function is >32 and/or evidence of hepatic encephalopathy
Acute spinal cord injury	30 mg/kg IV methylprednisolone bolus followed by 5.4 mg/kg/h for 23 h	Practice guidelines suggest this as optional therapy
Others (cardiac surgery, end-stage liver disease, hepatoadrenal syndrome, severe pancreatitis, community-acquired pneumonia)	Variable	Consensus is lacking, data is limited

ACTH, adrenocorticotropic hormone; IV, intravenous; kg, kilogram; mg, milligram.
*Side effects of steroids, including hyperglycemia, poor wound healing, hypertension electrolyte abnormalities, volume overload, neuromuscular weakness are numerous and should be considered in a risk-benefit fashion for every decision to use corticosteroids.
†Doses, duration of therapy, and choice of particular corticosteroid are largely empiric or based on expert opinion.

TABLE 153-6 Characteristics of Commonly Used Steroids

	Glucocorticoid Activity	Mineralocorticoid Activity	Half-life (h)	Approximate Equivalent Dose (mg)
Hydrocortisone	1	1	6-8	20
Prednisone	4	0.1-0.2	18-36	5
Methylprednisolone	5	0.1-0.2	18-36	4
Dexamethasone	30	<0.1	36-54	0.75
Fludrocortisone	0	20	18-36	0.05-2

- Has the patient been instructed to wear a medical alert bracelet or necklace or carry a steroid emergency card?
- Has the patient been given a prescription for an emergency hydrocortisone kit with prefilled syringes?
- Have follow-up appointments been arranged with the patient's primary-care provider and/or endocrinologist?

SUGGESTED READINGS

Bancos I, Hahner S, Tomlinson J, Arlt W. Diagnosis and management of adrenal insufficiency. *Lancet Diabetes Endocrinol.* 2015;3:216-226.

Bornstein SR. Current concepts: predisposing factors for adrenal insufficiency. *N Engl J Med.* 2009;360:2328-2339.

Charmandari E, Nicolaides NC, Chrousos GP. Adrenal insufficiency. *Lancet.* 2014;383:2152-2167.

Coursin DB, Wood KE. Corticosteroid supplementation for adrenal insufficiency. *JAMA.* 2002;287:236-240.

Dellinger RP, Levy MM, Rhodes A, et al. Surviving sepsis campaign: international guidelines for management of severe sepsis and septic shock: 2012. *Crit Care Med.* 2013;41:580-637.

Marik PE. Critical illness-related corticosteroid insufficiency. *Chest.* 2009;135:181-193.

Marik PE, Pastores SM, Annane D, et al. Recommendations for the diagnosis and management of corticosteroid insufficiency in critically ill adult patients: consensus statements from an international task force by the American College of Critical Care Medicine. *Crit Care Med.* 2008;36:1937-1949.

Meduri GU, Marik PE, Annanne D. Prolonged glucocorticoid treatment in acute respiratory distress syndrome: evidence supporting effectiveness and safety. *Crit Care Med.* 2009;37:1800-1803.

CHAPTER 154

Pituitary Disease

Shilpa H. Jain, MD
Laurence Katznelson, MD

Key Clinical Questions

1 How and when do you evaluate pituitary hormonal function?

2 How do you treat patients with excess or deficient pituitary hormonal function?

3 How do you classify pituitary tumors?

4 Which patients with pituitary disease require hospital admission?

5 What are the indications for consultation with endocrinology and/or neurosurgery?

6 What are the complications associated with neurosurgical resection of pituitary tumors?

EPIDEMIOLOGY

Pituitary disease is more common than popularly supposed. In unselected autopsies, the prevalence of pituitary adenomas averages about 14%. However, the prevalence of clinically significant pituitary adenomas is much lower, about 94 per 100,000 people. Pituitary adenomas can present clinically due to excessive secretion of hormones, impairment of normal pituitary function, neurologic changes due to local compressive mass effects, or hemorrhage. Approximately 30% of survivors of traumatic brain injury and subarachnoid hemorrhage have chronic anterior hypopituitarism; therefore, clinicians must consider this diagnosis in populations at risk, such as wounded combat veterans. Hypopituitarism is also frequent after cranial irradiation, and may complicate pituitary disease of any cause.

PITUITARY ANATOMY AND PHYSIOLOGY

The pituitary gland is located at the base of the brain within the sella turcica, which is the bony roof of the sphenoid sinus. It lies outside the dura mater. The pituitary stalk, containing neurovascular bundles, extends from the hypothalamus through a dural opening to the pituitary gland. This anatomical arrangement renders the pituitary stalk vulnerable to traumatic injury. The optic chiasm is located above the pituitary gland and anterior to the pituitary stalk. The pituitary gland is bordered on the sides by the cavernous sinuses, which consist of vascular lakes containing cranial nerves III, IV, V, and VI and a portion of the carotid artery. The pituitary gland consists of two lobes—anterior and posterior (**Figure 154-1**).

The anterior lobe, or adenohypophysis, is made up of secretory cells that manufacture at least six hormones: adrenocorticotropic hormone (ACTH), thyroid-stimulating hormone (TSH), growth hormone (GH), follicle-stimulating hormone (FSH), luteinizing hormone (LH), and prolactin (PRL). Secretion of the first five hormones is triggered by hypothalamic-releasing factors that travel down the pituitary stalk through a portal venous system. In contrast, anterior pituitary secretion of prolactin, which promotes lactation, is tonically inhibited by hypothalamic secretion of dopamine. Any disorder that compresses or interferes with the pituitary stalk can elevate prolactin levels.

In contrast, the posterior lobe, or neurohypophysis, is comprised of axons of cell bodies arising in the hypothalamus. These axons store and secrete vasopressin (antidiuretic hormone, or ADH) and oxytocin. Vasopressin has a key role in fluid and electrolyte balance, by promoting retention of water by the kidney. Oxytocin stimulates uterine contractions at parturition.

HYPOPITUITARISM

■ CAUSES

The most common cause of hypopituitarism is a **pituitary adenoma**. Other causes include **nonpituitary sellar masses**, such as craniopharyngiomas and meningiomas, damage to normal pituitary tissue during **neurosurgery** for pituitary adenoma, and sudden hemorrhage into a pituitary adenoma (**pituitary apoplexy**). **Sheehan syndrome** is pituitary necrosis related to postpartum hemorrhage and hypotension; presumably, the pituitary is at greater risk of ischemic injury in this setting because of its normal increase in volume during pregnancy. Patients usually present with failure of lactation, followed by slowly progressive symptoms and signs of hypopituitarism. **Cranial irradiation** causes hypopituitarism in approximately

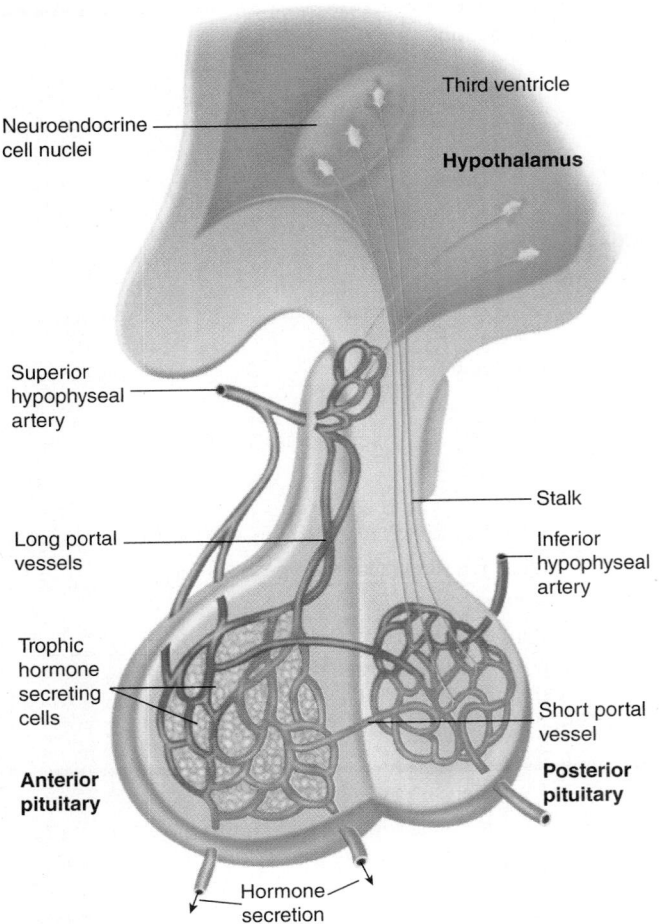

Figure 154-1 *The hypothalamic-pituitary axis. Hypothalamic nuclei secrete hormones in a pulsatile fashion into a portal venous system, which perfuses anterior pituitary secretory cells and regulates its activity. Posterior pituitary hormones are derived from direct neural extensions from the hypothalamus.* (Reproduced, with permission, from Fauci AS, Braunwald E, Kasper DL, et al. *Harrison's Principles of Internal Medicine,* 17th ed. New York, NY: McGraw-Hill, 2008. Fig. 333-2.)

40% of patients over a 10-year period, with the precise risk depending on the total radiation dose and length of time after exposure. The prevalence of hypopituitarism after **traumatic brain injury** and **subarachnoid hemorrhage** has been reported to be approximately 30% and 50%, respectively. Growth hormone deficiency is the most common endocrine abnormality following both traumatic brain injury and subarachnoid hemorrhage. **Developmental and genetic causes** of hypopituitarism are rare, and include pituitary aplasia or hypoplasia, hypothalamic defects, mutations in transcription factors, and genetic conditions such as Kallman syndrome and Prader-Willi syndrome. Other rare causes include metastatic disease from breast, lung, or skin cancer, histiocytosis X, and sarcoidosis.

■ PRESENTATION AND DIAGNOSIS

Specific tests are used to assess each hormonal axis (**Table 154-1**).

Central or secondary adrenal insufficiency, caused by decreased pituitary ACTH release, is associated with anorexia, orthostasis, arthralgias, fatigue, vomiting, and hyponatremia. Hyperpigmentation is absent and serum potassium is normal, unlike Addison disease (primary adrenal insufficiency). The evaluation of central adrenal insufficiency is somewhat controversial, as the criteria for diagnosis depend on the severity of the patient's condition. In a stable, noncritically ill patient, a fasting serum cortisol > 15 μg/dL

is considered normal. Central adrenal insufficiency is clearly present when the morning serum cortisol is < 3 μg/dL and ACTH is low or inappropriately normal. If the serum cortisol is between 3 and 15 μg/dL, then further testing is appropriate. Such testing may include a standard 250 μg ACTH (cosyntropin)stimulation test, in which serum cortisol is measured at baseline and 30 and 60 minutes after intravenous cosyntropin administration. Alternatively, serum cortisol may be measured 45 to 60 minutes after an intramuscular injection of cosyntropin. A peak serum cortisol of >18 μg/dL is considered normal in this test. An important limitation of cosyntropin stimulation testing in central adrenal insufficiency is that it may be normal in acute pituitary disease (such as following pituitary surgery) because the adrenal gland can respond normally to cosyntropin in the first few weeks following a pituitary insult. Over time, ACTH deficiency leads to adrenal atrophy, and at that point, the response to cosyntropin stimulation is blunted. It is also possible that the pharmacologic dose of cosyntropin may overshadow mild central adrenal insufficiency, and a normal result may give a false sense of security that adrenal function is intact. Other measures of ACTH reserve, such as insulin-induced hypoglycemia testing, may be more reliable as they measure integrity of the entire axis, but requires physician supervision and is therefore less commonly used in clinical practice. The diagnosis of central adrenal insufficiency in the presence of physiologic stress is less clear, as a normal cortisol value may be inappropriately low for the setting. Change in serum cortisol following cosyntropin has been used as a marker for adrenal function in the intensive care unit, but there is controversy as to the interpretation of such tests.

The symptoms of **central hypothyroidism** are similar to those of primary hypothyroidism, and include cold intolerance, fatigue, mild weight gain, dry skin, alopecia, and constipation. Findings include delayed tendon reflexes, facial puffiness and coarsening, bradycardia, slowed mentation, nonpitting edema, pleural effusions, and carpal tunnel syndrome. Hyponatremia in patients with sellar masses may reflect either central adrenal insufficiency or central hypothyroidism. Diagnosis is based on the presence of a low serum free T4 with low or normal TSH, in contrast to the elevated TSH seen in primary hypothyroidism. However, low free T4 can be the first thyroid abnormality associated with nonthyroidal illnesses (sick euthyroid), common in the inpatient setting. Therefore, the definitive diagnosis of central hypothyroidism may sometimes be delayed until the subject recovers from acute illness.

Hypogonadism (testosterone and estrogen deficiency) cannot be reliably diagnosed in the inpatient setting, as levels of both hormones decline markedly during acute illness. In men, secondary hypogonadism is associated with decreases in sexual function, libido, and muscle mass. In women, secondary hypogonadism is associated with secondary amenorrhea and symptoms of estrogen deficiency, such as hot flashes, vaginal dryness, or decreased libido. In the outpatient setting, secondary male hypogonadism is diagnosed based on low levels of testosterone and low or normal FSH and LH. In women, secondary hypogonadism is suggested by irregular or absent menses and low or normal FSH and LH.

Growth hormone deficiency in children is characterized by short stature, and in adults by increased body fat, reduced muscle mass and bone density, and diminished quality of life. GH is secreted in pulsatile fashion, and most secretion is nocturnal. During the day, GH levels in normal subjects may be low or undetectable. Therefore, random daytime GH levels are of little clinical utility. As GH stimulates production of insulin-like growth factor-1 (IGF-1) by the liver, IGF-1 is a surrogate marker of recent GH levels. A low serum IGF-1 level supports the diagnosis of GH deficiency, especially in the setting of other pituitary disease. Further evidence of GH deficiency may be provided by an insufficient GH response to insulin-induced hypoglycemia or to glucagon administration.

TABLE 154-1 Hormonal Profile in Excessive and Insufficient Anterior Pituitary Function

Pituitary Hormone	End-Organ and its Hormone	Criteria for Hormonal Excess	Criteria for Hormonal Deficiency
ACTH	Adrenal glands: Cortisol	↑ Cortisol • 24-h urine cortisol >3 times upper limit of normal × 2 collections • Overnight 1 mg dexamethasone suppression test with serum cortisol >1.8 µg/dL Normal/↑ ACTH	↓ Cortisol • 8 AM serum cortisol <3 µg/dL Normal/↓ ACTH
TSH	Thyroid gland: T4, T3	↑ T4, T3 Normal/↑ TSH	↓ T4 Normal/↓ TSH
Growth hormone (GH)	Liver: IGF-1	↑ IGF-1 • Serum IGF-1 > age and gender specific upper limit of normal ↑ GH • Oral glucose tolerance test with nadir GH >1 µg/L	↓ IGF-1 • Serum IGF-1 < age and gender specific upper limit of normal ↓ GH • Insulin-induced hypoglycemia, with peak GH <5.1 µg/L Glucagon stimulation with peak GH <3 µg/L
FSH, LH	Testes: testosterone	↑ Testosterone Normal/↑ FSH, LH	↓ Testosterone Normal/↓ FSH, LH
	Ovaries: estradiol, progesterone	Abnormal/absent menses Normal/↑ FSH, LH	Abnormal/absent menses Normal/↓ FSH, LH
Prolactin	Mammary glands	↑ Prolactin	↓ Prolactin (rare)

Central diabetes insipidus (DI) due to ADH deficiency presents with polyuria and polydipsia. The physical examination is normal unless dehydration has developed. If hypernatremia is present, the patient may be obtunded, but most patients are able to maintain eunatremia with a high fluid intake. The diagnosis is confirmed with a carefully supervised fluid deprivation test, demonstrating the inability to appropriately concentrate urine osmolality despite rising plasma sodium and osmolality. Patients with central DI will subsequently increase their urine osmolality more than 50% with desmopressin administration, whereas patients with nephrogenic DI will not.

PITUITARY TUMORS

Pituitary tumors are classified based on hormonal secretion and size. Tumors that secrete excessive amounts of pituitary hormones are referred to as functional or secretory tumors, and tumors that do not produce biologically active hormone are known as nonfunctioning or nonsecretory tumors. Pituitary tumors are classified as microadenomas if the diameter is less than 10 mm, and macroadenomas if the diameter is greater than 10 mm.

■ PRESENTATION

Patients with functioning pituitary adenomas present with classic manifestations specific to each hormone (**Table 154-2**). These benign tumors usually secrete in order of decreasing incidence excessive quantities of prolactin, growth hormone, ACTH, and rarely thyrotropin or gonadotropin.

Pituitary macroadenomas that extend beyond the sella may compress local structures, leading to temporal visual loss and hypopituitarism. The overwhelming majority of pituitary tumors are benign pathologically. Rarely, however, adenocarcinoma may arise in the pituitary.

Prolactinomas account for approximately 30% to 40% of all pituitary tumors. Symptoms in women include amenorrhea or oligomenorrhea, infertility, and galactorrhea. Postmenopausal women with prolactinomas are unlikely to develop galactorrhea, as their estrogen levels are usually very low. Men with prolactinomas may present with decreased libido, erectile dysfunction, and infertility.

The second most common functional pituitary tumor is a growth-hormone-secreting adenoma (approximately 10%), which results in **acromegaly**. Clinical manifestations of acromegaly include enlargement of soft tissues, cartilage and bones in face, hands, and feet and

TABLE 154-2 Clinical Presentations of Pituitary Tumors

1. Functioning tumors
   a. Prolactinoma
   b. Acromegaly
   c. Cushing disease
   d. Hyperthyroidism
2. Mass effects
   a. Hypopituitarism
      i. Adrenal insufficiency
      ii. Hypothyroidism
      iii. Hypogonadism
      iv. Growth hormone deficiency
   b. Headaches
   c. Neurological deficits
      i. Visual changes: decreased visual acuity, visual field deficits, ophthalmoplegia
      ii. Ptosis
      iii. Facial sensory syndromes
   d. Cerebrospinal fluid leakage ± meningitis
   e. Nasopharyngeal obstruction
3. Pituitary apoplexy
4. Asymptomatic
   a. Nonfunctioning tumors

enlarged viscera (heart, liver, thyroid). Cutaneous symptoms include excessive sweating, oily skin, and skin tags. Patients may also note changes in ring, hat, and shoe size over many years. Patients may have arthralgias, arthritis, carpal tunnel syndrome, hyperglycemia, obstructive sleep apnea, and congestive heart failure. On physical examination, they have signs of hypertension, enlarged hands and feet, with characteristically enlarged finger pulps and heel pads, jaw prognathism, gaps between teeth, frontal bone bossing, macroglossia, and coarse, soft, doughy skin. Acromegaly is associated with an increased risk of early mortality, primarily from cardiovascular disease.

Cushing disease, or hypercortisolemia due to an ACTH-secreting pituitary tumor, can present with truncal obesity, violaceous striae, moon facies, facial plethora, dorsocervical and supraclavicular fat deposition, bruising, proximal muscle weakness and wasting, edema, hirsutism, acne, mood disorders, hyperglycemia, hypokalemia, hypertension, increased susceptibility to infections, thromboembolism, and fractures related to osteoporosis. **TSH-secreting adenomas**, characterized by TSH-induced hyperthyroidism, are very rare, accounting for approximately 1% to 2% of pituitary tumors.

Nonfunctioning pituitary tumors, the most common type of pituitary adenoma accounting for up to 40% of all tumors, commonly stem from pituitary cells that produce the gonadotropins LH and FSH. They may be diagnosed during evaluation of headache, visual loss, or hypopituitarism. They may also be detected incidentally. Approximately, 10% of the normal adult population has a clinically unsuspected microadenoma on brain magnetic resonance imaging (MRI). While these patients may not have symptoms, subtle hormonal or neurological abnormalities may be present, and they should be evaluated for hormonal excess and deficiency, and carefully examined for visual field defects and other neurologic abnormalities.

COMPLICATIONS

■ MASS EFFECTS

Compression of the native pituitary gland may lead to hypopituitarism. The presence of a sellar mass and diabetes insipidus points to a nonpituitary lesion, as pituitary tumors rarely present with diabetes insipidus. Extension into the adjacent cavernous sinus can lead to diplopia, ophthalmoplegia, ptosis, and facial sensory syndromes due to cranial nerve involvement. Superior tumor extension may impinge upon the optic chiasm, leading to visual field deficits, classically bitemporal hemianopsia (**Figure 154-2**).

PRACTICE POINT

- The finding of temporal visual field loss may suggest that a lesion is compressing the optic chiasm, which is closely associated with the pituitary fossa. Involvement of the upper quadrants first, a sign of compression of the optic chiasma from below, suggests pituitary adenoma, nasopharyngeal carcinoma, or sphenoid sinus mucocele. Involvement of the lower quadrants first, signaling compression of the optic chiasma from above, suggests a craniopharyngioma or third ventricular tumor.
- Some pituitary tumors may expand laterally, compressing nerves lying within the walls of the cavernous sinus, especially cranial nerve III. Rarely, vertical expansion obstructs the foramen of Munro, leading to hydrocephalus and/or hypothalamic compression.

■ PITUITARY APOPLEXY

Rarely, patients may present with pituitary apoplexy, or acute hemorrhagic infarction of a pituitary adenoma. This is an endocrine

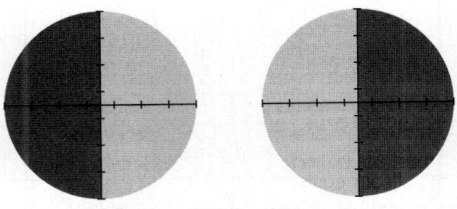

Bitemporal hemianopia

Figure 154-2 *Magnetic resonance imaging scan, coronal view, of a pituitary macroadenoma (solid arrow) with superior extension and compression of the optic chiasm (dashed arrow).*

emergency because of frequent associated acute adrenal insufficiency. Patients with apoplexy may present with severe headaches, visual field deficits, opthalmoplegia, and altered consciousness. Immediate management includes glucocorticoid coverage, intravenous fluids, and neurosurgical consultation. Predisposing factors include hemodynamic instability and anticoagulation.

EVALUATION

The approach to a patient with a pituitary tumor is outlined in **Figure 154-3**.

Patients with suspected pituitary tumors should be asked about headaches, visual changes, and symptoms of hormonal excess and deficiency. Patients with suspected acromegaly should be asked about surreptitious GH use for athletic purposes or purported antiaging effects. Signs of special interest on physical examination include abnormalities of blood pressure readings with orthostatics, heart rate, cranial nerves with visual field testing, and signs of hormone excess and deficiency.

The initial endocrine laboratory evaluation for patients with suspected hypersecretory syndromes includes measurements of serum prolactin, IGF-1, free T4, and TSH (**Figure 154-4**). Either 24-hour urinary-free cortisol or overnight 1 mg dexamethasone suppression test should be performed to exclude Cushing disease. Patients with suspected hypopituitarism should have measurements of serum 8 AM cortisol, ACTH, free T4, TSH, FSH, LH, testosterone (in men), IGF-1, and a cosyntropin-stimulation test.

All patients should have a brain MRI, with thin sections through the pituitary gland, with and without contrast enhancement.

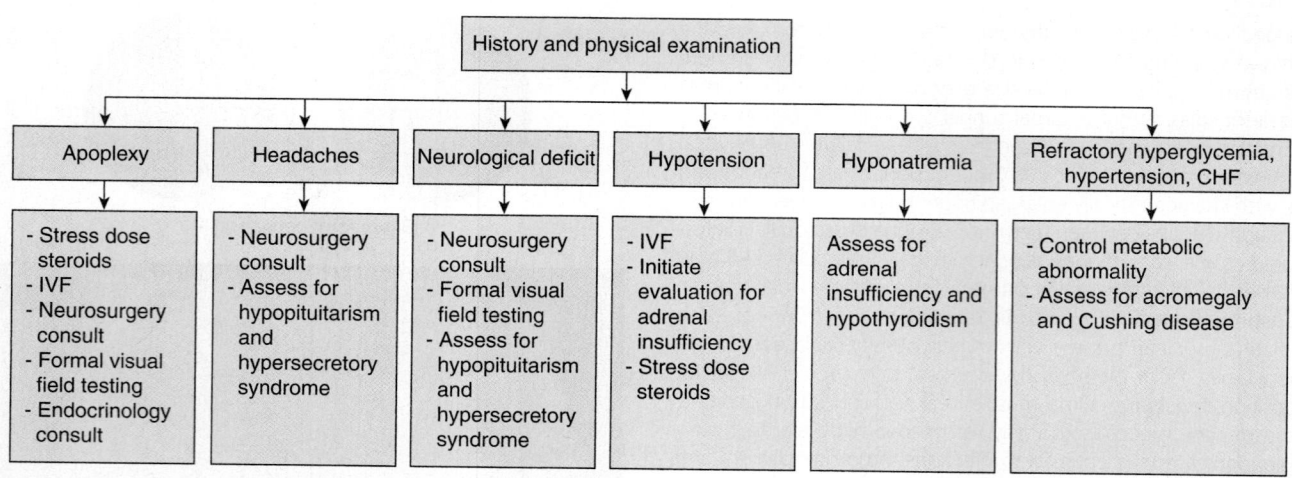

Figure 154-3 *Approach to the patient with a pituitary tumor.*

Neuro-opthalmological examination with formal visual field testing should be performed, especially in the presence of visual symptoms or compression of optic chiasm.

CONSULTATION

Endocrinology consultation is indicated for patients with suspected hypersecretory syndromes, hypopituitarism, sellar masses, pituitary apoplexy, and postoperative diabetes insipidus or syndrome of inappropriate ADH secretion. Neurosurgery consultation is indicated for patients with pituitary apoplexy, neurological deficits from pituitary disease, acromegaly, Cushing disease, TSH-secreting adenoma, cerebrospinal fluid leak, nasopharyngeal obstruction, and resistance or intolerance of medical therapy for prolactinoma.

DIAGNOSIS

Prolactinomas are diagnosed on the basis of an elevated serum prolactin, exclusion of other causes of hyperprolactinemia, and pituitary imaging confirming the presence of a pituitary adenoma. Macroprolactinomas (tumors >10 mm in greatest diameter) usually produce prolactin levels >150 ng/mL. When the serum prolactin is only mildly elevated (ie, up to 40 ng/mL), it should be repeated, as transient factors such as food, exercise, stress, and chest wall stimulation may cause modest hyperprolactinemia. Modest hyperprolactinemia is also caused by pregnancy, primary hypothyroidism, renal failure, cirrhosis, and medications such as metoclopramide, calcium-channel blockers, phenothiazines, selective serotonin reuptake inhibitors, and risperidone. Any sellar mass may compress the

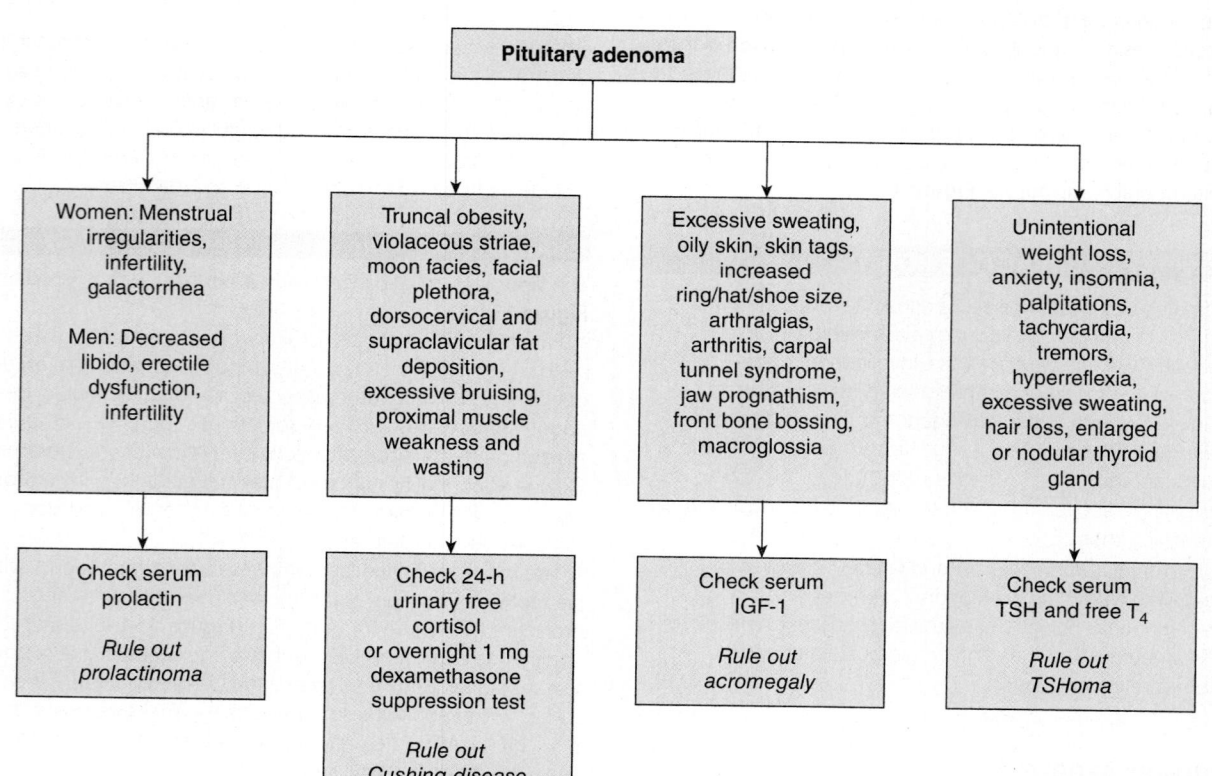

Figure 154-4 *Diagnostic algorithm for pituitary hypersecretory syndromes.*

pituitary stalk, reduce dopamine delivery to the pituitary, and lead to elevations in prolactin levels of up to approximately 150 ng/mL. For this reason, imaging studies should be performed in any patient with unexplained, modest hyperprolactinemia.

Acromegaly is a chronic, debilitating disease characterized by episodic hypersecretion of GH and continuously elevated levels of IGF-1. The best screening test for acromegaly is measurement of a random IGF-1 level, which shows less normal variability than serum GH. If IGF-1 is elevated after adjustment for age and gender, then a 75-g oral glucose tolerance test should confirm the diagnosis, with measurement of GH levels at baseline and 1 and 2 hours after glucose ingestion. The diagnostic value for acromegaly is a nadir GH level >1 µg/L. Most tumors are macroadenomas at diagnosis.

In **Cushing disease**, an ACTH-secreting tumor of the pituitary gland leads to overproduction of cortisol. Demonstration of an elevated 24-hour urinary-free cortisol or an abnormal dexamethasone suppression test is diagnostic of Cushing syndrome. The urine collection should be confirmed to be complete with a urine creatinine measurement. The urine-free cortisol excretion is usually at least two to four times normal in true Cushing disease. The urine cortisol can be mildly high in severe obesity, depression, anxiety, and alcoholism; these conditions are referred to as pseudo-Cushing states. The low-dose dexamethasone suppression test is performed by giving dexamethasone 1 mg at 11 PM, and measuring serum cortisol at 8 AM the following day. A morning serum cortisol > 1.8 µg/dL suggests Cushing syndrome. False positives can result from decreased dexamethasone absorption, increased dexamethasone clearance, and in pseudo-Cushing states. An elevated midnight salivary cortisol level, primarily used in the outpatient setting, can also help diagnose Cushing syndrome. After Cushing syndrome has been diagnosed, serum ACTH should be measured. A normal or increased ACTH level confirms ACTH-dependent Cushing syndrome. If a sellar mass >6 mm is present, a tentative diagnosis of Cushing disease (pituitary tumor) is made. If the source of the ACTH-dependent hypercortisolism is unclear, additional tests such as high-dose dexamethasone suppression testing, corticotropin-releasing hormone stimulation, or inferior petrosal sinus sampling may be necessary to determine whether ACTH secretion is pituitary or ectopic in origin.

As both nonfunctional and functional pituitary adenomas may compress the normal pituitary gland leading to hypopituitarism, adrenal insufficiency and hypothyroidism should be excluded in these patients.

DIFFERENTIAL DIAGNOSIS

The differential diagnosis of a pituitary adenoma includes several other sellar lesions. Meningiomas in or near the sella may affect pituitary function and compress the optic chiasm. Remnants of Rathke pouch, the embryological origin of the anterior pituitary lobe, may form a nonneoplastic cyst (Rathke cleft cyst) or low-grade tumor (craniopharyngioma). Rathke cleft cysts are typically asymptomatic, but can present with hypopituitarism and headaches. They may be differentiated from pituitary adenomas based on imaging features. Craniopharyngiomas most often present during childhood and adolescence with headaches, anterior pituitary deficiencies, and diabetes insipidus, which is rare in pituitary adenoma. Lymphocytic hypophysitis, or autoimmune inflammation and destruction of the pituitary gland, is a rare condition that is seen most often in young women, and may present in pregnancy. Up to 25% of patients also have autoimmune thyroid disease. Infiltrative diseases such as sarcoidosis and hemochromatosis may involve the pituitary. Rarely, lymphoma involves the pituitary stalk and hypothalamus. Metastases, especially from breast, lung, and gastrointestinal tract, can spread to the pituitary, particularly to the posterior lobe. Any sellar mass may have compressive effects, including hypopituitarism. The presence of diabetes insipidus and a sellar mass usually points away from a diagnosis of a pituitary tumor.

INPATIENT MANAGEMENT

■ PITUITARY APOPLEXY

Hemorrhagic infarction of the pituitary gland may lead to acute panhypopituitarism, visual loss, thunderclap headache, and shock. If hypotension is present, adrenal insufficiency should be presumed, and treated with intravenous fluids and stress dose glucocorticoids (eg, intravenous hydrocortisone 50-100 mg every 8 hours; dexamethasone may be preferred due to its lesser interference with tests of adrenal function). Formal visual field testing should be performed. Neurosurgery should be consulted for possible urgent surgical decompression. Endocrinology should also be consulted to assist with the diagnosis and management of hypopituitarism.

■ NEUROLOGICAL DEFICITS

Visual difficulties, such as visual field cuts and diplopia, are the most common neurological symptom of pituitary neoplasms. Transsphenoidal tumor resection may decompress cranial nerves and improve vision or restore it to normal. If surgery is not feasible, medical therapies or radiation may help shrink the tumor and alleviate the neurological deficit.

■ HYPOTENSION AND CENTRAL ADRENAL INSUFFICIENCY

Hypotension in the presence of a pituitary adenoma strongly suggests central adrenal insufficiency. Ideally, serum should be collected for diagnostic workup of adrenal insufficiency prior to initiation of treatment. However, if the patient is hemodynamically unstable, stress dose steroids should be started prior to confirmation of adrenal insufficiency. As hydrocortisone and prednisone are detected in the serum cortisol assay, the serum cortisol value is not informative while the patient is taking these medications. As dexamethasone is not detected by this assay, it may be used while evaluation of the hypothalamic-pituitary-adrenal axis is ongoing. After recovery from the acute illness, the glucocorticoid dose can be tapered to hydrocortisone 20 to 30 mg/d or prednisone 5 to 7.5 mg/d. Some patients may require repeat testing on an outpatient basis to confirm the diagnosis of adrenal insufficiency.

■ CENTRAL HYPOTHYROIDISM

Central hypothyroidism is treated with levothyroxine, with typical oral starting doses of 25 to 50 μg, depending on the patient's age and cardiovascular status. Over time, levothyroxine can be increased to full replacement dose, which is usually 1.6 μg/kg. The levothyroxine dose should be titrated until the free T4 is within the normal range. Serum TSH should not be used for dose titration, as the TSH concentration is not an appropriate marker of thyroid function in patients with hypothalamic or pituitary disease. If the patient cannot take oral medications, then levothyroxine can be administered as a daily intravenous dose of 70% to 80% of the oral dose. In central hypothyroidism, glucocorticoids should be administered when thyroid hormone replacement is initiated, as levothyroxine increases the metabolism of cortisol, and can precipitate an adrenal crisis if borderline adrenal function is present.

■ PITUITARY ADENOMA

Indications for treatment of prolactinoma include macroadenoma or enlarging microadenoma, headache, amenorrhea, infertility, acne, hirsutism, undesired galactorrhea in women, and gynecomastia and testosterone deficiency in men. Dopamine agonists are the primary mode of therapy for prolactinoma. These agents rapidly reduce prolactin secretion and adenoma size in most subjects. The dopamine agonists indicated for prolactinoma treatment in the United States are bromocriptine and cabergoline. Bromocriptine is less expensive, but is more often associated with nausea than cabergoline. It is typically started at a dose of 1.25 mg at bedtime, and then slowly titrated to a maximum dose of 2.5 mg twice daily. Cabergoline, a longer-acting dopamine agonist, may be more effective and better tolerated than bromocriptine, but it is more expensive. Cabergoline is started at a dose of 0.25 mg once weekly, and increased up to a maximum of 1 mg twice a week. High doses of cabergoline used in Parkinson disease are associated with an increased risk of cardiac valvular regurgitation, possibly due to stimulation of $5-HT_{2B}$ receptors on myofibroblasts. There is currently no definite evidence that this occurs with the lower doses of cabergoline used in the treatment of prolactinoma.

Serum prolactin levels should be monitored to determine the dose of the dopamine agonist being used. Patients with macroadenomas should be intermittently followed with pituitary MRI. Transsphenoidal surgery is offered for prolactinoma when medical therapy fails or is poorly tolerated, or when there is a significant cystic component that does not respond fully to dopamine agonist therapy. Radiotherapy is an option in patients who fail pharmacological and surgical therapy. Because prolactinomas may enlarge with gestation, serial visual field testing should be performed during pregnancy.

Aggressive treatment of **acromegaly** is essential, as it is associated with increased mortality and multiple morbidities. Transsphenoidal surgery is preferred for most patients, because it leads to the most rapid fall in serum GH levels, it is necessary for tumor debulking if there are local mass effects, and it is more often associated with biochemical cure than medical therapy. Approximately, 70% to 80% of patients with microadenomas and <50% of patients with macroadenomas attain biochemical normalization after surgery. Medical therapy is largely used as adjuvant therapy in patients who have failed surgery. Somatostatin analogs (octreotide and lanreotide) are available in monthly depot preparations, and control GH and normalize serum IGF-1 levels in approximately 50% to 70% of cases. Dopamine agonists, including cabergoline and bromocriptine, are less effective than somatostatin analogs. The GH receptor antagonist pegvisomant is highly effective in

reducing serum IGF-1 levels, and is often utilized as a secondary agent for subjects with incomplete or lack of response to somatostatin analogs. Radiation therapy is an adjuvant option for patients who have failed surgery and are unresponsive to or intolerant of medical therapy.

The primary therapy for **Cushing disease** is transsphenoidal resection. Remission rates in patients with a microadenoma undergoing selective adenomectomy by an expert pituitary surgeon are in the range of 65% to 90%. However, recurrence rates approach 20% at 10 years and may reflect dura mater invasion. In patients with persistent disease despite surgery, further options include radiation therapy, medical adrenalectomy, and surgical adrenalectomy. Medical therapy uses inhibitors of adrenal cortisol synthesis, such as ketoconazole and metyrapone. Novel medications recently approved by the Food and Drug Administration include pasireotide depot (a novel somatostatin analog) and mifepristone (an oral glucocorticoid receptor blocker). Medications are largely utilized in patients who have failed primary pituitary surgery, as a temporizing option during radiotherapy or while further surgery is being planned. Bilateral surgical adrenalectomy is a definitive treatment that provides immediate control of hypercortisolism, though the resultant adrenal insufficiency will require lifelong glucocorticoid and mineralocorticoid replacement therapy. Unfortunately, up to 25% of patients who undergo bilateral adrenalectomy develop Nelson syndrome, characterized by high serum ACTH levels, hyperpigmentation, and progressive pituitary enlargement with aggressive, often invasive tumor behavior. Surgical resection may be difficult. Directed radiotherapy may be indicated.

The primary therapy for **nonfunctioning adenomas** is surgery. Because they are often detected incidentally and diagnosis may be delayed, nonfunctioning tumors tend to be macroadenomas with extrasellar extension at diagnosis, and surgery is utilized for decompression of adjacent structures and is usually subtotal in extent. Medical therapies, including somatostatin analogs, are of limited use for these tumors. Radiation therapy is utilized in an adjuvant role for residual tumors following surgery, particularly in adenomas involving the cavernous sinus.

DIABETES INSIPIDUS, ADRENAL INSUFFICIENCY, AND OTHER COMPLICATIONS OF PITUITARY SURGERY

Transsphenoidal endonasal surgery is used to remove the majority of pituitary tumors. Rarely, craniotomy is required for a large pituitary tumor with suprasellar and extrasellar extension. Outcome depends on surgical expertise, tumor size, degree of invasiveness, preoperative hormone levels, and prior pituitary surgery. There is a robust relationship between transsphenoidal surgery complication rates and experience. Operators who have performed <200 procedures have complication rates two or three times higher than operators who have performed >500 procedures. The most common complications are anterior pituitary insufficiency (7%-21% of procedures) and diabetes insipidus (8%-19%). The endonasal approach may lead to sinusitis and nasal septum perforation. Cerebrospinal fluid leak occurs in 1.5% to 4% of transsphenoidal surgeries, and is typically corrected via reconstruction of the sellar floor with subcutaneous fat harvested from the abdomen or thigh. A temporary lumbar drain may be required if the CSF leak is persistent. Other complications, including carotid artery injury, intracranial hemorrhage, epistaxis, visual deficits, meningitis, and other central nervous system injuries occur in < 1% of cases when surgery is performed by a highly experienced neurosurgeon. Mortality rates range from 0.2% to 1.2%.

As acute adrenal insufficiency is a common complication, patients are either treated with stress dose glucocorticoids perioperatively or closely monitored for steroid sufficiency. The glucocorticoid dose is tapered based on the patient's hemodynamic status after surgery. If steroids can be successfully weaned to physiologic doses (prednisone 5 mg or hydrocortisone 20-30 mg daily), then a morning serum cortisol should be obtained prior to discharge to determine optimal dosing. Steroids can be stopped if the serum cortisol is > 10 μg/dL. However, if the morning serum cortisol is <10 μg/dL, then glucocorticoids should be continued and a morning serum cortisol repeated 1 week postoperatively.

Within 24 to 48 hours of surgery, reduction in ADH secretion may lead to diabetes insipidus. Approximately 7 to 12 days postoperatively, this may be followed by the syndrome of inappropriate ADH secretion (SIADH), presumably because of release of preformed ADH from the posterior pituitary. If damage to the hypothalamus or pituitary stalk is permanent, then posterior pituitary stores of ADH are not replenished, and diabetes insipidus may relapse. This postsurgical response has been called the triple phase response: diabetes insipidus, SIADH, and diabetes insipidus again. Close monitoring of electrolytes is therefore imperative following surgery. Patients with acromegaly often have significant polyuria following surgery, reflecting appropriate diuresis of the associated volume overload. However, if polyuria and hypernatremia develop in acromegaly patients postoperatively, this suggests diabetes insipidus, not physiologic diuresis.

Diabetes insipidus is characterized by polyuria (>3 L/d) and polydipsia. It is diagnosed based on a low urine osmolality (<250 mosmol/kg) in the setting of a high serum osmolality (>290 mosmol/kg) in the absence of hyperglycemia. When fluids are withheld or the thirst mechanism is impaired, then hypernatremia can also occur. Treatment consists of intravenous fluid replacement and administration of desmopressin (DDAVP) to control polyuria. Urine output, urine osmolality, and serum sodium should be closely monitored to help adjust fluids and DDAVP dosing. As diabetes insipidus may be a transient postoperative phenomenon, the need for continued DDAVP should be reassessed on an ongoing basis.

SIADH is diagnosed when hyponatremia is associated with a low plasma osmolality and an inappropriately normal to high urine osmolality (at least >100 mosmol/kg). Typically, the urine sodium concentration exceeds 40 mEq/L. Other causes of hyponatremia in the postoperative setting include central adrenal insufficiency, central hypothyroidism, over-replacement with hypotonic fluids, and possibly cerebral salt wasting. Mild hyponatremia (eg, 130-135 mmol/L) due to SIADH may be managed by restriction of free water. However, if the patient has symptomatic or severe hyponatremia (ie, <125 mmol/L), then more aggressive management with hypertonic saline or vasopressin antagonists (vaptans) may be required. Vasopressin receptor antagonists can increase the plasma sodium more rapidly than hypertonic saline and therefore may be considered in selected patients.

DISCHARGE CHECKLIST FOR PITUITARY DISEASE

- Follow-up appointments: Does the patient with a hypersecretory syndrome or hypopituitarism have a follow-up appointment with endocrinology? Does the patient who underwent neurosurgery have follow-up arranged with neurosurgery and endocrinology?
- Follow-up laboratory tests: If the patient is being discharged on DDAVP, has the patient been advised to have a serum sodium checked in 1 to 2 weeks?
- Patient education: Has the patient with adrenal insufficiency been counseled on adrenal sick day rules? Does the patient have extra glucocorticoid tablets and medic alert identification?

SUGGESTED READINGS

Agha A, Sherlock M, Brennan S, et al. Hypothalamic-pituitary dysfunction after irradiation of nonpituitary brain tumors in adults. *J Clin Endocrinol Metab*. 2005;90:6355-6360.

Dumont AS, Nemergut EC 2nd, Jane JA Jr, Laws ER Jr. Postoperative care following pituitary surgery. *J Intensive Care Med*. 2005;20:127-240.

Fish LH, Schwartz HL, Cavanaugh J, Steffes MW, Bantle JP, Oppenheimer JH. Replacement dose, metabolism, and bioavailability of levothyroxine in the treatment of hypothyroidism. *N Engl J Med*. 1987;316:764-770.

Freda PU, Beckers AM, Katznelson L, et al. Pituitary incidentaloma: an endocrine society clinical practice guideline. *J Clin Endocrinol Metab*. 2011;96:894-904.

Grinspoon SK, Biller BM. Laboratory assessment of adrenal insufficiency. *J Clin Endocrinol Metab*. 1994;79:923-931.

Jahangiri A, Wagner J, Tran MT, et al. Factors predicting postoperative hyponatremia and efficacy of hyponatremia management strategies after more than 1000 pituitary operations. *J Neurosurg*. 2013;119:1478-1483.

Katznelson L, Laws ER, Melmed S, et al. Acromegaly: an endocrine society clinical practice guideline. *J Clin Endocrinol Metab*. 2014;99:3933-3951.

Melmed S, Casanueva FF, Hoffman AR, et al. Diagnosis and treatment of hyperprolactinemia: an endocrine society clinical practice guideline. *J Clin Endocrinol Metab*. 2011;96:273-288.

Nieman LK, Biller BM, Finding JW, et al. The diagnosis of Cushing's syndrome: an Endocrine Society clinical practice guidelines. *J Clin Endocrinol Metab*. 2008;93:1526-1540.

Schneider HJ, Kreitschmann-Andermahr H, Ghigo E, Stalla GK, Agha A. Hypothalmopituitary dysfunction following traumatic brain injury and aneurysmal subarachnoid hemorrhage: a systematic review. *JAMA*. 2007;298:1429-1438.

SECTION 5

Gastroenterology

155

GERD and Esophagitis

Walter W. Chan, MD, MPH
Robert Burakoff, MD, MPH

Key Clinical Questions

❶ What is the approach to patients presenting with reflux, heartburn, or noncardiac chest pain?

❷ How should patients with esophagitis and gastroesophageal reflux disease (GERD) be managed in the inpatient setting?

❸ What are the possible complications resulting from esophagitis and GERD?

INTRODUCTION

Gastroesophageal reflux disease (GERD) and other esophageal disorders account for a significant number of physician office visits, hospital admissions, and endoscopic procedures each year. Annual management costs for GERD alone have been estimated to exceed $9 billion and continue to escalate. Gastroesophageal reflux disease results from the backflowing of gastroduodenal contents into the esophagus, leading to a variety of symptoms including heartburn, chest discomfort, regurgitation, and dysphagia. Compromise in the physiological barrier of reflux at the gastroesophageal junction is believed to be the primary mechanism of reflux. Esophagitis is defined as the presence of signs of inflammation of the esophageal mucosal surfaces, both macroscopically and microscopically. Gastroesophageal reflux disease is the most common cause of esophagitis, followed closely by medication-induced and infection-induced inflammation. Symptoms of esophagitis may range from mild chest discomfort to significant dysphagia and odynophagia.

EPIDEMIOLOGY

Epidemiological studies have shown that approximately 25% of the Western population report having symptoms of heartburn at least once a month, with up to 5% noting daily symptoms. While the prevalence of heartburn symptoms appears to be similar in both genders, female patients less likely possess objective findings of reflux on physiological studies. Moreover, numerous clinical studies have shown a lower response rate to antireflux treatment for female patients. No definite relationship between age and GERD has been concluded. At least one study has suggested less reflux symptoms in older individuals. However, elderly also seem to possess more severe esophagitis, suggesting a higher prevalence of asymptomatic reflux. An increase in body mass index both causes reflux and exacerbates existing symptoms.

PRESENTATION

Gastroesophageal reflux disease most typically presents as heartburn, regurgitation, and dysphagia. Patients often describe heartburn as a retrosternal, "burning" discomfort in the lower chest or epigastric region that often travels up toward the neck region. Symptoms often worsen after meals or when patients are in a supine position. As a result, patients may complain of symptoms or exacerbation of symptoms at night that may wake them up from sleep. Physiological studies suggest that gastric distention caused by meals and sleep can each induce transient relaxation of the lower esophageal sphincter (LES), leading to episodes of reflux. Dysphagia is a common symptom of GERD, and it is often a result of refluxate-induced esophageal mucosal inflammation or dysmotility. However, it is also one of the "alarming" signs of GERD that indicate the need for further evaluation to exclude possible underlying malignancy. Other "alarming" signs of GERD include odynophagia, weight loss, signs of gastrointestinal (GI) bleeding, advanced age, and a family history of upper GI tract malignancy. When one or more of the "alarming" signs are present, further evaluation with endoscopy or other radiographic imaging should be considered.

- "Alarming" signs of GERD include dysphagia, odynophagia, weight loss, signs of gastrointestinal bleeding, advanced age, and a family history of upper GI tract malignancy. When any is present, further evaluation with endoscopy or other radiographic imaging is indicated.

In addition to the typical esophageal presentation, GERD may also cause a variety of atypical, extraesophageal manifestations. Coexisting pulmonary disease with GERD occurs commonly, with the diagnosis established in 40% to 80% of asthmatics. Although airway irritation resulting from microaspiration of refluxed contents has been implicated as a possible trigger for asthma, certain medications used for asthma, such as bronchodilators, may also cause transient LES relaxation. Consistent treatment benefit for asthma has not been demonstrated using acid-suppression medications or anti-reflux surgery. Nevertheless, GERD likely plays a role in the pathogenesis of pulmonary disorders such as asthma, chronic bronchitis, bronchiectasis, aspiration pneumonia, and pulmonary fibrosis, as well as upper airway manifestations such as pharyngitis, laryngitis, or postnasal drip. Some studies have shown worsened clinical course of these pulmonary and airway disorders in patients with GERD. Oral problems such as dental erosions, halitosis, and aphthous ulcers have also been linked to GERD.

Patients with GERD or esophagitis may also present with noncardiac chest pain, often described by patients as nonspecific retrosternal discomfort. Such chest discomfort may be a result of direct irritation by the refluxate, mucosal inflammation, or esophageal spasm or dysmotility. Gastroesophageal reflux disease may mimic other causes of chest pain such as acute coronary syndrome or pulmonary disorders. Noncardiac chest pain resulting from esophageal disorders is a common presentation leading to emergency room visits and hospital admission for further workup.

PATHOPHYSIOLOGY

GERD

The lower esophageal sphincter, a tonic smooth muscle located in the lower esophagus around the gastroesophageal junction, serves as the major barrier to reflux of gastric content into the esophagus. Disruption in the tonic contractile pressure of the LES may result in the backflowing of gastric content into the esophagus. Such a disruption may present in the form of a general decrease in the tonic pressure of the LES (hypotensive LES) or inappropriate relaxation of the LES not during swallowing (pathologic transient LES relaxation). Many factors have been associated with disruption of the tonic contraction of the LES. For example, a hiatal hernia leads to anatomic disruption of the gastroesophageal junction and is associated with an increased risk of transient LES relaxation. Certain medications such as sedatives, food items such as caffeine and chocolate, and lifestyle behavior including alcohol and tobacco use can also lead to increased LES relaxation, resulting in GERD symptoms. In addition to LES relaxation, the barrier between the stomach and esophagus may also be pathologically overcome if the intragastric pressure exceeds the tonic contractile pressure of the LES. Most commonly, this situation results from obesity, delayed gastric emptying, or certain postoperative states, such as gastric bands for weight loss.

While GERD symptoms are often thought to be a result of the presence of acidic gastric content in the esophagus, leading to burning sensation and inflammation, the backflow of nonacidic contents such as bile may also generate similar symptoms. Since certain diagnostic modalities including pH study and the use of acid-suppression medications for treatment of GERD targets the presence of acid in the esophagus, nonacid reflux should be considered in patients who do not respond to common medical therapy for GERD symptoms.

ESOPHAGITIS

Esophagitis presents with inflammatory changes in the esophageal mucosa, with or without signs of erosion. The inflammatory reactions in the esophagus can be elicited by direct caustic injury, most commonly by acid, trauma, infection, or autoimmune processes. In the case of reflux-induced esophagitis, the diffusion of hydrogen ions into the esophageal mucosa leads to cellular acidification and necrosis. As a result, erosion and inflammatory cells infiltration ensue. Caustic injuries may also be caused by direct erosion or chemical reactions between the substance and the esophageal mucosa.

- Sedative medications, caffeine, chocolate, alcohol, or tobacco each can lead to LES relaxation, resulting in GERD symptoms. Medications that can cause a decrease in LES pressure include beta adrenergic agonists, -adrenergic antagonists, anticholinergics, benzodiazepines, calcium channel blockers, narcotics, progesterone, estrogens, and tricyclic antidepressants.

DIFFERENTIAL DIAGNOSIS

GERD

A variety of risk factors have been linked to GERD. Certain medications may cause a decrease in LES pressure, including β-adrenergic agonists, α-adrenergic antagonists, anticholinergics, benzodiazepines, calcium channel blockers, narcotics, progesterone, estrogens, and tricyclic antidepressants. Lifestyle behaviors such as smoking, alcohol ingestions, and food ingestion prior to incumbency have been linked to GERD symptoms. Some food items and beverages can also cause heartburn symptoms by reducing LES pressure. Examples include fatty food, chocolate, citrus fruits, tomato-based products, peppermint, vinegar, carbonated drinks, and caffeinated beverages.

In addition to lifestyle behavior and ingestions, other known risk factors for GERD include obesity, gastroparesis, certain surgical procedures, and hiatal hernia. Obesity may lead to an increase in intra-abdominal pressure that can cause LES relaxation. Gastroparesis causes intragastric distention, which may in turn activate stretch receptors of the stomach, resulting in decrease in LES pressure.

ESOPHAGITIS

Inflammation of the esophagus is most commonly related to GERD. Other risk factors for the development of esophagitis include medication, infection, radiation, or less common causes such as autoimmune disorders. Medication-induced esophagitis ("pill esophagitis") results from direct, caustic injury to the esophageal mucosa. Common examples include alendronate, aspirin, nonsteroidal anti-inflammatory drugs, iron salts, potassium chloride tablets, quinidine, and tetracycline. However, any medication or foreign object can lead to direct injury and erosion into the esophageal mucosa if its transit through the esophagus is prolonged.

Infectious esophagitis usually occurs in immunocompromised hosts such as patients with acquired immune deficiency syndrome, post-transplantation, or undergoing chemotherapy. The most common etiologies for infectious esophagitis are fungal and viral infections. Esophageal candidiasis is one of the most common opportunistic infections in immunocompromised patients (**Figure 155-1**). Often, it represents the initial presentation leading

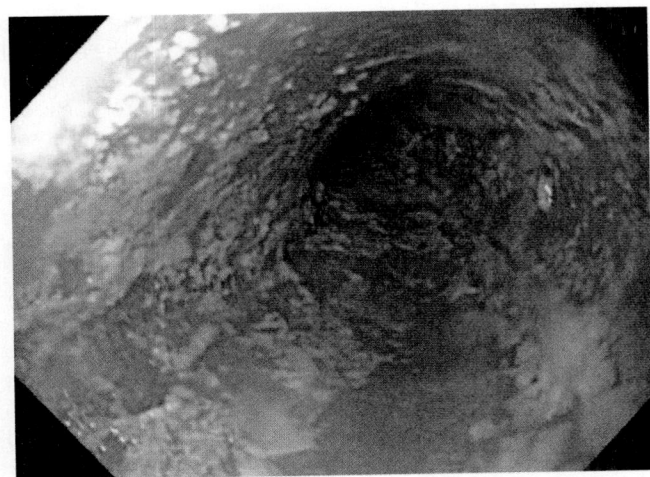

Figure 155-1 *Endoscopy revealing candida esophagitis.*

to the diagnosis of HIV infection, and candida esophagitis (unlike simple thrush alone) is an acquired immune deficiency syndrome defining illness. Patients with esophageal candidiasis usually complain of dysphagia and occasionally odynophagia. Esophageal candidiasis typically appears as whitish plaques on the esophageal mucosa that are easily scrapped off and oropharyngeal disease (thrush) often coexist. Therefore, in immunosuppressed patients who present with dysphagia, an oral examination may provide clues to possible esophageal candidiasis. Empiric treatment with antifungals may be considered in these high-risk patients. The most common agents causing viral esophagitis are human herpes simplex virus (HSV) and cytomegalovirus (CMV). Similar to fungal candidiasis, HSV and CMV esophagitis often present with dysphagia and odynophagia, although odynophagia presents more commonly in these cases. Concomitant oropharyngeal disease often occurs. Diagnosis requires endoscopic visualization of the typical HSV or CMV ulcers.

■ CANDIDA ESOPHAGITIS

Cancer patients with prior chest radiation therapy may also develop radiation-induced esophagitis. Symptom-onset can be immediate (within 3 weeks) or delayed (usually 3 or more months), with significant variation in the severity often unrelated to the dosage of radiation received. Symptoms range from mild dysphagia to severe odynophagia or stricturing requiring enteral tube feeding. As these patients are often also immunocompromised from chemotherapy, infectious esophagitis may coexist and must first be ruled out or treated.

Patients with a history of hematologic malignancy who have undergone bone marrow transplantation may develop graft-versus-host disease, which can involve any part of the gastrointestinal tract. Graft-versus-host disease of the esophagus often leads to significant inflammation and ulceration, resulting in symptoms of dysphagia, odynophagia, or bleeding. Therefore, this diagnosis must be considered in bone marrow transplant patients presenting with upper gastrointestinal bleeding or new-onset dysphagia symptoms, and mucosal biopsies should be obtained to establish the diagnosis. Similar to other cancer patients, infectious esophagitis is also very prevalent in this population and may coexist with graft-versus-host disease due to chronic immunosuppression.

Autoimmune disorders remain an uncommon cause of esophagitis. Inflammatory diseases such as Crohn's disease or Behçet's disease may involve the esophagus, leading to inflammation and often ulcerations. Eosinophilic esophagitis, another immune-mediated esophageal disorder, appears to be increasing in incidence in recent years. It is characterized by the infiltration of large numbers of eosinophils (>15 per high-powered field) in the esophageal

mucosa. Etiology of eosinophilic esophagitis remains unclear; however, it is often linked to other allergic disorders such as asthma or dermatitis. Patients with eosinophilic esophagitis are often young and they often first present with an episode of food impaction. While eosinophilic esophagitis can be associated with characteristic endoscopic appearances, its diagnosis requires histopathologic confirmation of eosinophilic infiltration. In recent years, a subset of patients with increased eosinophilic infiltration in the esophageal mucosa has been found to respond, both clinically and histologically, to proton pump inhibitor (PPI) therapy. This condition is now separately classified as PPI-responsive esophageal eosinophilia (PPI-REE). The etiology of PPI-REE is unclear, as most patients do not report GERD symptoms. Patients with PPI-REE are clinically, endoscopically, and histologically indistinguishable from patients with eosinophilic esophagitis, with response to PPI therapy being the only differentiating factor. Therefore, the most recent management guidelines from the American College of Gastroenterology suggest that patients found to have esophageal eosinophilia should first undergo a PPI trial of at least 8 weeks in duration. Repeat endoscopy with biopsies should then be performed to assess response to the PPI and classify patients into PPI-REE versus eosinophilic esophagitis.

DIAGNOSIS

■ ACID SUPPRESSION AS A DIAGNOSTIC TOOL

Gastroesophageal reflux disease diagnosis is most frequently achieved through history of classic symptoms combined with response to empiric antacid medical therapy, most commonly a PPI. A meta-analysis of studies on the diagnostic value of PPI response in GERD revealed a pooled sensitivity of 78% and specificity of 54% (likelihood ratio 1:70). In most cases, no further diagnostic testing is needed in patients with typical GERD symptoms who have no alarming signs that resolve with a therapeutic trial. However, patients who fail to respond to a trial of PPI or report alarm signs should undergo further diagnostic workup, including endoscopy, radiographic imaging, or physiologic testing such as manometry, impedance, and pH studies.

■ UPPER ENDOSCOPY

Upper endoscopy or esophagogastroduodenoscopy serves as an appropriate initial evaluation of GERD as it allows direct visualization

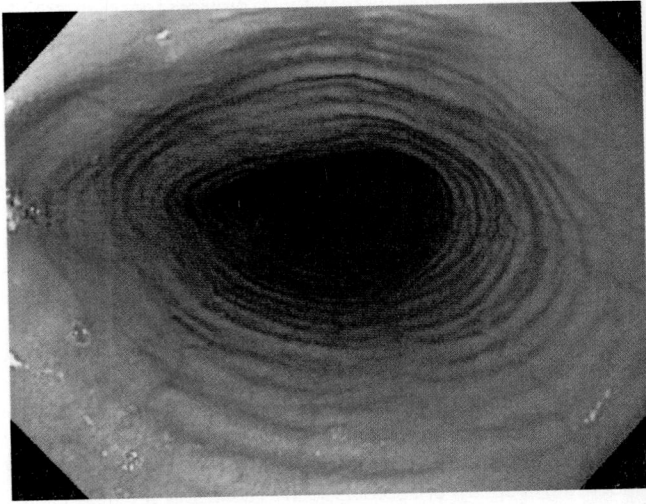

Figure 155-2 *Eosinophilic esophagitis. Findings of longitudinal markings and concentric rings in the middle third of the esophagus ("feline esophagus") consistent with eosinophilic esophagitis. Biopsies obtained revealed infiltration of >40 eosinophils/hpf.*

of the esophageal mucosa to exclude the presence of other diseases such as tumors and evaluate for signs and severity of GERD-induced esophagitis. The Los Angeles classification, the most commonly used system in the endoscopic grading of severity of reflux esophagitis, measures the length and circumferential involvement of mucosal breaks and assigns the findings into four different grades (A-D). In addition to evaluation of esophagitis, endoscopy also allows the diagnosis of complications from GERD, including strictures or the presence of Barrett's esophagus. Endoscopic dilation may be performed at the time of identification of strictures. Overall, endoscopy has been shown to exhibit high specificity (>90%) for the diagnosis of GERD but only a moderate sensitivity (~50%). The lack of endoscopic signs of GERD does not exclude its diagnosis. Previous studies have shown that many symptomatic patients with negative initial studies develop mucosal lesions during follow-up endoscopic examinations. Therefore, symptomatic patients with negative endoscopies should undergo further diagnostic workup.

■ RADIOGRAPHIC STUDIES

Radiographic studies such as barium swallow or upper GI series can also be used to detect esophagitis, hiatal hernias, esophageal strictures, or tumors. The primary goal of these studies is to exclude other significant diseases in patients with low clinical suspicion for them. Although they have the advantage of being noninvasive, inexpensive, and widely available, they are less sensitive and specific and should only be used over upper endoscopy if no endoscopist is available or if the patient cannot tolerate an endoscopic procedure.

■ MOTILITY STUDIES

Several kinds of motility studies have been used for the workup of reflux disease. **Ambulatory esophageal pH monitoring** records the distal esophageal pH continuously using a transnasal probe or a pill-sized capsule (Bravo capsule) placed 5 cm above the LES. A battery-powered device carried by the patient records data from the probe, as well as the time of meals and symptom-onset. This allows correlation between patient-reported symptoms and objective signs of acid exposure in the distal esophagus, described as symptom association probability (SAP) or symptom index (SI). SAP > 95% or SI > 50% indicates significant association between symptoms and acid exposure. A pH < 4 measured by the probe is defined as acid exposure. In normal individuals, the total amount of time with esophageal pH < 4 (total acid exposure time) over a day should be less than 4%. Although esophageal pH monitoring provides the most sensitive test for identifying presence of acid in the esophagus, its use should be reserved for selected patients: those with symptoms refractory to therapy, atypical symptoms unresponsive to acid suppression, or history of antireflux surgery, or those undergoing preoperative evaluation for antireflux surgery or lung transplantation.

Esophageal manometry measures the strength, duration, and sequential nature of esophageal smooth muscle contraction. An array of pressure sensors along a small catheter passed through the nose into the esophagus and stomach measures the esophageal body contraction, as well as the resting pressure and relaxation of the LES. With each swallow, different pattern of muscle contraction along the probe allows identification of the presence of any motility abnormalities, LES hypotension, or transient relaxation. This test is particularly important as a part of the preoperative evaluation for antireflux surgery. In addition to obtaining valuable information regarding LES pressure, manometry also identifies patients with underlying esophageal disorders such as achalasia or diffuse esophageal spasm that would be a contraindication to fundoplication.

Impedance monitoring is a technique in measuring bolus transit through the esophagus. Similar to manometry, it contains a small, flexible catheter placed through the nose into the esophagus.

In GERD patients, impedance can identify fluid bolus refluxing into the esophagus, regardless of its acidity, and measure the extent of reflux. The combined impedance-pH monitoring device can further classify the refluxed fluid bolus as acidic, weakly acidic, or nonacidic. Newer versions of these catheters may also have additional sensors located more proximally, up to the oropharynx, to help identify proximal or pharyngeal reflux.

TRIAGE AND HOSPITAL ADMISSION

Although GERD and esophagitis can cause significant morbidity for patients, they are still generally managed in the outpatient setting. In rare instances, patients who cannot tolerate oral diet due to significant dysphagia or odynophagia caused by severe esophagitis may require hospitalization for nutritional support. These patients may demonstrate clinical signs of significant dehydration, including hypotension and tachycardia. In the setting of prolonged poor nutritional status, clinical signs related to deficiency of other nutritional elements such as folate and certain vitamins may also be present. In these cases, intravenous hydration need to be initiated, and other forms of nutritional support such as tube feeding or total parenteral nutrition may need to be considered.

Hospital admission in patients presenting with GERD or esophagitis-related symptoms may be required to rule out other significant illnesses. Certain GERD and esophagitis symptoms may mimic more significant cardiovascular diseases such as acute coronary syndrome. Patients presenting with chest discomfort should undergo careful cardiac evaluation, and the diagnosis of GERD and esophagitis should not be assumed until cardiac causes can be ruled out.

MANAGEMENT
■ SYMPTOMATIC MANAGEMENT

Treatment of patients with GERD or esophagitis should control the symptoms as well as heal esophageal inflammation. Management of GERD and reflux esophagitis focuses on eliminating acid exposure to the esophagus using both pharmacological (antacid and antisecretory agents) and surgical means. Over-the-counter antacids neutralize refluxed gastric acid, are inexpensive and convenient, and may be used as short-term treatment for patients with occasional symptoms.

H_2 blockers inhibit gastric acid secretion by competitively binding the H_2 receptors on gastric parietal cells. They prevent heartburn symptoms when taken before meals and relieve postprandial heartburn if taken after meals. In patients with frequent GERD symptoms, twice daily H_2 blockers may be required for maximal effects. H_2 blockers offer a 10% to 24% therapeutic gain over placebo in healing mild-to-moderate esophagitis, but are not effective in healing moderate to severe esophagitis. No differences in efficacy among the different H_2 blockers have been found. If a patient remains symptomatic after 6 weeks of standard dose, twice daily H_2 blocker therapy, increased dose or prolonged therapy do not appear to provide additional relief.

Proton pump inhibitors directly block the hydrogen-potassium ATPase on the apical surface of the parietal cells and act on a more downstream pathway than H_2 blockers to decrease acid secretion. Compared to H_2 blockers, PPIs have greater effectiveness in treating esophagitis after 4 to 8 weeks of therapy. All first-generation PPIs (all except esomeprazole) have similar effects on healing of esophagitis and gastric acidity. Esomeprazole has been shown to have a statistically significant advantage in average gastric pH and percentage of time with nonacidic pH when compared to other PPIs after 5 days of therapy. However, no objective evidence has demonstrated any significant benefit of esomeprazole over other PPIs in symptoms-control or esophagitis healing. The timing of PPI use is important as its efficacy depends on the presence of proton pumps on the parietal cells. Therefore, PPIs should be taken during fasting state approximately 30 minutes before meals to allow for maximal effects.

While short-term side effects associated with PPI use are rare and relatively mild, increasing evidence have emerged over the past few years suggesting that prolonged use of PPI may have long-term, systemic consequences. Malabsorption, including vitamin B12 and vitamin D, osteoporosis, *Clostridium difficile* colitis, community-acquired pneumonia, and symptomatic small intestinal bacterial overgrowth have all been linked to chronic PPI use. Concerns regarding absorption and treatment effects of certain medications have also been raised in patients with concurrent PPI use. In particular, the concomitant use of PPI and clopidogrel has been under intense scrutiny given the large number of cardiac patients taking clopidogrel who also require PPI therapy. Several in vitro studies have demonstrated evidence of a decrease in efficacy of clopidogrel with PPI using serum markers for platelet response, leading the Food and Drug Administration (FDA) to issue a warning advising the avoidance of certain PPI and clopidogrel coadministration. A large number of nonrandomized, observational clinical studies have been published, with the results ranging from no clinical effect to a mild-to-moderate increase in clinical events such as recurrent MI or hospitalization. The only large, randomized trial studying the effect of PPI (omeprazole) versus placebo on clinical outcome in 3761 patients taking clopidogrel (COGENT) demonstrated no difference in cardiovascular events (HR 1.02, 95% CI: 0.70-1.51), but a significant decrease in GI events (HR 0.55, 95% CI: 0.36-0.85). Furthermore, a meta-analysis published in April, 2010 showed no significant association between concomitant PPI-clopidogrel use and overall mortality (RR 1.09, 95% CI: 0.94-1.26). A more recent systematic review and meta-analysis published in January, 2015 demonstrated higher ischemic event rates with coadministration of clopidogrel with PPI (as a class) among observational studies, but no increase in ischemic events among four randomized controlled trials studying omeprazole-clopidogrel coadministration. Given the short half-life of both PPI and clopidogrel, some experts have suggested that separating their intake by 12 to 20 hours (eg, one taken before breakfast and the other before bedtime) should, in theory, minimize any potential clinical interaction. Regardless, the use of PPI should be judicious in light of evidence of potential long-term side effects, and dose-reduction or discontinuation should be considered after symptom-control or mucosal healing has been achieved.

Other pharmacological agents studied for the management of GERD, especially in those with nonacidic or weakly acidic reflux, include baclofen, which has been found to be effective in inhibiting transient lower esophageal sphincter relaxation, thereby decreasing acid reflux. However, the use of baclofen has been limited by its short half-life and poor patient tolerability.

While most patients achieve adequate treatment response with pharmacotherapy, some may experience symptoms refractory to acid suppression or wish to discontinue medication use. In these cases, barrier enhancing antireflux therapy either surgically or endoscopically can be attempted. Antireflux surgeries have been safely performed since the 1950s, and the advance of laparoscopic approach further decreases the complication rate and postoperative hospital stay. Nissen fundoplication, either open or laparoscopic, involves enhancing the pressure at the LES region by wrapping and attaching part of the gastric fundus around the distal esophagus. Studies have shown a symptom response of 80% to 90% postoperatively. However, long-term studies demonstrated that the majority of patients experience recurrent symptoms and require acid-suppression medications again

within 10 years. Complication rate of fundoplication ranges from 5% to 20%, most commonly due to dysphagia, chest pain, gas-bloat syndrome, flatulence, and vagal nerve injuries. Dysphagia remains the most commonly encountered complication from fundoplication. It may occur early in 0% to 20% of patients, or late in up to 6% of patients at 2 years. Preoperative physiologic studies including manometry and pH testing can help identify patients with higher likelihood of positive or negative outcomes. Increased LES relaxation and positive pH testing results are positive predictors of fundoplication outcome, while patients with normal pH testing or normal LES pressure are less likely to respond to fundoplication. In addition, patients with advanced spastic esophageal disorders or signs of achalasia on manometry are contraindicated for surgery given the high risk of postoperative dysphagia.

A new surgical antireflux procedure has been approved by the FDA involving the placement of a bracelet with magnetic beads at the gastroesophageal junction. Magnetic force approximates the beads and tightens the bracelet, thereby enhancing the barrier at the gastroesophageal junction against refluxing of gastric contents. These magnetic beads are separated by the propulsive force from esophageal peristalsis during swallows, allowing the opening of the bracelet and passage of ingested food bolus through the gastroesophageal junction. Clinical studies have demonstrated this procedure to be effective and a safe alternative to traditional fundoplication in selected patients, although further studies are needed to assess the long-term efficacy and safety of this procedure.

Obesity has been increasingly recognized as an etiologic factor in GERD. Weight loss, through both surgical and nonsurgical strategies, has been shown to improve GERD and related symptoms. Therefore, in obese patients, weight loss surgery with Roux-en-Y gastric bypass may be preferred over traditional antireflux surgery in management of GERD symptoms. The selection of the type of bariatric surgery in GERD patients should be careful, as certain strategies, particularly gastric banding, have been associated with increased reflux.

NUTRITIONAL SUPPORT

In rare cases of patients with significant esophagitis causing severe dysphagia or odynophagia, nutritional support may be needed due to their inability to tolerate adequate oral diet or hydration. Enteral feeding and hydration through a gastrostomy or jejeunostomy tube may be required. Intravenous hydration or parenteral nutrition may be needed in certain patients with severe malnutrition or other concurrent gastrointestinal disorder. Clinicians should pay particular attention to any signs of deficiency of specific elements such as vitamin B12, vitamin D, and calcium and the need for replacement.

LONGITUDINAL/OUTPATIENT THERAPEUTICS

Outpatient care of patients with GERD or esophagitis focuses on medical treatment of underlying disorders as well as lifestyle modification. Acid-suppression medications, such as PPI or H_2 receptor antagonists, are the mainstay of therapy as described above. Once symptoms resolve or esophagitis heal, dosages of acid-suppression medications may be slowly tapered as tolerated. Lifestyle modifications remain a cornerstone of GERD treatment. Avoiding foods and acid-containing beverages that exacerbate their symptoms should be advocated. Patients should be educated about not lying down after eating for at least 3 hours to avoid refluxing of ingested food. Similarly, eating smaller and frequent meals can help decrease GERD symptoms. For patients with significant nocturnal reflux, elevation of the head of the bed to 30° to 45° angle can help reduce nocturnal symptoms. Such elevation may be achieved by placing blocks underneath the front feet of the bed or triangular wedge underneath the mattress. In addition, avoidance of alcohol or tobacco use may reduce GERD symptoms or esophagitis. Weight loss in overweight or obese patients is also a significant part of GERD management.

■ INFECTIOUS ESOPHAGITIS

Treatment strategy for infectious etiologies of esophagitis can be broadly divided into acute eradication and prevention of recurrence. In patients with acute, symptomatic infectious esophagitis, antimicrobial therapy should be initiated and targeted toward the organism responsible. Determination of the duration of therapy, mode of administration (oral vs parenteral), and choice of antimicrobial agent should depend on a combination of factors including the patients' symptoms, other medical comorbidities, and underlying immune function. Intravenous administration may be needed in those with significant odynophagia or patients who are acutely ill or severely immunosuppressed. Increased treatment duration and more potent agents should also be considered in these patients.

Patients with suspected or diagnosed esophageal candidiasis may be initially treated with a 14-day course of fluconazole (400 mg loading dose on first day followed by 200 mg daily on subsequent days), administered orally or intravenously. Fungal esophagitis unresponsive to fluconazole may require more potent antifungals such as amphotericin and should be managed with input from infectious diseases specialists. First-line therapy for HSV esophagitis in immunosuppressed patients involves a course of acyclovir (5 mg/kg IV every 8 hours for 7-14 days or 400 mg PO five times daily for 7-10 days), while CMV esophagitis requires the use of ganciclovir (5 mg/kg IV every 12 hours or 900 mg daily or twice daily) for 3 to 6 weeks. More potent antivirals such as foscarnet may be necessary in cases unresponsive to first-line agents and infectious diseases specialists should be involved in management of these cases. Herpes simplex virus or CMV esophagitis in immunocompetent hosts usually resolve without treatment after 1 to 2 weeks. Experience with orogenital HSV suggests that antiviral treatments may hasten symptom recovery. Therefore, some clinicians suggest treating immunocompetent patients with a shorter course of therapy.

■ COMPLICATIONS AND PROGNOSIS

Complications from chronic GERD can be divided by the sites of manifestations: esophageal versus extra-esophageal. Esophageal complications include ulcers, erosions, strictures, Barrett's esophagus, and malignancy. Extra-esophageal complications mainly involve upper airway or pulmonary manifestations of aspirated gastric contents.

Esophageal ulcers may result from esophagitis caused by chronic GERD or impacted foreign bodies. They may account for up to 2% of all upper GI bleeding. However, the vast majority heal completely with acid suppressive medications. Chronic GERD and esophagitis may also lead to peptic esophageal strictures, which have been described in up to 10% of patients seeking medical attention for reflux symptoms. Patients with strictures usually present with dysphagia to solid food but can tolerate fluid without difficulties. Weight loss is uncommon and malignancy needs to be ruled out when present. Treatment for peptic strictures involves a combination of acid-suppression therapy and endoscopic dilation. Food and foreign body impaction is another common complication for patients with esophageal strictures or significant esophagitis. In addition to reflux esophagitis, another form commonly associated with food impaction is eosinophilic esophagitis. Treatment strategies for eosinophilic esophagitis include the use of topical steroids (swallowed fluticasone or budesonide slurry) or an elimination diet.

Chronic GERD may also predispose patients to the development of Barrett's esophagus and esophageal adenocarcinoma. Barrett's esophagus is the metaplastic change of the esophageal lining due to chronic reflux injury and esophagitis. It involves the replacement of the normal squamous epithelium of the distal esophagus with specialized intestinal metaplasia. Such metaplastic change may protect the esophagus against further injury by gastric acid, but it also increases the risk for esophageal adenocarcinoma. The prevalence of Barrett's esophagus in GERD patients is approximately 5% to 10%. Caucasians, male, and middle-aged patients are more commonly affected. Other risk factors for Barrett's esophagus include tobacco and alcohol use. The exact risk of esophageal adenocarcinoma in patients with Barrett's esophagus remains debated, but is believed to be around 0.5% to 1%. The use of esophagogastroduodenoscopy to screen for Barrett's inpatients with a history of GERD symptoms remains controversial, as there is no direct clinical data to support the utility of screening. The American Gastroenterological Association recommended against screening of the general population with GERD for Barrett's in its most recent medical position statement published in 2014. However, it suggested screening for Barrett's among GERD patients with multiple risk factors for esophageal adenocarcinoma (male, age >50, white race, chronic GERD, hiatal hernia, elevated body mass index, and intra-abdominal distribution of body fat). Surveillance for signs of dysplastic changes should be performed periodically if a diagnosis of Barrett's has been confirmed on biopsy. Conservative treatment with continued surveillance remains the mainstay of therapy for Barrett's without dysplasia. For those with high-grade dysplasia present on biopsies, treatment strategy includes endoscopic ablative therapy or surgical resection. Treatment strategy for low-grade dysplasia remains controversial but involves ablative therapy or conservative surveillance. Acid control should be continued as part of medical therapy for Barrett's esophagus.

Extraesophageal complications of GERD may manifest in many forms, mainly resulting in pulmonary or upper airway abnormalities. GERD is believed to play a role in the pathogenesis of pulmonary disorders such as asthma, chronic bronchitis, bronchiectasis, aspiration pneumonia, and pulmonary fibrosis. Studies have also linked GERD to upper airway manifestations such as pharyngitis, laryngitis, or postnasal drip. Oral problems such as dental erosions, halitosis, and aphthous ulcers have also been associated with GERD. However, despite evidence of increased prevalence of these disorders in patients with GERD, treatment with acid-suppression medications has not consistently demonstrated clinical improvement in patients with these manifestations. Despite the lack of clear evidence, current clinical practice usually involves a workup for GERD in patients presenting with these disorders of unclear etiology or refractory to standard treatment.

The main goal of GERD and esophagitis treatment is to keep patients symptom-free with the least amount of acid-suppression medications that abates symptoms. Therefore, in patients who have responded to medical therapy or lifestyle changes, a trial of tapering and withdrawing medications should be attempted. In general, symptoms relief should be sustained for at least 2 to 3 weeks prior to the start of dosage tapering. Tapering should involve the sequential decrease in dosage or frequency for PPI, which may ultimately be switched to H_2 receptors antagonists. Abrupt withdrawal of PPI should be avoided as "rebound hypersecretion" may ensue when parietal cells secrete an elevated amount of acid after prolonged blockade. Adhering to lifestyle or dietary choices that decrease symptoms usually allows most motivated GERD patients to wean off medications. However, in patients with erosive esophagitis, relapse of symptoms and mucosal damage occurs in more than 80% of patients when therapy is stopped.

Patients with infectious esophagitis often respond well to first-line antimicrobial therapy. Those at highest risks of nonresponse are usually patients with profound immunosuppression. Clinical studies have demonstrated a decrease in Candida-, CMV-, or HSV-related diseases in immunosuppressed patients receiving respective prophylactic therapy. However, given the high acute treatment response rate, ease and low cost of therapy, and risk for development of drug resistance and sensitivity, long-term maintenance or secondary prophylaxis is not routinely recommended for infectious esophagitis, even in immunosuppressed patients. Some experts suggest consideration for maintenance therapy only in immunosuppressed patients with severe or frequent relapses of their infectious esophagitis.

■ DISCHARGE PLANNING

In the rare instances where patients were admitted for complications from their GERD or esophagitis, discharge planning mainly involves ensuring proper follow-up with a gastroenterology specialist, continuation of medical therapy, and patient education for secondary prevention. For patients with significant nutritional deficits requiring feeding tube placement, discharge planning should also include education on the proper use of the feeding tube, home nursing care or transfer to skilled nursing facilities, adequate equipment for continuation with tube-feeding after discharge, and instructions regarding caloric count. Follow-up for these patients should also include visits with a nutritionist for continued management of tube-feeding regimen. Educational materials regarding the prevention of recurrent GERD and esophagitis such as lifestyle modification strategies should be given, targeting their underlying etiologies.

■ QUALITY IMPROVEMENT

Secondary prevention

Secondary prevention plays a big role in the outpatient management of patients with GERD and esophagitis. Lifestyle modifications such as dietary and sleeping habits have been shown to be effective in decreasing symptoms in patients with GERD. In addition to providing educational materials, assistance from nutritionists and social workers may help patients achieve their lifestyle modification goals. Continued use of medications such as acid-suppression drugs may help prevent recurrent symptoms or development of complications. However, patients who adhere to lifestyle changes and achieve symptom relief should attempt a trial of medication weaning to allow maintenance on the lowest dose of medications possible. In patients with esophagitis, endoscopic surveillance to evaluate for mucosal healing aid in adjustment of medical therapy and in the evaluation of treatment efficacy, especially in other forms of esophagitis.

Transition of care

Patients with an initial diagnosis of GERD or esophagitis should continue care with a gastroenterology specialist for management of their diseases until symptoms resolve or condition stabilizes. Continued consultation with nutrition specialists may be needed for selected patients with ongoing GERD symptoms or difficulties adhering to lifestyle modifications. Certain underlying causes of esophagitis may require further care by other specialists, for example, patients found to have infectious esophagitis such as candidiasis or HSV may require further workup for underlying immunosuppression. Consultation with an allergy/immunology specialist should also be considered in patients diagnosed with eosinophilic esophagitis.

Outcomes to monitor

Symptoms resolution remains the main outcomes for monitoring in patients with GERD and esophagitis. Esophageal mucosal healing in patients with esophagitis, or endoscopic and pathologic evidence of resolution of underlying disease in patients with eosinophilic esophagitis, or Barrett's esophagus serve as other outcomes for monitoring and surveillance.

Costs and resource utilization

As the most common gastrointestinal disease, GERD also represents the most costly digestive disorder. The annual management cost of GERD has been estimated to exceed $9 billion. Much of the costs may be related to overuse of acid-suppression medications or unnecessary endoscopic or other diagnostic procedures. In both the primary care and inpatient settings, there have been signs of PPI overuse in the treatment of nonspecific gastrointestinal complaints. In addition, inappropriate use of high-dose PPI and lack of tapering or withdrawal strategies result in many patients being kept on more acid suppressive medications than they require. As stated above, empiric PPI should be used only in patients with signs and symptoms suggestive of GERD or esophagitis. Atypical symptoms or complaints should be thoroughly evaluated before PPI therapy is started. PPI tapering and withdrawal should be attempted in all patients with controlled symptoms. Lifestyle modification should be better promoted as its success often complements the tapering of medications. Endoscopic and other diagnostic procedures should be reserved for patients with atypical or alarming symptoms, or those who failed empiric PPI therapy (**Table 155-1**). Adherence to this strategy allows the delivery of the most cost-effective care for one of the most common and costly disorders today.

TABLE 155-1 Evidence-based Medicine Key References for GERD and Esophagitis

Study	Methodology	Results	Limitations	Bottom Line
Khan M, et al. *Cochrane Database Syst Rev.* 2007;2:CD003244	Cochrane review	• 137 treatment trials (36,978 patients) included • PPI superior to placebo (83% vs 18% at 8 wk, NNT = 1.7) and H2RA (84% vs 52%, RR = 0.51) for esophagitis healing • PPI superior to placebo (56% vs 8% at 4 wk, NNT = 2-3) and H2RA (77% vs 48% at 4-12 wk) for heartburn resolution	Pooled data with significant heterogeneity	PPI is superior to H2RA in the treatment of reflux esophagitis and heartburn symptoms
Locke GR, et al. *Gastroenterology.* 1997;112: 1448-1456	Population-based, observational, cohort	• 2200 Olmsted county residents aged 25-74 • 19.8% experienced at least weekly heartburn or acid regurgitation • Heartburn and acid regurgitation significantly associated with noncardiac chest pain (OR = 4.2), dysphagia (OR = 4.7), dyspepsia (OR = 3.1), and globus (OR = 1.9)	Single county patient population, questionnaire based	GERD is an important cause of noncardiac chest pain symptoms. Dysphagia, dyspepsia, and globus sensation are other manifestations of reflux

(Continued)

TABLE 155-1 Evidence-based Medicine Key References for GERD and Esophagitis (*Continued*)

Study	Methodology	Results	Limitations	Bottom Line
Bhatt DL, et al. *N Engl J Med*. 2010; 363(20):1909-1917	Randomized, placebo-controlled trial	• 3873 patients with indication for dual antiplatelet therapy • Randomized to clopidogrel with omeprazole or placebo • Omeprazole decreased GI bleeding rate compared to placebo (1.1% vs 2.9%, HR 0.18-0.63) • No difference in rate of cardiovascular event (4.9% vs 5.7%, HR 0.68-1.44)	Trial prematurely terminated due to loss of financing (planned enrollment = 5000 patients)	When used with clopidogrel, omeprazole decreased GI bleeding rate but showed no difference in cardiovascular event compared to placebo
av-Citrin O, et al. *Aliment Pharmacol Ther*. 2005;21:269-275	Prospective, controlled, observational	• 345 pregnant PPI users and 787 pregnant controls • No difference in rate of major congenital abnormalities: omeprazole (3.6%), lansoprazole (3.9%), and pantoprazole (2.1%) vs controls (3.8%)	Different doses of PPI	PPI does not represent a major teratogenic risk in humans
Mastronarde, et al. *N Engl J Med*. 2009 Apr 9;360(15):1487-1499	Randomized, placebo-controlled trial	• 412 patients with minimal to no reflux symptoms and inadequately controlled asthma randomly assigned to receive esomeprazole 40 mg BID or placebo for 24 wk • No difference in episodes of poor asthma control, pulmonary function, airway reactivity, symptoms score, nocturnal awakening, and quality of life.		PPI does not improve outcome of inadequately controlled asthma in patients with minimal to no reflux symptoms
Vakil, et al. *Aliment Pharmacol Ther*. 2003 Sep 15;18(6):559-568	Systematic review	• 32 trials comparing efficacy of different doses and formulations of PPI in the treatment of GERD and peptic ulcer disease • For GERD symptoms, all five PPI demonstrated similar efficacy after 1-2 wk of treatment, but lansoprazole and esomaprazole demonstrated faster symptom relief • Esomeprazole is superior in esophagitis healing	Pooled data with significant heterogeneity, inclusion of low-quality trials	All five PPIs are equally efficacious in treatment of GERD symptoms. Esomeprazole demonstrated slight superiority in healing esophagitis. Overall, there is insufficient evidence to establish the superiority of one agent over the others across all GERD-related complications

SUGGESTED READINGS

Bhatt DL, Cryer BL, Contant CF, et al. Clopidogrel with or without omeprazole in coronary artery disease. *N Engl J Med*. 2010;363(20):1909-1917.

Dellon ES, Gonsalves N, Hirano I, et al. ACG clinical guideline: evidenced based approach to the diagnosis and management of esophageal eosinophilia and eosinophilic esophagitis (EoE). *Am J Gastroenterol*. 2013;108(5):679-692.

Inadomi JM, Jamal R, Murata GH, et al. Step-down management of gastroesophageal reflux disease. *Gastroenterology*. 2001;121:1095-1100.

Kahrilas PJ. GERD pathogenesis, pathophysiology and clinical manigestations. *Cleve Clin J Med*. 2003;70(Suppl 5):S4-S19.

Kahrilas PJ, Shaheen NJ, Vaezi M. American Gastroenterological Association Medical Position Statement On The Management Of Gastroesophageal Reflux Disease. *Gastroenterology*. 2008;135:1383.

Katz PO, Gerson LB, Velas MF. American College of Gastroenterology. Guidelines for the diagnosis and treatment of gastroesophageal reflux disease. *Am J Gastroenterol*. 2013;108:308-328.

Klok RM, Postma MJ, van Hout BA, et al. Meta-analysis: comparing the efficacy of proton pump inhibitors in short-term use. *Aliment Pharmacol Therapeut*. 2003;17(10):1237-1245.

Numans ME, Lau J, de Wit NJ, et al. Short-term treatments with proton pump inhibitors as a test for gastroesophageal reflux disease: a meta-analysis of diagnostic test characteristics. *Ann Intern Med*. 2004;140:518-527.

Richter JE. Diagnostic tests for gastroesophageal reflux disease. *Am J Med Sci*. 2003;326:300-308.

Spechler SJ, Lee E, Ahnen D, et al. Long-term outcome of medical and surgical therapies for gastroesophageal reflux disease: follow-up of a randomized controlled trial. *JAMA*. 2001;285:2331-2338.

CHAPTER 156

Upper Gastrointestinal Bleeding

Stephen R. Rotman, MD

John R. Saltzman, MD

INTRODUCTION

Upper gastrointestinal (GI) bleeding is responsible for over 300,000 hospitalizations per year in the United States. An additional 100,000 to 150,000 patients develop upper GI bleeding during hospitalizations. The annual cost of treating nonvariceal acute upper GI bleeding in the United States exceeds $7 billion.

Upper GI bleeding is defined as a bleeding source in the GI tract proximal to the ligament of Treitz. The presentation varies depending on the nature and severity of bleeding and includes hematemesis, melena, hematochezia (in rapid upper GI bleeding), and anemia with heme-positive stools. Bleeding can be associated with changes in vital signs, including tachycardia and hypotension including orthostatic hypotension. Given the range of presentations, pinpointing the nature and severity of GI bleeding may be a challenging task.

The natural history of nonvariceal upper GI bleeding is that 80% of patients will stop bleeding spontaneously and no further urgent intervention will be needed. In contrast, only 50% of patients with a variceal hemorrhage stop bleeding spontaneously. Following cessation of active variceal bleeding, there is a high risk of recurrent bleeding within 6 weeks.

The mortality rate for nonvariceal upper GI bleeding is 2% to 14%. This mortality rate has improved because of the development of new medications, endoscopy (both diagnostic and therapeutic), intensive care units (ICUs), and advances in surgical management. The mortality remains high since patients with GI bleeding now are older, have more comorbidities, and are taking more medications, including nonsteroidal anti-inflammatory drugs (NSAIDs), anticoagulants, and antiplatelet agents. For variceal bleeding, mortality is between 15% and 50% for each bleeding episode, and 70% to 80% in those with continuous bleeding. Variceal hemorrhage is responsible for one-third of all deaths due to cirrhosis.

DIFFERENTIAL DIAGNOSIS

■ NONVARICEAL BLEEDING

Peptic ulcer disease

Diagnosis: Peptic ulcer disease is a common condition stemming from an imbalance of protective and disruptive factors of the GI mucosa. Ulcers are most commonly found in the stomach and proximal duodenum (**Figures 156-1** and **156-2**). Peptic ulcer disease is the most common cause of upper GI bleeding and accounts for up to 50% of total cases and over 100,000 hospital admissions per year in the United States. The annual incidence of peptic ulcer disease in patients infected with *Helicobacter pylori* is about 1% per year, which is six to ten times higher than patients who are uninfected. Diagnosis is made by endoscopy performed when symptoms prompt endoscopic investigation. An initial step in management is to identify *H. pylori* infection and users of NSAIDs. These two risk factors account for the vast majority of ulcers in the upper GI tract.

Disruptive factors that can damage the mucosa of the GI tract include acid, pepsin, bile salts, ischemia, and *H. pylori*. Exogenous causes are predominately medications (NSAIDs, aspirin, and SSRIs). Stress-induced ulcers are a common cause of bleeding in patients hospitalized for other severe illnesses. Risk factors for stress-induced ulcers include respiratory failure (especially intubated patients), coagulopathy (international normalized ratio [INR] > 1.5 or platelets <50,000/μL), trauma, sepsis, renal failure, burns, ICU admission, and surgery.

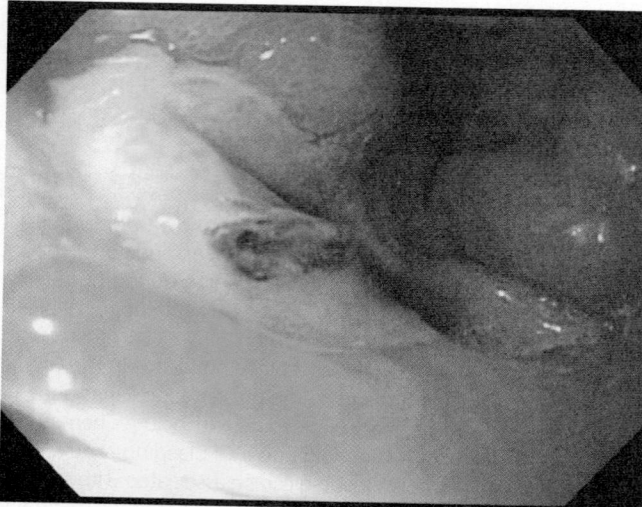

Figure 156-1 *Duodenal ulcer.*

Pathophysiology: The defensive forces of the esophagus include esophageal motility with clearance of refluxed materials, the lower esophageal sphincter to prevent reflux, and salivary secretions that contain bicarbonate. Gastric protective factors include the mucous layer as well as tissue mediators. *H. pylori* is a flagellated bacterium with several unique attributes that aid in its ability to break down gastric mucosa. These factors include its production of urease, which neutralizes the acidic gastric environment. NSAIDs inhibit cyclooxygenase, thus decreasing mucosal protective prostaglandin levels in the stomach. They also increase gastric vascular endothelial adhesion molecules, thus leading to neutrophil adherence and mucosal injury.

Clinical findings: Peptic ulcer disease presents in a variety of ways. Patients can experience epigastric pain, melena, hematochezia, dyspepsia, bloating, or can be asymptomatic with or without anemia. On examination, pain may be epigastric and reproducible, but many patients have right-sided pain or no pain at all.

Prognosis: Response to treatment and outcomes vary for peptic ulcer disease. Treatment is with proton-pump inhibitor (PPI) therapy until asymptomatic and/or mucosal healing is demonstrated via an esophagogastroduodenoscopy (EGD) and/or antibiotics where indicated and removal of offending agents (eg, NSAIDs) leads to mucosal healing (**Table 156-1**). Chronic, nonhealing gastric ulcers should prompt consideration of underlying illness or an alternative diagnosis, such as malignancy, and thus should be biopsied.

TABLE 156-1 Recommended Treatment Regimens for *H. Pylori* Infection

- **Three-drug regimens**
  - Proton-pump inhibitor (PPI) orally twice daily + clarithromycin 500 mg orally twice daily + amoxicillin 1 g orally twice daily. Eradication 85%-90%. Duration 10-14 days.
  - Proton-pump inhibitor orally twice daily + clarithromycin 500 mg orally twice daily + metronidazole 500 mg orally twice daily. Eradication 75%-85%. Duration 10-14 days. This regimen is generally used for PCN allergic patients.
- **Four-drug regimen**
  - Proton-pump inhibitor orally twice daily + bismuth subsalicylate 525 mg 4 times daily + Tetracycline 500 mg 4 times daily + metronidazole 500 mg orally 3-4 times daily. Eradication 75%-90%. Duration 2 weeks.

Mallory-Weiss tears

Diagnosis: Mallory-Weiss tears occur at the gastroesophageal junction, in the distal esophagus, or proximal stomach (**Figure 156-3**). Typically, these tears form after repeated and severe vomiting or retching. The tears may extend into the underlying blood vessels. Acute upper GI bleeding is the major clinical finding, which may be associated with epigastric pain, which may radiate to the back. Endoscopy is used to document the presence of a gastroesophageal tear and allows the possibility of therapeutic intervention.

Bleeding occurs when the tear involves the underlying esophageal venous or arterial plexus. Patients often have a history of nonbloody vomiting or retching before the onset of hematemesis. The tears are located at the esophagogastric junction, and can be within a hiatal hernia. Tears can extend downward into the cardia or, less commonly, upward into the esophagus.

Pathophysiology: Mallory-Weiss syndrome is characterized by longitudinal mucosal lacerations in the distal esophagus and proximal stomach, which are usually associated with forceful retching.

Prognosis: Although 40% to 70% of patients with bleeding Mallory-Weiss tears require blood transfusions, most tears heal spontaneously within 24 to 48 hours of presentation. Risk factors for rebleeding include portal hypertension and coagulopathy. Patients with active or ongoing bleeding can be treated with endoscopic hemostatic methods. For the rare patient with ongoing bleeding unresponsive to endoscopic control, intravenous (IV) infusions of octreotide, arterial embolization via angiography, and esophageal

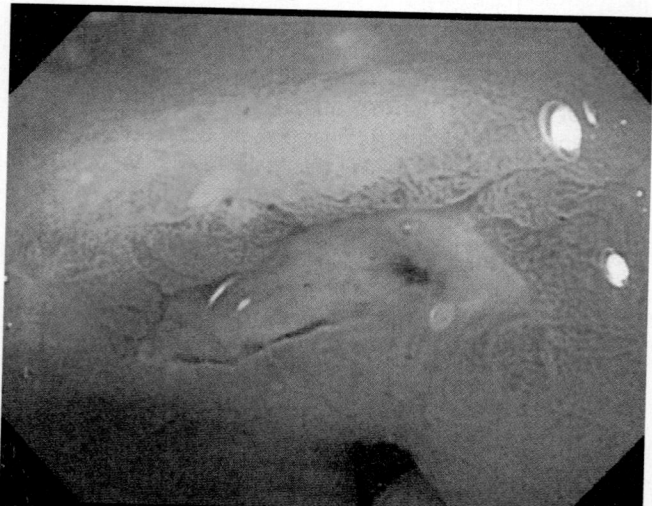

Figure 156-2 *Gastric ulcer.*

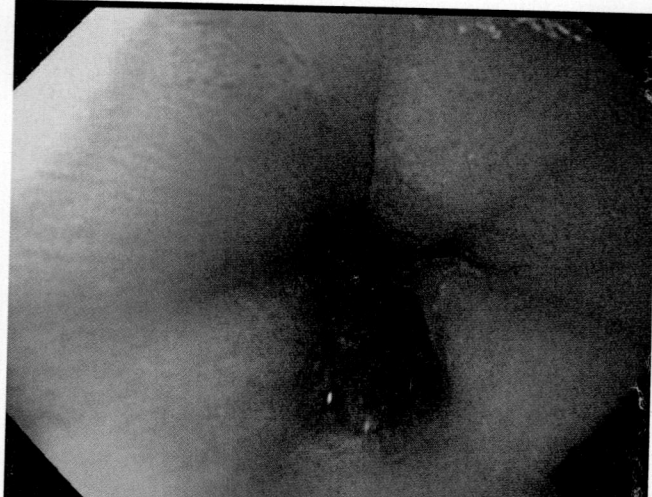

Figure 156-3 *Mallory-Weiss tear.*

balloon tamponade have been used. In refractory bleeding, surgery with over-sewing of the bleeding vessel may be required.

Dieulafoy lesion

Essentials of diagnosis: A Dieulafoy lesion is a dilated, aberrant submucosal vessel that erodes through normal epithelium and is not associated with an ulcer (**Figure 156-4**). Dieulafoy lesions are typically located just below the gastroesophageal junction on the lesser curvature of the stomach but can be found in areas throughout the GI tract, including the esophagus, duodenum, and colon. When a Dieulafoy lesion bleeds, massive arterial bleeding can occur. In the absence of active bleeding, the lesion is difficult to see as it may appear as a small and subtle raised area, such as a nipple or visible vessel without an associated ulcer. In patients with massive bleeding and no obvious cause, the lesser curvature of the stomach within 6 cms of the gastroesophageal junction should be carefully inspected endoscopically for evidence of a Dieulafoy lesion.

The typical patient with a Dieulafoy lesion is a man, with multiple comorbidities, already hospitalized for other problems. Diagnosis is confirmed with finding a visible vessel or active arterial pumping, without an associated ulcer or mass. The diagnosis can be difficult, as bleeding may be massive such that the area may be covered with blood and the source may not be visualized. It is especially challenging to diagnose Dieulafoy lesions that are not bleeding as the absence of an associated ulcer makes detection of the vessel difficult.

Pathophysiology: The cause of a Dieulafoy lesion is unknown. The arteries are 1 to 3 mm in size, which is approximately 10 times the caliber of mucosal capillaries. The typical location is in the upper stomach along the high lesser curvature, within 6 cm of the gastroesophageal junction.

Clinical findings: A Dieulafoy lesion often presents with a massive acute upper GI bleed, although the bleeding may be self-limited in nature. The diagnosis is confirmed with finding a visible vessel or with active arterial pumping without an associated ulcer or mass.

Prognosis: Endoscopic treatment is the mainstay for bleeding control of a Dieulafoy lesion via cautery, clips or the combination of epinephrine injection and one of these two treatment modalities. The risk of recurrent bleeding following endoscopic treatment is relatively high due to the size of the underlying artery. In patients with recurrent bleeding, repeat endoscopic therapy is often the next step; however, IR angiography or surgical therapy may be necessary and consultation by a surgeon and interventional radiologist early on is recommended.

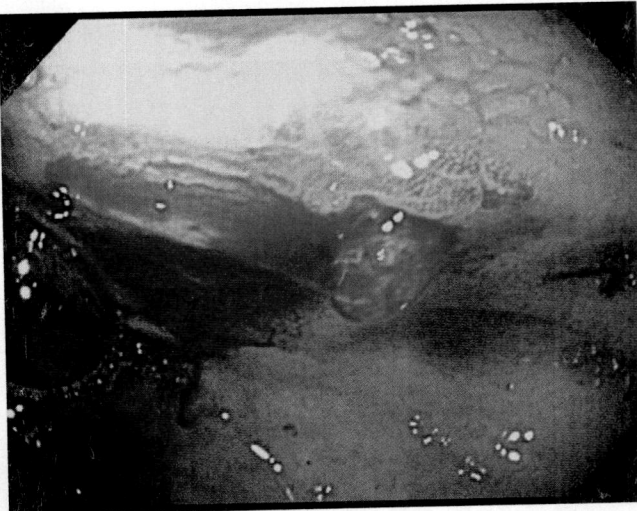

Figure 156-4 *Dieulafoy lesion.*

■ VASCULAR MALFORMATIONS

Angiodysplasia

Diagnosis: Angiodysplasias may occur throughout the GI tract, may be multiple in one gastrointestinal region, or coexist in several different gastrointestinal locations. Although angiodysplasias are a relatively common source of small bowel bleeding, they are a rare source of massive bleeding from the stomach. Bleeding from an upper GI vascular malformation is typically intermittent and low grade in nature, although it can be acute and overt.

Pathophysiology: The cause of most vascular malformations is unknown. Vascular malformations can be present at birth, although they do not appear to be hereditary. They occur equally in both sexes and in different races. Vascular malformations may be caused by a rupture or clotting of a blood vessel during fetal development, although not associated with other problems at birth.

Clinical findings: Bleeding from upper GI vascular malformations is typically intermittent and low grade in nature, although it can be acute and overt. The endoscopic appearance may be variable, but includes a superficial collection or tuft of blood vessels.

Prognosis: Endoscopic therapy with thermal coagulation is the treatment of choice with cautery applied first to the periphery and then to the center of the lesion. Argon plasma coagulation is most commonly used to treat vascular malformations and is an effective therapy. Certain medications have been utilized in an attempt to treat vascular malformations in the upper gastrointestinal tract. Combination estrogen/progesterone therapy has been widely used, as has octreotide. Angiography or surgery may be offered for failures of endoscopic and medical therapy, but is rarely necessary.

Gastric antral vascular ectasia

Diagnosis: Gastric antral vascular ectasia (GAVE), also known as "watermelon stomach," is an idiopathic condition often associated with portal hypertension. Gastric antral vascular ectasia is a relatively unusual cause of upper GI bleeding. The bleeding that occurs is typically chronic and low grade, often associated with iron deficiency anemia and occult bleeding. It is unusual to have acute or massive upper GI bleeding from GAVE.

Pathophysiology: The etiology of watermelon stomach is not known; however, it has been theorized to be due to gastroduodenal prolapse and occurs in patients with cirrhosis, portal hypertension, and systemic sclerosis. Patients with concomitant portal hypertension have bleeding that is more difficult to control, requiring treatment of the underlying portal hypertension.

Clinical findings: During endoscopy, vascular malformations occur in rows of reddish stripes that radiate outward from the pylorus, in a pattern that resembles the stripes on a watermelon; hence, this entity has been referred to as "watermelon stomach." These stripes represent rows of vascular malformations and the entity is easy to recognize in the classic form. However, GAVE may have a less organized appearance especially in patients with portal hypertension. Although the diagnosis is by endoscopy, it can be confirmed by biopsies obtained during endoscopy. GAVE histology shows areas of vascular ectasia associated with spindle cell proliferation and fibrohyalinosis.

Prognosis: Most patients will respond to endoscopic therapy most commonly with argon plasma coagulation. Several such endoscopic treatment sessions may be required. Radiofrequency ablation may be used to treat refractory cases. However, surgery with an antrectomy may be required for patients who have persistent bleeding despite endoscopic management.

Aortoenteric fistula

Diagnosis: Aortoenteric fistulas occur when there is a direct communication between the aorta and the gastrointestinal tract and can lead to massive bleeding. Patients may have a "herald" bleed with initial hematemesis or hematochezia, which may spontaneously remit. This might then be followed by torrential bleeding, including exsanguination, making it important to quickly diagnose this condition. Intermittent bleeding can occur if a blood clot overlies a fistulous connection. There may be abdominal or back pain (which occurs in about half of patients), or signs of fever and infection. On physical examination, a bruit may be heard and a pulsatile mass may be palpable at any point along the midabdomen representing the course of the abdominal aorta.

A high index of suspicion is needed to promptly diagnose a patient with an aortoenteric fistula for successful management. In a patient who has a known risk factor such as previous aortic grafting, this diagnosis should be considered early in the course. In fact, it should always be suspected in patients with massive bleeding from the second to third portion of the duodenum. The diagnosis can be confirmed by computed tomography with angiography or with traditional angiography. Diagnostic tests need to be done in an expeditious manner along with prompt vascular surgical evaluation as the management of an aortoenteric fistula is surgical. The mortality rate of an unrecognized fistula is 100%, whereas the mortality for a recognized fistula is 30%.

Hemobilia

Diagnosis: Hemobilia is a rare cause of acute upper GI bleeding that occurs from the hepatobiliary tract in less than 1% of patients who undergo a procedure to the biliary tree (endoscopic retrograde cholangiopancreatography [ERCP], surgery, or CT-guided procedures) and almost never spontaneously with the rare exception of invasive tumors. **The classic triad of hemobilia is biliary colic, obstructive jaundice, and gastrointestinal bleeding.** The diagnosis of hemobilia can be difficult by upper endoscopy, which may not clearly visualize the ampulla. A side-viewing duodenoscope is often utilized to visualize and access the ampulla directly or to perform ERCP.

Hemobilia should be considered in patients who have had a recent history of hepatic or biliary tract injury. This includes trauma to the area, percutaneous (or transjugular) liver biopsies, percutaneous transhepatic cholangiograms, ablations of liver tumors or biopsies. Hemobilia can also occur secondary to gallstones, cholecystitis, hepatobiliary tumors, hepatic abscesses, and aneurysms. Obstructive jaundice may be associated with biliary sepsis. Patients with these findings should be considered as potentially having hemobilia. Treatment is directed at the primary cause of bleeding, although ERCP may also be needed to remove clot from the bile duct causing obstruction. While treatment may occasionally be performed endoscopically, it usually needs to be done angiographically (such as by arterial embolization) or surgically.

Hemosuccus pancreaticus

Diagnosis: Hemosuccus pancreaticus is another rare cause of upper GI bleeding that occurs due to bleeding from the pancreatic duct. This can be secondary to chronic pancreatitis, pancreatic pseudocysts, and pancreatic tumors. This can also occur after a therapeutic endoscopy of the pancreas, including pancreatic sphincterotomy or stone removal. Hemosuccus pancreaticus can be difficult to detect by routine endoscopy; thus, a side-viewing duodenoscope and ERCP may be needed to reveal the source of the bleeding. The diagnosis may be confirmed by abdominal CT scan, angiography, or intra-abdominal exploration.

Bleeding occurs when there is erosion into a vessel, forming a direct communication with the pancreatic duct. Angiography is important for diagnosis and treatment, often with coil embolization to control the acute bleeding. For persistent or massive bleeding, surgery with resection of the bleeding area or ligation of a bleeding vessel may be required.

Cameron lesion

Diagnosis: Cameron lesions are erosions or ulcers that occur in the distal aspect of a hiatal hernia. Although this may be an incidental

finding on upper endoscopy, these lesions can be responsible for iron deficiency anemia or acute or chronic upper GI bleeding.

The mechanism of formation of a Cameron lesion is not well understood. Potential etiologies include gastroesophageal reflux and mechanical trauma of the area. Management of a Cameron lesion depends on the clinical situation. Patients with acute bleeding can be treated by endoscopic methods. Patients who do not have acute bleeding, but have chronic blood loss may be treated with medical therapy, such as a proton-pump inhibitor and iron repletion. Surgical repair of the hiatal hernia is curative, but rarely necessary.

Upper gastrointestinal tumors

Diagnosis: Neoplasms of the upper GI tract are a rare cause of upper GI bleeding. These tumors may be esophageal squamous carcinomas, malignant lymphomas or adenocarcinomas (primary or metastatic often from lung or breast), or benign lesions such as leiomyeiomas or gastrointestinal stromal tumors. The symptoms that suggest bleeding may be from a gastrointestinal tumor include symptoms that may be attributable to the primary tumor such as dysphagia from esophageal cancer, but symptoms may be nonspecific including cachexia, weight loss, and early satiety. If the diagnosis of a tumor is not previously known, it may be detected at the time of endoscopy and confirmed by brushings or biopsies. Endoscopic ultrasound may be needed to evaluate submucosal masses.

Bleeding from an upper gastrointestinal tumor may be from mucosal erosions or ulcerations, or from invasion of the tumor into an underlying vessel. Typically, endoscopic treatments are a temporizing measure prior to more definitive measures such as surgery because rebleeding will frequently occur after endoscopy. Medical therapy is often ineffective in this setting, although palliative measures may be provided including chemotherapy and radiation of the primary tumor. Patients who have bleeding due to an upper GI malignancy have a very poor prognosis. The majority of patients (>60%) will die within 3 months. However, patients who have a benign upper gastrointestinal tumor that bleeds will be cured by surgical resection.

■ VARICEAL BLEEDING

Gastroesophageal varices

Diagnosis: Varices are dilated venous collaterals that have a tendency to rupture and can bleed massively. Esophageal and gastric varices develop as a result of portal hypertension usually due to advanced liver disease and cirrhosis (**Figures 156-5** and **156-6**). Varices may be isolated to the stomach if they are due to splenic vein

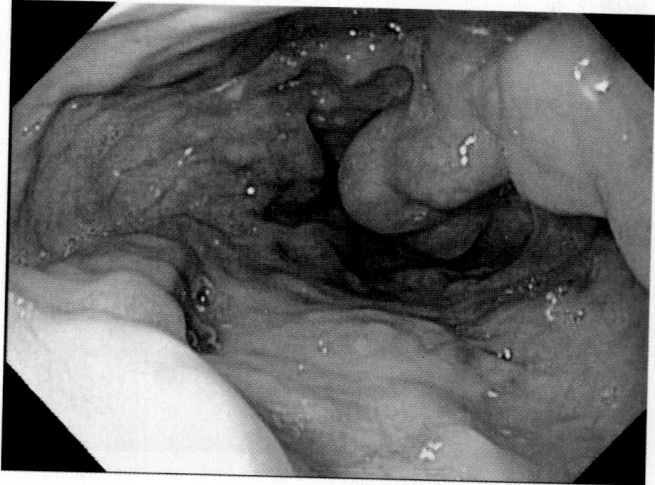

Figure 156-5 *Esophageal varices.*

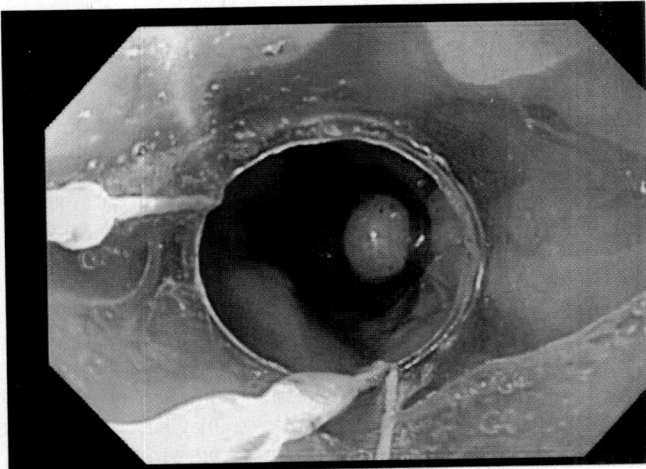

Figure 156-6 *Banded esophageal varix.*

thrombosis, acute pancreatitis, or a pancreatic tumor. Esophageal and gastric varices may occur without any clinical symptoms.

Acute variceal bleeding is different from nonvariceal bleeding in many respects. Upper endoscopy is the primary diagnostic modality and allows for direct visualization of columns of esophageal varices. Endoscopy should be performed quickly (within 24 hours) for potential intervention if varices are suspected as the source of upper GI bleeding. Abdominal CT and ultrasound may show the presence of collateral veins. Portal vein angiography may also demonstrate the presence of collaterals or recanalization of the umbilical vein.

Variceal hemorrhage is responsible for one-third of all deaths due to cirrhosis. Mortality is between 15% and 50% for each bleeding episode, and 70% and 80% in those with continuous bleeding. Following cessation of active variceal bleeding, there is a high risk of recurrent bleeding within 6 weeks (>50%). The time of greatest risk is within the first 48 to 72 hours (90% of rebleeds will occur in this time period), and over half of all subsequent rebleeding episodes occur within the first 10 days. Recurrent variceal bleeding may occur in up to 70% of patients within 6 weeks of the index bleed if preventive measures are not performed.

Survival during the 6 weeks following the index bleed is directly related to rebleeding. Risk factors include age greater than 60 years, large varices, severe initial bleed (hemoglobin <8 g/dL on admission) and renal failure. Patients with acute variceal bleeding are typically treated with multiple modalities simultaneously, including medical therapies and endoscopic management. Over-resuscitation should be avoided as overly vigorous volume repletion has been associated with precipitation of further bleeding. The target hemoglobin goal during resuscitation should be 7 g/dL. While early intervention in the form of transfusions (for low hemoglobin) and intravenous fluids may be warranted in the setting of hypotension, patients who are suspected to have variceal bleeding should undergo endoscopy within 12 hours of presentation and after resuscitation. In addition, radiologic and surgical treatments may be needed. Endoscopic variceal band ligation is a commonly applied therapy. This is a method of placing elastic bands over varices, similar to the technique of banding hemorrhoids. Varices are suctioned into a banding device and the bands are released around the base of the varices. It is typically performed in the distal 5 cm of the esophagus.

Pathophysiology: Normal pressure in the portal vein is 5 to 10 mm Hg. An elevated portal venous pressure of greater than 10 mm Hg (due to obstruction) increases capillary pressure. The connection between the portal and systemic circulation may enlarge to allow blood to bypass the obstruction and pass directly into the systemic circulation. One of the known sites of such confluence is the distal esophagus. Studies have demonstrated the role of endothelin-1 and nitric oxide in the pathogenesis of portal hypertension and esophageal varices.

Endothelin-1 is a powerful vasoconstrictor synthesized by sinusoidal endothelial cells, that has been implicated in the increased hepatic vascular resistance of cirrhosis and in the development of liver fibrosis. Nitric oxide is a vasodilator substance that is synthesized by sinusoidal endothelial cells. In the cirrhotic liver, the production of nitric oxide is decreased, and endothelial nitric oxide synthase activity and nitrite production by sinusoidal endothelial cells are reduced.

Clinical findings: Symptoms of variceal bleeding are nonspecific and include hematemesis, melena, and hematochezia. Patients may feel light-headed and dizzy; and those with severe liver disease may have hepatic encephalopathy, which may be the sole presenting feature in a cirrhotic patient who is bleeding from the upper GI tract. Other associated signs and symptoms are the clinical manifestations of cirrhosis including the laboratory abnormalities associated with cirrhosis (see **Chapter 160 [Cirrhosis and its Complications]**). The objective of upper endoscopy is to find and define the source of bleeding and to treat it. Varices are evaluated for signs of either active bleeding or markers of recent bleeding. These markers include large tortuous varices with red wale marks (longitudinal red streaks on varices that resemble red, corduroy wales), cherry-red spots (discrete cherry-red spots that are flat on a varix) and hemocystic spots (raised discrete red spots that overlie varices that appear as "blood blisters"). Platelet or fibrin plugs are white nipple-like projections that project from a varix indicative of a site with recent bleeding and with a very high risk of bleeding.

Prognosis: Variceal bleeding is a significant cause of rebleeding and mortality. Variceal bleeding will stop in approximately 50% of patients, but those who have continued bleeding have a mortality that approaches 80%. Patients have a high risk of rebleeding (up to 70%) until the gastroesophageal varices are obliterated. If a patient survives the initial bleeding episode, repeated courses of band ligation are performed approximately every 2 weeks until the varices are obliterated. This is combined with medical therapy using nonselective β-blockade to reduce portal pressures. Current data support the use of nonselective β-blockers for medium and large varices prophylactically and for any grade of varix found to bleed. The prognosis for patients with bleeding gastroesophageal varices is poor even with control of bleeding varices as this is indicative of progressive liver disease. Patients die from hepatic decompensation, rebleeding, infections, renal failure, and other complications. Bacterial infections occur in up to 20% of cirrhotics with GI bleeding and subsequently develop in an additional 50% of patients during hospitalization for variceal bleeds. These include spontaneous bacterial peritonitis, pneumonia, sepsis, and skin infections. The use of prophylactic antibiotics in patients with acute variceal bleeding has been shown to decrease the rates of subsequent infection, spontaneous bacterial peritonitis, bacteremia, and death. Data for the use of fluoroquinolones as the prophylactic antibiotic of choice is supported by frequent clinical use, but a growing resistance of organisms to this class must be considered in choosing an antibiotic and alternatives include third-generation cephalosporins.

PRACTICE POINT

- Management of acute variceal bleeding:
  - Volume repletion with a target hemoglobin goal during resuscitation of 7 g/dL
  - Upper endoscopy following resuscitation within 12 h of presentation
  - Prophylactic nonselective β-blockers for large varices and for any grade of varix identified as the source of bleeding
  - Prophylactic antibiotics to decrease the rates of subsequent infection, spontaneous bacterial peritonitis, bacteremia, and death

Portal hypertensive gastropathy

Diagnosis: In patients with cirrhosis and portal hypertension, gastric mucosal blood flow is increased, leading to congestion and hyperemia of the stomach. Portal hypertensive gastropathy occurs when edema and capillary venous dilatation in the stomach causes friability. This may subsequently result in bleeding with rupture of ectatic vessels. The endoscopic appearance is a mosaic-like pattern of pink mucosa, with a characteristic "snakeskin" appearance. Overall, this is a rare cause of acute upper GI bleeding, although it may be a source of chronic blood loss in patients with cirrhosis.

Portal hypertensive gastropathy may develop after treatment of esophageal varices. A proposed mechanism following treatment of varices is increased backpressure into the stomach vasculature, leading to the development of gastric congestion. Thus, the goal of treatment of portal hypertensive gastropathy is to decrease portal pressures. The affected area is diffuse and pharmacologic agents, such as octreotide, may be used acutely to decrease blood flow. Nonselective β-blockers (nadolol and propranolol) are often given, with the dose increased and adjusted if side effects occur. Endoscopic treatments are ineffective in this disorder. Patients with uncontrolled bleeding may need transjugular intrahepatic portal systemic shunt therapy or a surgical shunt in order to reduce portal pressure. In patients with decompensated liver disease, liver transplantation is indicated.

DIAGNOSIS

Upper GI bleeding may be life threatening. Factors that portend a favorable or a poor prognosis in patients with nonvariceal upper GI bleeding may be used to appropriately triage and manage patients. The role of nasogastric (NG) tube aspiration is controversial, and we do not routinely support its use. NG tube aspirates may be falsely negative; false-negatives most commonly occur in patients with bleeding from duodenal ulcers due to spasm of the pylorus, and may occur in other conditions, including gastric ulcers and rarely esophageal varices (if the tube is positioned in a nondependent area of the stomach).

■ HISTORY TO AID DIAGNOSIS

Similar to utilizing laboratory values to aid in diagnosis, a comprehensive history may help to predict a source of bleeding and prognosticate outcomes. An alcoholic with cirrhosis who has not recently undergone variceal screening endoscopy and presents with a large volume upper GI bleed should be managed as a variceal bleed until proven otherwise, including administration of octreotide and prophylactic antibiotics, and undergo urgent endoscopy. A patient with no history of liver disease or physical stigmata of cirrhosis probably presents with a nonvariceal source of bleeding. A patient with an extensive NSAID use history most likely has peptic ulcer disease.

■ LABORATORY TESTING TO ESTABLISH GI BLEEDING SOURCE

Although laboratory values cannot predict a source of bleed, they help to define the clinical status of the bleeding patient. The BUN will be elevated out of proportion to the creatinine due to digestion of blood in most patients with upper GI bleeding. In variceal bleeding, abnormalities of the liver enzymes (ALT, AST) are seen in patients with active hepatocellular damage. Patients may have hyperbilirubinemia and poor synthetic function, with hypoalbuminemia and an elevated INR indicating impaired liver function. Patients with bone marrow suppression from alcohol may have pancytopenia or those with hypersplenism may have low platelet counts. In patients with liver failure, hypoglycemia may be detected. Low albumin states may predict worse outcomes from bleeding.

TRIAGE/HOSPITAL ADMISSION

■ RISK ASSESSMENT: CLINICAL PREDICTORS AND GUIDELINES

Clinical guidelines have been developed to help optimize the management of patients with nonvariceal upper GI bleeding. The aim of guidelines is to identify low-risk patients who can be discharged either directly from the emergency room or at an early stage of hospitalization, and to identify high-risk patients who will need more resources. Several such guidelines include both clinical data and information obtained at the time of endoscopy. Newer guidelines focus on clinical data to determine which patients bear increased mortality risk and therefore merit urgent endoscopy and/or ICU level care.

Three main prognostic scores for upper GI bleeding have been used clinically. The Rockall score (**Table 156-2**) is a postendoscopy scoring system used to predict rebleeding and mortality in patients with nonvariceal upper GI bleeding. In this scoring system, scores of zero to three are assigned to the factors of age, the presence of shock, comorbidity, diagnosis, and endoscopic stigmata. A low-risk patient has a score of two or less, and about 30% of patients will belong to this category. In this low-risk group, there was a 4.3% risk of rebleeding and 0.1% mortality. Patients with Rockall scores of three to five have intermediate rates of rebleeding and mortality (2.0%-7.9%), whereas patients with a score of six or greater have a high rebleeding and mortality rate (15.1%-39.1%). Limitations of this scoring system include that it was derived from a relatively small number of patients and the full score requires both clinical and endoscopic information to calculate.

TABLE 156-2 The Components and Score Assignments of the Rockall Risk Assessment Score for Upper GI Bleeding

Variable	Score			
	0	1	2	3
Age (y)	<60	60-79	>79	
Shock	• BP >100 mg Hg • Pulse <100 bpm	• BP >100 mg Hg • Pulse >100 bpm	• BP <100 mg Hg • Pulse >100 bpm	
Comorbidity	None		Cardiac disease, any other major comorbidity not listed in next column	• Renal failure, liver failure • Disseminated malignancy
Endoscopic diagnosis	Mallory-Weiss tear, no lesion	All other diagnoses	Upper GI tract malignancy	
Major stigmata of recent hemorrhage	None, or dark spots only		Blood in upper GI tract, adherent clot or spurting vessels	

BP, blood pressure; GI, gastrointestinal. Max score = 11; low risk ≤2; high risk ≥5 (although this varies in the literature).

TABLE 156-3 The Components and Interpretation of the Blatchford Scoring System

Variables	Points
Systolic blood pressure (mm Hg)	
100-109	1
90-99	2
<90	3
Blood urea nitrogen (mmol/L)	
6.5-7.9	2
8.0-9.9	3
10.0-24.9	4
>25	6
Hemoglobin: Men (g/dL)	
12.0-12.9	1
10.0-11.9	3
<10	6
Hemoglobin: Women (g/dL)	
10.0-11.9	1
<10	2
Other variables	
Pulse >100	1
Presentation with melena	1
Hepatic disease	2
Cardiac failure	2
Total	—

A score of >1 is considered "high risk" while ≤1 is "low risk" in terms of predicting need for intervention.

A scoring system that only uses clinical information (and not endoscopic data) obtained at the time of presentation prior to endoscopy, developed by Blatchford and colleagues (**Table 156-3**), helps to determine urgency of endoscopy and need for intervention. The clinical information incorporated into this scoring system includes hemoglobin, BUN, heart rate, systolic blood pressure, the presence of syncope, melena, liver disease, and heart failure. A new scoring system that also only uses information available at the time of initial presentation is the AIMS65 score. This score includes five factors: albumin <3.0 g/dL, INR >1.5, altered mental status, systolic blood pressure <90 mm Hg, and age >65 years. In this score, each factor is assigned a score of 1 and high-risk patients have an AIMS65 score >1.

MANAGEMENT

■ INITIAL HOSPITAL TREATMENT

While the early goals of treatment for GI bleeding include identification of the bleeding source and facilitation of bleeding cessation, the *primary task is stabilization of the patient*. Patients need to have at least two large bore peripheral intravenous access catheters (18 gauge or larger). Supplemental oxygen should be administered routinely. Crystalloid fluids should be initially administered to maintain an adequate blood pressure. Patients who are not able to adequately protect their airways (including patients with ongoing, severe hematemesis) should be considered for elective endotracheal intubation.

Patients who are high risk, such as the elderly or those with active coronary artery disease, should be transfused to maintain hemoglobin above 10 g/dL. Young and healthy patients should be transfused to maintain hemoglobin of 7 g/dL. Any coagulopathy should be

corrected if possible with transfusion of fresh frozen plasma (initially 1 unit, followed by additional units based on subsequent INR) or administration of vitamin K (preferably 10 mg orally if at all possible). In patients with a low platelet count (<50,000/mL), it is recommended to transfuse platelets with a target platelet count goal >50,000/mL, initially with one or two units of platelets, followed by additional units based on subsequent platelet count.

Medications

Medications useful for management of acute upper GI bleeding include proton-pump inhibitors and octreotide. Other medications including H_2 blockers have not been demonstrated to favorably influence the natural history of acute GI bleeding.

Proton-pump inhibitor therapy

Proton-pump inhibitors help stop bleeding and prevent rebleeding in patients with significant nonvariceal GI bleeding. Endoscopic therapy is considered the standard of care for patients with active bleeding and nonbleeding visible vessels. Patients with peptic ulcer and successful endoscopic therapy have less rebleeding with the addition of intravenous PPI therapy (**Table 156-4**). In patients initially treated in the emergency room with a bolus infusion of omeprazole followed by a continuous infusion, active bleeding lesions found at endoscopy decreased and clean-based ulcers at endoscopy increased. A recent review and meta-analysis suggests that outcomes with an intermittent PPI dosing strategy is comparable to the previously recommended bolus and continuous infusion PPI dosing for patients with high-risk bleeding ulcers that are treated endoscopically. Patients who remain stable for 72 hours may then transition to standard dose oral PPIs.

Octreotide

The somatostatin analogue octreotide can be used to treat patients with both variceal and nonvariceal upper GI bleeding. This medication is indicated in patients with variceal bleeding or acute upper GI bleeding thought secondary to varices, using a loading dose of 25 to 50 μg followed by an intravenous infusion of 25 to 50 μg/h. Octreotide may also be helpful in patients with nonvariceal bleeding. While a useful adjunctive treatment in patients with non-variceal upper GI bleeding, octreotide should not be prescribed routinely to patients with nonvariceal upper GI bleeding. For all suspected etiologies of upper GI bleeding, the use of octreotide should be considered in patients who have persistent bleeding on optimal medical management, including PPIs, who are poor surgical risks (such as those with multiple comorbidities already in the hospital).

Endoscopic treatments

Endoscopic therapy for upper GI bleeding has been demonstrated to yield significant improvement in hemostasis, number of units

TABLE 156-4 Commonly Used Oral Proton Pump Inhibitors (PPIs) and Their Recommended Dose Regimen for Acute Upper Gastrointestinal (GI) Bleeding

PPI Name	Initial Bolus Dose	Continuous IV Infusion Dose	Duration
Lansoprazole (Prevacid)	60 mg	6 mg/h	Up to 72 h
Pantoprazole (Protonix)	80 mg	8 mg/h	Up to 72 h
Esomeprazole (Nexium)	80 mg	8 mg/h	Up to 72 h

of blood transfused, number of emergency interventions, hospital length of stay, and hospital costs. Endoscopic therapy is the standard of care for patients with the high-risk stigmata of recent hemorrhage of active bleeding or a nonbleeding visible vessel. The management of adherent clots has been controversial with recent data suggesting a possible role for endoscopic therapy.

For many conditions including active bleeding, visible vessels, and esophageal varices, endoscopic techniques are the mainstay of treatment. The timing and occasion for endoscopic treatment often depends on the clinical presentation and/or findings at time of endoscopy. An upper endoscopy examination is indicated within 24 hours of presentation for patients with suspected nonvariceal upper GI bleeding. Conditions that warrant rapid triage and planned endoscopy include bleeding in the setting of known varices, persistent hypotension requiring pressors, and increasing transfusion requirement. However, hemodynamic stability, protection of the airway (if necessary), and platelets, FFP, or vitamin K administration when applicable may be necessary steps prior to endoscopic evaluation regardless of the urgency. In addition, data support endoscopic evaluation within 24 hours and do not support a need for more urgent endoscopy in most patients with nonvariceal upper GI bleeding.

PRACTICE POINT

- Upper endoscopy is indicated within 24 hours of presentation for patients with suspected upper GI bleeding but most patients do not require more urgent endoscopy. Hemodynamic stability is necessary prior to endoscopy.

Optimization of visualization

One of the challenges of managing patients with GI bleeding is visualization during endoscopy due to blood within the gastrointestinal tract. This problem may be overcome by the use of a variety of techniques or a combination of endoscopic techniques including the use of double-channel or large-channel endoscopes and vigorous irrigation.

In addition to endoscopic techniques, intravenous erythromycin (250 mg IV bolus or 3 mg/kg over 30 minutes) can be used for its prokinetic properties to increase gastric emptying and clear the stomach of blood. The erythromycin is given intravenously 30 to 120 minutes prior to endoscopy as a useful adjunctive treatment in patients with large gastrointestinal bleeds. It can be used either initially or after an endoscopy shows large amounts of blood remaining in the stomach with withdrawal of the endoscope and the use of erythromycin before proceeding again with endoscopy. Metoclopramide may also be used similarly, although there are less available data about its effectiveness in patients with upper GI bleeding.

Methods to control bleeding

The current endoscopic modalities to treat nonvariceal GI bleeding include the use of injection therapies (primarily with dilute epinephrine), contact thermal therapies including heater and bipolar probes, noncontact thermal methods (predominantly argon plasma coagulation), mechanical treatments including a variety of clips including larger over-the-scope clips and band-ligation techniques, and a combination of the above treatment modalities (typically, injection therapies combined with one of the other modalities) (**Table 156-5**). For nonvariceal upper GI bleeding, combination therapy or use of hemoclips improves outcomes and decreases recurrent bleeding. For esophageal variceal bleeding, band ligation to tamponade blood flow offers effective treatment and outcomes. Success with injection of glues in the treatment of gastric varices

---

TABLE 156-5 Available Modalities for Endoscopic Therapy

- **Injection therapy**
  a. Epinephrine
  b. Hypertonic saline
  c. Sclerosant (absolute alcohol, polidoconol)
  d. Tissue adhesives: cyanoacyralate, thrombin/fibrin glue
- **Thermal therapy**
  a. Contact: HP, bipolar (gold probe, BICAP)
  b. Noncontact: APC, Nd: YAG laser
- **Mechanical therapy**
  a. Endoclips
  b. Endoscopic band ligation

Dual therapy (combination of above modalities)

APC, argon plasma cautery; BICAP, bipolar probe; HP, heater probe.

---

has been demonstrated. Decompression of portal pressures when possible is the optimal therapy.

While endoscopic injection sclerotherapy and banding ligation in conjunction with pharmacologic treatment are the primary methods for controlling acute variceal bleeding, tamponade with a Sengstaken-Blakemore tube may be indicated when these methods fail or before endoscopy if a rapid bleed occurs. The use of these tubes is indicated for acute bleeding from esophageal or gastric varices unresponsive to medical therapy, tears at the gastroesophageal junction, Mallory-Weiss tears unresponsive to medical therapy, or esophageal exclusion to manage distal esophageal perforation. The Sengstaken-Blakemore tube is absolutely contraindicated for patients in whom bleeding has stopped and in those with recent surgery of the gastroesophageal junction or known esophageal stricture.

CASE 156-3

A 62-year-old man with a history of NSAID use and tobacco abuse sought medical attention for intermittent hematemesis for 1 day. His vital signs revealed a heart rate of 114 beats/min and a low-normal BP (100/60 mm Hg). Laboratory studies reported anemia with a hematocrit of 21% (baseline 45%). His physicians administered erythromycin intravenously and initiated an IV PPI. After stabilization with two large bore IVs, and initiation of blood transfusions, a gastroenterologist performed an upper endoscopy, which identified a visible bleeding vessel in a deep duodenal ulcer. The ulcer was injected with dilute epinephrine, and clips were placed to achieve hemostasis. The patient was monitored in an intensive care unit and had an uneventful postprocedure course.

◼ CONSULTATION

Hospitalists should involve a gastroenterologist early in the course of upper GI bleeding. Emergent consultation is appropriate with rapid bleeds in the setting of hypotension, a very low hematocrit, known varices, or other instances when urgent endoscopy might be required. In most cases, however, patient stabilization is a crucial first step before gastroenterology intervention can be considered (**Figure 156-7**). A gastroenterology consultant can provide diagnostic and therapeutic advice early in the course of treatment and may be called as soon as a suspected upper GI bleeding patient is identified. In addition, IR angiography and surgery consultations are indicated in certain circumstances including patients requiring the ICU, those who require multiple blood transfusions or those who

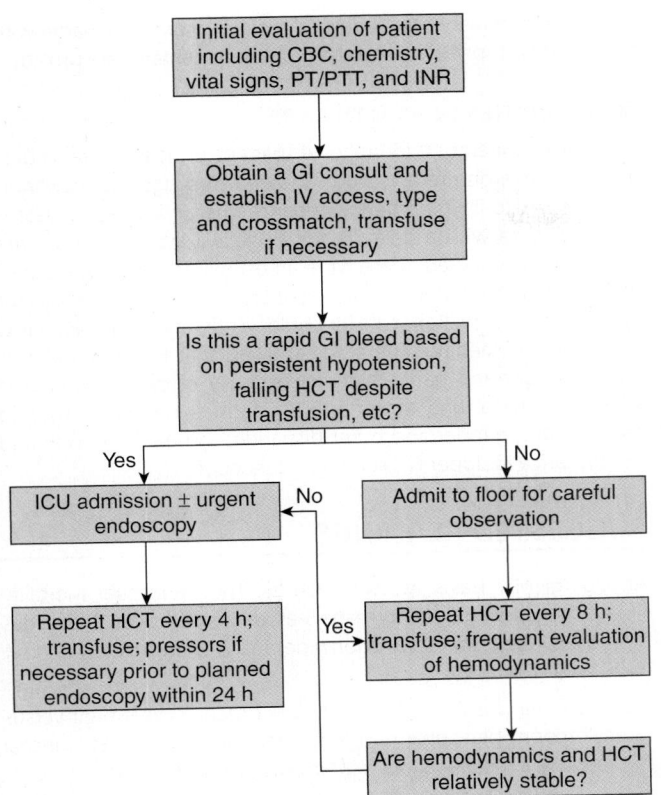

Figure 156-7 *Initial diagnostic algorithm for upper GI bleeding. (CBC, complete blood count; HCT, hematocrit; ICU, intensive care unit; INR, international normalized ratio; IV, intravenous; PT, prothrombin time; PTT, partial thromboplastin time.)*

undergo endoscopy without identification of a source of bleed or ability to stop the bleeding. In small bowel or lower GI bleeding patients, the patient may benefit from a tagged red blood cell scan and subsequent angiography. **The key to consultation is to involve the consultant early and to communicate any significant clinical changes.**

COMPLICATIONS AND PROGNOSIS

■ COMPLICATIONS OF GI BLEEDING

The reported mortality of upper GI bleeding generally ranges from 2% to 14%. Complications of GI bleeding include hypotension and subsequent shock, which can lead to organ failure and death if not addressed in a timely manner. Aspiration of blood contents and subsequent hypoxemia and respiratory failure represents another adverse outcome. Tachycardia in the setting of pre-existing coronary heart disease can lead to ischemia. Anemia can also further lead to underperfusion of vital organs and some patients die of complications subsequent to inadequate resuscitation with blood and fluids as discussed above.

■ COMPLICATIONS OF TREATMENT

The majority of the complications associated with treatment of upper GI bleeding stem from endoscopic treatments. Major complications include myocardial infarction, perforation, aspiration, hemorrhage, and death. Minor complications of endoscopy include mucosal tears, medication reactions, and hypoxemia. In addition, a small risk exists of infection or bleeding from the endoscopic intervention itself. As sedatives are utilized for the procedure, the individual risks of each medication are added to the overall risk of the procedure. Many of the complications of GI endoscopy are cardiopulmonary in origin.

The initial evaluation of patients with upper GI bleeding should include risk assessment to triage patients to appropriate levels of care and perform resuscitation measures. Elective endotracheal intubation should be considered in patients at high risk of aspiration, such as those with massive upper GI bleeding. Attention must be given to provide the proper level of sedation required to perform the procedure.

Epinephrine is a vasoconstrictor that can lead to local ischemia and can also cause tachycardia. Large doses of injected epinephrine during endoscopic therapy especially in the region of the esophagus and upper stomach are associated with significant elevations of systolic blood pressure and tachycardia. The use of cautery can lead to direct tissue injury, which may further damage the GI tract. The use of cautery may lead to perforation, especially if excessive pressure is exerted on the site of therapy. The depth of penetration of tissue injury may be lessened by the use of injection therapy that lifts the tissue and provides a safety barrier.

■ PROGNOSIS

In patients presenting with upper GI bleeding, a number of clinical prognostic factors have been shown to be helpful in predicting a poor outcome. These include older age (age >60 years), the presence of shock, hematemesis and/or hematochezia, onset of bleeding in a patient hospitalized for other reasons, bleeding from malignancies of the upper GI tract or varices, increasing comorbid diseases, and patients with severe coagulopathies.

DISCHARGE PLANNING

■ RESTARTING ANTICOAGULATION IN UPPER GI BLEEDING

Patients who require anticoagulants (eg, warfarin) or platelet function inhibitors (eg, clopidogrel, aspirin) may develop signs of upper GI bleeding. Most GI bleeding episodes on antiplatelet agents or anticoagulants occur within the first year of therapy. Once a source of bleeding is identified, the timing of restarting anticoagulants represents a difficult decision. Part of the decision-making process is evaluating the benefit of the anticoagulant or platelet inhibitor compared to the risk of bleeding. A patient with high-risk thromboembolic disease should have careful consideration of reversal of anticoagulation in consultation with the prescribing cardiologist or neurologist before endoscopy. A patient with low-risk thromboembolic disease can have complete reversal of anticoagulation followed by endoscopy. When to resume anticoagulation depends on the source and severity of bleeding as well as the underlying condition being treated. After hemostasis is achieved, patients who need to be restarted on anticoagulants have to be monitored carefully for subsequent bleeding.

■ OUTPATIENT SYMPTOM MONITORING

Patients discharged after upper GI bleeding require education about signs and symptoms to help identify any early bleeding. Patients should look for the return of black stool as a sign of a developing bleed. However, for the first 24 to 48 hours following active bleeding, patients can expect to see subsequent passage of blood, which may be maroon or black. Resting heart rate with evaluation for tachycardia can be measured by patients themselves. In addition, patients require education about over-the-counter medications to avoid that may affect GI bleeding, including drugs that contain NSAIDs, aspirin, or SSRIs. Bismuth subsalicylate (eg, Pepto-Bismol) should also be avoided as it causes the stool to appear dark and the stool color can be confused with melena.

■ OUTPATIENT LAB MONITORING

Patients who had bleeding related to supratherapeutic levels of warfarin need careful monitoring of the INR if the medication is subsequently resumed. Clinics that specialize in anticoagulation can reduce bleeding outcomes. In addition, anemic patients should have hemoglobin levels checked in the outpatient setting 1 to 2 weeks following discharge, as asymptomatic recurrent bleeding can present with worsening anemia. For upper GI bleeding, an elevated BUN can be a useful marker of recurrent bleeding. Patients with *H. Pylori*–related bleeding should have an *H. pylori* breath test or stool antigen performed if upper endoscopy is not scheduled to confirm that *H. pylori* has been successfully eradicated.

QUALITY IMPROVEMENT TO ADDRESS PERFORMANCE GAPS

■ PREVENTION

Primary and secondary prevention of upper GI bleeding requires careful evaluation of a patient's underlying medical problems and current medications. NSAID use should be minimized whenever possible and, if necessary, one should monitor frequently for symptoms and signs of GI bleeding, which may indicate peptic ulcer disease, esophagitis, gastritis, or duodenitis, which can follow NSAID use. β-blocker therapy with propranolol or nadolol should be used in patients with cirrhosis and a prior history of esophageal variceal bleeding (secondary prophylaxis) regardless of grade, or large esophageal varices without previous hemorrhage (primary prophylaxis). The comparison of nonselective β-blockers and placebo in several randomized controlled trials demonstrates a greater than 20% absolute risk reduction in subsequent bleeding from esophageal varices. Prevention of GI bleeding in admitted patients requires careful monitoring of medications (eg, anticoagulants and antiplatelet agents) and comorbidities. Patients at high risk for stress ulcer bleeding (eg, mechanical ventilation) benefit from prophylactic PPI dosing.

■ TRANSITIONS OF CARE

As patients transition from in-hospital care to outpatient management, several factors must be considered. Medications must be adjusted from the inpatient setting to appropriate outpatient regimens. For example, although patients with upper GI bleeding are often managed with high-dose proton-pump inhibitors in the hospital, at discharge, most patients can be managed on a once daily standard dose oral proton-pump inhibitor or twice daily for high-risk bleeding lesions.

Findings at endoscopy may require changes in the medical regimen or subsequent endoscopies. In patients with peptic ulcer disease, biopsy results positive for *H. pylori* infection indicate a necessary outpatient antibiotic regimen. Most patients with significant gastric ulcers will require repeat endoscopy examinations in 8 to 12 weeks to confirm healing of the ulcer and for biopsy to exclude malignancy.

Communication of in-hospital caregivers with outpatient physicians is critical to the successful management of patients with significant upper GI bleeding. Follow-up with a primary physician should take place for repeat blood draws and physical examination within 7 to 14 days of hospital discharge, and follow-up with a gastroenterologist either for a planned repeat endoscopy or office visit should take place within 2 to 4 weeks depending on the source of bleeding. For example, variceal bleeding may require a 2-week follow-up endoscopy for further banding and assessment of healing. Outpatient planning for follow-up with gastroenterology, general

surgery, and primary care should take place prior to discharge with the consulting specialists and the outpatient primary care provider.

■ DISPARITIES IN HEALTH CARE

While scarce literature identifies disparities in health care in gastroenterology, one recent study showed that significant proportion of visits to US emergency departments for acute GI illnesses are associated with a delay in initial clinical assessment. Of the patient visits analyzed, there were an estimated 1.6 million emergency department visits for acute pancreatitis, 2.2 million visits for appendicitis, 1.2 million visits for cholecystitis, and 3.9 million visits for upper GI bleeding. The study showed that Hispanic patients waited longer and had a higher frequency of delays compared with other racial and ethnic groups. Future investigations into racial, ethnic, gender and other disparities in health delivery and performance in upper GI bleeding are needed.

SUGGESTED READINGS

Abougergi MS, Travis AC, Saltzman JR. The in-hospital mortality rate for upper GI hemorrhage has decreased over 2 decades in the United States: a nationwide analysis. *Gastrointest Endosc.* 2015;81(4):882-888.

Banares R, Albillos A, Rincon D, et al. Endoscopic treatment versus endoscopic plus pharmacologic treatment for acute variceal bleeding: a meta-analysis. *Hepatology.* 2002;35:609-615.

Barkun AN, Bardou M, Kuipers EJ, et al. International Consensus Upper Gastrointestinal Bleeding Conference Group. International consensus recommendations on the management of patients with nonvariceal upper gastrointestinal bleeding. *Ann Intern Med.* 2010;152(2):101-113.

Bjorkman DJ, Zaman A, Fennerty MB, et al. Urgent vs. elective endoscopy for acute non-variceal upper-GI bleeding: an effectiveness study. *Gastrointest Endosc.* 2004;60(1):1-8.

Blatchford O, Murray WR, Blatchford M. A risk score to predict need for treatment for upper-gastrointestinal hemorrhage. *Lancet.* 2000;356:1318-1321.

Gralnek IM, Barkun AN, Bardou M. Management of acute bleeding from a peptic ulcer. *N Engl J Med.* 2008;359(9):928-937.

Laine L, Jensen DM. Management of patients with ulcer bleeding. *Am J Gastroenterol.* 2012;107:345-360.

Pfau PR, Cooper GS, Carlson MD, et al. Success and shortcomings of a clinical care pathway in the management of acute nonvariceal upper gastrointestinal bleeding. *Am J Gastroenterol.* 2004;99:425-431.

Rockall TA, Logan RFA, Devlin HB, et al. Steering Committee of the National Audit of Acute Upper Gastrointestinal Haemorrhage. Risk assessment after acute upper gastrointestinal hemorrhage. *Gut.* 1996;38:316-321.

Sachar H, Vaidya K, Laine L. Intermittent vs continuous proton pump inhibitor therapy for high-risk bleeding ulcers. A systematic review and meta-analysis. *JAMA Intern Med.* 2014;174(11):1755-1762.

Wolf AT, Wasan SK, Saltzman JR. Impact of anticoagulation on rebleeding following endoscopic therapy for non-variceal upper gastrointestinal hemorrhage. *Am J Gastroenterol.* 2007;102(2):290-296.

CHAPTER 157

Acute Pancreatitis

Julia McNabb-Baltar, MD

Peter A. Banks, MD

Key Clinical Questions

1 What are the criteria for the diagnosis of acute pancreatitis?

2 What efforts should be made to determine the etiology during hospitalization, and what is the optimal timing of diagnostic and/or intervention studies in acute pancreatitis?

3 What are the key components of early management?

4 What is the management of late complications?

5 When should consultation with gastroenterology, surgery, or interventional radiology be considered?

6 When are specific interventions such as endoscopic retrograde cholangiopancreatography, fine-needle aspiration, or antibiotics indicated?

EPIDEMIOLOGY

Acute pancreatitis is a common cause for hospitalization in the United States. Recent data from the National Center for Health Statistics have indicated a rising frequency of admissions for acute pancreatitis attributed to the increase in gallstone-related disease. Annually, more than 300,000 hospital admissions for acute pancreatitis present in the United States at a direct cost of more than $2 billion. Although acute pancreatitis is typically a mild, self-limited disease, a wide range of severity exists. Fifteen to twenty percent of patients experience a more severe form of disease with overall in-hospital mortality estimated to range between 2% and 5% of cases.

Risk factors for acute pancreatitis include both genetic susceptibility and environmental exposures. Genes involving mutation in the cystic fibrosis transmembrane conductance regulator, cationic trypsinogen gene (*PRSS1*), and secretory trypsin inhibitor (SPINK1) have been identified in patients with recurrent acute pancreatitis. Other patient-related factors such as obesity have also been demonstrated to be associated with increased severity of disease.

The most common etiology for acute pancreatitis is now gallstone-related disease, followed by alcohol and idiopathic pancreatitis (**Table 157-1**). Additional etiologies include metabolic derangements (hypercalcemia, hypertriglyceridemia) and medications (**Table 157-2**). Less common etiologies include autoimmune and hereditary forms of pancreatitis. Whether pancreas divisum itself is a cause for acute pancreatitis remains controversial.

Obstructive causes for pancreatitis secondary to pancreatic mass or cystic lesions, such as intraductal papillary mucinous neoplasms are increasingly recognized due to improvements in imaging techniques.

RISK STRATIFICATION

Given the wide variation in morbidity and mortality in acute pancreatitis, risk stratification is essential. In 2012, the Atlanta Classification was revised and stratifies patients as mild, moderately severe, and severe pancreatitis. Mild acute pancreatitis is characterized by absence of organ failure and local or systemic complications, moderately severe acute pancreatitis is characterized by transient organ failure and/or local and/or systemic complications, and severe acute pancreatitis is characterized by persistent organ failure (≥48 hours).

Prognostic scoring systems have also been developed. Systemic inflammatory response syndrome (SIRS) has been associated with severe course. Systemic inflammatory response syndrome is defined as the presence of two or more of the following: temperature less than 96.8°F or more than 100.4°F, heart rate greater than 90 beats/min, respiratory rate greater than 20 breaths/min or $PaCO_2$ less than 32 mm Hg, white Blood Cell count greater than 12,000 cells/mL or less than 4000 cells/mL. The bedside index of severity in acute pancreatitis (BISAP) assigns points for each of the following: blood urea nitrogen (BUN) >25, impaired mental status, SIRS, age > 60, and pleural effusion. The presence of three or more of these findings signals a substantially increased risk of mortality. Other stratification tools such as APACHE-II score ≥8, laboratory findings such as BUN >20 or rising, hematocrit >44% or rising, CRP level at 48 to 72 hours >150 mg/dL, and risk factor including BMI ≥ 30 are also associated with a more severe course. Recent guidelines recommend the use of risk stratification.

TABLE 157-1 Etiologies of Acute Pancreatitis

	Examples
Gallstone	
Alcohol	
Autoimmune	
Hereditary	PRSS1, CFTR, SPINK1, CTRC
Iatrogenic	Post-ERCP, postsurgery
Infectious	
• Viral	Mumps, Cytomegalovirus, Coxsackievirus
• Parasite	Toxoplasma
• Bacterial	Legionella, *Salmonella*, Aspergillus
• Fungal	
Metabolic	Hypercalcemia, hypertriglyceridemia
Medication	See Table 157-2
Obstructive	Pancreatic or ampullary tumors, pancreas divisum
Toxic	Scorpion venom, organophosphate poisoning
Trauma	Abdominal injury
Vascular	Vasculitis, ischemia, embolism
Idiopathic	

PRACTICE POINT

- A BISAP score in the first 24 hours of 0 to 1 point ≤ 1% mortality, 2 points = 2% mortality, 3 points = 5% to 8% mortality, 4 points = 13% to 19%, 5 points ≥ 20% mortality.

DISORDER: EVALUATION, INPATIENT MANAGEMENT

■ EVALUATION

Patients with acute pancreatitis usually complain of sudden onset unrelenting epigastric pain that is sharp in nature. This pain often

TABLE 157-2 Drug-Induced Pancreatitis

Class I	Class II
Amiodarone	Didanosine
Azathioprine	Acetaminophen
Cannabis	Clozapine
Valproic acid	Estrogen
Mercaptopurine	Propofol
Mesalamine	Hydrochlorothiazide
Omeprazole	Tamoxifene
Metronidazole	
Lamivudine	
Furosemide	
Simvastatin	
Dexamethasone	
Sulindac	

Class I Medications: Case reports of acute pancreatitis with at least one documented case following re-exposure.
Class II Medications: Case reports of acute pancreatitis with consistent latency.
Adapted from Badalov N, Baradarian R, Iswara K, et al. Drug-induced acute pancreatitis: an evidence-based review. *Clin Gastroenterol Hepatol.* 2007;5:648-661.

radiates to the back. Nausea and vomiting are common as is anorexia. Patients may present with signs of volume depletion in the setting of decreased oral intake as well as potential third-space losses. Signs of systemic inflammation are common at the time of presentation including fever, tachycardia, and leukocytosis. Rarely, physical examination findings may include evidence of hemorrhagic pancreatitis such as flank (Grey-Turner sign) or periumbilical (Cullen sign) ecchymosis.

The presence of epigastric pain with an elevation in amylase/lipase ≥3 times normal is highly accurate for the diagnosis of acute pancreatitis. Additional considerations should include acute cholecystitis or ascending cholangitis (both of which may be concurrent with an attack of biliary pancreatitis). Less common considerations include a penetrating duodenal ulcer, bowel ischemia, renal colic, or diabetic ketoacidosis. Further potentially life-threatening conditions include a perforated viscus, bowel obstruction or myocardial infarction. Serum amylase may also be elevated in salivary disorders, ectopic pregnancy, or macroamylasemia.

The diagnosis of acute pancreatitis requires at least two of the following: (1) typical epigastric abdominal pain, (2) amylase/lipase evaluation ≥3 times upper limit of normal, and/or (3) confirmatory findings on cross-sectional imaging. Findings on abdominal ultrasound in conjunction with liver function tests have very high sensitivity for the detection of gallstone-related illness. Specifically, an elevated ALT level > 2 to 3 times normal has been found to have a 95% positive predictive value for gallstone-related illness. More recently, magnetic resonance cholangiopancreatography (MRCP) has emerged as a highly accurate, noninvasive means to evaluate for the presence of biliary pancreatitis (**Figure 157-1**).

PRACTICE POINT

- The diagnosis of acute pancreatitis requires at least two of the following: (1) typical epigastric abdominal pain, (2) amylase/lipase evaluation ≥ 3 times upper limit of normal, and/or (3) confirmatory findings on cross-sectional imaging.

The finding of hypercalcemia in the setting of acute pancreatitis should prompt a thorough evaluation for the potential underlying etiology such as hyperparathyroidism or occult malignancy.

Autoimmune pancreatitis is a rare cause of acute pancreatitis that has recently gained increasing attention in the medical literature. An otherwise unexplained episode of acute pancreatitis in a patient with computed tomography (CT) scan findings of an enhancing "rim" or diffusely enlarged pancreas or pancreatogram

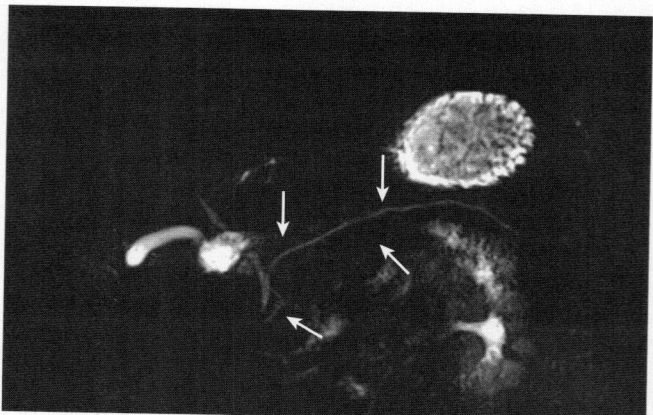

Figure 157-1 *Secretin-enhanced MRCP image demonstrating normal pancreatic duct anatomy (arrows).*

features of an irregularly narrowed pancreatic duct are suggestive of autoimmune pancreatitis on imaging. A serum IgG4 level greater than two times the upper limit of normal may be useful to establish the diagnosis in type 1 autoimmune pancreatitis, which rarely presents as acute pancreatitis. Type 2 autoimmune pancreatitis, which is IgG4 negative, presents in 18% to 31% of cases as acute pancreatitis.

■ INPATIENT MANAGEMENT

Patients with confirmed acute pancreatitis should be managed as inpatients because they need vigorous intravenous fluid resuscitation and intravenous analgesia. A possible exception includes patients with a Harmless Acute Pancreatitis Score, which is defined as absence of rebound tenderness or guarding, normal serum creatinine, and normal hematocrit on presentation. These patients may be considered for a short hospital stay of less than 24 hours.

Persistent or worsening organ dysfunction after initial fluid resuscitation or patients with significant comorbid or concurrent illness (eg, congestive heart failure and/or chronic kidney disease) should be considered for hemodynamic monitoring in an intensive care setting. Also, patients with a rise in either hematocrit or BUN after initial resuscitation efforts should strongly be considered for hemodynamic monitoring to guide further resuscitation efforts.

Persistent multiorgan dysfunction and infection are two major complications that can develop in the patient hospitalized for acute pancreatitis. Patients with organ dysfunction are best managed in an intensive care setting. In addition to extrapancreatic infection, infected necrosis and persistent multiorgan failure are associated with a high morbidity and mortality. These patients are best managed in a multidisciplinary setting involving gastroenterology, surgery, and interventional radiology services.

Initial management of acute pancreatitis should include determination of etiology, assessment of severity, fluid challenge, and analgesia (**Figure 157-2**). Etiology may guide subsequent management, as in the case of gallstone pancreatitis. Clinical practice guidelines recommend abdominal ultrasound in the early assessment of patients with acute pancreatitis. Further assessment should include routine laboratory tests (liver profile, calcium, complete blood count). The use of CT scan of the abdomen in the initial 48 to 72 hours should be restricted to if the diagnosis of acute pancreatitis is uncertain. Fluid resuscitation is the cornerstone of initial treatment for acute pancreatitis. Clinical practice guidelines recommend vigorous initial fluid resuscitation with the thought of potentially preventing complications such as necrosis. Although aggressive fluid resuscitation has not been demonstrated to directly prevent specific complications, a rise in hematocrit or BUN in the setting of intravenous hydration has been associated with necrosis and in-hospital mortality, respectively. Specifically, an elevated BUN at admission >25 mg/dL and/or a rise in BUN during the initial 24 hours in the setting of volume resuscitation indicate an increased risk for in-hospital mortality (**Figure 157-3**). Therefore, patients with a rise in either hematocrit or BUN during initial resuscitation efforts should strongly be considered for hemodynamic monitoring to guide further resuscitation efforts. Aggressive fluid resuscitation

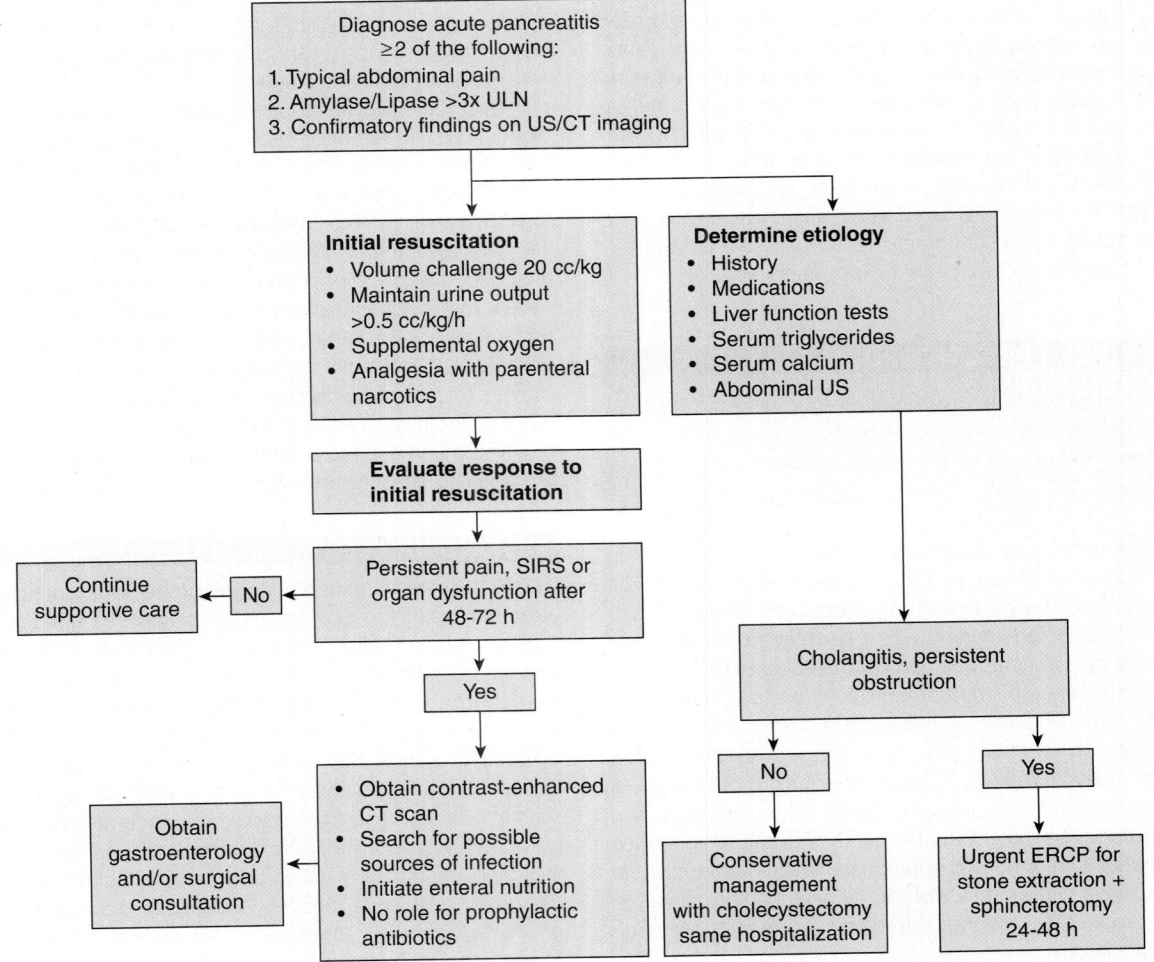

Figure 157-2 *Suggested initial management algorithm for acute pancreatitis (CT, computed tomography; ERCP, endoscopic retrograde cholangiopancreatography; ULN, upper limits of normal; US or U/S, ultrasound; SIRS, systemic inflammatory response syndrome).*

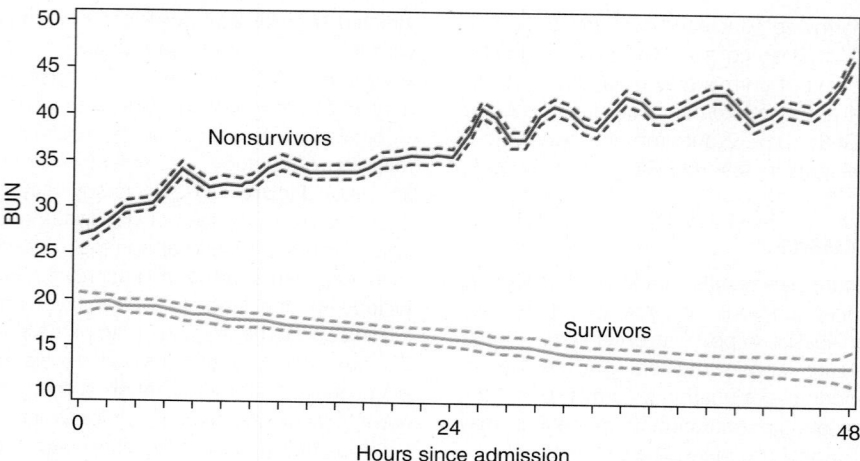

Figure 157-3 *Plot of early BUN changes among survivors versus nonsurvivors of acute pancreatitis. Data from 5819 cases of acute pancreatitis from 69 US hospitals. Solid lines represent mean BUN values and dashed lines indicate 95% confidence limits.*

should be focused in the initial 12 to 24 hours of presentation; continued aggressive hydration at 48 and 72 hours may be detrimental and associated with higher rate of SIRS and organ failure.

Adequate analgesia is central to patient comfort and recovery. Limited data are available regarding treatment options for pain in acute pancreatitis. However, there is no evidence to suggest a contraindication to morphine-related compounds due to sphincter of oddi spasm.

Recent studies have called attention to extensive use of imaging associated with acute pancreatitis. In an attempt to standardize use of imaging services, the American College of Radiology has issued appropriateness criteria for imaging tests in acute pancreatitis. Current recommendations are for the use of abdominal ultrasound early in the disease course to evaluate for biliary-related complications. Computed tomography is generally reserved for patients with evidence of systemic inflammation (SIRS) after 48 hours of illness or signs of clinical deterioration. If suspicion for biliary disease is high then MRCP may be considered as a noninvasive alternative to ERCP. Recent data also recommend the judicious use of contrast-enhanced CT scans to reduce patient exposure to radiation.

PRACTICE POINT

● Clinical practice guidelines recommend abdominal ultrasound (in preference to abdominal computed tomography) in the early assessment of patients with acute pancreatitis.

Endoscopic retrograde cholangiopancreatography is indicated within 24 hours when there is suspicion for ascending cholangitis. It is also indicated electively in the setting of persistent biliary obstruction (stone visualized on imaging with persistent elevation in liver function tests), or in patients deemed poor candidates for cholecystectomy. Fine-needle aspiration of pancreatic necrosis is indicated in a patient with evidence of persistent systemic inflammation in the absence of alternative source of infection (generally after 7-10 days of illness). Prophylactic antibiotics for the prevention of infected pancreatic necrosis are currently not recommended based on results from several recent double-blind randomized controlled trials. Antibiotics are considered appropriate while awaiting culture results in a patient with evidence of clinical deterioration. However, most experts advocate tailoring or removing antibiotics once culture results are known.

Gastroenterology should be consulted when gallstone pancreatitis is suspected, in the setting of a patient with persistent (>48 hours

duration) SIRS or in the setting of acute pancreatitis complicated by necrosis and/or organ failure. Surgical consultation is indicated in the setting of gallstone pancreatitis in order to arrange for appropriate timing of cholecystectomy. Recent data have indicated that routine ERCP prior to cholecystectomy is not indicated. Interventional radiological services can assist in the identification of infected necrosis through CT-guided fine-needle aspiration and Gram stain of necrosis in a patient with ongoing fever or systemic inflammation. A multidisciplinary team approach is indicated for the management of infected necrosis as care may need to be individualized. In general, a multidisciplinary care can help optimize use of procedures, antibiotics, and imaging studies.

In mild acute pancreatitis, oral nutrition with clear liquids or low fat diet may be initiated once pain is controlled with analgesic. A recent randomized controlled trial showed that even in severe pancreatitis, oral nutrition started at 72 hours after admission was safe compared to early enteral nutrition started at 24 hours and was not associated with increased rate of infection or death. Nutritional support services may be required for initiation of enteral or parenteral nutrition in a patient that is not anticipated to begin oral feeding within 7 days of hospitalization. In addition, both consultation with gastroenterology and interventional radiology may assist in placement of a nasojejunal catheter for purposes of enteral nutrition in a patient that is not anticipated to begin oral feeding within 7 days. Enteral route should always be favored and parenteral nutrition should be reserved for patients unable to tolerate enteral feeding, or if enteral nutrition is not available.

POSTACUTE CARE

During the convalescent or recovery phase from acute pancreatitis, attention should focus on prevention of future recurrence and management of long-term complications. Recent data from a randomized controlled trial have indicated that repeated alcohol counseling can reduce the recurrence of alcohol-associated pancreatitis when compared to a single, one-time intervention. In addition, cases of "idiopathic" pancreatitis should be further evaluated with either repeat abdominal ultrasound (which may detect abnormalities such as biliary sludge often missed in the context of acute illness) or secretin enhanced MRCP to evaluate for anatomical anomalies including intraductal papillary mucinous neoplasm and pancreas divisum. More invasive interventions such as endoscopic ultrasound or ERCP are generally reserved for patients with recurrent episodes of idiopathic acute pancreatitis.

Long-term sequelae that may arise in the setting of acute pancreatitis include both local and systemic complications. *Local complications*

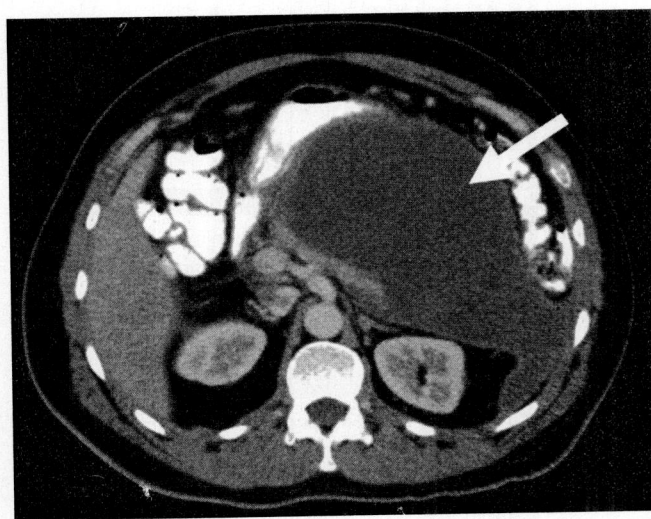

Figure 157-4 *Contrast-enhanced abdominal computed tomography demonstrating large heterogeneous postnecrotic collection (arrow) arising in a patient with necrotizing pancreatitis (8 weeks after initial episode).*

include development of fluid collections that may either comprise a pseudocyst (homogeneous fluid-filled collection) or a postnecrotic collection (heterogeneous cavity filled with fluid and necrotic debris) (**Figure 157-4**). The distinction can be important given that it may influence approach to treatment. In general, intervention in fluid collections that arise in the setting of acute pancreatitis is only indicated in the setting of symptoms or infection. A symptomatic or infected fluid collection following an episode of acute pancreatitis is an indication for consultation with gastroenterology and surgical services. Although far less common, an additional potentially serious local complication is development of a pseudoaneurysm. Hemorrhage from a pseudoaneurysm can be life threatening and is best managed by angiography with surgical treatment reserved for failure to achieve hemostasis by alternative measures.

PRACTICE POINT

- A rise in hematocrit or BUN in the setting of intravenous hydration has been associated with necrosis and in-hospital mortality. Specifically, an elevated BUN at admission >25 mg/dL and/or a rise in BUN during the initial 24 hours in the setting of volume resuscitation indicate an increased risk for in-hospital mortality.

PRACTICE POINT

- For pancreatic pseudocysts (homogeneous fluid-filled collections) or a postnecrotic collections (heterogeneous cavity filled with fluid and necrotic debris), intervention is only indicated in the setting of symptoms or infection. A symptomatic or infected fluid collection following an episode of acute pancreatitis is an indication for consultation with gastroenterology and surgical services.

Additional long-term *systemic complications* that can result from acute pancreatitis include both exocrine and endocrine insufficiency of the pancreas. Patients with symptoms of steatorrhea or signs of fat-soluble vitamin deficiency should be evaluated with a fecal elastase on a solid stool to screen for pancreatic exocrine insufficiency. If the diagnosis is unclear, referral to a pancreas center for direct pancreatic function testing may confirm the diagnosis. This procedure consists of endoscopic collection of duodenal secretions after injection of intravenous secretin, which stimulates the pancreas to produce a bicarbonate-rich fluid. Once the diagnosis of exocrine insufficiency is confirmed, treatment with pancreatic enzyme supplementation is indicated (generally at least 48,000 IU lipase with each meal). Patients suffering necrotizing pancreatitis and especially those who have undergone pancreatic debridement are at increased risk of worsening or new-onset diabetes. Fasting glucose or hemoglobin A1C can be useful to screen for development of diabetes in this high-risk category of patients. Patients may develop brittle diabetes in the setting of extensive necrosis in which case referral to endocrinology may be useful in order to optimize glycemic control.

DISCHARGE CHECKLIST

Goals of discharge planning for acute pancreatitis include (1) arrangement for adequate follow-up, (2) prevention of disease recurrence, and (3) initiation of appropriate secondary evaluation. Although follow-up interval should be based on an individual patient's needs, a 2-week interval has been routinely utilized. Patients with severe disease complicated by necrosis or fluid collections should be referred for outpatient follow-up with gastroenterology services. The two most important interventions for secondary prevention are cholecystectomy for gallstone-related acute pancreatitis and alcohol and smoking cessation counseling for patients with alcohol-associated disease. In the case of mild gallstone pancreatitis, cholecystectomy is strongly recommended during the same hospitalization to reduce the likelihood of recurrent episode of biliary complications while awaiting surgery. Prior studies have also shown this to be a cost-effective strategy for the prevention of gallstone pancreatitis. In the case of alcohol-associated disease, longitudinal alcohol cessation therapy is recommended.

SUGGESTED READINGS

Bakker OJ, van Brunschot S, van Santvoort HC, et al. Early versus on-demand nasoenteric tube feeding in acute pancreatitis. *N Engl J Med.* 2014;371(21):1983-1993.

Banks PA, Bollen TL, Dervenis C, et al. Classification of acute pancreatitis 2012: revision of the Atlanta classification and definitions by international consensus. *Gut.* 2013;62:102-111.

Dellinger EP, Tellado JM, Soto NE, et al. Early antibiotic treatment for severe acute necrotizing pancreatitis: a randomized, double-blind, placebo-controlled study. *Ann Surg.* 2007;245(5):674-683.

Gaisano HY, Gorelick FS. New insights into the mechanisms of pancreatitis. *Gastroenterology.* 2009;136(7):2040-2044.

Tenner S, Baillie J, DeWitt J, et al. American College of Gastroenterology Guideline: management of acute pancreatitis. *Am J Gastroenterol.* 2012;108(9):1400-1415.

van Santvoort HC, Besselink MG, Bakker OJ, et al. Dutch Pancreatitis Study Group. A step up approach or open necrosectomy for necrotizing pancreatitis. *N Engl J Med.* 2010;362(16):1491-1502.

Wu BU, Banks PA. Clinical management of patients with acute pancreaitits. *Gastroenterology.* 2013;144:1272-1281.

Wu BU, Johannes RS, Sun X, et al. The early prediction of mortality in acute pancreatitis: a large population-based study. *Gut.* 2008;57(12):1698-1703.

CHAPTER 158

Jaundice, Obstruction, and Acute Cholangitis

Allison R. Schulman, MD
Kunal Jajoo, MD

Key Clinical Questions

1 What causes jaundice?

2 How are biliary obstruction and cholangitis diagnosed?

3 What are the best imaging modalities?

4 What treatment strategies should be employed in patients with biliary obstruction or cholangitis?

5 When should procedure or surgical intervention be considered in patients with cholangitis?

INTRODUCTION

This chapter describes clinical conditions manifested as a result of acute or subacute biliary disease. Particular attention is paid to those conditions that frequently present to the inpatient setting, including jaundice, obstruction, and acute cholangitis.

JAUNDICE

Jaundice, from the French *jaune*, refers to the yellowish discoloration of the skin, sclera, and mucus membranes that reflects deposition of bilirubin in tissues. While jaundice is often used interchangeably with hyperbilirubinemia, this discoloration is only apparent when the serum bilirubin level exceeds at least two times the upper limit of normal (0.5-1.0 mg/dL), or over 2 mg/dL. Jaundice is typically recognized earliest in the oral mucus membranes (under the tongue and hard palate) and in the sclera, the latter of which has a high elastin content and a strong binding affinity for bilirubin.

PATHOPHYSIOLOGY

Jaundice results from a pathologic process that interferes with the normal metabolism and excretion of bilirubin (**Figure 158-1**). Physiologically, bilirubin is the product of hemoglobin breakdown formed during the elimination of senescent red blood cells. Macrophages, a component of the reticuloendothelial system, separate hemoglobin molecules into proteins (globulin) and heme. Splitting of the four pyrrole ring of heme produces biliverdin, which is then reduced to bilirubin. This type of bilirubin is unconjugated, and insoluble in water. As a result, it must be attached to albumin for transport to the liver for excretion.

Once in the liver, the bilirubin is rendered more water soluble by conjugation to glucuronic acid. Conjugated bilirubin is excreted into bile and subsequently enters the small intestine and colon. Exposure to oxidizing enzymes in the gut leads to the greenish color of bile. A portion of the bilirubin is deconjugated and reabsorbed into the circulation. The remaining segment is broken down by bacteria into urobilinogen, a fraction of which is converted into stercobilinogen and excreted in the stool, and the rest of which is excreted in the urine. Obstruction of the biliary system can hinder excretion of bilirubin into the gut and simultaneously exceed the processing ability of the kidneys, leading to pale stools and dark urine.

The amount of bilirubin in the serum is determined through measurement of light absorbance of the specimen following chemical treatment. Prior to examination, these specimens must be shielded from light to prevent excessive breakdown and falsely low results. The quantification of bilirubin is reported as direct (ie, conjugated), indirect (ie, unconjugated), and total (sum of conjugated and unconjugated forms). An increase in conjugated bilirubin is often the result of intra- or extrahepatic cholestasis. Elevations in unconjugated bilirubin, on the other hand, can occur as the result of three different pathophysiologic mechanisms including overproduction of bilirubin, impaired bilirubin uptake by the liver, or abnormalities of bilirubin conjugation.

■ CAUSES OF JAUNDICE

Prehepatic

Prehepatic jaundice occurs as a result of a pathologic process occurring outside the liver. The most common cause of prehepatic jaundice is hemolysis, whereby red blood cells are destroyed at an

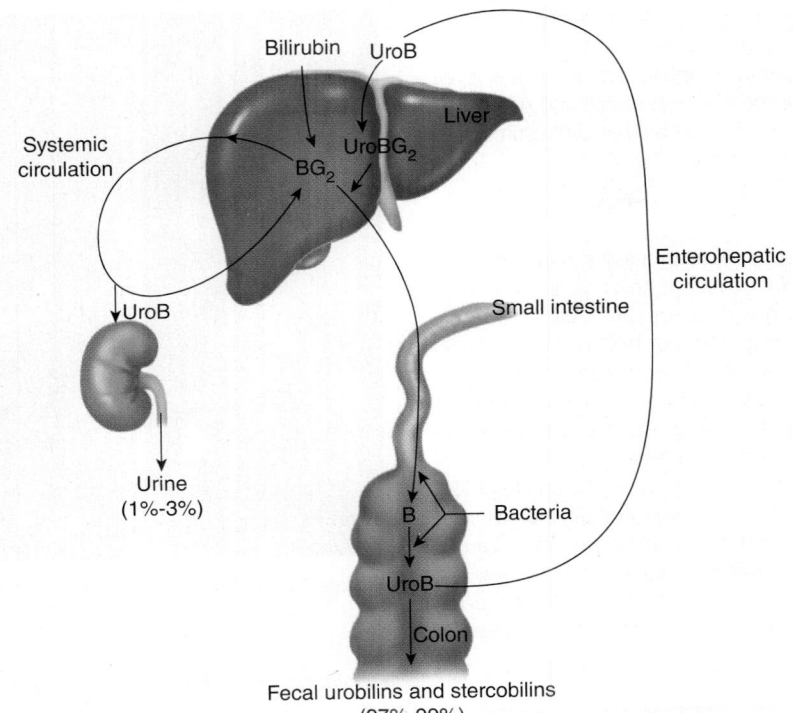

Figure 158-1 *Cycling of bilirubin and its products through the liver, intestines, portal and systemic circulations, and kidneys. (B, bilirubin; G, glucuronide; UroB, urobilinogen).*

increased rate, thereby leading to excessive breakdown of hemoglobin. Fractionation of bilirubin in the serum of patients with prehepatic jaundice will typically show a predominance of unconjugated, or indirect, bilirubin. Other laboratory findings suggestive of hemolysis include a decreased serum haptoglobin level and an elevated peripheral blood reticulocyte count.

Causes of hemolysis are subdivided into those that are intrinsic (intracorpuscular) and those that are extrinsic to the red blood cell. The majority of intrinsic causes are inherited, and typically involve a defect in one or more of the red blood cell components including the hemoglobin protein, the red blood cell membrane, or the metabolic machinery required to generate adenosine triphosphate (ATP). Examples of these abnormalities include defective production of either alpha or beta globin chains in thalassemia, unstable or missing red blood cell membrane proteins as in spherocytosis, and defective defense mechanisms against oxidant challenge as in glucose-6-phosphate dehydrogenase (G6PD) deficiency, the latter of which is the most common genetic deficiency in the world.

Extracorpuscular causes of hemolysis are largely acquired and occur in a variety of contexts. Antibodies directed against the membrane components of red blood cells can lead to hemolysis, and occur in conditions such as autoimmune hemolytic anemia, transfusion reactions, and drug-induced processes. The mechanisms of and predispositions to drug-related liver injury are complex. However, many of these reactions result in drug-cholestasis, which is often reversible when the drug is withdrawn.

Infection may also cause extrinsic hemolysis through a variety of mechanisms including direct parasitization as seen in malaria and bartonellosis, damage from the release of bacterial products as seen in *Clostridium* and *Haemophilus influenzae* type b, and the induction of hypersplenism that leads to trapping and subsequent destruction of red blood cells, as seen in malaria. Malfunctioning cardiac hardware or disseminated intravascular coagulation (DIC) cause hemolysis, similarly leading to an indirect hyperbilirubinemia.

Hepatic

Intrahepatic mechanisms of jaundice result from an abnormality in the metabolism of bilirubin by the liver including problems with uptake from the circulation, intracellular storage, conjugation with glucuronic acid, or biliary excretion. The type of hyperbilirubinemia that arises with hepatic jaundice depends on whether or not conjugation has occurred, and therefore can present as an elevation in either direct or indirect bilirubin. Uptake of unconjugated bilirubin by liver cells is partly due to passive diffusion, and partly requires transport proteins. If the liver is unable to take up the unconjugated bilirubin for processing, levels will increase in the plasma. Furthermore, various forms of intrinsic liver disease and genetic polymorphisms can impair the liver's ability to conjugate bilirubin, or alter the ability to subsequently secrete it into the bile. An example of this is in neonates, where immaturity of the liver may lead to jaundice because conjugation pathways are not fully functional.

Viral hepatitis, alcoholic hepatitis, drug or chemical toxicities, and autoimmune disease can lead to hepatocyte swelling or necrosis, which ultimately interferes with the aforementioned steps of bilirubin metabolism and results in jaundice. Replacement of normal liver parenchyma by either primary malignancy or metastatic disease can also cause jaundice by compressing normal adjacent tissue or bile canaliculi.

In the absence of other indicators of liver disease, genetic factors should be considered as a cause of jaundice. The most common inherited disorder of bilirubin glucuronidation, Gilbert syndrome, results from a defect in the promoter of the gene that encodes the enzyme uridine diphosphoglucuronate-glucuronosyl transferase 1A1 (*UGT1A1*), which is responsible for the conjugation of bilirubin with glucuronic acid. With the exception of intermittent episodes of jaundice, most patients with Gilbert syndrome are asymptomatic. Laboratory testing reveals unconjugated hyperbilirubinemia, with total bilirubin levels that are usually less than 3 mg/dL.

Crigler-Najjar syndrome is a rare, autosomal recessive disorder of bilirubin metabolism. It is due to a defect in the gene that encodes

UGT1A1. Unlike Gilbert's syndrome, which is the result of a defect in the promoter of this gene, these mutations lead to the production of an abnormal protein, resulting in complete loss or very low levels of *UGT1A1*. The phenotype can be severe jaundice and neurologic impairment due to bilirubin encephalopathy that can result in permanent neurologic sequelae (kernicterus).

Posthepatic

Several of the aforementioned disease processes may also contribute to posthepatic bilirubin elevations through inflammation or fibrosis of the intrahepatic bile ducts or canaliculi. As a result, these entities can potentiate obstruction of bile flow, also known as cholestasis. Extrahepatic mechanical obstruction to bile flow similarly causes a posthepatic obstruction and resultant jaundice, and is often the consequence of stones in the bile duct (choledocholithiasis), benign biliary strictures (eg, postsurgical, those associated with chronic pancreatitis, primary sclerosing cholangitis [PSC]), infiltrating tumors, or compression from adjacent carcinomas such as malignancy involving the head of the pancreas. Rarer causes include pancreatic pseudocysts, bile duct parasites, biliary varices, and inflammatory pseudotumor. As a result of backflow of conjugated bilirubin, serum direct bilirubin concentration increases in obstructive processes.

BILIARY OBSTRUCTION AND ACUTE CHOLANGITIS

Biliary obstruction refers to the blockage of any duct that carries bile from the liver to the gallbladder or from the gallbladder to the small intestine. Intrahepatic cholestasis generally occurs at the level of the hepatocyte or biliary canalicular membrane. Extrahepatic obstruction to the flow of bile, on the other hand, may occur within the ducts or secondary to external compression.

As detailed above, a variety of conditions can lead to obstruction of bile flow. In the setting of biliary obstruction, intrabiliary pressure rises, leading to increased permeability of the bile ductules and predisposing to translocation of bacteria from the portal circulation into the biliary tract. When the biliovenous pressure exceeds about 40 mm Hg, bacteria can migrate into the bloodstream. This increase in pressure also alters a variety of host-defense mechanisms including Kupffer cells, bile flow, and IgA production. With disruption of these barrier mechanisms, biliary bacteria are able to access the venous system.

Biliary obstruction and stasis are the most important predisposing factors leading to the development of biliary infection, known as acute cholangitis. In developed countries, the common causes of acute cholangitis include bile duct stones, which can be subdivided into primary (eg, intrahepatic stones), secondary (from gallbladder), and complicated stones (eg, Mirizzi syndrome), in addition to benign biliary strictures (eg, postsurgical, chronic pancreatitis, primary sclerosing cholangitis) and obstructed biliary stents and drains (catheters). Malignant biliary strictures from cholangiocarcinoma, and cancers of the gallbladder, ampulla and pancreas, less commonly present with acute cholangitis, but if unrelieved, can lead to biliary sepsis and liver abscesses (**Figure 158-2**). Parasites (eg, *Clonorchis sinesis, Fasciola hepatica*), viruses (eg, AIDS cholangiopathy), and fungal infections (eg, candida), may cause biliary obstruction and cholangitis. Additionally, interventions such as endoscopic retrograde cholagniopancreatography (ERCP), percutaneous transhepatic cholangiography (PTC) and surgery may result in the loss of the physiologic barrier between the bile duct and intestine, and facilitate entry of bacteria into the obstructed biliary system.

Inciting organisms typically ascend from the duodenum, although hematogenous spread from the portal vein has also been reported. These organisms are typically Gram-negative bacteria including

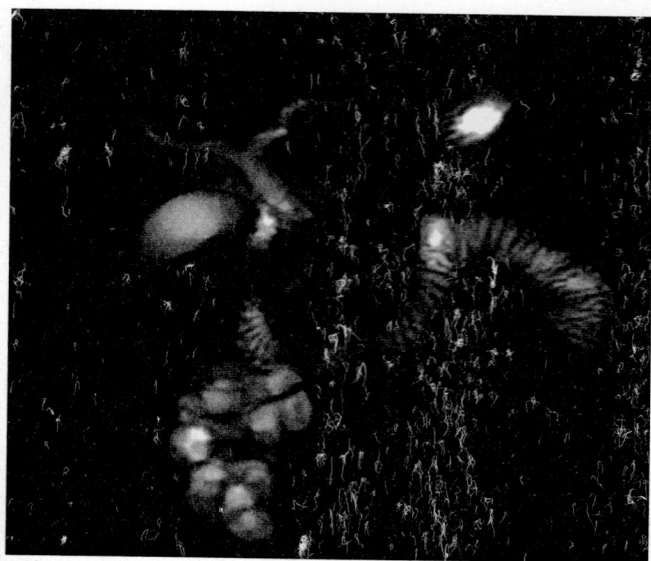

Figure 158-2 *Biliary obstruction from mass in the pancreatic head.*

Escherichia coli, Klebsiella, and *Enterobacter,* although infection with *Enterococci,* a Gram-positive bacterial species, is not uncommon. Unrelieved, acute cholangitis carries close to 100% mortality. Even when the biliary tree is decompressed, the mortality of acute cholangitis is not insignificant.

■ PRESENTATION AND DIAGNOSIS

Physical findings

The major signs and symptoms of biliary obstruction result directly from the failure of bile to reach its proper destination. Acute cholangitis, also referred to as ascending cholangitis, is characterized by a clinical syndrome known as Charcot's triad, which consists of pain, jaundice, and fever. The addition of hypotension and confusion to Charcot's triad suggests sepsis, and the combination of five symptoms makes up Reynolds Pentad. Diaphoresis and tachycardia also commonly occur, although these may be absent in elderly patients who may instead present with confusion or hypotension as the only sign.

Since Charcot reported a patient with severe acute cholangitis as a case of "hepatic fever" in 1877, Charcot's triad has been widely regarded as one of the most important diagnostic criteria. However, despite its high specificity, it has extremely low sensitivity. Moreover, only half to three-quarters of patients with acute cholangitis have all three findings of Charcot's triad. As a general rule, the diagnosis of acute cholangitis should be suspected if a patient has fever or shaking chills and laboratory evidence of an inflammatory response, in addition to either jaundice or abnormal liver function tests. Biliary dilation on imaging or evidence of an etiology such as a stone, stricture, or stent that is visualized confirms the diagnosis.

The most common presenting symptoms of acute cholangitis are fever and abdominal pain. Typically, the abdominal pain is either localized to the right upper abdomen or more diffuse. Surgical signs, such as abdominal rigidity and rebound tenderness, are absent, unless there is concurrent acute cholecystitis. Jaundice is a less common presenting sign, but when it is present, it tends to first occur in the sclera of the eyes or sublingually.

Unless a patient has concurrent chronic liver disease, he or she will not exhibit stigmata of chronic liver disease at the time of presentation, such as spider nevi, palmar erythema, or finger clubbing. Furthermore, the liver and spleen should not be enlarged, and no masses should be present. The one exception to this is palpation of an acutely distended gallbladder, which can occur in mechanical obstruction. This is rare in benign disease, but is the cause of *Courvoiser sign* in malignant obstructive jaundice.

Laboratory findings

Appropriate blood tests on presentation include a complete blood count, a comprehensive metabolic panel (including a liver panel), and basic coagulation studies. Typically, laboratory studies will reveal a leukocytosis with neutrophil predominance, in addition to a cholestatic pattern of liver test abnormalities including an elevation in both conjugated bilirubin and alkaline phosphatase.

Aerobic and anaerobic blood cultures should be drawn before the institution of antibiotics, and treatment modified as necessary when results are available. Bile is normally sterile; however, in the presence of gallbladder calculi or common bile duct (CBD) stones, the incidence of bactibilia increases.

Gram-negative bacteria cause the majority of cases of acute cholangitis. The most common organisms isolated in bile are *E. coli* (27%), *Klebsiella* species (16%), *Enterococcus* species (15%), *Streptococcus* species (8%), *Enterobacter* species (7%), and *Pseudomonas aeruginosa* (7%). Cultures should also be obtained from bile or stents removed at the time of endoscopic retrograde cholangiopancreatography. Organisms isolated from blood cultures are similar to those found in bile. The most common pathogens isolated in blood cultures are *E. coli* (59%), *Klebsiella* species (16%), *P. aeruginosa* (5%), and *Enterococcus* species (4%). In addition, polymicrobial infection is commonly found in bile cultures (30%-87%) and less frequent in blood cultures (6%-16%).

Imaging

Transabdominal ultrasonography may show dilatation of the common bile duct (normal diameter ≤8 mm), with or without the presence of stones in patients with choledocholithiasis (**Figure 158-3**). Biliary dilation greater than 8 mm in a patient with an intact gallbladder is usually indicative of biliary obstruction. A stone in the common bile duct seen on ultrasound is the most reliable predictor of choledocholithiasis at subsequent endoscopic retrograde cholangiopancreatography or surgery. Ultrasonography also provides useful information about the gallbladder in regard to cholelithiasis or cholecystitis.

Transabdominal ultrasonography may be falsely negative when only small stones (<6 mm) are present in the bile ducts or in patients with acute obstruction when the bile duct has not yet started to dilate. In this situation, magnetic resonance cholangiopancreatography (MRCP) is recommended to exonerate the bile duct of stones or

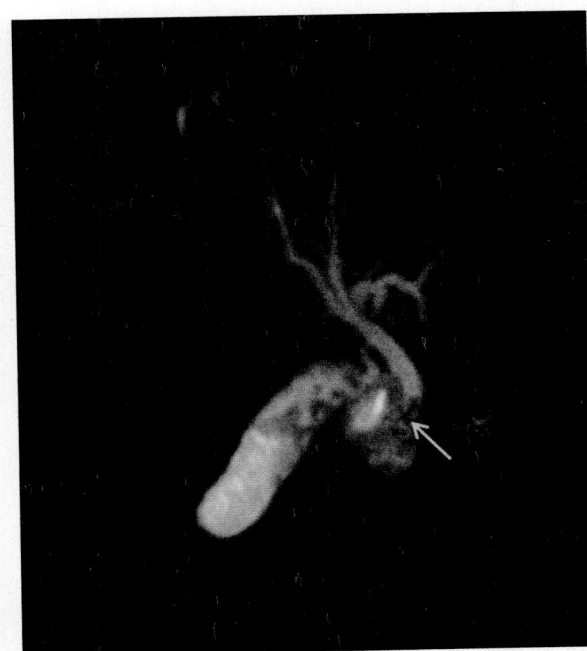

Figure 158-4 *Magnetic resonance cholangiopancreatography (MRCP) demonstrating dilation of common bile duct and obstructing stone (marked by arrow).*

other missed diagnoses (**Figure 158-4**). In patients who have a contraindication to MRI, ERCP is often performed if the clinical picture and laboratory studies suggest biliary obstruction. Cholangiography performed during ERCP may confirm the presence of biliary obstruction from choledocholithiasis, in addition to benign or malignant strictures (**Figure 158-5**). Endoscopic ultrasound (EUS) is also of great utility in patients who have more equivocal presentations for acute cholangitis or in whom ERCP is high risk. The use of EUS to determine if ERCP is indicated may avoid a significant number of ERCPs and result in fewer complications.

In early stages of acute gallstone pancreatitis, commonly used clinical predictors of biliary obstruction, such as cholestatic liver enzymes and imaging demonstrating a dilated CBD, are less reliable in predicting the presence of CBD stones. As a result, MRCP and/or EUS may be warranted in selecting patients for therapeutic ERCP. Furthermore, when the suspicion of acute gallstone pancreatitis is low to moderate, in equivocal presentations for acute cholangitis, and in patients who are high risk for ERCP, these alternative imaging modalities can be useful for exonerating the bile duct of stones or other missed diagnoses.

■ DIFFERENTIAL DIAGNOSIS

Patients with a variety of other disorders may also present with symptoms such as fever and abdominal pain, and a broad differential should be entertained in those with either atypical presentations or normal abdominal imaging. The differential ranges from biliary leaks to diverticulitis to liver abscesses to intestinal perforation, and even includes intrathoracic processes that can mimic right upper quadrant abdominal pain such as right lower lobe pneumonia or empyema.

■ MANAGEMENT

Initial hospital treatment

Acute cholangitis requires rapid relief of biliary obstruction by endoscopic, percutaneous, or surgical intervention. Patients who present with signs and symptoms of acute cholangitis should have liver and biliary imaging and basic blood work (complete blood count, comprehensive metabolic panel, blood cultures) performed without

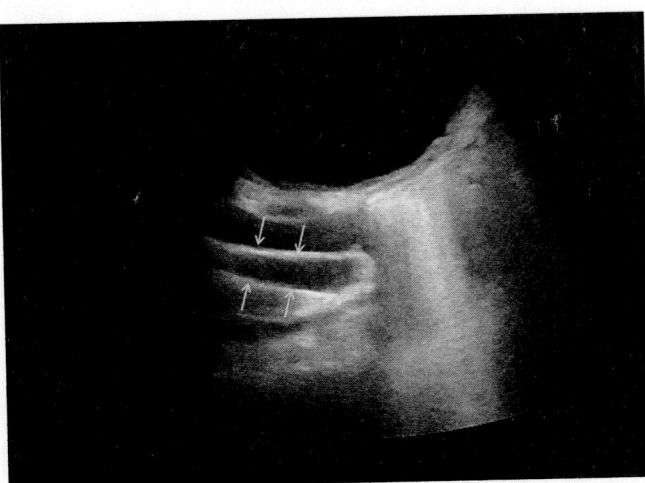

Figure 158-3 *Abdominal ultrasound demonstrating dilation of common bile duct.*

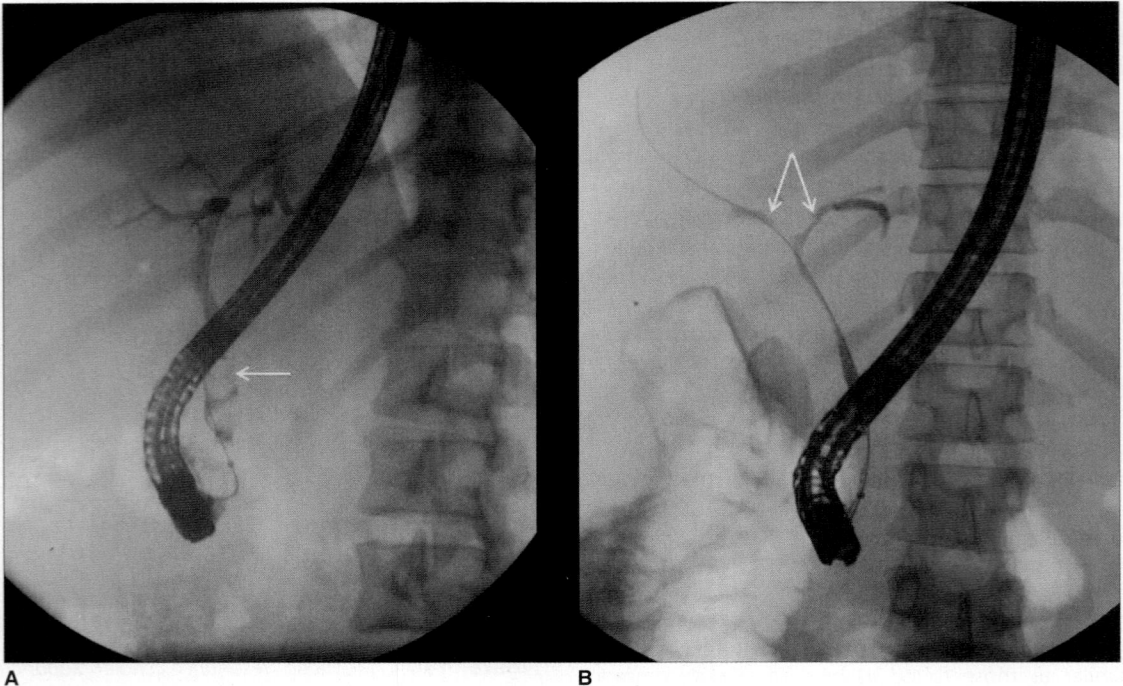

Figure 158-5 *Fluoroscopic imaging during endoscopic retrograde cholangiopancreatography (ERCP) in patients with acute cholangitis due to cholelithiasis (A, marked by single arrow) and benign strictures secondary to primary sclerosing cholangitis (PSC) (B, marked by multiple arrows).*

delay to support the diagnosis. Early initiation of antibiotics is also crucial in the management of patients with acute cholangitis.

Although there is no single accepted scoring system, the American Society for Gastrointestinal Endoscopy (ASGE) provides a proposed strategy to assign risk of choledocholithiasis in patients with symptomatic cholelithiasis. Very strong predictors of choledocholithiasis include a CBD stone on transabdominal ultrasonography, ascending cholangitis, or a bilirubin of over 4 mg/dL. Strong predictors include a dilated CBD on ultrasound or a bilirubin elevation of 1.8 to 4 mg/dL. Moderate predictors include abnormal liver biochemical tests other than bilirubin, age older than 55 years, or clinical gallstone pancreatitis. The probability of choledocholithiasis is categorized as high (>50%) when any of the very strong predictors or both of the strong predictors are present, low (<10%) when no predictors are present, and intermediate (10%-50%) for all other patients.

Typically, patients with a high probability of choledocholithiasis based on clinical presentation and noninvasive imaging are best served by proceeding directly to ERCP. Exceptions include patients in whom prior attempts at ERCP were unsuccessful or in whom the risk of pancreatitis and/or radiation exposure would make confirmatory testing desirable (eg, gallstone pancreatitis, pregnant women).

The majority of patients will respond favorably to antibiotic therapy. If a response to antibiotics is seen, it is reasonable to wait until arrangements can be made to perform an ERCP in the endoscopy suite with experienced staff, provided the procedure can be done within 24 to 48 hours. If ERCP is delayed and the patient has not improved over the first 24 hours with conservative management, urgent biliary decompression is required. In patients who develop signs of worsening disease or biliary sepsis (including hypotension despite adequate fluid resuscitation, fever greater than 102°F, or mental confusion), or in patients with acute gallstone pancreatitis and coexisting cholangitis, urgent biliary decompression is indicated given the observed benefits in morbidity and mortality.

Endoscopic sphincterotomy with stone extraction and/or stent insertion (depending on the cause of the obstruction) is the treatment of choice for establishing biliary drainage in acute cholangitis, and resolves nearly all episodes (**Figure 158-6**). In patients with large stones (>1.5-2 cm) or narrow distal bile ducts relative to the size of

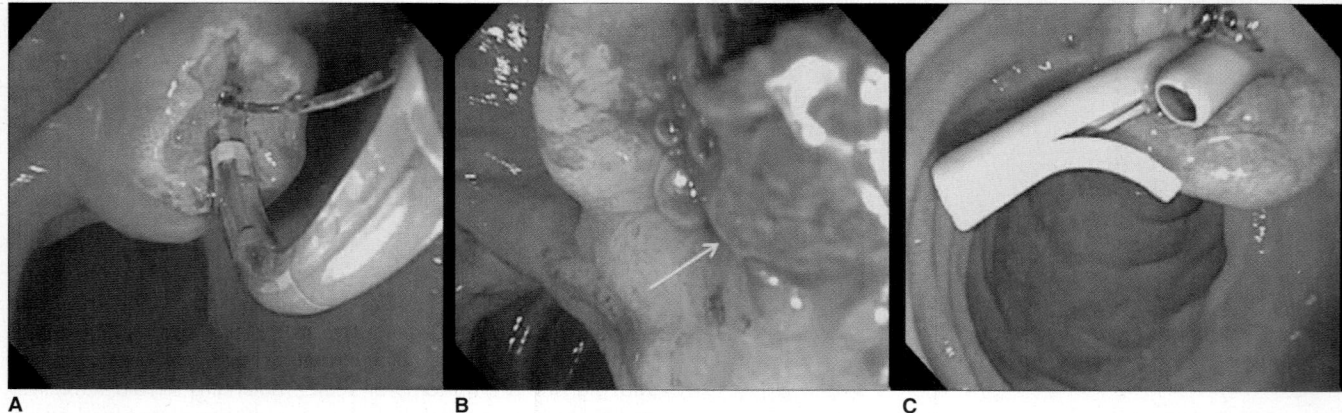

Figure 158-6 *Endoscopic sphincterotomy (A), stone extraction (B), (marked by arrow), and stent placement (C) in patient with acute cholangitis.*

the stone, large diameter endoscopic balloon dilatation immediately after sphincterotomy reduces the need for lithotripsy techniques. In general, an impacted ampullary stone can make biliary deep cannulation difficult and necessitate the need for precut sphincterotomy.

Acute cholangitis should be regarded as a medical emergency and treated aggressively. If ERCP is not technically feasible or fails to adequately re-establish bile drainage, PTC or open surgical decompression are the next steps at achieving biliary drainage. PTC allows external access to the biliary tree. Once access has been obtained, a percutaneous drain can be inserted for decompression. If the obstruction can be traversed, an internal-external drain is placed, with the distal end left in the duodenum (though the duodenal papilla) (**Figure 158-7**). The drain is usually held in position at the skin access site by a suture. Initially, the bile is allowed to drain externally into a bag. After the sepsis has resolved, the drain is internalized (capped at skin level), so that bile flows into duodenum through the catheter. To maintain patency, the internalized drain is typically flushed with sterile water two or three times a day.

It is unusual for surgery to be performed to manage cholangitis alone. In the setting of acute cholecystitis with acute cholangitis, open cholecystectomy with common bile duct exploration may be performed, with simultaneous placement of a T-tube for biliary drainage. However, it is preferable to have preoperative biliary decompression via ERCP if obstruction and sepsis are present. If acute cholecystitis is identified complicating acute cholangitis, the placement of a cholecystostomy tube under radiologic guidance is a useful temporizing maneuver until resolution of the infectious cholangitis. Elective cholecystectomy may then be considered. Additionally, in postsurgical strictures that fail endoscopic or percutaneous stenting, as evidenced by progressive liver damage and/or recurrent episodes of acute cholangitis, surgical bypass (eg, choledocho-jejunostomy) can reduce recurrence and worsening organ dysfunction. Furthermore, in a small subset of patients with primary sclerosing cholangitis, liver transplantation may be necessary to manage progressive deterioration due to recurrent cholangitis and cirrhosis. Patients who have chronic biliary sepsis are generally considered unsuitable for liver transplantation, and therefore, aggressive treatment of acute cholangitis episodes is paramount in the management of their disease.

Medical management in acute cholangitis includes fluid resuscitation, correction of electrolyte abnormalities, correction of infection-related complications (eg, disseminated intravascular coagulation), and administration of antibiotics. Patients with severe sepsis or shock should be managed in an intensive care setting, with aggressive diagnostic and therapeutic measures including central venous catheterization and vasopressors when needed. While there is no consensus regarding the best initial antibiotic regimen for cholangitis, patients are typically given broad-spectrum parenteral antibiotics aimed at colonic bacteria, taking into account local patterns of resistance. Regardless of initial drug regimen, therapy should be modified to reflect any organism(s) recovered in blood cultures.

PREVENTING RECURRENCE

Patients who develop acute cholangitis due to gallstones are at risk for recurrence. As with other complications of gallstone disease, cholecystectomy is generally recommended. If the obstruction is due to a benign stenosis, as is seen following bile duct injuries, endoscopic therapy or surgical repair may be required. Recurrent obstruction is common in patients with malignant stenosis. Management is typically with stent placement, though the specific therapy chosen will depend on the patient's life expectancy and the likelihood of stent occlusion.

Furthermore, patients with recurrent cholangitis from primary sclerosing cholangitis may also benefit from cycling oral antibiotics, although no standard guidelines exist for antibiotic regimens to maintain bile sterility. One week on and 2 weeks off, oral ciprofloxacin 500 mg twice daily may be considered. Metronidazole may be added for anaerobic coverage, although it frequently causes a metallic taste and nausea. Length of cyclical therapy does not have supporting studies to guide practice. A trial of 3 to 6 months may be reasonable before a trial off of cycling antibiotics, and clinicians should monitor and record episodes of recurrence while on and off preventive antimicrobial therapy. Episodes of cholangitis while on oral antibiotic therapy suggest unrelieved biliary obstruction or antibiotic resistance, or both. A different antibiotic regimen should be substituted if there is recurrence or concern for resistance while on prophylactic therapy.

■ PROGNOSIS

Biliary sepsis should be regarded as a medical emergency and managed with appropriate urgency. Acute cholangitis without adequate biliary drainage is associated with mortality approaching 100%. Since the introduction of antibiotics effective against Gram-negative bacteria and nonsurgical means of decompressing the biliary tree (ERCP and percutaneous drainage), the mortality has decreased dramatically. However, severely ill patients with cholangitis who have major comorbidities still may not survive, even if effective biliary drainage can be re-established.

Unrelieved chronic biliary obstruction is often associated with a low-grade cholangitis, typically seen in the setting of strictures of the biliary tree. Eventually, the part of the liver affected by the obstruction may undergo atrophy or develop secondary biliary cirrhosis. Chronic obstruction may also lead to the development of multiple abscesses within the liver.

■ DISCHARGE PLANNING

Discharging clinicians should assure adequate biliary drainage for patients leaving the hospital. Patients who have undrained or inadequately drained bile ducts are likely to return to hospital with recurrent cholangitis, even if maintained on the appropriate antibiotic regimen. Occasionally, the most effective form of biliary drainage is external, especially in patients with complex malignant hilar strictures. These patients often leave the hospital with internal-external biliary catheters. Biliary drains need to be flushed with sterile water several times a day. Discharging physicians should arrange for

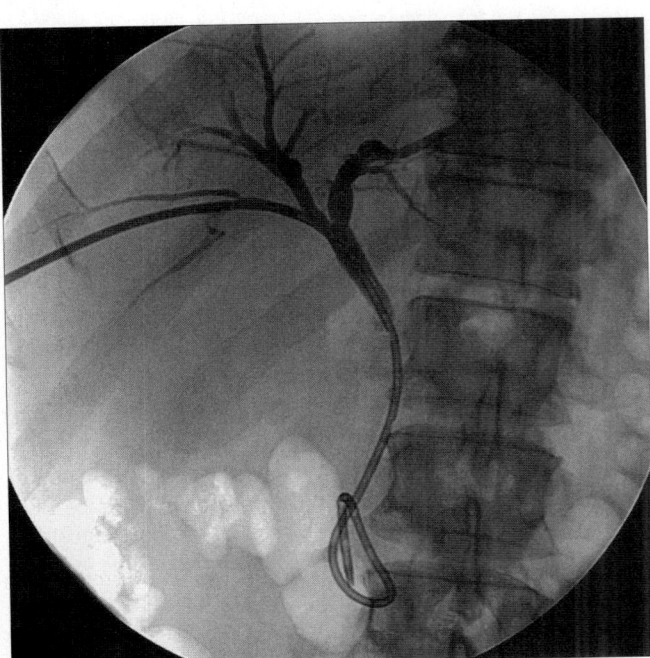

Figure 158-7 *Internal-external percutaneous biliary drain for managing a biliary stricture.*

home health nursing staff to assist with these drains and also teach patients how to care for these drains themselves.

Patients with recurrent cholangitis should be referred to and followed by a physician who understands the natural history of the disorder, including a gastroenterologist or surgeon with interest and expertise in the management of hepatobiliary disorders. Patients who may require surgery should be jointly managed by a gastroenterologist and a surgeon. Patients with chronic liver disease related to biliary obstruction and cholangitis should also be followed by a transplant hepatologist who will coordinate evaluation and listing for liver transplantation when indicated. Physicians managing patients on cyclical antibiotics often should consult infectious disease colleagues who will advise on the choice of antibacterial agents and their rotation, if needed. Patients at risk for recurrent cholangitis, who do not receive long-term antibiotics, should be provided with standing prescriptions for antibiotics, which they should start at the first sign of infection.

■ DISPARITIES IN HEALTH CARE

Patients who lack medical insurance frequently delay seeking care for symptoms of cholangitis, leading to increased mortality among this population. Indigent patients with comorbidities, such as chronic viral hepatitis or human immunodeficiency virus, have particular risk for overwhelming sepsis in the setting of cholangitis. The underinsured and uninsured typically lack outpatient health care providers in the community, and rely on emergency department care when they become seriously ill. Such patients should be identified when they present to health care facilities, so that social services and related resources are applied to find longitudinal care by appropriate physicians and other care providers.

■ OUTCOMES TO MONITOR

Patients with acute cholangitis do not always present with the classic symptoms described above. Rather, symptoms may be quite subtle, such as vague abdominal pain with or without shaking chills or a flu-like illness. This is especially true for patients with chronic cholangitis, and modified by intermittent courses of antibacterial agents. In some patients, the only symptom signaling biliary obstruction or cholangitis may be pruritus.

Patients at risk for recurrent attacks of cholangitis should be educated to recognize the early clinical signs, and encouraged to seek medical care as soon as they do. Cholangitis may be asymptomatic, and lead insidiously to chronic liver disease. One clue to asymptomatic cholangitis includes a progressive increase of liver alkaline phosphatase. When liver disease is established, decompensation accompanying biliary sepsis may present as confusion due to hepatic encephalopathy. Other complications of cirrhosis, especially bleeding from esophageal varices, may supervene. Regular clinic appointments and monitoring liver tests may help to identify those patients who have inadequate biliary drainage and are at risk for recurrent cholangitis and cirrhosis.

■ COSTS AND RESOURCE UTILIZATION

Early, aggressive management of acute cholangitis will help avoid costly complications, and reduce overall mortality. Tertiary care center referral for acute cholangitis is indicated if the admitting hospital is not equipped to perform ERCP or other necessary testing and interventions. Late transfer of a very ill patient to a specialist or referral center likely worsens morbidity and mortality.

CONCLUSION

The management of jaundice requires integration of bilirubin metabolism physiology with the pathologic processes that may interfere with this complex metabolic process (prehepatic, hepatic, and posthepatic mechanisms). Biliary obstruction and stasis are the

most important predisposing factors leading to the development of biliary infection, known as acute cholangitis. This entity should be suspected if a patient has abdominal pain, fever or shaking chills, and laboratory evidence of an inflammatory response, in addition to either jaundice or abnormal liver function tests. Confirmation of the diagnosis is made when the patient also has biliary dilation on imaging or evidence of an etiology such as a stone, stricture, or stent that is visualized. Unrelieved biliary obstruction can be fatal. Early recognition of acute cholangitis and the prompt re-establishment of biliary drainage is the key to successful management. ERCP is the treatment of choice. However, if ERCP is not technically feasible or fails to adequately re-establish bile drainage, PTC or open surgical decompression are the next steps at achieving biliary drainage. As elderly and immunosuppressed patients often fail to exhibit the classic signs and symptoms of acute cholangitis, a high index of suspicion is necessary to make the diagnosis.

SUGGESTED READINGS

Abdallah AA, Krige JE, Bornman PC. Biliary tract obstruction in chronic pancreatitis. *HPB (Oxf)*. 2007;9(6):421-428.

Addley J, Mitchel RM. Advances in the investigation of obstructive jaundice. *Curr Gastroenterol Rep*. 2012;14:511-519.

Attasaranya S, Fogel EL, Lehman GA. Choledocholithiasis, ascending cholangitis, and gallstone pancreatitis. *Med Clin North Am*. 2008;92(4):925-960.

ASGE Standards of Practice Committee, Maple JT, Ben-Menachem T, Anderson MA, Appalaneni V, Banerjee S, Cash BD, Fisher L, Harrison ME, Fanelli RD, Fukami N, Ikenberry SO, Jain R, Khan K, Krinsky ML, Strohmeyer L, Dominitz JA. The role of endoscopy in the evaluation of suspected choledocholithiasis. *Gastrointest Endosc*. 2010;71(1): 1-9. doi: 10.1016/j.gie.2009.09.041.

Bassari R, Koea J. Jaundice associated pruritis: a review of pathophysiology and treatment. *World J Gastroenterol*. 2015;21(5):1404-1413.

Catalano OA, Sahani DV, Forcione DG, et al. Biliary infections: spectrum of imaging findings and management. *Radiographics*. 2000;29(7):2059-2080.

de C Ferreira LE, Baron TH. Acute biliary conditions. *Best Pract Res Clin Gastroenterol*. 2013;27:745-756.

Kiriyama S, Takata T, Strasberg S, et al. TG13 guidelines for diagnosis and severity grading of acute cholangitis (with videos). *J Hepatobiliary Pancreat Sci*. 2013;20:24-34.

Lee JG. Diagnosis and management of acute cholangitis. *Nat Rev Gastroenterol Hepatol*. 2009;6(9):533-541.

Leung JW, Yu AS. Hepatolithiasis and biliary parasites. *Baillieres Clin Gastroenterol*. 1997;11(4):681-706.

Rösch T, Meining A, Frühmorgen S, et al. A prospective comparison of the diagnostic accuracy of ERCP, MRCP, CT, and EUS in biliary strictures. *Gastrointest Endosc*. 2002;55(7):870-876.

Rosing DK, De Virgilio C, Nguyen AT, et al. Cholangitis: analysis of admission prognostic indicators and outcomes. *Am Surg*. 2007;73(10):949-954.

Scheiman JM, Carlos RC, Barnett JL, et al. Can endoscopic ultrasound or magnetic resonance cholangiopancreatography replace ERCP in patients with suspected biliary disease? A prospective trial and cost analysis. *Am J Gastroenterol*. 2001;96:2900-2904.

Sharma BC, Kumar R, Agarwal N, Sarin SK. Endoscopic biliary drainage by nasobiliary drain or by stent placement in patients with acute cholangitis. *Endoscopy*. 2005;37(5):439-443.

van Erpecum K. Gallstone disease. Complications of bile-duct stones: acute cholangitis and pancreatitis. *Best Pract Res Clin Gastroenterol*. 2006;20(6):1139-1152.

CHAPTER 159

Acute Liver Disease

Rahul Maheshwari, MD
Ram M. Subramanian, MD
Ryan M. Ford, MD

Key Clinical Questions

1. How is acute liver failure (ALF) defined and diagnosed, and how does it differ from acutely decompensated cirrhosis?

2. Which causes of decompensated chronic liver failure can also be classified as "acute" failure with respect to transplant candidacy?

3. How should clinicians acutely evaluate, triage, and manage ALF patients, including initial diagnostic and follow-up testing?

4. What clinical and laboratory parameters should be frequently monitored?

5. What complications of ALF lead to high mortality, and how are they managed?

6. How is intracranial hypertension and cerebral edema managed medically?

7. What prognostic measures best identify ALF patients who will require liver transplant in order to survive?

8. What evidence-based interventions improve outcomes in patients with acute liver failure? Are they etiology specific?

INTRODUCTION

◼ DEFINITION

Acute liver failure (ALF) is a rare clinical syndrome that is defined by coagulopathy, usually an international normalized ratio (INR) >1.5, and any degree of mental alteration (encephalopathy) that occurs over a span of less than 26 weeks in a patient without pre-existing liver disease. Based on the time to encephalopathy from the onset of jaundice, three types of ALF have been described: hyperacute (0-7 days), acute (8-21 days), and subacute (>21 days and <26 weeks).

Patients with subacute liver failure often pose a clinical challenge, as they may show signs suggesting chronic liver disease, such as ascites or prolonged encephalopathy. Also, patients with subacute liver failure (eg, drug induced) may follow a variable and unpredictable course, often leading to heightened anxiety for the patient, family, and medical providers.

As an exception to the definition of ALF, patients with Wilson disease, reactivation/superinfection of chronic hepatitis B, or autoimmune hepatitis may be considered to have ALF despite the presence of underlying chronic liver disease.

◼ EPIDEMIOLOGY

Approximately 2000 cases of ALF occur each year in the United States. ALF can affect people of all ages and is associated with high morbidity and mortality. Multiorgan failure (MOF) is the most common cause of death (>50% of cases), with infection and intracranial hypertension (ICH) responsible for most of the remaining deaths. With recent improvements in care, spontaneous recovery and overall survival now exceed 40% and 65%, respectively. Over the past 25 years in the United States, overall mortality from ALF has decreased from more than 80% to 33%.

PATHOPHYSIOLOGY

Acute liver failure involves massive hepatocellular necrosis and liver dysfunction. A resulting cytokine storm leads to oxidative stress and a systemic inflammatory response syndrome. Anti-retroviral medications, Wilson disease, and acute fatty liver of pregnancy may uniquely cause severe mitochondrial dysfunction with resulting lactic acidosis. Ultimately, multiorgan dysfunction occurs.

Intracranial hypertension and cerebral edema may result from elevated ammonia levels that cause direct astrocyte toxicity and loss of cerebral blood flow autoregulation. Loss of cerebral autoregulation in ALF leads to ICH, and intracranial contents are rapidly damaged by both hydrostatic and osmolar shifts. Noncardiogenic pulmonary edema (acute respiratory distress syndrome [ARDS]) and renal failure may result from cytokine-induced damage and hemodynamic derangements. Cardiovascular collapse can be seen with a severe depression of systemic vascular resistance, another process that is driven by cytokines and derangements in vasoactive substances. Loss of the normal synthetic function of the liver also leads to both a coagulopathy and prothrombotic state. Metabolism of medications and other physiologic mechanisms, such as biliary excretion, are also disrupted in the setting of ALF.

Acute liver failure *differs* from acute-on-chronic liver failure. Although there are some examples of overlap (eg, Wilson disease, autoimmune hepatitis, acute-on-chronic hepatitis B), the pathophysiology of the two clinical syndromes differ with respect to physiologic adaptation. For instance, patients with ALF are at risk for elevated intracranial pressure (ICP) because neuronal adaptation does not have time to occur as the ammonia levels rapidly rise.

DIFFERENTIAL DIAGNOSIS

In the setting of possible ALF, clinicians must exclude chronic liver disease. Only a few chronic hepatic conditions may present with true ALF: (1) Wilson disease, (2) autoimmune hepatitis, and (3) acute-on-chronic viral hepatitis B.

A nodular-appearing liver on imaging studies can be misleading, as an irregular contour may represent regenerative nodules interspersed with areas of acute injury and necrosis. Similar to acute alcoholic hepatitis, acute portal hypertension and ascites may also be seen with ALF. Finally, sepsis with disseminated intravascular coagulation in a patient who has cirrhosis can also mimic ALF, as such a patient can present with altered mental status, coagulopathy, and jaundice.

■ CAUSES OF ALF

In the United States, acetaminophen toxicity is the number one cause of ALF (39%). Approximately 20% to 25% of these patients undergo orthotopic liver transplantation. Whereas most cases of acetaminophen-induced ALF involve ingestions exceeding 10 g/d, severe liver injury can occur with doses as low as 3 to 4 g/d, as is seen with therapeutic misadventure. Therapeutic misadventure, referring to therapeutic doses of acetaminophen in the setting of alcohol, malnutrition, or cytochrome p450-inducing medications, occurs in nearly half of acetaminophen toxicity cases (**Table 159-1**).

In addition to acetaminophen, multiple other causes can lead to ALF, and in the United States, approximately 20% of ALF cases have no discernible cause (**Table 159-2**). Non-acetaminophen drug or toxin-induced liver injury accounts for 13% of cases (**Table 159-3**). Toxins may include *Amanita phalloides* (mushrooms), sea anemone sting, or carbon tetrachloride. Acute hepatitis A and B account for 4% and 7% of ALF cases, respectively. The remainder of cases may be due to other viruses (herpes simplex virus [HSV], Epstein-Barr virus [EBV], cytomegalovirus [CMV]), Wilson disease, Budd-Chiari syndrome, sinusoidal obstruction syndrome, acute fatty liver of pregnancy, autoimmune hepatitis, malignant infiltration, or ischemia.

DIAGNOSIS

■ PRESENTATION

A patient can present at any point along the disease severity spectrum. Multiorgan failure may rapidly ensue and manifest with

TABLE 159-1 Cytochrome P450-inducing Medications

Cytochrome P450 Inducers
Ethanol
Isoniazid
Rifampin or rifabutin
Phenobarbital
Glucocorticoids
Phenytoin
Pioglitazone
Omeprazole
Insulin
Carbamazepine
Nafcillin
HIV antiretrovirals (efavirenz, nevirapine)
St John wort

TABLE 159-2 Causes of Acute Liver Failure

Category	Examples
Drug induced	See Table 159-3
Acute viral	Hepatitis A
	Hepatitis B
	Hepatitis D (superimposed on Hepatitis B)
	Hepatitis E
	Hepatitis C
	Herpes simplex virus
	Varicella zoster virus
	Cytomegalovirus
	Epstein-Barr virus
Indeterminate	
Toxin exposure	*Amanita phalloides* (mushrooms)
	Organic solvents
	Herbal medicines
	Bacterial toxins (eg, *Bacillus cereus*)
	Sea anemone sting
	Carbon tetrachloride
Wilson disease	
Pregnancy related	Acute fatty liver of pregnancy
	HELLP syndrome
Autoimmune hepatitis	
Malignancy	Lymphoma
	Diffuse metastatic disease
Hepatic ischemia	Shock
	Acute arterial thrombosis/injury
Vascular	Acute Budd-Chiari syndrome (hepatic vein thrombosis)
Heat stroke	
Postextensive hepatic resection	

HELLP, hemolytic anemia, elevated liver enzymes, and low platelet counts.

abrupt clinical decompensation. Some patients, such as those who recently ingested an acetaminophen overdose, or those with sub-acute liver failure, may initially present asymptomatically, despite having markedly abnormal bloodwork. Nonspecific symptoms may include nausea, vomiting, abdominal pain, fever, malaise, fatigue, arthralgias, itching, bleeding, headache, and diarrhea. Nonspecific clinical signs may include abdominal pain, altered mental status, jaundice, or ascites.

■ HISTORY

A detailed history, including a comprehensive review of possible exposure to viruses, drugs, or toxins, may help uncover a possible cause of liver failure. Clinicians must question about over-the-counter medications, alternative therapies, herbs, and supplements (Table 159-3). If the patient is encephalopathic, a collateral history from friends or family is important, as identifying a cause can be paramount in the management of ALF.

Acetaminophen toxicity may involve intentional overdose or may involve high doses over an extended period of time. For example, a patient who takes over-the-counter acetaminophen in addition to prescribed acetaminophen-containing pain medications may

TABLE 159-3 Drug-Induced Hepatotoxicity

Category	Drug Name
Prescription medications	
Antimicrobials	Ampicillin-clavulanate
	Trimethoprim-sulfamethoxazole
	Fluoroquinolones
	Macrolides
	Nitrofurantoin
	Tetracycline
	"-azole" antifungals (eg, fluconazole, voriconizole, etc)
Anticonvulsants	Isoniazid
	HIV antiretroviral drugs
	Valproic acid
Lipid-lowering drugs	Phenytoin
	Carbamazepine
	Statins
Antihypertensive drugs	Niacin
	Antiotensin-converting enzyme inhibitors
	Methyldopa
Diabetic drugs	Metformin
Antidepressants	Thioglitazones (eg, pioglitozone, rosiglitazone)
Hormonal therapy	Tricyclic antidepressants
Chemotherapy agents	Tamoxifen
Other	Propylthiouracil
	Amiodarone
	Allopurinol
Over-the-counter medications	Acetaminophen
	Nonsteroidal anti-inflammatory drugs
	Niacin
Recreational drugs	Cocaine
	MDMA (ecstasy)
	Methamphetamines

TABLE 159-4 Historical Clues to ALF Etiology

Historical Clue	Potential Etiology
Witnessed or confessed overdose	Acetaminophen or other drug-induced liver injury
History of polysubstance abuse, including intravenous drug use	Drug-induced, toxin (eg, mushrooms), hepatitis B, hepatitis D, hepatitis C
Travel to Russia, Pakistan, India, Mexico, or other endemic regions	Hepatitis E
Immunosuppressed state	Herpes simplex virus, varicella zoster virus, cytomegalovirus
Third trimester of pregnancy	Acute fatty liver of pregnancy, HELLP syndrome, herpes simplex virus, or any other cause of ALF
History of autoimmune disease (eg, Hashimoto thyroiditis, type 1 diabetes mellitus, Addison disease, lupus, vitiligo)	Autoimmune hepatitis
Hemodynamic instability (heart failure, arrhythmia, myocardial infarction)	Shock liver
History of hypercoagulable state	Budd-Chiari syndrome, shock liver from arterial thrombosis, malignant infiltration
History of chemotherapy	Sinusoidal obstruction syndrome
History of chronic Hepatitis B	Acute hepatitis B flare, superinfection with hepatitis D
Northwestern United States	*Amanita phalloides* (mushroom toxicity)
History of malignancy	Diffuse hepatic metastases
Hemolytic anemia, renal failure, low-normal alkaline phosphatase, or low uric acid	Wilson disease

HELLP, hemolytic anemia, elevated liver enzymes, and low platelet counts.

exceed a critical daily dose that leads to severe liver injury. Alcoholics and malnourished patients are at greater risk for acetaminophen-induced liver injury.

Most idiosyncratic drug-induced liver injuries are not dose related and tend to occur within the first 6 months of drug initiation (Table 159-3).

PRACTICE POINT

- Most idiosyncratic **drug-induced liver injuries** are not dose related and tend to occur within the first 6 months of drug initiation.
- Mechanisms of injury include hepatocellular necrosis, cholestasis, a mixed pattern, steatosis, autoimmune, hypersensitivity, phospholipidosis, mitochondrial toxicity, and sinusoidal obstruction syndrome.
- If suspected, immediate withdrawal of the offending agent is paramount.
- If autoimmune or hypersensitivity is suspected, steroids may be beneficial.

A history of IV drug abuse may indicate risk for infections such as acute hepatitis B and D. Travel to endemic regions (eg, Russia, Pakistan, India, Mexico) may place a patient at risk for acute hepatitis E infection. Immunosuppressed patients and women in their third trimester of pregnancy are at increased risk for herpes simplex infection. A history of preeclampsia in a pregnant woman increases the risk of acute fatty liver of pregnancy, which also occurs in the third trimester. Previous or coexisting autoimmune diseases (thyroiditis, insulin-dependent diabetes, lupus, vitiligo, etc) may indicate an increased risk for autoimmune hepatitis. Cardiac disease (congestive heart failure, myocardial infarction, arrhythmia) or hemodynamic instability may lead to "shock liver" from hypoperfusion. Documented hypotension is not always found with ischemic liver injury. A history of malignancy or hypercoagulable state may raise concern for malignant infiltration or Budd-Chiari syndrome (hepatic vein thrombosis), which often presents with acute abdominal pain, ascites, and striking hepatomegaly. A history of chemotherapy may place a patient at risk for sinusoidal obstruction syndrome, formerly known as veno-occlusive disease, which can present in a similar manner as Budd-Chiari syndrome (**Table 159-4**).

■ PHYSICAL EXAMINATION

With ALF, the most important step in the physical examination is assessing mental status and performing frequent neurological examinations. Clinicians must closely examine for any signs of chronic liver disease including spider angiomata, telangiectasias, Terry nails (fingernails and/or toenail appear white with a characteristic "ground-glass" appearance, with no lunula), palmar erythema, asterixis, splenomegaly, caput medusa, collateral venous patterns, and gynecomastia. Whereas ascites and varices are classically seen with chronic liver disease, these signs of portal hypertension can be seen with acute liver disease as well (eg, alcoholic hepatitis, venous thrombosis, presinusoidal portal hypertension).

In patients suspected of Wilson disease, a slit-lamp examination of the eye should be performed to assess for the presence of Kayser-Fleischer rings. In patients with intracranial hypertension from cerebral edema, Cushing triad—hypertension, bradycardia, irregular respirations—may or may not be present. Pupillary dilation or signs of decerebrate posturing typically occur late in the course of ALF and indicate a grave prognosis.

■ LABORATORY

A standard protocol of laboratory testing for patients admitted with ALF may facilitate a thorough evaluation, since the initial lab survey

is extensive. Even if a diagnosis seems clear, evaluating for concomitant diseases such as viral hepatitis or human immunodeficiency virus is important in a patient who may require a liver transplant. Frequent hepatic function testing often necessitates indwelling vascular access (central venous catheter or arterial catheter) for serial blood draws and other clinical management (**Table 159-5**). No consensus guidelines recommend specific laboratory testing in the setting of probable ALF; however, laboratory testing is necessary in anticipation of possible liver transplantation.

Upon presentation, very high transaminase levels (AST and ALT levels >1000 U/L) may limit the differential to a few possible etiologies: acute viral infection, acetaminophen-induced injury, shock liver, or autoimmune hepatitis. AST and ALT levels exceeding 3500 U/L are highly correlated with acetaminophen poisoning. Whereas transaminase levels may be helpful initially, they do not add much information once the diagnosis of ALF is established. Transaminase levels that appear to be normalizing may indicate an obliterated liver, especially if associated with hypoglycemia and an unabated rise in the international normalized ratio. Alternatively, normalizing liver enzymes may also indicate improving hepatic

TABLE 159-5 Initial Comprehensive and Serial Laboratory Tests to Order for Patients with Acute Liver Failure*

Initial (Comprehensive)	Laboratory Tests to Consider Ordering Initially	Laboratory Tests to Monitor Serially
Complete blood count with differential	24-h urine copper level	Complete blood count with differential every 6-8 h
Comprehensive metabolic profile	Coombs test	Comprehensive metabolic profile every 6-8 h
Coagulation studies (INR/PT/PTT)	Peritoneal fluid analysis (if ascites is present)	Coagulation studies (INR/PT/PTT) every 6-8 h
Arterial blood gas	Lactate dehydrogenase	Arterial blood gas every 6-8 h
Arterial lactate	Haptoglobin	Coagulation factor levels (factor V, VII) once or twice a day
Acetaminophen level	Uric acid	Fibrinogen daily
Coagulation factor levels (factors V, VII, VIII)	Serum ferritin	Serum osmolarity every 6 h (if patient is receiving IV mannitol therapy)
Urinalysis with microscopy	Arterial ammonia	
Urine drug screen for cocaine, amphetamines, opiates, barbiturates, benzodiazepines, and marijuana	Quantitative serum immunoglobulins	
Fibrinogen	EBV quantitative PCR	
Hepatitis B quantitative DNA	HIV viral load	
Hepatitis C quantitative RNA	D-dimers	
Hepatitis A IgM antibody	Blood cultures	
Hepatitis B surface antigen	Urine culture	
Hepatitis B core antibody (IgM and IgG)		
Hepatitis B surface antibody		
CMV IgG antibody		
CMV quantitative PCR		
EBV serologic panel		
HSV quantitative PCR		
HIV antibody		
Rapid plasma regain (RPR)		
Ceruloplasmin		
Alpha-1-antitrypsin level and phenotype		
Antinuclear antibody		
Antismooth muscle antibody		
Antimitochondrial antibody		
Serum osmolarity		

*Based on expert opinion of the authors; not based on any consensus guidelines.

injury facilitated by removal of a toxic exposure, natural history of a virus, or a treatment response (eg, autoimmune hepatitis, herpes simplex, hepatitis B). A bilirubin level on presentation carries prognostic significance, especially with drug-induced liver injury (*Hy's law*, a prognostic indicator that suggests that drug-induced liver injury leading to jaundice, without hepatic transplantation, has a case fatality rate of 10%-50%). Initial INR and creatinine also provide prognostic information.

■ IMAGING

Ordering a multitude of imaging tests that require patient transport and movement may present unnecessary risk for a critically ill patient with ALF. Nevertheless, imaging—when safe to perform—may provide diagnostic information to direct management. All patients with ALF should undergo an abdominal ultrasound with Doppler to assess for signs of chronic liver disease and to assess the hepatic vasculature (hepatic veins, portal vein, hepatic artery). Computed tomography (CT) scan of the abdomen without contrast is preferred if the patient's body habitus (eg, obesity, ascites, bowel distension) precludes an adequate ultrasound examination. Avoidance of IV contrast is important since many patients with ALF are at risk for developing acute kidney injury. Magnetic resonance imaging (MRI) of the abdomen with IV gadolinium is an alternative imaging modality that is center specific and depends on radiologic expertise.

> **PRACTICE POINT**
>
> ● Clinicians should avoid use of iodinated IV contrast in patients presenting with ALF as many of these patients bear high risk for developing acute kidney injury.

In a patient with worsening mental status, a noncontrast brain CT will help to evaluate for intracranial hemorrhage or cerebral edema. Whereas cerebral edema, while prognostically ominous if seen on CT, may indicate the need for placement of an intracranial pressure monitor, recent studies suggest that this does not confer a significant mortality benefit, and in certain cases (nonacetaminophen ALF), it may be associated with worse outcomes. In a patient with suspected brain damage, transcranial Doppler ultrasounds or continuous electroencephalograms (EEGs) may provide prognostic information. To assess heart function and valves, a transthoracic echocardiogram may be necessary, especially if a patient is a possible liver transplant candidate. Plain films, such as chest x-rays and abdominal radiographs, may also be ordered as clinically indicated but are generally performed at the patient bedside (portable machine) to avoid unnecessary patient transport.

■ LIVER BIOPSY

When specific diseases such as autoimmune hepatitis, Wilson disease, HSV hepatitis, or lymphoma are suspected, a liver biopsy may be useful in assisting with diagnosis. A liver biopsy may also help determine the extent of necrosis and regeneration in cases of subacute liver failure. *For the majority of ALF cases, a liver biopsy is not necessary and may even lead to complications such as hemorrhage or infection.* In cases of severe ALF, a biopsy will most likely show extensive necrosis and "ghosts" of hepatocytes.

TRIAGE AND HOSPITAL ADMISSION

Any patient with suspected ALF should be admitted to the hospital for a thorough evaluation and consideration for liver transplant. If a patient is being admitted to a hospital that is not a transplant center, early transfer to a transplant center should be considered, especially if both encephalopathy and coagulopathy are present. Rapid

TABLE 159-6 Grades of Encephalopathy

Grade	Clinical Picture
I	Mood instability
	Shortened attention span
	Insomnia
	Mild confusion
II	Lethargy
	Personality changes
	Moderate confusion/disorientation
III	Marked confusion
	Somnolence
	Incoherent
IV	Coma (unresponsive to verbal or noxious stimuli)

deterioration in clinical and biochemical status following an initial stable presentation can occur. Some centers may use prognostic models to determine who should be transferred. At the present time, there are no validated criteria that dictate when to transfer a patient. Prior to transfer, a detailed communication between the receiving and transferring facility should address the existing neurologic, cardiopulmonary, hepatic, hematologic, and renal status. Prior to transfer, it may be necessary to electively intubate a patient for airway protection, as advancing encephalopathy can occur unexpectedly during transit.

> **PRACTICE POINT**
>
> ● Acute liver failure patients admitted to a nontransplant center should be considered for early transfer to a transplant center, especially in patients with both encephalopathy and coagulopathy. Prior to transfer, it may be necessary to electively intubate a patient for airway protection, as advancing encephalopathy may occur unexpectedly in transit.

Patients that develop grade II, III, or IV encephalopathy should be managed in an ICU (**Table 159-6**). Patients with grade III or IV encephalopathy may require both intubation for airway protection and possible ICP monitoring. Even though a patient may appear stable, rapid changes in clinical status may occur and should be dealt with in an urgent manner. Frequent neurologic evaluation, serial laboratory testing, and 24-hour monitoring in an ICU together provide the best opportunity to detect clinically significant changes in status.

MANAGEMENT

■ INITIAL MANAGEMENT (OVERVIEW)

A directed history and physical examination, extensive laboratory panel, and relevant imaging should be performed as quickly and safely as possible. A comprehensive history and physical examination needs to focus on the potential causes of liver injury, and any evidence of chronic liver disease that would preclude a diagnosis of ALF. Any barriers to potential liver transplant (comorbidities, lack of social support, active neoplastic or infectious processes) should be assessed.

In known or suspected cases of acetaminophen toxicity, acetaminophen nomograms are unreliable if the time from ingestion is not known, or if a single large ingestion was not taken. Activated charcoal may be given to patients within the first 4 hours of intentional acetaminophen overdose. Serial measurements of liver

TABLE 159-7 Overview of Management in Patients with Acute Liver Failure

Rapid assessment and stabilization	Mental status?
	Adequate IV access?
	Need for intubation?
Directed history and physical exam	Cause of acute liver failure?
	Grade of encephalopathy?
	Medical comorbidities?
Activated charcoal within 4 h of known acetaminophen overdose	
Initiation of N-acetylcysteine	Intravenous or enteral, depending on patient stability
Full panel of lab tests	See Table 159-5
	Assess coagulopathy
Abdominal imaging study	Is there evidence of chronic liver disease?
Head imaging study (based on mental status)	Any evidence of cerebral edema?
Multiple consultations	Transplant hepatology
	Transplant surgery
	Pulmonary/critical care
	Nephrology
	Hematology
	Infectious disease
	Social services
	Psychiatry
	Anesthesiology
	Ethics?
Admission to ICU	
Organ-specific management of complications	See Table 159-8
Assessment of transplant candidacy (may include collateral history from family and friends)	Usually a multidisciplinary assessment based on consultations
Estimate prognosis of survival without transplant	King's College criteria (see Table 159-9)
	MELD score
	APACHE score

enzymes, coagulation parameters (INR and factor V levels), arterial pH, and arterial lactate will help to prognosticate the extent of liver damage. Serial assessments of mental status help determine stage of encephalopathy and direct further intervention (eg, head CT, ICP monitor) (**Table 159-7**).

■ ROLE OF N-ACETYL-CYSTEINE (NAC)

The administration of N-acetyl-cysteine (NAC) can provide protection from hepatotoxicity, especially if given within 12 hours of nonstaggered ingestion of acetaminophen. The main effects of NAC are to increase hepatic glutathione production and act as an antioxidant. The first dose of NAC may still be beneficial up to 48 to 72 hours following acetaminophen ingestion.

N-acetyl-cysteine may also offer benefit in non-acetaminophen causes of liver failure, as it seems to improve overall hemodynamic status and oxygen delivery to peripheral tissues. A recent trial randomized patients with non-acetaminophen ALF to intravenous

NAC or placebo. Transplant-free survival improved in patients who received NAC. N-acetyl-cysteine also improved 1-year overall survival in the subset of patients with mild (grades 1 and 2) encephalopathy.

Based on available evidence, all patients with ALF, regardless of etiology, should receive NAC. In the absence of significant upper GI symptoms, NAC may be given orally or by NG tube as follows: 140 mg/kg (5% dextrose solution) loading dose followed by 70 mg/kg every 4 hours for 17 doses. Oral NAC has several potential side effects that include nausea, vomiting, rare urticaria, and bronchospasm. N-acetyl-cysteine may also be administered intravenously as follows: 150 mg/kg (5% dextrose solution) loading dose over 15 minutes, followed by 50 mg/kg given over 4 hours, followed by 100 mg/kg given over 16 hours. Intravenous NAC may lead to rare anaphylaxis, ECG abnormalities, bronchospasm, and false improvements in INR. The US Food and Drug Administration has not yet approved the intravenous use of NAC for ALF. N-acetyl-cysteine therapy can be stopped when the patient proceeds to liver transplantation, or when there is evidence that hepatic dysfunction is resolving, defined by improved encephalopathy and coagulopathy (INR < 1.5).

PRACTICE POINT

- All patients with ALF, regardless of etiology, should receive N-acetyl-cysteine therapy to improve transplant-free survival.

■ CONSULTATION

Depending on the severity and extent of multiorgan involvement, patients with ALF often require multiple consultations (Table 159-7). A multidisciplinary approach is also very important for patients who may be candidates for liver transplantation. Consultations may include providers from critical care medicine, transplant hepatology (surgical and medical), anesthesiology, cardiology, nephrology, infectious diseases, pulmonary, psychiatry, social services, and possibly the ethics committee.

COMPLICATIONS AND PROGNOSIS

Since patients with advanced ALF present with multiorgan system failure, management should follow a system-based, goal-directed approach. Management of ALF in an organ-system-based manner requires multiple disciplines and coordinated care (**Table 159-8**).

■ CEREBRAL EDEMA AND INTRACRANIAL HYPERTENSION

Intracranial hypertension and cerebral edema remain serious complications of ALF, often leading to fatal herniation. Intracranial hypertension develops in approximately 20% to 30% of patients with ALF. Cerebral edema occurs more often in patients with a short time interval (28 days or less) between the development of jaundice and the onset of encephalopathy. Younger patients, with less cerebral atrophy than older patients, may not tolerate rapid shifts in ICP. Young age and high arterial ammonia correlate with increased risk of death from herniation. Cerebral edema is rarely seen in patients with mild (grades I and II) encephalopathy. Risk factors for progression to encephalopathy and cerebral edema include the presence of systemic inflammatory response syndrome, the need for vasopressors, the need for continuous renal replacement therapy (CRRT), or the presence of infection.

The exact mechanisms underlying elevated ICP in patients with ALF are not fully understood and are likely multifactorial. Both retrospective and prospective studies have shown that higher arterial ammonia levels portend a higher risk of cerebral herniation and death. An arterial ammonia >124 micromoles/L predicts mortality

TABLE 159-8 Organ-Specific Management of Acute Liver Failure

Organ System	Complication(s)	Management
Neurologic	Cerebral edema and intracranial hypertension	1. Consider placing an intracranial monitor 2. Maintain a cerebral perfusion pressure of 60-80 mm Hg 3. Maintain an ICP <25 mm Hg 4. Maintain head of bed somewhat elevated (45°) 5. Medical management of elevated ICP 6. Avoid stimulation of patient 7. Serial neurologic examinations 8. Consider EEG
Pulmonary	Mechanical ventilation for either airway protection from altered mental status or due to respiratory failure from ALI/ARDS	1. Lidocaine IV or endotracheal during intubation 2. Propofol for sedation 3. Consider cis-atracurium paralysis 4. Either volume or pressure-controlled ventilation 5. Low tidal volumes of 6 mL/kg of ideal body weight 6. Maintain maximal plateau pressure <30 cm H_2O 7. Avoid bronchoscopy
Cardiovascular	Hypotension (hemodynamic collapse)	1. Arterial catheter for direct measurement 2. Fluid resuscitation (often less volume than is required with sepsis) 3. Vasopressor support with norepinephrine as first choice 4. Avoid alpha-adrenergic agents 5. Consider a pulmonary artery catheter 6. Monitor mixed or central venous oxygen saturation
Renal	Acute kidney injury, volume overload, and metabolic disturbances	1. Early initiation of renal replacement therapy with CRRT preferred over HD 2. Nephrology consultation 3. Bicarbonate buffered hemofiltration 4. Renal ultrasound
Hematology	Thrombocytopenia and coagulation abnormalities involving both a bleeding and thrombosis risk	1. Vitamin K 10 mg SQ × 3 days 2. Avoid FFP unless there is bleeding, and monitor serial INR/PT/PTT 3. Transfuse platelets based on Practice Point recommendations (page 1293) 4. Subcutaneous heparin for DVT prophylaxis 5. Consider recombinant factor VII if placing an intracranial pressure monitor
Infectious Disease	Bacterial and fungal infections; acute viral causes of ALF	1. Maintain a low clinical threshold to culture and start empiric antimicrobials 2. Follow hospital protocols to reduce iatrogenic infections from central lines and catheters 3. Early antiviral therapy for acute hepatitis B, HSV, CMV, or VZV
Endocrine	Relative adrenal insufficiency	1. Maintain a low clinical suspicion if hypotension seems refractory 2. Consider stress dose steroid therapy
Electrolytes	Hypoglycemia, hypophosphatemia, hyponatremia, hypo- or hyperkalemia, low magnesium levels, metabolic acidosis	1. Frequent serum glucose checks; dextrose-containing fluids 2. Bicarbonate buffered solutions with CRRT 3. Replete phosphorous, potassium, and magnesium 4. Treat hyperkalemia 5. Early CRRT
GI/Nutrition	Stress ulcerations, severe catabolic state	1. Early enteral feedings should be considered 2. TPN if enteral feeds not possible (ileus, etc) 3. H_2 blocker or PPI therapy

ALI/ARDS, acute lung injury/acute respiratory distress syndrome; CMV, cytomegalovirus; CRRT, continuous renal replacement therapy; DVT, deep vein thrombosis; EEG, electroencephalogram; HD, hemodialysis; HSV, herpes simplex virus; ICP, intracranial pressure; PPI, proton pump inhibitor; TPN, total parenteral nutrition; VZV, varicella zoster virus.

with a 77.5% diagnostic accuracy (sensitivity 78.6%, specificity 76.3%). Elevated ammonia levels lead to osmotic shifts that negatively affect astrocytes. When ammonia levels rise in subacute or chronic liver disease, there is time for adaptation. In ALF, the rapidity of the rise in serum ammonia is thought to limit the time for adaptation.

ICP MONITORING

Intracranial pressure monitoring is controversial. It allows measurement of cerebral perfusion pressure (CPP) and detection of ICH that is otherwise clinically silent. This may facilitate timely and rational use of ICP-lowering therapies, and allow optimization of ICP before and during liver transplantation. However, insertion of ICP monitors risks intracranial hemorrhage, and no mortality benefit has been demonstrated. A recent retrospective cohort study found that ICH was common in patients with ICP monitors, and hemorrhagic complications were rare (7%), but there was no 21-day mortality benefit in acetaminophen-related ALF and a worse prognosis in the nonacetaminophen group.

The utility of ICP monitors is extrapolated from the neurointensive care literature regarding management of traumatic brain injury. Clinical signs of elevated ICP are not always present, and pupillary dilation, decerebrate posturing, or changes on brain CT scans are often discovered late in the course. Therefore, a more accurate and potentially objective measure of ICP using a monitoring device may enable determination of ICH and guide decisions of therapy, prognosis, and candidacy for liver transplantation.

Significant ICH is defined as a sustained (>10 minutes) elevation of ICP >25 mm Hg. In addition to the ICP, the cerebral perfusion pressure—defined as the difference between the mean arterial pressure (MAP) and ICP (ie, CPP = MAP − ICP) with optimal CPP 60 to 80 mm Hg—guides patient management. Augmentation of MAP with vasoactive agents in order to maintain adequate CPP in the setting of an elevated ICP may be necessary.

Refractory ICH or decreased CPP are considered contraindications to liver transplantation in many centers. One study showed that prolonged high ICP (>25 mm Hg) and low CPP (<40 mm Hg) for greater than 2 hours portended poor neurologic recovery and should preclude liver transplantation. However, absolute pressure thresholds predicting irreversible neurologic damage or precluding transplantation should be used with caution, since such pressure thresholds have been challenged by reports of complete neurologic recovery after prolonged (>24 hours) ICH (ICP > 35 mm Hg) with low CPP (<50 mm Hg). For patients with ALF who are listed for transplantation, ICP monitoring may help with ICU management of cerebral edema and ICH prior to transplantation. Furthermore, since elevated ICP can persist perioperatively, ICP monitors can also be useful both during and after the liver transplant surgery. Given the absence of large randomized controlled trials, the use of ICP monitors currently remains center dependent.

The major risks involved with placing an intracranial device include infection and bleeding, with mortality from bleeding reported to be 1% to 3%. Intraventricular catheters bear greater risk than intraparenchymal or subdural catheters, which in turn bear greater risk than epidural devices. The intraparenchymal location appears to offer the optimal balance between accuracy and safety. Aggressive correction of coagulation parameters, along with the use of recombinant activated factor VII, may reduce bleeding risk and allow wider use of ICP monitoring devices.

MEDICAL MANAGEMENT OF ELEVATED ICP

Patients with ALF can progress rapidly from grade 1 to 4 encephalopathy. Frequent and detailed neurological examinations are vital, as subtle changes of increasing ICP can be missed. Once a head CT has ruled out any other process, patients with suspected ICH should have as little stimulation as possible. Chest physiotherapy and endotracheal suctioning may need to be minimized. Visitors, lights, and noises should be reduced. The head of the bed should be elevated to 30°. Cerebral perfusion pressure should be maintained at 60 to 80 mm Hg, and this may require cautious titration of MAP to compensate for increasing ICP. Trendelenburg position, head flexion, head rotation, and sudden change of position to supine should be avoided except when necessary for placement of a central venous catheter. Clinicians should avoid the placement of bilateral internal jugular lines for access, as this may collectively compromise intracranial venous drainage.

Lactulose may be used with early encephalopathy, but it lacks long-term benefit. Lactulose may also lead to gaseous distension of the bowel, which can complicate subsequent transplant surgery. The role of nonabsorbable antibiotics, such as rifaximin, has not been demonstrated.

Patients with grade III or IV encephalopathy should be intubated for airway protection. Endotracheal or intravenous lidocaine prior to intubation may be helpful in reducing spikes of ICP. For intubation, small doses of propofol may be used with caution, as the half-life of propofol is prolonged in hepatic failure. Propofol may also cause a decrease in MAP, thus compromising CPP.

Nonconvulsive seizure activity has been documented in a high proportion of patients with ALF and advanced stages of hepatic encephalopathy (HE). Seizure activity should be treated with phenytoin or fosphenytoin; however, there are insufficient data to recommend prophylactic anticonvulsants in all patients with ALF. It should be noted that propofol or benzodiazepine infusions used for sedation also provide potent antiseizure prophylaxis.

With ALF, the ICP should be maintained below 25 mm Hg in order to improve CPP. Treatment of elevated ICP is usually instituted when there is either a sustained rise in ICP (>10 minutes) or if clinical signs suggest ischemia or herniation. Increased sedation with propofol may be used for transient spikes of ICP due to agitation.

In the past, patients were mechanically hyperventilated in order to reduce the serum partial pressure of carbon dioxide (pCO_2) and cause cerebral vasoconstriction, thus reducing both cerebral blood flow and ICP. This effect is very transient, perhaps only lasting several minutes. Out of concern for cerebral hypoxia with reduced cerebral blood flow, hyperventilation is no longer a mainstay of therapy. Short-term hyperventilation has not been shown to improve outcome in ALF, but it does prolong survival in the ICU; therefore, it may occasionally be used as bridge therapy in selected patients who await a liver transplant.

The choice of pharmacologic agent for treatment of ICH is not standardized across transplant centers. Osmotic diuresis with IV mannitol effectively reduces cerebral edema and improves survival, based on a prospective, controlled study performed at King's College in London. A bolus dose of 0.5 to 1 g/kg may be repeated once or twice as needed, as long as the serum osmolarity does not exceed 320 mOsm/L. Since mannitol is cleared by the kidneys, there is risk of intravascular hypervolemia and high-pressure pulmonary edema in the setting of renal failure. As mannitol is removed by dialysis, it may be used in patients on CRRT. Serum osmolarity and sodium level should be monitored every 6 to 8 hours when mannitol is used. In the absence of ICH, prophylactic mannitol is not indicated.

In recent years, hypertonic saline solution has become the more popular osmotic agent for hyperosmolar therapy. This growing popularity has come about in response to the complications associated with the use of mannitol, in particular acute renal failure and ICP rebound. Although an initial dose of mannitol may still be useful for acute control of elevated ICP, many centers move quickly to hypertonic saline as the mainstay of therapy. Induction and maintenance of hypernatremia may be used to prevent rising ICP. The efficacy of hypertonic saline in the prevention and treatment of ICH has been demonstrated in the neurologic intensive care literature. The goal of therapeutic hypernatremia is serum sodium of 145 to 155 mmol/L, which can be obtained by using 30% hypertonic saline in boluses of 20 mL. In contrast to mannitol, boluses of hypertonic saline have less tachyphylaxis to multiple doses. In the presence of CRRT, achieving the desired level of therapeutic hypernatremia may be a challenge, since a relatively hyponatremic replacement fluid is often used in the CRRT circuit.

Therapeutic cooling might protect against cerebral edema by various mechanisms: normalization of cerebral blood flow, decreased cerebral metabolic rate, decreased cytokine production, and decreased conversion of glutamate to glutamine, the compound that may precipitate cerebral edema in astrocytes. Decreased intracranial pressure and cerebral blood flow and increased cerebral perfusion pressure have been demonstrated with moderate (32-35°C) hypothermia. Patients may be iatrogenically hypothermic from transfusions or a CRRT circuit. Cooling blankets can be added to further reduce core temperature. Hypothermia can also prevent ICP spikes during liver transplant surgery. Despite the potential utility of therapeutic hypothermia (TH), there is the concern that lowering the core temperature might lead to increased bleeding events, microbial infections, cardiac dysrhythmias, and potentially reduced hepatic regeneration. Currently, there are no controlled data on the effects of TH in ALF and no evidence-based guidelines for its use in these patients. A recent retrospective cohort study of ALF patients in the US Acute Liver Failure Study Group concluded that TH was not significantly associated with a 21-day spontaneous survival in non-APAP (acetaminophen) ALF patients. In APAP patients, TH may potential be associated with benefits in patients younger than 26 years of age. Additionally, the study concluded TH was not associated with increased bleeding or infection. The avoidance of hyperthermia is clearly a goal in management of ALF patients; however, a prospective trial is required to clarify the utility of TH in these patients.

In cases of elevated ICP refractory to osmotherapy (ie, mannitol and hypernatremia) and hypothermia, induction of a barbiturate coma using thiopental or pentobarbital can be considered. Significant myocardial depression and systemic hypotension may limit the use of a barbiturate coma. Some ICUs have incorporated the use of neuromuscular paralysis to optimize patient-ventilator synchrony to prevent any ICP surges due to patient-ventilator dyssynchrony.

A continuous electroencephalogram can monitor burst suppression, the primary goal of either coma induction or paralysis with sedation.

Finally, intravenous indomethacin induces cerebral vasoconstriction and may temporarily reduce ICP; however, this medication is not easily prepared and it may be quite expensive for only a transient benefit.

■ AIRWAY AND VENTILATION

Patients with ALF who reach grades III to IV encephalopathy require intubation and mechanical ventilation. When intubating, a clinician skilled in the procedure should maintain adequate preoxygenation, prevention of hypercapnea, and avoidance of hypotension. Propofol sedation and lidocaine (endotracheal or intravenous) may help to minimize spikes in ICP. Pre-intubation, clinicians may utilize neuromuscular blockade. When indicated, cis-atracurium—a nondepolarizing agent, metabolized independently of liver or renal function—is the paralytic of choice and permits neurologic assessment 40 to 60 minutes after the bolus. No consensus drives practice regarding the specific mode of mechanical ventilation; therefore, either volume or pressure controlled mode can be utilized. Initial ventilator settings should include a low tidal volume strategy of 6 mL/kg of ideal body weight and a maximum plateau pressure of 30 cm H_2O, in order to minimize the effects of mechanical ventilation-induced barotrauma. If a low tidal volume strategy increases pCO_2, this may lead to cerebrovascular dilation and increase in ICP. Therefore, clinicians should strictly manage pCO_2 through minute ventilation and adjust respiratory rate accordingly.

Optimal patient-ventilator synchrony with adequate sedation and analgesia helps to prevent spikes in ICP. Critical care physicians should employ paralysis if patient-ventilator asynchrony occurs despite aggressive sedation and analgesia. While mechanical hyperventilation does not improve outcomes, spontaneous hyperventilation should not be inhibited, as it does result in mild hypocapnia and cerebrovascular constriction, thus reducing ICP. Whenever possible, to avoid any spikes in ICP, bronchoscopy should be avoided in patients with ALF.

■ CIRCULATION

Circulatory changes associated with ALF can resemble changes seen with endotoxinemia-induced septic shock. The pattern observed depends on the etiology and rapidity of ALF. In hyperacute liver failure due to acetaminophen overdose, patients can develop fulminant peripheral cardiovascular collapse that can lead to early death. Early hemodynamic changes in ALF include increased portal pressures, splanchnic sequestration of blood, and decreased central venous return. Fluid resuscitation and vasopressor support may be necessary, but fluid requirements in ALF may be less than in patients with septic shock. Some experts recommend placement of a pulmonary artery catheter to aid in assessing volume status. NAC benefits hemodynamic stabilization and improves oxygen consumption in patients with ALF.

In order to maintain an adequate CPP, systemic vasopressor support may be necessary, especially if the patient is hypotensive from ALF-induced vasodilation. Clinicians should maintain close monitoring and titration of oxygen delivery while using vasoconstrictors. A mixed, or central, venous oxygen saturation can guide the institution and titration of vasoactive agents.

Careful pressor selection facilitates adequate blood flow to the liver and brain. Norepinephrine serves as the vasopressor of choice in cases of ALF. It increases hepatic blood flow in parallel with cardiac output, and has less tachycardia than dopamine. Norepinephrine also leads to less lactate production than epinephrine. Alpha-adrenergic agents (epinephrine, high-dose vasopressin, terlipressin) can worsen peripheral oxygen delivery and lead to splanchnic ischemia. Terlipressin increases both cerebral blood flow and ICP, due to breakdown of autoregulation.

Relative adrenal insufficiency can occur with ALF, and stress dose steroids (hydrocortisone up to 200-300 mg daily) have been shown to reduce norepinephrine requirements. Intravenous steroids should be given to patient with ALF who develop persistent hypotension despite adequate IV fluids and vasopressor support.

Hemodynamics and intracranial hypertension frequently improve after removal of the native liver during liver transplant surgery. Therefore, ALF patients who are listed for transplantation but who have persistent circulatory dysfunction despite maximal medical measures, should be considered for a bridging, last-resort hepatectomy.

■ RENAL FAILURE

Acute renal failure occurs frequently in the setting of ALF, with an incidence up to 70%, and portends a poor prognosis. Causes of renal failure may include a prerenal insult (systemic vasodilation, hypovolemia, sepsis), direct renal injury (acute tubular necrosis from hypoperfusion, acetaminophen, or other toxins), or postrenal obstruction. The nephrotoxic effects of acetaminophen usually reverse spontaneously, but whether NAC contributes has not been proven.

Based on randomized trials, early initiation of CRRT improves outcomes over intermittent hemodialysis in order to reduce dramatic fluid shifts and avoid spikes in ICP. High-volume hemofiltration improves laboratory (lactate, base deficit) abnormalities and reduces vasopressor requirements, but may not affect survival in ALF. Because patients with ALF do not tolerate a lactate load, bicarbonate buffered hemofiltration is recommended.

■ BLEEDING AND CLOTTING

Coagulation abnormalities, due to both decreased synthesis and increased consumption, occur frequently in patients with ALF. Thrombocytopenia occurs in 50% to 70% of patients, but only 5% of patients with ALF experience significant bleeding. Variceal bleeding almost never occurs, as chronic portal hypertension is absent. Spontaneous intracranial bleeding (in the absence of an ICP monitor) is rare as well. Practice-based recommendations for platelet transfusion in ALF include (1) all patients with platelet count < 10,000/mm³, (2) patients with sepsis and platelet count < 20,000/mm³, or (3) patients with a planned invasive procedure or active bleeding and a platelet count < 50,000/mm³. Patients with ALF also bear increased thrombosis risk due to reduced protein C and protein S production; therefore, venous thromboembolism prophylaxis with subcutaneous heparin may be instituted.

PRACTICE POINT

Platelets and coagulation factors

- Platelet transfusion recommendations in ALF:
  1. All patients with platelet count <10,000/mm³
  2. Sepsis with platelet count <20,000/mm³, or
  3. Planned invasive procedure or active bleeding with platelet count <50,000/mm³
- Hepatically synthesized factors (factor V, factor VII) and INR provide the most sensitive biochemical indicators of hepatic synthetic function and recovery
- Administration of fresh frozen plasma—which can obscure the picture of endogenous coagulation factor production—should be avoided in the absence of active bleeding
- Vitamin K (5-10 mg subcutaneously daily for 3 days) can help eliminate any component of malnutrition as a source for coagulopathy

---

Hepatically synthesized factors (factor V, factor VII) and INR provide the most sensitive biochemical indicators of hepatic synthetic function and recovery. Therefore, administration of fresh frozen plasma (FFP)—which can obscure the picture of endogenous coagulation factor production—should be avoided in the absence of active bleeding. Vitamin K (5-10 mg subcutaneously daily for 3 days) can help in eliminating any component of malnutrition as a source for coagulopathy. Fresh frozen plasma transfusion and plasmapheresis carry additional risks of volume overload and transfusion-related acute lung injury. If an invasive procedure, such as an ICP monitor, is planned, activated recombinant factor VII can temporarily correct the INR. A minimum dose of 40 µg/kg is recommended in order to achieve a transient (therapeutic window

of 60-90 minutes) reversal of coagulopathy. Repeat dosing can be administered as necessary. Factor VIIa has been associated with rare cases of thromboembolism and cerebrovascular accident. Bleeding rarely poses a major problem with transplant surgery itself, and the preoperative degree of coagulopathy does not predict post-transplant outcome.

■ INFECTION

Patients with ALF have altered immune function and, in the setting of multiple intravenous lines, catheters, and devices, have moderate-to-high risk for bacterial and fungal sepsis. Up to 80% of ALF patients develop bacterial infections, and 30% of patients develop fungal infections. Most infections are diagnosed within 72 hours of hospital admission and are commonly localized to the respiratory tract, urinary tract, or bloodstream. Gram-positive infections with *Staphylococcus* or *Streptococcus* species occur more commonly than Gram-negative or *Candida* infections.

Clinicians should maintain a low threshold to evaluate for infection since the usual signs of infection may be absent in nearly one-third of individuals with ALF. Because active infection may preclude liver transplantation, some centers advocate starting empiric antimicrobial therapy upon hospital admission. While antibiotic prophylaxis reduces the incidence of infection and may reduce the risk of ICH and cerebral edema, such prophylaxis has not shown an overall survival benefit. Empiric antibacterial and antifungal therapy should be administered in the setting of shock, and may be considered in advanced encephalopathy or in patients listed for transplantation.

■ METABOLIC ABNORMALITIES AND NUTRITION

Metabolic derangements are common in patients with ALF. Alkalosis and acidosis may both occur and are best managed by identifying and treating the underlying disorder. Hypoglycemia should be managed with continuous glucose infusions and frequent serum glucose checks. Sodium, potassium, and magnesium levels are often low and should be supplemented. Hypophosphatemia is common and, while necessitating supplementation, may be a good prognostic sign, as it may reflect the consumption of ATP in a regenerating liver. High or normal phosphate levels may indicate a lack of hepatic regeneration and renal impairment. ALF patients frequently have increased energy expenditure and a catabolic state. Therefore, in order to reduce infectious complications, early enteral feedings should be initiated, including 60 g of protein per day. Enteral feedings may also reduce the risk of GI bleeding due to stress ulcerations in critically ill patients.

■ LIVER SUPPORT SYSTEMS AND AUXILIARY GRAFTS

The MARS® (Molecular Adsorbent Recirculating System) device is approved by the Food and Drug Administration for use in the US in the treatment of acute liver failure from drug overdose and poisonings as well as HE due to a decompensation of a chronic liver disease. MARS combines traditional continuous renal replacement therapy technology with large protein-bound particle removal via albumin dialysis. It removes ammonia, bilirubin, bile acids, aromatic amino acids, nitric oxide, tryptophan, copper, creatinine, protoporphyrin, urea, and diazepam. Human albumin cleans protein-bound toxins, while the bicarbonate-based dialysate binds other water-soluble elements. This reduces plasma toxicity, improves patient clinical conditions (hemodynamics, hepatic encephalopathy, urine output), enhances the regeneration of liver cells and may help to recover native liver functions.

TABLE 159-9 King's College Criteria—Prognostic Model for Determining Poor Outcome without Liver Transplantation in Acute Liver Failure (ALF)

For Acetaminophen-Induced ALF	For non–acetaminophen-Induced ALF
Arterial pH < 7.3	INR > 6.5
OR	OR
All 3 of the following	3 out of 5 of the following criteria
INR > 6.5	Age <11 or >40
Serum creatinine > 3.4 mg/dL	Serum bilirubin > 18 mg/dL
Grade III or IV encephalopathy	Time from jaundice to coma >7 days
	INR > 3.5
	Etiology non-A or non-B viral hepatitis OR drug-induced liver injury

For patients in whom a liver graft donor has been identified, total hepatectomy may be considered, as it removes the major source of proinflammatory cytokines that contribute to cerebral vasodilation. Auxiliary liver transplants refer to reduced size graft from living or deceased donor. They have been used in Europe to provide temporary hepatic function as a bridge to recover of the native liver. The best outcome has been seen in patients younger than 40 years of age with either acute viral hepatitis or acetaminophen toxicity.

■ PROGNOSIS

Regardless of the acuity, the etiology of ALF best predicts the likelihood of spontaneous recovery without transplantation. Patients with ALF due to acetaminophen, hepatitis A, shock liver, or pregnancy-related disease have > 50% transplant-free survival, whereas patients with other etiologies have a < 25% transplant-free survival. Patients with autoimmune hepatitis, acute hepatitis B, or acute HSV may improve with specific therapy and not require a liver transplant.

Clinicians should use accepted prognostic models to evaluate patients with ALF. The King's College prognostic criteria separate patients with acetaminophen-induced ALF from those with non–acetaminophen-induced ALF (**Table 159-9**).

The King's College model has high specificity (92%) in determining who will need a liver transplant, but low sensitivity (69%). If a patient fulfills the King's College criteria, the likelihood ratio positive for a poor prognosis without transplant is 8.63. On the other hand, the likelihood ratio negative for a patient with unfulfilled King's College criteria is 0.34. Therefore, the King's College criteria may misclassify a substantial number of patients who will die without a liver transplant. A recent meta-analysis found that the King's College criteria and a pH < 7.30 were both fairly specific in predicting a poor outcome.

One small study showed that an APACHE II score > 15 on admission for patients with acetaminophen-induced ALF shows a specificity of 92% and a sensitivity of 81% (likelihood ratio positive 10.1, likelihood ratio negative 0.21) for predicting need of liver transplant. The Model for End Stage Liver Disease (MELD) score may eventually prove to be superior to the King's College criteria in cases of non–acetaminophen-induced ALF. A single study in Argentina showed a MELD score of greater than 30 to be superior to the King's College criteria in predicting poor prognosis without transplant in patients with non–acetaminophen-induced ALF. The positive predictive value and negative predictive value of a MELD > 30 was found to be 91% and 100%, respectively (diagnostic accuracy 95%). Further studies are needed for validation.

Finally, multiple clinical predictors correlate with poor outcome in the absence of transplant. Encephalopathy at the time of admission predicts a worse prognosis. Patients presenting with grade III or IV encephalopathy die or require transplant in 60% to 90% of cases. Age, renal failure, and severity of coagulopathy are also independent predictors of mortality without transplant. Even the King's College criteria lack the sensitivity to replace an experienced transplant physician's clinical judgment.

DISCHARGE PLANNING

If a patient recovers from ALF with or without transplant, he or she should receive education about the disease and ways to prevent future injury. Depending on the etiology of ALF, ongoing treatment and follow-up may be necessary. For example, a patient with autoimmune hepatitis will need close hepatology follow-up and treatment with immunosuppressant medications. Also, a patient with acute-on-chronic hepatitis B will require hepatology follow-up, not only for antiviral treatment but also for hepatocellular carcinoma screening. The need for rehabilitation depends on overall performance and details of the hospitalization.

If a patient undergoes a liver transplant, a strong social network is vital, and close follow-up in the transplant center must be arranged. Rehabilitation or a skilled nursing facility may be necessary for some patients, especially if social support becomes a limitation. In contrast to patients transplanted for chronic liver disease, social support breakdown occurs more commonly when a patient undergoes liver transplantation for ALF, likely due to less time for education and a comprehensive assessment.

QUALITY IMPROVEMENT

Since fatal outcome occurs frequently in ALF without liver transplant, and because liver transplant is not always an option (eg, organ availability, poor candidate), public health measures should focus on prevention of ALF. Controlling distribution of acetaminophen could reduce overdoses. Some countries limit acetaminophen access by regulating the number of blister packs that can be purchased. Education about unintentional acetaminophen overdose, and education about drug and alcohol interactions, may help to reduce acetaminophen-related ALF in the United States. Finally, early recognition of drug-induced hepatoxicity, along with cessation of offending agents, may prevent some cases from progressing to liver failure.

In some cases, patients with ALF who are good candidates for liver transplant die before a donor liver becomes available. Increasing organ donation will lead to more lives saved, and additional education and outreach programs to increase liver donation are needed. Also, other creative ways to increase the donor pool (eg, extended criteria donors, paired exchanges, and partial-liver living donors) may augment the pool of available transplant organs.

Due to the low incidence of ALF, there are few controlled trials that can help to guide management (**Table 159-10**). Standards of intensive care in this patient population have not been well established and are mostly guided by expert opinion. Management may differ from center to center. Multicenter collaborations and prospective trials may improve future management of patients with ALF.

TABLE 159-10 Evidence-based Medicine Key References for Acute Liver Failure (ALF)

Reference	Methodology	Results	Limitations	Bottom Line
Epidemiology and Diagnosis				
Ostapowicz G, et al. *Ann Intern Med.* 2002;137:947-954.	Multicenter prospective cohort from 17 tertiary centers (United States Acute Liver Failure Study Group)	308 consecutive patients over 41 mo; 73% women, median age 38; acetaminophen-induced ALF most common etiology and with best prognosis; 29% of all patients underwent transplant, 43% of patients survived without transplant	Liver transplant not always available	Important multicenter study to define etiology, clinical features, and short-term outcomes in patients with ALF
N-acetylcysteine (NAC)				
Prescott L, et al. *BMJ.* 1979;2:1097-1100.	Outcome data of 102 patients with acetaminophen overdose who were treated with IV NAC as compared to a retrospective control group (n = 57) without NAC	IV NAC within 8 h of acetaminophen ingestion offers complete protection; within 10 h, only 1 of 62 patients developed severe hepatotoxicity	Not a randomized controlled trial	Give IV NAC asap with acetaminophen overdose
Smilkstein MJ, et al. *N Eng J Med.* 1988;319:1557-1562.	Analysis of a national multicenter study (1976-1985); outcome data from 2540 patients treated with investigational oral NAC for acetaminophen overdose	If given within 8 h of ingestion, oral NAC confers complete protection from severe hepatotoxicity (regardless of acetaminophen level); 72 h oral NAC protocol is as effective as 20 h IV regimen	Not a randomized controlled trial; no control group	Oral NAC is equivalent to 20 h IV NAC if a patient can take oral dosing
Smilkstein MJ, et al. *Ann Emerg Med.* 1991;20:1058-1063.	Nonrandomized multicenter study of 179 patients with acetaminophen overdose and IV NAC over 48 h	If given within 10 h of ingestion, 10% risk of severe hepatotoxicity; 14% of patients developed mild urticaria or rash during loading dose	Not a randomized controlled trial	48 h IV NAC protocol is safe and effective, especially if given within 10 h of acetaminophen ingestion
Keays R, et al. *BMJ.* 1991;303:1026-1029.	Prospective randomized controlled trial of 50 patients with acetaminophen-induced ALF; 25 patients received IV NAC until recovery or death; 25 patients received 5% dextrose (England)	IV NAC group had 48% survival vs 20% survival in control group (P = 0.037); IV NAC group had a lower incidence of cerebral edema and less hypotension requiring pressor support	Single center; 25 patients in each arm	IV NAC has survival benefit in patients with acetaminophen-induced ALF; give IV NAC regardless of time from acetaminophen ingestion
Prognosis and complications				
Clemmesen JO, et al. *Hepatology.* 1999;29:648-653.	Retrospective study of 44 patients with ALF (Denmark)	Patients with cerebral herniation (n = 14) had higher arterial ammonia levels than patients who did not herniate (P < 0.001)	Retrospective study	Higher arterial ammonia levels in patients with ALF portend a higher risk of cerebral herniation/death
Bhatia V, et al. *Gut.* 2006;55:98-104.	Prospective study of 80 patients admitted with ALF over 2 y (New Delhi)	42 patients died (median arterial ammonia level of 175); median ammonia level was 105 in survivors	Single center in India	Arterial ammonia > 124 predicted mortality with a sensitivity of 79% and specificity of 76%
Bailey B, et al. *Crit Care Med.* 2003;31:299-305.	Meta-analysis of prognostic criteria determining need for transplant in acetaminophen-induced ALF	King's College criteria (9 studies); sensitivity 69%, specificity 92%; APACHE II score >15 had LR+ of 16.4 and a LR– of 0.19 (1 study)	Only one study evaluated APACHE II score	KCH criteria and possibly APACHE II scores are useful but not perfect in predicting need for transplant in patients with acetaminophen-induced ALF
Yantorno SE, et al. *Liver Transpl.* 2007;13:822-828.	Retrospective cohort of 120 patients with non-acetaminophen causes of ALF (Argentina)	MELD > 30 predicted need for transplant with diagnostic accuracy of 95%, PPV 91%, NPV 100%	Single center; did not include acetaminophen-induced cases of ALF	MELD score > 30 may better predict need for transplant in non–acetaminophen-induced cases of ALF when compared to King's College

(Continued)

TABLE 159-10 Evidence-based Medicine Key References for Acute Liver Failure (ALF) *(Continued)*

Reference	Methodology	Results	Limitations	Bottom Line
Katoonizadeh A, et al. *Liver Int.* 2007;27:329-334.	Retrospective analysis of prospective cohort; 99 patients with non–acetaminophen-induced ALF	King's College criteria and MELD > 30 had similar NPV (91%-92%) and low PPV (52%-56%); MELD > 35 had sensitivity 86%, specificty 75%	Excluded acetaminophen-induced cases of ALF	Both King's College criteria and MELD score may have similar prognostic value in cases of non-acetaminophen ALF
Management				
Lidofsky SD, et al. *Hepatology.* 1992; 16:1-7.	Retrospective cohort study of 20 adults and 3 children with ALF who had intracranial pressure monitors placed (UCSF)	10 patients required medical therapy for sustained elevation of ICP, 6 had refractory ICH and died	Not a randomized controlled trial	ICP monitors may have a role in diagnosis and treatment of ICH in patients with ALF
Blei AT, et al. *Lancet.* 1993;341:157-158.	Survey of US centers; 262 patients with ALF who received an ICP monitor	Epidural most common and lowest risk (1% fatal bleed) compared to other types (4%–5% fatal bleed)	Survey data	If using an ICP monitor, an epidural device is most common and preferred for safety
Vaquero J, et al. *Liver Transpl.* 2005;11: 1581-1589.	Retrospective data from US ALF Study Group centers (24 sites)—332 patients	28% of patients underwent ICP monitor placement (center dependent); 30-d survival post liver transplant was equal with or without ICP monitor; pts with ICP monitor required more medical therapy and vasopressor support	Variation among centers	ICP monitors may be useful in patients who are potential transplant candidates, but this remains controversial
Shami VM, et al. *Liver Transpl.* 2003;9:138-143.	Comparative trial assessing FFP (8 patients) vs FFP/recombinant activated factor VII (7 patients) in 15 patients with poor prognosis based on King's College criteria	100% of patients who received FFP and recombinant activated factor VII could undergo placement of ICP monitor (vs 38% in FFP alone group)	Not a prospective, randomized controlled trial	Recombinant activated factor VII facilitates placement of an ICP monitor by reducing risk of bleeding
Canalese J, et al. *Gut.* 1982;23: 625-629.	Controlled trial comparing mannitol (17 patients) to no mannitol (17 patients) for treating cerebral edema in 34 patients with ALF	IV mannitol group had a 47% survival compared to 6% in the control group ($P = 0.008$)	Single center (all patients had an ICP monitor and were given IV dexamethasone)	IV mannitol treats ICH/cerebral edema and confers a survival benefit
Murphy N, et al. *Hepatology.* 2004;39:464-470.	Randomized controlled trial of 30 patients with ALF and severe (grade III–IV) encephalopathy; 15 patients with hypertonic saline; 15 patients with standard care	30% saline with a goal serum sodium of 145-155 mmol/L reduces the incidence and severity of ICH	Single center; all patients had an ICP monitor (Camino subdural)	Hypertonic saline is indicated in cases of ALF and advanced encephalopathy
Jalan R, et al. *Lancet.* 1999;354: 1164-1168.	Retrospective analysis of moderate hypothermia in 7 consecutive patients with elevated ICP not responding to mannitol or ultrafiltration	4 patients who underwent transplant had good outcomes	Not a randomized controlled trial	Moderate hypothermia should be used in cases of ALF with elevated ICP that does not respond to mannitol
Rolando N, et al. *Hepatology.* 1990;11:49-53.	Retrospective study of a prospective cohort of 50 consecutive patients with ALF and grade II encephalopathy	53 bacterial infections in 40 patients (47% respiratory, 23% urinary, 4% CVC related); 70% Gram-positive; 32% of patients developed fungal infections (15 *Candida*, 1 *Aspergillus*, and all had concominant bacterial infections; all deaths after 7 d were from infection; fever and leukocytosis absent in 30% of infections	Single center data	Maintain a high suspicion for bacterial and fungal infections in patients who present with ALF
Kjaergard LL, et al. *JAMA.* 2003;289: 217-222.	Meta-analysis for artificial and bioartificial support systems in acute (2 studies) and acute-on-chronic (10 studies) liver failure	No effect on mortality	Only 2 studies looking at acute liver failure	No role for artificial support systems at the present time, more studies needed

SUGGESTED READINGS

Farmer DG, Anselmo DM, Ghobrial RM, et al. Liver transplantation for fulminant hepatic failure: experience with more than 200 patients over a 17-year period. *Ann Surg*. 2003;237:666-675; discussion 675-676.

Hoofnagle JH, Carithers RL Jr, Shapiro C, Ascher N. Fulminant hepatic failure: summary of a workshop. *Hepatology*. 1995;21:240-252.

O'Grady JG, Alexander GJ, Hayllar KM, Williams R. Early indicators of prognosis in fulminant hepatic failure. *Gastroenterology*. 1989;97:439-445.

Ostapowicz G, Fontana RJ, Schiodt FV, et al. Results of a prospective study of acute liver failure at 17 tertiary care centers in the United States. *Ann Intern Med*. 2002;137:947-954.

Polson J, Lee WM. AASLD position paper: the management of acute liver failure. *Hepatology*. 2005;41:1179-1197.

Shakil AO, Kramer D, Mazariegos GV, et al. Acute liver failure: clinical features, outcome analysis, and applicability of prognostic criteria. *Liver Transpl*. 2000;6:163-169.

Stravitz RT, Kramer DJ. Management of acute liver failure. *Nat Rev Gastroenterol Hepatol*. 2009;6:542-553.

van Hoek B, de Boer J, Boudjema K, et al. Auxiliary versus orthotopic liver transplantation for acute liver failure. EURALT Study Group. European Auxiliary Liver Transplant Registry. *J Hepatol*. 1999;30:699-705.

CHAPTER 160

Cirrhosis and Its Complications

Patrick Avila, MD
Norman D. Grace, MD

INTRODUCTION

Cirrhosis of the liver is a chronic illness that progresses at a variable rate, dependent on the etiology and the activity of the offending toxin. It is a dynamic process, which is potentially reversible in the earlier stages if the offending agent is either removed or modified. Classically, cirrhosis has been defined histologically as architecturally abnormal nodules separated by bands of fibrous tissue. The diagnosis has usually been based on clinical suspicion, confirmed by radiologic studies and a liver biopsy as the gold standard. However, sampling error on biopsy may lead to incorrect staging of the disease, where the transition from severe fibrosis to cirrhosis is misinterpreted. Therefore, advanced chronic liver disease has been proposed as a more encompassing definition for the transitional stages. However, in this chapter, we will continue to use cirrhosis as the term to characterize this entity.

Patients with cirrhosis may be further classified as compensated or decompensated. Decompensation is defined as the appearance of ascites, variceal bleeding, hepatic encephalopathy or jaundice. A prognostic classification consisting of five stages has been proposed to account for the increasing mortality with progressive decompensation (**Figure 160-1**). Stage one includes patients with compensated cirrhosis that do not have any complications such as ascites or esophageal varices. In stage two, patients have developed nonbleeding esophageal varices but are still considered compensated. Stage three describes patients who have transitioned to decompensation, characterized by the development of hemorrhage from esophageal varices. Patients may further progress to stage four which is characterized by the development of nonbleeding complications, including the development of ascites, hepatic encephalopathy or the hepatorenal syndrome. Stage five includes patients who have developed a second decompensating event. In a recent study by D'Amico et al that included 494 patients with alcoholic, viral or cryptogenic cirrhosis, the initial decompensating event was ascites (33%), variceal bleeding (10%), and hepatocellular carcinoma (9%), while encephalopathy or jaundice as the first decompensating event was rare. In this study, the 5-year mortality was 1.5% for patients in stage one compared to 88% for patients in stage five. In addition to describing the natural history of the disease process, a potential benefit of this staging system is the ability to target specific therapy based on the prognosis at a given stage. For example, patients who presented with variceal bleeding without ascites had a significantly better survival than those in whom ascites was present at the onset of the bleeding event and would be less likely to be considered as candidates for liver transplantation.

PATHOGENESIS

The major complications of cirrhosis are secondary to the development of portal hypertension. The initiating event is an increase in intrahepatic and portocollateral resistance, followed by an increase in portal venous flow. The increase in intrahepatic resistance has relatively fixed components including sinusoidal encroachment, collagen deposition, vascular tree pruning and nodular formation. Dynamic components of intrahepatic resistance are governed by an overexpression of endogenous vasoconstrictors, especially endothelin, and a diminished expression of vasodilators, primarily nitric oxide. The increase in portal blood flow is related to systemic vasodilation secondary to increased systemic production of vasodilators, primarily nitric oxide but also including increased production

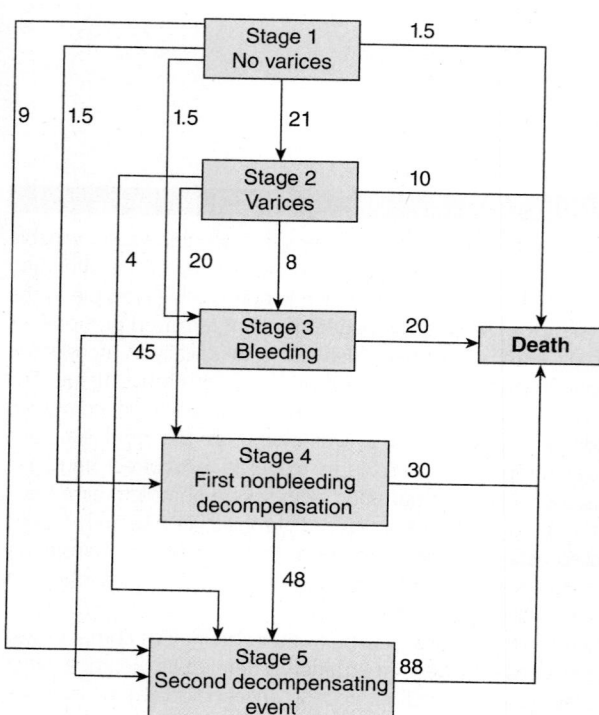

Figure 160-1 *Schematic representation of 5-year transitioning rate across stages and to death for the whole series of patients. Arrows represent transitions and the numbers close to each arrow are the relevant transition rates. A fairly steady increase in death rate was found across stages. (From D'Amico G, et al. Competing risks and prognostic stages of cirrhosis: a 25-year inception cohort study of 494 patients.* Aliment Pharmacol Ther. *2014;39(10):1180-1193.)*

of glucagon, tumor necrosis factor, prostaglandins and other cytokines. The resulting hyperdynamic circulation leads to an increase in portal venous blood flow against intrahepatic resistance, resulting in portal hypertension. Portal hypertension is further aggravated by an increase in angiogenesis which exacerbates the increase in portal pressure and promotes the development of a portosystemic collateral circulation including the development of esophageal varices.

CLINICAL PRESENTATION

Presenting symptoms of cirrhosis are nonspecific and include the development of fatigue and lethargy. Physical findings include jaundice, peripheral muscle wasting, splenomegaly, spider angiomata, abdominal collateral vessels and an altered mental status. However, patients presenting initially with cirrhosis often have none of these findings.

Laboratory findings include an increase in serum bilirubin, a decrease in serum albumin, increases in AST, ALT and alkaline phosphatase and prolongation of the prothrombin time. A decrease in platelet count in the presence of cirrhosis suggests the development of portal hypertension but the variability of this finding makes it unreliable as a screening test.

DIAGNOSIS OF CIRRHOSIS

Although liver biopsy remains the gold standard for the diagnosis of cirrhosis, the test is invasive, often limited by inadequate sample size and prone to sampling error. Recently, there is increased interest in noninvasive means for diagnosing cirrhosis. Most prominent of the noninvasive methods is the use of transient elastography (TE) (fibroscan) as a means of identifying patients with cirrhosis who are at risk of developing clinically significant portal hypertension.

The technique is easy to perform at bedside, has excellent reproducibility, and has very good correlation with invasive measurements of portal pressure (eg, the hepatic venous pressure gradient [HVPG]), especially in patients in the compensated stages of cirrhosis. Limitations include occasional false positives and unreliability in obese patients, patients with clinically evident ascites and patients with acute liver failure. The fibroscan has recently received Food and Drug Administration (FDA) approval and has become a standard diagnostic test in liver centers throughout Europe and North America.

Other noninvasive methods for the diagnosis of cirrhosis include serum biomarkers (eg, Fibrotest) which have gained popularity in Europe, more so than in the United States. A number of radiologic approaches are under investigation including MR elastography, ultrasound elastography and measurements of splenic stiffness but these should still be considered experimental techniques.

Portal pressure as measured by the HVPG provides excellent information for diagnosis, prognosis and management of portal hypertension. Hepatic venous pressure gradient measurements are excellent in predicting the development of esophagogastric varices, ascites, esophageal variceal hemorrhage, hepatic decompensation and the development of hepatocellular carcinoma. Hepatic venous pressure gradient measurements are especially useful in assessing response to pharmacologic therapy of portal hypertension. However, because of the invasive nature of these measurements, they are primarily used in clinical research studies and have limited usage in clinical practice.

PRACTICE POINT

- Patients with cirrhosis can be classified as compensated or decompensated.

- Decompensation is defined as the appearance of ascites, variceal bleeding, hepatic encephalopathy or jaundice.

- A prognostic classification consisting of five stages has been proposed to account for the increasing mortality with progressive decompensation. The 5-year mortality is 1.5% for patients in stage one compared to 88% for patients in stage five.

ESOPHAGOGASTRIC VARICES

Patients with cirrhosis develop esophageal varices at a rate of 8% per year. The risk of hemorrhage from varices is 5% to 15% per year, with patients having large varices at greater risk. Variceal hemorrhage is associated with a 15% to 20% 6-week mortality. If the index bleed is controlled and no further treatment to prevent rebleeding is initiated, the risk of recurrent hemorrhage is 60% to 70% with most episodes occurring within 1 year of the index bleed.

■ SCREENING FOR ESOPHAGEAL VARICES

Current practice guidelines recommend screening by esophagogastroduodenoscopy (EGD) for the presence of varices in all patients with the diagnosis of cirrhosis. In patients with compensated cirrhosis and no varices on the initial screening EGD, the EGD should be repeated in 2 to 3 years unless there is evidence of clinical progression of the disease. In patients with decompensated cirrhosis and no varices on the initial examination, EGD should be repeated yearly. Once varices have been detected, further EGD is not indicated unless there is evidence of gastrointestinal bleeding. Because of cost and patient preference considerations, there is considerable interest in noninvasive techniques that might identify patients with cirrhosis at low risk for the development of varices. Noninvasive serum markers combining a number of biochemical tests may identify patients at low risk for developing varices but their positive and negative predictive values are insufficient to avoid screening endoscopy. A low platelet count (<100,000/mm²) has been suggested for screening patients at risk for varices but the predictive accuracy is insufficient to defer patients from endoscopic screening. The platelet count/spleen diameter ratio as measured by abdominal ultrasound is somewhat better at identifying patients at risk. The best noninvasive test for identifying patients at low risk for the development of varices is the measurement of liver stiffness by transient elastography. In patients with TE values <10 kPa in the absence of clinical signs of portal hypertension, the risk of developing esophageal varices is extremely low and screening endoscopy may be avoided. Until more data are available, patients with a TE value >10 kPa should be screened by endoscopy for varices. If the TE value is >15 kPa, patients are at high risk for developing varices. Wireless capsule endoscopy has 85% to 95% accuracy in determining the presence of varices, variceal size and endoscopic red color signs. However, this technique is not widely available and it has not replaced endoscopic screening as the standard diagnostic procedure.

■ RISK STRATIFICATION FOR VARICEAL HEMORRHAGE

With rare exceptions, patients with cirrhosis require an HVPG >10 mm Hg for the development of esophageal varices and an HVPG >12 mm Hg for variceal hemorrhage to occur. Risk factors for variceal hemorrhage as identified by endoscopy include the size of varices (large varices are at greater risk than small varices) and the endoscopic red color signs. The latter include red wale marks that appear as longitudinal red streaks on varices, hematocystic spots which look like small varices on the surface of larger varices and cherry red spots. In addition, the worse the Child-Pugh score, the greater the risk of bleeding. In patients with alcoholic cirrhosis, active alcohol consumption increases the risk of hemorrhage.

TREATMENT OF ESOPHAGEAL VARICES AND VARICEAL HEMORRHAGE

Options for the treatment of esophageal varices include pharmacologic agents that decrease portal pressure, endoscopic techniques that obliterate the varices and TIPS (transjugular intrahepatic portosystemic shunt) or surgical shunts that achieve a major reduction in portal pressure.

■ PHARMACOLOGIC THERAPY

The goal of pharmacologic therapy is to reduce portal venous blood flow and/or intrahepatic and portocollateral resistance in order to achieve a decrease in portal pressure. The primary drugs to achieve this goal on a long-term basis are the nonselective β-blockers (propranolol, nadolol, and timolol) and the long acting nitrate, isosorbide-5-mononitrate (ISMN).

β-Blockers act by decreasing cardiac output via blockade of the β1 receptors and by blockade of the β2 receptors, leaving unopposed alpha adrenergic activity which causes vasoconstriction of the splanchnic vessels. These drugs are given orally and should be titrated to the maximally tolerated dose. Unfortunately, only 35% to 40% of patients treated with β-blockers achieve a clinically significant hemodynamic response, defined as a 20% reduction in HVPG or a reduction in HVPG to below 12 mm Hg. Carvedilol, a nonselective β-blocker with intrinsic anti-alpha-1 adrenergic activity has been shown to produce a greater reduction in HVPG than the nonselective β-blockers when given as monotherapy.

Isosorbide-5-mononitrate increases the delivery of nitric oxide to the intrahepatic circulation, thus decreasing intrahepatic resistance. It also decreases cardiac output by decreasing cardiac preload and enhances systemic vasodilation and venous pooling which causes a reflex splanchnic arterial vasoconstriction. When given together with nonselective β-blockers, there is an incremental reduction in HVPG. Isosorbide-5-mononitrate is clinically ineffective when given as monotherapy.

Simvastatin has been shown to produce an incremental decrease in the HVPG when combined with nonselective β-blockers and prospective trials are currently underway to determine its clinical efficacy.

The major side effects of nonselective β-blockers include hypotension, fatigue, lethargy, depression and dyspnea in patients with pulmonary disease. Their use is contraindicated in patients with restrictive airway disease, congestive heart failure, bradycardia and heart block. Their use in insulin dependent diabetics needs to be monitored carefully. As a result, 15% to 20% of patients with cirrhosis have contraindications to the use of β-blockers, and an additional 15% develop severe side effects leading to discontinuation of the drug. The major side effects of ISMN are systemic arterial hypotension and headaches.

The drugs used in the management of acute variceal bleeding include the vasopressin analog, terlipressin and somatostatin and its analogs, octreotide, vapreotide and lanreotide. The goal of these drugs is to reduce portal venous blood flow and portal pressure. Terlipressin achieves a greater reduction in portal pressure than the somatostatin analogs. The drugs are safe with minimal side effects (**Table 160-1**).

TABLE 160-1 Drugs Used in the Management of Portal Hypertension

Drug	Class of Drug	Starting Dose	Maximum Dose
Propranolol	Nonselective β-blocker	40 mg twice daily	640 mg/d
Nadolol	Nonselective β-blocker	40 mg daily	320 mg/d
Timolol	Nonselective β-blocker	10 mg daily	40 mg/d
Carvedilol	Nonselective β-blocker with intrinsic anti-α adrenergic activity	6.25 mg	12.5 mg/d
Isosorbide mononitrate	Long-acting nitrate	20 mg daily	240 mg/d
Spironolactone	Aldosterone antagonist	25 mg daily	400 mg/d
Furosemide	Loop diuretic	40 mg daily	160 mg/d
Octreotide	Splanchnic vasoconstrictor	50 μg bolus, followed by 50 μg/h or subcutaneously 100-200 mg three times daily	50 μg/h
Norfloxacin	Quinolone antibiotic	400 mg twice daily	—
Midodrine	Oral alpha-1 agonist	5 mg three times daily	52.5 mg/d
Terlipressin	Intravenous vasopressin analog	1-2 mg every 4-6 h	12 mg/d
Norepinephrine	Intravenous alpha 1 and beta 1 agonist	0.5 mg/h	3 mg/h

Unfortunately, none of these drugs (mostly generic) have received FDA approval specifically for the treatment of esophageal varices and variceal hemorrhage. The nonselective β-blockers and octreotide are used off label. Terlipressin is widely used in Europe but as yet, has not received FDA approval for use in the US.

■ ENDOSCOPIC VARICEAL LIGATION (EVL)

Endoscopic variceal ligation involves the placement of rubber bands on the variceal columns via an endoscope that causes mucosal and submucosal necrosis leading to the formation of scar tissue and the obliteration of the varix. It is a local treatment and does not significantly alter portal hypertension. The most serious side effects are possible perforation of the esophagus and the formation of mucosal ulcers that can lead to significant hemorrhage. Endoscopic variceal ligation has replaced sclerotherapy as the endoscopic treatment of choice.

■ TRANSJUGULAR INTRAHEPATIC PORTOSYSTEMIC SHUNT (TIPS)

The TIPS procedure involves placement of a catheter into the right internal jugular vein and advancing it via the hepatic vein through the liver to form a tract connecting to the portal vein. This transhepatic tract is then dilated and a flexible coated metallic stent is placed, resulting in a shunt between the hepatic and portal veins and a significant decrease in portal pressure. The procedure is performed by interventional radiologists and has replaced portosystemic shunt surgery in most institutions.

Short-term complications of the TIPS procedure include fever, infection, renal dysfunction, intrahepatic and intraperitoneal hemorrhage and progressive hepatic failure. The major long-term complication is the development or worsening of hepatic encephalopathy, which has an incidence of approximately 30% to 35%. Risk factors for the development or worsening of hepatic encephalopathy after TIPS include increasing age, the presence of minimal hepatic encephalopathy at the time of TIPS placement, and a history of overt hepatic encephalopathy. The severity of encephalopathy correlates with the diameter of the shunt. With the advent of coated stents, shunt occlusion is much less of a problem. Doppler sonography is a noninvasive method to monitor shunt patency and is usually performed at 6-month intervals for the first 2 years after TIPS placement.

PREVENTION OF FIRST VARICEAL HEMORRHAGE (PRIMARY PROPHYLAXIS)

Based on the results of a large, long-term, multicenter randomized controlled trial (RCT), there was no benefit for the use of nonselective β-blockers in the prevention of the development of esophageal varices or other complications of portal hypertension in patients with compensated cirrhosis and an elevated HVPG.

Because of the high risk of bleeding and the associated mortality, treatment to prevent initial variceal hemorrhage is mandatory. Current practice guidelines (AASLD, ACG, Baveno) recommend the use of either nonselective β-blockers or EVL for the prevention of variceal hemorrhage in patients with large varices or small varices in patients with Child-Pugh class C cirrhosis or in patients with small varices when red color signs are present on endoscopy.

In other patients with small varices, β-blockers may be used, but more data are needed to establish their efficacy. A meta-analysis of 11 RCTs totaling 1190 patients showed a reduction in first variceal hemorrhage in patients with large varices from 30% in the control groups to 14% in the treatment groups. Randomized controlled trials showed similar results when comparing EVL to control groups. Neither treatment has been shown to improve survival. In well-designed RCTs with reasonable sample sizes, β-blockers and EVL were equally effective. As they are comparable in efficacy, the choice should be based on local expertise, side effects of the treatment and patient preference. In patients in whom varices have been eradicated with EVL, surveillance endoscopy should be performed because of the risk of recurrent variceal formation. However, EVL only reduces the risk of variceal bleeding while nonselective β-blockers reduce the risk of other complications of portal hypertension (ie, ascites) in addition to variceal bleeding.

TREATMENT OF ACUTE VARICEAL HEMORRHAGE

In patients with acute upper gastrointestinal bleeding, the source of bleeding should be determined by endoscopy. If varices are suspected in patients with cirrhosis, the patient should be started on a vasoactive drug (eg, terlipressin, octreotide). The vasoactive drugs should be continued for up to 5 days. Intubation to protect the airway is recommended in patients with active bleeding or altered mental status. In the absence of contraindications (eg, QT prolongation), infusion of erythromycin 250 mg IV 30 to 120 minutes prior to endoscopy should be considered (**Figure 160-2**).

A hemoglobin of 8.0 g/dL or a hematocrit of 25% should be the goal of transfusion in order to avoid an increase in portal pressure and exacerbation of the bleeding episode associated with overtransfusion. If the platelet count is greater than 50,000, platelet transfusions are not warranted. If the platelet count is lower, the use of platelet transfusions is controversial and their use has not been shown to affect the bleeding episode. The use of fresh frozen plasma (FFP) or recombinant factor VII transfusions is also controversial without clear evidence of their efficacy.

In patients with acute variceal bleeding, infection has been associated with early rebleeding and a high mortality rate. Based on the results of several RCTs, the short-term use of prophylactic antibiotics is mandatory. Preferred antibiotics include norfloxacin (400 mg twice daily for 7 days) or quinolone antibiotics (eg, levofloxacin, ciprofloxacin). In patients with decompensated cirrhosis, intravenous ceftriaxone (1.0 g/d) has been shown to be superior to norfloxacin. As there is increasing hospital based drug resistance to quinolones, this should be considered in the choice of antibiotics. If there is evidence of hepatic encephalopathy, institution of lactulose or rifaximin is recommended.

Once esophageal varices have been established as the source of bleeding, esophageal variceal ligation should be instituted to control the bleeding episode, EVL is successful in up to 90% of patients. If the bleeding remains uncontrolled or if there is severe early rebleeding, TIPS should be considered as the next intervention. Balloon tamponade with the Sengstaken-Blakemore tube or the placement of an esophageal stent can be used for temporary control of bleeding as a bridge to TIPS. Balloon tamponade should be

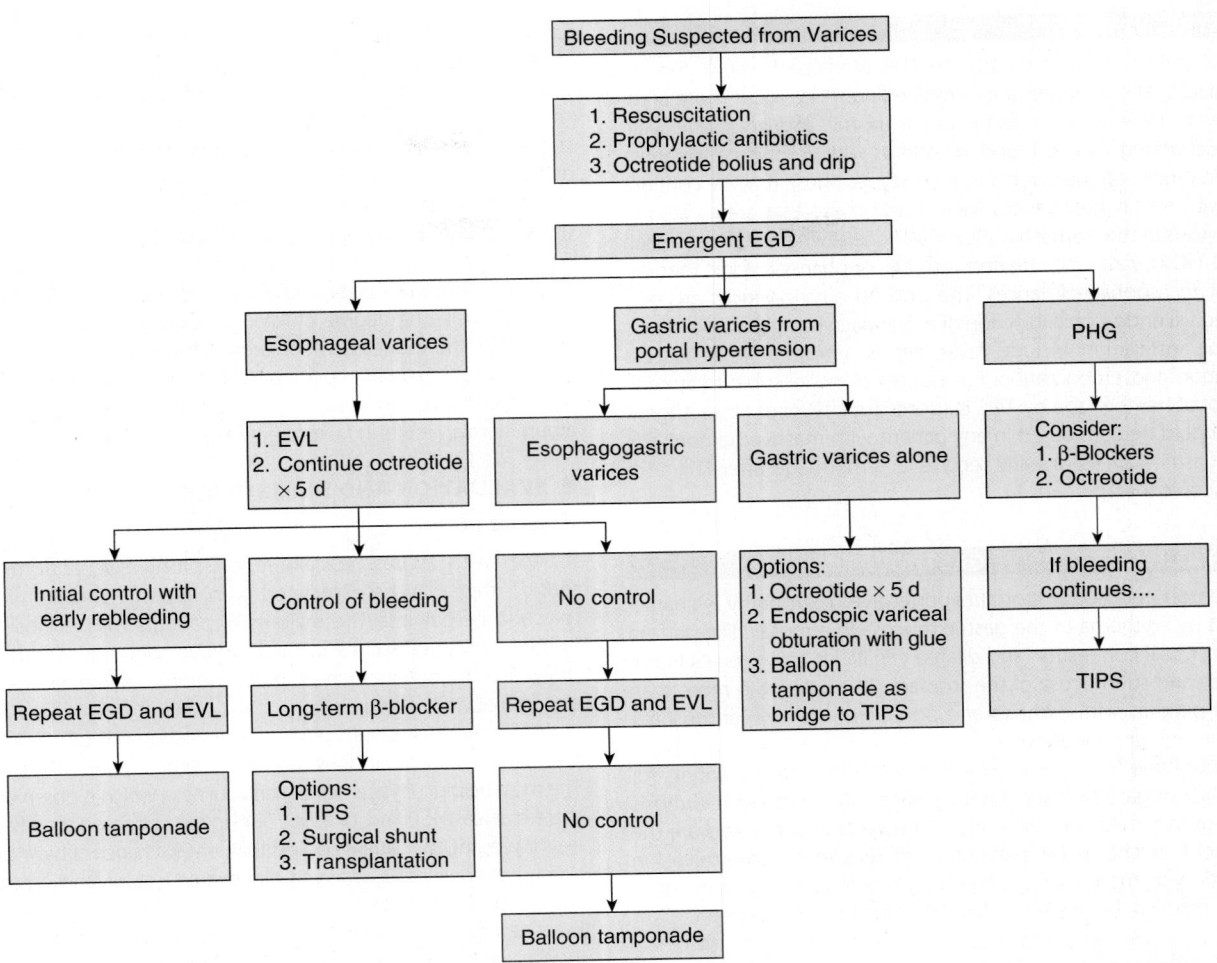

Figure 160-2 Management algorithm for acute variceal hemorrhage. EGD, esophagogastroduodenoscopy; EVL, endoscopic variceal ligation. (From Grace ND, Minor MA. Portal hypertension and variceal hemorrhage. In: Greenberger NJ, Blumberg RS, Burakoff R (eds). *Current Diagnosis and Treatment: Gastroenterology, Hepatology and Endoscopy.* New York, McGraw Hill Education Medical, 2016.)

limited to 24 hours as the complication rate increases significantly with longer use. Esophageal stents may be used for a longer period and are generally safer.

In patients with Child-Pugh class C cirrhosis or Child-Pugh class B with active bleeding, the placement of TIPS within the initial 24 hours from the onset of bleeding has been shown in a large multicenter RCT to be superior to medical therapy with EVL and vasoactive drugs and is associated with better control of the bleeding episode and improved survival.

PREVENTION OF RECURRENT VARICEAL HEMORRHAGE (SECONDARY PROPHYLAXIS)

As there is a 60% chance of recurrent hemorrhage after control of the acute bleeding episode, treatment to prevent recurrent hemorrhage is mandatory. Current practice guidelines recommend a combination of nonselective β-blockers and EVL as the treatment of choice. The addition of ISMN may offer a slightly lower rebleeding rate but has the risk of increased side effects. EVL should be performed every 1 to 2 weeks until varices have been obliterated. Endoscopy should be repeated every year to screen for recurrent varices. A meta-analysis of 23 RCTs comparing combination therapy to endoscopic monotherapy shows a reduction in recurrent variceal bleeding from 37.5% for endoscopic monotherapy to 25.3% for combination treatment. There is also a modest improvement in survival. If bleeding continues to recur, TIPS is the next option. Transjugular intrahepatic portosystemic shunt is very effective in preventing recurrent hemorrhage but is associated with an increased risk of hepatic encephalopathy. Surgically performed shunts are still an option in a few centers, but their use has declined significantly with the availability of TIPS. Variceal bleeding by itself is not an indication for liver transplantation.

GASTRIC VARICES

Gastric varices account for 10% to 15% of variceal bleeds and are associated with a higher rate of rebleeding. They occur more commonly in patients with extra-hepatic portal and/or splenic vein obstruction (eg, can be found in patients with chronic pancreatitis). Gastric varices can be divided into two types, those that are contiguous with esophageal varices (GOV1) and those that are located in the fundus of the stomach (GOV2, IGV1) or elsewhere in the stomach (IGV2). GOV1 varices are treated with EVL or pharmacologic therapy, similar to esophageal varices. The isolated gastric varices are best treated via endoscopic injection of a cyanoacrylate glue. Side effects of glue installation include fever, sepsis, retroperitoneal abscess formation and embolization. For failures of endoscopic treatment, control of hemorrhage by TIPS is successful in 90% of cases. Urgent TIPS should be considered in any patient with massive hemorrhage from gastric varices or early recurrent hemorrhage after failure of endoscopic therapy.

PORTAL HYPERTENSIVE GASTROPATHY

As seen on endoscopy, portal hypertensive gastropathy is characterized by erythema of the gastric mucosa in a mosaic like pattern with mucosal congestion and dilated capillaries and venules in the mucosa and submucosa of the stomach. It is present in more than half of patients with cirrhosis and portal hypertension and usually presents as a chronic anemia.

Hemorrhage from portal hypertensive gastropathy accounts for about 8% of gastrointestinal hemorrhage in patients with cirrhosis and is usually mild and self-limited. Nonselective β-blockers are the treatment of choice for prevention of recurrent hemorrhage. In patients with more massive bleeding requiring transfusions or in whom medical therapy has failed, TIPS should be considered.

PORTAL VEIN THROMBOSIS

Patients with portal vein thrombosis as the cause of portal hypertension should be evaluated for inherited and acquired thrombophilic factors, paroxysmal nocturnal hemoglobinuria, autoimmune disorders and myeloproliferative neoplasia. This is best managed in conjunction with a hematologist. For patients with acute primary thrombosis of the portal vein and/or the splanchnic venous circulation, anticoagulation is safe and recommended. Low molecular weight heparin and vitamin K antagonists are the treatment of choice. There is limited data on the use of long-term anticoagulation but it is probably safe.

ASCITES

Ascites is the pathologic accumulation of fluid within the peritoneal cavity. The most common cause of ascites is cirrhosis, which accounts for approximately 80% of cases. Other common causes include malignancy and congestive heart failure. Approximately 5% of patients with ascites have "mixed ascites" defined as ascites formation from two or more causes.

Ascites represents both the most common complication of portal hypertension and the leading cause for hospitalization in cirrhotic patients. Within 10 years after the diagnosis of compensated cirrhosis, about 50% of patients will have developed ascites. Approximately 15% of patients with cirrhosis die within 1 year of forming ascites, and 50% die within 5 years.

■ PATHOPHYSIOLOGY OF ASCITES

In patients with cirrhosis, progressive portal hypertension leads to the activation of endogenous vasoconstrictors and retention of sodium and water which then increases renal vasoconstriction. Cirrhotic vasodilation results in effective volume depletion. This is sensed as reduced pressure at the carotid and renal baroreceptors and activates sodium-retaining neurohumoral mechanisms. These mechanisms include the renin-angiotensin-aldosterone system, sympathetic nervous system and antidiuretic hormone. The net effect is avid sodium and water retention even though extracellular sodium stores and plasma volume are increased. Patients with ascites and urinary sodium below 10 mEq/d have a mean survival as low as 5 to 6 months in comparison to those who have a higher rate of sodium excretion. Similarly, the degree of water retention parallels the severity of cirrhosis. The degree of hyponatremia, as a result of increased antidiuretic hormone secretion, correlates with worsening survival. Over time, the expanded plasma volume and resulting lymph formation, in combination with decreased oncotic pressure from hypoalbuminemia, results in fluid retention within the peritoneal cavity.

■ EVALUATION AND DIAGNOSIS OF ASCITES

Physical exam

Patients with ascites typically report progressive abdominal distension that may be associated with abdominal discomfort, but may also be painless. The majority of patients with cirrhosis severe enough to cause ascites formation have stigmata of cirrhosis on physical examination, such as spider angioma, palmar erythema and abdominal wall collaterals.

Confirming ascites with physical examination can be challenging if the patient is obese or does not have a large amount of ascitic fluid. The most helpful physical sign is flank dullness, which is observed when there is at least 1500 mL of ascitic fluid in the abdomen. If no flank dullness is present, the patient has less than a 10% chance of having ascites. When flank dullness is observed, one should test for "shifting dullness," which has 83% sensitivity and 56% specificity in detecting ascites. Examination of the jugular veins should be performed since an elevated jugular venous pressure suggests ascites from heart failure or constrictive pericarditis. An abdominal ultrasound confirms that ascitic fluid is present and can determine where a diagnostic paracentesis can be safely performed. Ultrasonography is also a safe and cost-effective modality to evaluate the liver parenchyma for evidence of cirrhosis or malignancy as well as to check the patency of the portal and hepatic veins.

Diagnostic paracentesis

A diagnostic paracentesis with appropriate ascitic fluid analysis is a quick and cost-effective method to determine the etiology of ascites and should be performed in the initial evaluation of all patients with new-onset or recurrent ascites or patients hospitalized with ascites. Infected ascitic fluid may cause or exacerbate complications of cirrhosis such as encephalopathy, fever, or renal insufficiency (**Table 160-2**). Abdominal paracentesis should not be delayed in the evaluation of patients with suspected spontaneous bacterial peritonitis (SBP) as it has been shown that mortality increases by 3.3% per hour of delay in performing paracentesis.

Complications of abdominal paracentesis are rare. The most common complication is leak of ascitic fluid, which may occur in up to 5% of patients. Leaks typically arise when a proper Z-track technique has not been used. More serious complications such as severe hemorrhage and infection have been found to occur less than 1% of the time. Death due to paracentesis is extremely rare.

The routine administration of blood products (fresh frozen plasma and/or platelets) in patients with cirrhosis is not recommended. Blood products, such as FFP and platelets, should be reserved for patients with clinically evident disseminated intravascular coagulation or clinically evident hyperfibrinolysis. Patients with hyperfibrinolysis may be treated with aminocaproic acid or intravenous tranexamic acid. In patients with disseminated intravascular coagulation, platelets, and in some cases, fresh frozen plasma may be given prior to paracentesis.

TABLE 160-2 Indications for Abdominal Paracentesis in a Patient with Ascites from Cirrhosis Admitted to the Hospital

New onset ascites
At the time of admission to the hospital
Clinical deterioration (at any time during admission)
Fever
Abdominal pain
Abdominal tenderness
Mental status change
Ileus
Hypotension
Laboratory abnormalities that may indicate infection
Peripheral leukocytosis
Acidosis
Worsening of renal function
Gastrointestinal bleeding

From Runyon BA, AASLD. Introduction to the revised American Association for the Study of Liver Diseases Practice Guideline management of adult patients with ascites due to cirrhosis 2012. *Hepatology*. 2013;57:1651.

■ ASCITIC FLUID ANALYSIS

Initial tests that should be performed on the ascitic fluid include the gross appearance of the fluid, cell count and differential, total protein concentration, and albumin concentration. Serum albumin should be obtained so that a serum-to-ascites albumin gradient determination (SAAG) can be calculated. Culture of ascitic fluid should be sent in patients admitted to the hospital with ascites as well as patients with signs of decompensation such as fever, abdominal pain, azotemia, acidosis, or confusion. Many laboratories save an aliquot of fluid in case further testing is necessary.

The gross appearance of the ascitic fluid can range from clear fluid typically seen in the setting of cirrhosis, turbid or cloudy fluid in the setting of infection, milky fluid in the setting of chylous ascites, and bloody fluid in the setting of malignancy or a traumatic paracentesis.

The SAAG is the most helpful test to identify the presence of portal hypertension. The SAAG is calculated by subtracting the ascitic fluid albumin value from the serum albumin value, obtained on the same day. The presence of a gradient ≥1.1 g/dL indicates that the patient has portal hypertension as the cause of ascites with 97% accuracy. In patients with cirrhosis and ascites, the SAAG reflects the degree of sinusoidal hypertension as it is assumed that a SAAG greater than 1.1 is equal or exceeds a sinusoidal pressure of 12 mm Hg. The SAAG is not specific to ascites due to cirrhosis, but will be elevated with any disorder that leads to portal hypertension. Patients with portal hypertension plus a second cause of ascites will also have a SAAG ≥1.1 g/dL. Importantly, the SAAG will remain accurate despite fluid infusion and diuretic use.

The cell count with differential is the most helpful test performed on ascitic fluid to evaluate for infection. It should be ordered with every paracentesis, as ascitic fluid infection is a potentially reversible cause of death in patients with cirrhosis and ascites. The sample should be sent in a tube containing an anticoagulant to avoid clotting. The white blood cell and neutrophil count need to be corrected in patients with bloody samples. To obtain corrected white blood cell and neutrophil counts one white blood cell should be subtracted for every 750 red blood cells and one neutrophil should be subtracted for every 250 red blood cells. Antibiotic treatment should be considered in any patient with a corrected neutrophil count ≥250/mm³.

TABLE 160-3 Analysis of Ascitic Fluid

Routine analysis
Total protein
Albumin
Cell count and differential
Optional tests (when there is suspicion of infection)
Culture (in blood culture bottles)
Gram stain
Glucose
Lactate dehydrogenase
Additional tests: performed as appropriate based on suspicion of underlying disease
Triglyceride (chylous ascites)
Cytology (malignant ascites)
Amylase (pancreatic ascites)
AFB culture, Adenosine deaminase, TB smear (Tuberculous peritonitis)
Unhelpful tests
pH
Lactate
Cholesterol
Fibronectin
Glycosaminoglycans

From Runyon BA, AASLD. Introduction to the revised American Association for the Study of Liver Diseases Practice Guideline management of adult patients with ascites due to cirrhosis 2012. *Hepatology*. 2013;57:1651.

In cirrhosis total ascitic fluid protein is usually low (<1 g/dL) and high (>2.5 g/dL) in most other causes of ascites. For example, both ascites from cirrhosis and cardiac ascites have a SAAG ≥1.1 g/dL, but in cirrhosis the total protein is <2.5 g/dL, whereas in cardiac ascites it is ≥2.5 g/dL.

Milky ascitic fluid may suggest lymphatic obstruction and should be tested for elevated triglyceride levels. Cytology should be ordered when there is a high pretest probability of peritoneal carcinomatosis. Patients with peritoneal carcinomatosis usually have a history of breast, colon, gastric, or pancreatic carcinoma. The cancer antigen 125 (CA 125) is nonspecific in the differential diagnosis of ascites and is not recommended. In patients at high risk for tuberculous peritonitis, it is appropriate to check an adenosine deminase level and AFB culture (**Table 160-3**).

PRACTICE POINT

- A diagnostic paracentesis should be performed in the initial evaluation of all patients with new-onset or recurrent ascites. Initial tests that should be performed on the ascitic fluid include the gross appearance of the fluid, cell count and differential, total protein concentration, and albumin concentration.

■ MANAGEMENT OF ASCITES

While there is no evidence that treatment of fluid overload in patients with cirrhosis improves survival, it has important benefits. Removing ascitic fluid volume provides important symptomatic relief to patients, including less abdominal discomfort and shortness of breath as well as improved mobility and appetite. Removal of fluid reduces the risk of cellulitis and abdominal wall hernia formation. It also concentrates ascitic fluid opsonins, which may reduce the risk of spontaneous bacterial peritonitis.

The treatment of ascites in patients with cirrhosis includes abstinence from alcohol, sodium restriction and diuretic therapy. In addition, patients with tense ascites should be treated with large-volume therapeutic paracenteses unless they have SBP, as it may precipitate renal injury. Removal of less than 5 L of fluid does not appear to have hemodynamic or hormonal consequences and is more rapid than diuretic therapy for ascitic fluid removal. For paracenteses over 5 L an albumin infusion of 6 to 8 g/L of fluid removed can be given and has been shown to have a survival advantage. The correct identification of the etiology of ascites is critical because patients with a low SAAG (<1.1 g/dL), such as ascites from peritoneal carcinomatosis, do not respond to sodium restriction and diuretic therapy.

The formation of ascitic fluid in a patient with portal hypertension is the result of avid renal retention of sodium and water. Therefore, a mainstay in the treatment of ascites is to restrict sodium intake. All patients with ascites should have sodium intake restricted to 88 mEq (2000 mg) per day. More stringent sodium restriction is not recommended because it is generally not tolerated, has poor compliance and may worsen malnutrition in patients with cirrhosis. Education about the importance of dietary sodium restriction is essential to the management of patients with portal hypertension related ascites as fluid loss and weight change are directly related to sodium balance.

Routine fluid restriction is not recommended in patients with cirrhosis and ascites. The chronic hyponatremia in patients with cirrhosis is rarely problematic and fluid restriction may worsen thirst and be uncomfortable for patients. Fluid restriction should be limited to patients with neurologic symptoms that may be due to severe hyponatremia (<120 mEq/L), which is an uncommon finding (1% in one series). The use of vaptans (vasopressin antagonists) in the treatment of severe hyponatremia in patients with cirrhosis is controversial and without clear evidence of a beneficial effect.

The majority of patients with cirrhosis and ascites will need diuretic therapy in addition to salt restriction to avoid fluid retention. The usual diuretic regimen consists of single morning doses of oral spironolactone and oral furosemide, which promote natruesis through different mechanisms. The starting doses are 100 mg of spironolactone and 40 mg of furosemide; this ratio generally maintains normokalemia. The doses of both oral diuretics can be increased every 3 to 5 days maintaining the 100 mg: 40 mg ratio to a maximum of 400 mg/d of spironolactone and 160 mg of furosemide. Diuretics should be initiated with a diuresis goal of 1 L/d. Spot urine sodium to potassium concentration greater than one indicates that a patient has effective aldosterone blockade and should respond to sodium restriction. All diuretics should be discontinued if there is severe hyponatremia (serum sodium concentration <120 mmol/L), progressive renal failure, worsening hepatic encephalopathy, or incapacitating muscle cramps. In addition, furosemide should be stopped if there is severe hypokalemia (<3 mmol/L) and aldosterone antagonists should be stopped if patients develop severe hyperkalemia (serum potassium >6 mmol/L). In hospitalized patients, diuretics should also be withheld in the setting active gastrointestinal bleeding, hepatic encephalopathy or renal dysfunction. Unlike patients with cardiac ascites, patients with cirrhotic ascites should not be treated with intravenous diuretics as this may lead to azotemia. The complete resolution of clinically apparent ascites is not a prerequisite for discharge.

Certain medications should be avoided or used with caution in patients with cirrhosis and ascites. In patients with cirrhosis arterial blood pressure independently predicts survival. Drugs that inhibit vasoconstrictors, such as angiotensin converting enzyme inhibitors and angiotensin receptor blockers should be avoided or used with caution because of the increased risk of renal impairment. Although propranolol has been shown to prevent variceal hemorrhage in patients with large varices, in patients with refractory ascites,

β-blockers may adversely affect the patient. In patients with advanced cirrhosis, the risks versus benefits must be carefully weighed in each patient. Prostaglandin inhibitors, such as nonsteroidal anti-inflammatory drugs, should be avoided in patients since they can reduce urinary sodium excretion, lead to azotemia and may precipitate upper gastrointestinal bleeding in the setting of cirrhosis. In patients with cirrhosis and ascites, aminoglycosides alone or in combination with other antibiotics should be avoided in the treatment of bacterial infections because they are associated with a high incidence of nephrotoxicity. In addition, in hospitalized patients with cirrhosis and renal failure the use of contrast media should be used with caution.

◼ REFRACTORY ASCITES

Approximately 10% of patients with ascites due to cirrhosis develop diuretic-resistant ascites, defined as refractory ascites. Refractory ascites in patients with cirrhosis is present when at least one of the following criteria is met: an inability to mobilize ascites despite confirmed adherence to the dietary sodium restriction and the administration of maximum tolerable doses of oral diuretics (400 mg/d of spironolactone and 160 mg/d of furosemide); rapid reaccumulation of fluid after therapeutic paracentesis; the development of diuretic-related complications, such as progressive azotemia, hepatic encephalopathy, or progressive electrolyte imbalances. In hospitalized patients spot urine sodium to potassium ratio is an efficient method to determine compliance and efficacy. A urine sodium greater than urine potassium with weight loss indicates the patient is diuretic responsive and adherent to the sodium restriction; a urine sodium less than urine potassium without weight loss is diuretic resistant at the current doses; a urine sodium greater than urine potassium without loss indicates that the patient is diuretic responsive, but not adherent to the sodium restriction. It is also critical to differentiate refractory ascites from causes of ascites such as malignant ascites or the Budd Chiari syndrome (hepatic vein thrombosis), which may be determined through ascitic fluid analysis and an abdominal ultrasound with Doppler.

The first step in the management of refractory ascites is to discontinue medications that decrease systemic blood pressure and lead to renal vasoconstriction, such as angiotensin converting enzyme inhibitors, angiotensin receptor II blockers, and nonsteroidal anti-inflammatory drugs. Although many patients with cirrhosis are on β-blockers, such as propranolol, to decrease the risk of variceal bleeding, the risks versus benefits of β-blockers must be weighed carefully in each patient. β-Blockers should be discontinued in patients with refractory ascites if the systemic blood pressure is less than 90 mm Hg, if hyponatremia (<130 mEq/L) is present, or if there is acute kidney injury. Oral midodrine, an oral vasopressor, which often increases blood pressure in advanced cirrhosis, may theoretically convert diuretic-resistant patients back to diuretic sensitive. Midodrine may be started at 5 mg orally three times daily with the dose adjusted by 2.5 mg every 24 hours up to a maximal dose of 17.5 mg to achieve a mean arterial pressure greater than 82 mm Hg.

Therapeutic options for patients who fail noninvasive treatments include serial therapeutic large-volume paracenteses (LVPs), transjugular intrahepatic portosystemic shunt, and liver transplantation. Liver transplantation is primarily based on the patient's MELD (model for end stage liver disease) score but should not be delayed in patients with refractory ascites as 21% of patients with refractory ascites die within 6 months. Serial paracenteses of 4 to 6 L per session may be effective for symptomatic relief. The use of albumin replacement in LVP to prevent circulatory dysfunction after paracenteses is controversial. Based on the available data, for paracenteses larger than 5 L, albumin (6-8 g/L of fluid removed) may be administered either during or immediately after the procedure.

Transjugular intrahepatic portosystemic stent-shunt (TIPS) reduces portal hypertension and decreases the development of cirrhotic ascites. There is increasing evidence that TIPS is more effective than large-volume paracentesis in controlling ascites and may be associated with a survival advantage. As an invasive procedure, TIPS should only be considered in carefully selected patients with diuretic-resistant ascites intolerant of repeated large-volume paracentesis or patients requiring very frequent paracentesis (eg, weekly). Patients with refractory ascites who are not good candidates for TIPS include those with Child-Pugh class C cirrhosis, a high MELD score (>18), alcoholic hepatitis, congestive heart failure, a history of severe, spontaneous hepatic encephalopathy or the absence of a caregiver in the home. Echocardiograms are typically performed to screen for heart failure prior to TIPS placement. Patients with cirrhosis and ascites usually have ejection fractions of 70% to 75% due to hyperdynamic circulation. A baseline ejection fraction of 60% is a usual minimum cutoff prior to TIPS because central pressure usually increases after TIPS and cardiac function can deteriorate.

HEPATIC HYDROTHORAX

Hepatic hydrothorax is defined as the presence of a pleural effusion in a patient with cirrhosis and ascites in the absence of other causes. Hepatic hydrothorax occurs in approximately 5% to 10% of patients with cirrhosis and ascites. The development of hepatic hydrothorax results from the passage of ascites from the peritoneal cavity into the pleural cavity through small diaphragmatic defects during the negative intrathoracic pressure generated during inspiration. The right hemidiaphragm is more susceptible to diaphragmatic defects and hepatic hydrothorax develops on the right side in approximately 73% to 85% of patients. Hepatic hydrothorax usually presents with dyspnea, a nonproductive cough, pleuritic chest pain, and hypoxemia. Patients with suspected hepatic hydrothorax should undergo thoracentesis with testing of the pleural fluid as well as additional imaging including a chest computed tomographic scan and echocardiogram to confirm the diagnosis and exclude other causes of the effusion. Pleural effusions from hepatic hydrothorax are transudative in nature; however, the protein concentration of the pleural fluid is usually higher than that of ascitic fluid due to the differences in hydrostatic forces between the abdomen and chest. If the diagnosis is uncertain, an intraperitoneal injection of technetium-radiolabeled sulfur colloid into the abdomen can be performed shortly after therapeutic thoracentesis to detect rapid passage of isotope into the chest cavity during reaccumulation.

Patients who are severely symptomatic from a large effusion should undergo a therapeutic thoracentesis. Usually no more than 2 L of fluid are removed because of the risk of pulmonary edema and hypotension. After thoracentesis, patients should be on a sodium restricted diet (<88 mEq or 2000 mg daily) and diuretics to prevent reaccumulation of fluid. Chest tubes are contraindicated in the treatment of hepatic hydrothorax as they can result in massive protein and electrolyte depletion, infection, renal failure, and bleeding, and may result in rapid deterioration or death. Spontaneous bacterial empyema (SBEM), is defined as the lack of evidence of pneumonia on chest imaging study and a positive pleural fluid culture and a polymorphonuclear leukocyte count (PMN) cell count >250 cells/mm³ or negative pleural fluid culture and a PMN cell count >500 cells/mm³. Spontaneous bacterial empyema has been reported in 13% to 16% of patients with hepatic hydrothorax. Spontaneous bacterial empyema should be treated with intravenous antibiotics used for SBP (eg, ceftriaxone 2 g every 24 hours) and may be tailored based on culture results. A repeat thoracentesis may be performed to document a patient's response to treatment.

Patients with refractory hydrothorax, defined as a persistent hydrothorax despite a sodium-restricted diet and diuretic therapy, may initially be managed with repeated thoracentesis every 2 to 3 weeks for symptom control. Transjugular intrahepatic portosystemic shunt is the second line treatment and may be recommended in patients with a Child-Pugh score <13 who are younger than 70 years old and do not have clinically significant hepatic encephalopathy. Pleurodesis or thorascopic repair of the diaphragmatic defects are technically difficult and have had variable results, but may be considered in patients with no other therapeutic options. Liver transplantation is the definitive treatment for appropriate candidates.

SPONTANEOUS BACTERIAL PERITONITIS (SBP)

Spontaneous bacterial peritonitis is defined by the presence of an elevated ascitic fluid absolute polymorphonuclear leukocyte count (PMN) count (>250 cells /mm³) or a positive culture without an evident intra-abdominal, surgically treatable source of infection. Spontaneous bacterial peritonitis often presents with fever, abdominal pain, or altered mental status, but patients can also be asymptomatic. A diagnostic paracentesis must be performed to diagnose or exclude SBP. Therefore, all patients hospitalized with ascites should undergo a diagnostic paracentesis. Patients should have a repeat paracentesis during their hospitalization if they develop clinical signs or symptoms suggesting infection. The paracentesis should be performed prior to the administration of any antibiotics. A single dose of a broad-spectrum antibiotic may inhibit culture growth in 86% of patients. Most cases of SBP have a single organism due to gut bacteria such as *E. coli* and *Klebsiella*, though streptococcal and staphylococcal infections may also occur. A positive ascitic fluid culture is not necessary for the diagnosis of SBP and culture negative, neutrophil positive ascites occurs commonly (15%-50%). Findings suggestive of a secondary peritonitis, such as perforated viscus, diverticulitis, or intra-abdominal abscess, include polymicrobial infection, anaerobes, high protein concentration (>1 g/dL), low glucose (<50 mg/dL) or high LDH (> serum upper limit of normal). Patients with secondary bacterial peritonitis should undergo abdominal computed tomography (CT) scanning and surgical evaluation as indicated.

Broad-spectrum therapy is warranted in patients with suspected SBP until the results of sensitivity testing has returned. The infection-related mortality from SBP in the absence of renal failure or shock is low, but up to 82% in patients with cirrhosis and SBP-associated septic shock. Antibiotics should be initiated immediately after diagnostic paracentesis, especially for patients who have developed septic shock. One series showed an adjusted odds ratio for mortality of 1.9 for every hour delay in administrating antimicrobial therapy. β-Blockers use among patients with SBP has been associated with increased risk of the hepatorenal syndrome and a probable increased mortality. Therefore, β-blockers should be discontinued in a hospitalized patient with SBP.

Uncomplicated SBP should be treated with a third-generation cephalosporin, such as cefotaxime. Intravenous cefotaxime 2 g every 8 hours produces excellent ascitic fluid penetration. Lower doses can be used in patients with impaired renal function. The main adverse drug reaction of cefotaxime is rash, which occurs in approximately 1% of patients. Levofloxacin may be used for patients with a penicillin allergy, although it has less penetration into ascitic fluid than cefotaxime. Oral ofloxacin (400 mg twice per day) may also be considered for SBP treatment in patients without shock, vomiting, or a serum creatinine greater than 3 mg/dL. Fluoroquinolones, however, should not be used in a patient who had been receiving a fluoroquinolone for SBP prophylaxis as resistance to the antibiotic may have developed. The choice of antibiotics for treating SBP should also take into account local resistance patterns and recent antibiotic use. Nephrotoxic antibiotics should be avoided because the underperfused kidneys in cirrhosis are very sensitive to injury.

PRACTICE POINT

- In patients suspected of having SBP antibiotics should be initiated immediately after diagnostic paracentesis. First line therapy is typically with a third-generation cephalosporin, but the choice of antibiotics for treating SBP should also take into account local resistance patterns and recent antibiotic use.

In most patien.ts, including those who are bacteremic, 5 days of therapy is usually sufficient and antibiotics can be discontinued without a routine repeat paracentesis if the patient has clinically improved. However, if after 5 days of therapy, fever or pain persists, paracentesis is repeated, and the decision to continue or discontinue antibiotics is determined by the PMN response. If the PMN count is <250 cells/mm³, treatment is stopped; if the PMN count is elevated, but less than the pretreatment value, antibiotics are continued for another 48 hours, and paracentesis is repeated. If the PMN count is greater than the pretreatment value, a search for secondary bacterial peritonitis is initiated. Only patients who grow an unusual organism (eg, pseudomonas), an organism resistant to standard antibiotic therapy, or an organism routinely associated with endocarditis (eg, Staphylococcus aureus or viridans group streptococci) are initially considered for longer treatment.

Renal failure develops in 30% to 40% of patients with SBP and is a major cause of death. This risk may be reduced with an infusion of intravenous albumin (1.5 g/kg body weight within 6 hours of diagnosis and 1.0 g/kg on day 3). Albumin infusion should be given if the creatinine is >1 mg/dL, the blood urea nitrogen is >30 mg/dL, or if the total bilirubin is >4 mg/dL.

It is reasonable to give empiric therapy to patients with alcoholic hepatitis who present with fever and/or leukocytosis, but have a PMN count <250 cells/mm³. Empiric therapy can be discontinued after 48 hours if ascitic fluid, blood, and urine cultures remain negative.

Recurrence of SBP has been reported to be 69% in 1 year. Risk factors for the development of SBP include ascitic fluid protein concentration <1.0, variceal hemorrhage, or a prior episode of SBP. The use of antibiotic prophylaxis for patients at high risk for SBP decreases the risk of bacterial infection and mortality. However, the use of antibiotic prophylaxis does select for resistant flora, which can result in recurrent infection. Therefore, antibiotic prophylaxis should be limited to patients with strict indications. These include an ascitic fluid total protein less than 1.5 g/dL with impaired renal function (creatinine ≥1.2, BUN ≥25 or serum Na ≤130) or liver failure (Child score ≥9 and bilirubin ≥3), patients with a previous episode of SBP, or in patients with cirrhosis and gastrointestinal bleeding. The antibiotic regimen used for SBP prophylaxis depends on the indication. For patients with an ascitic fluid total protein less than 1.5 g/dL and with impaired renal function (creatinine ≥1.2, BUN ≥25 or serum Na ≤130) or liver failure (Child score ≥9 and bilirubin ≥3) or patients with a previous episode of SBP, prolonged therapy with norfloxacin 400 mg/d, orally, is preferred. Ciprofloxacin 750 mg/wk or trimethoprim-sulfamethoxazole (800 mg sulfamethoxazole and 160 mg trimethoprim, daily, orally) are acceptable alternatives if norfloxacin is not tolerated. In patients with cirrhosis and gastrointestinal bleeding, intravenous ceftriaxone 1 g daily is initiated and can be switched to oral norfloxacin (400 mg orally twice daily) for a total course of 7 days once bleeding has been controlled and the patient is stable.

In addition to antibiotic prophylaxis, general measures may be taken to prevent SBP in hospitalized patients with cirrhosis and ascites. The early recognition and aggressive treatment of localized infections (eg, cystitis and cellulitis) as well as the judicious use of urinary catheters can prevent bacteremia and SBP. Diuretic therapy, if not contraindicated, concentrates ascitic fluid and raises opsonic activity, which may help prevent SBP. Protein pump inhibitors have been associated with an increased risk of SBP and should be restricted to patients with a clear indication for their use (**Figure 160-3**).

HEPATORENAL SYNDROME

The hepatorenal syndrome is defined as the occurrence of renal failure in a patient with cirrhosis and ascites in the absence of other causes of renal failure, shock or hypovolemia. Hypovolemia is excluded by the absence of response defined as no sustained improvement of renal function (creatinine decreasing to <133 µmol/L) following at least 2 days of volume expansion with intravenous albumin (1 g/kg of body weight per day up to 100 g/d) and/or the discontinuation of diuretics. Other apparent causes for acute kidney injury should be excluded including current or recent treatment with nephrotoxic drugs, and the ultrasonographic evidence of obstruction or parenchymal disease. A kidney biopsy is often helpful in excluding pre-existing renal disease, especially if liver transplantation is being considered. The diagnosis is based on an increase in serum creatinine of 0.3 mg/dL or more within 48 hours, or an increase from baseline of 50% or more within 7 days. In hospitalized patients, repeat measurements of creatinine are helpful in the early diagnosis of hepatic renal syndrome (HRS). Additional clinical criteria include urine red cell excretion of less than 50 cells per high power field (in the absence of a urinary catheter) and protein excretion less than 500 mg/d The hepatorenal syndrome occurs in approximately 20% of patients with cirrhosis and ascites at 1 year and up to 40% at 5 years and is associated with a high mortality rate. There are two forms of hepatorenal syndrome based on the rate of decline in renal function. Type 1 hepatorenal syndrome is the more serious form and is defined as at least a twofold increase in serum creatinine to a level greater than 2.5 mg/dL during a period of less than 2 weeks. Precipitating conditions include infection, especially SBP, and severe alcoholic hepatitis. The median survival for untreated type 1 HRS is 1 month. The early diagnosis and treatment of infection can reduce the risk of HRS and is associated with an improved survival. Type 2 hepatorenal syndrome is defined as renal impairment that is less severe than in patients with the type 1 form. It is important to note that diuretics do not cause hepatorenal syndrome but can lead to diuretic-induced azotemia, which improves with the cessation of therapy and fluid repletion. Patients with relative adrenal insufficiency have greater impairment of circulatory and renal function and a higher probability of type 1 HRS and severe sepsis when compared to patients with decompensated cirrhosis but normal adrenal function.

■ TREATMENT OF HRS

The goal of medical therapy is to improve renal function by reversing portal hypertension induced arterial vasodilation in the splanchnic circulation. In patients with HRS who are admitted to the intensive care unit, careful monitoring of urine output, fluid balance, arterial pressure and vital signs is imperative. Initially, all diuretics should be discontinued. In patients with tense ascites, paracentesis may be helpful in alleviating abdominal discomfort.

Medical therapy is aimed at improving the severely impaired circulatory function by inducing vasoconstriction of the dilated vascular bed and increasing arterial pressure. Based on results of many randomized controlled trials, the use of vasoconstrictive drugs, especially terlipressin, has been associated with improvement in up to 50% of patients. Terlipressin in combination with albumin is the treatment of choice. Terlipressin is given as an intravenous bolus of 1 to 2 mg every 4 to 6 hours, and albumin is given for 2 days as an intravenous bolus of 1 g/kg/d (100 g maximum), followed by 25 to 50 g/d until

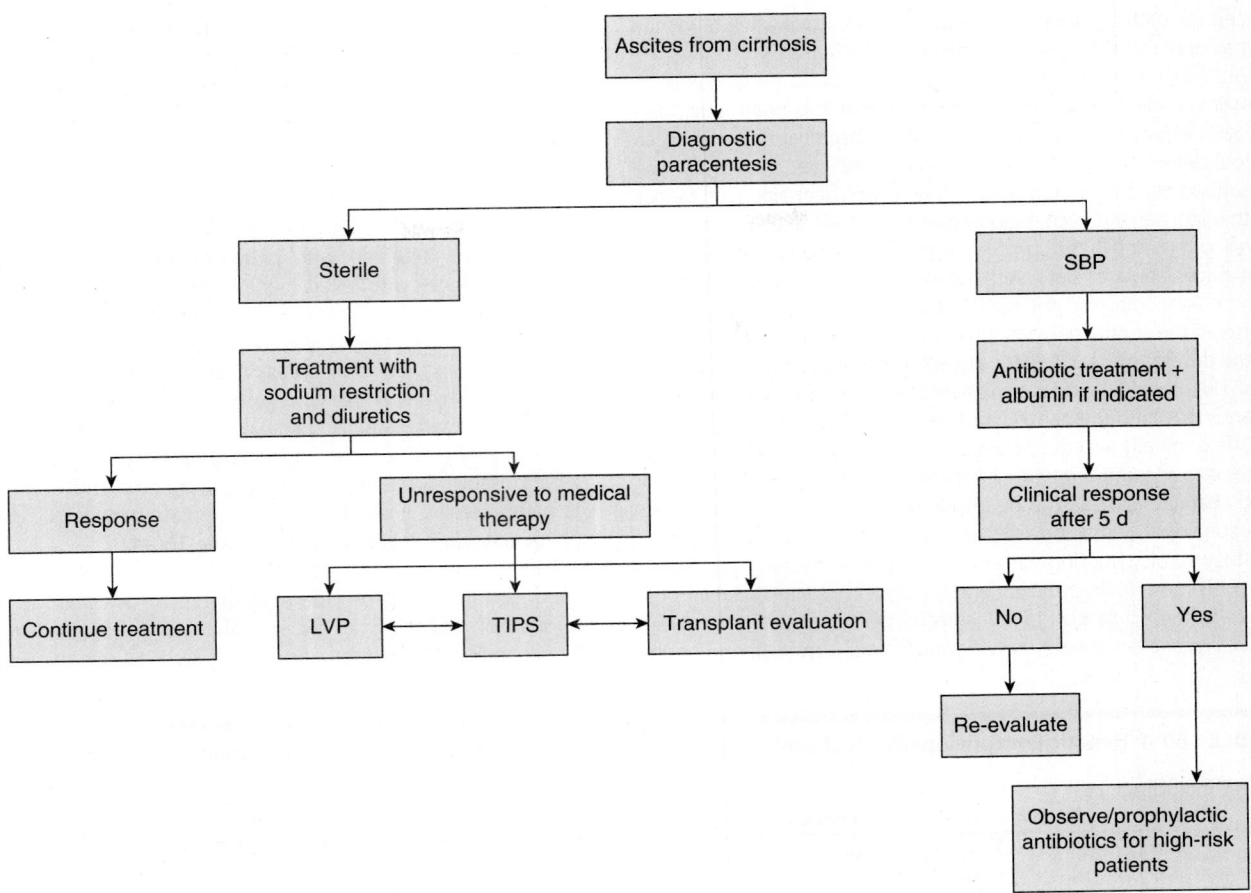

Figure 160-3 Approach to management of ascites.

terlipressin therapy is discontinued. Contraindications to terlipressin therapy include ischemic cardiovascular diseases. Patients treated with terlipressin should be carefully monitored for development of cardiac arrhythmias or signs of splanchnic or digital ischemia. Terlipressin is currently unavailable in the United States. Alternative treatments include noradrenaline and midodrine, a selective alpha-1 adrenergic agonist, plus octreotide, a somatostatin analog, in addition to albumin infusion. Midodrine is given orally at a starting dose 7.5 mg three times daily, uptitrated to 15 mg three times per day. The midodrine dose should be uptitrated with each consecutive dose to raise the mean arterial pressure by approximately 10 to 15 mm Hg. Octreotide is either given as a continuous intravenous infusion of 50 µg/h or subcutaneously 100 to 200 mg three times daily. Albumin is given for 2 days as an intravenous bolus of 1 g/kg (100 g maximum), followed by 25 to 50 g/d until midodrine and octreotide therapy is discontinued. Norepinephrine is administered as a continuous infusion (0.5-3 mg/h) with the goal of raising the mean arterial pressure by 10 to 15 mm Hg.

Patients treated with norepinephrine, terlipressin, or octreotide are typically treated for 2 weeks. The duration may be extended, however, if after 2 weeks there is some, but not complete improvement in renal function. In patients who respond to therapy, treatment with oral midodrine to maintain higher mean arterial pressure can be continued at discharge until resolution of liver injury or liver transplantation in appropriate candidates. If a patient has no improvement in renal function after 2 weeks then medical therapy is discontinued as the outcome is usually futile. In a recent study, patients with type 1 HRS associated with infection, HRS was not reversible despite treatment with vasoconstrictive drugs in two thirds of patients. Therefore, these patients must be treated immediately with antibiotics if there is suspicion of infection.

Options for patients who fail to respond to medical therapy include TIPS and hemodialysis. The use of TIPS in patients with hepatorenal syndrome may provide short-term benefit in selected patients but data to its applicability is very limited and many of these patients have contraindications to TIPS placement. Given the risks associated with the procedure, TIPS should be limited to patients who are well enough to tolerate the procedure and are awaiting liver transplantation. In patients who fail medical therapy and are not considered candidates for TIPS, hemodialysis or continuous venous hemofiltration can be considered as treatment for severe metabolic abnormalities such as metabolic acidosis and hyperkalemia but there is very limited data as to their efficacy. Studies are currently underway investigating artificial liver support systems in the management of HRS. In appropriate candidates, liver transplantation is the treatment of choice for both type 1 and type 2 HRS, with survival rates of approximately 65% in type 1 HRS.

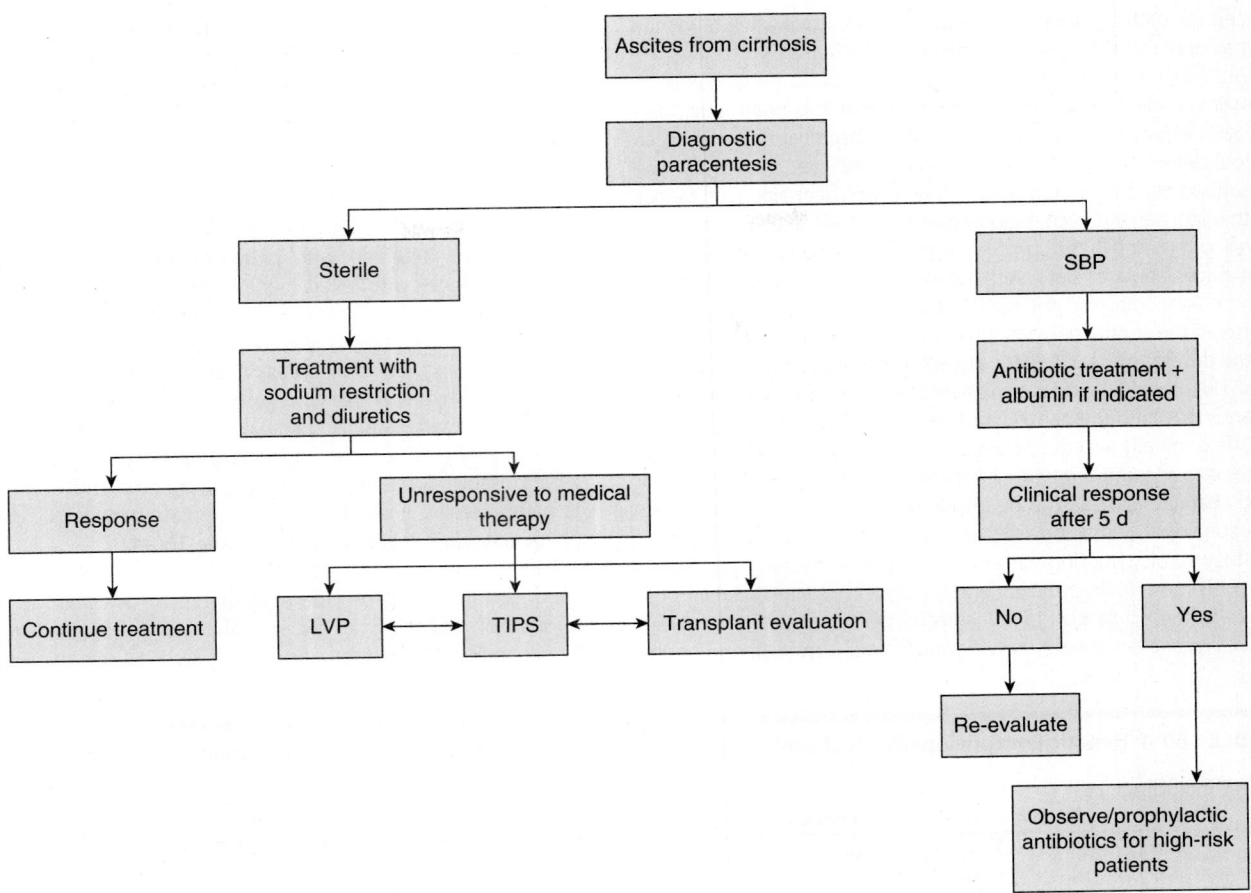

PRACTICE POINT

● Because of the poor prognosis in patients with type 1 hepatic renal syndrome, urgent evaluation is mandatory and treatment should be initiated as soon as possible.

■ HEPATIC ENCEPHALOPATHY

Hepatic encephalopathy represents a spectrum of neuropsychiatric disturbances in patients with impaired hepatic function. In patients with cirrhosis, overt hepatic encephalopathy develops in 30% to 45% of patients. Neuropsychiatric findings range from subtle abnormalities that are not apparent without specialized testing to overt coma. Important factors that determine the severity of hepatic encephalopathy include level of consciousness, cognitive function, behavioral disturbances, and neuromuscular features.

Although the exact pathogenesis of hepatic encephalopathy remains unclear, most theories suggest that the brain is exposed to toxic substances that are produced by bacterial flora, which are incompletely cleared by the compromised liver. The most well described neurotoxic substance is ammonia. The majority of patients with overt hepatic encephalopathy will have elevated arterial blood levels of ammonia, though the degree of ammonia elevation does not necessarily correlate with degree of hepatic encephalopathy. Gamma-aminobutyric acid (GABA), the primary inhibitory neurotransmitter in the central nervous system, may also play an important role in the development of hepatic encephalopathy. It has been theorized that gut bacteria produce increased endogenous benzodiazepine ligands that bind the benzodiazepine site of GABA receptors.

The generally accepted classification for hepatic encephalopathy takes into account the type of hepatic abnormality and the duration and characteristics of the neuropsychiatric manifestations. Hepatic encephalopathy may be associated with acute liver failure (type A), portosystemic shunting without intrinsic liver disease (type B), and cirrhosis (type C). Hepatic encephalopathy associated with cirrhosis is characterized as episodic, recurrent, persistent, or minimal. Episodic hepatic encephalopathy develops over a short period of time and is further classified based on whether it was precipitated or has developed spontaneously. Recurrent encephalopathy is defined as bouts of hepatic encephalopathy that occur within a time interval of 6 months or less. Patients with persistent encephalopathy exhibit continuous overt neurologic or behavioral abnormalities, which are interspersed with episodes of overt hepatic encephalopathy. Patients with minimal hepatic encephalopathy often appear asymptomatic and have subtle neuropsychiatric abnormalities that may only be detected with psychomotor or electrophysiologic testing. Patients with overt hepatic encephalopathy have signs and symptoms that can be detected clinically. The severity of overt hepatic encephalopathy is graded from I to IV. Grade I: patients have changes in behavior, mild confusion, slurred speech, and disordered sleep (both hypersomnia and insomnia); Grade II: patients have increasing lethargy and moderate confusion; Grade III: patients have marked confusion (stupor), incoherent speech, and often sleeping yet arousable; Grade IV: patients are in a coma and unresponsive to pain. In reality, it is difficult to differentiate between Grade II and Grade III hepatic encephalopathy (**Table 160-4**).

Patients with mild hepatic encephalopathy (Grade I) may be managed as outpatients, provided caregivers are available to monitor for signs of worsening hepatic encephalopathy. Patients with Grade II encephalopathy may be admitted to hospital depending on the

TABLE 160-4 Hepatic Encephalopathy in Chronic Liver Disease 2014 Practice Guideline WHC and Clinical Description

WHC Including MHE	ISHEN	Description	Suggested Operative Criteria	Comment
Unimpaired		No encephalopathy at all, no history of HE	Tested and proved to be normal	
Minimal		Psychometric or neuropsychological alterations of tests exploring psychomotor speed/executive functions or neurophysiological alterations without clinical evidence of mental change	Abnormal results of established psychometric or neuropsychological tests without clinical manifestations	No universal criteria for diagnosis Local standards and expertise required
Grade I	Covert	• Trivial lack of awareness • Euphoria or anxiety • Shortened attention span • Impairment of addition or subtraction • Altered sleep rhythm	Despite oriented in time and space (see below), the patient appears to have some cognitive/behavioral decay with respect to his or her standard on clinical examination or to the caregivers	Clinical findings usually not reproducible
Grade II		• Lethargy or apathy • Disorientation for time • Obvious personality change • Inappropriate behavior • Dyspraxia • Asterixis	Disoriented for time (at least three of the following are wrong: day of the month, day of the week, month, season, or year) ± the other mentioned symptoms	Clinical findings variable, but reproducible to some extent
Grade III	Overt	• Somnolence to semistupor • Responsive to stimuli • Confused • Gross disorientation • Bizarre behavior	Disoriented also for space (at least three of the following wrongly reported: country, state [or region], city, or place) ± the other mentioned symptoms	Clinical findings reproducible to some extent
Grade IV		Coma	Does not respond even to painful stimuli	Comatose state usually reproducible

All conditions are required to be related to liver insufficiency and/or PSS.
From Vilstrup H, Amodio P, Bajaj J, et al. Hepatic encephalopathy in chronic liver disease: 2014 Practice Guideline by the American Association for the Study of Liver Diseases and the European Association for the Study of the Liver. *Hepatology.* 2014;60:715.

degree of lethargy and confusion. Patients with more severe hepatic encephalopathy (Grades III and IV) require hospital admission for treatment, typically in an intensive care unit as they may require intubation for airway protection.

The diagnosis of hepatic encephalopathy is largely clinical. There are no specific signs, symptoms, laboratory, or imaging tests diagnostic of hepatic encephalopathy. Therefore, it is critical to rule out other etiologies of altered mental status, such as hypoglycemia, intracranial pathology, or uremia. The history should focus on changes in mental status, including subtle changes, such as changes in sleep patterns, and impaired work or driving performance. The physical examination should look for signs of chronic liver disease and neuromuscular impairment, which include bradykinesia, hyperreflexia, rigidity, myoclonus, and asterixis. Focal neurologic deficits such as hemiplegia, hemiparesis, and seizures are not commonly observed in patients with hepatic encephalopathy and warrant further central nervous system evaluation. Although elevated arterial blood levels of ammonia are commonly seen in hepatic encephalopathy, their diagnostic value remains controversial. Ordering of ammonia levels can be helpful, however, to determine the likelihood of hepatic encephalopathy in patients where another etiology for encephalopathy is reasonably likely. In patients whom minimal encephalopathy is suspected, psychometric testing, such as the number connection test (Reitan Test), can be helpful. The NCT is a timed connect-the-numbers test. Patients without hepatic encephalopathy should finish the test in a number of seconds less than or equal to their age in years (eg, a 40-year-old patient should finish the test in 40 seconds). Electroencephalogram testing in patients with overt hepatic encephalopathy is always abnormal, but the observed changes are not specific.

Common precipitating factors in patients with episodic hepatic encephalopathy associated with cirrhosis include gastrointestinal bleeding, infection, azotemia, hypokalemia, acute hepatitis, and sedative and diuretic drug side effects. It is critical to identify and treat any possible precipitating factors as this will often result in resolution or improvement of hepatic encephalopathy.

Gastrointestinal bleeding is the most common precipitant of episodic hepatic encephalopathy in patients with cirrhosis as a result of decreased hepatic perfusion and increased production of nitrogenous byproducts from the digestion of blood proteins. The most common infection that triggers hepatic encephalopathy in hospitalized patients is SBP. Therefore, all patients with hepatic encephalopathy and ascites should undergo a diagnostic paracentesis. If there is a high index of suspicion for infection, antibiotics should be initiated after cultures are drawn. Intravascular volume depletion results in reduced renal perfusion and increased ammonia production. Hypokalemic alkalosis also results in increased renal ammonia production. Common medications that can precipitate hepatic encephalopathy include sedatives and analgesics, especially benzodiazepines (**Table 160-5**).

In addition to correcting precipitating factors, patients admitted to the hospital with acute, overt hepatic encephalopathy, should be treated with pharmacologic therapy to lower the blood ammonia concentration. Initial therapy is with the nonabsorbable disaccharides, lactulose or lactitol (not available in the United States). These medications theoretically increase ammonia clearance through catharsis as well as decreasing intestinal ammonia through the lowering of the colonic pH, favoring the formation of nonabsorbable NH_4^+ from NH_3 and trapping NH_4^+ in the colon. Although there is limited evidence from large randomized controlled trials showing their efficacy, patients often show improvement in symptoms within hours of lactulose administration. The dose of medication should be titrated to achieve two to three soft stools per day. Typically, lactulose is given as 30 to 45 mL (20-30 g) two to four times per day. An equivalent dose of lactitol is approximately 67 to 100 g lactitol powder diluted in 100 mL of water. Lactulose and lactitol can also be given as enema in patients who are unable to take them

TABLE 160-5 Common Precipitants of Hepatic Encephalopathy

Drug side effects
- Benzodiazepines
- Narcotics
- Alcohol

Increased ammonia production, absorption or entry into the brain
- Gastrointestinal bleeding
- Infection
- Electrolyte disturbances such as hypokalemia
- Constipation
- Metabolic alkalosis
- Excess dietary intake of protein

Dehydration
- Vomiting, diarrhea, hemorrhage
- Diuretics
- Large volume paracentesis

Vascular occlusion
- Hepatic vein thrombosis
- Portal vein thrombosis

Portosystemic shunting

orally. Treatment is usually well tolerated and the main side effects are abdominal cramping, diarrhea, and flatulence.

Orally administered poorly absorbed antibiotics likely improve hepatic encephalopathy by decreasing toxin production by gut flora. For patients who have not improved within 48 hours of starting lactulose or lactitol, or who cannot take lactulose or lactitol, rifaximin is the nonabsorbable antibiotic of choice for treating hepatic encephalopathy. Rifaximin is a derivative of rifamycin and has broad-spectrum activity against Gram negative-rods and Gram-positive cocci. The dose of rifaximin is 550 mg orally twice daily or 400 mg three times daily. The cost of rifaximin ($1-2000 per month) may limit its use. Neomycin, an aminoglycoside, had been used in the past, but should be avoided due to the risk of ototoxicity and renal failure. Other antibiotics, such as vancomycin and flagyl have been shown to be effective in treating hepatic encephalopathy in limited trials, but are not used commonly given the risk of neuropathy with flagyl and concerns about bacterial resistance.

Other therapies that enhance ammonia clearance include sodium benzoate, and L-ornithine L-asparate (LOLA). Sodium benzoate reduces ammonia levels by reacting with glycine to form hippurate, which is excreted by the kidneys. A recent RCT found that 5 gm twice daily resulted in improvement in encephalopathy similar to that seen with lactulose. L-ornithine L-asparate increases hepatic conversion of ammonia and has been shown to perform better than placebo at lowering plasma ammonia as well improving the hepatic encephalopathy grade. Flumazenil, a benzodiazepine receptor antagonist, has been shown to improve the hepatic encephalopathy grade, but data are conflicting and it should not be used as routine therapy. Oral branched-chain amino acids, which are available in several different formulations, improve symptoms in patients who are protein-intolerant, and can be used in patients who do not respond to lactulose, lactitol, or rifaxmin and who are severely protein-intolerant. Probiotics reduce substrate for other gut bacteria and have been shown to reduce ammonia levels and improve psychometric hepatic encephalopathy scores.

Patients hospitalized with hepatic encephalopathy may be agitated and may be a hazard to themselves or caretakers and require physical use of restraints. It is important to remember that patients with advanced liver disease are more prone to oversedation, particularly with the use of benzodiazepines. If pharmacologic treatment is needed, haloperidol is a safer option.

High dietary protein intake may be associated with hepatic encephalopathy. In theory, dietary protein results in increased nitrogenous toxin production in the gut. However, while dietary protein restriction may improve symptoms in some patients, its efficacy has been difficult to establish in randomized controlled trials. Moreover, patients with cirrhosis are often malnourished and protein restriction is associated with increased mortality. Therefore, routine protein restriction is not recommended. Nutritional support should include maintaining an energy of 35 to 40 kcal/kg/d with a protein intake of 1.2 to 1.5 g/kg/d.

Patients with recurrent hepatic encephalopathy that has resolved during admission should be continued on lactulose, lactitol, and/or rifaximin at time of discharge. Prior to discharge patients admitted with overt hepatic encephalopathy should have an assessment regarding driving risk. It is also critical to determine if patients admitted with hepatic encephalopathy have an adequate outpatient support system.

ACUTE-ON-CHRONIC LIVER FAILURE

Acute-on-chronic liver failure (ACLF) is a recently recognized syndrome characterized by acute decompensation of cirrhosis and organ/system failure and is associated with a high-short-term mortality (estimated 28-day mortality rate of 23%-74% depending on the number of organ failures). Acute decompensation refers to the development of ascites, encephalopathy, gastrointestinal hemorrhage and/or bacterial infections. Acute decompensation develops in many cirrhotic patients in the absence of any other significant feature, but its development in association with organ failure with high mortality rates led to the recognition of acute-on-chronic liver failure as a distinct clinical entity. The prevalence of acute-on-chronic liver failure in patients hospitalized with acute decompensation is 30%.

In a large multicenter European study by Yiu et al involving 392 patients, acute decompensation and a single entity for liver failure and no evidence of acute kidney failure or hepatic encephalopathy, the short-term mortality was very low. However, if there was evidence of organ failure, especially acute kidney failure or bacterial infection, the mortality rate was 15 times higher than patients with uncomplicated acute decompensation (**Table 160-6**). Interestingly, ACLF occurred in half of the patients in whom there was no prior history of AD or in whom AD developed within a few weeks of hospitalization. Acute-on-chronic liver failure patients were younger (<55 years), often had alcoholic cirrhosis and were less likely to have hepatitis C as the cause of cirrhosis. Common precipitating events were bacterial infection or active alcoholism. Half of the patients had kidney injury as the primary organ failure. Predictors of ACLF and ACLF related mortality were a high leukocyte count and a prior history of AD although, somewhat surprisingly, patients without a prior history of AD had a more severe form of ACLF and a higher mortality.

Acute-on-chronic liver failure may develop at any time during the course of the disease in a patient from compensated cirrhosis to a patient with long-standing cirrhosis and history of acute decompensation. The severity of acute-on-chronic liver failure correlates with the number of organ failures. The development of acute-on-chronic liver failure occurs in the setting of a systemic inflammation although in 40% of cases no precipitating event can be identified. While the pathophysiology of acute-on-chronic liver failure is not well understood, it is thought that systemic inflammation may cause acute-on-chronic liver failure through complex mechanisms that include an

TABLE 160-6 Etiology of Precipitating Events for All Diagnosed ACLF Patients

Items	Frequency
With hepatic insults (N = 180)	
Hepatic insults alone	
Flare-up or exacerbation of HBV, no. (%)	145 (35.8)
Superimposed HAV or HEV infection, no. (5)	26 (6.4)
Hepatotoxic drugs, no. (%)	10 (2.5)
Active drinking, no. (%)	25 (6.2)
Flare-up of AIH or Wilson's disease, no. (%)	6 (1.5)
More than one hepatic insult, no. (%)	28 (6.9)
Mixed with extrahepatic insults	
Bacterial infection, no. (%)	28 (6.9)
UGIB, no. (%)	4 (1.0)
Extrahepatic insults alone (N = 142)	
Bacterial infection, no. (%)	113 (27.9)
UGIB, no. (%)	36 (8.9)
Surgery, no. (%)	1 (0.2)
More than one extrahepatic insult, no. (%)	8 (2.0)
Unknown (N = 83)	83 (20.5)

Data are expressed as number (percent).
Abbreviation: AIH, autoimmune hepatitis.
From Shi Yu, Yang Ying, Hu Yaoren, et al. Acute on chronic liver failure precipitated by hepatic injury is distinct from that precipitated by extrahepatic insults. *Hepatology*. 2015;62:232.

exaggerated inflammatory response and systemic oxidative stress to pathogen and/or alteration of tissue homeostasis to inflammation caused either by the pathogen itself or through dysfunction of tissue tolerance. Patients with acute-on-chronic liver failure have high leukocyte count and plasma-C reactive protein concentrations.

To further clarify the definition of ACLF, a division into three categories has been proposed by Jalen et al. which takes into account whether or not there is underlying cirrhosis, and whether there is a history of previous decompensation in patients with cirrhosis. Type A ACLF refers to noncirrhotic ACLF and includes as examples, patients with reactivation of hepatitis B, hepatitis A or hepatitis E, infection superimposed upon chronic hepatitis B, autoimmune hepatitis or patients with fatty liver and superimposed drug-induced liver injury. Type B ACLF is seen in patients with compensated cirrhosis who deteriorate rapidly after a major insult such as acute viral, drug or alcoholic hepatitis, infection or surgery. Type C ACLF refers to patients with a prior episode of decompensation and an acute precipitating event.

Various prognostic scores have been proposed to aid in the recognition, stratification, and management of patients with acute-on-chronic liver failure depending on whether the patient has hepatic or extrahepatic ACLF. Hepatic ACLF is precipitated by primarily hepatic insults while extrahepatic ACLF is exclusively precipitated by extrahepatic insults. The MELD score may be a better predictor for hepatic ACLF while the CLIF-SOFA score, which includes measurements of six organ systems including respiratory cardiovascular, renal, neurologic, liver and coagulation, appears to be more useful for extrahepatic organ failure. The EASL-Chronic Liver Failure consortium has recently proposed an algorithm using prognosis scores to aid in the management of patients with, or at risk for the development of, ACLF.

The general management of acute-on-chronic liver failure includes early identification and treatment of potential triggers and supportive care. Patients with acute-on-chronic liver failure should be managed in an intensive care unit for frequent monitoring and treatment of organ failure. Although not all patients with acute-on-chronic liver failure are transplant candidates, those that are should be transferred to a liver transplant center. Although data are limited, the 1-year survival after liver transplant is approximately 80%. Current therapies being explored further are extracorporeal liver support systems, bioartificial support, and stem cell therapy.

CONCLUSION

In addition to the patients' primary care physician and/or hospitalist, treatment of these patients usually requires input from specialists in hepatology, endoscopy, interventional radiology and, occasionally, surgery. This team approach has resulted in a significant reduction in the morbidity and mortality associated with the management of the complications of cirrhosis and portal hypertension.

SUGGESTED READINGS

■ ESOPHAGEAL VARICES

Castera L, Chan HLY, Arrese M, et al. EASL-ALEH Clinical practice guidelines: Non-invasive tests for evaluation of liver disease severity and prognosis. *J Hepatol*. 2015;63:237.

D'Amico GD, Garcia_Tsao G, Pagliaro L. Natural history and prognostic indicators of survival in cirrhosis: a systematic review of 118 studies. *J Hepatology*. 2006;44:217.

D'Amico G, Pasta L, Morabito A, et al. Competing risks and prognostic stages of cirrhosis: a 25-year inception cohort study of 494 patients. *Aliment Pharmacol Ther*. 2014;39:1180.

DeFranchis R. Expanding consensus in portal hypertension. Report of the Baveno VI consensus workshop: stratifying risk and individualizing care for portal hypertension. *J Hepatol*. 2015;63:743.

Garcia-Pagan JC, Caca K, Bureau C, et al Early use of TIPS in patients with cirrhosis and variceal bleeding. *N Engl J Med*. 2010;362:2370.

Garcia-Tsao G, Sanyal AJ, Grace ND, et al. Prevention and management of gastroesophageal varices and variceal hemorrhage in cirrhosis (AASLD and ACG practice guideline). *Hepatol*. 2007;46:922.

Gonzalez R, Zamora J, Gomez-Camarero J, et al. Meta-analysis: combination endoscopic and drug therapy to prevent variceal rebleeding in cirrhosis. *Ann Intern Med*. 2008;149:109.

Grace ND, Minor MA. Portal Hypertension and Variceal Hemorrhage. In: Greenberger NJ, Blumberg RS, Burakoff R (eds). *Current Diagnosis and Treatment: Gastroenterology, Hepatology and Endoscopy*. New York, NY: McGraw Hill Education Medical; 2015 (In press).

Groszmann RJ, Garcia-Tsao G, Bosch J, et al. Beta blockers to prevent gastroesophageal varices in patients with cirrhosis. *N Engl J Med*. 2005;353:2254.

Singh S, Fujii LL, Murad MH et al. Liver stiffness is associated with risk of decompensation, liver cancer, and death in patients with chronic liver disease: a systematic review and meta-analysis. *Clin Gastroenterol Hepatol*. 2013;11:1573.

■ ASCITES

Arroyo V, Ginés P, Rimola A, Gaya J. Renal function abnormalities, prostaglandins, and effects of nonsteroidal anti-inflammatory drugs in cirrhosis with ascites. An overview with emphasis on pathogenesis. *Am J Med*. 1986;81:104.

Bernardi M, Caraceni P, Navickis RJ, Wilkes MM. Albumin infusion in patients undergoing large-volume paracentesis: a meta-analysis of randomized trials. *Hepatology*. 2012;55:1172.

EASL clinical practice guidelines on the management of ascites, spontaneous bacterial peritonitis, and hepatorenal syndrome in cirrhosis. *J Hepatol*. 2010;53(3):397.

Kim JJ, Tsukamoto MM, Mathur AK, et al. Delayed paracentesis is associated with increased in-hospital mortality in patients with spontaneous bacterial peritonitis. *Am J Gastroenterol*. 2014;109:1436.

Orman ES, Hayashi PH, Bataller R, et al. Paracentesis is associated with reduced mortality in patients hospitalized with cirrhosis and ascites. *Clin Gastroenterol Hepatol*. 2014;12:496.

Peltekian KM, Wong F, Liu PP, et al. Cardiovascular, renal, and neurohumoral responses to single large-volume paracentesis in patients with cirrhosis and diuretic-resistant ascites. *Am J Gastroenterol*. 1997;92:394.

Runyon B. Management of adult patients with ascites due to cirrhosis: an update (AASLD practice guideline). *Hepatology*. 2009;49:2087.

Runyon BA, AASLD. Introduction to the revised American Association for the Study of Liver Diseases Practice Guideline management of adult patients with ascites due to cirrhosis 2012. *Hepatology*. 2013;57:1651.

Runyon BA, Antillon MR, McHutchison JG. Diuresis increases ascitic fluid opsonic activity in patients who survive spontaneous bacterial peritonitis. *J Hepatol*. 1992;14:249.

Runyon BA, Montano AA, Akriviadis EA, et al. The serum-ascites albumin gradient is superior to the exudate-transudate concept in the differential diagnosis of ascites. *Ann Intern Med*. 1992;117:215.

Sort P, Navasa M, Arroyo V, et al. Effect of intravenous albumin on renal impairment and mortality in patients with cirrhosis and spontaneous bacterial peritonitis. *N Engl J Med*. 1999;341:403.

■ SPONTANEOUS BACTERIAL PERITONITIS (SBP)

Chavez-Tapia NC, Soares-Weiser K, Brezis M, Leibovici L. Antibiotics for spontaneous bacterial peritonitis in cirrhotic patients. *Cochrane Database Syst Rev*. 2009;CD002232.

Fernández J, Ruiz del Arbol L, Gómez C, et al. Norfloxacin vs ceftriaxone in the prophylaxis of infections in patients with advanced cirrhosis and hemorrhage. *Gastroenterology*. 2006;131:1049.

Mandorfer M, Bota S, Schwabl P, et al. Nonselective β blockers increase risk for hepatorenal syndrome and death in patients with cirrhosis and spontaneous bacterial peritonitis. *Gastroenterology*. 2014;146:1680.

Rasaratnam B, Kaye D, Jennings G, et al. The effect of selective intestinal decontamination on the hyperdynamic circulatory state in cirrhosis. A randomized trial. *Ann Intern Med*. 2003;139:186.

Runyon BA, Hoefs JC, Canawati HN. Polymicrobial bacterascites. A unique entity in the spectrum of infected ascitic fluid. *Arch Intern Med*. 1986;146:2173.

Runyon BA, McHutchison JG, Antillon MR, et al. Short-course versus long-course antibiotic treatment of spontaneous bacterial peritonitis. A randomized controlled study of 100 patients. *Gastroenterology*. 1991;100:1737.

Sort P, Navasa M, Arroyo V, et al. Effect of intravenous albumin on renal impairment and mortality in patients with cirrhosis and spontaneous bacterial peritonitis. *N Engl J Med*. 1999;341:403.

Such J, Runyon BA. Spontaneous bacterial peritonitis. *Clin Infect Dis*. 1998;27:669.

■ HEPATORENAL SYNDROME

Acevedo J, Fernandez J, Prado V, et al. Relative adrenal insufficiency in decompensated cirrhosis: relationship to short-term risk of severe sepsis, hepatorenal syndrome, and death. *Hepatology.* 2013;58:1757.

Arroyo V, Ginès P, Gerbes AL, et al. Definition and diagnostic criteria of refractory ascites and hepatorenal syndrome in cirrhosis. International Ascites Club. *Hepatology.* 1996;23:164.

Barreto R, Fagundes C, Guevara M, et al. Type-1 hepatorenal syndrome associated with infections in cirrhosis: natural history, outcome of kidney function and survival. *Hepatology.* 2014;59:1503.

Cavallin M, Kamath PS, Merli M, et al. Terlipressin plus albumin versus midodrine and octreotide plus albumin in the treatment of hepatorenal syndrome: a randomized trial. *Heaptology.* 2015;62:567.

Ginès A, Escorsell A, Ginès P, et al. Incidence, predictive factors, and prognosis of the hepatorenal syndrome in cirrhosis with ascites. *Gastroenterology.* 1993;105:229.

Ginès P, Schrier RW. Renal failure in cirrhosis. *N Engl J Med.* 2009;361:1279.

Nassar Junior AP, Farias AQ, D' Albuquerque LA, et al. Terlipressin versus norepinephrine in the treatment of hepatorenal syndrome: a systematic review and meta-analysis. *PLoS One.* 2014;9:e107466.

Singh V, Dhungana SP, Singh B, et al. Midodrine in patients with cirrhosis and refractory or recurrent ascites: a randomized pilot study. *J Hepatol.* 2012;56:348.

■ HEPATIC ENCEPHALOPATHY

Basile AS, Jones EA. Ammonia and GABA-ergic neurotransmission: interrelated factors in the pathogenesis of hepatic encephalopathy. *Hepatology.* 1997;25:1303.

Córdoba J, López-Hellín J, Planas M, et al. Normal protein diet for episodic hepatic encephalopathy: results of a randomized study. *J Hepatol.* 2004;41:38.

Ferenci P, Lockwood A, Mullen K, et al. Hepatic encephalopathy—definition, nomenclature, diagnosis, and quantification: final report of the working party at the 11th World Congresses of Gastroenterology, Vienna, 1998. *Hepatology.* 2002;35:716.

Jiang Q, Jiang XH, Zheng MH, et al. Rifaximin versus nonabsorbable disaccharides in the management of hepatic encephalopathy: a meta-analysis. *Eur J Gastroenterol Hepatol.* 2008;20:1064.

Kircheis G, Knoche A, Hilger N, et al. Hepatic encephalopathy and fitness to drive. *Gastroenterology.* 2009;137:1706.

Manish KL, Sharma BC, Sharma P, et al. Probiotics prevent hepatic encephalopathy in patients with cirrhosis: a randomized controlled trial. *Clin Gastroenterol Hepatol.* 2014;12:1003.

Ong JP, Aggarwal A, Krieger D, et al. Correlation between ammonia levels and the severity of hepatic encephalopathy. *Am J Med.* 2003;114:188.

Riggio O, Amodio P, Farcomeni A, et al. A model for predicting development of overt hepatic encephalopathy in patients with cirrhosis. *Clin Gatroenterol Hepatol.* 2015;13:1346.

Vilstrup H, Amodio P, Bajaj J, et al. Hepatic encephalopathy in chronic liver disease: 2014 Practice Guideline by the American Association for the Study of Liver Diseases and the European Association for the Study of the Liver. *Hepatology.* 2014;60:715.

Weissenborn K, Ennen JC, Schomerus H, et al. Neuropsychological characterization of hepatic encephalopathy. *J Hepatol.* 2001;34:768.

■ HEPATIC HYDROTHORAX

Cardenas A, Kelleher T, Chopra S. Review article: hepatic hydrothorax. *Aliment Pharmacol Ther.* 2004;20:271.

Gurung P, Goldblatt M, Huggins JT, et al. Pleural fluid analysis and radiographic, sonographic, and echocardiographic characteristics of hepatic hydrothorax. *Chest.* 2011;140:448.

Huang PM, Chang YL, Yang CY, Lee YC. The morphology of diaphragmatic defects in hepatic hydrothorax: thoracoscopic finding. *J Thorac Cardiovasc Surg.* 2005;130:141.

Xiol X, Castellví JM, Guardiola J, et al. Spontaneous bacterial empyema in cirrhotic patients: a prospective study. *Hepatology.* 1996;23:719.

■ ACUTE-ON-CHRONIC LIVER FAILURE

Angeli P, Gines P, Wong F, et al. Diagnosis and management of acute kidney injury in patients with cirrhosis: revised consensus recommendations of the International Club of Ascites. *J Hepatology.* 2015;62:968.

Gustot T, Fernandez J, Garcia E, et al. Clinical course of acute-on-chronic liver failure syndrome and effects on prognosis. *Hepatology.* 2015;62:243.

Jalan R, Yurdaydin C, Bajaj JS, Acharya SK, Arroyo V, Lin HC, Gines P, Kim WR, Kamath PS. Toward an improved definition of acute-on-chronic liver failure. *Gastroenterology.* 2014;147:4–10.

Moreau R, Jalan R, Gines P, et al. Acute-on-chronic liver failure is a distinct syndrome that develops in patients with acute decompensation of cirrhosis. *Gastroenterology.* 2013;144:1426.

Shi Yu, Yang Ying, Hu Yaoren, et al. Acute on chronic liver failure precipitated by hepatic injury is distinct from that precipitated by extrahepatic insults. *Hepatology.* 2015;62:232.

Wong F, O'Leary JG, Reddy KR, et al. New consensus definition of acute kidney injury accurately predicts 30 day mortality in patients with cirrhosis and infection. *Gastroenterology.* 2013;145:1280.

Clinical Conditions in the Inpatient Setting

CHAPTER 161

Acute Lower Gastrointestinal Bleeding

Linda S. Lee, MD

Key Clinical Questions

① What risk factors increase the severity of lower gastrointestinal (GI) bleeding?

② What are the indications for tagged red blood cell scan and angiography in the setting of lower GI bleeding?

③ What are the indications for surgery in patients with diverticular bleeding and ischemic colitis?

④ What medical treatment options are available to treat recurrent lower GI bleeding from angiodysplasias?

⑤ What is the pathophysiology of ischemic colitis?

INTRODUCTION

Lower gastrointestinal (GI) bleeding refers to bleeding that occurs from a source in the colon, rectum, or anus. There are about 36 hospitalizations per 100,000 adults in the United States due to lower GI bleeding. Lower GI bleeding accounts for about 20% of major gastrointestinal bleeding and is less common and generally less severe than upper GI bleeding. It affects the older population with a mean age between 63 and 77 years old, and incidence of lower GI bleeding is increasing in the elderly especially over age 80. Nearly 80% of all GI bleeding, including lower GI bleeding, stops spontaneously. The overall mortality rate of lower GI bleeding is 1.5%. Patients who begin lower GI bleeding as an outpatient have a significantly lower mortality rate (3.6%) than in patients who develop lower GI bleeding (23%), which is similar to upper GI bleeding.

■ PRESENTATION

Definitions of bleeding

Hematochezia refers to bright red blood per rectum and often implies a left colonic source, although it can be caused by a more brisk, proximal source of bleeding. Maroon stools are stools mixed with maroon-colored blood that are usually associated with a right colonic source of bleeding; however, they can also result from a more brisk, proximal source of bleeding. Melena is black, tarry, foul smelling stool that results from bacterial degradation of hemoglobin over at least 14 hours. It implies an upper GI source of bleeding, although it may occur from a right colonic bleeding source. Occult blood refers to small quantities of blood in the stool that does not change its color and can only be detected by performing a stool guaiac card test. The gastrointestinal tract normally loses about 0.5 to 1.5 mL of blood per day, which is not detected by guaiac tests. A threshold blood loss of at least 5 to 10 mL/d is necessary before detection by stool guaiac card tests.

PRACTICE POINT

● Ingestion of iron, bismuth, charcoal, and licorice should be excluded as they all can turn stool black.

■ SIGNS AND SYMPTOMS

History in these patients should focus on factors associated with potential etiologies (**Table 161-1**). A differential diagnosis should be developed based on presenting complaints and physical examination. Patients should be asked about symptoms that might indicate hemodynamic compromise including dyspnea, chest pain, lightheadedness, and fatigue.

The physical examination should focus on

1. **Vital signs.** Orthostatic hypotension with decrease of 20 mm Hg in the systolic blood pressure within 2 to 5 minutes of standing implies at least a 15% loss of blood volume.
2. **Abdominal examination** for tenderness, masses, liver span, and splenomegaly.
3. **Rectal examination** including inspection of the anus, characterization of the stool color, and stool guaiac card test.

TABLE 161-1 History Features Based on Bleeding Etiology

Etiology of Lower GI Bleeding	Historical Features
Hemorrhoidal bleeding	Blood coating the stool
	Pain with defecation
Proximal large bowel bleeding	Blood mixed in the stool
IBD	Bloody diarrhea
	Tenesmus
	Abdominal pain
Infectious colitis	Bloody diarrhea
	Fever
	Abdominal pain
	Recent travel history
Anal fissure	Pain with defecation
Colon cancer	Change in stool caliber
	Weight loss
Ischemic colitis	Abdominal pain
	Pain out of proportion to exam
Diverticulosis	Painless bleeding
	NSAID use
AVM	Painless bleeding
Radiation proctitis	Painless bleeding
Colon ulcer	NSAID use
Postpolypectomy bleed	Recent colonoscopy

TRIAGE/HOSPITAL ADMISSION

APPROACH TO PATIENTS WITH ACUTE LOWER GASTROINTESTINAL BLEEDING

When patients initially present with acute lower GI bleeding, they should be triaged and managed based on the severity of the hemorrhage (**Figure 161-1**).

INITIAL CLINICAL ASSESSMENT AND MANAGEMENT

During the initial clinical evaluation of patients with suspected acute lower GI bleeding, resuscitation should proceed simultaneously with the placement of two large-bore (18-gauge or larger) peripheral catheters or a large bore central line (eg, cordis) followed by administration of intravenous fluids including normal saline and/or packed red blood cells (RBCs). Goal hematocrit is ≥7 g/dL or ≥9 g/dL in patients at increased risk of adverse events from anemia. **Blood tests** should be performed including complete blood count, prothrombin time, partial thromboplastin time, electrolytes, and typing and cross-matching for blood products. Coagulopathy and thrombocytopenia should be corrected immediately. Platelets should be maintained above 50,000/mL and coagulopathy reversed with vitamin K, fresh frozen plasma, or kcentra for goal INR <1.5 in active bleeding although endoscopic procedures can be performed once the INR falls below 3. Rapid reversal requires fresh frozen plasma or kcentra as the full effect of vitamin K takes 12 to 24 hours to occur. Vitamin K should be taken orally with the subcutaneous route preferred in patients with cirrhosis or biliary obstruction; the intravenous route should be used in severe bleeding. The effects of fresh frozen plasma last about 3 to 5 hours and large volumes

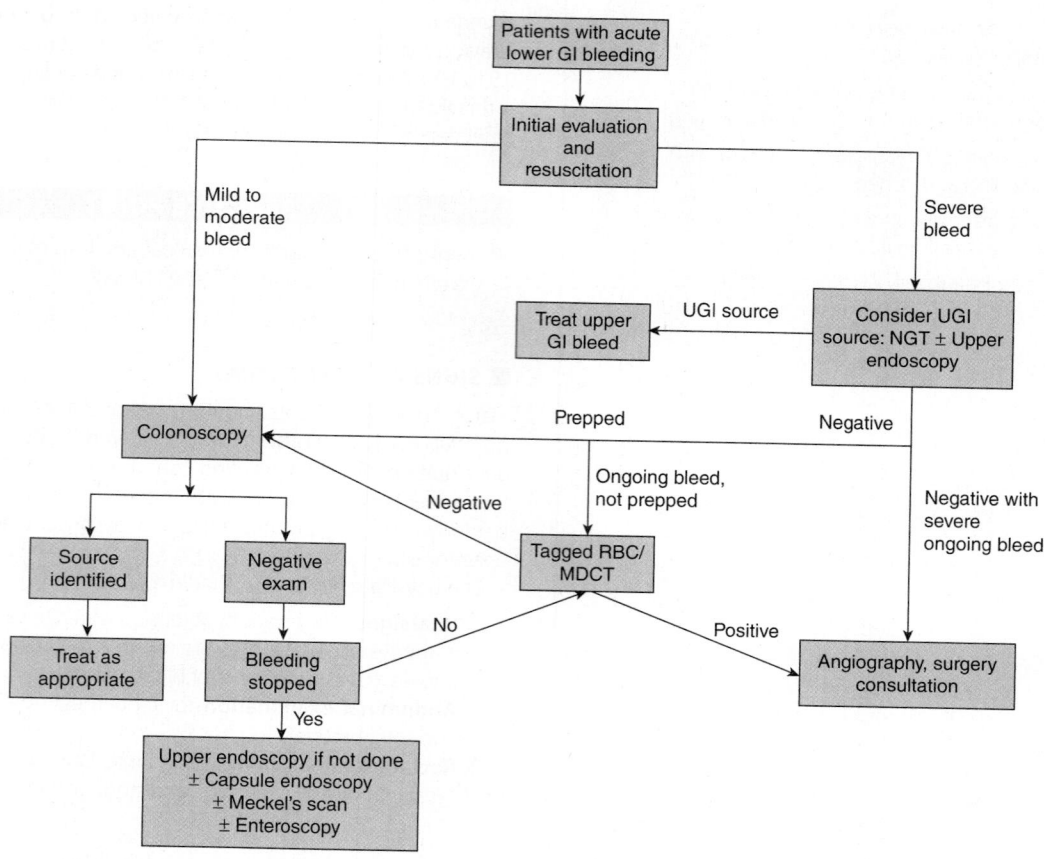

Figure 161-1 *Algorithm for management of patients with suspected lower GI bleeding.*

(over 2-3 L) may be required to completely reverse coagulopathy depending on the initial INR. Kcentra is a complex of factors II, VII, IX, X, protein C and S derived from fresh frozen human blood plasma. Advantages of kcentra include that approximately 85% less volume is required compared to fresh frozen plasma and rapid correction of INR <1.3 occurs in less than 30 minutes. However, it is nearly six times as expensive as fresh frozen plasma. Recombinant activated factor VII has been approved for use in patients with hemophilia A and B with factor VIII and IX inhibitors. Evidence of possible benefit in patients with cirrhosis and gastrointestinal bleeding has been demonstrated, although the optimal dose is unclear and recombinant activated factor VII is very expensive with a single 90 mcg/kg dose costing at least $4500.

■ PREDICTION OF MORBIDITY AND MORTALITY

Multiple validated scoring systems help predict the probability of rebleeding, surgery, and mortality in upper GI bleeding. These scoring systems enable appropriate triage and aggressive management of high-risk patients and potentially early discharge of low-risk patients. Few studies stratify patients by severity in lower GI bleeding. The strongest predictors of mortality include age over 70, ischemic colitis, and presence of at least two comorbidities.

> ### PRACTICE POINT
>
> Increased severity of lower GI bleeding is associated with the following risk factors (RF):
> - Heart rate greater than 100 beats/min
> - Systolic blood pressure less than 115 mm Hg
> - Syncope
> - Nontender abdomen
> - Rectal bleeding within 4 hours of presentation
> - Aspirin use
> - More than two comorbidities
>
> Zero RFs equate to a low incidence (6%) of severe bleeding.
> One to three RFs equate to a moderate incidence (43%) of severe bleeding.
> More than three risk factors equate to a high risk (79%) of severe bleeding.

■ OUTPATIENT VERSUS INPATIENT EVALUATION

Patients who have minor bleeding with scant hematochezia represent 75% to 90% of all patients with lower GI bleeding and may be evaluated as outpatients. For patients over the age of 50 years, colonoscopy should be performed to evaluate the source and to screen for colon cancer. In younger patients with rectal bleeding, there is debate regarding the necessity of a colonoscopy versus flexible sigmoidoscopy. Several studies demonstrate that 10% to 30% of patients with rectal bleeding had proximal lesions, which would have been missed by a flexible sigmoidoscopy. Other studies found that no cancers and only a very few polyps would have been missed by flexible sigmoidoscopy in patients with "outlet-type bleeding," defined as blood seen during or after defecation on the toilet paper or in the toilet bowl without symptoms or special risk factors for colorectal neoplasia. Physicians are unable to reliably predict based on history alone which patients with rectal bleeding will have significant pathology. As patients grow older, it becomes cost-effective to perform a full colonoscopy. Patients in their mid-30s or older should likely be evaluated with a colonoscopy while patients in their 20s with "outlet-type bleeding" may have a flexible sigmoidoscopy. If no lesion is discovered to explain the hematochezia, those patients should then undergo a full colonoscopy.

Another category of patients presents with chronic, intermittent bleeding, which manifests as guaiac positive stool and/or iron deficiency anemia. Evaluation of these patients can usually occur in the outpatient setting; however, if the patients are severely anemic with cardiopulmonary symptoms and/or disease, inpatient admission should be considered for further monitoring, evaluation, and management. All of these patients must be evaluated with colonoscopy. About 25% to 41% of these patients will have abnormalities on upper endoscopy. Therefore, if no source is identified on colonoscopy or if the patient has upper gastrointestinal symptoms, an upper endoscopy should be performed. Asymptomatic patients may also harbor upper gastrointestinal abnormalities, and those with iron deficiency anemia should undergo an upper endoscopy.

Other patients with lower GI bleeding include those with episodic, severe bleeding, and continuous active bleeding who must be evaluated in the hospital. Approximately 10% to 20% of initially suspected lower GI bleeding cases ultimately have an upper gastrointestinal source.

> ### PRACTICE POINT
>
> - Approximately 10% to 20% of initially suspected lower GI bleeding cases ultimately have an upper gastrointestinal source. Clues to a possible upper gastrointestinal source include hematochezia with hemodynamic instability, melena, history of upper GI bleeding, and elevated blood urea nitrogen.

DIAGNOSIS

Diagnostic evaluation must be performed after patients have been adequately resuscitated. If an upper GI source is suspected, an upper endoscopy should be performed first. Lower GI evaluation can be performed with anoscopy, flexible sigmoidoscopy, colonoscopy, rarely barium enema, and various radiologic studies.

■ ANOSCOPY

Anoscopy is useful only for diagnosing bleeding sources from the anorectal junction and anal canal including internal hemorrhoids and anal fissures. This requires an anoscope, which is a tube about the width of an average to large bowel movement and 3 to 4 in long through which a light may be shone. Anoscopy may be performed quickly in the office or at the bedside as an adjunct to flexible sigmoidoscopy and colonoscopy.

■ FLEXIBLE SIGMOIDOSCOPY

Flexible sigmoidoscopy uses a 65 cm long sigmoidoscope that visualizes the left colon. It may be performed without sedation and only minimal preparation with enemas. However, the diagnostic yield of flexible sigmoidoscopy in acute lower GI bleeding is only 9%. The role of anoscopy and flexible sigmoidoscopy in patients with acute lower GI bleeding is limited as most patients should undergo colonoscopy. Specific situations where sigmoidoscopy may be indicated include patients with suspected postpolypectomy bleeding after resection of a left-sided polyp and bleeding with evidence of left-sided colitis on imaging.

■ COLONOSCOPY

Colonoscopy is the test of choice in the majority of patients with acute lower GI bleeding as it may be both diagnostic and therapeutic. The diagnostic accuracy of colonoscopy in lower GI bleeding ranges from 48% to 90% and urgent colonoscopy appears to increase diagnostic yield. This wide range in yield is partially explained by different criteria for diagnosis, as often if no active bleeding, nonbleeding visible vessel, or adherent clot is found, bleeding is attributed to a lesion if blood is present in the area. The presence of fresh blood in the terminal ileum is presumed to indicate a noncolonic source of bleeding.

The overall complication rate of colonoscopy in acute lower GI bleeding is 1.3% with 0.3% risk of perforation. Bowel preparation is safe and well-tolerated in most patients. The complication rate of colonoscopy in an unprepped colon may be higher. About 2% to 6% of colonoscopy preparations in acute lower GI bleeding are poor. Between 4 and 8 L (1-2 gallons) of Golytely should be administered orally or via nasogastric tube until the effluence is clear. Antiemetics and prokinetics such as metoclopramide 10 mg should be given as needed during the preparation. In patients at risk of aspiration or fluid overload, the preparation should be cautiously administered, although complication rates are low with polyethylene glycol (PEG)-based preparations. Colonoscopy may be performed within 1 to 2 hours after the stool clears. There is no role for enemas in colonoscopy preparation.

Aggressive management with urgent colonoscopy does not clearly improve outcomes in patients with severe lower GI bleeding. There are two prospective randomized trials to date of patients with significant lower GI bleeding who were randomized to standard care or urgent colonoscopy. Patients in the standard care arm underwent elective colonoscopy within 4 days of admission while patients undergoing urgent colonoscopy were administered 4 to 6 L of a balanced electrolyte-PEG prepared solution orally or via a nasogastric tube over 3 to 4 hours and underwent colonoscopy within 8 to 12 hours of hospitalization or diagnosis of hematochezia. More bleeding sources were identified in the urgent colonoscopy group in one study, but there was no difference in early or late rebleeding, length of hospital stay, surgery, mortality, or complications in either study. A recent retrospective propensity score matched study confirmed these findings.

■ BARIUM ENEMA

There is no role for barium enema in acute lower GI bleeding. It may impede the performance of a colonoscopy or subsequent angiography due to the presence of barium in the colon. In young patients with minor hematochezia who have a negative flexible sigmoidoscopy, barium enema can be an alternative to colonoscopy.

■ TAGGED RED BLOOD CELL SCAN

Tagged red blood cell scan and angiography may be the tests of choice in patients with massive lower GI bleeding that prevents colonoscopy, in those with ongoing bleeding and a negative colonoscopy, or in patients who have not yet been prepared for a colonoscopy. Although tagged RBC scan is solely a diagnostic exam, angiography, like colonoscopy, may be both diagnostic and therapeutic.

Tagged RBC scan requires a bleeding rate of at least 0.1 to 0.5 mL/min. An injected radiotracer circulates in the blood and extravasation of blood into the gastrointestinal lumen is identified on a series of static images captured after injection or on multiple sequential dynamic images obtained at 15- or 30-second intervals (**Figures 161-2A, B**). Two radiotracers have been used for tagged RBC scan: technetium (Tc) 99 m sulfur colloid and technetium 99 m-labelled RBC, which involves labeling the patient's red blood cells **in vitro** and then reinjecting them into the patient. Sulfur colloid is rapidly cleared by the reticuloendothelial system and leaves the blood pool within minutes, which provides an approximate 10-minute window to detect extravasation. Red blood cells labeling is superior because the red blood cells persist at least 24 hours in the circulation. This allows for longer imaging and repeated imaging if the patient rebleeds during this time window. Typically, a 90-minute imaging period is used as the diagnostic yield plateaus at this time.

Accuracy of localization of the bleeding site ranges from 24% to 91%. Scans that are positive within 2 hours were 95% to 100% accurate in identifying the bleeding site compared to 57% to 67% accurate for scans positive after 2 hours. Because of the relatively high rate of false localization, confirmatory studies are required before proceeding to surgery.

A positive tagged RBC scan increases the diagnostic yield of subsequent angiography 2.4 times by removing patients who are not actively bleeding at the time of tagged RBC scan and allowing a more targeted angiography with decreased contrast load. Following a positive tagged RBC scan, urgent angiography should be performed ideally within 1 hour. Delaying angiography may lead to increased negative results, as lower GI bleeding is often episodic and intermittent.

■ ANGIOGRAPHY

A more rapid rate of bleeding of at least 0.5 to 1.5 mL/min is necessary to be detected during angiography compared to tagged RBC scan (**Figure 161-3**). Patients who are massively bleeding and hemodynamically unstable should be resuscitated and proceed directly to angiography without tagged RBC scan. The diagnostic yield of angiography ranges from 27% to 77%; sensitivity and specificity are 47% and 100%, respectively. Complications of angiography occur in 10% to 20% and include renal failure, hematoma, ischemia, and infarction. Provocative testing using anticoagulants (eg, intravenous heparin and intra-arterial tPA) and vasodilators (intra-arterial tolazoline) may increase diagnostic yield although concern for significant complications exist. This approach must only occur in very select situations after extensive discussion with the patient, gastroenterologist, surgeon, and radiologist. Further studies are necessary to optimize the efficacy and prove the safety of this approach.

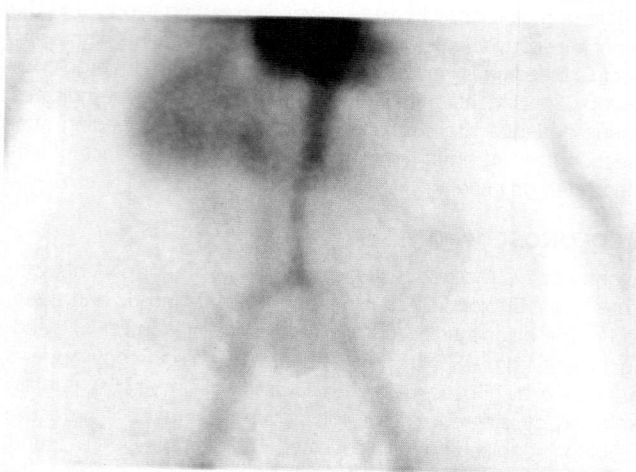

A

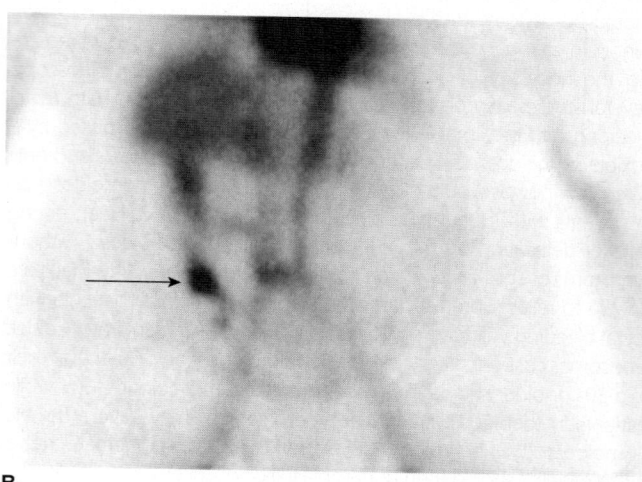

B

Figure 161-2 (A) *Baseline tagged RBC scan.* (B) *Tagged RBC scan with active bleeding from right colon (arrow).*

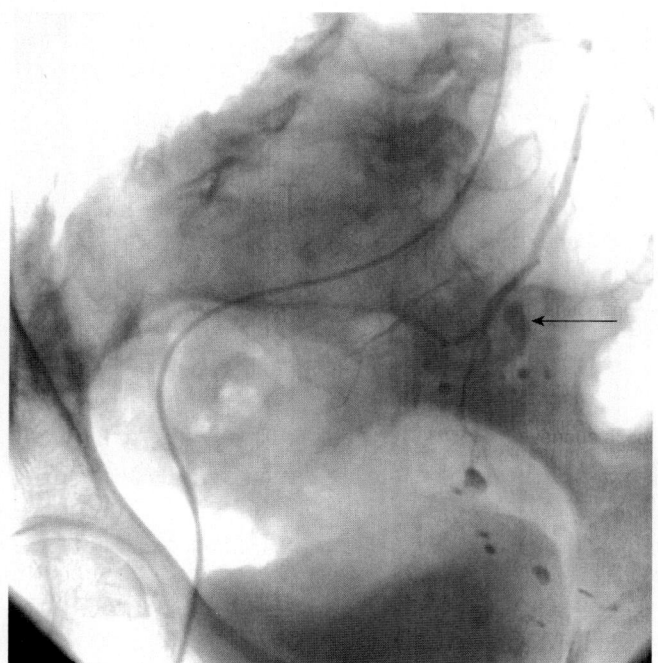

Figure 161-3 *Angiography with active bleeding from right colon (arrow).*

■ MULTIDETECTOR ROW COMPUTED TOMOGRAPHY

Multidetector row computed tomography (MDCT) offers another noninvasive modality for diagnosing lower GI bleeding and incorporates several improvements that allow enhanced delineation of mesenteric vessels: faster scanning time, more accurate acquisition of images in arterial and venous phases, and improved 3D display. Patients do not ingest any oral contrast and after an initial unenhanced computed tomography (CT) scan, images are obtained during the arterial phase to identify extravasation of contrast into the bowel lumen. A bleeding rate of at least 0.3-0.5 mL/ minute is necessary for detection by MDCT. Studies suggest over 90% sensitivity and specificity for detecting sources of bleeding. Preliminary evidence suggests that MDCT may be more accurate for detecting and localizing a bleeding source than tagged RBC.

■ MAGNETIC RESONANCE ANGIOGRAM

Magnetic resonance (MR) angiogram is not typically used in acute lower GI bleeding because it lacks the resolution to detect hemorrhage from small blood vessels. A new blood pool MR contrast agent may help localize bleeding to a bowel segment. This contrast agent remains in the intravascular space for many hours and subsequent imaging could identify extravascular contrast.

DIFFERENTIAL DIAGNOSIS

The differential diagnosis for lower GI bleeding is broad although the vast majority is due to diverticulosis, ischemic colitis, angiodysplasia, neoplasia and hemorrhoids (**Table 161-2**). Following initial evaluation, the cause of lower GI bleeding remains uncertain in about 12% of cases.

■ DIVERTICULOSIS

Diverticulosis is the most common etiology of lower GI bleeding. It is more prevalent in developed countries and older patients. While 5% to 10% of people under the age of 40 have diverticulosis, it affects nearly two-thirds of people older than 80 years.

TABLE 161-2 Common Sources and Prevalence of Lower Gastrointestinal Bleeding*

Source	Prevalence (%)
Diverticulosis	17-44
Colonic Angiodysplasia	2-30
Ischemia	9-21
Malignancy	4-14
Hemorrhoids/Anorectal	4-11
Postpolypectomy	6
Unknown	8-12

*Data from Longstreth GF. *Am J Gastroenterol.* 1997;92:419; Strate L. *Arch Int Med.* 2003;163:838; Zuccaro G. *Am J Gastroenterol.* 1998;93:1202; Barnert J. *Nat Rev Gastroenterol Hepatol.* 2009;6:637-646.

Presentation and pathophysiology

About 75% to 80% of people with diverticulosis are asymptomatic; however, 3% to 20% experience diverticular bleeding. Massive bleeding can occur in 3% to 5% of patients. Risk factors for diverticular bleeding include use of NSAIDs (nonsteroidal anti-inflammatory drugs), advanced age, and right colon location. Bleeding occurs where the vasa recta stretches over the dome of the diverticula resulting in segmental wall weakness and predisposing to abrupt painless rupture. Mild lower abdominal cramping may occur before passage of blood due to the cathartic nature of blood in the intestines. Melena is unusual from diverticular arterial bleeding. Guaiac positive stool alone and iron deficiency anemia are not consistent with diverticular bleeding.

Diagnosis

More than 75% of diverticula are located in the left colon, although about 60% of bleeding diverticula detected during angiography occur in the right colon compared to during colonoscopy with 60% in the left colon. The vast majority of diverticular bleeding stops spontaneously. Colonoscopy is often the initial diagnostic procedure performed to rule out other lesions and determine the bleeding site, which is found in less than 22% of cases. If bleeding without a clear source persists or recurs, tagged RBC scan or MDCT can be performed followed by immediate angiography if positive. If tagged RBC scan or MDCT is negative, repeat colonoscopy may be considered.

Management

Endoscopic options: There are multiple endoscopic options if a bleeding diverticulum is identified, including epinephrine injection, bipolar coagulation, combination therapy, or mechanical therapy. Epinephrine injection in four quadrants may control bleeding or close the mouth of the diverticulum by tamponade. The majority of bleeding vessels or nonbleeding visible vessels identified during colonoscopy are located on the neck of the diverticulum. Thermal therapy should be avoided at the dome of the diverticulum. Mechanical therapy with hemoclips or endoscopic band ligation may also be used to treat bleeding diverticula (**Figure 161-4**). A small study suggested that endoscopic treatment is successful long term with no recurrent bleeding over a median of 30 months, while 53% of patients treated conservatively rebled.

Interventional radiology options: Continuous, selective intra-arterial vasopressin infusion during angiography stops bleeding in about 90% of cases with up to 50% rebleeding after discontinuing the infusion. Vasopressin infusion may help allow bowel preparation before a semi-elective definitive surgical procedure. Vasopressin should be avoided in patients with known coronary artery disease.

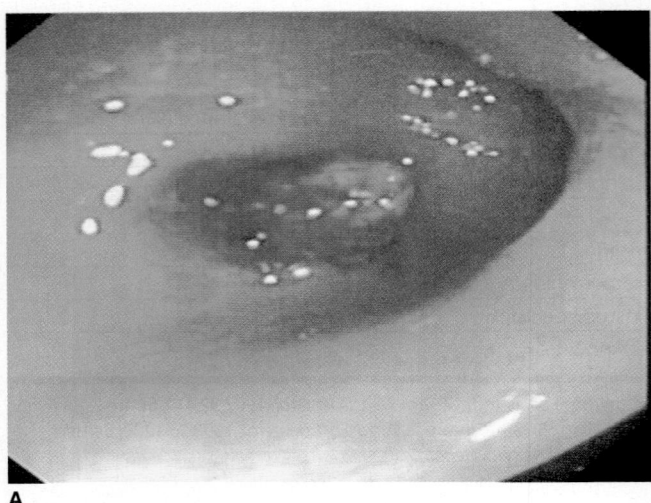
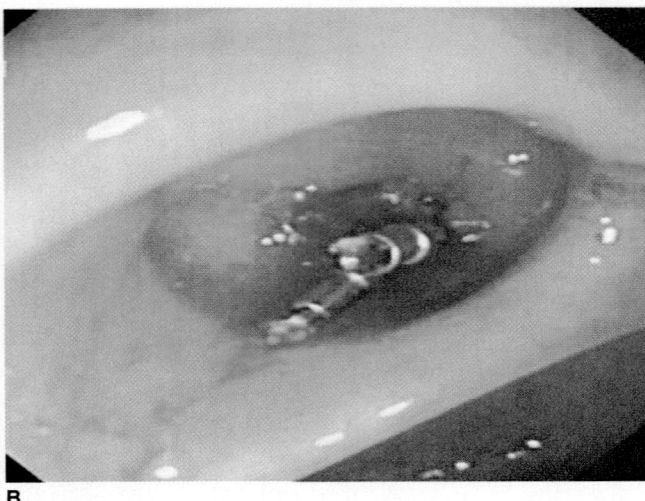

Figure 161-4 *(A) Diverticulum with large, oozing visible vessel. (B) Posttreatment of diverticulum with two endoclips.* (Reproduced, with permission, from Greenberger N, Blumberg R, Burakoff R. *Current Diagnosis & Treatment: Gastroenterology, Hepatology, and Endoscopy.* New York, NY: McGraw-Hill; 2008. Plates 64-65.)

Superselective embolization: uses 2.5 to 3 French microcatheters, which are advanced through conventional five French catheters to access smaller, more distal vessels. Various embolic agents are used, including gel foam, polyvinyl alcohol, and microcoils. Recurrent bleeding 1 month after embolization occurs in less than 15% of diverticular hemorrhage compared to more than 40% of nondiverticular causes such as angiodysplasia. Major complications leading to surgery or death occur in about 17% of patients.

Surgical options: Persistent massive hemorrhage, transfusion requirement over four units in 24 hours, and recurrent diverticular bleeding meet potential indications for surgery, necessary in up to 25% of people requiring transfusions. Mortality rate remains relatively high at 10% even following directed segmental resection with a 14% rebleeding rate at 1-year follow-up. Blind segmental resection should be avoided due to rebleeding rates as high as 33% with mortality rates ranging from up to 50% or more. Blind total colectomy yields the lowest rebleeding rates near 0% but mortality rates range from 0% to 33%. Therefore, aggressive efforts should be made to localize a bleeding site preoperatively.

Repeat diverticular bleeding occurs in 25% to 35%, while 50% of these people experience a third episode of diverticular hemorrhage. NSAID use is a potential risk factor. Whether avoiding NSAIDs reduces rebleeding is unclear, however, should be recommended in patients with diverticular bleeding.

■ ANGIODYSPLASIA

Angiodysplasias are the reported source of lower GI bleeding in 3% to 40% of patients, which are usually congenital and occur in 1% to 2% of colon autopsy specimens.

Presentation and pathophysiology

Angiodysplasias are degeneration of submucosal venules. Over half are located in the right colon and 47% of patients experience painless hematochezia similar to diverticular hemorrhage. Bleeding angiodysplasias can present with chronic, intermittent bleeding. Risk factors for bleeding include advanced age (> age 60 years), right-sided location, and possibly certain conditions (aortic stenosis and chronic renal failure).

Diagnosis

Angiography is considered the gold standard in diagnosing angiodysplasias with findings including ectatic slowly emptying veins, vascular

tufts, or early filling veins. The diagnostic sensitivity of colonoscopy is 80% to 90% with the characteristic finding of a 2 to 10 mm, red fern-like flat lesion with ectatic vessels radiating from a central vessel. Poor bowel preparation and use of meperidine, which transiently decreases mucosal blood flow, could potentially hinder the identification of angiodysplasias.

Management

Bleeding angiodysplasias discovered during colonoscopy can be treated with a variety of thermal therapies. Contact electrocautery can begin with the outer feeder vessels and progress toward the central vessel (**Figure 161-5**). Argon plasma coagulation (APC) has become a popular noncontact method with approximately 80% success rate. Nonbleeding angiodysplasias without evidence of GI bleeding should not be treated. However, if there is a history of guaiac positive stool or iron deficiency anemia, angiodysplasias should be treated even if not actively bleeding.

There is a potential role for medical treatment of angiodysplasias. Case series and reports have suggested the benefit of octreotide administered subcutaneously in doses ranging from 100 to 500 mcg two times a day decreasing the need for transfusions. Long-term estrogen-progesterone treatment for 1 year did not decrease rebleeding from angiodysplasias in a randomized trial. Another study that suggested benefit from hormone therapy included 50% of patients with Osler-Weber-Rendu disease. A randomized study supported the role of thalidomide taken orally at 100 mg daily for 4 months in stopping bleeding from angiodysplasias.

■ ISCHEMIC COLITIS

Colonic ischemia, which most commonly occurs in the elderly with multiple comorbidities, is caused by a reduction in colonic blood flow due to vasospasm, occlusion, and/or hypoperfusion, and must be distinguished from mesenteric ischemia that affects the small intestine. Eighty-five percent of patients with colonic ischemia have a benign course called nongangrenous ischemia with transient ischemia that resolves without sequelae. However, life-threatening complications occur in 15% of patients who develop gangrenous colonic ischemia.

Presentation and pathophysiology

The potential causes of colonic ischemia are varied (**Table 161-3**). However, the majority of patients with colonic ischemia have no

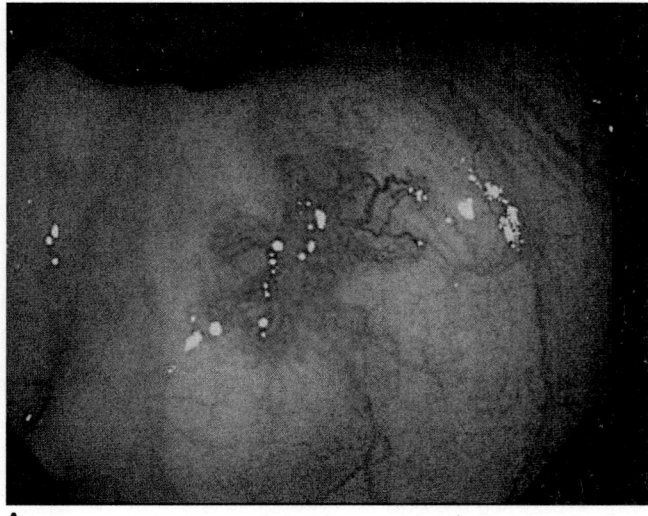
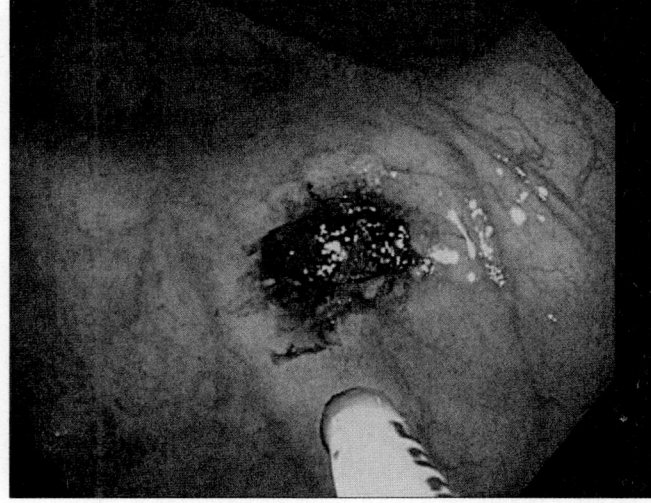

A

B

Figure 161-5 *(A) Angiodysplasia in patient with lower GI bleeding. (B) Posttreatment of angiodysplasia with argon plasma coagulation.*

identifiable cause. The colonic circulation is supplied by three arterial sources: the superior mesenteric artery (SMA) branches into the ileocolic (supplies terminal ileum, appendix, cecum, and proximal ascending colon), right colic (supplies distal ascending colon and

hepatic flexure) and middle colic arteries (supplies proximal transverse colon); the inferior mesenteric artery (IMA) branches into the left colic (supplies distal transverse and splenic flexure), sigmoid (supplies descending and sigmoid colon) and superior rectal arteries (supplies majority of rectum); and the internal iliac artery branches into the internal pudendal and middle rectal arteries (supplies remainder of rectum). Colonic blood supply helps determine the areas of weak blood supply due to narrow terminal branches. Watershed areas of the large colon occur at the splenic flexure (SMA) and at the rectosigmoid junction (IMA) and are most vulnerable to systemic hypotension leading to colonic ischemia.

This occurs with the SMA in the area of the splenic flexure and with the IMA in the area of the rectosigmoid junction. These are called the watershed areas, which are most vulnerable to systemic hypotension.

Colonic ischemia usually results from a sudden reduction in colonic blood flow due to local or systemic compromises of the circulation. Nonocclusive ischemia commonly affects the watershed areas of the colon, with the left colon involved in about 75% of cases, including 25% at the splenic flexure. A common cause of colonic ischemia is aortoiliac surgery with an incidence of colonic ischemia of 1% to 7%. The most commonly affected area is the distal left colon and risk factors for developing this complication postsurgery include older age, prior colectomy, surgeon experience, renal disease, cross-clamping time, and ligation of both iliac arteries.

The clinical manifestations of colonic ischemia vary depending on the cause of the ischemia and the clinical setting. The onset of symptoms is typically rapid with pain over the affected area of bowel, often on the left side. Within 24 hours, patients may develop rectal bleeding and bloody diarrhea. There are three progressive clinical stages. The hyperactive phase occurs soon after injury with abdominal pain and frequent bloody diarrhea. As most patients have injury confined to the mucosal and submucosal layers, symptoms will respond to conservative therapy in more than 80% of patients with resolution of symptoms and no long-term sequelae. The paralytic phase is characterized by less severe but more generalized abdominal pain along with a distended bowel and decreased bowel sounds. The last phase, found in 10% to 20% of patients, is called the shock phase associated with gangrenous bowel and the clinical manifestations of shock. Patients who develop metabolic acidosis and white blood cell counts greater than 20,000 μL may require rapid progression to surgery.

TABLE 161-3 Causes of Colonic Ischemia

Vascular occlusion	Iatrogenic
Mesenteric artery thrombosis	Cardiopulmonary bypass
Aortic reconstruction	Aortoiliac reconstruction
Aortic dissection	Colonoscopy
Cholesterol emboli	Renal transplant
Venous thrombosis	**Drugs**
Hypercoagulable state	Alosetron
Portal hypertension	Carboplatin
Pancreatitis	Cocaine
Sickle cell disease	Digitalis
Shock	Diuretics
Cardiac failure	Danazol
Anaphylaxis	Estrogens
Pancreatitis	NSAIDs
Mechanical	Paclitaxel
Adhesion	Simvastatin
Strangulated hernia	Sumatriptan
Colon cancer	Tegaserod
Rectal prolapse	**Miscellaneous**
Small vessel disease	Hemodialysis
Diabetes	Long distance running
Amyloidosis	Airplane flight
Rheumatoid arthritis	Neurogenic
Takayasu arteritis	Spontaneous (young adults)
Wegener arteritis	
Systemic lupus erythematosus	
Buerger disease	
Polyarteritis nodosa	
Vasculitis	

Diagnosis

The diagnosis of colonic ischemia is established by a combination of clinical setting, physical diagnosis, and diagnostic studies. The differential diagnosis includes infectious colitis, inflammatory bowel disease, diverticulitis, radiation enteritis, and colon cancer. In hospitalized patients, *Clostridium difficile* infection must be excluded. Although there are no specific blood tests for colonic ischemia, elevations may be noted in the white blood cell count, amylase, CPK (creatine phosphokinase), and serum lactate. Most plain x-rays in colonic ischemia have nonspecific findings with thumb printing due to submucosal edema and pneumatosis seen typically in patients with more advanced disease.

Diagnostic testing with CT scans may reveal segmental thickening of the involved colon. Endoscopic evaluation with sigmoidoscopy or colonoscopy may be used to confirm the diagnosis when unclear in patients who do not have signs of peritonitis or perforation. Care must be taken to avoid overdistension with air during the examination to prevent worsening of ischemic damage. Endoscopic findings typically occur in a segmental distribution and vary depending on the degree of damage, ranging from pale mucosa with petechial bleeding to cyanotic, necrotic bowel. **Figure 161-6** demonstrates a focal area of erythema with superficial ulceration in a patient with mild ischemic colitis. Angiography is usually not indicated in colonic ischemia as the blood flow to the colon returns to normal by the time of clinical presentation. Angiography will not detect specific occluding lesions because most patients have nonocclusive ischemia. Angiography is usually not indicated as the blood flow to the colon returns to normal by the time of clinical presentation.

Management

Treatment of colonic ischemia is supportive in the absence of signs of colonic gangrene or perforation. Patients are placed on bowel rest and supported with intravenous fluids. Antibiotics are recommended only for patients with moderate to severe disease. In patients with clinical deterioration—manifested by high leukocytosis, persistent fever, peritoneal signs, and ongoing GI bleeding—despite supportive measures, surgery with segmental resection is indicated. Patients with mesenteric venous thrombosis or hypercoagulability should be treated with anticoagulants.

Prognosis

The natural history of patients with ischemic colitis is that most patients with nonocclusive colonic ischemia will improve in 1 to 2 days with complete resolution within 2 weeks. Patients with more severe disease may develop segmental colitis or strictures. Most patients will not experience a recurrence, especially if potentially predisposing factors are identified and corrected.

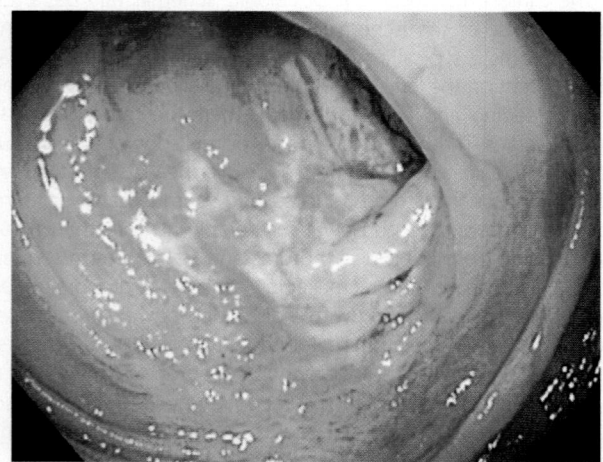

Figure 161-6 *Area of colonic ischemia.*

■ NEOPLASM

Colonic neoplasms may present with GI bleeding. In patients over the age of 50, rectal bleeding is due to a neoplasm in about 10% of cases; however, neoplasms are an uncommon source of rectal bleeding in persons younger than age 50.

Presentation and pathophysiology

Although most bleeding from colonic neoplasms tends to be low grade and occult, bleeding may be brisk and overt at times. Bleeding occurs due to erosion or ulceration of the lesion. Distal lesions (left side and rectum) are more likely to present with bright red blood per rectum, whereas more proximal lesions tend to present with maroon stool, melena, or occult blood.

Diagnosis

The diagnosis of a neoplasm as the source of lower GI bleeding is typically accomplished by colonoscopy with biopsies. Larger neoplasms may be detected on CT scans.

Management

The therapeutic options for those patients with bleeding neoplasms are limited. Standard endoscopic therapies have marginal effectiveness. The use of fibrin glue has been reported to be effective anecdotally and in small studies (**Figure 161-7**). The treatment for most patients with bleeding colonic neoplasms is surgical resection.

■ HEMORRHOIDS

Hemorrhoids and other anorectal disorders (solitary rectal ulcers and anal fissures) are an important source of lower GI bleeding.

Presentation and pathophysiology

Hemorrhoids are dilated submucosal vessels in the anus, which are considered internal if above the dentate line (**Figure 161-8**) and external if below. Hemorrhoids are extremely common and usually asymptomatic, but can present with pruritus, thrombosis, or hematochezia. Bleeding from hemorrhoids occurs when the blood vessel ruptures.

Clinical manifestations of bleeding hemorrhoids include painless hematochezia with the stool coated with bright red blood or on the toilet paper. Further bleeding may occur with blood dripping into the toilet bowl or staining underwear. Although hemorrhoidal bleeding is usually low-grade, high volume or massive bleeding may rarely occur. Severe bleeding from hemorrhoids may occur in patients with a coagulopathy.

Management

Acute treatment for most patients with bleeding hemorrhoids is not needed as most episodes are mild and resolve spontaneously. Topical medical treatments, such as hydrocortisone cream or hydrocortisone acetate/pramoxine cream, help decrease inflammation, and surgery is rarely needed for those with persistent or massive bleeding.

■ POSTPOLYPECTOMY

Postpolypectomy bleeding occurs after 1% to 6% of polypectomies and is the leading major complication following colonoscopy with polypectomy. Acute hemorrhage occurring at the time of polypectomy accounts for less than 50% of cases. Although bleeding usually occurs within 7 days, delayed bleeding can occur up to 29 days following polypectomy when the eschar falls off the site.

Risk factors for postpolypectomy bleeding include removal of large polyps (>1 cm in diameter), age over 65 years, cardiovascular or chronic renal disease, platelet dysfunction, and coagulopathy. Multiple studies have tried to identify techniques to reduce the risk of postpolypectomy bleeding. Submucosal injection of saline has

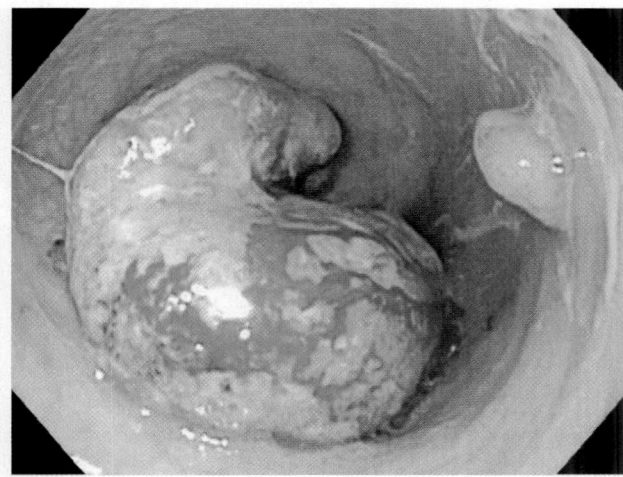

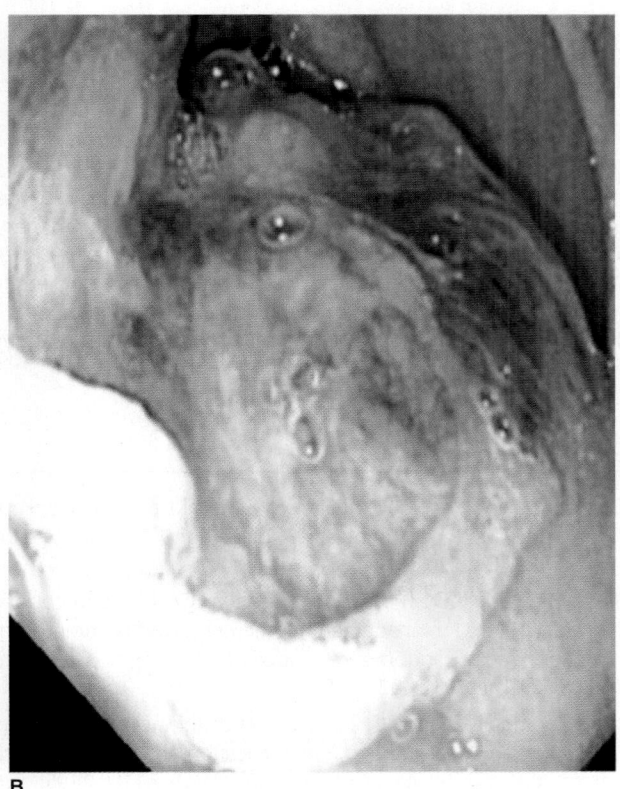

Figure 161-7 (A) *Colon cancer.* (B) *Posttreatment with Tisseel fibrin glue.* (Reproduced, with permission, from Greenberger N, Blumberg R, Burakoff R. *Current Diagnosis & Treatment: Gastroenterology, Hepatology, and Endoscopy.* New York, NY: McGraw-Hill; 2008. Plates 68-69.)

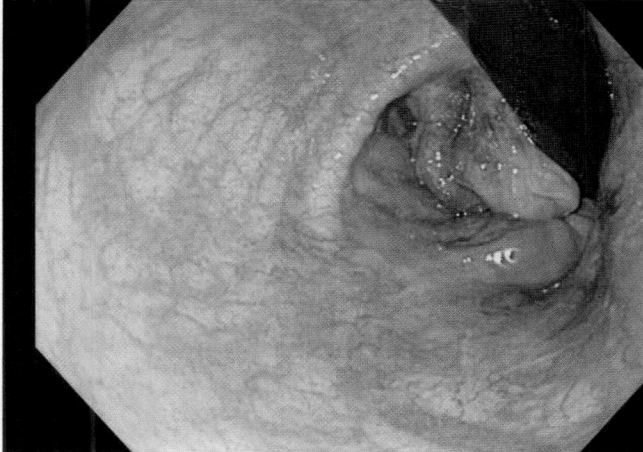

Figure 161-8 *External hemorrhoids seen during retroflexion with colonoscope in the rectum.*

proven useful in large polyps, while it is unclear whether the type of electrical current (blended vs cutting) or use of an endoloop decreases the risk of bleeding. Placement of prophylactic endoclips following removal of large (>2 cm) polyps may decrease postpolypectomy bleeding although further prospective studies are needed.

Management

Polypectomy bleeding is usually self-limited with more than 70% resolving with supportive care. Therapeutic options for persistent bleeding include resnaring the stalk of the polypectomy site to apply pressure, injection therapy with epinephrine, contact or

noncontact thermal treatment with bipolar coagulation or APC, and endoclip application (**Figure 161-9**).

■ NSAID-INDUCED BLEEDING

Similar to its effect on the upper GI tract, NSAIDs may also damage the large intestine and cause lower GI bleeding. Characteristic endoscopic findings include single or multiple well-defined ulcers with normal intervening mucosa classically located in the terminal ileum and proximal colon and single or multiple diaphragm-like strictures with normal intervening mucosa. Only 21% of patients with colonic ulcers have simultaneous gastric ulcers. Clinical presentation varies and includes guaiac positive stool, iron deficiency anemia, hematochezia, crampy abdominal pain, weight loss, and change in bowel habits. NSAID-induced colonic ulcers may also be an incidental finding in asymptomatic patients.

NSAID-induced colonic ulcers have nonspecific pathology and are diagnosed after excluding other potential causes of colonic ulcers including infectious, ischemic, and inflammatory. Symptomatic patients usually respond within a few days after stopping NSAIDs. If NSAIDs cannot be discontinued, concomitant therapy with misoprostol, sulfasalazine, or metronidazole may protect the mucosa from damage and help heal ulcers.

■ RADIATION PROCTITIS

Pelvic radiation can cause both acute and chronic radiation proctitis.

Presentation

Acute damage presents within 3 months of radiation therapy with diarrhea, tenesmus and rarely, bleeding. Chronic radiation proctitis affects up to 20% of patients and usually occurs 9 to 14 months following radiation, but can present years later (**Figure 161-10**). Bleeding is the main symptom and arises from mucosal atrophy and fibrosis leading to chronic mucosal ischemia.

Management

Endoscopic therapy appears superior to medical treatment in reducing severe bleeding with nearly 75% success following endoscopic treatment compared to 33% undergoing medical therapy. Multiple oral and topical therapies have been investigated (mainly in small clinical trials or case series), and a few may be effective including sucralfate enema, short-chain fatty acid enema, and topical formalin therapy.

Endoscopic management with heater probe and bipolar coagulation effectively controls bleeding following a mean of four treatment

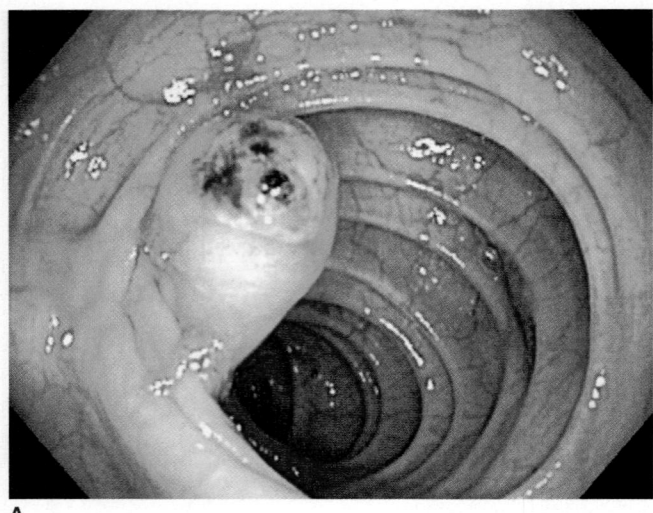

A

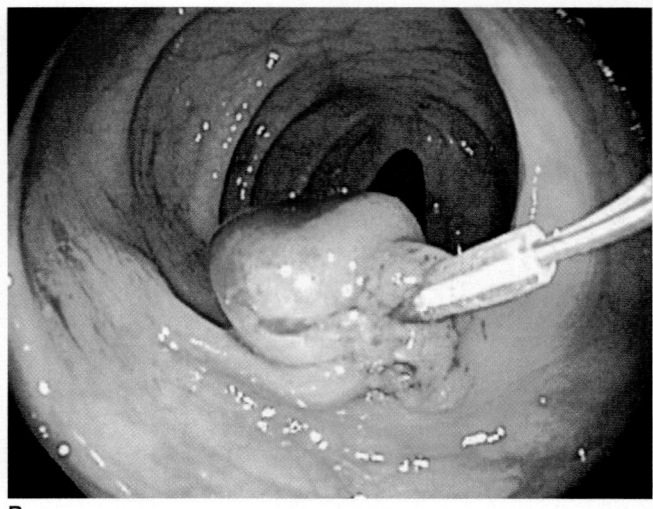

B

Figure 161-9 (A) *Visible vessels at polypectomy site.* (B) *Bleeding controlled with placement of endoloop.* (Reproduced, with permission, from Greenberger N, Blumberg R, Burakoff R. *Current Diagnosis & Treatment: Gastroenterology, Hepatology, and Endoscopy.* New York: McGraw-Hill; 2008. Plates 71-72.)

sessions performed every 4 to 6 weeks. Argon plasma coagulation has received more attention recently with 85% to 100% success in reducing or stopping bleeding after a mean of two to three treatments every 1 to 2 months. During long-term follow-up over 1 to 5 years, recurrent bleeding occurred in 0% to 8% of patients. Case reports of successful endoscopic treatment with radiofrequency ablation and cryoablation have been published.

All visible telangiectasias are obliterated at each session while rectal ulcers resulting from previous treatments are avoided. Short-term complications occur in 7% including rectal pain or fever. Rare major complications include rectovaginal fistula, anal/rectal stricture, and perforation, presumed secondary to accumulation of combustible gas. A full bowel preparation is necessary to avoid explosions of gas during APC when an enema preparation was used. Hyperbaric oxygen may present another therapeutic option, and is believed to promote angiogenesis and collagen formation leading to reepithelialization. Published case series have selected patients who had failed previous medical or endoscopic therapy for hyperbaric oxygen treatment, and report a 75% to 100% decrease or cessation

of bleeding. A randomized trial confirmed complete or partial healing of radiation proctitis in 89% treated with hyperbaric oxygen compared with 63% in the control group. The treatment regimen is rigorous with patients in a hyperbaric chamber at a pressure of 2.4 atmospheres with 100% oxygen for 90 minutes 5 days per week for 30 to 40 sessions. Hyperbaric oxygen therapy may be considered in patients refractory to standard medical and endoscopic treatment before proceeding to surgery.

SUGGESTED READINGS

Czymek R, Kempf A, Roblick UJ, et al. Surgical treatment concepts for acute lower gastrointestinal bleeding. *J Gastrointest Surg.* 2008;12:2212-2220.

Green BT, Rockey DC, Portwood G, et al. Urgent colonoscopy for evaluation and management of acute lower gastrointestinal hemorrhage: a randomized controlled trial. *Am J Gastroenterol.* 2005;100(11):2395-2402.

Laine L, Yang H, Chang SC, Datto C. Trends for incidence of hospitalization and death due to GI complications in the United States from 2001 to 2009. *Am J Gastroenterol.* 2012;107:1190-1195.

Maleux G, Roeflaer F, Heye S, et al. Long-term outcome of transcatheter embolotherapy for acute lower gastrointestinal hemorrhage. *Am J Gastroenterol.* 2009;104:2042-2046.

Pasha SF, Shergill A, Acosta RD, et al. ASGE Guideline: the role of endoscopy in the patient with lower-GI bleeding. *Gastrointest Endosc.* 2014;79(6):875-885.

Strate LL, Ayanian JZ, Kotler G, Syngal S. Risk factors for mortality in lower intestinal bleeding. *Clin Gastroenterol Hepatol.* 2008;6:1004-1010.

Strate LL, Naumann CR. The role of colonoscopy and radiological procedures in the management of acute lower intestinal bleeding. *Clin Gastroenterol Hepatol.* 2010;8:333-343.

Strate LL and Gralnek IM. ACG clinical guideline: management of patients with acute lower gastrointestinal bleeding. *Am J Gastroenterol.* 2016;111(4):459-474.

Theodoropoulou A and Koutroubakis IE. Ischemic colitis: clinical practice in diagnosis and treatment. *World J Gastroenterology.* 2008;14:7302-7308.

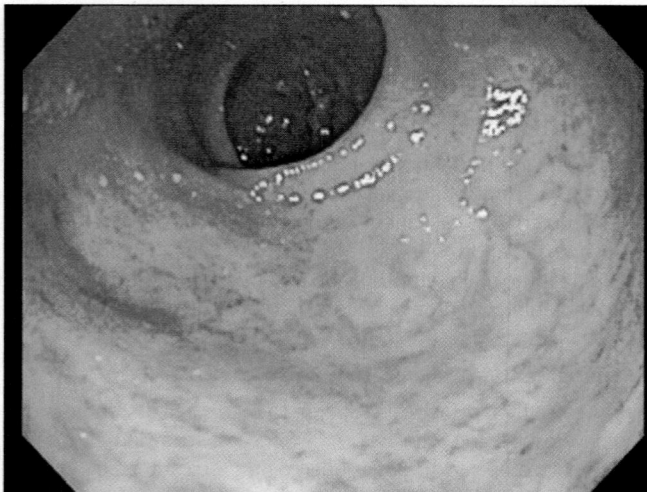

Figure 161-10 *Chronic radiation proctitis.* (Reproduced, with permission, from Greenberger N, Blumberg R, Burakoff R. *Current Diagnosis & Treatment: Gastroenterology, Hepatology, and Endoscopy.* New York, NY: McGraw-Hill; 2008. Plate 73.)

CHAPTER 162

Small Bowel Disorders

Anne C. Travis, MD, MSc
John R. Saltzman, MD

Key Clinical Questions

Malabsorption and Celiac Disease

1 Does this patient have malabsorption?

2 Is the malabsorption due to celiac disease?

3 What other diseases need to be considered?

4 What are the consequences of malabsorption?

5 How is malabsorption managed?

Small Bowel Obstruction

1 How do patients present with small bowel obstruction?

2 When do patients with small bowel obstruction need to go to surgery and when can they be managed medically?

Small Bowel Ileus

1 How is small bowel ileus treated?

2 When can a patient resume oral intake?

Acute Mesenteric Ischemia

1 Does this patient have acute mesenteric ischemia?

2 How does mesenteric ischemia differ from colonic ischemia?

3 Is emergent surgery necessary?

MALABSORPTION AND CELIAC DISEASE

■ EPIDIEMIOLOGY

Numerous causes lead to malabsorption and maldigestion, ranging from the common to the obscure. Causes of malabsorption and maldigestion include celiac disease, small bowel bacterial overgrowth, Crohn disease with small bowel involvement, chronic pancreatitis, short bowel syndrome, protein losing enteropathy, intestinal lymphangiectasias, amyloid, small bowel lymphoma, eosinophilic gastroenteritis, common variable immunodeficiency, lactose intolerance and other disaccharidase deficiencies, and Zollinger-Ellison syndrome (**Table 162-1**).

Lactose intolerance is a common cause of maldigestion. It is present in 7% to 20% of Caucasian adults, 50% of Hispanics, 65% to 75% of African Americans, and 90% of some East Asian populations. Celiac disease is most commonly seen in whites of northern European ancestry. In a large screening study from the United States, the prevalence of celiac disease in average risk individuals was 1:133. The prevalence was highest in first-degree relatives of a patient with celiac disease (1:22). Other disorders, such as primary intestinal lymphangiectasias, occur so rarely that it is difficult to estimate their true prevalence.

■ RISK STRATIFICATION

While generally managed as outpatients, patients with severe malnutrition or dehydration may need admission for nutritional support, volume repletion, and to correct electrolyte abnormalities. Significant weight loss (>10%) is associated with increased morbidity and mortality and should be treated aggressively.

■ EVALUATION

Malabsorption should be suspected in patients with weight loss, diarrhea, anorexia, flatulence, borborygmi, and/or greasy, foul smelling, voluminous pale stools. Patients may also have symptoms related to specific micronutrient deficiencies (**Table 162-2**). Some patients, however, are asymptomatic.

History

Taking a comprehensive history is the first step in diagnosing malabsorption. In addition to eliciting symptoms that are suggestive of malabsorption, the history can also help identify possible causes of malabsorption (eg, short bowel syndrome in a patient who has undergone a partial small bowel resection or chronic pancreatitis in a patient with a history of recurrent pancreatitis), as well as guide further testing. Conditions associated with celiac disease include dermatitis herpetiformis, diabetes mellitus, selective IgA deficiency, Down syndrome, liver disease, and thyroid disease.

Physical exam

The physical examination may give clues about underlying conditions that predispose to malabsorption, such as an abdominal scar in the case of a patient who has had a small bowel resection. The examination may also show evidence of nutritional deficiencies, such as pallor in the setting of anemia and neurologic abnormalities in the setting of vitamin B12 deficiency (Table 162-2).

TABLE 162-1 Disorders Associated with Malabsorption

Disorder	Affected Nutrient(s)	Mechanism(s)
Chronic pancreatitis	Fat	Lipase and colipase deficiencies
	Carbohydrate	Pancreatic amylase deficiency
	Protein	Protease deficiencies
Cystic fibrosis	Protein	Impaired protease excretion
Zollinger-Ellison syndrome	Fat, protein	Digestive enzyme inactivation
Cirrhosis	Fat, fat-soluble vitamins	Decreased bile salt production
Chronic cholestasis	Fat, fat-soluble vitamins	Impaired bile salt secretion
Bacterial overgrowth	Fat, fat-soluble vitamins	Bile salt deconjugation
	Carbohydrate	Damage to brush border enzymes
	Protein, carbohydrate, vitamin B12	Consumption of nutrients by bacteria
Lactose intolerance	Lactose	Lactase deficiency
Celiac disease, tropical sprue, common variable immunodeficiency	Carbohydrate	Decreased brush border enzyme activity due to villous damage
	Carbohydrate, protein, fat	Decreased absorptive surface area
Short bowel syndrome	Fat, carbohydrate, protein, vitamin B12	Decreased absorptive surface area
Pernicious anemia	Vitamin B12	Impaired production of intrinsic factor
Ileal disease (eg, Crohn, lymphoma, amyloid)	Vitamin B12	Decreased absorptive surface
Intestinal lymphangiectasia	Fat, fat-soluble vitamins	Impaired transport into lymphatics

TABLE 162-2 Symptoms and Laboratory Abnormalities Associated with Nutrient Deficiencies

Nutrient	Symptoms of Malabsorption	Laboratory Abnormalities
Fat	Pale, voluminous stool	Steatorrhea
	Diarrhea without flatulence	Stool fat >6 g/d on diet of 100 gm of fat/d
Carbohydrates	Watery diarrhea	Acidic stool
	Flatulence	Increased stool osmotic gap
	Dairy intolerance	
Protein	Edema	Hypoalbuminemia
	Muscle atrophy	Hypoproteinemia
	Amenorrhea	
Vitamin B12	Fatigue	Macrocytic anemia
	Dyspnea on exertion	Low serum B12 level
	Pallor	Elevated homocysteine and methylmalonic acid
	Ataxia	
	Paresthesias	
	Loss of vibration and position sense	
Folate	Fatigue	Macrocytic anemia
	Dyspnea on exertion	Decreased serum and red blood cell folate
	Pallor	Elevated homocysteine
Iron	Fatigue	Microcytic anemia
	Dyspnea on exertion	Low serum iron and ferritin
	Pallor	Increased total iron binding capacity
	Glossitis	
	Pagophagia (ice consumption)	
Calcium and vitamin D	Paresthesias	Hypocalcemia
	Tetany	Increased alkaline phosphatase
	Pathologic fractures	Low vitamin D
	Positive Chvostec and Trousseau signs	Low bone density
Vitamin A	Follicular hyperkeratosis	Decreased serum carotene
	Night blindness	
B Vitamins	Chelosis	Decreased serum levels
	Painless glossitis	
	Acrodermatitis	
	Angular stomatitis	
Vitamin K	Hematomas	Prolonged prothrombin time
	Bleeding disorders	Decreased vitamin K dependent clotting factors (II, VII, IX, X)

Laboratory evaluation

Various routine laboratory tests may suggest malabsorption (**Table 162-3**). To test for fat malabsorption, the initial test often obtained is a Sudan stain of the stool. This test will identify more than 90% of patients with clinically significant steatorrhea. However, its overall sensitivity and reliability are limited by variability in the performance and interpretation of the test. If fat malabsorption is suspected, a 72-hour fecal fat determination serves as the gold standard. Normal individuals will absorb 94% of the fat that is ingested. The stool should be collected and refrigerated for 72 hours with the patient on a 100 g of fat per day diet. Excretion of more than 6 g of fat is abnormal, though values up to 14 g/d have been seen in volunteers in whom diarrhea was induced and in patients with a stool weight of greater than 1000 g/d (normal is <200 g/d). Patients with true steatorrhea typically have fecal fat excretion of more than 20 g of fat per day.

While testing for protein malabsorption is not generally performed, enteral protein loss can be demonstrated by measuring alpha-1 antitrypsin clearance. In this test, stool is collected for 24 hours, along with a serum measurement of alpha-1 antitrypsin. Clearance is calculated by dividing the product of the fecal alpha-1 antitrypsin and the stool volume by the serum concentration of alpha-1 antitrypsin. In protein losing enteropathy, the value is typically greater than 100 mg/mL.

Laboratory testing may be particularly useful in the evaluation of celiac disease. In addition to nonspecific findings, such as iron

TABLE 162-3 Laboratory Abnormalities in Malabsorption

Decreased	Increased
Hemoglobin, iron, ferritin, total iron binding capacity	Urine oxalate
Folate (serum or red blood cell)	Prothrombin time
Vitamin B12	Stool fat
Calcium	
Magnesium	
Cholesterol	
Carotene	
Albumin	

deficiency, specific tests for celiac disease include antibodies to tissue transglutaminase (anti-TTG), which are highly sensitive and specific (95% and 94%, respectively). Tests can detect both IgA and IgG individually, which is important, since celiac is associated with selective IgA deficiency.

If celiac disease is suspected, serologic testing should be obtained for anti-TTG (with testing to confirm normal IgA levels if the suspicion for celiac disease is >5%). If IgA levels are low, IgG-based testing for anti-TTG or antigliadin antibodies should be obtained. An IgA endomysial assay is highly specific, but only moderately sensitive for detecting celiac disease in untreated patients, and will frequently be falsely negative in patients with celiac disease who are on a gluten free diet. Antigliadin antibody testing has only moderate sensitivity and specificity and the positive predictive value in a general population is poor.

PRACTICE POINT

- In the diagnosis of celiac disease, anti-TTG are highly sensitive and specific (95% and 94%, respectively). Celiac disease is associated with selective anti-TTG IgA deficiency. Antigliaden antibodies have poor sensitivity and specificity for celiac disease.

Endoscopic evaluation

Upper endoscopy

Some causes of malabsorption will be apparent on upper endoscopy. In the case of celiac disease, the duodenal mucosa may appear scalloped with a mosaic pattern and decreased duodenal folds (**Figure 162-1**). In Crohn disease, the mucosa may have a cobblestone appearance (see Chapter 164 [Inflammatory Bowel Disease]). Biopsies should always be obtained, as the findings may be subtle and not discernable to the endoscopist. Biopsies in celiac disease will demonstrate villous blunting with crypt elongation and an increase in intraepithelial lymphocytes. However, not all villous blunting is due to celiac disease. Other conditions that may result in villous blunting include bacterial overgrowth, common variable immunodeficiency, autoimmune enteropathy, Crohn disease, eosinophilic gastroenteritis, giardiasis, lymphoma, peptic duodenitis, gastroenteritis, tropical sprue, Zollinger-Ellison syndrome, and other immunodeficiency states.

Colonoscopy

Colonoscopy with intubation and biopsy of the terminal ileum may aid in making a diagnosis of Crohn disease. Additionally, random biopsies obtained from the colon may help to exclude alternative diagnoses, such as microscopic colitis.

Wireless capsule endoscopy

An advantage of wireless capsule endoscopy over standard endoscopy is that it allows for visualization of the entire small bowel. While generally not required to make a diagnosis of celiac disease (which typically involves the proximal small bowel), the procedure can be helpful in diagnosing other small bowel disorders with mucosal involvement, such as Crohn disease and lymphoma. It is also useful in patients with known celiac disease who are not responding to a gluten free diet. In these patients, considerations include inadvertent gluten ingestion, enteropathy associated T-cell lymphoma, ulcerative jejunitis and refractory celiac disease (ie, celiac disease that does not respond to strict gluten restriction). A disadvantage of wireless capsule endoscopy is that it does not allow for biopsies to be obtained. Additionally, it is contraindicated in patients with suspected small bowel obstructions.

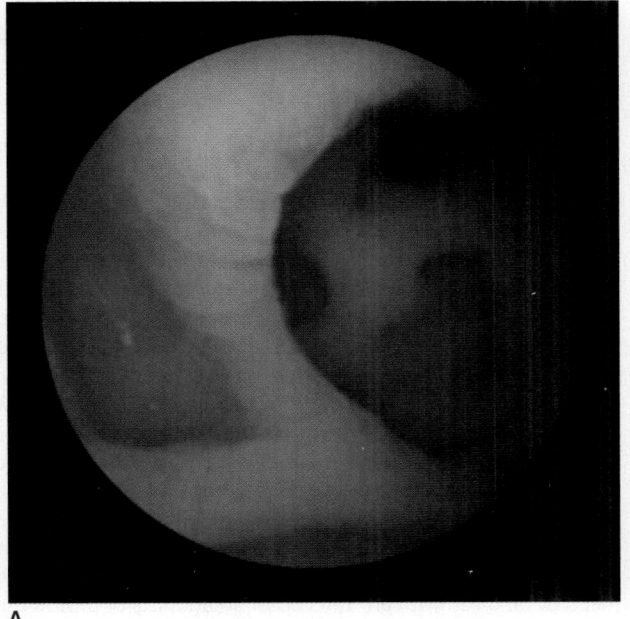
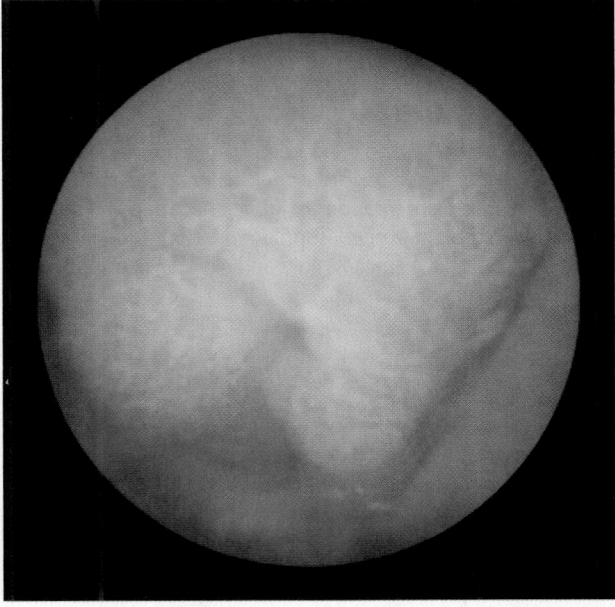

A   B

Figure 162-1 *Celiac disease. (A) Scalloping of the mucosa. (B) Mosaic mucosal pattern.*

Endoscopic retrograde cholangiopancreatography (ERCP) and endoscopic ultrasound (EUS)

Endoscopic retrograde cholangiopancreatography and EUS are sometimes employed to help make a diagnosis of chronic pancreatitis. Findings on ERCP include a dilated, irregular pancreatic duct and stones within the pancreatic duct. However, a normal ERCP does not exclude the diagnosis of chronic pancreatitis. Findings on EUS include both parenchymal and ductal abnormalities. The parenchymal abnormalities of chronic pancreatitis seen on EUS include hyperechoic (white) foci and strands, lobularity, atrophy, cysts, and calcifications. The ductal changes include ductal dilation, irregularity, visible side branches, hyperechoic walls, and pancreatic duct stones. However, the most sensitive finding for chronic pancreatitis is pancreatic function testing, with a reported sensitivity of 80% to 90%. At the time of endoscopy, samples of pancreatic juice are obtained from the duodenum following secretin stimulation. In the setting of chronic pancreatitis, the bicarbonate concentration will be low.

Radiologic evaluation

Radiologic testing has only limited value in the evaluation of malabsorption. Small bowel barium studies may show small bowel diverticula that can be associated with small bowel bacterial overgrowth, or mucosal disease that is not easily reached endoscopically (though capsule endoscopy is superior to small bowel follow-through [SBFT] for detecting mucosal disease). Computed tomography (CT) and magnetic resonance cholangiopancreatography (MRCP) may aid in the diagnosis of chronic pancreatitis.

Breath testing

Bacterial fermentation of undigested carbohydrates is the basis for breath testing. The fermentation results in increases in breath hydrogen, or in the elaboration of radiolabeled carbon dioxide. The tests commonly help diagnose bacterial overgrowth (in which case bacteria digest the carbohydrates within the small bowel) and lactose intolerance. Tests also exist for fructose, sucrose, and isomaltose malabsorption.

■ INPATIENT MANAGEMENT

Treatment of malabsorption is aimed at correcting nutritional deficiencies and, when possible, correcting the underlying disorder resulting in malabsorption (eg, antibiotic treatment for bacterial overgrowth). Consultation with a dietician is frequently helpful in managing patients with malabsorption. In complicated cases, however, a physician who specializes in nutrition support should be consulted. Patients with significant weight loss (>10%) should be treated aggressively and may need total parenteral nutrition. Vitamin and mineral deficiencies should be corrected if present. Typically, oral supplementation is sufficient. Patients with significant steatorrhea may need supplementation with fat-soluble vitamins (A, D, E, and K). Similarly, fluid and electrolyte abnormalities should be corrected if present.

Agents that may be helpful in controlling diarrhea include loperamide, diphenoxylate with atropine, deodorized tincture of opium, and bile acid binding agents such as cholestyramine (see Chapter 82 [Diarrhea]).

■ POSTACUTE CARE

Patients with celiac disease need to avoid all gluten-containing foods. Patients should receive counseling from a nutritionist to help them understand what foods to avoid. In the case of celiac disease, some patients believe they are following a gluten free diet because they are avoiding bread products, not realizing that gluten is present

TABLE 162-4 Sources of Gluten

Grains/Flours Containing Gluten	Foods Easier to Identify as Containing Gluten	Foods and Products That May Contain Hidden Gluten
Barley	Biscuits	Baked beans
Bulgur	Bread and rolls	Blue cheese
Farina	Cakes	Bran
Graham flour	Cereal	Chutney
Kamut	Communion wafers	Curry powder
Matzo	Cookies	Dry mustard powder
Oats*	Couscous	Gravy powders
Rye	Malted beverages	Hydrolyzed vegetable protein
Seitan	Muffins	Imitation bacon
Semolina	Pancakes	Imitation crab meat
Spelt	Pasta	Inexpensive chocolate
Triticale	Pastries and pie crust	Instant coffee
Wheat	Pizza	Licorice
Wheat germ	Pretzels	Lipstick
Wheat grass	Scones	Luncheon meat
	Stuffing	Malt vinegar
	Yorkshire pudding	Marinades
		Meat and fish pastes
		Meat loaf
		Monosodium glutamate
		Pickles
		Potato chips
		Salad dressing
		Sausages
		Self basting turkeys
		Soups/broths
		Soy sauce
		Stock cubes
		Supplements and pills
		Toothpaste
		White pepper

*May be contaminated with gluten.

in numerous other foods and products (eg, soy sauce, soups, lunch meats, some toothpastes) (**Table 162-4**).

For patients with isolated carbohydrate maldigestions (such as lactose intolerance), foods containing the offending carbohydrate should be avoided. Additionally, patients with celiac disease or bacterial overgrowth will often have lactose intolerance until their villi return to normal, and therefore should minimize intake of lactose-containing food products until adequately treated. Patients with steatorrhea should restrict their intake of long-chain fatty acids to below 40 g/d. Some patients may require supplementation with medium-chain triglycerides to maintain adequate caloric intake.

In the case of chronic pancreatitis, patients should follow a low-fat diet and receive pancreatic enzyme supplements. A typical dose is 30,000 IU of pancreatic lipase per meal. Some pancreatic enzyme supplements are enteric coated. Because pancreatic enzymes are inactivated at an acidic pH, non-enteric coated formulations need to be given with an H_2-receptor antagonists or proton pump inhibitor.

DISCHARGE CHECKLIST

- Fluid and electrolyte disorders have been corrected.
- Vitamin and mineral deficiencies have been addressed.
- Diarrhea has resolved.
- The patient is able to take adequate nutrition orally or arrangements have been made for outpatient parenteral nutrition.
- Specific treatments have been initiated if appropriate (eg, antibiotics for bacterial overgrowth or pancreatic enzyme supplements for chronic pancreatitis).
- The patient has been educated about and understands any necessary dietary restrictions.

SMALL BOWEL OBSTRUCTION

■ EPIDEMIOLOGY

Small bowel obstructions account for 15% of emergency admissions for abdominal pain (more than 300,000 hospitalizations per year in the United States). Mortality rates are significant, with an estimated 30,000 deaths per year.

Small bowel obstructions can be due to mechanical causes (eg, adhesions) or may be functional (pseudo-obstruction). In the case of mechanical obstructions, clinicians must differentiate between complete obstructions and partial obstructions, as the former generally require urgent surgical treatment, whereas the latter may be managed medically.

Adhesions

In adults, adhesions are responsible for 75% of SBOs, and the incidence of SBO from adhesions has increased over time due to an increasing number of laparotomies and laparoscopies. Approximately 5% of abdominopelvic surgeries are complicated by SBOs, with rates of up to 10% for colorectal surgery. The risk of SBO from adhesions is highest in the first few years following surgery, but can occur decades later.

PRACTICE POINT

- Approximately 5% of abdominopelvic surgeries are complicated by SBOs, with rates of up to 10% for colorectal surgery. The risk of SBO from adhesions is highest in the first few years following surgery, but may occur decades later.

Hernias

Hernias are another common cause of SBOs. Previously, hernias accounted for 30% of SBOs, but the proportion of SBOs due to hernias has decreased to 15% because of an increase in the rate of prophylactic herniorraphy. Hernias can be external (femoral, inguinal, midventral, periumbilical, and incisional hernias) or internal. Internal hernias can be subdivided further into congenital (obturator, paraduodenal, transmesenteric, and transomental hernias) or acquired (due to surgery).

Tumors

Tumors account for 5% to 10% of SBOs. The most common mechanism is extrinsic small bowel compression by gastrointestinal (GI) or gynecologic malignancies (especially colon and ovarian cancer). Small bowel cancer is a much less common cause.

Other causes

Other causes of SBOs occur much less frequently and include strictures (due to small bowel Crohn disease, medications such as nonsteroidal anti-inflammatory drugs, radiation enteritis, or ischemia), gallstone ileus, phytobezoars, foreign bodies, intussusception, and infection (peritoneal tuberculosis, actinomycosis, and enteric parasites). In children, common causes of SBOs include intussusception, intestinal atresia, and meconium ileus.

■ RISK STRATIFICATION

All patients with suspected SBO should be admitted to the hospital. Patients with confirmed or highly suspected complete obstruction should be admitted to a surgical team, while patients with a partial obstruction that has a reasonable likelihood of resolving with medical management alone, may be admitted to a hospital medicine or internal medicine team with surgical consultation. Failure to pass flatus is suggestive of a complete small bowel obstruction, whereas rigors, high fever, or systemic toxicity suggest possible intestinal necrosis or peroration. Patients with partial obstructions may not have typical presentations.

Patients with SBOs will often complain of colicky abdominal pain, nausea and vomiting, abdominal distension, and progressive obstipation. The pain is frequently sharp with a sudden onset. As the bowel fatigues, the pain may diminish. In addition, vomiting may temporarily relieve the pain by decompressing the distended bowel. Once ischemia or perforation develops, the pain becomes more severe and constant. Since closed-loop obstructions may be associated with mesenteric ischemia, the pain in these cases may be out of proportion to the examination (see section on mesenteric ischemia, below).

Patients with proximal obstructions typically complain of epigastric pain that occurs every 3 to 4 minutes. They also frequently have associated bilious emesis. By contrast, distal obstructions typically result in periumbilical pain that occurs every 15 to 20 minutes. Feculent emesis may also occur with distal obstructions, though it is infrequent.

Small bowel obstructions are complicated by strangulation in 30% of cases and necrosis in 15%. Intestinal ischemia may result in lactic acidosis, a marked leukocytosis with a left-shift, and hyperamylasemia. Patients with strangulation are at much higher risk for mortality (up to 31%) compared with patients who have a simple mechanical obstruction. Postoperative morbidity is 23% and mortality is 5%. Old age, comorbidities, nonviable strangulated bowel, and a delay in surgery are risk factors for mortality.

■ EVALUATION

History

In addition to determining if patients have a prior history of SBO, clinicians should inquire about conditions that predispose to SBO, such as a history of abdominal surgery, abdominal or pelvic radiation, abdominal cancer, symptoms of hernias, inflammatory bowel disease, or pelvic inflammatory disease. Clinicians should inquire of female patients about the timing of their last menstrual period.

Physical examination

While findings will vary based on the degree of obstruction, in severe cases patients appear acutely ill, restless, and are febrile. Signs suggestive of intravascular volume depletion may be present, including tachycardia, orthostatic hypotension, dry mucous membranes, and poor skin turgor. The abdomen is moderately distended in the case of proximal obstruction, whereas it may be severely distended with distal obstruction. Bowel sounds are high-pitched and hyperactive initially, with audible rushes or borborygmi that coincide with episodes of abdominal pain. As time progresses, the bowel sounds become progressively hypoactive and softer, eventually disappearing as a result of bowel fatigue. On percussion tympani may be present. Peritoneal signs (eg, rebound tenderness, guarding) are generally absent, unless necrosis or perforation has occurred.

Signs that may point to a possible etiology for the obstruction include jaundice in the case of obstruction due to a pancreatobiliary malignancy or gallstone ileus. Other signs of malignancy include a palpable abdominal mass, hepatomegaly, splenomegaly, and lymphadenopathy. Abdominal scars suggest possible adhesions, whereas external hernias should be examined for signs of incarceration. A rectal examination should be performed to rule out fecal impaction or a rectal malignancy.

Laboratory testing

Laboratory testing is generally nonspecific. Third-spacing of fluids may lead to electrolyte imbalances, azotemia, and hemoconcentration. Intestinal ischemia may result in lactic acidosis. Other signs of possible ischemia include a marked leukocytosis with a left-shift and hyperamylasemia. However, laboratory findings of ischemia may develop late, so their absence should not be seen as an indication of adequate perfusion. Because surgery may be indicated, a coagulation profile as well as platelet count should be obtained. Women of childbearing potential should have a serum pregnancy test.

Radiographic evaluation

Radiologic examination significantly aids the diagnosis of SBO since the physical examination and laboratory findings are nonspecific. A plain upright and supine abdominal x-ray is diagnostic in 50% to 70% of cases. The x-ray reveals a dilated, gas-filled proximal small bowel, with collapsed, gasless small bowel distal to the obstruction (**Figure 162-2**). The finding of a transition zone is highly specific for an SBO, but has poor sensitivity. Gas may not be present in cases of a closed-loop obstruction, resulting in a normal x-ray. The accuracy of plain films is highly dependent upon the experience of the radiologist interpreting the study.

PRACTICE POINT

- A plain upright and supine abdominal x-ray is diagnostic in 50% to 70% of SBO cases. The x-ray reveals a dilated, gas-filled proximal small bowel, with collapsed, gasless small bowel distal to the obstruction. The finding of a transition zone is highly specific for an SBO, but has poor sensitivity.

In cases where an x-ray is inconclusive, additional imaging is required, typically with abdominal computed tomography (CT) or abdominal magnetic resonance imaging (MRI). Other options include abdominal ultrasound and small bowel follow-through (SBFT). While abdominal ultrasound is as sensitive as an x-ray, with higher specificity, it is infrequently used for suspected SBO due to the availability of more accurate tests.

In patients with suspected partial SBOs, a small bowel follow-through may provide prognostic information, changing the diagnosis in about half of cases. Water-soluble contrast is given and followed through the small bowel with serial x-rays. The presence of contrast within the colon is highly sensitive (97%) and specific (96%) for predicting resolution without surgery. The disadvantages of SBFT include the time required for completion of the test and the lack of mucosal detail due to dilution of the contrast in the fluid-filled small bowel.

Abdominal CT allows for rapid and accurate diagnosis (**Figure 162-3**). Like SBFT, the presence of contrast in the colon suggests a partial SBO, with a sensitivity of 92% and a specificity of 93% for diagnosing a complete SBO. When intravenous contrast is used, CT can help identify the cause of the SBO, diagnose strangulation, and identify other pathology that may mimic an SBO (eg, superior mesenteric artery [SMA] or vein thrombosis causing an ileus). Computed tomography is 60% sensitive for identifying a closed-loop obstruction. Where available, CT enteroclysis or multidetector row CT improves the accuracy in identifying the cause of SBO.

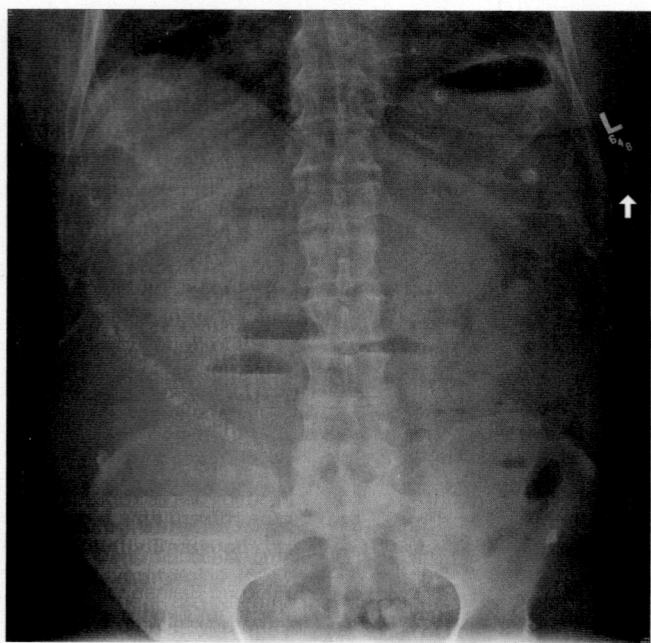

Figure 162-2 *Upright abdominal radiograph of small bowel obstruction (SBO). Eighty-seven-year-old man with early SBO from adhesions due to prior surgery.*

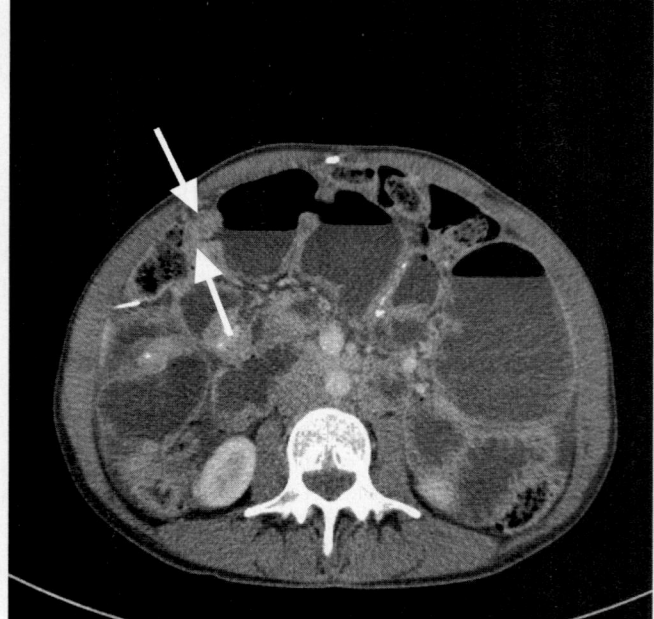

Figure 162-3 *Computed tomography (CT) image of small bowel obstruction (SBO). Computed tomography shows the transition point (arrows) of an SBO in a 49-year-old woman with metastatic ovarian cancer.*

Magnetic resonance imaging with T2-weighted images is more accurate than contrast-enhanced helical CT for identifying the point of obstruction (96% vs 93%) and in identifying the cause (88% vs 57%). Magnetic resonance imaging enterography is another alternative for diagnosing SBO.

Wireless capsule endoscopy is contraindicated in patients with suspected SBO (partial or complete) because of a very high risk of capsule retention at the site of obstruction.

■ DIFFERENTIAL DIAGNOSIS

Nonobstructive intestinal motility disorders (eg, paralytic ileus, intestinal pseudo-obstruction) should be considered in patients suspected of having an SBO (see section on small bowel ileus, below). Paralytic ileus is present to some degree in most patients who have undergone open abdominal surgery and may be exacerbated by electrolyte disorders and pain medications.

■ INPATIENT MANAGEMENT

Initial treatment in all cases of SBO includes aggressive intravenous volume repletion and bowel rest. Liberal use of antiemetics can provide symptomatic relief to patients with nausea and vomiting.

Nasogastric tube (NGT) decompression is used to clear gastric contents, decompress the proximal small bowel, and prevent aspiration. This may be done with a soft, lubricated 14 Fr tube. It is placed with the patient in an upright position. Ideally, the tip of the tube should be in the most dependent portion of the stomach. Once the tube is in proper position it should be taped to the nose, taking care to avoid pressure on the nares. The tube should then be placed on intermittent low wall suction and its output recorded. If the gastric aspirate is feculent, it is suggestive of a distal small bowel obstruction.

When the obstruction resolves (indicated by symptomatic improvement, low residual volumes of gastric aspirate, and resumption of the passage of stool and flatus), the tube can be removed and the patient's diet can be advanced, starting first with liquids. The rate at which the diet is advanced will depend upon the patient's tolerance of oral intake. If obstruction resolution is uncertain, the NGT can be clamped for 4 hours at a time. If the patient does not report nausea and the gastric residuals are less than 100 mL, the tube can be removed and the patient's diet advanced.

Conservative therapy will lead to resolution of a partial SBO in about 90% of cases. Any patients being managed conservatively require serial examinations to look for evidence of worsening obstruction. Surgery is required emergently if there is evidence of complete obstruction, peritonitis, pneumatosis intestinalis, or strangulation. In addition, surgery is indicated in patients with partial SBOs who have not shown signs of improvement after 24 to 72 hours. Patients requiring surgery should receive preoperative antibiotic therapy to cover anaerobic and Gram-negative bacteria.

PRACTICE POINT

- Conservative therapy will lead to resolution of a partial SBO in about 90% of cases. Medically managed patients require serial abdominal examinations to look for evidence of worsening obstruction. Surgery is required emergently if there is evidence of complete obstruction, peritonitis, pneumatosis intestinalis, or strangulation. In addition, surgery is indicated in patients with partial SBOs who have not shown signs of clinical improvement after 24 to 48 hours.

During surgery, ischemic, necrotic, or poorly viable small bowel is resected. It is important that only viable small bowel be left to decrease the risk of an anastomotic leak, intra-abdominal abscess,

or chronic stricturing. Viable bowel should not be removed due to the risk of increased operative mortality and short bowel syndrome. Bowel viability can be assessed at the time of surgery by inspection, palpation, and the use of vital dyes and/or Doppler flowmetry. In some cases, a second-look laparotomy is performed 24 hours after the initial surgery to ensure that no ischemic bowel was left in place.

While most patients who require surgery undergo open laparotomy, laparoscopic approaches are occasionally appropriate (eg, for an incarcerated inguinal hernia).

■ POSTACUTE CARE

Patients who respond to conservative therapy should have their diet slowly advanced as tolerated.

■ DISCHARGE CHECKLIST

- Patient is free of pain, nausea, and vomiting
- Patient is taking in adequate oral nutrition and hydration
- Electrolyte abnormalities have been corrected
- Patient is passing stool and flatus

SMALL BOWEL ILEUS
■ EPIDEMIOLOGY

Postoperative ileus (POI) occurs commonly following both abdominal and nonabdominal surgery. It occurs almost universally after abdominal surgery, but also develops following major nonabdominal surgery, such as knee or hip arthroplasty (2.1%) and infrarenal endovascular aneurysm repair (3.9%). Normal gut function typically returns following surgery within 0 to 24 hours for the stomach, 24 to 48 hours for the small intestine, and 48 to 72 hours for the colon. More recent data suggest that the recovery of normal gut function may be shorter, with gastric and small intestinal activity returning to normal within hours of surgery, and the colon in 1 to 2 days. In some cases, however, prolonged (3-5 days) postoperative ileus results in increased pain, decreased mobility, and continued hospitalization.

PRACTICE POINT

- Normal gut function typically returns following surgery within 0 to 24 hours for the stomach, 24 to 48 hours for the small intestine, and 48 to 72 hours for the colon. In some cases, postoperative ileus is prolonged (3-5 days), resulting in increased pain, decreased mobility, and prolonged hospitalization.

Multiple factors predispose to prolonged postoperative ileus (**Table 162-5**).

■ RISK STRATIFICATION

The primary element in risk stratification is to rule out small bowel obstruction (SBO; see section on small bowel obstruction, above). Many of the diagnostic tests employed in the evaluation of POI are aimed at ruling out small bowel obstruction. The signs and symptoms can be similar, which can make differentiation difficult.

■ EVALUATION
History and physical examination

Postoperative ileus often presents with nausea and/or vomiting; abdominal distension and bloating; diffuse, persistent abdominal pain; inability to pass flatus; and inability to tolerate oral intake.

The history should be reviewed to look for medical illnesses, medications, and prior surgeries that could predispose to POI or SBO. Patients with POI typically have abdominal distension along

TABLE 162-5 Factors that Predispose to Prolonged Postoperative Ileus

Abdominal surgery
Mechanical ventilation
Increased intracranial pressure
Burns
Infections/sepsis
Abdominal compartment syndrome
Volume overload
Hypotension
Use of vasoactive drugs
Electrolyte disorders
Hypokalemia
Hyponatremia
Hypomagnesemia
Hypermagnesemia
Hypocalcemia
Hypercalcemia
Use of opioids
Uremia
Diabetic ketoacidosis
Hypoparathyroidism

with mild, poorly localized abdominal pain. Patients may report the lack of passage of flatus or stool, intolerance of oral intake, or nausea and vomiting. Because many patients with POI are critically ill, they may be unable to communicate their symptoms.

The examination may reveal abdominal distension and tympani, hypoactive or absent bowel sounds, and mild, diffuse abdominal tenderness. Signs of volume depletion (tachycardia, orthostatic hypotension, dry mucous membranes) may also be present.

Patients with postoperative ileus typically develop symptoms immediately after surgery, whereas patients with SBO develop symptoms at variable times after surgery. Additionally, patients with SBO tend to have more severe symptoms, progress more rapidly, and appear more ill overall.

Laboratory evaluation

Laboratory testing may identify contributing factors such as electrolyte disturbances (sodium, potassium, magnesium, calcium) or evidence of metabolic acidosis suggesting alternative diagnoses (mainly SBO). An elevated white blood cell count should raise suspicion for a possible perforation, whereas evidence of hemoconcentration (elevated hematocrit, elevated blood urea nitrogen, elevated creatinine) suggests volume depletion.

Radiographic evaluation

Plain abdominal radiographs often demonstrate dilated loops of small bowel. While air-fluid levels are typically thought of as signs of SBO, they can also be seen in patients with postoperative ileus. If the diagnosis remains in question after obtaining the history, performing a physical examination, and obtaining plain abdominal radiographs, an abdominal computed tomographic scan can distinguish postoperative ileus from a complete SBO, with sensitivity and specificity of 90% to 100%. Computed tomography is less reliable in distinguishing postoperative ileus from a partial SBO. Upper GI contrast studies with water-soluble radio-opaque contrast can further elucidate the diagnosis if it is still uncertain after CT.

■ DIFFERENTIAL DIAGNOSIS

Small bowel obstruction occurs in up to 1% of patients within 30 days of abdominal surgery. Acute colonic pseudo-obstruction (Ogilvie syndrome) is often seen following surgery.

■ INPATIENT MANAGEMENT

Initial management of postoperative ileus is conservative and largely supportive. Patients should receive intravenous fluids and correction of any electrolyte abnormalities. Underlying conditions that may be contributing should be sought and treated (eg, antibiotics for sepsis), and drugs that promote GI dysmotility should be discontinued if possible.

Traditionally, oral intake was restricted until patients started passing flatus or stool. More recent studies, however, suggest that early enteral feeding is not only safe, but it also decreases the duration of POI and hospital stay. In cases of severe or protracted vomiting, a nasogastric tube may be required.

PRACTICE POINT

- In postoperative ileus, early enteral feeding should be employed as it decreases the duration of POI and hospital length of stay.

Peripheral opiate antagonists (eg, methylnaltrexone; available orally, subcutaneously, or intravenously) for the treatment of postoperative ileus block the peripheral antimotility effects of opioids without interfering with their analgesic effects. They act on the mu-opioid receptor and have limited to no ability to cross the blood-brain barrier.

Gum chewing may prevent prolonged postoperative ileus. Strategies for treating prolonged postoperative ileus with little or no supporting evidence for benefit include bran/fiber, metoclopramide, erythromycin, neostigmine, and early ambulation (though it has other benefits in the postoperative patient).

■ POSTACUTE CARE

When postoperative ileus is prolonged, patients may have compromised nutrition, leading to increased catabolism, poor wound healing, increased rates of infection, and the need for parenteral nutrition. Patients often will also have decreased mobility as a result of pain. Each of these factors may result in prolonged hospitalization. Additionally, these patients have increased risk of pulmonary complications and nosocomial infections.

■ DISCHARGE CHECKLIST

- Patient is free of pain, nausea, and vomiting
- Patient is taking in adequate oral nutrition and hydration
- Electrolyte abnormalities have been corrected
- Patient is passing stool and flatus

ACUTE MESENTERIC ISCHEMIA
■ EPIDEMIOLOGY

Acute mesenteric ischemia is an uncommon, but frequently catastrophic, vascular emergency. In the United States, it occurs in 1 in 1000 patients admitted to acute care hospitals, but its incidence is increasing as the population ages. Even with surgical intervention, it has a high mortality rate, ranging from 60% to 70%. Recognizing acute mesenteric ischemia quickly is critical, as delays in diagnosis and intervention portend a poor outcome.

Acute mesenteric ischemia occurs when prolonged reduction in the splanchnic blood flow occurs. There are four types of acute mesenteric ischemia, categorized based on their cause: arterial embolism, arterial thrombosis, nonocclusive, and venous thrombosis. The most common cause is arterial embolism, which accounts for 50% of cases, a third of which will have a history of a prior embolic event. The emboli most commonly originate from a cardiac source. Risk factors for developing the mural thrombi that embolize to the mesenteric arteries include myocardial ischemia/infarction, atrial arrhythmias (specifically atrial fibrillation and atrial flutter), valvular disorders, cardiomyopathies, endocarditis, and ventricular aneurysms. A mesenteric artery embolus can also occur following coronary or cerebral angiography. Most emboli lodge in the superior mesenteric artery because of the angle from which it takes off from the aorta.

Arterial thrombosis accounts for 15% to 25% of acute mesenteric ischemia cases. Like arterial emboli, arterial thrombosis most commonly involves the SMA. Almost all cases occur in the setting of severe atherosclerotic disease. Patients with arterial thromboses often have developed collateral blood flow due to the slow progression of atherosclerosis. These patients therefore frequently tolerate obstruction of a major visceral artery. Ischemia or infarction occurs when there is occlusion of the last remaining major visceral artery or of an essential collateral artery. Because of this, the extent of ischemia or infarction is much more extensive than is seen with arterial embolization (duodenum to transverse colon).

Nonocclusive mesenteric ischemia is seen in 20% to 30% of cases and is poorly understood. It often occurs in the setting of decreased cardiac output with diffuse mesenteric vasoconstriction. Splanchnic vasoconstriction occurs in response to decreased cardiac output, hypotension, hypovolemia, and vasopressors. Intestinal hypoxia results from the low-flow state. While not all patients will have clear risk factors for nonocclusive mesenteric ischemia, some predisposing factors include age greater than 50 years, myocardial infarction, aortic insufficiency, congestive heart failure, cardiopulmonary bypass, renal disease, liver disease, and major cardiovascular or abdominal surgery.

Mesenteric venous thrombosis is the cause of acute mesenteric ischemia in 5% of cases. The majority are due to primary clotting disorders, though in 10% no cause is found. The thrombi typically originate in the venous arcades and propagate to the arcuate channels. Occlusion of the intramural vessels results in hemorrhagic infractions. The superior mesenteric vein is the most commonly involved vessel, whereas involvement of the inferior mesenteric vein is uncommon. Predisposing conditions include primary clotting disorders (up to 75% of cases) and a history of deep vein thrombosis, inflammatory bowel disease, right-sided heart failure, pancreatitis, malignancy, hepatosplenomegaly, hepatitis, recent abdominal surgery or infection, estrogen use, sickle cell disease, and polycythemia.

■ RISK STRATIFICATION

Diagnosis of acute mesenteric ischemia requires a high clinical suspicion, especially in patients with risk factors. Due to its high mortality, any patient with suspected mesenteric ischemia should be admitted to the hospital for prompt evaluation and treatment.

Survival in acute mesenteric ischemia depends on expediency of diagnosis. Diagnosis within 24 hours of symptom onset portends a 50% survival, while further delays can lead to less than 30% survival.

■ DIAGNOSIS

Clinical presentation

The presentation of acute mesenteric ischemia is variable, depending on the underlying cause. The classic description includes rapid onset of severe abdominal pain, often out of proportion to findings on physical examination. Some patients will also report forceful bowel evacuation coinciding with the onset of pain. However, in patients with mesenteric venous thrombosis, the onset of symptoms may be insidious, occurring over weeks to months. These patients may complain of nausea, vomiting, and nonspecific abdominal pain.

Delays in the diagnosis of acute mesenteric ischemia may occur due to the nonspecific clinical presentation. Patients frequently complain of severe abdominal pain, but have few objective clinical findings. Mental status changes occur commonly (~one-third of cases) in elderly patients with mesenteric ischemia.

In cases of arterial embolism, symptoms typically have a sudden onset, with patients often complaining of severe periumbilical abdominal pain associated with nausea, vomiting, and diarrhea, which may turn bloody. The sudden onset of symptoms occurs because these patients often lack developed collateral circulation. These patients classically have "pain out of proportion to examination." As ischemia and infarction progress, these patients can become dehydrated, with massive third-spacing of fluids. These patients may present with mental confusion, tachycardia, and ultimately circulatory collapse.

PRACTICE POINT

- Acute mesenteric ischemia due to arterial embolism presents with sudden onset severe periumbilical abdominal pain ("pain out of proportion to examination"), associated with nausea, vomiting, and diarrhea (sometimes bloody). As ischemia and infarction progress, patients may have massive third-spacing of fluids, mental confusion, tachycardia, and ultimately circulatory collapse.

The presentation of patients with arterial thrombosis is frequently subacute. In the case of patients with SMA thromboses, prodromal symptoms include postprandial pain, nausea, and weight loss. Once acute ischemia has occurred, however, these patients develop symptoms like those seen with arterial embolism.

The presentation of nonocclusive mesenteric ischemia can be particularly difficult to recognize, as many of these patients are elderly and critically ill prior to the onset of the ischemia, which may overshadow the signs of mesenteric ischemia. In patients who are intubated and sedated, the indication that mesenteric ischemia is present may be an unexplained worsening of their clinical status or a failure to improve as anticipated.

Mesenteric venous thrombosis, unlike arterial causes of acute mesenteric ischemia, typically presents late. One to two weeks after the onset, patients will complain of diffuse, nonspecific abdominal pain, anorexia, and diarrhea. Signs on examination include fever, abdominal distension, and hemoccult positive stool. These patients have fewer prodromal symptoms compared with those with arterial thrombosis. Additional findings include bloody ascites and third-spacing of fluid with dehydration and hypotension.

Regardless of the cause, once infarction has occurred, patients develop peritoneal signs, hemodynamic instability, sepsis, and multiorgan failure.

Laboratory evaluation

Laboratory findings do not generally aid in diagnosis, as the findings are nonspecific; patients with acute mesenteric ischemia may have normal laboratory values. Abnormalities may include leukocytosis with a left shift, hemoconcentration, and metabolic acidosis. Other laboratory abnormalities include elevated serum lactate, elevated serum amylase, elevated aspartate aminotransferase (AST), elevated phosphate, elevated potassium, elevated creatinine kinase-BB isoenzyme (but not total creatinine kinase), and elevated lactate dehydrogenase. Many of these laboratory abnormalities occur late, once infarction has occurred.

Radiographic evaluation

Plain abdominal radiographs may be normal in 25% of patients with early acute mesenteric ischemia. If abnormal, the findings, while nonspecific, may include thumb-printing, thickening of the bowel loops (<40%) or ileus. Pneumatosis intestinalis and air in the portal vein are late findings and associated with a poor prognosis. The primary role for plain radiographs is to exclude other causes for the patient's symptoms.

Abdominal computed tomography is frequently employed in the evaluation of patients with abdominal pain. Unfortunately, in the case of acute mesenteric ischemia, CT has poor sensitivity and specificity for making the diagnosis. The ability to make the diagnosis is increased if multidetector row CT angiography or MRI angiography are used. Computed tomography angiography is estimated to have a sensitivity of 94% for acute mesenteric ischemia, with a sensitivity of 95%. Computed tomography is generally preferred over MRI because it is widely available. Oral contrast should not be used for CT angiography because it can obscure visualization of the mesenteric vessels and bowel wall enhancement and may delay the diagnosis.

Findings on CT include focal or segmental bowel wall thickening, intestinal pneumatosis with portal vein gas, lack of enhancement of the arterial vasculature (due to arterial occlusion), and liver or splenic infarcts. Findings in patients with mesenteric venous thrombosis included venous filling defects or the absence of flow.

If the diagnosis remains in doubt despite CT or MRI angiography, conventional catheter-based arteriography should be performed. Angiography is the gold standard for diagnosing acute mesenteric ischemia but it is less sensitive than CT for detecting mesenteric venous thrombosis. Angiography in both anteroposterior and lateral views are needed to obtain adequate visualization. In cases of arterial emboli or thrombosis, findings include lack of visualization distal to the obstruction. In nonocclusive mesenteric ischemia, areas of narrowing and irregularity in the major arteries may be seen, with decreased or absent flow in the smaller vessels. In the case of mesenteric venous thrombosis, venous filling defects or absent flow may be seen during the venous phase of the examination.

■ DIFFERENTIAL DIAGNOSIS

The differential diagnosis for acute mesenteric ischemia is broad and includes gastrointestinal, gynecologic, pulmonary, and cardiovascular considerations (**Table 162-6**).

TABLE 162-6 Differential Diagnosis of Acute Mesenteric Ischemia

Gastrointestinal	Gynecologic	Cardiovascular
Cholangitis	Ectopic pregnancy	Abdominal angina
Cholecystitis	Ovarian torsion	Abdominal aortic aneurysm
Choledocholithiasis	**Pulmonary**	
Cholelithiasis	Pneumonia	Aortic dissection
Colonic obstruction	Pneumothorax	Myocardial infarction
Diverticulitis		**Other**
Gastric volvulus		Boerhaave syndrome
Ileus		
Intestinal perforation		Intra-abdominal abscess
Intestinal pseudoobstruction		Porphyria
Pancreatitis		Pyelonephritis
Small bowel obstruction		Sepsis
		Testicular torsion

- The gold standard for diagnosing acute mesenteric ischemia is angiography, though it is less sensitive than CT for detecting mesenteric venous thrombosis. CT angiography has a sensitivity of 94% and a specificity of 95% for diagnosing acute mesenteric ischemia. Findings on CT include focal or segmental bowel wall thickening, intestinal pneumatosis with portal vein gas, lack of enhancement of the arterial vasculature, and liver or splenic infarcts. Findings in patients with mesenteric venous thrombosis included venous filling defects or the absence of flow.

■ INPATIENT MANAGEMENT

Once the diagnosis is made, treatment should be initiated immediately. The goals of treatment are to resuscitate the patient, treat the underlying condition if possible, reduce vasospasm, prevent propagation of intravascular clotting, prevent infection, and minimize reperfusion injury.

Initial management

Management starts with administration of intravenous fluids and blood products. Crystalloid intravenous fluid volume replacement up to 100 mL/kg will support patients who may have significant third-spacing of fluid. A nasogastric tube should be placed for gastric decompression. Patients should receive broad-spectrum antibiotics immediately. In the absence of contraindications, intravenous heparin is indicated, with a goal activated partial thromboplastin time of twice the upper limit of normal. Long-term anticoagulation may be indicated, based on the etiology of the ischemia, other interventions performed, and whether the patient continues to have risk factors for recurrent mesenteric ischemia.

Vasoconstrictors and digitalis should be avoided since they can worsen mesenteric ischemia. If patients require pressor agents or inotropes in their management, low-dose dopamine, dobutamine, or milrinone affect mesenteric profusion less than the other agents, and may be considered.

Angiographic therapies

Patients undergoing angiography, both for diagnosis and for treatment, must be hemodynamically stabilized prior to the procedure, since mesenteric vasoconstriction is a normal response to hypotension or hypovolemia, potentially leading to a false-positive result in a patient who has not been adequately resuscitated. Angiography allows for the administration of intra-arterial vasodilators or thrombolytic agents, angioplasty, stent placement, and embolectomy. Papaverine is used to prevent vasoconstriction in both occlusive and nonocclusive acute mesenteric ischemia. The specific treatments employed will depend on the underlying cause of the ischemia. Consideration of angiographic therapies should be done in consultation with vascular surgery and interventional radiology.

Surgery

If intestinal infarction or perforation is suspected (based on clinical, laboratory, or radiographic findings) emergency laparotomy is required. Even in patients without infarction, surgery is often required. The exception is in patients with nonocclusive acute mesenteric ischemia, where patients are managed medically in the absence of infarction (treatment of underlying condition if possible, infusion of papaverine). The goal of surgery is to re-establish blood flow via revascularization (embolectomy, thrombectomy, endarterectomy, or bypass). Once revascularization has been performed, infarcted bowel is resected. Determining intestinal viability at the time of surgery may be difficult, and some patients will require a "second-look" laparotomy to ensure that all infarcted bowel was removed.

■ POSTACUTE CARE

Recurrence is not uncommon and carries with it a poor prognosis. Patients who undergo significant small bowel resections are at risk of developing short gut syndrome and could require long-term total parenteral nutrition or small bowel transplantation.

The approach to preventing recurrences of acute mesenteric ischemia depends upon the cause of the ischemia. For patients with mesenteric arterial emboli, treatment is typically aimed at preventing future emboli using an anticoagulant (eg, a nonvitamin K antagonist oral anticoagulant). An anticoagulant may also be used for patients with mesenteric venous thrombosis. In patients with mesenteric venous thrombosis, anticoagulation is typically continued for 6 months, but long-term treatment may be warranted in patients with coagulation disorders. Antiplatelet agents such as aspirin may help prevent recurrent acute mesenteric ischemia that is due to mesenteric arterial thrombosis or nonocclusive mesenteric ischemia, though data are limited.

■ DISCHARGE CHECKLIST

- Patient is free of pain.
- Patient is taking in adequate oral nutrition and hydration.
- Treatment with an antiplatelet agent or an anticoagulant has been initiated, if indicated.

SUGGESTED READINGS

Batke M, Cappell MS. Adynamic ileus and acute colonic pseudo-obstruction. *Med Clin N Am*. 2008;92:649-670.

Brandt LJ, Boley SJ. AGA technical review on intestinal ischemia. *Gastroenterol*. 2000;118:954-968.

Cappell MS, Batke M. Mechanical obstruction of the small bowel and colon. *Med Clin N Am*. 2008;92:575-597.

Eltarawy IG, Etman YM, Zenati M, et al. Acute mesenteric ischemia: the importance of early surgical consultation. *Am Surg*. 2009;75:212-219.

Hogenauer C, Hammer H. Maldigestion and Malabsorption. In: Feldman M, Friedman L, Brandt L, eds. *Sleisenger and Fordtran's Gastrointestinal and Liver Disease*, 9th ed. Philadelphia, PA: Saunders, 2010;1735-1768.

Kehlet H, Holte K. Review of postoperative ileus. *Am J Surg*. 2001;182:3S-10S.

Kumar S, Saar MG, Kamat PS. Mesenteric venous thrombosis. *N Engl J Med*. 2001;345:1683-1688.

Oldenburg WA, Lau LL, Rodenberg TJ, et al. Acute mesenteric ischemia: a clinical review. *Arch Intern Med*. 2004;164:1054-1062.

Rubio-Tapia A, Hill ID, Kelly CP, et al. ACG clinical guidelines: diagnosis and management of celiac disease. *Am J Gastroenterol*. 2013;108:656-676.

Short V, Herbert G, Perry R, et al. Chewing gum for postoperative recovery of gastrointestinal function. *Cochrane Database Syst Rev*. 2015;2:CD006506.

Zeinali F, Stulberg JJ, Delaney CP. Pharmacological management of postoperative ileus. *Can J Surg*. 2009;52:153-157.

Large Bowel Disorders

Mitchell S. Cappell, MD, PhD

Key Clinical Questions

❶ When should you suspect and how do you evaluate ischemic colitis?

❷ What medications should be avoided, if possible, in patients with suspected ischemic colitis, and in suspected colonic pseudo-obstruction?

❸ How does the presentation of acute appendicitis in the older adult differ from that of younger individuals?

❹ How do you evaluate and treat diverticulitis, colonic obstruction, and colonic pseudo-obstruction?

INTRODUCTION

Large bowel disorders (LBD) impose a substantial burden on Americans, accounting for more than 1% of all inpatient admissions, contributing as comorbidities to other hospitalizations, and resulting in expenditures of more than 30 billion dollars annually, which is likely to increase as the population ages. This chapter describes disorders of ischemic colitis, diverticulitis, acute appendicitis, colonic obstruction, and colonic pseudo-obstruction. Other disorders, including lower gastrointestinal bleeding, inflammatory bowel diseases, tumors and cancer of the colon, and diarrhea are described in chapters dedicated to those disorders. **Table 163-1** describes key diagnostic tests and therapeutic options for important large bowel disorders, while **Table 163-2** describes the colonoscopic findings.

COLONIC ANATOMY

The colon is a tubular structure approximately 30 to 40 cm in length at birth, but grows to nearly 150 cm in adulthood. It has a much larger diameter than that of the small bowel. The colon extends from small bowel at the ileocecal valve to terminate at the anal verge. The longitudinal muscle fibers coalesce around the colonic circumference to form three discrete bands called *teniae*. The colon is divided into cecum, ascending colon, hepatic flexure, transverse colon, splenic flexure, descending colon, sigmoid colon, and rectum. The first portion of the ascending colon, called the *cecum*, is a sacculated structure 6 to 8 cm in length and breadth that generally lies in the right iliac fossa and projects downward as a blind pouch below the entrance of the ileum. The large diameter of the cecum makes it particularly vulnerable to rupture from distal colonic obstruction. Its large diameter also provides ample space for cecal tumors to grow before producing colonic obstruction. The mobility of the cecum is normally restricted by a small mesocecum, but 10% to 20% of people lack this mesocecum and are thereby predisposed to cecal volvulus. The *vermiform appendix* is a blind, digitiform outpouching of the cecum that begins inferior to the ileocecal valve. The *ascending colon* extends about 20 cm along the right side of the peritoneal cavity from the cecum to the hepatic flexure. The colon turns medially and anteriorly at the hepatic flexure to emerge as the *transverse colon*, which drapes itself across the anterior abdomen for 40 to 50 cm between the hepatic and splenic flexures. This is the most mobile colonic segment. This segment may dip down into the pelvis in the upright posture. The temporary festooned arrangement of transverse colon can become entrenched by adhesions, such as adhesions after hysterectomy. Such adhesions can result in a technically difficult colonoscopy. The *descending colon*, about 30 cm in length, continues as the S-shaped *sigmoid colon* in the retroperitoneum. The colonic diameter is narrowest (2.5 cm) in the sigmoid colon. The sigmoid colon does not provide ample space to accommodate local tumors or strictures and therefore tumors or strictures of the sigmoid colon produce early obstruction. The shape, tortuosity, mobility, and spasticity of the sigmoid colon create challenges for the colonoscopist, as well as render it susceptible to volvulus.

Despite individual anatomic variations, the colon generally has a specific vascular arrangement. The *superior mesenteric artery* (SMA) in addition to supplying nearly the entire small intestine, supplies the entire right colon, including the cecum, ascending colon, hepatic flexure, and most of the transverse colon. The *inferior mesenteric*

TABLE 163-1 Key Diagnostic Tests and Therapies for Important Large Bowel Diseases in Hospitalized Patients

Disease or Disorder	Key Diagnostic Tests	Major Therapeutic Options
Lower gastrointestinal bleeding	Colonoscopy—localizes site and determines etiology of bleeding. Nuclear scintigraphy using radiolabeled erythrocytes—locates approximate site of bleeding. Mesenteric angiography—can determine site & cause if lesion is actively bleeding. CT enterography or capsule endoscopy—second-line tests if other tests are unrevealing.	Colonoscopy—injection, ablation, or mechanical therapy to stop the bleeding. Angiography—intra-arterial vasopressin infusion or gelfoam or coil embolization to stop the bleeding. Surgery—for ongoing bleeding refractory to colonoscopic or angiographic therapy.
Ischemic colitis	Colonoscopy with colonoscopic biopsies—highly sensitive and specific. Mesenteric angiography—can be diagnostic and therapeutic, test mandatory for involvement of major branches of superior mesenteric artery. Abdominal computed tomography—important to exclude other conditions and often helps suggest the diagnosis.	Medical therapy—usually supportive, including bowel rest, intravenous fluids, antibiotic therapy, and reversal of precipitating factors. Surgery—required for frankly infarcted bowel, colonic perforation, impending peritonitis, and sepsis refractory to antibiotic therapy.
Inflammatory bowel disease (IBD)	Blood tests—complete blood count, erythrocyte sedimentation rate (ESR) or C-reactive protein. Stool tests—for bacterial culture, fecal leukocytes, ova and parasites, C. difficile toxin. Abdominal computed tomography—helpful to suggest IBD and to diagnose alternative conditions. Colonoscopy—highly diagnostic in combination with colonic biopsies; examination of terminal ileum recommended for Crohn's disease.	General therapy—bowel rest, intravenous hydration, correct electrolyte disorders. Medications—typically first corticosteroids, consider biologic anti-tumor necrosis factor (TNF) alpha therapy, antibiotics for abscesses or fistulas. Surgery—for large or refractory abscesses, refractory toxic megacolon, severe disease refractory to medical therapy.
Diverticulitis	Abdominal computed tomography—radiologic test of choice for diagnosis and evaluating complications. Colonoscopy—avoided in the setting of acute diverticulitis.	Medical therapy—bowel rest, intravenous antibiotics, intravenous hydration. Percutaneous drainage—for large, walled-off abscess. Surgery—multiple recurrent attacks, advanced Hinchey stage III or IV disease, severe abscesses, refractoriness to medical therapy, colonic perforation.
Acute appendicitis	Abdominal computed tomography—inflamed, distended appendix that fails to fill with contrast or air, appendicolith, mural thickening, pericecal fluid collection, periappendiceal fat stranding. Abdominal ultrasound—valuable only in certain circumstances: pediatric patients, pregnant women, and thin adults.	Preoperative resuscitation—intravenous hydration, antibiotics, replete electrolytes. Surgery—either open or laparoscopic appendectomy.
Acute diarrhea	Stool studies—for bacterial culture and sensitivity, for ova and parasites, for C. difficile toxin, stool for lactoferrin or fecal leukocytes, stool for fecal occult blood. Abdominal CT—helpful to exclude other diseases and can help define extent of colitis. Colonoscopy—generally only indicated if stool studies do not reveal a cause and if patient is still having diarrhea despite medical therapy.	Supportive therapy—bowel rest, intravenous fluids, replete missing electrolytes. Antibiotic therapy—indicated for certain specific infections or for systemic toxicity.
C. difficile colitis	PCR (polymerase chain reaction) or other assay for C. difficile toxin in stool. Colonoscopy—sometimes required to detect characteristic pseudomembranes. Generally superceded by noninvasive PCR test of stool.	Established therapy—discontinue offending antibiotic, treat with flagyl or vancomycin. Novel or experimental therapies—immunoglobulin, rifaximin, cholestyramine, nitazoxanide.
Colonic obstruction	Radiologic tests—obstructive series, abdominal computerized tomography, occasionally barium enema or CT colonography. Small bowel series or small bowel enterography—for suspected small bowel obstruction.	Supportive therapy—complete bowel rest, antibiotics, intravenous hydration, replete lost electrolytes. Treatment—depends upon etiology. Malignant obstruction or any complete obstruction refractory to medical therapy requires surgery. Sigmoid volvulus often initially responds to sigmoidoscopy or colonoscopy.

(Continued)

TABLE 163-1 Key Diagnostic Tests and Therapies for Important Large Bowel Diseases in Hospitalized Patients (*Continued*)

Disease or Disorder	Key Diagnostic Tests	Major Therapeutic Options
Colonic pseudo-obstruction	Daily abdominal flat plates—to monitor cecal and transverse colon diameters. Abdominal CT—helpful to exclude other disorders causing colonic distention. Colonoscopy—mostly for therapeutic decompression, but helpful diagnostically to exclude other disorders such as mechanical obstruction (eg, volvulus), and detect severity of colonic involvement (especially secondary colonic ischemia).	General measures—bowel rest, replete lost electrolytes, correct underlying reversible etiologic factors, discontinue narcotics. Nasogastric tube suction, rectal tube, and antibiotics are used in selected circumstances. Neostigmine—generally administered in an ICU. Colonoscopic decompression—usually done on an unprepared colon, emphasis on aspirating intraluminal air. Surgery—for pseudo-obstruction refractory to general measures, neostigmine therapy, and colonoscopic decompression.

artery (IMA) supplies most of the left colon including the descending colon, sigmoid colon, and part of the rectum. The rectum is also supplied by the inferior and middle rectal (hemorrhoidal) arteries derived from the internal pudendal and internal iliac arteries. Ischemia of the rectum is rare because it is supplied by both the IMA and the systemic circulation, via the internal pudendal and internal iliac arteries. On the contrary, the splenic flexure is vulnerable to ischemia because it lies at a watershed area that is supplied by end arteries of the SMA and the IMA, which have a low perfusion pressure. The splenic flexure can become ischemic when the systemic blood pressure declines in shock.

Extensive anastomotic and collateral circulations exist individually within the SMA and within the IMA, and between these two arteries. A series of arcades interconnect neighboring branches of the SMA, while a similar series of arcades interconnect neighboring branches of the IMA. The marginal artery of Drummond provides additional arterial collaterals. These extensive collateral pathways protect against intestinal ischemia because they immediately open up when one branch of a major vessel is occluded.

The venous system generally parallels the arterial system. The superior mesenteric vein (SMV) drains the cecum, ascending colon, hepatic flexure, and transverse colon, whereas the inferior

TABLE 163-2 Colonoscopic Findings with Large Bowel Disorders in Hospitalized Patients

Disease or Disorder	Colonoscopic Findings
Colonic diverticular bleeding	Stigmata of recent hemorrhage: active bleeding, feeding vessel, adherent clot. Blood pooling in area around diverticulum. No other significant lesion detected at colonoscopy.
Internal hemorrhoids	Purplish lesions just proximal to dentate line bulging into the rectal lumen detected by anoscopy or by rectal retroflexion during colonoscopy.
Angiodysplasia	Macular, intensely erythematous, reticular lesions with an internal structure (eg, "starburst pattern" or "fern tree"). Must distinguish true angiodysplasia from colonoscopic trauma.
Colon cancer	Irregular, exophytic mass with induration and superficial ulceration; or irregular, asymmetric stricture.
Dieulafoy lesion	Raised, pigmented (visible) vessel without surrounding ulceration. Most common in proximal stomach but can occur in colon or rectum.
Radiation colitis	Acute—sloughed off mucosa, mucosal exudate, and edema in colonic segment exposed to radiotherapy. Chronic—irregular telangiectasias, mucosal friability, active bleeding, mucosal pallor, fibrotic strictures.
Ischemic colitis	Colonic abnormalities of mottled, gray, or dusky bowel, mucosal friability, mucosal edema, mucosal erythema, superficial ulcers, abrupt transition from normal colon to colitis, rectal sparing, hemorrhagic nodules, de novo colitis, colonoscopic changes rapidly disappear.
Ulcerative colitis	Colonoscopic findings of mucosal granularity, erythema, blunting of normal vascular pattern, mucosal friability or bleeding, mucopus, superficial ulcers, pseudopolyps, rectum involved, continuous involvement without skip lesions.
Crohn disease	Deep linear ulcers, cobblestoning, fistulas, fibrotic strictures, rectal sparing, terminal ileal involvement, skip lesions.
Diverticulitis	Colonoscopy not recommended in the setting of acute diverticulitis due to increased risk of colonic perforation because of colonic spasm and tortuosity. Colonoscopy generally recommended about 6 wk after episode of acute diverticulitis to exclude colon cancer in the elderly.
Pseudomembranous colitis	Characteristic raised, yellow-to-green, densely adherent, plaques that are 2-8 mm wide and are randomly scattered over colonic mucosa with normal intervening mucosa.
Colonic pseudo-obstruction	Highly dilated, air-filled, compliant colon with minimal or no muscular activity and no demonstrable mechanical obstruction or stricture. At colonoscopy, evaluate colon for mucosal ischemia, and if dusky or frankly necrotic bowel encountered must abort colonoscopy.

mesenteric vein (IMV) drains the descending colon, sigmoid colon, and proximal rectum. The IMV drains into the splenic vein that then joins the SMV to form the portal vein.

ISCHEMIC COLITIS

Ischemic colitis (IC) is defined as inflammation of the colon secondary to diminished blood perfusion that leads to bowel wall ischemia. The colon is the most common site of gastrointestinal ischemic injury. Ischemic colitis encompasses numerous clinical entities that produce insufficient blood perfusion to a colonic segment or the entire colon, and result in variably severe ischemic necrosis ranging from superficial mucosal involvement to full-thickness transmural necrosis. The term *ischemic colitis* describes the phenomenology of colonic ischemic injury, especially as observed on colonoscopy, but lacks specificity because it fails to specify the obstructed vessel, mechanism, and etiology. The physician should not accept ischemic colitis as a final diagnosis but should assiduously analyze the cause to determine the *site* of occlusion, including colonic branches of the SMA, SMV, IMA, and IMV; to determine the *mechanism* of occlusion, including embolus, thrombus, or vasospasm; and to determine the *cause* of occlusion, including atherosclerosis, vasculitis, low flow states, and hypercoagulable states.

■ ETIOLOGY

Ischemic colitis is caused by diminished colonic perfusion due to a decrease in systemic perfusion or an anatomic occlusion, which is so severe that colonic metabolic demands are not met. Anatomic factors predisposing to colonic ischemia include the narrow caliber of the IMA and occasional vascular variations that lack the normally present collaterals between the SMA and IMA. Predisposing physiologic factors include the low perfusion pressure at the splenic flexure, a watershed area, a decrease in perfusion associated with colonic motility, and sustained mesenteric vasospasm associated with systemic hypotension or other severe physiologic stress produced by sympathetic activity. **Table 163-3** lists various conditions associated with ischemic colitis.

Ischemic colitis most often occurs in the older adult; the average age is 70 years. Age-related tortuosity of colonic arteries as well as cumulative atherosclerotic disease increases vascular resistance and contributes to colonic ischemia in elderly patients. Mesenteric arterial emboli, thrombi, or trauma may lead to occlusive vascular disease and impaired colonic perfusion. Colonic hypoperfusion due to congestive heart failure, transient perioperative hypotension, strenuous physical activity, or shock from various causes, such as hypovolemia or sepsis, can result in IC. About 10% to 15% of patients with ischemic colitis have colonic obstruction from colon cancer, benign colonic stricture, or colonic diverticulitis.

A hypercoagulable state is often a significant factor in the pathogenesis of IC in young patients. Vasculitidies can cause thrombosis and occlusion of small vessels perfusing the colon, resulting in IC (Table 163-3). Medications that predispose to colonic ischemia are listed in **Table 163-4**. Rare causes of ischemic colitis include spontaneous aortic dissection, inferior mesenteric artery trauma during aortic surgery, intra-abdominal inflammatory disease, and colonic infections, such as schistosomiasis or cytomegalovirus. Severe constipation is a risk factor for ischemic colitis. Constipation, however, is an exceedingly common complaint so that patients with mild-to-moderate constipation without other risk factors rarely develop ischemic colitis.

Infectious colitis and ischemic colitis may present similarly with acute abdominal pain. Characteristics that help differentiate ischemic colitis from infectious colitis are reviewed in **Table 163-5**.

TABLE 163-3 Etiologies of Ischemic Colitis

Primary circulatory abnormalities

Atherosclerosis with thrombosis of the IMA or SMA

Systemic hypotension with a low-flow state (non-occlusive mesenteric ischemia, NOMI)

  Shock

  Hypovolemia or dehydration

  Long distance running

Emboli of SMA or IMA

Aortic injury

Aortic surgery (intraoperative injury to IMA)

Aortic dissection

Extrinsic disease compressing the vasculature

Cancer infiltrating the mesentery

Retroperitoneal fibrosis

Vasculitis

Behcet's disease

Buerger's disease (thromboangiitis obliterans)

Polyarteritis nodosa

Rheumatoid arthritis with vasculitis

Systemic lupus erythematosus with vasculitis

Takayasu's disease

Wegener's granulomatosis

Hypercoagulopathy/blood dyscrasia

Anticardiolipin antibodies

Antithrombin III deficiency

Factor V Leiden mutation

Protein C deficiency

Protein S deficiency

Sickle cell disease

Extrinsic compression of bowel vasculature associated with intestinal obstruction

Incarcerated hernia

Sigmoid volvulus

Cecal volvulus

Intussusception

Bowel adhesions

Colonic obstruction with colonic distention

Colon cancer with stricture

Benign colonic stricture

Colonic diverticular stricture

Toxic megacolon

Colonic pseudo-obstruction (Ogilvie syndrome)

Drug induced injury

See Table 163-4

Other

Amyloidosis

IMA, inferior mesenteric artery; SMA, superior mesenteric artery.

■ CLINICAL PRESENTATION

The clinical presentation varies with the underlying cause, extent of vascular obstruction, rapidity of ischemic insult, degree of collateral circulation, presence of comorbidities, and time of presentation.

TABLE 163-4 Drugs Associated with Colonic Ischemia

Well-established associations—proposed mechanisms

Cocaine—vasoconstriction due to noradrenergic stimulation

Ergotamine—vasospasm

Estrogen (with progesterone) contraceptives—thrombosis due to hypercoagulability

Pseudoephedrine—α-adrenergic vasoconstrictor

Sodium polystyrene (kayexalate) —electrolyte shifts due to medication

Vasopressin—vasospasm

Probable associations—proposed mechanisms

Amphetamines—sympathetic vasoconstriction

Digitalis—mesenteric vasoconstrictor at toxic drug levels

Dopamine—potent vasoconstrictor

Epinephrine or norepinephrine—potent vasoconstrictors

Methysergide—mesenteric vascular compression from retroperitoneal fibrosis

Nonsteroidal anti-inflammatory drugs—decreased synthesis of local prostaglandins that promote intestinal vasodilation

Possible associations—proposed mechanisms

Alosetron—unknown mechanism related to 5-HT [5-hydroxy tryptophan]-(3) antagonism, induced constipation may play a role

α-interferon—unknown mechanism

Danazol—ischemia from constipation and bowel dilatation

Diuretics—cause volume depletion and decreased colonic perfusion

Tegaserod—serotonin 5HT(4) antagonist that may cause severe diarrhea and ischemic colitis

Tricyclic antidepressants—may decrease colonic perfusion

Modified from Cappell MS. Colonic toxicity of administered drugs and chemicals. *Am J Gastroenterol.* 2004;99(6):1175-1190 and Cappell MS. Intestinal (mesenteric) vasculopathy: II. Ischemic colitis and chronic mesenteric ischemia. *Gastroenterol Clin North Am.* 1998;27(4):827-860.

Patients typically present with a sudden onset of crampy abdominal pain, diarrhea, and an urge to defecate. The pain is commonly localized to the left lower quadrant because the left colon is most commonly affected, but localized ischemia to other areas of the colon will often lead to pain localized within the corresponding area of the abdomen. Gastrointestinal bleeding, manifesting as bright red or maroon blood mixed with stool, frequently occurs. The bleeding is generally mild and does not cause hemodynamic instability or require blood transfusion. Other symptoms include anorexia and nausea and vomiting from an associated ileus.

Signs include mild-to-moderate tenderness over the involved intestinal segment, abdominal distention, low-grade pyrexia, tachycardia, and fecal occult blood. The symptoms are generally more severe than the abdominal signs in early IC. In 10% to 20% of cases, marked tenderness with peritoneal signs may be present on physical examination accompanied by metabolic acidosis and septic shock due to severe ischemia, especially with transmural infarction. Advanced IC often presents with lactic acidosis and leukocytosis.

■ DIAGNOSIS

Because mild-to-moderate IC is nonspecific and variable, the diagnosis largely depends on a high index of clinical suspicion, often based on predisposing conditions (Table 163-3).

Plain abdominal roentgenogram shows nonspecific findings in about 20% of cases such as distended, air-filled (exhausted) bowel loops, colonic aperistalsis, and mural thickening, but is often valuable to exclude other abdominal disorders. Computed tomography (CT), usually the initial diagnostic test to assess patients presenting with abdominal pain, can reveal segmental mural thickening, thumbprinting from submucosal hemorrhage and edema, and pericolonic fat stranding, with or without peritoneal fluid. Mural thickening with IC is typically concentric, symmetric, and smooth.

Colonoscopy is usually performed on relatively stable patients with suspected IC, but emergency abdominal surgery is required on unstable patients with suspected colonic perforation or peritonitis. Colonoscopy is the best diagnostic test because of high sensitivity; the ability to obtain mucosal biopsy specimens to exclude other pathologic entities; and the ability to perform subsequent angiography, which is indicated for suspected superior mesenteric arteriopathy. Flexible sigmoidoscopy is adequate to evaluate colonic ischemia after aortic surgery or aortic aneurysm rupture because in these situations the ischemia almost always involves the distal colon, and colonoscopy is inadvisable in such critically ill patients. Colonoscopy may reveal bluish hemorrhagic nodules that represent submucosal edema and hemorrhage and correspond to the thumbprints present at abdominal CT (**Figure 163-1A**). Hemorrhagic nodules localized to the ascending colon suggest SMA occlusion and a need for angiography. Colonoscopy should be performed early because the hemorrhagic nodules usually disappear within several days. Segmental erythema, with or without ulcerations and bleeding, may be subsequently observed (**Figure 163-1B**). With severe ischemia, the mucosa may appear gray, dusky, or black from transmural infarction. The colonoscopist should discontinue colonoscopic intubation when encountering frankly necrotic bowel because of a high risk of colonic perforation. Colonoscopic evidence favoring the diagnosis of ischemic colitis rather than inflammatory bowel disease includes a segmental distribution of colonic injury, abrupt transition between injured and uninjured mucosa, rectal sparing, de novo colitis, occurrence in the elderly, and rapid mucosal healing on repeat colonoscopy. Pathologic examination of colonoscopic biopsies may demonstrate extensive colonic mucosal injury, with acute inflammatory cell infiltration, ghost cells, granulation tissue, mucosal hemorrhage, and capillary thrombosis.

■ TREATMENT

Treatment depends on etiology, disease severity, timing of presentation, and presence of comorbidities. Most cases of IC are transient and are treated expectantly with medical therapy. Patients should be placed on bowel rest and administered intravenous fluids to replete intravascular volume and reduce intestinal oxygen requirements. Patients with malnourishment, profuse diarrhea, or a prolonged clinical course should receive parenteral hyperalimentation. Empiric broad-spectrum intravenous antibiotics,

TABLE 163-5 Distinguishing Ischemic Colitis from Infectious Colitis

Clinical Characteristic	Ischemic Colitis	Infectious Colitis
Symptoms		
Acuity of symptoms	Often sudden	Often gradual
Abdominal pain	Predominant symptom, may be severe	Secondary symptom
Diarrhea	May occur early as minor symptom	Predominant symptom
Gastrointestinal bleeding	Frequent, mild blood per rectum	Sometimes bloody diarrhea
Risk factors		
Risk factors for atherosclerosis	Frequent	Sometimes
Prior manifestations of vascular disease	Frequent	Occasionally
Risk factors for ischemic colitis (Table 163-3)	Frequent	Occasionally
Physical examination		
Physical findings of dehydration (eg, dry mucous membranes)	Occasional	Frequent with severe diarrhea
Bowel sounds	Early hyperactive, then hypoactive	Hyperactive bowel sounds
Lab tests		
Serum bicarbonate level	Often low	Often normal
Serum lactate	Often elevated	Usually normal
Fecal leukocytes or lactoferrin	Often present	Often present
Stool culture	Nondiagnostic	Often diagnostic
Plain abdominal roentgenogram		
Thumbprinting	Characteristic later finding	Uncommon
Thickened colonic wall	Common	Common
Colonoscopy		
Gray or dusky bowel	Characteristic of colonic infarction	Rare
Rectal involvement	Rectum spared due to dual blood supply	Rectum often involved
Splenic flexure	Frequently involved due to "watershed" effect	Sometimes involved
Segmental involvement	Characteristic	Frequently widespread colitis
Skip lesions	Uncharacteristic	Occasionally occurs
Abrupt transition from normal to abnormal colon	Characteristic	Uncommon
Hemorrhagic nodules	Fairly characteristic finding	Rare

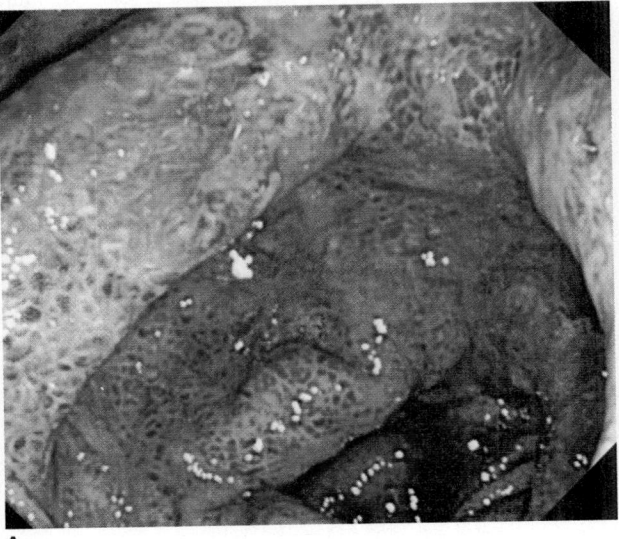
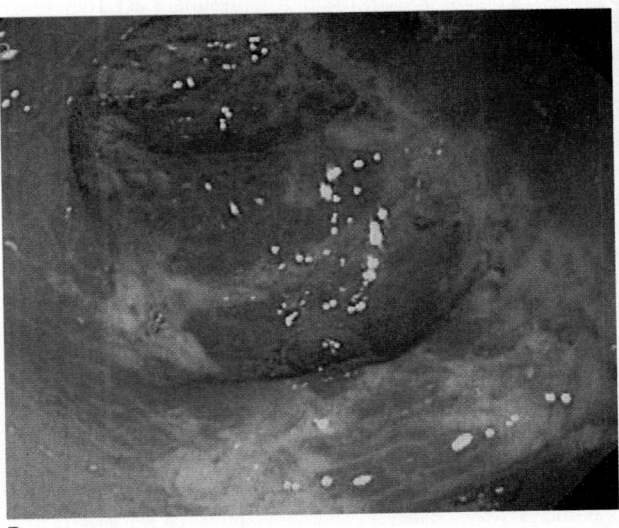

Figure 163-1 *(A) Colonoscopic videophotograph showing submucosal edema and hemorrhage (hemorrhagic nodules) in a patient with colonic ischemia. The patient presented with acute lower abdominal pain and rectal bleeding. (B) Colonoscopic videophotograph showing segmental erythema and ulcerations which developed in ischemic colitis several days after clinical presentation, as the hemorrhagic nodules disappeared.*

such as piperacillin/tazobactam, ceftriaxone plus metronidazole, ciprofloxacin plus metronidazole, or imipenem, are recommended to minimize bacterial translocation and sepsis due to the loss of mucosal integrity. A nasogastric tube should be placed if ileus is present. A rectal tube may help decompress a distended colon. Antiplatelet agents have not been evaluated in the treatment of IC and are generally not administered. Signs and symptoms often remit within 24 to 48 hours, and colonoscopic and roentgeno-graphic abnormalities often completely resolve within several weeks. Colonoscopy should be repeated several weeks after the initial presentation to verify disease recovery and thereby confirm the diagnosis.

> ### PRACTICE POINT
>
> ● Vasopressors should be discontinued or avoided whenever possible in ischemic colitis. Narcotic analgesics should be withheld early in treatment because these agents blunt the signs of peritonitis and promote abdominal distention. Cathartics are relatively contraindicated because they can precipitate colonic perforation.

About 20% of patients with acute IC require surgery because of signs or laboratory findings of peritonitis. The intraoperative appearance of the serosal surface of infarcted colon ranges from that of wet tissue paper to mottled or dusky bowel. It is important at surgery to resect all devitalized bowel to ensure viable surgical margins. Primary anastomosis is usually not performed because of the increased risk of anastomotic dehiscence. The proximal colonic loop is exteriorized to form a colostomy, and the distal loop is either exteriorized to form a mucous fistula or closed to form a Hartmann pouch. Selected patients can be treated by interventional radiology using vasodilators, such as papaverine, or by vascular surgery, using revascularization or endarterectomy.

DIVERTICULITIS

Diverticula are small mucosal herniations of colonic mucosa and submucosa through the smooth muscle layers of the intestines via the openings of vasa recta or nutrient vessels. Although diverticula may occur throughout the gastrointestinal tract, they most commonly occur in the colon, especially the sigmoid colon, which experiences much higher intraluminal pressures than the rest of the gastrointestinal tract. Diverticula are common, are frequently asymptomatic, and are associated with a low-fiber diet, obesity, and constipation. Exaggerated segmental colonic contractions may contribute to local mucosal herniation and diverticular formation due to increased pressures in focal colonic segments. Diverticulosis denotes the presence of uninflamed diverticula. Its incidence increases with age, from less than 5% before age 40 years to greater than 50% by age 85 years.

About 10% to 15% of patients with diverticulosis develop diverticulitis, defined as inflammation of one or more diverticula (**Figure 163-2**). While generally a disease of the older adult, 20% of cases occur in patients less than 50 years old. The pathogenesis is unclear. Inspissated food particles or fecaliths may abrade the mucosal wall of diverticula, resulting in focal inflammation, necrosis, and microperforation. Alternatively, fecal material or undigested food particles may collect in a diverticulum, cause diverticular obstruction, and result in distension of a diverticulum. This process leads to vascular compromise and colonic microperforation of the thin diverticular wall and inflammation of the adjacent colonic wall and paracolonic tissues. Typically, microperforations are walled off

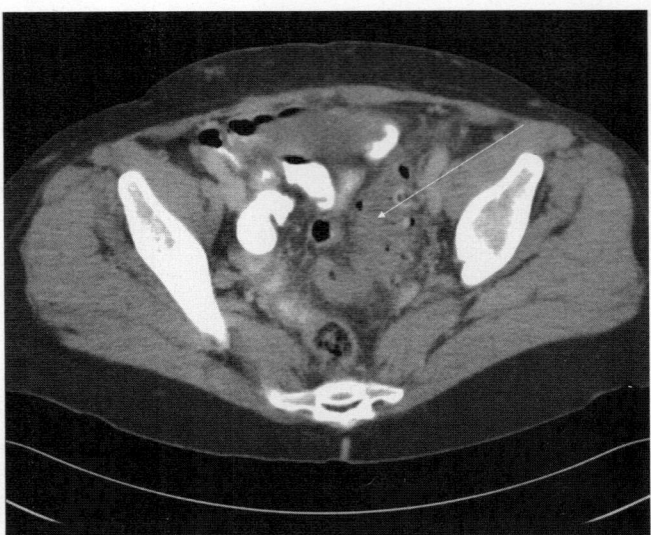

Figure 163-2 *Computed tomography of abdomen in a 60-year-old female presenting with left lower quadrant abdominal pain showing sigmoid colon mural thickening, several colonic diverticuli, and associated mesocolic fat infiltration, findings consistent with acute diverticulitis.*

by pericolonic fat and mesentery, and the inflammation remains contained and mild. However, macroperforations, from extensive disease, lead to abscess formation and, rarely, intestinal rupture or peritonitis. Fistulae or abscesses are complications of diverticulitis. Frank bacterial peritonitis is a rare, life-threatening complication. Multiple episodes of diverticulitis may lead to scarring, clinically manifesting as a colonic stricture.

■ CLINICAL PRESENTATION

Patients typically present with crampy, left lower quadrant abdominal pain and low-grade pyrexia. The pain may be intermittent or constant, and may be associated with a change in bowel habits, either diarrhea or constipation. Other symptoms include anorexia, nausea, and vomiting. Patients may complain of urinary symptoms, such as dysuria, urgency, and frequency due to bladder irritation from the inflamed adjacent sigmoid colon.

Signs reflect the severity of inflammation and the presence of complications. Common signs with uncomplicated diverticulitis are pyrexia and localized abdominal tenderness. The tenderness is usually located in the left lower quadrant where the sigmoid colon is located. Right lower quadrant tenderness, mimicking acute appendicitis, can occur with right-sided diverticulitis. Guarding, localized rebound tenderness, and a tender, palpable mass can occur with diverticulitis complicated by abscess formation. The abdomen may be distended and tympanitic. Bowel sounds are typically hypoactive, but may be normoactive in mild cases or hyperactive if obstruction occurs. If a fistula forms, the findings vary depending on the type of fistula. Colovesicular fistulas may present with suprapubic, flank, or costovertebral angle tenderness. Female patients with colovaginal fistulas may present with purulent vaginal discharge. Complicated diverticulitis is classified according to Hinchey's classification based on clinical findings, imaging studies, and presence of complications (**Table 163-6**).

■ LABORATORY EVALUATION

Laboratory studies are often nonspecific. A hemogram may reveal leukocytosis, neutrophilia, and a shift to immature neutrophil

TABLE 163-6 Classification and Treatment of Complicated Diverticulitis According to Hinchey's Classification

Stage	Description	Treatment
O	Uncomplicated diverticulitis	Treatment as outlined under stage I.
I	Small or confined pericolic or mesenteric abscess	An immunocompetent and reliable patient who can tolerate a diet, has no systemic symptoms, and no diffuse peritoneal signs can be managed as an outpatient with a clear liquid diet and oral antibiotics. Contraindications for outpatient management include immunocompromised state, corticosteroid therapy, severe comorbidities, and patient age >85 y old. Patients failing outpatient management should be hospitalized for bowel rest, intravenous antibiotics, and surgical consultation.
II	Large abscess, often confined to the pelvis	Hospitalization for intravenous antibiotics, bowel rest, CT-guided percutaneous drainage, and surgical consultation.
III	Generalized peritonitis due to rupture of a pericolic or pelvic abscess (noncommunicating with the colonic lumen because of obliteration of the diverticular neck by inflammation)	Urgent surgical intervention after patient resuscitation in an ICU.
IV	Feculent peritonitis due to free perforation of a diverticulum (communicating with colonic lumen)	Urgent surgical intervention after patient resuscitation in an ICU.

ICU, intensive care unit.

forms, indicating acute infection. An absence of leukocytosis does not, however, exclude diverticulitis. Urinalysis may reveal sterile pyuria if the bladder is adjacent to and irritated by the inflamed colonic segment. Electrolyte abnormalities may be present in patients with vomiting or diarrhea. Blood cultures should be obtained prior to empiric administration of parenteral antimicrobial therapy in patients who are febrile, severely ill, or have complicated disease.

Further studies are needed if the diagnosis is unclear or if complications are suspected. Upright and supine abdominal films are recommended in patients with significant abdominal pain. An upright chest radiograph should be obtained to exclude pneumoperitoneum or lower-lobe pneumonia. Abdominal radiographs are abnormal in 30% to 50% of patients with acute diverticulitis, with findings of bowel dilation, from obstruction or ileus, or findings of a soft tissue density suggesting an abscess.

Abdominal CT, preferably with oral and intravenous contrast, is the radiologic test of choice, with a sensitivity and specificity of about 95%. It is superior to intraluminal examinations, such as barium enema. Computed tomography can image mural and extramural disease. CT findings include colonic diverticulosis, pericolonic fat infiltration or "fat stranding," and mural thickening. CT can visualize complications of a colonic phlegmon, or pericolonic abscess. Ultrasonography (US) is a low cost, convenient, noninvasive, alternative diagnostic modality for acute diverticulitis, but it has limitations. Supportive findings include diverticulosis, mural thickening, mural hyperechogenicity, and abscesses. It is a second-line diagnostic tool because it is highly operator-dependent.

Colonoscopy or sigmoidoscopy is generally avoided in the initial evaluation of suspected acute diverticulitis because of the risk of colonic perforation, from the colonoscope or from intracolonic air insufflation due to colonic spasticity, tortuosity, and inflammation. If the diagnosis of diverticulitis is unlikely, a limited flexible sigmoidoscopy with minimal air insufflation may help exclude alternative diagnoses, such as inflammatory bowel disease or ischemic colitis. A colonoscopy should be electively performed about 6 weeks after initiating therapy, after the acute disease has resolved, to evaluate the extent of diverticulosis and to exclude colonic neoplasia in patients who have not undergone screening colonoscopy for several years.

■ TREATMENT

Patients with acute diverticulitis typically present with signs and symptoms sufficient to justify the clinical diagnosis and the institution of empiric therapy. The diagnosis should, however, be confirmed by abdominal CT; this CT can also detect complications of diverticulitis and exclude other intra-abdominal disorders. **Figure 163-3** shows an algorithm for the management of acute diverticulitis. Acute diverticulitis is treated according to Hinchey stage (Table 163-6).

Medical Management: Patients hospitalized for acute diverticulitis should have complete bowel rest (NPO) and receive intravenous hydration and intravenous broad-spectrum antibiotics, with coverage for common anaerobic microorganisms, such as *Bacteroides fragilis*, *Peptostreptococcus* and *Clostridium*, as well as aerobic microorganisms, such as *Escherichia coli*, *Klebsiella*, *Proteus*, *Streptococcus*, and *Enterobacter*. Recommended antibiotic regimens include anaerobic antibiotic coverage with metronidazole, and Gram-negative antibiotic coverage with an aminoglycoside, monobactam, or third-generation cephalosporin. Single-agent coverage, with second-generation cephalosporins or combined beta-lactamase inhibitors such as ampicillin/sulbactam or ticarcillin/clavulanate, is a reasonable alternative. Morphine is preferred over meperidine for pain control because of less toxicity. Nonsteroidal anti-inflammatory drugs (NSAIDs) and corticosteroids should be avoided because these drugs increase the risk of colonic perforation.

Once the diagnosis is established and the patient has been stabilized, patients hospitalized with moderate disease should undergo daily abdominal examinations to monitor the illness. With appropriate treatment, symptomatic improvement should occur within 2 to 3 days, at which time the diet may be advanced. If improvement continues, the patient may be discharged with instructions to complete a 7 to 10 days course of oral antibiotics. If pyrexia and leukocytosis do not resolve after 2 to 3 days of therapy, or serial examinations reveal worsening signs or new peritoneal findings, repeat abdominal CT is recommended to exclude complications.

Percutaneous Drainage: About one-sixth of patients with acute diverticulitis develop a peridiverticular abscess without peritonitis. CT-guided percutaneous drainage is indicated for a peridiverticular abscess that is *more than 4 cm in diameter* (Hinchey stage II disease, Table 163-6). The abdominal pain, pyrexia, and leukocytosis

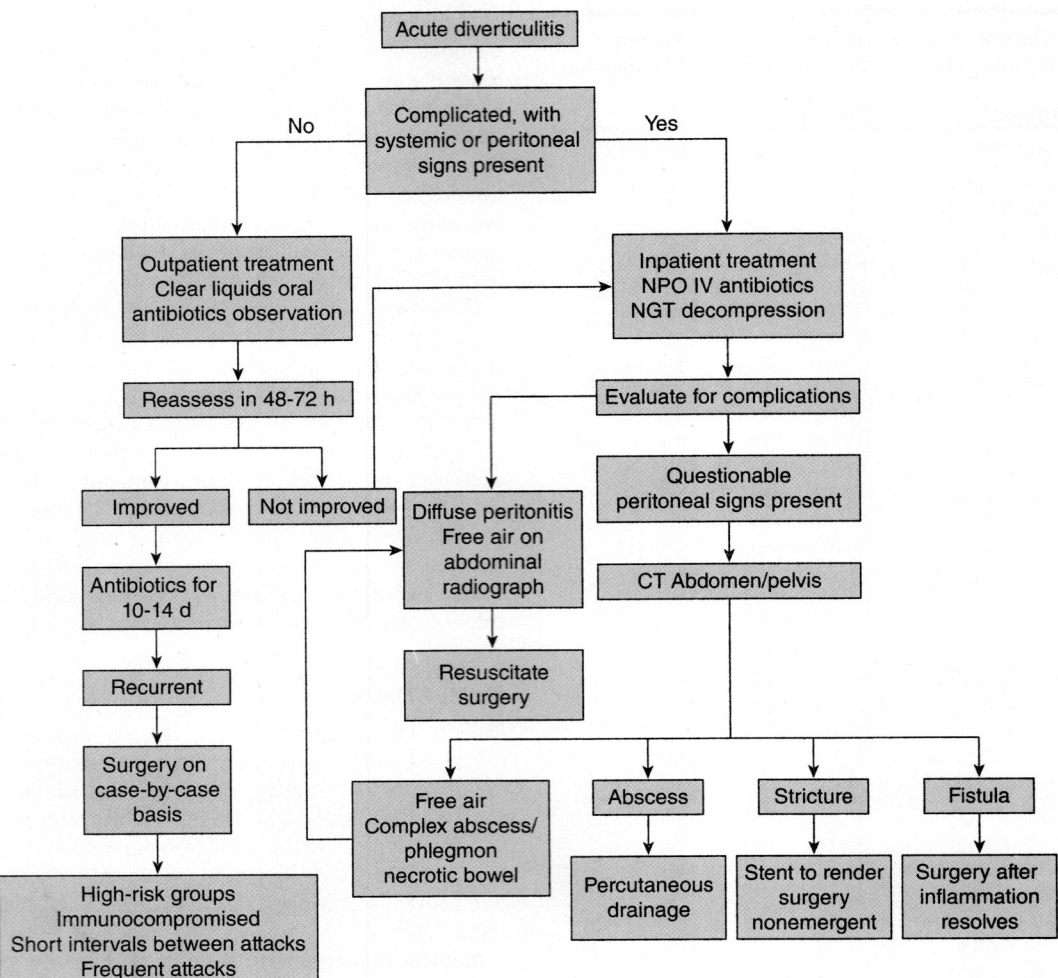

Figure 163-3 *An algorithm for the management of acute diverticulitis, depending on severity and presence of complications. (IV, intravenous; NGT, nasogastric tube; NPO, nothing per os.)*

usually promptly decrease after percutaneous drainage. Percutaneous drainage has eliminated the need for a multistage procedure with initial colostomy, and instead permits temporary palliative drainage with subsequent single-stage resection. The timing of surgery following drain placement depends upon resolution of the local inflammatory response. Follow-up CT scan is recommended 6 to 8 weeks after percutaneous drainage to plan elective surgical intervention. Colonoscopy to exclude other colonic pathology may be safely performed at this time, as long as the inflammation has resolved. Rarely the percutaneous drains inadequately control the local infection and urgent surgical intervention is required.

Elective Surgery: The American Society of Colon and Rectal Surgeons currently recommends consideration of elective colon resection on an individual basis for recurrent, uncomplicated diverticulitis to prevent further recurrences. Considerations regarding elective surgery include patient age, comorbidities, severity and frequency of the attacks, residual symptoms after resolution of the acute attack, and immunocompromised state.

Emergency Surgery: Urgent surgical intervention is required for patients who present with Hinchey stages III or IV, uncontrolled perforation, failed medical therapy, or unsuccessful percutaneous drainage of a clinically significant abscess (Table 163-6). Early identification of peritonitis is critical. A CT scan can confirm the diagnosis in ambiguous cases, but an abdominal series showing pneumoperitoneum together with a high clinical suspicion is sufficient to justify laparotomy. The surgical approach in an

emergent setting is a two-stage procedure: primary resection of diseased bowel with proximal end colostomy and oversewing of the distal stump (Hartmann pouch), followed by takedown of the colostomy and reanastomosis after the inflammation has resolved, usually 3 to 6 months later. Single-stage resection with primary anastomosis is the standard elective surgery for uncomplicated diverticulitis. After excluding colonic perforation, bowel preparation is essential before single-stage surgery, using either a 1-day polyethylene glycol electrolyte lavage or 2 to 3 days of mechanical preparation. For urgent or emergent surgery when free perforation is a concern, bowel lavage may be performed on the operating table, to permit a single stage, primary anastomosis.

ACUTE APPENDICITIS

Appendicitis is the most common abdominal surgical emergency in the United States, with more than 250,000 appendectomies per annum. The peak incidence occurs in the second and third decades of life; it is relatively rare at the extremes of age. However, perforation is more common in infancy and old age. Mortality is highest among older adults. Males and females are affected equally. Appendicitis may result from appendiceal luminal obstruction due to fecaliths, lymphoid hyperplasia, parasites, or tumors. Venous engorgement, with consequently impaired arterial flow, leads to ischemia and necrosis of mucosa and then muscularis propria. Mucosal necrosis, erosions, and ulcers permit bacterial invasion that produces a local inflammatory response.

CLINICAL PRESENTATION

Acute appendicitis presents initially with vague, mild-to-moderate, epigastric, or periumbilical discomfort. The periumbilical abdominal pain is visceral, resulting from distention of the appendiceal lumen. This pain sensation is transmitted by slow-conducting C nerve fibers and is usually poorly localized in the periumbilical or epigastric region, and is generally mild and crampy, visceral pain. After the inflammation spreads to parietal peritoneum, the pain migrates to the right lower quadrant, and becomes somatic, steady, more severe, and aggravated by motion or cough. Parietal afferent nerves are A delta fibers, which are fast-conducting and unilateral. These nerve fibers localize the pain to the right lower quadrant. This classic sequence occurs in two-thirds of patients.

Physical findings vary according to time after onset and location of the appendix, which may be situated deep in the pelvic cul-de-sac, in the right lower quadrant, or occasionally in the right upper quadrant (especially during pregnancy). Localized right lower quadrant tenderness is an important finding when present, but its absence does not exclude appendicitis. Tenderness is sometimes absent early in the visceral stage of appendicitis, but ultimately always develops at locations that correspond to the appendiceal location. Point tenderness typically occurs at McBurney's point, anatomically located on a line one-third of the distance between the anterior superior iliac spine (ASIS) and the umbilicus. Abdominal tenderness may be absent if a retrocecal or pelvic appendix is present, in which case the tenderness may occur in the flank or on rectal or pelvic examination. Rebound tenderness often manifests late in appendicitis. Flexion of the right hip and guarded movement by the patient are due to parietal peritoneal involvement. Cutaneous hyperesthesia of the right lower quadrant and the psoas or obturator signs are late findings. Tachycardia is uncommon with simple appendicitis, but common with complications. Most patients with simple appendicitis have a temperature less than 38°C; temperature greater than 38°C is commonly associated with perforated or gangrenous appendicitis. The diagnosis is challenging in older adults. They often lack the classic pattern of pain migration, right lower quadrant tenderness, pyrexia, and leukocytosis and often present later than young patients. For these reasons, the complication and perforation rates may be as high as 50% in the older adult.

PRACTICE POINT

- Psoas sign: Passive right hip flexion elicits right lower quadrant pain and may cause the patient to draw up the right knee. This sign indicates an inflamed (retrocecal) appendix lying against the psoas muscle.
- Obturator sign: Passive flexion of the right hip and knee, followed by internal rotation of the right hip, elicits right lower quadrant pain. This sign indicates an inflamed (pelvic) appendix that lies against the right obturator internus muscle.

EVALUATION

All patients with potential appendicitis should have urgent surgical consultation. Laboratory abnormalities include markers of acute inflammation, such as leukocytosis and a shift to immature neutrophil forms. Leukocytosis of >20,000 cells/μL suggests appendiceal perforation. A modified Alvarado scale provides a semiquantitative clinical diagnostic aid. In this scale, patients are assigned 1 point for each of the following: migratory right lower quadrant pain; anorexia;

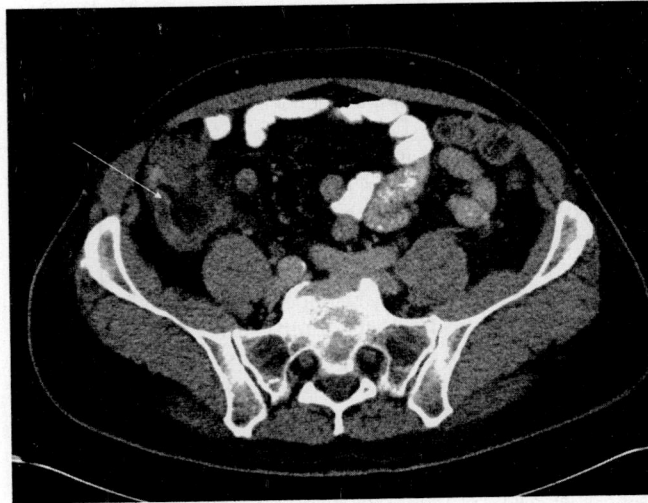

Figure 163-4 *Computed tomography of abdomen in a 24-year-old male presenting with an acute abdomen reveals massive dilation of the appendix with mural thickening, and severe periappendiceal inflammatory changes consistent with acute appendicitis.*

nausea and vomiting; rebound tenderness in the right lower quadrant; and temperature >37.5°C. Patients are assigned 2 points for each of the following: tenderness in the right lower quadrant, and leukocytosis. An Alvarado score <5 generally excludes appendicitis, whereas a score >7 strongly suggests appendicitis.

Abdominal radiographs are rarely helpful. Only 5% have an opaque fecalith in the right lower quadrant. Consequently, abdominal radiographs are obtained only if other conditions, such as intestinal obstruction or ureteral calculus, are in the differential diagnosis. Contrast-enhanced or nonenhanced abdominopelvic CT is superior to abdominal ultrasound and abdominal radiographs. CT findings include an inflamed, distended (>6 mm wide) appendix that fails to fill with contrast or air (**Figure 163-4**); an appendicolith (defined as a fecalith or calcified concretion of stool visible in the appendix by abdominal radiography); appendiceal mural thickening (>2 mm wide); periappendiceal inflammation (detected as fat stranding); cecal apical thickening; and pericecal fluid collections. Pneumoperitoneum is uncommon, even in perforated appendicitis. Computed tomography visualization of a normal appendix, containing air or contrast in its lumen; nonvisualization of the appendix altogether; or demonstration of alternative intra-abdominal pathology constitutes a negative study for appendicitis. The positive predictive value of CT is 95% to 97%, and accuracy is 90% to 98%.

The diagnostic role of abdominal ultrasound is controversial. A shadowing appendicolith, pericecal inflammation, or localized pericecal fluid collection suggest appendicitis. Appendicitis is excluded by ultrasonographic visualization of a normal appendix, but a study in which the appendix is nonvisualized does not exclude acute appendicitis. Unfortunately, a normal appendix is demonstrated by ultrasonography less than 50% of the time when there is no appendicitis. Ultrasound is more sensitive and specific in children (>90% sensitivity and specificity in children) than in adults. Abdominal ultrasound is an alternative first imaging study for appendicitis, especially for institutions with experienced ultrasonographers, in pregnant women, thin adult patients, and pediatric patients.

TREATMENT

Patients are administered intravenous antibiotics preoperatively to prevent bacterial invasion and to decrease the risk of postoperative wound infection or intra-abdominal abscess; intravenous fluids to correct intravascular volume depletion; and intravenous electrolytes to correct electrolyte imbalances. Common antibiotic regimens for nonperforated appendicitis include cefoxitin, ampicillin/sulbactam, or cefazolin plus metronidazole. Appendectomy is uniformly recommended, even though appendicitis sometimes spontaneously resolves. Patients highly suspected to have acute appendicitis by an expert clinician can go directly to surgery after emergency resuscitation without undergoing abdominal CT or other radiologic studies. Both open and laparoscopic appendectomies are safe and effective for nonperforated appendicitis. Laparoscopic appendectomy may be superior to open appendectomy for uncomplicated appendicitis, but this has not been definitively proven. Laparoscopic appendectomy takes more operative time and is more expensive, but patients require less pain medication, have a shorter hospitalization, and have a lower rate of wound infection after laparoscopic appendectomy compared to open appendectomy. Yet, patients experience an increased rate of intra-abdominal abscesses after laparoscopic appendectomy. Laparoscopic appendectomy is preferable for patients who need to rapidly return to work or who have an uncertain preoperative diagnosis. Colonoscopy should be performed in elderly patients about 6 weeks after appendectomy for acute appendicitis to exclude cecal cancer.

Patients with perforation and a palpable right lower quadrant mass usually have extensive periappendiceal inflammation or an abscess. In patients without diffuse peritonitis or systemic toxicity, initial management can be operative or nonoperative. With initial nonoperative management, patients are placed at bowel rest, and administered intravenous fluids and antibiotics. A CT scan of the abdomen is obtained. If a single abscess greater than 3 cm is discovered, percutaneous drainage of the abscess under CT guidance is performed. If multiple abscesses are found or if the patient does not improve within 24 to 48 hours of conservative therapy, operative drainage of the abscess(es) is/are performed. Success rates of 90% to 95% have been reported with initial nonoperative management. Interval appendectomy, after 6 to 12 weeks, when the acute inflammation has resolved is recommended, but the role of interval appendectomy remains controversial because the rate of recurrent appendicitis is less than 20% at 1 year.

COLONIC OBSTRUCTION

Colonic obstruction may occur as the primary problem requiring hospitalization or as a secondary complication during hospitalization. Common causes of colonic obstruction include malignancy, volvulus, diverticular stricture, and colonic adhesions. Infrequent causes include hernias, Crohn disease, endometriosis, intussusception, extrinsic tumors, and fecal impaction. Colonic obstruction is more common in the elderly because the incidence of neoplasms and other causative diseases is higher in this population.

Adenocarcinoma: Malignant neoplasms, nearly always adenocarcinomas, cause more than 50% of all cases of colonic obstruction (**Figure 163-5**). About 20% of patients with colorectal cancer present with obstructive symptoms, and half of these require emergency operative decompression. Three-fourths of obstructing adenocarcinomas occur distal to the splenic flexure, many within reach of a flexible sigmoidoscope. Carcinomas of the left colon can manifest as a scirrhous tumor causing progressive stenosis of the lumen, whereas cancers of the right colon typically grow as a polypoid or fungating mass (**Figure 163-6**) that obstructs the colon only upon reaching a large size that occludes the lumen, or, rarely, by acting as a lead point for a colonic intussusception.

Volvulus: Colonic volvulus is an axial twist of the colon on its vascular pedicle. It causes 10% to 15% of colonic obstructions. Anatomic factors promoting volvulus include a redundant, highly mobile, colonic segment that has two closely adjacent points of

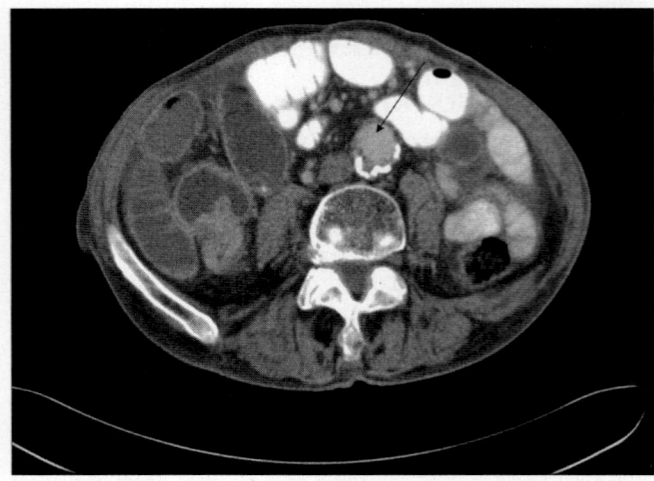

Figure 163-5 *Computed tomography of abdomen in an 89-year-old male with an intraluminal mass lesion (see arrow) in ascending colon. The mass almost totally obstructs the lumen, with only a thin margin of contrast medium seen circumferentially. Contrast is present in bowel proximal to the mass. The colon is decompressed distally via a patent rectum. Note the shift of the ascending colon from its normal position in the left lower quadrant to the central pelvis due to the dilated bowel proximal to the obstructing lesion.*

fixation to peritoneal structures. In sigmoid volvulus, the redundant sigmoid colon is fixed across a narrow base by the lateral peritoneal attachments proximally and the rectum distally. Failure of fusion of parietal peritoneum to the cecum and ascending colon permits formation of cecal volvulus in which the distal ileum, cecum, and ascending colon rotate and twist or fold. In the variant of a *cecal bascule*, the cecum folds upward without undergoing an axial twist. Volvulus typically produces a closed-loop obstruction with ischemia from occluding the vascular pedicle and from increased wall tension due to rapid distention. The ischemia rapidly leads to gangrene and perforation. Volvulus of the transverse colon is uncommon and is related to a congenital or surgical absence of supporting ligaments and tissues.

Benign Colonic Strictures: Benign colonic strictures occur most commonly from diverticulitis and less commonly at the site of a surgical anastomosis. Benign colonic strictures account for less than 10% of cases of colonic obstruction. Postoperative colonic adhesions can cause a kink or acute angulation in the colon that totally obstructs colonic flow.

■ EVALUATION

Mechanical obstruction must be differentiated from acute colonic pseudo-obstruction, which is characterized by clinical and radiological findings resembling that of large bowel obstruction in the absence of a mechanical blockage. Colonic pseudo-obstruction may result from impaired function of gastrointestinal muscle, innervating neurons, or pacemaker cells. This condition usually affects elderly people with underlying comorbidities, and early recognition and appropriate management are essential to prevent life-threatening complications. Colonic obstruction is subclassified into partial versus complete obstruction. Unrelieved, complete, colonic obstruction generally progresses rapidly and requires urgent therapy.

Symptoms of colonic obstruction include abdominal distention, abdominal pain that is commonly infraumbilical and colicky, and obstipation. The abdomen is typically diffusely distended and tympanitic. Pyrexia, tachycardia, hypotension, and rebound tenderness suggest colonic ischemia or impending

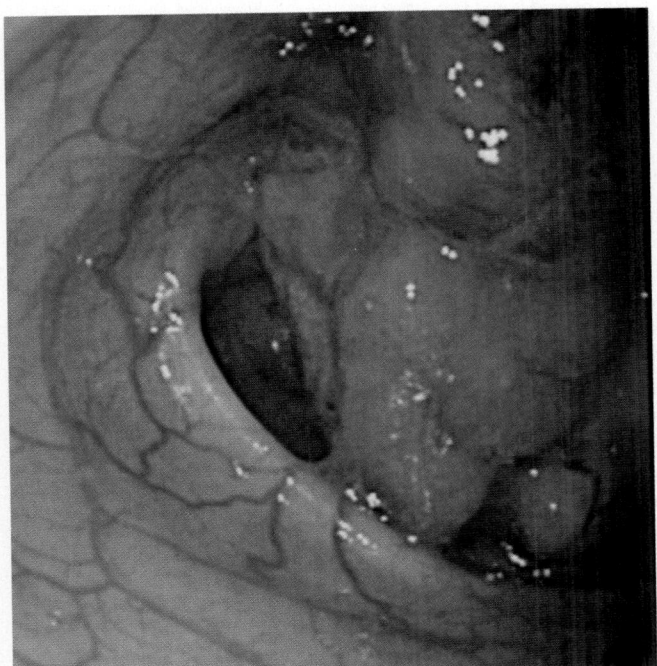

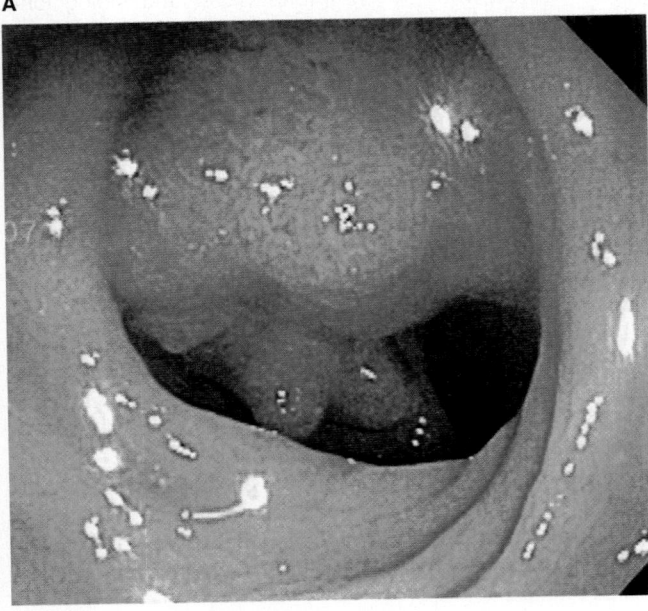

Figure 163-6 *Colonoscopic videophotographs of a multinodular mucosal mass mostly obstructing the lumen of the colon illustrated in two different patients (A and B) presenting with symptoms of colonic obstruction.*

colonic perforation. Routine laboratory studies may demonstrate prerenal azotemia, reflected by an elevated serum creatinine level and more highly elevated serum blood urea nitrogen level, from dehydration; and leukocytosis with a left shift from impending colonic necrosis.

PRACTICE POINT

- Upright chest and abdominal radiographs and supine abdominal radiographs constitute the standard "obstruction series" that should be obtained in every patient with suspected bowel obstruction.

Flat and upright abdominal radiographs demonstrate dilation of the small and/or large bowel and air-fluid levels. An upright chest radiograph is also ordered to exclude pneumoperitoneum, a radiologic sign of gastrointestinal perforation. Abdominal CT is very helpful in localizing the site and etiology of the colonic obstruction. Computed tomography can also identify extracolonic lesions, including metastases from malignant colonic obstruction. An abrupt cutoff in colonic air suggests the anatomic location of an obstruction. A dilated, air-filled colon without air in the rectum is more consistent with obstruction than pseudo-obstruction. The presence of air in the rectum is consistent with obstipation, pseudo-obstruction, or partial obstruction. This finding can, however, be misleading, particularly if the patient has undergone rectal examinations or enemas.

The classic radiologic feature of sigmoid volvulus on abdominal radiographs is a distended and ahaustral U-shaped sigmoid loop ("bent inner-tube" appearance), the apex of which is often directed toward the patient's right shoulder (**Figure 163-7**). Abdominal CT scan may also demonstrate a whirl pattern formed by a dilated sigmoid colon wrapped and constricted distally by its mesocolon and vessels. The classic radiologic features of cecal volvulus include (1) a massively dilated cecum located in the epigastrium or left upper quadrant; (2) a coffee-bean appearance of distended cecum; (3) distended loops of small bowel suggesting small bowel obstruction (SBO); and (4) a single, long air-fluid level present on upright or decubitus radiographs. Computed tomography or magnetic resonance imaging is not always required to detect colonic volvulus.

■ TREATMENT

General Treatment: Resuscitation of patients with colonic obstruction includes restoration of intravascular volume, correction of electrolyte disorders, and nasogastric aspiration for intestinal decompression. The need and urgency for surgical decompression depends upon the degree of obstruction (partial vs complete) and the presence versus absence of strangulation.

Benign and Malignant Colonic Strictures: The goals of surgery include: (1) prompt decompression of the obstructed colon; (2) definitively treating the obstructing lesion; and (3) re-establishing intestinal continuity. All these goals may not be achieved with one operation. Patients with partially obstructing benign or malignant strictures and no evidence of peritonitis may undergo semielective resection of the stricture after resuscitation and nasogastric aspiration. Conversion of an emergent to a semielective operation permits preparation of the colon for primary anastomosis and thereby lowers the operative risk. Complete, unremitting, colonic obstruction necessitates emergency operative decompression.

Obstruction proximal to the splenic flexure is most frequently due to adenocarcinoma and can usually be treated with right hemicolectomy and primary ileocolonic anastomosis. Acute colonic obstruction from advanced colonic malignancy is a surgical emergency. Obstructed patients who are medically unable to withstand resection should undergo tube cecostomy, colostomy, or loop ileostomy. Obstruction at or distal to the splenic flexure may be from either adenocarcinoma or diverticular stricture, differentiation of which may be difficult during laparotomy. Patients who are medically fit with relatively small tumors or inflammatory masses of the left colon or sigmoid may undergo left hemicolectomy or sigmoid colectomy with an end colostomy and closure of the distal bowel or the creation of a distal mucous fistula. Recently, self-expanding metallic stents have been successfully deployed at colonoscopy to relieve malignant colonic obstruction prior to definitive resection or to palliate obstructive symptoms in patients with advanced, unresectable cancer. This approach permits subsequent mechanical

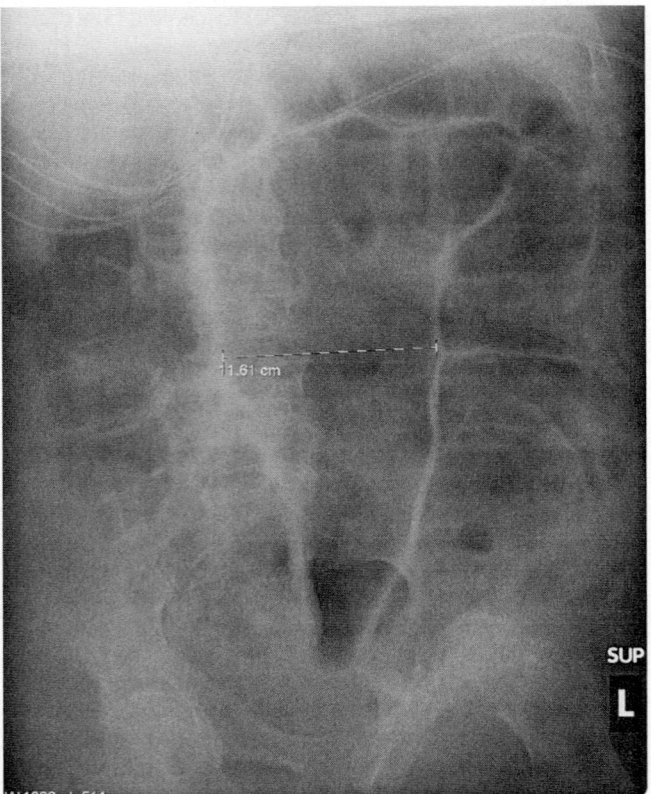

A

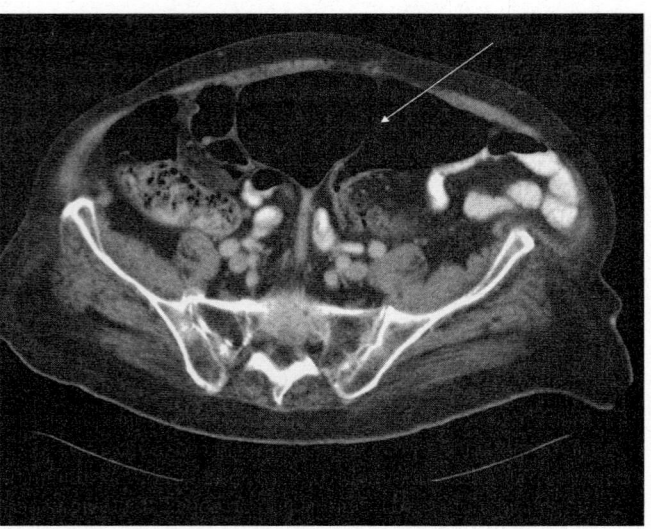

B

Figure 163-7 *(A) Upright abdominal radiograph of an 80-year-old male showing massively dilated loops of sigmoid colon measuring 11.6 cm maximally, findings consistent with sigmoid volvulus. (B) CT of abdomen in the same patient showing a massively dilated segment of sigmoid colon filled with air from sigmoid volvulus.*

bowel preparation and primary colo-colonic anastomosis, after treatment of significant concomitant medical illnesses.

Sigmoid Volvulus: The initial management of sigmoid volvulus without peritonitis is sigmoidoscopic or colonoscopic decompression and placement of a rectal tube beyond the point of obstruction. The procedure may, indeed, detort the volvulus. Colonoscopy must, however, be performed carefully with minimal insufflation of air (or preferably with insufflation of carbon dioxide) to minimize the risk of perforation of the distended, thin-walled, and inflamed

bowel. Endoscopic reduction of sigmoid volvulus is associated with a 25% to 50% recurrence rate, so elective sigmoid resection and coloproctostomy, or in medically compromised patients, end colostomy, is recommended after endoscopic decompression and bowel preparation. This approach reduces recurrence rates to 3% to 6%. Patients requiring emergency laparotomy for strangulated sigmoid volvulus require sigmoid resection with end colostomy and a Hartmann pouch.

Cecal Volvulus: The role of initial nonsurgical management of patients with cecal volvulus is poorly defined. Although colonoscopy has been successfully employed to reduce cecal volvulus, the risk of perforation of the thinned, often ischemic cecum is substantial, as is the danger of missing a short segment of necrotic bowel at colonoscopy with delay in definitive resection. Surgery is therefore the primary therapy. Surgical options for cecal volvulus include cecopexy, cecostomy, and colonic resection including either right colectomy or ileocolonic resection. Detorsion alone, or in combination with appendectomy, is associated with a high recurrence rate.

COLONIC PSEUDO-OBSTRUCTION

Acute colonic pseudo-obstruction, or Ogilvie syndrome, is a clinical disorder with the symptoms, signs, and radiographic appearance resembling those of acute large bowel obstruction but without mechanical obstruction (**Figure 163-8**). Colonic pseudo-obstruction typically occurs in a setting of a recent serious medical illness or surgical procedure. Narcotic administration for postoperative pain may aggravate the usual postoperative ileus and precipitate acute intestinal pseudo-obstruction. Patients with colonic pseudo-obstruction typically present with severe abdominal distention, without passage of stool or gas. Some patients with intestinal pseudo-obstruction, however, still pass some gas or even have limited bowel movements. Nausea and vomiting can be present.

Evaluation of these patients is similar to that discussed for colonic obstruction. A complete blood count and serum electrolytes are obtained. A serum lactate level is determined to help exclude colonic ischemia, which may occur consequent to severe colonic dilation from colonic pseudo-obstruction. Abdominal CT is useful to diagnose this condition, exclude other etiologies, and determine complications. The degree of colonic, especially cecal, dilatation as determined by abdominal CT is important because a maximal cecal diameter >12 cm significantly increases the risk of cecal necrosis and perforation.

■ TREATMENT

PRACTICE POINT

- The mainstay of treatment of colonic pseudo-obstruction is correction of underlying reversible etiologic factors, such as infection, hypotension, hypoxemia, and electrolyte imbalances, especially of potassium and calcium. Antikinetic agents such as narcotics or anticholinergics should be promptly discontinued.

Electrolyte abnormalities and dehydration are corrected by intravenous administration of electrolytes and fluid, as necessary. Medications that decrease colonic motility, such as opiates, calcium-channel antagonists, and anticholinergic medications, should be discontinued. Patients should receive nothing per os. Nasogastric suction may be helpful but does not produce major

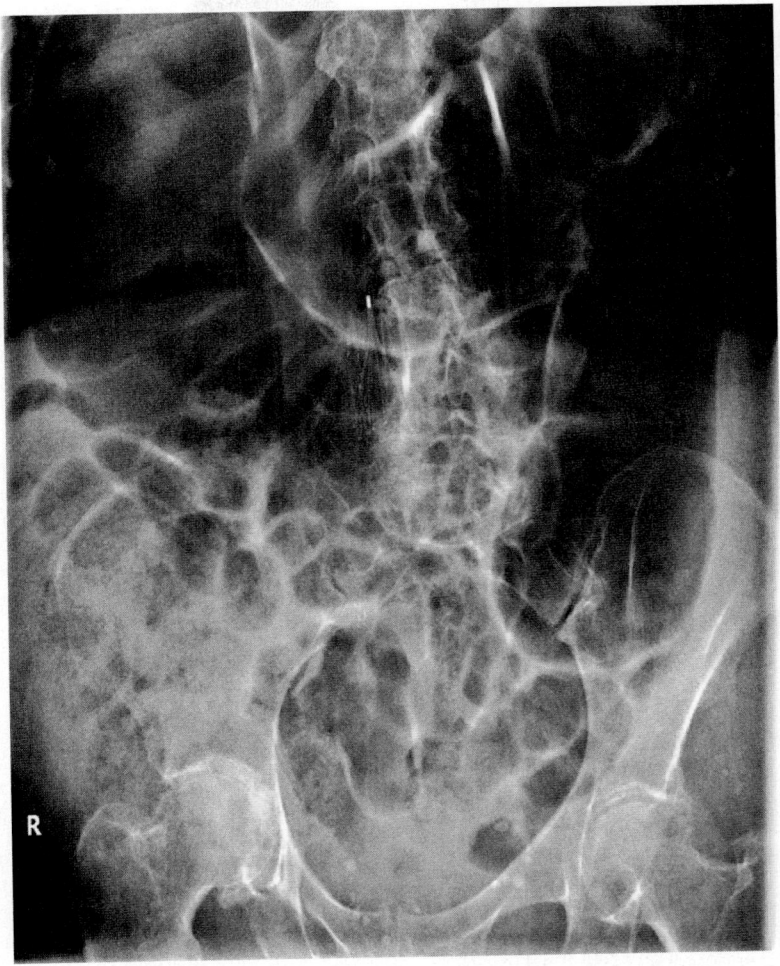

Figure 163-8 *Upright abdominal radiograph of a 90-year-old female showing dilation of both small and large bowel loops, including the rectum. This pattern of dilation throughout the bowel without a transition point from dilated to nondilated bowel is characteristic of colonic pseudo-obstruction.*

intestinal decompression because the functional obstruction is primarily colonic. Rectal tube decompression can be effective for sigmoid colon involvement. Morbidity and mortality from this condition is reduced by careful daily monitoring of abdominal radiographs, leukocyte counts, and serum electrolytes. Increasing abdominal pain and tenderness associated with leukocytosis warrants urgent surgical consultation to exclude bowel perforation.

If after 72 hours of conservative measures, the cecal diameter is still >9 cm, neostigmine (1-2 mg) can be rapidly infused intravenously. Contraindications to neostigmine include bradycardia, hypertension, severe renal insufficiency, signs of bowel perforation, and active bronchospasm. If neostigmine is ineffective or contraindicated, colonoscopic decompression is strongly considered. A decompression tube can be inserted in the transverse colon during colonoscopy via a guidewire. Colonoscopic decompression with placement of a decompression tube is therapeutic in about 75% or more of cases. The main risk of colonoscopic decompression is cecal perforation.

Patients occasionally require surgery. Tube cecostomy may be performed for colonic venting. Percutaneous cecostomy may also be performed under CT guidance, but this procedure entails significant morbidity. Surgical decompression by cecostomy, colostomy, or resection, is associated with a poor outcome, possibly because it is performed in patients with more severe disease in whom less invasive measures have failed. Surgery is essential for suspected perforation or peritonitis.

CONCLUSION

Inpatients are increasingly evaluated and treated by hospitalists who must be knowledgeable about inpatient medicine. In particular, large bowel diseases constitute an important cause of hospitalization, encompassing more than 1% of all hospitalizations and contributing as comorbid conditions to other hospitalizations. This chapter reviews many important inhospital large bowel diseases, including ischemic colitis, diverticulitis, acute appendicitis, colonic obstruction, and colonic pseudo-obstruction. This chapter emphasizes the inpatient evaluation and treatment of these diseases and deemphasizes the outpatient management of these diseases. This work also excludes or deemphasizes many important colonic disorders primarily diagnosed and medically treated in the outpatient setting, such as colon cancer, chronic diarrhea, and irritable bowel syndrome. **Table 163-7** summarizes data from key recent studies on the discussed colonic disorders using an evidence-based approach.

ACKNOWLEDGMENTS

I thank Dr. Mihaela Batke, Attending, Division of Gastroenterology & Hepatology, Department of Internal Medicine, William Beaumont Hospital, for providing the colonoscopic photographs; and Dr. Kristin Evans, Resident, Department of Radiology, William Beaumont Hospital, for providing the radiographs and CT images included in this chapter.

TABLE 163-7 Evidence-Based Medicine: Key References for Colonic Disorders

Study	Methodology	Results	Limitations	Bottom Line
Ischemic colitis				
Midian-Singh R, et al. *South Med J.* 2004;97:120-123.	Case series of prospective evaluation for hypercoagulopathy in 18 of 28 patients who presented with "idiopathic" ischemic colitis during a 2-y period. Hypercoagulopathy panel included 11 blood tests.	Five of 18 patients with "idiopathic" ischemic colitis had significant hypercoagulopathies, including factor V and protein C resistance, protein S deficiency, prothrombin mutation, and anticardiolipin antibody.	Small study. Potential selection bias because 10 of the 28 patients did not undergo hypercoagulopathy testing. Case series approach with no control group.	Hypercoagulopathy syndromes can frequently underlie otherwise "idiopathic" ischemic colitis. Tests for hypercoagulopathy should be performed in patients with "idiopathic" ischemic colitis who lack other risk factors.
Mosele M, et al. *Scand J Gastroenterol.* 2010;45:428-433.	Retrospective chart review at one hospital during a 6-y period of 46 elderly patients diagnosed with ischemic colitis based on computerized identification of discharge diagnoses vs elderly controls (without vascular gastrointestinal insufficiency or gastrointestinal inflammatory or infectious diseases).	Independent risk factors for ischemic colitis included: constipation (odds ratio = 4.8, 95%-CI: 1.1-20.1), vasculopathy (odds ratio = 4.9, 95%-CI: 1.4-16.6), hepatitis C virus infection (OR = 9.9, 95%-CI: 1.1-92.90), and cancer (odds ratio = 7.5, 95%-CI: 1.6-56.5).	Retrospective study, only moderate size of study and control populations. Potential selection bias when patients selected according to discharge diagnoses.	Constipation, vasculopathy, hepatitis C virus infection, and cancer appear to be strong risk factors for ischemic colitis in the elderly.
Won Chung J, et al. *Dis Colon Rectum.* 2010;53:1287-94.	Retrospective analysis of 153 of 173 patients who were diagnosed with ischemic colitis. Univariate and multivariate analysis to identify clinical, laboratory, and endoscopic parameters associated with a poor prognosis.	The following were independent predictors of severe ischemic colitis: tachycardia (OR = 4.6, 95% CI: 1.4-14.7), early shock (OR = 6.5, 95%-CI: 2.0-21.2), and endoscopic evidence of colonic ulceration (OR = 9.9, 95%-CI: 2.0-48.8).	Small size of subgroup with severe ischemic colitis (20 patients), retrospective analysis, potential selection bias due to 20 patients unavailable for retrospective analysis.	Tachycardia, early shock, or endoscopic evidence of colonic ulceration may be early predictors of a severe or complicated clinical course. Patients with these findings may require intensive care unit monitoring, aggressive diagnostic testing, and aggressive therapy.
Diverticulitis				
Andeweg C, et al. *World J Surg.* 2008;32:1501-1506.	Retrospective, observational study of 183 patients studied over 18-y period. Patients identified by a computerized pathology database.	Recurrence rate of diverticulitis after limited colon resection for diverticulitis was 8.7% over a mean of 7.2 y of follow-up. Only identified risk factors for postoperative recurrence of diverticulitis: younger age (mean age with recurrence = 54 y, mean age no recurrence = 64 y, $p < .02$), persistent postoperative abdominal symptoms (recurrence rate = 22.2% with symptoms vs 5.4% without symptoms, $P < .01$).	Retrospective, observational study. Computerized identification of study patients from a pathology database may not have captured all treated patients.	Younger age and persistent postoperative abdominal complaints may identify subgroups at high risk of recurrent diverticulitis after surgery.

(Continued)

TABLE 163-7 Evidence-Based Medicine: Key References for Colonic Disorders (*Continued*)

Study	Methodology	Results	Limitations	Bottom Line
Morris CR, et al. *Br J Surg*. 2008;95:876-881.	Retrospective observational study of incidence, mortality, and risk factors for mortality of perforated diverticulitis at 5 hospitals over a 5-y period. Patients identified by computerized search of discharge diagnostic codes.	Incidence of diverticular perforation for adults was 3.9 per 100,000 per annum. Mortality was 24.3%. Risk factors for mortality included: age >65 y (odds ratio = 10.3, 95%-CI: 3.0-35.4, *P* < .001), renal disease (odds ratio = 13.6, 95%-CI: 1.5-124, *P* = .02), prior NSAID use (odds ratio = 2.8, 95% CI: 1.4-5.7, *P* = .004), and ASA (American Society of Anesthesiologists) score > II (odds ratio = 8.9, 95%-CI: 3.8-20.7, *P* <.001).	Retrospective, observational study. Computerized identification of patients may have biased study toward more severe episodes of diverticulitis.	High mortality of diverticulitis associated with colonic perforation. Yet, most patients recover with early, aggressive surgical therapy, even in presence of high-risk factors.
Appendicitis				
Ingraham AM, et al. *Surgery*. 2010;148:625-635.	Retrospective observational study of patient outcomes after laparoscopic vs open appendectomy using a large multicenter database maintained by the American College of Surgeons that includes more than 200 hospitals.	Of 32,683 analyzed patients, 76.4% underwent laparoscopic appendectomy and 23.6% underwent open appendectomy. Patients undergoing laparoscopic appendectomy had less overall morbidity (4.5% vs 8.8%, odds ratio = .60, 95%-CI: .54-.68), had less frequent site-specific infections (3.3% vs 6.7%, odds ratio = .57, 95%-CI: .50-.65), and had less frequent serious morbidity or mortality (2.6% vs 4.3%, odds ratio = .87, 95%-CI: .74-1.01).	Retrospective study. Clinical parameters not collected in database were unstudied. Study results may not apply to community hospitals that did not participate in this database.	Laparoscopic appendectomy is a relatively low-risk procedure for acute appendicitis and may have generally superior outcomes compared to open appendectomy.
Lugo JZ, et al. *J Surg Res*. 2010;164:91-94.	Retrospective observational study of 46 patients undergoing interval laparoscopic appendectomy after nonoperative management of complication of right lower quadrant abscess or phlegmon from acute appendicitis during a 6-y period.	84% of operated patients had persistent or chronic appendicitis, complicated inflammatory bowel disease, or neoplasm and therefore likely benefited from surgical exploration.	Retrospective, observation. Limited study size. Method to identify study patients not described, but apparently based on computerized review of computed tomographic reports. Analysis may not have captured all treated patients. No comparison to unoperated control group.	Interval appendectomy following conservative management for complicated acute appendicitis is justified due to the otherwise high rate of problems requiring surgical therapy.
Colonic obstruction				
Vemulapalli R, et al. *Dig Dis Sci*. 2010;55:1732-1737.	Retrospective, observational study comparing 53 patients undergoing self-expanding stent placement vs 70 patients undergoing palliative surgery for obstructing, incurable colon cancer. Patients identified by a computerized pathology database.	Success rate at relieving obstruction: 94% for stent vs 100% for surgery. Median hospital stay: 2 d for stent vs 8 d for surgery. Complication rate: 8% for stent vs 30% for surgery. In-hospital mortality 0% for stent vs 8.5% for surgery.	Retrospective study, nonrandomized treatments, single center study. Computerized analysis of pathology database may not have captured all treated patients.	Self-expanding metal stents may be a highly effective and safe therapy when compared to surgery for palliation of incurable, obstructing colon cancer.

(Continued)

TABLE 163-7 Evidence-Based Medicine: Key References for Colonic Disorders (*Continued*)

Study	Methodology	Results	Limitations	Bottom Line
Larkin JO, et al. *Ann R Coll Surg Engl*. 2009;91: 205-209.	Retrospective study comparing nonoperative vs operative management of acute sigmoid volvulus. Patients identified by operating room registry and admissions office records.	27 patients treated for sigmoid volvulus during 11 y at one hospital, including 11 patients managed with colonoscopic decompression alone vs 15 requiring surgery. Of 11 patients undergoing only colonoscopy, 4 died and 5 were readmitted with recurrent volvulus, whereas only 1 of 15 patients initially undergoing surgery died. There was no mortality in 8 patients with ASA scores of IV undergoing surgery.	Retrospective study, nonrandomized treatments, small study size. Nonrandomized treatment may have led to bias of nonsurgical treatment for sickest patients, who then had a higher mortality.	Given the high risk of recurrence of sigmoid volvulus treated colonoscopically and the relatively low surgical mortality, all patients should be strongly considered for definitive surgery after successful colonoscopic detorsion and decompression of sigmoid volvulus.

Colonic pseudo-obstruction

Study	Methodology	Results	Limitations	Bottom Line
Loftus CG, et al. *Am J Gastroenterol*. 2002;97: 3118-22.	Retrospective, observational study of 18 patients receiving neostigmine for acute colonic pseudo-obstruction, which did not respond to conservative therapy. Patients identified using computerized database of patients classified according to diagnosis.	Only 18 of 151 patients presenting with colonic pseudo-obstruction received neostigmine. Among the 18 patients receiving neostigmine, 11 (61%) had a sustained therapeutic response. The remaining 7 (39%) required colonoscopic decompression or surgery for persistent colonic dilatation. Neostigmine responders were more likely to be older (mean age: 76 vs 54 y, $P = .03$), and had faster resolution of colonic pseudo-obstruction than patients treated conservatively (without neostigmine or colonoscopy) (mean resolution 2 vs 4 d, $P = .038$).	Retrospective study, nonrandomized treatments, limited number of patients treated with neostigmine. Computerized analysis may not have captured all treated patients.	Neostigmine was effective in resolving acute colonic pseudo-obstruction in the majority of treated cases. Neostigmine is likely underutilized.
Mehta R, et al. *J Gastroenterol Hepatol*. 2006;21: 459-461.	Prospective study of factors predicting successful outcome in 19 patients treated with neostigmine for colonic pseudo-obstruction.	Of 19 treated patients, 16 (84%) had an initial response with neostigmine and 10 (63%) had a sustained response. Of 9 patients retreated with neostigmine, 5 had a sustained response. Neostigmine responders were more likely to be postoperative patients (73% vs 25%, $P = .07$), less likely to have electrolyte disturbances (20% vs 100%, $P = .01$), and less likely to be on anti-motility agents (13% vs 100%, $P = .003$).	Small study size. Lack of control group to compare outcome in patients not receiving neostigmine.	Neostigmine leads to about a 65% sustained response in patients with acute colonic pseudo-obstruction. For neostigmine to be effective electrolyte imbalances should be corrected and anti-motility agents (eg, opiates) should be discontinued.

(Continued)

TABLE 163-7 Evidence-Based Medicine: Key References for Colonic Disorders *(Continued)*

Study	Methodology	Results	Limitations	Bottom Line
Valle RG, et al. *Ann Med Surg.* 2014;3:60-64.	Meta-analysis of 4 published randomized controlled studies evaluating 127 patients including 65 patients treated with neostigmine and 62 controls treated with placebo. Quality of each incorporated clinical trial was assessed by standard established criteria.	Among the 127 analyzed patients, neostigmine treatment was successful in 89.2% of cases vs 14.7% in untreated controls. Side effects of neostigmine therapy in treated patients included: abdominal pain >50% (from powerful intestinal smooth muscle contractions), sialorrhea >30%, and vomiting >15%. Bradycardia, the most severe side effect, occurred in 6.5% of treated patients.	Limited number (only 4) randomized clinical trials incorporated into meta-analysis. Substantial heterogeneity of analyzed clinical trials because of different study designs. Time to resolution of acute pseudo-obstruction after neostigmine therapy not analyzed because this data was reported in only 1 clinical trial. Insufficient data on etiologies of colonic pseudo-obstruction in all 4 analyzed clinical trials.	Neostigmine is a relatively safe and effective therapy for acute colonic pseudo-obstruction (up to 90% efficacy). The most important serious side effect is bradycardia that occurs in about 6.5% of cases. It is a first-line therapy for patients failing conservative therapy for acute colonic pseudo-obstruction, after correction of reversible risk factors for acute colonic pseudo-obstruction.

SUGGESTED READINGS

Antolovic D, Reissfelder C, Koch M, et al. Surgical treatment of sigmoid diverticulitis: analysis of predictive risk factors for postoperative infections, surgical complications, and mortality. *Int J Colorectal Dis.* 2009;24:577-584.

Byrnes MC, Mazuski JE. Antimicrobial therapy for acute colonic diverticulitis. *Surg Infect (Larchmt).* 2009;10:143-154.

Cappell MS, Friedel D. The role of sigmoidoscopy and colonoscopy in the diagnosis and management of lower gastrointestinal disorders: technique, indications, and contraindications. *Med Clin North Am.* 2002;86:1217-1252.

Cappell MS. Colonic toxicity of administered drugs and chemicals. *Am J Gastroenterol.* 2004;99:1175-1190.

De Giorgio R, Knowles CH. Acute colonic pseudo-obstruction. *Br J Surg.* 2009;96:229-239.

Dorn S, Lembo A, Cremonini F. Opioid-induced bowel dysfunction: epidemiology, pathophysiology, diagnosis, and initial therapeutic approach. *Am J Gastroenterol.* 2014;102:31-37.

Kaushik M, Bhullar JS, Bindroo S, Singh H, Mittal VK. Minimally invasive management of complicated diverticular disease: current status and review of literature. *Dig Dis Sci.* 2016;61:663-672.

Moriwaki Y, Sugiyama M, Toyoda H, et al. Lethal obstructive colitis: how and when patients with colonic obstruction should be prevented from falling into a lethal condition. *Hepatogastroenterology.* 2009;56:659-662.

Morris AM, Regenbogen SE, Hardiman KM, Hendren S. Sigmoid diverticulitis: a systematic review. *JAMA.* 2014;311:287-297.

Theodoropoulou A, Koutroubakis IE. Ischemic colitis: clinical practice in diagnosis and treatment. *World J Gastroenterol.* 2008;14:7302-7308.

Xu M, Zhong Y, Yao L, et al. Endoscopic decompression using a transanal drainage tube for acute obstruction of the rectum and left colon as a bridge to curative surgery. *Colorectal Dis.* 2009;11:405-409.

164

Inflammatory Bowel Disease

Joseph D. Feuerstein, MD
Kenneth R. Falchuk, MD

Key Clinical Questions

① When should you suspect inflammatory bowel disease (IBD) as the cause of a newly admitted patient with abdominal pain and diarrhea?

② How do differences between ulcerative colitis (UC) and Crohn disease (CD) impact hospital management?

③ What is the gastroenterologist's approach to induce and maintain remission?

④ What are the indications for surgical consultation?

⑤ What should be the hospitalist's approach while co-managing these patients?

⑥ How can clinicians minimize adverse events related to IBD, its medications, and related surgeries?

INTRODUCTION

Inflammatory bowel disease is a chronic inflammatory bowel condition that includes both ulcerative colitis (UC) and Crohn disease (CD). The underlying pathophysiology of disease remains unclear. The mainstay of therapy for both conditions is pharmacologic management. Ulcerative colitis is cured with surgical resection of the colon, while CD recurs even after surgical resection. This chapter will review the epidemiology of disease, diagnosis and workup of patients hospitalized with IBD, management of the hospitalized patient with IBD, and discharge planning.

EPIDEMIOLOGY

The peak age of onset of CD and UC is between 15 and 40 years old with a second possible peak between 50 and 80 years old. The disease is more common among Jewish ethnic groups, but is seen in other ethnic groups.

Only 10% to 25% of patients with IBD have a first degree relative with the disease. Genetic testing is not sufficient at this time to make a diagnosis or predict the likelihood of developing IBD.

Epidemiologic studies have identified multiple potential risk factors for developing IBD, including changes in the gut microbiome and/or disruption of the intestinal mucosa from gastrointestinal infections, antibiotics or medications such as nonsteroidal anti-inflammatory drugs. Other risk factors may include hormone replacement therapy and oral contraceptives. Tobacco usage is a risk factor for CD while protective against UC. Other factors that may be protective against IBD include increased physical activity, breast fed infants, and appendectomy (UC only).

■ UC

The overall incidence rate for UC in North America ranges from 2.2 to 19.2 cases per 100,000 person-years. In Europe the incidence rate varies with highs of 10 to 16.8 in Iceland, Denmark, United Kingdom, Netherlands, and Hungry, while ranging lower in Romania (0.97), Czech Republic (1.5), Estonia (1.7), and Poland (1.8). The overall incidence rates for Central and South America, Caribbean, Middle East, and Asia range from 0.74 to 6.02 cases per 100,000 patient years.

■ CD

Overall CD appears to have a higher incidence in industrialized countries and higher rates in the West compared to the East geographically. Crohn disease is more common in the North compared to the South in individual countries and in degrees latitude. In North America, it ranges from 6.3 to 13.4 cases per 100,000 person-years. In contrast, the incidence in Europe ranges from 0.1 in Poland to 10.1 in Denmark. Similar ranges are seen in the Middle East and Asia from 0.28 to 4.3 cases per 100,000 person-years.

CLASSIFICATION OF DISEASE ACCORDING TO ANATOMIC LOCATION

■ UC

Ulcerative colitis is categorized based on the segments of involved colonic disease:

- *Proctitis:* disease involving only the rectum
- *Proctosigmoiditis:* diseases involving the rectum and sigmoid colon

- *Left sided colitis:* disease involving up to the splenic flexure
- *Extensive colitis:* disease involving the colon beyond the splenic flexure

■ CD

Crohn disease has additional sub-categorizations given the differences in the location of disease and subtypes of disease.

- *Disease location:* colonic (localized to colon), ileal (localized to ileum), ileo-colonic (most common form), jejunal (localized to jejunum), upper gastrointestinal, peri-anal (localized to the perineum or present with any of the sub-types).
- *Disease activity descriptors:*
  - *Nonpenetrating and nonstricturing:* isolated inflammation
  - *Stricturing:* areas of narrowing that has resulted from fibrostenotic (scarring) changes in the mucosal wall
  - *Penetrating:* fistula or sinus tracts penetrating through the mucosal wall

PRESENTATION

Both diseases often present with abdominal pain and diarrhea that happens both during the day and overnight. **Table 164-1** for presenting symptoms and findings related to UC and CD.

■ SIGNS AND SYMPTOMS OF UC

Ulcerative colitis presents with inflammation that typically starts in the rectum and can involve the colon in a continuous fashion. In some cases of proctitis, proctosigmoiditis, or left-sided colitis there may also be inflammation in the cecum or around the appendix, termed cecal patch colitis. This is not considered a "skip lesion" and the diagnosis is still UC.

Ulcerative colitis classically presents with bloody diarrhea, urgency, tenesmus, and abdominal pain. Less frequently, patients will have more systemic symptoms of weight loss and low grade fevers. The symptoms typically develop over the course of weeks (see Table 164-1).

■ SIGNS AND SYMPTOMS OF CD

Crohn disease can involve any portion of the gastrointestinal tract from mouth to anus. The presenting symptoms are based on the variable locations and transmural involvement of the inflammation. Typically the disease spares the rectum, involves the gastrointestinal tract in a discontinuous fashion with intervening areas of normal mucosa (termed *skip lesions*), and is transmural which is the key differentiating factor from UC. Fifty percent of CD affects the terminal ileum and colon, 20% have isolated colonic disease, and 30% have only small bowel disease. Up to one-third of patients may develop perianal as well luminal disease. The disease can result in isolated inflammation, strictures, and/or fistulous tracts to other parts of the gastrointestinal tract, genitourinary organs, or skin.

Crohn disease typically presents with abdominal pain and diarrhea. When the colon is involved, bloody diarrhea may also be present. In contrast, if the small bowel is involved with stricturing disease, then patients will present with abdominal pain, weight loss, nausea, vomiting, and symptoms of complete or partial bowel obstructions. When fistulas develop, which occur in up to 45% of individuals at time of diagnosis, disease presentation is dependent on the location of the fistula and may include diarrhea, abscess, urinary tract infection, passage of stool from genitourinary organs or skin, and weight loss. A less frequent presentation of CD includes upper gastrointestinal involvement which may lead to dysphagia, odynophagia, and severe oral pain from oral ulcers (see Table 164-1).

TABLE 164-1 Presenting Symptoms Related to Ulcerative Colitis and Crohn Disease

	Common	Less common
Ulcerative colitis	Bloody diarrhea	Weight loss
	Abdominal pain	Fevers
	Urgency	
	Tenesmus	
Crohn	Diarrhea (can be bloody)	Fevers
	Weight loss	Nausea
	Abdominal pain	Vomiting
		Urgency (in colonic CD)
		Tenesmus (in colonic CD)
		Anal fissures
		Peri-anal fistula
Fistulizing Crohn disease	Abdominal pain	
	Diarrhea	
	Weight loss	
	Drainage to skin (enterocutaneous fistula)	
	Drainage to bladder (entero-vesicular fistula)	
	Drainage to vagina (entero-vaginal)	
	Drainage to perianal area (perianal fistula)	
	Diarrhea (entero-enteric fistula)	
	Fevers	
	Pain over fistula site	
Stricturing Crohn disease	Abdominal pain	Feculent vomitus
	Weight loss	No flatus
	Nausea	No bowel movements
	Vomiting	
Upper gastrointestinal Crohn disease	Abdominal pain	Dysphagia
	Reflux	Odynophagia
	Dyspepsia	
	Vomiting	
	Weight loss	

EXTRAINTESTINAL MANIFESTATIONS

The most commonly extraintestinal manifestations of IBD involve the skin, joints, eyes, and liver in up to one-third of patients. Erythema nodosum (EN) and pyoderma gangrenosum (PG) are immunologic related skin disorders that vary in presentation. Erythema nodosum presents as painful raised subcutaneous lesions on the anterior surfaces of the lower extremities and typically follows luminal disease activity. Pyoderma gangrenosum appears as shallow ulcers that coalesce into deeper ulcers on the lower extremities with no relationship to colonic disease activity. The development of arthritis can be peripheral or axial and involve the large or small joint symmetrically or asymmetrically. Axial involvement classically presents as ankylosing spondylitis and/or sacroileitis. Both conditions can range from being asymptomatic and noted only on imaging to severely debilitating pain with limited spinal flexion. Pain and stiffness typically improve with exercise. Type 1 peripheral arthropathy

TABLE 164-2 Summary of Common Extraintestinal Manifestations of IBD

Parallel course	Peripheral arthritis	5%-20%
	Aphthous stomatitis	25%
	Erythema nodosum	10%-20%
	Episcleritis	1.6%-6.3%
	Uveitis	0.5%-9%
Independent course	Ankylosing spondylitis	5%-10%
	Sacroileitits	3%-5%
	Primary sclerosing cholangitis	2.4%-7.5%
	Uveitits	1.6%-6.3%
	Pyoderma gangrenosum	1%-10%
Metabolic manifestations	Nephrolithiasis	7%-10%
	Osteopenia, osteoporosis	23%-59%

develops acutely following disease flares and classically involves less than six joints. Usually self-limited symptoms improve with treatment of the luminal disease. Type 2 peripheral arthropathy differs by not specifically following the luminal disease course, involving more than six joints, including the metacarophalangeal joints. Patients may describe chronic symptoms, such as a migratory arthritis with synovitis that persists for months.

Primary sclerosing cholangitis (PSC) can develop in both UC and CD but is significantly more common in UC. A chronic cholestatic disease involving the liver and bile ducts, PSC can progress to cirrhosis and necessitate liver transplantation. Additional extraintestinal manifestations include uveitis, scleritis, optic neuritis, sweet syndrome, aphthous stomatitis, venous thromboembolism, and impaired growth in children. Other manifestations specific to CD include renal stones, B12 deficiency, osteoporosis, osteopenia, and amyloidosis (see **Table 164-2**).

CLINICAL COURSE

UC

Periods of remission and flares characterize UC. At time of initial diagnosis, a majority of patients have mild-moderate disease with less than 10% presenting with severe disease. Approximately 15% of patients will develop severe flares of UC during their lifetime and may necessitate colectomy. Relapses of UC are unpredictable, but if a flare develops, then there is a 70% to 80% chances of a subsequent flare the following year. The presence of a flare within 2 years of diagnosis is predictive of subsequent relapse in the ensuing 5 years. During years three to seven following diagnosis, 25% will be in remission, 57% will have intermittent relapses, and 18% have annual disease flares. Patients who experience flares do not have an increased risk of mortality compared to the general population.

CD

Cycles of flares, remission, and relapse characterize CD. Population-based data from Scandinavia reports that 50% of patients with CD will relapse within 1 year. Over 4 years, 53% of patients develop a fluctuating course of flares and remission, 25% have ongoing chronic active symptoms, and only 22% are in remission. The majority of patients with CD will experience progressive disease with the development of strictures or penetrating disease. Up to a third of patients will also develop perianal complications. Many patients require surgical management with reports as high as 50%at 10 years after initial diagnosis and up to 80% at 20 years. Approximately 50% will relapse again within 5 years following the

first surgery and 30% will need a second procedure within 10 years. In contrast to UC, mortality is slightly increased compared to the general population.

DIAGNOSIS

UC

The diagnosis of UC is made in individuals with symptoms consistent with UC (eg, bloody diarrhea) and endoscopic evidence showing continuous colonic inflammation (eg, erythema, granularity, friability, ulcers) that starts in the rectum and extends proximally without skip lesions (**Figure 164-1**). The diagnosis is confirmed with biopsies showing findings of chronic histological changes with paneth cell metaplasia as well as varying degrees of inflammatory infiltrates in the mucosal layers including lymphocytes, plasma cells, and granuolycytes. Additional changes are present in the crypt architecture with shortening and disarray of the crypts, atrophy, abscesses, and branching (**Table 164-3**).

CD

The diagnosis of CD is made in individuals with classic symptoms of CD and confirmed with either endoscopic evidence of active disease or imaging of small bowel lesions with classic findings consistent with CD. The presence of fissures, fistula, mass, or larger skin tags may all suggest a diagnosis of CD. When the disease involves the colon or terminal ileum, colonoscopy with terminal ileum intubation is classically confirmatory with the findings of perianal involvement but relative rectal sparing with discontinuous (skip lesions), granularity, erythema, friability, aphthous ulcers or serpiginous ulcers (**Figure 164-2**). Biopsies confirm the diagnosis of CD with deep involvement through mucosal layers. In addition, biopsy may identify the rare, pathognomonic finding of a granuloma (Table 164-3). Magnetic resonance enterography (MRE) and MR pelvis can display features of chronic fibrostenotic disease as well as fistulous involvement further confirming the diagnosis. Computed tomography (CT) enterography has similar sensitivity to MRE for small bowel lesions but requires the use of iodinated contrast and exposes patients to radiation (**Figure 164-3**). Wireless capsule endoscopy can be used with very high sensitivity for

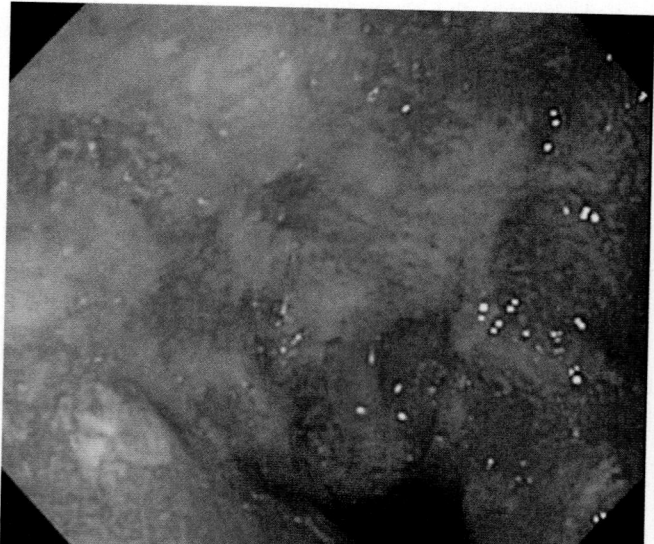

Figure 164-1 *Endoscopic image of inflamed colon in a patient with UC. Macroscopic features supporting a diagnosis of UC are loss of vascularity and granularity.*

TABLE 164-3 Endoscopic Features of UC and CD

UC	CD
Continuous inflammation progressing proximally in the colon	Rectum spared
	Perianal involvement
Rectal involvement	Discontinuous areas of involvement (*skip lesions*)
Ulcers	Aphthous ulcerations
Loss of vascular pattern	Linear and/or serpiginous ulcerations
Mucosal granularity	Mucosal granularity
Mucosal edema	Mucosal edema
Mucosal friability	Mucosal friability
Spontaneous bleeding	Spontaneous bleeding
	Fistulae
	Strictures
	Aphthae in terminal ileum

findings small bowel lesions in CD, but should be used with caution given the risk of capsule retention when strictures are present.

■ SEROLOGIC MARKERS

There is no serologic marker that is sensitive or specific enough to exclude the diagnosis or confirm the diagnosis. Anti-*Saccharomyces cerevisiae* (ASCA) is positive in patients with CD in 50% to 70% of cases and has a specificity of 92% if perinuclear antineutrophil cytoplasmic antibodies (pANCA) testing is negative. Perinuclear antineutrophil cytoplasmic antibody is positive in patients with UC in 40% to 80% of cases with a specificity of 98% if ASCA is negative. Other serologic markers like an elevated C-reactive protein (CRP) and/or erythrocyte sedimentation rate (ESR) can be helpful to indicate the presence of inflammation. However, a normal ESR and CRP does not have adequate negative predictive value to rule out active inflammation. Fecal lactoferrin, and fecal calprotectin have sensitivities and specificities over 90% for the presence of inflammation. However, a positive result cannot differentiate infection from IBD or differentiate UC from CD.

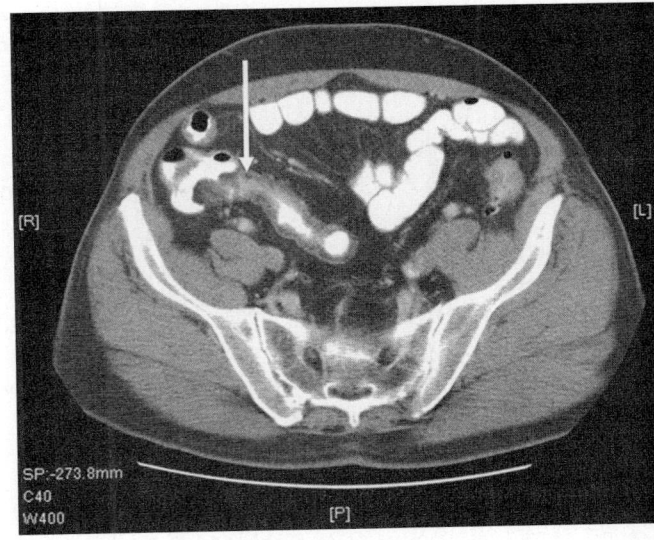

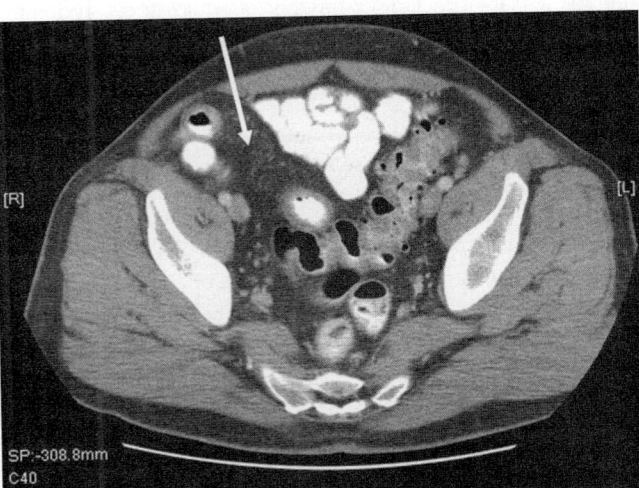

Figure 164-3 *Characteristic CT manifestations of CD involving the terminal ileum. (A) Inflamed terminal ileum and ileocecal valve resulting in irregular contrast enhancement and bowel wall thickening (arrow). (B) Encasement of terminal ileum by fat tissue, termed "creeping fat."*

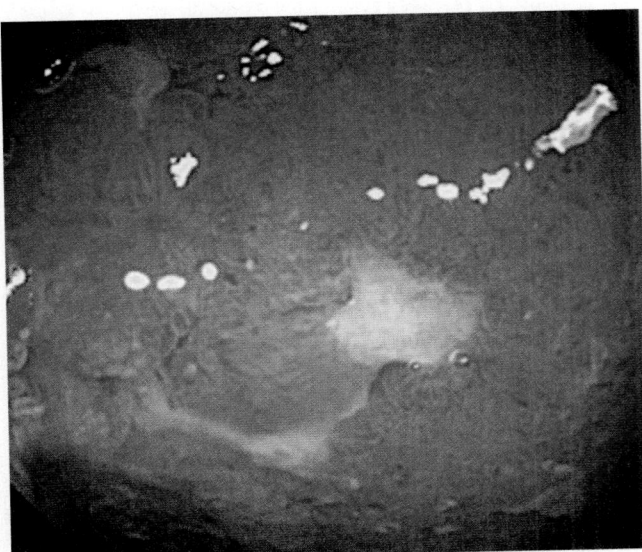

Figure 164-2 *Endoscopic findings during colonoscopy of a patient with CD. Large serpiginous ulceration on the ileocecal valve in a patient with CD.*

CRITERIA FOR GENERAL ADMISSION

The classic criteria for patients necessitating admission for a flare of UC were established by Truelove and Witts in 1955 (**Table 164-4**). The criteria include: greater than six stools per day, frequent blood in the stool, temperature greater than 37.8°C, heart rate greater than 90 per minute, hemoglobin less than 75% normal value, ESR greater than 30 mm/h, radiographic findings of air, edematous wall, or thumb printing, and abdominal tenderness on examination. Other indications for admission include failure of outpatient medical therapy, toxic megacolon, complications related to the disease (eg, thromboembolism), or complications related to pharmacologic management (eg, opportunistic infection).

In CD, patients with colonic involvement will usually present similarly to patients with UC. Patients with stricturing or fistulizing CD will present with more systemic symptoms related to bowel obstruction (eg, nausea, vomiting, lack of flatus, abdominal pain) or systemic infection (eg, nausea, vomiting, abdominal pain, fevers, chills) from abscess formation. Less frequently, patients may also present with severe malnutrition related to severe CD. One

TABLE 164-4 Truelove and Witts Classification of Ulcerative Colitis Disease Activity (Calculated on Day 3)

Disease severity	Mild	Severe	Fulminant
Number of bowel movements per day	<4	>6	>10
Blood in stool	Intermittent	Frequent	Always present
Temperature °C	Normal	Elevated (>37.5)	Elevated (>37.5)
Pulse	Normal	Elevated (>90 beats/min)	Elevated (>90 beats/min)
Hemoglobin	Normal	<75% normal	Transfusion required
Erythrocyte Sedimentation rate, mm/h	≤30	>30	>30
Radiographic features of colon	Na	Edematous wall, thumbprinting, air	Dilatation of bowel wall
Clinical exam findings	Na	Abdominal tenderness	Abdominal tenderness and distention

Abbreviation: Na, not applicable.
Note: moderate disease is an overlap of mild and severe findings.

scoring system that can be used to assess disease severity is the Crohn Disease Activity Index (CDAI) (**Table 164-5**). The CDAI uses multiple variables including: number of liquid stools, abdominal pain, general well-being, extraintestinal complications, antidiarrheal drug usage, abdominal mass, hematocrit, and body weight

to calculate a score. Scores greater than 450 points indicate severe disease.

Rapid evaluation, ICU monitoring, and early surgical consultation should be considered for patients with sepsis and multiorgan failure. These complications are associated with mortality rates of 70%.

TABLE 164-5 Crohn Disease Activity Index

Variable	Description	Score	Multiplier
Number of liquid stool	Sum of 7 d		2
Abdominal pain	Sum of 7 d	0 = none	5
		1 = mild	
		2 = moderate	
		3 = severe	
General well being	Sum of 7 d	0 = generally well	7
		1 = slightly under par	
		2 = poor	
		3 = very poor	
		4 = terrible	
Extraintestinal complications	Number of listed complications	Arthritis	20
		Arthralgias	
		Iritis	
		Uveitis	
		Erythema nodosum	
		Pyoderma gangrenosum	
		Aphthous stomatitis	
		Anal fissure/fistula/abscess	
		Fever >37.8°C	
Antidiarrheal drugs	Use in the prior 7 d	0 = no	30
		1 = yes	
Abdominal mass		0 = no	10
		2 = questionable	
		5 = definite	
Hematocrit	Expected minus observed level	Male: 47% – observed	6
		Female: 42% – observed	
Body weight	Checked in the last 7 d	1 – (ideal observed) × 100	1 (not if <10)

CDAI <150 = remission.
CDAI reduction of >70 or >100 (depending on study) = response.
CDAI 220-450 = moderate to severe disease.
CDAI >450 = severe disease.

INFECTION

Hospitalists should always perform a comprehensive history, physical examination, and assessment to identify any concurrent conditions that can mimic or trigger a flare of IBD or alter management. All patients admitted with a flare of IBD with diarrhea should be tested for *Clostridium difficle*. *Clostridium difficile* is more common in patients with IBD, especially those with colonic involvement. This infection is associated with increased mortality, (four times greater than when *C. difficile* arises in the absence of IBD or when an IBD flare arises in the absence of this infection), and with significant morbidity, (resulting in colectomy in up to 20% of cases). One study reported that nearly 40% of the patients admitted with *C. difficile* did not have any prior antibiotic exposure (see Chapter 82 [Diarrhea] and Chapter 190 [*C. difficile* Associated Diseases]).

Patients receiving immunosuppressive therapy should undergo endoscopy to obtain colonic biopsies to exclude cytomegalovirus (CMV) infection. Serologic testing for CMV viral load can be done, but low-grade viremia does not necessarily indicate CMV colitis and colonic biopsies are still required to diagnose CMV Colitis (see Chapter 198 [Viral Infections, Including MERS]). Any patient with IBD can also develop other gastrointestinal infections as well as systemic diseases concurrent with their IBD.

MANAGEMENT

Patients hospitalized for severe UC have a 27% rate of colectomy and 1% mortality rate. All cause 30-day readmission rates are as high as 25%. Patients with severe disease or requiring intensive unit care management may require transfer to a tertiary care hospital. Early transfer to a tertiary care center should also be considered in any patient who has already failed outpatient biologic therapy (eg, infliximab, adalimumab, golimumab, certolizumab pegol, vedolizumab, natalizumab), or has a flare of the disease complicated by *C. difficile* or CMV. These patients are at high risk of needing surgical management.

Initial management begins with fluid resuscitation and objective assessment of disease activity. The need for both an ESR and CRP is that some patients only trigger an elevation in one of the two inflammatory markers and if either area elevated, then they can be used to predict response to therapy. If there is concern for systemic toxicity, blood cultures should also be obtained. Additionally, when diarrhea is present, stool studies should be obtained including testing for *C. difficile*, *Escherichia coli*, *salmonella*, *shigella*, and in selected patients, ova and parasite and giardia and cryptosporidium. Patients presenting with a UC flare should have a plain abdominal x-ray to assess for signs of toxic megacolon. In cases of concern for systemic toxicity which may alter management, CT scan is preferred over MRI given the widespread availability and rapid imaging technique. If imaging can be delayed than MRE or MR pelvis is preferable given the enhanced image quality and lack of radiation exposure.

■ VTE PROPHYLAXIS

Patients with IBD have a two- to threefold increased risk of venous thromboembolism (VTE) compared to the general population with 8- to 15-fold higher risk during flares of IBD. Mortality is 2.5-fold higher in patients with VTE and IBD compared to IBD alone. VTE occurs most commonly in patients with more extensive disease but does not have an age or sex predominance.

All patients should receive pharmacologic prophylaxis with low molecular weight heparin or at least unfractionated heparin. Bloody diarrhea alone is not a contraindication to heparin prophylaxis. Only in rare cases of profuse hemorrhage necessitating aggressive resuscitation in the intensive care unit and red cell transfusions, contraindication to heparin, or significant thrombocytopenia should heparin prophylaxis be avoided and instead mechanical prophylaxis is used. However, in general, mechanical prophylaxis alone does not appear to be adequate to prevent VTE in patients with IBD. Ordering VTE prophylaxis does not ensure adequate prophylaxis without patient and nursing education about the indication of VTE prophylaxis and a notification system in place if patients decline injections.

(See Chapter 252 [VTE Prophylaxis in Hospitalized Medical Patients].)

■ INDUCTION OF REMISSION IN PATIENTS WITH UC

The mainstay of therapy for moderate to severe flares of UC is systemic corticosteroids. Even if oral steroids were used as an outpatient, still two thirds of individuals will respond to systemic corticosteroids. The usual dose is methylprednisolone 20 mg three times a day or equivalent administered intravenously. There is no benefit to higher doses or continuous infusion of steroids. Up to 30% of individuals will fail and necessitate salvage therapy with infliximab or cyclosporine or colectomy. From the onset of hospitalization narcotic usage should be minimized as this portends a poorer prognosis with increased morbidity (**Figure 164-4**).

Many experts advocate that patients should also undergo tuberculosis testing with a Quantiferon Gold assay and hepatitis B screening (hepatitis B antibody, hepatitis B surface antigen, hepatitis B core antibody) to assess the safety of using infliximab if steroids fail and salvage therapy is necessary. A serum cholesterol and magnesium should be obtained in patients hospitalized at institutions with expertise in the use of cyclosporine as an alternative rescue therapy option. The cost-effectiveness of this approach has yet to be established. Other experts advocate that this should be done once it is determined that steroids are not working.

Admission day
- Assess for triggers of flare (eg, NSAIDs, noncompliance with medications)
- History and Physical examination
- Labs/Stool tests: CBC, LFTS, ESR, CRP, *Clostridium difficle* with PCR
- Optional labs to consider:
  - If considering infliximab rescue therapy: TB testing with quantiferon gold or PPD with control, hepatitis B serologies
  - If considering cyclosporine rescue therapy: Magnesium, total cholesterol, and TPMT
- Abdominal KUB
  - Consider CT abdomen pelvis if severe abdominal pain or systemic symptoms like fevers, nausea, vomiting or if severe abdominal tenderness is present
- Flexible sigmoidoscopy to rule out CMV infection (ideally within 48 h)
- Start methylprednisolone 20 mg TID (or equivalent)

Day 2
- Continue IV steroids
- Abdominal exam
- Assess stool output in last 24 h
- If stool output reduced by 75% and no blood skip to day 5

Day 3
- Continue IV steroids
- Abdominal exam
- Assess stool output in last 24 h
- Labs: CBC, LFTS, ESR, and CRP
- Utilize clinical prediction rule Travis or Ho Index to determine risk of failing IV steroids
- If high risk for steroid failure:
  - If testing for safety of salvage therapy has not been done it should be done at this time
  - Review risks of salvage therapy
  - Initiate colorectal surgery consultation for complete discussion with patient prior to starting salvage therapy
  - Initiate salvage therapy with infliximab or cyclosporine based on centers experience

Day 4
- Continue IV steroids
- If high risk of failing IV steroids then either infliximab or cyclosporine therapy should have been initiated or surgical management of disease
- Abdominal examination
- Assess stool output in last 24 h

Day 5/ Discharge
- Patient has responded to therapy as determined by:
  - 1-2 bowel movements OR
  - ≤4 bowel movements with no blood
- Arrange follow-up appointment in 2 wk
- Provide adequate prescription for oral steroids—Prednisone usually dosed at 40-60 mg for 2 wk and then tapered by 10 mg/wk or 5 mg/wk until 20 mg and then by 5 mg/wk
- For those patients on rescue therapy, continue to assess on a daily basis. If not improved after 3-7 d of rescue therapy then consider colectomy at that time

Figure 164-4 *Management of inpatient flare of ulcerative colitis.*

In patients who present on admission already on immunosuppressive drugs (eg, steroids, thiopurines, antitumor necrosis factor, anti-integrin molecules) should undergo a flexible sigmoidoscopy with biopsies to rule out CMV colitis.

On a daily basis, patient should have the total number of bowel movements over the preceding 24 hours quantified.

There is disagreement regarding the optimal nutrition order for patients. Some experts recommend that for patient comfort, to reduce the overall volume of diarrhea, to initiate either nothing by mouth or liquid diet. In contrast, others argue that this may falsely reduce the overall number of bowel movements and does nothing to actually heal the disease and instead a regular diet should be provided to patients.

On day 3 of admission, the ESR and CRP should be repeated and an assessment using either the Travis index or Ho index should be used to determine the likelihood of failing steroids and requiring escalation of therapy (**Table 164-6**). The Travis index is used most often. The assessment is greater than eight bowel movements per day or greater than two bowel movements per day and a CRP greater than 45mg/L has an 85% positive predictive value of necessitating colectomy.

If predictors suggest response to steroids then continue management up to 5 to 7 days of intravenous steroids. The goal is to reduce the number of bowel movements to one to two bowel movements

per day or at least to achieve less than or equal to four nonbloody bowel movements over a 24-hour period.

■ SALVAGE THERAPY

In patients who are failing corticosteroids, a decision on day 3 of the hospitalization should be made regarding the likelihood of steroid failure (**Table 164-7**). In consultation with the patient's gastroenterologist, surgical consultation should proceed if the scoring system used predicts a high likelihood of colectomy. Sigmoidoscopy should be performed prior to initiation of salvage therapy to exclude any other infections that may be contributing to steroid failure (eg, CMV colitis) if not already performed during this hospitalization. Patients should be offered either colectomy which is a definitive therapy for UC, or consideration for salvage therapy with infliximab or cyclosporine. Both cyclosporine and infliximab have similar outcomes and are equal in efficacy. Given the ease of use of infliximab relative to cyclosporine, most centers have opted to use infliximab.

If a decision is made to attempt salvage therapy, patients should be counseled regarding the risks and benefits of each drug. There are very few long-term studies assessing the success rate of salvage therapy with some reporting rates of colectomy at 5 years upwards of 40%.

TABLE 164-6 Travis and Ho Indices

Travis index	Either >8 bowel movements per d OR >2 bowel movements per d and CRP > 45 mg/L	Ho index	Mean stool frequency	<4 = 0 points 4 ≤ 6 = 1 point 6 ≤ 9 = 2 points >9 = 4 points
			Colonic dilation	None = 0 points Present = 4 points
			Hypoalbuminemia (<3.0 g/dL)	Normal = 0 points <3.0 g/dL = 1 point
Interpretation if positive:	85% positive predictive value of needing colectomy		Scores	0-1 = low risk of steroid failure 2-3 = intermediate risk for steroid failure ≥4 = high risk for steroid failure

Abbreviation: CRP, c-reactive protein.

INFLIXIMAB

Prior to initiating infliximab therapy, patients need to be assessed for exposure and presence of latent tuberculosis and hepatitis B. In many patients, the Quantiferon Gold test may be equivocal due to anergy from active disease or use of steroids. In low-risk individuals a negative chest x-ray is likely adequate. In those who have possible exposures to tuberculous, an infectious disease consult should be obtained prior to starting infliximab. Adverse events associated with infliximab include: infusion reactions, hepatitis, infection, reactivation of tuberculosis or hepatitis B, melanoma, psoriasis, eczema, drug induced lupus, and other rarer side effects.

Infliximab is bound to albumin and secreted into the gut. In patients with a severe UC flare, the albumin is often low and a significant amount of infliximab is likely excreted into the gut resulting

TABLE 164-7 Salvage Therapy for Ulcerative Colitis

Medication	Dose	Mechanism	Lab Testing prior to Initiating Therapy	Relative Contraindication	Side Effect	Response in 7 d	Treatment failure at 98 d*
Cyclosporine	2-4 mg/kg dosed to goal drug level of 150-300 ng/ml	Calcineurin mediated T-cell suppression	Magnesium Total cholesterol	Uncontrolled infections Uncontrolled hypertension Low cholesterol <100 mg/dL	Hypertension Hypertrichosis Nephrotoxicity Hyperkalemia Infection Lymphoma Skin cancer Seizures Hepatitis Diabetes	86%	38%
Infliximab	5-10 mg/kg	anti TNF-α	Tuberculosis testing (recommend a Quantiferon gold assay) or PPD with control given risk of anergy Latent hepatitis B infection	Uncontrolled infections Severe heart failure Active/latent TB (may require cotreatment of TB) Latent hepatitis B (may require cotreatment of hepatitis B) Hypersensitivity to murine products	Infusion reaction Infection Non-Hodgkin lymphoma Melanoma Reactivation of latent TB Reactivation of latent hepatitis B Drug induced lupus Psoriaform reactions Worsening of severe CHF Demyelinating disease	84%	30%

*Relapse, lack of remission, unable to withdraw steroids.
Abbreviations: CHF congestive heart failure; TB tuberculosis; TNF tumor necrosis factor.

in suboptimal dosing of infliximab in the hospitalized patient with severe colitis. The optimal dosing strategy for inpatient induction with infliximab is unclear. A recent study has indicated that a more rapid induction than the classic 5 mg/kg dosing at week 0, 2, and 6 is necessary. Some experts utilize a dose of 5 mg/kg with a reassessment in 72 hours and if still not optimized then a second dose of 5 mg/kg is administered. Others administer 10 mg/kg initially and then reassess again in 72 hours. In patients who show no response in 72 hours, a discussion regarding aborting therapy and proceeding to colectomy is necessary. Once the patient responds to therapy, then most will follow the subsequent loading at week 2 and week 6 at whatever dose the patient initially responded to.

Some experts utilize combination therapy with a thiopurine to prevent antibody formation to infliximab if the drug is underdosed at this induction phase. If such a treatment is planned, testing for thiopurine methyltransferase (TPMT) should be obtained prior to starting the thiopurine. Patients should be counseled about the increased risk of side effects with combination therapy, specifically, the rare risk of hepatosplenic T-cell lymphoma that is 100% fatal.

Patients should be continued on a routine induction protocol at week 0, 2, and 6 followed by maintenance with infliximab every 8 weeks if salvage therapy succeeds. Most centers will still utilize a prednisone taper on discharge despite failure of systemic steroids.

CYCLOSPORINE

Cyclosporine was the initial drug of choice for salvage therapy. A relative contraindication to use of cyclosporine is a serum cholesterol less than 100 mg/dL. Side effects of cyclosporine include seizures, nephrotoxicity, tremor, hypertension, nausea, vomiting, headaches, anaphylaxis, infection, and paresthesias. Cyclosporine is not as effective orally, and all patients should have a TPMT level checked with the plan to bridge them to mercaptopurine or azathioprine. Any patient who already failed thiopurines, may not be an ideal candidate for cyclosporine therapy.

The initial dose of cyclosporine is a continuous infusion that ranges from 2 to 4 mg/kg. Drug levels need to be checked frequently starting on day 2 of administration with a goal level of 150 to 300 ng/mL. Patients should ideally respond within 7 days. Those failing to respond should be referred for urgent colectomy. Many experts recommend prophylaxis *Pneumocystis (carinii) jiroveci* pneumonia with trimethoprim-sulfamethoxazole for patients being discharged on cyclosporine requiring triple immunosuppressive therapy (ie, steroids, cyclosporine and thioprine). Serum concentrations of magnesium and cholesterol should be episodically monitored as a low level for both increases the likelihood of seizures with the use of cyclosporine. Cyclosporine levels should be checked every 1 to 2 weeks following discharge to the outpatient setting.

SURGERY

Indications for surgical consultation include signs of systemic toxicity, instability, and lack of response to systemic corticosteroids.

Urgent colectomy should be performed for toxic megacolon. Toxic megacolon should be considered in patients who on imaging have a transverse colon diameter greater than 6 cm. A colorectal surgeon should be consulted to discuss surgical treatment options when salvage therapy is under consideration.

Colectomy is the only definitive treatment for UC and current data regarding the long-term benefits of salvage therapy is limited. Cyclosporine does not appear to increase the postoperative complication rates if concomitant salvage therapy is administered. The data on infliximab and postoperative complication rates are equivocal at this time.

THIRD-LINE SALVAGE THERAPY

Third-line salvage therapy refers to the use of a third-line salvage therapy with infliximab after failure of cyclosporine salvage therapy or cyclosporine after infliximab salvage therapy. This option is associated with a 20% to 30% risk of significant adverse events and mortality and most gastroenterologists do not recommend this approach.

PRACTICE POINT

Interventions with no benefit in the management of severe UC include:

- The routine use of antibiotics (except in impeding perforation)
- Nutritional support with total parenteral nutrition (TPN)
- Administrion of antidiarrheals, opioid analgesics, and/or anticholinergics

---

INDUCTION OF REMISSION IN PATIENTS WITH CD

The inpatient management of patients with a flare of CD is dictated more based on the location of the CD and the resultant presenting symptoms. Colonic CD presents and is treated similarly to UC. Patients with symptoms of partial or small bowel obstruction require imaging, usually abdominal CT to diagnose stricturing CD. Once the diagnosis is established, fibrostenotic disease should be differentiated from active inflammation. Recent studies have supported the efficacy of MRI in differentiating active from chronic fibrostenotic inflammation.

When active inflammation has been identified as the source of obstruction, mechanical and pharmacologic treatment is necessary. Bowel rest (best achieved by the combination of nothing by mouth and nasogastric tube suction) facilitates bowel decompression. Medications include intravenous corticosteroids (ie, methylprednisolone 20 mg three times a day), and antibiotics (ie, ciprofloxacin and metronidazole or similar agents).

When fibrostenotic disease has been identified as the source of obstruction, the mainstay of therapy is initially bowel rest. Patients will not benefit from systemic corticosteroids and/or antibiotics unless there is a component of active inflammation.

When steroids or conservative measures fail to induce remission, strictures necessitate surgical management with limited bowel resection or in rarer cases stricturoplasty. The goal of surgery is to perform the most limited resection while removing the strictured area and ideally inducing surgical remission.

The benefits of systemic corticosteroids are less clear in the treatment of fistulizing CD, perianal fistula, and perianal abscess. Fistula rarely heal quickly; up to one-third of complex fistula fail to heal even with antitumor necrosis factor therapy. Fistulizing disease will often lead to secondary abscess formation. Antibiotics with ciprofloxacin and metronidazole (or similar agents) should be initiated to treat secondary abscess and corticosteroids and immunosuppressing drugs avoided. Any abscess amenable to drainage with interventional radiology or surgery should be drained to facilitate healing. Only once the abscess is resolved or clearly resolving as noted by improving in both systemic symptoms, laboratory values, and imaging, then immunosuppressive medications can be restarted in select cases. Surgical management with resection of the affected area may be necessary if an abscess fails to heal despite bowel rest and prolonged courses of antibiotics.

Patients with CD can present with severe malnutrition related to any subtype of CD. The mainstay of therapy for severe malnutrition is nutrition consultation and supplementation with high protein caloric drinks and/or TPN (see Chapter 58 [Nutrition and Metabolic Support]).

TABLE 164-8 Rutgeerts Scoring System to Predict Postoperative Clinical Recurrence of Crohn Disease

Endoscopic findings	Score
No Aphthous ulcers	0
Less than 5 aphthous ulcers	1
More than 5 aphthous ulcers with normal intervening mucosa, skip areas of larger lesions or lesions confined to the ileocolonic anastomosis (ie, <1 cm in length)	2
Diffuse aphthous ileitis with diffusely inflamed mucosa	3
Diffuse inflammation with larger ulcers, nodules, and or narrowing	4

■ PREVENTION OF POSTOPERATIVE RECURRENCE IN CD

Endoscopic recurrence of CD at the anastomotic site recurs in 90% of patients within 1 year of surgery. Majority of patients will develop symptomatic recurrence within 5 years and 70% will require additional surgical procedures for their CD. Factors most highly associated with early disease recurrence include smoking, perforating disease phenotype, perianal disease, prior surgical resections, young age at diagnosis (<25 years old), and disease involving greater than 50 cm of bowel.

Patients are assessed 6 to 12 months after their resection with colonoscopy using the Rutgeerts scoring system to assess the likelihood of clinical recurrence. The system is scored from I_0 to I_4 (Table 164-8). In patients with an I_0 or I_1, 80% to 85% will be asymptomatic 3 years after surgery. In contrast, patients scoring an I_2 or higher are deemed higher risk of clinical recurrence of over 90% at 3 years and postoperative prophylaxis to reduce the risk of clinical recurrence should be considered. Similarly, those patients with multiple risk factors for recurrence may be initiated on therapy immediately postoperatively given their high risk of clinical recurrence.

Multiple medications have been assessed to prevent disease recurrence but with overall limited success.

Mesalamine has minimal benefit when compared to placebo and generally has no role is postoperative prophylaxis. In contrast, metronidazole 20 mg/kg/d—when started within 7 days postoperatively and continued for 3 months—results in a significant but limited reduction of severe endoscopic recurrence. Unfortunately, however, few patients can tolerate 3 months of metronidazole at such a high dose due to the development of side effects (eg, metallic taste, peripheral neuropathy, inability to drink alcohol).

Data regarding the use of thiopurines and biologics is also limited but more robust relative to the other medications. Azathioprine and 6-mercaptopurine are more effective in comparison to mesalamine in decreasing postoperative recurrence of CD but provide a very modest prevention. In one study, those on placebo reported recurrence rates of 69% compared to 44% on thiopurine.

The best data though is with using either infliximab or adalimumab postoperatively or combining anti-TNF with a thiopurine., The long-term data on the efficacy of preventing clinical recurrence is limited to a few years and it is unclear if these options provide for long-term prevention of clinical recurrence.

Other medications and treatments that have very limited data include probiotics (VSL#3), budesonide, and fecal microbiota transplant.

■ OUTPATIENT MEDICATIONS FOR CD AND UC (TABLE164-9)

Once the patient has achieved clinical remission as defined by either one to two bowel movements or less than or equal to four bowel movements without blood, medications can be transitioned to outpatient regimens. Steroids can be changed to oral prednisone at doses from 40 to 60 mg daily. The steroids are tapered by 5 to 10 mg/wk. Those who taper by 10 mg/wk will slow the taper down to 5 mg/wk after reducing the dose to 20 mg. At the same time, mesalamine can be administered orally and/or rectally as an enema/suppository. If immunosuppressive agents are considered, then TPMT level should be checked and then either mercaptopurine or azathioprine can be commenced. Often, this medication will take up to 12 weeks to achieve its full effect. Methotrexate is dosed subcutaneous once a week if there are concerns about absorption due to small bowel disease absorption. Otherwise, it can be administered orally once a week. Prior to initiating any biologic drugs, the patient's hepatitis B status and exposure to tuberculosis must be assessed with hepatitis B serologies and Quantiferon Gold assay. Infliximab is an infusion that is dosed based on the patient's weight ranging from 5 to 10 mg/kg at weeks 0, 2, 6 and then every 8 weeks. There is some data indicating that this standard induction dosing protocol may need to be changed in acutely ill patients who may require both a higher dose and more frequent dosing of the drug. Adalimumab, golimumab, and certolizumab pegol are all set doses that are subcutaneous injections. Adalimumab is dosed every other week while golimumab, and certolizumab pegol are dosed monthly. Some experts advocate that hepatitis B and tuberculosis testing is necessary if

TABLE 164-9 American Gastroenterological Association IBD Quality Measures

Measure	Location of Care
1. IBD: type, anatomic location and activity all assessed	Outpatient
2. IBD preventive care: corticosteroid sparing therapy	Outpatient
3. IBD preventive care: corticosteroid related iatrogenic injury—bone loss assessment	Outpatient
4. IBD preventive care: influenza immunization	Outpatient
5. IBD preventive care: pneumococcal immunization	Outpatient
6. Testing for latent tuberculosis prior to starting anti-TNF therapy	Outpatient
7. Assessment of hepatitis B virus prior to starting anti-TNF therapy	Outpatient
8. Testing for Clostridium difficile	Inpatient
9. Prophylaxis for venous thromboembolism	Inpatient
10. IBD preventive care: tobacco—screening and cessation intervention	Outpatient

Abbreviations: IBD inflammatory bowel disease; TNF tumor necrosis factor.

vedolizumab is used. The drug is dosed at similar intervals to infliximab but at a set dose of 300 mg.

■ COMPLICATIONS AND PROGNOSIS

UC adverse outcomes

There are multiple adverse events associated with UC flare. One of the most ominous events is toxic megacolon (dilation of the transverse colon beyond 6 cm), which can develop in up to 10% of patients presenting with acute severe UC. The relatively low mortality rate (0.2%) is likely related to the use of abdominal x-ray on admission and emergent colectomy when toxic megacolon is present. Other complications include thromboembolism.

CD adverse outcomes

More frequently, intestinal obstruction develops as a complication of CD related to underlying stricturing or severe inflammatory small bowel CD. When fistulizing CD is present, abscess formation is a complication to be cognizant of. Similarly, even after attempted antibiotic therapy and/or drainage or surgical therapy of an abscess, the abscess can still recur necessitating further therapy. Less frequently, toxic megacolon develops in CD with a prevalence of only 2.3% and usually only with underlying colonic CD. Other complications include thromboembolism.

■ DISCHARGE PLANNING

In UC or colonic CD, discharge planning can be initiated once a patient has one to two bowel movements per day or at least less than or equal to four bowel movements without blood. In cases of stricturing CD, discharge planning is initiated once the patient is able to transition to an oral diet without symptoms. If a patient is unable to transition to an oral diet then usually surgery is necessary and will be performed prior to discharge. In cases of abscess formation, oral antibiotics are ideal. However, in certain situations, a decision will be made to continue intravenous antibiotics if the patient fails to improve when transitioning to oral antibiotics. These patients usually require infectious disease consultation, a peripherally inserted central catheter (PICC) line, provision of antibiotics through an infusion company, and laboratory monitoring.

The ability to prevent readmissions related to IBD is unclear. Few studies have assessed predictors of readmission and predictive variables have been identified consistently. Ideally, patients should have follow up with gastroenterology 2 weeks after discharge. There is also some data that patients with more complex underlying IBD may be best served by seeing a gastroenterologist who specializes in IBD.

PRACTICE POINT

- Patients exposed to corticosteroids for a total of 90 days or more should be assessed for iatrogenic bone loss with a bone density scan.
- Patients on prolonged courses of prednisone should be assessed for possible adrenal insufficiency prior to stopping the steroids.

■ QUALITY IMPROVEMENT TO ADDRESS PERFORMANCE GAPS

In 2011, the American Gastroenterological Association (AGA) established 10 quality metrics for the care of patients with IBD (**Table 164-10**). Two of the 10 measures are specifically applicable to the hospitalized patient. The 10 measures include:

- Testing for *C. difficile* (hospitalized patient)

- Thromboprophylaxis to reduce the risk of VTE (hospitalized patient)
- Assessment of disease activity
- Use of corticosteroid sparing medications when applicable
- Assessment for iatrogenic bone loss
- Screening for latent hepatitis B and tuberculosis, if antitumor necrosis factor is considered
- Vaccination for influenza, pneumococcal infection
- Assessment for tobacco abuse

The risk of osteopenia and osteoporosis in CD is quite significant. Studies report prevalence of osteopenia and osteoporosis ranging from 22% to 55% and 3% to 58%, respectively. Similar rates are noted in UC with osteopenia ranging from 32% to 67% and osteoporosis from 4% to 50%. The rates for both conditions are higher during active disease compared to when the disease is stable and in remission. Whenever steroids are utilized for 3 months or for severe, untreated active disease, a bone density scan is warranted. If osteoporosis is present, a low threshold for an endocrinology referral is acceptable. To help mitigate this complication, steroid sparing medications with either thiopurine, biologic, or anti-integrin drugs should be considered for patients receiving systemic steroids.

The goal of optimizing vaccination status is to reduce the risk of any preventable infections especially when utilizing immunosuppressive agents. Some experts argue that all vaccinations should be optimized including: hepatitis A, hepatitis B, pneumovax, prevnar 13, influenza, and when appropriate human papilloma virus, tetanus diphtheria and acellular pertussis, varicella, and zoster vaccine if not on immunosuppressive or biologic therapy.

■ DISPARITIES IN HEALTH CARE

Comparing African American and Caucasian, both ethnicities were similar with respect to age of CD onset, time to diagnosis, and number of gastrointestinal related hospitalizations and surgeries. Medication usage patterns were also similar.

After adjusting for age, sex, health insurance, comorbidities, median income, and hospital characteristics, the relative rate ratio of undergoing bowel resection for African Americans, Hispanics, and Asians compared to Caucasians was 0.68 (95% CI 0.61-0.76), 0.70 (95% CI 0.60-0.83), and 0.31 (95% CI 0.16-0.59), respectively. Compared to those with private insurance, the relative risk of surgery for those with Medicare was 0.48 (95% CI 0.44-0.54), Medicaid 0.52 (95% CI 0.46-0.59), and self-pay 0.67 (95% CI 0.58-0.77). Women were less likely than men to undergo bowel resection (incidence rate ratio = 0.80; 95% CI 0.76-0.85).

Approximately 25% of all IBD-related hospitalizations are for patients older than 65 years of age. This population was less likely to be hospitalized with fistulizing (4.0% vs 8.8%, $p < 0.001$) or stricturing (4.0% vs 5.8%, $p = 0.001$) disease. Even after adjusting for comorbidities, patients over the age of 65 years had higher in-hospital mortality (OR 3.91, 95% CI 2.50-6.11). In addition, older patients with fistulas are more likely to undergo surgery (OR 1.55, 95% CI 1.00-2.40) and have a longer postoperative stay.

CONCLUSION

Early recognition of IBD flares is critical to prevent unforeseen complications and surgery. In all cases, standardized protocols should be instituted consistent with the AGA core measures to minimize disease complications and optimize overall medical therapy. Ideally, both CD and UC can be treated medically with surgery reserved to only cases that fail medical therapy or present with serious complications.

TABLE 164-10 Medications for Maintenance of Remission Following Hospitalization (Excluding Steroids)

Medication	Disease Use	Route of Delivery	Mechanism	Contraindication	Side Effect	Routine Testing
Antibiotics Metronidazole Ciprofloxacin	CD	Oral	Antibacterial	Metronidazole Hypersensitivity to imidazole derivatives Ciprofloxacin Hypersensitivity to quinolones	Metronidazole: Nausea Antabuse effect Metallic taste Peripheral neuropathy Ciprofloxacin: Rash Spontaneous tendon rupture	
Azathioprine/ 6-MP	CD/UC	Oral	Inhibition of DNA synthesis in lymphocytes	Absent TPMT activity	Nausea Vomiting Hepatitis Bone marrow suppression Pancreatitis Infection Non-Hodgkin lymphoma Nonmelanoma skin cancer Abnormal pap smear	TPMT prior to initiation CBC LFT Yearly skin exam Yearly pap smear
Infliximab Adalimumab Certolizumab Pegol Golimumab	UC (except for certolizumab pegol) CD (except for golimumab)	Infusion Subcutaneous Injection	Neutralization of TNF-α	Untreated infection (TB, hepatitis B), Severe heart failure Hypersensitivity to murine products (infliximab only)	Infusion/injection site reaction Non-Hodgkin lymphoma Melanoma Reactivation of latent TB Reactivation of latent hepatitis B Drug induced lupus Psoriaform reactions Worsening of severe CHF Demyelinating disease	CBC LFT Yearly skin exam
Mesalamine	UC (limited data on use in CD not recommended in societal guidelines)	Oral or rectal	Control of peroxisome proliferator-activated receptor-γ resulting in modification of inflammatory and cytokine response	Hypersensitivity to aminosalicylates	Headache Nausea Diarrhea Interstitial nephritis Hemolytic anemia Leukopenia Hepatitis	Creatinine BUN
Methotrexate	CD	Oral or Subcutaneous injection	Inhibition of dihydrofolate reductase, resulting in decreased nucleic acid production	Pregnancy	Nausea Abdominal pain Loose stool Hepatitis Rash Headache Fatigue Anemia, bruising Stomatitis	CBC LFT
Vedolizumab	UC CD	Infusion	Anti-integrin	Hypersensitivity reaction to vedolizumab	Headache Arthralgias Nasopharyngitis Hepatitis Infection	

Abbreviations: BUN blood urea nitrogen; CBC complete blood count; LFT liver function test; TB Tuberculosis.

SUGGESTED READINGS

Baumgart DC, Sandborn WJ. Crohn's disease. *Lancet*. 2012;380: 1590-1605.

Bernstein CN. Treatment of IBD: where we are and where we are going. *Am J Gastroenterol*. 2015;110:114-126.

Doherty GA, Cheifetz AS. Management of acute severe ulcerative colitis. *Expert Rev Gastroenterol Hepatol*. 2009;3:395-405.

El-Hachem S, Regueiro M. Postoperative Crohn's disease: prevention and treatment. *Expert Rev Gastroenterol Hepatol*. 2009;3: 249-256.

Feuerstein JD, Cheifetz AS. Ulcerative colitis: epidemiology, diagnosis, and management. *Mayo Clin Proc*. 2014;89(11):1553-1563.

Pola S, Patel D, Ramamoorthy S, et al. Strategies for the care of adults hospitalized for active ulcerative colitis. *Clin Gastroenterol Hepatol*. 2012;10:1315-1325.e4.

Talley NJ, Abreu MT, Achkar J-P, et al. An evidence-based systematic review on medical therapies for inflammatory bowel disease. *Am J Gastroenterol*. 2011;106:S2-S25.

ONLINE RESOURCES

For Patients:

www.ccfa.org

http://patients.gi.org/topics/inflammatory-bowel-disease/

http://www.youandibd.com/en/home.aspx

SECTION 6

Geriatrics

CHAPTER 165

Principles of Geriatric Care

Margarita Sotelo, MD
William L. Lyons, MD

Key Clinical Questions

1. How do differences between hospitalized older adults and younger individuals alter the approach to this patient population?

2. What are the risk factors for functional decline and the development of geriatric syndromes during hospitalization?

3. What are the essential components of the initial hospital evaluation and how is this information used to trigger preventative measures? What are the essential components of daily rounds?

INTRODUCTION

From 2010 to 2030, the total US population is expected to grow by 20%, while the segment of population aged 65 years and older is projected to increase by 79%. Older adults account for a disproportionate fraction of hospital discharges. In 2008, they made up 35% of hospital discharges while accounting for only 13% of the total population. As a result of aging demographics and greater utilization of hospital care by this age group, hospitalists will be caring for an increasing number of older patients.

Optimal geriatric hospital care uses a dedicated systematic approach that takes into account key differences between older and younger patients regardless of the admitting diagnosis. This chapter begins with a description of clinically significant differences between older and younger hospital patients; describes the importance of self-care function among older adults; summarizes key features of well-studied acute geriatric interventions; provides tips for care of the older patient on admission day, daily work rounds, and discharge; and finishes with information about prognosis.

DECREASED PHYSIOLOGIC RESERVE

Physiologic changes of normal aging affect all organ systems (**Table 165-1**). Aging is the consequence of varying genetic, environmental, and lifestyle influences, and age alone is not an accurate predictor of outcomes of hospitalization. Aging results in a loss of physiological resilience, a reduced ability of the body to maintain normal function when confronted with an external stressor.

Chronic diseases like heart failure (HF), Alzheimer dementia, or emphysema detract further from physiological reserve. Geriatricians have long noted the "weakest link principle" whereby an elder's illness presentation will reflect failure of that physiological system with the least reserve, rather than the system that is the locus of the acute ailment. Hence, the elder with an impaired circulatory system may present with syncope when afflicted by a respiratory viral infection.

PRESENTATION OF DISEASE

As a result of age- and disease-associated decrements in physiologic reserves of multiple systems, older adults do not tolerate acute illness as well as younger individuals. In a cohort of predominantly older patients hospitalized with pneumococcal pneumonia, for example, 19% had a concurrent acute cardiac event, such as myocardial infarction, new-onset arrhythmias, and/or new-onset HF.

PRACTICE POINT

The admitting clinician should consider a wide range of incipient illnesses and conduct a correspondingly comprehensive evaluation of the older adult presenting with delirium or a fall.

- Avoid the pitfall of trying to uncover a unifying diagnosis for multiple symptoms and signs (Occam's razor).
- Recognize that the older adult with chronic comorbidities will have atypical presentations and commonly, have more than one contributing diagnoses.
- Do not overlook a coexistent condition due to age- and disease-associated decrements in physiologic reserve.

Common diseases present differently in older adults. Ill younger patients generally present with complaints and findings referable to the diseased organ. In a large community database, 90% of patients

TABLE 165-1 Selected Physiological Changes That Occur with Normal Aging

System	Changes
Nervous	Brain perfusion shows impaired autoregulation
	Slowed reaction time
	Impaired balance from reduced vestibular responsiveness
Circulatory	Decreased maximal HR and CO
	Impaired diastolic filling, greater dependence on atrial systole
	Reduced pacemaker cells in SA node
	Reduced response to beta-adrenergic stimulation
	Reduced elasticity of large arteries (increased systolic BP)
Respiratory	Reduced FEV1 and FVC
	Impaired ciliary clearance
	Reduced PaO_2 from V/Q mismatch
	Lungs less elastic
	Chest wall stiffer
Musculoskeletal	Reduced muscle mass with age
	Reduced bone mass
Renal/Urinary	Steady drop in GFR with age
	Reduced ability to concentrate or dilute urine
	Reduced ability to excrete acid load
	Renal perfusion more dependent on local prostaglandins
	Impaired bladder emptying
Sensory	Reduced contrast sensitivity (vision)
	Impaired dark adaptation (vision)
	Loss of high-frequency tones (hearing)
Immune	Diminished cell-mediated immunity
	Chronic low grade inflammation from innate immune activation
	Antibodies have lower affinity
Hematologic	Reduced erythropoietic response to EPO
	Increased procoagulant state predisposing to venous thromboembolic disease

BP, blood pressure; CO, cardiac output; EPO, erythropoietin; FEV1, forced expiratory volume in 1 second; FVC, forced vital capacity; GFR, glomerular filtration rate; HR, heart rate; PaO_2, arterial partial pressure of oxygen; SA, sinoatrial; V/Q, ventilation-perfusion ratio.

younger than 65 years with ST-elevation myocardial infarction presented with chest pain, compared with only 57% of those older than 85 years. Older patients with infarction were more likely to present with acute heart failure than their younger counterparts. Older patients are less likely to report cough, other respiratory and non-respiratory symptoms due to pneumonia than younger patients.

FUNCTIONAL DECLINE

Older patients are more likely to develop acute functional decline or a geriatric syndrome in the context of acute illness. Acute functional decline refers to the sudden loss of self-care capability, such as independence in bathing or dressing.

Function refers to the set of behaviors needed to remain independent in daily life. Functional capacity is a potent predictor of outcomes in older patients. Poor function has been shown to predict

length of stay, cost of care, institutional placement, caregiver burden, mortality, and quality of life. Functional domains include

- Basic activities of daily living (ADLs): bathing, dressing, toileting, transferring, continence, and feeding.
- Instrumental activities of daily living (IADLs): the ability to use the telephone, shop, prepare food, perform housekeeping, wash clothes, manage medications and finances, and handle the responsibility of transportation.
- Mobility: the ability to safely ambulate in the home or community and negotiate stairs.

The trajectories of physiological and functional measures often differ greatly during hospitalizations, while physiological markers (vital signs, laboratory assessments) typically improve by discharge, functional measures frequently worsen. Studies have shown that 20% to more than 30% of older patients admitted to general medical inpatient services lose independence in one or more ADLs by the time of discharge. One study of almost 2300 elders on the general medical service of two hospitals found that 35% were discharged with worse-than-baseline function. Twelve percent showed decline in the hospital only, 18% had prehospital decline from baseline but failed to recover, and 5% demonstrated both prehospital and in-hospital decline.

ADLs reflect more than simply physical function, but the overall match between a patient's physical abilities and the environment (including social support). As people age, ADLs are typically lost in a predictable fashion: the ability to bathe independently is lost first, the ability to feed oneself last. ADL loss progresses through predictable stages: first, one can do the ADL without difficulty; later, one can do it, but with difficulty; still later, one can do it only with assistance; and finally, one cannot do it at all. Performance of IADLs requires higher-order cognitive skills, and with most conditions (especially dementia), IADLs are lost before ADLs.

Patients' mobility often follows a different trajectory than their ADL or IADL function. Cognitively impaired patients, in particular, commonly maintain their mobility while suffering ADL and IADL losses.

HEALTH CARE GOALS

Health care goals of older adults may differ from than those of younger persons. Most younger patients seek rescue or life prolongation as a consequence of hospital care. Many older patients have the same desires; however, a substantial number consider maintenance of independence or achievement of symptomatic relief as equally important. One study of the treatment preferences of 226 older persons with life-limiting diagnoses of cancer, COPD, and HF reported that burden of treatment and likelihood of outcome were significant influences on the patients' decision making. While almost all would choose a low-burden treatment that would likely restore current health, almost 90% of participants would not choose a low-burden treatment associated with a likely outcome of severe cognitive impairment.

ABUSE

An estimated 2% to 10% of older adults in the United States suffer abuse each year. Many conditions common in older age present with signs and symptoms that mimic abuse. The fragile skin of an older adult, particularly with concurrent use of anticoagulants, is predisposed to ecchymoses from mild, accidental trauma. While there are no pathognomonic signs of physical abuse, characteristics of injury may be suggestive: bruising >5 cm in size in unusual locations, imprints caused by objects (belts, shoes), or ligature marks suggestive of physical restraint. Accidental bruising is uncommon in the neck, ears, buttocks, or soles of feet; if noted, they should raise the suspicion of intentional injury. Injuries in the genitals and inner thighs are highly suspicious for sexual abuse. Burns in stocking or glove distribution may suggest forced immersion. While pressure ulcers may develop even with the best care, evidence of suboptimal care raises the question of neglect. No distribution of injury reliably distinguishes accidental from nonaccidental mechanisms but clinicians should look for clinical findings that are discordant with the reported mechanism of injury. Clinicians are ethically and, in most states, legally mandated to report suspected elder abuse cases (see Chapter 167 [Elder Mistreatment]).

COMPLICATIONS OF HOSPITALIZATION

The syndrome of *frailty* **refers to** particularly diminished reserve and increased vulnerability to stressors. Most frailty indices involve measures in domains of mobility, physical activity, strength, cognition, mood, and nutrition. Frail patients appear to be at increased risk of hospitalization and eventual discharge to a nursing facility, and generally experience worse outcomes when subjected to surgical or chemotherapeutic treatments.

■ FUNCTION

Functional loss in the hospital probably reflects complex interactions between diseases, age, intrinsic frailty, and hospital care itself. **Table 165-2** lists factors that have been found in various studies to increase the risk of in-hospital functional decline. A validated clinical index identified the following risk factors for new-onset disability in hospitalized patients ≥70 years old: age, number of dependencies in IADL, mobility 2 weeks before admission, number of ADL dependencies on admission, metastatic cancer or stroke, severe cognitive impairment, and hypoalbuminemia. Higher-risk scores predicted more severe disability, greater likelihood of nursing-home placement, and worse survival.

The use of a cane or walker prior to admission has been shown to be a strong predictor of low in-hospital mobility. For patients without premorbid ambulatory impairment or acute conditions such as bone fracture that directly impair walking, illness severity is the predominant factor affecting mobility. Recent hospitalization is an independent risk factor for hip fracture among older adults. Restricted activity or bed rest predicts the development of disability. Older patients admitted to the hospital should be encouraged to ambulate (with assistance if necessary) several times a day, or at least spend time out of bed in a chair if they cannot ambulate. One research group found that older hospitalized patients are less likely to recover baseline ADL function lost prior to admission, and

are more likely to develop new functional impairments during hospitalization. Others have reported that cognitive impairment present at hospital admission predicts failure of functional recovery at 3 months following hospital discharge.

■ GERIATRIC SYNDROMES

A geriatric syndrome (such as delirium, fall, or new-onset urinary incontinence) refers to a health condition where the accumulated effects of impairments in multiple physiological systems render an individual vulnerable to external insults and stressors.

Risk factors for the development of geriatric syndromes in the hospital have been established. One group found the following predictors (a familiar list of markers of low resilience; see Table 165-2) of four specific geriatric syndromes (pressure sores, urinary incontinence, fecal incontinence, and falls): cognitive impairment, advanced age, prolonged hospital length of stay, and severe ADL disability.

Dementia is a risk factor for the development of delirium, as well as for difficulty adhering to therapy, and patients in early stages commonly go undiagnosed. Delirium should be suspected in the inattentive patient with acute onset and fluctuating course of mental status change, with altered level of consciousness, or with evidence of disorganized thoughts (see Chapter 166 [Agitation]).

Vulnerable older adults (due to a history of dementia, functional dependence, and vision impairment) are at greater risk for incident delirium and for decline in their ability to perform activities of daily living when exposed to precipitating factors in the hospital (eg, use of psychoactive drugs, physical restraint, lack of sleep).

■ ADVERSE DRUG EVENTS

Medications frequently contribute to the development of geriatric syndromes. Sedatives or antipsychotics will increase the risk of falling for a frail older person with baseline impaired balance (eg, from prior stroke and neuropathy). Withdrawal of specific classes of medications reduces falls in community-dwelling older adults. Hospitalists should assess the risk and benefit of continuing such medications at admission, and confer with the outpatient care provider.

Older hospitalized patients suffer almost twice the incidence of preventable adverse events related to medical procedures, drug effects, and falls than do younger counterparts, likely due to interacting and additive factors of frailty, multimorbidities, and hospital processes of care.

■ DEPRESSION

Depression among hospitalized older adults is associated with increased risk of death, ADL dependence, and need for institutional placement. The Geriatric Depression Scale (available in 15- and 30-item versions) has been shown to perform well as a screening measure in this setting. Patients identified on screening should be evaluated more thoroughly either in the inpatient or outpatient setting.

■ MALNUTRITION

Malnutrition in older hospitalized patients has been shown to predict increased risk for mortality, dependence in ADLs, and institutionalization, even after accounting for comorbid and acute illnesses. Some 15% of elders have severe protein-calorie malnutrition at admission, and 25% of older patients suffer nutritional decline during the course of their hospital stay. Patients with weight loss should be assessed for reversible causes, such as oral cavity disease, dysphagia, medication adverse effects, and impaired access to food. Food choices should be liberalized as much as possible to stimulate intake, and encouragement and assistance provided during mealtimes if needed. Dietary consultation and oral nutritional supplementation should be considered for malnourished patients (see Chapter 168 [Malnutrition and Weight Loss in Hospitalized Older Adults]).

TABLE 165-2 Risk Factors for In-Hospital Functional Decline in Older Patients

Age over 75
Presence of preadmission ADL disability
Presence of preadmission IADL disability
Cognitive impairment at admission
Delirium, including subsyndromal delirium
Pressure sores
Depression symptoms
Low body mass index
Longer hospital length of stay
Mobility impairment (use of assistive device) or bed rest
Institutional residence
Lower social activity level
Certain diagnostic categories (ICD-9 codes)

- Functional decline associated with hospitalization begins within 48 hours of admission.
- "Bed rest" activity orders are generally appropriate only for patients whose care goals are palliative.
- Essential components of the initial admission evaluation include a geriatric assessment of baseline function so that early interventions can be instituted to maintain or improve function.

COMPREHENSIVE GERIATRIC ASSESSMENT DURING HOSPITALIZATION

A shared feature of most of the approaches to improve hospital care processes for geriatric inpatients requires a comprehensive geriatric assessment (CGA) at the time of admission. CGA is defined as a multidimensional diagnostic process that uncovers medical, psychological, and functional vulnerabilities and develops a coordinated, integrated plan for treatment and long-term follow-up. In one model of CGA, a specialty multidisciplinary team delivers care in a discrete unit (such as the Geriatric Evaluation and Management (GEM) unit and the Acute Care for Elders (ACE) unit). Another model, a team (such as the Hospital Elder Life Program) carries its care processes to older adults wherever they are admitted in the hospital. In another model (the Hospital Elder Life Program [HELP]) a mobile team carries its care processes to older adults wherever they are admitted in the hospital.

Rubenstein and coworkers demonstrated the benefits of an inpatient GEM unit to which older adults are admitted after stabilization in another acute ward. In a later multicenter, randomized trial conducted at 11 Veterans Affairs medical centers, GEM units were demonstrated to improve ADL function and physical performance relative to usual hospital care.

The ACE system, in contrast to GEM units, allows for direct admission of acutely ill patients to the special inpatient ward without prior stabilization. ACE employs a proactive, "prehabilitative" approach, designed to help hospitalized elders maintain or achieve functional independence. Key elements of the ACE program are summarized in **Table 165-3**. ACE was shown, in a randomized controlled trial set in an academic medical center, to result in greater ADL independence at the time of hospital discharge, and less frequent need for nursing-home placement. A follow-up study performed at a community hospital showed a more modest difference in function between ACE and control patients. The performance of ACE (and other special geriatric acute care systems) is probably sensitive to factors that depend on interdisciplinary team function.

A systematic review and meta-analysis examined seven studies in which older hospital patients were randomized to either usual care or inpatient geriatric assessment and management. This meta-analysis found that specialized geriatric inpatient programs (two studies of ACE units, studies of Veteran Affairs GEM units, and a number of European programs) showed statistically significant improvements in both functional status at discharge and need for institutionalization at 1 year. Nonsignificant trends toward improvement were found in readmission risk and mortality. Another meta-analysis looking specifically at CGA for older adults admitted to hospitals reported favorable outcomes only from CGA delivered in discrete units, such as ACE and GEM, but not in mobile teams.

HELP is a multicomponent intervention designed to prevent incident delirium in hospitalized elders. Enrolled patients are admitted to wherever open beds exist, rather than to specialized inpatient wards. The program makes extensive use of well-trained and committed volunteers. At the time of admission, older patients are assessed for the presence of six risk factors for delirium (cognitive impairment, sleep deprivation, immobility, vision impairment, hearing impairment, and dehydration), and protocols are triggered to manage identified risks. In a randomized controlled study, delirium incidence in the intervention patients was 9.9%, significantly less than 15% in the control group. Both severity and duration of delirium appeared to be unaffected by the intervention. A meta-analysis of 14 studies of multicomponent nonpharmacologic delirium prevention interventions, nine of which were HELP adaptations, reported significant reductions in incident delirium. A compelling finding was a reduction in the rate of falls in the intervention groups of the four studies that reported falls as an outcome.

Leaders of such specialized hospital geriatrics programs typically establish admission criteria in order to exclude older patients who are either too vigorous or too functionally dependent to benefit (eg, profoundly demented, or terminally ill).

THE DAY OF ADMISSION

The history and physical examination guide diagnosis and treatment of acute illness. Systematically incorporating key features of a comprehensive geriatric assessment into the traditional history and physical examination will facilitate formulating an individualized assessment and plan that can trigger a multidisciplinary approach and appropriate discharge planning.

TABLE 165-3 Key Components of Acute Care for Elders ("Ace") Units

Component	Description
Prepared environment for mobility and orientation	Carpeting, abundant grab bars, raised toilet seats, low beds, clocks, and calendars
Nursing-initiated protocols for patient-centered care	Targeted at independence in self care, nutrition, sleep hygiene, skin care, mood, cognition
Planning for home	Early involvement of social services
Medical care review	Geriatrician advises about optimal medication prescribing, risk assessment of procedures, and so on.

The Medical History
Chief Complaint

- Clarify the patient's understanding of their illness with open-ended questions:
  "Tell me what you understand about your illness."
- Elicit the patient's hopes, fears, and concerns: "As you look ahead what worries you the most?"
- Allow patients time to enunciate concrete goals of care.

History of Present Illness

- Corroborate illness stories (especially in patients with chronic cognitive impairment or delirium) with primary caregivers: family, friends, nursing facility staff.
- Inquire about new functional problems that have arisen as a result of illness: trouble walking, transferring, bathing, shopping, managing medications.

Past Medical History

- Inquire and formulate an assessment about functional impairment attributable to comorbid illness: *"Gait impairment and frequent falls, secondary to Parkinson disease and knee osteoarthritis,"* or *"Dysphagia secondary to a cerebrovascular accident in 2002."*
- Inquire about complications from previous hospitalizations: prior delirium should prompt preventative measures during current hospitalization.

Medications

- Do not simply copy the outpatient drug list in the admitting orders: A patient's as-taken medication regimen often deviates substantially from the theoretical one listed in the outpatient medical record.
- Confirm medications with the patient's pharmacy: the complete outpatient regimen of many patients often includes a blend of pills ordered by multiple prescribers and bought at multiple pharmacies, as well as over-the-counter agents and herbal or nontraditional remedies.
- Ask about the patient's method for remembering to take doses and for an estimate of how often doses are missed.

Family History

- Ask about the health of people living with the patient: genetic predispositions to various diseases are less relevant to the patient's care than in the case of a younger adult.
- Listen to an older person's narrative of a family member's grave illness to catalyze further discussions about the patient's own global health care goals: *"My mother required a ventilator following a massive stroke. We made the difficult decision of withdrawing the life support."*

Social History

Ask the following questions:

- What is the extent of **social support**? Who lives in the patient's home, and how much of the time? Who is in the extended social network and would be able and willing to help in the event of prolonged illness or functional dependence? Is the patient a caregiver of a frail spouse; if so, who has taken over this responsibility?
- Discuss goals of care: In the event of lost decisional capacity, who is the patient's surrogate?

Review of Systems

Inquire about the following:

- ADLs: Does the patient have difficulty with bathing, dressing, toileting, transferring, continence, feeding?
- IADLs: Does the patient have difficulty using the telephone, shopping, preparing food, performing housekeeping, washing clothes, managing medications and finances, and arranging for transportation? Has the patient lost weight in the last 3 months and if so, how much? Does the patient receive regular dental care or require dentures for eating?
- Mobility: Does the patient have difficulty walking up or down stairs, walking several blocks, or walking across a room? Has the patient fallen in the past year? Does the patient use a cane or walker?
- Depression: Has the patient been feeling sad, depressed, or hopeless, or lost his or her usual interest or pleasure in doing things?
- Hearing and vision: Does the patient have a problem with hearing or vision?
- Who provides the assistance with ADLs and IADLs, and what do they do?

■ MEDICATION REVIEW

Explicit and implicit criteria are two strategies for minimizing the use of high risk and inappropriate medications in older adults. Implicit criteria require patient-specific information, published data, and clinical judgment in the assessment of medication appropriateness. In contrast, explicit criteria are lists of potentially inappropriate medications (PIMs) derived through an expert panel's review of the literature; of these, the Beers criteria is the most commonly referenced. PIMs are medications or classes of medications deemed more risky than beneficial particularly when safer alternatives are available. The Beers criteria designates 53 medications as PIMs that should generally be avoided in older adults, PIMs to avoid in older adults with certain conditions (to minimize drug-disease interactions), or medications to be used with caution. PIM lists are increasingly used as measures of quality of pharmacologic care of older adults. Pharmacoepidemiologic studies have reported associations between PIM use and adverse outcomes such as unplanned hospitalization.

PRACTICE POINT

The Physical Examination

Vital signs, including baseline weight

- Abnormal or unstable vital signs may limit the examiner's ability to perform a comprehensive evaluation on the day of admission.

General appearance

- Does the patient exhibit vitality or frailty when moving in bed?
- Is there an odor of incontinence or poor hygiene?
- Does the patient appear malnourished? That is, BMI < 20, loss of subcutaneous fat, concave temporal fossae, squared-off shoulders, atrophic intrinsic hand muscles.

Vision and hearing

- Use a pocket Snellen chart to evaluate vision, the whispered voice test to assess hearing.
- Ask the family to bring in from home assistive devices such as glasses or hearing aids.

Oral cavity

- Assess the health of teeth and gums.
- Does the patient wear dentures and if so, does the patient have them, and do they appear to fit?

Skin

- Inspect bony prominences: occiput, scapulae, sacrum, ischial tuberosities, greater trochanter, posterior calcaneus for nonblanching erythema (the earliest stage of pressure ulcer).
- Consider the possibility of abuse if the explanation provided for injury is not consistent with its appearance.

Mental status

- The medical history provides key information regarding patients' ability to pay attention, recall key information, and communicate goals of care.
- Try to engage the patient in a discussion of something that is familiar to them (such as a hobby).

Mobility

- Observe ability to arise from a seated position without the use of arms (inability typically reflects quadriceps weakness).
- Observe gait: speed, symmetry, stride length, truncal posture, arm swing.

DAILY WORK ROUNDS

While there are several disease-specific and technological issues that physicians are faced with when caring for hospitalized older

TABLE 165-4 Tips for Daily Work Rounds

1. ADL status and trajectory: Is the patient approaching baseline function?

2. Oral intake: How much of each meal is being eaten? Consider between-meal supplements.

3. Bowel function: When was the last bowel movement? Consider a laxative.

4. Mobility: Has the patient been out of bed? Encourage ambulation, consider physical therapy.

5. Physical examination: Document attachments (central lines, bladder catheters, etc) and discontinue them when possible.

6. Physical examination: Check mental status daily to identify incident delirium.

7. Physical examination: In the mobility-impaired patient, check high risk sites for pressure ulcers.

8. Pharmacotherapy: Practice good drug list hygiene by reviewing the medication list and discontinuing nonessential agents.

9. Discharge planning: Discharge destination identified? Family and Social Services recruited to help with arrangements?

adults, certain "low-tech" considerations should not be overlooked, as they are essential to achieving good outcomes. A suggested checklist of items to review daily when seeing older patients on hospital rounds is provided in **Table 165-4**.

The items in this table reflect lessons learned from specialized inpatient geriatric programs (such as ACE units), in which patients are frequently assessed for ADL status and mobility, nutrient intake and bowel function, mental status, skin health, polypharmacy, and determination of a discharge plan.

Known precipitating risk factors for incident delirium should be avoided or mitigated, and these include psychoactive medication use, physical restraints, bladder catheters, and dehydration. Sleep deprivation is associated with increased risk of delirium and over one-third of older patients have difficulty sleeping in the hospital. The sources of sleep disruption in hospitalized older adults include intrinsic (eg, pain, anxiety, medications) and extrinsic factors (eg, noise, processes of care such as phlebotomy, medication administration). Despite the associated risks of sedative use in older adults, including psychomotor and cognitive adverse events, at least one-third of older patients are prescribed these medications in the hospital. Pharmacologic treatment of insomnia has a poor benefit-to-harm ratio; the NNT for improved sleep quality is approximately 13, while the NNH for any adverse effect was 6. Therefore, sleep deprivation in the hospital is best managed nonpharmacologically (eg, use of warm beverages, soft music, or bundling of nighttime care).

Pain is frequently underdiagnosed and undertreated in people with dementia due to the patient's inability to communicate symptoms and the care provider's failure to recognize nonverbal signs. Challenging behavior in dementia may be secondary to untreated pain. Scheduled analgesia (such as acetaminophen 650 mg four times daily in patients without contraindications) should be considered, especially if pain is expected to occur frequently. The efficacy of NSAIDs in treating acute pain should be weighed against heightened renal, cardiovascular, and gastric toxicity in older adults. Older adults demonstrate increased sensitivity to opiates and pharmacokinetic changes with aging may lead to a prolonged half-life; a "start low and go slow approach" when using opiates is recommended. Comorbidities, renal function, and coprescribed medications should

be considered to minimize adverse drug events. Nonpharmacologic approaches to pain should be part of the care plan.

DISCHARGE OF THE OLDER PATIENT

Almost 20% of Medicare patients discharged from the hospital are readmitted within 30 days. Factors predicting rehospitalization include older age, the presence of certain medical diagnoses (cardiovascular disease, diabetes, and cancer), psychosocial considerations (depression, inadequate social support, Medicaid eligibility), previous hospital use, worse self-rating of health, and failure of the hospital team to provide discharge education.

The complex process of discharging patients requires the collaborative effort of various disciplines, ideally beginning on the day of admission. Discharge planning involves individualized planning prior to a patient leaving the hospital for home. In pooled data from randomized controlled trials, older medical inpatients allocated to discharge planning had reduced hospital length of stay and readmission rates (see Chapter 14 [Care Transitions at Hospital Discharge]).

The older hospitalized patient should be discharged to the least restrictive environment that will support functional, rehabilitative, and clinical needs. The discharge check list should include an assessment of the patient's ADL and mobility function; determination of the capabilities and willingness of family and other caregivers, as well as the patient's physical home environment; clarification of the needed rehabilitative disciplines (physical therapy, occupational therapy, speech therapy) and the intensity of their anticipated programs; and technical components of the patient's treatment plan (intravenous therapy, wound and ostomy care, etc). The availability of insurance benefits and community services may also determine discharge destination (see Part III [Rehabilitation Options and Skilled Nursing Care]).

Services that were in place prior to hospitalization generally need to be reinstated. Assessment of decisional capacity may be necessary when a patient demonstrates lack of insight into her needs following discharge and declines recommended assistance. ADL disability, particularly when onset was within 3 months of a hospitalization, predicts readmission in community-dwelling older adults.

Medicare provides funding for home health care deemed reasonable and necessary, provided that it is difficult for the patient to leave the home. There must be a "skilled need," meaning a need for a registered nurse, physical therapist, or speech pathologist. After a patient has been admitted to an agency's service under the care of one of these three disciplines, other disciplines (occupational therapy, medical social work) may be involved as needed. Potential "red flags," findings or symptoms that suggest that a clinical condition is worsening, should be routinely communicated to the patient and caregiver before discharge. Further, it is important to clarify *who* (the hospitalist? or primary care provider?) should be called in the event that a problem arises, and to provide necessary contact information.

Hospitalization is frequently associated with significant changes in an already complex medication regimen. In a prospective study of older adults discharged following an admission for heart failure, acute coronary syndrome, or pneumonia, 87% received at least one new medication and 22% of admission medications were stopped or redosed. Of the latter group of medications, 22% may have been unintended medication modification. During a postdischarge interview, patients demonstrated lack of understanding of two-thirds of intended changes or new medications. Cognitively impaired patients are at risk of medication nonadherence, and may benefit from implementation of reminder systems.

Communication between hospital-based and postacute clinicians includes a well-constructed and timely discharge summary, a telephone call to the receiving provider and/or e-mail communication (that assures HIPAA compliance). Essential information to help ensure a safe transition include notification of a pending, but critical laboratory result, changes in high-risk medications (anticoagulants, opiates), and the gist of any discussion with the patient or family about shifting health goals. Transfer of delicate psychosocial context is often best provided by telephone, rather than by written discharge summary.

PROGNOSIS

Recognition that a patient has limited life expectancy may prompt revision of treatment goals and consideration of referral to a palliative care service for optimized symptom management and provision of psychosocial support (see Chapter 214 [Principles of Palliative Care]).

Although not a substitute for clinical judgment, prognostic indices may lend objectivity to the task of clinically estimating mortality risk. A review of non–disease-specific prognostic indices for older adults identified functional level and comorbidities as the most commonly used factors. Walter and coworkers, in a study of hospitalized older patients on a general medical service, created and validated a prognostic index for 1-year postdischarge mortality and identified the following factors as predictors of greater risk: male sex, ADL dependence, heart failure, cancer, elevated creatinine, and hypoalbuminemia (see Chapter 105 [Using Prognosis to Guide Treatment]).

Patients with advanced, end-stage dementia commonly undergo invasive treatments that are not beneficial or pose significant burdens, such as tube feeding or use of physical restraints. Hospice care recipients with advanced dementia typically receive better symptom palliation for pain and dyspnea, and their health care proxies report fewer unmet needs, The US National Hospice Palliative Care Organization (NHPCO) guidelines for determining eligibility for hospice care requires functionally advanced dementia (based on a rating scale of 7C or greater on the Functional Assessment Scale) and the presence of medical complications (eg, aspiration pneumonia, pyelonephritis, sepsis, pressure ulcers). Despite the NHPCO endorsement, the Functional Assessment Scale 7C criterion was found in a recent review to be a poor predictor of 6-month mortality. Indicators found to be associated with 6-month mortality pertained to nutritional status, functional decline, and comorbidities. Regardless of our ability to accurately predict life expectancy, many older adults prefer care focused on quality of life and symptom relief, not longevity (see Chapter 74 [Hospice]).

CONCLUSION

Older patients often present with atypical manifestations of common diseases, necessitating wide-ranging diagnostic workups. They are at greater risk of injury and functional decline in the hospital, and optimal outcomes result from adopting a systematic approach to their care, regardless of admitting diagnosis. Approaches that have demonstrated improved outcomes for older adults employ comprehensive geriatric assessment of patients at admission, and those patients found to have predetermined risk factors for functional decline or geriatric syndromes reliably undergo targeted treatments designed to reduce those risks. The challenge for the hospitalist caring for older patients is to attend to the technical, disease-focused issues that prompt admission in the first place without neglecting the "prehabilitative" orientation that can prevent discharge to a nursing home.

SUGGESTED READINGS

Brown MA, Sampson EL, Jones L, Baron AM. Prognostic Indicators of 6-month mortality in elderly people with advanced dementia. *Palliat Med.* 2012;27:389-400.

Ellis G, Whitehead MA, Robinson D, O'Neill D, Langhorne P. Comprehensive Geriatric Assessment for Older Adults admitted to the Hospital: metaanalysis of randomized controlled trials. *BMJ.* 2011;343:d6553.

Fried TR, Bradley EH, Towle VR, Allore H. Understanding the treatment preferences of seriously ill patients. *N Engl J Med.* 2002;346:1061-1066.

Gibbs LM. Understanding the medical markers of elder abuse and neglect: physical exam findings. *Clin Geriatr Med.* 2014;30:687-612.

Hshieh TT, Yue J, Oh E, et al. Effectiveness of multicomponent nonpharmacological delirium interventions. *JAMA Intern Med.* 2015;175:512-520.

Shepperd S, Lannini NA, Clemson LM, Cameron ID, Barras SL. Discharge planning from hospital to home. *Cochrane Database Syst Rev.* 2013;1:CD000313.

Yourman LC, Lee S, Schonberg MA, Widera EW, Smith AK. Prognostic indices for older adults. *JAMA.* 2012;307:182-192.

ONLINE RESOURCES

Directed by the US administration on Aging, NCEA is a resource for policy makers, social service, health care practitioners, the justice system, researchers, advocates and families. Retrieved from http://www.ncea.aoa.gov on July 7, 2015.

CHAPTER 166

Agitation in Older Adults

Caroline N. Harada, MD
Heather Herrington, MD

Key Clinical Questions

❶ When is agitation due to delirium versus dementia?

❷ What are the most common causes of agitation in hospitalized older patients?

❸ What are the best nonpharmacologic techniques to manage agitation in older patients?

❹ Which medications are best for treating agitation in older patients?

❺ What are the potential complications of agitation?

❻ How can agitation due to delirium or dementia be prevented?

INTRODUCTION

It is horrible to see an agitated patient in the hospital, even worse to try to care for one, and probably worst of all to *be* an agitated patient. There is often significant internal and external pressure on hospital staff to "control the patient," and this can lead to thoughtless action. But the best (and often the only) way to address the agitation is to think carefully about the problem before acting. This chapter will attempt to present a thoughtful approach to agitation in hospitalized older adults.

Agitation in an older patient can take multiple forms: aggression, psychomotor agitation, and psychosis. ***Aggression*** refers to verbal or physical hostility, often involving resistance to care. ***Psychomotor agitation*** includes restless motor activity such as pacing, rocking, or other purposeless movement, as well as sleep disturbances, and repetitive vocalizations. ***Psychosis*** includes delusions, hallucinations, and misidentifications. Patients can experience any combination of these symptoms.

■ EPIDEMIOLOGY OF AGITATION IN OLDER HOSPITALIZED PATIENTS

Agitation is a common symptom in older hospitalized adults. It may be present on admission, or develop during the hospital stay. Reports of the incidence of agitation in this population vary widely, but may be as high as 50% or more in older ICU patients. The risk of behavioral disturbance is highest for patients who have cognitive impairment on hospital admission.

■ IMPACT OF AGITATION IN HOSPITALIZED PATIENTS

Agitation causes significant distress for patients, caregivers, and hospital staff. Hallucinations and delusions have been associated with the highest levels of anguish for patients, but agitation and aggression were most disturbing for hospital staff.

In addition to psychological distress, agitation in hospitalized patients is associated with higher risks of death and institutionalization, longer length of hospital stay, and increased health care costs. It increases the risk of injury to patients and staff, as well as the risk of complications such as falls, restraint-related injuries, and unintended removal of indwelling catheters and tubes.

If delirium is the cause of a patient's agitation, outcomes are particularly poor. Delirium increases mortality rates for ICU patients two- to four-fold, and 1.5-fold for general medicine patients. Multiple studies have also shown a risk of prolonged or permanent cognitive impairment after an episode of delirium, raising significant concerns about the possibility that delirium may actually lead to dementia in some cases.

DIFFERENTIAL DIAGNOSIS

Agitation can have multiple causes in an older hospitalized patient. The most common causes are delirium, dementia, and psychiatric disorders.

■ DELIRIUM

Delirium occurs in 29% to 64% of hospitalized patients on general medicine or geriatric wards, and up to 50% of surgical patients. The prevalence of delirium increases with age. Among older adults, a change in mental status due to delirium can be the sole presenting symptom of medical illnesses such as infection or cardiac ischemia.

The diagnosis of delirium is made from bedside observation. Key features include an acute change in cognition that results in inattention, altered level of consciousness, and disorganized thinking, usually with a fluctuating course. There is significant heterogeneity in the clinical presentation of delirium. Many patients develop the hypoactive form of delirium, which does not involve agitation, and is often overlooked. Other patients have agitation, which may include delusions or hallucinations in 30% of cases.

Delirium tends to occur in people with predisposing factors, such as advanced age, dementia, vision impairment, functional impairment, history of alcohol abuse, and multiple coexisting medical conditions. It usually is triggered by one or multiple precipitating factors, including medications, medical illness, neurologic disease, surgery, or environmental stressors.

■ DEMENTIA

Dementia affects approximately 13.9% of the US population over age 70. Prevalence increases with age, and in the population of adults age 90 and older, prevalence approaches 40%. It is estimated that by 2050, over 9 million people in the United States will have dementia. Most patients with dementia have agitation at some point during the course of their disease. It typically occurs in the moderate and severe stages of the disease, and symptoms are often transient. When these patients are admitted to the hospital with acute medical illness, it is common for these symptoms to persist or worsen.

PRACTICE POINT

- In patients with dementia, it can be difficult to distinguish between delirium superimposed on dementia, and agitation due to dementia, also known as behavioral and psychiatric symptoms of dementia (BPSD). The key differences are that delirium has an acute onset and usually results in inattention. In BPSD, on the other hand, agitated behaviors are often longstanding, and are usually not associated with a change in the level of attentiveness.

Alzheimer disease is the most common type of dementia, followed by cerebrovascular dementia and dementia with Lewy bodies (DLBs). Other forms of dementia such as frontotemporal dementia, Creutzfeldt-Jakob disease, and Parkinson dementia are less common. Agitation can accompany any type of dementia. Patients with DLB commonly suffer from visual hallucinations. Those with frontotemporal dementia often exhibit impulsiveness, lack of judgment, and personality changes that can result in agitated behaviors.

The diagnosis of dementia is best made when patients are medically stable in the outpatient setting. Unfortunately, dementia is commonly overlooked by primary care providers, who fail to document cognitive problems in up to two-thirds of cases. If dementia is suspected, it is prudent to defer the full diagnostic workup until the patient is truly at his or her medical and cognitive baseline, since even mild delirium interferes with accurate diagnosis and staging. It is appropriate, however, to perform a thorough neurologic examination, and check for reversible causes of cognitive impairment such as thyroid disease, vitamin B12 deficiency, and normal pressure hydrocephalus. Laboratory tests such as thyroid stimulating hormone (TSH), and vitamin B12 levels, as well as possibly brain imaging can be done while the patient is hospitalized to facilitate the outpatient workup. A complete discussion of the evaluation of cognitive impairment is beyond the scope of this chapter.

■ PSYCHIATRIC DISORDERS

Psychiatric disorders such as depression with psychotic features, acute mania, and schizophrenia are significantly less common causes of agitation in hospitalized older adults, but should be considered, particularly in patients with a history of psychiatric disease. In patients without such history, new onset bipolar disorder with mania could be considered as it does occur in older patients, although this is quite rare. Depression is common in older adults, so depression with psychotic features should also be considered.

PATHOPHYSIOLOGY

The pathophysiology of agitation in hospitalized older adults varies based on the underlying cause of the agitation, and it is poorly understood for most dementias and delirium. In both cases, cholinergic deficiency plays a key role. For this reason, drugs with anticholinergic properties often cause increased confusion and agitation in patients with dementia and delirium. Other neurotransmitters have been implicated in the pathophysiology of delirium, including dopamine, glutamate, serotonin, and melatonin. Mediators of inflammation such as interleukins, tumor necrosis factor alpha, interferon, cytokines, and cortisol also tend to be elevated in delirium and many types of dementia, and these may also play a role in agitation.

DIAGNOSIS: WHAT IS THE CAUSE OF THIS PATIENT'S AGITATION?

As discussed above, it is not always easy to distinguish between delirium and dementia. Many agitated patients suffer from both simultaneously. Yet no matter what the diagnosis, the key is the same: to identify and address the underlying trigger for the agitation. Because there is often no test to definitively determine if a particular factor is causing the patient's agitation, the diagnosis is sometimes achieved by correcting as many factors as possible and observing for improvement in symptoms (**Table 166-1**).

TRIAGE/HOSPITAL ADMISSION

Older patients with new onset agitation require hospitalization, usually on a general medicine ward, since medical illness is a common cause of agitation and one that must be identified and addressed in a timely manner. In addition, hospitalization is often required to control the agitated behaviors and keep the patient from harming themselves and others. Figure 166-1 outlines the approach to agitation in hospitalized older adults.

For patients who have undergone thorough medical evaluation without findings of acute medical or surgical illness, admission to a geriatric psychiatry unit is preferable in patients with a history of dementia-related agitation that has recently escalated. For patients of this type, a geriatric psychiatry unit is ideal because the staff is experienced in both pharmacologic and nonpharmacologic management of agitation. During the hospitalization, staff and family can determine the best living arrangement for the patient in the future. Many of these patients will require nursing home or other placement.

Patients who develop symptoms of agitation while hospitalized for medical or surgical illness can often stay in the ward to which they were originally admitted. If the patient is complex, consultation with geriatrics, geriatric psychiatry, or neurology can also be considered.

Some hospitals have created specialized medical care units for older patients. These units are designed to minimize stressful hospital stimuli. They offer structured activities and therapy during the day, open access to family caregivers, and nurses who are specially trained to deal with behavioral disturbances. These units are associated with lower rates of agitation and delirium among patients.

TABLE 166-1 Causes of Agitation in Older Patients

Acute medical illness
- Infection
- Acute coronary syndrome
- Hypoxia
- Shock
- Fever or hypothermia
- Dehydration
- Metabolic derangements
- Stroke
- Intracranial bleeding
- Other intracranial lesions (eg, brain tumors, NPH)
- Surgery

Drugs
- Sedative-hypnotics
- Narcotics
- Anticholinergic drugs
- Alcohol or drug withdrawal
- Illicit drugs

Basic needs
- Hunger or thirst
- Pain
- Boredom or immobilization
- Fatigue or sleep deprivation
- Wet or soiled
- Unable to hear or see
- Constipation or urinary retention

Environmental triggers*
- Unfamiliar environment
- Intensive care unit
- Physical restraints
- Bladder catheter
- Multiple procedures
- Change in daily routine
- Too cold/hot

Interpersonal issues*
- Strain in relationship with caregiver
- Grief/bereavement

*Cause agitation primarily in people with dementia—less likely to cause agitation in those who are cognitively intact.

MANAGEMENT OPTIONS

■ NONPHARMACOLOGIC MANAGEMENT OF AGITATION

Management of agitation should begin with nonpharmacologic treatments (**Table 166-2**). Identifying and removing causes of agitation is often the only treatment necessary. Agitation should be recognized for what it is: a response to an unpleasant situation. A patient who is constantly throwing off his hospital gown and bed sheets may simply be attempting to cool off in an overly-warm room. Nursing staff education is essential to the effective treatment of agitation; the Suggested Reading section contains a list of helpful articles and web-based resources.

Family members can be extremely helpful in calming and reorienting an agitated patient, but they often require education about the patient's symptoms and their role in the treatment plan. Using

the term delirium when applicable, and explaining that in many cases the only predictable feature of delirium is that it is unpredictable, may help family members and others better understand this condition. It may be helpful to educate family members that a delirious patient will respond to others' emotions, so it is of the utmost importance for caregivers to remain calm and reassuring. Ask the family to assist with calming reorientation and cognitive activities during the daytime, and to encourage sleep at night. The Hospital Elder Life Program (HELP) has nonpharmacologic recommendations for promoting sleep, and a recent study in the ICU suggests that use of earplugs at night may be helpful in this regard.

TABLE 166-2 Nonpharmacologic Management of Agitation*

Review medication list carefully and discontinue or taper possible contributors
- Ask about nonprescription medications (over-the-counter medications, herbal medications, alcohol, and illicit drug use)

Address basic needs
- Maintain hydration and nutrition
- Encourage use of hearing aids, glasses, and dentures to avoid sensory deprivation and improve orientation
- Avoid unnecessary nighttime interruptions to promote normal sleep-wake cycles (vital sign checks, blood draws, bathing, and turning)
- Physical therapy or nursing to mobilize patient as soon as it is safely possible

Keep the environment calm
- Avoid physical restraints
- Use sitters, bed alarms, low beds, move the patient to a room closer to the nurses' station for closer monitoring
- Consider removing other irritants/barriers to mobility such as urinary catheters, supplemental oxygen, telemetry monitors, continuous intravenous infusions
- Encourage family members to stay at the bedside as much as possible
- Educate family members so they can help calm and reorient the patient
- Encourage family members to place familiar items (photos, blankets, etc) at the bedside
- Keep clocks and calendars visible to assist with orientation
- Minimize staff and room changes
- Minimize excess noise, especially at night
- Ensure adequate lighting during the day (but avoid overly bright light in patients with cataracts)
- Ensure relative darkness at night
- Complementary therapy: music, art, pet, and massage therapy†
- Create a dayroom for activities (this will help motivate patients to stay awake and mobile during the day)
- Enlist hospital volunteers to provide companionship, activities, frequent reorientation

Promote helpful interpersonal interactions
- Frequent reorientation: "Mrs Smith, today is Thursday and you are in the hospital with pneumonia."
- Reassuring statements: "Mrs Smith, you are in the hospital and we are here to help you."

*These strategies should be employed for ALL older patients, not just those with agitation, as many have been shown to prevent delirium.
†Complementary therapies can worsen agitation in some patients, so use should be individualized.

Untreated pain may cause or exacerbate agitation, and it is essential to evaluate for, recognize, and treat pain. Patients who are agitated and confused may not be able to adequately or appropriately communicate their experience of pain, but various nonverbal assessments of pain can help identify pain in these patients. Standard pain protocols and training to help doctors, nurses, and other staff recognize nonverbal indicators of pain (such as grimacing or moaning) may help reduce agitation. Also, it is important to recognize that the older patient with agitation may not be able to reliably ask for pain medication, so it may be necessary to order scheduled analgesic medications for these patients.

Agitation and delirium are often accompanied by use of physical restraints. Though restraints are presumed to prevent falls and other safety problems, there is little evidence to support this notion, and quite a lot to refute it. Restraints are problematic because they prevent early mobility, which is associated with a decreased incidence of delirium in several studies of hospitalized older adults. Restraints, including bedside rails, can also lead to deconditioning and a higher fall risk. They are also associated with entrapment and asphyxiation. Restraints often worsen agitation. Nurses may also be distressed by the use of restraints, even though (and perhaps because) they requested that restraints be placed. Again, staff education is essential. Recognize the person's strengths. Can you redirect the agitated person who is pulling at the bed sheets by giving her towels to fold? A patient with dementia who can still play the piano may soothe herself and others by doing just that. Consider asking a family member or sitter to stay with the patient to help redirect the patient toward safer activities. Ensure that the patient gets out of the bed to a chair daily, and have him or her ambulate if possible; physical therapists may need to be involved if the patient has significant impairment. Employ all available resources to encourage mobility and avoid the use of physical restraints.

In addition, discontinue urinary catheters, supplemental oxygen, telemetry monitors, continuous intravenous infusions, and other barriers to mobility as soon as these treatments are no longer necessary, as these tethers act both as barriers to mobility and irritants that add to the stress of hospitalization. Automatic reminders and protocols in the electronic health record can help minimize the use of these interventions and improve outcomes.

Finally, review all medications, paying particular attention to medications that are known to be high risk for causing agitation in older adults. Potentially inappropriate medications to avoid in the older adult include antihistamines such as diphenhydramine, anticholinergics such as promethazine, muscle relaxants such as cyclobenzaprine, and benzodiazepines and other sedatives. Withdrawal, in particular from alcohol or benzodiazepines, can also result in agitation in hospitalized older adults. Review the patient's home medication list, review the actual medications and bottles if they are available, and inquire specifically about the use of anxiolytic medications, over-the-counter medications, and alcohol. Institutional protocols, such as automatic electronic reminders, should appear when clinicians try to order potentially inappropriate medications in older patients, as these have been demonstrated to be effective in decreasing rates of use.

■ PHARMACOLOGIC MANAGEMENT OF AGITATION

Agitated patients who are at acute risk of harming themselves or others may require immediate pharmacologic treatment. Pharmacologic treatment can also be considered for patients whose symptoms seem to cause them significant psychological distress. Medications to reduce agitation should be avoided in other cases, given the lack of data demonstrating effectiveness and the considerable risks of these medications. Some, but not all, studies of medications to treat delirium show reduction in delirium rates, but none show reduction in key outcomes such as complications, hospital length of stay, or mortality.

There is no FDA-approved drug for the treatment or prevention of agitation in patients with dementia, so all drugs discussed here are used off-label. In spite of limited evidence for efficacy, antipsychotic medications are often considered first-line therapy for psychotic and aggressive forms of agitation. They are less effective for psychomotor forms of agitation. Antipsychotic medications may cause adverse effects including sedation, tardive dyskinesia, and extrapyramidal symptoms. In addition, antipsychotics have been associated with increased mortality in patients who have co-existing dementia.

PRACTICE POINT

Antipsychotics and increased mortality in dementia

- Antipsychotics now come with a black box warning from the FDA advising that these drugs should not be used for patients with dementia due to the risk of increased mortality.
- It is essential to discuss the risks and benefits of treatment with health care surrogates prior to administration of these medications. Surrogates will often agree that the slightly increased risk of death is outweighed by the potential benefit of relief from distressing psychiatric symptoms.

If antipsychotic medications are prescribed, it is essential to identify the target symptoms and use the lowest possible dose for the shortest possible time. For example, starting doses of haloperidol should be 0.25 to 0.5 mg intravenous or by mouth. For quetiapine, 12.5 to 25 mg by mouth every 12 hours is appropriate. Monitor the patient carefully for the target symptoms, and as they resolve, taper and discontinue these medications.

Other medications have been used to treat agitation. Dexmedetomidine has been shown, in several studies, to reduce delirium when used prophylactically in mechanically ventilated patients, although it did not decrease length of ICU stay or affect mortality. In dementia patients whose agitation is chronic, studies suggest that cholinesterase inhibitors and memantine may have some efficacy for reduction of behavioral disturbances. There is insufficient evidence to support using these drugs as primary pharmacologic treatments for agitation, but they should certainly be continued when patients are already taking them at the time of admission. Antidepressants such as citalopram may also be modestly efficacious in the prevention of agitation, and one study found no difference in the efficacy of citalopram and risperidone when treating chronic agitation in patients with dementia. Mood stabilizers and anticonvulsants such as valproate preparations and carbamazepine are also used as second-line therapies for dementia patients with chronic agitation, but evidence to support their efficacy is still lacking.

PRACTICE POINT

Avoid benzodiazepines, except in the setting of withdrawal

- Benzodiazepines are rarely indicated for agitation in older patients as they may cause unintended side effects, particularly paradoxical agitation. However, in patients with alcoholism or chronic benzodiazepine use, benzodiazepines are often essential therapy to prevent withdrawal syndromes. Benzodiazepines may also be used in the treatment of dying patients, when delirium is terminal and nonreversible.

COMPLICATIONS

The agitated patient is at high risk for complications. Possible complications of agitation and recommended preventive strategies are summarized in **Table 166-3**.

DISCHARGE CHECKLIST

- Does the patient have a support network able to care for him or her at home? Many patients with delirium in the hospital setting can safely be discharged home with mild delirium, as long as they have 24-hour supervision and caregivers who are physically and cognitively able to provide the needed care.
- If patient cannot be cared for at home in his or her current state, would he or she qualify for skilled rehabilitation? During this rehabilitation period, patients will be reevaluated with respect to long-term nursing home care versus a more independent setting. Behavioral symptoms are one of the most common reasons for nursing home placement.
- Were antiagitation medications used in the hospital? If so, these generally should be discontinued or tapered.
- Have accepting providers been informed of the patient's current and prior cognitive baseline and functional status? They will need this information to keep the patient safe and set rehabilitation goals.

TABLE 166-3 Preventing Complications of Agitation

Complication	Preventive Strategy
Adverse drug reactions	Avoid drugs that can cause confusion or oversedation, especially benzodiazepines[1]
Aspiration	Protect the patient's airway, avoid over sedation
Deconditioning	Encourage mobilization (even if just out of bed to chair)
Deep vein thrombosis or pulmonary embolus	Encourage mobilization, avoid restraints
Dehydration or malnutrition	Monitor for signs of each and intervene early, offer water often, ensure patient can access water when thirsty, food when hungry
Injuries	Avoid restraints, avoid falls
	Promote night-time sleep
	Enlist a sitter or encourage family to stay with patient
Pain	Careful observation for signs of pain, empiric treatment may be necessary
Pressure ulcers	Avoid restraints, encourage early mobilization or frequent repositioning if patient is bedbound

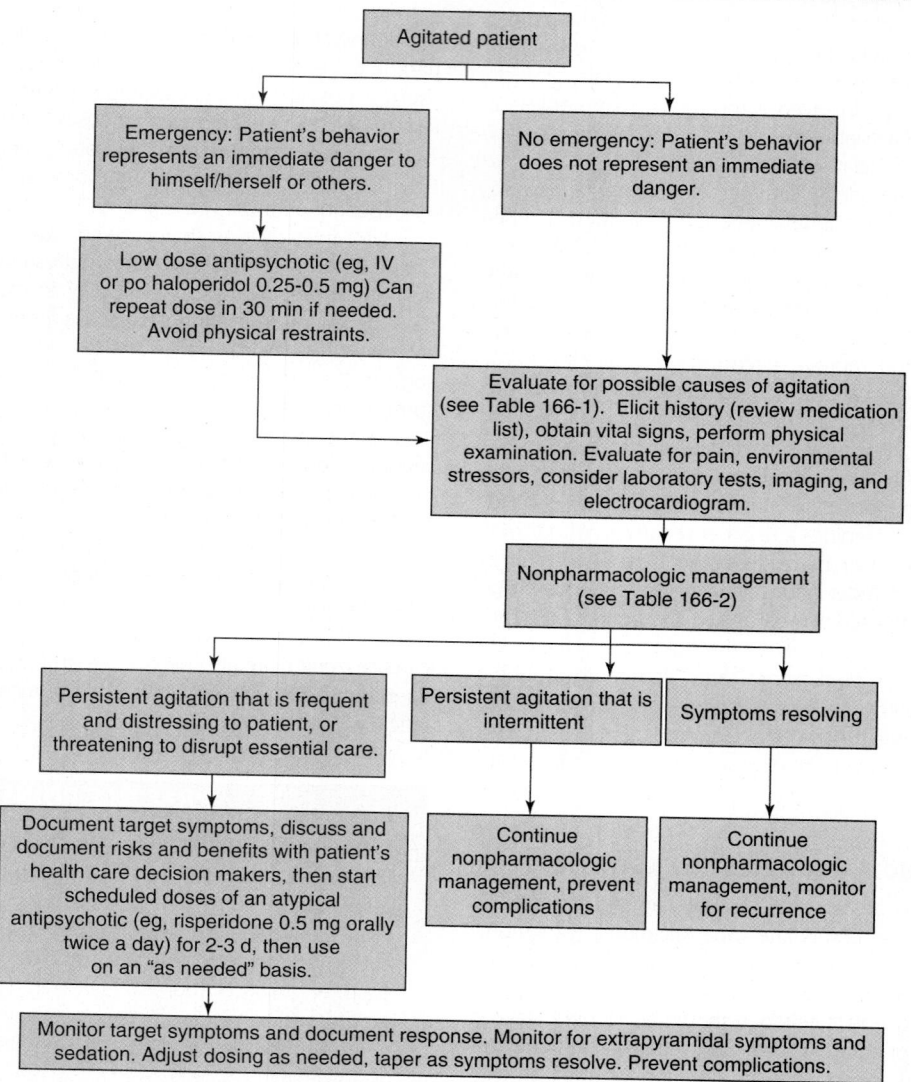

Figure 166-1 *Approach to agitation in older adults.*

PRACTICE POINT

Antipsychotics and hospital discharge

- Due to the risk of increased morbidity and mortality, antipsychotics initiated to treat agitation in hospitalized older adults should be discontinued or tapered at discharge if possible. A plan regarding taper of any continued psychoactive medications should be clearly communicated to both the patient's family and the clinician who will be assuming care at the time of discharge.

SUGGESTED READINGS

Ballard CG, Gauthier S, Cummings JL, et al. Management of agitation and aggression associated with Alzheimer disease. *Nat Rev Neurol.* 2009;5:245-255.

Blass DM, Rabins PV. In the clinic: dementia. *Ann Intern Med.* 2014;161(3):ITC1-16.

Fick D, Semla T, Beizer J, et al. American Geriatrics Society updated Beers Criteria for potentially inappropriate medication use in older adults. *J Am Geriatr Soc.* 2012;60:616-631.

Inouye SK, Bogardus ST Jr, Baker DI, Leo-Summers L, Cooney LM Jr. The Hospital Elder Life Program: a model of care to prevent cognitive and functional decline in older hospitalized patients. *J Am Geriatr Soc.* 2000;48:1697-1706.

Inouye SK, Westendorp RGJ, Saczynski JS. Delirium in elderly people. *Lancet.* 2014;383(9920):911-922.

Rivosecchi RM, Smithburger PL, Svec S, Campbell S, Kane-Gill SL. Nonpharmacological interventions to prevent delirium: an evidence-based systematic review. *Crit Care Nurse.* 2015;35:39-51.

Salzman C, Jeste DV, Meyer RE, et al. Elderly patients with dementia-related symptoms of severe agitation and aggression: consensus statement on treatment options, clinical trials methodology, and policy. *J Clin Psychiatry.* 2008;69:889-898.

ONLINE RESOURCES

Helpful websites for nurse education:

http://consultgerirn.org/

http://www.nicheprogram.org/

http://www.hospitalelderlifeprogram.org/

CHAPTER 167

Elder Mistreatment

Karin Ouchida, MD
Mark S. Lachs, MD, MPH

Key Clinical Questions

1. When should you suspect elder mistreatment?
2. How do you assess for elder mistreatment and what should you document in your assessment?
3. Who should you consult and what are the reporting requirements if you suspect elder mistreatment?
4. How do you create a safe discharge plan to ensure a smooth transition to the next setting?

INTRODUCTION

Elder abuse and neglect represent a growing public health problem with the potential for serious morbidity and mortality. A clinician will likely encounter at least one victim of elder abuse for every 20 to 40 older adults seen. As hospitalists assume care for an increasing proportion of older adults in acute care settings, they need to know which older adults are at greatest risk for elder mistreatment and how to properly assess them. Elder mistreatment is an independent risk factor for death. A prospective cohort study of 2800 community-dwelling adults age 65 and older by Lachs, et al. reported that the mortality rate was three times higher in the elder mistreatment group and 1.7 times greater in the self-neglect group. In the group with any elder mistreatment, the survival rate was 9% versus 40%. Every emergency room visit and admission represent critical opportunities for medical providers to positively impact the lives of both elder mistreatment victims and their caregivers.

Elder mistreatment occurs among men and women of all racial, ethnic, and socioeconomic groups. Older adults are at greater risk for mistreatment if they are dependent on others due to cognitive impairment, physical frailty or mental illness. Other risk factors for physical and psychological abuse include a shared living situation and lack of social support. In cases of financial abuse, however, the older adult more often lives alone. The perpetrators of abuse are most likely to be male and an adult child or spouse. Financial abuse may be the fastest growing yet least recognized form of elder mistreatment. In 2009, the direct cost of financial exploitation in the United States was an estimated $2.9 billion. Other characteristics that appear more frequently amongst perpetrators of elder mistreatment include mental illness, substance abuse, emotional or financial dependency on the older adult, a history of violence or antisocial behavior, and external stressors (medical illness, financial stress, caregiver burnout). In long-term care settings, abuse of older residents by other residents is becoming an alarming trend. The so-called resident-to-resident aggression takes the form of physical abuse, verbal abuse, or sexual aggression, and is actually more common than abuse of residents by nursing home staff.

In clinical practice, risk factors that create an imbalance between the older adult's needs and the ability of the caregiver/support system to meet those needs led to increased vulnerability. Three key risk factors leading to this critical imbalance include cognitive impairment, physical frailty, and social isolation. Despite being ideally suited to detect, manage, and prevent elder mistreatment, a 2004 study conducted by the National Center on Elder Abuse found that physicians are one of the least likely groups of individuals to report abuse and neglect. Barriers to physician reporting include insufficient knowledge of assessment protocols and mandatory reporting guidelines, concerns about a negative effect on relationships with patients and caregivers, reluctance to get involved with the legal system, and time constraints. Time constraints are a valid concern. An assessment for elder abuse and neglect is rarely a quick and simple endeavor. It often requires taking a detailed history from the patient and other caregivers and a thorough physical examination that includes a cognitive evaluation. A comprehensive evaluation may conflict with pressures to manage length of stay by focusing solely on the diagnosis and treatment of the acute medical issues. We will discuss how to utilize an inter-disciplinary team as well as expert consultants to lessen the burden on any one provider. Hospitalists may also make use of time-based billing in order to maximize reimbursement for managing these complex cases. Elder mistreatment cases often unfold, over the course of a single lengthy admission or multiple admissions, and hospitalists commonly "hand off" these complex patients to their colleagues in subacute, home care, or ambulatory settings. Because we understand the limitations of what may be reasonably accomplished in an acute care setting, we have devoted portions of this chapter to "hand offs" and how to ensure safe transitions between care providers.

This chapter will help hospitalists recognize the signs of elder abuse and neglect and provide them with the skills to perform an assessment and devise appropriate multidisciplinary interventions. We will detail the components of assessment, intervention, and follow-up.

DEFINITIONS

The American Medical Association (AMA) classifies elder abuse and neglect as "acts of commission or omission that result in harm or threatened harm to the health or welfare of an older adult." This broad description reminds the clinician to look beyond the image of the bruised and battered victim for the often subtle signs of neglect and other types of abuse. Both the World Health Organization and the US National Academy of Sciences definitions add that the "perpetrators" of abuse and neglect are typically persons whom the older adult holds in a position of trust. These responsible individuals may either cause the mistreatment or fail to prevent it. The AMA emphasizes that mistreatment may be intentional or unintentional. Unintentional mistreatment is often due to a caregiver's ignorance, inexperience, or inability, often stemming from his or her own medical or mental health problems. Despite the varying definitions of abuse and neglect, agreement exists for the following six types of mistreatment (listed in order of frequency substantiated by Adult Protective Services [APS] in the 1998 National Elder Abuse Incidence Study [NEAIS]).

1. **Neglect:** The refusal or failure of a designated caregiver to meet needs necessary for an older adult's physical and mental well-being. Neglect includes, but is not limited to, the failure to provide basic necessities like food, water, clothing, shelter, and medicine. It also encompasses the failure to ensure an older adult's comfort, safety, and personal hygiene.

2. **Self-neglect:** The refusal or failure of an older adult to meet his or her own physical and mental needs resulting in threats to personal health or safety. Self-neglect includes, but is not limited to, an elder's failure to take medications, adhere to medical treatment or maintain adequate nutrition, personal hygiene, and shelter. In its most extreme form, self-neglect is manifested by domestic squalor, social withdrawal, hoarding behaviors, lack of shame, and refusal to accept help. While self-neglect is a fundamentally different phenomenon than elder abuse by another actor, hospitalists may confront it even more frequently than elder abuse when neglected health problems cause or contribute to the reasons for hospital admission. Additionally, the same community resources (ie, adult protective services) are often called upon to address self-neglect.

3. **Psychological abuse:** Verbal or nonverbal acts intended to cause anguish, pain, or distress. Psychological abuse includes, but is not limited to verbal assaults, insults, threats (including threat of abandonment or institutionalization), intimidation, humiliation, harassment, infantilization and social isolation of an older adult.

4. **Financial or material exploitation:** The illegal or improper use of an elder's funds, property, or assets. Financial abuse includes, but is not limited to, cashing an older adult's checks without permission, forging an older adult's signature, stealing money or possessions, coercing or deceiving an older adult into signing documents (eg, contracts, wills, or property deeds), and improper use of conservatorship, guardianship, or power of attorney status.

5. **Physical abuse:** Acts intended to cause impairment, physical pain, or bodily injury. Physical abuse includes, but is not limited to, acts of violence such as striking (with or without an object), pushing, shoving, shaking, kicking, pinching, and burning. Additional examples include the inappropriate use of drugs or physical restraints, force feeding, and physical punishment of any kind.

6. **Sexual abuse:** Any type of nonconsensual sexual contact including situations in which an older adult is unable to consent.

Previously reported frequencies of elder mistreatment varied depending on the definition employed and the setting(s) examined. Extrapolating from the best available evidence, the overall prevalence of elder mistreatment in community settings is approximately 10% but this almost certainly underestimates the true extent of abuse and neglect that occurs. The original 1998 National Elder Abuse Incidence Study compared Adult Protective Services records and reports from "sentinels" at community agencies who frequently worked with elderly clients. The NEAIS found nearly 80% of incidents were never reported to Adult Protective Services, the major agency tasked with receiving and investigating reports of abuse and neglect.

UNIQUE CHALLENGES AND OPPORTUNITIES FOR HOSPITALISTS

■ POTENTIAL FOR POSITIVE INTERVENTION

While we acknowledge the challenges of performing assessments for elder mistreatment in an acute care setting, the stakes are high when it comes to elder mistreatment. The acute care admission may signal a crisis coming to a head or the first sign that an older adult is being abused or neglected. For example, the elderly woman with dementia admitted with a fall in the setting of hypoglycemia is being cared for by her increasingly frail husband who left her alone while he went to his doctor's office. She did not feel well and assuming it was her "sugar" took an extra dose of her oral diabetes medications. The husband's decision to leave his wife alone at home is most likely unintentional neglect but the resulting hospitalization provides an opportunity to intervene. Perhaps the patient's medication regimen can be simplified and short-term home care services ordered for nursing and physical therapy visits. While she is receiving home health care, a social worker may also visit the home to explore whether the patient qualifies for Medicaid or other entitlements that will ensure long-term supervision for the patient and support for her husband.

Hospital-based providers may be the only individuals who come into contact with the abused or neglected older adult. Physicians have the authority and expertise to (1) document the presence or absence of mistreatment using the physical examination, laboratory and other studies, (2) recommend admission or transfer to another setting, and (3) order critical services such as home health care. For known cases of ongoing abuse in the community, an acute care admission can provide vital opportunities to assess and counsel victims away from the influence of abusers and their environments, and to bring new resources to bear on the problem that would prove difficult in other settings (eg, psychiatric consultation, physical therapy, and social services).

■ POTENTIAL FOR HARM WITH INACTION

If the hospital-based clinician fails to recognize the signs of abuse or neglect and misses an opportunity for intervention, significant harm may come to the patient and his/her caregivers. For example, the frail bed-bound elderly female with multiple sclerosis admitted with several worsening pressure ulcers may confide in the physician that her son frequently yells and shakes his fist at her. Recently he broke her hospital bed and would not allow her aides to turn and reposition her. If the patient's report was dismissed and she was not asked, in private, whether she wanted to return home or go to a subacute facility for wound care, she could suffer increasing morbidity or mortality if violence at home escalates. Her son might "refuse" subacute rehabilitation because he actually is dependent on the patient for his housing. Furthermore, if the inpatient provider "fumbles the hand off" and fails to properly document the assessment and planned intervention, the patient and the health care system could pay the consequences. If the example patient was discharged to a subacute facility that was unaware of the patient's fears of her son, the receiving clinicians might inadvertently discharge the patient home several weeks later. Or, should the patient be readmitted to the acute care setting under a different hospitalist, that physician might also unknowingly involve the patient's son in discharge planning. The "social admission" and frequent admissions may on the surface appear to be "routine" admissions but subtle red flags should prompt consideration of elder mistreatment in the differential diagnosis.

HOW TO CONDUCT AN ASSESSMENT FOR ELDER MISTREATMENT

■ WHEN TO ASSESS

Hospitalists should adopt the practice of "universal precautions" for elder mistreatment. This entails maintaining a high index of suspicion, especially when a patient's caregiver and support system is clearly inadequate to meet his or her needs. The risk factors for elder abuse and neglect that most often lead to an imbalance between needs and supports are cognitive impairment, physical frailty, and social isolation. If one type of abuse or neglect is suspected, the hospitalist should screen for all other forms. The American Medical Association considers certain signs "red flags" indicating potential elder neglect or abuse (**Table 167-1**).

Often medical providers must act like detectives, putting together the smallest of details to form a larger picture. The presence of any one or a combination of these indicators should trigger an assessment for elder mistreatment (**Figure 167-1**).

■ WHAT TO ASSESS

The presence of any one of the red flags in Table 167-1 should prompt a full assessment for elder mistreatment. A comprehensive assessment similar to any admission or consultation includes a thorough history and physical exam.

In obtaining the history, the hospitalist should address and document the following:

- History from the older adult
- History from the suspected abuser/neglector
- History from any collateral sources (eg, caregivers, outpatient physicians, home care personnel)
- Assessment of functional status
- Assessment of social and financial resources

In performing a full physical exam the hospitalist should note and document the following:

- General appearance (hygiene, cleanliness, and appropriateness of attire)
- Vital signs (orthostatic blood pressure and pulse) and weight
- Head and neck exam (fit of dentures, dental hygiene, venereal lesions, deviated septum)
- Full skin examination (ecchymoses, burns, lacerations, abrasions, pressure ulcers)

TABLE 167-1 Red Flags or Indicators of Possible Elder Neglect and Abuse

Neglect and self-neglect
- Inappropriate dress for season
- Poor hygiene
- Dehydration
- Malnutrition
- Hypothermia or hyperthermia
- Pressure ulcers
- Lack of assistive devices
- Nonadherence with medications
- Nonadherence with recommendations for services (eg, refusal of home care services)
- Abandonment

Emotional or psychological abuse
- Depression
- Anxiety
- Agitation
- Passivity
- Evasiveness
- Fear
- Confusion

Financial or material exploitation
- Nonadherence with medications
- Nonadherence with recommendations for services (eg, refusal of home care services)
- Frequent emergency department visits
- Frequent hospital admissions
- Unpaid bills or rent; impending eviction
- Abrupt changes in an older adult's will or financial documents
- Unexplained or frequent withdrawals from bank accounts
- Disappearance of funds or possessions
- Unauthorized credit card charges

Physical abuse
- History inconsistent with injuries
- Delay in presentation
- Repeated emergency department or office visits
- Frequent hospital admissions
- Suspicious pattern or bruising or burns (eg, circumferential abrasions consistent with wrist restraints)
- Changes in demeanor or activity level
- Caregiver refusal to leave older adult alone
- Drug levels consistent with overdosing or underdosing of medications (eg, warfarin, antiepileptic drugs)

Sexual abuse
- Difficulty walking or sitting
- Vaginal or urinary symptoms
- Bruising around the breasts, genital area, and/or inner thighs
- Torn or stained undergarments
- Unexplained sexually-transmitted diseases
- Behavioral changes including withdrawal, depression, insomnia, aggressive behavior, sexual behavior

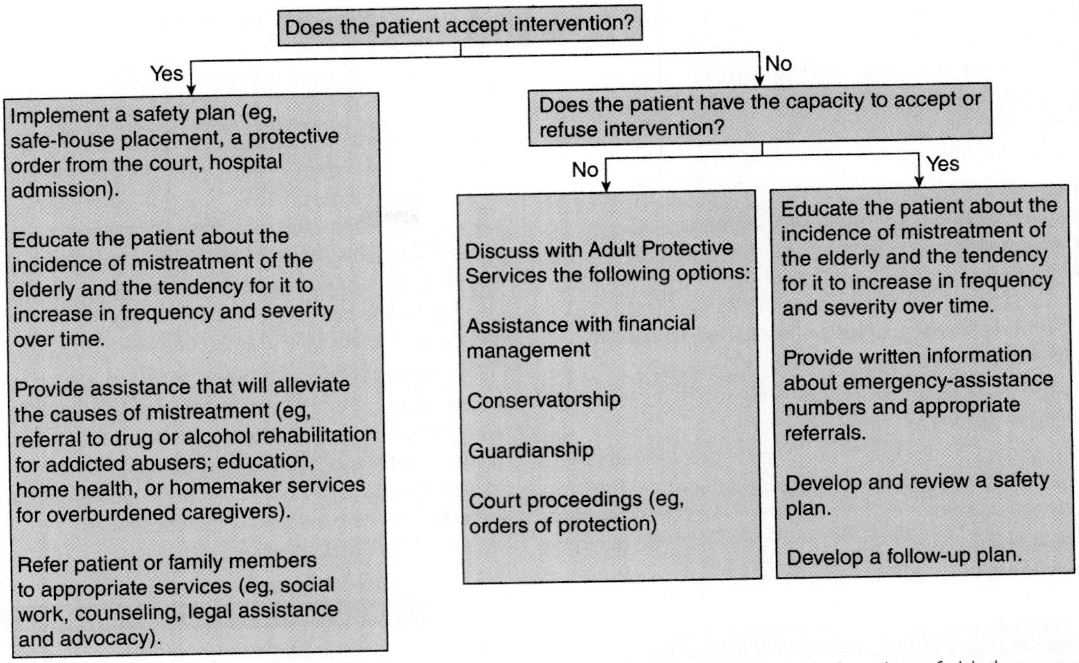

Does the patient accept intervention?

Yes

Implement a safety plan (eg, safe-house placement, a protective order from the court, hospital admission).

Educate the patient about the incidence of mistreatment of the elderly and the tendency for it to increase in frequency and severity over time.

Provide assistance that will alleviate the causes of mistreatment (eg, referral to drug or alcohol rehabilitation for addicted abusers; education, home health, or homemaker services for overburdened caregivers).

Refer patient or family members to appropriate services (eg, social work, counseling, legal assistance and advocacy).

No

Does the patient have the capacity to accept or refuse intervention?

No

Discuss with Adult Protective Services the following options:

Assistance with financial management

Conservatorship

Guardianship

Court proceedings (eg, orders of protection)

Yes

Educate the patient about the incidence of mistreatment of the elderly and the tendency for it to increase in frequency and severity over time.

Provide written information about emergency-assistance numbers and appropriate referrals.

Develop and review a safety plan.

Develop a follow-up plan.

Figure 167-1 *Approach to patient.* (Reproduced, with permission, from Lachs MS, Pillemer K. Abuse and neglect of elderly persons. *N Engl J Med.* 1995(332):437-443. Copyright Massachusetts Medical Society. All rights reserved.)

- Musculoskeletal examination (fractures or signs of previous fractures)
- Genitorectal examination (bruising, venereal lesions, inguinal rash, fecal impaction) including rape kit if indicated
- Mood and affect
- Assessment of cognitive function and decision-making capacity
- Gait

■ HOW TO ASSESS

When assessing for elder mistreatment, it is imperative to interview the older adult and suspected perpetrator separately. The older adult's willingness to accept help will ultimately determine the intervention strategies employed (Figure 167-1). The hospitalist can matter-of-factly inform the caregiver or family member that the hospital's policy requires the physician interview each patient privately and provide assurance that time will be allotted for the caregiver's questions/concerns to be addressed as well. For efficiency, another member of the interdisciplinary team (eg, the social worker, a resident, or fellow) can elicit the history from the caregiver or family member while the hospitalist completes the patient interview and physical examination. If the caregiver or suspected abuser/neglector refuses to allow the older adult to be interviewed alone, it should raise the examiner's suspicions and should be documented in the medical record. Special attention should be paid to how the older adult acts in the caregiver's presence. Note any comments or glances the person gives to the older adult conveying a message to "keep your mouth shut or else." Subtle changes in the older adult's demeanor when being interviewed alone can also signal abuse or neglect. The older adult may appear withdrawn or depressed, speak in low tones or make poor eye contact.

Older adults with cognitive impairment and/or sensory impairments can pose an additional challenge during the assessment. Providers, in a rush to obtain the history may ignore the older adult completely and allow the caregiver to provide all of the details. Remember, however, that older adults with cognitive deficits are more vulnerable to mistreatment. Do not assume that these individuals cannot adequately describe the mistreatment. When interviewing older adults with cognitive impairment, helpful tips for the hospitalist include the following:

- Allot extra time for the interview or break the interview up over several encounters
- Ensure that the patient has his/her assistive devices (eg, eyeglasses, hearing aid, dentures)
- Minimize background noise when possible (eg, draw the curtain, close the door)
- Position yourself so that you are at eye level (eg, raise head of the patient's bed, sit in a chair)
- Speak slowly and clearly; avoid shouting, which may come across as confrontational
- Assure the patient of privacy and confidentiality
- Repeat and clarify the patient's responses

For all suspected elder mistreatment victims, hospitalists can build rapport and collect key information by beginning with open-ended questions about the living environment and functional status and then progressing to more specific questions recommended by the American Medical Association.

Examples of general questions to begin an interview:

- Who lives with you?
- Who, if anyone, helps you with your activities of daily living? (eg, transfers, bathing, toileting, feeding, grooming)
- Who, if anyone, helps you with your instrumental activities of daily living (eg, meal preparation, shopping, medications, bills)?

Examples of specific questions suggested by the American Medical Association:

- Do you feel safe in your home?
- Does anyone ever threaten you or verbally assault you?
- Has anyone ever touched you without your consent?
- Has anyone ever asked you to sign documents you do not understand?
- Has anyone ever taken your things without your permission?
- Are you afraid of anyone in your home?
- Are you alone a lot?
- Has anyone ever failed to help you when you were unable to help yourself?

When interviewing caregivers or suspected perpetrators, the health care provider should remain nonjudgmental and avoid confrontation. One should also try to provide empathy for the burden of caregiving. Pay attention to inconsistencies in the explanations provided or frequently changing stories.

Helpful questions for caregivers or suspected perpetrators include the following:

- How long have you been caring for (the patient)?
- What are your primary caregiving responsibilities?
- Do you feel you have adequate support? Why or why not?
- How are you coping with your responsibilities?
- What is your understanding of the patient's medical conditions and needs?
- Can you tell me in your words what happened? (if physical signs of injury or history of injury)

If elder mistreatment is disclosed, be prepared to validate the patient's experience and listen supportively as you might be the first person the victim has confided in. It may take several conversations with a provider or providers before the victim reveals information about elder mistreatment.

PRACTICE POINT

- The evaluation and documentation of decision-making capacity in a potential elder mistreatment victim are critical. The description "alert and oriented times three" is insufficient documentation of a patient's decision-making capacity. To demonstrate capacity, the individual must be able to understand the relevant information or choices being presented, articulate a choice, and provide a reasonable explanation for that choice. Cognitive impairment does not automatically indicate a lack of capacity. The assessment of capacity must be decision-specific. For example, does this patient have capacity to participate in discharge planning?

Some victims choose not to disclose or refuse assistance. There are many reasons why a victim might refuse help, including a fear of escalating abuse or neglect if the nature of the relationship is altered or exposed. An abuser may not demonstrate aggression in front of the medical providers, often because he or she does not want any outsider to detect a problem. A caregiver who is neglecting an older adult may attribute signs of neglect like malnutrition, dehydration, uncontrolled chronic diseases, or mood disorders to the patient (eg, "she refuses to eat or take her medications") or to the aging process (eg, "would anyone not be depressed in this situation?").

OBTAINING HISTORY FROM ADDITIONAL SOURCES

While the older adult and the reported perpetrator of the abuse or neglect can provide critical history, it is often insufficient. The hospitalist and other members of the inpatient team may be approached by individuals wanting to share "their side of the story" or conversely may need to seek out other critical sources of information. Caution should be taken to avoid believing any one source without trying to corroborate the validity of the information being presented. The patient who reports her niece came in the middle of the night and stole thousands of dollars from her may be the victim of theft or may be suffering from cognitive impairment and paranoia. The patient's outpatient or community medical providers can be especially helpful by providing information about the patient's chronic illnesses, baseline cognitive status, compliance with medications and office visits, and caregivers. Home health providers who have visited patients at home can provide critical environmental history for example, is there evidence of clutter or

hoarding, is the neighborhood safe, and is there sufficient food in the kitchen?

Collateral history is frequently required and potential sources include

- The patient's primary care physician or other medical providers
- Individuals who live with the older adult (eg, relatives, friends, personal care workers)
- Home health care providers (eg, visiting nurse, physical or occupational therapist, social worker, home health aide)
- Neighbors, friends, additional family members
- Apartment superintendent or landlord
- Bank or financial institution officials

The responsibility to gather collateral information should be shared amongst members of the inpatient team. The hospitalist must interview and examine the patient but can and should engage physician assistants, nurses, medical trainees (residents and medical students), social work, physical and occupational therapy, nutrition, and others to help assess the patient's functional and psychosocial status and to elucidate any reports of abuse or neglect.

INDICATIONS FOR HOSPITAL ADMISSION

Most indications for admission of a suspected victim of elder mistreatment are the same as for all geriatric patients and include

- Hemodynamic instability
- New diagnoses requiring acute hospital care such as acute myocardial infarction or cerebrovascular accident
- Exacerbations of chronic illnesses requiring acute hospital care such as uncontrolled diabetes with hyperosmolarity or worsening of chronic obstructive pulmonary disease
- Change in mental status
- Trauma with major fracture, inability to ambulate, or uncontrolled pain

■ APPROACH TO THE "SOCIAL ADMISSION" AND THE "FREQUENT FLIER"

Less clear are those situations in which the hospitalist is called by the emergency department to admit a patient who is unsafe to return to the previous care setting. If coming from home, a concerned neighbor, family member or home care agency may have referred these patients. Older adults may also be transferred out of institutional settings such as rehabilitation facilities or nursing homes by caregivers dissatisfied with the care being provided. While there is a tendency for hospital-based physicians to dread these "social admits," any reports of abuse or neglect must be carefully and systematically addressed.

It may be easier to conceptualize a set of conditions or parameters for safe discharge from the emergency department rather than to list criteria for hospital admission. Patients sent from postacute settings such as rehabilitation facilities or nursing homes with any allegation of abuse or neglect will require admission and workup before transfer back to a postacute setting. Patients coming to the emergency department from home settings (private homes, assisted livings, etc) can be safely transitioned back if their functional status is accurately assessed and measures to ensure their safety can be put into place.

While the indication for acute hospital admission may not be disputed for patients frequently readmitted for exacerbation of chronic diseases, sometimes referred to as "frequent fliers," hospitalists should take the extra time to investigate the reasons behind the failed hospital-to-home transitions. In this case clinicians should look for red flags that may suggest elder neglect, including the reasons behind frequent admissions for decompensated chronic disease and medication noncompliance (implied by rapid recovery due to medications provided in the hospital). Much may be gained from interviewing the patient separate from the caregiver.

PRACTICE POINT

Red flags that may suggest elder neglect include
- Multiple admissions for repeated falls, discontinuation of home care services, the inability to reach the primary caregiver
- Signs of poorly controlled chronic illness
- Medication issues: missed doses or noncompliance (subtherapeutic international normalized ratio [INR] in patients on warfarin, poorly controlled blood pressure, diabetes, heart failure easily managed in the hospital setting)
- Presence of malnutrition, dehydration, evidenced by low albumin and renal insufficiency

Any one of these "medical diagnoses" could be used to "medically justify" an acute care admission and further evaluation for neglect.

Consider an elderly man with a history of dementia and diabetes brought in by his daughter for a fall at home and worsening confusion. The patient has a mild forehead laceration and abrasions on his knees but a negative computed tomography scan of the brain. The emergency department staff describes him as "belligerent and agitated." He is given a benzodiazepine in the emergency department, he has a bladder catheter placed to obtain a urinalysis, and he is placed in wrist restraints. The daughter appears overwhelmed by his care and the emergency department feels he is "unsafe to return home."

Clinicians must consider neglect in the differential and be prepared to investigate whether the patient was inappropriately left alone for an extended period of time, whether there is evidence of uncontrolled chronic illness, malnourishment or dehydration, and whether the patient reports any abuse or neglect. However, the hospitalist may also recognize delirium and simultaneously explore etiologies and remove exacerbating factors such as the urinary catheter and restraints. Perhaps the patient has a urinary tract infection and dehydration with a sodium level of 148. Once the benzodiazepine wears off and with some intravenous free water, it is possible that his mental status will improve and he will be able to demonstrate an ability to eat and drink on his own. The hospitalist must confirm that the patient has appropriate access to food and medications, follow-up medical care, and supervision. He could qualify for short-term home health care with a visiting nurse and physical therapist plus a few hours of a home health aide. Depending on the amount of supervision needed and how involved his daughter and other caregivers are, he could be discharged home. A safe transition home will require interdisciplinary coordination with social work, the home health agency, and the patient's outpatient provider.

The hospitalist's role consists of evaluating the patient's understanding of his medical problems, explaining his current health status, and assessing his functional status.

- What is his current health status? Does he understand his medical problems?
- Does he have regular follow-up with an outpatient physician?
- Does he have sufficient medications at home and is he getting them every day as directed?
- Why is he falling? Does he need assistance with toileting and transfers? Who is present to help with these activities of daily living while his primary caregiver is at work?
- Does he have home services and if not, why not?

Similar questions could be directed toward his relatives. As caregiver neglect may be due to ignorance, inexperience or inability, perhaps the son or daughter does not understand the importance of adhering to a diabetic diet or is unaware of what foods this patient should or should not eat. Family members may not be comfortable administering insulin or believe that the patient does not require it every day. Family members may not understand the impact of his poorly controlled illnesses on her functional status.

DIFFERENTIAL DIAGNOSIS

■ DIFFERENTIATING SIGNS OF ABUSE AND NEGLECT FROM "NORMAL" AGING

Some signs of abuse and neglect can be indistinguishable from "normal" changes associated with aging. Other signs of mistreatment may mimic the symptoms or consequences of medical conditions common to the older adult population. For example, bruising or skin tears may be due to thinning skin or use of blood-thinning medications. Multiple fractures may be a consequence of falls, osteoporosis, or underlying malignancy. Pressure ulcers may occur in the absence of neglect in a patient with end-stage dementia, malnutrition, and immobility. Changes in mood and behavior can reflect depression or anxiety independent of elder mistreatment.

A 2005 study by Mosqueda, et al in the *Journal of the American Geriatrics Society* examined the life cycle of bruises in older adults and found that 90% of accidental bruises occurred on the extremities and no accidental bruises occurred on the neck, ears, genital area, or soles of the feet. Murphy et al. reviewed the physical findings associated with elder abuse, found that two-thirds of abuse injuries are located on the upper extremities and maxillofacial region. However, location of bruising and injuries alone are usually insufficient to prove that abuse has occurred. Unlike child abuse, there are no pathognomonic signs of elder mistreatment. Therefore, obtaining a comprehensive history from the older adult, involved caregivers, and other collateral sources remains paramount. When documenting signs of skin breakdown or injury on physical examination, it is critical to describe the location, color, shape, and size of what is visualized as opposed to an overall impression or judgment. For example, bruises can be marked on a standard body diagram with notations for the color, shape, and exact size instead of being interpreted and documented in the medical record as "old," "fading," or "resolving." Mosqueda's study looking at the life-cycle of bruises in the elderly found that the color of the bruise did not predict its age (ie, some bruises were predominantly yellow during the first 24 hours after onset).

TREATMENT AND INTERVENTION STRATEGIES

■ CLEAR DOCUMENTATION

When conducting an elder mistreatment assessment, the hospital-based provider should adopt a "forensic approach" to documentation. This entails being mindful of the potential legal implications of one's findings.

The following should be clearly detailed in the medical record:

- Names of individuals present during the interview and examination and relationship to the patient
- The patient's demeanor and any observed reactions to caregivers
- Verbatim descriptions of events from the patient and caregivers in quotes
- Timeline of events
- Functional status
- Hygiene and dress
- Physical examination
- Cognitive evaluation
- Referrals made (eg, social work, home care, adult protective services)

- Education provided to the patient and/or caregivers
- Safety plan discussed

PHOTOGRAPHS AND PHYSICAL EVIDENCE

If possible, use photographs (with victim's consent) or body diagrams to document injuries. Photographs should be taken before any medical treatment is given (without jeopardizing health of patient). Photographs should be labeled with the victim's name, the location of the injury, the date and time, and the name of the photographer. Take photographs from several angles and use a coin or ruler to provide a sense of scale. Preserve all physical evidence (eg, torn or stained clothing, broken eyeglasses, or damaged assistive devices) as this might be used in court.

ENLIST THE HELP OF AN INTERDISCIPLINARY TEAM

Cases of suspected elder mistreatment can be both complex and time-consuming. Hospitalists should involve their interdisciplinary colleagues as soon as possible to benefit from their expertise in safety planning and development of interventions and to share responsibility for various components of the assessment. Formal interprofessional groups called "Multidisciplinary Teams" or MDTs are increasingly emerging as a critical intervention strategy to address the complex and multidimensional needs of elder

mistreatment victims. Multidisciplinary teams bring together representatives from medicine (often a geriatrician, neuropsychologist and mental health providers), Adult Protective Services, law enforcement, the district attorney's office, and victim advocacy groups (see **Table 167-2**).

SOCIAL WORK

In the acute care setting, hospitalists will most often collaborate with social workers to assess and treat victims of abuse and neglect. Inpatient social workers can be instrumental by obtaining collateral information from the patient's caregivers and/or family members, clarifying the patient's current level of social support, and investigating financial resources. Without sound knowledge of the patient's insurance coverage and potential entitlements, a safe discharge plan cannot be developed. For example, the hospitalist may want to discharge a patient with 24-hour supervision at home to ensure his safety but most insurances, including Medicare and state Medicaid plans, will not cover this level of personal care and the patient may not have the financial resources to pay out-of-pocket for a caregiver. Hospitalists should also be aware the home health care agencies often employ social workers who can relay critical information about the suspected victim's psychosocial functioning, resources, and entitlements prior to hospitalization.

TABLE 167-2 Groups Involved in Interprofessional Assessment and Intervention in Cases of Suspected Elder Abuse

Group	Role	Comments
Adult protective services	Receives mandatory reports of suspected abuse in most states	May serve as guardians in some states
Home health care agencies and personnel	Important in both detection and mitigation of abuse	Staff members may be abusers in some situations
Community nongovernmental or nonprofit services and programs for older adults	Provide a variety of programs and services that can mitigate all forms of abuse, including senior centers and home visitation to promote social integration	Some community-service agencies have programs exclusively devoted to preventing elder abuse or dealing with its manifestations (eg, daily money management and caregiver support)
Police	Often the first responders in cases of elder abuse	Awareness of the importance of training law-enforcement personnel to be sensitive to the needs of older persons is increasing
District attorney's office	Prosecutes cases of elder abuse	Some offices have dedicated units that focus on elder abuse and are separate from domestic-violence units
Housing authority	Handles issues involving eviction, squatting, or misuse of housing for older persons, which are common in cases of elder abuse	Eviction and homelessness can be manifestations of financial exploitation
Legal services agencies	Handle the myriad legal issues that are raised in cases of elder abuse, including decision-making capacity, living wills, and guardianship	Guardians may be financial abusers
Physicians	Play a critical role in identifying mistreatment and making appropriate referrals	Physicians are mandatory reporters of elder abuse in all states that have mandatory-reporting laws
Hospital personnel	Need to be prepared to identify cases of elder abuse	Medical personnel often fail to identify elder abuse, because of clinical and time pressures. The Joint Commission on Accreditation of Healthcare Organizations has guidelines with respect to elder abuse; accreditation may be jeopardized if protocols are absent or inadequate
Nursing homes	Can use excess capacity to house victims safely and provide services, as part of the growing movement in the United States to provide shelter to abused older persons	Elder abuse can occur in long-term care facilities; resident-to-resident abuse is increasingly recognized as the most common form of abuse in such settings
Banks and financial services industry	Critical to the detection of financial exploitation	Institutions in some communities train tellers and other employees to detect exploitation of older persons' finances

From Lachs MS, Pillemer KA. Elder abuse. *N Engl J Med*. 2015;373(20):1947-1956.

PHYSICAL AND OCCUPATIONAL THERAPY

Physical and occupational therapists can assist the hospitalist in assessing the suspected victim's functional and cognitive status. Knowing the patient's current level of function and the extent of decline is essential for setting goals for medical therapy and determining the appropriate discharge destination. It can also be helpful when trying to substantiate history provided by a caregiver or the patient. For example, if the caregiver reports the patient sustained a head laceration and periorbital bruising by falling out of bed, the physical therapist's assessment of the patient's ability to transfer in and out of bed and to ambulate will be critical. Similarly, if a patient is admitted with profound dehydration and reports she is able to perform her own shopping and feed herself, the occupational therapist's evaluation of the patient's ability to perform activities of daily living will become significant. Some occupational therapists can assess cognition using the Montreal Cognitive Assessment or MOCA.

CONSULT EXPERTS

The hospitalist who suspects elder mistreatment may also benefit from specialty consultations from geriatrics, psychiatry, geriatric psychiatry if available, and ethics. While a geriatrician may have experience in performing a complete assessment for elder abuse and/or neglect, the hospitalist should be prepared with a specific question or questions when calling the consultant. Geriatricians can assess functional status and assist with clarifying goals of care. Psychiatrists and geriatric psychiatrists can be especially particularly helpful in assessing a patient's decision-making capacity or determining whether cognitive impairment or a mood disorder is impacting the patient's care. Elder mistreatment cases often involve ethical dilemmas, so if the hospital utilizes an ethicist or ethics committee, a formal consultation can prove invaluable. For example, when treating the self-neglecting patient who puts himself at risk by refusing home services or not using assistive devices, the hospitalist must weigh the patient's autonomy against the duty to avoid harm (nonmaleficence). In extreme cases of self-neglect that are associated with hoarding, patients may put other roommates, neighbors, or even pets at risk as well. In these situations, physicians must also consider the impact of the patient's choices and behaviors on the safety of the surrounding community.

INVOLVE RISK MANAGEMENT AND LEGAL DEPARTMENTS

Risk management and the hospital's legal department can also be especially helpful to the hospitalist. The primary role of risk management is to minimize potential liability through continuous monitoring and evaluation of the processes and outcomes of patient care. Risk management teams are often composed of a combination of clinicians (nurses, physicians) and quality management experts. Elder mistreatment cases may reveal gaps in quality of care and/or inefficient processes. The hospitalist should involve risk management in cases in which the discharge plan may be disputed by the patient or caregivers, when the discharge plan is complicated by a patient who lacks decision-making capacity and no surrogate or proxy exists, and when the hospitalist suspects an ongoing or imminent threat to patient safety. Risk management will often guide the hospitalist as to whether the legal department's assistance is required. The legal department is frequently consulted in cases in which the patient lacks decision-making capacity due to cognitive impairment or psychiatric illness and a court-appointed guardian is needed to establish a safe discharge plan.

As with all members of the interdisciplinary team, hospitalists should contact risk management and legal as early as possible.

ACCESS COMMUNITY RESOURCES

In addition to the interdisciplinary and expert services available to the hospitalist in the acute care setting, extensive community resources should be utilized to create safe discharge plans for elder mistreatment victims. These organizations can also be valuable sources of collateral information if already involved with the victim prior to hospitalization.

HOME HEALTH CARE

The term home health care may refer to an extensive range of services provided in patients' homes from certified home health agencies providing short-term skilled care from nurses and physical therapists to privately hired personal care workers providing assistance with activities of daily living. Multiple types of home care services are often utilized as a critical intervention in elder mistreatment situations because it increases the number of "eyes and ears" on the patient and his/her caregivers. Especially in cases in which mistreatment is suspected but not confirmed, added supervision and monitoring can help clarify what is actually occurring in the patient's home. Here we will focus primarily on Medicare-certified home health care programs. Following a hospitalization for acute illness, elder mistreatment victims often meet the criteria for skilled services, that is, they need a visiting nurse or physical therapist. The hospitalist must also certify that the patient is homebound (ie, leaving home requires a considerable and taxing effort), requires short-term intermittent care, and has an outpatient physician to supervise home care services in order for the patient to quality for home health care postdischarge.

While the home health nurse's primary role may be to monitor a wound and instruct a caregiver to perform dressing changes, he or she can also report back to the outpatient physician on the caregiver's ability and willingness to provide appropriate care, the sanitary conditions in the home, and the patient's overall medical status. The physical therapist's orders may be to perform gait training and muscle strengthening exercises, but he or she can also alert the outpatient physician to red flags for mistreatment such as the patient/caregiver refusing visits, the patient's prescriptions going unfilled, and signs of uncontrolled medical illness.

While home health agencies can and do play a vital role in increasing the short-term supervision and monitoring of elder mistreatment victims, the hospitalist should know that agencies must also maintain the safety of their employees and will not accept patients whose home environments are compromised by extreme disrepair, bug or vermin infestation, or the presence of occupants who are suspected of engaging in criminal activity.

ADULT PROTECTIVE SERVICES

In most states, Adult Protective Services represents the first responders to reports of abuse, neglect, and exploitation of vulnerable adults. Established in 1975 under Title XX of the Social Security Act, APS exists in all 50 states. Because little or no federal funding was allotted, each state has developed its own program based on the state's individual laws and regulations. States may differ in their definitions of mistreatment, types of abuse and neglect addressed by state law, eligibility criteria, and settings covered. For example, California APS agencies investigate reports of abuse in private homes as well as in hospitals, whereas in New York, APS cannot evaluate clients in an acute care setting.

Similarities exist across state APS agencies in terms of the services provided, for example, receipt and investigation into reports of mistreatment, evaluation of client risk and capacity to consent to services, development and implementation of a case plan, client counseling, assistance with services and benefits, and monitoring of ongoing service delivery. Despite state differences, certain basic principles shape APS practice. These include the client's right to self-determination, the use of the least restrictive alternative, the maintenance of the family unit when possible, and the use of community-based services instead of institutions. A referral to APS can be a key component of ensuring a safe discharge plan but if the patient has decision-making capacity and refuses to allow APS representatives to perform an evaluation of the home or investigate potential entitlements, they cannot force the client to accept their services.

■ LAW ENFORCEMENT/DISTRICT ATTORNEY'S OFFICE

In cases of elder mistreatment in which the hospitalist suspects a crime has been committed and the victim wishes to press charges against the responsible party (eg, physical, financial, and/or sexual abuse), the hospitalist should file a report with law enforcement by contacting 911. The hospital's risk management and legal teams should also be immediately consulted. In accordance with the hospital's policies, they will provide further direction about involving law enforcement and involving the appropriate district attorney's office. In situations in which the hospitalist is unsure whether a crime has been committed, it can be helpful to contact the district attorney's office directly. Each office may have an attorney specifically assigned to an elder mistreatment unit and/or a community liaison who can offer guidance to the hospitalist. For example, the elderly gentleman who discloses to the nursing staff that he cannot afford his medications because he loaned his much younger girlfriend $25,000 for her dress business and she has failed to pay him back may be ambivalent about whether to press charges so the hospitalist can contact the district attorney's office to obtain advice for the patient should he decide he wants legal assistance.

■ MANDATORY REPORTING GUIDELINES

At the time of this writing, New York is the only state without a mandated reporting law. Social service employees such as Adult Protective Services workers are mandated reporters even in states like New York where physicians are not. "Good faith reporting" provisions typically protect physicians from liability for having informed Adult Protective Services or other investigative agencies of their suspicions even if the reports are not substantiated. Even in the absence of legal mandates, health and mental health professionals have an ethical and moral obligation to report elder mistreatment. Hospitalists need only have a reasonable suspicion of mistreatment to report. In cases in which abuse or neglect occurs in the community, APS is typically the agency tasked with investigation. For patients who reside in a nursing home or long-term care setting, the hospitalist and/or social worker may be required to alert the state Department of Health, APS, and/or the ombudsman.

■ TESTIFYING IN COURT

Concerns about being called to testify in court can pose a barrier to screening and assessment for elder mistreatment. In many cases, thorough documentation in the medical record can avert the need for in-court testimony by the physician. In other cases, the hospitalist's testimony may be required either as an expert witness or as a layperson to present general observations of behavior or statements made. When called as an expert witness, the physician may be asked to render opinions about the signs of neglect, the patient's decision-making capacity, and whether an explanation given is consistent with the victim's injuries.

The American Medical Association advises physicians providing testimony to

- Meet with the attorney presenting you as a witness before the trial to practice
- Suggest questions for the attorney to ask you if acting as an expert witness

- Propose questions for the opposing expert if acting as an expert witness
- Make sure you understand both the legal and factual issues and how they relate to your testimony
- Determine what evidence (ie, photographs) should be part of your testimony
- Answer only the questions asked; do not volunteer additional information
- Ask for questions to be repeated if necessary
- Explain when a one-word answer is insufficient
- Calmly correct an attorney who incorrectly reports prior testimony

PREVENTION

Just as an acute care stay may provide hospitalists with the chance to stop the cycle of abuse and neglect, hospitalization may also represent a critical window to intervene on an at-risk patient and prevent mistreatment from occurring in the first place. Prevention begins with knowing the risk factors for abuse and neglect so that hospitalists can identify the most vulnerable patients and gather an interdisciplinary team to devise a safety plan. Remember that the "vulnerable" patient is not always the one who is admitted with bruising or trauma but also the patients who are admitted monthly for uncontrolled chronic illness and have been nonadherent with their medications, the patients who come with worsening wounds or signs of poor nutrition, and the patients whose caregivers appear overwhelmed by their responsibilities. The same interventions for active abuse and neglect cases detailed above (eg, the early and intense involvement of an interdisciplinary team during the hospitalization and establishment of links to postdischarge community resources) may prevent situations from escalating into mistreatment.

SYSTEMS ISSUES

The hospitalist model has been associated with reduced length of stay, lower inpatient costs, and improved patient care in multiple complex conditions. However, the use of hospitalists also complicates the care coordination process by increasing the number of hand offs amongst providers and muddying lines of accountability to ensure safe transitions. Elderly patients at risk for abuse and neglect or victims of frank mistreatment represent a highly complex group of patients, and hospitalists may truly dread the potential for these patients to increase their workload and their average length of stay. We argue, however, that medical, financial, and ethical incentives exist for providing extra attention to the care transitions of suspected or confirmed elder mistreatment victims. All physicians have an ethical obligation to protect victims of elder abuse and neglect. Ethical dilemmas that arise when attempting to establish a safety plan for elder mistreatment victims typically involve weighing the need to protect patient autonomy against the physician's duty to promote beneficence and nonmaleficence.

Medically, the hospitalist who recognizes that ongoing abuse or neglect underlies the uncontrolled diabetes, congestive heart failure, or major depression will not only treat the victim's acute exacerbations but will introduce the supports and supervision necessary to give the patient an improved chance of success in controlling his or her illness. This strategy of addressing both the acute medical issue and the psychosocial factors contributing to it also makes financial sense if the inpatient team's interventions prevent unnecessary health care utilization, especially hospital readmissions. Elder mistreatment, especially psychological abuse, financial exploitation and caregiver neglect are associated with a twofold increase in emergency department use and increased rated of hospitalization. As Medicare begins to limit reimbursements to hospitals for readmissions for the same diagnosis, hospitals will also have an incentive to end the revolving door phenomenon. Contrary to the belief that bringing elder mistreatment victims into the medical system will result in a dramatic, downstream increase in health care utilization, in their 2008 study in the *Journal of the American Geriatrics Society*, Franzini and Dyer found that self-neglectors were no more expensive to the system than matched controls. Self-neglectors by definition are nonadherent to medical interventions and typically refuse services they are entitled to, putting themselves at risk for serious mental and physical decline. Yet after undergoing a comprehensive geriatric assessment and when given access to longitudinal primary care, these patients were not hospitalized more or for a significantly greater length of stay.

The essential components of transitional care for all hospitalized patients include physician-to-physician communication across care sites, medication reconciliation, patient education to encourage self-efficacy, and assurance of appropriate social supports. Ensuring a safe transition for hospitalized elder mistreatment victims starts with an accurate assessment of baseline and current functional status to determine the appropriate discharge destination and requires communication between the sending (hospitalist and inpatient team) and receiving providers (primary care physician, home health agency, APS). The transfer of information between the inpatient and outpatient providers is especially imperative in elder mistreatment cases because often there is a suspicion of abuse or neglect but no confirmation. In these situations, patients will often be discharged to short-term rehabilitation facilities or to their homes with referrals for home health care and an APS referral. Hospitalists should communicate directly with the patient's primary care provider or the nursing home to alert the receiving physician about abuse and/or neglect concerns. When home health care is part of the intervention for a victim, the agency should be made aware of the concerns about mistreatment and should know how to contact the outpatient physician if one of its employees witnesses abuse and/or neglect.

CONCLUSION

Identifying and treating victims of elder abuse and neglect can be a daunting challenge but each inpatient admission should be viewed by the hospitalist as an opportunity to have a potentially life-saving impact of the life of the elder mistreatment victim. The hospitalist may be the first individual to notice the medical consequences of abuse or neglect or may be viewed as a trusted individual in whom the patient confides. In either case, the hospitalist possesses the capacity to guide the inpatient workup and management, document his or her assessment, and enlist the help of an interdisciplinary team to devise a safety plan.

SUGGESTED READINGS

Acierno R, Hernandez MS, Amstadter AB, et al. Prevalence and correlates of emotional, physical, sexual, and financial abuse and potential neglect in the United States: The National Elder Mistreatment Study. *Am J Public Health*. 2010;100:292-297.

Ahmad M, Lachs MS. Elder abuse and neglect: what physicians can and should do. *Cleve Clin J Med*. 2002;69:801-808.

American Medical Association Diagnostic and Treatment Guidelines on Elder Abuse and Neglect. Chicago, IL: American Medical Association; 1992.

Franzini L and Dyer CB. Healthcare costs and utilization of vulnerable elderly people reported to adult protective services for self-neglect. *J Am Geriatr Soc*. 2008;(56):667-676.

Lachs MS, Pillemer KA. Elder abuse. *N Engl J Med*. 2015;373:1947-1956.

Lachs Ms, Williams CS, O'Brien S, et al. ED use by older victims of family violence. *Ann Emerg Med*. 1997;30:448-454.

Lachs MS, Williams CS, O'Brien S et al. The mortality of elder mistreatment. *JAMA*. 1998;280:428-432.

Mosqueda L, Burnight K, Liao S. The life cycle of bruises in older adults. *J Am Geriatr Soc*. 2005;53:1339-1343.

Murphy K, Waa S, Jaffer H, et al. A literature review of findings in physical elder abuse. *Can Assoc Radiol J*. 2013;64:10-14.

National Research Council. *Elder Mistreatment: Abuse, Neglect, and Exploitation in an Aging America*. Washington, DC; National Academy Press: 2003.

Navarro AE, Wysong J, DeLiema M, et al. Inside the black box: the case review process of an elder abuse forensic center. *Gerontologist*. 2015;60:1-11.

Peterson JC, Burnes DP, Caccamise PL, et al. Financial exploitation of older adults: a population-based prevalence study. *J Gen Intern Med*. 2014;29:1615-1623.

Pillemer K, Chen EK, Van Haitsma KS, et al. Resident-to-resident aggression in nursing homes: results from a qualitative event reconstruction study. *Gerontologist*. 2012;52:24-33.

ONLINE RESOURCES

Liao S, Smith S. Reporting elder mistreatment. ACP Pier. October 30, 2006. [Online] http://pier.acponline.orgphysicians/ethical_legal/el056.html. Accessed September 29, 2008.

MetLife Mature Market Institute. The MetLife Study of elder financial abuse: crimes of occasion, desperation, and predation against America's elders. New York, NY: The Institute; 2011. [Online] https://www.metlife.com/assets/cao/mmi/publications/studies/2011/mmi-elder-financial-abuse.pdf. Accessed December 3, 2015.

National Centre on Elder Abuse (NCEA). National Elder Abuse Incidence Study: Final Report 1998. Administration on Aging and American Public Human Services Association [on-line]. http://aoa.gov/AoA_Programs/Elder_Rights/Elder_Abuse/docs/ABuseReport_Full.pdf. Accessed December 3, 2015.

National Centre on Elder Abuse (NCEA). National Elder Abuse Incidence Study: Final Report 1998. Administration on Aging and American Public Human Services Association [on-line]. http://aoa.gov/AoA_Programs/Elder_Rights/Elder_Abuse/docs/ABuseReport_Full.pdf. Accessed December 3, 2015.

Otto, JM. National Adult Protective Services Association. History of NAPSA: The role of Adult Protective Services in Addressing Abuse. [Online] http://www.apsnetwork.org/About/history.htm. Accessed March 20, 2010.

The American Bar Association Commission on Law and Aging. Laws Related to Elder Abuse. [Online] http://new.abanet.org/aging/Pages/elderabuse.aspx. Accessed February 9, 2010.

The National Center on Elder Abuse. The 2004 Survey of State Adult Protective Services: Abuse of Vulnerable Adults 18 Years of Age and Older [Online]; http://www.ncea.aoa.gov/Resources/Publication/docs/APS_2004NCEASurvey.pdf Accessed on December 3, 2015.

Under the Radar: New York State Elder Abuse Prevalence Study. Lifespan of Greater Rochester, Weill Cornell Medical Center of Cornell University, New York City Department for the Aging [online]. http://nyceac.com/wp-content/uploads/2011/05/UndertheRadar051211.pdf. Accessed December 3, 2015.

CHAPTER 168

Malnutrition and Weight Loss in Hospitalized Older Adults

Grace Farris, MD
Melissa Mattison, MD

Key Clinical Questions

❶ What interventions can be employed to improve nutrition in older adults?

❷ What are the recommendations for nutrition supplementation in patients with advanced dementia?

DEFINITIONS

Weight loss can be classified as acute, subacute or indolent, and long-term. Weight loss is defined as a 2% loss from baseline body weight over 1 month, or a 5% loss over 3 months, or 10% loss over 6 months. In patients who reside in long-term care, weight loss is defined as 5% loss from baseline body weight over 30 days. Weight loss is associated with increased mortality as well as discharge to a skilled nursing facility (SNF).

Malnutrition has long eluded a strict and unifying definition, but the most common and generally agreed upon definition is one authored by the American Society for Parenteral and Enteral Nutrition (ASPEN) (**Table 168-1**). The ASPEN definition of malnutrition requires two of the following six attributes: "Insufficient energy intake, weight loss, loss of muscle mass, loss of subcutaneous fat, localized or generalized fluid accumulation, diminished functional status (measured by handgrip strength)."

The term 'failure to thrive' is a vivid catch-all that has been used historically to describe a patient with malnutrition, weight loss and diminished functional status. In the geriatric population, failure to thrive likely evokes frailty and diminished functioning, but presentations can vary. The Institute of Medicine describes failure to thrive in older adults as "a syndrome of weight loss, decreased appetite and poor nutrition, and inactivity, often accompanied by dehydration, depressive symptoms, impaired immune function, and low cholesterol." However, some have argued that the term 'failure to thrive' is too vague and nonspecific, and should be abandoned in favor of investigating the four syndromes usually associated with failure to thrive that are known to contribute individually to adverse outcomes in the older adult: functional decline, malnutrition, depression and cognitive impairment. This chapter will focus on malnutrition.

EPIDEMIOLOGY

In hospitalized adults over the age of 65, 40% are estimated to be malnourished, although various studies have found the range to be 20% to 50% depending on the nutrition assessment tool used, whether billing information (ICD-9 coding) was assessed, and hospital demographics. Studies based on ICD-9 codes likely underestimate the true burden of malnutrition in the elderly, since ICD-9 malnutrition codes have notoriously been divorced from etiologies of malnutrition and largely register the degree of malnutrition based on serum albumin level, which is no longer thought to be a reliable indicator of the severity or duration of malnutrition. Increasingly, physicians have used the ICD-9 code 263.9 Protein-Calorie Malnutrition, NOS (not otherwise specified) in order to skirt the issue of serum albumin. However, studies performed in Western Europe, South America, and Australia have found similar prevalence rates for malnutrition in the acutely hospitalized elderly.

In US emergency departments, at least 15% to 20% of elderly patients will present with malnutrition, while almost 60% will be malnourished or at risk for malnutrition. Multiple studies performed in various countries have found malnutrition in the hospitalized elderly to be an independent risk factor for increased length of stay (3-6 days), increased polypharmacy, and increased morbidity and mortality. Malnutrition also likely increases the odds of discharge to a skilled nursing facility, is associated with an increased risk of infections, impaired wound healing, and increased risk of developing pressure ulcers. There is also ample evidence that malnutrition in

TABLE 168-1 ASPEN Malnutrition Definition (2 out of 6 Signs)

Insufficient energy intake	Localized or generalized fluid accumulation
Weight loss	Diminished functional status (measured by handgrip strength)
Loss of muscle mass	Loss of subcutaneous fat

the elderly is under-evaluated and under-documented, with some studies finding rates of malnutrition to be 40%, but only 10% with documentation of malnutrition in the medical chart.

RISK STRATIFICATION

Inadequate dietary intake may be due to the following:

- Anorexia: age related physiologic changes of decreased taste and smell, delayed gastric emptying
- Social factors: isolation, poverty, lack of transportation or access to food, lack of community supports
- Psychological factors: alcohol and substance abuse, depression, dementia, delirium
- Sarcopenia: loss of muscle mass and functional ability
- Medications: antidepressants and anticholinergics (affect salivation, taste, appetite, swallowing dysfunction, sedation); alendronate and nonsteroidal anti-inflammatory agents (esophagitis)
- Mechanical factors: edentulous, dysphagia, paralysis, hand tremor, severe arthritis
- Medical and surgical illnesses, including hyperthyroidism, malignancy, end-stage disease, chronic infection, intestinal obstruction
- Cachexia: inflammatory disease states

Studies estimate that almost half of patients older than 65 are edentulous, which complicates mastication of some foods. Older adults produce less saliva and have a reduced sense of taste and smell, which makes certain foods unpalatable. There is evidence that older adults have increased secretion of enteric peptides Cholecystokinin and Pancreatic Polypeptide that result in longer periods of satiety and slower gastric emptying. Finally, underlying medical disorders may contribute to weight loss and malnutrition by causing mechanical obstructions, anorexia, increased metabolic activity (cachexia) and cognitive impairments that reduce an older person's ability to eat or tolerate feeding. Often these various mechanisms of weight loss with resultant malnutrition may overlap, such that a multidisciplinary approach is best to evaluate and manage the patient with malnutrition (**Figure 168-1**).

A number of screening tools are available to determine an older patient's likelihood of developing significant weight loss or malnutrition. The two screening tests with the highest sensitivity and specificity are the Malnutrition Screening Tool and the Mini Nutritional Assessment (MNA). The Malnutrition Screening Tool has been validated in acutely ill hospitalized older adults, and uses two questions: "Have you been eating poorly because of a decreased appetite?" and "Have you lost weight recently without trying?" Sensitivity for this tool is 74% to 100% in hospitalized adults. The Mini Nutritional Assessment is a questionnaire that takes 10 minutes and has been validated in the hospital setting as well. The MNA scale has been found to be predictive of mortality and hospital cost and can be used to identify patients at risk for malnutrition who might benefit from nutritional intervention.

EVALUATION

If a patient meets a definition of weight loss or malnutrition, the timeline should be established. The hospitalist should clarify if the weight loss was intentional, if there were any changes in activity level or medication changes that might have contributed, and if there is underlying substance abuse or depression (**Table 168-2**).

Once it has been established that an older adult suffers from malnutrition (based on ASPEN criteria), the evaluation of the cause of the malnutrition should include a comprehensive history and physical examination. The inpatient evaluation of malnutrition includes a full review of the patient's home medications. Older adults frequently suffer from "polypharmacy" in which the proliferation of home medications may produce side effects and medication interactions that cause anorexia, reduced sense of taste, or sedation, resulting in worsening oral intake. A patient's diet should also be reviewed to clarify whether a patient has been following a restricted diet (ie, a diabetic diet, heart healthy diet or renal diet) that has inadvertently resulted in a reduced intake of calories and protein. Discussion of alcohol use should be broached, as elderly patients with substance abuse frequently have underlying malnutrition.

The hospitalist should pay particular attention to the following signs on physical examination:

- Hair, skin, and nail changes that may reveal a micronutrient or vitamin deficiency (**Table 168-3**)
- Inability to chew, poor dental hygiene, need for dentures
- Evidence of heart failure and chronic respiratory disease that are known to be associated with cachexia
- Sigmata of liver disease
- Edema that may reflect low protein levels and/or fluid overload

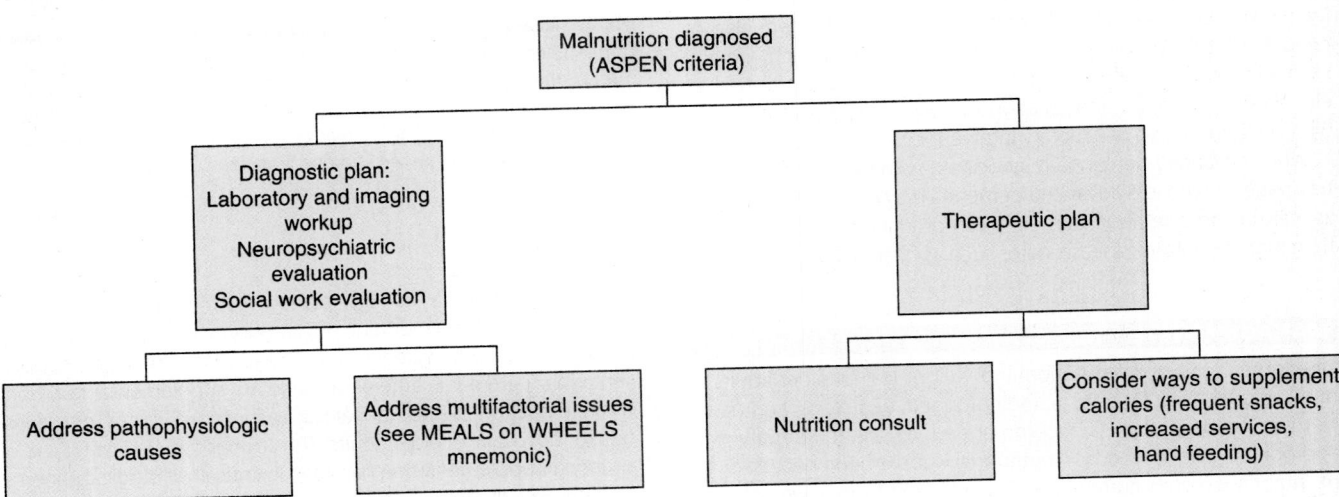

Figure 168-1 *Approach to the patient with malnutrition.*

TABLE 168-2 Causes of Weight Loss in the Elderly

M: medications (digoxin, theophylline, fluoxetine)

E: emotional (depression) A: alcohol, or elder abuse

L: late life paranoia, late life mania

S: swallowing problems (dysphagia, candidiasis, webs, tardive dyskinesia)

O: oral or dental problems (xerostomia, edentulousness)

N: nosocomial infections (TB, *C. difficile*, *Helicobacter pylori*) or no money (poverty)

W: wandering, dementia problems

H: hyperthyroidism, hypercalcemia, hypoadrenalism

E: enteric problems (gluten entropathy, pancreatic insufficiency)

E: eating problems (institutional food, loss of taste, monotony, tremor)

L: low salt, low fat diets (diabetic, renal and other therapeutic diets)

S: shopping and food preparation problems

Adapted from Morley JE. Anorexia of aging: physiologic and pathologic. *Am J Clin Nutr.* 1997;66(4):760-773. The 'Meals on Wheels' mnemonic for treatable causes of weight loss (table was developed by JEM with copyright held by US Government).

In addition to routine blood work as part of the hospital admission (ie, complete blood count, metabolic profile, liver biochemical and functional tests), thyroid function and vitamin levels (B12, iron, thiamine) should be measured. There is evidence that if folate deficiency is suspected, it is more cost-effective to replete the patient's folate and forgo serum folate level testing. Additional imaging depends upon the reason for admission, prior testing, and prognosis (see Chapter 105 [Using Prognosis to Guide Treatment]).

If a patient may have developed malnutrition due to financial or social obstacles, a social work consultation may be helpful to clarify any barriers to obtaining food and whether a patient requires additional community resources (such as Meals on Wheels or outpatient social work and case management) to improve access to food. If a patient resides in an institutional setting the approach to feeding may need to be altered (such as hand feeding or altering the consistency of food).

Nursing staff may be able to confirm that the patient has evidence of dysphagia on exam that may contribute to difficulty with oral intake. If dysphagia is noted, further investigations into the etiology of the dysphagia should be undertaken to clarify whether it is related to dental issues, upper airway or esophageal dysmotility, stroke, pseudobulbar problems, dementia, or the sequelae of radiochemotherapy to throat structures. Bedside speech therapy evaluation and videofluoroscopy evaluation can be performed to elucidate the severity and location of dysphagia, which can help with the formulation of a dietary intervention.

While advanced dementia is associated with swallowing difficulties, patients with less advanced dementia may develop weight loss as well. In some settings, dementia can produce more weight loss than highly catabolic disease states such as heart failure and cancer.

MANAGEMENT

Often, the cause of malnutrition and weight loss in older adults is multifactorial, and requires a multipronged treatment approach. Nutrition consultation is recommended to try to identify the appropriate caloric need or nutritional supplement necessary to maintain a patient's current weight and avoid further weight loss. The possible social and nonmedical barriers to weight gain should

TABLE 168-3 Clinical Signs and Nutritional Deficiencies

System	Sign or Symptom	Nutrient Deficiency
Skin	Dry scaly skin	Zinc/essential fatty acids
	Follicular hyperkeratosis	Vitamin A, C
	Petechiae	Vitamin C, K
	Photosensitive dermatitis	Niacin
	Poor wound healing	Zinc, vitamin C
	Scrotal dermatitis	Riboflavin
Hair	Thin/depigmented	Protein
	Easy pluckability	Protein, zinc
Nail	Transverse depigmentation	Albumin
	Spooned	Iron
Eyes	Night blindness	Vitamin A, zinc
	Conjunctival inflammation	Riboflavin
	Keratomalacia	Vitamin A
Mouth	Bleeding gums	Vitamin C, riboflavin
	Glositis	Niacin, piridoxin, riboflavin
	Atrophic papillae	Iron
	Hypogeusia	Zinc, vitamin A
Neck	Thyroid enlargement	Iodine
	Parotid enlargement	Protein
Abdomen	Diarrhea	Niacin, folate, vitamin B12
	Hepatomegaly	Protein
Extremities	Bone tenderness	Vitamin D
	Joint pain	Vitamin C
	Muscle tenderness	Thiamine
	Muscle wasting	Protein, selenium vitamin D
	Edema	Protein
Neurological	Ataxia	Vitamin B12
	Tetany	Calcium, magnesium
	Parasthesia	Thiamine, vitamin B12
	Ataxia	Vitamin B12
	Dementia	Vitamin B12, niacin
	Hyporeflexia	Thiamine

From Ahmed T, Haboubi N. Assessment and management of nutrition in older people and its importance to health. *Clin Interv Aging.* 2010;5:207-216. © 2010 Ahmed and Haboubi, publisher and licensee. Dove Medical Press Ltd. This is an open access article that permits unrestricted noncommercial use, provided the original work is properly cited.

be investigated, and a multidisciplinary treatment plan may include social work, case management, nursing home staff and family.

There is minimal evidence that any form of nutritional supplementation (parenteral, enteral or voluntary supplemental nutrition) has an impact on the nutritional status, functional status, or survival rates for hospitalized older adults. The strongest evidence for use of nutritional supplementation has been in critically-ill surgical patients, but true benefits from nutritional supplements (shakes, puddings, tube feedings) have not been proven in elderly adults hospitalized for medical reasons. This may be due to a number of mechanisms: it is well-documented that supplements are often not consumed, the supplements may not contain the correct micronutrients to provide medical benefit, or the risks of nutritional supplementation may offset their benefit. For an elderly patient hospitalized with a medical condition who is found to be malnourished, a less costly approach to optimizing nutrition and weight gain may be encouraging small frequent meals and snacking, providing foods that the patient enjoys, and confirming that the patient is able to consume the foods provided by ensuring that dentures are at the bedside, the food is the right consistency, and that staff is able to help with feeding.

It is unclear whether appetite stimulants, such as megestrol acetate, dronabinol and mirtazapine, are effective in older hospitalized adults. Megestrol acetate can exacerbate edema and congestive heart failure, and should be avoided in patients with these conditions. The few studies of dronabinol and mirtazapine have failed to demonstrate benefits in the older adult population.

Management of malnutrition in patients with dysphagia

Eating problems and dysphagia are widespread in older adults. Dietary modifications including alterations in food consistency, providing many snacks, changing inpatient diet to an unrestricted diet may mitigate weight loss and malnutrition due to swallowing difficulties. However, there is scant evidence for oral supplements as they do not seem to improve survival or quality of life, but may result in slight weight gain and minimal improvement in length of stay. Order a swallowing study only if it would change management.

If a patient is unable to tolerate oral nutrition due to recent stroke or esophageal obstruction, enteral nutrition is recommended. A trial of nasogastric tube feeding may be considered if deemed mechanistically safe and a patient is expected to improve within a month. Alternatively a percutaneous gastrostomy tube ("PEG" tube) may be placed if it is anticipated that the patient will require more than 30 days of supplemental enteral nutrition (see Chapter 58 [Nutrition and Metabolic Support] and Chapter 119 [Feeding Tube Placement]).

In patients with dementia, eating problems and dysphagia are common as the disease worsens in severity and the patients approach the end of life. In these patients, tube feeding via nasogastric tube or PEG has not been found to reduce infections or aspiration events, reduce the incidence of pressure ulcers, improve wound healing, functional status, patient comfort, or survival. For this reason, the American Geriatrics Society does not recommend initiation of tube feeding for patients with advanced dementia, and instead encourages hand-feeding patients with dementia, and offering frequent small meals and snacks. Unfortunately, patients with dementia often reside in institutional settings, where reimbursement rates are higher if a patient has a PEG tube placed. Caretakers and family members may feel pressure to allow for the placement of feeding tubes in order to facilitate administration of medications that patients are no longer able to take orally. In this setting, a hospitalist can provide essential education about the patient's prognosis, the options for nutrition and can help a patient's family explore goals of care.

Failure to thrive

The inpatient management of failure to thrive is complex, due to the intricate interplay of social, medical and cognitive components that are all difficult to "fix." The evaluation of the older adult with failure to thrive should begin with a review of all medications, a discussion with caregivers, an assessment of social support, review of prior testing, and basic metabolic laboratory testing. A physical therapist should assess physical functioning. Patients with failure to thrive may be slow to improve, and require intense attention in the postacute care setting to reverse the decline. See Part III (Rehabilitation

and Skilled Nursing Care) and Chapter 165 (Principles of Geriatric Care).

Postacute care

In the postacute care setting, a multidisciplinary approach should be arranged to manage malnutrition, weight loss and failure to thrive. If a patient is discharged home, home services include a visiting nurse and social worker to evaluate home safety, continued weight loss, and social barriers that may contribute to malnutrition, as well as physical therapy visits, which can help mitigate the functional decline implicit in "failure to thrive."

If a patient is discharged to a postacute care setting such as a skilled nursing facility or long-term acute care, the discharge plan should include instructions for hand feeding (if deemed appropriate), frequent monitoring of weight, and neuropsychiatric evaluation (if not obtained during the hospitalization). (See Section III [Rehabilitation and Skilled Nursing Care].)

> **PRACTICE POINT**
>
> - The ASPEN definition of malnutrition requires two of the following six attributes: "Insufficient energy intake, weight loss, loss of muscle mass, loss of subcutaneous fat, localized or generalized fluid accumulation, diminished functional status (measured by handgrip strength)."
>
> - Malnutrition is frequently under documented.
>
> - Serum albumin is not a reliable indicator of the severity or duration of malnutrition.
>
> - Cognitive impairments can frequently be associated with malnutrition, weight loss and failure to thrive.

Discharge Checklist for Malnutrition, Weight Loss, and Failure to Thrive Discharge summary checklist: key components relating to weight loss and malnutrition:

- Instructions on how to increase patient's oral intake (feeding techniques, supplements, home services)?
- A plan formulated by social work that will address issues with cost, access to food and transportation?
- Pending test results?
- Medication reconciliation: possible contributing unnecessary medications (either reduced or eliminated) with plan for further modification?
- Pending issues that the primary care physician will need to address such as reduction of polypharmacy, referral to other specialists, ongoing nutrition counselling?
- Goals of care discussions with family, and whether ongoing discussions are required, if advanced dementia has resulted in weight loss?
- Instructions on how to maximize oral intake and stabilize weight if the patient is being discharged to a facility?

SUGGESTED READINGS

Ahmed T, Haboubi N. Assessment and management of nutrition in older people and its importance to health. *Clin Interv Aging.* 2010;5:207-216.

Morley JE. Anorexia of aging: physiologic and pathologic. *Am J Clin Nutr.* 1997;66(4):760-773.

Morley JE. Undernutrition in older adults. *Fam Pract.* 2012; 29(Suppl 1):i89-i93.

SECTION 7

Hematology

Abnormalities in Red Blood Cells

Madeleine Verhovsek, MD, BSc
Andrew McFarlane, MLT, ART

Key Clinical Questions

Anemia

1. How does peripheral blood smear aid in the diagnosis of anemia?

2. How do I interpret iron studies?

3. What are the best tests to diagnose hemolytic anemia?

4. How do I determine the cause of hemolytic anemia?

5. When should I investigate for hemoglobinopathy?

6. What factors suggest the need for bone marrow examination?

7. What is the most effective way to administer oral iron?

8. When and how should I use erythropoietin (EPO) in anemia of renal dysfunction or anemia of chronic disease? (How is it dosed and when should I expect a response?)

Polycythemia and Secondary Erythrocytosis

1. How do I distinguish primary and secondary erythrocytosis in a patient who smokes or has chronic lung disease?

2. When should I be concerned about carbon monoxide poisoning?

3. How do I manage secondary erythrocytosis?

4. What tests should I do to rule out a myeloproliferative disorder?

5. What complications can occur in patients with myeloproliferative disorders?

6. When is phlebotomy indicated?

(continued)

ANEMIA

■ INTRODUCTION

Anemia is one of the most common blood disorders worldwide and, in developed countries, commonly affects older adults. The primary function of a red blood cell is to deliver oxygen to the tissues. Red blood cells are made in the bone marrow and must contain adequate amounts of hemoglobin to perform this function. Normal production is dependent on the availability of the required "ingredients" (ie, iron, folic acid, vitamin B12), a normal functioning bone marrow, and erythropoietin for stimulation of red cell production. Anemia can result from defects affecting hemoglobin production, dozens of disease states, including renal impairment and chronic inflammatory conditions, and may also be caused by other external or internal factors influencing the circulatory survival of red blood cells through premature destruction or blood loss. This chapter will provide a framework for investigation in order to navigate the many diagnostic tests and treatment options.

Anemia is defined as a reduction in the number of circulating red cells that results in a hemoglobin level lower than an age- and sex-matched population (**Table 169-1**).

In addition to the RBC count, hemoglobin, and hematocrit, which make the diagnosis of anemia possible, the complete blood count (CBC) provides essential information that helps tailor the investigation. One of the RBC indices, the mean corpuscular volume (MCV), permits classification of hypoproliferative anemias into hypochromic microcytic anemia (MCV <80 fl), normocytic anemia (MCV 80-100 fl), or macrocytic anemia (MCV > 100 fl). An increase in the reticulocyte count by 1% will increase the MCV by approximately 2 fl. The red cell distribution width (RDW) reflects the variation in RBC size or anisocytosis. Useful in distinguishing between certain hypoproliferative anemias, it is normally 11.5% to 14.5%. Normally between 0.5% and 2.5%, the reticulocyte count is calculated as a percentage of the total RBC; therefore, it must be corrected in the presence of anemia. The reticulocyte production index (RPI) is one method frequently used. The RPI = % reticulocytes × (patient Hct/45)/maturation time. With increasingly severe anemia, more reticulocytes are released from the marrow. The maturation time equals 1 if the patient's Hct is 45. Each 10-point drop in the patient's Hct increases the maturation time by 1.5 days. A low reticulocyte count suggests an underlying defect in RBC production; an elevated reticulocyte count suggests an underlying problem in RBC survival. Likewise, an RPI less than 2.5 suggests that the anemia stems from a hypoproliferative process; an RPI greater than 2.5 suggests that the anemia is due to bleeding or hemolysis. Examination of the peripheral smear may reveal morphologic abnormalities of the RBC that permit an accurate and timely diagnosis (**Table 169-2**).

■ PATHOPHYSIOLOGY

Although there are many causes of anemia, clinicians most commonly encounter iron-deficiency anemia, thalassemia trait, and anemia of chronic disease.

Acute anemia results from bleeding or hemolysis. In someone who has been injured or who has suffered complications of surgery, the source of acute bleeding is normally clear. Hemolysis-related anemia due to increased destruction of red blood cells occurs by various mechanisms and can be broadly categorized as intrinsic red cell defects or extrinsic processes (**Figure 169-1**).

Key Clinical Questions

7 How frequently should phlebotomy be performed and what are the monitoring parameters?

8 Is there a role for antiplatelet agents and anticoagulants in patients with a myeloproliferative disorder?

Thalassemia and Hemoglobinopathies

1 Which hemoglobinopathies are considered to be clinically significant?

2 How is thalassemia differentiated from iron deficiency anemia?

3 When should one investigate for hemoglobinopathies?

4 When should transfusion therapy be considered?

5 What are the common complications in patients with thalassemia?

Sickle Cell Disease

1 What are triggers for admission in a patient with sickle cell disease?

2 What is appropriate hydration for acute chest syndrome or painful crisis?

3 What clinical presentations benefit from red blood cell transfusion or red cell exchange?

4 What is an appropriate transfusion threshold?

5 How is pain optimally managed?

6 What are special considerations in management of sickle cell disease in pregnancy or in labor?

7 What are special considerations perioperatively?

8 When should hydroxyurea be used?

Internally, problems of the red cell membrane (hereditary spherocytosis), the hemoglobin (eg, sickle cell anemia) or the deficiency of glycolytic pathway enzymes (glucose-6 phosphate dehydrogenase [G6PD] and pyruvate kinase [PK]) result in shorter life span. External mechanisms can be further classified as immune-mediated or nonimmune resulting from infection, drugs, or mechanical injury. Hemolysis can occur intravascularly or extravascularly (ie, via the reticuloendothelial system), although many times it may be difficult to determine the site of cell destruction due to overlap in overwhelming acute cases.

The differential diagnosis of chronic anemia, whether microcytic, normocytic, or macrocytic, is broad. One of the most common causes of chronic blood loss is occult blood loss, particularly from the GI tract, or in younger women through menses, leading to iron-deficiency

TABLE 169-1 World Health Organization's Hemoglobin Threshold Used to Define Anemia

Age or Gender Group	Hb Threshold (g/dL)
Children (0.5-5.0 y)	11.0
Children (5-12 y)	11.5
Children (12-15 y)	12.0
Women, nonpregnant (>15 y)	12.0
Women, pregnant	11.0
Men (>15 y)	13.0

anemia. Once the bone marrow receives the signal from erythropoietin, it requires building blocks from which to assemble the components of the red blood cell. Iron deficiency is one of the most common causes of anemia, often due to dietary deficiency or occult blood loss.

Underproduction of RBC results from a number of chronic diseases. The bone marrow, which produces the majority of red cells, relies on erythropoietin secreted by the kidneys to signal the need for new red blood cell production. In renal impairment, a decreased erythropoietin level leads to chronic anemia. In bone marrow failure states, underproduction may be caused by a decrease of precursor cells (eg, aplastic anemia, pure red cell aplasia), crowding out of normal RBC precursors by malignant cells (eg, leukemia, metastatic cancer) or abnormal maturation (eg, myelodysplastic syndrome, vitamin B12, or folate deficiency). Inflammatory conditions can also cause chronic anemia by a combination of mechanisms due to pro-inflammatory cytokines that produce a "functional" iron deficiency in which iron is trapped in storage (eg, inside macrophages) instead of being available for hemoglobin production, abnormal proliferation of RBC progenitors in the bone marrow, insufficient erythropoietin, and reduced RBC life span.

■ DIAGNOSIS: HOW DO I DETERMINE THE CAUSE OF ANEMIA?

A complete blood count is the backbone for the evaluation of anemia. The World Health Organization (WHO) defines anemia in an adult as a hemoglobin < 13 g/dL for men and < 12 g/dL for women. A patient with chronic, mild, stable anemia can comfortably be evaluated in an outpatient setting. However, any patient with acute and/or severe anemia will benefit from the intensive investigations, monitoring, and treatment offered in the hospital. Anyone who is hemodynamically unstable due to blood loss should receive care in a monitored setting. After the diagnosis of anemia is confirmed, the next step is to determine why so that appropriate treatment can be administered (Figure 169-1).

Since the potential causes of anemia are numerous, a thorough and broad history should include query about:

- Any associated symptoms, in particular, bleeding (gastrointestinal, including melena, menses, hematuria) and constitutional B symptoms
- Past medical history, in particular, autoimmune/inflammatory disorder, chronic infection, liver disease, renal impairment, thyroid dysfunction, previous diagnosis, and treatment of anemia
- Medication history
- Social history, in particular, dietary intake, alcohol use, risk of sexually transmitted infections
- Family history of anemia
- Full review of systems, which may uncover symptoms of previously undiagnosed inflammatory disorders or organ dysfunction

Most prominent symptoms in severe anemia include fatigue, dizziness, palpitations, or breathlessness on physical exertion. Information about the onset of symptoms may help to determine whether the anemia is acute or chronic. The patient should also be questioned as to whether he or she has had a recent complete blood count.

PRACTICE POINT

- The average red blood cell survives for 120 days after it is released into circulation. If anemia is due to underproduction alone, the hemoglobin should decrease by less than 25% in a 30-day period (roughly 0.1 g/dL/d).

TABLE 169-2 The Peripheral Smear

RBC Size and Hemoglobin Content		Etiology
Hypochromic microcytic anemia with 1. RDW > 15% 2. RBC < 4.6 × 10^{12} 3. Smear—anisocytosis, poikilocytosis	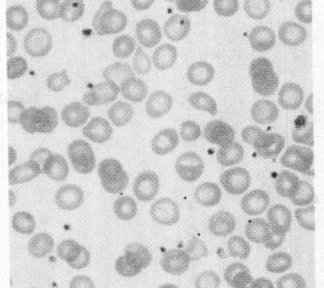	**Iron-deficiency anemia** (low serum ferritin <12 μg/L; low iron, high TIBC, <9% TS, high RDW) **Anemia of chronic disease** (normal/high ferritin, low serum iron, low TIBC, >9% TS, normal RDW) **Sideroblastic anemia** (Dimorphic population of hypochromic and normochromic cells, normal/high ferritin, high serum iron, normal TIBC, normal RDW)
Hypochromic microcytic anemia with 1. RDW < 15% 2. RBC > 4.6 × 10^{12} 3. Smear—uniform RBCs with basophilic stippling and target cells	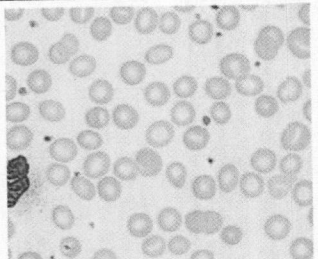	**Thalassemia** (normal/high ferritin, normal/high serum iron, normal TIBC, normal/high RDW—check Hb electrophoresis and HbA$_2$ quantitation) **Anemia of chronic disease** (normal pattern, increased iron stores, <15% ringed sideroblasts RS) **Aplastic anemia, myelofibrosis, anemia from metastatic cancer** (normal to increased iron stores, <15% RS) **Refractory anemia with RS, lead poisoning** (>15% RS)
Normochromic normocytic anemia with 1. Immature myeloid cells 2. Nucleated RBCs 3. Teardrop cells and/or 4. Elliptocytes	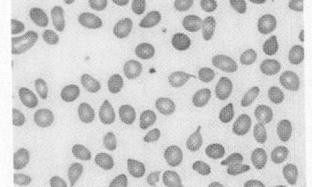	**Early iron deficiency** **Secondary BM failure; due to liver disease, hypothyrodism, inflammation or renal impairment**
Normochromic normocytic anemia without abnormal cells on smear	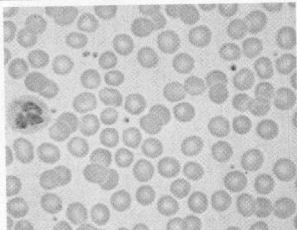	**Early iron deficiency** **Secondary BM failure from liver disease, hypothyroidism, inflammation, uremia**
Macrocytic anemia with hypersegmented neutrophils (one six-lobed nucleus or five-lobed nucleus in >5% of neutrophils)	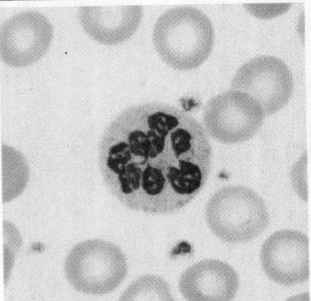	**Megaloblastic anemia** (check serum B12, serum folate, RBC folate; if all normal, BM for myedysplastic syndrome and myeloproliferative disorder)
Macrocytic anemia without macroovalocytes and hypersegmented neutrophils	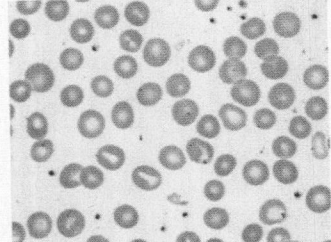	**Reticulocytosis** **Liver disease** **Thyroid disease** **Cold agglutinin disease** **Drugs**

(continued)

TABLE 169-2 The Peripheral Smear (*continued*)

RBC Size and Hemoglobin Content		Etiology
Abnormal cell type		
Basophilic stippling		Hemolytic anemias, thalassemias, lead poisoning
Bite cells (Heinz bodies removed by splenic macrophages)		G6PD deficiency, oxidative drugs or unstable hemoglobin
Burr cells, spur cells (acanthocytes)		Liver disease, uremia, hypersplenism
Elliptocytes		Iron-deficiency anemia Hereditary elliptocytosis
Hemolysis of RBC		Hemolytic anemia
Howell-Jolly bodies		Postsplenectomy or functional asplenia

(*continued*)

TABLE 169-2 **The Peripheral Smear** (*continued*)

RBC Size and Hemoglobin Content		Etiology
Abnormal cell type		
Nucleated RBC		Microangiopathic or macroangiopathic hemolysis eg, DIC, TTP
Schistocytes (fragmented RBCs)		
Sickled forms		Sickle cell disease
Spherocytes (RBCs lack central pallor)		Immune-mediated hemolysis, hereditary spherocytosis, hypersplenism
Target cells		Thalassemias, hemoglobin C, hemoglobin E, hemoglobin S, liver disease, postsplenectomy
Teardrop cells		Myelopthisis, hypersplenism

BM, bone marrow; CML, chronic myelogenous leukemia; DIC, disseminated intravascular coagulation; G6PD, glucose-6-phosphate dehydrogenase; RBC, red blood cell; RDW, red cell distribution width; RS, ringed sideroblasts; TIBC, total iron binding capacity; TS, transferrin saturation; TTP, thrombotic thrombocytopenic purpura.

The physical examination may reveal evidence of decompensation as in acute blood loss (eg, unstable vital signs) or chronic extreme anemia (eg, congestive heart failure), signs of severe anemia (eg, pallor of the skin, conjunctivae, tongue, nail beds, and palmar creases, or tachycardia and the presence of a flow murmur), or help to identify previously unknown systemic disease (eg, signs of chronic liver disease).

Recent blood tests showing a previously normal hemoglobin level may confirm that the anemia is acute. Elevated reticulocyte count or reticulocyte percent is suggestive of acute or ongoing blood loss or hemolysis. If the anemia is not acute, workup can be guided by the peripheral blood smear and the mean corpuscular volume of the red blood cells—small (microcytic), large (macrocytic), or normal size (normocytic). It is also important to

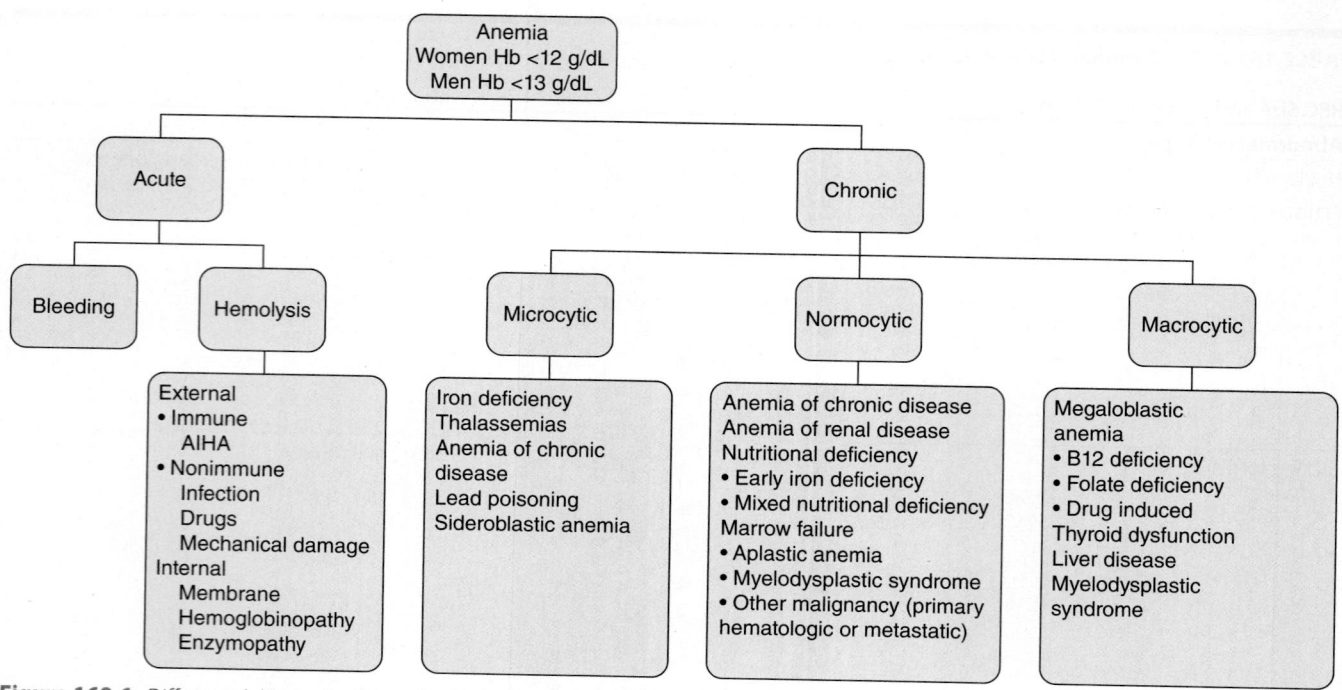

Figure 169-1 *Differential diagnosis of anemia. AIHA, autoimmune hemolytic anemia.*

note the white blood cell and platelet counts. Pancytopenia can be seen in aplastic anemia, vitamin B12 deficiency, myelodysplastic syndrome, primary bone marrow malignancies, or in liver disease with portal hypertension and splenomegaly. A normal white blood cell and platelet count with isolated anemia is unlikely to be due to marrow failure, with the exception of pure red cell aplasia. The reticulocyte count may also be useful to distinguish conditions associated with hyporegenerative anemia having low values of $< 50 \times 10^9$/L (aplastic anemia, pure red cell aplasia, or marrow infiltration) from a regenerative anemia seen with hemolysis or hemorrhage.

The appearance of the red cells in a peripheral blood film can be associated with the different causes of anemia, and offers suggestions for relevant subsequent investigations (Table 169-2).

PRACTICE POINT

- The first question to ask in the evaluation of anemia is whether the anemia is due to acute or chronic blood loss, decreased production of red blood cells, or increased destruction. The first step is a complete history and physical examination, followed by a review of the complete blood count, the reticulocyte count, and the peripheral blood smear. The objective is to make the correct diagnosis without subjecting the patient to unnecessary laboratory tests and invasive procedures.

■ MICROCYTIC ANEMIA

Peripheral blood smear in iron-deficiency anemia (IDA) shows small ("microcytic" or low MCV) red blood cells that are very pale ("hypochromic") containing less hemoglobin as indicated by a reduced mean corpuscular hemoglobin (MCH). Other changes of note may include anisocytosis (variable size of red blood cells) and poikilocytosis (variable shape of RBCs, eg, target cells and pencil cells). Based on

the blood smear alone it is difficult to discern IDA from a thalassemia trait. Therefore, further laboratory testing to investigate iron status and for exclusion of a possible hemoglobinopathy may be required.

Serum ferritin is considered a good measure of iron stores; levels below 30 mg/L in otherwise healthy patients are reflective of iron deficiency. However, ferritin is an acute phase reactant and may be higher in iron deficient patients with other medical problems. For this reason, the ferritin threshold may need to be increased. If the diagnosis is unclear, bone marrow examination, which is considered the "gold standard" test to confirm iron-deficiency anemia, should be considered. Other tests that may be useful for the confirmation of a diagnosis in microcytic anemia include serum iron, total iron-binding capacity (TIBC), serum transferrin receptor, and measurement of zinc protoporphyrin (ZPP) and free erythrocyte protoporphyrins (FEP) (**Table 169-3**).

TABLE 169-3 Typical Patterns of Iron Investigations in Iron Deficiency Anemia and Anemia of Chronic Disease

Biochemical Marker	Iron-Deficiency Anemia	Anemia of Chronic Disease/ Inflammation
Serum ferritin	Decreased	Normal or increased
Serum iron	Decreased	Deceased or normal
Total iron-binding capacity	Normal to increased	Decreased or normal
Transferrin saturation	Decreased	Decreased or normal
Serum transferrin receptor	Increased	Normal
ZPP or FEP	Increased	Increased

FEP, free erythrocyte protoporphyrin; ZPP, zinc protoporphyrin.

- Stages of iron deficiency are
  1. Storage iron depletion (decrease in serum ferritin levels, a reflection of total iron body stores).
  2. Iron-deficient erythropoiesis (a transferrin saturation <9%, an indicator of impaired iron supply for the developing RBC).
  3. Microcytic hypochromic RBCs (RDW > 15% and variation in RBC shape, poikilocytosis, unlike Thalassemia).
- The bottom line: The MCV, serum iron, total iron-binding capacity, and percentage of transferrin saturation can predict the presence or absence of bone marrow iron in most patients without requiring a bone marrow examination.

A hemoglobinopathy should be considered if the patient is healthy, not iron deficient, has a family history of microcytic anemia or thalassemia, or if the patient's ethnic group is known to commonly have thalassemia or variant hemoglobins associated with microcytosis (HbE). Initial hemoglobinopathy investigations will quantify normal and abnormal hemoglobins to identify beta-thalassemia trait, homozygous beta-thalassemia, and HbE. However, further DNA analysis may be required for diagnosis of alpha-thalassemia or may be useful to confirm the presence of other globin gene deletions or mutations. Pregnant women with microcytosis should always be considered for hemoglobinopathy testing regardless of iron status due to the risk of genetic transmission of a severe form of hemoglobinopathy or thalassemia to the fetus.

■ NORMOCYTIC ANEMIA

Normocytic anemia is the most frequently encountered category of anemia, and is often the most difficult to workup because it can result from many disparate disorders; it can be due to decreased RBC production, either primary (eg, aplastic anemia, acute leukemia) or secondary (eg, renal failure, anemia of chronic disease). Hemolytic anemia, both immune and nonimmune, and acute bleeding can also present as normocytic anemia.

Hemolytic anemia: increased red cell destruction

Hemolytic anemia may present in many ways; it can be acute and uncompensated or chronic and well compensated, or anything in between. Therefore most patients presenting with anemia of unclear etiology should be screened for hemolysis. The red cells in hemolytic anemia often vary in appearance depending on the underlying process. Examination of the peripheral smear is a useful tool for the differential diagnosis. Spherocytes can be present in autoimmune hemolytic anemia (AIHA) or in hereditary spherocytosis when the patient has a negative Coombs test. Sickle cell anemia manifests with characteristic sickle-shaped cells. Schistocytes are a hallmark of red cell destruction and can be correlated with platelet numbers for differentiating a microangiopathic hemolytic anemia from macroangiopathic hemolytic conditions caused by heart valves. Decreased platelets are seen in disseminated intravascular coagulation (DIC), thrombotic thrombocytopenic purpura (TTP), and hemolytic uremic syndrome (HUS). Platelets are normal in macroangiopathic hemolytic conditions caused by heart valves.

Screening tests that suggest the possibility of hemolysis include elevated lactate dehydrogenase, elevated unconjugated bilirubin, and elevated reticulocyte count. The level of haptoglobin, a protein that binds free hemoglobin in the circulation,

may be a useful indicator for hemolysis. A low level or absence of haptoglobin, along with the presence of free hemoglobin in circulation, is suggestive of hemolysis. However, low haptoglobin can also be seen in liver disease. Haptoglobins are an acute phase reactant and therefore may be falsely elevated during any inflammatory process.

Often further specialized testing is required to confirm and identify the cause of hemolytic anemia. This can include direct antiglobulin test (DAT or Coombs test), hemoglobinopathy testing, and/or enzymopathy testing, as indicated. The DAT identifies IgG and/or complement on the RBC surface and can be positive in AIHA, drug-induced anemia, or a hemolytic transfusion reaction. A hemoglobinopathy investigation separates and quantifies the expected hemoglobins (HbA, A2, and F) but will also identify many variant hemoglobins (eg, HbS, C, or E) or other rarer unstable hemoglobin variants (eg, Hb Köln, Hb Hasharon) known to cause hemolysis. To assess for enzyme deficiencies, quantitative testing of red cell pyruvate kinase and G6PD is performed. More recently, flow cytometry has been used to identify paroxysmal nocturnal hemoglobinuria (PNH) using the GPI-anchored antigens CD55 and CD59 on red cells or neutrophils. The osmotic fragility (OF) test is useful for confirmation of hereditary spherocytosis. However, the eosin-5-maleimide (EMA) dye binding test by flow cytometry has shown to have higher specificity and sensitivity than OF for red cell cytoskeleton disorders causing hemolysis.

Decreased red blood cell production

If anemia is due to decreased RBC production, the reticulocyte count will be low or "inappropriately normal." Serum erythropoietin level can be helpful but it is nondiagnostic; if it is high, it may indicate a primary bone marrow problem, which could be confirmed with a bone marrow aspirate and/or biopsy. Serum erythropoietin level will be low or inappropriately normal in any of the secondary causes of normocytic anemia, particularly in renal dysfunction. Moderate renal impairment can present with anemia, therefore renal function testing is essential, regardless of serum EPO level.

Anemia of chronic disease (ACD) is a difficult diagnosis to pin down. Essentially it is a clinical diagnosis in a patient who has had a sufficient and negative workup for other causes of anemia, and who has an underlying inflammatory condition. Measurement of iron indices or inflammatory markers (eg, erythrocyte sedimentation rate or C-reactive protein) may be a useful adjunct in testing. Bone marrow examination should reveal normal or increased amounts of stored iron and decreased iron staining in erythroid precursors, reflecting impaired iron utilization.

■ MACROCYTIC ANEMIA

B12 deficiency

Vitamin B12 (also known as cobalamin) is obtained by intake of animal products, including red meat, poultry, fish, dairy, and eggs. The total body store of vitamin B12 is 2 to 5 mg, primarily stored in the liver. Approximately 2 to 5 mcg of B12 is lost daily, most of which is excreted in the bile.

Although a typical Western diet contains 5 to 20 mcg/d of vitamin B12, which is more than sufficient to replace daily losses, B12 deficiency can occur in individuals following a strict vegan diet.

In patients with gastritis, gastric atrophy, or history of gastrectomy, absence of gastric acid and pepsin prevents release of cobalamin from the protein to which it is bound. Furthermore, production of gastric intrinsic factor (IF), a molecule that binds free cobalamin in the gastrointestinal tract and facilitates cobalamin absorption in the terminal ileum, may be impaired. Malabsorption can also occur if there is inadequate absorption at the terminal ileum, due to prior resection or Crohn disease.

One of the most common causes of B12 deficiency is pernicious anemia, in which there is a deficiency of IF due to presumed autoimmune destruction of gastric parietal cells or the IF itself.

Vitamin B12 deficiency presents most commonly with hematologic abnormalities and/or neuropsychiatric signs and symptoms. Macrocytic anemia, with macro-ovalocytes on peripheral blood smear, is the classic hematologic abnormality. Neutrophils have hypersegmented nuclei. There may also be leukopenia and/or thrombocytopenia. Bone marrow examination reveals megaloblastosis.

The classic neurological manifestation is subacute combined degeneration of the spinal cord, resulting in sensory and motor disturbances that cause ataxia. Peripheral and cranial neuropathies may also be seen. In severe cases, patients may present with stroke or dementia-like syndromes. Physical examination may reveal classic findings such as glossitis and jaundice.

A serum B12 level <200 ng/L (148 pmol/L) is very sensitive (97%) for the diagnosis of B12 deficiency. Because some patients with normal or low-normal serum B12 levels may be truly deficient and benefit from vitamin replacement, elevated methylmalonic acid (MMA) and homocysteine can help to clarify the diagnosis. Elevated MMA and hemocysteine are both sensitive early markers of B12 deficiency. Elevated levels should, however, be interpreted in the context of individual patients: homocysteine is also elevated in folate deficiency and hereditary homocyteinemia. Methylmalonic acid may be elevated in renal insufficiency and methylmalonic aciduria, and in some patients with folate deficiency. Serum MMA may be lowered in B12-deficient patients receiving antibiotic treatment. A Schilling test, involving oral administration of radiolabeled cocyanocobalamin, has historically been used to assess vitamin B12 absorption. Unfortunately, the Schilling test is not widely available. Anti-intrinsic factor antibodies are highly specific for pernicious anemia (specificity >95%) and therefore, if positive, help to confirm the diagnosis; however sensitivity is poor (50%-70%).

Folate deficiency

Folate is found in animal products and leafy green vegetables. As such, the most common cause of folate deficiency is inadequate nutritional intake. With universal folate supplementation, folate deficiency has become increasingly rare. However, patients with alcohol abuse remain at risk due to folate malabsorption and impaired folate metabolism in the liver. Individuals with increased folate requirements are also at increased risk. This includes pregnant women (for whom folate deficiency is associated with an increased risk of fetal spina bifida) and patients with chronic hemolytic anemia. The widespread use of routine, prophylactic folic acid supplementation in these groups can prevent deficiency. Use of some drugs has been linked to folate deficiency, including trimethoprim, pyrimethamin, methotrexate, and phenytoin.

Similar to vitamin B12 deficiency, folate deficiency can result in megaloblastic anemia. However, folate deficiency has no neurologic sequelae.

Diagnosis is made when the serum or red blood cell folate is below the normal range. Serum folate concentration may be normal in approximately 5% of individuals with folate deficiency; therefore if there is still a high index of suspicion, red blood cell folate should be tested.

Drug-induced anemia

A number of drugs can cause macrocytosis or macrocytic anemia. These include the following:

- Pyrimidine and purine analogs that inhibit DNA synthesis (eg, 5-FU, azathioprine)
- Antifolates (eg, methotrexate)
- Hydroxyurea
- Zidovudine

Other causes of macrocytic anemia

Occasionally, an exceptionally brisk reticulocytosis in response to anemia results in the average red blood cell being larger, thus increasing the MCV measurement. Other causes of macrocytosis that should be considered include liver disease, hypothyroidism, alcohol abuse, and myelodysplastic syndrome.

PRACTICE POINT

- Many anemias in their early stages have a normal MCV and then become either microcytic or macrocytic.
- The peripheral smear may provide important clues such as a myelopthisis (elliptocytes, teardrop cells, immature myeloid forms, nucleated RBCs), sickle cell disease (sickled RBCs), infectious disease (malaria).

■ TREATMENT

Iron-deficiency anemia

The goal of treatment for IDA is to improve the hemoglobin level and replenish iron stores. This typically requires 150 to 200 mg elemental iron per day for 4 to 6 months, or until serum ferritin has increased to approximately 50 mg/L. Iron is given orally unless the patient has severe gastrointestinal intolerance, malabsorption, or uncontrolled blood loss. The relative amounts of elemental iron in different preparations are listed below:

Ferrous gluconate:	300 mg	35 mg elemental iron
Ferrous sulfate:	300 mg	60 mg elemental iron
Ferrous fumarate:	300 mg	100 mg elemental iron
Polysaccharide iron complex:	150 mg	150 mg elemental iron

In the absence of ongoing blood loss, hemoglobin should increase by 1 to 2 g/dL within 3 weeks of starting adequate oral replacement, and iron stores should be replete in 3 months. Failure to respond may be due to nonadherence, poor iron absorption, or an incorrect diagnosis. If instead the patient has thalassemia, iron supplementation could be harmful, in that it will increase iron overload.

To improve iron absorption, the iron tablets should be taken on an empty stomach or with orange juice or a tablet of ascorbic acid. Concurrent administration of antacids should be avoided. Many patients complain of nausea or dyspepsia 30 to 60 minutes following a dose. This often subsides with ongoing treatment but, if it is an ongoing issue, night time dosing or administration of higher doses with food may improve symptoms and maintain adequate absorption.

Intravenous iron is an option for patients who are intolerant of or who do not respond to oral iron. These must be administered in a medically supervised area because of risks of hypotension, allergic, or anaphylactic reactions. Several iron preparations are available for intravenous administration, of which iron dextran has the highest risk of adverse reactions.

B12 deficiency

Vitamin B12 replacement can be divided into initial management (designed to quickly build up the tissue stores) and long-term maintenance treatment. A common initial regimen consists of intramuscular cyanocobalamin 1000 mcg/d for 1 or 2 weeks, followed by 1000 mcg/week for 1 month. Hematologic response should be evident 1 week after the first dose. In particular, there should be a noticeable increase in the reticulocyte count. If reticulocytosis is mild or absent, the original diagnosis should be questioned. By the eighth week, the MCV should have returned to the normal range.

Maintenance treatment can be given parenterally or orally. Parenteral cyanocobalamin may be given at a dose of 1000 mcg/month until the cause of deficiency is corrected, or lifelong in pernicious anemia. Oral therapy for pernicious anemia is 1000 mcg/d. Lower doses (eg, 125-500 mcg/d) can be given for other causes of deficiency; however the cost and risk of a higher dose are negligible and a standard dose of 1000 mcg/d is commonly prescribed.

Folate deficiency

Treatment is with oral folic acid (1-5 mg/d) until complete hematologic recovery. Patients with an ongoing cause of folate deficiency (eg, chronic hemolytic anemia or pregnancy) should continue on long-term supplementation. Because treatment with folic acid can partially reverse the hematologic abnormalities seen in vitamin B12 deficiency, but do not attenuate the progression of neurologic sequelae, serum vitamin B12 levels should be measured prior to therapy.

Anemia of chronic renal disease

As the glomerular filtration rates decline, anemia becomes increasingly common in patients with chronic renal disease. Erythropoiesis-stimulating agents (ESAs) are widely used in treatment. Other options include red blood cell transfusions or androgens.

ESAs may be started if the hemoglobin level is ≤ 10 g/dL for predialysis and peritoneal dialysis patients, and if the hemoglobin is ≤ 11 g/dL in dialysis patients. Adequate iron stores should be confirmed, and other causes of anemia should be ruled out. Epoetin alpha or darbepoeitin may be used with a target hemoglobin of 10 to 12 g/dL. Levels above 13 g/dL have been associated with increased risk of thrombotic events. Epoetin alpha can be started at a dose of 10,000 units subcutaneously once weekly or 20,000 units subcutaneously every other week. Lower starting doses may be appropriate for smaller patients or those with higher pretreatment hemoglobin. For dialysis patients, EPO can be administered intravenously during hemodialysis sessions. Throughout ESA therapy, iron supplementation should be used to maintain a transferrin saturation of 20% to 50% and a serum ferritin level of 100 to 500 ng/mL. Ongoing clinical trials are evaluating the precise determinants of cardiovascular risk and the optimal hemoglobin target. Updated clinical practice guidelines should be consulted.

Hemolytic anemia

Any hemolysis caused by an underlying disorder (eg, AIHA due to a lymphoproliferative disorder) is treated in the long term by bringing the disease under control. A short-term treatment may include high-dose oral corticosteroids. Hemolytic anemia caused by cold agglutinins typically improves with avoidance of cold exposure.

Myelodysplastic syndromes

The anemia of myelodysplatsic syndromes (MDS) is typically treated with chronic transfusions or erythropoiesis-stimulating agents (ESAs). Patients with MDS-related anemia with serum EPO level < 100 to 200 mU/mL and lower-risk disease are most likely to respond to ESAs. Relatively high doses of epoetin alpha or darbepoetin are usually required. Patients who do not qualify for or respond to ESAs are likely to require chronic red blood cell transfusions. Unfortunately, transfusion-dependent MDS patients have decreased overall survival, especially those in lower-risk categories. Decreased overall survival in these individuals is linked to elevated ferritin levels, indicating that transfusional iron overload is at least partially responsible for worsened outcomes. Serum ferritin and transferrin iron saturation should be monitored in transfusion-dependent MDS patients. T2-weighted magnetic resonance imaging (MRI) may be used to evaluate for cardiac and liver iron deposition. Chelation therapy should be considered in patients with evidence of iron overload.

■ COMPLICATIONS

Bone marrow examination may aid diagnosis if anemia is apparently due to underproduction, or if anemia is associated with leukopenia, thrombocytopenia, and/or other morphologic abnormalities suggesting bone marrow disease. Rarely, bone marrow examination is necessary to help quantify iron stores in a patient with normal serum ferritin but microcytic anemia is felt to be due to iron deficiency.

Consultation with a hematologist should be considered in complex cases and for patients with thalassemia, sickle cell disease, other variant hemoglobins, bone marrow failure syndromes, or autoimmune hemolytic anemia. Patients with anemia due to end-stage renal disease may be best managed by a renal specialist.

■ RARE CAUSES FOR CONSIDERATION

Thrombotic thrombocytopenic purpura (TTP) is caused by impaired cleavage of ultra large multimers of von Willebrand factor, causing increased platelet aggregation in small vessels. Thrombotic thrombocytopenic purpura presents with hemolytic anemia and thrombocytopenia. Other features can include fever, neurologic symptoms (headache, seizures, or coma), and acute renal impairment. Blood film shows red blood cell fragments (schistocytes) that result from damage to red cells in the microvasculature.

When a cause of microcytic or normocytic anemia is not found, remember to test for paroxysmal nocturnal hemoglobinuria (PNH), which typically presents with episodes of intravascular hemolysis and red urine. As a result of chronic and recurrent hemoglobinuria, patients can become iron deficient. Paroxysmal nocturnal hemoglobinuria is a clonal disorder that can result in aplastic anemia or acute leukemia. Patients with PNH are at increased risk of thromboembolism. The diagnosis of PNH is made when flow cytometry shows a clone of WBCs (PB or BM) lacking cell markers CD55 or CD59 or by FLAER (flourescein-labeled proaerolysin).

There are several rare congential bone marrow failure syndromes that result in lifelong anemia. These include Diamond-Blackfan anemia, Fanconi anemia, Schwachman-Diamond syndrome, and congential dyserythropoietic anemia. These disorders will typically present in early childhood and require ongoing follow-up. First diagnosis in adulthood is rare but does occur.

■ QUALITY IMPROVEMENT

Anemia is a common finding in hospitalized patients. Typically, low hemoglobin is caused by one or more of the numerous underlying problems describe above. However, daily in-hospital blood testing can exacerbate anemia. As a result, in all hospital patients, in particular those with preexisting anemia, blood sampling should be minimized by careful use of laboratory investigations. In any patient diagnosed with anemia, discharge planning should include a plan for routine monitoring of hemoglobin. The frequency and duration of follow-up will be tailored to the cause and severity of anemia.

POLYCYTHEMIA AND SECONDARY ERYTHROCYTOSIS

■ INTRODUCTION

Erythrocytosis is the term used to describe unusually high hematocrit, hemoglobin, and/or red blood cell count. An increased red blood cell count is a medical concern for two reasons: (1) It can be the "red flag" for some underlying medical problem that needs attention and (2) erythrocytosis itself can cause problems with sluggish blood flow and subsequent ischemic phenomena, particularly neurologic signs and symptoms. Investigations to determine the cause of erythrocytosis enable proper classification (ie, primary or secondary process), which guides the therapeutic strategy.

■ PATHOPHYSIOLOGY

True erythrocytosis (as opposed to spurious erythrocytosis, see below) is defined as having both an increased hematocrit and an increased red cell mass that can be classified as either primary or secondary. Primary erythrocytosis is due to a group of clonal bone marrow disorders known as myeloproliferative disorders (MPD) that include polycythemia rubra vera resulting in autonomous production of too many red blood cells, essential thrombocythemia in which the platelet counts are elevated, and primary myelofibrosis. The MPDs are discussed in Chapter 174 [Hematologic Malignancies].

Secondary erythrocytosis can occur by three mechanisms, all involving increased erythropoietin (EPO) signaling in the bone marrow.

1. **"Appropriate" increase in EPO production:** In healthy homeostasis, the kidneys make and secrete EPO based on the oxygen tension (PO_2) in the renal blood vessels. If oxygen delivered to the kidneys decreases, the kidneys release more EPO as a signal to the bone marrow that the blood needs increased oxygen-carrying capacity in the form of hemoglobin. Oxygen delivery to the body tissues may be decreased as a result of hypoxemia or anemia. Hypoxemia may be due to reasons listed in **Table169-4**. Relative renal hypoxia due to renal artery stenosis will cause increased EPO by the same mechanism.

2. **Autonomously produced erythropoietin:** Several types of neoplasm are known to produce excess EPO, including renal cell carcinoma, uterine fibroids, hemangioblastoma, and hepatocellular carcinoma. EPO production can also be increased following renal transplant, although this dysregulated EPO production effect is not completely understood. Inherited causes of upregulated EPO production due to defects in the oxygen-sensing pathway have been described with genetic mutations in the von Hippel-Lindau (VHL) gene including the Chuvash polycythemia (VHL 598C > T) mutation.

3. **Exogenous EPO:** Patients with anemia of renal disease or anemia that is associated with cancer may be on erythropoietin-stimulating agents. If the prescribed dose is too high or the patient takes the medication incorrectly, it can result in erythrocytosis.

EPO production is also increased with elevated testosterone levels. Elevated testosterone levels stimulate EPO release, and also increase bone marrow activity and iron incorporation into RBCs. This is why the hemoglobin reference range for men is higher than

TABLE 169-4 Classification of Absolute Erythrocytosis

Primary erythrocytosis
Polycythemia vera (and other myeloproliferative neoplasms)
Secondary erythrocytosis
Congenital
    Chuvash polycythemia (*VHL* mutation)
    Other defects in oxygen sensing pathway (eg, *PHD2* or *HIF*-2α mutations)
    EPO receptor mutation
    High oxygen-affinity hemoglobin
    2,3-Biphosphoglycerate mutase deficiency
Acquired
    EPO Mediated
        Central hypoxia
            High altitude
            Right-to-left cardiopulmonary vascular shunts
            Chronic lung disease
            Obstructive sleep apnea
            Carbon monoxide poisoning
            Smoking
        Local renal hypoxia
            Renal artery stenosis
            Renal cysts
            Post-renal transplant erythrocytosis
        Pathologic EPO production
            Renal cell carcinoma
            Hepatocellular carcinoma
            Cerebellar hemangioma
            Meningioma
            Uterine fibroids (leiomyomas)
            Pheochromocytoma
        Drugs
            Testosterone administration
            EPO agonist administration
        Idiopathic erythrocytosis

EPO, erythropoeitin.
Data from McMullen MF, et al. Guidelines for the diagnosis, investigation and management of polycythaemia/erythrocytosis. *Br J Haematol.* 2005;130:174-195.

that for women. Exogenous androgen administration (eg, "blood doping" by some body builders and athletes) or increased endogenous testosterone (eg, germ cell tumors) can result in increased hemoglobin.

Spurious erythrocytosis

Spurious erythrocytosis occurs when either the patient or the patient's blood sample has reduced plasma volume, giving a false increase in hemoglobin concentration. Common causes of dehydration should be excluded (eg, illness, diuretic medications, caffeine-containing beverages, smoking).

■ DIAGNOSIS: WHY DOES THIS PATIENT HAVE POLYCYTHEMIA?

The detection of erythrocytosis is largely based on laboratory findings of increased hemoglobin, hematocrit, and red cell counts; however, some findings on history and physical examination can suggest a primary polycythemia. As well, a good clinical evaluation of the patient may direct the clinician to the underlying cause of erythrocytosis.

History should include:

- History of prior polycythemia
- Date and results of most recent CBC
- Questions about possible causes of secondary polycythemia
- Symptoms and complications resulting from polycythemia, which can include:
- Thromboembolic—transient ischemic attack (TIA) or stroke, myocardial infarction, venous thromboembolism
- Hyperviscosity—headache, dizziness, tinnitus, dyspnea, chest pain
- Erythromelalgia (painful paresthesias in the hands and feet)
- Aquagenic pruritus (itch after skin exposure to water [eg, after a bath])
- Gout

Physical examination should be performed, with particular attention to vital signs, cardiac, and respiratory examinations. Low oxygen saturation on pulse oximetry may suggest hypoxemia as the cause of polycythemia. Polycythemia can lead to chronic hypertension. True polycythemia will commonly be accompanied by "plethora," a ruddy appearance of the skin, particularly apparent on the face. If cyanosis is present, it may be due to polycythemia alone (increased red blood cell mass and relatively increased deoxygenated hemoglobin) or may reflect an underlying hypoxemic condition. Presence of splenomegaly suggests a myeloproliferative disorder.

■ BLOOD TESTS

As per WHO guidelines, polycythemia is suspected when complete blood count results show a hemoglobin of > 16.5 in women or > 18.5 g/dL in men or other evidence of increased red cell volume (eg, hematocrit >99th percentile of method-specific reference range for age, sex, and altitude of residence). A patient with polycythemia may also have an elevated red blood cell count. However, this may not be reliable as it also occurs in patients with thalassemia minor or having high O_2 affinity hemoglobin variants.

When polycythemia is suspected, spurious polycythemia should be ruled out. Repeat CBC may be done to rule out transient clinical dehydration or laboratory error.

To classify absolute polycythemia as primary or secondary (Table 169-1), a serum erythropoietin level is essential. Evidence of chronic respiratory disease or hypoxemia on physical examination should be followed up with arterial blood gas to confirm low arterial oxygen saturation. Co-oximetry of arterial blood can also quantify carboxyhemoglobin, which will be elevated in polycythemia caused by chronic carbon monoxide exposure. Other laboratory investigations should be guided by clinical assessment of the most likely underlying cause of polycythemia, but may include screening tests for renal and liver function, serum ferritin level, hemoglobin electrophoresis, hemoglobin oxygen-affinity (p50) testing, and *JAK2* mutation analysis (see MPD in Chapter 174 [Hematologic Malignancies]).

■ IMAGING

Chest x-ray and/or computed tomography (CT) scan may be used to confirm findings on clinical evaluation or to exclude occult disease. Ultrasound can evaluate for splenomegaly (associated with MPDs), local renal vascular disease, or neoplastic processes causing increased EPO or testosterone production.

■ OTHER INVESTIGATIONS

A formal sleep study is indicated if the patient has clear signs and symptoms of obstructive sleep apnea. Bone marrow exam is rarely indicated in the workup of polycythemia.

■ TRIAGE AND HOSPITAL ADMISSION

Many of the conditions causing secondary polycythemia can present with acute illness and these cases should be triaged accordingly. Polycythemia in and of itself is not an indication for hospital admission, but it can be associated with severe symptoms and complications (see Diagnosis earlier in this chapter), which may necessitate acute medical attention.

■ TREATMENT

Goals of treatment in primary polycythemia include decreasing chronic symptoms due to hyperviscosity and increased RBC turnover, and reducing the long-term risk of thrombotic complications. Reduction of hemoglobin concentration may be achieved by a program of repeated phlebotomies and/or cytoreductive agents, such as hydroxyurea. A randomized trial showed lower rates of cardiovascular and thrombotic complications in polycythemia vera patients who were kept at a target hematocrit of less than 45%. Acetylsalicylic acid has been shown to reduce the risk of thrombotic events in polycythemia vera with minimal increase in risk of bleeding. Traditional risk factors for vascular disease should be managed as appropriate.

For patients with secondary erythrocytosis, the main principle of management is treatment of the underlying disorder.

■ COMPLICATIONS

Complications of primary polycythemia can include venous or arterial thrombotic events. Over time, a small percentage of patients develop myelofibrosis or, more rarely, acute myeloid leukemia. Bone marrow examination should be performed if progression of marrow disease is suspected.

■ RARE CAUSES FOR CONSIDERATION

In rare instances, primary or secondary polycythemia can be congenital. Congenital mutation of the EPO receptor can result in the EPO receptor being chronically "switched on." Congenital low 2,3-bisphosphoglycerate is associated with less off-loading of oxygen by hemoglobin at the peripheral tissues, and a compensatory increase in endogenous EPO.

■ DISCHARGE CONSIDERATIONS

In any patient diagnosed with polycythemia, discharge planning should include a plan for routine monitoring of hemoglobin and hematocrit. The frequency and duration of follow-up will be tailored to the cause and severity of polycythemia.

THALASSEMIA AND HEMOGLOBINOPATHIES

■ INTRODUCTION

The hemoglobinopathies are genetic disorders affecting the production, structure, or function of the globin chains that form hemoglobin contained within red cells. These are one of most common genetic diseases known, with worldwide estimates of 270 million carriers, and more than 300,000 infants born each year with clinically severe abnormalities. The hemoglobin tetramer is made from two pairs of globin chains, each attached to a heme group. Normally three types are of hemoglobin can be detected by electrophoretic techniques: HbA ($\alpha_2\beta_2$), the predominant adult form; HbF ($\alpha_2\gamma_2$), found at high levels in newborns; and a minor amount of HbA_2 ($\alpha_2\delta_2$). The genes responsible for producing these globin proteins are found on two gene clusters; chromosome 16p13.3 is the location for two alpha (α) globin genes, and on chromosome 11p15.5 are the beta (β), delta (δ), and gamma (γ) globin genes. Currently more than 1400 mutations have been described in the α, β, δ, and γ globin genes, which are categorized and listed on the

World Wide Web (http://globin.cse.psu.edu) with novel mutations continually being discovered. Heterozygous carriers of globin gene mutations are typically asymptomatic but can present with microcytosis, hemolysis, anemia, cyanosis, or erythrocytosis, depending on the underlying defect. Individuals who are homozygous or compound heterozygous for specific types of globin gene mutations can present with serious disease states ranging from thalassemia major, a condition that requires lifelong transfusion therapy, to severe sickling syndromes presenting with chronic hemolysis and periodic painful sickle cell crises. The detection and diagnosis of the hemoglobinopathies largely relies on a good clinical history and the correlation of physical findings, such as splenomegaly, with results of diagnostic laboratory tests. The most common hemoglobin disorders—sickle cell disease and thalassemia—can be diagnosed easily in most clinical laboratories; however, complex unusual cases may require further more sophisticated investigations including DNA-based procedures. Sickle cell disease is covered in more detail in this chapter.

◼ PATHOPHYSIOLOGY

The hemoglobin (Hb) tetramer contains four subunits, each containing a globin attached to a molecule of heme, a protein structure that transports oxygen efficiently. The major hemoglobin found in individuals older than 6 months is HbA, or adult hemoglobin, consisting of two α- and two β-globin subunits. The hemoglobin disorders are genetic mutations in these globin chains that can be divided into two broad categories: the "variants," in which qualitative changes in the globin chain structure may result in an abnormal function or electrophoretic properties, and the "thalassemias," in which reduced production of globin chains leads to a decrease in hemoglobin, resulting in a microcytic, hypochromic anemia. Hemoglobin disorders are most commonly found in people from malaria-endemic regions, where high gene prevalence has been attributed to a survival advantage for carriers. However, due to global population migration, these disorders are now found in all regions, including North America and northern Europe. Thus, consideration for an individual's ethnicity may be useful, but should not be the sole criterion to determine if a search for a hemoglobin disorder is indicated.

◼ HEMOGLOBIN VARIANTS

Most hemoglobin variants are due to single nucleotide point mutations in the globin genes that change the amino acid sequence. A variant hemoglobin can also result from deletions or gene rearrangements that lead to fusion of two globin genes, changes in the stop codon of the globin gene resulting in extending globin chains, or multiple nucleic acid substitutions at two different positions in the globin gene. Although most mutations are rare and of no clinical consequence, some can cause severe or lifelong conditions. Examples are HbS (β codon 6 GAG > GTG Glu > Val) causing sickle cell disease or HbC (β codon 6 GAG > AAG Glu > Lys), which, when combined with HbS, also causes a significant sickling disorder; and HbE (β codon 26 GAG > AAG or Glu > Lys), which can contribute to severe β-thalassemia syndromes. Other common variants are HbD, Hb Lepore, HbO, and Hb Constant Spring.

◼ THALASSEMIA

The most important thalassemia syndromes are those that affect either the α- or β-globin chains. Thalassemias can be caused by point mutations that reduce or eliminate the globin gene production. Thalassemia may also be the result of insertions or deletions in the gene itself that downregulate gene expression, or from a total deletion of the globin gene. Abnormalities affecting α-globin chain production are termed α-thalassemia and those affecting β-globin production are called β-thalassemia. Some mutations that affect globin gene expression may also produce detectable hemoglobin variants. The most common variants that present with a thalassemia phenotype are HbE (β codon 26 GAG > AAG or Glu →Lys), Hb Lepore (caused by a δ-β fusion globin chain), or Hb Constant Spring (α2 codon 142 TAA > CAA or Ter →Gln).

◼ CLINICALLY SIGNIFICANT HEMOGLOBINOPATHIES

The most common clinically significant hemoglobinopathies can be divided into three distinct syndromes: the sickle cell syndromes, the α-thalassemia syndromes, and the β-thalassemia syndromes. They are normally inherited as autosomal recessive abnormalities (ie, heterozygous individuals are asymptomatic), whereas homozygous or compound heterozygous individuals are severely affected. Other rare globin gene mutations may be inherited as autosomal dominant expression. These include the unstable hemoglobins (implicated in Heinz body-induced hemolysis), the high oxygen affinity hemoglobins (presenting with secondary compensated erythrocytosis), the low oxygen affinity hemoglobins, and HbM variants.

Therefore, reasons to correctly diagnose the hemoglobinoapthies are:

1. Diagnosis of serious or life-threatening hemoglobin abnormalities to plan for appropriate preventative management (eg, penicillin prophylaxis and pneumococcal vaccination in infants with sickle cell disease) and medical treatment (eg, chronic transfusion program and chelation therapy in β-thalassemia major).
2. Investigation of microcytic anemia to identify individuals with thalassemia trait so that unnecessary investigations (eg, endoscopy) and treatment for presumed iron deficiency can be avoided.
3. Identification of individuals of reproductive age who are carriers of clinically significant hemoglobin mutations to initiate proper genetic counseling and guide future reproductive decisions.

α-Thalassemia syndromes

Normally, individuals have four α globin genes—two on each chromosome 16. Carriers of α thalassemia have deletions of one (α/αα) or two (-/αα or α/-α) of the α globin genes. Deletion of three α globin genes results in hemoglobin H disease (HbH: -/-α). Deletion of all four α globin genes typically results in hydrops fetalis, which is not compatible with life unless antenatal diagnosis is followed by in utero transfusion. Rarely, α-thalassemia syndromes are caused by nondeletional mutations, such as Hb Constant Spring, which have the same effect as a single α gene deletion. Deletion of one α globin gene (referred to as α⁺-thalassemia) is often seen in individuals of African, Mediterranean, and Southeast Asian ethnic backgrounds, while deletion of two α globin genes in cis (- -αα; referred to as α⁰-thalassemia) is most often seen in the Southeast Asian population. The most commonly reported α-thalassemia genotypes are presented with the clinical presentation and reproductive significance in **Table 169-5**.

β-Thalassemia syndromes

Normally, individuals inherit two β-globin genes, one on each chromosome 11. β-Thalassemia syndromes are most often a result of point mutations, or small deletions or insertions in the β-globin gene. These mutations either reduce the β-globin chain production (β⁺-thalassemia mutations) or completely eliminate β-globin production from the affected gene (β⁰-thalassemia mutations). Also some β-chain variants can present as thalassemia phenotypes that are clinically severe when inherited as compound heterozygous (eg, HbE/β-thalassemia and Hb Lepore/β-thalassemia). There is a high prevalence of β-thalassemia in the African, Mediterranean, Middle Eastern, Indian, and Southeast Asian ethnic populations. Hemoglobin E is most commonly found in Southeast Asian populations, while Hb Lepore is found in Mediterranean, African, and Southeast Asian populations. These most commonly detected β-thalassemia

TABLE 169-5 The Clinical Presentation, Genotypes, and Reproductive Significance of the Various α–Thalassemia Syndromes

Hemoglobinopathy	Clinical Presentation	Genotypes	Reproductive Significance
α^+-Thalassemia heterozygous	Normal to mild microcytosis	$-\alpha/\alpha\alpha$ or $\alpha^T\alpha/\alpha\alpha$	Carrier for Hb H disease
Hb Constant Spring	Normal to mild microcytosis	$\alpha^{CS}\alpha/\alpha\alpha$	Carrier for Hb H/Hb Constant Spring Disease
Homozygous α^+-thalassemia	Microcytosis, normal Hb or mild anemia	$-\alpha/-\alpha$	Carrier for Hb H disease
α^0-Thalassemia trait	Microcytosis, normal Hb or mild anemia	$--/\alpha\alpha$	Carrier for Hb Bart Hydrops fetalis, and Hb H disease
Hb H disease, Hb H/Hb Constant Spring disease	Mild to moderate microcytosis with hemolytic anemia	$--/-\alpha$ or $\alpha^T\alpha/--$ or $\alpha^{CS}\alpha/--$	Carrier for Hb Bart hydrops fetalis and Hb H disease
Hb Bart hydrops fetalis	High-risk pregnancy with fetal death without *in utero* transfusion interventions	$--/--$	Carrier for Hb Bart hydrops fetalis and Hb H disease

$-\alpha/\alpha\alpha$, a thalassemia caused by a single-gene deletion; $\alpha^T\alpha/\alpha\alpha$, a thalassemia caused by a point mutation; $--/\alpha\alpha$, $\alpha\alpha$ thalassemia caused by a two-gene deletion in *cis*; α^{CS}, Constant Spring mutation of alpha gene.
Adapted, with permission, from Lafferty JD, Waye JS, Chui DH, et al. Good practice guidelines for laboratory investigation of hemoglobinopathies. *Lab Hematol.* 2003;9(4):237-245.

genotypes are presented with the clinical presentation and reproductive significance in Table 169-5. "β-thalassemia major" is used to describe patients who are transfusion dependent from infancy or early childhood (usually due to homozygosity or compound heterozygosity for β⁰-thalassemia), whereas "β-thalassemia intermedia" refers to patients with anemia that is more severe than that of someone with β-thalassemia trait, but less severe than typical β-thalassemia major (**Table 169-6**).

■ DIAGNOSIS: DOES THIS PATIENT HAVE A CLINICALLY SIGNIFICANT HEMOGLOBINOPATHY?

A patient who has an ethnic background with a high prevalence of hemoglobinopathies and a positive family history of anemia, chronic transfusions, painful sickle cell crises, or hydrops fetalis should alert the physician to the possibility of congenital hemoglobin disorders. However, heterozygous carriers of most hemoglobinopathies are asymptomatic and clinically well. A good clinical history is important, including demographic information.

The laboratory diagnosis of hemoglobinoapthies begins with a CBC and peripheral blood smear, specifically looking at the appearance of the RBCs, the hemoglobin level, and erythrocyte indices (**Figure 169-2**).

A low mean corpuscular volume and mean corpuscular hemoglobin (MCH) are associated with microcytosis and hypochromasia. These values may be indicative of thalassemia but need to be differentiated from iron-deficiency anemia or anemia of chronic disease (ACD), which may also present with microcytic, hypochromic anemia (see the Anemia section earlier in this chapter). Individuals with uncomplicated α- or β-thalassemia trait will usually have normal iron studies. However, a diagnosis of IDA or ACD does not rule out coexisting thalassemia trait.

Hemoglobin separation

Separation of the hemoglobin fractions are used to detect variant hemoglobins. In a normal adult, HbA, HbA₂, and HbF should all be present. Traditionally, hemoglobin separation has been done using

TABLE 169-6 The Clinical Presentation and Reproductive Significance of the Various β-Thalassemia Syndromes

Hemoglobinopathy	Clinical Presentation	Genotypes	Reproductive Significance
β-Thalassemia trait	Microcytosis with normal Hb or mild anemia, elevated HbA2	β^A/β^0, β^A/β^+	Carrier for β-thalassemia major or β-thalassemia intermedia or HbS/β-thalassemia
δ-β-Thalassemia trait	Microcytosis with normal Hb or mild anemia, normal HbA2 and elevated HbF	$\beta^A/\delta\beta$ Thal	Carrier for β-thalassemia intermedia
HbE trait or homozygous HbE	Normal to microcytosis, normal Hb or mild anemia	β^A/δ^E or β^E/β^E	Carrier for β-thalassemia intermedia or major
Hb Lepore trait	Microcytosis with normal Hb or mild anemia	β^A/β^{Lepore}	Carrier for β-thalassemia intermedia or major
β-Thalassemia intermedia	Moderate microcytosis with anemia sometimes requiring intermittent transfusion	β^+/β^E or β^+/β^+ or β^+/β^0 or β^+/β^{Lepore} or $\beta^0/\delta\beta$, or $\beta^+/\delta\beta$ or $\delta\beta/\delta\beta$ or β Thal with excess α globin genes	Carrier for β-thalassemia intermedia or major or HbS/β⁺ or HbS/β⁰-thalassemia
β-Thalassemia major	Transfusion-dependent microcytic anemia	β^0/β^0 or β^0/β^E or β^0/β^{Lepore} or $\beta^{Lepore}/\beta^{Lepore}$	Carrier for β-thalassemia intermedia or major

β^A, normal β-globin gene; β^0, beta-zero mutation (no β-globin gene produced); β^+, beta-zero mutation (reduced β-globin gene production); δ-β, delta-beta thalassemia deletion; β^E, HbE; β^{Lepore}, Hb Lepore.
(Adapted, with permission, from Lafferty JD, Waye JS, Chui DH, et al. Good practice guidelines for laboratory investigation of hemoglobinopathies. *Lab Hematol.* 2003;9(4):237-245.)

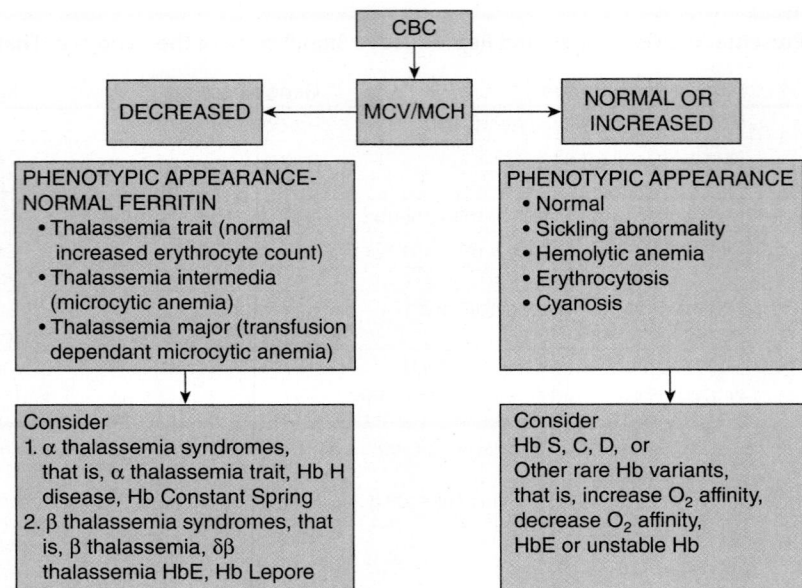

Figure 169-2 *Preliminary hemoglobinopathy considerations based on the MCV/MCH. (A normal RDW is not a reliable indicator of the thalassemia trait as it can be normal in some genotypes of thalassemia and abnormal in others.) MCV, mean corpuscular volume; MCH, mean corpuscular hemoglobin. (Adapted, with permission, from Lafferty JD, Waye JS, Chui DH, et al. Good practice guidelines for laboratory investigation of hemoglobinopathies.* Lab Hematol. *2003;9(4):237-245.)*

alkaline and acid electrophoresis. Although these methods are still used in some laboratories as initial screening for variant hemoglobin identification, automated methods are available that not only separate the hemoglobin fractions but also provide accurate quantification of the hemoglobin fractions.

1. **High performance liquid chromatography (HPLC):** One of the automated systems commonly used for hemoglobinopathy screening is a cation-exchange HPLC, a method based on elution of hemoglobin fractions on a chromatography column. The HPLC system quantifies the hemoglobin fractions, provides accurate levels of HbA, HbA$_2$, and HbF, and has good resolving power to detect many of the variant hemoglobins.

2. **Capillary electrophoresis (CE):** Capillary electrophoresis is an automated system available for hemoglobin separation and quantification. A hemoglobin solution migrates through a buffer solution contained in fine capillary tubes when an electrical current is applied. These automated systems have excellent resolving power, providing a rapid and sensitive method of hemoglobin separation and quantification.

Functional investigations

1. **P$_{50}$ analysis:** Hemoglobins that have changed oxygen affinity can be identified by performing a P$_{50}$ analysis or oxygen dissociation curve. Some variant hemoglobins will have a high O$_2$ affinity resulting in erythrocytosis or low oxygen affinity causing anemia or cyanosis. Several of these hemoglobin variants will show no differences in electrophoretic mobility from HbA.

2. **Stability testing:** Hemoglobin instability can be demonstrated by exposing hemoglobin to excessive heat or incubating it with a buffered isopropyl alcohol. These unstable hemoglobin variants may also be identified by increased Heinz body detection and the presence of bite cells and dense fragments in the peripheral red cell morphology.

3. **HbM testing:** Some variants will produce a methemoglobinemia that can be identified through performing a unique absorption spectral scan. These are a specific group of variant hemoglobins that produce methemoglobin called the HbMs.

4. **Molecular diagnostics:** Molecular diagnosis and DNA analysis are used for positive characterization of variant hemoglobins or confirmation of thalassemia. These are performed on DNA and include polymerize chain reaction (PCR), direct nucleotide sequencing, southern hybridization and multiplex ligation-dependent probe amplification (MLPA) techniques.

■ INTERPRETATION OF LABORATORY INVESTIGATIONS

In the setting of a suspected hemoglobin disorder, one must correlate laboratory findings with the patient's age, gender, ethnicity, and reproductive status. Standard investigations cannot definitively diagnose all clinically important variant hemoglobins. Interpretation of hemoglobinopathy investigations can be challenging. Therefore guidance from a knowledgeable laboratory professional can be helpful in determining if a clinically significant hemoglobin disorder is present.

Alpha-thalassemia syndromes are associated with microcytosis (see Table 169-5). Silent carriers (-α/αα) may have microcytosis without significant anemia, whereas individuals with two α genes deleted (-/αα or -α/-α) generally have a mild microcytic anemia. HbH disease (-/-α) is associated with moderate microcytic anemia that becomes more severe during pregnancy or acute illness. Unfortunately, hemoglobin separation methods do not always add additional information when α-thalassemia syndromes are suspected; it is most common to find normal proportions of HbA, HbF, and HbA$_2$. If HbH (β^4) is detected, it can aid in diagnosis. However, this hemoglobin is fast moving on gel electrophoresis, and may run off the gel prior to completion of the test. Furthermore, HbH is not always present in sufficient quantities for detection by standard methods. In practice, DNA analysis is often required to confirm α-thalassemia syndromes. After sufficient investigations have ruled out other common causes of microcytic anemia (eg, IDA, ACD), DNA analysis for α-thalassemia may be required to confirm most α-thalassemia syndromes. DNA testing for α thalassemia is advised in all pregnant women with unexplained microcytic anemia.

β-thalassemia trait is also associated with a microcytic anemia (see Table 169-6). Furthermore, HbA$_2$ is characteristically elevated (>3.5%) (**Table 169-7**). In cases in which there is δβ-thalassemia

TABLE 169-7 Typical Adult Hemoglobin Patterns*

	HbA	HbA2	Other Hemoglobins
Normal	95%-98%	<3.5%	—
α-Thalassemia—all types	95%-98%	<3.5%	—
β-Thalassemia trait	95%	>3.5%	—
δ-β-Thalassemia trait	80%-90%	<3.5%	Will have elevated HbF (5%-15%)
HbE trait	~70%	<5%	HbE = 25%-30%
HbE homozygous		<5%	HbE = 85%-95%

*HbF will also be present in small quantities with all of the above genotypes. Proportion varies, based on several genetic modifiers but typically represents <2%.

trait or β-thalassemia trait with a coexisting δ-globin mutation, HbA₂ level may be normal. In β-thalassemia major, the patient, by definition, is making very little or no HbA. In practice, because these patients require routine transfusion of donor blood, hemoglobin separation methods will show normal proportions of HbA, HbF, and HbA₂ expected from donor RBCs. Thalassemias can also be diagnosed in patients that have an elevated HbF quantity in the presence of a low MCV and MCH. Alternately, elevated HbF can be seen in individuals with hereditary persistence of fetal hemoglobin (HPFH), who are clinically well, with a normal MCV and MCH.

HbE is another cause of microcytic anemia. Heterozygous HbE is asymptomatic and is not associated with anemia, but RBCs can be slightly microcytic (MCV 80 ± 5 fL). Homozygous HbE is also asymptomatic, with most individuals having a mild anemia (11.4 ± 1.8) and microcytosis (MCV 70 ± 4 fL). Target cells represent 20% to 80% of RBCs. Typical adult hemoglobin patterns are presented in Table 169-7.

Homozygosity for the HbS mutation (HbSS), or compound heterozygosity for HbS and other β-globin mutations (eg, β-thalassemia, HbC, HbO, HbD) are associated with important clinical complications (see Sickle Cell Disease section of this chapter). Most other variant hemoglobins are not clinically significant and do not cause disease. An individual who is heterozygous for a β-globin gene mutation will present with one variant hemoglobin in a quantity slightly less in amount than HbA (eg, HbE in Table 169-7). When a patient is heterozygous for an α-globin gene mutations, he or she will usually have one variant hemoglobin in a quantity of approximately 10% to 25%, and the majority of the remaining hemoglobin will be normal HbA.

■ TRIAGE AND HOSPITAL ADMISSION

The thalassemias and hemoglobinopathies can present in diverse ways. Heterozygosity for globin gene deletions and mutations is usually asymptomatic or may be associated with mild anemia. These patients can be investigated as an outpatient.

Individuals with clinically significant disorders of hemoglobin, including β-thalassemia major, are usually diagnosed in early childhood and require close medical care and follow-up. Illness requiring inpatient treatment may develop due to acute worsening of anemia or transfusion related complications, including organ dysfunction due to chronic iron overload (see Complications below).

■ TREATMENT

Patients with β-thalassemia major (also referred to as transfusion-dependent thalassemia) require routine, chronic transfusion of RBCs (eg, every 3 to 4 weeks). For most patients, a target pretransfusion hemoglobin of 9 to 11 g/dL is appropriate. Higher levels (11-12 g/dL) may be necessary for patients with cardiorespiratory disease. Post-transfusion hemoglobin should not exceed 14 to 15g/dL.

As a result of the frequency and volume of RBC transfusions, most patients develop significant iron overload early in childhood and require lifelong chelation therapy. Care of these patients is optimally provided by a specialized, multidisciplinary, comprehensive care clinic.

■ COMPLICATIONS

Complications of thalassemia can be divided into complications of the disease itself, and complications of transfusion therapy. Historically, patients who have received inadequate chronic transfusion develop diffuse bone marrow expansion. Expansion of marrow production in atypical sites (eg, skull and maxillary bones) leads to the characteristic "thalassemic facies," with frontal bossing and prominent maxillae. Expansion of bone marrow in the pelvis and long bones leads to thinning of the bony cortex, high risk of fractures, and delayed growth.

With modern practices of regular RBC transfusion, many of these historical complications are now avoided. However, RBC transfusion is associated with risks that may include hemolytic transfusion reactions, alloimmunization, febrile nonhemolytic transfusion reaction, or transfusion-transmitted infection. All patients who are on a program of chronic transfusion should be vaccinated for hepatitis B virus.

Iron overload is an expected complication in all chronically transfused patients, since each milliliter of RBC transfusion contains 1 mg of iron—at least 200 mg of iron per unit of RBCs transfused. Since the human body has no mechanism for excreting excess iron, once body iron stores are replete, unnecessary free iron is deposited in the tissues, leading to organ dysfunction. Serum ferritin and transferrin saturation are easy tests to screen for iron overload. Although there is no widely accepted target for serum ferritin, it is well understood that increasing serum ferritin concentrations are associated with increased risk of iron deposition in the liver. Over time, significant iron overload of the heart, pancreas, and pituitary will follow if chelation is not initiated. Current practice in patients with β-thalassemia major is to start chelation after the first 20 transfusion or when the serum ferritin level rises above 1000. Chelation treatment usually commences at 2 to 3 years of age and continues throughout life. Three chelating agents are currently available: deferoxamine (parenteral), deferasirox (oral), and deferiprone (oral) (**Table 169-8**).

■ RARE CAUSES FOR CONSIDERATION: DETECTION AND DIAGNOSIS OF RARE HEMOGLOBIN VARIANTS

To date more than 1400 globin chain mutations have been described. The majority is not clinically significant and can be detected by routine testing. Variants found in patients who are clinically well and hematologically normal are unlikely to be clinically significant. However, some rare variants that are clinically significant are difficult to detect through conventional hemoglobin separation techniques and may require further specialized analysis as outlined in **Table 169-9**. Deoxyribonucleic acid investigation may be the only analysis that can definitively identify these hemoglobins and should be considered in patients who have pertinent symptoms.

■ THE UNSTABLE HEMOGLOBINS

Rare hemoglobin variants may denature readily, causing chronic hemolysis and anemia. The denatured globin precipitates in the RBC, producing Heinz bodies that are removed from the red cells by the spleen. Peripheral blood smear shows bite cells, irregularly contracted erythrocytes, or dense fragments. Other laboratory findings provide supporting evidence for active hemolysis (eg, elevated reticulocyte count, reduced haptoglobin). Unstable hemoglobins can fall into two categories: spontaneously unstable variants that result in congenital Heinz body hemolysis (eg, Hb Köln) or milder

TABLE 169-8 Dosing, Administration, and Possible Adverse Effects with Iron Chelating Agents

	Common Starting Dose and Administration	Maximum Daily Dose	Possible Adverse Effects
Deferoxamine	20 mg/kg administered by subcutaneous infusion over 8-12 h, 5-7 nights/wk (up to a maximum of)	60 mg/kg	Infusion site reactions; vision or hearing abnormalities; skeletal and growth abnormalities; zinc deficiency; Yersinia enterocolitica infection
Deferasirox	20-40 mg/kg administered by mouth daily (suspended in water)	40 mg/kg	Rash, GI symptoms; mild elevation in transaminases; hearing impairment; nonprogressive elevation in serum creatinine
Deferiprone	75 mg/kg/d in three divided doses	100 mg/kg	Agranulocytosis; arthalgias, zinc deficiency; mild GI symptoms and mild aminotransferase elevations

forms that present with hemolysis after ingestion of oxidative drugs. The unstable hemoglobins can be difficult to detect using conventional hemoglobin variant detection techniques and the diagnosis may rely on the erythrocyte morphology, Heinz body count, specialized tests to demonstrate in vitro instability, and DNA investigations.

■ HIGH OXYGEN AFFINITY HEMOGLOBIN VARIANTS

Hemoglobin variants that hold on to oxygen more avidly than HbA are called "high oxygen affinity" hemoglobins. Increased oxygen affinity results in tissue hypoxia that stimulates the production of erythropoietin leading to an erythrocytosis. These patients tend to be asymptomatic but can present with symptoms of increased blood viscosity. Since many of these variants do not separate by routine hemoglobin separation techniques, specialized analysis to measure oxygen equilibration curve and the partial pressure of oxygen at 50% saturation (called the P_{50} value) can be used in diagnosis. Alternately the P_{50} can be calculated by venous blood gas values. DNA analysis can confirm and characterize high oxygen affinity variants.

■ LOW OXYGEN AFFINITY HEMOGLOBIN VARIANTS

Some hemoglobin variants have a lower affinity for oxygen and therefore release oxygen more readily than HbA. This can suppress the production of erythropoietin, leading to a lower hemoglobin level. Like the unstable and high oxygen affinity variants, many hemoglobins with a low oxygen affinity will not separate from HbA using conventional Hb-separation techniques. The detection of an abnormal low oxygen affinity often relies on the clinical presentation correlated with the P_{50} value and a DNA investigation.

■ THE M HEMOGLOBINS

Patients presenting with cyanosis can also have an HbM. These hemoglobin variants have an accumulation of methemoglobin in the circulating red cells that causes a pseudocyanosis or brownish/slate pigmentation of the skin. The M hemoglobins also can be difficult to detect using conventional Hb variant-detection techniques. Detection relies on demonstration of abnormal absorption spectra followed by DNA investigation.

■ DISCHARGE CONSIDERATIONS

Close follow-up should be arranged for patients with complications of hemoglobinopathy. For patients with clinically symptomatic thalassemia syndromes, follow-up with a comprehensive care clinic is suggested.

SICKLE CELL DISEASE
■ INTRODUCTION

Sickle cell disease (SCD) is characterized by atypical red cells that assume a sickle shape when deoxygenated. The inheritance of a single sickle cell gene (heterozygous HbS, or sickle cell trait) offers a survival advantage against malaria, which has contributed to the high gene prevalence of HbS in many regions of Sub-Saharan Africa, the Middle East, India, and the Mediterranean. In part due to global immigration patterns, sickle cell disease has become one of the most common hemoglobinopathies seen worldwide. Patients with sickle cell disease are homozygous for the sickle gene (HbSS) or compound heterozygous for the HbS gene mutation and another β-globin gene mutation. Individuals with SCD have a decreased life expectancy and may present with severe clinical complications that can lead to death if not properly treated. Screening for this disorder has been the focus for many newborn screening programs across most of North America and Europe to ensure early prophylaxis is given for reduced mortality and morbidity.

■ PATHOPHYSIOLOGY

Hemoglobin S is the result of a substitution of valine for glutamic acid at the sixth amino acid of the β-globin chain that decreases the solubility of the hemoglobin molecule in the deoxygenated state

TABLE 169-9 Detection and Diagnosis of Clinically Significant Rare Hemoglobinopathy Syndromes

Rare Syndrome	Presentation	Detection	Hb Variant Identification
Unstable hemoglobins	Chronic or sporadic hemolytic anemia	• Abnormal erythrocyte morphology • Elevated Heinz body counts • Abnormal Hb instability testing (heat or isopropanol) • Suspicious HbH inclusion bodies	DNA sequencing
High oxygen affinity	Erythrocytosis	Hb oxygen affinity analysis -(p50)	DNA sequencing
Low oxygen affinity	Anemia, cyanosis	Hb oxygen affinity analysis -(p50)	DNA sequencing
Hemoglobin M	Cyanosis	Methemoglobin absorption spectrum	DNA sequencing

(Adapted, with permission, from Lafferty JD, Waye JS, Chui DH, et al. Good practice guidelines for laboratory investigation of hemoglobinopathies. *Lab Hematol.* 2003;9(4):237-245.)

TABLE 169-10 The Genotypes, Clinical Presentation, and Reproductive Significance of the Sickle Cell Syndromes

Hemoglobinopathy	Clinical Presentation	Genotypes	Reproductive Significance
HbS trait	None	β^A/β^S	Carrier for all sickling disorders
HbC trait	None	β^A/β^C	Carrier for HbSC disease and HbC disease
HbC disease	Occasional mild hemolytic anemia	β^C/β^C	Carrier for HbSC disease and HbC disease
HbD trait	None	β^A/β^D	Carrier for HbSD disease
HbO^Arab trait	None	β^A/β^{OArab}	Carrier for HbSO disease
β-Thalassemia trait	Microcytosis with normal Hb or mild anemia	β^A/β^0 or β^A/β^+	Carrier for HbS/β-thalassemia
Sickle cell disease	Severe sickling abnormality	β^S/β^S	Carrier for all sickling disorders
HbSβ⁰-thalassemia,	Microcytosis, severe sickling abnormality	β^S/β^0	Carrier for all sickling disorders or HbSβ⁰-thalassemia or thalassemia intermedia or major
HbSD disease	Severe sickling abnormality	β^S/β^D	Carrier for HbSD or all sickling disorders
HbSβ⁺-thalassemia	Microcytosis, mild to moderate sickling abnormality	β^S/β^+	Carrier for all sickling disorders or HbSβ⁺-thalassemia or β-thalassemia intermedia
HbSC disease, HbSO disease	Mild to moderate sickling abnormality	β^S/β^C or β^S/β^{OArab}	Carrier for all sickling disorders

β^A, normal β globin gene; β^S, HbS gene; β^C, HbC gene; β^D, HbD gene; β^{O-Arab}, HbO^Arab gene; β^0, beta-zero mutation (no β globin gene produced); β^+, beta-zero mutation (reduced β globin gene production).
(Adapted, with permission, from Lafferty JD, Waye JS, Chui DH, et al. Good practice guidelines for laboratory investigation of hemoglobinopathies. *Lab Hematol.* 2003;9(4):237-245.)

causing hemoglobin polymerization and sickle cell formation. The homozygous expression of HbS and the corresponding absence of HbA cause a severe sickling disorder, in which hemoglobin polymerization initiates an elaborate pathophysiological cascade involving RBC injury, release of free hemoglobin into the blood, and adhesive interactions among sickle RBCs, endothelial cells, and other blood cells. Damaged RBCs initiate vessel occlusion and ischemia. Furthermore, the ongoing premature destruction of these sickle cells leads to chronic anemia.

The compound heterozygous inheritance of HbS with other β-globin chain variants (HbC, HbD, HbO^Arab, or β-thalassemia trait) may also result in an absence of HbA and a severe sickling syndrome. These genotypes are detailed in **Table 169-10**. Sickle cell disease is associated with an increased risk of death from sepsis, acute chest syndrome or stroke, and chronic complications that accumulate with age.

■ DIAGNOSIS: DOES THIS PATIENT HAVE ACUTE COMPLICATIONS OF SICKLE CELL DISEASE?

Evaluation of a patient with sickle cell disease will begin with a thorough history and physical. History should include details of clinical symptoms (eg, bony pain, chest pain, or shortness of breath) and a history of previous complications and medical care. In patients with pain, it is critical to determine whether the pain is due to a vaso-occlusive crisis (pain related to sickling of RBCs) or whether another process may be responsible (eg, abdominal pain due to acute cholecytitis). As the patient is likely to have had numerous sickle painful episodes in his or her lifetime, asking the patient, "Is this your typical sickle cell pain?" can help guide whether further investigations are required.

Vital signs should be measured, including pulse oximetry. Hypoxemia can suggest an underlying acute chest syndrome, pneumonia or pulmonary embolism. Hypoxemia is also a risk factor for worsened RBC sickling.

Adult patients are usually aware of their diagnosis of sickle cell disease. However, if the diagnosis or the genotype is in question, further testing may be performed. A CBC will show variable degrees of anemia. Peripheral blood smear should show sickled RBCs. Target cells and Howell-Jolly bodies suggest functional asplenia, associated with splenic autoinfarction—a common complication of sickle cell disease in childhood. Reticulocytes are elevated due to hemolysis

of sickle cells. White blood cell count may be elevated if infection is present.

The sickle solubility test

The HbS solubility test is a simple screening test able to detect HbS. When reduced with sodium dithionite, HbS is insoluble and precipitates in high molarity phosphate buffer at neutral pH. An HbS solubility test is useful as a screening test for HbS in adult patients and as a confirmatory test when HbS is detected by either electrophoresis or HPLC, helping to distinguish HbS from other variants with similar migrating mobility as HbS. The sickle solubility test cannot distinguish between sickle cell trait, sickle cell disease, or HbS/β-thalassemia. The test is negative when the concentration of HbS is less than 15%, and thus it is not used to test blood samples from infants or patients who have received RBC transfusion. Importantly, the test cannot detect hemoglobin variants such as HbS, C, D Punjab, and O^Arab, which can cause a sickling disorder in combination with HbS. Thus, HbS solubility tests should not be used for assessment of potential reproductive risk, for genetic counseling, or as a primary diagnostic test.

Hemoglobin separation and molecular diagnostics

Methods such as gel electrophoresis, HPLC, and CE are effective for identifying the presence of HbS and/or other variant hemoglobins involved in compound heterozygous sickle cell disease. For more details on these methods, see Hemoglobin Separation in Thalassemia and Hemoglobinopathies section of this chapter. Molecular diagnostics and DNA analysis are used for positive characterization of the variant hemoglobin(s). Methods used include PCR, direct nucleotide sequencing, and southern hybridization.

■ TRIAGE AND HOSPITAL ADMISSION

Painful episodes are the most frequent complication in sickle cell disease. Patients who have had recurrent episodes may be treated at home with oral analgesics (acetaminophen, NSAIDs, or opiates). If the episode is more severe, they may require higher-dose therapy in a hospital-based setting. Severe pain requiring repeated doses of IV analgesia is best treated as an inpatient. Other supportive care should include judicious administration of intravenous fluid. Supplemental oxygen is indicated if the SpO_2 or SaO_2 are low. Painful episodes may take several days to a week or more to resolve.

Other indications for admission include acute chest syndrome, sepsis, stroke, and hyperhemolysis. These complications are best managed in an intensive care setting.

■ TREATMENT

Outpatient treatment of sickle cell disease can be divided into preventative care and symptom management. Preventative care includes penicillin prophylaxis in children, immunizations (especially against encapsulated organisms such as *Streptococcus pneumoniae*, *Hemophilus influenzae*, and *Neisseria meningitides*) and patient education to avoid extremes of heat, remain hydrated, and seek rapid medical attention in case of symptoms. In pediatric populations, there is evidence that chronic RBC transfusion is effective at preventing stroke in certain high-risk groups.

Hydroxyurea is increasingly used to prevent vaso-occlusive crises and hemolysis. There is good evidence in patients with HbSS that hydroxyurea leads to significantly fewer painful episodes, fewer episodes of chest syndrome, and reduced need for transfusion and hospitalization, with few side effects. Long-term follow-up data suggest that there is also a decrease in mortality proportional to the number of years on hydroxyurea therapy. The exact mechanism of improved clinical outcomes with hydroxyurea in SCD is unknown, although it is known that hemoglobin level and HbF percentage improve while on the medication, both of which are associated with less severe sickle cell disease phenotype. Hydroxyurea also results in reduced leukocyte count, which may have an anti-inflammatory effect.

The goal of hydroxyurea is to titrate to the maximal tolerated dose for each patient, based on maintaining safe blood counts. Laboratory testing of CBC, reticulocyte count, HbF levels, renal, and liver function tests should be performed prior to initiating hydroxyurea and should be repeated at regular intervals thereafter. Although the expected decrease in WBC and platelets and increase in HbF can be seen within weeks to months, a clinical response may not be seen until after 3 to 6 months of treatment. In addition to laboratory monitoring and dose adjustment, follow-up appointments should be used to assess symptoms and to encourage continued adherence. Because of increased rates of leukemia and skin cancers in patients who have taken hydroxyurea for myeloproliferative disorders, there has been concern about the risk of malignancy after long-term use of hydroxyurea in SCD. However, rates of cancer do not seem to be elevated in adults or children who have taken hydroxyurea for SCD. Although unsubstantiated in human studies, concern remains about possible teratogenesis and impaired spermatogenesis based on animal studies. As a result, contraception is advised for both men and women taking hydroxyurea, and hydroxyurea is contraindicated during pregnancy or breastfeeding.

Other preventative care in SCD disease involves monitoring for end-organ complications, including proliferative sickle retinopathy, pulmonary hypertension, renal impairment, avascular necrosis, and iron overload.

Inpatient treatment may be required for management of acute complications, the diagnosis and treatment of which are discussed in the proceeding section.

■ COMPLICATIONS

Anemia

Patients with SCD will be anemic at baseline, even during periods of good physical health. The anemia in sickle cell disease is caused by red cell destruction or hemolysis. Red cell survival is only 10 to 20 days, compared with 120 days in individuals without SCD. The bone marrow increases RBC production dramatically, but it is unable to keep pace with the destruction. Red cell production increases by 5- to 10-fold in most patients with sickle cell disease.

However, anemia in SCD may become more severe acutely, due to acute-on-chronic hemolysis, sepsis, hyperhemolysis, or aplastic crisis (eg, pure red cell aplasia due to parvovirus B19), or patients may become more symptomatic due to hypoxemia or increased oxygen demand. Red cell transfusions increase the oxygen-carrying capacity of blood, decrease the percentage of sickle RBCs, and improve microvascular perfusion. Simple transfusion is used when the patient has symptoms of anemia and the therapeutic goal is an increase in hemoglobin level. Transfusion is not advised in uncomplicated painful episodes.

Exchange transfusion involves removing the patient's RBCs and replacing them with HbS-negative donor RBCs. The main advantage of exchange transfusions over simple transfusions is avoidance of hyperviscosity and volume overload, while reducing the percentage of sickle hemoglobin. Acute chest syndrome and stroke are two indications for exchange transfusion. Exchange transfusion requires the availability of skilled staff to perform the procedure as well as adequate vascular access in the patient. For automated exchange transfusion (erythrocytapheresis), specialized equipment is also required. Any patient who is expected to need RBC transfusion should be vaccinated for hepatitis B virus.

Painful episodes

Painful episodes (sometimes referred to as "painful crises" or "vaso-occlusive crises") are the most frequent complication in sickle cell disease, and are presumed to be due to vaso-occlusive ischemia in bones and other tissues. Triggers may include hypoxia, dehydration, cold, or fever. The frequency and duration of the vaso-occlusive crisis may vary considerably between patients but it is the most common cause of morbidity and mortality in sickle cell disease. Patients who have had recurrent episodes should have a supply of appropriate oral analgesics (acetaminophen, NSAIDs, or opiates) at home so that pain can be treated quickly and effectively. If the episode is more severe, patients may require higher-dose therapy in a hospital-based setting. Often parenteral therapy (eg, NSAIDs or opiates) is most effective. Patients should be taken at their word about the severity of their pain. There is no objective measure of severity of a vaso-occlusive episode, and undertreatment or delays in analgesic administration lead to unnecessary suffering and weakening of the patient-provider relationship.

Acute chest syndrome

Acute chest syndrome (ACS) is an acute complication of SCD that may be defined as fever and respiratory symptoms in the presence of a new pulmonary infiltrate on chest x-ray. Acute chest syndrome is a leading cause of hospitalization in patients with SCD and a significant risk factor for early mortality. The incidence of ACS is highest in patients with HbSS genotype. Causes of ACS include pulmonary infections (eg, influenza, bacterial, or viral pneumonia), pulmonary infarction, or fat embolism from necrotic bone marrow. Sickle cell disease patients who have undergone abdominal surgery are at risk of developing ACS in the immediate postoperative period. Sickle cell disease patients with asthma are twice as likely to develop ACS as SCD patients who do not have asthma. The most frequent symptoms at diagnosis of ACS include fever, cough, chest pain, shortness of breath, and tachypnea. Acute chest syndrome requires admission to the hospital. If signs and symptoms are severe, patients should be treated in an intensive care setting. Supplemental oxygen should be administered to maintain oxygen saturation of ≥ 95%. Adequate analgesia is required for pain. Complete blood count, CXR, arterial blood gases, blood cultures (if febrile), sputum cultures, RBC blood grouping, and crossmatch should be done rapidly. Regardless of the etiology, management of ACS includes intravenous broad-spectrum antibiotics, bronchodilators, incentive spirometry, and careful hydration. Patients who are hypoxemic (SaO$_2$ < 80 mm Hb) should receive supplemental oxygen. Transfusion can be an important adjunct, especially if the patient is hypoxemic. There have been no randomized trials comparing simple and exchange transfusions in this setting. It is generally accepted that in severe acute chest syndrome, the goal of transfusion is to maintain a hemoglobin concentration > 10 g/dL and a HbS level of < 30%.

Stroke

Individuals with SCD are at higher risk of stroke than the general population. Patients with the homozygous form of SCD, HbSS, have the highest risk, with an 11% chance of developing a first stroke by the age of 20 years, compared with a 2% risk for patients with HbSC disease. Those age 2 to 5 years have the highest incidence of first stroke followed by those between 6 and 9 years of age. Most strokes in children with SCD are ischemic. Clinical features of ischemic stroke include focal weakness (usually hemiparesis); seizures; altered consciousness and mentation; confusion; and visual, speech, and sensory disturbances. In children, symptoms may be transient.

Known risk factors include low hemoglobin levels, high white cell count, hypertension, and a recent history of acute chest syndrome. Genetic factors and nocturnal hypoxemia may also contribute to stroke risk. Transcranial Doppler ultrasonography (TCD) is used as a screening tool for stroke prevention in children with SCD. Children with abnormal TCD receive prophylactic blood transfusion, based on the results of a randomized trial showing a 92% reduction in stroke risk with a chronic RBC transfusion strategy versus observation.

No large studies of stroke prevention have been done in adults with SCD. Early detection is important. Although treatment of acute stroke in children focuses on hydration and exchange transfusion, there is less consensus on SCD-specific interventions for adults with stroke. Practice guidelines from the National Institutes of Health (NIH) and the National Heart, Lung, and Blood Institute (NHLBI) are based on current recommendations for prevention and management of stroke in adults without SCD.

Sepsis

Patients with sickle cell disease are at increased risk of infection and bacteremia. Increased incidence of infection is partially explained by functional asplenia—immunization against encapsulated organisms should help to decrease the risk. Sickle cell disease patients with fever should receive an appropriate septic workup, with consideration of their immunization status and past history of sickle cell complications. Acute chest syndrome, osteomyelitis, and skin and soft tissue infections should be ruled out, as appropriate.

Priapism

Priapism occurs in 30% to 45% of male patients with SCD and it is defined as a prolonged, unwanted, and uncomfortable or painful erection. Priapism occurs when sickle veno-occlusion causes a pathologic decrease in venous outflow from the penile vascular chambers. Minor episodes can be uncomfortable but tolerable and self-limited, lasting up to several hours. Major episodes can last a few hours to several days and are often extremely painful. Prolonged priapism (>4 hours) can lead to ischemia and fibrosis and is considered a medical emergency. Prolonged or recurrent priapism can result in impotence.

Initial self-treatment by patients has some reported benefit, including analgesia, oral hydration, and exercise. However, for some patients the duration of the episode seems unresponsive to conservative measures. If a patient presents for medical attention, he should be treated rapidly and in a sensitive manner. First-line intervention includes supportive care measures such as intravenous hydration and narcotic analgesia. If the episode persists for more than 2 hours, additional measures must be considered. Use

of exchange transfusion in this setting is controversial because of conflicting evidence for efficacy and reports of ASPEN syndrome (association of sickle cell disease, priapism, exchange transfusion, and neurologic events). If the episode does not resolve rapidly, a urology specialist should become involved.

Bone and soft tissue complications

In SCD patients presenting with bone pain, clinicians must distinguish between common causes, including acute vaso-occlusive crisis, osteomyelitis (OM), and avascular necrosis, while also considering more rare complications such as abscesses or septic arthritis. It is useful to know that bone pain in sickle cell disease is much more likely to be due to vaso-occlusion than to OM; in one pediatric series, VOC was at least 50 times more likely.

A thorough evaluation begins with assessing historical features of the pain. If the onset of symptoms was acute, it may be suggestive of vaso-occlusion or OM versus the chronic pain and disability caused by AVN. Concurrent infectious symptoms (eg, fever, rigors) may be present in OM. Any prior history of bony complications can also guide further investigations.

Physical examination should include a musculoskeletal examination, targeting the joint or other location of symptoms. Elevated temperature may be suggestive of OM or other infectious etiology, while other abnormalities in vital signs (eg, tachycardia, hypotension) would be late signs and potentially indicative of progression to sepsis.

Leukocytosis and increased erythrocyte sedimentation rate (ESR) are nonspecific findings that may be present in both infectious and noninfectious processes. If infection is suspected, blood cultures should be drawn. Cultures of the suspected site of infection also aid in diagnosis (eg, joint aspiration, abscess drainage, bone aspirate, or bone biopsy), as indicated by clinical suspicion and results of imaging.

Plain radiography, radioisotope bone scanning, and radio-labeled leukocyte scanning are not always useful in the routine diagnostic evaluation of bone pain in SCD as these modalities can detect acute infarction but changes are often difficult to distinguish from those seen in OM. Ultrasonography is a rapid, simple, and noninvasive modality that is moderately sensitive for detecting acute osteomyelitis. The main ultrasonographic finding in OM is subperiosteal fluid. Magnetic resonance imaging can be useful in the diagnosis of OM. As with other imaging modalities, there is overlap between the changes seen in infection and infarction. Although still not 100% specific for differentiating OM from VOC, gadolinium enhancement improves the accuracy of MRI.

Management of bone pain may include oral, intravenous, or subcutaneous opiates, depending on severity of pain. More specific management should be tailored to the underlying process.

Perioperative complications

Surgical procedures such as splenectomy, cholecystectomy, or orthopedic surgery are commonly required in patients due to complications of their SCD. In addition, patients with SCD may require surgeries due to unrelated medical problems during their lifetimes. Patients with SCD have a higher risk of perioperative complications than the general population for several reasons. First, patients with SCD are already anemic and any procedural bleeding will further drop hemoglobin levels, leading to more severe anemia and decreased oxygen-carrying capacity. Second, intraoperative hypoxia, postoperative atelectasis, and decreased oral intake can trigger sickling of red blood cells. Sickling of red blood cells can lead to painful crisis or acute chest syndrome, among other SCD-related complications. All patients should undergo consultation with an anesthesiologist prior to surgery. Patients undergoing medium- and high-risk surgery should receive prophylactic red blood cell transfusions to target hemoglobin of 100 mg/L. If preoperative baseline hemoglobin level is 90 or higher, partial manual exchange transfusion should be performed to achieve a target HbS <60%. Red cell exchange apheresis can be considered prior to very high-risk procedures (eg, orthopedic surgery requiring tourniquet, vascular surgery requiring arterial clamping) or in patients with a history of postoperative complications. Cross-matched units of red blood cells should be on hold in the blood bank. Importantly, all patients should receive adequate hydration prior to surgery. If the patient is required to remain in NPO status prior to surgery, he or she should be admitted for intravenous hydration with isotonic solution during the NPO period. Postoperatively, isotonic intravenous fluids should be administered until the patient is drinking and eating well. Supplemental oxygen should be used as needed. Deep breathing exercises and/or incentive spirometry may be used to reduce the risk of postoperative atelectasis.

An in-depth discussion of chronic complications of SCD is beyond the scope of this chapter. An excellent resource for further information is the NIH/NHLBI Guidelines (2014) (The Evidence-Based Management of Sickle Cell Disease: Expert Panel Report, 2014). Full document available at https://www.nhlbi.nih.gov/health-pro/guidelines/sickle-cell-disease-guidelines. Close follow-up should be arranged for patients with complications of SCD.

CONCLUSION

Discharge considerations: Patients admitted for complications od sickle cell disease require close monitoring of symptoms and laboratory parameters during their hospital stay. If they are being treated for a painful episode, doses of pain medication should be carefully titrated downward as pain symptoms improve. Intravenuos opiates should be switched over equianalgesic doses of oral medication prior to discharge. Eligibility for discharge will depend on stable clinical status and ability of the patient to manage symptoms effectively at home. Follow-up with a comprehensive care clinic is suggested.

SUGGESTED READINGS

Brawley OW, Cornelius LJ, Edwards LR, et al. National Institutes of Health Consensus Development Conference statement: hydroxyurea treatment for sickle cell disease. *Ann Intern Med.* 2008;148(12):932-938.

Chui DHK, Fucharoen S, Chan V. Hemoglobin H disease: not necessarily a benign disorder. *Blood.* 2003;101:791-800.

Clement FM, Klarenbach S, Tonelli M, Johnson JA, Manns BJ. The impact of selecting a high hemoglobin target level on health-related quality of life for patients with chronic kidney disease: a systematic review and meta-analysis. *Arch Intern Med.* 2009;169(12):1104-1112.

Dhaliwal G, Cornett PA, Tierney LM Jr. Hemolytic anemia. *Am Fam Physician.* 2004;69(11):2599-2606.

Howard J, Malfroy M, Llewelyn C, et al. The Transfusion Alternatives Preoperatively in Sickle Cell Disease (TAPS) study: a randomised, controlled, multicentre clinical trial. *Lancet.* 2013;381(9870):930-938.

Lanzkron S, Strouse JJ, Wilson R, et al. Systematic review: hydroxyurea for the treatment of adults with sickle cell disease. *Ann Intern Med.* 2008;148(12):939-955.

Marchioli R, Finazzi G, Specchia G, et al. Cardiovascular events and intensity of treatment in polycythemia vera. *N Engl J Med.* 2013;368(1):22-33.

McMullin MF, Bareford D, Campbell P, et al. Guidelines for the diagnosis, investigation and management of polycythaemia/erythrocytosis. *Br J Haematol.* 2005;130(2):174-195.

Platt OS, Brambilla DJ, Rosse WF, et al. Mortality in sickle cell disease. Life expectancy and risk factors for early death. *N Engl J Med.* 1994;330(23):1639-1644.

TIF Non-Transfusion-Dependent Thalassemia guidelines (2014). http://www.ncbi.nlm.nih.gov/books/NBK190457/?report=reader. Accessed August 10, 2016.

TIF Transfusion-Dependent Thalassemia guidelines (2013). http://www.thalassaemia.org.cy/wp-content/uploads/eBook-publications/guidelines-for-the-management-of-transfusion-dependent-thalassaemia/. Accessed September 14, 2016.

Yawn BP, et al. Management of Sickle Cell Disease. Summary of the 2014 Evidence-Based Report by Expert Panel Members. *JAMA.* 2014;312(10):1033-1048.

Zempsky WT. Treatment of sickle cell pain: fostering trust and justice. *JAMA.* 2009;302(22):2479-2480.

CHAPTER 170

Disorders of the White Cell

Blair J. N. Leonard, MD, PhD, FRCP
Brian Leber, MD, FRCP(C)

Key Clinical Questions

1. What are the most common causes of leukocytosis in the hospital inpatient setting?
2. Which medications can cause neutropenia and agranulocytosis?
3. What are the most common causes of eosinophilia?
4. What key white blood cell (WBC) findings indicate an impending medical emergency and warrant immediate action?
5. What are the indications for a bone marrow biopsy and aspirate?
6. What is the role of molecular testing in the diagnostic workup of common WBC disorders?
7. What is the role for granulocyte colony-stimulating factors (GCSF) in nonmalignant hematologic disorders?

INTRODUCTION

Deviation from the normal range in the leukocyte count is one of the most common laboratory abnormalities in the inpatient setting and frequently indicates the onset of clinical conditions that significantly impact hospitalized patients. Individual laboratory values may vary from day to day depending on fluid status and other factors, Hence, a "normal" white blood cell (WBC) or differential count has a typical distribution of values (**Table 170-1**).

A natural response to the physiologic fluctuations of the host's hormonal and cytokine milieu, WBC counts also vary with the time of day and the season of the year. Typically, the hormonal variation associated with pregnancy will also increase the absolute WBC count due to an increase in circulating neutrophils.

There is also a significant genetic component to the ranges expressed on a WBC count, as neutrophil counts have been shown to vary considerably among ethnic groups. People of African descent, Yemenite and Ethiopian Jews, and people of Middle Eastern decent all have been shown to possess WBC counts with medians well below those established in predominantly Caucasian populations. Typically, these values do not fall below the threshold of mild neutropenia ($<1.5 \times 10^9$) for any significant period of time, and thus are not usually associated with significant infection risk. In fact, these physiologic deviations are not known to result in any clinically measurable increase in morbidity or mortality, and do not require any specific intervention once underlying pathology has been ruled out.

Recognizing abnormalities of the complete blood count (CBC) and, more specifically, the composition of the differential count are critical for formulating a differential diagnosis of disorders involving the WBC lineages. Valuable time and resources can be saved and best directed if careful attention is paid to these simple tests in the context of a good history and physical examination performed when abnormalities are first detected. As a general rule of thumb, malignant causes should always be considered in the differential diagnosis when red blood cell (RBC) or platelet lineages are also abnormal, or if there is a history of unexplained weight loss, anorexia, lymphadenopathy, or other systemic symptoms. This chapter will review each WBC lineage and the common nonmalignant conditions associated with their abnormalities. Hematologic malignancies will be addressed in Chapter 174.

EPIDEMIOLOGY OF WHITE BLOOD CELL ABNORMALITIES

In one recent large retrospective study of over 45,000 hospitalized patients, leukocytosis had a prevalence of 31.2% and leucopenia was prevalent in 6.1%. Underlying bacterial infection is the most common reason for both leukocytosis and leukopenia in the inpatient setting, and thus the overwhelming majority of these variations in WBC counts are due to disorders involving neutrophils. Therefore, practically speaking, the terms *leukocytosis* and *neutrophilia* are commonly interchanged in the medical literature. While disorders involving other components of the WBC differential are far less common, they can represent vastly different pathological processes, and thus require different diagnostic investigation. Not all leukocytoses are neutrophilias, and thus the timely identification of the cell lineage involved in a WBC abnormality can have a significant impact on clinical outcome.

TABLE 170-1 The Normal White Blood Cell Count

White Blood Cell Type	Typical Range of Values
Neutrophils	$4\text{-}11 \times 10^9/L$
Lymphocytes	$1.5\text{-}3.5 \times 10^9/L$
Monocytes	$0.2\text{-}0.8 \times 10^9/L$
Eosinophils	$0.05\text{-}0.4 \times 10^9/L$
Basophils	$0.01\text{-}0.1 \times 10^9/L$

■ PROGNOSIS

The WBC count can be thought of as equilibrium, with deviations above or below the normal distribution correlating with adverse outcomes in patients. Large, retrospective, population-based analysis of abnormalities in WBC magnitude has indicated that absolute WBC count correlates with all-cause mortality in an otherwise healthy population. As might be expected, this association is J-shaped, with both increasing leukopenia and increasing leukocytosis correlating with increased mortality. In hospitalized patients the presence of either abnormality has been shown to correlate with an increase in 30-day overall mortality. White blood cell deviations correlate with morbidity and mortality not only across patient settings, such as the intensive care unit and emergency department, but also across disease states.

Leukocystosis is a robust prognostic indicator of overall mortality in the hospitalized patient with underlying infection, such as profound sepsis, with several studies confirming that the absolute magnitude of the leukocytosis directly correlates with the overall mortality rate. Leukocytosis is also prognostic in cardiac conditions, including coronary artery disease and acute coronary syndrome. Though it is unclear if WBC abnormalities have an active or passive role in mortality of these pathologies, it is clear that abnormalities in WBC count herald a poorer outcome in such patients.

> ### PRACTICE POINT
>
> - An abnormal WBC count is a clear indicator of failing health in a broad spectrum of patient settings and, thus, is an important laboratory result that requires further investigation to ascertain etiology.

The bulk of experience with morbidity and mortality in leukopenic patients comes from patient populations with malignancies, where there is a direct correlation between depth of neutropenia and infection and mortality rates. However, patients without malignancy or primary bone marrow pathology can also develop significant leukopenia. In this setting, leukopenia may represent a myriad of pathologic mechanisms, such as direct cytokine suppression of marrow precursors or bone marrow infiltration, and is an ominous sign of profound compromise of the patient's immunity. Such patients typically require specialized clinical care as well as intensive support and monitoring. Despite the widespread availability of WBC growth factors, these medications have not shown significant efficacy in septic patients who are otherwise not immunocompromised and are not routinely recommended for septic hospitalized patients.

DISORDERS OF THE NEUTROPHIL
■ NEUTROPHILLIA

Infection and physiologic stress cause the overwhelming proportion of neutrophillia and, thus, leukocytosis (**Table 170-2**).

TABLE 170-2 Differential Diagnosis of Leukocytosis in the Hospitalized Patient

Diagnosis	Incidence
Infection	52%
Physiologic stress	38%
Medications or drugs	11%
Hematologic condition	6%
Necrosis/inflammation	6%
Unknown	4%

Data from Wanahita A, Goldsmith EA, Musher DM. Conditions associated with leukocytosis in a tertiary care hospital, with particular attention to the role of infection caused by clostridium difficile. *ClinInfect Dis.* 2002;34:1585-1592.

Common sources of infection include the pulmonary, urinary, and gastrointestinal tracts, as well as soft tissue infections. A burgeoning infective etiology in hospitalized patients in the era of widespread antibiotic use is *Clostridium difficile* colitis, and this diagnosis should be considered in the workup of an unexplained leukocytosis in a hospitalized patient, especially if there is a history of recent exposure to systemic antibiotic therapy.

> ### PRACTICE POINT
>
> - Given the importance of timely intervention with goal-directed therapy in septic patients, this paradigm underscores the need for initial consideration of infection in all hospitalized patients with an unexplained leukocytosis.

Both pathologic and physiologic stressors can cause glucocorticoid hormone release, and the elevated circulating cortisol will liberate neutrophils from the endothelium where they are normally marginalized. Thus, any state causing stress can potentially cause an elevated neutrophil count in hospitalized patients. Common causes of the neutrophilia that is associated with stress include the presence of a hyperdynamic cardiac output state from cardiorespiratory exertion, or a prolonged state of extreme anxiety. Though initially differentiating infection from physiologic stress as a cause of neutrophilia can be challenging, a few key elements may be more suggestive of the likely cause. Stress-related neutrophilia is typically characterized by an antecedent initiating event, followed by a transient process, such as seizure, rigors, hyperthermia, or hyperemesis, that commonly reverses within hours after the initiating stimulus. In addition, stress-hormone-mediated neutrophil demarginalization does not typically cause the characteristic morphologic findings of the activated neutrophil, such as toxic granulation of the cytoplasm or the presence of Dohle bodies. A history, physical examination, and review of the peripheral smear often identifies an obvious etiology and saves time and resources in the diagnostic workup.

Less commonly than infection or stress, some medications frequently cause neutrophilia in the hospitalized patient. These medications include systemic corticosteroids, anesthetic agents, β-agonists, and epinephrine. As there is often no easy way to confirm a medication-induced neutrophilia, it is a diagnosis of exclusion and should only be considered when infection has been essentially ruled out. Much like stress-induced neutrophilia, a drug-induced cause is less likely to show toxic changes to neutrophils on morphologic examination, and the presence of such changes or other concerning symptoms should lead the hospitalist to further investigate the possibility of infection as a cause.

■ NEUTROPENIA

Neutropenia is often classified into mild ($<1.5 \times 10^9$/L neutrophils), moderate ($<1.0 \times 10^9$/L), or severe ($<0.5 \times 10^9$/L), with infection risk and mortality highest in the severely neutropenic patient. Such patients are at high risk of death, and specialty care and consultation with a hematologist should be sought. In contrast to the outpatient setting where primary hematologic and "unknown" causes predominate, the most common causes of acquired neutropenia in the hospitalized setting include infection (both bacterial and viral), medication, and autoimmune and systemic inflammation. From a causal standpoint, neutropenia is relatively nonspecific for bacterial infections, and is more likely a reflection of the depth of immunocompromise rather than a reflection of any specific organism. Acute viral infections, such as with parvovirus B19, may give rise to a transient isolated neutropenia, typically associated with nonspecific viral infection symptoms and reticulocytopenia. Some chronic viral infections are also classically associated with an isolated neutropenia, including human immunodeficiency virus (HIV) and hepatitis C infection, and should be considered in the differential diagnosis of a persisting neutropenia if the history or physical examination is suggestive.

After infection, other benign causes of neutropenia are less common. A hypersplenic state can sequester neutrophils much like RBCs, causing a mild chronic neutropenia. Dietary insufficiency can cause megaloblastosis, which may initially manifest as neutropenia with classic megaloblastic changes of hypersegmented neutrophils indicating nuclear-cytoplasmic maturation dyssynchrony. Serum B12 and RBC folate levels are important to investigate if this abnormality is observed, as deficiencies in these nutrients are a common reversible cause of megaloblastosis. These findings may appear before a macrocytic anemia is present. Prevalence of B12 deficiency has been noted in the 10% to 15% range in older patients in the community, however, and perhaps as high as 30% to 40% in hospitalized patients. Metformin-related B12 deficiency is an underappreciated cause, and positively correlates with both the dose and duration of metformin therapy. In addition, common medications interfering with cellular metabolism, such as methotrexate or hydroxyurea, may also give rise to neutropenia with a megaloblastic picture, though without B12 or folate deficiency.

Acquired autoimmune neutropenia may occasionally be seen in hospitalized patients, and is associated with autoantibodies generated toward antigens on the neutrophil's surface. In elderly hospitalized patients, these antibodies are typically secondary to systemic inflammatory conditions such as systemic lupus erythematosus (SLE) or rheumatoid arthritis, though they may also be associated with a recent transfusion or the presence of a thymoma. Diagnosis is largely based on supportive history, physical, and diagnostic testing for the underlying systemic diseases, as the antineutrophil antibodies are often nonspecific and have not been validated for diagnosis. The course may be complicated with other autoimmune phenomena such as hemolytic anemia, antiphospholipid antibody syndrome, or Felty syndrome. Patients are at risk of overwhelming infection when profoundly neutropenic and need to be closely monitored for infection, with rapid initiation of therapy should infection arise. Treatment is largely supportive and aimed at treating the underlying condition, though occasionally granulocyte colony-stimulating factor (GCSF) may be used in selected patients. It is advisable to avoid fresh unwashed fruits and vegetables or flowers during the neutropenic period due to the potential increased risk of infection associated with such exposures.

A large population-based cohort study identified several drugs that have been associated with medication-induced agranulocytosis—a failure of bone marrow to produce neutrophils. Many of these medications are commonly used in hospitalized patients (**Table 170-3**).

TABLE 170-3 List of Drugs Causing Agranulocytosis in Hospitalized Patients

Medication	Attributable Risk
Metamizole sodium	16.29
Beta-lactam antibiotics	12.01
Ticlopidine	11.19
Antithyroid drugs	7.21
Sulfonamides	5.44
Calcium dobesilate	5.02
Diclonfinac	4.19
Spironolactone	3.22
Carbamazepine	2.57

Data from Ibáñez L, Vidal X, Ballarín E, Laporte JR. Population-based drug-induced agranulocytosis. *Arch Intern Med.* 2005;165(8):869-874.

Cyclic neutropenia, chronic benign neutropenia, and congenital bone marrow failure syndrome such as Kostmann disease can also occasionally present with asymptomatic neutropenia in a hospitalized patient. These patients typically will have a history of such a condition and given the rarity of these diagnoses, should be considered only when the more common etiologies have been ruled out.

■ ACQUIRED NEUTROPHIL DYSFUNCTION

Outside of absolute number, neutrophils can also be functionally impaired by conditions such as poorly controlled diabetes, chronic iron overload states, and chronic renal insufficiency. Typically these patients are more susceptible to bacterial infections secondary to neutrophil dysfunction, often with uncommon organisms such as *Vibrio vulnificus* or *Yersenia enterocolitica* as in the case of chronically iron-overloaded patients. Neutrophil dysfunction can occur as a result of the underlying condition as well as from instituted therapies, such as hemodialysis in renal failure patients. Treatment paradigms involve appropriate antimicrobial and supportive therapies, as well as control or resolution of the underlying condition if possible.

DISORDERS OF LYMPHOCYTES

Lymphocytes are generated in the bone marrow from a common precursor. They can differentiate in the bone marrow (B-cells) and become involved in antibody, or humoral, immunity, or they can differentiate in the thymus (T-cells) and become involved in cell-mediated immunity. Abnormalities of the lymphocyte are the next most common nonmalignant WBC abnormality encountered in the hospital after those involving the neutrophil. These can be broadly categorized as inherited or related to acquired lymphocyte abnormalities; the acquired variety will predominate in the hospitalist setting.

■ INHERITED LYMPHOCYTE DISORDERS

Inherited lymphocyte abnormalities are relatively infrequent, and typically the care of such patients would lie beyond the scope of the practicing hospitalist with few exceptions. However, selective immunoglobulin A (IgA) deficiency is a relatively common abnormality seen in the Caucasian population (~1 in 600) and, thus, will likely be encountered in the course of practice. Awareness for selective IgA deficiency should be raised when patients report recurrent pyogenic infections, typically involving skin and/or lungs. Appropriately focused antibiotic therapy is the treatment of choice in these patients, and there is no role for intravenous immunoglobulin (IVIG) supplementation, as IVIG does not contain IgA. Importantly, adverse reactions can occur upon transfusion of IgA-deficient patients with blood products, including life-threatening anaphylactic reactions. This is due to the presence of preformed IgA antibodies in IgA-deficient patients that react to contaminating IgA in the administered blood products. Autoimmune conditions such as systemic lupus erythematosus or rheumatoid arthritis are also commonly associated with IgA deficiency, and a further workup for these conditions in newly diagnosed patients would be prudent.

■ ACQUIRED LYMPHOCYTE DISORDERS: LYMPHOCYTOSIS

Acquired nonmalignant lymphocytosis is a relatively common finding in the hospitalized population, and typically represents a reactive process secondary to infection, most commonly of a viral nature. Mononucleosis syndromes, typically associated with characteristic morphologic changes to lymphocytes on the peripheral blood film (atypical lymphocytes), suggest viral etiologies such as acute cytomegalovirus or Epstein-Barr virus. Potential bacterial etiologies for lymphocytosis would be a less common finding, but would include such bacterium as *Bordetella pertussis* and *Toxoplasmosis gondii*.

Less common causes of an acquired lymphocytosis include a reactive process secondary to administration of a drug or medication such as a corticosteroid. Reactive lymphocytosis can also occur secondary to a variety of underlying systemic conditions such as Graves disease, Hodgkin lymphoma, or SLE. These less common etiologies should be considered if the lymphocytosis persists once infectious etiologies have been ruled out.

Monoclonal B-cell lymphocytosis (MBL) is an increasingly appreciated cause of chronic, persisting lymphocytosis in the elderly hospitalized patient with no obvious underlying etiology. Monoclonal B-cell lymphocytosis is similar to the monoclonal gammopathy of unknown significance in that a clonal population of cells is apparent with increasing age, with an unknown clinical significance. While MBL in and of itself does not require specific treatment, these patients are more likely to develop chronic lymphocytic leukemia (CLL) and, thus, would benefit from closer monitoring for the development of features of CLL. A lymphocytosis less than 5000/mm³ but greater than the normal range without clinical features of CLL would suggest MBL, whereas persistent lymphocyte counts of greater than 5000/mm³ would suggest a diagnosis of CLL. A diagnosis of MBL can be made on flow cytometry; does would not require a bone marrow aspirate or biopsy unless associated cytopenias are involved and the diagnosis of symptomatic CLL with bone marrow involvement is being considered.

■ ACQUIRED LYMPHOCYTE DISORDERS: LYMPHOCYTOPENIA

In the general population, the acquired immune deficiency syndrome is the most common cause of an acquired nonmalignant lymphocytopenia, typically skewing the CD4:CD8 ratio by selectively depleting the CD4 T-cell subpopulation. A persistent unexplained lymphocytopenia warrants further investigation, as occult chronic HIV infection would be high on the differential diagnosis and requires prompt recognition and treatment.

Other less common causes include hypersplenism, a reactive response to active inflammatory conditions, or concomitant corticosteroid use. Similar to chronic alcohol consumption, malnutrition may present with other findings, such as a transient lymphocytopenia, Serum immunoglobulins should be quantified in persistently lymphocytopenic patients, as IgG-deficient patients will be more susceptible to bacterial infections, such as pneumonia or sinusitis, and may respond well to IVIG supplementation. The reverse is not always true, however, and IgG-deficient patients may not be lymphocytopenic at all, with the diagnosis of IgG deficiency only suspected with a history of repeated unexplained infections in an otherwise healthy patient.

DISORDERS OF MONOCYTES AND MACROPHAGES

Monocytes are typically released into circulation once generated in the marrow and are sequestered in the red pulp of the spleen then released into the bloodstream to differentiate into functional macrophages at their destination. These WBCs are involved in phagocytosis, cytokine release, and appropriate antigen presentation at sites of infection. Benign abnormalities include monocytosis and monocytopenia, the dysregulation of function associated with the hemophagocytic syndromes, and the rare heterogeneous histiocytic diseases, which are beyond the scope of this review.

■ MONOCYTOSIS

The benign causes of a monocytosis are reactive processes and are numerous (**Table 170-4**), including infection, malignancy, and autoimmune processes.

■ MONOCYTOPENIA

Monocytopenia is less common and is associated with neoplastic processes such as hairy cell leukemia or autoimmune processes like SLE. Systemic corticosteroid use can cause a transient monocytosis, as can an associated thermal insult.

■ HEMOPHAGOCYTIC SYNDROMES

Hemophagocytic syndromes are characterized by a highly dysregulated immune response toward an underlying stimulus and may be associated with infection, products of host tissue damage, or underlying autoimmune or malignant conditions. They can be acquired or familial, and the presence of activated macrophages that consume host RBCs (hemophagocytosis) is the cardinal feature of these rare, but potentially fatal syndromes. The timely identification of a hemophagocytic syndrome is important, as death can occur rapidly due to the associated hyperinflammatory state. Clinical suspicion should be raised for this condition in any patient with cytopenias, splenomegaly, and a recurring or prolonged fever without any organism isolated and that is unresponsive to empirical antimicrobial therapy. No specific blood tests confirm hemophagocytic syndrome, though an elevated ferritin and fasting triglyceride with decreased fibrinogen levels accompanying the clinical findings are highly suggestive and are part of the diagnostic criteria. The hemophagocytic syndrome associated with fulminant Epstein-Barr virus infection is particularly concerning due to the high mortality associated with it, and urgent hematologic consultation should always be sought when the diagnosis is considered.

TABLE 170-4 Differential Diagnosis of Secondary Causes of Monocytosis

Infection
CMV infection, bacterial endocarditis
Tuberculosis, syphilis
Malignancy
Hodgkin disease, multiple myeloma
Systemic inflammatory conditions
Ulcererative colitis, connective tissue diseases
Sarcoidosis
Alcoholic hepatitis

DISORDERS OF EOSINOPHILS

Eosinophils are highly granular cells capable of producing a multitude of destructive enzymes, reactive oxygen species, and cytokines to combat parasitic and viral infections. Benign abnormalities of eosinophils, typically manifested as an eosinophilia, are a relatively rare abnormality of WBC. However, its timely identification in the hospitalized patient can help to appropriately direct the inquisition for an underlying etiology. Common causes of peripheral blood eosinophilia are listed in **Table 170-5**.

Classically, the diagnostic pathway of eosinophilia branches with the initial identification of a primary or clonal process versus a reactive or secondary process. For example, eosinophilia defined as an absolute eosinophil count of greater than 500/mm³ (or range 400-600/mm³) can be associated with HIV infection, syphilis, tuberculosis, parasitic infections, new medications, allergic bronchopulmonary aspergillosis, adrenal insufficiency, and hematologic malignancies such as Hodgkin disease. If an appropriate history and physical examination do not reveal an obvious reactive cause such as an acute inflammatory state, infection, or malignancy, further investigations should include a bone marrow biopsy with testing for eosinophilic clonality. Tests for clonality include conventional G-banding cytogenetics and molecular testing for clonal markers such as the X-linked *HUMARA* gene in females, the mutated *c-Kit* gene, or the FIP1L1-PDGF fusion protein. This latter molecular target is important to look for, as its presence portends a high likelihood of response to oral tyrosine kinase therapy, such as imatinib. If established as a clonal disorder, primary eosinophilic processes include the myelodysplastic/myeloproliferative disorders and acute or chronic eosinophilic leukemia. The idiopathic hypereosinophilic syndrome is a diagnosis of exclusion and should only be made in the absence of identification of either a primary clonal or secondary reactive process.

Drug reactions should also be considered in the differential diagnosis of a reactive eosinophilia, with common candidates including antibiotics such as the penicillins and cephalosporins, angiotensin-converting enzyme inhibitors, and anticonvulsants such as phenytoin.

The immediate danger of eosinophilia is that eosinophils are highly granular cells, possessing a variety of toxic proteins, such as peroxidase, and major basic protein; an excess can lead to indiscriminate and widespread tissue infiltration and damage. Regardless of etiology, eosinophils are exquisitely sensitive to large doses of corticosteroids. Other potential treatments include interferon alpha and selected tyrosine kinase inhibitors. Specialized consultation should be sought and treatment should be initiated promptly in cases of a severe eosinophilia to minimize the extensive tissue damage that can accompany this condition.

DISORDERS OF BASOPHILS AND MAST CELLS

Basophils and mast cells are related cells, sharing functional properties (such as histamine release) that help protect the host from parasitic infection. They also play a role in the innate immune system of the host against bacterial infection and are involved in the IgE-mediated hypersensitivity reaction. Benign abnormalities involving basophils or mast cells are very uncommon; typically, abnormalities of absolute number, as functional disorders of basophils, are rare.

■ BASOPHILIA

Primary basophilia is highly suggestive of chronic myelogenous leukemia (CML), and investigations should be initiated to rule out this condition when basophilia is found. Secondary basophilia can be seen in allergic reactions such as those accompanying drug or food hypersensitivity. In addition, it can accompany underlying infections such as varicella and/or autoimmune conditions, the classic being ulcerative colitis. Endocrine dysfunction such as that observed in hypothyroidism can also cause basophilia. In children and, less frequently, in adults, cutaneous mastocytosis typically presenting as urticarium pigmentosum may be seen, with characteristic lesions that become intensely pruritic when stroked. Though clonal in nature, in children this condition is not considered malignant and often resolves spontaneously. In adults the malignant counterpart, systemic mastocytosis, is more frequently found.

■ BASOPHILOPENIA

Basophilopenia is a relatively nonspecific finding associated with increased levels of stress and glucocorticoid levels, such as may be seen in sepsis, systemic inflammation conditions, and acute hemorrhage. Endocrine fluctuations such as those occurring in hyperthyroidism or ovulation can also be associated with a transient basophilopenia.

LEUKEMOID REACTIONS

Leukemoid reactions are elevated WBC counts (typically >50.0 × 10⁹/L) characterized by the presence of immature cell types, such as promyelocytes and metamyelocytes, in the peripheral blood—the so-called left shift along the flow of leukocyte differentiation (**Figure 170-1**).

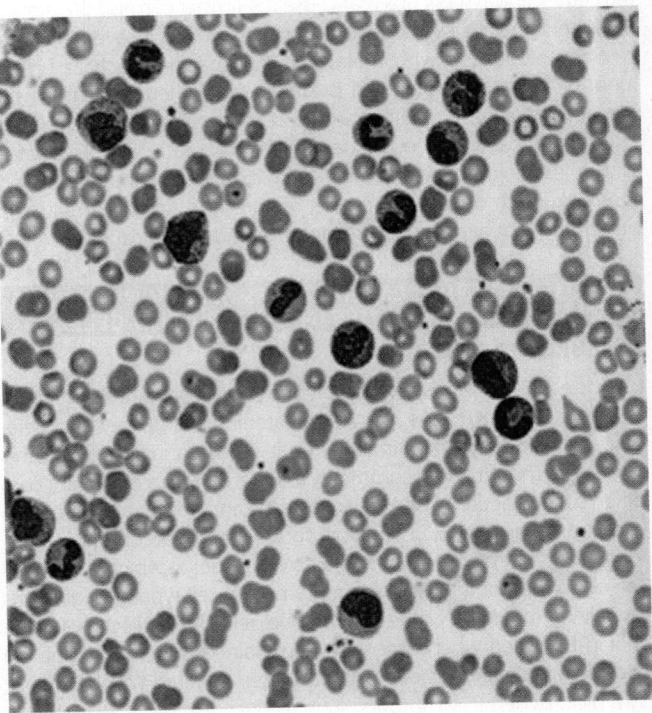

Figure 170-1 *Left-shifted peripheral blood film.*

TABLE 170-5 Differential Diagnosis of Secondary Causes of Eosinophilia

Allergic disorders
Helmenthitic parasitic infections
Drug hypersensitivity reactions
Pulmonary syndromes (eg, Loeffler syndrome)
Tuberculosis
Primary causes (eg, chronic eosinophilic leukemia)
Neoplastic process (eg, Hodgkin disease)
Hypereosinophilic syndrome
Myeloproliferative disorders (eg, chronic myelomonocytic leukemia)

These represent the pool of stored polymorphonuclear neutrophils typically harbored in the bone marrow. Unlike the similar presentation of CML, the leukemoid reaction is reactive and not of clonal origin. Historically, the elevated leukocyte alkaline phosphatase (LAP) score was more suggestive of the functional leukocytes of a leukemoid reaction than the suppressed LAP observed in CML. With the higher sensitivity and specificity of polymerase chain reaction (PCR) testing of peripheral blood samples for the breakpoint cluster region (BCR)-Abelson leukemia (ABL) virus transcript of CML, the LAP is largely of historical note only.

The leukemoid reaction can be seen in hospitalized patients secondary to several acute medical conditions, all of which appear to essentially "shock" the bone marrow into mobilizing its cellular components via cytokine- and growth-factor-mediated processes. Such conditions include the massive hemorrhage that can accompany trauma or a gastrointestinal bleed or the profound immunosuppression of severe sepsis. Infrequently, leukamoid reactions can be related to the administration of certain medications such as corticosteroids. Leukemoid reactions typically occur suddenly and can result in startling and impressive acute increases in the WBC count. Though reflective of the severity of the pathologic stress, leukemoid reactions are not known to be dangerous to the patient and will typically resolve with appropriate treatment and resolution of the underlying cause.

LEUKOERYTHROBLASTIC REACTION

The leukoerythroblastic reaction has a similar presentation to that of the leukemoid reaction. However, the presence of circulating RBC precursors, or nucleated red cells, as well as teardrop-shaped RBCs will also be noted. The presence of the leukoerythroblastic reaction is indicative of an infiltrative process involving the bone marrow, with displacement of bone marrow contents by extramedullary cells such as those of a malignant tumor or of granulomatous disease. Infiltration of the bone marrow with fibroblastic tissue can also present in this fashion (eg, the marrow fibrosis that accompanies myeloproliferative disorders such as primary myelofibrosis). However, the line between the leukemoid reaction and the leukoerythroblastic reaction is not a rigid one from an etiologic standpoint, and many of the acute clinical scenarios that cause the former can also precipitate the latter if the challenge to the bone marrow itself is severe enough.

When associated with metastatic malignancies such as breast, lung, or prostate cancer, the presence of the leukoerythroblastic reaction indicates advanced and disseminated metastatic disease. Thus, prognostically the leukoerythroblastic reaction is associated with a less favorable outcome. Much like the leukemoid reaction, the leukoerythroblastic response requires no specific treatment other than that aimed at addressing the underlying cause.

LIFE-THREATENING EMERGENCIES INVOLVING NONMALIGNANT ABNORMALITIES IN WHITE BLOOD CELLS

■ LEUKOSTASIS

Leukostasis is a hematologic condition that demands emergent action to prevent the severe life-threatening pulmonary and cerebral sequelae that will ultimately result if this condition progresses untreated. Though more commonly associated with a malignant condition such as acute leukemia, leukostasis can also occur as a sequela of a nonmalignant WBC condition, such as might accompany a profound reactive eosinophilia. Absolute WBC values at which leukostasis can occur are not rigid and differ among the cell type of origin, thus guidelines for cutoff values cannot be reliably applied. Suspicion should be raised when otherwise unexplained ischemic symptoms occur in a patient in the context of a grossly elevated WBC count.

Typical ischemic symptoms, such as dyspnea and chest pain, or both focal and general neurologic findings, such as a decreased level of consciousness, are often present. Fluid hydration and acute leukocytoreduction with leukapheresis are the mainstays of treatment, with the later shown in retrospective studies to have a significant impact on mortality at presentation for these patients. Hydroxyurea as a form of cytochemical reduction can be used initially if timely access to leukapheresis is an issue. Maintaining a high index of suspicion and recognizing the signs and symptoms are of the utmost importance in making the diagnosis quickly to allow for timely intervention.

PATHOBIOLOGY OF NONMALIGNANT WHITE CELL DISORDERS

■ EXAMINATION OF THE PERIPHERAL BLOOD SMEAR

Microscopic examination of the peripheral blood smear is a simple, expedient, and widely available analytical method that can be of tremendous diagnostic significance for the hospitalist in unexplained cases of WBC abnormalities. A preliminary examination of the peripheral smear can identify several obvious pathologic findings, such as the previously mentioned leukemoid reaction or the hypersegmented neutrophils of megaloblastosis (**Figure 170-2**).

In addition, several subtle but classic features of the peripheral blood smear can be readily identified and can aid the hospitalist in directing further investigations.

The presence of *toxic granulation*, seen as dark and dense azurophilic granules on Wright staining, can also be observed in the cytoplasm of activated neutrophils (**Figure 170-3**). These granules contain a variety of antimicrobial enzymes and mediators, and their presence is strongly suggestive of underlying infection. They can also be seen upon administration of colony-stimulating factors (CSFs) such as GCSF. When due to infection, the magnitude of the level of toxic granulation observed in leukocytes can be informative, as it has been shown to roughly correlate with sensitive serum markers of inflammation such as serum levels of C-reactive protein.

Dohle bodies, light blue-gray ovular inclusions seen typically on the periphery of activated neutrophils (see Figure 170-3), are thought to be caused by clumping of ribosomes and endoplasmic reticulum. These accumulate when the neutrophil is metabolically active, such as when fighting active infection. Cytoplasmic vacuolization of the neutrophil is another microscopically visible sign of an

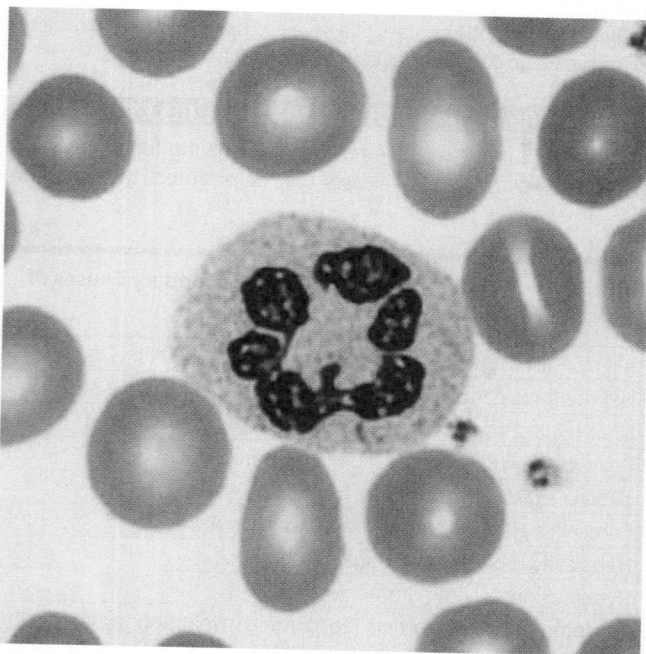

Figure 170-2 *Hypersegmented neutrophil of megaloblastosis.*

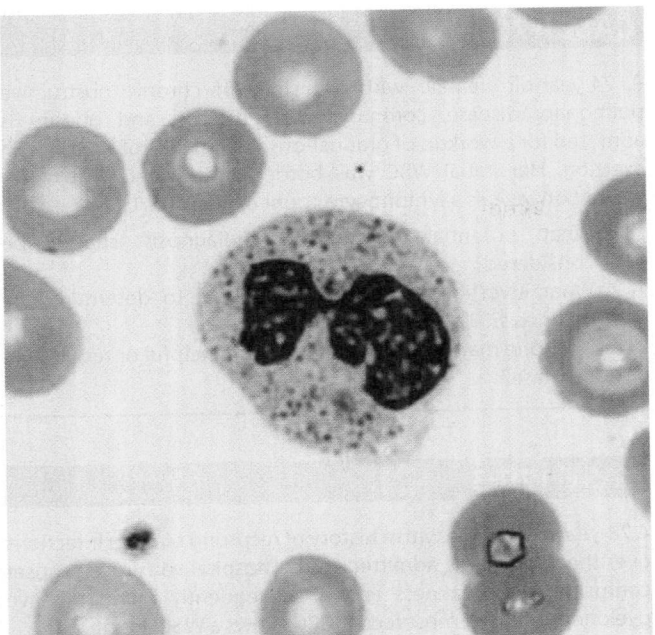

Figure 170-3 *Activated neutrophil with toxic granulation and Dohle bodies.*

activated neutrophil and, thus, the presence of underlying infection. Vacuolization correlates with the extent of lysosomal function and autophagy and is considered strongly suggestive for the presence of more severe sepsis and systemic bacteremia.

Leukoagglutination, another morphologic finding, is a possible cause of spurious leucopenia and the characteristic clumping of WBCs are easily diagnosed on examination of the peripheral blood smear. Leukoagglutination is a nonspecific finding and may be associated with malignancy, hepatic disorders, and infections; the associated infections are typically Gram-negative septicemia. However, leukoagglutination may be associated with the ethylenediaminetetraacetic acid anticoagulation used on blood sample collection similar to that seen with platelets, and recollection of the sample in alternate anticoagulants such as citrated or heparinized container may be enough to unmask the etiology.

Occasionally the presence of *reactive* or *atypical* lymphocytes, large lymphocytes with abundant basophilic cytoplasm and polymorphic nucleoli, can be noted in the peripheral blood. These are thought to represent antigenically stimulated lymphocytes responding to underlying active infection. Classically associated with viral infections such as cytomegalovirus and Epstein-Barr virus, the atypical lymphocyte is somewhat nonspecific and can also be associated with bacterial infections, drug reactions, and endocrinopathies such as Addison disease. These cells may be mistaken for the blasts of acute leukemia, especially in the context of a severe acute infection with marrow suppression. Thus, if there is any ambiguity on history and physical examination, more aggressive investigation, such as flow cytometry on a peripheral blood sample, should be performed to help elucidate the etiology.

PRACTICE POINT

- Microscopic examination of the peripheral blood smear is a simple, expedient, and widely available analytical method that can be of tremendous diagnostic significance in unexplained cases of WBC abnormalities.

■ FLOW CYTOMETRY ANALYSIS

Flow cytometry is an extremely useful investigational tool that allows simultaneous multiparametric analysis of the physical characteristics defining WBC types using the principles of light scattering, excitation, and fluorochrome emission. As such, it can allow for the rapid identification and quantification of populations of WBC in any given patient sample based on the characteristic immunophenotype of the population subset. This is an important characteristic, as conventional cell counters used in the CBC identify cell types based on size alone and can easily misidentify atypical cell types.

Flow cytometry can be a vital investigational tool for the hospitalist; for example, it can be used in the initial workup of a new leukocytosis to identify a malignant versus a benign reactive cause. Flow cytometry also has direct uses in nonmalignant hematologic conditions, such as in the determination of CD4/CD8 count ratios in HIV-associated lymphocytopenia or in the diagnosis of rarer conditions such as paroxysmal nocturnal hemoglobinuria and Langerhans cell histiocytosis. Unfortunately, flow cytometry cannot reliably determine clonality, and further molecular techniques, such as T-cell receptor or B-cell light chain sequencing, would be required to confirm clonality.

■ EXAMINATION OF THE BONE MARROW ASPIRATE AND BIOPSY

Bone marrow aspiration and biopsy can be exceedingly helpful in the diagnosis and management of hematologic malignancies as well as in ascertaining overall bone marrow function when investigating the etiology of unexplained cytopenias. It is important in the diagnosis and management of the myelodysplastic syndromes and acute leukemia. It also has a role in the investigation of certain infections, such as tuberculosis, and is central in the diagnostic workup of a fever of unknown origin. It is the gold standard for determining body iron stores and helpful for the diagnosis of cellular storage disorders such as Gaucher disease and infiltrative conditions such as sarcoidosis or amyloidosis.

Samples of bone marrow are typically taken under local anesthetic from the posterior superior iliac crest, as it is the easiest accessible site. The anterior superior crest and the sternum are alternative accessible sites when the posterior crest cannot be accessed; the sternum is an option only for aspiration because biopsy is contraindicated at this site. A bone marrow aspirate is typically sent for flow cytometry, morphologic, conventional G-banded cytogenetic, and specialized molecular studies, as the diagnostic question requires. Molecular testing with PCR-based assays or fluorescent in situ hybridization can only be performed if the molecular targets being looked for are previously known. A trephine biopsy of the trabecula should also be taken to appropriately assess bone marrow cellularity and morphologic cellular associations; the morphologic cellular associations may be characteristic of the underlying condition and, thus, of significant aid in establishing the diagnosis.

■ ROLE OF SUPPORTIVE MOLECULAR TESTING

After a complete history and physical examination and examination of the peripheral blood smear and bone marrow biopsy and aspirate, there are a few specific molecular tests that can be helpful in the workup of a WBC abnormality. These tests are of utility in the initial workup to differentiate between a malignant and a benign cause of a hematologic abnormality, thus facilitating the timely and appropriate request for a hematologic consultation.

Examples of molecular tests widely available on peripheral blood samples include PCR analysis for the presence of the BCR-ABL fusion transcript in granulocytes in the diagnostic workup of an unexplained left shift. Other common tyrosine kinase mutations such as those found in the Janus kinase 2 (Jak2) or myeloproliferative leukemia virus can be tested for, as a persisting leukocytosis can accompany myeloproliferative disorders such as essential thrombocythemia. Platelet-derived growth factor (PDGF) fusion proteins on fluorescent in situ hybridization of peripheral blood or marrow aspirate samples in eosinophilia can both identify clonality and establish the role of tyrosine kinase inhibitor therapy, as can *c-kit* mutations in mastocytosis. PCR-based sequencing of the T-cell receptor on T lymphocytes and the kappa and lamda light chain genes in B lymphocytes can also be done to confirm a clonal population of lymphocytic cells such as that in MBL or CLL.

Molecular testing will become more widespread and will gain prominence for identifying clonal disorders that may respond to targeted therapy in the future, so a working knowledge of the basics of molecular testing can be of great benefit to the hospitalist in the workup of hospitalized patients. Currently, however, the majority of molecular tests are specific for malignant conditions and, thus, of limited utility for benign abnormalities.

■ CLINICAL USE OF COLONY-STIMULATING FACTORS IN BENIGN HEMATOLOGIC CONDITIONS

The cornerstone of treatment for benign causes of WBC disorders is identification and removal of the underlying etiology whenever possible. However, the clinical development of colony-stimulating factors has enabled the practitioner to augment transient periods of neutropenia when elimination of the underlying cause in a timely fashion is not feasible.

The two clinically available CSFs are granulocyte macrophage colony-stimulating factor, which stimulates production of neutrophils, monocytes, and eosinophils, and granulocyte colony-stimulating factor, which stimulates production only of neutrophils. Administration of these CSFs not only augments the magnitude of the total WBC pool, but also appears to improve mature neutrophil function as well. Currently, only GCSF (Filgrastim) has approval for use in benign WBC conditions, specifically for reducing both the incidence and the duration of complications in patients with congenital, cyclic, and idiopathic neutropenia.

Despite the limited licensed indication, several off-label uses for GCSF in benign leukopenic conditions have also been reported in the literature. These include minimizing the sequelae of neutropenia associated with HIV disease or HIV-drug-associated neutropenia, as well as supporting neutropenia in benign conditions that require myelosuppresive drugs such as methotrexate. Case reports have also described usage for treating prolonged neutropenia related to autoimmune neutropenia as well as drug-induced agranulocytosis. Although efficacious and promising, the overall safety profile of these medications in such settings has not been completely determined, and, thus, their use remains largely investigational and should only be employed in conjunction with specialty consultation.

CASE 170-1

An 82-year-old male with a medical history of type 2 diabetes, hypertension, and coronary artery disease with triple bypass surgery 4 years ago is admitted to hospital for a workup of falls. On the medical ward he wakes with new-onset confusion. A routine CBC drawn that morning shows a WBC count of 38,000.

1. What things might be helpful on history? On physical examination? From the peripheral blood film?
2. What investigations would be the next ones to order?
3. What role for molecular testing, if any, exists here?

CASE 170-2

A 74-year-old female with a history of chronic obstructive pulmonary disease, coronary artery disease, and obesity is admitted for a workup of gradual-onset shortness of breath with exertion. Her initial WBC was borderline elevated, but closer inspection reveals a lymphocyte count of 4.2×10^9/L.

1. What potential nonmalignant diagnosis should be considered?
2. What investigations would be helpful to determine the diagnosis?
3. Is a bone marrow biopsy and aspirate helpful or required in this case?

CASE 170-3

A 78-year-old female with a history of recurring bladder infections over the past year is admitted to the hospital with recent-onset confusion and weakness and is subsequently found to have pyelonephritis. Her most recent CBC shows a WBC count of 1.8.

1. What aspect of the CBC would be directly related to her mortality risk?
2. Does she require a bone marrow biopsy and aspirate? What features of the peripheral smear may make you want to perform this test?
3. Is there a role for granulocyte colony-stimulating factor in the care of this patient?

CONCLUSION

Recognizing the composition of the differential white blood cell count and associated abnormalities is critical for formulating a differential diagnosis of disorders involving the WBC lineages and for initiating potentially life-saving treatment. Although benign causes should resolve with treatment of the underlying cause, the severity of the deviation of the WBC provides important prognostic information that may influence triage decisions and management. The WBC count may also provide important clues to previously undiagnosed underlying congenital and acquired disorders such as HIV or immunoglobin deficiency so that directed therapy can be initiated during hospitalization. Valuable time and resources can be saved and best directed if careful attention is paid to these simple tests in the clinical context of the acutely ill patient.

SUGGESTED READINGS

Hoffbrand AV, Moss PAH, Pettit JE. *Essential Haematology*, 5th ed. Oxford, UK: Blackwell Publishing.

Ibáñez L, Vidal X, Ballarín E, Laporte JR. Population-based drug-induced agranulocytosis. *Arch Intern Med*. 2005;165(8):869-874.

Kho AN, Hui S, Kesterson JG, McDonald CJ. Which observations from the complete blood cell count predict mortality for hospitalized patients? *J Hosp Med*. 2007;2(1):5-12.

Wanahita A, Goldsmith EA, Musher DM. Conditions associated with leukocytosis in a tertiary care hospital, with particular attention to the role of infection caused by clostridium difficile. *Clin Infect Dis*. 2002;34:1585-1592.

Quantitative Abnormalities of Platelets: Thrombocytopenia and Thrombocytosis

Theodore E. Warkentin, MD

Key Clinical Questions

Thrombocytopenia

1. Does the patient have true thrombocytopenia or pseudothrombocytopenia?

2. What is the timing of onset, progression, and severity of the thrombocytopenia?

3. Is the thrombocytopenia isolated, or is there concomitant anemia, leukopenia, or both?

4. What are the findings of the peripheral blood film?

5. What tests and studies are useful to evaluate each etiology?

6. What is the frequency of specific causes of thrombocytopenia in defined clinical circumstances?

7. Is the thrombocytopenia a marker of bleeding risk, thrombosis risk, or adverse prognosis?

8. What treatments are available for each etiology?

Thrombocytosis

1. Is the thrombocytosis newly acquired during the hospitalization?

2. Is there concomitant splenomegaly and/or abnormalities in hemoglobin or white blood cell levels?

3. Does the thrombocytosis predate the hospitalization?

4. Is the red cell size (mean corpuscular volume) increased or decreased?

THROMBOCYTOPENIA

■ INTRODUCTION

The normal platelet count range is approximately 150 to 400×10^9/L (150,000-400,000/mm³). An individual's platelet count usually remains relatively constant during life. The platelet count decreases normally during pregnancy (gestational thrombocytopenia). The platelet count increases to above the usual value following an acute self-limited thrombocytopenia. For example, after major surgery, an early postoperative platelet count nadir is observed; subsequently, thrombocytosis occurs, with the peak platelet count reached approximately 2-week postsurgery, with a late postoperative platelet count nadir occurring 2 weeks later (ie, approximately 1-month postsurgery) (**Figure 171-1**). As discussed later in this chapter, these postsurgery platelet count changes are expected, and reflect physiological consequences of changes in thrombopoietin-induced (TPO-induced) platelet production triggered by the initial acute surgery-associated platelet count fall.

PRACTICE POINT

- Evaluation of thrombocytopenia should include review of the peripheral smear. The timing of onset of thrombocytopenia is a valuable clue regarding its possible etiologies. Identification of the cause of the thrombocytopenia determines next steps, including identification of those patients with low platelet counts who are likely to benefit from platelet transfusions in select circumstances.

Many clinicians equate thrombocytopenia with increased bleeding risk. Indeed, severe immune-mediated thrombocytopenia does pose increased bleeding risk. But certain other thrombocytopenic disorders are associated with greatly increased risk of thrombosis (eg, heparin-induced thrombocytopenia [HIT], antiphospholipid syndrome, cancer-associated hypercoagulability), or increased mortality (thrombocytopenia complicating septicemia or multiorgan system dysfunction).

The various explanations for thrombocytopenia differ depending on the clinical setting. For patients who present to the emergency room with acute, severe thrombocytopenia, certain life-threatening disorders must be considered, such as thrombotic thrombocytopenia purpura (TTP), drug-induced immune thrombocytopenic purpura (D-ITP), and acute leukemia. In postoperative patients, the timing of onset of thrombocytopenia is important since early, transient thrombocytopenia (due to postoperative hemodilution) is expected, whereas later-onset thrombocytopenia suggests heparin-induced thrombocytopenia, septicemia, or other postoperative complications. Thrombocytopenia in the intensive care unit is often due to poorly defined platelet consumption complicating multiorgan system dysfunction.

The hospitalist may be the first physician called upon to evaluate a thrombocytopenic patient, especially when the platelet count decline begins during hospitalization. The hospitalist needs to appreciate the circumstances when referral to a hematologist is appropriate.

■ PHYSICAL EXAMINATION

The physical examination should focus on the presence of signs of bleeding (petechiae, purpura), fever, or chills (infection,

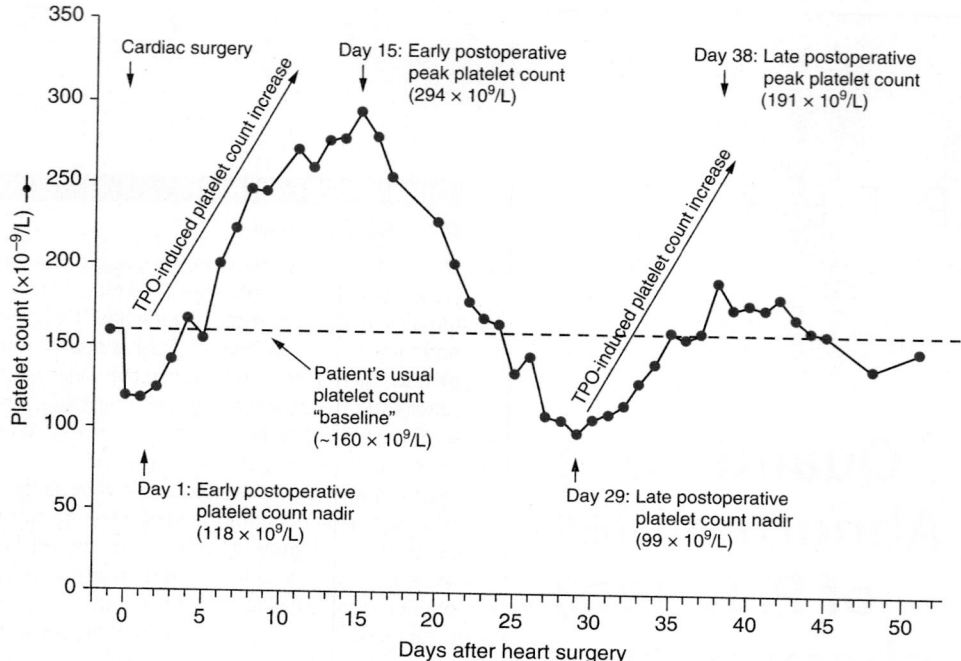

Figure 171-1 *Serial platelet counts in an 81-year-old male who underwent coronary artery bypass surgery (day 0). The patient's usual platelet count ("baseline") was ~160 × 10⁹/L. Following acute surgery-associated thrombocytopenia (early postoperative platelet count nadir, day 1), the platelet count rose, peaking by day 15 at 294 × 10⁹/L (ie, almost twice the preoperative value). The platelet counts then progressively declined, resulting in a late postoperative platelet count nadir (99 × 10⁹/L) observed on day 29, with a second, much less marked, platelet count peak (191 × 10⁹/L) reached on day 38. The platelet count value of 99 approximately 1-month postcardiac surgery prompted a hematology consultation. The hematologist's opinion was that these postoperative platelet count fluctuations were expected, reflecting physiological increases and subsequent later decreases in blood thrombopoietin (TPO) concentrations (as blood TPO levels correspond inversely with platelet count levels), with corresponding increases and decreases in platelet production by the bone marrow megakaryocytes. The over- and undershooting of the platelet counts—in relation to the patient's baseline platelet count value—are explained by the lag time of several days required for changes in TPO levels to produce corresponding changes in marrow platelet production. As predicted by the hematology consultant, the platelet counts began to recover, indeed overshooting the baseline platelet count one more time (days 38-44).*

anaphylactoid reaction secondary to acute HIT), the presence of invasive catheters and the integrity of the surrounding skin (source of infection), ventilator status (risk for pneumonia, indicator of multiorgan system failure), hemodynamic status (shock with risk of multiorgan failure-associated thrombocytopenia and disseminated intravascular coagulation [DIC]), pulses and distal limb ischemia (HIT-associated arterial or venous thrombosis), lymphadenopathy (lymphoproliferative disorders), hepatosplenomegaly (hypersplenism), and miscellaneous skin lesions (necrotizing skin lesions at heparin injection sites). Note that acral (distal extremity) tissue ischemic necrosis—despite palpable or Doppler-identifiable pulses—is a hallmark of disturbed procoagulant-anticoagulant balance and associated microvascular thrombosis that underlies several hematologic disorders such as overt (decompensated) DIC and HIT-associated venous limb gangrene (usually caused by warfarin).

The hallmark of severe thrombocytopenia is mucocutaneous bleeding, particularly pinpoint intradermal hemorrhages known as *petechiae*. These are nonpalpable, nonblanching, and indicate bleeding from capillaries. Petechiae are most evident in dependent areas (eg, the legs and feet in outpatients and the back and posterior thighs in bedridden patients) because of the effects of hydrostatic pressure. Generalized "oozing" from mucosal sites (eg, nose and genitourinary and gastrointestinal tracts) can be seen in severe thrombocytopenia. A classic finding is "blood blisters" (hemorrhagic vesicles of the oral mucosa or tongue) when the platelet count is less than 10 × 10⁹/L in the setting of autoimmune, alloimmune, or drug-induced immune thrombocytopenia. *Ecchymosis* denotes intradermal hemorrhage greater than 2 mm (ie, larger than petechiae); however, ecchymoses are less specific than petechiae for thrombocytopenic bleeding.

■ PATHOPHYSIOLOGY

Table 171-1 lists the five general mechanisms of thrombocytopenia, plus a sixth category of spurious thrombocytopenia ("pseudothrombocytopenia").

Pseudothrombocytopenia

A key question when evaluating a patient for thrombocytopenia is: Does the patient have true thrombocytopenia or pseudothrombocytopenia? Platelet clumping that occurs ex vivo (ie, only after the blood has been drawn into an anticoagulant) can be caused by naturally occurring antibodies that bind to platelets, resulting in platelet agglutination, but only in the presence of anticoagulant. This is most often seen when blood is collected into the purple tube (containing ethylenediaminetetraacetic acid [EDTA]) for determination of the complete blood count (CBC) (ie, EDTA-induced pseudothrombocytopenia). The thrombocytopenia is spurious because the electronic particle counter fails to detect the clumped platelets. Examination of the blood film reveals platelet clumping. Usually, platelet clumping does not occur, or is less marked, when blood is collected into another anticoagulant (eg, citrate, heparin). Pseudothrombocytopenia is clinically insignificant except when inappropriate treatment results from a wrong diagnosis of thrombocytopenia.

Hemodilution

A decline of 20% to 70% occurs universally in patients following major surgery, a phenomenon that is most dramatic in postcardiac surgery patients. The platelet count nadir usually occurs between postoperative days 1 and 4 (median, day 2), with a subsequent rise

TABLE 171-1 Six General Explanations for Thrombocytopenia

Explanation	Comment	Examples
Pseudothrombocytopenia	Antibody-mediated platelet clumping that occurs ex vivo (spurious thrombocytopenia)	EDTA-induced pseudothrombocytopenia
Hemodilution	Abrupt platelet count fall due to administration of fluids or blood products	Early postoperative thrombocytopenia
Hypersplenism	Splenomegaly may require imaging studies to detect; concomitant leukopenia and (to lesser extent) anemia are usually present	Cirrhosis-associated portal hypertension
Decreased platelet production	Usually there is concomitant leukopenia and anemia (a notable exception is certain types of hereditary thrombocytopenia)	Myelodysplasia; aplastic anemia; marrow infiltration by metastatic cancer; MYH9-associated thrombocytopenia
Platelet consumption	Accelerated platelet clearance due to pathologically increased thrombin generation or other poorly defined mechanisms of increased platelet clearance	Disseminated intravascular coagulation; septicemia; multiorgan system failure
Platelet destruction	Accelerated platelet clearance due to pathologic mechanisms that target platelets, especially due to autoantibodies	Autoimmune thrombocytopenic purpura; HIT; drug-induced immune thrombocytopenia; TTP/HUS

EDTA, ethylenediaminetetraacetic acid; HIT, heparin-induced thrombocytopenia; HUS, hemolytic uremic syndrome; MYH9, myosin heavy chain 9 (nonmuscle); TTP, thrombotic thrombocytopenic purpura.

in the platelet count that peaks at approximately day 14, at levels that are usually two to three times the patient's preoperative baseline (postthrombocytopenia thrombocytosis). The platelet count decline is roughly proportional to the amount of crystalloid, colloid, or blood products administered, plus some component of platelet consumption. Dilutional coagulopathy generally accompanies the thrombocytopenia, accounting for the minor increases in prothrombin time (PT) and activated partial thromboplastin time (aPTT) that are commonly seen immediately after surgery. Hemodilution occurs universally after major surgery and represents the most common explanation for thrombocytopenia in the early postoperative period.

The diagnosis of dilutional thrombocytopenia is a good example of considering the key question: What is the timing of onset, progression, and severity of the thrombocytopenia? Here, the timing is abrupt in onset (directly follows surgery), the thrombocytopenia progresses to its usual nadir at approximately day 2 (range, days 1-4), and is mild to moderate in severity depending on the nature of the surgery and the amount of fluids and blood products administered. In the case of cardiac surgery utilizing extracorporeal circulation (cardiopulmonary bypass), the maximum decline in platelet count averages 50%, but can be as high as 70%. Furthermore, the natural history of dilutional thrombocytopenia is for the platelet count—after attaining its nadir—to progressively increase to peak levels at approximately day 14 that are considerably greater than the preoperative baseline.

Hypersplenism

When approaching the diagnosis of hypersplenism, consider the following question: Is the thrombocytopenia isolated, or is there concomitant anemia and/or leukopenia? Whereas isolated thrombocytopenia usually indicates consumption or destruction of platelets (eg, DIC or immune thrombocytopenia) or hereditary thrombocytopenia (eg, MYH9-associated thrombocytopenia), thrombocytopenia associated with anemia and leukopenia can indicate hemodilution (discussed previously), hypersplenism, or marrow failure (eg, leukemia, marrow infiltration by metastatic cancer), or the combination of anemia and thrombocytopenia (eg, a disorder such as TTP).

Normally, about one-third of the circulating platelets are exchangeably sequestered within the spleen. Increased spleen size leads to greater splenic pooling (as high as 70%-90%) and, thus, thrombocytopenia ("hypersplenism"). Two factors determine the extent of splenic pooling: splenic blood flow and splenic transit time. The most important determinant of splenic blood flow is spleen size, and the most important determinant of splenic transit time is splenic perfusion (spleen blood flow/spleen volume). However, since disorders that alter splenic transit time (eg, congestive heart failure, rheumatologic disorders) usually have counterbalancing effects on splenic blood flow, in practical terms, spleen size itself correlates well with the degree of splenic platelet pooling. Hence, radiologic imaging of spleen size can assess whether thrombocytopenia is caused by hypersplenism. A more recent concept is that reduced hepatic production of thrombopoietin also contributes to thrombocytopenia of hypersplenism, in the setting of severe liver disease.

Decreased platelet production

Decreased platelet production can be caused by congenital or acquired bone marrow disorders, often manifesting as pancytopenia. However, isolated thrombocytopenia is seen in the MYH9-associated thrombocytopenias. Suspicion of decreased marrow production is often based on the answer to the question: What are the findings of the peripheral blood film? The blood film often points to a diagnosis of a primary bone marrow disorder, for example, primitive cells such as leukoblasts (acute leukemia) or abnormal lymphoid cells (neoplastic lymphoproliferative disorders), dysplastic white cells (myelodysplasia), tear-drop red cells (infiltrative marrow disorders such as carcinoma metastatic to the bone marrow, myeloproliferative neoplasms with increased marrow fibrosis), and large red and white cells (megaloblastic anemia of vitamin B12 deficiency). The presence of very large platelets, together with neutrophil inclusions, is suggestive of MYH9-associated thrombocytopenia. **Table 171-2** lists some of the findings of the peripheral blood film in patients with decreased platelet production, as well as some other disorders.

Demographic trends, particularly increasing numbers of elderly patients, suggest that clonal marrow disorders such as myelodysplasia ("preleukemia") and chronic lymphoid leukemia will become more common. These are often "incidental" findings when patients are admitted for nonhematologic problems, and a routine CBC can lead to detection of thrombocytopenia.

Platelet consumption

Pathological activation of the coagulation system, often termed *disseminated intravascular coagulation* (DIC) or *consumptive coagulopathy*,

TABLE 171-2 The Blood Film in The Evaluation of Thrombocytopenia

Feature	Suggested Diagnosis	Comment
Platelet clumping; platelet rosetting around neutrophils and/or monocytes (rare)	Pseudothrombocytopenia	Clinically insignificant (other than potential for false diagnosis of thrombocytopenia)
Neutrophilia; "toxic" white cells (increased granules, vacuoles)	Septicemia or other marked proinflammatory conditions	Blood cultures should be ordered, as bacteremia/fungemia is common cause of thrombocytopenia
Giant platelets; neutrophil inclusions	MYH9-associated macrothrombocytopenia	Inclusions may be difficult to discern without special stains
Red cell macrocytosis, "target" red cells, acanthocytes (spur cells), pancytopenia	Liver disease with portal hypertension and hypersplenism	Thrombocytopenia and neutropenia usually parallel one another in severity
Hypogranular leukocytes, left shift, Pelger-Huët anomaly (*pince-nez* appearance)	Myelodysplasia, myeloid leukemia	*Pince-nez* (French: "eyeglasses clipped to the bridge of the nose") appearance of leukocyte nuclei
Red cell fragments (schistocytes, eg, "helmet" cells); polychromasia	Microangiopathic hemolysis (TTP, HUS), DIC	Red cell fragments more prominent in TTP and HUS than in DIC
Red cell microbial inclusions	Malaria, babesia, *Cryptococcus* (rarely seen in red cells)	Type of malaria can be determined, eg, "ring forms" of *Plasmodium falciparum*

DIC, disseminated intravascular coagulation; HUS, hemolytic uremic syndrome; MYH9, myosin heavy chain 9; TTP, thrombotic thrombocytopenic purpura.

is usually accompanied by thrombocytopenia. Underlying problems can include shock, trauma/burns, septicemia, multiorgan system failure, malignancy, envenomations, severe hemolysis, certain complications of pregnancy (eg, placental abruption, retained products), and so forth. Sometimes, thrombocytopenia due to increased platelet consumption occurs even when the global coagulation assays (PT, aPTT) are not markedly elevated; this can be seen in some infections or in multiorgan system failure, and might reflect nonthrombin-mediated mechanisms of accelerated physiologic platelet clearance.

A key question is: What tests and studies are useful in evaluating each etiology? Testing for DIC should include the global coagulation assays (PT, aPTT) in addition to fibrinogen and one or more markers of fibrin formation, such as the fibrin D-dimer, fibrin(ogen) degradation products (FDPs), or fibrin monomer. Blood cultures should be

done because bacteremia is a common explanation for consumptive thrombocytopenia (with or without laboratory evidence for DIC) in hospitalized patients; when a consumptive thrombocytopenia occurs in a patient who has received antibiotics for a prolonged period, fungemia becomes an increasingly plausible explanation for a consumptive thrombocytopenia. **Table 171-3** lists some of the laboratory tests that can be helpful in evaluating thrombocytopenia.

Platelet destruction

The term *platelet destruction* (or *destructive thrombocytopenia*) refers to disorders in which pathologic factors destroy platelets in a nonphysiologic manner, most often as a direct or indirect result of antibodies. **Table 171-4** lists different antibody-mediated thrombocytopenic disorders. Heparin-induced thrombocytopenia (HIT)

TABLE 171-3 Laboratory Tests Used to Investigate a Patient with Thrombocytopenia

Test	Comment
Complete blood count (CBC)	Electronic particle counters; detects thrombocytopenia
Review of blood film	See Table 171-2
Blood cultures	Bacteremia, fungemia
Antinuclear antibody test	Systemic lupus erythematosus (associated with immune thrombocytopenia)
Direct antiglobulin test (if anemic)	Combined immune hemolysis and immune thrombocytopenia (Evan syndrome)
Coagulation tests: PT/INR, aPTT, TCT	Screen for deficiency of coagulation factor (or factors), or detect presence of inhibitor (anticoagulant or antibody inhibitor)
Coagulation tests: fibrinogen; fibrin D-dimer, FDPs, fibrin monomer	Low fibrinogen and presence of other markers can indicate DIC or hyperfibrinolysis (caveat: fibrinogen levels can be normal in DIC)
Coagulation assays: "nonspecific inhibitor"; anticardiolipin; anti-β2-glycoprotein I	APS suggested by positive tests for antiphospholipid antibodies detected either by functional (coagulation) or immunologic assays
Serum protein electrophoresis; quantitative immunoglobulin levels	Plasma cell or lymphoproliferative disorders (usually monoclonal) or chronic hepatitis/hypersplenism (polyclonal hypergammaglobulinemia)
HIV serology	HIV-associated thrombocytopenia
Bone marrow aspirate and biopsy	Assess megakaryocyte numbers and morphology; evaluate for primary or secondary (eg, metastatic neoplasm) bone marrow disorder

APS, antiphospholipid syndrome; aPTT, activated partial thromboplastin time; DIC, disseminated intravascular coagulation; FDPs, fibrin degradation products; HIV, human immunodeficiency virus; PT/INR (prothrombin time/international normalized ratio); TCT, thrombin clotting time.
Note: This table excludes certain specialized tests, such as those for antibodies that cause heparin-induced thrombocytopenia, flow cytometry-based immunophenotyping, and cytogenetic studies of peripheral blood or marrow blood cells.

TABLE 171-4 Antibody-Mediated Thrombocytopenia

Disorder	Comment
Platelet count often <20 × 10⁹/L	
(Auto) immune thrombocytopenic purpura	Primary (idiopathic) or secondary (eg, associated with systemic lupus erythematosus, lymphoproliferative disorders, viral hepatitis, HIV infection)
Posttransfusion purpura	Severe thrombocytopenia 5-10 d after blood transfusion
Drug-induced immune thrombocytopenia	See Table 171-5
Thrombotic thrombocytopenic purpura–hemolytic uremic syndrome	Idiopathic thrombotic thrombocytopenic purpura in many cases is caused by autoantibodies that bind to the von Willebrand factor–cleaving metalloprotease, ADAMTS13; "typical" HUS is usually triggered by enterohemorrhagic *E. coli*, whereas "atypical" HUS is often associated with congenital or acquired (autoimmune) abnormalities in the alternative complement system
Platelet count often >20 × 10⁹/L	
Heparin-induced thrombocytopenia	Prothrombotic adverse drug reaction characterized by high risk of venous and arterial thrombosis; risk factor for warfarin-associated microthrombosis

overlaps the differing concepts of destructive and consumptive thrombocytopenia: it arises from pathologic platelet-activating antibodies (destructive thrombocytopenia) and, in its severe form, can also feature overt DIC (consumptive thrombocytopenia).

A key question is: What is the frequency of specific causes of thrombocytopenia in defined clinical circumstances? For example, when a patient has very severe thrombocytopenia (platelet count <20 × 10⁹/L), destructive thrombocytopenia is the likely problem (eg, ITP [autoimmune], D-ITP [drug-induced], TTP, and occasionally, very severe HIT or DIC) as it is unusual for consumptive thrombocytopenia or hypersplenism to produce such severe thrombocytopenia. Severe thrombocytopenia due to primary bone marrow disorders is usually clinically obvious (eg, pancytopenia

with circulated myeloblasts). The next section deals with some of the possible explanations for thrombocytopenia when it occurs following the patient's admission to hospital, particularly in the postsurgery context.

■ ONSET OF THROMBOCYTOPENIA AFTER HOSPITALIZATION

In hospitalized patients, the timing of onset of thrombocytopenia is a valuable clue regarding its possible etiologies. **Figure 171-2** shows the typical evolution of platelet counts after surgery: after an early postoperative decline, the platelet count increases steadily, reaching levels that are usually two to three times the preoperative baseline, peaking at postoperative day 14, before gradually

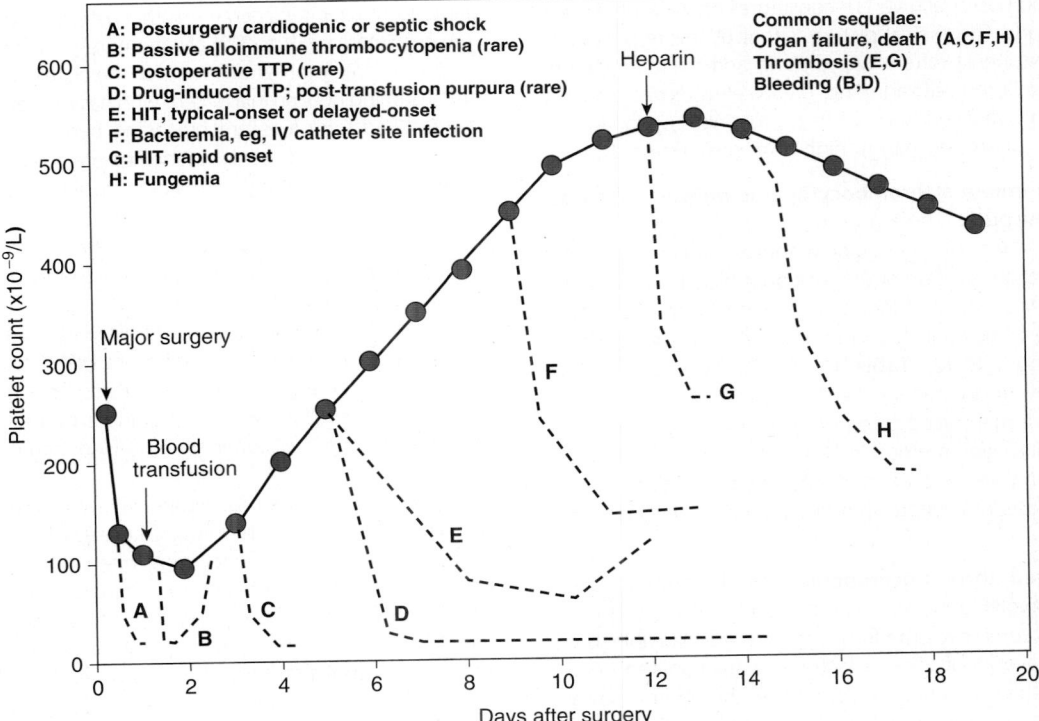

Figure 171-2 *Timing of onset of thrombocytopenia in a postoperative patient: diagnostic implications. The circles connected by a solid line indicate the typical evolution of postoperative thrombocytopenia (usual nadir, day 2) to postoperative thrombocytosis (usual peak, day 14). The dashed lines indicate various temporal profiles of unexpected postoperative thrombocytopenia and associated diagnostic considerations. In profile D, it is assumed that the responsible drug or blood product was started (or given) in the intra- or perioperative period. Note: For profile G, thrombosis is the usual reason why heparin is given, leading to rapid-onset HIT.*

declining over the third and fourth weeks. The figure also shows the usual timing of onset of several common (and rare) explanations for thrombocytopenia.

Diagnostic considerations

Hemodynamic compromise and circulatory or septic shock:
Thrombocytopenia with or without overt DIC is a common finding in patients with early postsurgery circulatory shock, such as resulting from cardiac failure or sepsis (see profile A in Figure 171-2). Hypotension and vasopressor use can contribute to acral limb ischemia, but there is usually also a prominent role of microvascular thrombosis, manifesting clinically as "symmetrical peripheral gangrene," that is related to failure of natural anticoagulants (protein C pathway, antithrombin III) to control pathologic thrombin generation. Recently, acute ischemic hepatitis ("shock liver") has been identified as a potential risk factor for acral limb ischemia (via compromised production of hepatically synthesized protein C and/or antithrombin III) in the setting of DIC.

Passive alloimmune thrombocytopenia:
Rarely, blood products contain cell-specific alloantibodies that cause life-threatening sequelae. Best known is transfusion-associated acute lung injury (TRALI), where transfusion of blood product—usually from a multiparous female donor—containing antigranulocyte alloantibodies causes life-threatening pulmonary edema. The platelet analogue of TRALI is passive alloimmune thrombocytopenia (PAT), which is characterized by severe thrombocytopenia that begins abruptly after administering a blood product (eg, fresh frozen plasma [FFP], red cell concentrates) containing platelet-reactive alloantibodies (see profile B in Figure 171-2).

Postoperative TTP:
Rarely, patients develop TTP in the early postoperative period, probably because postoperative proinflammatory factors trigger someone already predisposed to TTP to develop overt disease (see profile C in Figure 171-2). TTP itself is a rare disease, and postoperative TTP constitutes only about 1% of all TTP presentations. The clinical picture is that of severe postoperative thrombocytopenia (often $<20 \times 10^9$/L) and microangiopathic hemolysis (anemia, red cell fragments, greatly elevated lactate dehydrogenase, negative direct Coombs test). Treatment is managed by a hematologist (plasma exchange, high-dose corticosteroids).

Drug-induced immune thrombocytopenic purpura and posttransfusion purpura:
The onset of severe thrombocytopenia (platelet count $<20 \times 10^9$/L) beginning approximately 1 week after the institution of a new drug or the receipt of blood products, suggests the diagnosis of drug-induced immune thrombocytopenic purpura (D-ITP) or posttransfusion purpura (PTP), respectively (see profile D in Figure 171-2). **Table 171-5** lists some of the drugs most frequently implicated in classic (typical) D-ITP, as well as other atypical drug-induced thrombocytopenic syndromes. Petechiae and purpura are common in D-ITP and PTP, and when such signs of bleeding are encountered, platelet transfusions with or without high-dose intravenous immunoglobulin G (IVIgG) may be appropriate.

Heparin-induced thrombocytopenia:
This immune-mediated drug reaction involving platelets is more common than all of the causes of D-ITP combined. The frequency is highly variable, but in patients who have all of the risk factors—unfractionated heparin use for more than 1 week, postoperative thromboprophylaxis, female sex—the frequency is 1% to 5%. The typical picture (~65% of patients; see profile E in Figure 171-2) is an otherwise unexpected platelet count fall that begins 5 to 10 days after beginning heparin, most often in the setting of postsurgical thromboprophylaxis. The frequency of HIT is approximately tenfold less with low-molecular-weight heparin (LMWH), and even less common (although reported)

TABLE 171-5 Drug-Induced Immune Thrombocytopenic Purpura: Implicated Drugs (Selected List)

Typical D-ITP
Quinine, quinidine
Antibiotics (ceftriaxone, levofloxacin, nafcillin, piperacillin, rifampin, sulfamethoxazole, trimethoprim, vancomycin)
Anti-inflammatory (acetaminophen*, ibuprofen*, naproxen)
Antineoplastic (oxaliplatin)
Cardiac (amiodarone, furosemide)
Neurologic (carbamazepine, phenytoin)
Atypical
GPIIb/IIIa antagonist–induced thrombocytopenia (abciximab, eptifibatide, tirofiban)†
HIT (see also Table 171-6)
TTP/HUS (quinine, cyclosporine, gemcitabine, mitomycin C)

D-ITP, drug-induced immune thrombocytopenic purpura; HIT, heparin-induced thrombocytopenia; HUS, hemolytic-uremic syndrome; TTP, thrombotic thrombocytopenic purpura.

Note: This is a partial list only. Readers should consult published lists (see Suggested Reading) or a website (www.ouhsc.edu/platelets/DITP.html) for additional drugs.

*Drug metabolites implicated.

†An atypical feature of D-ITP caused by GPIIb/IIIa antagonists is that ~1% of patients who receive one of these agents for the first time develop abrupt-onset D-ITP because of naturally occurring antibodies.

with the pentasaccharide anticoagulant, fondaparinux. Rarely, an illness clinically and serologically indistinguishable from HIT can occur in the absence of a preceding exposure to heparin; triggers for so-called "spontaneous HIT syndrome" include orthopedic surgery (particularly, knee replacement surgery) or infection.

Approximately 25% to 30% of patients (see profile G in Figure 171-2) present with rapid-onset HIT, in which the platelet count falls abruptly after resuming heparin in a patient who has circulating HIT antibodies that resulted from a recent preceding heparin exposure. Heparin-induced thrombocytopenia antibodies are transient (median time of detectability, 50-80 days, depending upon the assay performed), which explains why recent—rather than remote—preceding exposure to heparin is a crucial factor in accounting for rapid-onset HIT. About one-quarter of patients who develop rapid-onset HIT following a heparin bolus evince an anaphylactoid reaction. It is increasingly recognized that patients can present with HIT several days after their last exposure to heparin (delayed-onset HIT); here, the patient can present to the emergency room with thrombosis and thrombocytopenia 1 or 2 weeks following a preceding exposure to heparin, which can be quite brief (eg, administered only during cardiac or vascular surgery).

Heparin-induced thrombocytopenia is a "clinicopathologic disorder," and its diagnosis rests on two criteria: (1) the presence of one or more clinically evident events (most often, thrombocytopenia with or without thrombosis) bearing a temporal relationship to a preceding immunizing heparin exposure and (2) detectability of heparin-dependent platelet-activating antibodies against PF4/heparin complexes. **Table 171-6** lists the various sequelae of HIT.

Two types of laboratory assays—platelet activation assays (eg, serotonin-release assay [SRA]) and PF4-dependent enzyme immunoassays (EIAs)—are very sensitive for HIT, and, thus, a negative assay generally rules out the diagnosis. Platelet activation assays have superior sensitivity-specificity tradeoffs compared with EIAs, and a positive SRA is more diagnostically specific for HIT than the EIA. The "strength" of an EIA (measured in optical density

TABLE 171-6 Heparin-Induced Thrombocytopenia: Clinical-Pathologic Criteria for Diagnosis

Clinical	Pathologic
At least one of the following: • **Thrombocytopenia*** • **Thrombosis** (eg, *venous*: deep-vein thrombosis, pulmonary embolism, venous limb gangrene, adrenal hemorrhage,† cerebral vein thrombosis, splanchnic vein thrombosis; *arterial*: limb artery thrombosis, stroke, myocardial infarction, mesenteric artery thrombosis, miscellaneous artery; *microvascular*) • Necrotizing skin lesions at heparin injection sites‡ • Acute anaphylactoid reactions§ Timing: Above event (or events) demonstrates temporal relation to a preceding immunizing heparin exposure¶ Absence of another more compelling explanation	Heparin-dependent, platelet-activating IgG** • Positive platelet activation assay (eg, serotonin-release assay [SRA]) • Positive anti-PF4/polyanion-IgG EIA (infers possibility of platelet-activating IgG††)

*Greater than 50% platelet count fall is seen in ~90% of patients; in 5%-10%, the platelet fall is 30%-50%.

†Adrenal hemorrhagic necrosis is a consequence of adrenal vein thrombosis.

‡Nonnecrotizing lesions (erythematous plaques) are less specific for heparin-induced thrombocytopenia (HIT).

§Usually occur 5-30 min after intravenous heparin bolus and, rarely, after subcutaneous heparin.

¶Typical onset is 5-10 d after immunizing heparin exposure (usually, given intra- or perioperatively); rapid-onset HIT can occur if heparin is given to a patient who already has circulating HIT-Abs, usually due to heparin given in the last 5-100 d.

**Acute serum or plasma should be used for testing, as HIT-Abs are transient.

††In the appropriate context, a strong-positive EIA (IgG-specific or polyspecific assay that detects IgG/A/M antibodies) can be used to infer presence of platelet-activating HIT-Abs.

(Reprinted, with permission, from Warkentin TE. Agents for the treatment of heparin-induced thrombocytopenia. *Hematol/Oncol Clin N Am.* 2010;24(4):755.)

units) corresponds strongly to the presence of platelet-activating antibodies and, hence, risk of HIT. Therefore, one should be skeptical about the diagnosis of HIT if the EIA is only weakly positive (eg, 0.4-1.0 units; usual cutoff, 0.4 U).

When HIT is strongly suspected or serologically confirmed, the heparin is stopped, and an alternative anticoagulant is given, usually in therapeutic doses (options include danaparoid [outside the United States], fondaparinux, lepirudin, argatroban, bivalirudin [note: dosing guidelines for these anticoagulants is outside the scope of this chapter]). *It is important not to give warfarin during the acute thrombocytopenic phase of HIT* for three reasons: (1) warfarin does not inhibit HIT-associated hypercoagulability; (2) warfarin causes depletion of protein C (vitamin K-dependent natural anticoagulant), a finding characteristic of devastating microthrombosis syndromes in HIT, such as venous limb gangrene (limb necrosis despite palpable pulses in the setting of deep-vein thrombosis); and (3) warfarin use leads to systematic underdosing of alternative anticoagulants that are usually monitored by the aPTT (lepirudin, argatroban, bivalirudin). Indeed, if warfarin has already been given when HIT is diagnosed, the warfarin should be reversed with intravenous vitamin K. Other tenets of HIT management include

avoiding, if possible, prophylactic platelet transfusions and insertion of inferior vena cava filters, and imaging for lower-limb deep-vein thrombosis (the most common complication of HIT).

For a patient with a previous history of HIT, repeat exposure to heparin can be considered in special circumstances, most often for cardiac or vascular surgery, provided that platelet-activating antibodies are no longer detectable (negative SRA), and a nonheparin anticoagulant (such as fondaparinux) is given for postoperative anticoagulation, if required. With these precautions, the risk of HIT recurrence is believed to be low.

The relative high frequency of HIT raises important issues regarding hospital quality control through platelet count monitoring for HIT. Recently, the American College of Chest Physicians (ACCP) evidence-based clinical practice guidelines (8th edition) opined that intensity of platelet count monitoring should reflect the risk of HIT in any given situation. Thus, for patients at highest risk (>1%), such as postoperative patients receiving antithrombotic prophylaxis with unfractionated heparin, platelet count monitoring should occur at least every other day between postoperative days 4 and 14 (or until UFH is stopped, whichever occurs first). For patients at intermediate risk (0.1%-1%) (eg, postoperative patients receiving LMWH or medical patients receiving UFH), monitoring should occurs "at least every 2 or 3 days from day 4 to day 14 (or until heparin is stopped, whichever occurs first), when practical" (Warkentin et al, 2008). However, when HIT risk is rare (<0.1%), such as with use of LMWH for medical or obstetric patients, or fondaparinux for any indication, routine platelet count monitoring for purposes of early detection of HIT is not advised. Of course, routine platelet count monitoring itself can be problematic if it leads to overdiagnosis of HIT and inappropriate cessation of heparin. Systematic platelet count monitoring for HIT is controversial, and was not endorsed by the 9th (2012) edition of the ACCP guidelines.

Bacteremia and fungemia: Infection is a relatively common explanation for thrombocytopenia in hospitalized patients, and usually indicates microbial invasion of the blood (hence, the importance of performing blood cultures in patients with unexplained thrombocytopenia). Supporting blood film abnormalities include leukocyte "left-shift" (bands, metamyelocytes) and "toxic" features (eg, cytoplasmic vacuolation, toxic granules). Coagulation assays for DIC should be performed, although in many cases there is elevation in fibrin D-dimer levels with normal INR, aPTT, and fibrinogen levels. In patients with overt DIC (elevated INR, reduced or low-normal fibrinogen), there is a risk for microvascular thrombosis (eg, acral ischemia) and special treatment approaches (eg, heparin anticoagulation) may be appropriate. (Fibrinogen is an acute phase reactant, and only one-quarter of patients with DIC have fibrinogen values below the normal range.) The pathogenesis of thrombocytopenia is multifactorial (thrombin-mediated, increased macrophage clearance of platelets, decreased marrow platelet production, effects of microbial toxins). Persistence of thrombocytopenia in sepsis is a poor prognostic factor. As a general rule, fungemia occurs later in the course of hospitalization than does bacteremia (compare profile H with profiles A and F in Figure 171-2).

■ CHRONIC THROMBOCYTOPENIA

Thrombocytopenia in a hospitalized patient can indicate the presence of a preexisting disorder of platelet number, such as hypersplenism, chronic (auto)immune thrombocytopenic purpura (ITP), or a primary bone marrow disorder, either congenital (eg, hereditary thrombocytopenia) or acquired (eg, myelodysplasia). Sometimes, there is an exacerbation of the chronic thrombocytopenia, such as a relapse of ITP or infection-associated worsening of thrombocytopenia in a patient with myelodysplasia.

Diagnostic considerations

Hypersplenism: Table 171-7 lists various explanations for splenomegaly. In North America, the most common cause is cirrhosis, and, thus, concomitant coagulopathy due to liver dysfunction is common. Often, incidentally detected mild or moderate thrombocytopenia is the first clue that a patient has cirrhosis due to alcohol abuse or chronic viral hepatitis.

Chronic autoimmune thrombocytopenia: Immune thrombocytopenic purpura, also known as autoimmune or idiopathic thrombocytopenic purpura, is an acquired, antibody-mediated disorder of adults and children characterized by persistent decrease of the platelet count ($<100 \times 10^9$/L) and, depending upon its severity, increased bleeding risk. Unlike children, most adults with acute ITP exhibit persistence of thrombocytopenia, that is, *chronic* ITP. When there is an associated illness (eg, systemic lupus erythematosus, HIV infection, monoclonal lymphoproliferative disorder), the ITP is called *secondary*; in their absence, the patient is said to have *primary* ITP. Although the role of autoantibodies in ITP is not disputed, there is no clear role for laboratory testing in the diagnosis of ITP.

Most patients are benefited at least transiently with therapies such as oral corticosteroids, intravenous IVIgG, or Rh immune globulin, although the last is only potentially effective if the patient is Rh(D) positive. Unfortunately, the thrombocytopenia often relapses during corticosteroid tapering, or 1 to 3 weeks following administration of IVIgG or Rh immune globulin. Thus, many patients will eventually undergo splenectomy, since durable remissions are observed in 60% to 70% of patients. The large number of third-line treatment approaches (immunosuppressives, danazol, rituximab, thrombopoietin analogues) speaks to the challenge in managing chronic ITP that is refractory to the first- and second-line treatment approach of corticosteroids followed by splenectomy. Two thrombopoietin receptor agonists, eltrombopag (oral agent) and romiplostim (administered by subcutaneous injection), are approved in the United States for treatment of chronic ITP, but their high cost and requirement for ongoing use are drawbacks. Platelet transfusions are usually indicated only to manage life-threatening bleeding.

Hereditary thrombocytopenia: Hereditary (or congenital) thrombocytopenia (eg, MYH9-associated macrothrombocytopenia) is more common than generally recognized. Although there are different syndromes, most common is MYH9-associated macrothrombocytopenia, so named because the defect is in the nonmuscle myosin heavy chain, and affected patients have very large platelets. Often, the platelet count is greater than that reported by the electronic particle counter, as it fails to count the largest sized platelets. Inheritance is autosomal dominant. Depending on the exact location of the mutation, patients can have one or more of the following features: leukocyte inclusions, sensorineural hearing loss, presenile cataracts, and renal disease. Most patients have no or minimal bleeding symptoms and signs. Many patients are misdiagnosed as having chronic ITP.

Myelodysplasia and other primary marrow disorders: Numerous primary marrow disorders can cause thrombocytopenia, usually with leukopenia and anemia (pancytopenia). If there are increased numbers of circulating neoplastic cells, leukocytosis can be seen (eg, acute or chronic myeloid or lymphoid leukemia). *Myelodysplasia* (preleukemia) refers to clonal disorders of myeloid cells in which the marrow "blast" count is less than 30%; diagnostic clues include anemia with elevated red cell size (macrocytosis), leukopenia/leukocytosis with dysplastic white cells changes (eg, Pelger-Huet appearance, hypogranular leukocytes), and thrombocytopenia; characteristic chromosomal abnormalities of affected blood and bone marrow cells are common. Sometimes, isolated thrombocytopenia is the presenting feature of myelodysplasia.

TABLE 171-7 Differential Diagnosis of Splenomegaly and Hypersplenism

Congestive splenomegaly
Intrahepatic
Cirrhosis*
Extrahepatic
Portal vein obstruction
Splenic vein obstruction
Hepatic vein occlusion (Budd-Chiari syndrome)
Chronic passive congestion
Heart failure
Infections
Acute
Viral (viral hepatitis, infectious mononucleosis, cytomegalovirus infection)
Bacterial (septicemia, salmonellosis, brucellosis, splenic abscess)
Parasite (toxoplasmosis)
Subacute and chronic
Subacute bacterial endocarditis
Tuberculosis
Malaria
Kala-azar
Fungal disease
Inflammation
Felty syndrome
Systemic lupus erythematosus
Serum sickness
Rheumatic fever
Sarcoidosis
Hematologic disorders
Red cell disorders: hemolytic anemias, thalassemia, sickle cell disorders
Neoplasia
Malignant
Myeloproliferative disorders
Myeloid metaplasia
Polycythemia rubra vera
Essential thrombocythemia
Chronic leukemia
Chronic myeloid leukemia
Chronic lymphocytic leukemia
Hairy cell leukemia
Lymphoma
Acute leukemia
Malignant histiocytosis
Benign
Hamartoma
Hemangioma
Lymphangioma
Fibroma
Storage diseases
Gaucher disease
Niemann-Pick disease
Miscellaneous
Amyloidosis
Cysts

*The most common cause of hypersplenism in North America.

Myelophthisis and other secondary marrow disorders: *Myelophthisis* refers to marrow replacement by tumor or fibrosis, yielding a characteristic peripheral blood picture known as *leukoerythroblastosis* (leukocyte left shift, circulating nucleated red blood cells) together with tear-drop red cells. When the cause of marrow infiltration is metastatic adenocarcinoma, there may also be red cell fragments and coagulopathy indicating overt DIC. In that setting, thrombocytopenia reflects both decreased marrow production and increased consumption.

◼ ACUTE THROMBOCYTOPENIA PRECIPITATING ADMISSION TO HOSPITAL

Sometimes, acute thrombocytopenia is *the* major feature of the patient's presentation, and the emergency room and early hospitalization period are aimed at establishing diagnosis and treatment. Many of these disorders are life threatening.

Diagnostic considerations

Drug-induced immune thrombocytopenic purpura: Certain drugs newly started in outpatients, such as sulfa antibiotics and carbamazepine, can cause severe immune thrombocytopenia (see Table 171-5). Always ask about possible exposure to quinine, as this component of "tonic water" is a relatively common cause of severe thrombocytopenia in patients presenting to the emergency room. Treatment includes stopping any suspected drugs, and administering one or more of the following: corticosteroids, high-dose IVIgG, or platelet transfusions. The presence of oropharyngeal blood blisters indicates a higher risk of life-threatening bleeding (intracranial, pericardial) than cutaneous purpura (petechiae, ecchymoses) alone.

Acute immune thrombocytopenic purpura: Most adults have chronic ITP, but the initial presentation of this disorder by definition is *acute*, as the natural history of persisting chronic thrombocytopenia is not yet known. Treatment with corticosteroids and/or IVIgG is usually given only if there are bleeding symptoms or signs, and platelet transfusions are reserved for life-threatening bleeding, as their therapeutic benefit is transient and sensitization to platelet antigens could develop.

Thrombotic thrombocytopenic purpura and hemolytic-uremic syndrome: Thrombocytopenia and microangiopathic (or schistocytic) hemolysis constitute the TTP duad. Affected patients can exhibit organ dysfunction due to platelet—von Willebrand factor (vWF) thrombi in small arteries and arterioles, most commonly involving the central nervous system (confusion, dysarthria, coma), kidneys (oliguric renal failure), and muscles (elevated creatine kinase, cardiac dysrrhythmias including sudden death). A useful diagnostic clue is measurement of lactate dehydrogenase: levels are typically markedly elevated in patients with TTP. TTP has female predominance and increased risk in African Americans. Most often, the disorder is idiopathic, although autoantibodies against the shear-dependent vWF-cleaving protease, known as ADAMTS13 (a disintegrin and metalloproteinase with thrombospondin motifs, member 13), have been identified in a high proportion of affected patients. TTP can also occur in association with autoimmune disorders (eg, systemic lupus erythematosus), with certain drugs (eg, quinine, cyclosporine, gemcitabine, mitomycin C), or soon after surgery or acute pancreatitis.

Untreated, the mortality of TTP approaches 100%. Even when successfully treated with corticosteroids and plasma exchange, there is a relatively high risk (at least one-third) of subsequent relapse, although this might occur months or years in the future. Rituximab appears to be an effective treatment for patients with refractory or relapsing TTP.

A related syndrome known as hemolytic-uremic syndrome (HUS) has prominent renal dysfunction, and in about 75% of patients occurs with a diarrheal prodrome, as a common precipitant is preceding infection with verotoxin-producing *Escherichia coli*. In the remaining 25% of (atypical or nondiarrheal) HUS, congenital abnormalities in the alternative complement pathway can often be implicated. Rarely, quinine can cause a syndrome that strongly resembles HUS.

Delayed-onset heparin-induced thrombocytopenia with thrombosis: Thrombocytopenia accompanying venous or arterial thrombosis, or adrenal hemorrhagic infarction (itself an indicator of adrenal vein thrombosis) in a recently hospitalized patient should prompt consideration of *delayed-onset HIT*. Patients have strong-positive tests for HIT antibodies and often concomitant DIC. Interestingly, some patients have not had any preceding exposure to heparin (eg, they received warfarin for postorthopedic surgery thromboprophylaxis ["spontaneous HIT syndrome"]). Thus, it appears that surgery itself can rarely precipitate the anti-PF4/heparin immune response that underlies HIT. Ideally, heparin should be avoided in patients with delayed-onset (or spontaneous) HIT, but if given, a further abrupt decline in platelet count–with or without an anaphyactoid reaction–is characteristic.

THROMBOCYTOSIS

◼ INTRODUCTION

Thrombocytosis (platelet count $>450 \times 10^9$/L) is often an unexpected abnormality detected by routine CBC. Usually, thrombocytosis arises *during* hospitalization as a physiologic response to preceding acute thrombocytopenia. When thrombocytosis is already apparent at the time of admission, it most often represents a *secondary* (or reactive) thrombocytosis, and usually does not pose thrombotic or other risks. In contrast, *primary* thrombocytosis indicates that the increase in platelets is caused by alterations targeting hematopoietic cells and can indicate risk of thrombosis and/or bleeding. **Table 171-8** classifies various explanations for thrombocytosis.

PRACTICE POINT

- Similar to thrombocytopenia, evaluation of thrombocytosis should include review of the peripheral smear and determination of whether other cell lines are abnormal. The timing of the onset of thrombocytosis is also an important clue to the cause. Thrombocytosis that arises *during* hospitalization is usually a physiologic response to preceding acute thrombocytopenia. Thrombocytosis already apparent at the time of admission most often represents a secondary (or "reactive") thrombocytosis, but sometimes a primary thrombocytosis (eg, myeloproliferative neoplasm).

◼ PHYSIOLOGIC THROMBOCYTOSIS

Platelet count regulation through constitutive production of thrombopoietin infers that any acute self-limited thrombocytopenia will naturally be followed by transient, self-limited thrombocytosis. Another physiologic tenet is that absence of a spleen (and associated splenic pooling) will yield approximately a 30% increase in the platelet count on a chronic basis.

Diagnostic considerations

Postthrombocytopenia thrombocytosis: Consider the key question: Is the thrombocytosis newly acquired during the hospitalization? If so, it is likely that there was a transient drop in the platelet count approximately 1 to 2 weeks earlier, as exemplified in Figures 171-1 and 171-2. Typically, the platelet count peaks approximately 2 weeks following any acute drop in platelet count and represents a physiologic response to increased TPO levels that occur as a

TABLE 171-8 Causes of Thrombocytosis

Physiologic

Postthrombocytopenia thrombocytosis (2nd and 3rd week post-any acute platelet count decline)

Postsplenectomy or congenital/acquired asplenia

Secondary or "reactive"

Inflammatory/infectious, eg, polymyalgia rheumatica (giant cell arteritis), rheumatoid arthritis, polyarteritis nodosa, inflammatory bowel disease, tuberculosis, other chronic infections), solid tumors, especially metastatic carcinoma

Iron deficiency

Hemolytic anemia

Primary

Hereditary or familial thrombocytosis

Neoplastic (myeloproliferative disorders, eg, polycythemia rubra vera, chronic myeloid leukemia, essential thrombocythemia, myeloid metaplasia, myelodysplasia [eg, 5q- syndrome, refractory anemia with ringed sideroblasts])

Spurious

Pseudothrombocytosis (eg, burns)

Postsplenectomy thrombocytosis: Greatly elevated platelet counts can occur following splenectomy. This is because physiologic thrombocytosis that follows acute surgery-associated thrombocytopenia is exacerbated by the lack of splenic sequestration of platelets. Thus, peak platelet counts as high as 1500 to 2000 × 10⁹/L can be seen approximately 2 weeks postsplenectomy, before returning to a "baseline" that is approximately one-third higher than the patient's usual presplenectomy platelet count.

■ SECONDARY (REACTIVE) THROMBOCYTOSIS

It is important to identify the underlying explanation for secondary thrombocytosis, as the causes can be life threatening (eg, giant cell arteritis, occult abscess, lung carcinoma, iron deficiency anemia secondary to colon cancer). Further, management of the thrombocytosis necessarily focuses on treatment of the underlying disease.

Diagnostic considerations

Inflammatory/infectious thrombocytosis: Answering yes to the key question, "Does the thrombocytosis predate the hospitalization?" suggests that the patient may have a subacute or chronic inflammatory/infectious cause of thrombocytosis (see Table 171-8 for representative disorders). Unlike neoplastic disorders, increased risk of thrombosis is not usually a feature of reactive thrombocytosis that represents a response to inflammatory cytokines, although exceptions to this general rule exist. For example, the author once encountered a patient who presented with cerebral venous (dural sinus) thrombosis who had an incidental finding of thrombocytosis; this proved to be one of

direct result of the preceding platelet count decline (**Figure 171-3**). In this author's opinion, the finding of thrombocytosis in this clinical setting does not require any additional antithrombotic measures over what would already be prudent in the same clinical situation, had thrombocytosis not been evident.

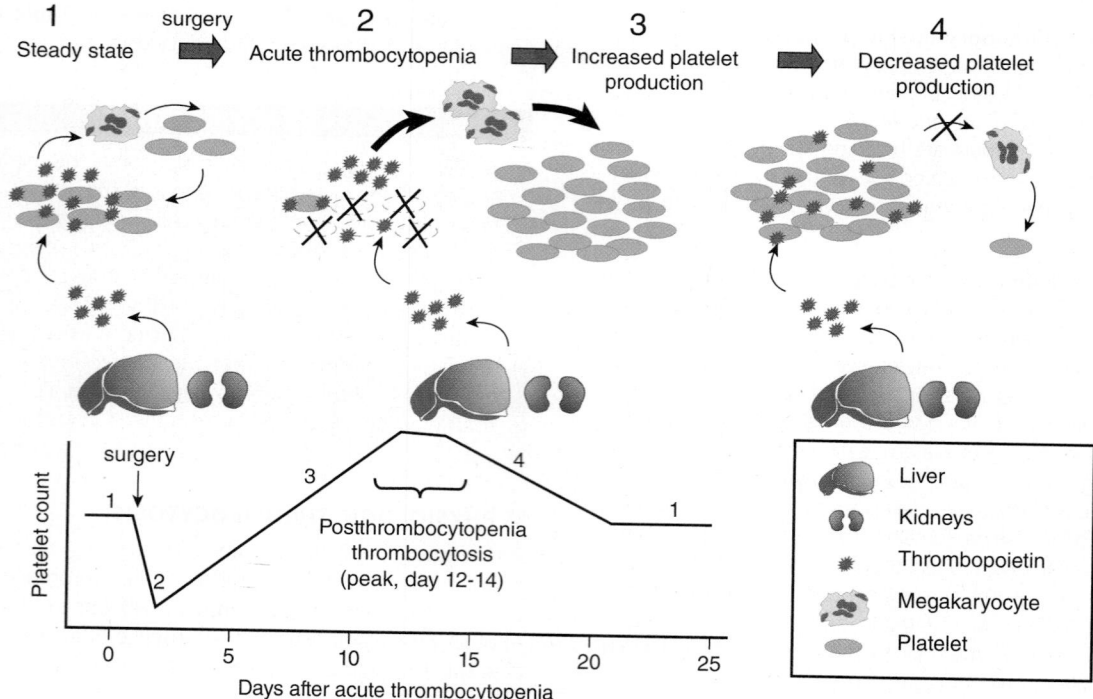

Figure 171-3 *Pathophysiology of postthrombocytopenia thrombocytosis. Thrombopoietin (TPO) binds to platelets and megakaryocytes via a specific receptor (c-Mpl, not shown). The receptor-bound TPO is removed from circulation and degraded. The level of circulating TPO is, thus, inversely related to the mass of platelets and megakaryocytes. In thrombocytopenia, fewer binding sites are available, and, consequently, free TPO levels are high, stimulating megakaryocyte proliferation and differentiation and leading to increased platelet production. In thrombocytosis, the high platelet mass acts as a "sink" for removing TPO, with decreased stimulus for platelet production. Thus, following acute thrombocytopenia, TPO levels rise about twofold, leading to increased platelet production that begins on days 3 to 4, with resulting thrombocytosis that generally peaks about days 12 to 14 (postthrombocytopenia thrombocytosis), and returns to baseline by approximately day 21.* (Reprinted, with permission, from Arnold DM, Warkentin TE. Thrombocytopenia and thrombocytosis. In: Wilson WC, Grande CM, Hoyt DB, eds. *Trauma: Critical Care* (vol. 2). New York, NY: Informa Healthcare USA; 2007:983-1005.)

the clues (along with mild diarrhea) that the patient had undiagnosed inflammatory bowel disease.

Iron deficiency anemia or hemolytic anemia: Anemia with microcytosis suggests iron deficiency anemia as the cause of thrombocytosis, whereas anemia with elevated mean corpuscular volume (MCV) suggests that acute or chronic hemolytic anemia should be ruled out (young red cells known as reticulocytes have MCV values of ~160 fL, and thus the MCV is usually elevated in patients with hemolysis). The key question should be: Is the MCV increased or decreased? Of course, elevated MCV is also a feature of many primary hematologic disorders, such as myelodysplasia, considered earlier.

■ PRIMARY THROMBOCYTOSIS

Primary thrombocytosis disorders are important to recognize as patients can be at increased bleeding or thrombotic risk, and sometimes both. Moreover, specialized care by a hematologic oncologist is standard.

Diagnostic considerations

Hereditary or familial thrombocytosis: The pathophysiologic explanation for hereditary thrombocytosis is usually unknown. However, in 10% to 20% of patients, an underlying genetic abnormality in thrombopoiesis has been identified (eg, mutations in thrombopoietin or its receptor).

Primary neoplastic disorders: The key question, "Is there concomitant splenomegaly and/or abnormalities in hemoglobin or white blood cell levels?," aims to address the possibility of a primary hematologic neoplasm. Any of the classic myeloproliferative neoplasms (MPN)—polycythemia vera (PV), chronic myeloid leukemia (CML), essential thrombocythemia (ET), or primary myelofibrosis (PMF)—can feature thrombocytosis, generally without significant dysmyelopoiesis. In such patients, the Jak2 mutation is often positive (eg, >99% in PV and 55% in ET), whereas the Philadelphia chromosome is usually present in CML. In contrast, myelodysplastic syndrome (MDS) is characterized by dysplastic bone marrow hyperplasia (sometimes, hypoplasia), with variable degrees of peripheral blood cytopenias. However, sometimes MDS features prominent elevations in blood count: the "5q syndrome" is a specific type of MDS that features severe anemia, thrombocytosis with dysmegakaryopoiesis, and a more benign clinical course.

The presence of thrombocytosis does not necessarily indicate increased thrombotic risk: for example, platelet counts >1500 × 10⁹/L can be associated with bleeding (due to acquired vWF syndrome from accelerated vWF clearance); further, platelet dysfunction is common in bone marrow neoplasia. Also, thrombotic risk factors besides elevated platelet count values per se are also important, such as elevated hematocrit in PV and possibly elevated WBC levels.

■ SPURIOUS THROMBOCYTOSIS

Pseudothrombocytosis

Sometimes, spurious thrombocytosis results when the electronic particle counter misclassifies tiny red cell fragments, which can result in burn victims, as platelets.

CONCLUSION

Quantitative platelet disorders, thrombocytopenia and thrombocytosis, have diverse causes. Clinicians should focus on determining the probable cause of the patient's abnormal platelet count, as this will direct the management approach and prognosis.

SUGGESTED READINGS

THROMBOCYTOPENIA

Arnold DM, Nazi I, Warkentin TE, et al. Approach to the diagnosis and management of drug-induced thrombocytopenia. *Transfus Med Rev.* 2013;27:137-145.

Balduini CL, Savoia A, Seri M. Inherited thrombocytopenias frequently diagnosed in adults. *J Thromb Haemost.* 2013;11:1006-1019.

Provan D, Stasi R, Newland AC, et al. International consensus report on the investigation and management of primary immune thrombocytopenia. *Blood.* 2010;115:168-186.

Rodeghiero F, Stasi R, Gernsheimer T, et al. Standardization of terminology, definitions and outcome criteria in immune thrombocytopenic purpura of adults and children: report from an international working group. *Blood.* 2009;113:2386-2393.

Tsai HM. A mechanistic approach to the diagnosis and management of atypical hemolytic uremic syndrome. *Transfus Med Rev.* 2014;28:187-197.

Warkentin TE. Drug-induced immune-mediated thrombocytopenia—from purpura to thrombosis. *N Engl J Med.* 2007;356:891-893.

Warkentin TE. Agents for the treatment of heparin-induced thrombocytopenia. *Hematol/Oncol Clin N Am.* 2010;24:755-775.

Warkentin TE. Heparin-induced thrombocytopenia in critically ill patients. *Semin Thromb Hemost.* 2015;41:49-60.

Warkentin TE. Ischemic limb gangrene with pulses. *N Engl J Med.* 2015;373:642-655.

Warkentin TE, Kelton JG. Temporal aspects of heparin-induced thrombocytopenia. *N Engl J Med.* 2001;344:1286-1292.

Warkentin TE, Kelton JG. Delayed-onset heparin-induced thrombocytopenia and thrombosis. *Ann Intern Med.* 2001;135:502-506.

Warkentin TE, Anderson JAM. How I treat patients with a history of heparin-induced thrombocytopenia. Blood. 2016;128:348-359.

Warkentin TE, Basciano PA, Knopman J, Bernstein RA. Spontaneous heparin-induced thrombocytopenia syndrome: 2 new cases and a proposal for defining this disorder. *Blood.* 2014;123:3651-3654.

Warkentin TE, Elavathil LJ, Hayward CPM, et al. The pathogenesis of venous limb gangrene associated with heparin-induced thrombocytopenia. *Ann Intern Med.* 1997;127:804-812.

Warkentin TE, Greinacher A, Koster A, Lincoff AM. Treatment and prevention of heparin-induced thrombocytopenia. American College of Chest Physicians evidence-based clinical practice guidelines (8th edition). *Chest.* 2008;133(6 Suppl):340S-380S.

Warkentin TE, Sheppard JI, Moore JC, Sigouin CS, Kelton JG. Quantitative interpretation of optical density measurements using PF4-dependent enzyme-immunoassays. *J Thromb Haemost.* 2008;6:1304-1312.

THROMBOCYTOSIS

Abou Zahr A, Saad Aldin E, Komrokji RS, Zeidan AM. Clinical utility of lenalidomide in the treatment of myelodysplastic syndromes. *J Blood Med.* 2014;6:1-16.

Skoda R. Thrombocytosis. *Hematology Am Soc Hematol Educ Program.* 2009:159-167.

Tefferi A, Barbui T. Polycythemia vera and essential thrombocythemia: 2015 update on diagnosis, risk-stratification and management. *Am J Hematol.* 2015;90:162-173.

CHAPTER 172

Approach to Patients with Bleeding Disorders

Kathryn Webert, MD, MSc, FRCPC
Catherine P. M. Hayward, MD, PhD

Key Clinical Questions

1. When should a bleeding disorder be suspected?
2. How should patients suspected of bleeding disorders be evaluated?
3. How does one interpret the results of hemostasis testing?
4. What is the general approach to management of an individual with a bleeding disorder?

INTRODUCTION

In general, severe bleeding disorders are uncommon, unlike mild bleeding problems, which can be more challenging to diagnose. Most episodes of clinically significant bleeding requiring medical attention result from local causes (eg, a duodenal ulcer), surgery, or trauma. However, it is important to recognize when bleeding problems are more serious or more frequent due to an underlying hemostatic abnormality.

Abnormal bleeding represents an important health care problem. For example, in the United States, it has been estimated that at least 5% to 10% of women of childbearing age seek medical care for menorrhagia and have bleeding severe enough to require medical intervention. Among the many defects that can cause abnormal bleeding, inherited and acquired von Willebrand disease (VWD) and platelet function disorders are much more common than defects in coagulation and fibrinolytic proteins.

PATHOPHYSIOLOGY

■ REVIEW OF NORMAL HEMOSTASIS

Hemostasis consists of the following steps: (1) initiation and formation of the platelet plug, also known as primary hemostasis; (2) propagation and amplification of the clotting "cascade" or secondary hemostasis, which involves activation of a series of coagulation factors resulting in the generation of thrombin that cleaves fibrinogen to fibrin; (3) cross-linking of fibrin; (4) termination of procoagulant response by antithrombotic control mechanisms; (5) removal of the clot by fibrinolysis; and (6) tissue repair and regeneration.

When a vessel is injured, platelets adhere to exposed collagen and other components of the subendothelium as the first defense against bleeding. This initial adhesion is dependent on von Willebrand factor (VWF) as well as specific platelet receptors (eg, glycoprotein IbIXV) for VWF and collagen. This adhesion leads to platelet activation and shape change as well as platelet aggregation, which promotes recruitment of additional platelets.

Coagulation is initiated in vivo when endothelial or vascular cells are damaged. This results in exposure of blood to tissue factor (TF), which binds to factor VII (FVII) and its activated form, factor VII (FVIIa). TF-FVIIa complexes (extrinsic tenase) then activates factors IX and X directly. Activated factor IX can also form a complex with factor VIIIa as well as phospholipids and calcium, called the *intrinsic tenase complex*, which promotes further conversion of factor X to factor Xa. The generated factor Xa associates with activated factor V, phospholipids, and calcium to form the prothrombinase complex that activates prothrombin to thrombin. Intrinsic and extrinsic tenase are needed to generate enough thrombin for normal hemostasis. Once thrombin is generated, it cleaves fibrinogen to fibrin, which leads to formation of a fibrin clot and promotes platelet activation and the generation of activated factors V and VIII. Thrombin also results in the formation of activated XIII, an enzyme that cross-links fibrin to make the clot more resistant to fibrinolysis (the cleavage of the fibrin clot).

When coagulation is activated, fibrinolysis is activated, leading to slow dissolution of the clot as part of wound healing. The process of fibrinolysis requires activation of plasminogen to plasmin, which is a serine protease that cleaves cross-linked fibrin. Fibrinolysis results in the formation of fibrin degradation products, including D-dimers. The generation of plasmin is controlled by both activators (ie, tissue-type and urinary-type plasmin activators) and inhibitors (ie, plasminogen activator inhibitor 1 and α2 plasmin inhibitor).

■ GENERAL CLASSIFICATION OF BLEEDING DISORDERS ACCORDING TO PATHOPHYSIOLOGY

Bleeding disorders may be classified according to whether they are inherited or acquired, and by their underlying pathophysiology. The latter classification is often divided into the following broad categories: vascular disorders (eg, hemorrhagic telangiectasia and diseases of the connective tissue in the vessel wall, which are often challenging to diagnose); disorders of primary hemostasis (eg, platelet and VWF deficiencies and defects); disorders of secondary hemostasis (eg, clotting factor defects and deficiencies); and disorders of fibrinolysis (see **Table 172-1**). Some disorders (eg, severe VWD) impair hemostasis by impairing both platelet adhesion and fibrin formation, due to the associated factor VIII deficiency. Drugs that inhibit platelet function (eg, aspirin, nonsteroidal anti-inflammatory drugs, serotonin reuptake inhibitors) and those that inhibit coagulation (eg, heparin, warfarin) are important causes to consider when evaluating and managing an individual with bleeding.

TABLE 172-1 Questions to Consider when Evaluating a Patient for a Possible Bleeding Disorder

What are the patient's bleeding symptoms?

- Is there a personal or family history of bleeding with trauma or procedures?
- What are the site(s) of bleeding?
- For women: Is there a history of prolonged, heavy periods or bleeding with childbirth?
- What is the severity of bleeding?
- What is the duration of bleeding events?
- Has the patient required any treatments for bleeding?

Does the history suggest a congenital or acquired problem?

- Note: For congenital bleeding disorders, the bleeding symptoms may date back to childhood and may affect other family members; acquired bleeding disorders should be considered when the bleeding problems are more recent, and a drug-induced defect should be excluded.

What is the timing of the bleeding?

- Is the bleeding immediate or delayed (onset one or more days after challenges)?

Is the bleeding systemic or local?

- Note: Local bleeding is suggestive of a local cause, although acquired or inherited bleeding disorders can make it worse.

Are there any aggravating or contributing factors?

- Note: The drug history (prescription, nonprescription, and other supplements) should be carefully reviewed.

What is the patient's general medical history?

- Does the patient have a history of liver, kidney, or thyroid diseases? The patient should also be questioned about relevant symptoms of these disorders.
- Does the patient have a history of pregnancy loss (may be associated with disorders of fibrinogen).
- Does the patient have a history of poor wound healing (can occur in a variety of bleeding disorders).

How many times has the patient experienced a significant hemostatic challenge, and how many of these were associated with abnormal bleeding?

- Note: A history of bleeding with only some challenges suggests a mild or acquired bleeding problem.

DOES THIS PATIENT HAVE A BLEEDING DISORDER?

■ WHEN TO SUSPECT A BLEEDING DISORDER

In general, a bleeding disorder should be suspected when bleeding occurs with minimal or no provocation, when it is more severe than expected for a given challenge, and when bleeding episodes occur repeatedly with challenges. Care should be taken to avoid asking very subjective questions about bleeding. For example, it is preferable to ask women about menstrual periods lasting longer than 7 days, with more than 2 to 3 days of heavy flow, and/or periods that interfere with their lifestyle than to ask if they experience "heavy" periods. Similarly, asking about bruises as big as or larger than oranges and/or bruises appearing without provocation is better than asking about "easy bruising."

While individuals with severe bleeding problems may report spontaneous bleeding and serious bleeding with major and minor hemostatic challenges, individuals with milder defects can report abnormal bleeding with some but not all significant hemostatic challenges. While inherited, severe bleeding problems typically present early in life, milder inherited bleeding problems and acquired bleeding problems often get diagnosed in adult life. The clinical assessment should be directed toward identifying the type and severity of bleeding problems experienced by an individual, in order to plan appropriate laboratory testing and therapy.

■ KEY COMPONENTS OF THE HISTORY

What are the patient's bleeding symptoms?

The patient should be questioned about his or her current bleeding symptoms and past bleeding symptoms and a family history of bleeding problems (**Table 172-2**). The following characteristics of the bleeding should be determined: association with trauma or procedures and if it occurred with some or all minor and major procedures; site(s) (including joint bleeds); severity (eg, bleeding resulting in additional interventions such as blood transfusions, intensive care unit admission, and/or prolongation of hospitalization stay); duration of bleeding; and any treatments that were given to control bleeding (types of drugs or blood products). It may be helpful to determine if the patient received anticoagulants or drugs that inhibit platelet function. Female patients should be asked questions about menstrual periods and abnormal bleeding with childbirth and pregnancy losses. Mucocutaneous bleeding (ie, abnormal bruising, gum bleeding, and epistaxis) is more suggestive of a defect in primary hemostasis. Some bleeding symptoms, such as deep tissue bleeding, joint hemorrhages, and spontaneous unexplained hematuria are uncommon but can occur in severe inherited coagulation protein deficiencies. Some bleeding problems, such as epistaxis, can be experienced by individuals without bleeding disorders. Bleeding after trauma should be considered but can be difficult to evaluate because it is not specific to individuals with bleeding disorders.

PRACTICE POINT

- The timing of the bleeding relative to the surgical or dental procedure may be an important clue to the etiology of the bleeding disorder. Patients with disorders of primary hemostasis will often describe abnormal bleeding during or within a few hours whereas disorders of secondary hemostasis (including defects in clot stabilization and fibrinolysis) typically manifest as delayed-onset bleeding evident days following trauma or surgery.

What is the timing of bleeding?

The bleeding history is often used to assess when abnormal bleeding occurred (eg, same day or days later) relative to invasive surgical

TABLE 172-2 General Classification of Bleeding Disorders According to Pathophysiology

Vascular disorders
- Congenital (eg, hereditary hemorrhagic telangiectasis, Ehlers-Danlos syndrome)
- Acquired (eg, secondary to steroid use, vitamin C deficiency)

Disorders of platelets and their function
- Thrombocytopenia
  - Acquired (eg, drug-induced, immune-mediated)
  - Congenital (eg, inherited platelet or bone marrow disorders)
- Disorders of platelet function
  - Congenital (secretion defects are the most common)
  - Acquired (eg, drug-induced, renal failure)
- von Willebrand disease
  - Congenital
  - Acquired

Disorders of coagulation
- Coagulation factor deficiencies
  - Congenital (ie, hemophilia A [factor VIII deficiency], hemophilia B [factor IX deficiency], deficiencies or defects of factors II, V, VII, X, XI, fibrinogen, or XIII)
  - Acquired (vitamin K deficiency, liver disease, anticoagulant therapy, massive blood loss [hemodilution], acquired coagulation factor inhibitors)

Disorders of fibrinolysis
- Congenital (ie, α-2 antiplasmin deficiency, plasminogen activator inhibitor-1 deficiency, Quebec platelet disorder)
- Acquired (ie, hyperfibrinolytic syndrome, disseminated intravascular coagulation)

Other
- Acquired bleeding secondary to other disorders such as renal failure, thyroid disease, or Cushing syndrome

or dental procedures. Bleeding during, immediately after, or on the same day as the challenge is suggestive of a disorder of primary hemostasis (see Disorders of Primary Hemostasis later in this chapter), whereas bleeding that becomes problematic one or more days after a challenge is more typical of a factor deficiency or a fibrinolytic defect.

Is the bleeding disorder congenital or acquired, and are there aggravating or contributing factors?

Inherited problems tend to present earlier in life than acquired problems unless they are mild. Inherited problems are often associated with a positive family history, which may be negative if the condition is recessive or X-linked. A thorough bleeding history should include questions about potential aggravating or contributing factors such as new medications (eg, aspirin or antidepressant therapy).

Individuals with acquired bleeding disorders often describe bleeding that is more recent in onset. Causes of an acquired bleeding disorder are listed in Table 172-2 and include liver disease, vitamin K deficiency, autoimmune-mediated conditions (eg, immune thrombocytopenic purpura), hypothyroidism, acquired factor VIII deficiency or acquired VWD, and other conditions such as Cushing syndrome.

It is important to emphasize that the patient's entire bleeding history must be assessed in order to determine if the problem is mild or severe and if it is likely congenital or acquired.

Has the patient experienced any hemostatic challenges?

Patients should be questioned about how many operative and invasive dental procedures they have undergone, and how many of these were associated with abnormal bleeding. It may be helpful to ask if the patient has experienced any unusually large ecchymosis around incisions when evaluating the surgical bleeding history. It is important to note that individuals who have undergone a number of common surgical and dental procedures (eg, tonsillectomy, wisdom tooth extraction) without experiencing abnormal bleeding might still have a mild bleeding problem (particularly if other aspects of their bleeding history are abnormal); however, they are unlikely to have a severe bleeding disorder. Alternately, it is important to recognize that sometimes abnormal bleeding occurs in healthy individuals undergoing a major procedure due to technical complications.

What is the patient's general medical history? Is there a systemic disease that is causing or contributing to the patient's bleeding symptoms?

An evaluation of a patient's general medical history for new or worsening bleeding, and other changes in health, is important for assessing undiagnosed liver, kidney, or endocrine disorders such as thyroid disease or Cushing syndrome. The manifestations of some bleeding disorders, such as severe fibrinogen deficiency, can include recurrent pregnancy losses (due to hemorrhagic abruptions) and poor wound healing. Intracranial hemorrhage is seen more frequently in severe bleeding disorders (such as severe congenital factor XIII deficiency, severe coagulation factor, or fibrinolytic protein deficiencies and/or defects). Anemia can make bleeding worse and a history of iron deficiency (with or without anemia) can suggest chronically increased blood loss (eg, due to menorrhagia). Sometimes the history can suggest a rare inherited syndrome such as a platelet disorder associated with albinism, hearing loss, renal insufficiency, or skeletal malformations.

Has the patient ingested any medications that may have caused or worsened bleeding?

It is helpful to obtain a list of all medications (including prescription, nonprescription, and herbal) that the patient was taking in order to determine what might have caused or worsened their bleeding. Drugs can cause or worsen bleeding by a variety of mechanisms inducing: thrombocytopenia (eg, quinine, penicillin); impaired platelet function (eg, due to nonsteroidal anti-inflammatory drugs such as aspirin, clopidogrel, serotonin reuptake inhibitors, or fish oil supplements); or defective coagulation (eg, due to heparin or warfarin).

■ PHYSICAL EXAMINATION

The physical examination is often not very informative in individuals with a bleeding disorder. An initial assessment of acute bleeding should determine the patient's hemodynamic status and if there are signs of anemia. Blood blisters in the mouth, hemorrhages on the bite margins in the mouth, and petechiae (tiny red-colored skin lesions that reflect small hemorrhages into the skin, particularly on dependent parts of the body and at sites of trauma) may suggest significant thrombocytopenia. Large bruises or purpura may suggest a defect in primary hemostasis or acquired hemophilia. Sometimes the purpuric skin lesions of severe anticoagulant protein deficiencies (eg, purpura fulminans due to severe congenital protein C deficiency) are mistaken for skin bleeding. Abnormalities in joints, lymph nodes, spleen, and liver should raise concern for the possibility of a secondary bleeding disorder.

TABLE 172-3 Distinction between Disorders of Primary and Secondary Hemostasis

	Disorders of Primary Hemostasis	Disorders of Secondary Hemostasis
Timing of bleeding	Immediate	Delayed (starts one or more days after trauma or surgery)
Petechiae	Common (especially with thrombocytopenia)	Not seen
Ecchymoses	Common	May occur (usually large)
Deep hematomas	Not common	Common in severe factor deficiencies
Joint bleeding (hemarthoses)	Not common	Common in severe factor deficiencies
Mucous membrane bleeding	Common	Uncommon
Epistaxis	Common, particularly in childhood	Uncommon
Menorrhagia	Common	May occur
Inheritance (if congenital)	Dominant or recessive	Most common cause (hemophilia) is X-linked

■ DIFFERENTIAL DIAGNOSIS BASED ON CLINICAL ASSESSMENT

Table 172-3 outlines the differences between disorders of primary and secondary hemostasis.

Disorders of primary hemostasis

Patients with disorders of primary hemostasis will often describe experiencing abnormal bleeding during or within a few hours of a surgical or dental procedure. These problems, with or without mucocutaneous bleeding symptoms, should raise questions about VWF and platelet abnormalities (both qualitative and quantitative) or, less commonly, blood vessel abnormalities. Defects in primary hemostasis can also present as troublesome epistaxis and/or gingival bleeding, petechiae, superficial bruising or ecchymosis, and menorrhagia. Petechiae are very suggestive of a platelet or vascular disorder.

Disorders of secondary hemostasis

Disorders of secondary hemostasis typically manifest as delayed-onset bleeding that becomes evident in the days following trauma or surgical procedure. When there is a severe factor deficiency, there can be spontaneous bleeding into joint spaces (hemarthroses) and into deep, soft tissues (eg, muscle hematomas). The most common inherited disorders of secondary hemostasis include hemophilia A (factor VIII deficiency) and hemophilia B (factor IX deficiency). Acquired hemophilia, due to an antibody directed against factor VIII, accounts for about 10% of all hemophilia. Factor XIII deficiency and fibrinolytic disorders can also present with delayed bleeding, but these conditions are less common. Acquired autoantibodies against coagulation proteins are important but infrequent causes of bleeding and most commonly affect factor VIII, VWF, factor XIII or factor V.

HOW SHOULD THIS PATIENT WITH A SUSPECTED BLEEDING DISORDER BE INVESTIGATED?

Investigations for bleeding problems need to consider the etiologies of mild and severe and common and rare disorders. **Figure 172-1** summarizes a stepwise approach to investigation, some of which may be performed at the time of a specialist evaluation. Often, a broad range of tests is needed to assess an individual with a suspected bleeding disorder (see Figure 172-1). A complete blood count is helpful to evaluate for thrombocytopenia and to determine if there are other hematologic abnormalities such as anemia (which may reflect acute or chronic bleeding), or white blood cell abnormalities that may suggest an underlying bone marrow disorder. An assessment for iron deficiency (which may be present without anemia) should be considered. A blood group and antibody screen should be done before surgery in individuals with a history of abnormal bleeding and can be helpful when interpreting VWD testing results.

When selecting tests of hemostasis to investigate a bleeding problem, it is helpful to consider that coagulation defects are generally much rarer than defects in platelets and VWF. Like the bleeding time, closure times measured by the platelet function analyzer (PFA)-100 are optional and cannot be used to exclude VWD or platelet disorders. While it is common practice to order a prothrombin time (PT, sometimes reported as an international normalized ratio [INR]) and an activated partial thromboplastin time (APTT) in individuals with bleeding problems, the results are often normal. A fibrinogen level and a thrombin time should be considered because the PT and APTT are insensitive to fibrinogen problems. **Table 172-4** lists the different causes of abnormal coagulation tests.

To assess for VWD, a VWF antigen, VWF ristocetin cofactor activity, or newer VWF activity assays, and a factor VIII level should be ordered. The VWF level can be mildly low in blood group O individuals.

Platelet disorders are typically evaluated by specialized tests of platelet aggregation and secretion assays, which may require referral to a bleeding disorder specialist.

Additional tests can be helpful to evaluate if there is a history of acquired bleeding, which could reflect liver or renal disease or an endocrine disorder such as hypothyroidism or Cushing syndrome. As fibrinolytic defects are uncommon, testing is rarely done except by specialists.

PRACTICE POINT

- In general, the patient's symptoms, not the laboratory values, should be treated. Local factors can be significant contributors to bleeding and should be considered in the plans for investigation and treatment, even in patients with documented coagulopathies. Always consider risks and benefits (including those of treating or not treating) when deciding on appropriate therapies as the risks of certain therapies include increased prothrombotic risks. Patients with congenital bleeding disorders are best managed in a multidisciplinary care setting to plan treatment and prevention of acute bleeding episodes and to deal with complications (eg, hemophilic arthropathy). Information on the patient's bleeding problem and the treatment plans must be communicated to both the patient and their health care providers.

HOW SHOULD THIS PATIENT WITH A BLEEDING DISORDER BE TREATED?

The management of each patient with a bleeding disorder depends on the cause and severity of their bleeding disorder.

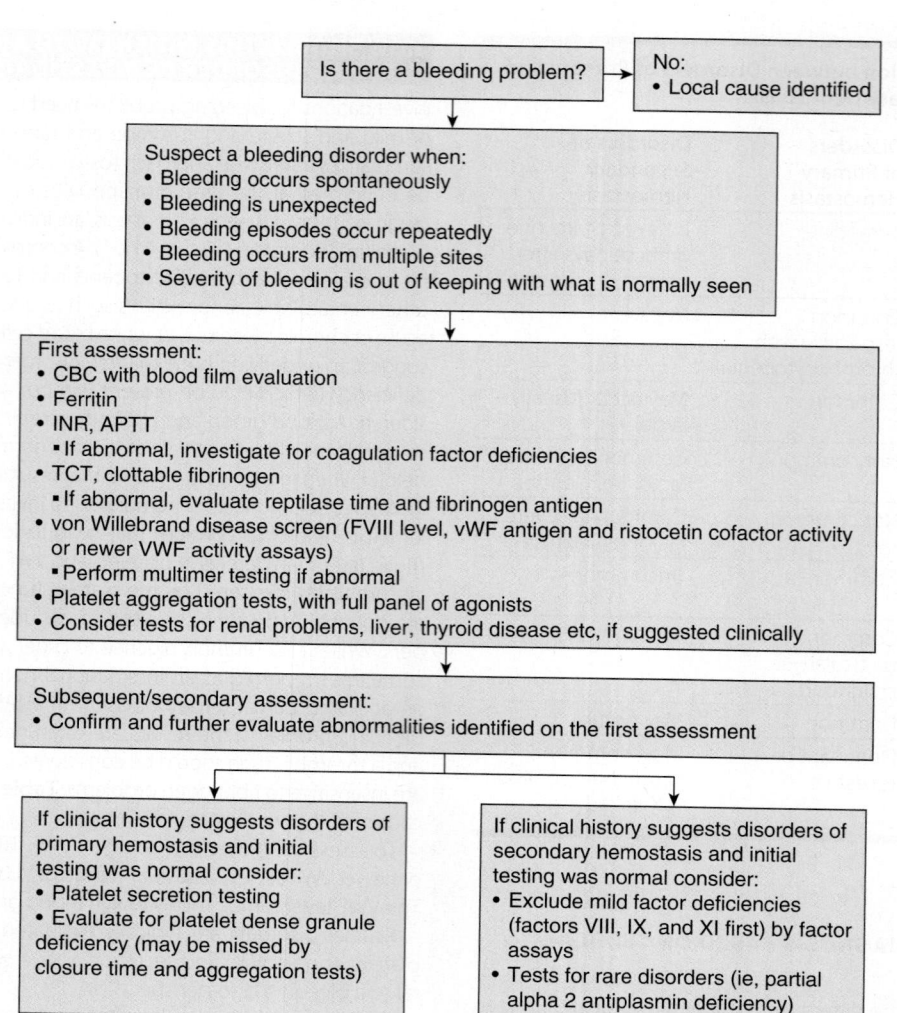

Figure 172-1 *A staged assessment to the diagnostic testing of bleeding disorders. (APTT, activated partial thromboplastin time; CBC, complete blood count; INR, international normalized ratio; TCT, thrombin clot time; VWF, von Willebrand factor.)*

■ GENERAL CONSIDERATIONS

- The patient's symptoms, not the laboratory values, should be treated. In general, treatment should be considered when the patient is bleeding or when the risk of bleeding is high (eg, if the patient is undergoing an invasive procedure).
- Local factors can be significant contributors to bleeding and should be considered in the plans for investigation and treatment, even in patients with documented coagulopathies.
- It is necessary to consider risks and benefits (including those of treating or not treating) when deciding on appropriate therapies, as the risks of certain therapies include increased prothrombotic risks. Other risks of hemostatic therapies (for treatment or propylaxis) include risks for viral transmission (ie, with blood products; recombinant products are generally preferred over blood-derived products to minimize these risks), and hyponatremia (with desmopressin acetate, if fluid restriction is not imposed for 12 hours post-therapy). In addition, treatment plans need to consider whether standard treatments (eg, use of intramuscular injections, postoperative anticoagulants, anti-inflammatory drugs that inhibit platelet function) should be modified because of the patient's bleeding problems.
- Information on the patient's bleeding problem and the treatment plans must be communicated to both the patient and his health care providers. Patients with congenital bleeding disorders must be "taught" that prophylactic treatment is required prior to invasive procedures.

- Patients with congenital bleeding disorders are best managed in a multidisciplinary care setting to plan treatment and prevention of acute bleeding episodes and to deal with complications (eg, hemophilic arthropathy).

■ OTHER ISSUES TO CONSIDER FOR TREATMENT OF CONGENITAL BLEEDING DISORDERS

Treatments for factor deficiencies

Individuals with moderate-to-severe clinically significant factor deficiencies often require factor concentrates (recombinant products generally preferred over plasma-derived products), although some conditions and circumstances (eg, mild hemophilia due to factor VIII deficiency with mild bleeding) may be managed with desmopressin. Fibrinolytic inhibitor drugs (aminocaproic acid and tranexamic acid) are often used as an adjunctive therapy for some procedures, such as dental and oral-nasal surgeries. Fibrinolytic inhibitor drugs are the treatment of choice for fibrinolytic disorders.

von Willebrand disease

The treatment of VWD depends on the type and severity of the disease. With mild VWD, which is more common, treatment with desmopressin acetate may be sufficient for many situations. In general, the treatment goal is to raise the levels of VWF (by giving the medication desmopressin acetate or VWF concentrates) to normal.

TABLE 172-4 Differential Diagnosis of Coagulation Test Abnormalities

	PT	APTT	Thrombin Time	Fibrinogen	Platelet Count
Reference Intervals	~ 10-13 s	Ranges Vary	Ranges Vary	150-400 mg/dL 1.5-4.0 g/L	150-400 × 10⁶/mL
Fibrinogen deficiency	N – ↑	N – ↑	↑	↓	N
Factor VII deficiency	↑	N	N	N	N
Factor VIII, IX, or XI deficiency	N	↑	N	N	N
Factor II, V, X deficiency	↑	↑	N	N	N
Factor deficiencies not associated with bleeding (factor XII, high-molecular-weight kininogen or prekallikrein deficiency)	N	↑	N	N	N
Acquired hemophilia and congenital hemophilia with inhibitors	N	↑*	N	N	N
Lupus anticoagulant	N – ↑	N – ↑†	N – ↑	N	N
Heparin therapy or sample contamination	N – ↑	↑	↑↑	N	N
Liver disease	N – ↑	N – ↑	N – ↑	↓ – N – ↑	↓ – N
Vitamin K deficiency	↑	N – ↑	N	N	N
Fibrinolytic therapy	↑	↑	↑	↓	N
Consumptive coagulopathy	N – ↑	↑	↑	↓	↓
Dilutional coagulopathy	N – ↑	N – ↑	N – ↑	↓ – N	↓
von Willebrand disease	N	N – ↑	N	N	N ↓ in type 2B and platelet type
Thrombocytopenia	N	N	N	N	↓
Platelet function disorders	N	N	N	N	↓ – N

↑, elevated; ↓, reduced; APTT, activated partial thromboplastin time; N, normal; PT, prothrombin time.

*An APTT of a 1:1 immediate mix of patient plasma containing a specific factor inhibitor and normal plasma can be N to ↑ depending on the features of their inhibitor. If a specific factor inhibitor is suspected, factor assays and tests for specific factor inhibitors should be performed.

†APTT reagents have different sensitivities to lupus anticoagulants. A lupus anticoagulant usually prolongs the APTT with a 1:1 mix of patient and normal plasma.

Platelet function disorders

Most platelet function disorders are mild bleeding disorders that respond to treatment with desmopressin acetate, which enhances platelet procoagulant activity in addition to increasing plasma VWF levels. Other options for therapy include fibrinolytic inhibitors (eg, for menorrhagia, oral-nasal surgery, or dental extractions), platelet transfusions (reserved for rare, severe disorders, such as Glanzmann thrombasthenia and Bernard Soulier syndrome and also given when bleeding is serious and not adequately controlled by desmopressin), and sometimes activated factor VII concentrate (generally reserved for situations where there is a wish to avoid platelet transfusions and other drug therapies, such as desmopressin, are not adequate).

■ GENERAL MANAGEMENT OF COMMON ACQUIRED BLEEDING DISORDERS

Liver disease

The coagulopathy related to liver disease is multifactorial, as the liver is the major source of all hemostatic proteins in plasma except for VWF and tissue plasminogen activator. Individuals with liver disease often have deficiencies of multiple coagulation factors, and in mild liver disease, there can be low levels of factors VII and, at times, factors XI and XII. Fibrinogen deficiency is typically only seen with severe liver disease. In fact, fibrinogen levels are often elevated in mild liver disease. Sometimes patients with liver disease have additional hemostatic defects such as vitamin K deficiency, thrombocytopenia, dysfibrinogenemia, platelet function abnormalities, and disseminated intravascular coagulation (DIC). If an individual with coagulopathy from liver disease requires treatment (ie, for active bleeding or, in some instances, before a procedure associated with a significantly increased risk of bleeding), one or more of the following treatment options should be considered: vitamin K replacement (if deficient), plasma infusion (typically requires four or more units to have measurable effects), fibrinogen replacement (with cryoprecipitate or fibrinogen concentrate), and/or platelet transfusion. The role of prothrombin complex concentrates in patients with liver disease is uncertain.

Anticoagulant medications

Treatment of serious bleeding due to anticoagulants may require reversal of the anticoagulant. Patients on an oral vitamin K antagonist, who require reversal to treat bleeding, should receive vitamin K, and when more rapid reversal is required (eg, to treat life-threatening gastrointestinal bleeding), prothrombin complex concentrate (if available) or plasma infusion should be considered. Protamine sulfate can be considered when there is a need to rapidly reverse unfractionated heparin or low-molecular-weight heparin because of bleeding. However, this treatment reverses only about 60% of the antifactor Xa activity of low-molecular-weight heparin. Unfortunately, agents are not currently available to rapidly reverse some of the newer, novel anticoagulants that are direct inhibitors of thrombin or factor Xa. However, specific antidotes for direct thrombin inhibitors and factor Xa inhibitors have been developed and are undergoing clinical testing. It is unclear whether bleeding from these newer agents is improved by treatment with desmopressin acetate, fibrinolytic inhibitor drugs, or other treatments, such as prothrombin complex concentrates and factor VIIa.

Vitamin K deficiency

Acquired bleeding due to vitamin K deficiency results from decreased gamma-carboxylation of the vitamin K-dependent factors II, VII, IX, and X and can be treated by administration of vitamin K.

CONCLUSION

Abnormal bleeding in an important health care problem that should be suspected when bleeding occurs spontaneously is more severe than expected or occurs on repeated occasions.

SUGGESTED READINGS

DeSimone N, Sarode R. Diagnosis and management of common acquired bleeding disorders. *Semin Thromb Hemost.* 2012;39:172-181.

Hayward CP. Diagnostic approach to platelet function disorders. *Transfus Apher Sci.* 2008;38:65-76.

Hayward CP, Moffat KA. Laboratory investigations for bleeding disorders: strategic uses of high and low yield tests. *Int J Lab Hematol.* 2013;35:222-333.

James AH. Guidelines for bleeding disorders in women. *Thromb Res.* 2009;123(Suppl 2):S124-S128.

Keeling D, Tait C, Makris M. Guideline on the selection and use of therapeutic products to treat haemophilia and other hereditary bleeding disorders. A United Kingdom Haemophilia Center Doctors' Organisation (UKHCDO) guideline approved by the British Committee for Standards in Haematology. *Haemophilia.* 2008;14:671-684.

Mannuci PM, Duga S, Peyvandi F. Recessively inherited coagulation disorders. *Blood.* 2004;104:1243-1252.

Nichols WL, Hultin MB, James AH, et al. von Willebrand disease (VWD): evidence-based diagnosis and management guidelines, the National Heart, Lung, and Blood Institute (NHLBI) Expert Panel report (USA). *Haemophilia.* 2008;14:171-232.

Rydz N, James P. Approach to the diagnosis and management of common bleeding disorders. *Semin Thromb Hemost.* 2012;38:711-719.

Rojas-Hernandez CM, Garcia DA. The novel anticoagulants. *Semin Thromb Hemost.* 2012;39:117-126.

Verhovsek M, Moffat KA, Hayward CP. Laboratory testing for fibrinogen abnormalities. *Am J Hematol.* 2008;83:928-931.

CHAPTER 173

Hypercoagulable States

Sam Schulman, MD, PhD
Karina Meijer, MD, PhD

Key Clinical Questions

1. Which hospitalized patients are at risk for venous thromboembolism (VTE)?
2. Who is at increased risk for complications from thromboprophylaxis?
3. How do we make sure that thromboprophylaxis is prescribed to all patients who should get it?

INTRODUCTION

The main question in most patient groups detailed below is whether they can expect a net benefit from pharmacological thromboprophylaxis, mainly low-molecular-weight heparins (LMWH). One has to balance the risk of venous thromboembolism (VTE) and the consequences of VTE with the risk of bleeding and other complications. Ideally, this balance is sought in every individual patient, also taking the values and preferences of that patient into consideration.

To facilitate this balancing process, institutions and national and international organizations have developed guidelines for the use of thromboprophylaxis. The use of these guidelines and local protocols has greatly improved patient outcomes, mainly by increasing the use of pharmacological thromboprophylaxis in patients at risk for VTE. We strongly advise the development and use of a local protocol.

THROMBOPHILIA AND VENOUS THROMBOEMBOLISM

■ DEFICIENCIES OF NATURAL INHIBITORS OF COAGULATION

Less than 1% of the general population has a congenital deficiency of one of the natural inhibitors of coagulation, antithrombin, protein C, and protein S. These deficiencies are associated with a high lifetime risk of VTE (60%-70% in a recent study) and with a high risk of recurrence after a first event (50% after 10 years). A limitation to these data is that they are derived from highly selected families, which might have led to an overestimation of risk. No population-based data are available.

Acquired deficiencies are seen with disseminated intravascular coagulation (DIC), extensive deep vein thrombosis (DVT), severe liver disease, infection, malignancy, adult respiratory distress syndrome (ARDS), the hemolytic uremic syndrome, thrombotic thrombocytopenic purpura (TTP), and following L-asparaginase therapy. The result of consumption or decreased synthesis of both pro- and anticoagulant factors, they may predispose the individual to bleeding or to thrombosis. This is often difficult to judge. In the case of liver disease, a convincing case has been made that the resultant is a new hemostatic balance, with no clearly increased risk of bleeding or thrombosis.

Total and free protein S decrease steadily during pregnancy, with the lowest levels at term. They are also somewhat decreased in patients who take the combined oral contraceptive pill. Protein C levels are lower before puberty, which should be born in mind when testing children in affected families. Antithrombin levels are increased with cholestasis.

Patients with a known congenital deficiency, primarily of antithrombin, but to some extent also protein C and protein S, have a strong indication for pharmacological thromboprophylaxis in any situation that increases the risk of thrombosis, including lower-limb immobilization, pregnancy, and bed rest as a medical patient. Given the high risk of recurrence, long-term anticoagulation should be considered in these patients after a first episode of VTE, especially if it was unprovoked (ie, not associated with a transient major risk factor for VTE, such as major surgery or trauma).

The utility of testing for a deficiency of a natural inhibitor is strongly debated, mainly because of its low prevalence. Testing in the context of thromboprophylaxis is not indicated. Even in patients who present with DVT, the prevalence of these deficiencies is so low that testing is rarely cost effective. Most centers limit thrombophilia testing to those patients who are young or to those who have recurrent VTE or a strong family history.

COMMON THROMBOPHILIC MUTATIONS

Heterozygous factor V Leiden (causing resistance to degradation by activated protein C) and prothrombin mutation (causing higher levels of prothrombin) occur in 5% and 2% to 3%, respectively, of the Caucasian population and rarely in other races. The lifetime risk of VTE associated with these mutations is 5% to 10% in unselected populations. While the risk of a first VTE is increased, these mutations hardly increase the risk of recurrence after a first event. Testing for factor V Leiden and prothrombin mutation is not recommended in routine clinical practice, as their (heterozygous) presence does not influence the indication for, or intensity of thromboprophylaxis, or the duration of treatment for VTE.

ANTIPHOSPHOLIPID SYNDROME

The antiphospholipid syndrome (APS) is defined as a combination of laboratory evidence—presence of lupus anticoagulant or antibodies against cardiolipin or β2-glycoprotein I—and clinical manifestations—at least one thrombotic event or obstetric complications. Thromboembolic events are more frequently venous than arterial and often involve unusual locations. The strongest laboratory association with thromboembolism is for lupus anticoagulant, followed by β2-glycoprotein I antibodies and then cardiolipin antibodies; combined serologic abnormalities result in even stronger associations. When the APS is secondary to systemic lupus erythematosus, the presence of lupus anticoagulant or antibodies against cardiolipin increases the risk of VTE sixfold and twofold, respectively.

Primary prophylaxis with anticoagulation in APS should be provided for high-risk situations (surgery, trauma, puerperium).

After a VTE event, secondary prophylaxis should be with the same intensity (warfarin with an international normalized ratio range of 2.0-3.0) as for other VTE. The duration of anticoagulation needs to be assessed after 3 to 6 months, taking into account whether the event was unprovoked, presence of multiple serologic abnormalities, the serologic titer, adherence, and patient preferences. The risk of recurrence, including fatal events is increased and some patients may experience recurrence in spite of anticoagulant therapy. This may be due to falsely prolonged coagulation times, and a switch from warfarin to long-term LMWH or to monitoring warfarin with a coagulation factor X method is then helpful. Patients with APS and arterial events should receive aspirin, since there is no evidence that warfarin is more effective. Pregnancy loss in APS is most typical in patients with systemic lupus or with previous pregnancy complications. For these patients, heparin in combination with aspirin provides the highest success rate

regarding live births. Low-molecular-weight heparin (LMWH) is generally preferred over unfractionated heparin (UFH) because it is not associated with bone loss. As patients with APS and pregnancy loss are also at increased risk of thrombosis, it seems reasonable to continue heparin for 6-week postpartum.

The catastrophic APS (cAPS, Asherson's syndrome) is characterized by microthrombi, anemia with schistiocytes and thrombocytopenia and is often triggered by an infection. The clinical course is rapid with multiorgan failure (usually pulmonary, cardiac, and renal) and about 50% mortality but this occurs only in 1% of patients with APS. Treatment with a combination of UFH intravenously, high-dose corticosteroids and plasma exchange results in the highest rate of recovery (78%). Addition of intravenous immunoglobulin does not seem to improve the prognosis. The survivors may sometimes develop additional APS manifestations but relapse of cAPS is very unusual.

MEDICALLY ILL PATIENTS

Medically ill patients have a moderately increased risk of VTE, depending on their conditions, age, and treatments (Table 173-1). In addition to potentially preventable mortality due to pulmonary embolism, VTE in medically ill patients prolongs hospitalization and increases costs. A growing body of evidence shows that thromboprophylaxis is underused in this patient group.

Pharmacological prophylaxis is recommended for all patients admitted with congestive heart failure, severe respiratory disease, and those in intensive care, unless there is an increased risk of bleeding. Patients who are confined to bed and have no contraindications should be prescribed pharmacological prophylaxis if they have additional risk factors for VTE, including previous VTE, known thrombophilic states (as explained above), pregnancy (see below), inflammatory diseases or malignancy and no contraindications. In case of recent, current or high risk of bleeding mechanical prophylaxis (graduated compression stockings or intermittent pneumatic compression of the legs) should be used. Extended pharmacological prophylaxis after discharge is not recommended due to difficulties in establishing a safe and effective dose.

The elderly have a higher risk of VTE but also a higher risk of bleeding. Clinicians tend to overestimate the risk of bleeding and to underestimate the risk (and consequences) of VTE, thus withholding thromboprophylaxis from patients who are likely to benefit. However, older patients are more likely than younger patients to have renal dysfunction, which increases the bleeding risk with any anticoagulant. A prophylactic dose of LMWH is unlikely to result in drug accumulation, even with severe renal dysfunction.

Sickle cell disease is associated with hypercoagulability, through activation of both plasma coagulation and platelets. Ischemic stroke, pulmonary hypertension, avascular joint necrosis, and leg ulcers are viewed

TABLE 173-1 Medical Patients to Consider for LMWH Prophylaxis

Indications		Contraindications	
Congestive heart failure		Risk of VTE outweighed by risk of bleeding	Concomitant (dual) antiplatelet therapy
Severe respiratory disease			Uncontrolled hypertension
Admission to intensive care			Recent or current bleed
Bedrest and	Previous VTE		Bleeding disorder, thrombocytopenia (<50)
	Known thrombophilic states		
	Pregnancy		
	Inflammatory diseases		
	Malignancy		
Sickle cell crisis			

LMWH, low-molecular-weight heparin; VTE, venous thromboembolism.

as thrombotic complications. The hypothesis that antiplatelet agents, warfarin and heparin, can prevent vaso-occlusive events and subsequent complications has been tested, results were not conclusive. At this point, maintenance antithrombotic therapy is not routinely given but additional studies are ongoing. Patients who are hospitalized with a sickle cell crisis should be given thromboprophylaxis to prevent VTE.

Patients with nephrotic syndrome have an increased risk of renal vein thrombosis, deep vein thrombosis, and pulmonary embolism. This is probably mediated by imbalances between pro- and antithrombotic factors. Estimates of the absolute risk vary from 2% to 40% of patients during their course of disease, with higher incidences in older studies. Randomized studies to guide prophylactic anticoagulant treatment in these patients have not been performed. Clinical practice is to consider vitamin K antagonists in patients with serum albumin below 20 to 25 g/L who do not have an increased risk of bleeding, especially when other risk factors including previous VTE, positive family history, and high body mass index are present.

POSTOPERATIVE PATIENTS

The risk of VTE and need for adequate thromboprophylaxis in postoperative patients is well established. Early ambulation is sufficient in low-risk patients who undergo minor or laparoscopic or arthroscopic procedures, and mechanical prophylaxis can be used in patients at increased risk of bleeding, but all others should receive pharmacological prophylaxis. This includes patients who undergo major general, orthopedic, gynecological, urological, and thoracic surgery. A prophylactic dose of LMWH is adequate for most patients, with fondaparinux as an alternative, and possibly subcutaneous UFH for patients with renal dysfunction. In most patients, thromboprophylaxis is given until discharge. For very high-risk patients (eg, abdominal or pelvic surgery for malignancy), extended thromboprophylaxis for about a month after surgery should be considered.

Patients after hip fracture surgery or hip- or knee arthroplasty are at very high risk of VTE. This is illustrated by the fact that the first phase three studies with new anticoagulants are almost always performed in these patient groups. They should receive pharmacological prophylaxis for at least 10, but preferably 35 days after surgery. The preferred agents are LMWH, direct oral anticoagulants (DOACs), and fondaparinux, with vitamin K antagonists for patients with renal dysfunction. Although aspirin is used in this setting, this is not generally considered as effective as anticoagulants.

The main challenge in postoperative patients, as in the medically ill patients, is to assure that thromboprophylaxis is prescribed for all patients who do not have contraindication. As stated in the introduction, every hospital should use a protocol or guideline, and adherence should be monitored.

PREGNANCY AND THE POSTPARTUM PERIOD

During pregnancy and the postpartum period, women have a four to five times increased risk of VTE. One to two per 1000 pregnancies are complicated by VTE, which is the cause of 20% to 30% of all maternal deaths in the developed world. The risk of VTE is equal in the three trimesters of pregnancy, but does increase postpartum. About one-third of all pregnancy-associated DVT and about half of all pregnancy-related pulmonary embolism occur during the 6-week postpartum, as compared to the 9-month antepartum. The increased risk of VTE during and after pregnancy is caused by both altered hemostatic balance and compromised venous flow.

The risk of VTE is higher in obese and older women, and after cesarian section as compared to vaginal delivery. Black women seem to be at higher risk than Caucasian women, while the risk is probably lower in Asian women.

Thromboprophylaxis is not indicated in healthy women during uncomplicated pregnancy or after uncomplicated vaginal delivery. There are no high-quality studies on routine thromboprophylaxis after cesarean section. The ACCP guidelines advise against it, while it is commonly used in European practice. Thromboprophylaxis should be used after cesarean section in patients with additional risk factors, such as emergency indication, delayed immobilization, and obesity (**Table 173-2**).

Antepartum thromboprophylaxis is indicated in women with a marked increased risk of VTE (Table 173-2). This includes women with a history of spontaneous or recurrent VTE and those with high-risk thrombophilia (deficiency of antithrombin, antiphospholid syndrome, and homozygous/compound heterozygous factor V Leiden or prothrombin mutation). Thromboprophylaxis should also be considered in hospitalized pregnant patients, if they are ill or bedridden. Thromboprophylaxis for 6-week postpartum is given at a lower threshold of risk than prophylaxis antepartum, as the daily risk of VTE is much higher. In addition to women with an antepartum indication, this includes women with any history of VTE and lower-risk thrombophilia (deficiencies of protein C or protein S). For asymptomatic patients with low-risk thrombophilia like heterozygous factor V Leiden or prothrombin mutation, thromboprophylaxis is usually not prescribed. In many cases of increased risk of VTE, the decision to give or withhold thromboprophylaxis is not clear cut and the pros and cons should be discussed with the patient.

In the setting of thromboprophylaxis in pregnant women, LMWHs are preferentially used. They do not pass the placenta and do not have the potential for teratogenicity or fetal bleeding. However, they are associated with hypersensitivity skin reactions. If these appear, patients can be switched to another brand of LMWH,

TABLE 173-2 Prophylaxis Against Venous Thromboembolism During and After Pregnancy

Condition	Pregnancy	In Hospital after Delivery	Puerperium
VTE during pregnancy or previous VTE with indefinite duration of VKA	LMWH, TD	LMWH, TD	LMWH, TD/VKA
Previous unprovoked VTE	LMWH, PID	LMWH, PID	LMWH, PID/VKA
No VTE but antithrombin deficiency; or previous VTE with antithrombin deficiency, APLA, homozygosity or compound heterozygosity for FVL and prothrombin mutation and not on VKA	LMWH, PID	LMWH, PID	LMWH, PID/VKA
Previous VTE in pregnancy or on estrogen or previous VTE with low-risk thrombophilia	LMWH, PID	LMWH, PID	LMWH, PID/VKA
Previous VTE and transient risk factor		LMWH, PID	LMWH, PID/VKA
Cesarian section and at least one additional risk factor		LMWH, PD	
APLA and recurrent pregnancy	LMWH, PD Plus aspirin	(LMWH, PD)	(LMWH, PD)

APLA, antiphospholipid antibodies; LMWH, low-molecular-weight heparin; PD, prophylactic dose; PID, prophylactic or intermediate dose; TD, therapeutic dose; UFH, unfractionated heparin; VTE, venous thromboembolism.

although the skin reactions tend to recur after a number of weeks. Fondaparinux or danaparoid can then be used as an alternative. The disadvantages of UFH is osteoporosis when used for long (>1 month) periods of time, heparin-induced thrombocytopenia (HIT) and inferior efficacy when used in nonpregnant populations. Warfarin is associated with teratogenicity when used between 6 and 12 weeks of gestation and with risk of fetal bleeding. If long-term use of LMWH is not feasible, warfarin might be an acceptable alternative between 12 and 36 weeks of gestation. Use of warfarin at the time of birth places the child at risk for intracranial bleeding. For postpartum prophylaxis, both LMWH and warfarin are good options. Warfarin can be safely used in breastfeeding women. The use of oral factor IIa- or Xa inhibitors is contraindicated in women who are pregnant or breastfeeding. Data in humans are not available, because these patients were excluded from the studies, but reproductive toxicity was shown in animals.

CANCER AND HYPERCOAGULABILITY

About 5% of patients with a first, unprovoked event of VTE have undiagnosed cancer. The neoplasm causes hypercoagulability via production and secretion of procoagulant substances, by endothelial injury, platelet and monocyte activation and by vascular occlusion. Multiple myeloma is associated with a high risk of VTE. Solid tumors with the greatest risk of associated VTE include gliomas and adenocarcinomas of the pancreas, stomach, biliary tree, breast, and lung. Many chemotherapeutic agents and growth factors increase the risk of thrombosis further and the risk also increases with the extent of the disease. In myeloproliferative disease, presence of the JAK2-mutation has been associated with increased risk for thrombosis. Screening for cancer in patients with VTE, beyond a careful history and physical examination, has very low utility and is not routinely recommended. **Table 173-3** lists the exceptional situations when screening is warranted. Routine prophylaxis for outpatients with malignancy is not recommended, except for patients with multiple myeloma. Primary prophylaxis should be given when any additional risk factor is present, for example, immobilization or surgery, usually with LMWH. If UFH is used, the dose should be 5000 units t.i.d. Prophylaxis should be given for at least a week after surgery and extension to 1 month is suggested. When a patient with cancer has developed VTE anticoagulant treatment is more challenging than in other patients. The risk of recurrence despite adequate treatment is paralleled with an increased risk of bleeding complications. LMWH is a better choice than warfarin for secondary prophylaxis and should be given at full therapeutic dose for at least 1 month and may then be reduced to three-fourth of that dose. Anticoagulation should

TABLE 173-3 Screening for Malignancy in Patients with VTE

When to be Alert for Underlying Malignancy	How to Screen
All unprovoked VTE	All patients with VTE: Careful history, physical examination.
Recurrence on therapeutic anticoagulation	Low degree of suspicion: Further testing without clues is not useful.
Multiple site VTE simultaneously	
Recurrent unprovoked superficial thrombosis (Trousseau sign)	Moderate degree of suspicion: CT of abdomen and pelvis.
	High degree of suspicion: Routine chemistry, CBC, CT of chest, abdomen and pelvis; mammography and gynecology consultation in females, PSA in males.

continue as long as there is active cancer but may be switched to warfarin (INR, 2-3) or a DOAC after 3 to 6 months.

DISSEMINATED INTRAVASCULAR COAGULATION

Disseminated intravascular coagulation is an acquired syndrome, caused typically by sepsis, trauma, organ destruction, cancer, obstetric complications, vascular malformations, severe liver failure, or severe toxic or immunologic reactions. Any of these may trigger excessive activation of the blood coagulation—with or without concomitant inflammation. The result is widespread fibrin formation in the microvasculature rather than the normal concentration of a clot to an injured locus. In severe, uncompensated DIC organ dysfunction will ensue. In the early phase, microthrombi will cause organ hypoxia but if the DIC is not controlled and the hemostatic components are consumed faster than they can be replaced the patient will develop bleeding tendency, which eventually becomes generalized. The International Society on Thrombosis and Hemostasis has proposed an algorithm for diagnosis of overt DIC. The underlying cause has to be identified and treated or removed. Other treatment modalities depend on whether the patient develops bleeding or thrombosis. In the case of bleeding replacement of coagulation factors with plasma or more specific components (fibrinogen or cryoprecipitate) might be necessary. UFH or LMWH in subtherapeutic doses are sometimes used to prevent thrombosis, but there are little data to support this practice. Activated protein C or antithrombin concentrates have not been proven effective.

THROMBOTIC THROMBOCYTOPENIC PURPURA

Thrombotic thrombocytopenic purpura is a disease defined by microangiopathic hemolytic anemia and thrombocytopenia, without an alternative explanation (for instance, DIC, malignancy, or obstetric disorders). Patients often present with fever and renal and neurological abnormalities, but these are not required for the diagnosis. The annual incidence is low, at about 4 per million.

Thrombotic thrombocytopenic purpura is caused by either a congenital deficiency of ADAMTS13 or acquired with autoantibodies directed against ADAMTS13. This protein cleaves and inactivates the large, very active, von Willebrand multimers that interact with platelets at the site of vascular injury. The absence of ADAMTS13 leads to unchecked accumulation of platelets and growth of thrombi, particularly microvascular thrombosis. Secondary forms of TTP can be associated with human immunodeficiency virus infection or certain drugs, including quinine.

ADAMTS13 levels can be measured, but turnaround times are commonly too long to help in making the acute diagnosis. A test result can be helpful to confirm the diagnosis though, especially when the response to therapy is not optimal.

The natural course of TTP is fatal in over 90% of patients. Observations in the 1960s and 1970 led to the conclusion that normal plasma contained a factor that could reverse TTP (with the present knowledge: ADAMTS13). A subsequent randomized trial showed that plasma exchange has even better results than plasma infusion: 78% versus 63% survival at 6 months. The current standard of care is that plasma exchange should be started the same day a clinical diagnosis of TTP is made. When plasma exchange is not immediately available, plasma infusion should be started first. A useful strategy is to continue daily exchanges of the patient's plasma volume until the neurological status, platelet count, and lactate dehydrogenase (LDH) have normalized. After this, plasma exchange on alternate days is continued for about a week. Some centers start low-dose aspirin (80 mg) and/or prophylactic dose of LMWH as soon as the platelet count rises above 50×10^9/L. Plasma exchange can be combined with steroids. Although most patients will respond to this

TABLE 173-4 Determination of Pretest Probability of HIT Using the 4T Model

4T's	2 Points	1 Point	0 Point
Thrombocytopenia	Platelet count fall >50% and platelet nadir ≥20 × 10⁹/L	Platelet count fall 30%-50% or platelet nadir 10-19 × 10⁹/L	Platelet count fall <30% or platelet nadir <10 × 10⁹/L
Timing of platelet count fall	Clear onset between days 5 and 10 or platelet fall ≤1 d (prior heparin exposure within 30 d)	Consistent with fall days 5-10, but not clear (eg, missing platelet counts); onset after day 10, or fall ≤1 d (prior heparin exposure 30-100 d ago)	Platelet count fall <4 d without recent exposure
Thrombosis or other sequelae	New thrombosis (confirmed); skin necrosis; acute systemic reaction postintravenous unfractionated heparin bolus	Progressive or recurrent thrombosis; non-necrotizing (erythematous) skin lesions; suspected thrombosis (not proven)	None
Other causes for thrombocytopenia	None apparent	Possible	Definite

Scores of 0-3, 4-5, and 6-8 indicate low, intermediate, and high pretest probability for HIT. From Lo GK, et al. Evaluation of pretest clinical score (4T's) for the diagnosis of heparin-induced thrombocytopenia in two clinical settings. *J Thromb Haemost*. 2006;4:759-765.

therapy, relapse is expected in about 30%. Nonresponding or relapsing patients can be treated with rituximab. Trials with recombinant ADAMTS13 are underway.

THE VASCULITIDES

The vasculitides have inflammation and fibroid necrosis in vessel walls as common denominators but they differ regarding the size and type of blood vessels affected, cellular reactions, and serologic manifestations. In systemic lupus erythematosus, both arterial disease with accelerated atherosclerosis, typically affecting the heart and the kidneys, and venous thrombosis are seen. Behçet's disease (oral ulcers, genital ulcers, uveitis, retinitis, cutaneous vasculitis, synovitis, meningoencephalitis) is also associated with arterial and venous thrombosis in up to 40% of the patients but pulmonary embolism is rare due to adherence to the vessel wall. Thromboembolic events may be the initial presentation of disease. In Buerger's disease, small arteries and veins distally in the extremities manifest occlusions. Conversely, in Kawasaki disease the systemic vasculitis has a predilection for the coronary arteries. In patients with antineutrophil cytoplasmic antibody-associated vasculitis, the incidence of venous thrombosis is high. The interaction between the inflammatory process and the hemostatic mechanisms appears in both directions and therefore the risk of thrombotic complications relates to the activity of the vasculitis.

Treatment with antiplatelet agents is recommended in giant cell arteritis and in Kawasaki disease and for the latter, anticoagulation and thrombolytic therapy are indicated in certain phases. Long-term anticoagulation is also required in association with the antiphospholipid syndrome (see above). In general, there is a lack of evidence-based guidelines on antithrombotic prevention and therapy in the vasculitides.

DRUG-INDUCED HYPERCOAGULABILITY: HEPARIN-INDUCED THROMBOCYTOPENIA (SEE CHAPTER 171 [THROMCYTOPENIA AND THROMBOCYTOSIS])

Patients receiving UFH for more than 5 days after surgery constitute a typical risk group for HIT, which is an antibody reaction with new epitopes exposed on platelet factor 4 when it is bound to heparin. Heparin-induced thrombocytopenia may, however, also occur in medical patients and occasionally with LMWH. Only a small proportion of patients with this antibody reaction develop symptoms of venous or arterial thromboembolism, but in those few patients, the hypercoagulability is pronounced and can result in loss of limb or life. Other symptoms indicative of HIT are necrotic skin reactions at

the site of heparin injection, adrenal necrosis and in case of intravenous injection of heparin, anaphylactoid reactions. Patients at risk of HIT should be monitored with platelet count every 2 to 3 days for the first 2 weeks while on UFH. Diagnosis using the 4T model is described in **Table 173-4**. When the platelet count falls by at least 50% or if a thrombotic event is observed within 2 weeks from starting treatment with heparin, even if since then discontinued, screening for HIT antibodies should be done. If a screening test (immunoassay testing for antiplatelet factor 4) is positive, heparin should immediately be replaced by a therapeutic dose of non-heparin parenteral anticoagulant and a definitive functional assay should be performed. Warfarin should be reversed with vitamin K to be resumed only when the platelet count has normalized or HIT is excluded. Alternative anticoagulants are lepirudin, argatroban, danaparoid, bivalirudin, and fondaparinux. Re-exposure to heparin within 100 days from HIT is likely to cause recurrent symptoms without any delay and must be avoided. Later re-exposure is probably safe since antibodies can no longer be demonstrated.

DRUG-INDUCED HYPERCOAGULABILITY: COUMARIN-INDUCED SKIN NECROSIS

Vitamin K antagonists may cause skin necrosis in approximately 1 of 5000 patients with 85% of the affected cases being women. The mechanism is an imbalance between the rapidly occurring, profound depression of the natural anticoagulants protein C and protein S and on the other hand a slower and mild reduction of the procoagulant vitamin K dependent coagulation factors. Therefore, pre-existing deficiency of protein C, protein S, or antithrombin is also a risk factor. Fibrin is then deposited in subcutaneous small veins and venules, typically in the breasts, thighs, or buttocks. The syndrome starts with localized pain and a maculopapular rash 3 to 10 days after initiation of coumarin therapy, then progresses within 24 to 48 hours to hemorrhagic lesions, hemorrhagic bullae, and finally necrosis. This develops into an eschar with slow healing but often requiring plastic surgery or mastectomy. Immediately upon recognition of the syndrome vitamin K should be given, warfarin stopped, replacement of the natural anticoagulants with plasma or a specific concentrate (protein C or antithrombin) and anticoagulation continued with heparin. After healing of the lesions, the vitamin K antagonist may be resumed extremely carefully (start dose 1-2 mg/d).

DRUG-INDUCED HYPERCOAGULABILITY: ESTROGENS

The combined oral contraceptive pill (COC) is associated with a three- to fivefold increased risk of VTE. This risk is attributed to the estrogen component, but modulated by the type of progestagen: the newer third and fourth generations of progestagens double the risk of second-generation pills containing levonorgestrel. Therefore, only second-generation COC should be routinely prescribed, also in women without additional risk factors. Oral estrogens for hormone replacement are also associated with an increased risk of VTE, but transdermal preparations seem safe. This difference is not seen for contraceptive agents: the VTE risk of patches and vaginal rings containing estrogen and third- or fourth-generation progestagens is similar to that of oral preparations. Women with a personal history of VTE or other strong risk factors should not be prescribed estrogens, except for transdermal administration of replacement doses.

SUGGESTED READINGS

Ortel TL, Erkan D, Kitchens CS. How I treat catastrophic thrombotic syndromes. *Blood*. 2015;126:1285-1293.

DEFICIENCIES OF NATURAL INHIBITORS OF COAGULATION

Crowther MA, Kelton JG. Congenital thrombophilic states associated with venous thrombosis: a qualitative overview and proposed classification system. *Ann Intern Med*. 2003;138:128-134.

ANTIPHOSPHOLIPID SYNDROME

Lim W. Antiphospholipid syndrome. *Hematology Am Soc Hematol Educ Program*. 2013;675-680.

HOSPITALIZED PATIENTS

Ataga KI, Key NS. Hypercoagulability in sickle cell disease: new approaches to an old problem. *Hematology Am Soc Hematol Educ Program*. 2007;91-96.

Cohen AT, Tapson VF, Bergmann J-F, et al. Venous thromboembolism risk and prophylaxis in the acute hospital care setting (ENDORSE) study: a multinational cross-sectional study. *Lancet*. 2008;371:387-394.

Gould MK, Garcia DA, Wren SM, et al. Prevention of VTE in non-orthopedic surgical patients: antithrombotic therapy and prevention of thrombosis, 9th ed: American College of Chest Physicians Evidence-Based Clinical Practice Guidelines. *Chest*. 2012;141(2 Suppl):e227S-e2277S.

Kahn SR, Lim W, Dunn AS, et al. Prevention of VTE in nonsurgical patients: antithrombotic therapy and prevention of thrombosis, 9th ed: American College of Chest Physicians Evidence-Based Clinical Practice Guidelines. *Chest*. 2012;141(2 Suppl):e195S-e226S.

PREGNANCY AND THE POSTPARTUM PERIOD

Bates SM, Greer IA, Middeldorp S, Veenstra DL, Prabulos AM, Vandvik PO. VTE, thrombophilia, antithrombotic therapy, and pregnancy: antithrombotic therapy and prevention of thrombosis, 9th ed: American College of Chest Physicians Evidence-Based Clinical Practice Guidelines. *Chest*. 2012;141(2 Suppl):e691S-e736S.

Marik PE, Plante LA. Venous thromboembolic disease and pregnancy. *N Engl J Med*. 2008;359:2025-2033.

DIC

Taylor FB, et al. Towards definition, clinical and laboratory criteria, and a scoring system for disseminated intravascular coagulation. *Thromb Haemost*. 2001;86;1327-1330.

TTP

Rock GA, Shumak KH, Buskard NA, et al. Comparison of plasma exchange with plasma infusion in the treatment of thrombotic thrombocytopenic purpura. Canadian Apheresis Study Group. *N Engl J Med*. 1991;325:393-397.

Sadler JE. Von Willebrand factor, ADAMTS13, and thrombotic thrombocytopenic purpura. *Blood*. 2008;112:11-18.

THE VASCULITIDES

Trifiletti A, et al. Hemostatic changes in vasculitides. *Thromb Res*. 2009;124:252-255.

HIT

Linkins LA1, Dans AL, Moores LK, et al. Treatment and prevention of heparin-induced thrombocytopenia: antithrombotic therapy and prevention of thrombosis, 9th ed: American College of Chest Physicians Evidence-Based Clinical Practice Guidelines. *Chest*. 2012;141(2 Suppl):e495S-e530S.

174

Hematologic Malignancies

Victor M. Orellana, MD

Eric S. Winer, MD

Key Clinical Questions

1. How do the most common hematologic malignancies present?
2. How do you definitively diagnose these malignancies?
3. How do you stage these diseases?
4. How do you determine prognosis for patients with each of these malignancies?
5. Which are the standard treatment options for these malignancies and what are their side effects?

INTRODUCTION

Hematologic malignancies represent a growing percentage of inpatient oncology admissions. Patients with these diseases may receive a significant portion of their cancer-specific treatment in the hospital under the supervision of hematology specialists. Admitting clinicians should be able to recognize common presentations, arrange for prompt hematology or oncology consultation, explain standard treatment protocols, and anticipate complications that may arise during their course.

The cellular origin of the various hematologic malignancies will dictate the downstream disease manifestations and treatment options. The cancer ultimately derives from a single cancer cell which has undergone a sufficient string of genetic mutations to allow for unchecked and exponential replication (a "clonal" process). Some pathologies may be "polyclonal," coming from multiple over replicating cells. This chapter will focus on "monoclonal" entities that may be traced back to mutations in a single cell which has copied itself prolifically.

Myeloid neoplasms, such as acute myeloid leukemia, myelodysplastic syndrome, and the myeloproliferative neoplasms, tend to arise from an aberrant primitive hematopoietic cell. In contrast, lymphoid neoplasms may arise from malignant transformation at various points along the maturation process of B or T lymphocytes. This may manifest as an acute lymphoblastic leukemia, chronic lymphocytic leukemia/small lymphocytic lymphoma, or one of the many other types of B- or T-cell lymphomas.

"Leukemia" generally refers to cancers more predominantly localized in the marrow and peripheral blood, whereas "lymphoma" refers to disease burden within the lymph nodes and lymphatic system. However, many hematologic malignancies may situate in either or both categories during their course.

TECHNIQUES USED IN THE EVALUATION OF HEMATOLOGIC MALIGNANCIES

■ BONE MARROW BIOPSY AND ASPIRATE

The most common study to evaluate hematologic malignancies is the bone marrow biopsy and aspirate. This two-step procedure includes bone marrow biopsy for examination of cellularity and morphology and bone marrow fluid aspiration for cytogentics and molecular studies. A core piece of bone marrow generally 0.2 cm in width and 1 to 1.5 cm in length is obtained using a Jamshidi needle, after which immunohistochemical staining may be performed to optimize elucidation of malignant cells. An additional 5 to 10 mL of marrow fluid is collected into an EDTA tube for smears and flow cytometry, and into a sodium heparin tube for cytogenetic analysis.

■ FLOW CYTOMETRY

Flow cytometry is critical in the diagnosis of leukemias. This laser-based analytical technique is used to evaluate the surface markers on individual cells. Cells from the given tissue sample are incubated with fluorescent-labeled tags and then run as a column through a device that uses these labels to chemically distinguish between the various protein surface markers on individual cells. For example, samples with a surface marker signature of CD5+/CD23+/CD20 dim would signify a chronic lymphocytic leukemia.

■ CYTOGENETICS

Fluorescent in situ hybridization (FISH) uses fluorescent probes specific to chromosomal sequences to detect disease-specific translocations. Studying the chromosomal components of malignant hematologic cells is vital for prognostic purposes and will frequently dictate treatment. For example, identification of or a chromosome 8 addition (trisomy 8 or +8) conveys a poor prognosis in acute myeloid leukemia. Cytogenetics has occasional diagnostic benefits as well. Identifying a translocation between chromosomes 9 and 22 [t(9:22)] is pathognomonic of chronic myeloid leukemia (CML), and there are many other findings seen in myelodysplastic syndrome (MDS), acute promyelocytic leukemia, and non-Hodgkin's lymphomas.

Molecular studies

Polymerase chain reaction (PCR) has become standard of care for diseases such as CML and acute promyelocytic leukemia. Genetic sequencing has identified mutations such as Fms-like tyrosine kinase 3 gene (FLT3) and Nucleophosmin 1 (NPM1), prognostic markers in acute myelogenous leukemia (AML).

■ ACUTE LYMPHOBLASTIC LEUKEMIA

Acute lymphoblastic leukemia (ALL) is a heterogeneous class of disorders arising from aberrant precursor B and T lymphocytes. Both the cellular origin and the age at diagnosis have major implications on the type of ALL pathophysiology involved and the treatment paradigm required; ALL is seen far more commonly in children, although it can affect patients of any age. As with any acute leukemia, bone marrow biopsy is essential in diagnosing ALL. Histology may resemble AML or various B-cell lymphomas; flow cytometry and cytogenetic evaluation help distinguish B- and T-ALL from other related disorders. The Philadelphia chromosome (Ph) may be expressed in some cases, which has major treatment implications. **Table 174-1** summarizes findings that may distinguish ALL from other hematologic malignancies.

These patients are intrinsically immunocompromised, due to their malignancy itself and any secondary neutropenia or treatment-related susceptibilities. While fevers and chills are common initial symptoms, any fever should be considered infectious until proven otherwise. Likewise, most patients experience significant fatigue during their course, but true focal weakness should still raise the concern for CNS involvement of ALL as this is a well-known complication. A subset of patients may present with a mass-like lesion more consistent with a lymphoma in the mediastinum (usually from thymic-originating T-cell disease) or in various lymph node chains and extranodal sites such as skin, bone, and gonads.

Treatment

ALL is an aggressive disease that requires equally aggressive and prolonged treatment. All patients receive induction chemotherapy; subsequent treatment may range from intensive consolidation and maintenance chemotherapy, to allogeneic hematopoietic stem cell transplant (HSCT), to palliative treatment.

Age at diagnosis will help discern which patients can tolerate more aggressive chemotherapy regimens. Adolescents and young adults (up to age 39) with ALL may also have slightly different disease pathology and thus may respond better to treatment paradigms resembling pediatric regimens. Both pediatric and adult regimens are multidrug combinations which often include anthracyclines, steroids, vincristine, cytarabine, asparaginase, and methotrexate and cytarabine intrathecally. **Table 174-2** describes common chemotherapies used in ALL and other hematologic malignancies.

Following induction, many patients will undergo an intensive *consolidation phase* in their treatment. High doses of systemic methotrexate, cytarabine, mercaptopurine, and asparaginase are commonly used, especially in younger patients. Following eradication of any residual disease, *maintenance chemotherapy* with mercaptopurine and weekly methotrexate is often continued for at least 2 years given the propensity for relapse. CNS prophylaxis is continued during all phases of treatment (ie, consolidation and maintenance).

Ph-positive disease or its equivalents have a poor prognosis when treated with conventional chemotherapy alone and may do better with upfront allogeneic HSCT after the first complete remission is achieved. Incorporation of tyrosine kinase inhibitors (TKIs) such as imatinib and dasatinib, frequently used in treating CML, is now part of induction therapy in Ph-positive disease, often allowing less toxic chemotherapy to be used in the induction treatment. They have been shown to be briefly effective even as single-agent therapy in relapsed Ph-positive ALL. However, any patient in this prognostic category who achieves complete remission following induction

---

TABLE 174-1 Acute Lymphoblastic Leukemia

Epidemiology	Most common childhood malignancy; only 24% >45 y of age, 20% adult leukemias
Clinical presentation (over weeks to months)	B symptoms: fever, chills, night sweats, weight loss; lymph node, liver, spleen enlargement in 50% of patients; CNS involvement; fatigue, easy bruisability
Laboratory	Cytopenia
Bone marrow biopsy	*B-ALL:* almost uniformly positive for CD19, cytoplasmic CD79a and CD22, and TdT. Depending on the differentiation stage of the malignant clone, CD10 may be positive. CD20 typically (but not uniformly) negative, as this disease arises from precursor cells prior to initiation of natural CD20 expression.

T-ALL: also positive for TdT, and generally positive for CD7 and cytoplasmic CD3, and may also express CD1a, Cd2, CD4, CD5, and CD8. |
| Cytogenetics and molecular studies | Various chromosomal and genetic abnormalities may be present, many of them more frequently documented in pediatric cases such as hyperdiploidy (ie, >50 chromosomes) or the t(12:21) translocation which carries a favorable prognosis. |
| Prognosis | Favorable: t(12:21) translocation

Very unfavorable: Presence of the Philadelphia (Ph) chromosome t(9:22) or expression of the BCR-ABL product as identified on RT-PCR; seen at any age (more frequently above age 60), may occur in progression from chronic lymphocytic leukemia to ALL or in *de novo* cases.

"Ph chromosome-like" mutations such as *Ikaros IKZF1* which do not demonstrate the classic Philadelphia translocation. |

TABLE 174-2 Common Chemotherapies Used in Hematologic Malignancies

Drug	Mechanism	Uses	Side Effects	Comments
Chemotherapy and targeted therapy				
All-trans retinoic acid (ATRA) and arsenic trioxide (ATO)	Differentiating agents	Acute promyelocytic leukemia	Life-threatening hyperleukocytosis Differentiation syndrome: weight gain and edema, progressing to dyspnea, interstitial pulmonary infiltrates, pleural and/or pericardial effusions, unexplained fevers, and acute renal insufficiency. ATRA: pseudotumor cerebri ATO: hyperglycemia, QT prolongation.	Start dexamethasone 10mg IV q12h at first sign of differentiation syndrome, even if other processes such as CHF or sepsis are present. Hold ATRA/ATO if acute renal failure develops or respiratory distress requiring ICU admission. Hold ATO if QTc >500 ms, or if syncope/palpitations develop.
Anthracyclines (daunorubicin, doxorubicin, idarubicin, epirubicin)	Intercalating agent (inhibits DNA synthesis)	Acute leukemias (daunorubicin in "7+3" induction); NHL (C**H**OP; H = hydroxydaunomycin, aka doxorubicin)	Myelosuppression, nausea/vomiting, alopecia, radiation recall. Secondary leukemias. Cardiotoxicity: early (presents usually as sinus tachyarrhythmias) or late (cardiomyopathy leading to CHF; dose dependent, based on lifetime exposure)	All patients require baseline echocardiogram prior to initiating treatment. Contraindicated if LVEF <45%, myocardial infarction within 3 mo, or significant arrhythmias present. Cumulative lifetime doses are limited to 450-550 mg/m² doxorubicin, 800 mg/m² daunorubicin, 150 mg/m² idarubicin.
5-Azacytidine and decitabine	Demethylating agent	Myelodysplastic syndromes; AML in elderly patients	Myelosuppression, nausea, diarrhea, constipation. *5-Azacytidine:* neuropathy, hepatotoxicity, rash, hypokalemia, acute renal failure.	Profound cytopenias may herald an eventual response to treatment rather than progressive disease.
Bendamustine	Alkylating agent	CLL; indolent NHL (incl. mantle cell); Multiple myeloma, Waldenström Macroglobulinemia	Cytopenias, fatigue, nausea/vomiting, decreased appetite. Tumor lysis may occur, less commonly acute renal, hepatic, and cardiac toxicities.	CBC, Creatinine, LFTs, should be followed. Hold if moderate to severe renal or hepatic impairment develops.
Bleomycin	Glycopeptide antibiotic; causes single- and double-stranded DNA breaks, interferes with DNA repair	HL; less commonly now for NHL	Fever and chills occur in half of patients within hours of treatment. Anaphylactoid reactions may occur. Interstitial pneumonitis and pulmonary fibrosis may be life threatening. The presentation may be subtle: nonproductive cough, dyspnea, unexplained fever. CXR usually shows bilateral reticular or nodular opacities without pleural effusions, but may be normal, and reduced DLCO is the first PFT abnormality. Flagellate erythema is a rare but distinctive rash that may appear from 1 d to several months following bleomycin administration. Bleomycin enhances radiation injury. Alopecia.	Bleomycin should be withheld if the DLCO falls to 30%-35% of the initial value, if the FVC falls significantly, or if there are clinical or radiographic features suggesting pulmonary toxicity. Prednisone 1 mg/kg should be employed in patients with pneumonitis. Since oxygen may synergize with bleomycin to produce fibrosis, supplemental oxygen administered during operative procedures and critical illnesses should be minimized.

(Continued)

TABLE 174-2 Common Chemotherapies Used in Hematologic Malignancies (*Continued*)

Drug	Mechanism	Uses	Side Effects	Comments
Bortezomib/ carfilzomib	Proteosome inhibitor	Multiple myeloma. Waldenström macroglobulinemia. Mantle cell NHL	Peripheral neuropathy that is sometimes painful, orthostatic hypotension, gastrointestinal upset, constipation, ileus, thrombocytopenia, herpes zoster, tumor lysis syndrome.	Zoster prophylaxis is advisable in VZV+ patients. The neuropathy may require dose reductions and usually improves or resolves within 2 y of discontinuing treatment.
Chorambucil	Alkylating agent	CLL, low-grade NHL	Myelosuppression. Pulmonary toxicity, rash, and toxic epidermal necrolysis are rare occurrences.	Monitor CBC closely, especially with continuous administration.
Cyclophosphamide	Alkylating agent	NHL, transplant conditioning	Myelosuppresion, hemorrhagic cystitis (10%-40%, more with higher doses), SIADH, alopecia, radiation recall. Secondary leukemias. Nasal stuffiness and facial discomfort are common complaints with rapid infusions. Pulmonary toxicity: uncommon, but frequently life-threatening when occurs. Transplant patients: main culprit drug for sinusoidal obstruction syndrome; cardiac necrosis can occur at high doses.	Maintain adequate hydration Hemorrhagic cystitis: aggressive hydration (goal 100 cc/h UOP) maintain plt >50k. If AKI develops, urine fails to clear, or pain persists, obtain renal u/s and start continuous bladder irrigation. May require cystoscopy if this is unsuccessful. Mesna may be used for prophylaxis.
Cytarabine	Pyrimidine analog	ALL, AML, MDS, NHL	Cerebellar toxicity. Myelosuppression, chemical conjunctivitis, palmar/solar rash (erythrodysesthesia; from cutaneous drug accumulations) Can provoke a generalized rash, fever, and myalgia 6-12 h after administration of high doses. Hepatotoxicity and pulmonary toxicity may occur.	Test for cerebellar dysfunction (include handwriting) before each high dose infusion used in consolidation therapy. If develops, stop all further doses. Steroids may be used to treat pulmonary toxicity, which may present as a capillary leak syndrome 2-21 d after the first dose. Give prophylactic steroid eye drops to prevent chemical conjunctivitis
Dacarbazine	Alkylating agent	HL	Myelosuppression, hepatotoxicity, nausea/ vomiting, alopecia	Dose reduce if renal impairment occurs.
Etoposide	Topoisomerase II inhibitor	ALL, AML; HL and NHL; multiple myeloma (treatment refractory)	Myelosuppression, hepatotoxicity, mucositis, dysgeusia, nausea/vomiting, diarrhea, alopecia	Hold for ANC <500. Dose-reduce by 50% if WBC <2k or Plt <75k, or if significant renal or hepatic impairment occur.
Fludarabine	Purine analog	CLL, lymphomas, AML (salvage tx), conditioning regimens in non-myeloablative HSCT	Myelosuppression may persist for many months. Profoundly reduces B and T lymphocytes, placing at risk for opportunistic infection with intracellular pathogens (*Pneumocystis*, **Listeria**) and transfusion-related graft-versus-host disease. Interstitial pneumonitis and dose-dependent irreversible neurotoxicity (including confusion, cortical blindness, and necrotizing leukoencephalopathy) rarely occur in current protocols. Autoimmune hemolytic anemia is common when used in DAT+ CLL patients.	Blood banks and patients themselves should be aware of the need to irradiate cellular blood products (transplant patients only). PCP prophylaxis is required.

(*Continued*)

TABLE 174-2 Common Chemotherapies Used in Hematologic Malignancies (*Continued*)

Drug	Mechanism	Uses	Side Effects	Comments
Ibrutinib	Bruton tyrosine kinase inhibitor	CLL, mantle cell NHL, Waldenström macroglobulinemia	Atrial fibrillation or flutter, which requires stopping treatment. Cytopenias and bleeding may occur. Fatigue, nausea, diarrhea are common. Rare severe renal impairment.	Baseline and daily EKG to watch for atrial fibrillation. Monitor for renal toxicity. CYP 3A4 cleared—reduce dose or hold for hepatic impairment, avoid grapefruit.
Imatinib (1st gen.), nilotinib, dasatinib (2nd gen.), ponatinib (3rd gen.)	Tyrosine kinase inhibitors with varying specificity for **BCR-ABL** and other kinases	CML, Ph+ ALL, subsets of CMML, chronic eosinophilic leukemia	Myelosuppression, hepatotoxicity; asymptomatic lipase elevations. Nausea/vomiting, diarrhea, rash. Fluid retention (I). Pericardial and pleural effusions (D, P). QT prolongation (N, D). *Ponatinib*: potentially cardiotoxic, increased risk for thrombosis-related events	Very different drug-drug interactions and side effect profiles for each agent. Toxicity from one TKI does not preclude switching to another.
Thalidomide, Lenalidomide, and Pomalidomide	Immunomodulators with antiangiogenic activity	Multiple myeloma; 5q- syndrome/MDS (lenalidomide)	Increased risk of thrombosis. Rash. Rare cases of toxic epidermal necrolysis. *Thalidomide*: Somnolence, constipation, peripheral neuropathy. *Lenalidomide/Pomalidomide*: myelosuppression, especially thrombocytopenia; renal insufficiency, rare pneumonitis.	The risk of thrombosis is augmented by concurrent glucocorticoids or erythropoietin. The optimal VTE prophylaxis is debated.
Melphalan	Alkylating agent	Low dose: elderly or unfit patients with myeloma. High-dose: conditioning for autologous HSCT in myeloma, NHL, HL	Myelosuppression, mucositis. Rarely, can cause pneumonitis and pulmonary fibrosis. Tissue necrosis with extravasation.	Prolonged alkylator exposure precludes subsequent autologous stem cell collection, which is why melphalan is avoided as initial therapy in transplant-eligible patients.
Methotrexate	Anti-folate	High-grade NHL, ALL, prevention of graft-versus-host disease in the transplant setting	Myelosuppression, stomatitis, mucositis, , hepatotoxicity, acute renal insufficiency, idiosyncratic pulmonary toxicity, radiation recall, chemical meningitis with intrathecal administration.	Many drugs (incl penicillins) can reduce renal clearance of MTX or displace MTX from albumin, increasing bioavailability. Drug will accumulate in effusions and edema fluid, which can lead to substantial toxicity. All effusions should be drained before starting MTX. Leucovorin rescue and hydration are the mainstays of treating MTX toxicity.
Vinca alkaloids (vincristine and vinblastine)	Antimicrotubule agents	ALL, NHL, HL, multiple myeloma	Neurotoxicity (esp w/ vincristine), may present as peripheral sensory impairment, paresthesias, and loss of deep tendon reflexes. Painful dysesthesia, motor impairment that includes foot drop and difficulty with fine finger movements, ataxia, cranial nerve palsies manifesting as hoarseness, ptosis, facial nerve palsies, or jaw pain, and in extreme cases paralysis can occur. Autonomic toxicity includes constipation and ileus.	Support with aggressive bowel regimens to prevent obstipation and ileus. Extravasation may be treated by infiltrating the area with 1-2 mL of hyaluronidase, 150 U/mL, then applying warm compresses for 72 h.

(Continued)

TABLE 174-2 Common Chemotherapies Used in Hematologic Malignancies (*Continued*)

Drug	Mechanism	Uses	Side Effects	Comments
Immunotherapy				
Rituximab/ Ofatumumab/ Obinutuzumab	Monoclonal anti-CD20 antibody	CLL, B-cell NHL	Common infusion reactions: fevers, rigors, urticaria, bronchospasm, hypotension. Incidence is highest with the first dose (77%) and diminishes with subsequent doses. Anaphylaxis may occur, usually at the second or subsequent infusion. Pulmonary reactions that manifest with dyspnea, bronchospasm, hypoxia, and lung infiltrates may occur acutely (1-2 h after initiation of the first infusion) or be delayed (one to 4 wk after infusion). Major risk for TLS. Risk for reactivation of TB and hepatitis; extremely rarely can precipitate a progressive multifocal leukoencephalopathy; risk of PML is likely augmented when rituximab is combined with chemotherapy.	Most infusion reactions are mild-to-moderate and can be managed by interrupting or slowing the infusion and supportive care (saline, antihistamines, methylprednisolone, acetaminophen, bronchodilators, ± epinephrine if severe). All patients should have PPD and hepatitis panel checked prior to initiating tx.

should be offered allogeneic transplant when an HLA-matched donor is available.

Post-treatment monitoring, including a comprehensive physical examination (with testicular exam) and a complete blood count (CBC), should be performed every 1 to 2 months during the first year, then decreased to every 3 months for the second year and 6 months for the third year.

Residual disease after treatment may be minimal, but any residual leukemic burden portends a high risk for relapsed disease and thus a very poor prognosis. These patients should be taken to transplant if possible. Relapsed disease is often treated with chemotherapy similar to the induction regimens used, or with the recently approved blinatumumab, a bispecific T-cell engager (BiTe) targeting CD19. Patients then should be treated with an allogeneic (preferred) or autologous transplant.

◼ ACUTE MYELOID LEUKEMIA

Acute myeloid leukemia (AML), the most common adult form of leukemia, most often arises *de novo* although myelodysplastic and myeloproliferative diseases may progress to AML. Current criteria through the WHO places increased reliance on cytogenetic and molecular markers to distinguish between various subtypes of myeloid leukemia. Cytochemistry is still useful in this setting, but at this point the FAB classification scheme is used mainly out of familiarity. For all patients with suspected AML, bone marrow biopsy is the *sine qua non* for establishing the diagnosis. Samples should be sent for flow cytometry and cytogenetic studies as well as standard pathology stains (including immunohistochemistry).

Virtually every organ system can be affected by AML, although clinical presentation is often predominantly driven by its effects in the bone marrow (see **Table 174-3** for clinical features that distinguish AML from other entities). When present, fever should be considered infectious even if the patient is not already neutropenic at the time of presentation.

Risk stratification and treatment

Once AML has been diagnosed, the patient's risk category is stratified based on age, functional status, cytogenetic profile (**Table 174-4**), and underlying etiology (if known). All treatment decisions including curative versus palliative intent are based on this risk assessment and the patient's wishes. Response to treatment and overall survival in AML is widely variable. Prognosis will depend largely upon patient risk factors (age, functional status, cytogenetic profile, comorbidities) and measured response to therapy. The natural history of untreated AML may be days to months, and when complete remission can be achieved with treatment, 5-year survival averages 15% to 20%.

Good risk—curative intent

For patients stratified as "good risk," the standard treatment aiming for cure of AML is a 7-day course of chemotherapy designed to rapidly achieve complete remission. The "7+3" regimen employs 7 days continuous infusion of cytarabine and daily infusions of an anthracycline (usually daunorubicin) for the first 3 days of treatment. Anthracyclines, in particular, have potential for cardiotoxicity; all patients receiving these medications require a baseline echocardiogram prior to starting treatment.

Following induction, a bone marrow biopsy is usually performed around day 14 of the treatment cycle with day 1 being the first day chemotherapy is administered. Further chemotherapy is immediately administered if there is persistent disease and the patient can tolerate treatment. If the bone marrow is aplastic (defined as <10% cellularity with <5% blasts), the patient is monitored to complete count recovery and a bone marrow biopsy is repeated. If a complete remission is achieved (<5% blasts on posttreatment marrow plus full cell-count recovery in the peripheral blood), consolidation therapy is administered with 3 to 4 cycles of single-agent high-dose cytarabine (HiDAC), given twice daily, every other day over 5 days. Doses used for this regimen may cause cerebellar toxicity in any patient, but more commonly in older patients and in those with

TABLE 174-3 Acute Myeloid Leukemia

Epidemiology	~3.5 people per 100,000, more common in men and in older individuals (median age 67).
	Risk factors include:
	• Chemotherapy for other malignancies
	▪ 1-3 y post topoisomerase-inhibitors
	▪ 5-10 y post alkylating agents
	• Radiation exposure
	• Down syndrome; congenital disorders with chromosomal instability
Clinical presentation	Symptoms: fatigue, anorexia, weight loss, easy bruising, poor wound healing, fever*, headache, shortness of breath over days to weeks (common)
	*Any fever should be considered infectious until proven otherwise, with or without neutropenia
	Exam: petechiae (common), hepatomegaly and splenomegaly (less common than other hematologic disorders), lymphadenopathy (rare)
Laboratory	Anemia, thrombocytopenia, myeloid precursors
	May present with high peripheral WBC; >50-100k may lead to leukostasis (*medical emergency*)
Bone marrow biopsy	Presence of >20% myeloid blasts
Cytogenetics and Molecular Studies	Presence of any characteristic cytogenetic abnormalities automatically upgrades the diagnosis to acute myeloid leukemia regardless of blast count
Prognosis	Good risk: favorable cytogenetics in a patient <60 y of age
	Intermediate risk: those fall in neither good or high risk category
	High risk: older patients, those with poor level of function, multiple comorbidities, or adverse cytogenetic profiles
	Unfavorable: duration of symptoms for >3 mo

renal impairment. All further cytarabine doses should be held if CNS symptoms occur.

If CR is not achieved, several regimens exist as second-line "re-induction" therapy. A modified "5+2" regimen employs the same chemotherapies as induction but for less duration. HiDAC or other salvage regimens may also be given. If CR is not achieved after two cycles of induction chemotherapy, most patients should be taken to transplant (HSCT).

Intermediate-/high-risk-transplant versus palliative treatment
For patients classified as intermediate- or high-risk on initial diagnosis, treatment attempting cure is usually directed toward achieving CR and then immediately proceeding to transplantation. Some intermediate patients will be offered HiDAC consolidation therapy prior to transplant. Allogeneic HSCT achieves better survival rates and allows for graft-versus-leukemia effects but may be associated with potentially fatal graft-versus-host disease. Autologous HSCT is not always an option and is associated with higher relapse rates (~20%). Salvage chemotherapy is sometimes used after unsuccessful induction to decrease the cancer burden before attempting transplant.

TABLE 174-4 Cytogenetic and Molecular Stratification in AML

Favorable risk cytogenetics

t(8;21)(q22;q22); *RUNX1-RUNX1T1* (previously *ETO-AML1*)

inv(16)(p13.1q22) or t(16;16)(p13.1;q22); *CBFB-MYH11*

Mutated *CEBPA* with normal karyotype

Mutated *NPM1* with no *FLT3*-ITD

Intermediate-I

Mutated *NPM1* and FLT3-ITD (normal karyotype)

Wild-type *NPM1* and *FLT3*-ITD (normal karyotype)

Wild-type *NPM1* without *FLT3*-ID (normal karyotype)

Intermediate-II

t(9;11)(p22;q23); *MLLT3-MLL*

Cytogenetic abnormalities not classified as favorable or adverse

Poor risk

Inv(3)(q21; q16.2) or t(3;3)(q21;q26.2); *RPN1-EVI1*

t(6;9)(p23;q34); *DEK-NUP214*

t(v;11)(c;q23); *MLL* gene rearrangement

-5 or deletion(5q)

-7

Abnormality in 17p

Complex karyotype

From Döhner H, Estey EH, Amadori S, et al. Diagnosis and management of acute myeloid leukemia in adults: recommendations from an international expert panel, on behalf of the European LeukemiaNet. *Blood.* 2010;115:453.

AML in the elderly

Elderly AML patients, defined here as age >60 years, have comorbidities and decreased physiologic reserve that often limit their ability to tolerate aggressive chemotherapy. The biology of their leukemia often differs from that of younger patients. Their cancer cells manifest multidrug resistant proteins (MDRs) at higher rates, and their outcomes with traditional chemotherapy regimens are consequently less favorable. Thus, modified regimens have been developed for the older adult with AML who is not likely to tolerate traditional intensive chemotherapy. These include lower doses of cytarabine with hypomethylating agents such as azacitidine and low-dose decitabine (which may be used in patients with poor risk cytogenetics). Not all older adults require this approach, and hematology consultation should direct appropriate therapy.

■ ACUTE PROMYELOCYTIC LEUKEMIA

AML patients found to have t(15;17) or expression of PML-RARα have a subtype of the disease known as acute promyelocytic leukemia (APML). These are usually younger patients (median age 31) whose disease frequently presents with a leukemia-related bleeding diathesis, evidenced by epistaxis, gastrointestinal bleeding, intracranial

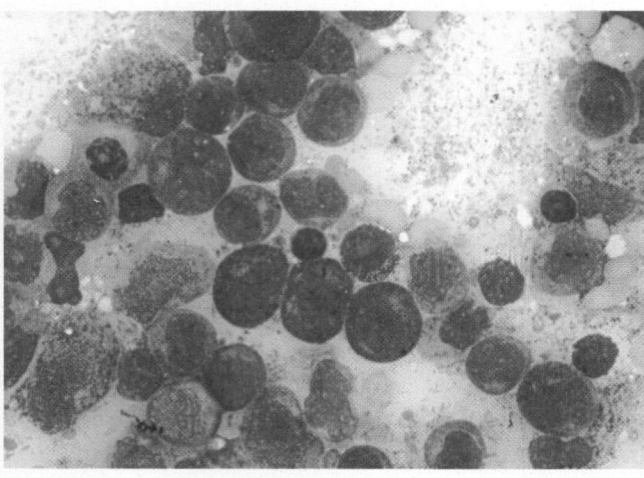

Figure 174-1 *Acute promyelocytic leukemia, 1000x magnification. Notable is the high nuclear to cytoplastmic ratio, nucleoli, and granules in the periphery. (Courtesy of Mark Legolvan, DO, Department of Pathology, Rhode Island Hospital.)*

hemorrhage, and disseminated intravascular coagulation (DIC). Bone marrow biopsy and peripheral smear demonstrate an abundance of promyelocytes (**Figure 174-1**).

Patients with good risk factors (defined as WBC <10k with good functional status and no elevations in creatinine or bilirubin) may receive induction regimens of all-trans retinoic acid (ATRA) and arsenic trioxide with exceptional results, while higher risk patients require the addition of anthracycline therapy.

Approximately 25% of patients receiving ATRA induction therapy develop "differentiation syndrome" due to massive cytokine release as the ATRA drives the arrested promyelocytes to mature. Manifestations may include dyspnea, peripheral edema, noninfectious fever, hypotension leading to shock, increasing WBC with falling RBC and platelet counts, and DIC. For this reason, some institutions will begin APML induction therapy in the intensive care setting, but decisions should be individualized for each patient.

■ MYELODYSPLASTIC SYNDROME

Myelodysplastic syndrome (MDS) is a malignant stem cell disorder that is characterized by ineffective hematopoiesis leading to dysplasia (Greek for "bad formation") in one or all of the white blood cell, red blood cell, and platelet lineages. The pathogenesis of MDS remains unclear but it is thought to be a clonal disorder. There are specific chromosomal translocations (associated with 50% of diagnoses) and genetic mutations that are common in MDS, but they are not pathognomonic for the disease.

Any or all cell lines may be affected, although anemia is most common. Patients may also present with a macrocytosis with or without a related anemia. Blast count in the bone marrow must be less than 20% to distinguish from AML. **Table 174-5** summarizes findings that may distinguish MDS from other hematologic malignancies.

The diagnosis of MDS requires both peripheral blood and bone marrow studies. If patients have cytopenias and no dysplasia evident on bone marrow biopsy, a diagnosis may still be made by identifying a cytogenetic abnormality associated with MDS. Other causes of dysplasia should be excluded; such as deficiencies in vitamin B12, iron, and copper levels and infection with HIV.

TABLE 174-5 Myelodysplastic Syndrome

Epidemiology	Incidence ~4 per 100,000 annually, increasing with age, reaching a peak of 89 per 100,000 in patients over the age of 80. ~14% rate of transformation rate from MDS to AML
Clinical presentation	Asymptomatic, identified on routine blood counts (common).
	Symptoms: fatigue due to anemia, infections from both the neutropenia and neutrophil dysfunction, and bleeding due to thrombocytopenia.
	Cutaneous abnormalities: Sweet syndrome [neutrophilic dermatosis] (uncommon)
	Autoimmune complications: vasculitis, rheumatoid arthritis, or pernicious anemia.
Laboratory	Cytopenias: • An absolute neutrophil count of < 1800/μL • Hemoglobin of <10 g/dL • Platelets of <100,000/ μL Peripheral blood smear: • WBCs ↓ segmentation, sometimes bilobed, pseudo-Pelger-Huet cells; ↓ granulation or agranular. • RBCs macrocytic, large ovalocytes along with RBC precursors showing dysplastic features such as abnormal nuclear inclusions, multinucleation, and karyorrhexis.
Bone marrow biopsy	Hypercellular; significant dysplasia, defined as ≥10% in either the white blood cell, red blood cell, or platelet lineage.
Cytogenetics and molecular studies	Unbalanced translocations include: -7/del(7q), -5/del(5q), del(13q), del(11q), del(12p) or t(12p), del(9q), idic(X)(q13), and t(17p) or i(17q). Balanced translocations include: t(11;16)(q23;p13.3), t(3;21)(q26.2;q22.1), t(1;3)(p36.3;q21), t(2;11) (q21;q23), inv(3)(q21;q26.2) and t(6;9)(p23;q34).
Prognosis	Prognostic indices in MDS: • WHO model • International Prognostic Scoring System (IPSS) • MD Anderson Cancer Center (MDACC) MDS model
	These all take into consideration blast percentage, cytogenetics, and cytopenias, while some consider transfusion requirements, age, and performance status. In most of these indices, the blast count and karyotype are weighted due to ↑influence on survival.

After MDS is diagnosed, classification of the disease into one of six categories establishes prognosis: refractory cytopenia with unilineage dysplasia, refractory anemia with ring sideroblasts, refractory cytopenia with multilineage dysplasia; refractory anemia with excess blasts; MDS with isolated del(5q), and MDS unclassified. Patients considered low risk may have a median survival over 13 years; patients with high-risk disease have a median survival of less than a year.

Treatment

There is no evidence that an asymptomatic patient benefits from treatment. These patients require close monitoring with serial CBCs and should maintain current vaccination. Commonly cited indications for treatment include symptomatic cytopenias or recurrent infections. Patients should be evaluated for HLA-DR15 to identify MDS susceptibility to immunosuppressive agents.

The patient's age and overall fitness guides treatment options:

- Unfit due to age and comorbidity: supportive care by transfusions or erythropoietin-stimulating agents in the setting of symptomatic anemia, monitoring iron status and the need iron chelation therapy for iron overload.
- Fit patients: evaluation for low- or high-intensity chemotherapy.

Low-intensity chemotherapy with either of the DNA hypomethylating agents like azacitidine and decitabine has been shown to decrease transfusion requirements and reduce the onset of transformation to AML. Combination chemotherapy is used to treat young and fit patients with poor prognostic scores with the ultimate goal of proceeding to HSCT. Patients who have deletion of the long arm of chromosome 5 (del5q-) receive treatment with lenalidomide, which leads to decreased transfusion requirements and complete cytogenetic responses.

◼ MYELOPROLIFERATIVE NEOPLASMS

Introduction

The myeloproliferative neoplasms (MPNs) are a group of neoplasms that involve both monoclonal and polyclonal proliferation. Although different pathognomonic genetic features are seen in these diseases (ie, BCR-ABL translocation, JAK-2 mutation, see below), all of the MPNs result in a proliferation of mature myeloid cells in both the marrow and peripheral blood. The 2008 WHO classification system separates these disease entities into classic and atypical. The most common of the classic MPNs include Chronic Myeloid Leukemia (CML), Polycythemia Vera (PV), Essential Thrombocythemia (ET), and Primary Myelofibrosis (PMF); less common variants include Chronic Neutrophilic Leukemia (CNL), Chronic Eosinophilic Leukemia (CEL), mast cell diseases, and Chronic Basophilic Leukemia. Atypical variants include Chronic Myelomonocytic Leukemia, Juvenile Myelomonocytic Leukemia, and Myelodysplastic/myeloproliferative (MDS/MPN) disorders not otherwise classified.

Although this is diverse group of disease, patients tend to present with elevated blood counts, with often more than one cell line affected and have splenomegaly. All of the classic myeloproliferative diseases can have a clonal evolutions and transformation to Acute Myeloid Leukemia; these patients tend to have lower response rates when treated with conventional AML regimens. Whereas CML is restricted to mutations in BCR-ABL, the mutations in the other myeloproliferative neoplasms are more promiscuous, with prominence of the JAK2, MPL, and Calreticulin (CALR) gene mutations.

◼ CHRONIC MYELOID LEUKEMIA (CML)

Virtually all of patients affected with CML have an abnormality in Chromosomes 9 and 22. The translocation creates a chromosome product dubbed the Philadelphia chromosome, labeled as t(9;22)(q34;q11). This chromosomal abnormality creates a fusion gene product and protein known as BCR-ABL1, which is a constitutively active tyrosine kinase. The fusion protein can be seen in three different sizes; p190 which occurs in two-thirds of patients with Philadelphia-positive ALL a small proportion of CML, p210 which occurs in most patients with CML, and p230 which is notable in chronic neutrophilic leukemia. The active tyrosine kinase from the BCR-ABL fusion protein leads to phosphorylation of multiple cellular pathways including but not limited to JAK/STAT, MAP kinase, and Ras. Diagnosis is made by a bone marrow biopsy evaluation and using both FISH and PCR to evaluate for the 9;22 chromosomal translocation and molecular presence of the BCR-ABL fusion protein.

There are three phases associated with CML: chronic phase, accelerated phase, and blast crisis. Chronic phase, the indolent initial phase, occurs in about 85% of patients with the disease (Figure 174-2). Accelerated phase, a more aggressive form, is associated with one or more of the following abnormalities (by WHO criteria):

- 10% to 19% blasts in the peripheral blood or bone marrow
- Platelets greater than 1000/mm^2 unresponsive to therapy
- Platelets <100/mm^2 unrelated to therapy
- Peripheral basophil count greater than 20%
- Cytogenetic evolution to a more aggressive karyotype
- Progressive splenomegaly or leukocytosis unresponsive to chemotherapy

Blast crisis, the most aggressive phase, is defined by greater than 20% blasts in the peripheral blood or bone marrow, or by extramedullary involvement. Blast crisis is most commonly myeloid in nature (80%), but may also be lymphoid in nature (20%). The evolution from chronic phase to either accelerated phase or blast crisis is a complex process that involves increased expression of BCR-ABL, cell differentiation arrest through acquisition of other mutations, or a loss of tumor suppressor genes.

Table 174-6 summarizes findings that may distinguish CML from other hematologic malignancies.

TABLE 174-6 Chronic Myeloid Leukemia

Epidemiology	Incidence of CML: 1-2 per 100,000, median age at diagnosis ~50 y of age.
Clinical presentation	Suspected by routine blood work (20%-50%); fatigue, weight loss, sweating, bleeding; abdominal pain, discomfort, or early satiety due to an enlarged spleen (48%-76%), hepatomegaly.
Laboratory	Median WBC ~100/mm^3 Left shift among myeloid line: neutrophils, bands, myelocytes, metamyelocytes, promyelocytes, rare blasts (usually <2%) (**Figure 174-2**). Absolute basophilia (100%) Anemia (40%-60%) Normal or ↑platelet count >600/mm^3 (15%-30%)
Bone marrow biopsy	Although commercial tests available to evaluate the BCR-ABL gene product by polymerase chain reaction (PCR), the standard of care is still to perform a bone marrow biopsy and aspirate to evaluate the phase of disease and perform cytogenetics to search for other chromosomal abnormalities.
Cytogenetics and molecular studies	FISH and PCR to evaluate for the 9;22 chromosomal translocation and molecular presence of the BCR-ABL fusion protein: a chromosome product dubbed the Philadelphia chromosome labeled as t(9;22)(q34;q11).
Prognosis	Chronic indolent phase (85% of patients) Accelerated phase Blast crisis

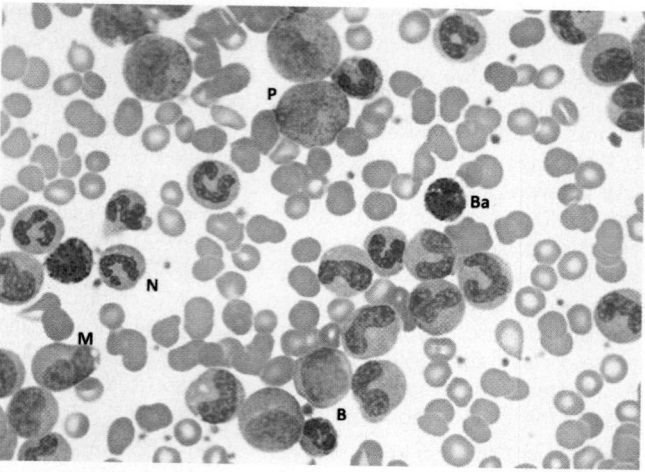

Figure 174-2 *Chronic myelogenous leukemia, 1000× magnification. Peripheral smear from a patient who presented with a white blood cell count of 400/mm³. This slide demonstrates expansion of the myeloid lineage, including blasts (B), promyelocytes (P), metamyelocytes (M), neutrophils (N) and Basophils (Ba).* (Courtesy of Mark Legolvan, DO, Department of Pathology, Rhode Island Hospital.)

Treatment

Tyrosine kinase inhibitors are the standard of care for chronic phase CML. Some of the second-generation TKIs, such as dasatinib and nilotinib, lead to faster and deeper responses, although a benefit in long-term survival has not been proven. Patients with accelerated or blast phase CML tend not to have profound responses with TKIs, and they tend to ephemeral. Patients with myeloid blast crisis are often treated with chemotherapy similar to AML regimens in combination with TKIs, whereas patients with lymphoid blast crisis are often treated with ALL induction protocols combined with a TKI. These patients should all undergo evaluation for HSCT.

Response to treatment is measured by hematologic response, cytogenetic response, and molecular response. Hematologic response pertains to a normal CBC level with a WBC<10/mm³ and no immature cells, and platelet count <450/mm³. Cytogenetic response, evaluated

by FISH studies for the BCR-ABL chromosomal translocation, is defined as complete (no Philadelphia chromosome cells), major (1%-35% Ph chromosome cells), minor (36%-65%), and minimal (66%-95%). A molecular remission is defined as a negative quantitative PCR for the BCR-ABL transcript. There are distinct criteria for evaluating response and time to reach response as published by the European LeukemiaNet (**Table 174-7**).

■ POLYCYTHEMIA VERA (PV)

Polycythemia vera is a clonal disease that arises from a single hematopoietic progenitor cell which leads to mature red blood cell proliferation. The causal gene involved with this process, the JAK2 mutation, is most commonly a single-nucleotide mutation changing a Valine (V) at site 617 to a Phenylalanine (F). This allows for a constitutively activated tyrosine phosphorylation which leads to STAT activation. The JAK2 mutation occurs in approximately 95% of patients with the disease; the remaining subset of the PV population has separate JAK2 mutations in exon 12.

The World Health Organization (WHO) diagnostic criteria include:

- Major criteria: hemoglobin >16.5 g/dL in men and >16.0 g/dL in women and the presence of a functional JAK2 mutation.
- Minor criteria: bone marrow biopsy showing hypercellularity for age with erythroid, granulocytic, or megakaryocytic proliferation; serum erythropoietin level below normal or endogenous erythroid colony formation in vitro.

The diagnosis of PV requires either two major criteria and one minor criteria or one major criteria and two minor criteria. The evaluation for PV must exclude other causes of secondary polycythemia, including chronic hypoxia from either chronic pulmonary disease or sleep apnea, left to right cardiac shunts, erythropoietin secreting neoplasms (such as renal cell carcinoma), familial genetic causes such as Chuvash Polycythemia, and elevated carboxyhemoglobin. Other secondary causes of polycythemia include patients living at high altitude, carbon monoxide poisoning, exogenous use of erythropoietin, and androgen or anabolic steroid use. **Table 174-8** summarizes findings that may distinguish PV from other hematologic malignancies.

With treatment, the median survival of patients with PV is over 13 years. Treatment targets complications from elevated blood volume

TABLE 174-7 Definition of CML Response to Tyrosine Kinase Inhibitors in First-Line Treatment

	Optimal	Warning	Failure
Baseline	N/A	High Risk or	N/A CCA/Ph+, major Route
3 mo	BCR-ABL1 <10% and/or Ph+ ≤35%	BCR-ABL >10% and/or Ph+ 36%-95%	Non-CHR and/or Ph+ >95%
6 mo	BCR-ABL1 <1% and/or Ph+ 0	BCR-ABL 1%-10% and/or Ph+ 1%-35%	BCR-ABL >10% and/or Ph+ > 35%
12 mo	BCR-ABL1 < 0.1% and/or	BCR-ABL 0.1%-1% and/or	BCR-ABL >1% and/or Ph+ > 0%
Any time after 1 y	BCR-ABL1 <0.1%	CCA/Ph- (-7 or 7q-)	Loss of CHR Loss of CCyR Confirmed loss of MMR New mutations CCA/PH+

CCA/PH+, clonal chromosomal abnormalities in Ph+ cells; CCA/Ph-, clonal chromosome abnormalities in Ph- cells; MMR, BCR-ABL1 ≤ 0.1%; NA, not applicable.

TABLE 174-8 Polycythemia Vera

Epidemiology	The median age of diagnosis: ~ 60 y.
	Incidence: ~1.9/100,000 per year, in males aged 70-79, 24/100,000 persons.
Clinical presentation	Symptoms: facial plethora, ruddiness; pruritus, stinging, or a burning sensation of the skin (especially following a warm shower); visual changes due to engorgement of veins of the optic fundus, arterial or venous thrombosis; gouty arthritis.
	Exam: palpable splenomegaly (> 33% of patients); serial exams used to monitor disease progression
Laboratory tests	↑↑hemoglobin and hematocrit; ↑leukocyte count and platelet count in some patients; low serum erythropoietin
Bone marrow biopsy	Hypercellularity for age with erythroid, granulocytic, or megakaryocytic proliferation
Cytogenetics and molecular studies	Functional JAK2 mutation
Prognosis	High risk defined as age > 60 or a history of thrombosis

TABLE 174-9 Essential Thrombocytosis

Epidemiology	Incidence of ET: ~2.5 new cases/100,000 population per year
Clinical presentation	Asymptomatic: elevated platelet counts found on routine blood work (50%)
	Symptoms: headache, lightheadedness, and syncope; erythromelalgia (burning in hands or feet); thrombosis due to ↑platelet count, or bleeding, due to an acquired von Willebrand disease; miscarriage, often a trigger to evaluate for the disease in women
	Exam: splenomegaly (25%-48%).
Laboratory tests	Platelet count of > 450/mm³
Bone marrow biopsy	No evidence of MDS or myelofibrosis
Cytogenetics and molecular studies	No evidence BCR-ABL by molecular or cytogenetic studies
Prognosis	International prognostic scoring system based on Age >60, WBC >11/mm³, and history of thrombosis

associated with PV, such as thromboses and cardiac sequelae. Other complications include postpolycythemic myelofibrosis and transformation to AML. The goal of treatment with phlebotomy is a hematocrit less than 45% in men and 42% in women. This requires serial monitoring of blood counts to avoid symptomatic anemia Patients become functionally iron deficient, and should not receive iron supplementation. Medications include:

- Aspirin to lower the risk of cardiac death and major or minor venous thrombosis
- Hydroxyurea for high-risk patients (defined as age > 60 years or a history of thrombosis)
- Antihistamines or serotonin reuptake blockers for pruritus
- Allopurinol for gout

■ ESSENTIAL THROMBOCYTHEMIA (ET)

ET causes a monoclonal or polyclonal elevation in the platelet count. The JAK2 gene mutation is seen in 50% to 64% of patients, and is associated with a higher incidence of thrombosis. An additional 15% to 25% of patients have been found to have calreticulin (CALR) gene mutations, and up to 4% of patients have mutations in MPL. The life expectancy of patients with ET is similar to the general population, although between 0.6% and 5% of cases transform to AML. The most commonly used diagnostic criteria for ET is the WHO criteria and includes: (1) a platelet count of >450/mm³, (2) no evidence BCR-ABL by molecular or cytogenetic studies, (3) no evidence of MDS or myelofibrosis, and (4) exclusion of all causes of reactive thrombocytosis, including iron deficiency anemia. Since between 10% and 35% of patients have no currently known mutation, ET remains a diagnosis of exclusion, with diagnostic attention to the following:

- Specific marrow-derived causes, such as myelodysplastic syndrome with 5q-, CML, or PV
- Reactive thrombocytosis
- Iron deficiency
- Asplenia
- Trauma (with or without acute blood loss)
- Infectious or inflammatory syndromes
- Other malignancies, particularly lymphoma or metastatic cancers

Rebound from myelosuppressive treatment or other drug suppression or alcohol

Table 174-9 summarizes findings that may distinguish ET from other hematologic malignancies.

Treatment

An international prognostic scoring system for ET is based on age > 60 years, WBC > 11/mm³, and history of thrombosis. Low-dose aspirin has demonstrated a decreased risk of thrombosis. In high-risk patients (ie, age > 60 years or history of prior thrombosis) hydroxyurea is generally the first treatment option. Anagrelide is a viable option in patients who cannot tolerate hydroxyurea. The goal of treatment with myelosuppressive agents is to maintain a platelet count between 100 and 400/mm³.

■ PRIMARY MYELOFIBROSIS

Primary myelofibrosis is a clonal proliferation of myeloid cells that create an inhospitable environment for normal hematopoiesis, thereby causing extramedullary hematopoiesis. **Table 174-10** summarizes findings that may distinguish primary myelofibrosis from other hematologic malignancies.

Myelofibrosis in the bone marrow is believed to be a stem cell disorder that has two components:

1. Myeloid proliferation that causes a megakaryocytic hyperplasia.
2. Release cytokines such as TGF-beta, platelet-derived growth factor (PDGF), epidermal growth factor (EGF), and fibroblast growth factor (FGF) by megakaryocytes, causing a polyclonal proliferation of fibroblasts in the marrow.

Like the other MPDs, PMF is diagnosed by the WHO criteria:

- The major criteria: presence of megakaryotype proliferation with reticulin and/or collagen fibrosis, no evidence of PV, CML, MDS, or other myeloid neoplasm, and a clonal mutation such as JAK2 or MPL, or in the absence of a mutation no evidence of an underlying inflammatory or neoplastic process.
- Minor criteria: leukoerythroblastosis, elevated lactate dehydrogenase (LDH), anemia, and palpable splenomegaly.

To make the diagnosis, all three major criteria and two minor criteria must be met.

TABLE 174-10 Primary Myelofibrosis

Epidemiology	Incidence: ~1.5/100,000 per year, median age of 67 y of age; ~3.9% transformation to AML
Clinical presentation	Fatigue caused by significant anemia (50% of patients); massive splenomegaly often the major site of extramedullary hematopoiesis; hepatomegaly (40%-70% of patients); dyspnea due to pleural or pulmonary involvement: abdominal pain due to gastrointestinal disease
Laboratory tests	Low hemoglobin (50% < 10 g/dL at presentation); variable platelet count, decreasing as the disease progresses; leukopenia or leukocytosis; often a leukoerythroblastic picture with an occasional myeloblast due to the extramedullary hematopoiesis
Bone marrow biopsy	Extensive fibrosis on core biopsy; difficult aspiration usually revealing a "dry tap"
Cytogenetics and molecular studies	JAK2 mutation in 50% of patients; MPL mutations in 5% of patients; CALR mutations in some patients
Prognosis	The Dynamic International Prognostic Scoring System (DIPSS) Plus: • 1 point for age >54, leukocyte count > 25/mm³, circulating blasts > 1%, and constitutional symptoms • 2 points added for a hemoglobin <10 g/dL This creates an initial grouping of risk to which further points are added for unfavorable karyotype, platelet count < 100/mm³, and need for transfusions. Median survival of 15.4 y in low-risk category; median survival of 1.7 y in highest risk category

Treatment

Treatment is aimed at symptom control if the patient is not a candidate for allogeneic hematopoietic stem cell transplant, the only curative treatment option. Ruxolitinib, the oral JAK2 inhibitor, has been shown to decrease spleen size in both JAK2-positive and -negative patients. Hydroxyurea may control splenomegaly, bone pain, and constitutional symptoms. Radiation and splenectomy may reduce pain from extramedullary sites. Androgens and danazol may be used to control anemia, and thalidomide and lenalidomide to manage constitutional symptoms.

■ CHRONIC LYMPHOCYTIC LEUKEMIA/SMALL LYMPHOCYTIC LYMPHOMA (CLL)

CLL is a chronic lymphoid neoplasm that is due to a monoclonal B-cell production of mature lymphocytes. The majority of cases occur sporadically. There does not appear to be a single genetic causal mutation responsible for the development of CLL. The diagnosis of CLL is either made by lymph node biopsy or flow cytometry of the peripheral blood. A bone marrow biopsy is not necessary to diagnose CLL. In order for the diagnosis of CLL to be made from the peripheral blood, there has to be at least 5000/mm³ clonal lymphocytes. If this threshold is not reached, then the diagnosis of monoclonal B-cell lymphocytosis is raised—this is thought to be a precursor to CLL with a rate of transformation at approximately 1% per year. Prolymphocytes (larger lymphocytes usually with a single eccentrically located nuclei) are seen in up to 55% of CLL cells. If more prominent, then the diagnosis becomes a different, more aggressive entity called prolymphocytic leukemia (PLL).

A direct antiglobulin (Coombs) test (DAT) is performed to evaluate anemia. A bone marrow may be required to make the diagnosis of CLL in patients with thrombocytopenia and is often warranted to evaluate marrow reserve. Current American Society of Hematology guidelines discourage staging CT scans at the time of diagnosis.

Hypogammaglobulinemia commonly occurs either at the time of diagnosis of CLL or as the disease progresses, making patients vulnerable to chronic bacterial infections or viral infections. Although chronic infections may lead to initiation of treatment, patients may also receive periodic intravenous immunoglobulin (IVIG) either at the time of a severe infection or prophylactically. Immune dysregulation leads to an increased incidence of skin malignancies, especially squamous cell skin cancer and melanoma, and lung, laryngeal, and colon cancers. **Table 174-11** summarizes findings that may distinguish CLL from other hematologic malignancies.

Treatment

Poor prognostic markers lead to close monitoring and aggressive initial treatments. None of the prognostic markers are an indication to initiate treatment. Multiple studies and meta-analyses have demonstrated that there is no survival advantage for immediate treatment of asymptomatic patients. Asymptomatic autoimmune cytopenia is not an indication for initiating chemotherapy, and patients are often treated with prednisone at 1 mg/kg/d with a taper over 2 to 3 months. Reasons for treatment include:

- Lymphocyte doubling time of less than 6 months
- Rapidly enlarging lymph nodes or organomegaly
- Symptomatic anemia and/or thrombocytopenia
- Repeat infections due to hypogammaglobulinemia
- Constitutional symptoms such as fevers, night sweats, weight loss, fatigue, and weakness

Chemotherapy choice for CLL is dependent on the performance status and to some extent the age of the patient afflicted. Young and healthy patients receive a chemoimmunotherapy regimen containing a purine analogue and a monoclonal antibody—most commonly fludarabine, cyclophosphamide, and rituximab (FCR). This regimen cause severe myelosuppression; therefore, patients should receive prophylaxis for *Pneumocystis jirovecii* and varicella zoster. Older but still considered fit patients use a less toxic yet slightly less effective chemoimmunotherapy (bendamustine and rituximab [BR]) than the purine analogues. Elderly or patients with poor performance may receive chlorambucil based regimens, either as a single agent or in combination with the novel anti-CD20 monoclonal antibody obinutuzumab.

New drugs, such as the novel Bruton's tyrosine kinase (BTK) inhibitor ibrutinib, the phosphoinositide 3-kinase (PI3K) inhibitor Idelalisib, and the selective BCL-2 inhibitor ABT-199 hold significant promise for the treatment of CLL with potential increased remissions and less toxicity.

■ HODGKIN'S LYMPHOMA

Hodgkin's lymphoma (HL) refers to a group of hematologic malignancies that account for 10% of lymphomas. Their etiologic agent is a binucleated clonal B-cell, referred to as the Reed--Sternberg cell (**Figure 174-3**). One of the hallmarks of Hodgkin lymphoma is the contiguous spread of the disease rather than a distant or random appearing distribution. Of the 4-5 subtypes of this disease, most cases are of the nodular sclerosis (70%) or mixed cellularity

TABLE 174-11 Chronic Lymphocytic Leukemia

Epidemiology	Incidence: 6.75/100,000 (men), 3.65/100,000 (women), median age at diagnosis: 70 y of age.
Clinical presentation	Asymptomatic, frequently diagnosed by routine CBC demonstrating a lymphocytosis.
	Lymphadenopathy, spread pattern not contiguous unlike Hodgkin's lymphoma, may wax and wane, often hyperreactive to infections, generally painless, nontender; splenomegaly (25%-55% of patients)
Laboratory studies	Lymphocytosis: ↑ in the absolute lymphocyte count (the product of the total WBC times the differential percent of lymphocytes) > 5000/mm³
	Peripheral smear: morphologically normal appearing mature lymphocytes with occasional "smudge cells".
	Anemia and thrombocytopenia due to marrow infiltration from the lymphocyte proliferation or due to an autoimmune process: autoimmune hemolytic anemia (11%) or idiopathic thrombocytopenia purpura (2%-3%).
	Hypogammaglobulinemia
Flow cytometry of peripheral blood	Classic immunophenotype of CLL cells: positive co-expression of CD5, CD19, CD23; dim ↑ expression of CD20; cells either κ or λ restricted.
Bone marrow biopsy	Not required to make the diagnosis of CLL
Prognosis	Staging (Rai system) directly related to overall survival:
	• Stage 0—lymphocytosis (median survival 150 mo)
	• Stage I—lymphadenopathy
	• Stage II—organomegaly
	• Stage III—anemia
	• Stage IV—thrombocytopenia
	Favorable: mutated immunoglobulin heavy chain variable (IGHV) genes
	Cytogenetics
	• Favorable: deletions in the long arm of chromosome 13 (13q), trisomy 12
	• Unfavorable: deletion of chromosome 11q, deletions in chromosome 17 (del17p)
	Surface marker from flow cytometry
	• Unfavorable: zeta chain associated protein 70 (ZAP-70), a tyrosine kinase; CD38

(20%-25%) variations. Somewhat distinct from other HL subtypes, nodular lymphocyte-predominant HL presents more commonly with axillary lymphadenopathy which may be accompanied or followed by a second, non-Hodgkin's lymphoma. **Table 174-12** summarizes findings that may distinguish HL from other hematologic malignancies.

Treatment

Determining limited versus extensive disease burden will have significant impact on treatment decisions. Asymptomatic stage I

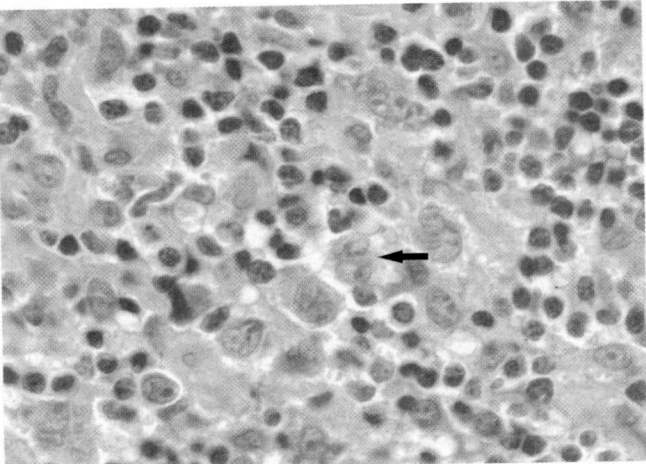

Figure 174-3 *Lymph node biopsy of Hodgkin lymphoma. The biopsy has an abundance of Reed-Sternberg cells (arrow).* (Courtesy of Mark Legolvan, DO, Department of Pathology, Rhode Island Hospital.)

disease or any stage II disease that is restricted to one side of the diaphragm and without any bulky sites fall under the "limited" category. Patients with limited disease and a favorable risk profile receive localized radiation plus two cycles of anthracycline-based chemotherapy, currently doxorubicin, bleomycin, vinblastine, and dacarbazine. This regimen is extended to four cycles with concurrent radiation for patients with a less favorable risk profile and limited disease. Extensive disease (bulky stage II or any stage III-IV) requires further extension of chemotherapy to six cycles. The role of radiation is limited to any bulky disease burden, as the necessary exposure to irradiate a diffusely spread HL disease carries significant increases in the risk of long-term complications. Lymphocyte predominant HL is approached slightly differently as this entity responds more avidly to rituximab-based chemotherapeutic regimens due to its expression of CD20 on the cell surface. This is reflective of its pathophysiologic overlap with the B-cell non-Hodgkin's lymphomas.

For relapsed HL, salvage chemotherapy using second-line regimens such as ICE (Ifosfamide, carboplatin, and etoposide) or DHAP (Dexamethasone, cytarabine, cisplatin) are often used as a bridge to autologous bone marrow transplantation. Other promising agents include the anti-CD30 agent brentuximab (resulting in upward of a 70% response rate in relapsed disease) and the PD-1 inhibitor nivolumab.

Post-treatment monitoring

As many cases of HL occur in younger patient populations, treatment-related toxicities and long-term complications become a much larger concern. Chest irradiation has been linked with increased incidences of heart disease (including ischemic and valvular etiologies), thyroid disease, and secondary malignancies such as breast cancer. This population requires yearly TSH monitoring,

TABLE 174-12 Hodgkin Lymphoma

Epidemiology	Bimodal distribution, with peak incidences in younger adults around age 20 and older adults around age 65, men slightly more than women
	Environmental risk factors, including Epstein-Barr virus infection; ↑ incidence with immunosuppression and HIV (not AIDS defining)
Clinical presentation	Lymphadenopathy, most commonly above the diaphragm and usually in the cervical or supraclavicular chains; axillary not uncommon; often non-tender, may present due to swelling from impaired lymphatic drainage rather than a discrete mass. Disease spreads contiguously.
	Classic B-symptoms in 30% of cases, typically low-grade and irregular fever.
	Various paraneoplastic phenomena may occur; direct CNS involvement of the lymphoma is rare.
Imaging	Intrathoracic disease (2/3 of patients): • Mediastinal involvement • Malignant pleural effusions • Compression of superior vena cava
Excisional biopsies of predominant lesion	Reed-Sternberg cell
Additional testing	PET-CT imaging to document the extent of disease (all patients) Echocardiography and PFTs before chemotherapy Bone marrow evaluation in selected patients with stage I-II disease. ESR: serial measurements a prognostic indicator, especially in patients with limited disease
Prognosis	The Hodgkin Prognosis Score (HPS) incorporates age, gender, disease stage, total WBC, total lymphocyte count, serum hemoglobin, and serum albumin. • Older patients, males, those with leukocytosis >15,000 or lymphopenia < 600, and patients with extensive disease burden tend to do more poorly. • These prognostic factors still apply in relapsed or treatment-refractory disease and can be useful when considering a patient for autologous HSCT. Favorable: ESR < 50, mediastinal mass ratio < 0.33 or less than 10 cm, and ≤ 3 nodal sites. Unfavorable: any extranodal burden or elevation in the mediastinal-mass ratio for thoracic disease on imaging

yearly breast exams starting 8 to 10 years after their course of radiation, and increased suspicion for cardiac and pulmonary diseases on routine screening.

■ NON-HODGKIN'S LYMPHOMA

Non-Hodgkin's lymphoma is a broad category of lymphomas that have a heterogeneous pathogenesis and presentation. Some non-Hodgkin's lymphomas are indolent, or slow growing, and may be monitored with a "watch and wait" philosophy, while others may be highly aggressive and require intensive regimens of intravenous and intrathecal chemotherapy. For this reason, it is imperative to obtain large samples of tissue at diagnosis, before any lymphoma changing medication, such as steroids, are given. Ideally, diagnostic biopsies are excisional, with incisional biopsies performed if that is not possible. In certain circumstances, such as abdominal lymph nodes, only a core biopsy is possible, and in this situation multiple cores should be obtained. *Fine needle aspirates should not be performed if lymphoma is suspected, as they do not allow any evaluation of nodal architecture.*

Staging for non-Hodgkin's lymphoma permeates all subsets. It is critical to fully stage the patient, either by CT of the neck, chest, abdomen and pelvis, or by a CT/PET scan. A bone marrow biopsy may be warranted to prove low stage disease, although its utility in stage III or IV disease is questionable. High-grade disease requires lumbar puncture to evaluate for CNS disease.

Staging is based on the Ann Arbor staging system. Stage I disease is defined by disease confined to one lymph node or one extranodal site (I_E). Stage II disease involves two or more lymph node groups on the same side of the diaphragm or a single group of lymph nodes that extend to an organ (II_E). Stage III disease involves lymph nodes on both sides of the diaphragm, including splenic involvement (III_S) or extension into an organ (III_E). Stage IV is defined as extension into a nonadjacent organ, bone marrow involvement, or CNS involvement.

■ INDOLENT NON-HODGKIN'S LYMPHOMAS

Indolent lymphomas are usually an insidious group of lymphomas that present with slowly enlarging lymphadenopathy, splenomegaly, or cytopenias. **Table 174-13** summarizes findings of two of the most common indolent lymphomas, marginal zone lymphoma and follicular lymphoma.

Marginal Zone Lymphoma or Mucosal-Associated Lymphoid Tissue (MALT) Lymphomas are thought to be antigen driven, and in many circumstances, a bacterial driver has been identified. Therefore, treating the underlying infectious driver may often cause remission in the cases of gastric (*H. pylori*), bladder (*E. coli*), skin (*B. burgdorferi*), and ocular (*C. psittaci*), although in cases other than gastric MALT the data is mostly anecdotal. Gastric MALT Lymphomas classified as stage I_E are initially treated with *H. pylori* regimens. If the lymphoma then persists, gastric radiation or single-agent rituximab is the standard of care.

Follicular lymphoma, the second most common type of non-Hodgkin's lymphoma, has a pathologic nodular growth pattern and a mixture of centrocytes and centroblasts. Grading, which usually correlates with clinical aggressiveness, ranges from grade I through IIIA.

Patients who are asymptomatic often fall into the category of "watch and wait." In this group, treatment is initiated when the patient becomes symptomatic from enlarged lymph nodes or when there is a potential for lymph node obstruction, that is, growth near the ureter or another vital structure. Treatment may either employ

TABLE 174-13 Marginal Zone Lymphoma and Follicular Lymphoma

Marginal zone lymphoma or mucosal associated lymphoid tissue (MALT) lymphoma	Nodal or extranodal disease
	Most common extranodal sites: gastric, skin, lung, ocular, adnexa, thyroid, head and neck, intestinal, salivary gland, bladder and breast
	Biopsy: usually small to medium sized cells, with abundant and pale cytoplasm.
	Immunohistochemical features: CD79a+, CD20+ CD5-, CD10- CD23-; generally express IgM, may be CD43-.
Follicular lymphoma	Cells demonstrate the pan-B cell antigens CD19, CD20, CD22, and CD79a; stain positive for BCL2+, BCL6+, CD10+, negative for CD5 and CD43.
	Chromosome 18 abnormalities (the site of the BCL2 oncogene) are often associated with FL, with over 85% of these involving the Ig Heavy Chain on chromosome 14 seen in the t(14:18) translocation.
	Follicular Lymphoma International Prognostic Index (FLIPI) 1 and 2:
	• FLIPI-1 5 adverse prognostic factors:
	■ Age > 60 y
	■ Stage III or IV
	■ Hemoglobin < 12 g/dL
	■ Number of involved nodal areas > 4
	■ ↑ serum lactate dehydrogenase
	• FLIPI-2
	■ Same age and hemoglobin criteria
	■ Bone marrow involvement
	■ Diameter of largest node > 6cm
	■ β-2 microglobulin > upper limit of normal

single agent rituximab, the monoclonal anti-CD20 antibody, or a chemoimmunotherapy combination of bendamustine and rituximab for a total of six cycles. This regimen has proven to be more effective and less toxic than the well-established R-CHOP. Patients with high risk FLIPI-1 or FLIPI-2 scores receive maintenance rituximab, dosed every 3 months for 2 years, following initial treatment. Patients with relapsed or refractory disease may receive other chemotherapy regimens such as R-CHOP, fludarabine-based regimens, or undergo autologous or allogeneic bone marrow transplantation. Grade IIIB, which is greater than 15 centroblasts seen in sheets, is treated similarly to a diffuse large B-cell lymphoma.

■ MANTLE CELL LYMPHOMA

Classified somewhere between the indolent and aggressive lymphomas, mantle cell lymphoma (MCL) is often unrecognized until the advanced stages and thus tends to behave aggressively by the time of clinical presentation. Cytogenetically it is characterized by the t(11:14) mutation, leading to overexpression of cyclin D1. However, this mutation alone does not appear sufficient to cause MCL and a number of other possible concurrent mutations have been identified which function as a "second hit" to produce MCL. One study related 25 genes, including Notch1, ATM, p53, and MLL2, that may play a role in the oncogenic potential of mantle cell lymphoma. The diagnosis of MCL is based on morphology, cytogenetics and immunohistochemistry. **Table 174-14** summarizes findings that may distinguish MCL from other hematologic malignancies.

Treatment

Survival after MCL diagnosis depends on the stage at diagnosis and overall functional status throughout treatment, if offered. Clinically it may be difficult to identify which patients will have more indolent disease and which will go on to have a more aggressively-behaving MCL. Patients with more indolent disease may be followed like a low-grade B-cell lymphoma. Advanced disease (bulky stage II or any stage III-IV) is customarily treated with chemotherapy. Many different regimens exist, and depending on the regimen used and the clinical

TABLE 174-14 Mantle Cell Lymphoma

Epidemiology	Incidence: older age, with median age 68, and approximately 2:1 male predominance.
Clinical presentation	B symptoms; abdominal pain and diarrhea, small bowel obstruction and bowel perforation (25% of patients); bone marrow involvement, at times a leukemic phase (50% of patients)
	Exam: spleen or liver enlargement (40% of patients)
Excisional biopsy of an affected lymph node	Variable histology: small cell, marginal zone-like, blastic, and pleomorphic with proliferation noted in the mantle zone of the lymph node or diffusely.
Additional testing	Localized disease uncommon and additional testing required to look for disease burden
	• Upper and lower endoscopy
	• CT scan of the chest, abdomen and pelvis or CT/PET scan
	Bone marrow biopsies reserved for cases where identified cytopenias are thought to be lymphoma-related or for patients with a markedly elevated white blood cell count.
	Lumbar puncture in patients with blastic sub-type
Cytogenetics and molecular studies	Cytogenetics: translocation between chromosomes 11 and 14 [t(11;14)(q13;q32)]; although this is not pathognomonic for MCL and is also seen in multiple myeloma.
	Flow cytometry and immunochemistry: B-antigens CD19, CD20, CD22, and CD5 but not CD23. Cells display high levels of IgM and IgD and often are λ restricted. Nuclear staining is highly positive for Cyclin D1.
Prognosis	Favorable: low Ki-67
	Unfavorable: ↑serum LDH, any cytopenia especially in the setting of a blastoid histologic variant
	Mantle cell lymphoma international prognostic index (MIPI) incorporates age, ECOG performance status, LDH, and white blood cell count. This and other prognostic models pre-date implementation of newer agents and treatment regimens into a constantly-evolving therapeutic approach with MCL

response, patients may be offered consolidation/maintenance chemotherapy, localized radiation for bulky disease, or autologous transplant. However, no single approach has been clearly established as standard of care, and any newly diagnosed patient should be considered for referral to a clinical trial.

The two most commonly used chemotherapy regimens in advanced MCL are R-CHOP (dosed similarly to DLBCL) and VcR-CAP (bortezomib, rituximab, cyclophosphamide, doxorubicin, prednisone). More aggressive regimens such as R-HyperCVAD and others which incorporate high dose cytarabine are also used, but toxicities and side effects from these regimens may outweigh any added therapeutic benefit. Newer evidence suggests bendamustine plus rituximab followed by rituximab maintenance may be better tolerated with longer progression-free survival, but randomized trial data remains limited.

Patients will typically receive consolidation dosing after their induction chemotherapy course, and depending on whether complete remission is achieved, they may be offered maintenance rituximab with or without autologous HSCT. Upper and lower endoscopy should be repeated prior to offering HSCT to exclude any progressive GI involvement while undergoing therapy.

When remission is not achieved, MCL may respond to fludarabine-based protocols or allogeneic HSCT, but this is best attempted at a center with specialized expertise and preferably in the setting of a clinical trial. More recently, ibrutinib has been used as second-line treatment, especially in elderly patients not eligible for HSCT.

■ DIFFUSE LARGE B-CELL LYMPHOMA

Diffuse large B-cell lymphoma (DLBCL) is the most common non-Hodgkin lymphoma (NHL) subtype, accounting for 25% to 30% of cases. Most arise de novo, although 1% to 3% of patients each with low-grade lymphomas will progress to DLBCL. DLBCL may be highly invasive and have a propensity for CNS involvement. Molecular genetics are increasingly being associated with prognosis and treatment decisions, especially c-myc, BCL-2, and BCL-6; these help distinguish between germinal center and activated B-cell subtypes of DLBCL, which respond differently to certain chemotherapies.

Table 174-15 summarizes findings that may distinguish DLBCL from other hematologic malignancies.

Treatment

DLBCL is an aggressive lymphoma which often responds well to treatment. Regimens are determined by extent of disease (see Table 174-15), presence of bulky or extranodal disease, whether relapsed and treatment refractory, and by the patient's IPI score (see **Table 174-16**) and goals of care.

Limited stage

Standard R-CHOP chemotherapy is typically offered upfront: Rituximab, Cyclophosphamide, Doxorubicin (Hydroxydaunomycin), Vincristine (Oncovin), and Prednisone. One of two approaches is used to treat Stage I or II DLBCL: 3 cycles of chemotherapy with adjuvant radiation, or 6 to 8 cycles of chemotherapy alone. Radiation alone is not usually offered as it is associated with more than a 70% risk of recurrence. Bulky and extranodal disease typically responds better to regimens that include radiation, and there is less local recurrence and less systemic side effects from chemotherapy with this approach. However, some individuals may have relative contraindications to XRT such as breast irradiation in young women.

CNS involvement is typically treated with systemic or intrathecal methotrexate, regardless of stage. Involvement of the spinal cord may represent a medical emergency and is unlikely to be cured by neurosurgical resection. These patients require emergent chemotherapy followed shortly by local irradiation.

Advanced stage

Advanced-stage lymphomas are treated primarily with systemic chemotherapy using R-CHOP dosed every 14 to 21 days for 6 to 8 cycles, with further cycles dependent on response to treatment. Addition of lenalidomide, bortezomib, or ibrutinib may improve disease-free survival for certain patients, including those with activated B-cell lymphoma phenotypes which are noted to be CD10 and BCL-6 negative on flow cytometry. Autologous HSCT is not

TABLE 174-15 Diffuse Large B-Cell Lymphoma

Epidemiology	Incidence ↑ with age, mean age 64 y, higher rates in HIV-positive and immunosuppressed patients
Clinical presentation	Common symptoms: classic B symptoms (fever, malaise, night sweats, weight loss); local effects from a single, rapidly-enlarging mass in the neck or abdomen compressing or otherwise interfering with organ function. Any organ system may be affected and not be limited to lymph nodes.
	Primary CNS disease (small subset)
Surgical excision of suspicious mass	Histopathology: diffuse proliferation of large lymphoid cells that generally efface the lymph node architecture. All samples should be sent for flow cytometry.
Flow cytometry and molecular studies	pan B-cell markers CD19, CD20, CD22 positive; CD10, MUM1, and CD30 expression in some cases.
	CD10 positive or BCL-6 positive cases classified as germinal center type, while other cases are considered non-germinal center type.
Additional testing	Imaging to establish stage and extent of disease in all patients: • "Limited" stage lymphomas: any stage I or II disease that falls within a single radiation field • "Advanced" stage: higher stage or spread beyond a single field (60%-70% of patients at initial presentation) Lumbar puncture (LP) for metastatic disease in any patient with focal neurologic signs, any involvement of specific sites (testes, marrow, paranasal sinuses), or an elevated serum LDH level Bone marrow to evaluate for marrow involvement in any patient with cytopenias (10%-20% of patients) and in any patient with advanced disease.
Prognosis	Revised International Prognostic Index (R-IPI; Table 174-4), factoring in patient's age, functional status, the stage and extent of their disease, and informative serum markers such as LDH.
	Poor response to standard treatments: "double hit" lymphomas with positivity for c-myc either by FISH or immunohistochemistry, along with positivity for either BCL-2 or BCL-6.

TABLE 174-16 Outcome According to International Prognostic Index (IPI) Factors in Patients Treated with RCHOP

Risk Group	No. of IPI factors*	%Patients	4-y PFS (%)	4-y OS (%)
Standard IPI				
Low	0,1	28	85	82
Low-Int	2	27	80	81
High-Int	3	21	57	49
High	4,5	24	51	59
Revised IPI				
Very Good	0	10	94	94
Good	1,2	45	80	79
Poor	3,4,5	45	53	55

*Factors include: Age > 60 y; ECOG performance status >2; Elevated LDH; >1 extranodal site; Stage III/IV.
From Sehn LH, Berry B, Chhanabhai M, et al. The revised International Prognostic Index (R-IPI) is a better predictor of outcome than the standard IPI for patients with diffuse large B-cell lymphoma treated with R-CHOP. *Blood.* 2007;109:1857-1861.

typically offered after achieving initial remission as studies do not show a significant survival benefit. However, some patients with high mortality risk as estimated by their R-IPI score may benefit from transplant once they are in remission without attempting any further chemotherapy or monitoring.

Chemotherapy with heart disease

For patients with preexisting cardiac disease, anthracyclines should not be used if the LVEF is less than 45%. Some regimens substitute gemcitabine or etoposide for the doxorubicin in R-CHOP, but none have been compared directly in major studies. All patients with cardiac disease should be monitored closely, even if chemotherapeutic agents with relatively less cardiotoxicity are used.

Treatment in the elderly

Older patients (age >60) should still receive standard dosing of chemotherapy unless there are limiting conditions like heart failure or side effects. Dose-reduced treatment regimens have been associated with poorer outcomes including mortality, even when accounting for higher chemotherapy-related toxicities. In fact, older adults with high IPI scores may benefit from additional doses of rituximab after all cycles of R-CHOP have been completed.

Treatment in patients with HIV/AIDS

DLBCL is an AIDS-defining illness in HIV-positive patients, as is Burkitt lymphoma, and these malignancies are often very advanced when found. These patients should receive antiretroviral therapy (ART) and appropriate antimicrobial prophylaxis prior to initiating standard chemotherapy. Rituximab should be held if CD4 count is less than 50, and zidovudine should be avoided if possible given its myelosuppressive effects.

"Double hit" diffuse large B-cell lymphoma

Lymphomas with certain specific cytogenetic profiles may respond poorly to the standard R-CHOP regimen. Translocations of the c-MYC gene at 8q24 and BCL-2 gene at 18q21, termed "double hit" DLBCL, occur in approximately six percent of cases. These changes overlap with Burkitt lymphoma and portend a poor prognosis compared to those with standard DLBCL or BL alone. Patients should be treated with a more aggressive regimen than R-CHOP, such as dose adjusted R-EPOCH (rituximab, etoposide, doxorubicin, cyclophosphamide, vincristine, prednisone).

Relapsed/treatment-resistant disease

Most patients with DLBCL will experience recurrence of their lymphoma, most commonly within the first 2 years after initial treatment. "Refractory" or treatment-resistant disease is defined as less than 50% decrease in size of the initially presenting tumor, while "progressive" or relapsing disease more typically presents with new masses. The standard approach is to use two to three cycles of second-line systemic chemotherapy, with adjuvant radiation if the disease is within a single field. Common regimens include R-GDP (rituximab, gemcitabine, dexamethasone, cisplatin), R-ICE (ifosfamide, carboplatin, etoposide), and R-DHAP (dexamethasone, high-dose cytarabine, cisplatin). Refractory lymphomas respond variably to these regimens, and these patients should be offered autologous HSCT if possible after achieving a second remission as further relapses are quite common (30%-60% vs 10%-20% with HSCT). If transplant is not possible or if remission cannot be achieved, third-line chemotherapy may be offered.

■ BURKITT LYMPHOMA

BL is a highly aggressive, rapidly growing malignancy with three distinct presentations being classically described: endemic (eBL), sporadic (sBL), and immunosuppression-related (irBL). A heavier burden of lymphatic, marrow, and CNS disease are seen in irBL, and a subset of patients with sBL and irBL may present with significant enough involvement of the marrow and peripheral blood to be considered a Burkitt leukemia. Symptoms are often related to the anatomic region involved; classic B symptoms are not a classic hallmark of BL but do occur in some cases. Diagnosing BL is identical for all three subtypes. Of note, when identified in HIV-positive patients, irBL is considered AIDS-defining, even though it is not necessarily seen with the same low CD4+ counts or high burden of opportunistic infections as with other malignancies in this population. **Table 174-17** summarizes findings that may distinguish BL from other hematologic malignancies.

Treatment

Prompt initiation of chemotherapy is essential given how rapidly and aggressively BL can proliferate. There is no single regimen which is used for all patients, but several of the regimens used initially in the pediatric setting have been carried over to adult tumors with good results. All regimens include CNS prophylaxis, as BL can readily infiltrate the brain and spinal cord. The timing of each given chemotherapy dose should be contingent on recovery from the previous dose rather than following a specific schedule as done with other B-cell lymphomas; waiting too long between cycles may allow the BL tumor burden to outgrow any therapeutic benefit from the chemotherapy being administered.

Three regimens are commonly used, each with a subset of BL patients for whom that combination tends to benefit most. None of these include concurrent radiation or surgical intervention. All include concurrent tumor lysis syndrome (TLS) prophylaxis with IV hydration, use of oral allopurinol and IV rasburicase if needed, as well as frequent monitoring of electrolytes. Studies investigating the addition of rituximab to these regimens show favorable results, although it is not currently considered standard of care. CODOX-M/IVAC is the most commonly used regimen in children, while dose adjusted R-EPOCH is more commonly used in elderly patients (**Table 174-18**).

In cases of known CNS disease, intrathecal cytarabine is commonly added, given as an alternating dose with intrathecal methotrexate if the latter is already being used. Patients with preexisting or drug-related cardiomyopathy may not be able to receive anthracycline-based regimens. A pretreatment echocardiogram should always be obtained, and any patient with an ejection fraction <30% should be considered for alternative therapies.

TABLE 174-17 Burkitt Lymphoma

Epidemiology	*Endemic BL (eBL):* predominantly in equatorial Africa, mostly in children, accounting for up to 50% of childhood cancer cases regionally; Epstein-Barr virus (EBV) often implicated
	Sporadic BL (sBL): mostly in the US and Europe, where again more commonly in children than adults with a mean age of 30 at diagnosis and peak incidence around age 11.
	Immunosuppression-related BL (irBL): any cause of immunosuppression is a risk factor, but mostly diagnosed in HIV-positive patients. AIDS-defining; incidence has decreased since advent of HAART regimens. EBV often implicated.
Clinical presentation	Fulminant growing mass; may show evidence of spontaneous tumor lysis at the time of diagnosis.
	• For endemic BL, this mass is commonly on the jaw or neck, but spread to various extranodal sites can occur.
	• Sporadic BL is more likely to involve the abdomen early on, though 25% of cases do involve the head and neck, and up to 15% may involve the CNS at diagnosis with higher prevalence in treatment resistant and recurrent disease.
Excisional biopsy of dominant mass lesion	Classic "starry sky" appearance on histology; reflects the high cell turnover rate with cell debris and macrophages interspersed among many basophilic, rapidly dividing tumor cells. Nearly 100% of these cells may be mitotic, showing a Ki-67 stain of 95%-100%.
Cellular and molecular markers	Immunophenotype: expression of B-cell antigens (CD19, CD20, CD22), CD10, BCL6, CD38; either negative or weakly positive for BCL2; negative for TdT.
	Cytogenetics: translocations involving the *c-MYC* oncogene on chromosome 8q24. The most common translocation pairing is with the Ig heavy chain at chromosome 14q32, but it can also pair with the λ gene on 22q11 or the λ gene on 2p12. These are not specific to BL, and is sometimes identified in so-called "double hit" diffuse large B cell lymphomas.
Additional studies	Bone marrow and lumbar puncture in all patients
Prognosis	Unfavorable: "overlap" lymphomas bearing features partially resembling BL and DLBCL

TABLE 174-18 Regimens Used for Burkitt Lymphoma

R-CODOX-M (cycles 1 and 3)	Intrathecal Treatment:
Rituximab 375 mg/m^2 on day 1	If no CNS involvement: Methotrexate 12 mg IT on days 1 and 5 cycles 4, 5, 6
Cyclophosphamide 800 mg/m^2 IV on day 1, 200 mg/m^2 IV days 2-5	If CNS involvement: Methotrexate 12 mg twice weekly × 4 wk, then weekly × 6 wk, then monthly × 4 mo
Doxorubicin 40 mg/m^2 IV on day 1	*If nadir ANC ≥ 500/µL, increase doses by 20% over preceding cycle
Vincristine 1.5 mg/m^2 IV (max 2 mg) IV on day 1, 8 C#1, days 1, 8, 15 C#2	
Methotrexate 3 g/m^2 IV total if <65, 1g/m^2 IV total if >65 on day 10 with leucovorin rescue	If ANC < 500/µL on 1 or 2 measurements, maintain dose
Neulasta 6 mg SC on day 12	If ANC < 500/µL on ≥3 measurements or platelets <25,000/µL, doses reduced by 20%
Intrathecal therapy	
Cytarabine 70 mg IT on days 1 and 3 if age >3	Doses of doxorubicin and etoposide are not reduced below starting dose
Methotrexate 12 mg IT on day 15 if age >3	HyperCVAD
If Positive CNS disease at presentation, cytarabine day 5 and methotrexate day 15	Odd cycles (1, 3, 5, 7)
R-IVAC (cycles 2 and 4)	Cyclophosphamide 300 mg/m^2 IV q 12 h days 1-3 (6 doses)
Rituximab 375 mg/m^2 IV on day 1	Mesna 600 mg/m^2/d IV continuous infusion days 1-3
Ifosfamide 1500 mg/m^2 IV if <65, 1000 mg/m^2 IV if >65 on days 1-5 with mesna	Vincristine 2 mg on days 4 and 11
Etoposide 60 mg/m^2 IV on days 1-5	Doxorubicin 50 mg/m^2 IV on day 4
Cytarabine 2 g/m^2 IV if <65 m 1 g/m^2 IV if >65 every 12 h days 1 and 2 (4 doses)	Dexamethasone 40 mg PO/IV daily days 1-4 and 11-14
Intrathecal methotrexate 12 mg IT if >3 y old on day 5 with oral leucovorin	Rituximab 375 mg/m^2 IV on days 1 and 11 of cycle 1 and 3
If Positive CNS disease at presentation, cytarabine day 7 and 9	Even cycles (2, 4, 6, 8)
Dose Adjusted R-EPOCH*	Methotrexate 200 mg/m^2 IV over 2 h then 800 mg/m^2 IV over 24 h day 1 with leucovorin rescue
Rituximab 375 mg/m^2 IV on day 0 or 1	Cytarabine 3 g/m^2 IV (patients < 60) or Cytarabine 1 g/m^2 (patients >60) ever 12 h for 4 doses on days 2 and 3
Etoposide 50 mg/m^2 IV + Doxorubicin 10 mg/m^2 IV + Vincristine 0.4 mg/m^2 IV infused over 24 h daily days 1-4	Rituximab 375 mg/m^2 IV on days 2 and 8 on cycles 2 and 4
Cyclophosphamide 750 mg/m^2 IV on day 5	Intrathecal treatment:
Prednisone 60 mg/m^2 IV days 1-5	Methotrexate 12 mg IT on day 2 of each cycle
Neulasta 6 mg SC on day 6	Cytarabine 100 mg IT on day 8 of each cycle

T-CELL LYMPHOMAS

T-cell lymphomas, a heterogeneous group of aggressive non-Hodgkin's lymphomas, make up less than 15% of all NHL. Incidence is markedly increased in the HIV population, and disease may have peripheral or cutaneous manifestations. *Peripheral T-cell lymphomas* include anaplastic large cell lymphoma, extranodal NK/T-cell lymphoma, angioimmunoblastic T-cell lymphoma, hepatosplenic T-cell lymphoma, subcutaneous panniculitis-like T-cell lymphoma, enteropathy-associated T-cell lymphoma, and peripheral T-cell lymphoma not otherwise specified. Patients may present with both nodal and extranodal disease.

Diagnosis is made by tissue histology from an enlarged lymph node or from extranodal sites such as skin, lung, or GI tract. The malignant cells demonstrate expression of one or more of the pan-T cell antigens (CD2, CD3, CD5, and CD7); there is often a downregulation of CD5 and CD7.

T-Cell lymphomas are often treated with the same CHOP or dose-adjusted EPOCH chemotherapy regimen as used in B-cell lymphomas, generally without use of rituximab as the T cells are CD20 negative. Other agents include brentuximab, a recently approved anti-CD30 monoclonal antibody, and the histone deacetylase inhibitors (HDACs), such as romidepsin, or pralatrexate. Some aggressive T-cell lymphomas that do not respond to chemotherapy alone, such as anaplastic large cell lymphoma, are consolidated with an autologous bone marrow transplant. The histone deacetylase inhibitors, such as romidepsin, are active in these diseases as well as pralatrexate, a folate inhibitor.

Cutaneous T-cell Lymphoma (CTCL) broadly describes T-cell lymphomas that involve the skin, but also blood, lymph nodes, or viscera. The most common type of CTCL, mycosis fungoides (MF), may appear with generalized erythroderma, scaly patches, plaques or tumors, and is often pruritic. The lesions may wax and wane over a period of years, and is often misdiagnosed as a form of psoriasis. Sezary syndrome, another subset of CTCL, involves a leukemic phase where the malignant T cells in the peripheral blood match the malignant cells in the skin. The incidence of MF is approximately 6 per million annually, with a median age of 55 to 60.

Specific diagnostic criteria for mycosis fungoides include a scoring system for size and shape of lesions, histopathology, clonal T-cell receptor gene rearrangement, and immunohistochemistry demonstrating aberrant T cells (ie, <50% of T-cells expressing CD2, CD3, or CD5). Staging of CTCL does not follow the typical Ann Arbor system; instead it uses a combined metric of skin evaluation, lymph node and visceral involvement, and blood involvement.

Treatment of CTCL depends on staging of disease. For early-stage disease, topical agents are the standard of care, including steroids, nitrogen mustards, bexarotene, or BCNU. Treatment of larger or more widespread lesions includes phototherapy and radiation therapy, often with electron beam treatment. There is no standard treatment for extensive disease, although systemic therapy is generally warranted. Patients with generalized erythroderma or desquamation may be treated with oral retinoids, histone deacetylase inhibitors (romidepsin and vorinostat) or an anti-CD52 monoclonal antibody alemtuzumab. Patients who receive alemtuzumab need prophylaxis for varicella zoster virus and *Pneumocystis jirovecii* due to marked T-cell immunosuppression. Systemic chemotherapy may be given as a single agent (oral methotrexate, pralatrexate, pegylated liposomal doxorubicin, or gemcitabine) or in combination (CHOP or another gemcitabine-based regimen). Hematopoietic stem cell transplant has the highest rate of cure in patients who have had a complete response to induction chemotherapy.

MULTIPLE MYELOMA

Multiple myeloma, smoldering myeloma (SMM) and monoclonal gammopathy of unknown significance (MGUS; also referred to as essential monoclonal gammopathy) exist on a spectrum with distinctly identified criteria for each category (**Table 174-19**). SMM and MGUS are precursors to MM; about 10% of smoldering myeloma and one percent of MGUS cases will progress to MM each year. Both MGUS and SMM may also develop into B-cell lymphomas or lead to secondary amyloidosis, the latter developing more often in full MM; however, most amyloidosis cases occur in the absence of myeloma.

Table 174-20 summarizes the features distinguishing these diseases from other hematologic malignancies.

End organ damage is necessary to distinguish MM from SMM or MGUS; Hyper**C**alcemia, **R**enal impairment, **A**nemia, and **B**ony (often painful) lytic lesions (CRAB) are present in some combination (CRAB). Anemia is the most common of these symptoms and is related to marrow infiltration, kidney disease, or in some cases to a myeloma-related B12 deficiency. Renal impairment may result from glomerular damage from free light chains (aka, myeloma kidney), prolonged or severe hypercalcemia, AL amyloidosis, or as a side effect from the multiple nephrotoxic medications needed to treat MM.

Hypercalcemia and bony pain often result from the cortical bone destruction that occurs in MM from unopposed osteoclast activity. Significant marrow involvement may cause bony pain independently.

TABLE 174-19 Multiple Myeloma, Smoldering Myeloma, and MGUS Criteria*

Definition of multiple myeloma

  Clonal bone marrow plasma cell ≥ 10% or biopsy proven bony or extramedulary plasmacytoma and any one or more of the following myeloma-defining events (End organ damage):

    Hypercalcemia: serum calcium >0.25 mm/L (>1 mg/dL) higher than the ULN or > 2.75 mmol/L (>11 mg/dL)

    Renal insufficiency: Creatinine clearance <40 mL/min or serum creatinine >177 μmol/L (>2 mg/dL)

    Anemia: Hemoglobin >20 g/L below LLN or a hemoglobin <100 g/L

    Bone lesions: one or more osteolytic lesions on skeletal radiography, CT or PET-CT

  Any one or more of the following biomarkers or malignancy

    Clonal bone marrow plasma cell ≥ 60%

    Involved:uninvolved serum free light chain ratio ≥ 100

    >1 focal lesion on MRI studies

Definition of Smoldering multiple myeloma

  Both criteria must be met:

    Serum monoclonal protein (IgG or IgA) >30 g/L or urinary monoclonal protein ≥ 500 mg per 24h and/or clonal bone marrow plasma cells 10%-60%

    Absence of myeloma defining events or amyloidosis

Definition of Monoclonal Gammopathy of Undetermined Significance (MGUS)

  Serum monoclonal protein < 30 g/L

  Clonal bone marrow plasma cells <10%

  Absence of end organ damage, ie., hypercalcemia, renal dysfunction, anemia, and bone lesions*

  Absence of amyloidosis

*In IgM MGUS, there also must be no evidence of hyperviscosity, lymphadenopathy, hepatosplenomegaly, or other end-organ damage attributed to a lymphoproliferative disorder.
Original table modified for from Rajkumar SV, Dimopoulos MA, Palumbo A, et al. International Myeloma Working Group updated criteria for the diagnosis of multiple myeloma. *Lancet Oncol.* 2014;15:e538.

TABLE 174-20 Multiple Myeloma, Smoldering Myeloma, MGUS

Epidemiology	MM 10% of adult hematologic malignancies, 1% of all adult cancers, in older individuals, median age 66; most sporadic
Clinical presentation	Symptoms reflect end-organ damage which distinguishes MM from SMM or MGUS
Laboratory tests	Hyper**C**alcemia, **R**enal impairment, **A**nemia, and **B**ony (often painful) lytic lesions (CRAB)
	All patients: CBC, comprehensive metabolic panel, serum albumin, β2- microglobulin, SPEP, UPEP, serum free light chains and immunofixation
	• An aberrant monoclonal spike on serum protein electrophoresis (SPEP) in most (97%), typically with a corresponding peak on 24-h urine protein electrophoresis (UPEP)
	• Malignant monoclonal plasma cells typically exhibit a restricted light chain phenotype for the antibodies they release, showing either κ or λ outnumbering the other by 100:1 (normal physiologic ratio is closer to 2:1).
	Serum osmolarity and viscosity in patients who have monoclonal IgM spikes, putting them at risk for hyperviscosity syndrome.
Bone marrow biopsy	Bone marrow biopsy for most patients:
	> 10% plasma cellularity raises diagnosis to SMM
	> 60% or greater is diagnostic of MM even without further evidence of end-organ damage.
	When peripheral biopsy (eg, bone or soft tissue mass) confirms the diagnosis of MM, deferring the bone marrow biopsy may be considered for some patients.
	Cytogenetics to establish prognosis and guide treatment decisions
Imaging	Skeletal survey with plain film radiography to screen for bony lytic lesions (alternatively, fractures or diffuse osteopenia may be seen).
	MRI to evaluate for bony disease in the setting of bone pain without visible bony lesions on x-ray
	Either MRI or PET/CT to confirm the absence of more than one focal lytic lesion in patients with suspected MGUS or SMM especially important, because more than one bony lytic lesion will automatically upgrade the diagnosis to MM. PET/CT is being used with increased frequency as part of the initial diagnostic work-up for MM, although not always standard procedure.
Prognosis	Cytogenetics: specific translocations and gene expression profiling signatures will help distinguish favorable vs intermediate vs high risk patients.
	Patients with serum LDH more than twice the upper limit of normal are automatically considered high risk, as are those with evidence of a primary plasma cell leukemia.
	The myeloma prognosis score (MPS) relies on albumin and beta-2 microglobulin. While still frequently used, the MPS predates most modern therapies for MM.

Neurologic symptoms develop in a minority of patients at some point during their course. A radiculopathy or peripheral neuropathy may be seen in the setting of amyloidosis. Cord compression, a rare complication, may result from infiltration of a paravertebral plasmacytoma or frank bony collapse of the spinal vertebrae. Cord compression is a medical emergency that requires immediate evaluation for chemotherapy, radiation, and possible surgical intervention. MM involving the CNS usually manifests from contiguous anatomical spread from bony lesions in the skull or as leptomeningeal disease, both of which are rare complications. Altered mental status should warrant consideration of hyperviscosity syndrome and hyperammonemia (with or without liver disease).

Treatment

Current treatment protocols rely heavily on chemotherapy followed by up-front autologous HSCT. Transplant eligibility should be determined at the time of diagnosis, as autologous HSCT features prominently in the treatment algorithm for MM. Higher-risk patients for transplantation include:

• Older individuals (>77 years) who tend to do more poorly with the myeloablative process
• Elevated direct bilirubin (>2.0), elevated creatinine (>2.0)
• Heart failure with NYHA class III/IV symptoms
• ECOG performance status of 3 or 4

Typical regimens include an immunomodulating agent such as lenalidomide (Revlimid) and a proteasome inhibitor such as bortezomib (Velcade) along with dexamethasone. Bortezomib containing regimens are preferred in patients with a high-risk cytogenetic profile. Cyclophosphamide in combination with bortezomib is another induction regimen often used in patients who present with renal damage. Melphalan is used for elderly myeloma patients in combination with a steroid, and should not be given to patients who are eligible for transplant.

Treatment response should be assessed after two cycles of chemotherapy. If tolerated, patients receive two additional induction cycles followed by autologous HSCT in most eligible patients. Following induction, with or without HSCT, all MM patients receive 4 to 6 cycles of consolidation chemotherapy with either lenalidomide (in favorable risk disease) or bortezomib (in intermediate-/high-risk disease). If HSCT is contraindicated or if a complete or very good partial response is not achieved, further cycles of consolidation chemotherapy may be indicated.

Most patients with multiple myeloma will relapse with recurrent CRAB-related symptoms (not necessarily the same constellation as on initial presentation) or a rise in paraprotein levels in either serum (by 1 g/dL) or 24-hour urine (by >500 mg) on two consecutive measurements. Each patient should be risk-stratified again once relapsed disease is recognized when deciding which therapeutic interventions should be attempted (HSCT, reinduction chemotherapy, second-line agents, etc.).

Adjunctive therapies

Hypercalcemia, bone pain, and bony lytic lesions are usually related to overactive osteoclasts. Therefore, patients with MM should receive intravenous *bisphosphonates* if possible. However, aggressive bisphosphonate administration may aggravate preexisting renal impairment, and all patients should receive hydration with intravenous fluids if necessary to preserve renal function and reduce serum calcium. Patients may benefit from orthopedic consultation if pathologic fractures develop.

■ APLASTIC ANEMIA

Aplastic anemia (AA) is a stem cell disorder of the bone marrow defined by decreased or absent hematopoietic progenitor cells in the bone marrow. The diagnosis of aplastic anemia is based on bone marrow findings and degree of peripheral cytopenias. See **Table 174-21** for disease features which distinguish AA from other hematologic malignancies.

Treatment

Treatment of aplastic anemia depends on the severity of disease. Any identified drug or toxin should be removed. Patients also should receive transfusion support as needed. There are minimal data on how or whether to treat patients with moderate aplastic anemia, and some patients with mild cytopenias may be monitored.

Treatment for patients with severe or very severe aplastic anemia varies according to patient age. For patients younger than age 20, the standard care is a sibling matched allogeneic bone marrow transplant. For patients over the age of 50 or patients without a sibling donor, immunosuppression is the standard of care, the most common regimen being anti-thymocyte globulin (ATG) and cyclosporine with or without steroids. Patients commonly develop a serum sickness-like reaction (fevers, rigors, arthralgias, and rash) during the first few days of infusion of ATG. Recent studies have found horse ATG to be superior to rabbit ATG. Patients who relapse or have refractory disease may be retreated with an ATG based regimen, using a different ATG, or receive the TPO receptor agonist eltrombopag, which has demonstrated effects on trilineage hematopoiesis.

TABLE 174-21 Aplastic Anemia

Epidemiology	Rare, incidence of ≈2-4 per million annually
	Two forms of AA: congenital and acquired
	Congenital
	Acquired due to exposure to:
	• Radiation
	• Drug
	▪ Anti-seizure medications (carbamazepine, hydantoins), sulfonamide antibiotics, and antithyroid medications (methimazole, propylthiouracil)
	▪ Rarely used: chloramphenicol, gold, phenalbutazone
	• Chemical exposure
	▪ Benzene, organic solvents, and blue vapors
	• Viral
	▪ Epstein-Barr virus (EBV0)
	▪ HIV
	▪ Herpes, particularly HHV6
	▪ Seronegative hepatitis
	• Autoimmune related to bone marrow lymphocytes causing damage to stem cells
	• Clonal associated with
	▪ Fanconi's anemia
	▪ Telomerase mutations and telomer length
	▪ Paroxysmal nocturnal hemoglobinuria (diagnosed by flow cytometry with a lack of CD55 and CD59 expression)
	▪ Abnormalities in either thrombopoietin or the thrombopoietin receptor, MPL
Clinical presentation	Symptoms: profound fatigue, dyspnea directly associated with progressive anemia: bleeding or bruising from thrombocytopenia; increased risk and rate of infections (bacterial, fungal)
Laboratory tests	Pancytopenia with a decreased number of reticulocytes
Bone marrow biopsy	Marked hypocellularity with a marrow composed mostly of fat cells and sparse stroma. Rare cells that are seen are morphologically normal without evidence of dysplasia
Additional testing to exclude other causes of pancytopenia	• Flow cytometry for CD55 and CD59: paroxysmal nocturnal hemoglobinuria
	• Cytogenetics: hypoplastic MDS
	• Chromosome fragility studies: Fanconi's anemia
Severity of disease	Moderate AA: bone marrow cellularity <30% and a depression of at least 2 of the 3 peripheral lines below the normal levels without evidence of severe pancytopenia
	Severe aplastic anemia: bone marrow cellularity <25% with cytopenias or a bone marrow biopsy demonstrating <50% cellularity with <30% hematopoietic cells and two of the following:
	• Absolute reticulocyte count <40,000/μL
	• Absolute neutrophil count (ANC; neutrophils + bands) <500/μL, or
	• Platelet count <20,000/μL
	Very severe aplastic anemia: defined as severe aplastic anemia with an ANC <200/μL

■ HEMATOLOGIC EMERGENCIES

Hematologic malignancies have numerous associated pathologic derangements at various points during their course; a small number of complications are true medical emergencies that require appropriate haste, consideration, and aggressive medical management.

Tumor lysis syndrome

Tumor cell breakdown, typically with administration of chemotherapy, may release toxic levels of intracellular contents into the circulation. Patients develop hyperkalemia, hyperphosphatemia, hyperuricemia, acute kidney injury due to precipitation of uric acid and calcium phosphate, and secondary hypocalcemia. With these derangements, they may experience various symptoms including nausea, vomiting, weakness, oliguria, bowel changes, weight gain, cramping, tetany, and seizures.

Hematologic malignancies tend to carry higher risk for TLS compared to most solid tumors. Screening and prophylactic treatment for TLS with intravenous fluids, low dose allopurinol, and daily electrolyte monitoring should be considered in patients with high tumor burden, high blast count (such as in AML with blast crisis), and rapidly growing tumors like Burkitt lymphoma. High-risk patients often receive prophylaxis with rasburicase (recombinant urate oxidase).

Treatment should be escalated at the time of diagnosis of TLS to avoid complications such as acute renal injury. This requires:

- Aggressive intravenous fluids
- High dose allopurinol or IV rasburicase
- Monitoring of metabolic parameters multiple times daily until levels normalize and chemotherapy has completed

Rasburicase is becoming standard of care despite limited evidence; unlike allopurinol, it can directly reduce serum uric acid levels. Contraindications include pregnancy and G6PD deficiency.

Hyperleukocytosis and leukostasis

Hyperleukocytosis is defined as any elevated WBC >50 to 100,000/L. *Leukostasis* specifically applies to hyperleukocytosis from an elevated blast count most commonly associated with AML, CML in blast crisis, or ALL, although the smaller size of blast cells in ALL typically requires a much higher cell count to produce the same symptoms. Regardless of the underlying etiology, leukostasis may be deadly if not recognized and treated immediately.

High numbers of culprit blast cells in these patients cause microvascular occlusion leading to decreased tissue perfusion. Neurologic and respiratory effects are the most frequently identified presenting features of leukostasis and the most concerning. Headache, dizziness, confusion, and depressed mental status ranging from somnolence to coma may occur, as well as dyspnea, hypoxia, and respiratory distress to the point of requiring mechanical ventilation. Inflammation related to the underlying malignancy or a concurrent infection causes fever in up to 80% of cases. Forty percent of patients will develop disseminated intravascular coagulation (DIC). Ten percent will undergo spontaneous TLS from the significant tumor blast burden; many more develop TLS during cytoreduction.

Treatment should focus on rapid cytoreduction, typically with emergent chemotherapy or hydroxyurea, and stabilization of hematologic and metabolic abnormalities. Tumor-specific chemotherapy (eg, cytarabine and daunorubicin induction for AML) is the only modality with proven survival benefit and should be started without delay when possible.

If treatment must be delayed, hydroxyurea may be used as a temporizing measure; however, it does not replace the need for chemotherapy. Leukapheresis should be reserved for patients who cannot undergo chemotherapy emergently, and the extensive preparation for this procedure should never delay definitive treatment. Because of the extensive disease-related coagulopathies in promyelocytic leukemia, APML patients should not be offered leukapheresis as it has been linked to significant complications.

Hyperviscosity syndrome

Very high concentrations of serum paraproteins, especially in the setting of high IgM levels in Waldenström macroglobulinemia, may lead to marked increases in serum viscosity. This in turn may bring about decreased tissue perfusion from red blood cell sludging, thrombosis or bleeding from platelet dysfunction. Patients may develop weakness, headache, dizziness, confusion, peripheral neuropathies, mucosal bleeding and congestive heart failure.

Seen most commonly in Waldenström macroglobulinemia, hyperviscosity has also been associated with polycythemia, essential thrombocytosis, IgG or IgA myeloma, and the acute leukemias (especially blast crisis). A serum viscosity greater than 4.0 Otswald units (normal 1.4-1.8) establishes the diagnosis in symptomatic patients, and these patients require emergent treatment with plasmapheresis to alleviate symptoms. Intravenous fluids and diuretics should also be used as a temporizing measure before plasmapheresis and to reduce symptom recurrence afterward. Chemotherapy should be administered as soon as it may be done safely to treat the underlying malignancy.

Spinal cord compression

Although less common than other cancers, hematologic malignancies account for 5% to 10% of malignant spinal cord compressions, most frequently non-Hodgkin lymphomas (especially DLBCL) and multiple myeloma. Patients most commonly present with localized back pain, often worse with supine position, which may precede onset of neurologic symptoms by days to months. Findings may include a tingling sensation along the back and extremities with neck flexion or extension ("Lhermitte's sign"), localized loss of sensory or motor function, ataxic gait, or loss of bladder or bowel continence. Deep tendon reflexes may be diminished or brisk, depending on the acuity and anatomic location of the cord compression. Symptoms of saddle anesthesia, bowel/bladder incontinence, and low back pain should raise the possibility of a *cauda equina syndrome*.

Suspected tumor-related cord compression should prompt immediate neurosurgery consultation. Patients should receive high dose dexamethasone (6-10 mg IV q6h) to help reduce inflammation and restore neurologic function. If possible in neurologically stable patients, a biopsy should be obtained prior to initiating dexamethasone since this treatment may change the pathology and make a definitive diagnosis more difficult. Full-length spinal MRI is the preferred imaging modality to evaluate suspected lesions; steroid administration should rarely, if ever, be delayed for MRI evaluation because symptomatic cord compression is a true medical emergency. Many patients may be treated with emergent chemotherapy and/or radiation, depending on the cancer type. Indications for surgery to relieve cord compression include mechanical instability, rapidly progressing neurologic deficits, compression from a bony fragment or other structure, unknown tissue diagnosis, and any compression from recurrent or progressive disease in a region already treated with maximal radiation therapy.

Neutropenic fever

Decreases in the absolute neutrophil count (ANC; total neutrophil count + total band cell count) below the threshold of 1500 is defined as neutropenia, a condition which predisposes patients to severe and opportunistic infections often with less warning signs by way of symptoms or physical exam findings than in an immunocompetent host. Neutropenia typically follows administration of cytotoxic chemotherapy or radiation by a few days but may present at any point in the patient's course depending on the underlying malignancy. Any fever, defined as a single oral temperature >38.4°C (101°F) or a temperature of 38°C (100.4°F) or greater for more than 1 hour should be considered an emergent situation.

High-risk patients are defined as patients with a neutropenia that is supposed to last more than 7 days, unstable hemodynamics, pulmonary infiltrates, gastrointestinal symptoms, neurologic changes, signs of a catheter infection, liver insufficiency, or progression of disease. Recent alemtuzumab use is also considered a high-risk feature. Low-risk patients have an expected duration of neutropenia of less than seven days and no active comorbidities or other organ dysfunction. Low risk patients may be treated with an oral fluoroquinolone such as levofloxacin, or an oral β-lactam agent such as amoxicillin-clavulanic acid.

High-risk patients with neutropenic fever need to be treated aggressively. Physicians should promptly obtain cultures from blood, urine, and sputum, as well as blood fungal cultures. Broad-spectrum antibiotics usually with β-lactam agents with *Pseudomonas* coverage should be given within 60 minutes of identifying fever. Most patients will require addition of vancomycin for improved gram-positive coverage, and if suspicion is high enough early on, antifungals may be given as part of the initial antimicrobial regimen. Physicians should have a low threshold for obtaining abdominal imaging if neutropenic enterocolitis (NEC; aka, *typhlitis*) is suspected, and additionally should avoid performing a digital rectal exam as the microinjuries sustained during this maneuver are thought to allow for translocation of gut flora and thus serve as a precipitant for infection.

Antifungal agents should be given after 4 to 7 days if fevers persist or recur, if no causative microorganism is identified, or if there is a high suspicion for fungal infection (see Chapter 204 [Infections in the Immunocompromised Host]).

Superior vena cava syndrome

SVC syndrome causing *airway obstruction* or *cerebral edema* is a true medical emergency. Any process causing compression of the superior vena cava (SVC) may precipitate an SVC syndrome, often secondary to tumor or lymphadenopathy-related SVC compression or related to thrombosis of central venous and portal catheters. Patients typically develop facial edema, dyspnea at rest, chest and referred shoulder pain, as well as prominent neck veins.

Tumor-related compression often requires either emergent chemotherapy or localized external beam radiation, with chemotherapy typically being the preferred approach (especially for lymphomas);

this is often combined with high-dose intravenous corticosteroids to reduce inflammation. As with cord compression, it is important to obtain tissue for diagnosis prior to steroids or radiation therapy as lymphomas may have a marked and rapid change in morphology after a single treatment. When secondary to thrombosis, any culprit device or indwelling line is usually removed if possible, and patients should receive therapeutic anticoagulation. Balloon dilatation or stenting may be required if residual stenosis leading to persistent SVC compression occurs.

SUGGESTED READINGS

Aukema SM, Siebert R, Shuuring E, et al. Double hit B-cell lymphomas. *Blood*. 2011;117(8):2319-2331.

Baccarani M, Deininger MW, Rosti G, et al. European LeukemiaNET recommendations for the management of chronic myeloid leukemia: 2013. *Blood*. 2013;122(6):871-884.

Byrd JC, Brown JR, O'Brien S, et al. Ibrutinib versus Ofatumumab in Previously treated Chronic Lymphoid Leukemia. *N Engl J Med*. 2014;371:213-223.

Cheson BD, Fisher RI, Barrington SF, et al. Recommendations for initial evaluation, staging, and response assessment of Hodgkin and Non-Hodgkin lymphoma: the Lugano classification. *JCO*. 2014;32:1-10.

Dunleavy K, Pitaluga S, Shovlin M, et al. Low-Intensity therapy in Adults with Burkitt's Lymphoma. *N Engl J Med*. 2013;369:1915-1925.

Grimwade D, Hills RK, Moorman AV, et al. Refinement of cytogenetic classifications in acute myeloid leukemia: determination of prognostic significance of rare recurring chromosomal abnormalities among 5876 younger adult patients treated in the United Kingdom Medical Research Council trials. *Blood*. 2010;116(3):354-365.

Lo-Coco F, Avvisati G, Vigneti M, et al. Retinoic acid and arsenic trioxide for acute promyelocytic leukemia. *N Engl J Med*. 2013;369:111-121.

Tefferi A, Thiele H, Orazi A, et al. Proposals and rationale for revision of the World Health Organization diagnostic criteria for polycythemia vera, essential thrombocythemia, and primary myelofibrosis: recommendations from an ad hoc international expert panel. *Blood*. 2007;110(4):1092-1097.

Younes A, Bartlet NL, Leonard JP, et al. Brenduximab Vedotin (SGN-35) for Relapsed CD30-Positive Lymphomas *N Engl J Med*. 2010;363:1812-1821.

SECTION 8

Oncology

CHAPTER 175

Overview of Cancer and Treatment

Jennifer Duff, MD

Merry Jennifer Markham, MD

Key Clinical Questions

1. What types of biopsies can aid in the diagnostic workup of cancer?
2. How is the cancer stage determined?
3. What are the goals of therapy in the neoadjuvant, adjuvant, and palliative setting?
4. What are the different types of systemic therapies commonly used in the treatment of cancer?
5. What are the approaches to treating chemotherapy-related nausea, vomiting and mucositis?
6. When are modified blood products recommended for cancer patients and what are the transfusion thresholds for anemia and thrombocytopenia?

EPIDEMIOLOGY

Cancer is a group of diseases characterized by uncontrolled proliferation of abnormal cells that invade surrounding tissue and carry the potential to metastasize. Environmental and lifestyle risk factors and genetic susceptibility all contribute to an individual's risk of developing cancer. In 2015, more than 1.6 million Americans will be diagnosed with cancer, and approximately 600,000 cancer-related deaths will occur. The most common cancers afflicting men and women are prostate and breast, respectively, followed by lung and colorectal. Overall, lung cancer is the leading cause of cancer-related mortality, followed by colorectal cancer. The incidence of lung and colon cancer in men is steadily declining, perhaps reflecting decreased tobacco use and emphasis on colorectal cancer screenings. Lung cancer incidence in women is finally starting to decrease after rising over the last few decades, reflecting the delayed uptake in smoking (and later, smoking cessation) by women compared to men.

DIAGNOSIS AND STAGING

Biopsy of a primary and/or metastatic site of a presumed malignancy is necessary to provide histologic confirmation of a cancer diagnosis. Involving a hematologist-oncologist early in the workup of a newly diagnosed cancer patient can be helpful in guiding the appropriate testing, biopsy sites, or biopsy techniques. For example, different biopsy techniques—including fine needle aspiration (FNA), core needle biopsy, excisional biopsy, or laparotomy—may be utilized depending on the type of cancer suspected. An FNA alone is inadequate in the diagnosis of lymphomas as the morphology of the nodal tissue is crucial in determining lymphoma subtype. Core needle biopsies and excisional or incisional biopsies provide a larger volume of tissue for pathologic evaluation of morphology and for molecular or genetic analysis. When a hematologic malignancy, such as lymphoma, is suspected, sending a fresh, not fixed, specimen for comprehensive immunophenotyping using flow cytometry is important in yielding the correct diagnosis. Finally, in addition to confirming a cancer diagnosis, the biopsied tissue specimen may guide therapeutic decisions. For example, molecular biomarkers, such as HER2Neu for breast cancer and KRAS/NRAS for colon cancer, have implications for the oncologist's choice of antineoplastic agents used during therapy.

Accurately staging patients to determine the extent of their disease is critical in determining prognosis and for guiding treatment decisions. Staging often involves radiographic imaging (such as computed tomography [CT] or positron emission tomography [PET] scans) or endoscopic or surgical visualization to determine local and distant organ involvement. Comprehensive radiologic imaging is not always necessary in the staging process when the cancer appears to be locally confined and has a low likelihood of distant involvement (eg, early stage breast cancer). Serum tumor markers have a role in the staging of some cancers, such as testicular and ovarian cancers. Bone marrow biopsy or lumbar puncture may be important in the staging of various hematologic malignancies. Decisions about type of staging studies needed for an individual patient should be made in conjunction with a consulting hematologist-oncologist.

Solid organ tumors are staged by the American Joint Committee on Cancer (AJCC) TNM classification system, where T refers to tumor size or degree of mucosal infiltration of the primary tumor, N describes lymph node involvement, and M refers to the presence or absence of metastatic disease. Lymphomas have their own unique staging systems and, as in solid tumors, prognosis and treatment options vary with stage.

Typically, early stage (stages I and II) solid tumors lack lymph node involvement and are curable. Stage III solid organ cancers are often referred to as locally advanced and typically involve regional lymph nodes. Metastatic, or stage IV, solid organ cancers are generally incurable but are often treatable. However, some solid tumors, including colorectal and breast cancers, and melanoma with limited metastatic sites, have curative potential with a multidisciplinary treatment approach.

TREATMENT

■ A CASE EXAMPLE

Ms J, a 55-year-old woman, presented with intermittent rectal bleeding and difficulty passing bowel movements. A colonoscopy revealed a friable, partially circumferential mass in the rectum. Biopsy of the mass confirmed a moderately well-differentiated adenocarcinoma. Staging with contrasted CT of the chest, abdomen, and pelvis, did not show any distant metastatic disease. Further staging with endoscopic ultrasound confirmed a stage IIIA (T3N1M0) rectal cancer. She was treated with neoadjuvant chemoradiation using oral capecitabine with daily radiation therapy for 5.5 weeks. After completing neoadjuvant treatment, she underwent a low anterior resection with an end-to-end anastomosis. The surgical pathology showed moderate treatment response with down-staging of the disease and no involved lymph nodes. She completed 3 out of 4 months of curative adjuvant systemic chemotherapy with fluorouracil, leucovorin, and oxaliplatin, stopping 1 month short due to side effects. For the next 3 years, she had no radiographic or clinical evidence of recurrent disease until she developed persistent right upper quadrant abdominal pain. Computed tomography imaging demonstrated innumerable hypodensities in the liver and scattered nodules in the lungs, all concerning for metastatic disease. A core biopsy of a liver lesion confirmed metastatic colorectal adenocarcinoma. Mutational testing of the tissue confirmed wild-type KRAS and NRAS genes. She was treated with palliative chemotherapy consisting of fluorouracil, leucovorin, irinotecan, and bevacizumab with good tumor response and relief of pain symptoms. However, restaging imaging after 8 months demonstrated peritoneal carcinomatosis, consistent with progressive disease. Her treatment was switched to irinotecan plus cetuximab. She tolerated this regimen poorly with a declining performance status. After two cycles, the chemotherapy was discontinued and she was enrolled in Hospice. She lived another 2.5 months without treatment, allowing her to travel with her family prior to her death.

This case illustrates the continuum of cancer care in an initially curable cancer that ultimately relapsed and progressed, resulting in death. In this example, neoadjuvant, adjuvant, and palliative treatment regimens were utilized, each intended to accomplish a specific goal. Neoadjuvant therapy was used to improve surgical outcomes and reduce the risk of local tumor recurrence. Adjuvant therapy was used to eradicate micrometastatic disease and reduce the likelihood of systemic recurrence. Palliative chemotherapy was used to improve disease control, survival, and to relieve cancer-related symptoms.

The optimal treatment of cancer patients often requires a multidisciplinary, team-based approach, with collaboration among all health care providers involved including surgeons, radiation oncologists, medical oncologists, radiologists, pharmacists, nursing, social workers, psychologists, and nutritionists. Providing patient-centric care for cancer patients extends beyond formulating treatment plans; it involves understanding patients' emotional well-being, their psychosocial needs, and recognition of socioeconomic barriers that may impede safe care. Early identification of depression or anxiety, inadequate support systems, or insufficient understanding of the diagnosis and treatment goals, is crucial in providing humanistic oncology care.

■ SURGERY, SYSTEMIC THERAPY, RADIATION THERAPY

Surgical resection of the tumor burden is the gold standard therapy for achieving cure in most solid-organ cancers. Lymphomas and other hematologic malignancies, small-cell lung cancer, locally advanced non–small-cell lung cancer, and prostate and cervical cancer are among those malignancies that have curative potential with chemotherapy or radiation therapy alone, or a combination of these treatment modalities. The extent of surgical resection depends on the operative risk, size and location of the primary tumor, involvement of surrounding tissues, and the degree of lymph node dissection indicated. For certain high-risk, complex surgeries, such as esophagectomy for esophageal cancer, surgeon and hospital experience and higher surgical volume yield improved outcomes for patients, and referral to an experienced surgeon in a high-volume center is important. Similarly, for the gynecologic cancers, outcomes are improved for women who have surgical resection by a gynecologic oncologist rather than a general surgeon or gynecologist.

Systemic therapy is an umbrella term encompassing a variety of cancer treatments, including chemotherapy, biologic (or targeted) therapy, immunotherapy, and hormonal therapy. Oncologists' choice of a chemotherapy regimen is based on current evidence-based national guidelines, the goals of treatment (curative vs palliative), and patient performance status. Multiagent chemotherapy regimens are often selected in the curative setting or when maximum disease control is preferred and feasible. Single-agent chemotherapy is often selected when palliation is desired. When chemotherapy agents are combined, they are often selected due to diverse mechanisms of action and nonoverlapping side effects in order to maximize efficacy while minimizing undesirable toxicity to the patient.

Cytotoxic chemotherapy drugs lead to cancer cell death through a variety of mechanisms that interfere with the cell growth cycle. Each class of chemotherapy drugs carries its own unique set of side effects, some of which are short term and only occur transiently during treatment, while others may occur during or after treatment and result in permanent morbidity (**Table 175-1**). The drugs in the vinca alkaloid, platinum, and taxane classes may result in varying degrees of motor or sensory neuropathy. Anthracyclines (eg, doxorubicin) are associated with a risk of cardiac toxicity in the short and long term, including cardiomyopathy and/or arrhythmias.

Systemic cancer therapies are continuously evolving and novel biologics and immunotherapies have an important and growing role in the treatment of malignancy. Biologic agents, also referred to as targeted therapies, are directed toward specific intracellular characteristics or pathways of tumors. One of the first targeted therapies was imatinib, the oral drug that inhibits the Bcr-Abl tyrosine kinase, the constitutive abnormal gene product of the Philadelphia chromosome in chronic myeloid leukemia. Monoclonal antibodies selectively target specific cell antigens found predominantly on tumor cells. For example, rituximab is an anti-CD20 monoclonal antibody which, when paired with chemotherapy, has substantially improved response rates and survival in B-cell non-Hodgkin lymphoma. Other monoclonal antibodies include bevacizumab, which binds to the vascular endothelial growth factor protein interfering with angiogenesis; cetuximab, which binds to the EGFR receptor to prevent downstream signals involved in tumor growth and proliferation; trastuzumab and pertuzumab, which work through targeting the HER2 receptor; and ado-trastuzumab (also known as T-DM1) which

TABLE 175-1 Chemotherapy Drug Classes and Usual Toxicities

Chemotherapy Class	Examples of Drugs	Side Effects
Alkylating agents	Cyclophosphamide Ifosfamide Dacarbazine Temozolomide Chlorambucil	Myelosupression Dose-related emesis Pneumonitis Syndrome of inappropriate ADH (SIADH) Secondary leukemias
Anthracyclines	Doxorubicin Daunarubicin Epirubicin	Myelosupression Mucositis Cardiotoxicity Vesicant
Antimetabolites	5-fluoruracil Capecitabine Pemetrexed Methotrexate	Myelosuppression Mucositis Gastrointestinal (nausea, vomiting, diarrhea)
Platinum agents	Carboplatin Cisplatin Oxaliplatin	Renal Toxicity Neuropathy Nausea/vomiting Myelosuppression
Taxanes	Docetaxel Paclitaxel	Myelosupression Hypersensitivity reactions Neuropathy
Topoisomerase I inhibitors	Irinotecan	Diarrhea Early onset (1-6 h from infusion), due to inhibition of acetylcholinesterase; treated with atropine Later onset, from mucosal damage; treated with aggressive loperamide dosing
Topoisomerase II inhibitors	Etoposide	Myelosuppression Nausea/vomiting Secondary acute myelogenous leukemia
Vinca alkaloids	Vincristine Vinblastine	Vesicant Peripheral neuropathy, motor and sensory Autonomic neuropathy (such as ileus) Cranial nerve palsies SIADH Myelosuppression with vinblastine

combines trastuzumab with a chemotherapeutic to target delivery of the cytotoxic agent specifically to cancer cells.

Immunotherapy refers to those agents aimed at stimulating the immune system to overcome the immune evasion triggered by the malignancy. For example, Sipuleucel-T, an autologous immunotherapy approved in advanced prostate cancer, primes a patient's antigen presenting cells to promote an immune response against their disease. Newer immunotherapy agents block immune checkpoints such as the cytotoxic T-lymphocyte-associated antigen 4 (CTLA-4) and the programmed death 1 (PD-1) receptor, thus enhancing antitumor immunity. Ipilimumab used in metastatic melanoma is an antibody directed against CTLA-4, and pembrolizumab and nivolumab are anti-PD-1 antibodies both used for metastatic melanoma. Nivolumab is also approved for use in metastatic squamous cell non–small-cell lung cancer.

Hormonal, or endocrine, therapy refers to agents that modulate hormones that are a driving factor in the growth and proliferation of a tumor. They function through several mechanisms, some of which include direct hormone receptor blockade, interfering with hormone production by the pituitary and adrenal glands and ovaries, and inhibiting peripheral hormone conversion. The treatment of breast and prostate cancers frequently incorporates hormonal therapies such as antiestrogenic agents including the aromatase inhibitors (eg, anastrazole, letrozole, and exemestane) and selective estrogen receptor modulators (eg, tamoxifen) and LHRH agonists (eg, goserelin).

Radiation therapy consists of delivering high-energy x-rays or other particles to a specified body region, resulting in DNA destruction and tumor death. Common radiation therapy techniques include external beam radiation, 3-D conformational radiation therapy (3-D CRT), intensity modulated radiation therapy (IMRT), stereotactic and proton beam radiation therapy. All of these methods have varying degrees of precision in targeting the tumor to minimize the impact on surrounding healthy tissue. Internal radiation therapy, or brachytherapy, involves placing radioactive material into or near the tumor tissue; this technique is often used in the treatment of prostate or cervical cancer. Radioimmunotherapy is a method to target radiation to a tumor site using monoclonal antibodies attached to radioactive substances.

Radiation therapy may be used as a neoadjuvant, adjuvant, or palliative therapy. More than half of all cancer patients will receive radiation at some point during their treatment course. Radiation therapy can be used to shrink the tumor burden, allowing for a less extensive surgical procedure and/or improved cosmesis (eg, performing a lumpectomy instead of a mastectomy for a breast mass). It may also be used to reduce the risk of local cancer recurrence or to palliate tumor-related symptoms, such as bleeding or pain. For some cancers, such as head and neck or cervical cancer, modified doses of chemotherapy may be administered simultaneously with radiation to enhance the radiation effect.

PRACTICE POINT

Workup and evaluation for cancer

- Involve a hematologist-oncologist early in the workup to advise on diagnostic studies or biopsy site/technique.
- A biopsy is necessary to confirm a histologic diagnosis.
- Consider a biopsy approach that will obtain the most tissue for diagnosis and allow for molecular analysis, if appropriate. Typically core needle biopsies are preferred over fine needle aspirates.
- Staging imaging should consist first of a contrasted CT chest, abdomen, pelvis.
- Not all stage IV malignancies are incurable. Some solid tumors, including colorectal and breast cancer with oligometastatic disease, may be cured using a multidisciplinary approach.
- Comprehensive cancer treatment utilizes a multidisciplinary team of physicians, often including medical oncologists, surgeons, and radiation oncologists.

■ INPATIENT MANAGEMENT OF COMMONLY ENCOUNTERED SCENARIOS

Cancer treatment can result in complications leading to hospitalization. Some of the commonly encountered inpatient scenarios include febrile neutropenia, nausea, vomiting, diarrhea, severe anemia or thrombocytopenia necessitating transfusion, and tumor lysis syndrome.

Nausea and vomiting

Prevention of nausea and vomiting is the most widely used supportive care measure in cancer treatment, and the development of new classes of antiemetics have had significant impact on the ability of patients to tolerate chemotherapy. Despite these efforts, nausea in the cancer patient may be encountered in the inpatient setting. It is important to consider potential reasons for nausea and vomiting other than cancer treatment, such as altered gut motility, bowel obstruction, electrolyte disturbance, brain metastases, narcotic use, or dyspepsia. Several antiemetics have been developed in the last decade that have substantially reduced the incidence of treatment-related emesis by interfering with the effect of endogenous neurotransmitters such as dopamine, histamine, and serotonin at the chemoreceptor trigger zone. The categories of available antiemetics include corticosteroids, benzodiazepines, cannabinoids, NK-1 receptor antagonists, serotonergic and dopaminergic receptors antagonists, and the atypical antipsychotic olanzapine. Antiemetics may be administered intravenously, orally, or per rectum, with rare use of intramuscular delivery due to discomfort and the risk of tissue fibrosis with repeated doses. Prior to administration of chemotherapy, one or more of these agents are administered depending on the emetogenic potential of the chemotherapy regimen. The 5HT3-receptor antagonists are among the most effective agents in preventing chemotherapy-related emesis. Benzodiazepines such as lorazepam are valuable in the prevention of anticipatory nausea triggered by the anxiety of receiving chemotherapy and are typically used simultaneously with other antiemetics. For patients who develop breakthrough nausea and vomiting despite these preventative efforts, treating with an antiemetic from a different class is helpful (**Table 175-2**) (see Chapter 97 [Nausea and Vomiting]).

Mucositis

Another potential consequence of both chemotherapy and radiation is damage to rapidly dividing epithelial cells of the mucosa lining the oropharynx and the gastrointestinal tract leading to mucositis. Oral mucositis is defined as painful inflammation of the oral mucosa manifesting as erythema, ulcerations, and soft white

patches. This particularly afflicts patients treated with 5-flurouracil, methotrexate, high-dose chemotherapy used prior to hematopoietic stem cell transplantation, or those undergoing radiation treatments to the head and neck. It typically develops within 7 to 10 days from initiation of chemotherapy and lasts several weeks. There are few remedies available to expedite recovery and supportive measures to minimize discomfort are the mainstay of treatment. Palifermin, a keratinocyte growth factor, is approved in patients receiving high-dose chemotherapy in the setting of hematopoietic stem cell transplant to decrease the incidence and duration of severe mucositis. Other management strategies include mouth rinses (avoiding alcohol based), topical anesthetics, mucosal coating agents, analgesics, and lubricants (**Table 175-3**). One effective regimen that is frequently prescribed is a mixture of a mucosal coating agent with a topical anesthetic. Opioids may be required for patients whose discomfort is not relieved with topical treatments.

Anemia and thrombocytopenia

Cancer patients may be hospitalized for symptomatic anemia necessitating red cell transfusion. The anemia may be directly related to chemotherapy myelosuppression or it may be multifactorial secondary to anemia of chronic disease, nutritional deficiencies, cancer infiltrating the marrow, or impaired erythropoietin production. The hemoglobin threshold at which to initiate red cell transfusion depends on the goals of care. Transfusion guidelines recommend that cancer patients be transfused in a manner similarly to other noncardiac, hospitalized patients, for example, transfusion is considered when the hemoglobin (Hgb) is between 7 and 8 g/dL, using the minimum number of units necessary. If the Hgb is less than 9 g/dL and the patient is symptomatic from the anemia, transfusion is also reasonable. For patients with advanced cancer and anemia, transfusion may provide palliation and subjective benefit according to small observational studies. For patients who would benefit from an increased hemoglobin but decline red cell transfusion, erythropoietin stimulating agents (ESAs) and iron infusions are alternative approaches to enhancing red cell production. Because studies using both available ESAs—epoetin and darbepoetin alfa—report a potential risk of increased tumor growth and chance of death from cancer, the use of ESAs are typically reserved for patients with incurable malignancies and not generally used when the goal of treatment is cure.

The threshold at which to transfuse platelets depends on a patient's risk of bleeding, need for invasive procedures, and whether they are critically ill versus clinically stable. Patients have been observed to be at increased risk of spontaneous bleeding with severe thrombocytopenia, defined as platelet counts less than 5000/μL. There has been no observed difference in bleeding risk between platelet counts of 10,000/μL versus 20,000/μL in clinically stable patients. Thus, it is recommended to consider platelet transfusion for all patients with platelets less than 10,000/μL. There are some clinical scenarios where different platelet triggers are recommended. For example, in patients with coagulopathy, on anticoagulation, or if there is an anatomic lesion at risk for bleeding, transfuse platelets if the platelet count is less than 20,000/μL. One may also consider transfusing platelets to achieve a platelet count over 50,000/μL if an invasive surgical procedure is planned or transfusing platelets to achieve a platelet count over 100,000/μL in the case of bleeding or surgery within the central nervous system.

Certain groups of cancer patients, such as those with neutropenia or those who have received or are being considered for stem cell transplant, may require certain modifications to transfused blood products. Leukoreduction is a common modification that depletes the blood product of leukocytes, thus minimizing the risk for alloimmunization against leukocyte antigens. Leukocyte contamination of red cell products results in febrile nonhemolytic transfusion reactions (FNHTR), and leukoreduction reduces the risk of this complication.

TABLE 175-2 Antiemetics Used for Breakthrough Nausea and Vomiting

Antiemetic Drug	Drug Class	Dose/Frequency
Dexamethasone	Steroid	4-12 mg PO/IV daily
Dronabinol	Cannabinoid	5-10 mg PO 3-6 h
Lorazepam	Benzodiazepine	0.5-2 mg PO/IV q 6 h
Metoclopramide	Prokinetic	10-40 mg PO/IV q 4-6 h
Olanzopine	Atypical antipsychotic	2.5-5 mg PO daily
Ondansetron	5-HT3 receptor antagonist	8-24 mg PO or 8-12 mg IV (max 32 mg/d)
Prochlorperazine	Phenothiazine	10 mg PO/IV q 6 h
Promethazine	Phenothiazine	12.5-25 mg PO/IV q 4-6 h
Scopolamine	Other	1 transdermal patch q 72 h

TABLE 175-3 Mucositis Management

Bland Rinses	Topical Anesthetics	Mucosal Coating	Lubricating Agents	Analgesia
0.9% normal saline - Mix 1 teaspoon of table salt in 32 ounces of water **Sodium bicarbonate solution** - Mix 0.5 teaspoon salt and 2 tablespoons sodium bicarbonate in 32 ounces water	**Lidocaine** -2% viscous **Benzocaine** Spray or gel **Diphenhydramine solution**	**Milk of Magnesia** **Kaopectate** **Amphojel** - **Cellulose film-forming agents** eg, Zilactin	**Artificial saliva**	**Opioids** - Patient controlled analgesia [PCA] - Elixir - Transdermal patches

Leukoreduction also substantially decreases the risk of cytomegalovirus (CMV) transmission by blood transfusion. Most health care facilities in the United States have adopted universal leukoreduction of blood products; however, in centers that have not implemented this, leukoreduced products should be considered for patients with the following characteristics: past history of FNHTR, prior history of solid organ or hematopoietic stem cell transplant, planned solid organ or hematopoietic stem cell transplant, immunocompromised CMV negative patients, and patients requiring chronic transfusions.

Irradiated blood products are recommended for immunocompromised patients at risk for transfusion-related graft versus host disease (GVHD), a condition with high mortality. The blood products are exposed to gamma irradiation, thereby inactivating the donor lymphocytes responsible for this phenomenon. Irradiated blood products should be considered in these specific patient scenarios: current or prior treatment with chemotherapy agents in the purine analog class (eg, fludarabine, cladribine); a diagnosis of Hodgkin lymphoma (compared to other lymphomas, patients with Hodgkin lymphoma are at higher risk for developing transfusion-related GVHD); previous hematopoietic stem cell transplantation; receiving blood products from a related donor; and patients needing HLA-matched platelets. Patients with acute leukemia do not require irradiated blood products unless they are receiving conditioning therapy in preparation for allogeneic stem cell transplant. In summary, the decision to transfuse blood products should be individualized for each patient and the risks of transfusion must be carefully considered.

Venous thromboembolism prophylaxis

Cancer itself is associated with a hypercoaguable state, and treatment with chemotherapy further contributes to the risk of thrombotic complications. Deep venous thrombosis (DVT) is the most common thrombotic complication seen in patients with cancer. Compared to patients without cancer, those with cancer are at a substantially elevated risk of thrombosis after surgical procedures and extended DVT prophylaxis beyond hospital discharge is sometimes considered. It is essential to be mindful of this elevated risk and to provide appropriate DVT prophylaxis to hospitalized cancer patients (see Chapter 252 [Venous Thromboembolism Prophylaxis for Hospitalized Medical Patients]).

PRACTICE POINT

Caring for a hospitalized cancer patient

- Cancer produces a state of hypercoagulability. All patients should be offered deep venous thrombosis prophylaxis while hospitalized.
- Breakthrough nausea/vomiting can be controlled with a variety of medications, including antiemetics, prokinetic agents, steroids, atypical antipsychotics, and benzodiazepines.
- First-line treatment for supporting mucositis includes saline washes and topical agents. Opioids may be necessary for pain relief.
- Certain populations of cancer patients are recommended to have leukoreduced blood products to minimize the risk of febrile nonhemolytic transfusions reactions and reduce the risk of CMV transmission. Irradiated blood products are reserved for patients at risk for transfusion related graft versus host disease.
- For most cancer patients, transfuse the minimum number of blood products necessary to maintain a hemoglobin between 7 and 8 g/dL and a platelet count greater than 10,000/μL.

SUGGESTED READINGS

Bensinger W, Schubert M, Ang KK, et al. NCCN Task Force Report: prevention and management of mucositis in cancer care. *J Natl Compr Canc Netw.* 2008;6(Suppl 1):S1-S21.

Edge SB, Byrd DR, Compton CC, Fritz AG, Greene FL, Trotti A, eds. *AJCC Cancer Staging Manual*, 7th ed. New York, NY: Springer; 2010.

Gerber DE, Chan TA. Recent advances in radiation therapy. *Am Fam Physician.* 2008;78(11):1254-1262.

Jordan K, Sippel C, Schmoll HJ. Guidelines for antiemetic treatment of chemotherapy-induced nausea and vomiting: past, present, and future recommendations. *Oncologist.* 2007;12(9):1143-1150.

Szczepiorkowski ZM, Dunbar NM. Transfusion guidelines: when to transfuse. *Hematology Am Soc Hematol Educ Program.* 2013;638-644.

Oncologic Emergencies

Kenneth D. Bishop, MD, PhD
Tina Rizack, MD, MPH

Key Clinical Questions

1. What is the initial management of tumor-related emergencies?

2. What is the initial management of cancer treatment related emergencies?

3. Which oncologic emergencies require an intensive care setting and which can be managed on a hospitalist service? What are the indications for emergent consultation with other specialists?

INTRODUCTION

Patients with cancer are at risk for potentially life-threatening medical complications. The possibility of rapid decompensation in cancer patients requires preventive strategies, prompt recognition, and treatment when complications occur. Emergent conditions encountered in the inpatient setting may be due to the presence of cancer itself or may be the result of anticancer therapy. They may be structural or metabolic in etiology.

TUMOR-RELATED EMERGENCIES

■ HYPERCALCEMIA

Elevation of the total serum calcium may be associated with drugs, malignancy, hyperparathyroidism, and other diseases (such as sarcoidosis, tuberculosis, and endocrine disorders). Total calcium reflects the free or ionized calcium (the biologically active form of calcium), calcium bound to organic and inorganic anions, and that bound to albumin. When protein concentrations, especially albumin, are abnormal, total calcium levels change in the same direction whereas ionized calcium remains relatively constant due to hormonal control. The biologically active calcium level can be estimated by calculating the corrected calcium for the serum albumin level or by measuring serum ionized calcium concentration (see Chapter 240 [Disorders of Calcium and Phosphorous]).

PRACTICE POINT

- Volume replacement with isotonic saline is the first line of therapy for symptomatic hypercalcemia.
- A single elevated serum calcium concentration should be repeated to confirm the diagnosis.
- **Corrected calcium = Serum calcium (mg/dL) + 0.8*(normal albumin level – patient's albumin level).**
- The ionized calcium level may provide a more accurate diagnosis of hypercalcemia, as the corrected total calcium level can be inaccurate in the setting of reduced GFR[CE12], in the presence of a paraprotein, or in the setting of acidosis.

Up to 30% of patients with cancer develop hypercalcemia. The most common associated malignancies are breast cancer, lung cancer, and myeloma. The mechanisms by which cancer causes hypercalcemia include osteolytic metastases and increased bone resorption, tumor secretion of parathyroid hormone-related protein (PTHrP), and increased production of 1,25-dihydroxyvitamin D.

Clinical presentation

The severity of symptoms from hypercalcemia typically correlates with the degree of calcium level elevation and the acuity of rise. Patients with moderate hypercalcemia (corrected calcium ≥12 mg/dL) develop constipation, fatigue, and depressed mood. Progressive symptoms of polyuria, polydipsia, anorexia, nausea, weakness, lethargy, confusion, and coma may occur as the calcium level rises (corrected calcium ≥14 mg/dL). Acute hypercalcemia can cause QT shortening that can result in cardiac arrhythmias. Profound muscle weakness may also be a sign of acute, severe hypercalcemia. In general, hypercalcemia associated with malignancy portends a poor prognosis, as it is often attributable to large tumor burden or metastatic skeletal disease.

Diagnosis

Hypercalcemia may be the presenting sign of a new malignancy. Hypercalcemia of malignancy is often associated with low PTH levels. Elevated PTHrP may indicate a paraneoplastic syndrome, and computed tomography (CT) scan with contrast should be performed to evaluate for a solid tumor. Elevated 1,25-dihydroxyvitamin D can be associated with sarcoidosis or lymphoma. When PTHrP and vitamin D levels are normal, serum protein electrophoresis with immunofixation, urine protein electrophoresis, and thyroid-stimulating hormone should be measured.

Management

Patients with calcium levels ≤11.5 mg/dL often have mild or no symptoms and may not require urgent correction. With calcium levels over 12 mg/dL, corrective therapy is indicated even if patients are only mildly symptomatic, as long-term complications such as soft-tissue calcium deposition are possible. When calcium levels exceed 14 mg/dL, urgent treatment is necessary as these patients are at high risk for complications such as hypovolemia, hypotension, acute kidney injury, obtundation, muscle weakness, and arrhythmia. Volume replacement with isotonic saline at a rate tolerated by patient's comorbidities (taking risk of congestive heart failure and pulmonary edema into consideration) is indicated and will often bring calcium levels down by 1 to 2 mg/dL. Patients with malnutrition or malignancy-associated hypoalbuminemia may also be less tolerant of rapid volume saline infusion given the high risk of third space fluid redistribution.

There is very little high-quality evidence to support the benefit of loop diuretic use (such as furosemide) to treat hypercalcemia. The theoretical benefit has historically been attributed to the ability of loop diuretics to drive calciuria by reducing Ca^{2+} reabsorption in the loop of Henle. More recent consensus recommends the use of loop diuretics only in the setting of volume overload due to overly rapid saline infusion, so as to avoid the risk of overdiuresis and clinically significant hypovolemia.

Calcitonin use is recommended for severe hypercalcemia. Calcitonin administered via the subcutaneous route is believed to be more effective than the intranasal formulation, and acts to lower serum Ca^{2+} levels primarily by inhibition of bone resorption. The effect of calcitonin tends to reflect in the serum calcium levels within the first several hours after administration, and can provide temporary benefit while waiting for longer-term treatments to take effect.

PRACTICE POINT

- Repeated calcitonin administration results in tachyphylaxis and use should be limited to a total of 48 hours.

Longer-term stabilization of bone resorption can be achieved by the administration of bisphosphonates, which can have profound effect on serum Ca^{2+} levels. Pamidronate and zoledronic acid are the most commonly used bisphosphonates for hypercalcemia of malignancy, with zoledronic acid being generally preferred due to more effective correction of Ca^{2+} and faster administration time. Bisphosphonates should be administered at the same time as calcitonin and the initiation of intravenous fluid, as their effect can be delayed up to 4 days after the dose is given. Denosumab use is largely based on case reports and should be reserved for patients refractory to zoledronic acid or for patients with severe renal failure precluding the use of bisphosphonates.

Hemodialysis can rapidly lower the serum calcium levels when medical management fails to reduce calcium levels. This option can also be considered in patients who have severe altered mental status or coma, cardiac arrhythmias, or in patients with heart failure or renal insufficiency who will not tolerate large volume fluid administration.

■ SPINAL CORD COMPRESSION

Malignant spinal cord compression (MSCC) has the potential to cause significant morbidity from cancer due to the high prevalence of pain, sensory loss, paralysis, and urinary or bowel dysfunction. MSCC caused by metastatic disease is significantly more common than symptoms caused by primary spine tumors, and has been reported to occur in approximately 2.5% of advanced cancer patients, with incidence varying widely depending on tumor type. The three cancers that most commonly cause MSCC are lung cancer, breast cancer, and myeloma.

Clinical presentation

Symptoms from MSCC depend on the anatomic level of spinal cord injury. Pain is present in up to 95% of patients with cord compression and often precedes other neurologic signs and symptoms. Pain often starts local to the site of cord injury and tends to increase in intensity as injury to the cord progresses. Pain can also present in a radicular pattern with radiation of pain down a limb; this tends to be more common with metastatic disease in the lumbar spine rather than other sites. Motor weakness is present in up to 85% of cases of MSCC, and is generally symmetric in distribution. Lesions above the thoracic spine can result in weakness of the upper extremities, and lesions in the thoracic spine and above the cauda equina tend to cause weakness in the lower-extremity flexors. Sensory deficits manifest between one and five anatomic levels below the site of compression. Saddle anesthesia is associated with cauda equina lesions.

PRACTICE POINT

- Magnetic resonance imaging (MRI) is the gold standard imaging modality for evaluation for malignant spinal cord compression.
- New onset of back pain in a cancer patient should always be evaluated given the potential for permanent skeletal or neurological damage from vertebral metastases.
- **Lhermitte's phenomenon** is a sensation of electricity traveling down the spine triggered by flexion of the neck muscles, and can be associated with malignant spinal cord compression.

MSCC can also cause autonomic symptoms such as urinary retention, though this rarely presents as an isolated symptom. Bowel and bladder dysfunction are typically late findings and rarely occur without associated pain and other neurologic dysfunction. Ataxia can be caused by sensory loss or spinocerebellar tract compromise (see Chapter 104 [The Neurologic Examination] and Chapter 106 [Weakness: How to Localize the Problem]).

Diagnosis

The presence of any symptom suggesting spinal cord compromise, especially in the setting of known malignancy, requires **immediate** evaluation with MRI. Evaluation of the entire epidural space and thecal sac is necessary as multilevel disease is often present. Prior to the validation of MRI as the gold-standard imaging modality, CT myelography was used to screen for MSCC. Patients with strong contraindications to MRI, such as those with incompatible hardware or a nonremovable foreign body can undergo CT myelography as an alternative to MRI. Computed tomography without myelography, plain radiograph, and bone scan are not sufficiently sensitive to rule out spinal cord compression, therefore, these should not be used in this setting.

Management

The detection of spinal cord ischemia on imaging requires prompt intervention given the risk of rapid progression. An 8- or 10-mg bolus of intravenous dexamethasone followed by dexamethasone 16-mg PO daily divided in two or four doses and tapered gradually once definitive therapy is underway is accepted practice. Some recommend a higher bolus dose (up to 100-mg IV) and higher maintenance doses (up to 96 mg/d PO for 3 days with taper over 10 days) for grade 3 paresis (defined as tumor impingement on the spinal cord) or higher, though this is not common practice given the relatively high complication rates relative to lower glucocorticoid doses.

PRACTICE POINT

- Prompt systemic glucocorticoids are indicated in any patient with neurologic deficits from malignant spinal cord compression unless these are medically contraindicated.

Depending on the tumor type, both radiation therapy and surgical resection can be effective in decompressing the spinal cord. Surgical intervention can be limited by patient performance status and tumor location but may be preferable in patients with a single site of disease, better overall prognosis, vertebral instability, and in patients with nonradiosensitive tumors (such as melanoma). Surgical decompression is typically followed by radiation. Intraspinal bony fragment, sphincter dysfunction, and no response to previous radiotherapy treatment are also indications for surgery. According to a recent review, decompressive surgery is only indicated in 10% to 15% of patients with MSCC, and the majority of patients undergo radiation therapy.

For patients with a poor prognosis, a single fraction of 8 Gray (Gy) of external-beam radiation therapy can confer symptomatic benefit. In patients with a better prognosis and performance status, higher doses of radiation such as 30 Gy given in 10 fractions can be considered.

Recurrence of MSCC occurs in up to 14% of cases. Surgical intervention is indicated for recurrences located within a previous radiation field, but for patients who are not good candidates for surgery, reirradiation can be considered. Precise radiation methods such as intensity-modulated radiation therapy, radiosurgery, stereotactic body radiotherapy, or proton-beam radiation therapy can be employed to minimize cumulative-dose-related toxicities.

■ SUPERIOR VENA CAVA SYNDROME

Superior vena cava (SVC) syndrome is a constellation of symptoms resulting from superior vena cava obstruction. It occurs in approximately 15,000 patients in the United States per year. Symptoms correlate to degree of tumor expansion and resulting vessel impingement, and onset tends to be subacute. Severity may range from mild, including neck swelling and engorgement of the neck and arm vessels, to severe, including cerebral edema, functional compromise of the larynx and pharynx, and coma. The majority of cases are malignant, most frequently due to lung cancer, lymphoma, or primary mediastinal tumors. The increased use of chronic intravascular catheters has resulted in an increasing proportion of SVC thrombus causing SVC syndrome, as well.

TABLE 176-1 Symptoms and Signs Associated with SVC Syndrome

Sign or Symptom	Frequency (%)
Facial edema	82
Arm edema	46
Distended neck veins	63
Distended chest veins	53
Facial plethora	20
Visual symptoms	2
Dyspnea	54
Cough	54
Hoarseness	17
Stridor	4
Syncope	10
Headaches	9
Dizziness	6
Confusion	4
Obtundation	2

Modified from Wilson LD, Detterbeck FC, Yahalom J. *N Engl J Med*. 2007;356: 1862-1869. Copyright © 2007. Reprinted with permission from Massachusetts Medical Society.

Clinical presentation

The most common presenting symptoms of SVC syndrome are head, neck, or arm edema (**Table 176-1**). Acuity of onset depends on the degree of SVC obstruction, rapidity of development of collateral vessels, and rate of growth of the culprit lesion. Other common signs and symptoms are cough, voice hoarseness, dyspnea, stridor, and dysphagia. Cerebral edema is rare but has been reported and can be fatal, but overall, SVC syndrome very rarely directly results in death.

PRACTICE POINT

- The urgency of intervention for SVC syndrome depends on the severity of symptoms and the underlying etiology.
- In a patient with mild symptoms, there are times when treatment may be delayed in order to first obtain a tissue diagnosis.
- Intramuscular injection in the arms should be avoided given the decreased rates of drainage and potential for delayed absorption in patients with the SVC syndrome.

Diagnosis

Duration of symptoms, presence of a known malignancy, and recent intravascular procedures are pertinent historical elements. Superior vena cava syndrome may be the presenting manifestation of a previously unknown malignancy, or may develop later in the disease course. Diagnosis is confirmed with a CT scan of the chest with intravenous contrast. If a patient cannot receive contrast, MRI can also be used to evaluate for SVC compression. Biopsy is warranted if the patient has no known cancer diagnosis, and bronchoscopy and mediastinoscopy can generally be performed with low risk of hemorrhage despite the presence of SVC syndrome. Superior vena cavogram is the gold standard for diagnosing SVC thrombosis.

Management

Treatment of malignant SVC syndrome includes direct relief of the obstructing process, and treatment of the underlying malignancy. Median life expectancy for patients with SVC syndrome is approximately 6 months, with wide variations in this depending on the culprit malignancy. It has been shown that this estimate is a function of the type of cancer and disease stage rather than the presence of SVC compression specifically.

Patients with lymphoma, small-cell lung cancer, and germ-cell tumors have been shown to respond to systemic chemotherapy more quickly than non–small-cell lung cancers. Radiation therapy is also an important component of SVC syndrome treatment, as the types of tumors commonly known to cause SVC syndrome are often radiosensitive. Improvement may be detectable as early as 72 hours after initiation of treatment, but complete relief of obstruction may take up to 2 weeks after onset of radiotherapy.

Intravascular stent placement is an option for patients who require urgent intervention, especially if there is a potential delay in obtaining a tissue diagnosis. It is also recommended in patients whose primary tumor does not respond well to chemotherapy, such as mesothelioma. Complications from stent placement include bleeding, perforation, infection, pulmonary embolism, and stent migration. Surgical bypass is a possible management option, but with improvement in stent techniques, it is less commonly used except in cases where resection is the primary treatment modality, such as with thymomas. The use of glucocorticoid therapy, loop diuretics, or patient positioning to relieve symptoms from SVC compression is not supported by high-quality evidence but in some cases may confer benefit.

■ SIADH

The syndrome of inappropriate secretion of antidiuretic hormone (SIADH) is a common paraneoplastic disorder often associated with small-cell lung carcinoma seen less commonly in other malignancies (**Table 176-2**). The hallmark finding is normovolemic hyponatremia due to excess arginine vasopressin. This results in the kidney's inability to eliminate free water due resulting in excess total body water. This is often exacerbated by a subsequent increase in urinary sodium excretion, further lowering the plasma sodium level.

Clinical presentation

The most common presenting symptoms of SIADH are nausea, vomiting, headaches, difficulty concentrating, delirium, and muscle cramping. In severe cases (serum sodium <125 mmol/L or onset <48 hours), patients may develop hallucinations, seizures, coma, or respiratory failure (see Chapter 242 [Disorders of Sodium and Water Balance]).

Diagnosis

A diagnosis of SIADH is made by serum and urinary testing (**Table 176-3**).

TABLE 176-2 Malignancies Associated with SIADH

Small-cell lung cancer
Brain (primary and metastatic)
Mesothelioma
Head and neck cancers
Gastric cancer
Melanoma
Pancreas cancer
Bladder cancer
Endometrial cancer
Endocrine thymoma
Non-Hodgkin Lymphoma
Ewing sarcoma

TABLE 176-3 Essential Features of SIADH

Lab Findings
Decreased effective osmolality (<275 mOsm/kg of water)
Urinary osmolality >100 mOsm/kg of water during hypotonicity
Urinary sodium >40 mmol/L with normal dietary salt intake
Normal thyroid and adrenal function

Clinical Findings
Clinical euvolemia
No clinical signs of volume depletion of extracellular fluid
No orthostasis, tachycardia, decreased skin turgor, or dry mucous membranes
No clinical signs of excessive volume of extracellular fluid
No edema or ascites
No recent use of diuretic agents

From Ellison DH, Berl T. *N Engl J Med*. 2007;356:2064-2072. Copyright © 2007. Reprinted with permission from Massachusetts Medical Society.

Urinary osmolality must exceed 100 mOsm/kg H_2O in the setting of low plasma osmolality, and the patient must be clinically euvolemic to make a diagnosis of SIADH. Low uric acid, low blood urea nitrogen, and urinary sodium level >40 mmol/L in the setting of hyponatremia are also suggestive of SIADH but are not diagnostic of the condition.

Management

Asymptomatic patients with long-standing or mild hyponatremia may not require treatment. If the diagnosis is uncertain, infusion of 2 L of normal saline over 24 to 48 hours will often result in some improvement of serum sodium if the etiology of hyponatremia is volume depletion. Symptomatic patients with severe hyponatremia or hyponatremia that develops over a short (<48 hours) period need rapid intervention. Treatment generally consists of short-term correction of serum sodium levels for symptom management, and longer-term treatment of the underlying cause to decrease the risk of recurrence.

The initial intervention to correct serum sodium levels should be restriction of fluid intake, with a goal of total intake of less than 800 to 1000 mL fluids/d. Hypertonic saline may be required in selected patients with neurologic symptoms or signs.

PRACTICE POINT

Indications for hypertonic saline in SIADH:
- Severe symptoms (seizure, obtundation, or coma) to prevent cerebral edema.
- Subarachnoid hemorrhage due to increased risk of cerebral vasospasm and infarction with fluid restriction.

Correction of serum sodium with hypertonic saline should be administered in the intensive care unit with frequent monitoring of sodium levels to avoid overly rapid correction.
- A correction rate faster than 10 mEq/L per 24 hours may result in osmotic demyelination with permanent neurologic sequelae.

An intravenous bolus of 100 mL of 3% saline may correct the serum sodium enough to avoid neurologic damage. If symptoms continue to worsen, this can be repeated twice more at 10-minute intervals. Upon improvement of symptoms, frequent monitoring of serum sodium is required to avoid correcting the sodium level too rapidly.

Maintenance of sodium levels can be achieved with ongoing fluid restriction (800-1000 mL/d), oral salt tablets, or loop diuretic therapy to impair urinary concentration. SIADH may improve with treatment of the underlying malignancy, therefore sodium levels should be monitored regularly over the course of systemic therapy.

TREATMENT-RELATED EMERGENCIES

■ TUMOR LYSIS SYNDROME

Tumor lysis syndrome (TLS) is the most common emergency associated with treatment of hematologic cancers. Complications are due to metabolic and electrolyte abnormalities resulting from release of intracellular contents of tumor cells. Recognition of the potential for TLS and preventative measures can mitigate the risk of complications.

Clinical presentation

A patient undergoing treatment for a hematologic malignancy or with a high tumor burden prior to treatment who develops oliguria (average urine output of <0.5 mL/kg/h for 6 hours) should raise suspicion for developing TLS. Signs and symptoms correlate to electrolyte and metabolic disturbances. These include cardiac arrhythmia, sudden cardiac death, seizure, neuromuscular irritability (including tetany, paresthesias[CE13], or carpopedal spasm), hypotension, and heart failure.

Diagnosis

Tumor lysis syndrome can be diagnosed by clinical or laboratory criteria (**Table 176-4**). Laboratory criteria include a uric acid >8 mg/dL, a phosphorus level over 4.5 mg/dL, potassium level >6 mEq/L, and corrected calcium <7 mg/dL or ionized calcium <1.12 mg/dL. These can also be associated with an increase in the creatinine level of 0.3 mg/dL or a single value >1.5 times the upper limit of age-related normal for a single measurement.

There is a higher risk of TLS in hematologic malignancies than in solid tumors, in patients with bulky tumor or extensive metastatic disease, organ infiltration by cancer cells, or bone marrow involvement. These cancers typically have a high proliferation rate, are highly sensitive to anticancer therapy, or require high intensity of therapy. Additional risk factors include the presence of renal outflow obstruction or infiltration of the kidney parenchyma. Patients are also more likely to develop TLS if they have pre-existing nephropathy, volume depletion, recent exposure to nephrotoxins, or inadequate hydration during treatment.

PRACTICE POINT

- Hydration to preserve kidney function and electrolyte management are primary goals of tumor lysis syndrome management.
- Patients should be placed on cardiac monitoring if tumor lysis syndrome is suspected.

TABLE 176-4 Cairo-Bishop Criteria for Tumor Lysis Syndrome

Clinical criteria
Creatinine ≥1.5 ULN
Cardiac arrhythmia/sudden death
Seizure
Laboratory criteria (2+ changes, within treatment day −3 or +7)
Uric acid ≥8 mg/dL (476 µmol/L) or 25% increase from baseline
Potassium ≥6 mEq/L (6 mmol/L) or 25% increase from baseline
Phos ≥4.5 mg/dL (1.45 mmol/L) or 25% increase from baseline
Calcium ≤7 mg/dL (1.75 mmol/L) or 25% decrease from baseline

Management

Intravenous hydration up to 3000 mL/m²/d is a mainstay of preventive treatment for TLS to optimize renal perfusion and glomerular filtration, as well as to minimize urinary acidosis. In patients with low urine output despite optimal hydration, use of a loop diuretic to achieve diuresis of at least 2 mL/kg/h is recommended. Reduction of uric acid level can preserve or improve renal function. Allopurinol prevents formation of uric acid but can take 2 or more days to take effect in the setting of hyperuricemia. Rasburicase is an enzyme that catalyzes the conversion of uric acid to allantoin, which is highly water soluble and does not precipitate in acidic solution. Rasburicase has been compared to allopurinol with regard to TLS prevention and its usage was found to result in lower uric acid levels, lower phosphorous levels, and better kidney function versus patients treated with allopurinol.

Potassium and phosphorous levels should be checked every 4 to 6 hours in patients at high risk for TLS, and continuous cardiac monitoring should be used. Hyperkalemia can be temporarily managed with insulin and beta-agonist therapy, and the use of calcium gluconate can reduce the risk of arrhythmia when hyperkalemia is present. In this setting, rapid removal of potassium with hemodialysis should be considered. Close monitoring of phosphate levels and prompt reduction can mitigate the risk of clinically significant hypocalcemia. Low calcium levels can lead to cardiac arrhythmias and neuromuscular irritability. If necessary, supplementation with calcium should be limited to the lowest dose that is effective in reducing symptoms as excess serum calcium drives precipitation of calcium-phosphate crystals. The duration of risk for TLS varies with the tumor type and selected treatment regimen, and monitoring may be necessary for up to 7 days after initiation of treatment.

■ INFUSION REACTIONS

Many chemotherapeutic agents are associated with a risk for systemic infusion reactions, ranging from mild flushing and itching to anaphylaxis. The risk of fatal reactions with these agents requires that care providers are familiar with the rates of reaction for each agent, the types of reactions associated with them, and how to promptly intervene. Patient education about what signs or symptoms are suggestive of an infusion reaction is also of paramount importance, as this can help with accurate and timely reporting of symptoms.

PRACTICE POINT

- Any signs or symptoms that suggest the development of an infusion reaction should prompt immediate discontinuation of the infusion.
- Orders for steroids, antihistamines, and bronchodilators should be in place at the start of the infusion so quick treatment can be delivered if necessary.

Clinical presentation

Though there are some chemotherapeutic agents that have idiosyncratic reactions associated with them, skin flushing, itching, or angioedema should prompt consideration of anaphylaxis. Often, respiratory symptoms present, such as cough, dyspnea, chest tightness, a sensation of the throat closing, or a change in voice quality due to laryngeal edema. Gastrointestinal symptoms associated with infusion reactions include abdominal cramping, nausea, vomiting, or diarrhea. Reactions can progress to include neurologic symptoms such as dizziness, seizure, or tunnel vision. Signs of an infusion reaction typically occur during or a few hours after the agent is administered, but it is important to recognize that some agents, including some monoclonal antibodies or platinum agents, are

TABLE 176-5 NCI-CTCAE v4.0 Infusion-Related Reactions

Grade 1	Grade 2	Grade 3	Grade 4	Grade 5
Mild transient reaction; infusion interruption not indicated; intervention not indicated	Therapy or infusion interruption indicated but responds promptly to symptomatic treatment (eg, antihistamines, NSAIDs, narcotics, intravenous fluids); prophylactic medication indicated for ≤24 h	Prolonged (ie, not rapidly responsive to symptomatic medication and/or brief interruption of infusion); recurrence of symptoms following initial improvement; hospitalization indicated for other clinical sequelae	Life-threatening consequences; urgent intervention indicated	Death

associated with delayed reactions or the development of reactions with repeated infusions (see Chapter 230 [Allergy and Anaphylaxis]).

The more common chemotherapeutic agents associated with systemic infusion reactions are platinum drugs, taxanes, cytarabine, etoposide, and monoclonal antibodies. Anaphylaxis is most commonly associated with platinum drugs and taxanes. Overall, severe systemic reactions are rare, occurring with ≤5% of infusions, provided patients receive appropriate prophylaxis and prompt treatment if signs of a reaction appear.

Diagnosis

Systemic infusion reactions are diagnosed clinically, with no strict diagnostic criteria to define them. The NCI[CE14] provides a grading system to classify reactions, making a distinction between hypersensitivity reactions and acute infusion reactions (**Table 176-5**).

Management

Prophylactic management of infusion reactions is specific to the chemotherapeutic agents being used, whereas the treatment of a developing infusion reaction follows a somewhat standard algorithm. Standing orders for medications such as epinephrine, diphenhydramine, hydrocortisone, and inhaled albuterol should be in place for any patient undergoing treatment with an agent known to cause hypersensitivity reactions so medications can be given promptly. At the onset of a reaction, the infusion should be stopped immediately, but in some grade I or II reactions with agents such as taxanes or some monoclonal antibodies, restarting the infusion at a slower rate can mitigate the likelihood of a recurrence and may facilitate completion of therapy.

■ FEBRILE NEUTROPENIA

Fever that occurs in a neutropenic patient is a true emergency given the high risk of developing fulminant systemic infection. Fevers in this patient population are common, occurring in 10% to 50% of patients with solid tumors, and over 80% of patients with hematologic cancers. Empiric and timely use of antibiotics in this setting results in decreased morbidity and mortality, even if no source of infection is identified. The Infectious Disease Society of America has generated guidelines based on high-quality evidence to steer management of these patients. Infections may be caused by Gram-negative and Gram-positive organisms, with the latter becoming more prevalent in the era of antibiotic prophylaxis and increasing use of indwelling catheters for cancer patients. Increasing rates of antibiotic resistance also need to be considered when selecting therapy for patients with febrile neutropenia. (See Chapter 204 [Infections of the Immunocompromised Host].)

Clinical presentation

Fever is defined as a single oral temperature of 101°F (38.3°C) or a temperature over 100.4°F (38°C) sustained for an hour. A specific source of infection is identified in only 20% to 30% of patients who develop febrile neutropenia, and often fever is the only presenting sign. It is important to recognize that patients with immune suppression from malignancy or chemotherapy may not mount as

robust a response as one with an intact immune system; therefore, severity of symptoms may not be proportional to the severity of infection.

Diagnosis

Neutropenia is defined as an absolute neutrophil count (ANC) of <500 cells/mm³ or an ANC that is expected to decrease below 500 cells/mm³ over the next 48 hours. The ANC is the percentage of the total white blood cell count comprised of polymorphonuclear cells/neutrophils and band forms combined. Evaluation should include a targeted history and physical examination to evaluate for a specific site of infection. Digital rectal examination should be avoided in patients with neutropenia, but a careful perianal examination may reveal a source of infection such as abscess or fissure.

Additional laboratory testing should also include creatinine, transaminases, bilirubins, and blood cultures (from a peripheral site and from a central catheter if present) and urine culture. Other infectious testing should be directed by clinical presentation or suspected site of infection. Imaging studies should also be directed by signs of symptoms at presentation.

> **PRACTICE POINT**
>
> - Antibiotic therapy should be started promptly in the setting of febrile neutropenia as delay in treatment has been associated with increased mortality.
> - Digital rectal examination should be avoided in patients with neutropenia, but a careful perianal examination may reveal a source of infection such as abscess or fissure.

Patients with febrile neutropenia can be risk stratified by the Multinational Association for Supportive Care in Cancer (MASCC) risk index (**Table 176-6**). The MASCC score stratifies patients who are at high risk for complications and require hospital admission for treatment.

TABLE 176-6 MASCC Score for Febrile Neutropenia

Category	Weight
Burden of illness: no or mild symptoms	5
No hypotension	5
No chronic obstructive pulmonary disease	4
Solid tumor or no previous invasive fungal infection	4
Outpatient status	3
Burden of disease: moderate symptoms	3
No dehydration	3
Age <60 y	2

A MASCC score ≥21 identifies low-risk patients.
From Klastersky J, Paesmans M. *Support Care Cancer.* 2013;21:1487-1495. With permission of Springer.

Management

Early studies reported mortality rates up to 70% with delay of antibiotics. In the setting of febrile neutropenia, antibiotics should be given immediately after blood cultures have been obtained and should not be delayed for any other reason. The goal of empiric treatment is to broadly cover rapidly fatal infections. Patients with a high-risk MASCC score (between 0 and 20 points) require hospital admission for intravenous antibiotics given a known increased risk of serious medical complications.

Initial therapy should be an antipseudomonal beta-lactam antibiotic (**Table 176-7**). These include cefepime, piperacillin-tazobactam, meropenem, or imipenem-cilastatin. Ceftazadime is included as an option for initial therapy in current guidelines but it is falling out of favor given limited Gram-positive coverage and rising resistance rates in many antibiograms. Institutional standards regarding antibiotic resistance and use should be utilized to guide therapy.

Vancomycin and other agents that target Gram-positive microbes are not currently recommended in the initial treatment regimen for all patients. Gram-positive coverage should be added in patients with skin or soft-tissue infection, pneumonia, suspected catheter-related infection, hemodynamic instability or if antimicrobial resistance is demonstrated. Anaerobic coverage should be included if there is suspicion for intra-abdominal infection, mucositis, typhilitis, or anaerobic bacteremia.

Patients with penicillin allergy who cannot tolerate cephalosporins due to a hypersensitivity reaction should be treated with combination therapy. Aztreonam and vancomycin or ciprofloxacin and clindamycin are acceptable alternatives to penicillin agents. Selection should be tailored to regional antibiotic resistance patterns. For patients who require broad Gram-positive therapy, linezolid can be used as an alternative but the risk of myelosuppression needs to be taken into consideration in some cancer patient populations. Daptomycin is another alternative for Gram-positive coverage in nonpulmonary infections.

Antifungal therapy should be considered in high-risk patients with persistent or recurrent fever after 4 to 7 days of antibacterial coverage.

TABLE 176-7 Antipseudomonas Dosing of Antibiotics

Cefepime	2 g IV every 8 h
Meropenem	1 g IV every 8 h
Imipenem-cilastatin	500 mg IV every 6 h
Piperacillin-tazobactam	4.5 g IV every 6-8 h
Ceftazidime	2 g IV every 8 h

CONCLUSION

There are a number of emergent conditions associated with malignancy and its treatment that can present with severe symptoms or can progress over a short period of time. Identifying and treating oncologic emergencies requires vigilance and often the need to consult appropriate services, such as radiation oncology or surgery, to preserve vital functions. Prevention and prompt treatment is imperative to prevent short- and long-term sequelae or death in this population.

SUGGESTED READINGS

Cairo MS, Bishop M. Tumour lysis syndrome: new therapeutic strategies and classification. *Br J Haematol*. 2004;127:3-11.

Ellison DH, Berl T. The syndrome of inappropriate antidiuresis. *N Engl J Med*. 2007;356:2064-2072.

Freifeld AG, Bow EJ, Sepkowitz K, et al. Clinical practice guideline for the use of antimicrobial agents in neutropenic patients with cancer: 2010 Update by the Infectious Diseases Society of America. *Clin Infect Dis*. 2011;52:e56-e93.

Howard SC, Jones DP, Pui CH. The tumor lysis syndrome. *N Engl J Med*. 2001;364:1844-1854.

Klastersky J, Paesmans M. The Multinational Association for Supportive Care in Cancer (MASCC) risk index score: 10 years of use for identifying low-risk febrile neutropenic cancer patients. *Support Care Cancer*. 2013;21:1487-1495.

Lenz, HJ. Management and preparedness for infusion and hypersensitivity reactions. *Oncologist*. 2007;12:601-609.

Loblaw DA, Mitera, G, Ford M, et al. A 2011 updated systematic review and clinical practice guideline for the management of malignant extradural spinal cord compression. *Int J Radiation Oncol Biol Phys*. 2012;84:312-317.

Lyman GH, Abellab E, Pettengell R. Risk factors for febrile neutropenia among patients with cancer receiving chemotherapy: a systematic review. *Crit Rev Oncol Hematol*. 2014;90: 190-199.

Rades D, Abrahm JL. The role of radiotherapy for metastatic epidural spinal cord compression. *Nat Rev Clin Oncol*. 2010;7: 590-598.

Rosner MW and Dalkin AC. Electrolyte disorders associated with cancer. *Adv Chronic Kidney Dis*. 2014;21:7-17.

Wilson LD, Detterbeck FC, Yahalom J. Superior vena cava syndrome with malignant causes. *N Engl J Med*. 2007;356:1862-1869.

CHAPTER 177

Approach to the Patient with Suspected Malignancy

Kerry Reynolds, MD

Aditya Bardia, MD, MPH

Key Clinical Questions

1 What are the next steps in evaluation and management priorities for patients admitted to the hospital with suspected cancer diagnosis, including carcinoma of unknown primary?

2 What are the common tests, including molecular tests, utilized for cancer diagnosis and their significance?

3 What are the key issues to consider before discharging a patient admitted with suspected/new cancer diagnosis?

INTRODUCTION

As an inpatient provider, one must adapt to each individual patient presentation of suspected malignancy, and expedite a workup with the goal of obtaining enough clinical, laboratory, and radiographic data for diagnosis. Most patients that are ill enough to require hospitalization with suspected malignancy present with either complications of their disease, paraneoplastic syndromes, or advanced stage of cancer. While it is important to obtain a comprehensive history and physical exam, every patient should be asked about the following:

- Details of symptom duration and chronology leading to admission.
- Comorbidities, any previous cancers, premalignant or spontaneously regressing lesions, and/or prior history of chemotherapy or radiation.
- Risk factors causing predisposition for certain malignancies such as alcohol, tobacco, drug use, occupations with notable exposures, use of hormone replacement therapy.
- Family history of any malignancies.

The next steps in assessment and management can be tailored to the particular patient presentation.

Knowledge of the incidence of common cancer across various age groups may help with the pretest probability when a patient is admitted with a suspected cancer diagnosis. Five cases highlight common presentations of suspected malignancy. These cases provide a diagnostic framework, but cannot be comprehensive due to the variety or patient characteristics and disease presentations.

PRACTICE POINT

- Important to assess for comorbidities, any previous cancers, premalignant or spontaneously regressing lesions, and/or prior history of chemotherapy or radiation.

EPIDEMIOLOGY

It is estimated that there will be more than 1.5 million new cases of cancer diagnosed in the United States in 2015. Breast cancer accounts for 29% of all newly diagnosed cancers in females, and it is the most common noncutaneous malignancy among females in the United States. In 2015, it is estimated that 231,840 women will be diagnosed with breast cancer. Among males, prostate cancer is the most common malignancy and accounts for 26% of new cancer cases in males. In 2015, it is estimated that 220,840 men will be diagnosed with prostate cancer. Lung cancer is second most common cancer among males and females followed by colorectal cancer.

While heart disease is the leading cause of death among all ages, cancer is actually the leading cause of death among adults between ages 40 to 59 and 60 to 79, with lung cancer being the most common among both sexes. It is estimated that approximately 86,380 men and 71,660 women will die of lung cancer in 2015. It should be noted that while pancreatic cancer is not in the top five most common cause of cancer among males (in sequence they include prostate, lung, colon, bladder, and melanoma) or females (in sequence they include breast, lung, colon, uterine, and thyroid), it is the fourth most common cause of death among both males and females, and thus portends a poor prognosis.

While breast cancer is the most common cancer among females and prostate cancer among males, this estimate is based on overall incidence across lifetime, and the probability of specific cancers varies across different age groups. Among adolescents, leukemia is the most common cancer in both boys and girls. Among young adults (20-39 years), the common cancers include breast cancer, cervical cancer, leukemia, lymphoma, lung, colorectal, and central nervous system neoplasms. Among the elderly, besides breast, prostate, lung, and colorectal, other common cancers include ovarian, esophageal, pancreatic, and bladder cancer. The probability of death due to cancer also varies across different age groups and patients admitted to the hospital are likely the ones who have a worse prognosis. **Figures 177-1 A and B** summarize the top five leading causes of cancer-related deaths across different age groups.

Carcinoma of unknown primary or occult primary account for approximately 5% all newly diagnosed cancers. In 2015, it is estimated that there will be 31,510 patients with newly diagnosed cancers from unspecified sites. The incidence of carcinoma of unknown primary has been decreasing over time, partly due to newer diagnostic techniques, but still a primary site is identified in less than one-third of patients who present with an unknown primary. In general, patients with carcinoma of unknown primary have a poor prognosis and identification of the primary tumor can potentially lead to better outcomes.

In this chapter, we will review the evaluation and management of five common clinical presentations including new bone lesions, liver lesions, lymphadenopathy, mediastinal mass, and brain lesion. We will also review commonly used tumor markers, immunohistochemical tests, and molecular profiling. Lastly, the chapter will cover risk stratification and postacute care.

PRACTICE POINT

- While heart disease is the leading cause of death among all ages, cancer is actually the leading cause of death among adults between ages 40 to 59 and 60 to 79.

EVALUATION AND MANAGEMENT

CASE 177-1

BONE PAIN

A 57-year-old female presented to the emergency department with worsening lumbar back pain. The back pain started about 8 weeks ago and was felt to be from lifting a heavy box at work. She was initially treated conservatively with a course of nonsteroidal anti-inflammatory drugs and physical therapy, with no improvement in her symptoms. Her review of systems was positive for bony pain, most notably in the lumbar region, and a 10 lb weight loss over 3 months. She had no lower-extremity motor weakness or sensory change, gait instability, sciatica, saddle anesthesia, or urinary/fecal incontinence. She had no prior operations, and her only medication was 0.3 mg Premarin. She did not use alcohol, tobacco, or drugs. Her examination was unremarkable. Laboratory tests were normal except for an alkaline phosphatase of 223 and calcium of 10.4. Imaging with a lumbar spine magnetic resonance imaging (MRI) revealed evidence of multiple lesions concerning for metastatic disease.

Bone metastases

Bone metastases are a common complication of advanced disease, and can be a cause of significant morbidity. Roughly 80% of cases with bone metastasis have an underlying diagnosis of breast, lung, prostate, or renal cell carcinoma. However, many types of malignancies can spread to the bone.

PRACTICE POINT

- For bone metastasis, the cannot-miss diagnoses are spinal cord compression, pathological fracture, and severe hypercalcemia.

Approach if malignancy involves skeletal metastases

History should include assessment of cancer risk factors. As breast cancer is one of the top differentials in a females presenting with bone metastasis, clinicians should ask questions pertaining to breast

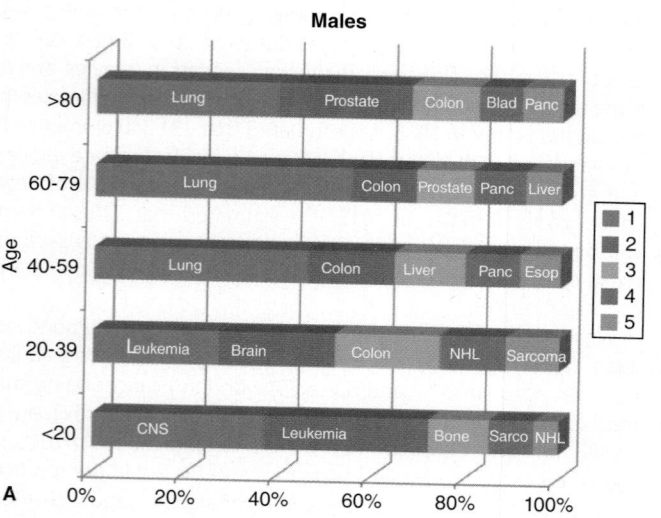

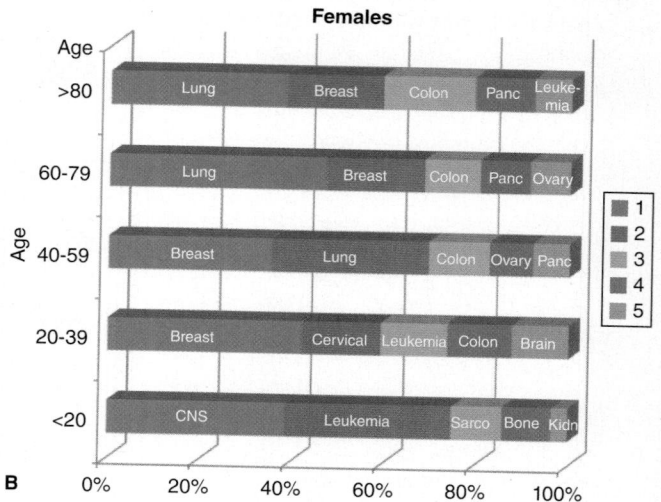

Figure 177-1 *The top five leading causes of cancer-related deaths across various age-groups among males (A) and females (B).* (Based on Siegel R, et al. *CA Cancer J Clin.* 2015;65[1]:5-29.)

cancer risk including date of last mammogram, prior abnormal mammograms or breast biopsies, family history of breast or ovarian cancer, parity, age at menopause, and whether any use of hormone replacement therapy.

A comprehensive physical exam should specifically include a breast exam, axillary lymph nodes (LNs), and in males a prostate exam including inguinal lymph nodes. Laboratory studies should include CBC with differential, metabolic panel, hepatic panel, lactic dehydrogenase, vitamin D level, serum protein electrophoresis, and serum-free light chains. If the patient is male over 40 years of age, prostate specific antigen (PSA) should be measured. The utility of other tumor markers is generally nonspecific, and therefore not helpful in the diagnostic workup. Specific radiographic studies should be performed for painful lesions and/or lesions in weight-bearing areas to rule out pathological fracture.

Imaging may reveal osteolytic or osteoblastic (sclerotic) lesions, or a mix of both. Plain films require 30% to 50% of bone mineral loss in order to visualize. Bone scan or computed tomography (CT) scan will identify bony metastasis, pathological fractures, and primary source of malignancy. Osteoblastic lesions are characterized by new bone formation and are best detected with the use of a nuclear medicine scan, such as a radionuclide bone scan. However, osteolytic lesions destroy normal bone and can be missed by bone scans. Osteolytic lesions, such as the ones seen in multiple myeloma, are often best picked up by skeletal survey (bone x-ray) or CT scans.

Differential if malignancy involves skeletal metastases

It is important to note that most types of cancer produce both osteolytic and osteoblastic lesions. However, there are specific tumor types that have a predilection for a certain presentation (see **Figure 177-2**).

Next step in evaluation

In Case 177-1, the highest malignancy on the differential would be breast cancer given her history of hormone replacement therapy, gender, age, and nulliparity. Therefore, a mammogram and breast ultrasound should be performed. In premenopausal female, particularly those with dense breasts, breast MRI should be considered if needed.

A biopsy is necessary to determine the histology and the site of origin of the cancer. Often, the oncology consult and interventionalist can assist with institution specific protocols and choosing the ideal site of biopsy. The general principles of choosing an optimal site for biopsy include:

- Choose the least invasive and safest modality of biopsy
- Core biopsy is preferred over fine needle aspirate
- Ensure there is an ability to get an adequate sample for further testing

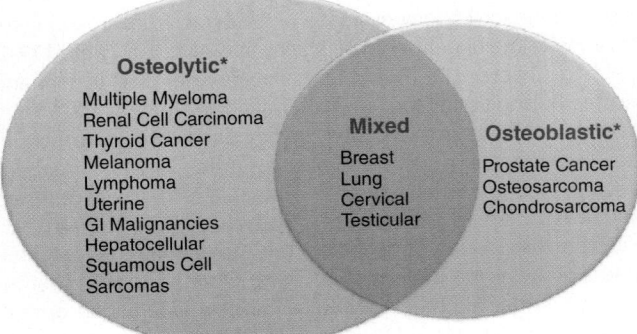

*Despite these cancers having a predilection for a certain type of bone metastasis, they can cause both types of lesions.

Figure 177-2 *Differential diagnosis according to type of bone lesion.*

Depending on institution and reagents used, a bone biopsy is less optimal due to the procedure of decalcification, which can alter DNA quality for subsequent molecular testing.

Management priorities

Management priorities in cases such as the one described above focus on pain relief and ruling out the "cannot-miss" diagnoses. In the case of painful bony metastasis, IV analgesics are often needed for immediate and effective pain relief in addition to adjuvant medications such as acetaminophen and NSAIDs.

The cannot-miss diagnoses are spinal cord compression, pathological fracture, and severe hypercalcemia. See **Table 177-1** for management of these conditions, or refer to Oncology Emergencies, Chapter 176 for additional details. Early diagnosis and intervention leads to decreased morbidity in this patient population.

CASE 177-2

LIVER METASTASIS

A 63-year-old male presents to the hospital with a 25 lb unintentional weight loss over the last 2 months, polydipsia, nocturia, right upper quadrant (RUQ) pain, pruritis, and jaundice. He had not sought medical attention previously, but his daughter brought him to the hospital because of his "yellowish hue." Review of systems was positive for the above, as well as fatigue and loss of appetite.

He had no prior surgical history, and was on no other medications. He had been a lifelong smoker with 40+ pack years, and consumed 4 to 5 alcoholic drinks per night, but no history of drug use. Past medical history is significant for alcohol related pancreatitis, chronic obstructive pulmonary disease (COPD), and gastroesophageal reflux disease (GERD), but no known inflammatory bowel disease (IBD), hepatitis B/C/NASH, or Barrett's esophagus. There was no family history of liver disease or cancer.

Exam: Notable for scleral icterus, jaundice, multiple excoriations of the skin, and midepigastric tenderness on deep palpation, but no murphy's sign or subcutaneous nodules in the para-umbilical area.

Labs: T Bili of 8.1, D Bili of 6.0, glucose of 360, AG 16, 2+ bilirubin in urinalysis.

Imaging: RUQ US—Large hypoechoic mass measuring 2.8 × 4.4 cm within the head of the pancreas, resulting in dilatation of the common bile duct to 10 mm. Extensive intrahepatic biliary ductal dilatation, with multiple liver lesions concerning for metastatic disease.

Liver metastases

The key step in the assessment of one or more liver lesions suspected to be malignant is to determine whether or not it is a primary liver or biliary tumor, versus a metastatic lesion from a cancer outside of the liver. Of note, it is much more common (18-40 ×) for liver lesions to represent metastatic disease rather than primary liver neoplasms.

Differential if suspected malignancy involves liver metastases

Nearly all metastatic solid malignancies have been reported to present with liver disease; however, the most common cancers are as follows:

- GI—pancreas, colon, esophageal, gastric, neuroendocrine
- Breast
- Lung
- GU (renal cell cancer, bladder, adrenal)
- GYN (ovary, endometrial)
- Melanoma
- Sarcoma

TABLE 177-1 Cannot-Miss Diagnosis in Patient Presenting with Persistent Back Pain

Diagnosis	Presentation	Evaluation	Management
Spinal cord compression	Progressive pain, worse when supine, proximal leg weakness, sensory changes or bowel/bladder incontinence	MRI for cord compression, CT myelography: used when MRI not available or accessible	IV Dexamethasone 10 mg followed by 4 mg IV q 6 h. STAT neurosurgical and radiation oncology consultations.
Pathological fracture	Localized musculoskeletal pain, persistent despite NSAIDS and/or narcotics	x-Ray followed by CT scan if suspicion is high enough	Pain relief, orthopedic and radiation oncology consultation for treatment and possible prophylactic fixation. Consideration of bisphosphonate (eg, zoledronic acid, pamidronate). Consideration of kyphoplasty or vertebroplasty for painful fractures.
Hypercalcemia	Confusion/altered mental status, fatigue, hypovolemia, abdominal pain, constipation, symptoms of nephrolithiasis	PTH, PTHrP, 1,25-Dihydroxyvitamin D	Normal saline to promote calciuresis. Bisphosophate with zolendronic acid or pamidronate. Consideration of calcitonin (2-8 U/kg SC every 6-12 h).

Even though the incidence is lower, a primary liver etiology must also be on the differential. There are three main categories of aggressive invasive carcinomas originating in the liver: hepatocellular carcinoma (HCC), cholangiocarcinoma, and gallbladder carcinoma.

Approach if suspected malignancy involves liver metastases

A complete physical exam should be performed, including digital rectal exam and guaiac fecal occult blood test for both sexes.

Laboratory studies include CBC with differential, with specific attention to platelet count (surrogate for portal venous hypertension), chemistry panel, serum levels of direct and indirect bilirubin, aspartate aminotransferase, alanine transaminatse, alkaline phosphatase, prothrombin time, international normalized ratio (INR), albumin, Ca, lactate dehydrogenase (LDH), and albumin. Tumor marker levels of carcinoembryonic antigen (CEA) and cancer antigen 19-9 (CA 19-9) should be sent if pancreatic biliary tract, or colon primary are suspected, and alpha-fetoprotein (AFP) if HCC is suspected. In a patient with known liver disease such as hepatitis C, a rising AFP is highly suggestive of HCC.

Further evaluation with imaging is usually needed. For patients with liver nodules on ultrasound, such as the patient presentation above, National Comprehensive Cancer Network guidelines recommend evaluation with a multiphase contrast-enhanced CT or MRI. A high-quality triple phase CT scan with intravenous and oral contrast medium provides an excellent assessment of disease extent in the liver, as well as elsewhere in the abdominal cavity. The three phases of the study allow for differentiation of metastatic lesions by their vascular nature. Colorectal, gastric, and lung metastases tend to be hypovascular lesions, and are best detected on portal venous phase contrast-enhanced images; renal cell carcinoma, melanoma, neuroendocrine, thyroid, and sarcoma are hypervascular, and enhance to a greater degree than normal liver parenchyma on arterial phase imaging.

Imaging can also be very useful in determining whether or not a biopsy is needed. The most common primary liver neoplasm in the United States is hepatocellular carcinoma, which appears as a hypodense mass on CT. Often, the HCC lesion receives direct blood flow from the hepatic artery, which lends it to having arterial hypervascularity on imaging in comparison to the liver parenchyma, which is fed by the portal vein. Again, a multiphase (unenhanced, arterial phase, portal venous phase, and delayed venous phase)

helical CT or dynamic contrast-enhanced MRI can be very suggestive of HCC. The characteristic finding is intense arterial update followed by contrast washout in the delayed venous phase. It is important to review the images with experts in abdominal radiology, because if there is a classical enhancement pattern for HCC, one can forego a biopsy.

Next step in evaluation

Besides imaging of the abdomen, a chest CT is also recommended to search of a primary and/or other evidence of metastatic disease.

If there is no evidence of a primary lesion, or if there is a suspected primary pancreatic mass such as in the case above, endoscopic evaluation can be useful for biopsy given that tissue must be obtained to complete the diagnostic workup. This may include endoscopic ultrasound, esophagodenoscopy, and/or colonoscopy. For women, a mammogram and breast ultrasound is also indicated in the search for the primary.

If there is concern for biliary obstruction in a patient presenting with jaundice and elevated bilirubin as in the case above, a gastroenterology consultation for consideration of MRCP or ERCP with biliary stenting should be strongly considered. For principles of obtaining a biopsy, see Case 177-1.

Management priorities

Management priorities in cases such as the one described above focus on identifying any evidence of biliary obstruction and identification of the underlying malignancy as outlined in **Table 177-2**. Refer to Chapter 158 (Biliary Disease: Jaundice, Obstruction, and Acute Cholangitis) for additional information.

In the case above, the patient had evidence of biliary obstruction and underwent successful biliary stenting with a subsequent decrease in the bilirubin levels. The pancreatic mass was biopsied and was found to be consistent with adenocarcinoma. Treatment in these cases depends on the tumor type, performance status, and overall patient preference. Often, systemic chemotherapy is the treatment of choice. Surgery is rarely an option, however there are exceptions—colorectal cancer, sarcomas, neuroendocrine (to palliate tumor-related pain or hormonal symptoms)—where a multidisciplinary team is assembled and surgery is considered.

TABLE 177-2 Management Priorities in Patient Presenting with Liver Lesions

Diagnosis	Presentation	Evaluation	Management
Biliary obstruction	Often painless jaundice, dark urine, and light-colored stools Fever, tachycardia, and possible hypotension if there is superimposed cholangitis	Labs including CBC with differential, chemistry panel including liver function tests, bilirubin, coags. Blood cultures if febrile Right upper quadrant ultrasound or abdominal CT scan as mentioned above often can identify the biliary obstruction If negative, consult gastroenterology for consideration of MRCP or ERCP	Urgent gastroenterology consultation for consideration of biliary stent to alleviate the obstruction Broad-spectrum antibiotics and IVF if febrile with concern of superimposed cholangitis

CASE 177-3

LYMPHADENOPATHY

A 56-year-old immunocompetent male presents to the hospital with painless "lumps" in his neck. In addition, he had been having difficulty breathing, dysphasia, and an altered voice for the past several days. Review of systems was negative for fevers, weight loss, or night sweats. He had not had any sore throat or viral illness recently. He took Ibuprofen, but his symptoms remained unchanged. He had no prior surgical history, and was on no other medications. He had been a lifelong smoker (2 packs/d) with a 60+ pack year history, and consumes 1 to 2 alcoholic drinks on a nightly basis, but had no history of drug use.

On examination, temperature was 98.1, blood pressure (BP) 130/85, heart rate (HR) 105 bpm. Notably, there were nontender, fixed lymph nodes measuring 1 to 3 cm in the cervical chain, bilaterally. The rest of the physical exam was unremarkable. Plain films of the chest and neck showed no evidence of tracheal deviation, foreign body, or extrinsic compression. ENT was called urgently since the symptoms were concerning for an upper airway obstruction.

Approach if suspected malignancy involves lymphadenopathy

Lymphadenopathy is defined as enlargement of lymph nodes, and is generally considered pathologic if >1 cm in adults, although this varies by lymph node basin involved. Unfortunately, there is not a clear definition of size for lymph nodes to be suspected of having a malignant etiology. There are data to suggest that an LN > 2 cm or an abnormal chest x-ray (CXR) increases the positive predictive value of the node being malignant, whereas recent ENT symptoms increases the negative predictive value. Other features suggestive of malignancy include progression over weeks to months, painless/nontender, matted or "hard," located in the supraclavicular, cervical/scalene, or isolated in the axillary region, or symptoms such as dysphagia/voice changes or B-type symptoms (fever, weight loss of >10%, and night sweats).

History is essential, and should include a thorough evaluation for any infectious or autoimmune signs or symptoms considering those, as opposed to malignancy, are the most common etiologies in a patient presenting with lymphadenopathy. Additional questions to determine the probability of an underlying malignancy include: any prior malignancy, HPV status, HIV/HHV8, history of organ transplant and EBV exposure, history of *H. pylori*, and use of tobacco and alcohol.

A complete physical exam should be performed. Further assessment (eg, ENT exam of tongue, buccal mucosa, gums, palate, full skin exam, evaluation of liver/spleen, breast exam) becomes necessary depending on the lymphatic region involved.

Basic laboratory studies include CBC with differential, chemistry panel, liver function tests, B-HCG if patient is of reproductive age,

and LDH. If there is concern for infectious, autoimmune, or granulomatous conditions, testing for EBV/CMV/HIV/viral panel/Toxo/Brucella/ANA/anti-ds DNA/ACE level is indicated.

Imaging techniques to aid in the determination as to whether an LN is malignant can begin with an ultrasound. The long axis (L)/short axis (S), or L/S ratio is a highly sensitive and specific test to differentiate between a benign or malignant LN. Over 95% of enlarged cervical nodes identified on US with an L/S ratio of greater than 2 are correctly diagnosed as benign. Similarly, patients with a rounder shape and L/S ratio of less than 2 are consistent with metastatic disease 95% of the time.

As long as there are no contraindications, additional imaging with CT scans and IV contrast is generally the next step in evaluating underlying malignancy. Given the high cost, use of positron emission tomography (PET) or PET-CT is generally limited to patients with neck lymphadenopathy suggestive of squamous-cell carcinoma or diffuse lymphadenopathy consistent with an aggressive lymphoma. Aside from those indications, the usefulness of PET-CT is less well defined, and should be discussed in consultation with oncology colleagues.

Differential of suspected malignancy with lymphadenopathy

The differential and the workup would vary according to the specific lymph node region involved (outlined in **Figure 177-3**):

- Cervical LN: Highest on the differential is head and neck cancer, workup includes PET/CT, pan-endoscopy with laryngoscopy, staging bilateral tonsillectomies, and bronchoscopy, and biopsy for immunohistochemistry (IHC).
- Supraclavicular LN: Highest on the differential is abdominal primary (however, lung, head and neck, breast, ovary, and prostate can metastasize to supraclavicular LN), workup includes CT of neck/chest/abdomen and pelvis, endoscopy with EGD and colonoscopy, and biopsy for IHC.
- Isolated axillary LN: Highest on the differential in females is breast cancer, workup includes mammogram, breast US, and biopsy for IHC.
- Inguinal LN: Highest on the differential is squamous cell of cervix/anus, workup includes CT of neck/chest/abdomen and biopsy for IHC.

Next step in evaluation

As noted above, it is important to rule out infection, autoimmune disorders, reactive causes, granulomatous diseases, etc. For the next steps in assessing a patient with lymphadenopathy, multiple factors must be considered, such as location of enlarged LN (see Figure 177-3), size, duration, and likelihood of malignancy when deciding what and how to attempt a diagnostic biopsy. In general, biopsy should be considered for LNs that are persistent (>4 weeks, or despite antibiotic treatment), hard, and fixed/matted.

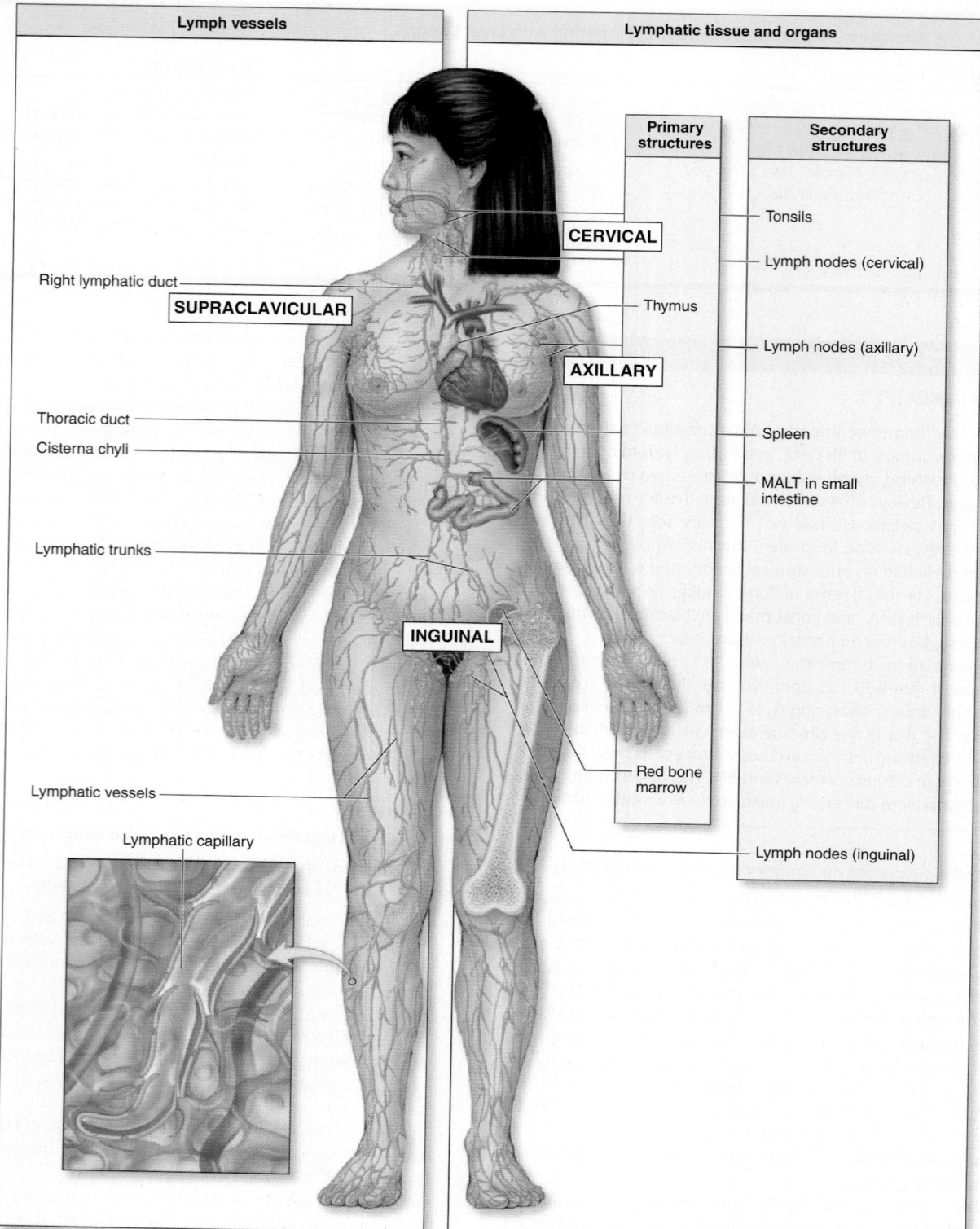

Figure 177-3 *Differential of lymphadenopathy by lymph node region.* (Adapted, with permission, from Mescher AL. *Junqueira's Basic Histology: Text and Atlas*, 14th ed. New York, NY: McGraw-Hill Education; 2016. Fig. 14-1.)

When considering a biopsy, the principals discussed in Case 177-1 apply here as well. However, with lymphadenopathy and any concern for lymphoma, an excisional biopsy is ideal to preserve architecture for an accurate diagnosis. Biopsy sites that have the highest yield include the supraclavicular and axillary, whereas the inguinal LNs have the lowest yield and are most often reactive.

Management priorities

Management priorities in cases such as the one described above focus on identifying any evidence of upper airway obstruction as a result of a head and neck primary, which is a life-threatening emergency that requires immediate diagnosis. Involve specialists such as ENT or anesthesia urgently to ensure airway is patent; if any concerns exist, the goal should focus on airway management with steroids, epinephrine, consideration of heliox, or even intubation if patient does not improve.

Other considerations for patients with diffuse lymphadenopathy concerning for an aggressive lymphoma is evaluation for tumor lysis syndrome. Often tumor lysis syndrome occurs after the start of treatment, but can occur spontaneously with aggressive cell turnover causing lysis and release of K, P, nucleic acids, which can lead to renal and cardiac complications. Key labs to evaluate for tumor lysis syndrome include uric acid, K, P, Ca, and Cr. Management focuses on aggressive hydration, treating hyperkalemia, hyperphosphatemia, symptomatic hypocalcemia, and elevated uric acid. Elevated uric acid can be managed with either allopurinol, which inhibits xanthine oxidase to decrease uric acid production, or Rasburicase in severe cases, which breaks down existing uric acid (see Chapter 176 [Oncologic Emergencies] for additional information).

CASE 177-4

MEDIASTINAL MASS

A 35-year-old male presents to the hospital with a history of feeling "congested" for several weeks. He also notes progressive shortness of breath with exertion and fatigue. He was treated initially with a 7-day course of antibiotics, and his symptoms improved slightly but have not resolved. In addition, he has noted progressive head/neck/arm swelling. The review of systems was negative. Specifically, he has no fevers, weight loss, night sweats, cough, or hemoptysis. He had no prior operations and was on no other medications. He did not use alcohol, tobacco, or drugs. There was no family history of malignancy.

On examination, temperature was 98.2, BP 120/71, HR 110 bpm. Notably, there was evidence of facial edema, upper extremity edema, distended veins over the chest wall, and a positive Pemberton's sign (worsening of his respiratory symptoms, cyanosis, and facial congestion after he elevated his arms in the air). The rest of the physical exam was unremarkable. Plain films of the chest and neck showed a widened mediastinum with concern for a large mediastinal mass.

Approach if suspected malignancy involves mediastinal mass

Mediastinal masses can be malignant or benign, and generally form in the membranous portion between the lungs where the heart, large arteries/veins, trachea and bronchi, and esophagus reside. This area is separated anatomically into the anterior, middle, and posterior mediastinum. Most patients with mediastinal masses are asymptomatic, however patients can present, such as in the example above, with symptoms related to extrinsic compression on the vessels, nerves, esophagus, or airways.

A comprehensive history is important, including an evaluation for any prior radiation, chemotherapy, and chemical exposure (asbestos/silica/diesel exhaust, etc), and a thorough physical exam should be performed.

Labs include β-HCG, AFP for men followed by testicular US if markers if elevated, PTH if parathyroid adenoma is suspected, and antiacetylcholine receptor antibodies if there is concern for thymic tumor with myasthenia gravis.

Initial imaging with a CXR is appropriate. Once a mediastinal mass is identified, or if suspicion remains despite a negative CXR, a CT scan with contrast is necessary, unless the use of contrast is contraindicated. CT scanning is the most appropriate and valuable imaging modality for evaluating mediastinal masses.

TABLE 177-3 Common Etiology of the Mediastinal Mass

Anterior Mediastinum	Middle Mediastinum	Posterior Mediastinum
Thymoma or thymic cyst	Lymphoma	Neurogenic tumor
Lymphoma	Metastatic disease to LN	Cysts
Teratoma/germ cell tumor	Granulomatous involvement of LN	Meningocele
Thyroid mass		Esophageal abnormalities
Intrathoracic goiter	Vascular abnormalities	Extramedullary hematopoiesis
Thoracic aneurysm	Bronchogenic cyst or tumor	
Metastatic carcinoma	Pericardial cyst	
Parathyroid adenoma		
Lipoma		
Hernia		

Differential diagnosis

The differential diagnosis for mediastinal masses is broad and largely based on age, symptoms, and anatomic location of the tumor. The initial step is to identify which compartment (anterior, middle, or posterior) the tumor is located, thus narrowing the differential, as summarized in **Table 177-3**.

The most common etiologies of an anterior mediastinal mass is a thymic mass (70% are benign, 30% are malignant) or a lymphoma (Hodgkin's or Non-Hodgkin's lymphoma/NHL). Others include germ cell tumors, thyroid masses, goiter, aneurysm, metastatic carcinoma, parathyroid adenoma, lipoma, or a hernia. The pneumonic 5Ts (Thymus tumor, Thyroid tumor, Teratoma, Terrible lymphoma, and Thoracic aorta aneurysm) is often used to remember the differential diagnosis of anterior mediastinal mass.

The most common etiology of a middle mediastinal mass is a lymphoma (Hodgkin's or NHL) or an enlargement of the lymph nodes as a result of malignancy or granulomatous disease. Others include vascular abnormalities such as aortic dissection or aneurysm, vascular masses, or benign growths from respiratory mucosa or pericardium, known as a bronchogenic or pericardial cysts.

The most common etiology of a posterior mediastinal mass is a neurogenic tumor (nerve sheath, ganglion cell, paraganglionic tumors) or a cyst. Others include meningocele, an extension of the meninges through an opening in the spine as a result of a congenital defect, esophageal abnormalities such as acalasia, hernia, or malignancy, cysts, or areas of bone marrow expansion used for extramedullary hematopoiesis.

Next step in evaluation

Although the diagnosis may be convincing based on the history and imaging, a tissue guided biopsy is normally the next step, however there are exceptions to this rule. For example, if imaging is suggestive of a thymoma, a biopsy is not necessary. It is important to consult with your surgical team and oncologists to determine if a biopsy is the next step, and what procedure is indicated.

Depending on the case scenario, a surgical biopsy may be preferred to FNA or core biopsies, in order to ensure the specimen has adequate architecture and quantity to make a diagnosis.

Often, for masses in the anterior and middle mediastinum, a diagnosis can be made with a biopsy via mediastinoscopy or anterior mediastinotomy. Alternative procedures that can achieve an adequate biopsy sample, depending on location of the mass, include endoscopic transesophageal or endobronchial ultrasound-guided biopsy, or video-assisted thoracoscopy, so it is important to organize a multidisciplinary team in these cases to determine the next step in evaluation.

Management priorities

As discussed above, in cases where mediastinal masses are causing symptoms, it is generally related to extrinsic compression on the vessels, nerves, esophagus, or airways, which can cause Horner syndrome, superior vena cava (SVC) syndrome, a pleural or pericardial effusion (possible tamponade), or phrenic nerve involvement. It is important to recognize these complications and manage them appropriately and in a timely fashion (see Chapter 176 [Oncologic Emergencies] for additional information).

CASE 177-5

BRAIN LESION

A 55-year-old right-handed female presented to the emergency department with complaints of word-finding difficulty for the past couple days. No weakness or sensory deficit. No falls. No aura like symptoms. No fever or chills. No history of seizures. She denied any trouble swallowing or hoarseness in voice. She denied any pain, changes in bowel/bladder pattern, SOB, chest pain. No nausea/vomiting. Besides the symptoms mentioned above, review of systems was positive for dull headaches, particularly on coughing for the past couple weeks.

Past medical history significant for hypercholesterolemia and gastro-esophageal reflux disease. No known history of malignancy or radiation exposure. Family history positive of coronary artery disease on paternal side. Excellent performance status (KPS = 90).

Examination was remarkable for slurred speech. No cranial nerve deficit noted. No sensory or motor weakness. Labs did not reveal any hematological or metabolic abnormality. She underwent a CT scan of the brain which revealed a 1.4 cm lesion in the left frontal lobe suggestive of brain metastasis. She was started on decadron and admitted to the inpatient hospitalist service for further workup and management.

Brain metastases

While brain metastasis usually present later in the course of malignancy, in about 10% of patients brain metastasis is the presenting feature of malignancy. The key step in the assessment is to distinguish brain metastasis from primary brain malignancy and other nonmalignant causes.

Differential if suspected malignancy involves brain metastases

While any malignancy can potentially cause brain metastasis, the common malignancies associated with brain metastasis include:

- Lung cancer (adenocarcinoma and small cell cancer)
- Breast cancer (particularly HER2+ and triple negative)
- Renal cell carcinoma
- Melanoma
- Ovarian carcinoma
- Colon cancer
- Choriocarcinoma
- Sarcoma

In general, majority of metastasis occur in the supratentorial region, usually in the vascular border and gray-white matter junction, but cerebellar metastasis can also occur.

Approach if suspected malignancy involves brain metastases

While clinical features from brain metastasis can mimic other neurological conditions, presence of headache that increases with cough

or bending (brain metastasis raise intracranial pressure), acute onset of focal neurological deficit in a patient with known history of malignancy, should raise the possibility of brain metastasis. A complete physical exam should be performed, including a breast and axillary exam specifically in females (to evaluate for breast lump and axillary lymphadenopathy). Laboratory studies include CBC with differential, chemistry panel, and relevant tumor markers (to help with differential diagnosis of malignancy).

While patients may have had brain metastasis diagnosed by CT scan, a dedicated MRI with contrast is usually required to (a) delineate the specific lesion better and (b) identify other sites of brain metastasis, particularly in the posterior fossa. Multiple brain metastases usually indicate spread from other sites as opposed to primary brain malignancy. Brain metastasis from renal cell carcinoma, melanoma, and choriocarcinoma usually tend to be hemorrhagic with tendency to bleed, as opposed to metastasis from other solid tumors, and therefore, anticoagulation should be considered in caution in patients with these malignancies.

Besides MRI with contrast, if brain metastasis is suspected (as opposed to primary brain malignancy), then obtaining restaging CT scans is often helpful in identifying the potential primary site of tumor origin. In particular lung cancer should be high on the differential, and if needed PET scan should be considered. If breast cancer is suspected, then mammogram and/or breast ultrasound (breast MRI in premenopausal women with dense breasts) should be considered.

Next step in evaluation

While brain biopsies can be technically challenging, whenever possible a brain biopsy should be obtained in a patient presenting with brain metastasis, particularly solitary brain metastasis without any systemic evidence of disease. The biopsy can help distinguish between primary brain malignancy, metastasis, or nonmalignant cause, such as infection, and can also help narrow down the primary site of tumor origin.

Sometimes, resection of a solitary brain lesion is preferred to a biopsy as it can be both diagnostic and therapeutic. Accordingly, neurosurgery should be consulted early in the admission of a patient admitted for brain metastasis.

Questions related to prognosis often come up in such admissions. A graded prognostic index called recursive partitioning analysis (RPA) can be helpful in this scenario. Class 1 RPA refers to young patients (<65 years) with good KPS (>70) and no/controlled systemic disease, while class 3 RPA includes patients with poor KPS (<70), and class 2 includes those who do not fall in class 1 or 3. Patients with class 1 RPA have a better prognosis as compared to those with class 3 (median 7.1 vs 2.3 months). However, the prognosis is also dependent on site of primary malignancy (in general patients with breast cancer do better than those with lung cancer), and the RPA score has been modified as diagnosis-specific graded prognostic index (DS-GPA) to account for the type of malignancy.

Management priorities

Management priorities in cases such as the one described above should focus on distinguishing brain metastasis from other diagnostic possibilities and identification of the primary site of malignancy, as outlined in **Table 177-4**.

In the case above, the patient had an MRI brain which demonstrated a left frontal enhancing circumscribed lesion measuring 1.5 cm in greatest dimension. No evidence of any other lesion. The patient underwent surgical resection of the brain lesion which demonstrated metastatic adenocarcinoma, ER/PR negative, HER2 positive, TTF-1 negative. Staging CT scans revealed no radiological evidence of disease. Mammogram and breast ultrasound revealed a 1.3 cm lesion in the left outer quadrant. Breast sore biopsy revealed adenocarcinoma,

TABLE 177-4 Management Priority for a Patient Presenting with Brain Lesion

Diagnosis	Presentation	Evaluation	Management
Brain lesion	Headache that increases with cough or bending, focal neurological deficit	MRI brain with contrast. Staging scans to identify primary site. Mammogram and/or breast ultrasound if breast cancer suspected.	Brain biopsy. In certain instances, surgical resection is preferred as it can be diagnostic and therapeutic. Avoid anticoagulation in hemorrhagic brain metastasis (usually melanoma, renal cell carcinoma, and choriocarcinoma).

ER/PR negative, HER2 positive, with histological features similar to the brain metastasis. The patient was referred to a medical oncologist and was started on systemic anti-HER2 based therapy.

RISK STRATIFICATION

Generally, patients with suspected malignancy do not require hospital admission, and most can be treated as outpatients with an expedited workup. Exceptions include patients with rapidly progressive disease that need urgent chemotherapy (eg, small cell carcinoma, lymphoma), oncological emergencies, or other medical concerns that require urgent evaluation and intervention, such as the following:

- Acute complications of malignancy, for example perforation, bleeding, or fistula
- Respiratory distress
- Hemoptysis
- Severe pain
- Biliary or bowel obstruction
- Cholangitis
- High-grade esophageal obstruction with inability to manage oral secretions or maintain hydration
- Protracted vomiting, inability to maintain hydration or nutrition

TUMOR MARKERS

The tumor marker name is a bit of a misnomer, as tumor markers are not specific to malignancy and may be present in benign conditions or falsely elevated with liver disease or renal failure, and therefore need to be interpreted with caution. Tumor markers are not 100% sensitive and negative tumor markers cannot rule out the possibility of malignancy. Similarly tumor markers are not 100% specific and positive tumor markers cannot replace a histological diagnosis.

The diagnostic utility of tumor markers is predominantly as an adjunctive test to aid in evaluating patients hospitalized with a clinical presentation of suspected advanced malignancy and should largely be confined to cases where a certain primary is favored (see **Table 177-5**). For example, a high or rising PSA, a marker of prostate cancer, is helpful in a male patient over 40 years of age with suspected malignancy presenting with osteoblastic metastases. The markers of a germ cell tumor, such as β-HCG and AFP, can be helpful in males presenting with midline masses. Similarly, in a patient with known liver disease, a rising AFP can be suggestive of hepatocellular carcinoma. Common tumor markers and the associated malignancies are outlined in Table 177-5.

PRACTICE POINT

- The diagnostic utility of tumor markers is predominantly as an adjunctive test to aid in evaluating patients hospitalized with a clinical presentation of suspected advanced malignancy and should largely be confined to cases where a certain primary is favored.

IMMUNOHISTOCHEMISTRY AND TISSUE DIAGNOSIS

Tissue diagnosis remains the goal-standard test in cases of suspected malignancy. The general principle is to acquire enough tissue to allow for diagnosis, accurately stage the patient, and perform the necessary molecular testing, including genomic testing for targetable mutations.

A core or excisional biopsy is preferred, considering fine needle aspiration often results in insufficient tissue and loss of the detailed histology needed for diagnosis. Inadequate tissue limits the number of special studies that can be done on the sample, and therefore can have major implications for treatment (see **Table 177-6** for examples of cancers with known targetable mutations and FDA approved treatments), or even necessitate a second biopsy. Often, determining the site to biopsy is a multidisciplinary discussion with radiology, the oncology consult, and interventional radiology or surgery.

The key to diagnosis is immunohistochemical classification, as it is reliable, inexpensive, and generally available. Cytokeratins (CKs), proteins in the intermediate filament protein family, in epithelial cells are particularly useful in the diagnosis of malignancy. Expression of these cytokeratins is often specific to tissue or organ, and can aid in correctly identifying the origin of the tumor. CK 7 generally involves tissue from the lung, ovary, endometrium, or breast, whereas CK 20 is usually expressed in the colon or Merkel cells. The combination of CK 7 and CK 20, either both present or both absent, also proves to be useful in identifying a primary site (see **Figure 177-4**). Once cytokeratin profiling by CK 7 and CK 20 have narrowed the possible tumor origin, additional IHC can also be informative. For example, certain cancers have specific profiles.

- Breast: Estrogen (ER) and Progesterone Receptor (PR) +, HER2 +, Mammaglobin +
- Lung Adenocarcinoma: TTF-1 +, NapsinA +
- Lung Squamous Cell Carcinoma: P63 +, CK5/6 +

TABLE 177-5 Common Tumor Markers Associated with Solid Tumors

Tumor Marker	Tumor Type
CEA	Colon adenocarcinoma, hepatocellular
CA 19-9	Pancreatic, biliary tract
NSE	Neuroendocrine tumors, small cell lung cancer (SCLC), carcinoid
CA 15.3, CA 27.29	Breast cancer
CA 125	Ovarian cancer
PSA	Prostate cancer
AFP	Hepatocellular carcinoma, germ cell tumor
β-HCG	Germ cell tumor, gestational trophoblastic disease

TABLE 177-6 List of Specific Genomic Alterations and Matched Targeted Therapy

Cancer	Genomic Alteration	Targeted Treatment(s)
Breast	HER2 (Human Epidermal Growth Factor Receptor 2)	• Trastuzumab (Herceptin) • Pertuzumab (Perjeta) • Ado-trastuzumab emtansine (Kadcyla) • Lapatinib (Tykerb)
Breast	ER (Estrogen Receptor)	• Tamoxifen • Aromatase inhibitors (anastrozole [Arimidex], letrozole [Femara], exemestane [Aromasin])
NSCLC (adenocarcinoma)	EGFR (Epidermal Growth Factor Receptor)	• Erlotinib (Tarceva) • Afatinib (Gilotrif)
NSCLC (adenocarcinoma)	ALK (Anaplastic lymphoma kinase fusion)	• Crizotinib (Xalkori) • Ceritinib (Zykadia)
Chronic myelogenous leukemia (Philadelphia chromosome +)	BCR-ABL	• Imatinib (Gleevec) • Nilotinib (Tasigna) • Dasatinib (Sprycel) • Bosutinib (Sosulif) • Ponatinib (Inclusig)
GI stromal tumor (GIST)	KIT	• Imatinib (Gleevec)
Melanoma	BRAF	• Vemurafenib (Zelboraf) • Dabrafenib (Tafinlar) • Trametinib (Mekinist)
Ovarian	BRCA (germline)	• Olaparib (Lynparza)
Medullary thyroid cancer	RET	• Vandetanib (Caprelsa)

- Lung Small Cell Carcinoma: TTF-1 +, Synaptophysin +
- Prostate: Prostate Specific Antigen +, Prostate Acid Phosphatase (PAP) +
- Melanoma: S100 +, Vimentin +, Melan-A +
- Neuroendocrine: Chromogranin +, Synaptophysin +, CD56 +
- Hepatocellular: Alpha-fetoprotein (AFP) +, HepPar-1 +
- Germ cell: HCG +, AFP +, Oct4 Transcription Factor +, PAP +

MOLECULAR PROFILING

In oncology, molecular profiling of the tumor is being increasingly utilized to select specific marched targeted therapies as outlined in Table 177-6. For example, breast cancer is no longer considered one disease and it is a routine practice to obtain the status of ER (estrogen receptor) and HER2 (Human Epidermal Growth Factor Receptor 2) to select specific targeted therapy. Similarly, lung cancer is divided by presence/absence of EGFR mutation, ALK fusion, and there are a few others in development. The key is to detect an actionable alteration that could guide therapy and potentially lead to better outcomes.

In addition, molecular profiling may have diagnostic benefit and could be considered in the workup of a patient with suspected malignancy in which the primary cannot be established. The tissue-of-origin molecular profiling assays take advantage of the fact that there are specific gene expression profiles, depending on the site of origin of the tumor. They can identify a probable primary site of origin up to 70% to 98% of the time. Historically, these cases of "cancer of unknown primary" represent 5% of all newly diagnosed patients with solid malignancies each year, and have a poor prognosis (approximately 9 months when treated with empiric chemotherapy). With tissue-of-origin molecular profiling and site-specific directed chemotherapy, or targeted therapy, this increased to 12.5 months in one study performed at Sarah Cannon Research Institute, which is a promising for the future investigation into the use of this tool. However, as of this publication, as the clinical utility of gene signature profiling has not been proven, routine gene signature profiling to identify tissue of origin is not routinely recommended as standard of care according to the National Comprehensive Cancer Network.

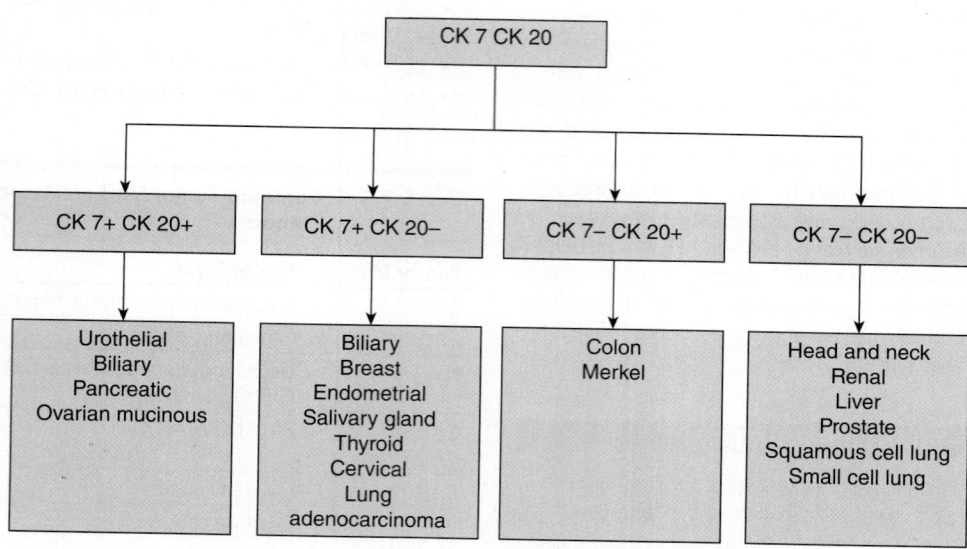

Figure 177-4 *Immunohistochemical features of common cancers.* (Adapted, with permission, from Varadhachary GR, Abbruzzese JL, Lenzi R. Diagnostic strategies for unknown primary cancer. *Cancer.* 2004;100:1776-1785.)

POSTACUTE CARE

The discharge planning process must ensure that the patient's care needs can be met once they leave the acute hospital setting. Following a hospitalization for a suspected malignancy, many patients require ongoing medical care, the details of which will be unique to each patient presentation. If any drains or catheters were placed during the hospitalization, it is important to ensure the patient is aware of the follow-up plan, has services scheduled or knows how to care for the drain or catheter, knows if they are safe to shower or bathe, and knows how to check for signs of infection.

Often a biopsy will be performed in the hospital, or scheduled on discharge. If the biopsy will be after discharge, consider notifying the patient to stop taking aspirin and NSAIDS 7 days before the procedure if appropriate, fast after midnight the day night before, and arrange a caregiver to drive them home and stay with them following the biopsy. Whether the biopsy is inpatient or outpatient, if results are not available it is helpful to set expectations and explain that the pathologist needs to process the sample, which can take 7 to 10 days or longer. Ensure the patient has a contact name/number in case they are not notified of any results within that timeframe.

Importantly, a quarter of patients become clinically depressed after a diagnosis of cancer, while others can suffer from extreme stress or anxiety. It is helpful to tell patients the signs and symptoms of these conditions, and encourage them to reach out to others such as their provider team after discharge, friends, family, and support groups (American Cancer Society programs may be offered in the area—1-800-227-2345). Early intervention with palliative care follow-up, focusing on psychological and physical symptoms, should be considered in certain circumstances, as there are adequate data to show a quality of life and possible survival benefit in patients with advanced disease. The Center to Advance Palliative Care and the American Cancer Society states "palliative care is appropriate at any age and at any stage in a serious illness, and can be provided together with curative treatment." Try to provide encouragement and instill that adequate sleep, eating, light exercise, and a daily schedule can be ways of ensuring they stay mentally and physically healthy to optimize the chances of success during cancer management.

DISCHARGE CHECKLIST FOR DISORDER

- If a biopsy occurred in the hospital, patient is aware of how to care for the site and has follow-up if required (eg, to remove stitches).
- Any necessary home medical equipment (oxygen, nebulizer, walker, etc) has been scheduled for delivery, and the patient has been provided education to ensure proper and safe use.
- Medications and management of side effects (eg, pain medication causes constipation so laxative use should be addressed) have been reviewed.
- Patient is aware of what to expect, and has a provider name/number to contact if he/she experiences any fever, infection, severe pain, bleeding, or other concerning symptoms.
- All follow-up tests and appointments have been scheduled, and patient is aware of date, location, and time of each, and can arrange necessary transportation to these visits.
- The patient or family have been asked if they require any documentation to address employment issues or family medical leave.

SUGGESTED READINGS

Bazemore A, et al. Lymphadenopathy and malignancy. *Am Fam Physician*. 2012;66:2103-2110.

Hainsworth J, et al. Molecular gene expression profiling to predict the tissue of origin and direct site-specific therapy in patients with carcinoma of unknown primary site: a prospective trial of the Sarah Cannon research institute. *J Clin Oncol*. 2013;31:217-223.

Longo DL. Approach to the patient with cancer. In: Kasper DL, et al, eds. *Harrison's Principles of Internal Medicine*, 19th ed. New York, NY: McGraw-Hill Education, 2015:467-475.

Molina R, et al. Utility of serum tumor markers as an aid in the differential diagnosis of patients with clinical suspicion of cancer and in patients with cancer of unknown primary site. *Tumour Biol*. 2012;33:463-474.

Namasivayam S, et al. Imaging of liver metastases: MRI. *Cancer Imaging*. 2007;7:2-9.

National Comprehensive Cancer Network. Occult Primary (Cancer of Unknown Primary) (Version 1.2015). http://www.nccn.org/professionals/physician_gls /pdf/occult.pdf. Accessed July 1, 2015.

Siegel R, et al. Cancer statistics, 2015. *CA Cancer J Clin*. 2015;65(1):5-29.

Varadhachary G, et al. Carcinoma of unknown primary site. *N Engl J Med*. 2014;371(21):2040.

Vassilakopoulos T, et al. Application of a prediction rule to select which patients presenting with lymphadenopathy should undergo a lymph node biopsy. *Medicine (Baltimore)*. 2000;79(5):338-347.

CHAPTER 178

Breast, Ovary, and Cervical Cancer

Evelyn Cantillo, MD, MPH

Katina Robison, MD

Ashley Stuckey, MD

Key Clinical Questions

❶ How do the different treatment modalities for cancers unique to women put patients at risk for future complications?

❷ What is the initial evaluation and treatment of these complications?

❸ Which complications require emergent consultation?

INTRODUCTION

While many cancers have similar medical complications that require hospitalizations, cancers specific to women, breast and gynecologic cancers, often have unique medical presentations. In this chapter, we will discuss common presentations, diagnostic workup, and treatment for complications that may arise during treatment or surveillance for breast and gynecologic cancers. Since many of the issues that impact ovarian and endometrial cancer patients are similar, the topic will speak mostly toward complications for women with ovarian cancer. In addition, since chemoradiation is a primary treatment for cervical cancer, complications related to cervical cancer treatment will be reviewed; these issues are relevant and similar for women treated for vulvar or vaginal cancers.

BREAST CANCER

In the United States, breast cancer is the most commonly diagnosed cancer among women and the second most common cause of cancer death. Generally, the mainstay of treatment is surgical, typically with breast conservation therapy (BCT) for women with early-stage disease, which consists of a lumpectomy followed by radiation therapy (x-ray therapy [XRT]). However, some women will undergo a modified radical mastectomy due to tumor size or patient preference. With rare exceptions, women with invasive carcinoma (and those women undergoing mastectomy for ductal carcinoma in situ [DCIS]), will have nodal evaluation.

Management of the axilla continues to evolve. Traditionally, patients with a positive sentinel lymph node would undergo an axillary lymph node dissection. Randomized clinical trials directly comparing BCT with mastectomy have shown equivalent survival between the two treatment approaches. The American College of Surgeons Oncology Group (ACOSOG) Z11 trial showed that in selected patients with one to two positive sentinel nodes, a sentinel lymph node biopsy (SLNB) can obviate the need for an axillary lymph node dissection (ALND). More recently, the EORTC (European Organization for Research and Treatment of Cancer) AMAROS trial reported that in patients with a T1-2 primary breast cancer, no palpable lymphadenopathy and with a positive sentinel node, axillary radiotherapy is noninferior to axillary lymph node dissection in controlling 5-year axillary node recurrence.

The use of postoperative (or adjuvant) systemic therapy is guided by the patient's clinical status, tumor characteristics, and more and more, the genomic characteristics of the tumor. Patients with hormone receptor (estrogen/progesterone)-positive malignancies are candidates for endocrine therapy such as the selective estrogen receptor modulator, tamoxifen, or aromatase inhibitors. However, genomic tests, such as the Recurrence Score, may be used to predict prognosis for women treated with endocrine therapy and therefore identify higher-risk patients who should be offered chemotherapy. Patients with human epidermal growth factor receptor 2 (HER2)-positive cancers should receive therapy that includes HER2-directed treatment (trastuzumab, pertuzumab). Patients with triple negative breast cancer will also receive cytotoxic chemotherapy. Febrile neutropenia as a complication of cytotoxic chemotherapy should be managed as outlined in Chapter 204 [Infections of the Immunocompromised Host].

- Chemotherapy regimens in breast cancer are considered high risk for febrile neutropenia.

■ CELLULITIS

The soft-tissue infection that characterizes cellulitis typically occurs in the context of breast surgery, lactation, or trauma. The XRT that accompanies BCT places the patient at further risk for developing a breast cellulitis. Cellulitis is a clinical diagnosis, in which women will present with pain, diffuse erythema, tenderness, and warmth in the affected breast. Beta-hemolytic *Streptococcus* and *Staphylococcus aureus*, including methicillin-resistant species (MRSA), have been identified as important pathogens. Most cases of breast cellulitis can be treated on an outpatient basis with clinical improvement seen between 48 and 72 hours after the initiation of antibiotics (**Table 178-1**) Options for outpatient management included icloxa-cillin, cephalexin, or clindamycin in the setting of a penicillin allergy. Indications for hospitalization and intravenous antibiotic therapy include lack of response to oral antibiotics in the outpatient setting, signs of hemodynamic instability and systemic toxicity, or neutropenia. Intravenous antibiotic options include oxacillin, cefazolin, clindamycin, or vancomycin, if there is a risk for MRSA infection. Neutropenic patients or those undergoing chemotherapy should receive broad spectrum antibiotics that include coverage for aerobic Gram-negative bacilli, including *Pseudomonas aeruginosa*.

If patients have not responded to antibiotics within 48 to 72 hours, ultrasound imaging of the breast should be pursued and other sources of infection should be explored.

■ INFLAMMATORY BREAST CANCER

Inflammatory breast cancer (IBC) is rare and aggressive—accounting for 1% to 5% of new cases. At the time of diagnosis, patients will present with diffuse erythema and/or edema—the hallmarks of IBC. The international expert panel on IBC developed minimum criteria required for diagnosis:

1. Rapid onset of breast erythema
2. Edema and/or peau d'orange, warm breast, with or without an underlying palpable mass
3. Duration of history no more than 6 months
4. Erythema occupying at least one-third of the breast
5. Pathological confirmation of invasive carcinoma

It can be difficult to distinguish IBC from cellulitis or mastitis. However, since IBC is not caused by an inflammatory process but rather lymphovascular tumor emboli, it should be considered if symptoms do not improve after a course of antibiotic treatment. A breast biopsy is required for definitive diagnosis.

■ LYMPHEDEMA

All women with a history of axillary lymph node sampling are at risk for lymphedema. However, women who have a history of a complete axillary lymph node dissection are at higher risk than women with a history of a sentinel lymph node biopsy alone. Lymphedema may present at any point in the postoperative or survivorship period. Radiation therapy can worsen lymphedema by further disrupting the lymphatic channels. Depending on the severity, chronic lymphedema can impact a woman's mobility, sensation, and overall quality of life. Furthermore, the affected extremity can undergo changes that make it more susceptible to infections. An overlying cellulitis should be treated as outlined above. Compression bandages or stockings should be applied to the affected extremity while patients are hospitalized. Referral to a lymphedema specialist can be arranged upon discharge and in some instances these resources are available during a hospital stay. There are case reports of lymphedema as an initial presenting symptom for invasive breast cancer. These patients will typically have significant tumor burden; a physical examination plus a mammogram may identify an underlying lesion.

■ RADIATION-INDUCED DERMATITIS

Women with a history of breast cancer who underwent radiation therapy often present with radiation-induced dermatitis (**Table 178-2**). This occurs due to direct tissue damage from high-dose radiation to the epidermis and underlying structures leading to an inflammatory response. Patients will present with erythema, edema, pigment changes, and/or skin desquamation. It may be differentiated from cellulitis by the lack of fever or leukocytosis. This process can be acute, occurring within 90 days of XRT exposure, or chronic, within months to years after XRT exposure. In the acute setting, epidermal necrosis can lead to blistering and sloughing that would manifest as moist desquamation. Dermal fibrosis and telangiectasias are characteristic of chronic dermatitis.

Women may require hospitalization for pain control or severe desquamation, but typically desquamation is treated as an outpatient. Moist desquamation as seen in Grade 2 and 3 acute dermatitis may benefit from treatments with petroleum-based products, topical emulsions, silicone foam bandages, or hydrocortisone cream, which can be added in a stepwise manner. Grade 3 dermatitis may require temporary cessation of XRT while Grade 4 dermatitis may require permanent discontinuation of XRT as well as consultation with a wound specialist, dermatologist, and/or radiation oncologist.

OVARIAN CANCER

In the United States, more women die from ovarian cancer each year than from any other gynecologic malignancy. Due to the vague

TABLE 178-1 Antibiotic Regimens for Treatment of Cellulitis

Outpatient	
Dicloxacillin	500 mg orally every 6 h
Cephalexin	500 mg orally every 6 h
Clindamycin	300 mg to 450 orally every 8 h
Trimethoprim-sulfamethoxazole	1 double-strength tab orally twice daily
Inpatient	
Oxacillin	2 g intravenously every 6 h
Cefazolin	1 g intravenously every 8 h
Clindamycin	600 mg intravenously every 8 h
Vancomycin	15-20 mg/kg/dose every 8-12 h
Neutropenic	
Piperacillin-tazobactam	4.5 g IV every 6-8 h
Cefepime	2 g IV every 8 h
Meropenem	1 g IV every 8 h

TABLE 178-2 Grading System for Acute Radiation Dermatitis

Grade	Clinical Description
1	Faint erythema or dry desquamation
2	Bright erythema, moist desquamation, moderate edema
3	Confluent moist desquamation in areas other than skin folds and creases, pitting edema
4	Ulceration, hemorrhage, necrosis
5	Death

symptomatology including abdominal bloating, early satiety, and fatigue, patients are often not diagnosed until the cancer has spread outside of the pelvis (Stage III). The majority of ovarian malignancies are epithelial in origin with the remaining minority being germ cell and sex cord-stromal tumors. This discussion will be limited to epithelial ovarian cancer (EOC) and will include fallopian tube and primary peritoneal, which are clinically similar.

■ ASCITES

Women may present to the emergency room/hospital with shortness of breath due to either pleural effusion(s) and/or ascites. Symptomatic treatment involves removal of the fluid via thoracentesis and/or paracentesis. The fluid should in turn be sent for cytologic evaluation. Malignant Müllerian cells on cytology suggest a diagnosis of EOC, and further evaluation with a computed tomography (CT) scan of the abdomen and pelvis should be pursued. For patients presenting to the emergency room/hospital with abdominal pain or signs of a bowel obstruction, CT scans are readily available in most hospitals and tend to be the imaging modality of choice. The finding of an adnexal mass is concerning for ovarian cancer and tumor markers such as CA125 and HE-4 should be drawn. It is important to note that woman with primary peritoneal cancer will not present with an adnexal mass; however, imaging may reveal peritoneal carcinomatosis.

■ VENOUS THROMBOEMBOLISM

Women may present to the hospital with a new diagnosis of a deep vein thrombosis or pulmonary embolism. Workup for an occult malignancy in a patient with a first episode of an unprovoked venous thromboembolism (VTE) should be limited to routine preventive care with additional follow-up based on abnormal clinical findings. Although an increased incidence of occult malignancy has been found in women presenting with a VTE, a survival advantage has not been confirmed by including routine malignancy workup in this setting. It is important to review the patient's age and history of appropriate screening such as mammograms and colonoscopies as gastrointestinal and breast malignancies may metastasize to the ovary. If concern for EOC exists, the patient should be referred to a gynecologic oncologist who is trained to perform comprehensive surgical staging and cytoreductive surgery as these patients have a better prognosis than those not comprehensively staged. Treatment for VTE with low-molecular-weight heparin over warfarin is preferred in patients with malignancy as studies have shown improved efficacy (see Chapter 173 [Hypercoagulable States] and Chapter 253 [Diagnosis and Treatment of Venous Thromboembolism]).

■ MALIGNANT BOWEL OBSTRUCTION

Malignant bowel obstruction (MBO) can occur during initial cancer presentation but is most common in the setting of recurrent ovarian cancer. Bowel obstruction due to adhesive disease should be ruled out. Computed tomography scan of the abdomen and pelvis may identify transition points, severity of obstruction and burden of disease. If a CT scan is not immediately available, a flat and upright x-ray may quickly confirm the diagnosis of bowel obstruction by identifying dilated loops of small bowel, air-fluid levels, and less commonly free air. The presence of free air mandates emergent surgical consultation.

Patients with clinical features of small bowel obstruction (SBO) who are diagnosed with acute mechanical SBO generally require admission to the hospital for initial management. Most patients will present with a several day history of nausea, emesis, and abdominal pain that may lead to dehydration and corresponding electrolyte abnormalities. Initial management of patients admitted for MBO includes intravenous fluid therapy with lactated ringers or normal saline and electrolyte replacement. Patients with an MBO should be made *nil per os* (NPO). Placement of a nasogastric tube should be considered for patients with large volume emesis and/or abdominal distention to allow for gastrointestinal decompression. If the MBO is partial, metoclopramide may relieve nausea and improve gastrointestinal motility. Metoclopramide should be avoided in patients with a complete obstruction; these patients will develop worsening symptoms. Emesis may be controlled with antiemetics. Somatostatin analogs, such as octreotide, rapidly reduces gastrointestinal secretions.

Malignant small bowel obstructions raise a distinct set of challenges. Small bowel obstructions that do not resolve with conservative management are sometimes not amenable to surgical intervention. A younger patient with a new diagnosis of cancer or a discrete transition point on imaging will likely benefit from surgery more than a patient with recurrent ovarian cancer, several comorbidities, or with extensive peritoneal disease, with limited life expectancy. A patient with an MBO that does not respond to conservative management should be evaluated by a surgeon or gynecologic oncologist, if available.

PRACTICE POINT

A multidisciplinary approach is required to address complex issues relating to malignant small bowel obstruction. Consultation with surgery and gynecology oncology should be taken to:
- Discuss goals of care and prognosis
- Determine the best approach for symptom relief
- Balance risk versus benefit of surgical intervention in patients whose bowel obstruction does not respond to conservative management
- Address nutritional issues
- Identify small bowel obstruction due to adhesions

For patients with a nonresolving MBO who are not surgical candidates, a gastric tube (G-tube) may be placed in a minimally invasive manner for palliation of symptoms. No consensus guidelines exist for the initiation of total parenteral nutrition which has not been shown to improve survival. Total parenteral nutrition may be a consideration in patients with minimal or no PO intake for a minimum of 7 to 14 days and in patients who have not yet received treatment of their cancer.

CERVICAL CANCER

The introduction of the papanicolaou (pap) test has dramatically decreased cervical cancer rates in industrialized nations. There were an estimated 266,000 deaths from cervical cancer worldwide in 2012, accounting for 7.5% of all female cancer deaths. Almost 9 out of 10 (87%) cervical cancer deaths occur in developing regions. In the United States, it is estimated that 12,900 new cases of invasive cervical cancer will be diagnosed and 4100 women will die from the disease in 2015. Women with early-stage disease can be treated successfully with surgery. Women with locally advanced cervical cancer (Stages IB2, IIB to IVA) will receive primary chemoradiation. Complications arise from the disease itself or its treatment.

■ RENAL INSUFFICIENCY

Cervical cancer spreads by extension to adjacent structures. Patients may present with clinical Stage IIIB disease, which involves extension to the pelvic side wall and/or hydronephrosis. These patients are at increased risk for urinary tract infections, including pyelonephritis. Physical examination may reveal costovertebral tenderness due to severe hydronephrosis or infection. Patients with a known diagnosis of cervical cancer or those in which there is a strong suspicion based on history and/or examination should be hydrated with intravenous fluids and urine output strictly monitored (oral and intravenous intake, urine output, daily weights). Laboratory tests include a basic metabolic panel, a complete blood count, and urinalysis.

A CT scan with IV contrast may be contraindicated if the serum creatinine is elevated; however, a renal ultrasound will usually demonstrate hydronephrosis unless the ureters are encased by tumor. Depending on the obstruction, these patients will benefit from either ureteral stenting or a percutaneous nephrostomy tube; urology should be consulted.

PRACTICE POINT

In patients with cervical cancer metastatic to adjacent structures:
- Ultrasound may not demonstrate hydronephrosis if the ureters are encased by tumor.
- Anuric or severely oliguric patients with renal insufficiency require emergent urologic consultation for ureteral stenting or consideration of percutaneous nephrostomy placement.

■ RADIATION PROCTITIS

Definitive XRT for a patient with an intact cervix includes external beam radiation therapy (EBRT) with brachytherapy for a total dose of 80 to 85 Gy and possibly more depending on tumor size. It is generally agreed that treatments <45 Gy cause very few side effects. Doses between 45 and 70 Gy cause more complications that tend to be of lesser intensity. Doses above 70 Gy can cause significant and long-standing injury to the surrounding area. Radiation proctitis should be suspected in any patient who has had pelvic radiation exposure presenting with diarrhea, nausea, cramps, tenesmus, urgency, mucus discharge, and minor bleeding.

Acute radiation proctitis is an inflammatory process involving only the superficial mucosa that occurs almost immediately after the initiation of therapy or up to 3 months after the onset of XRT. Symptoms will develop in up to 20% of patients necessitating an interruption in treatment. Since it is a self-limiting process, supportive medical management is usually the only treatment required and includes hydration and antidiarrheals. The discontinuation of the radiation therapy is the definitive treatment.

Chronic radiation proctitis occurs when the blood supply to the rectal wall is compromised resulting in full-thickness ischemia and fibrotic changes that may not become apparent until months to years after the cessation of therapy (median 8-12 months after the completion of therapy). Patients will have pain and may experience

TABLE 178-3 Management of Radiation Proctitis

Acute	Cessation or adjustment of XRT regimen
Chronic	
Grade 0	No intervention
Grade 1 and 2	First-line: anti-inflammatories
	If persistent, sucralfate, hyperbaric oxygen treatment
Grade 3	Anti-inflammatories, sucralfate, hyperbaric oxygen treatment
	If persistent, laser or argon plasma coagulation
Grade 4	Surgical intervention

electrolyte abnormalities secondary to excessive diarrhea and the corresponding fluid losses. Gastroenterology (GI) should be consulted to perform a colonoscopy, which can assess the severity of proctitis. For patients who do not respond to antidiarrheals, minimally invasive techniques may be employed. Some patients will require surgery as indicated in **Table 178-3**.

CONCLUSION

The malignancies discussed in this chapter are quite variable and their complications reflect the unique disease processes. A multidisciplinary approach to hospitalized women initially presenting with one of these malignancies or with complications of treatment is advisable to relieve suffering and to provide the best outcome for the patient.

SUGGESTED READINGS

Common Terminology Criteria for Adverse Events (CTCAE), Version 4.0, June 2010, National Institutes of Health, National Cancer Institute.

Dawood S, Merajver SD, Viens P, et al. International expert panel on inflammatory breast cancer: consensus statement for standardized diagnosis and treatment. *Ann Oncol.* 2011;22(3):515-523.

Donker M, van Tienhoven, G, et al. EORTC 10981-22023 AMAROS): a randomised, multicentre, open-label, phase 3 non-inferiority trial. *Lancet Oncol.* 2014;15(12):1303-1310.

Giuliano AE, Hunt KK, Ballman KV, et al. Axillary dissection vs No axillary dissection in women with invasive breast cancer and sentinel node metastasis: a randomized clinical trial. *JAMA.* 2011;305(6):569-575.

CHAPTER 179

Men's Cancers

Nazli Dizman, MD
Sumanta K. Pal, MD

Key Clinical Questions

① What is the current landscape of treatment for advanced prostate cancer?

② Which treatments for advanced prostate cancer are more likely to result in hospital admission?

③ What is the current landscape of treatment for advanced testicular cancer?

④ What treatments for advanced testicular cancer are more likely to result in hospital admission?

⑤ What are some commonly used strategies to mitigate the risk of hospital admission in the context of therapy for advanced prostate cancer and advanced testicular cancer?

⑥ What are some of the disease-related sequelae of prostate and testicular cancer that can result in inpatient admission?

PROSTATE CANCER

DISEASE OVERVIEW

Prostate cancer is the most common cancer in men, with an estimated 233,000 cases diagnosed in 2014. Due to the therapeutic advances outlined herein, the death rate for prostate cancer has been declining over the past decade—nonetheless, approximately 29,480 deaths were still attributable to the disease in 2014. Screening for prostate cancer is controversial and largely beyond the scope of the current chapter. Briefly, widespread screening in the mid-1990s led to a dramatic rise in the incidence of prostate cancer. Given that many of the detected prostate cancers might be indolent and not result in prostate-cancer-related mortality, the utility of screening has been called into question. Current recommendations suggest individual counseling of patients, with consideration of risk factors (eg, family history) and consideration of risks associated with screening (eg, infection and pain secondary to prostatic biopsies performed in response to an elevated prostrate-specific antigen [PSA]).

For the vast majority of patients (>90%), prostate cancer is diagnosed when still localized to the pelvis. For these individuals, a risk-adapted approach is often employed. This approach entails utilizing clinical factors (including clinical stage, Gleason grade, and baseline PSA) to determine the potential risk of metastatic recurrence. Similar emphasis is also placed on ascertaining the patients' projected life expectancy, utilizing Social Security Life Indices and other tools. Patients with low-risk disease who have a shorter anticipated life expectancy may be considered for conservative measures, such as active surveillance (repeat assessment of the PSA and intermittent prostatic biopsies), while younger individuals with higher-risk disease might be considered for more definitive strategies such as surgery or radiation. Typically, radiation therapy to the prostate is conducted in the outpatient setting in multiple daily fractions over several weeks. Surgery for prostate cancer typically entails removal of the prostate and adjacent lymph nodes. Prostatectomy is typically followed by a 1- to 2-day postoperative stay prior to discharge.

TREATMENT OF METASTATIC PROSTATE CANCER

In the management of prostate cancer, the hospitalist will more likely be called upon to care for the patient with metastatic disease. The treatment of metastatic disease has evolved markedly over the past decade, and some familiarity with the wide range of agents used in this setting may be helpful. In the ensuing section, these treatments will be described.

For some time, it has been known that prostate cancer is a disease driven by testosterone. This understanding dates back to the 1940s, when Nobel laureate Charles Huggins observed that surgical castration led to regression of advanced prostate cancer. Testosterone activates the androgen receptor, a nuclear receptor which drives growth and proliferation of prostatic tissues. Surgical castration has been largely supplanted by chemical castration, using luteinizing hormone releasing hormone (LHRH) agonists (eg, leuprolide) or antagonists (eg, degarelix). These agents are frequently complemented by androgen receptor antagonists, such as bicalutamide, nilutamide, and flutamide.

The combination of LHRH agonists with or without androgen receptor antagonists is often used as an adjunct to radiotherapy for more aggressive localized prostate cancer and for the front-line management of metastatic disease. The most common side effects incurred with these agents include fatigue, hot flashes, insomnia, decreased libido, and mood changes or irritability. These hormonal therapies also compromise bone density, and therefore, contingent on the duration of therapy, bone strengthening agents (eg, denosumab or zoledronic acid) are prescribed. Bearing this in mind, the practicing hospitalist should be keen to prevent not just pathologic fractures incurred from metastatic prostate cancer, but osteoporotic fractures that occur as a consequence of hormonal therapy. An emerging literature also suggests that hormonal therapy for prostate cancer may increase the long-term risk of cardiovascular events.

For patients with metastatic prostate cancer, the prognosis typically spans several years. However, primary therapy with androgen receptor antagonists and LHRH analogues inevitably fail after a period of time. Failure of these therapies gives rise to a state that has been termed metastatic castration resistant prostate cancer (mCRPC). Until recently, scant options were available for this disease state. One of the first agents to obtain Food and Drug Administration (FDA) approval in this state is the chemotherapeutic agent mitoxantrone. This approval came on the basis of data suggesting that mitoxantrone therapy led to an improvement in pain (notably, the agent did not significantly prolong survival).

In 2005, the agent docetaxel was approved for advanced prostate cancer. The agent was rigorously tested in two phase III trials. Ultimately, docetaxel-based chemotherapy was shown to prolong survival as compared to active comparators. Docetaxel was also recently shown to improve survival in a phase III study in patients with newly diagnosed metastatic disease. Given these data, a trend toward earlier use of docetaxel chemotherapy is anticipated. The principal side effects of docetaxel chemotherapy include fatigue, myelosuppression, fluid retention, and neuropathy. In selected patients, docetaxel is administered in concert with growth factor support (filgrastim or pegfilgrastim) to mitigate the rate of neutropenia. Without use of such agents, a higher rate of febrile neutropenia and neutropenic sepsis might be anticipated. Management of neutropenic sepsis requires prompt hospital admission with empiric antibiotic therapy while investigations are underway to determine the source of infection.

From 2009 onward, a steady stream of agents has been approved for the management of mCRPC. The agent cabazitaxel was approved on the basis of a phase III trial comparing the agent to mitoxantrone in patients with prior docetaxel therapy. Cabazitaxel is similar to docetaxel in chemical structure with the exception of two hydroxyl side chains. Despite the subtle difference in chemical structure, the phase III trial evaluating cabazitaxel noted a survival improvement over conventional therapy in patients previously receiving docetaxel. The side effect profile of cabazitaxel differs somewhat from docetaxel. The agent is myelosuppressive, and therefore, use of growth factor support is strongly encouraged. Cabazitaxel tends to cause a lesser degree of alopecia and neuropathy as compared to docetaxel, although the rate of diarrhea appears to be much higher. Diarrhea associated with cabazitaxel can be quite severe, and the practicing hospitalist may occasionally see patients admitted for dehydration secondary to this phenomenon. Management entails administration of vigorous fluids and standard antimotility agents.

Beyond the cytotoxic agents used in metastatic prostate cancer (docetaxel, cabazitaxel, and mitoxantrone), there are three novel classes of agents that have been developed for mCRPC: (1) vaccine therapies, (2) next generation hormonal treatments, and (3) radiation particle-based therapies. Sipuleucel-T is an FDA-approved vaccine therapy for mCRPC. As opposed to conventional, "off-the-shelf" vaccines, sipuleucel-T is an autologous dendritic cell vaccine. Generation of the vaccine entails sequestration of leukocytes from the patient and subsequent ex vivo stimulation of these cells in the presence of prostate cancer antigens. The vaccine is administered as a subcutaneous injection every 2 weeks for a span of 6 weeks.

Side effects from the vaccine itself tend to be minimal, including mild infusion reactions and chills. Hickman catheters are frequently placed in the process of generating the vaccine product as many patients do not have sufficient venous access to allow for pheresis and sequestration of leukocytes. These catheters are prone to clotting and infection. Catheter-related complications may give rise to inpatient admission. For catheter-related sepsis, prompt removal of the catheter (with culture of the catheter tip) and aggressive antibiotic therapy should be employed (see Chapter 188 [Intravascular Catheter-Related Infections]).

Two next generation hormonal treatments have also been approved for the treatment of mCRPC. The first, abiraterone, is a CYP17-lyase inhibitor, a potent androgen synthesis inhibitor that may serve to abrogate intratumoral androgen production. The agent is administered orally daily. The toxicity profile of the agent is mild and typically entails mild electrolyte abnormalities. The agent also can cause transaminitis, and thus, labs are typically checked on a monthly basis. In about 3% to 5% of patients receiving abiraterone, transaminase levels may elevate to above 5 × the upper limit of normal. Immediate discontinuation of the drug and close monitoring until resolution is warranted under these circumstances. Notably, patients receiving abiraterone should receive concomitant therapy with prednisone to compensate for potential drops in serum cortisol caused by the drug. The hospitalist should be mindful that patients taking abiraterone without prednisone may therefore present with adrenal insufficiency (see Chapter 153 [Adrenal Insufficiency]).

Another second-generation hormone therapy for mCPRC, enzalutamide, is administered orally daily, and importantly, coadministration of prednisone is not required. Like bicalutamide, enzalutamide is a competitive antagonist for the androgen receptor. However, enzalutamide binds to the androgen receptor with greater affinity, and has also been demonstrated to inhibit nuclear translocation of the protein complex. In broad terms, the agent is very well tolerated, with fatigue representing the most frequent adverse event. In earlier trials of the drug, there was concern for several occurrences of seizure in a small proportion of patients. In the pivotal trials leading to the approval of enzalutamide, the rate of seizure appears to be minimal (<3%). Nonetheless, the hospitalist should be mindful of this potential adverse effect and the drug should be used cautiously in patients with a lowered threshold for seizure.

The most recent drug approved for mCRPC is radium-223, an alpha-emitting radioparticle administered as six monthly injections. Radioparticles have a long history in the management of advanced prostate cancer—beta-emitting radioisotopes such as strontium or samarium have been administered to many patients with the intent of palliative. These radioparticles localize to the bone, delivering a radiation dose to adjacent tumor tissue. As beta-emitters, strontium and samarium emit a radiation dose over a long range in contrast to the alpha-emitting radium-223. Furthermore, while strontium and samarium have been shown to reduce pain, neither has convincingly improved survival for patients with mCRPC. In a study including patients who were not fit for chemotherapy or who had progressed beyond it, radium-223 was shown to improve survival relative to placebo. The drug was well tolerated and did result in improvement in pain-related measures. The hospitalist should be aware, however, of potent myelosuppression seen in some patients receiving the drug. There has been some discordance in who delivers the agent, with medical oncologists, nuclear medicine specialists, radiologists, and radiation oncologists representing potential administering physicians.

■ NOTABLE COMPLICATIONS OF ADVANCED PROSTATE CANCER

In addition to understanding the toxicities associated with therapies for advanced prostate cancer, the hospitalist should be aware of complications associated with the underlying disease. Perhaps the most important oncologic emergency associated with prostate cancer is spinal cord compression. Neurologic manifestations of spinal cord compression (eg, severe back pain, loss of function/sensation in extremities) should prompt immediate evaluation with magnetic resonance imaging. If cord compression is observed, steroids should be administered and consultations with neurosurgery and radiation oncology obtained. Surgery or radiation therapy may reverse (either partially or completely) the symptoms of cord compression if implemented quickly enough.

Fortunately, the rate of cord compression associated with prostate cancer is declining as a consequence of use of bisphosphonate therapies (eg, zoledronic acid) and Receptor Activator of Nuclear Factor Kappa-B ligand inhibitors (eg, denosumab) to reduce cancer-associated bone loss. The most severe toxicity associated with these drugs is osteonecrosis of the jaw, a challenging entity to treat. Often, surgical correction is attempted in association with adjunctive therapies such as hyperbaric oxygen.

TESTICULAR CANCER

■ DISEASE OVERVIEW

In contrast to prostate cancer, testicular cancer has a relatively low incidence, with an estimated 8430 cases in 2015. Testicular cancer accounts for just 1% of cancer in males, but is the most common solid cancer in men aged 20 to 34. The greatest risk factor for developing testicular cancer is a previous history of the disease. In addition to this, men with undescended testes or Klinefelter's syndrome are also at risk. The disease presents typically as an enlarging testicular mass, although more advanced disease may present with site-specific symptoms (eg, shortness of breath in the context of lung metastases).

In terms of diagnosis, testicular ultrasound is helpful in clarifying the nature of a testicular mass. A radical inguinal orchiectomy should be performed for suspicious lesions. The staging of testicular cancer is unique in that it incorporates tumor markers, namely the alfa-fetoprotein (AFP), beta-human chorionic gonadotropin (beta-hCG) and lactate dehydrogenase (LDH) (see **Table 179-1**). These labs should be ordered prior to orchiectomy and should also be followed thereafter. Imaging including abdominal and pelvic computerized tomography should be performed; chest tomography should also be performed if there are suspicious lesions seen on chest x-ray.

The management of testicular cancer differs widely by histologic subtype. The two predominant subtypes of testicular cancer are seminoma and nonseminoma. The management of both seminoma and nonseminoma is nuanced and is highly dependent on clinical stage and marker status. For a comprehensive overview

of management, the reader is encouraged to refer to the National Comprehensive Cancer Network guidelines (available at http://www.nccn.com). The current section will focus on advanced stage testicular cancer.

■ TREATMENT OF METASTATIC TESTICULAR CANCER

Both patients with seminoma and nonseminoma with advanced disease are risk-stratified using three characteristics: (1) tumor marker levels, (2) the presence of a testicular or retroperitoneal primary tumor (as opposed to a mediastinal tumor), and (3) the presence or absence of nonpulmonary visceral metastases (eg, liver or brain metastases). Patients with nonseminoma are characterized as having good, intermediate, or poor risk on the basis of these characteristics, while patients with seminoma are either characterized as having good- or intermediate-risk disease (no poor-risk stratum exists).

Across both subtypes, patients with good-risk disease may receive either three cycles of bleomycin, etoposide, and cisplatin (BEP), or four cycles of etoposide and cisplatin (EP). Each of these drugs is administered intravenously. Cisplatin and etoposide are given for five consecutive days at the start of a 3-week cycle, while bleomycin is given once weekly during the 3-week cycle. Many oncologists prefer to admit patients for the first week of therapy, as the combination of cisplatin and etoposide requires a lengthy infusion time. The choice between BEP and EP for good-risk disease is predicated on patient preference related to (1) length of the regimen (BEP is given for 9 weeks total, while EP is given for 12 weeks total) and (2) bleomycin-related toxicities. A randomized trial demonstrated similar efficacy with four cycles of EP and three cycles of BEP.

Notable toxicities with bleomycin include myelosuppression and pulmonary fibrosis. Myelosuppression is typically ameliorated with use of growth factors, such as filgrastim or pegfilgrastim. With use of these agents, the incidence of febrile neutropenia is quite low. Pulmonary fibrosis associated with bleomycin typically presents with cough, shortness of breath, and possibly pleuritic chest pain. Diagnosis typically requires high-resolution computerized tomography of the chest. If infectious etiologies are suspected, these should be first ruled out using bronchoscopy and lavage. If infection is thought to be unlikely, treatment can be implemented with high-dose steroids if the patient is severely symptomatic. Treatment with bleomycin should be discontinued, as well. Several risk factors for bleomycin-induced lung injury exist, including a history of cigarette smoking and other underlying pulmonary fibrosis. For this reason, pulmonary function tests should be obtained at baseline. The

---

TABLE 179-1 Risk Stratification of Advanced Testicular Cancer

Classification	Seminoma	Nonseminoma
Good risk	Any primary site *and*	Testicular/retroperitoneal primary tumor *and*
	No nonpulmonary visceral metastases *and*	No nonpulmonary visceral metastases *and*
	Normal AFP with any beta-hCG or LDH	Tumor markers including AFP < 1000,* beta-hCG <5000 and LDH <1.5 × ULN
Intermediate risk	Any primary site *and*	Testicular/retroperitoneal primary tumor *and*
	Nonpulmonary visceral metastases *and*	No nonpulmonary visceral metastases *and*
	Normal AFP with any beta-hCG or LDH	Tumor markers including AFP 1000-10,000, beta-hCG 5000-50,000 and LDH 1.5-10 × ULN
Poor risk	*(Poor-risk category does not exist for advanced seminoma)*	Mediastinal primary site *or*
		Nonpulmonary visceral metastases *or*
		Tumor markers including AFP >10,000, beta-hCG > 50,000 and LDH > 10 × ULN

Note that the tumor markers used for risk stratification reflect postorchiectomy markers. *Units for AFP and beta-hCG are ng/mL and iu/L, respectively. **ULN, upper limit of normal. (Table adapted from the 2015 National Comprehensive Cancer Network Guidelines for Testicular Cancer, available at http://www.nccn.org.)

diffusing capacity for carbon monoxide (DLCO) is the most critical parameter to follow. An impaired baseline DLCO might suggest underlying lung disease. A drop in the DLCO by 30% or greater would suggest bleomycin-related toxicity and should prompt discontinuation.

For patients with intermediate- or high-risk disease, a total of four cycles of BEP are recommended. In addition to the toxicities typically associated with bleomycin, the hospitalist should be aware of toxicities related to cisplatin and etoposide administered during this regimen. Cisplatin may cause nephrotoxicity, and the agent is typically not administered to patients with a creatinine clearance less than 60 mL/min. To mitigate the risk of nephrotoxicity, cisplatin is accompanied by vigorous fluid hydration before and after administration. Cisplatin may also cause a spectrum of other toxicities, including nausea, vomiting, hearing loss, and neuropathy. Etoposide is well known to cause myelosuppression. As noted previously, coadministration of growth factors may mitigate this toxicity.

Fortunately, the cure rates for advanced testicular cancer are quite high. For instance, with three cycles of BEP or four cycles of EP, the cure rate for good-risk nonseminoma is in excess of 90%. However, curability varies with risk status—for patients with poor-risk disease, approximately half of patients will experience relapse. Relapsed testicular cancer is managed through one of two principle strategies—either salvage chemotherapy or high-dose chemotherapy (HDCT) with autologous peripheral autologous cell transplant (PSCT). High-dose chemotherapy with autologous PSCT results in durable remissions in a large proportion of patients. Considerations for autologous PSCT are complex and are discussion in other chapters of this textbook. Two distinct salvage chemotherapy regimens may also be considered in the same clinical setting: (1) vinblastine, ifosfamide, and cisplatin (VelP) or (2) paclitaxel, ifosfamide, and cisplatin (TIP). Both regimens are comprised of intravenous agents administered in the inpatient setting. Common to both of these regimens are ifosfamide and cisplatin. Toxicities associated with cisplatin have previously been reviewed. The hospitalist should be aware of several toxicities associated with ifosfamide. In addition to causing profound myelosuppression, ifosfamide is known to cause hemorrhagic cystitis. Urine should be monitored for the presence of microscopic hematuria. Furthermore, ifosfamide should be administered with mesna, which reduces the risk of bladder injury. If hemorrhagic cystitis is encountered, a urology consultation should be obtained and continuous bladder irrigation should be instituted. In patients receiving VelP, vinblastine can cause substantial myelosuppression. In patients receiving TIP, paclitaxel can cause myelosuppression, neuropathy, fluid retention, and fatigue.

There is currently equipoise as to whether HDCT with autologous PSCT or salvage chemotherapy represents a superior choice for first relapse of testicular cancer. A randomized trial is planned which will directly juxtapose these options. Beyond these options, there are few effective systemic therapy options available for patients with metastatic testicular cancer. Patients should be referred for clinical trials when possible.

NOTABLE COMPLICATIONS OF ADVANCED TESTICULAR CANCER

Bony metastases occur far less frequently in the context of testicular cancer as compared to prostate cancer. In the rare event of spinal cord compression, management is similar to that described in the context of prostate cancer. A second potential disease-related complication from testicular cancer is superior vena cava (SVC) syndrome. Superior vena cava syndrome occurs in the context of bulky lymphadenopathy often associated with testicular cancer. Occlusion of the SVC can lead to engorgement of proximal vessels and pain. If such symptoms are noted, a prompt consultation with a radiation oncologist or interventional radiologist should be considered. Radiotherapy is highly effective in this context, and endovascular stents can serve as a temporizing measure. For patients with newly diagnosed disease presenting with SVC syndrome, bear in mind that advanced testicular cancer tends to be chemosensitive. Thus, prompt initiation of systemic therapy may aid in relieving symptoms quickly.

SUMMARY

The hospitalist should be aware of site-specific complications of advanced prostate and testicular cancer (eg, spinal cord compression, SVC syndrome), as well as potential treatment-related adverse effects. The landscape of therapy in prostate cancer has changed markedly in recent years (see **Figure 179-1**). Chemotherapy with docetaxel is often combined with androgen synthesis inhibitors and androgen receptor antagonists in the front-line setting. As castration-resistant disease evolves, multiple new treatments have been approved by the US FDA over the past decade, including (1) second-generation hormone treatments (abiraterone and enzalutamide), (2) novel cytotoxics (cabazitaxel), (3) vaccine therapies (sipuleucel-T), and (4) radioparticles (radium-223). Each has a distinct profile of adverse effects, summarized in *"Practice Point: Agents for mCRPC and Notable Side Effects."* In contrast to prostate cancer, relatively few changes to the systemic management of testicular cancer have been observed over the past decade. However, existing chemotherapy strategies result in a high cure rate, even in the context of metastatic disease. Toxicities associated with these agents are summarized in *"Practice Point: Agents for Testicular Cancer and Notable Side Effects."* It is important to bear in mind that a subset

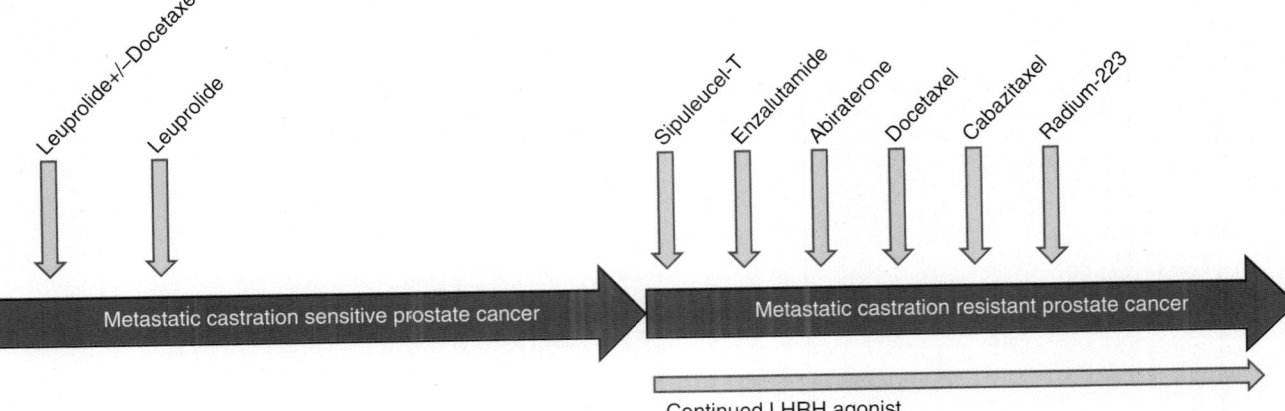

Figure 179-1 *Available agents for the treatment of mCRPC. Note that there is substantial debate regarding the appropriate sequencing of therapies.*

of patients does not respond to conventional chemotherapy regimens such as BEP, and these patients with a poor prognosis may be overrepresented in the inpatient setting. Thus, the hospitalist should have some familiarity with salvage chemotherapy regimens (eg, TIP or VeIP) or HDCT with autologous PSCT as discussed previously. Further research is needed to identify viable strategies for patients that progress beyond these modalities.

PRACTICE POINT

Agents for mCRPC and notable side effects

There are now a total of six FDA-approved agents for the treatment of mCRPC, with the following toxicities relevant to the practicing hospitalist:

- Sipuleucel-T, an autologous dendritic cell vaccine, often requires central catheter placement for pheresis to facilitate generation of the vaccine product. Catheter-based complications (eg, thrombosis or infection) may occur.
- Enzalutamide is a second-generation androgen receptor antagonist. Rare reports of seizure have been identified with the agent.
- Abiraterone decreases androgen synthesis through inhibition of CYP17 lyase. If not taken with prednisone, adrenal insufficiency may arise.
- Docetaxel is a cytotoxic agent that can cause potent myelosuppression. If growth factors are not administered, patients may be at risk for neutropenic sepsis.
- Cabazitaxel is a cytotoxic agent that is structurally related to docetaxel. It also carries a risk of myelosuppression, and a higher rate of diarrhea has been observed with the agent.

PRACTICE POINT

Agents for testicular cancer and notable side effects

Several of the common agents used in advanced testicular cancer are noted below, along with side effects relevant to the practicing hospitalist:

- Bleomycin may cause lung injury, manifesting as pulmonary fibrosis. Prompt consultation with a pulmonary specialist should be considered. If infectious etiologies are ruled out and the patient remains symptomatic, corticosteroids may be administered.

- Etoposide is given with bleomycin in the context of the BEP chemotherapy regimen. Both agents cause potent myelosuppression. The risk of febrile neutropenia and neutropenic sepsis can be mitigated with use of growth factors.
- Cisplatin may cause nephrotoxicity. Vigorous hydration should accompany administration to mitigate this risk.
- Ifosfamide is given as a component of several salvage chemotherapy regimens for advanced testicular cancer. In addition to the risk of potent myelosuppression, the hospitalist should be aware of the risk of hemorrhagic cystitis. Hemorrhagic cystitis can possibly be prevented with coadministration of Mesna. Urology consultation should be obtained and continuous bladder irrigation should be considered.

SUGGESTED READINGS

Albers P, Albrecht W, Algaba F, et al. Guidelines on Testicular Cancer: 2015 Update. *Eur Urol.* 2015;68(6):1054-1068.

Beer TM, Armstrong AJ, Rathkopf DE, et al. Enzalutamide in metastatic prostate cancer before chemotherapy. *N Engl J Med.* 2014;371:424-433.

Kantoff PW, Higano CS, Shore ND, et al. Sipuleucel-T immunotherapy for castration-resistant prostate cancer. *N Engl J Med.* 2010;363:411-422.

National Comprehensive Cancer Network (NCCN) Guidelines for Management of Prostate Cancer. Available at http://www.nccn.org Accessed September 26, 2015.

National Comprehensive Cancer Network (NCCN) Guidelines for Management of Testicular Cancer. Available at http://www.nccn.org. Accessed September 26, 2015.

Parker C, Nilsson S, Heinrich D, et al. Alpha emitter radium-223 and survival in metastatic prostate cancer. *N Engl J Med.* 2013;369:213-223.

Scher HI, Fizazi K, Saad F, et al. Increased survival with enzalutamide in prostate cancer after chemotherapy. *N Engl J Med.* 2012;367:1187-1197.

Sweeney CJ, Chen YH, Carducci M, Liu G, et al. Chemohormonal therapy in metastatic hormone-sensitive prostate cancer. *N Engl J Med.* 2015;373:737-746.

CHAPTER 180

Cancers of the Kidney, Renal Pelvis, and Ureter

Joseph Brito, MD
Dragan Golijanin, MD
Jodi Layton, MD

Key Clinical Questions

① What are the most common presenting signs of renal tumors?

② How are renal tumors diagnosed?

③ How do renal pelvis and ureteral tumors present?

④ Which specialists should be involved in the care of renal tumors and their complications?

RENAL TUMORS

■ EPIDEMIOLOGY

Renal masses may represent renal cell carcinoma, metastasis from other malignancies, lymphoma, or benign tumors such as angiomyolipoma (AML), oncocytomas, benign complex cystic structures or adenomas. Occasionally, focal pyelonephritis or infiltration of a renal pelvis malignancy may mimic the appearance of a primary renal mass on imaging studies and must be considered in the appropriate clinical setting. Renal masses of one form or another can be found in an estimated 50% of all patients over age 50. Small renal masses, defined generally as those <4 cm in size (see **Figure 180-1**), represent a large proportion of incidentally discovered renal neoplasms and can present a management dilemma for the urologist and oncologist given a sometimes unclear natural history.

Renal cell carcinoma (RCC) accounts for approximately 3% of all adult malignancies in the United States with approximately 65,000 cases per year and accounts for approximately 14,000 deaths per year. This incidence represents a doubling in the rate of newly diagnosed RCC over the past 10 years and likely reflects an increased rate of detection due to increased utilization of ultrasound and high-resolution computed tomography (CT) scan for the evaluation of abdominal complaints.

According to the Surveillance, Epidemiology and End Results (SEER) database from 2008 to 2012, RCC occurs more commonly in men than women (approximately 2:1), with a median age of 64 years and is found to be metastatic in approximately 17% of patients at time of diagnosis. Of patients diagnosed with kidney-confined disease (approximately 65% at diagnosis), 92% will have a 5-year survival rate.

The most common type of RCC is clear cell carcinoma comprising approximately 80% of all RCCs. Other subtypes include papillary (types I and II), chromophobe, collecting duct, medullary, and translocation tumors. Some tumors develop more aggressive features and can have sarcomatoid or rhabdoid histological features. Poorly differentiated tumors often act very clinically aggressive.

While the majority of cases of RCC are sporadic, approximately 2% to 3% are felt to be genetic in origin. Many familial syndromes involving RCC have been described in the literature. The most common among these is von Hippel-Lindau syndrome which is characterized by hemangioblastomas of the central nervous system, retinal angiomas, pheochromocytoma, and RCC of the clear cell subtype. Other familial syndromes include hereditary papillary RCC, familial leiomyomatosis and RCC, and Birt-Hogg-Dube syndrome. Patients with a strong family history of renal malignancies warrant a comprehensive history and physical to screen for associated disease processes.

Risk factors for the development of RCC include tobacco exposure, which confers a relative risk of 1.4 to 2.5 times the unexposed population. More recently obesity has become recognized as a significant risk factor, rising in proportion to patient BMI. Finally, hypertension appears to be an independent risk factor for RCC development, possibly related to the resultant renal injury and subsequent inflammation.

■ PRESENTATION

The discovery of renal masses has risen with increasing use of radiographic studies such as abdominal ultrasounds, computed tomography, and magnetic resonance imaging (MRI) studies utilized to

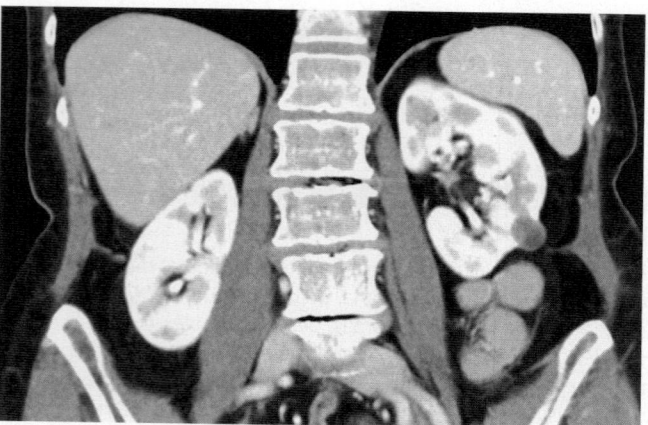

Figure 180-1 *Exophytic small renal mass of the left kidney highly suspicious for primary renal cell carcinoma.*

evaluate often unrelated symptoms. Most commonly, the diagnosis of kidney cancer is made incidentally and patients are completely asymptomatic.

The classic triad of flank pain, hematuria and a palpable mass are rarely presenting symptoms in the modern era. Among symptomatic patients, back or flank pain are common presenting signs owing to local growth and mass effect of the tumor. Gross hematuria is less common unless the tumor communicates or affects the collecting duct system but can be seen in up to 50% of symptomatic patients. Amongst all patients with gross or microscopic hematuria, approximately 10% will have a renal carcinoma while the remaining 90% will be composed of patients with nephrolithiasis, infectious processes, medical renal disease, or malignancies of ureters or bladder. Constitutional symptoms such as unintentional weight loss, fatigue, or night sweats suggest advanced or metastatic disease at diagnosis. Renal cell carcinomas are associated with paraneoplastic syndromes approximately 20% of the time and can include the production of excess erythropoietin causing erythrocytosis or hypercalcemia from parathyroid hormone-related peptide (PTHrP) overproduction. Stauffer Syndrome is a paraneoplastic syndrome characterized by hepatic dysfunction, elevated alkaline phosphatase and hypoalbuminemia.

■ INPATIENT MANAGEMENT

Workup necessary for kidney tumors depends on size of the tumor, radiographic characteristics of the tumor, and whether advanced disease is suspected based on laboratory, radiographic and physical examination findings. Small renal tumors with classic characteristics for RCC can sometimes be safely monitored with surveillance imaging in appropriately selected patients.

Inpatient consultation with urology should be obtained for any newly found renal mass for assistance in workup and management. Oncology input may be beneficial for the workup of any large kidney mass (≥7 cm) or signs of systemic disease. A multidisciplinary approach is useful in determining treatment options. Unlike other solid-organ malignancies, needle biopsy is not often necessary to diagnose renal cell carcinomas given characteristic imaging findings. Needle biopsy may be of assistance in cases where clinical findings suggest either the presence of lymphoma or the possibility of metastatic disease. Historically, percutaneous needle biopsy was felt to confer a risk of tumor seeding along biopsy tract; however, more recent studies suggest that this risk is minimal. Biopsy should generally be preserved for select cases where tissue diagnosis is absolutely necessary to determine course of treatment. Biopsy can also be performed at the time of a planned ablative procedure, which is often done in a percutaneous fashion.

In general, CT with and without IV contrast incorporating delayed imaging should be obtained in all candidate patients. Patients unable to tolerate IV contrast may benefit from noncontract CT scanning with or without ultrasound adjunct or MRI to characterize renal parenchyma and surrounding structures. As a rule, patients with hematuria should undergo cystoscopy prior to surgical planning in order to rule out a concurrent bladder tumor, but this may be completed as a part of the outpatient workup. Patients unable to tolerate contrast may undergo cystoscopy with retrograde ureteral contrast instillation to ensure no ureteral or renal pelvis component to the mass. Full staging should be obtained for large tumors, radiographic findings suggestive of tumor thrombus or extension to the inferior vena cava, regional lymphadenopathy, or the presence of constitutional or localizing symptoms suggesting metastatic disease such as weight loss or focal bone pain. Full body cat scans and nuclear medicine bone scan in addition to baseline laboratory evaluation should be considered in these cases.

Need for ongoing inpatient care depends on presenting signs and symptoms at time of diagnosis. Metabolic derangements and severe anemia should be corrected prior to discharge. Asymptomatic patients can be safely worked up on an outpatient basis unless there is concern for inadequate follow-up with urology, oncology or issues related to the patient's resources and availability of imaging studies and possible surgical intervention.

Although more common in patients with primary bladder malignancies, gross hematuria and evidence of urinary retention warrant urgent urology consultation and may require urethral catheterization with manual irrigation of obstructing clots from the bladder. Correction of pharmacologic or other coagulopathy is especially important in this population.

Patient's overall health, life expectancy and size of tumor at time of diagnosis help determine appropriateness and timing of definitive intervention. Renal cell carcinoma staging follows the TNM system, with stage 1 and 2 tumors confined to the kidney and stage 3 and 4 tumors involving local and distant sites, respectively. Five-year survival rates are highest for stage 1 tumors at 81% and poorest for stage 4 tumors at 8%. In very selected patients, small tumors can be managed with outpatient routine surveillance scans for which surveillance protocols are being developed. Ablative techniques can be considered for tumors upward of 4 cm or for patients in whom definitive surgical intervention is not an option.

Surgical resection via total or partial nephrectomy is the gold standard for definitive treatment for larger tumors or symptomatic tumors. Laparoscopic partial or total nephrectomies have equivalent cancer control and side effect profiles when performed by experienced urologists. Partial nephrectomy has overtaken radical nephrectomy as the gold standard in management for small tumors as it allows for better preservation of long-term renal function. This is especially important given increasing rates of chronic kidney disease and diabetes with a concomitant need for nephron sparing options.

Patients diagnosed with metastatic disease upon presentation may still benefit from surgical resection of the primary mass, termed "cytoreductive" nephrectomy. This decision should be made by oncology and urology consultants to determine sequence and timing of systemic and surgical interventions. Patients found to have advanced disease should have additional laboratory workup including total calcium levels, complete blood counts and metabolic panels. Systemic options for management of metastatic disease include both oral and intravenous chemotherapeutics. Current regimens include interleukin-2 (IL-2) and interferon-alpha (INFα), tyrosine kinase inhibitors (TKIs), vascular endothelial growth factor receptor inhibitors (VEGF-R), and mammalian target of rapamycin (mTOR) inhibitors each of which has demonstrated modest benefit in clear cell carcinomas (**Table 180-1**). The efficacy of these agents in non–clear cell tumors remains under investigation and clinical trial

TABLE 180-1 Standard of Care Agents Utilized to Treat Metastatic Renal Cell Carcinoma

Treatment	Mechanism of Action	Route
Sunitinib	Multikinase inhibitor	Oral
Pazopanib	Multikinase inhibitor	Oral
Axitinib	Second-generation VEGFR-1, 2, 3 inhibitor	Oral
Sorafenib	Multikinase inhibitor	Oral
Everolimus	mTOR inhibitor	Oral
Temsirolimus	mTOR inhibitor	Intravenous
Interferon-α	Immunomodulator	Intravenous
Interleukin-2	Immunomodulator	Intravenous
Bevacizumab	Anti-VEGF monoclonal antibody	Intravenous
Nivolumab	PD1 inhibitor	Intravenous

mTOR, Mammalian target of rapamycin; VEGFR, vascular endothelial growth factor receptor.

enrollment is recommended where available. The choice of chemotherapeutic regimen should be made by the oncologist in conjunction with the patient, taking comorbidities, performance status, and side effect profiles into account. IL-2 and INFα require specific monitoring and management and are offered at only a small number of institutions. TKI, VEGF inhibitors, and mTOR inhibitors demonstrate similar efficacy as IL-2 and INFα and are now more readily used as first-line therapy in metastatic disease. Despite benefit in treating patients with advanced disease, systemic therapy does not offer any proven benefit in the adjuvant setting in nonmetastatic disease.

■ COMPLICATIONS

In-hospital complications are rare on presentation but may include hematuria, retroperitoneal bleeding, or thromboembolic events. New onset atrial fibrillation has been reported and may represent sequela of either metabolic derangements or rapid fluid shifts in the setting of transfusion. Patients undergoing surgical extirpation with either radical or partial nephrectomy are at risk for various postoperative complications of which the hospitalist should have a basic awareness. Complications of radical nephrectomy include surgical site infections, bleeding, or worsening renal function due to a poorly functioning solitary kidney, prerenal insult due to dehydration, nephrotoxic medications resumed postoperatively, or postrenal obstruction such as acute urinary retention. Patients undergoing partial nephrectomy are at increased risk of bleeding from the tumor bed as well as the unique risk of urine leak from an inadequately sealed collecting system. Such patients warrant urology involvement and may require percutaneous or retrograde ureteral stent placement. Patient undergoing either ablation procedures or partial nephrectomy are also at risk for pseudoaneurysm formation within the renal parenchyma which may require interventional radiology embolization.

■ POSTACUTE CARE

Postdischarge care should focus on completion of staging with any outstanding laboratory and imaging studies. Follow-up consultation with urology and or oncology should be established prior to discharge. Additionally, patients with medical comorbidities may benefit from subspecialist evaluation to elucidate candidacy for surgical intervention and or chemotherapeutics. Definitive management, either through surgical planning or chemotherapy initiation, should begin soon after discharge to impart the best survival potential. Postintervention follow-up will be managed by the Urologist or

Oncologist and generally includes periodic CT imaging to assess for response to therapy and any evidence of recurrence.

■ DISCHARGE CHECK LIST

- Laboratory workup completed
- Imaging studies completed
- Appropriate follow-up (urology, oncology) established

RENAL PELVIS and URETERAL TUMORS

The renal pelvis, ureters, and bladder all share the same histologic lining comprising of a thin layer of urothelium. These cells are classically known as "transitional cells" due to their change in histologic appearance in various physiologic states. Therefore, malignancy of the renal pelvis, ureter or bladder is known as either urothelial carcinoma or transitional cell carcinoma. Urothelial carcinomas of the renal pelvis and ureter have similar risk factors for development and likewise share many presenting symptoms.

■ EPIDEMIOLOGY

Urothelium along the entire genitourinary tract is exposed to carcinogens during urinary excretion and is at risk for multifocal tumor development due to field cancerization effect. Accordingly, people who develop upper tract tumors are at increased risk for developing bladder tumors and contralateral upper tract disease, with 15% to 75% of patients with upper tract urothelial tumors developing bladder tumors over a 5-year period. Approximately 3000 new cases of upper tract tumors are diagnosed each year with the incidence increasing slightly over the past two decades. Fortunately due to improved management strategies patients have experienced an improvement in survival over this same time period. The vast majority of ureteral tumors occur in the distal ureter, with only about 5% occurring in the proximal ureter and renal pelvis. Urothelial cancers of the upper tract (renal pelvis and ureters) are twice as common in men than women.

Rarely, metastatic tumors from other cancers, primary adenocarcinoma or squamous cell carcinoma arise from the renal pelvis.

Cigarette smoking is a well-established risk factor for upper tract urothelial carcinoma, with a relative risk of up to 7 for smokers of >45 pack years. Occupational exposure to industrial plastics, petroleum, coal, asphalt and tar are also at an elevated risk. Analine dye, benzidine and B-naphthylamine exposures also represent occupational exposure risks and can have long latency periods. A mild increase in risk has been characterized for coffee consumption, analgesic abuse, and arsenic exposure. Lynch syndrome represents a genetic predisposition to upper tract malignancy.

■ PRESENTATION

Hematuria is a common presenting sign in upward of 90% of people with upper tract cancers. In patients with gross or microscopic hematuria, approximately 5% of people will have a malignancy of the renal pelvis or ureter. Flank pain may be present if malignant ureteral obstruction or renal pelvis distension from hydronephrosis or hemorrhage is present. A palpable abdominal mass can sometimes be present but is rare.

Depending on site of tumor growth, chronic obstruction can occur leading to hydronephrosis and progressive loss of renal function (**Figures 180-2 and 180-3**). Because such obstruction generally occurs gradually over time, patients may not present with the same type of acute ureteral obstructive symptoms as seen with renal colic. Malignant hydronephrosis can be a setup for infection due to poor kidney drainage and as such patients may present with systemic inflammatory response syndrome or sepsis.

Constitutional symptoms such as unintentional weight loss, fatigue, and cachexia often indicate advanced or metastatic disease

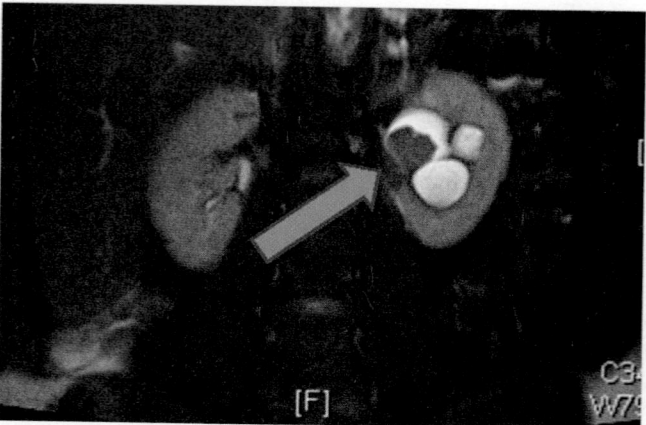

Figure 180-2 *Left renal pelvis tumor of urothelial origin.*

at diagnosis. Location of the primary tumor in the renal pelvis may delay metastatic spread as the renal parenchyma appears to provide some degree of containment. Tumors arising from the thin-walled ureter allow earlier local extension and subsequent metastasis.

■ INPATIENT MANAGEMENT

Inpatient management is often determined by complications caused by primary tumor location. If a tumor is found incidentally by imaging and without acute complications, urology consult can be obtained and outpatient workup can be pursued. Generally such imaging should be CT scan with and without IV contrast with delayed ureteral imaging to evaluate for a filling defect and further characterization of the tumor. Patients who cannot tolerate IV contrast media but for whom there exists a high index of suspicion should undergo noncontrast CT with or without ultrasound or MRI and may require cystoscopy with retrograde ureteropyelogram to characterize the tumor. Initiation of diagnosis can be helpful by obtaining urine sample for urine cytology. Historically, urine samples from three different voided specimens were recommended in order to increase sensitivity, however more recent data suggest that a single specimen provides adequate disease detection for high-grade lesions. Notably, upper tract urothelial carcinomas are less likely to be diagnosed via urine cytology compared to primary bladder or lower ureteral tumors.

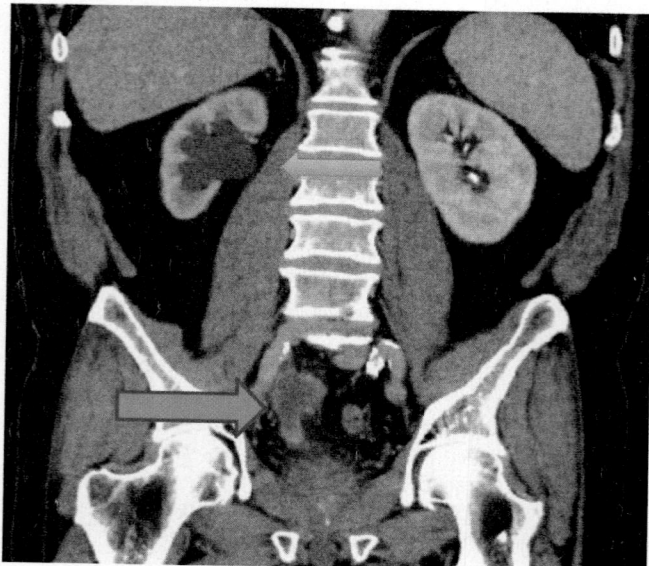

Figure 180-3 *Hydronephrosis (small arrow) caused by right distal ureteral mass (large arrow).*

Patients presenting with signs and symptoms of ureteral obstruction with hydronephrosis generally require acute intervention. Emergent renal decompression should be pursued for patients for patients presenting with sepsis. Options include cystoscopy with ureteral stent placement by urologists or percutaneous nephrostomy placement via interventional radiologists. Percutaneous decompression is preferred in the setting of large bladder or distal ureteral tumors which can obscure visualization of the ureteral orifice and bladder trigone anatomy. Urology consult should be obtained to determine the best method for decompression for these patients. Stable patients without evidence of sepsis but with acute kidney injury or flank pain should be decompressed in a timely fashion but generally do not require emergent procedures. The presence of renal insufficiency and/or hydronephrosis will often dictate need for hospital admission and acuity of management.

Patients undergoing renal decompression for sepsis often require monitoring in an acute care unit such as an intermediate care "stepdown" unit or intensive care. As is the case with renal decompression for obstructive ureterolithiasis, such patients may experience worsening septic physiology following renal decompression due to seeding of bacteria into the bloodstream via the highly vascularized renal parenchyma during nephrostomy tube placement. Broad spectrum antibiotics to cover urinary flora as well as aggressive intravenous fluid resuscitation should be initiated.

While ureteral stents placed in a retrograde fashion require no maintenance care, percutaneous nephrostomy tubes are prone to external disturbances and require daily cleaning and maintenance. Newly placed tubes will generally display bloody output for the first 12 to 24 hours with expected progressive clearing thereafter. Periodic flushing of the tube with small quantities of normal saline during this period can prevent clot formation and obstruction. Both nephrostomy tubes and indwelling ureteral stents require regular exchange. Patients who undergo either procedure will need firmly established urology and or interventional radiology follow-up.

Once acute management of renal decompression has been addressed, patients with suspected upper tract urothelial carcinoma will require definitive diagnosis via either antegrade (via nephrostomy tract) or retrograde (via bladder and distal ureteral orifice) ureteroscopy with biopsy. If patients are otherwise stable or must complete an antibiotic course due to septic presentation, this diagnostic procedure may be accomplished on an outpatient basis. If outpatient follow-up cannot be reliably established, diagnostic procedures should be completed prior to discharge.

Patients with physical, constitutional or radiographic findings suggestive of metastatic disease (such as regional lymphadenopathy) should undergo full staging imaging with CT scans of the chest, abdominal, pelvis, and nuclear bone scans. Once acute care is completed to address any issues from the primary tumor, further management for metastatic disease can be accomplished on an outpatient basis.

■ COMPLICATIONS

Complications of upper tract urothelial malignancies beyond presentation are most often related to postprocedural issues after renal decompression, following endoscopic biopsy or ablative interventions. Complications resulting from ureteral stent placement include infection, bleeding, bladder spasm due to stent irritation, and stent migration or failure requiring replacement or additional procedures. Percutaneous nephrostomy placement avoids the problems of bladder irritation but confers a similar infectious risk. Bleeding from nephrostomy tube placement is generally minimal but occasionally can be severe requiring tube replacement or angiography with embolization.

Ureteroscopy with biopsy puts patients at risk for ureteral perforation, retroperitoneal bleeding and stent discomfort. Patients undergoing nephroureterectomy are also at risk of bleeding and require transfusion in less than 2% of cases. Due to manipulation of the distal ureter and bladder cuff excision these patients are at risk for bladder perforation or continued urinary extravasation postoperatively. Generally this can be managed with prolonged indwelling Foley catheter but occasionally requires return to the operating room for bladder closure. Incisional hernia is a risk in patients undergoing open nephroureterectomy and can also be seen after robotic assisted or laparoscopic approaches albeit at much lower rates.

■ POSTACUTE CARE

Posthospital care of upper tract ureteral and renal pelvic malignancies depend on many factors including aggressiveness of disease, presence of a functional and uncompromised contralateral renal unit, patient comorbidities and life expectancy. Low-grade, low-volume ureteral or renal pelvic tumors may be amenable to endoscopic ablation with periodic surveillance thereafter to assess for disease recurrence. Higher-grade, multifocal or large volume lesions generally require en bloc excision of the kidney and ureter with incorporation of a small cuff of bladder to ensure clean surgical margins. A subset of patients with isolated distal ureteral tumors may benefit from distal ureterectomy with ureteral reimplantation into the native bladder. All patients will require periodic follow-up involving imaging as well as cystoscopy with or without ureteroscopy depending on the intervention performed. Such follow-up occurs at decreasing intervals if no disease recurrence is detected.

Systemic chemotherapy may be recommended for some patients with advanced tumors noted after surgical resection. Patients presenting with metastatic disease should be evaluated for the appropriateness of systemic chemotherapy. There is minimal role for surgical resection of ureteral tumors for patients with metastatic disease at time of diagnosis. First-line treatment for both adjuvant and first-line treatment in metastatic urothelial cancer utilizes a platinum-based chemotherapy and is most commonly administered in an outpatient setting. Patients undergoing chemotherapy for urothelial carcinoma are at risk for readmission for febrile neutropenia, symptomatic anemia, bleeding risks from thrombocytopenia and acute renal failure. Oncology consultation is recommended for patients admitted while receiving chemotherapy.

■ DISCHARGE CHECK LIST

- Laboratory workup completed
- Imaging workup completed
- Ensure close follow-up with urologist and or oncologist
- Ensure patient is familiar with care of and plan for nephrostomy and or ureteral stent

---

PRACTICE POINT

A Multi-Disciplinary Approach to GU Malignancies is Key

1. A multidisciplinary approach with urology, oncology, and interventional radiology is often key to determine appropriate course of workup and treatment for kidney, renal pelvis, and ureteral tumors.
2. Transition from inpatient to outpatient workup and treatment should be established prior to discharge.
3. Referral to genitourinary specialists (both urology and medical oncology) is preferred when possible.

PRACTICE POINT

Hematuria is Never Normal

1. Hematuria is never normal and should prompt initiation of workup upon discovery as this can be the only sign of underlying genitourinary malignancy.
2. Common causes of hematuria include: urinary tract infections, renal stones, medical renal disease.

PRACTICE POINT

Reducing the Risk of PCN Infections

1. Newly inserted nephrostomy tubes require routine flushing with small volumes of normal saline to ensure patency. Difficulty with tube irrigation, poor or scant drainage and or excessive bleeding should be assessed by interventional radiology for proper positioning. Chronic indwelling ureteral stents and percutaneous nephrostomy tubes require regular maintenance and exchanges; patients are at increased risk of infectious complications and often require inpatient attention.
2. If there is suspicion for urinary infection, cultures should be taken from all reservoirs of urine (ie, bilateral PCN and urethral samples when possible) to help improve culture sensitivity and direct antibiotic management when necessary.
3. Chronic indwelling percutaneous nephrostomies often become colonized over time. Colonization does not warrant antibiotic treatments unless a patient demonstrates signs of systemic infection.

SUGGESTED READINGS

Audenet F, Yates DR, Cussenot O, Rouprêt M. The role of chemotherapy in the treatment of urothelial carcinoma of the upper tract (UTT-UCC). *Urol Oncol.* 2010;31(4):407-413.

Campbell SC, Lane BR. Malignant renal tumors. In: McDougal WS, et al, eds. *Campbell-Walsh Urology*, 10th ed. Philadelphia, PA: Elsevier, 2012.

Huang SY, Philip A, Richter MD, et al. Prevention and management of infectious complications of percutaneous interventions. *Semin Intervent Radiol.* 2015;32(2):78-88.

Kunkle D, Uzzo RG. Cryoablation or radiofrequency ablation of the small renal mass: a meta-analysis. *Cancer.* 2008;113: 2671-2680.

Leibovich BC, Lohse CM, Crispen PL, et al. Histological subtype is an independent predictor of outcome for patients with renal cell carcinoma. *J Urol.* 2010;183:1309-1315.

Leow JJ, Orsola A, Chang SL, Bellmunt J. A contemporary review of management and prognostic factors of upper tract urothelial carcinoma. *Cancer Treat Rev.* 2015;41(4):310-319.

Stewart S, et al: Evaluation of the National Comprehensive Cancer Network and American Urological Association Renal Cell Carcinoma Surveillance Guidelines. *J Clin Oncol.* 2014;32(36): 4059-4065.

CHAPTER 181

Oncologic Issues of the Aerodigestive Tract

Adeel M. Khan, MD, MPH

Tobenna Nwizu, MD

Key Clinical Questions

1. What complications of cancers of the aerodigestive tract often cause hospital admission?

2. What consultant services should be pursued for specific clinical syndromes?

3. Which cancer types are the most prone to emergencies of the aerodigestive tract?

INTRODUCTION

The aerodigestive tract, also called the mixed airway/gastrointestinal tract, constitutes the organs of the oral cavity, nasal cavity and pharynx, larynx and vocal cords, bronchi and small airways, and the esophagus. Cancers of the upper aerodigestive tract constitute approximately 4% of all malignancies, and chiefly include head and neck cancers, lung cancers, esophageal cancers, and lesser common cancers such as nasopharyngeal carcinomas and salivary gland cancers. Thyroid cancers, skin cancers of the head and neck, lower gastrointestinal tract cancers, and non–bronchoalveolar-mediastinal cancers are generally not included in this category. The two primary histologic varieties of aerodigestive tract cancers include squamous cell carcinoma and adenocarcinoma and common etiologies include tobacco use, alcohol use, human papilloma virus infection, and gastroesophageal reflux disease (GERD)—all of which are at least partially modifiable risk factors.

Admissions related to the treatment of aerodigestive tract cancers, rather than the cancers themselves, such as febrile neutropenia or chemotherapy-associated nausea are largely not included here with the notable exceptions of dysphagia and mucositis (see Chapter 97 [Nausea and Vomiting] and Chapter 204 [Immunocompromised Host]). Patients with aerodigestive tract neoplasia often present with complaints of the airway, breathing, or swallow function. Spinal cord compression and superior vena cava (SVC) syndrome are the two causes for admission that are considered oncologic emergencies (see Chapter 176 [Oncologic Emergencies]).

PRACTICE POINT

- Patients should be counseled about the health risks of tobacco and excessive alcohol use. Clinicians must be proactive in referring patients who smoke and/or those who may be drinking too much for counseling or other programs. Similarly, all patients with GERD should be on an antireflux regimen, preferably a proton-pump inhibitor, or initiate diet modification.

EPIDEMIOLOGY

Lung cancer is one of the most common cancers worldwide, with 225,000 new cases annually in the United States alone. Despite numerous advances in therapies, its mortality exceeds that of breast, prostate, and colon cancers combined, amounting to 160,000 deaths annually in the United States. Esophageal cancer carries an even worse fatality rate but is a much rarer disease. It represents 1% of all new cancer cases in the United States with approximately 17,000 new cases occurring annually and 15,500 deaths. Head and neck cancers constitute 3% of all malignancies in the United States and approximately 12,000 will die from the disease in a given year. In total, the combined burden of aerodigestive tract cancers is sizable and although no published data exists on admission frequency, it is likely that any given patient with such a cancer would present to the hospital numerous times during the course of their illness. See **Table 181-1** for incidence and mortality rates.

■ MALIGNANT AIRWAY OBSTRUCTION

A number of malignant conditions of the aerodigestive tract can progressively occlude the large tracheobronchial airways resulting

TABLE 181-1 Crude Incidence Rate and Mortality Rates (per 100,000 per year) of Different Aerodigestive Tract Cancers in the United States from 2008 to 2012

Cancer Site	Crude Incidence	Crude Death Rate
Lung and bronchus	69.2	51.1
Oral cavity and pharynx	12.5	2.7
Larynx	5.2	1.2
Esophagus	4.1	4.6

Data from Centers for Disease Control and Prevention, http://wonder.cdc.gov/cancer.html.

in potentially life-threatening suffocation. Less serious obstructions may still significantly impact quality of life and lead to hospital admission by causing subjective dyspnea and reducing activity tolerance. Lung cancers, particularly bronchial squamous cell carcinomas and adenocarcinomas, are the most frequent culprits of malignant airway obstruction followed by head and neck cancers of the larynx and vocal cords. Metastatic processes can behave similarly but are less common.

Airway obstruction may be classified by location: upper airway obstruction, which involves the portion of the airway that extends from the mouth and the upper trachea including the nasopharynx and larynx; central airway obstruction, which involves the lower trachea and mainstem bronchi; and lower airway obstruction, which involves the smaller bronchi in the distal airways further from the mainstem bronchi and is typically affected more by chronic obstructive pulmonary disease and parenchymal disease.

Clinical presentation

The clinical presentation for malignant airway obstruction depends upon the location, degree of luminal obstruction, and chronicity. Cough and dyspnea are the most common presenting symptoms but are nonspecific. Stridor, if present, signals significant airway occlusion, typically of the upper or central airways, and may be found in advanced disease. Accessory muscle use, tachycardia, diaphoresis, restlessness, and eventual hypercapnia and hypoxia with cyanosis may also be noted on examination. Auscultation may either reveal prolonged inspiratory and expiratory phases with profound wheeze and stridor or it may reveal relative silence indicating total upper airway obstruction or central obstruction to the affected lung lobe.

Inpatient management

The severity of the occlusive lesion and its location dictates care. Urgent stabilization of the airway is the goal. Definitive airway placement is the immediate necessity in proximal upper airway obstruction. Upper airway cancers such as tongue base, pharyngeal, pyriform fossa, epiglottis, or vocal cords may require tracheotomy or cricothyrotomy to bypass the lesion, particularly with large tumor burden. Intubation must be undertaken very cautiously since these lesions can distort the airway and bleed profoundly. In lower and distal airway obstruction, intubation or other advanced airway placement may not be of much use since the lesion is farther in the respiratory tract, beyond the reach of what an endotracheal tube could bypass. Lung cancers are the most frequent cause of this scenario and may arise originally from anywhere in the bronchial tree.

If the patient shows signs of instability, immediate rigid bronchoscopy should be pursued since it allows ventilation while the obstructing lesion can be found and managed via stenting. Arterial blood gases are not particularly useful in initial evaluation since they are frequently normal. Chest radiography is typically more revealing but only if the obstructing lesion is of the large airways, that is, trachea or main stem bronchus. Computed tomography (CT) scan is much more sensitive and can differentiate between extraluminal and intraluminal obstructions by tumors. The procedure of choice is prompt bronchoscopy (either rigid or flexible) as it allows both diagnostic and therapeutic benefit. In cases of unclear aerodigestive tract neoplasm, bronchoscopy also allows for tissue diagnosis. It should be cautioned however that flexible bronchoscopy may further occlude the airway resulting in hypoxia. And, restless patients may require sedation, which may depress ventilation. An advanced airway kit should always be present if one has not already been placed.

For patients with airway obstruction from an intraluminal mass, bronchoscopic ablative techniques such as argon plasma coagulation (APC), electrocautery, laser, cryosurgery, endobronchial brachytherapy, and phototherapy are available options. More mechanical options include airway dilation and/or stenting or surgical resection with airway debridement and coring.

In the case of extraluminal lesions, options are more limited and include dilation and stenting, external beam radiation therapy (EBRT), or surgery. For extraluminal lesions causing severe life-threatening disease, dilation and stenting is the procedure of choice as it can result in immediate airway patency. This is typically followed with EBRT for a more sustained effect. EBRT alone is the procedure of choice if the obstruction is not life threatening and the patient is clinically stable. Pulmonology and radiation oncology consultation is recommended in all cases and treatment should be individualized to the patient's tumor histology and radiosensitivity, accessibility via bronchoscopy, and clinical presentation. Other ablative techniques may also require thoracic surgery consultation.

Vocal cord obstruction and paralysis

Infiltration of the recurrent laryngeal nerve by malignancy or interference in the patient's vocal cord mobility may lead to vocal cord obstruction and paralysis. Disruption of the vocal cords may result in hoarseness and may be the first clinical manifestation of a laryngeal tumor. In patients with a known smoking history, this should lead to a thorough workup for malignancy. Bilateral vocal cord paralysis often results in airway compromise and tracheotomy should be considered. The absence of airway compromise suggests unilateral paralysis. Referral to otolaryngology (ENT) is warranted for laryngoscopy and evaluation.

Postacute care

Once the airway is stabilized and the patient is deemed stable, definitive therapy of the underlying malignancy can be pursued. This will depend on the nature of the aerodigestive tract cancer and whether the lesion is intraluminal or extraluminal. Radiation oncology referral should be considered for EBRT candidacy. Furthermore, surgical and pulmonary consultation is necessary for expert opinion on ablative and resection therapies such as laser resection, electrocautery, or mechanical resection. In the interim, transfer to higher level of care should be considered since airway reocclusion is possible.

PRACTICE POINT

- As with all acute airway obstruction cases, stabilization and security of the airway is the first priority. Signs such as trouble speaking, cyanosis, accessory muscle use, and a silent chest on auscultation warn of impending respiratory crisis which early invasive management may avoid.

◼ DYSPHAGIA AND MUCOSITIS

Nearly 1 million patients in the United States are diagnosed with some sort of dysphagia annually but no data exists on what fraction of those has an underlying aerodigestive tract malignancy. Dysphagia or difficulty swallowing may be as a result of the malignancy itself or due to treatment. Dysphagia can be the first presenting sign of esophageal or tongue base cancers. It may also be the result of any esophageal procedure or manipulation.

Mucositis or inflammation and ulceration of the mucous membranes lining the digestive tract is usually an adverse effect of chemotherapy and radiotherapy. Mucositis alone occurs in a high percentage of patients with head and neck and esophageal cancer undergoing concurrent chemoradiation. It is often exquisitely painful and exposes the patient to infection. The combined impact of dysphagia and mucositis on quality life is severe and its effects on performance status and poor oral intake make these symptoms essential to treat.

Clinical presentation

Dysphagia in patients with unknown aerodigestive tract malignancy is slowly progressive, causing first difficulty in swallowing solids then progressively to liquids. Weight loss is common and may be due to underlying cancer or to deteriorating oral intake. In cases of known aerodigestive tract malignancy and active treatment, dysphagia may present at any time and has been associated with frequent hospital readmissions and other prolonged health care costs. A bedside swallow test may reveal drooling, gagging, or coughing with ingestion of food or liquid.

See Chapter 70 (The Role of Speech/Language Pathologists in Dysphagia Management).

Mucositis on the other hand typically occurs 4 to 5 days after receiving chemotherapy and typically peaks around day 10. In patients receiving radiotherapy, it typically appears around the end of the second week. Patients typically present with markedly painful swallowing with prominent sensitivity to spicy or acidic foods. Dysgeusia, which is defined as a distortion of the sense of taste, is also frequent amongst these patients, especially in those receiving concomitant chemoradiation. Red sores or ulcers appearing as burn-like lesions with white patches are commonly seen on physical examination in the oral cavity and may extend distally down the esophagus beyond visualization.

Inpatient management

Patients presenting with dysphagia should undergo a CT scan to assess for an obstructing lesion or diverticulum. The CT may suggest a nonmalignant etiology, such as neurogenic esophagus, if no mass or pocket is identified. Any lesion suggesting malignancy should be followed up with gastroenterology referral and endoscopy for biopsy and possible placement of a temporary feeding tube for nutritional support while the patient is being properly diagnosed. Endoscopic stenting or surgical management should not be immediately pursued until histologic diagnosis is made. Esophageal stenting is typically reserved for patient with severe dysphagia from an esophageal malignancy when local therapy is not an option. Oncology referral for staging and prognostication is indicated if a new esophageal or head and neck cancer is found. Laboratory testing particularly on nutrition markers such as albumin, prealbumin, and hemoglobin are helpful in characterizing the patient's degree of malnutrition (see Chapter 58 [Nutrition and Metabolic Support]).

For patients with mucositis, treatment is largely supportive, consisting of optimizing oral hygiene and offering medication for pain control. Water-soluble jelly solutions may aid in lubrication and lidocaine-containing mouthwash may desensitize the inflamed mucosa. Specific mouthwashes formulated for mucositis may be institution specific. Benzydamine is a nonsteroidal anti-inflammatory oral rinse with topical anti-inflammatory, analgesic, anesthetic, and antimicrobial activity.

"Miracle" or "magic" mouthwashes are usually a combination of a topical anesthetic combined with an antacid suspension and/or diphenhydramine (for local drying effect) with or without nystatin in a "cocktail"; the formulation may also include steroids and antibiotics. One example is equal parts 2% viscous lidocaine, diphenhydramine, and Maalox. For severe cases, opiates may be required to achieve pain control. For patients with severe mucositis an infection of the oral cavity should be excluded. In particular, fungal infections, such as candidiasis, are very common and are amenable to antifungals, including fluconazole and nystatin. Empiric antibiotic therapy may be indicated when there is suspicion for bacterial superinfection.

For patients with cancer treatment-related dysphagia and mucositis, temporary discontinuation of antineoplastic therapy may be necessary and if not already involved, the oncology team should be consulted. These situations often call for a temporary means of nutrition, and in such cases, placement of a nasogastric tube is favored since they are easily placed and removed. However, if the patient cannot tolerate nasogastric insertion or presence (such as when mucositis is severe) or the tube cannot be passed beyond the esophageal obstruction, a gastrostomy tube (such as a percutaneous endoscopic gastrostomy tube) should be performed.

Patients not amenable to cancer therapy

For most patients with malignancy-associated dysphagia, the primary treatment remains the treatment of the cancer. Therapeutic plans will be based on histologic diagnosis, stage of the aerodigestive tract cancer, and performance status. The final plan is often based on multidisciplinary input from surgery, medical oncology, and radiation oncology. However, for patients who are not candidates for anticancer treatment, an esophageal stent may be placed for palliative nutrition purposes. For mucositis, the clinician should offer a supportive treatment plan incorporating oral hygiene and adequate pain control that will carry forward to discharge.

◼ SVC SYNDROME

The superior vena cava syndrome results from obstruction of blood flow through the superior vena cava from any malignant or benign process. Obstruction may be caused by either thrombosis of blood within the SVC or invasion/external compression of the SVC by a pathologic process from adjacent structures, that is, right lung, lymph nodes, or mediastinal structures. Malignancy is the most common cause and is reported to account for 90% of all cases, with lung cancer being the culprit in 70% of all cases. The SVC syndrome is caused by nonneoplastic processes in up to 30% of cases, including vasculitis, pericarditis, and infections such as histoplasmosis, tuberculosis, and syphilis. The increased use of intravascular devices such as central vein catheters and pacemaker wires has, however, led to an increase incidence in SVC syndrome secondary to thrombosis.

Clinical presentation

The onset of symptoms and signs depends on the rate at which complete obstruction of the SVC occurs in relation to the development of venous collaterals. Patients with malignant disease typically present early, because rapid tumor growth does not allow adequate time for the formation of collateral blood flow. These patients may present as an oncologic emergency with stridor due to central airway obstruction or severe laryngeal edema or coma from cerebral edema.

Dyspnea is the most common symptom of SVC syndrome, noted in 63% of patients. Other respiratory symptoms include orthopnea, hoarseness, cough, and stridor, which are caused by interstitial edema of the head and neck resulting in narrowing of the nasal lumen passages, pharynx, and larynx. The classic association for SVC syndrome is facial swelling that is worse in the mornings and improved in the evenings. Other symptoms include head fullness, nasal or sinus congestion, and neck or arm swelling. On physical examination, distention of the neck veins, facial edema, plethora, and papilledema are common. Bending forward or laying supine chiefly worsens symptoms and is strongly suggestive of SVC syndrome.

Inpatient management

Immediate imaging is not necessary to confirm SVC syndrome in cases of clear physical examination. However imaging does rule out other causes such as pneumothorax and may be the initial revelation of an aerodigestive tract tumor. Chest radiography is an appropriate initial study and may note right-sided primary aerodigestive tract tumors or metastasis, a widened mediastinum, or may be grossly normal. However, radiography is not diagnostic in any of these cases. CT scanning is the test of choice for SVC syndrome and would be expected to reveal an obstructing mass, thrombosis, or other mechanism of compression against the SVC. Advanced imaging such as magnetic resonance imaging (MRI) or gold standard invasive venography is typically unnecessary.

The goal of management of SVC syndrome is to reduce immediate symptoms and treat the underlying condition and is thus based heavily on the underlying condition's anticipated response to treatment. Most patients report improvement of symptoms with symptomatic measures such as supplemental oxygen and elevation of the head of the bed. Definitive therapy for SVC syndromes caused by cancers of the aerodigestive tract requires radiation that provides symptomatic relief in the majority of patients and relieves 70% of cases resulting from lung cancer. Needle biopsy of the obstruction mass should be obtained prior to treatment if there is no known histologic diagnosis. Some oncologists may advocate for reduction via chemotherapy in known chemo-sensitive tumors such as small cell lung cancer instead of radiotherapy. Surgical referral for bypass and stenting can be made, although recent evidence suggests that this is best for SVC syndrome of benign origin or as an appropriate option for palliation.

Postacute care

Establishing the patient on an appropriate antineoplastic regimen is vital after SVC syndrome is noted. Appropriate biopsy and oncology referral will guide definitive therapy. This may involve any combination of chemotherapy or radiation but in cases where these therapies are not possible due to advanced disease, poor performance status, or other contraindication, surgical referral should be undertaken for palliative stenting.

■ SPINAL CORD COMPRESSION

Malignant spinal cord compression (MSCC) occurs in 5% to 30% of the cancer patient population and typically arises from breast, prostate, renal cell, and hematologic malignancies. In the case of the aerodigestive tract, non–small cell lung cancer is a frequent cause either by metastatic or locally advanced disease due to its propensity to invade bone. From indentation, displacement, or encasement of the spinal cord, the resultant injury results in neurological compromise which is the hallmark of MSCC.

Clinical presentation

In MSCC, the presenting signs and symptoms vary with location of the tumor (**Table 181-2**). A focal neurological deficit corresponding with the level of the compression would be seen such as foot drop or bladder incontinence.

TABLE 181-2 Common Symptoms of Malignant Spinal Cord Compression Divided by Expected Location of the Compressing Tumor

Cervical Spine	Thoracic Spine	Lumbosacral Spine
Loss of sensation in neck, shoulder, arms, or hands	Loss of sensation below level of the tumor	Loss of sensation in legs or feet
Paralysis of neck, shoulder, arms, or hands	Paralysis below level of tumor	Paralysis in legs or feet
Breathing difficulty	Pain in chest and/or back	Foot drop
Headache or pain in neck, shoulder, arm, or hand	Difficulty with balance or truncal instability	Bowel incontinence
		Bladder incontinence
		Sexual dysfunction
		Decreased reflexes in legs

Pain arising from vertebral destruction by the tumor occurs in 83% to 95% of patients at the time of initial diagnosis. Pain typically precedes the onset of neurological symptoms by several weeks. Usually, a band-like pain or paresthesia develops in a dermatomal distribution due to compression of the spinal cord. Radicular pain may travel down an affected extremity, particularly a leg. Unexplained loss of sensation, burning, or tingling in a similar distribution is also very suspect for MSCC. Motor dysfunction, particularly foot drop or rapidly progressive limb weakness occurs in 80% of cases. A thorough neurologic examination including digital rectal examination will characterize the patient's deficits and be useful for tracking progress to resolution.

Very often, MSCC patients have symptoms that are insidious and described as a soreness, discomfort, or vague weakness. This may be misattributed to nonspecific causes such as old injury or musculoskeletal strain. However, these symptoms rapidly progress to neurological compromise and may become permanent if not intervened upon immediately.

Cauda equina syndrome

The tip of the spinal cord lies at the level of L1 vertebral body in adults. Below this level, the lumbrosacral nerve roots form the cauda equina, which floats in cerebrospinal fluid (CSF). Compression of this part of the spinal cord leads to cauda equina syndrome. Autonomic dysfunction resulting in urinary incontinence, bowel incontinence, or urinary retention is suggestive of cauda equina syndrome. Perianal numbness (saddle anesthesia) with absent anal reflex and bulbocavernosus reflex is essentially diagnostic and indicates especially urgent treatment necessary in less than 48 hours. Intrathecal metastasis from lung cancer is the most common malignant cause and its association with cauda equina syndrome portends a poor prognosis with a mean survival of 3 months.

Inpatient management

Once suspected, MRI should be obtained of the entire spine, not just where symptoms have been localized to on examination, since 10% to 30% of MSCC patients have multiple lesions. In cases where MRI is not possible, CT myelography is an acceptable alternative but this involves invasive administration of radiographic contrast into the intrathecal sac. Spinal radiographs are rarely diagnostic of MSCC but may be useful in rapidly showing lytic or sclerotic lesions of the vertebra. In cases of advanced disease, x-ray may even show large tumors. Notably, lumbar puncture is typically contraindicated in MSCC because removal of cerebrospinal fluid may worsen the condition.

Once the diagnosis has been established, corticosteroid therapy should be administered intravenously to relieve the edema that exacerbates symptoms of MSCC. Dexamethasone is typically the steroid of choice. Additionally, referral to both radiation oncology and neurosurgery should be immediate for antineoplastic treatment. Therapy is tailored to the specific patient and could be surgery, EBRT, or stereotactic body radiotherapy (SBRT) or a combination. Surgery typically entails mechanical decompression and spine stabilization and is followed with EBRT. Lung cancers are usually very radiosensitive and this modality usually provides relief typically within days to weeks. However in those patients with large, rapidly progressing, or radioresistant tumors, surgery alone may be indicated.

Postacute care

Whether radiation or surgery, treatment in MSCC is almost always palliative since its presence indicates advanced disease. As such, radiation oncology and medical oncology referral and prognostication is essential for establishing duration of corticosteroid therapy, duration of radiotherapy, and expectations for recovery. For those patients who underwent surgery, all standard postoperative measures should be in place particularly vigilance for venous thromboembolism due to such cancer's hypercoagulability. In cases of CT myelography, specific postprocedure care is necessary such as lying at 30°, avoiding strenuous activity, monitoring for headaches, and possibly performing blood patch injection for cerebrospinal fluid leak.

■ MALIGNANT PLEURAL EFFUSION

Malignant effusion is the most common pleural manifestation of cancers of the aerodigestive tract. Approximately 1.5 million cases of pleural effusion occur in the United States per year and of those, approximately 150,000 are malignant pleural effusions. The most common etiologies are lung and breast cancers, which account for 50% to 65% of malignant pleural effusions. They tend to be more common in women and their presence portends a poor prognosis.

Clinical presentation

The main presenting symptom of malignant pleural effusion is dyspnea, which may begin insidiously. The patient may first note breathlessness on exertion and gradually progress to feel the inability to inspire deeply. Accompanying this may be nonproductive cough and commonly pleuritic chest pain since the exudative nature of malignant pleural effusions causes direct pleural irritation. The chest pain may be very mild or overwhelming and typically does not localize well to the area of the effusion other than ipsilaterality. A lack of chest pain may indicate a large volume effusion since the lack of contact of pleural surfaces diminishes sensation.

Signs of consolidation, tactile fremitus, decreased breath sounds, and pleural friction rub may all be noted on auscultation. The lack of findings, however, does not rule out pleural effusions since it may be that the volume of fluid is inadequate to cause audible signs. Tachycardia and increased respiratory rate, partly due to the subjective breathlessness are common. Oxygen saturations tend to be well preserved until the effusion becomes very advanced.

Inpatient management

Chest radiography is an excellent initial test for any pleural effusion. The presence of more than 200 mL is usually noted as costophrenic angle blunting (meniscus sign) and has high specificity. Combining upright films with lateral films increases the sensitivity of the imaging to show layering with gravity. However, this change with positioning will not be seen on radiography in cases of loculated malignant pleural effusions. Ultrasound is typically best done at the time of thoracentesis to localize the effusion and to identify adjacent structures. Ultrasound may also reveal pleural tumors, which

TABLE 181-3 Basic Fluid Analysis Relevant for Pleural Effusions*

Pleural Fluid Type	Pleural Fluid/Serum Protein Ratio	Pleural Fluid/Serum LDH Ratio	Pleural Fluid LDH (U/L)
Transudative	<0.5	<0.6	<2/3 of URL
Exudative	≥0.5	≥0.6	≥2/3 of URL

*Any of the following parameters, if met, suggests an exudative process which is necessary to establish an effusion as malignant. URL, upper reference limit of serum LDH.

essentially confirms the diagnosis of a malignant pleural effusion even without fluid analysis.

The decision for thoracentesis is based on the need to relieve symptoms and the need for diagnosis. Malignant pleural effusions tend to recur and thus should be drained when symptomatic, not simply when fluid is noted. A therapeutic thoracentesis generally should not remove more than 1 to 1.5 L since it runs the risk of re-expansion pulmonary edema and pneumothorax. Pleural fluid should be sent for any of the following studies as appropriate: cell count with differential, pH, protein content, glucose, lactate dehydrogenase (LDH), Gram stain and culture. Blood tests of total protein, complete blood count with differential, and LDH are also helpful. Cytology should also always be sent with suspicion of malignant pleural effusion but its interpretation must be done cautiously. Cytology has essentially 100% specificity but a low (around 60%) sensitivity. Thus, a negative cytologic evaluation does not exclude malignancy as the cause, especially when the pretest probability is high in a patient with known aerodigestive tract cancer. In such cases, a negative cytologic evaluation is very possibly a false negative. Fluid analysis that reveals a hemorrhagic exudative process in the context of known cancer is very suggestive of malignant pleural effusion (see **Table 181-3**). Thoracentesis will immediately relieve symptomatology and if it does not, other etiologies of dyspnea and/or chest pain should be sought.

The decision to treat a malignant effusion with a pleural intervention depends upon the presence of respiratory symptoms, although untreated malignant pleural effusion will invariably lead to symptoms. In cases of severe effusion or loculations, surgical consultation is necessary to place chest tubes after manual breaking of the pleural pockets. This commits the patient to a prolonged hospital stay and thus should be pursued conservatively.

PRACTICE POINT

- Malignant pleural effusions are the most common type of pleural effusions seen in cancer patients. However, other etiologies such as reduced oncotic pressure, inflammation, and trauma may still be the underlying etiology. Infection should remain on the differential for any cancer patient who is relatively immunosuppressed from chemotherapy, steroids, or other reasons. History and thoracic fluid analysis are the most clinically useful ways in determining what type of pleural effusion is at hand, not fluid cytology (see Table 181-3).

Postacute care

Malignant pleural effusions tend to recur in over 90% of patients. Thus, once relieved by thoracentesis, the patient should be evaluated for preventive or definitive therapy. If slowly evolving, management with repeated thoracenteses is a reasonable option.

However, if the episode of malignant pleural effusion at hand or the pattern of repeated effusions suggest a history of rapid reaccumulation, surgical consult for pleurodesis with talc may be most appropriate for the patient. A low pleural pH tends to be associated with decreased survival and poor pleurodesis efficacy so indwelling tunneled catheters may be an option since they allow the patient to self-drain at home as a palliative measure. Malignant pleural effusions usually indicate advanced, incurable disease so palliative measures are appropriate.

■ DISCHARGE CHECKLIST

The discharge checklist revolves around appropriate oncologic follow-up and pursuit of definitive therapy.

1. Outpatient referral to medical oncology with established tissue diagnosis, with or without complete staging.
2. Addition referral to radiation oncology in cases of SVC syndrome and MSCC.
3. Establishment of treatment plan for dysphagia and mucositis to relieve symptoms and provide nutrition.

4. Securing airway with minimal threat of persistent obstruction for malignant airway obstruction.
5. Adequate, ongoing pain control where necessary.

SUGGESTED READINGS

Bagley CA, Gokaslan ZL. Cauda equine syndrome caused by primary and metastatic neoplasms. *Neurosurg Focus.* 2004;16(6):11-18.

Rice TW, Rodriguez RM, Light RW. The superior vena cava syndrome: clinical characteristics and evolving etiology. *Medicine (Baltimore).* 2006;85(1):37-42.

Rizvi AZ, Kalra M, Bjarnason H, Bower TC, Schleck C, Gloviczki P. Benign superior vena cava syndrome: stenting is now the first line of treatment. *J Vasc Surg.* 2008;47(2):372-380.

Sahn SA. Malignant pleural effusions. *Semin Respir Crit Care Med.* 2001;22(6):607-616.

Zarogoulidis K, Zarogoulidis P, Darwiche K, et al. Malignant pleural effusion and algorithm management. *J Thorac Dis.* 2013;5(Suppl 4): S413-S419.

CHAPTER 182

Gastrointestinal Cancers

Lauren Colbert, MD
Andrew S. Epstein, MD

Herein, we delineate and describe some of the most common issues encountered by clinicians caring for hospitalized patients with gastrointestinal cancers. These issues arise from the cancers themselves or as complications of the oncologic treatment.

MALIGNANT BOWEL OBSTRUCTION

Malignant bowel obstruction in patients with gastrointestinal malignancies is a common problem and is most commonly due to peritoneal carcinomatosis. Other etiologies include obstruction from the primary malignancy, or metastatic lesions other than peritoneal carcinomatosis. Patients with a history of prior abdominal surgery may also develop obstruction from surgical adhesions. Bowel obstruction may also be the presenting symptom of a gastrointestinal malignancy and is not uncommonly diagnosed at surgical resection. Management is dependent on the etiology of obstruction, severity of obstruction, and the patient's overall prognosis.

Small bowel obstruction generally presents with symptoms of abdominal distension, nausea, vomiting, and occasionally with hiccups or belching. Signs can include high-pitched, "tinkling" bowel sounds and a distended and/or tympanic abdomen on examination. Laboratory abnormalities may include hypochloremic hypokalemic metabolic alkalosis from repeated vomiting and increased blood urea nitrogen (BUN) and creatinine from dehydration. An elevated serum lactic acid or peritoneal signs on abdominal examination should raise concern for bowel strangulation or perforation, and the patient should receive immediate surgical evaluation (see Chapter 162 [Small Bowel Disorders]).

Small bowel obstruction may be diagnosed on abdominal imaging, most commonly by plain radiograph or abdominal computed tomography (CT). Plain radiograph will likely diagnose the obstruction, and CT may be useful in further characterizing the obstruction, such as in determining whether the obstruction is due to primary malignancy or peritoneal disease (see Chapter 116 [Basic Abdominal Imaging] and Chapter 117 [Advanced Abdominal Imaging]).

Initial management should include bowel rest and bowel decompression with placement of nasogastric tube (NGT), particularly if the patient has nausea and vomiting. Intravenous (IV) fluids should be administered and adjusted accordingly if electrolyte abnormalities exist from persistent vomiting. In the absence of signs of bowel strangulation or perforation, it is reasonable to continue with conservative management for 48 to 72 hours. After this time, if the obstruction does not resolve with conservative management, surgical evaluation is warranted.

Whether surgical intervention is warranted depends on several factors, including the patient's overall prognosis and goals of care, medical suitability for surgery, and location and type of obstruction. Obstruction due to peritoneal carcinomatosis often results in multifocal obstruction, which is not amenable to surgical resection. If the obstruction is due to primary malignancy or a single metastatic site, a surgical bypass procedure, or resection of that site may provide symptomatic relief. In patients with obstruction from primary malignancy who are not surgical candidates, radiation therapy may be an option.

In patients for whom surgical intervention is not indicated, interventional procedures by interventional radiology or endoscopy may provide relief of symptoms. In certain instances, stenting may provide temporary or partial relief in the obstruction is in a location amenable to stenting, such as at the gastric outlet or gastroesophageal junction. For small bowel obstruction or gastric outlet obstruction, placement of a drainage (or "venting") percutaneous endoscopic gastrostomy (dPEG) or percutaneous endoscopic jejunostomy (dPEJ) tube may allow for oral intake without symptoms of obstruction. The tube may be intermittently clamped to allow modest absorption, or left to drainage in the event of complete, unremitting obstruction. It is important to emphasize to patients that the primary goal of placement of a dPEG or dPEJ tube in setting of distal bowel obstruction primarily is to prevent the noxious sequelae of oral intake (eg, vomiting, belching, pain, and reflux) and to allow pleasure feeding, and that there will be minimal if any absorption of oral hydration or nutrition. It is entirely appropriate to discuss hospice transitioning with patients in whom a dPEG tube has been or will be placed, as these bowel obstructions are associated with a poor prognosis and an inability to gain benefit from further cancer-directed treatment (see Chapter 123 [Feeding Tube Placement]).

For large bowel obstructions not amenable to immediate surgical intervention, once again, interventional management or radiation therapy may be appropriate depending on patient circumstances. Rectal stenting may serve to palliate symptoms from obstructing rectal cancers, or to allow the patient to move past the acute phase of obstruction and allow for chemotherapy, radiation or surgical resection. Previous studies have shown success rates between 70% and 100% for this intervention although there are risks of stent perforation (5%), migration (2%), and obstruction (2%). In certain cases, placement of a cecostomy tube may be considered as a last resort. This serves to provide drainage in a similar fashion to the dPEG tube approach discussed above.

Medical management of unfixable obstruction primarily includes symptomatic management of pain, distension, nausea, vomiting, and constipation. In addition to standard antiemetics including 5-HT3 receptor antagonists, phenothiazines and other antipsychotic agents and promotility agents, other agents to consider include octreotide, which may decrease bowel secretions, and low-dose dexamethasone, which may help with appetite in addition to nausea. Benzodiazepines may be useful particularly in patients with an anxiety associated with their nausea. As we discuss below, opiates are a mainstay of pain management in patients with cancer, including in situations of bowel obstruction (see Chapter 216 [Palliation of Common Symptoms]).

MALIGNANT ASCITES

Malignant ascites is also a common presenting symptom in hospitalized patients with gastrointestinal malignancies. Care should be taken to rule out other causes of ascites, such as underlying cirrhosis, as malignant ascites only accounts for approximately 7% of patients with ascites. A diagnostic paracentesis could be performed to evaluate for serum albumin/ascites gradient and cytology.

Malignant ascites is often a sign of peritoneal carcinomatosis, but gastrointestinal malignancy may cause ascites through a variety of other mechanisms, including portal hypertension from significant liver metastatic burden (neoplastic pseudocirrhosis), primary liver malignancies, portal vein involvement, and hepatic vein occlusion causing Budd-Chiari syndrome. Therefore, treatment of malignant ascites should take into account the underlying mechanism.

Patients may present with rapidly increasing abdominal girth, bilateral lower extremity swelling, shortness of breath due to upward pressure on the diaphragm and/or development of pleural effusion, abdominal pain, nausea and vomiting, decreased appetite, or constipation. Patients with a pseudocirrhosis picture may present with orthostasis due to intravascular depletion. Signs on examination include a bulging umbilical mass, palpable fluid wave, decreased sounds at the lung bases, and dullness to percussion. A bedside ultrasound can quickly determine the volume of ascites and the amenability to paracentesis (see Chapter 126 [Paracentesis]).

The overall prognosis in patients with malignant ascites is poor, with a median survival of a small number of months. Patients presenting with malignant ascites should always be counseled regarding supportive and palliative care and hospice care. Despite a patient's overall philosophy regarding hospice care, management should be directed toward patient comfort. The primary management of recurrent ascites is therapeutic paracenteses. For patients who quickly accumulate fluid, an indwelling peritoneal dialysis, or Tenckhoff, catheter may provide better quality of life. Compared to patients with cirrhotic liver disease, rates of peritonitis for patients with primary malignant ascites are relatively low. Catheters should be avoided in patients with underlying hepatitis, and instead, these patients should undergo repeat therapeutic paracenteses as necessary for comfort. For patients preferring conservative management, or with slow accumulation of ascitic fluid, diuretics may be the considered as an alternate therapy. Diuretic therapy should be monitored carefully for electrolyte abnormalities and hypotension.

PAIN MANAGEMENT

Unfortunately, it is not infrequent that patients with gastrointestinal malignancies are hospitalized for pain management. Patients with pancreatic cancers may have locally advanced disease, and may have significant back and abdominal pain despite narcotic use. Patients with metastatic liver disease or primary liver cancers can have visceral pain due to stretch of the liver capsule. General concepts of cancer pain management apply to these patients. Additionally, patients with refractory pain due to liver capsule stretch often respond very well to steroids, and so this should be considered as a treatment option. Many patients with gastrointestinal cancer have significant hepatic dysfunction; however, this does not indicate that pain medication should be avoided in these patients. Generally, acetaminophen is acceptable in lower dosages (up to 2 g daily) as long as liver function tests are stable. Regular use of nonsteroidal anti-inflammatory medications should be avoided due to increased risk of gastrointestinal bleeding in these patients. Opioids may still be used safely in patients with hepatic dysfunction, and remain the mainstay on the WHO pain ladder in patients with moderate to severe pain, with the caveat that opioid clearance is reduced in these patients due to both reduced hepatic blood flow and limited first pass metabolism, in addition to decreased CYP450 enzyme activity. Low serum albumin and ascites also may significantly affect the volume of distribution (V_d) and rate of absorption of these drugs. Fentanyl is preferable regarded as the preferable drug for hepatic and/or renal dysfunction, but cost considerations may preclude its prolonged use. Hydromorphone and oxycodone can be used safely at reduced doses (such as 50%) and frequency, with careful monitoring. The first pass 3-glucoronide metabolite of morphine has no analgesic effects, but may accumulate and cause neurotoxicity with primarily neuro-excitatory effects. Codeine and morphine should generally be avoided in patients with hepatic and renal impairment due to accumulation of metabolites with analgesic and toxic effects.

Select patients may also be benefitted by interventional pain management techniques, including celiac plexus block (in patients where the majority, if not all, of the disease burden, such as in patients with locally advanced pancreas cancer, is localized to the region of the celiac plexus), select nerve blocks, and epidural anesthesia. Interventional pain management should be consulted in these instances of localized pain. Palliative radiation therapy can also be used in patients with locally advanced tumors, and may provide better pain control and a decrease in narcotic pain medication requirements.

HEMATOLOGIC DISORDERS

Patients with gastrointestinal tumors are prone to both gastrointestinal bleeding and thrombosis, which may create unique therapeutic challenges. Patients with colorectal cancers may present with lower gastrointestinal tract bleeding from the primary lesion, either occult or frank bleeding, and should be treated according to the guidelines established for lower gastrointestinal tract bleeding (see Chapter 161 [Acute Lower Gastrointestinal Bleeding]). Patients with gastric, esophageal, and pancreatic tumors may present with (potentially brisk in the case of pancreas tumors and their associated arterial vasculature eroding into the duodenum) upper gastrointestinal tract bleeding. The risk of severe anemia is increased due to the fact that these patients may already be at increased risk of coagulopathy such as cases of significant liver disease burden (ie, insufficient coagulation factors, thrombocytopenia), leading to increased bleeding risk. Chemotherapy-induced thrombocytopenia and anemia may also be present.

Upper gastrointestinal tract bleeding should be treated with intravenous proton-pump inhibitors, the establishment of bilateral large bore IVs, supportive red blood cell, platelet and coagulation factor transfusions (as necessary), and immediate endoscopic evaluation when clinically stable. If bleeding is due to primary tumor, endoscopic interventions may be limited, and in this case patients should be evaluated by interventional radiology for potential embolization and radiation oncology for radiation therapy. Patients with lower gastrointestinal tract bleeding should also be treated with supportive transfusions and endoscopic, interventional, or radiation oncology evaluation (see Chapter 156 [Upper Gastrointestinal Bleeding]).

The rate of malignancy-associated venous thromboembolism (VTE) is relatively high in gastrointestinal cancers, with pancreatic cancer as the most common culprit. This may be due to increased inflammatory cytokines in these patients. Prophylactic anticoagulation is controversial, but once these patients develop thromboses, they will likely require lifelong anticoagulation in the absence of contraindications. Low-molecular-weight heparin (LMWH) has been shown to be superior to warfarin in cancer patients for recurrent VTE prevention and also has less potential interactions with chemotherapy. The newer oral anticoagulants are more convenient for patients but there efficacy in secondary VTE prevention in cancer patients is not yet known and these agents require gastrointestinal absorption and sufficient liver function (see Chapter 252 [Venous Thromboembolism Prophylaxis for Hospitalized Medical Patients]).

CHAPTER 183

Immune-Related Adverse Events (irAEs) in Cancer Patients

Kerry Reynolds, MD

Ashwin Ananthakrishnan, MD

Michael Dougan, MD, PhD

Aditya Bardia, MD, MPH

Key Clinical Questions

1. When should immune-related adverse events (irAEs) be suspected in acutely ill hospitalized oncology patients?

2. How do you evaluate an oncology patient who may have an irAE related to immunotherapy treatment?

3. How do you manage patients with irAEs?

4. What should you consider when discharging a patient that has been treated for an irAE?

BACKGROUND

The function of the immune system is to protect the host tissues, recognized as "self," against foreign organisms, recognized as "nonself." Upon recognition as "nonself" an antigen, shown in red in **Figure 183-1**, is captured and presented on an antigen presenting cell (APC), which then displays that antigen to the immune effector T-cell. T-cells predominantly recognize peptide antigens derived from "nonself" proteins displayed on major histocompatibility complex (MHC) class I/II. The T-cell is activated to generate a response against the specific antigen. Activation requires two signals directed by the APC: (a) the presentation of the antigenic peptide to stimulate the T-cell receptor (TCR), and (b) the binding of CD28 on T-cells to B7.1 (CD80) or B7.2 (CD86) on the APC. This process of T-cell activation of the host plays a critical role in mediating immune surveillance.

To counter the possibility of unregulated activation of T-cells, two molecules, CTLA-4 (cytotoxic T-lymphoctye-associated-protein-4) and PD-1 (programmed death receptor-1) play a critical role. Once the T-cell is activated, CTLA-4, a molecule present on the activated T-cell that can bind with greater avidity to B7 than CD28, is upregulated to shut down the system and mute the immune response, avoiding an uncontrolled inflammatory cascade of events. Besides CTLA-4 inhibition, there are other mechanisms to inhibit the inflammatory signaling that occurs in the periphery. One pathway, of particular importance in tumors, that down regulates the T-cell response is the programmed death 1 (PD-1) receptor: PD-Ligand (PD-L) pathway. The PD-1 receptor on the surface of the activated T-cell binds to one of two ligands expressed on the surface of antigen presenting cells, PD-L1 or PD-L2, to limit the activity of the already activated T-cells. When PD-1 binds to the ligand, an "off" signal is sent to the T-cell to suppress expansion and stop the attack. These inhibitory checkpoints are essential in a delicate system of checks and balances to ensure there is not overactivation of the immune system and protect the body from a chronic inflammatory state.

A number of tumors develop complex mechanisms that allow them to specifically evade the immune system and ensure their survival within a host. Despite having tumor antigens that may be recognized as "nonself," they develop an ability to dampen this normal antitumor response by taking full advantage of the inhibitory checkpoint pathways, creating an immunosuppressive environment that allows it to hide from the immune system. Certain malignancies express PD-L1 on their cell surface (melanoma and non–small cell lung cancer being the classical examples), while others are able to dampen the immune responses via mechanisms that are not well understood.

Over the past decade, deeper understanding of tumor biology as well as a spurt in the development of developmental therapeutics has ushered in a new era of "immuno-oncology." Preclinical animal models demonstrating that blockade of CTLA-4 and PD-1 by monoclonal antibodies could lead to major responses against tumors in a variety of malignancies led to the clinical testing of humanized CTLA-4 and PD-1 immune checkpoint antibodies in clinical trials and demonstrated improvements in response rate and durability of response in comparison to standard care. In 2011, the Food and Drug Administration (FDA) approved Ipilimumab, a CTLA-4 antibody, based on a phase 3 clinical trial that demonstrated a statistically significant overall survival benefit (10.1 vs 6.4 month) in advanced melanoma. In 2014, the FDA approved Nivolumab and Pembrolizumab, both PD-1 antibodies, for advanced melanoma. In 2015, the approval was extended for squamous non–small cell lung cancer, and it is anticipated that these drugs will be approved for other solid tumors in the near future.

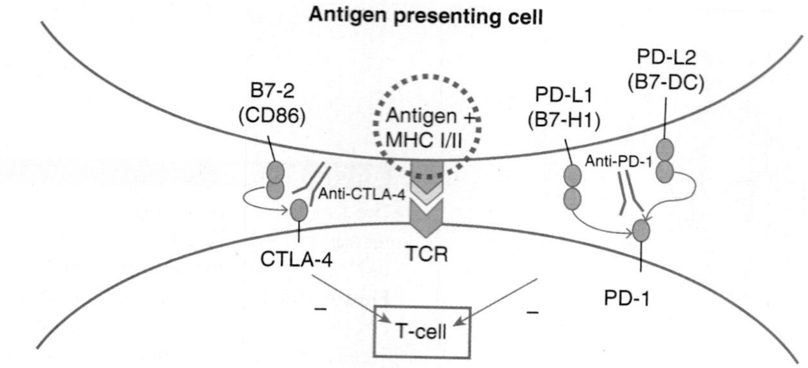

Figure 183-1 *T-cell regulation by CTLA-4 and PD-1 pathways.* (From Kasper DL, et al, eds. *Harrison's Principles of Internal Medicine*, 19th edition. New York, NY: McGraw-Hill Education Medical; 2015.)

TARGETING THE IMMUNE SYSTEM FOR ANTITUMOR PURPOSES

Immunotherapy does not target the cancer, but instead directly targets the immune system to alter it in a way that allows the immune system to develop a specific antitumor response in a wide variety of tumors. The main goal of the monoclonal antibodies being developed is to interfere with this adaptation by cancer cells and reinstate the antitumor immune response, in order to hone the patient's immune system to target the specific cancer cells.

Targeting the host immune system is an exciting strategy that has been shown to have clinical activity in a wide variety of cancers and all data suggests that targeted immunotherapy is going to be the next major breakthrough for solid tumors. The first immune checkpoint inhibitor, a monoclonal antibody against CTLA-4, was approved for metastatic melanoma in 2011, and since that time two monoclonal antibodies directed at PD-1 have been approved, and a number of other agents are in clinical development (see **Figure 183-2**). Accordingly, use of immunotherapies and immunotherapy based combinations will exponentially increase over the coming years. However, significant immune-related adverse events (irAEs) have been associated with these agents, some of which can be fatal. As the use of these therapies becomes more prevalent and the numbers of individuals experiencing these toxicities increases, it is anticipated that inpatient admission will also increase and the hospitalist community will face the challenge of managing patients admitted specifically for irAEs.

The most common irAEs requiring hospitalization include diarrhea/colitis, endocrinopathies (hypophysitis, thyroiditis, adrenalitis),

hepatitis, and pneumonitis. These can be severe and even fatal. **Figure 183-3** outlines the common toxicities and their incidence. While most irAEs appear within first few months of immunotherapy, generally, dermatologic irAEs occur early (within first month), followed by gastrointestinal and hepatic toxicities (second month), and endocrine toxicities (third month and beyond).

While the first generation of immunotherapy clinical trials utilized checkpoint inhibitors as single agents, clinical trials are now combining immune checkpoint inhibitors. For example, in the checkMate 067 trial, ipilimumab and nivolumab were used in combination in patients with melanoma, showing an impressive response rate (57.6%) and significant improvement in median progression free survival (11.5 months), however this was also associated with increased toxicity. Nearly 54% of patients who received the combination of ipilimumab and nivolumab experienced grade 3 or 4 toxicity (see **Figure 183-4**).

The following discussion will focus on the irAE's associated with the novel FDA-approved immunomodulatory treatments approved in melanoma and lung cancer.

■ GASTROINTESTINAL TOXICITY

Assessment of grade and severity of the gastrointestinal symptoms guides evaluation and management (see **Table 183-1**). Most patients with mild toxicity (grade 1 or 2 irAEs) may be treated successfully as outpatients unless there are other medical concerns or significant comorbidities that should prompt hospital admission. The management of patients with grade 1 or 2 irAEs includes holding immune checkpoint inhibitors and close follow-up. If the symptoms do not

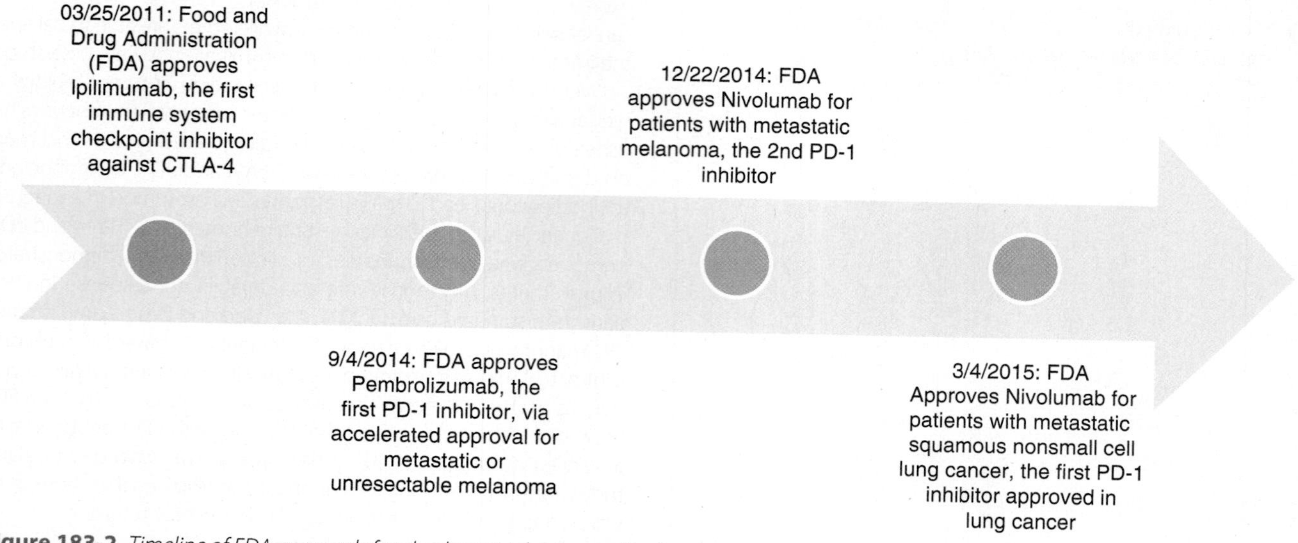

03/25/2011: Food and Drug Administration (FDA) approves Ipilimumab, the first immune system checkpoint inhibitor against CTLA-4

12/22/2014: FDA approves Nivolumab for patients with metastatic melanoma, the 2nd PD-1 inhibitor

9/4/2014: FDA approves Pembrolizumab, the first PD-1 inhibitor, via accelerated approval for metastatic or unresectable melanoma

3/4/2015: FDA Approves Nivolumab for patients with metastatic squamous nonsmall cell lung cancer, the first PD-1 inhibitor approved in lung cancer

Figure 183-2 *Timeline of FDA approvals for checkpoint inhibitor antibodies.*

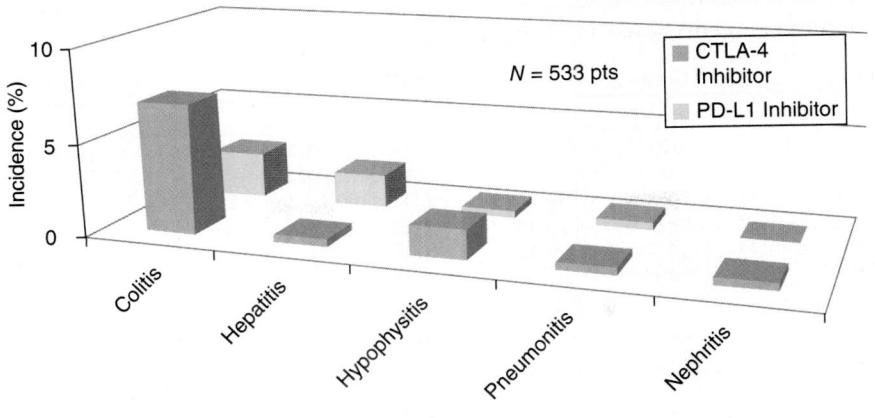

Figure 183-3 *Incidence of severe toxicities from CTLA-4 and PD-L1 inhibitor.* (Data from Postow MA, Chesney J, Pavlick AC, et al. Nivolumab and ipilimumab versus ipilimumab in untreated melanoma. *N Engl J Med.* 2015;372(21):2006-2017.)

improve to grade 1 or less within 1 week, then oral prednisone (0.5-1 mg/kg/d) is typically prescribed in the outpatient setting. Patients with grade 3 or 4 irAEs require more intensive management, usually in the hospital setting.

DIARRHEA/COLITIS

Treatment with CTLA-4 inhibitors such as ipilimumab is associated with unique adverse events due to the medication's immune upregulation. The most common adverse effects of CTLA-4 inhibitors in ≥5% of patients are diarrhea and colitis. The monoclonal immune checkpoint inhibitors are an effective way to harness the body's natural antitumor immune response. However, these agents can induce immune-mediated inflammation of healthy tissues, most commonly in the gastrointestinal tract leading to diarrhea or colitis.

The diarrhea usually starts with loose, watery stools, and can progress to clinically significant colitis with abdominal pain, blood, or mucus in the stool, with or without fever. The diarrhea is graded depending on stool frequency, as mild/grade 1 toxicity (<4 stools/d over baseline), moderate/grade 2 toxicity (4-6 stools/d over baseline), severe/grade 3 toxicity (>7 stools/d over baseline), or life-threatening/grade 4 toxicity (see Table 183-1). The colitis is graded as mild/grade 1 colitis (no symptoms but radiographic evidence of

colitis), moderate/grade 2 colitis (abdominal pain, blood or mucus in the stool), severe/grade 3 colitis (abdominal pain, change in bowel habits, or peritoneal signs) or life-threatening/grade 4 colitis. Although, the standard toxicity grading criteria separate these entities, clinically they are one and the same (see Table 183-1).

The CTLA-4 inhibitors, such as Ipilimumab, cause gastrointestinal toxicity with grade 3 and 4 diarrhea/colitis occurring in up to 15% of patients receiving the drug, generally within 1 to 2 months of starting the medication, whereas this occurs in less than 3% of patients treated with a PD-1 or PD-L1 inhibitor (see Figure 183-3).

PRACTICE POINT

Documentation includes the following basic components:
- Severity, grade, chronology, and duration of symptoms
- Immunotherapy: dose, frequency, number of treatments, last dose
- Complications of treatment
- Prior history of organ specific diseases
- Risk factors for infectious complications
- Oncologic history including response to treatment

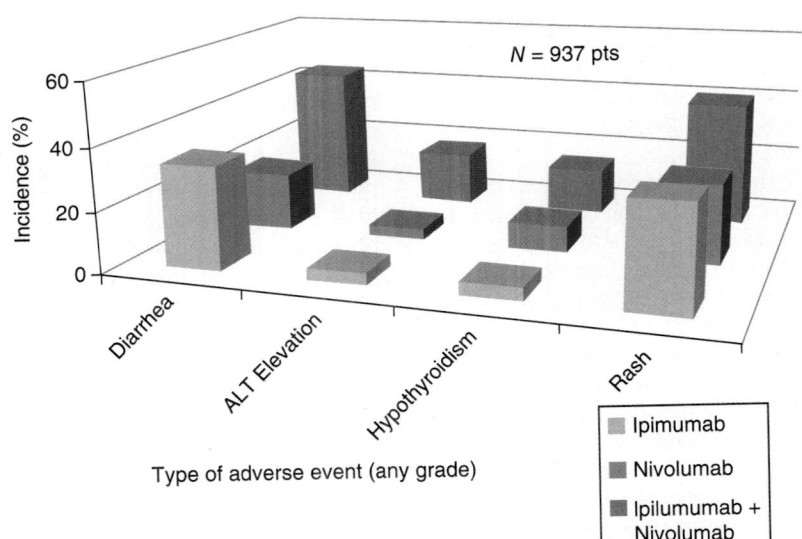

Figure 183-4 *Incidence of adverse events from CTLA-4 inhibitor, PD-1 inhibitor, and combination.* (Data from Postow MA, Chesney J, Pavlick AC, et al. Nivolumab and ipilimumab versus ipilimumab in untreated melanoma. *N Engl J Med.* 2015;372(21):2006-2017.)

TABLE 183-1 Severity of Adverse Events Based on CTCAE Criteria

Adverse Event	Grade 1	Grade 2	Grade 3	Grade 4	Grade 5
Gastrointestinal toxicity					
Diarrhea	Increase of <4 stools per day over baseline; mild increase in ostomy output compared to baseline	Increase of 4-6 stools per day over baseline; moderate increase in ostomy output compared to baseline	Increase of ≥7 stools per day over baseline; incontinence; hospitalization indicated; severe increase in ostomy output compared to baseline; limiting self-care ADL	Life threatening	Death
Colitis	No symptoms; radiographic evidence only	Abdominal pain; blood or mucus in stool	Severe abdominal pain; change in bowel habits; peritoneal signs	Life threatening	Death
ALT	>ULN-3.0 × ULN	>3.0-5.0 × ULN	>5.0-20.0 × ULN	>20.0 × ULN	
AST	>ULN-3.0 × ULN	>3.0-5.0 × ULN	>5.0-20.0 × ULN	>20.0 × ULN	
ALP	> ULN-2.5 × ULN	>2.5-5 ULN	> 5-20 ULN	> 20.0 × ULN	
Bilirubin	>ULN-1.5 × ULN	> 1.5-3 × ULN	> 3.0-10 × ULN	> 10 × ULN	
Endocrine toxicity					
Endocrine disorders	Asymptomatic; clinical or diagnostic observations only	Moderate symptoms; minimal, local, or noninvasive intervention indicated; limiting ADLs	Severe or medically significant but not immediately life-threatening; hospitalization or prolongation of existing hospitalization indicated; disabling; limiting self-care ADLs	Life-threatening consequences; urgent intervention indicated	Death
Pulmonary toxicity					
Pneumonitis	Asymptomatic; clinical or diagnostic observations only	Symptomatic; medical intervention indicated; limiting instrumental ADLs	Severe symptoms; limiting self-care ADL; oxygen indicated	Life-threatening respiratory compromise; urgent intervention indicated (eg, tracheotomy or intubation)	Death
Derm toxicity					
Maculo-papular rash	Covers <10% body surface area	Covers 10%-30% body surface area	Covers >30% body surface area		
Renal toxicity					
Creatinine	>1-1.5 × baseline; >ULN-1.5 × ULN	>1.5-3.0 × baseline; >1.5-3.0 × ULN	>3.0 baseline; >3.0-6.0 × ULN	>6.0 × ULN	
Neurological toxicity					
Peripheral Neuropathy	Asymptomatic	Moderate symptoms, limiting instrumental ADLs	Severe symptoms, limiting self-care ADLs	Life-threatening, Urgent intervention needed	

Based on the National Cancer Institute's Common Terminology Criteria for Adverse Events (CTCAE), Version 4.0. Published: May 28, 2009. US Dept of Health and Human Services.

A comprehensive history and physical examination should assess volume status, severity of illness, extent of disease, and functional status. The clinician should identify risk factors for infectious complications, including country of origin, travel, foods (meats/dairy, rewarmed meats, undercooked meats, fried rice), recent antibiotics or hospitalizations, sick contacts, interaction with daycare children, or exposure to unpurified water.

Routine admission laboratory tests include complete blood count with differential, basic metabolic profile, hepatic biochemical tests, urinalysis, Clostridium difficile assay, stool culture for enteric pathogens, and stool ova and parasites, as well as blood cultures and stool enzyme-linked immunosorbent assay (ELISAs) for viruses and Giardia in patients with relevant history.

The patient should have the following tests in anticipation that further immunosuppression beyond steroids may be required to control symptoms: T-spot or purified protein derivative (PPD), hepatitis B surface antigen, surface antibody, and core antibody.

Imaging includes an initial abdominal kidneys ureter bladder (KUB) film and upright film in all patients, and an abdominal computed tomography (CT) in patients with persistent, severe, progressive symptoms.

In general, the gastrointestinal symptoms are reversible and stopping the CTLA-4 or PD-1 blockade leads to an improvement in the diarrhea/colitis. For a summary of the evaluation and management of diarrhea and colitis related to the novel monoclonal checkpoint inhibitors (see **Figure 183-5**).

The first critical decision point in inpatient management of diarrhea/colitis is to evaluate whether the patient has any indicators or radiographic evidence of serious complication, as outlined in Figure 183-5. After it is clear that there is no perforation, a flexible sigmoidoscopy or colonoscopy can be considered on a case by case basis. In general, patients are nothing by mouth initially and then placed on a low residue diet once they are pain free.

For treatment of the grade 3 or 4 diarrhea/colitis related to the immunotherapy agent, the immunotherapy should be held and 1 to 2 mg/kg methylprednisolone or equivalent (see **Table 183-2**) should be started, as outlined in Figure 183-5. Antidiarrheals and medications with anticholinergic side effects are avoided until a definitive diagnosis, and opiates are used sparingly in order to avoid masking symptoms of perforation. Antibiotics should be initiated if infectious workup is positive and therapy is indicated. (See Chapter 82 [Diarrhea] and Chapter 190 [Clostridium difficile].)

For uncomplicated cases, continue steroids until the patient's symptoms have returned to grade 1, and taper steroids over

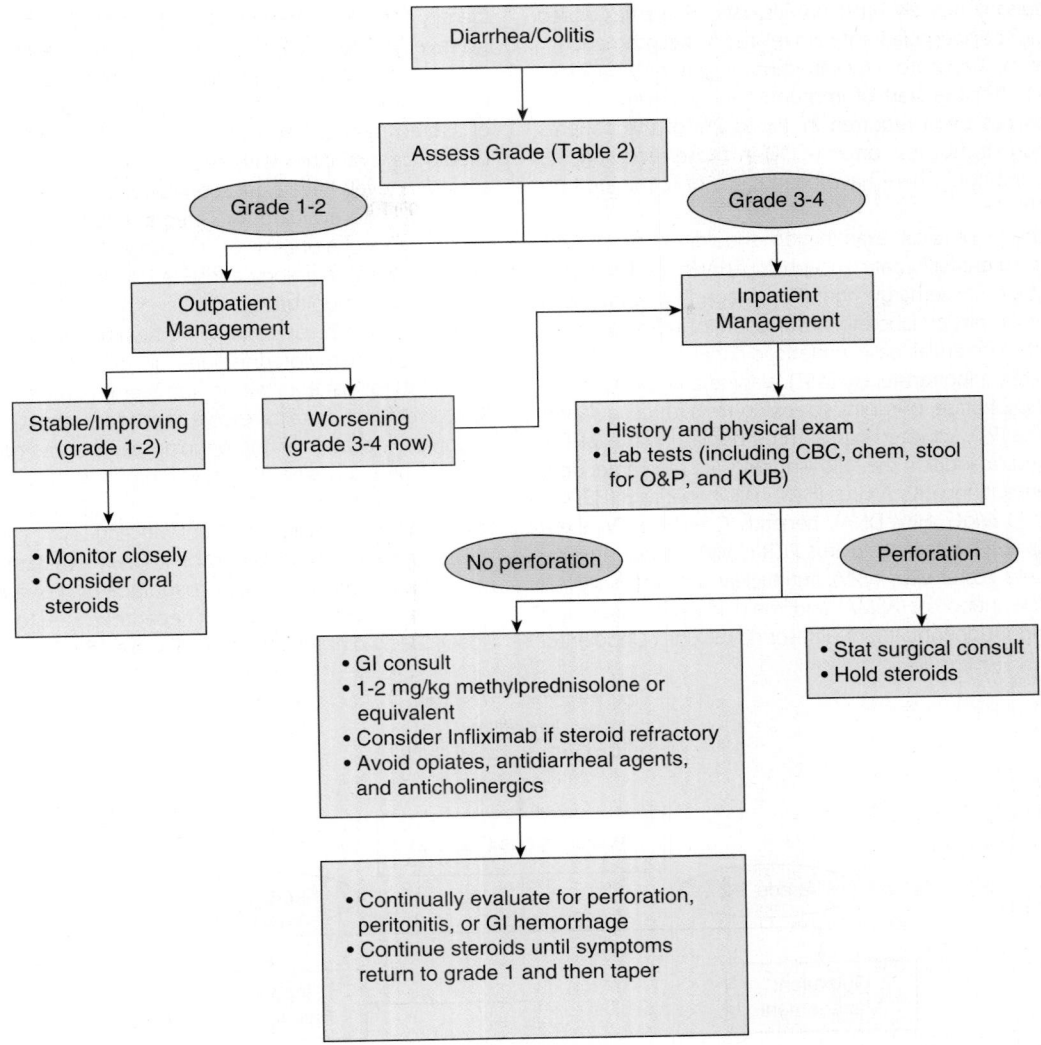

Figure 183-5 *Summary of evaluation and management for diarrhea, colitis.*

1 month. However, endoscopy or repeat endoscopy may be necessary if symptoms persist or progress. One should consider, under the direction of a gastrointestinal (GI) consultant, a single dose of infliximab 5 mg/kg (anti-TNF agent) for immunosuppressive therapy for patients with severe, fulminate colitis that are not responding to steroids after 48 hours or those with less severe colitis for which there is no improvement after prolonged course of steroids. Note that infliximab is contraindicated in bowel perforation and sepsis. Tuberculosis (by PPD skin test or quantiferon as per institute policy) and chronic hepatitis B are necessary before starting infliximab. Rarely, up to three doses of infliximab (or another anti-TNF agent) may be required. Long-term maintenance treatment is never needed in this setting.

HEPATITIS

The hepatitis induced by immunotherapy is similar to autoimmune hepatitis, and biopsies from patients during the acute episode have shown a diffuse T-cell infiltrate, supporting the mechanism being immune-related.

Patients may have mild/grade 1 elevated LFTs and bilirubin, moderate/grade 2 toxicity, severe/grade 3, or life-threatening/grade 4 toxicity (see Table 183-1). The clinical presentation varies from individual to individual. Some develop elevated alanine aminotransferase, aspartate aminotransferase, and/or hyperbilirubinemia without any symptoms, while others may experience anorexia, nausea/vomiting,

TABLE 183-2 Commonly Used Steroids and Their Relative Potencies

Generic Name	Duration	Half-Life	GC Potency	MC Potency	Equiv Dose (mg)
Hydrocortisone	Short	8-12 h	1	1	20.0
Prednisone	Intermediate	18-36 h	3	0.75	5.0
Prednisolone	Intermediate	18-36 h	3	0.75	5.0
Methylprednisolone	Intermediate	18-36 h	6.2	0.5	4.0
Dexamethasone	Long	36-54 h	26	0	0.75

GC, glucocorticoid; MC, mineralocorticoid.

fatigue, jaundice/conjunctival icterus, pruritis, dark urine, pale colored stools, or even right upper quadrant pain related to hepatomegaly.

The timing of the hepatotoxicity varies, but is generally between 8 and 12 weeks after the start of immunotherapy. Severe inflammatory hepatitis has been reported in 1% to 2% of the patients receiving Ipilimumab, but less often (<1%) in those receiving the PD-1 or PD-L1 inhibitors. There have been cases of fulminate liver failure and death.

A comprehensive physical examination should be performed, including an assessment for hepatic encephalopathy (stage 1 = altered mental status, stage II = lethargy, confusion, stage III = stupor, and stage IV = coma). Admission laboratory evaluation includes complete blood count with differential, basic metabolic panel, liver biochemical tests (aspartate aminotransferase (AST), alanine aminotransferase (ALT), alkaline phosphatase, bilirubin), screening tests for coagulation (prothrombin time (PT), activated partial thromboplastin time (aPTT), and platelet count). In addition the following tests are recommended: toxicology screen, antihepatitis A virus (HAV IgM), hepatitis B (HBsAg, HBsAb, anti-HBc IgM/IgG, HBV DNA), hepatitis C virus (HCV RNA), Epstein-Barr virus (EBV), cytomegalovirus PCR (CMV), herpes simplex virus (HSV), varicella zoster virus (VZV), antinuclear antibodies (ANA), antismooth muscle antibodies (ASMA), and iron studies (Fe/TIBC ratio). Imaging with a right upper quadrant ultrasound includes Doppler to identify thrombus, abdominal CT scan to distinguish between progressive liver disease and immune-mediated hepatitis.

The immune-mediated hepatitis is reversible and stopping the CTLA-4 or PD-1 blockade leads to an improvement. The presence of altered mental status that may signify hepatic encephalopathy should be evaluated with serum ammonia, with the caveat that ammonia levels have a questionable role in the diagnosis, and head CT imaging to evaluate for cerebral edema. If evidence of severe hepatic encephalopathy exists, consider transfer to an intensive care unit with neurology consultation for possibility of intracranial pressure (ICP) monitoring.

The immunotherapy should be held and systemic corticosteroid (2 mg/kg/d methylprednisolone qd or BID or equivalent) should be started for patients with grade 3 or 4 immune-related hepatitis. Once liver function tests resolve, taper corticosteroids over 1 month.

Consult hepatology for ongoing symptoms, not responsive to steroids, and consider alternative immunosuppressive therapy after 48 hours with mycofenolate mofetil (500 mg BID). Note, there is also a case report of successful treatment with anti-thymocyte globulin (ATG).

Throughout hospitalization continually evaluate for evidence of hepatic encephalopathy and coagulopathy. For a summary of the evaluation and management of hepatitis related to the novel monoclonal checkpoint inhibitors (see **Figure 183-6**).

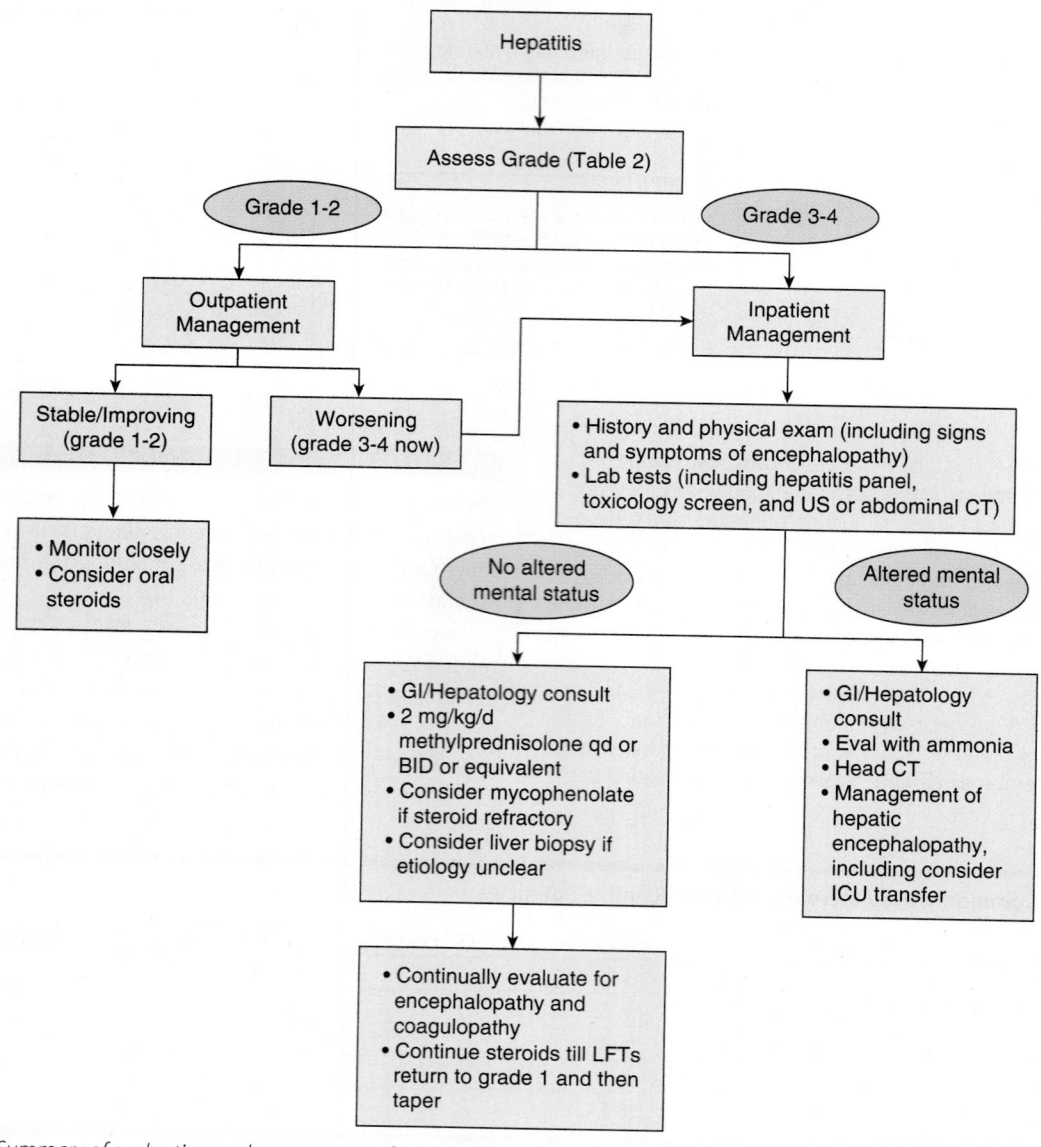

Figure 183-6 *Summary of evaluation and management for hepatitis.*

ENDOCRINE TOXICITY

The decision for inpatient versus outpatient management depends on the grade and severity of the endocrinopathy. Most patients with grade 1 (asymptomatic) endocrine irAEs generally do not require hospital admission and can be managed with close monitoring on appropriate endocrine replacement without having to stop immunotherapy. However, grade 2 (symptomatic) endocrinopathies requires cessation of the immune checkpoint inhibitor, endocrine replacements as needed, and initiation of steroids (1-2 mg/kg/d of prednisone or equivalent), usually as an outpatient. Patients who do not improve or those with more severe symptoms (grade 3 or 4 endocrine irAEs [see Table 183-1]) often need admission to the hospital, and require more intensive management based on the specific condition as outlined below.

■ ENDOCRINOPATHIES

Endocrine irAE's can present in a variety of ways. The most common endocrinopathies reported in association with the immune checkpoint inhibitors are hypophysitis and thyroiditis. Of note, the thyroiditis can present with an initial hyperthyroid phase, but is generally followed by subsequent hypothyroidism. Adrenalitis causing primary adrenal insufficiency is much rarer. Depending on specific organ involved and severity, patients may have a subtle presentation or a more florid, classic presentation of the endocrinopathy.

For hypophysitis, infiltration of T-lymphocytes leading to pituitary destruction is the proposed mechanism of inflammation of the *anterior* pituitary, which leads to decreased production of thyroid stimulating hormone (TSH), adrenocorticotropic hormone (ACTH), luteinizing hormone (LH), follicle stimulating hormone (FSH), and prolactin. Similarly, thyroiditis and adrenalitis are thought to be a result of off-target inflammation, although the exact mechanisms are not clearly understood. Interestingly, *posterior* pituitary inflammation, which causes diabetes insipidus, is not a common presentation and is case reportable.

The CTLA-4 inhibitors cause hypophysitis (all grades) in 10% to 15% of cases, but thyroiditis is less common, and adrenalitis is case reportable. Dose-dependent grade 3 and 4 symptomatic endocrinopathies are reported in less than 3% of patients receiving the drug, generally within 2 to 3 months of starting the medication, whereas these severe, endocrine irAEs requiring hospitalization, occur in less than 1% in patients treated with a PD-1 inhibitor. The PD-1 inhibitors more commonly cause mild to moderate thyroid function abnormalities (5%-10%) but it is rare to have a grade 3 or 4 reaction with this class of drug.

Hypotension, nausea, vomiting, abdominal pain, and fatigue may suggest adrenal crisis (see Chapter 153 [Adrenal insufficiency]). Hypophysitis causes headaches and fatigue. Mass effect as a result of compression of the optic chiasm with visual field changes and cranial nerve palsy are not reported with immune checkpoint inhibitors. Myxedema crisis is also unlikely (see Chapter 152 [Thyroid Emergencies]).

Admission laboratory evaluation includes complete blood count with differential, platelet, basic metabolic profile, liver biochemical tests, urinalysis. In addition, endocrine studies TSH, free thyroxine (T4), ACTH, am cortisol, cosyntropin stimulation test, LH, FSH, prolactin, and testosterone (for men) should be obtained to distinguish primary versus secondary endocrinopathy (see **Table 183-3**), an 8 AM cortisol level less than 3 µg/dL diagnostic for AI. The cosyntropin stimulation test (ie, a baseline am cortisol followed by a standard 250 µg dose of cosyntropin, a recheck cortisol level 60 minutes after ACTH) can be normal in acute central AI. If repeat cortisol is less than 18 µg/dL diagnostic for AI. Follicle stimulating hormone and luteinizing hormone can be decreased in acute illness, so the results may be difficult to interpret during the hospitalization. IGF-1 is not thought to be an adequate surrogate to detect growth hormone (GH) deficiency, and therefore might not add much value but can be helpful in confirming the presence of hypopituitarism in the context of the other values.

Imaging should include a pituitary protocol magnetic resonance imaging (MRI) if there is concern for hypophysitis and compared to any prior brain MRI for relative pituitary enlargement. If there is evidence of pituitary inflammation causing compression of optic chiasm on imaging, the patient should be referred to ophthalmology for full visual field testing.

Unlike other irAE's the endocrinopathies are not always reversible by stopping the CTLA-4 or PD-1 inhibitors. The first critical decision point for management of the endocrine axis is to recognize and treat patients with both adrenal insufficiency and hypothyroidism correctly, otherwise an adrenal crisis can be precipitated (see Chapter 152 [Thyroid Emergencies] and Chapter 153 [Adrenal Insufficiency]). Start treatment with steroids, and follow with thyroid hormone. The hypothyroidism can cause an SIADH presentation with hyponatremia which should be recognized and treat appropriately (see Chapter 242 [Disorders of Sodium and Water Balance]). For grade 3 or 4 toxicity associated with immunotherapy, start with high-dose intravenous corticosteroids (1-2 mg/kg/d methylprednisolone or equivalent) and consult your endocrinology colleagues to aid with further evaluation and hormone replacement therapy.

PRACTICE POINT

- For patients with thyroiditis, hypothyroidism can cause hyponatremia due to a profound SIADH.

TABLE 183-3 Characteristic Lab Results of Primary vs Secondary Endocrinopathies

	TSH	Free T4	Prolactin	ACTH	Cort stim	FSH/LH	Testosterone
Central hypophysitis	⇓	⇓	⇓	⇓	●	⇓	⇓
Adrenal insufficiency				⇓	●		
Hypothyroidism	⇓	⇓					
Hypogonadism						⇓	⇓
Primary hyperthyroidism	⇓	⇑					
Primary hypothyroidism	⇑	⇓					
Primary adrenal insufficiency				⇑	⇓		

Key ⇓ - Indicates low or inappropriately normal value.
⇑- Indicates high or inappropriately normal value.
● - Indicates abnormal value.

■ HYPOPHYSITIS

Once the diagnostic studies have confirmed hypophysitis, high-dose steroids (1-2 mg/kg/d methylprednisolone or equivalent) should be initiated. In addition, the deficient hormones should be replaced. The steroid and thyroid replacement are often essential, however sex hormones are considered on a case by case basis and generally only replaced if levels do not normalize after steroids and resolution of pituitary inflammation. Note that administering growth hormone in the setting of malignancy is generally contraindicated. Once replacement is started, subsequent titration of dose is based on repeat lab values and/or symptoms. It should be noted that hypopituitarism can be permanent, and very few patients are able to discontinue steroid replacement, therefore this is one of the few irAEs that does not recover after discontinuation of immunotherapy (see Chapter 154 [Pituitary Disease]).

■ THYROIDITIS

In addition to the 1 to 2 mg/kg/d methylprednisolone as discussed above, patients diagnosed with grade 3 or 4 thyroiditis and initial thyrotoxicosis benefit from a nonselective β-blocker such as propranolol to control tachycardia. Propranolol also decreases T4 → T3 conversion. The starting dose is generally 10 to 20 mg every 6 hours, and can be increased until symptoms are under optimal control.

Those patients with hypophysitis and low TSH, or thyroiditis and hypothyroidism, require thyroxine replacement. While myxedema coma is exceedingly rare, severe hypothyroidism requires intravenous loading of thyroxine if there is evidence of bradycardia or hypothermia. In severe cases of both thyrotoxicosis and hypothyroidism, the starting dose of thyroxine should be discussed with the endocrine consultant. Use caution with doses of thyroid replacement in elderly patients or those with heart arrhythmias (see Chapter 152 [Thyroid Emergencies]).

■ ADRENALITIS (PRIMARY ADRENAL INSUFFICIENCY)

If patients present with severe dehydration, hypotension, and shock, an infectious source should be ruled out in addition to a full endocrine workup for adrenal crisis. It is much more common with the immune checkpoint inhibitors to have hypophysitis than adrenalitis (case reportable) causing primary adrenal insufficiency. In the latter cases, unlike in hypophysitis and central adrenal insufficiency, ACTH will be increased, and because aldosterone secretion is no longer intact, this condition can often be associated with hyperkalemia or salt cravings.

For individuals with primary adrenal insufficiency, steroids are essential along with volume resuscitation with normal saline. If replacing with hydrocortisone at stress doses there will be adequate mineralcorticoid activity; however, if using another agent (eg, dexamethasone) you may need to discuss adding fludrocortisone in primary adrenal insufficiency with your endocrine consultant.

PULMONARY TOXICITY

Patients with asymptomatic grade 1 pneumonitis do not require hospital admission or corticosteroids. However, for moderate grade 2 pneumonitis the immune checkpoint inhibitor should be held, and corticosteroids administered with consideration of hospitalization, for observation, even at this early stage. Severe grade 3 or 4 pneumonitis is a rare but serious adverse event, and these patients should be hospitalized and managed intensively with a multi-disciplinary care team including general medicine, medical oncology, pulmonology, and consideration of infectious disease.

■ PNEUMONITIS

The clinical presentation of pneumonitis can be acute or sub-acute with new onset of cough, dyspnea on exertion, progressive shortness of breath, and worsening fatigue. Although it is rare to develop drug-related pneumonitis, with an incidence of <1% with PD-1 inhibitors and even less in CTLA-4 directed therapies, it is very important that it is recognized early in these patients. A higher suspicion should be in individuals with lung cancer, prior chest well radiation, or a smoking history. The time to onset in the cases that have been reported ranges from 25 days to 9.9 months.

The admission history and physical assesses the grade and severity of pulmonary symptoms and guide the hospital workup, including consideration of other diagnostic possibilities such as infection, heart failure, or progression of disease (see Table 183-1). Other risk factors should be documented, including recent travel, occupation, exposures, tobacco use, and prior treatments, such as chemotherapies, and any history of ionizing radiation to the lung, with exact Gy and volume of lung irradiated if that information can be obtained.

Admission laboratory evaluation includes a complete blood count with differential, basic metabolic panel, liver biochemical tests, and urinalysis. In addition, consider measurement of arterial blood gas, cultures including sputum to identify typical or atypical bacterial, fungal, or mycobacterial infections, a viral panel, and brain natriuretic peptide (BNP) if any evidence of heart failure. Imaging should include an initial chest x-ray (posteroanterior (PA) and lateral) or high-resolution chest CT to diagnose other possibilities and to restage disease. Pneumonitis is a rare complication of these therapies, and immune based therapies can be associated with "pseudo-progression", that is, disease can appear worse on initial scans. The hospitalist should review the films with the interpreting radiologist, consult with the patient's oncologist, and consider early pulmonary consultation.

The clinical presentation may be similar to that of a patient presenting with infection (eg, Pneumocystic jiroveci) or other causes of pneumonitis so a comprehensive laboratory evaluation can assist in sorting through the differential diagnosis. Urgent workup is necessary to establish a diagnosis because early and aggressive management with corticosteroids is paramount to the treatment of acute, drug-induced pneumonitis. Recommendations for grade 3 to 4 pneumonitis include treatment with 2 to 4 mg/kg/d IV methylprednisolone, and consideration of bronchoscopy to exclude infection. In addition, lung biopsy to determine underlying histology of lung pathology should be considered if cause remains unclear. For those cases that are steroid refractory, other immunosuppressive agents such as infliximab, mycophenolate, or cyclophosphamide have been used on a case by case basis. For patients who improve with IV methylprednisolone, and symptoms improve to grade 1 or less, the steroids could be tapered slowly over 6 to 8 weeks.

PRACTICE POINT

- Drug-related pneumonitis should be considered in individuals at higher risk due to lung cancer, prior chest well radiation, or a smoking history.

DERMATOLOGIC TOXICITY

■ DERMATITIS

Immune-mediated dermatitis is the most common toxicity associated with the immune checkpoint inhibitors, and generally presents as a rash, pruritis, or vitiligo.

■ RISK STRATIFICATION

Most of the skin reactions seen with immune checkpoint inhibitors are mild to moderate, and respond to topical moisturizers and corticosteroids, oatmeal baths, and antihistamines. If there is no improvement, oral corticosteroid therapy (prednisone 1 mg/kg qD or equivalent) is started. However, 2% of the reactions result in grade

3 or 4 toxicity, covering >30% of the body surface area and require intensive management. Careful attention must be paid to look for evidence of full thickness ulceration, bullous disease, or necrosis, considering Stevens-Johnson syndrome (SJS) (<10% BSA has epidermal detachment) and toxic epidermal necrolysis (TEN) (>30%), both life-threatening conditions, have been reported. The onset of the dermatologic irAEs is generally within 2 to 3 weeks.

■ EVALUATION

The examiner should perform an ocular examination, examine the skin and the mucosa for erythema, blistering, necrosis, or ulceration.

Admission laboratory tests include a complete blood cell count with differential, total eosinophil count, basic metabolic panel, hepatic biochemical tests, urinalysis, and blood and skin cultures.

■ MANAGEMENT

In general, the immune-mediated dermatitis is reversible, and stopping the CTLA-4 or PD-1 blockade leads to improvement. If there is any clinical evidence of extensive BSA involvement, vesicobullous lesions, ocular/oral/genital involved, or rapid progression, urgent dermatology consult for skin biopsy and assistance in management is necessary, along with ophthalmology, ENT, gynecology, or urology, depending on mucosal surfaces involved. Unless there is a clear diagnosis, immune-mediated dermatitis should be the default, and potent topical steroid creams plus systemic steroids (prednisone 1-2 mg/kg/d or equivalent) and antihistamines should be initiated.

The immune checkpoint inhibitors are permanently discontinued for any of the generalized exfoliative, full thickness dermal ulceration, ulcerative or bullous dermatitis, skin necrosis, SJS, or TEN patients. Once dermatitis has resolved to grade 1, steroids could be tapered over 1 month.

RENAL TOXICITY
■ ACUTE KIDNEY INJURY

Acute kidney injury related to lupus nephritis, immune-mediated nephritis, or interstitial nephritis, is a rare toxicity (<1% incidence) associated with the immune checkpoint inhibitors; but it could require hospitalization and management on the inpatient service.

The severity is determined by level of creatinine, with higher grade toxicity being >3 × baseline or ULN (see Table 183-1). Corticosteroids should be administered for grade 2 or greater nephritis.

The prognosis for the patients that developed acute kidney injury as a complication of immune checkpoint inhibitors thus far in clinical trials has been good, with the majority fully recovering renal function after steroids.

The differential diagnosis of acute kidney injury remains broad because this is such a rare side effect of the immune checkpoint inhibitors (see Chapter 239 [Acute Kidney Injury]). Admission laboratory tests include complete blood count with differential, basic metabolic profile, hepatic function panel, and urinalysis, urine sediment. Plasma and urine electrolytes may be measured to calculate fractional excretion of sodium FE_{Na} in oliguric patients (see Chapter 111 [Urinalysis and Urine Electrolytes]). Additional workup includes uric acid, urine eosinophils, antinuclear antibody (ANA), antineutrophil cytoplasmic antibody (ANCA), anti–glomerular basement membrane antibody (anti-GBM), antistreptolysin O (ASO), cryoglobulins (C3/C4), and serum protein electrophoresis (SPEP)/serum free light chains in the right clinical context. Imaging should include a renal ultrasound to rule out obstruction.

In general, the immune-mediated nephritis is reversible, and stopping the CTLA-4 or PD-1 blockade leads to an improvement. A critical decision point in inpatient management of acute kidney injury is to evaluate whether there is a need for hemodialysis which can be made in collaboration with a nephrologist.

In general, management includes avoiding nephrotoxins (NSAIDs, contrast, ACEi/ARB), renal dosing of medications, correcting volume status, and in the case of immune checkpoint inhibitor induced nephritis, administration of corticosteroids with IV methylprednisolone 0.5 to 1.0 mg/kg/d or oral equivalent. In cases of grade 4 nephritis, higher doses of IV methylprednisolone have been used in certain circumstances.

If the acute renal failure progresses despite steroids, renal biopsy should be considered. A number of patients who are on immune-based therapies have advanced disease with guarded prognosis, and therefore it is critical to involve the primary oncologist about goals of care and prognosis before a nephrologist initiates dialysis. Throughout the hospitalization, the clinician should continually evaluate for acidemia, electrolyte disarray, volume overload, and uremia. Once renal function improves to grade 1 or less, then steroids can be tapered over 4 to 6 weeks.

> **PRACTICE POINT**
>
> - Assess severity and grade of the Immune Related Adverse Event (see Table 183-1).

NEUROLOGICAL TOXICITY

In general, the initial step in evaluation and management is assessment of grade and severity of the neurological symptom. While patients with grade 1 or 2 irAEs can usually be successfully treated as an outpatient with drug interruption and oral steroids, those with grade 3 or 4 often need inpatient admission for intravenous steroids, plasmapheresis, intravenous immunoglobulin (IVIG), based on the specific neurological symptom (see Table 183-1).

The neurological adverse effects from immunotherapy can range from peripheral neuropathies like Gullian-Barre Syndrome (GBS), autoimmune multifocal neuropathy, to spinal cord lesions such as transverse myelitis, to central nervous system disorders such myelitis or aseptic meningitis, cranial nerve paralysis, myasthenia gravis, or even Posterior Reversible Encephalopathy Syndrome (PRES). Peripheral neuropathy is the most common neurological irAE from immunotherapy and even that is infrequent with incidence less than 2%.

Immunotherapy can cause a myriad of neurological irAEs, but given that these are very rare, it is important to give thoughtful consideration to the diagnosis in a patient presenting with neurological symptoms. For example, it is important to distinguish immunotherapy mediated neuropathy from neuropathy due to other causes such as chemotherapy. The common chemotherapy agents associated with peripheral neuropathy include platinums (cisplatin, carboplatin), taxols (paclitaxel, docetaxel), and vinca alkaloids (vinctristine, vinblastine). In general chemotherapy induced neuropathy is cumulative, dose-dependent, has a subacute clinical presentation, and does not respond to steroids. Similarly, in a patient presenting with seizure, it is important to consider brain metastasis as a differential diagnosis along with rare irAEs such as PRES. However, this does not mean that the possibility of neurological irAEs should be ignored. Clinical presentation of immune mediated occlusive enteric neuropathy may mimic that of immune mediated colitis, and immune mediated phrenic nerve paralysis may mimic acute onset of dyspnea due to pulmonary embolism.

Admission laboratory tests include complete blood count with differential, basic metabolic panel, hepatic function panel, urinalysis, thyroid stimulating hormone, vitamin B12, folate, relevant infectious workup, electromyogram and nerve conduction studies to evaluate the etiology of the neuropathy. Additional studies include CT or MRI brain to evaluate for brain metastasis as well to evaluate for presence of PRES. Cerebrospinal fluid analysis may be appropriate in selected patients.

Grade 3/4 neurological symptoms require permanent discontinuation of the immune agent, initiation of intravenous steroids and consideration of plasmapheresis, IVIG, or other immunosuppressive therapies as clinically appropriate. However, as neurological irAEs are a rare side effect, the scientific literature is scarce and it is important to consider expert opinion from neurology.

The first critical decision point in inpatient management of patients with neurological irAEs, is identification of patients who require plasmapheresis and/or intravenous immunoglobulin (IVIG), such as those with GBS. Unlike classical GBS in which steroids should be avoided, patients with GBS secondary to immunotherapy may respond to high-dose intravenous steroids with a complete recovery in 4 to 6 weeks.

Patients with grade 3/4 peripheral neuropathy require high-dose intravenous steroids (methylprednisolone 2 mg/kg qd or equivalent). Throughout the hospitalization close monitoring of the respiratory status is important, particularly in patients with GBS and myasthenia gravis, as they could develop respiratory compromise needing mechanical ventilation. Once the symptoms improve to grade 1 or less, the steroids could be tapered over 6 to 8 weeks. In general, discontinuation of the immunotherapy and steroids results in complete recovery in the majority of patients.

DISCHARGE CHECKLIST

Following a hospitalization for an irAEs, many patients require ongoing medical care with prolonged immunosuppression, such as oral steroids. Generally, the steroid taper is done over at least 1 month in order to prevent recurrence of the irAE.

■ PCP PROPHYLAXIS

- Patients should be educated regarding the risk of infection while on steroids. The National Comprehensive Cancer Network (NCCN) guidelines suggest that *Pneumocytis jiroveci* prophylaxis be considered for patients treated with 20 mg of prednisone daily for at least 4 weeks.

■ ADRENAL SUPPRESSION

- Patients and care providers must be aware of signs of adrenal insufficiency (fatigue, nausea, vomiting, abdominal pain, myagias/athralgias) as steroids taper to physiologic levels and ensure they have a plan if they become ill (fever >100°, GI illness, infection, other illness or injury) for increasing steroids.

■ HYPERGLYCEMIA

- Patients with prediabetes or existing diabetes will need to check frequent blood sugars, and will need to adjust their diabetes medications as the tapering progresses.

■ VOLUME OVERLOAD

- Patients on long-term steroids, especially those with a history of CHF or renal insufficiency, can have issues with volume overload resulting in edema and weight gain. They must be educated to notify their treatment team if this is occurring so that it can be addressed before hospital admission becomes necessary.

■ GASTRIC ULCERS AND GI BLEEDING

- Patients on steroids are at increased risk of gastric and ulcer development. They should be counseled not to use NSAIDS, and should be prescribed a proton pump inhibitor to decrease this risk. In addition, they should notify their treatment team immediately if they experience abdominal pain or black tarry stools.

FINAL CHECKLIST

- Has the patient been counseled regarding postacute care (see above) issues?

- Patient is now immunosuppressed with corticosteroids and is at risk for developing opportunistic infections. Was PCP Prophylaxis with Bactrim, Atovaquone, or Pentamidine considered if 20 mg prednisone, or equivalent, is planned for at least 4 weeks?
- Is the patient scheduled for follow-up appointments with the oncologist and any consulting specialty teams?
- Does the patient have transportation to those appointments?
- Have they been provided with educational materials? Advise the patient to read the FDA-medication guide (http://www.fda.gov/Drugs/DrugSafety/ucm085729.htm).
- Have instructions been provided as to when to call the MD?
  - Pneumonitis: Contact your physician immediately or seek medical attention if you develop new or worsening shortness of breath, cough, or chest pain.
  - Colitis: Contact your physician immediately or seek medical attention if you develop new or worsening diarrhea or abdominal pain.
  - Hepatitis: Contact your physician immediately, or seek medical attention if you develop new or worsening yellowing of the skin, nausea, vomiting, bruising, or bleeding.
  - Hypophysitis: Contact your physician immediately, or seek medical attention if you develop new or worsening headache, weakness, dizziness, or fainting.
  - Nephritis: Contact your physician immediately, or seek medical attention if you develop new decreased urine output, blood in your urine, facial puffiness, or lower-extremity swelling.
- Have females of reproductive age been advised to inform their health care provider of any possible pregnancy? Advise highly effective contraception during treatment with immune checkpoint inhibitors and for 4 to 5 months after last dose, and no breastfeeding

SUGGESTED READINGS

Hodi FS, et al. Improved survival with ipilimumab in patients with metastatic melanoma. *N Engl J Med*. 2010;363:711-723.

Lake D. Immunopharmacology, in Katsung B, et al, eds. *Basic & Clinical Pharmacology*, 13th ed. New York, NY: McGraw-Hill Education Medical; 2014.

Naidoo J, et al. Immune checkpoint blockade. *Hematol Oncol Clin North Am*. 2014;28:585-600.

Postow MA, et al. Nivolumab and ipilimumab versus ipilimumab in untreated melanoma. *N Engl J Med*. 2015;372:2006-2017.

Robert C, et al. Nivolumab in previously untreated melanoma without BRAF mutation. *N Engl J Med*. 2015;372:320-330.

Weber JS, et al. Management of immune-related adverse events and kinetics of response with ipilimumab. *J Clin Oncol*. 2012;30:2691-2697.

Weber JS, et al. Toxicities of immunotherapy for the practitioner. *J Clin Oncol*. 2015;33:2092-2099.

YERVOY (ipilimumab). *Risk Evaluation and Mitigation Strategy*. Princeton, NJ: Bristol-Myers Squibb Company; 2015.

HIGHLIGHTS OF PRESCRIBING INFORMATION

- YERVOY (ipilimumab). Princeton, NJ: Bristol-Myers Squibb Company; 2015.
- OPDIVO (nivolumab). Princeton, NJ: Bristol-Myers Squibb Company; 2015.
- KETRUDA (pembrolizumab). Whitehouse Station, NJ: Merck & Co, Inc; 2015.

SECTION 9

Infectious Diseases

CHAPTER 184

Fundamentals of Antibiotics

Matthew E. Falagas, MD, MSc, DSc
Ioannis A. Bliziotis, MD, MSc, PhD

Key Clinical Questions

1. What resistance patterns are associated with major nosocomial pathogens?

2. When should empiric antibiotic therapy be initiated? When is it permissible to delay empiric antibiotic therapy, if ever?

3. What impact do pharmacokinetics and pharmacodynamics have on antibiotic choice?

4. In what circumstances is combination antibiotic therapy appropriate?

5. What are the major adverse effects of antibiotics?

INTRODUCTION

In this chapter, we will use the terms antibacterial agents and antibiotics interchangeably. The term antibiotic has sometimes been defined as a substance, produced by microbes, that inhibits the growth of other microbes, especially bacteria. More broadly, it is used to characterize any agent with antibacterial properties, whether found in nature or synthesized artificially. Antibiotics are prescribed to approximately one-third of all hospitalized patients, and account for greater than 10% of hospital pharmacy expenditures. Up to one-half of antibiotic orders may be unnecessary, poorly chosen, or dosed incorrectly. Indiscriminant use of broad-spectrum agents is also believed to be a key contributor to emerging worldwide antimicrobial resistance. The estimated additional hospital costs associated with drug-resistant hospital-acquired bacterial infections in the United States is estimated to several billions of dollars. Hospitalists should be familiar with the currently available antibiotics, their penetration into various tissues, their major adverse effects, and their spectrum of activity relative to local patterns of antibacterial resistance. Antimicrobial prescribing should also take into account issues of cost and the potential for the emergence of resistance.

ANTIBIOTIC CATEGORIES AND SPECTRUM OF ACTIVITY

Major categories, subdivisions, and some individual antibacterial agents are summarized in **Table 184-1** according to their mode of action, and side effects and drug-drug interactions are listed in **Table 184-2**. Antibacterial spectrum often overlaps between different antibiotic groups. However, few antibiotics are active against multidrug- or highly resistant bacteria. Thus, the clinician may sometimes have several choices of potentially appropriate antibiotics, but at other times may only have only one, or even none.

When choosing antibacterial therapy in the hospital setting, it is crucial to know local patterns of antibiotic susceptibility and resistance. Prevalence, virulence, and susceptibility patterns of pathogens should affect the choice of antibiotic therapy. For example, most isolates of pneumococci are still sensitive to amoxicillin, and especially to ceftriaxone. However, since pneumococcal infections are very common, even a small percentage of resistant isolates results in a large absolute number of infections with them. In addition, penicillin or ceftriaxone-resistant pneumococci, although rare, are highly virulent and associated with potentially lethal lower respiratory tract or central nervous system infections. High-dose vancomycin is often used empirically when such infections are suspected. Vancomycin-resistant enterococci (VRE) are common in specific hospital settings such as in hematologic and intensive care units. VRE are not virulent for most immunocompetent patients, however they are highly transmisible, cause serious infections in debilitated and immunocompromised patients, and are resistant to most antimicrobials.

Methicillin-resistant *Staphylococcus aureus* (MRSA), by contrast, is both virulent and increasingly common in both the hospital and community settings. The susceptibility patterns of nosocomial strains of MRSA differ from those of community-acquired *Staphylococcus aureus* (cMRSA). Hospital-acquired MRSA is usually susceptible only to vancomycin, teicoplanin (available in Europe, but not the United States), and agents such as linezolid, tigecycline, daptomycin, and the new lipoglycopeptide antibiotics. However, cMRSA is often susceptible to trimethoprim-sulfamethoxazole (TMP-SMX), fluoroquinolones, and clindamycin.

TABLE 184-1 Categories of Antibacterial Agents, with Spectrum of Activity and Modes of Action

Antibiotic Category	Subdivisions (Individual Substances)	Spectrum of Antibacterial Activity
Antibiotics acting on bacterial cell wall		
A. Beta-lactams		
1. Penicillins	Naturally occurring (penicillin G, penicillin V)	Gram-positive cocci, excluding staphylococci and most enterococci. Gram-positive rods, including anaerobes. Spirochetes.
	Penicillinase-resistant antistaphylococcal (methicillin, oxacillin, nafcillin, dicloxacillin)	Methicillin-susceptible staphylococci (MSS). Gram-positive cocci, but not many enterococci.
	Aminopenicillins (ampicillin, amoxicillin)	All the above plus enterococci, *Listeria monocytogenes*, *Hemophilus influenzae*, *Moraxella catarrhalis*, and some enteric Gram-negative rods.
	Carboxy-penicillins and ureido-penicillins (ticarcillin, piperacillin)	All the above plus *Enterobacter*, *Klebsiella*, *Pseudomonas*, *Acinetobacter* species, and anaerobes.
2. Cephalosporins	First generation (cefadroxil, cefazolin, cephalexine, cephradine)	Gram-positive cocci including MSS, excluding enterococci. Some strains of *Escherichia coli*, *Klebsiella*, *Proteus mirabilis*. Not active against indole-positive *Proteus* and *Serratia*.
	Second generation (cefamandole, cefaclor, cefprozil, cefuroxime, cefotetan, cefoxitin, loracarbef)	Similar to first generation, plus *Hemophilus influenzae*, *Enterobacter* species, indole-positive *Proteus* and *Serratia*, *Neisseriae*. Cephamycins (cefotetan, cefoxitin) have good anaerobic activity against *Bacteroides fragilis* but poor against Gram-positive cocci and *Enterobacter* species.
	Third generation (cefotaxime, ceftriaxone, ceftazidime, cefoperazone, cefixime)	Enhanced activity against Gram-negative rods. Ceftazidime has good, cefoperazone moderate, and the rest poor activity against *Pseudomonas aeruginosa*. Good against Gram-negative cocci. Variable activity against Gram-positive cocci, with cefotaxime and ceftriaxone being excellent for pneumococci. Poor anaerobic activity.
	Fourth generation (cefepime, cefpirome)	Good activity against Gram-positive cocci, with enhanced activity against *P. aeruginosa* and other Gram-negative rods.
3. Monobactams	(Aztreonam)	Gram-negative rods including *P. aeruginosa* and some strains of *Acinetobacter baumannii*. Poor against Gram-positive bacteria and anaerobes.
4. Carbapenems	(Meropenem, imipenem/cilastatin, ertapenem)	Excellent activity against Gram-negative rods, including *Enterobacter* species, as well as multidrug-resistant *Klebsiella pneumoniae*, *P. aeruginosa*, and *A. baumannii* (not ertapenem). Good Gram-positive activity. No advantage over ampicillin for enterococci. Compared to imipenem, meropenem has better Gram-negative but worse Gram-positive activity. Ertapenem has narrower spectrum than the other two.
B. Glycopeptides	(Vancomycin, teicoplanin)	Excellent activity against Gram-positive cocci, including MRS, highly resistant pneumococci, and enterococci.
Antibiotics acting on bacterial cell membrane		
C. Polypeptides		
1. Bacitracin		Used only topically against Gram-positive bacteria
2. Polymyxins	(Polymyxin B and polymyxin E also known as colistin)	Gram-negative microbes including multidrug-resistant *K. pneumoniae*, *P. aeruginosa*, and *A. baumannii*. Naturally inactive against *Proteus*. Poor Gram-positive activity
D. Lipopeptides	(Daptomycin)	Similar activity to glycopeptides. Good against vancomycin-resistant enterococci
E. Lipoglycopeptides	(telavancin, oritavancin. dalbavancin)	Semisynthetic derivatives of glycopeptides (act also against bacterial cell wall). Similar *in vitro* activity to glycopeptides and lipopeptides. Very long half-life. Approved for use in skin and soft tissue infections
Antibiotics acting on bacterial protein synthesis		
E. Macrolides	(Erythromycin, clarithromycin, azithromycin)	Good against Gram-positive cocci (excluding many staphylococci and most enterococci), *Mycoplasma* and *Chlamydia* species, *Legionella pneumoniae*, and nontuberculous mycobacteria.
F. Tetracyclines	(Tetracycline, minocycline, doxycycline)	Similar to macrolides plus rickettsiae, *Brucella* species and spirochetes
G. Glycylcyclines	(Tigecycline)	Gram-positive cocci, including MRS, highly resistant pneumococci, and enterococci. Gram-negative bacteria, including multidrug-resistant *K. pneumoniae* and *Acinetobacter baumanii*, but not *P. aeruginosa*. Good anaerobic activity
H. Aminoglycosides	(Streptomycin, gentamicin, tobramycin, amikacin, netilmicin, kanamycin)	Gram-negative bacteria including multidrug-resistant *K. pneumoniae*, *A. baumannii* and *P. aeruginosa*. Moderate activity against Gram-positive cocci. Poor anaerobic activity

(Continued)

TABLE 184-1 Categories of Antibacterial Agents, with Spectrum of Activity and Modes of Action (Continued)

Antibiotic Category	Subdivisions (Individual Substances)	Spectrum of Antibacterial Activity
I. Chloramphenicol		Gram-positive and negative cocci including MRS and *Neisseria meningitidis*. Enterobacteriaceae. Not active against *P. aeruginosa* and *Enterobacter* species. Good anaerobic activity
J. Lincosamides	(Clindamycin)	Activity against Gram-positive cocci, including some MRS. Excellent anaerobic activity
K. Mupirocin		Topical antistaphylococcal agent active against MRS
L. Oxazolidinones	(Linezolid)	Similar activity to glycopeptides. Good against vancomycin-resistant enterococci (VRE)
M. Streptogramins	(Quinupristin/dalfopristin, pristinamycin)	Similar activity to glycopeptides. Good against vancomycin-resistant *Enterococcus faecium* but not *Enterococcus faecalis*. Good activity against Gram-positive anaerobes
N. Fusidic acid		Gram-positive cocci, active against many MRS but not enterococci. Gram-negative cocci. Poor activity against Gram-negative rods except *Moraxella* and *Legionella* species
Antibiotics acting against cell metabolism		
O. Sulfonamides	(Sulfamethoxazole, sulfacetamide, sulfasalazine, sulfadiazine)	Moderate antistaphylococcal activity, also against some MRS. Poor against streptococci and enterococci. Good Gram-negative activity, including *Haemophilus influenza*, *Moraxella*, enteric Gram-negative rods, *Stenotrophomonas maltophilia* and *Acinetobacter* species. Poor anaerobic activity. Good against nocardiosis, *Pneumocystis jiroveci*, toxoplasmosis
Antibiotics acting on DNA synthesis		
P. Quinolones		
1. First-generation quinolones (nonfluorinated)	(Nalidixic acid, cinoxacin,[†] enoxacin,[†] norfloxacin)	Gram-negative activity, mainly Enterobacteriaceae
2. Second generation, fluoroquinolones	(Ofloxacin, ciprofloxacin, levofloxacin[*])	Wide Gram-negative activity. Additional activity against intracellular microbes. Ciprofloxacin and (to a lesser degree) levofloxacin have good antipseudomonal activity. Moderate activity against Gram-positive cocci
3. Third generation, respiratory quinolones	(Levofloxacin,[*] moxifloxacin, sparfloxacin,[†] gatifloxacin[†])	Added good activity against streptococci, especially pneumococcus
4. Fourth generation	(Clinafloxacin,[§] trovafloxacin,[†] prulifloxacin)	Wide spectrum of activity with additional Gram-positive (including MRS, highly resistant pneumococci, and enterococci) and anaerobic activity to the previous categories
Q. Rifampin		Specific Gram-positive and Gram-negative microbes (staphylococci including MRS, Neisseriae, Brucella). First-line antimycobacterial. Always used combined with other antibiotics
R. Nitroimidazoles	(Metronidazole, tinidazole)	Excellent antianaerobic activity
Various mechanisms of action		
S. Beta-lactamase inhibitors	(Clavulanic acid, sulbactam, tazobactam)	Enhance the spectrum and activity of aminopenicillins and carboxypenicillins. Sulbactam used as monotherapy against highly-resistant *A. baumannii* in ICUs

[*]Can be classified to more than one category.
[†]Withdrawn from US market.
[§]Currently tested in clinical trials.

Gram-negative rods encountered in the hospital may have characteristic susceptibility phenotypes. Resistance to ampicillin and trimethoprim-sulfamethoxazole is rising among *Escherichia coli*, limiting the role of these antibiotics when used as empiric therapy for urinary tract infections (UTIs) in the community. This has led to increased use of wide spectrum beta-lactams in the community. As a result, urine isolates of enteric Gram-negative rods in hospitalized patients, especially *E. coli* and *Klebsiella pneumoniae*, commonly produce various types of beta-lactamases. Extended-spectrum beta-lactamases (ESBLs) are of particular significance. They confer resistance to all penicillins and commonly to all cephalosporins, and they are often accompanied by resistance to TMP-SMX, aminoglycosides, and fluoroquinolones. Carbapenems are at present the best choice for infections caused by ESBL-producing Gram-negative organisms.

Enterobacter cloacae and *Enterobacter aerogenes* commonly exhibit multidrug resistance due to the broad-spectrum AmpC beta-lactamase. AmpC confers resistance to second- and third-generation cephalosporins, monobactams, and many beta-lactam/beta-lactamase inhibitor combinations. However, *Enterobacter* species are often susceptible to TMP-SMX or fluoroquinolones, as well as carbapenems and fourth-generation cephalosporins, such as cefepime, which are considered the last line of antibiotics active against Gram-negative infections, and should be withheld from use as much as possible.

Pseudomonas aeruginosa and *Acinetobacter baumannii* often cause nosocomial infections in patients with multiple comorbidities,

TABLE 184-2 Major Adverse Effects and Partial List of Drug-Drug Interactions of Antibiotics

Antibiotics	Major Adverse Effects	Interactions
Penicillins	Allergic and hypersensitivity reactions, including fever, rash, anaphylaxis; high intravenous doses may be associated with sodium load and edema, as well as central nervous system toxicity in patients with renal insufficiency; hepatitis (especially oxacillin)	Nafcillin decreases the effect of warfarin and cyclosporine; the combination of ampicillin and allopurinol is associated with a higher risk of rash; oral absorption of β-blockers is diminished in patients taking amoxicillin or ampicillin; risk of anaphylaxis may be increased in patients taking β-blockers
Cephalosporins	C. difficile colitis; less often associated with allergy than penicillins; cefepime associated with mental status change in elderly patients with renal insufficiency	Minimal
Carbapenems	Seizures, especially when doses not properly adjusted for renal function; seizure risk is highest with imipenem, and lowest with meropenem; C. difficile colitis	Decreased levels of valproic acid
Aminoglycosides	Nephrotoxicity, ototoxicity, neuromuscular blockade in critically ill patients	Increased risk of nephrotoxicity with use of other nephrotoxic agents, such as cyclosporine, cisplatin, NSAIDs, and vancomycin; increased ototoxicity when administered with diuretics
Sulfa drugs	Rash, fever, hyperkalemia, cytopenias, crystalluria (at high doses or with impaired renal function)	Increased anticoagulation with warfarin
Macrolides	Gastrointestinal upset, hepatitis, cholestatic jaundice, pancreatitis, QT interval prolongation	Increases the levels of many drugs by inhibiting hepatic cytochrome P450 metabolism, including cyclosporine, tacrolimus, theophylline, ergot alkaloids, carbamazepine, antihistamines, cisapride, warfarin, statins, class I antiarrhythmics, and some benzodiazepines and neuroleptics
Lincosamides (eg, clindamycin)	Diarrhea, including C. difficile colitis; rash	May potentiate the effect of warfarin
Fluoroquinolones	C. difficile colitis; tendinopathy; mental status changes; rash	Oral absorption inhibited by antacids, ferrous sulfate, cimetidine
Tetracyclines	Diarrhea, photosensitivity, hepatitis, pill esophagitis	Oral absorption inhibited by antacids, ferrous sulfate, calcium supplements, tube feedings
Glycopeptides (eg, vancomycin)	Infusion-related flushing (red person syndrome), nephrotoxicity, ototoxicity	Use with caution when patient taking other potentially nephrotoxic agents, such as aminoglycosides, cisplatin, or colistin
Oxazolidinones (eg, linezolid)	Nausea, diarrhea, cytopenias, neuropathy	Serotonin syndrome in patients also taking selective serotonin reuptake inhibitors (SSRIs)
Lipopeptides (eg, daptomycin)	Gastrointestinal upset, creatine kinase elevations	Rhabdomyolysis in patients also taking statin therapy
Lipoglycopeptides	Nausea, headache, rare renal or liver toxicity with currently approved dosing. Increased incidence of osteomyelitis with oritavancin.	Minimal
Polymixins (eg, colistin)	Nephrotoxicity (20%), neuropathy (7%)	May potentiate neuromuscular blockade associated with aminoglycosides and curariform muscle relaxants
Polyene antifungals (amphotericin B)	Febrile infusion reaction (nearly universal side effect); renal tubular injury with severe potassium and magnesium wasting, metabolic acidosis, and nephrogenic diabetes insipidus; electrolyte imbalances and possibly direct cardiotoxicity may lead to life-threatening arrhythmias; cytopenias	Renal toxicity more common and severe with concomitant use of other nephrotoxins, such as cisplatin and diuretics
Azole antifungals	QT prolongation and hepatotoxicity possible with all azoles Voriconazole: transient blurring of vision (unknown mechanism) Fluconazole: generally well tolerated; less hepatotoxic than other azoles because of major renal route of excretion Posaconazole: gastrointestinal upset	Azoles inhibit the cytochrome P450 system, leading to extensive drug interactions, including cyclosporine, oral hypoglycemic agents, antiretroviral therapy, phenytoin, rifabutin, rifampin, theophylline, and warfarin; dose adjustment of other medications may be necessary

prolonged hospitalizations, prior antibiotic exposure, and intensive care unit (ICU) admission. These two bacteria are almost universally multidrug resistant. In many countries, a large proportion of isolates are susceptible only to carbapenems, polymyxins, and tigecycline (the later being active only against *Acinetobacter*). Isolates of *P. aeruginosa*, *A. baumannii*, and *K. pneumoniae* resistant to all commercially available antibiotics have been described in recent literature, primarily in ICU settings. Carbapenems, antipseudomonal penicillins, and the relatively toxic aminoglycosides and polymyxins in various combinations have been the main agents used against such isolates.

INITIATION OF EMPIRIC ANTIBACTERIAL THERAPY

■ PROPER DIAGNOSIS

A high degree of **clinical suspicion** for possible bacterial infection should always constitute the basis for initiation of antibiotic therapy. Unnecessary use of antibacterial agents can harm both the patient and the hospital environment. First, initiation of antibiotics without adequate documentation of infection can obscure or delay the correct diagnoses. Second, antibiotics may cause toxicity, including life-threatening *Clostridium difficile* colitis. Third, when administering an antibiotic to a patient, the clinician should consider this antibiotic inactive against future infections in the same patient and avoid using it again for at least 3 months. Finally, antibiotic use leads to emergence of resistant microorganisms in the hospital environment.

As with most diseases, a carefully taken and complete medical history should always be the mainstay of diagnosis. Patients should be questioned about exposure to the health care system, vaccination, living conditions, animal exposure, travel history, sexual practices, chronic diseases, immunodeficiency, recent surgery, and foreign bodies such as heart valves and joint prostheses. While the physical examination is similar to that performed in other patients, hospitalists examining patients with suspected infection should pay special attention to aspects that are sometimes neglected, such as the skin, lymph nodes, surgical wounds, decubitus ulcers, intravenous line sites, and genitals. Laboratory investigations should include complete blood count, indices of inflammation, such as erythrocyte sedimentation rate, C-reactive protein, and perhaps procalcitonin, serology, urinalysis, and pharyngeal swabs with rapid testing for group A streptococcus or influenza A. Cultures from the infected site remain the gold standard for diagnosis, allowing definite identification of the responsible pathogen and optimization of antibiotic therapy. Finally, clinicians should distinguish between true infection and situations mimicking infections that need only limited or no antibiotic therapy (eg, UTI vs asymptomatic bacteriuria, pneumonia versus exacerbation of chronic obstructive pulmonary disease).

■ TIMING OF THERAPY

Once the diagnosis of a possible infection is made, the clinician has to decide on the appropriate timing of antibiotic administration. **Early initiation** of antibiotic therapy is the rule for all severe infections. Patients with sepsis have better outcomes, including reduced mortality, when antibiotic therapy is initiated as soon as possible. A large retrospective study of 2700 ICU patients with septic shock revealed that mortality was proportional to the time to initiation of appropriate antimicrobial therapy. Timely administration of antibiotics has a positive impact on a variety of serious infections. When central nervous system infection is suspected, antibiotic therapy should be administered well before the definitive documentation of infection. Thus, only a few minutes' delay is acceptable between the clinical suspicion of meningitis and lumbar puncture. When longer delays are expected, antibacterial therapy should be administered immediately, despite the consequent decreased diagnostic yield of lumbar puncture. Similarly, pneumonia-associated in-hospital morbidity and mortality is significantly reduced by prompt antibacterial therapy.

Delays in administering antimicrobial therapy are justified only in specific clinical settings. As a rule, antibiotic therapy is only withheld when patients are hemodynamically stable, bacterial infection is doubtful, or an infection is suspected which requires definitive identification of the responsible pathogen for appropriate treatment. Examples of clinical scenarios in which it is appropriate to delay antibiotics include a young adult with tonsillitis while awaiting the results of heterophile antibody testing, patients with possible endocarditis, in whom therapy should be delayed for at least an hour to perform three sets of aerobic and anaerobic blood cultures, and patients with suspected chronic infections due to brucellosis, syphilis, and other

pathogens with nonspecific symptoms and signs, which require specific therapy that differs from most empiric antibacterial regimens.

Antibiotic therapy begun prior to identification of the causative infecting agent is termed **empiric**, a Greek word meaning derived from experience. Empiric antibiotics are chosen based on knowledge of the microbes commonly causing infection at a specific body site, antibiotic penetration into this site, local patterns of antimicrobial susceptibility, and antibacterial side effect profile. Empiric antibiotic therapy usually has a broad spectrum of activity, including resistant organisms prevalent in relevant clinical settings. For example, the emergence of cMRSA has led to the increasing use of vancomycin (considered a last-line antibiotic in other situations) or costly newer agents in the empiric therapy of skin and soft tissue infections. Similarly, the rise of multidrug-resistant Gram-negative organisms such as *K. pneumoniae*, *Acinetobacter baumanii*, and *P. aeruginosa* has led to the use of last-line antibacterials such as meropenem or colistin as empiric therapy in certain ICUs. When culture results become available, the broad spectrum of activity of the empiric regimen should be narrowed as much as possible (stepdown therapy).

PHARMACOKINETICS AND PHARMACODYNAMICS

■ PHARMACOKINETICS

Antibiotic **pharmacokinetics**, or the effects of the body on the antibiotic, depend on drug absorption, tissue distribution, metabolism, and excretion. Antibiotic **absorption** is most relevant to the oral administration of antibiotics. Some antibiotics, such as linezolid or levofloxacin, are nearly entirely absorbed from the gut. By contrast, oral vancomycin achieves negligible serum levels, but this route is best when high intraluminal concentrations of the drug in the gastrointestinal tract are desired, such as when treating *C. difficile* colitis. **Tissue distribution** plays a significant role in the success or failure of antibiotic therapy. For example, an antibiotic with poor distribution to the lungs is unlikely to be effective for pneumonia. Some antibiotics reach useful levels in one tissue compartment, but not another; for example, tigecycline is distributed widely in the body but serum concentrations may be inadequate to treat bacteremias and endocarditis. In general, it is harder to achieve therapeutic antibiotic concentrations in the central nervous system, bones, pleural cavity, prostate, and poorly vascularized infected foci, such as abscesses. Fluoroquinolones often penetrate tissues that other antibiotics fail to reach, including bone and prostate. Local factors may also interfere with tissue distribution. Infections on foreign bodies often fail to respond to treatment because of the difficulty in penetrating the bacterial biofilms formed on their surfaces. Rifampin may be active in staphylococcal infections forming biofilm on foreign bodies.

Drug **metabolism** also affects antibiotic levels. Patients with hepatic or renal insufficiency may accumulate drugs, putting them at higher risk of toxicity, and need corresponding dose adjustment. Hepatic metabolism in particular is affected by genetic characteristics (pharmacogenetics) and drug-drug interactions. For example, isoniazid is metabolized by liver acetylation. About 50% of Europeans and Americans are slow acetylators, and will have higher isoniazid levels, increasing the risk for polyneuropathy and other toxicities. In addition, many antibiotics are metabolized by hepatic cytochrome P450 enzymes, resulting in numerous drug-drug interactions, as discussed below in the section on antibiotic toxicity.

■ PHARMACODYNAMICS

Antibiotic **pharmacodynamics**, or the effect of the antibiotic on the bacteria, are related to antibiotic concentrations in blood and tissues, time, and bacterial inhibition or killing. Based on pharmacodynamic characteristics, antimicrobial agents can be divided into those that exhibit primarily **concentration-dependent** bacterial killing or **time-dependent** bacterial killing. Concentration-dependent agents, such as aminoglycosides and fluoroquinolones, achieve greater bacterial killing at higher drug concentrations. Time-dependent agents, such as beta-lactams and vancomycin, accomplish maximal killing at concentrations four times higher than the minimum inhibitory concentration (MIC), with no extra bacteriocidal effects at higher concentrations.

For concentration-dependent agents, the main parameters predictive of successful clinical outcomes are the peak concentration achieved over MIC ratio (Cmax/MIC) and the area under the concentration-time curve to MIC ratio (AUC/MIC). Thus, one or two high daily doses are considered optimal for aminoglycosides and fluoroquinolones. For time-dependent agents such as beta-lactams, the time with achieved concentrations above the MIC ($t > MIC$) is the pharmacodynamic parameter most predictive of bacterial killing and clinical efficacy. Thus, beta-lactam antibiotics are optimally administered in three or four doses daily, with some evidence supporting continuous administration. However, some beta-lactams antibiotics, such as ceftriaxone and ertapenem, have half-lives long enough to allow for once-daily dosing, without compromising concentrations in blood and tissues during the 24-hour period.

PRACTICE POINT

Concentration-dependent and time-dependent bacterial killing

- Antibiotic pharmacodynamics, or their effects on bacteria, determine how they should be dosed for maximal effectiveness.
- Aminoglycosides and fluoroquinolones kill more bacteria when they are present in higher concentrations (concentration-dependent killing). Therefore, once- or twice-daily dosing is optimal, to ensure high peak concentrations.
- Beta-lactam antibiotics, such as penicillins and cephalosporins, display maximal killing at concentrations four times over the MIC, with no additional killing at higher concentrations. Therefore, beta-lactam antibiotics should ideally be dosed three or four times daily, unless they have especially long half-lives.

COMBINATION ANTIMICROBIAL THERAPY

Combination antibiotic therapy is indicated when (1) broader empiric coverage is desired than can be accomplished with a single agent; (2) infection is proven or suspected to involve bacteria with a high potential to develop resistance against a single agent, such as *Mycobacterium tuberculosis*; (3) when the infection site interferes with the ability of certain antibiotics to reach satisfactory concentrations (eg, aminoglycosides do not penetrate the lungs adequately to be used alone in pneumonia); (4) when infections are expected to be polymicrobial, as in intra-abdominal or pelvic infections; and (5) when a drug combination results in synergy, with a considerable decrease in the MIC of each drug when tested together against a pathogen in vitro, as seen with the use of ampicillin and gentamicin in enterococcal endocarditis. However, this in vitro increase in activity does not always translate into superior clinical results, for reasons that are not always clear. Various synergistic combinations of beta-lactams with aminoglycosides have not been shown to be better than beta-lactam monotherapy in serious infections causing sepsis, according to a large meta-analysis of 64 trials including 7586 patients. Similarly, the development of several broad-spectrum beta-lactam agents, such as antipseudomonal penicillins combined with beta-lactamase inhibitors, fourth-generation cephalosporins, and carbapenems, has led to the widespread use of beta-lactam monotherapy in febrile neutropenia, a clinical setting in which combinations of beta-lactams with aminoglycosides had once been standard.

Antibiotic combinations, especially beta-lactams with aminoglycosides, were often considered to prevent the development of resistance until recently. These two drug categories have different mechanisms of action, often exhibit synergy in vitro, and provide a wide spectrum of antibacterial activity. Animal studies in the 1980s provided some evidence that this combination could forestall the emergence of resistance, but meta-analyses in patients have not shown a clear benefit. **Table 184-3** shows common indications for using antibiotic combinations in everyday clinical practice, as well as commonly used antibiotic combinations according to indication.

TABLE 184-3 Commonly Used Antibiotic Combinations, According to Indication

Infection-Clinical Setting	Antibiotic Combinations Commonly Used	Comments
Endocarditis by staphylococci, enterococci, or relatively resistant streptococci	Beta-lactam or vancomycin *plus* an aminoglycoside	Rifampin added in cases of prosthetic valve endocarditis
Enterococcal bacteremia	Gentamicin *plus* a beta-lactam or vancomycin	
Tuberculosis	Rifampin plus isoniazid plus ethambutol plus pyrazinamide	Various combinations are used as second-line therapy in infection by resistant mycobacteria
Brucella infections	Tetracycline plus streptomycin *or* rifampin plus doxycycline	Combinations of fluoroquinolones and rifampin have also been used
Empirical antibiotic therapy of:		
Community-acquired pneumonia	Beta-lactam *plus* a macrolide	Alternative to monotherapy with respiratory fluoroquinolones
Hospital-acquired pneumonia	Ampicillin/sulbactam *or* antipseudomonal penicillin *plus* aminoglycoside	Alternative to monotherapy with respiratory fluoroquinolones *or* antipseudomonal penicillin *or* third generation cephalosporin
Meningitis	Third generation cephalosporin *plus* vancomycin	Ampicillin added to therapy in patients >50 y old at risk for infection with *Listeria monocytogenes*
Intra-abdominal infections	Beta-lactams *or* ciprofloxacin *plus* metronidazole	
Skin and soft tissue infections (especially diabetic foot)	Ciprofloxacin *plus* metronidazole *or* clindamycin	Alternatively cephalosporin *plus* metronidazole *or* clindamycin

TOXICITY

Antibiotic toxicity may occur when drug levels rise due to impaired drug metabolism, as in renal failure, hepatic insufficiency, or drug-drug interactions (dose-dependent toxicity). In other cases, reactions to antibiotics occur despite acceptable or even low drug levels. **Beta-lactams** are mainly metabolized in the kidneys, and thus dose adjustment is needed in renal failure. An important exception is ceftriaxone, which is primarily metabolized in the liver. Gastrointestinal discomfort and mild diarrhea are the most common side effects of beta-lactams, with severe diarrhea or pseudomembranous colitis occurring occasionally. Up to 10% of patients report a penicillin allergy, but the true prevalence is probably closer to 1%, as most of these patients will not have a reaction if rechallenged. Possible reactions include skin rash, drug fever, nephritis, Coombs-positive hemolytic anemia, leukopenia, and even contact dermatitis. Interstitial nephritis usually results in mild, reversible renal failure, and is mainly associated with antistaphylococcal penicillins. Seizures may occur with high doses of imipenem or penicillins. Penicillin-induced anaphylaxis occurs with approximately 1 out of 10,000 administrations. Skin testing predicts penicillin IgE-mediated allergy and anaphylaxis, but not toxic epidermal necrolysis and Stevens-Johnson syndrome. Allergic reactions are much less common with cephalosporins. Fewer than 10% of patients with penicillin allergy are also allergic to cephalosporins or carbapenems. Monobactams, such as aztreonam, do not cross react with penicillin, having a substantially different chemical structure (**Figure 184-1**).

Aminoglycosides are excreted by the kidneys, reaching high concentrations in the urinary tract. However, they are nephrotoxic in 10% to 25% of patients, leading to acute kidney injury from tubular necrosis, mesangial damage, and renal vasoconstriction. This is more common in elderly, severely ill, or dehydrated patients. Serum creatinine should be closely monitored in patients at risk for aminoglycoside-related nephrotoxicity. If possible, the concomitant use of other nephrotoxic agents such as loop diuretics, vancomycin, and amphotericin B should be avoided, as these may potentiate aminoglycoside nephrotoxicity. The nephrotoxicity of aminoglycosides is usually ameliorated by dose adjustment or drug withdrawal. Once-daily administration and short treatment duration (≤7 days) may reduce the risk of nephrotoxicity. Ototoxicity with sensorineural deafness is the other major adverse effect of aminoglycosides. It manifests initially with high-frequency hearing loss, which may be irreversible in some cases. It is more common with prolonged administration, as with streptomycin use for tuberculosis or brucellosis, or gentamicin use in endocarditis. Neuromuscular blockade may occur when aminoglycosides are erroneously given by rapid intravenous push, or when they are administered to ICU patients receiving other inhibitors of the neuromuscular junction. Aminoglycoside use is generally avoided during pregnancy, since these antibiotics cross the placenta. Trough levels should be measured in patients receiving aminoglycosides for longer than 1 week, to ensure that drug accumulation is not occurring. Peak levels are measured in few cases, to ensure adequate drug concentrations in serious infections such as endocarditis.

Glycopeptides such as vancomycin commonly exhibit mild nephrotoxicity, which may become worse if dose adjustments are not performed based on renal clearance, similar to aminoglycosides. Serum levels of vancomycin are helpful in preventing toxicity in patients with pre-existing renal failure, unstable renal function, and the elderly. There is no contraindication to coadministration with other nephrotoxic agents such as aminoglycosides, but this should be performed with great caution, and only when necessary. Red man syndrome is a mild anaphylactoid reaction that causes flushing of the upper trunk and head of the patient. It is most common with the first dose of vancomycin, diminishes with subsequent doses,

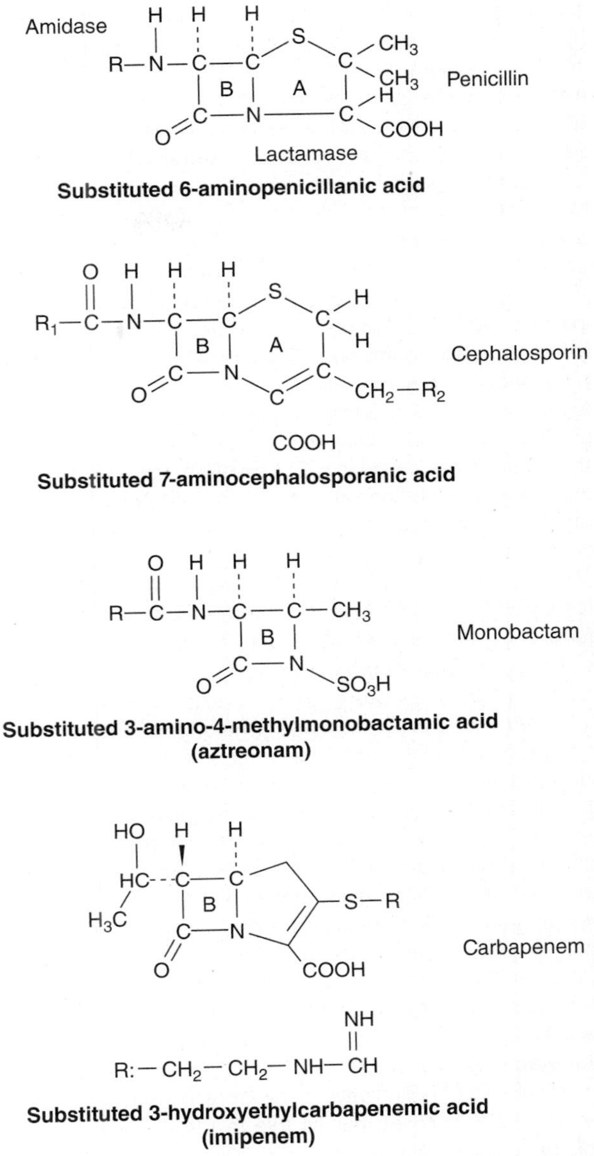

Figure 184-1 Core structures of four beta-lactam antibiotic families. The ring marked B in each structure is the beta-lactam ring. The penicillins are susceptible to bacterial metabolism and inactivation by amidases and lactamases at the points shown. Note that the carbapenems have a different stereochemical configuration in the lactam ring that apparently imparts resistance to beta-lactamases. (Reproduced, with permission, from Katzung BG, Masters SB, Trevor AJ. Basic & Clinical Pharmacology, 11th ed. New York, NY: McGraw-Hill; 2009. Fig. 43-1.)

and can be prevented by slow administration over 2 hours. Some patients require premedication with antihistamines to minimize symptoms. True allergic skin rash may also occur occasionally with glycopeptide use. Ototoxicity may occur in patients with pre-existing renal impairment and prolonged exposure.

Macrolides generally have mild side effects. Gastrointestinal upset due to increased motility is common and is most marked with erythromycin. This side effect is the basis for using erythromycin to treat patients with gastroparesis and pseudo-obstruction syndromes. Macrolides may also cause mild hepatotoxicity and QT interval prolongation. However, the most important macrolide adverse effect is drug interactions. Macrolides inhibit the CYP3A4 enzyme of the cytochrome P450 (important for widely used clarithromycin) of the liver, leading to decreased metabolism and potentially toxic levels of several substances, including statins, warfarin, digoxin, carbamazepine, valproic acid, benzodiazepines, ergotamine, theophylline, vinca alkaloids, and cyclosporine. Polymorphic ventricular tachycardia (torsades de pointes), often preceded by QT prolongation, may occur when a macrolide is administered with other potent P450 inhibitors, such as cisapride, terfenadine, or astemizole.

Gastrointestinal upset is common with **tetracyclines**. Esophageal irritation and ulceration may occur with oral administration. This may be minimized by drinking generous amounts of water with pills and avoiding ingestion at bedtime. Phototoxicity is very common. Hepatotoxicity may occur with large intravenous doses. Use of tetracycline, and to a lesser degree doxycycline, is contraindicated in patients with pre-existing renal failure, because tetracyclines may worsen renal insufficiency. Teteracyclines should be avoided in pregnancy, as they may cause fulminant hepatic failure in the mother, and skeletal deformities and dental discoloration in the fetus. Drug interactions with digoxin, warfarin, theophylline, and statins are similar to macrolides, but usually milder. Carbamazepine and phenytoin induce hepatic metabolism of tetracyclines, reducing their activity. Antacids, cimetidine, and milk decrease tetracycline absorption.

Diarrhea is the most frequent side effect of **fluoroquinolones**. Unfortunately, *C. difficile* colitis is common with respiratory fluoroquinolones such as levofloxacin and moxifloxacin; it may occur less often with older fluoroquinolones, such as ciprofloxacin. All fluoroquinolones may cause QT prolongation, although this is less marked with ciprofloxacin and other older fluoroquinolones. Other important, occasional side effects include phototoxicity, tendon rupture, especially involving the Achilles tendon, seizures, and confusion. Tendinopathy and central nervous system side effects are more common in the elderly. Fluoroquinolone use should generally be avoided in patients younger than 18 years old because of their epileptogenic potential and adverse effects on developing joints. Fluoroquinolones may be teratogenic and are contraindicated in pregnancy. Ciprofloxacin inhibits theophylline metabolism; this interaction does not occur with respiratory fluoroquinolones. Fluoroquinolones require dose adjustment in severe renal failure.

Lincosamides, such as clindamycin, most commonly cause gastrointestinal distress. Clindamycin was once considered the major cause of *C. difficile* colitis, but its role in the epidemiology of *C. difficile* has declined due to a rise in *C. difficile* infections related to beta-lactams and fluoroquinolones. **Sulfonamides** may cause nephrotoxicity from crystalluria, especially with the use of high doses in the treatment of conditions such as nocardiosis and toxoplasmosis. Patients receiving high-dose sulfonamides should be adequately hydrated, and dose adjustments should be made for patients with renal failure. Sulfa antibiotics may trigger hemolysis in patients with G6PD deficiency, and rarely lead to toxic epidermal necrolysis/Stevens-Johnson syndrome. Sulfonamides decrease the metabolism of phenytoin, warfarin, and digoxin. In combination with **trimethoprim**, they may act as antimetabolites and cause marrow aplasia.

INTRAVENOUS VERSUS ORAL ANTIBIOTICS

Initial intravenous therapy is essential for all serious infections and critically ill patients, for various reasons, including pharmacokinetics. On the other hand, oral antibiotic therapy is generally less expensive than intravenous therapy. As well, the greater ease of administration, improved mobility, and avoidance of adverse events associated with parenteral therapy, such as bacterial and fungal line infections or postinfusion phlebitis, may result in decreased hospital length of stay. Thus, oral antibiotics are often appropriate in patients tolerating oral medications or nasogastric feeding. Certain agents are especially suited for oral administration. The bioavailability of oral levofloxacin and oral metronidazole approaches 100%, and oral

fluconazole is 90% bioavailable. The ease of administration should not, however, lead to indiscriminate use of these and newer agents. For example, overuse of linezolid, an expensive drug active against most strains of VRE and MRSA, may promote resistance in these Gram-positive organisms.

ANTIMICROBIAL RESISTANCE AND ITS PREVENTION

In recent decades, the prevalence of nosocomial antibacterial resistance has been rising, with increased in-hospital morbidity and mortality. Acute care hospitals should take steps to reduce the inappropriate use of antibiotics. This may require developing antibiotic guidelines, educational strategies, and computer support. Specific practices are necessary to combat antibacterial resistance. Hospitals must have **surveillance systems**, involving physicians, infection control practitioners, nurses, and the microbiology laboratory, to identify increases in the incidence of infections caused by resistant pathogens. This surveillance also includes monitoring of antibiotic consumption, and correlating usage with patterns of antibiotic resistance. When specific antibiotics appear to be linked to the emergence of resistance, **local antibiotic policies** may be needed to limit use. In most cases, antibiotic use is itself the main factor promoting resistance. Antibiotic use may also be reduced by **infection control measures**, such as hand washing, isolation precautions, and immunization.

The principle of "hit hard, hit fast" or the prompt use of **high and appropriately divided antibiotic doses** should be applied to most hospital infections. Depending on an antibiotic's mode of action and pharmacodynamic characteristics, low antibiotic concentrations favor the development of bacterial resistance, mainly by means of stepwise mutations. Thus, for example, development of resistance to fluoroquinolones is linked to low areas under the concentration-time curve to MIC ratio (AUC/MIC), while beta-lactam resistance is linked to low time with achieved concentrations above the MIC ($t >$MIC). The risk of emergence of resistance is highest in organisms with MICs close to susceptibility breakpoint.

Prolonged, intense antibiotic pressure eventually selects for resistant organisms, which may heavily colonize both the affected patient and the hospital environment in general, including other hospital patients not receiving antibiotics. Thus, antibiotic therapy should be as **brief** as possible in order not to compromise overall efficacy, with rapid **de-escalation**, or narrowing the spectrum of antibiotic therapy, as soon as antimicrobial sensitivity data are available. Other suggested measures to limit antibiotic resistance, such as periodic cycling or "crop rotation" of antibiotic classes, or antibiotic combination therapy, have inadequate evidence to support their use at this time.

PRACTICE POINT

- The accelerating pace of antibiotic resistance threatens to leave clinicians with no viable therapeutic options for nosocomial infections.

- Measures to slow down the development of antibiotic resistance in hospitals include: treating infections with adequate antibiotic doses, to forestall the development of stepwise resistance mutations, tailoring therapy to narrow-spectrum antibiotics once culture results are available (de-escalation), giving antibiotics for the minimum adequate duration, restricting the use of broad-spectrum antibiotics in hospitals, monitoring and surveillance of antimicrobial resistance, and enforcing infection control measures to prevent the spread of resistant pathogens between patients.

SUGGESTED READINGS

Bliziotis IA, Samonis G, Vardakas KZ, Chrysanthopoulou S, Falagas ME. Effect of aminoglycoside and beta-lactam combination therapy versus beta-lactam monotherapy on the emergence of antimicrobial resistance: a meta-analysis of randomized, controlled trials. *Clin Infect Dis*. 2005;41:149-158.

Dellinger RP, Levy MM, Rhodes A, et al. Surviving sepsis campaign: international guidelines for management of severe sepsis and septic shock: 2012. *Crit Care Med*. 2013;41:580-637.

Kasiakou SK, Sermaides GJ, Michalopoulos A, Soteriades ES, Falagas ME. Continuous versus intermittent intravenous administration of antibiotics: a meta-analysis of randomised controlled trials. *Lancet Infect Dis*. 2005;5:581-589.

Kumar A, Roberts D, Wood KE, et al. Duration of hypotension before initiation of effective antimicrobial therapy is the critical determinant of survival in human septic shock. *Crit Care Med*. 2006;34:1589-1596.

Maragakis LL, Perencevich EN, Cosgrove SE. Clinical and economic burden of antimicrobial resistance. *Expert Rev Anti Infect Ther*. 2008;6:751-763.

Paul M, Lador A, Grozinsky-Glasberg S, Leibovici L. Beta lactam antibiotic monotherapy versus beta lactam-aminoglycoside antibiotic combination therapy for sepsis. *Cochrane Database Syst Rev*. 2014;1:CD003344.

Poulikakos P, Tansarli GS, Falagas ME. Combination antibiotic treatment versus monotherapy for multidrug-resistant, extensively drug-resistant, and pandrug-resistant *Acinetobacter* infections: a systematic review. *Eur J Clin Microbiol Infect Dis*. 2014;33:1675-1685.

CHAPTER 185

Antibiotic Resistance

L. Silvia Munoz-Price, MD, PhD

Key Clinical Questions

❶ What are the most frequent types of antibiotic resistance?

❷ Which patients are at risk for infections with antibiotic-resistant organisms?

❸ How are antibiotic-resistant organisms transmitted among patients?

❹ What types of genes confer antibiotic resistance?

❺ What types of isolation precautions exist, and when are they indicated?

INTRODUCTION

Antibiotic resistance was described at the dawn of the antibiotic era. In Alexander Fleming's initial report of the antibacterial action of penicillin in 1929, he noted that it was usually inactive against enteric Gram-negative bacteria. In 1940, while engaged in isolating and purifying penicillin, Edward Abraham and Ernst Chain incidentally discovered that *Escherichia coli* produced penicillinase. While the global explosion and dissemination of antibiotic resistance in recent decades is alarming, perhaps it should not be too surprising. As most antibiotics are derived from substances produced by molds and bacteria to inhibit the growth of rival microorganisms, mechanisms of antibacterial resistance evolved before humans harnessed these compounds for medicinal use.

When antibiotics reduce populations of nonresistant organisms, resistant organisms are able to proliferate. Rates of invasive infections with drug-resistant bacteria increase after recent antibiotic exposure. Conversely, reduced use of antibiotics has been shown to decrease the prevalence of antibiotic-resistant organisms. Certain bacterial infections are now resistant to all antibiotics, with a limited number of promising antibiotics in the developmental pipeline.

Highly antibiotic-resistant organisms are usually thought of as exclusively hospital-acquired pathogens. However, community acquisition of resistant pathogens is on the rise, including methicillin-resistant *Staphylococcus aureus* (MRSA) and extended-spectrum beta-lactamase-producing *E. coli*. This chapter reviews resistant bacteria of importance to the hospitalist, including the ESKAPE pathogens, for which there may be no effective drug therapy in the near future (**Table 185-1**).

METHICILLIN-RESISTANT *STAPHYLOCOCCUS AUREUS* (MRSA)

The medically important staphylococci may be divided into two main groups based on the rapid coagulase test, a measure of the ability of a staphylococcal colony to produce a clot in a tube of rabbit serum. Coagulase-negative staphylococci (principally *Staphylococcus epidermidis*) have little virulence aside from biofilm production, and generally only cause infections of medical devices, such as central venous catheters and joint prostheses. By contrast, *S. aureus* (coagulase-positive) is innately pathogenic, and is one of the few bacteria that cause severe infection in both community and health care settings. An important exception to this rule is *Staphylococcus lugdunensis*, which despite being a coagulase-negative staphylococcus, clinically resembles *S. aureus*.

PRACTICE POINT

- A major strategy to reduce antibiotic resistance is to prescribe the narrowest spectrum antibiotic. For example, for documented methicillin-sensitive *S. aureus* infection, preferred drugs for intravenous therapy are nafcillin, oxacillin, and cefazolin. Drugs such as vancomycin, daptomycin, linezolid, and tigecycline should be reserved for infection with methicillin-resistant *S. aureus*, or cases of allergy or intolerance to other antibiotics.

Although methicillin is no longer used in clinical practice, methicillin resistance is still used as marker of staphylococcal resistance

TABLE 185-1 ESKAPE Pathogens: Multidrug-Resistant Bacteria Most Likely to have no Effective Drug Therapy in the Immediate Future

*E*nterococcus faecium (VRE)

*S*taphylococcus aureus (MRSA)

*K*lebsiella pneumoniae

*A*cinetobacter baumannii

*P*seudomonas aeruginosa

*E*nterobacter species

Data from Boucher HW, et al. *Clin Infect Dis.* 2009;48:1-12.

to beta-lactams. Methicillin-resistant *Staphylococcus aureus* isolates are also resistant to oxacillin, nafcillin, cefazolin, and all other beta-lactams. Contact precautions are required for hospitalized patients with MRSA (**Table 185-2**). While many clinical isolates of coagulase-negative staphylococci are methicillin-resistant, contact precautions are not required for these organisms because of their minor clinical and epidemiological implications.

HOSPITAL VERSUS COMMUNITY-ACQUIRED MRSA

Hospital-associated MRSA (HA-MRSA) tend to cause invasive disease in debilitated or immunocompromised individuals, including pneumonia, bloodstream infections such as endocarditis, deep wound infections, and osteomyelitis. Patients are usually treated with vancomycin, with daptomycin and tigecycline as newer, more expensive alternatives. Tigecycline does not achieve good serum concentrations, and should not be used for bacteremias; daptomycin is inhibited by pulmonary surfactant, and should not be used to treat pneumonia. Vancomycin is sometimes combined

TABLE 185-2 Isolation Precautions for Hospitalized Patients with Infection, in Addition to Standard Precautions, Hand Hygiene, and use of Dedicated Medical Equipment

Type of Isolation	Components of Isolation	Most Common Examples
Contact	Gowns and gloves upon room entry	VRE
		MRSA
		ESBL-producing Gram-negatives, and other highly resistant Gram-negative bacteria
		Clostridium difficile with active diarrhea
Droplet	Surgical mask upon room entry	Influenza
		Meningococcal meningitis
		Rubella
		Pertussis
		Mycoplasma
Airborne	Negative pressure room	Pulmonary tuberculosis
	N95 mask upon room entry	Varicella zoster
		Herpes zoster (shingles) or disseminated herpes simplex infection in an immunocompromised patient
		Measles

ESBL, extended-spectrum beta-lactamases; MRSA, methicillin-resistant Staphylococcus aureus; VRE, vancomycin resistant enterococci.

with rifampin (for prosthetic joint infection), or with gentamicin and rifampin (for prosthetic valve endocarditis), based on somewhat limited clinical data.

Since the late 1990s, community-acquired MRSA (CA-MRSA) strains have spread across the United States, and in Europe to a lesser degree. Populations at greatest risk include children, military personnel, prisoners, and athletes, although CA-MRSA infections are increasing among otherwise healthy adults. CA-MRSA most commonly causes pyogenic skin and soft tissue infection in the form of boils, deep abscesses, and cellulitis. CA-MRSA is also capable of causing potentially lethal infections, such as necrotizing fasciitis, necrotizing pneumonia, and bacteremia. When skin infection is well localized (boil < 3 cm diameter), incision and drainage seem to suffice. Antibiotic treatment with either trimethoprim-sulfamethoxazole or other active oral agents can be used for more extensive skin involvement. Clindamycin should be considered as a treatment option only if the D-test for inducible resistance is negative. If this test is not locally available, clindamycin should only be used for strains that are erythromycin-susceptible. Recurrent soft tissue infections are frequent with CA-MRSA. These patients usually require decolonization (see below).

Despite its name, CA-MRSA may be emerging as a nosocomial pathogen. It has been predicted that CA-MRSA will eventually replace HA-MRSA as the dominant hospital strain. Differentiating between CA- and HA-MRSA strains solely on epidemiological grounds may not be possible in the future. Molecular testing is definitive, but this is not practical for most clinical laboratories. The antibiogram may be helpful in differentiation: CA-MRSA strains are usually still susceptible to non–beta-lactam antibiotics, such as fluoroquinolones and trimethoprim-sulfamethoxazole.

Patients with MRSA infection or colonization at any site should be placed on contact precautions (gowns and gloves upon room entry) to prevent horizontal spread. Some institutions add droplet precautions (surgical masks) for patients with MRSA in the sputum. Active screening, using nasal cultures or rapid PCR, and reporting are currently mandatory in some states, such as Illinois; however, the impact of this intervention is still under debate. As above, decolonization can be accomplished using intranasal mupirocin twice daily and daily chlorhexidine baths. The length of this intervention varies depending on the study (range 3-14 days). Additionally, some patients might not respond or relapse after decolonization. Application technique is critical point for the success of decolonization with chlorhexidine. If the 2% liquid formulation is used, which is available in most drugstores, the product should be applied from the neck all the way to the toes, including the axillae, pubic and perianal area. The solution should not be applied to mucosae, such as the mouth, eyes, ears, rectum, or vagina. Chlorhexidine is a long-acting antiseptic that has up to 24 hours of activity. The skin should *not* be rinsed off after application; excess solution may be patted dry with a sterile gauze.

VANCOMYCIN-RESISTANT ENTEROCOCCI (VRE)

Enterococci are not highly virulent organisms, but they are important hospital pathogens because of their high degree of innate drug resistance, and their environmental persistence and resistance to degradation. The two predominant enterococci causing hospital-acquired infections are *Enterococcus faecalis* and *Enterococcus faecium*. Vancomycin-resistant enterococci (VRE) were first described in Europe in the late 1980s, and rapidly spread within the United States in the late 1990s. More than 50% of *E. faecium* in the United States are VRE. *E. faecalis* tends to be susceptible to vancomycin.

Risk factors for VRE acquisition include prolonged hospitalization, use of antibiotics, acuity of illness, and surgery. Patients may become colonized with VRE on skin, wounds, and rectum. Vancomycin-resistant enterococci colonization does not require treatment, and there is currently no effective means of eliminating the carrier state. The most frequent site of VRE infection is the urinary tract. However, some VRE isolates in urine may represent asymptomatic bacteriuria, and do not necessarily require treatment. Other foci of VRE infection include bacteremias, especially in setting of hemodialysis, parenteral nutrition or central venous access for other reasons, chemotherapy, and postoperative intra-abdominal sepsis.

Treatment options include daptomycin, linezolid, and tigecycline. Susceptible strains may be treated with ampicillin, with or without aminoglycosides. Cephalosporins should not be used for treatment of VRE infections, regardless of susceptibility reports.

Screening for VRE is performed using rectal swab cultures. Contact isolation (gowns and gloves) should be instituted if surveillance or clinical cultures are VRE-positive, or if there is recent history of positive VRE cultures. Active decolonization for VRE is not standardized at this time.

Contamination of the environment with VRE (fecal patina) has been previously described. The degree of contamination increases with rectal carriage, as well as with diarrhea. A room previously occupied by a VRE-positive patient significantly increases the risk of VRE acquisition of the subsequent patient. As with MRSA, *Clostridium*

difficile, and resistant Gram-negative rods, terminal room disinfection is critical to reducing nosocomial transmission.

RESISTANT GRAM-NEGATIVE RODS

Gram-negative antibiotic resistance has multiple mechanisms, including porin mutations, overexpression of efflux pumps, penicillin-binding protein mutations, and production of inactivating beta-lactamase enzymes (**Figure 185-1**). In most cases, clinical laboratories will be able to identify beta-lactamase production based on automated susceptibility testing. The two main mechanisms of high-level resistance are production of either extended spectrum beta-lactamases (ESBLs) or carbapenemases.

■ EXTENDED SPECTRUM BETA-LACTAMASES (ESBLS)

Extended spectrum beta-lactamases are a heterogenous group of enzymes that belong to different families, and thus express different phenotypes. These enzymes tend to confer resistance to most beta-lactams, including cephalosporins, without hydrolyzing carbapenems. In recent years, there has been a worldwide increase in the prevalence of ESBLs of the CTX-M family, as well as a worrisome

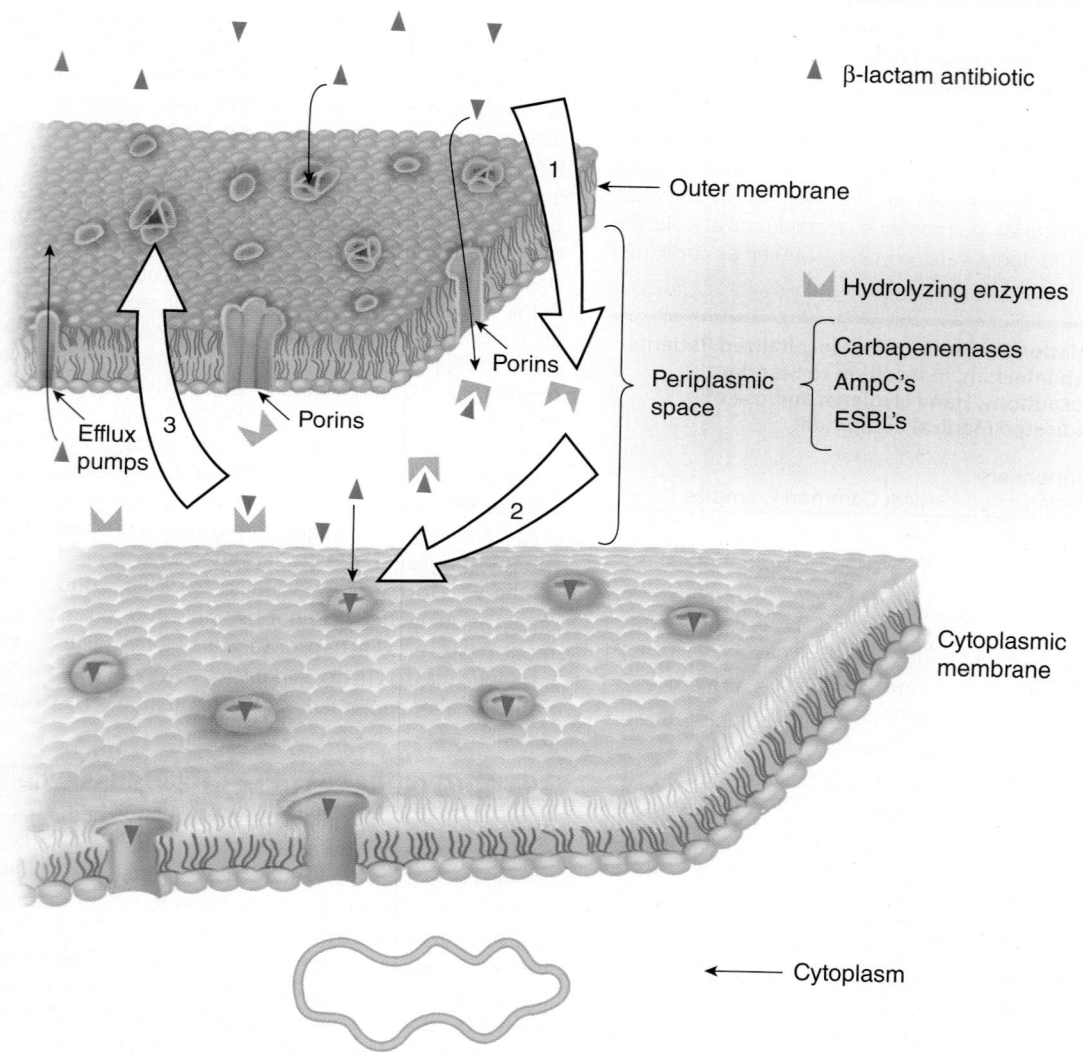

Figure 185-1 *Multiple resistance mechanisms may be present in Gram-negative bacteria, including (1) mutations leading to decreased function or loss of the porin channels that provide antibiotics with access to the periplasmic space; (2) production of inactivating beta-lactamase enzymes, or mutations in penicillin-binding proteins, leading to decreased antibiotic activity in the periplasmic space; (3) overexpression of efflux pumps, leading to rapid antibiotic expulsion via the outer membrane.*

rise in community-acquired urinary tract infections due to CTX-M-positive *E. coli*.

In 2010, the Clinical and Laboratory Standards Institute (CLSI) eliminated the requirement for American clinical laboratories to determine or report ESBL production. One clue to the presence of an ESBL-producing organism is an antibiogram showing resistance to third-generation cephalosporins, but susceptibility to cephamycins, such as the second-generation cephalosporins cefoxitin and cefotetan. (Although ESBL-producing organisms may appear sensitive to cephamycins, resistance may develop in practice.) Another clue is the partially restoration of beta-lactam susceptibility in vitro by clavulanic acid.

Severe infections due to ESBL-producers should be treated with a carbapenem, such as imipenem, meropenem, doripenem, or ertapenem. Although some strains may test susceptible to some cephalosporins in the antibiogram, these antibiotics should be considered inactive against ESBL-producing organisms. Piperacillin/tazobactam may be considered for nonlife-threatening infections, such as urinary tract infections, in apparently susceptible strains. Patients found to harbor ESBL-positive organisms should be placed on contact isolation (gowns and gloves).

■ CARBAPENEMASES

The prevalence of carbapenemases has risen alarmingly in recent years, probably due to the widespread use of carbapenem. The distribution of different carbapenemases varies depending on the country. In the United States, *Klebsiella pneumoniae* carbapenemases (KPCs) are the most frequently found carbapenemases. As the name suggests, these enzymes are most often expressed in *K. pneumoniae*, but may also be found in *E. coli*, *Enterobacter* spp., *Pseudomonas* spp., and *Salmonella*. *K. pneumoniae* carbapenemase have rapidly spread across the United States since early 2000, and they are currently endemic in areas of New York and New Jersey. They tend to colonize and infect patients with multiple comorbidities, intensive care unit stays, and prolonged hospitalization.

PRACTICE POINT

- *Acinetobacter baumannii* has emerged as a major opportunistic pathogen, able to survive and thrive in the hospital environment because of its tolerance of a wide range of physical conditions and high degree of innate resistance to antibiotics and disinfectants. Infection has become common in intensive care units and among repatriated combat casualties, who perhaps acquired infection in contaminated field hospitals. For multidrug resistant *Acinetobacter* strains, carbapenems are preferred treatment for sensitive isolates, with ampicillin-sulbactam as a second option. Strains resistant to these antibiotics may be treated with colistin, both systemically and also by aerosol in patients with *Acinetobacter* pneumonia. Inhaled colistin is not systemically absorbed. Tigecycline is a drug of last resort. Due to concerns about inferior outcomes in patients with nosocomial pneumonia treated with tigecycline, higher doses may be considered if it must be used for lower respiratory tract infection.

Infections caused by KPC-producing Gram-negatives have 40% to 50% mortality. Treatment options are limited to polymyxins, and in some cases tigecycline. Mortality may be reduced in bacteremias caused by KPC-producing Gram-negative bacilli by treating with three or four drug combinations, including colistin and even carbapenems (despite being resistant on susceptibility panels). Patients found to carry carbapenemase-producing Gram-negative bacilli should be placed on contact isolation.

Isolates of *E. coli* and *Klebsiella* producing a novel carbapenemase, New Delhi metallo-beta-lactamase 1 (NDM-1), have become prominent in India. These bacteria are resistant to all beta-lactams, fluoroquinolones, and aminoglycosides. Most isolates were sensitive to tigecycline and colistin, although a few were resistant. NDM-1 may be widespread in the community in India, where antibiotics are readily available over the counter. A few cases of infections with NDM-1 have been reported in Western travelers to India and Pakistan, often in patients seeking medical care abroad. Although the "NDM-1 superbug" has attracted much media attention, presumably because of its somewhat exotic origins, the equally resistant and increasingly endemic KPC-positive Gram-negatives represent a more imminent threat to hospitalized patients in Western countries. During the past couple of years, isolated outbreaks of NDM-1 in the United States have been associated with returning travelers with asymptomatic carriage.

PRACTICE POINT

When first-line antibiotic therapy can be avoided in normal hosts

Urinary tract infections:

- Asymptomatic bacteriuria should not be treated unless patients are pregnant or undergoing urinary tract instrumentation.
- Candiduria may represent vaginal flora or colonization.
- Urine cultures are usually positive in the presence of a Foley catheter, and should not be treated in the absence of symptoms. If treatment is necessary, remove the Foley and treat for 7 days. Treatment of bacteriuria or candiduria with a Foley catheter in place is usually ineffective, and may select for resistant microbes.

Skin and soft tissue infections:

- Drainage of abscess (<3 cm) without cellulitis

Pulmonary infections:

- Bronchitis usually does not require antibiotic treatment, with some exceptions, such as COPD exacerbations. Sputum cultures with yeast usually represent colonization or thrush.

QUALITY IMPROVEMENT

Control of antimicrobial resistance in the hospital requires multidisciplinary efforts, involving physicians, nurses, infection control practitioners, microbiologists, and pharmacists. Recommended components include heightened compliance with hand hygiene, environmental disinfection, active and passive surveillance for antibiotic resistance, prompt isolation precautions for patients with proven or suspected infection or colonization with resistant organisms, and antibiotic restriction and stewardship.

Working with their infectious disease colleagues, hospitalists may lead quality improvement efforts that include education about antibiotic overuse, appropriate prescribing based on local antibiotic sensitivity data, and optimal dosing and monitoring of antibiotics. Timely infectious disease consultation may facilitate changing empiric coverage to narrow-spectrum antibiotics, based on laboratory analysis of sensitivities. Hospitalists should also bear in mind that preventive measures that decrease the burden of infection, such as pneumococcal and influenza vaccination, may also reduce antibiotic use and alleviate the spread of resistance.

ISOLATION PRECAUTIONS

Most facilities routinely employ contact precautions for patients infected or colonized with multidrug-resistant organisms, such as MRSA, VRE, or highly resistant Gram-negative rods. However, in recent years, some hospitals with good compliance with horizontal infection control interventions, such as hand hygiene and environmental disinfection, have opted to forego contact precautions for patients colonized or infected with MRSA or VRE.

Additionally, a new guideline released by the Society of Hospital Epidemiology of America in 2015 addresses contact precautions for visitors. In general, visitors to rooms occupied by MRSA or VRE patients are not required to wear gowns and gloves. Visitors to rooms occupied by *C. difficile*, ESBL or carbapenemase-producing Gram-negatives should continue to wear gowns and gloves upon room entry.

SUGGESTED READINGS

Garnacho-Montero J, Amaya-Villar R. Multiresistant *Acinetobacter baumanii* infections: epidemiology and management. *Curr Opin Infect Dis.* 2010;23:332-339.

Jacoby G, Munoz-Price LS. The new beta-lactamases. *N Engl J Med.* 2005;352:380-391.

Kumarasamy KK, Toleman MA, Walsh TR, et al. Emergence of a new antibiotic resistance mechanism in India, Pakistan, and the UK: a molecular, biological, and epidemiological study. *Lancet Infect Dis.* 2010;10:597-602.

Morgan DJ, Kaye KS, Diekema DJ. Reconsidering isolation precautions for endemic methicillin-resistant *Staphylococcus aureus* and vancomycin-resistant *Enterococcus. JAMA.* 2014;312:1395-1396.

Munoz-Price LS, Banach DB, Bearman G, et al. Infection precautions for visitors. *Infect Control Hosp Epidemiol.* 2015;36(7): 747-758.

Munoz-Price LS, Hayden MK, Lolans K, et al. Successful control of an outbreak of carbapenemase-producing K. pneumoniae at a long term acute care hospital. *Infect Control Hospital Epidemiol.* 2010;31:341-347.

Munoz-Price LS, Poirel L, Bonomo RA, et al. Clinical epidemiology of the global expansion of *Klebsiella pneumoniae* carbapenemases. *Lancet Infect Dis.* 2013;13:785-796.

Munoz-Price LS, Quinn JP. Deconstructing the infection control bundles for the containment of carbapenem-resistant Enterobacteriaceae. *Curr Opin Infect Dis.* 2013;26:378-387.

Pitout JD, Nordmann P, Laupland KB, Poirel L. Emergence of Enterobacteriaceae producing extended-spectrum beta-lactamases (ESBLs) in the community. *J Antimicrob Chemother.* 2005; 56:52-59.

Popovich KJ, Weinstein RA. The graying of methicillin-resistant *Staphylococcus aureus. Infect Control Hosp Epidemiol.* 2009; 30:9-12.

Popovich KJ, Weinstein RA, Hota B. Are community-associated methicillin-resistant *Staphylococcus aureus* (MRSA) strains replacing traditional nosocomial MRSA strains? *Clin Infect Dis.* 2008;46: 787-794.

CHAPTER 186

Community-Acquired Pneumonia

Daniel M. Musher, MD

Key Clinical Questions

1 How is pneumonia diagnosed?

2 How should the decision be made to hospitalize the patient?

3 What are the major infectious causes of community-acquired pneumonia?

4 What empiric antibiotic therapies are appropriate in community-acquired pneumonia?

5 What steps should be taken for patients not responding to usual therapy for community-acquired pneumonia?

INTRODUCTION

More than one million episodes of community-acquired pneumonia (CAP) occur each year in adults in the United States. While most clinicians are familiar with CAP, its diagnosis remains imprecise, its microbiology is often elusive, and management is usually empiric. Pneumonia is defined as a lung infection, characterized by cough, fever, and a pulmonary infiltrate, often with sputum production. If this sounds obvious, the reader is too easily deceived. Patients with pneumonia may not cough, a variable proportion have sputum, elderly patients are often afebrile when first evaluated, and infiltrates may be hard to detect, especially in high-risk adults with chronic lung disease, the obese, or those for whom only a portable chest radiograph is available.

To complicate matters, certain noninfectious illnesses are also characterized by cough, fever, and pulmonary infiltrates. Many patients with these conditions are admitted with a diagnosis of community-acquired pneumonia; the best example is patients with pulmonary edema. Some of these conditions are even called pneumonia, such as cryptogenic organizing pneumonia, sarcoid pneumonia, and lupus pneumonitis, and they may in every way mimic pneumonia as already defined. Taken together, all these infectious and noninfectious conditions cause what could be called a pneumonia syndrome. The more experienced physician recognizes the diverse etiologies of the pneumonia syndrome and should be unhappy about pigeonholing a patient under the rubric of CAP without considering other etiologies.

PATHOGENESIS

NORMAL HOST DEFENSES

An array of host factors protects the lower respiratory tract against inhaled or aspirated organisms. The predisposition to pneumonia increases to the extent that these factors are altered or bypassed.

The configuration of the upper airways ensures that a thin, laminar flow of air passes close to hairs and sticky surfaces that can trap potentially infectious particles. Secretory immunoglobulin A (IgA), which constitutes 10% of the protein in nasal secretions, neutralizes viruses. These and other immunoglobulins appear to prevent bacterial colonization, probably by blocking binding sites on bacterial surfaces. Closure of the epiglottis prevents food particles from passing into the trachea during swallowing. The larynx prevents the passage of secretions into the trachea and allows the generation of intrapulmonic pressure needed for an effective cough. If potentially infective particles bypass these mechanisms, ciliary action of epithelial cells moves them steadily upward toward the larynx; the cough reflex propels them more rapidly in the same direction.

When infective agents bypass these mechanisms and reach the alveoli, several innate (nonspecific) and specific defenses come into play. Cells that line the respiratory tract produce substances that kill microorganisms or opsonize them for phagocytosis, including lysozyme, lactoferrin, beta-defensins, and surfactant. Bacterial cell wall components, such as lipopolysaccharide in Gram-negative and peptidoglycan in Gram-positive bacteria, activate the alternative complement cascade, leading to opsonization and killing of bacteria. They also upregulate toll-like receptors, with subsequent activation of humoral and cellular immune mechanisms. Antibodies to bacterial cell wall components greatly enhance the host defense response; serotype-specific antibodies are especially important in host defenses against the pneumococcus.

One way of putting these defense mechanisms into perspective is to consider animal models of infection. Some strains of *Streptococcus pneumoniae* are lethal if a few viable organisms are injected into the peritoneal cavity, but in order to produce infection by inhalation, an inoculum of 10^3 or 10^4 colony-forming units may be required. Other microorganisms resist all defense mechanisms. For example, a single inhaled *Mycobacterium tuberculosis* organism that lodges in an alveolus establishes infection in guinea pigs and is thought to do the same in humans.

■ RISK FACTORS FOR PNEUMONIA

Extremes of age may be the most important risk factor for pneumonia (**Table 186-1**).

Pneumonia is most common among children under the age of 2 and the elderly. Not only is bacterial pneumonia, exemplified by pneumococcal infection, more common in the elderly, it is also more severe, with the risk of death rising steadily through adulthood (**Figure 186-1**).

Factors predisposing the elderly to pneumonia include diminished gag and cough reflexes, poor glottal function, diminished toll-like receptor responses, and less robust antibody responses. Pneumococcal pneumonia generally does not affect perfectly healthy young adults. Most adults with pneumonia have one or more predisposing underlying conditions. Even when outbreaks of pneumococcal pneumonia occur among presumably healthy young adults, as in military camps, concurrent viral infection and physical and emotional stress are all thought to play a contributory role. In contrast, viral pneumonia occurs when organisms are transmitted to immunologically naïve hosts, with the presence or absence of humoral antibody as the principal determinant of immunity, rather than age.

■ HOST RESPONSE

In bacterial pneumonia, the host inflammatory response causes most of the disease manifestations. The presence of bacteria and the accumulation of inflammatory cells and cytokines in alveoli initiate a vicious cycle in which additional inflammatory cells are attracted

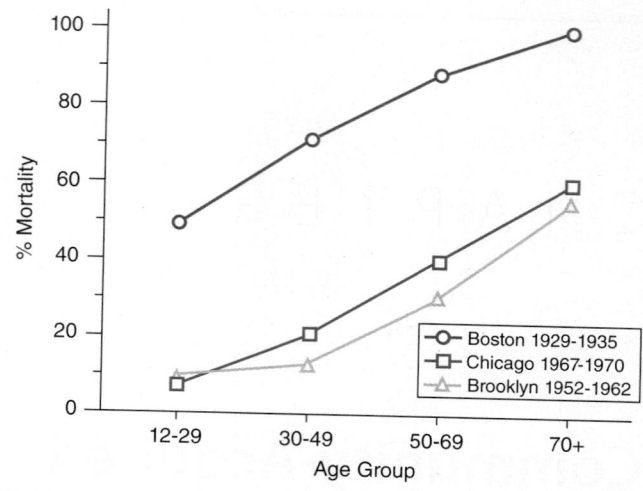

Figure 186-1 *Death from bacteremic pneumococcal pneumonia, although much lower than in the preantibiotic era, still rises with age.* (Adapted, with permission, from Musher DM. In: Mandell GL, Bennett JE, Dolin R, eds. *Principles and Practice of Infectious Diseases*, 6th ed. Philadelphia, PA. Elsevier. 2004:2392-2411.)

and further cytokine release is stimulated. These substances cause capillary leakage with exudation of plasma into the alveoli, leading to a progressive inflammatory exudate that is detected radiologically as pneumonia.

Microorganisms other than bacteria cause pneumonia by other means. Influenza virus directly invades columnar epithelium cells, resulting in pathologic changes that range from vacuolization of some respiratory epithelial cells to desquamation of the entire epithelial layer. These changes are diffuse, leading to an interstitial pattern on chest radiograph. Further, influenza virus damages the phagocytic function of polymorphonuclear leukocytes. Taken together, these factors predispose to secondary bacterial invasion, which is thought to have caused the staggering death rate during the influenza outbreak of 1918–1919. Although other viral infections also predispose to bacterial pneumonia, influenza seems to have a particularly high propensity to do so. *Chlamydophila pneumoniae* adheres to specific receptors and replicates within cells, producing microcolonies that stimulate an inflammatory response upon release, with a resulting focal pneumonia. Mycoplasmas also damage respiratory epithelial cells. Rather than invading cells, they adhere to the cell surface, impairing ciliary activity and generating toxic substances. Secondary bacterial pneumonia is uncommon, perhaps because mycoplasmas do not adversely affect phagocytic cells as influenza viruses do. Fungal and mycobacterial pneumonia are dealt with elsewhere in this volume.

ETIOLOGY

If pneumonia is defined as an acute or subacute condition characterized by a pulmonary infiltrate accompanied by systemic symptoms, fever, and cough, the list of possible causes infectious and noninfectious is great (**Tables 186-2** and **186-3**).

The prudent physician should consider these causes before concluding that a supposed case of typical CAP merits treatment with recommended empiric therapy.

In prospective studies to identify an etiologic agent in CAP, when every available modern technique is applied, a causative organism is still not identified in more than 50% of cases. In one such study of 259 consecutive patients admitted to a veterans hospital with a diagnosis of CAP (Table 186-2), 44 (17%) were found not to be infected, including 24 with pulmonary edema, 14 with lung cancer 12 of whom had no evidence for infection, and 6 with

---

TABLE 186-1 Conditions Predisposing to (Bacterial) Pneumonia

A. Multifactorial: extremes of life, prior hospitalization, malnutrition, alcoholism

B. Decreased pulmonary clearance
   1. Chronic lung disease
   2. Cigarette smoking
   3. Alcohol, opiates
   4. Viral respiratory infection
   5. Pollution

C. Diminished neutrophil function (chemotaxis, ingestion, or killing)
   1. Diabetes mellitus
   2. Corticosteroids
   3. Renal insufficiency
   4. Cirrhosis
   5. Alcohol
   6. Genetic defects of neutrophil function

D. Defective IgG production
   1. Congenital
   2. Acquired: myeloma, lymphoma, common variable immunodeficiency
   3. HIV infection

TABLE 186-2 A Study of 259 Consecutive Patients Admitted to a Veterans Hospital with a Diagnosis of Community-Acquired Pneumonia

Noninfectious cause		44
Pulmonary edema	24	
Lung cancer, uninfected	14	
Other	6	
Bacterial		64
Pneumococcus	20	
Haemophilus	12	
Staphylococcus aureus		11
Pseudomonas	7	
Other	12	
Legionella	2	
Mycobacteria		4
Nocardiosis		2
Fungi (Pneumocystis)		6
Viruses		44
Coronavirus	7	
Human metapnv	3	
Influenza	1	
Parainfluenza	4	
RSV	3	
Rhinovirus	26	
No etiology found		119

**PCR technology to detect Mycoplasma or Chlamydophila was not available at the time this study was done.
Modified from Musher DM, Roig I, Cazares G, et al. Can an etiologic agent be identified in adults who are hospitalized for community-acquired pneumonia? J Infect. 2013;67:11-18.

TABLE 186-3 Causes of a Syndrome of Pneumonia Leading to Hospital Admission (See Text)*

Common	Less Common	Uncommon
Streptococcus pneumoniae	Pulmonary infarction	Nontuberculous mycobacteria
Haemophilus influenzae	Klebsiella	Adenovirus
Staphylococcus aureus	Pseudomonas	Nocardia
Influenza virus	Other Gram-negative rods	Legionella[†] Chlamydophila
Other respiratory viruses	Mycobacterium tuberculosis	Mycoplasma
Pulmonary edema	Moraxella catarrhalis	Anaerobic bacteria[†]
Lung cancer	Non-TB mycobacteria	Cryptogenic organizing pneumonia
Pneumocystis jiroveci*	Cryptococcus	Eosinophilic pneumonia
		Other noninfectious pneumonias
		Sarcoidosis
		Kaposi sarcoma*
		Q fever[‡]
		Coccidioides[‡]
		Histoplasma[‡]

*Chiefly in association with HIV infection or other immunosuppressive conditions
[†]Situational: eg, seen in patients who have specific exposures and/or predisposing factors
[‡]Regional; where they are endemic these may be relatively common causes of admission for pneumonia

miscellaneous, noninfectious causes of pulmonary infiltrates. In the remaining 215 cases, no etiologic agent was identified in 119 (55%). Sixty patients (28% of those with infection) had a bacterial infection. Although *S. pneumoniae* was the most commonly identified, it was responsible for only 9% of those with an identified pathogen. Large multicenter studies, one conducted by the Centers for Disease Control and Prevention (CDC) and another in the Netherlands, found similar results (**Table 186-4**). The proportion of cases of CAP attributable to pneumococcus has steadily declined since the beginning of the antibiotic era; recent studies in the US have implicated this organism in only 8% to 16% of all cases, although a higher proportion is found in Europe. Among other bacterial causes, *Haemophilus influenzae* and *Staphylococcus aureus* are the next most common. *H. influenzae* and *Moraxella catarrhalis* generally cause pneumonia only in persons with pre-existing lung disease. *S. aureus* pneumonia presents in one of two forms: either as a segmental or lobar pneumonia or as a multiple, small cavitating emboli secondary to an intravascular infection. *Pseudomonas aeruginosa* and other Gram-negative rods cause pneumonia in persons with extensive chronic lung disease on treatment with corticosteroids, as well as in immunocompromised hosts, patients with cystic fibrosis, and infrequently in severe alcoholics. The multicenter CDC study, which only accepted isolation from a sterile site (usually blood) as indicating bacterial pneumonia, found no more than 1% of CAP was due to Gram-negative bacilli, and this results was supported by the Houston VAMC and the Netherlands studies. These results suggest that pneumonia due to Gram-negative rods receives excessive and

inappropriate emphasis when empiric antibiotic therapy is selected for patients hospitalized for CAP. In many of the cases for which no etiology is found it seems likely that microaspiration of mixed respiratory flora is responsible.

Evidence for viral infection is found in 20% to 25% of adults hospitalized for CAP. Identification of a virus by polymerase chain reaction (PCR) does not mean that antibiotic therapy need not be given, because up to one-quarter may have a concurrent bacterial infection; influenza virus appears to be more likely to predispose to a secondary bacterial pneumonia than other respiratory viruses. As patients with influenza pneumonia might benefit from antiviral treatment, even if initiated > 48 hours after the onset of symptoms, clinicians should consider diagnostic testing for influenza in the presence of suggestive features and treating if results are positive. Rhinovirus, respiratory syncytial virus and human metapneumovirus are common viruses causing hospitalization for pneumonia and even leading to intensive care unit (ICU) admission, but are currently untreatable. Although *Mycoplasma* and *C. pneumoniae* may be common in the ambulatory setting, these organisms are implicated in fewer than 3% of adults hospitalized for pneumonia. Older literature, based on questionable serologic studies, overemphasizes their importance and should be disregarded. Clinical presentation may suggest viral rather than bacterial pneumonia. Patients with viral pneumonia often have exposure to someone (usually a child) with a respiratory infection. Their disease is generally not as serious, cough is prominent but is not productive of sputum, and the white blood cell (WBC) count is likely not to be elevated. A low serum procalcitonin level in these circumstances supports the diagnosis of viral pneumonia.

Epidemiologic clues may suggest other causes of a pneumonia syndrome. *Coccidioides immitis*, found in arid regions of the Americas, or *Histoplasma capsulatum*, found worldwide but especially in river basins of North America, cause a variable proportion of CAP in endemic regions. Exposure to livestock or late summer

TABLE 186-4 Causative Organisms in CAP: Summary of Three Recent Studies*

	VAMC 2013[a]	CDC 2015[b]	Holland 2015[c]
Bacteria	29	15	30
Pneumococcus	9	5	16
Haemophilus	6	<1	7
Staph aureus	5	2	3
Pseudomonas	3	<1	2
Legionella	1	1	1
Mycoplasma, Chlamydia	—	<3	1
Other	6	3	3
Mycobacteria	2	1	<1
Nocardia	1	0	0
Fungi (Pneumocystis)	3	1	2
Viruses	20	27	ND
Rhinovirus	13	9	—
Coronavirus	3	2	—
Human metapneumovirus	2	4	—
Influenza	2	6	—
Parainfluenza	2	3	—
RSV	2	3	—
No cause identified	55	62	66

*Data presented as percentage of patients studied.
[a]VAMC, Musher DM, Roig I, Cazares G, et al. Can an etiologic agent be identified in adults who are hospitalized for community-acquired pneumonia? *J Infect.* 2013;67:11-18.
[b]CDC, Jain S, Self WH, Wunderink RG, et al. Community-acquired pneumonia requiring hospitalization among U.S. adults. *N Engl J Med.* 2015;373(5):415-427.
[c]Holland Postma, DF, van Werkhoven CH. van Elden LJ. Antibiotic treatment strategies for community-acquired pneumonia in adults. *N Engl J Med.* 2015;372:1312-1323.

residence in a hot and dry ranching area suggests *Coxiella burnetii* (Q fever), especially if severe headache and abnormal liver enzymes are associated. Exposure to sick birds raises concern for *Chlamydia psittaci*. A mild illness with prolonged cough, low-grade fever, and a pulmonary infiltrate in a parent whose children have similar symptoms suggests *Mycoplasma*. *Mycobacterium avium*, a well-known cause of pneumonia in patients with bronchiectasis or extensive lung scarring, has increasingly been recognized as a cause of chronic pneumonia in thin but otherwise healthy postmenopausal women. Tuberculosis should be suspected in persons from endemic areas, the immunocompromised, and those who have served time in prison or been homeless. Patients with AIDS are prone to opportunistic infection with *Pneumocystis, Histoplasma, M. avium,* or *Cryptococcus,* all of which tend to present, in such patients, with diffuse interstitial infiltrates. AIDS patients are also highly susceptible to pneumococcal disease; the age-related incidence of pneumococcal pneumonia may be increased 50- to 100-fold in young adults with HIV infection. For this reason, patients with CAP should be asked about HIV risk factors and screened if appropriate. Table 186-3 shows the breadth of causes of CAP, and should always be kept in mind during evaluation and empiric treatment of patients admitted with a consistent clinical picture.

CLINICAL PRESENTATION

In younger patients with pneumonia, acute severe malaise and subjective fever are common, often with chills, cough, and sputum production, or at least a sensation of needing to produce sputum. When sputum is produced, it may be flecked with blood. Middle-aged men with underlying lung disease nearly always have increased sputum production. Elderly subjects tend to have much less prominent symptoms; they produce lower levels of cytokines and may respond to them less vigorously than younger adults. A common presentation of pneumonia in very old adults is that they are less communicative than usual, or "not acting themselves." Much has been made of the classical presenting symptoms of pneumonia, as described by Osler: the sudden onset of rigors, followed by high fever, cough, pleuritic chest pain, and production of tenacious blood-tinged sputum. This presentation is uncommon today, perhaps because the incidence of CAP in otherwise healthy young adults is much lower now than in the preantibiotic era. Diarrhea is common in Legionnaires disease, but it is also frequent in pneumococcal pneumonia, probably reflecting a nonspecific gastrointestinal response to circulating cytokines.

In patients who have chronic lung disease, fever, cough, and increased sputum production without a new pulmonary infiltrate is often referred to an exacerbation of chronic obstructive pulmonary disease, although acute purulent tracheobronchitis might be a better descriptive term. A respiratory virus or, *H. influenzae,* is most often implicated. In cases where a cause is not identified, allergens, air pollutants, changes in humidity, or other unrecognized factors may be responsible. Persistent cough of several weeks' duration without fever or sputum suggests pertussis or a postviral infection syndrome, for example, due to adenovirus. Several prediction rules for pneumonia exist, but they all have shortcomings, and cannot be allowed to replace clinical judgment.

PHYSICAL EXAMINATION

Younger patients with bacterial or influenza pneumonia appear acutely ill. In contrast, elderly and frail persons may simply seem listless. Young patients nearly always have fever and cough, often with chest pain, whereas these symptoms are often absent in the elderly. Younger adults with viral, *Mycoplasma,* or *Chlamydophila* pneumonia generally do not look as acutely ill, and those with tuberculosis or other more chronic forms of pneumonia may appear chronically ill or may look relatively well. Vital signs other than fever are of great prognostic importance. Physicians should personally determine the respiratory rate and pay close attention to elevated pulse and respiratory rate or low blood pressure.

In bacterial pneumonia, crackles and increased tactile fremitus (which many young physicians forget to do) are generally present over the affected area. Dullness to percussion is detectable in about one-half of cases. Bronchial breath sounds and egophony strongly suggest pneumonia when present but are not sensitive for diagnosis. The failure to detect excursion of the diaphragm by percussion suggests that an effusion is present. Unfortunately, the overall sensitivity of the physical examination for pneumonia is fairly low, and pneumonia is usually diagnosed not by physical findings but by chest radiograph, with the absence of an infiltrate on a high-quality chest radiograph with posteroanterior and lateral views excluding the diagnosis. The problem, as noted above, is that obesity and dependence upon portable x-rays render the images less reliable, thereby increasing the importance of the physical examination.

RADIOGRAPHIC FINDINGS

In the great majority of cases, the radiographic appearance of a pulmonary infiltrate provides only limited insight into the etiology. Dense consolidation of a segment or lobe is usually bacterial; when due to pneumococcus, such an infiltrate tends to be associated with bacteremia (**Figure 186-2**).

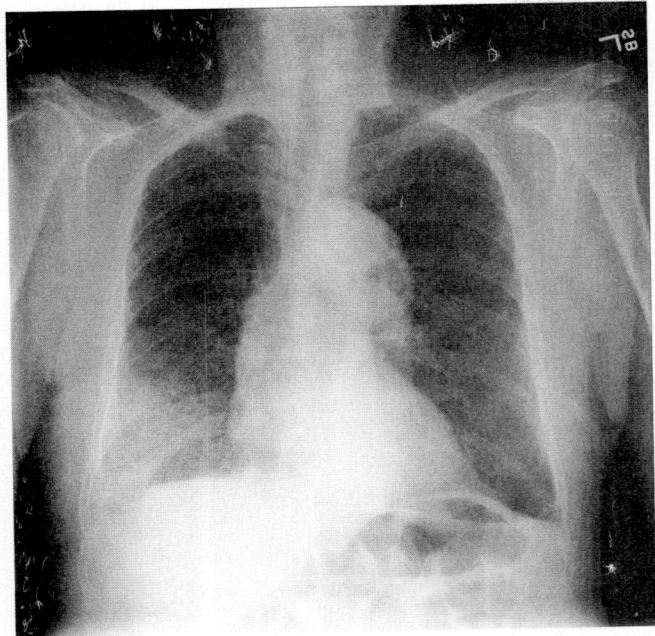

Figure 186-2 *Pneumococcal lobar pneumonia. A 78-year-old man with chronic lung disease had subjective fever, right-sided pleuritic chest pain, and greatly increased shortness of breath for 2 days. He was afebrile, and his WBC count was 10,600/mm³ with 40% band forms. Blood cultures were positive for S. pneumoniae. A sputum submitted for culture more than 24 hours after antibiotics were begun yielded no pneumococci.*

When *S. aureus* causes pneumonia via aspiration or inhalation, infiltrates resemble those caused by any other bacterial pneumonia. When hematogenous, as with endocarditis or an infected intravascular source, staphylococcal pneumonia presents with one or more round lesions, 2 to 3 cm in diameter, which are likely to cavitate (**Figures 186-3A, B**).

Subsegmental or "patchy" pneumonia may be due to bacteria, viruses, *Mycoplasma*, and *Chlamydophila*. Patchy involvement of multiple areas suggests a nonbacterial cause (**Figure 186-4**).

Pneumocystis causes a diffuse interstitial infiltrate that may be mistaken for prominent pulmonary markings in the earlier clinical stages. Mixed anaerobic, microaerophilic, and facultative organisms may cause a lung abscess with a thick wall, a fluid level, and surrounding consolidation (**Figure 186-5**); the superior segments of a lower lobe (right more commonly than left) are the most likely places for these to appear.

Cavitary lesions of the upper lobes without a fluid level, especially if confined to the posterior segment, suggest tuberculosis, but other infections, including those due to nontuberculous mycobacteria or *Nocardia* may be responsible. Occasionally, more acute presentations of tuberculosis may mimic CAP (**Figure 186-6**).

In one of several presentations for *Aspergillus* pneumonia, organisms grow as a mass within a cavity, causing the distinctive appearance of an intracavitary mycetoma (fungus ball) surrounded by an arc or halo of air (crescent sign).

Pneumonia of any cause, especially when rapidly progressive, may cause diffuse pulmonary infiltrates consistent with the acute respiratory distress syndrome. Although it is sometimes said that infiltrates progress after hospitalization because of correction of dehydration, animal studies suggest that the commonly observed progression of infiltrates during treatment in the hospital may be due to the ongoing inflammatory response, rather than to fluid replacement.

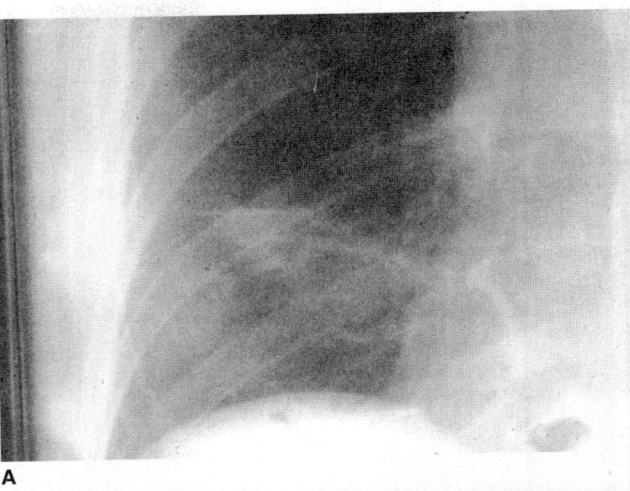

A

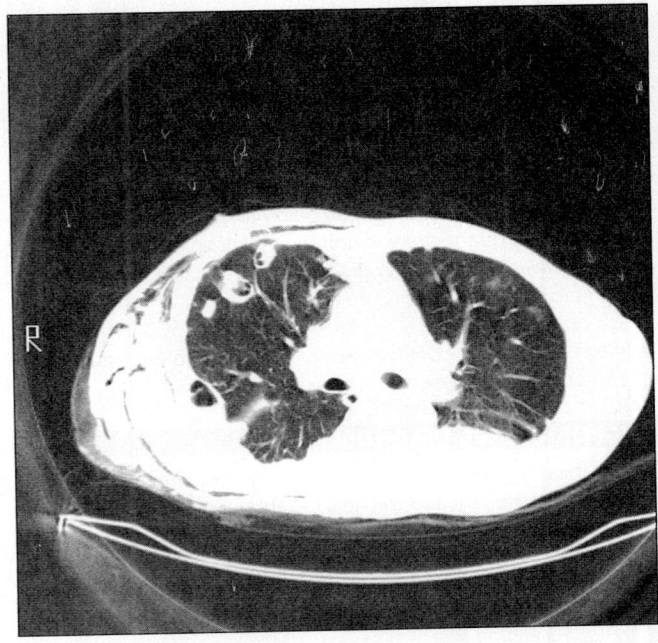

B

Figures 186-3 *(A and B) Hematogenous S. aureus pneumonia. A 47-year-old drug user who presented with 3 days of fever and chest pain and was found to have S. aureus endocarditis. Chest radiographs showed characteristic round lesions with cavitation, confirmed by computed tomographic scan.*

Chest computed tomography may help clarify the nature of an infiltrate and determine if an effusion or mass is present, but it is usually not necessary at hospital admission for patients in whom a good-quality chest radiograph can be obtained.

LABORATORY FINDINGS

Most patients with bacterial pneumonia have a WBC count greater than 12,000/mm³. In one-quarter of cases, the WBC count is within normal limits, although this should not be interpreted as reassuring. A low WBC count, for example, ≤ 6000/mm³, may be seen in overwhelming infection; in patients with pneumococcal pneumonia, this finding is associated with > 65% mortality. Thrombocytopenia also indicates serious infection. A serum sodium < 130 mEq/L, elevated blood urea nitrogen (BUN), or serum glucose > 250 mg/dL (13.9 mmol/L) in a nondiabetic patient is also associated with a poor prognosis. Serum bilirubin may be mildly increased, and lactate dehydrogenase (LDH) and liver transaminases may be slightly elevated.

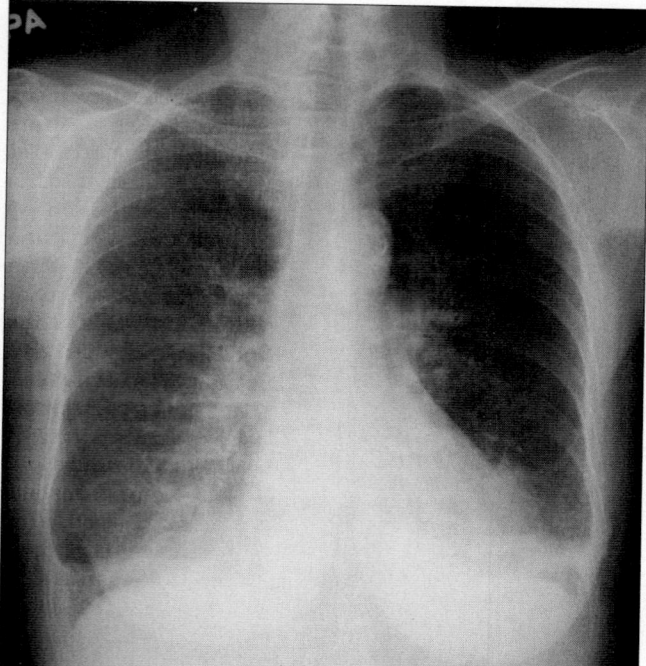

Figure 186-4 *Patient with pneumonia proven to be due to human metapneumovirus; chest radiograph shows patchy involvement of right and left lower lobes.* (Courtesy of Dr. Thomas J. Marrie.)

Marked elevations of LDH are seen in *Pneumocystis* and *Histoplasma* pneumonia in AIDS patients.

MICROBIOLOGIC DIAGNOSIS

The respiratory tract clears inflammatory exudate by the ciliary action of the bronchi and trachea, together with cough. Sputum is made up of this exudate, with a greater or lesser admixture of saliva.

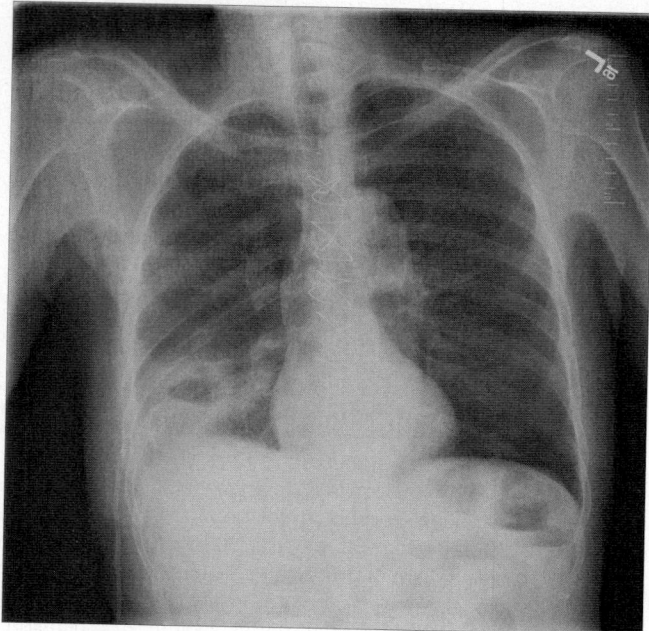

Figure 186-5 *Typical lung abscess due to aspiration of anaerobic and microaerophilic mouth organisms, generally occurring in patients with poor dentition, malnutrition, excess alcohol ingestion, and cigarette smoking.*

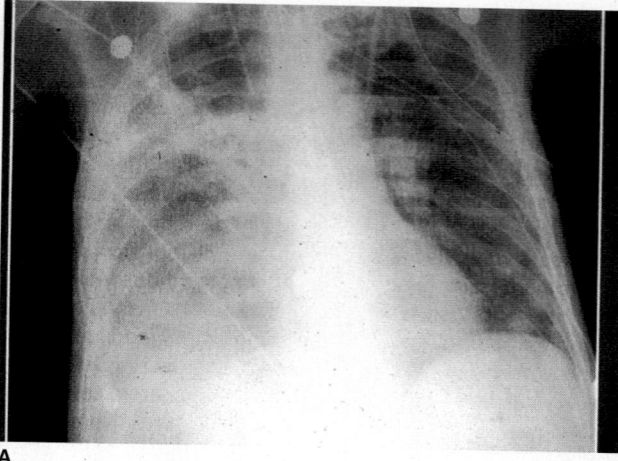

A

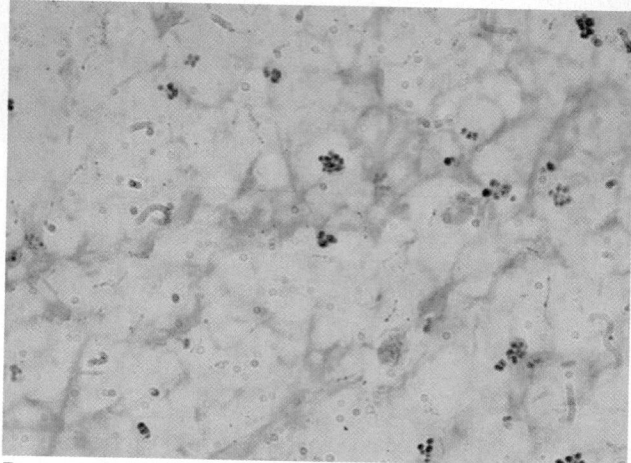

B

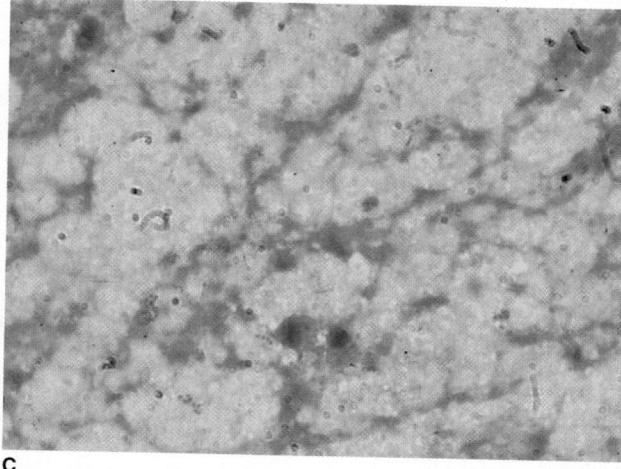

C

Figure 186-6 *(A) This homeless man was admitted to a general medical service with a diagnosis of "community-acquired pneumonia" and begun on ceftriaxone and azithromycin. No sputum sample was obtained. Blood cultures drawn on admission were negative. The patient rapidly deteriorated and was transferred to intensive care where he was intubated. (B) Microscopic examination of Gram stained tracheal secretions showed proteinaceous material with many staphylococci and almost no white blood cells, indicating an overwhelming pneumonia. (C) Also visible on the Gram stain are faint, beaded gram indeterminate rods; acid fast stain was strongly positive for mycobacteria. The patient died, perhaps due in part to delay in diagnosis; many medical personnel were exposed to tuberculosis, which was certainly due to delay in diagnosis.*

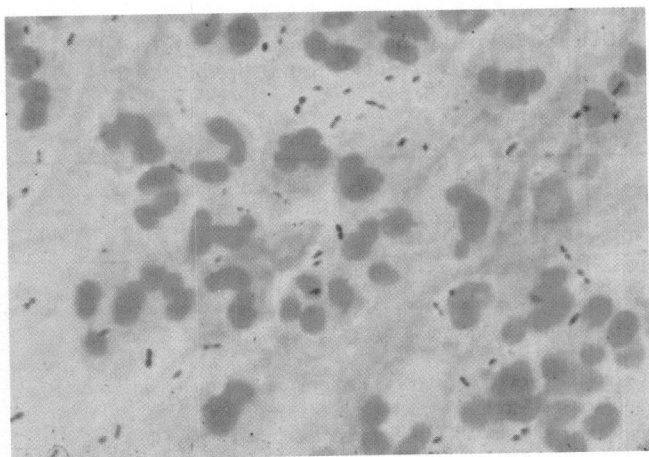

Figure 186-7 *Gram stain of sputum from a patient with pneumococcal pneumonia showing large numbers of polymorphonuclear leukocytes and many lancet-shaped Gram-positive cocci with no epithelial cells, indicating that this specimen originated in the lower airways. Such a specimen is diagnostic of pneumococcal pneumonia, although it cannot exclude coexisting infection by organisms which are not seen by Gram stain, such as influenza virus.*

If microscopic examination of a Gram-stained sputum specimen identifies areas with inflammatory cells and few or no epithelial cells, such a sample should be a reliable indicator of the microbial flora in the infiltrate. The presence of large numbers of a single type of bacterium in an inflammatory specimen strongly suggests this organism as the etiologic agent of the pneumonia (**Figure 186-7**).

The absence of visible organisms in an inflammatory specimen suggests certain bacteria that do not accept Gram stain (*Legionella* or *Mycobacteria*), or other organisms such as *Mycoplasma*, *Chlamydophila*, *Coxiella*, and viruses.

Reports of the poor sensitivity of sputum to detect bacteria largely reflect the inclusion of patients who do not provide a specimen, provide inadequate specimens, or have already been treated with antibiotics. In patients with proven (bacteremic) pneumococcal pneumonia who provide sputum that is judged to be good quality by the laboratory and who have not received antibiotics for >12 hours, the Gram stain is about 90% sensitive in detecting pneumococci. *Haemophilus*, *Moraxella*, and Gram-negative rods are even more distinctive in their microscopic appearance. Clinicians are urged to pay more attention to Gram stain results than they have done traditionally. The finding of *S. aureus* or Gram-negative rods by culture when they have not been seen microscopically in a good-quality sputum suggests that these are contaminating mouth flora, perhaps explaining the overemphasis in the medical literature on Gram-negative organisms as a cause of CAP.

Bacterial cultures in most laboratories will readily yield pneumococcus, *Haemophilus*, *Moraxella*, *S. aureus*, or Gram-negative bacilli when these organisms cause pneumonia. Preliminary results are likely to be available after 12 to 16 hours of culture, and laboratory technologists are generally happy to discuss cases with clinicians and give early results by telephone. Cultures for *Mycobacteria* and fungi take much longer, although most large hospital laboratories now follow CDC recommendations and do a PCR for TB on at least one sputum that is submitted for mycobacterial culture.

Additional techniques are available to establish the cause of pneumonia. An enzyme-linked immunosorbent assay (ELISA) detects pneumococcal cell wall polysaccharide in the urine of up to 75% of patients with bacteremic pneumococcal pneumonia, and a smaller proportion of those with nonbacteremic disease. An ELISA for urinary *Legionella* antigen detects only the most common *Legionella*

serotype, but is positive in about 70% of cases, with greatest sensitivity in more severe disease. *Histoplasma* urine and *Cryptococcus* serum antigen tests are positive in patients with disseminated disease, but less likely so in those with discrete pulmonary infiltrates.

The largest diagnostic advance in recent years has been in real-time PCR. This can now be performed directly on sputum to detect *M. tuberculosis*, or on nasal secretions to detect most respiratory viruses. Sensitivity and specificity are very high compared to culture results. PCR is not used to detect bacteria in sputum because, unlike *M. tuberculosis* or respiratory viruses, most of the bacteria that cause pneumonia may also colonize the upper airways in normal adults, so a highly sensitive technique may detect colonization rather than infection. However, quantitative PCR techniques may soon be perfected enabling PCR to be done directly on sputum. PCR for influenza virus is currently the gold standard for diagnosis. By comparison, viral culture is positive in 90% to 95% of cases, and rapid influenza tests in 30% to 70%. PCR also detects respiratory syncytial virus (RSV), parainfluenza virus, human metapneumovirus, coronavirus, and rhinovirus.

In several studies have that systematically applied the most up-to-date technology to determine an etiologic diagnosis for CAP, no causative organism has been identified in more than one-half of all cases. Gram stains often reveal large numbers of mixed Gram-positive flora, and cultures yield mouth organisms. These findings suggest that an important cause of CAP is microaspiration of normal oral flora, that is, the mixed streptococci and microaerophilic organisms that normally inhabit the upper airways.

Blood cultures yield *S. pneumoniae* in 20% to 25% of adult patients hospitalized for pneumococcal pneumonia. At present, in many hospitals, blood cultures are positive in about 50% of all patients diagnosed with pneumococcal pneumonia, but that is because fewer adequate sputum cultures are obtained, and the diagnosis is more often made on the basis of positive blood cultures. Blood cultures are probably positive in 20% to 25% of patients with inhalation or aspiration pneumonia due to *S. aureus* or Gram-negative rods, in a lower proportion of those with pneumonia caused by nontypable *H. influenzae*, and only rarely in pneumonia due to *Moraxella catarrhalis*. In contrast, patients with hematogenous *S. aureus* pneumonia virtually always have positive blood cultures.

DIFFERENTIAL DIAGNOSIS

Many noninfectious conditions mimic pneumonia and also present with pulmonary infiltrates, leukocytosis, and fever; the most important of these are listed in Table 186-3. Lung cancer, pulmonary edema, and pulmonary infarction are the most common, with other noninfectious causes of pulmonary infiltrates such as eosinophilic pneumonia or cryptogenic organizing pneumonia also being responsible.

Patients with lung cancer commonly present with fever and a pulmonary infiltrate. Despite the frequent diagnosis of postobstructive pneumonia, it is unclear whether infection is involved, and antibiotics are generally given, often to no avail. Patients who do not respond to the first course of antibiotics may have repeat sputum cultures, which reveal new and different flora; antibiotics selected on this basis are virtually never of benefit, and fever may persist until cancer chemotherapy is begun. Tumor necrosis may also cause fever in this setting.

Pulmonary embolus with infarction produces pulmonary infiltrates with sputum containing neutrophils, but few or no bacteria. Pleuritic chest pain may be prominent. Pulmonary edema and acute respiratory distress syndrome are often indistinguishable from pneumonia; establishing the diagnosis is especially problematic in an intensive care setting.

Cryptogenic organizing pneumonia, acute interstitial pneumonia, and other interstitial pneumonias are less common, but are noteworthy because they are almost always initially misdiagnosed as

CAP. Attention to the patient's history and careful review of earlier chest radiographs may reveal a longer history of symptoms and subtle prior radiologic abnormalities, more consistent with a non-infectious process.

Patients with septic pulmonary emboli should be assessed for other foci of infection, such as an infected heart valve or intravascular device. In acute aspiration of gastric contents, pneumonia results from the presence of acid; antibiotic treatment is not indicated. Pulmonary hemorrhage and vasculitis may also cause pulmonary infiltrates and fever. In vasculitis, these infiltrates may also be associated with cavitary lesions, as in antineutrophil cytoplasmic antibody (ANCA)-associated granulomatous vasculitis. The CURB-65 score (**Table 186-7**), although easy to calculate, is less sensitive and less specific than the PORT score.

MANAGEMENT

■ HOSPITAL ADMISSION

Scoring systems have been designed to help physicians decide whether a patient with pneumonia requires hospitalization. The most widely cited is the Pneumonia Outcomes Research Trial (PORT) score, sometimes called the Pneumonia Severity Index (PSI) (**Tables 186-5** and **186-6**).

TABLE 186-5 Pneumonia Outcomes Research Trial (PORT) Severity Index*

Age (subtract 10 for women)	—
Nursing home	10
Neoplasm (active, not skin)	30
Cirrhosis or chronic hepatitis	20
CHF, CVA, chronic renal disease	10
Altered mental status	20
Respiratory rate >30	20
Systolic BP <90	20
Temp < 35 or > 40°C	15
Pulse >125/min	10
Arterial pH <7.35	30
BUN >30 mg/dL (11 mmol/L)	20
Serum sodium <130	20
Glucose >250 mg/dL (13.9 mmol/L)	10
Hematocrit <30	10
pO_2 <60 or O_2 sat <90%	10
Pleural effusion	10

BP, blood pressure; BUN, blood urea nitrogen; CHF, congestive heart failure; CVA, cerebrovascular accident.
*Points assigned for each criterion.
Data from Fine MJ, Auble TE, Yealy DM, et al. A prediction rule to identify low-risk patients with community-acquired pneumonia. *N Engl J Med.* 1997;336:243-250.

TABLE 186-6 Pneumonia Outcomes Research Trial (PORT) Severity Index: Prognostic Value of the PORT Score

Point Score	Class	CAP*	Mortality VAMC†
≤ 70	II	< 1%	–
71-90	III	3%	3%
91-130	IV	8%	21%
> 130	V	29%	35%

CAP, community-acquired pneumonia; VAMC, Veterans Affairs Medical Center, Houston.
*Original calculation in patients with community acquired pneumonia report of PORT score.
†Results in patients with proven pneumococcal pneumonia.
Data from Fine MJ, Auble TE, Yealy DM, et al. A prediction rule to identify low-risk patients with community-acquired pneumonia. *N Engl J Med.* 1997;336:243-250.
Data from Musher DM, Alexandraki I, Graviss EA, et al. Bacteremic and nonbacteremic pneumococcal pneumonia: a prospective study. *Medicine (Baltimore).* 2000;79:210-221.

TABLE 186-7 CURB-65 Scoring System

One point for each of the following:
Confusion
Urea >19 mg/dL (7 mmol/L)
Respiratory rate >30
Blood pressure <90/60 (either systolic or diastolic value)
≥ 65 y of age

Score of ≥ 2 indicates need for hospitalization.
Data from Lim WS, van der Eerden MM, Laing R, et al. Defining community acquired pneumonia severity on presentation to hospital: an international derivation and validation study. *Thorax.* 2003;58:377-382.

TABLE 186-8 SMART-COP Scoring System*

Low **s**ystolic blood pressure (2 points)

Multilobar involvement (1 point)

Low **a**lbumin (1 point)

High **r**espiratory rate (1 point)

Tachycardia (1 point)

Confusion (1 point)

Poor **o**xygenation (2 points)

Low arterial **p**H (2 points)

*In one study, a SMART-COP score of ≥ 3 points identified 92% of patients who required intensive respiratory and/or vasopressor support and correctly identified 84% of patients who did not need immediate admission to the intensive care unit. In another study, SMART-COP performed better than PSI or CURB-65 but still stratified 15% of patients incorrectly.
Data from Chalmers JD, Singanayagam A, Hill AT. Predicting the need for mechanical ventilation and/or inotropic support for young adults admitted to the hospital with community-acquired pneumonia. *Clin Infect Dis.* 2008;47:1571-1574.

The immediate decision whether to hospitalize must ultimately depend upon physician judgment, but it is strongly recommended that all PORT score factors be considered in reaching a decision; before it was developed, many of these factors, such as the low serum sodium, elevated BUN/creatinine, and elevated blood sugar in a nondiabetic, were not well recognized as indicating a poor prognosis. Because the PORT score is so age-dependent, a moderately elevated score in a young adult should be regarded with alarm.

A corollary decision is whether a patient needs admission to an intensive care unit. The SMART-COP score (**Table 186-8**), based on systolic blood pressure, multilobar involvement, serum albumin level, respiratory rate, tachycardia, confusion, oxygenation, and arterial pH, may be more reliable than PSI or CURB-65 at predicting which patients will require ICU transfer for intensive respiratory or vasopressor support, being 92% sensitive compared to 74% and 39%, respectively, for the other two scoring systems. Other indicators of overwhelming infection requiring ICU admission include relative leukopenia in bacterial pneumonia (WBC count ≤ 6000/mm³), thrombocytopenia, and hypothermia.

■ ANTIBIOTIC THERAPY

Fortunately or unfortunately, guidelines have been developed for treatment of community-acquired pneumonia: fortunately, because there is now some evidence-based uniformity in the approach to treating pneumonia; unfortunately, because some physicians remain satisfied with a diagnosis of CAP, without understanding that this is a broadly descriptive term that does not address an etiological diagnosis. Such physicians may reflexly adhere to guidelines without considering the full range of possible diagnoses. As a result, patients with noninfectious causes of fever and pulmonary infiltrate may receive inappropriate therapy with antibiotics, delaying correct diagnosis and appropriate treatment.

Guidelines published jointly by the Infectious Disease Society of America and the American Thoracic Society (IDSA/ATS) focus on common bacterial causes of pneumonia. It is difficult to know how to apply these guidelines in light of new data, presented in Tables 186-2 and 186-4, showing that a bacterial cause is identified in only a minority of patients hospitalized for CAP. The full guidelines document is detailed, listing epidemiologic clues that might raise consideration of less common causes and giving approaches to evaluating

TABLE 186-9 Recommended Empiric Antimicrobial Treatment for Presumed Bacterial Pneumonia, Hospitalized Patients

Non-ICU patients

Respiratory fluoroquinolone

OR

β-lactam (cefotaxime, ceftriaxone, or ampicillin/sulbactam) plus macrolide

ICU patients

β-lactam (cefotaxime, ceftriaxone, or ampicillin/sulbactam) PLUS azithromycin or a respiratory fluoroquinolone

For *Pseudomonas,* antipneumococcal, antipseudomonal β-lactam (piperacillin/tazobactam, cefepime, imipenem, or meropenem) plus a quinolone (ciprofloxacin or levofloxacin)

OR

Antipneumococcal, antipseudomonal β-lactam as above with an aminoglycoside and azithromycin

For possible *Staphylococcus aureus,* presume methicillin resistance and add vancomycin or linezolid

Data from Mandell LA, Wunderink RG, Anzueto A, et al. Infectious Diseases Society of America/American Thoracic Society consensus guidelines on the management of community-acquired pneumonia in adults. *Clin Infect Dis.* 2007;44 (Suppl 2):S27-S72.

and treating them. Physicians who utilize the recommendations are urged first to read the document in its entirety.

Recommended antimicrobial treatment for non-ICU hospitalized patients who are presumed to have a bacterial pneumonia (**Table 186-9**) includes a respiratory fluoroquinolone (levofloxacin or moxifloxacin, but not ciprofloxacin) or a beta-lactam (cefotaxime, ceftriaxone, ampicillin, or ampicillin/sulbactam) together with a macrolide. The reasoning is that this regimen will treat pneumonia due to pneumococcus, *Haemophilus, Moraxella, Legionella, Mycoplasma,* and *Chlamydophila,* as well as some less common organisms, although a recent study showed no difference in outcome when patients were treated with ceftriaxone alone versus ceftriaxone plus azithromycin. A major problem is that none of these regimens is likely to be effective in methicillin-resistant *S. aureus* (MRSA) pneumonia, currently a relatively common cause of bacterial pneumonia in the United States; this emphasizes the importance of Gram stain and culture of sputum at the time of admission. Two studies have suggested that patients who do not have nasal colonization by MRSA are unlikely to have MRSA pneumonia, so hospitals that routinely test admitted patients for nasal colonization and find a negative study will be able to predict that this organism is not responsible. If patients have a Gram stain showing Gram-positive cocci in clusters, or clinical risk factors for MRSA infection, such as injection drug use, chronic renal failure, influenza, or prior antibiotics, vancomycin or linezolid should be added. Preliminary data suggest that ceftaroline, which is very much like ceftriaxone but is active against MRSA in vitro, may be effective in this setting.

For ICU patients, a beta-lactam (cefotaxime, ceftriaxone, or ampicillin/sulbactam) should be given, plus either azithromycin or a respiratory fluoroquinolone. When *Pseudomonas* is a consideration, as in patients with Gram-negative rods on Gram stain, prior failed antibiotic treatment, bronchiectasis and other structural lung disease, or chronic obstructive pulmonary disease requiring frequent antibiotics or glucocorticoids, patients should receive an antipneumococcal, antipseudomonal beta-lactam (piperacillin/tazobactam, cefepime, imipenem, or meropenem) plus a respiratory fluoroquinolone (ciprofloxacin or levofloxacin). Once again, Gram stain of sputum at admission may rule out *Pseudomonas* pneumonia if a good quality sputum specimen fails to show large numbers of Gram-negative rods. If *Pseudomonas* pneumonia is present, some experts recommend double coverage (treatment with two anti-pseudomonal antibiotics). However, the evidence for this recommendation is very weak unless there is a reason to believe that the organisms might be resistant to one of the antibiotics chosen.

In patients without an indication for a fluoroquinolone, some authorities suggest that a macrolide should be selected because of modest evidence for a beneficial immunomodulatory effect. However, a recent study comparing a beta-lactam alone to a beta-lactam plus a macrolide or a quinolone in non-ICU admissions showed no difference, suggesting that a beta-lactam alone may be appropriate therapy. Clinicians should also bear in mind that azithromycin use has been associated with sudden cardiac death, which needs to be balanced against the fact that the mortality of CAP is as high as 10%.

Recommendations for empiric therapy are problematic unless they emphasize that therapy should be begun pending definitive determination of an etiologic agent, or as a fallback position if appropriate specimens cannot be obtained. The IDSA/ATS guidelines clearly recommend diagnostic testing in all hospitalized patients to help determine the etiologic agent of the infection. However, in the rush to treat empirically, many physicians tend to overlook this recommendation. In the author's experience, ICU patients who are intubated for pneumonia—thereby providing a ready source for specimen culture—are often begun on treatment with three antibiotics (eg, piperacillin/tazobactam, azithromycin, and vancomycin) *without a specimen being obtained for culture.* If the patient improves, it is unclear which, if any, of these drugs may be discontinued. Often, one or two drugs are arbitrarily discontinued in the absence of new evidence, raising questions about whether all were needed in the first place. Later in the hospitalization, if the patient deteriorates, a culture may be obtained which, by this point, will provide misleading results. In the absence of a microbiological proof of cause, all three drugs may alternatively be given to complete a 7 to 10 days course of therapy, although they may well not be needed. The administration of such broad spectrum antibiotics to ICU patients with pneumonia, which certainly contributes to the rate of *Clostridium difficile* infection and antibiotic-resistant hospital flora, is especially ironic since pneumococcus remains the most commonly identified cause of pneumonia leading to ICU admission, perhaps followed next by viral infection. Initial therapy is best selected in light of Gram stain of tracheal secretions, PCR on a nasal swab for respiratory viruses and urine antigen tests for pneumococcus and *Legionella.* Treatment for other organisms may be considered, depending upon epidemiologic factors, medical history, and the index of suspicion.

The time lag between arrival in the emergency department (ED) for symptoms of pneumonia and the administration of effective antibiotics has been a subject of controversy. The Joint Commission, the body responsible for hospital accreditation in the United States, mandated that antibiotics be initiated within 4 hours of arrival in the ED in pneumonia patients. This policy, based on limited evidence, led to possible pneumonia patients being seen before others who might have had more urgent conditions, and also to unnecessary antibiotics being administered to patients who eventually were found not to have pneumonia. The IDSA/ATS committee has dropped the 4-hour rule from its recommendations, but now states that antibiotics should be given as soon as possible after the diagnosis of pneumonia is considered likely. Recognizing that long delays may occur during transfer from the ED to a hospital bed, the committee specifically recommended that the first dose of antibiotics be given at the site where the diagnosis of pneumonia is first made.

The optimal duration of therapy for pneumonia is uncertain. In the case of pneumococcal pneumonia, organisms are no longer readily visible by microscopic examination of sputum or detectable by culture 24 hours after the administration of an effective antibiotic. Experience from early in the antibiotic era showed that 5 to 7 days of therapy sufficed to treat pneumonia. During the Korean War, a single dose of procaine penicillin, which maintains an effective antimicrobial level for as long as 24 hours, was shown to cure otherwise healthy young adults. Nevertheless, many physicians now treat pneumonia for 10 to 14 days, despite the absence of data for additional benefit. One study showed that patients who received treatment for ≤7 days did just as well as patients who were treated for longer periods of time. In the author's opinion, 2 to 3 days of close observation with parenteral therapy for pneumococcal pneumonia and a final few days of oral treatment, in all not exceeding 7 days may be the best approach. In pneumococcal pneumonia, the documentation of bacteremia need not alter this recommendation.

The proper duration of therapy for pneumonia due to other bacteria is even less clear. *Haemophilus* and *Moraxella* pneumonia probably respond similarly, and treatment should not exceed 7 days. In contrast, pneumonia due to *S. aureus* or Gram-negative bacilli tends to be destructive, and concern that small abscesses have formed in the lung parenchyma might require 10 to 14 days of treatment. When *S. aureus* bacteremia is documented in a patient with pneumonia, most authorities will treat for 4 weeks. Data purporting to show that ventilator-associated pneumonia can be treated with shorter courses of antibiotics probably speak more to the uncertainty of diagnosis than to the responsiveness of true Gram-negative pneumonia to therapy. Relapses of *Legionella* pneumonia have been documented when treatment is discontinued too soon. Suggested duration of treatment is 5 to 10 days of azithromycin, which has a prolonged tissue half-life, 14 days with a fluoroquinolone, and 3 weeks recommended in immunocompromised patients.

■ ADJUNCTIVE THERAPY

Two prospective randomized control studies have recently been published on adjunctive glucocorticosteroids in patients hospitalized for CAP. One showed that the time to clinical stability was shortened by about 24 hours, which might prompt earlier discharge. The other showed a higher rate of treatment failure in patients who did not receive steroids, but the failures were nearly all related to a predetermined definition of failure as radiographic progression at 72 hours, rather than other clinical outcome parameters. In the opinion of the present author, the evidence does not strongly favor adjunctive therapy with glucocorticosteroids.

Several retrospective studies have shown that patients who are taking statins at the time of admission for CAP have better outcomes, even when the so-called healthy patient effect is excluded. A prospective study in ventilator-associated pneumonia showed no benefit.

■ FAILURE TO RESPOND TO THERAPY

The expected response to therapy includes defervescence, return of the WBC count to normal, and disappearance of systemic signs of acute infection within 5 to 7 days after antibiotics have been begun. Cough and fatigue may persist for weeks. The failure to respond may have a number of possible explanations (**Table 186-10**).

If the patient simply does not improve, the antibiotic therapy may not be appropriate for the infecting organism or an infection may not be responsible. Admitting cultures and antibiotic susceptibilities should be reviewed to ensure that the patient has received an adequate dose of an appropriate antibiotic. The patient may have received appropriate antimicrobial therapy, but there may be a loculated infection, such as empyema, or infection lurking behind an obstruction, such as lung cancer or a foreign body. The diagnosis of bacterial pneumonia may be incorrect; an organism from another class (mycobacterium, fungus) may be responsible, or the syndrome may be noninfectious in origin. Initial improvement followed by

TABLE 186-10 Some Reasons for Failure of Antimicrobial Therapy in Community-Acquired Pneumonia

Inappropriate antibiotic choice or dose
    Organism not susceptible
    Wrong dosage (eg, morbidly obese patient)
    Antibiotic not given
Correct antibiotic but loculated infection
    Empyema
    Obstruction (eg, lung cancer)
Unidentified causative organism responsible
Noninfectious cause
    Malignancy
    Inflammatory infiltrate

persistent lower-grade fever and leukocytosis strongly suggests an empyema. Additional diagnostic measures that should be considered in patients with an inadequate response to initial therapy include thoracentesis of significant effusions, chest computed tomography, and bronchoscopy with bronchoalveolar lavage and possibly transbronchial biopsy.

QUALITY IMPROVEMENT

The most recent IDSA guidelines target four key performance indicators for quality improvement, monitoring of guideline adherence, and educational efforts:

1. Empiric antibiotic administration that conforms to guidelines; if administered antibiotics diverge from recommended regimens, the reasons for this should be clearly stated in the medical record.
2. The first antibiotic dose should be given in the emergency room; in the current guidelines, an explicit time frame is not mandated, but the suggested range is within 6 to 8 hours of presentation.
3. Mortality data for all patients admitted with CAP should be collected, monitored, and compared to severity-specific norms; as well, the proportion of patients with severe CAP that are not admitted to ICUs should also be tracked.
4. The proportion of eligible patients receiving influenza and pneumococcal vaccination should be monitored (see later discussion).

The expected adherence to the key indicators is expected to be in the 80% to 95% range, except for influenza and pneumococcal vaccination, where adherence is expected to be > 90% in patients over the age of 65 years.

PREVENTION

Pneumococcal vaccination is recommended for all patients ≥ 65 years, and for patients 19 to 64 years of age with predisposing conditions, including smoking, asthma, chronic lung disease, heart failure, diabetes, alcoholism, cerebrospinal fluid leaks, chronic liver disease, functional or anatomic asplenia, and compromised immunity. There are two available pneumococcal vaccines: the traditional one marketed as Pneumovax® or Pnu-immune®, based on vaccination with relatively purified capsular polysaccharides (PPSV23) and the conjugate pneumococcal vaccine that contains 13 capsular polysaccharies (Prevnar13®) (PCV13). Recommendations have changed. For patients who are immunocompromised or asplenic or who have a cochlear implant, and for all patients >65, a first dose of PCV13 is recommended to be followed 8 weeks later by PPSV23. Patients who have previously received PPSV23 should receive a dose of PCV13, provided that at least 1 year has passed since the PPSV23. Cigarette smokers, patients with heart disease, diabetes kidney, or liver disease of any age should receive PPSV23 alone. Multiple revaccinations are not currently recommended, except for asplenic patients who should be revaccinated at 7-year intervals with PPSV23.

Patients over 50 years of age, younger patients with comorbid medical conditions at risk for influenza complications, household contacts of high-risk persons, and all health care workers should receive inactivated influenza vaccine annually. Smoking cessation guidance should be provided to smokers.

DISCHARGE CHECKLIST

- Can the patient tolerate oral medications? (It is traditional to observe patients in the inpatient setting for up to 24 hours after switching from intravenous to oral therapy, when clinical stability has been achieved, but this author favors an additional 24 hours of observation prior to discharge.)
- Is the patient clinically stable? Suggested markers of clinical stability include temperature ≤ 37.8°C, heart rate ≤ 100 beats/min, respiratory rate ≤ 24 breaths/min, systolic blood pressure ≥ 90 mm Hg, arterial oxygen saturation ≥ 90% or pO_2 ≥ 60 mm Hg on room air (for patients not previously dependent on supplemental oxygen), and mental status at baseline.
- Has the patient's pneumococcal and influenza vaccination status been assessed?
- Has counseling regarding smoking cessation been given, where appropriate?
- Does the patient have a safe home environment?

SUGGESTED READINGS

Chalmers JD, Singanayagam A, Hill AT. Predicting the need for mechanical ventilation and/or inotropic support for young adults admitted to the hospital with community-acquired pneumonia. *Clin Infect Dis.* 2008;47:1571-1574.

Charles PG, Wolfe R, Whitby M, et al. SMART-COP: a tool for predicting the need for intensive respiratory or vasopressor support in community-acquired pneumonia. *Clin Infect Dis.* 2008;47:375-384.

Jain S, Self WH, Wunderink RG, et al. Community-acquired pneumonia requiring hospitalization among U.S. adults. *N Engl J Med.* 2015;373:415-427.

Johnstone J, Majumdar SR, Fox JD, Marrie TJ. Viral infection in adults hospitalized with community-acquired pneumonia: prevalence, pathogens, and presentation. *Chest.* 2008;134:1141-1148.

Mandell LA, File TM Jr. Short-course treatment of community-acquired pneumonia. *Clin Infect Dis.* 2003;37:761-763.

Mandell LA, Wunderink RG, Anzueto A, et al. Infectious Diseases Society of America/American Thoracic Society consensus guidelines on the management of community-acquired pneumonia in adults. *Clin Infect Dis.* 2007;44(Suppl 2):S27-S72.

Musher DM, Alexandraki I, Graviss EA, et al. Bacteremic and nonbacteremic pneumococcal pneumonia: a prospective study. *Medicine (Baltimore).* 2000;79:210-221.

Musher DM, Roig I, Cazares G, et al. Can an etiologic agent be identified in adults who are hospitalized for community-acquired pneumonia? *J Infect.* 2013;67:11-18.

Musher DM, Thorner AT. Community-acquired pneumonia. *N Engl J Med.* 2014;371:1619-1628.

Postma DF, van Werkhoven CH, van Elden LJ, et al. Antibiotic treatment strategies for community-acquired pneumonia in adults. *N Engl J Med.* 2015;372:1312-1323.

Wunderink RG. Corticosteroids for severe community-acquired pneumonia: not for everyone. *JAMA.* 2015;313:673-674.

CHAPTER 187

Health Care and Hospital-Acquired Pneumonia

Michael Klompas, MD, MPH

Key Clinical Questions

1. What are common mimickers of hospital-acquired pneumonia (HAP)?
2. Is an invasive sampling procedure necessary for accurate diagnosis?
3. Which pathogens typically cause HAP?
4. Which antibiotics are indicated for treatment?
5. For how long should patients be treated?
6. What can be done to prevent HAP?

INTRODUCTION

More than 100 years ago, Sir William Osler noted the frequent mismatch between clinical and postmortem diagnoses of pneumonia. The disparity ran both ways: clinicians both overdiagnosed and underdiagnosed the disease. Despite profound advances in the tools available to clinicians, including computed tomography (CT) scans, bronchoscopy, and advanced microbiological diagnostics, the diagnosis of hospital-acquired pneumonia (HAP), or pneumonia acquired more than 48 hours after hospital admission, continues to be elusive, partly because it has many mimickers, and partly because the population at risk tends to be very complex.

Misdiagnosis has three serious consequences: failure to treat truly infected patients is associated with increased mortality; inappropriate use of antibiotics in uninfected patients promotes antibiotic resistance and *Clostridium difficile* colitis; and premature closure may result in alternative diagnoses being missed.

The selection of appropriate antibiotic regimens for patients with hospital-acquired pneumonia is hampered by limitations in both diagnostic tools and the evidence base. Guidelines published in 2005 recommended rapid, empiric broad-spectrum coverage for all patients with HAP and health care associated pneumonia (HCAP), given observational data suggesting that delayed treatment is associated with increased mortality, inappropriate treatment is associated with increased mortality, and that HAP and HCAP can be caused by pathogens resistant to the typical agents used to treat community-acquired pneumonia. While this strategy may be appropriate for some patients, overtreatment may result, leading to *C. difficile* colitis, adverse drug reactions, and excess costs. The HCAP concept in particular has come under scrutiny, because more recent case series suggest that only a fraction of HCAPs are due to resistant pathogens. A consensus has yet to emerge on how to best stratify patients into those who require early and aggressive broad-spectrum regimens versus those in whom it is safe to observe, treat using narrower spectrum agents, or await the results of further diagnostic testing.

This chapter will focus primarily on ventilator-associated pneumonia (VAP), since mechanically ventilated patients are at greater risk and better studied than other populations. However, many of the treatment principles for VAP can inform the approach to other kinds of HAP.

EPIDEMIOLOGY

VAP rates have dropped dramatically over the past 20 years. Older literature suggested incidence rates of 10% to 15% of ventilated patients, but more recent series report VAP in 5% or fewer of ventilated patients. The risk of VAP is primarily related to the duration of mechanical ventilation. Consequently, the risk of VAP tends to be higher in burn and trauma units, and lower in medical and cardiac units. On meta-analysis, an episode of VAP appears to extend intensive care length of stay by about 6 days, and doubles the risk of dying. The attributable cost of VAP is approximately $10,000 per episode. Data on HAP are more limited. The incidence is lower than VAP, about 0.3% to 0.5% of hospitalized patients, but the absolute number of cases is higher than VAP, given that there are so many more nonventilated patients than ventilated patients in most hospitals.

PATHOPHYSIOLOGY

The histological hallmark of HAP is heterogeneity. The lungs of ventilated patients tend to have multiple patchy areas of inflammation and infection, in various stages of recovery and progression.

Cultures of these different areas often yield different organisms. These findings arise because patients tend to repeatedly aspirate small amounts of secretions that either resolve spontaneously, or progress to clinical pneumonia. In intubated patients, organisms enter the lungs through leakage around the endotracheal tube cuff. Factors that increase the risk of aspiration increase the risk of HAP. These include sedation, delirium, impaired consciousness, intubation, vomiting, and abnormal swallowing. Proton pump inhibitors are also associated with an increased risk of pneumonia, presumably because they facilitate greater microbial colonization of the upper gastrointestinal tract.

Causative organisms mirror the microbiome of the mouth. They vary according to how long patients have been hospitalized. Early infections tend to be caused by the same organisms that cause community-acquired pneumonia, namely *Streptococcus pneumoniae*, *Haemophilus influenzae*, *Moraxella catarrhalis*, and respiratory viruses such as influenza. Later infections are typically caused by *Staphylococcus aureus* and Gram-negative organisms such as *Pseudomonas*, *Klebsiella*, *Enterobacter*, and *Acinetobacter*. The longer patients remain in hospital, the greater the risk of colonization and infection with multidrug-resistant bacteria, including methicillin-resistant *S. aureus*, extended-spectrum beta-lactamase-resistant Gram negatives, and carbapenem-resistant Enterobacteraciae.

DIAGNOSIS

There are no pathognomonic findings of VAP. The cardinal signs sought by clinicians (fever, hypoxemia, purulent sputum, leukocytosis, and new radiographic infiltrates) are all insensitive, with positive and negative likelihood ratios near one (**Table 187-1**). Even when present in combination, these signs have a low positive likelihood ratio.

The limited diagnostic value of these signs is due to the complexity of the patient population at risk for VAP. Hospitalized patients in general, and ventilated patients in particular, tend to be at risk for a wide array of complications. The clinical signs associated with pneumonia have a broad differential diagnosis, including noninfectious aspiration pneumonitis, thromboembolic disease, sepsis, atelectasis, pulmonary edema, hemorrhage, contusion, and acute respiratory distress syndrome. Typically, only about a third of patients with the clinical syndrome of VAP (fever, purulent sputum, leukocytosis, and a new infiltrate) have confirmed pneumonia if they undergo intensive investigation or autopsy. Instead, two or more alternative processes are often present that alone or in combination mimic the clinical picture of VAP (eg, atelectasis and line-associated bacteremia).

Laboratory analysis of pulmonary secretions is critical to aid diagnosis and guide treatment, but considerable judgment is still required to make sense of microbiology results, as their predictive power is nuanced (**Table 187-2**). False-positive and false-negative cultures are common. False-positive cultures usually reflect contamination of the specimen with oral or endotracheal tube colonizers.

TABLE 187-1 Likelihood Ratios of Clinical Signs in Ventilator-Associated Pneumonia

Sign	Positive LR	Negative LR
Fever	1.2	0.86
Hypoxemia	1.1	0.91
Purulent sputum (macroscopic)	1.3	0.63
Leukocytosis	1.3	0.74
New radiographic infiltrate	1.7	0.35
Two or more of fever, leukocytosis, and/or purulent sputum	2.8	0.41

TABLE 187-2 Likelihood Ratios of Laboratory Findings in Ventilator-Associated Pneumonia

Sign	Positive LR	Negative LR
>50% neutrophils in BAL fluid	2.0	0.09
Organisms seen on Gram stain		
Blind bronchial aspirate	2.1	0.60
Blinded BAL fluid sampling (mini-BAL)	5.3	0.50
Fiberoptically guided BAL fluid sampling (regular BAL)	18	0.56
Quantitative cultures		
Blind bronchial aspirate (>10⁵ CFU/mL)	9.6	0.42
Fiberoptically guided BAL fluid sample (>10⁴ CFU/mL)	1.4	0.78
Protected specimen brush (>10³ CFU/mL)	1.6	0.81

BAL, bronchoalveolar lavage; CFU, colony-forming units.

False-negative cultures are due to sampling an uninfected lung segment, inhibition of bacterial growth by prior antibiotic exposure, or failure to cross an arbitrarily set quantitative growth threshold.

The absence of neutrophils in bronchoalveolar lavage (BAL) fluid helps rule out VAP, but their presence is not diagnostic. By extension, a Gram stain of good quality expectorated sputum or endotracheal aspirate with few or no neutrophils probably makes HAP unlikely. Visualizing organisms on a BAL Gram stain is suggestive of VAP, and can provide clues about etiology. Organisms on Gram stain from blind bronchial aspirates and expectorated sputum are less reliable, since these specimens are more prone to contamination. While cultures tend to magnify small amounts of contamination, the converse is true when looking at quantitative culture data. Positive quantitative cultures from BAL specimens, which have low growth thresholds for positivity, are often contaminants, but exuberant growth from a bronchial aspirate, which has a high growth threshold for positivity, is predictive of VAP, presumably because bona fide disease has a very high bioburden that is able to outgrow bystander bacteria contaminating the specimen.

Meta-analysis of randomized controlled trials comparing routine BAL to endotracheal aspirates for the diagnosis of suspected VAP suggests no differences in mortality, length of stay, appropriateness of antibiotic choices, or total amount of antibiotic usage between invasive and noninvasive diagnostic techniques. As such, bronchoscopy should be reserved for patients who are failing initial therapy.

Radiographic studies contribute to diagnosis, but they are also imprecise. Chest radiographs have low sensitivity and positive predictive values for pneumonia relative to computed tomography. Portable radiographs often suffer from technical factors that limit interpretation, such as poor inspiration, patient rotation, and obscuring of the lung fields by overlying support tubes and lines. As these patients are prone to fluid shifts, uneven ventilation, barotrauma, and alveolar damage, new radiographic opacities may represent pulmonary edema, pleural effusions, or atelectasis, rather than infectious infiltrates. Computed tomography can help distinguish between these entities, but even this modality is imperfect. Atelectasis, pneumonitis, edema, and hemorrhage can resemble consolidation, particularly on noncontrast studies, and it is difficult to distinguish new from resolving infiltrates with a single study. Radiographic findings always need to be interpreted with the patient's clinical picture in mind.

Given the absence of definitive signs, laboratory studies, or radiographic evidence for the diagnosis of HAP, identification and management of HAP is a dynamic process that requires repeatedly integrating findings from clinical examination, sputum findings, and serial radiography to make a presumptive diagnosis. Both diagnosis and management demand great humility, frequent revaluation, and a low threshold to alter therapy or look for diseases other than pneumonia if initial presumptions are not borne out by a patient's clinical trajectory.

DIFFERENTIAL DIAGNOSIS

Most ventilated patients with fever, purulent sputum, and radiographic infiltrates do not have pneumonia. These patients often have abnormal underlying lungs, and are prone to an array of complications that collectively or individually mimic VAP. For example, hypoxemia and an abnormal chest radiograph might be due to atelectasis or pulmonary edema. Fever, leukocytosis and purulent secretions might be due to tracheobronchitis or sinusitis, or the combination of pulmonary edema with simultaneous infection outside the lungs, such as central venous catheter-associated bloodstream infection or *C. difficile* colitis. In addition, lungs undergoing mechanical ventilation are in a state of flux due to fluid shifts, mucus plugging, segmental variations in ventilation pressures, and endotracheal tube interference with the clearance of secretions. These changes can lead to the transient appearance of pulmonary syndromes which resemble VAP, but often resolve spontaneously without antibiotics. Changes in the quality or quantity of pulmonary secretions do not necessarily indicate infection, but may be due to impaired clearance of normal pulmonary secretions due to a weak cough or the disruptive presence of an endotracheal tube.

Several serious conditions also mimic VAP. Pulmonary embolism, aspiration pneumonitis, vasculitis, pulmonary hemorrhage, pneumothorax, organizing pneumonia, and acute respiratory distress syndrome may all present with fever, leukocytosis, hypoxemia, abnormal pulmonary secretions, and radiographic infiltrates. True lung infections may also be secondary to other processes, such as right-sided endocarditis. Depending on the clinical scenario, clinicians may consider a variety of other tests, such as CT angiography, bronchoscopy with or without biopsy, rheumatologic tests, echocardiography, measurement of pulmonary capillary wedge pressures, and video-assisted thorascopic biopsy.

TRIAGE/HOSPITAL ADMISSION

Outpatients with possible health care associated pneumonia should be assessed for clinical stability. Mortality prediction scores such as the Pneumonia Severity Index (PSI), CURB-65, and Severe Community-Acquired Pneumonia (SCAP) scores were developed and validated for patients with community-acquired pneumonia. Their applicability to patients with HAP is unknown. However, they are still helpful to the extent that they highlight clinical signs that most likely portend a poor prognosis in all pneumonias: age ≥65, confusion, tachypnea, hypotension, hypoxemia, uremia, and multilobar involvement. Outpatients with these signs are more likely to require admission. Inpatients with these signs require close observation for deterioration that might necessitate ICU transfer. Persistent hypoxemia, hypercapnia, and hypotension are indications for ICU admission. Blood and sputum specimens should be obtained for culture and sensitivities to expedite detection of antibiotic-resistant strains.

Patients with illness of intermediate severity may be candidates for noninvasive strategies to avoid intubation, such as high-flow oxygen by nasal cannula or noninvasive positive pressure ventilation. Both approaches appear to be beneficial in selected populations. High-flow oxygen by nasal cannula is useful in patients with hypoxemic respiratory failure, while noninvasive positive pressure ventilation is more appropriate for patients with exacerbations of chronic obstructive lung disease or congestive heart failure. However, noninvasive strategies carry risk if they delay intubation in severe disease. Practitioners are therefore advised to discuss their use with pulmonary, critical care, and respiratory therapy colleagues.

TREATMENT OPTIONS

Inappropriate or delayed treatment is associated with increased mortality. The push for early aggressive treatment has to be balanced against the many conditions that mimic pneumonia, the risks of antibiotic therapy, and the inadequacy of clinical signs, microbiology, and radiography to definitively confirm pneumonia in this population. Broad-spectrum agents should be started as soon as possible in vulnerable patients and those with multiple negative prognostic signs. Equivocal cases may merit narrower spectrum therapy, or even close observation alone. In all cases, it is critical to deliberately re-evaluate patients at 24 hours and daily thereafter to assess whether pneumonia seems more or less likely, whether investigation for other disorders is warranted, and whether antibiotics ought to be tailored, broadened, or stopped.

Reassessment should take into account the clinical course, the results of sputum or endotracheal aspirate cultures, and follow-up radiographs. A patient whose pulmonary syndrome has resolved or whose radiography has substantially improved in the space of a single day most likely did not have pneumonia, and antibiotics can safely be stopped. However, if the patient's syndrome is just starting to show signs of improvement, it is reasonable to continue treatment.

Antibiotics should be tailored according to culture results at this point. Patients who fail to improve or worsen despite antibiotics merit evaluation for organisms resistant to current antibiotics, for complications such as a lung abscess or empyema, or for alternative diagnoses such as viral pneumonia, pulmonary embolism, cryptogenic organizing pneumonia, pulmonary vasculitis, or acute respiratory distress syndrome. Bronchoscopy and directed fungal, mycobacterial, and viral studies are warranted in failing patients whose sputum or endotracheal aspirate cultures are unrevealing.

Initial treatment choice depends upon the timing of the pulmonary syndrome relative to admission, and patient risk factors for resistant organisms. Previously healthy patients who develop HAP within the first 3 to 5 days of admission (typically due to an aspiration event immediately preceding or following admission) are usually infected with the same relatively susceptible organisms that cause community-acquired pneumonia: pneumococcus, *Haemophilus*, *Moraxella*, *Legionella*, *Mycoplasma*, and respiratory viruses. A respiratory fluoroquinolone such as levofloxacin or moxifloxacin, or combination therapy with a third-generation cephalosporin with or without a macrolide, is usually adequate for this population. Suggested dosing for patients with normal renal function is shown in **Table 187-3**.

Antibiotic choices should be modified in light of each patient's presenting history, epidemiologic risks, prior infections, recent antibiotic exposure, and the local microbial ecology. Patients that report a biphasic respiratory illness with transient improvement, followed by severe symptoms, may have bacterial superinfection following a respiratory virus. *S. aureus* is a frequent pathogen in this setting and should be covered with the initial empiric regimen. MRSA coverage, such as vancomycin or linezolid, is prudent for patients with severe illness or a history of recent exposure to IV antibiotics. Patients with structural lung disease and prior infections are more likely to be infected with antibiotic-resistant nonenteric Gram negatives, such as *Pseudomonas* or *Stenotrophomonas*. Patients that have recently been exposed to fluoroquinolones are more likely to be colonized with fluoroquinolone-resistant organisms.

Patients who have been in hospital for more than 5 days, who have recently been exposed to antibiotics, who have a history of

TABLE 187-3 Suggested Doses of Antibiotics Commonly Used to Treat Health Care Associated, Hospital-Acquired, and Ventilator-Associated Pneumonia

Antibiotic	Suggested Dose (Normal Renal Function)	Dose Modification for Renal Dysfunction?
Antibiotics appropriate for patients more at risk for community-acquired pathogens		
Ceftriaxone	2 g IV every 24 h	No
Levofloxacin	750 mg orally or IV every 24 h	Yes
Moxifloxacin	400 mg orally or IV every 24 h	No
Azithromycin	500 mg orally every 24 h	No
Antibiotics active against MRSA pneumonia		
Vancomycin	15-20 mg/kg IV every 8-12 h In seriously ill patients, begin with a loading dose of 25-30 mg/kg; goal trough 15-20 mg/L	Yes
Linezolid	600 mg orally or IV every 12 h	No
Antipseudomonal agents		
Ceftazidime	2 g IV every 8 h	Yes
Cefepime	2 g IV every 8 h	Yes
Ciprofloxacin	500-750 mg orally every 12 h or 400 mg IV every 12 h	Yes
Imipenem	500 mg IV every 6 h	Yes
Meropenem	1-2 g IV every 8 h	Yes
Piperacillin-tazobactam	4.5 g IV every 6 h	Yes
Aztreonam	2 g IV every 8 h	Yes
Gentamicin	7 mg/kg IV every 24 h Goal trough <1 µg/mL	Yes
Tobramycin	7 mg/kg IV every 24 h Goal trough <1 mcg/mL	Yes
Amikacin	20 mg/kg IV every 24 h Goal trough <4-5 mcg/mL	Yes

drug-resistant infections, or who have a history of regular contact with health care facilities (including acute care hospitals, skilled nursing and rehabilitation facilities, dialysis and infusion centers) are at higher risk of harboring drug-resistant organisms.

PRACTICE POINT

Antibiotic selection in nursing home pneumonia

- There is a paucity of data to guide treatment of pneumonia in patients admitted to the hospital from nursing homes. According to the joint guidelines of the American Thoracic Society and the Infectious Diseases Society of America, these patients should be considered to be at risk for multidrug-resistant pathogens, such as MRSA and *Pseudomonas*, and treated accordingly. However, for many patients who acquire pneumonia while in a nursing home, the microbiology is similar to that of community-acquired pneumonia. The nursing home patients at highest risk for antibiotic-resistant pathogens are those with severe illness, immune suppression, hospitalization within the past 3 months, antibiotic therapy within the past 6 months, poor functional status, and who live in a locale with a high prevalence of multidrug-resistant organisms.

Empiric treatment in this population should include coverage for MRSA and multidrug-resistant Gram negatives such as *Pseudomonas*, *E. coli*, *Enterobacter*, and *Klebsiella*, particularly in hospitals with high prevalence of drug-resistant pathogens. It is wise to include two Gram-negative agents in empiric therapy for patients with serious infections, given the increasing frequency of extended-spectrum beta-lactamases, carbapenemases, and other modes of resistance. Early treatment with two agents increases the likelihood that at least one agent will be active against the causative pathogen. Reasonable empiric coverage combinations include the following:

- Gram-positive coverage:
  - Vancomycin or linezolid
- Gram-negative coverage:
  - Two anti-Pseudomonal agents (choose one agent from each column):

Antipseudomonal cephalosporin (ceftazidime, cefepime)	Antipseudomonal quinolone (ciprofloxacin, levofloxacin)
Antipseudomonal carbapenem (meropenem, imipenem)	Antipseudomonal aminoglycoside (amikacin, tobramycin, gentamicin)
Piperacillin-tazobactam	
Aztreonam	

Suggested doses for patients with normal renal function are shown in Table 187-3. Aztreonam has a narrow spectrum of activity compared to most other Gram-negative agents in this list. It should therefore generally be reserved for patients with beta-lactam allergy and for combination therapy. Daptomycin is not recommended for respiratory infections, because it is inactivated by pulmonary surfactant. Doripenem and tigecycline have been associated with poor outcomes in patients with VAP.

PRACTICE POINT

Central nervous system (CNS) side effects of antimicrobials

- The elderly patients at high risk for health care associated pneumonia are also prone to CNS side effects from antibiotics. Carbapenems lower the seizure threshold, cefepime may cause delirium, and fluoroquinolones may both cause confusion and reduce the seizure threshold.
- The risk of these side effects may be reduced by using appropriate doses for age and renal function.

Once culture and susceptibility results are available, the regimen should be trimmed to the most parsimonious regimen possible, ideally a single agent. In most settings, there is little benefit to double coverage once antimicrobial susceptibilities of the causative pathogen are known.

Therapy should be continued until patients' physiological parameters (temperature, respiratory rate, oxygen saturation, and white blood cell count) are clearly normalizing. In uncomplicated cases, this usually requires less than a week. Randomized controlled trial data suggest that outcomes are similar for patients treated with 8 versus 15 days of antibiotics. Short courses are therefore preferred to minimize selection for drug-resistant pathogens and other adverse effects. Patients who fail to show signs of improvement within 48 to 72 hours merit further investigation for alternative diagnoses, drug-resistant pathogens, pyogenic complications, or underlying structural lung disease.

COMPLICATIONS

Patients with pneumonia occasionally develop septic complications such as empyema or pulmonary abscess. These are best detected on computed tomography. Some pathogens, such as *S. aureus*, *Pseudomonas*, and *Klebsiella* may cause necrotizing infections with pulmonary hemorrhage or cavitation. Anaerobes are also frequently implicated in abscesses and cavitating lesions. Patients with severe pneumonia, chemical aspiration, or barotrauma from mechanical ventilation are at risk for the acute respiratory distress syndrome. Clinicians need to be vigilant for complications of antibiotic therapy including *C. difficile*, drug fever, renal toxicity, hepatitis, bone marrow suppression, hemolysis, hypersensitivity reactions, and delirium. Patients may also suffer complications from intravascular antibiotic delivery devices, such as central lines and peripherally inserted central catheter lines, since they are loci for infection and thrombosis.

PREVENTION

In the intensive care setting, quality advocates recommend (and some states mandate) a bundle of measures to prevent VAP. These bundles vary, but usually include some or all of the following:

- Elevation of the head of the bed above 30°
- Oral care with an antiseptic such as chlorhexidine
- Daily assessment of readiness to extubate (spontaneous breathing trials)
- Daily cessation of sedative medications to determine the minimum necessary amount of sedation (spontaneous awakening trials)
- Deep vein thrombosis (DVT) prophylaxis
- Stress ulcer prophylaxis

However, these recommendations are controversial, as the evidence base underlying each bundle component varies considerably. The connection between DVT prophylaxis and pneumonia is unclear. Stress ulcer prophylaxis may paradoxically increase pneumonia rates. Aspiration of oral antiseptics may precipitate the acute respiratory distress syndrome. Although many hospitals have reported dramatic decreases in VAP rates after implementing these bundles, these reports need to be interpreted with caution. HAP and VAP definitions are highly subjective. Desires for lower rates may lead surveyors to subconsciously interpret subjective clinical signs more strictly and thereby detect fewer cases. Nonetheless, the plethora of reports suggesting lower VAP rates after implementing ventilator bundles have helped elevate ventilator bundles to be a de facto standard of care.

Minimizing sedation, daily sedative interruptions, and spontaneous breathing trials are probably the most powerful strategies within the bundle, since they have consistently been shown to decrease duration of mechanical ventilation and length of stay. Selective digestive decontamination with intravenous and topical antibiotics is associated with lower mortality rates but is rarely practiced in North America due to fears of nurturing multidrug-resistant bacteria. Early physical therapy and ambulation, even in ventilated patients, is emerging as a potent strategy to shorten length of stay, prevent delirium, and improve long-term outcomes.

DISCHARGE PLANNING

- Have antibiotic choices been reviewed in light of final culture data? If the pathogen is susceptible to an oral agent with high bioavailability, such as a fluoroquinolone or linezolid, then an oral agent to complete therapy is adequate. Otherwise, the patient will require a central line for IV therapy, with attendant implications for discharge.

- Has primary care or pulmonary follow-up been arranged to assess resolution of symptoms and to obtain repeat chest radiography? Chest imaging should be repeated 1 to 3 months following the infection to document clearance of lesions, and to assess the underlying parenchyma for occult lesions (this can be deferred if the patient had normal chest imaging immediately prior to developing HAP). Patients with persistent infiltrates require evaluation for endobronchial lesions causing postobstructive pneumonia, disorders that impair ciliary clearance of secretions such as cystic fibrosis, or alternative sources of pulmonary infiltrates such as congestive heart failure, cryptogenic organizing pneumonia, and vasculitis.
- For patients on acid suppressant medication, has the need for this been reassessed? Acid suppressants, particularly proton pump inhibitors, increase the risk of pneumonia, so these medications should be reserved for individuals at high risk for gastrointestinal bleeding.
- Have the patient, family, and other caregivers been educated about the need for aspiration precautions, where applicable?
- Have smokers been counseled regarding medications and behavioral strategies to facilitate smoking cessation?
- Is the patient up to date with vaccinations against influenza and pneumococcus?

SUGGESTED READINGS

Chastre J, Wolff M, Fagon JY, et al. Comparison of 8 vs 15 days of antibiotic therapy for ventilator-associated pneumonia in adults: a randomized trial. *JAMA*. 2003;290:2588-2598.

de Smet AM, Kluytmans JA, Cooper BS, et al. Decontamination of the digestive tract and oropharynx in ICU patients. *N Engl J Med*. 2009;360:20-31.

Girard TD, Kress JP, Fuchs BD, et al. Efficacy and safety of a paired sedation and ventilator weaning protocol for mechanically ventilated patients in intensive care (Awakening and Breathing Controlled trial): a randomised controlled trial. *Lancet*. 2008;371:126-134.

Heyland D, Dodek P, Muscedere J, Day A. A randomized trial of diagnostic techniques for ventilator-associated pneumonia. *N Engl J Med*. 2006;355:2619-2630.

Heyland D, Dodeck P, Muscedere J, Day A, Cook D. Randomized trial of combination versus monotherapy for the empiric treatment of suspected ventilator-associated pneumonia. *Crit Care Med*. 2008;36:737-744.

Kalil AC, Metersky ML, Klompas M, et al. Management of adults with hospital-acquired and ventilator-associated pneumonia: 2016 Clinical Practice Guidelines by the Infectious Diseases Society of America and the American Thoracic Society. *Clin Infect Dis*. 2016;63(5):e61-e111.

Klompas M. Does this patient have ventilator-associated pneumonia? *JAMA*. 2007;297:1583-1593.

Rothberg MB, Zilberberg MD, Pekow PS, et al. Association of guideline-based antimicrobial therapy and outcomes in healthcare-associated pneumonia. *J Antimicrob Chemother*. 2015;70:1573-1579.

Society for Healthcare Epidemiology of America and Infectious Disease Society of America. Strategies to prevent ventilator-associated pneumonia in acute care hospitals: 2014 Update. *Infect Control Hosp Epidemiol*. 2014;35:915-936.

CHAPTER 188

Intravascular Catheter-Related Infections: Management and Prevention

Saima Aslam, MD, MS

Key Clinical Questions

1 How are catheter-related infections diagnosed?

2 What are the potential complications of catheter-related infection?

3 What is the appropriate management of catheter-related infection?

4 When is it appropriate to attempt salvage of an infected intravascular catheter?

5 How can catheter-related infections be prevented?

EPIDEMIOLOGY

Indwelling vascular catheters are the most common cause of nosocomial bloodstream infections. They are particularly common among critically ill patients, hemodialysis-dependent patients, and persons receiving chemotherapy or total parenteral nutrition. In the United States, approximately 41,000 central line associated bloodstream infections (CLABSI) occurred in 2009, of which 18,000 were in the intensive care units (ICUs). Although these numbers represent an almost 50% reduction from the previous decade, CLABSIs are still associated with prolonged hospitalization up to 3 weeks, cost about $50,000 per episode, and continue to have an attributable mortality of 14% to 40%. CLABSI rates are now publically reported in the United States, and may be used as a basis to deny payment claims by the Centers for Medicare and Medicaid Services (CMS).

Staphylococci, including *Staphylococcus epidermidis* and *Staphylococcus aureus*, cause more than two-thirds to 90% of all CLABSI. Other infecting organisms include enteric Gram-negative rods, *Pseudomonas aeruginosa*, and *Candida* species. Less common pathogens include *Serratia marcescens*, *Enterobacter* species, *Burkholderia cepacia* complex, *Citrobacter freundii*, atypical mycobacteria, among others.

PATHOPHYSIOLOGY

Infections of vascular catheters arise from bacterial biofilm, comprised of bacteria embedded within an extracellular polysaccharide matrix on the catheter surface (**Figure 188-1**). Bacterial biofilm may develop as early as 24 hours after catheter placement. As shown by electron microscopy, biofilm forms on the external surface of short-term catheters that have been in place for <10 days, and may be found on the luminal surface of long-term catheters that have been in place for ≥10 days.

The first step in biofilm formation is the binding of free-floating, or planktonic, organisms to the catheter surface by cell-wall–associated adhesins. This is facilitated by the formation of a film of host fibrin and fibronectin on the catheter surface. Other factors favoring attachment include hydrophobic and electrostatic forces, cell surface structures such as pili or fimbriae, platelet binding, and shear stress from the fluid environment. Attached organisms multiply to form microcolonies, and secrete an extracellular polysaccharide matrix that forms the architectural structure of the biofilm. Bacteria embedded in biofilm typically have a lower metabolic rate and can demonstrate resistant phenotypes, making them less susceptible to the effects of antibiotics; the minimal inhibitory concentrations of microorganisms in biofilm can be up to 1000-fold higher than for planktonic organisms. Additionally, some antibiotics have difficulty penetrating biofilm and others are not effective in the relatively hypoxemic biofilm environment. This explains why biofilm-based infections are difficult to eradicate without removal of the infected device.

Catheter infection may arise by several routes. The external catheter may become colonized by skin flora during insertion, or by subsequent migration of skin organisms along the catheter surface. Luminal colonization occurs when microorganisms are introduced through the hub of the catheter. The risk of luminal infection increases with frequent manipulation of the hub. Hematogenous seeding of the catheter may occur during bloodstream infection from another source. Rarely, contaminated intravenous fluids or drugs can cause CLABSI, sometimes leading to outbreaks. **Table 188-1** lists factors associated with development of CLABSIs.

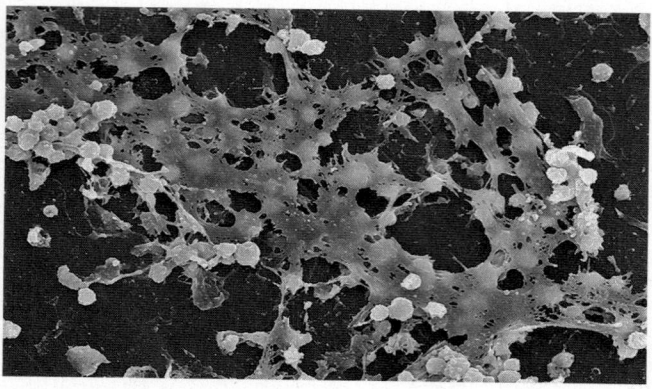

Figure 188-1 *Electron micrograph showing S. aureus bacteria embedded in biofilm on the luminal surface of an intravenous catheter.* (Public Health Image Library, Centers for Disease Control and Prevention, Rodney M. Donlan, PhD and Janice Carr.)

EVALUATION

The clinician must accurately make a diagnosis of catheter-related infection to appropriately treat the patient and reduce the rate of unnecessary procedures. The most common presenting manifestation of catheter-related infection is fever. Erythema and purulence at the catheter site are only present in a minority of patients. Sicker patients may have hypotension and tachycardia. Leukocytosis is usually present. Diagnosis can be established by either performing blood cultures from the catheter in situ or removing the catheter and sending the tip for culture.

■ DIAGNOSTIC TECHNIQUES NOT REQUIRING CATHETER REMOVAL

Diagnostic techniques that do not require catheter removal are not widely used. Quantitative blood cultures allow a comparison of the number of microorganisms in blood collected simultaneously via the lumen of the catheter and from a peripheral vein. A central-to-peripheral blood culture colony count ratio of 5 to 10:1 is indicative of the catheter being the source of the bacteremia. Although this technique is useful in diagnosing CLABSIs, it is not routinely

TABLE 188-1 Factors Associated with Increased Risk of Catheter-Related Bloodstream Infection

Size of catheter

Greater number of catheter lumens

Frequency of hub manipulation

Type of catheter (plastic > steel)

Location of catheter (central > peripheral; femoral > jugular > femoral > subclavian; lower extremity sites > upper extremity sites)

Type of placement (cutdown > percutaneous; nontunneled > tunneled)

Duration of catheter placement

Urgency of placement (emergent > elective)

Skills of person performing venipuncture (others > IV team)

Type of skin antisepsis (povidone-iodine > chlorhexidine)

Patient factors (neutropenia, immunosuppression, end-stage renal disease, burns)

Data from Beekmann SE, Henderson DK. Bacteremia due to percutaneous intravascular devices. In: Mandell GL, Bennett JE, and Dolin R, eds. *Principles and Practice of Infectious Diseases*, 6th ed. New York, NY: Churchill Livingstone; 2005:3347-3361.

performed in most hospitals. A single bacterial count of > 100 colony-forming units (CFU)/mL in the catheter blood specimen is also suggestive of CLABSI, in the presence of a positive peripheral blood culture.

Differential time to positivity (DTP) compares the time it takes for a blood culture to become positive when drawn from the catheter versus peripheral blood. The underlying assumption is that blood drawn via the lumen of an infected catheter will have higher number of bacterial colonies than that obtained from a peripheral blood draw, and thus will become positive earlier. When catheter cultures become positive ≥2 hours earlier than peripheral blood, DTP is quite sensitive for the diagnosis of CLABSI. The specificity of DTP is dramatically reduced in patients receiving antibiotics at the time cultures were drawn. Most hospitals have automated blood culture machines, making information on time to positivity readily available in the microbiology laboratory.

Endoluminal brushing of the catheter while still in place and subsequent culture is very sensitive for the diagnosis of catheter-related infection in patients with peripheral bacteremia. However, adverse events such as cardiac arrhythmias, embolization, and subsequent bacteremia have been reported.

■ DIAGNOSTIC TECHNIQUES REQUIRING CATHETER REMOVAL

The most commonly employed method in clinical microbiology laboratories is semiquantitative culture of the catheter tip, the so-called roll-plate method. This technique consists of rolling the distal 4 cm of the catheter tip on an agar plate for culture. A yield of ≥ 15 CFU of bacteria distinguishes catheter colonization from infection. A major limitation is that only microorganisms from the external surface of the catheter are cultured, potentially underdiagnosing catheters with primarily intraluminal infection. Rapid diagnosis of CLABSI may also be achieved by direct microscopic examination of the catheter tip stained with Gram stain or acridine orange.

A more sensitive technique involves sonication of the catheter tip to dislodge biofilm-embedded organisms, with culture of the resultant sonicate. This technique is much more sensitive than the roll-plate method, with a cutoff limit for infection of ≥10^2 to 10^3 CFU/catheter segment. This culturing technique retrieves organisms from both the external and internal surfaces of the catheter. **Table 188-2** shows the relative sensitivity and specificity of the methods outlined above.

■ DIFFERENTIAL DIAGNOSIS

Positive blood cultures must be distinguished from asymptomatic catheter colonization, as well as bacteremia from another source. Potentially life-threatening conditions that may masquerade as a CLABSI include infective endocarditis and septic thrombophlebitis.

COMPLICATIONS OF CATHETER-RELATED INFECTION

Complicated bacteremia should be suspected in patients with persistent bacteremia or fever. Potential complications of CLABSIs include infective endocarditis, septic thrombophlebitis, osteomyelitis, septic arthritis, meningitis, epidural abscess, metastatic abscess, catheter or venous thrombosis, prosthesis infection, various embolic phenomenon, and septic shock.

S. aureus bacteremia is associated with an especially high risk of complications, ranging from 25% to 43%. In one study, the strongest predictor of complicated bacteremia was a positive follow-up blood culture result at 48 to 96 hours. A scoring system based on the presence or absence of four risk factors (community acquisition, skin findings suggesting acute systemic infection, persistent fever at 72 hours, and positive follow-up blood culture at 48-96 hours) accurately identified complicated *S. aureus* bacteremia.

TABLE 188-2 Accuracy of Various Methods for the Diagnosis of CRBSIs

	Diagnostic Criteria	Accuracy		Disadvantages
		Sensitivity	Specificity	
Techniques without CVC removal				
Simultaneous quantitative blood cultures	Quantitative blood culture drawn through CVC yields CFU count fivefold higher or more than CFU count from simultaneously drawn blood from peripheral vein	93%	97%-100%	Labor intensive, costly
Differential time to positivity	Blood culture drawn from CVC becomes positive ≥2 h before simultaneously drawn blood culture from peripheral vein	89%-90%	72%-87%	Hard to interpret when patient is taking antibiotics through the CVC
CVC-drawn quantitative blood culture	Quantitative blood culture from CVC is ≥ 100 CFU/mL	81%-86%	85%-96%	Cannot differentiate between CRBSI and high-grade bacteremia
Acridine orange leucocyte cytospin	Presence of any bacteria	87% (96% if followed by Gram stain)	94% (92% if followed by Gram stain)	Not widely tested or used
Endoluminal brush	Quantitative culture with > 100 CFU/mL	95%	84%	May induce bacteremia, arrhythmia, embolization
Techniques requiring CVC removal				
Semiquantitative CVC tip culture, roll plate	≥ 15 CFU/mL from CVC tip	45%-84%	85%	Unable to culture organisms embedded intraluminally
Quantitative CVC culture: centrifugation, vortexing, sonication	≥ 10³ CFU from CVC tip	82%-83%	89%-97%	The cut-off point of ≥10³ CFU vs ≥10² CFU is not well defined
Microscopy of stained CVC: Gram stain and acridine orange staining	Direct visualization of the microorganisms	84%-100%	97%-100%	Labor intensive, impractical

CFU, colony forming units; CRBSI, catheter-related bloodstream infection; CVC, central venous catheter.
From Raad I, Hanna H, Maki D. Intravascular catheter-related infections: advances in diagnosis, prevention and management. *Lancet Infect Dis.* 2007;7:645-657. Reprinted with permission from Elsevier.

Another study evaluated all cases of central venous catheter (CVC) related *S. aureus* bacteremia in order to determine host and pathogen factors that were associated with hematogenous complications. On multivariable analysis, symptom duration, hemodialysis dependence, presence of a long-term intravascular catheter or a noncatheter device, and infection with methicillin-resistant *S. aureus* (MRSA) were significantly associated with complications. Thus, at least in patients with *S. aureus* CLABSI the above mentioned factors should prompt providers to remove the infected catheter as soon as possible.

Vascular catheter infections can be associated with thrombosis and septic thrombophlebitis. This may be manifested by evidence of peripheral emboli distal to the site of catheter insertion, or swelling in an extremity. In one study, thrombosis was a common complication of CVC-related *S. aureus* bacteremia (71%), with poor sensitivity of physical examination findings.

Many cases of infective endocarditis are not suspected clinically and therefore are not detected. Studies using transesophageal echocardiogram (TEE) to identify endocarditis in patients with *S. aureus* bacteremia have shown high rates of valvular vegetations (25%-32%). TEE is more sensitive than transthoracic echocardiogram, and is most sensitive when performed 5 to 7 days after the onset of bacteremia. Clinically, endocarditis is seen in 17% to 20% of cases of *S. aureus* bacteremia. In general, patients with *S. aureus* bacteremia have a high 90-day mortality rate of 25% to 30%.

TEE should be considered in patients with CLABSI who have a prosthetic heart valve, pacemaker, or implantable defibrillator, persistent bacteremia or fungemia, or fever more than 3 days after

catheter removal and initiation of appropriate antibiotic therapy. TEE should also be obtained for any case of *S. aureus* CLABSI in which a duration of therapy less than 4 to 6 weeks is being considered. Depending on the clinical scenario, it may be reasonable to seek other metastatic foci of *S. aureus* infection, such as vertebral osteomyelitis in patients with back pain.

Some experts believe that a TEE is not required for patients without intravascular hardware who have rapid resolution of *S. aureus* bacteremia after initiation of appropriate antimicrobial therapy.

INPATIENT MANAGEMENT

The Infectious Diseases Society of America last published guidelines for the management of catheter-related infections in 2009. **Figure 188-2** describes the approach to a patient with an infected catheter. Treatment differs depending on the type of vascular catheter used.

■ PERIPHERAL CATHETER

Infection of peripheral catheters is generally associated with local manifestations such as erythema, tenderness, or suppuration. Systemic signs such as fever or leukocytosis may be present. In general, infected peripheral catheters should be immediately removed. Local symptoms may be alleviated with warm compresses. If suppuration is present, the exudate should be cultured in order to provide appropriate therapy. Most of these infections are caused by Gram-positive skin flora, and empiric therapy against these organisms may be started. In the absence of bacteremia, 7 to 10 days of oral

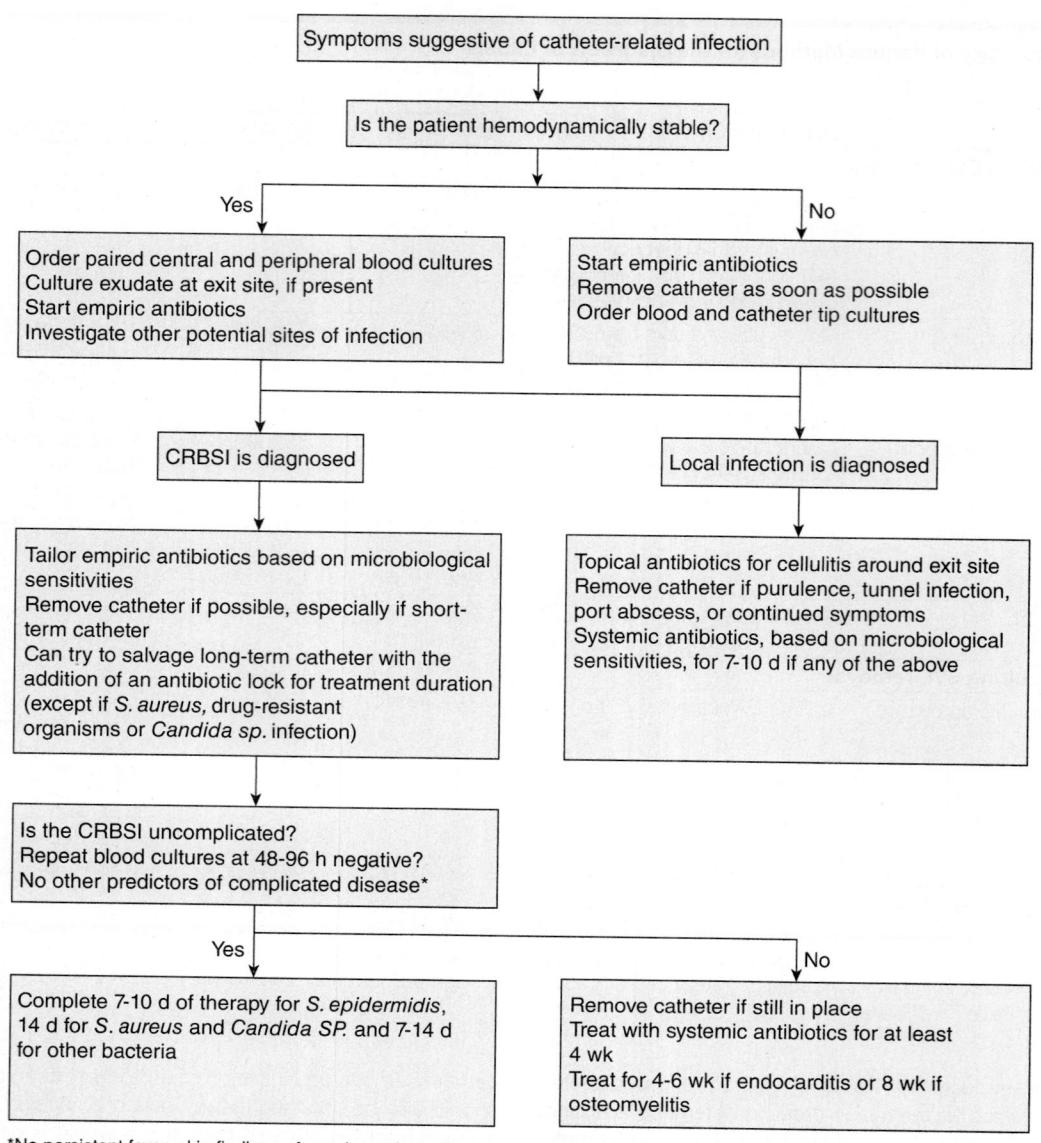

Figure 188-2 *Approach to suspected catheter-related infection.*

Contents of figure:

Symptoms suggestive of catheter-related infection

Is the patient hemodynamically stable?

Yes

Order paired central and peripheral blood cultures
Culture exudate at exit site, if present
Start empiric antibiotics
Investigate other potential sites of infection

No

Start empiric antibiotics
Remove catheter as soon as possible
Order blood and catheter tip cultures

CRBSI is diagnosed

Tailor empiric antibiotics based on microbiological sensitivities
Remove catheter if possible, especially if short-term catheter
Can try to salvage long-term catheter with the addition of an antibiotic lock for treatment duration (except if *S. aureus*, drug-resistant organisms or *Candida sp.* infection)

Local infection is diagnosed

Topical antibiotics for cellulitis around exit site
Remove catheter if purulence, tunnel infection, port abscess, or continued symptoms
Systemic antibiotics, based on microbiological sensitivities, for 7-10 d if any of the above

Is the CRBSI uncomplicated?
Repeat blood cultures at 48-96 h negative?
No other predictors of complicated disease*

Yes

Complete 7-10 d of therapy for *S. epidermidis*, 14 d for *S. aureus* and *Candida SP.* and 7-14 d for other bacteria

No

Remove catheter if still in place
Treat with systemic antibiotics for at least 4 wk
Treat for 4-6 wk if endocarditis or 8 wk if osteomyelitis

*No persistent fever, skin findings of sepsis, endocarditis, suppurative thrombophlebitis, metastatic infection, or intravascular hardware, and lack of community-onset bacteremia for *S. aureus*.

antibiotic are recommended. The risk of bacteremia from such an infection is low.

PRACTICE POINT

Septic thrombophlebitis

- Septic (suppurative) thrombophlebitis should be suspected in patients with bacteremia or fungemia that persists despite 72 hours or more of adequate antimicrobial therapy, and who have no evidence of endocarditis. The diagnosis is made on the basis of positive blood cultures plus evidence of a clot by ultrasound, CT scan, or another imaging study. Treatment consists of catheter removal, followed by a minimum of 2 weeks of intravenous antibiotic therapy when a peripheral vein is involved; this should be increased to at least 4 weeks when a central vein is infected. Patients are often anticoagulated, although no randomized controlled trials have been performed to support this practice. Rarely, the infected vein needs to be ligated and removed for failure to respond to conventional therapy.

◼ NONTUNNELED CENTRAL VENOUS CATHETER

CVCs in patients with unexplained fever should not routinely be removed unless there is a local infection at the site of insertion. Catheter removal is only indicated when CLABSI is documented, local infection at the site of catheter insertion is present, or if the patient is hemodynamically unstable and the catheter is suspected as the source of infection. The tip of the removed catheter should be sent for culture. If a catheter is to be removed for suspected infection, guidewire exchange of the catheter can decrease the risk of mechanical complications. However, if culture of the removed catheter is positive, the newly inserted catheter should be replaced a second time *at a new site.* **Table 188-3** describes pathogen-specific antibiotics that can be used in the treatment of CLABSI.

◼ TUNNELED OR IMPLANTED CATHETER

Tunneled catheters with uncomplicated exit site infections (ie, those without systemic signs of infection, positive blood culture results, or purulence) can be managed with topical antimicrobial agents. If an uncomplicated exit site infection fails to resolve with topical therapy, or is accompanied by purulent drainage, systemic antibiotics

TABLE 188-3 Intravenous Antimicrobial Therapy for Catheter-related Bloodstream Infections

Pathogen	Preferred Antimicrobial Agent	Example, Dosage*	Alternative Antimicrobial Agent	Comment
Gram-positive cocci				
Staphylococcus aureus				
Methicillin- susceptible	Penicillinase-resistant Pen[?]	Naf or Oxa, 2 g every 4 h	Cfaz, 2 g every 8 h; or Vm, 15 mg/kg every 12 h	Penicillinase-resistant Pen or Csps are preferred to Vm.[§] For patients receiving hemodialysis, administer Cfaz 20 mg/kg (actual weight), round to nearest 500 mg increment, after dialysis
Methicillin- resistant[©]	Vm	Vm,15 mg/kg every 12 h	Dapto, 6-8 mg/kg/d, or linezolid; or Vm plus (Rif or Gm); or TMP-SMZ alone (if susceptible)	Strains of *S. aureus* with reduced susceptibility or resistance to Vm have been reported; strains resistant to linezolid and strains resistant to Dapto have been reported
Coagulase-negative staphylococci				
Methicillin susceptible	Penicillinase-resistant Pen	Naf or Oxa, 2 g every 4 h	First-generation Csp or Vm or TMP-SMZ (if susceptible)	Vm has dosing advantages over Naf and Oxa, but the latter are preferred because of concerns about increasing Vm resistance
Methicillin- resistant	Vm	Vm, 15 mg/kg IV every 12 h	Dapto 6 mg/kg/d, linezolid, or Quin/Dalf	For adults <40 kg linezolid dose should be 10 mg/kg; strains resistant to linezolid have been reported
Enterococcus faecalis/ Enterococcus faecium				
Amp susceptible	Amp or (Amp or Pen) ± aminoglycoside	Amp, 2 g every 4 h or every 6 h; or Amp ± Gm, 1 mg/kg every 8 h	Vm	Vm may have dosing advantages over Amp, but there are concerns about Vm resistance
Amp resistant, Vm susceptible	Vm ± aminoglycoside	Vm, 15 mg/kg IV every 12 h ± Gm, 1 mg/kg every 8 h	Linezolid or Dapto 6 mg/kg/d	Quin/Dalf is not effective against *E. faecalis*
Amp resistant, Vm resistant	Linezolid or Dapto	Linezolid, 600 mg every 12 h; or Dapto 6 mg/kg/d	Quin/Dalf 7.5 mg/kg every 8 h	Susceptibility of Vm-resistant enterococci isolates varies; Quin/Dalf is not effective against *E. faecalis*
Gram-negative bacilli**				
***Escherichia coli* and *Klebsiella* species**				
ESBL-negative	Third-generation Csp	Ctri, 1-2 g/d	Cipro or Atm	Susceptibility varies
ESBL-positive	Carbapenem	Erta,1 g/d; Imi, 500 mg every 6 h; Mero, 1 g every 8 h; or doripenem, 500 mg every 8 h	Cipro or Atm	Susceptibility varies
Enterobacter* species and *Serratia marcescens	Carbapenem	Erta, 1 g/d; Imi, 500 mg every 6 h; Mero, 1 g every 8 h	Cefepime or Cipro	Susceptibility varies
***Acinetobacter* species**	Amp/Sulb or carbapenem	Amp/Sulb, 3 g every 6 h; or Imi, 500 mg every 6 h; Mero, 1 g every 8 h	—	Susceptibility varies
Stenotrophomonas maltophilia	TMP-SMZ	TMP-SMZ, 3-5 mg/kg every 8 h	Tic and Clv	—
Pseudomonas aeruginosa	Fourth-generation Csp or carbapenem or Pip and Tazo with or without aminoglycoside	Cefepime, 2 g every 8 h; or Imi, 500 mg every 6 h; or Mero, 1 g every 8 h; or Pip and Tazo, 4.5 g every 6 h, Amik, 15 mg/kg every 24 h or Tobra 5-7 mg/kg every 24 h	—	Susceptibility varies
Burkholderia cepacia	TMP-SMZ or carbapenem	TMP-SMZ, 3-5 mg/kg every 8 h; or Imi, 500 mg every 6 h; or Mero, 1 g every 8 h	—	Other species, such as *B acidovorans* and *Burkholderia (Ralstonia) pickettii*, may be susceptible to same antimicrobial agents

(Continued)

TABLE 188-3 Intravenous Antimicrobial Therapy for Catheter-related Bloodstream Infections (*Continued*)

Pathogen	Preferred Antimicrobial Agent	Example, Dosage*	Alternative Antimicrobial Agent	Comment
Fungi				
Candida albicans or other *Candida* species	Echinocandin or fluconazole (if organism is susceptible)	Caspo, 70 mg/kg loading dose, then 50 mg/kg/d; micafungin,100 mg/d; anidulafungin, 200 mg loading dose followed by 100 mg/d; or fluconazole, 400-600 mg/d	Lipid AmB preparations	Echinocandin should be used to treat critically ill patients until fungal isolate is identified
Uncommon pathogens				
Corynebacterium jeikeium (group JK)	Vm	Vm, 15 mg/kg every 4 h	Linezolid (based on in vitro activity)	Check susceptibilities for other corynebacteria
Chryseobacterium (Flavobacterium) species	Fluoroquinolone, such as Lvfx	Lvfx 750 mg every 24 h	TMP-SMZ or Imi or Mero	Based on in vitro activity
Ochrobacterium anthropi	TMP-SMZ or fluoroquinolone	TMP-SMZ, 3-5 mg/kg every 8 h; or Cpfx, 400 mg every 12 h	Imi, Mero, Erta, or Dori plus aminoglycoside	—
Malassezia furfur	AmB	—	Voriconazole	Intravenous lipids should be discontinued; some experts recommend removal of catheter
Mycobacterium species	Susceptibility varies by species	—	—	Different species have wide spectra of susceptibility to antimicrobials [256, 257]

Note: AmB, amphotericin B; Amp, ampicillin; Atm, aztreonam; Cfaz, cefazolin; cfur, cefuroxime; Clv, clavulanate; Cpfx, ciprofloxacin; Csp, cephalosporin; Ctri, ceftriaxone; Czid, ceftazidime; Erta, ertapenem; Gm, gentamicin; Imi, Imipenem; iv, intravenous; Ket, ketoconazole; Lvfx, levofloxacin; Mero, meropenem; Meth, methicillin; Mez, mezlocillin; Naf, nafcillin; Oxa, oxacillin; Pen, penicillin; PenG, penicillin G; po, by mouth; Pip, piperacillim; Quin/Dalf, quinupristin/dalfopristin; Rif, rifampin; Sulb, sulbactam; Tic, ticarcillin; Tm, tobramycin; TMP-SMZ, trimethoprim-sulfamethoxazole; Vm, vancomycin.

*Initial antibiotic dosages for adult patients with normal renal and hepatic function and no known drug interactions. Fluoroquinolones should not be used for patients <18 y of age.

?Pen, if the strain is susceptible.

§Some clinicians will add an aminoglycoside for the first 5 d of therapy.

**Pending susceptibility results for the isolate.

From Mermel LA, Allon M, Bouza E, et al. Clinical practice guidelines for the diagnosis and management of intravascular catheter-related infection. *Clin Infect Dis.* 2009;49:1-45. Reprinted with permission from the University of Chicago Press.

should be given based on the antimicrobial susceptibility of the causative pathogen. The catheter should be removed if treatment with systemic antibiotics fails.

When tunneled or implanted catheters are associated with bacteremia, it is preferable to place a new catheter at a new location once the bacteremia has resolved, as documented by negative blood cultures. If other vascular access sites are unavailable, or the patient is at high risk for bleeding in the setting of CLABSI not complicated by an exit site or tunnel infection, exchange of the infected catheter over a guidewire can be performed. Guidewire exchange can also be considered for patients whose symptoms resolve after 2 to 3 days of IV antibiotic therapy and who do not have evidence of metastatic infection.

Catheter salvage can be considered if the patient is hemodynamically stable, does not have bacteremia complicated by emboli, endocarditis, or thrombophlebitis, and is infected with an organism that is readily treatable. Catheter salvage may be attempted with systemic antibiotics and simultaneous antibiotic lock solution (ALS; high dose of antibiotics instilled locally in the catheter lumen) for the duration of systemic therapy. If the infection is due to *S. aureus*, drug-resistant organisms, or *Candida* species, catheter salvage should not be attempted due to the high rates of failure, recurrence, and complications.

■ HEMODIALYSIS CATHETER

A substantial proportion of patients with CLABSI who receive hemodialysis can be managed on an outpatient basis, given the ease of antibiotic administration and the frequency of access to the health care system. Since the risk of Gram-negative infections appears to be higher in this population than in nonhemodialysis patients, empiric antibiotics should always include coverage against both Gram-positive and Gram-negative organisms. Once a CLABSI is identified, catheter salvage may be attempted if the infection is due to an organism with low virulence and the patient is hemodynamically stable. This can be attempted using an antibiotic lock solution, in addition to systemic antibiotics. In the case of hemodialysis catheters, the antibiotic is mixed with an anticoagulant, and instilled locally within the catheter lumen when it is not in use.

An alternative to catheter exchange is replacement of the infected catheter with a new temporary catheter, either over a guidewire or at a new location, or prompt catheter removal with placement of a new long-term catheter once the bacteremia has resolved.

Vancomycin is less effective than nafcillin, oxacillin, or cefazolin in patients with bloodstream infection with methicillin-sensitive *S. aureus* (MSSA). Hemodialysis-dependent patients with MSSA bacteremia treated with vancomycin are at a higher risk of treatment failure than those who receive cefazolin. In the absence of allergy to beta-lactams, vancomycin should not be continued beyond empiric therapy for hemodialysis-dependent patients with MSSA bacteremia.

A recent meta-analysis comparing outcomes of various management strategies for hemodialysis CLABSI demonstrated a trend toward higher cure rates with guidewire exchange versus catheter salvage (67% vs 57%), although this was not statistically significant. The study also noted that cure rates were highest for coagulase-negative staphylococci, followed by Gram-negative rods and *S. aureus*. Among *S. aureus* infections specifically, guidewire exchange led to a higher cure than use of an antibiotic lock solution.

PRACTICE POINT

- Vancomycin is inferior to oxacillin, nafcillin, and cefazolin for the treatment of bloodstream infections due to MSSA. When MSSA is known to be the cause of bacteremia, empiric therapy with vancomycin should be switched to one of these beta-lactam agents, unless the patient has a beta-lactam allergy.

■ COMPLICATED VERSUS UNCOMPLICATED CLABSI

In general, patients with CLABSI due to *S. aureus* should receive at least 4 weeks of intravenous antibiotic therapy after catheter removal. However, selected patients with uncomplicated CLABSI due to *S. aureus* and a negative TEE may be considered for a 2-week antibiotic course after catheter removal. If patients have risk factors or clinical predictors of a complication, including persistent fever or positive blood cultures at 48 to 96 hours, a more aggressive approach to identify and treat potential complications should be pursued. The catheter must always be removed in such a case due to concern for persistent seeding of the bloodstream. Delay in removing the catheter increases the risk of complications. Even if a distinct complication is not uncovered, such patients should be treated with at least 4 weeks of IV antibiotics.

WHEN MAY SALVAGE OF AN INFECTED CATHETER BE ATTEMPTED?

Catheter salvage may be attempted for long-term catheters with intraluminal infection in hemodynamically stable patients with uncomplicated bacteremia. In catheter salvage, systemic antibiotics are given, in addition to an antibiotic lock solution. Lock therapy counters the inherent antimicrobial resistance of bacteria in biofilm by achieving a local antibiotic concentration within the catheter lumen that is 100- to 1000-fold higher than can be obtained by systemically administered antibiotics. Catheter salvage without ALS is not recommended, as it is associated with poor rates of success.

In small open-label trials, catheter salvage without relapse occurred in 77% of episodes with the use of ALS. However, success is much lower when the infecting organism is *S. aureus*. In hemodialysis catheters, the antibiotic is combined with an anticoagulant and instilled into each catheter lumen at the end of each dialysis session. In small uncontrolled studies with short-term follow-up, the success rate was 87% to 100% for infection due to Gram-negative pathogens and 75% to 84% for infection due to *S. epidermidis*, but only 40% to 55% for *S. aureus* infection. The overall success rate for catheter salvage was 57%, according to a recent meta-analysis involving only hemodialysis catheters. A small pilot trial showed improved success rates up to 83% when an antibiofilm agent, *N*-acetylcysteine, was added to the ALS in hemodialysis patients. Antibiotics that have been used in studies include vancomycin, cefazolin, linezolid, tigecycline, fluoroquinolones, and aminoglycosides. Generally, these are mixed with heparin, trisodium citrate, or sodium ethylenediaminetetraacetic acid (EDTA) as the anticoagulant.

PREVENTION

■ SITE OF CATHETER INSERTION

Catheter site influences the subsequent risk for infection and phlebitis. This is related in part to the risk for thrombophlebitis and density of local skin flora. Internal jugular catheters are more likely to become infected than subclavian catheters due to proximity of oropharyngeal secretions, higher skin temperature, and difficulties in immobilizing the catheter and maintaining an optimal dressing. Femoral catheters generally have rates of colonization, infection, and thrombosis that greatly exceed both subclavian and internal jugular catheters. More recent studies have demonstrated no difference in infection risk between the three sites when experienced operators placed CVCs with maximal sterile precautions and trained staff performed catheter care. Current guidelines recommend avoidance of femoral catheters whenever possible.

■ ASEPTIC TECHNIQUE

For short-term peripheral catheters, standard hand hygiene before catheter insertion or maintenance, combined with proper aseptic technique during catheter manipulation, protects against infection. Hand hygiene should be achieved with either a waterless, alcohol-based product or antibacterial soap and water with adequate rinsing. However, given the higher risk of infection with CVCs, more stringent antisepsis is recommended. Maximal sterile barrier precautions during insertion of CVCs, including sterile gloves, gown, cap, mask, and a large drape, lead to decreased rates of CLABIs, and are now a basic tenet of CLABSI prevention. Use of maximal barrier precautions prior to insertion of arterial lines has not been shown to be beneficial. The Healthcare Infection Control Practices Advisory Committee (HICPAC) and Infectious Diseases Society of America (IDSA) guidelines strongly recommend the use of maximum sterile barrier precautions during the insertion of all CVCs and pulmonary artery catheters.

■ CUTANEOUS ANTISEPSIS PRIOR TO CATHETER INSERTION

Multiple studies and meta-analyses demonstrated an almost 50% reduction in the rates of CLABSIs when site preparation with chlorhexidine was used, compared with 10% povidone-iodine or 70% alcohol. The alcohol-based preparation of chlorhexidine combines the rapid onset of killing by alcohol with the delayed antisepsis of chlorhexidine. Use of >0.5% chlorhexidine with alcohol for skin antisepsis prior to arterial catheter and CVC insertion is now included in the standard guidelines. Any skin antiseptic, such as povidone-iodine, 70% alcohol, tincture of iodine, an iodophor or chlorhexidine may be used prior to insertion of peripheral catheters.

■ TOPICAL ANTISEPTICS AND DRESSINGS AFTER CATHETER INSERTION

Routine use of povidone-iodine ointment at the catheter insertion site of hemodialysis catheters reduces the incidence of exit-site infections, catheter-tip colonization, and CLABSIs when compared with no ointment. Mupirocin ointment applied to the catheter insertion site also decreases the rate of CLABSIs. However, there are concern regarding the development of mupirocin-resistant organisms and the possible loss of integrity of polyurethane catheters. More recently, randomized trials using topical chlorhexidine or chlorhexidine-impregnated sponges applied to the catheter site have noted about 50% reduction in the rate of CLABSI, compared with topical povidone-iodine. A cost-benefit analysis based on the experience of Philadelphia-area hospitals estimated the potential annual United States net benefits to range from $275 million up to approximately $1.97 billion. Mortality analyses showed that nationwide use of chlorhexidine dressings might lead to up to 3906 fewer deaths annually in the United States.

Current guidelines recommend use of topical antibiotic ointment or cream only for hemodialysis catheters. Chlorhexidine-impregnated sponges at the catheter exit site are recommended for temporary short-term catheters if the institutional rate of CLABSI is high despite adherence to basic infection prevention measures.

The use of transparent dressings versus gauze dressings does not seem to affect the rate of CLABSI. However, transparent dressings permit continuous visual inspection of the catheter site, allow patients to bathe and shower without saturating the dressing, and require less frequent changes than do standard gauze and tape dressings. The choice of dressing can thus be a matter of preference. The data on frequency of dressing changes are not conclusive.

■ CATHETER SECUREMENT DEVICES

Compared with skin sutures, sutureless securement devices may decrease the rate of CLABSI by decreasing skin trauma, as well as decreasing bacterial colonization of the skin around the catheter. These devices increase catheter dwell time and decrease the overall rate of complications, and are now recommended instead of sutures to secure intravascular catheters.

■ ANTIMICROBIAL AND ANTISEPTIC CATHETERS

Several randomized controlled trials and two meta-analyses demonstrated that minocycline/rifampin-coated catheters significantly reduced CLABSIs, compared with placebo or chlorhexidine/silver sulfadiazine silver-coated catheters. Minocycline/rifampin-coated catheters have shown success in the hemodialysis population as well. In vitro studies demonstrate superior and prolonged activity of minocycline/rifampin-coated CVCs against staphylococci, compared with first-generation chlorhexidine/silver sulfadiazine-coated catheters, without the emergence of resistant organisms.

Chlorhexidine/sulfadiazine silver-coated catheters (both first-generation catheters with coating of only the external catheter surface, and second-generation catheters with coating of both the external and internal lumens) reduce catheter colonization, but not the clinical endpoint of CLABSI. A platinum/silver/carbon-impregnated catheter that allows ionic silver release has demonstrated variable decrease in catheter colonization, but no effect on the rate of CLABSIs.

The decision to use antimicrobial or anti-infective catheters should be based on the need to enhance prevention of CLABSI after standard procedures have been implemented, including staff education, use of maximal sterile barrier precautions, and use of >0.5% chlorhexidine preparation with alcohol for skin antisepsis during CVC insertion. The benefits of anti-infective catheters must be balanced against the risk of emergence of resistant pathogens and the higher costs of antimicrobial catheters.

■ ANTIBIOTIC LOCK SOLUTIONS

Catheter lock solutions have been used not only for treatment of infections but also for prevention. A recent meta-analysis of oncology patients demonstrated decreased rate of Gram-positive sepsis when long-term CVCs were locked or flushed with antibiotic-heparin combinations, compared to catheter locks using heparin alone. Antibiotics used included vancomycin, amikacin, and taurolidine. Further data from large prospective studies are required to address concerns regarding development of antibiotic resistance, though this has not been borne out thus far in observational and retrospective studies. Chelators such as EDTA or citrate have an anticoagulant activity similar to heparin, and enhance the activity of antimicrobial drugs against organisms embedded in biofilm. Other antimicrobial catheter lock solutions that may reduce catheter infection include minocycline and EDTA, gentamicin, and ethanol, at concentrations ranging between 25% and 40%.

A meta-analysis of randomized controlled trials showed that antibiotic catheter lock solutions in hemodialysis patients significantly reduced CLABSIs by 44% and catheter removal rates by 35%, compared with heparin lock alone. Use of citrate instead of heparin as an anticoagulant solution used for hemodialysis catheters has also demonstrated reduced rate of infections. Other agents associated with reduced hemodialysis catheter infections are taurolidine-citrate-heparin and gentamicin-citrate combinations.

Currently, use of antibiotic lock solutions is recommended in patients with long-term catheters who have had multiples episodes of CLABSI despite aseptic technique.

■ SCHEDULED REPLACEMENT OF CATHETERS

There are no convincing data that demonstrate decreased infection risk with scheduled changing of pulmonary artery catheters or CVCs. Peripheral catheters can be changed every 72 to 96 hours to reduce the risk of phlebitis.

■ EDUCATION MEASURES

Education of staff can reduce the risk of vascular catheter-related infections. A prospective, multicenter, observational study demonstrated that education of health care workers based on the Centers for Disease Control and HICPAC recommendations, followed by feedback about compliance, significantly reduced the risk of CLABSI. The baseline infection rate significantly decreased from 45.9/1000 to 17.1/1000 device-days in the education phase, and fell further to 9.9/1000 device-days in the compliance feedback phase. Another study demonstrated that the use of a self-study module to educate physicians and nurses decreased the rate of CLABSIs by 43%.

A quality improvement initiative that included rigorous measurement, feasible interventions, and cultural change was associated with a decrease in the rate of CLABSIs by almost 50% in 103 ICUs in the United States. Interventions included hand washing, using full barrier precautions during the insertion of CVCs, skin cleansing with chlorhexidine, avoiding femoral catheters whenever possible, and removing unnecessary catheters. Both technical and cultural aspects of implementing the intervention were addressed through engagement, education, execution, and rigorous evaluation. This effect on CLABSIs was sustained to at least 4 years from the implementation of the protocol, and highlighted the critical role that bundling of preventive approaches has on the rate of infection.

■ ADEQUATE STAFFING

Adequate nurse staffing has also been identified as a factor integral to preventing CRBSI. Observational studies suggest that a higher proportion of pool nurses or an elevated patient-to-nurse ratio is associated with CRBSI in ICUs. Additionally, several studies have found that the use of dedicated teams for placement of vascular catheters, including peripherally inserted central catheters (PICCs), decreases the rate of infection. **Table 188-4** highlights various preventive measures to decrease the rates of catheter-related infections.

DISCHARGE CHECKLIST

- Have catheters been removed from patients with infection due to *S. aureus* or *Candida* species?
- Have catheters been removed from patients with > 72 hours of bacteremia or fungemia, despite administration of antimicrobial agents to which the pathogens were susceptible?
- Has prolonged antibiotic therapy (≥4 weeks) been arranged for patients with *S. aureus* bacteremia persisting for > 72 hours after catheter removal, despite appropriate antibiotic therapy?
- Has sterilization of blood cultures been documented?

TABLE 188-4 Recommendations to Decrease Rates of Vascular-Catheter-Related Infection

Educate health care workers regarding the indications for intravascular catheter use, and proper procedures for the insertion and maintenance of intravascular catheters.
Use maximal barrier precautions for CVC insertion.
Use 2% chlorhexidine for cutaneous antisepsis prior to catheter insertion.
Use a subclavian site (rather than a jugular or a femoral site) in adult patients to minimize infection risk for nontunneled CVC placement. Place catheters used for hemodialysis and pheresis in a jugular or femoral vein rather than a subclavian vein to avoid venous stenosis.
If adherence to aseptic technique is not ensured, replace catheter within 48 h.
Change peripheral short-term catheters every 72-96 h.
Topical antimicrobials only recommended for hemodialysis catheters.
Clean hubs with 70% ethanol prior to use.
Use an antimicrobial or antiseptic impregnated CVC in adults whose catheter is expected to remain in place > 5 d if, after implementing a comprehensive strategy to reduce rates of CLABSI, the CLABSI rate remains above the goal set by the individual institution based on benchmark rates and local factors.
Designate trained personnel for the insertion and maintenance of intravascular catheters.
Promptly remove a catheter that is no longer required.
Conduct surveillance in ICUs and other patient populations to determine CLABSI rates, monitor trends, and assist in identifying lapses in infection-control practices.

Data from O'Grady NP, Alexander M, Dellinger EP, et al. Guidelines for the prevention of intravascular catheter-related infections. *Clin Infect Dis.* 2002;35:1281-1307.

- Is a beta-lactam antibiotic being used in preference to vancomycin in CLABSI due to MSSA, among patients without a beta-lactam allergy?
- Has a follow-up clinic appointment been arranged for patients being discharged on intravenous antibiotics (preferably while the patient is still on antibiotics)?
- For patients being discharged on intravenous antibiotics, has weekly laboratory testing been arranged, including complete blood count, blood urea nitrogen and a serum creatinine at a minimum? These results should be sent to the physician who has agreed to follow-up with the patient. For patients being discharged on daptomycin, weekly creatine phosphokinase levels should also be monitored.

SUGGESTED READINGS

Aslam S, Vaida F, Ritter M, Mehta RL. Systematic review and meta-analysis on management of hemodialysis catheter-related bacteremia. *J Am Soc Nephrol.* 2014;25(12):2927-2941.

Darouiche RO, Raad II, Heard SO, et al. A comparison of two anti-microbial-impregnated central venous catheters. *N Engl J Med.* 1999;340:1-8.

Fowler VG, Olsen MK, Corey GR. Clinical identifiers of complicated *Staphylococcus aureus* bacterermia. *Arch Intern Med.* 2003;163:2066-2072.

Mermel LM, Allon M, Bouza E, et al. Clinical practice guidelines for the diagnosis and management of intravascular catheter-related infection. *Clin Infect Dis.* 2009;49:1-45.

O'Grady NP, Alexander M, Burns LA, et al. Guidelines for the prevention of intravascular catheter-related infections. *Am J Infect Control.* 2011;39(4 Suppl 1):S1-S34.

Pronovost PJ, Needham D, Berenholtz S, et al. An intervention to decrease catheter-related bloodstream infections in the ICU. *N Engl J Med.* 2006;355:2725-2732.

Raad I, Hanna HA, Alakech B, et al. Differential time to positivity: a useful method for diagnosing catheter-related bloodstream infections. *Ann Intern Med.* 2004;140:18-25.

Raad I, Hanna H, Maki D. Intravascular catheter-related infections: advances in diagnosis, prevention and management. *Lancet Infect Dis.* 2007;7:645-657.

Vassallo M, Dunais B, Roger PM. Antimicrobial lock therapy in central-line associated bloodstream infections: a systematic review.*Infection.* 2015;43:389-398.

CHAPTER 189

Infective Endocarditis

Thomas A. Owens, MD
Vance G. Fowler Jr., MD, MHS
Edward F. Pilkington, III, MD

Key Clinical Questions

❶ Does the patient have symptoms consistent with infective endocarditis?

❷ What tests and studies are indicated to evaluate infective endocarditis?

❸ What infectious etiologies should be considered?

❹ What treatments should be considered?

❺ What complications should be expected?

INTRODUCTION

Infective endocarditis (IE) is a relatively common infection in the hospital setting, with an inpatient mortality rate of about 18%. The incidence of IE rises linearly with age, from around 1 case per 100,000 person-years among young adults to over 10 cases per 100,000 person-years among those older than 75 years. The hallmark lesion of IE is the endocardial vegetation. Although the heart valves are affected most commonly, IE also may involve septal defects, mural endocardium, or prosthetic cardiac structures. Vegetations may result in valvular regurgitation or obstruction, myocardial abscess, or mycotic aneurysm. Definitive diagnosis requires identification of the causative organism in blood, cardiac structures, or emboli. Cure requires prolonged antimicrobial treatment and often valve replacement surgery, leading to substantial expense.

EPIDEMIOLOGY

Historically, IE was a disease of younger patients with rheumatic heart disease, and mainly involved viridans group streptococci. In the past two decades, a new form of the disease, health care associated IE, has emerged. This new form of IE is distinct in its microbiology (predominantly *Staphylococcus aureus*) and risk factors (eg, intravenous catheters, hyperalimentation lines, pacemakers, dialysis shunts). The incidence of *S. aureus* IE has significantly increased over the last decade, such that it is now estimated to be the most common causative organism of IE in the developed world.

■ RISK FACTORS FOR IE

Almost any type of structural heart disease may predispose to IE, especially when the defect results in turbulent blood flow. Right-sided IE is primarily an infection of injection drug users and patients with indwelling transvenous pacemakers. In developed countries, the proportion of cases related to rheumatic heart disease has declined to 5% or less in the past two decades, while in developing countries, rheumatic heart disease remains the most common predisposing cardiac condition. Congenital bicuspid aortic valve is the underlying lesion in more than 15% of IE cases in patients (especially men) older than 60 years, and is associated with a poor prognosis, despite rapid valve replacement. Degenerative cardiac lesions (eg, calcified mitral annulus, calcific nodular lesions secondary to arteriosclerotic cardiovascular disease, and postmyocardial infarction thrombus) assume the greatest importance in the 30% to 40% of IE patients without any demonstrable underlying valvular disease. Marfan syndrome, when associated with aortic insufficiency, also has been associated with IE. Intravascular infections involving cardiac devices (eg, permanent cardiac pacemakers, defibrillators) also have increased significantly since the 1990s. Injection drug users are at high risk for recurrent and polymicrobial IE.

PATHOGENESIS AND PATHOPHYSIOLOGY

Mitral and aortic valvular involvements are most common in IE. Distributions of valvular involvement range from 28% to 45% of cases for isolated mitral valve IE, 5% to 36% for isolated aortic valve IE, and 0% to 35% for combined aortic and mitral valves IE. In the absence of injection drug use, the tricuspid valve rarely is involved (0%-6% of cases). Pulmonary valve IE is rare (< 1%) in any clinical circumstance.

The development of IE probably requires several independent events. The normal myocardial endothelial lining is relatively resistant to infection, and constant blood flow thwarts bacteria and fungi from settling on an endocardial surface. The initiation of IE requires the simultaneous presence of both a predisposing endocardial abnormality and microorganisms in the bloodstream (bacteremia). Occasionally, massive bacteremia or particularly virulent microorganisms—especially *S. aureus*—may cause IE on normal valves.

Bacteremia may occur whenever a mucosal surface heavily colonized with bacteria is traumatized, such as with dental extractions and invasive procedures, as well as gastrointestinal, urologic, and gynecologic procedures. The degree of bacteremia is proportional to the trauma produced by the procedure and to the number of organisms inhabiting the surface.

■ ORGANISMS RESPONSIBLE FOR IE

Many microorganisms have been identified in IE, but streptococci and staphylococci account for 80% to 90% of the cases in which an organism is isolated. The most common etiologic agents are outlined in **Table 189-1**.

S. aureus is the most common cause of native valve IE, prosthetic valve IE, and injection-drug use associated IE. It is associated with aggressive disease, extracardiac metastatic infections, and a high

mortality rate. **Group A, C, and G streptococci** cause aggressive IE with high mortality (up to 70%). **Group B streptococci** also lead to acute disease with high mortality, often requiring valve replacement. It is more common in elderly or immunosuppressed patients. *Streptococcus pneumoniae* is no longer common, but is notable for its acute and destructive course. A classical, often lethal presentation was Austrian's triad (simultaneous pneumococcal pneumonia, meningitis, and IE). *Pseudomonas aeruginosa* and **enteric Gram-negative rods** cause acute IE, and require surgery for cure. Although traditionally thought to be primarily an infection of injection drug users, recent studies have demonstrated that the primary risk factor for Gram-negative IE is health care contact.

Viridans group streptococci are the most common cause of community-acquired, subacute IE. **Enterococci** also usually present in subacute fashion, and comprise about 10% of IE. **Coagulase-negative Staphylococcus species** are typically associated with subacute disease, accounting for 20% of IE associated with prosthetic valves and 8% of cases of native valve IE. **HACEK organisms** (*Haemophilus* species, *Aggregatibacter* species, *Cardiobacterium hominis*, *Eikenella corrodens*, *Kingella* species) cause subacute disease, causing about 5% of all IE. **Fungal organisms such as Candida and Aspergillus species** are uncommon pathogens in IE, but devastating when they occur. They frequently present subacutely, with bulky, destructive, and recalcitrant vegetations, and almost always require surgery for cure.

CLINICAL PRESENTATION

The clinical presentation of IE is nonspecific, and the differential diagnosis is broad (**Table 189-2**). The diagnosis of IE may be delayed or occasionally missed entirely because of its protean manifestations. Thus, the clinician must maintain a high index of suspicion for this potentially lethal infection. Factors contributing to the overall clinical picture of IE include local cardiac complications, embolization, which may involve any organ and is frequently clinically underappreciated, persistent bacteremia, often leading to metastatic infection, and immunopathologic factors.

Traditionally, IE was classified as acute or subacute. Acute IE is associated with *S. aureus*, *Streptococcus pyogenes*, or *S. pneumoniae*. Fever is almost always present. Patients often appear toxic and occasionally exhibit septic shock. Untreated cases are rapidly fatal. Although most patients with subacute IE will develop valvular dysfunction, only half of patients with acute IE will have a detectable cardiac murmur on initial examination. In right-sided endocarditis, septic pulmonary emboli may cause cough, pleuritic chest pain, and sometimes hemoptysis.

Subacute IE (death occurring in 6 weeks to 3 months) and chronic IE (death occurring later than 3 months) often occur in the setting of prior valvular disease, with viridans streptococci as a frequent pathogen. Symptoms are vague: low-grade fever (< 39°C), night sweats, fatigue, malaise, and weight loss. Chills and arthralgias may occur. Symptoms and signs of valvular insufficiency may be present.

TABLE 189-1 Etiologic Agents in Infective Endocarditis

Cause of Endocarditis	Percentage of Patients		
	Drug Users	Nondrug Users	Prosthetic Valve
Staphylococcus aureus	68	28	23
Coagulase-negative *Staphylococcus*	3	9	17
Viridans group streptococci	10	21	12
Streptococcus bovis	1	7	5
Other streptococci	2	7	5
Enterococcus species	5	11	12
HACEK	0	2	2
Fungi/yeast	1	1	4
Polymicrobial	3	1	0.8
Negative culture findings	5	9	12
Other	3	4	7
Surgical therapy	38	48	49
In-hospital mortality	10	17	23

Data from Murdoch DR, Corey GR, Hoen B, et al. International Collaboration on Endocarditis-Prospective Cohort Study (ICE-PCS) Investigators. Clinical presentation, etiology, and outcome of infective endocarditis in the 21st century: the International Collaboration on Endocarditis-Prospective Cohort Study. *Arch Intern Med*. 2009;169:463-473.

TABLE 189-2 Clinical Admission Findings in Patients with Definitive Endocarditis

Findings	% Patients
Examination	
Fever (>38°C)	96
New murmur	48
Worsening of old murmur	20
Vascular embolic event	17
Splenomegaly	11
Splinter hemorrhages	8
Conjunctival hemorrhage	5
Janeway lesions	5
Osler nodes	3
Roth spots	2
Laboratory studies	
Elevated C-reactive protein	62
Elevated erythrocyte sedimentation rate	61
Hematuria	26
Elevated rheumatoid factor	5

Data from Murdoch DR, Corey GR, Hoen B, et al. International Collaboration on Endocarditis-Prospective Cohort Study (ICE-PCS) Investigators. Clinical presentation, etiology, and outcome of infective endocarditis in the 21st century: the International Collaboration on Endocarditis-Prospective Cohort Study. *Arch Intern Med.* 2009;169:463-473.

Initially, up to 15% of patients have fever or a murmur, but eventually almost all develop both.

Physical examination is often entirely normal, especially in patients with a short duration of symptoms. Findings, when present, may include pallor, fever, change in a prior murmur or development of a new regurgitant murmur, and tachycardia. Retinal emboli can cause round or oval hemorrhagic retinal lesions with small white centers (Roth spots). Cutaneous manifestations include petechiae (on the upper trunk, conjunctivae, mucous membranes, and distal extremities), nontender hemorrhagic macules on the palms or soles (Janeway lesions; **Figure 189-1**), painful erythematous subcutaneous nodules

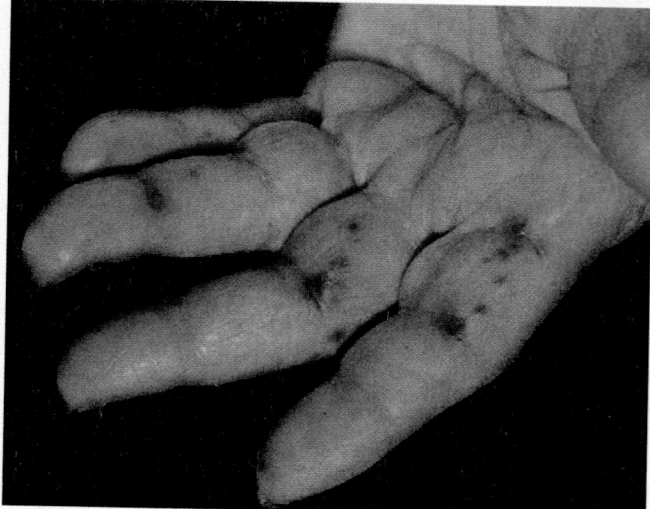

Figure 189-1 *Janeway lesions: nontender, hemorrhagic lesions on the palms and sole, from cardiac microemboli.* (Reproduced, with permission, from Wolff K, Johnson RA, Suurmond D. *Fitzpatrick's Color Atlas & Synopsis of Clinical Dermatology,* 5th ed. New York, NY: McGraw-Hill; 2005. Fig. 24-46.)

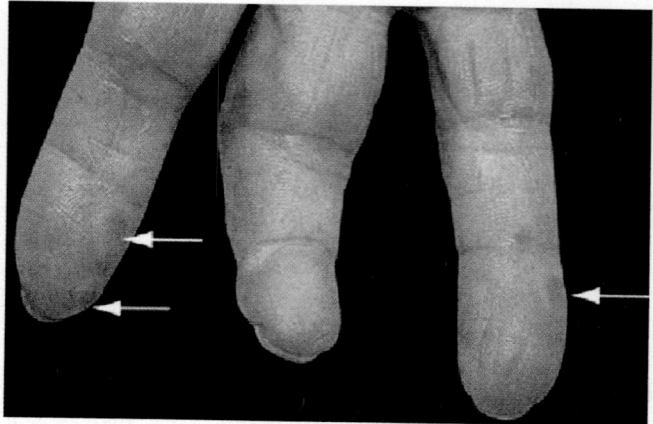

Figure 189-2 *Osler nodes: painful nodules in the fingers and toes, now rarely observed in endocarditis. Formerly thought to be immune-complex related, but probably have a similar pathogenesis to Janeway lesions, except that the microemboli are lodged in more sensitive dermal tissue.* (Reproduced, with permission, from Wolff K, Goldsmith LA, Katz SI, et al. *Fitzpatrick's Dermatology in General Medicine,* 7th ed. New York, NY: McGraw-Hill; 2008. Fig. 151-11.)

on the tips of digits (Osler nodes; **Figure 189-2**), and splinter hemorrhages under the nails. Approximately one-third of IE patients have neurologic disease which may include transient ischemic attacks, stroke, toxic encephalopathy, brain abscess, or subarachnoid hemorrhage associated with mycotic aneurysm rupture. Renal emboli may cause flank pain or gross hematuria, while splenic emboli cause left upper quadrant pain. Prolonged infection may cause splenomegaly or clubbing of fingers and toes.

This historical classification ignores the frequent overlap in manifestations of infection by specific organisms, such as the enterococci, and the fact that most IE in the 21st century are acute infections. Therefore, classification based on the etiologic causes for IE is more useful as it has implications for the expected clinical course, the likelihood of preexisting heart disease, and the appropriate antimicrobial therapy.

DIFFERENTIAL DIAGNOSIS

The differential diagnosis of IE includes other diseases with complex and varied manifestations, including noninfectious cardiac conditions such as marantic endocarditis, atrial myxoma, and other cardiac neoplasms; systemic infections such as septic thrombophlebitis, tickborne febrile illness, tuberculosis, brucellosis, and syphilis; and rheumatologic conditions such as antiphospholipid syndrome, polymyalgia rheumatica, reactive arthritis, systemic lupus erythematosus, and temporal arteritis.

DIAGNOSTIC TESTING

■ BLOOD CULTURES

The blood culture is the most important laboratory test performed in a diagnostic workup for IE. Identification of the organism and its antimicrobial susceptibility is vital to guide treatment. Documentation of continuous bacteremia (>30 minutes in duration) is pivotal for establishing the diagnosis of IE. Multiple positive blood cultures, especially if *S. aureus* is isolated, is an important clue for the presence of IE or other endovascular infections, such as septic thrombophlebitis or mycotic aneurysm. The presence of heart valve disorders, recent invasive procedures or intravascular catheters, or a history of injection drug use all increase the probability of endovascular infection. Patients with documented bacteremia should be examined thoroughly and repeatedly for signs and symptoms suggesting IE or other infectious complication.

Blood cultures should be obtained before starting antibiotics. To reduce false-positive blood cultures, site preparation must be carefully performed and obtained by peripheral venipuncture whenever possible. At least three blood culture sets (no more than two bottles per venipuncture) should be obtained in the first 24 hours. While three blood cultures are generally sufficient for the initial diagnosis of most forms of IE, more specimens may be necessary if the patient has received antibiotics in the preceding 2 weeks. Additional blood cultures drawn at regular intervals are important to document resolution of bacteremia. At least 10 mL of blood should be injected into each culture bottle. When IE is present and no prior antibiotic therapy was given, multiple blood cultures are usually positive because the bacteremia is continuous; at least one culture is positive in 99%. Premature use of empiric antibiotics is discouraged, to avoid culture-negative endocarditis. If prior antimicrobial therapy has been given, blood cultures should still be obtained, but they may be negative.

As many as 50% of positive clinical blood culture results have been estimated to be falsely positive, and one such result can lead to 4 days of unnecessary patient hospitalization. The interpretation of positive blood cultures depends on several factors, including the virulence of the organism. Positive blood cultures for *S. aureus* and fungal organisms are always significant; the risk of IE in patients with positive blood cultures for *S. aureus* is 10% to 12%. Blood cultures growing *Corynebacterium* species (diphtheroids) or *Bacillus* species (except *B. anthracis*) are rarely significant. Coagulase-negative staphylococci are most often contaminants, except in the setting of patients with prosthetic valves. Blood cultures have greater significance with increasing numbers of cultures positive for the same organism, a shorter time to culture positivity (implying higher bacterial load), and more severe clinical illness. The probability of IE is also increased by cardiac prosthetic material, absence of an alternative explanation for bacteremia, community acquisition, clinical evidence of IE, persistent fever, or persistent bacteremia.

Blood cultures are negative in only 5% of patients with IE confirmed by strict diagnostic criteria. In most cases, culture-negative IE is caused by the receipt of antibiotics prior to blood cultures. In a minority of patients, blood culture-negative IE is caused by fastidious organisms. The most commonly encountered true culture-negative pathogens in the United States are *Bartonella* species. Two species predominate. *Bartonella quintana* is a louseborne infection associated with homelessness. *Bartonella henselae* is generally fleaborne, and associated with cat exposure. *Coxiella burnetti* (Q fever) is a common cause of culture-negative IE in Europe, and is associated with exposure to livestock, especially sheep and goats, as well as birthing animals. *Tropheryma whipplei*, the agent of Whipple disease, and *Chlamydia* species are rare causes of chronic IE. Although improvements in blood culture platforms have significantly increased the ability to successfully isolate yeast (eg, *Candida*) from blood, IE with molds such as *Aspergillus* continue to present with apparently sterile blood cultures. HACEK bacteria and other fastidious organisms, such as *Abiotrophia* and *Granulicatella*, formerly caused a modest proportion of culture-negative endocarditis, but these may be isolated without difficulty in most contemporary blood culture systems.

OTHER LABORATORY FINDINGS

Aside from positive blood cultures, laboratory findings in IE are nonspecific. A normocytic anemia is often seen in established infections, as are an elevated WBC count, increased erythrocyte sedimentation rate, hypergammaglobulinemia, circulating immune complexes, and rheumatoid factor, but these findings are not helpful diagnostically. Urinalysis routinely shows microscopic hematuria and, occasionally, red blood cell casts, pyuria, or bacteriuria. *S. aureus* in the urine of a patient without an indwelling urinary catheter suggests staphylococcal bacteremia as the source.

PRACTICE POINT

Enterococcal endocarditis

- Enterococci may be tolerant to the bactericidal action of ampicillin and vancomycin. Cure rates are higher in enterococcal endocarditis when a cell wall active agent, such as ampicillin or vancomycin, is combined with an aminoglycoside. The microbiology laboratory should be asked to test enterococcal isolates from patients with endocarditis for synergy with gentamicin and streptomycin.
- For patients with enterococcal endocarditis with strains resistant to both gentamicin and streptomycin, or who are at particularly high risk of aminoglycoside toxicity, double beta-lactam therapy with ampicillin and ceftriaxone may be an option.

ECHOCARDIOGRAPHY

Echocardiography should be performed on all patients with suspected IE. Echocardiography is unnecessary in patients in whom IE is very unlikely based on clinical features, or in bacteremia with organisms that rarely cause IE (eg, *Escherichia coli*). In patients with suspected IE, transthoracic echocardiography (TTE) is obtained first. Due to conditions such as obesity, chest wall abnormalities, history of prior thoracic surgery, or chronic obstructive pulmonary disease, TTE may be technically inadequate in up to 20% of American adults. The sensitivity of TTE for vegetations is only about 60%, so a negative study does not rule out disease. TTE is more sensitive in right-sided IE than left-sided IE, as it visualizes the pulmonic and tricuspid valves particularly well. Specificity of TTE is excellent, and false-positive studies are rare. A negative TTE in patients without the typical constellation of clinical or laboratory features suggestive of IE should prompt clinicians to broaden their differential and consider other causes of fever and sepsis.

In patients with at least intermediate suspicion of IE, and negative or inconclusive results on TTE, transesophageal echocardiography (TEE) should be pursued. TEE should be obtained as quickly as possible after TTE in patients with high-risk clinical features, such as prosthetic heart valves, congenital heart disease, prior endocarditis, new heart murmurs, heart failure, and stigmata of endocarditis. TEE is more sensitive than conventional TTE for detecting intracardiac vegetations (95% sensitivity), particularly in prosthetic valve endocarditis. While TEE is better than TTE in the diagnosis of prosthetic valve endocarditis, both TEE and TTE are somewhat less sensitive and specific in imaging prosthetic valves, due to echogenic artifact from the sewing ring and support structures, and the difficulty of distinguishing sterile thrombus and degenerative changes from vegetations.

Patients with *S. aureus* bacteremia have a high risk of underlying IE (10%-12%). Cost-effectiveness studies suggest that in the setting of *S. aureus* bacteremia, TEE should be the first examination in patients with suspected IE. If TEE cannot be performed for clinical reasons, or must be delayed, then TTE should be performed promptly.

PRACTICE POINT

- The risk of endocarditis in patients with *S. aureus* bacteremia is high, up to 12%. A negative transthoracic echocardiogram does not exclude endocarditis in this setting. Cost-effectiveness studies suggest that it is reasonable to proceed with transesophageal echocardiogram as the initial echocardiographic study, if available.

Echocardiography is invaluable in assessing local complications of IE. Several echocardiographic findings, such as congestive heart failure (CHF), severe valvular regurgitation, paravalvular abscesses, and flail or perforated valve leaflets, indicate a need for surgical intervention. Larger and more mobile vegetations pose a greater risk of embolization. Most studies suggest that mitral valve vegetations (particularly those involving the anterior leaflet) are associated with higher rates of embolization than are noted with aortic valve vegetations. However, visualization of large vegetations by echocardiography, in the absence of clinical embolic episodes, is not sufficient to prompt early surgery. The risk of embolization drops rapidly after the first week of effective antibiotic therapy.

DIAGNOSTIC CRITERIA

The Duke criteria are the basis for establishing the diagnosis of IE. The Duke criteria use major and minor criteria to group patients as having definite or possible IE, or to reject IE in patients unlikely to have the disease. There are three ways of diagnosing definite IE: on a microbiologic basis (eg, isolation of microorganisms from cardiac tissue or a thromboembolus), on a pathologic basis (eg, evidence of active IE on histopathologic examination), and on a clinical basis (**Table 189-3A**). Major clinical criteria include echocardiographic evidence of IE (eg, vegetations or paravalvular complications of IE) and the isolation of typical IE pathogens from blood cultures. In addition, fever, predisposing cardiac conditions, physical examination findings of IE, and active injection drug use are included as minor criteria (**Table 189-3B**).

Fungal IE has a low rate of positive blood culture results. At best, only 50% of *Candida* species are associated with positive blood culture results. *Histoplasma* and *Aspergillus* are almost never retrieved from the bloodstream. Thus, fungal IE must always be considered in the clinical setting of culture-negative IE that fails to respond to appropriate antibiotic therapy.

The diagnosis of pacemaker IE may be difficult as its clinical presentation is often subtle. For this reason, fever or a positive blood culture without a primary source in patients with pacemakers or implantable cardioverter-defibrillators represents device-associated IE until proven otherwise.

TABLE 189-3A Definition of Infective Endocarditis According to the Modified Duke Criteria

Definite Infective Endocarditis

Pathological criteria

Microorganisms demonstrated by culture or histological examination of a vegetation, a vegetation that has embolized, or an intracardiac abscess specimen; or

Pathological lesions; vegetation or intracardiac abscess confirmed by histological examination showing active endocarditis

Clinical criteria

2 major criteria; or

1 major criterion and 3 minor criteria; or

5 minor criteria

Possible IE

1 major criterion and 1 minor criterion; or

3 minor criteria

Rejected

Firm alternative diagnosis explaining evidence of IE; or

Resolution of IE syndrome with antibiotic therapy for 4 d; or

No pathological evidence of IE at surgery or autopsy, with antibiotic therapy for 4 d; or

Does not meet criteria for possible IE as above

Data from Li J, Sexton DJ, Mick N, et al. Proposed modifications to the Duke criteria for the diagnosis of infective endocarditis. *Clin Infect Dis.* 2000;30:633-638.

TABLE 189-3B Definition of Terms Used in the Modified Duke Criteria for the Diagnosis of Infective Endocarditis

Major Criteria

Blood culture positive for IE

Typical microorganisms consistent with IE from 2 separate blood cultures: Viridans streptococci, *Streptococcus bovis*, HACEK group, *Staphylococcus aureus*; or community-acquired enterococci in the absence of a primary focus; or

Microorganisms consistent with IE from persistently positive blood cultures defined as follows: at least 2 positive cultures of blood samples drawn >12 h apart; or all of 3 or a majority of 4 separate cultures of blood (with first and last sample drawn at least 1 h apart)

Single positive blood culture for *Coxiella burnetii* or antiphase 1 IgG antibody titer > 1:800

Evidence of endocardial involvement

Echocardiogram positive for IE (TEE recommended for patients with prosthetic valves, rated at least "possible IE" by clinical criteria, or complicated IE [paravalvular abscess]; TTE as first test in other patients) defined as follows: oscillating intracardiac mass on valve or supporting structures, in the path of regurgitant jets, or on implanted material in the absence of an alternative anatomic explanation; or abscess; or new partial dehiscence of prosthetic valve; new valvular regurgitation (worsening or changing or preexisting murmur not sufficient)

Minor criteria

Predisposition, predisposing heart condition, or IDU

Fever, temperature > 38°C

Vascular phenomena, major arterial emboli, septic pulmonary infarcts, mycotic aneurysm, intracranial hemorrhage, conjunctival hemorrhages, and Janeway lesions

Immunologic phenomena: glomerulonephritis, Osler nodes, Roth spots, and rheumatoid factor

Microbiological evidence: positive blood culture but does not meet a major criterion as noted above* or serological evidence of active infection with organism consistent with IE

Echocardiographic minor criteria eliminated

---

*Excludes single positive cultures for coagulase-negative staphylococci and organisms that do not cause endocarditis.
TEE, transesophageal echocardiography; TTE, transthoracic echocardiography, IDU, injection drug user.
Data from Li J, Sexton DJ, Mick N, et al. Proposed modifications to the Duke criteria for the diagnosis of infective endocarditis. *Clin Infect Dis.* 2000;30:633-638.

TREATMENT

The diagnosis of IE should be made rapidly to initiate antibiotic therapy and identify patients at high risk for complications who may benefit from early surgery. The response to antimicrobial therapy for IE is unique among bacterial infections. While organisms may exhibit exquisite in vitro susceptibility to antibiotics, eradication takes many weeks, and relapses and medical failures may occur. There are two possible explanations for these findings. First, the vegetation is a privileged site of impaired host defenses. Bacteria are encased in a fibrin meshwork which hinders the penetration of both neutrophils and antibiotics. Second, bacteria in these vegetations reach tremendous population densities, and exist in a state of diminished metabolic activity and cell division. This reduces their susceptibility to antimicrobial therapy.

General principles have been accepted that provide the framework for the current recommendations for treatment of IE.

- Parenteral antibiotics are preferred over oral drugs because of the importance of sustained antibacterial activity. Erratic and unpredictable enteral absorption with many antimicrobials makes oral therapy less desirable.

- Short-term therapy is associated with relapse, and most guidelines emphasize prolonged drug administration.
- Bacteriostatic antibiotics are less effective in the treatment of bacterial IE, and their use has been associated with relapses, a failure to control the infection, or both.
- The selection of antibiotics should be based on antimicrobial susceptibility tests, and treatment should be monitored with antimicrobial blood levels (when indicated) and clinical response to therapy.
- In antimicrobial regimens which include multiple agents, antibiotics should be administered simultaneously or consecutively when possible.
- At least two sets of blood cultures should be obtained every 24 to 48 hours during the early phase of therapy to ensure clearance of the bacteremia, and also in the setting of persistent or recurrent fever despite appropriate antimicrobial therapy.

- Surveillance blood cultures should be obtained immediately before a patient's next scheduled antibiotic dose.
- When calculating the total duration of antimicrobial therapy, the date on which the first set of negative blood cultures are drawn should be assigned as "Day 1".
- If intraoperative cardiac tissue cultures return positive, it is reasonable to designate the time at which antibiotics are started postoperatively as "Day 1" of antimicrobial therapy.

A summary of recommended antimicrobial therapies is outlined in **Table 189-4**. Recommendations for antimicrobial treatment of IE caused by other pathogens may be found in the 2015 American Heart Association guidelines for diagnosis, antimicrobial therapy, and management of complications in IE. Consultation with an infectious diseases specialist is recommended in all cases of IE.

Hospitalized patients with newly diagnosed IE should be placed on cardiac telemetry and receive daily electrocardiograms to monitor for P-R interval prolongation, cardiac arrhythmias, myocardial infarctions (due to emboli showering the coronary artery,

TABLE 189-4 Definitive Therapy of Bacterial Endocarditis*

Organism/Regimen	Comments
PCN-susceptible viridans streptococci and *S. gallolyticus* (*bovis*) (MIC ≤ 0.12 µg/mL) native valve IE	
1. PCN 12-18 million U/24 h IV either continuously or in 4 or 6 equally divided doses × 4 wk	1. Also effective for other PCN-susceptible nonviridans streptococci
2. Ceftriaxone 2 g/24 h IV/IM in 1 dose × 4 wk	2. Uncomplicated infection with viridans streptococci, candidate for outpatient therapy; also PCN allergy
3. PCN 12-18 million U/24 h IV either continuously or in 6 equally divided doses × 2 wk or ceftriaxone 2 g/24 h IV/IM in 1 dose *plus* gentamicin 3 mg/kg IV every 24 h × 2 wk	3. Uncomplicated infection without the following features: renal insufficiency, eighth cranial nerve deficit, prosthetic valve infection, severe heart failure, known cardiac or extra cardiac abscess, CNS complications or age > 65. Also should not be used for *Abiotrophia*, *Granulicatella*, or *Gemella* species
4. Vancomycin 30 mg/kg per 24 h IV in 2 equally divided doses × 4 wk	4. Recommended only for patients unable to tolerate PCN or ceftriaxone. Goal vancomycin trough co concentration range 10-15 µg/mL
Relatively PCN-resistant viridans group Streptococci and *S. gallolyticus* (*bovis*) (MIC > 0.12 to < 0.5 µg/mL) native valve IE	
1. PCN 24 million U/24 h IV either continuously or in 4-6 equally divided doses × 4 wk or ceftriaxone 2 g/24 h IV/IM in 1 dose × 4 wk *plus* gentamicin 3 mg/kg per 24 h IV/IM in 1 dose × 2 wk	1. Ampicillin, 2 g/4 h IV is a reasonable alternative if a penicillin shortage exists
2. Vancomycin 30 mg/kg per 24 h IV in 2 equally divided doses not to exceed 2 g/24 h unless serum concentrations are low × 4 wk	2. For PCN allergy recommended only for patients unable to tolerate PCN or ceftriaxone. Goal vancomycin trough 15-20 µg/mL
Enterococci sensitive to PCN†, *Abiotrophia*, *Granulicatella*, and *Gemella* species, and PCN-resistant viridans group streptococci (MIC ≥ 0.5 µg/mL)	
1. Ampicillin 12 g/24 h IV in 6 equally divided doses or PCN 18-30 million U/24 h IV either continuously or in 6 equally divided doses × 4-6 wk *plus* gentamicin 3 mg/kg per 24 h IV/IM in 3 equally divided doses × 4-6 wk‡	1. Increase duration of both drugs to 6 wk for prosthetic valve or prosthetic material infection or symptoms longer than 3 mo in enterococcal infection
2. Ampicillin 2 g/4 h IV × 4-6 wk *plus* ceftriaxone 2 g/12 h × 4-6 wk	2. For patients with initial CrCl of ≤50 mL/min, patients who develop CrCl of ≤50 mL/min during treatment with a gentamicin-containing regimen, or patients with strains resistant to both gentamicin and streptomycin
3. Vancomycin 30 mg/kg per 24 h IV in 2 equally divided doses × 6 wk *plus* gentamicin 3 mg/kg per 24 h IV/IM in 3 equally divided doses × 6 wk§	3. For PCN allergy; PCN desensitization is also an option. Goal vancomycin trough 10-20 µg/mL; high risk of nephrotoxicity with this regimen
4. Linezolid 600 mg IV or orally every 12 h *or* daptomycin 6-10 mg/kg IV once daily × > 6 wk⊕	4. For NVE/PVE due to *Enterococcus* species caused by strains resistant to penicillins, aminoglycosides, and vancomycin; involvement of multidisciplinary team including infectious disease, cardiology, and cardiothoracic surgery specialists recommended
Staphylococcal Native Valve IE	
1. Nafcillin or oxacillin 12 g/24 h IV in 4-6 equally divided doses × 6 wk	1. For left-sided and complicated right-sided IE with oxacillin-susceptible strain; consider longer duration of therapy for patients with IE complications including perivalvular abscess formation and septic metastatic complications

(Continued)

TABLE 189-4 Definitive Therapy of Bacterial Endocarditis* (Continued)

Organism/Regimen	Comments
2. Vancomycin 30 mg/kg per 24 h IV in 2 equally divided doses × 6 wk	2. PCN allergy (immediate hypersensitivity or anaphylaxis) or oxacillin-resistant strain. Goal vancomycin trough 10-20 µg/mL. Daptomycin is a possible alternative, although additional study is required to define optimal dosing
3. Nafcillin 2 g IV every 4 h × 2 wk; or daptomycin 6 mg/kg IV once daily for 2-4 wk; or nafcillin 2 g IV every 4 h × 2-4 wk	3. Right-sided IE due to oxacillin-susceptible strain; 2-wk regimen only for use in IV drug abuser with infection limited to the tricuspid valve with normal renal function and no extrapulmonary infection; adjunctive gentamicin no longer recommended
4. Cefazolin 6 g/24 h IV in 3 equally divided doses × 6 wk	4. PCN allergy other than immediate hypersensitivity
Staphylococcal prosthetic valve IE	
1. Vancomycin 30 mg/kg 24 h in 2 equally divided doses × > 6 wk *plus* wk *plus* gentamicin§§ 3 mg/kg per 24 h IV/IM in 2 or 3 equally divided doses × 2 wk *plus* rifampin 900 mg per 24 h IV or orally in 3 equally divided doses × > 6 wk	1. Infection with methicillin-resistant staphylococci (or immediate-type hypersensitivity reaction to beta-lactam antibiotics); goal vancomycin trough 10-20 µg/mL
2. Nafcillin or oxacillin 2 g/24 h IV in 6 equally divided doses × >6 wk *plus* gentamicin§§ 3 mg/kg per 24 h IV/IM in 2 or 3 equally divided doses × 2 wk *plus* rifampin 900 mg per 24 h IV or orally in 3 equally divided doses × >6 wk.	2. Prosthetic valve infection with methicillin-susceptible staphylococci; cefazolin may be substituted for nafcillin in non–immediate-type hypersensitivity reactions to penicillins Careful monitoring for IE complications, including, perivalvular extension of infection and extra-cardiac foci of infection, is recommended for patients with IE due to *S. lugdunensis*
HACEK strains	
1. Ceftriaxone 2 g/24 h IV/IM in 1 dose × 4 wk; 6 wk for prosthetic valves	
2. Ampicillin-sulbactam 12 g/24 h IV in 4 equally divided doses × 4 wk; 6 wk for prosthetic valves	2. HACEK strains increasingly may produce beta-lactamase
3. Ciprofloxacin 1000 mg/24 h orally or 800 mg/24 h IV in 2 equally divided doses × 4 wk	

*Dosages for patients with normal renal function; adjustments must be made for renal insufficiency for all drugs except nafcillin, rifampin, and ceftriaxone. Gentamicin doses should be adjusted to achieve a peak serum concentration of ~ 3-4 µg/mL 30 min after dosing, and a trough gentamicin level of < 1 µg/mL.
†These recommendations are for enterococci sensitive to penicillin, gentamicin, and vancomycin. Testing for susceptibility to daptomycin and linezolid should be done for strains that are resistant to beta-lactams and vancomycin, and/or aminoglycosides.
‡Recent observational data supports 2 wk instead of the previously recommended 4-6 wk of synergistic gentamicin in patients with *Enterococcus faecalis* IE without high-level aminoglycoside resistance.
§Need for addition of aminoglycoside has not been demonstrated for PCN-resistant streptococci. The combination of vancomycin and gentamicin is only recommended for patients with Enterococcal infection unable to tolerate penicillin or ampicillin or for *E. faecalis* isolated that are resistant to penicillin.
ΦLinezolid use may be associated with potentially severe bone marrow suppression, neuropathy, and numerous drug interactions.
§§For Staphylococcal species resistant to gentamicin substitute an aminoglycoside to which the isolate is susceptible. For Staphylococcal species resistant to all aminoglycosides, substitute a fluoroquinolone for isolates susceptible to fluoroquinolones.
HACEK, *Haemophilus* species, Aggregatibacter species, *Cardiobacterium hominis, Eikenella corrodens,* and *Kingella* species; MIC, minimum inhibitory concentration; MRSA, methicillin-resistant *Staphylococcus aureus*; PCN, penicillin.
Data from Baddour LM, Wilson WR, Bayer AS, et al. Infective endocarditis: diagnosis, antimicrobial therapy, and management of complications. *Circulation.* 2015;132(15):1435-1486.

especially in patients with aortic IE), and myocardial abscesses or hemodynamic fistulae. An emerging atrioventricular block on electrocardiogram is an ominous finding, and suggests a paravalvular abscess eroding into the conduction system. Patients with IE may have associated myocarditis with heart failure and cardiac arrhythmias. These patients require close monitoring in an intensive care unit.

Anticoagulation during therapy for IE is controversial. Most experts agree that anticoagulants in patients with native valve IE are contraindicated, as fatal subarachnoid hemorrhage and other bleeding complications are associated with anticoagulation in this setting. In patients with mechanical valve IE who have had a recent central nervous system embolic event, guidelines suggest discontinuation of anticoagulation for at least the first 2 weeks of antibiotic therapy.

Anticoagulation should be reintroduced cautiously in these patients with close monitoring. In prosthetic valve IE in patients without evidence of significant vascular emboli, many clinicians continue therapeutic anticoagulation.

SURGICAL INTERVENTION

Approximately half of all patients with IE ultimately require cardiac surgery, and up to one-third of patients with left-sided IE will require surgical intervention during the acute stages of infection, either for valve replacement or metastatic infection. Heart failure, perivalvular extension, and embolic events represent the most common indications for early surgery.

Given that the need for emergent surgery can arise rapidly, especially in patients with hemodynamic or perivalvular complications, it is recommended that patients with IE be treated in centers with appropriate surgical expertise. Early involvement of a multispecialist heart valve team, which should include a cardiologist, a cardiothoracic surgeon, a radiologist, and an infectious disease specialist, is also essential in guiding the provision of optimal early management and treatment, and determining the need for and timing of surgical intervention in patients with IE. Telecommunication with a referral-center heart valve team may also be reasonable for management of stable IE patients at smaller centers without immediate access to multispecialty care.

Patient factors such as location of infected valves (left- vs right-sided IE), vegetation size, symptomatic valvular dysfunction, onset of conduction system abnormalities, persistent fevers or bacteremia, type of infecting organism, recurrent emboli, hemodynamic status, age and other medical comorbidities are crucial determinants in the timing of valve replacement.

Early surgery, defined by the American Heart Association/American College of Cardiology (AHA/ACC) as surgery during initial hospitalization and prior to completion of a full course of antibiotics, is currently indicated in patients with left-sided native valve IE that is complicated by the development of heart failure, heart block, annular or aortic abscesses, destructive penetrating lesions, or persistent fever or infection (>5-7 days). Early surgery should also be considered in patients with IE caused by fungi or highly resistant organisms, such as multidrug-resistant Gram-negative rods or vancomycin-resistant *Enterococcus*, or that is complicated by severe valvular dysfunction, recurrent emboli, or enlarging or mobile vegetations >10 mm in length despite appropriate antibiotic therapy, particularly when large vegetations involve the anterior leaflet of the mitral valve.

PRACTICE POINT

Indications for early surgical intervention in left-sided IE
- New onset or worsening congestive heart failure
- New onset or worsening heart block
- Annular or aortic abscess or other destructive penetrating intracardiac lesions
- Persistent fever or septicemia (>5-7 days) despite appropriate antimicrobial therapy

Recommendations for early surgery in patients with prosthetic valve IE are similar to those for native valve IE with an additional consideration being relapsing infection (defined as recurrence of bacteremia after completing an appropriate course of antibiotic therapy). Although 1-year mortality is higher in patients with prosthetic valve IE due to *S. aureus*, compared to prosthetic valve IE due to other organisms, the decision to perform valve surgery should be individualized in these patients, as early valve surgery is not associated with better outcomes, after adjustment for patient factors.

The majority of the above recommendations are based on data derived from observational studies including an analysis of a large, prospectively ascertained, international cohort of patients with native valve IE, which revealed that early surgery was associated with significantly lower in-hospital mortality than medical therapy. This benefit was most significant in patients with indications for surgical intervention, including paravalvular complications, systemic embolization, stroke, or *S. aureus* infection. A dual-center, prospective randomized control trial was also recently conducted which showed that early surgery (within 48 hours of diagnosis of IE) in patients with left-sided IE with severe valvular dysfunction and associated vegetations >10 mm in diameter resulted in a statistically significant decrease in systemic embolism.

The timing of valve surgery in patients with stroke or hemorrhage due to emboli in IE is controversial. There are data to suggest worse outcomes with early surgery in IE patients with major stroke or hemorrhage. The 2015 AHA/ACC guidelines state that it is reasonable to delay valve surgery for 4 weeks in patients with major ischemic

stroke or intracranial hemorrhage, but that valve surgery without delay may be considered in patients with mild and subclinical stroke and no evidence of intracerebral hemorrhage on imaging studies.

In contrast to left-sided IE, in which CHF is the usual indication for surgical intervention, persistent infection with resistant or difficult-to-treat organisms is the most common indication for surgery in patients with right-sided IE. As most cases of right-sided IE are secondary to intravenous drug use (IVDU), conservative management with antibiotics and medical therapy directed against heart failure is favored over surgical intervention in these patients. Placement of valvular prostheses are generally avoided in right-sided IE given that continued IVDU places many patients at risk for prosthetic valve infection. Surgery may be considered in patients with the following complications from right-sided IE: symptomatic tricuspid valvular dysfunction that is refractory to medical therapy, tricuspid valve vegetations ≥20 mm in size, or persistent infection or recurrent pulmonary embolism despite appropriate antimicrobial therapy. If surgical intervention is required, valve repair should be pursued in place of valve replacement whenever possible.

COMPLICATIONS

Complications are part of the natural history of IE. Changes in clinical status or persistent signs and symptoms of active infection should prompt evaluation for myocardial or valve abscesses, embolic phenomena, heart failure, metastatic infection, including vertebral osteomyelitis and mycotic aneurysms, conduction defects, and especially valvular dysfunction. Valvular regurgitation in endocarditis sometimes presents in abrupt and catastrophic fashion.

PROGNOSIS

Cure rates of native valve IE due to viridans streptococci are 80% to 90%, compared to 60% to 90% for *S. aureus*. Cure rates are higher in injection drug users with right-sided involvement. Cure rates in fungal endocarditis are less than 50%, even with aggressive medical and surgical therapy. For prosthetic valve IE, cure rates are about 10% less for each etiology, and surgery is needed more frequently.

DISCHARGE PLANNING/TRANSITIONS OF CARE

To receive prolonged intravenous antibiotics, patients need early planning for long-term vascular access (after the initial bacteremia has cleared), home antimicrobial administration (once medically stabilized), and close medical outpatient follow-up. Peripherally inserted central catheters, which have relatively low secondary local and bloodstream infection rates, have facilitated home parenteral antibiotic therapy in many patients.

Careful monitoring of antimicrobial levels and renal function (when indicated), as well as other clinical signs and symptoms of infection, should be arranged. Outpatient follow-up should include the primary care provider, infectious disease specialist, and cardiologist. Cardiothoracic surgery should be involved in the follow-up of patients with valvular damage which may require surgery after completion of antimicrobial treatment. Outpatient providers should be informed about diagnosis, therapeutic decisions and duration, required monitoring, and plans for possible surgical intervention. Finally, patients with newly diagnosed IE should be educated about dental prophylaxis (see below).

Active injection drug users are of special concern in discharge planning for IE. Acute infection accounts for approximately 60% of hospital admissions for this population; IE is implicated in 5% to 15% of these episodes. Nonadherence to treatment plans, central catheter care, and follow-up in this population may be particularly challenging; these patients are poor candidates for discharge home with central catheters. Secondary catheter-related bloodstream infections may be more common in this population. Successful management of IE in this population requires treatment of substance abuse and psychiatric comorbidities, if present.

PRIMARY AND SECONDARY PREVENTION

Recent guidelines for antibiotic prophylaxis before procedures associated with bacteremia have recommended prophylaxis for far fewer procedure types and cardiac conditions. The proportion of cases of IE that are preventable are probably few, and the risk of IE after dental procedures is probably low compared to the cumulative risk from such daily activities as tooth brushing and chewing food. As well, no large, prospective randomized trials of the use of prophylactic antibiotics prior to procedures causing bacteremia have been carried out.

The administration of prophylactic antibiotics solely to prevent endocarditis is no longer recommended for patients undergoing genitourinary or gastrointestinal tract procedures. Antibiotic prophylaxis may be considered for patients at high risk for IE who undergo an invasive procedure of the respiratory tract that involves incision or biopsy of the respiratory mucosa (eg, tonsillectomy, adenoidectomy). With regard to dental procedures, the number of cardiac conditions for which prophylaxis is still recommended is now reduced to four settings:

- Prosthetic heart valves, including bioprosthetic and homograft valves
- Prior history of IE
- Certain congenital heart defects, including (a) unrepaired cyanotic congenital heart disease, including palliative shunts and conduits; (b) completely repaired congenital heart defects with prosthetic material or devices, whether placed by surgery or by catheter intervention, during the first 6 months after the procedure; or (c) repaired congenital heart disease with residual defects at the site or adjacent to the site of the prosthetic device
- Cardiac valvulopathy in a transplanted heart

The choice of antibiotics for prophylaxis is unchanged from previous iterations of the guidelines. Antibiotics should be effective against the organisms most likely to be released into the bloodstream by the procedure. Thus, primarily oral flora should be covered by antibiotics given before dental, oral, and respiratory tract procedures. The standard regimen in patients able to take oral medications is amoxicillin 2 g 30- to 60-minute preprocedure, with regimens in patients with penicillin allergy including cephalexin 2 g, clindamycin 600 mg, or azithromycin 500 mg.

DISCHARGE CHECKLIST

- Does the patient have long-term vascular access for outpatient antibiotic therapy, and have support and patient education been arranged for line care and antibiotic infusion?
- Have patients with intravenous drug use been referred to addiction treatment and counseling?
- Has a dental evaluation been performed or arranged to address potential sources of oral infection?
- Have patients been educated regarding signs or symptoms suggestive of endocarditis recurrence or metastatic complications, such as fevers and chills, dyspnea and edema suggestive of new

heart failure, palpitations or dizziness suggestive of cardiac arrhythmias, or neurological events suggestive of systemic emboli?
- Have patients been educated regarding the need for antibiotic prophylaxis prior to certain dental procedures?
- Has close follow-up been arranged with primary care, cardiology, infectious diseases, and cardiothoracic surgery?
- Has monitoring of serum antimicrobial levels, complete blood counts, creatinine, and liver enzymes been arranged?

SUGGESTED READINGS

Baddour LM, Wilson WR, Bayer AS, et al. American Heart Association Scientific Statement. Infective endocarditis: diagnosis, antimicrobial therapy, and management of complications. *Circulation*. Published online before print September 15, 2015. Available at http://circ.ahajournals.org/content/early/2015/09/15/CIR.0000000000000296.full.pdf+html.

Chirouze C, Alla F, Fowler VG Jr, et al. Impact of early valve surgery on outcome of *Staphylococcus aureus* prosthetic valve infective endocarditis. *Clin Infect Dis*. 2015;60:741-749.

Dahl A, Rasmussen RV, Bundgaard H, et al. *Enterococcus faecalis* infective endocarditis: a pilot study of the relationship between duration of gentamicin treatment and outcome. *Circulation*. 2013;127:1810-1817.

Fernández-Hidalgo N, Almirante B, Gavaldà J, et al. Ampicillin plus ceftriaxone is as effective as ampicillin plus gentamicin for treating enterococcus faecalis infective endocarditis. *Clin Infect Dis*. 2013;56:1261-1268.

Kang DH, Kim YJ, Kim SH, et al. Early surgery versus conventional treatment for infective endocarditis. *N Engl J Med*. 2012;366:2466-2473.

Lalani T, Cabell CH, Benjamin DK, et al. Analysis of the impact of early surgery on in-hospital mortality of native valve endocarditis: use of propensity score and instrumental variable methods to adjust for treatment-selection bias. *Circulation*. 2010;121:1005-1013.

Li J, Sexton DJ, Mick N, et al. Proposed modifications to the Duke criteria for the diagnosis of infective endocarditis. *Clin Infect Dis*. 2000;30:633-638.

Murdoch DR, Corey GR, Hoen B, et al. Clinical presentation, etiology, and outcome of infective endocarditis in the 21st century. *Arch Intern Med*. 2009;169:463-473.

Task Force on the Prevention, Diagnosis, and Treatment of Infective Endocarditis of the European Society of Cardiology. Guidelines on the prevention, diagnosis, and treatment of infective endocarditis. *Eur Heart J*. 2009;30:2369-2413.

Tleyjeh IM, Abdel-Latif A, Rahbi H, et al. A systematic review of population-based studies of infective endocarditis. *Chest*. 2001;132:1025-1035.

Tleyjeh IM, Steckelberg JM, Georgescu G, et al. The association between the timing of valve surgery and six-month mortality in left-sided infective endocarditis. *Heart*. 2008;94:892-896.

Wilson W, Taubert KA, Gewitz M, et al. Prevention of infective endocarditis: guidelines from the American Heart Association. *Circulation*. 2007;116:1736-1754.

CHAPTER 190

Clostridium difficile–Associated Disease (CDAD)

Danielle B. Scheurer, MD, MSCR, SFHM

Key Clinical Questions

① Which factors are associated with an increased risk of primary or recurrent *Clostridium difficile*–associated disease (CDAD)?

② What factors affect the accuracy of diagnostic testing of CDAD?

③ What are the most common complications of CDAD?

④ What therapies are most efficacious for primary, recurrent, or refractory CDAD?

⑤ What system improvements can reduce the incidence of CDAD?

INTRODUCTION AND EPIDEMIOLOGY

Clostridium difficile was first described in 1935 by pediatricians studying the acquisition of bowel flora in newborns and was termed "difficult" because of its resistance to growth on conventional media. It was not until 1978 that it was found to be associated with toxins in the stools of patients with colitis. *Clostridium difficile*–associated disease (CDAD) has now become a major nosocomial problem, affecting three million inpatients yearly in the United States. Acquisition of *C. difficile* occurs in up to 30% of hospitalized patients, although only 30% to 60% have symptoms. Patients with symptomatic disease stay an average of 3.6 days longer in hospital than expected, at a cost of over $3.2 billion annually in the United States.

Normal gut flora confers resistance to *C. difficile* colonization; only 1% to 4% of healthy adults carry *C. difficile* in their bowel flora. Loss of normal colonic flora, usually from antibiotics, allows *C. difficile* proliferation (clindamycin, cephalosporins, and fluoroquinolones are common offenders). *C. difficile* colitis is also associated with other events that disturb gut flora or host immunity, such as bowel preparations, cytotoxic agents, and colonic inflammation due to inflammatory bowel disease.

CDAD was first described in frail or elderly hospitalized patients after antibiotic exposure, but it is now occurring in younger, healthy individuals with no apparent exposure to health care environments or antibiotics. Up to ~20% of CDAD cases are now community-acquired. *C. difficile* and its spore form are easily transmitted from person-to-person or by contact with objects in the hospital environment, such as stethoscopes, clothing, and toilets. The spore form is ubiquitous in the hospital environment, is resistant to alcohol-based treatment and other disinfectants, and can survive for months. Even after routine cleaning, 10% to 50% of room surfaces still contain spores.

PATHOPHYSIOLOGY

C. difficile is an anaerobic spore-forming bacterium that produces two exotoxins (A and B) that adhere to intestinal epithelial cells, causing cell death. These toxins are transcribed from a locus composed of five genes (two toxin genes and three regulatory genes). The epidemic strain of *C. difficile* (BI/NAP1/027) has several factors that increase its virulence. A mutation in one of the regulatory genes results in a massive increase in toxin production. This strain also shows high-level fluoroquinolone resistance, giving it a competitive advantage in environments where fluoroquinolone use is widespread. This strain also produces an additional toxin (binary toxin), which is of uncertain clinical significance.

Patient risk of acquiring CDAD and severity of clinical illness are variable (**Table 190-1**). The clinical spectrum of CDAD ranges from minor diarrhea to fulminant colitis with toxic megacolon. Most patients present with some combination of acute, nonbloody, watery diarrhea, lower abdominal pain, and leukocytosis. A minority of patients present with obstipation, especially when there is right colon involvement or paralytic ileus; these patients may have severe illness. Fever is relatively uncommon, being present in less than one-third of patients. Mimickers of CDAD include bowel obstruction, fecal impaction, or toxic megacolon.

DIFFERENTIAL DIAGNOSIS

The differential diagnosis of acute diarrhea in hospitalized patients is extensive, and less than a third of cases of nosocomial diarrhea are

TABLE 190-1 Factors Associated with Higher Incidence and Severity of CDAD

	Host Factors	Medications	Other Factors
Higher incidence	Older age Comorbidities • COPD • Cancer • Immuno-suppression • Tube feeds High colon toxin receptors Low antitoxin IgG	Antibiotics • Fluoroqu-inolones • Clindamycin Proton pump inhibitors H_2-blockers	
Higher severity	Older age Comorbidities • COPD • Cancer • Renal failure Low cognitive score High colon toxin receptors Low antitoxin IgG	Antiperistaltics Clindamycin Immuno-suppressants	Recurrence Recent endoscopy Albumin < 3 g/dL Pain/peritonitis Hemocon centration WBC < 1.5 K/µL WBC > 25 K/µL

COPD, chronic obstructive pulmonary disease; IgG, immunoglobulin G; WBC, white blood cell.

due to CDAD. Non-CDAD causes of diarrhea should be considered in all patients, especially those for whom *C. difficile* testing is negative, or those who do not respond to appropriate treatment. Common benign conditions causing nosocomial diarrhea include medications (including stool softeners or laxatives as part of standardized order sets), foods (including tube feedings), oral contrast from computed tomographic scans, and antibiotic-induced alterations of bowel flora. Less common microbial causes of diarrhea include *Klebsiella oxytoca*, *Klebsiella pneumoniae*, and *Staphylococcus aureus*. For a full discussion of the approach to nosocomial diarrhea, see Chapter 82.

PRACTICE POINT

- A growing body of evidence suggests that proton pump inhibitors (PPIs) increase the risk of *C. difficile* acquisition and recurrence in hospitalized patients. Loss of the gastric acid barrier may make it easier for *C. difficile* spores acquired in the hospital environment to reach the colon. PPIs also have adverse effects on the gut microbiome. Much PPI use in the hospital setting is not evidence-based, and PPIs can be discontinued or tapered in many hospitalized patients with ill effects.

DIAGNOSIS

The diagnosis should be made on the combination of symptoms and microbiologic data. Testing for *C. difficile* is imperfect but improving (**Table 190-2**). The cytotoxic assay is the gold standard, with excellent sensitivity (94%-100%) and specificity (99%), but it is expensive and time-consuming, and requires specialized equipment and trained personnel. Hence, most medical centers no longer routinely perform it. There are several types of enzyme immunoassay (EIA) tests for toxins. Most detect both toxin A and B, but some only detect toxin A. EIA tests have the advantage of being quicker and cheaper, but have a sensitivity of only 70% to 90%. Sensitivity is reduced in strains that do not produce toxin A (or have mutant toxin A), as well as in patients that have already received antibiotic treatment for CDAD. False-positive tests are rare, and any symptomatic patient with a positive test should be treated. Rapid EIA tests are also available to detect glutamate dehydrogenase (GDH), but this is present in both toxigenic and nontoxigenic strains (about half of strains are nontoxigenic). PCR tests to detect the genes for the toxin production are also available. PCR for toxin genes is very sensitive and specific, and is often used as a confirmatory test when the results of EIA or GDH testing are equivocal. Hospitalists need to know which *C. difficile* tests are offered at their hospital and their sensitivity and specificity, in order to interpret test results in the context of the patient's clinical presentation. *C. difficile* cultures are not routinely available, lack sensitivity and specificity, and are best reserved for outbreak investigations.

Severe colitis with pseudomembranes is virtually pathognomonic for *C. difficile* (**Figure 190-1**). It is diagnosed endoscopically by the appearance of raised yellow or white plaques scattered over the colonic mucosa.

TABLE 190-2 Diagnostic Tests for *Clostridium difficile*

	What It Tests	Advantages	Disadvantages	False Positive	False Negative
EIA	Exotoxins A, B, or both	Time (h) Low cost High specificity	Low sensitivity (70%-90%)	Rare	Prior treatment Mutant strain Toxin A deficient strain Low toxin density
EIA	Glutamate dehydrogenase enzyme (expressed by *C. difficile*)	Time (hours) Low cost	Low sensitivity (58%-68%)	Rare	Prior treatment Low *C. difficile* density
Cytotoxic assay	Characteristic cytopathic effect on cell monolayer	High sensitivity and specificity	Time (d) High cost	Rare	Rare
Organism culture	*C. difficile* organism culture on selective medium	Epidemiological tracking Genotyping Performing susceptibilities	Needs confirmation of toxigenic strain	Rare	Rare
Nucleic acid amplification testing	Genes that express toxin	Time (hours) High sensitivity and specificity	High cost	Rare	Rare

EIA, enzyme immunoassay.

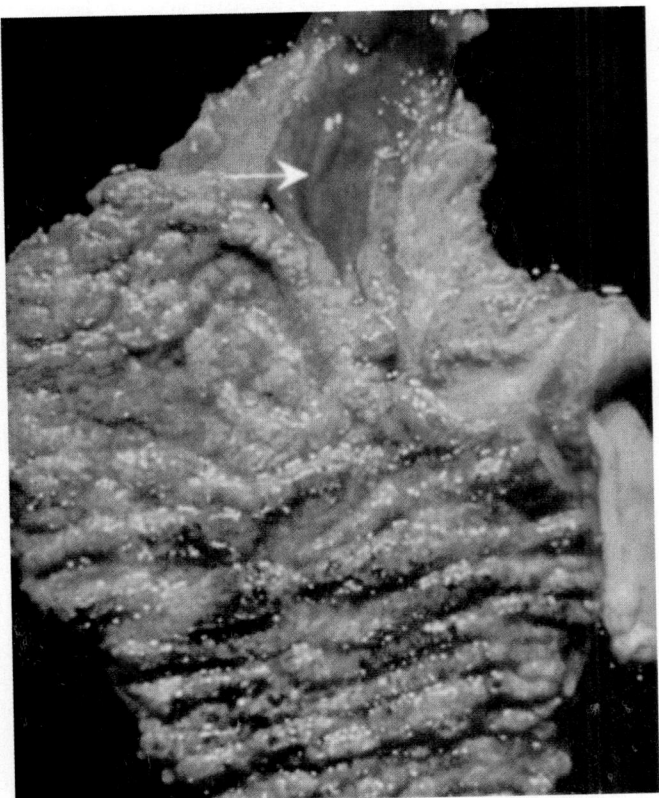

Figure 190-1 *Autopsy specimen with confluent pseudomembranes covering the cecum of a patient with pseudomembranous colitis. Note the sparing of the terminal ileum (arrow).* (Reproduced, with permission, from Fauci AS, Braunwald E, Kasper DL, et al. *Harrison's Principles of Internal Medicine*, 17th ed. New York, NY: McGraw-Hill; 2008. *Fig. 123-1*.)

In summary, 20% to 30% of hospitalized patients are colonized with *C. difficile*, but some strains fail to produce toxins, and some patients do not develop symptoms from the toxin when it is present. Patients without diarrhea should not be tested for *C. difficile* (except in suspected severe cases with ileus or megacolon). Some patients with symptomatic *C. difficile* will have a negative test and should be treated if clinical suspicion is high. Symptomatic patients with a positive test should always be treated.

TRIAGE/HOSPITAL ADMISSION

Patients with mild CDAD usually do not require hospital admission, but those with severe CDAD usually do. To protect other patients, contact precautions should be instituted immediately for any patient with proven or suspected *C. difficile* infection. This includes gowns and gloves for patient contact, and dedicated equipment in each room, such as blood pressure cuffs and stethoscopes. Strict handwashing before and after all patient contact is required, as *C. difficile* spores are resistant to alcohol-based treatment.

TREATMENT

Treatments depend on the severity of the disease at presentation and the response to initial therapy (**Table 190-3**). The offending antibiotic should be stopped whenever feasible. Symptomatic improvement is likely in mildly ill patients after antibiotics are ceased. It is also recommended to discontinue all antiperistaltic agents (although data showing worse outcomes with these agents are retrospective only). These include loperamide, diphenoxylate with atropine (Lomotil), bismuth subsalicylate (Pepto-Bismol), and tincture of opium.

TABLE 190-3 First-line Treatment for CDAD Based on Severity of Illness and Initial Clinical Response

Clinical Categories	Clinical Criteria	Treatment
Mild	WBC < 15,000 *and*	Oral metronidazole 500 q8
	Serum creatinine <1.5 times premorbid	If no clinical response at 5-7 d, escalate to severe CDAD treatment
Severe	WBC > 15,000 *or*	Oral vancomycin 125 q6
	Serum creatinine >1.5 times premorbid	
Severe complicated	Hypotension, shock, ileus, or megacolon	Oral vancomycin 125 q6 *and* IV metronidazole 500 q8
		For ileus, megacolon, distention:
		Oral vancomycin 500 q6 *and* rectal vancomycin q6 *and* IV metronidazole 500 q8 *and* surgical consultation

CDAD, *Clostridium difficile*–associated disease; IV, intravenous.

PRACTICE POINT

- Fidaxomicin was approved for the treatment of *C. difficile* colitis by the US Food and Drug Administration in 2011. In a randomized clinical trial of 629 patients, a 10-day oral course of fidaxomicin 200 mg twice daily produced rates of clinical cure equivalent to a 10-day course of oral vancomycin 125 mg four times daily. Overall, rates of relapse were lower in the fidaxomicin group. However, rates of relapse were similar in the subgroup of patients with the hypervirulent BI/NAP1/027 epidemic strain of *C. difficile*. Side effects of fidaxomicin were generally mild and comparable to oral vancomycin. Rash, dizziness, elevated uric acid, and elevated liver transaminases were more common in the patients receiving fidaxomicin.

First-line treatment with either oral vancomycin or metronidazole is usually successful (~20% will recur). A recent Cochrane review concluded that no single antibiotic was superior in symptomatic or bacteriologic outcomes for unselected patients. However, a more recent randomized, controlled trial of 172 patients found that vancomycin and metronidazole had equivalent cure rates in low-risk patients, but that vancomycin had higher rates of cure in high-risk patients. If intravenous therapy is required, metronidazole is more effective than vancomycin. Treatment should be continued for at least 14 days (or at least 10 days after the symptoms have abated).

There are few antibiotic therapies available other than vancomycin and metronidazole. In a Cochrane review, vancomycin and metronidazole were compared to several other agents, including teicoplanin, fusidic acid, bacitracin, rifaximin, and nitazoxanide. None of the comparisons showed a significant advantage or disadvantage, other than bacitracin, which appeared inferior to vancomycin for initial bacteriologic response. As well, teicoplanin, which is not currently available in the United States, appeared superior to vancomycin for initial bacteriologic response and cure.

There is some evidence that adding probiotics to standard antibiotic regimens may enhance treatment of CDAD. One study found that adding the probiotic *Saccharomyces boulardii* to a standard antibiotic regimen improved symptoms and reduced the risk of recurrence compared to placebo. However, these over-the-counter preparations are not regulated, and there have been case reports of fungemia in elderly and debilitated patients. Therefore, they cannot be recommended for routine use in all CDAD cases, but may be appropriate for immunocompetent patients at high risk of recurrence.

C. difficile colitis is partly driven by a deficiency of the normal gut flora. Fecal microbiota transplantation, the transfer of healthy donor stool into the GI tract of an infected patient, is a promising therapy. It has had good clinical outcomes in small trials, with resolution of disease in ~90% of patients. This is much higher than the cure rates achieved with conventional therapy in patients with relapsing *C. difficile*, which are typically only 30%. Fecal transplantation can be accomplished via a variety of mechanisms including nasogastric tube installation, colonoscopy, and frozen fecal capsules. Human feces are considered to be an investigational new drug by the Food and Drug Administration (FDA), because of the potential for transfer of stool and bloodborne pathogens. Fecal bacteriotherapy is at present only available in a limited number of medical centers.

Few data exist to support other therapies. The toxin binder tolevamer appeared to be equivalent to vancomycin in phase 2, but failed to reach noninferiority to vancomycin or metronidazole in a phase 3 study. Therapies studied in uncontrolled settings or case series include intravenous immunoglobulin, active and passive immunization, and anion binding resins, none of which can be recommended for routine use.

In patients with refractory or fulminant disease unresponsive to metronidazole or vancomycin, second-line therapies should be considered, including vancomycin enemas (especially for patients with ileus), fecal transplant, or subtotal colectomy.

RECURRENCE

Recurrence of CDAD occurs in about 20% of patients. Relapses probably result from persistent colonization with *C. difficile* spores, which revert to toxin-producing forms after antibiotics are stopped, and not antibiotic resistance. Recurrences usually present within 5 days of cessation of treatment, but can be delayed up to a month later. Risk factors include the number of prior episodes, resumption or continuation of antibiotics, poor antibody response, female gender, and diverticular disease. If the patient has more than one recurrence, the chance of another is more than 60%. Noncompliance and other causes of diarrhea should also be considered as possible explanations for continued symptoms.

The first recurrence should receive the same treatment as the first occurrence. The second recurrence should be treated with a pulsed vancomycin regimen. If there is a third recurrence after a pulsed vancomycin regimen, fecal microbiota transplant should be considered if available. The pulsed vancomycin regimen should be tapered over several weeks; one small study used a tapering vancomycin regimen over the course of 6 weeks. The regimen started with vancomycin four times daily for a week, then twice daily for a week, then daily for a week, then every second day for a week, then every third day for 2 weeks. Of the 22 patients treated in this study, all were disease free at 6 months. Oral rifaximin (200 mg twice daily for 10 days) following traditional treatment has also been effective in reducing subsequent recurrences in trials.

PREVENTION

Preventing primary or recurrent CDAD is of paramount importance, but there is little evidence that lactobacilli or other agents are effective in primary or secondary prevention. There is also no evidence that routine use of vancomycin or metronidazole in patients starting antibiotics for other conditions reduces the incidence of CDAD.

COMPLICATIONS

Refractory or fulminant CDAD develops in some patients, leading to systemic inflammatory response (characterized by leukocytosis, hypotension, anasarca, and renal failure). The most devastating complication of CDAD is toxic megacolon. In this condition, the large bowel becomes massively dilated (>7 cm) with characteristic thumbprinting due to submucosal edema. These patients are at high risk of perforation and need surgical consultation to be assessed for emergent colectomy. Mortality is high, approximately 50%. Unfortunately, atypical presentations of toxic megacolon are not unusual. In one study of patients requiring colectomy, 20% had a negative *C. difficile* antigen test, and almost 40% had no diarrhea. Therefore, CDAD should be entertained in any patient with colonic dilation.

SYSTEMS IMPROVEMENT

Four major areas of system improvement can decrease the hospital prevalence of *C. difficile*.

1. **Antibiotic stewardship.** Several studies have shown that antibiotic restrictions can decrease rates of *C. difficile* infection. This should be part of a systemwide attempt to reduce unnecessary antibiotics by the use of automatic stop days and formulary restriction. Shorter course of antibiotics and narrow-spectrum antibiotics should be used whenever possible; hospitalists should bear in mind that most cases of *C. difficile* caused by antibiotics given in the hospital develop after hospital discharge.

2. **Early diagnosis and isolation.** Early diagnosis, treatment, and immediate contact isolation of patients are essential in curbing the nosocomial spread of *C. difficile*. Rapid turnaround time of diagnostic testing is essential, and immediate provider notification of positive tests should be built within the laboratory notification system. Systematic, reproducible protocols should exist for initiating contact precautions as soon as a *C. difficile* test is ordered.

3. **Hand hygiene.** Handwashing is essential; *C. difficile* spores are environmentally hardy and resistant to alcohol-based hand rubs. A hand hygiene program with active surveillance and provider feedback should be part of a systemwide attempt to reduce all hospital-acquired infections, including *C. difficile*.

4. **Environment.** Appropriate environmental cleaning and surveillance are crucial to ensure patient and workplace areas are not contaminated.

DISCHARGE CHECKLIST

- Is the patient able to walk, eat, and toilet? Transitional care may be needed in patients unable to perform these elements of self-care.
- For patients not being discharged to home, is the accepting facility aware of the *C. difficile* diagnosis? Continued infection control practices (contact isolation and hand hygiene) should generally remain in effect wherever the patient is being discharged; it can be presumed that patients remain infectious for the duration of the diarrhea (and possibly for some poorly defined time after resolution of diarrhea).
- Does the patient have the financial and functional wherewithal to obtain and complete the full course of antibiotics prescribed? Oral vancomycin capsules may be expensive, and often require prior authorization and hefty copayments from patients. Vancomycin suspension may be formulated more cheaply by hospital pharmacies or compounding pharmacies in the community, although this is not FDA-approved for *C. difficile* colitis.
- Is there a contingency plan if the diarrhea recurs or worsens after discharge? Patients should have a designated physician to contact to arrange for repeat stool testing in the event of recurrent diarrhea.

SUGGESTED READINGS

Bagdasarian N, Rao K, Malani PN. Diagnosis and treatment of *Clostridium difficile* in adults; a systematic review. *JAMA*. 2015;313:398-408.

Cohen SH, Gerding DN, Johnson S, et al. Clinical practice guidelines for clostridium difficile infection in adults: 2010 update by the society for healthcare epidemiology of America (SHEA) and the infectious diseases society of America (IDSA). *Infect Control Hosp Epi*. 2010;31(5):431-455.

Dubberke ER, Gerding DN, Classen D, et al. Strategies to prevent *Clostridium difficile* infections in acute care hospitals. *Infect Control Hosp Epidemiol*. 2008;29(suppl 1):S81-S92.

Kelly CP. A 76-year-old man with recurrent *Clostridium difficile*–associated diarrhea: review of *C. difficile* infection. *JAMA*. 2009;301:954-962.

Lessa FC, Mu Y, Bamberg WM, et al. Burden of *Clostridium difficile* infection in the United States. *N Engl J Med*. 2015;372:825-834.

McDonald EG, Milligan J, Frenette C, Lee TC. Continuous proton pump inhibitor therapy and the associated risk of recurrent *Clostridium difficile* infection. *JAMA Intern Med*. 2015;175:784-791.

Monaghan T, Boswell T, Mahida YR. Recent advances in *Clostridium difficile*-associated disease. *Gut*. 2008;57:850-860.

Surawicz CM, Brandt LJ, Binion CD, et al. Guidelines for diagnosis, treatment, and prevention of *Clostridium difficile* infections. *Am J Gastroenterol*. 2013;108:478-498.

CHAPTER 191

Peritonitis and Intra-Abdominal Abscess

Shira Doron, MD
David R. Snydman, MD, FACP

Key Clinical Questions

❶ How is spontaneous bacterial peritonitis diagnosed?

❷ What is the optimal duration of treatment of spontaneous bacterial peritonitis?

❸ How is secondary peritonitis diagnosed and treated?

❹ When should tuberculous peritonitis be suspected?

❺ How are intra-abdominal abscesses diagnosed and treated?

EPIDEMIOLOGY

Peritonitis and intra-abdominal abscesses are much feared because of the high frequency of associated septic shock and multisystem organ failure. Both primary and secondary peritonitis have an in-hospital mortality rate of approximately 20%. Intra-abdominal infections are the second leading cause of infectious death in the intensive care unit. Although the precise incidence of peritonitis is unknown, it is encountered with some regularity by physicians caring for inpatients. Spontaneous bacterial peritonitis (SBP), or primary peritonitis, occurs in up to 30% of all patients with liver cirrhosis and ascites. Secondary peritonitis and intra-abdominal abscesses are important complications of common conditions on general medical wards, such as diverticulitis, peptic ulcer disease, pancreatitis, and cholecystitis. Classic symptoms and signs of intra-abdominal infection may be blunted in older or immunosuppressed patients, increasing the challenge for clinicians.

PERITONITIS

Peritonitis is inflammation of the peritoneal surface, caused by microorganisms or irritants such as foreign bodies, bile, and barium. Peritonitis is classified as primary (or spontaneous), secondary, or tertiary. In primary peritonitis, there is inflammation of the peritoneal surface without another intra-abdominal process. Secondary peritonitis develops as a result of inflammation of another structure within the abdomen. Tertiary peritonitis refers to persistent inflammation after treatment for secondary peritonitis.

■ SPONTANEOUS (PRIMARY) PERITONITIS

Primary peritonitis, or spontaneous bacterial peritonitis (SBP), is most commonly seen in cirrhotic patients with ascites, and less often in patients with ascites from other causes, such as heart failure or systemic lupus erythematosus. Bacteria may gain access to the peritoneal fluid from hematogenous or lymphogenous spread, traversing the intact intestinal wall from the gut lumen, or by passing through the fallopian tubes from the vagina in women.

Presentation

The classic signs and symptoms of peritonitis are fever, abdominal pain, and rebound tenderness. These may be mild or completely absent in cirrhotic patients. Spontaneous bacterial peritonitis should be suspected in all cirrhotic patients with clinical decompensation, such as the development of hepatic encephalopathy or hepatorenal syndrome.

Bacteriology

Most episodes of SBP are caused by enteric Gram-negative rods, such as *Escherichia coli* and *Klebsiella* species. An important minority are caused by Gram-positive organisms, especially *Streptococcus pneumoniae*. Infections are rarely polymicrobial, and generally do not involve anaerobic bacteria. **Table 191-1** shows the relative frequencies of common organisms isolated from ascitic fluid in patients with SBP.

Diagnosis

The diagnostic approach to peritonitis is summarized in **Figure 191-1**. Fluid should be obtained by paracentesis and sent for Gram stain, culture, cell count with differential, and albumin. Paracentesis is generally safe, even in the setting of grossly abnormal coagulation tests and

TABLE 191-1 Microbiology of Spontaneous Bacterial Peritonitis

Organism	Percent of Isolates
Escherichia coli	43-49
Klebsiella pneumonia	11-20
Other enteric Gram-negative rods	4-5
Streptococcus pneumoniae	3-9
Other streptococci	6-19
Staphylococcus sp.	3-6
Pseudomonas aeruginosa	1-3
Miscellaneous	8-10

Data from Heo J, et al. *Gut Liver*. 2009;3:197-204, and McHutchison JG, Runyon BA. Spontaneous bacterial peritonitis. In: Surawicz CM, Owen RL eds. *Gastrointestinal and Hepatic Infections*. Philadelphia, PA: WB Saunders; 1995:455.

low platelets. Peritoneal fluid should be inoculated into blood culture bottles at the bedside, after changing the needle on the paracentesis syringe to a sterile needle. At least 10 cc of fluid should be inoculated into the bottle if possible. A separate syringe, tube, or container of fluid should be sent for immediate Gram stain. Fluid should also be injected into purple and red top tubes for cell count and chemistries, respectively.

Gram stain is positive in only a minority of cases. In SBP, the cell count is generally greater than 300 white blood cells/mm³, and is usually more than 1000 cells/mm³, with neutrophils predominating on differential. An absolute polymorphonuclear (PMN) leukocyte count of greater than or equal to 250 cells/mm³ in conjunction with a positive culture is diagnostic of peritonitis. A small percentage of patients, such as those with neutropenia, will have fewer cells with active infection. A traumatic procedure can result in entry of blood into the fluid being analyzed, artifactually raising red and white cell counts. To correct for extraneous blood, one can subtract one PMN for every 250 red blood cells present. In appropriately treated SBP, ascitic fluid cell count should start to decline within 48 to 72 hours. If a decline is not seen, an evaluation for secondary peritonitis should be undertaken, beginning with imaging of the abdomen. Repeat paracentesis is not necessary in a patient who is responding well clinically.

It can be difficult to distinguish secondary peritonitis from SBP. Some clues that the infection is secondary to an intra-abdominal process include failure to respond rapidly to antibiotic therapy, serum ascites-albumin gradient less than 1.1 g/dL, indicating the absence of portal hypertension, ascitic total protein greater than 1 g/dL, ascitic fluid glucose concentration less than 50 mg/dL, lactate dehydrogenase greater than the upper limit of normal for serum, and polymicrobial culture. If any of these findings are present, the patient should be imaged with flat and upright abdominal x-rays and an abdominal computed tomography (CT) with oral and intravenous contrast.

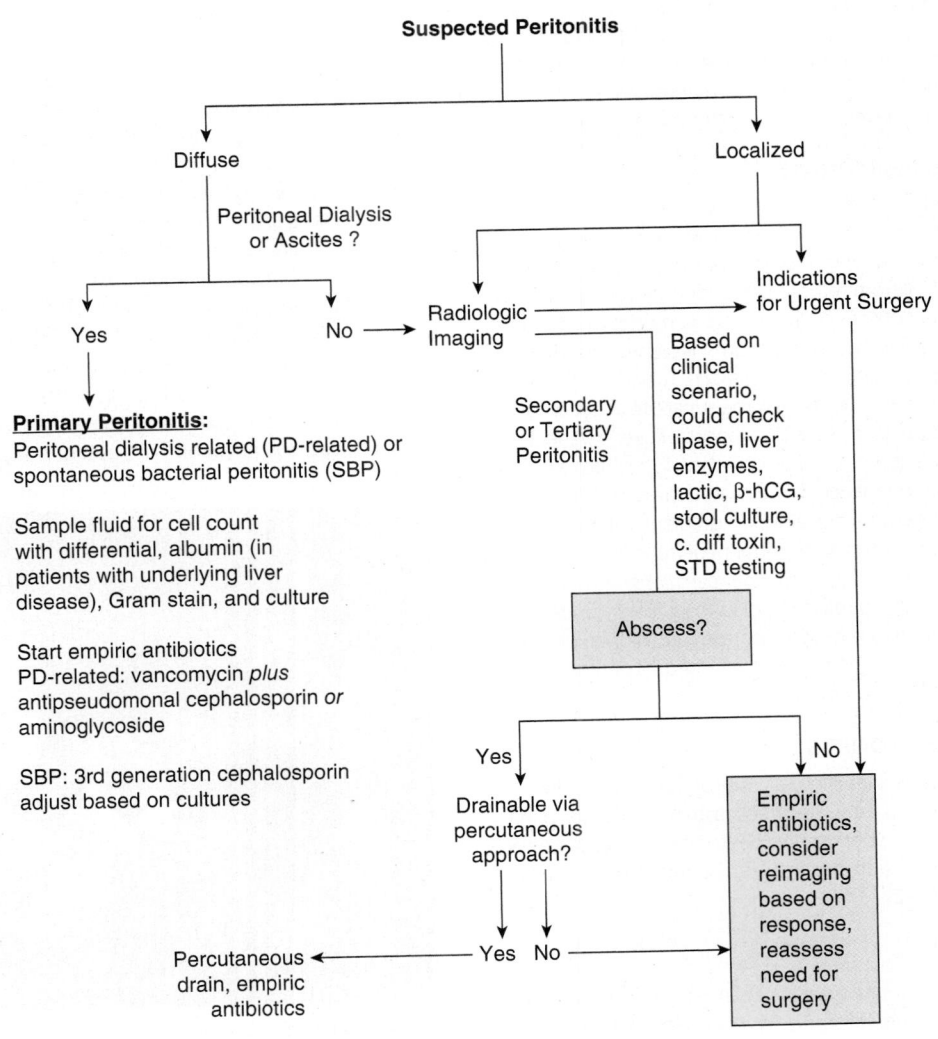

Figure 191-1 *Diagnostic algorithm for suspected peritonitis.*

Treatment

When SBP is suspected, treatment should not be delayed while awaiting the results of laboratory tests. Third-generation cephalosporins are preferred for initial therapy. It is not necessary to empirically cover *Enterococcus* or anaerobic bacteria. Historically, there has been reluctance to use ceftriaxone due to fear of provoking cholestasis in patients with liver failure, but this has not been supported by clinical experience. Due to increasing resistance, fluoroquinolones such as ciprofloxacin should not be used for empiric therapy. However, if culture results reveal a fluoroquinolone-susceptible organism, the high bioavailability of these drugs makes them a good option for oral therapy. Fluoroquinolones should never be used empirically in patients that have received fluoroquinolone prophylaxis for SBP. In patients with a good clinical response, 5 days of therapy is adequate. In patients with an incomplete response after 5 days (eg, persistent pain, fever, or altered mental status), paracentesis should be repeated. If the white blood cell count in ascitic fluid is less than 250 cells/mm³, treatment may be stopped. If the white blood cell count is in excess of 250 cells/mm³, but improved compared to the pretreatment value, treatment should continue, and repeat paracentesis should be considered in a few days. If the white blood cell count remains high, evaluation for secondary peritonitis is indicated. Bacteremia associated with SBP does not require a longer course of therapy, unless it is due to an organism with a robust association with endocarditis, such as *Staphylococcus aureus* or *Enterococcus*.

Prevention

Oral antibiotics are recommended as prophylaxis against SBP in patients with an ascitic fluid protein concentration less than 1.0 g/dL, a prior history of SBP, and recent variceal bleeding. Ciprofloxacin, norfloxacin, and trimethoprim/sulfamethoxazole are all effective and cost effective. Daily dosing is preferred to intermittent dosing, due to the lower likelihood for the development of antibiotic resistance.

■ TUBERCULOUS PERITONITIS

Tuberculous peritonitis is often confused with other conditions. In alcoholic patients, it may mimic SBP, and in women, it may be mistaken for ovarian carcinoma. It results from hematogenous dissemination of tuberculosis (TB) from remote foci of disease such as the lung, or from direct inoculation of bacilli into the peritoneum from intraabdominal lymph nodes. The peritoneum becomes studded with tubercles that exude fluid, and ascites develops. Tuberculous peritonitis should be suspected in patients with the subacute onset of ascites, abdominal pain, and risk factors for TB exposure. Fever is variable. On paracentesis, there will generally be greater than 150 white cells/mm³, with lymphocytic predominance and elevated protein. If the patient is not cirrhotic, the serum ascites-albumin gradient will be less than 1.1 g/dL, indicating the absence of portal hypertension. Ascites fluid culture is rarely positive for *Mycobacteria tuberculosis*, and peritoneal biopsy is usually necessary to make the diagnosis. Biopsy under direct visualization, ideally via laparoscopy, has a much higher yield than blind percutaneous biopsy. Therapy for confirmed TB peritonitis is the same as that given for pulmonary TB.

■ SECONDARY PERITONITIS

Secondary peritonitis is classified as perforation peritonitis and nonperforation peritonitis. Any ruptured gastrointestinal or genitourinary organ may result in perforation peritonitis. Causes of perforation include trauma, infection, peptic ulcer, ischemia, neoplasm, and surgery (see **Table 191-2**).

Presentation

Abdominal pain is almost universal in secondary peritonitis. Nausea, vomiting, and anorexia are common. Fever and leukocytosis are frequently present. Alteration in bowel function may also be present.

TABLE 191-2 Common Causes of Secondary Peritonitis by Source

Esophagus	Perforation (eg, Boerhaave syndrome, tumor)
Stomach	Perforation (eg, from peptic ulcer, tumor)
Duodenum	Perforation (eg, from peptic ulcer, tumor)
Biliary tract	Cholecystitis
	Perforation
Small intestine	Appendicitis
	Ischemic bowel
	Incarcerated hernia
	Crohn's disease
	perforation
Large intestine	Diverticulitis
	Perforation
	Ulcerative colitis, Crohn's disease
	Ischemic colitis
	Infectious colitis
Female reproductive organs	Pelvic inflammatory disease
Urinary tract	Perinephric abscess
Other	Necrotizing pancreatitis
	Perihepatic abscess

The specific character, location, and progression of the abdominal pain depend on the etiology of the peritonitis. Ruptured peptic ulcer pain has a sudden onset and is worse in the epigastric region, while appendicitis pain has a gradual onset and classically begins as a diffuse pain that localizes to the right lower quadrant, sometimes with periappendiceal abscess formation (**Figure 191-2**).

Peritoneal signs are used by clinicians to distinguish peritonitis that may require surgery from other types of abdominal pain. These signs include rebound tenderness, which indicates the presence of parietal peritoneal inflammation, and muscular rigidity of the abdominal wall (including both voluntary guarding and reflex muscle spasm). In general, peritoneal signs are specific but not sensitive for the diagnosis of peritonitis. Patients with peritonitis may lack peritoneal signs due to lax abdominal musculature (eg, postpartum women), ascites, glucocorticoid use, or the presence of an abscess

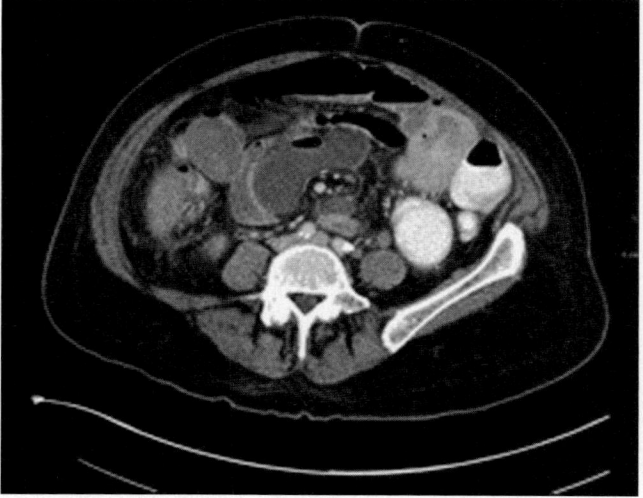

Figure 191-2 *Abdominal CT scan with oral and intravenous contrast demonstrating periappendiceal abscess in the right lower quadrant.*

that is not in contact with the anterior abdominal wall. Carnett sign may help distinguish pain arising from the abdominal wall from that of visceral origin. The patient is examined while he or she tenses the abdominal muscles by raising the head and shoulders off the bed. If the abdomen becomes more tender during this maneuver, Carnett sign is positive, and a pain source in the abdominal wall, such as a hernia or rectus sheath hematoma, should be suspected.

Bacteriology

Infection in perforation peritonitis is usually polymicrobial, featuring *E. coli*, other Gram-negative rods, and anaerobic bacteria (**Table 191-3**). The bacteria involved vary depending on the organ perforated. Different segments of the gastrointestinal tract have different microbial ecologies, and these may be further altered by hospitalization, surgery, acid blockers, or antibiotics.

Diagnosis

Initial evaluation of a patient with suspected peritonitis should always include flat and upright abdominal films and a chest x-ray. These may reveal free air in the abdomen in the case of perforated viscus (**Figure 191-3**), and also help to rule out a thoracic or pulmonary process masquerading as peritonitis.

Abdominal CT scan is the next step, unless the disease is suspected to be in the right upper quadrant, retroperitoneum, or pelvis, in which case ultrasound is often more helpful diagnostically. It is currently rare for a patient to be taken to the operating room without a CT or ultrasound. Laboratory studies that may be helpful include complete blood count, urea nitrogen, creatinine, liver enzymes, lipase, urinalysis, and pregnancy test in women of childbearing potential. Blood cultures, if positive, are helpful in determining appropriate regimen and duration of therapy in patients with health care associated or severe infection, or those at high risk for treatment failure (**Table 191-4**).

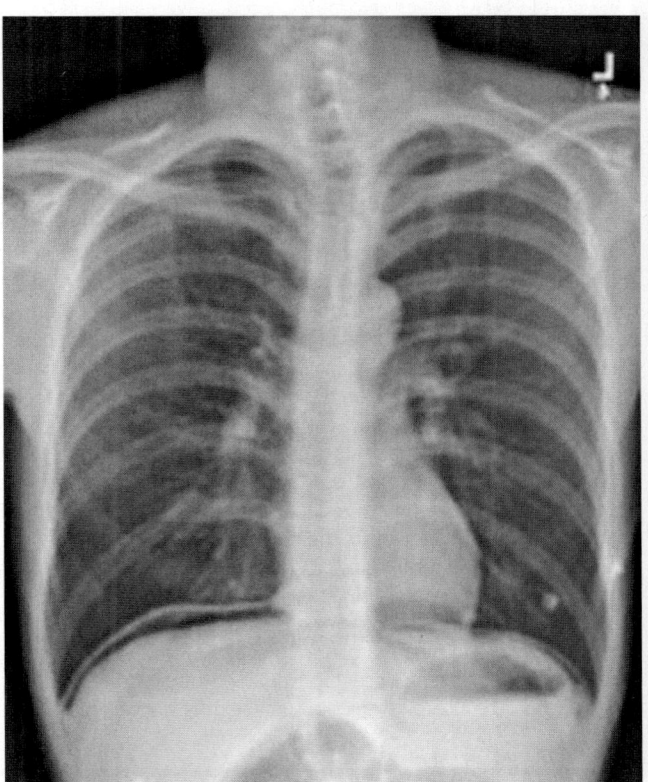

Figure 191-3 *Chest radiograph demonstrating free air under both hemidiaphragms due to perforation of a hollow viscus.* (Reproduced, with permission, from Fauci AS, Braunwald E, Kasper DL, et al. *Harrison's Principles of Internal Medicine,* 17th ed. New York, NY: McGraw-Hill; 2008, Fig. 121-2.)

Intra-abdominal specimens should be sent for culture in health care associated infection and severe infection. Intra-abdominal culture should also be obtained in community-acquired infection of mild to moderate severity when there is a substantial local prevalence of antimicrobial resistance to drugs such as fluoroquinolones or ampicillin-sulbactam. At least 1 mL of fluid or tissue from the infection site should be transported to the laboratory. In order to isolate anaerobic organisms, an anaerobic transport tube should be used.

Treatment

In most cases, definitive therapy for secondary peritonitis involves either surgical or percutaneous drainage. Perforated organs usually

TABLE 191-3 Organisms in Complicated Intra-abdominal Infection

Organism	Percent of Isolates
Facultative and aerobic Gram-negative	
E. coli	48-71
Klebsiella species	14
Pseudomonas aeruginosa	7-14
Proteus mirabilis	5
Enterobacter species	5
Anaerobic	
Bacteroides fragilis	7-35
Other *Bacteroides* species	71
Clostridium species	29
Prevotella species	12
Peptostreptococcus species	17
Fusobacterium species	9
Eubacterium species	17
Gram-positive aerobic cocci	
Streptococcus species	4-38
Enterococcus faecalis	12
Enterococcus faecium	3
Enterococcus species	8
S. aureus	1-4

Data from Solomkin JS, et al. *Clin Infect Dis.* 2010;50:133-164. Chen Z, et al. *BMC Infect Dis.* 2010;10:217.

TABLE 191-4 Clinical Factors Predicting Treatment Failure in Intra-Abdominal Infection

Delay in initial intervention (>12 h)

High severity of illness (APACHE II score 15 or higher)

Advanced age

Comorbidity and degree of organ dysfunction

Low albumin level

Poor nutritional status

Degree of peritoneal involvement or diffuse peritonitis

Inability to achieve adequate debridement or control of drainage

Presence of malignancy

APACHE, Acute Physiology and Chronic Health Evaluation.
Reproduced from Solomkin JS, Mazuski JE, Bradley JS, et al. *Clin Infect Dis.* 2010;50:133-164 by permission of Oxford University Press.

need closure or removal, and fecal spillage requires washout. Focal collections generally are not cured without drainage. Fluid resuscitation should be initiated when the diagnosis of secondary peritonitis is made. Antimicrobial therapy should be initiated as soon as possible, while awaiting a procedure and before culture data are obtained. Many broad-spectrum antibiotics and antibiotic combinations provide good empiric coverage for the Gram-negative enteric organisms and gut streptococci usually involved in intra-abdominal infection. Antibiotics active against obligate anaerobes such as *Bacteroides* and *Clostridium* species are necessary when infection arises from the distal small bowel or colon, or from a more proximal source in the setting of obstruction or ileus. Cefotetan and clindamycin are no longer acceptable empiric agents for coverage of *Bacteroides* due to rising resistance. Empiric coverage for *Pseudomonas* is generally unnecessary in patients with mild to moderate community-acquired peritonitis. Infections arising from the biliary tract are treated similarly to proximal small bowel infections, unless they occur after a bilio-enteric anastamosis, which should be treated with regimens used for severe or high-risk peritonitis. It is unnecessary to treat every organism identified on culture. *Enterococcus* and *Candida*, in particular, can often be left untreated without compromising the resolution of the infection. Therapy for these organisms should be considered if they are isolated from blood, are the predominant organism on culture, or persist as the sole organism after treatment. Acceptable antibiotic regimens are listed in **Table 191-5**. The use of ampicillin-sulbactam is discouraged in the

TABLE 191-5 **Antibiotic Regimens for Secondary Peritonitis**

Infection	Regimen
Community-acquired, mild to moderate severity, infection of gastric or proximal small bowel source, including cholecystitis without bilio-enteric anastomosis	Cefazolin, cefuroxime, or ceftriaxone
Community-acquired, mild-to-moderate severity, patient not high risk (see Table 191-4), source distal small bowel or colon	Cefoxitin, ertapenem, tigecycline, or ticarcillin-clavulanic acid alone OR metronidazole plus either cefazolin, cefuroxime, ceftriaxone, cefotaxime, ciprofloxacin, levofloxacin, or moxifloxacin
Community-acquired, high risk (see Table 191-4) or severe, source distal small bowel or colon, or cholecystitis after bilio-enteric anastomosis	Imipenem-cilastatin, meropenem, doripenem, or piperacillin-tazobactam alone OR metronidazole plus cefepime or ceftazidime (in many communities resistance to the fluoroquinolones ciprofloxacin and levofloxacin is too high to make these agents acceptable for empiric therapy of severe infections)
Health care associated	Use local microbiologic data to guide empiric therapy: Imipenem-cilastatin, meropenem, doripenem, or piperacillin-tazobactam alone OR metronidazole plus cefepime or ceftazidime Add vancomycin to cover methicillin-resistant *S. aureus* (MRSA)

2010 Infectious Diseases Society of America guidelines, due to increasing resistance among *E. coli*. In late 2014 and early 2015, two new drugs with activity against multidrug-resistant Gram-negative organisms, ceftolozane-tazobactam and ceftazidime-avibactam, were approved by the Food and Drug Administration for treatment of intra-abdominal infection. Similar products are in the pharmaceutical pipeline.

PRACTICE POINT

- When treating an intra-abdominal abscess, it is not necessary to target antibiotic therapy to every organism isolated. Likewise, if a patient is responding clinically to an antibiotic regimen, and culture data show that there is an organism that is not being covered, it is not imperative to change the regimen.

In most cases, when good source control is achieved within 24 hours, only perioperative antibiotics are needed as therapy. This includes appendicitis, cholecystitis, and penetrating bowel trauma. Infections requiring a longer course are generally adequately treated after 4 to 7 days. Patients with clinical evidence of persistent infection after 4 to 7 days should be assessed for possible ongoing intra-abdominal infection, an extra-abdominal source of infection, or antibiotic resistance.

■ TERTIARY PERITONITIS

Tertiary peritonitis refers to recurrent intra-abdominal infection after therapy with antibiotics and drainage for secondary peritonitis. Abscess formation is expected in this setting. The predominant organisms reflect exposure to antimicrobials and the hospital environment and are therefore commonly resistant to first-line antibiotics. Examples include yeast, *Enterococcus*, and resistant Gram-negative bacteria such as *Pseudomonas* and *Enterobacter*. Most patients with tertiary peritonitis require one or more additional operative procedures to achieve control of their infection.

■ PERITONEAL DIALYSIS-RELATED

Many patients with renal failure prefer home peritoneal dialysis (PD). Unfortunately, peritonitis is an exceedingly common complication, and the major reason that PD patients have to switch to hemodialysis. Gram-positive bacteria cause the majority of infections, Gram-negative bacteria cause about one-quarter, and fungal peritonitis accounts for less than 5% of episodes. International Society of Peritoneal Dialysis guidelines recommend empiric coverage for both Gram-positive (including methicillin-resistant *S. aureus* where this organism is prevalent) and Gram-negative organisms. This is usually achieved with a combination of vancomycin plus a cephalosporin or aminoglycoside. Antifungal therapy should be initiated only if the Gram stain reveals yeast. Antibiotics may be given intraperitoneally. Antimicrobial therapy should be narrowed based on culture results. A minimum treatment duration of 2 weeks is appropriate for uncomplicated infections. Three weeks of therapy are advised if response to treatment is slow, especially when the infection is caused by *S. aureus*, *Enterococcus* or Gram-negatives.

Peritoneal dialysis catheter removal is an important part of therapy under certain circumstances. Clinical scenarios that should prompt catheter removal include relapse of infection within 4 weeks after completing antibiotic therapy, infection not responding to appropriate antibiotics, exit site or tunnel infection, fungal peritonitis, and possibly tuberculous peritonitis.

Recommended measures to reduce the risk of PD-related peritonitis include the use of prophylactic antibiotics at the time of catheter insertion, training of the patient or caregiver in meticulous catheter care, and use of topical antibiotics either at the catheter exit site, intranasally or both.

■ PERITONITIS IN THE IMMMUNOCOMPROMISED PATIENT

In the immunocompromised or elderly patient, signs of peritoneal inflammation may be blunted or absent, so a low threshold is needed to evaluate the abdomen for peritonitis. Many intra-abdominal conditions preferentially affect the patient weakened by drugs or disease, such as typhlitis (necrosis of the bowel wall related to breakdown of microbial defenses) in the postchemotherapy neutropenic patient, or cytomegalovirus colitis in the post-transplant or AIDS patient. Patients who have been hospitalized or who have received antibiotic courses are at high risk of developing *Clostridium difficile* colitis.

PRACTICE POINT

- *C. difficile* colitis without diarrhea can mimic SBP or intra-abdominal abscess. Suspect *C. difficile* in any patient with abdominal symptoms and recent antibiotic use or hospitalization, especially if the serum white blood cell count is high, or if colitis is seen on CT scan.

INTRA-ABDOMINAL ABSCESSES

Abscesses can be classified by cause, like peritonitis, into primary or secondary, or by location, as intraperitoneal, retroperitoneal, or visceral. Primary abscesses develop for unknown reasons. Secondary abscesses develop near an infected organ, after a perforation or trauma, as a postoperative complication, as in anastamotic leak, or after primary peritonitis. The location of an abscess is generally related to the site of origin of the infection and the direction of dependent drainage. Abscesses may also extend and erode. They can track from the abdomen down into the thigh, or up into the pleural space. They can form fistulae, or erode into blood vessels and cause hemorrhage.

Abscesses are typically polymicrobial and involve normal bowel flora. Most have an anaerobic component, although the anaerobic bacteria are often not successfully grown on culture. Increasingly, *S. aureus* is found as a cause of intra-abdominal abscesses. **Table 191-6** lists common associated organisms and features of abscesses in various visceral locations.

■ PRESENTATION

Presenting features vary widely, depending on location and source. Anorexia and nausea are common. Fever and leukocytosis are usually present. The course can be acute or subacute, or even chronic in the case of some subphrenic abscesses. There is usually tenderness and possibly fullness over the abscess. Abscesses eroding into or near the thoracic cavity may cause chest and respiratory signs and symptoms. Abscesses adjacent to the colon may cause diarrhea, and those adjacent to the bladder may cause urinary symptoms.

■ DIAGNOSIS

Computed tomography scan of the abdomen is usually the first step in diagnosis. Findings consistent with abscess include low-density tissue mass, capsule formation, and extraluminal gas. Oral contrast helps to distinguish intraluminal contents from abscess, and intravenous contrast helps to enhance the abscess for identification. **Figure 191-4** shows a CT scan of a liver abscess with typical ring enhancement.

Ultrasound is generally not used for diagnosis of intra-abdominal abscess, except for those in the right upper quadrant and female reproductive structures, as its sensitivity is reduced by overlying bowel gas, and it is difficult to perform in the setting of abdominal wounds and drains. Occult abscesses can sometimes be detected on radionuclide scan using radiolabeled leukocytes in a patient undergoing workup for prolonged fever or leukocytosis of unknown origin.

■ TREATMENT

Drainage (source control) is necessary for cure in all but the smallest abscesses. Antibiotics are used as adjunctive therapy. Percutaneous drainage is suitable when there is only one or a few abscess cavities, ideally with communication between them, so that only a minimal number of passes with the catheter is needed for drainage; the catheter does not need to traverse bowel or other organs on its route from the skin to the abscess; and the infected fluid is not too viscous to drain through the catheter. If percutaneous drainage cannot be achieved, a surgical procedure is usually necessary. Abscess material should always be sent for culture. Drains placed percutaneously must be closely followed to ensure that the desired result, resolution of the abscess, is achieved. This generally requires periodic follow-up imaging and may also include injection of contrast material to confirm placement of the catheter in the appropriate space or to

TABLE 191-6 Visceral Abscesses

Organ	Causes	Microbiology	Other Features
Pancreas	Complication of pancreatitis Secondary infection of pancreatic pseudocyst	Polymicrobial, enteric; occasionally *S. aureus*	Serum amylase frequently elevated
Liver	Complication of cholecystitis, appendicitis or diverticulitis Complication of liver transplantation Chronic granulomatous disease	Polymicrobial, enteric Increasingly monomicrobial due to *Klebsiella*, especially in Asia *Entamoeba histolytica* Occasionally *S. aureus* Rarely *Yersinia enterocolitica* *Candida* in immunocompromised hosts	Alkaline phosphatase is the most frequently deranged laboratory value Amoebic abscess does not require drainage for effective treatment
Spleen	Trauma Bacteremia, especially in IV drug users Hematogenous spread to infarcted tissue in sickle cell patients Embolic from bacterial endocarditis	*S. aureus* and streptococci if due to endocarditis *Salmonella* in sickle cell disease Occasionally polymicrobial, enteric *Candida* in immunocompromised hosts	May experience referred pain in left shoulder (Kehr sign) Splenic rub

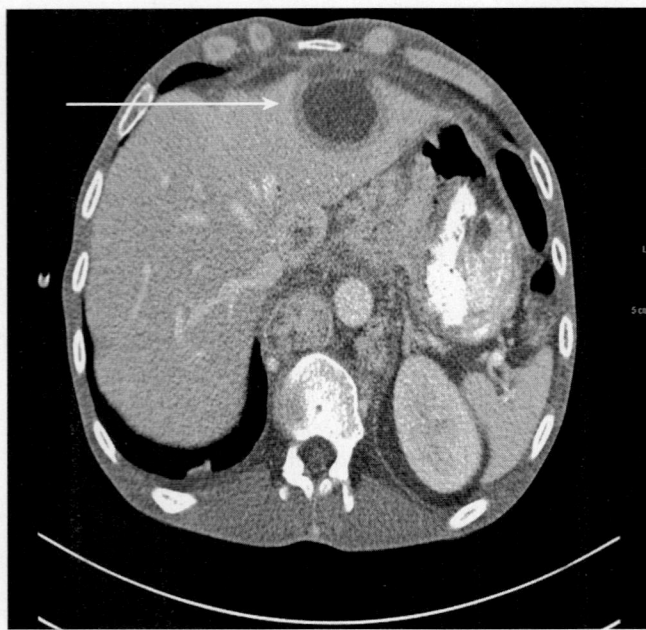

Figure 191-4 *Abdominal CT scan with intravenous and oral contrast demonstrating abscess in the left lobe of the liver; ring enhancement is present.*

assess the size of the cavity. Adjunct drainage maneuvers such as catheter flushing and upsizing of the tubing may be necessary in some circumstances. The catheter should be removed promptly upon documentation of resolution of infection, as it can be a cause of secondary infection.

Empiric antibiotic choice should follow the same principles as in secondary peritonitis, except that anaerobic coverage is essential. Treatment should be targeted to culture results when they become available. The 2015 STOP-IT trial evaluated the efficacy of fixed-duration antibiotics (4 days following source control procedure) versus extended therapy (given for 2 days after resolution of physiologic abnormalities consisting of fever, leukocytosis and difficulty eating; the median duration of treatment in this group was 8 days). There was no difference between groups in the outcomes of surgical site infection, recurrent intra-abdominal infection, or death. Given global efforts to minimize antibiotic use due to resistance, cost, and adverse effects including risk of *C. difficile* infection, these conclusions should be reassuring that a short antibiotic course after adequate drainage is a very reasonable option. If a catheter is left in for prolonged drainage, experts generally recommend that antibiotics continue for as long as the catheter is in place.

SUGGESTED READINGS

Koulaouzidis A, Bhat S, Saeed AA. Spontaneous bacterial peritonitis. *World J Gastroenterol.* 2009;15:1042-1049.

Li PK, Szeto CC, Piraino B, et al. Peritoneal dialysis-related infections recommendations: 2010 update. *Perit Dial Int.* 2010;30:393-423.

Piraino B, Bernardini J, Brown E, et al. ISPD position statement on reducing the risks of peritoneal dialysis-related infections. *Perit Dial Int.* 2011;31:614-630.

Sawyer RG, Claridge JA, Nathens AB, et al. Trial of short-course antimicrobial therapy for intraabdominal infection. *N Engl J Med.* 2015;372:1996-2005.

Solomkin JS, Mazuski JE, Bradley JS, et al. Diagnosis and management of complicated intra-abdominal infection in adults and children: guidelines by the Surgical Infection Society and the Infectious Diseases Society of America. *Clin Infect Dis.* 2010; 50:133-64.

CHAPTER 192

Meningitis and Encephalitis

Karen L. Roos, MD
Jared R. Brosch, MD, MS

Key Clinical Questions

1. Is the classic triad of fever, headache, and stiff neck reliable for bacterial meningitis?
2. What signs and symptoms distinguish meningitis from encephalitis?
3. What is appropriate empiric antimicrobial therapy?
4. When should a computed tomography (CT) scan be done before lumbar puncture, and is magnetic resonance imaging (MRI) or CT the better study to obtain?
5. What cerebrospinal fluid (CSF) studies are essential, and which ones should be done if the initial studies do not yield a diagnosis?
6. Which MRI abnormalities are classic for a specific viral etiology of encephalitis?
7. How soon can the patient be discharged, and how long to continue antimicrobial therapy?
8. When should a neurology consult be obtained?

INTRODUCTION

Meningitis and encephalitis may be the most terrifying diseases in medicine. Bacterial meningitis and viral encephalitis may be rapidly fatal, even in healthy persons. Survivors may suffer lasting neurological sequelae, including memory loss and seizures. Cases of meningococcal meningitis spark great anxiety in both caregivers and casual contacts. Viral meningitis, by contrast, gives patients a bad headache and a stiff neck, but uneventful recovery is the rule.

In the United States, bacterial meningitis affects 1.4 to 2.0 per 100,000 population annually, viral meningitis approximately 14 per 100,000 annually, and encephalitis 7 per 100,000 annually. Encephalitis generally implies viral encephalitis, although bacteria, parasites, spirochetes, and fungi may all cause encephalitis. In this chapter, encephalitis refers specifically to viral encephalitis.

CLINICAL PRESENTATION

■ MENINGITIS

Is the classic triad reliable?

The classic triad of meningitis is fever, headache, and stiff neck (nuchal rigidity). Patients with bacterial meningitis may also have an altered level of consciousness. Almost all patients with bacterial meningitis have at least two of these features, so the absence of all four makes bacterial meningitis unlikely. Patients may also complain of photophobia, nausea, and vomiting.

It is difficult, if not impossible, to exclude bacterial meningitis based on the physical examination. Findings may include nuchal rigidity (pain on passive flexion of the neck), Kernig's sign, and Brudzinski's sign. Kernig's sign is elicited with the patient in the supine position. The thigh is flexed on the abdomen with the knee flexed. Attempts to passively extend the leg cause pain when meningeal irritation is present. Brudzinski's sign is elicited with the patient in the supine position, and is positive when passive flexion of the neck results in flexion of the hips and knees. Patients with bacterial meningitis may also have focal neurological deficits or seizures.

Less than 50% of children with bacterial meningitis have nuchal rigidity. The possibility of bacterial meningitis should be considered in every child with fever, vomiting, photophobia, lethargy, or altered mental status. Many cases of bacterial meningitis in children are preceded by upper respiratory tract infections or otitis media. Signs of meningitis in the neonate are nonspecific, and include irritability, lethargy, poor feeding, vomiting, diarrhea, temperature instability (fever or hypothermia), respiratory distress, apnea, seizures, and a bulging fontanel.

Patients with viral meningitis complain of fever, headache, stiff neck, photophobia, nausea, and vomiting, but are awake and alert.

PRACTICE POINT

- Patients with viral meningitis are awake and alert. They are not lethargic or confused. The patient with a febrile illness, CSF lymphocytic pleocytosis, and lethargy or confusion has encephalitis, not viral meningitis.

Tuberculous meningitis presents as either a slowly progressive illness with persistent and intractable headache that has been present for weeks, followed by confusion, lethargy, meningismus, focal neurological deficits, and cranial nerve deficits, or an acute

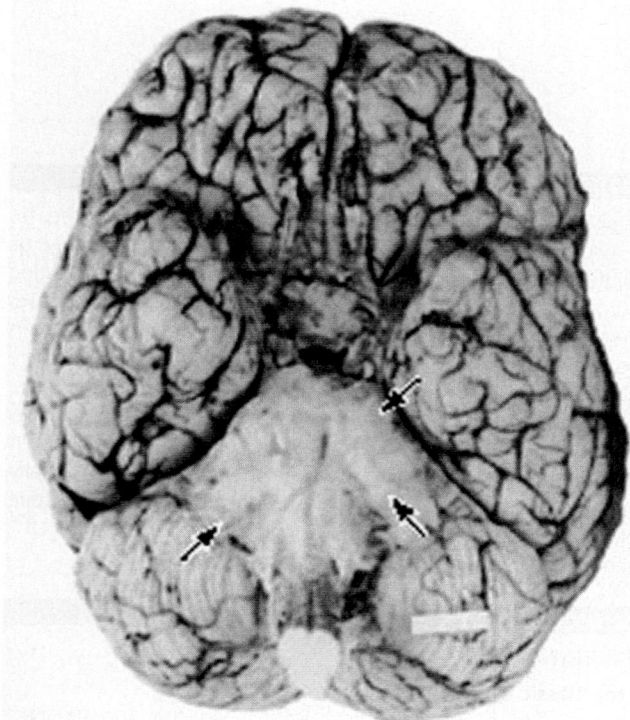

Figure 192-1 *Autopsy specimen in a patient with tuberculous meningitis, with prominent basilar exudate (arrows).* (Reproduced, with permission, from Waxman SG. *Clinical Neuroanatomy*, 26th ed. New York, NY: McGraw-Hill; 2010. Fig. 25-17.)

meningoencephalitis characterized by coma, raised intracranial pressure, seizures, and focal neurological deficits. The basilar meninges are predominantly involved (**Figure 192-1**). Fungal meningitis clinically resembles tuberculous meningitis. Patients complain of headache, fever, and malaise, followed by meningeal signs, altered mental status, and cranial nerve palsies.

■ ENCEPHALITIS

Patients with encephalitis have fever and headache and at least one of the following: altered level of consciousness, confusion, or abnormal behavior, new onset seizures, and focal neurological deficits.

ETIOLOGY

■ BACTERIAL MENINGITIS

Pathogens causing meningitis depend upon age and predisposing or associated conditions (**Table 192-1**). *Streptococcus pneumoniae* is the most common cause of meningitis in adults older than 20 (45%-50% of cases). Infection may begin with pneumonia, otitis media, or sinusitis. Meningococci are directly spread by large droplet respiratory secretions, and tend to infect adolescents who share cigarettes, cokes, and kisses. *Listeria monocytogenes* (about 8% of cases) is a food-borne infection found in sources as diverse as processed meats, unpasteurized cheeses, cheese balls, hot dogs, and raw vegetables.

■ VIRAL MENINGITIS

The most common etiological agents of aseptic meningitis are viruses. Enteroviruses have been found in more than 75% of cases in which a specific pathogen has been identified. Enteroviruses include the coxsackieviruses, echoviruses, poliovirus, and numbered enteroviruses (such as EVD68, associated with severe respiratory illness, and EVD71, the cause of hand, foot, and mouth disease).

TABLE 192-1 Bacterial Etiology for Meningitis Based on Predisposing Condition

Predisposing Condition	Bacterial Pathogen
Neonate	Group B streptococcus, *Escherichia coli, Listeria monocytogenes*
Healthy children and adults with community acquired disease	*Streptococcus pneumoniae, Neisseria meningitidis*
Otitis, mastoiditis, sinusitis	Streptococci sp, Gram-negative anaerobes (*Bacteroides* sp, *Fusobacterium* sp), Enterobacteriaceae (*Proteus* sp, *E. coli, Klebsiella* sp), staphylococci, *Haemophilus influenzae*
Adults over age 55 or with chronic illness	*S. pneumoniae, N. meningitidis,* Gram-negative bacilli, *L. monocytogenes, H. influenzae*
Postneurosurgical or intraventricular device	Staphylococci, Gram-negative bacilli
Endocarditis	Viridans streptococci, *Staphylococcus aureus, Streptococcus bovis,* HACEK group, enterococci

HACEK group, *Haemophilus* sp, *Actinobacillus actinomycetemcomitans, Cardiobacterium hominis, Eikenella corrodens,* and *Kingella kingae.*

Herpes simplex virus-2 (HSV-2) and HIV are also common etiological agents of viral meningitis. Approximately 25% of women and 11% of men develop meningitis during the primary episode of genital herpes, with up to 20% of these patients having recurrent attacks of meningitis (Mollaret's meningitis). Arthropod-borne viruses (arboviruses), such as West Nile, can cause meningitis or encephalitis. Lymphocytic choriomeningitis virus causes a prolonged lymphocytic meningitis syndrome.

■ VIRAL ENCEPHALITIS

Viral encephalitis is an acute febrile illness. Herpes simplex virus-1 (HSV-1) is the most important cause of sporadic encephalitis in immunocompetent adults, and the most common cause of viral encephalitis in developed countries. The arboviruses are viruses transmitted by the bite of a mosquito or tick. The most common arboviruses causing encephalitis in North America are West Nile virus, St. Louis encephalitis virus, and La Crosse virus.

Varicella zoster virus may cause encephalitis in association with shingles, months after shingles, and in the absence of shingles. Epstein-Barr virus may cause encephalitis as an acute complication of mononucleosis. Cytomegalovirus causes encephalitis in the immunocompromised.

PRACTICE POINT

- *L. monocytogenes*, herpes simplex virus-1, flaviviruses (West Nile virus, St. Louis encephalitis virus, Japanese encephalitis virus), enterovirus-71, and rabies may cause a rhombencephalitis, or brainstem encephalitis, often with a prodrome of several days of headache, vomiting, and fever, followed by cranial nerve palsies, cerebellar, and long-tract motor and sensory deficits.

DIFFERENTIAL DIAGNOSIS

■ BACTERIAL MENINGITIS

The differential diagnosis of bacterial meningitis includes viral meningitis, fungal meningitis, tuberculous meningitis, viral encephalitis, and an infectious mass lesion. Subarachnoid hemorrhage may also present with headache and stiff neck.

■ VIRAL MENINGITIS

The differential diagnosis of viral meningitis includes partially treated bacterial meningitis, fungal meningitis, tuberculous meningitis, Lyme disease, drug-induced meningitis (NSAIDs, intravenous immunoglobulin, cephalosporins, penicillins, sulfa drugs, isoniazid, and muromonab-CD3), carcinomatous meningitis, lymphomatous meningitis, and sarcoidosis.

■ VIRAL ENCEPHALITIS

The differential diagnosis of viral encephalitis includes the other etiological agents of encephalitis: bacteria, mycobacteria, fungi, *Rickettsia*, protozoa, and parasites. Encephalitis may also be an autoimmune illness, such as nonvasculitic autoimmune inflammatory meningoencephalitis (steroid responsive encephalopathy associated with autoimmune thyroiditis [SREAT]), a paraneoplastic encephalitis, or a para- or postinfectious disorder, such as acute disseminated encephalomyelitis.

DIAGNOSIS

■ MENINGITIS

The diagnostic approach to the patient with fever and headache is summarized in **Figure 192-2**. The first step in the diagnosis of meningitis is physical examination, followed by CBC with differential, C-reactive protein, and blood for Gram stain and culture.

Antimicrobial therapy is initiated at this step. When bacterial meningitis is suspected, always start empiric and adjunctive therapy immediately after obtaining CBC and blood cultures. Do not wait for the results of spinal fluid analysis to initiate antimicrobial therapy.

Serum procalcitonin, if available, is one of the most sensitive labs for distinguishing between bacterial and viral meningitis. Serum procalcitonin and C-reactive protein (>40 mg/L) are significantly higher in patients with bacterial meningitis than in those with viral meningitis.

When is a CT scan needed before an LP?

Although every patient with suspected meningitis or encephalitis needs an LP for spinal fluid analysis, not every patient needs a CT prior to an LP. **Table 192-2** lists the indications for CT prior to LP. In hospital practice, nearly every patient gets neuroimaging, either CT or MRI prior to LP. If empiric antimicrobial therapy has been initiated, MRI is the more sensitive study for meningitis and encephalitis. If MRI is obtained after LP, the meninges may enhance with the administration of gadolinium, thus it is preferable to obtain MRI prior to LP.

Although CT and MRI scans do not diagnose increased intracranial pressure, they do demonstrate mass lesions with associated edema and brain parenchymal shifts that potentially can cause herniation following lumbar puncture. Even with a normal CT or MRI scan, there is a risk of cerebral herniation in bacterial meningitis, and lumbar puncture is often not the cause of the herniation. One indication for CT scan or MRI, although not often discussed, may be simply to demonstrate that lumbar puncture was safe to perform in the event that cerebral herniation occurs.

What are the best tests on cerebrospinal fluid (CSF) to make the diagnosis?

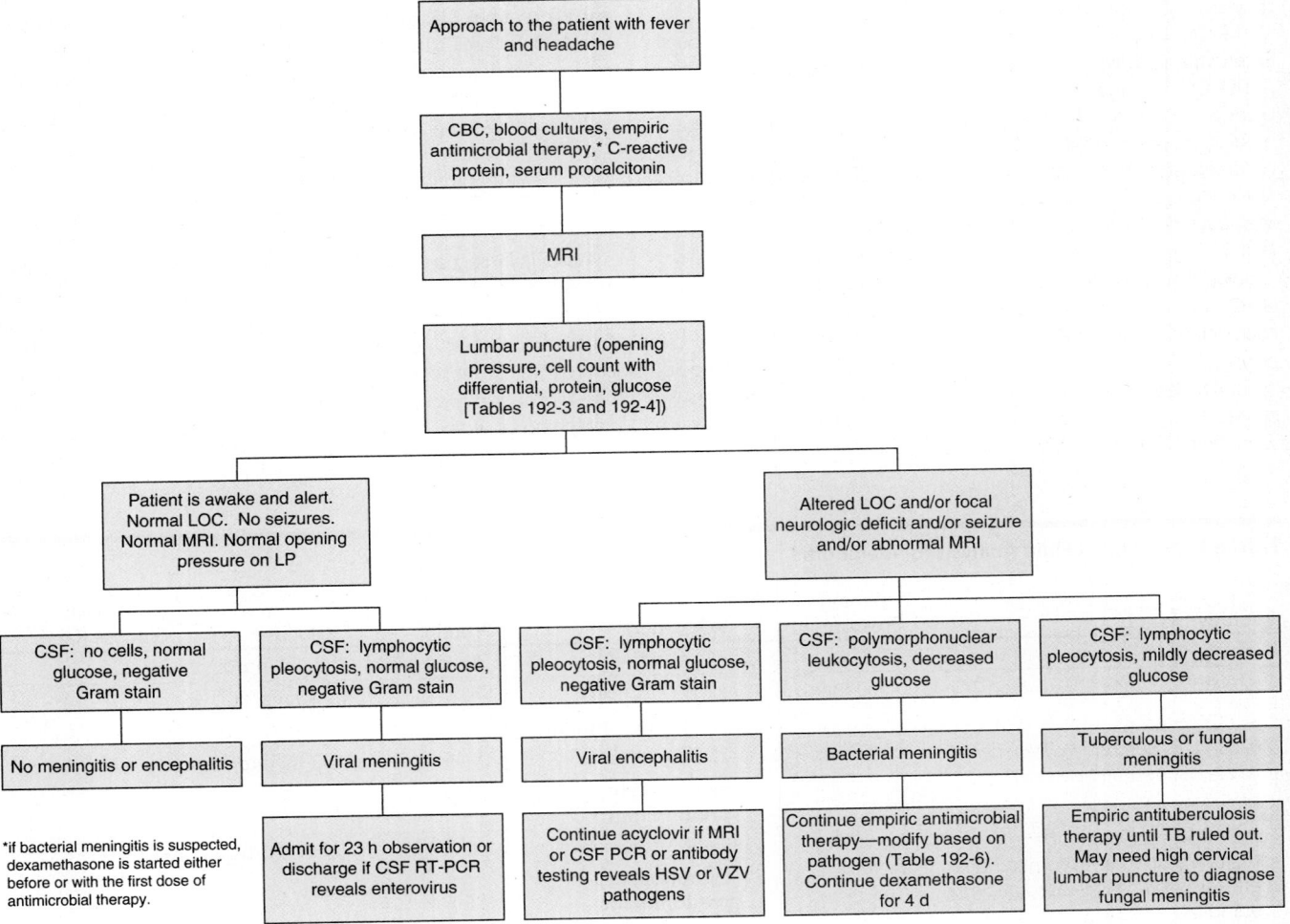

Figure 192-2 *The diagnostic approach to the patient with fever and headache.*

TABLE 192-2 Indications for CT Prior to LP

Abnormal level of consciousness	New onset seizure
Focal neurological deficit	Immunocompromised state
Papilledema	Poorly visualized fundi

Table 192-3 provides a list of the expected results for opening pressure, cell count with differential, glucose concentration, and protein concentration in normal and infected CSF. **Table 192-4** lists the CSF diagnostic tests for meningitis. There are several important exceptions to the expected CSF values shown in Table 192-3. In enteroviral meningitis and arboviral infections, there may be a predominance of polymorphonuclear leukocytes early in the disease. In enteroviral infection, the transition to a lymphocytic pleocytosis usually occurs over the course of 24 hours. For arboviruses, the transition to a CSF lymphocytic pleocytosis may take a week or more, and the transition may never occur in West Nile virus infection.

The CSF white blood cell count is affected by the amount of time between collection and laboratory analysis. Polymorphonuclear leukocytes have a half-life of approximately 2 hours. Therefore, it is important that the spinal fluid is analyzed within 90 minutes of collection to obtain an accurate result.

In cases of suspected bacterial meningitis, CSF Gram stain allows for rapid identification of the meningeal pathogen, and culture allows for specific identification and antimicrobial susceptibility testing. There is both a broad-range bacterial 16S ribosomal DNA PCR (polymerase chain reaction) and a meningeal pathogen-specific PCR, but their sensitivity and specificity have not been defined, and they are not routinely available.

The CSF RT-PCR for enteroviruses is usually available in 4 hours. Enteroviruses grow in CSF culture; HSV-2 typically does not.

The CSF in tuberculous meningitis typically has a lymphocytic pleocytosis of 200 to 500 cells/mm^3, and a mildly decreased median glucose concentration of 40 mg/dL. The last tube of CSF collected should be sent for acid-fast bacilli smear and culture. The nucleic acid amplification test (NAAT) to detect nucleic acid of *Mycobacterium tuberculosis* in spinal fluid is available, and should be sent, but the sensitivity and specificity is unknown.

Spinal fluid in fungal meningitis typically displays a normal or slightly elevated opening pressure, lymphocytic pleocytosis, elevated protein concentration, and decreased glucose concentration. The cryptococcal polysaccharide antigen is a highly sensitive and specific test, and should be performed on all CSF specimens when fungal meningitis is suspected. Histoplasma polysaccharide antigen should be performed in suspected fungal meningitis in patients who reside in or have traveled to the Ohio and Mississippi River valleys. *Coccidioides immitis* is a dimorphic fungus that is endemic to the desert areas of California, Arizona, New Mexico, and Texas. The CSF complement fixation antibody test is reported to have a specificity of 100% and a sensitivity of 75% in the setting of an active *Coccidioides* infection. *Cryptococcus neoformans*, *Histoplasma capsulatum*, and *C. immitis* may also be identified by India ink stain of CSF, and will grow in fungal culture. If culture obtained from a lumbar puncture fails to yield the diagnosis, consider obtaining CSF from a high cervical puncture.

Aspiration or biopsy of rashes may aid the diagnosis of meningococcal disease. The rash of meningococcemia begins as a diffuse erythematous maculopapular rash resembling a viral exanthema, but the lesions rapidly become petechial. Petechiae are found predominantly on the trunk and lower extremities, but also in the mucous membranes and conjunctiva and occasionally on the palms and soles. Purpura fulminans and skin necrosis occasionally develop (**Figure 192-3**). The characteristic rash due to enteroviruses consists of erythematous macules and papules on the face, neck, trunk, and to a lesser degree the extremities.

Patients with meningitis due to *Borrelia burgdorferi* complain of headache and fatigue, and often have myalgias and arthralgias. Unilateral or bilateral facial nerve palsy may be present, or a painful radiculopathy. Diagnosis typically begins with a serum ELISA (enzyme-linked immunosorbent assay) for antibody to *B. burgdorferi*. A positive result is confirmed with a Western blot. The Western blot IgM is often over-interpreted, resulting in false-positive results. A positive IgM should be associated with a positive IgG. CSF examination demonstrates a lymphocytic pleocytosis with normal glucose, and a mild to moderately elevated protein concentration. Intrathecal anti-*B. burgdorferi* antibodies can be detected. Because Lyme disease antibodies can be passively transferred from blood to CSF and persist in the CSF for years, demonstration of anti-*B. burgdorferi* antibodies in the CSF is not definitive evidence of neurologic Lyme disease. Instead, one must calculate the *B. burgdorferi* antibody index, which is positive when >1.3 to 1.5.

B. burgdorferi antibody index:

$$\frac{\text{Anti-Borrelia IgG in CSF/anti-Borrelia IgG in serum}}{\text{Total IgG in CSF/total IgG on serum}}$$

Arboviral infection is defined by the Centers for Disease Control as a febrile illness with mild neurological symptoms during a period of likely arboviral transmission, plus at least one of the following: a fourfold or greater increase in serum antibody titer between acute and convalescent sera, viral isolation from tissue/blood/CSF, or specific IgM antibody to an arbovirus in the CSF.

Meningitis from neurosarcoidosis is diagnosed by excluding infectious meningitis, with histologic documentation of sarcoidosis

TABLE 192-3 Spinal Fluid Analysis for Meningitis

Etiology	Opening Pressure	WBC Count	Protein	Glucose	CSF/Serum Glucose Ratio
Normal	<180 mm H$_2$O	≤5 cells/mm^3	15-45 mg/dL	45-80 mg/dL	0.6-0.7
Bacterial	>180 mm H$_2$O	>100 cells/mm^3 **PMNs predominant**	>45 mg/dL	<40 mg/dL	<0.4
Viral, *Borrelia burgdorferi*, *Treponema pallidum*, *Bartonella henselae*	<180 mm H$_2$O	25-500 cells/mm^3 **Lymphocyte predominant**	15-45 mg/dL	45-80 mg/dL	0.6-0.7
Fungi, *Mycobacterium tuberculosis*, sarcoid, lymphoma, leptomeningeal metastases, partially treated bacterial meningitis	Normal or increased	25-500 cells/mm^3 **Lymphocyte predominant**	>45 mg/dL	<40 mg/dL	<0.6

TABLE 192-4 Cerebrospinal Fluid Diagnostic Tests in Meningitis

Stain and culture

Gram stain and culture

India ink and fungal culture

Acid-fast bacilli and *M. tuberculosis* culture

Antibody

Coccidioides immitis complement fixation

West Nile virus CSF-IgM

B. burgdorferi

Antigen

Histoplasma polysaccharide antigen

Cryptococcal polysaccharide antigen

Polymerase chain reaction

Broad-range bacterial 16S ribosomal DNA

S. pneumoniae

Herpes simplex virus types 1 and 2

Epstein-Barr virus

M. tuberculosis

N. meningitidis

Reverse transcriptase for enteroviruses

West Nile virus

Varicella zoster virus

HIV RNA

Other

Cytology and flow cytometry for metastases

IL-10 (lymphoma), IL-6 (infection, inflammation)

elsewhere, such as a lymph node, skin lesion, salivary gland, or from the conjunctiva. CSF angiotensin-converting enzyme is not useful.

■ VIRAL ENCEPHALITIS

The diagnosis of viral encephalitis is *suggested by the clinical presentation* and *supported* by spinal fluid analysis and neuroimaging abnormalities. The spinal fluid analysis has similar characteristics to viral meningitis: lymphocytic pleocytosis and a normal glucose

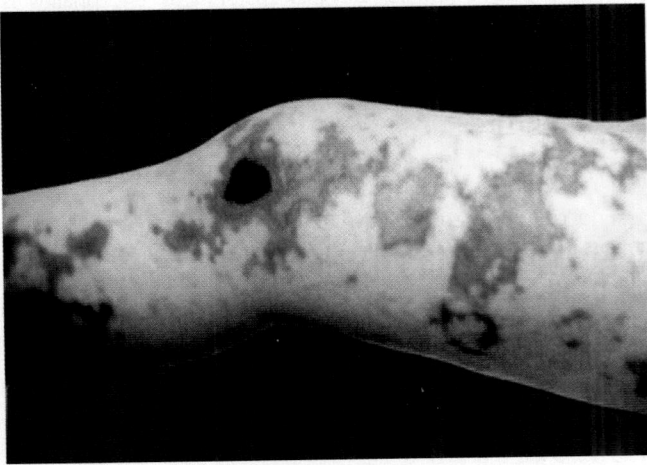

Figure 192-3 *Purpura fulminans: disseminated intravascular coagulation with cutaneous hemorrhage and necrosis in meningococcal disease.* (Reproduced, with permission, from Wolff K, Goldsmith LA, Katz SI, et al. *Fitzpatrick's Dermatology in General Medicine*, 7th ed. New York, NY: McGraw-Hill, 2008. Fig. 180-1C.)

concentration. CSF PCR has become the primary diagnostic test for encephalitis due to HSV-1. A negative test does not exclude the disease, as the PCR can be falsely negative in the first 72 hours of symptoms, and after day 10. CSF and serum should be sent to determine if there is intrathecal synthesis of HSV antibodies. A serum:CSF ratio of less than 20:1 is diagnostic of HSV encephalitis. CSF-IgM for West Nile virus is more sensitive than PCR, with PCR only being positive in approximately 60% of cases.

The characteristic abnormalities of HSV encephalitis on neuroimaging are hyperintensity in the frontotemporal, cingulate, or insular regions of the brain on T2-weighted, diffusion-weighted images (DWIs), and fluid-attenuated inversion recovery (FLAIR) sequences. MRI may be normal in the early stages of HSV-1 encephalitis, but the majority of patients will have MRI abnormalities on FLAIR and DWI within 48 hours of symptom onset. In both West Nile virus encephalitis and St. Louis encephalitis, MRI may reveal hyperintense lesions in the basal ganglia and thalami on T2 and FLAIR sequences. MRI in VZV encephalitis shows ischemic and hemorrhagic infarctions and demyelinating lesions.

PRACTICE POINT

● In 90% of adults with HSV-1 encephalitis, FLAIR and diffusion-weighted MRI sequences will be abnormal within 48 hours of symptom onset.

TRIAGE/HOSPITAL ADMISSION

Patients with suspected bacterial meningitis or encephalitis should be admitted for close observation and frequent neurological assessment, as they are at risk for the development of cerebral edema, increased intracranial pressure, and seizures. Patients with suspected viral meningitis should be monitored or admitted for 24-hour observation and treated with empiric antimicrobial therapy until results of the spinal fluid analysis are available.

Neisseria meningitidis is the only bacterial meningitis that requires respiratory isolation. Patients with a suggestive rash or a CSF Gram stain showing Gram-negative diplococci should be immediately placed in respiratory isolation. Close contacts should be treated with chemoprophylaxis (see below).

When should a neurology consult be obtained?

Neurology consultations are important for many cases of meningitis and encephalitis. Straightforward cases of viral meningitis can be managed without a consult. All patients with an altered level of consciousness, new onset seizure, or focal neurological symptoms or signs should be evaluated by a neurologist. All hospitalized patients should be followed by a neurologist, and monitored closely for signs of increased intracranial pressure and the development of focal neurological deficits.

TREATMENT

■ EMPIRIC THERAPY

Meningitis and encephalitis are neurologic emergencies. Empiric therapy should begin within 60 minutes of arrival in the emergency room. Significant increases in mortality are found with treatment delayed more than 6 hours from presentation. Empiric therapy includes antimicrobial agents and adjunctive dexamethasone. The specific antimicrobial agents chosen depend on the patient's predisposing conditions, and the time of the year (**Table 192-5**). In patients with suspected bacterial meningitis, dexamethasone (adult dose: 10 mg every 6 hours for 4 days) either prior to antibiotic therapy or with the first dose of antibiotics is recommended. Acyclovir (10 mg/kg every 8 hours) is added to the empiric regimen for HSV encephalitis. Doxycycline (100 mg every 12 hours) is added for tick-borne infection, if ticks are prevalent and in season in the patient's part of the country.

TABLE 192-5 Empiric Therapy

Patient Population	Empiric Treatment
Neonate	Ampicillin plus cefotaxime or an aminoglycoside
Healthy children and adults with community-acquired disease	Third- or fourth-generation cephalosporin + vancomycin [+metronidazole if otitis, mastoiditis, sinusitis are predisposing conditions]
Adults over age 55 or with chronic illness or immunosuppressed patients	Third- or fourth-generation cephalosporin + vancomycin + ampicillin
Postneurosurgical	Vancomycin + meropenem
All patients	Dexamethasone + acyclovir (if illness compatible with HSV encephalitis) + doxycycline (during tick season)

■ BACTERIAL MENINGITIS SPECIFIC THERAPY

Modify antimicrobial therapy based on specific bacterial pathogen antimicrobial sensitivity testing (**Table 192-6**). The length of treatment is dependent on the specific pathogen. Meningitis due to *S. pneumoniae, Haemophilus influenzae,* and group B streptococci is treated with intravenous antibiotics for 10 to 14 days. Patients with *S. pneumoniae* meningitis should have repeat spinal fluid analysis, if safe to do so, after 48 hours of treatment to ensure the culture is sterile. Bacterial meningitis due to *L. monocytogenes* and *Enterobacteriaceae* is treated for 3 to 4 weeks. Meningitis caused by *N. meningitidis* requires treatment for 5 to 7 days. Respiratory isolation must be continued for at least 24 hours after the initiation of antimicrobial therapy. Chemoprophylaxis for meningococcal meningitis is typically rifampin 600 mg every 12 hours for 2 days (four doses total). A single injection of intravenous or intramuscular ceftriaxone (250 mg for adults; 125 mg for children) is recommended for pregnant women and for children, as rifampin should not be given to children. Meningococcal meningitis patients should also receive rifampin prophylaxis before discharge from the hospital.

Lyme meningitis is treated with either intravenous ceftriaxone 2 g/d for 14 to 28 days, or oral doxycycline, which is likely as effective, given as 200 to 400 mg twice daily for 10 to 14 days for adults and children >8 years old. There are currently no indications to treat Lyme disease for longer than 28 days, despite cases of patients with subjective symptoms beyond that point.

■ VIRAL MENINGITIS

Viral meningitis is treated symptomatically with antipyretics, antiemetics, and analgesics. Amytriptyline and NSAIDs are often required for months to treat headache from viral meningitis. Patients with HSV-2 meningitis can be treated with acyclovir 800 mg five times daily, famciclovir 500 mg three times daily, or valacyclovir 1000 mg three times daily for 7 to 14 days.

■ FUNGAL MENINGITIS

The treatment of cryptococcal meningitis includes a combination of either intravenous amphotericin B (0.7-1.0 mg/kg/d), amBisome 4 mg/kg/d, or abelcet 5 mg/kg/d, *plus* oral flucytosine (25 mg/kg four times daily). This combination is typically used for 2 weeks or until the CSF culture is sterile. This induction therapy is followed by fluconazole 400 to 800 mg/d, which is continued for 8 to 10 weeks. CNS histoplasmosis is treated with intravenous amphotericin B (0.7-1.0 mg/kg/d). A total dose of 30 mg/kg is recommended.

A course of amphotericin B is followed by oral itraconazole 200 mg twice daily for 6 months to a year. *C. immitis* meningitis is treated with either high-dose fluconazole (1000 mg daily) as monotherapy, or a combination of intravenous and intrathecal amphotericin B (0.25-0.75 mg/d three times weekly). High-dose fluconazole therapy as induction therapy can be followed by lower doses of fluconazole (200-400 mg daily) indefinitely. Treatment of fungal meningitis requires frequent examination of CSF for culture.

The management of increased intracranial pressure is as critical to a successful outcome from fungal meningitis as antifungal therapy. Intracranial pressure should be measured at the initial lumbar puncture and at the completion of induction therapy, and any time during the course of the illness when the patient has a change in mental status or a change in the neurological examination. Increased intracranial pressure is best managed with a ventriculostomy during acute infection, followed by a ventriculoperitoneal shunt. The practice of daily lumbar punctures to decrease CSF pressure by 50% and maintain CSF pressure at <300 mm/H$_2$O is impractical. Shunt revision should be done quickly in patients with deteriorating consciousness. The longer the duration of symptoms at presentation, the less impact shunting will have on reversing neurological complications.

■ TUBERCULOUS MENINGITIS

Patients with tuberculous meningitis are treated with isoniazid, rifampin, and pyrazinamide for 2 months, followed by isoniazid and rifampin for an additional 10 months. Present recommendations are that HIV-negative patients are treated with dexamethasone for the first 3 to 4 weeks of therapy, and then the patient is switched to prednisone therapy for an additional 4 weeks. Previous practice had been to use corticosteroid therapy only in patients who developed hydrocephalus or coma.

■ VIRAL ENCEPHALITIS

There are very few antiviral agents for viral encephalitis. Encephalitis due to HSV-1 is treated with intravenous acyclovir 30 mg/kg/d divided every 8 hours, and infused over 60 minutes. Slow acyclovir infusion prevents renal tubular crystal formation and renal insufficiency. Oral antivirals have not been adequately studied in this setting; therefore, patients should be maintained on intravenous acyclovir for 3 weeks. Patients who are not responding to acyclovir and those in whom a definitive agent cannot be identified can be treated with foscarnet. The recommended dose is 60 mg/kg every 8 hours. Varicella zoster virus encephalitis is treated with intravenous acyclovir.

COMPLICATIONS
■ MENINGITIS

The mortality rate for bacterial meningitis is between 10% and 20%. Up to 25% of survivors have serious neurologic sequelae, including hearing loss, impaired executive functioning, seizure disorders, and deficits from ischemic stroke or intraparenchymal hemorrhage. Patients with viral meningitis often complain of headache for weeks to months.

■ ENCEPHALITIS

Complications from HSV encephalitis include impaired memory and seizure disorder.

DISCHARGE PLANNING
■ MENINGITIS

- Have patients with bacterial meningitis completed a course of appropriate parenteral antibiotic therapy? (Patients with fungal

TABLE 192-6 Recommended Specific Antibacterial Treatment and Dosing

Microorganism	Antibiotic	Dose
S. pneumoniae Penicillin susceptible (MIC <0.1 mg/L)	Penicillin G	Neonates: 0.15-0.2 mU/kg/d (every 8-12 h) Infants and children: 0.3 mU/kg/d (every 4-6 h) Adult: 24 million units/d (every 4-6 h)
	or ceftriaxone	Infant or child: 80-100 mg/kg/d (every 12 h) Adult: 4 g/d (every 12 h)
	or cefepime	Infants and children: 150 mg/kg/d (every 8 h) Adult: 6 g/d (every 8 h)
	or cefotaxime	Neonate: 100-150 mg/kg/d (every 8-12 h) Infant or child: 225-300 mg/kg/d (every 6-8 h) Adult: 8-12 g/d (every 4-6 h)
Penicillin tolerant (MIC 0.1-1.0 mg/L)	Ceftriaxone *or* cefepime *or* cefotaxime	As above
Penicillin resistant (MIC >1 mg/L or Cefotaxime/ceftriaxone MIC ≥1 mg/L)	Cefepime (*or* cefotaxime *or* ceftriaxone)	As above
	plus vancomycin	Neonates: 20-30 mg/kg/d (every 8-12 h) Infant and child: 60 mg/kg/d (every 6 h) Adults: 45-60 mg/kg/d (every 6-12 h)
N. meningitidis	Penicillin G	as above
	or ampicillin	Neonate: 150 mg/kg/d (every 8 h) Infant and child: 300 mg/kg/d (every 6 h) Adult: 12 g/d (every 4-6 h)
Penicillin resistant	Ceftriaxone *or* cefotaxime	As above
L. monocytogenes	Ampicillin	As above
Critically ill patients	*plus* gentamicin	Neonate: 5 mg/kg/d (every 12 h) Infant and child: 7.5 mg/kg/d (every 8 h) Adult: 5 mg/kg/d (every 8 h)
Streptococcus agalactiae (group B streptococci)	**Ampicillin** *or* penicillin G *or* cefotaxime	As above
E. coli or other Enterobacteriaceae	Ceftriaxone *or* cefepime *or* cefotaxime	As above
Pseudomonas aeruginosa	**Meropenem** *or*	Infant and child:120 mg/kg/d (every 8 h) Adult: 6 g/d (every 8 h)
	ceftazidime	
S. aureus Methicillin susceptible	Nafcillin *or* oxacillin	Neonates: 75 mg/kg/d (every 8-12 h) Infants and children: 200 mg/kg/d (every 6 h) Adult: 9-12 g/d (every 4 h)
Methicillin resistant	Vancomycin	As above
Staphylococcus epidermidis	**Vancomycin**	As above
	or linezolid	Neonates: 20 mg/kg/d (every 8-12 h) Infant and child: 30 mg/kg/d (every 8 h) Adult: 600 mg (every 12 h)
H. influenzae	Ceftriaxone *or* cefepime *or* cefotaxime	As above

Recommended agents are in **bold**.
Intraventricular vancomycin administration: children 10 mg/d, adults 20 mg/d.

meningitis and tuberculous meningitis may be discharged to continue antimicrobial therapy at home when they are stable. Patients with viral meningitis can be managed primarily as outpatients, although observation is required until CSF tests results are available.)

- Has chemoprophylaxis been provided for close contacts of patients with meningococcal meningitis?

■ ENCEPHALITIS

- For patients with HSV encephalitis, have they received 2 weeks of inpatient parenteral acyclovir therapy? Patients who are stable after 2 weeks of parenteral therapy can complete the last week of therapy in an outpatient setting. A recent clinical trial found no benefit of prolonged acyclovir therapy (90-day duration) in HSV encephalitis survivors.

SUGGESTED READINGS

Day JN, Chau TT, Wolbers M, et al. Combination antifungal therapy for cryptococcal meningitis. *N Engl J Med*. 2013;368:1291-1302.

Hasbun R, Abrahams J, Jekel J, Quagliarello VJ. Computed tomography of the head before lumbar puncture in adults with suspected meningitis. *N Engl J Med*. 2001;345:1727-1733.

Lindsey NP, Lehman JA, Staples JE, Fischer M. West Nile virus and other arboviral diseases—United States, 2013. *MMWR Morb Mortal Wkly Rep*. 2014;63:521-526.

Nigrovic LE, Fine AM, Monuteaux MC, et al. Trends in the management of viral meningitis at United States children's hospitals. *Pediatrics*. 2013;131:670-676.

Thigpen MC, Whitney CG, Messonnier NE, et al. Bacterial meningitis in the United States 1998-2007. *N Engl J Med*. 2011;364:2016-2025.

Tunkel AR, Glaser CA, Bloch KC, et al. The management of encephalitis: clinical practice guidelines by the Infectious Diseases Society of America. *Clin Infect Dis*. 2008;47:303-327.

Tunkel AR, Hartman BJ, Kaplan SL, et al. Practice guidelines for the management of bacterial meningitis. *Clin Infect Dis*. 2004;39:1267-1284.

CHAPTER 193

Osteomyelitis and Septic Arthritis

Laura K. Certain, MD, PhD
Yonatan H. Grad, MD, PhD

Key Clinical Questions

Osteomyelitis

1. How does bone become infected?
2. What parts of the history and physical examination are most helpful in diagnosis?
3. What treatment options should be considered?
4. How is the response to treatment monitored?

Septic Arthritis

1. How should possible acute bacterial (septic) arthritis be evaluated?
2. When should empiric antibiotics be used in suspected septic arthritis? Which antibiotics?
3. What are the key elements of treatment of septic arthritis?

OSTEOMYELITIS

EPIDEMIOLOGY

Osteomyelitis is infection of bone, with accompanying inflammation and destruction. In healthy adults, osteomyelitis is rare. Bone infection usually requires predisposing factors. These include adjacent soft-tissue infections, such as diabetic foot ulcers and stage IV pressure sores, hematogenous seeding, as may occur in endocarditis, or direct inoculation of bone during trauma or surgery.

Once microbes invade bone, they attach to host cells and extracellular matrix, as well as prosthetic biomaterials, if present. Bacteria in bone may produce biofilm, a slimy polymer that acts as a physical barrier against both antibiotics and the host immune system. Bacteria embedded in biofilm are less metabolically active, making them even less susceptible to antibiotics. Inflammation associated with bacterial toxins and the host immune response leads to bone lysis. Over time, as infection becomes chronic, suppuration leads to vascular congestion, raised intraosseous pressure, and ischemia of infected bone. The necrotic bone separates from healthy bone to form a sequestrum, a diagnostic finding of chronic osteomyelitis. If the dead bone cannot be resorbed, healthy new bone may form around it, encasing the sequestrum in an involucrum. The walled-off sequestrum may act like an abscess, with bacterial growth continuing in a pocket of necrotic tissue inaccessible to immune policing and antibiotics. As pressure in the sequestrum builds, infection may erupt through the involucrum, leading to subperiosteal or soft-tissue abscesses, or a sinus tract through overlying soft tissue.

RISK STRATIFICATION

Bone resists infection under normal circumstances. Factors that influence the establishment and progression of osteomyelitis include pathogen virulence, inoculum size, bone health, presence of foreign objects, host immunity, and duration of infection. Patients should be asked about risk factors for osteomyelitis, such as diabetes, vascular disease, intravenous drug use, sickle cell disease, and recent trauma or surgery.

In osteomyelitis, regardless of cause, cure often requires both medical and surgical intervention, with prolonged antibiotics as well as debridement of infected bone and soft tissue. When debridement is extensive, reconstructive surgery may be necessary, including bone grafts and muscle and skin flaps. Sufficient vascular supply is a critical element to healing; revascularization procedures may be necessary. Because of the multispecialty approach required for diagnosis and treatment, patients with suspected osteomyelitis should be admitted for further evaluation. Infectious disease and orthopedic surgery consultation is recommended, and input from vascular surgery and plastic surgery may also be indicated.

OSTEOMYELITIS—GENERAL EVALUATION AND MANAGEMENT

EVALUATION

Physical findings of osteomyelitis may include sinus tracts, wounds, and ulcers that probe to bone, and evidence of associated peripheral vascular disease or diabetes. However, the examination is often unrevealing, especially in hematogenous osteomyelitis of deep sites, such as the spine. Laboratory evaluation includes blood cultures, white blood cell (WBC) count with differential, erythrocyte sedimentation rate (ESR), and C-reactive protein (CRP) level. The WBC count is usually nonspecific and more often elevated in acute than chronic osteomyelitis. ESR and CRP can be elevated in many conditions and may also be normal early in osteomyelitis. If ESR and CRP are elevated due to osteomyelitis, they can be used to assess patient response to treatment. CRP may drop within 1 to 2 weeks of starting appropriate therapy, while ESR falls more slowly. Other serum markers associated with bone disease, such as calcium, phosphate, and alkaline phosphatase, are usually normal in osteomyelitis.

The initial radiographic study in suspected osteomyelitis should be plain films of the affected area. These may show soft-tissue swelling, narrowing or widening of joint spaces, bone destruction, and periosteal reaction. If plain radiographs are suggestive and blood cultures are positive, a presumptive diagnosis of osteomyelitis can be made, and no further evaluation is required. When plain films are not diagnostic, magnetic resonance imaging (MRI) should be obtained next. Both MRI and computed tomography (CT) are useful in revealing medullary and cortical destruction, periosteal reaction, articular damage, and soft-tissue involvement. MRI is better for diagnosing soft-tissue involvement, and CT is more sensitive for detecting cortical and medullary sequestra. Overall, MRI is more sensitive than CT, and also does not expose the patient to radiation. Bone marrow edema on MRI may be seen as early as 3 days into the course of osteomyelitis. However, MRI is not helpful in assessing the response to therapy, as bone marrow edema persists for months after microbiological cure. Another limitation is that bone marrow edema on MRI is not specific for osteomyelitis: it may also be caused by trauma, Charcot arthropathy, and surgery. Radionuclide bone scans have similar sensitivity to MRI, but they suffer from poor specificity, and have a much lower spatial resolution. They may be useful in the presence of orthopedic devices, which create artifacts on CT and MRI.

Bone biopsy is the preferred procedure for bacteriologic diagnosis in osteomyelitis. Superficial cultures of overlying wounds or sinus tracts are of relatively low utility. Microbes cultured from superficial samples are often nonpathogenic, and correlate poorly with those responsible for the bone infection, with the exception that identification of *Staphylococcus aureus* from a draining sinus tract usually correlates with deep infection.

Isolation of a pathogen from a bone biopsy, with histologic confirmation of inflammation and osteonecrosis, is the gold standard for the diagnosis of osteomyelitis. Unless the patient is prohibitively ill, antibiotics should be held before biopsy to optimize culture results. Percutaneous bone sampling should be pursued when feasible, but is limited by sampling error. Larger needles increase the diagnostic yield. Bone biopsy should be performed through healthy tissue under direct imaging guidance. If percutaneous biopsy and blood cultures are negative, and clinical suspicion of osteomyelitis remains high, then percutaneous biopsy should be repeated, or an open biopsy performed. Open bone biopsy provides the highest yield, but is more morbid.

■ INPATIENT MANAGEMENT

Initial inpatient management should focus on establishing the diagnosis, as described above. Most patients with osteomyelitis are not septic, and therefore antibiotics should be withheld until after adequate tissue and blood samples have been collected for microbial analysis. The diagnostic and therapeutic approach varies depending on the mode of infection. However, as treatment for osteomyelitis is long, complex, expensive, and not always successful even when management is optimal, proper diagnosis and pathogen identification is of great importance in all cases.

Empiric antibiotic therapy should begin after collecting samples for Gram stain, culture, and histology, or sooner if the patient's clinical status mandates immediate treatment, and should be targeted

to the most common pathogens in the clinical scenario. Empiric regimens typically include vancomycin for Gram-positive coverage, with a second drug, such as ciprofloxacin, ceftazidime, or cefepime, with activity against *Pseudomonas* and other Gram-negative bacilli. Once culture and susceptibility data are available, empiric therapy should be narrowed as much as possible. Treatment usually lasts 6 weeks, but may be lengthened depending on the extent of surgical debridement, vascular supply, presence of foreign material, and immune function. Additionally, if evidence of infection persists through antibiotic therapy, and the antibiotic was selected based on reliable microbiological data, then complications such as sequestra or abscesses should be sought.

In cases of chronic osteomyelitis in which the patient or the clinical context favor a nonsurgical approach, oral antibiotics can be given to treat intermittent flares. If a foreign body such as an internal fixation device is present at the area of osteomyelitis, then the goal may be to perform limited interventions and provide antimicrobial treatment until sufficient healing that the bone is strong enough to sustain definitive intervention.

OSTEOMYELITIS FROM ADJACENT SOFT-TISSUE INFECTION

■ EVALUATION

Individuals with diabetes and peripheral vascular disease are at high risk of this type of osteomyelitis, especially in the feet. Peripheral neuropathy predisposes to foot ulceration, and vascular disease impairs the immune response and wound healing. Foot ulceration and soft-tissue inflammation lasting a week or longer should raise suspicion of underlying osteomyelitis, even though fever may be absent, and signs of inflammation scant. A significant percentage of these patients ultimately require amputation due to chronic soft tissue and bone infection.

Physical examination should include the evaluation of pulses and Doppler ultrasound measurement of vascular flow, as well as characterization of neuropathy. If necessary, arteriography and nerve conduction studies may be considered.

One of the most useful tests for osteomyelitis in patients with soft-tissue wounds is the "probe-to-bone" test, which involves advancing a sterile surgical probe through the ulceration. If the probe reaches bone, then the bone is almost certainly infected. In patients with diabetic foot ulcers, an ulcer measuring more than 2 cm² strongly suggests osteomyelitis (**Table 193-1**). If suspicion remains high in the absence of convincing data from clinical examination and plain films, MRI is a sensitive and specific tool to assist in confirming infection.

TABLE 193-1 Likelihood Ratios (LR) for Diagnosing Lower-Extremity Osteomyelitis in Patients with Diabetes Mellitus

Risk Factors/Findings	Positive LR	Negative LR
Probe to bone	6.4	0.39
Bone exposure	9.2	0.70
Ulcer area >2 cm	7.2	0.48
Ulcer inflammation	1.5	0.84
Clinical gestalt	5.5	0.54
Erythrocyte sedimentation rate >70	11	0.34

Adapted from Butalia S, Palda VA, Sargeant RJ, Detsky AS, Mourad O. Does this patient with diabetes have osteomyelitis of the lower extremity? In: Simel DL, Rennie D, eds. *The Rational Clinical Examination*. New York, NY: McGraw-Hill; 2009.

■ INPATIENT MANAGEMENT

As with other causes of osteomyelitis, initial management should focus on diagnosis and specialty consultation. These infections are chronic processes; initiation of antibiotics is rarely urgent, and should generally wait until after the diagnosis is established. Since most of these patients require surgical debridement, antibiotics should be withheld until surgical bone biopsies are obtained for culture.

These infections are frequently polymicrobial, and include aerobic and anaerobic Gram-positive and negative bacteria, with staphylococcal and streptococcal species commonly involved. Treatment usually requires broad-spectrum antimicrobial treatment and surgical debridement or amputation. Revascularization may be critical, as debridement and antibiotics will fail to clear infection if the vascular supply is inadequate. Antimicrobial treatment should continue at least 6 weeks after surgical debridement. (Amputation should be curative, if carried out one joint above the infected bone.) Some argue that antimicrobial therapy should continue until complete resolution of the skin and soft-tissue defects.

OSTEOMYELITIS FROM HEMATOGENOUS SEEDING

■ EVALUATION

Any bone may be seeded by the hematogenous spread of microbes, but in adults the spine is most often affected. Vertebral osteomyelitis, or spondylodiscitis, most often involves the lower thoracic or lumbar spine, and presents with low back pain. Cervical spine involvement is less common; it may present as torticollis. Vertebrae are well perfused, and neighboring vertebrae share segmental arteries. Infection therefore often involves adjacent vertebrae with their intervertebral disc (**Figure 193-1**). Epidural or psoas abscesses are common complications. The source of bacteremia may include skin and soft-tissue infections, urinary tract infections, dental abscesses, and central venous catheter-associated infections, but it is often unidentified.

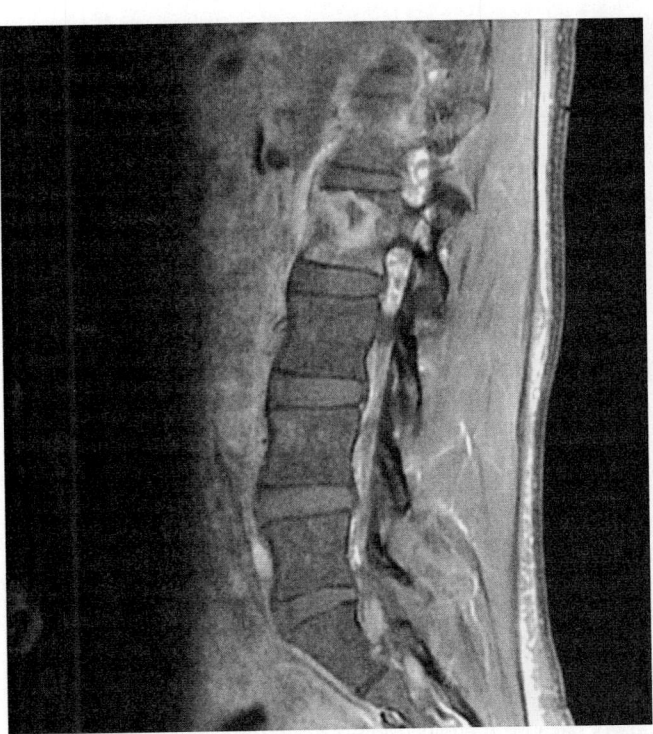

Figure 193-2 *Sagittal T1 postcontrast images demonstrating rim-enhancing lesion in the L2 vertebral body, suggestive of intraosseous abscess. Bone biopsy was positive for tuberculosis.*

Fever is present in fewer than half of cases. Motor and sensory deficits from spinal cord or nerve root compression are found in only a small percentage of patients. As the presentation of vertebral osteomyelitis is nonspecific, a high clinical suspicion is necessary for timely diagnosis. Physical examination may reveal tenderness over the affected area of the spine, with paraspinal muscle spasm.

Most cases of vertebral osteomyelitis are monomicrobial. The most common pathogen is *S. aureus*, but many organisms may be responsible, including *Mycobacterium tuberculosis* and *Brucella* in endemic areas, *Salmonella* in patients with sickle cell disease, and Gram-negative organisms and fungi in immunosuppressed patients and intravenous drug users. *M. tuberculosis* typically involves the thoracic spine. Tuberculosis may produce intravertebral lesions with a characteristic radiographic appearance, which it shares with brucellosis (**Figure 193-2**). Plain radiographs are often unrevealing, but MRI has high sensitivity for disk space infection, cord compression, and paraspinal abscess. As blood cultures are positive in less than half of cases, CT-guided biopsy is the diagnostic procedure of choice. Open surgical biopsy should be considered when percutaneous biopsy fails to provide a diagnosis, or patients fail to improve on empiric or directed treatment. If blood cultures are positive, bone biopsy is unnecessary, but infectious endocarditis must be ruled out.

■ INPATIENT MANAGEMENT

As above, initial inpatient management should focus on bacteriologic diagnosis. Except in unstable patients, antibiotics should be withheld until a microbial diagnosis can be made, or at least until after adequate specimens have been collected. In patients with vertebral osteomyelitis, a careful neurologic history and examination is crucial. Neurologic signs or symptoms should prompt urgent neuroimaging (MRI preferred) and neurosurgical consultation. Neurologic status should be reassessed daily while in the hospital.

The mainstay of treatment is antimicrobial therapy for at least 6 weeks. Many infectious diseases physicians treat for 8 weeks or

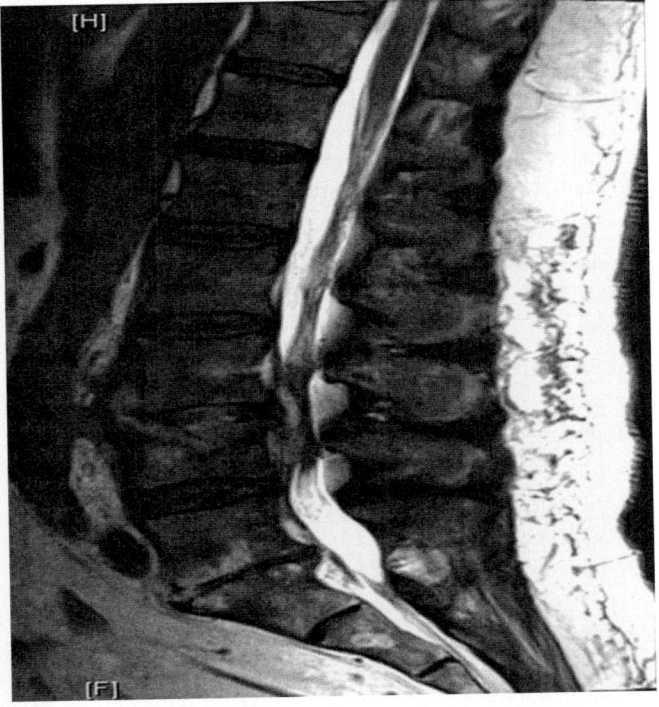

Figure 193-1 *Sagittal T2-weighted image demonstrating increased signal in the disc space and soft-tissue posterior to the vertebral bodies suggestive of discitis in a patient with blood cultures positive for Staphylococcus aureus.*

more, depending on the extent of disease and the virulence of the infecting organism, although this has not been shown to improve outcomes in clinical trials. As the vertebrae are more vascular than other bones, surgical debridement is less often required. However, epidural or paraspinal abscess, spine instability, neurologic symptoms, and failure to improve on appropriate antimicrobial therapy should prompt neurosurgical consultation. Clinical examination and the inflammatory markers ESR and CRP are helpful in following response to treatment. Follow-up MRI may be misleading, giving a false impression of progressive osteomyelitis, despite clinical improvement; MRI results should be cautiously interpreted in the broad clinical context.

OSTEOMYELITIS FROM DIRECT INOCULATION

■ EVALUATION

Direct inoculation of bone tissue by pathogens may take place during surgery or orthopedic trauma. The risk of osteomyelitis after an open fracture depends on the type of fracture, the degree of contamination, the extent of surrounding soft-tissue injury, and the timing of local or systemic antibiotics after contamination. Commonly involved organisms include staphylococci, Gram-negative bacilli, and skin flora and soil organisms. As these patients often undergo multiple surgical procedures, they are also at risk for nosocomial pathogens.

Acute trauma-associated osteomyelitis can often go undiagnosed, because the initial signs can be mistaken for inflammation associated with trauma. As untreated acute osteomyelitis progresses to chronic osteomyelitis, signs and symptoms indicative of chronic osteomyelitis may appear: fracture nonunion, poor wound healing, and sinus tract formation. Plain radiographs are often unhelpful, as traumatic and postoperative changes confound interpretation. MRI is sensitive, but less specific in this setting. It is reasonable to pursue another imaging modality, such as CT or radionuclide bone scan, prior to surgical intervention.

■ INPATIENT MANAGEMENT

The management principles for open fracture include early surgical debridement and a short course of antimicrobial prophylaxis to prevent osteomyelitis. When osteomyelitis develops, the practice principles are microbe identification, surgical debridement, and tailored antibiotic therapy. The presence of foreign objects, such as fixation devices, requires long-term oral antimicrobial therapy until fractures have healed and fixation devices can be removed. When oral suppression fails to result in fracture healing, definitive therapy with removal of foreign objects, further surgical debridement, and additional directed antimicrobial therapy should be considered.

PRACTICE POINT

- Management of osteomyelitis hinges on making an accurate microbiological diagnosis. Unless patients are unstable, antibiotics should be held until after a bone biopsy can be performed, as it is critical to confirm the diagnosis of osteomyelitis and identify the infectious agent and its antibiotic susceptibilities.
- Vertebral osteomyelitis may be complicated by epidural abscess and neurologic compromise; ongoing evaluation of these patients should include regular neurologic examination.

POSTACUTE CARE

Patients should be monitored for side effects of treatment and treatment failure. Prolonged antibiotic treatment poses a risk of *Clostridium difficile* infection. Antibiotic-specific reactions may include

renal failure, hepatitis, and cytopenias. Peripherally inserted central catheters may lead to catheter-associated infection and thrombosis. Failure of therapy may require further surgery and antibiotics.

Patients discharged on parenteral antibiotics should have routine, usually weekly, monitoring of complete blood count (CBC), electrolytes, and antibiotic levels if vancomycin or aminoglycosides are used, as well as ESR and CRP to monitor response to therapy. A single health care provider should be identified as responsible for review of laboratory results. Outpatient management should be pursued in conjunction with an infectious diseases specialist.

DISCHARGE CHECKLIST FOR OSTEOMYELITIS

- Has the infected site been adequately debrided and revascularized if necessary?
- Have antibiotics been narrowed as much as possible?
- Has a baseline ESR and CRP been obtained?
- Is there a plan in place for long-term monitoring of parenteral antibiotic therapy?

SEPTIC ARTHRITIS

■ EPIDEMIOLOGY

Native joint septic arthritis occurs at a rate of 2 to 10 cases per 100,000 per year in the general population, and as high as 38 cases per 100,000 per year among patients with rheumatoid arthritis. The most important risk factor for the development of septic arthritis is preexisting joint disease, with up to half having a history of joint inflammation or injury (**Table 193-2**). Systemic illness and other conditions, such as immunosuppression, diabetes mellitus, renal and liver insufficiency, and intravenous drug abuse, also predispose to septic arthritis. Rheumatoid arthritis places individuals at particularly high risk through the combination of joint damage, immunosuppressive medications, and poor skin quality.

Bacteria enter the joint space primarily through hematogenous spread, and occasionally through direct inoculation and spread from a contiguous infection in soft tissue or bone. Synovial capillaries lack a basement membrane, facilitating translocation of bacteria during episodes of bacteremia. The resulting inflammatory response of the synovium is intensely neutrophilic. Bacterial toxins and neutrophil proteases break down cartilage, and the increased intra-articular pressure leads to ischemic injury through vascular thrombosis and obstruction. In acute bacterial septic arthritis, injury happens quickly; significant joint damage can take place within 1 to 2 days.

TABLE 193-2 Likelihood Ratios (LR) for Diagnosing Septic Arthritis

Risk Factors/Findings	Positive LR	Negative LR
Age >80 y	3.5	0.86
Diabetes mellitus	2.7	0.93
Rheumatoid arthritis	2.5	0.45
Recent joint surgery	6.9	0.78
Skin infection	2.8	0.76
HIV-1 infection	1.7	0.47
Fever	0.67	1.7
Abnormal WBC count	1.4	0.28
ESR >30 mm/h	1.3	0.17
CRP >100 mg/L	1.6	0.44

Adapted from Margaretten ME, Kohlwes J, Moore D, Bent S. Does this adult patient have septic arthritis? In: Simel DL, Rennie D, eds. *The Rational Clinical Examination.* New York, NY: McGraw-Hill; 2009.

TABLE 193-3 Organisms Isolated in 2407 Cases of Septic Arthritis

Organism	Number of Isolates (% Total)
Gram positive	
Staphylococcus aureus	1066 (44)
Staphylococci, coagulase negative	84 (3)
Streptococci	
Streptococcus pyogenes	183 (8)
Streptococcus pneumoniae	156 (6)
Streptococcus agalactiae	69 (3)
Other streptococci	104 (4)
Gram negative	
Escherichia coli	91 (4)
Haemophilus influenzae	104 (4)
Neisseria gonorrhoeae	77 (3)
Neisseria meningitidis	28 (1)
Pseudomonas aeruginosa	36 (1)
Salmonella spp	25 (1)
Other Gram-negative rods	110 (5)
Miscellaneous (including anaerobes)	136 (6)
Polymicrobial	33 (1)

Adapted from Ross JJ, Saltzman CL, Carling P, et al. Pneumococcal septic arthritis: review of 190 cases. *Clin Infect Dis.* 2003;36:319-327.

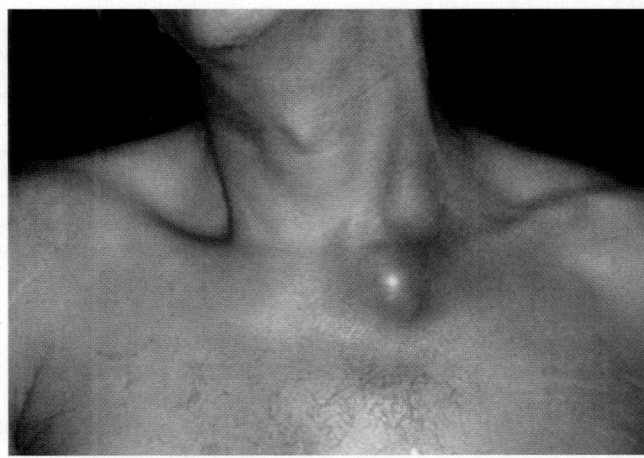

Figure 193-3 *Sternoclavicular septic arthritis accounts for 17% of septic arthritis in intravenous drug users, but only 1% of septic arthritis in the general population. Osteomyelitis, chest wall abscess, and mediastinitis are serious and common complications that require surgical debridement. Staphylococcus aureus is usually responsible.* (Reproduced, with permission, from Fauci AS, Braunwald E, Kasper DL, et al. *Harrison's Principles of Internal Medicine,* 17th ed. New York, NY: McGraw-Hill; 2008, Fig. 328-1.)

All microbial pathogens can infect synovium. *S. aureus* is the most common pathogen overall (**Table 193-3**). Certain bacteria are correlated with certain demographics. Intravenous drug users are at risk for staphylococcal and streptococcal infections, as well as pseudomonal and other Gram-negative infections. Polymicrobial infections are usually seen after contaminated open injuries. Animal bites, particularly from cats, are associated with *Pasteurella* infection, and human bites with *Eikenella corrodens* and other human oral flora. TNF-inhibitors predispose to mycobacterial infections. Disseminated gonococcal infection (DGI) may present as septic arthritis.

■ RISK STRATIFICATION

A painful, warm, swollen joint has many possible causes, including infection, trauma, osteoarthritis, crystal disease, or systemic disease. Of these, acute bacterial septic arthritis results in the most rapid joint destruction, and it is primarily for this reason that the joint must undergo prompt evaluation. Patients with septic joints should be admitted to hospital for orthopedic and infectious disease consultation, consideration of joint debridement and irrigation, and initiation of parenteral antibiotics. Approximately half of the cases of septic arthritis result in impaired joint function, and mortality rates range from 10% to 15% in normal hosts and up to 30% in patients with comorbidities.

NONGONOCOCCAL ACUTE BACTERIAL ARTHRITIS

■ EVALUATION

Septic arthritis classically presents with a swollen, painful joint with limited range of motion. Typical features of infection, including fever and leukocytosis, are frequently absent, especially in patients with rheumatoid arthritis, renal or hepatic disease, or immunosuppression. Most cases present as monoarticular arthritis, with up to half affecting the knee; most other cases involve other large peripheral joints. Involvement of small joints of the hand usually reflects direct inoculation or bite, and involvement of the joints of the feet usually

arises with progression of contiguous soft-tissue infection or osteomyelitis, as seen in patients with diabetes and vascular insufficiency. Intravenous drug users are more prone to sacroiliac and sternoclavicular involvement (**Figure 193-3**). Polyarticular arthritis is more common among patients with impaired immunity, and with gonococcal, pneumococcal, group B streptococcal, and Gram-negative infection.

The differential diagnosis of septic bacterial arthritis includes rheumatoid arthritis, crystal-induced joint diseases, reactive arthritis, osteoarthritis, trauma, viral arthritis, Lyme disease, and other systemic diseases. Joint warmth, pain, swelling, and restricted motion suggest septic arthritis and mandate arthrocentesis (**Figure 193-4**). When bedside joint aspiration cannot be accomplished, the procedure should be done by CT or ultrasound guidance. Synovial fluid should be evaluated for cell count and differential, Gram stain, aerobic and anaerobic culture, and crystals. Pathogen identification via Gram stain and culture of synovial fluid are the gold standard for diagnosis for septic arthritis, with cultures being informative in >90% of cases of nongonococcal bacterial septic arthritis. Arthrocentesis should be performed prior to the administration of antibiotics, unless the patient's clinical status does not allow a delay in empiric treatment. Inoculating the synovial sample into blood culture bottles offers a theoretical improvement in sensitivity. A synovial fluid white blood cell count of more than 50,000 cells/mm³ and neutrophil predominance is traditionally taken as indicative of infection. However, this is neither specific nor sensitive for septic arthritis. Crystalline arthropathy commonly causes synovial white blood cell counts in this range, while immunosuppressed patients may not be able to mount synovial leukocytosis in response to infection. As well, atypical joint pathogens such as *M. tuberculosis* or fungi may be associated with synovial white blood cell counts of lower magnitude. Synovial protein and glucose studies are neither sensitive nor specific, and should not be checked.

Serum studies should include blood cultures, peripheral white blood cell count with differential, and inflammatory markers (ESR and CRP). None of these tests are specific, but a leukocytosis with left shift, or an elevated ESR and CRP, at the beginning of treatment may be helpful to track response to treatment. Serologic studies for Lyme disease should be considered in patients from endemic areas with evidence of inflammatory arthritis but negative Gram stain and culture.

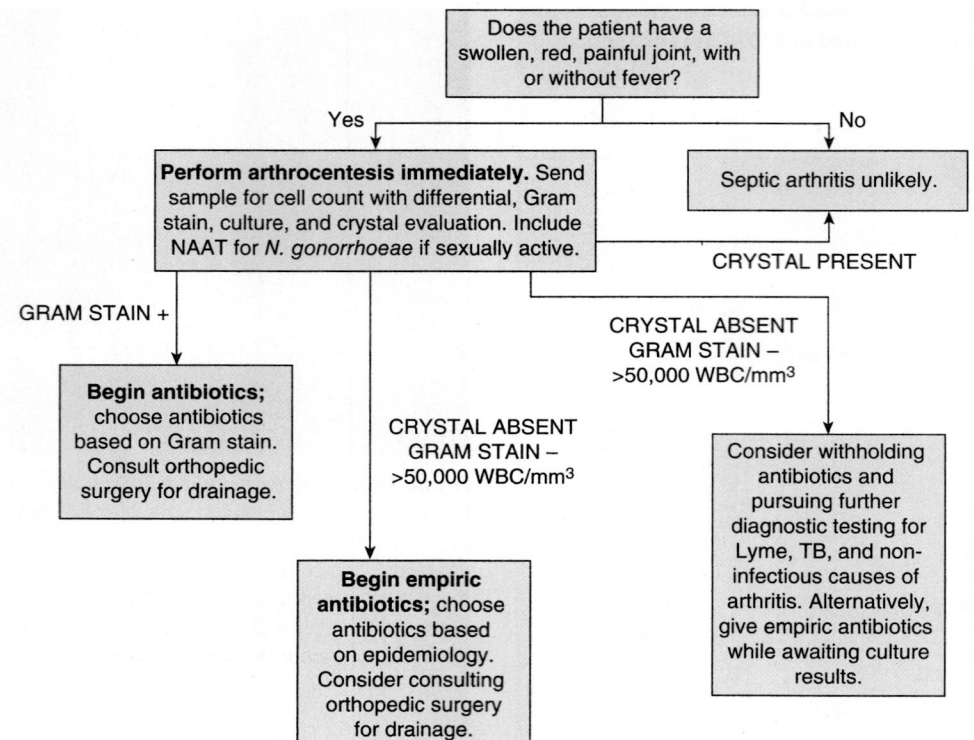

Figure 193-4 *Diagnostic approach to suspected septic arthritis.*

Radiographic studies are not essential in uncomplicated septic arthritis, but may help to diagnose complicating factors. Plain films can demonstrate foreign bodies, adjacent osteomyelitis, periarticular soft-tissue swelling in early septic arthritis, joint space loss, periosteal reaction, marginal and central erosions, and destruction of subchondral bone. CT and MRI can demonstrate nonspecific joint inflammation, effusion, subchondral cysts, and articular cartilage destruction.

■ INPATIENT MANAGEMENT

Antibiotics and joint drainage are essential. Empiric broad-spectrum antibiotics can be considered once arthrocentesis has been performed, or without delay if indicated by the clinical situation, such as septic physiology. Antibiotic selection should be guided by the Gram stain of the synovial fluid and the patient's epidemiology and clinical history. In the absence of informative microbiological data, epidemiological data can assist in directing empiric antibiotic selection. Vancomycin may be used as monotherapy for otherwise healthy patients with septic arthritis. In intravenous drug users and patients with underlying illness at higher risk for infection with Gram-negative rods, vancomycin plus an antipseudomonal beta-lactam or ciprofloxacin may be used. If the Gram stain shows Gram-positive cocci, vancomycin alone can be used. Once culture and antibiotic susceptibility data become available, antimicrobial therapy should be tailored appropriately. If the Gram stain is negative and the patient is hemodynamically stable, antibiotic treatment should be held pending culture data and investigation of alternative diagnoses.

Antibiotics should be administered in conjunction with joint drainage. The goal of drainage is to decrease the bacterial burden, remove necrotic debris, and disrupt loculated fluid. Drainage can be performed by arthrocentesis if the joint is readily accessible and the clinical context appropriate, or by arthroscopy or arthrotomy, combined with joint irrigation. Large joints, including axial joints, shoulders, and hips, should preferentially undergo arthroscopy or open drainage. Treatment of smaller joints may include initial aspiration, followed by more invasive procedures if treatment fails.

Serial drainage procedures should be repeated until resolution of effusions and demonstration of negative Gram stain and cultures.

Though definitive data regarding duration of antibiotics are lacking, common practice is to treat for 3 to 4 weeks. Antibiotics are often administered parenterally initially, followed by oral therapy in good responders with infections sensitive to oral antibiotics. Treatment duration and route should be adjusted based on local or systemic factors contributing to immune impairment, the antibiotic susceptibility of the organism, concomitant bacteremia or other infection, and the overall clinical picture. Physical therapy and rehabilitation of the joint are critical to maintaining joint function, and in their absence loss of joint function may ensue.

GONOCOCCAL SEPTIC ARTHRITIS

■ EVALUATION

Arthritis is a prominent symptom of disseminated gonococcal infection. Disseminated gonococcal infection classically consists of dermatitis, tenosynovitis, polyarthralgias, and suppurative arthritis; however, patients often have only a subset of these features. Genitourinary symptoms are often absent at the time of presentation with septic arthritis, and—particularly in women—the initial genitourinary infection may have been asymptomatic. Gonococcal arthritis yields positive synovial fluid cultures in fewer than half of cases. Diagnosis is usually based on the combination of finding gonococci in genitourinary, rectal, or oropharyngeal samples, and a clinical syndrome suggestive of disseminated gonococcal infection (**Figure 193-5**). It is also possible to diagnose gonococcal arthritis by performing nucleic acid amplification tests (NAAT) on joint fluid; however, this method of diagnosis does not allow for susceptibility testing. An attempt to culture the organism should always be made.

■ INPATIENT MANAGEMENT

Arthrocentesis should be performed to confirm the diagnosis, to rule out infection with nongonococcal organisms, and to drain the

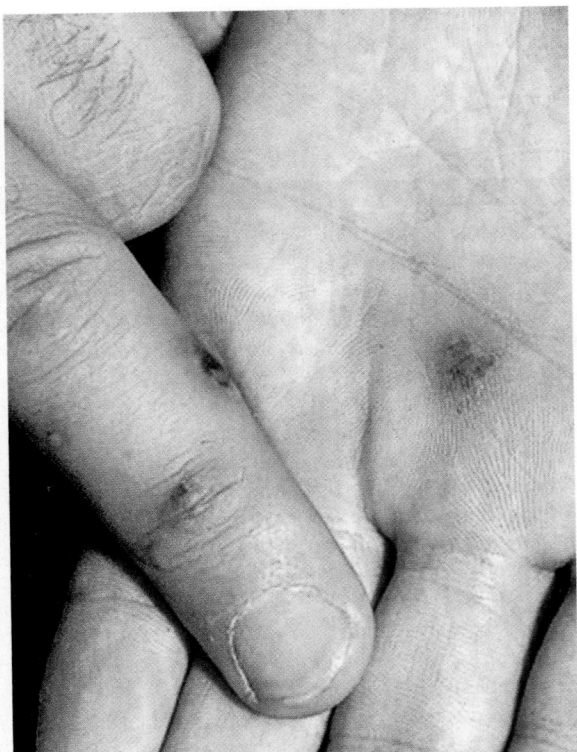

Figure 193-5 *Skin lesions of disseminated gonococcal infection (DGI): the classic triad of DGI includes tenosynovitis, arthritis, and dermatitis, often in the form of scattered hemorrhagic pustules, more often found on the extremities than the trunk. Most patients with DGI do not have all components of the syndrome. (Reproduced, with permission, from Wolff K, Goldsmith LA, Katz SI, et al. Fitzpatrick's Dermatology in General Medicine, 7th ed. New York, NY: McGraw-Hill; 2008. Fig. 205-4.)*

joint of purulence. The initial inpatient treatment of DGI is ceftriaxone 1 g IV q24h. Once symptoms have resolved for >24 to 48 hours, the patient may be discharged to complete an antibiotic course of 7 to 14 days. Given the emergence of resistance to extended-spectrum cephalosporins, the regimen should consist of ceftriaxone 250 mg IM or IV daily, unless the organism has been cultured and antibiotic susceptibilities are available. Depending on antibiotic susceptibilities, regimens could include oral antibiotics such as cefixime 400 mg PO BID, ciprofloxacin 500 mg PO twice daily, doxycycline 100 mg PO twice daily, or amoxicillin 500 mg PO four times daily. Patients with DGI should receive empiric treatment for *Chlamydia*, testing for other sexually transmitted infections, and counseling about safe-sex practices. Patients with recurrent episodes of DGI should be screened for complement deficiency.

PRACTICE POINT

- Septic joints should be followed for recurrent signs and symptoms of infection, as they may require repeat irrigation and drainage even after appropriate antibiotic therapy and initial drainage.
- In patients with bacteremia and septic arthritis, endocarditis should be considered as an underlying diagnosis.

POSTACUTE CARE

Patients with septic arthritis may be discharged once there is significant improvement in symptoms and follow-up has been arranged with orthopedic surgery and, when comanaged, with the infectious diseases service. Depending on the clinical scenario, the patient may require continued parenteral antibiotics via a peripherally inserted central catheter or, if tolerating oral medications and sufficiently clinically improved, may be discharged with oral antibiotics. All patients with septic arthritis need aggressive physical therapy. If functional status is poor at discharge, the patient may require a stay in a short-term rehabilitation facility.

DISCHARGE CHECKLIST FOR SEPTIC ARTHRITIS

- Has the joint been adequately drained? Have signs and symptoms of infection subsided?
- Has antibiotic therapy been narrowed as much as possible?
- If the patient will be on parenteral antibiotic therapy, has a specific provider been identified to monitor weekly lab tests?
- If necessary, has follow-up with orthopedic surgery and/or infectious disease been arranged?
- If the patient had gonococcal arthritis, has she/he been treated for *Chlamydia* and screened for other sexually transmitted infections?

SUGGESTED READINGS

■ OSTEOMYELITIS

Bernard L, Dinh A, Ghout I, et al. Antibiotic treatment for 6 weeks versus 12 weeks in patients with pyogenic vertebral osteomyelitis: an open-label, non-inferiority, randomized, controlled trial. *Lancet.* 2015;385(9971):875-882.

Butalia S, Palda VA, Sargeant RJ, Detsky AS, Mourad O. Does this patient with diabetes have osteomyelitis of the lower extremity? In: Simel DL, Rennie D, eds. *The Rational Clinical Examination.* New York, NY: McGraw-Hill; 2009.

Calhoun JH, Manring MM. Adult osteomyelitis. *Infect Dis Clin N Am.* 2005;19:765-786.

Jeffcoate WJ, Lipsky BA. Controversies in diagnosing and managing osteomyelitis of the foot in diabetes. *Clin Infect Dis.* 2004;39:S115-S122.

Lipsky BA, Berendt AR, Deery HG, et al. Diagnosis and treatment of diabetic foot infections. *Clin Infect Dis.* 2004;39:887.

■ SEPTIC ARTHRITIS

Coakley G, Mathews C, Field M, et al. BSR & BHPR, BOA, RCGP and BSAC guidelines for management of the hot swollen joint in adults. *Rheumatology.* 2006;45:1039-1041.

Dubost JJ, Couderc M, Tatar Z, et al. Three-decade trends in the distribution of organisms causing septic arthritis in native joints: single-center study of 374 cases. *Joint Bone Spine.* 2014;81:438-440.

Margaretten ME, Kohlwes J, Moore D, Bent S. Does this adult patient have septic arthritis? In: Simel DL, Rennie D, eds. *The Rational Clinical Examination.* New York, NY: McGraw-Hill; 2009.

Ross JJ, Saltzman CL, Carling P, Shapiro DS. Pneumococcal septic arthritis: review of 190 cases. *Clin Infect Dis.* 2003;36:319-327.

CHAPTER 194

Prosthetic Joint Infections

Geoffrey Tsaras, MB, ChB, MPH

Elie F. Berbari, MD

Key Clinical Questions

❶ How is prosthetic joint infection (PJI) diagnosed, and distinguished from aseptic failure of the joint?

❷ How and why does the diagnosis and treatment of PJI differ from native joint septic arthritis?

❸ What are the medical and surgical treatment options for infected prosthetic joints?

❹ Can an infected prosthetic joint be effectively treated with retention of the prosthesis?

❺ How should patients with PJIs on long-term antibiotics be monitored and followed up?

EPIDEMIOLOGY

Joint replacement surgery (arthroplasty) is a cost-effective intervention for alleviating pain and improving mobility and quality of life in patients with debilitating joint disease. Over a million prosthetic joints are implanted each year in the United States. It is projected that more than 4 million primary arthroplasties will be performed annually by 2030. Hips and knees are the most commonly replaced joints, but shoulder, elbow, ankle and other small joint arthroplasties are not uncommon. Most prosthetic joints last 10 to 15 years, but 1 in 10 may need revision sooner. Of those that need revision, the majority are due to mechanical problems, such as loosening, fracture, or dislocation. Overall, the incidence of prosthetic joint infection (PJI) is about 1% to 2%. Total knee arthroplasties (TKAs) have a higher incidence of infection compared with total hip arthroplasties (THAs) (2.5% vs 1.5%). The incidence of infection in revised prosthetic joints is higher, compared to primary arthroplasties. About two-thirds of PJIs occur within the first 2 years of implantation or index arthroplasty.

Despite the relatively lower proportion of joint failure attributable to infection, the rising number of joints replaced every year and the exponential increase in existing arthroplasties have caused an upsurge in the cumulative numbers of PJI. Infection remains the most devastating and costly complication of arthroplasty. Potential dire consequences of PJI may include multiple surgeries on the index joint (with the attendant risks of anesthesia and surgery), permanent removal of the prosthesis, large skeletal defects after surgery, prolonged courses and associated adverse effects of antimicrobial therapy. Patients may be left with severe functional impairment and persistent joint pain. Rarely, PJIs result in loss of limb or life. The cost of treatment of PJIs is in excess of $50,000 per episode, with an estimated total expenditure of over $566 million per year in the United States, in 2009. This is projected to reach $1.62 billion by 2020.

RISK STRATIFICATION

Factors that predispose a prosthetic joint to infection can be classified as host factors, arthroplasty factors, perioperative factors, and postoperative factors. Host characteristics include advanced age, morbid obesity (BMI > 35), diabetes mellitus (and perioperative hyperglycemia), immunosuppression (malignancy, HIV seropositivity), and the use of immunomodulating agents such as systemic corticosteroids. Arthroplasties in patients with rheumatoid arthritis are four times more likely to be infected compared to those performed for degenerative osteoarthritis. Prior PJI is an independent risk factor for infection.

The incidence of infection following joint revision, regardless of indication, is higher than primary arthroplasties, presumably due to longer operating time, abnormal surrounding soft tissue, or recrudescence of unrecognized infection at the time of surgery. Primary arthroplasty undertaken due to trauma or fracture or prior septic arthritis of the native joint are also risk factors for infection. Perioperative factors such as American Society of Anesthesiologists score greater than 2, duration of surgery longer than 3 hours, allogeneic blood transfusion, postoperative superficial surgical site infection, and wound drainage or hematoma increase the risk of joint infection. Distant nonarticular infections such as respiratory infections, urinary tract infections (UTIs) and soft tissue infection increase the risk for PJI, presumably due to transient bacteremia seeding the prosthesis during this high-risk period. Asymptomatic pyuria or bacteriuria in the absence of UTI does not appear to be associated with the development of PJI. Preoperative screening for *Staphylococcus aureus* and decolonization in carriers, the use of systemic perioperative antimicrobial prophylaxis, and the use of antimicrobial therapy in the fixation of impregnated bone cement reduce the risk of PJI in patients undergoing joint arthroplasty.

PRACTICE POINT

- Routine preoperative screening of asymptomatic patients by urinalysis would results in added expense, potential antimicrobial exposure, and a delay in surgery, without improving outcomes. Patients should instead be carefully evaluated for historical symptoms or signs suggestive of urinary tract infection at the preoperative assessment, and managed accordingly.

PATHOPHYSIOLOGY

There are three mechanisms by which prosthetic joints become infected. The device can become colonized with microorganisms during the index surgery or immediately thereafter; organisms may spread from contiguous skin and soft tissue infections, penetrating trauma, or pre-existing osteomyelitis; or infection may spread hematogenously from distant foci. PJIs are classified by their onset relative to the date of implantation. Infections are categorized as early (within 3 months), delayed (3 months-2 years), or late (after 2 years). Generally, early and delayed infections are acquired at the time of implantation. Postoperative wound healing complications, especially superficial surgical site infections, have been the most significantly and consistently identified risk factor for PJIs. Late infections, on the other hand, occur predominantly from the hematogenous route. Bacteremia arising from respiratory tract infection, urinary tract infection, or cellulitis can hematogenously seed a well-fixed prosthesis and cause a PJI. This is particularly true of *S. aureus* and beta-hemolytic streptococci. Patients with prosthetic joints with *S. aureus* bacteremia, regardless of the primary source, should be thoroughly evaluated and treated aggressively, as they are at high risk of developing *S. aureus* PJI.

▄ THE FOREIGN BODY AND ROLE OF BIOFILM

The presence of a foreign body and the production of bacterial biofilm make it extremely difficult to cure prosthetic joint infection. The prosthetic implant is a foreign body devoid of microcirculation. This prevents adequate delivery of antibiotics to the site of infection. Furthermore, the implant is nonphagocytosable, and renders granulocytes around the prostheses functionally defective. Local immunity is thus further impaired. A low innoculum of micro-organisms is needed to establish infection in the presence of prosthetic material. Less than 100 colony-forming units (CFUs) of *S. aureus* are sufficient to infect a hip hemiarthroplasty in a rabbit model, compared to >10,000 CFU when no implant is placed.

The first phase of PJI is adherence of microorganisms to the surface of the implant. These microorganisms then elaborate a glycocalyx of highly hydrated exopolysaccharides, better known as slime. Biofilm refers to both slime and the bacteria embedded within. Bacteria in biofilm form organized and complex communities, with structural and functional heterogeneity, resembling multicellular organisms. Bacteria in biofilm even communicate by a signaling process known as quorum sensing. Bacteria in biofilms (sessile/attached forms) are protected from antimicrobial agents and host immune responses, compared with free-living (planktonic) bacteria. Biofilm acts as a physical barrier to antibiotics and white

TABLE 194-1 Common Pathogens in Infected Hip and Knee Arthroplasty

Pathogens	% Frequency
Staphylococcus aureus	27
Coagulase-negative staphylococci	27
Streptococcus sp.	8
Enterococcus sp.	3
Aerobic Gram-negative bacilli	9
Propionibacterium acnes, other anaerobes	4
Culture-negative	14
Polymicrobial	15
Other (fungal, mycobacterial)	3

Data from Tande AJ, Patel R. *Clin Microbiol Rev*. 2014;27:302-345.

blood cells (WBCs). As well, microorganisms in biofilms are in a low metabolic state (stationary phase) due to poor availability of nutrients such as glucose and oxygen. This renders them less susceptible to growth-dependent antibiotics, such as beta-lactams. Infections are therefore difficult to diagnose (low inoculum, few planktonic bacteria, mild inflammatory reaction), difficult to cure (poor access of antimicrobials to bacteria), and persist or recur after discontinuing antibiotics (reversion to planktonic state after antibiotic pressure has been released).

MICROBIOLOGY OF PROSTHETIC JOINT INFECTION

The major pathogens causing infection of prosthetic hips and knees are listed in **Table 194-1**. Empiric antimicrobial therapy should cover common organisms causing PJI such as staphylococci, streptococci, and aerobic Gram-negative bacteria. Overall, staphylococcus species account for the majority (50%-60%) of PJIs. Infections in the early postoperative period, or those presenting with sudden joint pain and effusion, are commonly due to virulent organisms such as *S. aureus* and aerobic Gram-negative bacilli. Polymicrobial infections are relatively more common in the early postoperative period, and often reflect poor wound healing and innoculation of mixed organisms at time of surgery. Coagulase-negative staphylococci are ubiquitous, and may present at any time after implantation. Chronic infections with subtle symptoms and signs are generally caused by less virulent bacteria such as coagulase-negative staphylococci, enterococci, and *Propionibacterium acnes*. Shoulder arthroplasties have a greater frequency of *P. acnes* infections, compared to lower-extremity joints (24% vs 4%). When PJIs are preceded by dentogingival processes or gastrointestinal manipulations, *viridans streptococci*, *Peptococcus* species, *Peptostreptococcus* species, and Gram-negative rods may be recovered. There is no evidence that routine antibiotic prophylaxis prior to dental procedures may reduce the risk of PJI. More than 10% of patients with PJI have no organisms isolated. The most common reason for culture-negative PJI is prior use of antimicrobial therapy. Unusual bacteria, fungi, and mycobacteria are rarely the cause of apparent culture-negative PJI.

DIFFERENTIAL DIAGNOSIS

▄ ASEPTIC FAILURE

Pain or malfunction in a prosthetic joint could be due to infection (septic failure) or biomechanical (aseptic) failure. Recent data suggest that infection is now the most common reason for revision knee arthroplasty, and the third most common cause of hip arthroplasty revision. The major mechanism of aseptic implant failure is osteolysis from particulate wear debris. Relative motion between opposed surfaces leads to loss of prosthetic material, with generation of particles that get deposited in the space between implant and bone. These are phagocytosed by macrophages, and a granulomatous reaction ensues. Inflammatory mediators are released, stimulating osteoclastic bone resorption. Biopsy specimens from tissues surrounding the osteolytic lesions may demonstrate this process, commonly referred to as *arthroplasty effect*. Misalignment of the arthroplasty can also result in inappropriate (eccentric) mechanical loads, and cause implant loosening and mechanical damage to the implant material or the bone-implant interface. Other reasons for aseptic failure include dislocation of the prostheses, periprosthetic fracture, fracture of the prosthetic material itself, and implant malposition.

■ SKIN AND SOFT TISSUE INFECTIONS

Patients who develop cellulitis overlying a prosthetic joint may present with pain, tenderness, differential warmth, and erythema over the joint. These features may be clinically indistinguishable from a PJI. If the localized pain is worse with movement, and a joint effusion with ballotable swelling is present, then the joint prosthesis is most likely infected. Nonetheless, clinical signs and symptoms are usually unreliable, with very low sensitivity and specificity. In the absence of concurrent joint infection, the risk of subsequent spread of subcutaneous tissue infection to the joint is quite high, so infectious diseases and orthopedic surgeon consultation should be promptly sought for appropriate evaluation and management.

PRACTICE POINT

- The possibility of prosthesis infection should be considered in all patients with wound infections after implantation of a prosthetic joint. A sinus tract to the prosthesis is diagnostic of prosthetic joint infection, but this is absent in most cases.

■ STERILE JOINT INFLAMMATION

Patients whose joints have been replaced due to rheumatoid arthritis or systemic lupus erythematosus occasionally experience inflammation of their prosthesis from activation of the underlying disease. Gout and pseudogout may also result in joint pain that may be clinically indistinguishable from a PJI. Aspiration of the joint looking for crystals may be needed to distinguish these conditions, although coexisting infection needs to be ruled out.

EVALUATION

■ DIAGNOSIS: DOES THIS PATIENT HAVE A PJI?

It is very important to make a distinction between an infected prosthesis and aseptic implant failure for appropriate preoperative planning. In the majority of cases, no single clinical feature, laboratory test, or imaging study can unequivocally establish a diagnosis of PJI before surgery. It requires careful synthesis of information from multiple investigations. Inadvertent placement of a new prosthesis into an infected surgical site without appropriate debridement, as well as inadequate local or systemic antimicrobial treatment, will lead to recrudescence of the infection and ultimately failure of the new implant. On the other hand, suspicion of PJI where there is none can result in delayed reimplantation, extended length of hospital stay, increased number of surgeries and anesthetic exposures, prolonged patient immobilization and rehabilitation, and increased overall costs. The tools available to clinicians and orthopedic surgeons in making a correct diagnosis, their accuracy and reliability, is the subject of discussion in the next section.

■ HISTORY AND PHYSICAL EXAMINATION

The symptoms and signs of PJIs may vary, and may vary depending on the onset of infection relative to time of implantation, and the mechanism of infection. Early infections often present with joint swelling, tenderness, erythema, and warmth. Systemic symptoms such as fever, chills, rigors, and malaise are uncommon. Wound dehiscence and purulent drainage in the early postoperative period should prompt suspicion for a PJI. The presence of a sinus tract communicating with the prosthesis is diagnostic of PJI, although this is uncommon. Late infections occur mostly from hematogenous seeding, and also tend to present with pain of acute onset, and an acute septic arthritis syndrome. Delayed infections are the most challenging, as the symptoms and local signs are often subtle or absent. Joint pain, when present, is insidious in onset, persistent and progressive, and may be associated with implant loosening and functional deterioration. Important information from the history includes the type of prosthesis, date of implantation, past surgeries on the joint, comorbid conditions, current or prior antimicrobial therapies, and drug allergies or adverse effects, as these affect prognosis and treatment. The elderly are disproportionately represented in total joint recipients and PJIs, and so a preanesthetic medical evaluation is almost always indicated.

■ LABORATORY TESTS

Inflammatory markers of prosthetic joint infections

The peripheral WBC count, percentage of segmented neutrophils and band neutrophils, erythrocyte sedimentation rate (ESR), and C-reactive protein (CRP) are routinely used to screen for PJIs. They are widely available, inexpensive, and have a rapid turnaround time in most laboratories. Each inflammatory marker alone may lack specificity to firmly rule out or establish the diagnosis, but a combination of results may be more helpful. The WBC count may be elevated in acute infections, but within the normal range in indolent infections due to the lack of a systemic inflammatory response. WBC may also be misleadingly elevated due to concurrent nonarticular infections. ESR tends to be elevated with infected joints, but relatively low in aseptic failure. However, the ESR is also a nonspecific acute inflammatory marker that may remain high for up to 3 months after joint replacement surgery in the absence of infection. Likewise, CRP may remain elevated up to 3 weeks after arthroplasty. Several studies have evaluated the performance characteristics and accuracy of these screening tests. In a meta-analysis from our group, CRP was found to have the best discriminative function of the three (**Table 194-2**). Other studies have shown that a combination of an elevated ESR and CRP has an enhanced sensitivity (96%), but either alone has a low specificity (56%). The finding of a normal ESR and CRP is therefore useful in ruling out the possibility of a PJI in patients with middle to low clinical suspicion. For infections occuring within 4 weeks of joint replacement, one large retrospective study revealed that these tests may still be of value, albeit with higher thresholds. ESR >55 mm/h had a sensitivity of 80% and specificity of 93%, whereas CRP >23.5 mg/L had a sensitvity of 87% and specificity of 94% for the diagnosis of very early PJI.

Newer cytokine markers of PJI, including IL-6 and procalcitonin, have been studied with promising results, but there is currently not enough evidence to justify their routine use in the preoperative diagnosis of PJI.

Synovial fluid analysis

Synovial fluid sampling for cell count and cultures of joint or periprosthetic fluid is extremely useful in the diagnosis of PJI. Aspiration of the prosthetic hip joint may be done under fluoroscopic or ultrasound guidance, whereas knee aspiration is easily done in the office, in the emergency room, or at the bedside by an experienced clinician. The optimal thresholds of nucleated cells for the diagnosis of PJI have

TABLE 194-2 Tests for the Preoperative Diagnosis of Prosthetic Joint Infection

Test	Sensitivity %	Specificity %	Positive LR	Negative LR
Peripheral blood*				
WBC >11,000 cells/mm³	45	87	2.6	0.7
ESR >30 mm/h	75	70	2.6	0.4
CRP >8 mg/L	88	74	3.3	0.2
IL-6 >10 pg/mL	97	91	10.8	0.0
Procalcitonin >0.3 ng/mL	33	98	16.5	0.7
Synovial fluid				
†WBC >1100 cells/mm³	91	88	7.6	0.1
¶WBC >4200 cells/mm³	84	93	12	0.2
Culture	72	95	14.4	0.3
Gram stain	< 26	> 97	>10.8	<0.8
Imaging studies	75	28	1.0	0.9
Plain radiograph				
⁶⁷Gal bone scan	50	78	>24	<0.6
⁹⁹Tc bone scan	100	< 23	>1.4	<0.5
¹¹¹Indium WBC scan	>38	>88	>1.9	<0.6
Bone and WBC scan	>64	>70	2.1	0.5
18-FDG PET scan	82.1	86.6	6.1	0.2

CRP, C-reactive protein; ESR, erythrocyte sedimentation rate; IL-6, interleukin 6; LR, likelihood ratio; WBC, white blood cell.

† = TKA.

¶ = THA.

*Cutoff may vary with laboratory.

Data from Berbari EF, Mabry T, Tsaras G, et al. *J Bone Joint Surg Am.* 2010;92:2102-2109; Lentino JR. *Clin Infect Dis.* 2003;36:1157-1161; Tande AJ, Patel R. *Clin Microbiol Rev* 2014;27:302-345.

varied between studies. In the largest study to date, a synovial fluid WBC count greater than 1100/mm³ and proportion of neutrophils more than 64% have a high degree of accuracy in distinguishing PJIs from aseptic failure of the knee (Table 194-2). Recent studies suggest that the threshold for the hip might be higher, at about 4200/mm³. In the very early postoperative period, hemarthrosis and inflammation increases the average baseline synovial fluid nucleated cell count. A threshold as high as 27,800/mm³ in one study had a sensitivity of 84% and specificity of 99% for infections occuring within 6 weeks of knee arthroplasty. A neutrophil percentage threshold of 89% has a similar sensitivity (84%), but lower specificity (69%). Most studied exclude patients with underlying inflammatory joint disease. Synovial fluid cell count results should be interpreted in context, and individualized to each case. These cutoffs are much lower than those used to suggest infection in native joint septic arthritis. Other synovial fluid markers such as leukocyte esterase, CRP, IL-6 and other cytokines are under study, but there are not yet adequate data to support their routine use.

Prosthetic joint fluid Gram stain is extremely helpful when positive (specificity >97%), but the absence of organisms on microscopy

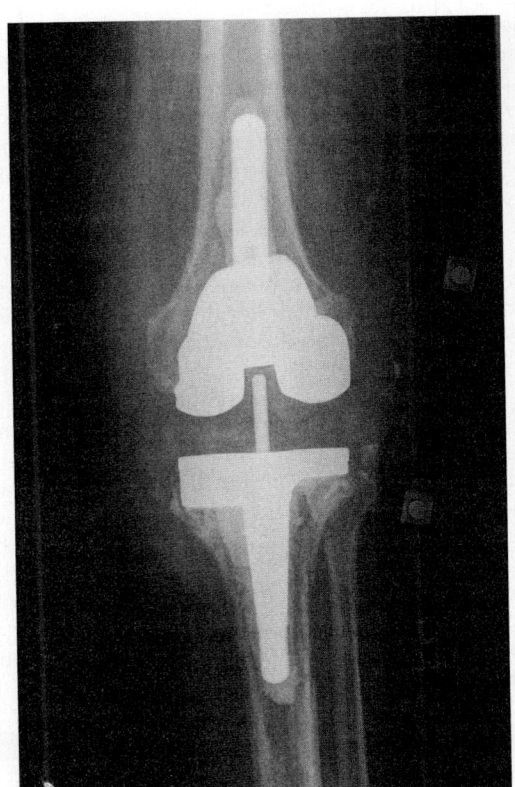

Figure 194-1 *Plain radiograph showing lucency at the bone-cement interface in a chronically infected left prosthetic knee.*

does not reliably rule out infection (sensitivity < 26%). Synovial fluid may be inoculated into blood culture bottles at the time of collection, or transported to the microbiology laboratory for inoculation into solid or liquid media. Ideally, synovial fluid culture provides a definitive diagnosis, and determines the type of surgery to be performed and the appropriate perioperative antimicrobial therapy, including antibiotics for impregnation into cement spacer or beads during surgery. For patients who are not candidates for surgery, cultures should facilitate the choice of a suppressive antibiotic regimen.

■ RADIOLOGIC STUDIES

Radiologic studies have a supportive role in the diagnosis of PJI. Imaging studies are useful for ruling out noninfectious processes, such as dislocation or fractures of periprosthetic material or the arthroplasty itself. Conventional radiograph findings that are suggestive, but not specific for infection, include periprosthetic lucency at the bone-cement interface and bony erosions (**Figure 194-1**). New subperiosteal bone growth is specific for infection, but often absent in early PJI (100% specific, but present in only 16% of cases). Imaging artifacts caused by metallic implants severely limit the use of CT scans. MRI has better resolution for soft tissue abnormalities and provides greater anatomic detail, but can only be used safely when implants are made of titanium or tantalum. In summary, plain radiographs are useful for diagnosing noninfectious causes of joint pain, while CT and MRI have serious technical limitations that preclude their routine use in the diagnosis of PJI.

■ NUCLEAR MEDICINE STUDIES

Radionucleotide imaging studies are quite sensitive and are not affected by metallic implants. However, results are limited by lack of specificity because of the increased periprosthetic bone remodeling that occurs up to a year after arthroplasty.

Bone scintigraphy with technetium-99m-labeled methylene diphosphonate has an almost 100% sensitivity, but is less than 23% specific. Sequential bone and gallium-67 scanning may improve the specificity of bone scintigraphy. Bone scans have also been combined with indium-111 oxyquinoline or 99-m Tc-hexamethylpropyleneamine-oxime–labeled white cell scans, 99m-Tc-labeled antigranulocyte monoclonal bodies and 99m-Tc ciprofloxacin scans to improve specificity. A recent systematic review and meta-analysis of four studies utilizing this combined bone/labeled WBC scanning showed a pooled sensitivity and specificity of 72% and 88%, respectively. The role of fluorine-18-fluorodeoxyglucose positron emission tomography (FDG PET) scans for diagnosis of PJIs is evolving. In a recent systematic review of 11 studies, the pooled sensitivity and specificity was 82% and 86%, respectively. The utility of hybrid imaging modalities like PET/CT scans is currently under study, but present data are inadequate to influence current practice. Generally, radionucleotide imaging studies are most useful in ruling out, rather than confirming PJIs. A negative study reduces the likelihood of a PJI significantly. A positive result requires additional investigation. Most patients with suspected PJI will not need radionucleotide studies. These studies may be used when there is medium to high likelihood of infection, but systemic and periprosthetic joint fluid laboratory tests are inconclusive.

INTRAOPERATIVE ASSESSMENT

When the diagnosis of PJI remains elusive after performing serum markers, synovial fluid assays, and radiologic studies, additional information may be obtained from gross examination of the open joint and additional testing of periprosthetic tissue at the time of surgery.

■ HISTOPATHOLOGY

Intraoperative frozen sections, sampled from multiple areas including the bone-cement or prosthesis-bone interfaces and abnormal appearing areas, should be subjected to histopathologic examination for the presence of acute tissue inflammation. A meta-analysis of 26 studies involving over 3000 patients by our group revealed that the presence of acute inflammation had a high positive likelihood ratio of 12 for infection. Absence of acute inflammation had a moderate negative likelihood ratio of 0.23. Frozen sections have better overall value to the orthopedic surgeon than the intraoperative Gram stain, but require an experienced pathologist.

■ INTRAOPERATIVE CULTURES

At least three and optimally five or six intraoperative samples should be sent for aerobic and anaerobic culture to optimize the diagnostic yield for PJI. In vitro antimicrobial susceptibility data should always be requested. Prolonged incubation, for up to 14 days, may be needed in certain circumstances, to isolate selected pathogens such as *P. acnes*. Fungal and mycobacterial cultures may be considered if bacterial cultures are negative in patients with apparent infection, but should not be routinely performed. Swab cultures from superficial wounds or sinus tracts tend to represent microbial colonization of surrounding skin, and may not be representative of the bacteriology of the deeper space. However, when deep cultures are delayed or not performed, swab cultures may be of marginal benefit, especially in the diagnosis of *S. aureus* or *Pseudomonas aeruginosa*. Ideally, antibiotics should be discontinued for at least 2 weeks before surgery when patient safety is not compromised. Despite these measures, intraoperative cultures could remain falsely negative. Possible causes of negative cultures include low organism burden, inappropriate culture medium, fastidious microorganisms, noninfectious processes such as crystalline or rheumatoid arthritis, or prolonged transport time to the microbiology laboratory.

■ NOVEL TECHNIQUES

Novel techniques to improve the detection of microorganisms include ultrasonication of the prosthesis or amplification-based analysis of bacterial 16S ribosomal DNA by polymerase chain reaction. Sonication of the explanted prosthesis to dislodge adherent bacteria for culture has better yields than conventional tissue cultures, especially in those who have received antimicrobial therapy within 2 weeks of surgery. As with sonication, molecular techniques to diagnose PJI may be most useful in patients with culture-negative PJI who have received recent antibiotics. There are two major techniques: broad range PCR that identifies many different bacteria, including unexpected pathogens, and multiplex (multiassay) PCR which is limited to those organisms for which primers are included. The advantages of PCR technology include rapid turnaround and high sensitivity (71%-91%) compared to cultures (44%-65%). Limitations include discordance between PCR results and conventional culture (as high as 17% in one study), and low specificity (false positives). Specificity may be enhanced by testing multiple tissue samples. Broad range PCR tests may miss polymicrobial infections if additional sequencing is not done. PCR electrospray ionized mass spectrometry (ESI-MS) has been evaluated on synovial fluid and sonicate fluid for diagnosis of PJI, but also has issues with specificity. Generally, these novel approaches involve highly specialized techniques, and are not routinely available in most hospitals. Utilization of these techniques should be discussed with the microbiology laboratory and infectious diseases physician before sampling and transport to the laboratory.

■ DEFINITIVE DIAGNOSIS OF PROSTHETIC JOINT INFECTIONS

According to the Infectious Diseases Society of America (IDSA) guidelines, fulfillment of any of these three criteria provides definitive evidence of PJI:

1. Presence of a sinus tract that communicates with the prosthesis, or
2. Purulence surrounding the prosthesis observed at the time of debridement or removal of the prosthesis, without another known etiology, or
3. Two or more cultures from joint aspirates or intraoperative cultures that yield the same microorganism.

Findings supportive or highly suggestive of PJI include:

1. The presence of acute inflammation seen on histopathologic examination of periprosthetic tissue at the time of surgical debridement or prosthesis removal, as defined by the attending pathologist, or
2. Growth of a virulent microorganism such as *S. aureus* in a single specimen of a tissue biopsy or synovial fluid.

The Musculoskeletal Infection Society has the same major criteria for definitive evidence of PJI, except purulence which is considered a minor (supportive) criterion. Other minor criteria by the MSIS are acute inflammation, single culture of any organism, elevated synovial fluid leukocyte count, elevated synovial fluid neutrophil percentage, and elevated ESR and CRP. Any combination of four of these six minor criteria is diagnostic of PJI. Both societies recommend the use of clinical judgment for consideration of the possibility of PJI even if the above criteria are not met. Validation of these definitions has not been perfomed.

TREATMENT OF PROSTHETIC JOINT INFECTIONS

The treatment of PJI usually requires both surgical and medical management. The goal of surgery is to remove all infected tissue and hardware, or to decrease the burden of biofilm if any prosthetic material is retained. Antimicrobial therapy is given to eradicate residual infection. Ideally, treatment of PJI cures the infection while retaining a painless, functional mechanical joint. In practice, one or both of these goals may not be achievable. The infected prosthesis may be retained in some instances, but may require removal in others, with or without eventual replacement. Palliation through conservative surgery or chronic suppressive antimicrobial therapy may offer a safer alternative than cure in selected cases. Factors influencing the preferred surgical and medical approach include duration of symptoms, implant age and condition, status of surrounding bone and soft tissue, pathogen virulence and antimicrobial susceptibility, comorbid conditions of the patient, technical aptitude of the surgical team, and patient preference. Patient priorities may vary as to the importance of pain relief, restoration of mobility, willingness to take long-term antimicrobial therapy, and willingness to undergo

further surgery. These wishes should be factored into the treatment plan.

TREATMENT OPTIONS

Various medical and surgical treatment strategies have been utilized in the management of PJIs. These include debridement and implant retention (DAIR), staged exchange arthroplasty, permanent removal of the prosthesis, or limb amputation. Surgical treatments may differ between individual centers, and among individual orthopedic surgeons, but certain general principles apply (**Figure 194-2**). The various surgical options, the patient characteristics that inform these choices, and their advantages and disadvantages are outlined in **Table 194-3**.

Antimicrobial therapy is usually an adjunct to surgery, or on rare occasions is the only modality for those who cannot undergo surgical intervention. Antibiotics should be withheld until multiple intraoperative specimens are obtained for microbiologic analysis, unless patient has systemic symptoms, or the culprit organism has been identified by preoperative blood or synovial fluid cultures. Antimicrobials should be targeted at the

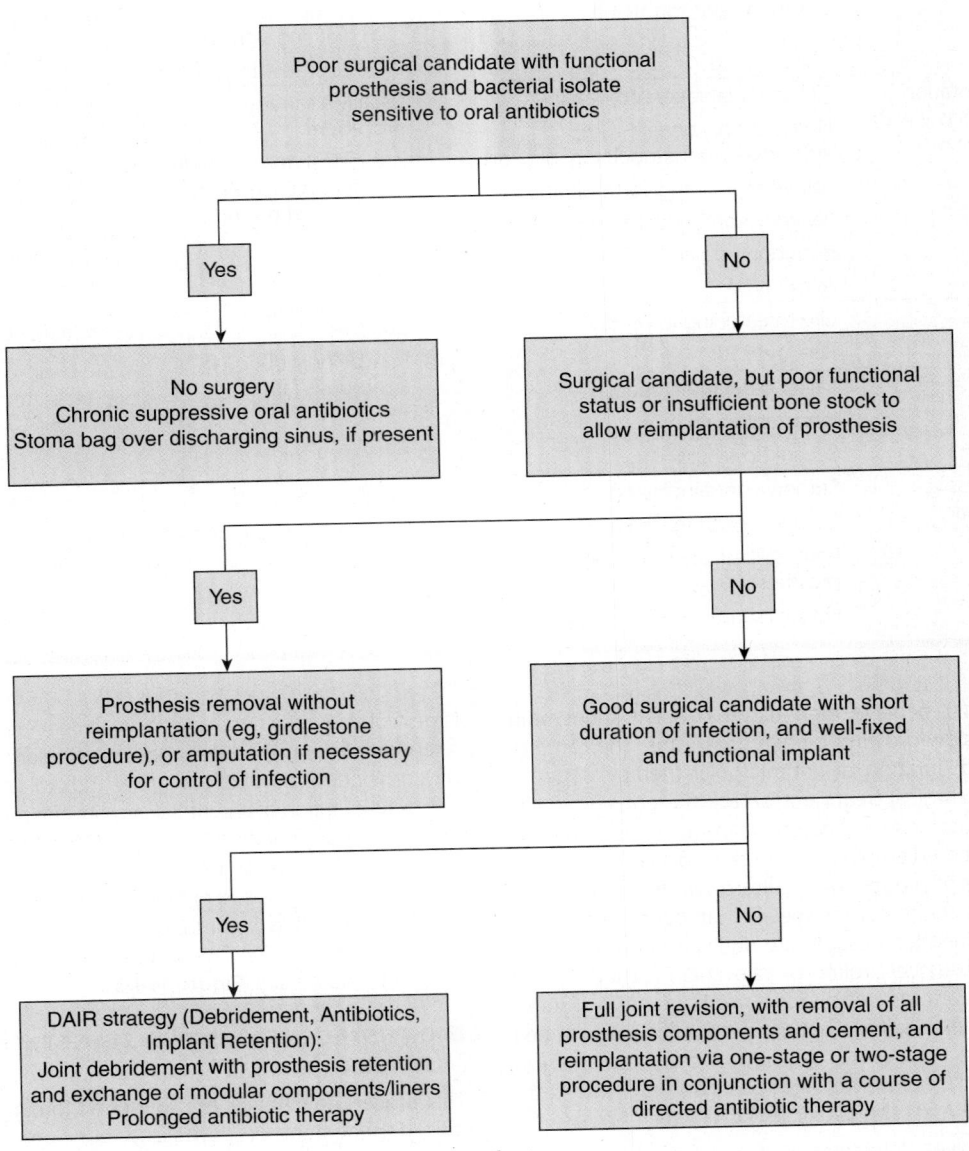

Figure 194-2 *Approach to treatment of patients with prosthetic joint infections.*

TABLE 194-3 Treatment Modalities for Prosthetic Joint Infections

Treatment	Patient Characteristics	Pros	Cons
Debridement and implant retention	Early postop infection (< 3 mo) Hematogenous infection Short duration of symptoms (< 3 wk) Well-fixed, stable prosthesis No sinus tract	Single surgery Preserves prostheses and bone stock Favorable response with susceptible streptococcal PJI	Leaving infected FB in place High failure rate with MRSA High failure rate with chronic infections, previous revision and arthroscopic debridement
One-stage revision arthroplasty	Healthy patient Adequate bone stock Intact soft tissue Low virulence, antibiotic sensitive organism Unable to tolerate second major surgery	Avoids second surgery with additional cost Low morbidity Early mobility Can be used with draining sinuses Can be used for GNB infection 86%-100% success with THA	Suboptimal for TKA infections Risk of reinfection with residual organism Poor outcomes if sinus tract present
Two-stage revision arthroplasty	Medically fit for ≥ 2 surgeries Adequate bone stock Compromised soft tissue	Treatment of choice for TKA Can be used for patients with draining sinus tracts 97% success with *S. aureus*	Restricted mobility Expensive Time consuming Risk of further tissue damage
Permanent explantation (resection arthroplasty with or without arthrodesis)	TKA reimplantation not feasible No functional benefit with arthroplasty(nonambulatory patient) Failure of exchange arthroplasty Severely immunocompromised Poor bone stock Active IVDA	Usually a salvage procedure Arthrodesis may provide excellent pain relief and stable leg when successful	Shortened limbs Poor functional outcome Decreased success with GNB or mixed infections Risk of pin tract infections and bone fracture following arthrodesis
Amputation	Life-threatening infections Recurrent PJI Failed other interventions Intractable pain Severe bone loss	Curative May be only option if arthrodesis fails	Functional limitation
Long-term suppressive antibiotics as primary therapy	Surgery contraindicated Severe coexisting illness Immobilized, does not need functional prostheses Refuses surgery	Symptomatic relief Maintain functioning joint Prevent sepsis	Success rate only 10%-25% Potential toxicities of antibiotics

isolated organism(s), achieve high tissue concentrations, and be active against slow-growing biofilm organisms. The route of administration and duration of antimicrobial therapy depends on the associated surgical treatment or lack thereof, and is discussed below. Intraoperatively, parenteral antimicrobial therapy may need to be initiated empirically based on local prevalence of resistant organisms, if preoperative cultures were not obtained. Commonly utilized antibiotics for specific pathogens, alternative agents, and recommended dosages are outlined in **Table 194-4**. Newer agents such as ceftaroline or televancin for MRSA, and ceftazidime-avibactam or ceftolazone-tazobactam for Gram-negative enterobacteriacea have not yet been sufficiently studied or validated for PJIs.

■ DEBRIDEMENT AND IMPLANT RETENTION

This procedure involves debridement of all infected tissue, with removal of fibrous membranes and devitalized bone and soft tissue,

large volume irrigation, and polyethylene liner exchange, with retention of the *original* prosthesis in one surgery. This is followed by a prolonged course of parenteral and oral antimicrobial therapy. The exact duration of parenteral and oral antimicrobial therapy may vary among practitioners. We recommend parenteral antimicrobial therapy for 4 to 6 weeks, followed by lifelong oral antimicrobial suppression. If a rifampin-susceptible *Staphylococcus* species is isolated, we recommend 3 to 6 months of a rifampin-based combination oral antibiotic regimen after THA and TKA infections respectively, before lifelong monotherapy (**Figure 194-3**).

■ ONE-STAGE VERSUS TWO-STAGE EXCHANGE SURGERY

This procedure involves excision of all foreign material, meticulous debridement of devitalized bone and soft tissues, and reimplantation of a *new* prosthesis. Reimplantation during the *same* surgery (one-stage revision or direct exchange) is mostly

TABLE 194-4 Initial Antimicrobial Treatment of Prosthetic Joint Infection Due to Commonly Occurring Organisms

Microorganism	Agents of Choice	Alternative Regimen(s)
S. aureus or CoNS, oxacillin-susceptible	Nafcillin (or oxacillin) 1.5-2 g IV every 4 h *or* Cefazolin 1-2 g IV every 8 h	Vancomycin 15-20 mg/kg IV every 12 h
S. aureus or CoNS, oxacillin-resistant	Vancomycin 15-20 mg/kg IV every 12 h	Linezolid 600 mg IV or orally every 12 h *or* Daptomycin 4-6 mg/kg every 24 h
Enterococcus species, penicillin susceptible	Penicillin G 20-24 million units every 24 h, by continuous infusion or in six divided doses *or* Ampicillin sodium 12 g IV every 24 h, by continuous infusion or in six divided doses	Vancomycin 15-20 mg/kg IV every 12 h
Enterococcus species, penicillin resistant	Vancomycin 15-20 mg/kg IV every 12 h	Linezolid 600 mg IV or orally every 12 h *or* Daptomycin 4-6 mg/kg every 24 h
Beta-hemolytic streptococci	Penicillin G 20-24 million units every 24 h, by continuous infusion or in six divided doses *or* Ceftriaxone 2 g IV every 24 h	Vancomycin 15-20 mg/kg IV every 12 h
P. acnes, Corynebacteria species	Penicillin G 20-24 million units every 24 h, by continuous infusion or in six divided doses *or* Ceftriaxone 2 g IV every 24 h	Vancomycin 15-20 mg/kg IV every 12 h *or* Clindamycin 600-900 mg IV every 8 h
Pseudomonas aeroginosa	Cefepime 1-2 g IV every 12 h *or* Meropenem 1 g IV every 8 h *or* Doripenem 500mg IV every 8 h *or* Imipenem 500 mg IV every 6-8 h	Ceftazidime 2 g IV every 8 h *or* Ciprofloxacin 750 mg orally every 12 h *or* Ciprofloxacin 400 mg IV every 12 h
Enterobacter species	Meropenem 1 g IV every 8 h *or* Imipenem 500 mg IV every 6-8 h *or* Doripenem 500mg IV every 8 h *or* Ertapenem 1g IV every 24 h	Ceftazidime 2 g IV every 8 h *or* Ciprofloxacin 750 mg orally every 12 h *or* Ciprofloxacin 400 mg IV every 12 h

*Dose adjustment necessary for renal impairment.

performed in Europe. This is followed by 4 to 6 weeks of parenteral antimicrobial therapy. Additional oral antimicrobial therapy is optional.

A two-stage replacement arthroplasty is preferred by most authorities, and is the method most commonly employed in the United States. Following resection of prosthetic components and debridement, reimplantation is carried out at a *second* surgery several weeks later. In the intervening period, patients receive 4 to 6 weeks of IV antibiotics. Patients may be observed off therapy for a brief period for evidence of residual infection, either clinically or by serial inflammatory markers, before reimplantation. Confirmation of successful joint sterilization is also required by histologic or microbiologic criteria prior to prosthesis reimplantation. Repeated debridement may thus be necessary. Typically, the new prosthesis is inserted 6 to 8 weeks after removal of a TKA, and 8 to 12 weeks after removal of a THA. Antibiotic-impregnated cement is often used to fix the prosthesis at the time of reimplantation.

■ PERMANENT PROSTHESIS REMOVAL (RESECTION ARTHROPLASTY, ARTHRODESIS)

This procedure consists of removal of the prosthesis and debridement without reimplantation. Resection is followed by 4 to 6 weeks of parenteral antibiotics. Arthrodesis of the knee (fusion of the tibia and fibula to facilitate weight bearing) can be done by external fixation at the time of resection, or delayed till completion of antibiotic course for internal fixation with intramedullary rods.

■ AMPUTATION

This is a procedure of last resort when all other limb salvage surgeries have failed. The infection is essentially cured by surgical removal. Antibiotics are administered perioperatively for only 24 to 48 hours to decrease surgical wound infection and perioperative bacteremia. In occasional patients with a long stem prosthesis, residual osteomyelitis may be present in the stump bone, and a 4- to 6-week course of pathogen-directed antimicrobial therapy may be warranted.

■ LONG-TERM ORAL SUPPRESSIVE ANTIBIOTICS

Indefinite, and possibly lifelong, oral antimicrobial therapy may be appropriate for patients treated with

- Debridement and retention of the prosthesis
- One-stage prosthesis exchange
- Revision arthroplasty, if residual acute inflammation is noted at the time of reimplantation

In addition, patients failing more than one two-stage procedure and/or those with significant comorbidities, where the risks of surgery outweigh the benefits, may also require indefinite, possibly lifelong, oral antimicrobial therapy.

POSTACUTE CARE

Hospitalists involved in the postoperative care of patients with PJI should optimize pre-existing medical conditions and monitor for complications, such as spread of the original infection to other sites, hematoma formation, persistent drainage from the surgical wound site, venous thromboembolism, nosocomial infections, or antibiotic side effects. Hospitalists should also ensure that patients are receiving adequate analgesia, and being mobilized early in the postoperative course, in conjunction with physical therapy. Patients with persistent severe pain should be assessed for prosthesis dislocation and periprosthetic fracture.

Most PJIs require intravenous antimicrobial therapy in the outpatient setting. Antibiotics can be administered at home by the patient

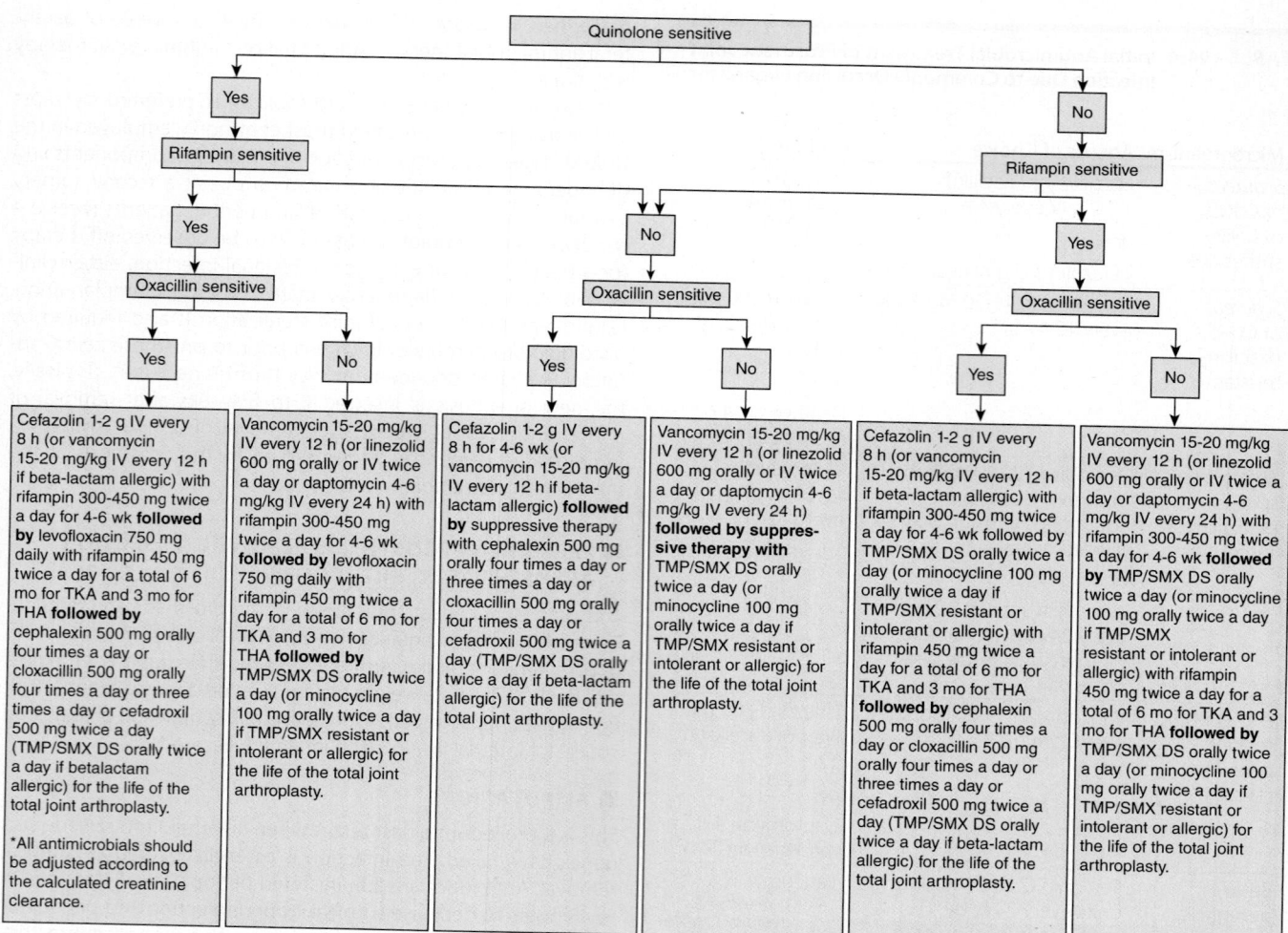

Figure 194-3 *Guidelines for the treatment of staphylococcal species prosthetic joint infection after debridement and retention of the joint prosthesis components. *TKA, total knee arthroplasties; THA, total hip arthroplasties; TMP/SMX DS, trimethoprim-sulfamethoxazole double strength.*

or visiting nurses, at outpatient infusion centers, or in extended care facilities. Infectious diseases consultation should be obtained early to define the choice and duration of antimicrobial therapy. Hospital discharge planners or care managers should also be involved early on during admission to coordinate with pharmacy, social services, and outpatient care providers. In preparation for outpatient parenteral antibiotic therapy (OPAT), most patients will require placement of a percutaneous intravascular central venous catheter (PICC). PICC complications include arrhythmias, bloodstream infection, and venous thrombosis. Patients should be monitored for antibiotic toxicity, both in the inpatient and outpatient settings. **Table 194-5** summarizes the potential adverse effects of commonly used parenteral and oral antimicrobial agents.

DISCHARGE CHECKLIST

- Has the diagnosis of PJI been confirmed through a review of operative findings, pathology, and microbiology reports? If these

reports are not finalized, has a provider been designated to follow-up on the results?
- Have the dose and duration of antibiotic treatment been defined, with specified end dates?
- Have arrangements been made for laboratory monitoring during therapy? Recommended laboratory parameters and frequency of monitoring are shown in Table 194-5.
- Has the most appropriate care setting at discharge been determined? Most patients will be expected to require inpatient rehabilitation after surgery for PJI.
- Have arrangements been made for follow-up with the outpatient primary care provider, infectious disease specialist, and orthopedic surgeon?
- Have patient and caregivers been provided with oral and written instructions on adverse effects of their antibiotics?
- Have the patient and caregiver been provided with instructions for wound care and central line care?

TABLE 194-5 Potential Side Effects and Suggested Laboratory Monitoring Parameters for Commonly Used Antimicrobial Agents for Prosthetic Joint Infections

Antimicrobial	Notable Side Effects	Caution	Laboratory Monitoring[*]
Beta-lactams	Maculopapular rash, antibiotic-associated diarrhea, reversible neutropenia, hepatic dysfunction	Hypersensitivity to beta-lactams	CBC, RFTs; liver enzymes (for nafcillin, oxacillin, carbapenems)
Vancomycin	Red person syndrome, reversible neutropenia, reversible nephrotoxicity, irreversible ototoxicity (rare)	Avoid in patients with previous severe hearing loss	CBC, RFTs, vancomycin levels (goal trough 10-15 μg/mL)
Daptomycin	GI side effects, myopathy	Caution with concurrent HMG-CoA reductase inhibitors	CBC, RFTs, liver enzymes, creatine kinase
Aminoglycosides	Irreversible ototoxicity, reversible nephrotoxicity	Caution in patients with preexisting renal failure, hearing loss	CBC, RFTs,[†] aminoglycoside levels[†]
Linezolid	Myelosuppression, peripheral and optic neuropathy	Avoid tyramine-containing foods and serotonergic agents	CBC (IV or orally)
Fluoroquinolones	GI side effects, phototoxicity, tendon rupture, arrhythmias (rare)	Do not take with antacids, monitor QTc with concurrent arrhythmogenic medications	Liver enzymes
Trimethoprim-sulfamethoxazole	GI upset, dermatological reactions, myelosuppression, nephrotoxicity	Avoid if hypersensitive to any sulfa drug	CBC, RFTs
Minocycline	Photosensitivity, hyperpigmentation of skin, drug-induced lupus, dizziness, vertigo	Do not take with antacids or iron, caution with concurrent anticoagulant therapy or OCP	CBC,[§] liver enzymes[§]
Rifampin	Orange discoloration of body secretions, hepatotoxicity	Should not be used as monotherapy, caution with concurrent anticoagulant therapy or OCP	CBC,[§] liver enzymes[§]
Clindamycin	Rash, hepatotoxicity, *C. difficile* colitis	History of *C. difficile* colitis	CBC, RFTs, liver enzymes

CBC, complete blood count; GI, gastrointestinal; OCP, oral contraceptive pill; RFTs, renal function tests.

[*]Laboratory tests for *parenteral antibiotics* should be done weekly unless otherwise stated (Infectious Diseases Society of America guidelines).

[†]Twice weekly.

[§]Frequency as clinically indicated.

SUGGESTED READINGS

Berbari E, Mabry T, Tsaras G, et al. Inflammatory blood laboratory levels as markers of prosthetic joint infection: a systematic review and meta-analysis. *J Bone Joint Surg Am*. 2010;92:2102-2109.

Osmon DR, Berbari EF, Berendt AR, et al. Diagnosis and management of prosthetic joint infection: clinical practice guidelines by the Infectious Diseases Society of America. *Clin Infect Dis*. 2013;56(1):e1-e25.

Parvizi J, Ghanem E, Menashe S, Barrack RL, Bauer TW. Periprosthetic infection: what are the diagnostic challenges? *J Bone Joint Surg Am*. 2006;88(Suppl 4):138-147.

Sia IG, Berbari EF, Karchmer AW. Prosthetic joint infections. *Infect Dis Clin North Am*. 2005;19:885-914.

Tande AJ, Patel R. Prosthetic joint infection. *Clin Microbiol Rev*. 2014;27:302-345.

Tice AD, Rehm SJ, Dalovisio JR, et al. IDSA practice guidelines for outpatient parenteral antimicrobial therapy. *Clin Infect Dis*. 2004;38:1651-1672.

Trampuz A, Osmon DR, Hanssen AD, Steckelberg JM, Patel R. Molecular and antibiofilm approaches to prosthetic joint infection. *Clin Orthop Relat Res*. 2003;414:69-88.

Tsaras G, Maduka-Ezeh A, Inwards CY, et al. Utility of intraoperative frozen section histopathology in the diagnosis of periprosthetic joint infection: a systematic review and meta-analysis. *J Bone Joint Surg Am*. 2012;94:1700-1711.

CHAPTER 195

Sexually Transmitted Infections

Clare Rock, MD, MS, MRCPI
Colm Bergin, MD, FRCPI, FRCP

Key Clinical Questions

❶ Which hospitalized patients should be screened for sexually transmitted infections?

❷ How should patients with vaginal or urethral discharge be diagnosed?

❸ What are the common causes of genital ulcers?

❹ What are the benefits of universal HIV screening in health care settings?

EPIDEMIOLOGY

In the United States, there are 15 million cases of sexually transmitted infections (STIs) yearly, including 4 million cases of *Chlamydia trachomatis* alone, and the current seroprevalence of herpes simplex virus type 2 (HSV-2) is 22%. The prevalence of genital chlamydia and HSV-2 is thought to be similar in Europe and in other developed nations. Worldwide, there are an estimated 90 million new cases of genital chlamydia per year and 60 million cases of gonorrhoea per year. Syphilis has recently re-emerged in many regions where it had become uncommon, including the United States, Europe, and China. All STIs increase the risk of HIV acquisition. Most, but not all, cases of STIs occur in young people, who may be oblivious or indifferent to the associated dangers, which include pelvic inflammatory disease, infertility, cervical cancer, a higher risk of HIV acquisition, and cardiac and neurologic complications of syphilis. Up to 40% of sexually active females aged 15 to 19 in the United States have an STI.

There are many barriers to care for patients with STIs. These include privacy concerns, fear of disclosure, lack of health care access and affordability, ongoing mental health or substance abuse problems, and denial. Adolescents are a particularly vulnerable group: symptomatic female teens may take up to 10 days before seeking medical attention, and many more do not present because of the absence of symptoms. For many patients, an emergency room visit or hospitalization, often for an unrelated reason, may be the only opportunity for medical personnel to screen for HIV and other STIs, and provide point-of-care diagnosis and treatment and sexual risk reduction counselling.

SEXUAL HISTORY

The most important element in the diagnosis of an STI is a complete sexual history. The sexual history should be obtained in a professional, nonjudgmental, and thorough fashion. The interview should be in a private setting, with the patient physically comfortable and at eye level with the physician. The physician should emphasize the confidential nature of the information obtained, and that the questions asked are part of routine medical care. There should be no physical barrier, such as a desk, between the patient and physician, and the physician's body language should suggest acceptance, with arms and legs uncrossed. The physician should make eye contact with the patient, nod encouragement, and employ strategic pauses when necessary. The physician should use terminology that the patient understands, and assess for comorbid mood disorders, alcohol, and drug abuse that may increase the patient's risk of STIs. A useful format for the sexual history interview is the five Ps: partners, prevention of STIs (if any), prevention of pregnancy (if any), practices, and previous STI history.

PRACTICE POINT

The five Ps: a structured approach to taking a sexual history
Partners

• Do you have sex with men, women, or both?
• In the past 2 months, how many partners have you had sex with?
• In the past 12 months, how many partners have you had sex with?

Prevention of pregnancy
- Are you or your partner trying to get pregnant?
- If not, what are you doing to prevent pregnancy?

Protection for sexually transmitted diseases (STDs)
- What do you do to protect yourself from STDs and HIV?

Practices
- To understand your risks for STDs, I need to understand the kind of sex you have had recently.
- Have you had vaginal sex, meaning "penis in vagina sex"?
- Have you had anal sex, meaning "penis in rectum/anus sex"?
- Have you had oral sex, meaning "mouth on penis/vagina/anus"?
- If yes, do you use condoms: never, sometimes or always?
- If never, why? If sometimes, in what situations?

Past history of STDs
- Have you ever had an STD?
- Have any of your partners ever had an STD?
- Have you or any of your partners ever injected drugs?
- Have you or any of your partners ever exchanged money or drugs for sex?
- Is there anything else about your sexual practices I need to know?

SEXUAL HEALTH ISSUES IN HOSPITALIZED PATIENTS

■ HIV SEROCONVERSION ILLNESS

Acute HIV infection may resemble a mononucleosis-like syndrome. Patients have high-level viremia and are highly infectious. Clinical features may include fever, sweats, malaise, lymphadenopathy, pharyngitis, aphthous ulcers, maculopapular rash on the trunk and extremities, and aseptic meningitis. Patients may also be asymptomatic. Benefits of early HIV diagnosis include establishment of ongoing HIV care and prevention of opportunistic infections (Table 195-1). A recent large randomized controlled clinical trial, Strategic Timing of AntiRetroviral Treatment (START) study, found that HIV-infected individuals have a considerably lower risk of developing AIDS or other serious illnesses if they start taking antiretroviral drugs sooner, when their CD4+ T-cell count is higher, instead of waiting until the CD4+ cell count drops to lower levels. Knowledge of HIV-positive status also discourages risky behaviour and facilitates partner testing. Although the possibility of acute HIV syndrome is an indication for obtaining HIV serology and viral load testing, clinicians should note that current guidelines recommend HIV screening in all health care settings in an opt-out capacity.

■ POSTEXPOSURE PROPHYLAXIS FOR HIV

Postexposure prophylaxis (PEP) with a 28-day course of antiretroviral treatment (ART) is recommended in sexual contacts of HIV-positive persons presenting within 72 hours of exposure. Receptive and insertive anal intercourse has an especially high risk of HIV acquisition. If the patient's contact is of unknown HIV status, as in sexual assault or anonymous sex, then the risk is weighed on

TABLE 195-1 Benefits of Early HIV Diagnosis

Awareness of diagnosis can decrease onward transmission

Opportunity to engage in services and education on prevention of other STIs

Prevention of complications of HIV for index patient

Contact tracing and testing of current and previous partners

individual basis. The possibility of surreptitious sexual assault should also be considered in patients who are brought to the hospital with alcohol or drug intoxication. A full medical and medication history should be obtained prior to commencement on PEP. Monitoring of complete blood counts and renal function on ART and outpatient HIV clinic follow-up are recommended. A full STI screen should also be performed.

■ UNIVERSAL HIV TESTING

Every person presenting with an STI or suspected STI should have an HIV test. This is particularly true for high-risk groups such as sex workers, drug users, men who have sex with men (MSM), and people with multiple sexual contacts or contacts from countries of high prevalence. The benefit of screening for HIV before symptoms develop includes decreased transmission, a greater likelihood of starting antiretroviral treatment in a timely manner, and a decreased risk of opportunistic infection. In 2006, the Centers for Disease Control and Prevention recommended that HIV screening be performed as part of routine medical care on all patients aged 13 to 64, some calling for extension of the upper age range to reflect sexual health practices in older populations. The demographics of HIV in the United States have changed over the past 20 years, with a higher prevalence in persons younger than 20 years, women, racial or ethnic minorities, and heterosexual men and women. As a result, the effectiveness of risk-based testing to identify HIV-infected persons has diminished.

■ SEXUALLY ACQUIRED VIRAL HEPATITIS

Sexual transmission of hepatitis B represents a major mode of acquisition, particularly among MSM. In the United States and other developed countries, hepatitis B vaccine is a routine childhood vaccination. Nonimmune groups who are potentially vulnerable to hepatitis B include persons who have not been vaccinated due to lack of health care access, vaccine nonresponders, or those with waning immunity to vaccine. Acute hepatitis B can present as an influenza-like illness with anorexia, fatigue, nausea, right upper quadrant pain, and jaundice. Blood tests can show very elevated alanine aminotransferase (ALT) and aspartate aminotransferase (AST) (often >1000 IU/L), with or without an elevated bilirubin. Fulminant disease with hepatic failure is unusual (0.1%-0.5%); risk factors include concomitant acetaminophen and alcohol intake. Initial treatment is supportive, although antiviral therapy may be considered in fulminant disease. Vaccination of household members and partners and screening of contacts is also important.

MSMs are also at risk of acquisition of hepatitis C through anal sexual intercourse. Those who are HIV infected are particularly at risk. It is recommended that HIV-infected MSMs have regular hepatitis C testing. Although acute hepatitis C is asymptomatic in 80% of cases, testing for hepatitis C should be performed in persons with risk factors and symptoms such as jaundice, fever, fatigue, abdominal pain, nausea, and vomiting. The average time for symptoms to occur is 6 weeks after exposure. Early identification of HCV infection will improve management and may facilitate interventions to limit transmission. Well-tolerated, highly effective, and short course oral treatments for hepatitis C have recently become available, such as ledipasvir/sofosbuvir. These represent a significant advance over older, poorly tolerated, and relatively ineffective therapies, such as interferon and ribavirin, although the expense may be an obstacle for many patients.

■ STIS THAT MAY MASQUERADE AS OTHER CONDITIONS

Syphilis is known as the great pretender because of its protean manifestations and ability to mimic a wide variety of other diseases.

Clinical findings may include indurated ulcers (chancres) or heaped-up lesions (condylomata lata) involving the genitals, oropharynx, or rectum, a wide variety of psoriasiform skin rashes, lymphadenopathy, alopecia, aseptic meningitis, uveitis, hearing loss, visual loss, bone pain (periostitis), aortic regurgitation, stroke, psychiatric disease, gait disorder, and dementia. Diagnosis and treatment are discussed in further detail below.

Lymphogranuloma venereum (LGV) is caused by serovars L1, L2, and L3 of *C. trachomatis*. It is endemic in Central and South America, Southeast Asia, Africa, and the Caribbean. It is uncommon in the United States and Europe, where most cases occur in MSM. Clinical manifestations include a primary stage, leading to a small, painless genital or anorectal ulcer that may not be recognized by the patient. In the secondary stage of infection, occurring days to weeks later, patients develop fever and tender inguinal and femoral lymphadenopathy, which may lead to formation of draining abscesses (buboes). Alternatively, patients may develop a painful anorectal syndrome with scanty rectal discharge, bleeding, pruritis, or constipation. Hemorrhagic proctitis due to LGV may be mistaken for inflammatory bowel disease; biopsy findings in LGV proctitis may be similar to those of Crohn disease. Laboratory diagnosis is difficult. It is traditionally based on *C. trachomatis* serology, although most tests lack specificity for the serovars causing LGV. Reference laboratories may be able to perform nucleic acid amplification tests (NAATs) on genital or rectal swab specimens. LGV is treated with doxycycline 100 mg twice daily for 3 weeks. When LGV is likely, presumptive treatment is recommended.

CARDINAL SYMPTOMS OF STIs

■ VAGINAL DISCHARGE

Vaginal discharge may be physiological or pathological. Physiologic discharge, comprised of vaginal secretions, exfoliated cells, and cervical mucus, varies with menstrual cycle, pregnancy, age, and use of oral contraceptives. It is usually minor in amount. The most common causes of vaginal discharge in premenopausal women are candidiasis, bacterial vaginosis, and trichomoniasis; trichomoniasis and perhaps bacterial vaginosis are acquired sexually. Atrophic vaginitis is a major additional cause in postmenopausal women. Other causes include allergy, chemical irritation, retained foreign body, and cervicitis from gonorrhoea or chlamydia. Vaginal candidiasis is especially common on general medical wards, due to the high prevalence of diabetes mellitus and the frequent use of antibiotics.

The diagnostic approach to vaginal discharge is summarized in **Figure 195-1**. Helpful historical features include a fishy odor, worse after sexual intercourse, which suggests bacterial vaginosis, and thick cottage cheese discharge without odor, which is consistent with vaginal candidiasis. Cervicitis on examination suggests trichomoniasis, chlamydia, or gonorrhoea. Testing should include:

- Measurement of **vaginal pH** (vaginal pH is normally ≤4.5; elevated pH suggests bacterial vaginosis or trichomoniasis)
- **Whiff test**, performed by mixing vaginal secretions with 10% potassium hydroxide; a subsequent fishy odor indicates production of volatizied amines, suggestive of bacterial vaginosis
- **Light microscopy** of vaginal secretions, looking for white cells, yeast, mobile trichomonads, and clue cells (vaginal epithelial cells studded with bacteria)

Additional tests that may be helpful include rapid card tests for bacterial vaginosis and trichomoniasis that may be performed at the bedside. A culture system is now available for *Trichomonas vaginalis*, which is much more sensitive than wet mount testing.

Vaginal candidiasis may be treated with several topical imidazoles, with single-dose treatment with oral fluconazole 150 mg being equally effective. *Trichomonas* is treated with a single 2-g dose of oral metronidazole; partners must also be treated to prevent reinfection. Bacterial vaginosis is treated with metronidazole 500 mg twice daily for 7 days.

■ URETHRAL DISCHARGE

Sexually transmitted pathogens associated with urethritis include *Neisseria gonorrhoeae*, *C. trachomatis*, *Mycoplasma genitalum*, *T. vaginalis*, and herpes simplex. The diagnostic approach to urethritis is summarized in **Figure 195-2**. If urethral discharge can be obtained, Gram stain should be performed. If more than five white blood cells are present per high-power field, patients should be empirically treated for both gonorrhea and chlamydia. Preferred therapy is single-dose intramuscular ceftriaxone 250 mg (for gonorrhea) and oral azithromycin 1 g (for chlamydia as well as gonorrhea). When no discharge is present, NAATs for gonorrhea and chlamydia should be obtained from urine specimens. These should be obtained at least 2 hours after last voided urine to optimize sensitivity. Empiric treatment may still be appropriate if clinical suspicion is high and adherence to follow-up uncertain. If empiric therapy is administered, culture and sensitivity testing for gonorrhea should also be obtained, due to concerns about emerging resistance (see below). Testing for *Mycoplasma* is not widely available,

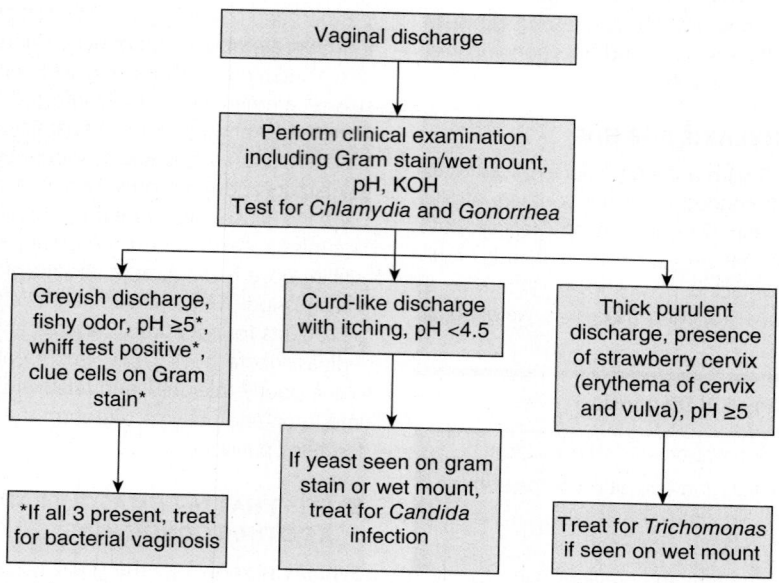

Figure 195-1 *Diagnostic approach to vaginal discharge.*

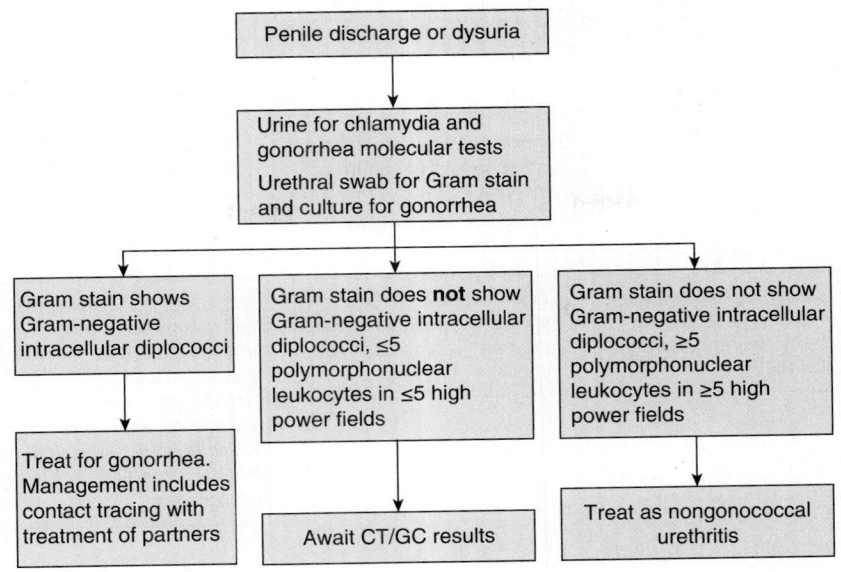

Figure 195-2 *Diagnostic approach to urethritis.*

and is usually not necessary, as empiric treatment for chlamydia with azithromycin is also effective against *Mycoplasma*. Patients with recurrent or persistent urethritis will require evaluation and treatment for *Trichomonas* and HSV.

GENITAL ULCERS

The most common cause of genital ulceration in the United States and Europe is herpes simplex virus (**Table 195-2**). HSV-2 predominates in genital herpes, although sexual transmission of HSV-1 has risen in recent years due to the increasing practice of oral sex. HSV-2 in particular causes painful genital ulcers and erosions, sometimes with fever and

TABLE 195-2   Etiology of Infectious Genital Ulcers in 801 Patients in the United States, France, and the Netherlands

Herpes simplex	72%
Syphilis	20%
Chancroid	5%
Mixed	2%
Other	1%

Data from Hope-Rapp E, Anyfantakis V, Fouéré S, et al. Etiology of genital ulcer disease. A prospective study of 278 cases seen in an STD clinic in Paris. *Sex Transm Dis.* 2010;37:153-158; Bruisten SM, Cairo I, Fennema H, et al. Diagnosing genital ulcer disease in a clinic for sexually transmitted diseases in Amsterdam, The Netherlands. *J Clin Microbiol.* 2001;39:601-605; Mertz KJ, Trees D, Levine WC, et al. Etiology of genital ulcers and prevalence of human immunodeficiency virus coinfection in 10 US cities. The Genital Ulcer Disease Surveillance Group. *J Infect Dis.* 1998;178:1795-1798.

other systemic features, especially aseptic meningitis. Most patients with genital herpes do not have pustular lesions by the time they present to medical attention. Syphilis also causes genital ulceration, which is usually but not always painless. Chancroid, caused by *Haemophilus ducreyi*, is a common cause of genital ulceration in developing countries, although it is uncommon in North America and Europe. Chancroid usually produces a deep ulcer with painful inguinal lymphadenopathy.

The diagnostic approach to genital ulcers is summarized in **Figure 195-3**. Evaluation of genital ulcers includes culture for HSV and serologic testing for syphilis. Polymerase chain reaction for HSV may be useful in patients with older genital ulcers, in whom the yield of culture is lower. The sensitivity of syphilis serology is as low as 50% in primary syphilis. Darkfield microscopy was traditionally used to diagnose primary syphilis. However, darkfield microscopes are no longer widely available, and clinical expertise in interpreting darkfield microscopy is wanting. When no pathogen has been identified, empiric treatment for both herpes simplex (eg, valacyclovir 1000 mg twice daily for 1 week) and syphilis (a single dose of intramuscular benzathine penicillin G 2.4 million U) should be administered. As the differential diagnosis of genital ulcers encompasses a variety of noninfectious conditions (**Table 195-3**), including malignancy, skin biopsy should be performed in patients with persistent unexplained genital ulcers.

POSTCOITAL BLEEDING

Postcoital bleeding (PCB) has many causes, including vaginitis, cervicitis, cervical dysplasia and malignancy, uterine lesions, and pregnancy. The assessment includes pregnancy testing and vaginal and cervical examination, with Papanicolaou testing, NAATs from cervical specimens for gonorrhea and chlamydia, and testing for *Trichomonas*. Diagnostic tests for vaginitis should be performed as above, in the presence of suggestive signs and symptoms. Uterine tenderness on examination suggests endometritis or adenomyosis.

ABDOMINAL AND PELVIC PAIN

The symptoms of pelvic inflammatory disease (PID) are highly variable, and include acute or chronic lower abdominal and pelvic pain, with or without fever. All women in their childbearing years presenting with abdominal pain should have pregnancy testing. Ectopic pregnancy commonly presents with acute abdominal pain; repeated episodes of PID are a major risk factor. Other causes of pelvic pain in women include endometritis, torsion or hemorrhage

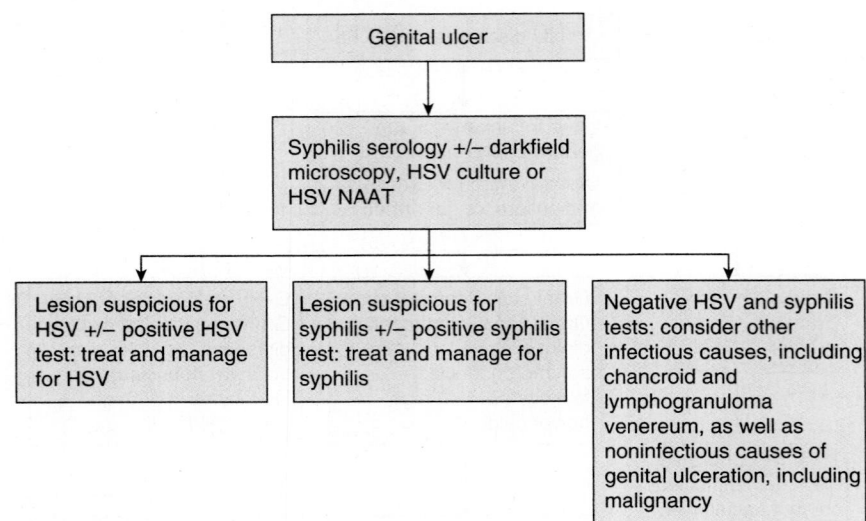

Figure 195-3 *Diagnostic approach to genital ulcers.*

of an ovarian cyst, endometriosis, appendicitis, inflammatory bowel disease, urinary tract infection, and nephrolithiasis. LGV should be considered when anorectal symptoms present, particularly in MSM.

COMMON SEXUALLY TRANSMITTED PATHOGENS

■ CHLAMYDIA TRACHOMATIS

C. trachomatis is the most common bacterial etiology of STDs, causing 50% to 70% of nonspecific urethritis. It is an obligate intracellular organism with an incubation period of 7 to 21 days. Genital chlamydia infection is currently at epidemic levels among young people in the United States. Women are asymptomatic in 75% of cases and men in up to 40% of cases, making case detection difficult and reinfection common. Symptoms in men include dysuria and urethral discharge. Symptoms in women include vaginal discharge, dysuria, postcoital bleeding, intermenstrual bleeding, dyspareunia, and abdominal pain. The major complications include pelvic inflammatory disease and sexually acquired reactive arthritis (SARA), in which urethritis is followed by polyarthritis, conjunctivitis, and mucocutaneous lesions. Sexually acquired reactive

TABLE 195-3 Differential Diagnosis of Genital Ulcers

Infectious

Herpes simplex

Syphilis (*Treponema pallidum*)

Chancroid (*Haemophilus ducreyi*)

Donovanosis (*Calymmatobacterium granulomatis*)

Noninfectious

Crohn disease

Behçet disease

Contact dermatitis

Squamous cell cancer

Pemphigus vulgaris

Erosive lichen planus

Pyoderma gangrenosum

Lipschutz ulcers (immunologic reaction to a distant source of infection)

Trauma

arthritis is predominantly is disease of men. Early recognition and treatment of *C. trachomatis* prevents these complications.

The most sensitive and specific test is NAAT, performed on first-void urine in males and endocervical or vaginal (self-testing) swab in females. Recommended treatment is single-dose oral azithromycin 1 g or doxycycline 100 mg twice daily for 7 days. Patients are often treated empirically. Requiring patients to return for results and treatment can result in loss to follow-up, a missed opportunity for therapy, and further propagation of infection.

■ NEISSERIA GONORRHOEAE

Approximately 335,000 cases of gonorrhea are reported annually in the United States, with a stable incidence over the past decade. The incubation period is 3 to 5 days. Infected men usually have urethritis with dysuria and purulent penile discharge, but infected women are usually asymptomatic. Invasive infections with *N. gonorrhoeae* may lead to disseminated gonococcal infection (DGI), with oligoarthritis, tenosynovitis, and a rash with purulent hemorrhagic pustules on the extremities (**Figure 195-4**). Gonorrhea in women may result in PID, infertility, ectopic pregnancy, and chronic pelvic pain.

Diagnosis is based on Gram stains of urethral or cervical discharge showing Gram-negative intracellular diplococci or NAATs from urine or cervical specimens. Cultures for *N. gonorrhoeae* should still be obtained, as these are useful both for management of individual patients as well as epidemiological surveillance of antibiotic resistance. For MSM, pharyngeal and rectal swabs for culture should also be obtained. However, Gram stains from these sites are of limited value due to the many nonpathogenic *Neisseria* species in these locations. Blood cultures should be performed in patients with suspected DGI, although the sensitivity may be as low as 30%.

Of worldwide public health concern is the rising level of antibiotic resistance in *N. gonorrhoeae*. Penicillins, tetracyclines, and fluoroquinolones are no longer recommended for treatment of gonorrhea. As well, there is a serious and very worrisome problem with emerging cephalosporin resistance. This has reinforced the need for routine gonorrheal culture and sensitivity testing prior to treatment in patients with positive NAATs for gonorrhea. As of July 2011, the Centers for Disease Control recommended that patients with uncomplicated gonorrhea should be treated with intramuscular ceftriaxone 250 mg and azithromycin 1 gm. As guidelines may change rapidly, providers are advised to consult local authorities prior to providing therapy. Patients with DGI require hospitalization and treatment with intravenous ceftriaxone 1 g daily for 7 days.

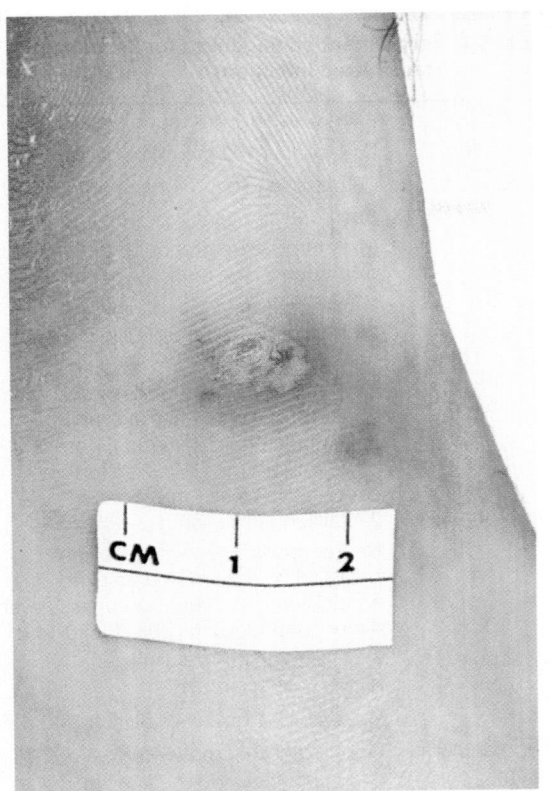

Figure 195-4 *Hemorrhagic pustule of disseminated gonococcal infection. When patients have skin lesions, only a few are typically present.* (Public Health Image Library, Centers for Disease Control and Prevention.)

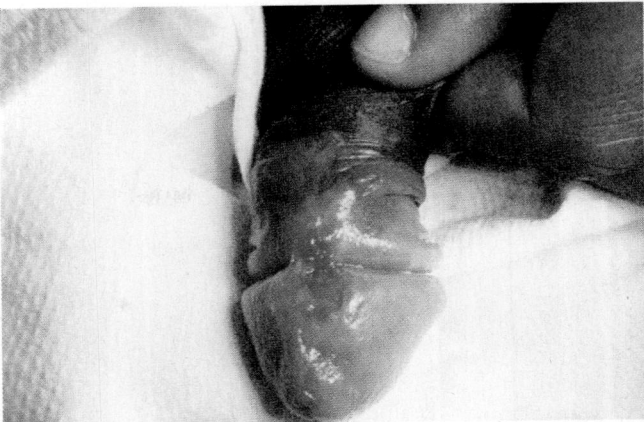

Figure 195-5 *Indurated ulcerative lesion (chancre) of primary syphilis on the ventral surface of the penis.* (Public Health Image Library, Centers for Disease Control and Prevention.)

■ HERPES SIMPLEX VIRUS

Genital herpes has been called "cold sores in a less obvious location." Patients may have associated fever, malaise, inguinal lymphadenopathy, and dysuria. While HSV-2 genital infection is currently more common, the incidence of genital HSV-1 infection has risen due to transmission via oral sex. Primary genital HSV-2 infection is more likely to be symptomatic and severe than primary genital HSV-1 infection. Recurrences of genital HSV are usually milder than the initial attack, and tend to abate over time.

Patients with primary genital HSV-2 infection are sometimes hospitalized due to extragenital manifestations. Up to 8% of patients develop aseptic meningitis, and up to 10% of women have urinary retention. Urinary retention may be due to painful vulval lesions, which may respond to sitz baths, or secondary to sacral nerve root involvement, which may require temporary urinary catherization. Systemic and topical analgesics may also be helpful. Diagnosis can be made clinically, but vesicles should be unroofed and contents sent to laboratory for viral culture. Early treatment (within 72 hours) can decrease length and severity of illness. Oral acyclovir, valacyclovir, and famciclovir are all effective. Patients with extragenital manifestations generally require therapy with parenteral acyclovir, at least initially. Patients with frequent recurrences may benefit from episodic or suppressive antiviral therapy.

■ SYPHILIS

Syphilis has increased in prevalence in the past decade. One to several weeks after infection with *Treponema pallidum*, patients develop primary syphilis, manifesting as an indurated ulcer (chancre) on the penis, mouth, rectum, or any mucosal surface (**Figure 195-5**). Chancres are usually single, but may be multiple. As lesions are usually painless, patients may not seek medical

attention. Patients with primary chancres are highly infectious to sexual contacts. Chancres heal without treatment in about 3 weeks. As spirochetes disseminate throughout the body, secondary syphilis ensues, typically days to weeks after the resolution of the primary chancre. Secondary syphilis is usually accompanied by systemic symptoms, such as fever, malaise, anorexia, arthralgias, and bone pain. A prominent generalized rash may occur, classically described as a scaly, copper-colored maculopapular rash involving the trunk and extremities, including the palms and soles (**Figure 195-6**). Alopecia may develop. Heaped-up lesions may appear on the genitals and perineum (condylomata lata) as well as the face and oropharynx (mucous patches). Other features may include lymphadenopathy, hepatosplenomegaly, uveitis, and aseptic meningitis. Tertiary syphilis develops after a latency of years to decades. Features may include destructive lesions in soft tissue and bone (gummas), thoracic aortic aneurysm with aortic regurgitation, and a wide variety of psychiatric and neurologic syndromes, including personality change, psychosis, strokes, ocular and otic disease, and degeneration of the dorsal columns of the spinal cord.

PRACTICE POINT

- In secondary syphilis, titers of nontreponemal tests may be very high. In fact, titers may be so high that the flocculation reaction does not occur, leading to a false negative result. This is known as the ***prozone phenomenon***. This may also occur with some treponemal tests. If secondary syphilis is suspected and syphilis serology is negative, the laboratory should be asked to dilute the specimen and repeat the test.

Diagnosis is based on serology. Traditionally, nontreponemal tests such as the rapid plasma reagin or Venereal Disease Research Laboratory were performed initially as screening tests, followed by specific treponemal antibodies. Increasingly, treponemal tests are being used as screening tests, as the treponemal enzyme immunoassay has become more widely available and may now be run in automated fashion. Nontreponemal tests are still important in assessing the response to antibiotic therapy. A major limitation of both treponemal and nontreponemal tests is their lower sensitivity in primary syphilis; treponemal tests are more sensitive than nontreponemal tests in this setting.

Primary syphilis, secondary syphilis, or early latent syphilis (patients within 1 year of developing secondary syphilis) is treated with a

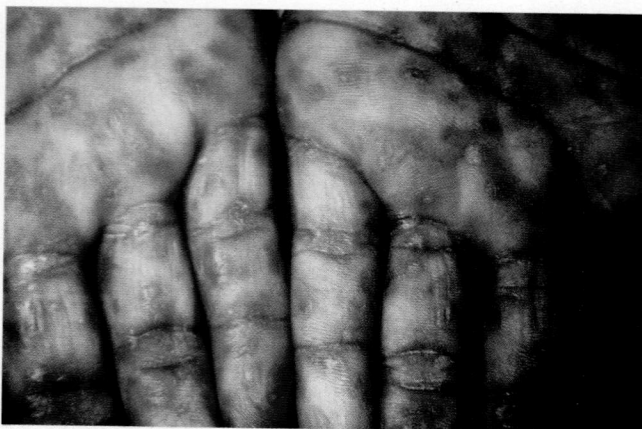

Figure 195-6 *Papulosquamous rash on the palms of a patient with secondary syphilis. Lesions are classically copper-colored in fair-skinned individuals and hyperpigmented in dark-skinned individuals.* (Public Health Image Library, Centers for Disease Control and Prevention.)

single dose of intramuscular benzathine penicillin G 2.4 million units. A transient acute febrile reaction (Jarisch-Herxheimer reaction) may develop after penicillin treatment. This is the result of treponemal lysis, and should be distinguished from an allergic reaction. Doxycycline 100 mg twice daily for 14 days may be used in patients with true penicillin allergy. For pregnant women at risk of mother-to-child transmission, or those with neurologic involvement, desensitization to penicillin may be appropriate. Patients with late latent syphilis or cardiovascular syphilis are treated with intramuscular benzathine penicillin G 2.4 million units weekly for 3 weeks. Neurosyphilis requires 10 to 14 days of intravenous therapy with 18 to 24 million units of penicillin G daily. All patients with syphilis should attend specialist STD clinics where contact tracing and treatment of partners can be undertaken.

■ CHANCROID

Chancroid is caused by *Haemophilus ducreyi*. It is the most common cause of genital ulcerative diseases in developing countries. It is rare in the United States and Europe, but increasing travel and migration may lead to an increased incidence. It should be suspected in a returned traveler from the tropics with a painful deep undermined ulcer and tender inguinal lymphadenitis. Diagnosis is difficult. Gram stain may reveal small, pleomorphic Gram-negative coccobacilli. Even with special media, the yield of culture is rather low. Polymerase chain reaction testing may be available at specialized reference laboratories. If chancroid is suspected, infectious diseases consultation is recommended to assist with diagnosis. Treatment options include azithromycin at 1 g orally as a single dose, ceftriaxone at 250 mg intramuscularly as single a dose, erythromycin at 500 mg orally thrice daily for 7 days, or ciprofloxacin at 500 mg orally twice daily bid for 3 days. Treatment recommendations for STIs are summarized in **Table 195-4**.

■ VACCINATION

Patients diagnosed with STIs may be candidates for vaccination against viral hepatitis and papillomavirus. Consideration should be given to administration of the first vaccine dose in the hospital, with outpatient follow-up for further doses and antibody testing, where appropriate.

Hepatitis A vaccine is indicated for susceptible MSM, patients with chronic liver disease, and injection drug users. Postvaccination hepatitis A antibody check is recommended only for those with advanced immunosuppression.

TABLE 195-4 Recommended Regimens for Sexually Transmitted Infections

Chlamydia	Azithromycin 1 gm × one dose OR
	Doxycycline 100 mg twice daily × 7 d
Gonorrhea	Ceftriaxone 250 mg IM × one dose PLUS
	Azithromycin 1 gm × one dose
	(presumptive treatment for *Chlamydia* is given due to the high rate of coinfection)
Syphilis	Primary, secondary, and early latent syphilis: benzathine penicillin G 2.4 million units IM (single dose)
	Late latent syphilis, syphilis of unknown duration, or cardiovascular syphilis: benzathine penicillin G, total dose of 7.2 million units IM, given as three consecutive weekly injections of 2.4 million units each
	Neurosyphilis: aqueous crystalline penicillin G 18-24 million units per day, administered as 3-4 million units IV every 4 h or continuous infusion, for 10-14 d
Herpes simplex	Acyclovir 400 mg three times daily × 7-10 d OR
	Valacyclovir 1 gm twice daily × 7-10 d
Lymphogranuloma venereum	Doxycycline 100 mg twice daily × 21 d
Chancroid	Azithromycin 1 gm po × one dose OR
	Ceftriaxone 250 mg IM × one dose

Based on Centers for Disease Control and Prevention. Sexually transmitted diseases treatment guidelines, 2015. *MMWR Recomm Rep.* 2015;64(RR-3):1-137.

Hepatitis B vaccine is indicated for susceptible MSM, HIV-infected patients, or those with risk factors for an STI. Routine vaccination series is 0, 1, and 6 months, with hepatitis B surface antibody check after the last vaccine dose. For HIV-infected patients, consider doubling the regular dose, or revaccination when CD4 counts are greater than 200.

Human papillomavirus vaccine should be considered for girls and women aged 9 to 26 years of age for prevention of HPV infection. Bivalent vaccine protects against HPV type 16 and 18, which cause 70% of cervical cancers. The quadrivalent vaccine protects against types 16 and 18, while also covering types 6 and 11, which are implicated in 90% of genital warts. HPV vaccination consists of three vaccine doses over a minimum of 24 weeks. Only the quadrivalent vaccine is licensed for use in males. HPV vaccination in men is somewhat controversial. The Amerian Committee on Immunization Practices recommends HPV vaccination for boys aged 12, up to 21 years of age if not previously vaccinated, and up to 26 years of age for MSMs and those that are HIV-infected or otherwise immunocompromised. Male vaccination for HPV provides a secondary benefit of decreasing the burden of HPV in the community, providing additional protection to females against cervical cancer and other HPV-related diseases. A specific benefit to the MSM population is to decrease HPV-related anogenital diseases, such as anal cancer, commonly seen in this group.

DISCHARGE CHECKLIST

- Have other STIs been excluded? Presence of one STI is a risk factor for others. Appropriate testing includes HIV serology (and possibly HIV viral load), nucleic acid amplification testing for chlamydia and gonorrhea, hepatitis C antibody, and hepatitis B surface antigen, surface antibody, and core antibody.

- Has the patient been assessed for appropriate vaccinations, including hepatitis A, hepatitis B, and human papillomavirus?
- Have patients been educated about barrier precautions? Consistent condom use is associated with decreased risk of HIV, chlamydia, gonorrhea, syphilis, human papillomavirus, chancroid, trichomoniasis, and genital herpes simplex virus.
- Has follow-up testing been arranged, when appropriate? Patients should be advised to have routine STI screens with each new partner. Those with ongoing risk factors should have more frequent STI testing.
- Is there a plan for identification and diagnosis of the patient's sexual contacts? Contact tracing may be difficult due to patient reluctance, and the anonymous nature of some sexual encounters. Sexual partners are often asymptomatic and if not treated will reinfect the index case. Partners of patients with chlamydia, gonorrhea, and early-stage syphilis should be treated empirically. Referral to sexual health services may facilitate counseling and tracing of previous partners.
- Have public health officials been notified, where appropriate? Public health officials may be able to assist in contact tracing.
- Has HIV acquisition prophylaxis been considered? HIV-negative persons with ongoing risky behaviors may be considered for pre-exposure or postexposure prophylaxis with antiretroviral drugs.

This should be done in conjuction with an infectious diseases specialist.

SUGGESTED READINGS

Branson BM, Handsfield HH, Lampe MA, et al. Centers for Disease Control and Prevention (CDC). Revised recommendations for HIV testing of adults, adolescents, and pregnant women in health-care settings. *MMWR Recomm Rep*. 2006;55(RR-14):1-17.

Centers for Disease Control and Prevention. Sexually transmitted diseases treatment guidelines, 2015. *MMWR Recomm Rep*. 2015; 64(RR-3):1-137. Available at http://www.cdc.gov/std/tg2015/toc.htm.

Dowell D, Polgreen PM, Beekmann SE, et al. Dilemmas in the management of syphilis: a survey of infectious diseases experts. *Clin Infect Dis*. 2009;49:1526-1529.

Janier M, Hegyi V, Dupin N, et al. 2014 European guideline on the management of syphilis. *J Eur Acad Dermatol Venereol*. 2014;28:1581-1593.

Miller WC, Ford CA, Morris M, et al. Prevalence of chlamydial and gonococcal infections among young adults in the United States. *JAMA*. 2004;291:2229-2236.

CHAPTER 196

Skin and Soft Tissue Infections

Cameron Ashbaugh, MD

Key Clinical Questions

❶ How does the presentation of skin and soft tissue infection help with diagnostic and therapeutic decisions?

❷ What are the common bacterial causes of cellulitis?

❸ What are the differences in bacterial etiology and therapeutic management between nonpurulent and purulent cellulitis?

❹ What features suggest more complicated infection?

❺ What are the strategies for patients with recurrent infections?

INTRODUCTION

Skin and soft tissue infections are distinguished by their pattern of presentation, tissues involved, microbiology, and response to therapy. Cellulitis is defined as inflammation involving the dermis and subcutaneous tissues. Cellulitis usually is due to an acute bacterial infection. Bacterial cellulitis may occur as rapidly spreading skin erythema without a purulent collection or may be associated with an abscess or infected wound. Occasionally, cellulitis is due to nonbacterial pathogens or noninfectious inflammatory conditions. An abscess is a contained dermal collection of pus. Necrotising fasciitis is rapidly progressive infection with destruction of subcutaneous soft tissue, muscle, and deep fascia. Beta-hemolytic streptococci cause the majority of nonpurulent cellulitis; *Staphyloccocus aureus* is responsible for most cellulitis cases with abscess formation or arising from infected wounds. Necrotizing fasciitis is commonly due to group A streptococci, or when occurring near the perineum, a mixture of bowel flora.

PATHOPHYSIOLOGY

A breach in skin integrity is usually required for the development of soft tissue infection. The skin injury may be obvious, or too subtle to detect. Tinea pedis is a common portal of entry for bacteria in nonpurulent lower-extremity cellulitis. Other local risk factors for cellulitis include lymphedema, inflammation and edema associated with venous insufficiency, and trauma, including skin injury from injection drug use and bites. Medical risk factors include diabetes, arterial insufficiency, cirrhosis, renal insufficiency, and neutropenia.

Less commonly, soft tissue infection arises from systemic bacteremia, with secondary seeding of the skin. In neutropenic patients, bacterial proliferation in the vessel wall leads to tissue ischemia and skin necrosis. Clinically, this presents as ecthyma gangrenosum, an area of inflamed skin with a hemorrhagic pustule that develops into a necrotic ulcer. In patients with cirrhosis, ingestion of shellfish contaminated with *Vibrio* species may lead to gastroenteritis, followed by bacteremia, and finally metastatic skin infection with hemorrhagic bullae.

■ PRESENTATION PATTERNS OF SOFT TISSUE INFECTION

A number of epidemiologic features in cellulitis put patients at risk for particular pathogens. These are summarized in **Table 196-1** and discussed in more detail later in this chapter.

NONPURULENT CELLULITIS (ERYSIPELAS)

The onset of nonpurulent cellulitis is sudden, with local pain and rapidly progressive erythema. Associated symptoms include fever, headache, nausea, and myalgias. The time from onset to fully developed cellulitis can be as short as a few hours. There is no associated wound or abscess. Inflammation in the dermis may lead to edema and dimpling of the skin about hair follicles, giving the appearance of an orange peel (peau d'orange) (**Figure 196-1**). Inflammation involving lymphatic drainage may present as erythematous lines directed to regional lymph nodes (lymphangitic streaking). The draining nodes may be enlarged and tender. The most typical laboratory abnormality is a polymorphonuclear leukocytosis. The microbiology is usually not determined. Serologic studies, molecular diagnostics, occasional positive blood cultures, and the observation

TABLE 196-1 Cellulitis Pathogens Associated with Particular Epidemiology*

Exposure	Pathogen
Dog bite	*Pasteurella multocida*, *Capnocytophaga* spp., mixed aerobic and anaerobic flora
Cat bite	*Pasteurella multocida*, mixed aerobic and anaerobic flora
Fish exposure	*Mycobacterium marinum*, *Erysipelothrix rhusiopathiae*, *Streptococcus iniae*
Salt water	*Vibrio vulnificus*
Fresh water	*Aeromonas hydrophilia*, *Edwardsiella tarda*, *Chromobacterium violaceum*, protothecosis
Cirrhosis	*Vibrio vulnificus* from raw seafood consumption; Gram-negative rods
Intravenous drug use	*Eikenella corrodens* and other oral flora, *Pseudomonas aeruginosa* and other Gram-negative rods, anaerobes including *Clostridium* spp.
Neutropenia	*Pseudomonas aeruginosa* and other Gram-negative rods, fungi

Staphylococcus aureus and group A streptococcus must be suspected in all patients with cellulitis, regardless of other exposures.

that penicillin is effective therapy lead to the conclusion that these infections are caused by beta-hemolytic streptococci. Group A and group G streptococci are responsible for most cases, with group C and group B streptococci accounting for the remainder. After a single episode of nonpurulent cellulitis there is a significant risk of

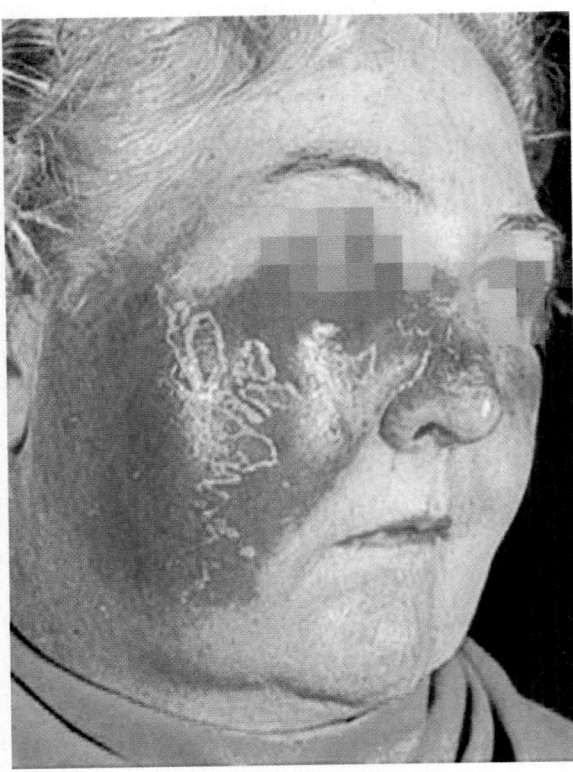

Figure 196-1 *Nonpurulent cellulitis (erysipelas) with typical clinical features (superficial, fiery-red, well-demarcated, indurated dermal cellulitis with peau d'orange). Most cases involve the cheeks or extremities. Beta-hemolytic streptococci are responsible.* (Reproduced, with permission, from Fauci AS, Braunwald E, Kasper DL, et al. *Harrison's Principles of Internal Medicine*, 17th ed. New York, NY: McGraw-Hill; 2008. Fig. 130-4.)

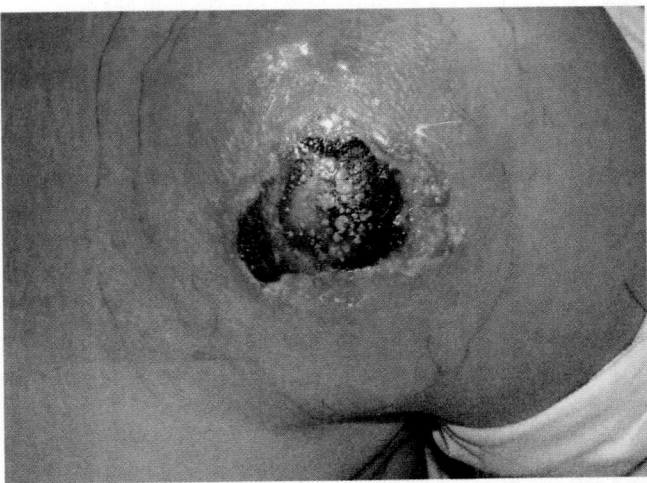

Figure 196-2 *Skin abscess (furuncle) due to methicillin-resistant Staphylococcus aureus.* (Courtesy of Gregory Moran, MD.)

future episodes in the same location. Recurrent cellulitis often is related to underlying anatomic abnormalities. Many patients have recurrent leg cellulitis in the setting of edema from chronic venous or lymphatic insufficiency or after saphenous vein removal for vascular grafting. Other common sites of recurrent nonpurulent cellulitis are the chest wall or ipsilateral arm after mastectomy.

CELLULITIS ASSOCIATED WITH SKIN ABSCESS

Skin abscesses (furuncles) develop in otherwise healthy individuals in the absence of recognized trauma. Onset is over days with progressive local swelling, erythema, and pain. Initially, there is focal induration. Later, as the abscess matures, the central area will suppurate and soften. Skin inflammation is most prominent over the abscess and extends circumferentially. Pain and tenderness are dominant features. Fever and malaise may occur with large abscesses, but constitutional symptoms are usually not prominent. Compared with streptococcal cellulitis, the evolution of skin abscess and skin erythema is slower, taking place over days rather than hours. *S. aureus* causes most skin abscesses. Recurrent furuncles (**Figure 196-2**) are a typical presentation of community-acquired methicillin-resistant *S. aureus* (MRSA). Perineal abscesses usually are due to either *S. aureus* or mixtures of aerobic and anaerobic bowel flora.

CELLULITIS WITH WOUNDS INCLUDING PATIENTS WITH BITES, DIABETES, OR ARTERIAL INSUFFICIENCY

Wound infection with associated cellulitis is common. Surgical sites, burns, bites, and lower-extremity ulcers associated with arterial or venous insufficiency or diabetes, are areas with impaired local immunity. Bacterial infection presents with worsening erythema of the surrounding skin and increased drainage from the wound. The cellulitis can be minimal or very extensive, as often seen with bite injury or infection of a pressure ulcer in a diabetic foot with arterial insufficiency. The diagnosis and management of diabetic foot infections are described in detail in Chapter 147. Cellulitis in the patient with peripheral vascular disease may be associated with rest pain, especially in the toes and forefoot, relieved by allowing the foot to hang down over the edge of the bed. The feet are cool and pulseless, with pallor on elevation and reddish-blue discoloration when dependent. Dry, necrotic, and nonhealing pedal ulcers may be present, especially on the tips of toes or pressure points such as the malleoli or metatarsal heads. The presence of infection in this setting may lead to rapidly progressive wet gangrene.

NECROTIZING SOFT TISSUE INFECTION

Necrotizing fasciitis is a rapidly progressive infection centered in the deep fascial tissues. Patients complain of severe pain at the site of involvement and frequently present with sepsis syndrome. Early in the course, the overlying skin may appear normal. Later, there is erythema with a waxy unhealthy congested appearance. In the final stages, after thrombosis of the underlying subcutaneous vessels, there is violaceous discoloration and blistering. The severe pain and critical illness of these patients differentiate them from those with more superficial infection.

PERIORBITAL AND ORBITAL CELLULITIS

The soft tissues around the eye are separated from the orbit by the septum, a tough membrane of protective connective tissue. Periorbital (preseptal) cellulitis is much more common than orbital (postseptal) cellulitis. Periorbital cellulitis arises from local skin breakdown and inoculation, as with cellulitis elsewhere. Orbital cellulitis may arise from sinusitis, eye surgery, trauma, periodontal infection, and occasionally preseptal cellulitis. Periorbital and orbital cellulitis may be difficult to distinguish at the bedside. Orbital cellulitis may be diagnosed if proptosis, diplopia, vision loss, and limitation of eye movement are present. The bacteriology of periorbital cellulitis is generally similar to that of other skin sites. By contrast, orbital cellulitis may involve Gram-negative rods and anaerobes, as well as staphylococci and streptococci, especially if it arises from a sinus or odontogenic source. Orbital cellulitis in neutropenic patients, or those with diabetic ketoacidosis, is frequently due to invasive fungal infection.

CELLULITIS ASSOCIATED WITH WATER EXPOSURE

The clinical presentation is local pain and tenderness and an enlarging area of skin erythema. Infection begins after water contaminates an area where there has been minor trauma. Beta-hemolytic streptococci and *S. aureus* remain the most common pathogens responsible for acute cellulitis that occurs after water exposure. However, *Aeromonas*, *Vibrio*, *Edwardsiella*, *Shewanella*, *Chromobacterium*, and *Erysipelothrix* species are responsible for a significant minority of infections. If a wound is present, culture can be helpful in identifying the microbiology. In the absence of a wound, a microbiologic diagnosis may not be achieved. In patients with cirrhosis and impaired reticuloendothelial bacterial clearance, ingestion of undercooked seafood contaminated with *Vibrio vulnificus* may result in enteritis with secondary bacteremia and metastatic skin involvement. Inflammation is severe and extensive, often with subcutaneous hemorrhage and the development of "blood lakes" (**Figure 196-3**).

CELLULITIS IN IMMUNOCOMPROMISED PATIENTS

Cellulitis in immunosuppressed patients poses special challenges. These patients are susceptible to the usual pathogens causing cellulitis, as well as unusual causes due to inoculation injuries (*Nocardia*, *Aspergillus*, atypical mycobacteria), or hematogenous dissemination after inhalation (pneumococcus, *Legionella*, *Cryptococcus*, *Aspergillus*, *Penicillium*, *Nocardia*). Faced with diverse possibilities, it is difficult to choose an empiric antimicrobial regimen with acceptable toxicities and be certain of activity. In stable patients, particularly those where the presentation is not typical, a preferred approach is to withhold therapy pending results of skin biopsy for culture and histopathologic examination.

■ DIAGNOSTIC TESTING

Complete blood count, electrolytes, blood urea nitrogen, creatinine, and glucose should be performed in sicker patients or those with comorbid conditions. Blood cultures are of low utility in healthy

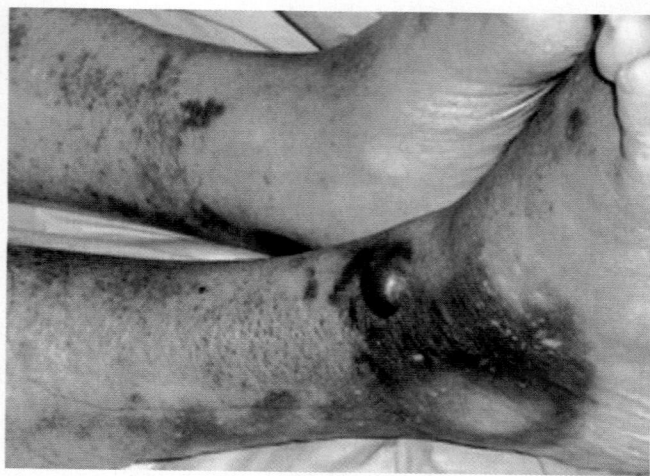

Figure 196-3 *Necrotizing cellulitis with hemorrhagic bullae due to Vibrio vulnificus in a diabetic patient with cirrhosis.* (Reproduced, with permission, from Wolff K, Goldsmith LA, Katz SI, et al. *Fitzpatrick's Dermatology in General Medicine*, 7th ed. New York, NY: McGraw-Hill; 2008. Fig. 183-4.)

patients with cellulitis. By contrast, blood cultures are often informative in patients with high fever, sepsis, or compromised immunity. If wounds or abscesses are present, material from these sites should be cultured to identify possible pathogens and obtain antibiotic susceptibilities to guide final therapeutic choices. Culture material obtained at the time of surgical debridement is superior to swab cultures, but swab cultures are acceptable if debridement is not anticipated. All, few, or only one species present in a wound may be pathogenic in a particular patient. In general, *S. aureus* and beta-hemolytic streptococci in wounds are most likely to be significant, Gram-negative rods may be significant, and enterococci, coagulase-negative staphylococci, *Corynebacterium* species, and *Candida* species are least likely to be pathogenic. In immunocompromised patients, tissue biopsies should be sent for routine aerobic and anaerobic bacterial, fungal, and mycobacterial culture; pathology should include special stains for microorganisms. In unstable patients suspected to have necrotizing fasciitis, emergent surgical exploration is critical; devitalized fascial planes are diagnostic by inspection, frozen section pathology is used in event of uncertainty. Imaging studies are sometimes helpful in the management of soft tissue infection. Plain radiographs may reveal a foreign body if there is a history of traumatic injury. In stable patients with a possible diagnosis of necrotizing fasciitis, plain film or computed tomography (CT) scan support the diagnosis if there is visible gas in the soft tissues; magnetic resonance imaging (MRI) is sensitive to fascial edema, but the finding is limited by lack of specificity. Ultrasound is useful in the detection of abscesses or infected fluid collections in patients not responding to antibiotic therapy. In patients with orbital cellulitis and concern for invasive fungal infection, CT imaging demonstrating soft tissue inflammation and adjacent osteolysis supports the diagnosis.

■ DIFFERENTIAL DIAGNOSIS

Lyme disease

Early Lyme disease commonly presents with erythema migrans—a focal rash with skin erythema extending circumferentially from the site of a tick bite. Most typically, erythema migrans is a target lesion with intense erythema peripherally and central pallor, but lesions with uniform erythema are common, and central blistering with necrosis occurs occasionally. Unlike streptococcal cellulitis, the erythema is circular or ovoid. Unlike cellulitis associated with skin abscess, there is no localized fluid collection.

Flu-like symptoms with fever, arthralgias, and myalgias are common in early Lyme disease, but do not help to distinguish it from cellulitis. In areas of high incidence, possible or confirmed tick exposure, and a typical rash are sufficient for a clinical diagnosis and initiation of antibiotic therapy.

NONINFECTIOUS PROCESSES MISTAKEN FOR INFECTIOUS CELLULITIS

Several noninfectious conditions may mimic cellulitis. These are summarized in **Table 196-2**.

Patients with *chronic venous insufficiency* may develop dermatitis and acute inflammation, most commonly in the lower leg. Both lower extremities are usually involved, although when the venous injury is due to antecedent trauma or venous clot, inflammation may be restricted to a single limb. Critical to the development of dermatitis is chronic edema. Over time, the skin becomes indurated and develops a characteristic nodular appearance, often with bronze or purple-brown hyperpigmentation from hemosiderin deposition. Inflammation may be sufficient to appear as uniform erythema. By contrast to bacterial infection, involvement is often bilateral, the site is not tender, systemic signs of infection are absent, and the erythema improves rapidly over 8 to 24 hours with limb elevation.

Gout presents as severe pain centered at a joint. Classically, the first metatarsal-phalangeal joint is involved (podagra). Midfoot, ankle, knee, wrist, and finger involvement are also common. Low-grade fever and periarticular erythema are typical. Rarely, joint inflammation extends beyond periarticular soft tissues. The periarticular location is helpful in distinguishing gout from isolated bacterial cellulitis, but does not exclude skin infection associated with septic arthritis. Joint fluid analysis is needed to distinguish a gout attack from an infected joint.

Insect bites can induce a local hypersensitivity reaction with edema and erythema. Cases are more common in the warm and wet seasons of the year when populations of mosquitoes and other biting insects are highest. Lesions are pruritic with circumferential erythema; abscess formation is unusual. Modest fever is possible, but high fever is unusual. Inflammation may be severe enough to merit treatment with a systemic corticosteroid.

Skin and soft tissue inflammation after *vaccine injection* can be confused with bacterial skin infection. Erythema, malaise, fever, and local tenderness usually are mild, but rarely can be substantial. Localization to the upper arm and vaccination within the past 72 hours, especially with pneumococcal vaccine, are highly suggestive. Bacterial infection at the injection site must be considered, but is less common than sterile inflammation.

◼ TRIAGE AND HOSPITAL ADMISSION

Patients presenting with fever, pain, and rapidly advancing erythema, patients failing outpatient therapy, patients with hemodynamic instability, patients with comorbidities such as peripheral vascular disease, diabetes, or chronic venous insufficiency that may complicate or delay recovery, and patients with immune deficiency are best admitted to the hospital. Other patients with cellulitis may be managed outside the hospital with oral antibiotics and careful observation, unless the patient has cognitive, compliance, or other

TABLE 196-2 Skin Conditions that Mimic Cellulitis

Condition	Distinguishing Features
Venous stasis	Erythematous, swollen, warm lower extremity with dermatitis and hyperpigmentation; typically bilateral in obese individuals, and unilateral when occurring after saphenous vein harvest or deep venous thrombosis; skin breakdown and ulceration may develop at the medial and lateral malleoli; if there is no bacterial superinfection, fever and leukocytosis will be absent, and clinical improvement occurs with limb elevation and other measures to reduce edema.
Arterial insufficiency	Nonhealing foot wounds with dependent rubor may mimic cellulitis; patients may also have claudication, rest pain, and diminished or absent pedal pulses; if suspected, noninvasive vascular studies, such as ankle-brachial index, should be performed.
Superficial thrombophlebitis	Swelling, induration, and erythema, typically at an intravenous site; palpable cord usually present; fever and leukocytosis absent if no superinfection.
Deep venous thrombosis	Unilateral swollen leg; low-grade fever may be present; superficial veins may be congested, and a cord may be palpable, but physical examination not sensitive; if suspected, obtain duplex ultrasonography.
Contact dermatitis	Weeping skin with vesicles and erythema; well-localized lesion, sometimes with pattern suggestive of irritant exposure; superinfection may occur.
Herpetic whitlow	Swollen painful finger with vesicles; patients are often health care workers, such as dental hygienists or intensive care nurses, who come into contact with the oral cavity and saliva of patients.
Pyoderma gangrenosum	Ragged undermined ulcer, typically on the lower extremity; cultures usually positive as heavily colonized with bacteria; common in inflammatory bowel disease; obtain dermatology consult and biopsy if suspected.
Insect bite	Rapid and sometimes impressive local swelling and erythema, without fever or systemic toxicity; good response to antihistamines; rarely, with spider bites, central necrosis develops.
Erythema nodosum	Hot, warm, tender plaques (panniculitis) involving the shins; seen with sarcoid, rheumatologic disease, fungal infection.
Sweet syndrome	Papules, plaques, and panniculitis involving the head, neck, upper trunk and arms; fever and neutrophilia often present; may be postinfectious syndrome in young person, or a harbinger of hematopoietic malignancy in an older one.
Gout	Exquisitely tender arthritis, often with prominent soft tissue inflammation, involving the great toe, midfoot, knee, and other joints; fever and leukocytosis often prominent; tophi may be present; may complicate hospital admission for other illness.
Calciphylaxis	Painful plaques on the extremities, which may become necrotic; typically occurs in hemodialysis patients with extensive atherosclerosis and high calcium-phosphate product.
Familial Mediterranean fever	Recurrent, brief, self-limited attacks of fever, serositis and erysipelas-like skin erythema; patients are typically of Mediterranean or Middle Eastern descent, and have a positive family history.

social issues that might jeopardize care. Infectious disease consultation should be considered in patients with immunodeficiency, severe cellulitis, or who fail to respond to the initial antibiotic regimen. Necrotizing soft tissue infection is life threatening, and requires surgical consultation at the time of presentation.

■ TREATMENT

In general, the first dose of the antibiotic should be promptly administered. Parenteral or oral agents with high bioavailabity are preferred early in treatment.

NONPURULENT CELLULITIS (ERYSIPELAS)

All beta-hemolytic streptococci remain susceptible to penicillin, cephalosporins, carbapenems, beta-lactam/beta-lactamase inhibitor combinations, vancomycin, and linezolid. Most strains are susceptible to fluoroquinolones with expanded activity against Gram-positive bacteria. Drug allergy, interactions with other medications, ease of administration, and cost all influence the choice of antibiotic in an individual patient. Penicillin remains appealing due to its narrow spectrum of activity. Symptomatic improvement with decrease in fever, malaise, and pain is expected in 24 to 48 hours. Skin erythema is slower to resolve, and often extends for the first 48 hours. Even after improvement, erythema will be more prominent when the affected area is dependent, or after bathing in warm water. The absence of a microbiologic diagnosis, the early progression of skin inflammation on therapy, and the situational changes in skin appearance commonly lead to escalation of antibiotic therapy. In this setting, drug allergies often further complicate management. The inclination to change therapy in the first few days of administration should be resisted unless there is additional evidence of clinical deterioration. Once improvement is clear, oral amoxicillin can be substituted for intravenous therapy. Antibiotics are continued for 5 to 10 days. Shorter courses are acceptable if the skin appearance is at a prior baseline.

PRACTICE POINT

- Erythema often increases in extent in the first 24 to 48 hours after admission, despite adequate antibiotic therapy.
- In morbidly obese patients, ensure that the antibiotic dose is adequate for the patient's body mass.
- Areas of cellulitis will appear more discolored when dependent or after bathing the area in warm water. Erythema under these conditions does not indicate treatment failure if other symptoms and signs of infection are improving.
- Avoid the temptation to modify antibiotic early in the course of therapy, particularly for erythema alone.

PRACTICE POINT

- Cellulitis in the setting of venous or lymphatic insufficiency may be slow to resolve, and aggressive measures to reduce edema, such as compression stockings and elevation of the extremity above the level of the heart, may speed resolution of infection.

CELLULITIS ASSOCIATED WITH SKIN ABSCESS

Early administration of an antibiotic before lesions reach the point of suppuration may be sufficient for cure, but usually clinical improvement only begins when an abscess drains, either from spontaneous rupture or incision. Community-acquired MRSA must be assumed when making empiric antibiotic choices. Doxycycline, trimethoprim-sulfamethoxazole, and linezolid are predictably

active oral agents against MRSA. Clindamycin and fluoroquinolones may be active, but should not be used in the absence of susceptibility data. Intravenous vancomycin or daptomycin or ceftaroline are additional options for sicker patients. Antibiotic therapy for patients presenting with a perineal abscess should include agents active against MRSA as well as bowel flora. Independent of the location, incision, and disruption of internal compartments within the abscess cavity is the most effective therapy. Small abscesses may be incised at the bedside. Adequate local anesthesia is difficult to achieve, so both patient and physician need to be prepared for some patient discomfort. Abscesses larger than several centimeters are best drained in the operating room. Purulent fluid recovered at abscess drainage should be cultured to provide a microbiologic diagnosis and susceptibility data. If the debridement is complete and the cellulitis is confined to several centimeters around the abscess, antibiotic therapy can be discontinued after the procedure. If pockets of infected fluid are left or the cellulitis is more extensive, antibiotics should be continued until erythema and induration improve. Antibiotic susceptibility information is used to refine empiric antibiotic choices. Oral administration is effective, unless the pathogen is only susceptible to an antibiotic that must be given intravenously. A typical duration of antibiotic would be 3 to 5 days.

NECROTIZING SOFT TISSUE INFECTION

Patients with suspected necrotizing fasciitis require prompt surgical exploration and debridement. In these critically ill patients, initial empiric antibiotic regimen should include agents active against MRSA, beta-hemolytic streptococci, enteric Gram-negative rods, and bowel anaerobes. Therapy should include one antibiotic that inhibits protein synthesis and toxin production. Clindamycin is most frequently used, but linezolid and aminoglycosides are also effective. Potential three-drug regimens include an intravenous agent active against MRSA (such as vancomycin, daptomycin, ceftaroline, or linezolid), plus an agent active against Gram-negative rods and anaerobes (a third- or fourth-generation cephalosporin, piperacillin-tazobactam, or a carbapenem), plus an agent that inhibits protein synthesis (clindamycin or linezolid preferred over aminoglycosides). The initial regimen should be tailored based on microbiology. For streptococcal or clostridial necrotizing fasciitis, penicillin and clindamycin combination therapy is continued until the patient is no longer critically ill, at which point pencillin alone is sufficient. In patients with necrotizing fasciitis and streptococcal toxic shock syndrome, intravenous immune globulin (IVIG) may decrease mortality by neutralizing streptococcal toxins.

CELLULITIS ASSOCIATED WITH WOUNDS

Prior to culture information, empiric antibiotic choices are influenced by the history of the wound and the stability of the patient. Infection in wounds of brief duration in stable patients without MRSA risk factors (**Table 196-3**) usually involves streptococcal species, methicillin-sensitive *S. aureus*, and sensitive *Enterobacteraciae*.

TABLE 196-3 Epidemiologic Risk Factors for Methicillin-Resistant *Staphylococcus Aureus* Colonization

- Prior colonization	- HIV infection
- History of boils	- Injection drug use
- Antibiotic use in the past 3 mo	- Incarceration in the past year
- Health care admission in the past year	- Chronic hemodialysis
	- Men who have sex with men

Either cefazolin or nafcillin plus a quinolone or ceftriaxone alone or ampicillin-sulbactam alone are appropriate for initial therapy, together with a quinolone, ceftriaxone, or ampicillin-sulbactam. In medically experienced patients at risk for infections with antibiotic-resistant bacteria, or in unstable patients with limb- or life-threatening infections, a drug with activity against MRSA, such as vancomycin, daptomycin, ceftaroline, or linezolid, should be combined with a drug active against multidrug-resistant Gram-negative pathogens and anaerobes, such as cefepime, imipenem, or piperacillin-tazobactam.

Infected bite wounds should be empirically treated with agents active against beta-hemolytic streptococci, MSSA, and the oral flora of the biting species: in humans, oral anaerobes such as *Eikenella corrodens*; in cats, *Pasturella multocida*; and in dogs, *Capnocytophaga canimorsus*. Ceftriaxone, cefepime, ampicillin-sulbactam, and imipenem are active against these pathogens.

When results of wound cultures are available, complex regimens should be simplified to minimize the risk of drug toxicity and the development of antibiotic resistance. Initial therapy is with intravenous antibiotic or oral agents with high bioavailability. After clinical improvement, oral antibiotics can be substituted for intravenous agents if the susceptibility data are favorable. Duration of antibiotic is usually between 7 and 14 days, with therapy being stopped when erythema and purulent wound discharge are resolved.

CELLULITIS ASSOCIATED WITH WATER EXPOSURE

Empiric treatment is directed at beta-hemolytic streptococci, MSSA, and environmental Gram-negative rods. Salt water exposure is associated with *Vibrio* infection, freshwater exposure with *Aeromonas*, *Shewanella*, *Chromobacterium*, *Edwardsiella*, and *Erysipelothrix*. Cefepime or an antipseudomonal carbapenems, such as imipenem or meropenem, are reasonable empiric agents. In patients with seawater exposure and possible *Vibrio* infection, the addition of doxycycline to cefepime or antipseudomonal carbapenem is recommended based on animal and limited human studies. In patients who are critically ill or who have risk factors for MRSA infection, an additional agent directed at MRSA is included. Empiric regimens should be simplified based on culture results.

CELLULITIS IN IMMUNOCOMPROMISED HOSTS

In stable patients with typical presentations, therapy may be identical to that described above for normal hosts. In odd and indolent presentations, therapy should be deferred until culture and pathologic data are available to inform the choice of agent. In unstable patients, antibiotic therapy is directed at MRSA, streptococci, and drug-resistant enteric and nonenteric Gram-negative rods, with vancomycin, daptomycin, ceftaroline, or linezolid, combined with cefepime, imipenem, or piperacillin-tazobactam.

■ COMPLICATIONS

Bacterial cellulitis should respond to antibiotic therapy after several days of treatment. Disease progression or failure to improve usually reflects infected fluid collections or involvement of tissue deep to the skin. Involvement of deeper tissues and structures should also be suspected in cases of systemic toxicity or disproportionate pain (necrotizing fasciitis), foot ulcers in diabetics (osteomyelitis), cellulitis overlying a joint replacement (infected prosthetic joint), or cellulitis of the abdominal wall (bowel inflammation or enterocutaneous fistula) (**Table 196-4**).

Ultrasound is helpful in identifying infected fluid collections. CT or MRI studies are useful for demonstrating deep tissue infection, with MRI being particularly helpful in the diagnosis of osteomyelitis. Surgical consultation should be obtained if these are abnormal. *Clostridium difficile* colitis may complicate any course of antibiotic therapy.

TABLE 196-4   Cellulitis: When to Consider Involvement of Deeper Tissues

- Assume necrotizing fasciitis if there is hypotension and cellulitis with severe site pain, especially if the pain is out of proportion to the examination.
- Evaluate for underlying osteomyelitis in diabetic patients with forefoot wounds of more than 2-wk duration, or if a probe can be passed to bone.
- Evaluate for infected orthopedic hardware for surgical site cellulitis after joint replacement or fracture fixation.
- Consider underlying bowel inflammation/infection as a cause of cellulitis localized to the abdominal wall.

PREVENTION OF RECURRENCE

■ RECURRENT NONPURULENT CELLULITIS (ERYSIPELAS)

Patients with recurrent nonpurulent cellulitis require a plan at hospital discharge to prevent future recurrence. Strategies include long-term prophylaxis or preemptive therapy. If episodes are frequent, prophylaxis with oral penicillin is effective in decreasing the number of episodes. The dose required needs to be determined empirically, and may range from 250 mg twice daily to 1 g four times daily. Patients with morbid obesity and edematous states are more likely to need higher doses. In patients with less frequent episodes or in those with breakthrough infection despite prophylaxis, administration of an antibiotic at the first typical symptoms and signs is effective in preventing hospitalization. A fluoroquinolone with extended Gram-positive activity or linezolid is effective. The first dose should be double the usual maintenance dose to rapidly achieve therapeutic concentrations. Tinea pedis is a risk factor for recurrent streptococcal cellulitis. Daily application of topical antifungal therapy to toe web spaces decreases the frequency of cellulitis. In patients with venous stasis disease, elevation, diuretic therapy, and compression stockings may reduce the frequency of infections.

■ RECURRENT CELLULITIS ASSOCIATED WITH BOILS

Patients with one episode of *S. aureus* skin abscess are prone to others in the future. Antibiotic therapy to eradicate carriage, or chronic suppressive antibiotics, may prevent recurrent staphylococcal abscesses. The optimal regimen for eradication of colonization has not been established. In patients without chronic wounds or dermatitis, the combination of 1 to 4 weeks of oral doxycycline 100 mg twice daily and rifampin 600 mg once daily, with topical mupirocin to the nares twice daily, and chlorhexidine oral rinse and skin baths twice daily during the final week of oral antibiotic therapy, has been successful. Isolates must be susceptible to the oral regimen for treatment to be effective. Rifampin has many problematic drug interactions, and should not be used before careful review of a patient's medications. When eradication is not feasible due to chronic wounds, drug interactions, or failure of therapy to eradicate colonization, then chronic antibiotic administration may decrease the frequency of episodes. Choice is guided by susceptibility, drug interactions, and side effects. Oral doxycycline, trimethoprim-sulfamethoxazole, fluoroquinolones, and clindamycin may all be effective. If therapy seems efficacious, it should be continued for several months and then discontinued, and the patient observed for recurrence.

■ DISCHARGE CHECKLIST

- Is it appropriate for the patient to transition to oral antibiotics? Clinical benchmarks of suitability for oral therapy include resolution of systemic symptoms, a white blood cell count which has fallen toward normal levels, and improvement in skin appearance. In more severe cases of cellulitis treated initially with a beta-lactam antibiotic, it may be safer to transition to oral therapy with a fluoroquinolone, clindamycin, or linezolid, if bacterial susceptibilities are favorable, as the bioavailability of these agents is superior to oral beta-lactams.

- Has outpatient follow-up been arranged within 10 to 14 days after discharge to confirm resolution of infection, assess for complications of antibiotic therapy, and education about preventive measures, including foot care?
- Has the management of predisposing factors, such as diabetes, arterial insufficiency, venous stasis, and fungal infection, been optimized?
- Have preventative antibiotics been considered in patients with recurrent cellulitis?
- Have measures to eradicate MRSA been considered in patients with recurrent staphylococcal skin abscesses?

SUGGESTED READINGS

Bernard P. Management of common bacterial infections of the skin. *Curr Opin Infect Dis*. 2008;21:122-128.

Finklestein R, Oren I. Soft tissue infections caused by marine bacterial pathogens: epidemiology, diagnosis, management. *Curr Infect Dis Rep*. 2011;13:470-477.

Hussein QA, Anaya DA. Necrotizing soft tissue infections. *Crit Care Clin*. 2013;29:795-806.

Lipksy BA, Peters EJG, Senneville E, et al. Expert opinion on the management of infections in the diabetic foot. *Diabetes Metab Res Rev*. 2012;28(Suppl 1):163-178.

Liu C, Bayer A, Cosgrove SE, et al. Clinical practice guidelines by the Infectious Diseases Society of America for the treatment of methicillin-resistant Staphylococcus aureus infections in adults and children. *Clin Infect Dis*. 2011;52:e18-e55.

Oehler RL, Velez AP, Mizrachi M, et al. Bite-related and septic syndromes caused by cats and dogs. *Lancet Infect Dis*. 2009;9: 439-447.

Stevens DL, Bisno AL, Chambers HF, et al. Practice guidelines for the diagnosis and management of skin and soft tissue infections: update by the Infectious Diseases Society of America. *Clin Infect Dis*. 2014;59:e10-e52.

CHAPTER 197

Urinary Tract Infections

John J. Ross, MD

EPIDEMIOLOGY

Over half of all women have at least one urinary tract infection (UTI) during their lifetime. In the United States, community-acquired UTIs lead to 7 million office visits, 1 million emergency room visits, over 100,000 hospitalizations, and costs of over $1.6 billion annually. The most common nosocomial infection is catheter-associated UTI, with over 1 million cases yearly in the United States alone.

The vast majority of UTIs arise by the ascending route. Most are caused by strains of *Escherichia coli* with surface filaments (fimbriae) that stick to urinary epithelium. UTIs occasionally arise from bacteremia. This is especially true of *Staphylococcus aureus*. While *S. aureus* may cause cystitis in patients with Foley catheters, when patients present with staphylococcal pyelonephritis from the community, beware of the possibility of underlying bacteremia and endocarditis.

Cystitis and pyelonephritis are 5 to 10 times more common in women, due to the short-female urethra. In women under the age of 50 years, the major risk factor for UTI is frequency of sexual intercourse, which facilitates passage of bacteria into the bladder. In healthy women, UTIs are also associated with new sexual partners, reflecting sexual acquisition of uropathogenic strains of *E. coli*, and use of spermicides, which promote periurethral *E. coli* colonization.

The normal urinary tract has robust anatomical, chemical, and immunological defenses against infection. These are all negated by the placement of an indwelling urinary catheter, which allows bacteria to migrate upward along the external and internal catheter surfaces. The rate of acquisition of bacteriuria after placement of a urinary catheter is 5% per day. Essentially 100% of patients have bacteriuria 1 month after placement of an indwelling urinary catheter. Other host abnormalities that predispose to UTI include diabetes mellitus and glucosuria, urinary stasis from obstruction, bladder diverticula, neurologic disease, vesicoureteral reflux, and urinary calculi (**Figure 197-1**), which may cause local irritation, obstruction, and serve as a nidus for persistent infection.

RISK STRATIFICATION

Patients with uncomplicated cystitis or infection limited to the urinary bladder do not require hospital admission unless there are other medical concerns, such as confusion, dehydration, and inability to take oral antibiotics. Reliable patients with kidney infection or pyelonephritis with mild illness, good oral intake, and anatomically normal urinary tracts may be treated as outpatients with oral fluoroquinolones. Conversely, patients with pyelonephritis who have moderate-to-severe illness, nausea and vomiting, renal insufficiency, structural abnormalities of the urinary tract, poor social situation, high risk for noncompliance, or who are pregnant require hospital admission and stabilization.

Predictors of poor outcome in pyelonephritis include infection with an antibiotic-resistant pathogen, diabetes mellitus, kidney stones, older age, male sex, renal insufficiency, sepsis, bedridden status, and immunosuppression. There are no clinical prediction models for hospital admission in pyelonephritis which have been prospectively validated. Laboratory predictors of higher risk in pyelonephritis may include segmented neutrophils greater than 90% of white blood cell differential, C-reactive protein greater than 10 mg/dL, and elevated levels of procalcitonin and proadrenomedullin. In one study, greater degrees of renal parenchymal involvement on computed tomography (CT) predicted longer hospital stay and duration of fever.

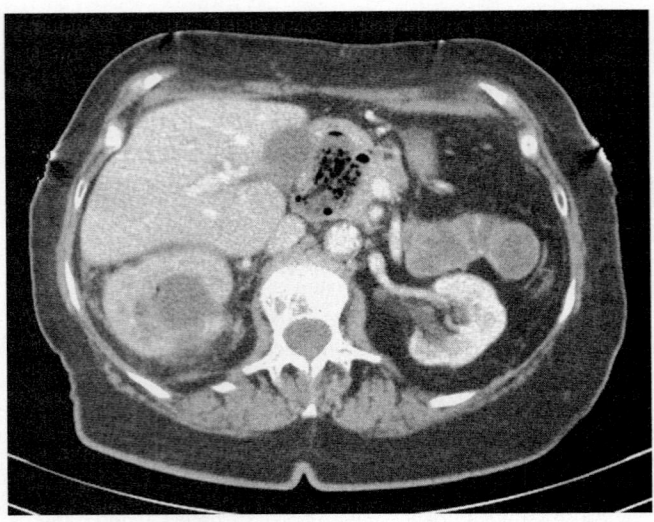

Figure 197-1 *CT scan of the abdomen, showing pyelonephritis in a patient with urinary tract obstruction from a stone at the ureteropelvic junction. The right kidney is significantly enlarged, with hydronephrosis and perinephric fat stranding.*

ASYMPTOMATIC BACTERIURIA

◼ EVALUATION

Asymptomatic bacteriuria is the presence of bacteria on cultures of voided midstream urine or catheter urine, without clinical symptoms. Asymptomatic bacteriuria is exceedingly common. It is found in 5% of healthy women, 50% of elderly patients in long-term care facilities, and in most patients with spinal cord injury. Rates of bacteriuria are essentially 100% in patients with chronic indwelling Foley catheters or permanent ureteric stents.

◼ INPATIENT MANAGEMENT

Asymptomatic bacteriuria is grossly overtreated. Even the presence of pyuria or cloudy urine by itself does not warrant antibiotic treatment. In almost all groups studied, treatment of asymptomatic bacteriuria is associated with antibiotic side effects, acquisition of antibiotic-resistant organisms, and no long-term benefits. Similarly, treatment of asymptomatic candiduria has not been associated with clinical benefit, and long-term eradication rates are disappointing. Therefore, most patients with asymptomatic bacteriuria should not be treated. There are three notable exceptions: pregnant women; patients undergoing transurethral resection of the prostate or other urologic procedures involving mucosal bleeding; and preschool children with vesicoureteral reflux. Pregnant women with asymptomatic bacteriuria should receive 3 to 7 days of antibiotic therapy, and should have urine cultures repeated later in pregnancy. Screening and treatment of asymptomatic bacteriuria has been studied and found not to be helpful in the following groups: premenopausal, nonpregnant women; diabetic women; older persons living in the community; elderly, institutionalized subjects; persons with spinal cord injury; and patients with chronic indwelling urinary catheters.

CYSTITIS (UNCOMPLICATED UTI)

◼ EVALUATION

The diagnosis of cystitis, or infection limited to the urinary bladder, is straightforward in women with dysuria, urinary frequency, or both, who also have positive leukocyte esterase or nitrites on urine dipstick, or pyuria on urine microscopy (defined as at least five white cells per high-power field on a centrifuged specimen). Vaginal irritation or discharge decreases the likelihood of UTI (**Table 197-1**);

TABLE 197-1 Likelihood Ratios for Urinary Tract Infection in Women

Symptom/Finding	Positive LR	Negative LR
Dysuria present	1.5	0.5
Frequency present	1.8	0.5
Vaginal discharge absent	3.1	0.3
Vaginal irritation absent	2.7	0.2
All of the above	23	—
Positive urine dipstick (either positive leukocyte esterase or positive nitrates)	4.2	0.3

Adapted from Bent S, Nallamothu BK, Simel DL, Fihn SD, Saint S. Does this woman have an uncomplicated urinary tract infection? In: Simel DL, Rennie D, eds. *The Rational Clinical Examination*. New York, NY: McGraw-Hill, 2009.

women with these symptoms should be assessed for other diagnoses, such as vaginal candidiasis and sexually transmitted diseases. Fever and flank pain are not expected in cystitis, and their presence should prompt consideration for pyelonephritis.

The vast majority of cases of acute cystitis in healthy women are caused by *E. coli*. Gram-positive bacteria such as enterococci and group B streptococci sometimes isolated from the urine in women with acute cystitis syndromes, but are usually found in conjunction with *E. coli*, and their significance as uropathogens in healthy women is probably overestimated.

◼ INPATIENT MANAGEMENT

In outpatients, urine cultures need not be checked in most cases of suspected cystitis. However, they should be obtained if the diagnosis is unclear, if symptoms are atypical, if symptoms persist or relapse after treatment, or if pyelonephritis is suspected (ie, if fever or back pain is present). In hospitalized patients, urine cultures should be obtained whenever UTI is suspected. If urine cultures demonstrate fewer than 10^5 organisms/mL, patients may have bacterial urethritis, without cystitis. Gonorrhea or chlamydia should be considered in this setting (**Figure 197-2**).

The preferred treatment regimens for uncomplicated, community-acquired cystitis are trimethoprim-sulfamethoxazole (TMP-SMX) 160/800 mg twice daily for 3 days, nitrofurantoin 100 mg twice daily for 5 days, or a single 3-g dose of fosfomycin (**Table 197-2**). TMP-SMX is preferred where local resistance rates in *E. coli* are low (ie, <20%), due to its lower cost, and the desire to forestall the emergence of resistance to fluoroquinolones from overuse.

Nitrofurantoin is a time-honored urinary anti-infective, whose active metabolites damage bacterial ribosomes and DNA. As resistance in the community to both TMP-SMX and fluoroquinolones increases, nitrofurantoin may be an increasingly important first-line therapy for cystitis. Nitrofurantoin is generally active against *E. coli* and *Citrobacter*, as well as many strains of vancomycin-resistant enterococci. However, it is less useful against many Gram-negative rods causing urinary catheter-associated UTI, including *Pseudomonas*, *Providentia*, *Serratia*, *Proteus*, *Enterobacter*, and *Klebsiella*. Nitrofurantoin is not effective against pyelonephritis. It should be avoided in patients with creatinine clearances of less than 40 mL/min, as therapeutic concentrations may not be achieved in the urinary tract.

Fosfomycin is an old, broad-spectrum urinary tract anti-infective, given as a single 3 gm dose. A structural analog of phosphoenolpyruvate, it inhibits the initial step in bacterial cell wall synthesis. Although it is more expensive than TMP-SMX and nitrofurantoin, it is a cost-effective treatment for uncomplicated urinary tract infection due to many strains of vancomycin-resistant enterococci

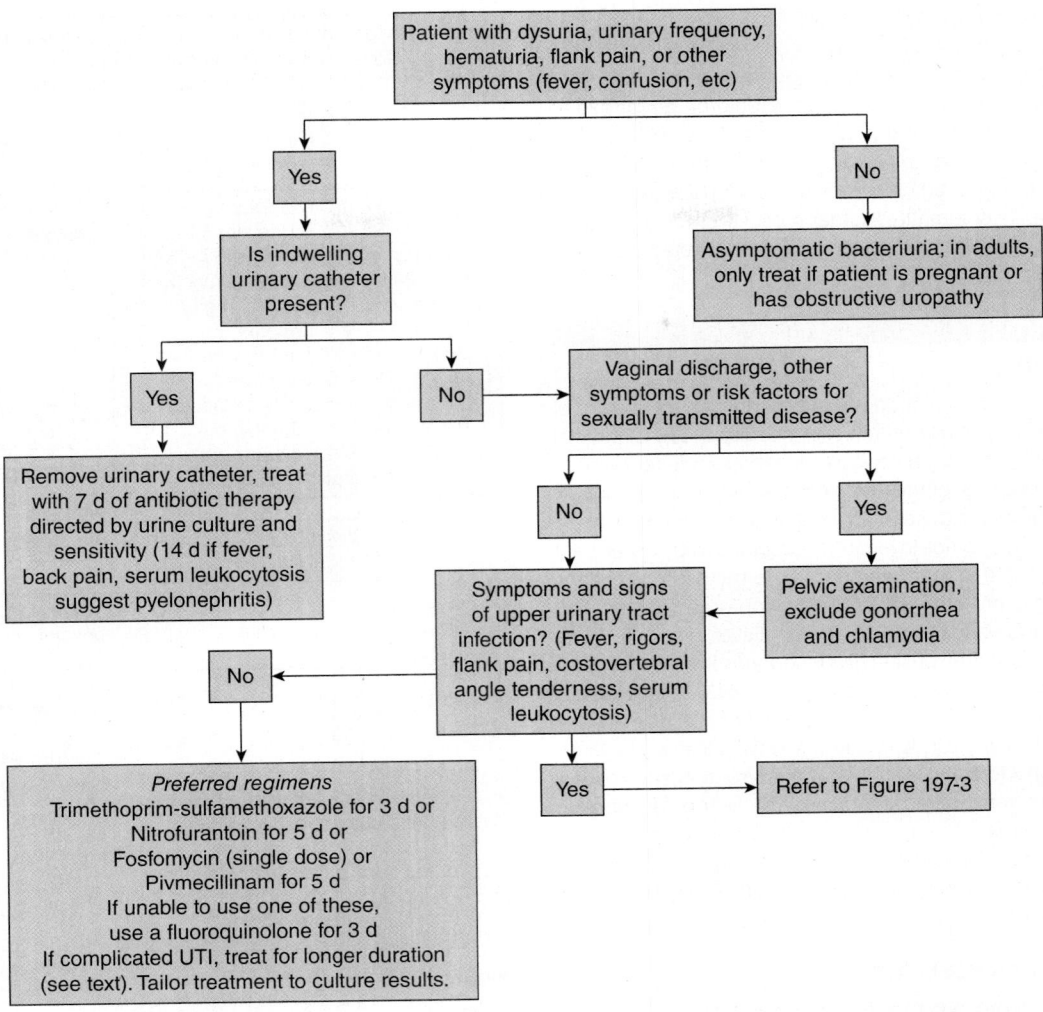

Figure 197-2 *Approach to the patient with urine culture, urine dipstick, or urine microscopy suggestive of urinary tract infection.*

and extended-spectrum beta-lactamase-producing *Klebsiella pneumoniae*.

Fluoroquinolones and beta-lactam antibiotics are no longer considered first-line treatments for uncomplicated cystitis. The risk of collateral damage to the human microbiota, such as acquisition of antibiotic-resistant organisms and *Clostridium difficile* colitis, is higher with fluoronquinolones than other antibiotics. As well, rates of fluoroquinolone resistance in the community have risen dramatically, and there is a desire to forestall the emergence of resistance to this class of agents, due to their usefulness in treating patients with serious infections. Beta-lactam antibiotics are less effective for cystitis than other available agents, and have a higher likelihood of relapse.

Patients with complicated UTI, or cystitis in the setting of intermittent catheterization, spinal cord injury, urinary tract abnormalities, or weakened immunity, should receive longer courses of antibiotic therapy. Studies support a 10-day course of conventional doses of oral ciprofloxacin (500 mg twice daily), or a 5-day course of high-dose oral levofloxacin (750 mg/d), for complicated UTI with fluoroquinolone-sensitive pathogens. Patients with severe illness

TABLE 197-2 Preferred Empiric Treatment of Uncomplicated Cystitis

Generic and Trade Names	Dosage and Duration	Comments
Trimethoprim-sulfamethoxazole (Bactrim, Septra)	160/800 mg (one DS tablet) twice daily for 3 d	Least costly option; consider another empiric regimen if patient exposed to TMP-SMX in past 6 mo; rash more common than with other alternatives
Nitrofurantoin monohydrate (Macrobid)	100 mg twice daily for 5 d	Not active in the upper urinary tract; avoid if early pyelonephritis suspected; pulmonary toxicity may occur with chronic use or repeated courses
Fosfomycin (Monurol)	3 g as a single dose (dispensed as sachet of powder which is mixed with water)	Expensive, despite being a single dose regimen; broad-spectrum anti-infective with activity against many strains of resistant uropathogens; similar to TMP-SMX and nitrofurantoin, has negligible effects on gut flora
Pivmecillinam (Selexid)	400 mg twice daily for 5 d	Not available in North America; may be less active than other first-line regimens

Based on Gupta K, et al. *Clin Infect Dis.* 2011;52:e103-e120.

or major urinary tract anomalies, or those treated with beta-lactam antibiotics, may require longer-antibiotic courses.

In women with vaginal discharge, a suggestive sexual history, or a negative urinalysis, a pelvic examination should be performed to exclude vaginitis, cervicitis, and pelvic inflammatory disease, with studies for gonorrhea and chlamydia. Other causes of dysuria in women include atrophic vaginitis, seen in postmenopausal women, interstitial cystitis, an enigmatic disorder most common in younger women, and irritant urethritis from tampons, contraceptive gel, and other substances.

PYELONEPHRITIS

■ EVALUATION

In healthy adults, kidney infection is diagnosed when all or most of the following findings are present: oral temperature ≥38°C or rectal temperature ≥38.5°C, flank pain or costovertebral angle tenderness, serum leukocytosis, and nitrites or leukocyte esterase on urinary dipstick or pyuria or white cell casts on urine microscopy. These findings are usually, but not invariably, combined with lower tract symptoms of urinary frequency and dysuria. In the geriatric patient, pyelonephritis may present with atypical symptoms, such as malaise, confusion, and vague abdominal pain. Fever is usually lower grade, and flank pain often absent. Pyelonephritis is the most common cause of Gram-negative bacteremia. Up to 61% of older adults with pyelonephritis are bacteremic at presentation.

Genitourinary tuberculosis is rare in the United States. However, it should be considered in patients with dysuria, sterile pyuria, calcification of the renal parenchyma, and risk factors for tuberculosis. Most patients lack fever, night sweats, or active pulmonary tuberculosis. Diagnosis is made on the basis of three early morning urine cultures for acid-fast bacilli. Treatment is similar to that of other forms of tuberculosis.

■ INPATIENT MANAGEMENT

Previously healthy women with mild pyelonephritis who are able to take oral fluoroquinolone therapy need not be admitted to the hospital (**Figure 197-3**). Patients with pyelonephritis who are ill enough to require hospital admission should generally receive 14 days of antibiotic therapy. Most, if not all, antibiotic therapy can be delivered orally. Initial therapy for patients from the community is directed against Gram-negative rods, and especially *E. coli*, as they predominate in the microbiology of pyelonephritis (**Table 197-3**). Preferred regimens include ampicillin plus an aminoglycoside, a fluoroquinolone, or a broad-spectrum cephalosporin such as ceftriaxone (**Table 197-4**). Regimens containing ampicillin have a minor advantage in that they are usually active against enterococci; fluoroquinolones and cephalosporins are not. Most antibiotics are excreted in the urinary tract, and achieve high concentrations in urine. As aminoglycosides and fluoroquinolones display concentration-dependent killing, compared to the time-dependent killing of beta-lactam antibiotics, they may be superior to beta-lactams in the treatment of pyelonephritis. Moxifloxacin has inferior urinary tract penetration, compared to other fluoroquinolones, and is not indicated for the treatment of UTIs.

When patients with prior UTI are admitted to hospital with pyelonephritis, antibiotic therapy should take into account prior culture and sensitivity data, and broader-empiric therapy should be prescribed if the patient has a previous history of antibiotic-resistant organisms. Patients who develop pyelonephritis in the hospital or chronic care setting may also require broader-empiric therapy, possibly with an antipseudomonal beta-lactam or carbapenem. Contrary to popular wisdom, there is no evidence that hydration is beneficial in treating or preventing UTI, unless patients also have prerenal azotemia or kidney stones. Hydration has been recommended as

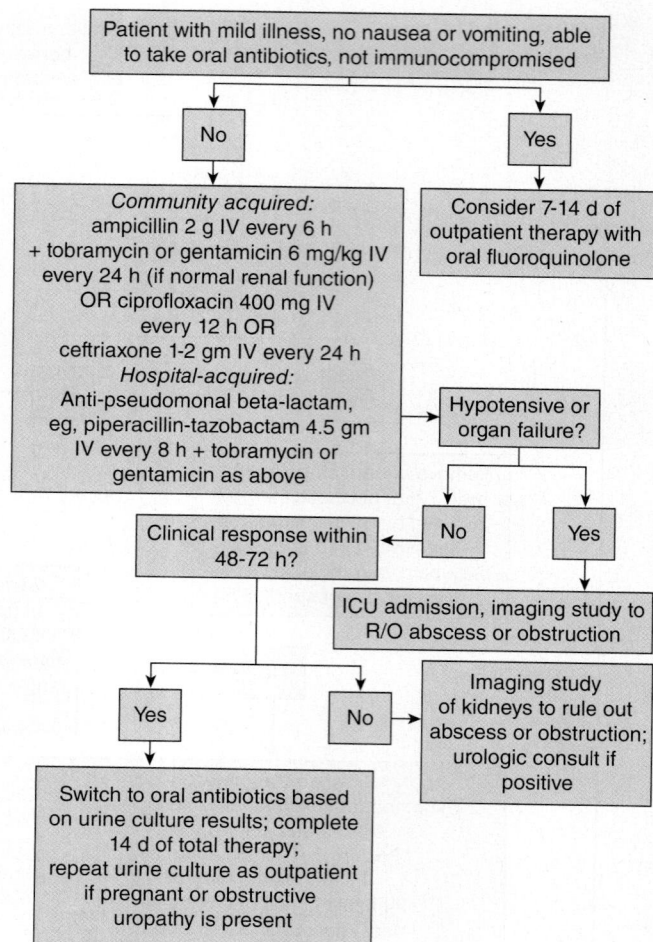

Figure 197-3 *Approach to the patient with upper tract urinary infection.*

a means of rapidly reducing bacterial counts by dilution. However, this is probably negated by dilutional effects on antibiotics and urinary antibacterial factors, such as Tamm-Horsfall protein. Hydration may be useful in minimizing the potential nephrotoxicity of aminoglycosides. Urinary analgesics, such as phenazopyridine (Pyridium)

TABLE 197-3 Bacteriology of Acute Pyelonephritis in 885 Patients

Pathogen	No. (%)
Gram negative	823 (93)
E. coli	707 (80)
Klebsiella spp.	39 (4)
Pseudomonas spp.	33 (4)
Enterobacter spp.	19 (2)
Proteus mirabilis	16 (2)
Citrobacter spp.	5 (0.5)
Acinetobacter spp.	4 (0.5)
Gram positive	62 (7)
Enterococcus spp.	38 (4)
S. saprophyticus	16 (2)
S. aureus	4 (0.5)
Group B streptococci	4 (0.5)

Data from Talan DA, et al. *JAMA.* 2000;283:1583-1590; Peterson J, et al. *Clin Ther.* 2007;29:2215-2221; Wi YM, et al. *Int J Clin Pract.* 2014;68:749-755.

TABLE 197-4 Empiric Treatment of Pyelonephritis in Hospitalized Patients

Drug and Dosage	Comments
Ciprofloxacin 400 mg IV q12h	Can step down rapidly to oral therapy in patients without nausea and vomiting
Ceftriaxone 1-2 g IV q24h	Active against most community-acquired Gram-negative bacilli in pyelonephritis
Cefepime 1-2 g IV q12h	Appropriate when *Pseudomonas* is suspected; may cause confusion in the elderly; dose adjust for renal insufficiency
Ampicillin 2 g IV q6h plus gentamicin 1 mg/kg IV q8h	Provides empiric coverage for enterococcal infection; avoid in renal insufficiency
Imipenem 500 mg IV q6h	Appropriate in patients with a history of infection with extended-spectrum beta-lactamase-producing organisms; use with caution and dose adjustment in renal insufficiency

Based on Gupta K, et al. *Clin Infect Dis*. 2011;52:e103-e120.

are generally unnecessary, and may cause gastrointestinal upset, headache, and rarely methemoglobinemia.

In healthy young women with appropriately treated pyelonephritis, fever may be impressive and sustained, taking up to 4 days to resolve. Older women with pyelonephritis tend to become afebrile more quickly than younger ones. This probably reflects a more vigorous inflammatory response in younger patients.

Imaging studies are not warranted in acute pyelonephritis when the diagnosis is straightforward and the patient is not critically ill. Renal ultrasound or CT should be performed in patients with presumed pyelonephritis when the diagnosis is unclear, when patients are severely ill or immunocompromised, when new or worsening renal insufficiency is present, when patients are not improved after 72 hours of antibiotics, when structural abnormalities or obstruction of the urinary tract are suspected, or when pyelonephritis is relapsing or recurrent (**Table 197-5**). Plain films of the abdomen may also be helpful in excluding nephrolithiasis. Some authorities also recommend obtaining renal imaging in diabetics with pyelonephritis, as these patients are at high risk of papillary necrosis, renal abscess, and other complications. If there is evidence of urinary tract obstruction on imaging studies, urologic consultation should be obtained (**Table 197-6**).

Imaging studies may reveal suppurative complications in patients who are critically ill or who fail to improve with standard therapy. **Perinephric abscess** may complicate pyelonephritis when urinary tract obstruction is present. The abscess is usually confined to the perinephric space by Gerota's fascia. Percutaneous

TABLE 197-5 Indications for Renal Imaging in Patients with Presumed Pyelonephritis

Uncertain diagnosis

Severe illness

Immunocompromise

Worsening renal function

Failure to improve after 72 h of antibiotics

Suspected kidney stone or urinary tract obstruction

Relapsing or recurrent pyelonephritis

Male gender

TABLE 197-6 Indications for Considering Urologic Consultation in Pyelonephritis

Urinary tract obstruction and/or high urinary postvoid residual volume

Nephrolithiasis

Perinephric abscess

Intrarenal abscess

Emphysematous pyelonephritis

Xanthogranulomatous pyelonephritis

Gross hematuria

catheter drainage is now standard, and avoids the need for surgery in most cases.

Intrarenal abscess may complicate systemic bacteremia, sometimes in the setting of staphylococcal endocarditis. Patients present with flank pain and fever, with a delayed response to antibiotics. Early in the course, contrast-enhanced CT scans may show intense focal inflammation in a lobe of the kidney (facetiously termed *lobar nephronia*, by analogy with lobar pneumonia). These patients may respond to antibiotics alone, but if frank suppuration is evident on CT scans, percutaneous catheter drainage is appropriate.

Emphysematous pyelonephritis is a life-threatening form of upper urinary tract infection in diabetics, associated with gas and tissue necrosis in the renal parenchyma and perinephric soft tissues, and is usually caused by *E. coli*. Emergent nephrectomy is the traditional treatment in septic patients. However, percutaneous catheter drainage with medical therapy has been successful in less severely ill patients in case reports and in the author's experience. Kidney function is often significantly reduced on the affected side.

Xanthogranulomatous pyelonephritis is a variant of pyelonephritis in middle-aged women, associated with chronic nephrolithiasis, obstruction, and prior symptomatic UTIs. Patients present with fever, malaise, and abdominal pain. The renal calyces are dilated, and the parenchyma replaced by necrotic inflammatory tissue, especially lipid-laden macrophages. Kidney stones are usually embedded in the inflammatory process. Involvement is usually unilateral. *E. coli* and *Proteus* are most often responsible. As the involved kidney is usually defunct at the time of diagnosis, nephrectomy is customary. Localized disease can be treated with partial nephrectomy and antibiotics.

PROSTATITIS

■ EVALUATION

Acute bacterial prostatitis presents with fever, rigors, perineal discomfort, dysuria, and urinary urgency and frequency. The prostate is swollen and often exquisitely tender on examination. Acute prostatitis is generally seen in older men, with *E. coli* as the most common culprit. Urinalysis and urine cultures should be sent. (Urinary cultures after vigorous prostate massage have fallen out of favor, due to concerns regarding provocation of bacteremia.) In the sexually venturesome, *Neisseria gonorrhoeae* should be entertained, and urethral swabs or urinary gene probes sent for gonococcus. Prostatic abscess is uncommon, but should be suspected in men with persistent fever and exquisite prostate tenderness. Human immunodeficiency virus (HIV) and diabetes mellitus are predisposing factors. Pelvic CT or transrectal ultrasound is diagnostic.

Chronic bacterial prostatitis presents with relapsing dysuria and other urinary symptoms. If perineal discomfort and prostatic tenderness are present, they are usually much milder than in acute prostatitis. *E. coli* and other Gram-negatives are usually responsible; rarely, *Cryptococcus neoformans* or other fungi are involved.

■ INPATIENT MANAGEMENT

Relapses of prostatitis are common because of poor-antibiotic penetration and the limited drainage of infected secretions from the prostate. Acute bacterial prostatitis is usually treated with 3 to 4 weeks of oral antibiotics, based on culture results, with needle drainage of abscesses if present. Chronic prostatitis may require 6 to 12 weeks of oral therapy; cure rates are often low because of microabscesses or small calculi, which enable infection to persist. TMP-SMX or fluoroquinolones are preferred for their superior penetration into the prostate. Prostatic abscesses should be drained transperineally or transrectally under ultrasound guidance. Men with chronic pelvic pain, sterile urine cultures, and no response to antibiotics may be suffering from the chronic pelvic pain syndrome. Alpha-blockers and nonsteroidal anti-inflammatories may be considered in these patients.

NOSOCOMIAL CATHETER-ASSOCIATED UTI

■ EVALUATION

The diagnosis of catheter-associated UTI is imprecise. Surveillance definitions use as criteria the presence of a positive urinary culture ($\geq 10^5$ colony-forming units per milliliter), with at least one of the following symptoms: fever >38°C, urgency, frequency, dysuria, and suprapubic tenderness. As urinary symptoms are usually absent in catheterized patients, catheter-associated UTI in the hospital is usually a diagnosis of exclusion, made on the basis of fever, a positive urine culture, and the absence of another infectious source.

While *E. coli* is still the most common microbe in catheter-associated UTI, enterococci, *Pseudomonas*, *Enterobacter*, *Providentia*, *Citrobacter*, and *Candida* each cause significant proportions of catheter-associated UTI. Bacteremia from catheter-associated UTI is uncommon, occurring in less than 1% of cases, but because of the large number of hospitalized patients with Foley catheters, up to 15% of nosocomial bacteremias may be urinary in origin.

■ INPATIENT EVALUATION

Removal of the urinary catheter is essential for successful treatment, as bacteria deposit biofilm (glycocalyx) on the catheter and bladder epithelium, protecting them from antibiotics and host defenses. Ideally, the urinary catheter should be removed permanently. Condom catheterization is an alternative to the indwelling urinary catheter in men with impaired mobility and no urinary obstruction. Most men prefer condom catheters from a comfort standpoint, and the incidence of bacteriuria is less than with indwelling urinary catheters. Clean intermittent catheterization (straight-catheterization) every 6 hours may also be considered, especially in the setting of neurologic disease such as spinal cord injury.

Data are lacking to make definitive recommendations regarding duration of therapy. However, 7 days of treatment is customary, based on culture and sensitivity data. If bacteremia is documented, or flank pain is present to suggest pyelonephritis, 14 days of total therapy is indicated.

Elderly patients with chronic Foley catheters and drainage bags occasionally develop purple urine due to bacterial breakdown of tryptophan to indirubin and indigo. Multiple Gram-negative bacteria are implicated, and urine cultures are usually polymicrobial. The condition is benign, and responds to antibiotics and removal of the urinary catheter and bag. If patients are asymptomatic, antibiotic treatment may not be necessary. However, many patients consider resolution of purple urine desirable.

Another complication of chronic Foley catheterization is infection with the diphtheroid *Corynebacterium urealyticum*. This urea-splitting Gram-positive rod may cause struvite stone formation in the bladder and encrusted cystitis. Clues include the presence of alkaline urine, and repeated urine cultures with Gram-positive rods, often misinterpreted as normal flora. Because microbiology laboratories usually assume that urinary diphtheroids are contaminants, the condition may not be diagnosed unless the clinician requests speciation of the isolate. Treatment involves bladder stone removal and intravenous vancomycin. Linezolid is a potential option for oral therapy.

POSTACUTE CARE

Several interventions may help prevent UTI recurrence. **Postcoital voiding** reduces UTI incidence in susceptible, sexually active women. **Postcoital antibiotics** (single-strength TMP-SMX or ciprofloxacin 100 mg) may also be helpful, and are as effective as daily prophylaxis in premenopausal women. **Continuous low-dose antibiotics** are also used as prophylaxis in women with frequent UTIs, particularly when infection is not related to coitus. TMP-SMX, fluoroquinolones, and nitrofurantoin have all been used in this setting. Clinicians should be aware that both short- and long-term use of nitrofurantoin are associated with uncommon but potentially severe reactions, including pulmonary hypersensitivity, hepatitis, hemolytic anemia, and peripheral neuropathy.

In acidic urine, **methenamine mandelate and methenamine hippurate** break down to ammonia and formaldehyde, which denatures proteins and act as broad-spectrum antibiotics active against Gram-positive bacteria, Gram-negative bacteria, and fungi. They are ineffective against *Proteus* and other urea-splitting bacteria that produce alkaline urine. Methenamine compounds may prevent UTI recurrences, and they are generally well tolerated, aside from occasional gastrointestinal upset. Administration of vitamin C (ascorbic acid) may help to ensure acidic urine. Methenamines should be avoided in patients with chronic renal failure. They are also not effective in patients with chronic indwelling urinary catheters, as formaldehyde cannot accumulate in the bladder.

Cranberry juice or tablets are perhaps modestly effective in UTI prophylaxis in ambulatory women. Polyphenols in cranberry juice prevent the fimbrial adhesion of uropathogenic strains of *E. coli*. Cranberry juice may potentiate warfarin. **Vaginal estrogens** in postmenopausal women reduce vaginal overgrowth with Gram-negative bacteria, promote protective colonization by lactobacilli, and reduced UTIs in small-clinical trials.

Impregnated urinary catheters, coated with silver alloy or minocycline and rifampin in combination, reduce the short-term risk of urinary tract infection in hospitalized patients, but the cost-benefit implications are hazy. There are no data on whether **suprapubic urinary catheters** reduce short-term infection rates in hospitalized patients, compared to Foley catheter insertion, although some patients may prefer them for reasons of comfort.

Not inserting a urinary catheter and promptly removing a urinary catheter that is not indicated are the most effective means of preventing UTIs and other complications of catheter insertion (**Table 197-7**). Foley catheters are widely overused in the inpatient setting; up to 50% of urinary catheter use is inappropriate. Even when insertion is appropriate, urinary catheters are often left in for too long. Accepted indications for urinary catheters are bladder outlet obstruction, urinary incontinence in patients with open sacral or perineal wounds, as a comfort measure in the terminally ill, at the patient's request, monitoring of urine output in the critically ill, and during prolonged surgical procedures with general or spinal anesthesia.

TABLE 197-7 Complications of Foley Catheter Insertion

Common

Asymptomatic bacteriuria

Urinary tract infection

Hematuria from traumatic insertion or bladder irritation

Bladder spasm

Diminished patient mobility

Encrustation and blockage by bacterial biofilm

Retained catheter due to nondeflating balloon

Less common

Urethral false passage

Balloon inflation in urethra

Urethral stricture or necrosis

Bladder stone formation around the balloon

Polypoid cystitis

Bladder perforation or peritonitis

Laceration or erosion of the glans penis

PRACTICE POINT

Reducing the risk of catheter-associated UTI

- Several interventions may reduce the risk of catheter-associated UTI:
- Stasis of urine in the tubing increases the risk of UTI. Continuous gravity flow should be maintained at all times. The tubing should not be kinked, elevated above the bladder, or allowed to droop below the collecting bag.
- Catheters should be inserted using sterile technique.
- A closed system should be used. The connection between the bag and catheter should not be disrupted, and hands should be washed before and after contact with the catheter and drainage bag.
- Consider the use of a toileting schedule and perineal underpads to wick away moisture as alternatives to the use of a urinary catheter.
- Condom catheters and intermittent catheterization are associated with lower infection risk than an indwelling urinary catheter.

PRACTICE POINT

UTI and delirium in the elderly

- It is widely accepted that urinary tract infection is a common cause of delirium in elderly patients. However, the evidence base for this assertion is slender. The association of delirium and UTI appears to be modest, after statistical adjustment for

risk factors for UTI and delirium. Asymptomatic bacteriuria is common in patients with cognitive impairment and high risk for delirium, and hospitalists should be judicious about the treatment of positive urine cultures in this setting. Serum markers for bacterial infection such as procalcitonin may provide additional information in these patients.

DISCHARGE CHECKLIST FOR URINARY TRACT INFECTION

- Is the patient being discharged with an appropriate antibiotic based on culture and sensitivity data? Is the patient able to take oral therapy? Has antibiotic therapy been narrowed, if possible?
- Is the treatment duration appropriate for the clinical syndrome? (ie, 7-10 days for catheter-associated UTI, 14 days for pyelonephritis requiring hospital admission)
- Does the patient have insurance coverage or other financial resources to pay for antibiotic therapy?
- Has the patient been counseled on prevention measures, such as postcoital voiding and avoidance of spermicides? Would the patient be an appropriate candidate for suppressive antibiotic therapy, vaginal estrogen therapy, or urinary anti-infectives such as methenamine?
- Has a follow-up urine culture been arranged? *(Only necessary for pregnant patients or if urinary tract obstruction is present.)*

SUGGESTED READINGS

Balogun SA, Philbrick JT. Delirium, a symptom of UTI in the elderly: fact or fable? A systematic review. *Can Geriatr J.* 2014;17:22-26.

Gupta K, Hooton TM, Naber KG, et al. International clinical practice guidelines for the treatment of acute uncomplicated cystitis and pyelonephritis in women: a 2010 update by the Infectious Diseases Society of America and the European Society for Microbiology and Infectious Diseases. *Clin Infect Dis.* 2011;52:e103-e123.

Hooton TM, Roberts PL, Cox ME, Stapleton AE. Voided midstream urine culture and acute cystitis in premenopausal women. *N Engl J Med.* 2013;369:1883-1891.

Hunter KF, Bharmal A, Moore KN. Long-term bladder drainage: suprapubic catheter versus other methods. *Neurourol Urodyn.* 2013;32:944-951.

Litke A, Bossart R, Regez K, et al. The potential impact of biomarker-guided triage decisions for patients with urinary tract infections. *Infection.* 2013;41:799-809.

Paick SH, Choo GY, Baek M, et al. Clinical value of acute pyelonephritis grade based on computed tomography in predicting severity and course of acute pyelonephritis. *J Comput Assist Tomogr.* 2013;37:440-442.

CHAPTER 198

Viral Infections

Stephen B. Greenberg, MD, MACP

Key Clinical Questions

Infectious Mononucleosis

1. What are the major complications of Epstein-Barr virus associated infectious mononucleosis ("mono")?
2. What other viruses cause a mononucleosis-type clinical syndrome?
3. What are the appropriate diagnostic tests for acute Epstein-Barr virus infections?
4. What are the current treatment recommendations for Epstein-Barr virus associated infectious mononucleosis?

Varicella-Zoster Virus

1. What are the complications of adult varicella-zoster virus infection?
2. What are the treatment options for varicella-zoster virus infections?
3. What is the best way to treat postherpetic neuralgia?
4. What are the indications for the varicella-zoster vaccine in adults?

Influenza

1. When should patients with influenza-like illness be hospitalized?
2. How good are rapid virus diagnostic tests for influenza virus?
3. How is influenza infection best treated with antiviral agents?
4. What are the major complications of acute influenza?

INTRODUCTION

Viruses may infect any organ system of the body, and present with common or rare clinical conditions. Viral infections may be trivial or life threatening. Any given clinical syndrome, such as pneumonia, may have a multitude of viral causes. Additionally, some viruses, such as human cytomegalovirus (CMV), have protean clinical manifestations, including pneumonitis, colitis, encephalitis, and a mononucleosis-like syndrome. This chapter will discuss three common viruses in hospitalized patients: Epstein-Barr virus (EBV), varicella-zoster virus (VZV), and influenza virus, along with their complications.

INFECTIOUS MONONUCLEOSIS

■ EPIDEMIOLOGY

Infectious mononucleosis, often referred to as mono or kissing disease, is spread by close physical contact with infected secretions. It is most often seen in adolescents and young adults, and is not serious in most individuals. However, it can lead to significant time away from school or work, and may be associated with persistent fatigue and prolonged convalescence in some individuals.

■ PATHOPHYSIOLOGY

Although other viruses produce a similar clinical syndrome, infectious mononucleosis is most often caused by acute EBV infection. Most people become infected with EBV before the age of 6 years. When EBV infection occurs early in life, it is usually asymptomatic or subclinical. Infection in young adulthood is more likely to lead to clinical mono, perhaps because of a more robust immune response. The major cell infected by EBV is the B lymphocyte; up to 20% of host B lymphocytes may be infected. Cellular immunity is heavily involved in containing EBV infection: the atypical lymphocytes seen in acute EBV infections are activated CD8+ T-cells. The humoral immune system produces antibodies directed against the virus. For unclear reasons, antibodies are also produced against unrelated antigens found on sheep and horse red cells. These antibodies are known as heterophile antibodies, and they form the basis for the mononucleosis spot (monospot) test.

■ CLINICAL PRESENTATION

Infectious mononucleosis usually presents with exudative pharyngitis, fever, and symmetrically enlarged cervical lymph nodes. Sore throat may cause severe discomfort. Tonsillitis is common; if massive, "kissing tonsils" may impinge on the airway. Fever lasts from a few days to 2 weeks. The cervical lymphadenopathy can become generalized, but usually subsides over 2 to 3 weeks. Splenomegaly, usually mild, is present in ~50%. Epstein-Barr virus needs to be distinguished from other causes of exudative pharyngitis, such as group A streptococcus, CMV, and acute human immunodeficiency virus (HIV) infection. Occasional complications (**Table 198-1**) include acute airway obstruction, spontaneous splenic rupture, rash, autoimmune hemolytic anemia, and neurologic syndromes such as meningoencephalitis, transverse myelitis, facial nerve palsy, optic neuritis, and Guillain-Barré syndrome.

■ DIAGNOSIS

Laboratory tests support the diagnosis of infectious mononucleosis, but are not definitive. Most patients have an absolute lymphocyte

TABLE 198-1 Complications of Epstein-Barr Virus Associated Mononucleosis

- Rash, including nonallergic rash to amoxicillin and other antibiotics
- Airway obstruction
- Splenomegaly and splenic rupture
- Splenic infarct
- Autoimmune hemolytic anemia
- Thrombocytopenia
- Aplastic anemia
- Hepatitis and cholestasis
- Meningoencephalitis or Guillain-Barré syndrome
- Hemophagocytic syndrome
- Malignancy (Hodgkin lymphoma; Burkitt lymphoma in Africa; nasopharygeal carcinoma in Asia; CNS lymphoma in AIDS; lymphoproliferative disease in transplant patients)

count over 4500/mm³ and more than 10% atypical lymphocytes on peripheral blood smear. Total white blood cell counts are often elevated. Mildly elevated aminotransferase levels are common. The monospot test is a rapid latex agglutination assay for heterophile antibodies. The sensitivity of infectious mononucleosis heterophile antibodies is >80%, and the specificity approaches 100%. Heterophile antibodies persist for up to 1 year after acute EBV infection.

Epstein-Barr virus specific antibody assays are useful in patients with negative heterophile antibodies (see **Figure 198-1**). The viral capsid antigen (VCA) antibody test measures either specific immunoglobulin G (IgG) or IgM antibodies. Epstein-Barr nuclear antigen antibody (EBNA) test measures IgG, which rises during convalescence and stays elevated for life. Early antigen antibody assay (EA–D)

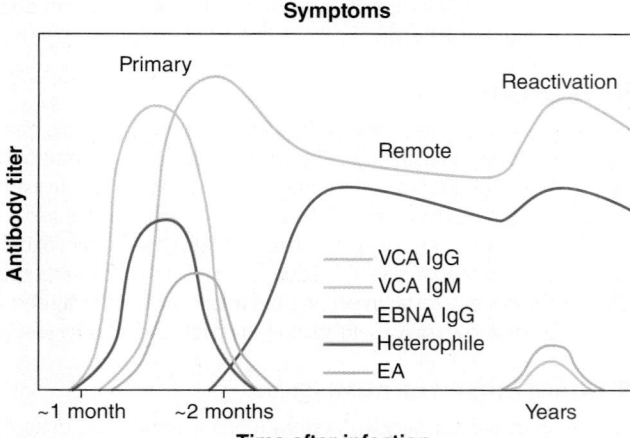

Figure 198-1 *Serologic titers distinguish primary infection from remote infection. Immunoglobulin G (IgG) anti-viral capsid antigen (VCA) and IgM anti-VCA rise in concert with symptoms of primary infection and a positive heterophile test. After symptoms resolve, remote infection is characterized by Epstein-Barr nuclear antigen (EBNA) and IgG anti-VCA without early antigen (EA), although EA and IgM may reappear with or without symptoms on viral reactivation or Epstein-Barr virus–related neoplasia.* (Reproduced, with permission from the American Society for Investigative Pathology, from Gulley M, et al. *J Mole Diagn. 2008;10:272-292.*)

is usually positive during acute infection. Polymerase chain reaction (PCR) assays are available, but rarely used in diagnosing infectious mononucleosis. Epstein-Barr virus does not grow in routine tissue culture.

■ TRIAGE/HOSPITAL ADMISSION

Most patients with infectious mononucleosis have a good prognosis and recover quickly. However, some cases can be severe and last for several months. A minority of patients develop chronic fatigue syndrome, which may be more common in women and in those with pre-existing mood disorders. If airway obstruction or difficulty breathing is observed, tracheotomy or endotracheal intubation should be considered. If splenic rupture has occurred, admission for attempted splenic preservation or splenectomy will be necessary.

■ TREATMENT OPTIONS

Supportive care with rest, fluids, and moderate doses of acetaminophen, ibuprofen, or other anti-inflammatories is the mainstay of care for infectious mononucleosis. Warm saltwater gargles may relieve the discomfort of sore throat. The use of steroids for EBV-associated infectious mononucleosis remains controversial. A recent meta-analysis suggests that there is insufficient evidence for its use in routine cases (**Table 198-2**). Many clinicians use corticosteroids in mononucleosis complicated by impending airway obstruction, autoimmune hemolytic anemia, thrombocytopenia, aplastic anemia, or neurologic complications, but the evidence to support its use in these settings is not robust.

Impending airway obstruction, as defined by difficulty breathing, mandates admission to the hospital and close observation. Otolaryngology consult should be considered in these patients. The clinical benefit of acyclovir for treating acute infectious mononucleosis remains unclear based on published studies.

■ COMPLICATIONS

Airway obstruction with acute infectious mononucleosis is rare but serious. It usually requires close observation, with the ability to do emergent tracheotomy or endotracheal intubation. Splenic rupture presents with acute abdominal pain (or, rarely, left-sided chest pain) and symptoms and signs of hypovolemia. Kehr's sign (radiation of pain to the left shoulder) is present in 50% of cases. Splenic rupture may be spontaneous or due to trauma, and usually occurs within 3 weeks after clinical symptoms have begun. Computed tomography of the abdomen and surgical consultation should be obtained if the diagnosis is suspected. Hemodynamically unstable patients should undergo splenectomy. In stable patients, close observation with nonoperative management or spleen-sparing interventions such as partial splenectomy, splenorrhaphy, and splenic artery embolization may be considered. Other complications that may require subspecialty consultation are autoimmune hemolytic anemia, encephalitis, and pneumonitis. Generalized rash may appear

TABLE 198-2 Infectious Mononucleosis and Corticosteroids

- Randomized trials: 6
- Number of children and young adult patients: 268
- Treatment: acyclovir/valacyclovir (2/6) Prednisone/prednisolone × 5-10 d
- Result: "modest" clinical benefit, no significant reduction in duration of illness or days missed from school or work, no difference in relapse rate

Data from McGee S, Hirschmann J. Use of corticosteroids in treating infectious diseases. *Arch Intern Med.* 2008;168(10):1034-1046.

following antibiotic administration. The most frequently reported antibiotics to result in a rash are the pencillins, especially amoxicillin.

■ DISCHARGE CHECKLIST

- Has the patient been counselled about physical activity? Individuals who play contact sports should avoid participation for at least 3 weeks, when they may resume noncontact training. Those who do weight lifting or strenuous contact sports should wait at least 1 month after their illness began. In selected cases, it may be useful to obtain an ultrasound at 3 weeks after the onset of illness to document resolution of splenomegaly and assess suitability to return to athletic activity, but this practice is not accepted by many individuals.
- Has the patient been counselled about prognosis? In most patients, energy level is back to normal by 1 month, but fatigue may take months to resolve in some patients.

VARICELLA-ZOSTER VIRUS

■ INTRODUCTION/EPIDEMIOLOGY

Varicella (chickenpox) is the primary infection with varicella-zoster virus (VZV). It usually occurs in childhood, in temperate climates, and in adolescence or young adulthood in the tropics. Before the introduction of the varicella vaccine in 1996, there were an estimated 4 million cases of chickenpox in the United States each year. Since the introduction and widespread use of the vaccine in childhood, the incidence of chickenpox has been reduced in many populations by as much as 90%.

■ PATHOPHYSIOLOGY

Primary infection with VZV occurs in the nasopharynx, with spread to lymphoid tissue and memory CD4+ T-cells. Skin involvement develops within the first few days following infection. Cell-free virus is present in skin vesicles, and can infect sensory nerves, resulting in virus latency in sensory ganglia. Latent VZV genomes are localized to <10% of sensory ganglia and neurons. Herpes zoster (shingles) increases with increasing age and with other causes of decreased cellular immunity. Susceptible children are more likely to develop chickenpox from exposure to virus of varicella patients than from exposure to herpes zoster lesions.

■ CLINICAL PRESENTATION

Primary varicella infection is an illness of 3 to 5 days in duration, associated with rash, malaise, and low-grade fever. The characteristic rash of varicella consists of macules and papules that evolve into vesicles and crust over. Lesions are usually in different stages of development at any given time. The vesicle sits atop an erythematous base and has been referred to as a "dewdrop on a rose petal" because of its appearance. Lesions may become superinfected with staphylococci or streptococci; necrotizing fasciitis is an occasional complication. Disseminated infection occurs in the immunocompromised patient. In adults, varicella pneumonia is common, occurring in at least 1 in 400 patients; asymptomatic radiologic infiltrates are even more common.

Following recovery from chickenpox, VZV remains latent in ganglion cells. Shingles, or herpes zoster, is caused by reactivation of latent VZV. It is usually limited to a dermatomal distribution (**Figure 198-2**), but it may disseminate in immunodeficient patients. Most often, shingles involves the trunk or face. A dreaded form of shingles is **herpes zoster ophthalmicus**, or involvement of the first division of the trigeminal nerve. It may be sight threatening if keratitis (corneal lesions) develops. Involvement of the nasociliary nerve, with vesicles at the tip or side of the nose (Hutchinson sign), is said to predict corneal involvement in herpes zoster opthalmicus. Another shingles variant is Ramsay Hunt syndrome, with involvement of nerves of the geniculate ganglion; findings may include facial nerve palsy and other cranial neuropathies,

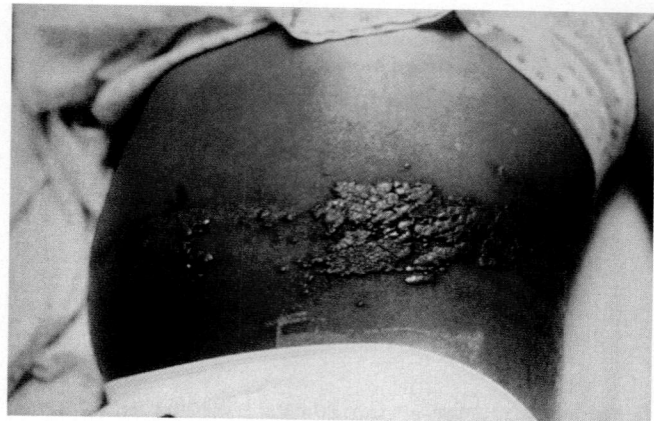

Figure 198-2 *Herpes zoster lesions in a thoracic dermatome.* (Courtesy of the Centers for Disease Control and Prevention, Public Health Image Library.)

as well as pain and vesicle formation involving some combination of the face, neck, external ear, tympanic membrane, anterior tongue, and soft palate. Vertigo, tinnitus, and hearing loss may also be present. Herpes zoster without skin lesions (*zoster sine herpete*) is sometimes invoked as a cause of acute and chronic radicular pain.

The incidence of shingles increases with increasing age. The median age in herpes zoster is ~64 years. As the population ages, the incidence of herpes zoster may well increase over the next few decades. Second episodes of herpes zoster occur in <5% of individuals. When zoster is severe and involves multiple dermatomes in a younger patient without known immunosuppression, HIV should be considered.

■ DIFFERENTIAL DIAGNOSIS

The differential diagnosis of chickenpox includes smallpox, in which skin lesions in the same area are at similar clinical stages, unlike varicella, and contact dermatitis secondary to poison ivy, which tends to form intensely pruritic crops of blisters in a linear distribution. Recurrent skin lesions mimicking a dermatomal distribution may be due to herpes simplex virus. Reactivation in the same location does not occur with herpes zoster.

■ DIAGNOSIS

Varicella-zoster virus infections can be identified using histologic staining of skin lesions, viral cultures, PCR, or serologic assays. Immunohistologic staining of skin scrapings is inexpensive, and 90% sensitive and 95% specific for the diagnosis of infections. Although viral cultures are specific, they take several days and appear to have a sensitivity of only 60% to 75%. Polymerase chain reaction is the most sensitive and specific test for varicella-zoster infections, but it takes at least 1 day and is expensive. Serology is only useful for screening for susceptibility to VZV.

■ TRIAGE/HOSPITAL ADMISSION

Patients with central nervous system (CNS) involvement, disseminated infection, high risk for dissemination, and those who require intravenous (IV) medications should receive inpatient care. Patients with herpes zoster ophthalmicus should be admitted to the hospital, and ophthalmology consultation obtained.

Varicella infection is highly contagious, and patients with primary varicella infection (chickenpox), disseminated herpes zoster, or immunocompromised patients with zoster at risk for disseminated infection may transmit infection via airborne virus from respiratory secretions. These patients should be placed in a negative pressure room on both airborne precautions and contact precautions until all lesions have dried and are crusted over. Only personnel who are immune to chickenpox should enter the room and care for the patient. Immunocompetent patients with uncomplicated herpes zoster and localized dermatomal involvement need only standard precautions, but they also should be cared for by health care workers who are varicella immune.

■ TREATMENT OPTIONS

Skin lesions of varicella and herpes zoster should be kept clean and dry. Topical antibiotics or dressings with tight adhesives should be avoided. Antivirals shorten the duration of infection in adults with primary varicella infection and shingles, and probably lower the risk of complications if started within 24 to 48 hours of new vesicle development. Medications approved for use in adults include acyclovir, valacyclovir, and famciclovir (**Table 198-3**). In shingles, each may reduce pain, time to skin lesion resolution, and duration of postherpetic neuralgia (PHN). Famciclovir and valacyclovir are oral prodrugs that are converted to the active form after ingestion. They have high oral bioavailability, and offer the advantage of three times daily dosing in herpes zoster, compared with five times daily for acyclovir. All three agents require dosage adjustment in renal insufficiency. The use of steroids in patients with herpes zoster is controversial. Although they may help reduce postherpetic neuralgia, controlled studies are inconclusive; therefore, they are not routinely indicated in herpes zoster infections (**Table 198-4**).

Postherpetic neuralgia is pain persisting for at least 120 days after the onset of herpes zoster. Poor quality of life, insomnia, and depression are often associated with PHN. Risk factors for PHN are older age, more severe initial pain, more severe rash on presentation, and painful prodrome. Postherpetic neuralgia has a variable response to treatment. Three medications are approved for treatment of PHN: gabapentin, 5% lidocaine patch, and pregabalin (**Table 198-5**). Tricyclic antidepressants and opioid analgesics are also efficacious. A proposed algorithm for treating PHN is given in **Figure 198-3**. Antivirals alone do not appear to be effective in treating or preventing the pain of PHN. Some patients appear to be refractory to all treatments.

■ COMPLICATIONS

Because VZV is able to replicate in nerve tissue and establish latency there, neurologic complications are not unusual. Primary varicella infection may be complicated by cerebellar ataxia (1 in 4000 cases) and encephalitis (1 in 1000 cases). Cerebral vasculitis may lead to late strokes.

TABLE 198-4 Herpes Zoster Infections and Corticosteroids

- Randomized trials: 5
- Number of patients: 780
- Treatment: acyclovir (3/5)
- Prednisone/prednisolone × 21 d
- Result: beneficial (3/5), failure (2/5), no effect on postherpetic neuralgia

Data from McGee S, Hirschmann J. Use of corticosteroids in treating infectious diseases. *Arch Intern Med.* 2008;168(10):1034-1046.

The most common complication of herpes zoster is PHN. Zoster may also be associated with aseptic meningitis. (Mild cerebrospinal fluid lymphocytosis may also be seen in herpes zoster in the absence of aseptic meningitis.) The syndrome of herpes zoster ophthalmicus with delayed contralateral hemiplegia is usually seen 6 weeks following a case of trigeminal nerve herpes zoster. Less common complications include hepatitis, pneumonitis, and myelitis (**Table 198-6**).

Varicella-zoster virus reactivation may occur in the absence of shingles, as in CNS vasculopathy and necrotizing retinitis. Varicella-zoster virus vasculopathy of the CNS presents with headache, fever, confusion, transient ischemic attacks, and strokes. Cerebral angiography reveals areas of arterial stenosis and occlusion. Diagnosis is made by finding VZV DNA by PCR, or VZV IgG, in spinal fluid. Necrotizing retinitis may present as acute retinal necrosis (ARN) or progressive outer retinal necrosis (PORN). Both conditions may lead to retinal detachment and blindness and are more common in AIDS. Acute retinal necrosis is caused by both varicella-zoster and herpes simplex viruses, whereas progressive outer retinal necrosis is caused almost exclusively by VZV.

■ DISCHARGE CHECKLIST

- Is there a pain relief plan in place for patients with herpes zoster? Continued pain relief will be needed in most cases as an outpatient. Patients who develop PHN must be seen at regular intervals to receive additional medical therapy and emotional support.
- Are family members and other caregivers aware of the patient's varicella status? Patients should preferentially have

TABLE 198-3 Oral Antiviral Medications for Herpes Zoster

Medication	Dosage	Duration of Treatment (d)	Most Common Adverse Effects	Precautions and Contraindications
Acyclovir	800 mg 5 times daily (every 4-5 h)	7-10	Nausea, headache	Dosage adjustment required for patients with renal insufficiency
Brivudine	125 mg once daily	7	Nausea, headache	Contraindicated for patients treated with 5-fluorouracil or other 5-fluoropyrimidines because of drug interaction associated with severe and potentially fatal bone marrow suppression
Famciclovir	500 mg 3 times daily (approved dosage in United States; in some other countries, 250 mg 3 times daily is approved)	7	Nausea, headache	Dosage adjustment required for patients with renal insufficiency
Valacyclovir	1000 mg 3 times daily	7	Nausea, headache	Dosage adjustment required for patients with renal insufficiency; thrombotic thrombocytopenic purpura/hemolytic uremic syndrome reported at dosages of 8000 mg daily in immunocompromised patients

Reproduced, with permission, from Dworkin RH, Johnson RW, Breuer J, et al. *Clin Infect Dis.* 2007;44:S1-S26. University of Chicago Press. © 2006 by the Infectious Diseases Society of America.

TABLE 198-5 Analgesic Medications Useful in the Treatment of Patients with Herpes Zoster

Medication	Beginning Dosage	Titration	Maximum Dosage	Most Common Adverse Effects
Opioid analgesics (dosages given are for oxycodone)*	5 mg every 4 h as needed; dosage can be converted to long-acting opioid analgesic combined with short-acting medication continued as needed	Increase by 5 mg 4 times daily every 2 d as tolerated	No maximum dosage with careful titration; consider evaluation by a pain specialist at dosages >120 mg daily	Nausea/vomiting, constipation, sedation, dizziness
or				
Tramadol*	50 mg once or twice daily	Increase by 50-100 mg daily in divided doses every 2 d as tolerated	400 mg daily (100 mg 4 times daily); for patients >75 y of age, 300 mg daily in divided doses	Nausea/vomiting, constipation, sedation, dizziness, seizures, postural hypotension
Gabapentin†	300 mg at bedtime or 100-300 mg 3 times daily	Increase by 100-300 mg 3 times daily every 2 d as tolerated	3600 mg daily (1200 mg 3 times daily); reduce if renal function is impaired	Sedation, dizziness, peripheral edema
or				
Pregabalin†	75 mg at bedtime or 75 mg twice daily	Increase by 75 mg twice daily every 3 d as tolerated	600 mg daily (300 mg twice daily); reduce if renal function is impaired	Sedation, dizziness, peripheral edema
Tricyclic antidepressants, especially nortriptyline†	25 mg at bedtime	Increase by 25 mg daily every 2-3 d as tolerated	150 mg daily	Sedation, dry mouth, blurred vision, weight gain, urinary retention§

*Consider lower starting dosages and slower titration for frail and elderly patients (eg, 5 mg twice daily for oxycodone); dosages given are for short-acting formulations.

†Consider lower starting dosages and slower titration for frail and elderly patients (eg, 10 mg at bedtime for tricyclic antidepressants).

§Consider a screening electrocardiogram for patients ≥40 y of age.

As adapted from Dworkin RH, et al. with permission from *Clin Infect Dis.* 2007;44:S1-S26. University of Chicago Press. © 2006 by the Infectious Diseases Society of America.

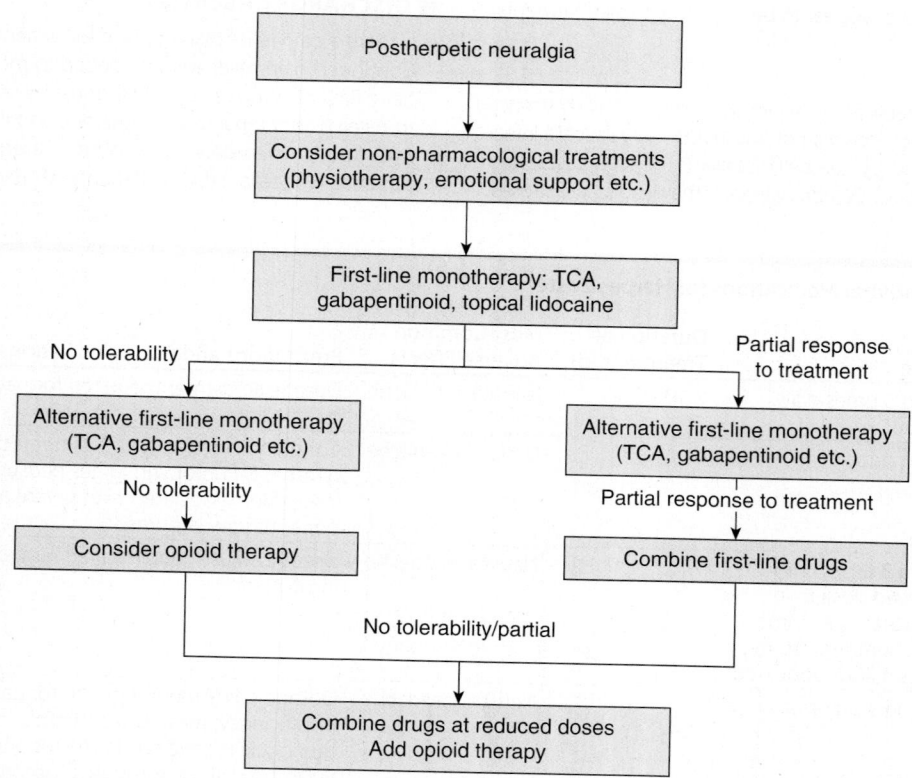

Figure 198-3 *Algorithm for treating postherpetic neuralgia (PHN).* (Reproduced from Galvez R, Redondo M. Evidence-based treatment of postherpetic neuralgia. In: Magel GD, ed. *Herpesviridae-A Look Into This Unique Family of Viruses.* InTech; 2012.) Available from http://www .intechopen.com/books/herpesviridae-a-look-into-this-unique-family-of-viruses/evidence-based-treatment-of-postherpetic-neuralgia.)

TABLE 198-6 Complications of Varicella-Zoster Virus Infections

Dissemination
Hepatitis
Pneumonitis
Encephalitis/CNS and peripheral vasculopathy
Postherpetic neuralgia

TABLE 198-8 Viral Causes of Pneumonia

- Influenza viruses A and B most common
- Respiratory syncytial virus, parainfluenza virus, and coronavirus/rhinovirus less common
- Increased frequency in elderly
- Cause up to 10%-30% of community-acquired pneumonia

varicella-immune caregivers until crusting occurs. Skin lesions take up to 3 weeks to heal, and may often look worse in the second and third week as they crust over. Viral shedding from skin lesions occurs until they become crusted over.

INFLUENZA

■ INTRODUCTION/EPIDEMIOLOGY

Influenza occurs worldwide in yearly outbreaks, mainly during winter months. It is caused by influenza A or B viruses. When significant changes occur in both surface proteins, hemagglutinin and neuraminidase, worldwide pandemics can occur, as recently observed with the novel A/H1N1 virus.

Once an outbreak begins, it usually spreads in a community over 8 to 12 weeks and becomes the major cause of acute upper and lower respiratory tract illnesses. Infection with epidemic strains is common in school-age children. However, increased mortality occurs primarily in the elderly. Transmission occurs by aerosols or droplets generated during coughing or sneezing. In the United States, an average of 20,000 to 40,000 deaths and 300,000 hospitalizations occur annually with influenza epidemics. In April 2009, the first case of novel H1N1 virus was recognized in Mexico. Over the next few months, 41 countries reported cases. The World Health Organization declared that a pandemic situation was in effect in June 2009 (see **Table 198-7**).

■ PATHOPHYSIOLOGY

There are three types of influenza viruses: A, B, and C. Only influenza A viruses have pandemic potential. Eight gene segments encode 10 or 11 proteins. Minor changes, or antigenic drift, occur in the surface proteins each year. Major changes, or antigenic shift, occur every 10 to 20 years in the viral surface hemagglutinin and neuraminidase. The updated yearly vaccine is based on the observed antigenic drift. Influenza viruses spread by respiratory secretions to susceptible hosts. Respiratory symptoms are secondary to dysfunction of cells and release of inflammatory mediators. The incubation period is from 18 to 72 hours.

■ CLINICAL PRSENTATION

The acute onset of fever and cough suggests influenza, but it is nonspecific, as other respiratory viruses may have a similar presentation.

TABLE 198-7 Pandemic H1N1 Influenza

- First reported case in Mexico, March 2009
- Pandemic declared by the World Health Organization in June 2009
- Novel H1N1 is quadruple reassortment of two swine strains, one human strain, and one avian strain of influenza
- Spread throughout the United States in fall 2009
- Monovalent vaccine developed and distributed in 2009

Pharyngitis and myalgias are common. Acute HIV syndrome can be mistaken for an influenza-like illness.

Primary influenza pneumonia is a serious complication in a minority of patients with acute influenza illness. Influenza can lead to secondary bacterial pneumonia, or a mixed picture of both viral and bacterial pneumonia (**Table 198-8**). *Streptococcus pneumoniae* is the most common bacterial pathogen isolated following acute influenza. However, *Staphylococcus aureus* pneumonia is diagnosed with increased frequency in patients following recent influenza infection. Other potentially life-threatening conditions associated with influenza infection include myositis, rhabdomyolysis, CNS involvement, and myocarditis.

■ DIAGNOSIS

Influenza-like illness is associated with fever, sore throat, cough, and systemic complaints. During an outbreak of influenza in a community, febrile acute respiratory tract illness can be assumed to be due to influenza virus. There are a number of rapid antigen tests that vary in sensitivity between 40% and 60% in adults. These rapid antigen tests are more sensitive in children because of the increased viral excretion in younger patients. Other diagnostic tests are indirect fluorescent antibody (IFA) and direct fluorescent antibody (DFA), as well as PCR and viral culture. Polymerase chain reactionis highly sensitive and specific, but it often requires at least a day for results and is not readily available in many laboratories. Viral cultures are also sensitive and specific, but they take several days before giving a positive result. Influenza serology is available, but is mainly of epidemiologic utility.

Who should be tested for influenza virus? During a communitywide outbreak of influenza, patients with underlying disease and influenza-like illness (ILI) should be tested for the presence of influenza virus. In individuals who are immunocompetent and present with an ILI, testing for the presence of virus is not usually indicated. However, all hospitalized patients with ILI should be tested for the presence of influenza virus. A positive rapid antigen test can be used to make decisions about specific antiviral therapy. A negative rapid antigen test does not exclude influenza in a patient with a high pretest probability. If a rapid antigen test is negative in a hospitalized patient is thought to have an ILI, then a specimen should be sent for further testing, such as viral culture or PCR, and empiric antiviral therapy should be initiated. If PCR results are negative, therapy can be discontinued.

■ TRIAGE/HOSPITAL ADMISSION

Patients with acute respiratory tract illness during an influenza outbreak should be considered for hospital admission if they are elderly or too weak to care for themselves at home, have an underlying condition such as chronic obstructive pulmonary disease or congestive heart failure, or there is a clinical suspicion for pneumonia. During an influenza epidemic, it is important to triage as many patients as possible for care at home.

■ TREATMENT OPTIONS

Several antiviral agents are currently approved for use in acute influenza illness. The adamantanes, amantadine and rimantadine, are only active against influenza A viruses. Because widespread

TABLE 198-9 Antivirals for Influenza Virus Infections

Antiviral	Activity	Dosage (5 d)	Side Effects
Amantadine	Influenza A only	100 mg/d orally	CNS, GI
Rimantadine	Influenza A only	100 mg/d orally	CNS, GI
Oseltamivir	Influenza A and B	75 mg twice/d orally	GI
Zanamivir	Influenza A and B	2 inhalations twice/d	Bronchospasm

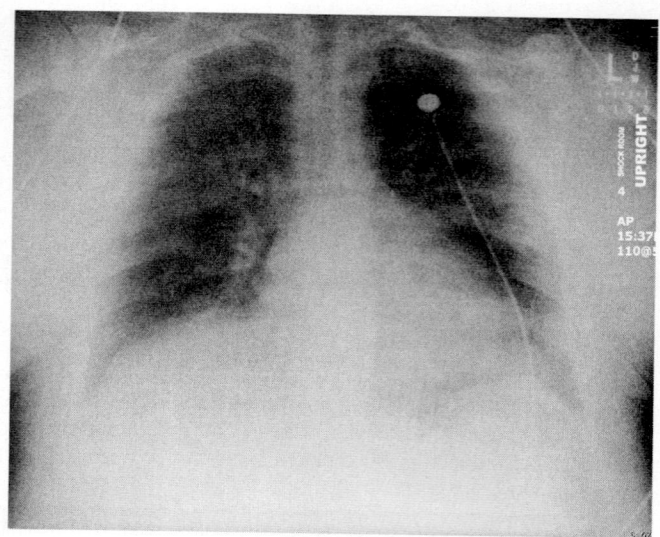

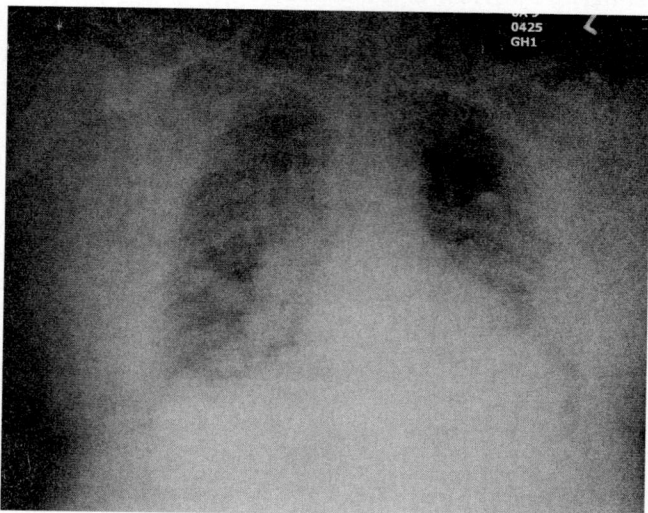

resistance to the adamantanes has emerged among recent isolates of influenza A, these antivirals are no longer used. The neuraminidase inhibitors oseltamivir and zanamivir are active against both influenza A and B viruses. Resistance to the neuraminidase inhibitors has been described in previous years. However, over 98% of recent H1N1, H3N2, and influenza B isolates are sensitive to oseltamivir (**Table 198-9**). Zanamivir resistance has been reported rarely.

■ COMPLICATIONS

Pneumonia is a serious complication of acute influenza infection. Primary influenza pneumonia, although rare, is a serious cause of increased mortality. Clinically, the patient presents with cough and dyspnea. A chest radiograph will reveal diffuse infiltrates or an acute respiratory distress syndrome (ARDS) pattern (**Figure 198-4**). Elderly patients and those with cardiovascular disease constitute the highest risk groups. The mortality rate in acute influenza pneumonia is high. Secondary bacterial pneumonia can occur 2 to 3 weeks after the onset of influenza symptoms. *S. pneumoniae* or *S. aureus* (including methicillin-resistant *S. aureus* [MRSA]) are the most commonly identified bacterial pathogens. Mixed viral and bacterial pneumonia has also been described following acute influenza.

Another uncommon complication of influenza infection is myositis (**Table 198-10**). This occurs more commonly with influenza B than with influenza A, and is more common in children. Myoglobinuria and rhabdomyolysis have also been reported following acute influenza infection. CNS complications are also rarely reported. These include encephalitis, transverse myelitis, and Guillain-Barré syndrome.

■ DISCHARGE PLANNING

- Patients should be cautioned that, although the prognosis is good in acute influenza, malaise and fatigue may persist for some time.
- If the patient is a nursing home resident, have nursing home personnel been contacted to take measures to protect other residents from an outbreak of acute influenza?

TABLE 198-10 Influenza Virus–Associated Myositis

- Influenza type A > B
- Mostly in school-age children
- Calf muscles commonly involved
- Increased creatine kinase levels
- Begins during convalescence
- Self-limited
- Antivirals

Figure 198-4 *Chest radiographs of a hospitalized patient with novel H1N1 pneumonia and acute respiratory distress syndrome over 48 hours.* (Courtesy of Venkata Bandi, Ben Taub Hospital, Houston, Texas.)

SUGGESTED READINGS

Bader MS. Herpes zoster: diagnositic, therapeutic, and preventive approaches. *Postgrad Med.* 2013;125:78-91.

Bruxelle J, Pinchinat S. Effectiveness of antiviral treatment on acute phase of herpes zoster and development of post herpetic neuralgia: review of international publications. *Med Mal Infect.* 2012;42:53-58.

Canadian Pain Society Study Day Participants. Safety and effectiveness of the herpes zoster vaccine to prevent postherpetic neuralgia. 2015;20:46-47.

Chiang F, Panyaping T, Tedesqui G, et al. Varicella zoster CNS vascular complications. A report of four cases and literature review. *Neuroradiol J.* 2014;27:327-333.

Chovel-Sella A, Ben Tov A, Lahav E, et al. Incidence of rash after amoxicillin treatment in children with infectious mononucleosis. *Pediatrics.* 2013;131:e1424-e1427.

Di Lernia V, Mansouri Y. Epstein-Barr virus and skin manifestations in childhood. *Int J Dermatol.* 2013;52:1177-1184.

Estabragh ZR, Mamas MA. The cardiovascular manifestations of influenza: a systematic review. *Int J Cardiol.* 2013;167:2397-2403.

Galvez R, Redondo M. Evidence-based treatment of postherpetic neuralgia. In: Magel GD, ed. *Herpesviridae-A Look Into This Unique Family of Viruses.* InTech; 2012. Available from http://www.intechopen.com/books/herpesviridae-a-look-into-this-unique-family-of-viruses/evidence-based-treatment-of-postherpetic-neuralgia.

Mertz D, Kim TH, Johnstone J, et al. Populations at risk for severe or complicated influenza illness: systematic review and meta-analysis. *BMJ.* 2013;347:f5061.

Muthuri SG, Myles PR, Venkatesan S, Leonardi-Bee J, Nguyen-Van-Tam JS. Impact of neuraminidase inhibitor treatment on outcomes of public health importance during the 2009-2010 influenza A (H1N1) pandemic: a systematic review and meta-analysis in hospitalized patients. *J Infect Dis.* 2013;207:553-563.

Viasus D, Oteo Revuelta JA, Martinez-Montauti J, Carratalà J. Influenza A(H1N1)pdm09–related pneumonia and other complications. *Enferm Infecc Microbiol Clin.* 2012;30(Suppl 4):43-48.

CHAPTER 199

Tickborne Infections

Roger P. Clark, DO

LYME DISEASE

■ EPIDEMIOLOGY

Poor land management prior to the 1920s resulted in massive deforestation in the Northeastern and upper Midwestern United States. The conservation movement and the decline in small family farms in these parts of the country have led to the return of forest and meadow land. With reforestation has come the large scale recovery of deer and other mammals, making for conditions in which Lyme disease and other tickborne illnesses can thrive. Since it was first described in 1977 in Lyme, Connecticut, Lyme disease has become the most common vectorborne disease in the United States. In 2013, the Centers for Disease Control and Prevention (CDC) reported over 36,000 confirmed or probable cases in the United States, with 95% of cases occurring along the eastern seaboard from Virginia to Maine, as well as in the upper Midwest states of Minnesota and Wisconsin.

Lyme disease is caused by the organism *Borrelia burgdorferi*, a spirochete, or corkscrew-shaped bacterium. The life cycle of this organism includes both invertebrate (tick) and vertebrate (mammalian) hosts. The major tick vector for Lyme disease in the United States is *Ixodes scapularis*, with *Ixodes pacificus* ticks transmitting the disease in areas along the West Coast. There is no transovarian spread of *B. burgdorferi*; ticks are not infected when they are hatched from eggs. Ticks must take a blood meal during each of its life stages (larvae, nymph, and adult), and acquire infection by feeding on an infected mammalian host.

The vast majority of Lyme disease cases are reported from May through August, but ticks may forage at any time the weather is warm enough for them to be active. A good rule of thumb is that if it is warm enough not to need gloves on while out of doors, it is warm enough for ticks to forage.

■ RISK STRATIFICATION

Lyme disease may usually be managed as an outpatient. However, there may be patients with acute complications which require hospitalization. These include those with meningitis, high-degree atrioventricular (AV) block, and systemic illness with possible coinfection with *Anaplasma*, *Ehrlichia*, or *Babesia* species.

■ EVALUATION

Lyme disease is often described as having three distinct phases: early localized disease, early disseminated disease, and late Lyme disease. This is a useful framework, but in reality Lyme may be more of a disease continuum, as there is often significant overlap of many features.

Early localized disease (Table 199-1). Patients with acute *B. burgdorferi* infection may experience a wide variety of symptoms. In a vaccine trial in states with the highest incidence of Lyme disease, approximately 10% of those who seroconverted were asymptomatic. The most common clinical manifestation is the erythema migrans (EM) rash (**Figure 199-1**). This erythematous rash initially occurs at the site of the tick bite, and is round or ovoid in shape. Over time, the lesion expands, sometimes to very large proportions (>50 cm in size in extreme cases). While classically it has the bullseye appearance, most EM rashes are uniformly erythematous, or have a darker center or slightly pronounced leading edge. It is usually painless, although sometimes it is described as pruritic. This rash was once held to be pathognomonic for Lyme disease, but it may also be seen in association with Southern tick-associated rash illness (STARI), following the bite of the *Amblyomma americanum*, the Lone Star tick. The rash of STARI does not appear to be caused by *B. burgdorferi* infection.

TABLE 199-1 Clinical Features of Early Localized Lyme Disease

Clinical Manifestation	Frequency
Any systemic complaint	68%-80%
Erythema migrans (single)	80%-90%
Fatigue	54%-80%
Arthralgia	42%-54%
Myalgia	44%
Headache	28%-68%
Fevers/chills	39%-50%
Neck stiffness	5%-44%
Localized lymphadenopathy	21%-41%
Generalized lymphadenopathy	4%-20%
Nausea/anorexia	3%-26%

Data from Nadelman RB, et al. *Am J Med.*1996;100:502-508; Shapiro ED. *N Engl J Med.* 2014;370:1724-1731; Steere AC. et al. *Ann Intern Med.* 1983;99:76-82, Logigian EL, et al. *N Engl J Med.* 1990;323:1438-1444.

With early localized infection, patients often develop systemic symptoms, including fatigue, malaise, arthralgias, myalgias, headaches, fevers, chills, and neck stiffness. These systemic symptoms also occur in **early disseminated Lyme infection**, along with additional clinical features which may provide clinical clues to the diagnosis—especially in those who did not develop (or notice) an erythema migrans rash.

PRACTICE POINT

- The classic bullseye rash occurs in only a minority of cases of erythema migrans. Most rashes of erythema migrans are uniformly erythematous, or have a leading edge of slightly accentuated erythema.
- Many patients with erythema migrans do not recall a tick bite.
- Erythema migrans often occurs in locations where it may not be seen by the patient, such as the groins, axillae, popliteal fossa, and gluteal cleft.

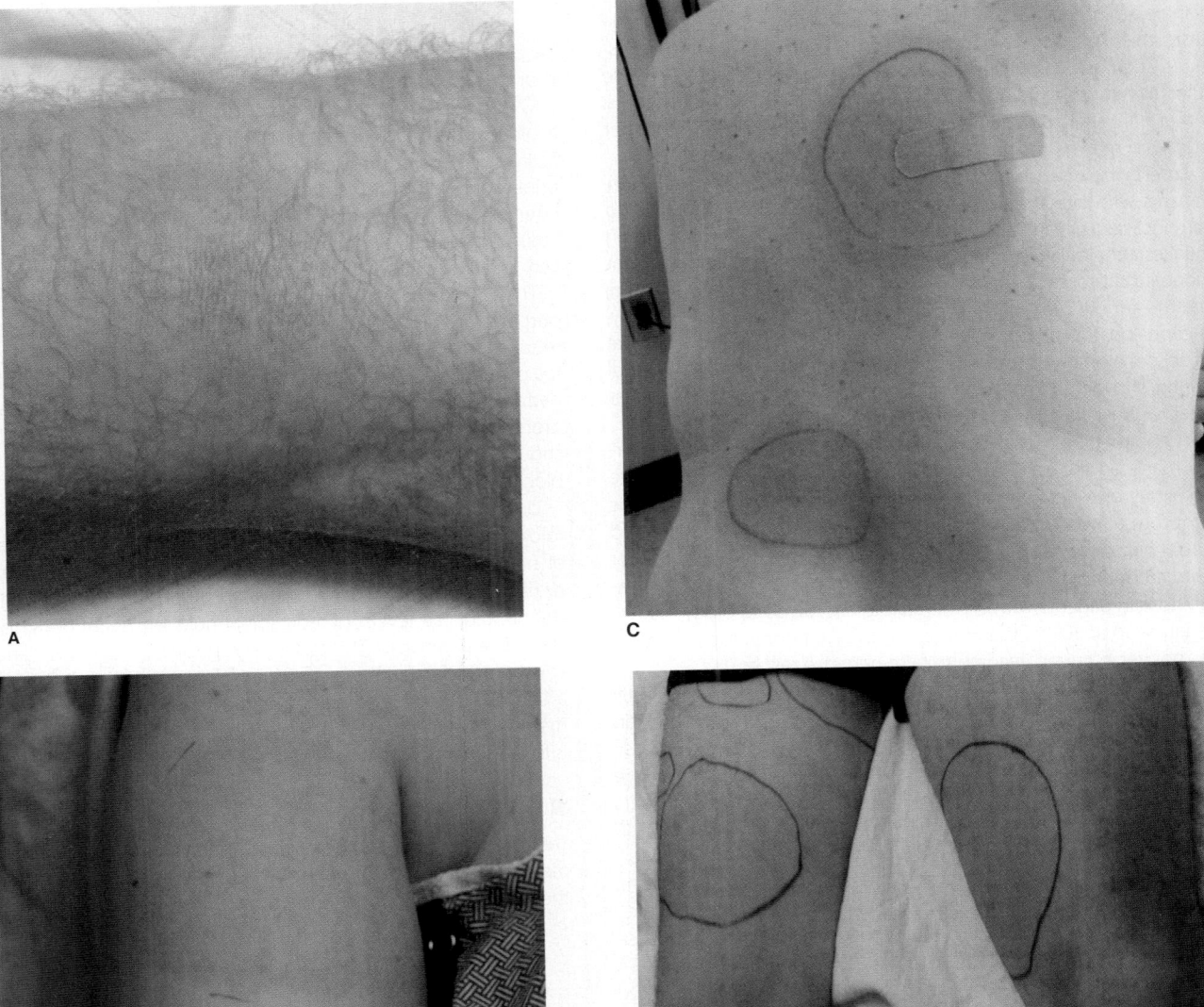

Figure 199-1 *(A) Classic bullseye lesion of erythema migrans. (B) Lesion of erythema migrans with accentuation of erythema at the leading edge. (C and D) Erythema migrans with secondary lesions.*

Patients with early disseminated Lyme disease may have **multiple erythema migrans rashes**. These are thought to arise from hematogenous spread of spirochetes. These lesions are similar in appearance to the primary lesion, but are generally smaller and do not have the central punctum which may arise as the result of the tick bite.

Carditis may occur during early disseminated Lyme disease. This may be manifest as disruption of the conducting system at any level, although first-, second-, and third-degree atrioventricular block are most commonly seen. This generally resolves within a week or so. Myocarditis and pericarditis may occur with Lyme, but are generally mild. Progressive cardiomyopathy resulting in heart failure is generally not seen in the United States. It may rarely occur in Europe, where other *Borrelia* species are found.

Neurologic manifestations of Lyme disease include lymphocytic meningitis and cranial nerve palsies. Facial nerve palsy is common, and when bilateral should strongly suggest Lyme disease as the etiology. Peripheral neuropathy, mononeuritis multiplex, and radiculopathy are also seen. Very rarely, encephalomyelitis or cerebellar ataxia may be encountered. **Eye involvement** has been described, with conjunctivitis being the most common manifestation. Iritis, choroiditis, and panophthalmitis are rare.

Mild elevations in serum aspartate aminotransferase (AST) and alanine aminotransferase (ALT) levels have been reported. In some cases this may be related to coinfection with other tickborne diseases such as *Babesia* spp. or *Anaplasma*. Generally, Lyme disease does not cause respiratory or gastrointestinal signs or symptoms. If these are seen, alternative diagnoses or coinfection with another organism may be suspected.

Late Lyme disease occurs from months to years after infection. Patients with late Lyme disease may have no history of preceding early localized or early disseminated Lyme disease. The most common manifestation of late Lyme disease in the United States is a large joint monoarthritis or oligoarthritis. The knee is most commonly affected, and the arthritis may be intermittent or chronic and persistent. Rarely, encephalopathy or polyneuropathy may be found. The presence of encephalopathy should be based on formal neuropsychological testing, showing objective evidence of cognitive changes, as well as cerebrospinal fluid (CSF) antibody positivity for *B. burgdorferi*.

In endemic areas, the diagnosis of early Lyme disease is generally made on the basis of possible tick exposure and the presence of solitary or multiple erythema migrans, with or without systemic symptoms. In order to become infected, exposure to ticks infected with *B. burgdorferi* is necessary. An infected tick must be attached for 36 to 48 hours before the organism can be passed to the mammalian host. In patients with erythema migrans, Lyme serology may be negative up to 50% of the time, as a robust antibody response often has not yet occurred, leading to false negative results.

When a typical EM rash is not present, but Lyme disease is still suspected, serologic testing may be useful. Care should be taken to select the most useful and accurate test for helping diagnose Lyme disease. Many available tests are not validated and may be misleading. To help avoid misleading test results, the CDC offers guidance on a validated procedure for testing, summarized in **Figure 199-2.**

First, a plausible clinical suspicion and exposure must be present. A serologic enzyme immunoassay (EIA) or immunofluorescence assay (IFA) should follow if definitive evidence of Lyme disease is lacking (such as erythema migrans rash). A negative EIA or IFA result should lead to a reanalysis of the diagnosis. If the suspected exposure was within the past 30 days, a repeat or convalescent test could be repeated.

Positive or equivocal tests should be confirmed with a western blot. For infections suspected to have taken place within the past 30 days, a western blot IgM and IgG should be performed. For infection with duration of greater than 30 days, only an IgG test should

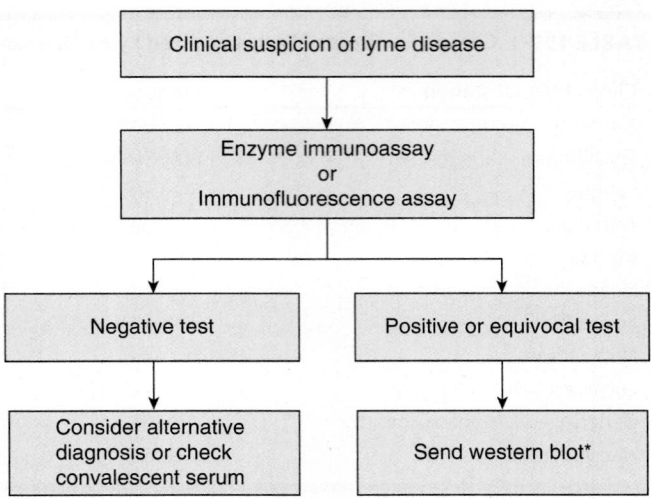

*Note: if signs or symptoms present ≤ 30 d, send IgM and IgG Western Blot
If signs or symptoms present >30 d, send IgG Western Blot only

Figure 199-2 *Algorithm for Lyme disease testing.*

be performed to avoid false positive results. Western blot testing should not be performed without a preceding EIA or IFA.

Other testing modalities have dubious validity and should be avoided. These include blood cultures for *B. burgdorferi*, assays for cell wall deficient forms of the organism, CD57 lymphocyte assays, urine antigen testing, and reverse western blot tests. Some labs offer in-house interpretation of immuoblots which are not validated. These in-house interpretations should be avoided, as most have very poor specificity.

The vast majority of cases of Lyme disease can be managed as an outpatient. If clinical signs and symptoms suggest that the patient requires hospitalization, further workup may be necessary. Testing for coinfection with *Babesia*, *Anaplasma*, and *Ehrlichia* should be performed, as well as a complete blood count, basic metabolic profile and liver function testing. An electrocardiogram (ECG) should be performed in hospitalized patients to assess for heart block and carditis.

Lumbar puncture should be performed if meningitis or other neurologic illness is suspected. Cerebrospinal fluid findings suggestive of neurologic Lyme disease include pleocytosis with lymphocyte or monocyte predominance, elevated protein, and normal or near normal glucose levels. Cerebrospinal fluid Lyme antibody testing should be performed. This test is very specific, but syphilis—another spirochete infection—may produce false positive results; therefore, a CSF VDRL should also be ordered. Cerebrospinal fluid Lyme polymerase chain reaction (PCR) is used in some research settings, but it is limited by poor positive and negative predictive values.

■ INPATIENT MANAGEMENT

Treatment is based on illness duration and organ system involvement. For acute (early) Lyme disease, including erythema migrans, the following oral options are available:

- Doxycycline 100 mg po bid × 10 to 21 days, or
- Amoxicillin 500 mg po tid × 14 to 21 days, or
- Cefuroxime axetil 500 mg po bid × 14 to 21 days.
- Neurologic Lyme disease is treated with either:
- Ceftriaxone 2 g once daily for 14 to 28 days, or
- Penicillin G 20 million units divided four times daily for 14 to 28 days.

Isolated facial nerve palsy may be treated with oral doxycycline for 2 to 4 weeks.

First-degree AV block is treated with the same oral regimens used for early Lyme disease, as above. More severe cardiac involvement requiring hospitalization is treated with

- Ceftriaxone 2 g once daily for 14 to 28 days, or
- Penicillin G 20 million units divided four times daily for 14 to 28 days.

Patients with third-degree AV block may require temporary pacing. Patients with Lyme arthritis and without neurologic disease may be treated with either

- Doxycycline 100 mg po bid × 28 days or
- Amoxicillin 500 mg po tid × 28 days.

Patients who have Lyme arthritis with neurologic symptoms, or patients with recurrent Lyme arthritis after oral therapy, may be treated with intravenous antibiotics, as follows:

- Ceftriaxone 2 g once daily for 14 to 28 days, or
- Penicillin G 20 million units divided four times daily for 14 to 28 days.

Occasionally, within 24 hours of initiation of treatment of Lyme disease, a patient may experience a Jarisch-Herxheimer reaction, with fever and rigors. Body aches and rash often occur, and rarely the patient will experience hypotension. Jarisch-Herxheimer reactions are caused by sudden treponemal lysis during the initiation of antibiotics. The patient should be advised about this possible complication prior to starting treatment. The Jarisch-Herxheimer reaction is not a drug reaction, and should not recur after the first dose of antibiotics. Nonspecific symptoms which occur weeks or months after treatment should not be ascribed to Jarisch-Herxheimer reactions.

■ POST-TREATMENT LYME DISEASE SYNDROME

While the vast majority of patients respond to treatment with complete resolution of symptoms in a timely manner, a minority of patients continue to have persistent fatigue, musculoskeletal symptoms, cognitive or memory complaints, or some combination of these. When these symptoms persist for several months, they are collectively often referred to as post-treatment Lyme disease syndrome or post-Lyme disease syndrome. There is no evidence that prolonged treatment with antibiotics alters the course of these symptoms, and several high-quality studies have demonstrated that longer than standard antibiotic courses do not improve outcomes and increase the likelihood of adverse effects.

PRACTICE POINT

- There is no high-quality evidence to support the prolonged administration of antibiotics in patients with the so-called chronic Lyme disease. Randomized, double-blind, controlled trials in patients with persistent symptoms after Lyme disease have shown that longer than standard courses of antibiotics are associated with an increased risk of side effects, with no improvement in outcomes.

■ POSTACUTE CARE

For mild to moderate Lyme disease not involving the nervous system, cardiovascular system, or musculoskeletal system, the patient may follow-up with their primary care provider. The patient should be advised that, as after any acute infection, they may experience mild fatigue, headache, myalgias, and arthralgias, which may persist for some time. It should be emphasized that this is not the result of chronic infection, but simply the residual effects of the body's response to infection. Patients with infection involving specific organ systems may require follow-up with specialists in these areas in order to demonstrate that the results of the infection have resolved.

■ DISCHARGE CHECKLIST: LYME DISEASE

- Is the patient being discharged with the appropriate antibiotic duration?
- Has appropriate follow-up care been arranged?
- For patients being discharged with intravenous antibiotics and a peripherally inserted central catheter (PICC), has proper care of the PICC line been arranged, with dressing changes at least weekly?
- Has the patient been counseled regarding side effects of medications and signs of PICC line infection or thrombosis?
- Is there a plan for PICC removal?
- For patients receiving long-term antibiotics, has periodic monitoring of complete blood counts, creatinine, and liver enzymes been arranged, and has a provider been designated to follow these lab tests?
- Has the patient been educated regarding measures to decrease or prevent tick exposures and bites, such as avoiding walking through tall grass, wearing light-colored clothing to better visualize ticks, and the using of N,N-diethyl-meta-toluamide (DEET) insect and tick repellants or acaricides such as permethrin on clothing?

BABESIA

■ EPIDEMIOLOGY

Babesia species are parasites with a life cycle involving asexual reproduction in mammals and sexual reproduction within the tick host. These organisms were discovered by Victor Babes in the 1888 and have long been important veterinary pathogens. While over 100 species have been identified, relatively few seem to cause human illness. These include *B. microti*, *B. divergens*, and *B. duncani* (formerly known as WA-1). The vast majority of infections in North America are with *B. microti*, while the major cause of babesiosis in Europe is *B. divergens*. There are scattered cases of a *B. divergens*-like babesiosis syndrome in Washington State, Missouri (the MO-1 strain), and Kentucky. *B. duncani* has been reported from patients in California and Washington State.

Babesia is transmitted by the same tick vectors responsible for Lyme disease. In the United States, the *I. scapularis* tick is largely responsible for spreading *Babesia* to humans, who are accidental hosts. Most cases of babesiosis occur during the summer months (June through September). Babesiosis is thought to be largely unreported or under-reported, as the signs and symptoms are less apparent than with Lyme infection. Most cases in the United States are due to *B. microti*, and occur in New York, New England, and the Upper Midwest. Travel to endemic areas is not always necessary for acquisition of babesiosis, as a small but significant proportion of *Babesia* infections occur from blood transfusion.

■ RISK STRATIFICATION

Babesia infections present with varying degrees of severity, depending on the host. In young, healthy adults, infection may be inapparent, or manifest as a mild, self-limited illness with fever, myalgia, and weakness, which may masquerade as a viral infection. However, in certain populations, babesiosis can be severe and even life threatening. Risk factors for severe babesiosis include age >50 years, splenectomy, and weakened immunity, as with HIV, transplantation, or malignancy.

■ EVALUATION

Babesia infections in humans can result in severe infections and even mortality, but up to one-third of patients are entirely asymptomatic. Most cases in healthy adults present as a mild flu-like illness, with onset within 7 to 42 days after being bitten by an infected tick. Patients experience fevers, chills, malaise, fatigue, myalgias, and arthralgias. Headache is not uncommon, especially during febrile episodes. Splenic or hepatic enlargement may lead to anorexia and abdominal fullness and discomfort.

Manifestations of severe disease include splenic infarction or rupture, acute respiratory failure, and liver or renal failure. The host immune response can lead to sepsis syndrome, including septic shock and multiorgan failure. Acute respiratory failure is generally due to immune-mediated noncardiac pulmonary edema.

Those who are coinfected with other tickborne illnesses, such as Lyme disease or *Anaplasma*, tend to experience more severe infections. Patients hospitalized with babesiosis should be evaluated for these coinfections, as treatment and potential complications would differ if these are present. In general, *B. divergens* and *B. duncani* present with more severe symptoms and complications than *B. microti*. With all species, higher parasitemia is associated with more severe illness and a greater risk of complications and death.

The diagnosis of babesiosis is generally made on a Giemsa stain of thick and thin blood smears. Polymerase chain reaction tests are now commercially available, either alone or as part of a tickborne illness panel, which are able to detect *Babesia* infection even at a very low parasitemia. PCR is more sensitive than smear. If babesiosis is still suspected after a negative smear, PCR testing should be pursued. PCR may also be useful in the setting of a returning traveler to an area where malaria is endemic. The microscopic appearance of these organisms is very similar, and accurate identification of the organism is important in making treatment choices. Serology can be used to diagnose *Babesia* infection even after the parasites have been cleared by the host's immune system.

■ TREATMENT

Treatment of *B. microti* varies depending upon the severity of illness. Those with mild or moderate infection can be treated with atovaquone 750 mg po bid and azithromycin 500 to 600 mg po daily, both for 7 to 10 days. This is generally better tolerated than the treatment usually reserved for more severe illness: clindamycin 600 mg po tid (or 1.2 g IV bid) plus quinine 650 mg po tid. The duration for this course is also 7 to 10 days.

For severe illness, or those with a parasite load of >10%, exchange transfusion should be employed. If a patient is admitted to a facility that does not offer exchange transfusion and has a high degree of parasitemia, or otherwise has severe illness, transfer to an institution that offers this treatment should be considered.

B. divergens and *B. duncani* are generally with oral quinine or IV quinidine, combined with clindamycin. Exchange transfusion may also be considered, especially in more severe cases or with high parasite loads. Most patients with babesiosis should be managed in conjunction with infectious diseases consultation, especially patients who are immunocompromised, as treatment can be lengthy and complex, with close follow-up being necessary.

PRACTICE POINT

Babesiosis

- Consider babesiosis in patients with febrile illness following transfusion.
- Patients with babesiosis should be evaluated for coinfection with Lyme disease and *Anaplasma*, which are spread by the same tick vectors.
- Immunocompromised patients may have much more severe illness, especially patients who are asplenic.
- Patients with severe illness or parasitemia >10% should be evaluated for exchange transfusion.
- Check an ECG to exclude QT prolongation in patients being treated with quinine or quinidine.

■ POSTACUTE CARE

Patients with risk factors for recurrence of babesiosis, such as HIV, rituximab therapy, and asplenia, should be monitored with serial

smears to demonstrate parasite clearance. Monitoring the complete blood count as well as hepatic and renal function may also be considered, especially in more serious disease.

■ DISCHARGE CHECKLIST: BABESIOSIS

- Has there been a substantial reduction in the percentage of infected red blood cells, to at least <5% parasitemia?
- Is the patient responding well to treatment and tolerating oral therapy?
- Are there barriers to clearance of infection that will require closer outpatient follow-up, such as use of rituximab and other immunosuppressive drugs or splenectomy?
- Has QTc prolongation been excluded in patients taking quinine?
- Has the patient been educated regarding measures to decrease or prevent tick exposures and bites, such as avoiding walking through tall grass, wearing light-colored clothing to better visualize ticks, and the using of DEET insect and tick repellants or acaricides such as permethrin on clothing?

ANAPLASMOSIS AND EHRLICHIOSIS

■ EPIDEMIOLOGY

Human granulocytic anaplasmosis (HGA) and human monocytic ehrlichiosis (HME) are caused by different organisms with similar clinical manifestations. As with Lyme disease, these were discovered to be human pathogens in the relatively recent past, with the first human case of ehrlichiosis identified in 1986 and the first human case of anaplasmosis being described in 1990.

Anaplasma and *Ehrlichia*, as well as *Rickettsia* spp., are all in the family Anaplasmataceae (order Rickettsiales), and are genetically closely related. These are obligate intracellular organisms which live within vacuoles (morula) in the cytoplasma of host cells. The vectors, reservoir hosts, and geographic distribution are all different for these organisms, simplifying presumptive diagnosis in most cases.

Human granulocytic anaplasmosis (previously referred to as human granulocytic ehrlichiosis) is caused by the organism *Anaplasma phagocytophilum*. This is spread to humans through the tick vector *I. scapularis*, the same vector responsible for Lyme disease and babesiosis. As such, the range of infection with this organism is the same as that for Lyme disease. The Atlantic coastal states from Pennsylvania northward and upper Midwest account for >90% of all cases reported in the United States. In 2012, 2389 anaplasmosis cases were reported to the Centers for Disease Control and Prevention. Fatality rates from human granulocytic anaplasmosis (HGA) are generally in the range of 0.5% annually. Cases occur throughout the year, but most cases occur between May and September, when ticks are most actively foraging for blood meals.

Human monocytic ehrlichiosis is caused by *Ehrlichia chaffeensis*. Most cases of human disease caused by *Ehrlichia* species is caused by this organism. *E. chaffeensis* infections have been found in a widespread geographic distribution, predominantly in the southeastern and central regions of the United States. This correlates to the distribution of the tick vector *A. americanum* (the Lone Star tick). While the majority of cases occur in the geographic areas mentioned above, the range of tick is widespread, and includes the East Coast states from Florida to coastal Maine, so there is some overlap between the ranges of *Anaplasma* and *Ehrlichia*. However, anaplasmosis is much more common in New England than ehrlichiosis. There were 1128 cases of ehrlichiosis reported to the CDC in 2012. Case fatality rates for ehrlichiosis in the United States are about 1%, slightly higher than for anaplasmosis. The seasonality of ehrlichiosis is nearly identical to that of anaplasmosis.

■ RISK STRATIFICATION

Patients with ehrlichiosis tend to be sicker than patients with anaplasmosis; about half of all symptomatic patients of ehrlichiosis are hospitalized. Patients with known or suspected coinfection with other tickborne illness, those with significant medical comorbidities, those who are immunocompromised, or those who have signs of end-organ damage or hemodynamic instability should be hospitalized.

■ EVALUATION

As with babesiosis, the spectrum of illness encountered with *Anaplasma* and *Ehrlichia* infection ranges from asymptomatic to multiorgan failure and death. After being bitten by a tick, the mean incubation period for both organisms is about 1 week (range 5-21 days). As with Lyme disease, it appears there is some processing of the organism within the tick before infection can be spread to the mammalian host. If the tick has been attached for less than 36 hours, the chance of a person being infected by that tick is negligible. Of course, in those with frequent outdoor exposure, many tick bites may go unnoticed, and these occult tick bites must be considered when regarding a patient with suspected *Anaplasma* or *Ehrlichia* infection.

Following the incubation period, virtually all patients experience fever. Most have malaise, fatigue, and myalgias, and a significant proportion have gastrointestinal complaints such as nausea, vomiting, and diarrhea. About a quarter of patients exhibit some degree of cough. Rash is found in perhaps a quarter of HME patients, but is rare in HGA (~5%). A small percentage of patients develop severe complications. These occur more commonly with *E. chaffeensis*, and include acute kidney injury, disseminated intravascular coagulation, meningoencephalitis, myocarditis, and adult respiratory distress syndrome (ARDS).

Patients who are immunocompromised are more likely to suffer complications, and symptomatic disease occurs more often in the elderly. The incidence of ehrlichiosis is age related, with the highest rate of infection reported in those in the 60 to 64 age group, while anaplasmosis is most commonly found in the 65+ age range. The mean length of stay in those who are hospitalized is about 1 week.

Common laboratory abnormalities include elevations in the liver transaminase levels (AST and ALT), low platelets, and anemia. A rise in the creatinine level is noted in roughly one-third of patients with *Ehrlichia* infections, and half of those with anaplasmosis.

HGA and HME should be suspected in patients with unexplained fever and exposure to ticks in areas where these diseases are endemic, especially in the months of May through August. The presence of elevated transaminase levels, leukopenia, and thrombocytopenia are strongly suggestive, but not necessary for diagnosis. A buffy coat smear demonstrating the presence of intracytoplasmic morulae can give a very rapid presumptive diagnosis (**Figure 199-3**). Morulae are much more likely to be present with HGA (25%-75%) than with HME (<10%).

Serologic assays are useful in retrospective diagnosis, with a fourfold rise in titer expected on convalescent sera. However, early in disease, elevated titers are often not found, and treatment should not be withheld either while awaiting results or because an early titer is negative. PCR from whole blood is becoming a useful tool in diagnosing HGA and HME, with high sensitivity and a relatively quick turnaround time. If suspicion is high for these illnesses, treatment should begin right away while awaiting results of confirmatory tests, as a negative result cannot entirely rule out the presence of disease.

Patients who test positive for HGA (but not HME, as different tick vectors are involved) should be tested for Lyme disease and babesiosis as well. The incidence of coinfection with HGA and Lyme disease in areas where both are endemic is estimated to be between 2% and 10%.

■ INPATIENT MANAGEMENT

Doxycycline is the treatment of choice for patients of all ages in those suspected of having anaplasmosis or ehrlichiosis. The adult

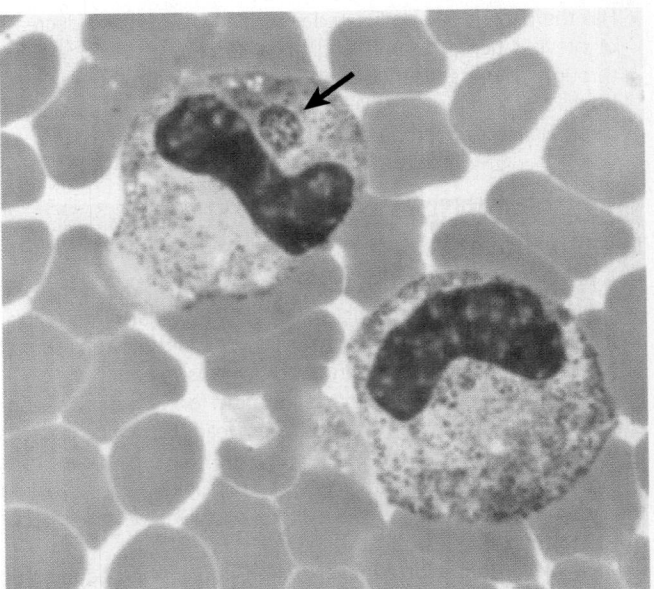

Figure 199-3 *Intracytoplasmic morula from infection with* Anaplasma *(arrow).*

dose of doxycycline is 100 mg po bid, generally for 7 to 10 days, and at least 3 days after clinical improvement and cessation of fever. In those who have a life-threatening allergy to doxycycline or in pregnant patients, rifampin has been used successfully.

PRACTICE POINT

Anaplasmosis and ehrlichiosis

- Consider *Anaplasma* and *Ehrlichia* infection in older patients with unexplained fever in endemic areas with tick exposure during the summer months.
- Treatment should begin immediately if infection is suspected.
- The treatment of choice is doxycycline, even in pediatric patients.

■ POSTACUTE CARE

Patients should be instructed that they may experience fatigue and malaise for an extended period following successful treatment. HGA and HME do not cause chronic infection, but any organ-specific damage experienced during hospitalization, such as acute kidney injury or ARDS, should be followed up after discharge from the hospital. All patients who experience tickborne illness should be instructed on measures to decrease or prevent tick exposures and bites. These include avoiding walking through tall grass, wearing light-colored clothing to better visualize ticks, and the use of DEET insect and tick repellants as well as the use of acaricides such as permethrin on clothing. Environmental treating of the yard may also decrease exposure.

■ DISCHARGE CHECKLIST: ANAPLASMOSIS AND EHRLICHIOSIS

- Have patients been assessed for the presence of concomitant tickborne infections?
- Has the patient been discharged to complete a minimum course of 7 to 10 days of doxycycline in total, to continue for at least 3 days after resolution of fever?
- Has appropriate follow-up care been arranged, with special attention to any end-organ damage suffered during hospitalization?
- Have local and state health departments been notified?

- Has the patient been educated regarding measures to decrease or prevent tick exposures and bites, such as avoiding walking through tall grass, wearing light-colored clothing to better visualize ticks, and the using of DEET insect and tick repellants or acaricides such as permethrin on clothing?

ROCKY MOUNTAIN SPOTTED FEVER

■ EPIDEMIOLOGY

Rickettsia rickettsii belongs to the same family as *Anaplasma* and *Ehrlichia*. Like these organisms, *Rickettsia* are obligate intracellular organisms which live within vacuoles (morula) in the cytoplasma of host cells. Once the host is bitten, the organisms spread to the circulatory system, where they have tissue tropism for the vascular endothelial cells. Disruption of the endothelium leads to varying degrees of vascular permeability. Vascular injury and the subsequent host immune response can lead to widespread tissue damage, involving the heart, lungs, central nervous system, skin, liver, gastrointestinal tract, and muscle.

Rocky Mountain spotted fever (RMSF) has a wide geographic range in the United States, and it is also found in Mexico and Central and South America. Multiple tick vectors are responsible for spreading this infection to humans. While most states have reported RMSF, 60% of cases are found in five states: North Carolina, Tennessee, Arkansas, Missouri, and Oklahoma. Similar to the other tickborne infections covered in this chapter, cases have been reported throughout the year, but most occur between May and August. Incidence of RMSF increases with age until the age range of 60 to 64, then drops off slightly in the 65+ age range.

Nationally, the incidence appears to increase and decrease in a cyclical manner. There was a peak in the mid-1930s through 1950, and another from 1970 through the mid-1980s. Starting in 2000, there was a dramatic sharp upturn in cases, to an all-time high of 2553 cases in 2008. Fortunately, over time there has been a corresponding decrease in the fatality rate from over 25% in 1944 to the current rate of less than 1%.

■ RISK STRATIFICATION

The greatest risk factor for death from RMSF is the failure to consider the diagnosis. Several factors may hinder early recognition. Patients may not be asked about possible tick exposure, and the rash of RMSF may be more difficult to recognize in persons of color. Glucose-6-phosphate dehydrogenase (G6PD) deficiency, male sex, age >40 years, and delay in treatment by 5 days or more are also associated with a higher risk of death.

■ EVALUATION

Unlike the organisms covered earlier in this chapter, transmission of *R. rickettsii* via the tick salivary glands may occur after as few as 6 to 10 hours of attachment. The incubation period of RMSF is 2 to 14 days, with a mean duration of 1 week. The initial presentation is generally one of nonspecific febrile illness, with the classic triad of fever, rash, and known tick exposure rarely being present at the initial physician visit. Fever is almost always present, and is often high, with temperatures exceeding 102°F (38.9°C) in two-third of cases at initial presentation. While rash is often lacking initially, it develops in an estimated 85% to 90% of cases. It often begins as a blanching, macular rash, starting at the ankles and wrists, then spreading to include the trunk, palms and soles. By this time, it is often petechial in nature. The presence of a rash on the palms and soles often alerts providers to consider RMSF as an etiology, as there are a limited number of disease states which cause rash in these areas. Headache and myalgia are usually present as well, and nausea and vomiting

TABLE 199-2 Clinical Features of Rocky Mountain Spotted Fever

Clinical Manifestation	Frequency
Fever	81%-100%
Headache	58%-93%
Myalgia	72%-92%
Rash	68%-90%
Rash on palms and soles	49%-82%
History of a tick bite	54%-66%
Classic triad (fever, headache, and rash)	32%-67%

Data from Thornier AR, et al. *Clin Infect Dis*. 1998;27:1353-1360; Traeger MS, et al. *Clin Infect Dis*. 2015;60:1650-1658.

are found about half the time. Patients may also exhibit conjunctival injection (**Table 199-2**).

Less common presentations include pneumonitis, severe abdominal pain, which may be mistaken for acute abdomen or appendicitis, hepatosplenomegaly, anorexia, diarrhea, altered mental status, ataxia, meningismus, and diffuse lymphadenopathy.

Complications arise from the endothelial damage caused by rickettsial invasion. These include adult respiratory distress syndrome (ARDS), cardiac arrhythmias, coagulopathy, encephalitis, skin necrosis (multiple cases of gangrene are reported in the literature), and gastrointestinal bleeding. Hemolysis may arise, especially in those with G6PD deficiency. Long-term sequelae include organ damage, neurologic deficits, or limb amputation.

A high index of suspicion must be maintained for RMSF, especially in highly endemic regions. Given the organism's widespread range, many providers may be unfamiliar with the disease, and it is often not considered when the rash is absent or nonpetechial. The classic triad of fever, tick bite, and rash is present only one-half to two-thirds of the time. Serology may be useful in confirming the diagnosis, but this is often only retrospective, as serology is often negative in the first 7 to 10 days. IgM is less specific than IgG, and as such may represent a false positive result. A fourfold rise in convalescent titers taken 2 to 4 weeks after initial titers is taken as strong evidence of infection.

Suggestive laboratory findings include thrombocytopenia, anemia, elevated transaminases (AST and ALT), hyperbilirubinemia, hyponatremia, and elevated creatine kinase levels. If a lumbar puncture is performed, pleocytosis with monocyte predominance may be noted. The Weil-Felix test has historically been used to diagnose rickettsial infections, but it suffers from poor sensitivity or specificity and should be avoided.

■ INPATIENT MANAGEMENT

Doxycycline is the treatment of choice for patients of all ages in those suspected of having infection with Rocky Mountain Spotted Fever. Infectious diseases consultation should be placed in cases of life threatening Rocky Mountain Spotted Fever, especially with a life threatening allergy to doxycycline, or if pregnant. The adult dose of doxycycline is 100 mg po bid, generally for 7 days, and at least 3 days after clinical improvement and cessation of fever. For those who have a life-threatening allergy to doxycycline or are pregnant, chloramphenicol 50 to 75 mg/kg/d given in four divided doses has been successfully used, but has a higher rate of failure and death than doxycycline.

■ POSTACUTE CARE

Appropriate follow-up will vary depending upon the severity of illness and the presence of complications. Barring organ damage or limb ischemia, patients who are discharged prior to completion of antibiotics should be impressed with the importance of finishing their course, and should be seen in close follow-up by their provider.

■ DISCHARGE CHECKLIST: ROCKY MOUNTAIN SPOTTED FEVER

- Has the patient been instructed to complete a minimum of 7 to 10 days of doxycycline, continuing for at least 3 days after resolution of fever?
- Has appropriate follow-up care been arranged, especially for patients with complications?
- Have local and state health departments been notified?
- Has the patient been educated regarding measures to decrease or prevent tick exposures and bites, such as avoiding walking through tall grass, wearing light-colored clothing to better visualize ticks, and the using of DEET insect and tick repellants or acaricides such as permethrin on clothing?

TICKBORNE ENCEPHALITIS VIRUSES

Powassan virus (POWV) and **deer tick virus (DTV)** are related viruses which are rare causes of encephalitis. Since Powassan virus was first described in Powassan, Ontario in 1958, fewer than 100 cases have been reported. Powassan and deer tick viruses cause similar manifestations, and have related genetic lineages with an 84% nucleotide sequence identity. Infections occur in the same general regions where Lyme disease is found. However, there is mounting evidence that cases in the Northeastern United States previously attributed to POWV are actually due to DTV. The enzootic cycle for POWV involves *Ixodes cookei*, with the usual mammalian hosts consisting of the groundhog (*Marmota momax*) and the striped skunk (*Mephitis mephitis*). The replication cycle for DTV is the same as that of Lyme disease, *Anaplasma*, and *Babesia*, involving the deer tick *I. scapularis* and the white-footed mouse *Peromyscus leukopus*.

In one case series of POWV/DTV in New York State, 12 of the 14 patients were admitted to the intensive care unit (ICU), and half required mechanical ventilation. The all-cause mortality rate was 36%. All patients had fever, 86% had generalized weakness, and 72% complained of lethargy. About half of the patients displayed confusion, seizures, headache, or rash. Cerebrospinal fluid analysis demonstrated a modest lymphocytic pleocytosis.

The CDC criteria for the diagnosis of neuroinvasive disease due to POWV/DTV requires meningitis, encephalitis, acute flaccid paralysis, or other acute signs of central or peripheral neurologic dysfunction, as documented by a physician, in the absence of a more likely clinical explanation, along with a confirmatory laboratory test, such as isolation of virus from CSF or blood, positive POWV/DTV IgM in CSF or serum, or a fourfold rise in POWV/DTV antibody titers between acute and convalescent sera. There is no specific treatment for POWV/DTV. Some data suggest that corticosteroids may be beneficial, but further studies are required.

BORRELIA MIYAMOTOI

Borrelia miyamotoi has been recently recognized as a human pathogen. First discovered in Japani in 1994, the initial human cases were described in Russia in 2011. Subsequently, a number of cases have now been found in the United States as well. While this organism is related *B. burgdorferi*, the causative agent of Lyme disease, its clinical features more resemble that of *B. recurrentis*, the agent responsible for tickborne relapsing fever.

B. miyamotoi usually presents as an undifferentiated febrile illness, with headache, often described as severe, malaise, and prominent myalgias and arthralgias (**Table 199-3**). Common laboratory findings include leukopenia, thrombocytopenia and mildly elevated

TABLE 199-3 Features of *Borrelia miyamotoi* Infection

Clinical Manifestation	Frequency
Laboratory findings	
Thrombocytopenia	60%
Elevated transaminases	68%-82%
Clinical signs/symptoms	
Fevers/chills	96%-98%
Headache	89%-96%
Malaise or fatigue	82%-98%
Myalgia	59%-84%
Arthralgia	28%-76%

Data from Platonov AE, et al. *Emerg Infect Dis*. 2011;17:1816-1823; Molloy PJ, et al. *Ann Intern Med*. 2015;163:91-98.

liver function tests. Symptoms recur in 4% to 10% of patients. This is likely higher in those not treated with antibiotics.

Currently available tests for *B. miyamotoi* include whole blood PCR and antibodies against GlpQ protein. Treatment is with doxycycline. Given the geographic distribution in areas where Lyme disease and *Anaplasma* are found, it is very likely that some patients started empirically on doxycycline for suspected tickborne illness may have unrecognized infection with *B. miyamotoi*.

SUGGESTED READINGS

Centers for Disease Control and Prevention. *Tickborne Diseases in the United States*. 3rd ed., 2015. Available at http://www.cdc.gov/lyme/resources/tickbornediseases.pdf.

Clark RP, Hu LT. Prevention of Lyme disease and other tick-borne infections. *Infect Dis Clin North Am*. 2008;22:381-396.

Dantas-Torres F. Rocky Mountain spotted fever. *Lancet Infect Dis*. 2007;7:724-732.

El Khoury MY, Camargo JF, White JL, et al. Potential role of deer tick virus in Powassan encephalitis cases in Lyme disease-endemic areas of New York, U.S.A. *Emerg Infect Dis*. 2013;19:1926-1933. http://www.ncbi.nlm.nih.gov/pmc/articles/PMC3840892/.

Horowitz HW, Aguero-Rosenfeld ME, Holmgren D, et al. Lyme disease and human granulocytic anaplasmosis coinfection: impact of case definition on coinfection rates and illness severity. *Clin Infect Dis*. 2013;56:93-99.

Klempner MS, Baker PJ, Shapiro ED, et al. Treatment trials for post-Lyme disease symptoms revisited. *Am J Med*. 2013;126:665-669.

Klempner MS, Hu LT, Evans J, et al. Two controlled trials of antibiotic treatment in patients with persistent symptoms and a history of Lyme disease. *N Engl J Med*. 2001;345:85-92.

Molloy PJ, Telford SR 3rd, Chowdri HR, et al. *Borrelia miyamotoi* disease in the Northeastern United States. *Ann Intern Med*. 2015;163:91-98.

Shapiro ED. Lyme disease. *N Engl J Med*. 2014;370:1724-1731.

Wormser GP, Dattwyler RJ, Shapiro ED, et al. The clinical assessment, treatment, and prevention of Lyme disease, human granulocytic anaplasmosis, and babesiosis: clinical practice guidelines by the Infectious Diseases Society of America. *Clin Infect Dis*. 2006;43:1089-1134. http://cid.oxfordjournals.org/content/43/9/1089.long.

Vannier EG, Diuk-Wasser MA, Ben Mamoun C, Krause PJ. Babesiosis. *Infect Dis Clin North Am*. 2015;29:357-370.

CHAPTER 200

Tuberculosis

Michael Gardam, MD, MSc, FRCPC
Susy Hota, MD, MSc, FRCPC

Key Clinical Questions

❶ When should tuberculosis be suspected in the inpatient setting?

❷ What diagnostic testing should be performed in patients with suspected tuberculosis?

❸ What precautions are necessary for patients with possible tuberculosis? When may they be discontinued?

❹ What treatment regimen should be begun for patients with newly diagnosed tuberculosis? What monitoring is appropriate in patients being treated for tuberculosis?

INTRODUCTION

A global pandemic of tuberculosis (TB) that began three centuries ago continues today, although globally, rates have begun to decline for the first time over the past few years. According to estimates from the World Health Organization, 9.4 million people developed active TB in 2013, and 1.5 million died. Tuberculosis remains the leading cause of death in the HIV-infected, accounting for 26% of acquired immunodeficiency syndrome (AIDS)-related deaths throughout the world. The incidence of TB is highest in Asia, Africa, Latin America, Russia, and Eastern Europe (**Figure 200-1**). Rates are substantially lower in developed countries, where TB is increasingly a disease of the foreign born. However, some populations in developed nations have a relatively high incidence of the disease, including homeless persons, injection drug users, incarcerated persons, and some aboriginal populations. Another group at risk in developed nations is the elderly. Rates of TB in the developed world 50 years ago were similar to rates in developing countries today. Older patients born and raised in developed nations therefore have a higher likelihood of developing active TB than younger patients, due to the risk of late reactivation of latent infection.

As TB in the developed world has become uncommon, the diagnosis is often overlooked, even when in retrospect it should have been fairly apparent. Unfortunately, because pulmonary TB may be highly contagious, delays in diagnosis may have disastrous implications not only for the patient, but also for family, friends, and other close contacts, including health care workers.

PATHOPHYSIOLOGY

Tuberculosis is caused almost exclusively by *Mycobacterium tuberculosis*. Rarely, it is caused by the related organism *Mycobacterium bovis*, acquired from infected cattle or contaminated milk products. *M. tuberculosis* is transmitted almost exclusively through the respiratory route by microscopic droplet nuclei. These particles are small enough to remain airborne for long periods of time and to be inhaled directly into the terminal alveoli, typically in the lower lung zones. Droplet nuclei are produced when a patient with pulmonary TB speaks, coughs, or sneezes. Rarely, droplet nuclei may arise from other activities, such as irrigation of TB-infected areas during surgery, dressing changes of draining wounds, or emptying of containers of infectious fluid.

M. tuberculosis has adapted to survive within alveolar macrophages, the cells that normally would be expected to eradicate it. Within the macrophage, the organism travels to the mediastinal lymph nodes. It then disseminates throughout the body via the bloodstream, with more vascular areas receiving more organisms. Microscopic foci of live bacteria are thus deposited throughout the body, including the lung apices. Typically, 3 to 8 weeks after infection, the cellular immune system responds by walling off the bacteria in granulomas. This process is paralleled by the development of a positive tuberculin skin test. Granulomas are not static structures; the organisms within them are alive, albeit dormant, and the cells forming the granuloma constantly turn over. At this stage, the infected individual has what is referred to as *latent tuberculosis infection*. Patients with latent infection are neither ill nor infectious to others. Roughly, 85% to 90% of otherwise healthy individuals in this state never develop symptoms throughout their lifetime, despite ongoing infection. Of the 10% to 15% who do go on to develop symptoms, most do so within the first few years of becoming infected. Once symptoms have developed, the patient is referred

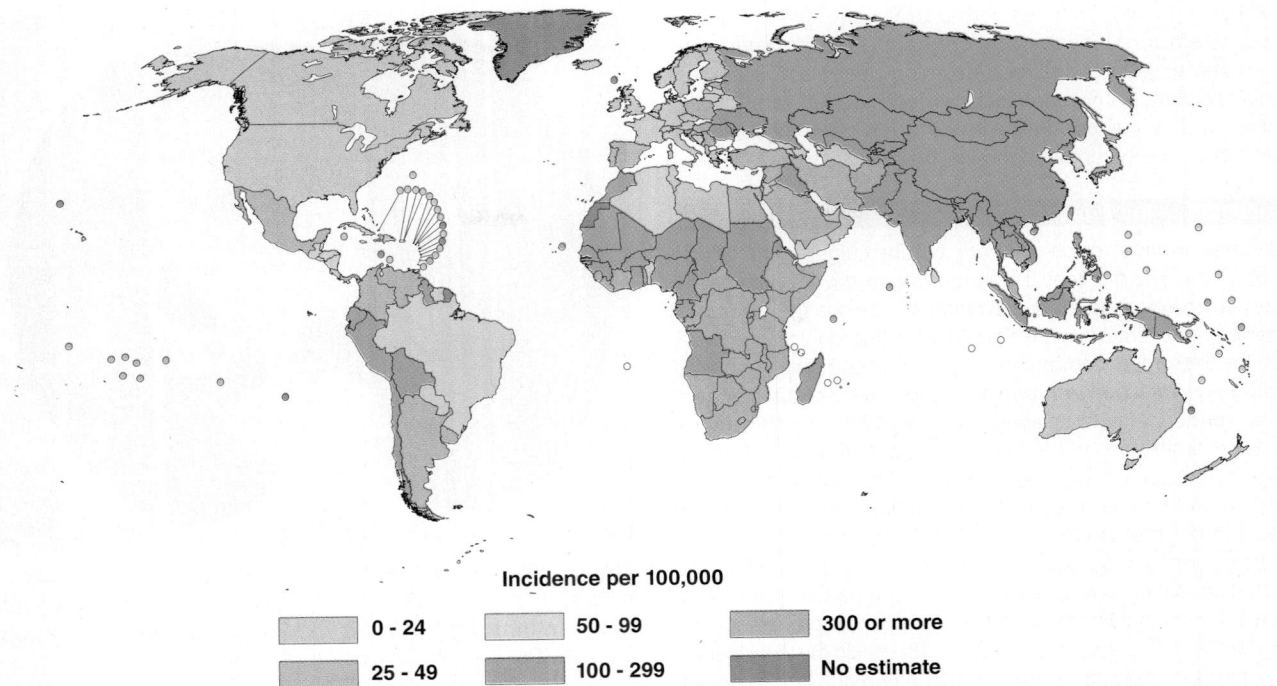

Incidence per 100,000

0 - 24	50 - 99	300 or more
25 - 49	100 - 299	No estimate

Figure 200-1 *Tuberculosis incidence in 2005, based on World Health Organization data.* (Courtesy of the Stop TB Department, WHO; with permission.)

to as having *active tuberculosis*. Although there is a predilection for disease to develop in the apices of the lungs, a large minority of patients will develop symptoms outside the lungs. Commonly involved extrapulmonary sites include regional lymph nodes, pleura, spine, bones and joints, and meninges. Patients with certain underlying medical conditions or receiving immunosuppressive therapy are at higher risk of developing active disease if infected (**Table 200-1**).

PRACTICE POINT

● About 25% to 50% of patients with extrapulmonary TB also have active pulmonary tuberculosis. Although extrapulmonary tuberculosis is not usually contagious, chest imaging is indicated in these patients to exclude concomitant contagious pulmonary disease.

CLINICAL PRESENTATION

Unfortunately, the symptoms of active TB are often vague and nonspecific, sometimes leading to initial misdiagnosis. It is common for a TB clinic to see patients who were initially investigated for malignancy. Patients typically report having had symptoms for weeks to months prior to being diagnosed. In some cases, symptom onset can be so gradual that patients realize the extent of their illness only after they have improved with treatment. Early cases can be entirely asymptomatic, having been detected on a chest radiograph performed for other reasons. Rarely, patients present with acute symptoms, mimicking more typical bacterial infections, or they may develop disseminated (miliary) TB, with a rapidly progressive febrile wasting illness, with or without pulmonary complaints.

Constitutional symptoms such as weight loss, fatigue, fever, night sweats, and rigors tend to be more common with pulmonary and pleural disease, together with a worsening productive cough. Massive hemoptysis was once common in the preantibiotic era, but hemoptysis is now rare, and if present, is typically minor. Constitutional symptoms may be absent in extrapulmonary TB, especially in patients with disease confined to lymph nodes. *Tuberculous*

lymphadenitis is the most common form of extrapulmonary TB. It usually presents as painless swelling of the posterior cervical or supraclavicular lymph nodes, although patients may also develop lymph node tenderness and fistula formation. *Pleural tuberculosis* may present with fever, dyspnea, and pleuritic chest pain if the effusion is sizable enough. *Genitourinary tuberculosis* may present with dysuria, urinary frequency, flank pain, and hematuria, although it may also often be asymptomatic until hydronephrosis and severe kidney damage have occurred. *Spinal tuberculosis* (Pott disease) most often presents with back pain from infection of the thoracic or lumbar spine, often with paravertebral cold abscesses involving the psoas muscle. *Tuberculous meningitis* presents as subacute or

---

TABLE 200-1 Risk Factors for Active Tuberculosis Among Persons Who Have Been Infected with Tuberculosis

Factor	Relative Risk/Odds
Recent infection (<1 y)	12.9
Fibrotic lesions (spontaneously healed)	2-20
Comorbidity	
HIV infection	100
Silicosis	30
Chronic renal failure/hemodialysis	10-25
Diabetes	2-4
Intravenous drug use	10-30
Immunosuppressive treatment	10
Gastrectomy	2-5
Jejunoileal bypass	30-60
Post-transplantation period (renal, cardiac)	20-70
Malnutrition and severe underweight	2

Reproduced, with permission, from Fauci AS, Braunwald E, Kasper DL, et al. *Harrison's Principles of Internal Medicine*, 17th ed. New York, NY: McGraw-Hill, 2008. Table 158-1.

chronic basilar meningitis, often with cranial nerve palsies; central nervous system (CNS) involvement may also produce a *tuberculoma*, leading to seizures and focal neurologic deficits. *Tuberculous peritonitis* presents with abdominal pain and ascites, with diffuse peritoneal implants on abdominal imaging. It is often mistaken for ovarian cancer or other intra-abdominal malignancies.

DIAGNOSIS

The greatest obstacle to the diagnosis of tuberculosis is the failure to consider it in the differential diagnosis. Patients with pulmonary TB may seek medical attention several times before the diagnosis is considered. Patients may be treated with fluoroquinolone antibiotics for presumed community-acquired pneumonia, resulting in temporary improvement and false negative sputum smears that may further delay the diagnosis and lead to potentially more contacts becoming infected. Patients with extrapulmonary TB often undergo diagnostic tests focused on detecting malignancy rather than TB. For example, patients with tuberculous lymphadenitis may have excisional lymph node biopsies to exclude lymphoma, without tissue being sent for mycobacterial culture. TB should be clinically suspected in patients who present with compatible symptoms and have epidemiologic risk factors for infection or progression to active disease. For example, pulmonary TB should be considered in a patient originally from an endemic area with chronic renal failure and a new cough. Once suspected, the diagnosis can usually be confirmed with appropriate testing without great difficulty, although there are exceptions as mentioned below.

■ RADIOLOGY

Basic chest radiography is useful in diagnosing pulmonary TB, especially if cavities (**Figure 200-2**) or evidence of prior TB infection is present, such as apical scarring or pleural thickening. Rarely, tiny miliary nodules are seen (**Figure 200-3**). Computed tomography (CT) and magnetic resonance imaging (MRI) scans are more appropriate for diagnosing spinal TB, meningitis, pericarditis, and TB of

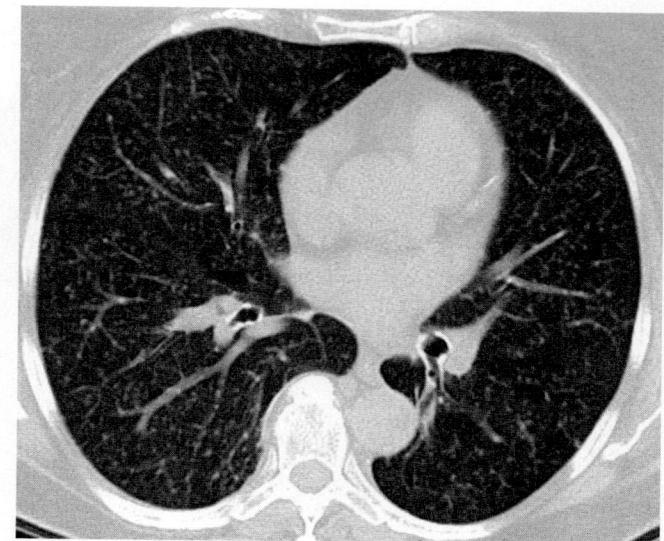

Figure 200-3 *Miliary tuberculosis: innumerable small pulmonary nodules, 1 to 3 mm in diameter, in a patient with rheumatoid arthritis treated with a tumor necrosis factor inhibitor.* (Courtesy of John J. Ross, MD.)

deep organs or organ spaces. Although radiographic findings can be typical for TB, such as tree-in-bud alveolar infiltrates, they are rarely pathognomonic. Hence, collection of fluid or tissue for histology and mycobacterial culture is essential to confirm the diagnosis.

■ MICROBIOLOGIC TESTING

Specimens for TB testing are concentrated, smeared on a slide, and then stained with fluorochrome and fuchsin to visualize acid-fast bacilli (**Figure 200-4**). Usually, these represent *Mycobacteria* species (but not necessarily *M. tuberculosis*). However, *Nocardia* and *Rhodococcus* species are weakly acid-fast, and may be detected with these stains as well. Rapid nucleic acid amplification tests (NAATs) that may be performed in 3 to 5 hours are now available to detect *M. tuberculosis* complex nucleic acids on smear-positive specimens. A positive smear with a positive NAAT is presumptive evidence that *M. tuberculosis* is present. A negative smear cannot rule out a diagnosis of TB, as the concentration of TB bacilli may simply have been below the limit of detection, or the specimen may have been inadequate. In such instances, if the clinical suspicion remains, it is best to wait for the mycobacterial culture result or consider repeat sampling.

M. tuberculosis takes up to 8 weeks for growth and identification, using traditional solid mycobacterial culture media. Many laboratories have adopted more rapid techniques, incubating the specimen in broth and using molecular methods or analysis of mycolic acids by chromatography for species identification. This usually allows for growth and identification of *M. tuberculosis* within 2 to 3 weeks. Drug susceptibility testing takes an additional 1 to 2 weeks.

Microbiologic identification of TB is affected by the type and quality of specimen submitted to the lab. In pulmonary TB, the most sensitive methods of isolating the organism are induced sputum collection and bronchoalveolar lavage. Induced sputum collection involves inhalation of a nebulized hypertonic saline solution to generate a hearty cough. Unfortunately, the process is labor intensive, and requires the supervision of a respiratory therapist. The alternative is to collect multiple spontaneously expectorated sputum specimens, ideally on three consecutive mornings. This ensures a deeper, more concentrated sample, especially if the patient is not terribly symptomatic with cough. For those who are very symptomatic, it may not be necessary to wait a day between specimens; they can be collected every 8 hours.

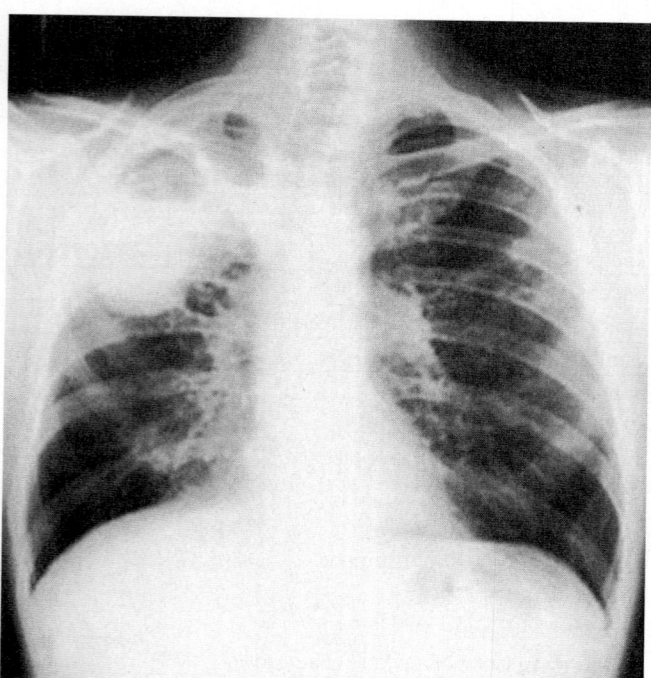

Figure 200-2 *Cavitary upper lobe tuberculosis.* (Reproduced, with permission, from Tintinalli JE, Kelen GD, Stapczynski JS. *Tintinalli's Emergency Medicine: A Comprehensive Study Guide,* 6th ed. New York, NY: McGraw-Hill; 2004. Fig. 70-2.)

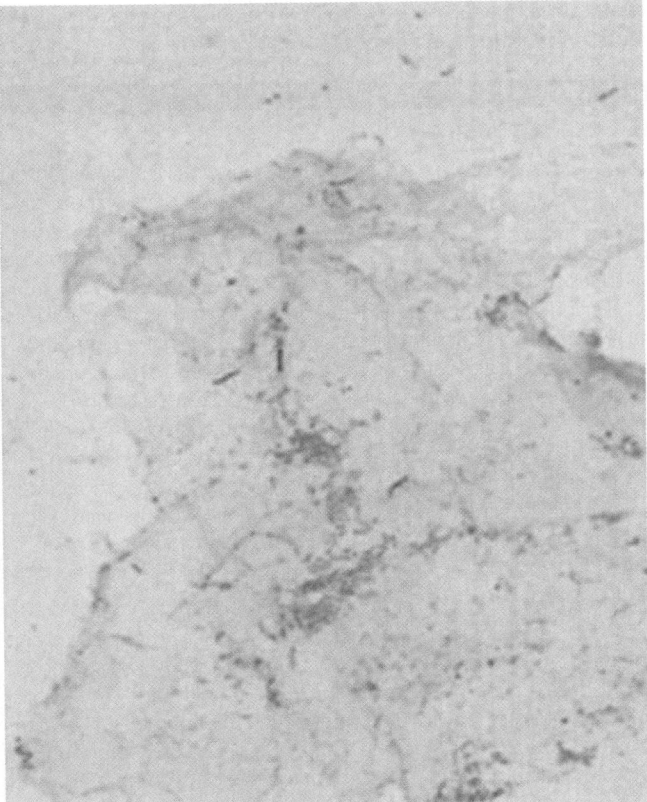

Figure 200-4 *Positive Ziehl-Neelsen sputum stain, with magenta-colored acid-fast bacilli on a blue background.* (Courtesy of the Centers for Disease Control and Prevention.)

PRACTICE POINT

- Tuberculosis is more common at all stages of HIV disease. In HIV-positive patients with relatively normal CD4+ counts, it usually presents with upper lobe fibrocavitary lung disease, similar to that seen in HIV-negative patients. Patients with AIDS and pulmonary TB have a variety of clinical presentations, from massive hilar and mediastinal lymphadenopathy to primary pneumonia and nodular and miliary patterns. Cavitation is typically absent. Extrapulmonary TB is seen in 50% of AIDS patients, compared with approximately 40% of HIV-negative patients. Diagnosis of TB is more difficult in AIDS, as sputum smears more often negative, perhaps because of the absence of chest cavities.

Identifying *M. tuberculosis* on smear and culture can be more difficult in cases of extrapulmonary TB. This is especially true for tuberculous meningitis, peritonitis, pericarditis, and pleural disease. In these cases, smears are typically negative, and cultures are also often negative, but the pathology may demonstrate granulomas or even acid-fast bacilli embedded in the tissue. Finding these in biopsy specimens may require a large number of tissue sections and a very dedicated pathologist, as acid-fast bacilli may be scant in extrapulmonary TB. Therefore, all biopsy specimens should be sent to both pathology and microbiology laboratories.

INFECTION CONTROL

Once the diagnosis of TB is considered in a hospitalized patient, it is critically important to immediately assess the risk of the organism spreading to patients and staff. The decision to initiate airborne isolation should precede obtaining sputum samples for smear and

---

TABLE 200-2 Indications to Initiate Isolation for Suspected Tuberculosis

Cough and chest radiograph suggestive of tuberculosis (apical infiltrate, cavitary lesion, military pattern, infiltrate with mediastinal adenopathy)

Positive smear for acid-fast bacilli

Known tuberculosis of uncertain status (ie, adequacy of treatment uncertain)

HIV infection with undiagnosed pulmonary condition

Patients with tuberculosis risk factors and undiagnosed pulmonary infiltrates

HIV, human immunodeficiency virus.

---

culture in a patient with compatible symptoms and epidemiologic risk factors (**Table 200-2**). For example, an HIV-positive homeless patient with pneumonia should be housed in a negative pressure airborne isolation room while being investigated, and staff should wear appropriately fit-tested respirators while in the room.

Airborne isolation may subsequently be discontinued in patients for whom an alternative diagnosis has been ruled in, initial testing for *M. tuberculosis* has been negative, and the case has been discussed with the hospital infection prevention and control department (**Table 200-3**).

The decision to discontinue airborne isolation in patients with known pulmonary TB must weigh several factors, including whether the patient is clinically improving; whether cough is still present or absent; whether a cavity is present on chest radiograph, which suggests greater contagiousness; whether repeat sputum smears; and whether drug sensitivities are known. In general, 2 weeks of treatment should be considered the absolute minimum duration of airborne isolation that is required. More typically, patients with pulmonary TB remain in airborne isolation for several weeks while in the hospital. Again, removal from isolation should be done in consultation with the infection prevention and control department.

■ LATENT TUBERCULOSIS

By definition, latent TB produces no symptoms. Screening for latent TB is most appropriate for patients with epidemiologic risks such as immigration from endemic areas, homelessness, intravenous drug use, incarceration, or close contact with a patient with active TB in the setting of medical risk factors for TB reactivation (see Table 204-1). Screening should generally not be performed in those at low risk for being infected, as this increases the risk that results will be falsely positive. An exception to this is the Food and Drug Administration requirement to screen all patients embarking upon

---

TABLE 200-3 Indications to Discontinue Isolation for Tuberculosis

- Patients admitted to rule out tuberculosis may be taken out of negative pressure isolation when three acid-fast bacteria smears on consecutive days are negative, including one early-morning specimen, or when the diagnosis of tuberculosis seems highly unlikely on clinical grounds (ie, resolution of pneumonia with antibiotic which is not active against tuberculosis)

- Patients with known tuberculosis may be removed from negative pressure isolation when clinical improvement has occurred (improvement in cough, fever, night sweats, anorexia) and three AFB smears are negative on consecutive days are negative, including one early-morning specimen

antitumor necrosis factor alpha therapy, regardless of epidemiologic risk factors.

Tuberculin skin test

The diagnosis of latent TB has traditionally been made by demonstrating a positive response to the tuberculosis skin test (TST). Planting, reading, and interpreting the TST is deceptively simple, and misinterpretation is common. Because of this, TSTs should be performed and interpreted by experienced personnel. In general, the TST is highly sensitive and specific for latent TB infection; however, false-positive and false-negative reactions may occur. False-positive reactions may occur due to cross-reactivity with other mycobacteria or to previous bacille Calmette-Guérin (BCG) vaccination, if the vaccine was given after the first year of life. Once a TST is positive, it should be considered positive for life and not repeated. False-negative reactions are common in the immunosuppressed, the chronically ill, and the elderly.

PRACTICE POINT

- The effects of bacille Calmette-Guérin (BCG) vaccination on the results of the tuberculin skin test (TST) depend on the age at time of vaccination. When BCG is given in infancy, as is now recommended by the World Health Organization, its effect on the TST is negligible more than 10 years after. Therefore, a TST with 10 mm or more of induration in an adolescent or adult with risk factors for infection who received BCG in infancy is indicative of tuberculosis infection. Individuals who received BCG as older children or adults are more prone to false-positive tuberculin skin test results, although this risk also diminishes with time. Use of an interferon-gamma release assay, which does not contain antigens present in BCG, may be useful to clarify the results of TST in these patients, and to exclude false-positive TST results.

Interferon-gamma release assays

Interferon-gamma release assays (IGRAs) are blood tests that can be used to diagnose latent TB infection. These tests have the advantage of not producing false-positive reactions from prior BCG vaccination. Whereas some guidelines have suggested that they can replace the TST, others have taken a more cautious approach, citing the difficulty in interpreting the sizable proportion of discordant results between the TST and IGRAs that cannot all be explained by BCG vaccination. IGRAs are most clinically useful when skin test-positive patients without obvious TB risk factors

are found to have a negative IGRA. In such cases, the IGRA likely represents a true negative result.

TREATMENT

■ LATENT TUBERCULOSIS

The treatment of choice for latent TB is isoniazid (INH) for 9 months. This has been shown to decrease the risk of developing active tuberculosis by 90%. INH is taken with vitamin B_6 (pyridoxine), which prevents the potential adverse effect of peripheral neuropathy. The major risk of INH is hepatotoxicity. Clinical hepatitis typically occurs in <1% of individuals; however, the chance of developing hepatotoxicity increases with age and in patients with pre-existing liver abnormalities. Therefore, before starting treatment, all patients should undergo screening blood work to ensure there is no baseline elevation in liver enzymes. Some guidelines recommend regular screening while on therapy. In those with underlying liver disease, consideration can be made for a second-line treatment, such as a 4-month regimen of rifampin. Treatment with rifampin may also be considered if the affected patient is in contact with someone with INH-resistant TB.

■ ACTIVE TUBERCULOSIS

Unlike latent TB infection, the treatment of active TB requires multiple drugs. Most patients with newly diagnosed TB will be started on a four-drug regimen of INH, rifampin, pyrazinamide, and ethambutol while awaiting sensitivity data, after which the regimen will be simplified (**Table 200-4**). Side effects may be significant, compounded by the need for prolonged treatment for at least 6 months. The most common adverse event is hepatotoxicity. The highest risk drug for hepatotoxicity is pyrazinamide, followed by INH and rifampin. Treatment is stopped if liver enzymes rise above five times the upper limit of normal in asymptomatic patients, or above three times normal levels in patients with symptoms compatible with hepatitis. Rash may develop due to sensitivity to one of the medications, usually rifampin or pyrazinamide. Rifampin may also interact with other medications metabolized by the liver, so careful attention should be paid to the patient's medication history. Patients on rifampin should be forewarned that a benign but invariable effect of being on this medication is an orange discoloration of tears, urine, and sweat. Ethambutol can lead to optic neuropathy, resulting in decreased visual acuity and loss of peripheral vision and color vision, so sight should be assessed during every follow-up visit while on the medication.

TREATMENT REGIMENS

There are four regimens for treatment of uncomplicated active TB approved by the American Thoracic Society, Centers for Disease Control, and Infectious Diseases Society of America. The most

---

TABLE 200-4 First-line Drugs for Tuberculosis, Typical Daily Dosages, and Major Side Effects

Drug	Typical Daily Dosage	Major Adverse Effects
Isoniazid (INH)	5 mg/kg, maximum 300 mg	Peripheral neuropathy, hepatitis, allergy
Rifampin	10 mg/kg, maximum 600 mg	Hepatitis, fever, rash, nausea; orange discoloration of sweat, urine, and tears, with staining of contact lenses; extensive drug interactions via hepatic cytochrome metabolism
Pyrazinamide	20-25 mg/kg, maximum 2 g	Hepatotoxicity, gout, arthralgias, rash, nausea
Ethambutol	15-20 mg/kg	Optic neuritis, typically presenting with loss of peripheral vision; periodic screening of visual fields, visual acuity, and red-green color discrimination recommended
Pyridoxine (vitamin B_6)	10-25 mg	Given to prevent INH-induced neuropathy in patients with predisposing conditions, such as diabetes, alcoholism, pregnancy and lactation, malnutrition, uremia, and HIV infection; pyridoxine supplementation also recommended in patients with seizures, as INH may increase seizure frequency

popular regimen is INH and rifampin for 6 months, combined with pyrazinamide for the first 2 months. Ethambutol is also given until sensitivity data are available. Treating TB is not like treating other bacterial infections. The antibiotics used are quite distinct, and for the most part are not interchangeable; each drug in the regimen fills a specific role. Because each drug has side effects that may require changes to the initial treatment regimen, expert advice should be sought when treating active TB, as inappropriate regimens can lead to treatment failure and the emergence of drug-resistant bacteria.

Fully drug-sensitive pulmonary and most extrapulmonary TB can usually be cured with 6 months of treatment. In extensive disease, treatment may be more prolonged. Meningeal and other forms of CNS TB require longer treatment courses. Corticosteroids may be beneficial to decrease the inflammatory component of TB meningitis, pericarditis, and adrenal disease.

Drug-resistant TB is a growing problem in many parts of the world, and it is expected to become more common in developed countries. Second-line agents, such as fluoroquinolones, aminoglycosides, cycloserine, ethionamide, and clofazime can be used to treat these cases. However, widely accepted guidelines for treatment of drug-resistant TB do not yet exist. In addition, many of these medications cause serious adverse events with prolonged use. Therefore, all cases of drug-resistant TB should be referred to and managed by a TB specialist.

Quinolone antibiotics require special mention as they are increasingly being used in the treatment of tuberculosis, even as replacements for front-line drugs in the absence of drug intolerance or resistance. It is important to note that the absence of clear clinical studies and guidelines, these drugs should not be used as first-line therapy.

DISCHARGE CONSIDERATIONS

- Have the patient and family been educated about the need for prolonged treatment, close outpatient follow-up, and screening of the patient's close contacts for TB?
- Have providers addressed potential obstacles to successful treatment, such as cultural and language barriers, denial, and perceived social stigma relating to TB?
- Has follow-up arranged with an outpatient treatment program, ideally one that uses directly observed therapy?
- Have public health authorities been notified?

- Has social work been involved, if there is any concern that the patient may not be adherent or lacks adequate social support?
- Have baseline liver enzymes been tested?
- If health care workers were exposed to the patient without appropriate protection, have arrangements been made to test their TB status?

SUGGESTED READINGS

Blumberg HM, Burman WJ, Chaisson RE, et al. American Thoracic Society/Centers for Disease Control and Prevention/Infectious Diseases Society of America: treatment of tuberculosis. *Am J Respir Crit Care Med.* 2003;167:603-662.

Centers for Disease Control and Prevention (CDC). Updated guidelines for the use of nucleic acid amplification tests in the diagnosis of tuberculosis. *MMWR Morb Mortal Wkly Rep.* 2009;58(1):7-10.

Farhat M, Greenaway C, Pai M, Menzies D. False-positive tuberculin skin tests: what is the absolute effect of BCG and non-tuberculous mycobacteria? *Int J Tuberc Lung Dis.* 2006;10:1192-1204.

Getahun H, Matteelli A, Chaisson RE, Raviglione M. Latent *Mycobacterium tuberculosis* infection. *N Engl J Med.* 2015;372:2127-2135.

Jensen PA, Lambert LA, Iademarco MF, Ridzon R. Centers for Disease Control. Guidelines for preventing the transmission of *Mycobacterium tuberculosis* in health-care settings, 2005. *MMWR Recomm Rep.* 2005;54(RR-17):1-141.

Mazurek M, Jereb J, Vernon A, et al. Updated guidelines for using interferon gamma release assays to detect *Mycobacterium tuberculosis* infection—United States, 2010. *MMWR Recomm Rep.* 2010;59(RR-5):1-25.

Taylor Z, Nolan CM, Blumberg HM. American Thoracic Society, Centers for Disease Control and Prevention, Infectious Diseases Society of America. Controlling tuberculosis in the United States. Recommendations from the American Thoracic Society, CDC, and the Infectious Diseases Society of America. *MMWR Recomm Rep.* 2005;54(RR-12):1-81.

World Health Organization. Companion handbook to the WHO guidelines for the programmatic management of drug-Resistant tuberculosis. Geneva: World Health Organization; 2014. http://www.ncbi.nlm.nih.gov/books/NBK247420/.

CHAPTER 201

Candida and *Aspergillus*

Dimitrios Farmakiotis, MD

John J. Ross, MD

Sophia Koo, MD

Key Clinical Questions

1. When should a positive urine culture for *Candida* species be treated?

2. When should invasive candidiasis be suspected? How is it diagnosed and treated?

3. What is the clinical significance of a positive sputum culture for *Aspergillus* species?

4. How useful are antigen detection tests for the diagnosis of infection with *Candida* and *Aspergillus* species?

5. When should infectious diseases be consulted?

CANDIDA INFECTIONS

■ EPIDEMIOLOGY

Candida species are normal commensal flora of the oropharynx, bowel, vagina, and skin. *Candida* overgrowth of these surfaces may arise in the setting of broad-spectrum antibiotics, corticosteroid exposure, diabetes mellitus, or HIV infection, resulting in oral thrush, *Candida* esophagitis, intertriginous candidiasis, and vaginal candidiasis. High estrogen states, such as pregnancy or oral contraceptive use, are an additional risk factor for vaginal yeast infection. Localized *Candida* skin infections (*Candida* intertrigo) are often seen in moist, macerated intertriginous folds, such as in the groin, perineum (diaper rash), pannus, axillae, and breasts.

While superficial candidiasis is common in both ambulatory and hospitalized patients, candidemia and disseminated candidiasis are usually seen in health care settings. Candidemia is the third most common bloodstream infection in hospitalized patients, and is associated with high mortality rates. Risk factors include critical illness, broad-spectrum antibiotic or corticosteroid exposure, intra-abdominal surgery, hemodialysis, central venous catheters, parenteral nutrition, intravenous drug use, and neutropenia.

■ MUCOCUTANEOUS *CANDIDA* (CUTANEOUS, THRUSH, ESOPHAGITIS, VAGINITIS)

Evaluation

The diagnosis of mucocutaneous *Candida* infections is usually made clinically. **Cutaneous candidiasis** has a typical distribution in intertriginous areas, with central erythema and maceration, surrounded by a collar of scale (**Figure 201-1**). Beyond this, there may be papular and pustular satellite lesions. Disseminated, hematogenous candidiasis can lead to a different, diffuse maculopapular rash (**Figure 201-2**).

Oral thrush presents with painless white plaques on the tongue and, sometimes, the hard palate and the oropharynx (**Figure 201-3**), that are easily scraped off. Fissures of the angles of the mouth (cheilitis) may also be present. Budding yeasts, hyphae, and pseudohyphae of *Candida* can be seen on microscopy when scrapings of skin or oral lesions are mixed with a drop of 10% potassium hydroxide, which digests host cells but not fungi.

Esophageal candidiasis presents with odynophagia. Oral thrush is sometimes also present. Endoscopy is required for confirmation in most patients. In AIDS patients with odynophagia, empiric treatment with fluconazole is reasonable. If symptoms do not subside in 3 to 4 days, endoscopy is indicated to exclude alternative causes, such as herpes simplex, cytomegalovirus, and malignancy.

Vulvovaginal candidiasis presents with vaginal itching, soreness, dysuria, and dyspareunia, frequently after a course of antibiotics. Vaginal discharge is often absent; when present, it may be thick and curdy, sometimes described by the patient as cheesy. Odor is usually absent, in contrast to bacterial vaginosis and *Trichomonas* infection, the two other most common causes of vaginitis. In addition to potassium hydroxide preparations, the usual investigations for the diagnosis of vaginitis should be performed, including the "whiff" test, vaginal pH measurement, and microscopy with saline (wet prep) for trichomonads, white cells, and clue cells.

Intertriginous candidiasis and *Candida* vaginitis can sometimes be the first manifestations of undiagnosed diabetes mellitus. Such patients should have their glucose levels tested.

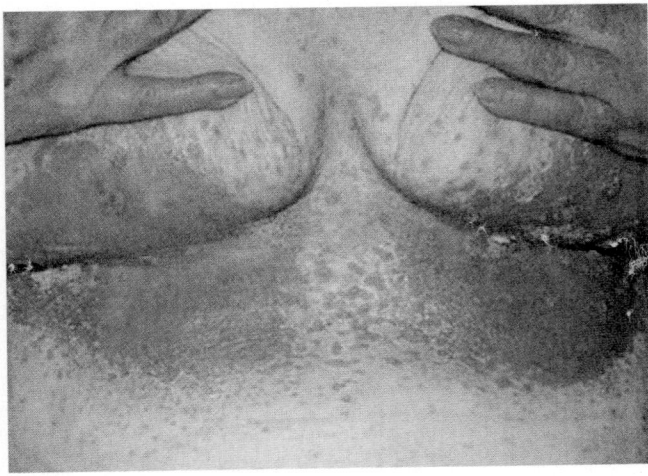

Figure 201-1 *Candida intertrigo, with prominent satellite lesions at the margins.* (Reproduced, with permission, from Wolff K, Goldsmith LA, Katz SI, et al. *Fitzpatrick's Dermatology in General Medicine*, 7th ed. New York, NY: McGraw-Hill; 2008. Fig. 189-4B.)

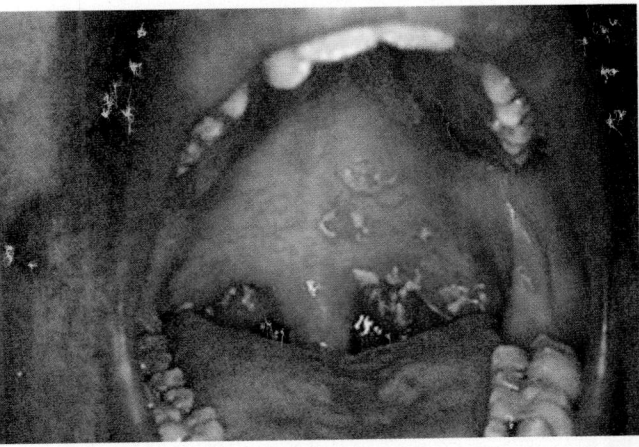

Figure 201-3 *Oral thrush, with characteristic plaques on the hard palate.* (Reproduced, with permission, from Wolff K, Goldsmith LA, Katz SI, et al. *Fitzpatrick's Dermatology in General Medicine*, 7th ed. New York, NY: McGraw-Hill; 2008. Fig. 189-2A.)

Inpatient management

The treatment of **Candida intertrigo** should include measures to improve aeration and drying of involved skin folds, correction of predisposing factors, such as hyperglycemia, and a topical antifungal agent, such as nystatin or an azole. Some authors argue that an antifungal cream or ointment should be used for the first several days, due to their superior skin penetration, followed by several days of a drying agent, such as nystatin powder. Antifungal powders may also be used as maintenance therapy in patients at high risk of relapse. Topical glucocorticoids should be avoided, as they reduce inflammation while allowing fungal infection to persist.

Mild cases of **oral thrush** may be treated topically with clotrimazole troches 10 mg five times daily, nystatin suspension (concentration of 100,000 U/mL) 5 mL four times daily, or nystatin pastilles (200,000 U each) four times daily for 7 to 14 days. Moderate-to-severe disease is treated with fluconazole 100 to 200 mg orally once daily for 7 to 14 days.

Esophageal candidiasis is treated with oral (or intravenous, in patients unable to swallow) fluconazole 200 to 400 mg daily, for 14 to 21 days. Patients with AIDS or other immunocompromising conditions and prior chronic fluconazole exposure may develop thrush and esophagitis from fluconazole-resistant strains. In those cases, further susceptibility testing, infectious diseases (IDs) consultation, and treatment with newer triazoles (voriconazole,

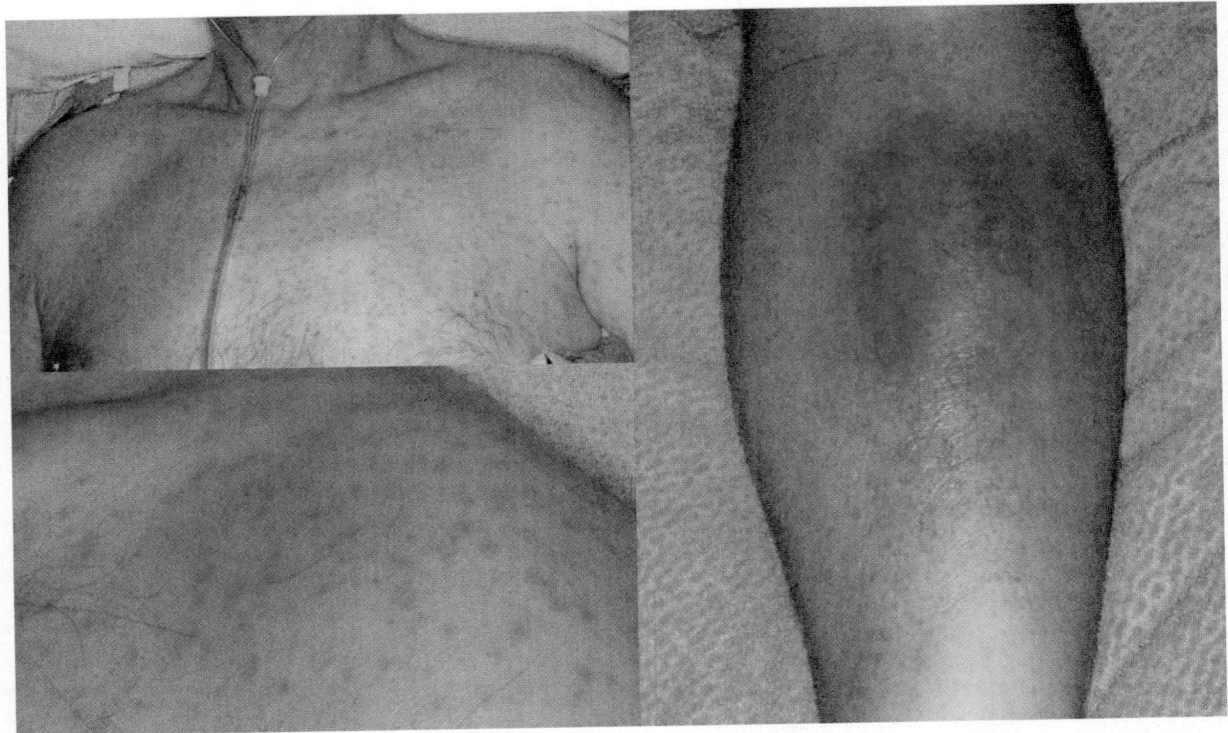

Figure 201-2 *Skin manifestations of disseminated fungal infections in neutropenic patients with leukemia: Candida tropicalis fungemia with skin dissemination (left) and cutaneous invasive aspergillosis mimicking bacterial cellulitis (right).*

posaconazole, or isavuconazole if the isolate is susceptible) or an echinocandin are indicated.

Vulvovaginal candidiasis may be successfully treated with many topical agents, including clotrimazole 100 mg vaginal tablet, or 5 g of 1% clotrimazole cream, intravaginally once daily for 7 days. Some patients prefer a single dose of 150 mg oral fluconazole for its ease of administration.

■ URINARY CANDIDIASIS

Evaluation

Candida species are readily grown from urine culture. Most patients with candiduria have underlying illness, such as recent surgery, diabetes mellitus, an abnormal urinary tract, or malignancy, have been treated with antibiotics in the preceding month, or have indwelling urinary catheters. On many occasions when candiduria is documented, urine cultures were performed for evaluation of cloudy urine, without symptoms or evidence of infection. The vast majority of patients with candiduria are asymptomatic, and funguria tends to clear spontaneously without treatment. Progression to candidemia is unusual. However, treatment should be considered in patients with urinary symptoms and positive urine cultures for *Candida*, especially in those with diabetes or other risk factors for candidiasis who have not recently received antibiotics.

Inpatient management

Asymptomatic urinary *Candida* infection does not require antifungal treatment, except in neutropenic patients, low birth weight neonates, or patients undergoing urologic procedures. When possible, predisposing factors should be eliminated, such as indwelling urinary catheters or stents, immunosuppressive drugs, or broad-spectrum antibiotics.

For symptomatic patients, oral fluconazole is the treatment of choice, because of high urinary tract concentrations and ease of administration. *Candida* cystitis is treated with fluconazole 200 mg once daily for 14 days, and *Candida* pyelonephritis with fluconazole 200 to 400 mg once daily for 14 days. The newer triazoles (voriconazole, posaconazole), the echinocandins, and the liposomal formulations of amphotericin B do not achieve high urinary concentrations, but can be used for parenchymal disease (pyelonephritis). Amphotericin B deoxycholate has adequate urine penetration, but is associated with significant nephrotoxicity and serious infusion side effects. Infectious diseases should be consulted for urinary tract infections caused by fluconazole-resistant *Candida* strains.

■ CANDIDEMIA AND DISSEMINATED CANDIDIASIS

Evaluation

Candidemia and disseminated candidiasis (*Candida* infection of usually sterile sites) should be suspected in febrile or septic patients with exposure to antibiotics, intravenous catheters, parenteral nutrition, immunosuppressive agents, or chemotherapy. *Candida* species, unlike many other fungi, are not fastidious, and can be grown without difficulty from blood cultures and subcultured onto regular blood agar plates. However, the diagnosis of disseminated candidiasis may be elusive, as only 50% to 80% of patients with disseminated candidiasis have documented candidemia. The *Candida* score (**Table 201-1**) has been proposed as a diagnostic tool to define a population of sick patients at high risk of disseminated candidiasis who would benefit from early antifungal therapy.

Measurement of serum 1,3-β-D-glucan is a useful, if imperfect, adjunctive test in the diagnosis of invasive candidiasis. This component of the cell wall of *Candida* and other fungi may be detected in the serum of patients with candidemia and disseminated candidiasis, sometimes at high levels. However, the 1,3-β-D-glucan test

TABLE 201-1 *Candida* Score for Discriminating Between *Candida* Colonization and Invasive Candidiasis in Non-neutropenic Patients

Risk Factor	Points
Multifocal candidal colonization	1
Recent surgery	1
Total parenteral nutrition	1
Severe sepsis	3

A *Candida* score of ≥ 3 in a critically ill patient is associated with an eightfold increased risk of disseminated candidiasis; early antifungal administration is warranted.

Data from Leon C, Ruiz-Santana S, Saavedra P, et al. Usefulness of the "*Candida* score" for discriminating between *Candida* colonization and -invasive candidiasis in non-neutropenic critically ill patients: a prospective multicenter study. *Crit Care Med*. 2009;37:1624-1633.

lacks specificity, and false positive results are common, especially for results close to the threshold of normal. Moreover, the sensitivity of 1,3-β-D-glucan testing for the diagnosis of candidemia can be limited. The most frequent causes of falsely elevated serum β-D-glucan levels are summarized in **Table 201-2**.

Patients with candidemia or possible disseminated candidiasis should be asked about focal complaints suggestive of metastatic *Candida* infection, such as eye pain and decreased visual acuity (endophthalmitis), back pain (vertebral osteomyelitis), and joint pain (septic arthritis).

An important if rare variant of disseminated candidiasis is hepatosplenic candidiasis, or chronic disseminated candidiasis. This syndrome typically occurs in patients with persistent fever after recovery from neutropenia, and has a strong host inflammatory component, similar to other clinical manifestations that fall within the immune reconstitution inflammatory syndrome (IRIS) spectrum.

TABLE 201-2 Usefulness and Limitations of 1,3-β-D-Glucan Assays

Fungal infections that may result in positive tests
Candidemia/invasive candidiasis
Aspergillosis
Cryptococcosis
Histoplasmosis
Blastomycosis*
Coccidioidomycosis
Pneumocystis jiroveci (formerly *Pneumocystis carinii*) pneumonia
Causes of false-positive tests
Bacteremia, including *Streptococcus pneumoniae* and *Pseudomonas aeruginosa*
Antibiotics (amoxicillin-clavulanic acid, piperacillin-tazobactam)
Hemodialysis with cellulose membranes
Immunoglobulin and albumin infusion with cellulose filters
Serosal exposure to gauze

*Blastomyces dermatitidis releases very little 1,3-β-D-glucan in its yeast phase, and may not be detected in clinical infections. Serum 1,3-β-D-glucan levels are also not elevated in *Cryptococcus neoformans* infections and mucormycosis.

Right upper quadrant pain and elevated liver enzymes, particularly alkaline phosphatase, are usually present. Abdominal computed tomography (CT) scan demonstrates hepatic, splenic, and occasionally, renal microabscesses.

Inpatient management

Candidemia can lead to septic shock and death, and early initiation of appropriate antifungal treatment is paramount. Antifungal susceptibility patterns differ among *Candida* species. *C. albicans* and *C. tropicalis* are usually sensitive to all antifungals (azoles, echinocandins, amphotericin B). *C. parapsilosis* demonstrates reduced in vitro susceptibility to echinocandins, but the clinical significance of this finding is uncertain. *C. krusei* is intrinsically resistant to fluconazole, but typically susceptible to voriconazole and posaconazole. *C. glabrata* isolates often show intermediate susceptibility or resistance to fluconazole. The vast majority of fluconazole-resistant *C. glabrata* isolates are also resistant to all other azole antifungals.

In nonneutropenic patients with candidemia and mild illness, fluconazole is reasonable initial therapy. Empiric echinocandin therapy is preferred in nonneutropenic patients with moderate-to-severe illness, and patients with neutropenia or recent azole antifungal exposure (**Figure 201-4**). Azole antifungals are preferred for *C. parapsilosis* infection, especially in cases of breakthrough fungemia in patients who are already receiving an echinocandin. Amphotericin B use has become much less common, due to the availability of less toxic agents.

Antifungal susceptibility testing is expensive and not routinely performed for most bloodstream *Candida* isolates, but should be obtained in *C. glabrata* isolates from blood, and in *Candida* isolates from sterile sites that fail to respond to therapy. Given the emergence of resistance to multiple antifungal classes in non*albicans Candida* species, particularly *C. glabrata*, we favor susceptibility testing in the hospital setting if local epidemiology shows an increasing frequency of non*albicans Candida* strains and high rates of antifungal agent use.

In nonneutropenic patients, candidemia should be treated for at least 2 weeks after blood cultures become negative and symptoms have resolved. Longer courses are indicated for metastatic disease, such as *Candida* endophthalmitis, meningitis, or osteomyelitis. *Candida* endocarditis usually requires valve replacement. Neutropenic patients with candidemia should be treated for at least 2 weeks after blood cultures become sterile, and symptoms and neutropenia have both resolved.

Intravenous catheters should be removed from patients with candidemia who are not neutropenic. Catheter removal should be considered in neutropenic patients, although the benefit is less marked in this patient population. In neutropenia, candidemia is more likely to arise from mucositis and gut overgrowth with translocation, rather than an indwelling catheter, and interrupting intravenous access may be more problematic in neutropenic patients. Infectious disease consultation is indicated in patients with suspected or proven candidemia or disseminated candidiasis.

■ COMPLICATIONS OF CANDIDEMIA

Ocular dissemination and endophthalmitis are common in candidemia. Ophthalmologic consultation and dilated retinal examination are recommended for all patients with candidemia, especially critically ill patients who cannot report symptoms. *Candida* endocarditis should be suspected in patients with persistent fever and fungemia, embolic manifestations, or cardiac murmurs, and an echocardiogram should be performed. Back pain suggests vertebral osteomyelitis. *Candida* meningitis presents with fever, headache, and neck pain, although confusion may predominate in debilitated patients. Chronic renal infection may result in formation of urinary fungus balls (*Candida* bezoars), which may require local amphotericin B instillation and surgical removal.

■ PREVENTION

Prophylaxis with fluconazole can be considered in populations at high risk of invasive candidiasis, such as neutropenic patients, solid organ transplant recipients, patients undergoing induction chemotherapy or stem-cell transplantation, and high-risk patients hospitalized in intensive care units with a high incidence of invasive candidiasis. However, it should be noted that in clinical trials, fluconazole or echinocandin prophylaxis in critically ill adults with risk factors for invasive candidiasis did not improve outcomes.

In women with a history of recurrent *Candida* vulvovaginitis, a 150-mg dose of fluconazole at the beginning and completion of antibiotic therapy may prevent the development of symptomatic vaginal yeast infection.

■ DISCHARGE CHECKLIST

- Is the patient tolerating antifungal therapy?
- Has the duration of antifungal therapy been defined?
- Has infectious diseases follow-up been arranged, if appropriate?
- If the patient is on long-term therapy with fluconazole or an echinocandins, such as caspofungin or micafungin, has monitoring of liver enzymes been arranged?
- If the patient is taking an azole antifungal, has the ECG been reviewed to exclude QT prolongation, and have other active medications been reviewed for possible drug-azole interactions?

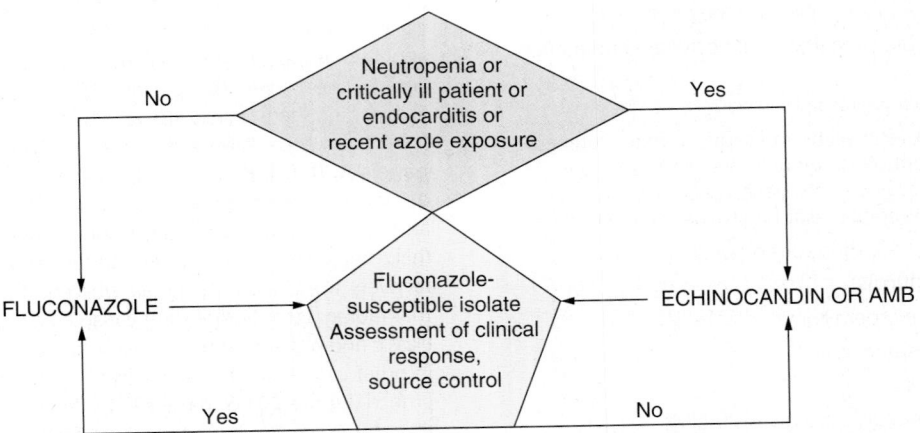

Figure 201-4 *Empiric treatment of candidemia. AMB, amphotericin-B. (Adapted from Brigham and Women's Hospital infectious diseases clinical guidelines.)*

(Azole antifungals are substrates and potent inhibitors of cytochrome P450 enzymes.)

- If discharge is considered in a patient receiving amphotericin B, which is associated with nephrotoxicity, hypokalemia and hypomagnesemia, is the accepting facility capable of closely monitoring serum creatinine, potassium, and magnesium?

ASPERGILLUS INFECTIONS

■ EPIDEMIOLOGY

Aspergillus species are ubiquitous molds that flourish in soil, decaying vegetation, and damp places, such as basements, at a wide range of temperatures. Human exposure to *Aspergillus* is common; it is not unusual to inhale hundreds of *Aspergillus* spores on a daily basis. Despite near-universal exposure and occasional bronchial colonization, symptomatic infection is exceedingly rare in immunocompetent hosts. Most cases are seen in immunocompromised patients, especially those with neutropenia or receiving high-dose glucocorticoid therapy, and patients with underlying lung disease, especially pre-existing lung cavities. Some patients with aspergillosis have low levels of mannose-binding lectin, a serum protein which is part of the innate immune system. It binds to carbohydrate residues of *Aspergillus* and other pathogens, enhancing phagocytosis by activating complement.

■ EVALUATION

Aspergillus-related disease can be thought of as a spectrum ranging from hypersensitivity (allergic bronchopulmonary aspergillosis [ABPA]), through colonization of pulmonary cavities (aspergillomas, or fungus balls), progressing to local invasion around pulmonary cavities (chronic necrotizing or semi-invasive aspergillosis), to frankly invasive aspergillosis (**Table 201-3**).

Allergic bronchopulmonary aspergillosis is an asthma syndrome driven by airway colonization with *Aspergillus*, which leads to severe and persistent bronchial inflammation and damage. Patients usually have a history of asthma, other atopic diseases, or cystic fibrosis (CF). Clinical features of asthma or CF that should increase the suspicion of ABPA include frequent wheezing, poor responses to medical therapy, fatigue, fever, fleeting pulmonary infiltrates,

TABLE 201-3 Aspergillosis Syndromes

Invasive Aspergillosis (IA)

Pulmonary:

— Invasive pulmonary aspergillosis

— Tracheobronchial aspergillosis (in patients with AIDS and lung transplant recipients, affecting the anastomotic sites)

— Chronic or subacute (semi-invasive) necrotizing pulmonary aspergillosis

— Cavitary (semi-invasive) aspergilloma

Extrapulmonary IA: osteomyelitis and septic arthritis, cutaneous aspergillosis, malignant otitis, sinonasal IA, central nervous system aspergillosis, endocarditis, pericarditis, myocarditis, endophthalmitis and keratitis, esophagitis, nephritis, hepatitis

Disseminated IA (≥2 noncontiguous organs)

Saprophytic aspergillosis

Single nonprogressive aspergilloma

Chronic pulmonary aspergillosis

Allergic aspergillosis

Allergic bronchopulmonary aspergillosis (ABPA)

Allergic *Aspergillus* sinusitis

hemoptysis, and expectoration of copious sputum with brown plugs. Patients with advanced ABPA may have central bronchiectasis on chest imaging. About 50% of ABPA patients have a positive sputum culture for *Aspergillus*. (*Aspergillus* grows on regular blood agar from sputum specimens within 1-3 days.)

The screening test for ABPA is a skin prick test with *Aspergillus* antigens. A negative result rules out ABPA. A positive result (a wheal-and-flare reaction) is not specific for ABPA, and should be confirmed with other tests, such as measurement of total serum IgE and *Aspergillus*-specific IgE or IgG.

Aspergillomas are masses of fungal material and cellular host debris in pre-existing lung cavities in patients with bullous emphysema, sarcoidosis, old tuberculosis, or other lung conditions. Isolated aspergillomas are often asymptomatic and picked up incidentally on chest radiography (**Figure 201-5, panels C-D**). Symptomatic aspergillomas present with cough, hemoptysis, malaise, weight loss, and occasionally fever. Bacterial superinfection may occur, and may be mistaken for a primary lung abscess. The diagnosis is usually made on the basis of the typical radiographic appearance of a fungus ball within a lung cavity. If the patient is rotated during chest CT scanning, the ball should be found to be mobile. Sputum and bronchoalveolar lavage cultures positive for *Aspergillus* species support the diagnosis, as do elevated levels of *Aspergillus*-specific IgG. Erythrocyte sedimentation rate and C-reactive protein are usually elevated, but these are nonspecific.

Chronic necrotizing (cavitary) aspergillosis may arise as an aspergilloma which gradually invades the surrounding lung parenchyma. Symptoms are similar to those of aspergillomas, but more severe. Patients have worsening cough, shortness of breath, and sometimes chest pain. Fever, malaise, and weight loss are often present. Hemoptysis may be massive, and is the most common cause of death in patients with chronic necrotizing aspergillosis. The definitive diagnosis of chronic necrotizing aspergillosis is based on the finding of fungal hyphae, usually with tissue invasion and infarction on lung biopsy. The yield from percutaneous biopsy is low, and thorascopic and open-lung biopsies are hazardous in these patients because of the risk of severe bleeding. If tissue is sent to microbiology for culture, it should be held for 4 weeks, as the inoculum may be very small. More often, the diagnosis is based on clinical findings. The radiographic findings are similar to those of an aspergilloma, but cavities tend to be larger and thicker walled (**Figure 201-5, panels E-I**). There may be pleural thickening adjacent to the cavity. *Aspergillus* IgG or IgE are usually elevated, but sputum cultures may be negative for *Aspergillus* species. Antigen tests (serum galactomannan and 1,3-β-D-glucan) may also be negative, even in cases with radiographic and clinical progression.

Invasive pulmonary aspergillosis (IPA) usually presents as acute pneumonia in a severely immunosuppressed patient, especially those with prolonged neutropenia, hematologic malignancy, and hematopoetic stem-cell transplantation), with cough, fever, and dyspnea. *Aspergillus* species often invade blood vessels, leading to bleeding, hemoptysis, tissue infarction, and hematogenous dissemination, especially to the central nervous system (**Figure 201-5, panels A, B, I, J, K**). High-resolution chest CT may show nodules, ground-glass changes, or peribronchial infiltrates. There may be low attenuation around lung nodules due to hemorrhage and infarction (halo sign), which may progress to formation of a lucent zone after recovery from neutropenia (air crescent sign). It should be noted that radiographic findings are variable and often nonspecific; even classic findings, including cavities and the halo sign, can be present in other clinical syndromes, such as bacterial pneumonia or septic emboli (**Figure 201-5, panels K, L**). While sputum cultures are negative for *Aspergillus* in up to 70% of patients with IPA, positive sputum cultures for *Aspergillus* in an immunosuppressed patient with pneumonia is strongly suggestive of IPA. The yield of bronchoscopy

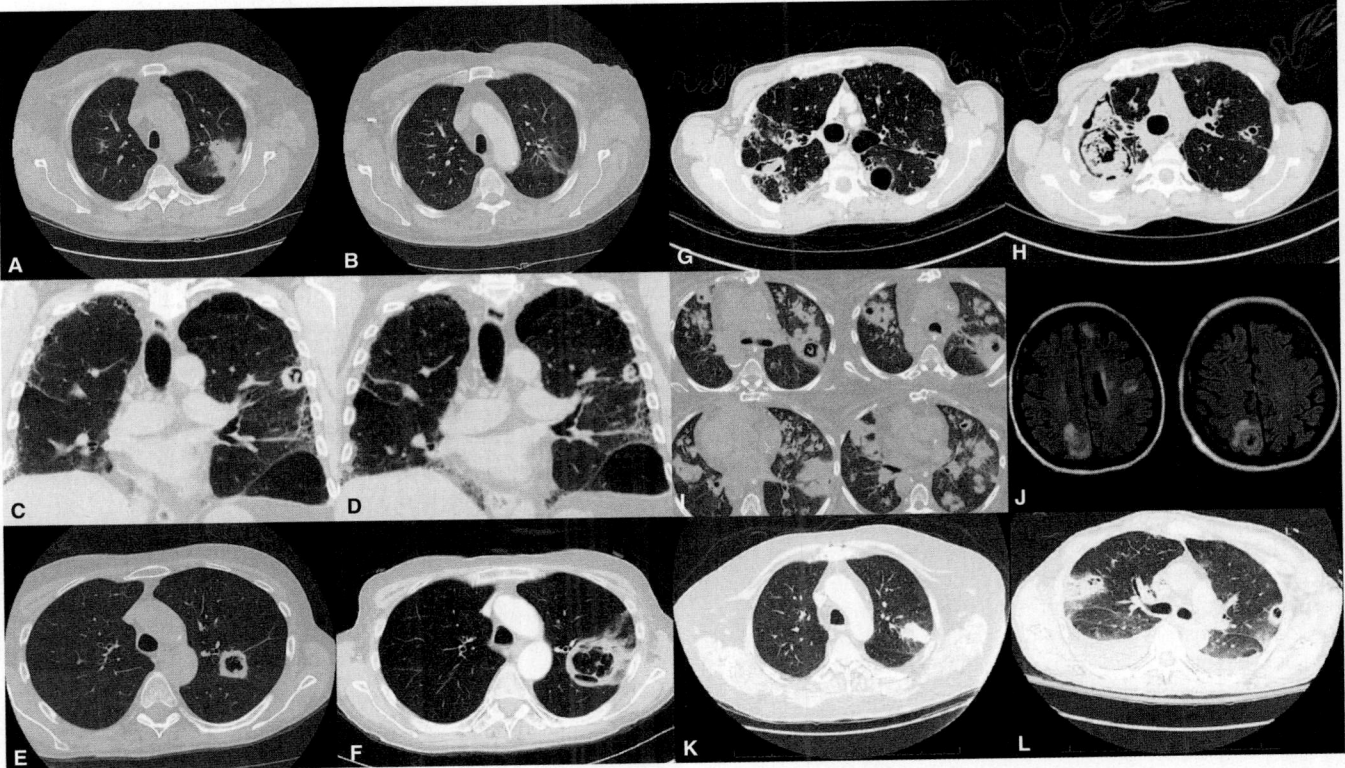

Figure 201-5 *Clinical spectrum of aspergillosis syndromes, chest computerized tomography (CT): (A and B) Invasive aspergillosis with halo sign in a patient with acute myeloid leukemia and prolonged neutropenia at presentation (A) and after 6 months of antifungal treatment and in remission with neutrophil recovery (B). (C and D) Single nonprogressive aspergilloma in a patient with idiopathic pulmonary fibrosis, slightly decreased in size after 1 year (D) without antifungal treatment. (E and F) Cavitary (semi-invasive) aspergilloma in a hematopetic stem-cell transplant (HSCT) recipient with graft-versus-host disease (GVHD), increased in size over 1 month (F). (G and H) Chronic cavitary pulmonary aspergillosis in a patient with bronchiectases, with progression after 2 years (H). (I and J) Disseminated (necrotizing cavitary pulmonary [I] and CNS [J]) aspergillosis in a patient on very high-dose chronic steroids. (K and L) The differential diagnosis for consolidated and cavitary lung lesions in the immunocompromised host is broad: invasive pulmonary aspergillosis in a HSCT recipient (K) and septic emboli with central cavitation in a solid tumor patient with MRSA bacteremia (L).*

with cultures of bronchoalveolar lavage fluid is about 50%. Tissue biopsies have a high yield, but may not be feasible due to thrombocytopenia. On biopsy specimens, *Aspergillus* species appear as filamentous fungi with frequent septations and acute-angle branching (other fungi have a similar appearance in biopsy specimens, including *Scedosporium*, *Pseudallescheria*, and *Fusarium* species).

Elevations in serum galactomannan, a cell-wall constituent of *Aspergillus* and other molds, support the diagnosis of IPA in high-risk populations, with limitations (**Table 201-4**). At the higher cutoff value

of 1.5 Optical Density Index (ODI), sensitivity is 64% and specificity is 95%. At a lower cutoff value of 0.5 ODI, sensitivity rises to 78%, but specificity falls to 81%. Serial measurements of serum galactomannan may to assess the response to therapy. Serum 1,3-β-D-glucan is less sensitive and specific than galactomannan for the diagnosis of IPA. Polymerase chain reaction for *Aspergillus* DNA in the blood and assays for *Aspergillus*-specific volatile metabolites in breath samples have shown promise as novel bedside diagnostic tests.

■ INPATIENT MANAGEMENT

High-dose glucocorticoids are the primary treatment of ABPA. Antifungal therapy is also helpful as it diminishes the burden of airway colonization with *Aspergillus*, improves clinical outcomes, and allows more rapid tapering of glucocorticoids. Oral itraconazole is the best studied agent so far, but voriconazole is also likely to be effective. Anti-IgE antibody (omalizumab) is a promising experimental treatment. Avoidance of damp areas where *Aspergillus* exposure is likely, and domestic use of high-efficiency particulate air (HEPA) filtration units, may also be beneficial.

Surgical therapy for aspergillomas and chronic necrotizing aspergillosis is potentially curative, and thoracic surgery consultation, as well as infectious diseases and pulmonology involvement, should be obtained for these patients. However, because of poor underlying lung function, surgery is risky and fraught with major complications, including bronchopleural fistulas, hemothorax, and *Aspergillus* empyema. Patients with asymptomatic aspergillomas may be observed. Patients with symptomatic aspergillomas,

---

TABLE 201-4 Usefulness and Limitations of Galactomannan Assays

Fungal infections that may result in positive tests

  Aspergillosis

  Other mold infections (*Penicillium, Paecilomyces, Alternaria, Geotrichia, Fusaria*, many others)

  Cryptococcosis

  Histoplasmosis

Causes of false-positive tests

  Antibiotics (amoxicillin-clavulanic acid, piperacillin-tazobactam, ticarcillin-clavulanic acid)

  Gluconate-containing intravenous fluids (eg, Plasmalyte)

  Graft-versus-host disease of the gastrointestinal tract

evidence of increase in size and progression on radiologic studies, or chronic necrotizing or cavitary aspergillosis may be treated with oral itraconazole or voriconazole, or intravenous voriconazole if they are acutely ill. Patients with chronic aspergillosis often require lifelong antifungal therapy.

Prior to the availability of voriconazole, the prognosis of invasive aspergillosis was extremely poor, with >50% mortality. Antifungal therapy should be initiated as soon as the disease is clinically suspected, and infectious diseases consultation should be obtained. Doses of immunosuppressive drugs, such as glucocorticoids, should be minimized. Intravenous voriconazole is recommended as primary therapy, with initial doses of 6 mg/kg IV every 12 hours for the first day, followed by 4 mg/kg IV every 12 hours thereafter. Six to 12 weeks is the minimum duration of therapy. The oral formulation has high bioavailability, and patients may be transitioned to the oral form (200 mg twice daily) once they are clinically stable and tolerating oral intake. Voriconazole directly stimulates the retina, resulting in blurring, light sensitivity, and other visual disturbances in up to 30% of patients; this phenomenon is reversible and generally mild. Liver enzymes should be monitored while on azole antifungal therapy. Long-term exposure to voriconazole is an independent risk factor for skin cancer. Because of its high fluoride content, prolonged voriconazole administration can lead to fluoride accumulation and periostitis, manifesting as diffuse bone, joint and muscle pains, along with elevated levels of bone-derived alkaline phosphatase. In patients with renal insufficiency, oral voriconazole is usually preferred for long-term use over the intravenous formulation, as the intravenous solubilizer of voriconazole (β-cyclodextrin) may accumulate and lead to worsening renal function. Alternative agents for the treatment of aspergillosis include caspofungin, micafungin, posaconazole, isavuconazole, or lipid formulations of amphotericin B. Amphotericin B is less effective against *Aspergillus terreus*.

■ COMPLICATIONS

If it is unclear whether patients are responding to voriconazole, an echinocandin may be added. (Note that pulmonary infiltrates in patients with IPA may worsen in the first week of therapy or after recovery from neutropenia.) Clinicians should monitor patients with IPA for symptoms and signs suggestive of hematogenous dissemination of *Aspergillus* to other organs. Patients with metastatic lesions may benefit from surgical debridement to reduce symptoms and increase the chance of cure. Patients with IPA and major hemoptysis, or pulmonary infiltrates adjacent to the great vessels or pericardium, may need surgery to prevent exsanguination. In patients with major hemoptysis and chronic necrotizing aspergillosis, bronchial artery embolization may be useful as a temporizing measure until medical therapy has time to be effective.

■ PREVENTION

In certain high-risk populations, such as stem-cell transplant recipients and patients undergoing induction chemotherapy for acute leukemia, posaconazole prophylaxis was shown to be beneficial in clinical trials, and has been adopted by many cancer centers. Antifungal prophylaxis should be tailored to the incidence of invasive fungal infections in local institutions and patient populations.

At-risk patients should also be cared for in special units with HEPA filters and other measures to minimize fungal exposure. Providers should educate their immunocompromised outpatients who are at risk for invasive mold infections and advise them to avoid activities that are associated with exposure to large mold inocula, such as construction or gardening.

■ DISCHARGE CONSIDERATIONS

- Is the patient medically stable for discharge on oral voriconazole therapy?
- Has outpatient infectious disease follow-up been arranged, with periodic monitoring of liver function tests and fungal markers?
- Has therapeutic drug monitoring (TDM) of voriconazole levels been arranged? The recommended target level is 1 to 5 mg/L; levels below 1 mg/L are associated with a higher risk of treatment failure, and levels above 5 mg/L with a higher risk of toxicity.

PRACTICE POINT

***Candida* and *aspergillus* in sputum cultures**

- *Candida* in a sputum culture rarely requires treatment. While some patients may have additional indications for antifungal therapy, such as oral thrush or disseminated candidiasis, antifungal therapy should not be initiated on the basis of a positive sputum culture alone.
- *Aspergillus* species are occasionally isolated from sputum cultures of elderly hospitalized patients. Most of these patients have underlying lung disease or other chronic illnesses. This usually represents bronchial colonization; less than 5% of these patients are found to have invasive pulmonary aspergillosis. More aggressive evaluation is warranted in patients with fever, pulmonary infiltrates, or weakened immunity. An important exception is recent lung transplantation, where *Candida* and *Aspergillus* can infect the anastomotic sites causing anastomotic breakdown and empyema. When sputum cultures are positive for *Candida* or *Aspergillus* in this patient population, prolonged antifungal treatment is usually indicated.

SUGGESTED READINGS

Kauffman CA. Diagnosis and management of fungal urinary tract infection. *Infect Dis Clin North Am.* 2014;28:61-74.

Leeflang MM, Debets-Ossenkopp YJ, Visser CE, et al. Galactomannan detection for invasive aspergillosis in immunocompromized patients. *Cochrane Database Syst Rev.* 2008;4:CD007394.

Leon C, Ruiz-Santana S, Saavedra P, et al. Usefulness of the "Candida score" for discriminating between Candida colonization and invasive candidiasis in non-neutropenic critically ill patients: a prospective multicenter study. *Crit Care Med.* 2009;37:1624-1633.

Marr KA, Schlamm HT, Herbrecht R, et al. Combination antifungal therapy for invasive aspergillosis: a randomized trial. *Ann Intern Med.* 2015;162:81-89.

Marty FM, Koo S. Role of (1→3)-beta-D-glucan in the diagnosis of invasive aspergillosis. *Med Mycol.* 2009;47(Suppl 1):S233-S240.

Pappas PG, Kauffman CA, Andes D, et al. Clinical practice guidelines for the management of candidiasis: 2009 update by the Infectious Diseases Society of America. *Clin Infect Dis.* 2009;48:503-535.

Segal BH. Aspergillosis. *N Eng J Med.* 2009;360:1870-1884.

Walsh TJ, Anassie EJ, Denning DW, et al. Treatment of aspergillosis: clinical practice guidelines of the Infectious Diseases Society of America. *Clin Infect Dis.* 2008;46:327-360.

Wheat JL. Approach to the diagnosis of invasive aspergillosis and candidiasis. *Clin Chest Med.* 2009;30:367-377.

CHAPTER 202

Histoplasmosis, Blastomycosis, Coccidioidomycosis, and Other Dimorphic Fungi

Donald C. Vinh, MD, FRCPC, FACP
John M. Embil, MD, FRCPC, FACP

Key Clinical Questions

❶ What are the dimorphic mycoses, and where are they endemic?

❷ What are the clinical manifestations of histoplasmosis?

❸ What is the most common extrapulmonary manifestation of blastomycosis?

❹ What patients are at greatest risk for disseminated coccidioidomycosis?

❺ What is the most common clinical presentation of sporotrichosis?

INTRODUCTION

The thermally-dimorphic mycoses are fungi which exist in the environment as a mold, but adopt a yeast-like form in the warmer conditions of the infected host. They include histoplasmosis, blastomycosis, coccidioidomycosis, penicilliosis, sporotrichosis, and paracoccidioidomycosis. With the exception of sporotrichosis, these fungi are found only in certain geographic regions. However, they may stay dormant in the host, and reactivate when the host is no longer in an endemic area, making recognition of these infections more challenging. The risk of serious infection with these pathogens is increased with iatrogenic immunosuppression, particularly tumor necrosis factor blockade.

HISTOPLASMOSIS

Histoplasma capsulatum is endemic to river basins of the United States and Canada, particularly the Mississippi, Missouri, Ohio, and St. Lawrence River valleys, as well as southwestern Ontario. It is also prevalent in Central America and the Caribbean, Southeast Asia (especially Vietnam, Thailand, Indonesia, and Malaysia), and the Mediterranean basin. In the environment, *H. capsulatum* is found in acidic, nitrogen-rich soil, conditions provided by bird or bat guano. Infections may occur when such soil is disrupted. Certain occupations, such as farming, landscaping, demolition, construction, or recreational activities, such as spelunking, may lead to high-inoculum exposures and outbreaks.

■ CLINICAL MANIFESTATIONS

In the vast majority of cases, persons infected with *H. capsulatum* are asymptomatic or have only a mild illness that is never recognized to be histoplasmosis. (These patients may be noted later in life to have pulmonary and splenic calcifications on imaging studies, consistent with remote histoplasmosis.)

A variety of clinical syndromes are seen in symptomatic patients. It is estimated that <1% of infected patients develop symptoms, although the manifestations can be diverse (**Table 202-1**). It typically presents as a self-limited pneumonic illness, characterized by chest discomfort and dry cough, with fever, fatigue, headache, myalgias, and arthralgias. Radiographically, patchy lung infiltrates involving one or more lobes is seen, frequently accompanied by mediastinal and hilar lymphadenopathy. In most patients, improvement is prompt even without treatment, although fatigue may persist. Most patients who seek medical attention are initially misdiagnosed with community-acquired pneumonia syndrome due to atypical organisms such as *Mycoplasma* or *Chlamydophila*. These patients usually improve without antifungal treatment. A minority of patients with acute self-limited pulmonary histoplasmosis develop extrapulmonary manifestations, such as erythema nodosum, self-limited symmetrical polyarticular arthritis, or sterile exudative pleural or pericardial effusions. Severe acute pulmonary histoplasmosis may occur, especially in patients with impaired cell-mediated immunity, and occasionally in healthy persons exposed to large inocula. It features the abrupt onset of fever, chills, cough, and dyspnea, with diffuse, bilateral reticulonodular or miliary infiltrates; intrathoracic lymphadenopathy may or may not be present. Acute respiratory distress syndrome may ensue.

Acute disseminated histoplasmosis occurs in patients with impaired cell-mediated immunity, such as AIDS. It manifests with

TABLE 202-1 Manifestations of Histoplasmosis

Acute pulmonary histoplasmosis syndromes

Asymptomatic/mild respiratory symptoms (most common)

Acute pneumonia, mimicking community-acquired atypical pneumonia

Severe, life-threatening pneumonia

Complications of acute pulmonary histoplasmosis

Cutaneous: erythema nodosum and erythema marginatum

Rheumatologic: myalgias, arthralgias, polyarticular symmetrical arthritis

Inflammatory pericarditis with or without pleural effusion

Granulomatous mediastinitis

Fibrosing mediastinitis

Chronic cavitary pulmonary histoplasmosis

May be accompanied by "marching cavity" or pleural thickening

Disseminated histoplasmosis

Acute disseminated histoplasmosis

Chronic progressive disseminated histoplasmosis

Endocarditis/endovascular histoplasmosis

Central nervous system histoplasmosis

relatively rapid onset of fever, chills, anorexia, malaise, and weight loss. Most patients also have pulmonary involvement, with dyspnea and cough, and diffuse reticulo-nodular, miliary, or interstitial infiltrates on chest imaging. Many other systems may be involved. Ulcers, nodules, or verrucous lesions may be present in the oral cavity. Patients may have skin ulcers, nodules, and umbilicated papules. There is usually hepatosplenomegaly and generalized lymphadenopathy. Bone marrow involvement may lead to pancytopenia. Granulomatous destruction of the adrenal glands may result in adrenal insufficiency. Gastrointestinal involvement is common in autopsy series, but is seldom symptomatic; it may occasionally produce abdominal discomfort and diarrhea. Culture-negative endocarditis, central nervous system (CNS) infection, septic arthritis, and osteomyelitis may also occur. The presentation of acute disseminated histoplasmosis can be dramatic, manifesting as severe sepsis, acute respiratory distress syndrome, multiorgan failure, disseminated intravascular coagulation, or reactive hemophagocytosis.

PRACTICE POINT

The presumed ocular histoplasmosis syndrome (POHS) causes vision loss and blindness due to chorioretinal scarring and macular choroidal neovascularization.

- Patients are typically aged 20 to 50 years, and present with sudden onset of blurred vision and loss of central visual acuity. Involvement is often bilateral.

- Most patients have resided in areas where histoplasmosis is endemic, and have pulmonary and lymph node calcification suggestive of past histoplasmosis infection.

- The histoplasmin skin test is usually positive. As antifungals are not beneficial, POHS probably represents an allergic reaction to histoplasma antigen trapped in the retina or choroidal vessels, rather than active infection.

- The prognosis was historically poor, but is much improved with contemporary therapies, including laser photocoagulation and monoclonal antibody to vascular endothelial growth factor.

Chronic progressive disseminated histoplasmosis typically occurs in older adults with no obvious immunosuppression. Patients present with fever, night sweats, weight loss, and fatigue over several months. Diffuse organ involvement similar to acute disseminated histoplasmosis is observed. Both forms of disseminated histoplasmosis are fatal if untreated.

Chronic cavitary pulmonary histoplasmosis presents in older adults with pre-existing pulmonary disease, usually emphysema. Patients have prolonged symptoms of cough, dyspnea, sputum production, and occasionally hemoptysis, resembling exacerbations of chronic obstructive pulmonary disease, but also accompanied by fatigue, fever, night sweats, anorexia, and weight loss. Radiologically, there are unilateral or bilateral cavitary upper lobe infiltrates with lower lobe fibrosis. Histoplasmosis infection of emphysematous bullae leads to wall thickening, fibrosis, and cavity formation. Ongoing necrosis can increase the size of the cavity, leading to the so-called marching cavity, with lobar destruction and progressive respiratory insufficiency. Pleural thickening adjacent to involved lung is usually seen. Fibrosis can lead to lung retraction and volume loss. Lymphadenopathy is uncommon, although calcified lymph nodes can be seen. This constellation of findings can be mistaken for tuberculosis or lung cancer, particularly in an older person with tobacco exposure.

Two rare chronic complications of histoplasmosis are worthy of mention. In most patients with acute pulmonary histoplasmosis, mediastinal lymph nodes enlarge but subsequently recede and calcify. However, in *granulomatous mediastinitis*, mediastinal and hilar lymph nodes become massive, matted, and occasionally necrotic, with enlargement persisting for months to years. In most patients, cultures are negative for *H. capsulatum*. Many patients are asymptomatic. Symptoms develop if the enlarged lymph nodes coalesce and compress adjacent structures, such as bronchi, causing recurrent postobstructive pneumonias, the superior vena cava, leading to the superior vena cava syndrome, or the esophagus, resulting in dysphagia, esophageal diverticula, or tracheoesophageal fistula. Fistulous tracts may result if the nodes drain spontaneously into adjacent structures, such as the airway or soft tissues of the neck. Most individuals have a protracted recovery over months to years, with ultimate calcification of the involved nodes.

Fibrosing mediastinitis is rare. Exuberant mediastinal fibrosis probably results from a reaction to *Histoplasma* antigens in predisposed individuals, rather than ongoing infection, as the organism is rarely seen in biopsies of involved tissue. Systemic symptoms are typically absent. The fibrotic response gradually encroaches on adjacent structures, compressing the great vessels, esophagus, heart, and the airways. It is often fatal.

■ DIAGNOSIS

The diagnosis of histoplasmosis is subject to several technical difficulties (**Table 202-2**). Definitive diagnosis requires the visualization of the yeast form in clinical specimens (**Figure 202-1**), or isolation of *H. capsulatum* in microbiological culture. However, *H. capsulatum* needs special media for recovery, and may take up to 4 weeks to grow. The sensitivity of culture is highest in chronic pulmonary histoplasmosis and disseminated histoplasmosis, where the fungal burden is large. Culture is less sensitive in milder forms of histoplasmosis with a low fungal burden. An additional limitation of culture is that the long turnaround time precludes its use for early diagnosis and initiation of treatment of histoplasmosis.

Nonculture methods have been developed to improve the diagnosis of histoplasmosis, primarily through antibody or antigen detection. For antibody detection, the two routine methodologies are complement fixation (CF) and immunodiffusion (ID). CF antibodies are more sensitive than immunodiffusion, and are the better screening test. Complement-fixing (CF) antibodies appear 2 to 6 weeks after infection and precede the ID response. A high titer

TABLE 202-2 Diagnostic Approach for Different Clinical Manifestations of Histoplasmosis

Manifestation	Diagnostic Tests
Mild acute respiratory symptoms	Serology (complement-fixation and immunodiffusion antibodies)
Acute pulmonary histoplasmosis	Bronchoalveolar lavage with antigen detection, fungal culture and stains
	Urine: antigen detection
	Serum: antigen detection; acute and convalescent serology
	Consider lung biopsy
Granulomatous mediastinitis or fibrosing mediastinitis	Serology
Chronic pulmonary histoplasmosis	Respiratory secretions: fungal stain and culture
	Serology
Disseminated histoplasmosis	Blood: fungal culture; antigen detection
	Urine: antigen detection
	Serology
	Bronchoalveolar lavage: antigen detection, fungal stain and culture
	Consider bone marrow biopsy, if patient has pancytopenia and other tests are negative
	When using antigen detection to monitor disease, serial testing should be performed before treatment, at 2 wk, 1 mo, and then every 3 mo during therapy, and for at least 6 mo after treatment is stopped

(1:32 or greater) or a fourfold increase in titer over time indicates active histoplasmosis. However, CF antibodies are less specific, often cross-reacting to *Histoplasma*-like antigens in patients infected with other fungi, such as blastomycosis, coccidioidomycosis, aspergillosis, candidiasis, and cryptococcosis. ID measures antibodies that precipitate (precipitins) to specific *Histoplasma* antigens. These antibodies appear 4 to 8 weeks after infection. While ID is more specific for histoplasmosis than CF, it is less sensitive. Limitations to serologic testing include delays of many weeks before seroconversion occurs,

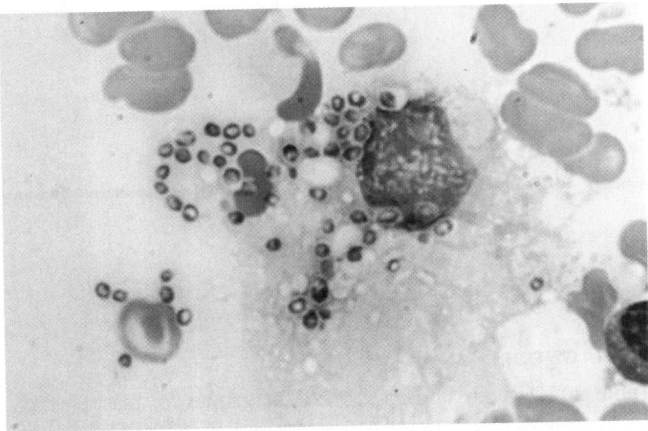

Figure 202-1 *Disseminated histoplasmosis. Bone marrow biopsy, demonstrating intracellular yeast forms in a macrophage.*

and the frequent absence of seroconversion in immunosuppressed patients with disseminated histoplasmosis. Positive serology results may also represent prior resolved infection, rather than active histoplasmosis.

Antigen detection allows histoplasmosis to be diagnosed more rapidly than traditional methods. It is most useful in patients with disseminated histoplasmosis, where its sensitivity is 95% to 98%. In patient with early acute pulmonary histoplasmosis, its sensitivity is 75% to 90%. The sensitivity of antigen detection is usually higher in urine, relative to serum. However, testing of both urine and serum provides the highest sensitivity. Antigen may also be detected in broncho-alveolar lavage fluid of patients with diffuse pulmonary infiltrates. Antigen levels can be serially followed to monitor response to therapy and diagnose relapse. Antigen testing is markedly less sensitive in the diagnosis of chronic cavitary pulmonary histoplasmosis.

■ TREATMENT

Treatment recommendations for histoplasmosis are summarized in (**Table 202-3**).

BLASTOMYCOSIS

Blastomycosis is caused by *Blastomyces dermatitidis* and *Blastomyces gilchristii*. In the United States, it is endemic in the states bordering the Great Lakes and in the Mississippi River basin. It is especially common in Wisconsin, Mississippi, Missouri, Kentucky, Tennessee, Arkansas, and Alabama. In Canada, blastomycosis is endemic in Manitoba and western Ontario, and has been occasionally reported from eastern Canada. It is also seen sporadically worldwide. Risk factors for blastomycosis infection include exposure to soil, especially disrupted or aerosolized soil, recreational or professional exposure to waterways, and immunosuppression.

Infections occur from inhalation of aerosolized conidia; rarely, infections result from animal bites or laboratory accidents. Inhaled conidia transform to the yeast phase at body temperature in the lungs. Initial infection may be asymptomatic or lead to symptomatic pneumonia. In either case, most patients contain *B. dermatitidis* infection in noncaseating granulomas. A few persons have progressive pneumonia, or develop extrapulmonary manifestations from dissemination beyond the lungs. The most common sites of involvement in blastomycosis, in descending order of frequency, are lung, skin, bone, genitourinary tract, and central nervous system. The median incubation period is 30 to 45 days, with a longer incubation period for extrapulmonary disease.

■ CLINICAL MANIFESTATIONS

Blastomycosis is one of the diseases that has been called "the great mimic." This is particularly true of **pneumonia** may cause lobar infiltrates indistinguishable from bacterial pneumonia, miliary disease that resembles pulmonary tuberculosis, nodules and mass lesions that are similar to pulmonary neoplasms, and cavities that mimic anaerobic lung abscesses or tuberculosis. Acute pneumonia presents with fevers, chills, dyspnea, and cough which is usually nonproductive initially. Chronic pneumonia may develop, with the clinical presentation of a nonresolving community-acquired pneumonia. It may be associated with additional symptoms of weight loss, productive cough, and hemoptysis. Occasionally, patients may develop respiratory failure and the acute respiratory distress syndrome.

Cutaneous lesions are the most common extrapulmonary form of blastomycosis. They result from dissemination of a primary pulmonary lesion or less often from direct inoculation, and are either verrucous or ulcerated in appearance. Other forms of extrapulmonary blastomycosis include osteomyelitis, with the long bones and axial skeleton

TABLE 202-3 Recommendations for the Treatment of Histoplasmosis

Manifestation	Primary Treatment	Alternative Treatment	Comments
Asymptomatic	None		
Mild/self-limited disease	None		
Acute pulmonary histoplasmosis	None usually required	If patient remains symptomatic for >1 mo: itraconazole 200 mg orally three times a day for 3 d, then 200 mg orally qd or twice a day for 6-12 wk	
Acute severe pulmonary histoplasmosis	Lipid-AmB 3-5 mg/kg IV qd for 1-2 wk, then itraconazole 200 mg three times a day for 3 d then 200 mg twice a day (for total 12 wk of itraconazole)	AmB deoxycholate 0.7-1 mg/kg IV qd in place of Lipid-AmB	If there is significant hypoxia or acute respiratory distress syndrome, consider concomitant methylprednisolone 0.5-1 mg/kg IV for the first 1-2 wk of antifungal therapy
Dermatologic/rheumatologic complications of acute pulmonary histoplasmosis	Nonsteroidal anti-inflammatory drugs	In severe cases, consider prednisone 0.5-1 mg/kg qd (max 80 mg qd) in tapering doses over 1-2 wk	If steroids are administered, itraconazole is recommended: 200 mg orally three times a day for 3 d, then 200 mg orally qd or twice a day for 6-12 wk
Granulomatous mediastinitis	Incidental findings do not usually require therapy	If symptomatic: itraconazole 200 mg orally three times a day for 3 d, then 200 mg orally qd or twice a day for 6-12 wk	
Fibrosing mediastinitis	None	Symptomatic support (eg, intravascular stents for vessel obstruction); airways stents should be approached cautiously because of high risk of granulation tissue leading to recurrent obstruction	If findings suggest more of an inflammatory process (rather than chronic fibrosis), consider antifungal treatment If clear distinction from granulomatous mediastinitis is not possible, consider antifungal treatment Corticosteroids are ineffective and are discouraged
Chronic cavitary pulmonary histoplasmosis	Itraconazole 200 mg orally three times a day for 3 d, then 200 mg orally qd or twice a day for ≥1 y (possibly 18-24 mo)		Continue treatment until pulmonary imaging reveals no further improvement at 4-6 mo intervals. Monitor for ≥ 1 y after treatment is stopped
Disseminated	Lipid-AmB (3-5 mg/kg) IV qd for 1-2 wk, then itraconazole 200 mg orally three times a day for 3 d, then 200 mg twice a day for ≥12 mo	AmB deoxycholate 0.7-1 mg/kg IV qd in place of Lipid-AmB; for mild-to-moderate disseminated disease, itraconazole 200 mg orally three times a day for 3 d, then 200 mg orally twice a day for ≥12 mo	In patients with irreversible immunocompromise, and in patients who relapse despite appropriate therapy, lifelong suppression with oral itraconazole 200 mg qd Monitor antigen level during therapy, and for 12 mo after therapy is ended
Endocarditis	AmB or Lipid-AmB	Surgical valve replacement	If valve surgery is not possible, consider lifelong suppression with itraconazole
Central nervous system	Liposomal AmB (5.0 mg/kg IV qd for a total of 175 mg/kg given over 4-6 wk) followed by itraconazole (200 mg orally 2 or 3 times qd) for ≥1 y and until resolution of cerebrospinal fluid abnormalities, including antigen levels		

AmB, amphotericin B; Lipid-AmB, lipid formulation of amphotericin B.
Because of insufficient data, all other available azoles are deemed alternatives to itraconazole.
When using itraconazole, random blood concentration of ≥ 1 μg/mL is recommended.

being most frequently affected, prostatitis, and central nervous system involvement, which may present with chronic meningitis, mass lesions, or brain abscess. Blastomycosis may be especially aggressive in immunocompromised hosts, who are prone to respiratory failure and disseminated disease, with mortality rates of 30% to 40%.

■ DIAGNOSIS

Table 202-4 summarizes diagnostic techniques for blastomycosis. The most reliable is recovery of *Blastomyces* sp in culture. Direct observation of the pathogen with wet preparations under light microscopy, calcofluor white stains under immunofluorescence microscopy, or

TABLE 202-4 Diagnostic Tests for Blastomycosis

Technique	Comments
Direct examination	A wet preparation of respiratory secretions or other tissues under light microscope may reveal characteristic forms of the pathogen, but have a low diagnostic yield; calcofluor white stains are more useful but require fluorescence microscopy
Histopathologic examination	The microorganism may be difficult to identify with standard hematoxylin and eosin stains; Gomori methenamine-silver stain should be performed if *B. dermatitidis* is suspected
Culture	Diagnostic yield is approximately 86% from sputum and 92% from bronchoscopic specimens. Growth of *B. dermatitidis* may require several weeks
Serology	Serology is neither sensitive nor specific
Nucleic acid detection	Detect genetic material in culture specimens where *B. dermatitidis* is suspected; may reduce the time required for identification of the pathogen in culture
Antigen detection	The only currently available antigen detection assay has its greatest sensitivity in urine, although antigens can be detected in serum and other body fluids. Cross-reaction with other antigens (eg, histoplasmosis) may occur. Probably most useful in following the efficacy of treatment response
Skin testing	Not currently available for clinical use

biopsy specimens may also be helpful. Serologic assays have limited sensitivity and specificity, and are not reliable in diagnosis. Urinary antigen assays are reasonably sensitive in diagnosis, especially when the burden of disease is high. Newer assays can reliably distinguish blastomycosis from nonfungal infections, but false positive tests may still be a problem in patients with histoplasmosis.

■ TREATMENT

Amphotericin B deoxycholate is recommended for severe blastomycosis or central nervous system involvement, based on the greater clinical experience with these agents compared to alternative drugs. Lipid preparations of amphotericin may also be effective, although clinical experience in blastomycosis is limited. After stabilization with amphotericin B, patients with severe disease or central nervous system involvement may be stepped down to oral itraconazole to complete the total duration of therapy. Although fluconazole is effective against *Blastomyces* sp., experience with this agent is limited. Fluconazole has excellent penetration into the central nervous system, and may be considered for step-down therapy of central nervous system blastomycosis. Voriconazole has also been used in central nervous system blastomycosis and in refractory blastomycosis. The echinocandins, such as caspofungin, micafungin and anidulafungin, have limited activity against *Blastomyces* sp., and should be avoided. Pulmonary, cutaneous, or musculoskeletal blastomycosis of mild to moderate severity may be treated with prolonged courses of oral itraconazole. Patients with irreversible immunosuppression may require lifelong suppressive itraconazole therapy at 200 mg/d, after completion of primary therapy (**Table 202-5**).

COCCIDIOIDOMYCOSIS

Coccidioidomycosis is caused by two morphologically indistinguishable but genetically distinct fungi, *Coccidioides immitis* and *Coccidioides posadasii*. *Coccidioides* species grow in nature as a mold composed of barrel-shaped arthroconidia that alternate with nonviable brittle cells. The brittle cells degenerate, allowing the arthroconidia to become airborne in the event of wind or soil disturbance. Infection occurs after inhalation of an arthroconidial spore. Within the lung, the arthroconidia develop into large multinucleated spherical structures called spherules. These undergo internal division to release infectious endospores, which may develop into new spherules.

Unlike most fungi, which thrive in damp conditions, *Coccidioides* species are endemic to hot, arid regions of the southwestern United States, particularly Arizona and the San Joaquin Valley of California. They may also be found in neighboring states (New Mexico, Texas, Utah, Nevada), Central America (Mexico, Guatemala, Honduras, Nicaragua) and South America (Venezuela, Colombia, Paraguay, Argentina). The incidence of coccidioidomycosis is increasing, probably because of environmental factors and population influx into endemic regions.

■ CLINICAL MANIFESTATIONS

The spectrum of illness due to *Coccidoides* is broad (**Tables 202-6** and **202-7**). While infection is common, disease is not. Determinants of disease state and severity reflect biological interactions between pathogen and host.

Asymptomatic. Approximately 60% of persons infected by *Coccidioides* spp., as evidenced by recent exposure and skin test conversion, are asymptomatic and identified primarily during epidemiological investigations. Virtually all persons with these subclinical infections are protected from second primary infections.

Symptomatic. The remaining 35% to 40% of infected patients are acutely or subacutely symptomatic. The most common presentation is a mild, influenza-like respiratory syndrome or a community-acquired pneumonia 1 to 3 weeks after exposure. Primary coccidioidal pneumonia cannot readily be distinguished from viral or bacterial pneumonia. High clinical suspicion is required for diagnosis, based on patient residence or travel history, and confirmed by specific laboratory testing. The most common chest radiographic finding is a nondescript pulmonary infiltrate. In up to 25% of cases, there may be ipsilateral hilar or paratracheal lymphadenopathy. Mediastinal adenopathy is associated with a higher risk of disseminated disease. Pleural effusions are present in 5% to 20% of symptomatic acute primary infections; these are typically small exudates with a predominance of mononuclear cells (usually lymphocytes), and a glucose concentration similar to that of serum. A mild increase in eosinophils may also be seen in pleural fluid.

Most cases of acute pneumonia resolve completely, either spontaneously or with treatment, within 3 weeks. However, some develop pulmonary or systemic sequelae. Approximately 5% of primary infections result in toxic erythema, erythema nodosum or erythema marginatum, with associated noninfectious arthritis; most of those patients have self-limited infection. Asthenia, or profound fatigue interfering with normal activities, is common and may last weeks to months. Approximately 5% to 10% of patients who present with respiratory symptoms, but without sepsis or extrapulmonary disease, develop residual lung complications, typically nodules or peripheral thin-walled cavities; cavities may be particularly more common in patients with diabetes mellitus. These manifestations may erroneously raise a suspicion of lung cancer, especially in nonendemic areas.

Occasionally, the pneumonic illness persists for greater than 3 months, progressing to a chronic pulmonary infection, with productive cough, hemoptysis, dyspnea, fever, night sweats, fatigue, and weight loss. In association with these symptoms, biapical fibronodular lesions with retraction are commonly seen radiographically; occasionally, cavitary lesions also occur.

TABLE 202-5 Treatment Regimens for Blastomycosis

Presentation	Treatment Suggestions	Comments
Pulmonary infection		
• Moderate to severe	• Amphotericin B deoxycholate 0.7-1 mg/kg/d for 1-2 wk until stable or lipid preparations of amphotericin B 3-5 mg/kg/d for 1-2 wk followed by oral itraconazole 200 mg twice a day for 6-12 mo	• An alternative approach is to use deoxycholate amphotericin B to complete a total dose of 1.5-2.5 g, however, amphotericin B toxicity can be attenuated by minimizing the duration of therapy and switching to oral therapy when the patient is stable.
• Mild to moderate	• Itraconazole 200 mg orally once daily or twice a day for 6-12 mo	• Alternative therapies that have been suggested are ketoconazole 400-800 mg/kg or fluconazole 400 mg-800 mg/d.
Disseminated infection, not involving central nervous system		
• Moderate to severe	• Amphotericin B deoxycholate 0.7-1 mg/kg/d or lipid preparations of amphotericin B 3-5 mg/kg/d for 1-2 wk followed by oral itraconazole 200 mg twice a day to complete 12 mo of therapy	• An entire treatment course can be completed with deoxycholate amphotericin B to achieve a total dose of 2 g. To minimize toxicity, however, switching to oral therapy once the patient is stable should be considered. Bone and joint infections are usually treated for 12 mo with itraconazole.
• Mild to moderate	• Itraconazole 200 mg orally once daily or twice a day for 6-12 mo	• It has been suggested that liposomal amphotericin B achieves higher central nervous system levels than other lipid formulations. Switching to oral fluconazole 800 mg orally once daily or itraconazole 200 mg orally twice a day or three times a day; or voriconazole 200-400 mg orally twice a day should be considered. Longer durations of therapy may be necessary for those who are immunocompromised. Bone and joint infections are usually treated for 12 mo with itraconazole.
• Involving central nervous system	• Lipid preparations of amphotericin B 5 mg/kg/d for 4-6 wk followed by an oral azole for at least 12 mo	
Special populations		
• Immunocompromised	• Amphotericin B deoxycholate 0.7-1 mg/kg/d or lipid preparation of amphotericin B 3-5 mg/kg/d for 1-2 wk followed by itraconazole 200 mg orally twice a day for 12 mo	• Lifelong suppression with itraconazole 200 mg orally once daily may be required for those in whom immunosuppression cannot be reversed.
• Pregnant	• If the newborn demonstrates evidence of infection, amphotericin B deoxycholate 1.0 mg/kg/d	• During pregnancy, azoles should be avoided because of potential teratogenicity.

Data from Chapman SW, Bradsher RW, Campbell GD, Pappas PG, Kauffman CA. Practice guidelines for the management of patients with blastomycosis. *Clin Infect Dis.* 2000;30:679-683; and Chapman SW, Dismukes WE, Proia LA, Bradsher RW, Pappas PG, Threlkeld MG, Kauffman CA. Clinical practice guidelines for the management of blastomycosis: 2008 update by the Infectious Diseases Society of America. *Clin Infect Dis.* 2008;46:1801-1812.

Although self-limiting respiratory symptoms are by far the most common presentation of pulmonary coccidioidomycosis, diffuse multilobar pneumonia may also occur. This presentation may occur during primary infection, typically from inhalation of an overwhelmingly large inoculum of arthroconidia in otherwise immunocompetent individuals. Alternatively, it may occur as a late manifestation from hematogenous dissemination in patients with underlying immunodeficiency. Typically, patients are severely ill and hypoxemic; respiratory failure or septic shock may develop. Radiographically, diffuse miliary or reticulonodular infiltrates are seen. As diffuse coccidioidal pneumonia usually results from hematogenous dissemination, patients should be evaluated for extrapulmonary disease.

TABLE 202-7 Symptoms of Acute or Subacute Pulmonary Coccidioidomycosis

Most common

Fever

Cough, with or without sputum production

Pleuritic chest pain

Dyspnea

Systemic

Fatigue, chills, weight loss, night sweats, headache

Associated findings

Toxic erythema: diffuse, erythematous, pruritic rash

Erythema nodosum: painful, erythematous nodules

Erythema multiforme: erythematous, raised patches with a target-like appearance

Arthralgias and myalgias ("desert rheumatism")

TABLE 202-6 Main Clinical Manifestations of Coccidioidomycosis

Acute pneumonia

Chronic progressive fibrocavitary pneumonia

Diffuse pneumonia

Pulmonary nodules and cavities

Extrapulmonary, nonmeningeal disease

Meningitis and other central nervous system disease

Pulmonary nodules or cavities may be the residua of acute coccidioidal pneumonia in patients with longitudinal follow-up and serial radiographs. It may also be the initial manifestation of coccidioidal infection, particularly in patients who were previously asymptomatic or subacutely ill. An exposure history and specific *Coccidioides* testing may elucidate the cause of the nodule or cavity. However, exclusion of other etiologies may also be necessary. While most coccidioidal nodules or cavities are asymptomatic, they may also be associated with cough, pleuritic chest pain, or hemoptysis, depending on the proximity of the lesions to adjacent structures. Peripheral or pleural-based lesions may even rupture into the pleural space, resulting in a hydropneumothorax.

Disseminated disease occurs via hematogenous dissemination, usually from a primary pulmonary source, and manifests weeks to months after initial infection. Disseminated coccidioidomycosis occurs in <1% to 5% of those infected, with Filipinos, African Americans, Latinos, pregnant women, and immunocompromised patients being at highest risk. The most common sites of involvement are the CNS, skin, bones, joints, and lymph nodes. Hepatosplenomegaly and miliary lung disease also occur. Most, but not all, patients with extrapulmonary coccidioidomycosis have disseminated disease.

Coccidioidal CNS disease primarily manifests as meningitis. The most common symptom is headache. Fever and altered mental status may or may not be present. Coccidioidal meningitis is typically basilar in location, and may lead to cranial nerve deficits. Meningismus is found in about 50% of cases. Examination of the cerebrospinal fluid (CSF) reveals lymphocyte-predominant pleocytosis, although neutrophil predominance may be seen. The presence of eosinophils, while uncommon, is highly suggestive of coccidioidal meningitis in a patient with appropriate risk factors. CSF protein is elevated and CSF glucose is depressed. Untreated coccidioidal meningitis is fatal. Even with treatment, patients are high risk for complications. Hydrocephalus is common, and may be either a presenting manifestation or a late complication. Ventriculoperitoneal shunt placement is often necessary. Late-onset hydrocephalus suggests active infection, even in patients on appropriate antifungal therapy. CNS vasculitis with endarteritis obliterans is a dreaded complication. It presents with rapidly evolving mental status changes and focal neurological deficits.

The skin is the most common site of disseminated disease. Cutaneous coccidioidal disease must be distinguished from immunologic reactions, such as erythema nodosum, accompanying primary pulmonary coccidioidomycosis. Dermatologic manifestations most commonly occur as papules, nodules, or verrucous plaques; lesions can progress to ulcers, with or without draining sinuses, and abscesses. Classically, skin lesions are seen on the nasolabial fold as well as the sternoclavicular area, although they may occur anywhere.

Musculoskeletal involvement occurs in 20% of patients with disseminated disease. Coccidioidal osteomyelitis most commonly affects the vertebral column. Spinal disease is frequently accompanied by retroperitoneal or paraspinal masses, but spares the intervertebral disks. Affected long bones demonstrate well-demarcated lytic lesions, while smaller bones usually have a moth-eaten appearance.

■ DIAGNOSIS

Definitive diagnosis requires visualization of the fungus in clinical specimens, or growth in fungal culture. The identification of spherules on mycological stains from tissues or fluids is pathognomonic for disease, although the sensitivity varies depending on the type of clinical specimen. Fungal culture is more sensitive than stains, but results are delayed. The availability of specific DNA probes allows earlier identification of positive cultures than traditional tests for dimorphism (mold-to-yeast conversion).

Serology is a mainstay of diagnosis, particularly when satisfactory specimens cannot be obtained for culture. Serology results

are also useful for monitoring response to therapy. Two major serologic assays are used. The tube precipitin-reacting antigen detects IgM antibodies, which are found in up to 75% of case of primary infection. These antibodies eventually disappear with resolution of the primary infection, and are not seen in chronic disease. The complement-fixing (CF) antigen detects IgG antibodies. In addition to indicating chronic infection, the IgG titer correlates with activity of disease. In coccidioidal meningitis, CSF can be tested for IgG by CF antigen to confirm diagnosis; IgG titers in CSF are useful for monitoring disease. Of note, serologic testing may produce false-negative results early in infection, as well as in immunosuppressed patients.

An enzyme immunoassay (EIA) for detection of *Coccidioides* galactomannan antigen has been developed. This assay performs relatively well in immunocompromised patients with severe coccidioidomycosis, and antigen levels correlate well with disease activity.

PRACTICE POINT

- *Coccidioides immitis* is especially hazardous to microbiology technicians, as arthroconidia are easily dispersed and aerosolized in the laboratory.
- Specimens from patients with suspected coccidioidomycosis should be sent to the clinical microbiology laboratory with explicit notification of this provisional diagnosis, to minimize the risk of inadvertent exposure to laboratory workers.

■ TREATMENT

Treatment is summarized in **Table 202-8**.

OTHER DIMORPHIC MYCOSES

■ PENICILLIOSIS

Penicillium marneffei is a dimorphic fungus endemic to tropical Asia, causing disseminated infections in HIV-positive and immunocompromised travelers and residents. It is most common in Vietnam, Thailand, Taiwan, China, Hong Kong, and northeastern India. The fungus is thought to be a primary pulmonary pathogen, with infection presumably via inhalation of conidia from the environment. Penicilliosis most often affects patients with advanced HIV (CD4+ lymphocyte counts ≤100 cells/µL). Most patients present with fever, weight loss, respiratory symptoms, skin findings, generalized lymphadenopathy, and hepatosplenomegaly. Definitive diagnosis of pencilliosis due to *P. marneffei* is made by identification of the fungus from smear, culture, or histopathological sections. Amphotericin B for 2 weeks, followed by itraconazole for 10 weeks, is effective primary therapy. After primary treatment, secondary prophylaxis with itraconazole is given to prevent relapse. HIV-positive patients may possibly discontinue secondary prophylaxis when there is sustained immune reconstitution.

■ SPOROTRICHOSIS

Sporotrichosis is caused by *Sporothrix schenckii*, a thermally dimorphic fungus with a worldwide distribution. It is ubiquitous in the environment, growing well in soil, sphagnum moss, and decaying vegetation. Gardeners, carpenters, farmers, and forestry workers become infected by traumatic inoculation of fungal spores through the skin, typically from rose and other plant thorns or wood splinters. Cutaneous or lymphocutaneous sporotrichosis is the most common presenting syndrome. After fungal inoculation into soft tissues, a papulonodular lesion develops 1 to 4 weeks later, followed by secondary erythematous nodular lesions ascending proximally along

TABLE 202-8 Management of Coccidioidomycosis

Syndrome	Antifungal Therapy		Comments
	Primary	**Alternative**	
Acute coccidioidal pneumonia			
Uncomplicated	Unclear if treatment necessary in most cases	Some authorities recommend treatment for all symptomatic patients: fluconazole or itraconazole 400 mg qd for at least 4-6 wk after active infection resolved	If no treatment, follow-up recommended every 3-6 mo for up to 2 y (history, physical examination, imaging, serology)
At-risk for disseminated disease*	Fluconazole (400-800 mg) or itraconazole (200-400 mg) qd for 3-6 mo		During pregnancy, amphotericin B is recommended, as azoles may be teratogenic
Severe illness†	Fluconazole (400-800 mg) or itraconazole (400-600 mg) qd for 3-6 mo		
Chronic progressive fibrocavitary pneumonia	Oral azole for at least 1 y	If no improvement with primary azole, consider alternate azole, increasing dose, or amphotericin B	For circumscribed refractory lesions, or if hemoptysis: consider resection
Diffuse pneumonia‡	Amphotericin B (0.5-1.5 mg/kg qd or alternate day) *or* lipid-formulation amphotericin B (≥ 2.0-5.0 mg/kg/d) or Fluconazole (400-800 mg) until clear evidence of improvement (usually weeks), then maintenance therapy	Maintenance therapy: oral azole for total duration of therapy of at least 1 y; or oral azole for duration of immunodeficiency (if one identified)	Evaluation for extrapulmonary disease should be performed
Pulmonary nodules	For stable nodules:§ antifungal therapy or resection not necessary	For completely resected lesion: antifungal therapy usually not required	For enlarging lesion, confirm diagnosis of coccidioidomycosis, exclude alternate diagnosis (eg, malignancy). Treat if active infection documented
Pulmonary cavities	If asymptomatic: no intervention	If present > 2 y later, if enlargement, if adjacent to pleura, if symptomatic (eg, hemoptysis): consider resection If rupture with pyopneumothorax: lobectomy with decortication	
Extrapulmonary, nonmeningeal disease	Oral azole, consider high-doses (eg, fluconazole up to 2000 mg qd, or itraconazole 800 mg qd)	Amphotericin B or lipid formulation amphotericin B	Consider surgical debridement or stabilization (eg, with vertebral body involvement)
Meningitis	Fluconazole 400 mg qd (up to 800-1000 mg qd)	Itraconazole 400-600 mg qd alone or with Intrathecal amphotericin B 0.1-1.5 mg /dose	Monitor for hydrocephalus, which may require shunt decompression (but not necessarily a change in antifungal agent); after resolution, lifelong azole therapy indicated

*Conditions associated with potential for severe or disseminated disease and thus warrant consideration of treatment include advanced HIV infection, diabetes mellitus, preexisting cardiac or pulmonary disease, pregnancy (especially 3rd trimester or immediate postpartum period), high-dose corticosteroids, tumor necrosis factor antagonists, and Filipino or African descent.
†Age > 55 y; weight loss > 10%; intense night sweats > 3 wk; symptoms > 2 mo; inability to work; infiltrates involving > ½ of one lung or portions of both lungs; prominent or persistent hilar lymphadenopathy; anticoccidioidal complement-fixing antibody > 1:16.
‡Bilateral reticulo-nodular or miliary infiltrates.
§Stable nodule defined as no change in size on serial radiologic imaging for 2 y.

lymphatic channels. This pattern is known as nodular lymphangitis (**Figure 202-2**). *Mycobacterium marinum* and other pathogens may also cause a similar clinical picture (**Table 202-9**). Diagnosis requires fungal isolation from tissue cultures. Itraconazole or terbinafine are used in treatment. Hot compresses may be a useful adjunctive therapy, as heat inhibits the growth of *S. schenckii*.

■ PARACOCCIDIOIDOMYCOSIS

Paracoccidioidomycosis is caused by *Paracoccidioides brasiliensis*, a dimorphic fungus endemic in South America, with most reported cases from Brazil, Colombia, Venezuela, Ecuador, and Argentina. It mainly affects men, and usually presents as an indolent systemic infection over several months, leading to skin nodules, mucosal ulcerations, ulcerative lymphadenitis, and chronic pneumonia of the lower lobes. Hematogenous dissemination may lead to visceral involvement, bone disease, and involvement of the CNS. Definitive diagnosis of paracoccidioidomycosis is based on the visualization of the gemmating (budding) "ship's wheel" yeast-like forms in biopsy specimens, as well as culture and serology. Prolonged treatment is required. Trimethoprim-sulfamethoxazole or itraconazole are used in non–life-threatening disease. Severe disease should be treated initially with amphotericin B.

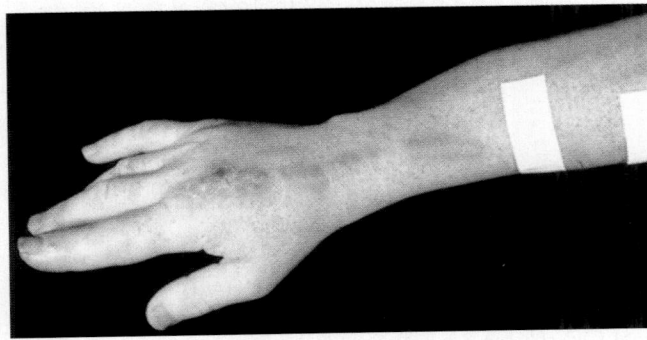

Figure 202-2 *Lymphangitic spread of nodular sporotrichosis.* (Reproduced, with permission, from Wolff K, Johnson RA, Suurmond D. *Fitzpatrick's Color Atlas & Synopsis of Clinical Dermatology*, 5th ed. New York, NY: McGraw-Hill, 2005. Fig. 25-44.)

TABLE 202-9 Differential Diagnosis of Nodular Lymphangitis

Sporothrix schenckii

Mycobacterium marinum

Francisella tularensis

Nocardia spp.

Leishmania brasiliensis

Other fungi: *Blastomyces dermatitidis*; *Histoplasma capsulatum*; *Cryptococcus neoformans*

Miscellaneous: *Bacillus anthracis*; cowpox virus

SUGGESTED READINGS

Assi MA, Sandid MS, Baddour LM, Roberts GD, Walker RC. Systemic histoplasmosis: a 15-year retrospective institutional review of 111 patients. *Medicine (Baltimore)*. 2007;86:162-169.

Chapman SW, Dismukes WE, Proia LA, et al. Clinical practice guidelines for the management of blastomycosis: 2008 update by the Infectious Diseases Society of America. *Clin Infect Dis*. 2008;46:1801-1812.

Galgiani JN, Ampel NM, Blair JE, et al. Infectious Diseases Society of America. Coccidioidomycosis. *Clin Infect Dis*. 2005;41:1217-1223.

Kauffman CA, Bustamante B, Chapman SW, Pappas PG. Infectious Diseases Society of America. Clinical practice guidelines for the management of sporotrichosis: 2007 update by the Infectious Diseases Society of America. *Clin Infect Dis*. 2007;45:1255-1265.

Luckett K, Dummer JS, Miller G, et al. Histoplasmosis in patients with cell-mediated immunodeficiency: HIV infection, organ transplantation, and tumor necrosis factor-α inhibition. *Open Forum Infect Dis*. 2015;2(1):ofu116.

Wheat LJ, Freifeld AG, Kleiman MB, et al. Infectious Diseases Society of America. Clinical practice guidelines for the management of patients with histoplasmosis: 2007 update by the Infectious Diseases Society of America. *Clin Infect Dis*. 2007;45:807-825.

CHAPTER 203

The Hospitalized Patient with HIV

Claire E. Farel, MD, MPH
Jonathan B. Parr, MD, MPH
Paul E. Sax, MD

Key Clinical Questions

1. What conditions cause symptoms in human immunodeficiency virus (HIV) patients?

2. How are opportunistic infections diagnosed and treated?

3. What noninfectious problems are common in HIV patients?

4. When should antiretroviral therapy be started?

INTRODUCTION

More than 1.2 million people are human immunodeficiency virus (HIV) seropositive in the United States. As survival with HIV has increased because of antiretroviral therapy (ART), the spectrum of illness affecting this population has expanded. Opportunistic infections (OIs) still occur in untreated patients and patients who do not adhere to therapy. However, in patients whose HIV infection is controlled by ART, noninfectious problems such as metabolic syndrome, coronary artery disease, pulmonary hypertension, and malignancy are increasing in prevalence. This chapter uses a symptom-based approach to guide differential diagnosis in HIV, and outlines the presentation, diagnosis, and treatment of common opportunistic infections. Other aspects of HIV therapy important to the hospitalist are discussed, including medication interactions and side effects.

PATHOPHYSIOLOGY AND NATURAL HISTORY

Most patients with acute HIV infection develop symptoms between 2 and 4 weeks after exposure. Some patients are asymptomatic, but many report an acute febrile illness resembling mononucleosis. Features may include rash, anorexia, mucocutaneous ulcerations, pharyngitis, lymphadenopathy, diarrhea, myalgias, and rarely meningoencephalitis. HIV antibody does not appear until 3 to 4 weeks after the symptoms of acute HIV syndrome develop. However, fourth-generation HIV immunoassays that detect both HIV antibody and p24 antigen can detect acute HIV as early as 2 weeks after infection. Current guidelines recommend routine initial testing with a fourth-generation HIV immunoassay followed by confirmatory testing. HIV RNA (viral load) testing can detect acute infection at as early as 5 days and should be obtained if there is concern for recent infection, fourth-generation immunoassay testing is unavailable, or initial results are indeterminate. Clinicians should bear in mind that patients with acute HIV infection may also have acquired other infections, such as viral hepatitis, syphilis, or cytomegalovirus (CMV), at the time of their HIV exposure.

Human immunodeficiency virus depletes CD4+ lymphocytes, also known as T-helper cells, leading to OIs. In acute HIV infection, CD4+ cells decline sharply, generally followed by a modest rebound, as HIV replication is brought under partial control. Over time, viremia rises, CD4+ cells are gradually depleted, and acquired immunodeficiency syndrome (AIDS) develops.

The tempo for progression to AIDS has great individual variability. Illnesses such as seborrheic dermatitis, cutaneous zoster, bacterial pneumonia, and cytopenias, while not specific to HIV, occur with increased frequency in patients with waning CD4+ cells and may be a clue to undiagnosed HIV.

TRIAGE/CONSULTATION

Admission of the patient with CD4+ count >500 cells/mm³, suppressed viral load, and admission for a non–HIV-related reason does not necessarily require infectious diseases consultation. By contrast, newly diagnosed HIV, acute opportunistic infections, undifferentiated illness in patients with more advanced HIV, or possible modification of ART warrant review by a specialist familiar with HIV disease and its management.

DIAGNOSTIC APPROACH: GENERAL PRINCIPLES

Along with whether the patient is currently taking ART, the most recent CD4+ cell count is critical in determining the likelihood of an

TABLE 203-1 HIV: Stages of Immunodeficiency and Commonly Associated Illnesses

CD4+ Count	Opportunistic Infections	HIV- or AIDS- Associated Conditions
<500 cells/mm³	• *M. tuberculosis* (seen at all stages of HIV infection)	• Candidal infection (oral, vaginal) • Herpes simplex infection (oral, genital) • Cutaneous zoster
<200 cells/mm³	• *P. jirovecii* pneumonia • *Candida* esophagitis • Cryptococcal infection	AIDS-associated malignancies: • Kaposi sarcoma • Non-Hodgkin lymphoma
<50 cells/mm³	• Disseminated *Mycobacterium avium* complex • Cytomegalovirus infection • Toxoplasmosis	• AIDS-associated wasting • AIDS-associated dementia

HIV-related complication (**Table 203-1**). If recent CD4+ counts are unavailable, there is controversy about the usefulness of CD4+ testing in the context of acute illness, which lowers the CD4+ below the patient's true baseline. Despite this caveat, we recommend measuring CD4+ cell count during hospital admissions, as markedly low values (eg, <100 cells/mm³) almost invariably indicate severe HIV-related immunosuppression, especially in a patient not prescribed or adherent to ART. Conversely, OIs are exceedingly unusual in patients with normal CD4+ cell counts and undetectable HIV viral loads. Although HIV RNA values do not provide as much information about a patient's immune status as CD4+ counts, they are excellent markers of ART medication adherence, as over 90% of patients faithfully taking appropriate ART will have HIV RNA levels below the limits of detection of available assays. One potential exception to this rule is that acute infections transiently raise HIV RNA levels, but usually not to high levels.

In general, admission of the HIV-positive patient on ART warrants a baseline check of renal and hepatic function, as well as a CBC. HIV therapy may result in signature laboratory abnormalities in some patients, such as the indirect hyperbilirubinemia seen in patients on atazanavir and the increased mean corpuscular volume (MCV) seen in those taking zidovudine (**Table 203-2**).

For patients with excellent medication adherence, suppressed HIV RNA, and immunologic recovery with CD4+ cell counts >200 cells/mm³, traditional AIDS-related illnesses are vanishingly rare. Individuals with these characteristics are generally admitted for similar reasons as HIV-negative patients. However, long-term

TABLE 203-2 Laboratory Abnormalities Associated with Selected Antiretroviral Agents

Drug	Laboratory Abnormality
Atazanavir Indinavir	Indirect hyperbilirubinemia
Zidovudine	Bone marrow suppression, macrocytic anemia
Tenofovir Cobicistat	Renal dysfunction

follow-up of treated HIV patients shows that they may have a higher risk of certain noninfectious complications than age-matched, HIV-negative controls. Cardiovascular, hepatic, and renal disease occurs more frequently in patients with HIV, probably due to a combination of ART-induced side effects and chronic inflammation. Malignancies are also increased, perhaps as a consequence of reduced immune tumor surveillance.

SYMPTOM-BASED DIAGNOSTIC APPROACH

■ RESPIRATORY ILLNESS

Causes of respiratory symptoms in HIV include bacterial, mycobacterial, viral, and fungal pathogens, as well as malignancy and cardiovascular disease (**Table 203-3**). Clues to the etiology of the illness include the symptoms, time course, and imaging. A careful history can narrow the differential diagnosis significantly. For example, a relatively acute illness with fever, chills, sputum production, and pleuritic chest pain suggests bacterial pneumonia. A subacute illness with progressive dyspnea, dry cough, low-grade fever, and weight loss suggests *Pneumocystis jirovecii* pneumonia (PCP). The social history may elicit risk factors for endemic fungal infections and tuberculosis (TB). In patients from highly TB endemic areas, or with known TB exposure, this is one of the most common presenting OIs, but is quite rare without these risk factors. Physical examination findings of cachexia or oral candidiasis should raise suspicion for more advanced HIV, as should a history of weight loss.

Initial studies in the hospitalized HIV-positive patient with respiratory illness should include measurement of oxygen saturation or an arterial blood gas measurement, complete blood count with differential, two sets of blood cultures, sputum culture, urine legionella antigen, chest radiograph, and serum lactate dehydrogenase (LDH), which is nonspecific, but often elevated in patients with PCP. A nasopharyngeal swab for respiratory viruses, such as influenza A and B, should be sent if local epidemiology and seasonality are appropriate (**Table 203-4**). Induced sputum should be ordered for PCP and acid-fast bacilli (AFB) staining, as well as bacterial culture. Serum testing for 1,3 beta-D-glucan—a component of many fungi, including *P. jirovecii*—can be quite useful, as most patients with HIV-related PCP have markedly elevated levels. A strongly positive test in a patient with a compatible clinical syndrome for PCP may obviate the need for invasive testing such as bronchoscopy.

If initial tests are unrevealing and the patient does not improve on empirical therapy, serum cryptococcal antigen and urine *Histoplasma* antigen should be considered. Other evaluation at this

TABLE 203-3 Causes of Respiratory Disease in HIV

Very Common	Less Common	Rare
• *P. jirovecii* pneumonia • *S. pneumoniae* • *H. influenzae* • *M. tuberculosis**	• Gram-negative rods, especially *Pseudomonas* • *Histoplasma capsulatum* • *C. neoformans* • *Aspergillus* spp. • Cytomegalovirus • Pulmonary lymphoma • Kaposi sarcoma • Heart failure	• *N. asteroides* • *Legionella* spp. • Mycobacterium avium complex • *Toxoplasma gondii* • Cryptosporidia • *Rhodococcus equii* • Primary pulmonary hypertension • Abacavir hypersensivity

*Dependent on local *M. tuberculosis* prevalence and patient risk factors (such as past or current residence in an endemic area).

TABLE 203-4 Diagnostic Studies for Respiratory Illness in the HIV-positive Patient

Nasopharyngeal Swab*	Bronchoalveolar Lavage
Influenza A and B (rapid testing and/or polymerase chain reaction)	Viral studies as listed under Nasopharyngeal Swab
H1N1 influenza	Varicella
Respiratory syncytial virus	Cytomegalovirus
Adenovirus	AFB stain and culture
Parainfluenza	Cytology
Metapneumovirus	*P. jirovecii* pneumonia
	Bacterial culture
	Fungal culture

*Although uncomfortable for the patient, this must be inserted 1 to 2 cm into the nasopharyngeal space to ensure diagnostic yield.

time may include bronchoscopy with bronchoalveolar lavage and possible transbronchial biopsy, cardiac evaluation including echocardiography, computed tomography (CT) guided biopsy, or potentially nodule or mass resection via video-assisted thoracoscopy.

■ CENTRAL NERVOUS SYSTEM ILLNESS

Central nervous system (CNS) disease in HIV may be caused by cryptococcal meningitis, cerebral toxoplasmosis, progressive multifocal leukoencephalopathy (PML), and many others (**Table 203-5**). Advanced AIDS may be complicated by HIV-related dementia. Another important HIV-related CNS process is non-Hodgkin lymphoma, which may present as a primary mass lesion in the brain, or as metastatic disease to the meninges in patients with high-grade lymphoma elsewhere.

Initial evaluation of the HIV-positive patient with neurologic or neuropsychiatric symptoms should include an assessment of medication adherence, possible use of illicit drugs, immunologic status, and complete physical examination, with special attention to sensory-motor and mental status assessments. Brain magnetic

TABLE 203-5 Causes of Central Nervous System Disease in HIV

Very Common	Less Common	Rare
• *C. neoformans*	• Cytomegalovirus	• *N. asteroides**
• *T. gondii**	• *M. tuberculosis*†	• *H. capsulatum*
• Drug reactions	• Bacterial brain abscess*	• *Coccidioides immitus*
• Psychiatric illness		• *Aspergillus* spp.*
• Progressive multifocal leukoencephalopathy*		• *Listeria monocytogenes*
• Lymphoma*		• Fungal brain abscess
• HIV		• Herpes simplex virus*
• Varicella zoster virus		• *Acanthamoeba* spp.*
		• *Trypanosoma cruzi*
		• *Treponema pallidum*

*Generally characterized by focal lesions on MRI or CT scan.
†Dependent on local *M. tuberculosis* prevalence and patient risk factors.

resonance imaging (MRI) should be performed (or head CT, if MRI is not available).

Lumbar puncture is usually indicated (after head imaging or ophthalmologic examination is performed to evaluate for increased intracranial pressure), even in the absence of nuchal rigidity, as many of the above processes induce a relatively indolent inflammatory response. Opening pressure should be obtained in all cases. Cerebrospinal fluid (CSF) should be sent for cell count and differential, glucose, protein, Gram stain and routine culture, as well as India ink stain (for *Cryptococcus*), fungal culture, and CSF cryptococcal antigen. If indicated, AFB stain and culture and VDRL may be sent as well. Leftover CSF (at least 5 cc) should be held for other potential studies including cytology, polymerase chain reaction (PCR) testing for other pathogens such as Epstein-Barr virus (EBV), varicella zoster virus, cytomegalovirus, herpes simplex viruses, JC virus, *Toxoplasma*, and quantitative HIV viral load.

Mass lesions that enhance with contrast

Mass lesions with enhancement occur more commonly in the setting of lower CD4+ counts (<200 cells/mm³), and are most often due to toxoplasmosis (discussed below), primary CNS lymphoma (PCNSL) or other malignancies, or rarely other infections, such as brain abscess or tuberculoma. If the patient has a history of positive *Toxoplasma* IgG serology and has multiple enhancing CNS lesions, empirical treatment for toxoplasmosis is appropriate. If the patient has a documented negative *Toxoplasma* serology, neurosurgical consultation for brain biopsy is usually appropriate. Serum *Toxoplasma* IgM or *Toxoplasma* antibody studies of the cerebrospinal fluid are not useful in this clinical setting, though CSF PCR for toxoplasmosis is a specific (but not sensitive) test for encephalitis due to this infection.

Patients with mass lesions and midline shift on imaging or evidence of increased intracranial pressure should receive adjunctive corticosteroids, usually dexamethasone. Symptoms and radiographic appearance of the lesion may improve on steroids, but this improvement should not shorten the anticipated course of antibiotic treatment.

Since combination ART became the standard of care, the incidence of all AIDS-defining malignancies in the United States has decreased significantly. However, PCNSL is still over 1000 times more common in patients with HIV than uninfected controls. PCNSL may present with symptoms ranging from mental status changes to seizures, and with a single lesion or multiple lesions. PCNSL is most common in patients with more advanced disease, especially with CD4+ cell counts <50 cells/mm³. Diagnostic workup includes MRI, CSF cytology, and, in most cases, stereotactic brain biopsy to confirm the diagnosis. CNS lymphoma in HIV usually involves B lymphocytes infected with EBV; PCR testing of CSF for EBV is sensitive, but not specific for this diagnosis.

The incidence of non–AIDS-defining primary CNS malignancies is not higher in the HIV-positive patient population. However, lung cancer, which sometimes presents with brain metastases, is increased in HIV patients.

Nonenhancing lesions

HIV encephalopathy: HIV-related dementia, or HIV encephalopathy, is usually a disease of advanced immunosuppression in patients not receiving ART. Characteristic findings include loss of memory, apathy, gait disturbance, and incontinence. Symptoms may be exacerbated by underlying psychiatric illness or substance abuse. There is often atrophy and nonenhancing white matter disease on MRI imaging. CSF examination may show mild lymphocytic pleocytosis, elevated protein, and detectable HIV RNA by viral load testing. Treatment with ART may lead to dramatic improvement, especially if the symptoms are of recent onset. However, the prognosis is highly variable, improvement may be delayed for months, and full recovery from severe cases is unusual. HIV encephalopathy, even when mild, may increase susceptibility of patients to the CNS side effects of antiretrovirals and other medications.

Progressive multifocal leukoencephalopathy: As with HIV encephalopathy, the incidence of PML has greatly declined with the advent of ART. PML is a demyelinating disorder caused by JC virus, a common polyomavirus that is usually asymptomatic in the immunocompetent. Symptoms of PML are gradual in onset, and may culminate in hemiparesis, mental status changes, and visual field deficits, depending on the areas of involvement, which may be single or multiple. These lesions are less symmetrical than in HIV encephalopathy and are usually nonenhancing on imaging studies. The diagnosis is made on the basis of PCR testing of the CSF for JC virus. While PML is most common in patients with CD4+ counts <200 cells/mm³, it may also be seen in patients initiating ART as an immune reconstitution inflammatory response to subclinical JC virus infection. There is currently no therapy that directly targets JC virus. One-third of patients with PML improve with effective ART; unfortunately, the remaining two-thirds have either long-term residual deficits or disease progression despite effective ART.

GASTROINTESTINAL ILLNESS

Gastrointestinal symptoms in HIV may result from infection or, more commonly, from side effects of antibiotics and antiretrovirals, especially the protease inhibitors. Chronic diarrhea with weight loss may be due to untreated HIV itself; this HIV enteropathy is a diagnosis of exclusion, and typically responds promptly to effective ART.

Diarrhea: Causes of diarrhea in HIV are summarized in **Table 203-6**. Evaluation of the HIV-positive patient with diarrhea should consist of a careful exposure history, including travel, food, drink, and sexual activity. The medication history should include both antiretrovirals as well as antibiotics. The quality, frequency, volume, and time course of the diarrhea are important, as is the presence or absence of fevers and weight loss.

Diagnostic evaluation includes assessment of electrolyte and hematologic status, as well as a stool sample for ova and parasites, AFB and trichrome stains for mycobacteria and protozoa (*Cryptosporidium, Cyclospora, Isospora,* and microsporidia), *Clostridium difficile* toxin, and enzyme immunoassay for *Giardia*. Multiplex PCR assays are increasingly available and allow for rapid testing for these and other common gastrointestinal pathogens. If these studies are unrevealing, endoscopic evaluation may be required for evaluation of intraluminal pathology and biopsy, especially in patients with low CD4+ counts who are at risk for additional processes such as CMV, lymphoma, and Kaposi sarcoma.

ART-related diarrhea is usually secondary to protease inhibitors. It is rarely associated with weight loss, and may in some cases be controlled with loperamide. For individuals with debilitating diarrhea due to these medications, an HIV specialist will often consider an alternative antiretroviral regimen. However, these changes should not be made without a thorough review of the patient's treatment history, including results of prior resistance testing.

Dysphagia: *Candida* esophagitis is by far the most common cause of dysphagia, and is often, but not always, accompanied by visible oral candidiasis (thrush) on examination. Empirical fluconazole is reasonable (200 mg daily for 7-14 days). If the diagnosis is correct, improvement often occurs within 24 to 48 hours. For patients who fail to respond to antifungal therapy, endoscopy is indicated to exclude other possible causes of dysphagia and odynophagia. These include idiopathic aphthous ulcers, CMV, herpes simplex, histoplasmosis, and lymphoma.

UNDIFFERENTIATED FEVER

The differential diagnosis for fever in HIV is broad and includes infection (either opportunistic or otherwise), inflammatory conditions (including immune reconstitution inflammatory syndrome [IRIS]), fever from medications or malignancy, or HIV itself (**Table 203-7**).

Helpful historical information includes fever duration and severity, prior opportunistic infections and hospitalizations, medication history, including new medications and adherence to prophylaxis, domestic and international travel, sexual history, intravenous drug use, and other substance use.

Differential diagnosis is highly contingent on the stage of HIV infection, based on the most recent CD4+ count. When such information is not immediately available, inferences about immune status can often be made based on physical examination findings such as cachexia or oral candidiasis that indicate advanced HIV; leukopenia and lymphopenia also suggest advanced immunosuppression. Causes of fever in HIV-positive patients with CD4+ counts >500 cells/mm³ are similar to those in immunocompetent patients. Patients with CD4+ counts between 200 and 500 cells/mm³ are more likely to have fever secondary to sexually transmitted infections (especially syphilis and hepatitis C among gay men) or respiratory infections, either bacterial (*Streptococcus pneumoniae* and *Haemophilus influenzae*) or viral (seasonal and H1N1 influenza). Patients with more advanced disease (CD4+ count <200 cells/mm³) are vulnerable to both opportunistic and nonopportunistic infections. Patients with

---

TABLE 203-6 Causes of Diarrheal Illness in HIV

Common	Less Common	Rare
• Cytomegalovirus	• *Shigella*	• Amebiasis
• *C. difficile*	• *Campylobacter*	• *Strongyloides stercoralis*
• *Salmonella*	• Microsporidia	• Enterotoxigenic *E. coli*
• Mycobacterium avium complex	• Cryptosporidia	
• *Giardia*	• *Isospora*	• GI lymphoma
• Norovirus	• *Cyclospora*	• Kaposi sarcoma
• Protease inhibitors		

GI, gastrointestinal.

TABLE 203-7 Causes of Undifferentiated Fever in HIV

Common	Less Common	Rare
• *Mycobacterium avium* complex	• *C. neoformans*	• Extrapulmonary PCP
• Cytomegalovirus	• *H. capsulatum*	• *Bartonella henselae*
• Drug fever*	• Endocarditis	• *C. immitis*
• Sinusitis	• Lymphoma	• Other nontuberculous mycobacteria
• Central line infection	• Mononucleosis	
• Early PCP	• Autoimmune disease	• *Penicillium marneffei*
• HIV	• Syphilis	• *Leishmania* spp.
• *M. tuberculosis*†		• Parvovirus
		• *T. gondii*

*If suspected, modification of antiretroviral regimen should be performed with the input of an expert in HIV treatment.
†Dependent on local *M. tuberculosis* prevalence and patient risk factors (such as past or current residence in an endemic area).

TABLE 203-8 Undifferentiated Fever in Persons with HIV: Diagnostic Evaluation

- Blood cultures: routine for endocarditis or line infections; isolators for mycobacteria (especially *M. avium*), *H. capsulatum*
- Urinalysis and urine culture
- Rapid plasma reagin
- Nasal swab for influenza A and B, H1N1 influenza, and respiratory viral panel
- Induced sputum or bronchoalveolar lavage: *P. jirovecii*, *M. tuberculosis*
- Serum cryptococcal antigen, serum/urine histoplasmosis antigen (latter if patient from endemic area), urine legionella antigen
- CT abdomen/pelvis: look for adenopathy, organomegaly
- Sometimes useful: bone marrow, liver, lymph node biopsy; cytomegalovirus viral load, parvovirus polymerase chain reaction

more advanced immunosuppression are also at risk for infections seen at earlier stages of disease. Diagnostic evaluation that may help to differentiate the source of fever in the absence of localizing signs or symptoms is summarized in **Table 203-8**.

■ IMMUNE RECONSTITUTION INFLAMMATORY SYNDROME (IRIS)

Recovery of immune function with ART is associated with a resurgence of pathogen-specific immunity. This can lead to IRIS, a brisk inflammatory reaction to pre-existing infections, which may have been subclinical or minimally symptomatic before ART. Virtually all HIV-related OIs have been reported in association with IRIS. The most common pathogens in IRIS are mycobacteria (both tuberculosis and atypical mycobacteria), herpes viruses, zoster, and CMV.

IRIS usually occurs in the first 3 months after starting ART. Rarely, delayed cases occur a year or more after starting therapy. In a typical scenario, a patient with severe immunosuppression (CD4+ cell count <100 cells/mm³) and/or high HIV RNA begins ART and then presents several weeks later with fever and cervical, mediastinal, and mesenteric adenopathy. Biopsy of involved nodes reveals mycobacteria and poorly formed granulomata, with cultures eventually yielding *Mycobacteria avium* complex (MAC). Other relatively common causes of IRIS include severe herpes zoster or herpes simplex, vitritis due to CMV, and worsening of cutaneous Kaposi sarcoma.

Treatment of IRIS is directed at the underlying pathogen. ART should be continued, if at all possible. If symptoms cannot be controlled with anti-infective therapy alone, or if the IRIS is life threatening, as can rarely occur with CNS diseases such as cryptococcal meningitis or toxoplasmosis, adjunctive corticosteroids should be given. A typical starting dose will be 60 mg of prednisone a day, with therapy continued for several weeks followed by a slow taper. Fortunately, prospective studies show that IRIS occurs in 10% of AIDS patients starting ART or less and is rarely fatal.

■ NONINFECTIOUS CAUSES OF FEVER

Drug fever

HIV-positive patients have a higher rate of drug hypersensitivity than the general population, including a higher incidence of severe systemic reactions such as Stevens-Johnson syndrome and toxic epidermal necrolysis. Common offending agents include sulfonamides

(including trimethoprim-sulfamethoxazole [TMP-SMX]), dapsone, clindamycin, and beta-lactam antibiotics.

Some antiretroviral agents cause drug hypersensitivity. The two most important are nevirapine and abacavir. The incidence of systemic hypersensitivity reactions to nevirapine—which is often accompanied by rash and hepatitis—is significantly higher in HIV patients who are female and immunologically healthier. As a result, nevirapine is not recommended in women with CD4+ cell counts >250 and men >400 cells/mm³. Abacavir may cause a multisystem hypersensitivity reaction shortly after initiation of the drug that may worsen after successive doses. Continued treatment, or rechallenge after cessation, may be fatal. This reaction is strongly associated with the HLA-B*5701 haplotype. Screening tests are widely available; abacavir is contraindicated in anyone testing positive for this allele. Several protease inhibitors, including darunavir, fosamprenavir, and tipranavir, contain a sulfonamide moiety, and can rarely induce systemic hypersensitivity. However, patients with prior allergic reactions to trimethoprim-sulfamethoxazole can usually receive these sulfonamide antiviral agents safely, though they should be avoided in patients with prior life-threatening sulfa reactions.

Malignancy

The incidence of malignancies is higher in HIV-positive patients than in the general population. While AIDS-associated malignancies (including Kaposi sarcoma and non-Hodgkin lymphoma) were previously the most common causes, the range of HIV-associated malignancies has expanded due to prolonged patient survival in the ART era. Of these, non-Hodgkin lymphoma is most often associated with fever, although Hodgkin lymphoma is also more common in HIV-positive patients and may also present with fever, night sweats, and weight loss. Malignancy should be considered in the differential diagnosis of lymphadenopathy in HIV.

SELECTED HIV-RELATED OPPORTUNISTIC INFECTIONS AND CONDITIONS

■ *PNEUMOCYSTIS JIROVECII* PNEUMONIA

P. jirovecii (formerly *carinii*) pneumonia is caused by a fungus ubiquitous in the environment, and nonpathogenic in the lungs of the normal host. Effective ART and chemoprophylaxis both markedly reduce the risk of PCP. As a result, cases today typically occur either in those who are unaware of their HIV status or not taking prescribed antiretroviral medications.

PCP most often presents as a respiratory illness progressing over weeks to months. Patients complain of dyspnea on exertion, first noticed when everyday tasks (climbing stairs, completing sentences, carrying household items) become difficult. Associated symptoms may include cough and chest tightness, and a sense that deep breathing is restricted. Constitutional symptoms including fever and weight loss are common, and physical examination may reveal other signs of immunosuppression, such as thrush and shallow respirations. Chest radiographs often show diffuse bilateral infiltrates, with CT scanning demonstrating characteristic patchy ground-glass opacities.

In the presence of a subacute respiratory illness with hypoxemia and a confirmed or suspected CD4+ count <200 cells/mm³, therapy for PCP should generally be initiated, regardless of the appearance of the chest radiograph. While diffuse interstitial infiltrates are classic—often seen as ground-glass opacities on CT scan—lobar infiltrates, nodular or cavitary disease, or rarely, a normal chest radiograph may be observed. The diagnostic procedure of choice is sputum induction with immunofluorescence staining for PCP, but sensitivity varies depending on patient ability to provide an adequate sample and laboratory expertise. Bronchoalveolar lavage has a reported sensitivity of >90% in patients with HIV infection, considerably higher than that reported in HIV-negative patients. When microscopy is negative or difficult to obtain, serum 1,3 beta-D-glucan, a cell wall component of many fungi (including *P. jirovecii*), and LDH can be useful adjuncts.

If pulse oximetry is low or the patient is tachypneic, an arterial blood gas should be performed. The degree of hypoxemia divides PCP into clinical classifications and guides the treatment course. Mild PCP is characterized as a partial pressure of arterial oxygen (PaO_2) >70 mm Hg, and an alveolar-arterial gradient (A-a gradient) of less than 35. Moderate to severe PCP is characterized by a partial pressure of arterial oxygen (PaO_2) of ≤70 mm Hg, and/or an alveolar-arterial gradient (A-a gradient) of greater than 35. In moderate to severe PCP, corticosteroid therapy should be initiated, preferably before or at the time of antimicrobial treatment. The preferred steroid regimen is prednisone 40 mg orally twice daily for 5 days, followed by 40 mg once daily for 5 days, then 20 mg once daily for 11 days, for a total 21-day course.

Patients often worsen after starting therapy for PCP, perhaps related to an enhanced inflammatory response to dying organisms, as well as the fluid load associated with intravenous trimethoprim-sulfamethoxazole. In the setting of deterioration on therapy, adjunctive corticosteroids should be started even for patients not initially deemed candidates.

First-line treatment for PCP is TMP-SMX dosed at 15 to 20 mg/kg of trimethoprim daily in three divided doses. Therapy should be continued for 21 days. As TMP-SMX is well-absorbed orally, therapy can be dosed at two double-strength tablets of coformulated TMP-SMX given three times daily. For sulfa-allergic patients, second-line therapy is clindamycin 600 mg orally or intravenously given every 8 hours, along with primaquine 30 mg given orally every 24 hours. In mild disease, atovaquone oral suspension 750 mg twice daily may be considered. For moderate-severe disease only, pentamidine 4 mg/kg/d IV may also be used, but should generally be avoided due to high rates of side effects such as renal dysfunction, electrolyte abnormalities, pancreatitis, and islet cell toxicity. Of note, sulfa allergy should be confirmed in this clinical setting by a careful review of the allergy history, as TMP-SMX is the preferred treatment. Rechallenge may be considered in cases of mild sulfa allergy or sulfa intolerance.

Creatinine elevation and hyperkalemia are often associated with high-dose TMP-SMX use. Elevated creatinine in patients on TMP-SMX usually reflects inhibition of the tubular secretion of creatinine, rather than renal injury. Rarely, TMP-SMX may cause acute renal failure as a result of interstitial nephritis. TMP-SMX–induced hyperkalemia—due to an amiloride-like effect of trimethoprim—can be life threatening and should be treated aggressively with sodium polystyrene sulfonate (Kayexalate) or by changing to an alternative PCP regimen.

If the patient is on ART, it should be continued throughout the PCP treatment course. If PCP occurs in the context of a new diagnosis of HIV, or if the patient is off ART, both prospective and observational studies have demonstrated a clinical benefit of starting ART before the completion of PCP treatment, preferably within 2 weeks of beginning PCP therapy.

BACTERIAL PNEUMONIA

While the incidence of bacterial pneumonia among HIV-positive patients has declined in recent years due to ART, it remains common in patients at all stages of the disease. Although vaccination against *S. pneumoniae* is now standard of care in HIV-positive patients, pneumococcal pneumonias remain common. Other frequent pathogens include *H. influenzae*, *Staphylococcus aureus*, both methicillin-sensitive and methicillin-resistant (MRSA), and

Gram-negative bacteria such as *Pseudomonas aeruginosa*. *Legionella* species, notably *L. pneumophila*, do occur at a higher rate than in negative controls, and hence coverage for atypical pathogens is also warranted.

As noted above, bacterial pneumonia in HIV-positive patients presents similarly to bacterial pneumonia in HIV-negative patients: the relatively acute onset of fever, chills, cough (often productive), anorexia, and pleuritic chest pain. As bacteremia is more common in bacterial pneumonia in HIV patients, obtaining blood cultures prior to institution of antibiotics is strongly recommended. Sputum Gram stain and culture may be useful if obtained prior to antimicrobial therapy; by contrast, urinary antigen testing for *S. pneumoniae* and *L. pneumophila* typically remain positive for days to weeks after starting therapy.

Treatment of suspected bacterial pneumonia in HIV patients is usually similar to those without HIV. Empirical initial therapy in most patients may be a third- or fourth-generation cephalosporin such as ceftriaxone (2 g IV daily) as well as azithromycin (500 mg daily, orally or IV). A fluoroquinolone (eg, levofloxacin or moxifloxacin, but not ciprofloxacin) may be used instead if TB seems unlikely. If the patient has a history of pseudomonal infection, consider antipseudomonal therapy such as ceftazidime or cefepime (in place of ceftriaxone) or adding ciprofloxacin. If MRSA colonization is documented, the patient is critically ill, or the pneumonia occurs during influenza season, vancomycin should be added to the regimen. Therapy should be given promptly upon evaluation, but blood and sputum cultures should be obtained prior to antibiotic administration if possible. Improvement is typically prompt, and changing to an oral regimen within days of hospitalization is usually possible. Duration of therapy is generally 5-7 days, depending upon clinical response.

TUBERCULOSIS

Tuberculosis disease should always be considered in the differential diagnosis of respiratory illness in the HIV-positive patient. Although overall incidence of TB in the United States is declining gradually both in the general population and in the HIV-positive population, TB remains a major cause of mortality among HIV-positive persons worldwide. In the United States, 7% of patients with TB tested for HIV were positive, while 12% of all patients with TB have unknown HIV status.

TB has wide-ranging clinical presentations. Patients with relatively intact immune status typically present much as HIV-negative patients do, with a subacute systemic and respiratory illness featuring constitutional symptoms, cough, and cavitary infiltrates of the upper lobes on chest radiograph. By contrast, AIDS patients are more likely to have pulmonary infiltrates without cavitation, mediastinal and other lymphadenopathy, extrapulmonary TB, and disseminated disease. Underlying tuberculosis should also be suspected in at-risk patients with slow-to-resolve pneumonia or characteristic lymphadenopathy on imaging. Diagnostic workup of TB should always include thoracic imaging.

The diagnostic approach to suspected TB should include serial sputa for AFB stain and culture, preferably obtained in the morning to maximize bacillary yield. Sputum acid-fast stains are most likely to be positive in patients with cavitary pulmonary disease. PCR or the Xpert MTB/RIF assay can be performed on smear-positive sputum samples to allow for rapid differentiation of tuberculous and nontuberculous mycobacterial disease. AFB blood cultures may yield the diagnosis as well, especially in patients with advanced HIV immunosuppression and disseminated disease. Biopsies of affected sites may be required if extrapulmonary disease is suspected, and should be sent for AFB stain and culture as well as for pathologic examination.

A practical management issue is whether HIV-infected patients with pneumonia require isolation in a negative pressure room. In patients with risk factors for TB, isolation is good clinical practice until an alternative diagnosis is obtained or there is clear clinical response to treatment of an alternative condition, such as bacterial pneumonia. TB risk factors include residence in an endemic area, homelessness or incarceration, or exposure to persons with TB (eg, a family member or in an occupational setting). Patients with a prior positive purified-protein derivative (PPD) test or interferon gamma release assay (IGRA) who do not have documented appropriate treatment should also be placed on precautions. Patients with suspected active TB should not receive a fluoroquinolone until TB is ruled out, as this drug class may have partial activity against TB, may confound diagnosis, and can limit future treatment options.

PRACTICE POINT

- Since antiretroviral drugs first became available, there has been a lively debate about the optimal timing of initiation of HIV treatment. Current US guidelines recommend starting ART for all HIV-infected patients, regardless of CD4+ count.

Of note, PPD testing may be falsely negative in patients with advanced immunosuppression, those on corticosteroids, or when the test is administered incorrectly (eg, intramuscularly, rather than intradermally). IGRA testing may also be negative in patients with advanced immunosuppression.

■ CRYPTOCOCCAL MENINGITIS

Cryptococcus neoformans meningitis is usually seen in patients with low CD4+ counts (<100 cells/mm^3). These patients often present with the gradual onset of meningitic symptoms, including headache, mental status changes, and fever. Meningeal signs and photophobia may be absent. Elevated intracranial pressure (>200 mm H$_2$O) may be observed. This is an ominous prognostic finding that must be monitored during treatment. CSF pleocytosis may be minimal. Modest elevations in CSF protein and reductions in CSF glucose are often present. CSF should be sent for routine culture as well as fungal culture: *C. neoformans* grows on most bacterial and fungal media within a few days. India ink stain of CSF is positive in 60% to 80% of AIDS patients with cryptococcal meningitis but is no longer performed in many labs. CSF and serum cryptococcal antigen tests are both highly sensitive due to high fungal burden in immunosuppressed patients. Serum cryptococcal antigen testing has nearly 100% sensitivity, and hence a negative test virtually excludes cryptococcal meningitis even without CSF sampling.

The treatment of cryptococcal meningitis consists of both antimicrobial therapy and serial lumbar punctures to lower raised intracranial pressure. The volume of CSF removed on initial lumbar puncture should be sufficient to lower closing pressure to <200 mm H$_2$O, or 50% of the opening pressure. Occasionally lumbar drains or shunts are required for refractory cases. Corticosteroids should be avoided. Cryptococcal meningitis is treated with a 2-week induction period of liposomal amphotericin B, dosed at 3-4 mg/kg/d, in combination with oral flucytosine (5-FC) 100 mg/kg/d divided over four doses. Flucytosine is associated with more rapid CSF sterilization and decreased risk of relapse but may be poorly tolerated, with common side effects including nausea and bone marrow suppression. After this 2-week induction period, patients who are clinically improved are switched to consolidation therapy with oral

fluconazole, 400 mg daily for an additional 8 weeks. After that time, the dose may be lowered to 200 mg daily for maintenance, and continued for at least 12 months and until the CD4+ cell count exceeds 100 cells/mm^3 and HIV viral load is undetectable for at least three consecutive months.

Timing of ART in cryptococcal meningitis is controversial. There are some data to indicate that early initiation of ART is associated with worse outcomes, perhaps because of IRIS leading to worsening intracranial pressure, although this has not been found in all studies. We recommend deferring ART at least until the initial induction phase of treatment of cryptococcal meningitis is complete (2 weeks) and there has been some clinical improvement.

■ TOXOPLASMOSIS

The prevalence of toxoplasmosis infection varies by geography and diet. The major risk factors are consumption of undercooked meat (lamb, pork, and beef) and kitten exposure. The prevalence of positive toxoplasma IgG in the general population (indicating past infection, often subclinical) ranges from 15% in the United States to 75% in some European countries.

Toxoplasmic encephalitis presents as a neurologic illness with systemic symptoms. Common complaints include headache, confusion, focal neurologic deficits, and fever. Brain imaging usually reveals multiple lesions with a surrounding ring of contrast enhancement and edema (**Figure 203-1**). CD4+ cell counts are typically below 100 cells/mm^3.

Toxoplasmosis in HIV most often arises from reactivation of latent subclinical disease. Most patients have serologic evidence of prior infection, with a positive serum toxoplasmosis IgG. Serum toxoplasma IgM and CSF toxoplasma antibody studies are rarely useful. In a patient with advanced HIV-related immunosuppression, a known positive toxoplasmosis IgG, and characteristic clinical presentation with suggestive imaging, empiric therapy directed at toxoplasmosis is warranted. If diagnostic CSF examination is possible, PCR positivity for *Toxoplasma gondii* confirms the diagnosis. In the absence of seropositivity, neurosurgical consultation should be obtained for a stereotactic brain biopsy to diagnose other possible causes of enhancing mass lesions, including primary CNS lymphoma, bacterial brain abscess, fungal infection, tuberculosis, or other malignancies.

Recommended regimens include pyrimethamine (200 mg loading dose given orally followed by 50-75 mg/d, depending on patient weight), with folinic acid (10-25 mg/d orally) to prevent drug-induced folate deficiency, plus sulfadiazine (4-6 g/d orally in four divided doses, depending on patient weight). In sulfa-allergic patients, clindamycin (600 mg IV or orally four times daily) may be substituted for sulfadiazine. Small studies have also suggested that TMP-SMX, dosed at 5 mg/kg of TMP component twice daily, may also be effective; this treatment is particularly useful in patients too ill to take oral therapy. Several other, less studied, alternative regimens are occasionally employed, involving various combinations of atovaquone, pyrimethamine, sulfadiazine, and/or azithromycin. Patients who have significant mass effect and associated symptoms (depressed level of consciousness or other signs) may require dexamethasone to reduce cerebral edema. Individuals with seizures should receive anticonvulsants, but these do not need to be given prophylactically.

Clinical improvement typically occurs within 7 to 14 days, more rapidly if adjunctive dexamethasone is used in the setting of mass effect or edema. Failure to improve over this time period suggests an alternative diagnosis, and neurosurgical consultation would be indicated to obtain a stereotactic brain biopsy. Timing of ART is uncertain, given the potentially catastrophic side effect of increasing inflammation in patients with focal brain lesions. Our practice is to

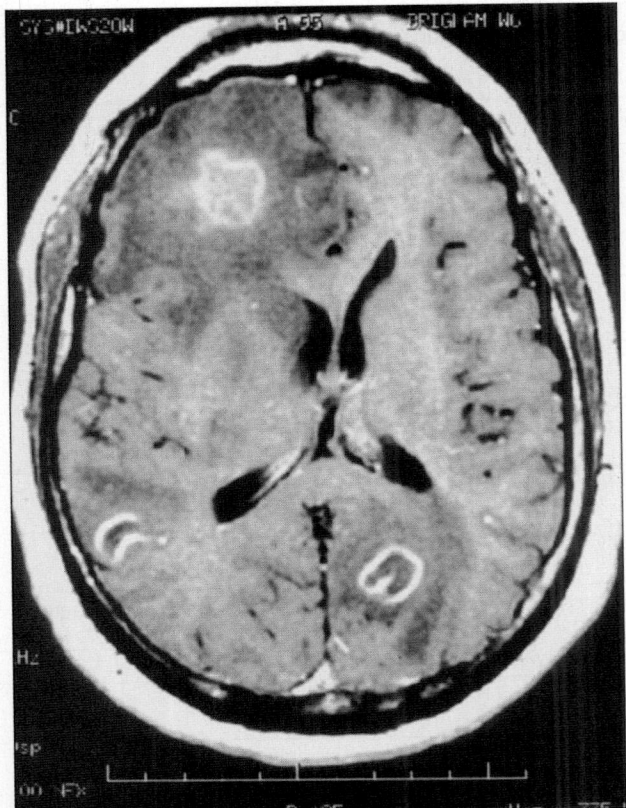

A

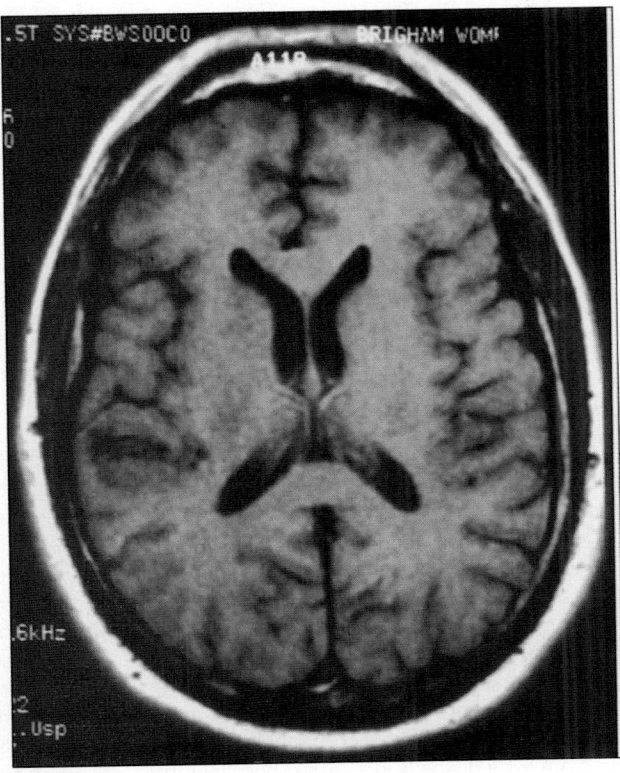

B

Figure 203-1 *Toxoplasma encephalitis in an AIDS patient.* (A) *Magnetic resonance imaging with gadolinium, demonstrating multiple ring-enhancing lesions.* (B) *Resolution of lesions after 8 weeks of therapy with pyrimethamine and sulfadiazine. On initial presentation, the patient was also given adjunctive corticosteroids for brain edema; combination anti-retroviral therapy was initiated 1 week later.*

start ART as soon as there is clinical improvement, typically after 7 to 14 days of antitoxoplasmosis therapy.

OTHER ISSUES IN THE CARE OF THE HOSPITALIZED PATIENT WITH HIV

■ ANTIRETROVIRAL THERAPY

Clinicians who specialize in HIV and follow a large volume of hospitalized patients with HIV should decide when to start ART and which regimen to use. As medication adherence is critical to the success of therapy, patients receiving ART who are hospitalized are often acutely aware that these acute illnesses or surgeries may interrupt their treatment. While 1 to 2 days of missed therapy is unlikely to influence outcome, every effort should be made to continue the same ART regimen that was being received prior to admission.

■ DRUG-DRUG INTERACTIONS

Drug-drug interactions involving antiretroviral agents are common. Antiretrovirals have complex interactions with the cytochrome P450 enzymes of the liver. Most HIV protease inhibitors, but especially ritonavir, have a potent inhibitory effect on cytochrome P450 3A4 (CYP3A4). Cobicistat, a component of the newer but popular once daily elvitegravir/cobicistat/emtricitabine/tenofovir, is also a potent cytochrome P450 3A inhibitor. This property dramatically boosts the levels of some common drugs, including statins, benzodiazepines, corticosteroids (including those given by inhalation or injection), calcium channel blockers, and digoxin. For example, simvastatin levels can be dangerously increased when given with protease inhibitors, and sedation from midazolam markedly prolonged. Another important drug-drug interaction is in the reverse direction: rifampin potently induces CYP3A4, significantly reducing plasma concentrations of all available protease inhibitors.

Because drug-drug interactions with ART are numerous and difficult to predict, some of the more important ones are summarized in **Table 203-9**. As a general rule, consultation with a clinician with expertise in HIV is the best approach to identify and avoid drug-drug interactions. Clinicians are encouraged to check updated resources when considering starting new medications in patients with HIV, especially those already known to have numerous drug interactions or narrow therapeutic safety ranges. Two good sources for this issue are the drug interaction tables of the HIV treatment guidelines (aidsinfo.nih.gov) and the site run by the University of Liverpool (www.hiv-druginteractions.org).

■ HIV AND AGING

Effective ART has led to a marked age increase among people with HIV in the United States, and it is estimated that more than half are now over 50 years of age. People with HIV are thus increasingly at risk for diseases of aging, such as cardiovascular and renal disorders. Age-based screening for common malignancies is especially important, as HIV-positive patients are at increased risk of developing many common cancers. There is also evidence that HIV itself may accelerate aging, due to chronic inflammation and immune activation. Older patients are at risk of neurocognitive decline due to HIV-associated dementia, in addition to the dementing diseases which are common in the general population.

■ CORONARY ARTERY DISEASE

HIV is associated with several risk factors for coronary artery disease (CAD), including hyperlipidemia, insulin resistance, a higher rate of

TABLE 203-9 Selected Interactions Between HIV Medications and Commonly Used Drugs

Drug	Interaction
Antacids and calcium supplements	Decreased absorption of some protease inhibitors (PIs) and integrase inhibitors
Anticonvulsants	Carbamazepine, phenytoin, and phenobarbital levels may be increased or decreased; levetiracetam not affected. Levels of some antiretrovirals may also be reduced
Antidepressants	Levels of selective serotonin reuptake inhibitors may be increased or decreased by PIs and cobicistat; levels of trazodone and tricyclic antidepressants may be increased by PIs and cobicistat
Benzodiazepines	Levels of alprazolam, midazolam, and triazolam increased by many antiretrovirals
Calcium channel blockers	Levels may be increased by ritonavir and cobicistat
Digoxin	Levels may be increased by ritonavir and cobicistat
Fluticasone	Levels increased by ritonavir and cobicistat; Cushing syndrome may result
H_2-blockers and proton pump inhibitors	May decrease absorption of PIs, especially atazanavir, and rilpivirine
Metformin	Potential increased adverse gastrointestinal effects from metformin, dose adjustment to 1000 mg or less should be considered
Methadone	Zidovudine increases methadone levels; abacavir, efavirenz, and ritonavir decrease methadone levels; ritonavir also reduces levels of other narcotics
Metronidazole	Tipranavir and lopinavir/ritonavir syrup contain alcohol, resulting in disulfiram reactions when administered with metronidazole
Oral contraceptives	Ethinyl estradiol levels decreased by ritonavir and cobicistat, increased by efavirenz
Sildenafil, tadalafil, vardenafil	Levels increased by PIs and cobicistat, decreased by efavirenz and etravirine
Statins (HMG-CoA reductase inhibitors)	Levels increased by PIs and cobicistat, decreased by efavirenz and etravirine; magnitude of interaction varies with statin

Adapted from Elke Backman, used with permission.

smoking than the general population, and chronic inflammation associated with the virus itself. Controlled studies consistently show that patients with HIV have higher rates of CAD than age-matched seronegative controls. Patients with HIV and CAD should be considered for the same risk factor modifications as HIV-negative patients, although new medications (such as statins) should be checked carefully for drug-drug interactions with the patient's ART.

■ PULMONARY HYPERTENSION

The prevalence of pulmonary hypertension in patients with HIV is 0.5%, several orders of magnitude higher than the prevalence of idiopathic pulmonary hypertension in the general population. Patients present with dyspnea and fatigue, and less commonly with chest pain, symptoms similar to those experienced by other patient populations with pulmonary hypertension. Diagnosis is made by physical examination, imaging (chest radiography, echocardiography), and more definitively via right heart catheterization. Treatment is similar to the HIV-negative patient.

■ ENDOCARDITIS

Infective endocarditis in patients with HIV is usually associated with injection drug use. *S. aureus* and other Gram-positive organisms are most often responsible, although a variety of organisms have been reported. The prevalence of endocarditis among HIV-positive intravenous drug users has been reported to be higher than in HIV-negative users. Patients with lower CD4+ counts have worse survival and higher complication rates.

■ MALIGNANCY

The incidence of cancer is increased in HIV-positive patients for many reasons, including lifestyle factors, faulty immune surveillance, and coinfection with cancer-causing viruses. Patients are at heightened risk for AIDS-defining malignancies such as Kaposi sarcoma, non-Hodgkin lymphoma, and cervical cancer, as well as several non–AIDS-defining cancers, including anal cancer associated with human papillomavirus (HPV), Hodgkin lymphoma, lung cancer, liver cancer, and squamous cell cancer of the head and neck. Providers should encourage risk factor reduction, such as smoking cessation and minimizing alcohol consumption. Women with HIV should have regular Pap smears with reflex HPV testing.

■ PSYCHOSOCIAL ISSUES

HIV remains one of the most politically charged diagnoses in medicine. Confidentiality issues surrounding the admission and treatment of HIV-positive patients can be challenging. It may surprise inpatient clinicians to learn that an HIV-positive patient has not disclosed his or her status to a partner or family member, despite having an HIV diagnosis for years. For many patients, the threat of inadvertent disclosure is a significant stressor of hospital admission. A rule of thumb in treating HIV-positive patients is to avoid discussing HIV or treatment related to HIV in front of any other person without the patient's express permission. In addition, every effort should be made to avoid such discussions in front of a patient's roommate, if he or she is in a shared hospital room or open emergency ward. A benefit of the advent of the Health Insurance Portability and Accountability Act is the clinician's ability to cite federal privacy regulations in interactions with a patient's employer, friends, or family members. With the patient's permission, discussion of the patient's illness can and should include family members, spouses, partners, and friends.

TABLE 203-10 Prevention of Selected HIV-associated Opportunistic Infections

OI	Indication	First Choice	Alternative
PCP	• CD4+ count <200 cells/mm³ • CD4+ <14% or history of AIDS-defining illness	TMP-SMX • 1 DS orally daily (if *Toxoplasma* IgG positive) *or* • 1 SS daily	• TMP-SMX 1 DS orally 3 times weekly • Atovaquone 1500 mg orally once daily • Dapsone 100 mg orally daily or 50 mg orally 2 times a day • Dapsone 50 mg orally daily + pyrimethamine 50 mg orally weekly + folinic acid 25 mg orally weekly • Aerosolized pentamidine 300 mg via Respigard II nebulizer monthly
T. gondii encephalitis	• Toxoplasma IgG positive patients with CD4+ count <100 cells/mm³ • Seronegative patients receiving PCP prophylaxis not active against toxoplasmosis should have toxoplasma serology retested if CD4+ count declines to <100 cells/mm³	• TMP-SMX 1 DS orally daily	• TMP-SMX 1 DS orally 3 times weekly • TMP-SMX 1 SS orally daily • Dapsone 50 mg orally daily + pyrimethamine 50 mg orally weekly + folinic acid 25 mg orally weekly • (Dapsone 200 mg + pyrimethamine 75 mg + leucovorin 25 mg) orally weekly
Disseminated MAC disease	• CD4+ count <50 cells/mm³ (after ruling out active MAC infection)	• Azithromycin 1200 mg orally once weekly *or* • Clarithromycin 500 mg orally 2 times a day	• Rifabutin 300 mg orally daily (dosage adjustment based on drug-drug interactions with ART); rule out active TB before starting rifabutin

ART, antiretroviral therapy; DS, double strength; MAC, *Mycobacterium avium* complex; PCP, *Pneumocystis jirovecii* pneumonia; SS, half strength; TB, -tuberculosis; TMP-SMX, trimethoprim-sulfamethoxazole.

PRACTICE POINT

• Some HIV-positive patients have not disclosed their status to partners or family members, despite having an HIV diagnosis for years. A rule of thumb in treating HIV-positive patients is to avoid discussing HIV or related diagnoses in front of any other person without the patient's express permission.

■ FACTITIOUS HIV

There are numerous case reports of patients claiming to have HIV infection, but ultimately found to be HIV seronegative on repeat testing. The most common explanation for this phenomenon is the secondary gain associated with an HIV diagnosis, such as eliciting a group of caring providers and access to community and health benefits. Clinicians should suspect factitious HIV whenever a patient is admitted with HIV to the hospital with a potential complication of HIV disease and found, on laboratory testing, to have a normal CD4+ cell count and undetectable HIV RNA, especially if the patient-provided history includes multiple manifestations of advanced immunosuppression. The management strategy of choice is repeat HIV testing and, if the test is negative, psychiatric consultation.

DISCHARGE CHECKLIST

• Does the patient have enough medications to last until scheduled outpatient follow-up? This is especially important for ART and OI prophylaxis. Many patients receive government-funded ART, and applications for these programs should be started in the hospital.

• Does the patient have appropriate prophylaxis for opportunistic infections? Depending on their CD4+ count, patients may need to be discharged with medications for prophylaxis against PCP, toxoplasma, and MAC disease (**Table 203-10**).

• Have patients been vaccinated against seasonal influenza and pneumococcal pneumonia? Both the PCV-13 and PPSV-23 vaccines are recommended, but these should not be administered simultaneously. They should be separated by at least 8 weeks, with the PCV-13 administered first in previously unvaccinated patients.

• Have medications been reviewed to exclude drug-drug interactions? This is especially important when new medications have been started during the hospitalization.

• For patients admitted with opportunistic infections, started on ART, or at high risk of nonadherence, has follow-up been arranged with the patient's primary HIV provider within 2 weeks of discharge? Loss to follow-up is a common and harmful occurrence, and linkage of the HIV-positive patient to care is a key step in increasing the chance of virologic suppression in the future. The HIV treatment cascade, a continuum beginning with HIV diagnosis, and progressing to linkage to care, retention in care, prescription of antiretroviral therapy, and finally plasma viral suppression, is a cornerstone of the National HIV/AIDS therapy. Unfortunately, only a small proportion of HIV patients in the United States have achieved viral load suppression (**Figure 203-2**).

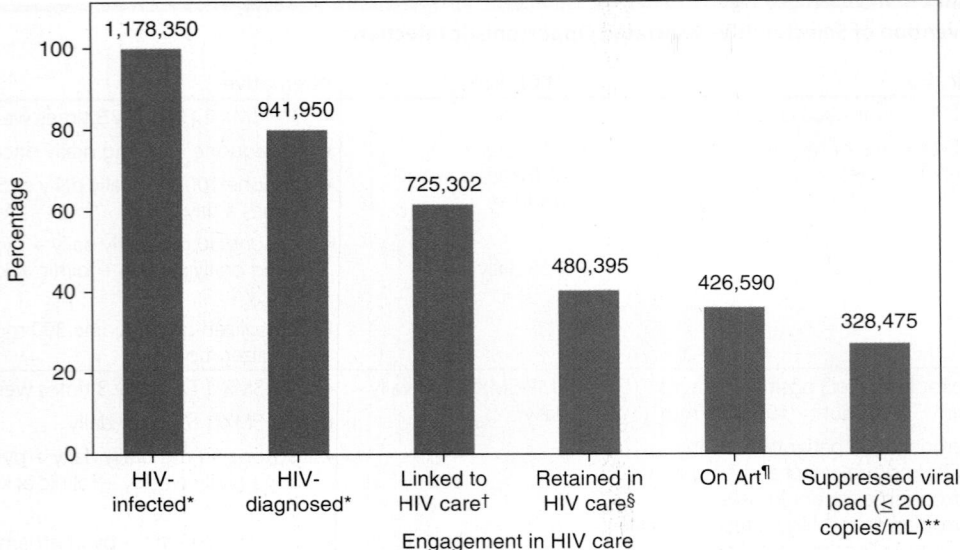

Abbreviations: ART, antiretroviral therapy; HIV, human immunodeficiency virus.

*HIV-infected, N = 1,178,350; HIV-diagnosed, N = 941,950. Source: CDC. HIV surveillance—United States, 1981-2008. MMWR 2011;60:689-693.

†Calculated as estimated number diagnosed (941,950) × estimated percentage linked to care (77%); n = 725,302. Sources: Marks G, Gardner LI, Craw J, Crepaz N. Entry and retention in medical care among HIV-diagnosed persons: a meta-analysis. *AIDS.* 2010;24:2665-2678; Torian LV, Wiewel EW. Continuity of HIV-related medical care, New York City, 2005-2009: do patients who initiate care stay in care? *AIDS Patient Care STDS.* 2011;25:79-88.

§Calculated as estimated number diagnosed (941,950) × estimated percentage retained in care (51%); n = 480,395. Sources: Marks G, Gardner LI, Craw J, Crepaz N. Entry and retention in medical care among HIV-diagnosed persons: a meta-analysis. *AIDS.* 2010;24:2665-2678; Torian LV, Wiewel EW. Continuity of HIV-related medical care, New York City, 2005-2009: do patients who initiate care stay in care? *AIDS Patient Care STDS.* 2011;25:79-88; Hall IH, Mahle KC, Tang T, Li J, Johnson AS, Shouse L. Retention in care of HIV-infected adults and adolescents in 13 U.S. areas. Presented at the National HIV Prevention Conference, Atlanta, GA, August 14-17, 2011; Tripathi A, Youmans E, Gibson JJ, Duffus WA. The impact of retention in early HIV medical care on viro-immunological parameters and survival: a statewide study. *AIDS Res Hum Retroviruses.* 2011;27:751-758.

¶Calculated as estimated number retained in HIV care (480,395) × percentage prescribed ART in MMP (88.8%); n = 426,590. Source: Data from the Medical Monitoring Project.

**Calculated as estimated number on ART (426,590) × percentage with suppressed viral load in MMP (77.0%); n = 328,475 (28% of the estimated 1,178,350 persons in the United States who are infected with HIV). Source: Data from the Medical Monitoring Project.

Figure 203-2 *Number and percentage of HIV-infected persons engaged in selected stages of the continuum of HIV care—United States.* (From *MMWR Morb Mortal Wkly Rep.* 2011;60(47);1618-1623.)

SUGGESTED READINGS

Boulware DR, Meya DB, Muzoora C, et al. Timing of antiretroviral therapy after diagnosis of cryptococcal meningitis. *N Engl J Med.* 2014;370:2487-2498.

Chu C, Selwyn PA. Complications of HIV infection: a systems-based approach. *Am Fam Phys.* 2011;83:395-406.

Grulich AE, van Leeuwen MT, Falster MO, Vajdic CM. Incidence of cancers in people with HIV/AIDS compared with immunosuppressed transplant recipients: a meta-analysis. *Lancet.* 2007;370:59-67.

Jones JL, Dargelas V, Roberts J, Press C, Remington JS, Montoya JG. Risk factors for *Toxoplasma gondii* infection in the United States. *Clin Infect Dis.* 2009;49:878-884.

Lederman MM, Sereni D, Simonneau G, Voelkel NF. Pulmonary arterial hypertension and its association with HIV infection: an overview. *AIDS.* 2008;22(Suppl 3):S1-S6.

Meintjes G, Scriven J, Marais S. Management of the immune reconstitution inflammatory syndrome. *Curr HIV/AIDS Rep.* 2012;9:238-250.

Mugavero MJ, Amico KR, Horn T, et al. The state of engagement in HIV care in the United States: from cascade to continuum to control. *Clin Infect Dis.* 2013;57:1164-1171.

Panel on Antiretroviral Guidelines for Adults and Adolescents. Guidelines for the use of antiretroviral agents in HIV-1-infected adults and adolescents. Department of Health and Human Services. Available at http://aidsinfo.nih.gov/contentfiles/lvguidelines/AdultandAdolescentGL.pdf.

Panel on Opportunistic Infections in HIV-Infected Adults and Adolescents. Guidelines for the prevention and treatment of opportunistic infections in HIV-infected adults and adolescents: recommendations from the Centers for Disease Control and Prevention, the National Institutes of Health, and the HIV Medicine

Association of the Infectious Diseases Society of America. Available at http://aidsinfo.nih.gov/contentfiles/lvguidelines/adult_oi.pdf.

Pisculli ML, Sax PE. Use of a serum beta-glucan assay for diagnosis of HIV-related *pneumocystis jirovecii* pneumonia in patients with negative microscopic examination results. *Clin Infect Dis.* 2008;46:1928-1930.

Pulvirenti JJ, Kerns E, Benson C, et al. Infective endocarditis in injection drug users: importance of human immunodeficiency virus serostatus and degree of immunosuppression. *Clin Infect Dis.* 1996;22:40-45.

Zolopa A, Andersen J, Powderly W, et al. Early antiretroviral therapy reduces AIDS progression/death in individuals with acute opportunistic infections: A multicenter randomized strategy trial. *PLoS One.* 2009;4(5):e5575.

CHAPTER 204

Infections of the Immunocompromised Host

Sarah P. Hammond, MD

Lindsey R. Baden, MD

Key Clinical Questions

❶ What is the approach to an immunocompromised patient with suspected infection?

❷ What are common infectious complications in patients receiving chronic corticosteroids, or recently treated with tumor necrosis factor inhibitors or rituximab?

❸ Should preventative measures be taken to prevent infectious complications in patients taking these medications?

❹ What infectious complications are common among patients who have undergone splenectomy?

❺ How should a transplant patient presenting with possible infection be evaluated?

INTRODUCTION

With the advent of newer immunosuppressive medications and the rise in organ transplantation internationally, the numbers of immunocompromised patients are increasing. The diagnosis and management of infection in this growing population is challenging. In immunocompromised patients, the usual signs and symptoms of infection may be obscured, and they often have a higher burden of pathogens and disseminated infection, leading to worse outcomes. These patients are also prone to infection with a broad array of less familiar pathogens, including opportunists such as *Listeria monocytogenes* and *Pneumocystis jiroveci*, and latent pathogens such as cytomegalovirus (CMV), toxoplasma, and *Mycobacterium tuberculosis*, as well as typical community-acquired and nosocomial microbes.

GUIDING PRINCIPLES

Two pieces of information are essential to the care of the patient with impaired immunity: the patient's epidemiologic exposures and overall state of immunosuppression.

The net state of immunosuppression is determined by the type, intensity, and duration of immunosuppression (including the dose and number of immunosuppressive agents or the presence of innate immunodeficiencies); anatomic factors causing a mechanical breakdown in the host defenses, such as abnormal lymphatic drainage at the site of previous surgery or radiation; and the presence or absence of immunosuppressive infections such as human immunodeficiency virus (HIV) or CMV.

Patients should be questioned about epidemiology that places them at risk for specific pathogens. These include recent events (sick contacts, animal exposure, travel, consumption of undercooked meat or unpasteurized dairy products), as well as remote residence in countries where tuberculosis is endemic, or regions of the United States and the world where histoplasmosis, blastomycosis, or coccidioidomycosis are endemic.

MEDICATION-RELATED IMMUNODEFICIENCY

Dozens of medications, used in a wide variety of medical conditions, may impair immunologic function; an abbreviated list is shown in **Table 204-1**. Some agents, such as corticosteroids and alemtuzumab, undermine several layers of host defenses. Others have a more targeted effect, such as tacrolimus and cyclosporine, which prevent normal T lymphocyte responses to immunologic stimuli. Understanding the impact of medications on immunity helps to predict which infections the host may develop. In particular, with the availability of novel immunosuppressive targeted or biologic agents such as ibrutinib, tocilizumab, eculizumab, and others, particular attention should be paid to the mechanism of the immunosuppressive agent in order to understand the potential effect on host immunity. For example, the infectious complication that has been most often linked to the C5 complement inhibitor eculizumab is meningococcal infection, similar to what is seen in patients with congenital C5 to C9 complement deficiencies.

■ CORTICOSTEROIDS

Corticosteroids are prescribed for rheumatologic conditions, inflammatory bowel disease, allergic disease, asthma, among others. The immediate impact of corticosteroids on host defenses includes depletion of circulating lymphocytes (particularly T lymphocytes)

TABLE 204-1 Selected Immunosuppressive Agents

Immunosuppressive Agent	Immunologic Effect	FDA-Approved Uses
Corticosteroids		
Prednisone, dexamethasone	Depletes circulating lymphocytes; suppresses phagocyte migration and function	Treatment of pulmonary and rheumatologic conditions
Antimetabolites		
Methotrexate	Inhibits dihydrofolate reductase; impairs cellular replication and repair	Treatment of RA, psoriasis, ALL, and several solid organ malignancies
6-mercaptopurine	Purine analogue; inhibits cellular DNA synthesis	Treatment of Crohn disease and ALL
Azathioprine	Disrupts purine metabolism	Treatment of RA; prevention of rejection in SOT
Mycophenolate mofetil	Inhibits inosine monophosphate dehydrogenase; inhibits B and T lymphocytes	Prevention of rejection in SOT
T lymphocyte active agents		
Tacrolimus, cyclosporin	Inhibits T lymphocyte activation	Prevention of rejection in SOT
Sirolimus, everolimus	Suppresses cytokine induction of T lymphocyte activity	Prevention of rejection in SOT
Monoclonal antibodies		
Infliximab, adalimumab, cetolizumab pegol, golimumab	Blocks effect of TNF-α, which mediates immunologic control of intracellular organisms and granuloma formation	Treatment of RA
Rituximab, Obinutuzumab, Ofatumumab	Monoclonal antibody to CD20; depletes B lymphocytes	Treatment of lymphoma and RA (rituxmab only)
Alemtuzumab	Monoclonal antibody to CD52; depletes B and T lymphocytes	Treatment of CLL
Basiliximab, daclizumab	IL-2 receptor antagonist; prevents IL-2 mediated lymphocyte activation	Induction of immunosuppression in SOT
Tocilizumab	IL-6 receptor antagonist	Treatment of RA
Biologic agents		
Etanercept	Blocks effect of TNF-α, which mediates immunologic control of intracellular organisms and granuloma formation	Treatment of RA
Anakinra	IL-1 inhibitor	Treatment of RA

ALL, acute lymphoblastic leukemia; CLL, chronic lymphocytic leukemia; RA, rheumatoid arthritis; SOT, solid organ transplantation.

and monocytes, and suppression of phagocyte migration and function. Long-term effects that increase infection risk include impaired skin and soft tissue healing.

Corticosteroid use increases susceptibility to common bacterial infections in a dose and duration-dependent manner (**Table 204-2**). Reactivation of latent tuberculosis is also increased among previously tuberculosis-infected patients started on corticosteroid therapy. Patients should be screened for latent tuberculosis before starting corticosteroid therapy. Chronic corticosteroid use also increases susceptibility to opportunistic infections. Infrequently, infection with invasive fungi such as *Aspergillus* and *Fusarium* occurs with chronic glucocorticoid use.

Two infection syndromes associated with corticosteroid use deserve special mention: *P. jiroveci* pneumonia (PCP) and *Strongyloides* hyperinfection syndrome.

PCP is associated with prolonged corticosteroid use; the risk for PCP rises with increasing steroid dose and duration. Clinically, PCP causes fever, dyspnea, and dry cough. It is characterized radiographically by diffuse bilateral pulmonary infiltrates (**Figure 204-1**). Patients with PCP may be profoundly hypoxic, particularly with ambulation. The mortality associated with PCP infection in non–HIV-infected patients is high—up to 50% in some case series. Therefore, suspected PCP should be treated empirically while the diagnostic workup is ongoing.

TABLE 204-2 Corticosteroid-Associated Infections

Infection	Preventative Strategy
Bacterial infections	
Increased susceptibility to all bacterial infections	Vigilance; routine vaccinations (including influenza and pneumonia vaccines)
Mycobacterial infections	
Tuberculosis	Check purified protein derivative or interferon-gamma release assay prior to steroid initiation; treat if indicated
Fungal infections	
P. jiroveci pneumonia	Prophylaxis when appropriate
Aspergillus	Rare, prophylaxis usually not warranted
Fusarium	Rare, prophylaxis usually not warranted
Parasitic infections	
Strongyloides hyperinfection syndrome	Screen with *Strongyloides* antibody before steroid initiation; treat if indicated

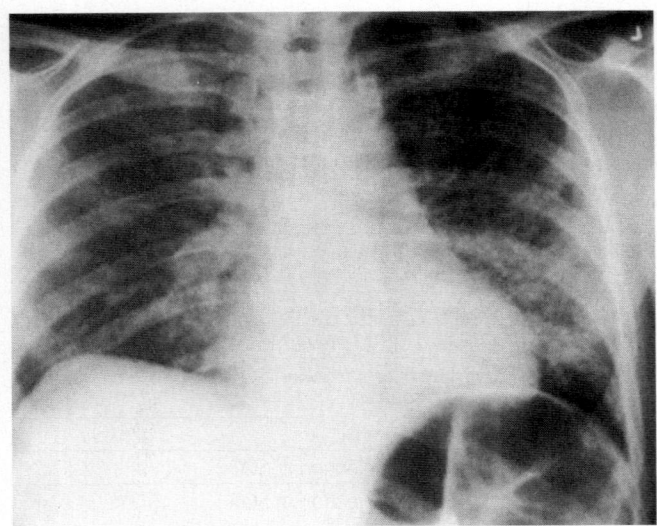

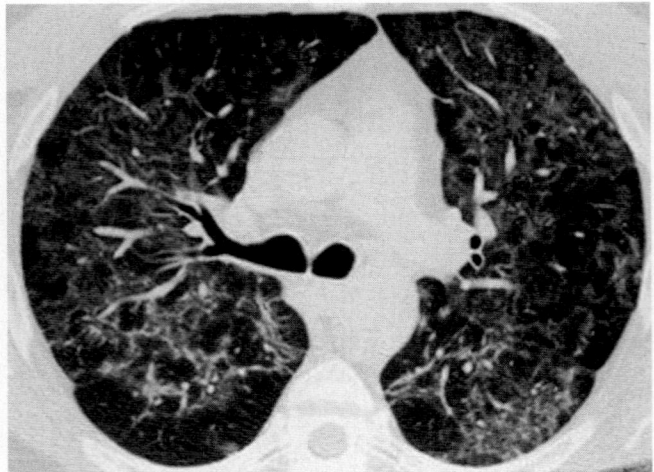

Figure 204-1 *Chest radiograph with diffuse interstitial infiltrates, and chest CT revealing ground glass infiltrates, in an HIV-positive patient with Pneumocystis carinii pneumonia (PCP). Radiographic findings in PCP may vary from impressive to quite subtle.* (Reproduced, with permission, from Fauci AS, Braunwald E, Kasper DL, et al. *Harrison's Principles of Internal Medicine*, 17th ed. New York, NY: McGraw-Hill 2008. Fig. 200-1.)

There are several methods of diagnosing PCP (**Table 204-3**). The gold standard is lung biopsy, with demonstration of characteristic cysts. More often, patients undergo bronchoscopy with bronchoalveolar lavage (BAL) or sputum induction, with testing of BAL fluid or sputum with direct fluorescent antigen or silver stain. A useful noninvasive test is the serum fungal marker 1→3, β-D-glucan, which may be very elevated in PCP, sometimes above the upper limit of the assay. (For the treatment of PCP in the non–HIV-infected population, see Practice Point.)

PRACTICE POINT

Treatment of PCP in the non–HIV-infected patient

- Trimethoprim-sulfamethoxazole (TMP-SMX) is the first-line agent for treating PCP. For patients with allergy or intolerance to TMP-SMX, alternatives include combination clindamycin and primaquine or intravenous pentamidine. Pentamidine

---

TABLE 204-3 Diagnosis of *P. Jiroveci* Pneumonia

Diagnostic Method	Advantage	Disadvantage
Lung biopsy	Gold standard for diagnosis	Invasive—requires transbronchial biopsy or surgical procedure
DFA of bronchoalveolar lavage fluid	Increased sensitivity compared to induced sputum	Requires invasive bronchoscopy
DFA of induced sputum	Less invasive than biopsy or bronchoalveolar lavage	Low burden of *Pneumocystis* in sputum leads to low sensitivity
β-D-glucan	Noninvasive; result characteristically greater than assay	Results often not rapidly available as it is usually a send-out test; false positive results possible in patients on hemodialysis, those who have received IVIg or albumin recently, or those with other invasive fungal infections

has numerous toxicities, including infusional cardiac toxicity, nephrotoxicity, and hypoglycemia, and is generally a drug of last resort. Mild cases of PCP can be treated with atovaquone. No randomized studies have assessed the use of adjunctive corticosteroids, in addition to antibiotics, to treat severe PCP infection in the non–HIV-infected patient. However, in severe cases with prominent hypoxia, or in patients requiring intubation, adjunctive steroids are often used.

Risk for PCP in patients on chronic steroids is predictable and therefore should be preventable. PCP has been reported in patients on less than 20 mg of prednisone per day for fewer than 8 weeks. Unfortunately, no formal study has assessed the corticosteroid dose and duration at which prophylaxis for PCP is necessary. Many providers add prophylaxis for PCP in patients receiving between 20 and 30 mg of prednisone (or prednisone equivalent) for over 20 to 30 days. Low-dose trimethoprim-sulfamethoxazole is the first-line agent for PCP prophylaxis. Alternative prophylaxis for patients with intolerance or allergy to trimethoprim-sulfamethoxazole includes dapsone, atovaquone, and monthly inhaled pentamidine. (Of note, breakthrough cases of PCP have been reported in patients on pentamidine prophylaxis, typically in the upper lobes.)

Corticosteroids are also associated with *Strongyloides* hyperinfection syndrome. The helminth *Strongyloides stercoralis* is found in soil in many parts of the world, including the Americas; in the United States, it is endemic in the Southeast. Initial infection occurs when larvae from soil penetrate the skin of a human host (often through bare feet) and travel to the gastrointestinal tract via the venous and pulmonary systems. Infection may be clinically silent for years to decades. Eosinophilia is variably present. The hyperinfection syndrome, an accelerated phase of infection with high morbidity and mortality, can be triggered by corticosteroids. This syndrome occurs when noninfectious *Strongyloides* larvae, hatched in the intestine of an infected patient, mature into infectious larvae prior to excretion, and subsequently invade the gastrointestinal tract of the host, leading to a large increase in the parasite burden and significant clinical illness. The hyperinfection syndrome is characterized by pulmonary infiltrates and diarrhea, due to the large burden of worms in transit in the gastrointestinal tract and lungs. In addition, associated Gram-negative sepsis and occasionally Gram-negative meningitis may occur, as bacteria use the larvae to hitchhike into the bloodstream from the gut.

Hyperinfection syndrome is diagnosed by finding characteristic larvae in BAL fluid or sputum. Patients recently initiated on steroids with appropriate epidemiologic history and unexplained Gram-negative sepsis, particularly meningitis, should be assessed for *Strongyloides* typically with stool and sputum ova and parasite assessment and serum antibody testing. Hyperinfection syndrome is treated with ivermectin or albendazole. Broad-spectrum antibiotics may be required for Gram-negative sepsis. To prevent *Strongyloides* hyperinfection syndrome in patients starting corticosteroid therapy, patients with eosinophilia or epidemiologic history consistent with possible exposure should be screened with serum *Strongyloides* antibody. If antibody is positive, antihelmenthic therapy should be given before steroid initiation.

■ TUMOR NECROSIS FACTOR-ALPHA (TNF-α) INHIBITORS

TNF-α is a cytokine produced by macrophages and T lymphocytes. It is important in granuloma formation and the immunologic control of intracellular organisms. Five TNF-α inhibitors are approved in the United States for the treatment of rheumatoid arthritis (RA), Crohn disease, and other conditions. These include infliximab, certolizumab pegol, adalimumab, and golimumab, monoclonal antibodies that bind to TNF-α, and etanercept, a soluble form of TNF-α receptor. These agents are also used in an off-label capacity to treat other inflammatory conditions.

Postmarketing studies of TNF-α inhibitors report an association between these agents and reactivation of granulomatous diseases, such as tuberculosis, histoplasmosis, and coccidioidomycosis, as well as opportunistic infection with nontuberculous mycobacteria and possibly the intracellular pathogen *Listeria*. TNF-α inhibitors may also increase the risk of serious bacterial infection in RA patients.

The association of TNF-α inhibitors and reactivation of dormant tuberculosis has been well documented. Reactivation of latent tuberculosis has been reported mostly during the first 6 months in patients treated with infliximab, and after 6 months in patients treated with etanercept. Many patients present with extrapulmonary tuberculosis, and a large proportion have disseminated disease and bad outcomes. Therefore, patients recently treated with TNF-α inhibitors presenting with a chronic febrile illness or unintentional weight loss and an appropriate epidemiologic history should be evaluated for tuberculosis, including careful assessment for extrapulmonary and disseminated disease. To prevent reactivation of latent tuberculosis in patients treated with TNF-α inhibitors, screening purified protein derivative testing or interferon-gamma release assay should be done. Patients with positive tests should begin treatment for latent tuberculosis before starting a TNF-α inhibitor.

Infection with *L. monocytogenes* may be more frequent in patients who have been treated with TNF-α inhibitors. Patients who have been treated with TNF-α inhibitors or other immunosuppressive drugs with signs and symptoms of meningitis or sepsis should be empirically treated with antibiotics active against *L. monocytogenes*, and blood and cerebrospinal fluid cultures should be obtained for definitive diagnosis.

■ RITUXIMAB

Rituximab is a monoclonal antibody to CD20, a marker found on B lymphocytes which makes it particularly useful for treating B-cell lymphomas. It is approved for use in non-Hodgkin lymphoma, RA, and chronic lymphocytic leukemia, and it is also used off-label for a variety of autoimmune disorders.

Rituximab depletes circulating B cells, leading to impaired antibody responses to new pathogens and vaccine antigens. Multiple studies have shown that patients treated with rituximab have significantly impaired humoral responses to new and recall vaccine antigens within a year after rituximab treatment. Furthermore, treatment with rituximab, particularly when given intermittently over long periods of time, has also been linked to development of hypogammaglobulinemia with associated risk for recurrent sinus and pulmonary infections, as is seen with common variable immunodeficiency (CVID) (see below).

In premarketing trials, there was no increased risk for infection among rituximab-treated patients, compared to those treated with other regimens for RA or lymphoma. However, since rituximab has been available commercially, it has been linked in case reports and case series to several uncommon infections, including progressive multifocal leukoencephalopathy caused by JC virus, reactivation of CMV, severe enterovirus infection, and pure red cell aplasia associated with parvovirus infection. Notably, the effect of rituximab alone is difficult to interpret in these anecdotal reports, because most of the reported patients have underlying immunonmodulatory conditions and have been treated with other immunosuppressive agents that independently increase infection risk, in addition to rituximab.

Rituximab is also linked to increased risk of severe manifestations of infection with *Babesia microti*, a tickborne parasitic infection endemic to the northeastern United States. (Other *Babesia* species are endemic to temperate regions of Europe.) Rituximab-treated patients with babesiosis tend to have high parasite burdens and severe clinical manifestations, including adult respiratory distress syndrome. Prolonged or repeated courses of therapy for babesia infection with atovaquone and azithromycin may be necessary to eradicate the infection in these patients. Fever, transaminitis, anemia, and thrombocytopenia suggest *Babesia* infection in patients in endemic areas treated with rituximab, and should trigger diagnostic testing with thick and thin blood smears.

Rituximab use has been definitively linked to severe hepatitis B virus reactivation. Specifically, rituximab use in patients who are hepatitis B surface antigen positive can result in development of fulminant hepatitis, with liver failure and death. In addition, hepatitis B reactivation has been reported in patients who have received rituximab with serologic evidence of resolved hepatitis B prior to rituximab (hepatitis B surface antigen negative and hepatitis B core antibody positive). Based on this association, patients being started on rituximab should be screened for hepatitis B before treatment. Patients treated with rituximab with liver function abnormalities, including florid hepatitis, should be assessed for active hepatitis B infection.

In addition to rituximab, ofatumumab, a newer monoclonal antibody approved for the treatment of chronic lymphocytic leukemia, also targets CD20. There is less clinical experience with this new agent, but it appears to have similar infectious complication risks to rituximab.

INNATE IMNUNODEFICIENCIES

Many innate immunodeficiencies, such as severe combined immunodeficiency and chronic granulomatous disease, are uncommon, require specialized care, and are beyond the scope of this chapter. However, CVID is not rare, and these patients are often cared for by hospitalists.

■ COMMON VARIABLE IMMUNODEFICIENCY

While many immunodeficiencies are diagnosed at an early age, CVID usually develops in adolescence or young adulthood. It is a disorder characterized by poor production of immunoglobulins in response to antigenic stimuli. This limited humoral response to antigens leads to recurrent sinus and pulmonary infections, often caused by *Streptococcus pneumoniae* and other bacterial pathogens. Recurrent pulmonary infections over time may lead to bronchiectasis, a common complication of CVID in adults. Patients with CVID may also have chronic enteric infection with *Giardia lamblia* and chronic meningoencephalitis due to enterovirus. Patients with CVID

TABLE 204-4 Infections Associated with Asplenia

Infection	Preventative Strategy
Encapsulated organisms (*Streptococcus pneumoniae, Haemophilus influenzae, Neisseria meningitidis*)	Vaccinate before or 2 wk after splenectomy
Capnocytophaga canimorsus	Thorough washing and medical evaluation for prophylactic antibiotics after dog bites
Babesia microti	Tick precautions when at risk for tick exposure in areas of risk (Northeast US)

may also suffer from allergic and autoimmune disorders, and are at increased risk of lymphoma.

While low quantitative total immunoglobulin levels suggest CVID, the diagnosis is made by evaluation of immunologic response to new or recall antigens. Patients with CVID fail to mount an appropriate antibody response to new or booster immunizations. Regular immunoglobulin infusions in patients with CVID may prevent recurrent infections and possibly limit the respiratory tract damage that can lead to bronchiectasis.

ASPLENIA

Splenectomy may be medically necessary in patients with trauma, malignancy, refractory idiopathic thrombotic purpura, and other hematologic disorders. Patients with sickle cell anemia are usually functionally asplenic early in life and become anatomically asplenic due to auto-infarction over time. Asplenic patients are at risk for overwhelming bacterial infection with encapsulated organisms,

including *S. pneumoniae, Haemophilus influenzae,* and possibly *Neisseria meningitidis* (**Table 204-4**). Progression of bacterial infection in asplenic patients may be rapid, and historically was associated with high mortality. In patients with surgical splenectomy, the risk for postsplenectomy sepsis due to an encapsulated organism is probably highest in the first few years after splenectomy. Sepsis may be more common in asplenic individuals with hematologic disease such as thalessemia than in those who underwent splenectomy for trauma. Asplenic patients with fever, chills, malaise, rigors, or other signs or symptoms of infection should be immediately treated with antibiotics directed at encapsulated organisms, and blood cultures must be obtained (**Figure 204-2**).

Asplenic patients are also at increased risk for severe infection due to *B. microti* and *Capnocytophaga canimorsus*. As in patients treated with rituximab, babesiosis is more severe in splenectomized patients. Treatment options include atovaquone and azithromycin, or clindamycin and quinine. Asplenic patients with babesiosis may also require multiple or prolonged treatment courses.

C. canimorsus is a Gram-negative organism that inhabits the oral cavity of dogs. Dog bites may lead to local inoculation, and in asplenic patients may progress rapidly to systemic infection. *C. canimorsus* has been associated with severe sepsis and digital (and occasionally nasal) necrosis. Asplenic patients should be instructed to carefully wash all dog bites and seek medical assessment regarding prophylactic antibiotics after animal bites, particularly dog bites. Oral amoxicillin-clavulanic acid is useful for prophylaxis; ampicillin-sulbactam, fluoroquinolones, or third-generation cephalosporins are options for patients requiring intravenous therapy or with penicillin allergy. Dog bite and animal exposure history should be obtained in all asplenic patients with sepsis.

Patients scheduled for splenectomy or who recently had an emergent splenectomy should be vaccinated for *S. pneumoniae, H. influenzae,* and *N. meningitidis*. When splenectomy is planned,

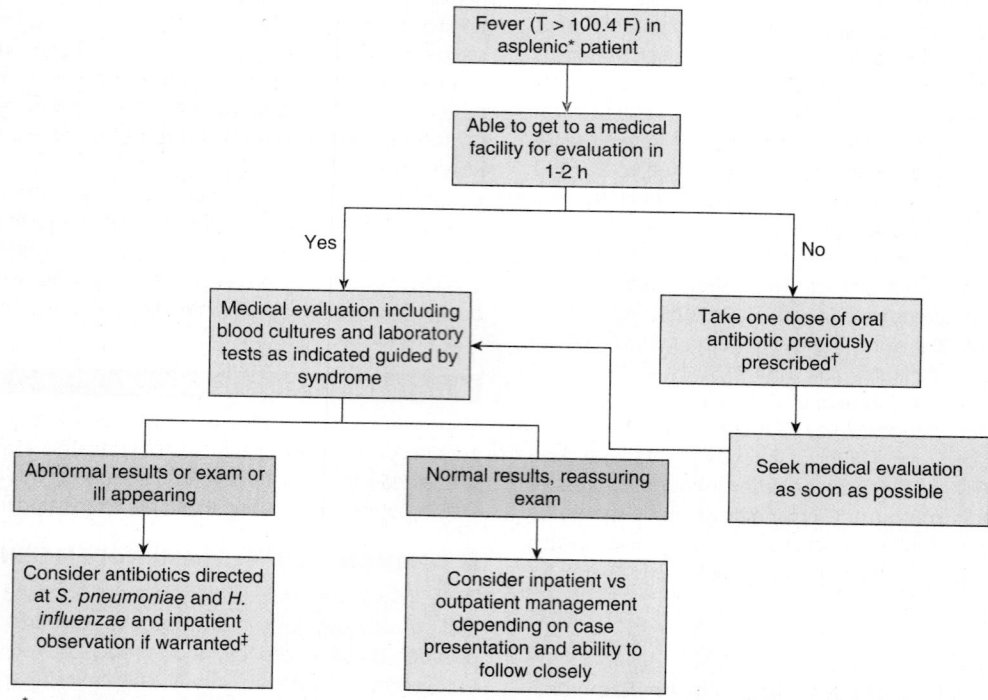

* Includes anatomic asplenia due to previous splenectomy, congenital disorder, or autoinfarction related to sickle cell disease.
† Appropriate oral antibiotics include amoxicillin-clavulanate, cefuroxime, levofloxacin, moxifloxacin depending on local antimicrobial resistance data.
‡ A special case includes patients with evidence of recent animal bite in whom empiric antibiotics should also be directed at *Capnocytophaga canimorsus*.

Figure 204-2 *How to manage fever in an asplenic patient.* (Adaptation from LG Rubin and W Schaffner. Care of the asplenic patient. *N Engl J Med.* 2014;371:349-356.)

TABLE 204-5 Evidence-based Medicine: Key References for Infections of Immunocompromised Hosts

Reference	Methodology	Results	Limitations	Bottom Line
Yale S, Limper A. *Mayo Clin Proc.* 1996;71:5-13.	Retrospective cohort study	Among 116 HIV-negative patients diagnosed with PCP, 91% received corticosteroids within the last month. Median steroid dose was 30 mg prednisone daily for 12 wk, but 25% of patients were on as little as 16 mg prednisone daily for as few as 8 wk	Examines the association between corticosteroids and PCP, but does not determine absolute risk	PCP in non-HIV infected patients was associated with corticosteroid use, even in patients on relatively low doses of prednisone for a short period of time. PCP prophylaxis should be considered in these circumstances
Sepkowitz KA, et al. *JAMA.* 1992;267:832-837.	Retrospective cohort study	Among 142 patients diagnosed with PCP at a cancer hospital, 87% were previously treated with corticosteroids. 49% of patients diagnosed with PCP premortem died	HIV testing only performed in 40 of 142 patients (all tested were negative)	PCP infection in patients with malignancy was commonly associated with corticosteroid use. Mortality was high
Cruz T, et al. *N Engl J Med.* 1966;275:1093-1096.	Case series	Description of 5 fatal cases of overwhelming *Strongyloides* infection in patients previously treated with corticosteroids. Common clinical findings included diarrhea, vomiting, abdominal pain, and shock	Uncontrolled case series	First description of overwhelming *Strongyloides* infection associated with steroids. *Strongyloides* hyperinfection can be a fatal complication of corticosteroid use
Bongartz T, et al. *JAMA.* 2006;295:2275-2285.	Meta-analysis	Meta-analysis that included 9 randomized trials of adalimumab or infliximab for the treatment of RA that found a pooled odds ratio of 2.0 for developing serious infection while on adalimumab or infliximab vs placebo	Because study is a metaanalysis, there is heterogeneity in study population in terms of RA and duration of treatment	This study suggests that there is increased risk of serious infection among patients with RA treated with adalimumab or infliximab
Keane J, et al. *N Engl J Med.* 2001;345:1098-1104.	Retrospective cohort study	From 1998-2001, 70 cases of tuberculosis in patients treated with infliximab were reported to FDA. 57% of cases were extrapulmonary, including 17 cases (24%) of disseminated infection. The rate of tuberculosis in patients treated with infliximab was higher than background rate	Small number of cases; this study depends on accurate reporting to the FDA	Development of active tuberculosis is a significant risk after initiation of infliximab. Screening for latent tuberculosis should be undertaken in all patients prior to initiation of infliximab
Slifman NR, et al. *Arthritis Rheum.* 2003;48:319-324.	Retrospective cohort study	From 1998-2001, 15 cases of listeriosis in patients treated with etanercept or infliximab were reported to FDA. All 15 were receiving other immunosuppressive agents in addition to TNF-α inhibitor. The rate of listeriosis among patients treated with TNF-α inhibitors was higher than the general US population reported to federal programs (FoodNet)	Tiny number of affected patients; this study depends on accurate reporting to the FDA	Listeriosis may be a serious risk to patients treated with TNF-α inhibitors, particularly those treated with other adjunctive agents concurrently
Yeo W, et al. *J Clin Oncol.* 2008;27:605-611.	Retrospective cohort study	In a cohort of 46 lymphoma patients with evidence of resolved HBV, 5/21 who received rituximab-based chemotherapy vs 0/25 who received non-rituximab based chemotherapy developed HBV reactivation	Small sample size limits interpretation	Receipt of rituximab among patient with resolved HBV treated for lymphoma predisposed to HBV reactivation
Krause PJ, et al. *Clin Infect Dis.* 2008;46:370-376.	Retrospective case-control study	Compared the immunologic status and clinical course of 14 patients with relapsing babesiosis to 46 controls with treatment-responsive babesiosis	May be limited by selection bias of cases which were from different centers	Patients with relapsing babesiosis had more complications and were more likely to have lymphoma, asplenia, or to have received rituximab

HBV, hepatitis B virus; PCP, *Pneumocystis jiroveci* pneumonia; RA, rheumatoid arthritis.

vaccination should be carried out at least 2 weeks before the procedure. For unplanned splenectomies, patients should be vaccinated 2 weeks after the procedure or prior to hospital discharge (whichever is first), so that it is not overlooked. Patients who have undergone splenectomy should be carefully educated about their increased risk for infection and the need to seek medical care during fever or after dog bites. Asplenic patients should also have oral antibiotics available at home for self-administration if fever develops (Figure 204-2).

TRANSPLANTATION

Recipients of solid organ transplantation (SOT) and stem cell transplantation (SCT) are at risk for infection with community and nosocomial pathogens, as well as reactivation of latent pathogens. A few distinctions between SOT and SCT are helpful when evaluating a transplant recipient with possible infection. Infections often localize to the transplanted organ and surrounding tissues in SOT recipients. For example, urinary tract infection and pyelonephritis are common after renal transplantation. Most SOT recipients require lifelong immunosuppressive therapy after transplant, and those who develop organ rejection require further immunosuppression and are at heightened risk for infection.

In contrast to SOT recipients, SCT recipients have often undergone extensive cancer treatment already, leading to immunosuppression even before the transplant procedure. Some SCT recipients have already had opportunistic infections prior to SCT. The donor stem cell type in SCT may be somewhat predictive of infectious risk after transplantation. While allogeneic stem cell recipients require immunosuppression after transplantation to prevent graft-versus-host disease (GVHD), autologous stem cell transplant recipients do not, and so are at lower risk for infectious complications after transplant. Unlike SOT recipients, allogeneic SCT recipients are often weaned off immunosuppressive medications months to years after transplantation, unless they develop GVHD, which requires increased immunosuppression analogous to rejection in SOT recipients.

When a transplant recipient presents with suspected infection, the differential diagnosis is broad. However, some infections tend to cluster during certain time frames after transplant.

During the first month after transplantation, most infections are related to the surgical procedure (in the case of SOT), the hospitalization during transplantation, conditioning chemotherapy-related neutropenia (in the case of SCT), or the donor tissue. Infections related to surgery (for SOT recipients) and hospitalization (for both SOT and SCT recipients) include wound infection, central venous catheter infection, and catheter-associated urinary tract infection. Stem cell transplantation recipients are also at significant risk for bacterial and fungal infection associated with neutropenia during this period of time. Bacterial infection during neutropenia often results from translocation from endogenous sources, such as the gastrointestinal tract. Mucositis from chemotherapy also increases the risk of endogenously derived bacterial infection in SCT recipients. Donor-derived infection is uncommon due to extensive donor pretransplant screening. Exotic pathogens may sometimes be encountered in this setting, such as lymphocytic choriomeningitis virus, rabies virus, and Encephalitozoon cuniculi (microsporidia). Donor-derived infection should be a consideration in SOT recipients when fever starts shortly after transplantation, and there is no evidence of nosocomial or surgical infection.

Infections in the early posttransplant period (between 2 and 6 months after transplant) are often due to opportunists, including PCP, aspergillosis, cryptococcosis, and reactivation of latent pathogens, such as CMV, varicella zoster virus (VZV), toxoplasma, and BK virus. SCT recipients with GVHD, and SOT recipients who develop rejection during this period, require aggressive immunosuppressive therapy, placing them at very high risk of infection, particularly for invasive mold infection in SCT recipients. In transplant patients with aspergillosis and other aggressive infections, reducing doses of corticosteroids and other immunosuppressive drugs should be strongly considered. PCP is also a significant risk during this time period; most transplant patients receive PCP prophylaxis for at least 3 to 12 months.

Herpes viruses, including CMV, VZV, and herpes simplex (HSV), commonly reactivate in previously exposed transplant recipients between 2 and 6 months posttransplant. Cytomegalovirus can cause pneumonitis, esophagitis, and colitis. Cytomegalovirus also has an intrinsic immunosuppressive effect, leading to increased susceptibility to other infections. Transplant recipients at risk for CMV reactivation include those who were CMV seropositive prior to transplant and those with CMV seropositive donors. Typically, SOT and SCT recipients are treated with prophylactic valganciclovir for 3 to 12 months, or are monitored for CMV reactivation weekly for 3 to 6 months after transplantation to prevent CMV end organ disease. VZV and HSV infection are also common during this time period, so patients who are not treated with prophylactic valganciclovir for CMV are typically treated with prophylactic acyclovir or valacyclovir to prevent VZV and HSV reactivation.

Patients more than 6 months out from transplantation remain at increased risk for infection with community-acquired pathogens, particularly from encapsulated organisms after SCT, and late reactivation of latent viruses such as hepatitis B. Transplant recipients who received prophylaxis for CMV or VZV for the first 6 months after transplant are also at risk for reactivation of these pathogens after prophylaxis is stopped. There is also a risk of transplant-associated malignancy, due to latent viruses such as Epstein-Barr virus and human papillomavirus, in this time period. Patients with rejection or GVHD more than 6 months after transplant may develop the same opportunistic pathogens seen earlier.

SUGGESTED READINGS

Cantini F, Niccoli L, Goletti D. Adalimumab, etanercept, infliximab, and the risk of tuberculosis: data from clinical trials, national registries, and postmarketing surveillance. *J Rheumatol Suppl.* 2014;91:47-55.

Chapel H, Cunningham-Rundles C. Update in understanding common variable immunodeficiency disorders (CVIDs) and the management of patients with these conditions. *Br J Haematol.* 2009;145:709-727.

Curtis JR, Patkar N, Xie A, et al. Risk of serious bacterial infections among rheumatoid arthritis patients exposed to tumor necrosis factor α antagonists. *Arthritis Rheum.* 2007;56:1125-1133.

Fishman JA. Infection in solid-organ transplant recipients. *N Engl J Med.* 2007;357:2601-2614.

Koo S, Marty FM, Baden LR. Infectious complications associated with immunomodulating biologic agents. *Infect Dis Clin N Am.* 2010;24:285-306.

Krause PJ, Gewurz BE, Hill D, et al. Persistent and relapsing babesiosis in immunocompromised patients. *Clin Infect Dis.* 2008;46:370-376.

Rubin LG, Schaffner W. Care of the asplenic patient. *N Engl J Med.* 2014;371:349-356.

Stuck AE, Minder CE, Frey FJ. Risk of infectious complications in patients taking glucocorticosteroids. *Rev Infect Dis.* 1989;11:954-962.

Yale SH, Limper AH. Pneumocystis carinii pneumonia in patients without acquired immunodeficiency syndrome: associated illness and prior corticosteroid therapy. *Mayo Clin Proc.* 1996;71:5-13.

CHAPTER 205

Fever in the Returning Traveler

Serena Koenig, MD, MPH

James H. Maguire, MD, MPH

Key Clinical Questions

1. What infections should be considered?
2. What questions should be asked in the travel history?
3. What diagnostic tests should be conducted?
4. Which patients should be hospitalized?
5. What clinical factors put patients at risk for serious complications?
6. When should an infectious disease physician be consulted?

INTRODUCTION

International travelers are commonly plagued by medical problems, particularly after travel to a resource-poor setting. About 8% of travelers to developing countries seek medical care while they are away or after they return. Although fever in the traveler may be caused by mild illnesses, it may also be a harbinger of potentially lethal infection. The evaluation of the febrile traveler is complicated by the wide array of possible etiologies. It is critical to consider the infections are endemic to the area visited, potential exposures, time between exposure and the onset of symptoms, and associated clinical findings. This chapter reviews the common causes of fever in returning travelers and the appropriate initial evaluation.

EPIDEMIOLOGY

GeoSentinel, a worldwide network of travel and tropical medicine clinics, provides the largest database for travel-related infections. From 1996 to 2004, the five most common diagnoses for patients with systemic febrile illnesses presenting to GeoSentinel clinics from the developing world were malaria, dengue, mononucleosis due to Epstein-Barr virus or cytomegalovirus, rickettsial infection, and typhoid fever. GeoSentinel clinic data from 2007 to 2011 were similar. Malaria was the top overall diagnosis, followed by dengue, typhoid and paratyphoid fevers, and rickettsial disease. The emerging infection chikungunya virus rounded out the top five.

Malaria remains the leading cause of systemic febrile illness in travelers returning from Sub-Saharan Africa, and it was one of the three top causes from all regions of the developing world. In the United States, more than 50% of cases of imported malaria occurred among immigrant families who had made recent visits to their country of origin. Dengue was the leading cause for fever in travelers to Southeast Asia, Latin America, and the Caribbean. Rickettsial infections were an important cause of fever in travelers to Sub-Saharan Africa, who often had *Rickettsia africae* (African tick-bite fever). Typhoid fever was most common in travelers to South Central Asia, especially in travelers to India, Pakistan, Bangladesh, and Nepal, but cases also occurred in travelers to other regions. Other notable diagnoses among febrile travelers with systemic illness included viral hepatitis, leptospirosis, tuberculosis, brucellosis, measles, and acute HIV.

Among patients with fever and diarrhea, the most common diagnoses were traveler's diarrhea, *Campylobacter*, nontyphoidal *Salmonella* species, and shigellosis. In those with fever and respiratory symptoms, nearly half were diagnosed with bronchitis or an acute unspecified respiratory infection. Other common diagnoses were bacterial pneumonia, tonsillitis, influenza or an influenza-like illness, and sinusitis.

WHAT INFORMATION SHOULD BE ELICITED FROM THE MEDICAL HISTORY?

It is critical to identify all regions that the traveler has visited in the past year, including layovers or short stops. The Centers for Disease Control and Prevention (CDC) website (www.cdc.gov) has a travel site that lists common infections by each country and region, as well as reports on disease outbreaks. The World Health Organization (WHO) website (www.who.int) also has information about disease outbreaks. The importance of this awareness was illustrated by the largest-ever outbreak of Ebola virus disease in West Africa that started in late 2013, and spread to distant countries. It is also particularly important to identify regions of travel where malaria and dengue are endemic.

It is also necessary to define the dates of travel and the timing of symptom onset, which may permit the estimation of the approximate incubation period. **Table 205-1** lists the incubation periods for several bacteria, viruses, fungi, and parasites that cause fever in returning travelers. Some infections can be excluded based

on an incubation period that is inconsistent with the timing of fever. For example, a traveler presenting with a systemic febrile infection 3 weeks after returning would be very unlikely to have dengue, which nearly always presents within 14 days. The duration of the trip can also be helpful. Malaria is more often reported in long-term (>6 months) than short-term travelers, though 5% of patients with malaria in the GeoSentinel database had traveled for

TABLE 205-1 Infectious Causes of Fever and Associated Incubation Periods in Returning Travelers

Infection	Incubation Period (Range)	Infection	Incubation Period (Range)
Bacteria		Cytomegalovirus	3 wk-3 mo
Plague (Yersinia pestis)	1-6 d	Hepatitis E	26-42 d (2-9 wk)
Anthrax (Bacillus anthracis)	1-7 d	Hepatitis A	28-30 d (15-50 d)
Meningococcemia (Neisseria meningitidis)	1-14 d	Epstein-Barr virus	4-6 wk
Meliodosis (Burkholderia pseudomallei)	1-21 d	Rabies	1-2 mo (9 d-years)
Shigellosis (Shigella species)	2-6 d (1-20 d)	Hepatitis B	60-90 d (45 d-9 mo)
Campylobacter enteritis (Camplyobacter jejuni)	2-6 d (1-20 d)	**Fungal infections**	
Salmonellosis (Salmonella species)	2-6 d (1-20 d)	Acute histoplasmosis (Histoplasma capsulatum)	7-14 d (3-21 d)
Yersinia enteritis (Yersinia enterocolitica)	4-6 d (1-14 d)	Acute coccidioidomycosis (Coccidioides immitis)	10-14 d (7-28 d)
Legionellosis (Legionella pneumophila)	5-6 d (2-10 d)	**Parasites**	
Human monocytic ehrlichiosis (Ehrlichia chaffeensis)	5-15 d	Trichinosis (Trichinella spiralis)	3 d to weeks
Human granulocytic anaplasmosis (Anaplasma phagocytophilum)	5-21 d	East African trypanosomiasis (Trypanosoma brucei rhodesiense and gambiense)	Acute: 5-16 d (3-21 d) Chronic illness: months to years
Leptospirosis (Leptospira interrogans)	7-12 d (2-26 d)	Toxoplasmosis (Toxoplasma gondii)	5-23 d
Spotted fever (Rickettsiae, spotted fever group)	About 1 wk (few days to 2-3 wk)	Visceral leishmaniasis (Leishmania species)	10 d-6 mo
Lyme disease (Borrelia burdorferi)	7-10 d (3-30 d)	Angiostrongyliasis meningitis (Angiostrongylus cantonensis)	2 wk (5 d-6 wk)
Typhoid and paratyphoid fever (Salmonella enterica serotype typhi and Salmonella paratyphi A, B, or C)	7-18 d (3-60 d)	Malaria (Plasmodium falciparum)	12-14 d (8-25 d)
Bartonellosis (Bartonella species)	7-21 d	Malaria (Plasmodium ovale)	14-16 d (10-20 d)
Scrub typhus (Orientia tsutsugamushi)	10 d (6-21 d)	Malaria (Plasmodium vivax)	14-15 d (10 d to, in rare cases, months)
Syphilis (Treponema pallidum)	10-90 d	Malaria (Plasmodium malariae)	18-20 d (15 d to, in rare cases, months to years)
Q fever (Coxiella burnetti)	14-21 d (2-29 d)		
Brucellosis (Brucella species)	2-4 wk (5 d-5 mo)	Acute schistosomiasis (Schistosoma species)	4-8 wk
Tuberculosis (Mycobacterium tuberculosis)	Primary: weeks Reactivation: years	Fascioliasis (Fasciola hepatica and gigantica)	Acute: days-3 mo Chronic: months to years
Viruses		Gnathostomiasis (Gnathostoma species)	3 wk-months
Influenza virus	1-3 d	Clonorchiasis (Clonorchis sinensis)	Acute: weeks-months Chronic: months to years
Chikungunya fever virus	3-7 d (2-12 d)	Amebic liver abscess (Entamoeba histolytica)	weeks-months
Viral hemorrhagic fevers (Hantavirus, Lassa fever virus, yellow fever virus, Ebola virus, Marburg virus, Rift Valley fever virus)	3-14 d (2 d-2 mo)	Visceral leishmaniasis (Leishmania donovani, L. infantum, L. chagasi, and others)	2-6 mo (10 d-years)
Arboviruses (many, such as Japanese encephalitis, tick-borne encephalitis, West Nile virus)	3-14 d (1-20 d)	Lymphatic filariasis (Wuchereria bancrofti and Brugia malayi)	3-6 mo-longer
Dengue fever	4-8 d (3-14 d)		
Poliomyelitis	7-14 d (3-35 d)		
Acute HIV infection	10-28 d (10 d-6 wk)		
Rubella	14 d (12-23 d)		

Data from Ryan ET, Wilson ME, Kain KC. Illness after international travel. *N Engl J Med.* 2002;347:505-516; and the Travelers' Health Yellow Book of the Centers for Disease Control and Prevention.

TABLE 205-2 Medical History for Fever in the Returning Traveler

- Region of travel
- Duration and timing of travel, incubation period, and duration of fever
- History of impaired immunity from disease (HIV, asplenia) or medications
- History of vaccinations, pretravel immunizations, and use of malaria chemoprophylaxis and compliance with the prescribed regimen
- Description of accommodations (including whether bed nets and air conditioners were used) and whether urban or rural areas were visited
- Possible tuberculosis exposures, such as history of working in a health care center
- History of treatment at a health center, particularly if the traveler received a blood transfusion, injection, or dental or surgical procedure
- Ingestion of untreated water, contaminated food, unpasteurized milk or cheese, or raw or undercooked meat or fish
- History of bites from mosquitoes, ticks, fleas, mites, or other biting arthropods
- Exposure to animals or animal products
- History of camping, hiking, safari expeditions, or walks through grassy or shrubby areas
- Exposure to freshwater from swimming, boating, or wading
- Sexual activity while traveling (number of partners and protection used, if any)
- Exposure to caves, construction, or excavation sites
- Other unusual activities or exposures

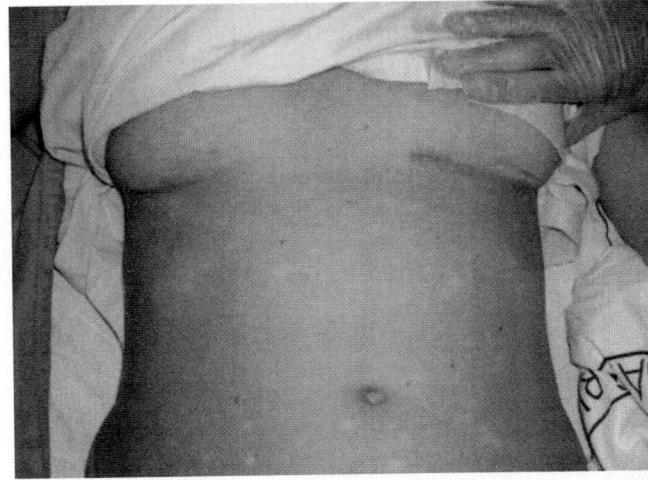

Figure 205-1 *Confluent maculopapular rash of dengue, with scattered petechiae and early bruising under the breasts.* (From Pinazo MJ, Muñoz J, Betica L, et al. *Emerg Infect Dis.* 2008;14:1329-1330.)

less than 1 week. Seasonal infections such as influenza may present at unusual times, given that peak seasons may differ in tropical climes.

The history should also elicit pertinent exposures for the traveler. Those who stay in houses may have more exposure to infection than those staying in tourist hotels. Camping, hiking, safari expeditions, and walking in grassy areas increase the risk of tick bites, which can cause rickettsial infections, Lyme disease, babesiosis, anaplasmosis, ehrlichiosis, and tickborne encephalitis. Malaria, dengue, yellow fever, and chikungunya fever are spread though mosquito bites. Fungal infections such as histoplasmosis may be acquired through inhalation of spores in caves or at excavation or construction sites. Coccidioidomycosis most often afflicts travelers to the American Southwest, but may be rarely seen in travelers to arid parts of Mexico, Guatemala, Honduras, Venezuela, Argentina, and Colombia.

Leptospirosis can be acquired through exposure to freshwater, including swimming, boating, or wading. A sexual history is also important. Sexually transmitted diseases that can cause fever include acute HIV infection, hepatitis B virus, syphilis, and herpes viruses. Certain infections such as hepatitis A and acute schistosomiasis are more likely to occur among short-term travelers than immigrants or long-term expatriates, who in turn are more likely to have tuberculosis. **Table 205-2** provides a list of pertinent information that should be elicited from the febrile traveler.

DIAGNOSIS AND MANAGEMENT: GENERAL CONSIDERATIONS

The differential diagnosis of fever in the returning traveler is broad, as outlined in Table 205-1. The initial diagnostic evaluation of fever in travelers should focus on infections that can be rapidly life

threatening, such as malaria and meningococcal meningitis, or highly contagious, such as hepatitis A, measles, and tuberculosis. Dengue, rickettsial diseases, chikungunya fever, and typhoid fever should always be considered in patients with compatible clinical and epidemiologic presentations. Noninfectious causes of fever such as pulmonary embolism from long flights and drug fever from prophylactic or empiric medical therapy for travel-related conditions are also possibilities. Febrile illnesses unrelated to travel or infections acquired after return from travel should also be considered.

A careful physical examination for the returning traveler is essential. The retina, lymph nodes, heart, lungs, abdomen (in particular, liver and spleen), genital area, and extremities should be carefully examined, and the patient should have a complete neurologic examination. The skin should be carefully examined for the presence of a maculopapular rash compatible with dengue fever (**Figure 205-1**) or chikungunya, for the rose spots of typhoid, and for petechiae and ecchymoses suggestive of dengue hemorrhagic fever (DHF), viral hemorrhagic fever, or meningococcemia.

The initial laboratory evaluation should include complete blood count with differential, creatinine, urea nitrogen, electrolytes, liver function tests, and cultures of blood and urine. The recommended diagnostic workup for the initial evaluation of returning patients with fever is outlined in **Table 205-3**.

In general, hospital admission is warranted for most travelers with an undiagnosed febrile illness, due to the possibility of a serious condition such as malaria or typhoid. Clinicians should not hesitate to seek infectious disease consultation before deciding to treat the traveler as an outpatient, since some infections can present with mild findings in the early stage of disease and rapidly progress over hours to days.

■ MALARIA

Evaluation

Malaria is the most common cause of fever in travelers returning from developing countries, and untreated falciparum malaria can lead to death within hours of presentation. Therefore, it is essential to consider malaria in persons with systemic symptoms who have recently traveled to an endemic area, even if they report taking chemoprophylaxis and do not complain of fever. Though most patients present with fever, rigors, and influenza-like symptoms, at least 10% of patients initially present without fever. Headache, respiratory symptoms, or gastrointestinal symptoms may predominate at presentation.

TABLE 205-3 Initial Diagnostic Tests to Evaluate Fever in the Returning Traveler

All travelers:
- Electrolytes, blood urea nitrogen, creatinine, glucose
- Complete blood count and differential
- Blood and urine cultures

Travelers with relevant exposure or compatible clinical presentation:
- Thick and thin smears for malaria; rapid diagnostic test for malaria
- Acute and convalescent serology for dengue, chikungunya virus, rickettsial infections, and other infections
- HIV antibody test and/or viral load
- Stool cultures and stool studies for fecal leukocytes and ova and parasites
- Chest radiograph; consider sputum Gram stain and culture, and testing for influenza and other respiratory viruses, agents of bacterial and atypical pneumonia
- Tuberculin skin test, sputum for acid fast bacilli and mycobacterial culture
- Histoplasma antigen in urine, blood or bronchoalveolar fluid, and test for complement-fixing-type anticoccidioidal antibodies
- Serologic tests for *Coxiella burnetii* (Q fever) if there is hepatitis and animal exposure history
- In persons with eosinophilia: microscopic examination of stool for ova and parasites and serological tests for strongyloidiasis, schistosomiasis, and helminthic infections

As malaria is notorious for its ability to mimic other conditions, malaria smears should generally be sent in all travelers with nonspecific febrile illnesses.

Thick and thin smears of peripheral blood should be performed immediately in possible malaria (**Figures 205-2** and **205-3**). Thick smears are performed on hemolyzed specimens and are more sensitive for the detection of parasitemia, but the parasite morphology is often distorted, and speciation may not be possible. Thin smears are better for species identification and for estimating parasitemia. Giemsa stains are preferred for thin and thick smears for malaria

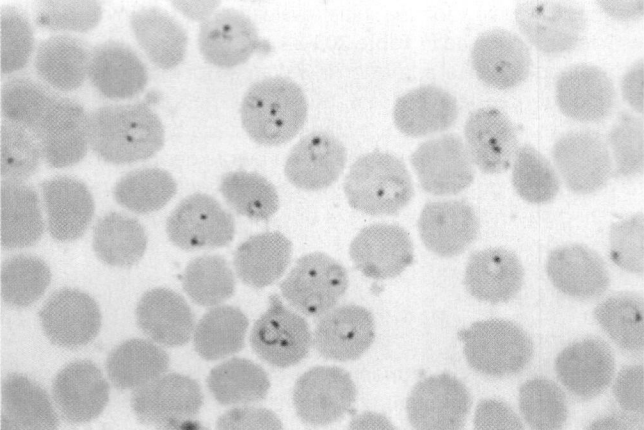

Figure 205-2 *Thin blood film with a monotonous population of small ring trophozoites, characteristic of Plasmodium falciparum; heavy parasitemia is present. Falciparum malaria is more lethal than other forms of malaria because of the high parasite burdens that may arise. Giemsa stain. (Public Health Image Library, Centers for Disease Control and Prevention.)*

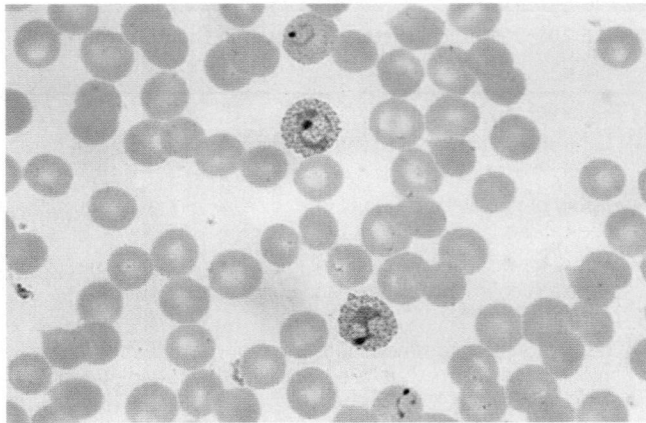

Figure 205-3 *Thin blood film with trophozoites of various ages covered in Schüffner dots, typical of Plasmodium vivax. Giemsa stain. (Public Health Image Library, Centers for Disease Control and Prevention.)*

detection. If Giemsa stains are unavailable or delayed, the Wright stain, commonly used to perform white blood cell differential counting in hematology laboratories, may be used as a somewhat inferior substitute. Rapid diagnostic tests are also available for centers without skilled microscopists. If the initial blood smears for malaria are negative but the diagnosis is still suspected, additional smears should be repeated within 12 to 24 hours.

Inpatient management

Travelers with falciparum malaria or malaria that has not been speciated should be admitted for urgent treatment and monitoring for potential complications. Patients at highest risk include nonimmune travelers, pregnant women, young children, and the elderly. Most deaths occur among patients with severe malaria within the first 48 hours after hospital admission. Those with severe malaria should be admitted to the intensive care unit.

Specific medications for the treatment of malaria vary based on the species of malaria, the risk of drug resistance (based on the region of travel), the age, pregnancy status, and comorbidities of the patient, and the degree of parasitemia and clinical severity of the disease. All nonimmune patients with falciparum malaria should be admitted for observation and urgent treatment, and an infectious disease specialist should be consulted for management. Consideration of hospitalization should be given even to persons who claim heavy prior exposure to falciparum malaria because it is difficult to assess acquired immunity, and immunity wanes without constant re-exposure.

The World Health Organization criteria for severe malaria include prostration, impaired consciousness, respiratory distress, repeated convulsions, circulatory collapse, pulmonary edema, abnormal bleeding, jaundice, hemoglobinuria, severe anemia, hypoglycemia, acidosis, renal impairment, elevated lactate, or hyperparasitemia. Patients meeting criteria for severe malaria should be admitted to an intensive care unit for parenteral therapy, management of volume status, identification and treatment of complications, and mechanical ventilation and dialysis if needed. Treatment of malaria is beyond the scope of this chapter, but is outlined in several recent reviews (see Suggested Readings). The Centers for Disease Control also provides up-to-date management guidelines on its website (www.cdc.gov/malaria).

■ DENGUE
Evaluation

Dengue should also always be considered in febrile travelers returning from endemic areas. The prevalence of dengue has risen in many areas; reported cases increased approximately fourfold from 1995 to

2005 in South America, Central America, Mexico, and the Caribbean. Dengue fever typically presents with fever, headache, retro-orbital pain, myalgia, joint pain, bone pain (breakbone fever), and fatigue, with or without a maculopapular or petechial rash. Classically, the fever has a biphasic or saddleback pattern, although this has been uncommon in recent series. Dengue is usually an asymptomatic or self-limited, if highly unpleasant, illness. However, patients that have previously been exposed to dengue may develop life-threatening DHF or dengue shock syndrome (DSS) on re-exposure.

The diagnosis of dengue infection is usually based on clinical findings. Acute and convalescent serology confirms the diagnosis, but testing is available only in specialized centers, and results do not return in time to impact decisions in care. Laboratory findings associated with dengue include thrombocytopenia, leukopenia, and elevated hepatic transaminases. The tourniquet test is a traditional diagnostic test for dengue, which indirectly measures both capillary fragility and thrombocytopenia. A blood pressure cuff is inflated to midway between systolic and diastolic pressures and left on the upper arm for 5 minutes. The resulting petechiae on the volar forearm just below the antecubital fossa are counted; a positive result is more than 20 petechiae per square inch. However, the tourniquet test is not very sensitive for the diagnosis of dengue, but it may indicate which patients are at risk of hemorrhagic complications.

Inpatient management

Patients with suspected dengue should be monitored for early signs of hemorrhage and vascular permeability. DHF and DSS are rare among short-term travelers, and more likely to occur among immigrants and others who were previously infected with another serotype. Nevertheless, all persons with dengue should be closely monitored for potential complications. DHF or DSS is a clinical diagnosis, suggested by a platelet count less than 100,000/mm³ and evidence of hemorrhage or plasma leakage (pleural effusion, ascites, or elevated hematocrit). All patients with suspected dengue meeting any of these criteria should be hospitalized.

Patients with dengue can develop hemorrhage and hypovolemic shock due to increased intravascular permeability, thrombocytopenia, and coagulopathy. Vital signs and hematocrit should be followed for signs of dehydration and hemoconcentration. Platelet counts should be monitored, and radiographic studies such as ultrasound should be performed to detect fluid accumulation in serosal cavities. Plasma leakage typically develops 4 to 7 days after the onset of symptoms, approximately coinciding with the resolution of fever. There is no specific therapy for dengue. Acetaminophen is the preferred agent for fever and myalgia. Nonsteroidal anti-inflammatory medications and aspirin should be avoided as they could increase the risk of bleeding. Intravascular hydration with fluids or colloids is essential for those with increased intravascular permeability. All patients with suspected dengue should be seen in consultation with an infectious disease specialist because early signs of increased vascular permeability and coagulopathy may be subtle, and patients may develop life-threatening shock and hemorrhage.

■ ENTERIC FEVER (TYPHOID AND PARATYPHOID)

Evaluation

Typhoid fever should be considered in any febrile traveler, particularly those returning from the Indian subcontinent, and those with a history of consuming unclean food or water. Typhoid presents as escalating fever, often without distinguishing features. There may be right lower quadrant pain from inflammation of Peyer patches of the ileum. Either constipation or diarrhea may be present. Rarely, rose spots are seen on the trunk of light-skinned persons. Pulmonary infiltrates, presumably arising from bacteremia, may be found in those with prolonged fever. Typhoid fever can be diagnosed by culturing blood, stool, and urine; serology is unreliable.

Inpatient management

Typhoid fever is treated based on antibiotic susceptibility testing. Because of the emergence of multidrug-resistant strains in recent years, some authors recommend starting an antibiotic combination initially, such as ceftriaxone and ciprofloxacin, until the results of susceptibility testing are available and therapy can be tailored.

■ CHIKUNGUNYA FEVER

Evaluation

The mosquitoborne chikungunya virus has emerged from West Africa in recent years to cause major outbreaks in Latin America, the Caribbean, and much of Asia. It presents with the abrupt onset of high fever after a relatively short incubation of about 3 days. Severe myalgias and arthralgias are characteristic. Joint pains may be severe and usually involve large joints of the legs and arms, as well as smaller joints. Ligamentous and periarticular pain and swelling may also occur. A maculopapular rash involving the trunk is common; the rash may also involve the palms, soles, face, and oddly enough, the ears.

Polymerase chain reaction is the most sensitive means of diagnosing chikungunya in acute infection. IgM antibody to Chikungunya is detectable 5 days into the course of infection. Lymphopenia, thrombocytopenia, and mild transaminitis may also be seen.

Inpatient management

Treatment for chikungunya fever is supportive, and includes nonsteroidal anti-inflammatory drugs for joint pain. Patients should be cautioned that joint pain and tenosynovitis may persist for months after resolution of fever. Cryoglobulinemia and Raynaud phenomenon may also occur in the recovery phase.

■ RICKETTSIAL DISEASE

Evaluation

Rickettsial diseases also present with fever, headache, and myalgia. In Sub-Saharan Africa, tick-bite fever due to *Rickettsia africae*, the most common rickettsial infection, should be considered for travelers with potential exposure to tick bites whilst on safari, camping, or hiking. On physical examination, a painless eschar with regional lymphadenopathy occurs frequently at the inoculation site; in some cases, multiple inoculation eschars may be noted. A maculopapular rash is usually not present. Rickettsial infections are primarily diagnosed clinically and confirmed by serologic tests.

Inpatient management

African tick bite fever and other rickettsial spotted fevers are treated with doxycycline 100 mg twice daily.

PRACTICE POINT

- Returning travelers with fever and hemorrhage, neurologic symptoms, respiratory distress, or other severe symptoms should be evaluated immediately. Because such infections may be rapidly fatal, urgent consultation with an infectious disease expert is advisable.

POTENTIAL COMPLICATIONS

Patients infected with falciparum malaria, particularly travelers who are nonimmune, can rapidly develop the life-threatening complications of severe malaria as defined by WHO (already described).

In contrast, travelers are less likely than foreign nationals to develop life-threatening dengue because severe disease is associated with a second infection with a different dengue serotype. Nevertheless, all travelers with suspected dengue should be evaluated for early signs of hemorrhage or plasma leakage.

Because the list of potential diagnoses in critically ill travelers is exceedingly long, infectious disease consultation should be urgently obtained for any traveler with danger signs, including high fever, mental status changes and other neurologic symptoms, respiratory distress, hemorrhage, and severe laboratory abnormalities, such as metabolic acidosis, renal failure, or profound anemia. Empiric treatment for possible diagnoses should be considered in such patients.

CONCLUSION

Malaria is common in the febrile traveler and may be rapidly lethal. When evaluating the febrile patient, it is critical to obtain a travel history and determine if the patient is at risk for malaria based on the region visited. Those at risk for malaria must be tested immediately, and those infected must be promptly treated. Severe malaria is a medical emergency, and delays in treatment increase the mortality rate. Despite this, the diagnosis of malaria is frequently missed initially, and delays in treatment are common. Malaria, dengue, typhoid fever, and other tropical and exotic diseases should be reported to public health authorities in the United States and other countries.

DISCHARGE CHECKLIST

Malaria:

- Has infectious diseases clinic follow-up been arranged? Has the patient had daily blood smears with documentation of clearance of parasitemia?
- Have patients been educated that malaria can recur, and that they should undergo repeat evaluation if they develop fever after discharge?
- Have patients been counseled about the importance of completing malaria medication, and potential side effects? Do patients have adequate financial resources to obtain medications?
- Have public health authorities been notified?

Dengue:

- Has infectious diseases clinic follow-up been arranged? Has follow-up laboratory monitoring been arranged to document resolution of cytopenias and abnormal liver tests, if present?

- Have patients been counseled to maintain fluid intake to avoid dehydration, and to take acetaminophen (and not aspirin or nonsteroidal anti-inflammatory drugs) for fever and myalgia?
- Have patients been educated about warning signs suggestive of severe dengue, including abnormal mental status, persistent vomiting, lethargy, severe abdominal pain, and bleeding?
- Have public health authorities been notified?

SUGGESTED READINGS

Centers for Disease Control and Prevention. *CDC Health Information for International Travel (Yellow Book 2016)*. Available at http://wwwnc.cdc.gov/travel/yellowbook/2016/table-of-contents.

Dengue: guidelines for the diagnosis, treatment, prevention, and control. World Health Organization, Geneva, Switzerland, 2009. Available at http://whqlibdoc.who.int/publications/2009/9789241547871_eng.pdf?ua=1.

Freedman DO, Weld LH, Kozarsky PE, et al. Spectrum of disease and relation to place of exposure among ill returned travelers. *N Engl J Med*. 2006;354:119-130.

Griffith KS, Lewis LS, Mali S, Parise ME. Treatment of malaria in the United States: a systematic review. *JAMA*. 2007;297:2264-2277.

Leder K, Torresi J, Libman MD, et al. GeoSentinel surveillance of illness in returned travelers, 2007–2011. *Ann Intern Med*. 2013;158:456-468.

Newman RD, Parise ME, Barber AM, Steketee RW. Malaria-related deaths among U.S. travelers, 1963–2001. *Ann Intern Med*. 2004;141:547-555.

Ryan ET, Wilson ME, Kain KC. Illness after international travel. *N Engl J Med*. 2002;347:505-516.

Wilder-Smith A, Schwartz E. Dengue in travelers. *N Engl J Med*. 2005;353:924-932.

Wilson ME, Weld LH, Boggild A, et al. Fever in returned travelers: results from the GeoSentinel Surveillance Network. *Clin Infect Dis*. 2007;44:1560-1568.

World Health Organization, Geneva, Switzerland, 2015. Guidelines for the treatment of malaria. Third edition. Available at http://apps.who.int/iris/bitstream/10665/162441/1/9789241549127_eng.pdf?ua=1.

206

Undiagnosed Fever in Hospitalized Patients

David A. Oxman, MD

Key Clinical Questions

1. What are the major categories of fever of unknown origin (FUO)?
2. What basic tests should be done in evaluating patients with FUO?
3. When is more specific laboratory testing or diagnostic imaging indicated?
4. Which patients should receive empiric therapy?
5. What is the prognosis of FUO?

INTRODUCTION

The classic definition of fever of unknown origin (FUO) by Petersdorf and Beeson in 1961 was a fever greater than 38.3°C (101°F) on several occasions, persisting without diagnosis for at least 3 weeks, despite 1 week of investigation in the hospital. In the 50 years since, medical practice has changed substantially, and much of the diagnostic evaluation for FUO can be accomplished on an outpatient basis. One proposed revision of the definition of classic FUO is a febrile illness that has not been diagnosed after at least three outpatient visits or 3 days of hospitalization (**Table 206-1**). In practice, while an exact definition is difficult, FUO can be thought of as a persistent febrile illness that has eluded diagnosis despite a thorough history, physical examination, and routine diagnostic testing. Additionally, several specific categories of FUO have been proposed, including nosocomial FUO, HIV-related FUO, and FUO in the returning traveler. Over 200 different causes of FUO have been reported, but all etiologies fall into four broad groups: infectious, neoplastic, rheumatologic, and miscellaneous. The incidence of each etiology will vary with different patient populations and geographic locations.

PATHOPHYSIOLOGY

■ PHYSIOLOGY OF FEVER

Fever is a complex common response to dissimilar diseases. The febrile response includes not only elevation of core body temperature but also activation of numerous physiological, endocrine, and immunologic systems. Although the neural regulation of body temperature involves several parts of the brain, the preoptic and anterior regions of the hypothalamus play the greatest role. Pyrogens—either endogenous or exogenous—stimulate pyrogenic cytokines such as interleukin (IL)-1, IL-6, tumor necrosis factor alpha (TNF-α), interferon gamma (IFN-γ), or act directly on hypothalamic neurons and decrease their firing rate, leading to physiological responses that decrease heat loss and increase heat production. Exogenous pyrogens include microbes and toxins, whereas endogenous pyrogens include antigen-antibody complexes, complement, tissue necrosis, and sensitized lymphocytes.

■ PATTERNS OF FEVER

Throughout medical history, clinicians have tried to link patterns of fever with specific diseases. In *saddleback* or *biphasic fever*, fever is present for several days, remits for a day, and then relapses for several days. This pattern has been associated with dengue, yellow fever, influenza, leptospirosis, ehrlichiosis, and tickborne relapsing fever. In *Pel-Ebstein fevers*, patients have days or even weeks of fever, followed by remission of equal duration, then another recurrence. Pel-Ebstein fevers are generally considered to suggest Hodgkin disease. However, with the exception of the tertian fever (recurring every 48 hours) of vivax malaria and the quartan fever (recurring every 72 hours) of *Plasmodium malariae*, fever patterns are not specific and are unreliable for diagnosis.

ETIOLOGIES OF FEVER OF UNKNOWN ORIGIN

■ MAJOR INFECTIOUS CAUSES

Since the 1950s the percentage of FUOs attributable to infections has decreased, but infection still makes up a large proportion of FUO cases. Tuberculosis—mostly reactivation of latent disease—is the

TABLE 206-1 Contemporary Definitions of Fever of Unknown Origin (FUO)

Type of FUO	Definition	Common Causes
Modified "classic" FUO	Fever ≥ 38.3°C (101°F) on several occasions for at least 3 wk	Infection, malignancy, vasculitis and other rheumatological conditions, drug fever
	No diagnosis after 3 d of hospitalization or three outpatient visits	In elderly patients in developed countries, often neoplastic; in young patients, often no diagnosis
Nosocomial FUO	Hospitalized patients with fever ≥ 38.3°C (101°F) on several occasions	*Clostridium difficile* enterocolitis, pneumonia, infection of central line and other devices, candidemia, urosepsis, acalculous cholecystitis, drug fever, thromboembolism, sinusitis, gout, pseudogout, central fever, stroke, myocardial infarction
	Fever not present or incubating at admission	
	Diagnosis uncertain after 3 d of appropriate investigations, including 48 h of incubating cultures	Dressler syndrome, malignant hyperthermia
Neutropenic FUO	Fever ≥ 38.3°C (101°F) on several occasions in a patient with an absolute neutrophil count of <500/mm³	Pneumonia, central line sepsis, *C. difficile* enterocolitis, mucositis, cellulitis, aspergillosis, candidiasis, fusariosis, herpes simplex virus, neutropenic enterocolitis (typhlitis)
	Diagnosis uncertain after 3 d of appropriate investigations, including 48 hours of incubating cultures	
HIV-related FUO	Patient with HIV infection and fever ≥ 38.3°C (101°F) on several occasions	Usually infectious, especially in patients not taking highly active antiretroviral therapy (HAART)
	Duration of at least 4 wk in outpatients or 3 d in inpatients	Most common cause worldwide is tuberculosis; others include *Pneumocystis jiroveci* pneumonia, *M. avium*, cytomegalovirus, toxoplasmosis, cryptococcosis, endemic mycoses, visceral leishmaniasis (Africa/Asia/Southern Europe)
	Diagnosis uncertain after 3 d of appropriate investigations, including 48 h of incubating cultures	Occasionally due to lymphoma, drug fever, Castleman disease, immune reconstitution inflammatory syndrome

most important infectious cause of FUO (**Table 206-2**). While PPD testing and chest x-ray are helpful for diagnosis, they may be falsely negative due to either anergy or extrapulmonary disease. Similarly, patients with advanced HIV disease and coinfection with tuberculosis may lack typical signs of TB infection.

Subacute bacterial endocarditis (SBE) was once a common cause of FUO, but it is now relatively uncommon. The diagnosis can typically be made by blood culture and echocardiography, but prior antibiotics may render blood cultures sterile. The classic physical findings associated with SBE—Roth spots, Janeway lesions, and splinter hemorrhages—are late findings seen in a small proportion of cases. True culture-negative endocarditis is less common in the United States than in Europe or the developing world. Organisms that cause

TABLE 206-2 Etiologies of FUO by Category

Infectious	*Bacterial:* **tuberculosis, subacute bacterial endocarditis,** intra-abdominal abscess, osteomyelitis, brucellosis, Lyme disease
	Viral: cytomegalovirus and Epstein-Barr virus
	Fungal: endemic mycoses
	Parasitic: malaria, babesia
Neoplastic	*Hematological:* **lymphoma,** leukemia, myelodysplastic disorders
	Solid organ: renal cell cancer, hepatocellular carcinoma, atrial myxoma, breast and colon cancer
Autoimmune	**Giant cell arteritis, Still disease** (adult juvenile rheumatoid arthritis), polyarteritis nodosa, familial Mediterranean fever, polymyalgia rheumatica, sarcoidosis, systemic lupus erythematosus
Miscellaneous	**Drug fever, factitious fever, thromboembolic disease,** Kikuchi necrotizing lymphadenitis, hyperthyroidism

Most common causes in bold.

culture-negative endocarditis include *Coxiella brunetti* (Q fever), *Bartonella* species, *Tropheryma whipplei* (the causative organism of Whipple's disease), *Brucella* species, and the so-called HACEK organisms, *Haemophilus parainfluenzae, Aggregatibacter aphrophilus, Aggregatibacter actinomycetemcomitans, Cardiobacterium hominis, Eikenella corrodens,* and *Kingella kingae.* Special microbiological techniques to facilitate the growth of fastidious organisms, as well as polymerase chain reaction (PCR), may help identify specific pathogens. When culture-negative endocarditis is suspected, the microbiology lab should be asked to hold blood cultures for up to 21 days.

Recurrent urinary tract infection, osteomyelitis, and occult intra-abdominal abscesses are other bacterial causes of FUO. Conditions that predispose to intra-abdominal abscess include inflammatory bowel disease, diverticular disease, and previous bowel surgery. Vertebral osteomyelitis is common in the elderly and should be considered in the patient with fever and back pain. Common viral causes of FUO causing a mononucleosis-like syndrome of fever, pharyngitis and lymphadenopathy include cytomegalovirus (CMV) and Epstein-Barr virus. Tickborne diseases such as Lyme disease, human monocytic ehrlichiosis, and human granulocytic anaplasmosis may be associated with prolonged fevers and nonspecific symptoms such as malaise, headache, and myalgias. Babesiosis often causes subclinical disease but may cause fever and in asplenic or otherwise immunocompromised patients can cause fulminant and life-threatening illness.

■ MAJOR NEOPLASTIC CAUSES

Fever associated with neoplasm or malignancy can result from either tissue necrosis or the release of pyrogenic cytokines. Lymphoma, myeloproliferative syndromes, and other hematopoietic malignancies are a common cause of FUO. Overall, with the advent of advanced diagnostic imaging and earlier detection, the percentage of solid-organ malignancies presenting as FUO has declined. Among solid organ tumors, renal cell carcinoma is most commonly associated with FUO, with hematuria notably absent in a large minority of patients. Other solid tumors occasionally associated with FUO are hepatocellular, breast, and colon cancer.

MAJOR AUTOIMMUNE AND INFLAMMATORY CAUSES

The relative percentage of FUOs in the developed world attributable to rheumatologic diseases has risen over time, in part due to the decline in undiagnosed infections and cancer, and also due to improved laboratory diagnostic techniques. Vasculitides, especially giant cell arteritis, are common causes of FUO in the elderly. Adult-onset Still disease is a common cause of FUO in young adults. The periodic fevers, of which familial Mediterranean fever (FMF) is the most common, are a group of inherited autoinflammatory disorders due to specific genetic mutations that cause recurrent fevers and often other symptoms such as serositis, splenomegaly, edema, and arthritis. Untreated FMF can lead to secondary amyloidosis and eventual renal failure.

PRACTICE POINT

- Giant cell arteritis (temporal arteritis) is the single most common cause of FUO in the elderly. It should be strongly suspected in any patient over the age of 50 with FUO and a high erythrocyte sedimentation rate (ESR). Classic manifestations include new headache, visual disturbances such as diplopia, tenderness and diminished pulsation of the temporal artery, and occasionally jaw claudication. However, the history and physical examination are not sensitive for giant cell arteritis (GCA). About 12% of GCA is silent or masked, presenting only with fever, weight loss, fatigue, and malaise.

MAJOR MISCELLANEOUS CAUSES

Many medications are associated with drug fever, but several cause it more frequently (**Table 206-3**). Common culprits include beta-lactam antibiotics, cardiac medications such as quinidine, amiodarone, or procainamide, antitubercular drugs such as isoniazid or rifampin, and anticonvulsants such as phenytoin and carbamazepine. Rash and eosinophilia may also be present, but often are not. Drug fever is more often observed with recently initiated medications but occasionally may develop in a patient that has been taking the offending agent chronically. Drug fever is a diagnosis of exclusion, and can only be confirmed when the fever resolves with cessation of the suspected agent. Factitious fever may be simulated by manipulation of thermometers or self-induced by the injection of pyogenic materials. One review of FUO put the incidence of factitious fever causing FUO as high as 10%. Typically, the patient is a young adult with experience working in health care. Thromboembolic disease should be considered as a possible cause of FUO in the right clinical setting (eg, hypercoagulable state or prolonged immobilization).

THE IMMUNOSUPPRESSED PATIENT

The percentage of FUOs caused by infections is high in this group. Decreased cell-mediated or humoral immune responses lead to an increased risk of acute infection, as well as reactivation of latent infections such as tuberculosis. Impaired immune responses may also lead to an absence of typical signs on physical examination or radiography. Transplant patients on antirejection medications or patients on high-dose steroids are at increased risk of disseminated fungal infection. Febrile neutropenic patients are at high risk for bacterial sepsis, and should receive empiric broad-spectrum antibiotics after appropriate cultures have been obtained. Immunosuppressed patients with FUO and pulmonary nodules should be considered for early bronchoscopy. Hepatosplenic candidiasis is typically seen after neutrophil counts have recovered and presents with abdominal pain, elevated alkaline phosphatase levels, and tiny hepatosplenic nodules on imaging studies. This condition is less often observed today because neutropenic patients receive antifungal therapy earlier in the course of illness.

THE PATIENT WITH HIV

The vast majority of FUOs in patients with advanced HIV (CD4 cell count < 200 cells/mm^3) are caused by infections, with mycobacterial infection, specifically *Mycobacterium. tuberculosis* and M avium-intracellulare (MAI), and *Pneumocystis jiroveci* pneumonia (PCP) being the most common in the United States. *Cryptococcus* and other fungi are also common. Endemic mycoses should be suspected in patients from certain geographic areas: histoplasmosis in those from the Ohio and Mississippi river valleys or the Caribbean, coccidioidomycosis in patients from arid regions of the Southwestern United States, Mexico, and South America. In Southern Europe, visceral leishmaniasis is common. An important noninfectious cause of FUO in patients with AIDS is lymphoma, especially non-Hodgkin lymphoma. Primary HIV infection often leads to a self-limited mononucleosis-like febrile illness and should be considered as a cause of FUO with an exposure history. AIDS patients with FUO should, in addition to standard blood cultures, have isolator bottles sent for fungus and mycobacteria. Serum cryptococcal antigen and sputum stains for *Pneumocystis* should also be performed. Urine histoplasmosis antigen can be done if the patient is from an endemic area.

FEVER AND THE INTRAVENOUS DRUG USER (IVDU)

Bloodstream and complicated intravascular infections such as endocarditis are common causes of fever in the IVDU. Additionally, bacteremia may lead to metastatic infections such as osteomyelitis, discitis, or septic arthritis. IVDUs are also at high risk for having undiagnosed HIV and are therefore subject to occult opportunistic infections. Acute viral hepatitis transmitted from shared needles may present with acute fever and liver function abnormalities.

NOSOCOMIAL FEVER OF UNKNOWN ORIGIN

Nosocomial FUO denotes a hospital-acquired fever with no identifiable cause lasting for at least 3 days. There is a scanty and dated literature on the causes of nosocomial FUO, summarized in **Table 206-4**. *Nosocomial pneumonia* is the most common cause, with many of these patients having impaired swallowing and recurrent aspiration. Recent medications should be carefully reviewed in any hospital patient with unexplained fever, as ***drug fever*** is the second most common cause of nosocomial FUO. Antibiotics and anticonvulsants (especially phenytoin) are the most frequent offenders. The drug history should also include a history of exposure to iodinated radiocontrast; thyroid storm is a rare cause of hospital-acquired fever, but may be precipitated by surgery or iodine exposure.

Serotonin syndrome is probably underdiagnosed in the hospital setting, and should be suspected in patients with fever, hyperautonomia, confusion, and myoclonus. Many drugs commonly prescribed in the hospital increase the risk for serotonin syndrome, such as selective serotonin reuptake inhibitors, serotonin-norepinephrine reuptake inhibitors, trazodone, bupropion, tramadol, linezolid, fentanyl,

TABLE 206-3 Medications Frequently Cited as Causes of Drug Fever

Antibiotics	β-lactams (penicillins, cephalosporins, carbapenems), nitrofurantoin, sulfonamides, amphotericin, isoniazid, rifampin
Anticonvulsants	Phenytoin, carbamazepine
Cardiac medications	Amiodarone, procainimide, quinidine, nifedipine, captopril, hydralazine
Anticholinergics	Phenothiazines (chlorpromazine, compazine)

TABLE 206-4 Causes of Nosocomial Fever of Unknown Origin in 241 Patients

Pneumonia	15%
Drug fever (including neuroleptic malignant syndrome)	12%
Urinary tract infection, including pyelonephritis and prostatitis	10%
Thromboembolic disease (including superficial thrombophlebitis, deep venous thrombosis, pulmonary embolism, and fat embolism)	7%
Bloodstream infection	4%
Device infection or procedural complication	4%
Clostridium difficile colitis	3%
Central nervous system process (including stroke, subarachnoid hemorrhage, subdural hematoma)	3%
Hematoma	3%
Gout	2%
Bowel perforation or ischemia	2%
Pancreatitis	1%
AIDS-related	1%
Undiagnosed	21%
Miscellaneous (includes upper respiratory tract infections, viral syndromes, tracheobronchitis, cellulitis and other soft tissue infections, various intra-abdominal infections, sickle cell crisis, cancer)	13%

Data from Arbo MJ, et al. *Am J Med.* 1993;95:505-512; Abolnik IZ, et al. *Infect Dis Clin Pract.* 1999;8:396-398.

oxycodone, triptans, ondansetron, metoclopramide, risperidone, and olanzapine. **Neuroleptic malignant syndrome** causes a similar clinical picture, with fever, rigidity, confusion, and autonomic instability in patient with recent use of neuroleptics or lithium. Leukocytosis is usually present, along with an elevated serum creatine kinase.

Nosocomial FUO often results from other iatrogenic causes, such as intravascular or urinary catheter-related infections, blood transfusions, and thromboembolic disease from prolonged immobilization. Postoperative fevers are common, and are often a normal physiologic response, not related to infection. **Clostridium difficile** infection is generally not subtle and usually leads to profuse diarrhea and leukocytosis. The diagnosis of *C. difficile* colitis may be more difficult when diarrhea is delayed, or completely absent due to ileus, or when false-negative tests for toxin occur. Disseminated candidiasis should be suspected in patients with malnutrition, chronic wounds, recent surgery, heavy antibiotic exposure, or receiving total parenteral nutrition. Patients who have recently been mechanically ventilated are at risk for sinusitis and mastoiditis.

Chronically ill patients are at risk for **acalculous cholecystitis**. Patients may have right upper quadrant tenderness and abnormal liver enzymes. Ultrasound reveals a distended gallbladder with wall thickening, with or without pericholecystic fluid. Other nosocomial complications that occur with some regularity in hospitalized patients and may result in fever include pressure ulcers, shingles (herpes zoster), herpes simplex, bowel ischemia, hematoma, and flares of gout and pseudogout.

As in all investigations of unexplained fever, the workup should be tailored to the clinical situation, but there are some tests that should be done routinely. Blood cultures and chest x-rays should be obtained in all newly febrile hospitalized patients. Urinalysis and urine culture may be useful, but must be interpreted with caution as pyuria and bacteruria are common in hospitalized patients without urinary tract infection. Similarly, Doppler ultrasound of the legs looking for deep venous thrombosis must be interpreted in context, for while occult deep venous thrombosis are common in hospitalized patients, they are only an occasional cause of fever. Chest CT may be useful in suspected nosocomial pneumonia, aspiration, or empyema when plain chest radiography is equivocal. CT abdomen should be performed in patients with histories, examinations or laboratory findings suggestive of a new intra-abdominal process, or in whom other workup has not been fruitful.

■ FEVER IN THE INTENSIVE CARE UNIT (ICU)

Fever is a common occurrence in the critically ill. A single temperature elevation greater than 101°F complicates up to 50% of all intensive care unit admissions. The majority of these fevers are benign and self-limited, but some can signal a new and significant process. Evaluation of the febrile ICU patient should primarily focus on distinguishing between infectious and noninfectious causes. Typical nosocomial causes of fevers, such as catheter-associated bloodstream infection, hospital-acquired pneumonia, drug fever, and transfusion reactions, are also common in the ICU. Other causes of hospital-acquired fever, such as acalculous cholecystitis, sinusitis, pancreatitis, and the acute respiratory syndrome (ARDS) are seen even more often in the ICU.

■ IMMIGRANTS AND RETURNING TRAVELERS

When travelers or immigrants present with FUO, fever may be due to common illnesses such as urinary tract infection or pneumonia, but careful consideration should be given to the infectious diseases endemic to the regions of recent travel. Malaria is potentially fatal if not diagnosed early, and should be suspected in any febrile traveler from an endemic area. Typhoid fever is common in most developing nations. Dengue and chikungunya are insectborne viral infections often accompanied by rash and may be seen in the returning traveler from South America, Africa, or Asia. Brucellosis is a bacterial infection transmitted by contact with animal carcasses, placentas, or contaminated milk and meat products. It is prevalent in the Middle East, Mediterranean basin, and parts of South America. Patients may have FUO as a manifestation of acute infection or reactivation of latent disease. Arthritis, spondylitis, sacroiliitis, and hepatitis are common manifestations of brucellosis. Q fever (caused by the bacterium *Coxiella burnetii*) is a common cause of culture-negative endocarditis in Australia, France, and Spain. Melioidosis (caused by the bacterium *Burkholderia pseudomallei*) may cause FUO in patients from Southeast Asia. Liver abscess, the most common extraintestinal manifestation of amebiasis caused by the protozoan *Entamoeba histolytica*, is seen in developing countries worldwide. HIV and syphilis should be suspected in sex tourists.

DIAGNOSIS

■ HISTORY AND PHYSICAL EXAMINATION

A comprehensive medical history and a physical examination are the most important parts of any FUO evaluation. Prior illnesses, past surgical procedures, medication lists, and vaccination histories should be thoroughly reviewed. Particular attention should be paid to travel and sexual history, recreational activities, occupational exposures, exposure to pets and other animals, and culinary habits, such as handling and consuming raw and unpasteurized foods. Physical examination may reveal rashes, poor dentition, oral or genital ulcers suggestive of herpes simplex, Behçet disease, or Crohn disease, lymphadenopathy, sinus tenderness, heart murmurs, hepatosplenomegaly, or stigmata of endocarditis that may direct further diagnostic workup. Rectal examination may reveal a perirectal abscess or prostatitis. Relative bradycardia, or pulse-fever dissociation (Faget sign) suggests intracellular infection, as in typhoid fever, legionellosis, and rickettsial infection. Repeating the history and physical examination over a period of time may unearth additional clues.

TABLE 206-5 Suggested Diagnostic Approach to FUO

All patients

Complete history and physical examination

Laboratory investigations: complete blood count and differential, erythrocyte sedimentation rate, C-reactive protein, urinalysis, liver function tests, creatine kinase, HIV antibody, rapid plasma reagin (RPR), HIV, cytomegalovirus IgM, monospot, antinuclear antibody, rheumatoid factor, serum protein electrophoresis, tuberculin skin test or interferon-gamma release assay, routine serum chemistries, serum ferritin, blood set aside for acute and convalescent serology

Microbiology: blood cultures (three sets, off antibiotics), urine culture, sputum, and other body fluid cultures as suggested by clinical scenario

Chest radiograph

CT scan of chest, abdomen, and pelvis

All patients, if above studies unrevealing or equivocal

Venous duplex imaging of lower extremities

Fluorodeoxyglucose positron emission tomographic scan, if available; if not, consider gallium-67 scintigraphy or indium-111 white blood cell scan

Selected patients

Tissue biopsy (if rash, lymphadenopathy, mass, or other target identified)

Consider temporal artery biopsy in older patients with high ESR and no other explanation for fever

■ ROUTINE TESTING

Diagnostic testing for FUO is summarized in **Table 206-5** and **Figure 206-1**. Routine diagnostic tests that should be ordered as part of most initial evaluations include complete blood cell count with differential, serum transaminases, blood cultures (ideally three sets drawn from different sites over a period of several hours or longer), erythrocyte sedimentation rate (ESR), and C-reactive protein. Additionally, urinalysis with urine culture, tuberculin skin testing (PPD), HIV testing, and chest x-ray should be performed.

Most of these studies are nonspecific, but they provide a starting point for refining the differential diagnosis and pursuing further testing. For example, lymphopenia is commonly seen with viral infections and neoplastic processes. Eosinophilia suggests a drug reaction, neoplasm, or parasitic infection, whereas basophilia, although uncommon, is associated with myeloproliferative disorders. The ESR and C-reactive protein are nonspecific measures of inflammation. The ESR measures the distance that red blood cells in an upright tube fall in an hour. In inflammatory states, the liver produces fibrinogen, which increases the stickiness of red blood cells and makes them settle faster. C-reactive protein (CRP) is an acute phase reactant produced by the liver in inflammatory states. CRP is generally more sensitive for inflammatory states than the ESR, because CRP levels in the blood rise more quickly after the onset of an inflammatory or infective process. Procalcitonin is a novel biomarker that has been used distinguish infection from inflammation. It is generally markedly elevated in acute infections, and much less so in noninfectious inflammatory states. It may be useful in some specific settings, but has little track record in the workup of FUO.

Given the frequency with which tuberculosis and other pulmonary processes cause FUO, all patients should undergo routine chest radiography and PPD testing. HIV testing was formerly only recommended in high-risk individuals, but should be done universally in patients presenting with FUO. If acute HIV is suspected, HIV viral load testing should be performed. Autoantibody tests such as antinuclear antibody (ANA) titers and rheumatologic factor (RF) have a high false-positive rate, but are useful when the clinical picture suggests rheumatological disease.

PRACTICE POINT

- HIV testing should be performed in all patients presenting with fever of unknown origin. If the history or epidemiology suggests acute HIV syndrome, HIV viral load should also be obtained.

■ IMAGING STUDIES

Computed tomographic scans of chest, abdomen, and pelvis have become a routine and high-yield component of the FUO workup. Computed tomographic scans may identify lymphadenopathy, pulmonary nodules, abdominal masses, and abscesses that are targets for biopsy or aspiration. Magnetic resonance imaging (MRI) is more sensitive for detecting central nervous system (CNS) causes of FUO, such as epidural abscess or cerebral vasculitis.

Radionuclide imaging may be a useful adjunct in FUO. Fluorine-18 fluorodeoxyglucose positron emission tomography (18F-FDG PET), sometimes performed in conjunction with CT scanning (18F-FDG PET/CT), is a particularly promising imaging modality in FUO that is able to localize sites of malignancy, inflammation, and infection. It may be more sensitive in FUO than radionuclide imaging with gallium-67 and radiolabeled leukocyte scanning with indium-111. Although nuclear medicine studies often contribute to diagnosis in FUO, lack of specificity and high false-positive rates may be a problem, and the results should be interpreted with caution.

■ BIOPSY

Examination of tissue is often required to diagnose an FUO. Localized abnormalities seen on physical examination or diagnostic imaging, such as enlarged lymph nodes or pulmonary nodules, may be targeted for biopsy. In general, biopsies should be directed toward an abnormal finding, and not be done routinely. The exception is in elderly patients with features suggestive of temporal arteritis, where temporal artery biopsy should be done despite the absence of physical findings. The role of bone marrow aspiration and liver biopsy in the diagnosis of FUO is debatable. We recommend pursuing bone marrow or liver biopsies only if there are suggestive abnormalities (cytopenias or abnormal peripheral smears, abnormal liver function tests) and a thorough diagnostic evaluation has been otherwise unrevealing.

TREATMENT

Specific treatment depends on the underlying cause of the FUO. Therapeutic trials without a diagnosis are generally not recommended. Undirected treatment may not only delay the diagnosis but can also cause considerable harm. Empiric antibiotics can obscure growth from blood cultures, and the routine administration of corticosteroids can worsen illness in such conditions as tuberculosis or parasitic disease. Exceptions to this rule are FUO in an immunocompromised patient or potentially septic immunocompetent patient. In these cases, empiric therapy with antimicrobials must be initiated. Similarly, when a patient is suspected to have temporal arteritis, early initiation of steroids may prevent blindness or other vascular complications and may be indicated before a definitive diagnosis can be made.

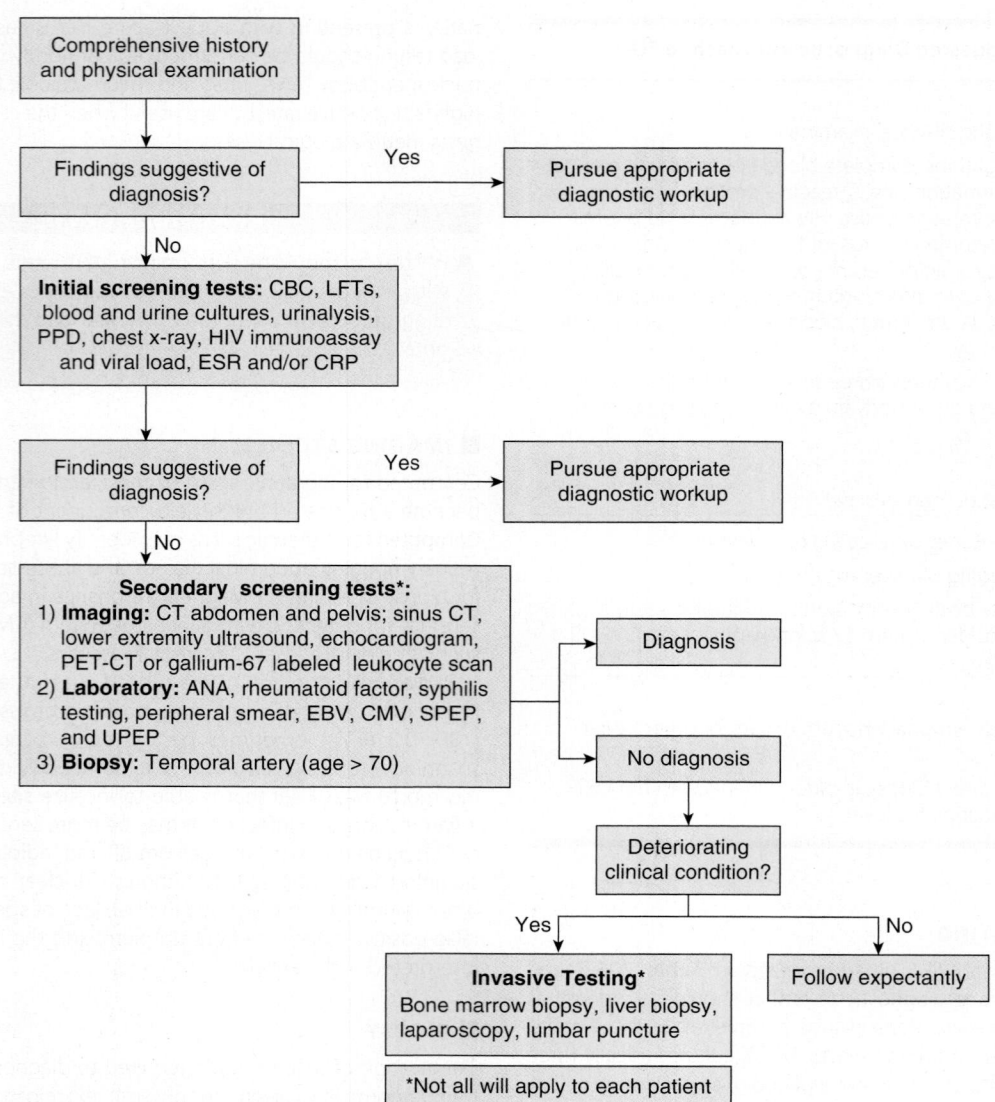

Figure 206-1 *Proposed algorithm for the management of fever of unknown origin.*

- Is the patient clinically stable for discharge? Persistent fever in a patient who is hemodynamically stable, ambulatory, and able to maintain oral intake does not necessarily mandate continued inpatient admission. Patients with continued fever who are otherwise stable may be discharged with close ambulatory follow-up. Up to 30% of patients with FUO are never definitively diagnosed. The prognosis in these patients is generally good. Fever resolves spontaneously in the vast majority, and mortality is low.
- Has a provider, such as an infectious disease physician, been designated to follow-up any cultures, serologies, biopsies, or other tests that are pending at the time of discharge?

SUGGESTED READINGS

Blockmans D, Knockaert D, Maes A, et al. Clinical value of [^{18}F] fluoro-deoxyglucose positron emission tomography for patients with fever of unknown origin. *Clin Infect Dis.* 2001;32:191-196.

Cunha BA. Fever of unknown origin: clinical overview of classic and current concepts. *Infect Dis Clin North Am.* 2007;21:867-915.

Knockaert DC, Dujardin KS, Bobbaers HJ. Long-term follow-up of patients with undiagnosed fever of unknown origin. *Arch Intern Med.* 1996;156:618-620.

Knockaert DC, Vanderschuerne S, Blockmans D. Fever of unknown origin in adults: 40 years on. *J Intern Med.* 2003;253:263-275.

Limper M, de Kruif MD, Duits AJ, Brandjes DP, van Gorp EC. The diagnostic role of procalcitonin and other biomarkers in discriminating infectious from non-infectious fevers. *J Infect.* 2010;60: 409-416.

Niven DJ, Leger C, Stelfox HT, Laupland KB. Fever in the critically ill: a review of epidemiology, immunity, and management. *J Intensive Care Med.* 2012;27:290-297.

Mackowiak P. Concepts of fever. *Arch Intern Med.* 1998;158: 1870-1881.

Mourad O, Palda V, Detsky AS. A comprehensive evidence-based approach to fever of unknown origin. *Arch Intern Med.* 2003;163:545-551.

Petersdorf RG, Beeson PB. Fever of unexplained origin: report of 100 cases. *Medicine (Baltimore).* 1961;40:1-30.

CHAPTER 207

Coma and Disorders of Consciousness

Liam Durcan, MD, FRCPC

Key Clinical Questions

1 Which historical features and examination findings are useful in the diagnosis of patients with an acutely altered level of consciousness?

2 How is acute coma in hospitalized patients managed?

3 How does vegetative state differ clinically from the minimally conscious state?

4 What prognostic information should be given to surrogate decision makers for patients with severe alterations of consciousness?

INTRODUCTION

Hospitalists are often required to assess patients with an abnormal level of consciousness, the most profoundly abnormal of which is coma. Coma is a state of unarousable unresponsiveness that may be produced by a number of acute or subacute central nervous system insults. The acute onset of coma is a medical emergency and requires urgent assessment, intervention, investigation, and specific therapy. Coma is distinct from vegetative state, minimally conscious state, and locked-in syndrome, conditions that are sometimes confused with it. The timing and probability of recovery from coma and the vegetative state and minimally conscious state differ considerably, depending on the nature of the underlying brain injury. This chapter will review the diagnosis and prognosis in disorders of consciousness, address ethical challenges arising in the care of these patients, and provide a guide to discussions with surrogate decision makers for the comatose or severely brain-injured patient.

COMA AND RELATED DISORDERS OF CONSCIOUSNESS

■ LETHARGY, OBTUNDATION, AND STUPOR

The terms lethargy, obtundation, and stupor have traditionally been used to denote mild, moderate, and severe disturbances in responsiveness respectively, but these terms pose a number of problems. Instead of specific states of brain function, these terms describe points on a spectrum of an abnormal level of consciousness. They are also poorly quantifiable and largely unvalidated in terms of their reliability, in contrast to other rating scales that may more reliably convey information about a patient's condition. Based on this, it is advisable to avoid these terms, as they may cause confusion and imply a precision that is unwarranted.

■ COMA

Coma is a pathological brain state, referring to patients who are completely unresponsive and cannot be aroused to demonstrate increased alertness or purposeful movements. It is distinguished from syncope, concussion, and other forms of transient unconsciousness by its time course of more than 1 hour. Although some comatose patients recover rapidly, especially when coma is due to a concurrent systemic illness, a more gradual recovery is often seen for patients with brain injuries sufficient to produce even a day of coma. In such patients, recovery will be marked by the patient's entering into a vegetative state or minimally conscious state, as defined below.

In its most basic neuroanatomical sense, coma requires disruption of either bilateral hemispheric functioning or the brainstem reticular activating system (**Figure 207-1**). Any process causing coma must disrupt either (or both) of these functional systems. Such causes include metabolic disturbances, drug intoxication, severe bilateral injuries to the cerebral hemispheres, and injuries to a small set of regions of the upper brainstem or thalamus resulting from stroke or herniation syndromes (**Table 207-1**).

Following a coma produced by severe brain injury, patients may either deteriorate, with progressive neuronal damage leading to brain death, or show some evidence of recovery, with evolution into the vegetative state, minimally conscious state, or other related clinical syndromes.

■ VEGETATIVE STATE

The term "vegetative state" suggests the presence of autonomic function and a partial recovery of arousal, with spontaneous periods

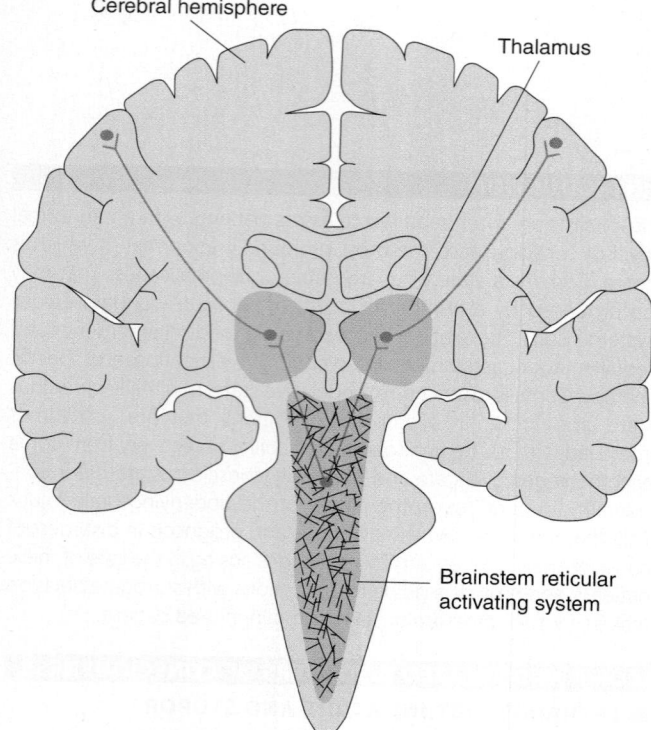

Figure 207-1 *Anatomical basis of coma. Consciousness is maintained by the normal functioning of the brainstem reticular activating system above the midpons and its bilateral projections to the thalamus and cerebral hemispheres. Coma results from lesions that affect either the reticular activating system or both hemispheres.* (Reproduced, with permission, from Simon RP, Greenberg DA, Aminoff MJ. *Clinical Neurology*, 7th ed. New York, NY: McGraw-Hill, 2009. Fig. 10-1.)

of eye opening and return of the sleep-wake cycle, reflecting some activity of the brainstem and reticular activating system, but without evidence of awareness of self or the environment. The vegetative state frequently arises following coma, and the structural injuries producing the vegetative state strongly overlap with those that produce coma. Common causes include diffuse axonal injury from brain trauma and anoxic brain injury from cardiac arrest. Autopsies of patients in the persistent vegetative state typically show widespread disconnection of the corticothalamic system, with extensive death of thalamic neurons and functional neuroimaging studies have demonstrated reduced brain activity in the fronto-temporal-parietal network, with activation limited to primary sensory cortex after noxious or auditory activation, suggesting an absence of integrated brain processing.

■ MINIMALLY CONSCIOUS STATE

The minimally conscious state is differentiated from the vegetative state by inconsistent but unequivocal evidence of awareness of self or the environment. Subtle behaviors may indicate responsiveness in the minimally conscious state. For example, a patient might be limited to tracking of objects in the visual field or localization of auditory stimuli, such as head turning to a ringing bell. Because these behaviors may be manifested only intermittently, the patient must be assessed over multiple examinations.

■ LOCKED-IN SYNDROME

The locked-in syndrome, which results from lesions ventral to the reticular activating system in the midpons, is characterized by patients who are conscious, but mute and quadriplegic. They usually retain control

TABLE 207-1   Causes of Acute Coma
Supratentorial lesions that cause raised intracranial pressure and may lead to herniation syndromes
Subdural hematoma
Epidural hematoma
Cerebral contusion
Intracerebral hemorrhage
Brain abscess
Cerebral infarction
Brain tumor
Subtentorial lesions affecting brainstem function
Basilar artery thrombosis or embolism
Pontine hemorrhage
Cerebellar hemorrhage or infarct
Metabolic abnormalities
Acid-base disturbances
Anoxia
Drug intoxications
Hepatic encephalopathy
Hyperosmolar states
Hypertensive encephalopathy/Posterior reversible encephalopathy syndrome (PRES)
Hyperthermia
Hypothermia
Hypoglycemia
Hyponatremia
Sepsis/systemic inflammatory response syndrome
Meningitis or encephalitis
Subarachnoid hemorrhage
Seizures, status epilepticus, and postictal state

over eye opening, vertical eye movements, and ocular convergence. The major cause is pontine ischemia due to basilar thrombosis in 60% of patients. Other less frequently encountered causes include pontine hemorrhage, central pontine myelolysis, tumor, and encephalitis.

DIAGNOSIS AND MANAGEMENT OF COMA AND STUPOR

■ HISTORY

Caregivers of patients in a coma may provide useful information about the tempo of coma onset. Precipitous onset suggests a brainstem stroke, subarachnoid hemorrhage, or other vascular calamity. The rapid evolution of hemiparesis and other hemispheric findings to coma over minutes or hours suggests intracerebral hemorrhage. A more indolent progression from localizing findings to coma over days to weeks suggests a more slowing evolving process such as tumor, abscess, or subdural hematoma. Coma preceded by delirium or other behavioral changes and lacking focal neurologic deficits suggests an intoxication or metabolic derangement.

■ GENERAL PHYSICAL EXAMINATION

Vital signs

The patient may have hypertension, which predisposes to intracerebral hemorrhage or stroke. Severe hypertension may also more directly cause coma due to hypertensive encephalopathy, or PRES (Posterior Reversible Encephalopathy Syndrome). Hypothermia may be associated with endogenous metabolic encephalopathies due to hypoglycemia, myxedema, hepatic encephalopathy, or drug intoxication. Hyperthermia may be seen in heatstroke, malignant hyperthermia from inhalational anesthetics, neuroleptic malignant syndrome, anticholinergic drug toxicity, or in the postictal phase after status epilepticus.

Trauma

Patients should be examined for signs of cranial trauma: soft tissue injury and skull irregularities accompanying depressed skull fracture, suggestive patterns of bruising such as the raccoon eyes sometimes seen in basilar skull fractures, Battle sign (bruising over the mastoid process), and hemotympanum, and cerebrospinal fluid leak from the nose or ear.

Meningeal irritation

Nuchal rigidity and the Brudzinski sign (involuntary flexion of the hip and knee in response to passive neck flexion) may be seen in meningitis and subarachnoid hemorrhage, but they may be absent in elderly, immunosuppressed, debilitated, or deeply comatose patients with these conditions.

■ NEUROLOGIC EXAMINATION

Key elements of the neurologic examination in stupor and coma include the pupillary response to light, whether eye movements occur in response to head rotation or cold caloric stimulation of the tympanic membrane, corneal reflexes, and the motor response to a painful stimulus. These signs are especially helpful in localizing the level of involvement in transtentorial herniation (**Figure 207-2**). The

Glasgow Coma Scale (GCS) (**Table 207-2**) and the Full Outline of UnResponsivenss (FOUR) Scale (**Table 207-3**) are used to summarize this information and assess changes in neurologic status over time.

Pupils

Normal pupils are 3 to 4 mm in diameter, and respond briskly and symmetrically to light. Pupils tend to be smaller in elderly persons. Minor pupillary asymmetry may be seen in some normal individuals, but does not exceed 1 mm. Pupillary size and reactivity may be affected by structural lesions (in which case additional localizing signs are present) or systemic processes (in which case additional localizing signs are absent). Lesions at specific levels of the central nervous system may cause characteristic pupillary abnormalities. Bilateral pinpoint pupils may be seen in pontine dysfunction; thalamic lesions result in small reactive pupils, perhaps because of loss of descending sympathetic pathways. Fixed dilated pupils may be seen in compression of the oculomotor nerve, transtentorial herniation of the medial temporal lobe, and intoxication with anticholinergic and sympathomimetic drugs. Fixed midsize pupils are indicative of brainstem damage. Pinpoint pupils are seen with narcotic overdose, organophosphate poisoning, pontine damage, and miotic eye drops for glaucoma.

Optic fundi

Fundoscopy may reveal papilledema or retinal hemorrhages in patients with raised intracranial pressure. Subhyaloid hemorrhages have been described in patients who have experienced rapid increases in intracranial pressure due to subarachnoid hemorrhage.

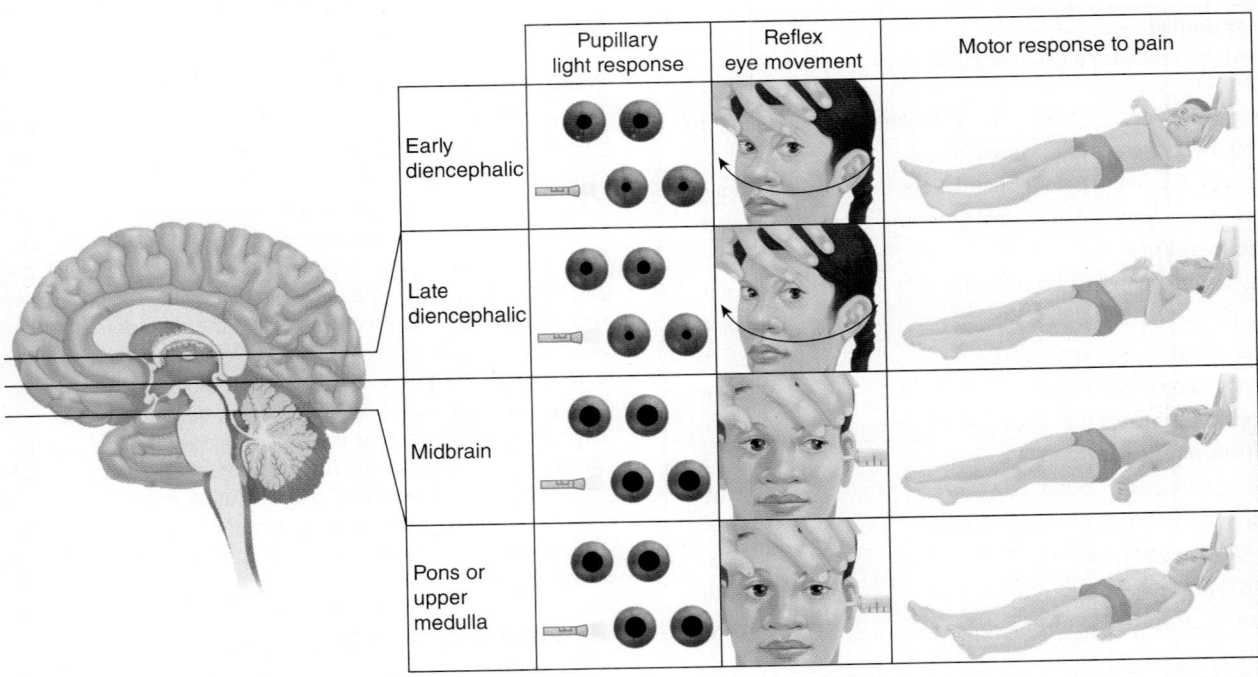

Figure 207-2 *Neurologic signs in coma with downward transtentorial herniation. In the early diencephalic phase, the pupils are small (~2 mm in diameter) and reactive, reflex eye movements are intact, and the motor response to pain is purposeful or semipurposeful (localizing) and often asymmetric. The late diencephalic phase is associated with similar findings, except that painful stimulation results in decorticate (flexor) posturing, which may also be asymmetric. With midbrain involvement, the pupils are fixed and midsize (~5 mm in diameter), reflex adduction of the eyes is impaired, and pain elicits decerebrate (extensor) posturing. Progression to involve the pons or medulla also produces fixed, midsize pupils, but these are accompanied by loss of reflex abduction as well as adduction of the eyes and by no motor response or only leg flexion upon painful stimulation. Note that, although a lesion restricted to the pons produces pinpoint pupils as a result of the destruction of descending sympathetic (pupillodilator) pathways, downward herniation to the pontine level is associated with midsize pupils. This happens because herniation also interrupts parasympathetic (pupilloconstrictor) fibers in the oculomotor (III) nerve. (Reproduced, with permission, from Simon RP, Greenberg DA, Aminoff MJ. Clinical Neurology, 7th ed. New York, NY: McGraw-Hill, 2009. Fig. 10-2.)*

TABLE 207-2 Glasgow Coma Scale*

I. Best motor response	
Obeys commands for movement	6 points
Purposeful movement to painful stimulus	5 points
Withdraws to painful stimuli	4 points
Abnormal flexion (decorticate posturing)	3 points
Extension (decerebrate posturing)	2 points
No response	1 point
II. Verbal response	
Oriented	5 points
Confused but able to answer questions	4 points
Inappropriate words	3 points
Incomprehensible speech	2 points
No response	1 point
III. Eye opening	
Spontaneous	4 points
To verbal stimuli, command, speech	3 points
To pain only (not applied to face)	2 points
None	1 point

*Total score is the sum of I + II + III (maximum 15 points).

TABLE 207-3 The Full Outline of UnResponsiveness (FOUR) Scale

Eye response	
Opens eyes spontaneously, tracks, blinks to commands	4 points
Opens eyes, does not track or blink to command	3 points
Eyes closed, open to loud voice	2 points
Eyes closed, open to painful stimulation	1 point
Eyes remain closed following painful stimulation	0 points
Motor response	
Obeys, makes sign, eg, "thumbs up"	4 points
Localizes painful stimulus	3 points
Flexes to painful stimulus	2 points
Extends to painful stimulus	1 point
No response/myoclonic status epilepticus	0 points
Brainstem reflexes	
Pupils+, Corneals+, Cough	4 points
1 pupil unreactive, Corneals+, Cough+	3 points
Pupils−, Corneals+, Cough N/A	2 points
Pupils+, Corneals−, Cough N/A	2 points
Pupils−, Corneals−, Cough+	1 point
Pupils−, Corneals−, Cough−	0 points
Intubation	
Not intubated, normal respirations	4 points
Not intubated, Cheynes-Stokes respirations	3 points
Not intubated, irregular respirations	2 points
Not intubate, apneic	0 points
Intubated, breathes above ventilator settings	1 point
Intubated, breathes below ventilator settings	0 points

*Total score is the score of subscales 1-4 (0-16).

Corneal reflex

Lightly touching the cornea with a thin wisp of sterile cotton should provoke involuntary closure of that eye, as well as closing of the opposite eye (consensual response). A normal corneal reflex implies intact afferent and efferent limbs, as well as integrity of the pontine structures on the side of the response.

Extraocular movements

In comatose patients, information about extraocular movements, and the integrity of brainstem structures that control them, is derived from testing two reflexes: the oculocephalic reflex and the oculovestibular reflex. The oculocephalic reflex requires that the patient's cervical spine be cleared. The patient's eyes are held open and the head is briskly turned from side to side, with the head briefly held still at the end of each movement. A positive response is seen when the eyes move in the direction opposite to head turning. With rapid flexion, a normal response is upward deviation of both eyes, with downward deviation seen in rapid extension. The oculovestibular reflex involves elevation of the head to 30° and, after ensuring the tympanum is intact, introducing ice water into the external auditory canal. In a comatose patient with an intact brainstem, coldwater irrigation should produce deviation of both eyes toward the side of irrigation. Both ears should be tested, with a pause of at least 5 minute between sides to allow re-equilibration. If comatose patients have conjugate horizontal eye movements spontaneously (roving eye movements), with oculocephalic or with cold caloric testing, the brainstem pathways for conjugate eye movement are intact.

Abnormalities in conjugate eye movements imply impaired brainstem function from structural lesions, but are sometimes seen in metabolic disorders or intoxications, and thus do not always imply irreversible damage.

Motor response to pain

The response to noxious stimuli is used to test motor function in comatose patients. Noxious stimulation is produced by carefully applying pressure to the brow ridges on both sides of the head, the sternum, and the nail beds of all extremities. Motor responses can be categorized as displaying localization, flexion, extension, or no response. When consciousness is only moderately depressed, patients may reach toward the site of painful stimuli (localization). In *decorticate posturing*, the arms flex and the shoulders are adducted, with extension of the leg and ankle. *Decerebrate posturing* includes extension of the elbow, with internal rotation of the shoulder and forearm and leg extension. Traditionally, decorticate posturing has been thought to indicate thalamic damage or compression, with decerebrate posturing implying midbrain dysfunction, although neither sign is precisely localizing. Posturing may be seen in reversible metabolic disorders and intoxications, as well as focal lesions. Unilateral posturing suggests a lesion of the contralateral cerebral hemisphere or brainstem.

■ ASSESSMENT SCALES

Elements of the neurological examination may be organized into scoring systems that assess level of consciousness and help to establish the diagnosis, either in the acute or chronic care setting.

The Glasgow Coma Scale (GCS) is the most widely used scale in acute care settings. The GCS consists of three subscales that assess level of arousal, motor function, and verbal abilities, with subscale scores yielding a total score ranging from 3 to 15. It has been validated and found to be reliable for patients with traumatic and non-traumatic causes of coma. Drawbacks of the GCS include a lack of brainstem evaluation, and difficulties deriving scores from patients requiring ventilatory support.

The Full Outline of UnResponsiveness scale (FOUR) is another scale used to assess unresponsive patients in the acute care setting. There are four subscales, assessing ocular responses, motor responses, brainstem reflexes, and breathing. Scores on each subscale range from 0 to 4 to yield a total score of 0 to 16. Although less widely used than the GCS, the FOUR scale, through its use of oculomotor signs and respiratory function, does offer the advantages of being better able to diagnose patients with locked-in syndrome, and those whose examinations may meet criteria for brain death.

The Coma Recovery Scale (CRS-R) was developed to assist with the differential diagnosis and prognosis of patients with disorders of consciousness in a nonacute setting. The CRS-R uses six subscales assessing auditory, visual, motor, oromotor, communication, and arousal functions. The CRS-R (**Table 207-4**) has been shown to be a valid and reliable tool to differentiate patients in a vegetative state from those in a minimally conscious state, and helps to establish prognosis and inform treatment decisions.

TABLE 207-4 CRS-R Response Profile

Auditory function scale
4-Consistent movement to command*
3-Reproducible movement to command*
2-Localization to sound
1- Auditory startle
0-None

Visual function scale
5-Object recognition*
4- Object localization: reaching*
3-Pursuit eye movements*
2-Fixation*
1-Visual startle
0-None

Motor function scale
6-Funcitonal object useᴱ
5-Automatic motor response*
4-Object manipulation*
3-Localization of noxious stimulation*
2-Flexion withdrawal
1-Abnormal posturing
0-None/flaccid

Oromotor/verbal function scale
3-Intelligible verbalization*
2-Voclaization/oral movement
1-Oral reflexive movement
0-None

Communication scale
<2-Functional: accurateᴱ
1-Nonfunctional: intentional*
0-None

Arousal
3-Attention*
2-Eye opening w/o stimulation
1-Eye opening with stimulation
0-Unarousable

*Denotes MCS.
ᴱDenotes emergence from MCS.

TABLE 207-5 Emergency Management of the Acutely Comatose Patient

Assess the adequacy of the patient's airway, breathing, and circulation.

Secure IV access and draw blood for serum glucose and electrolytes, hepatic and renal function, coagulation studies, and complete blood count.

Administer IV glucose (typically as 50 mL of 50% dextrose), thiamine 100 mg, and naloxone 0.4-1.2 mg.

Obtain arterial blood gas and pH measurements to assess for acid-base disturbances.

Treat seizures, if present.

Detailed physical and neurologic examination.

CT scan of the head, especially if signs suggestive of mass lesion or subarachnoid hemorrhage are present.

Lumbar puncture if signs of meningeal irritation are present.

Blood and urine toxicology screens.

■ INVESTIGATIONS AND MANAGEMENT

Urgent general steps in the diagnosis and management of the patient with coma and stupor are summarized in **Table 207-5**. Specific treatment is directed at the underlying cause.

PROGNOSIS IN COMA, MINIMALLY CONSCIOUS STATES, AND VEGETATIVE STATES

Coma is an inherently precarious condition. The short-term mortality of patients with coma after brain trauma is 40% to 50%, rising to 54% to 88% for patients comatose after a cardiac arrest. Patients with traumatic brain injuries have a higher likelihood of significant recovery than those who have sustained a cardiac arrest. This may be partly due to the fact that patients with traumatic brain injury are typically younger and have fewer comorbid medical conditions than patients who sustain cardiac arrest. Recovery after prolonged traumatic coma is well described. Unlike coma from anoxic brain injury, unconsciousness for 1 month after trauma does not necessarily preclude significant recovery. However, outcome in traumatic brain injury is highly unpredictable, due to delayed neuronal death following axonal disconnection and variable degrees of neuroregeneration. Prognosis in nontraumatic coma is influenced by etiology. Mortality is highest in coma due to cerebral anoxia and stroke, and lowest in metabolic causes and drug intoxications.

Traditionally, the prognosis of patients with anoxic brain injury who do not meet brain-death criteria has been related to the duration of neurologic impairment. If brainstem functions, such as pupillary, corneal responses, and motor responses, such as the withdrawal to noxious stimuli, were still absent 3 days after cardiac arrest, there was felt to be no likelihood for recovery beyond the vegetative state. Prospective studies that involved use of controlled hypothermia (cooling to 32°C-34°C) in the treatment of patients in coma following anoxic damage have called into question the validity of absent motor function at 72 hours as a valid prognostic indicator. The absence of pupillary light or corneal responses is still considered to be reliable indicators of a poor prognosis in cooled patients at 72 hours.

Prognosis in vegetative state is highly dependent on the underlying mechanism of brain injury. Patients who remain in the vegetative state for 3 months after anoxic brain injury are highly likely to remain in a permanent vegetative state. However, the time frame for recovery following post-traumatic vegetative state is considerably longer, with recovery occurring as late as 1 year. Recovery thereafter is rare and restricted to the minimally conscious state.

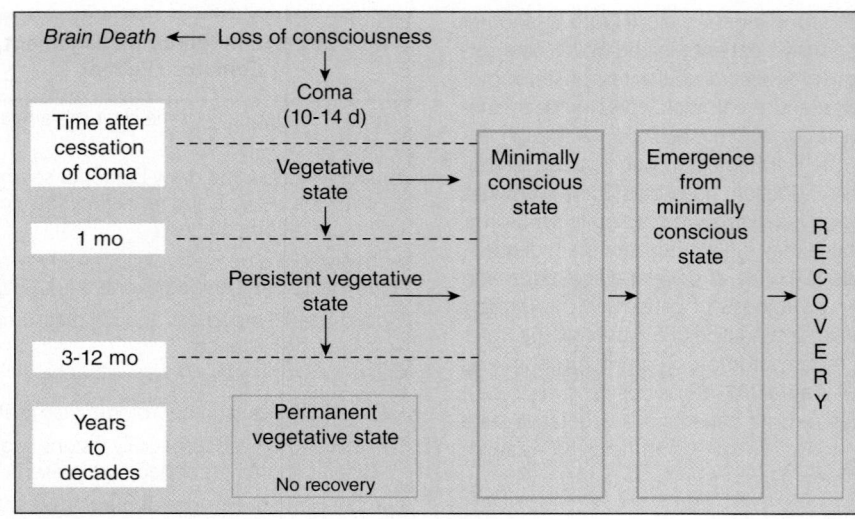

Figure 207-3 *Outcomes after the development of a vegetative state.* (Adapted from Fins JJ. Neuroethics and neuroimaging: moving towards transparency. *Am J Bioeth.* 2008;8[9]:46-52, http://www.informaworld.com.)

Prognosis in the minimally conscious state is another rapidly evolving area. Patients in the minimally conscious state for months may recover above the level of severe disability. In addition, the rare examples of very late recovery of communication in severely brain-injured patients have invariably been in patients in the minimally conscious state. Patients in the minimally conscious state have faster rates of recovery within the first year after either traumatic or nontraumatic injury, compared with patients in the vegetative state (**Figure 207-3**). It is critical for the clinician to distinguish between the vegetative and minimally conscious states when evaluating the postcomatose patient, as even small signs of consciousness identified by hospitalists on rounds may have a major bearing on prognosis.

ENGAGING SURROGATE DECISION MAKERS

Decisions about ongoing care or its withdrawal in patients with severe disorders of consciousness necessarily involve surrogates. A surrogate decision maker is a legally-designated person, such as a spouse, partner, family member, or friend, who directs care when the patient is incapacitated. Surrogate decision makers face multiple challenges, including unfamiliarity with coma and related conditions. The hospitalist can help surrogates make informed decisions by educating them about the distinctions between these disorders of consciousness and, informed by etiology, their likely outcomes.

Discussions with surrogates can be structured around *time-delimited prognostication*. The hospitalist provides guidance on possible outcomes, based on the patient's current status and evolution over time. For example, it is justified to provide an early and definitive diagnosis of brain death when patients meet clinical criteria (**Table 207-6**). For other patients, prognostication is more difficult. It would be inappropriate and premature to offer a definitive prognosis in a comatose patient with traumatic brain injury who has begun to regain brainstem function and appears to be moving quickly into the vegetative state. Clinicians should explain to surrogates that prognosis depends on etiology, and whether the patient reaches certain milestones over time.

If patients remain in the vegetative state for 1 month, they are classified as being in a persistent vegetative state. Although some patients may still improve to the minimally conscious state and above, the prognosis for recovery becomes less favorable at this point. The vegetative state is considered permanent if it persists at 3 months after anoxic brain injury, 12 months after traumatic brain injury.

The minimally conscious state indicates at least some awareness, with the potential to regain consistent consciousness, and sometimes even the ability to communicate. The prognosis of the minimally conscious state is variable and less well defined. Instances of recovery of personality and speech, albeit with persisting severe disability, have arisen even after years in the minimally conscious state. When patients enter the minimally conscious state, surrogates should be updated but cautioned to temper expectations, although not extinguish them. The distinction between the vegetative and minimally conscious states is critical during care hand-offs and transitions, such as hospital discharge, so that a patient does not

---

TABLE 207-6 Criteria for the Diagnosis of Brain Death

Cessation of brain function

Unresponsiveness to all sensory input, including pain and speech

Absent brainstem reflexes: absent papillary, corneal, and oropharyngeal responses; no eye movement with oculocephalic (doll's eye) and vestibulo-ocular (caloric testing) maneuvers; no ventilatory effort when the patient's Pco_2 is permitted to rise to 60 mm Hg

Irreversibility of brain dysfunction

The cause of coma must be known, adequate to explain the clinical picture, and irreversible.

Sedative drug intoxication, hypothermia, neuromuscular blockade, and shock must be ruled out, as neurologic recovery may still be possible in these conditions.

Persistence of brain dysfunction

These criteria must persist for an appropriate length of time, as follows:

1. Six hours with a confirmatory isoelectric (flat) electroencephalogram (EEG)

2. Twelve hours without a confirmatory isoelectric EEG

3. Twenty-four hours for anoxic brain injury without a confirmatory isoelectric EEG

Additional confirmatory tests

Demonstration of the absence of cerebral blood flow confirms brain death without a waiting period. Cerebral angiography provides the most unequivocal assessment; Doppler techniques and technetium imaging are used in some centers.

become erroneously labeled as permanently vegetative, when in fact he or she is transitioning into a minimally conscious state. A failure to inform accepting physicians about ongoing evolution of brain states may adversely affect a patient's chances for improvement.

DISCHARGE CHECKLIST

- If the patient is being transferred to a facility, has the accepting physician been informed of the patient's neurologic status and prognosis, and the status of communications with surrogate decision makers?
- Has neurologic follow-up been arranged, if appropriate?

PRACTICE POINT

- Reactive pupils in the presence of otherwise impaired brainstem function suggests metabolic encephalopathy.

ACKNOWLEDGMENT

Nicholas D. Schiff and Joseph J. Fins contributed to this chapter in the first edition and some material from that chapter has been retained here.

SUGGESTED READINGS

Bouwes A, Binnekade JM, Kuiper MA, et al. Prognosis of coma after therapeutic hypothermia: A prospective Cohort study. *Ann Neurol.* 2012;71:206-212.

Fins JJ. Neuroethics and neuroimaging: moving towards transparency. *Am J Bioeth.* 2008;8:46-52.

Hannawi Y, Lindquist MA, Caffo BS, Sair HI, Stevens RD. Resting brain activity in disorders of consciousness: a systematic review and meta-analysis. *Neurology.* 2015;84:1272-1280.

Lammi MH, Smith VH, Tate RL, Taylor CM. The minimally conscious state and recovery potential: A follow-up study 2 to 5 years after traumatic brain injury. *Arch Phys Med Rehabil.* 2005;86:746-754.

Laureys S, Owen AM, Schiff ND. Brain function in coma, vegetative state, and related disorders. *Lancet Neurol.* 2004:3:537-546.

Laureys S, Boly M. What is it like to be vegetative or minimally conscious? *Curr Op Neurol.* 2007;6:609-613.

Rossetti AO, Oddo M, Logroscino G, Kaplan PW. Prognostication after cardiac arrest and hypothermia: A prospective study. *Ann Neurol.* 2010;67:301-307.

Stender J, Gosseries O, Bruno MA, et al. Diagnostic precision of PET imaging and functional MRI in disorders of consciousness: a clinical validation study. *Lancet.* 2014;384:514-522.

Intracranial Hemorrhage and Related Conditions

Alexander E. Ropper, MD

Allan H. Ropper, MD

Key Clinical Questions

1. What are the types of intracranial hemorrhage, and how are they identified?

2. How is anticoagulation reversed and when can it be reinstituted?

3. What is the appropriate management of blood pressure after cerebral hemorrhage?

4. What medical treatments bear on the management of intracranial hemorrhage?

5. How is raised intracranial pressure managed?

6. Is anticoagulation safe after an intracranial hemorrhage?

7. What tests should be obtained in patients with ventriculoperitoneal shunts and fever?

INTRODUCTION

Intracranial hemorrhages, increasingly frequent in practice as a result of anticoagulation, are of three main types. They are categorized as spontaneous intracerebral hemorrhage (bleeding within the brain parenchyma), subarachnoid hemorrhage from aneurysm rupture, and intracranial bleeding from cranial trauma. Intracerebral hemorrhage accounts for 10% of strokes, with rates in the United States of approximately 10 cases per 100,000 persons yearly, and a higher incidence in African Americans and Hispanics than in whites. The highest incidence globally is found in Japan, where rates approach 60 cases per 100,000.

SPONTANEOUS INTRACEREBRAL HEMORRHAGE

■ PATHOPHYSIOLOGY

The most common underlying causes of intracerebral hemorrhage are hypertension and therapeutic anticoagulation. Other associated conditions include acquired coagulopathy, bleeding into a cerebral tumor, cerebral venous thrombosis, vascular malformations, hemorrhagic transformation of ischemic stroke, and amyloid angiopathy. The frequency of chronic hypertension in patients with cerebral hemorrhage had been ~75% in population studies, but the proportion of bleeds related to anticoagulant and antiplatelet medications has been increasing. Hypertensive patients at high risk for intracranial hemorrhage are those with poorly controlled disease, those younger than 55 years, smokers, and especially those who have recently stopped taking chronically administered antihypertensive medications. Spontaneous intracerebral bleeding with the use of adrenergically active medications and toxins such as cocaine should be suspected in young individuals. Acquired coagulopathy from underlying systemic disease is a well-known cause of primary intracerebral hemorrhage, particularly when caused by cancer or chemotherapy-related bone marrow suppression, uremia, or liver failure.

■ PRESENTATION

The clinical features that distinguish cerebral hemorrhage from other forms of stroke are headache, nausea, vomiting, confusion, acute and severe hypertension, and with large clots, decreased level of consciousness, hemiplegia, and enlargement of the pupils. The most common location for spontaneous intracerebral hemorrhage is the basal ganglia, accounting for ~65% of cases. Thalamic hemorrhage manifests similarly, usually with hemiplegia and hemianesthesia. Pontine hemorrhage causes rapid coma, quadriplegia, pinpoint pupils, and loss of extraocular movements. Cerebellar hemorrhage has special significance because of the benefits from surgical evacuation; vomiting, vertigo, dizziness, gait ataxia, and progressive coma from hydrocephalus are typical. Lobar hemorrhages confined to one subcortical region cause signs referable to the area affected and simulate ischemic stroke.

■ DIAGNOSIS

Computed tomography (CT) scan without contrast is the primary diagnostic tool. Conventional or CT angiogram or magnetic resonance imaging (MRI) may be required in special cases to establish the diagnosis of an underlying aneurysm, vascular malformations, or bleeding from an intracranial neoplasm. Patients with suspected intracranial hemorrhage should have coagulation parameters checked, specifically partial thromboplastin time (PTT), international normalized ratio (INR), and platelet count. History should be obtained regarding use of anticoagulants, aspirin, clopidogrel, other antiplatelet agents, and recent cranial trauma.

■ TREATMENT

Initial considerations include correction of coagulopathy, seizure prophylaxis, control of hypertension, and treatment of brain swelling. The majority of oral anticoagulant-related hemorrhages occur with INR under three, but higher levels confer a greater risk. Head injury and the use of antiplatelet agents with anticoagulation are additional risks. Acutely, there is concern for hematoma expansion, cerebral edema, and secondary compression of the brainstem. It is now appreciated that approximately one-quarter of spontaneous cerebral hemorrhages enlarge in the first several hours. In subsequent days, medical complications related to coma and immobilization, such as aspiration and pulmonary embolism, become the focus of treatment.

Reversal and restarting of anticoagulation

Patients receiving chronic warfarin therapy require correction of the INR, preferably to a level ≤1.3 to 1.4. This is typically accomplished with vitamin K 10 mg IV, which reverses coagulopathy over hours, as well as more rapid means of reversal, with either infusion of fresh frozen plasma, prothrombin complex concentrate, or activated factor VII. There are no directive studies comparing these options. If emergency neurosurgical intervention or other surgery is required in patients on warfarin, concentrated recombinant factor VII or factor IX may be used, with the understanding that these may subsequently increase systemic clotting risk.

Prothromin complex concentrates or newer agents such as adnexanet are used to reverse the effects of the newer anticoagulants, such as the factor Xa inhibitors apixaban and rivaroxaban. Activated prothrombin complexes' concentrates may have a particular role in the management of bleeding due to the direct thrombin inhibitor dabigatran. Dabigatran, unlike apixiban and rivaroxaban, may be removed by hemodialysis, although this may be a logistical challenge in a critically ill, unstable patient.

Patients receiving antiplatelet medications, probably including low-dose daily aspirin, may receive six units of platelets, but no benefit to this approach has been demonstrated. In thrombocytopenic patients with cerebral hemorrhage, it is probably advisable to correct the platelet level to >100,000 if feasible.

Several studies have shown that resuming warfarin after intracerebral hemorrhage, for example, in patients with atrial fibrillation or prosthetic heart valves, carries a small to moderate risk of recurrence of bleeding. This risk is often equivalent to the risk of an embolic event from not restarting medication, but the evidence is of low quality, and only an approximate estimate for rebleeding of 5% to 10% can be given after restarting anticoagulation at various intervals after the hemorrhage. If possible, based on the risk of withholding anticoagulation in particular patients, we wait at least 3 months before resuming warfarin.

PRACTICE POINT

- Anticoagulation should be reversed with vitamin K and faster-acting agents such as factor concentrate.
- The risk of repeat hemorrhage after resumption of anticoagulation is low, and may be similar to the risk of ischemic stroke due to omission of anticoagulation. The optimal interval for restarting medication has not been established, and may need to be decided on the basis of risks and benefits for individual patients.

Unfractionated heparin is reversed with protamine 1 mg per 100 units of heparin administered in the previous 6 hours, with monitoring to establish that PTT has been reduced below 1.5 times the upper limit of normal. There is limited guidance on the reversal of unfractionated heparins, as they are known to be partially or totally resistant to protamine; nonetheless, protamine is used in larger doses than for heparin reversal.

Blood pressure management

Most patients with cerebral hemorrhage are acutely hypertensive from the effect of raised intracranial pressure (ICP) on barosensitive areas in the medulla. A trial has demonstrated that lowering systolic blood pressure intensively, to below 140 mm Hg within 1 hour, was not deleterious and had similar clinical outcomes to a target of lowering to 180 mm Hg; furthermore, it may have resulted in less expansion of the hematoma and improved functional outcome (INTERACT2) and ATACH-2. A reasonable approach is to keep mean arterial pressure between 70 and 100 mm Hg, which balances the risks of expansion of the clot from hypertension, and decreased cerebral perfusion from hypotension. Nicardipine and labetalol are generally used as antihypertensive drugs in neurologic practice, as they are short acting and easily titrated. Patients who are chronically hypertensive may be maintained on their home medications. After the acute stage, β-blockers or angiotensin-converting enzyme inhibitors may be instituted, but the choice is determined by local practice and other medical factors.

PRACTICE POINT

- Mean arterial pressure at normal heart rates may be estimated as (diastolic blood pressure × 2/3) + (systolic blood pressure × 1/3).
- Systolic blood pressure may be safely lowered to 140 mm Hg after cerebral hemorrhage.

Seizure prophylaxis

In most centers, antiseizure drugs are administered for several weeks or until resolution of the clot, although this practice has not been studied adequately. The preferred anticonvulsant varies between institutions. We use levetiracetam, given its favorable side effect profile and predictable kinetics. Phenytoin use has been associated with worse outcomes after intracerebral hemorrhage in some series.

Surgical evacuation

There is evidence from several trials (STICH) that surgical evacuation of spontaneous intracerebral hemorrhage does not improve outcome. However, there may be exceptions for smaller lobar clots that are close to the cortical surface. Hydrocephalus accompanies some hemorrhages, and may require intraventricular drainage or surgical evacuation of the clot. The exception to these statements relates to moderate and large cerebellar hemorrhages (generally considered to be >3 cm in diameter), which often require evacuation to prevent brainstem compression and were not included in the main surgical trials. Several trials also suggest that corticosteroids do not improve outcome.

■ DISCHARGE CHECKLIST FOR CEREBRAL HEMORRHAGE

- Is the neurologic examination stable? Has gait safety been established by physical therapy?
- Have INR, PTT, and platelet count normalized?

- Has a plan been established for reinstitution of anticoagulation in patients with atrial fibrillation, pulmonary embolism, or mechanical heart valves?
- Is blood pressure adequately controlled?
- Has a decision been made on institution and duration of antiepileptic medication?

ANEURYSMAL SUBARACHNOID HEMORRAGE

■ PRESENTATION

The typical presentation of this disorder is sudden, extreme headache described as "the worst of my life," often associated with vomiting and variable degrees of neck stiffness. Approximately 75% of spontaneous (nontraumatic) subarachnoid hemorrhages are due to rupture of intracranial aneurysms (**Figure 208-1**), and another 10% are attributed to arteriovenous malformations (AVMs). Patients may be alert or become suddenly comatose. Systemic hypertension and meningismus are common on examination. The sudden rise in ICP may produce bleeding in the posterior compartment of the eyes, most characteristically subhyaloid (Terson syndrome). The clinical state is graded by the Hunt and Hess scale (**Table 208-1**), casually referred to as the "H and H" score. Common complications of subarachnoid hemorrhage include acute and delayed hydrocephalus, vasospasm with resultant ischemic stroke, and rerupture of the aneurysm, which is often fatal. Management is therefore geared to securing the aneurysm and treating any hydrocephalus at the earliest possible time, and subsequently to assuring adequate cerebral perfusion to prevent stroke from vasospasm.

■ DIAGNOSIS

The initial test is a noncontrast head CT scan, which demonstrates 95% of subarachnoid hemorrhages within 24 hours of aneurysm rupture (**Figure 208-2**) (although the sensitivity of head CT falls to <75% by 72 hours). If the CT scan fails to demonstrate hemorrhage

TABLE 208-1 Hunt and Hess Scoring System for Subarachnoid Hemorrhage

Grade	Description
I	Asymptomatic or with slight headache
II	Moderate to severe headache, nuchal rigidity; cranial nerve palsy
III	Confusion, drowsiness, and mild focal deficit
IV	Persistent stupor or semicoma, early decerebrate rigidity
V	Deep coma and decerebrate rigidity

in a case with compatible clinical features, lumbar puncture is performed to detect blood and blood products in the spinal fluid. Xanthochromia of the supernatant demonstrates that blood in the cerebrospinal fluid (CSF) space has been present for some time and is not the result of a traumatic puncture; this coloration persists for up to 2 weeks, but may not present in CSF collected in the first hours after hemorrhage. A substantial decline in the number of red blood cells in serial tubes is expected from a traumatic lumbar puncture, whereas the red blood cell count and xanthochromia remain consistent across tubes in subarachnoid hemorrhage. CT angiogram, MR angiogram, or conventional angiogram is used to identify the site of aneurysm or other vascular malformation.

■ TREATMENT

General measures in the treatment of subarachnoid hemorrhage include intensive care unit monitoring of blood pressure and neurological state, bed rest, analgesia, provision of a quiet environment, and hydration. The risk of rebleeding from a single aneurysm following rupture is ~4% within the first 24 hours, and 1.5% each day through the first 2 weeks. As the cumulative risk of rebleeding is

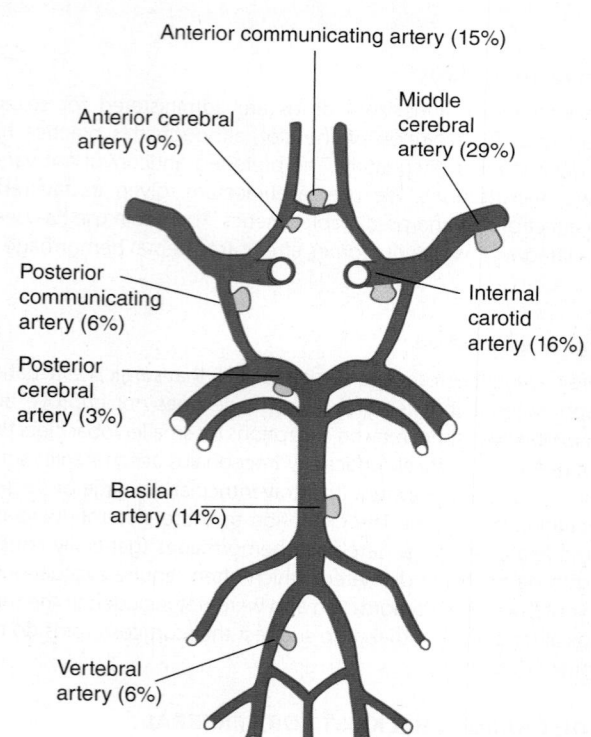

Figure 208-1 *Frequency and distribution of intracranial aneurysms.* (Reproduced, with permission, from Simon RP, Greenberg DA, Aminoff MJ. *Clinical Neurology*, 7th ed. New York, NY: McGraw-Hill; 2009.)

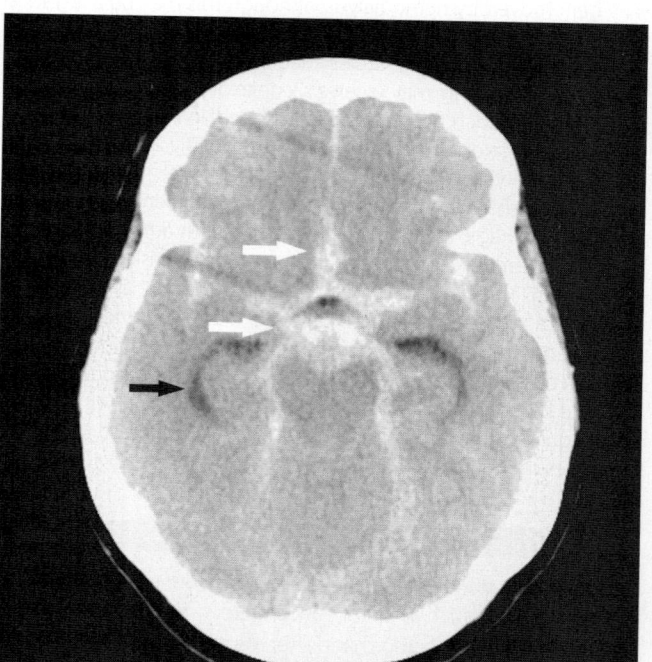

Figure 208-2 *Subarachnoid hemorrhage from a ruptured basilar artery aneurysm. Blood appears as a white signal diffusely in the subarachnoid spaces (white arrows), and incipient hydrocephalus is demonstrated by enlarged temporal horns of the lateral ventricles (black arrow).*

20%, and the outcome of rebleeding is poor, craniotomy with placement of titanium clips across the aneurysm neck (clipping), or endovascular obliteration of the aneurysm with platinum coils or other embolic material (coiling) is planned within the first 24 hours after presentation in most centers. The decision to clip or coil is individualized, and depends on factors such as aneurysm size, morphology, and location, as well as patient's age and clinical status. As the risk of rebleeding is lower with AVMs, surgical removal, or endovascular reduction is less urgent and can be undertaken electively at a later date. One large trial (ARUBA), albeit widely criticized, has suggested that interventional therapy results in worse outcome than medical measures. Further studies may be necessary before accepting these results uncritically.

Vasospasm

Blood in the subarachnoid space leads to delayed spasm of the vessels of the circle of Willis. The incidence of vasospasm peaks between the fourth and seventh days after hemorrhage, but may occur as late as 3 weeks. The conventional management of vasospasm has been to induce hypervolemia and hypertension with vasopressors such as phenylephrine. Because of the risk of rerupture of the aneurysm, clipping or coiling of the aneurysm is first required. Nimodipine has been shown to be protective for ischemic stroke from vasospasm, and is instituted at 60 mg every 4 hours, orally or by nasogastric tube. If mean arterial pressure is below 70 mm Hg, the medication is held, or the dose is reduced to 30 mg every 2 hours. Nimodipine is continued for 21 days following hemorrhage or at least for the duration of the inpatient stay. The use of antiepileptics and corticosteroids in subarachnoid hemorrhage is controversial and center dependent.

CEREBRAL HEMORRHAGE IN TRAUMATIC BRAIN INJURY

Traumatic brain injury (TBI) comprises a spectrum of clinical entities, most of which include intracranial bleeding. Management of patients with traumatic intracranial hemorrhages includes correction of coagulopathy, blood pressure regulation, and antiseizure medication. The clinical examination of brain-injured patients is best performed before sedation or paralytic agents are administered. The Glasgow Coma Scale (GCS) is widely used to grade the severity of traumatic brain injury. It incorporates verbal response (1-5), eye opening (1-4), and best motor response (1-6) with the highest score being 15, signifying normal alertness and responsiveness, and the lowest score of three indicating deep coma.

Initial radiographic evaluation of TBI patients is with a cranial CT scan, which detects most skull fractures, acute and chronic hemorrhages, hydrocephalus, and intraventricular and subarachnoid blood. The cervical spine should initially be considered to be injured until demonstrated otherwise by clinical features (lack of pain and full mobility in an awake patient), or radiographic demonstration of stability. It has become standard practice in many institutions to leave the patient in a cervical collar until these findings have been established.

■ EPIDURAL HEMATOMA

Epidural hematomas usually result from rupture of the middle meningeal artery underlying a fracture, leading to bleeding between the dura and the inner table of the skull (**Figure 208-3**). The temporal course has traditionally been described as a brief loss of consciousness followed by a lucid interval, then progressive neurologic deterioration; however, this sequence is not common. Most epidural hematomas present with progressive hemiplegia and variably reduced consciousness from the time of injury. Although most cases require surgery, patients who remain awake and without focal neurologic signs for approximately 6 hours after the injury can be

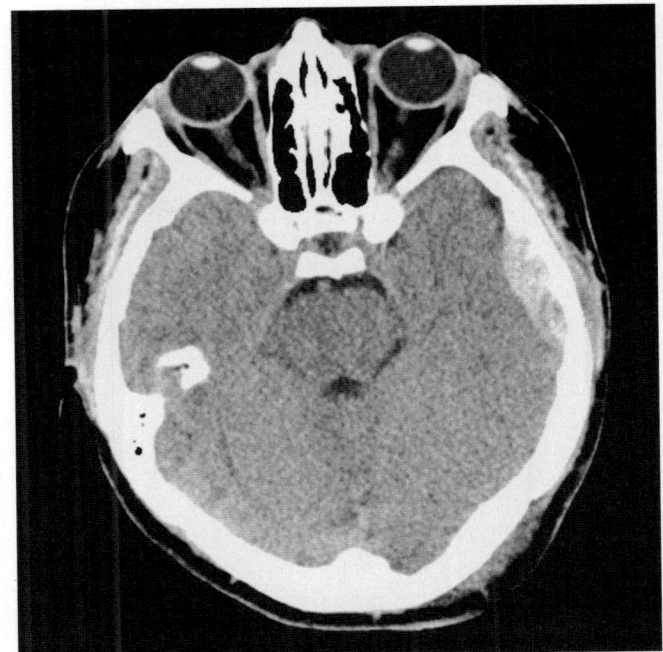

Figure 208-3 *Acute epidural hematoma in a 31-year-old woman who was hit by a truck.*

observed. Because epidural hematomas are infrequently epileptogenic, antiseizure medications are usually not given unless there is an underlying brain contusion.

■ SUBDURAL HEMATOMA

Subdural hematomas are most common in the elderly as a result of the expanded spaces produced by brain atrophy, the prevalence of anticoagulation and antiplatelet agents, and falls. Bleeding usually results from the rupture of veins that bridge the dura and the cortex. There may be acute, subacute, or chronic hemorrhage, as well as combinations of these. CT scan without contrast detects hematoma size, and can assist in estimating hemorrhage age (**Figure 208-4**). There is a variety of presentations with subdural hematoma but many are asymptomatic. Clinical features may include headache, often unilateral, mental dullness that may fluctuate, seizure and mild hemiparesis.

As with other cerebral hemorrhages, the decision regarding surgical evacuation depends on the patient's age, neurologic deficits, the estimated age of the hemorrhage, and its size. There is often difficulty in differentiating a chronic hematoma with low radiologic density from a subdural hygroma, which is a subdural CSF collection due to a small rent in the arachnoid membrane, also common in patients with brain atrophy. Hygromas rarely cause symptoms, and generally do not require surgery.

Antiseizure medications are advised, as subdural blood or the underlying brain contusion is epileptogenic, although the appropriate duration of treatment has not been established. Levetiracetam is used commonly, with no particular evidence favoring it over other drugs, but it has the advantage of not requiring a loading dose or monitoring of serum concentration. Larger doses are used if the patient has posttraumatic seizures. The clinician should be aware of the potential for this antiepileptic drug to cause depression and suicidal ideation.

Management strategies for correction of coagulopathy are as discussed in the previous section on intracerebral hemorrhage. There is no generally accepted interval after subdural hemorrhage during which anticoagulant or antiplatelet drugs are interdicted; the risks must be weighed by the hospitalist for each patient. We generally

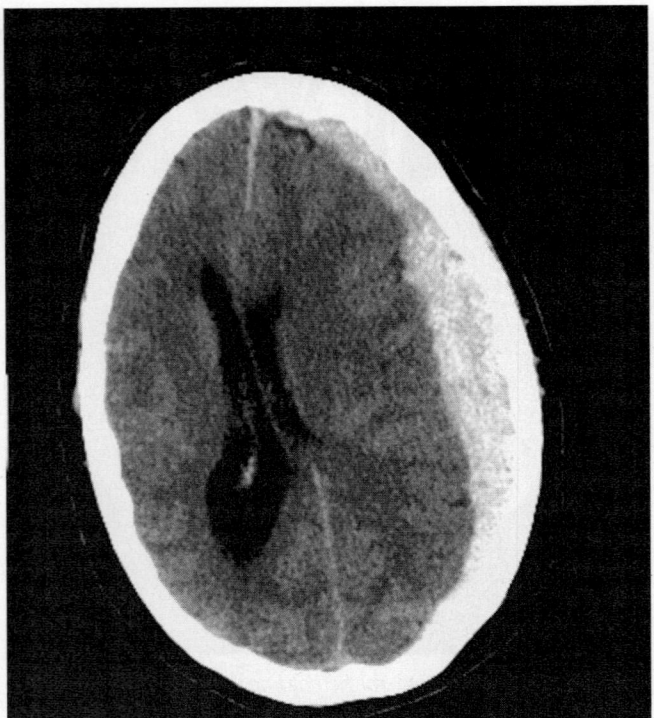

Figure 208-4 *Acute left hemispheric subdural hematoma in a 52-year-old man following a fall.*

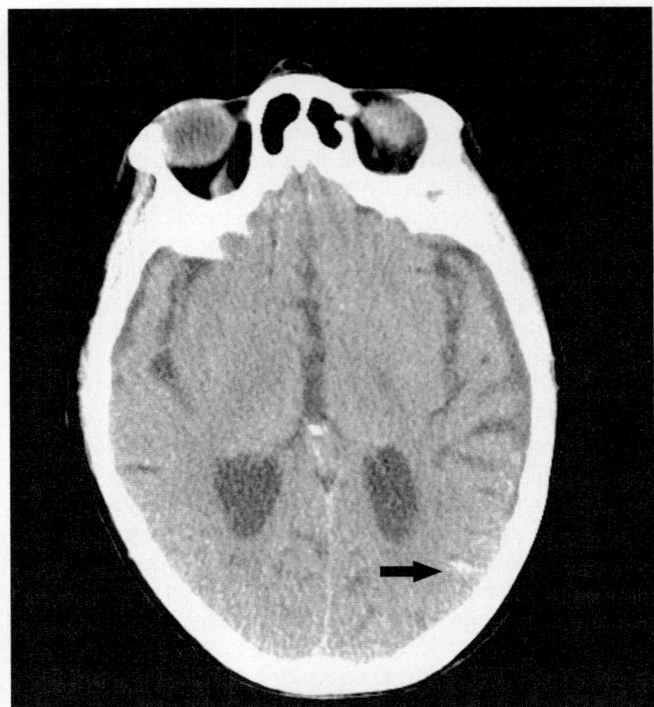

Figure 208-5 *Traumatic subarachnoid hemorrhage. Subarachnoid blood is collected in the sulci of the left parietal lobe (arrow); this is a common occurrence and does not require surgical intervention.*

withhold these drugs for a minimum of 1 month, unless there is an absolute requirement related to mechanical heart valves, recently placed stents, or other apparatus.

■ TRAUMATIC CEREBRAL HEMORRHAGE

Traumatic hemorrhages are managed similarly to the previously discussed spontaneous intracerebral hemorrhages. They may be difficult to distinguish from a brain contusion. Traumatic brain contusions tend to occur in the anterior frontal or temporal lobes and may enlarge and cause surrounding swelling with secondary brainstem compression, especially if the patient had been receiving anticoagulants. Patients with large traumatic contusions may benefit from surgical decompression to allow for brain swelling, but this condition only rarely requires direct removal of damaged brain tissue.

Traumatic subarachnoid hemorrhage is also common after moderate and severe head injury. Although it can occur anywhere in the subarachnoid space, it is most common over the convexities of the cerebral hemispheres (**Figure 208-5**), whereas aneurysmal rupture usually leads to a characteristic distribution of blood in the basal cisterns and Sylvian fissures (compare to Figure 208-2). The amount of blood resulting from traumatic hemorrhage is also less than from aneurysmal rupture. If the history is not entirely clear, as in cases in which a patient has fallen and reports a headache before or after the fall, a CT or conventional angiogram of the cerebral vessels or other vascular imaging may be required in order to exclude an aneurysm.

For patients with minimal or mild TBI (loss of consciousness <5 minute, Glasgow Coma Scale score of 14-15, and minimal blood on CT scan), we perform a repeat CT scan 6 hours following the original scan to detect further bleeding, observe for 24 hours, and administer levetiracetam for 7 days. These choices are based on our stylistic approach and have little evidence-based support. Most patients with mild and moderate brain injury are discharged home with appropriate physical and psychological (cognitive) therapy. Repeat outpatient imaging is generally not required, unless there has been a clinical change. Individuals with severe residual motor or

cognitive difficulties are discharged to specialized units that provide comprehensive head trauma rehabilitation, including family support and instruction.

■ DISCHARGE CHECKLIST FOR CERERBAL TRAUMA

- Has the appropriate care level been established for the patient's motor, cognitive, and sensory needs?
- Has a plan been established for antiepileptic and prophylactic anticoagulant medications?
- If ventriculoperitoneal shunt has been placed, has a baseline head CT been performed prior to discharge, and has outpatient follow-up been arranged for establishment of shunt continuity and pressure level assessment?

RELATED TOPICS IN ACUTE NEUROLOGY

■ PHYSIOLOGY OF INTRACRANIAL PRESSURE (ICP)

The fixed space of the cranial vault allows for only a small amount of added volume. Elevation in ICP is thus expected with all cerebral mass lesions, including intracerebral hemorrhage, large ischemic strokes with edema, herpes simplex encephalitis, and global brain swelling after hypoxia. Intracranial hypertension may also be associated with acute hepatic failure, uremia, and medications such as retinoids and tetracyclines.

As volume-buffering mechanisms fail, ICP rises exponentially and eventually reaches levels that approximate the mean blood pressure in the arteries at the base of the brain, compromising cerebral blood flow. This relationship can be approximated as cerebral perfusion pressure (CPP) = mean arterial blood pressure (MAP)—ICP. The result of greatly reduced CPP is ultimately brain death.

Intracranial pressure can be measured directly with one of several devices, including external ventricular drains (EVD) or intraparenchymal fiberoptic wires. The normal ICP in a resting adult is ~5 to 10 mm Hg. Elevations >20 mm Hg generally require treatment.

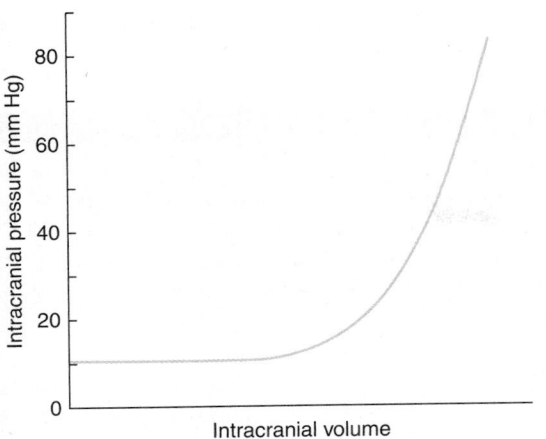

Figure 208-6 *Intracranial compliance curve. Minor changes in intra-cranial volume lead to alarming increases in intracranial pressure once an intracranial pressure of 20 mm Hg has been reached.* (Reproduced, with permission, from Morgan GE, Mikhail MS, Murray MJ. *Clinical Anesthesiology*, 4th ed. New York, NY: McGraw-Hill; 2006.)

Although pressures at this level do not compromise cerebral perfusion, the exponential shape of the intracranial compliance curve causes any additional mass to produce a marked and precarious rise in ICP (**Figure 208-6**).

■ TREATMENT OF ELEVATED INTRACRANIAL PRESSURE

Several treatments and maneuvers are effective in reducing ICP, among them sedation, elevation of the head of the bed, and control of fever. Most patients who require ICP treatment are drowsy, stuporous, or unresponsive. There is no reason to withhold pain medications or sedating drugs such as benzodiazepines once a clinical examination has been performed. These medications are withdrawn at regular intervals in order to re-examine the patient. For patients who are more awake, short-acting alternatives such as dexmedetomidine may be used for sedation.

Increases in core body temperature elevate cerebral blood flow and cerebral blood volume, thereby increasing ICP. Treating febrile episodes aggressively with acetaminophen, cooling blankets, appropriate antibiotics, and, if necessary, neuromuscular paralysis, are all effective in reducing ICP. Induced hypothermia is also effective in reducing ICP, but several trials have failed to show a benefit for TBI. Hypothermia as a component of resuscitation after cardiac arrest has, in contrast, improved neurological outcome but only to the extent that recent trials suggest that assiduously maintaining core temperature at 36°F gives equivalent outcomes to 33°F.

Levels of blood pressure that are appropriate for each configuration of head trauma have not been determined. Management is guided by direct measurement of ICP, allowing calculation of cerebral perfusion pressure. In general, individuals who are chronically hypertensive are allowed to retain a degree of moderate hypertension. However, mean arterial blood pressure >100 mm Hg is generally treated with rapid-acting, titratable IV medications such as labetalol or nicardipine. In addition, hypotension is avoided in these patients, and systolic blood pressures should generally be maintained above 90 mm Hg. Blood pressure targets may be guided by CPP that is calculated from the difference between ICP and mean blood pressure and is maintained between 50 and 70 mm Hg.

The mainstay of medical treatment for raised intracranial pressure has been hyperosmolar therapy. Hyperosmolarity of the blood establishes a gradient for water movement from the interstitial space of the brain into the vasculature. Any agent that raises serum osmolarity is effective in proportion to its ability to remain in the blood and not move into the brain (measured as its reflection coefficient), the degree of dehydration achieved, and its duration of action. Serum sodium concentration or serum osmolarity can be used as a guide to treatment, as these broadly reflect the degree of dehydration produced by a hyperosmolar agent.

Saline has a reflection coefficient of 1, meaning that it does not transgress into the brain, thus making it an ideal agent to reduce brain swelling. Normal saline has an effective osmolarity of 309 mOsm/L and creates only mild hyperosmolarity. High osmolarity is achieved more quickly by infusing boluses of mannitol, 3% saline, or 23.4% saline which act over minutes to hours. Subsequent infusion of normal saline may be used to maintain elevated osmolarity. Furosemide may also be used for this purpose, but has a delayed effect. Hypertonic saline infusions risk causing intravascular volume overload and congestive heart failure, whereas furosemide or mannitol may produce volume depletion and hypotension. Several trials have indicated that corticosteroids do not improve outcome in head injury or cerebral hemorrhage, and they are generally not used.

Serum sodium concentrations of ~145 to 154 mEq/L or serum osmolarity levels of ~310 to 325 mOsm/L are appropriate targets for treatment of raised ICP. Once a target level of hyperosmolarity has been achieved, a return to normal sodium levels is allowed only slowly to avoid rebound brain swelling. When syndrome of inappropriate antidiuretic hormone (SIADH) or diabetes insipidus is part of the clinical illness, management with hyperosmolar agents becomes complex, and nephrology consultation may be helpful.

■ ACQUIRED DISORDERS OF WATER AND SODIUM BALANCE IN BRAIN INJURY

Many acute and chronic cerebral diseases produce SIADH. However, hyponatremia may also result from the "cerebral salt wasting" observed in subarachnoid hemorrhage and cerebral trauma. This is the result of release of natriuretic peptides from either the brain or cardiac atria. Hyponatremia from either SIADH or cerebral salt wasting can exaggerate brain edema and cause convulsions; it is therefore appropriate to treat low serum sodium aggressively in patients with cerebral injury. The distinction between the two disorders is difficult but may be made by assessing intravascular volume and urinary electrolytes. Patients with SIADH are euvolemic, whereas those with cerebral salt wasting become volume depleted. Fluid restriction for acute hyponatremia from SIADH is usually initiated when serum sodium is below 132 mEq/L. If unsuccessful, 3% saline is infused. In salt wasting, normal saline and hypertonic solutions are used. Some centers also add fludrocortisone. Overly rapid correction of hyponatremia should be avoided, as this may lead to pontine and extrapontine myelinolysis.

> ### PRACTICE POINT
> - Hyponatremia after cranial injury or hemorrhage may be due to inappropriate ADH secretion, cerebral salt wasting, or both simultaneously.
> - Hypertonic saline can be used to reverse hyponatremia from all these circumstances but it causes volume expansion, and should be accompanied by assessment for intravascular overload.

Diabetes insipidus is also encountered after cerebral injury from trauma or surgery. The diagnosis should be suspected in the presence of polyuria, hypernatremia, and urine that is dilute in comparison to serum. Treatment is by allowing patients to drink *ad libitum* to satisfy their thirst, with the goal of a neutral fluid balance. For comatose patients or refractory cases, fluid and sodium replacement is given intravenously in proportion to urine output, and DDAVP (desmopressin) is added.

■ PROPHYLACTIC ANTICOAGULATION AFTER HEAD INJURY, INTRACRANIAL HEMORRHAGE, AND NEUROSURGERY

A common question asked in the management of neurosurgical patients is the safety of prophylactic anticoagulation for the prevention of venous thromboembolism. Patients with brain lesions are at high risk for thrombosis as a result of prolonged immobility and paralyzed extremities. We use both compression stockings and sequential compression devices on the legs of operative and nonoperative patients. Early ambulation is also important, and early involvement of physical and occupational therapists is advocated.

There are few adequate studies regarding the use of prophylactic unfractionated heparin or low-molecular-weight heparins to reduce venous thromboembolism in neurosurgical patients. The consensus has been that the potential risk of intracranial bleeding is outweighed by the benefit of prevention of thromboembolism in an immobilized patient. However, this is a discussion that the hospitalist and neurosurgeon should individualize for each patient. It is advisable to monitor PTT and platelets to avoid excessive anticoagulation and thrombocytopenia.

■ VENTRICULAR SHUNTS

Placement and revision of permanent ventricular shunts are common neurosurgical procedures. Hydrocephalus is the usual indication for diverting CSF from the ventricles. Hydrocephalus results from overproduction or underabsorption of CSF or from blockage of the ventricular outflow pathways. A shunt redirects CSF from the ventricular system to the peritoneum, pleural space, or right atrium. Many of these shunts have valves inserted that allow for adjustment of the opening pressure by a magnet placed over the device.

Fever in patients with shunts is a common problem faced by hospitalists. Shunt infection as a cause of fever is uncommon after the immediate postoperative period, and certainly much less common than mundane causes such as urinary tract infections and pneumonia. Attribution of fever or systemic leukocytosis to shunt infection is a last resort. Recently operated patients are at greater risk of shunt infection than those who had shunts inserted months or years previously.

Patients with acute shunt malfunction from infection or mechanical disruption generally have gait deterioration and somnolence, or headache, nausea and vomiting from hydrocephalus. A noncontrast head CT may be obtained if there is no other source of fever, as ventricular enlargement is commonly but not always seen in acute shunt malfunctions, as well as a shunt series. This consists of a total of four plain films, including PA and lateral films of the skull, PA or AP chest film, and flatplate of the abdomen, to assess the continuity and proper placement of shunt tubing, and including an image of the valve to determine its setting.

PRACTICE POINT

- Shunt infection is not a common source of fever and becomes less common after the immediate postoperative period.
- An x-ray shunt series can be used to assess the mechanical continuity of a shunt from the ventricular to the peritoneal spaces and to determine the pressure setting of an adjustable valve.

When shunt malfunction is suspected, a shunt tap may be performed to assess catheter patency, measure pressure, and obtain CSF for analysis. If CSF is needed to exclude meningitis, it is prudent to consider a lumbar puncture rather than a shunt tap because of the lower risk of shunt contamination with lumbar puncture.

SUGGESTED READINGS

Epstein NE. A review of the risks and benefits of differing prophylaxis regimens for the treatment of deep venous thrombosis and pulmonary embolism in neurosurgery. *Surg Neurol.* 2005;64:295-301.

Hamilton MG, Yee WH, Hull RD, Ghali WA. Venous thromboembolism prophylaxis in patients undergoing cranial neurosurgery: a systematic review and meta-analysis. *Neurosurgery.* 2011;68:571-581.

Mendelow AD, Gregson BA, Fernandes HM, et al. Early surgery versus initial conservative treatment in patients with spontaneous supratentorial intracerebral haematomas in the International Surgical Trial in Intracerebral Haemorrhage (STICH): a randomised trial. *Lancet.* 2005;365:387-397.

Mohr JP, Parides MK, Stapf C, et al. Medical management with or without interventional therapy for unruptured brain arteriovenous malformations (ARUBA): a multicentre, non-blinded, randomised trial. *Lancet.* 2014;383:614-621.

Naidech AM, Garg RK, Liebling S, et al. Anticonvulsant use and outcomes after intracerebral hemorrhage. *Stroke.* 2009;40:3810-3815.

Poli D, Antonucci E, Dentali R, et al. Recurrence of ICH after resumption of anticoagulation with VK antagonists. *Neurology.* 2014;82:1020-1026.

Qureshi AI, Palesh YI, Barsan WG, et al. Intensive blood-pressure lowering in patients with acute cerebra hemorrhage. *New Engl J Med.* 2016; June 8 epub.

Roberts I, Yates P, Sandercock I, et al. Effect of intravenous corticosteroids on death within 14 days in 10008 adults with clinically significant head injury (MRC CRASH trial). *Lancet.* 2004;364:1321-1328.

Ropper AH. Hyperosmolar therapy for raised intracranial pressure. *N Engl J Med.* 2012;367:746-752.

CHAPTER 209

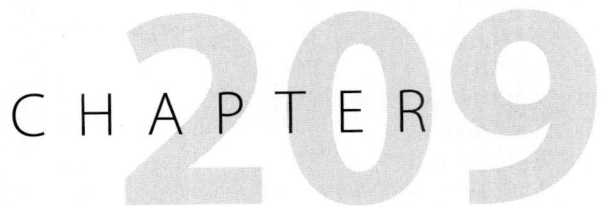

Transient Ischemic Attack and Stroke

Galen V. Henderson, MD

Key Clinical Questions

❶ How are stroke and transient ischemic attack differentiated?

❷ Who is eligible for IV recombinant tissue plasminogen activator?

❸ What is the best cerebral imaging modality?

❹ What is the optimal blood pressure in hospitalized patients with stroke?

❺ What is the best antiplatelet therapy for secondary prevention of transient ischemic attack and stroke?

❻ Should every patient be started on a statin?

INTRODUCTION

Stroke is the third leading cause of death in the United States. There are more than 700,000 strokes in the United States each year, resulting in more than 160,000 deaths annually. Although there was a 60% decline in stroke mortality between 1968 and 1996, the rate of decline began to slow in the 1990s and has plateaued in several regions of the country. The incidence of stroke may actually be increasing. From 1988 to 1997, the age-adjusted hospitalization rate for stroke grew by 19%, and total stroke hospitalizations increased by 39%. In 2004, the cost of stroke in the United States was estimated at $53.6 billion (direct and indirect costs), with a mean lifetime cost estimated at $140,048. Stroke is also a leading cause of functional impairments, with 20% of survivors requiring institutional care after 3 months, and 15% to 30% being permanently disabled. Utility analyses show that a major stroke is viewed by more than half of those at risk as being worse than death.

CAUSES OF STROKE

The most common cause of stroke is atherosclerosis of large- and medium-sized vessels of the neck and base of the brain (**Figure 209-1**). Risk factors for atherosclerosis include hypertension, diabetes, hyperlipidemia, cigarette smoking, and family history. Hypertension and diabetes also predispose to lacunae, which result from blockage of small perforating branches of the large cerebral arteries, with a predilection for the basal ganglia, thalamus, internal capsule, and pons. Patients with giant cell arteritis, systemic lupus erythematosus, and other vasculitides are at increased risk of stroke. Fibromuscular dysplasia is a cause of stroke in younger patients and is more common in women. Atrial fibrillation and valvular heart disease predispose to embolic stroke. Cocaine use predisposes to stroke for several reasons, including vasospasm, platelet activation, and rupture of arteriovenous malformations and aneurysms with acute elevations in blood pressure. Intravenous (IV) drug users may develop embolic stroke from bacterial endocarditis. Stroke may also result from dissection of the carotid or vertebral arteries. Moyamoya syndrome results from bilateral narrowing of the distal internal carotids and adjacent anterior and middle cerebral arteries (MCAs), with the development of fragile collateral vessels on angiography (**Figure 209-2**). It may be inherited as an autosomal recessive disorder or acquired in the setting of atherosclerosis, sickle cell disease, or basilar meningitis. Children present with ischemic stroke, whereas adults tend to develop intracranial hemorrhage (ICH). Hypercoagulability from genetic abnormalities in coagulation factors, leukemia, myeloproliferative disorders, antiphospholipid antibody syndrome, oral contraceptives (OCs), and sickle cell disease also predispose to stroke. Causes of stroke are summarized in **Table 209-1**.

CLINICAL PRESENTATION

Strokes and transient ischemic attacks (TIAs) present with the abrupt onset of neurologic deficits. In stroke, the duration of symptoms is longer than 24 hours. In TIA, symptoms resolve completely within 24 hours, usually within 30 minutes to 1 hour. However, if patients with clinical TIA have evidence of ischemia on magnetic resonance imaging (MRI) with diffusion-weighted sequences, the lesion is considered to be a stroke. The distinction between TIA and ischemic stroke has become less important in recent years, as measures for

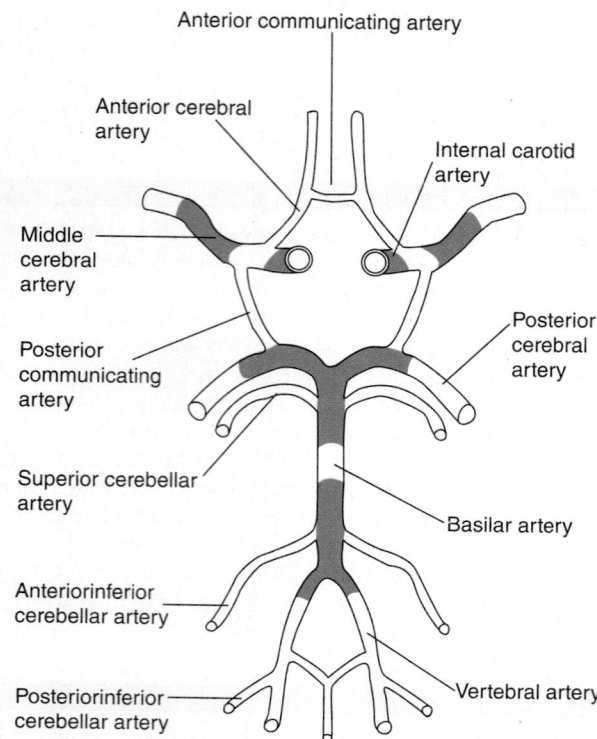

Figure 209-1 *Sites of predilection (shaded areas) for atherosclerosis in the intracranial arterial circulation.* (Reproduced, with permission, from Greenberg DA, Aminoff MJ, Simon RP. *Clinical Neurology*, 5th ed. McGraw-Hill; 2002. Fig. 9-4.)

secondary prevention are similar in each group. Moreover, TIA is a robust short-term predictor of stroke: the 90-day stroke risk after TIA is as high as 10.5%, with the greatest risk in the first week.

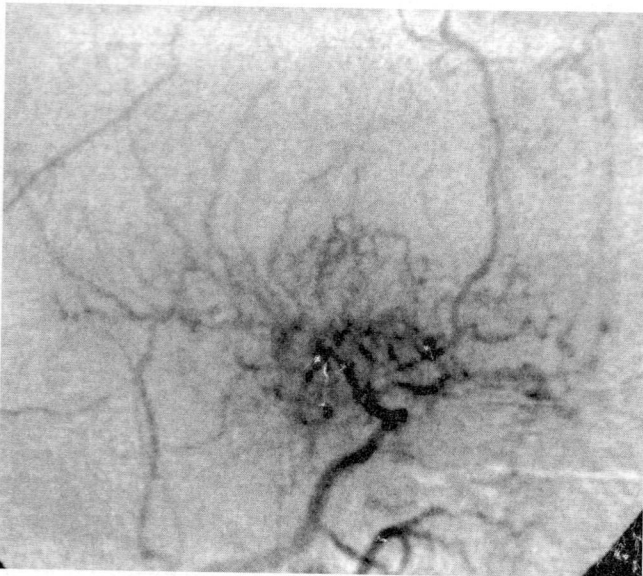

Figure 209-2 *Right carotid angiogram in moyamoya syndrome, lateral view. The middle cerebral artery and its branches are replaced by a diffuse capillary pattern that resembles a puff of smoke (moyamoya is Japanese and means "smoke" or "haze").* (Reproduced, with permission, from Greenberg DA, Aminoff MJ, Simon RP. *Clinical Neurology*, 5th ed. McGraw-Hill; 2002. Fig. 9-7B.)

TABLE 209-1 Conditions Associated with Stroke

Vascular disorders
Atherosclerosis
Lacunar infarction
Carotid or vertebral artery dissection
Fibromuscular dysplasia
Vasculitis and infections
  Giant cell arteritis
  Systemic lupus erythematosus
  Behçet disease
  Primary angiitis of the CNS
  Syphilis
  Varicella zoster
  HIV/AIDS
Cocaine, amphetamines, and other drugs of abuse
Moyamoya syndrome (multiple progressive intracranial occlusions)
Venous and sinus thrombosis

Embolism
Atrial fibrillation
Mural thrombus
Prosthetic heart valves
Rheumatic heart disease
Infectious endocarditis
Marantic endocarditis
Patent foramen ovale
Atrial septal defect
Atrial myxoma

Hypercoagulable states
Antiphospholipid antibody syndrome
Thrombocytosis
Polycythemia
Sickle cell disease
Leukemia
Waldenström macroglobulinemia
Oral contraceptives
Activated protein C resistance
Deficiency of protein C, protein S, or antithrombin III
Thrombotic thrombocytopenic purpura
Disseminated intravascular coagulation

Miscellaneous
Fabry disease
CADASIL
MELAS

AIDS, acquired immunodeficiency syndrome; CADASIL, cerebral autosomal dominant angiopathy with subcortical infarcts and leukoencephalopathy; HIV, human immunodeficiency virus; MELAS, mitochondrial encephalopathy with lactic acidosis and strokelike episodes.

Stroke may be produced by thrombosis, embolism, and hemorrhage. In embolic stroke, lesions are characteristically maximal at onset, whereas symptoms of thrombotic stroke evolve over minutes to hours. In subarachnoid hemorrhage, patients may present with the sudden onset of "the worst headache of my life" or with a sudden extreme pressure sensation in the head or neck. For parenchymal hemorrhages, symptoms occur suddenly and progress over 30 minutes to 1 hour. Many conditions may mimic ischemic or hemorrhagic stroke (**Table 209-2**). It is important to determine anterior versus posterior circulation stroke to tailor imaging and intervention. In addition, posterior circulation strokes are more likely to produce complications related to altered consciousness. Large cerebellar strokes pose a risk of herniation and may require emergent neurosurgical decompression, especially if >3 cm in size or if there is evidence of edema or hemorrhagic transformation. Recognition of progressive brainstem and cerebellar symptoms due to thrombosis of the basilar artery may allow for early intervention to prevent the devastating morbidity from infarct due to complete occlusion.

Lesions in the *anterior cerebral artery* are uncommon. Patients present with paralysis and sensory loss of the contralateral leg. Patients may have urinary urgency and incontinence from the failure to inhibit reflex bladder contractions.

The *middle cerebral artery*, the largest branch of the internal carotid artery, is the vessel most commonly affected in ischemic stroke. The clinical picture depends on the location of the damage (ie, whether all cortical branches are affected vs individual cortical branches) and whether the dominant or nondominant hemisphere is affected. Strokes affecting the *superior division* of the MCA lead to hemiparesis affecting the contralateral face, hand, and arm but sparing the leg, with accompanying sensory deficits; if the dominant hemisphere is involved, expressive (Broca) aphasia may develop, with loss of speech production but preserved speech comprehension. *Inferior division MCA* strokes may lead to contralateral homonymous hemianopia, hemineglect, loss of graphesthesia and stereognosis, and apraxias. Involvement of the dominant hemisphere also produces Wernicke (receptive) aphasia, with speech consisting of fluent but meaningless babble. Lesions at the bifurcation of the MCA may lead to deficits in both superior and inferior vascular territories. Leg weakness may also ensue if the occlusion is proximal to the lenticulostriate branches of the MCA.

Internal carotid artery occlusion may be asymptomatic if collateral circulation is adequate, or it may produce strokes similar to middle cerebral artery syndromes if collateral circulation is poor. About 15% of cases of incipient carotid occlusion are heralded by episodes of transient monocular blindness (amaurosis fugax).

TABLE 209-2 Conditions that Mimic Thromboembolic Stroke

Sudden onset of persistent focal deficit

Partial seizure with postictal (Todd) paralysis

Abscess with seizure

Tumor with bleeding or seizure

Toxic-metabolic insult superimposed on old cerebral lesion

Hypoglycemia

Subdural hematoma (acute)

Multiple sclerosis

Cerebritis

Sudden onset of transient focal deficit

Partial seizure

Migraine with aura

Arteriovenous malformations (may also present with symptoms of partial seizure or migraine)

PRACTICE POINT

- In acute stroke, it is important to determine whether the patient's speech is fluent, whether the patient understands speech, and whether the patient can repeat simple phrases. In acute global aphasia, the patient will not have fluent speech, will not comprehend speech, and will be unable to repeat phases. It is not possible at this point to localize the site of damage.
- Expressive or receptive aphasia from anterior circulation strokes may present acutely as global aphasia, but then become productive or receptive as the patient recovers.
- If the patient does not have fluent speech and cannot repeat phrases, but can comprehend speech, the patient has an expressive (Broca) aphasia localizing to the inferior frontal gyrus.
- If the patient's speech becomes fluent without the ability to comprehend speech or repeat phrases, the patient has a receptive (Wernicke) aphasia localizing to the superior temporal gyrus.
- It is also important to distinguish a language disorder (aphasia) from a purely motor disorder (dysarthria).

Posterior cerebral artery strokes produce contralateral homonymous hemianopia. If the vascular lesion is near the origin of the posterior cerebral artery in the midbrain, vertical gaze palsy, oculomotor (III) nerve palsy, and internuclear ophthalmoplegia may occur. If the dominant hemisphere is affected, patients may also have anomia, alexia without agraphia, or visual agnosia.

Strokes involving the *vertebrobasilar* circulation may lead to a variety of symptoms from brainstem ischemia, such as ipsilateral cranial nerve palsies with contralateral hemiplegia, ipsilateral cerebellar ataxia, nystagmus, vertigo, vomiting, dysphagia, dysarthria, Horner syndrome, and hiccup.

PRACTICE POINT

Horner syndrome is characterized by

- Ptosis, usually slight
- Miosis (pupillary constriction), more marked in the dark
- Anhidrosis (absence of facial sweating), if the lesion is proximal to the carotid arteries

Horner syndrome may result from sympathetic damage at any of the following locations:

- Brainstem, especially lateral medullary infarction (Wallenberg syndrome)
- Cervical spinal cord
- Anterior roots of C8 and T1
- Cervical sympathetic chain (carcinoma of the apex of the lung)
- Trauma, occlusion, aneurysm, or dissection of the internal carotid artery

Horner syndrome may thus result from either anterior or posterior (vertebrobasilar) cerebrovascular disease. If accompanied by vertigo and ataxia, it suggests cerebellar or medullary stroke from a vertebral artery lesion.

Lacunar infarcts occur from degenerative changes in small penetrating arteries deep in the brain from hypertension. They are often clinically silent. When symptomatic, they may have an acute or subacute onset and may produce distinctive syndromes, such as pure motor hemiparesis (the most common type of lacunar infarct), pure sensory loss, dysarthria/clumsy hand syndrome, and ataxic hemiparesis, with incoordination out of proportion to motor weakness.

ASSESSMENT

■ PHYSICAL EXAMINATION

Areas of special interest on general examination include vital signs (hypertension, irregular pulse); funduscopic examination, which may reveal retinal emboli (Hollenhorst crystals) in carotid disease; presence of carotid pulses or bruits; temporal arteries, which may be nodular, thickened, or pulseless in giant cell arteritis; and the cardiac examination, for evidence of atrial fibrillation, cardiomegaly, and valvular disease. Blood cultures should be obtained in febrile patients to exclude endocarditis.

■ NEUROLOGIC FINDINGS

The neurologic examination attempts to identify the site of the lesion and the likely culprit vessel. Certain findings are helpful in localizing a stroke to either the anterior circulation (the internal carotid artery and its major branches, the anterior cerebral, middle cerebral, and anterior choroidal arteries) or the posterior circulation (the vertebral arteries and basilar artery, their cerebellar branches, and their termination in the posterior cerebral arteries). Aphasia indicates a lesion in the anterior circulation, rather than posterior, and makes lacunar infarction unlikely. Hemianopia also makes lacunar infarct unlikely. Although hemianopia may be present in either anterior or posterior circulation lesions, isolated hemianopia indicates a posterior cerebral artery lesion. Ocular palsies, nystagmus, and internuclear ophthalmoplegia indicate a posterior circulation lesion affecting the brainstem. Hemiparesis can be produced by a wide variety of lesions. However, hemiparesis of the face, hand, and arm, with relative sparing of the leg, suggests an MCA lesion. Hemiparesis that affects the face, hand, arm, and leg equally suggests a lesion in the internal carotid, stem of the MCA, a lacuna in the internal capsule or basal ganglia, or a brainstem stroke. Crossed hemiparesis (affecting the face and contralateral side of the body) suggests a brainstem lesion, as does a crossed sensory deficit. An isolated hemisensory deficit is likely due to a lacunar infarct.

The neurologic examination is discussed in detail in Chapter 104.

■ BLOOD TESTS

Routine blood tests in stroke should assess for potentially treatable causes of stroke: complete blood count (thrombocytosis, polycythemia, sickle cell disease, leukemia), erythrocyte sedimentation rate (giant cell arteritis and other vasculitides, endocarditis), serum glucose (to exclude hypoglycemia masquerading as stroke), serologic tests for syphilis, and lipid panel.

■ ELECTROCARDIOGRAM

Electrocardiogram should occur as soon as possible after TIA or stroke to exclude atrial fibrillation or flutter. Inpatient telemetry monitoring may be useful to exclude paroxysmal atrial fibrillation.

■ NEUROIMAGING

Imaging of the brain is recommended before therapy for acute ischemic stroke. Magnetic resonance imaging, with diffusion-weighted imaging (DWI) and apparent diffusion coefficient (ADC) sequences, is the most sensitive imaging modality (**Figure 209-3**). Acute infarct appears bright on DWI and dark on ADC; these changes correlate with the presence of cytotoxic edema. The relative intensities of DWI and ADC change over time, and are helpful in dating the infarct if this is unclear from the history. Changes may be apparent on MRI with DWI/ADC 30 minutes after the onset of symptoms, whereas noncontrast computed tomography (CT) is insensitive in the first several hours after infarction.

If MRI is not immediately available, head CT should be performed. Despite the diagnostic superiority of MRI, CT remains the most practical initial brain-imaging test. In most instances, CT provides the necessary information to make decisions about emergency management, particularly thrombolysis. A physician skilled in assessing CT or MRI studies should be available to interpret the initial scan.

Echocardiography is reasonable in the evaluation of patients with TIA or stroke of possible embolic cause, especially in patients in whom no other cause has been identified. Transesophageal echocardiography is particularly useful in identifying patent foramen ovale, aortic arch atherosclerosis, and endocarditis and is reasonable when identification of these conditions will alter management.

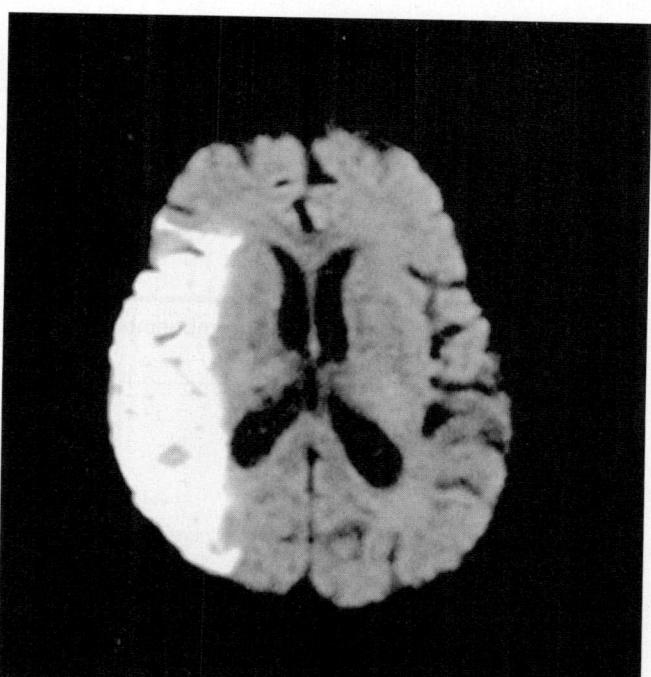

Figure 209-3 *Magnetic resonance imaging (MRI) with diffusion-weighted image (DWI) showing a large right middle cerebral artery infarction. The DWI bright signal changes are evident well before and more clearly than alterations in the computed tomography (CT) scan or conventional MRI.* (Reproduced, with permission, from Ropper AH, Samuels MA. *Adams & Victor's Principles of Neurology*, 9th ed. New York, NY: McGraw-Hill; 2009. Fig. 34-3A.)

■ VASCULAR IMAGING

Noninvasive imaging of the extracranial vessels should be performed routinely as part of the evaluation of patients with suspected TIA or stroke. Initial assessment may involve carotid duplex ultrasound, MR angiogram, or CT angiogram, depending on local availability and expertise. Transcranial Doppler ultrasound is especially helpful in the serial assessment of vasospasm after subarachnoid hemorrhage. Catheter angiography is the most sensitive and specific vascular imaging test; it is used to confirm abnormalities detected on non-invasive imaging or to further define unusual pathology, such as suspected vasculitis (**Figure 209-4**). Imaging of the intracranial or extracranial vasculature in the emergency assessment of patients with suspected stroke is useful at institutions providing endovascular recanalization therapies.

INDICATIONS FOR HOSPITALIZATION ON FIRST EVALUATION OF

■ TRANSIENT ISCHEMIC ATTACK

The ABCD^2 (age, blood pressure, clinical symptoms, duration of symptoms, and diabetes) is the most useful prediction score for stroke risk after TIA. Patients presenting with TIA score points (indicated in parentheses) for each of the following factors: age ≥ 60 years (1), blood pressure 140/90 mm Hg on first evaluation (1), clinical symptoms of focal weakness with the spell (2) or speech impairment without weakness (1), symptom duration ≥ 60 minutes (2) or 10 to 59 minutes (1), and diabetes (1). In combined validation cohorts, the 2-day risk of stroke was 0% for scores of 0 or 1, 1.3% for 2 or 3, 4.1% for 4 or 5, and 8.1% for 6 or 7.

It is reasonable to hospitalize patients with TIA if they present within 72 hours of the event and any of the following criteria are present:

1. ABCD^2 score ≥ 3.
2. ABCD^2 score = 0 to 2, and uncertainty that diagnostic workup can be completed within 2 days as an outpatient.
3. ABCD^2 score = 0 to 2 and other evidence to indicate that the patient's event was caused by focal ischemia.

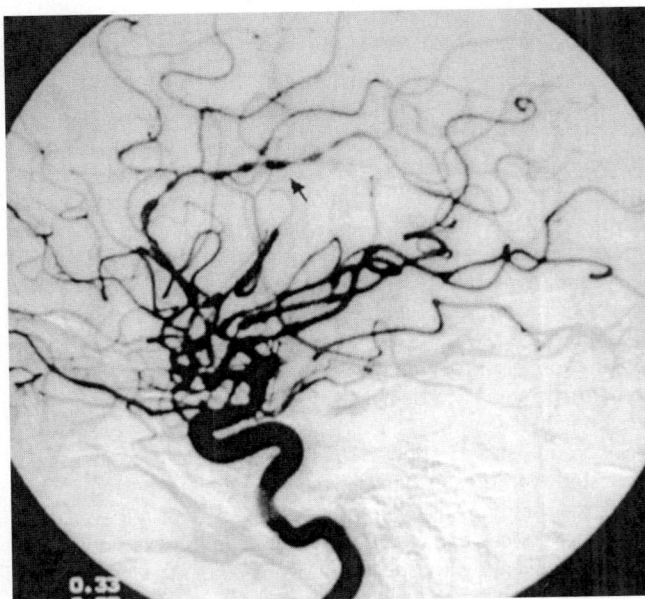

Figure 209-4 *Cerebral angiogram from a 32-year-old man with CNS vasculitis. Dramatic beading (arrow) typical of vasculitis is seen.* (Modified, with permission, from Fauci AS, Braunwald E, Kasper DL, et al. *Harrison's Principles of Internal Medicine*, 17th ed. New York, NY: McGraw-Hill; 2008. Fig. 364-5.)

In general, I recommend treating patients with a suspected neu-rovascular event with similar urgency as patients with chest pain and possible myocardial infarction. Rapid evaluation and treatment of TIA may avert the devastating consequences of stroke in many patients.

■ STROKE CENTERS

Ideally, patients with stroke should be cared for in certified stroke centers, which have been shown to improve patient outcomes and reduce complications. In many states, emergency medical services are directed to bring patients with suspected stroke directly to stroke centers, bypassing facilities that are not able to provide specialized care. However, this may not be feasible in some areas due to low population densities.

Key elements of *primary stroke centers* include acute stroke teams, stroke units, stroke care protocols, and an integrated emergency response system. Essential support services include the ability to obtain and interpret head CT scans 24 hours daily and rapid laboratory testing. Administrative support, strong leadership, and continuing medical education are also important elements for stroke centers. Most stroke patients may be appropriately cared for in primary stroke centers.

Comprehensive stroke centers are capable of caring for seriously ill stroke patients with complex cerebrovascular disease. The components of comprehensive stroke centers include expertise in neurosurgery, vascular neurology, and neuroradiology; advanced neuroimaging capabilities, such as MRI and cerebral angiography; the ability to perform clipping and coiling of intracranial aneurysms, carotid endarterectomy, and intra-arterial thrombolytic therapy; and specialized infrastructure elements, such as a neurologic intensive care unit and stroke registry.

SELECTION CRITERIA FOR ADMISSION TO THE INTENSIVE CARE UNIT

Triage to an intensive care unit (ICU) setting for monitoring and treatment is appropriate for patients with

- Cerebellar strokes >3 cm. Because cerebral edema is usually maximal in ischemic stroke 3 to 5 days after the event, large cerebellar strokes may lead to serious delayed complications, such as brainstem compression or hydrocephalus from obstruction or compression of the fourth ventricle or the cerebral aqueduct.
- Strokes involving >50% of the MCA circulation in patients younger than 60. These patients are at risk of malignant cerebral edema and may eventually require decompressive hemi-craniectomy, with temporary removal of the overlying skull, which is either frozen or inserted in the patient's peritoneal cavity, and incision of dura to allow the brain to swell outward.

MANAGEMENT OF TRANSIENT ISCHEMIC ATTACK AND STROKE

■ GENERAL SUPPORTIVE MEASURES

Hypoxia and the increased metabolic demands associated with fever may be deleterious to patients with stroke, as they may lead to infarct extension. Hypoxic patients with stroke should receive supplemental oxygen. Airway support and ventilatory assistance are recommended for patients with acute stroke with decreased consciousness or bulbar dysfunction causing compromise of the airway. The source of fever should be sought and antipyretic medications given to lower body temperature in febrile stroke patients. Other factors that may reduce neuronal viability, such as hypoglycemia, hypovolemia, and cardiac arrhythmias, should be corrected. Cardiac monitoring should be performed to screen for atrial fibrillation during the first 24 hours after onset of ischemic stroke.

■ IV THROMBOLYSIS

Intravenous recombinant tissue plasminogen activator (rtPA) is the only Food and Drug Administration (FDA)-approved therapy for acute ischemic stroke. It improves outcomes for a broad spectrum of patients treated within 3 hours of stroke onset. Treatment within 90 minutes is most likely to result in a favorable outcome, although treatment at 90 to 180 minutes is also beneficial. Patients with major strokes, determined by a National Institutes of Health Stroke Scale (NIHSS) (http://www.ninds.nih.gov/doctors/NIH_Stroke_Scale.pdf) score >22, have a very poor prognosis, but some positive treatment effect with rtPA has been documented. Patients with large strokes with substantial edema, mass effect, or midline shift on CT scan, as well as patients of advanced age, are at higher risk of hemorrhage, and the decision to treat with rtPA should be made with caution. Treatment with rtPA is associated with symptomatic intracranial hemorrhage in ~6% of cases, which may be fatal. The use of anticoagulants and antiplatelet agents should therefore be delayed for 24 hours after treatment.

Intravenous rtPA (0.9 mg/kg, maximum dose 90 mg) is recommended for selected patients within 3 hours of onset of ischemic stroke. Physicians should review the criteria used in clinical trials to determine the eligibility of the patient (**Table 209-3**). Significant risks include bleeding complications and angioedema. Patients whose blood pressure can be lowered safely with antihypertensive agents may be eligible for treatment, and the physician should assess blood pressure stability before starting rtPA (see below). A patient with a seizure at the time of onset of stroke may be eligible for treatment, as long as the physician is convinced that residual impairments are secondary to stroke and not a postictal phenomenon.

Intravenous streptokinase for the treatment of stroke is not recommended, and ancrod, tenecteplase, reteplase, desmoteplase, urokinase, or other thrombolytic agents should not be used outside the setting of a clinical trial. American Stroke Association guidelines suggest that thrombolysis may be considered for patients between 3 and 4.5 hours after stroke onset, provided patients are younger than 80 years, have NIHSS ≤25, are not taking oral anticoagulants, and do not have a history of both prior stroke and diabetes. However, clinicians should bear in mind that rtPA is not FDA-approved for use in this patient population.

■ THROMBOLYSIS BEYOND 3 HOURS AFTER ONSET OF STROKE

Thrombolysis in stroke is most effective when administered as early as possible after the onset of symptoms. Based on the European Cooperative Acute Stroke Study (ECASS-3), there is a modest benefit of thrombolysis given between 3 and 4.5 hours after stroke, although this seems to be less than the benefit observed with thrombolysis between 0 to 3 hours after stroke onset. The eligibility criteria for treatment are similar to those for persons treated at earlier time periods. However, patients who meet any of the following additional criteria should be excluded:

- Patients older than 80 years
- Baseline NIHSS >25
- Patients with a history of both stroke and diabetes
- All patients receiving an oral anticoagulant are excluded, regardless of their international normalized ratio (INR)

The safety and efficacy of treatment with rtPA within 3 to 4.5 hours after stroke in patients with these exclusion criteria have not been established and require further study. Additionally, the relative utility of rtPA in this time window compared with other methods of thrombus dissolution or removal has not been established. Patients should be informed that use of rtPA between 3 and 4.5 hours after stroke is considered off-label or investigational by the FDA.

■ ENDOVASCULAR TREATMENT

Unfortunately, thrombolytic therapy for large-vessel ischemic stroke is successful in only a minority of patients. Endovascular treatments have emerged as a successful strategy to reduce the clot burden and restore vessel patency. In a recent large meta-analysis of high-quality clinical trials, functional independence was markedly improved with endovascular treatment, rising from 31% in those receiving tissue plasminogen activator (tPA) alone to 45% in those also given endovascular therapy. Rates of intracranial hemorrhage and all-cause mortality were similar between the two groups at 90 days.

Subgroup analysis showed that endovascular treatment was associated with greater benefit when given after tPA rather than alone, that better results were achieved with stent retrievers than with other devices, and that functional outcomes were significantly better in patients with angiographic imaging showing proximal arterial occlusion.

Patients eligible for intravenous rtPA should receive intravenous rtPA, even if endovascular treatment is being considered. Observing patients after intravenous rtPA to assess for clinical response prior to endovascular therapy is not necessary to achieve beneficial outcomes and is not recommended. Patients should receive

---

TABLE 209-3 Administration of IV Recombinant Tissue Plasminogen Activator (rtPA) for Acute Ischemic Stroke*

Indications	Contraindications
Clinical diagnosis of stroke with disabling deficit	Sustained blood pressure > 185/110 mm Hg despite treatment
Onset of symptoms to time of drug administration ≤ 3 h	Platelets < 100,000; hematocrit < 25%; glucose < 50 or > 400 mg/dL
	Use of heparin within 48 h and prolonged PTT, or elevated INR > 1.7
CT scan showing no hemorrhage,	Rapidly improving symptoms
well-established infarct, or alternative explanation for the focal deficit	Prior stroke or head injury within 3 mo; prior intracranial hemorrhage
	Major surgery in preceding 14 d
Age ≥ 18 y	Minor stroke symptoms
	GI bleeding in preceding 21 d
Consent by patient or surrogate	Recent myocardial infarction
	Coma or stupor

Administration of rtPA

IV access with two peripheral IV lines (avoid arterial or central line placement)

Review eligibility for rtPA

Administer 0.9 mg/kg IV (maximum 90 mg) IV as 10% of total dose by bolus, followed by remainder of total dose over 1 h

Frequent cuff blood pressure monitoring

No other antithrombotic treatment for 24 h

For decline in neurologic status or uncontrolled blood pressure, stop infusion, give cryoprecipitate, and reimage brain emergently

Avoid urethral catheterization for 2 h

---

*See Activase (tissue plasminogen activator) package insert for complete list of contraindications and dosing.

CT, computed tomography; INR, international normalized ratio; PTT, partial thromboplastin time.

Modified, with permission, from Fauci AS, Braunwald E, Kasper DL, et al. *Harrison's Principles of Internal Medicine*, 17th ed. New York, NY: McGraw-Hill; 2008, Table 364-1.

endovascular therapy with a stent retriever if they meet all the following criteria:

- Prestroke modified Rankin score (mRS) score of either 0 (no symptoms) to 1 (symptoms without disability)
- Acute ischemic stroke receiving intravenous rtPA within 4.5 hours of onset according to guidelines from professional medical societies
- Causative occlusion of the ICA or proximal MCA
- Age ≥18 years
- NIHSS score of ≥6
- Alberta stroke program early CT score (ASPECTS) of ≥6, and
- Treatment can be initiated (groin puncture) within 6 hours of symptom onset

As with intravenous rtPA, reduced time from symptom onset to reperfusion with endovascular therapies is highly associated with better clinical outcomes. To ensure benefit, reperfusion to TICI (Thrombolysis in Cerebral Infarction) grade 2b/3 should be achieved as early as possible and within 6 hours of stroke onset. Use of salvage therapy, including intra-arterial fibrinolysis, may be reasonable to achieve these angiographic results if completed within 6 hours of symptom onset.

When treatment is initiated beyond 6 hours from symptom onset, the effectiveness of endovascular therapy is uncertain for patients with acute ischemic stroke with occlusion of the ICA or proximal MCA. Additional clinical trial data are needed.

In carefully selected patients with anterior circulation occlusion who have contraindications to intravenous rtPA, endovascular therapy with stent retrievers completed within 6 hours of stroke onset is reasonable. Endovascular therapy with stent retrievers may also be considered for carefully selected patients with acute ischemic stroke in whom treatment can be initiated within 6 hours of symptom onset and who have causative occlusion of the M2 or M3 portion of the MCAs, anterior cerebral arteries, vertebral arteries, basilar artery, or posterior cerebral arteries.

Although benefits are uncertain, the use of endovascular therapy with stent retrievers may be reasonable for patients with acute ischemic stroke in whom treatment can be initiated (groin puncture) within 6 hours of symptom onset and who have prestroke mRS score >1, ASPECTS <6, or NIHSS score <6 and causative occlusion of the ICA or proximal MCA. Additional randomized trial data are needed.

Intra-arterial fibrinolysis is beneficial for carefully selected patients with major ischemic strokes of <6 hours duration caused by MCA occlusion. However, these data are derived from clinical trials that no longer reflect current practice including the use of fibrinolytic drugs that are not available. The optimal dose of intra-arterial rtPA is not established, and rtPA does not have US Food and Drug Administration approval for intra-arterial use. Therefore, endovascular therapy with stent retrievers is recommended over intra-arterial fibrinolysis as first-line therapy. Intra-arterial fibrinolysis within 6 hours of stroke onset in carefully selected patients who have contraindications to the use of intravenous rtPA may be considered, but the risks and benefits are unknown.

If endovascular therapy is contemplated, a noninvasive intracranial vascular study such as CTA or MRA is strongly recommended during the initial evaluation of the acute stroke patient, but should not delay intravenous rtPA if indicated. For patients who are candidates for intravenous rtPA, initiating intravenous rtPA before noninvasive vascular imaging is recommended for patients who have not had noninvasive vascular imaging as part of their initial imaging assessment for stroke. Noninvasive intracranial vascular imaging should then be obtained as quickly as possible.

Endovascular therapy should be performed in an experienced stroke center with rapid access to cerebral angiography and qualified neurointerventionalists. Air medical transport and hospital bypass may be necessary for optimal and timely stroke management.

■ BLOOD PRESSURE MANAGEMENT

The management of arterial hypertension in acute stroke remains controversial, as data are inconclusive or conflicting. Many patients have spontaneous declines in blood pressure during the first 24 hours after onset of stroke. Until more definitive data are available, a cautious approach is recommended.

Patients with hypertension who are otherwise eligible for treatment with rtPA may have their blood pressure lowered so that their systolic blood pressure is ≤185 mm Hg and diastolic blood pressure ≤110 mm Hg before lytic therapy is begun. The clinician should be sure that the blood pressure is stabilized at the lower level before treating with rtPA and maintained below 180/105 mm Hg for at least the first 24 hours after IV rtPA treatment. Because the maximum interval from stroke onset until treatment with rtPA is short, many patients with sustained hypertension above the recommended levels cannot be treated with IV rtPA.

It is generally agreed that patients with markedly elevated blood pressure may have their blood pressure lowered. A reasonable goal would be to lower blood pressure by ~15% in the first 24 hours after onset of stroke. In the CATIS trial of over 4000 patients with acute ischemic stroke, a target blood pressure reduction of 10% to 25% within the first 24 hours of presentation was associated with similar rates of death and disability compared to the untreated control group.

Evidence from one clinical trial indicates that initiation of antihypertensive therapy within 24 hours of stroke is relatively safe. Thus, antihypertensive medications should be restarted at ~24 hours for patients with pre-existing hypertension who are neurologically stable, unless there is a specific contraindication to restarting treatment.

■ STATIN THERAPY

Patients suffering from ischemic stroke or TIA with elevated cholesterol, coronary artery disease (CAD), and evidence of atherosclerosis should be managed with lifestyle and diet modification and medications. Statins are indicated for these patients, with a low-density-lipoprotein cholesterol (LDL-C) goal of <100 mg/dL. An LDL-C <70 mg/dL is recommended for patients with multiple risk factors. In the Stroke Prevention by Aggressive Reduction in Cholesterol Levels (SPARCL) trial, therapy with atorvastatin 80 mg/d also reduced the risk of stroke and cardiovascular events in patients with atherosclerotic ischemic stroke or TIA but without known CAD. In this group, it is recommended to treat to a target LDL-C <70 mg/dL or an absolute reduction in LDL-C of at least 50%, as the greatest benefits of statin therapy were seen in patients who achieved these goals. Ischemic stroke or TIA patients with low high-density-lipoprotein cholesterol may be considered for treatment with niacin or gemfibrozil.

■ ANTICOAGULANTS

Urgent anticoagulation with heparin to prevent early recurrent stroke, halt neurologic worsening, or improve outcomes is not recommended for patients with acute ischemic stroke. Urgent anticoagulation should not be used in lieu of IV thrombolysis for treatment of otherwise eligible patients, and it is not recommended for patients with moderate to severe strokes because of an increased risk of serious intracranial hemorrhage. Although anticoagulation is indicated in patients with stroke due to embolism from atrial fibrillation or prosthetic heart valves, it should be avoided within 24 hours of treatment with IV administered rtPA. In contrast, anticoagulation is recommended for patients with TIA from cardiac embolism in the setting of atrial fibrillation.

■ ANTIPLATELET THERAPY IN ACUTE ISCHEMIC STROKE

Administration of aspirin (initial dose 325 mg) within 24 to 48 hours after stroke onset is recommended for most patients. Aspirin should not be considered a substitute for other acute interventions for treatment of stroke, including IV rtPA. Aspirin use should be avoided within 24 hours of thrombolytic therapy. The administration of clopidogrel alone or in combination with aspirin is not recommended for the treatment of acute ischemic stroke. Outside the setting of clinical trials, the IV administration of antiplatelet agents that inhibit the glycoprotein IIb/IIIa receptor is not recommended.

ANTIPLATELET THERAPY FOR SECONDARY PREVENTION

Patients with stroke or TIA are at high risk of recurrent stroke and other vascular events. In-hospital initiation of secondary stroke prevention avoids gaps in care, promotes better adherence, and leads to better short-term vascular outcomes. For patients with noncardioembolic ischemic stroke or TIA, antiplatelet agents, rather than oral anticoagulation, are recommended to reduce the risk of recurrent stroke and other cardiovascular events. Aspirin (50-325 mg/d) monotherapy, aspirin combined with extended-release dipyridamole, and clopidogrel monotherapy are all acceptable options for initial therapy. The combination of aspirin and extended-release dipyridamole is recommended over aspirin alone. Clopidogrel is preferred in patients with aspirin allergy. The combination of aspirin and clopidogrel increases the risk of major hemorrhage, and it is not routinely recommended for patients with ischemic stroke or TIA unless they have a specific indication, such as a coronary stent or acute coronary syndrome. Clopidogrel was compared with aspirin plus extended-release dipyridamole in the Prevention Regimen for Effectively Avoiding Second Strokes (PRoFESS) trial and found to have similar efficacy in the prevention of recurrent stroke. For patients who have an ischemic cerebrovascular event while taking aspirin, there is no evidence that increasing the dose of aspirin provides additional benefit. These patients are often changed to other antiplatelet regimens, although no clinical trials have been performed to validate this strategy.

HYPERGLYCEMIA

Persistent hyperglycemia (>140 mg/dL) in the first 24 hours after stroke is associated with poor outcomes. Serum glucose concentrations >140 to 185 mg/dL probably should trigger insulin administration. Glucose concentrations should be closely monitored with adjustment of insulin doses to avoid hypoglycemia.

HYPERBARIC OXYGEN AND HYPOTHERMIA

Data on the utility of hyperbaric oxygen are inconclusive, and some data imply that it may be harmful. Thus, with the exception of stroke secondary to air embolization, this intervention is not recommended for treatment of patients with acute ischemic stroke. Although data demonstrate the efficacy of hypothermia for improving neurologic outcomes after cardiac arrest, the utility of induced hypothermia for patients with ischemic stroke is not established.

CAROTID DISEASE

The treatment of symptomatic carotid stenosis is evolving. Best medical therapy in major published trials of carotid endarterectomy did not include statin therapy, newer antiplatelet agents, or optimized control of hypertension. Ongoing trials are comparing carotid endarterectomy (CEA) with the newer technique of carotid angioplasty and stenting (CAS) using embolic protection devices. Current recommendations are that patients with recent TIA or stroke within the past 6 months and ipsilateral severe (70%-99%) carotid stenosis should undergo CEA if the estimated morbidity and mortality are <6%. Carotid endarterectomy is also recommended for patients with recent TIA or stroke and ipsilateral moderate (50%-69%) carotid stenosis, provided that estimated morbidity and mortality are <6%, although the benefit is less marked in this group, particularly in women, for reasons that are unclear but may relate to the smaller caliber of carotid vessels in women. Carotid endarterectomy is not indicated for carotid stenosis <50%. Many patients benefit from early revascularization (performed within 2 weeks of TIA or stroke). Carotid endarterectomy performed by experienced operators with morbidity and mortality rates known to be <6% is an alternative to CEA in patients who are not favorable surgical candidates.

DEEP VENOUS THROMBOSIS PROPHYLAXIS

Patients with an ischemic stroke or a hemorrhagic stroke who are nonambulatory should start receiving deep venous thrombosis (DVT) prophylaxis by the end of hospital day 2. Stroke patients with a paretic or paralyzed lower extremity are at very high risk of developing DVT. One study noted proximal DVT in more than a third of patients with moderately severe stroke. Nonpharmacologic approaches include early mobilization and use of intermittent pneumatic compression stockings. Pharmacologic approaches include subcutaneous unfractionated heparin, low-molecular-weight (LMW) heparins, or direct thrombin inhibitors in patients with heparin-induced thrombocytopenia.

ANTICOAGULATION FOR ATRIAL FIBRILLATION/FLUTTER AND OTHER CAUSES OF CARDIOGENIC EMBOLISM

Patients with an ischemic stroke of cardiogenic origin due to atrial fibrillation, atrial flutter, or rheumatic mitral valve disease should be discharged on lifelong anticoagulation therapy with warfarin with a target INR of 2.5 (range 2-3). Aspirin is an alternative agent for patients with contraindications to warfarin. Anticoagulation for at least 3 months is recommended for patients with stroke due to myocardial infarction with mural thrombus with an INR target of 2.5. Antithrombotic therapy with warfarin, aspirin, clopidogrel, or aspirin-dipyridamole may be considered in patients with cardiomyopathy and a left ventricular ejection fraction ≤35%. Patients with mechanical prosthetic heart valves should be treated with warfarin to maintain an INR target of 3 (range 2.5-3.5). Patients with prosthetic valves who develop embolic stroke despite a therapeutic INR may be treated with low-dose aspirin in addition to warfarin. Although the risk of thromboembolism in patients with biomechanical heart valves is low, warfarin anticoagulation with an INR target of 2 to 3 may be considered if they develop otherwise unexplained ischemic stroke.

CONTROL OF OTHER RISK FACTORS

Hypertension

Treatment of hypertension is indicated in all patients with TIA or stroke more than 24 hours after presentation. Although optimal blood pressure after stroke is uncertain, normal blood pressure has recently been redefined by the seventh report of the Joint National Committee on Prevention, Detection, Evaluation, and Treatment of High Blood Pressure (JNC 7) as <120/80 mm Hg. A comprehensive blood pressure reduction plan includes sodium restriction, weight loss, regular aerobic exercise, and a diet rich in fruits and vegetables. Drug therapy should be individualized, but diuretics and angiotensin-converting enzyme (ACE) inhibitors are reasonable initial choices. Reduction in stroke risk is strongly correlated with the absolute magnitude of blood pressure reduction.

Diabetes

Diabetic patients with stroke should be treated with diet, exercise, oral hypoglycemic drugs, and insulin to achieve conventional targets for glycemic control, such as hemoglobin A1c (HbA1c) <7%.

Alcohol

Heavy alcohol consumption increases stroke risk, whereas light consumption of alcohol, especially wine, reduces the overall risk of stroke. However, there is a linear increase in the risk of hemorrhagic stroke with all degrees of alcohol consumption. Heavy drinkers should curtail or stop alcohol use. For those who choose to drink alcohol, consumption should be limited to a maximum of two drinks per day for men and one drink per day for nonpregnant women. Several drugs of abuse, including cocaine, amphetamines, and heroin, increase stroke risk through their effects on vessels, platelets, and the endothelium. Referral for counseling is appropriate in these patients.

Obesity

Weight loss is recommended for the obese, as increased body weight and abdominal fat are directly associated with stroke risk, and weight reduction may also assist in the control of hypertension, diabetes, hyperlipidemia, and metabolic syndrome. Obesity also increases the risk of sleep-disordered breathing, which has been independently associated with increased stroke risk. Physical activity reduces the risk of stroke. Ideally, patients should engage in aerobic exercise of at least 30 minutes' duration three times weekly. Patients with disabilities after stroke benefit from physical therapy and occupational therapy consultation for specialized exercise and rehabilitation programs.

Oral contraceptives

The incremental risk of stroke associated with low-dose OCs in women without additional risk factors appears to be low, if it exists. It is suggested that OCs be discouraged in women with additional risk factors, such as cigarette smoking or prior thromboembolic events. For those who elect to assume the increased risk, aggressive therapy of stroke risk factors may be useful.

Hyperhomocysteinemia

Hyperhomocysteinemia is associated with a twofold increase in the risk of stroke. Following guidelines for daily intake of folate, vitamin B6, and vitamin B12 by consumption of vegetables, fruits, legumes, meats, fish, and fortified grains and cereals may reduce the risk of stroke, particularly for primary prevention. However, the efficacy of folate, vitamin B6, and vitamin B12 supplementation in the secondary prevention of stroke has not been demonstrated.

■ REHABILITATION

Patients with stroke should be assessed for rehabilitation services. Forty percent of stroke patients are left with moderate functional impairment and 15% to 30% with severe disability. More than 60% of those with stroke never receive rehabilitation. The primary goal of rehabilitation is to prevent complications, minimize impairments, and maximize function. Stroke rehabilitation should begin as soon as the diagnosis of stroke is established and life-threatening problems are under control. Patients should be mobilized and encouraged to resume self-care activities as soon as possible. Substantial evidence indicates better clinical outcomes when patients with stroke are treated in a setting that provides coordinated, multidisciplinary stroke-related evaluation and services. Effective rehabilitation interventions initiated early after stroke can enhance the recovery process and minimize functional disability (see Chapter 68: [Post-Acute Care Rehabilitation Options]).

■ DISCHARGE CHECKLIST

- Is the patient being discharged on an antiplatelet agent? Patients with a noncardioembolic ischemic stroke or TIA should be discharged on aspirin monotherapy (50-325 mg daily), aspirin 25 mg/extended-release dipyridamole 200 mg twice daily, or clopidogrel 75 mg daily, as long as no contraindications exist.
- For patients with cardioembolic stroke and no contraindications to anticoagulation, is warfarin being prescribed? (Warfarin is not recommended for secondary stroke prevention in patients presumed to have a noncardioembolic stroke.)

- Is a statin being prescribed for patients with ischemic stroke or TIA who have atherosclerosis and an LDL-C level ≥100 mg/dL?
- Has the patient had dysphagia screening? Patients with stroke should undergo screening for dysphagia with an evidence-based bedside testing protocol before being given food, fluids, or medication by mouth. Up to 50% of stroke patients develop dysphagia, and are at risk for increased length of hospital stay, malnutrition, and aspiration pneumonia. Patients with abnormal screening results should be referred for a complete examination by a speech and language pathologist or other qualified individual.
- Have the patient and family been counseled about risk factors for stroke, warning signs of stroke, need for follow-up and lifestyle modification, and new medications? Have prognosis, rehabilitation potential, and health care access been addressed?
- Has smoking cessation counseling been addressed? Smoking nearly doubles the risk of ischemic stroke. Patients who receive even brief smoking cessation advice from their physicians are more likely to quit than those receiving no counseling at all. Nicotine products and medications such as sustained-release bupropion or varenicline may be helpful for smoking cessation and should be considered.
- Is there a treatment plan for risk factors such as hypertension, diabetes, alcohol and drug use, and obesity?
- Has the patient been assessed for rehabilitation?

SUGGESTED READINGS

Amarenco P, Bogousslavsky J, Callahan A III, et al. High-dose atorvastatin after stroke or transient ischemic attack. *N Engl J Med.* 2006;355:549-559.

Arima H, Chalmers J, Woodward M, et al. Lower target blood pressures are safe and effective for the prevention of recurrent stroke: The PROGRESS trial. *J Hypertens.* 2006;24:1201-1208.

Badhiwala JH, Nassiri F, Alhazzani W, et al. Endovascular thrombectomy for acute ischemic stroke: a meta-analysis. *JAMA.* 2015;314:1832-1843.

Del Zoppo GJ, Saver JL, Jauch EC, Adams HP Jr. American Heart Association Stroke Council. Expansion of the time window for treatment of acute ischemic stroke with intravenous tissue plasminogen activator: a science advisory from the American Heart Association/American Stroke Association. *Stroke.* 2009;40:2945-2948.

Easton JD, Saver JL, Albers GW, et al. Definition and evaluation of transient ischemic attack: a scientific statement for healthcare professionals from the American Heart Association/American Stroke Association Stroke Council. *Stroke.* 2009;40:2276-2293.

Furie KL, Kasner SE, Adams RJ, et al. Guidelines for the prevention of stroke in patients with stroke or transient ischemic attack: a guideline for healthcare professionals from the American Heart Association/American Stroke Association. *Stroke.* 2011;42:227-276.

Goldstein LB, Bushnell CD, Adams RJ, et al. Guidelines for the primary prevention of stroke: a guideline for healthcare professionals from the American Heart Association/American Stroke Association. *Stroke.* 2011;42:517-584.

He J, Zhang Y, Xu T, et al. Effects of immediate blood pressure reduction on death and major disability in patients with acute ischemic stroke: the CATIS randomized clinical trial. *JAMA.* 2014;311:479-489.

Powers WJ, Derdeyn CP, Biller J, et al. 2015 American Heart Association/American Stroke Association focused update of the 2013 guidelines for the early management of patients with acute ischemic stroke regarding endovascular treatment. *Stroke.* 2015;46:3020-3035.

Sacco RL, Diener HC, Yusuf S, et al. Aspirin and extended-release dipyridamole versus clopidogrel for recurrent stroke. *N Engl J Med.* 2008;359:1238-1251.

CHAPTER 210

Parkinson's Disease and Related Disorders

Joseph Rudolph, MD
Ruth H. Walker, MB, ChB, PhD

Key Clinical Questions

❶ Does the patient meet diagnostic criteria for idiopathic Parkinson's disease (PD)?

❷ What is the differential diagnosis of a patient with parkinsonian symptoms?

❸ What is the pathophysiology of Parkinson's disease?

❹ What treatments are available, and how do they relate to the underlying pathophysiology?

❺ What are the short- and long-term side effects that may occur in a PD patient on medication?

❻ What are typical complications that may occur when a PD patient is admitted to the hospital?

EPIDEMIOLOGY

Parkinson's disease (PD) appears in 12 to 20/100,000 people per year, approaching a prevalence of 1 in 2000 people. Quality of life can be markedly affected due to a wide variety of factors, some of which have only recently been recognized, such as autonomic dysfunction.

The economic burden of Parkinson's disease is high. On average, $4000 to $5000 can be spent per patient/year, and of that amount, roughly 33% to 40% may be indirect costs, such as lost productivity. On average, PD-affected patients are unable to work full time 3.4 years after diagnosis, and most file for disability by 5 years. In addition, having PD is a risk factor for nursing home placement.

PATHOPHYSIOLOGY

Parkinson's disease is caused by the loss of midbrain dopaminergic neurons in the substantia nigra pars compacta (SNc). How dopamine loss disrupts normal functioning of the basal ganglia is not fully understood, but it appears to result in pathological synchronization of neuronal firing throughout the region, which interferes with the production of both voluntary and involuntary movements.

Parkinson's disease also has many nonmotor symptoms, with effects on cognition, behavior, and sleep. There is emerging evidence of a more widespread neurodegenerative process in PD, affecting brainstem, midbrain, and cortical structures, and probably involving neurotransmitters other than dopamine.

In most cases, the cause of PD is unknown. Mutations of genes associated with PD, such as *parkin, DJ-1, GBA,* and *LRRK2,* have recently been identified, although these still make up a minority of cases. The relationship of these mutations to dopaminergic neuron death is not known.

The pathological hallmark of PD is the presence of Lewy bodies in the neurons of the SNc. These are intracellular clumps of proteins, which include alpha-synuclein, ubiquitin, and others. Alpha-synuclein is thought to be a phospholipid-binding protein that helps vesicles dock with the plasma membrane. It is not known whether these inclusion bodies kill the neurons in which they develop, or more likely, whether they represent a "waste-basket" keeping damaged proteins out of the way of normal cellular functioning. In addition to being found in the brainstem, particularly in the SNc, in PD, Lewy bodies can be more widely distributed, and are found specifically in the cortex in the related disorder known as dementia with Lewy bodies (see below).

Patients who are early in their clinical course of PD have already lost about 80% of the SNc neurons, implying that the degenerative process begins long before symptoms are first seen, and that the basal ganglia can compensate until there is significant dopamine loss.

DIFFERENTIAL DIAGNOSIS OF PARKINSONISM

Parkinsonism refers to the presence of the slowness of movement (bradykinesia), absence of movement (akinesia), increased tone (rigidity), resting tremor, and impairment of postural reflexes. Some or all of these features may be seen in idiopathic PD, but they may also be due to a variety of other causes. These include several other neurodegenerative disorders known as the Parkinson-plus syndromes or atypical parkinsonism. Secondary parkinsonism refers to cases in which another etiology has been identified, such as medication or cerebrovascular disease.

■ PARKINSON-PLUS SYNDROMES

Multiple system atrophy (MSA)

Multiple sytem atrophy may manifest as a spectrum of symptoms and can look similar to PD, especially in the early stages. Patients may have different combinations of parkinsonism, cerebellar findings, and autonomic problems.

MSA-parkinsonism (MSA-P) involves striatonigral degeneration, rather than the nigrostriatal degeneration seen in PD. Multiple system atrophy affects neurons postsynaptic to dopaminergic neurons, although MSA-P patients may be at least partially responsive to levodopa therapy. MSA-cerebellar (MSA-C) involves the olivo-cerebellar connections, with disproportionate involvement of the middle cerebellar peduncles, which carry fibers from the pon to the cerebellar cortex. MSA-autonomic (also known as Shy-Drager syndrome) is characterized by degeneration of the locus coeruleus, the dorsal motor nucleus of the vagus nerve, and the catecholamine-producing neurons of the ventrolateral medulla.

Pathologically, alpha-synuclein inclusions are found in glial cells, rather than neurons, as in PD. The locations of the inclusions determine the clinical spectrum of disease, and can include the SNc, locus coeruleus, putamen, inferior olives, pontine nuclei, cerebellar Purkinje cells, and the intermediolateral columns in the spinal cord.

The cause of MSA is not known, and it tends not to be inherited. There is no disease-modifying therapy; treatment is symptomatic. Parkinsonian MSA patients may have some response to levodopa, which should be increased to the maximum tolerated dose, which may be in grams of levodopa/day. Autonomic dysfunction can be managed with vasoconstrictors such as midodrine, and mineralocorticoids such as fludrocortisone to increase blood pressure. Urinary incontinence may be treated with antispasmodics and catheterization.

Physical and speech therapies may be useful. As with all parkinsonian disorders, swallowing is often affected, and should be evaluated to reduce the chances of aspiration, a major cause of morbidity and mortality.

Progressive supranuclear palsy (PSP)

Progressive supranuclear palsy (PSP) can be indistinguishable from PD in the early stages, but axial symptoms such as gait and balance impairment usually occur earlier and with greater severity than in PD. The name PSP refers to abnormal eye movements, classically affecting vertical gaze, and especially downward gaze. Mild dementia, particularly with frontal features, is more common in PSP. Dysarthria and dysphagia are typical, and early involvement of a speech therapist is important. Progressive supranuclear palsy, as with most atypical parkinsonian syndromes, shows a poor response to levodopa, but this should be tried as one of the few available pharmacotherapeutic options. The cause of PSP is not known, and it does not appear to be inherited.

PRACTICE POINT

Patients with PSP tend to have a surprised appearance, with excessive eyelid retraction

Dementia with Lewy bodies (DLB)

Patients have features identical to idiopathic PD, with early dementia and behavioral abnormalities out of proportion to the accompanying motor symptoms. Visual hallucinations, which are usually benign and nondistressing, are a typical early feature. Pathologically, DLB resembles PD in that affected cells have the same cytoplasmic inclusion bodies, Lewy bodies, but these are more widely distributed, and the affected area includes the cerebral cortex, in addition to the SNc. Cognitive symptoms are treated with acetylcholinesterase inhibitors, similar to Alzheimer's disease. Motor symptoms may improve with levodopa, although this may worsen confusion.

PRACTICE POINT

Patients with DLB are hypersensitive to antipsychotics, and may get very sedated or parkinsonian when they receive them

Corticobasal degeneration (CBD)

Corticobasal degeneration is a tauopathy that manifests with parkinsonian symptoms and dementia, but has unique neuropathological characteristics. Recent studies have shown that the typical corticobasal syndrome can be due to many pathologies, including Alzheimer's disease and PSP, in addition to CBD. The neurologic symptoms are related to the distribution of the tau-immunoreactive inclusion bodies in the cortex and basal ganglia. There may be cortical symptoms, such as apraxia or aphasia, higher order sensory loss, or alien hand syndrome, in which one hand performs complex, involuntarily movements, such as picking at the hair or clothes. There may be asymmetric parkinsonism or limb dystonia. Imaging may show asymmetric atrophy of the frontoparietal cortex. Ballooned, achromatic neurons are seen on pathology.

■ SECONDARY PARKINSONISM

Vascular parkinsonism

Atherosclerosis and microvascular disease may lead to disruption of the fibers of the basal ganglia, causing parkinsonian symptoms without degeneration of the dopamine-producing cells. This is usually due to typical vascular risk factors, such as hypertension, diabetes, hyperlipidemia, smoking, or age. Patients may present with parkinsonian symptoms, but generally with early gait problems, including falling and freezing. There may also be marked postural tremor. Levodopa therapy should be attempted, although vascular parkinsonism patients are less responsive to levodopa than PD patients. The mainstay of treatment is physical therapy. Treatment is also geared toward minimizing future ischemic events by improving reversible risk factors (smoking cessation, lowering blood pressure, controlling blood sugar and cholesterol, etc) and treating with antiplatelet agents.

Medication-induced parkinsonism

Numerous agents can block dopaminergic neurotransmission, resulting in parkinsonian symptoms. Classical antipsychotics, such as haloperidol, thioridazine, and perphenazine, work by blocking dopamine receptors. A predictable side effect of these medicines is the development of tremor, rigidity, and slowness of movement, indistinguishable from idiopathic PD. Some patients, particularly when hospitalized, are unaware of the nature of the drugs with which they have been treated. For example, if an elderly person who was recently discharged from hospital has new parkinsonian symptoms, it may be that he or she was given haloperidol to treat sundowning. In these cases, symptoms are usually, though not necessarily, bilateral. Treatment begins with discontinuing the offending agents. If symptoms persist for several months and interfere with activities of daily living, cautious, gradually increasing therapy with levodopa may be warranted. In this scenario, it is likely that the medication unmasked underlying idiopathic PD.

If absolutely essential for the management of psychosis or agitation, atypical antipsychotics with fewer parkinsonian side effects can be used, such as quetiapine and clozapine, starting at very low doses. Patients on clozapine need to have frequent blood tests to monitor for agranulocytosis.

Drug-induced parkinsonism may also be a side effect of antiemetics, such as metoclopramide, promethazine and prochlorperazine. These drugs work by blocking peripheral dopamine receptors, but they may cross the blood-brain barrier and block dopamine receptors in the central nervous system, causing parkinsonism. As with antipsychotics, these drugs are often prescribed too liberally to hospitalized patients and outpatients. Use of an antiemetic with a different mechanism of action, such as ondansetron, may be appropriate.

PRACTICE POINT

Although newer, atypical antipsychotics, such as risperidone and olanzepine, are not widely recognized as causing parkinsonism, they can certainly have this effect, especially in the older patient with frank or incipient dementia.

DIFFERENTIAL DIAGNOSIS: NON-PARKINSONIAN DISORDERS

Problems with walking, especially in the older patient, can be due to a wide variety of causes. These include pain, orthopedic problems, arthritis of the foot and ankle, fear of falling, and other neurologic causes such as peripheral neuropathy, in addition to the nonbasal ganglia disorders discussed here.

■ ESSENTIAL TREMOR

A condition that frequently brings patients to the neurologist for evaluation for possible PD is essential tremor (ET), previously known as benign familial tremor. However, it is often neither familial nor benign, as it may be very debilitating. In ET, the hand tremor is typically bilateral rather than unilateral, although it can be asymmetric. In contrast to the tremor of PD, it is absent at rest, and brought on by activity. There is little stiffness or postural instability, although severe tremor can affect walking and balance. Tremor in the neck may lead to head shaking. Tremor is worsened by stress and improved by relaxation. Alcohol can reduce the symptoms.

The diagnosis is made on clinical grounds. About 50% of ET cases are familial; an affected family member supports the diagnosis. If the tremor is not apparent on examination, the patient should be asked to do whatever brings the tremor out, such as writing or pouring water from one cup to another (over a sink!). Drawing a spiral is useful to bring out subtle tremor and to document tremor severity.

Reversible causes of tremor should be excluded, specifically hyperthyroidism and medications such as lithium, valproate, theophylline, cyclosporine, and caffeine. If tremor improves with alcohol intake, an alcoholic beverage might be useful in cases of embarrassment during social dinners (care should be taken that patient does not develop tolerance or dependence on alcohol). The two first-line medications are primidone, a once popular antiepileptic, and propranolol. Other anticonvulsants, such as gabapentin, levetiracetam, and topiramate, have been tried, with varying success. Deep brain stimulation (DBS) (surgical implantation of electrodes) in the motor nuclei of the thalamus can be an effective therapy.

PRACTICE POINT

Head tremor is not generally seen as a feature of PD. Its presence is strongly suggestive of ET. Conversely, rigidity and bradykinesia are not seen in patients with ET.

■ NORMAL PRESSURE HYDROCEPHALUS

Another condition causing gait difficulty which may be confused with PD is normal pressure hydrocephalus (NPH). This diagnosis is often raised in the parkinsonian patient by family members who have heard of impressive cures following ventriculoperitoneal shunt placement. The gait in NPH is characterized by a wide base, with slow, short steps, and the patient has difficulty lifting each foot off the ground, often referred to as magnetic gait. By contrast, PD patients usually do not have frozen steps with each step, and the stance is not widened.

The gait disorder in NPH is caused by dysfunction or destruction of the periventricular fibers from the leg region of the motor cortex. This syndrome is frequently misdiagnosed, leading to unnecessary placement of ventriculoperitoneal shunts. Nevertheless, the presence of the complete triad of cognitive dysfunction, urinary problems, and gait dysfunction supports this diagnosis. Although the diagnosis is primarily clinical, it may be suggested if neuroimaging demonstrates ventricular enlargement out of proportion to cortical atrophy of the cortex. The ideal diagnostic study is the short-term placement of a lumbar drain, with careful monitoring of gait. However, placebo effects can occur with this procedure, and care should be taken to avoid false positive interpretations, as placement of a ventriculoperitoneal shunt is not a benign procedure.

■ CEREBELLAR DISEASE

Cerebellar dysfunction causes a wide-based, ataxic gait, distinct from the shuffling, parkinsonian gait. However, the basal ganglia may be involved in cerebellar disorders, and parkinsonian symptoms may be seen in some of the autosomal dominantly inherited spinocerebellar ataxias and in the cerebellar form of MSA. The diagnosis is supported by the presence of abnormalities of eye movements and limb or truncal ataxia.

■ SPINAL STENOSIS

Narrowing of the cervical canal with compression of the spinal cord may cause spasticity and interfere with walking. This may be detected as a clasp-knife increase in tone of the lower extremities, distinguishable from the lead-pipe rigidity of PD (see below). Increased activity of the deep tendon reflexes at the knees and ankles, with positive Babinski signs, helps to localize the lesion to the cervical spinal cord. In some cases, PD may be responsible for structural abnormalities in the spine, causing increased wear and tear on the vertebra from abnormal posture. Scoliosis and other spinal abnormalities are recognized sequelae of longstanding PD.

PRACTICE POINT

Atrophy of the small muscles of the hands due to cervical radiculopathy can be a sign of cervical spine disease.

DIAGNOSIS

There is no definitive test for PD prior to autopsy. The diagnosis is determined by the presence of major clinical criteria, as delineated by the UK Brain Bank, namely bradykinesia with resting tremor, rigidity, or postural instability, not related to another known etiology. Nonmotor symptoms, such as REM sleep behavior disorder, depression, anxiety, impaired cognition, muscle aches, insomnia, daytime somnolence, impaired olfaction, and constipation may precede the onset of motor symptoms (**Figure 210-1**).

Unilateral tremor is the most common initial motor symptom (**Table 210-1**). Despite subsequent involvement of the contralateral side, the disease usually continues to be somewhat asymmetric. The tremor is present at rest, and is often observed when the patient is distracted and relaxed. There may be a component of action tremor

Pathology

Brainstem and cortex	Hippocampus and basal forebrain
Lewy Protofibrils, fibers bodies	**Cholinergic pathology**

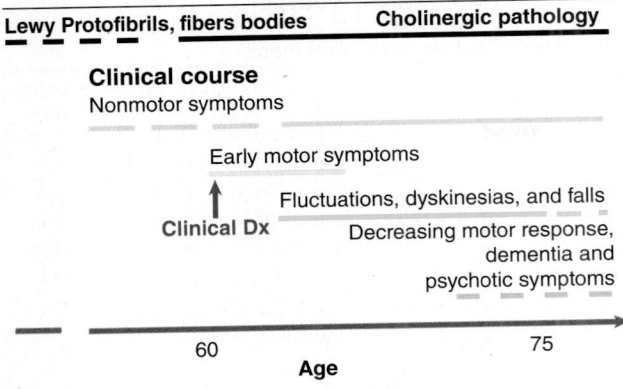

Figure 210-1 *Natural history of Parkinson disease, with neuropathologic correlation.* (Reproduced, with permission, from Fauci AS, Braunwald E, Kasper DL, et al. *Harrison's Principles of Internal Medicine,* 17th ed. New York, NY: McGraw-Hill 2008. Fig. 366-2.)

or of postural tremor, but if either of these is the major symptom in the absence of parkinsonian signs, then another diagnosis, such as ET, should be considered. The postural tremor of PD tends to manifest after patients have held their hands outstretched for a few seconds, known as an emergent tremor, rather than immediately as in ET. However, PD and ET are both common conditions, and may occasionally coexist.

PRACTICE POINT

The resting tremor of PD increases with walking and when the opposite hand performs repetitive movements.

For diagnosis of PD, exclusion of the atypical and secondary parkinsonism is required. Early falling (within 5 years of disease onset), prominent autonomic dysfunction, early dementia, and visual hallucinations suggest atypical parkinsonism. Patients should be asked about the use of neuroleptics and antiemetics.

The neurologic examination focuses on parkinsonian features. The limbs and neck are examined for rigidity. Spasticity may be

TABLE 210-1 Initial Symptoms in Patients with Parkinson Diseases

Symptom	Percentage of Patients
Tremor	70
Gait disturbance	11
Stiffness	10
Slowness	10
Muscle aches	8
Loss of dexterity	7
Handwriting disturbance	5
Depression, nervousness, other psychiatric disturbance	4
Speech disturbance	3

Modified from Ropper AH, Samuels MA. *Adams and Victor's Principles of Neurology,* 9th ed. New York, NY: McGraw-Hill; 2009.

difficult to distinguish from rigidity. Spasticity, the increase in tone that appears following an upper motor lesion such as a stroke or spinal cord injury, is velocity-dependent, being almost minimal when the limb is moved slowly, and becoming highly resistant when force is applied suddenly. This is known as clasp-knife rigidity. In parkinsonian rigidity, the muscle tone is unchanged regardless of the velocity with which force is applied. This is known as lead-pipe rigidity.

Bradykinesia, slowness of movement, is evaluated by having the patient perform repetitive tasks using one limb at a time: tapping the index finger on the thumb, opening and closing fists, pronating-supinating the hand on the knee, and tapping each heel on the ground. (It is not necessary to tap all the fingers to the thumb in sequence—this requires frontal lobe function and can confuse the examination.) There is usually an asymmetry between the speed of each side. A positive glabellar tap test, where the patient continues to blink with repetitive tapping between the eyebrows, is seen in PD.

PRACTICE POINT

Mild bradykinesia is often dismissed as being due to age, but this is not seen in normal aging. If possible, compare the patient's spontaneous facial movements and hand gesticulations to those of someone of similar age.

Postural stability and gait are evaluated in several ways. The patient is asked to stand up without the use of his or her arms (these may be crossed over the chest). Walking is observed, with attention to arm swing, stride length, posture (either forward or sideways tilt), and the ability to pivot and turn. If the patient cannot pivot and requires multiple little steps in order to turn, this is referred to as turning "en bloc." Patients may freeze, especially on turning or in doorways, and be unable to take a step without help. Festination (hurrying) may occur, with patients taking rapid small steps without being able to stop, until they fall forward. Balance is tested using the pull test. The patient is told to stand with feet at shoulder width, warned what is to come and instructed to take a couple of steps to try and stop themselves from falling. The patient is then pulled firmly backward from the shoulders (the physician should position the hands either side of the patient in order to be prepared to catch him or her if necessary). If the patient requires more than 2 to 3 steps backward to restore balance, or would fall if not caught by the examiner, then postural reflexes are impaired.

There are no blood tests or brain scans which confirm the diagnosis of PD. At present, in the absence of molecular therapies, genetic testing is not clinically useful. Similarly, brain imaging is not useful for diagnosing PD, although a brain MRI may have features that raise the possibility of MSA, PSP, or vascular parkinsonism. Cerebellar or pontine atrophy is more consistent with MSA, while midbrain atrophy would indicate PSP. Iron deposition in the striatum may be seen in MSA.

Imaging of the dopamine transporters localized on the presynaptic nigrostriatal axon terminals, marketed as DaTscan, can be used to determine whether a tremor is due to PD or ET. However, this imaging modality does not reliably distinguish between PD and other causes of parkinsonism. It is currently approved only to support the diagnosis of PD, and does not replace clinical evaluation. Fluoro-deoxy-glucose positron emission tomography (FDG-PET) scans are sometimes used in a research setting to refine the diagnosis.

The diagnosis of PD becomes more evident over time, as the clinical progression and response to medication can be observed. While atypical parkinsonian disorders often respond partially to levodopa, a sustained motor response to levodopa over several years supports the diagnosis of idiopathic PD.

The most widely used scale for evaluating the severity of PD is the Unified Parkinson's Disease Rating Scale (UDPRS), which has recently been refined and revised. This rating scale has sections dedicated to cognitive and psychiatric symptoms, activities of daily living, physical examination, and medication-related and autonomic symptoms. The scale is used to measure severity of disease as well as progression, and scores can be compared at serial visits. Disease severity may also be evaluated in the setting of a medication trial, both for clarifying the diagnosis and for estimating medication effect.

HOSPITAL ADMISSION

Parkinson's disease is usually not the primary reason for hospital admission, unless the presenting complaint relates to falls and gait disorder. Up to 80% of PD patient admissions are due to comorbid issues. Tremor, stiffness, or otherwise unexplained gait problems are sometimes recognized in patients admitted for other reasons, leading to a new diagnosis of PD.

■ ACUTE WORSENING

Parkinson's disease is a characterized by slow, gradual progression, and any sudden deterioration is always due to another cause. As with many neurologic conditions, any metabolic derangement can exacerbate the symptoms of the underlying disorder. The health care provider must exclude acute infections, specifically of the urinary or respiratory tract, or electrolyte disturbances, with dehydration being the most common. Adverse effects from new medications should be excluded. New neurological signs may indicate a stroke, or subdural hematoma or cord injury following a fall.

Patients who have deep brain stimulation electrodes implanted will acutely deteriorate if their DBS batteries wear out, and they may become extremely rigid and unable to walk. They may even have a clinical appearance that resembles neuroleptic malignant syndrome, with severe rigidity and rhabdomyolysis. These patients should be treated with aggressive dopaminergic therapy and hydration. Contact should be made with a neurosurgeon as soon as possible to schedule a battery replacement. This situation should be avoided by calculation of battery life and monitoring.

■ MEDICATION ADMINISTRATION

To minimize the chance of complications due to under- or overtreatment while in hospital, it is vital that patients continue to take their medications as they did at home. Careful attention must be paid to dosage and timing. Undertreatment results in impaired mobility with the risk of falls, aspiration, deep venous thrombosis, constipation, and decubiti. It can also worsen confusion. Overtreatment causes dyskinesia, falls, agitation, confusion, and hallucinations.

As timing of PD medications is critical for patients with more than mild disease, it is essential that medications are taken on time. In the hospital this may be difficult, as medication every 3 hours or even less is a departure from typical administration schedules. If a patient with PD is admitted to the ward, nursing staff must be educated that PD medications should be given on a schedule closest to the patient's home schedule (but that the patient should not be woken during the night to take the next dose). In extreme cases, when the patient takes medication every 3 hours or more frequently, it may be helpful for pharmacy to become involved. Medication errors frequently arise due to the different formulations available for carbidopa-levodopa (**Table 210-2**). The pharmacy should be made aware of which formulation is desired, especially when different ones are taken by the same patient.

Although drug holidays were previously utilized to manage medication complications, these are a thing of the past, with risks and

TABLE 210-2 Some Available Formulations of Carbidopa–Levodopa

Drug Name (Trade Name)	Comment
Carbidopa-levodopa(Sinemet)10/100*	75 mg daily of carbidopa is required to inhibit dopa-decarboxylase; thus, three times daily dosing of this formulation is inadequate
Carbidopa-levodopa(Sinemet) 25/100	This is the most commonly used formulation. In most patients, it can be started at one-half tablet three times daily and increased to one tablet three times daily
Carbidopa-levodopa(Sinemet) 25/250	Highest strength formulation
Carbidopa-levodopa orally disintegrating (Parcopa) 10/100, 25/100, 25/250	Sublingual formulation can be useful in patients with dysphagia. There is no improvement in efficacy or release time
Carbidopa/levodopa(Sinemet) CR 25/100	With the controlled-release formulation, patients often report that they do not feel the medication "kicking in" as they do with regular-release tablets. Serum levels can be erratic. This formulation is most useful for overnight or early morning symptoms
Carbidopa/levodopa(Sinemet) CR 50/200	

*The first number indicates milligrams of carbidopa, the second, milligrams of levodopa. An additional formulation contains entacapone (Stalevo). There are also several newer time-release formulations of carbidopa/levodopa, marketed as "Rytary", however, conversion from standard carbidopa/levodopa can be complex.

little benefit. Amantadine should never be suddenly stopped as this can cause a withdrawal syndrome.

> ### PRACTICE POINT
> Another cause for emergency room visits is caregiver burnout. The decompensation may not be in the patient, but rather in the home situation.

■ DECONDITIONING

Elderly patients may become deconditioned after even a short hospital stay. This is especially true of parkinsonian patients, and may be compounded by disruptions in medication administration. Parkinsonian patients admitted to the hospital should receive physical and occupational therapy as soon as possible. They may also benefit from a posthospital rehabilitation course prior to returning home.

TREATMENT OPTIONS

■ PHARMACOTHERAPY

Current American Academy of Neurology guidelines suggest starting patients on an MAO-B inhibitor such as selegiline, which provides mild symptomatic benefit. When dopaminergic therapy is required, it is controversial whether patients should be started on levodopa, which is more effective for motor symptoms, but which may hasten the appearance of levodopa-induced dyskinesia (see below), or on dopamine agonists (ropinirole and pramipexole), which are slightly less efficacious.

We prefer to use dopamine agonists in younger patients in an attempt to delay the onset of dyskinesia. Younger patients are more likely to tolerate the necessary slow titration of these medications, and have fewer side effects. When functioning is no longer adequately treated, levodopa should be added. Levodopa should be used in older patients, particularly if gait and balance are already compromised by other factors, including normal aging, and effective treatment needs to be instituted quickly for safety reasons. Drugs used in PD are summarized in **Table 210-3** and a treatment algorithm is suggested in **Figure 210-2**.

■ LEVODOPA

Levodopa, the biochemical precursor to dopamine, has been the mainstay of treatment since the early 1970s. Levodopa is metabolized in plasma by dopa decarboxylase to dopamine. Dopamine, a polar molecule, cannot cross the blood-brain barrier. As a result, only a limited amount of ingested levodopa is transported into the brain. In addition, dopamine produced in the periphery leads to severe nausea. To combat this problem, carbidopa, a dopa decarboxylase inhibitor, is coformulated with levodopa. This minimizes peripheral metabolism of levodopa, reducing nausea, and enables more of it to cross the blood-brain barrier via the large neutral

amino acid transporter. Extra carbidopa (25 mg) taken with each dose can help reduce peripheral side effects.

Other levodopa side effects include hypotension, arrhythmias, vivid dreams, hallucinations, and somnolence. There may be effects upon mood, including emotional lability, increased libido, or anxiety. Confusion and loss of mental acuity can also occur. Unfortunately, decreased mental acuity and orthostatic hypotension tend to be late features of PD itself, so it may be difficult to distinguish between disease-related and medication-induced symptoms.

As PD progresses, higher doses of levodopa are required for functioning, and in most patients involuntary choreiform movements known as levodopa-induced dyskinesia will appear. These are often more troubling to caregivers than to patients, and do not require dose modification, but can sometimes be violent and disabling.

The long-acting form of carbidopa-levodopa (brand name Sinemet CR) can be useful in certain situations, although the term "controlled release" is something of a misnomer. Given the erratic bioavailability of this formulation, as compared with the standard preparation, it is most useful when given at bedtime for overnight symptoms, when attempting to maintain some drug in the system

TABLE 210-3 Drugs Commonly Used in the Treatment of Parkinson Disease

Medication	Starting Dose	Target Dose	Main Benefit	Side Effects
Levodopa				
Carbidopa-levodopa (Sinemet)	12.5-50 mg three times daily	Up to 50-200 mg every 3 h	Reduction of tremor and bradykinesia; less effect on postural difficulties	Nausea, dyskinesias, orthostatic hypotension, hallucinations, confusion
Controlled release carbidopa–levodopa	25-100 mg once daily	Up to 50-200 mg every 4 h	May prolong levodopa effects	
Dopamine agonists				
Ropinirole	0.25 mg three times daily	9-24 mg daily	Moderate effects on all aspects; reduced motor fluctuations of levodopa	Orthostatic hypotension, excessive and abrupt sleepiness, confusion, hallucinations
Pramipexole	0.125 mg three times daily	0.75-3 mg daily	As above	As above
Glutamate antagonist				
Amantadine (Symmetrel)	100 mg daily	100 mg twice or three times daily	Smoothing of motor fluctuations	Leg swelling, congestive heart failure, prostatic outlet obstruction, confusion, hallucinations, insomnia
Anticholinergics				
Benztropine (Cogentin)	0.5 mg daily	Up to 4 mg daily	Tremor reduction, less effect on other features	Atropinic effects: dry mouth, urinary outlet obstruction, confusion, psychosis, sedation
Trihexyphenidyl (Artane)	0.5 mg twice daily	Up to 2 mg three times daily	As above	As above
COMT inhibitors				
Entacapone	200 mg with levodopa	Up to 8 times a day	Prolonged effect of levodopa	Urine discoloration, diarrhea, increased dyskinesias
MAO-B inhibitors				
Rasagiline	0.5 mg	1 mg daily	Reduced "off" time, questionable neuroprotection	Hallucinations, confusion
Selegiline	5 mg	5 mg twice daily	Questionable neuroprotection	Nightmares, agitation
			Mild symptomatic effect, reduced off time, mild psychomotor stimulation, antidepressant effect	

COMT, catechol-O-methyltransferase; MAO-B, monoamine oxidase type B. Newer medications include the dopamine agonist rotigotine patch (Neupro) and a multiple time-release formulation of carbidopa/levopoa (Rytary).
From Ropper AH, Samuels MA. *Adams and Victor's Principles of Neurology*, 9th ed. New York, NY: McGraw-Hill; 2009.

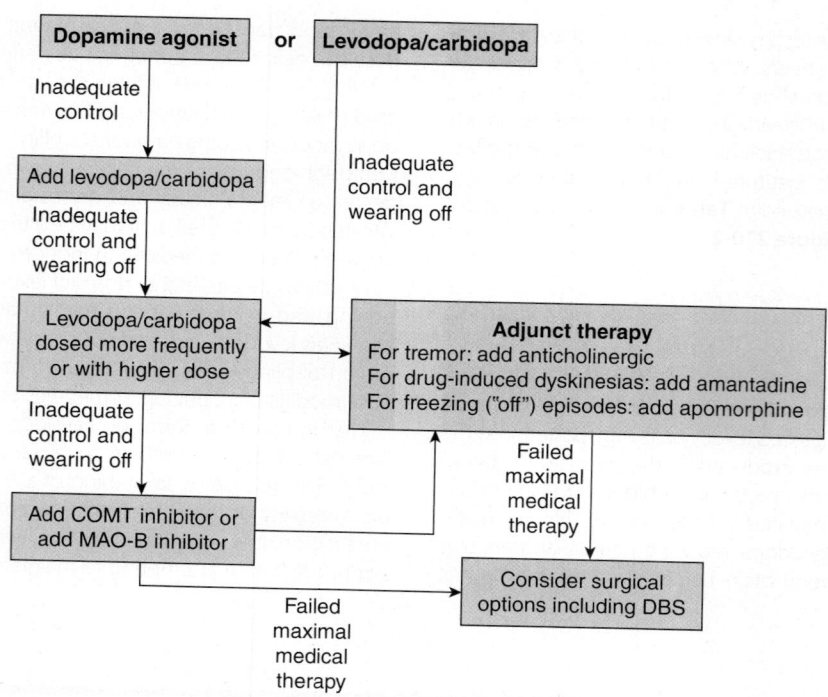

Figure 210-2 *Suggested treatment algorithm for symptomatic Parkinson disease.* (Reproduced, with permission, from Fauci AS, Braunwald E, Kasper DL, et al. *Harrison's Principles of Internal Medicine,* 17th ed. New York, NY: McGraw-Hill 2008. Fig. 366-4.)

until morning. Although many patients experience sleep benefit, this formulation can be useful for those who experience early-morning foot cramps or motor difficulties prior to their first morning medication dose.

> **PRACTICE POINT**
>
> Although often prescribed by non-specialists, controlled-release levodopa/carbidopa rarely gives the same motor benefits as regular levodopa/carbidopa. It is equivalent to about two-thirds of the equivalent regular dose, and does not provide the kick to switch on and improve motor symptoms.

■ INHIBITORS OF DOPAMINE METABOLISM

An alternative to taking exogenous levodopa is to inhibit metabolism of dopamine. There are two primary pathways for dopamine breakdown, each utilizing either monoamine oxidase (MAO) or catechol-O-methyl transferase (COMT). Medications that inhibit either of these enzymes result in delayed metabolism of dopamine. Monoamine oxidase inhibitors can be taken alone or along with levodopa. COMT inhibitors are only prescribed as adjuncts to levodopa. One agent from each class may be combined for a synergistic effect. This may be queried by pharmacies, but use of these medications in combination is both safe and effective. Taken as an adjunct to carbidopa-levodopa, these medicines permit the dosing interval to be lengthened slightly and improve quality of life, as the patient is less bound to the clock and does not have to take pills as frequently. It may also be possible to lower the dose of levodopa with COMT inhibitor use. The earliest COMT inhibitor, tolcapone, carries the risk of liver toxicity, but is more effective as it inhibits both peripheral and central COMT. Liver enzymes should be monitored regularly in patients on this drug. The more recently developed COMT inhibitor, entacapone, is better tolerated, although less effective, as it inhibits only peripheral COMT. Entacapone is available formulated with

carbidopa-levodopa to reduce pill burden, although it also increases the expense.

There are two versions of MAO, and both break down dopamine equally. MAO-A inhibitors have been used primarily as antidepressants, and require compliance with a low-tyramine diet to avoid increased norepinephrine levels and hypertensive crisis, and avoidance of SSRI antidepressants which can lead to serotonin syndrome. MAO-B inhibitors, which are currently used for treatment of PD, have a lower risk of this occurring, except at high doses. Dietary restriction or avoidance of SSRIs or SNRIs is not required with MAO-B inhibitors, despite the information provided by the manufacturer.

Initial evidence suggested a neuroprotective effect of the first MAO-B inhibitor, selegiline, but this was subsequently questioned. Selegiline has a mild symptomatic effect, and may improve depression and fatigue. However, its metabolic products include methamphetamine, and it should be taken early in the day to reduce the likelihood of insomnia and nightmares. Rasagiline has a mild symptomatic effect, but has not been shown conclusively to slow disease progression. Either of these medications may help reduce motor fluctuations in more advanced disease.

> **PRACTICE POINT**
>
> Warning patients that entacapone will turn their urine orange may save a call to your office.

■ DOPAMINE AGONISTS

Rather than replacing missing dopamine in the presynaptic nerve terminal, dopamine agonists act directly upon the postsynaptic dopamine receptor. Pramipexole and ropinirole are oral formulations, while rotigotine is used in transdermal form. The dopaminergic ergot derivatives (pergolide and bromocriptine) are no longer widely used, as they may cause pulmonary or cardiac valve fibrosis.

This class of medications should be started at a low dose and increased slowly to reduce the likelihood and severity of side effects such as confusion, sedation, and hallucinations. They should be used with particular caution in the elderly. Other side effects of dopamine agonists are lower extremity edema, impulse control disorders, and sleep attacks. Sleep attacks occur more frequently in people who are already sleep deprived, as is often seen in PD. Impulse control disorders, such as shopping, cleaning, gambling, internet use, or hypersexuality, usually occur in individuals with predispositions to these behaviors. Patients should be asked about these behaviors, as the connection to medication use may not be recognized.

Apomorphine is an injectable dopamine agonist that can be used in situations when the patient needs to have a rapid response and cannot wait for the effect of carbidopa-levodopa. Typically, patients still in the workforce are the ones who utilize this option.

■ ANTICHOLINERGIC MEDICATIONS

These medications, which include benztropine and trihexyphenidyl, were used prior to the discovery of levodopa. These agents are believed to be most useful when used in younger patients with a chief complaint of tremor, although studies have yet to show this unequivocally. Anticholinergics should be used with caution, particularly in the elderly, who are particularly susceptible to side effects including hallucinations, cognitive impairment, and urinary retention. These effects are usually reversible when the drug is discontinued.

■ AMANTADINE

The antiviral drug amantadine was noted to reduce the symptoms of PD prior to the levodopa era. It is effective both for primary PD symptoms and for levodopa-induced dyskinesias. It acts by blocking glutamatergic NMDA receptors. Glutamate hyperfunction may be seen both in the setting of dopamine depletion and parkinsonism, and as part of the pathophysiology of dyskinesia. As would be predicted from blockade of glutamate receptors, amantadine can cause confusion and hallucinations.

■ NEUROSURGERY

Neurosurgical options are now state of the art for the treatment of PD in selected patients whose symptoms are no longer controlled by optimal medical therapy. Historically, surgical destruction of specific structures in the basal ganglia (lesioning or ablative therapy) predated the development of levodopa, but became obsolete after this medication was discovered. Currently, stimulation of basal ganglia targets via deep brain stimulation (DBS) is preferred to ablative therapy, as having fewer side effects and being less destructive. However, ablation may be indicated in patients who require surgery, but who cannot have DBS electrodes implanted for medical or logistical reasons, such as residence remote from programming sites.

Deep brain stimulation delivers electrical impulses directly to a nucleus in the basal ganglia that partially reverses the effects of dopamine depletion. It is unclear exactly how DBS works, but while the original hypothesis was that it inhibited the target area, recent evidence suggests that it may alter the excitatory outputs of the target zone. Both inhibitory and stimulatory effects have been reported. DBS may also work by normalization of pathological hypersynchronization in the setting of dopamine depletion.

Most DBS patients experience improvement at least in terms of motor symptoms and side effects. DBS appears to be equivalent to levodopa, in that the optimal effect is as good as the patient's best on-medication state, but not better. Patients are able to decrease the amount of medication they take, typically by 50% to 70%, and no longer experience severe motor fluctuations. What DBS does not improve, and may indeed worsen, are the nonmotor effects, including depression, apathy, and impaired cognition. Speech may also be adversely affected. Some of these effects may be attributable to decreased doses of dopaminergic medication.

Brain MRI can generally be performed on patients with DBS, but body MRI scans should be avoided due to the higher energy levels and greater risk of thermal injury from heating up of electrodes. When brain MRIs are performed, the voltage should be set to zero and the stimulation switched off. Patients undergoing tests involving electricity, such as electrocardiograms, should turn their DBS off temporarily, which they can do using their own remote control on/off device. Any change of stimulation settings should be performed by a trained DBS programmer. More specific issues, such as the safety of electrocautery for dental or surgical procedures, should be directed to the patient's neurosurgeon or to the device company.

PRACTICE POINT

DBS performed on patients without PD, such as patients with atypical parkinsonism syndromes, do not have good outcomes. Patients should be evaluated for DBS by a movement disorders specialist for appropriate patient selection.

■ NONMEDICAL THERAPIES

Nonpharmacologic treatments are an essential part of care of the PD patient. A multidisciplinary team approach can be utilized to provide effective comprehensive care for the PD patient. In PD, speech can be severely hypophonic and challenging to a hearing-impaired caregiver. Speech therapists can provide exercises, such as the Lee Silverman Voice Therapy (LSVT), to optimize speech output. A swallowing evaluation should be considered in patients who have progressed to the stage of balance impairment, even if they do not report coughing when they drink water. Use of thickened liquids may reduce the likelihood of a fatal pneumonia. Severe dysphagia may eventually warrant percutaneous gastrostomy tube placement.

Early attention to posture and mobility is vital. Evaluation by physical and occupational therapists is invaluable. Assistive walking devices including canes, walkers and wheelchairs should be used appropriately. Patients should be encouraged to stay active, with all the attendant medical and psychological benefits this entails. Data from animal models suggest that exercise has a beneficial effect upon brain chemistry. Music therapy may be very helpful as people with PD can move better to the external stimulus provided by music.

Patients with PD lose weight for reasons which are not entirely explained by motor difficulties and dysphagia. Malnutrition may worsen PD symptoms, and increases the risks of falls and infection. Diets high in vitamins E and C may reduce risk of PD, probably due to their antioxidant properties. Dietary vitamins appear to be more beneficial than vitamins in nutritional supplements. Adequate calcium and vitamin D intake is important for bone health, as PD patients are at high risk for falls.

High protein meals can interfere with the effects of medication, as amino acids compete with levodopa for uptake in the gut. However, taking medication on an empty stomach can cause nausea. Some patients find it helpful to ingest most of their daily protein at the evening meal, when the need for motor function is decreased.

Older patients with impaired mobility tend to drink less fluid to reduce urinary frequency and the risk of incontinence, putting them at risk for dehydration. This can aggravate orthostatic hypotension, which may be a feature of PD and may also be exacerbated by medications, thus contributing to fall risk. Constipation is a common PD symptom, and is also relieved with increased fluid intake, as well as a high fiber diet and regular physical activity. Despite these measures, regular administration of a stool softener is usually required.

ISSUES IN HOSPITALIZED PD PATIENTS

■ WEARING OFF

In advanced disease, the therapeutic effects of levodopa wear off more quickly. After excluding decompensation due to metabolic disturbances and infection there are several potential strategies to follow. Drug dosage or frequency may be increased, or an inhibitor of dopamine metabolism such as entacapone, rasagiline, or selegiline may be prescribed. These choices are guided by efficacy of the current dose, medication side effects, and patient preference.

■ LEVODOPA-INDUCED DYSKINESIA

Choreiform or dystonic movements may occur at peak blood levels of dopaminergic medications (peak-dose dyskinesia), but can also occur when medication is taking effect or wearing off (on-off dyskinesia). Dyskinesia occurs more typically with levodopa, but may be seen with dopamine agonists. It may manifest in any part of the body, and may include behavior that appears to be restless fidgeting or facial twitches. More severe forms may include toe-curling dystonia, violent limb movements, or even difficulty breathing due to involvement of the diaphragm. These symptoms usually resolve as the levodopa dose wears off, and the patient is often left with a window of time during which their PD symptoms are controlled and their dyskinesia is less severe. This window is soon followed by medication off time, as PD symptoms return. In some cases, motor fluctuations can involve nonmotor features, such as sweating, cardiac arrhythmias, and anxiety. The temporal relationship of these symptoms to medication intake suggests the diagnosis and management.

For most patients, the dyskinesia is mild enough that they prefer the medication on-state to the rigid, akinetic off-state. In many cases, the spouse or caregiver is more bothered by the abnormal dyskinetic movements more than the patient. Patients generally prefer dyskinesia to being undermedicated. Amantadine may be helpful in controlling dyskinesia, most likely due to its antiglutamatergic actions.

Dysphagia

As PD progresses, pharyngeal muscle dysfunction may develop, and the patient may have trouble swallowing. The risk of aspiration is increased by undertreatment while hospitalized. Management in hospitalized patients may include limiting the diet to avoid thin liquids and eating meals while sitting in a chair, but ideally should include a formal speech and swallowing evaluation.

Falling

Falling is a frequent PD symptom and reason for emergency room visits. However, a sudden increase in falls should not be blamed on PD alone. As discussed above, PD does not rapidly progress, and secondary causes should be sought, such as infections, metabolic derangements, spinal cord injury, stroke, and subdural hematoma.

Cognitive Impairment

Cognition and behavior are frequently affected in moderate to advanced stages of PD. With more sensitive testing, deficits can be detected even in relatively early stages. The typical deficits that develop are dysfunction in executive function and decision making (frontal type dementia). There is also slowing of information processing, known as subcortical dementia. This is in comparison to the memory dysfunction and other cortical functions typical of Alzheimer's disease. Along with these changes can appear personality changes such as disinhibition or apathy. Poor judgment, increased risk taking, and lack of insight may contribute to increased falls.

Individuals with, and even without, cognitive decline may have visual hallucinations. These often consist of animals and people, especially children, and are usually non-threatening, at least in the initial stages. Hallucinations may be worsened by many PD medications, in particular the dopamine agonists.

Elderly patients admitted to the hospital, regardless of diagnosis, often become more confused in the evenings and may become prone to sundowning and agitation. Exposure to daylight during daytime may be helpful. Typical antipsychotic medications should not be used, as these may worsen parkinsonism. Atypical antipsychotics such as quetiapine may be given in very low doses, but may cause sedation or hypotension. Benzodiazepines tend to worsen confusion in this population.

Depression

Depression in PD is more than a predictable response to a chronic, progressive illness. It seems to be an organic depression, and responds to antidepressants. The older, less selective, antidepressants may be more effective, rather than selective serotonin reuptake inhibitors, although they may also have more side effects. Some patients are prone to anxiety, which may worsen with disease progression, and can exacerbate motor symptoms. In addition, anxiety may be a feature of either the off-state, or peak-dose dyskinesia. Apathy and fatigue appear to be distinct features in PD, without good therapies at present. MAO-B inhibitors can have a mild stimulant effect in some patients.

Sleep Problems

Parkinson's disease patients may be caught in a vicious cycle of sleep difficulties. PD and associated medications may contribute to nocturnal awakenings and insomnia, while daytime somnolence may exacerbate neurologic symptoms. REM sleep behavior disorder can occur particularly in men with PD, and often predate the development of frank motor symptoms. In this disorder the sufferer acts out his dreams, and may kick and thrash during sleep, resulting in injury to the patient and to the bed partner. This can be effectively treated with low doses of clonazepam, possibly through reduction of REM sleep.

In the hospital, it is important for night staff to be aware of this sleep dysregulation, as the patient may request a sleep aid. The patient may try to walk to the nursing station or bathroom if he or she cannot sleep, with the danger of falling, especially if medication has not been given recently. Parkinson's disease patients with gait dysfunction should be classified as fall risks and therefore need to be accompanied to the bathroom, or instructed to use a urinal, or bedside commode especially at night.

Autonomic Nervous System Problems

Marked autonomic dysregulation suggests the diagnosis of MSA, but it can also occur in idiopathic PD. Orthostatic drops in blood pressure can result in unsteadiness, lightheadedness, and even loss of consciousness. Use of antihypertensive medications should be reassessed, and dose reduction or even cessation may be necessary. Patients should stay hydrated, liberalize salt intake, wear compression stockings, and sleep with the head of the bed raised by 30°. If these measures do not work, a blood pressure raising agent such as fludrocortisone or midodrine may be used. These drugs should not be used late in the day, due to the risk of nocturnal hypertension.

Parkinson's disease patients may develop neurogenic bladder, leading to nocturia and sleep disturbance. Giving an anticholinergic agent at bedtime may improve nocturia, in addition to promoting sedation and having mild antiparkinsonian effects. Unfortunately, anticholinergics have cognitive and hallucinatory side effects, and may result in nocturnal falls. In addition, bladder dysfunction may make patients prone to urinary tract infections.

Patients may complain of excess salivation, due to impaired swallowing. This can be cautiously treated with peripherally-acting anticholinergic agents, such as propantheline, or with botulinum toxin injections into the salivary glands. Rimabotulinum toxin B is preferred, as it appears to have a stronger anticholinergic effect.

Constipation is very common in PD and may predate the diagnosis. Unfortunately, levodopa therapy is often unhelpful in resolving constipation, and entacapone may even make it worse. For hospitalized PD patients, it should be ensured that they have regular bowel movements, as limited mobility will worsen their pre-existing constipation. Nausea should be treated with nondopamine blocking antiemetics.

■ END OF LIFE CARE

Parkinson's disease continues to respond to medications even in advanced disease. However, higher and more frequent dosing may be required, and the results are less predictable, with dose failures and sudden off periods. The medication schedule is often simplified as the disease progresses, until only levodopa/carbidopa is given. It is important to ensure that PD medications continue to be given despite impaired swallowing, as inadequate treatment can result in significant pain and worsened bradykinesia. Levodopa/carbidopa can be administered ground up in apple sauce. An orally-disintegrating formulation of levodopa/carbidopa, marketed as Parcopa, may also be useful.

The terminal phase of PD and other parkinsonian disorders is similar to that of other neurodegenerative conditions such as Alzheimer's disease, with progressive debility and vulnerability to pneumonia and urinary tract infections. Constipation and falls are common. Aspiration is a particular risk due to dysphagia, kyphosis, and hypokinesia. Weight loss is typical, and a feeding tube may be considered to facilitate safe and adequate nutrition. It has not yet been determined whether feeding tubes enhance quality of life, or reduce mortality, in advanced PD. Patients, families, and physicians should consider early planning of advanced directives regarding difficult issues such as gastrostomy tube placement and preferred place of death, as patients with severe PD may be physically and cognitively unable to engage in such decision making. Palliative care physicians may help facilitate these discussions.

■ DISCHARGE PLANNING CHECKLIST

- Do the patient and caregiver understand changes to medications?
- Has follow-up with the treating neurologist been scheduled in the next 2 to 4 weeks?
- Home safety evaluation: are additional items required, for example shower chair, bathroom railings, hospital bed? Should a visiting nurse assess the home situation?

- Is outpatient physical therapy indicated? Are new assistive devices required?
- Has the caregiver been educated on the appropriate consistency diet and any new nutritional needs, such as high-calorie supplements?
- Have the needs of the caregiver been addressed? Have mechanisms of support been discussed, including home health aides and support groups? Have future respite admissions been considered?

SUGGESTED READINGS

Braga M, Pederzoli M, Antonini A, et al. Reasons for hospitalization in Parkinson's disease: a case-control study. *Parkinsonism Relat Disord.* 2014;20:488-492.

Connolly BS, Lang AE. Pharmacological treatment of Parkinson disease: a review. *JAMA.* 2014;311:1670-1683.

Gerlach OH, Broen MP, van Domburg PH, et al. Deterioration of Parkinson's disease during hospitalization: survey of 684 patients. *BMC Neurol.* 2012;12:13.

Goetz CG, Tilley BC, Shaftman SR, et al. Movement Disorder Society UPDRS Revision Task Force. Movement Disorder Society-sponsored revision of the Unified Parkinson's Disease Rating Scale (MDS-UPDRS): scale presentation and clinimetric testing results. *Mov Disord.* 2008;23:2129-2170.

Schuepbach WM, Rau J, Knudsen K, et al. Neurostimulation for Parkinson's disease with early motor complications. *N Engl J Med.* 2013;368:610-622.

van der Marck MA, Klok MP, Okun MS, et al. Consensus-based clinical practice recommendations for the examination and management of falls in patients with Parkinson's disease. *Parkinsonism Relat Disord.* 2014;20:360-369.

Walker RW. Palliative care and end-of-life planning in Parkinson's disease. *J Neural Transm.* 2013;120:635-638.

ONLINE RESOURCES

For patients and caregivers.

National Parkinson Foundation: www.parkinson.org

Parkinson's Disease Foundation: www.pdf.org

Michael J. Fox Foundation: www.michaeljfox.org

American Parkinson Disease Association: www.apdaparkinson.org

CHAPTER 211

Seizures

Claire S. Jacobs, MD, PhD
Tracey A. Milligan, MD

Key Clinical Questions

1. How can clinicians distinguish between seizures, syncopal events, and other seizure mimics?
2. What historical features are helpful? What diagnostic tests are appropriate?
3. Which patients with new-onset seizures require an antiepileptic drug?
4. How should patients with status epilepticus be managed?

INTRODUCTION

A *seizure* is defined as a sudden attack of involuntary behavior or sensory experiences resulting from abnormal cortical neuronal activity. About 10% of the population of the United States will experience a seizure at some point during their lifetime, and seizure accounts for 1% to 2% of emergency room visits in the United States each year. *Epilepsy* is a disease of the brain defined by any of the following conditions: (1) at least two unprovoked (or reflex) seizures occurring greater than 24 hours apart; (2) one unprovoked (or reflex) seizure and a probability of further seizures similar to the general recurrence risk (at least 60%) after two unprovoked seizures, occurring over the next 10 years; (3) diagnosis of an epilepsy syndrome. Epilepsy is the fourth most common neurological disorder in the United States, and has a lifetime prevalence of 3%. The World Health Organization (WHO) reports that in primary care settings worldwide, epilepsy is the second most common neurologic condition, after headache.

TRIAGE AND HOSPITAL ADMISSION

Epilepsy and seizures are also common in the inpatient setting. In a large multicenter study in both community and academic hospital emergency departments, 1.2% of 31,508 patient visits were related to seizures. Overall, 27% of these patients were admitted. Of those patients suspected of having new-onset seizures, 63% were admitted. Reasons for admission of patients with seizures include diagnostic evaluation, uncontrolled seizures, toxicity from antiepileptic drugs (AEDs), and injuries sustained during a seizure.

CLASSIFICATION AND CLINICAL FINDINGS

Seizures are classified into two broad categories, based on whether the primary onset is focal or generalized (**Table 211-1**). The terminology has recently been updated, so both the updated and the former terms will be presented. *Focal seizures* (formerly known as *partial seizures*) start with abnormal neuronal discharges from a seizure focus limited to one cerebral hemisphere. The abnormal electrical activity may remain limited to that hemisphere, or can generalize to involve both hemispheres. Focal seizures are further subdivided based on whether there is an associated change in mental status or awareness. During a *focal seizure without dyscognitive features* (previously called a *simple partial seizure*), the patient remains awake and aware throughout and does not experience a change in cognition. In contrast, a *focal seizure with dyscognitive features* (previously termed a *complex partial seizure*) arises from abnormal electrical activity in one cerebral hemisphere and is accompanied by alteration in awareness or consciousness during the event. This change in consciousness may manifest as inattentiveness, blank staring, or unresponsiveness to questions or stimulus, but unless the seizure secondarily generalizes, it does not involve loss of consciousness.

The area of cortex and networks involved in the abnormal electrical activity of a seizure dictate the clinical symptoms, or the *semiology*, of the seizure. As seizures in epilepsy patients arise from the same seizure focus or foci, the seizure semiology is stereotyped, that is, the semiology does not vary drastically from seizure to seizure for individual patients. Patients with a temporal lobe seizure focus may report subjective symptoms such as nausea, anxiety, a feeling of "epigastric rising," visual distortion, déjà vu, or auditory or olfactory hallucinations (typically involving an unpleasant smell). Witnesses to a focal seizure with dyscognitive features may report that the patient was staring, walking aimlessly, or engaging in stereotyped,

TABLE 211-1 Seizure Types in Adults

Focal	Primary Generalized
Without dyscognitive features (simple partial)	Absence
With dyscognitive features (complex partial)	Myoclonic
With secondary generalization	Tonic
	Clonic
	Tonic-clonic
	Atonic
	Myoclonic-astatic
	Other idiopathic generalized

purposeless automatisms such as lip smacking or picking at clothes or bedsheets. Focal seizure duration is typically 1 to 3 minutes. Following a focal seizure without dyscognitive features that does not generalize, patients will immediately return to their cognitive baseline, while patients may be confused or somnolent for up to 30 minutes after a focal seizure with dyscognitive features.

The other broad category of seizures is that of *generalized seizures*, which are due to abnormal neuronal electrical discharges originating within and rapidly spreading throughout bilaterally distributed networks. Generalized seizures often have an underlying genetic etiology. *Absence seizures* are typically brief staring spells lasting seconds, and *atypical absence seizures* may also include automatisms. Absence seizures usually begin in early childhood and remit in adolescence, but can persist into adulthood. It is very rare for an adult to develop *de novo* absence seizures. Patients with *myoclonic epilepsy* experience quick jerking movements, most often in the morning after awakening. Diagnosis often does not occur until these patients progress to a generalized tonic-clonic seizure. *Generalized tonic-clonic seizures,* also known as convulsions, are characterized by tonic extension, followed by rhythmic clonic jerking of the extremities (**Figure 211-1**). Variations of these include generalized seizures with either a primarily tonic or clonic component. *Atonic seizures* are characterized by sudden loss of tone. These patients are especially prone to injuries as a result of falling without warning.

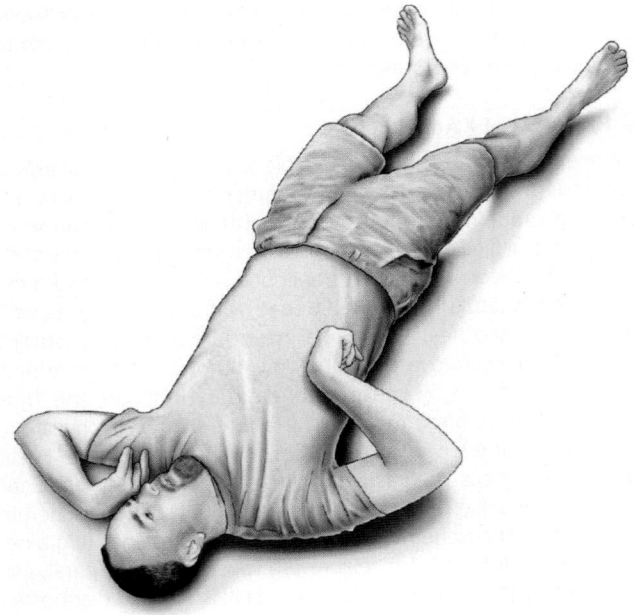

Figure 211-1 *Generalized tonic-clonic seizure.*

EVALUATION OF A POSSIBLE EPILEPTIC SEIZURE

When called upon to care for a patient with a reported seizure, the first question the hospitalist must ask is whether the "seizure" was an epileptic seizure (ie, due to abnormal cerebral electrical activity) or a seizure mimic. Many physiologic events are characterized by changes in awareness or abnormal motor movements. Common conditions that can mimic seizure are listed in **Table 211-2**. Obtaining a thorough clinical history from the patient and from any witnesses to the event is crucial. Important points of the history include: *Was the event paroxysmal?* Epileptic seizures are always sudden in onset. This is also true of some, but not all, seizure mimics, and this information alone cannot distinguish epileptic seizures from nonepileptic events.

1. *Was the event provoked?* Common triggers for epileptic seizures include sleep deprivation, systemic illness, drug intoxication or withdrawal, introduction or discontinuation of pharmacologic agents, and flashing lights. Syncope often follows a change in posture, micturition, or sudden fright.

2. *Was there a clinical prodrome?* A seizure may begin with an aura of focal neurologic symptoms or signs. The aura may consist of obvious behavior changes, such as focal motor jerking or staring into space with oral automatisms, or it may be a purely internal experience for the patient consisting of visual or olfactory hallucinations, focal sensory changes, déjà vu, or a subjective feeling that patients often find difficult to put into words. A seizure aura is stereotypic for any given patient, and is typically short in duration, lasting seconds to 1 to 2 minutes. Conversely, the prodrome of many seizure mimics, if present, is usually described as feeling lightheaded or unwell, and can last minutes to hours.

3. *What were the clinical features of the event?* The appearance and actions of the patient during and following the event are critical pieces of information. Clinical features that may help differentiate epileptic seizures from seizure mimics are noted in **Table 211-3**. Some are more specific than others. For example, tonic posturing is often seen in focal seizures emanating from the frontal lobe, but is rare in nonepileptic events. Tongue biting, traditionally considered a reliable sign of a generalized seizure, occurs in less than 30% of convulsions, and may also occur during nonepileptic events. Similarly, urinary incontinence is not specific to epileptic seizures. Bizarre behavior, such as bicycling, pelvic thrusting, flailing or thrashing movements, or highly emotional outbursts, is often ascribed to nonepileptic, or psychogenic, events. These presentations, however, can be seen in physiologic events, such as frontal

TABLE 211-2 Seizure Mimics

Syncope (cardiac, vasovagal, hypovolemic, orthostatic)
Transient ischemic attack
Transient global amnesia
Migraine, with or without aura
Metabolic disturbances
Movement disorder (tremor, tics, paroxysmal dyskinesias, choreoathetosis)
Postanoxic myoclonus
Sleep disorders (narcolepsy, parasomnias, night terrors, somnambulism, paroxysmal nocturnal dystonia)
Benign nocturnal myoclonus
Panic or anxiety attack
Psychogenic nonepileptic events

TABLE 211-3 Clinical Characteristics in Epileptic vs Psychogenic Nonepileptic Spells

Clinical Sign or Symptom	Epileptic	Nonepileptic
Appearance	Flushed or cyanotic	Pale, diaphoretic
Motor movements	Rhythmic tonic-clonic jerks	Complex tonic posturing
	Tonic extension	Myoclonus
	Sudden onset flailing/thrashing, repetitive rocking	Nonrhythmic jerking
	Lip smacking, oral automatisms	
	Nonpurposeful picking/slapping	Nonsudden onset flailing/thrashing
	Versive/head turning	Head shaking
	Eye deviation	Eye closure
	Fencing posture	
Subjective experience	Stereotypical olfactory, gustatory, visual, or aural (rare) hallucination	Tunnel vision
	Fear or anxiety	Light-headedness
	Epigastric rising	Palpitations
	Déjà vu	
Tongue biting	Can occur but < 50%	Rare but can occur
Urinary incontinence	Can occur	Can occur
Sensory changes	Positive symptoms (eg, paresthesias, dysesthesias)	Negative symptoms (eg, numbness)
Postevent state	Unresponsiveness usually < 1 h	Unresponsiveness < 5 min (nonepileptic events may sometimes be followed by prolonged unresponsiveness)
	Agitation	
	Confusion	
	Headache	
	Extreme fatigue	

lobe epileptic seizures and some sleep disorders, as listed in Table 211-2. Fear or anxiety, the hallmark of panic disorder, is common in focal seizures with dyscognitive features emanating from the amygdala. Hallucinations, especially visual, are common in migraine, but hallucinations are also common auras in temporal lobe focal seizures with dyscognitive features. A change in mental status can occur during and after both epileptic seizures and some mimickers. The duration of the event and postevent confusion may be helpful in making the distinction. Postevent unresponsiveness is typically briefest with syncope (seconds to 1 minute), longer in epileptic seizures (up to 30-60 minutes), and longest with psychogenic nonepileptic events where "unresponsiveness" can last hours and can fluctuate in intensity. In cases of prolonged unresponsiveness, however, subclinical or nonconvulsive status epilepticus (SE) is on the differential diagnosis, and must be ruled out.

4. When trying to decide whether a spell is an epileptic seizure or a nonepileptic event, remember that not all that shakes or jerks are epileptic. Myoclonus, characterized by quick, sudden jerks, is common after cerebral hypoxia and anoxia, and patients who suffer syncope may suffer brief convulsions immediately after loss of consciousness (convulsive syncope). Metabolic derangements may cause myoclonus or tremor. Myoclonus, tremor, and convulsive syncope are seldom epileptic, and should be recognized as symptoms of an underlying medical condition rather than due primary epileptic seizures.

PRACTICE POINT

- Confusion following a spell strongly suggests seizure. Recovery of full orientation is rapid after syncope, but typically takes 10 to 30 minutes after a seizure.

---

5. *Was this the first such event?* Careful history from the patient and those living with them may reveal previous similar episodes. A report of highly stereotyped events raises the suspicion for epileptic seizures. The risk of seizure recurrence and a diagnosis of epilepsy increases if there have been prior events, so this information affects management and prognosis.

6. *What is the patient's medical history?* A history of diabetes, renal failure, or liver disease should raise the clinician's suspicion that the event in question was a seizure provoked by a systemic metabolic disturbance. A patient with a cancer history who has an episode of altered awareness should be evaluated for brain metastases causing a focal or generalized seizure. Cardiac or vascular disease favors the diagnosis of syncope. In patients with psychiatric disease, it should not be assumed that the presenting episode is a nonepileptic (psychogenic) event. Adult patients with mood disorders are 1.7 to 7 times more likely to develop epilepsy than those without a psychiatric history. In addition, seizures can be provoked by certain antidepressants and antipsychotic medications, or by medication withdrawal. Thus, it is incumbent on the hospitalist to exclude other physiologic conditions before a diagnosis of nonepileptic seizure is made.

The value of an accurate history and description of an episode concerning for seizure cannot be overemphasized. This information is often elusive when a patient is cognitively impaired or postictal. The hospitalist must be dogged in the pursuit of history from family or witnesses to the event, in order to avoid a misdiagnosis and to provide the most appropriate treatment.

◼ PHYSICAL EXAMINATION

When evaluating a patient for possible seizure, the physical examination is most helpful during or immediately after the event. Ongoing subtle motor movements (particularly eye movements and unilateral face and hand movements) should prompt consideration of nonconvulsive status epilepticus. Elevated blood pressure or tachycardia is commonly seen with convulsions as well as with focal seizures. An irregular heart rate is more consistent with a primary cardiovascular etiology. Although seizures arising from certain foci may cause autonomic dysfunction, this dysautonomia more often manifests as a rate change (tachycardia, bradycardia, or even asystole) rather than an arrhythmia. Focal neurologic deficits such as hemiparesis or hemiparesthesias are common sequelae of focal cerebral ischemia, such as ischemic stroke, transient ischemic attack (TIA) or hemiplegic migraine, but can also follow focal seizure (eg, postictal Todd paralysis). Thus, although the examination by itself is seldom diagnostic, when combined with the clinical history, it can help distinguish epileptic seizure from its mimics.

■ ELECTROENCEPHALOGRAPHY

Electroencephalography (EEG) is the gold standard to distinguish epileptic seizures from nonepileptic events and other seizure mimics. The study is most diagnostic if the patient has an event during EEG recording, as only approximately 30% of patients with chronic unprovoked seizures show epileptiform activity on routine interictal EEG. If done within 24 to 48 hours of a seizure, some studies have shown that the yield of scalp EEG increases to up to 70%. About 2% to 3% of healthy adults have a false-positive EEG. Overall, a positive EEG may be helpful in ascertaining whether an event was epileptic, especially if done within 24 to 48 hours of the spell. A negative study is not helpful, as some focal seizures will not be detected on scalp EEG, and an interictal EEG has a low sensitivity.

■ SYNCOPE VERSUS SEIZURE

Perhaps the most vexing diagnostic problem for the hospitalist faced with a patient with an episode of altered consciousness is distinguishing a syncopal event from an epileptic seizure. Overall, syncope is much more common than seizure, especially in elderly patients, who comprise a large portion of the hospitalist's practice. A thorough history of the paroxysmal event provides the most reliable data in differentiating seizure from syncope. Clinical features useful in drawing this distinction are presented in **Table 211-4**. Findings on physical exam may help in the differential diagnosis. Abnormal cardiac findings or orthostatic changes in vital signs are more consistent with syncope, while focal neurologic signs are more suggestive of seizure. Beyond the history and physical, diagnostic tests are surprisingly of low yield. An electrocardiogram (ECG) is abnormal in only approximately 7% of patients who present to the emergency department with syncope. Despite this statistically low yield, it is recommended that all adult patients who present with an episode of altered consciousness have an ECG and, if admitted, be placed on telemetry monitoring.

EEG is of less diagnostic value than ECG. When ordered as part of a syncope workup, EEGs are abnormal in up to one-quarter of patients, but most of these abnormalities are nonspecific. Less than 2% of EEG studies show epileptiform discharges, the definitive EEG finding in seizures. Thus, an EEG is most helpful if clinical features of the patient's event raise suspicion of epileptic seizures.

DIAGNOSTIC EVALUATION FOR SEIZURES

Once the hospitalist has decided that their patient did experience an epileptic seizure, diagnostic testing should be pursued to evaluate the underlying cause and guide treatment decisions. Seizures may be idiopathic or provoked by a systemic problem, such as electrolyte disturbances, medication, drug or alcohol withdrawal, or infection. Provoked seizures are usually generalized tonic-clonic convulsions, but may be focal, particularly in patients with a prior stroke or other focal neurologic injury. A provoked seizure is managed by treating the underlying cause; prolonged treatment with an antiepileptic drug is usually not indicated.

■ LABORATORY STUDIES

In general, laboratory studies are low yield, but the decision to order laboratory studies must also be informed by the overall clinical presentation. Routine laboratory studies, including electrolytes, calcium, magnesium, and glucose, are often performed, as seizures may be seen with hyponatremia or hypernatremia, hypoglycemia or hyperglycemia, hypocalcemia, and hypomagnesemia. Altered potassium levels are not associated with seizures. The yield of these studies is generally low, and the American Academy of Neurology (AAN) guidelines cite insufficient evidence to make a recommendation either for or against laboratory studies. However, as uncorrected metabolic disturbances can result in ongoing seizures and even status epilepticus, these studies are often included in the evaluation of patients presenting with seizures. Particularly important are measurements of sodium and glucose, as hypoglycemia and hyponatremia are two of the most common causes of provoked seizures. Blood urea nitrogen and creatinine should be obtained to exclude uremia, as well as liver function tests and ammonia levels, if hepatic dysfunction is possible. Complete blood count is of low yield; meningoencephalitis may present with a normal or only marginally elevated white blood cell (WBC) count, while an epileptic seizure can itself cause a mild leukocytosis. Serum lactate and creatine kinase are often transiently elevated following seizure, but may also be elevated in the setting of other medical conditions, including nonepileptic events. Serum prolactin level may be elevated if measured within 20 minutes of a focal seizure with dyscognitive features or a generalized tonic-clonic seizure, but not following a nonepileptic spell. The AAN guidelines, however, warn against using a normal serum prolactin level to diagnose nonepileptic events or to rule out epileptic seizure due to the low sensitivity and low negative predictive value of serum prolactin.

There are insufficient data to support routine lumbar punctures on patients presenting with seizures. The decision on whether a lumbar puncture is indicated must be made on a case-by-case basis, and lumbar puncture should only be performed after imaging to evaluate for herniation is complete. Metabolic disturbances and systemic disorders that provoke seizures are summarized in **Table 211-5**.

■ DRUG SCREEN AND TOXICOLOGY

Alcohol-related seizures account for up to one-half of patients with new-onset seizures in some emergency departments. An

TABLE 211-4 Clinical Features in Syncope vs Seizures

Favors Seizures	Favors Syncope
Flushed, cyanotic	Pallor, diaphoresis
Head turning	Lightheadedness, dizziness
Unusual posturing	Occurs with prolonged standing sitting, micturition, defecation, cough
Unusual behavior	Feeling hot
Tongue biting	Vertigo
Prodromal deja-vu	Nausea
Prodromal rising epigastric sensation, prodromal hallucinations, prodromal mood changes	Tinnitus
Focal neurologic deficit on exam	Palpitations
Postevent headache	Chest pain
Postevent confusion	History of hypertension
Lesion on brain MRI	Orthostatic hypotension
Abnormal EEG	Abnormal EKG

TABLE 211-5 Metabolic Disturbances and Systemic Disorders Associated with Seizures

Hypoglycemia
Hyponatremia
Hyperosmolar states, including hypernatremia and hyperosmolar nonketotic hyperglycemia
Hypocalcemia
Hypomagnesemia
Uremia
Hepatic encephalopathy
Porphyria
Drug overdose or withdrawal
Global cerebral ischemia
Hypertensive encephalopathy, aka posterior reversible encephalopathy syndrome (PRES)
Eclampsia
Hyperthermia

alcohol level is appropriate when there is clinical suspicion of excessive use, though alcohol-related seizures typically occur in the setting of alcohol withdrawal, and the blood alcohol level may be normal or only slightly elevated. Other recreational drugs, particularly stimulants such as cocaine, methamphetamine, MDMA (3,4-methylenedioxymethamphetamine, also known as Ecstasy), bath salts (which often contain derivatives of the hallucinogen cathinone or methylenedioxypyrovalerone, a compound structurally related to MDMA), or synthetic cannabinoids, can cause seizures. Benzodiazepine withdrawal is another drug-related cause of seizures. A multitude of other drugs, especially when taken in excess, are associated with seizures (**Table 211-6**).

Exposure to some toxins can trigger generalized tonic-clonic seizures. Carbon monoxide poisoning does not usually cause seizures unless the carboxyhemoglobin level is greater than 50%. Ethylene glycol or methanol can cause severe neurologic dysfunction, including seizures. These substances are often not included in routine toxicology screens, so the diagnosis may easily be missed.

There are no prospective studies of the yield and utility of drug screens in new-onset seizures, and AAN guidelines state that current data are insufficient to recommend either for or against routine toxicology testing. However, the failure to diagnose drug intoxication can lead to inappropriate and potentially harmful anticonvulsant treatment, as well as a missed opportunity for intervention in a patient's substance abuse problem. Hence, drug screens are usually included in the evaluation of new-onset seizures.

TABLE 211-6 Drugs Associated with Seizure Occurrence

Bupropion
Tricyclic antidepressants
Tramadol
Diphenhydramine
Venlafaxine
Antipsychotics
Theophylline
Metronidazole
Penicillins
Fluoroquinolones (levofloxacin, ciprofloxacin)

Serum AED levels may sometimes be useful, but the results must be interpreted with caution. In a patient with known epilepsy, a low AED level does not always reflect nonadherence with medications. Some patients maintain seizure control on doses of medications that result in low measured levels. Likewise, a drug level above the recommended therapeutic range is not cause for immediate reduction in medication dose, unless the patient is clinically toxic. Serum levels of many of the newer AEDs are not available for at least 48 to 72 hours, and are thus of limited use in the acute care of the patient with seizures.

■ NEUROIMAGING

When evaluating a patient with an unprovoked first seizure, brain imaging with CT or MRI should be considered. Neuroimaging is more likely to be positive in patients presenting with altered mentation, focal seizures, or focal deficits on neurologic examination. MRI is the preferred neuroimaging modality for detecting structural abnormalities associated with some epilepsy syndromes. If present, these structural abnormalities portend a high risk of recurrent seizures. Consultation with a neurologist and neuroradiologist may be appropriate to decide on the most appropriate MRI sequence. CT imaging may be appropriate for patients who are not sufficiently stable for a lengthy MRI, or in whom there is suspicion of an intracerebral hemorrhage. Although studies report that 34% to 52% of CT scans done in the emergency department after a seizure are abnormal, the findings changed acute management in only 9% to 17% of patients. Significant abnormalities include cerebral hemorrhage, stroke, subdural hematoma, tumor, and brain abscess. The AAN recommends consideration of brain imaging, especially in the presence of an abnormal neurologic exam or focal seizure onset, as it may reveal underlying structural abnormalities or findings that may alter treatment.

In patients with known epilepsy who present with seizure, acute brain CT is indicated if the presenting seizure (1) has a different semiology than their usual seizures, (2) is prolonged (lasting > 5 minutes), or (3) is followed by a prolonged postictal period of altered mentation. New findings on neurologic exam are also a clear indication for acute brain imaging. If the CT scan is negative, MRI should be done once the patient is stable to look for a new cerebral lesion to explain the altered seizure presentation. Follow-up MRI is also indicated when a lesion is suggested but not well defined on CT scan. A patient who presents with a focal seizure or has focal neurologic deficits on exam should have an MRI if the CT scan is negative.

MRI brain is indicated for patients who suffers a seizure in the setting of human immunodeficiency virus (HIV) infection or who are otherwise immunocompromised. MRI is more sensitive than CT in detecting opportunistic infections, such as toxoplasmosis, progressive multifocal leukoencephalopathy (PML), cytomegalovirus (CMV), tuberculosis, *Cryptococcus neoformans*, and primary central nervous system (CNS) lymphoma. Seizures can be the initial presentation of these conditions, and early detection can improve the patient's prognosis.

■ ELECTROENCEPHALOGRAM

For patients admitted with a first unprovoked seizure, a routine EEG may help estimate the risk of seizure recurrence; epileptiform activity on EEG doubles the risk of seizure recurrence. In a meta-analysis of early studies, patients with epileptiform activity on EEG were more likely to have seizure recurrence, with a relative risk of 2. Similar results were found in a more recent analysis, where the probability of seizure recurrence in patients with these EEG abnormalities was 49.5% versus 27.4% in patients with normal EEGs. Common, nonspecific EEG abnormalities, such as focal or diffuse slowing, have not been shown to be associated with an increased risk of seizure recurrence. For the patient with chronic seizures, it is important to obtain an EEG when there is a concern for ongoing subclinical seizures. This is especially true for patients admitted in clinical status epilepticus, as discussed below.

INPATIENT MANAGEMENT

■ PATIENTS WITH A FIRST SEIZURE

In a patient with a first unprovoked seizure, the hospitalist is faced with the difficult decision of whether to start treatment with an AED. Probably, the most important consideration in this decision is the risk of a recurrent seizure, which can be estimated and stratified on the basis of clinical factors. The AAN recommends that adults presenting with an unprovoked first seizure be informed that: (1) the chance for a recurrent seizure is greatest within the first 2 years after a first seizure (21%-45%); (2) clinical factors associated with a higher risk for seizure recurrence include a prior brain insult such as a stroke or trauma and an EEG with epileptiform abnormalities; and (3) clinical factors associated with an increased risk for seizure recurrence include a significant brain-imaging abnormality and a nocturnal seizure.

Does treatment with an AED reduce the risk of seizure recurrence? The answer to this question is complex. In large studies, the initiation of AED treatment immediately after a first seizure is associated with a 34% reduction in the risk of a second seizure within the next 1 to 2 years. At 5 years, however, there was no significant difference in seizure remission rate between patients treated with an AED and those who were untreated. Thus, after a single seizure, treatment with an AED reduces the short-term risk of seizure recurrence, but does not affect long-term prognosis for the development of epilepsy. The AAN recommends that patients be advised that immediate AED therapy is likely to reduce the risk for seizure recurrence in the 2 years after a first seizure, but over the long term (>3 years) immediate AED treatment is unlikely to improve the prognosis for sustained seizure remission, and may not improve quality of life. The AAN guideline cites a risk of adverse events with AED treatment of 7% to 31%, which are predominantly mild and reversible. The only study appraising the incidence of sudden unexplained death after an unprovoked first seizure demonstrates no advantage with immediate AED therapy.

Given all this, the decision about whether to initiate AED treatment should be based on the available statistical evidence, as well as patient lifestyle, occupation, anxiety level, and other personal circumstances. The optimum AED balances tolerability of side effects with efficacy in treating seizures, and will vary from patient to patient.

PRACTICE POINT

- Factors that predict seizure recurrence in patients with new-onset seizures include prior brain insults, such as stroke or trauma, abnormal findings on brain imaging, and nocturnal seizures. The risk of a recurrent seizure is highest in the first 2 years after a seizure episode.

■ PATIENTS WITH EPILEPSY

The most common reason for hospital admission in patients with known epilepsy is breakthrough seizures. Common triggers for breakthrough seizures include missed medication doses, chronic nonadherence, sleep deprivation, and concurrent medical illness. In adherent patients, the prescribed AED dose may be inadequate, and require upward titration, if tolerated. Dosage adjustment should be based primarily on patient response rather than serum drug levels. AED titration should be done in consultation with a neurologist.

Breakthrough seizures in epilepsy patients may be due to the loss of efficacy of the prescribed AED. In this case, transition to a different AED or addition of a second drug is usually required. These treatment decisions are complicated, and referral to an epileptologist is suggested, particularly for patients on multiple AEDs.

■ MEDICATIONS

Since the mid-1990s, the number of available AEDs has doubled, and the hospitalist needs to be familiar with their efficacy and side effects. **Table 211-7** lists current AEDs, with recommended daily doses for otherwise healthy adults, as well as common side effects. Patients with renal or hepatic dysfunction may require dose adjustment. Drug–drug interactions are not addressed in the table. Several AEDs have major drug interactions, notably phenobarbital, phenytoin, carbamazepine, and valproic acid.

In female patients of childbearing age, the hospitalist must be aware that phenobarbital, phenytoin, carbamazepine, valproic acid, topiramate, and oxcarbazepine reduce the efficacy of oral contraceptives. Patients should be made aware of this and educated about additional or alternative contraceptives. In contrast, estrogen lowers the level of lamotrigine, and patients taking oral contraceptives may require higher doses of lamotrigine to prevent seizures.

The hospitalist is often faced with expeditiously stabilizing a patient with acute seizures. In this setting, the choice of AEDs will be limited to those that can be tolerated in relatively high initial doses, so that a therapeutic level is reached quickly. Medications that best meet this criterion include phenytoin, valproic acid, levetiracetam, and lacosamide, all of which are available for IV administration, and benzodiazepines such as clonazepam and lorazepam.

PRACTICE POINT

- Older AEDs, including phenobarbital, phenytoin, and carbamazepine, are associated with low vitamin D levels and early bone loss. Sodium valproate is also associated with premature bone loss. There are currently insufficient data about newer AEDs and bone health. Vitamin D levels should be followed in all patients treated with an AED, and it is reasonable to give prophylactic vitamin D supplementation to patients on AEDs.

■ MEDICATION TOXICITY

A frequent reason for hospital admission in patients on AEDs is drug toxicity. Symptoms of toxicity with commonly prescribed AEDs are listed in Table 211-7. The most common are gait ataxia, gastrointestinal (GI) upset, and somnolence. These toxicities are usually dose-related. Other toxicities, particularly organ dysfunction or failure, are not dose-related. Idiosyncratic allergic reactions, including Stevens-Johnson syndrome, have been reported with all AEDs, as have mood changes and suicidal ideation. In general, treatment is discontinuation of the AED until symptoms have resolved, particularly in idiosyncratic reactions or organ dysfunction. However, holding AEDs results in subtherapeutic drug levels and increases the risk of recurrent seizures. A benzodiazepine bridge may be used temporarily to minimize the risk of recurrent seizures. AED toxicity presents a complicated treatment challenge. Appropriate treatment requires knowledge of the pharmacokinetics of AEDs, and may best be done in consultation with a neurologist.

SPECIAL CONSIDERATIONS IN WOMEN OF CHILDBEARING AGE

Women with epilepsy of childbearing age deserve special consideration. As discussed above, hepatic P450 enzyme inducers may affect bone density and efficacy of oral contraceptive agents.

TABLE 211-7 Antiepileptic Drugs: Recommended Daily Dosing for Healthy Adults, Side Effects, and Contraindications

Drug	Dosing	Common Side Effects	Serious Side Effects	Contraindications
Broad Spectrum Agents				
Valproic acid	15 mg/kg/d dosed bid Increase by 5-10 mg/kg/d weekly to max 60 mg/kg/d	Weight gain Alopecia Peripheral edema Nausea/vomiting, constipation Nystagmus, diplopia Ataxia, tremor	Agranulocytosis SJS/TEN Aplastic anemia Hepatic failure Hyperammonemia Pancreatitis Polycystic ovary syndrome Thrombocytopenia Ototoxicity	Urea cycle disorders Significant hepatic impairment Mitochondrial disorders Women of childbearing age
Levetiracetam	500-1500 mg bid	Somnolence Nasopharyngitis Nausea/vomiting Irritability/mood changes	Pancyctopenia Hepatic failure Suicidal behavior SJS/TEN	
Lamotrigine	100-400 mg/d daily or bid, depends on other drug therapy	Ataxia Dizziness Abdominal symptoms Dysmenorrhea Incoordination Diplopia Tremor Insomnia	Renal failure Hepatic failure DIC Aseptic meningitis Rare life-threatening SJS (increased risk with rapid titration or valproic acid co-therapy)	
Zonisamide	100 mg daily, increase by 100 mg q2wk to goal 400 mg daily	Loss of appetite Dizziness Ataxia Confusion Diplopia, nystagmus Fatigue	Aplastic anemia Agranulocytosis SJS/TEN Schizophreniform d/o	Sulfonamide hypersensitivity
Phenobarbital	2-3 mg/kg/d	Somnolence Dizziness Irritability Nausea/vomiting Hyperactivity in children	Agranulocytosis SJS/TEN Hepatic failure Dermatitis/rash Thrombophlebitis Megaloblastic anemia Thrombocytopenia Serum sickness Osteopenia, rickets	Porphyria Significant liver disease Respiratory disease (dyspnea, obstruction)
Phenytoin	100,200 mg tid	Encephalopathy Ataxia GI upset Gingival hyperplasia Coarsening of facial features Osteoporosis	Agranulocytosis SJS/TEN Aplastic anemia Hepatic failure Lupus syndrome Dermatitis Serum sickness Adenopathy Pseudolymphoma Neuropathy Hirsutism	
Felbamate	400 mg tid, increase by 600 mg/d q2wk to max 3600 mg tid	Anorexia, weight loss Abdominal symptoms Photosensitivity Purpura HA, insomnia	Aplastic anemia Hepatic failure Seizures	History of blood dyscrasia History of liver disease

(Continued)

TABLE 211-7 Antiepileptic Drugs: Recommended Daily Dosing for Healthy Adults, Side Effects, and Contraindications (*Continued*)

Drug	Dosing	Common Side Effects	Serious Side Effects	Contraindications
Perampanel	2 mg qHS, increase by 2 mg/d weekly, max 12 mg/d	Dizziness Somnolence Headache Nausea Weight gain Gait disturbances Irritability, mood changes	Serious neuropsychiatric effects Aggression	Severe hepatic impairment Severe renal impairment
Topiramate	25 mg bid, increase 50 mg/d weekly to goal 200 mg bid	Anorexia, weight loss Cognitive impairment Parasthesias Somnolence Mood changes	Renal calculi Metabolic acidosis Open-angle glaucoma Hepatic failure Hyperammonemia Oligohydrosis Hyperthermia	
Narrow Spectrum Agents				
Carbamazepine	200 mg bid, increase by 200 mg/d weekly to max 800 mg bid	Hyper- or hypotension Nausea, vomiting Dizziness Nystagmus, diplopia somnolence	AV block, CHF SJS/TEN Aplastic anemia Agranulocytosis Angioedema Hepatitis Acute renal failure Acute intermittent porphyria Hypocalcemia Hyponatremia	History of bone marrow suppression MAOI within 14 d TCA hypersensitivity Prior to initial dose, test for HLA-B*1502 allelic variant (typically in patients of Asian descent)
Oxcarbazepine	300 mg bid, increase 300 mg/d q3d to goal 600-1200 bid	Abdominal symptoms Ataxia Diplopia, nystagmus vertigo	Hyponatremia SJS/TEN Angioedema Multiorgan hypersensitivity Pancytopenia	
Esclicarbazepine	400 mg daily, increase q7-14d to max 1200 mg daily	Dizziness Somnolence Nausea Headache Diplopia, blurred vision Vertigo Ataxia tremor	Hyponatremia Prolonged PR interval AV block Abnormal LFTs SJS/TEN	Severe hepatic impairment Prior hypersensitivity reaction to oxcarbazepine or carbamazepine
Pregabalin	75 mg bid, increase to max 600 mg/d given bid or tid	Weight gain Constipation Peripheral edema Xerostomia Ataxia Dizziness Diplopia, blurred vision	Angioedema Rhabdomyolysis Hypersensitivity reactions	
Gabapentin	300 mg tid, up to max 3600 mg tid	Somnolence Dizziness Nystagmus Peripheral edema Myalgias Rarely, myoclonus	SJS Seizures Coma	

(Continued)

TABLE 211-7 Antiepileptic Drugs: Recommended Daily Dosing for Healthy Adults, Side Effects, and Contraindications (*Continued*)

Drug	Dosing	Common Side Effects	Serious Side Effects	Contraindications
Tiagabine	4 mg/d, increase 4-8 mg/d weekly to max 56 mg/d divided bid or qid	Increase appetite Abdominal symptoms Parasthesias Pruritus Pharygnitis Confusion	Seizures Status epilepticus Sudden death SJS/TEN	
Ezogabine	100 mg tid, increase by 50 mg tid weekly to 200-400 mg tid	Dizziness Somnolence Weight gain	Urinary retention Retinal abnormalities and vision loss UTI Withdrawal seizures QT interval changes Behavioral changes	
Primidone	100-125 mg qHS × 3 d, increase 100-125 mg/d q3d to goal 250 mg tid	Ataxia Nausea/vomiting Dizziness Somnolence	Agranulocytosis Thrombocytopenia Megaloblastic anemia Hepatic failure SJS/TEN	Porphyria Barbiturate hypersensitivity
Vigabatrin	500 mg bid, increase by 500 mg weekly to max 1500 mg bid	Drowsiness Headache Dizziness Mood changes Weight gain	Permanent concentric visual field loss MRI abnormalities Angioedema Hypersensitivity reactions	
Clobazam	5 mg/d, increase q5d to max 40 mg/d. Doses above 30 mg/d should be divided	Excessive salivation Somnolence, insomnia Ataxia Dizziness Seizures Behavioral changes	Respiratory depression SJS/TEN	Significant hepatic failure Acute narrow angle glaucoma
Lacosamide	50 mg bid, increase 100 mg/d weekly to 200-400 mg/d	Diplopia Headache Dizziness	Prolonged PR interval AV block Syncope Hypersensitivity reactions Suicidal behavior	Severe hepatic impairment Severe cardiac disease AV block
Ethosuximide	500 mg/d, increase by 250 mg/d q4-7d to goal 20-30 mg/kg/d	Anorexia Abdominal symptoms Ataxia Dizziness Headaches Hiccups	Aplastic anemia Agranulocytosis SJS/TEN Hepatic failure Seizures	
Rufinamide	400-800 mg bid, increase by 400-800 mg/d q2d to max 1600 mg bid	Shortened QT interval Nausea/vomiting Dizziness Headache Lethargy	Suicidal behavior Dermatitis SJS/TEN	Familial short QT syndrome

AV, atrioventricular; DIC, disseminated intravascular coagulopathy; GI, gastrointestinal; LFTs, liver function tests; SJS, Stevens-Johnson syndrome; TEN, toxic epidermal necrolysis.

Sodium valproate, phenobarbital, and topiramate should be avoided if possible. Folate 1 mg daily is recommended, with an increase to 4 mg daily during pregnancy and prior to pregnancy, if pregnancy is planned or likely.

Hormonal fluctuations during puberty, pregnancy, menopause, and even during the menstrual cycle affect seizures. Catamenial seizures may occur just before or at the onset of menses, due to the drop in progesterone, or with ovulation due to the estrogen surge. No specific AED has been shown to have superior efficacy in the prevention of catamenial seizures. A patient experiencing severe breakthrough catamenial seizures merits consultation with an epileptologist.

Epilepsy may reduce fertility in women with epilepsy, and there is a higher rate of polycystic ovarian syndrome and anovulatory cycles in this population. Some AEDs increase the risk of major congenital malformations following *in utero* exposure. The risk of malformations is related to the individual AED as well as other factors, and the benefit of ongoing treatment with an appropriate AED is felt to outweigh the increased risk of congenital malformations. AEDs that affect folic acid metabolism or are enzyme inducers have the greatest increased risk of congenital malformations. Carbamazepine, phenytoin, phenobarbital, and topiramate are associated with an increased incidence of midline congenital malformations, such as cleft lip, cleft palate, and hypospadias.

Valproic acid confers the greatest risk of major congenital malformations, as well as cognitive impairment and behavioral changes, and it is now labeled pregnancy Category X. The risk of cognitive impairment or congenital malformation increases with polypharmacy, particularly if the polypharmacy includes valproic acid. The mean IQ of children exposed *in utero* to AEDs was higher among those whose mothers took folic acid supplementation, so a prenatal vitamin is especially important in this patient group. Rates of congenital malformations and neurocognitive outcomes appear to be low for levetiracetam and lamotrigine. However, the dose of lamotrigine may require frequent adjustment by an epileptologist during the course of the pregnancy and in the postpartum period.

Although AEDs are expressed in breastmilk, concentrations in breastmilk are lower than they are in maternal serum, and the serum levels in the child are significantly lower than the maternal paired serum concentrations. Recent data suggests that in children born to women with epilepsy, the overall cognitive benefit of breastfeeding that is conferred on all children outweighs any adverse impact of consumption of maternal AED while breastfeeding. It is recommended that women attempt to breastfeed, as with any child, and that they continue AED therapy during this time.

For 53% to 64% of women with epilepsy, their seizure frequency does not change during pregnancy, and for 16% to 23% it decreases. In the remaining 17% to 24% of pregnant women with epilepsy, their seizures increase in frequency or severity, typically due either to nonadherence or pharmacokinetic changes associated with pregnancy. As many pregnancies are not planned, the best maternal and fetal outcomes result from working with women with epilepsy to select an appropriate regimen prior to pregnancy, with education on the risk of major congenital malformations, the importance of contraception, and drug interactions with AEDs. Women with epilepsy should be told to contact their physician once they realize they are pregnant prior to making any medication changes. Some women with epilepsy may benefit from referral to an epileptologist or a neurologist specializing in caring for women with neurological issues during their pregnancy.

SPECIAL CONSIDERATIONS IN THE ELDERLY

The most common identifiable cause of new-onset seizures in the elderly is cerebrovascular disease, which accounts for up to one-half of acute seizures in older patients. Seizures are more likely in large hemorrhagic strokes with cortical involvement. Alzheimer dementia and other neurodegenerative disorders are another important cause of seizures in geriatric patients. Older patients are often prescribed antidepressants and antipsychotics, which may lower the seizure threshold. Other causes of new-onset seizures in the elderly include metabolic disturbances, trauma, and tumors. Seizures in this patient population are often focal in onset, with or without secondary generalization. Focal seizures with dyscognitive features in the elderly most often originate in the temporal lobe and manifest as episodes of confusion and staring into space; oral and motor automatisms are usually absent, which makes them difficult to detect. Older patients often have prolonged postictal confusion and sedation. The geriatric patient is more vulnerable to sedation, hyponatremia, drug-drug interactions, and other side effects of AEDs. Drug clearance may be reduced in the setting of age-related renal or hepatic failure.

STATUS EPILEPTICUS

The traditional definition of SE is a prolonged seizure, or cluster of seizures, without a return to baseline, lasting longer than 30 minutes. A revised operational definition is any seizure lasting more than 5 minutes or two or more seizures without return to baseline. This reflects the fact that spontaneous termination is less likely in any seizure lasting longer than 5 minutes, and that aggressive treatment should be initiated to reduce morbidity and mortality. Status epilepticus may feature focal seizures, with or without dyscognitive features, generalized tonic-clonic seizures, absence seizures, or may be nonconvulsive (ie, subclinical). Up to 50% of cases of SE occur in patients with epilepsy due to recent changes in AEDs or nonadherence. The remainder of cases in adults are most often secondary to stroke.

SE is a medical emergency, with mortality ranging from 7% to 40%. Predictors of mortality include generalized seizure, increased patient age, anoxic brain injury, stroke, CNS infection or tumor, and duration of SE. Adverse consequences of SE include hypoxia, hypotension, acidosis, hyperthermia, rhabdomyolysis, and neuronal injury. Successful outcomes require early and aggressive treatment. The discussion that follows provides guidelines for the treatment of generalized SE (summarized in **Figure 211-2**).

■ SUPPORTIVE TREATMENT

Once the diagnosis of SE is made, treatment should start immediately. Initial treatment consists of stabilization of airway, breathing, and circulation and administration of oxygen while blood is drawn for laboratory studies. It is recommended that the patient be treated empirically with IV thiamine 100 mg and 50 mL of 50% glucose.

■ PHARMACOLOGIC TREATMENT

First line

IV benzodiazepines are the first-line drug treatment of SE. Diazepam, midazolam, and lorazepam have all been used successfully. Lorazepam is more effective than diazepam, with no difference in adverse events. Midazolam has not been adequately evaluated in comparative studies. Therefore, lorazepam is recommended, with an initial 1 to 2 mg IV bolus, followed by sequential boluses at intervals of 5 minutes, up to a total of 0.1 mg/kg. If there is no IV access, alternative therapy with diazepam 20 mg PR or midazolam 10 mg intranasally, intrabuccally or IM may be considered, though these formulations may not be available or may be impractical.

Second line

While benzodiazepines are being given, a long-acting AED should also be given IV. Phenytoin has traditionally been used. Fosphenytoin is now recommended, as it can be administered more quickly and has a lower risk of cardiovascular complications. Fosphenytoin is dosed in phenytoin equivalents (PE); 75 mg of fosphenytoin is

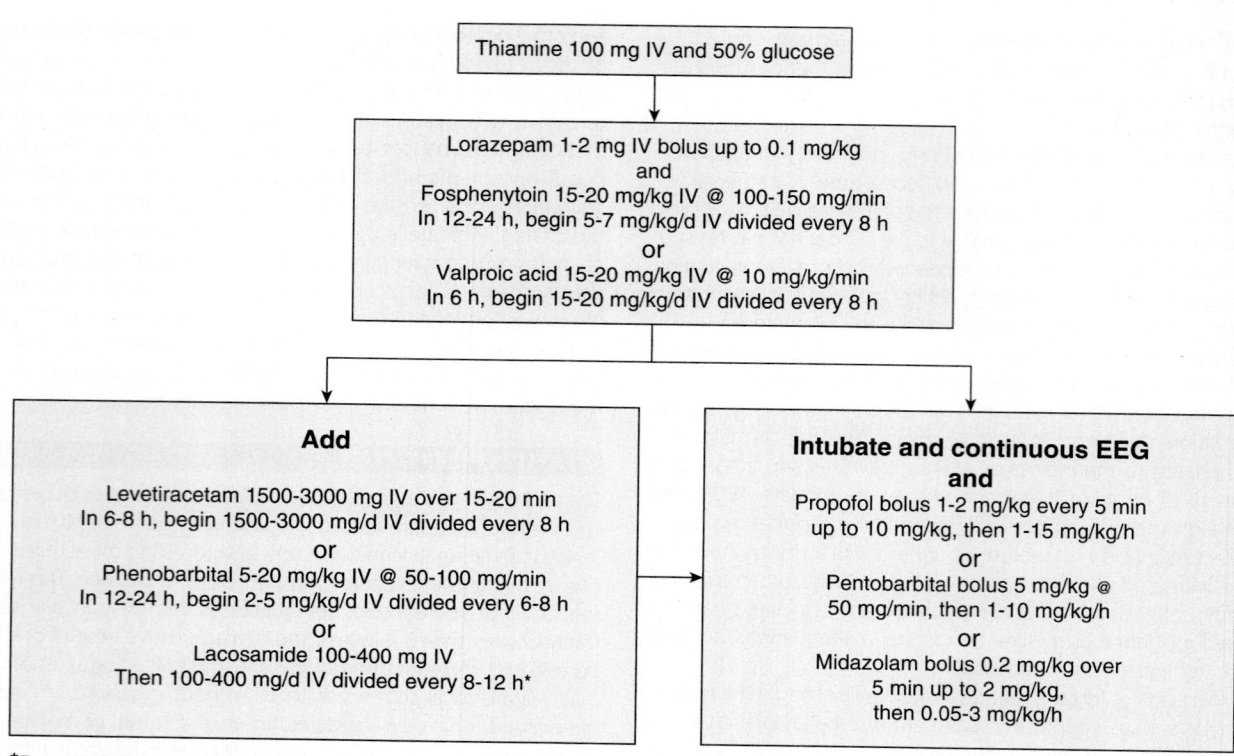

Figure 211-2 *Treatment protocol for status epilepticus. (EEG, electroencephalogram; SE, status epilepticus.)*

equivalent to 50 mg of phenytoin. The loading dose of fosphenytoin is 15 to 20 mg PE/kg, at a rate of 100 to 150 mg PE/min, with careful attention to the patient's blood pressure and heart rate. Maintenance therapy can be started 12 to 24 hours after the initial load, at 5 to 7 mg PE/kg/d divided into doses administered every 8 hours.

A reasonable alternative is IV valproic acid. The initial loading dose is 20 to 30 mg/kg given IV over ~15 minutes. A maintenance dose of 15 to 20 mg/kg/d given in 8-hour intervals should be started within 6 hours of the initial load. Serum AED levels should be followed, and extra doses should be given as necessary to maintain levels at the high end of the therapeutic range. Although levetiracetam is not, strictly speaking, indicated as monotherapy for treatment of partial seizures or primary generalized epilepsy, it is frequently used in treating first-time seizures as well as SE due to the fact that an IV formulation exists, it has few drug-drug interactions, and is generally well tolerated by patients. An initial loading dose is levetiracetam 20 to 30 mg/kg, and maintenance dosing as per Table 211-7 may be started 12 hours later.

Third line

There is currently debate about the next line of therapy if seizures continue after treatment with benzodiazepines and an AED. Conventional algorithms recommend IV loading doses of a second AED, such as valproic acid, phenobarbital, levetiracetam, and lacosamide. Phenobarbital is known to be very effective in SE, but it must be given slowly to minimize the risks of hypotension and cardiac side effects. In addition, it causes severe respiratory depression, and most patients treated with phenobarbital require intubation. Levetiracetam and lacosamide are both available in IV formulations and can be given rapidly with few adverse side effects. However, there is little published data regarding efficacy of either drug in SE.

More aggressive treatment protocols for SE have been proposed recently, in which SE that persists after treatment with two AEDs,

including a benzodiazepine, is classified as refractory SE. At this stage, it may be difficult to ascertain on exam alone if a patient is experiencing ongoing seizures, as there may be no visible motor movements, so evaluation with an EEG is recommended. The rationale for this proposal is based on evidence that neuronal cell death begins after 30 minutes of continuous seizures. From a practical point of view, 30 minutes will have elapsed by the time a patient in SE has been stabilized and treated with benzodiazepines and one AED. Hence, these schemes recommend that the administration of a second AED should be skipped and aggressive treatment for refractory SE started.

Refractory status epilepticus

Treatment of patients in refractory SE involves intubation and coma induction with an anesthetic agent in the intensive care unit (ICU). Continuous EEG monitoring is required. Anesthesia is given continuously, with the dose titrated to cause suppression of the background activity on EEG. Agents used most often are propofol, midazolam, and pentobarbital or phenobarbital. In a literature review, pentobarbital was reported as most effective in stopping seizures, but also more likely to cause hypotension and prolonged hospitalization. No difference in mortality was found. Coma is typically maintained for 24 to 48 hours, after which the anesthetic is weaned. If seizures recur, other treatments can be attempted, such as the addition of other AEDs, ketamine, lidocaine, or electroconvulsive therapy. The prognosis in this situation is very poor.

Partial status epilepticus

SE due to focal seizure with dyscognitive features is not as clinically dramatic as generalized SE. Patients often present in a twilight state or with persistent confusion. An EEG should be obtained in such patients to avoid a misdiagnosis of psychiatric disease. Aggressive medical therapy is recommended for SE due to focal seizure with dyscognitive features. SE due to focal seizure without dyscognitive features usually manifests as repetitive focal motor seizures (epilepsia partialis continua) and typically reflects an acute cortical injury, cerebral inflammatory process or mass lesion. Epilepsia partialis continua is often resistant to treatment with AEDs, but the morbidity and mortality of focal seizure without dyscognitive features SE are relatively low. The risks and benefits of medical therapy must be carefully assessed when deciding how aggressively to treat this entity.

Nonconvulsive status epilepticus

Ongoing seizure activity on EEG in the absence of clinical seizures is termed *nonconvulsive status epilepticus (NCSE)*, also known as subclinical status. It is often unrecognized, especially in comatose patients in the ICU. NCSE is most common after clinical generalized SE appears to have resolved, with a reported incidence of 14% to 20%. In studies, NCSE was found on EEG in 8% to 17% of patients in coma without signs of clinical seizures during hospitalization. This evidence highlights the importance of obtaining an EEG in patients with SE after it appears that clinical seizures have stopped, and in critically ill patients in coma of unclear etiology. As with SE, ongoing NCSE may cause lasting neuronal injury or cell death, so prompt recognition and treatment of NCSE affects prognosis.

■ EDUCATION, SAFETY, AND PREVENTION

Patients with epilepsy and a first-time seizure are often keen to learn their prognosis and how their daily life may be affected. It is often helpful to explain seizures in order to frame a conversation with patients and families about patient safety and seizure prevention.

Seizures can be scary to witness, and family members and friends often are confused about what they should do when they witness the patient having a generalized seizure. The hospitalist should educate them on how to protect the patient, including turning the patient on his or her side and cushioning the head, arms, and legs. Families and friends should be reminded that forcibly restraining the patient or placing something in the mouth to prevent swallowing or severing the tongue is inappropriate and may cause unintentional harm to the patient.

Patients with a first seizure as well as patients with chronic epilepsy should be reminded to avoid risk factors for seizure recurrence, including sleep deprivation, alcohol and recreational drugs, medication noncompliance, and severe stress. Patients should be counseled on the importance of taking medications as scheduled and common side effects of any AEDs. For patients with chronic epilepsy, a seizure calendar may be helpful for future medication adjustments. Other recommendations for patient protection are the avoidance of activities that could result in injury or even death of the patient or those around them should they have a seizure while participating in that activity. Typical examples of such activities include heights, unsupervised baths, operating heavy machinery or power tools, swimming without close supervision, and driving. Patients should be educated on when they should seek further medical help after they return home, and should be provided with a contact number if appropriate.

The hospitalist must discuss driving restrictions with a patient who has had a seizure. This conversation is often unpleasant, as these limitations invariably distress the patient. To correctly advise the patient, the hospitalist should be aware that driving laws and recommendations vary from state to state. Regulations for each state can be found on the Epilepsy Foundation website at www.epilepsyfoundation.org.

DISCHARGE CHECKLIST

- Have the patient and family been educated about protective measures in the event of a future seizure, including putting the patient on a flat surface on his or her side, avoiding restraining the patient or putting anything in the patient's mouth, and recording the time of the onset of the seizure?
- Have restrictions on driving and avoidance of hazardous activities and situations been discussed with the patient?
- Has the patient been cautioned to avoid triggers, such as drugs, alcohol, and sleep deprivation?
- Does the patient have a medical alert bracelet or pendant indicating their seizure history?
- Has follow-up been arranged with the patient's primary care provider and neurologist?
- Have referrals to other providers, such as a psychiatrist or psychologist for counseling, been considered? Mood disorders are a common comorbidity of epilepsy, and the stress of living with epilepsy can precipitate or exacerbate mood disorders. Neuropsychological evaluation may be useful for patients with epilepsy who complain of memory loss. Social services are often helpful for patients with epilepsy and difficulty with employment, housing, and cost of medications. Finally, referral to an epileptologist should be considered for patients with recurrent seizures or where the diagnosis remains unclear.

SUGGESTED READINGS

Bayrlee A, Ganeshalingam N, Kurczewski L, Brophy GM. Treatment of super-refractory status epilepticus. *Curr Neurol Neurosci Rep.* 2015;15:589.

Berg AT. Risk of recurrence after a first unprovoked seizure. *Epilepsia.* 2008;49(Suppl 1):13-18.

Brophy GM, Bell R, Claassen J, et al. Guidelines for the evaluation and management of status epilepticus. *Neurocrit Care.* 2012;17:3-23.

Claassen J, Hirsch LJ, Emerson RG, et al. Treatment of refractory status epilepticus with pentobarbital, propofol, or midazolam: a systematic review. *Epilepsia.* 2002;43:146-153.

Claassen J, Mayer SA, Kowalski RG, et al. Detection of electrographic seizures with continuous EEG monitoring in critically ill patients. *Neurology.* 2004;62:1743-1748.

DeLorenzo RJ, Waterhouse EJ, Towne AR, et al. Persistent nonconvulsive status epilepticus after control of convulsive status epilepticus. *Epilepsia.* 1998;39:833-840.

Glauser T, Ben-Menachem E, Bourgeois B, et al. Updated ILAE evidence review of antiepileptic drug efficacy and effectiveness as initial monotherapy for epileptic seizures and syndromes. *Epilepsia.* 2013;54:551-563.

Krumholz A, Wiebe S, Gronseth G, et al. Practice parameter: evaluating an apparent unprovoked first seizure in adults (an evidence-based review). *Neurology.* 2007;69:1996-2007.

Marson A, Jacoby A, Johnson A, et al. Immediate versus deferred antiepileptic drug treatment for early epilepsy and single seizures: A randomized controlled trial. *Lancet.* 2005;365:2007-2013.

Prasad K, Krishnan PR, Al-Roomi K, et al. Anticonvulsant therapy for status epilepticus. *Br J Clin Pharmacol.* 2007;63:640-647.

Rossetti A, Lowenstein D. Management of refractory status epilepticus in adults: still more questions than answers. *Lancet.* 2011;10:922-930.

Treiman DM, Meyers PD, Walton NY, et al. A comparison of four treatments for generalized convulsive status epilepticus. *N Eng J Med.* 1998;339:792-798.

Wiebe S, Tellez-Zenteno JF, Shapiro M. An evidence-based approach to the first seizure. *Epilepsia.* 2008;49(Suppl 1):50-57.

CHAPTER 212

Multiple Sclerosis

John J. Ross, MD, CM, FIDSA

Allan H. Ropper, MD, FRCP

Key Clinical Questions

❶ What are the major disease manifestations and complications of multiple sclerosis?

❷ How are exacerbations of multiple sclerosis treated?

❸ What are treatment options for complicating symptoms of multiple sclerosis, such as fatigue, bladder dysfunction, and spasticity?

❹ What disease-modifying agents are available to treat multiple sclerosis? What are their major toxicities and long-term risks?

INTRODUCTION

Multiple sclerosis (MS) in its most typical form is an autoimmune, T-cell-driven disease of the central nervous system characterized initially by demyelination and, eventually, by axonal destruction and neuronal loss. It is the most common neurologic disease of young adults.

EPIDEMIOLOGY

The peak age of onset is between 20 and 40 years with a twofold higher incidence in women. It has long been observed that latitude of residence in childhood is a risk factor for the development of the disease. Multiple sclerosis is rare in equatorial areas, and the prevalence rises sharply with increasing distance from the equator. Potential explanations for this phenomenon include geographical clustering of susceptibility genes, effects of ultraviolet light exposure in childhood on immune development, and latitudinal variation in vitamin D levels. Low vitamin D levels early in the course of multiple sclerosis are associated with increased size and number of lesions on MRI, and a higher risk of relapse and disability.

Genetic factors play a major role in the development of MS, and a family history is present in 15% of patients and 3% to 5% in first degree relatives. The major histocompatibility complex alleles, among them HLA-DRB1*1501, and two cytokine receptor genes, the interleukin 7 receptor alpha chain gene (IL7RA) and the interleukin 2 receptor alpha chain gene (IL2RA), have been implicated. Susceptibility to MS is likely polygenic, with the contribution of any single locus being small. Clusters of MS cases have suggested an infectious trigger, with limited data to implicate EBV. Smoking, obesity, and high salt intake have inconsistently been implicated as MS risk factors.

CLINICAL PRESENTATION

■ SYMPTOMS

Multiple sclerosis is characteristically a relapsing and remitting disease, but there is great variation in its course. Common presenting symptoms of MS are summarized in **Table 212-1**. Weakness, numbness, or both in one or more limbs are common first symptoms. Patients may have paresthesias in the extremities or a band-like tightness around the trunk or limbs. The legs may feel heavy or difficult to control. Neck flexion may cause a sensation of electric shocks in the shoulders, back, and occasionally in the thighs. This finding, known as the Lhermitte sign, may also be present in cervical spondylosis, vitamin B12 deficiency, radiation myelopathy, and other conditions affecting the cervical spine.

Certain acute or subacute clinical syndromes are particularly characteristic of MS, although they also occur in association with other diseases of the nervous system. *Optic neuritis* most often presents with a deep aching sensation in the eye for a day or two, followed by rapid visual loss over several days or less. It is usually unilateral, but may be bilateral or sequential. Swelling of the optic nerve head (papillitis) is seen in 10% of patients; the majority of cases are retrobulbar and show a normal disc head. In *acute myelitis*, patients develop paraparesis or paraplegia over hours to days, with extensor plantar responses, ascending paresthesias, a sensory level on the trunk, and impaired sphincter function. *Cerebellar ataxia* and *brainstem syndromes* with vertigo or diplopia are also frequent. Sphincter dysfunction, especially urinary urgency, is common as the disease progresses.

TABLE 212-1 Predominant Presenting Symptoms of Multiple Sclerosis

Paresthesias and other sensory disturbances	37%-45%
Motor weakness	20%-27%
Disturbance of gait or balance	13%-35%
Vision loss or optic neuritis	15%-17%
Diplopia and/or vertigo	10%-13%

Data from Swanson JW. *Mayo Clin Proc.* 1989;64:577-586; Weinshenker BG, Bass B, Rice GP, et al. *Brain.* 1989;112(Pt 1):133-146.

■ SIGNS

Common examination findings include hyperreflexia, extensor plantar responses, lower-extremity ataxia, impaired rapid alternating movements, and loss of distal vibration and proprioceptive sensation. Evidence of optic neuropathy may be present, either obvious (visual loss) or subtle (afferent pupillary defect). Previous episodes of optic neuritis cause optic nerve atrophy. Less frequent findings include nystagmus, intention tremor, spasticity, dysarthria, and paraparesis. Unilateral internuclear ophthalmoplegia is another characteristic finding but is not common.

NATURAL HISTORY

Most patients (85%) initially fall into the category of relapsing-remitting MS, undergoing symptomatic flares (relapses) with incomplete recovery (remission). Emotional stress and infections have tentatively been associated with flares. The postpartum period is another frequent time of relapse; MS often abates during pregnancy. In 10% of patients, the disease has little response to treatment and progresses inexorably from the onset (primary progressive MS). A minority (5%) have "benign" MS, with few relapses and little disease progression 10 to 15 years after diagnosis. Most patients with relapsing-remitting MS eventually develop a secondary progressive course characterized by steady neurologic deterioration and pathologically, by a progression from demyelination to axonal loss. The cervical cord is particularly prone to disease in these cases. Cerebral atrophy is found in a large proportion of patients with longstanding disease.

DIAGNOSIS

The diagnosis of MS requires evidence of dissemination of disease in both space and time, although the time-honored requirement for clinical relapses has been replaced by imaging evidence of lesions of varying ages and in several central nervous system locations (**Table 212-2**). The major diagnostic test for MS is now magnetic resonance imaging (MRI). Typical lesions on MRI are bright on T2-weighted and fluid-attenuation inversion recovery images, consistent with high water content (**Figure 212-1**). Early lesions are isodense on T1-weighted images and display enhancement with gadolinium, but more advanced ones may be T1 isodense, indicating necrosis ("black holes"). Typical locations, often asymptomatic, are the periventricular regions, corpus callosum, cerebellar peduncles, and cervical spinal cord.

Lumbar puncture is helpful but not mandatory for the diagnosis of MS. The cerebrospinal fluid (CSF) may display a minimal increase in lymphocytes (usually < 20/mm³) and in total protein content. Levels of myelin basic protein may be increased during disease flares. Elevations of the IgG fraction of protein and oligoclonal bands on electrophoresis are the most sensitive CSF tests for MS, but these may also be present in infectious and inflammatory conditions, such

TABLE 212-2 The 2010 Revised McDonald Criteria for the Diagnosis of MS

The diagnosis of multiple sclerosis requires demonstration of dissemination of lesions in both time and space, as follows:

Dissemination in time	Dissemination in space
≥ 2 attacks	Objective clinical evidence of ≥ 2 lesions
OR	OR
Simultaneous gadolinium-enhancing and non-enhancing lesions on MRI at any time	≥ 1 T2 lesion in at least 2 of 4 typical locations (periventricular, juxtacortical, infratentorial, spinal cord)
OR	
A new T2 and/or enhancing lesion on follow-up MRI, in addition to a previously documented MRI lesion	

The diagnosis of primary progressive MS requires 1 y of insidious neurological progression, plus 2 of 3 of the following:

1. ≥ 1 T2 lesions in at least 1 area characteristic for MS (periventricular, juxtacortical, or infratentorial);
2. ≥ 2 T2 lesions in the cord;
3. Positive CSF (isoelectric focusing evidence of oligoclonal bands and/or elevated IgG index)

CSF, cerebrospinal fluid; MRI, magnetic resonance imaging; MS, multiple sclerosis.
Data from Polman CH, Reingold SC, Banwell B, et al. *Ann Neurol.* 2011;69:292-302.

as Lyme disease, HIV, and neurosarcoidosis. Abnormal visual-evoked potentials support the diagnosis of MS by demonstrating otherwise inevident optic nerve damage.

PRACTICE POINT

- The diagnosis of multiple sclerosis should be made with caution if a patient's symptoms and signs can be explained by a single lesion. A definitive diagnosis of multiple sclerosis requires demonstration of multiple lesions with evolution over time (dissemination in space and time), either clinically or on MRI. Imaging can show lesions of different ages, thereby fulfilling these diagnostic criteria.

PRACTICE POINT

- Multiple sclerosis may begin as a clinically isolated syndrome, such as optic neuritis, acute myelitis, or acute brainstem syndrome, without definite evidence of disseminated MS. Treatment of patients with clinically isolated syndromes using disease-modifying agents may reduce the risk of evolution to clinically definite MS.

DIFFERENTIAL DIAGNOSIS

A number of infectious, inflammatory, vascular, and genetic conditions may mimic MS, both clinically and radiologically (**Table 212-3**). The diagnosis is most difficult early in the course of the disease, when evidence for dissemination in space and time are lacking, or when the disease runs a progressive course without periodic

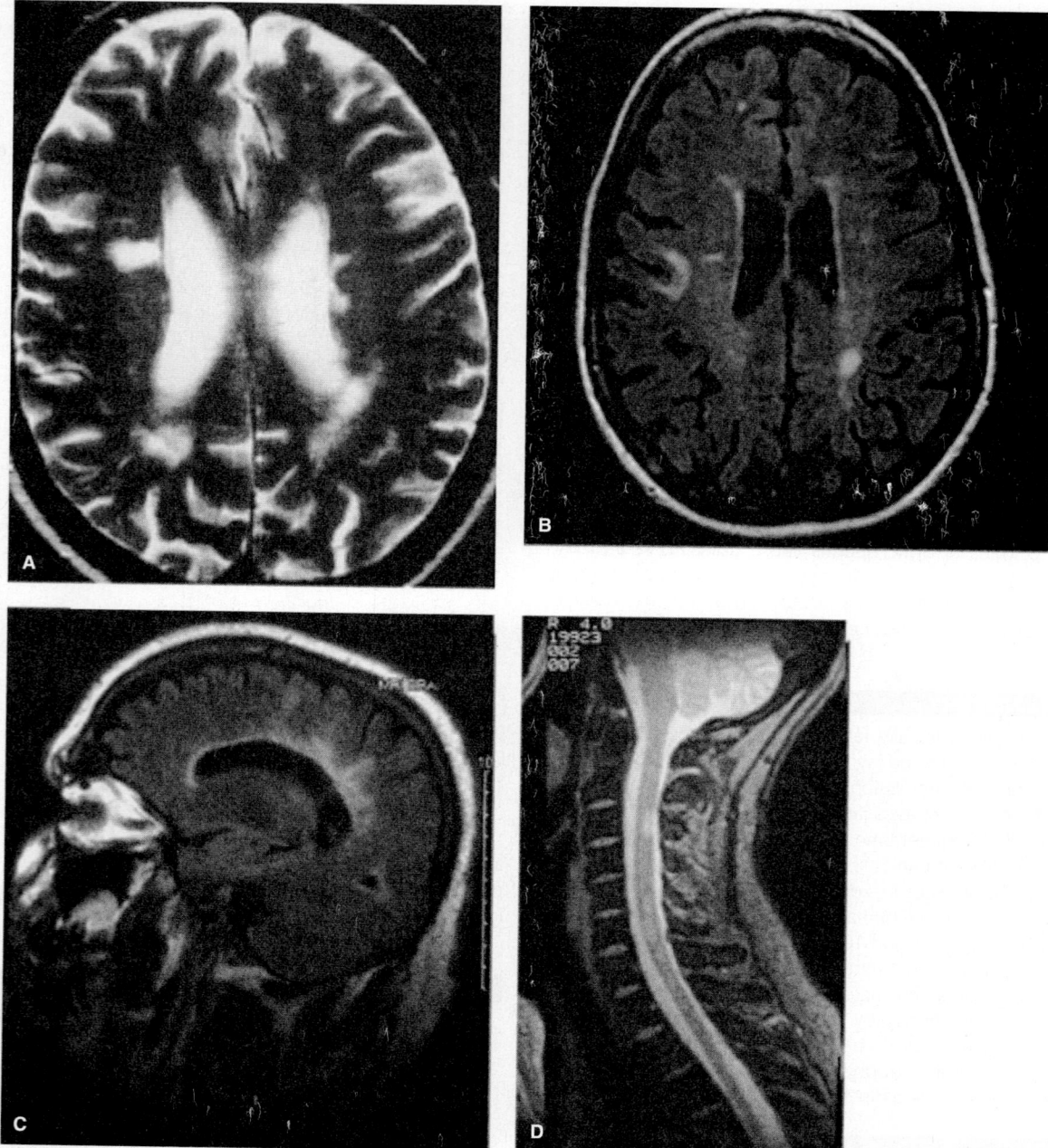

Figure 212-1 *Multiple sclerosis. T2-weighted and fluid-attenuated inversion recovery (FLAIR) sequence MRIs demonstrating multiple plaques in the periventricular white matter (A), emanating radially from the corpus callosum ("Dawson fingers"; B), a "C-like"–shaped lesion in the right subcortical white matter that is created by interruption of the lesion by the adjacent cortex (C) and cervical spinal cord (D) . The radial orientation and periventricular location of cerebral lesions are typical of MS. (Reproduced, with permission, from Ropper AH, Samuels MA. Adam's & Victor's Principles of Neurology, 9th ed. New York, NY: McGraw-Hill; 2009. Fig. 36-1.)*

exacerbations. Connective tissue diseases, particularly lupus and Sjögren syndrome, may cause multifocal inflammatory lesions in the cord or brain that mimic MS ("lupus sclerosis"). The presence of systemic features (eg, fever, sweats, or rigors) or involvement of other organ systems (eg, arthritis, rash, sicca syndrome, or peripheral neuropathy) suggests an underlying systemic disorder that is causing secondary lesions in the nervous system, rather than MS.

TREATMENT

■ DISEASE-MODIFYING TREATMENT

Treatments for multiple sclerosis and their major toxicities are summarized in **Table 212-4**. In the majority of patients, MS is an initially

relapsing and remitting disease that eventually becomes progressive. The early form of disease is treated with "disease modifying agents," which reduce the number of relapses and may improve long-term outcome, including retention of cognitive ability. If one treatment is not tolerated, or fails as evidenced by disease progression or frequent relapses, another is substituted. There are differences in the approach to treatment between specialized MS centers, both in the choice of the first drug to be tried and in subsequent treatments. The recent inception of oral agents, generally but not uniformly preferred by patients has produced even wider variability in practice. Beyond disease modification, aggressive treatment with monoclonal antibodies or immunosuppression is reserved for patients with rapid progression and threatening deficits. There are

TABLE 212-3 Differential Diagnosis of Multiple Sclerosis

Infections

Neurosyphilis

HIV

Lyme disease

Progressive multifocal leukoencephalopathy (PML)

Human T-cell lymphotropic virus 1 (HTLV-1, tropical spastic paraparesis)

Neurobrucellosis

Inflammatory conditions

Systemic lupus erythematosus

Sjögren syndrome

Mixed connective tissue disease

Systemic sclerosis

Behçet disease

Neurosarcoidosis

Central nervous system vasculitis

Toxic-metabolic disturbances

Vitamin B12 deficiency

Vascular conditions

Cerebrovascular disease

Vascular malformations with recurrent bleeding

Antiphospholipid antibody syndrome

Microinfarcts due to polycythemia vera or thrombocytosis

Subacute bacterial endocarditis with recurrent emboli

Cerebral autosomal dominant arteriopathy with subcortical infarcts and leukoencephalopathy (CADASIL)

Genetic disorders

Adrenoleukodystrophy

Mitochondrial diseases

Spinocerebellar ataxias

Structural conditions and mass lesions

Central nervous system lymphoma

Syringomyelia

Tumors of the foramen magnum and posterior fossa

Platybasia

Chiari malformation

Cervical spondylosis

Herniated disc

Other demyelinating diseases

Acute disseminated encephalomyelitis

no clearly effective therapies for MS that is primarily progressive from the outset, and it has been hypothesized that this represents a different form of the disease. It is uncertain if therapy is effective in delaying or preventing a secondary phase of relapsing-remitting disease or affecting the course of secondarily progressive disease.

Glatiramer acetate (subcutaneous) and the beta-interferons (subcutaneous or intramuscular) have similar efficacy as disease modifiers, reducing the yearly risk of relapse by about 30%. Until recently, these have been the most widely used agents for MS. Glatiramer is a preferred first nonoral agent in some centers, partly because autoantibodies to the drug are not problematic, as they may be with interferon. Glatiramer may cause anxiety and panic attacks,

and interferons may elicit depression. Both produce an acute flu-like syndrome that abates with time in most patients, and is mitigated by premedication.

Dimethyl fumarate is a newly available agent with a relatively favorable safety profile. Flushing and gastrointestinal symptoms are common, but usually limited in duration. Dimethyl fumarate leads to lymphopenia, and it should be used with caution in patients with reduced lymphocyte counts. Rare cases of progressive multifocal leukoencephalopathy (PML) (see below) have occurred. Fingolimod, another oral agent, is more effective at reducing relapse rates than interferon beta-1a. Adverse effects include transient bradycardia in the first few days of therapy, macular edema, and hepatitis. Rates of serious infections appear to be increased, including pneumonia, disseminated varicella zoster infection, and herpes simplex encephalitis. Patients should have documentation of varicella immunity prior to initiation of fingolimod.

Among several available monoclonal antibodies, rituximab, ocrelizumab, and alemtuzumab, are moderately to highly effective in reducing relapse rates. The target antigen for rituximab and ocrelizuman is CD20. The target antigen for alemtuzumab is CD52, an antigen found on both lymphocytes and monocytes. As a result, it depletes T cells, B cells, and natural killer cells, and may lead to both opportunistic infections such as cytomegalovirus disease and PML, and autoimmune disorders, such as Graves disease and immune thrombocytopenic purpura. Patients on alemtuzumab should be on antibiotic prophylaxis against both *Pneumocystis jiroveci* and herpes viruses.

Intravenous monthly natalizumab is among the most effective agents for aggressive relapsing-remitting MS, reducing relapse rates by over 60%. However, its use in 0.1% of cases is complicated by progressive multifocal leukoencephalopathy, caused by reactivation of John Cunningham (JC) virus. The risk of PML is highest in patients with positive JC virus titers and prior treatment with immunosuppressive therapies. Natalizumab is currently reserved for patients who have failed or are intolerant of other disease-modifying therapies, or those who have rapid progression of MS with an abundance of active lesions on MRI. Multiple sclerosis patients who develop new neurologic symptoms on natalizumab should have an MRI. If it is not possible to exclude PML based on MRI (**Figure 212-2**), a lumbar puncture should be performed, and cerebrospinal fluid should be sent for polymerase chain reaction for JC virus. PML in most clinical settings is usually fatal. However, patients with PML due to natalizumab may recover if the drug is stopped immediately and patients undergo plasma exchange, immunoadsorption, or both to rapidly remove natalizumab, which may otherwise persist for many months. Patients may experience worsening of symptoms and enlarging lesions on MRI days to weeks after cessation of natalizumab, a phenomenon that is likely attributable to immune reconstitution inflammatory syndrome (IRIS), as seen more commonly in HIV-infected patients treated with highly active antiviral therapy. Patients with IRIS benefit from corticosteroid therapy to reduce inflammation and prevent immune-inflicted neurologic damage.

A number of other drugs such as methotrexate, azathioprine, and mycophenylate have been used sporadically and mainly in Europe. Mitoxantrone has been used in limited fashion in the secondary progressive phase of MS, but it has cardiac toxicity with cumulative doses.

■ **ACUTE RELAPSES**

Acute symptomatic relapses of MS may be treated with pulses of high-dose corticosteroids. A typical regimen is methylprednisolone 1 g intravenously daily for 3 to 5 days. Some authorities recommend following this with a short course of tapering doses of oral prednisone. Prior to treatment, MRI is generally performed to assess for

TABLE 212-4 Typical Drug Therapy of Multiple Sclerosis

Drug	Dosage and Route	Mechanism	Side Effects
Primary progressive multiple sclerosis			
No therapies with proven efficacy at present			
Relapsing-remitting multiple sclerosis			
Alemtuzumab (Lemtrada)	12 mg intravenous infusion daily for 5 d, followed by 12 mg infusion daily for 3 d 1 y later	Monoclonal antibody directed against CD52, an antigen found on the cell surface of mature lymphocytes, monocytes, and dendritic cells	"AIDS in a bottle": robust, long-lasting immune suppression due to depletion of B-cell and T-cell lymphocytes; increased risk of infection with fungi, viruses, tuberculosis, *Listeria*, and *Legionella*; risk of autoimmune disease increased, especially autoimmune thyroid disease and immune thrombocytopenic purpura, because of shift from Th1 to Th2 immune responses; infusion reactions such as rash, fever, and headache are also common
Dimethyl fumarate (BG-12, Tecfidera)	240 mg orally twice daily	Exact mechanism of action unclear; may downregulate Th1 immune responses and enhance neuronal resistance to oxidative damage	Flushing, headache, GI upset; risk of opportunistic infection in patients with lymphopenia
Fingolimod (Gilenya)	0.5 mg orally once daily	Sphingosine 1-phosphate receptor modulator; blocks egress of lymphocytes from peripheral lymph nodes, indirectly leading to decreased lymphocyte migration into the central nervous system	Transient bradycardia and decreased atrioventricular node conduction with first few doses, monitor for bradycardia for at least six hours after the initial dose; macular edema, cough, altered pulmonary function tests, headache, diarrhea, altered liver enzymes, back pain, infections, especially reactivation of varicella and herpes simplex
Glatiramer (Copaxone)	20 mg subcutaneously once daily	Polypeptide mixture with structural resemblance to myelin basic protein; produces bystander suppression, activates anti-inflammatory Th2 cells, blocks autoreactive T cells, and induces anergy; onset of action is delayed for several months	Injection site reactions, flulike symptoms, chest pain, tachypnea, facial erythema, urticaria, fat necrosis at recurrent injection sites
Interferon beta-1a (Avonex)	30 µg intramuscularly once weekly	Do not cross blood-brain barrier; may act by blocking peripheral T-cell activation and proliferation, and by inducing apoptosis of autoreactive T cells	Fatigue, fever, flulike symptoms, injection-site reactions, neutropenia, liver function test elevations, depression; efficacy may be hindered by the formation of anti-interferon antibodies in some patients, especially with more frequent dosing regimens some patients, especially with more frequent dosing regimens
Interferon beta-1a (Rebif)	44 µg subcutaneously three times weekly		
Peginterferon beta-1a (Plegridy)	125 µg subcutaneously every 2 wk		
Interferon beta-1b (Betaseron)	250 µg subcutaneously every other day		
Natalizumab (Tysabri)	300 mg intravenously every 4 wk	Monoclonal antibody against the lymphocyte α4-β1 integrin receptor; prevents lymphocyte binding to vascular endothelial cells and inhibits lymphocyte migration into the central nervous system	Headache, fatigue, arthralgias, infections, and infusion reactions, including anaphylaxis; about 0.1% of patients develop progressive multifocal leukoencephalopathy (PML)
Teriflunomide (Aubagio)	7 or 14 mg orally once daily	Active metabolite of leflunomide; inhibits pyrimidine synthesis; disrupts the interaction of antigen-presenting cells and T cells	Diarrhea, nausea, vomiting, hair loss, rash, hypertension, peripheral neuropathy, interstitial lung disease, elevated liver enzymes (avoid in known liver disease)
Secondary progressive multiple sclerosis			
Mitoxantrone	12 mg/m^2 intravenously every 3 months, to a maximum lifetime dose of 140 mg/m^2	Topoisomerase inhibitor; impairs DNA synthesis and repair; broad-spectrum immunosuppressive agent	Cardiac toxicity, nausea, alopecia, neutropenia, anemia

Agents with limited supporting evidence: Azathioprine, cyclophosphamide, methotrexate, mycophenolate mofetil, simvastatin.

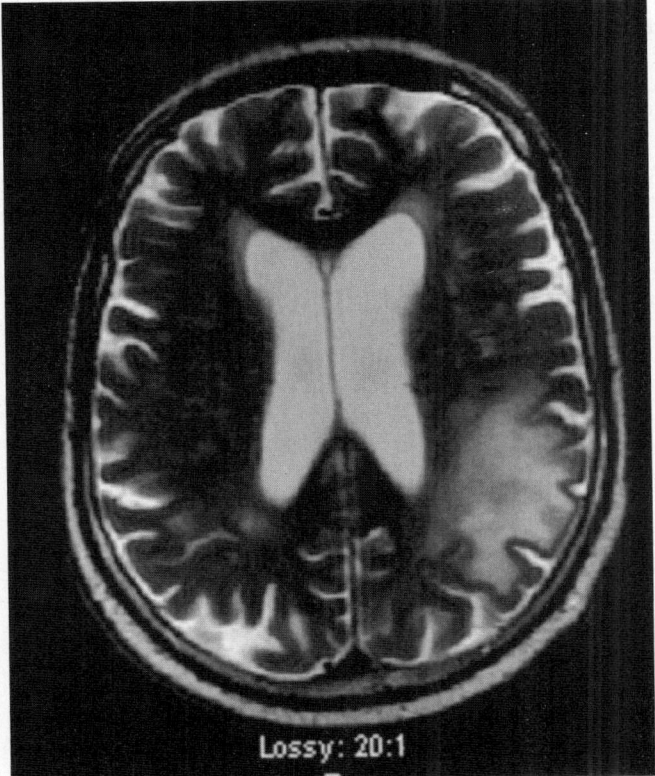

Figure 212-2 *Compared with multiple sclerosis (MS), progressive multifocal leukoencephalopathy (PML) is more likely to produce large, confluent lesions on T2-weighted magnetic resonance imaging (shown). Clinically, PML more often presents with hemiparesis and mental status changes, whereas MS is more likely to produce optic neuritis, brainstem syndromes, and spinal cord lesions. However, it is often impossible to distinguish a relapse of MS from PML based solely on clinical and radiologic findings, and a lumbar puncture with PCR for JC virus is usually required for definitive diagnosis. (Reproduced, with permission, from Ropper AH, Samuels MA. Adam's & Victor's Principles of Neurology, 9th ed. New York, NY: McGraw-Hill; 2009. Fig. 33-4B.)*

new T2 and enhancing lesions. The possibility of "pseudorelapse" due to infection, fever of any source, psychoactive medications, and other medical conditions should be considered, and a urinalysis, urine culture, and chest radiograph should be performed to exclude urinary tract infection (UTI) and pneumonia.

■ SYMPTOMS DUE TO PROGRESSION OF NEUROLOGIC DISEASE

The management of common symptoms complicating MS is summarized in **Table 212-5**. *Bladder management* is of particular relevance to the hospitalist. Urologic symptoms are present in up to 75% of patients with MS. These may result from bladder (detrusor) overactivity, leading to urgency, frequency, and urge incontinence; detrusor insufficiency, with incomplete bladder emptying; or detrusor-sphincter dyssynergia, causing hesitancy and interrupted urinary stream. It is not unusual for MS patients to suffer from all three conditions.

MS patients with urinary urgency and frequency should be evaluated for urinary tract infection with urinalysis and urine culture. A postvoid residual volume (PVR) of the bladder should also be obtained, either by portable ultrasound or catheterization. If the PVR is greater than 100 ml, patients should be educated in clean intermittent bladder self-catheterization. Urgency often responds to

urinary antispasmodics such as oxybutynin or tolterodine; patients taking these medications may need to perform intermittent self-catheterization as well, as they may aggravate concomitant urinary retention. Pelvic floor exercises and bladder retraining may alleviate urinary urgency by enhancing the ability of the pelvic floor muscles to counteract detrusor contraction. Treatment of constipation is thought to improve bladder function, although there are little data to support this contention. Patients with pure detrusor insufficiency may benefit from bethanecol to promote bladder emptying.

Although urinary tract infections are common in MS patients with bladder dysfunction, asymptomatic bacteriuria should not be treated. Cystoscopy and renal ultrasound should be performed in patients with frequent UTIs to assess for bladder stones, nephrolithiasis, and anatomic lesions that may predispose to infection. Cranberry juice may have modest efficacy in the prevention of UTIs.

Depression and fatigue are ubiquitous in MS and may be the most disabling symptoms in some patients. They deserve attention with both psychotherapy and medications. Changing from interferon to an alternative drug should be considered. Spasticity in the legs may be more prominent than weakness and can be treated with baclofen or tizanidine. Selective injection of botulinum toxin into adductor muscles of the legs may be helpful. Extreme cases benefit from an implantable intrathecal pump for infusion of baclofen. *Impotence* responds variably to phosphodiesterase inhibitors.

Cognitive decline has been recognized as an important but variable accompaniment of longstanding MS and correlates roughly with cerebral atrophy on imaging studies. Neuropsychological testing and cognitive rehabilitation techniques may prove helpful.

Dalfampridine has been introduced as an agent that improves walking speed in MS. Excessive doses may cause seizures.

PRACTICE POINT

- The symptoms of MS may transiently worsen in response to elevated body temperature (*Uhthoff phenomenon*). This may be due to the adverse effects of heat on conduction in demyelinated nerves. Fever, infection, saunas, hot baths, and vigorous exercise may all lead to pseudoexacerbations of MS. Pseudoexacerbations or pseudorelapses may also be caused by medications, metabolic derangements, and the premenstrual phase of the menstrual cycle.

DISCHARGE CHECKLIST FOR MULTIPLE SCLEROSIS

- Has the patient been screened for common symptoms associated with multiple sclerosis, such as anxiety, constipation, depression, falls, fatigue, sexual dysfunction, and spasticity?
- Has the patient been screened for bulbar symptoms and signs, such as dysarthria, dysphagia, and absent gag reflexes? If present, has a speech therapist been consulted for formal swallowing assessment?
- Has the patient been screened for bladder dysfunction? Has a postvoid residual volume been measured?
- Does the patient have scheduled follow-up with both neurology and primary care? Is the patient currently on or being considered for therapy with a disease-modifying agent?
- Is the patient up to date on influenza and pneumococcal vaccines?
- Has the patient been screened for decubitus ulcers? Would the patient benefit from preventive measures such as gel seat cushions and pressure-reduction mattresses?
- If the patient has disabilities, he has or she been evaluated by physical therapy, occupational therapy, and social work?

TABLE 212-5 Treatment of Associated Symptoms in Multiple Sclerosis

Symptom	Therapy	Possible Side Effects
Bladder urgency	Oxybutynin 5 mg two or three times daily (immediate release), 5 mg daily (extended release) Tolterodine 2-4 mg twice daily	Anticholinergic side effects (dry mouth, constipation, confusion, somnolence), exacerbation of glaucoma, urinary retention
Cognitive dysfunction	No drug therapy with proven benefit; treatment of associated fatigue and depression and cognitive behavior therapy may helpful	
Depression	Selective serotonin reuptake inhibitors (SSRIs)	Generally well tolerated; may cause sexual dysfunction; possible risk of suicidality in younger patients
	Selective serotonin and norepinephrine reuptake inhibitors	Useful alternative to SSRIs in patients who suffer side effects
	Tricyclic antidepressants	Limited by anticholinergic side effects; may be useful in patients with insomnia and urinary urgency
Fatigue	Amantidine 100 mg two or three times daily	Hallucinations, ankle swelling, skin mottling, anticholinergic side effects
	Modafinil 100-200 mg twice daily	Anxiety, insomnia, anorexia, palpitations, severe dermatologic reactions
	Methylphenidate 5-10 mg/d	Anxiety, insomnia, anorexia
Pain	Gabapentin 100 mg three times daily; may be slowly titrated upward to maximum dose of 3600 mg/d	Fatigue and somnolence are usually dose-limiting
	Carbamazepine 100 mg twice daily, titrated to a maximal dose of 400-1000 mg/d	Rash, hepatitis, drowsiness, nystagmus, nausea, cytopenias; hypothyroid patients may need higher levothyroxine doses due to accelerated T4 metabolism
	Amitriptyline 25-75 mg/d at bedtime	Anticholinergic side effects are common, including dry mouth, urinary retention, and confusion
Spasticity	Baclofen 10 mg two or three times daily, titrate to a maximal dose of 100 mg/d	Somnolence, fatigue, hypotonicity
	Tizanidine 2 mg at bedtime, titrate up to a maximum dose of 16-20 mg/d	Somnolence, fatigue
	Gabapentin 100 mg three times daily, titrate to 300-900 mg three times daily	Somnolence, fatigue
	Nabiximols (Sativex) oromucosal spray, typical dose four to eight times daily	Topical cannabinoid; approved in Europe and Canada, not yet available in United States; oral irritation, dizziness, intoxication, altered mood, disorientation, impaired cognition

SUGGESTED READINGS

Ascherio A, Munger KL, White R, et al. Vitamin D as an early predictor of multiple sclerosis activity and progression. *JAMA Neurol.* 2014;71:306-314.

Calabresi PA, Radue EW, Goodin D, et al. Safety and efficacy of fingolimod in patients with relapsing-remitting multiple sclerosis (FREEDOMS II): a double-blind, randomised, placebo-controlled, phase 3 trial. *Lancet Neurol.* 2014;13(6):545-556.

Confavreux C, O'Connor P, Comi G, et al. Oral teriflunomide for patients with relapsing multiple sclerosis (TOWER): a randomised, double-blind, placebo-controlled, phase 3 trial. *Lancet Neurol.* 2014;13:247-256.

Fox RJ, Miller DH, Phillips JT, et al. Placebo-controlled phase 3 study of oral BG-12 or glatiramer in multiple sclerosis. *N Engl J Med.* 2012;367:1087-1097.

Hedström AK, Hillert J, Olsson T, Alfredsson L. Alcohol as a modifiable lifestyle factor affecting multiple sclerosis risk. *JAMA Neurol.* 2014;71:300-305.

Polman CH, Reingold SC, Banwell B, et al. Diagnostic criteria for multiple sclerosis: 2010 revisions to the McDonald criteria. *Ann Neurol.* 2011;69:292-302.

CHAPTER 213

Peripheral Neuropathy

Megan Ann Waldrop, MD
Annabel Kim Wang, MD

Key Clinical Questions

1 What are the symptoms and signs of peripheral neuropathy?

2 Which patients with peripheral neuropathies require hospitalization?

3 Which peripheral neuropathies are seen in the inpatient setting?

4 What are the common causes of peripheral neuropathies?

5 How are peripheral neuropathies evaluated?

6 What are the best treatment options for peripheral neuropathy?

INTRODUCTION AND EPIDEMIOLOGY

Nontraumatic peripheral neuropathy is present in ~3% of the general population and in as many as 8% of individuals over the age of 55. Diabetes is the most common cause in developed nations, with vitamin B12 deficiency, thyroid dysfunction, and monoclonal gammopathy as other common causes. At least 60% of diabetics have objective evidence for peripheral neuropathy. Overall, diabetic neuropathy ranks third behind macrovascular disease and nephropathy in lifetime expenditures associated with diabetic complications. Neuropathy is responsible for more hospital admissions than all the other diabetic complications combined, and is a causative factor in up to 75% of all nontraumatic amputations.

PATHOPHYSIOLOGY AND CLINICAL FEATURES

Peripheral neuropathy is classified by the level of anatomical involvement (**Table 213-1**).

Radiculopathy affects the spinal root, leading to pain, paresthesias, and weakness in the distribution of the nerve root. It is most often caused by herniation of an intervertebral disk. Other causes include Lyme disease and neoplasia.

Plexopathy involves either the brachial plexus or the lumbosacral plexus, with symptoms involving multiple nerves. Causes include trauma, tumor infiltration, bony or vascular compression, radiation injury, and viral infection. Plexopathy may occur acutely in-hospital as a procedural complication, as in lumbosacral plexopathy due to groin hematoma after cardiac catheterization, or brachial plexopathy from stretch injury after cardiothoracic surgery.

Mononeuropathy is dysfunction of a solitary peripheral nerve. This is typically due to trauma (as in foot drop from peroneal nerve palsy after fibular fracture), compression (as in "Saturday night palsy," compression of the radial nerve in the axilla from falling asleep with the arm draped over a hard surface, as seen in alcoholics), or entrapment (median nerve in carpal tunnel syndrome or ulnar nerve in cubital tunnel). Involvement of several noncontiguous individual nerves is referred to as *multiple mononeuropathies* or *mononeuropathy multiplex*; vasculitis is the most common cause.

Polyneuropathy affects many peripheral nerves simultaneously, with distal and more or less symmetric involvement. Symptoms typically begin in the feet, before ascending to involve the legs and hands. It may involve sensory, motor, and autonomic nerves, either in isolation or varying combinations. Sensory symptoms may be persistent or intermittent. Positive sensory symptoms (dysesthesias or paresthesias) are described as tingling, burning, freezing, and electric-like sensations. Negative sensory symptoms include numbness and anesthesia. Allodynia or dysesthesia occurs when innocuous stimuli are perceived as being painful. Loss of balance, impaired coordination, and gait difficulty may also occur with sensory neuropathies. Weakness, when present, is also generally distal and symmetric. Symptoms of autonomic neuropathy (**Table 213-2**) include lightheadedness or orthostatic hypotension, diminished sweating and heat intolerance, and diarrhea. They may be mistaken for non-neurologic illness. Autonomic neuropathy may be prominent in diabetes mellitus, Guillain-Barré syndrome, uremia, porphyria, and systemic or inherited amyloidosis. Autonomic neuropathy without polyneuropathy can be seen in Chagas disease.

Polyneuropathy is classified by the temporal onset of symptoms (**Table 213-3**): acute (<4 weeks in duration), subacute (4-8 weeks in duration), or chronic (>3 months in duration). Polyneuropathy may

TABLE 213-1 Patterns of Peripheral Neuropathy

Pattern	Example
Radiculopathy	Cervical, thoracic, lumbar, sacral
Plexopathy	Brachial, lumbosacral
Mononeuropathy	Median, ulnar, radial, axillary, femoral, peroneal, tibial, sciatic
Multiple mononeuropathies	Mononeuritis multiplex
Polyneuropathy	Motor, sensory, autonomic

further be subclassified as axonal, demyelinating, or mixed injury, based on the results of nerve conduction studies. Clinical evaluation of polyneuropathy is often approached by classification of temporal onset and presentation of symptoms: focal, multifocal/asymmetric, or symmetric (**Figure 213-1**).

■ ACUTE POLYNEUROPATHY

Acute or subacute polyneuropathies tend to be inflammatory, infectious, or postinfectious in origin. Acute symmetric polyneuropathy with the rapid onset of ascending paralysis is usually due to *acute inflammatory demyelinating polyradiculoneuropathy (AIDP),* also known as *Guillain-Barré syndrome*. AIDP results from an autoimmune attack on peripheral nerves. It is preceded by recent *Campylobacter jejuni* infection in up to one-third of cases. AIDP also occurs after viral infections, such as cytomegalovirus and Epstein-Barr virus. The diagnosis is based on the development of symmetric and ascending weakness of the limbs, hyporeflexia or areflexia, with variable sensory and cranial nerve involvement. Autonomic failure with fluctuating blood pressure and heart rate occurs in one third of patients and is a significant cause of morbidity. An elevated cerebrospinal fluid (CSF) protein without cells (albuminocytologic dissociation) is diagnostic. AIDP has also been reported in the setting of recent human immunodeficiency virus (HIV) infection, viral hepatitis, Lyme disease, lymphoma, and systemic lupus erythematosus. Miller-Fisher syndrome is a GBS subtype which presents with ataxia, ophthalmoplegia, and areflexia. Other causes of acute polyneuropathy are porphyria, diphtheria, vasculitis, paraneoplastic syndromes, drugs, and toxins such as arsenic. Other causes of acute flaccid paralysis are listed in **Table 213-4**.

TABLE 213-2 Symptoms of Autonomic Neuropathy

Type	Cause	Symptom
Parasympathetic		
Pupillomotor	Lack of pupillary constriction	Glare/blurred vision
Secretomotor	Decreased lacrimation	Dry eyes
	Decreased salivation	Dry mouth
Gastrointestinal	Dysmotility	Bloating, early satiety, diarrhea, constipation
Genitourinary	Dysfunction	Urinary retention, sexual dysfunction
Sympathetic		
Adrenergic	Orthostatic hypotension	Lightheadedness, shoulder pain
Sudomotor	Decreased sweating	Hypohidrosis, anhidrosis, heat intolerance
Vasomotor	Impaired vasoconstriction	Cold extremities

TABLE 213-3 Classification of Polyneuropathies

Acute polyneuropathies

Acute inflammatory demyelinating polyradiculoneuropathy (AIDP) or Guillain-Barré syndrome

Acute motor axonal neuropathy (AMAN)

Acute motor and sensory axonal neuropathy (AMSAN)

Acute autonomic neuropathy

Miller Fisher syndrome

Chronic polyneuropathies	Examples
Inflammatory	Chronic inflammatory demyelinating polyneuropathy, vasculitis
Infectious	Hepatitis C, HIV, diphtheria, leprosy
Inherited	Familial amyloid polyneuropathy, Charcot-Marie-Tooth disease, Refsum disease
Metabolic	Diabetes, hypothyroidism, uremia, liver failure
Toxic	Alcohol, amiodarone, cisplatin, ethambutol, isoniazid, lead, linezolid, metronidazole, dapsone, nitrofurantoin, pyridoxine, fluoroquinolones
Nutritional deficiencies	Vitamins B1, B6, B12, and E deficiencies
Systemic disorders	Rheumatoid arthritis, sarcoidosis, Sjögren syndrome, cryoglobulemia
Monoclonal gammopathy	Monoclonal gammopathy of undetermined significance, systemic amyloidosis, Waldenström macroglobulinemia, cryoglobulinemia, POEMS (polyneuropathy, organomegaly, endocrinopathy, M protein, skin), Castleman disease
Malignancies and associated treatment	Small cell lung cancer, breast cancer, lymphoma, chemotherapy

Polyneuropathies with autonomic symptoms

AIDP or Guillain-Barré syndrome

Paraneoplastic neuropathy (acute and chronic)

Diabetes

Amyloidosis (familial and systemic)

Fabry disease

Porphyria

Hereditary and sensory autonomic neuropathies

HIV-associated polyneuropathy

Sjögren neuropathy

Neuropathies associated with chemotherapy (cisplatin, paclitaxel, vincristine) and toxins (arsenic, acrylamide, organophosphates)

PRACTICE POINT

Critical illness polyneuropathy

- Critical illness polyneuropathy is a common and often unrecognized cause of hospital-acquired polyneuropathy. Risk factors include sepsis or systemic inflammatory response syndrome, prolonged intensive care unit stay, renal failure, low serum albumin, parenteral nutrition, hyperglycemia, and hyperosmolarity; the relationship between glucocorticoid exposure and critical illness polyneuropathy is unclear. In mild cases, some improvement may occur within weeks. In more severe cases, improvement may take months and be incomplete or absent. Therapy is supportive, and includes

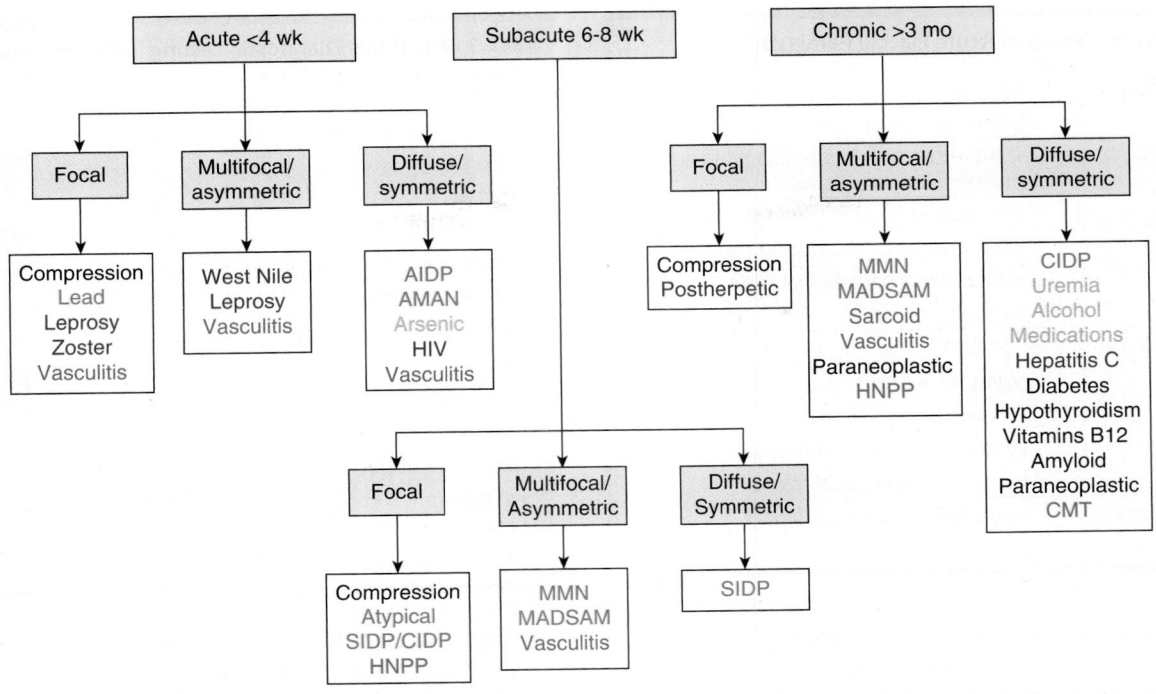

AIDP: acute inflammatory demyelinating polyneuropathy; AMAN: acute motor axonal neuropathy; CMT: Charcot Marie Tooth; CIDP: chronic inflammatory demyelinating polyneuropathy; HNPP: hereditary neuropathy pressure palsies; MADSAM: multifocal acquired demyelinating sensory and motor neuropathy; MMN: multifocal motor neuropathy; SIDP: subacute inflammatory demyelinating polyneuropathy

Red = demyelinating; Blue = autoimmune; Green = hereditary; Orange = toxic; Purple = infectious

Figure 213-1 *Approach to the patient with peripheral neuropathy.*

attention to nutritional status, early mobilization, and physical and occupational therapy to prevent contractures and maintain range of motion of the extremities.

■ CHRONIC POLYNEUROPATHY

Chronic symmetric polyneuropathy is the most common form of polyneuropathy. Axonal involvement is usual. Causes include metabolic, toxic, inherited, infectious, and inflammatory etiologies (Table 213–3). In the hospital setting, diabetes mellitus, uremia, alcohol, and HIV are especially prevalent causes. Many drugs are associated with neuropathy, including cisplatin, vincristine, amiodarone, isoniazid, ethambutol, metronidazole, and nitrofurantoin. Vitamin B12 and copper deficiency may cause polyneuropathy, as well as myelopathy. Vitamin B6 deficiency causes neuropathy, while excess can cause neuropathy or ganglionopathy.

PRACTICE POINT

Chronic neuropathy

● In the hospital setting, diabetes mellitus, uremia, alcohol, and HIV are common causes of chronic polyneuropathy. Many drugs are associated with neuropathy, including cisplatin, vincristine, amiodarone, isoniazid, ethambutol, metronidazole, and nitrofurantoin. Hospitalists can take steps to educate patients, especially diabetics, about foot care and to avoid medications which may exacerbate their problem. Measures to improve outpatient glucose control should begin in the hospital, as these have been shown to have sustained effects on long-term diabetic complications such as neuropathy, nephropathy, retinopathy, and cardiovascular disease.

Chronic neuropathy is occasionally demyelinating in nature. *Chronic inflammatory demyelinating polyneuropathy (CIDP)* resembles Guillain-Barré syndrome, with predominantly motor symptoms and a progressive or relapsing course over 3 months or more. *Multifocal motor neuropathy* presents with wasting and weakness, predominantly in the upper extremities, and may be mistaken for motor neuron disease (amyotrophic lateral sclerosis [ALS]). *Paraproteinemia* may cause a progressive, predominantly sensory polyneuropathy, in which the paraprotein is often an immunoglobulin M (IgM) antibody directed against myelin-associated glycoprotein. Some variants of *Charcot-Marie-Tooth disease* are demyelinating. Classically, these patients have a positive family history of neuropathy, foot drop, "stork" legs or "inverted champagne bottle" legs with calf wasting, high arches, and palpable peripheral nerves, but the clinical picture is highly variable. Patients with unrecognized inherited neuropathies, such as Charcot-Marie-Tooth disease, are at risk for a devastating acute polyneuropathy after chemotherapy or other neurotoxic drug administration.

DIAGNOSIS

The evaluation of peripheral neuropathies always begins with a detailed medical history, followed by both complete general and neurologic physical examinations. Past medical history, associated symptoms, medications, drug and alcohol use, toxin exposures, and family history may provide insight. The pattern of onset (eg, distal, proximal, and symmetric), the temporal onset (eg, acute, subacute, and chronic), and associated symptoms and signs are useful clues. The general physical examination may provide clues to the etiology of neuropathy (**Table 213-5**). Neurologic examination should include examination of major sensory modalities, including

TABLE 213-4 Causes of Acute Flaccid Paralysis

Localization	Diagnosis
Brain	Brainstem stroke, infection
Spinal cord	Transverse myelitis, arteriovenous dural malformation, tumor, abscess
Anterior horn cell	Infection (poliovirus, West Nile virus)
Muscle	Inflammatory or necrotizing myopathy
	Hypokalemia periodic paralysis
	Hypophosphatemia
Neuromuscular junction	Botulism
	Myasthenia gravis
	Tick bite paralysis
	Lambert-Eaton myasthenic syndrome
	Industrial or biological toxins
Sodium channel blockade	Neurotoxic marine poisoning

TABLE 213-6 Initial Diagnostic Testing in Polyneuropathy

Complete blood count

Erythrocyte sedimentation rate or C-reactive protein

Vitamin B12

Folate

Serum electrolytes, blood urea nitrogen, and serum creatinine

Serum glucose and hemoglobin A1c

Liver function tests

Thyroid-stimulating hormone

Urinalysis

Serum and 24-h urine protein electrophoresis and immunofixation

HIV antibody

Hepatitis C antibody

Chest radiograph (for pulmonary malignancy as a cause of paraneoplastic neuropathy)

Nerve conduction studies/needle electromyography

light touch, pinprick and temperature, vibration, and joint position sense. Romberg test, motor bulk and tone, strength, and deep tendon reflexes should also be evaluated. Mental status changes are unusual in peripheral neuropathies but may occur with West Nile virus, porphyria, and acute heavy metal poisoning.

Nerve conduction studies are helpful in delineating the relative contributions of axonal and demyelinating disease and the degree of motor and sensory involvement. However, such studies cannot evaluate the small nerve fibers that carry pain and temperature sensation, which are often involved in diabetic neuropathy. Absent sensory responses with normal motor studies are consistent with a sensory ganglionopathy. Abnormal motor responses with normal sensory studies are suggestive of motor neuropathy, such as multifocal motor neuropathy with conduction block or a motor neuronopathy, including causes such as polio, West Nile Virus, and ALS. *Needle electromyography (EMG)* is helpful in determining the chronicity of the peripheral neuropathy, but it can also identify concomitant

nerve root (radiculopathy) or muscle (myopathy) involvement. Both nerve conduction studies and needle electromyography should be performed as a two-part study and are collectively referred to as an EMG. Electrodiagnostic testing in the inpatient setting can often be fraught with technical difficulties, but it is helpful in the diagnosis and prognosis of AIDP, botulism, myasthenia gravis, and critical care neuromyopathy.

Small nerve fibers are preferentially affected in distal painful neuropathies. Small fiber neuropathy can be diagnosed using quantitative sensory testing of cold and heat/pain sensation, autonomic testing, or skin biopsy. *Autonomic testing*, which evaluates heart rate, blood pressure, and sweating, can provide further information about small fiber and autonomic nerve function. However, autonomic testing of cardiovagal, adrenergic, and postganglionic sudomotor function may not be readily available in the inpatient setting.

Suggested initial tests in peripheral neuropathy are listed in **Table 213-6**. Common causes of peripheral neuropathy should be excluded, including hypothyroidism (thyroid-stimulating hormone), diabetes (fasting glucose and hemoglobin A1c), and vitamin B12 deficiency. In addition to B12 levels, methylmalonic acid and homocysteine may help to diagnose vitamin B12 deficiency in patients with low-normal B12 levels. Erythrocyte sedimentation rate and C-reactive protein are helpful screening tests for autoimmune disorders. Rheumatoid factor, antinuclear antibodies, antineutrophil cytoplasmic antibodies, antibodies to Sjögren syndrome antibodies A and B (SS-A and SS-B), copper, as well as vitamin B1, B6, and E levels may be indicated in select patients. HIV antibody, hepatitis C antibody, and syphilis serology screen for neuropathy related to infection. Systemic causes of polyneuropathy can be evaluated with routine complete blood count and metabolic panel to assess for anemia, uremia, and liver disease. Monoclonal gammopathies may be excluded with serum and 24-hour urine for immunofixation.

Nerve biopsy can be useful when diagnoses such as vasculitis, amyloidosis, lymphoma, leprosy, and sarcoid are being considered. *Punch skin biopsy* may identify isolated small fiber neuropathy through diminished epidermal nerve fiber density. *Chest radiograph* is useful in screening for neoplasms, especially when there is a smoking history and a possible paraneoplastic disorder.

TABLE 213-5 Findings on Physical Examination Associated with Specific Peripheral Neuropathies

Unusual Findings	Associated Peripheral Neuropathy
Orange tonsils	Tangier disease (deficiency of high-density lipoproteins)
Retinitis pigmentosa, hearing loss, ichthyosis	Refsum disease (peroxisomal disorder/phytanic acid)
Papilledema	POEMS
Hearing loss	Inherited neuropathy, mitochondrial disorders
Bilateral facial palsy	Guillain-Barré syndrome, sarcoid, lymphoma
Enlarged tongue, petechiae	Systemic amyloidosis
Severe autonomic failure	Diabetes, amyloidosis (Systemic or Familial)
High arches, hammer toes, palpable nerves	Inherited neuropathy (eg, Charcot-Marie-Tooth Disease)
Angiokeratomas	Fabry disease
Alopecia, Mees lines	Arsenic, thallium

POEMS, polyneuropathy, organomegaly, endocrinopathy, M. protein, skin changes.

DIFFERENTIAL DIAGNOSIS

Disorders of the spinal cord, anterior horn cells, and neuromuscular junction can all mimic peripheral neuropathy. *Cervical spondylosis* may present as quadriparesis, whereas *thoracic or lumbosacral spinal cord lesions* may lead to paraparesis. Deep tendon reflexes may be diminished, and bladder dysfunction may occur acutely. *Transverse myelitis,* secondary to multiple sclerosis, collagen vascular disease, infections, and paraneoplastic disorders, can present with motor, sensory, and autonomic symptoms, which vary depending on the size and location of the spinal cord lesion. Cerebrospinal fluid analysis demonstrates inflammation with moderate lymphocytic pleocytosis, and elevated protein and IgG index. A spinal sensory level and a focal area of increased T2 signal on spinal magnetic resonance imaging (MRI) are often present. *Spinal dural arteriovenous malformations* may present in a similar fashion. *Subacute combined degeneration* of the spinal cord due to vitamin B12 or copper deficiency may present as a neuromyelopathy. Upper motor neuron signs, such as increased deep tendon reflexes, are often masked by the superimposed polyneuropathy.

The anterior horn cells of the spinal cord may be involved in degenerative conditions, such as motor neuron disease and infections, such as poliomyelitis. West Nile virus is a mosquito-borne illness with peak transmission in late summer. Infection usually results either in no symptoms or a mild flu-like illness. West Nile virus occasionally leads to meningitis, encephalitis, or a poliomyelitis-like, rapidly progressive febrile paralytic illness from damage to the anterior horn cells. Weakness is usually asymmetric and ranges from flaccid monoplegia to disabling quadriplegia. Cerebrospinal fluid and serum IgM antibodies against West Nile virus are positive. Treatment is supportive.

Pre- and postsynaptic neuromuscular junction disorders should also be considered. In *myasthenia gravis,* caused by antibodies that block the postsynaptic acetylcholine receptors, weakness is fluctuating, worse in the evening, and usually proximal and fatigable. The ocular, pharyngeal and laryngeal muscles are often involved, leading to ptosis, diplopia, dysphagia, and a nasal voice. The diagnosis may be overlooked in the setting of acute respiratory failure. *Lambert-Eaton myasthenic syndrome (LEMS)* results from antibody-mediated blockade of presynaptic acetylcholine release. It is usually related to underlying small cell lung cancer or autoimmune disease. The hallmark of LEMS is proximal weakness of the limbs, which increases in power with sustained contraction; the ocular muscles are spared.

Botulinum toxin blocks presynaptic release of acetylcholine, leading to a descending flaccid paralysis with blurry vision, ptosis, dysphagia, dysarthria, and eventually respiratory compromise. Patients are often intubated, but careful examination may reveal dilated pupils with a normal sensory examination. *Botulism* usually occurs after ingestion of contaminated food. It may also be acquired from open wounds, use of black tar heroin, or inhalation of aerosolized toxin, as in bioterrorism. Diagnosis is made by assay of stool, serum and food (if available) for botulinum toxin. Later in the course, neurotoxin assays are less sensitive, but anaerobic cultures of wounds and stool for *Clostridium botulinum* may still be positive. Nerve conduction studies reveal small compound motor action potential amplitudes that increase with exercise. Antitoxin therapy is most effective when administered within 24 hours. Treatment is otherwise supportive with special attention to the respiratory status.

In patients with foot pain, it may be difficult to distinguish small fiber neuropathy from peripheral vascular disease, arthritis, or plantar fasciitis. Small fiber neuropathy is often unrecognized because the distal pain and temperature loss can be subtle, and the presence of ankle reflexes and normal nerve conduction velocities are misleading. As noted above, punch skin biopsy may be helpful in these instances.

TRIAGE/HOSPITAL ADMISSION

Peripheral neuropathy is often diagnosed in patients who are admitted to the hospital for other reasons, but rarely does it justify hospital admission on its own. There are a few major exceptions. Sudden flaccid paralysis warrants immediate admission with close monitoring for respiratory compromise in a step-down unit or intensive care unit. Patients who present with the acute asymmetric onset of weakness have vasculitis, which is potentially life-threatening until proven otherwise.

Hospitalization for chronic polyneuropathy is unusual. Admission is reasonable for complications of chronic polyneuropathy, such as infection, fracture, or threatened amputation, or for treatment of intractable pain. Patients with inflammatory, or demyelinating, chronic polyneuropathies may require hospital admission for IV immunoglobulin or plasmapheresis.

TREATMENT

Most forms of neuropathy have no specific treatment, aside from identification and correction of the underlying cause. For example, glucose control should be optimized in diabetics, vitamin B12 and thyroxine should be repleted in those who are deficient, alcoholics should receive thiamine and encouragement to abstain from drinking, and medications responsible for neuropathy should be stopped. In the setting of chemotherapeutic agents, discontinuation may not be feasible. In this setting, alternative dosing schedules or modification of treatment may be possible. For example, when using oxaliplatin, the stop and go strategy as opposed to continuous use has shown the same tumor response rate, with less resultant chemotherapy induced peripheral neuropathy. Patients with entrapment neuropathies, such as carpal tunnel syndrome, may benefit from surgical release.

Neuropathic pain may be diminished by therapy with antiepileptic drugs (gabapentin, pregabalin, or carbamazepine), serotonin-norepinephrine reuptake inhibitors (venlafaxine and duloxetine), or a tricyclic antidepressant (amitriptyline or nortriptyline).

Patients with allodynia and dysesthesias may obtain relief from a metal frame to raise the bedclothes off the feet. Focal pain may respond to capsaicin or topical lidocaine ointment or lidocaine patch.

Specific treatments for acute demyelinating polyneuropathies include IV immunoglobulin or plasmapheresis. Acute flaccid paralysis requires supportive care with aggressive attention to rehabilitation. Continuous pulmonary, blood pressure, and heart rate monitoring is required. Respiratory deterioration, as indicated by a negative inspiratory pressure <−15 cm H_2O, should prompt intubation. Mechanical ventilatory assistance is required in about one-third of patients with AIDP. Tracheostomy is recommended if mechanical ventilation will be required for more than 2 to 3 weeks. Enteric nutrition is necessary for patients on mechanical ventilation. Heparin and graduated pressure stockings should be started to prevent deep venous thrombosis. Prevention of pressure sores is necessary. Patients should be treated by a multidisciplinary rehabilitation team.

Patients with autonomic neuropathy and orthostatic hypotension may be managed by liberal salt and fluid intake, small, and frequent meals. Fludrocortisone or midodrine may also be helpful. At night, patients with orthostatic hypotension should sleep in a semirecumbent position, with the head of the bed elevated at 30°, to facilitate salt and water retention and avoid supine hypertension. Gastroparesis may respond to prokinetic agents such as metoclopramide and erythromycin. Pressure stockings and abdominal binders may reduce pooling of blood and mitigate orthostatic hypotension.

COMPLICATIONS

Hospital complications in patients with peripheral neuropathies are related to immobility and invasive treatments and may include skin breakdown, nosocomial pneumonia, urinary tract infection, central venous catheter sepsis, deep vein thrombosis, and pulmonary embolism. Death may occur from respiratory insufficiency, infection, or severe dysautonomia. Complications of IV immunoglobulin may include headache, rash, stroke, renal failure, or anaphylaxis, especially in individuals with IgA deficiency. Large fluid volume shifts can lead to myocardial infarctions, and complications from line placement can occur in patients receiving plasmapheresis. Superimposed compressive neuropathies may occur in immobile patients. Undertreated anxiety, depression and pain may increase morbidity. Those with underlying neuropathy (diabetes, Charcot-Marie-Tooth) have increased risk of potential iatrogenic causes of neuropathy. Alcohol withdrawal may be seen in patients with polyneuropathy secondary to alcohol abuse. In-hospital injuries from falls or orthostatic hypotension can occur.

DISCHARGE CHECKLIST

- Evaluation for assistive devices has been completed, if needed, and delivery arranged.
- Home safety and modification evaluation has been completed or arranged.
- Outpatient referrals have been placed to podiatry and physical and occupational therapy, if indicated.
- Follow-up with primary care and neurology has been scheduled.
- The primary care provider has been updated regarding new care recommendations and the potential for future complications, such as falls, pain, fatigue, and dysautonomia.
- Periodic blood work has been ordered, if the patient is taking immunosuppressive medication for autoimmune forms of neuropathy.
- The patient with limited mobility has been educated about DVT prevention.
- The patient has adequate insurance and financial resources to fill new prescriptions.

PRACTICE POINT

Preventable complications of neuropathy

- Preventable complications in the hospitalized patient with peripheral neuropathy are primarily related to their limited mobility. These patients should be recognized at being at

high risk of decubitus ulcers and placed on preventive nursing measures. Pressure, friction, and shear forces should be minimized by frequent turning and positioning and avoidance of excessive bed rest. The use of pressure-relieving devices, such as dynamic air mattresses, should be strongly considered in patients with severe polyneuropathy. Nutritional status should be assessed. Physical therapy, occupational therapy, and wound care consultations may be of benefit. Thermal injury such as from hot water baths is likely and thus temperature of bathing water should be monitored closely. Prevention measures should be in place for deep vein thrombosis, nosocomial pneumonia, and falls. Patients with diabetes should have their glycemic regimen reassessed if their hemoglobin A1c indicates suboptimal glucose control. Social work/psychology consultations may be of use in patients who are experiencing difficulty adapting to their change in functional status.

SUGGESTED READINGS

Beutler AS, Kulkarni AA, Kanwar R, et al. Sequencing of Charcot–Marie–Tooth disease genes in a toxic polyneuropathy. *Ann Neurol.* 2014;76:727-737.

Hammond N, Wang Y, Dimachkie MM, Barohn RL. Nutritional neuropathies. *Neurol Clin.* 2013;31:477-489.

Latov N. Diagnosis and treatment of chronic acquired demyelinating polyneuropathies. *Nat Rev Neurol.* 2014;10:435-446.

Mauermann ML, Burns TM. Pearls and oysters: evaluation of peripheral neuropathies. *Neurology.* 2009;72:e28-e31.

Miltenburg NC, Boogerd W: Chemotherapy-induced neuropathy. *Cancer Treat Rev.* 2014;40:872-882.

van den Berg B, Walgaard C, Drenthen J, et al. Guillain-Barré syndrome: pathogenesis, diagnosis, treatment and prognosis. *Nat Rev Neurol.* 2014;10:469-482.

Ziegler D, Fonseca V. From guideline to patient: a review of recent recommendations for pharmacotherapy of painful neuropathy. *J Diabetes Complications.* 2015;29:146-156.

SECTION 11
Palliative Care

CHAPTER 214

Principles of Palliative Care

Irene M. Yeh, MD, MPH
Rachelle E. Bernacki, MD, MS

Key Clinical Questions

1 What are the primary palliative care skills that every hospitalist should know?

2 What is specialty palliative care and how does it differ from hospice?

3 How do you identify patients in need of a palliative care assessment in a hospital setting?

INTRODUCTION

Palliative care focuses on effective management of pain and other distressing symptoms, and integrates psychosocial and spiritual care by considering a patient's and family's needs, preferences, values, beliefs, and culture (see **Table 214-1**). The palliative care approach works to improve quality of life for the patient and family by reducing a patient's symptom burden, providing clear communication about what to expect in the future, and aligning realistic treatment options with patient- and family-determined goals of care (see **Table 214-2**).

Unlike hospice, which requires that a physician endorse a 6-month prognosis in order for a patient to qualify for hospice services, palliative care (sometime referred to as supportive care), is provided in conjunction with curative treatment at any point in the disease trajectory from the time of diagnosis (see **Figure 214-1**). Palliative treatment options may become a greater focus for the patient and the care team when the burden of curative treatment outweighs the benefits, or when there are no longer effective disease-modifying treatments. Provision of palliative care in the course of serious illness occurs across multiple care settings, and requires communication across the varied settings to maintain continuity of care (**Table 214-3**).

ROLE OF HOSPITALISTS IN PALLIATIVE CARE

Modern palliative care is no longer considered brink-of-death care. Timely palliative care consultations provided alongside disease-directed therapies have demonstrated improvement in quality of care, reduction of costs, and sometimes an increase in longevity. An interdisciplinary team is a key component to palliative care, where the focus is not only on the patient's needs but also the needs of the family, which includes any person the patient identifies as part of his or her support network.

However, challenges in the delivery of effective palliative care remain. In 2014, the Institute of Medicine released a report entitled, "Dying in America: Improving Quality and Honoring Individual Preferences near the End of Life." Key findings highlight the deficiencies and challenges in the universal delivery of high-quality palliative care, including

- Slow, widespread adoption of timely referrals to palliative care
- Multiple transitions between and within health care settings for patients with advanced serious illness
- Increasing demand for family caregivers for patients
- Surrogate decision making about treatment decisions without a clear understanding of prognosis

Hospitalists play a key role in ensuring that patients receive quality palliative care. Beyond disease management related to acute exacerbations of chronic illness, hospitalists are able to take advantage of crucial moments to address and document a patient's understanding of prognosis, treatment options and goals of care at various points along a disease course. Unlike the outpatient primary care clinician who may have the benefit of developing a close relationship with the patient and family members over time, hospitalists can assess a patient's condition from a fresh perspective. Because hospitalists need to elicit a patient's and/or family's understanding of a patient's overall condition quickly without the benefit of a long-term relationship, this can allow an opportunity for open discussion and more accurate prognostication.

TABLE 214-1 Palliative Care Services

- Provides relief from pain and other distressing symptoms
- Will enhance quality of life and may also positively influence the course of illness
- Is applicable early in the course of illness, in conjunction with other therapies that are intended to prolong life, such as chemotherapy or radiation therapy
- Includes those investigations needed to better understand and manage distressing clinical complications
- Integrates the psychological and spiritual aspects of patient care
- Offers a support system to help patients live as actively as possible until death
- Affirms life and regards dying as a normal process
- Intends neither to hasten or postpone death
- Offers a support system to help the family cope during the patient's illness and in their own bereavement
- Uses a team approach to address the needs of patients and their families, including bereavement counseling, if indicated

Reproduced with permission from World Health Organization's Definition of Palliative Care. http://www.who.int/cancer/palliative/definition/en. Accessed April 7, 2015.

PRIMARY AND SPECIALIST PALLIATIVE CARE

Training in palliative care for hospitalists caring for patients with serious advanced illness has become an urgent priority. Data from the Dartmouth Atlas show that more than 70% of Americans who die of a chronic illness each year are admitted to a hospital during the last 6 months of life. Existing palliative care needs continue to outstrip the availability of the palliative care workforce: a shortage of approximately 11,000 clinicians to staff existing hospital-based palliative care programs was found in 2010 and this gap is expected to widen as the population ages.

Because of the scope of work and volume of patients seen, hospitalists are primed to achieve palliative care competencies in effective symptom management, skilled and nuanced communication, and

TABLE 214-2 Areas of Palliative Care

Area	Examples
Physical	Pain, shortness of breath, nausea, fatigue, weakness, anorexia, insomnia, confusion, constipation, treatment side effects, functional capacities, treatment efficacy and alternatives (and patient and family preferences)
Psychological/ psychiatric	Anxiety, depression, care-giving needs or capacity of family; stress; grief and bereavement risks for the patient and family (ie, depression and comorbid complications); coping strategies
Social	Family structure and geographic location; cultural concerns and needs; finances; sexuality; living arrangements; caregiver availability; access to transportation; access to prescription and over-the-counter medicines
Spiritual/ religious/ existential	Spiritual background, beliefs, and practices of the patient and family; hopes and fears; life completion tasks; wishes regarding care setting for death

Data from National Consensus Project for Quality Palliative Care. 2009. *Clinical Practice Guidelines for Quality Palliative Care,* 2nd ed.

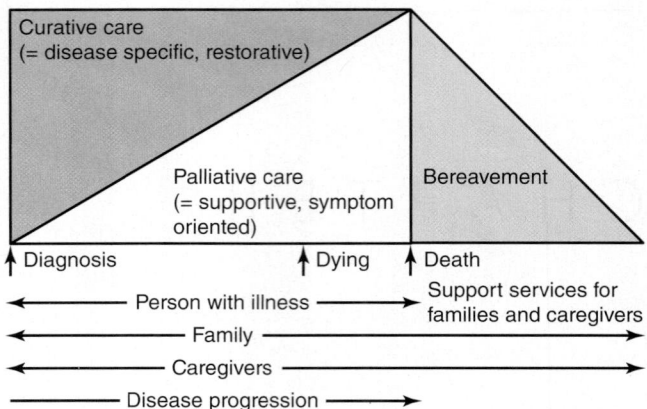

Figure 214-1 *Palliative care model.* (Courtesy of the United States Department of Health and Human Services.)

interdisciplinary teamwork. This is considered "primary" or generalized palliative care, as compared to specialized palliative care. Core components of primary palliative care include: (1) skills in symptom assessment and management, such as the safe use of opioids in pain relief, adjuvant approaches to pain management, and treatment of nonpain symptoms and treatment side effects, (2) skills in effective and emphatic communication, such as how to communicate bad news and address strong emotions and how to clarify a patients' wishes and build consensus among treatments teams and patients/ families, and (3) skills in interdisciplinary teamwork, such as knowing how to work together with an interdisciplinary team to provide an effective and appropriate care management plan upon discharge.

Patients with complex needs may require a referral to a specialized palliative care team, which can provide assistance with difficult-to-control symptoms and conflict resolution regarding goals and treatments with families, between staff and families, and among treatment teams.

TRIGGERS FOR PALLIATIVE CARE ASSESSMENT

Hospital teams are using specified triggers to help initiate assessment for palliative care needs. One trigger, the surprise question— "Would you be surprised if the patient died within 12 months?" has been successfully utilized to identify patient populations in need of advance care planning (ACP) discussions. Worsening disease status, rapid functional decline, or repeat hospitalizations over a short period of time may also signal a need for a more in-depth conversation with the patient and family. Other triggers may be

TABLE 214-3 Palliative Care Models

Model	Care Setting
Consultation service team	Usually in a hospital or nursing home; often includes social work evaluations
Combined hospice program and palliative care program	Hospital, nursing home, freestanding hospice inpatient facilities
Dedicated inpatient unit	Acute hospitals, nursing homes
Hospice-based palliative care in the home	Home
Outpatient palliative care practice or clinic	Hospital or private practice

Data from National Consensus Project for Quality Palliative Care. 2009. *Clinical Practice Guidelines for Quality Palliative Care,* 2nd ed.

based on events, such as device placement (eg, feeding tube, tracheostomy, left ventricular assist device [LVAD], automatic implantable cardioverter defibrillator [AICD]), or when initiation of dialysis, bone-marrow transplantation, or solid-organ transplantation are being considered.

By building a collaborative relationship between the hospitalist team and consulting palliative care team, one can foster mutual learning to improve the care of the patient. Hospitalists can gain knowledge about the components of a palliative care consultation and continue their education and development of palliative care skills; palliative care clinicians can learn more about new approaches to care management for specific illnesses. Joint visits can help alleviate a patient's fear of abandonment by the hospital team and provide a greater sense of support. Implementation of palliative care consult triggers at time of admission and palliative care team participation in interdisciplinary rounds with hospitalists are other potential areas of collaboration.

To improve access to palliative care, delivery models of specialized palliative care have been developed in the hospital beyond consultation care services. Increasingly, hospitals are opening inpatient palliative care units, which specialize in the management of severe to refractory symptoms and the delivery of medical-surgical hospital care in a combined fashion. These inpatient palliative care units can also provide an inpatient level of hospice care for eligible patients that choose to elect these services.

> ### PRACTICE POINT
> - To address the fear that a palliative care consultation may signal to the patient that the hospital team is 'giving up,' hospitalists could state:
>
>   *"We want to make sure we are doing everything possible to help you feel as best as you possibly can. We will be asking the palliative care team to visit and provide an extra layer of support for you and your family. They will help us make sure that your symptoms are well controlled, and we will continue to be your primary doctors during this hospitalization." (Adapted from Lindvall et al. 2014)*

CARDIOPULMONARY RESUSCITATION (CPR) DISCUSSIONS

Discussions around preferences regarding cardiopulmonary resuscitation, often referred to as "code status discussions," are frequently obtained early in the hospitalization, typically on the first day of admission. These sensitive conversations can be challenging, especially if there have been no prior discussion about the patient's values and goals of care during past hospitalizations or in the outpatient setting. Patients and/or families may be unaware of how the increasing frequency of acute exacerbations of a chronic illness or the gradual decline in functional and nutritional status may signify a poorer prognosis. Moreover, a clinician's desire to promote a patient's self-determination and an institutional pressure "to get an answer" can lead to ineffective "procedure-focused" discussions that feel "scripted and depersonalized" to the patient, particularly if these conversations occur without context. Poorly-led conversations can lead to anxiety, misunderstanding and distrust in the patient-physician relationship and create unfertile ground for future communication.

Ideally, discussions about preferences in cardiopulmonary resuscitation are part of a larger advance care planning process and highlight the importance of patient-centered and family-centered care. Successful "CPR discussions" are not dependent on the outcome of the discussion but the process itself. These complex discussions involve the care team assessing the patient's values and goals and sharing likely outcomes and recommendations, with the final 'code status' decision made jointly between the medical team and the patient and family.

> ### PRACTICE POINT
> - *After exploring a patient's values and goals, incorporate this information when transitioning the discussion from goals to recommendation regarding resuscitation measures. Discussion as to whether the patient would be able to regain previous functional status, accomplish their goals, and/or maintain their current quality of life following resuscitation attempts are critical.*
> - *Avoid framing "code status" as a solely patient decision, for example. "We want to know what you would like us to do." Instead, discussions should occur in the context of shared decision making, for example. "It is important that we start talking about this so that if things should become worse, we are prepared and that you can be comfortable with the decisions we have made together."*
> - *Realistic recommendations should be based on a patient's values and goals, not the physician's own preferences.*
> - *Language is critical; patients may misunderstand the term "Do not resuscitate/do not intubate (DNR/DNI)" and may fear they will not continue to receive usual treatment for their medical condition. For this reason, some prefer using the phrase "Full care without resuscitation" as an alternative.*
>
> *(Adapted from Sharma et al. 2014)*

See Chapter 105 (Using Prognosis to Guide Treatment).
See Chapter 215 (Communication Skills for End of Life Care).

GOALS OF CARE DISCUSSIONS

Hospitalists face challenges and barriers to goals of care discussions, which include patient and family difficulty in accepting a poor prognosis, poor understanding of the limitations and consequences of life-sustaining treatment, and a lack of clinician training on how to conduct these discussions. Learning how and when to elicit patient disclosures of emotional distress and explore such distress has been likened to a "delicate dance." Navigating difficult conversations in the context of challenges in a patient's illness and/or treatment and responding to the emotional reactions of patients and families is a skill set that requires practice and training.

> ### PRACTICE POINT
> *Do*
> - *Give a direct and honest prognosis*
> - *Provide prognostic information as a range (eg, hours to days, days to weeks, weeks to months), acknowledging uncertainty*
> - *Allow for silence so patients and families can process information*
> - *Acknowledge and explore emotions*
> - *Focus on the patient's quality of life, fears, and concerns*
> - *Make a recommendation (eg, "Based on x medical situation and y goals and values with z treatment options, I recommend")*
>
> *Don't*
> - *Talk more than half the conversation*
> - *Fear silence*
> - *Give premature reassurance*
> - *Provide facts in response to strong emotions*
> - *Focus on medical procedures*
>
> *(Adapted from Bernacki & Block 2014)*

See Chapter 105 (Using Prognosis to Guide Treatment).
See Chapter 215 (Communication Skills for End of Life Care).

CLINICAL PRACTICE OF PALLIATIVE CARE

The National Consensus Project (NCP) published initial guidelines in 2004 entitled "Clinical Practice Guidelines for Quality Palliative Care." These guidelines directed the "development and structure of both new and existing palliative care teams; established uniform definitions of essential elements of palliative care, including generalized and specialty palliative care; established national goals for access to palliative care; promoted performance measurement and quality improvement initiatives in palliative care services; and fostered continuity of palliative care across settings, including home, hospital, and hospice."

The key aspects of palliative care are divided into eight domains, including Structure and Processes of Care, Physical Aspects of Care, Psychological and Psychiatric Aspects of Care, Social Aspects of Care, Spiritual, Religious and Existential Aspects of Care, Cultural Aspects of Care, Care of the Patient at the End of Life, and Ethical and Legal Aspects of Care, based on the 3rd edition of the Clinical Practice Guidelines (2013). In 2006, the National Quality Forum developed the following guidelines to delineate the optimal practice of palliative care that corresponds to each of the eight domains:

■ DOMAIN 1: STRUCTURE AND PROCESSES OF CARE

Recommended practices include provision of palliative care by an interdisciplinary team and access to palliative care that is responsive to the patient and family that is 24 hours a day, 7 days a week.

For general processes of care, a care plan based on comprehensive interdisciplinary assessment of the values, preferences, goals, and needs of the patient and family is formulated, utilized, regularly reviewed, and communicated to all professionals involved in the patient's care in a timely fashion. Upon transfer between health care settings, timely and thorough communication of a patient's goals, preferences, values, and clinical information to ensure continuity of care and follow-up is recommended.

Health care professionals should begin discussing hospice as an option to all patient and families when death within a year would not be surprising, and reintroduce the hospice option as the patient declines with an estimated prognosis of less than 6 months. Furthermore, an assessment of a health care practitioner's ability to discuss hospice as an option should be standard. By educating patients on the process of their disease, prognosis, and the benefits and burdens of potential interventions, health care practitioners can enable patients to make informed decisions about their care. Family support and education is also recommended to assure safe and appropriate care of the patient.

See Chapter 105 (Using Prognosis to Guide Treatment).
See Chapter 215 (Communication Skills for End of Life Care).

■ DOMAIN 2: PHYSICAL ASPECTS OF CARE

Assessment, measurement and documentation of pain, nausea/vomiting, dyspnea, constipation, and other symptoms is essential to quality palliative care and using available standardized scales is recommended. The assessment and management of symptoms and side effects in a timely, safe, and effective manner to a level acceptable to the patient and family is essential to providing quality care to patients with advanced serious illness. Palliative Care Fast Facts provide concise, peer-reviewed and evidence-based summaries on key palliative care topics, accessible at https://www.mypcnow.org/fast-facts/ or in the Journal of Palliative Medicine.

See Chapter 80 (Constipation).
See Chapter 85 (Dyspnea).
See Chapter 96 (Sleep Disturbance in the Hospitalized Patient).
See Chapter 97 (Nausea and Vomiting).
See Chapter 99 (Pain).
See Chapter 216 (Domains of Care: Physical Aspects of Care).

■ DOMAIN 3: PSYCHOLOGICAL AND PSYCHIATRIC ASPECTS OF CARE

As with physical aspects of care, the measurement and documentation of anxiety, depression, delirium, behavioral disturbances, and other common psychological symptoms is recommended using available standardized scales, with the assessment and management of these symptoms in a timely, safe and effective manner. In addition, addressing potential emotional and functional impairment and loss requires regular ongoing assessment and management of the psychological reactions of patients and families. This includes assessment for anticipatory grief, coping and stress. The development of a grief and bereavement care plan should occur prior to and after the death of a patient.

See Chapter 166 (Agitation in Older Adults).
See Chapter 216 (Domains of Care: Physical Aspects of Care).
See Chapter 223 (Mood and Anxiety Disorders).
See Chapter 228 (The Difficult Patient).

■ DOMAIN 4: SOCIAL ASPECTS OF CARE

Regular patient and family care conferences with physicians and other appropriate members of the interdisciplinary team is a recommended best practice to provide information, discuss goals of care, disease prognosis, advance care planning, and offer support. A comprehensive social care plan addresses the social, practical, and legal needs of the patient and caregivers, which include but is not limited to: relationships, communication, existing social and cultural networks, decision making, work and school settings, finances, sexuality/intimacy, caregiver availability/stress, and access to medicines and equipment.

See Chapter 167 (Elder Mistreatment).

■ DOMAIN 5: SPIRITUAL, RELIGIOUS, AND EXISTENTIAL ASPECTS OF CARE

Beliefs surrounding illness and death are profoundly influenced by a patient's and family's religious and spiritual values. The salient spiritual needs of patients encompass questions of meaning, value, and relationship. Existential questions can include: What is the meaning of my life? How will I be remembered? Who do I need to forgive?

A plan based on an assessment of religious, spiritual, and existential concerns using a structured instrument is integral to the palliative care plan. The four-question FICA Spiritual History Tool is one such instrument to assess for spiritual needs and concerns (see **Table 214-4**). Patients and their family should be provided information about the availability of spiritual care services. Spiritual care should be made available through hospital chaplaincy, spiritual counseling or through the patient's own clergy relationships. Specialized palliative care teams should include spiritual care professionals that are appropriately trained and certified in palliative care.

TABLE 214-4 FICA Spiritual History Tool

F—Do you have a spiritual belief or **F**aith? Do you have spiritual beliefs that help you cope with Stress?

What gives your life meaning?

I—Are these beliefs **I**mportant to you? How do they influence you in how you care for yourself?

C—Are you part of a spiritual or religious **C**ommunity?

A—How would you like your health care provider to **A**ddress these issues with you?

Data from GW Spirituality Institute of Spirituality and Health 2015. FICA Spiritual History Tool, developed by Dr. Pulchalski. http://smhs.gwu.edu/gwish/clinical/fica/spiritual-history-tool. Accessed April 8, 2015.

These professionals help to build partnership with community clergy and provide education and counseling related to end-of-life care.

■ DOMAIN 6: CULTURAL ASPECTS OF CARE

Cultural assessment incorporated as a component of comprehensive palliative care assessment includes but is not limited to: locus of decision making including preferences regarding disclosure of information, truth telling and decision making; dietary preferences; language and interpreter preferences; family communication preferences; desire for support measures such as palliative and complementary and alternative medicines; perspectives on death, suffering, and grieving; and funeral/burial rituals. Professional interpreter services and culturally sensitive materials should be provided in the patient's and family's preferred language.

See Chapter 37 (Cultural Competence).

■ DOMAIN 7: CARE OF PATIENT AT THE END OF LIFE

Health care practitioners should be able to recognize and document the transition to the active dying phase and communicate to the patient, family, and staff the expectation of imminent death. Families need education on a timely basis regarding the signs and symptoms of imminent death in a developmentally, culturally, and age-appropriate manner. As part of the ongoing care planning process, patient and family's wishes about the care setting for the site of death, should be documented. During the active dying phase, adequate dosages of analgesics and sedatives as appropriate to achieve patient comfort is provided, with fears and concerns about use of narcotics and analgesics hastening death appropriately addressed. Postdeath, the body should be treated with respect according to the cultural and religious practices of the family and in accordance with local law. Effective grieving is facilitated by implementing a bereavement care plan in a timely manner after the patient's death, with the family remaining as the focus of care.

See Chapter 74 (Hospice).
See Chapter 215 (Communication Skills for End of Life Care).
See Chapter 217 (Care of the Dying Patient).

■ DOMAIN 8: ETHICAL AND LEGAL ASPECTS OF CARE

For advanced care planning, the designated surrogate/decision maker should be documented in accordance with state law, as well as the patient and surrogate preferences for goals of care, treatment options, and setting of care; documentation should occur at first assessment and at frequent intervals as a patient's clinical condition changes. Advance care planning is a process that supports people in identifying personal values, in setting goals and plans with respect to future medical care, and in decision making over time. It brings together the individual, surrogates, families, and clinicians to develop a coherent care plan that aligns with the person's goals, values, and preferences based on a shared understanding of the person's evolving medical condition, prognosis, and potential future treatment options. When appropriate, conversion of the patient's treatment goals into medical orders, with the completion of Physician Orders for Life-Sustaining Treatments (POLST) forms, will help to ensure that the information is transferable and applicable across care settings, including long-term care, emergency medical services, and between hospitals.

Advance care planning documentation, POLST forms, and surrogacy designations should be available across care settings. Community collaborations can help promote advance care planning and completion of advance directives for all individuals. When ethical conflicts arise at the end of life, ethics consultation should be available across care settings.

See Chapter 33 (Common Indications for Ethics Consultation).
See Chapter 34 (Advance Directives and Surrogate Decision Making).

QUALITY IMPROVEMENT

The development of standards and guidelines in palliative care continues at a steady pace. In 2012, the American Hospital Association issued two reports on advanced illness management strategies that stressed the importance of patient and family understanding of advance illness planning and management, encouraged education and training of all health professionals to provide care over the continuum of health and decline, and suggested hospitals and care systems to improve the support and delivery of care for patients with serious and terminal illnesses.

The Joint Commission currently has an Advanced Certification for Palliative Care for hospitals that "demonstrate exceptional patient- and family-centered care that optimizes the quality of life for patients with serious illness." In 2015, the American Academy of Hospice and Palliative Medicine, in conjunction with the Hospice and Palliative Nurses Association, published 10 key quality indicators in palliative care as part of the Measuring What Matters project. Three criteria had to be met for each quality indicator, ensuring that each: (1) was meaningful for patient and families, (2) was able to be implemented by clinicians, and (3) can significantly improve the quality of care for patients and families (see **Table 214-5**).

Health care organizations are beginning to utilize palliative care more frequently to improve quality because it has been shown to be an effective approach to reducing symptoms and improving patient and family satisfaction. In addition, the use of palliative care services can improve transitions of care, support timely and successful discharge, avert unnecessary readmissions, and contribute to efficient use of health care resources. Many hospitals now use palliative care

---

TABLE 214-5 Ten Quality Indicators of Palliative Care

1. Palliative care and hospice patients receive a comprehensive assessment (physical, psychological, social, spiritual, and functional) soon after admission.

2. Seriously ill palliative care and hospice patients are screened for physical symptoms (eg, pain, shortness of breath, nausea, and constipation) during the admission visit.

3. Seriously ill palliative care and hospice patients who screen positive for at least moderate pain receive treatment (medication or other) within 24 h.

4. Patients with advanced or life-threatening illness are screened for shortness of breath and, if positive to at least a moderate degree, have a plan to manage it.

5. Serious ill palliative care and hospice patients have a documented discussion regarding emotional needs.

6. Hospice patients have a documented discussion of spiritual concerns or preference not to discuss them.

7. Seriously ill palliative care and hospice patients have documentation of the surrogate decision-maker's name (such as the person who has health care power of attorney) and contact information, or absence of a surrogate.

8. Seriously ill palliative care and hospice patients have documentation of their preferences for life-sustaining treatments.

9. Vulnerable elders with documented preferences to withhold or withdraw life-sustaining treatments have their preferences followed.

10. Palliative care and hospice patients or their families are asked about their experience of care using a relevant survey.

Data from AAHPM & HPNA Consensus Project: Measuring What Matters Project. 2015. http://aahpm.org/quality/measuring-what-matters and http://www.futurity.org/palliative-care-858232/. Accessed Feb 28, 2015.

programs to help meet pain management and other quality accreditation standards.

CONCLUSION

Today's hospitalist needs primary palliative care skills to provide quality care to patients with serious illness. Ongoing assessment and management of a patient's physical, emotional, social, and spiritual well-being is essential, with the referral to expert-level palliative care and/or hospice for refractory symptoms and complex psychosocial needs. Hospitalists will need to demonstrate proficiency in initiating conversations about difficult treatment choices with patient and families, particularly when medical interventions no longer improve health or restore a quality of life that is acceptable to the patient.

SUGGESTED READINGS

Abrahm JL. *A Physician's Guide to Pain and Symptom Management in Cancer Patients.* Baltimore, MD: Johns Hopkins University Press; 2014.

Anderson WG, Kools S, Lyndon A. Dancing around death: hospitalist-patient communication about serious illness. *Qual Health Res.* 2013;23(1):3-13.

Bernacki RE, Block SD. Communication about serious illness care goals: a review and synthesis of best practices. *JAMA Intern Med.* 2014;174(12):1994-2003.

Center to Advance Palliative Care. *A State-by-State Report Card on Access to Palliative Care in Our Nation's Hospitals.* 2012; http://www.capc.org/reports/card/. Accessed April 7, 2015.

Palliative Care Network of Wisconsin. *Palliative Care Fast Facts and Concepts.* https://www.mypcnow.org/fast-facts/. Accessed August 29, 2016.

Institute of Medicine. *Dying in America: Improving Quality and Honoring Individual Preferences Near the End of Life.* Washington, DC: The National Academies Press; 2014.

Lin RJ, et al. The sentinel hospitalization and the role of palliative care. *J Hosp Med.* 2014;9:320-323.

Lindvall C, Hultman TD, Jackson VA. Overcoming the barriers to palliative care referral for patients with advanced heart failure. *J Am Heart Assoc.* 2014;3(1):e000742.

National Consensus Project for Quality Palliative Care. *Clinical Practice Guidelines for Quality Palliative Care,* 3rd ed; Washington DC: NQF, 2013; http://www.nationalconsensusproject.org. Accessed March 30, 2015.

National Quality Forum. *A National Framework and Preferred Practices for Palliative and Hospice Care Quality: A Consensus Report.* 2006; http://www.qualityforum.org/Publications/ 2006/12/A_National_Framework_and_Preferred_Practices_for_Palliative_and_Hospice_Care_ Quality.aspx. Accessed March 30, 2015.

Quill TE, Abernathy AP. Generalist plus specialist palliative care-creating a more sustainable model. *N Engl J Med.* 2013;368(13):1173-1175.

Sharma RK, Jain N, Peswani N, et al. Unpacking resident-led code status discussions: results from a mixed methods study. *J Gen Intern Med.* 2014;29(5):750-757.

Temel J, Greer J, Muzikansky A, et al. Early palliative care for patients with metastatic non-small cell lung cancer. *N Engl J Med.* 2010;363:733-742.

Weissman DE, Meier DE. Identifying patients in need of a palliative care assessment in the hospital setting: a consensus report from the Center to Advance Palliative Care. *J Palliat Med.* 2011;14(1):17-23.

You JJ, Downar J, Fowler RA, et al. Barriers to goals of care discussions with seriously ill hospitalized patients and their families, a multicenter survey of clinicians. *JAMA Intern Med.* 2015;175(4):549-556.

CHAPTER 215

Communication Skills for End-of-Life Care

Amanda Caissie, MD, PhD, FRCPC
Camilla Zimmermann, MD, PhD, FRCPC

Key Clinical Questions

1. What are some practical methods of breaking bad news at any stage of disease?

2. How do you maintain hope while discussing goals of care in the context of a poor prognosis?

INTRODUCTION

Palliative care requires excellent communication skills. Clinicians navigate difficult situations including prognostication, breaking bad news, discussing hospice, and planning for the end of life, while acknowledging and addressing physical, psychological and spiritual distress for both the patient and family. Before focusing on details for each of these situations, physicians must establish basic goals of care. Communication strategies may vary based on individual preferences of the patient and family, cultural norms, the context of the situation, and the patient's stage of disease. The latter may be divided broadly into the time of diagnosis, the transition toward palliative care, and the time leading up to and including the patient's death. This chapter will describe approaches to communication for situations that arise commonly in the treatment of patients with life-threatening illnesses.

GENERAL COMMUNICATION SKILLS

Communication skills are essential for all physicians, as they develop rapport, gather and relay information, and help patients make informed decisions. It is important to keep in mind that the parties involved often have divergent perspectives, stemming from diverse generational, educational, socioeconomic, cultural, and spiritual backgrounds, which can have a profound effect on physician-patient/family interactions. Thus, diverse viewpoints may coexist within any one seemingly similar group. For this reason, it is essential to elicit individual communication preferences, rather than assuming that these fall neatly into a specific category.

All clinical interactions have emotional as well as informational elements. The exploration of a patient's previous experiences may add invaluable information or insight to the conversation, as certain experiences, such as having been a caregiver for a dying family member, increase the patient's readiness to have his or her own end-of-life discussions. Effective communication requires that clinicians recognize their own emotions in addition to those of patients and families. Likewise, communication has verbal and nonverbal components and it is important to recognize and respond to nonverbal cues in addition to listening for verbal ones and eliciting concerns. Respect and empathy are paramount, and both can be expressed verbally or nonverbally in very little time. In contrast to entering a room looking at the chart instead of the patient, the simple gesture of making introductions to everyone present speaks volumes as one begins the clinical relationship.

■ COMMUNICATION PRACTICES

While each encounter between clinician, patient, and family will be unique, there are basic communication skills that may facilitate difficult conversations. Open-ended questions promote greater understanding and are used to start the "Ask-Tell-Ask" approach, which lends itself to almost any clinical interaction (Back et al, 2008). When first communicating with a patient about a particular issue, such as diagnosis or prognosis, start by asking what the patient understands about her illness. After assessing what the patient knows (and identifying and acknowledging any associated emotions), tell the patient any additional information and/or clarify misconceptions. Perhaps most importantly, follow-up by asking another question to both ensure that the patient understands and that you have understood the emotional impact on the patient. When in doubt, it is useful to ask, "Do you have any questions?"

While open-ended questions are often an excellent beginning to a conversation while developing rapport, they rarely provide responses that delve into more difficult topics such as disease progression, prognosis or death. Indirectness, linking questions, and hypothetical talk are communication practices that are commonly used in these situations (Parry et al, 2014). While indirect, allusive or euphemistic talk makes it easy for patients to deflect or avoid difficult topics, it allows clinicians to gauge whether a patient is ready to engage and may act as a first step to more direct discussions. For example, to begin by saying "The biopsy results were not what we hoped." can gently open the door to further dialogue. To encourage communication about future issues, it is helpful to link questions with what patients have said or hinted at (eg, "You mentioned you were afraid of the future. Do you think it might help to plan for the worst case scenario, so that you don't have to deal with that later?"). Hypothetical questions are also useful in this situation; for example, "I know it's hard to think about, but say in the future you got so ill you couldn't make decisions for yourself. Have you thought about who you would like to make decisions for you?"

As a means of encouraging patients to talk, it is often helpful for clinicians to leave gaps of silence once a difficult topic has been raised, and allow the patient to continue the dialogue. Such nonverbal communication strategies are often overlooked but may be the most effective at relaying empathy or sensitivity through the touch of a hand or the passing of a tissue. By simply providing delays or hesitations within the conversation, clinicians may convey the seriousness of the topic.

■ POTENTIAL BARRIERS TO COMMUNICATION

Potential barriers to communication include clinician, system or institution and patient-related factors (Bernacki et al, 2014). Many experienced clinicians struggle with a comfort level during end-of-life discussions and feel inadequately prepared to deal with their own or the patient's emotional reaction. Communication skills training has been shown to be effective, and may use didactic approaches as well as standardized role-play. The benefit of mentorship and teachable moments in clinical situations should not be underestimated; observation of role models may be the first step in graduated comfort with difficult conversations. Both supervisors and trainees need to recognize their own limitations and comfort levels, with awareness that patients' perceptions of their disease, their treatment decisions and the patient-physician relationship will depend on the way that bad news is communicated.

Patients' emotions such as anxiety and denial are often described as affecting communication. It is important to identify patients with severe anxiety in order to offer counseling and support. While some clinicians avoid difficult subjects in an effort to limit anxiety, it is important to recognize that some level of anxiety is usual for patients with a life-threatening illness and that avoidance of end-of-life issues may limit the patient's ability to plan for the future. Patients generally expect health care providers to initiate discussions about advance care planning and will not take the initiative themselves if clinicians are reluctant to broach the subject.

System barriers to communication include diffusion of responsibility or ambiguity of responsibility for difficult conversations. Patients may receive mixed messages from different members of the health care team, or may receive no information if the responsibility for discussions of future planning is unclear. Care may be optimized by choosing one member of the health care team who assumes primary responsibility for timely end-of-life discussions, and maintaining a unified message among the health care professionals who are involved. Consistent, clear written communication and documentation in health records of patient wishes and goals of care discussions is essential. The culture of life-sustaining treatment as a default or systematic underuse of palliative care services is an institutional barrier to end-of-life communication that will hopefully be overcome with increasing evidence for the effectiveness of early palliative care in improving quality of life and satisfaction with care (Zimmermann et al, 2014).

■ CLINICIAN-FAMILY COMMUNICATION

Although communication in medicine often involves the family as well as the patient, this is particularly the case in palliative care. In the last days to hours of life or in the situation of patients who are no longer competent, clinician-family communication becomes critical. Good physician-family communication requires awareness of the roles of various family members as well as an appreciation for the wide array of emotions and conflicts that may arise in difficult times. Poor communication resulting from an intention to protect the patient or family from bad news may have the opposite and negative impact of increasing family conflict. End-of-life conversations that include caregivers or bereaved family members allow dialogue about personal relationships and memories; facilitate planning for the future, and enable expressions of important thoughts and sentiments including gratitude, love, forgiveness, and farewell.

BREAKING BAD NEWS

The communication of bad news is initially difficult for both clinician and patient and emotions at the time may be uncomfortable for all parties. However, contrary to common fears, honest communication is not associated with subsequent psychological distress or hopelessness. Breaking bad news allows for discussion of goals of care and patient care consistent with such goals, while increasing quality of life for patients and caregivers. Therefore, timely discussions are encouraged. Although most studies regarding strategies for breaking bad news have focused on the time of diagnosis, there are various stages in the disease trajectory where these strategies may be useful. For patients with cancer, for example, this may include each successive time that the cancer progresses on a certain treatment, the news that no further chemotherapy is indicated, and the news that the prognosis is short. While each situation will be different, it is useful to develop a core communication strategy that can be tailored to the circumstances.

The SPIKES protocol is a practical method for breaking bad news at any stage of disease (**Table 215-1**, Baile et al, 2000). It is easy to use and applicable to almost any clinical communication situation. Addressing the patient's emotions is typically the most difficult aspect for physicians. It is important for patients to feel that the emotional impact of the news is acknowledged; this can be achieved by the use of a simple statement such as "I know that this is very difficult news for you." A mnemonic that is helpful in this regard is NURSE: Name the emotion, Understand and Respect the emotion, Support the patient, and Explore the emotion.

The dreaded phrase "nothing else can be done" is a fallacy and should not be used. In addition to supportive medical treatments, emotional and social supports can always be offered and are interventions in themselves. Indeed, one may argue that the physician-patient/family relationship is one of the most valuable components of therapy regardless of disease stage.

■ THE REQUEST TO WITHHOLD BAD NEWS

Requests to withhold bad news about a diagnosis or prognosis may come directly from the patient or, more often, from the family. In survey studies, most patients report a desire to know information about their disease and prognosis, even if it is bad news. If a family requests nondisclosure, one should attempt to identify possible reasons for this request and whether it reflects the desire of the patient. Reasons may range from cultural norms regarding family-based decisions, to beliefs that discussing a poor prognosis will

TABLE 215-1 SPIKES Protocol for Delivering Bad News

Setting up the interview:
  Arrange for privacy
  Involve significant others
  Sit down
  Make connection with the patient
  Manage time constraints and interruptions

Assess the patient's *perception*:
  What does the patient know?

Obtain the patient's *invitation*:
  How much does the patient want to know?

Give *knowledge* and information to the patient:
  Warn the patient that bad news is coming (eg, "Unfortunately, I have some bad news to tell you.")
  Start at the level of comprehension and vocabulary of the patient
  Use nontechnical words
  Avoid excessive bluntness
  Give information in small portions, and check for the patients understanding

Address the patient's *emotions* with empathic responses

Summarize and *strategize*:
  Check the patient's understanding
  Ask if the patient is ready at that time to discuss a plan
  Make a treatment plan

Adapted from Baile WF, Buckman R, Lenzi R, et al. SPIKES–a six-step protocol for delivering bad news: application to the patient with cancer. *Oncologist*. 2000;5:302-311.

make it come true or destroy a patient's hope. At times the family is concerned about disclosure when in reality the patient already knows or would want to know if given the option.

According to the principle of autonomy, the patient should have the right to choose whether or not to be told information about his or her illness. Thus, the first step in communicating bad news is to assess how much information a patient would like to know. For patients who do not speak English, a translator should be present, rather than relying on the family for translation. Patients should be asked if they would like family or friends to be present during important discussions. Family meetings allow a shared awareness among all those affected by the illness, and allow family members to better understand the patient's perspective should they eventually act as power of attorney. In the initial discussion, it is helpful to begin with an opening statement about information that is known to the patient, such as "As you know, we have performed a number of tests." Further dialogue may proceed as follows: "Would you like to know detailed information about your illness, or are there aspects that you would prefer not to know?" If the patient requests the information, one may wish to add a confirmatory statement such as "I unfortunately have bad news for you. Would you like me to continue?"

The amount of information patients want may depend on social factors such as cultural background and level of assimilation, as well as individual factors such as not being ready to cope with the information. For the minority of patients who do not want to know their diagnosis and/or prognosis, one must respect this and try to understand their decision. Permission may then be obtained from the patient to discuss the situation and treatment plan with an appointed family member. It is important, however, to stress that

disclosure to the patient may be necessary for informed consent for certain treatments and procedures. If there is conflict about disclosure, a hospital ethics consultation should be sought. Patients who do not want to know clinical information at a given time should be given the invitation to ask questions at any point in the future.

PROGNOSTIC DISCLOSURE

The question, "How long do I have Doctor?" is both difficult and important to answer, as it will help patients and families to prioritize and plan for the limited time ahead. Prognostication involves the discussion of the probable course and outcome of an illness. This is not limited to a discussion of the likely duration of survival, but includes discussion of the symptoms and situations that may occur as a result of the illness, and an explanation of the goals, benefits, and risks of possible treatments.

Communication of prognosis is central to patient education, and is necessary for informed consent and shared decision making. Patients may make different choices regarding investigations or active treatments if they are properly informed rather than relying on their own preconceptions. In the Study to Understand Prognoses and Preferences for Outcomes and Risks of Treatment (SUPPORT), where explicit prognostic information was provided, patients were more likely to discuss advance directives and less likely to desire cardiopulmonary resuscitation (CPR) if they felt prognosis was "poor" (Covinsky et al, 2000). Disclosure of prognosis is important not only because it respects patient autonomy in terms of medical decisions, but also because it affords the patient and family an opportunity to fulfill plans such as attending a family member's wedding, traveling to see friends or family, or saying goodbyes, and to deal with practical issues such as assigning power of attorney, making a will and preparing funeral arrangements.

Physicians are constantly formulating a prognosis when making treatment decisions, but often do not communicate this information explicitly to the patient. Although clinical predictions are often optimistic, physicians are generally able to identify patients with less than 3 to 6 months to live. Barriers to disclosing the prognosis may include a focus on diagnosis or treatment, lack of formal education around prognostication, lack of self-confidence, beliefs in a self-fulfilling prophecy, attempts to maintain patient hope, difficulty dealing with emotional issues, time constraints, and fear regarding medical-legal implications of predictions. Given the importance that patients place on timely and empathic disclosure of prognosis, it is important to be aware of these barriers so that they may be addressed.

There are many tools available to assist with prognostication. These range from performance status scales such as the Karnofsky performance status scale and Eastern Cooperative Oncology Group scale, to detailed tools incorporating information such as age, gender, performance status, comorbidity, symptoms, diagnosis, and laboratory results. For patients with cancer, visceral and brain metastases are poor prognostic factors, as are symptoms such as dyspnea, anorexia, and delirium, and laboratory values such as hypercalcemia, leukocytosis, and hypoalbuminemia. Although these tools are useful for clinicians in determining prognosis, they must be supplemented and individualized with clinical experience and knowledge (see Chapter 105 [Using Prognosis to Guide Treatment]).

Communication of the prognosis is not a one-time occurrence, but a dynamic process that continues on an ongoing basis throughout the disease trajectory. While the SPIKES protocol may be used as a general framework for communicating prognosis; specific guidelines are presented in **Table 215-2**. It is likely that the patient already has some perception of the prognosis, which may be based on conversations with other clinicians, friends, or on information from the Internet or other sources. Sometimes the patient has a sound understanding, and other times expectations appear to be

TABLE 215-2 Discussing Prognosis

Determine the patient's understanding of the prognosis
Ask the patient how much information she wants to know about prognosis
Explain that any prognosis is an estimate and that exact information is not possible
Explain that the prognosis is dynamic and changes with time
Give a prognosis that is not too exact or too vague (eg, "measured in months" rather than "6 mo")
Present the information honestly while demonstrating empathy
Discuss what may occur in the future regarding symptoms and what arrangements should be made
Emphasize the clinician-patient connection and resources available to the patient and family
Book a follow-up appointment to address outstanding questions
Document the discussion in the chart
Ensure consistency of information communicated by various members of the clinical team

entirely unrealistic. It is important to elicit and acknowledge the patient's understanding of the situation as well as to gauge how much prognostic information she wants to know and to what level of detail. Some patients desire very little prognostic information and this should be respected provided that the goals of care are discussed and appropriate plans are made for the patient and family. Although some patients desire exact information, it should be emphasized that a prognosis is always an estimate and that the situation may change with time. Median survivals are just that and do not represent the outcome for every patient. Nonabandonment should be emphasized while developing an action plan and establishing goals of care.

■ ESTABLISHING GOALS OF CARE

The discussion of prognosis is inextricable from the discussion of goals of care. These should be readdressed frequently throughout the patient's disease course and individualized based on the stage of disease and unique characteristics of the patient. An individual's values will influence how they prioritize goals of care, and two patients with a similar prognosis may desire very different courses of treatment. For example, whether or not a patient will accept or decline life-prolonging treatment will depend on how he prioritizes the goals of prolonged duration of life compared with minimization of treatment side effects, symptom control, and quality of life. Illness may also change one's perceptions and treatment preferences. One study found that patients with advanced cancer were more likely to accept second-line chemotherapy treatments with only slight potential benefit and substantial potential side effects, compared to what oncologists or healthy counterparts might imagine accepting in the patient's situation (Balmer et al, 2001).

What physicians think they convey in terms of information is not always what the patient perceives. MacKillop and colleagues (1998) showed that while over 90% of physicians felt they had accurately conveyed the extent of disease and intent of treatment, almost one-third of patients with metastatic disease thought their disease was localized, and almost one-third of patients on palliative treatment thought the intent was curative. This may result from a misunderstanding of medical information: terms such as *curable*, *controlled*, or *terminal* disease need to be explained to avoid miscommunication. Other patients and families may understand the palliative nature of the medical treatment, but hope for a miracle or cure. It is important

for clinicians to realize that such seemingly contradictory thinking is common and is a manner of coping with the illness. Often patients or families will ask several clinicians the same questions about prognosis; it is therefore important that all members of a clinical team are communicating the same information in a consistent fashion.

Many physicians are concerned about destroying hope when discussing goals of care in the context of poor prognosis. If the physician is honest in informing patients when they are passing through various stages of their disease, there is a wide spectrum of realistic hopes that patients may have depending on the situation, ranging from cure or prolonged life to finding meaning in life, quality of life, symptom control, spending time with loved ones, and dying peacefully with dignity. A clinical pearl of communication is "Hope for the best, prepare for the worst," which acknowledges that hope can be sustained while also planning for the occurrence of clinical situations that may evolve quickly (Back et al, 2008).

END-OF-LIFE PLANNING DISCUSSIONS

Most patients in Western countries would like to be involved in their health care decisions. Although the focus of end-of-life discussions is often on code status or on planning for a crisis situation, there are many other decisions that need to be made. These include preferences about the extent of investigations, aggressiveness of treatment, hospice enrollment, place of death, organ donation, and religious rites to be performed prior to or after death. As important as what to do in the case of incompetence is how to proceed with care while the patient is competent and able. This requires that the patient understand the nature of the underlying illness and the consequences of treatment at any given time. For example, there is a time in the course of illness when treatment of hyperkalemia can be lifesaving and another when it will produce added suffering without appreciably increasing life expectancy. In order for discussions about end-of-life preferences to be effective, the patient needs to gain an appreciation for the extent of his or her underlying illness, and the physician needs to understand the cultural and individual preferences of the patient. Thus end-of-life discussions are always conversations, rather than information sessions.

■ ADVANCE DIRECTIVES

Advance directives provide an opportunity for patients to state their preferences for care while they are capable of doing so. The Patient Self Determination Act (PSDA) became effective in the United States in 1991, and requires that Medicare and Medicaid providers (eg, hospitals, nursing homes, and home health agencies) provide information to patients at the time of enrolment on their rights regarding advance directives. These include the right to participate in their health care decisions, the right to accept or refuse treatment, the right to prepare an advance directive, and the right to information on providers' policies regarding these rights. Unlike other legally binding documents, advance directives can be completed without an attorney, which facilitates their implementation (see Chapter 34 [Advanced Directives and Surrogate Decision Making]).

Advance directives typically consist of a living will and the assignment of a substitute decision maker, or durable power of attorney, who will make decisions for a patient in the case of incompetence. Although the number of patients with completed advance directives has increased substantially since the passage of the PSDA, approximately half of all severely or terminally ill patients still lack advance directives. This may be due to a patient's lack of understanding of his prognosis, a lack of awareness of the existence and process for completion of advance directives, or a perceived lack of relevance to the patient's situation. Physicians should be honest with patients regarding their prognosis, inform them about the availability of advanced directives and their importance, and indicate their willingness to discuss any medical issues that arise during or after the completion of the advanced directive.

■ LIVING WILL

The living will states the patient's preferences for care and serves not only to maintain patient autonomy, but also to minimize the burden of decision making on families faced with the emotionally charged situation of a loved one who is near death. Typically, the directive has instructions regarding whether or not life-sustaining treatment should be given, and may have specific directions regarding the use of CPR, mechanical ventilation, tube feeding, and use of antibiotics. In order for these directives to be meaningful, it is important to explain to patients what these various life-sustaining procedures are, and how they would or would not contribute to quality and/or quantity of life in the patient's situation. Many patients do not inform their physicians that they have an advance directive or living will, and this needs to be specifically asked about, so that physicians can discuss patients' answers and clarify any misinterpretations. As the patient's situation changes, the living will may need to be updated.

■ DURABLE POWER OF ATTORNEY

Regardless of whether or not a living will is completed, it is important for patients to assign a durable power of attorney. If patients have not made such an assignment, the law in Canada and in certain areas of the United States outlines a hierarchy of substitute decision makers for patients who are incapacitated (**Table 215-3**). However, the first person on a hierarchy list may not be the one the patient would have chosen, and may not share similar view points or values. At times, a patient may want to protect his loved ones and prefers not to discuss his medical situation with them. This becomes problematic when a person who has not been involved in the care of the patient is later acting as a substitute decision maker. In addition, substitute decision makers may inaccurately predict the patient's wishes (eg, believing that a patient would want more interventions than they actually would). For these reasons, it is useful for physicians to meet with patients and their assigned power of attorney to clarify wishes for care. The documentation of these wishes in the living will as well as in the patient's chart can avoid misunderstandings and ensure that future care proceeds as the patient desires.

■ CODE STATUS

Studies have shown that physicians are concerned about futile interventions at the end of life, and that most patients want to be involved decisions about CPR. In a study focusing on

TABLE 215-3 Substitute Decision Maker in Approximate Order of Priority*

1. Durable power of attorney for health care
2. Spouse
3. Legal guardian
4. Adult child (18 y or older)**
5. Parent
6. Sibling (18 y of age or older)**
7. Close friend (only in certain states)

*Order may vary from state to state; if it is not clear who should make decisions, consult with the hospital ethics board.

**If there are several family members with the same priority, then decisions are made by consensus, by majority, or by choosing one member who is responsible for making decisions on behalf of the group.

TABLE 215-4 A Framework for Discussions of Code Status and End-of-Life Care with Families

Determine whether the patient has an advance directive
Schedule a family meeting to discuss the patient's condition and clarify the family's understanding of the illness
If there is no durable power of attorney, determine who is the substitute decision maker (SDM)
Remind the SDM of his obligation to act in the person's best interest, taking into account the patient's values rather than the SDM's own preferences
Explain the patient's underlying condition and prognosis
Explain the nature and outcome of cardiopulmonary resuscitation
Explain and discuss specific procedures and treatments
Summarize what will or will not be done and answer any questions
Assure the family that the patient's comfort and dignity will be respected, and that appropriate management of symptoms will continue
Inform the family of how to contact you if they have further questions
Document the discussion and outcome in the patient's medical record
Continue to review and revise the plan as needed

Adapted from Lang F, Quill T. Making decisions with families at the end of life. *Am Fam Physician*. 2004;70:719-723.

American veterans who had died from cancer, families reported higher satisfaction with end-of-life care when the patient had a do-not-resuscitate (DNR) order at the time of death. However many physicians are uncomfortable initiating discussions about code status, and patients generally do not spontaneously ask about this subject. Although the majority of patients are competent when admitted to hospital, DNR orders are usually either not written at all, or written when the patient is no longer competent to make medical decisions. Discussions regarding code status therefore often occur with the family and with substitute decision makers rather than with patients themselves. **Table 215-4** outlines a framework for these types of discussions. Family involvement at end-of-life is associated with higher likelihood of DNR order and palliative care consultation. While early advanced care planning is advisable for all patients with a life-threatening illness, patients without family or social support should be considered in particular need of early advance care planning (Sudore et al, 2014).

The approach to discussing code status is important and may dictate the outcome. If one approaches a code discussion with the question "Would you want everything done in the event of…" then most patients and family members understandably request a full code. Ideally, code status preferences are already indicated in a living will and it is important to ask on admission to hospital whether or not an advance directive exists. If so, then the advance directive should be reviewed and the patient's preferences documented. If there is no advance directive, then a discussion needs to take place with the patient and/or power of attorney to review the patient's underlying condition and overall prognosis, explain what is involved in CPR, and outline what the outcomes typically are for patients in a similar situation. Success rates of CPR are low with a chance of survival to hospital discharge of approximately 15%. Conditions such as metastatic cancer, renal failure, sepsis, or reduced performance status diminish the prognosis considerably. This may not be understood by patients or families, whose impression of the outcome of CPR may be founded on overly optimistic scenarios typically depicted in movies or on television.

At times, orders are written which are variations of the "full code" or DNR orders. This is not ideal as confusion may arise in the midst of a code when an order such as "chest compressions, and defibrillation but no intubation" exists. The actions taken at the time of a code are stepwise and often automatic, potentially resulting in unwanted interventions if DNR orders are not clear or if a variation on the order exists. Increasingly hospitals and other health care institutions have protocols regarding code status, including which exact order should be written. Conversely, one should not assume that because a DNR order exists, the patient does not desire any other therapeutic interventions. Specific treatments should be discussed in detail with the patient or substitute decision maker, so that a complete understanding can be reached of what is desired. This also serves to allay patients' fears that their care will be inferior if a DNR order exists. Finally, it is important to emphasize that the patient will not be abandoned, and care will continue for pain and symptom management as well as support for the patient and family.

DISCUSSING HOSPICE AND PALLIATIVE CARE

Communicating the roles of hospice and palliative care to patients and families is a challenge in itself. When the hospice and palliative care movements were established in the 1960s and 1970s, the focus was mainly on care at the end of life. The role of palliative care has since broadened, as indicated by the most recent World Health Organization definition. Contemporary palliative care focuses on quality of life as well as dignity in death and is complementary to, not exclusive of, therapies directed at the underlying illness. Hospice is more limited, due to what is or is not covered by the Medicare hospice benefit. The Medicare hospice benefit was established in 1983 and is available to patients with a prognosis of 6 months or less and the desire to receive the benefits of hospice services while foregoing disease-directed treatment. Both palliative care and hospice employ an interdisciplinary approach with expertise from fields such as medicine, nursing, social work, physiotherapy, occupational therapy, and spiritual care, and provide support to both the patient and the family. Hospice also includes services such as homemakers, medications, supplies and equipment; care may occur at home or in a hospice facility, nursing home or hospital.

■ HOSPICE

Referrals to hospice typically occur very late, and only approximately one-third of Americans die under hospice care (Glare & Sinclair, 2008). This may be due to a lack of understanding of the prognosis on the part of the clinician or patient, and/or the lack of coverage by many hospices of costly services such as palliative chemotherapy, palliative radiation, and blood transfusions. For patients who are not willing to forego such treatments, the prognosis and goals of care should be clarified. If these are understood and a patient still refuses referral to hospice, then another option is simultaneous palliative care or a hospice bridge program, if available. The involvement of palliative care services prior to the discussion of hospice may help with the difficult communication issues that arise at this transition point. As with communicating other types of difficult news, it is important to acknowledge the emotional aspect of these discussions. Multiple discussions over time may be necessary before a patient will agree to a hospice referral.

■ PALLIATIVE CARE

While palliative care referrals can be placed at any time, early referral (eg, at the diagnosis of metastatic disease for patients with cancer) can optimize management of physical and psychological symptoms,

link the patient with services that will be available in acute crises, and facilitate communication regarding end-of-life planning. Some patients are able to acknowledge their prognosis and are active participants in advance care planning. Such patients are generally appreciative of early referral to palliative care services, and may even initiate the referral themselves. For others who have difficulty coming to terms with their prognosis, explicit discussions about palliative care may not be possible; for these patients, the referral may be better introduced in terms of management of specific symptoms or as a "safety net" for dealing with future concerns. Paradoxically, it is often the latter group of patients who benefit most from specialized palliative care, as the palliative care team is able to support them through the psychological and physical distress that they are experiencing. It is important to emphasize to the patient that unlike hospice, palliative care is not restricted to those with a limited prognosis. Patients can and should receive palliative care support if needed for symptom control during disease-directed treatments such as chemotherapy.

COMMUNICATION IN THE LAST DAYS AND HOURS OF LIFE

In the last days and hours of life, the patient's desire for information inevitably lessens compared to their need for emotional support. The family, on the other hand, requires a great deal of communication and information to prepare for the patient's death. If possible, the family will need forewarning that death is imminent, to prepare emotionally as well as practically for issues such as time spent with the patient and preferences regarding religious or cultural practices. It is important to obtain contact information from loved ones who would like to be with the patient in their last days to hours, so that they can be informed when death is near. If feasible, arranging for more privacy at this time will help not only the patient and family but also surrounding patients.

Even in the last days and hours of life, some families find it difficult to accept that the end of life is near. If the patient is imminently dying, and the cause is irreversible, it is important to meet formally with the family to address any outstanding concerns and emphasize the goals of care. Once the patient and family have acknowledged that the prognosis is short and the goal of care is comfort, they will need explicit guidance regarding what to expect during the dying process. It is important to explain that patients will likely stop eating and drinking and that verbal communication will likely cease as sleep increases. The family may feel helpless at this point and will take comfort in knowing that they are helping simply with their presence or with small gestures such as assistance with the patient's mouth care.

A pain-free and peaceful death is an obvious goal of palliative care, but bereavement care should not be overlooked. The family is integral to the therapeutic relationship throughout, and will retain memories of the patient's illness, and of the day of death, long after their loved one has died. The support and preparation of the family by the health care team can make a large difference in rendering these memories as positive as possible.

CONCLUSION

Communication is important in any clinical discipline but particularly in palliative care, as the information conveyed often involves bad news and evokes emotions in all participants of the clinical interaction. These emotions need to be acknowledged and addressed with empathy in order for a therapeutic relationship to ensue. This is a stage when many important decisions are made, not only for palliative treatment and advance care planning, but also for personal projects and goals. Patients and families appreciate honest, open communication that leaves room for hope and promises nonabandonment. Although these discussions are often difficult, they are also meaningful and will have a lasting impact on all involved.

PRACTICE POINT

1. In palliative care discussions, address not only the medical needs of the patient but also the psychosocial concerns of patient and family.
2. Determine what the patient understands and how much this individual would like to know before communicating new information.
3. During and after clinical interactions, ensure that the patient understands the plan and that you have understood the emotional impact on the patient.
4. Avoid expressions such as "nothing else can be done." Instead, emphasize what can be done in terms of palliation, and reassure the patient and family that they will not be abandoned.
5. Initiate conversations about advance care planning, palliative care and hospice early in the course of illness.
6. Ensure that there is consistency in the clinical team when discussing prognosis and the treatment plan.
7. Respect a patient's hopes while encouraging plans for the future: "Hope for the best; prepare for the worst."

SUGGESTED READINGS

Back AL, Anderson WG, Bunch L, et al. Communication about cancer near the end of life. *Cancer.* 2008;113(S7):1897-1910.

Balmer CE, Thomas P, Osborne RJ. Who wants second-line, palliative chemotherapy? *Psychooncology.* 2001;10(5):410-418.

Bernacki RE, Block SD, for the American College of Physicians High Value Care Task Force. Communication about serious illness care goals. A review and synthesis of best practices. *JAMA Intern Med.* 2014;174(12):1994-2003.

Covinsky KE, Fuller JD, Yaffe K, et al. Communication and decision-making in seriously ill patients: findings of the SUPPORT project. The Study to Understand Prognoses and Preferences for Outcomes and Risks of Treatments. *J Am Geriatr Soc.* 2000;48(5 Suppl):S187-S193.

Ehlenbach WJ, Barnato AE, Curtis JR, et al. Epidemiologic study of in-hospital cardiopulmonary resuscitation in the elderly. *N Engl J Med.* 2009;361:22-31.

Emanuel EJ, Emanuel LL. Proxy decision making. *JAMA.* 1992;267:2221-2226.

Emanuel LL, Ferris FD, von Gunten CF, et al. EPEC-O: Education in Palliative and End-of-Life Care for Oncology. Participant's Handbook Module 9: Negotiating goals of care. Chicago, IL: The EPEC Project, 2005.

Finlay E, Casarett D. Making difficult discussions easier: using prognosis to facilitate transitions to hospice. *CA: Cancer J Clin.* 2009;59:250-263.

Glare PA, Sinclair CT. Palliative medicine review: prognostication. *J Pall Med.* 2008;11(1):84-103.

Parry R, Land V, Seymour J. How to communicate with patients about future illness progression and end of life: a systematic review. *BMJ Support Pall Care.* 2014;4:331-341.

Saraiya B, Bodnar-Deren S, Leventhal E, et al. End-of-life planning and its relevance for patients' and oncologists' decisions in choosing cancer therapy. *Cancer.* 2008;113(S12):3540-3547.

Sudore RL, Casarett D, Smith D, Richardson DM, Ersek M. Family involvement at the end-of-life and receipt of quality care. *J Pain Symptom Manage.* 2014;48(6):1108-1116.

Wallace CL. Family communication and decision making at the end of life: A literature review. *Palliat Support Care.* 2014;28:1-11.

Zimmermann C, Swami N, Krzyzanowska M, et al. Early palliative care for patients with advanced cancer: a cluster-randomised controlled trial. *Lancet.* 2014;383(9930):1721-1730.

CHAPTER 216

Domains of Care: Physical Aspects of Care

Cindy Lien, MD

PAIN

■ INTRODUCTION

Studies of patient perspectives on end-of-life care consistently report pain control as a major priority. Nonetheless, the literature shows that many patients experience poor pain control. In one well-known study (SUPPORT trial: Study to Understand Prognoses and Preferences for Outcomes and Risks of Treatments), approximately 40% of hospitalized patients experienced severe pain in the last 3 days before death.

When the focus of care is quality of life and comfort, any poorly controlled symptom should be treated urgently. Many patients already fear that pain will be an inevitable part of their disease process and that "nothing can be done." Hospitalists play a vital role in correcting this misconception and ensuring that patients with advanced illnesses receive adequate pain control.

■ PATHOPHYSIOLOGY

Pain can be described as nociceptive or neuropathic in origin. In nociceptive pain, peripheral nociceptors in the skin, musculoskeletal system, or viscera detect noxious stimuli and send impulses via afferent A-delta or C fibers to the dorsal horn of the spine. These signals are transmitted through ascending spinothalamic tracts to the thalamus and then to the cortex. Neuropathic pain occurs when the peripheral or central nervous system itself suffers damage or develops pathologic changes in sensitization. Neuropathic pain is generally more difficult to control than nociceptive pain. In reality, however, any type of chronic pain can significantly alter the sensory pathways and cause pathologic activation of the nervous system even after the initial pain stimulus has dissipated. The mechanisms of activation are quite complex and can involve central sensitization pathways, including multiple neurotransmitters (substance P, amino acid ligands), receptors (mu opioid, neurokinin-1, N-methyl-D-aspartate [NMDA]), and intracellular pathways (nitric oxide, protein kinase C).

The patient ultimately experiences pain not just as a physical phenomenon, but as an emotional experience. The International Association for the Study of Pain (IASP) has defined *pain* as "an unpleasant sensory and emotional experience associated with actual or potential tissue damage, or described in terms of such damage. While it is unquestionably a sensation in part or parts of the body, it is always unpleasant and, therefore, an emotional experience." Patients with life-threatening illness are especially vulnerable to emotional and cognitive factors that can influence their experience of pain.

■ EVALUATION

Assessment of pain begins with a thorough history, including location, onset, duration, intensity, quality, and aggravating or ameliorating factors. The evaluation should also include a history of any associated functional decline, a psychosocial assessment (including exploration of any associated fears and concerns about disease progression), and a careful physical exam. The clinician should formulate a differential diagnosis of the clinical etiology of pain, which may include processes unrelated to the patient's known terminal disease. For example, chest pain in a patient with breast cancer could be due to bony metastases, postradiation skin

Terminal Delirium

❶ How do I evaluate an agitated dying patient?

❷ How do I identify terminal delirium and distinguish it from other kinds of delirium?

❸ What medications are useful for treating terminal delirium?

Nutrition and Hydration

❶ How do I counsel family members who are upset that the patient is no longer eating?

❷ Are there any clinical situations in which artificial nutrition and hydration may be helpful for patients with advanced disease?

Complementary Medicine

❶ Is there data to support the use of complementary therapy to relieve common symptoms such as pain and nausea?

❷ How do I advise a patient who asks me about a therapy with which I am unfamiliar?

- Neuropathic pain can result from injury to any part of the nervous system, such as the peripheral nerves or spinal cord. Examples include postherpetic neuralgia, radiation-related brachial plexus injury, post-thoracotomy pain, and phantom limb pain. Neuropathic pain is frequently described as *burning, tingling, stabbing, electric,* or *shooting*. It may also be described as *aching*. Physical findings may include allodynia, which is pain caused by a normally painless stimulus such as light touch. Neuropathic pain may also radiate.
- Some pathologic processes can cause a mixed pain syndrome with both nociceptive and neuropathic pain. One example is bone metastases to the spine, which may incite nociceptive, somatic bone pain as well as neuropathic pain from nerve root compression.

When a patient is unable to communicate, the clinician must then rely on the family or caregiver's report and careful observation for nonverbal cues, such as guarding or grimacing with movement, to assess pain. One common misconception is that a patient who exhibits no physiologic signs of discomfort (such as tachycardia or hypertension) is unlikely to be experiencing pain. In fact, patients with chronic pain rarely show these signs of sympathetic arousal. These physiologic changes are more typically seen in acute pain, though even some patients with acute pain do not exhibit these signs.

Several pain scales have been developed to monitor pain intensity and efficacy of treatment (**Figure 216-1**). Some patients may have no difficulty with the numerical pain scale, whereas others find it easier to report simplified categories of mild, moderate, or severe pain. Patients with mild cognitive deficits may be able to utilize the Faces Pain Scale, which was originally developed for pediatric patients.

Diagnostic tests should be tailored appropriately to a patient's overall goals of care. Generally, if a study has good potential to lead to therapies (such as radiation) that would enhance a patient's comfort, then the study may be indicated even in the setting of advanced disease.

changes, cardiac ischemia, pulmonary embolism, costochrondritis, or gastroesophageal reflux disease.

The clinician should also determine the type of pain a patient is experiencing, as this will guide the appropriate treatment strategy.

- Nociceptive pain can be categorized as somatic or visceral. Somatic pain includes skin, musculoskeletal, or bone pain. It may be described as *sharp, constant, throbbing, aching,* and *exacerbated by movement*. It is usually well localized. Unlike somatic pain, visceral pain is generally poorly localized and arises from injury to organs or the lining of body cavities. It may be described as *cramping, aching, tearing, deep,* or a *pressure sensation*. Examples of visceral pain include symptoms from bowel obstruction, cholecystitis, or cardiac ischemia.

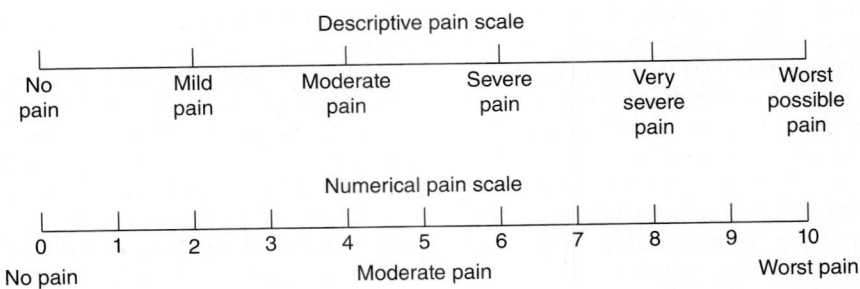

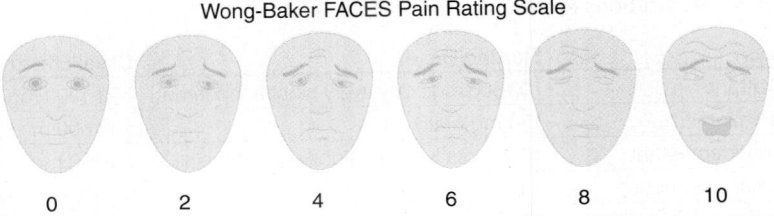

Figure 216-1 *Pain intensity scales*. (From Hicks CL, von Baeyer CL, Spafford P, van Korlaar I, Goodenough B. Faces Pain Scale-Revised: Toward a Common Metric in Pediatric Pain Measurement. *Pain*. 93:173, 2001. Wong-Baker FACES Foundation (2015). Wong-Baker FACES® Pain Rating Scale. Retrieved [Date] with permission from http://www.WongBakerFACES.org.)

■ TREATMENT

General principles

The World Health Organization (WHO) has developed a well-known analgesic ladder that recommends nonopioid analgesics such as nonsteroidal anti-inflammatory drugs (NSAIDs) or acetaminophen for mild pain, with the addition of opioids for moderate and severe pain. The WHO ladder also recommends consideration of adjuvant therapies such as antidepressants and anticonvulsants at any level of pain if appropriate. One should keep in mind that many patients with terminal illness have at least moderate to severe pain and thus will need an opioid immediately in addition to nonopioid analgesics.

Medication choice should also be guided by the type of pain. Opioids are generally effective for nociceptive pain, including both somatic and visceral types. Somatic pain such as musculoskeletal or bone pain may also be quite responsive to NSAID therapy. Bone pain may require a combination of additional therapies including bisphosphonates, corticosteroids, calcitonin, or radiation therapy. Visceral pain from bowel obstruction may warrant an antisecretory agent such as a somatostatin analogue (octreotide) or an anticholinergic agent with antispasmotic activity (hyoscyamine, glycopyrrolate, scopolamine). Neuropathic pain is often less responsive to opioids and requires the addition of adjuvant medications. **Table 216-1** shows common adjuvant medications for neuropathic pain.

The mainstays in neuropathic pain therapy include anticonvulsants (gabapentin, pregabalin) and antidepressants (tricyclic antidepressants, serotonin-norepinephrine reuptake inhibitors). Topical agents such as lidocaine and capsaicin can be helpful. Depending on the etiology of pain, second-line agents such as corticosteroids and autonomic drugs (clonidine, prazosin, terazosin) may have a role. NMDA receptor antagonists such as ketamine can be considered for intractable pain but would require administration by a pain specialist.

The side-effect profile may greatly influence one's choice of pain medication. NSAIDs are not recommended for those with significant risk of renal compromise, including patients who are elderly or have chronic kidney disease. Patients with multiple myeloma and a normal creatinine still carry a substantial risk for renal failure with NSAIDs. NSAIDs may also be contraindicated in patients at risk for gastrointestinal bleed or those on concomitant blood-thinning agents. Tricyclic antidepressants should be used cautiously in the elderly due to anticholinergic side effects. Nortriptyline is well studied and is generally considered the best-tolerated tricyclic agent for the elderly, as it has the least anticholinergic activity. Opioids have some well-known side effects including constipation and sedation.

However, because many patients with terminal illness will eventually need an opioid for adequate pain control, the clinician should become adept at dosing opioids and managing their side effects.

Opioid analgesics

Many clinicians have received little formal training in pain management and do not feel fully confident selecting and dosing opioids. This discomfort may be exacerbated by misconceptions about opioids on the part of both clinicians and patients. Opioids rarely cause respiratory depression when dosed appropriately for pain. Studies have shown that patients with underlying lung disease such as chronic obstructive pulmonary disease (COPD) can safely use opioids if dosed appropriately.

True opioid addiction is uncommon in terminally ill patients. Providers sometimes mistake behaviors like clock-watching or irritability as signs of addiction, but usually these are manifestations of an inadequate pain regimen. These apparent drug-seeking behaviors (termed *pseudoaddiction*) tend to cease when patients are given adequate doses at regular intervals.

Some patients and family members may not readily articulate their fears of opioid addiction. They may also worry that their disease is progressing or that they are "giving up" if they take opioids. Many patients directly associate morphine with dying. Clinicians should be attuned to these fears and educate their patients accordingly. It is also important to emphasize that pain medications will not advance one's disease, and may in fact improve function by reducing pain.

Selecting an opioid

Commonly used opioids include morphine, oxycodone, hydromorphone, fentanyl, and methadone. For most patients being initiated on opioids, there is not a compelling reason to choose, for example, hydromorphone over morphine. For certain patient populations, however, the choice of opioid does matter. Patients with significant renal failure should generally avoid morphine. The metabolites of morphine can accumulate in renal failure and cause neurotoxic side effects including myoclonus and delirium. Fentanyl and methadone are the safest opioids to use in renal failure patients including those on dialysis. Hydromorphone and oxycodone may be used cautiously in those with mild to moderate renal failure, with consideration of a reduction in dose or decrease in frequency. Similarly, patients with liver failure may need dose and frequency adjustments, but it is not clear that one particular opioid is significantly safer than the others in this setting.

Methadone may be effective for patients with severe pain who have responded poorly to other opioids or who have developed intolerable side effects. In addition to its opioid receptor activity, methadone is also believed to act as an NMDA receptor antagonist. It has good bioavailability and no known active metabolites (thus accounting for its safety in renal failure). However, due to its long half-life and complexities in dosing, it should generally be initiated by clinicians with prior training or in consultation with a specialist.

TABLE 216-1 Common Adjuvant Medications for Neuropathic Pain

Drug	Drug Class	Starting Dose	Usual Effective Dose
Gabapentin	Anticonvulsant	100-300 mg orally every night at bedtime*	300-1200 mg orally three times a day
Pregabalin	Anticonvulsant	150 mg orally daily	300-600 mg orally twice a day
Nortriptyline	Tricyclic antidepressant	10 mg orally every night at bedtime	50-150 mg orally every night at bedtime
Lidocaine 5% patch	Topical local anesthetic	1 patch 12 h/d	1-3 patches 12 h/d
Capsaicin cream	Topical substance P modulator	0.025% cream three times a day	0.025%-0.075% three to four times a day

*Use low dose of gabapentin initially to minimize sedation, titrate every 3-7 d as tolerated. Maximum dose in renal impairment ~300 mg/d. Discuss dialysis dosing with pharmacy.

TABLE 216-2 Equianalgesic Opioid Doses*

Drug	Oral	Intravenous
Morphine	30 mg	10 mg
Oxycodone	20 mg	—
Hydromorphone	7.5 mg	1.5 mg
Fentanyl#	—	0.1 mg (100 mcg)

*These values are intended as estimates for conversion calculations, not as starting doses.

#To convert oral morphine equivalents to fentanyl patch: Divide the morphine oral total 24-h dose by 2 to reach an approximate dose of fentanyl transdermal in mcg/h. See sample calculation in Figure 216-2.

Certain opioids are almost never recommended. Both meperidine and propoxyphene should be avoided because their metabolites can accumulate with repeated dosing and cause serious neurotoxicity such as seizures. Codeine should not be used for severe pain because it has a "ceiling effect" whereby further titration results only in increased side effects without improved pain relief. Furthermore, codeine must first be metabolized to morphine to provide analgesia, and approximately 10% of the population lacks the appropriate hepatic enzyme. These patients derive no benefit from codeine.

Principles of opioid dosing
Equianalgesic doses:

Different opioids have different potencies (ie, dose required to achieve a certain effect). Equianalgesic doses of two different opioids should achieve a similar degree of pain relief for most patients, although some patients may have idiosyncratic responses to different opioids due to genetically determined variations in metabolism. **Table 216-2** shows equianalgesic doses of commonly used opioids. Looking at the table, morphine 10 mg intravenously should achieve similar pain relief as morphine 30 mg orally and oxycodone 20 mg orally. Misconceptions that "morphine does not work but hydromorphone does" may arise from a lack of knowledge of equianalgesic doses. A patient who finds no relief with morphine 4 mg intravenously but responds well to hydromorphone 1 mg intravenously may have in fact needed a higher dose of morphine (hydromorphone 1 mg intravenously is equianalgesic to approximately morphine 6.6 mg intravenously).

General opioid dosing guidelines:

- **Table 216-3** lists reasonable starting doses and dosing intervals for moderate to severe pain in opioid-naïve patients.
- **Figure 216-2** demonstrates opioid conversions using simple mathematical ratios.
- Many clinicians find it helpful to consult an opioid calculator program. One commonly used opioid calculator is available through Global RPh: www.globalrph.com/narcotic.cgi.

TABLE 216-3 Commonly Used Opioids: Moderate to Severe Pain in Opioid-Naïve Patients

Drug	Initial Oral Dose*	Initial Intravenous Dose*
Morphine	7.5-15 mg every 4 h	2-5 mg every 2 h
Oxycodone	5-10 mg every 4 h	—
Hydromorphone	2-4 mg every 4 h	0.25-0.75 mg every 2 h

*Use the lower end of the dose range for elderly patients or patients with renal/liver compromise. Morphine is not recommended in patients with significant renal failure.

- When switching between different opioids, most experts recommend a 25% to 50% dose reduction after one has calculated the equianalgesic dose. This is to account for *incomplete cross tolerance*. A patient who has developed some tolerance to the old opioid may not have the same degree of tolerance to the new opioid. The dose reduction is intended to reduce the risk of undesired side effects.
- Patients with chronic pain will generally need a long-acting pain medication (eg, sustained-release oxycodone or morphine, fentanyl patch, or methadone), not just short-acting medications. Figure 216-2 demonstrates the initiation of a long-acting opioid in a patient with metastatic bone pain. If unable to use a long-acting pain medication, chronic pain patients should at least receive a standing pain regimen with additional as-needed availability.
- Patients on sustained-release medications should also have a short-acting medication for breakthrough pain. Each dose of breakthrough opioid should be approximately 10% to 20% of the total daily requirement of the sustained-release opioid.
- If greater than three doses of breakthrough pain medications are needed in a 24-hour period, one may consider increasing the amount of sustained-release opioid. An appropriate increase would be 50% to 100% of the total amount used for breakthrough pain in 24 hours.

Acute pain crisis

Patients with terminal illness, particularly those with cancer, may suffer severe exacerbations of pain from bone metastases, pathologic fractures, bowel obstruction, or other manifestations of progressive disease. When a patient presents with severe, uncontrolled pain (7-10 intensity), this is considered an acute pain crisis or palliative care emergency. Clinicians should treat these symptoms aggressively while determining the underlying cause. The National Comprehensive Cancer Network has published guidelines for rapid titration of opioids to treat severe pain (Figures PAIN-4 and PAIN-5 in NCCN Clinical Practice Guidelines in Oncology: Adult Cancer Pain. To access: www.nccn.org/professionals/physician_gls/f_guidelines.asp).

> **PRACTICE POINT**
> - Severe pain should be treated as a palliative care emergency.

> **PRACTICE POINT**
> - Consider a pain or palliative consult in patients with uncontrolled pain or intolerable side effects. Also consider a consult in patients with unusual dosing needs due to a history of chronic opioid use, illicit drug use, or methadone maintenance. Such patients are at great risk of undertreatment due to high opioid tolerance and psychosocial or behavioral issues.

Opioid infusions

Infusions can be useful in certain settings but require a good understanding of basic principles.

- Opioid infusions should be used only when there is a specific indication. They should not be automatically started in a dying patient who is "comfort care" unless the patient has symptoms of discomfort and has demonstrated an ongoing need for opioids.
- Patients who were previously on sustained-release oral regimens but are now unable to take pills (eg, surgery, bowel obstruction) will need another means of fulfilling their baseline opioid requirement. For most inpatients, an opioid infusion is appropriate. The total daily opioid requirements should be

Your patient has been receiving hydromorphone 0.5-1 mg IV every two hours PRN during this hospitalization for pain due to bone metastases. You would like to initiate an appropriate oral regimen of both long-acting and short-acting medications.

Step 1: Determine the patient's total daily opioid requirement:
In this example, you review the record and calculate that your patient has been using an average of 6 mg IV hydromorphone per 24 h for several days now.

Step 2: Convert to oral morphine equivalents using equianalgesic ratios:
You know that 1.5 mg IV hydromorphone is equianalgesic to 30 mg orally morphine. Thus, convert 6 mg IV hydromorphone to oral morphine equivalents using this ratio:

$$\frac{1.5 \text{ mg hydromorphone IV}}{30 \text{ mg orally morphine}} = \frac{6 \text{ mg hydromorphone IV}}{x \text{ mg orally morphine}}$$

$$x = 120 \text{ mg orally morphine}$$

Step 3: Reduce by approximately 25% for incomplete cross tolerance:
120 mg orally morphine – (25% x 120 mg orally morphine) → 90 mg orally morphine

Step 4: Determine a long-acting regimen that approximates the total oral morphine requirement.
A reasonable option is sustained release morphine 45 mg orally every 12 hours which will yield 90 mg orally morphine/day.
(Constraints will include what doses are available commercially. Sustained release morphine is available in 15, 30, 60, 100, 200 mg tablets.)

Step 5: Determine a breakthrough dose that reflect 10%-20% of the total daily requirement of sustained-release opioid
15% of 90 mg orally morphine →13 mg orally morphine → select morphine immediate release 15 mg orally every 4 hours PRN

Suppose your patient is unable to take sustained release morphine due to inability to swallow whole pills (sustained release morphine is not crushable). One option is to use a fentanyl transdermal patch instead.

From Step 3: You have determined that the goal is approximately 90 mg orally morphine equivalents per day, which reflects a 25% reduction for incomplete cross tolerance.

Divide by 2 to calculate an approximate dose of fentanyl mcg/hr transdermal
90 mg ÷ 2 → approximately fentanyl 45 mcg/h transdermal → select fentanyl 50 mcg/h patch

An appropriate breakthrough dose is still morphine 15 mg orally every 4 h PRN. Your patient can either crush the immediate release morphine tablets or use liquid formulations. A concentrated elixir form is also available commercially in 20 mg/mL concentration for patients who cannot swallow.

Figure 216-2 *Opioid equianalgesic conversion example.*

converted into intravenous morphine or hydromorphone equianalgesic units, then divided by 24 hours for an hourly infusion rate. Consider a 25% to 50% dose reduction for incomplete cross-tolerance if switching between opioids. Fentanyl patch (discussed later) may be an option for those without intravenous access, but it is not appropriate for acute pain due to the time required to reach peak effect.

- Patients with severe pain who have required multiple opioid doses to control their symptoms may also be potential candidates for an opioid infusion. The initial infusion rate should be calculated based on the prior total documented 24-hour needs, or if in an acute pain crisis, projected from their needs over the past 4 hours.
- Opioid infusion orders should not be written as broad ranges of "morphine 2 to 20 mg/h, titrate to comfort." This type of order places the patient at risk for inappropriate titration of the infusion. Many clinicians do not realize that it takes at least 8 to 12 hours to achieve new steady-state blood levels of morphine or hydromorphone after a change in the basal infusion rate. If

one simply continues titrating up an infusion in a symptomatic patient without administering as-needed boluses, this patient is at risk for undertreatment of symptoms in the immediate setting, as well as overdose in several hours once the opioid reaches a new steady state. Many experts therefore recommend that opioid infusions be written as a specific rate without any range, with an additional order for as-needed boluses, either nurse-administered or through patient-controlled analgesia (PCA).

- Bolus orders can be rapidly titrated for poorly controlled pain. Peak effect for morphine and hydromorphone boluses occurs within 15 to 30 minutes. If a particular bolus dose is inadequate, the dose can be safely increased every 15 to 30 minutes without needing to rapidly titrate up the basal infusion rate.
- The basal infusion rate should be reassessed every 8 hours but not more frequently. The infusion rate can be increased based on the amount of boluses required, but generally should not be increased by more than 100% at a time.
- When using an opioid infusion to treat a patient who is not at the final stages of illness, the clinician should be attuned to

TABLE 216-4 Patient-Controlled Analgesia (PCA): Opioid-Naïve Patients

Drug	Loading Dose	Initial PCA Dose*	Typical Lockout
Morphine	2 mg	1 mg	6 min
Hydromorphone	0.4 mg	0.2 mg	6 min
Fentanyl	20 mcg	10 mcg	6 min

*Elderly patients and those at risk for sleep apnea should be monitored closely for symptoms of somnolence and respiratory depression. Consider reducing initial PCA dose by 25%-50% for these patients.

potential fears that the patient may be actively dying. Many people associate a "morphine drip" with dying.

- Seek the advice of a pain expert before starting an infusion for a patient who is opioid-naïve.

Patient-controlled analgesia

Patient-controlled analgesia (PCA) may be used for patients with significant pain who are alert and able to use the equipment appropriately. PCAs should not be used by patients who have delirium, dementia, or other cognitive deficits. **Table 216-4** shows commonly used PCA doses and lockout intervals in opioid-naïve patients. Higher doses may be needed in patients who have previously been on opioids. PCA pumps can be programmed to deliver patient-controlled boluses, a basal infusion, or both, although opioid-naïve patients generally should not be started on a basal infusion without the advice of a pain expert.

Fentanyl patches

The fentanyl transdermal patch is another option for patients who cannot reliably take pills, but it is important to understand appropriate dosing and limitations of use:

- Equianalgesic dosing for the fentanyl patch compared with oral morphine appears earlier in this chapter (Table 216-2). Note that the commonly used fentanyl 25 mcg/h patch is equianalgesic to approximately 50 mg oral morphine per day. Elderly or opioid-naïve patients should not be initiated on the 25 mcg/h dose unless there is demonstrated need for this quantity of opioid. A 12 mcg/h patch is available for patients with lesser needs, but in general fentanyl patches should only be initiated in patients with chronic pain and well-documented opioid requirements.
- The patch can take greater than 24 hours to reach peak effect. It is not appropriate for acute pain or if frequent titration is needed.
- Fentanyl patches are not recommended for patients with significant cachexia. The patch requires subcutaneous fat for effective absorption and release of drug.
- Fentanyl patches generally should not be used in febrile patients, as the uptake of medication may increase with temperature and cause unexpected side effects (such as sedation) or poor analgesia if the patch runs out early.

■ COMPLICATIONS

Concerns about side effects from opioids often lead to undertreatment of pain. Clinicians should make it a priority to recognize and treat opioid-induced side effects.

Sedation

Many patients complain about mild sedation or "fogginess" when initiating opioids or immediately after dose titration, but the effect

usually wanes after 2 to 7 days. If a patient complains of persistent symptoms and other causes of sedation have been ruled out (eg, other medications, metabolic disturbances, or central nervous system processes), one can consider several options:

- Reduce opioid dose (10%-25%) if pain symptoms allow. Consider adding nonopioid adjuvant pain medications to facilitate dose reduction.
- Rotate to another opioid.
- Add a psychostimulant such as methylphenidate, with a starting dose of 2.5 mg orally twice a day and titrate up to a maximum of 1 mg/kg/d in divided doses. Psychostimulants should be avoided in patients with significant anxiety, arrhythmias, delirium, or psychosis.

Nausea

Like sedation, opioid-induced nausea usually improves after the first week. This symptom is discussed in greater detail in the nausea section of this chapter. First-line therapies for opioid-induced nausea include dopamine antagonists such as prochlorperazine and haloperidol.

Constipation

Unlike other opioid side effects, constipation does not wane with time. Patients taking opioids should be given a standing bowel regimen. Even patients with regular bowel movements should have a bowel regimen in place to prevent future constipation. The combination of docusate sodium (stool softener) with senna (laxative) is one option. Many patients will need an additional laxative, such as polyethylene glycol or lactulose, to maintain regular bowel function. Methylnaltrexone, a selective opioid antagonist, can be considered for more severe cases of opioid-induced constipation that have not responded to laxatives and enemas. Unlike naloxone, methylnaltrexone does not cross the blood-brain barrier and provides effective relief of constipation without opioid withdrawal or reduction in analgesia. Methylnaltrexone can be given subcutaneously every other day as needed.

Delirium

Any mental status change in a patient taking opioids should be taken seriously. Delirium can cause a myriad of complications including patient and family distress, uncertainty in overall prognosis, injury, and a delay in discharge. Delirium can be particularly distressing because it compromises a patient's sense of self. Patients may find this quite frightening, and families often struggle with a heightened sense of loss, feeling like they are losing their loved one even before death.

However, one should not automatically blame opioids for every new mental status change, especially if a patient has been on a stable dose for some time. Workup for delirium should include an evaluation for other reversible causes, including other medications, infection, central nervous system disease, hypoxemia, metabolic/electrolyte disorders, and renal or liver failure.

If the delirium ultimately seems attributable to opioids but the patient needs continued pain control, consider the following options:

- Reduce opioid dose (10%-25%) if pain symptoms allow. Use nonopioid adjuvants if needed.
- Treat concurrently with an antipsychotic such as haloperidol or olanzapine.
- Rotate to a different opioid.
- Use nonpharmacologic strategies, including environmental cues for day and night, glasses and hearing aids, and family presence.

Neurotoxicity

Patients on chronic opioids can develop neurotoxic side effects from opioid metabolites, especially in the setting of high opioid doses, dehydration, or renal failure. Myoclonus is a common manifestation of this neuroexcitatory state. Symptoms may be mild, such as an occasional jerking of extremities, but with continued opioid administration patients may develop frequent twitching of muscle groups in the extremities and face. Other signs of neurotoxicity include delirium, hyperalgesia (increased sensitivity to pain), and allodynia (pain from non-noxious stimuli). In severe neurotoxicity, patients may even develop generalized seizures. Hyperalgesia is particularly confusing because clinicians may mistake this as worsened pain from an underlying disease process. Further opioid escalation actually worsens the hyperalgesia.

Treatment strategy depends on both the severity of symptoms and overall prognosis. In an imminently dying patient with mild myoclonus, it may be appropriate to simply monitor the patient for any worsening symptoms. For patients with ongoing need for opioids and concerning manifestations of neurotoxicity, consider several strategies:

- Reduce opioid dose (10%-25%) if neurotoxic symptoms are mild (only occasional myoclonus). Consider adding nonopioid adjuvant pain medications to facilitate opioid dose reduction.
- Rotate to another opioid if there are signs of significant neuroexcitation, including myoclonus, allodynia/hyperalgesia, delirium, or hallucinations. The new opioid should be initiated at 25% of the equianalgesic dose. Methadone and fentanyl are particularly good options in severe neurotoxicity because they do not have active metabolites. Clinicians without specific training in pain management should consult an expert for any cases of significant neurotoxicity and when initiating methadone or fentanyl, due to complexities of dosing in this setting.
- Add medications to reduce myoclonus. Options include benzodiazepines (lorazepam, clonazepam, midazolam) and muscle relaxants (baclofen, nifedipine).

PRACTICE POINT

- Consider opioid neurotoxicity in patients with worsening pain despite rapidly increasing doses of opioids.

Respiratory depression

Though respiratory depression remains a commonly feared side effect, clinically significant respiratory depression is actually quite rare when opioids are dosed appropriately. Respiratory depression is a late effect, and patients should exhibit signs of somnolence before their respiratory function is compromised. Naloxone should be reserved for those with life-threatening respiratory depression. To prevent sudden reversal of analgesia (and almost certain pain crisis), an incremental dosing approach is recommended. Mix 0.4 mg (1 mL ampule) of naloxone into 9 mL of saline to make a diluted 0.04 mg/mL naloxone solution. Administer 1 to 2 mL of this diluted solution intravenously approximately every 1 to 2 minutes until respiratory depression resolves. Repeated doses may be necessary due to the short duration of naloxone, and a continuous infusion may be required if the patient was on long-acting opioids.

■ DISCHARGE CHECKLIST

- Does the patient understand how to use pain medications appropriately, including the difference between long-acting and breakthrough medications? Create a written pain management plan, review it with the patient and family members, and confirm that they know who to contact for uncontrolled symptoms.

- Is your patient on a standing bowel regimen to prevent opioid-induced constipation?
- Is the responsible outpatient clinician aware that you have initiated opioids or changed doses during this hospitalization? Has the outpatient provider agreed to continue writing for these controlled substances?
- Have you communicated with the case manager and home care agency (visiting nurse agency, hospice agency) about the current pain medication plan? Have you considered a contingency plan if the patient is no longer able to take oral medications?

NAUSEA

■ INTRODUCTION

Symptoms of nausea and vomiting are common in patients with advanced illnesses, including cancer, congestive heart failure, end-stage renal disease, and AIDS. For patients and families facing a life-threatening illness, nausea and vomiting can cause substantial distress due to concerns about maintaining adequate nutrition and worries that these symptoms indicate disease progression.

■ EVALUATION

Evaluation should include a thorough history and physical exam, with careful attention to common causes of nausea in the terminally ill, including medications (chemotherapy, opioids), constipation, electrolyte abnormalities, liver and kidney failure, radiation therapy, central nervous system lesions, bowel obstruction, and anxiety. It is important to try to identify the likely mechanism or pathway responsible for a patient's nausea, as this can guide the therapeutic approach.

Nausea and vomiting can be triggered by activation of any of four general pathways:

- Cortex: Activation can occur due to meningeal irritation, increased intracranial pressure, or cognitive/emotional factors such as anxiety.
- Chemoreceptor trigger zone: This area is located in the floor of the fourth ventricle and lacks a blood-brain barrier. It is easily activated by metabolic abnormalities, toxins, and medications present in the cerebrospinal fluid (CSF). Activation of the chemoreceptor trigger zone is mediated primarily by the dopamine (D2) receptor, but others include neurokinin-1 (NK1) and serotonin (5HT3).
- Vestibular system: Motion or inner ear disease can activate the vestibular apparatus via histamine (H1) and muscarinic acetylcholine (ACh) receptors.
- Peripheral pathways: Activation can occur through mechanoreceptors and chemoreceptors in the gastrointestinal tract and heart, as well as 5HT3 receptors in the gastrointestinal tract. These signals are then transmitted along afferent tracts including the vagus, glossopharyngeal, splanchnic, and sympathetic nerves.

Each of these four pathways can then activate the vomiting center, a specific area of the medulla that coordinates the final act of vomiting via the parasympathetic system and gastrointestinal tract. Activation of the vomiting center is believed to be mediated by H1 receptors or muscarinic ACh receptors.

■ INPATIENT MANAGEMENT

Nonpharmacologic treatment

Nonpharmacologic strategies may be helpful for many patients. Patients should avoid strong smells and eat small, frequent meals as they are able. Relaxation techniques may be useful for patients with significant anxiety or anticipatory nausea (nausea that occurs prior to chemotherapy sessions due to a conditioned response). Acupuncture appears to be helpful for chemotherapy-related nausea and vomiting. Although further research is needed, there have been a few randomized controlled trials demonstrating that acupuncture-point stimulation reduces the incidence of acute chemotherapy-induced vomiting.

Pharmacologic treatment

Most patients with nausea or vomiting will need some type of pharmacologic therapy. **Table 216-5** shows common clinical etiologies of nausea and recommended first-line pharmacologic therapies based on likely mechanisms and receptors. **Table 216-6** lists common antiemetics, doses, and side effects.

TABLE 216-5 Common Causes of Nausea and First-line Pharmacologic Therapies

Etiology	Probable Mechanism and Receptors	First-line Treatment
CNS lesion	Increased ICP, meningeal irritation	Dexamethasone
Opioid-induced	Stimulation of CTZ (D2) Gastroparesis Constipation	D2 antagonists: haloperidol, metoclopramide, prochlorperazine Consider opioid rotation
Metabolic/uremia/liver failure	Stimulation of CTZ (D2)	Treat reversible causes (electrolytes, meds) D2 antagonists: see above
Chemotherapy-induced	Gut release of 5HT3 → stimulation of peripheral pathways Stimulation of CTZ (D2, 5HT3, NK1) Anticipatory nausea	5HT3 antagonist: ondansetron Dexamethasone NK1 antagonist: aprepitant Anxiolytics: lorazepam (see also guidelines from American Society of Clinical Oncology)
Radiation-associated	Gut release of 5HT3 → stimulation of peripheral pathways	5HT3 antagonist: ondansetron
Bowel obstruction	Gut mechano/chemoreceptors → stimulation of peripheral pathways Toxins, inflammatory agents → CTZ (D2)	Metoclopramide (if incomplete obstruction) or haloperidol Dexamethasone Octreotide Nasogastric tube, venting gastrostomy
Constipation	Gut mechanoreceptors	Aggressive scheduled bowel regimen
Gastroparesis	Gut mechanoreceptors	Promotility: metoclopramide
Motion, vestibular disease	Stimulation via vestibulocochlear nerve (H1, ACh)	Anticholinergic: scopolamine H1 blockers: promethazine, diphenhydramine

ICP, intracranial pressure; CTZ, chemoreceptor trigger zone; D2, dopamine type 2 receptor; 5HT3, 5-hydroxytryptamine type 3 receptor (serotonin); NK1, neurokinin type 1 receptor; ACh, acetylcholine receptor; H1, histamine type 1 receptor; CNS, central nervous system.

Opioid-induced nausea

Opioid-induced nausea warrants further discussion because it is particularly common and troublesome in this population. Opioids cause nausea through multiple mechanisms, including decreased gut motility (constipation, gastroparesis), stimulation of the chemoreceptor trigger zone via dopamine receptors, and enhanced vestibular sensitivity. Symptoms of opioid-induced nausea usually improve after the first week of opioid use. One strategy is to use a dopamine antagonist such as prochlorperazine, haloperidol, or metoclopramide on a scheduled basis for several days. The antiemetic may be subsequently be tapered as the patient develops tolerance to the opioid side effects. Another effective agent is olanzapine, which has mixed dopamine, acetylcholine, histamine, and serotonin activities. Patients with persistent nausea may require an opioid dose reduction (10%-20%) or rotation to another opioid. Patients taking opioids should be on a scheduled bowel regimen to prevent constipation.

Malignant bowel obstruction

Malignant bowel obstruction is a common complication in patients with advanced abdominal and pelvic malignancies. In patients who are not surgical candidates, medical management should include several concurrent mechanical and pharmacologic strategies:

- Pain control is a priority and generally requires the use of opioids.
- Decompression with a nasogastric tube may provide rapid relief of nausea and abdominal distension. A percutaneous gastrostomy tube may be considered in patients with persistent obstruction since patients can be transitioned home with a gastrostomy tube in place.
- Patients should be given a scheduled antiemetic to relieve associated nausea. Metoclopramide is recommended for patients with partial obstruction, but it should be discontinued if the patient develops worsened abdominal pain or cramping. It should not be used in patients with complete bowel obstruction. Haloperidol may be used for nausea in patients

TABLE 216-6 Common Antiemetics

Antiemetic	Class	Dosage	Major Adverse Effects
Haloperidol	D2 antagonist (CTZ)	0.5-2 mg orally or intravenously every 4-6 h	EPS
Metoclopramide	D2 antagonist (GI, CTZ)	5-20 mg orally or intravenously every 6 h	EPS, GI colic
Prochlorperazine	D2 antagonist (CTZ)	5-10 mg orally or intravenously or 25 mg by rectum every 6 h	EPS, sedation
Olanzapine	Multiple: D2, ACh, H1, 5HT3 antagonist	2.5-5 mg orally or sublingually every night at bedtime and every 6 h	Sedation, dizziness
Promethazine*	H1 blocker, Anticholingergic	12-25 mg orally or intravenously or 25 mg by rectum every 6 h	EPS, sedation, delirium
Diphenhydramine*	H1 blocker	25-50 mg orally or intravenously every 6 h	Sedation, delirium, dry mouth, urinary retention
Ondansetron	5HT3 antagonist	4-8 mg orally or intravenously every 8 h	Constipation
Dexamethasone	Anti-inflammatory Central activity unknown	4-20 mg orally or intravenously once or twice a day	Delirium, anxiety, insomnia, GI mucosal irritation
Lorazepam*	Anxiolytic	0.5-2 mg orally or intravenously every 6 h	Sedation, delirium
Scopolamine*	Anticholinergic	1.5 mg patch every 72 h	Dry mouth, blurred vision, delirium, urinary retention

*Use with particular caution in elderly patients due to adverse effects.

EPS, extrapyramidal symptoms; CTZ, chemoreceptor trigger zone; D2, dopamine type 2 receptor; 5HT3, 5-hydroxytryptamine type 3 receptor (serotonin); NK1, neurokinin type 1 receptor; ACh, acetylcholine receptor; H1, histamine type 1 receptor; GI, gastrointestinal.

with complete obstruction or those with symptoms of colic. Dexamethasone 4 mg orally or intravenously two to three times a day may be useful for both its antiemetic and anti-inflammatory properties, including treating tumor-associated inflammation and potentially reducing the obstruction.

- Anticholinergic agents may be helpful for reducing abdominal distension and cramping. Hyoscyamine can be given 0.125 to 0.25 mg sublingually four times a day or scopolamine can be administered through a patch.
- Octreotide is a somatostatin analogue that inhibits motility and reduces gastrointestinal secretions. It can be administered subcutaneously 50 to 150 mcg three times a day. Patients who respond well to subcutaneous octreotide may be candidates for a monthly depot injection of octreotide for longer-term palliation of bowel obstruction.
- Studies have demonstrated successful symptom management of malignant bowel obstruction using a combined regimen of metoclopramide, octreotide, and dexamethasone, including the recovery of bowel transit in some patients with partial obstruction.

■ COMPLICATIONS

Antiemetics may cause a number of side effects. Sedation is common with antihistamines and neuroleptic agents, including dopamine antagonists and atypical antipsychotics. Sedation may be a desired effect for some patients nearing the end of life, but a dose adjustment or medication change may be necessary for patients who find this problematic. Almost all classes of antiemetics can cause delirium, including antihistamines, benzodiazepines, anticholinergics, corticosteroids, and cannabinoids. The elderly are especially vulnerable and should be monitored closely. Patients on dopamine antagonists may develop extrapyramidal symptoms such as akathisia and dystonia. Management includes treatment with diphenhydramine or benztropine and discontinuation of the

offending agent. Serotonin antagonists such as ondansetron may cause constipation and patients may need prophylactic laxatives. Clinicians should also be aware that many antiemetics (such as haloperidol, metoclopramide, ondansetron) may prolong the QT interval. EKG monitoring may be warranted, depending upon the patient's clinical situation and overall goals of care.

Patients with persistent nausea and vomiting often develop dehydration and electrolyte disturbances, which can further exacerbate symptoms of nausea. It may be reasonable to consider intravenous hydration, even in patients with a limited prognosis, with the goal of relieving symptoms. Consider referring patients with persistent bowel obstruction for surgical evaluation, depending on the stage of illness and overall prognosis. Additionally, patients and families may struggle with news that disease-modifying therapies (such as chemotherapy) are no longer possible due to intractable symptoms, poor functional status, or advanced disease. Their psychosocial distress should be addressed with the assistance of the primary outpatient clinician, palliative care clinician, social worker, or chaplain.

DYSPNEA

■ INTRODUCTION

Dyspnea, defined as the subjective experience of difficult or uncomfortable breathing, is a very common and distressing symptom for patients. Dyspnea has been reported in up to 78% of cancer patients, 70% of patients with congestive heart failure, 70% of patients with dementia, 56% of COPD patients, and 62% of patients with AIDS. Of note, studies show that patients with higher dyspnea scores report decreased quality of life indices. Despite its prevalence and impact on quality of life, dyspnea often goes untreated. One study reported that over 60% of patients with advanced cancer had dyspnea for greater than 3 months, yet most had not received any treatment for their symptoms.

■ PATHOPHYSIOLOGY

The pathophysiology of dyspnea is complex and not yet fully understood. The respiratory center, located in the medulla and pons, coordinates the movements of the diaphragm and chest wall muscles during breathing. The respiratory center receives sensory input from several sources, including pulmonary vagal afferents, peripheral and medullary chemoreceptors, and peripheral mechanoreceptors from respiratory muscles and joints. The pulmonary vagal afferents include pulmonary stretch receptors, alveolar C fibers that respond to interstitial and capillary pressure, and pulmonary irritant receptors.

Several mechanisms appear to trigger the sensation of dyspnea:

- Increased work of breathing: This can be caused by increased airway resistance, such as in COPD or asthma, or weakened musculature, as occurs in neurodegenerative disorders or severe cachexia.
- Chemoreceptor activity: Receptors in the medulla primarily detect hypercapnia, and those in the carotid and aortic bodies detect hypoxemia. Hypercapnia appears to have a greater role in triggering dyspnea than hypoxemia.
- Neuromechanical dissociation: Researchers have described an important relationship between the brain's efferent motor output for respiration and the afferent information it receives in response to these efforts. Dyspnea can occur when there is a mismatch, or neuromechanical dissociation, between what the brain desires from respiration and the sensory feedback from pulmonary vagal afferents and peripheral mechanoreceptors. A patient with amyotrophic lateral sclerosis (ALS) may experience dyspnea because the brain is not receiving the expected feedback in chest wall expansion. In another example, normal subjects became dyspneic when researchers limited the inspiratory flow rate despite no change in respiratory work or oxygenation status.

■ EVALUATION

The gold standard for diagnosis is always the patient's report of symptoms. Studies have demonstrated that there is no clear correlation between symptoms of dyspnea and respiratory rate, oxygen saturation, and accessory muscle use. Interestingly, some patients feel dyspneic despite normal oxygen saturations, while others do not feel dyspneic even though they are hypoxemic. It is therefore important to screen all patients for dyspnea, since patients may have no obvious signs of respiratory compromise or distress.

Common etiologies should be considered, including pneumonia, pleural effusion, space-occupying lung lesions, bronchospasm, pulmonary embolism, COPD, cardiac ischemia, congestive heart failure, anemia, and ascites. Patients with cancer may also have disease-specific processes such as radiation or chemotherapy-induced pneumonitis, malignant pericardial effusion, superior vena cava syndrome, or lymphangitic spread of tumor. Patients with primary neurologic or neuromuscular disorders may have symptoms of dyspnea associated with progressive muscle weakness.

The decision of whether to pursue diagnostic studies should take into account the patient's overall goals of care, disease trajectory, and the likelihood that the study results will enhance management of dyspnea symptoms. For some patients, workup to rule out pneumonia, pleural effusion, or pulmonary embolism may still be appropriate as there are specific treatments that can help their symptoms. Sometimes no clear etiology for dyspnea can be found. The National Hospice Study, which followed terminal cancer patients during their last 6 weeks of life, found that 24% of patients with dyspnea had no signs of lung involvement or cardiac disease.

■ INPATIENT MANAGEMENT

Treatment of dyspnea should be directed at the etiology, if known. Patients with advanced illness may still be considered candidates for procedures like thoracentesis for a large pleural effusion and pleural catheter for recurrent effusions. The ultimate goal in all cases should be the subjective relief of symptoms rather than the correction of any single parameter, such as oxygen saturation or respiratory rate. Patients may need further nonpharmacologic and pharmacologic therapies if treatment of the underlying etiology of dyspnea does not fully relieve their symptoms.

Nonpharmacologic treatment

Placing patients in an upright position improves the mechanics of the intercostal muscles and lessens the work of breathing. A cool fan or moist cloth over the face can improve symptoms, possibly through stimulation of the V2 branch of the trigeminal nerve, which may then inhibit dyspnea perception centrally. The presence of a family member or volunteer at the bedside can help relieve anxiety associated with dyspnea. Cognitive and behavioral interventions, similar to those used in pulmonary rehabilitation for COPD patients, can also improve symptoms of dyspnea. Several trials of nursing-led interventions, which included relaxation techniques, breathing control, activity pacing, and psychosocial support, demonstrated a reduction in dyspnea scores.

Oxygen is frequently used in patients with dyspnea, though evidence to support its use is mixed. There is strong evidence to support oxygen use in COPD patients, for both symptomatic relief and improved survival. However, the role of oxygen in cancer patients with dyspnea is less clear. A meta-analysis of cancer-related dyspnea did not demonstrate any clear symptom improvement with oxygen compared to air. In the palliative care population, a trial of supplemental oxygen seems reasonable if the patient has had insufficient relief with other approaches. The potential benefits and risks of oxygen therapy should be considered before discharging a patient with home oxygen. Considerations include the degree of symptom relief, the risk of falls with tubing, and the presence of smokers in the home.

Pharmacologic treatment

Opioids

Opioids are the first-line agents in pharmacologic therapy for dyspnea near the end of life. Their exact mechanism is not fully understood, but opioids are believed to decrease the chemoreceptor response to hypercapnia and increase preload through cardiovascular vasodilation. Opioids have been shown to reduce dyspnea in patients with advanced cancer, congestive heart failure, and COPD, and can also increase exercise tolerance in patients with COPD and congestive heart failure. Doses required to control dyspnea are usually lower than those required for pain (**Table 216-7**). A reasonable starting dose of morphine for an opioid-naïve patient is morphine 1 to 2 mg intravenously every 2 hours or 2 to 5 mg orally every 4 hours. For patients already on opioids for pain, consider a 25% increase in their usual opioid dose to treat dyspnea. Other opioids

TABLE 216-7 Opioids for Dyspnea

Drug	Oral	Parenteral
Opioid-naïve patients		
Morphine	3-5 mg orally every 4 h	1-2 mg intravenously every 2 h
Oxycodone	2.5-5 mg orally every 4 h	—
Hydromorphone	1-2 mg orally every 4 h	0.2 mg intravenously every 2 h
Opioid-tolerant patients		
Increase baseline opioid dose by 25%		

TABLE 216-8 Anxiolytics for Dyspnea

Drug	Dose
Lorazepam	0.5-1 mg orally or intravenously every hour until dyspnea controlled; then every 4-6 h
Clonazepam	0.25-0.5 mg orally every 12 h
Midazolam	0.2-0.5 mg intravenously slowly every 15 min until dyspnea controlled; consider infusion

TABLE 216-9 Anticholinergics for Secretions

Drug	Dose
Hyoscyamine	0.125-0.25 mg sublingually every 6-8 h
Glycopyrrolate	0.1-0.2 mg intravenously every 8 h
Scopolamine	1.5 mg patch every 72 h*
Atropine (1% ophth)	1-2 gtt sublingually every 6 h

*Scopolamine patch takes approximately 12 h for onset of action (24 h to reach steady state). Consider other agents if more rapid effect is desired.

such as hydromorphone and oxycodone can be used. There is no evidence to suggest any substantial differences in efficacy between opioids in the treatment of dyspnea. Patients who require frequent opioid doses may need initiation of either long-acting opioids or an opioid infusion. Principles for ordering and titrating infusions can be found in the section on pain management.

PRACTICE POINT

- Opioids can be used safely for dyspnea even in patients with underlying lung disease.

Anxiolytics

Dyspnea can be closely associated with anxiety, with each symptom exacerbating the other. Anxiolytics may be a helpful adjunct to opioids for treating dyspnea (**Table 216-8**). Lorazepam can offer rapid relief and is available in oral concentrate form. Clonazepam can be beneficial for chronic dyspnea due to its longer half-life. One trial has shown that midazolam can improve dyspnea control when added to a morphine regimen, though in practice its use is generally reserved for severe symptoms. Midazolam can be given 0.2 to 0.5 mg intravenously slowly for severe dyspnea or for refractory symptoms of panic or anxiety.

■ COMPLICATIONS

Respiratory depression

Some clinicians or patients may be hesitant to use opioids due to fears that they will cause respiratory depression and hasten death. These fears are largely unfounded. Many studies have shown that opioids improve dyspnea without compromising respiratory function when dosed appropriately. One meta-analysis that included COPD, congestive heart failure, cancer, and interstitial lung disease patients reported statistically significant improvement in dyspnea with no deaths attributable to opioids. It is also important to recognize that major changes in respiratory status such as apnea or periodic breathing may be indicative of imminent death from natural disease progression, rather than opioid-induced.

In the rare instance of respiratory depression due to accidental opioid overdose, naloxone can be used, but it should be diluted to avoid complete reversal of analgesia in palliative care patients. One ampule (0.4 mg in 1 mL) should be diluted with 9 mL saline to create a 0.04 mg/mL solution and then given in 1 mL doses every 1 to 2 minutes until respiratory depression is reversed. Further doses may be needed if long-acting opioids were used. If the only manifestation of opioid overdose is somnolence with intact respiratory function, naloxone should not be given and the patient should just be monitored closely.

SECRETIONS

■ EVALUATION AND MANAGEMENT

As their level of consciousness diminishes, many dying patients lose the ability to clear oropharyngeal secretions and develop noisy respirations, also known as the "death rattle." Some family members and providers may find the noise distressing, though patients are generally obtunded and are thought to be undisturbed by it.

Management strategies include placing the patient in a lateral or semiprone position to promote drainage of secretions. Gentle suctioning may be helpful for secretions that are easily accessible, but deep suctioning is generally ineffective and may cause discomfort to the patient. Intravenous fluids can increase the production of secretions and should be minimized or discontinued.

Anticholinergic agents are often used in an attempt to reduce oropharyngeal secretions, though studies have not shown any clear benefit. **Table 216-9** lists commonly used agents. Anticholinergics may cause significant side effects including sedation, delirium, urinary retention, constipation, and dry mouth. Patients receiving anticholinergic agents should receive scheduled mouth care including lip balm and mouth swabs.

Noisy secretions may be difficult to control despite the above interventions, and family education is paramount to minimize emotional distress. Clinicians should explain that as patients become less alert, the oropharyngeal muscles relax and patients are no longer able to swallow secretions. The loud respirations occur when air moves past the pooled secretions and relaxed muscles. Some family members may need reassurance that the patient is receiving adequate air and that this is not a sign of drowning. It is especially important to emphasize that these symptoms are normal and an expected part of the dying process.

TERMINAL DELIRIUM

■ EVALUATION AND TREATMENT

Nearly half of all dying patients will display signs of restlessness or agitation in their last days of life due to delirium. Symptoms include grimacing, moaning, mumbling speech, hallucinations, twitching or jerking, and changes in the level of arousal. Because delirium is common in hospitalized patients both with and without terminal illness, it is important to recognize other physiologic signs that may indicate a patient is in the dying phase. Manifestations can include decreased perfusion with cool extremities or cyanosis, tachycardia or bradycardia, hypotension, respiratory changes such as Cheyne-Stokes breathing or apnea, decreased urine output, and progressive somnolence.

Many of the general principles of delirium assessment and treatment still apply in the dying patient. Medications such as anticholinergic drugs (antiemetics, antisecretion agents, tricyclic antidepressants), opioids, sedatives, and corticosteroids are common precipitants for delirium in this population. The offending medications should be discontinued or weaned if possible, keeping in mind that delirious patients should not be left with undertreated pain, dyspnea, or other symptoms. Certain drugs such as opioids may need to be rotated (ie, a patient with severe renal insufficiency and signs of opioid neurotoxicity from morphine may need to be rotated

TABLE 216-10 Antipsychotics for Terminal Delirium

Drug	Dose
Haloperidol	0.5-2 mg orally, intravenously, or subcutaneously every 6 h and every hour as needed (maximum 20 mg in 24 h)
Olanzapine	2.5-5 mg orally or sublingually every 12 h and every 4 h as needed (maximum 30 mg in 24 h)
Chlorpromazine	25-50 mg orally, by rectum, or intravenously every 8 h and every 4 h as needed

to fentanyl or methadone). Other common and reversible causes of delirium include untreated pain, full bladder, or fecal impaction. If a patient appears to be nearing the end of life, it is often appropriate to forgo a full evaluation of delirium and transition instead to comfort-focused care.

Nonpharmacologic interventions for delirium may be helpful, including family presence at the bedside, gentle reminders to help with reorientation, hearing or visual devices, and psychosocial/spiritual support. Antipsychotic medications are the primary pharmacologic treatment for terminal delirium. Common medications are listed in **Table 216-10**. Antipsychotics can cause varying levels of sedation, with haloperidol causing the least sedation and chlorpromazine causing the most sedation.

Most clinicians recognize that benzodiazepines are generally discouraged in delirious patients due to the potential for paradoxical worsening of symptoms and agitation. One exception is the dying patient with significant agitation despite treatment with strong doses of antipsychotic medications. In this situation, benzodiazepines may be added for their sedative effect. Lorazepam can be given 0.5 to 2 mg intravenously, orally, or subcutaneously every 2 hours as needed. Diazepam is available rectally and can be given 10 mg rectally 6 hours. If these measures prove ineffective, consider contacting a palliative care specialist to discuss the possibility of further sedating medications.

NUTRITION AND HYDRATION

INTRODUCTION

Patients and families can experience tremendous emotional distress when nutritional issues arise. For many, nutrition may become a symbolic battleground of the fight against death. Many families express their love through food. When patients do not eat, well-intentioned family members may struggle with feelings of rejection or fear that their loved one has "given up." Clinicians are sometimes pressed with questions about artificial nutrition and hydration (ANH) in the setting of advanced illness.

ANOREXIA-CACHEXIA SYNDROME

Patients may show signs of anorexia-cachexia, a complex wasting syndrome mediated by cytokine and neurohormonal factors. This syndrome is well recognized in cancer and AIDS patients, but is also seen in patients with advanced chronic illnesses such as congestive heart failure and COPD. It is important to explain to patients that this decline is a natural part of the disease process and not due to any deficiency on their part. Patients or family members may focus on weight loss as a sign that they have not done enough to ensure adequate calories. Although patients appear malnourished, this catabolic condition is generally not reversible even with aggressive nutrition.

Clinicians should screen for treatable causes of poor intake that may masquerade as anorexia-cachexia. These conditions include oral mucositis or candidiasis, esophagitis, reflux disease, gastrointestinal dysmotility, constipation, nausea, chronic pain, or depression. If a reversible

cause for anorexia is not found, management of the anorexia-cachexia syndrome includes behavioral and pharmacologic strategies.

Referral to a nutritionist may provide guidance to patients and families. Patients should be empowered to determine their own eating habits, including eating the foods that are most appealing and deciding the quantity and frequency of intake. Patients who are easily nauseated or have early satiety should eat small portions only as they are able. Families should be advised to refrain from any comments and behavior that pressure the patient to consume more. Patients can liberalize dietary restrictions, including those that were previously important for management of long-standing conditions such as diabetes or hyperlipidemia, provided that doing so will not cause uncomfortable symptoms such as edema. Some patients and family members may need tremendous support and education as they make this transition. Many have spent years doing everything "right" to fight their illness, maintaining their caloric intake, eating specific foods while undergoing chemotherapy, or carefully adhering to a diabetic diet. Patients and family members may find themselves having to acknowledge for the first time that the disease is advancing and incurable. Clinicians should be attuned to these psychosocial concerns and may need to facilitate appropriate support systems for their patients, such as social work, chaplaincy, palliative care, and hospice.

Patients or family members may ask if there is a role for appetite stimulants. Pharmacologic agents can be considered, but appetite stimulants have demonstrated only modest or limited benefit at best, and all have certain contraindications and side effects. Before starting an agent, it is important to discuss specific goals (such as a small amount of weight gain or increased appetite) and a clear timeframe in which to assess whether the goals are being met. If there is no obvious benefit after 2 or 3 weeks, the drug should be discontinued. **Table 216-11** lists common appetite stimulants and doses. These include the following:

- Megestrol acetate (Megace) is a synthetic progestational agent that has been shown to increase appetite and weight in randomized control trials of patients with cancer and AIDS. Weight gain manifests as increased fat stores but not lean muscle mass. The data for improved quality of life indices is less clear than the effects on appetite and weight. Potential adverse effects include fluid retention, adrenal insufficiency, hypertension, and thromboembolic events. Megestrol should not be used in patients with a history of thromboembolism and is generally not recommended for patients with congestive heart failure.
- Corticosteroids such as dexamethasone and prednisone have been shown in randomized controlled trials to improve subjective appetite and overall sense of well-being, though patients did not demonstrate any significant weight gain. Corticosteroids are most appropriate for patients with a shorter life expectancy or for those who cannot receive megestrol due to history of thromboembolism. They should not be used longer

TABLE 216-11 Appetite Stimulants

Drug	Dose
Megestrol*	400 mg orally twice a day
Prednisone	5 mg orally three times a day
Dexamethasone	4-8 mg daily in divided doses
Dronabinol	2.5-7.5 mg orally three times a day

*Liquid form of megestrol is associated with better compliance and ease of administration than tablets.

than a few weeks due to the potential for significant side effects including peptic ulcer disease, cushingoid changes, and myopathy.

- Dronabinol (Marinol) is a synthetic cannabinoid that has demonstrated modest benefit in appetite stimulation in AIDS patients, but unconvincing effect on weight gain. For cancer patients with anorexia, studies have not demonstrated any improvement in appetite or weight gain. Adverse effects of dronabinol are primarily central nervous system related and include dizziness, euphoria, and confusion. Cannabinoids should be avoided in elderly patients, as they are particularly sensitive to the side effects.

Other agents that are still undergoing study as potential appetite stimulants include mirtazapine, thalidomide, COX-2 inhibitors, and L-carnitine.

■ ARTIFICIAL NUTRITION AND HYDRATION

When patients and families inquire about a feeding tube or TPN, clinicians should explore their specific concerns and goals. Many people hope that artificial nutrition and hydration (ANH) will improve strength or lengthen survival. For the vast majority of patients with advanced illness, ANH does not improve survival or quality of life.

ANH can lengthen survival of patients with certain conditions including extreme short-bowel syndrome, amyotrophic lateral sclerosis, acute phases of stroke or head injury, and those in a permanent vegetative state. The data for cancer patients is more varied due to the heterogeneity of the population. Most clinicians would consider ANH appropriate for patients whose disease location interferes with their ability to swallow or transit food (eg, head and neck cancer, esophageal cancer, proximal bowel obstruction) but who otherwise have good functional status. Some studies suggest that ANH may be useful in patients who are actively undergoing chemotherapy or radiation, while other studies do not support this finding. Patients with cancer-related anorexia-cachexia do not gain weight even when given aggressive calories. When a patient's disease is no longer responding to disease-modifying treatments, experts agree that the risks of ANH, such as infection, aspiration, or volume overload, generally outweigh the benefits.

The literature does not support the use of ANH in patients with advanced dementia. Enteral tube feeds have been shown to increase the risk of aspiration, diarrhea, and gastrointestinal discomfort. Patients with dementia are at risk for pulling on feeding tubes, and studies have shown that the presence of a feeding tube increases the likelihood that patients will be physically restrained. Advanced dementia patients receiving ANH and adequate caloric intake still demonstrate continued weight loss or depletion of lean body mass. There is no evidence to suggest improved healing of pressure ulcers.

If a decision is made to pursue ANH, the clinician should discuss

- Specific goals with the patient and family, such as weight gain or maintenance.
- Designate a timepoint at which they will reassess whether ANH is still meeting these goals.
- Indications for discontinuing ANH, including any significant complication, such as infection when the risks of ongoing ANH outweigh any potential benefits.

Patients, families, and clinicians may have their own deeply rooted beliefs about the role of ANH at the end of life. Cultural or religious traditions may influence an individual's beliefs, even when medical providers feel that the data does not support the use of ANH. If significant concerns arise, clinicians should include a palliative care clinician, chaplain or clergyperson, social worker, or ethics support staff in these discussions.

> ### PRACTICE POINT
>
> - Define specific and measurable goals before initiating patients on appetite stimulants or artificial nutrition and hydration.

■ EDUCATING PATIENTS AND FAMILIES

Clinicians play a key role in educating patients and families on nutritional issues at the end of life. Although families may express great concern that their loved one will suffer from hunger, patients in the last stage of life rarely report feeling hungry. Many patients can live comfortably for weeks with minimal food and water. Forcing patients to eat may cause emotional distress, nausea, and aspiration. Many patients and families are also unaware that artificial nutrition and hydration may cause complications including infection, aspiration, and fluid overload with worsened pulmonary edema or ascites, all of which can shorten lifespan.

Conversely, families of patients at risk for aspiration may have been instructed not to offer any food or liquids by mouth. In the context of limited prognosis or imminent death, these restrictions may be lifted as long as there are not obvious symptoms of discomfort. Measures such as sitting upright, tucking the chin when swallowing, and using a thickening agent with fluids, may enable patients at risk for aspiration to eat and drink small quantities for pleasure.

Palliative care includes helping family members learn other ways of nurturing their loved ones at the bedside. Families may be encouraged to interact with patients through conversation, reading, or music. Thirst is a common complaint at the end of life, and intravenous fluids have not been shown to affect the sensation of thirst. Visitors can learn how to moisten the mouth and provide ice chips to alleviate thirst. Small sips of fluid and candy lozenges can be appropriate if patients are alert and do not show signs of discomfort.

COMPLEMENTARY MEDICINE
■ INTRODUCTION

The National Center for Complementary and Alternative Medicine (NCCAM), an agency of the National Institutes of Health, has defined complementary and alternative medicine as "a group of diverse medical and health care systems, practices, and products that are not generally considered to be part of conventional medicine." The term *complementary medicine* refers to therapies that are used together with conventional medicine. *Alternative medicine* describes practices that are used in place of conventional medicine. The field of complementary and alternative medicine (CAM) includes a wide variety of practices, some of which do not conform to usual biomedical and scientific principles.

The NCCAM groups complementary and alternative medicine into several domains:

- Whole medical systems: These practices are built on complete systems of theory and practice that have evolved separately from conventional medicine. Some have existed longer than Western medical practices. Examples include homeopathy, traditional Chinese medicine, and Ayurveda (practiced on the Indian subcontinent). Systems such as traditional Chinese medicine may incorporate other domains below such as biologically based practices (herbal therapies) and energy-based therapies (acupuncture).
- Mind-body medicine: These techniques utilize the mind to affect bodily function and control symptoms. Examples include meditation, guided imagery, music therapy, and hypnosis. Some would include patient support groups and cognitive-behavioral therapies in this category.
- Biologically based practices: These therapies are based on substances found in nature including food, herbs, vitamins, and minerals.

- Manipulative and body-based practices: These treatments are based on movement of specific body parts. Examples include chiropractic and massage therapy.
- Energy-based therapies: These practices focus on energy fields such as electromagnetic fields or biofields, which purportedly surround and penetrate the body. Examples include qi gong, reiki, acupuncture, and magnetic therapy.

The use of CAM is very common in the general population. The Centers for Disease Control and Prevention's (CDC's) National Center for Health Statistics conducted a National Health Interview Survey in 2012 and found that an estimated 34% of adults had used CAM therapy in the past 12 months. CAM use appears to be particularly high in oncology patients, with studies reporting CAM use in 48% to 88% of patients.

■ ROLE OF THE CLINICIAN

Despite the widespread use of CAM in the general public, most medical providers have limited knowledge about these practices. They may not even be aware that their patients are pursuing CAM. Studies have found that most patients do not mention the use of CAM to their providers unless specifically asked. Clinicians may also struggle with how best to advise patients about certain unproven therapies without alienating those with different personal, cultural, or religious belief systems. Clinicians may encounter patients whose family members or friends are actively encouraging them to use CAM therapies. Studies have shown that friends, families, and mass media are very common sources of information for patients who decide to use CAM.

Clinicians can play a key role in advising patients who are considering the use of CAM therapies. Patients should be counseled that overall, research suggests that CAM therapies are most useful when used for alleviation of symptoms and enhancement of quality of life. There is no compelling scientific evidence at this time to support the use of alternative approaches in lieu of conventional therapies. Patients should carefully consider the potential risks and benefits of CAM therapies using reliable sources, including their medical provider and government-sponsored websites that detail current research findings and potential adverse effects.

Clinicians should advise patients and their families to consider the following questions before pursuing a CAM therapy:

- Is there research to support the use of this particular therapy?
- Does the therapy require that you stop conventional medical treatments?
- Are there substantial side effects that can interfere with your ongoing medical treatments?
- Does the treatment or practitioner make unfounded claims such as the ability to cure cancer?
- Does the treatment require travel to another country?
- Is the treatment available to the general public or is it promoted as a secret, exclusive therapy?
- Is the CAM practitioner licensed by the state to provide that specific therapy?
- Is the treatment offered by an established medical institution or is it offered only by one individual?
- How expensive is the treatment and does it require substantial out-of-pocket expense?

A full review of the different CAM therapies is beyond the scope of this discussion, but clinicians should familiarize themselves with the following:

- Commonly used therapies that might benefit palliative care patients
- CAM therapies with potential safety issues
- Resources for further education of providers and patients

■ COMPLEMENTARY AND ALTERNATIVE THERAPIES WITH POTENTIAL BENEFIT

There is some clinical data to support the use of CAM in palliative care patients, but the body of evidence is not extensive. Research challenges include small sample sizes, difficulty creating an appropriate control arm, difficulty standardizing the delivery of intervention, short trial duration, and limited funding.

Acupuncture has been studied for its potential role in the management of symptoms, including nausea, vomiting, and pain. There has been some positive evidence for its use in chemotherapy-induced nausea and vomiting. Some trials have suggested that acupuncture may also be useful in the treatment of pain, but systematic reviews have concluded that further studies are still needed. The risks of adverse events from acupuncture are minimal, and most complications have been related to lack of sterility of needles. Patients should be advised to only seek treatment from qualified, licensed practitioners who use disposable single-use needles. Although bleeding events are generally minor and localized, it is probably best to advise patients with bleeding disorders or on anticoagulation to avoid acupuncture. There have been case reports of rare serious events such as pneumothorax, but in general acupuncture is a safe complementary therapy.

Massage therapy can provide relief of anxiety and fatigue, based on several trials in cancer patients, though the duration of effect is not well established. Massage therapy has also been studied for its effect on pain, with several trials showing statistically significant reductions in pain measures in the immediate setting. Of note, however, pain reduction was not sustained over time. One particular form of massage, manual lymph drainage, was found in a few limited trials to reduce symptoms of lymphedema when used with compressive measures. Massage therapy is generally safe, but clinicians should advise patients with bleeding disorders or bony metastases to exercise caution and avoid all but the gentlest massage techniques.

Mind-body therapies such as hypnosis, meditation, guided imagery, and relaxation techniques have increasingly become integrated into the care of palliative care patients. Studies of mind-body interventions demonstrate potential to improve mood, relieve emotional distress, and enhance overall quality of life. Randomized control trials of relaxation training and guided imagery support their use in the treatment of anxiety. Some mind-body interventions also show promise in the treatment of physical symptoms. Hypnosis may have a role in pain and nausea treatment, based on several small randomized controlled trials. Additionally, nursing-led interventions such as breathing and relaxation techniques reduced dyspnea scores in several studies. If a patient reports benefit from mind-body therapies, clinicians can generally support their continued use as long as there is no clear interference with conventional treatments.

■ SAFETY CONCERNS

Clinicians should advise their patients that certain practices carry potential risks. Patients should not initiate any CAM therapies without carefully researching and considering the risks.

Quality control for herbal preparations is not standardized, and there is real potential for harm through inconsistencies in preparation and contamination. Clinicians should counsel patients that claims of "natural" ingredients do not necessarily guarantee safety. Patients have developed renal failure necessitating dialysis and even renal transplant after taking herbal preparations containing a nephrotoxic Chinese herb, *Aristolochia fang chi*. One case series reported a manufacturing error resulted in the substitution of *Aristolochia fang chi* for the herbal preparation intended for weight loss. Patients taking herbal remedies for eczema also have developed end-stage renal failure due to contamination from *Aristolochia fang chi.* This herb is implicated in the development of urothelial cancer. In another example, PC-SPES ("PC" stands for prostate cancer; "spes" means "hope" in Latin), a product containing eight herbs, initially showed promise in the treatment of patients with advanced prostate cancer including decreased serum prostate-specific antigen, but it was recalled due to toxicity and contamination with conventional medications including warfarin and indomethacin. A report of a severe acquired bleeding diathesis after PC-SPES use suggested possible anticoagulant effect from warfarin contamination. The FDA subsequently issued a warning to discontinue use of PC-SPES, and this product is no longer available.

Additionally, many agents are pharmacologically active and carry the potential to interact with important conventional therapies. St. John's wort is an inducer of cytochrome P450 (CYP3A4) and has been found to reduce levels of chemotherapeutic agents including irinotecan. Experts in CAM therapies advise against the use of St. John's wort with concurrent chemotherapy. Ginseng and ginkgo biloba can also increase cytochrome P450 activity. Green tea (polyphenols) and grapefruit juice are known inhibitors of the cytochrome P450 system. Further information about drug interactions can be found in the resources listed below.

Patients at risk for malnutrition should avoid macrobiotic and other highly restrictive diets. Macrobiotic diets are mainly vegetarian, high in grains and low in fat. Some macrobiotic diets are also high in phytoestrogens and may pose some risk for patients with estrogen-positive breast or endometrial cancer. Similarly, the literature recommends that these patients avoid large quantities of soy products and ginseng, as some preparations of ginseng have been found to contain phytoestrogens.

Many patients take high doses of vitamins with the hope of slowing cancer progression, but there is no reliable evidence to support this. Additionally, vitamin C has some anticoagulant effect and vitamin E can diminish platelet function. Patients who are thrombocytopenic or taking anticoagulants should avoid high doses of these vitamins.

One of the most serious consequences of CAM therapies is the delay of conventional treatment in favor of alternative therapies. Clinicians should strongly caution their patients against pursuing any CAM therapies that interfere with the initiation of recommended conventional therapies.

PRACTICE POINT

- Many herbal therapies are pharmacologically active and can interact with conventional treatments such as chemotherapy.

ONLINE RESOURCES FOR PATIENTS AND CLINICIANS

Further information is available for both patients and providers on a variety of reputable websites (**Table 216-12**).

SUGGESTED READINGS

PAIN

Abrahm JL. A Physician's Guide to Pain and Symptom Management in Cancer Patients. Baltimore: John-Hopkins; 2014.

NCCN Clinical Practice Guidelines in Oncology: Adult Cancer Pain; 2014 http://www.nccn.org/professionals/physician_gls/f_guidelines.asp.

Moryl N, Coyle N, Foley KM. Managing an acute pain crisis in a patient with advanced cancer: "This is as much of a crisis as a code." *JAMA.* 2008;299:1457-1467.

Principles of Analgesic Use in the Treatment of Acute Pain and Cancer Pain. Glenview: American Pain Society; 2008.

NAUSEA

Abrahm JL. A Physician's Guide to Pain and Symptom Management in Cancer Patients. Baltimore: John-Hopkins; 2014.

Basch E, Prestrud AA, Hesketh PJ, et al. Antiemetics: American Society of Clinical Oncology clinical practice guideline update. *J Clin Oncol.* 2011;29:4189-4198.

Wood GJ, Shega JW, Lynch B, et al. Management of intractable nausea and vomiting in patients at the end of life: "I was feeling nauseous all of the time…nothing was working." *JAMA.* 2007;298:1196-1207.

DYSPNEA

Ben-Aharon I, Gafter-Gvili A, Leibovici L, et al. Interventions for alleviating cancer-related dyspnea: a systematic review and meta-analysis. *Acta Oncologica.* 2012;51:996-1008.

Luce JM, Luce JA. Management of dyspnea in patients with far-advanced lung disease: "Once I lose it, it's kind of hard to catch it…" *JAMA.* 2001;285:1331-1337.

Thomas JR, von Gunten CF. Management of dyspnea. *J Support Oncol.* 2003;1:23-32.

SECRETIONS

Lokker M, van Zuylen L, van der Rijt C, et al. Prevalence, impact, and treatment of death rattle: a systematic review. *J Pain Symptom Manage.* 2014;47:105-122.

TERMINAL DELIRIUM

Breitbart W, Alici Y. Agitation and delirium at the end of life: "We couldn't manage him." *JAMA.* 2008;300:2898-2910.

White C, McCann MA, Jackson N, et al. First do no harm…terminal restlessness or drug-induced delirium. *J Palliat Med.* 2007;10:345-351.

TABLE 216-12 Online Resources

General information on CAM

National Center for Complementary and Alternative Medicine

nccam.nih.gov

NIH Office of Dietary Supplements

ods.od.nih.gov

NIH Dietary Supplements Label Database

dsld.nlm.nih.gov/dsld

Natural Medicines

naturalmedicines.therapeuticresearch.com

Cancer websites

National Cancer Institute (NCI) Office of Cancer Complementary and Alternative Medicine

cam.cancer.gov/cam

Memorial Sloan-Kettering Cancer Center

Mskcc.org/aboutherbs

Reporting of adverse events

Any adverse events from dietary or herbal supplements should be reported to the US Food and Drug Administration

FDA Medwatch: 1-800-FDA-1088 www.fda.gov/medwatch/how.htm

NUTRITION AND HYDRATION

Casarett D, Kapo J, Caplan A. Appropriate use of artificial nutrition and hydration—fundamental principles and recommendations. *N Engl J Med.* 2005;353:2607-2612.

Goldstein N, Morrison R. *Evidence-Based Practice in Palliative Medicine.* Philadelphia: Elsevier; 2013.

COMPLEMENTARY MEDICINE

Bardia A, Barton DL, Prokop LJ, et al. Efficacy of complementary and alternative medicine therapies in relieving cancer pain: a systematic review. *J Clin Oncol.* 2006;24:5457-5464.

Weiger WA, Smith M, Boon H, et al. Advising patients who seek complementary and alternative medical therapies for cancer. *Ann Intern Med.* 2002;137:889-903.

ADDITIONAL SUGGESTED READINGS

Abrahm JL. *A Physician's Guide to Pain and Symptom Management in Cancer Patients.* Baltimore: John-Hopkins; 2014.

Center to Advance Palliative Care: Fast Facts and Concepts (peer-reviewed, evidence-based summaries of key palliative care topics). Accessed at www.capc.org/fast-facts.

Goldstein N, Morrison R. *Evidence-Based Practice in Palliative Medicine.* Philadelphia: Elsevier; 2013.

Pantilat S, Anderson W, Gonzales M. *Hospital-Based Palliative Medicine: A Practical, Evidence-Based Approach.* Harrisonburg: Wiley-Blackwell; 2015.

CHAPTER 217

Care of the Dying Patient

Lindy H. Landzaat, DO, FAAHPM
Christian T. Sinclair, MD, FAAHPM

Key Clinical Questions

❶ What are the signs that death is approaching?

❷ How does the clinician decide what medications are still needed at the end of life?

❸ How does the clinician address end-of-life concerns?

INTRODUCTION

Caring for dying patients is an integral role of hospitalists; recent data show that approximately 25% of medicare beneficiaries die in hospitals. This chapter will focus on the imminently dying patient with an expected life expectancy in the range of a few weeks or less. In the United States, the most common causes of dying include heart disease, cancer, and chronic lower respiratory disease, followed by accidents, stroke, and Alzheimer's disease. The mere thought of dying can invoke great distress, and it is a natural response that people often try to disregard the universal inevitability of death. Not confronting end-of-life risks compounds suffering: unwanted medical interventions, impaired family bereavement, and unfulfilled life closure tasks. Physical, emotional, spiritual, and existential suffering are all possible, though not guaranteed. Health care providers need to remain sensitive to the many ways that patients and families may suffer near end of life.

Any illness that cannot be cured and contributes to a short life expectancy is a terminal illness. Most, though not all, stage IV cancers are terminal. Heart failure, chronic obstructive pulmonary disease, Alzheimer's dementia progress from chronic to terminal illness, although these are less commonly thought of as terminal illnesses compared to cancers.

The dying process may be categorized as "acute" due to a sudden event, "chronic" due to progressive disease and/or acute exacerbations of chronic disease, or "acute-on-chronic" due to a catastrophic complication of the chronic illness. Terminal illness generally creates a negative trend in functional abilities over time with an "active dying" phase that spans a few days to a week. Active dying in the final days includes withdrawing from the world and shutting down of body organ functions. Sometimes an additional acute process complicates the signs which otherwise would have pointed to a longer, though limited, prognosis. The presence of several characteristics dying signs and symptoms mark a transition to "active" or "imminently dying" (see **Table 217-1**). These may be witnessed in the final minutes, hours, or days of life. Acute dying processes are less predictable; clinicians may suddenly bear witness to active dying with minimal notice during a sudden terminal event.

MOST VALUED ELEMENTS OF END-OF-LIFE CARE

A systematic review looked at the most valued elements of end-of-life care according to patients and families from United States, Canada, and UK. The top five ranked value categories were described in **Table 217-2**. "Effective communication and shared decision making" include honest communication, ability to prepare for life's end, being prepared for what to expect about one's future physical condition, not being placed on life support when there was little hope for recovery, and having an opportunity to nominate a decision maker. "Expert care" included good physical care (including being kept clean), symptom management (especially pain and agitation), and integrated care (coordination related to discharge planning, etc). "Respectful and compassionate care" which included preservation of dignity and "trust and confidence in care" were third and fourth priorities for all. Finally, families rated having "financial affairs" in order as fifth most important while patients were split in ranking "adequate environment for care" and "minimizing burden" (ie, not being a burden either physically or emotionally) as their next priority. Optimizing care within these categories will help hospitalists meet the end-of-life needs for their patients and families.

TABLE 217-1   Common Signs Associated with the Dying Process

Dying Patients Typically Have a Constellation of These Symptoms, Not Just One

Sign	Comments
Weeks-Months	
Anorexia	Nearly universal in final days
Increasing weakness and debility	
Days-Weeks	
Sleeping most of the day	
Decreasing urine output	
More starring, withdrawing from the world	
Worsening dysphagia	
Near-death awareness	Eg, seeing or interacting with deceased friends/family
Transient clinical improvement, a "rally"	Eg, family reports unexpected "really good day"
Confusion, disorientation, delirium	Sometimes "terminal delirium"
Hours-Days (Active Dying)	
Disordered or irregular breathing	Caution with pre-existing sleep apnea, neuro injury associated Cheyne-Stokes
Audible oral secretions	Sometimes called "death rattle"
Skin mottling (livedo reticularis)	may fluctuate
Ileus	
Minimal to no urine output	Unless progressing neuro dysregulation with diabetes insipidus and polyuria
Eyes open, decreased blinking	
Minutes-Hours	
Abnormal terminal patterned breathing	Low tidal volume with agonal type respiratory pattern and/or jaw thrusting

TABLE 217-2   Elements of End-of-Life Care That Patients and Families Rank Most Important

Rank	Patients	Families
1	Effective communication and shared decision making	Expert care
2	Expert care	Effective communication and shared decision making
3	Respectful and compassionate care	Respectful and compassionate care
4	Trust and confidence in clinicians	Trust and confidence in clinicians
5	Adequate environment for care (tied)	Financial affairs
	Minimizing Burden (tied)	

Virdun C, et al. Dying in the hospital setting: a systematic review of quantitative studies identifying the elements of end-of-life care that patients and their families rank as being most important. *Palliat Med.* 2015;29:774-796.

END-OF-LIFE PROGNOSTICATION

The patient's prognosis is a strong driver of goals of care, and yet many clinicians lack formal training on how to best estimate prognosis and hesitate to have these discussions with patients. If one overestimates or underestimates by a significant margin, a patient may make major choices which impact their last few days with family and friends. The accuracy of prognostication diminishes with the longer time scales, and there are multiple tools with variable validation behind them for many major diseases. Hospice eligibility guidelines are used to help identify if patients have less than 6 months to live and therefore eligible for hospice; however, these guidelines lack accuracy (see Chapter 105 [Using Prognosis to Guide Treatment]).

Formulating a prognosis for the hospitalized patient begins with a fundamental understanding of the patient's current clinical status, functional trajectory, medications, life-sustaining treatments, and the expected course for the patients' primary disease along with their co-morbidities. Reaching out to specialists familiar with the disease and patient's history may also help add prognostic information. However, some research has shown providers with longstanding close relationships have historically overestimated prognosis (see **Figure 217-1**).

PRACTICE POINT

- Functional status could be considered a vital sign, because of its primary role in prognosis: the lower the function, the poorer the prognosis. The change in functional status over time may be a helpful indicator to define the likely trajectory if the disease runs a natural course without intervention.
- Major organ failure may be the most significant factor in making predictions, because it may trump the primary disease as the primary cause of death. If major organ failure is present, the prognostic estimate should be based on the progression of the organ failure.
- Communicating prognostic information with patients and families includes a discussion of how functional status, comorbidities, and major organ insufficiency has deteriorated over time.

Some prognostic tools use signs and symptoms like anorexia, cachexia, dyspnea, and confusion when looking at prognosis in the days to weeks range. These symptoms may be amenable to treatment interventions which may then alter the prognostic course. Any one symptom has not been shown to be indicative of a defined prognostic time frame.

■ COMMUNICATING A PROGNOSIS

Multiple surveys show *most* patients want information about their prognosis, be it good news or bad. The clinician should ask patients and families about their understanding of the medical problem, and then clarify key elements (medical facts, functional status, and disease trajectory) to set the tone for the prognostic revelation. Asking the patient how much they would like to know and whether they have questions about the time frame, helps ensure they are not pushed past what they can handle. "Some patients I've care for are worried about what the time ahead looks like. Is that something you'd like to discuss? Can you first tell me what information would be most helpful?" Patients or families may find evasiveness or inconsistencies to be distressing and unhelpful (see Chapter 215 [Communication Skills for End of Life Care]).

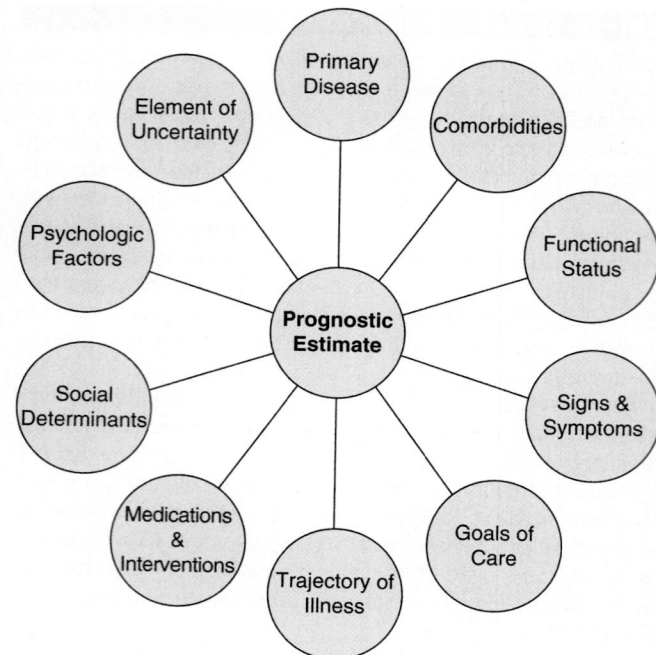

Figure 217-1 *Determinants in estimating prognosis.*

- Communication of a poor prognosis is often desired.
- Prognostic estimates should always be delivered with compassion.
- To acknowledge uncertainty, clinicians should avoid broad ranges (hours to months) that do not help patients and family plan for death; clinicians should also avoid narrow ranges (8 hours) that risk the physician's credibility or increase patient and family anxiety. What ultimately is needed may not so much an accurate prediction of time but an acknowledgement of the possibility of dying.

CODE STATUS

Patients wanting "everything to be done" often translates into "everything helpful," and "everything" with a reasonable chance of getting the patient back to an acceptable quality of life. Discussing code status is significantly easier if the goals of medical care have already been discussed. When providers have a good understanding of the patient's priorities for their care, it is easier to offer a medical recommendation for a code status that aligns. "We have heard you say that your goal is to ensure that your remaining days are peaceful and as pain free as possible. Given that, we recommend that we protect you from invasive medical procedures such as a code blue. It is our medical opinion that attempting resuscitation with a code blue procedure in your final moments would create pain and suffering and is contrary to your goal of being peaceful and pain free." If there is an agreement for a do not resuscitate (DNR) order, it may be important to summarize and close the conversation with the institutionally appropriate next steps that will follow the code status change. "So we will place a doctor's order in your chart to protect you from a code blue, and the nurse will place a band on your wrist with the initials DNR." Accidently forgetting this step may lead to confusion when the nurse comes in to apply an indicator, prompting unnecessary clarification calls and distress.

Patients and families fear DNR labels will preclude them from receiving equal medical treatments independent of code blue

resuscitative efforts. Clinicians should not overinterpret a DNR order. Just because a patient would not want CPR performed, does not mean that an ICU transfer is automatically out of the question. Discussions about precode interventions such as blood pressure support, intensive care unit level of care, and ventilation support is not always possible on the same encounter. Patients and families may not have the stamina to make more emotional decisions; others may prefer a decision happen after an assessment of the specific medical circumstances emerge since such a wide range exists.

- Focus on clarifying the patient's priorities for their care first, then align and recommend a code status.
- A medical recommendation for a DNR is often more appreciated than entirely placing the burden of decision making on a loved one.

COMFORT CARE

When goals have been shifted to comfort care only, the medical team should reassess all interventions such as daily labs and imaging, telemetry, finger sticks, waking the patient up for vital signs, and other technology driven data for their utility. The daily physical examination may eventually be curtailed or limited to the key aspects which may inform prognosis or guide comfort plans. A physical examination, even if limited, may help support the expectations of patient and family that the team continues to be directly involved with the care of the patient. Skipping the examination all together may be perceived by some as uncaring or disengaged and a minor threat of abandonment.

Weighing a decision to transition the patient to another setting at the end of life.

Sometimes a patient may urgently request to "get home" when time is short. The medical team should respect this request if a safe discharge plan consistent with goals of care can be implemented. **Table 217-3** offers a matrix for decision making about transferring a patient near end of life.

■ END-OF-LIFE MEDICATION

During their final days and weeks patients will have more difficulty with swallowing and taking oral medication becomes burdensome. Consider the goals of each medication, the associated burden, the risks and the benefits of continuing or discontinuing each medication (**Table 217-4**). Prioritize which medications take highest priority when it is not possible for patients to take all of their medications. Their decreasing ability to successfully ingest their medication sometimes offers a natural weaning phenomenon. Proactively starting to wean some medications may help avoid withdrawal.

- Patients and families often anticipate that stopping medications, dialysis or a ventilator may lead to a rapid decline and death within hours. Patients who seek comfort care will not always have a shorter lifespan; this presupposes that every medical intervention is always helpful and without harm or side effect. It is not uncommon for someone to live longer than expected when therapies are de-escalated.
- Helping patients and families prepare for a potential longer time course is important to help prevent them from second guessing the decision to focus fully on comfort care.

TABLE 217-3 Weighing a Decision to Discharge a Patient Nearing Death

	Lower-Risk Transport	Higher-Risk Transport
Low patient/ surrogate motivation to transition to alternative care setting	• Assess for underlying worries/concerns contributing to desire not to change location • Work toward developing safe and agreeable discharge plan	• Advocate for continued inpatient care • Document findings to suggest need for ongoing hospitalization and reasons for concern about moving patient
High patient/ surrogate motivation to transition to alternate care setting	• Work on expediting a reasonable discharge plan that maximize time outside the acute care setting • Sometimes negotiation needed as patient and family may want to move faster than system can • Realize patient's and family's time together is short, try to prioritize	• Educate about risks of transport, and ensure contingency plans are understood (ie, what happens if patient were to die in transport) • Anticipate and acknowledge provider angst about moving a high-risk patient, cite the patient/ family priorities

In all cases where DNR has been established, recommend continuation of these orders with any required outside the hospital forms for the transporters and next site of care (ie, POLST/DNR forms).

■ IMPLANTABLE CARDIOVERTER DEFIBRILLATORS (ICD)

The 2013 ABIM's Choosing Wisely List for Evidence Based Recommendations in Hospice and Palliative Medicine list includes deactivating ICDs when consistent with goals of care so that patients may be spared unnecessary painful defibrillation shocks as they near end of life. Patients and caregivers can be reassured that the pacing component can be continued despite disabling the shocking mechanism. Consider addressing this possibility prior to discharge home, as it is much easier to have an ICD deactivated inside a health care setting than following discharge.

TABLE 217-4 An Approach to Evaluating End-of-Life Medications

Consider the Goals of Care	
Benefits	**Risk**
What are the Benefits of continuing?	What are the Risks of continuing?
What are the Benefits of discontinuing?	What are the Risks of discontinuing?
Also	
Will the medication require a taper?	
Will the medication require a change in administration route?	
Will the patient continue to have access to the medication in another care setting?	

Communicate the ICD status, whether active or disabled, to the hospice or next physician caring for the patient. Caregivers of a patient with an active ICD should discuss with their cardiologist and hospice team an emergency plan for management at the end of life to minimize suffering.

■ PACEMAKERS

It is generally not necessary to deactivate pacemakers at the end of life. Palliative care consultation should be considered when these discussions take place. For a patient who is dependent on their pacemaker, discontinuing may invoke a host of sudden symptoms such as dyspnea and chest pain that require aggressive symptomatic palliation. Many patients die with pacemakers firing, they just fail cardiac capture. Rarely, pacemakers can be burdensome and undesired in dying patients, and, it is ethically permissible to discontinue a pacemaker.

THE DYING PROCESS

The heart, lungs, and brain are generally the three most critical organs with regards to time estimates and symptom control in the last days and weeks. As the whole body weakens, these three organs start to work toward their lowest effective rate manifesting as tachycardia, hypotension, short shallow breaths, and increasing somnolence and confusion. These findings may be incorrectly ascribed to comfort medications. Key physical examination findings and their possible prognostic significance are noted in Table 217-1. The presence or absence of a single symptom on this list is not enough to confidently define a survival time frame.

■ GRIEF

It is normal and natural for patients to have anticipatory grief as they grapple with their own impending death. Grief in terminal illness may relate to loss of lifestyle, identify, dreams now destined to go unfulfilled, independence, dignity, and being separated from loved ones. When clinicians recognize anticipatory grief, it may be therapeutic to name or verbalize the loss and to normalize, not minimize, the loss. "Losing the ability to care for yourself as you once could is a real loss. It's normal to grieve this." Providers should avoid statements such as "I understand what you are going through." These statements are presumptuous and will more often distance rather than foster connections. Even when providers share similar experiences, it is impossible for them to be identical. Many terminally ill patients will still enjoy some of their interests, including spending time with loved ones. A patient's hope typically shifts during terminal illness but does not evaporate. Acceptance of death and open discussion of dying happens by some and should not be mistaken for suicidal ideation.

PRACTICE POINT

- Sadness and grief are normal during end of life. Significant emotional or behavioral symptoms with impairment in social functioning (adjustment disorder) and anhedonia, utter hopelessness, and suicidal ideation (depression) are not automatically part of dying.
- Involving mental health professionals, interdisciplinary team members, education, and interventions are encouraged for adjustment disorders and depression, even near end of life. These disorders may be amenable to interventions such as psychotherapy, support groups and improving coping skills. Psychostimulants may be helpful in terminal illness due to their short onset of action.

■ REQUESTS FOR HASTENED DEATH

Patients and family members sometimes ask medical providers for aid in dying. The legality and physician protections for physician-assisted suicide vary in different areas of the country. Euthanasia, the intentional ending of the life of another suffering individual, is illegal in the United States. Physician-assisted suicide, sometimes referenced as "Death with Dignity Acts," first requires that a series of conditions be met. These steps include patient initiated verbal and written requests, a psychiatric evaluation, proof of terminal illness and state residency, and mandated waiting periods. If criteria are properly met, the physician provides a lethal prescription for medication that the patient being of sound mind administers to him or herself. Sometimes prioritizing symptom control, stopping artificial life prolongation efforts and medications will lead to a shortened lifespan. This differs from euthanasia because of the intent; removing burdensome treatments that a patient does not want any longer, compared to intending the death of the patient.

A request for aid in dying should be handled gently as it typically stems from love, concern, personal suffering, or wishes to spare another from suffering. Family members may feel guilty for asking. Sharing that other family members ask for the same and recognizing that the request stems from compassion, may assuage some guilt. The family members may be aware that the patient would not want to linger and that existing in some intermediate condition ('not really living, but not dead either') feels purposeless to them. The family member may be exhausted and sometimes project their own suffering on the patient. Clinicians are encouraged to listen to patient and family concerns and try to understand the suffering that likely prompted the request. Be gentle, honest, and clear in your limits. Sometimes family members just need to be reminded that this phase of illness will not continue forever. Give permission for them to take breaks and care for themselves. Offer reassurance that symptoms will not go untreated. Reach out to other interdisciplinary team members (nurses, chaplains, social workers, palliative care) to help support family Sometimes another clinician's assessment of the patient's suffering may help both providers and family.

Palliative sedation is intended to control symptoms and reduce suffering, not to hasten death when all other efforts have been exhausted. This option requires informed consent and discussion with the interdisciplinary team, and possibly including palliative care specialists.

■ TERMINAL DELIRIUM

Many patients experience delirium (waxing and waning altered sensorium) as the body and systems are shutting down. At any given point in time it may be difficult to know if the delirium will be reversible or not (terminal delirium) near end of life. Clinicians should set expectations and prepare the family that delirium may not be reversible in a dying patient. Treatment of terminal delirium is guided by the goals of care (see Chapter 216 [Domains of Care: Physical Aspects of Care]).

■ NEAR DEATH AWARENESS

Patients may possess a sense of near death awareness when their body is failing and their existence is getting short. Physicians often come to respect the "impending doom" sign when a patient presents with a catastrophic sense that something is changing in their body. Family members may report that the patient is talking to or seeing deceased acquaintances or loved ones. Often these experiences are not fearful and may provide comfort. Redirection or medication for agitation may be necessary if the patient is distressed. The clinician should focus on listening to the patient's needs, optimize comfort, and reassure the family that this normally happens near death.

■ ARTIFICIAL NUTRITION AND HYDRATION

Dying patients with failing physiology often distribute fluid ineffectively contributing to anasarca, ascites, pulmonary edema and eventually respiratory distress. Forcing food and fluids (artificially or naturally) on a dying body can add to patient discomfort. Artificial nutrition and hydration may cause increased secretions, nausea and vomiting, and patients may develop an ileus as the body shuts down. Often when artificial nutrition and hydration have been discontinued in a dying patient, some of the third spaced fluid may remobilize into the intravascular space and secretions and congestion often improve.

Most of the time dying patients are not interested in eating; some foods have transient appeal and the patient may be satiated after just a few bites. This often prompts family distress, worried their loved one is "giving up" or "starving". Despite popular misconceptions, there is not a definite, defined, number of days after which the patient will expire from not eating or drinking. Helping family members recall the last time they were ill and not interested in eating can add insight. Assisting family members in finding alternative ways to "nourish" the patient such as reading, massage, music, etc. can prove patient-centered. For some withdrawing artificial fluid and nutrition provokes distress. Input from palliative and hospice consultants, ethics committees, chaplains, or relevant community spiritual leaders may help minimize harm and discomfort to the dying patient.

■ DYSPHAGIA AND SECRETIONS

A dying patient's swallow function becomes less effective and their innate ability to manage even their own oral secretions worsens. In the final stages, these secretions may pool in the back of the throat near the vocal cords and as air moves past, these secretions make noise and rattle. This is sometimes called the "death rattle." Typically, when secretions are present, the patient is near comatose and unaware of the phenomenon. Education is the first line of intervention for families, explaining the noise, and reassurance that the patient is not suffering (provided that aligns with the examination) or sharing the plan for making the patient more comfortable.

For excessive and noisy secretions, repositioning the patient in a lateral decubitus position to facilitate postural drainage may help. If oral secretions then drain from the mouth, keeping a washcloth tucked under the cheek allows for quick and easy changes. Often the secretions are too deep to be comfortably suctioned and other interventions are preferred. For extreme cases, suctioning might be trialed. If a rigid suction device is not feasible, than limited attempts of a small, flexible nasotracheal suction catheter may be applied orally or nasally. Anticholinergics may reduce new secretions but risk making them more thick and tenacious. Anticholinergics do not "dry up" secretions through reabsorption. Awake patients who have difficulty clearing thick, mucous secretions may find attempts to thin secretions more helpful. For secretions that correlate with clinical signs of pulmonary edema, clinicians may hesitate over whether or not to diurese a patient with a marginal blood pressure, but recalling the goals of care, will help guide that decision (see Chapter 216: [Domains of Care: Physical Aspects of Care]).

■ FEVER

Patients may experience fever at the end of life from a variety of infectious sources and sometimes from central nervous system dysregulation. As the body changes its hemodynamics and skin perfusion, thermometer readings may be less reliable. Palliating fever may help with tachypnea and excessive work of breathing. Remove any sources of excessive heat sources, electric blankets or bulky covers, and consider acetaminophen rectal suppositories.

■ ORGAN DONATION

Hospitalists are encouraged to reach out to their local organ and tissue procurement organization for specific questions related to donation of organ and tissues. Some states have restrictions on who may discuss aspects of donation with patients and family members. Most hospitals have protocols regarding how this should be done.

TABLE 217-5 Elective Removal of Life Support Checklist

- Invested health care providers are up to date about change in plan of care (ie, transplant attending, primary care provider, others actively involved in care)
- Confirm no outstanding labs/tests that would significantly change prognosis or therapy
- Confirm correct patient and procedure
- Place DNR if not already done
- Deactivate defibrillator therapies for a patient that has an ICD
- Confirm patient has not been pharmacologically paralyzed, do not proceed unless paralytics have worn off
- Remove unnecessary attachments to the patient, monitor leads, restraints
- Confirm that all family and others who need or wanted to be present at the time of removal of life support
- Review with family next steps, probable prognosis but allow for uncertainty
- Based on the goals of care, and anticipated symptom needs, consider premedicating patients with opiate for work of breathing and a benzodiazepine for anxiety. For medication naive patients, suggest opiate premedication doses of morphine 2-10 mg or fentanyl 25-100 mcg IV and benzodiazepine of midazolam 1-2 mg or lorazepam 1-2 mg IV. Allow medication to take effect and re-dose if patient shows symptoms of discomfort as appropriate. A continuous infusion may be necessary for comfort if symptoms recur frequently.
- Discontinue unnecessary medications and tests
- Ask RN/RT to suction oral cavity, lungs prior to removal of the ETT
- Monitor and intervene depending on symptoms in the postextubation period

■ REMOVAL OF LIFE SUPPORT

A stepwise checklist for removal of life support is provided in **Table 217-5**. The clinician may check for paralysis with a patient's ability to over-breathe the set respiratory rate on the ventilator, motor movements, and/ or use a train-of-four stimulator where 4 of 4 stimuli produce muscle contraction. For most patients the endotracheal tube (ETT) may be fully withdrawn and removed unless airway collapse is anticipated. If the ETT is serving as an airway stent (ie, tumor compression, severe inhalation injuries with edema) patients may be more comfortable leaving the ETT in place but disconnecting the ETT from the ventilator tubing. For patients on high ventilator support, it may be more peaceful to incrementally decrease support to room air settings, medicating for comfort as needed prior to removal of the endotracheal tube. Consider minimizing monitor alarms, detaching monitor leads, easing visitor restrictions to create a better ambiance. Listen to family members concerns and provide education about the process.

THE PATIENT'S FAMILY
■ CAREGIVER STRESS

Even individuals and family units with normal coping skills may do poorly in the setting of caregiver exhaustion and intense emotions. Family members typically need information, sometimes repeated, to allow time for processing and acceptance. Empathetic and clear communication is essential to prepare patients and families and to optimize care. When signs of caregiving stress are present, engaging interdisciplinary team members such as chaplains, palliative care consultants, and social workers can be very helpful. Encourage the family member to reach out to their personal physician (or offer to do yourself with their permission) to provide an update. Encourage

the family member to take breaks and care for themselves too, chances are the patient would wish that for them.

"DON'T TELL"

A patient's biggest worry may not be for themselves but for the wellbeing of their family members. The patient may wish to try to "protect" loved ones by avoiding difficult truths and conversations. Family members may hope to protect the patient when they fear emotional pain, are concerned that the patient will "give up", or other reasons. Sometimes family members accurately know that their loved one is not able to integrate the information. Clinicians should listen to the family members' concerns. Patients have the right to hear medical information about their condition if they so wish, but also to defer decision making and information sharing to others. Before divulging difficult information, the clinician should assess how the patient wants information to flow (ie, directly to the patient, or through an appointed family member, or surrogate) and explain to the concerned family member that the patient will not be forced to hear unwanted information.

Set expectations with the concerned family member that it not acceptable to deceive the patient if the patient asks for information. If the patient does not want information, and the family wants to maintain pretenses, it is best not to promise that the system can maintain the same pretenses. When patients say in private one thing, but in the presence of family express contradictory wishes, consider whether the patient is trying to protect others, is ambivalent, second-guessing, intimidated, or just prioritizing someone else's wishes above their own. Family members accept decisions better if they know it originated from the person they love.

POSTACUTE CARE

For dying patients discharging from the acute hospital setting to a different level of care for end of life (usually either to home with hospice, long-term care nursing facility with hospice, or inpatient hospice unit), **Table 217-6** offers a checklist for discharge to facilitate a smoother transitions. Sample language addressing families' concerns is included in **Table 217-7**. Proper preparation for discharge includes involving hospice. Not only will hospice assist with care

TABLE 217-6 Discharge Checklist for Dying Patient Transitioning Care Settings

- Goals of care are clear by patient (or surrogate)
- Support services: resources for end-of-life care have been arranged (ie, hospice)
- Medication reconciliation: medications have been reviewed for burden/benefit ratio and those that will not contribute to comfort or to the goals of care have been discontinued
- Code status: outside the hospital DNR, POLST form, or equivalent has been completed. Persons assisting with transportation and next site of care are aware
- If patient has an ICD: relay ICD status and whether an offer to deactivate the defibrillator component has been extended
- Education: if patient will be discharging with hospice, avoid an unnecessary hospital readmission by reminding caregivers to call hospice with questions, concerns, and emergencies, instead of 911
- Contingency planning with those persons transporting the patient if there is risk of dying en route
- Prescriptions supplied: a new set of prescriptions with patients active medications and particularly controlled substance prescriptions is often required (hospice may have preferred pharmacy; receiving facility may not carry some drugs)
- Communication to next attending physician: receiving facility clinician, PCP, patient's oncologist, or hospice attending that will follow the patient

TABLE 217-7 Common Patient/Family End-of-Life Concerns

Common Concern	Education	Potential Response
"Doctor, How long?"	Before answering, consider: • Does everyone present want to hear that information? • Recognize variability in the dying with some degree of uncertainty, even if you are fairly certain • Communicate ranges such as days to weeks, weeks to months	"I can never know for sure, but I will give you my best educated guess. Does everyone gathered want to hear this information?" "Naturally, something sudden could always happen that I can't predict. Based on my experience, the time may be in the range of hours to days"
"Am I starving my mother?"	Prepare the family for what is normal and expected at the end of life Remind family members of the underlying cause (ie, cancer, heart failure, etc) Prepare family for what the plan will be if the patient expresses hunger or thirst, guided by the goals of care and what the plan will be when the patient is not awake	"Many family member worry about this. What we know is: • Dying patients almost universally lose their appetite; her dying is a result of cancer • The body does not process food and drink the same at this stage of illness • A failing body typically starts to third space fluids; this can add to symptoms and discomfort • Commonly, artificial fluids start to accumulate in the wrong places such as the skin, lungs, abdomen, making her feel worse If she becomes alert enough and wants something by mouth, we're happy to start with sips and bites of whatever sounds good since our first priority is her comfort If she is not awake, it's not safe to put food in her mouth. We will continue to provide oral care for her comfort."
"But he wanted to die at home"	Family members may carry guilt when a patient cannot die at home Explain why care in a setting other than home better helps meet the patient's goals	"Due to his current symptoms that require close monitoring and frequent adjustments of medications, we think right now he is better served by remaining here for the time being. Most patients tell us that they want to be at home, but that wish often includes being able to be aware of their surroundings and not being in pain or a burden on their family. We think managing his care needs would be very high at home. Are there ways we can make his hospital room more home-like?"
"His breathing seems noisy. Is he having discomfort?"	In the absence of coughing, choking, gagging, work of breathing, the secretions are not known to cause discomfort. Most of the time the patient is stuporous and the noise is more distressing to family than patient Positional maneuvers and medications may be attempted to help	"The noise you are hearing is caused by a small amount of drainage in his throat" "We don't have any reason to believe he is uncomfortable from this pooling of secretions that he cannot swallow"
"She had a good day, and she doesn't seem to be dying as fast as we thought. Did we make the wrong decision?"	Patients sometimes have a surprising "rally" in the days preceding death much to the surprise of families and providers. Sometimes dying doesn't happen in the expected timeframe. Reviewing the medical circumstances that lead to the goals of care can be helpful for family and providers. [Revisit goals if medical circumstances have significantly changed]	"I'm so glad that he had a good day yesterday; often that can cause some families to second guess earlier decisions. If you remember, he said he did not want any more transfusions because they did not help him feel any better. With his leukemia that continues to progress, I still expect that time is short"
"Isn't there anything you can do to speed this dying process along?" (Other variations, "can't you give him a shot, a pill?")	This request is typically coming from a place of compassion, possibly coupled with caregiver fatigue Sometimes family members just need to be reminded that this phase of illness will eventually end. Give permission to take breaks and care for themselves Be gentle but be clear in your limits, and be honest Reassure that you will respond to signs of patient suffering when you see them Reach out to other team members to help support family, nursing, chaplains, social workers	"Families sometimes ask me this when their loved one is dying. Are you worried he is suffering? Tell me what you've noticed I cannot intentionally hasten your loved one's dying process, and we WILL watch for signs of suffering and treat those Currently he appears quite peaceful to me. This state will not continue indefinitely. Are you able to get breaks and take care of yourself? I'm guessing he would want you to take care of yourself"

for patient and family unit, they also offer important bereavement (grief) support to family members (if desired) for the 13 months following the patient's death (see Chapter 74 [Hospice]). The EMS crew transporting near-death patients should be prepared for the possibility of death en route and be provided a completed POLST (Physician Orders for Life Sustaining Treatment) or DNR form. In addition, some ambulance crews may prefer a physician order directing that if the patient should expire it is acceptable to continue to the planned destination. Some protocols require the ambulance to pull over to the side of the road and await the arrival of the police or coroner or to transport the patient to the nearest Emergency Room for death pronouncement. Prior to discharge consider if the patient will need medications as they travel to their destination, what the local transportation services can provide, and what prescriptions are requested by hospice.

HOSPITAL DEATH

■ HOLISTIC NEEDS OF THE DYING

Religious, spiritual, or cultural beliefs may play an important role in meeting the holistic needs of the dying. Practices that may be important in the dying and postmortem care include the presence of a spiritual leader for end-of-life rituals, the presence of someone of the same faith with the body at all times, restrictions on who may touch the body after death. Beliefs may vary significantly even within a particular faith or cultural belief. Some families will create a reverent atmosphere in the dying patient's environment and others may prefer lighthearted festivity. The variation may be a result of tradition, coping styles, patient's personality, lifestyle, or family tradition based on prior deathbed exposures. Team members should remain vigilant to any hints about end-of-life needs, and as opportunities arise, make sensitive inquiries. "Some families have important traditions or customs surrounding the time of death, is there anything that our team should know to best respect and care for you and the person you love?"

Family members will commonly ask "So what happens afterward?" Clinicians may respond by asking if the family member has a particular concern and then outline their institution's process for handling a death, including formal death pronouncement, notification of family, and death certification. The nursing staff usually provide information about the duration of time the family may remain with the deceased, where the body is moved and stored, when and how the body leaves the hospital.

■ DEATH PRONOUNCEMENT

The clinician performing the death pronouncement should:

- Gather key information from the chart and nurse before entering the room to determine if death was expected
- Ask if the nurse (or chaplain) would like to accompany the physician as they likely have a relationship with the patient and family
- Introduce him or herself with an explanation of why the clinician is there and what the clinician is going to do
- Listen for heart sounds, breath sounds, and pupillary responses

- Clearly and compassionately state that the patient has died
- Offer condolence statements which feel natural
- Document the patient's death in the medical record
- Inform attending of record and primary care physician of death
- Complete the death certificate

Testing for response to painful stimuli is not necessary in an expected death. Families may have questions or they may often choose to have time alone.

■ THE DEATH CERTIFICATE

Timely attention to completing the death certificate is required so that family members have proof of the death in order to attend to the deceased's affairs such as planning burial or cremation and accessing funds for these services. Funeral directors will complete most of the information about the deceased with help from family. Attending physicians are expected to complete the medical aspects of the death certificate. Experience in completing death certificates varies in training programs yet this crucial role deserves close attention. For more information on physician certification of death certificates, see the Suggested Reading.

■ AFTER DEATH

Physicians may wish to send a condolence card or call and express their sympathies to a family member after a patient has died. Hospitalists are encouraged to explore their own responses during such intense times. The death of a patient with whom you have developed a meaningful relationship can have a lasting impact, depending on how one copes with loss.

SUGGESTED READINGS

Block SD. Assessing and managing depression in the terminally ill patient. *Ann Intern Med*. 2000;132:209-218.

Gurschick L, Mayer DK, Hanson LC. Palliative sedation: an analysis of international guidelines and position statements. *Am J Hosp Palliat Care*. 2015;32:660-671.

Hoyert D, et al. Physicians' Handbook on Medical Certification of Death. Department of Health and Human Services, Center for Disease Control and Prevention, National Center for Health Statistics. 2003. DHHS Publication No. (PHS) 2003-1108. http://www.cdc.gov/nchs/data/misc/hb_cod.pdf.

Lampert R, Hayes DL, Annas GJ, et al. HRS Expert Consensus Statement on the Management of Cardiovascular Implantable Electronic Devices (CIEDs) in patients nearing end of life or requesting withdrawal of therapy. *Heart Rhythm*. 2010;7:1008-1026.

Palliative Care Network of Wisconsin: Fast Facts and Concepts. Edited by Sean Marks. http://www.mypcnow.org/fast-facts.

Virdun C, Luckett T, Davidson PM, Phillips J. Dying in the hospital setting: a systematic review of quantitative studies identifying the elements of end-of-life care that patients and their families rank as being most important. *Palliat Med*. 2015;29:774-796.

SECTION 12
Pregnancy

Overview of Physiologic Changes of Pregnancy

Meghan Hayes, MD

Lucia Larson, MD

Key Clinical Questions

1. What are normal physiologic adaptations during pregnancy?
2. What are abnormal, concerning findings during pregnancy?
3. How does pregnancy affect laboratory values?

INTRODUCTION AND EPIDEMIOLOGY

Pregnancy and delivery require amazing maternal adaptation, with nearly every organ system altered by hormonal and/or mechanical means. Physiologic changes begin at conception and continue throughout pregnancy and the postpartum period. Such changes may impact the manifestation and course of a disease process as well as have implications for treatment. Maternal vulnerabilities, such as increased risk of thrombosis, hypertension, or diabetes, may also be revealed during pregnancy. Since any woman of reproductive age has the potential to be pregnant, their care must occur in the context of an understanding of normal and abnormal pregnancy physiology.

PHYSIOLOGY BY SYSTEM

■ CARDIOVASCULAR

A healthy heart adapts well to the marked demands of pregnancy, but congenital or acquired heart disease may present or worsen in the gravid woman due to the cardiovascular changes associated with increased cardiac workload. Estrogen mediates an increase in cardiac output (CO) by 6-week gestation via increased preload and stroke volume. Blood volume rises by 30% to 40% during pregnancy, peaking at the end of the second trimester. Cardiac output peaks in the third trimester, typically 30% to 50% above baseline. Total peripheral resistance declines by 20%. Systolic and diastolic blood pressures drop by 10 to 15 mm Hg in the first trimester then return to baseline in the second half of pregnancy; diastolic blood pressure declines more than systolic, so pulse pressure widens. The cardiac axis is shifted leftward, anterior and cephalad.

Blood flow distribution changes during pregnancy such that up to 25% of CO is directed to the uteroplacental unit (a new "end-organ") and up to 20% to the kidneys. An increased proportion of CO supplies breast tissue, but cerebral blood flow remains at baseline proportions.

Cardiovascular adaptations lead to common complaints in pregnant women: palpitations, decreased exercise tolerance, and dizziness. A shift of the heart toward the chest wall may contribute to the experience of palpitations by the gravida, but palpitations may also represent increased sensitivity to mild sinus tachycardia, premature atrial or ventricular systoles, or, less likely, supraventricular tachycardia. It is postulated that the increase in blood volume may be associated with stretching of the myocardium, thereby potentially increasing myocardial irritability and predisposing to arrhythmias. While this is not clearly proven, both atrial and ventricular arrhythmias may occur in pregnancy just as they occur in the nonpregnant patient. By late pregnancy there is attenuated ability to increase cardiac output with exercise, and this combined with normal weight gain of pregnancy can lead to decreased exercise tolerance. Beyond midpregnancy the gravid uterus causes aortocaval compression in the supine position, decreasing CO by 30%, and venous return, leading to dizziness and dyspnea (termed *supine hypotensive syndrome*) in some women. Pertinent exam findings include systolic flow murmur by midpregnancy, mammary soufflé, point of maximal impulse displaced leftward and cephalad, and mild bilateral lower-extremity edema. Heart rate increases but is not generally above 100 beats/min. While the neck veins may appear full, jugular venous pulsation is not elevated. Electrocardiograms of pregnant women often will show left axis deviation, atrial enlargement and nonspecific ST-T wave changes, but such findings should be carefully interpreted within clinical context. The cardiac silhouette may be generous on chest radiograph. Increased cardiac output and volume of distribution in pregnant women necessitate careful attention to timing of intravenous contrast dye bolus for computed tomography pulmonary angiography, in order to avoid radiation exposure for an inconclusive study. *Care should be taken to position pregnant woman in the left lateral decubitus (or at least with hip elevation to displace the pregnant uterus off the vena cava) when performing medical investigations or treating ill pregnant women to minimize such adverse hemodynamic effects.*

■ RESPIRATORY

Pregnancy contributes to mechanical changes as well as progesterone-mediated physiologic adaptations in the respiratory system. In the upper airway, hyperemia, glandular hyperactivity, increased edema, and friability occur, related to elevated plasma volume and estrogen. Chest wall circumference increases by 5 to 7 cm due to elevated relaxin levels, and, eventually, the uterus elevates the diaphragm by about 4 cm though diaphragmatic excursion remains unchanged or even increased.

During pregnancy, oxygen consumption increases by 30% to 60% due to increased metabolic demands. Elevating progesterone levels increase respiratory drive early in pregnancy with continued effect throughout. Minute ventilation (tidal volume multiplied by breaths/min) increases by up to 50% through increased tidal volume; respiratory rate should remain unchanged. Vital capacity remains unchanged while functional residual capacity declines by up to 25%. Overall, pulmonary function testing interpretation remains unchanged, as forced expiratory volume in 1 second (FEV1), FEV1/forced vital capacity ratio, and peak expiratory flows remain stable.

Compensated respiratory alkalosis is expected on arterial blood gas testing, with PaO_2 elevated to 100 to 105 mm Hg, and $PaCO_2$ expected at 28 to 32 mm Hg. Clinically, pregnant women may complain of mild exertional dyspnea because of increased respiratory drive and physiologic anemia; however, this should not limit activities of daily living nor worsen with progressing pregnancy. Pertinent chest radiographic findings include generous cardiac silhouette, increased anteroposterior diameter, and prominent pulmonary vasculature.

PRACTICE POINT

- Clinical implications of respiratory anatomic changes in pregnancy include common complaints of gestational rhinitis (nasal congestion), epistaxis, and snoring, increased difficulty with intubation, and effect on needle insertion site for thoracentesis by the elevated diaphragm. It is recommended that the most experienced provider available perform intubation since failure rates are far higher in pregnant women. Maternal oxygen saturation of 95% or greater is desirable to maintain PaO_2 greater than 70 mm Hg for optimal placental oxygen diffusion.

■ RENAL/URINARY

Anatomic changes in the genitourinary system begin early in pregnancy, with kidneys increasing in size by about 1 cm in length and 30% in volume by midpregnancy, related to elevated blood volume and enlarging vasculature. The renal collecting system dilates due to progesterone- and prostaglandin-mediated smooth muscle relaxation initially and mechanical obstruction by the uterus later, so that mild to moderate hydronephrosis is expected on imaging. As a standard ultrasound parameter, ultrasound imaging should visualize ureteral jets in the absence of true obstruction. Ureteral peristalsis decreases, increasing the risk for ascending infection.

Early pregnancy vasodilatation due to surging progesterone and relaxin lead to increased glomerular filtration rate and renal plasma flow by 6 weeks. Glomerular filtration rate increases by 50%, and renal plasma flow increased by an even greater percentage. Medication metabolism is therefore accelerated, such that medications may require more frequent dosing (eg, twice daily rather than once daily) and higher doses (eg, when using antimicrobials with dosing ranges) for efficacy. Creatinine clearance rapidly increases by 25%, so that serum creatinine values average 0.5 mg/dL and blood urea nitrogen and uric acid levels decline. Bicarbonate excretion is accelerated, related to respiratory changes; pregnant women therefore have decreased buffering capacity and increased susceptibility to acidosis.

Altered glomerular membrane charge selectivity increases excretion of protein, albumin, and glucose. Up to 300 mg of protein on 24-hour urine collection is considered normal during pregnancy. Correlation between spot urine protein-to-creatinine ratios and 24-hour urine protein collection values has been variable, therefore only very low or very high urine protein-to-creatinine values are useful; and, although cumbersome, 24-hour urine protein collection remains the gold standard.

Progesterone markedly stimulates the renin-angiotensin system. Renin is produced by the placenta, thus there is an increase in maternal sodium absorption and potassium excretion. Between 6 and 8 L of water are retained to sustain normal pregnancy. Erythropoietin levels also increase, in order to meet red blood cell demands.

PRACTICE POINT

- Clinical implications of renal physiologic adaptations include increased susceptibility to urinary tract infections including pyelonephritis, nephrolithiasis, and acidosis.

See Chapter 219 (Medication Management for a discussion of the implications of medication prescribing).

■ GASTROINTESTINAL

Progesterone mediates gastrointestinal (GI) smooth muscle relaxation, decreasing motility. As pregnancy progresses, the mechanical impact of the gravid uterus alters GI function. The majority of pregnant women experience nausea and vomiting early in pregnancy, attributed to high human chorionic gonadotropin (hCG) levels plus estrogen and progesterone. Constipation is common, related to decreased motility and delayed gastric emptying; absorption may be delayed. Not surprisingly, gastroesophageal reflux is reported by up to half of pregnant women and is related to progressive uterine enlargement, decreased lower esophageal sphincter tone and increased intra-abdominal pressure.

Hepatic physiology is generally stable during pregnancy. The high estrogen state of pregnancy may mimic liver disease findings, with palmar erythema and telangiectasias, in the absence of hepatic pathology. Alkaline phosphatase levels rise due to placental production. Dilution causes serum albumin and total protein levels to decline, which may impact pharmacokinetics of protein-bound medications. It is therefore preferable to obtain free drug levels rather than total levels when clinically indicated.

The gallbladder increases in size, although emptying capacity declines. Bile is more lithogenic during pregnancy and more saturated with cholesterol. Biliary sludge is common and may spontaneously resolve after delivery. Gallstones are more likely to be symptomatic than sludge and less likely to resolve spontaneously. Thus, there is an increased incidence of symptomatic gallstones both during pregnancy and postpartum.

HEMATOLOGIC

Marked adaptation allows increased blood flow to the uterus and developing placenta and preparation for delivery's hemostatic challenge. Blood volume increases by 50% to 100% beginning by the 6th week of gestation. Plasma volume increases by 50% with an initial rapid rise, then gradual increase to peak at the 30th week. Erythrocyte mass rises less significantly, leading to the physiologic anemia of pregnancy, with typical Hgb levels of 10 to 12 g/dL by term. Neutrophilic leukocytosis may be seen, typically not beyond 16×10^9/L. Platelet count typically remains stable in pregnancy. Isolated mild thrombocytopenia (115-150 $\times 10^9$/L) occurs in approximately 10% of pregnancies by term. Pregnant women are hypercoagulable due to increased estrogen effects on clotting factors as well as increased venous stasis. There is a marked increase in venous thromboembolic risk continuing through 6 to 8 weeks postpartum. Levels of the following may double by the third trimester: fibrinogen, factors V, VII, VIII, X, von Willebrand factor, and thrombin activation. D-dimer increases by the second trimester and remains elevated to the postpartum period. Protein S level and activity decline during pregnancy, as does sensitivity to activated protein C (APC). Protein C level and activity and antithrombin remain stable in normal pregnancy, but decreased antithrombin may be seen in association with pre-eclampsia and/or proteinuria.

PRACTICE POINT

- D-dimer is not a useful test to rule out venous thromboembolism in pregnancy since it is elevated in most pregnancies by term. Although thrombocytopenia can occur during pregnancy, it should not be forgotten that pre-eclampsia, sepsis, disseminated intravascular coagulation, and abruption are important causes of decreased platelet counts in pregnancy.

ENDOCRINE

Pancreas

Early normal pregnancy is characterized by accelerated starvation, with mildly decreased fasting plasma glucose and increased ketogenesis, which leads to risk of starvation ketosis after prolonged fasting. By mid to late pregnancy, insulin resistance increases, heralded by large volumes of dilute urine and generally tolerated unless fluid is restricted via human placental lactogen (hPL), human placental growth hormone (hPGH), and likely tumor necrosis factor-alpha (TNF-α). This adaptation supplies the fetoplacental unit with 50 to 100 g of glucose daily by the third trimester. Insulin sensitivity returns to baseline within 48 hours of delivery. Thus, the insulin needs of type 1 and type 2 diabetics may decrease early in pregnancy (particularly if there is significant "morning sickness" causing nausea and vomiting), causing an increased risk of nocturnal hypoglycemia. Insulin doses generally need to be increased later in pregnancy in response to increasing insulin resistance. This physiology is also responsible for the development of gestational diabetes in some women. There is a higher incidence of fetal loss with diabetes, both due to an increase in congenital anomalies related to the teratogenic effect of glucose in patients with elevated hemoglobin A1C and to the renal and vascular complications of the disease itself. Management with a multidisciplinary team that includes specialists with expertise in diabetes in pregnancy is important.

Thyroid

Maternal thyroid hormone production increases by 50%. Hepatic production of thyroid hormone-binding globulin increases by two- to threefold, driven by elevated estrogen levels. Free levels of T4 and T3 remain stable but total levels rise. Maternal iodine requirements increase in order to fulfill T4 production, with increased renal iodine clearance. The fetal thyroid begins to function by 12 weeks and is fully functional by 18 weeks, so it is essential that maternal levels are sufficient for early development. Multidisciplinary collaboration enhances maternal and neonatal outcomes.

In the first trimester, b-hCG levels peak at 8 to 12 weeks and stimulate thyrocytes, which causes transient T4 production and thyroid-stimulating hormone (TSH) suppression. This may be exaggerated in molar pregnancy or hyperemesis gravidarum. If the mother is iodine replete, by the third trimester, there is a mild decrease in T4 and mild increase in TSH.

PRACTICE POINT

- Mild increase in TSH and decrease in T4 often result in the need to increase levothyroxine doses during pregnancy as compared with the prepregnancy dose. Recommendations are to increase doses by 25% to 30% in all patients on thyroid replacement in the third trimester.
- Patients may develop mild diabetes insipidus (DI) during pregnancy. Clinicians should monitoring of volume and electrolyte status in these patients, and confirm that the DI is due to a benign process and not to posterior pituitary disease.

Parathyroid

Maternal mineral hemostasis is challenged by fetal skeletal formation then further challenged during lactation. Total serum calcium declines slightly due to decline in serum albumin; ionized calcium remains unchanged. Urinary calcium levels rise by 12-week gestation. Parathyroid hormone (PTH) is key to calcium homeostasis in the nonpregnant state, acting directly via renal and bone effects and indirectly via intestinal absorption. Levels of PTH decline during pregnancy, and it would be expected that 1,25 $(OH)_2$ vitamin D levels would drop as well, but 1,25 $(OH)_2$ vitamin D levels rise. It is likely that the placenta may contribute 1,25 $(OH)_2$ vitamin D. Prenatal vitamins provide adequate vitamin D supplementation.

Pituitary

The size of the pituitary increases by up to 70% by the third trimester largely due to hyperplasia of lactotrophic cells in the anterior lobe. Prolactin levels increase due to estrogen and progesterone stimulation of lactotrophic cells, and the placenta also produces prolactin by late pregnancy. Adrenocorticotropic hormone (ACTH) levels rise due to placental corticotropin-releasing hormone (CRH), which is not suppressed by dexamethasone. ACTH levels rise further during labor. Oxytocin levels rise throughout pregnancy, eventually facilitating parturition. Vasopressin levels decline due to placental production of vasopressinase, which may be a cause of transient diabetes insipidus (DI) during pregnancy.

LABOR AND DELIVERY-PERTINENT PHYSIOLOGY

A complex biochemical cascade, beyond the scope of this discussion, culminates in parturition. During labor, cardiac output further increases by one-third from the already augmented output of pregnancy, and systemic vascular resistance increases up to 25% with contractions. With each contraction, 300 to 500 mL of blood is "autotransfused" from the uteroplacental to the maternal circulation. Valsalva maneuvers while pushing increase myocardial oxygen consumption and may increase maternal blood pressure. These changes may be important in patients with underlying cardiac disease who are unable to tolerate increased volume and increased cardiac work.

Regional anesthesia for pain control during delivery, either spinal, epidural, or combined spinal-epidural, may lead to acute vasodilatation and resulting hypotension. Spinal anesthesia has been associated with greater hypotension than epidural anesthesia, however, it can be administered more rapidly if needed urgently. An epidural catheter offers the opportunity to provide continued pain relief after delivery with neuraxial opioids. Hypotension from neuraxial anesthesia may be reduced by preloading with crystalloid, or occasionally colloid, decreased dose, and slower administration.

CONCLUSION

This chapter reviews the physiologic changes that begin at conception and continue throughout pregnancy and the postpartum period, how such changes impact the manifestation and course of a disease process, and maternal vulnerabilities. An understanding of normal and abnormal pregnancy physiology is central to providing optimal care for this population of patients.

SUGGESTED READINGS

Hill CC, Pickinpaugh DO. Physiologic changes in pregnancy. *Surg Clin N Am.* 2007;88:391-401.

Rosene-Montella K, Keely E, Barbour LA, Lee RV, eds. *Medical Care of the Pregnant Patient*, 2nd ed. Philadelphia, PA: American College of Physicians; 2008.

Smith R. Parturition. *N Engl J Med.* 2007;356:271-283.

CHAPTER 219

Medication Management

Raymond O. Powrie, MD, FRCP, FACP
Karen Rosene-Montella, MD, FACP

Key Clinical Questions

❶ What key questions should the practitioner ask to ensure safe use of medication during pregnancy?

❷ What are the limitations of the Federal Drug Administration drug classification?

❸ How should the physiologic changes in pregnancy that affect pharmacokinetics influence prescribing of medication?

INTRODUCTION

Until the middle of the last century there was a widespread belief among both clinicians and patients that the human fetus grew in a protected environment that minimized any potential effects of substances ingested by the mother. This misperception ended dramatically when the effects of thalidomide became widely known in the late 1960s. Ever since this tragedy, a primary driver for both patients and providers of the approach the use of medications in pregnancy is fear of causing adverse fetal effects. Despite this, use of medications during pregnancy remains widespread throughout the world. Therefore, it seems that a dichotomy exists: a widely perceived fear regarding the ingestion of medication during pregnancy juxtaposed against the practical reality that medications are necessary and continue to be used during the course of gestation.

This chapter aims to provide a helpful evidence-based approach to guide hospitalists who may be asked to consult on or care for pregnant women. **Table 219-1** lists some references that discuss the safety of particular agents in pregnancy. **Table 219-2** makes some clinically based recommendations about which medications are preferred for specific indications during pregnancy. The remainder of this chapter will provide a general approach to prescribing in pregnancy that should guide the reader in the informed use of the information contained in both the listed references and the provided summary table.

KEY CONCEPTS FOR APPROPRIATE USE OF MEDICATIONS IN PREGNANCY

■ MOST MEDICATIONS "CROSS THE PLACENTA"

With few exceptions, no placental barrier exists for medications that can be administered orally. Drug levels in the fetus may be the same, lower, or higher than in the mother. In general, lipophilic drugs, drugs that are nonionized at physiologic pH, and drugs of low molecular weight cross the placenta more efficiently than other drugs, but the fetus will have exposure to almost any medication that can be administered orally to the mother.

■ MEDICATION USE DURING PREGNANCY CAN CAUSE A WIDE RANGE OF ADVERSE EFFECTS

Teratogenesis is more than just "missing parts." Although the thalidomide tragedy drew attention to medication-associated malformations such as limb reduction defects, drugs may have other, perhaps more subtle, effects during pregnancy such as intrauterine growth restriction (eg, atenolol), intrauterine fetal demise (eg, possibly cyclophosphamide), long-term cognitive or behavioral toxicities (eg, valproic acid and mental retardation), and neonatal toxicities (eg, neonatal abstinence syndrome such as may be seen with narcotics and benzodiazepines).

PRACTICE POINT

Potential teratogenic effects of medications in pregnancy
- Malformations
- Intrauterine death due to either embryotoxicity or fetotoxicity
- Intrauterine growth restriction
- Behavioral toxicity
- Neonatal toxicities

TABLE 219-1 Resources for Helping to Determine which Medication to Use when Treating Medical Illness in Pregnancy

Publication	Authors	Publisher	Format
Drugs in Pregnancy and Lactation: A Reference Guide to Fetal and Neonatal Risk	Briggs GS, Freeman RK, Yaffe SY	Lippincott Williams & Wilkins; 8th ed., 2008	Hardcover 2144 pages
Teratogenic Effects of Drugs: A Resource for Clinicians (TERIS)	Friedman JM, Polifka JE	John Hopkins University Press, 2nd ed., 2000	Hardcover 793 pages
Medication Safety in Pregnancy and Breastfeeding: The Evidence-Based, A to Z Clinician's Pocket Guide	Koren G	McGraw-Hill Professional, 1st ed., 2006	Paperback 312 pages
Medication Safety in Pregnancy and Breastfeeding	Koren G	McGraw-Hill Professional, 1st ed., 2007	Hardcover 623 pages
Drugs for Pregnant and Lactating Women	Weiner CP, Buhimschi C	Churchill Livingstone, 1st ed., 2004	Hardcover 1101 pages
Drugs During Pregnancy and Lactation	Schaefer C, Peters PWJ, Miller RK	Academic Press, 2nd ed., 2007	Hardcover 904 pages
Prescribing in Pregnancy	Rubin PC, Ramsey M	BMJ Books, 4th ed., 2008	Paperback 256 pages
Catalog of Teratogenic Agents	Shepard TH, Lemire RJ	John Hopkins University Press, 12th ed., 2007	Hardcover 656 pages
Medications & Mothers' Milk: A Manual of Lactational Pharmacology	Hale T	Pharmasoft Medical Publishing, 13th ed., 2008	Conveniently sized paperback 1172 pages
Online computer databases			
REPRORISK	Produced and marketed by Thomson Reuters Micromedex Inc. Module available at http://thomsonreuters.com		Online data base or diskette contains TERIS, REPROTOX, REPROTEXT, and Shepard's Catalog of Teratogenic Agents
TERIS	Information available at http://depts.washington.edu/terisweb/teris		Online subscription or diskette
Reprotox	Thomson Reuters Micromedex Inc. Module available at www.REPROTOX.org		Online subscription or diskette PDA version available

Reprinted, with permission, from Powrie RO and Wiley-Blackwell Publishers. Prescribing in Pregnancy: A Practical Approach. In deSwiet's *Medical Disorders in Obstetric Practice*, 5th ed. London: UK, 2010:636-640. Table 30-1 and Table 30-2.

TABLE 219-2 Suggested Medications in Pregnancy by Indication

Condition or Product Type	Data Suggests Use Justifiable when Indicated	Data Suggests Use may be Justifiable in Unique Circumstances	Data Suggests Rarely Justifiable for Indication Listed	Useful Review Articles and Comments
Acne	Topical erythromycin$_B$ Topical benzoyl peroxide$_C$ Topical clindamycin$_B$	Oral erythromycin$_B$	Tetracycline$_D$ Doxycycline$_D$ Topical tretinion$_C$	PMID: 2971690 PMID: 16487888
Analgesics	Acetominophen$_A$ Codeine$_C$ Meperidine$_C$ Morphine$_C$	All NSAIDS$_{B/C}$ (Intermittent use of NSAIDs in the first two trimesters for anti-inflammatory purposes may be justifiable but repeated use after 28 wk is to be avoided.) ASA$_D$ (Low-dose ASA < 100 mg/d does appear to be safe in pregnancy.)		These review article details issues surrounding the use of NSAIDs in pregnancy including case reports of constriction of the ductus arteriosus, renal dysfunction and hemostatic abnormalities in the fetus and neonate. Malformations associated with NSAIDs have not been reported however PMID: 16638921 PMID: 16194696 PMID: 15013926

(Continued)

TABLE 219-2 Suggested Medications in Pregnancy by Indication (Continued)

Condition or Product Type	Data Suggests Use Justifiable when Indicated	Data Suggests Use may be Justifiable in Unique Circumstances	Data Suggests Rarely Justifiable for Indication Listed	Useful Review Articles and Comments
Antihistamines	Diphenhydramine$_B$ (but avoid in first trimester) Chlorpheniramine Dimenhydrinate$_B$ Loratidine$_B$ Cetirizine$_B$	Fexofenadine$_C$		These 2006 review articles systematically and critically review the literature on the treatment of allergic rhinitis in pregnancy. PMID: 16579874 PMID: 16443148
Antimicrobials	Erythromycin$_B$ base, ethyl succinate or stearate (not estolate) Penicillins$_B$ Cephalosporins$_B$ Azithromycin$_B$ Vancomycin$_C$ Nitrofurantoin$_B$ Metronidazole$_B$ (after first trimester) Isoniazid$_C$ Acyclovir$_C$ AZT$_C$ and other antiretrovirals except for Efavirenz$_D$ (sustiva)	Antifungals: (all$_C$ exceptamphotericin$_B$ nystatinclotrimazole and terbinafine, which are$_B$) The following agents are commonly used in pregnancy but are best reserved for use when alternate agents are less effective: Clarithromycin$_C$ Aminoglycosides$_D$ Trimethoprim$_C$ Sulfonamides$_C$	Tetracycline$_D$ Fluoroquinilones$_C$ despite very concerning animal data; increasing human data suggests fluoroquinolones might warrant their placement in the "use may be justified in rare circumstances" category: erythomycin estolate$_B$ efavirenz$_D$	Two 1997 and one 2006 review article on the use of antimicrobials in pregnancy are: PMID: 9266582 PMID: 9067781 PMID: 16648419
Asthma	Beta-agonists: Albuterol$_C$ Metaproterenol$_C$ Salmeterol$_C$ Pirbuterol$_C$ Formeterol$_C$ Inhaled steroids: Budesonide$_B$ Beclomethasone$_C$ Flunisolide$_C$ Fluticasone$_C$ Triamcinolone$_C$ Systemic steroids$_C$: Ipatropium$_B$ Cromolyn$_B$	Zafirlukast$_B$ Montelukast$_B$ Omalizumab$_B$		New national recommendations for the management of asthma in pregnancy were published in early 2005 and can be obtained through the NHLBI at *http://www.nhlbi.nih.gov/ health/prof/lung/asthma/ astpreg.htm*. Most medications commonly used to treat asthma (aside from the leukotriene antagonists) have considerable clinical experience with their use in pregnancy that suggests their safety and particularly justifies their use to control asthma in pregnancy. PMID: 17363831 PMID: 17181448 PMID: 16946229 PMID: 16443145 PMID: 17889809
Constipation	Bisacodyl$_C$ Docusate Glycerin Psyllium Sodium biphosphate Magnesium hydroxide Sorbitol Mineral oil			

(Continued)

TABLE 219-2 Suggested Medications in Pregnancy by Indication (Continued)

Condition or Product Type	Data Suggests Use Justifiable when Indicated	Data Suggests Use may be Justifiable in Unique Circumstances	Data Suggests Rarely Justifiable for Indication Listed	Useful Review Articles and Comments
Cough	Guaifenesin$_C$ Dextromethorphan$_C$ Albuterol$_C$ Codeine$_C$			This review article discusses the treatment of the common cold in pregnancy PMID: 18474699
Depression	Amitriptyline$_D$ Nortriptyline$_D$ Fluoxetine$_C$ Sertraline$_C$	Sertraline$_C$ Fluvoxamine$_C$ Escitalopram$_C$ Citalopram$_C$ Venlafaxine$_C$ Mirtazapine$_C$ Paroxetine$_C$ (Increasing data suggests this agent may fall into the category to the right because of a small risk of both teratogenicity and neonatal syndromes.)		General review of behavioral health: PMID: 18378767 Bipolar affective disorder: PMID: 17764378 Depression: PMID: 18760228 Anxiety: PMID: 17955910 Schizophrenia: PMID: 12553132
Diabetes	Insulin (human, beef or pork, lispro)	Glyburide$_B$ has a developing role in the management of gestational diabetes as an alternative to insulin with comparable outcomes. PMID: 18622055 Metformin$_B$ *glucophage*™: Use of this agent in early pregnancies of women with polycystic ovary syndrome is increasing. PMID: 19084097	Chlorpropamide$_C$ Tolbutamide$_D$ Glipizide	PMID: 19104375 PMID: 18297574 PMID: 17596473
Diarrhea	Loperamide$_B$ Diphenoxylate/atropine			PMID: 12635420 PMID: 16673005
Dyspepsia	Ranitidine$_B$ Famotidine$_B$ Nazitidine$_C$ Cimetidine$_B$ Sulcrafate$_C$ Antacids$_B$: Al(OH)$_3$, Mg(OH)$_2$, CaCO$_3$	Omeprazole$_B$ Lansoprazole$_C$ Esomeprazole$_B$	Misoprostol$_X$	Despite placing proton pump inhibitors in the second category here, they are widely used in pregnancy and published data suggest they are not a major teratogenic risk in humans. We recommend their use if agents in the first column are ineffective in controlling symptoms. PMID: 12635419 PMID: 11430180
Headache	Acetaminophen$_A$ Codeine$_C$ Meperidine$_C$ Morphine$_C$ Metoclopramide$_B$ Caffeine$_C$ For prophylaxis: Amitryptiline$_B$ Nortiptyline$_D$ Beta-blockers$_{B\text{ and }C}$	All NSAIDs $_{B/C}$ (Intermittent use of NSAIDs in the second trimester may be justifiable.) Butalbital$_C$ in *fioricet* and *esgic*.	Sumatriptan$_C$ Noratriptan$_C$ Rizatriptan$_C$ Zolmatriptan$_C$ A growing literature about the use of these agents (particularly sumatriptan) in human pregnancies may eventually support their use as a second-line agent in pregnancy.	These review articles summarize the data about the treatment of migraine in pregnancy PMID: 18583683 PMID: 18345969 PMID: 18332840 An effective role for nonpharmacologic management with biofeedback, physical

TABLE 219-2 Suggested Medications in Pregnancy by Indication *(Continued)*

Condition or Product Type	Data Suggests Use Justifiable when Indicated	Data Suggests Use may be Justifiable in Unique Circumstances	Data Suggests Rarely Justifiable for Indication Listed	Useful Review Articles and Comments
			This article reports on the data presently available from the drug manufacturer's pregnancy registry for sumatriptan and cautiously reports no demonstrable teratogenic effect at this time. PMID: 10649172 Ergotamine$_x$ (Although unlikely to be a teratogen this agent is concerning for its potent vasoconstrictive and uterotonic effects.)	Therapy and relaxation is suggested in this small trial PMID: 8682668
Hypertension	Labetalol$_C$ Methyldopa$_B$ Pindolol$_B$ Other beta-blockers: Acebutalol$_B$ All others (may want to avoid atenolol because of an association with intrauterine growth restriction) Nifedipine$_C$ Hydralazine$_C$	Calcium channel blockers other than Nifedipine$_C$ Clonidine$_C$ Prazosin$_C$ Hydrochlorothiazide$_B$ Diazoxide$_C$	ACE inhibitors D Accupril, perindopril, ramipril, captopril, benazepril, trandolapril, fosinopril, lisinopril, moexipril, enalapril Angiotensin II Antagonists D eprosartan, telmisartan, valsartan, candesartan, irbesartan, valsartan	PMID: 15805801 PMID: 18259046
Nasal Congestion	Oxymetazoline$_C$ Nasal steroids Nasal cromolyn$_B$ Nasal ipratropium$_B$	Pseudoephedrine$_C$		PMID: 16579874 PMID: 16443148
Nausea Vomiting	Metoclopramide$_B$ Prochloperazine$_C$ Dimenhydrinate$_B$ Promethazine$_C$ Doxylamine plus pyridoxine	Ondansetron$_B$		PMID: 17967157 PMID 18077743 PMID: 17889806 Although ondansetron is commonly used o treat nausea and vomiting in pregnancy, the published experience is limited and the authors view it as a second-line agent
Pruritus	Topical: Moisturizing creams and lotions, Oatmeal cream or powder Calamine lotion, Topical glucocorticoids$_C$ Systemic: Hydroxyzine$_{C'}$ Chlorpheniramine$_B$ Diphenhydramine$_B$			PMID: 2289340 PMID: 10396430 PMID: 12031026

(Continued)

TABLE 219-2 Suggested Medications in Pregnancy by Indication (Continued)

Condition or Product Type	Data Suggests Use Justifiable when Indicated	Data Suggests Use may be Justifiable in Unique Circumstances	Data Suggests Rarely Justifiable for Indication Listed	Useful Review Articles and Comments
Thrombosis	Heparin (both low molecular weight and unfractionated)	Fibrinolytics such as streptokinase$_C$ and tPA Altepase$_{C8}$	Warfarin$_x$ coumadin™ This agent is believed by some to have a role in the management prosthetic heart valves after the first trimester as it may be associated with a lower risk of prosthetic valve thrombosis PMID: 10647757	PMID: 1918847 PMID: 18987370
Vaccines	Diptheria$_C$ Tetanus$_C$ Hepatitis A$_C$ Hepatitis B$_C$ Influenza$_C$ Immune globulin$_C$ Inactivated polio vaccine$_C$ Tuberculin test$_C$		Live vaccines: MMR Sabin polio vaccine (oral) varicella	General PMID: 14719841 Influenza and pertussis: PMID: 18677141 Pertussis, tetanus, diphtheria: PMID: 18509304 For travelers: PMID: 18760249

Letter designations are US FDA Pregnancy Categories from individual product package inserts.

References in the final column of this table are listed by their PubMed identification number. The citation and abstract can be obtained by going to www.pubmed.gov and entering this number into the search function.

Note: Every patient and circumstance is different and the literature on medication use in pregnancy is continually evolving. This table does not constitute specific therapeutic recommendations, and the reader is referred to the resources in in this table as a guide to therapeutic decisions.

Reprinted, with permission, from Powrie RO and Wiley-Blackwell Publishers. Prescribing in Pregnancy: A Practical Approach. In deSwiet's *Medical Disorders in Obstetric Practice*, 5th ed. London: UK, 2010:636-640. Table 30-1 and Table 30-2.

■ THE LIST OF KNOWN HUMAN TERATOGENS IS SHORT

Despite all the potential effects of medication use during pregnancy, there are really only about 30 known human teratogens that could be prescribed by physicians. Many of these known teratogens are not commonly used in medical practice. The most commonly prescribed human teratogens are listed in the Practice Point on page 1833.

■ MEDICATION EFFECTS MAY VARY DEPENDING ON THE GESTATIONAL AGE AT WHICH THEY ARE ADMINISTERED

Human gestation can be divided into specific periods, and each of these periods may be associated with distinctive medication-use risks.

The first 14 days after conception (the 2-week period between conception and the first missed menstrual period) are often called the "all or nothing period." During this time frame, drug effects are likely to be nil or result in miscarriage. At this point, the conceptus has not interfaced significantly with maternal circulation and drug exposures are likely to be only at a very low level. At this same time, all cells in the conceptus are nonspecialized (pluripotential) and are generally believed either to experience lethal effects of drugs (resulting in pregnancy loss) or no effect at all.

Between days 14 and 60 after conception (the *embryonic period*—a 7-week time frame following the first missed menstrual period) organogenesis is occurring, and drug exposure during these weeks can lead to major or minor malformations. This high-risk period accounts for only 5% of the 280-day human gestation. In fact, most human teratogens probably have even shorter specific periods when

the developing embryo is specifically susceptible to their toxicities. For example, thalidomide effects were seen only if the drug was taken between days 21 and 36. Valproic acid, which can cause neural tube defects, will not do so if taken after day 27 because the neural tube has completely closed by this date.

An important consequence of unique vulnerabilities of the embryonic period is that some significant toxicities may have already occurred before a woman or her provider is aware of her pregnancy. Therefore, the onus is on all providers prescribing medication to women of reproductive age to speak to these patients about the potential effects of their medications during pregnancy and the potential for harm even before the pregnancy is clinically apparent.

During the period between days 60 and 280 of gestation, progressive fetal growth and neurologic development is occurring. Toxicities during this period may cause impaired growth (eg, atenolol), neurologic or behavioral abnormalities (eg, valproic acid and mental retardation), or specific organ toxicities (eg, angiotensin converting enzyme [ACE] inhibitors and renal dysfunction). There is, therefore, no period in a pregnancy during which a medication can be considered completely safe. Rather, each distinct period in gestation represents unique potential vulnerabilities.

MEDICATION PREGNANCY SAFETY DATA: SOURCES AND THEIR LIMITATIONS

Much of the data that exist about the effects and safety of drug use in pregnancy are on the basis of animal studies. Before drugs are released on the market in the United States and Canada, animal testing looking for drug-related malformations needs to have occurred. Human data, however, are not required. This is because new drug testing on pregnant women is felt to be unethical and (aside from the important exception of thalidomide) most human teratogens have been found to be teratogenic in laboratory animals as well. However, two major problems with the use of animal data exist. First, animal data cannot always be confidently extrapolated to humans. There is considerable variability between species and even between strains of a species regarding the effects of the medication on a developing fetus. Second, behavioral and intellectual effects of medications are very difficult to recognize in animals. Much of human gestation is a time of progressive neurologic development. Medications that do not cause gross malformations may still have effects on developmental milestones, intelligence, and behavioral health that will not be readily discernable in animal models.

In general, the best use of animal data is when it is paired with human data and the findings suggest a common and biologically plausible association. However, most of the human data we presently have have their own challenges. One of the most significant problems with human data is that there is a large background risk of congenital abnormalities making it difficult to differentiate abnormalities that are caused by medications from those due to other causes. Between 2% and 4% of infants are born with some defect, and of these 20% are due to chromosomal abnormalities. Five percent are due to gene mutations and 65% of these defects remain unexplained. Likely, no more than 10% of identified human malformations are due to teratogenic agents. Because most human teratogens have their effect in only 0.1% to 30% of exposed fetuses, large numbers of exposures need to be studied to clearly identify an increase against the background risk of anomalies. The best evidence for teratogenic effects would be from prospective studies in humans, but these are done infrequently because they are difficult, lengthy, and expensive. Most studies determining effects of drugs in pregnancy are either case-control or cohort studies. In case-control studies, infants with anomalies are paired with infants without a particular anomaly. The number of infants exposed to the studied agent in each group is then compared. In cohort studies, the incidence of a particular anomaly among infants exposed to a particular agent is compared with the incidence of that anomaly among infants not exposed to that agent. In a case-control study, 220 cases and 220 controls must be studied to find a relative risk of 2.5 with a power of 80%.

The problems with such retrospective data are many. Most importantly, associations attributed to medication effects may simply reflect the reason the mother was on the medication rather than the medication itself. One must be cautious about ascribing anomalies to medication effects when in fact the anomaly may be caused by the underlying maternal condition that is being treated, or consider that an untreated maternal condition may also result in an anomaly.

Human case reports and registries are another flawed source of human data. There is substantial recall bias among women with a difficult pregnancy outcome. Women who bear children with an anomaly are much more likely to recall medication use in pregnancy and so are their providers. An illustration of this is the fact that the incidence of teratogenesis of isotretinoin was felt to be 80% with voluntary reporting to a registry at the pharmaceutical company but has been subsequently found to be only 36% in prospective studies.

PRACTICE POINT

Some known human teratogens
Commonly used agents
- Carbamazepine
- Cyclophosphamide
- Diethylstilboestrol
- Isotretinoin
- Lithium
- Methimazole
- Methotrexate
- Mycophenolate Mofetil
- Penicillamine
- Phenobarbital
- Phenytoin
- Tetracyclines
- Valproic Acid
- Warfarin
- ACE inhibitors (eg, captopril) and angiotensin receptor blockers (eg, losartan)

Less commonly used agents
- Androgenic hormones and high-dose norprogesterones
- Busulfan
- Iodides
- Thalidomide

Agents generally no longer in use as medication
- Mercury
- Trimethadione
- Acitretin/etretinate

Another difficulty with human data is that there is a difference in the response of individual human fetuses to different medications much in the same way as there is in adults. A classic example of such a phenomenon is seen with phenytoin. Many teratologists believe that phenytoin can cause something known as fetal hydantoin syndrome in 10% of infants exposed in utero. Fetal hydantoin syndrome (FHS) is a combination of features of intrauterine growth restriction, mild mental deficiency, a large anterior fontanel, a metopic ridge, ocular hypertelorism, depressed nasal bridge, short antevertal rise, bowed upper lip, cleft lip and palate, and nail and distal phalangeal hypoplasia. The risk of this syndrome increases dramatically in subsequent pregnancies if the mother has previously borne a child with FHS. One theory for this phenomenon is that the teratogenic risk of phenytoin varies with the activity of the enzyme epoxide hydrolase in mother and fetus. Decreased activity of this enzyme in patients taking phenytoin may lead to increased levels or toxic arene oxide intermediates, which some investigators suspect may be the direct teratogen in some cases of FHS.

Another problem with human data is that most cautionary information about medication use in pregnancy is related to anatomic defects identified in newborns on the initial exam at birth. Rarely are there studies that examine behavioral, functional, developmental, and/or delayed effects. The logistics and expense of carrying out such studies are daunting. This is especially true if one considers the potential for medications to affect the offspring of offspring through toxicities of a medication on the gametes in utero. Such effects are very unlikely to ever be uncovered.

An illustration of the complexity of drug pregnancy safety data is found in the history of the ACE inhibitors. Captopril was the first ACE inhibitor marketed in the United States and was initially released to market as an FDA category C drug on the basis of animal studies suggesting it is unlikely to be a teratogen. (See the discussion of the FDA pregnancy drug classification later in this chapter.) Postmarketing surveillance of this drug revealed an association with ogliohydramnios, fetal calvarial hypoplasia, fetal pulmonary hypoplasia, intrauterine growth restriction, intrauterine fetal death, and neonatal anuria. Most teratologists believed that the effect of ACE inhibitors was not a direct effect on organogenesis but rather a fetal toxicity. They hypothesized that high levels of angiotensin are probably physiologically necessary to maintain glomerular filtration at the low perfusion pressure seen inside the fetus. Therefore, use of ACE inhibitors in pregnancy is associated with poor perfusion of the kidneys, followed by renal failure and atrophy of the kidneys. Poor urine output contributes to the oligohydramnios, fetal calvarial hypoplasia, and fetal pulmonary hypoplasia seen in infants exposed to the drug. Since this association was made, ACE inhibitors were classified as class C drugs for the first trimester but as class D drugs for second and third trimesters. Subsequent population-based studies of ACE inhibitors, however, have suggested that there may also be a first trimester effect on organogenesis in addition to the later effects on fetal renal function and have led to recommendations to avoid the use of these agents completely during pregnancy, although the FDA has not yet changed the pregnancy safety classification for these agents.

Another example of the complexity of drug safety data in pregnancy is metronidazole. Metronidazole was long considered a human teratogen because it was found to be mutagenic in bacteria, carcinogenic in mice, and associated with congenital anomalies in several case reports in the medical literature. Therefore, this important agent for the treatment of bacterial vaginosis was often not used or used only with hesitation by obstetricians. However, this changed when a series of publications demonstrated no increased human risk associated with the use of metronidazole during pregnancy. Therefore, a drug that was withheld from pregnant women is now widely used during gestation with no evidence of untoward effects.

PRACTICE POINT

Four questions to ask in guiding medication use in pregnancy
- **Question 1:** Is the symptom to be treated self limited and/or amenable to nonpharmacologic management?
- **Question 2:** If the medication is *not* administered, what are the possible outcomes for mother and fetus?
- **Question 3:** What data are available on the safety of this medication in pregnancy and is there a similar drug with better safety data available that could be used instead?
- **Question 4:** How is the patient's (and the provider's) understanding and belief system affecting decisions about the use of this medication in pregnancy?

How then should the clinician sensibly approach this flawed and limited data? Neither the clinician nor the patient should believe that any drug can be called completely safe in pregnancy any more than we would believe that any drug can be called completely safe outside of pregnancy. At the same time, the provider and the patient should not feel that any drug is absolutely contraindicated in pregnancy. A more evidence-based approach is to consider whether benefits of a particular agent warrant any known or theoretical risks. Likewise, it is worth discarding the concept that there are any "safe" periods for medication use in pregnancy; again, a more evidence-based approach is to talk of "more vulnerable" and "less vulnerable" times during the pregnancy.

How then should the clinician approach the problem of deciding what drugs should or can be used during pregnancy? A useful approach is to address this question in four separate parts, listed in the Practice Point and discussed in the proceeding section.

■ QUESTION 1: IS THE SYMPTOM TO BE TREATED SELF LIMITED AND/OR AMENABLE TO NONPHARMACOLOGIC MANAGEMENT?

It is important when approaching medication use in pregnancy to have the patient (and the provider) understand that pregnancy is

a time when unnecessary or unhelpful medications that do not significantly affect the course of an illness should be avoided. As well, the option of nonpharmacologic management should always be considered in pregnancy. Treatment such as biofeedback or relaxation techniques for tension headaches might be preferable to analgesics in some cases.

■ QUESTION 2: IF THE MEDICATION IS NOT ADMINISTERED, WHAT ARE THE POSSIBLE OUTCOMES FOR THE MOTHER AND THE FETUS?

Many providers incorrectly entertain the idea of there being a central conflict regarding medication use in pregnancy in which the fetal and maternal needs are at odds. This is rarely the case. Fetal well-being is dependent on maternal well-being, and, therefore, treatment of maternal disease to maintain maternal health is generally very much in the interest of the fetus. For this reason, when deciding whether use of a particular medication is justifiable in pregnancy, it is important to consider the possible outcomes for the mother and fetus of *not* instituting (or continuing) pharmacologic treatment. It is often the case that withholding treatment will place the fetus and mother at greater risk than any potential effects of the medication, such as with antiepileptic drugs.

■ QUESTION 3: WHAT DATA IS AVAILABLE ON THE SAFETY OF THIS MEDICATION IN PREGNANCY, AND IS THERE A SIMILAR DRUG WITH BETTER SAFETY DATA AVAILABLE THAT MIGHT BE USED INSTEAD?

This is the question that many clinicians find the most challenging. **Table 219-1** lists several of the most helpful references available to assist in the answering of this question. Table 219-2 also offers a symptom- and disease-based list summarizing which agents are generally justifiable, sometimes justifiable, and almost never justifiable for a particular indication during pregnancy.

PRACTICE POINT

Food and drug administration pregnancy drug classification
- *The US FDA Pregnancy Drug Classification system was put in place in 1979. In 1997, the FDA advised that the system be revised to address its limitations and in 2008 a proposal was put forward to eliminate the letter-based categorization and rely solely on prose summaries of available pregnancy safety data. When and if this proposed change will be adapted remains unclear.*

Category A: controlled studies show no risk
- Controlled studies in women fail to demonstrate a risk to the fetus in the first trimester, there is no evidence of a risk in later trimester, and therefore, the possibility of fetal harm appears remote.

Category B: no evidence of risk in humans
- Either animal reproduction studies have not demonstrated a fetal risk but there are no controlled studies in pregnant women, or animal-reproduction studies have shown an adverse effect (other than decrease in fertility) that was not confirmed in controlled studies in women in the first trimester (and there is no evidence of a risk in later trimester).

Category C: risk cannot be ruled out
- Either studies in animals have revealed adverse effect on the fetus (teratogenic) or appropriate animal data is not available. Drugs should be given only if the potential benefit justifies the potential risk to the fetus.

Category D: positive evidence or risk
- There is positive evidence of human fetal risk, but the benefits from use in pregnant women may be acceptable despite the

risk (eg, if the drug is needed in a life-threatening situation or for a serious disease for which safer drugs cannot be used or are ineffective). There will be an appropriate statement in the "warnings" section of the labeling.

Category X: contraindicated in pregnancy

● Studies in animals or human beings have demonstrated fetal abnormalities or there is evidence of fetal risk based on human experience, or both, and the risk of the use of the drug in pregnant women clearly outweighs any possible benefit. The drug is contraindicated in woman who are or may be pregnant.

Perhaps somewhat unfortunately, the most commonly used resource in the United States with which question 3 is answered is the US Food and Drug Administration's (FDA's) pregnancy categories. These classification categories are found in most prescription medication package inserts and in the Physician's Desk Reference (PDR). The categories are summarized in the Practice Point and listed as subscripts following each agent in Table 219-2. The intent of the FDA classification was to help the clinician briefly summarize available data about the potential toxicities of an agent in pregnancy. Clinicians tend to use the letter categories as an order of safety, although a drug may be in category B when there are no human data available. Problems result from the fact that the complexity of the data is not fully considered and that the classification of agents rarely changes even after decades of accumulated data.

Even within medications from both the same drug class and pregnancy safety category, it is worth being cautious about the use of the newest agents during pregnancy unless there have been significant human pregnancy data. Many fetal toxicities such as the first trimester effects of ACE inhibitors have been identified in the years following release onto the market. Therefore, even an older drug with a less favorable pregnancy safety category may at times be preferable to a newer agent with an apparently more favorable pregnancy classification. An example of this would be the use of amitriptyline (an FDA pregnancy category D drug) to initially treat depression rather than newer agents such as venlafaxine (an FDA category C drug) given the lack of published human data about the use of venlafaxine in pregnancy.

■ QUESTION 4: HOW DOES THE PATIENT'S AND THE PROVIDER'S UNDERSTANDING AND BELIEF SYSTEM AFFECT DECISIONS ABOUT THE USE OF MEDICATION IN PREGNANCY?

Studies suggest that women believe that medications ingested in pregnancy end in significant malformations in a significant number of cases. Misinformation can come from media, friends, family, and even nurses, pharmacists, and physicians. Therefore, it is important for the provider to know what the patient's understanding of the potential toxicities are and work with her to clarify and address her concerns. The physician should determine how the patient understands her illness, what the patient's specific fears are, and what the patient can tolerate in terms of outcome. Often irrational fears can be allayed by exploring these questions. A woman at 20 weeks may want to avoid taking medication for fear that her baby will be born with a missing arm or leg, an outcome that the provider can reassure her could hardly be attributed to any drug taken that late in gestation. These same questions should also be asked of the providers. The provider's understanding of the patient's illness, his or her own sense of the patient's capability of tolerating the symptoms, and what outcomes he or she fears may significantly effect willingness to prescribe medication in pregnancy. Providers need to be cognizant of these issues to avoid being too paternalistic or having their own fears or prejudices guide decision making that should be

based on evidence and the patient's preference rather than the physician's anxieties. In the end, providers should work with our patients to make a judgment based on the available data, the indication of a particular agent and an awareness of the patient's belief system to determine whether the available information justifies or warrants the risk inherent in the use of all medication in pregnancy.

Once the best medication choice has been made in conjunction with the patient, the provider should consider pregnancy-related changes in pharmacokinetics that can affect drug dosing and response during pregnancy. A 30% to 50% increase in gastric emptying time during pregnancy may delay absorption of oral agents. An increase in gastric pH related to a 40% decrease in gastric acid secretion that occurs in pregnancy may also affect medication absorption. Renal clearance of medication is increased in pregnancy because glomerular filtration rates increase to 150% of nonpregnant values. Therefore, medications that are cleared renally, such as penicillin, digoxin, and lithium, may require shortened dosing intervals or significant dosage changes in pregnancy. Hepatic clearance of pharmacologic agents may be altered in pregnancy. Progesterone increases hepatic metabolism of some drugs such as phenytoin (Dilantin) but may also decrease metabolism of agents such as theophylline and caffeine through competitive inhibition of microsomal oxidases. The cholestatic effect of estrogen during pregnancy may affect clearance of drugs such as rifampin that are excreted in the biliary system.

The commonly used agent labetalol has an elimination half-life (t1/2) of 102 minutes in patients with pregnancy-induced hypertension as opposed to its t1/2 of 160 to 480 minutes in nonpregnant controls. The nifedipine elimination half-life is 1.35 hours in pregnancy versus 3.4 hours in controls.

Substantial changes in the volume of distribution also occur in pregnancy. Plasma volume increases to 150% of prepregnancy values by 24 to 28 weeks' gestation so that the volume of distribution for medication is increased and drugs may require dosage increases. At the same time the physiologic dilutional hypoalbuminemia that occurs in pregnancy combined with the displacement of bound drugs by the hormones of pregnancy may lead to an increase in free drug level for a particular serum level.

PRACTICE POINT

Physiologic changes in pregnancy that can affect medication pharmacokinetics

● Increased blood volume
● Increased glomerular filtration rate
● Dilutional hypoalbuminemia
● Slowing of gastric and intestinal motility

The main practical applications of the above physiologic and pharmacokinetic changes are as follows:

1. Serious consideration should be made to monitoring of medication levels and adjustment of medication dose during pregnancy.
2. Free drug levels in general are better guides than total serum levels in pregnancy because of altered protein binding.
3. Dosing intervals may need to be shortened in pregnancy.
4. Inadequate dosing frequency always needs to be considered as a possible cause for failure of medications during pregnancy.

The last and perhaps most important issue to be aware of when prescribing in pregnancy is that medication compliance is a significant challenge. Drug labeling warnings, pharmacists, and an unrealistically high perception of teratogenic risks all contribute to this phenomenon. One small study from Wales found that 15% of women with epilepsy who claimed to be taking antiepileptic drugs in pregnancy showed no evidence of having done so on testing of their hair. One of the patients with an absent drug level died suddenly at 30 weeks' gestation. Providers need to work with their patients to increase understanding about the important interdependence of maternal and fetal health and the justifiable and "healthful" use of indicated medications during pregnancy.

CONCLUSION

All providers prescribing medication to women of reproductive age should speak to these patients about the potential effects of their medications during pregnancy and the potential for harm even before the pregnancy is clinically apparent. The acute hospitalization presents an opportunity to evaluate all medications, adjust dosages, and educate patients and families about their indication and safety profile.

SUGGESTED READINGS

Brent RL. How does a physician avoid prescribing drugs and medical procedures that have reproductive and developmental risks? *Clin Perinatol.* 2007;34(2):233-262.

Briggs GS, Freeman R, Yaffe S. *Medication in Pregnancy and Lactation*, 8th ed. Philadelphia, PA: Lippincott Williams & Wilkins; 2008.

Buhimschi CS, Weiner CP. Medications in pregnancy and lactation: part 1. Teratology. *Obstet Gynecol.* 2009;113(1):166-188.

Buhimschi CS, Weiner CP. Medications in pregnancy and lactation: part 2. Drugs with minimal or unknown human teratogenic effect. *Obstet Gynecol.* 2009;2(1):417-432.

Cooper WO, Hernandez-Diaz S, Arbogast PG, et al. Major congenital malformations after first-trimester exposure to ACE inhibitors. *N Engl J Med.* 2006;354(23):2443-2451.

Einarson A, Ho E, Koren G. Can we use metronidazole during pregnancy and breastfeeding? Putting an end to the controversy. *Can Fam Physician.* 2000;46:1053-1054.

Friedman JM, Polifka JE. *Teratogenic Effects of Drugs: A Resource for Clinicians (TERIS)*, 2nd ed. Baltimore, MD: Johns Hopkins University Press; 2000.

Koren G. *Medication Safety in Pregnancy and Breastfeeding.* New York, NY: McGraw-Hill Professional; 2007.

Koren G, Levichek Z. The teratogenicity of drugs for nausea and vomiting of pregnancy: perceived versus true risk. *Am J Obstet Gynecol.* 2002;186(5, part 2):S248-S252.

Kyle PM. Drugs and the fetus. *Curr Opin Obstet Gynecol.* 2006;18(2):93-99.

Pavek P, Ceckova M, Staud F. Variation of drug kinetics in pregnancy. *Curr Drug Metab.* 2009;10(5):520-529.

Prevost RR, Akl SA, Whybrew WD, Sibai BM. Oral nifedipine pharmacokinetics in pregnancy-induced hypertension. *Pharmacotherapy.* 1992;12(3):174-177.

Rayburn WF, Amanze AC. Prescribing medications safely during pregnancy. *Med Clin North Am.* 2008;92(5):1227-1237, xii.

Rogers RC, Sibai BM, Whybrew WD. Labetalol pharmacokinetics in pregnancy-induced hypertension. *Am J Obstet Gynecol.* 1990;162(2):362-366.

Rosene-Montella K, ed. Medical Management of the Pregnant Patient. *A Clinician's Handbook.* New York, NY: Springer Science+Business Media; 2015.

Rosene-Montella K, Keely E, Barbour LA, Lee RV. *Medical Care of the Pregnant Patient*, 2nd ed. Philadelphia, PA: American College of Physicians-American Society of Internal Medicine; 2008.

Rubin PC, Ramsey M. *Prescribing in Pregnancy*, 4th ed. London, U.K.: BMJ Books; 2008.

Schaefer C, Peters P, Miller RK. *Drugs During Pregnancy and Lactation*, 2nd ed. London, U.K.: Academic Press; 2007.

Shehata HA, Nelson-Piercy C. Drugs in pregnancy. Drugs to avoid. *Best Pract Res Clin Obstet Gynaecol.* 2001;15(6):971-986.

Webster WS, Freeman JA. Prescription drugs and pregnancy. *Expert Opin Pharmacother.* 2003;4(6):949-961.

Weiner CP, Buhimschi CS. *Drugs for Pregnant and Lactating Women.* Philadelphia, PA: Churchill Livingstone; 2004.

CHAPTER 220

Critical Care of the Pregnant Patient

Meghan Hayes, MD
Ghada Bourjeily, MD

Key Clinical Questions

1. What are physiologic changes of pregnancy pertinent to critical care?
2. What are common reasons for pregnant women to require critical care?
3. What factors impact airway intubation during pregnancy?
4. What issues arise in hemodynamic monitoring during pregnancy?
5. What vasopressors can and should be used during pregnancy?
6. Are there special considerations for resuscitation during pregnancy?

INTRODUCTION

The majority of critical care admissions for pregnant and peripartum women are for obstetric disorders, primarily hypertensive complications (particularly hemorrhagic stroke) or hemorrhage. Medical indications, such as sepsis, respiratory failure, cardiomyopathy, or ischemic stroke are less common. Maternal mortality in developed nations remains rare (650 in the United States annually); however, the proportion attributable to medical disorders has been increasing as women with underlying medical conditions and older women conceive, perhaps with assisted reproductive technology. Standard scoring systems, such as APACHE scores, overestimate mortality in pregnant and peripartum women, particularly if they have an obstetric indication for critical care. Delivery or surgery may contribute to rapid improvement. A small proportion of obstetric patients, approximately 12 per 1000, require critical care. Hospitalists and intensivists may have limited experience managing these patients.

■ PHYSIOLOGIC ADAPTATIONS

Virtually every organ system adapts to accommodate pregnancy and delivery. Hemodynamic alterations prepare for blood loss of one-half to 1 L at delivery. Blood volume increases by 50% (**Table 220-1**).

Cardiac output increases by 30% to 50% and total peripheral resistance decreases by 20%, leading to blood pressure declining by 10 to 15 mm Hg in the first half of pregnancy, then returning to baseline in the second half. Diastolic blood pressure decreases more than systolic; pulse pressure is widened. Central venous pressure (CVP) and pulmonary capillary wedge pressure (PCWP) remain unchanged. Blood flow distribution is altered such that up to 25% of maternal cardiac output is directed to the uterus, 20% to kidneys, with an increase in breast flow. When supine, women in the second half of pregnancy experience aortocaval compression (termed supine hypotensive syndrome), in which cardiac output may drop by 30%. Left lateral decubitus positioning relieves aortocaval compression and improves venous return and cardiac output.

Maternal respiratory adaptations help optimize fetal oxygenation. Initial changes are progesterone mediated with diaphragmatic elevation contributing to changes later in pregnancy. Minute ventilation increases 30% to 60% by increased tidal volume; respiratory rate remains unchanged. Tachypnea is abnormal and warrants investigation! Diaphragmatic elevation leads to a 20% reduction in functional residual capacity by late pregnancy. Given that diaphragmatic excursion is usually unchanged in pregnancy, this drop in functional residual capacity is counterbalanced by an increase in inspiratory capacity and the resultant effect is no significant change in total lung capacity. On the other hand, oxygen consumption is significantly increased during pregnancy and rises further during labor and delivery. For those reasons, oxygen reserve is reduced in pregnancy. Arterial blood gas testing reveals a compensated respiratory alkalosis due to the above described changes and enhanced renal bicarbonate excretion. PaO_2 is typically 100 to 105 mm Hg during pregnancy and $PaCO_2$ decreases to 28 to 32 mm Hg. Maternal pulse oximetry greater than 95% is desirable in order to maintain a PaO_2 greater than 70 mm Hg and optimize placental oxygen diffusion.

Hematologic changes also occur in pregnancy with a progressive activation of the hemostatic system to prepare the parturient for the hemostatic challenge of delivery. The anticoagulant

TABLE 220-1 Cardiac, Respiratory and Hematologic Physiologic Changes in Pregnancy

	Direction of Change	Percentage of Change or Normal Range in Pregnancy
Blood volume	↑	30%-40% increase
Heart rate	↑	Increases by 10-20 bpm
Cardiac output	↑	30%-60% increase
Systemic vascular resistance	↓	25%-30% decrease
Blood pressure	↓	10-15 mm Hg decrease in first two trimesters
Colloid oncotic pressure	↓	10%-15% decrease
Total lung capacity	↓	4%-5% decrease
Functional residual capacity	↓	20% decrease
Diffusion capacity	↔	No change
Tidal volume	↑	Increased
Respiratory rate	↔	No change
Minute ventilation	↑	50% increase
PaO_2	↑	Average 100-105
$PcaCo_2$	↓	Average 28-32
pH	↑	Mild respiratory alkalosis
A-a gradient	↑	Increase in late gestation to approximately 20
Protein S	↓	
Activated protein C resistance, fibrinogen, factor V, VIII, IX, X	↑	
Plasminogen activator inhibitor type 1 and 2	↑	
Activity of tissue plasminogen	↓	

Modified from Miller MA, Bourjeily G. Management of the critically ill pregnant patient. Pulmonary and Critical Care Update (PCCU). April 2009, 23 (Lesson 8); with permission.

activity of protein S is reduced and activated protein C resistance rises. Procoagulant activity is increased, with higher concentrations of fibrinogen and factors V, VIII, IX, and X, leading to enhanced thrombin production. On the other hand, fibrinolysis is decreased as a result of increased activity of plasminogen activator inhibitor type 1 and type 2 and decreased activity of tissue plasminogen. Shortcomings of these changes are an increase in the risk of venous thromboembolism (VTE) antepartum until 6 weeks, postpartum.

■ INDICATIONS FOR CRITICAL CARE DURING PREGNANCY/PERIPARTUM

Obstetric indications include preeclampsia and related complications: eclampsia, HELLP (hemolysis, elevated liver enzymes, low platelets), hypertensive crisis, pulmonary edema, oliguric renal failure, and cerebral hemorrhage. All of these complications would meet criteria for severe preeclampsia and would warrant urgent delivery. Specific indications for when a patient needs to be transferred to an intensive care unit have been described in a practice bulletin published by the American College of Obstetricians and

Gynecologists. Close collaboration with obstetrics is essential for optimal maternal (and fetal/neonatal) outcome. Although often maternal manifestations of preeclampsia are quickly reversible with delivery and judicious fluid and blood pressure management, they may persist or even worsen in the postpartum period, requiring ongoing vigilance. While still pregnant, blood pressure goals must minimize maternal hypertensive complications, which are more likely above 160 mm Hg systolic and 110 mm Hg diastolic, while maintaining sufficient uteroplacental flow. Blood pressure reduction should be attempted promptly with caution in pregnant women given the potential for impaired uteroplacental flow and fetal compromise. Options include intravenous labetalol or hydralazine, noting that hydralazine has been associated with greater hypotension in this setting. Short-acting oral nifedipine may be useful if intravenous access is delayed but may also precipitously lower the blood pressure. Magnesium sulfate infusion is superior to phenytoin and benzodiazepines for preventing seizures in preeclampsia and reducing recurrence of eclamptic seizures. Given that most seizures are self-limited, there are limited studies comparing different drugs; however, benzodiazepines may be helpful for acute seizure treatment, noting risk of neonatal respiratory depression.

Additional obstetric conditions warranting critical care include acute fatty liver of pregnancy, peripartum cardiomyopathy, amniotic fluid embolism, and placental abruption and hemorrhage. Acute fatty liver of pregnancy (AFLP) is rare, estimated to occur in 1 in 13,000 deliveries, but carries a high mortality. Manifestations may include fulminant hepatic failure with hypoglycemia, coagulopathy, and renal failure; about half of cases are associated with preeclampsia. It may initially be difficult to differentiate AFLP from HELLP syndrome (defined as transaminases greater than twice the upper limit of normal and platelet count <100,000 per mm^3), but AFLP should be suspected in patients with otherwise unexplained hypoglycemia and severe hepatic dysfunction. Liver transplantation may be necessary. Recurrence rates are significant in subsequent pregnancies.

Peripartum cardiomyopathy is defined as dilated cardiomyopathy with no other known cause, with onset in the last month of pregnancy or within 5 months postpartum. Rates vary markedly across the world, with highest rates reported in Africa. The etiology has not fully been defined. Risk factors include advanced maternal age, multiple gestations, preeclampsia, and African descent. Treatment includes standard congestive heart failure management, including vasodilators, diuretics, and sodium restriction. Prior to delivery, hydralazine and nitrates should be used rather than angiotensin converting enzyme inhibitors, which have adverse fetal renal effects at all stages of gestation. After delivery, enalapril and captopril are considered compatible with breastfeeding. Anticoagulation should be initiated if ejection fraction is less than 35%, mural thrombus is present on imaging, or atrial fibrillation is observed, as thrombosis is a major cause of mortality in these patients. Up to half of women recover ventricular function to baseline levels within 6 months, with variable persistent dysfunction ranging from mild to fatal in the other half. Recurrence rates are high, and women warrant careful counseling and surveillance regarding future pregnancies.

Amniotic fluid embolism (AFE) remains exceptionally rare, described as occurring in between 1 to 8000 and 1 to 80,000 deliveries, with high maternal morbidity and mortality. Reported risk factors include prolonged labor, multiparity, increased maternal age, and oxytocin administration. The pathophysiology remains in question. Some propose terming AFE "the anaphylactoid syndrome of pregnancy," with maternal response to miniscule amounts of amniotic fluid's vasoactive and procoagulant factors. This theory remains debatable as amniotic fluid has been found in the maternal circulation in patients without signs or symptoms of AFE. Sudden decline in maternal and/or fetal status intrapartum or maternal status postpartum is the most common presentation, with hypotension, respiratory symptoms, coagulopathy, and cardiac arrest occurring in the majority. Early recognition of the syndrome and initiation of supportive measures, including aggressive blood products, are essential. If onset is antepartum, rapid delivery improves perinatal and maternal outcome. Novel interventions such as the use of recombinant factor VII administration, cardiopulmonary bypass, ventricular assist devices, and ECMO have been reported.

Medical conditions requiring critical care for pregnant and peripartum women include sepsis, pneumonia, acute respiratory distress syndrome (ARDS), venous thromboembolism, status asthmaticus/asthma exacerbations, sepsis, pneumonia, and myocardial infarction. Pyelonephritis is of particular concern during pregnancy, with maternal complications including ARDS and sepsis due to reduced buffering capacity and decreased oncotic pressure. Pregnant women with pyelonephritis warrant inpatient management given potential maternal complications plus risk of preterm labor and premature delivery. Careful fluid administration and ongoing monitoring are essential for these women to ensure they are adequately fluid resuscitated but do not progress to fluid overload. Extensive discussion of medical conditions is outside the scope of this chapter and is reviewed in more detail in the chapter on medical disorders in pregnancy.

Trauma also leads to critical care admissions for pregnant and peripartum women, with the majority of cases due to motor vehicle accidents (MVAs). Falls, particularly in the third trimester, and domestic violence are the next leading causes in this population. Improper seat belt positioning contributes to maternal and fetal injury in MVAs; the lap belt should be placed below the gravid uterus and shoulder belt between the breasts. Obstetric complications of traumatic injuries include placental abruption, uterine rupture, and preterm delivery. The gravid uterus upwardly displaces abdominal organs so that bowel may be involved in upper abdominal trauma. Fetal instability often precedes maternal instability. Uteroplacental flow will be compromised to maintain maternal blood pressure. Multidisciplinary care for pregnant trauma patients that includes fetal monitoring will lead to optimal outcome for both mother and fetus.

■ AIRWAY

In addition to the usual causes of respiratory failure in the nonpregnant population, there are a number of pregnancy-specific conditions that might lead to acute respiratory failure. These causes include preeclampsia, amniotic fluid embolism, peripartum cardiomyopathy, and hemodynamic instability related to massive obstetric hemorrhage. Ovarian hyperstimulation related to hormonal manipulation surrounding assisted reproduction may also be associated with ARDS. Although indications are quite similar, the threshold for intubation might be different in the pregnant population since $PaCO_2$ is normally decreased and PaO_2 increased in pregnancy and a $PaCO_2$ of 38 and a PaO_2 of 70 are indications of acute respiratory failure. Arterial oxygen saturation ≥95% is desirable for fetal and maternal well being.

Noninvasive ventilation (NIV)

Case series are accumulating regarding use of NIV for acute respiratory failure in the obstetric population. Successful use of NIV has been described in pregnancy in chronic, stable settings such as in obstructive sleep apnea or chronic respiratory failure from neuromuscular disease. The use of NIV may be suboptimal in acute settings given airway edema and the increased risk of aspiration

in pregnancy. However, in patients with a preserved mental status and no other contraindications who may not require assisted ventilation for prolonged periods of time, short trials of NIV may be attempted prior to endotracheal intubation.

Endotracheal intubation

Anesthesia-related mortality ranks seventh in maternal mortality in the United States. This is in part due to the fact that failure rate for endotracheal intubations in pregnant patients is 1 in 250 compared to 1 in 2330 in the general surgical population. Failure to intubate may be associated with a higher risk for cardiac arrest and aspiration.

A number of factors complicate endotracheal intubation in pregnancy. Reduced airway patency is one of the factors. Higher blood volume and estrogen levels in pregnancy cause capillary engorgement and mucosal edema leading to difficult visualization of the landmarks of the upper airway. Mallampati scores, a measure of upper airway patency, increase progressively in pregnancy and upper airway size as measured by acoustic reflectance method is reduced in the supine position. Airway edema may be further exaggerated in patients with a prolonged second stage of labor, excessive intravenous fluids, and preeclampsia. Preeclampsia is associated with lower oncotic pressures with possible coagulopathy worsening airway edema. Weight gain and the increase in breast size can lead to difficulty in manipulating the upper airway and reduced chest compliance. Obesity is also one of the major risk factors for maternal mortality in a review of anesthesia-related maternal mortality.

Pregnant women are also at a higher risk for aspiration related to a progesterone mediated relaxation of the lower esophageal sphincter, an increase in intra-abdominal pressure (due to the enlarging uterus), and delayed gastric emptying. The use of aspiration precautions is advisable.

An important consideration during sedation and paralysis of a pregnant woman is the reduced oxygen reserve given the 20% reduction in functional residual capacity (which is likely more pronounced in the supine position) and the increase in oxygen consumption. Sedation and paralysis eliminate the rise in minute ventilation that usually occurs to compensate for these changes/demands and rapid desaturation and hypoventilation occur.

Therefore, preoxygenation with 100% oxygen should be done before and between intubation attempts during pregnancy and lower doses of sedatives may be needed. This should be done with caution as prolonged manual ventilation may distend the stomach increasing the risk of aspiration even further. Manual left uterine displacement also helps improve venous return in patients with a tenuous hemodynamic status, since cardiac output may be reduced by 25% to 30% in the supine position in the late stages of pregnancy.

An additional complicating factor is the urgent nature of airway intubation in the obstetric population.

Because of the increased risk of morbidity and mortality associated with airway intubation in pregnancy, airway intubation should be performed by providers with the most extensive experience. Airway assessment according to the American Society of Anesthesiology practice guidelines is critical in pregnancy, even in cases of urgent intubation. The management of the difficult airway should follow the American Society of Anesthesiology practice guidelines. In this algorithm, the laryngeal mask airway (LMA) is recognized as the tool of choice for "cannot ventilate, cannot intubate" (CVCI) patients. Video laryngoscopy has been successful in failed direct laryngoscopy in obstetric patients.

A chest radiograph to ensure proper placement of the endotracheal tube carries only a negligible risk of fetal radiation exposure and should be done as in the nonpregnant patient.

■ HEMODYNAMIC MONITORING

Profound hemodynamic changes occur in pregnancy to prepare for the needs of the growing feto-maternal unit and to compensate for the expected losses during pregnancy. These changes are summarized in Table 220-1. Indications for hemodynamic monitoring specific for obstetric patients include severe preeclampsia with either refractory hypertension, oliguric renal failure, or unclear intravascular volume status. Hemodynamic monitoring may also be needed in obstetric patients with severe structural heart disease in the peripartum period, or cardiovascular collapse such as in the setting of an acute amniotic fluid embolism.

Monitoring may be done either invasively or noninvasively. Echocardiography has been shown to correlate with invasive monitoring in the measurement of cardiac output, ventricular filling pressures, stroke volume, and pulmonary artery pressures.

Echocardiography interpretation should be performed with caution in pregnancy given that physiologic chamber dilatation and the increase in flow may overestimate pulmonary artery pressures. Patients with refractory hypertension and oliguria were successfully managed in a small series with echocardiography suggesting that this test may be an effective alternative to pulmonary artery catheterization during pregnancy in specific circumstances.

Invasive monitoring may be needed in cases of severe stenotic valvular disease, severe cardiomyopathy, sudden cardiovascular collapse, ARDS/indeterminate fluid status, refractory oliguria, and unclear volume status despite fluid resuscitation and refractory septic shock. Invasive monitoring may occasionally be indicated for labor and delivery in high-risk patients. Invasive monitoring has somewhat fallen out of favor with recent trials not showing any clear benefit compared to central venous catheters. There are no randomized controlled trials evaluating the clinical usefulness of pulmonary artery catheters in pregnancy in general. Available data suggest that although there is a modest correlation between central venous pressures (measured with a central venous catheter) and a pulmonary capillary wedge pressure in the management of patients with untreated preeclampsia, this correlation may lessen after initial interventions.

■ VASOPRESSORS

Acute hypotension requiring vasopressor support in the pregnant woman most commonly results from vasodilatation in the setting of neuraxial anesthesia. Additional vasodilatation on top of the physiologic vasodilatation of pregnancy is poorly tolerated. Hemodynamic compromise may also be precipitated by hypovolemia, sepsis, anaphylaxis, and cardiogenic shock. A pregnant woman has an additional end organ, the fetus, with uteroplacental flow receiving 20% to 30% of maternal cardiac output. Maternal hypotension risks fetal and neonatal acidosis. It is critical to restore intravascular volume first, as uteroplacental flow is compromised further by vasoconstriction in addition to hypovolemia.

Limited data are available comparing vasopressors during pregnancy, so physician familiarity and drug availability have roles in vasopressor choice. All vasopressors have potential to impair uteroplacental flow. There is minimal information regarding developmental toxicity. Currently, phenylephrine and ephedrine are the most commonly used vasopressors in this population. Phenylephrine is a short-acting alpha agonist with potent vasoconstricting effect that may be easily titrated. It does not act on beta receptors thus does not lead to maternal tachycardia; however, reflex bradycardia due to increased venous return may occur, requiring atropine administration. Ephedrine has been used extensively by obstetric anesthesiologists. It is a direct alpha and beta agonist and also indirectly releases norepinephrine. Maternal cardiac output increases by increased heart rate and contractility. Alpha effect causes peripheral vasoconstriction and increased blood pressure. Titration is difficult due to its slow onset and tachyphylaxis develops after repeated doses.

Reports comparing ephedrine to phenylephrine infusion at cesarean delivery show that ephedrine is associated with more maternal nausea and vomiting, higher heart rate, and a higher incidence of fetal acidosis but comparable effects on blood pressure. A meta-analysis comparing the two drugs reported similar findings including a higher fetal pH associated with phenylephrine. In summary, if hypotension persists after an adequate intravascular volume has been restored, phenylephrine is the drug of choice in pregnant patients with circulatory collapse, unless a clear benefit in restoring hemodynamics is expected from another drug.

■ CARDIAC ARREST AND RESUSCITATION

The incidence of cardiac arrest in pregnancy has been estimated at 1 in 30,000, causing about 10% of maternal deaths. It remains a rare and potentially catastrophic event for mother and fetus. Outcomes for both depend on the underlying cause of arrest and rapidity of resuscitation. The mnemonic BEAU-CHOPS allows rapid assessment of potential causes for arrest in the parturient: Bleeding/disseminated intravascular coagulation (DIC), embolism: coronary/ pulmonary/amniotic fluid, anesthetic complications, uterine atony, cardiac disease (myocardial infarction (MI)/ischemia, aortic dissection, cardiomyopathy), hypertension (preeclampsia/eclampsia), other (differential diagnosis per standard ACLS guidelines), placenta: abruptio/ previa, sepsis.

Prompt initiation of cardiopulmonary resuscitation protocols is essential, with attention to a few additional details. Maternal and neonatal resuscitation teams must be activated urgently. Pregnant women are at increased risk of aspiration during resuscitation and desaturate rapidly, therefore immediate intubation with 100% oxygen administration and cricoid pressure is advised in this population. Manual left uterine displacement relieves aortocaval pressure. Hand position for compressions is advised a few centimeters higher on the sternum due to breast engorgement and diaphragmatic elevation but no studies are available to demonstrate that higher compressions result in better cardiac output. Defibrillation energy and locations are unchanged. Any fetal monitoring devices must be removed prior to defibrillation to avoid the possibility of arcing.

Drug administration generally proceeds as usual, with note of potential issues with amiodarone and vasopressin. Alternatives to amiodarone, such as lidocaine and procainamide, would be preferable given concern for its fetal thyroid impact; however, if resuscitation team members are most familiar with amiodarone and it is most quickly available, antiarrhythmic administration should not be delayed as the risk of untreated ventricular arrythmias by far outweighs the risk of fetal thyroid dysfunction. The placenta produces vasopressinase, which could degrade vasopressin, thus epinephrine is preferable.

If the fetus is viable (24 weeks or greater), it is strongly recommended to perform cesarean delivery by 5 minutes into resuscitation to improve maternal and fetal outcomes. In 1986, Katz, et al, recommended perimortem cesarean delivery and in 2005 published data revealing intact neurologic outcome in neonates delivered within 5 minutes of arrest. Maternal chest compressions should continue throughout delivery efforts. Immediately after uterine evacuation, maternal cardiac output increases due to autotransfusion from uterine circulation and relief of aortocaval compression; chest compressions are more effective after delivery as well. Data are lacking regarding therapeutic hypothermia for maternal benefit. Regular maternal cardiac arrest drills are recommended to ensure all pertinent disciplines are prepared for this uncommon event.

CONCLUSION

As women with underlying medical conditions and older women conceive, the proportion of critically ill, pregnant women with medical disorders may increase. This chapter briefly reviews common obstetric disorders that may require critical care and aspects of resuscitation that are unique to pregnancy.

SUGGESTED READINGS

ACOG Practice Bulletin No. 100: Critical care in pregnancy. *Obstet Gynecol.* 2009;113(2 Pt 1):443-450.

Baskett TF, O'Connell CM. Maternal critical care in obstetrics. *J Obstet Gynaecol Can.* 2009;31(3):218-221.

Bourjeily G, Miller M. Obstetric disorders in the ICU. *Clin Chest Med.* 2009;30(1):89-102, viii.

Gaffney A. Critical care in pregnancy-is it different? *Semi Perinatol.* 2014;38(6):329-340.

Gist RS, Stafford IP, Leibowitz AB, Beilin Y. Amniotic fluid embolism. *Anesth Analg.* 2009;108(5):1599-1602.

Katz V, Balderston K, DeFreest M. Perimortem cesarean delivery: were our assumptions correct? *Am J Obstet Gynecol.* 2005;192:1916-1920.

Katz VL, Dottes DJ, Droegemuller W. Perimortem cesarean delivery. *Obstet Gynecol.* 1986;68:571-576.

Lipman S, Cohen S, Einav S. The Society For Obstetric Anesthesia and Perinatology consensus statement on the management of cardiac arrest in pregnancy. *Anesth Analg.* 2014;118(5):1003-1016.

Miller MA, Bourjeily, G. Management of the critically ill pregnant patient. Pulmonary and Critical Care Update (PCCU). April 2009; 23 (Lesson 8) www.chestnet.org/education/online/pccu/vol23/lessons07_08/index.php.

Neligan PJ, Laffey JG. Clinical review: Special populations- critical illness and pregnancy. *Crit Care.* 2011;15(4):227.

Reidy J, Douglas J. Vasopressors in obstetrics. *Anesthesiol Clin.* 2008;26(1):75-88, vi-vii.

Saving Mothers' Lives: Reviewing maternal deaths to make motherhood safer: 2006–2008. *BJOG.* 2011;118:1-203.

Stevens TA, Carroll MA, Promcene PA, Seibel M, Monga M. Utility of Acute Physiology, Age, and Chronic Health Evaluation (APACHE III) score in maternal admissions to the intensive care unit. *Am J Obstet Gynecol.* 2006;194:e13-e15.

Vasquez DN, Estenssoro E, Canales HS, et al. Clinical characteristics and outcomes of obstetric patients requiring ICU admission. *Chest.* 2007;131(3):718-724.

Zeemany GG. Obstetric critical care: a blueprint for improved outcomes. *Crit Care Med.* 2006;34(9 Suppl):S208-S214.

CHAPTER 221

Common Medical Problems in Pregnancy

Niharika D. Mehta, MD

Kenneth K. Chen, MD, FRACP

Carmen Monzon, MD

Karen Rosene-Montella, MD, FACP

Key Clinical Questions

1 How do common diseases and their treatment impact on pregnancy?

2 How might pregnancy impact on common illness?

INTRODUCTION

Although women of childbearing age represent a younger and generally healthy population, currently 40% of women entering pregnancy have chronic medical conditions such as obesity and type 2 diabetes mellitus. Modern medical technology has facilitated pregnancy in older and sicker women. Diseases and their treatment may impact pregnancy and pregnancy may affect certain diseases.

CARDIAC DISEASES

During pregnancy, blood volume and cardiac output rise, and systemic vascular resistance decreases. Later in pregnancy the gravid uterus may compress the inferior vena cava (IVC), thereby significantly decreasing preload in the supine position. Cardiac output increases 40% by mid-pregnancy until labor and delivery when it increases further. Increased blood volume and left atrial dimensions may contribute to the increase in palpitations and supraventricular tachycardia. If the heart is damaged either by congenital heart disease or by cardiomyopathy, the increase in cardiac work cannot occur as effectively. In addition, just after delivery, with a uterine contraction a liter of blood can be shunted from the uterus into the general circulation. Cardiac lesions associated with a fixed cardiac output will not tolerate this sudden increase in volume. Hence, the most common complications in late pregnancy or immediately after delivery include pulmonary edema and, less commonly, right heart failure. In addition, the risk of a fetus developing congenital heart disease is increased if the mother has the same problem (eg, 1:4 in tetralogy of Fallot and 1:15 in atrial septal defects). Patients with severe pulmonary hypertension and/or Eisenmenger syndrome characterized by a reversed right-to-left shunt have increased mortality rates, especially during the first 48 to 72 hours postpartum.

Systemic vascular resistance decreases about 25%, which may improve any cardiac condition that benefits from after-load reduction such as aortic insufficiency. When compression of the inferior vena cava decreases venous return to the heart, patients with preload-dependent cardiac conditions such as aortic stenosis or poor left ventricular function may experience hypotension, especially when supine. Because the increased cardiac demands peak at 24 to 28 weeks of gestation, cardiac decompensation may become evident at the end of the second trimester.

Labor and delivery may be associated with cardiac decompensation when one to two units of blood leave the uteroplacental circulation during contraction. When the contraction ceases, the blood returns to the uteroplacental circulation.

Patients with peripartum cardiomyopathy that occurs in the third trimester and up to 6 months following delivery have symptoms and signs consistent with congestive heart failure. Approximately, one-third of these patients will completely recover, one-third will have chronic congestive heart failure, and one-third may have a progressive cardiomyopathy that may require cardiac transplantation in severe cases.

Postpartum fluid shifts occur during involution of the uterus and the low-resistance circulation of the placenta, postpartum blood loss, and increase in preload when the uterus no longer compresses the inferior vena cava.

Acute myocardial infarction is a rare complication during pregnancy. Coronary dissection with normal coronary arteries on angiography is more common in the peripartum or postpartum period.

Patients with longstanding diabetes may develop myocardial ischemia during pregnancy. Antiphospholipid antibody-associated arterial thrombosis and arterial vasospasm and cocaine ingestion may also result in myocardial infarction.

Women with artificial heart valves who receive anticoagulant treatment will need to continue to do so during pregnancy. Decision about type of anticoagulation requires a risk-benefit discussion, monitoring to achieve consistently therapeutic levels of anticoagulation, and should not include warfarin during the first trimester or toward term. Ideally these patients should receive care and obstetric at a tertiary medical center that can provide combined cardiac and obstetric antenatal care.

INFECTIOUS DISEASES

■ THE FEBRILE PREGNANT FEMALE

Pregnancy may alter the course of some infections while certain infections are more likely to occur in a pregnant woman. Clinicians need to consider maternal-fetal transmission and the impact of antimicrobial therapy upon the fetus.

A primary systemic infection with toxoplasmosis, rubella, cytomegalovirus, herpes simplex virus, syphilis, and parvovirus (TORCH infections) can be associated with congenital malformations and disease. Primary infection with coccidiomycoses, which is especially common in the southwestern United States, can be complicated by fungal meningitis in a pregnant woman, which would otherwise be a rare complication in a normal host.

Fever, uterine tenderness, and contractions may suggest chorioamnionitis or infection of the amniotic sac and fluid. The diagnosis is made by consultation with an obstetrician and consideration of amniocentesis (positive Gram stain, amniotic fluid glucose usually <15 mg/dL). Treatment may require delivery.

Infection of the endometrium, an ascending polymicrobial infection, occurs in the postpartum period. Risk factors include prolonged rupture of membranes, delivery requiring instrumentation, and cesarean section, especially unplanned or emergent. Obstetricians can advise on the best antibiotic regimen depending on early postpartum endometritis (within the first 48 hours) and later endometritis (more than 1-week postpartum). Septic pelvic thrombophlebitis may be considered when a patient has persistent fevers despite an appropriately treated postpartum endometritis. Consider alternative diagnoses such as abscess, hematomas, and necrotizing fasciitis in a postpartum febrile patient, if computed tomography (CT) or magnetic resonance venography (MRV) of the pelvis rules out pelvic thrombosis.

■ PYELONEPHRITIS

Acute pyelonephritis complicates 1% to 2% of all pregnancies and can be associated with significant maternal and fetal morbidity, including the development of acute respiratory distress syndrome (ARDS) in up to 10% of patients. It is more common in patients with pyelonephritis and preterm labor who are being treated with beta-agonist tocolysis. Acute pyelonephritis during pregnancy is also associated with preterm delivery, with reported incidence between 6% and 50%, depending upon gestational age at presentation. Asymptomatic bacteriuria in a pregnant patient should always be treated because it is associated with a 25% incidence of pyelonephritis.

Pyelonephritis is most common during the second half of the pregnancy as a result of increased ureteral obstruction and urinary stasis, which result from both mechanical and hormonal factors. Usually unilateral, it affects the right kidney more frequently, because of uterine dextrorotation. Prior history of pyelonephritis, urinary tract malformations, and calculi put patients at a higher risk for development of an acute episode of pyelonephritis.

■ DIAGNOSIS

Pyelonephritis most commonly presents with systemic signs and symptoms including flank pain, fever, costovertebral angle tenderness, shaking chills, nausea, vomiting, and less often with features of cystitis, such as dysuria and frequency. Laboratory findings generally include a positive urine culture and pyuria on urinalysis. Additional laboratory studies should include a complete blood cell count and serum chemistry evaluation. Transient renal insufficiency with as much as 50% decrease in creatinine clearance is observed in about a quarter of all patients. Although blood cultures are often obtained in these patients, their utility is limited. Pathogens isolated from blood cultures rarely differ from those found in the corresponding urine culture. Blood cultures are recommended in cases that are complicated by sepsis, temperature of at least 39°C, or respiratory distress syndrome. Ovarian vein thrombosis may present as fever and flank pain and should be considered in patients suspected of having pyelonephritis who have normal urinalysis.

■ MANAGEMENT

Early aggressive treatment of pyelonephritis is important in preventing complications. The current standard of care includes hospitalization and parenteral antibiotics. Several equally efficacious antibiotic regimens are summarized in **Table 221-1**. Most patients respond within 72 hours. Therapy with the best oral agent, according to culture and sensitivity testing, should be continued to complete a 2-week course. Most experts recommend that suppressive therapy should be continued until delivery for all pregnant patients with a single episode of pyelonephritis. Prophylactic regimens include nitrofurantoin 100 mg once daily or cephalexin 250 mg once daily taken by mouth.

■ LISTERIOSIS

The incidence of listeriosis in pregnancy is 12 per 100,000, compared with a rate of 0.7 per 100,000 in the general population. In contrast to maternal illness, fetal and neonatal infection is severe and frequently fatal, with a case fatality rate of 20% to 30%. Neonatal listerial infection can cause pneumonia, sepsis, or meningitis. A characteristic severe in utero infection, granulomatosisi infantiseptica, may result from transplacental transmission, characterized by widespread abscesses and/or granulomas in multiple internal organs. Most infants with this condition are either stillborn or die soon after birth.

Diagnosis

Although severe maternal illness from listeriosis has been reported, it is rare. In most cases, maternal illness is mild and sometimes even asymptomatic. Fever, chills, back pain, and flu-like symptoms

---

TABLE 221-1 Suggested Antimicrobial Regimens for the Treatment of Pyelonephritis in Pregnancy

Ampicillin (+) Gentamicin 2 g IV every 6 h

Gentamicin 2 mg/kg load, then 1.7 mg/kg in 3 divided doses (once daily dosing is also acceptable)

Ampicillin-sublactam 3 g IV every 6 h

Ceftriaxone 1 g IV/IM every 24 h

Cefuroxime 0.75-1.5 g IV every 8 h

Cefazolin 1-2 g IV every 6-8 h

Mezlocillin 3 g IV every 6 h

Piperacillin 4 g IV every 8 h

IM, intramuscularly; IV, intravenously.

are most commonly reported. Illness can resolve spontaneously and the diagnosis be missed if cultures are not obtained. Patients with comorbidities, such as a history of splenectomy, human immunodeficiency virus (HIV) infection, steroid use, diabetes, or use of immunosuppressive medications, are at increased risk for severe maternal illness, which includes meningitis and meningoenchepalitis.

Diagnosis of listerial infection can only be made by culturing the organism from a sterile site such as blood, amniotic fluid, or spinal fluid. Vaginal or stool cultures are not helpful in diagnosis because some women are carriers but do not have clinical disease. Gram stain is useful in only about 33% of cases, both because *Listeria* is an intracellular organism and can be entirely missed, and because the organism can resemble pneumococci (diplococci), diphtheroids (*Corynebacteria*), or *Haemophilus* species.

Management

Pregnant women with isolated listerial bacteremia can be treated with ampicillin alone (2 g IV every 4 hours). Patients who are allergic to penicillin can be skin tested and desensitized, if necessary, or treated with trimethoprim-sulfamethoxazole (5 mg/kg of the trimethoprim component IV every 6 hours). Vancomycin has also been used in case reports of listerial infection.

■ ACUTE BRONCHITIS

Acute bronchitis usually refers to a self-limited respiratory illness characterized by the predominance of a productive cough in a patient with no history of chronic obstructive pulmonary disease and no evidence of pneumonia.

No studies have particularly looked at the course of acute bronchitis in pregnancy. A retrospective cohort study found an association between placental abruption and acute respiratory illnesses including acute bronchitis among white women.

■ MANAGEMENT

Most pregnant patients with acute cough syndromes require no more than reassurance and symptomatic treatment with inhaled beta-agonists. Most cases of acute bronchitis have a viral etiology; however, atypical bacteria including *Bordetellapertussis*, *Chlamydia pneumoniae*, and *Mycoplasma pneumonia* may cause acute bronchitis. The etiologic pathogen is isolated from the sputum in only a minority of patients. A chest x-ray should be performed if clinically indicated. Antimicrobial therapy may be considered in patients when a treatable pathogen is identified or in epidemic settings to limit transmission. **Table 221-2** includes suggested antimicrobial regimens for pregnant patients.

There are no compelling data suggesting improved outcomes of acute bronchitis as a result of treatment with antibiotics.

■ PNEUMONIA

Pregnancy is associated with reduction in cell-mediated immunity, which places pregnant women at an increased risk of severe pneumonia and disseminated disease from some atypical pathogens such as herpes virus, influenza, varicella, and coccidioidomycosis. Mothers who develop pneumonia are more likely to have coexisting medical problems including asthma, drug abuse, anemia, and HIV infection. The use of corticosteroids for enhancement of fetal lung maturity and tocolytic agents has also been associated with antepartum pneumonia.

The incidence of pneumonia requiring hospitalization in pregnancy is between 2.6 to 15.1 per 10,000 deliveries, a rate comparable to that seen in nonpregnant women of a similar age. Pregnancy increases the risk of maternal complications from pneumonia, including the need for mechanical ventilation. Respiratory

TABLE 221-2 Recognized Causes of Acute Bronchitis and Treatment Options

Pathogen	Comments	Treatment Options in Pregnancy
Influenza virus	Precipitous onset with fever, chills, headache, cough and myalgias	Antiviral agents recommended for treatment of influenza have either very little or concerning pregnancy safety data. With the H1N1 pandemic, pregnant women have been found to be at increased risk of complications and treatment with oseltamivir 75 mg orally twice daily is recommended
Parainfluenza virus	Epidemic may occur in fall. Croup in a child at home suggests the presence of this organism	No treatment available
Respiratory syncytial virus	Outbreaks occur in winter or spring. Approximately 45% of adults exposed to an infant with bronchiolitis become infected	No treatment available
Coronavirus	Severe respiratory symptoms may occur	No treatment available
Adenovirus	Infection is clinically similar to influenza, with abrupt onset of fever	No treatment available
Rhinovirus	Fever is uncommon, infection is generally mild.	No treatment available
Bordetella pertussis	Incubation period is 1-3 wk. Post-tussive vomiting may be present. Fever is uncommon	Azithromycin for 5 d (500 mg on day 1, 250 mg days 2-5) or Erythromycin for 14 d (500 mg 4 times daily) or Trimethoprim/ Sulfamethoxazole for 14 d (160/800 mg twice daily)
Mycoplasma pnemoniae	Gradual onset over 2-3 d of headache, fever malaise, and cough. Wheezing may occur. Dyspnea is uncommon	Azithromycin for 5 d (500 mg on day 1, 250 mg days 2-5) or no therapy
Chlamydia pneumoniae	Gradual onset of cough with preceding hoarseness	Azithromycin for 5 d (500 mg on day 1, 250 mg days 2-5) or no therapy

Data from Wenzler RP, Fowler AA. Clinical practice. Acute bronchitis. *N Engl J Med.* 2006;355(20):2125-2130.

failure due to pneumonia is the third leading indication for intubation in pregnancy. Other maternal complications include pulmonary edema, bacteremia, empyema, pneumothorax, and atrial fibrillation. Pregnancies complicated by acute respiratory illnesses, including viral and bacterial pneumonia have been shown to be associated with placental abruption. Increased rates of preterm labor and delivery before 34 weeks of gestation have also been described.

The neonatal mortality rate due to antepartum pneumonia ranges from 1.9% to 12%, with most mortality attributable to complications of preterm birth. Although most cases of pneumonia in pregnancy are caused by organisms that do not affect the fetus except through their effects on maternal status, some organisms, such as varicella and CMV may present specific risks to the fetus. The fetus may also be at risk from maternal conditions that predispose to pneumonia.

The etiology of pneumonia in pregnancy is similar to the non-pregnant population, with streptococcus pneumoniae being the most commonly isolated organism (see Chapter 186 [Community Acquired Pneumonia]).

Diagnosis

Pregnant women with pneumonia present no differently than nonpregnant women and pneumonia should be considered in any woman presenting with fever, cough, sputum production, chills, rigors, dyspnea, and pleuritic chest pain. Occasionally, non-respiratory symptoms such as vomiting, abdominal pain, and fever may predominate. Pulmonary embolism (PE), aspiration, chemical pneumonitis, amniotic fluid embolism, and pulmonary edema related to sepsis, tocolysis, or preeclampsiacan present similarly to an acute pneumonia with dyspnea, cough, chest pain, fever, and chest x-ray infiltrates.

A chest radiograph should be performed in all patients suspected to have pneumonia. Laboratory data should include a complete blood count, serum chemistries for hepatic, renal, glucose evaluation, assessment of oxygenation, and two sets of blood cultures; however, blood cultures may be positive only 7% to 15% of the time. The American Thoracic Society (ATS) does not recommend routine performance of sputum culture and Gram stain. However, if a drug-resistant pathogen oran organism not covered by usual empiric therapy is suspected, sputum culture should be obtained. HIV status should be reviewed for all pregnant women with pneumonia and testing should be offered if it has not previously been done. Testing for pneumocystis carinii infection should occur in all HIV-positive women.

Management

While no specific guidelines exist to help assess severity and the need for hospitalization in pregnant women, it is best to ensure adequate maternal oxygenation (oxygen saturation $\geq$ 95% or $pO_2 \geq$ 70 mm Hg) and fetal well-being before considering outpatient treatment.

Several recommendations exist for treatment of pneumonia in pregnancy. **Table 221-3** summarizes some suggested recommendations based upon ATS guidelines. Although levofloxacin and doxycycline are often recommended in the treatment of pneumonia in the nonpregnant population, these drugs should be avoided in pregnancy. Clarithromycin has shown to have adverse effects in animal trials at doses equivalent to 2 to 17 times the maximum recommended human dose. It is therefore best avoided in pregnancy, with use limited to those cases in which no alternative therapy is appropriate.

With appropriate therapy, an improvement can be expected in 72 hours, after which the regimen can be changed to an oral medication to complete 10 to 14 days therapy.

■ VIRAL HEPATITIS

In general, pregnancy does not affect the diagnosis or clinical course of viral hepatitis. It has been reported, however, that acute hepatitis

TABLE 221-3 Recommendations for Treating Pneumonia in Pregnancy

Type of Pneumonia	Recommended Antibiotics Acceptable for Use in Pregnancy	Comments
Community-acquired pneumonia Organisms: S. pneumoniae Respiratory viruses M. pneumoniae H. influenza C. pneumoniae Legionella Unknown	Ceftriaxone (2 g IV daily) or cefotaxime or ampicillin/ sulbactam (3 g IV every 6 h) **PLUS** Macrolide (azithromycin, erythromycin) If concern for MRSA, add vancomycin (15 mg/kg every 12 h)	Avoid tetracycline and doxycycline in pregnant or breastfeeding mothers Antipneumococcal fluoroquinolone may be used in nonpregnant patient but generally avoided in pregnancy or breastfeeding mothers
Hospital-acquired pneumonia/health care-associated pneumonia/ ventilator-associated pneumonia Organisms: Aerobic Gram-negatives (P. aeruginosa, Escherichia coli, Klebsiella pneumoniae, Acinetobacter spp.) Gram-positive cocci Staphylococcus aureus, especially methicillin resistant (MRSA) Oropharyngeal commensals (viridans group strep, coagulase negative staph, Neisseria spp., Corynebacterium spp.)	Ceftriaxone (2 g IV daily) or ampicillin/ sulbactam (3 g IV every 6 h) If concern for MDR: Ceftazidime (2 g IV every 8 h) or cefepime (2 g IV every 8 h) or imipenem (500 mg every 6 h) or piperacillin/ tazobactam (4.5 every 6 h) or aztreonam (2 g every 6-8 h) **PLUS** Gentamycin or tobramycin **PLUS** Vancomycin (15 mg/kg every 12 h)	Efficacy of once daily dosing for gentamycin in pregnancy not well established
Aspiration pneumonia Organisms: Oropharyngeal commensals (viridans group strep, coagulase negative staph, Neisseria spp., Corynebacterium spp.)	Clindamycin or Penicillin	
Varicella pneumonia	Acyclovir IV 10 mg/kg every 8 h	

may be more severe with hepatitis E. The differential diagnosis includes other common causes of liver dysfunction such as biliary obstruction, drug-induced liver disease, as well as liver diseases uniquely associated with pregnancy such as acute fatty liver, preeclampsia or HELLP (**h**emolysis, **e**levated **l**iver enzymes, and **l**ow **p**latelets), and cholestasis of pregnancy.

Herpes simplex virus (HSV) hepatitis

As a form of disseminated primary herpes infection, usually Herpes simplex type 2, HSV has been reported in the second and third trimester. Pregnant patients may have characteristic mucocutaneous lesions and anicteric liver failure due to severe hepatocyte injury with extreme elevations of serum transaminases, an increased prothrombin time, and only mildly elevated serum bilirubin. If prescribed early in the course of illness, acyclovir may be effective in ameliorating the course of illness.

PULMONARY DISEASE

■ SHORTNESS OF BREATH

Normal pregnancy is characterized by an increase in minute ventilation, due to an increase in tidal volume but not respiratory rate.

Dyspnea of pregnancy usually begins in the middle of gestation as the patient's increased perception of dyspnea. These patients should have a completely normal physical examination, oxygenation, chest x-rays, and pulmonary function testing.

If shortness of breath occurs at 24 to 48 weeks when blood volume reaches its maximum, underlying heart disease should be considered. Pregnant women have an increased risk for pulmonary edema due to an increase in blood volume that is predominantly achieved through an increase in plasma-free water and a lower oncotic pressure during pregnancy. Pyelonephritis, medications that are used to stop preterm labor and preeclampsia may precipitate pulmonary edema. Pregnancy-associated pulmonary edema often responds to withdrawal of the precipitating cause and a low diuretic dose. Other causes of dyspnea include venous thromboembolism (VTE) and respiratory illness (see Chapter 85 [Dyspnea]).

A rare cause of dyspnea unique to pregnancy is amniotic fluid embolism occurring during the third trimester but usually during delivery. Rapid and progressive respiratory failure may be associated with hemodynamic instability and disseminated intravascular coagulopathy. This is a diagnosis of exclusion and treatment is supportive care.

Management

The average PaO_2 in pregnancy 100 mm Hg at sea level and PCO_2 in the range of 28 and 32 mm Hg. An arterial blood gas (ABG) with a PaO_2 of 79 mm Hg and a PCO_2 of 40 mm Hg, considered within normal limits for a nonpregnant patient, is very abnormal in a pregnant female. Because fetal hemoglobin has a different oxygen dissociation curve from adult hemoglobin, in order to adequately oxygenate fetal tissue, maternal oxygen saturation needs to remain greater than 95% or $PaO_2 > 70$ mm Hg.

■ ASTHMA

Asthma affects 3.7% to 8.4% of all pregnancies and is one of the most common serious medical complications encountered in pregnancy in the United States. Asthma may develop during gestation triggered by an upper respiratory infection with persistent bronchospasm or be triggered due to reflux or sinusitis, both increased during pregnancy.

The course of asthma is usually unpredictable in pregnancy and numerous studies have suggested that a third of the patients improve, a third remain the same, and another third worsen. Factors contributing to improvement may be the pregnancy-associated rise in serum cortisol or the increase in progesterone that acts as a potent smooth muscle relaxant. Several factors may be responsible for worsening. Gestational rhinitis, bacterial sinusitis, and gastroesophageal reflux disease, all of which occur at an increased incidence in pregnancy, may worsen asthma control in the gravid state.

Most studies have shown that well-controlled pregnant patients with asthma do not have a significantly higher rate of adverse outcomes than those without asthma. However, patients with poorly controlled asthma are more likely to have miscarriages or therapeutic abortions, infants with low birth weight, and intrauterine growth restriction, and are more likely to undergo cesarean section. Preterm delivery and maternal hypertension have also been noted in poorly controlled women with asthma, but these risks have not been shown consistently and may partly be related to use of systemic steroids in these patients. Preeclampsia has also been associated with severe asthma in some studies.

Management

Management of asthma in pregnancy does not significantly differ from the nonpregnant patient. **Table 221-4** discusses the use and safety of commonly used asthma medications in pregnancy. While dealing with an acute asthma exacerbation in a pregnant woman, it is of vital importance to recognize that normal CO_2 in pregnancy is 28 to 32 mm Hg, which is lower than the nongravid state. Therefore, a tachypneic pregnant patient with a $PaCO_2$ above this range might be in impending respiratory failure. **Figure 221-1** shows the recommendations for assessment and management of acute asthma exacerbation in the hospital setting. These are based on the NAEP guidelines for asthma management in pregnancy.

While asthma exacerbations are rare in labor and delivery, it is important to ensure that asthma medications are not discontinued through labor and delivery. Most drugs used for asthma treatment can be safely used in breastfeeding women. Whether breastfeeding decreases the likelihood of the development of asthma in offspring is as yet controversial, but it does appear to decrease atopy.

■ PLEURAL EFFUSION IN PREGNANCY

Pleural effusions can be caused by a variety of conditions, both specific and unrelated to pregnancy. Physiologic changes of pregnancy, including an increased blood volume and decreased colloid osmotic pressure, promote transudation of fluid into the pleural space. Benign postpartum pleural effusions have been noted on chest radiographs and ultrasound studies after normal vaginal delivery with an incidence of about 25%. Pregnancy-specific conditions that predispose to pulmonary edema such as preeclampsia, amniotic fluid embolism, chorioamnionitis, or endometritis, may also result in pleural effusion.

Diagnosis

Diagnostic approach is largely guided by findings on history and physical examination and conditions being considered in the differential. A diagnostic thoracocentesis should always be considered in the presence of fever, hemoptysis, weight loss, or when hemothorax or emphysema is suspected.

Management

Management usually involves treatment of the underlying condition. Rarely, a therapeutic thoracentesis may be necessary, particularly in case of a large (eg, TB) or rapidly accumulating effusion (eg, malignancy). Presence of blood, pus, or chylous effusion warrants placement of a thoracostomy tube. While performing these procedures in pregnancy, it is important to remember that the diaphragm is about 4 to 5 cm elevated and a higher approach with ultrasound guidance is advisable.

■ PNEUMOTHORAX IN PREGNANCY

Primary spontaneous pneumothorax (PSP) usually resolves satisfactorily with simple observation, aspiration, or tube drainage.

TABLE 221-4 Safety of Asthma Medications in Pregnancy

Medication Type	Data Suggests Use Justifiable When Indicated	Data Suggests Use Justifiable in Rare Circumstances	Data suggests Use Almost Never Justifiable	Useful Review Articles and Comments
Short-acting inhaled beta-2 adrenergic agonists	Albuterol$_C$ Bitolterol$_C$ Pirbuterol$_C$ Metaproterenol$_C$ Terbutaline$_C$			Published experience with these drugs in animals and humans suggests that beta-sympathomimetics do not increase the risk of congenital anomalies. Albuterol is the most studied of these agents. Metaproterenol is the second most studied. NAEP guidelines for the management of asthma in pregnancy can be obtained through the NHLBI at http://www.nhlbi.nih.gov/health/prof/lung/asthma/astpreg.htm
Long-acting inhaled beta-2 adrenergic agonists	Salmeterol$_C$ Formoterol$_C$			Of the few studies that have examined pregnancy outcomes with prenatal exposure to long-acting beta-2 agonists, no adverse events were found. However, due to small numbers in the studies, and because animal models have shown delayed ossification, use of this agent should be reserved for patients who have failed low potency steroids and/or cromolyn alone
Xanthines	Theophylline$_C$ Aminophylline$_C$			These drugs do not appear to be human teratogens. The clearance of aminophylline and theophylline is increased in pregnancy but may be variable. If daily dose exceeds 700 mg, blood levels should be checked for optimal dosing
Inhaled corticosteroids	Low potency: beclomethasone dipropionate$_C$ Medium potency: trimacinolone acetonide$_C$ High potency: fluticasone propionate$_C$ budesonide$_B$ flunisolide$_B$			Beclomethasone and budenoside are the most widely studied of the inhaled corticosteroids in pregnancy and should be considered the preferred inhaled steroids in pregnancy. Relatively little of these agents are absorbed and human data has not suggested any teratogenic effects of these agents

Triamcinolone is the next most studied inhaled steroid in pregnancy, with this limited experience suggesting no adverse pregnancy effects

Fluticasone has not been studied in pregnancy; however its minimal systemic absorption and the safety of the other steroids in pregnancy make its use in pregnancy generally felt to be justifiable |
| Systemic steroids | prednisone$_C$ methylprednisolone$_C$ dexamethasone$_C$ hydrocortisone$_C$ | | | Most data suggest that systemic steroids do not present a teratogenic risk in human pregnancy. In doses equivalent to prednisone 25 mg/d, they do not cross the placenta because of placental metabolism (the same is not true for betamethasone or dexamethasone). Even in higher doses, the effect of hydrocortisone or prednisone on the fetus in terms of suppression of the hypothalmo-pituitary-adrenal axis is minimal

Several case control studies have found a significant association with first trimester steroid use and oral clefts; however this was not seen in cohort studies. Even if this association is real, the risk is still small. For every 1000 embryos exposed during the susceptible days of first trimester, probably no more than three will develop an oral cleft. The background risk in the general population is 1 per 1000. Therefore, the benefits of controlling a life-threatening disease make steroid use when indicated in the first trimester still generally justifiable |
| Mast cell stabilizers | Cromolyn sodium$_B$ Nedocromil$_B$ | | | Human and animal data suggest these agents are not teratogens. These agents are virtually not absorbed through mucosal surfaces and the swallowed portion is largely excreted in the feces |

(Continued)

TABLE 221-4 Safety of Asthma Medications in Pregnancy (*Continued*)

Medication Type	Data Suggests Use Justifiable When Indicated	Data Suggests Use Justifiable in Rare Circumstances	Data suggests Use Almost Never Justifiable	Useful Review Articles and Comments
Inhaled anticholinergics	Ipratropium$_B$			Although animal studies are reassuring, no published human data exists. These drugs are poorly absorbed by the bronchial mucosa so fetal exposure is likely minimal
Leukotriene inhibitors		Zafirlukast$_B$ Montelukast$_B$ Omalizumab$_B$	Zileuton$_B$	Although these agents have reassuring animal data and are widely used in pregnancy because of the FDA category B rating, published safety data in human pregnancy is limited at this point. Their use should be limited in pregnancy to those cases in which a woman has had significant improvement in asthma control with these medications prior to becoming pregnant that was not obtainable through other methods. Zileuton is different than other agents in this class as there is some animal data to suggest association with adverse pregnancy outcomes
Antihistamines	Diphenhydramine$_B$ (but avoid in first trimester) Chlorpheniramine Dimenhydrinate$_B$	Cetirizine$_B$ Fexofenadine$_C$ Loratidine$_B$		While the newest generation antihistaminic agents are widely used in pregnancy and have not had any concerning animal data associated with them, we still consider them to be second-line agents in pregnancy because of the lack of published human pregnancy safety data about them
Cough	Guaifenesin$_C$ Dextromethorphan$_C$ Albuterol$_C$ Codeine$_C$			
Nasal congestion	Pseudoephedrine$_C$ Oxymetazoline$_C$ Nasal steroids Beconase$_C$ Rhinocort$_C$ Flonase$_C$ Nasacort$_C$ Nasal cromolyn$_B$ Nasal ipratropium$_B$			

Adapted, with permission, from Mehta N, Newstead-Angel J, Powrie RO. Prescribing in Pregnancy and Lactation. In: Bourjeily G, Rosene-Montella K, eds, Pulmonary Problems in Pregnancy, Respiratory Medicine, Humana Press, a part of Springer Science+Business Media, LLC. 2009;71-88.

Recurrence occurs more frequently in pregnant patients. Majority of these recurrences occur during the same pregnancy or in the postpartum period.

Management

Observation may suffice for a small pneumothorax (<2 cm) in patients without shortness of breath. Further intervention should be considered in patients with difficulty breathing or if the pneumothorax is larger than 2 cm. Chest tube drainage would be indicated in patients with persistent air leak. Surgical correction may be considered in the postpartum period to prevent recurrence in subsequent pregnancies.

Risk of recurrence may be increased in labor and delivery due to the repeated Valsalva maneuvers during vaginal birth, with resulting increase in intrathoracic pressures. Therefore in a pregnant woman with a past history of PSP, vaginal delivery should be assisted with forceps or vacuum to limit Valsalva breathing. Should a cesarean section be necessary, it is best performed under regional anesthesia to avoid intrathoracic pressure increases associated with intubation and general anesthesia.

■ ACUTE RESPIRATORY DISTRESS SYNDROME (ARDS)

Acute respiratory distress syndrome is an acute, diffuse, inflammatory lung injury that leads to increased pulmonary vascular permeability, increased lung weight, and a loss of aerated tissue. Although no studies clearly elucidate the frequency of ARDS in the obstetric population, the incidence is felt to be similar to the general population (see Chapter 142 [ARDS]).

Pregnancy does not change total lung capacity, nor does it increase the A-a gradient. Noncardiogenic pulmonary edema is

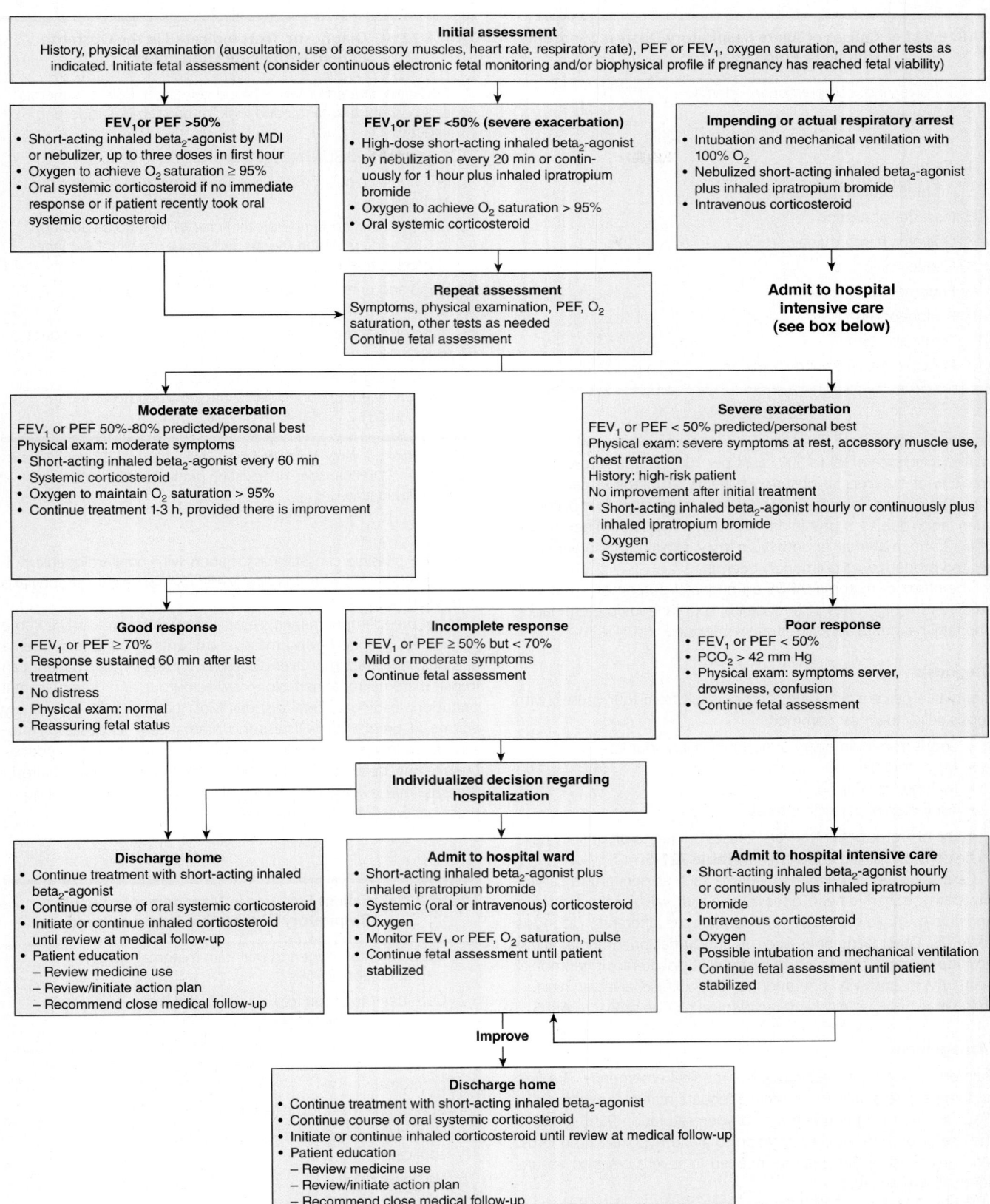

Figure 221-1 *Management of asthma exacerbations during pregnancy and lactation: Emergency department and hospital-based care. FEV$_1$, forced expiratory volume in 1 second; MDI, metered-dose inhaler; PCO$_2$, carbon dioxide partial pressure; PEF, peak expiratory flow. (From the Asthma and Pregnancy Report. NAEPP Report of the working group on Asthma and Pregnancy. NIH publication No. 93-3279. Bethesda, MD: U.S. Department of Health and Human Services; National Institutes of Health; National Heart, Lung, and Blood Institute 1993. Available from URL: http://www.nhlbi.nih.gov/health/prof/lung/asthma/astpreg.txt.)*

TABLE 221-5 Causes of Acute Respiratory Distress Syndrome Unique to Pregnancy

1. Tocolytic induced pulmonary edema
2. Preeclampsia
3. Acute fatty liver of pregnancy
4. Gastric aspiration
5. Amniotic fluid embolism
6. Placental abruption
7. Obstetric hemorrhage
8. Chorioamnionitis
9. Endometritis
10. Pyelonephritis
11. Septic abortion
12. Retained products of conception

TABLE 221-6 Diagnostic Tests Indicated in the Obstetric Patient with Acute Lung Injury

1. CBC with differential white blood cell count: Rule out anemia as a contributing factor and look for bandemia, suggesting infection
2. Creatinine and BUN: rule out renal failure
3. PTT, fibrinogen, and FDP: Look for evidence of amniotic fluid embolism
4. AST, uric acid, and urine protein creatinine ratio (in addition to CBC and creatinine mentioned above): Look for evidence of preeclampsia
5. Blood and urine cultures in all patients with fever or bandemia
6. Urine drug screen: Look for evidence of cocaine or narcotics as a cause
7. Echocardiogram: Rule out underlying cardiac cause for pulmonary edema or evidence of cardiac compromise in preeclampsia

AST, aspartate transaminase; BUN, blood urea nitrogen; CBC, complete blood count; FDP, fibrinogen degradation products; PTT, partial thromboplastin time.

known to occur more frequently in pregnant women with an estimated incidence of 80 to 500 cases per 100,000 and is responsible for 25% of transfers of obstetric patients to intensive care units. Both the normal decrease in serum oncotic pressure that occurs in pregnancy due to a physiologic dilutional hypoalbuminemia and changes in maternal endothelium may explain this pregnancy-related propensity to pulmonary edema.

The effect of maternal ARDS on neonatal outcomes is not well studied, but high rates of fetal death, spontaneous preterm labor, and fetal heart rate abnormalities are reported.

Diagnosis

Eighty-five percent of all ARDS cases result from four causes, with sepsis being the most common:

- Sepsis from pulmonary or nonpulmonary sources
- Major trauma
- Multiple transfusions
- Aspiration of gastric contents

In the obstetric patient, several causes unique to pregnancy have to be considered. These are listed in **Table 221-5**.

Cardiac causes of pulmonary edema such as peripartum cardiomyopathy, ischemic heart disease, or occult valvular heart disease and fluid overload should be considered in the differential diagnosis of ARDS. Other conditions such as interstitial pneumonia, acute eosinophilic pneumonia, acute bronchiolitis obliterans pneumonia, acute hypersensitivity pneumonitis, and diffuse alveolar hemorrhage may have a clinical and radiological picture similar to ARDS.

Management

Pulmonary edema in pregnancy is a medical emergency. The first and immediate goal is to maintain adequate maternal oxygenation ($PaO_2 \geq 70$ mm Hg equivalent to oxygen saturation 95%) through the use of oxygen supplementation to avoid hypoxia in the fetus. Mechanical ventilation may be needed in severe cases to ensure adequate oxygenation.

Tables 221-6 and **221-7** list the salient features of investigation and management of ARDS in the pregnant patient.

When pulmonary edema is suspected to be related to preeclampsia, initial management consists of oxygen supplementation, fluid restriction, and blood pressure (BP) control while plans are made for delivery. Intravenous magnesium is used as a first-line agent for seizure prophylaxis and treatment in preeclampsia/eclampsia, based on two randomized controlled trials that confirm superiority over dilantin. However, its use in the setting of ARDS may not be justified

given the possible causative association with noncardiogenic pulmonary edema. Dilantin may be preferable for seizure prophylaxis in this setting.

Many preeclamptic patients are relatively intravascularly volume contracted, despite having massive amounts of peripheral edema and pulmonary edema. Over-diuresis of a preeclamptic patient can impair maternal renal perfusion, cardiac output, and uteroplacental perfusion, leading to fetal distress. Most patients with pulmonary edema in pregnancy will respond dramatically to doses of furosemide as low as 10 mg IV especially if renal function is normal. Despite the need for careful fluid restriction and gentle diuresis, there is little evidence that central hemodynamic monitoring in these patients improves outcomes.

TABLE 221-7 Salient Features in Management of Acute Respiratory Distress Syndrome in Pregnancy

1. Supplemental oxygen to maintain maternal oxygen saturation above 95%
2. Consider intubation for $PaO_2 < 70$ mm Hg or $PaCO_2 > 45$ mm Hg on 100% oxygen
3. Look for precipitating causes listed in Table 221-5 in addition to sepsis, massive transfusion, aspiration of gastric contents, or trauma
4. Appropriate diagnostic testing as listed in Table 221-6
5. Immediate discontinuation of tocolytic therapy when applicable
6. Fluid restriction
7. IV furosemide 10-20 mg
8. IV antibiotics if infection suspected
9. Echocardiogram to rule out cardiac cause for pulmonary edema
10. Consider afterload reduction with sodium nitroprusside or hydralazine if patient is pregnant, and angiotensin converting enzyme inhibitors or angiotensin-receptor blockers in the postpartum patient

Whether delivery has a positive impact on maternal condition in patients with ARDS is unclear. There are case reports describing improvement in maternal oxygenation after delivery in patients with ARDS, but the mechanism for this is not well understood and may be partly related to resultant decreased cardiac work.

For the most part, patients with ARDS secondary to chorioamnionitis, placental abruption, amniotic fluid embolism and preeclampsia need immediate delivery, while those with pyelonephritis or varicella pneumonia can often recover without delivery.

RENAL DISEASE

■ NEPHROLITHIASIS

Renal stones are commonly encountered in pregnancy, complicating about 1 in 200 pregnancies. While some data suggests an increased risk of preterm labor in patients with stones, most available reports do not suggest a significant increase in obstetric complications.

Pregnancy is associated with physiologic dilatation of the ureters, resulting from smooth muscle relaxation induced by progesterone. This may occur as early as the first trimester. Furthermore, there is decreased peristalsis and anatomic dilatation resulting from mechanical obstruction of the collecting system from the gravid uterus. With the resultant urinary stasis, there is increased propensity for infection and crystal aggregation. In addition, increases in glomerular filtration rate (GFR) lead to higher concentration of urinary calcium that further predisposes to stone formation.

Diagnosis

Pregnant patients with urolithiasis present no differently from nonpregnant patients, usually with renal colic or severe pain associated with complete or partial obstruction of the ureters. The diagnosis of urolithiasis may be challenging in pregnancy due to the physisologic changes in the renal system in the gravid state.

Ultrasonography (USG) is the preferred initial test, as opposed to abdominal CT scan, to avoid fetal radiation exposure. Bilateral hydronephrosis may be seen on ultrasound (US) due to physiologic changes. It is therefore important to identify the presence of ureteral jets in the bladder, which would rule out a ureteral obstruction by stone.

The sensitivity of ultrasound in confirming urolithisis ranges from 34% to 86%. If a stone is clinically suspected despite ultrasound findings, a single shot IVP may be performed. If diagnosis still remains in question, magnetic resonance urography may be helpful. Whenever possible, the stone should be collected for analysis.

Management

The initial management plan for urinary stones in pregnancy is conservative (hydration, analgesics, and antibiotics if infection is present). Opioid analgesics can safely be used in pregnancy. Nonsteroidal anti-inflammatory drugs (NSAIDs) should be avoided due to oligohydramnios and premature narrowing or closure of the patent ductusarteriosis. Most patients will spontaneously pass the stone with conservative management. Urology consult may be appropriate in patients with prolonged or recurrent symptoms in which ureteral stents may be needed. Indications for a diversion procedure, stenting, or percutaneous nephrostomy, include persistent pain, infection or high-grade hydronephrosis beyond normal pregnancy-related dilatation.

■ ACUTE RENAL FAILURE

By definition, acute renal failure (ARF) is a syndrome of rapid decrease in glomerular filtration rate, increasing serum creatinine,

TABLE 221-8 Severity Ranges of Creatinine in Pregnancy

Severity	Creatinine Range (mg/dL)
Mild	0.9-1.4
Moderate	1.4-2.9
Severe	3.0 or greater

and urea levels and oliguria or anuria (see Chapter 239 [Acute Kidney Injury]).

Acute renal injury is rare in pregnancy, but transient mild to moderate renal dysfunction is more common. Adverse fetal outcomes associated with acute renal insufficiency are typically due to altered uteroplacental hemodynamics. It is therefore crucial to maintain volume and maternal acid-base balance and prevent further renal deterioration. If delivery is imminent in these patients, the neonate may be subject to rapid dehydration as a result of increased solute load in fetal circulation leading to osmotic diuresis.

Diagnosis

The physiologic increase in GFR leads to lower serum creatinine and BUN during pregnancy. Renal dysfunction in pregnancy is therefore defined as creatinine above 0.8 mg/dL (**Table 221-8**).

Acute renal injury can result from prerenal, intrarenal, or postrenal causes (see **Table 221-9**).

Management

Initial management of ARF commences with identification and treatment of underlying causes. Judicious fluid management and avoidance of nephrotoxins are important. Care should be taken to adjust dosing of medications that are renally cleared. Low-dose dopamine has not been found to be effective and is not recommended. Loop diuretics may be helpful in treatment of volume overload; however, there is no data to support the use of diuretics in patients with oliguric renal failure from preeclampsia, a disease of hemoconcentration and vasospasm. Renal replacement therapy should be considered in the case of volume overload, hyperkalemia refractory to medical management, metabolic acidosis, or symptomatic uremia (mental status changes, pericarditis, neuropathy).

Dialysis

Although uncommon, pregnancy does occur in women on chronic dialysis. Conversely, dialysis may become necessary in a pregnant

TABLE 221-9 Causes of Renal Failure in Pregnancy

- Blood loss resulting from abrution, postpartum hemorrhage, placenta previa
- Volume contraction: preeclampsia, eclampsia, hyperemesis
- Infection: sepsis resulting from pyelonephritis, chorioamnionitis, endometritis, septic abortion
- HELLP; acute fatty liver of pregnancy, TTP; HUS; amniotic fluid embolism
- Drug reactions
- Obstruction from pelvic hematoma, damage to ureters during cesarean section, ureteral stones or strictures, compression by gravid uterus or tumor
- Related to underlying disease: Lupus nephritis, scleroderma crisis, antiphospholipid antibody syndrome

HELLP, hemolysis, elevated live enzymes, and low platelets; HUS, hemolytic uremic syndrome; TTP, thrombotic thrombocytopenic purpura.

woman with ARF from worsening underlying renal disease or de novo causes. There is no difference in outcomes with peritoneal or hemodialysis. In general, an increased dose of dialysis is recommended for pregnant patients to achieve a target predialysis blood urea nitrogen of less than 50 mg/dL.

HYPERTENSIVE DISORDERS

Hypertensive disorders represent one of the most common medical problems in pregnancy and encompass the diagnoses of chronic hypertension, gestational hypertension, and preeclampsia.

■ CHRONIC HYPERTENSION

Chronic hypertension in pregnancy is defined as a blood pressure of 140/90 or greater on two separate occasions before 20 weeks' gestation or persisting beyond 12 weeks' postpartum. It is associated with a 20% risk of developing preeclampsia. While essential hypertension is the most common cause, consideration of secondary causes is necessary in this young population.

Physiologic changes in the cardiovascular system during pregnancy allow for a decrease in blood pressure in the first two trimesters, with a return toward baseline in the third trimester. In the second half of pregnancy, inferior vena cava compression from a gravid uterus in the supine position may falsely lower blood pressure readings, so it is important to measure blood pressure in a pregnant woman in the seated position.

Treatment of mild to moderate hypertension in pregnancy neither benefits the fetus nor prevents preeclampsia. In addition, excessive lowering of blood pressure may result in adverse fetal outcomes from decreased placental perfusion. Oral agents that are commonly used to treat hypertension in pregnancy include labetalol, nifedipine, and methyldopa. Clonidine has also been used in pregnancy without increased risk of congenital malformations; however, an effect on offspring behavior has been suspected based on human and animal studies. Other oral agents that are reasonably safe for pregnancy but with limited efficacy include hydralazine and hydrochlorthiazide. Angiotensin-converting enzyme (ACE) inhibitors and angiotensin receptor blockers are contraindicated at any gestational age in pregnancy. **Table 221-10** outlines the pharmacologic management of hypertensive urgency in a pregnant woman.

■ GESTATIONAL HYPERTENSION

Gestational hypertension is defined as elevation in blood pressure developing after 20 weeks' gestation without proteinuria. Women with gestational hypertension progress to preeclampsia in 15% to 45% of cases and often require early delivery. Surveillance for development of preeclampsia and close fetal monitoring is recommended.

■ PREECLAMPSIA

Preeclampsia is a pregnancy-specific complication that occurs in 5% to 10% of all pregnancies. It is defined as a BP ≥ 140/90 accompanied by proteinuria of > 300 mg per 24 hours after the 20th week of gestation in a previously normotensive patient. When it is diagnosed in a patient with pre-existing chronic hypertension, it is referred to as chronic hypertension with superimposed preeclampsia. Most cases of preeclampsia occur close to term.

Risk factors for development of preeclampsia include first pregnancy or pregnancy with a new partner, age less than 18 years or older than 35, past history of preeclampsia, chronic hypertension, renal disease, diabetes mellitus (type I, II, or gestational), obesity, systemic lupus erythematosus (SLE), thrombophilia, multiple gestation, and molar pregnancy.

Etiology of preeclampsia is unclear. On a pathophysiologic level, preeclampsia is characterized by systemic endothelia dysfunction brought about by an imbalance between proangiogenic (VEGF, PlGF) and antiangiogenic factors (sFlt-1) resulting in various inflammatory responses leading to hypertension, hemoconcentration, and vasospasm.

Diagnosis

The main symptoms of preeclampsia include headache, visual disturbance, epigastric or right upper quadrant abdominal discomfort, edema, and rapid weight gain. Signs include hypertension, retinal vasospasm, right upper quadrant tenderness, and clonus. Lab studies supporting the diagnosis of preeclampsia are outlined in **Table 221-11**.

Severe preeclampsia is defined as the presence of one of the following symptoms or signs in the presence of preeclampsia (1) systolic BP of ≥ 160 mm Hg or diastolicBP of ≥ 110 mm Hg on two

---

TABLE 221-10 Pharmacologic Treatment of Hypertensive Urgency in a Pregnant Woman

Medication	Onset of Action and Duration of Action	Acute Dosing for Severe Hypertension	Maintenance Dose
Labetalol	Begins to work in 5-10 min Lasts 3-6 h	Labetalol is given as a series of boluses until BP comes down to the desired level: • 10 mg IV push • Then in 10 min, 20 mg IV push • Then in 10 min, 40 mg IV push • Then in 10 min, 80 mg IV push • Then in 10 min, 80 mg IV push up to a total dose of no more than 300 mg total • Then followed with oral labetalol or a labetalol drip	• Oral labetalol 100-200 mg 2-3 times a day (100-600 mg 2-3 times a day; maximum 2400 mg/d) • IV labetalol infusion 0.5-2.0 mg/min (Labetalol comes in vials of 100 mg/20 mL) • Put 5 vials (100 mL) of labetalol into 150 mL of IV fluid (D5W/LR/NS) to get a solution of 2 mg/mL • Start at 15 mL/h (0.5 mg/min) • Titrate up to as high as 60 mL/h (2 mg/min)
Nifedipine	Begins to work in < 30 min Lasts 4-5 h	10-20 mg orally every 30 min to a maximum of 50 mg	Maintenance 10-20 mg orally 3 times a day of the short-acting or 30-120 mg once daily of long-acting formulation
Hydralazine	Begins to work in 10-20 min Lasts for 3-6 h	2.5-10 mg IV every 30 min	Maintenance dose starts at 10 mg orally 4 times a day and can be gradually increased to 50 mg orally 4 times a day

D5W, dextrose 5% in water (solution); LR, lactated Ringer (solution); NS, normal saline.

TABLE 221-11 Lab Abnormalities in Pre-eclampsia

1. Hemoglobin > 12 g/dL (normally near 10 g/dL in pregnant women near term)
2. Platelet count < 150,000/mm³
3. Elevated liver enzymes (AST and ALT)
4. Creatinine > 0.8 mg/dL (normal for pregnancy 0.5-0.7 mg/dL)
5. Uric acid > 0.5 mg/dL
6. 24-h urine collection with > 300 mg of protein

ALT, alanine transaminase; AST, aspartate transaminase.

occasions at least 6 hours apart; (2) proteinuria of more than 5 g in 24-hour period; (3) pulmonary edema; (4) oliguria (< 400 mL in 24 h); (5) persistent headaches and/or seizures (eclampsia); (6) epigastric pain and/or impaired liver function; (7) thrombocytopenia; and (8) intrauterine growth restriction. HELLP syndrome characterized by **h**emolysis, **e**levated **l**iver **e**nzymes and **l**ow **p**latelet count is a variant of severe preeclampsia occurring in about 20% of cases of severe preeclampsia.

Treatment

The only known treatment of preeclampsia once it occurs is delivery as soon as obstetrically feasible. Despite this, it is important to note that preeclampsia can present postpartum, and both preeclampsia and eclampsia have been reported for up to 21 days following delivery. Management of preeclampsia includes treatment of hypertension, seizure prophylaxis, and limitation of fluids due to the risk of pulmonary edema. **Table 221-12** outlines the management of a pregnant woman hospitalized with severe preeclampsia.

ENDOCRINE DISORDERS

■ DIABETES

Insulin requirements often decrease by 10% to 20% in the first trimester of pregnancy due to increased insulin sensitivity. The risk of overall and nocturnal hypoglycemia during this time is further compounded if the patient has hyperemesis or pre-existing gastroparesis.

Rising human placental lactogen and human placental growth hormone levels from the beginning of the second trimester then cause an increase in insulin resistance, and insulin requirements rise gradually until approximately 36 weeks of gestation. Women with pre-existing type 2 diabetes controlled with diet and exercise will usually require pharmacologic treatment by mid–second trimester. A sudden decrease in insulin requirements in the third trimester needs to be taken very seriously, as it may be a signal of placental failure, and close fetal surveillance is required.

All metabolic processes are accelerated during pregnancy and the threshold of starvation ketoacidosis occurring after a prolonged fast is much lower. This coupled with hyperemesis in early pregnancy and subsequent increased insulin resistance in later pregnancy increases the risk of diabetic ketoacidosis (DKA) in pregnant women.

It is recommended that a baseline eye check occur as part of preconception counseling as pre-existing diabetic retinopathy has been shown to progress more quickly during pregnancy due to the increased production of growth factors as well as the hypercoagulable state of pregnancy. Laser therapy during pregnancy is as effective as outside pregnancy and can be safely used if required.

In women with pre-existing diabetic nephropathy, pregnancy may worsen the degree of proteinuria, cause progression of renal sufficiency, and aggravate hypertension. Discontinuation of ACE

TABLE 221-12 Labor and Delivery Sample Admission Orders for Severe Pre-eclampsia

Bed rest with seizure precautions

Vital signs (blood pressure, pulse, respiration); deep tendon reflexes; and mental status every 15-60 min until stable, then every 60 min while on magnesium sulfate

Accurate intake and output; Foley catheter if needed

Administer lactated Ringer solution at 75 mL/h IV to maintain urine output of 30-40 mL/h; total intake (IV and oral) should not exceed 125 mL/h or 3000 mL/d

Continuous fetal heart rate monitoring

Laboratory tests:

Dipstick urine collection for protein level on admission

24-h urine collection for total protein level

CBC with platelets, peripheral blood smear

BUN, creatinine, uric acid

AST, ALT, LDH

Fetal evaluation: nonstress test on admission; obstetric ultrasonography for estimated fetal weight, amniotic fluid volume, and umbilical artery Doppler measurements

Medications:

Magnesium sulfate

Loading dose of 4-6 g diluted in 100 mL of normal saline, given IV over 15-20 min, followed by a continuous infusion of 2 g/h

Assess serum magnesium level if urine output is < 30 mL/h or there is a loss of deep tendon reflexes, decreased respiratory rate, or altered mental status

Therapeutic range for serum magnesium is 4-7 mg/dL

Corticosteroids (if between 24 and 34 wk of gestation and not previously administered)

Betamethasone (Celestone), 12 mg IM initially, then repeat in 24 h

or

Dexamethasone, 6 mg IM initially, then repeat every 12 h for three additional doses

For systolic blood pressure > 160 mm Hg or diastolic > 110 mm Hg, one of the following should be given to achieve a systolic measurement of 140-155 mm Hg and/or a diastolic measurement of 90-105 mm Hg

Hydralazine, 5-10 mg IV every 15-30 min (maximal dose: 30 mg)

or

Labetalol, 20 mg IV initially; if the initial dose is not effective, double the dose to 40 mg and then 80 mg at 10-min intervals until target blood pressure is reached or a total of 220 mg has been administered; the maximal dose of IV labetalol is 220 mg in a 24-h period

Calcium gluconate, 1 g IV; keep at bedside in case of respiratory depression from magnesium sulfate use

ALT, alanine transaminase; AST, aspartate transaminase; BUN, blood urea nitrogen; CBC, complete blood count; IM, intramuscularly; IV, intravenously; LDH, l-lactate dehydrogenase.

Reprinted, with permission, from Hypertensive disorders of pregnancy, July 1, 2008, American Family Physician. Copyright 2008, American Academy of Family Physicians. All rights reserved.

inhibitors or angiotensin II receptor blockers before conception together with an increase in GFR are the main reasons for a physiologic increase in proteinuria during pregnancy. Although pregnancy may accelerate the progression of nephropathy, postpartum renal function usually returns to prepregnancy levels in most cases. In women with moderate renal insufficiency, pregnancy has been estimated to shorten the time to end-stage renal failure by 36 months.

Hypertension occurs in 30% of women with diabetic nephropathy in the first trimester and in 75% by the third trimester. Deteriorating renal function and superimposed preeclampsia are responsible for the high rates of preterm delivery, low birth weight, and operative delivery. Differentiating preeclampsia from worsening nephropathy can be very difficult as proteinuria and worsening hypertension occur in both situations.

Women with pre-existing types 1 and 2 diabetes are at increased risk of preeclampsia, operative delivery, and antenatal infections (such as urinary tract and respiratory). These risks are further increased if the mother has premorbid obesity as well.

The rate of early pregnancy loss or congenital anomalies is increased for women with poor preconception glycemic control. Glucose is a potent teratogen and there is a linear increase in rates of congenital anomalies with rising HgbA1C levels. Late pregnancy losses are also increased in women with poor glycemic control during pregnancy. It is thought that oxidative stress resulting from oxygen depletion caused by hyperglycemia is the underlying mechanism for these findings. It has been shown that the overall rate of adverse pregnancy outcome is much lower in women who receive preconception counseling and are euglycemic at conception and during organogenesis.

The incidence of macrosomia is increased in diabetic pregnancies. Excess fetal growth is due to fetal hyperinsulinemia in response to maternal hyperglycemia. Macrosomic babies (> 4000 g) are at increased risk for traumatic or surgical delivery, shoulder dystocia, and brachial plexus injury. Neonatal hypoglycemia due to fetal hyperinsulinemia and neonatal hyperbilirubinemia are metabolic complications that are more common in babies born to diabetic mothers.

Gestational diabetes mellitus

Gestational diabetes mellitus (GDM) is defined as glucose intolerance of variable severity that is first detected during pregnancy. It is the leading endocrine condition in pregnancy and continues to rise in the face of the obesity epidemic. Pregnancy is effectively a stress-test in which the insulin-resistant hormones of pregnancy trigger overt hyperglycemia in women who have a background of previously undiagnosed insulin resistance and/or decreased pancreatic beta-cell reserve.

It is usually diagnosed at the end of the second trimester via a diagnostic glucose tolerance test. Treatment needs to begin immediately as there is only a short window of opportunity to achieve euglycemia in order to minimize its impact on the fetus. If the following targets are not met with diet and exercise therapy alone (fasting blood glucose level or BGL < 5.3 mmol/L or 95 mg/dL and/or 1-hour postprandial BGL < 7.8 mmol/L or 140 mg/dL and/or 2-hour postprandial BGL < 6.7 mmol/L or 120 mg/dL), insulin therapy is commenced though glyburide, or metformin therapy may be recommended if the patient refuses insulin therapy and/or the degree of hyperglycemia is only mild. Glyburide has traditionally been the preferred agent as it does not cross the placenta, but more recent studies have emerged regarding the safety and efficacy of metformin use beyond the first trimester.

Glucose tolerance returns to normal immediately after delivery of the placenta and so treatment can be ceased. Women with GDM are at much greater risk of developing type 2 diabetes in the future and so they should be tested for such on a regular basis by their primary care physicians.

The use of oral hypoglycemic agents, subcutaneous insulin regimes, and insulin pumps

Insulin is considered the gold standard of treatment for both pre-existing and gestational diabetes. However, there has been a trend toward increasing use of glyburide and metformin in recent times. There is currently no data to suggest that the use of either in the first trimester is associated with an increase in congenital anomalies. Glyburide does not cross the placenta and can be used throughout the second and third trimesters as well.

Metformin is frequently used as an ovulation induction agent in women with polycystic ovarian syndrome and for these women, continuing its use during the first trimester has been shown to reduce miscarriage rates. Its use during the second and third trimesters had been questionable in the past given that significant placental transfer does take place (cord blood levels similar to maternal levels) but recent data suggests that there is no long-term deleterious effects on the fetus and it may in fact reduce the risk of the offspring developing type 2 diabetes in the future.

None of the other oral hypoglycemic agents currently on the market are recommended or approved for use during pregnancy.

All the insulin types available on the market are safe for use in pregnancy. These include the newer insulin analogs, which are more rapid in onset (Humalog, Novolog) and longer in action (Lantus, Levemir) compared with the traditional recombinant human insulins (Humulin-R, Humulin-NPH).

An increasing number of women of childbearing age with type 1 diabetes are using insulin pumps that provide a continuous subcutaneous infusion of insulin for glycemic control. The main caveat here is that they need to recognize potential problems such as a blockage or kink in the infusion set that can precipitate an episode of diabetic ketoacidosis more quickly in pregnant patients.

Management of diabetic ketoacidosis

The presentation of DKA is similar in the nonpregnant and pregnant patient, but the acidosis tends to be more pronounced at a lower serum glucose level in the pregnant patient. This is due to the combination of the accelerated starvation state of pregnancy, lower buffering capacity due to the physiologic respiratory alkalosis of pregnancy that leads to lower serum bicarbonate levels and the increased GFR in pregnancy that leads to increased renal excretion of glucose.

Treatment requires prompt recognition and maternal stabilization with rehydration, intravenous insulin therapy, and electrolyte replacement. Infections such as those of the urinary tract should be excluded. As starvation ketosis is often the main component of ketoacidosis, the mother needs to receive adequate dextrose (with the insulin infusion) in order to meet fetal-placental glucose needs until she is eating normally. Ketone bodies and glucose cross the placenta readily and so there is high fetal morbidity and mortality associated with DKA. Fetal compromise will improve once the metabolic acidosis reverses. An urgent C-section while the mother is still acidotic is not generally recommended because of high maternal risk.

Management at time of labor and delivery

It is recommended that an insulin plan for the time of labor and delivery be provided to all patients well before the expected due date so that there is no confusion between the patient and various medical and nursing caregivers. It is important to avoid maternal blood glucose levels more than 9.0 mmol/L (162 mg/dL) in the intrapartum period as this has been associated with an increased risk of neonatal hypoglycemia (which may require NICU admission), but it is also important to avoid hypoglycemia for maternal safety and well-being during this strenuous process.

In early labor, subcutaneous insulin use should be continued while the woman is still eating but these doses will need to be reduced if oral intake is decreased. When the woman is in active labor and no longer eating, an intravenous insulin and dextrose infusion should be commenced to keep the blood glucose levels in the desired range of 4.0 to 8.0 mmol/L (72-144 mg/dL).

For patients with active proliferative retinopathy, using the Valsalva maneuver repeatedly in the second stage of labor is a concern as there is an increased risk of retinal hemorrhage.

Management in the immediate postpartum period

With delivery of the placenta, insulin requirements rapidly decrease back to prepregnancy levels. The target range of blood glucose levels postpartum in the pre-existing diabetic is much more relaxed compared with during pregnancy, with levels between 6.0 and 10.0 mmol/L (108-180 mg/dL) all being acceptable. Breastfeeding will lower blood glucose levels and having extremely tight glycemic control may increase the risk of hypoglycemia in a lactating woman. The usual postpartum insulin requirement is approximately two-thirds of the prepregnancy insulin dosage.

Women with type 2 diabetes may be able to discontinue insulin therapy and use diet and exercise and/or oral hypoglycemic agents in the postpartum period. The two oral hypoglycemic agents that have been documented to be safe in breastfeeding are glyburide and metformin. The former does not enter breast milk at all and infant exposure to the latter has been estimated to be only approximately 0.5% of the maternal dose.

ACE-inhibitors or angiotensin II receptor blockers can also be recommended in lactating women, though it is recommended that a preterm infant not be exposed to it until he has reached an age equivalent to full term.

◼ OBESITY IN PREGNANCY

The prevalence of obesity worldwide has increased dramatically over the past 25 years. It affects 26% of the population in the USA. Of concern is the fact that the majority of the obese population tend to be women of reproductive age, according to the WHO.

Overweight and obese women are at increased risk of maternal, fetal and peripartum complications. Maternal complications include gestational diabetes mellitus, gestational hypertension, preeclampsia, cesarean delivery, and postpartum weight retention. It is also well recognized that obesity is an independent risk factor for spontaneous abortion among women who conceive naturally or undergo infertility treatment, and hence it is recommended that obese women be provided with counseling for weight reduction prior to conception. Nutrition and exercise counseling should be provided at this time as well as continuing throughout the pregnancy, in the postpartum period and subsequently before attempting another pregnancy. Institute of Medicine guidelines published in 2009 recommend that overweight women (BMI 25.0-29.9) should put on no more than 15 to 25 lbs and obese women (BMI >30.0) no more than 11 to 20 lbs during the entire pregnancy.

Associated fetal risks include an increased rate of congenital anomalies (eg, neural tube defects), lower detection rate of fetal anomalies during prenatal ultrasonography, macrosomia, prematurity, stillbirth, as well as subsequent childhood and adolescent obesity.

At the time of delivery, the use of regional anesthesia is preferred as the rate of failed or difficult intubation is as high as one in three for obese pregnant women. It is recommended that anesthesiology consultation occurs early on during the laboring process in order to better identify strategies to reduce the failure rate of administering epidural or spinal anesthesia. The presence of obstructive sleep apnea may further complicate airway and postoperative management. Obese women who require cesarean deliveries have increased rates of excessive blood loss, operative time greater than 2 hours, wound infection and endometritis. Postoperative wound disruption is thought to be less prevalent with the use of suture closure of the subcutaneous layer. Consideration should be given to using a higher dose of preoperative antibiotics for surgical prophylaxis. Obesity is also an additional risk factor for thromboembolic events and hence the routine use of pneumatic compression devices following cesarean deliveries is recommended. Prophylactic anticoagulation for 2 weeks is also recommended in obese individuals with additional risk-factors. Obese women are less likely to initiate and sustain breastfeeding.

The number of obese reproductive-aged women undergoing bariatric surgery is increasing. The two most common procedures currently performed are gastric bypass and sleeve gastrectomy (about 50% each). It is generally recommended that pregnancy be delayed for 12 to 18 months postoperatively. With gastric bypass patients, there is an increased risk of failure in absorption of medications (eg, oral contraceptive pill, extended release formulations such as metformin). Care should be taken to monitor and supplement these patients with micronutrients such as iron, folate, vitamin B12, calcium and vitamin D. Oral glucose tolerance tests may not be well tolerated due to the dumping syndrome and so routine blood glucose monitoring is often recommended in these patients.

◼ THYROID

Hypothyroidism

Management of thyroid diseases during pregnancy requires special considerations because pregnancy induces major changes in thyroid function, and maternal thyroid disease can have adverse effects on the pregnancy and the fetus. Avoiding maternal (and fetal) hypothyroidism is of major importance because of potential damage to fetal neural development, an increased incidence of miscarriage, and preterm delivery. However, universal screening of pregnant women for thyroid disease is not yet supported by adequate studies, but case finding targeted to specific groups of patients who are at increased risk is currently strongly supported.

Both overt and subclinical hypothyroidism can have an adverse impact on the course of pregnancy or fetal development. Overt hypothyroidism should be corrected before initiation of pregnancy and preconception thyroxine (T4) dosage should bring the thyroid-stimulating hormone (TSH) level < 2.6 mU/L. Women with subclinical hypothyroidism (serum TSH above the upper reference limit but free T4 [fT4] within the reference limits) should also be treated with T4 replacement. This recommendation is based on observational evidence demonstrating that women suffering from overt or subclinical hypothyroidism deliver babies with an average intelligence quotient (IQ) score seven points below the mean IQ score of children born to healthy women and women on T4 replacement. The importance of maternal thyroid hormone replacement is emphasized by the fact that the fetal thyroid does not develop until the second trimester of pregnancy and fetal thyroid hormone production does not become optimal until mid-gestation.

Maintaining a serum TSH < 3.0 mU/L is acceptable in the second and third trimesters of pregnancy. After delivery, the dose of T4 therapy can usually be reduced back to the preconception dosage after checking a repeat set of thyroid function tests at the 6-week postpartum visit.

Hyperthyroidism

If a suppressed TSH is detected during pregnancy, hyperthyroidism must be distinguished from normal physiology (gestational thyrotoxicosis) and hyperemesis gravidarum because of the potential adverse effects on the mother and fetus.

Hyperthyroidism in pregnancy is not rare; estimated prevalence is 0.1% to 0.4% with Graves disease accounting for 85% of cases and toxic solitary or multiple nodules plus thyroiditis accounting for most of the rest. Hydatidiform molar disease is a very uncommon cause these days due to the advent of dating ultrasounds.

Gestational thyrotoxicosis presents in the mid- to late first trimester, often with hyperemesis. Classical hyperthyroid symptoms are absent or minimal apart from weight loss, which is often the result of malnutrition secondary to vomiting. The suppression in TSH is mediated by rising human chorionic gonadotropin (hCG) levels and therefore it will usually self-resolve by mid-gestation at the latest. Approximately 50% of women suffering from hyperemesis have a subnormal TSH and elevated fT4 level. In this setting, the assessment of free triiodothyronine (fT3) level and thyroid-stimulating immunoglobulin (TSI) level are helpful as 90% of hyperemesis cases have normal fT3 and most cases of Graves disease will be TSI positive.

If Graves disease or hyperfunctioning nodules are diagnosed, propylthiouracil is preferred to methimazole because of the association with congenital abnormalities with the latter medication. Therapy should be adjusted to maintain maternal fT4 in the upper non-pregnant reference interval. Though rare, the possibility of neonatal Graves disease needs to be entertained if the maternal TSI levels are high in the third trimester. Women with well-controlled Graves disease during pregnancy should be warned about the possibility of postpartum flare-up, which usually occurs between 6-weeks and 6-months postpartum. It is not recommended that radioactive iodine therapy be used during pregnancy and lactation.

Postpartum thyroiditis

Postpartum thyroiditis may occur in up to 10% of all pregnancies, usually between 6 weeks and 6 months after delivery, but it can occur up to 1 year later (see Chapter 222 [Postpartum Consultation for Common Complaints]). A hypothyroid phase often follows the hyperthyroid phase and is occasionally permanent. Monitoring is necessary, as women may be hypothyroid at the time of any subsequent pregnancy.

■ PARATHYROID

Hypercalcemia

Primary hyperparathyroidism is usually diagnosed during pregnancy through routine blood testing following prolonged or extremely severe hyperemesis gravidarum or else the serendipitous finding of nephrocalcinosis, renal calculi, or excessive calcification of the placenta during fetal ultrasonography. It may frequently be part of the multiple endocrine neoplasia (MEN-1 or MEN-2a) syndrome. Urinary calcium excretion is typically not used as part of the diagnostic evaluation as it is increased in normal pregnancy.

Symptomatic hyperparathyroidism is best treated by minimally invasive surgical removal of the parathyroid adenoma during the second trimester, after embryogenesis is complete and before such time that premature labor may be stimulated. In skilled hands, the procedure takes no more than 30 minutes.

Surgery can also be offered in late pregnancy (after 35 weeks' gestation) if the patient becomes profoundly symptomatic, as the neonatal outcome is much improved with surgery. This is due to the reduced risk of stillbirth, intrauterine growth restriction (IUGR), premature labor, and especially neonatal hypocalcemictetany, which can frequently cause prolonged neonatal intensive care unit admissions especially if fetal parathyroid suppression takes a long time to recover.

Hypocalcemia

Hypoparathyroidism is very rare in pregnancy and is usually part of the autoimmune polyglandular syndrome, which would frequently be associated with mucocutaneous candidiasis and adrenal insufficiency. Maintenance of normocalcemia involves substantial oral supplementation with calcium and activated vitamin D (calcitriol). The doses of supplementation usually have to be increased, particularly in the third trimester, as there is high fetal uptake of calcium into the skeleton.

TABLE 221-13	Causes of Hypopituitarism in the Pregnant Patient
Pre-existing before Pregnancy	
Pituitary adenoma	
Vasculitis	
Infiltrative disorders (hemochromatosis, sarcoidosis, amyloidosis)	
Hypothalamic tumors (craniopharyngiomas, germinoma, meningioma, glioma)	
Eosinophilic granuloma (histiocytosis X)	
Pituitary apoplexy	
Prior surgical or radiotherapy treatment	
During Pregnancy or Postpartum	
Lymphocytic hypophysitis/infundibulohypophysitis	
Sheehan syndrome (peripartum necrosis)	

■ PITUITARY

Pituitary insufficiency

The differential diagnosis of pituitary insufficiency in the pregnant patient is diverse and is listed in **Table 221-13**.

The management of the pregnant woman with pre-existing pituitary insufficiency centers on adequate hormonal replacement. In general, thyroid hormone and cortisol requirements increase throughout pregnancy due to increased hepatic production of thyroxine-binding globulin (TBG) and cortisol-binding globulin (CBG). It is vital that fT4 rather than TSH level is monitored as the latter will always be low in patients with hypopituitarism. Hydrocortisone is generally the preferred glucocorticoid replacement therapy of choice as there is minimal transplacental passage to the fetus.

Mineralocorticoid replacement is not required in pituitary insufficiency as the renin-angiotensin-aldosterone axis is intact. Regular obstetrical follow-up with serial ultrasounds to detect IUGR is recommended.

Stress doses of glucocorticoids must be given at the time of labor and delivery; please refer to the section on Primary Adrenal Insufficiency for recommended doses.

See Chapter 222: Postpartum Consultation for Common Complaints on lymphocytic hypophysitis and Sheehan syndrome.

■ PROLACTINOMAS

It is uncommon for pregnancy to occur in women with untreated prolactinomas because hyperprolactinemia is associated with infertility. However, the ability of dopamine agonists to reduce prolactin levels to the normal range restores ovulation in about 90% of patients, many of whom are then able to achieve pregnancy.

Rising estrogen levels during pregnancy have a stimulatory effect on prolactin secretion that can cause the growth of the lesion. The risk is much higher for macroadenomas compared with microadenomas. For this reason, dopamine agonists are always discontinued once pregnancy is confirmed in someone with a microadenoma.

With macroadenomas, dopamine agonists are frequently continued throughout pregnancy in order to prevent tumor growth. Numerous studies have shown that there are no adverse effects on the fetus with the use of bromocriptine. There is much less data on cabergoline, but it is thought to be safe as well, though it is not favored in any case due to its longer half-life.

It is recommended that prepregnancy baseline visual field testing and MRI imaging of the pituitary be done for women with macroadenoma and that they be reviewed on a regular basis (every 4-6 weeks) throughout gestation for evidence of tumor expansion.

There is no role for measuring prolactin levels throughout pregnancy as the levels increase in any case.

In the postpartum period, lactation has not been shown to increase the size of adenomas and is strongly encouraged.

Diabetes insipidus

The development of new-onset diabetes insipidus in the third trimester is usually due to increased vasopressinase activity either due to increased placental production or decreased hepatic vasopressinase metabolism due to liver damage from various causes including preeclampsia, acute fatty liver of pregnancy, or HELLP, syndrome. This phenomenon is called transient vasopressin-resistant diabetes insipidus (DI) of pregnancy.

Pre-existing central diabetes insipidus often worsens during pregnancy due to the increased clearance of endogenous vasopressin by increasing levels of vasopressinase. Subclinical central DI can also be unmasked for the first time during pregnancy due to this mechanism.

DDAVP is the treatment of choice for both central DI and transient vasopressin-resistant DI of pregnancy as it is not degraded by vasopressinase. Thiazide diuretics, which are used for the treatment of nephrogenic diabetes insipidus, are safe to be continued during pregnancy. Transient vasopressin-resistant DI of pregnancy tends to resolve a few days to weeks after delivery.

■ ADRENAL

Adrenal insufficiency

The most common cause is immune-mediated destruction of the adrenal cortex (Addison disease). This diagnosis should always be entertained in patients who have irretractable lethargy, nausea, and vomiting that is out of keeping with normal symptoms of pregnancy. A normal pregnancy outcome should be expected as long as the patient takes the appropriate dosages of glucocorticoids and mineralocorticoids; these doses often need to be increased slightly throughout pregnancy as rising progesterone levels act as antagonists to the glucocorticoid and mineralocorticoid receptors.

Hydrocortisone and prednisone are the preferred glucocorticoid replacement agents as their placental passage to the fetus is much lower compared with dexamethasone or betamethasone. Stress doses must always be administered in times of severe hyperemesis or physical stress as well as at the time of labor and delivery; please refer to **Table 221-14** for a suggested protocol of the latter.

Pheochromocytoma

This condition can have profound effects on both mother and fetus and so it is important that it be considered as part of the differential

---

TABLE 221-14 Stress Dose Steroids During Surgery or Delivery

1. Hydrocortisone 100 mg IV on call to operating room or at onset of labor
2. Hydrocortisone 100 mg IV every 8 h over course of surgery or labor and delivery
3. Hydrocortisone 50 mg IV every 8 h day 1 postoperative or postpartum
4. Hydrocortisone 25 mg orally every 8 h day 2 postoperative or postpartum
5. Usual preadmission doses of hydrocortisone orally from day 3 postoperative or postpartum

---

diagnosis for hypertension in the pregnant woman, particularly in the first half of pregnancy.

Fasting plasma metanephrine levels are the most sensitive and specific diagnostic test, though it should be noted that the levels are slightly increased in pregnancy. Falsely elevated levels can be caused by pharmacologic agents such as tricyclic antidepressants, labetalol, and methyldopa.

Anatomic localization is required for definitive treatment once a biochemical diagnosis has been made. In pregnancy, the modality of choice to achieve this is MRI. Nuclear scanning with metaiodobenzylguanidine (MIBG) is contraindicated in pregnancy.

Medical therapy in the form of alpha-blockade should be initiated once a biochemical diagnosis is made; and the patient should be counseled that the benefits of alpha-blockade in pregnancy far outweigh any potential unknown effects. Beta-blockade is then instituted after alpha-blockade is achieved to avoid tachyarrhythmias; the dose should be titrated to achieve a maternal heart rate of 80 to 100 beats/min.

Surgery, in the form of laparoscopic adrenalectomy, can be considered once adequate medical therapy and localization of the lesion have been achieved. If the lesion is diagnosed during the first two trimesters, the best time to operate is during the second trimester, and if the lesion is diagnosed during the third trimester, surgery should be delayed until delivery though the timing of this will need to be brought forward if the mother remains symptomatic despite the medical blockade. An elective C-section is the delivery method of choice as the process of labor exacerbates the catecholamine surges.

Primary hyperaldosteronism

This condition is frequently unmasked in the postpartum period as the high progesterone levels during pregnancy antagonize the action of mineralocorticoids on their own receptors. Hypertension with hypokalemia is the classic presentation, though often the potassium level may be normal.

Both renin and aldosterone levels are increased during pregnancy. Therefore a suppressed renin level may be useful in diagnosing this condition during pregnancy. Medications that suppress renin levels such as β-blockers and calcium channel blockers need to be discontinued for at least 2 weeks before formal testing of renin and aldosterone levels.

It is recommended that spironolactone not be used in pregnancy due to its antiandrogenic effects; there is a theoretical risk that feminization of a male fetus may occur. Calcium channel blockers are regarded to be the most effective antihypertensive agent, as they have some effect in reducing aldosterone synthesis and release. If the hypertension and/or hypokalemia cannot be controlled medically, laparoscopic removal of the affected adrenal gland during the second trimester may be warranted.

DEPRESSION

Depressive disorders affect at least 12% of women at some time in their lives. In the United States, depression is the leading cause of nonobstetric hospitalization among women age 18 to 44 years. The peak period for onset of depression occurs during the childbearing years and its impact extends to the offspring and the families involved. Unfortunately, perinatal depression remains underdiagnosed and undertreated in ob-gyn and primary care settings. Furthermore, the diagnosis of depression in pregnant women can be challenging because there is great overlap between the diagnostic symptoms of depression and the symptoms of normal pregnancy.

A systematic review found prevalence rates of depression that vary from trimester to trimester: 7.4% in the first, 12.8% in the second, and 12% in the third trimester. Risk factors for depression in pregnancy include a previous depressive episode, recent negative life events, adolescence, unmarried status, financial disadvantage, African American or Hispanic ethnicity, and poor social support. Untreated depression can lead to harmful prenatal health behaviors such as poor nutrition, poor prenatal medical care, smoking, alcohol, and other substance use. The fetus of untreated depressed women may demonstrate abnormal neurobehavioral responses such as altered heart rate reactivity.

Obstetric complications associated with depression include preeclampsia, preterm delivery, low birth weight, miscarriage, small-for-gestational age babies, low Apgar scores, neonatal complications, and high neonatal cortisol levels at birth. Exposure to higher cortisol levels is thought to be the mechanism of the effect on later childhood development that may include language and cognitive impairment, sleep problems, impulsivity, attention deficit disorders, behavioral dyscontrol, and psychopathology.

ANTIDEPRESSANT USE AND PREGNANCY

How can depressive symptoms be treated during pregnancy? Depression in nonpregnant patients is mostly treated with selective serotonin reuptake inhibitors (SSRIs) and serotonin-norepinephrine reuptake inhibitors (SNRI). Up to 9% of women have taken an antidepressant at some point during gestation, given that at least one-half of pregnancies are unplanned. Most of these exposures will be to one of the newer antidepressant medications. The odds ratio of 1.7 for spontaneous miscarriage with SSRI exposure, and reports of a 1.45 relative risk are within the range of the normal population.

Most meta-analyses report that newer antidepressants do not increase the risk of malformation rates above the 1% to 3% population baseline risk. The teratogenicity data from Denmark reports a 1.34 increased relative risk, but it does not control for underlying maternal psychiatric disorders. Small increased risk in omphalocele, craniosynostosis, and anencephaly with all SSRIs, and right ventricular outflow tract obstruction with paroxetine have been found in some other studies, but these findings were not replicated in other studies. Nevertheless, the Food and Drug Administration issued a public health advisory in 2005 regarding paroxetine and the FDA pregnancy category was changed from C to D.

Neonatal adaptation symptoms with maternal SSRI exposure have been reported. The syndrome described includes transient and usually mild jitteriness, poor muscle tone, weak or absent cry, respiratory distress, hypoglycemia, low Apgar scores, and possible seizures. The drugs with the highest association with the neonatal adaptations syndrome include paroxetine, fluoxetine, and venlafaxine, with one study reporting on citalopram as well. Long-term sequelae have not been systematically studied and an accurate blinded infant assessment as well as a neonatal behavioral symptom scale should be helpful in examining this syndrome more accurately.

A case control study published in 2006 showed an increased risk of persistent pulmonary hypertension of the newborn (PPHN) from a baseline of 1 to 2 per 1000, to 6 to 12 per 1000 for infants exposed to SSRI after 20 weeks of gestation. The authors of the study suggest that SSRIs may promote pulmonary artery constriction after birth by inhibiting nitric oxide or by a direct effect on pulmonary smooth muscle cells. These theories have been challenged, and furthermore, SSRI use before week 20 seemed to be a somewhat protective factor against PPHN, so it is difficult to advise patients about the absolute risk.

Other psychotropic medications and pregnancy

Benzodiazepines are used during pregnancy for management of anxiety or insomnia. Meta-analyses have identified a small increased risk of oral cleft with in utero exposure, though a case-control study failed to confirm this teratogenic risk. Pyloric stenosis and alimentary

tract atresias have also been reported, as well as low birth weight and floppy infant syndrome.

If benzodiazepines need to be used, consider delaying treatment until after oral cleft closure and choose medications with shorter half-lives at the lowest possible dose.

Mood stabilizers are the most widely used medications for management of mood instability (mania, depression, and psychosis in bipolar patients) and include lithium and the antiepileptic medications. The main concern with first trimester exposure to lithium is an increased risk (0.1%) in Ebstein anomaly, which has a risk of 0.05% in the unexposed population. Lithium remains one of the preferred treatments for bipolar disorder and this increased risk needs to be weighed against the risk of a mood decompensation. Stable serum levels may require increase in dosages as the pregnancy progresses due to the normal changes in blood volume in pregnancy. Careful monitoring of dosage and lithium level at delivery is recommended to avoid toxicity.

Valproate has an increased risk of neural tube defects of 5% to 9% with first trimester exposure and a fetal valproate syndrome that includes cardiovascular abnormalities and developmental delays, and craniofacial abnormalities have been described. There is newer information that exposure to valproate later in gestation may be associated with neurobehavioral changes as well. Toxicity at birth with valproate may include decreased fibrinogen levels, liver toxicity, hypoglycemia, deceleration in heart rate, abnormal muscle tone, and lower IQ. Women of reproductive age who are planning to have children should be switched from valproate to another agent prior to pregnancy so that the disease can be controlled by an alternative agent before gestation.

Exposure to carbamazepine in the first trimester carries an increased risk of craniofacial abnormalities, fingernail hypoplasia, growth restriction, and a risk of neural tube defect of 0.5% to 1%.

Lamotrigene is associated with an increased risk of congenital malformations similar to the general population (2%-3%). Some studies have suggested an increased risk of cleft palate deformity and it is worth noting that infants with antigen characteristics that differ from the mother may be at increased risk for skin rash and liver toxicity.

Haloperidol is the most commonly used antipsychotic in pregnancy because several studies have not found increased risks of congenital malformations. Chlorpromazine has a poor side-effect profile in pregnancy due to orthostasis and sedation and has an increased risk of malformations of 2.4% and so should generally be avoided.

Newer antipsychotics are better tolerated than the above mentioned medications, but the data regarding safety with these is limited. Some studies have shown no increased risk of major malformations with olanzapine, risperidone, quetiapine, and clozapin but have found lower birth weight. Side effects of these medications can also be problematic in pregnancy, particularly weight gain and glucose intolerance.

Postpartum blues, depression, and psychosis

Between 15% and 85% of normal postpartum women may experience the blues (postpartum blues), which present within the first 10 days after giving birth with a peak incidence at the fifth day. It can be difficult to distinguish from a true depressive disorder given that symptoms include mood swings, mild elation, irritability, tearfulness, fatigue, and confusion. Women who experienced postpartum blues may have a history of premenstrual dysphoria and depression. No treatment is required other than improved sleep and support, but it can be a risk factor for postpartum depression.

The DSM IV classifies postpartum depression as a major depressive disorder with a specifier of postpartum onset within 1 month after childbirth. Screening with a specific tool such as the Edinburgh Postnatal Depression Scale (EPDS) is important since it emphasizes clinical domains of depression and may help differentiate from normal postpartum findings. Risk factors for postpartum depression include depression during or prior to the pregnancy, previous premenstrual dysphoria, stressful life events during the pregnancy, poor social support, marital conflict, low income, immigrant status, and young maternal age. It is thought that the etiology may be related to hormonal fluctuations, either as a direct influence in mood or due to their affect on sleep patterns in the postpartum period.

Postpartum psychosis is a true psychiatric emergency that occurs in 1 to 2 per 1000 births. The onset usually occurs within the first 4 weeks after delivery, although manifestations of the clinical picture can be present in the first 3 days postpartum. The cognitive disorganization that occurs with postpartum psychosis may result in a mother's neglect of her infant's needs and unsafe practices. It is highly associated with bipolar disorder and most of the time requires inpatient psychiatric hospitalization for rapid stabilization and decreased risk of suicide or infanticide. Patients present with acute confusion, delusions, and grossly disorganized behavior.

The use of antidepressants during lactation for treatment of PPD or other psychiatric disorders such as obsessive-compulsive disorder and panic disorder is an important clinical issue. The evidence on the effects of antidepressants during breastfeeding consists of small sample studies and case reports. It is important to take into account the amount of medication present in the breast milk, the reported adverse events, and the infant serum level of the drug to discuss recommendations with patients. Pooled analyses indicate that sertraline and paroxetine tend to have undetectable infant serum drug levels. Fluoxetine and citalopram were more likely to result in elevated breast milk levels. Of the tricyclic antidepressants, nortriptyline and imipramine have the largest serum level data showing levels that are not detectable. Doxepin, on the other hand, has been associated with sedation and respiratory depression and is considered contraindicated in breastfeeding women.

Antipsychotics and breastfeeding

Studies of the safety of both first- and second-generation antipsychotics are quantitatively insufficient to make specific recommendations regarding breastfeeding. Risperidone and chlorpromazine have the lowest degree of excretion in breast milk and there is only one case report of drowsiness with chlorpromazine. One antipsychotic, clozapine, is considered contraindicated with breastfeeding due to high infant-relative dosage and reported adverse effects.

The available data suggests that the amount of medications (anxiolytics) to which newborns are exposed is not very high; it is important to note that neonates metabolize these medications more slowly than adults and accumulation may occur, causing infant sedation, nausea, and poor feeding. Therefore, long-acting medications are not recommended, and the lowest possible dose of a short-acting benzodiazepine should be used if these medications are needed while breastfeeding.

NEUROLOGY

■ HEADACHES

In general, pregnancy does not have a consistent impact on the frequency or severity of migraine headaches and the onset of migraines may begin during pregnancy. Migraine that presents for the first time after 20 weeks' gestation should prompt an investigation for preeclampsia. Pseudotumorcerebri is an unusual cause of headache that is more frequently seen in pregnant women. The fundoscopic examination will reveal papilledema but otherwise the neurologic examination will be normal. Increased intracranial pressure on the optic nerve may cause progressive visual loss. The postpartum period (defined as 6 weeks after delivery) but not pregnancy is associated with an increased risk of stroke and intracerebral hemorrhage, which may be related to thrombosis and/or preeclampsia.

■ EPILEPSY

Seizure disorders complicate approximately 1% of all pregnancies, and up to 10% of epileptic women will present for the first time during pregnancy. Not all seizures result from epilepsy. Both patients with and without known seizure disorders may have seizures as a consequence of preeclampsia or eclampsia, so investigation for preeclampsia is necessary for all third-trimester seizures.

Although most antiepileptic drugs have teratogenicity of various degrees, epileptic women have an increased risk of fetal malformations even without their administration. The maternal and fetal risk of uncontrolled seizures resulting in hypoxemia and acidosis must be part of any risk-benefit assessment of withdrawing effective treatment. If a patient has been seizure free for greater than a year, holding treatment first trimester in consultation with a neurologist could be considered.

The dosage of antiepileptic medications may be influenced by the increased volume of distribution and by increases in hepatic and renal clearance.

Valproate and carbamazepine are preferred in breastfeeding women, given the low degree of excretion in breast milk and limited reported adverse effects in infants. Lamotrigene has its own particular set of concerns. Even though only 60% of the drug is transferred to the breast milk, infants present with higher-than-expected drug levels when breastfed.

GASTROINTESTINAL DISEASE

■ ABDOMINAL PAIN

Gastroesophageal reflux disease occurs due to delayed gastric emptying and decreased gastroesophageal sphincter tone from progesterone effects on smooth muscle. Constipation is also common and related to the effects of progesterone upon the smooth muscle of the bowel. The differential of abdominal pain is broad and includes contractions, pain from adhesions interfering with expansion of the uterus into the abdomen, urinary retention, degenerating fibroid, ectopic pregnancy, ovarian torsion, stress on the round ligaments as the uterus expands, rupture of an ovarian cyst, and bleeding into a corpus luteal cyst. Late in pregnancy, uterine contractions, abruption placentae, pelvic arthropathy, and rarely rectus hematoma may occur.

Vomiting, pyelonephritis, appendicitis, cholecystitis, and rarely volvulus of the large bowel may also be seen during pregnancy.

■ CHOLELITHIASIS

Pregnancy is a risk factor for the development of cholesterol gallstones and biliary sludge. Higher estrogen levels increase biliary cholesterol secretion and higher progesterone levels decrease gallbladder smooth muscle motility. Preexisting gallstones are more likely to cause symptoms.

■ BUDD-CHIARI SYNDROME

Pregnancy-associated hypercoagulability is also a risk factor for hepatic vein thrombosis or the Budd-Chiari syndrome. Typically, patients suddenly develop abdominal pain and ascites after delivery.

■ JAUNDICE

Common causes of jaundice during pregnancy include cholestasis from raised estrogen levels, acute fatty liver of pregnancy, disseminated intravascular coagulopathy, severe preeclampsia, hyperemesis, and severe septicemia in late pregnancy. Drug effects (chlorpromazine, tetracycline, steroids), chronic liver disease, gall stones, and chronic hemolysis should also be considered.

■ LIVER DISEASE

Pregnancy-associated changes

Some of the physiologic changes of pregnancy can simulate laboratory abnormalities seen with liver disease. For example, serum albumin concentrations typically decrease from a mean of 4.2 g/dL in nonpregnant women without liver disease to 3.1 g/dL at the end of gestation due to an increase in plasma volume. Due to leakage of placental alkaline phosphatase into the maternal blood during the fifth month, typically serum alkaline phosphatase levels rise. Hepatosplenomegaly should not be found in the normal pregnancy and bilirubin, AST, ALT, and 5'nucleotidas, and γ-glutamyl levels should be normal. Telangiectasis of the chest, back, and face and palmar erythema may occur in up to 60% of normal pregnant women but should disappear after delivery. Acute fatty liver of pregnancy (AFLP) can lead to jaundice, liver failure, and death.

Diagnosis

The week of gestation may provide an important clue to the diagnosis. Liver diseases specifically associated with pregnancy occur at certain times. In the first trimester, nausea and vomiting with jaundice is consistent with hyperemesis gravidarum and AFLP has not been reported to occur during this time. Cholestasis of pregnancy typically presents at 30 weeks, usually with generalized pruritis, malaise, and fatigue due to symptoms being worse at night. Jaundice may develop in one-third to one-half of patients after the onset of pruritis. In 5% to 10% of pregnancies, liver diseases may develop with preeclampsia and eclampsia in the third trimester. In approximately 1 in 13,000 pregnancies, AFLP occurs in the third trimester.

The pattern of serum liver enzyme abnormalities may be helpful in establishing the diagnosis. The jaundice of cholestasis of pregnancy is usually not severe, less than 6 mg/dL along with elevated alkaline phosphatase levels three to four times the upper limit of normal in pregnancy and elevated serum bile acids. With preeclampsia and eclampsia, the liver injury is due to hepatocellular injury or ischemia so aminotransferase levels are more elevated than alkaline phosphatase or bilirubin. When patients develop abdominal pain, hypotension, fever, leukocytosis, nausea, and vomiting with abnormal liver tests in the third trimester, hepatic infarction, subcapsular hematoma, and hepatic rupture are rare complications of preeclampsia and eclampsia. AFLP is a disease of acute hepatocyte failure so laboratory tests may be initially unimpressively abnormal. If the serum transaminases rise to more than 10 times the upper limit of normal, alternative diagnoses should be considered. The prothrombin time and rising bilirubin are the most reliable indicators of hepatic failure.

Treatment

For patients with AFLP, supportive care and early delivery are critical due to the high fetal and maternal mortality. If hepatic failure is present, patients should be referred to a transplant unit early in the course. Likewise, the preferred treatment of patients with severe preeclampsia-related liver diseases is delivery.

Effect of chronic liver disease on pregnancy

Pregnancy does not alter the progression of chronic liver disease, but the outcome of the pregnancy may be influenced by the patient's overall health, resulting in a higher incidence of miscarriage and prematurity.

HEMATOLOGIC CONDITIONS

■ SICKLE CELL DISEASE

Rates of severe preeclampsia, chest and urinary infections, and biliary disease are higher in pregnant patients with sickle cell disease.

Even in high-risk perinatal clinics, the perinatal mortality rate and maternal mortality rate is increased.

VENOUS THROMBOEMBOLISM IN PREGNANCY

■ INCIDENCE

There is a five-fold increase in the incidence of venous thromboembolism in pregnancy that occurs at an incidence of 0.5 to 3 per 1000 pregnancies. VTE continues to be the leading nonobstetric cause of maternal death in the developed world. Thromboembolic events are evenly distributed throughout the three trimesters and the postpartum period, although more recent studies suggest a slightly higher incidence in the first trimester. In addition, because the postpartum period is by definition shorter (6 weeks, as compared to 12 weeks in a trimester), the day-to-day risk of VTE in the postpartum period is higher. The incidence of fatal pulmonary embolism is also higher in the postpartum period.

Pregnancy is a hypercoagulable state, characterized by an increase in levels of clotting factors, decrease in anticoagulant activity (lower levels of protein S and increased activated protein C resistance), and decreased fibrinolytic activity. In addition, stasis induced by venous compression by the gravid uterus and hormonal influence on vasculature further adds to the coagulant risk.

Risk factors that may contribute to the development of VTE in pregnancy include prolonged bed rest, cesarean section, obesity, parity >3, underlying thrombophilia, prior VTE, or preeclampsia.

The genetic predisposition to VTE may be identified by a positive family history in those patients for whom pregnancy is an additional risk factor.

Diagnosis

Clinical features of deep vein thrombosis (DVT) include pain and swelling in the affected leg, but it is important to remember that lower-extremity edema in pregnancy is common and is often asymmetric. Anatomy of the pelvic vasculature is such that the right iliac artery crosses over the left iliac vein. With the cardiovascular changes of pregnancy, there is compression of the left iliac vein by the right iliac artery, resulting in asymmetric lower-extremity edema (left greater than right) and the finding that the vast majority of DVTs occur in the left leg.

Symptoms of pulmonary embolism include dyspnea, chest pain that may be pleuritic, syncope, hemoptysis, and apprehension. Shortness of breath is a very common complaint in pregnancy, but tachypnea is always an abnormal finding. The diagnosis of PE should be considered in a dyspneic pregnant woman who is tachycardic and tachypneic.

Clinical diagnosis of DVT and PE in pregnancy is unreliable. Compression of pelvic veins by the gravid uterus can make interpretation of results difficult. In addition, isolated iliac vein thrombosis may not be picked up by routine methods of detection. D-dimers are known to be elevated in pregnancy. Clinical prediction rules for PE have not been validated in pregnancy. Pregnant patients with PE are younger and less likely to have comorbid conditions compared with nonpregnant patients, and generally appear "well" and in more than 60% of cases have normal arterial blood gases.

Doppler ultrasound is the noninvasive test of choice in the pregnant woman with suspected DVT. In symptomatic patients with a high pretest probability but a negative test, serial Dopplers should be done and an MRV of the pelvis should be considered to look for an isolated iliac clot. A recent study found that 60% of DVT in pregnancy is found in the proximal veins without evidence of calf thrombosis, suggesting that propagation from calf vein clots may not be the mechanism of proximal thrombosis in pregnancy. Chest x-ray and ECG are helpful in a patient with suspected PE to rule out other causes. Both ventilation-perfusion lung scan

TABLE 221-15 Fetal Radiation Exposure with Maternal Testing

Study	Radiation Exposure (RADS)
Chest x-ray	<.001
Lung scan	0.01-0.02 ventilation
	0.01-0.03 perfusion
Pulmonary angiogram	<.050 via brachial route
	0.2-0.3 via femoral route
CT angiogram	0.2-0.3
Ultrasound	None
MRI/MRA/MRV	None
Upper GI series	0.1
Lumbar spine series	0.9
Barium enema	1
Complete IVP	0.5
Head CT	<0.01
CT abdomen	2.0-3.0

(V/Q scan) and CT angiogram can be safely used in pregnancy for diagnosis of PE. Fetal radiation exposure with either of these tests is minimal (**Table 221-15**). In the majority of cases of fatal PE in the UK. Confidential Enquiry into Maternal Mortality, the diagnosis was not made antemortem because of the mistaken belief that diagnostic testing would be harmful to the fetus. Pulmonary angiogram is usually reserved for severe cases in which localization of embolus is necessary prior to embolectomy.

Management

Treatment of VTE in pregnancy involves anticoagulation with low-molecular-weight heparin (LMWH) or unfractionated heparin (UFH). Dosing is weight based, and may require increases with increasing gestation. Warfarin is a known human teratogen and its use in pregnancy is contraindicated for this indication. **Table 221-16** lists medications for treatment of acute DVT and PE in pregnancy.

Most centers maintain patients on full therapeutic anticoagulation for the rest of their pregnancy until 6 weeks postpartum or at least 6 months, whichever is longer. Trials investigating lowering the intensity of anticoagulation after 4 to 12 weeks are currently

TABLE 221-16 Medications for Treatment of Venous Thromboembolism in Pregnancy

Drug	Dose	Route	Frequency
Unfractionated heparin	80 units/kg bolus, then 18 units/kg/h	Intravenous	Continuous, with dose adjustment using a PTT values
Enoxaparin	1 mg/kg	Subcutaneous (SQ)	Every 12 h. Due to increased clearance once daily dosing at 1.5 mg/kg may not be adequate
Tinzaparin	175 units/kg	SQ	Every 24 h
Dalteparin	200 units/kg	SQ	Every 24 h

TABLE 221-17 Suggested Regimens for Thromboprophylaxis in Pregnancy

1. Enoxaparin 40 mg SQ once daily until 20 wk gestation, then 40 mg twice daily. At 36-wk gestation, switch to UFH 10,000 units SQ twice daily until delivery
2. UFH 5000 units SQ twice daily in the first trimester, 7500 units SQ twice daily in the second trimester, and 10,000 units SQ twice daily in the third trimester

Suggested regimens for postpartum prophylaxis

1. Enoxaparin 40 mg SQ once daily
2. Warfarin, with target INR of 1.5-2

UFH 5000 units SQ twice daily

INR, international normalized ratio; SQ, suncutaneously; UFH, unfractionated heparin.

underway, but this practice has not yet been validated in pregnancy. LMWH is the preferred agent in pregnancy, and has been associated with less thrombocytopenia and osteoporosis. Weight gain, increased blood volume, and increased clearance with pregnancy progression may require change in dosing, but this is usually guided by checking peak anti-Xa levels, which are done monthly.

Peripartum management of anticoagulation can be challenging. Epidural analgesia for pain control during labor or spinal anesthesia may be necessary for an operative delivery. Guidelines from the American society of Regional Anesthesia and Pain management (ASRA) recommend that in patients on therapeutic doses of LMWH, regional anesthesia be delayed at least 24 hours after last dose of LMWH injection to decrease the risk of spinal hematoma. This may be possible in a patient undergoing an elective induction of labor, but in most cases, the onset of labor cannot be predicted. We therefore switch the patient over to subcutaneous unfractionated heparin in the last month of pregnancy, two or three times a day, at a dose sufficient to keep the mid-interval aPTT approximately twice normal. The patient is instructed to stop heparin injections at the first sign of labor and aPTT is monitored closely once the patient is admitted to the hospital. Provided the aPTT is normal, regional anesthesia can be used with no contraindication. Following delivery, LMWH can be resumed 24 hours after removal of epidural or spinal catheter. In the postpartum period, warfarin can be safely used, even in breastfeeding mothers. Anecdotal evidence suggests that there is increased incidence of bleeding from surgical sites during the overlap of warfarin and LMWH. In patients who have had an operative delivery, we usually start warfarin 2 weeks after delivery, to avoid the risk of surgical bleeding.

Women with prior VTE are believed to have a higher risk of recurrent VTE in a subsequent pregnancy. There is evidence to suggest that this is especially true in patients whose first event was related to pregnancy, puerperium, or oral contraceptive use. An underlying thrombophilia and a family history of VTE are considered additional risk factors. Thromboprophylaxis is therefore recommended in these patients in subsequent pregnancies. **Table 221-17** lists some anticoagulant prophylaxis regimens in pregnancy and the postpartum period. Prophylaxis needs to be continued for 6 weeks postpartum.

CONCLUSION

Any hospitalized patient of childbearing age contemplating children should have optimal medical management and counseling prior to becoming pregnant. Clinicians should take steps to identify coexisting diseases in the pregnant patient and complications of pregnancy before they become more severe. Optimally, management of medical problems requires prevention strategies to reduce progression of illness that would otherwise necessitate multiple medications, emergency treatment, and readmissions to the hospital. Team management of these patients with obstetric internists, high-risk obstetricians, and appropriate subspecialty consultation is recommended to achieve optimal medical status and function. Care of this unique population also requires optimal communication among team members so that it is clear who will be responsible for monitoring treatment and patient and family education.

SUGGESTED READINGS

Bourjeily G, Paidas M, Khalil H, Rosene-Montella K, Rodger M. Pulmonary embolism in pregnancy. *Lancet*. 2010;375(9713):500-512.

Brito V, Niederman MS. Pneumonia complicating pregnancy. *Clin Chest Med*. 2011;32(1):121-132.

Cole DE, Taylor TL, McCullough DM, Shoff CT, Derdak S. Acute respiratory distress in pregnancy. *Crit Care Med*. 2005;33(suppl 10):S269-S278.

Gammill HS, Jeyabalan A. Acute renal failure in pregnancy. *Crit Care Med*. 2005;33(suppl 10):S372-S384.

Janakiraman V. Listeriosis in pregnancy: diagnosis, treatment, and prevention. *Rev Obstet Gynecol*. 2008;1(4):179-185.

Joshi D, James A, Quaglia A, Westbrook RH, Heneghan MA. Liver disease in pregnancy. *Lancet*. 2010;375(9714):594-605.

Lal A, Anderson G, Cowen M, Lindow S, Arnold AG. NAEP Guidelines. *Chest*. 2007;(132)3:1044-1048.

Macejko AM, Schaeffer AJ. Asymptomatic bacteriuria and symptomatic urinary tract infections during pregnancy. *Urol Clin North Am*. 2007;34(1):35-42.

Mantel GD. Care of the critically ill parturient: oliguria and renal failure. *Best Prac Res Clin Obstet Gynecol*. 2001;15(4):563-581.

Mittal P, Wing DA. Urinary tract infections in pregnancy. *ClinPerinatol*. 2005;32(3):749-764.

Munnur U, Bandi VD, Guntupalli KK. Management principles of the critically ill obstetric patient. *Clin Chest Med*. 2011;32(1):53-60.

Nwoko R, Plecas D, Garovic VD. Acute kidney injury in the pregnant patient. *Clin Nephrol*. 2012;78(6):478-486.

Reddy SS, Holley JL. Management of the pregnant chronic dialysis patient. *Advances in chronic kidney disease*. 2007;14(2):146-155.

Semins MJ, Matlaga BR. Kidney stones in pregnancy. *Nat Rev Urol*. 2014;11(3):163-168.

Sheffield JS, Cunningham FG. Urinary tract infection in women. *Obstet Gynecol*. 2005;106(5 Pt 1):1085-1092.

CHAPTER 222

Postpartum Consultation for Common Complaints

Courtney Bilodeau , MD
Karen Rosene-Montella, MD

Key Clinical Questions

1. What are the common causes of postpartum fever?
2. What antibiotics are recommended for common postpartum infections?
3. What is the differential diagnosis for a postpartum headache?
4. When does a postpartum headache require radiologic imaging?
5. What are the common postpartum neuropathies?

INTRODUCTION

The postpartum period, lasting 6 months, is a unique time during which there is a physiological return to the prepregnancy state. Night sweats, mood disturbance, urinary frequency, perineal and vaginal discomfort, and breast engorgement are all common complaints from postpartum women. Clinicians treating postpartum patients in the hospital setting must be able to differentiate these normal changes from disease states.

POSTPARTUM FEVER

■ EPIDEMIOLOGY AND RISK STRATIFICATION

Low-grade fever frequently occurs in the first 24 hours after delivery. Postpartum fever is defined as a temperature of ≥ 38.0°C (100.4°F) on any two of the first 10 days postpartum exclusive of the first 24 hours. Infection is the leading cause of postpartum fever in the United States; the overall postpartum infection rate is around 6%, with the incidence in planned cesarean deliveries up to 10%, and higher in unplanned deliveries. Endometritis is the most common infection in the postpartum period, followed by urinary tract infection, lower genital tract infection, wound infection, pulmonary infection, thrombophlebitis, cholecystitis, and breast infections. Mastitis and abscess are rare in women who do not breastfeed but occur in 2% to 3% of breastfeeding women. A recent pregnancy also increases the risk for pneumonia, appendicitis, and cholecystitis.

EVALUATION AND INPATIENT MANAGEMENT

■ POSTPARTUM ENDOMETRITIS

Postpartum endometritis is typically a polymicrobial infection with lower genital tract flora infecting the upper genital tract. The prevalence of endometritis has been greatly reduced with the standard use of antibiotic prophylaxis with cesarean deliveries. The risk of endometritis is increased by various factors listed in **Table 222-1**.

The criteria for diagnosis of endometritis include fever and uterine tenderness. Other signs and symptoms include foul lochia and chills. The postpartum uterus should be firm, nontender, and below the umbilicus; with endometritis a soft, subinvoluted uterus may lead to excessive vaginal bleeding.

When endometritis is suspected, laboratory or imaging data are rarely needed before initiating treatment. If despite treatment, a patient has persistent fever or unusually severe or localized pain, further studies may be helpful. A white blood cell with differential, blood cultures (which are positive in 10%-20% of patients), and endometrial cultures may be diagnostic and can help direct antimicrobial therapy. Endometrial cultures should be acquired with a double or triple lumen technique to prevent vaginal and cervical contamination. Pelvic ultrasonography can identify retained products of conception, which need to be removed by dilatation and curettage because they are an ongoing nidus of infection. Computed tomography (CT) or magnetic resonance imaging (MRI) is used to diagnose alternative causes of persistent pain and fever including ovarian vein thrombosis, abscess, or hematoma. Please refer to a full discussion of ovarian vein thrombosis in Chapter 221 (Common Medical Problems in Pregnancy).

The most common infectious agents when endometritis is suspected in the first 24 to 48 hours postpartum are Gram-positive cocci (predominantly group B streptococci, *Staphylococcus epidermidis,* and *Enterococcus* spp.) or Gram-negative bacteria

TABLE 222-1 Risk Factors of Endometritis

Prolonged labor

Prolonged rupture of membranes

Multiple vaginal examinations

Operative vaginal delivery

Bacterial vaginosis

Chorioamnionitis

Cesarean section (especially nonelective)

Antepartum isolation of group B streptococci, Chlamydia, or mycoplasma

(predominantly *Gardnerella vaginalis, Escherichia coli, Klebsiella pneumoniae,* and *Proteus mirabilis*). After 48 hours, involvement of anaerobic bacteria (predominantly *peptostreptococci, Bacteroides* spp., and *Prevotella* spp.) is likely, and by 7 days, *Chlamydia trachomatis* is often found. The treatment regimen for postpartum endometritis includes broad-spectrum parenteral antibiotics. In the first 48 hours after delivery, the recommended regimen is clindamycin (900 mg every 8 hours) plus gentamicin (1.75 mg/kg every 8 hours or 5 mg/kg every 24 hours). If there is persistent fever or enterococcus is suspected, ampicillin or vancomycin in penicillin allergy should be added. Alternative regimens include cefotetan, cefoxitin, piperacillin/tazobactam, and ampicillin/sulbactam. Treatment continues until a patient has been afebrile for 48 hours and uterine tenderness has resolved. Oral therapy after parenteral therapy is not recommended as there is no evidence for improved outcome or decreased risk of recurrence. However, patients with bacteremia confirmed by positive blood cultures should complete a 7- to 10-day course of antibiotics. Late postpartum endometritis (48 hours-6 weeks postpartum) may be treated with oral metronidazole and doxycycline (100 mg IV or orally every 12 hours) for 14 days.

■ BREAST INFECTION

The majority of postpartum patients experience breast discomfort with swollen, firm, and tender breasts. Simple engorgement causes low-grade fevers without any other clinical signs of infection and typically resolves within 48 hours. The patient with a breast infection may describe chills, flu-like symptoms, and have high fevers (102°F-104°F). Mastitis causes localized erythema and swelling with a cellulitic appearance. A breast abscess is characterized by fluctuance and diffuse erythema, with a localized area of tenderness.

The most frequent pathogen in postpartum breast infection is *Staphylococcus aureus* and toxic shock has been reported with mastitis in the postpartum period. Other less common pathogens include β-hemolytic streptococci, *Haemophilus influenzae, Haemophilus parainfluenzae, E. coli,* and *K. pneumoniae.*

Clinical evaluation includes culture of expressed breast milk and aspirated fluid if there is a fluctuant mass. Prompt antibiotic treatment is required and should continue for 7 days or until resolution of infection. Recommended antibiotic coverage includes clindamycin 300 mg orally three times a day, dicloxacillin 500 mg orally every 6 hours, or cephalexin 500 mg orally every 6 hours. Alternative regimens include amoxicillin/clavulanate 875 mg orally every 12 hours or azithromycin 500 mg orally initially, then 250 mg orally daily. If methicillin-resistant *S. aureus* (MRSA) is suspected then TMP-SMX-DS orally every 12 hours or vancomycin 1 g IV every 12 hours are recommended.

For mastitis, the patient should be encouraged to avoid milk stasis by continuing to nurse or pump expressed milk. Hot compresses also aid in comfort and expression of milk. Patients should be closely followed as an abscess can develop even after antibiotics have begun. If a patient has a breast abscess, then incision and drainage or needle aspiration may be warranted. Patients with breast abscesses should be advised to discontinue breastfeeding until after drainage is performed, if indicated, and signs of infection are resolved. In communities with a high rate of MRSA, it is found in up to 50% of women with postpartum breast abscesses.

PRACTICE POINT

- Pregnant patients have decreased buffering capacity, increased cardiac output, and decreased systemic vascular resistance so patients with sepsis related to postpartum infection may decompensate quickly. Prompt action with close follow-up is recommended.

■ POSTACUTE CARE AND DISCHARGE CHECKLIST

Once diagnosis is confirmed and treatment established the febrile postpartum patient should have postdischarge follow-up with an outpatient provider. The patient should be aware of the medication instructions and expected course of the infection. A patient should also be warned of the symptoms such as recurrent fever, pain or intolerance to medications that prompt immediate medical attention.

POSTPARTUM HEADACHE
■ RISK STRATIFICATION

Hormonal fluctuations, sleep deprivation, and anxiety all contribute to the increased frequency of headaches in the postpartum period. The differential diagnosis of headache varies from minor to life-threatening causes and therefore warrants a prompt and thorough clinical evaluation. Alarm symptoms that warrant emergent evaluation with neurologic imaging include headache of acute onset, abnormal or focal neurologic findings, seizure, and/or decreased level of consciousness. If a postpartum patient has a new Horner's syndrome, the anterior and posterior circulation should be imaged at the same time to rule out dissection. The hypercoagulable state present during pregnancy and postpartum is a significant risk factor for thrombosis, including cerebral venous thrombosis. Additional risk factors include thrombophilia, cesarean section, anemia, dehydration, and infection.

■ EPIDEMIOLOGY

Migraines have an increased predominance in the postpuberty years of females over males, suggesting a role of ovarian sex hormones in their pathogenesis. It is thought that migraines may be trigged by the decline of estrogen levels after a period of elevated estrogen, which occurs during the menstrual and postpartum periods. The majority of women who suffer from migraines have an improvement during pregnancy, and 30% to 50% of women experience a recurrence postpartum. Tension-type headaches (TTHSs) are the most common type of headaches in adulthood. Similar to migraines, there is a female predominance in TTHS prevalence, suggesting a female sex hormone contribution to their pathophysiology. There are fewer studies on TTHS in pregnancy compared with migraines, but remission in pregnancy and recurrence in postpartum has been suggested. The accidental dural puncture (ADP) rate with epidural insertion is rare amongst practiced obstetric anesthesiologist (<2%). However when ADP occurs the headache incidence is 60% to 80%. The incidence of cerebral vein thrombosis (CVT), subarachnoid hemorrhage, and posterior reversible encephalopathy syndrome (PRES), especially in association with preeclampsia, increases in the postpartum period. In adulthood, CVT is more common in women than men, with 75% of cases found in women.

■ EVALUATION AND INPATIENT MANAGEMENT

Table 222-2 summarizes the differential diagnosis of postpartum headache along with common features, and modes of evaluation or treatment.

PRACTICE POINT

- Women with a history of headaches outside of pregnancy often have an increased frequency in the postpartum. Most common treatments for migraine, tension and cluster headaches are safe in the postpartum, including with lactation. Preeclampsia and a cerebrovascular event should always be considered in a postpartum patient with a severe headache.

■ POSTACUTE CARE AND DISCHARGE CHECKLIST

Depending on the nature of the headache in postpartum, a patient may warrant follow-up with a headache specialist for long-term management and prevention. A patient should be warned of the risk for medication overuse headaches if treatments such as acetaminophen or NSAIDs are used on a daily basis.

POSTPARTUM NEUROPATHIES

■ EPIDEMIOLOGY AND RISK STRATIFICATION

Neuropathies are common in the postpartum period. An inpatient postpartum woman with new neurologic complaints warrants a thorough history and physical exam to rule more ominous causes of neurologic changes such as a stroke.

■ EVALUATION AND INPATIENT MANAGEMENT

Bell's palsy

Bell's palsy, facial nerve palsy, is caused by compression or ischemia to the nerve. Bell's palsy is most commonly seen in the third trimester, but can be seen in the postpartum period. After careful examination, treatment includes reassurance, as the majority of patients gradually improve within 3 months. Corticosteroids and antivirals should be considered for treatment to shorten the course and limit long-term sequelae. Both have been used safely in pregnancy. Bell's palsy may be a presenting feature of preeclampsia, probably related to edema. All patients with Bell's palsy are at risk for eye dryness and corneal injury, therefore artificial tears during the day and a lubricant at night is recommended.

Carpal tunnel syndrome (CTS)

The edema from fluid retention in pregnancy can predispose women to median nerve entrapment causing CTS. The symptoms can first present in the postpartum period and may last until after weaning in breastfeeding women. Due to the transient nature of CTS in the postpartum period, conservative management is recommended. This includes wrist splints, modifications of daily activities that exacerbate symptoms, and NSAIDs. As in nonpregnant patients, hypothyroidism should be excluded.

de Quervain tenosynovitis

Stenosing tenosynovitis of the first dorsal compartment of the wrist, known as de Quervain tenosynovitis, may occur during the postpartum period due to repetitive activities in newborn care. Ice and NSAIDs and physical and/or occupational therapy may be used for symptomatic relief.

TABLE 222-2 Postpartum Headache

Cause of Headache	Common Features	Treatment/ Evaluation
Migraine	Bifrontal, prolonged, and pulsatile Other: nausea, vomiting, and aversion to loud noise, bright light, and physical activity	Acetaminophen, NSAIDS, caffeine, opiods, triptans Severe: intravenous hydration, antiemetics, and steroids
Tension-type	Bifrontal, bioccipital or neck with squeezing and aching Other: nausea, light, and sound sensitivity	Acetaminophen, NSAIDS, caffeine, opiods Alternative therapies: relaxation techniques, biofeedback, and physical therapy
Cluster	Unilateral, orbito-temporal and nonthrobbing, penetrating Other: ptosis, conjunctival injection, or lacrimation	Oxygen, intranasal lidocaine, triptans
Postdural puncture	Severe, postural (worse with sitting up or standing)	Blood patch, intravenous fluid
Cerebral vein thrombosis	Severe headache (gradual or acute) Other: focal neurological signs (motor, sensation, aphasia), disordered consciousness, seizure, papilledema, nuchal rigidity, intracranial hypertension	MRI/V, CT venography, cerebral angiography. Treatment may include intravenous mannitol, neurosurgical intervention, anticoagulation, or thrombolysis
Subarachnoid hemorrhage (Arteriovenous malformation or aneurysm)	Mild to severe sudden, diffuse headache Other: nausea and vomiting, confusion, focal neurologic deficit, nuchal rigidity, intraocular hemorrhages, hypertension, hypoxemia, ECG changes	Head CT or MRI, Lumbar puncture Treatment includes blood pressure and pain control, possible neurosurgical intervention
Posterior reversible encephalopathy syndrome (PRES)	Severe diffuse headache, confusion, seizure, and visual abnormalities	MRI Blood pressure management
Preeclampsia	Vascular headache Visual complaints Sudden, severe headache	PRES Intracerebral bleed Laboratory findings of preeclampsia, hypertension

---

Lumbosacral spine and lower-extremity nerve injuries

While rare, stretch and compression nerve injuries may occur during vaginal and cesarean section deliveries. Risk of these injuries is increased by prolonged labor and fetal macrosomia or malposition. Lateral femoral cutaneous nerve injury (also known as meralgiaparesthetica) is a sensory-only deficit of the anterolateral thigh that is a common postpartum complaint. Femoral nerve injury can cause decreased sensation in the anterolateral thigh and medial calf along with impaired knee extension. Common peroneal nerve injury causes decreased sensation at the anterloateral calf and dorsum of the foot and foot drop. Obturator nerve injury causes decreased sensation to the medial thigh and decreased adduction of the leg. Prognosis from these injuries is typically good, and physical therapy may play a role in recovery.

PRACTICE POINT

- Postpartum patients commonly experience neuropathies. A thorough physical exam is typically sufficient to diagnose a neuropathy. However, a low threshold for further studies and specialist consultation is warranted when alarm symptoms develop. A neuropathy may occur as a secondary complaint in a more severe condition, such as Bell's palsy in an edematous preeclamptic patient.

■ POSTACUTE CARE AND DISCHARGE CHECKLIST

The postpartum patient should be advised of the expected duration for their neuropathy symptoms and told when to seek medical attention if symptoms worsen or fail to resolve. If medication is needed for symptom relief, clinicians should consider medication metabolism as the patient returns to the prepregnancy state, and how these and any new medications may impact the breastfed infant.

SUGGESTED READINGS

Berg CJ, MacKay AP, Qin C, et al. Overview of maternal morbidity during hospitalization for labor and delivery in the United States 1993–1997 and 2001–2005. *Obstet Gynecol.* 2009;113:1075-1081.

Jahanfar S, Ng CJ, Teng CL. Antibiotics for mastitis in breastfeeding women. *Cochrane Database Syst Rev.* 2013.

Katz VL. Postpartum care. In: Gabbe SG, Niebyl JR, Simpson JL, eds. *Obstetrics: Normal and Problem Pregnancies*, 5th ed. Philadelphia, PA: Churchill Livingstone; 2007:566-576.

Ko ML, Pan HS, Huang LW. Posterior reversible encephalopathy syndrome in a pregnant woman. *Taiwan J Obstet Gynecol.* 2008;47(1):98-100.

Pearce CF, Hansen WF. Headache and neurological disease in pregnancy. *Clin Obstet Gynecol.* 2012;55:810-828.

Rosene K, Eschenbach DA, Tompkins LS, et al. Polymicrobial early postpartum endometritis with facultative and anaerobic bacteria, genital mycoplasmas, and chlamydia trachomatis: treatment with piperacillin or cefoxitin. *J Infect Dis.* 1986;153(6):1028-1037.

Yokoe DS, Christiansen CL, Johnson R, et al. Epidemiology of and surveillance for postpartum infectious. *Emerg Infect Dis.* 2001;7(5):837-841.

SECTION 13

Psychiatry

CHAPTER 223

Mood and Anxiety Disorders

Martha C. Ward, MD
Steven Garlow, MD, PhD

Key Clinical Questions

Depression

❶ What are the signs and symptoms of a major depressive episode (MDE)?

❷ What is the pathophysiology of major depression?

❸ What medications, intoxicants, and diseases cause depressed mood?

❹ What is adjustment disorder?

❺ What is the appropriate diagnostic workup for a patient with depressive symptoms?

❻ What is the treatment for major depressive disorder (MDD)?

❼ What are the complications of antidepressant use?

Bipolar Disorder

❶ What are the signs and symptoms of bipolar disorder?

❷ What medical conditions and substances can induce mania?

❸ What is the appropriate diagnostic workup for a patient with mania?

❹ How is bipolar disorder treated?

Anxiety Disorders

❶ What are the signs and symptoms of anxiety?

❷ What are the common anxiety disorders?

❸ How does generalized anxiety disorder (GAD) differ from major depression?

❹ What medical conditions present with symptoms of anxiety?

❺ What studies should be ordered for the acutely anxious patient?

❻ What is the treatment for anxiety?

MAJOR DEPRESSIVE DISORDER

■ INTRODUCTION

Major depressive disorder (MDD) is widespread and devastating, with lifetime prevalence greater than 17% in the general population. Total costs exceed $44 billion annually, including hospitalization, medications, and loss of productivity. In medically ill patients, mood disorders are even more common; 6-month prevalence increases from 5.8% to 9.4% with at least one chronic medical condition. Despite this, many physicians fail to address depressive symptoms, believing them to be appropriate in illness ("I would be depressed too, if I were that sick"). This misconception leads to poor outcomes, as physical recovery is impeded by affective disorders.

CASE 223-1

A 66-year-old man with a history of type-2 diabetes, hypertension, and tobacco use was admitted for non-ST elevation myocardial infarction (MI) and cardiac catheterization with stent placement. During morning rounds, his care team noted that the patient ate only about 10% of his breakfast and appeared to have a blunted affect. He had a history of multiple episodes of depressed mood, insomnia, and anhedonia over the years. The patient reported feeling "worthless" and sometimes wishing that he had "just gone ahead and died." Though initially reluctant because of worries about dependence, Mr G agreed to try an antidepressant, sertraline. At his 6-week posthospitalization appointment he is free of mood symptoms, engaged in cardiac rehabilitation and feels hopeful about the future.

PATHOPHYSIOLOGY

The primary etiology of major depression remains obscure. Dysregulation of central nervous system (CNS) monoamine neurotransmitters (including norepinephrine, serotonin, and dopamine) occurs in MDD. Newer theories focus on broader neuroregulatory circuits involving cholingeric activation, GABA hypoactivity, and chronically elevated hypothalamic-pituitary-adrenal activity. Immune system abnormalities and increased inflammation likely play a role, particularly in medically ill individuals.

■ DIAGNOSIS

Major depressive disorder

Major depressive disorder is defined by the occurrence of one or more major depressive episodes (see **Table 223-1**). Though many patients will readily admit to feeling "sad" or "down," others may initially deny dysphoria, imagining this to reflect a weakness of character. Direct confrontation may not be fruitful, though observational statements made in a neutral tone might aid with patient disclosure ("you're upset"). In such cases, mood changes can also be determined by the presence of tearfulness or blunted effect. Depressed mood may also manifest as irritability, particularly in adolescence. However, caution must be taken not to label the angry patient "depressed" in the absence of other signs of MDD. There is a distinct quality and severity of mood in MDD that differs from mere sadness, and the patient who is simply despondent should likewise not be diagnosed with this disorder.

Loss of interest, or anhedonia, is the most common presenting symptom in MDD (particularly in the elderly). This may be difficult to

TABLE 223-1 Major Depressive Episode

A. Five (or more) symptoms present for 2 wk with either (1) depressed mood or (2) loss of interest or pleasure:

1. Depressed mood most of the day
2. Diminished interest or pleasure in all, or almost all, activities
3. Significant weight loss or gain (change in 5% body weight in 1 mo or decrease or increase in appetite)
4. Insomnia or hypersomnia
5. Psychomotor agitation or retardation (observable by others)
6. Fatigue or loss of energy
7. Feelings of worthlessness or excessive guilt (not merely self-reproach about being sick)
8. Diminished ability to think or concentrate or indecisiveness
9. Recurrent thoughts of death (not just fear of dying), recurrent suicidal ideation with or without a plan, or suicide attempt

B. The symptoms cause significant distress or impairment.

C. The symptoms are not due to the effects of a substance or a general medical condition.

D. The occurrence of the major depressive episode is not better explained by schizoaffective disorder or another psychotic disorder.

E. There has never been a manic episode or a hypomanic episode.

TABLE 223-2 Distinguishing Grief from a Major Depressive Episode

Grief	Major Depressive Episode
Feelings of emptiness and loss	Persistent depressed mood and the inability to anticipate happiness or pleasure
Decreases in intensity over days to weeks and occurs in waves, associated with thoughts or reminders of the loss of health or function	Persistent and not tied to specific thoughts or preoccupations
Dysphoria may be accompanied by positive emotions and humor	Pervasive unhappiness and misery
Thought content features a preoccupation with thoughts of loss and memories of life before the loss	Thought content features self-critical or pessimistic ruminations
Self-esteem is preserved; if self-derogatory ideation is present, it typically involves perceived failings vis-à-vis the loss	Feelings of worthlessness and self-loathing are common
Does not involve suicidal ideation	May entail thoughts of ending one's own life because of feeling worthless, undeserving of life, or unable to cope with the pain of depression

identify in the context of hospitalization, where the patient's usual pleasurable activities are curtailed. Lack of engagement with family members or other visitors, as well as refusal to participate in physical therapy, may indicate anhedonia. Anorexia, fatigue, insomnia, and poor concentration may be easily attributed to the direct effects of medical illness. However, if a patient also shows depressed mood and lack of interest, these qualities should be counted toward the diagnosis of MDD. Assessment of insomnia should focus on pattern of sleep and activities during nighttime awakening, as sleeplessness in the hospital may be due to poorly controlled pain or frequent visits by caregivers. Middle insomnia (waking in the night and not being able to return to sleep) and early awakening are more typical of depression, and patients often ruminate on negative thoughts. Guilt about illness is a common symptom. Patients may express concern about not meeting financial and interpersonal obligations or about being a burden to their loved ones.

Assessment of suicidality must be direct and avoid euphemisms such as "hurting yourself." Questions should elicit increasing levels of intent. First ask about passive ideation ("do you ever feel so bad that you wish you were not alive?"). When an affirmative is given, questioning should then focus on active suicidal thoughts and designs. If the patient has access to firearms or potentially toxic medications, a plan should be made for securing them prior to discharge.

Though not explicitly delineated in the Diagnostic and Statistical Manual of Mental Disorders (DSM) criteria, somatic complaints may be a manifestation of depression. Individuals with psychiatric pathology may experience physical discomfort out of proportion to the severity of medical disease. Patients may also have functional pain, consciously or unconsciously converting depressed mood into more culturally sanctioned symptoms.

Medical illness or disability may represent a significant loss to the patient, and can include feelings of intense sadness as well as other symptoms consistent with a depressive episode. Recognition of a major depressive episode in addition to a normal grief response may

be challenging, and the individual's history and the cultural norms for the expression of distress should be taken into account. **Table 223-2** highlights some differences between a major depressive episode and a grief response that may aid in distinguishing these diagnoses.

Substance/medication-induced depressive disorder

Medications and intoxicants can both cause depressive symptoms (see **Table 223-3**). Defining the temporal relationship between onset of mood disturbance and start of a new drug can help

TABLE 223-3 Substance/Medication-Induced Depressive Disorder

A. A prominent and persistent disturbance in mood predominates in the clinical picture and is characterized by either

1. depressed mood, or
2. markedly diminished interest or pleasure in all, or almost all, activities.

B. There is evidence from the history, physical examination, or lab findings that the symptoms in Criterion A developed during or soon after substance intoxication or withdrawal or after exposure to a medication, and the involved substance/medication is capable of producing the symptoms in Criterion A.

C. The disturbance is not better accounted for by another depressive disorder.

D. The disturbance does not occur exclusively in the context of a delirium.

E. The symptoms cause clinically significant distress or impairment in social, occupational, or other important areas of functioning.

TABLE 223-4 Pharmacological Causes of Depression

1. Interferon and other immunomodulators
2. Corticosteroids and hormones
3. Antineoplastic agents (antiestrogens, antiandrogens; to a lesser extent, vincristine, vinblastine, procarbazine, and asparaginase)
4. Neurological agents, such as levodopa and acetylcholinesterase inhibitors, as well as antiepileptics
5. Antipsychotics
6. Sedative-hypnotics
7. Analgesics (particularly opioids and NSAIDs)
8. Antibacterials (especially sulfonamides) and antifungals
9. Cardiovascular drugs: antihypertensives, digoxin

determine this correlation. **Table 223-4** lists commonly prescribed offending medications.

Chronic alcohol use leads to depressed mood. Forty percent of patients with an alcohol-related disorder meet criteria for MDD at some point in their lives. Diagnosis of major depression in the context of active alcohol use is difficult at best, and treatment with antidepressants in this situation can be deleterious and even dangerous. Abuse of other sedative-hypnotics (benzodiazepines [BZDs] and barbiturates), as well as opiates, can similarly produce a mood disturbance. Stimulants (cocaine and amphetamines) potentiate monoamine neurotransmitters, leading to depletion and subsequent depressed mood. Effects of stimulants on the brain linger for months to years following cessation.

Addicts usually downplay their drug and alcohol use. Inquiries into the frequency of ingestion and the amount consumed should always be overestimated, and clues must be obtained, including collateral from friends and family. Objective measures, such as a urine drug screen and serum ethanol level, may also provide further insight.

Depressive disorder due to another medical condition

To meet criteria for depression due to another medical condition, it is not necessary to have symptoms for any duration of time or to exhibit a certain number of characteristics. Patients must simply display anhedonia or depressed mood that interferes with function and is directly caused by medical illness. When direct causality is not definite, patients should be diagnosed with MDD. However, this is purely a semantic differentiation and should not affect treatment decisions.

Heart disease and major depression are frequently comorbid. In hospitalized patients who have suffered an MI, 65% show depressive symptoms and 30% meet criteria for MDD. Depression in the post-MI period imparts a four- to sixfold increased risk of cardiac mortality at 6 and 18 months (independent of epidemiologic factors, medications, or severity of disease). Despite this, only 10% of post-MI patients are diagnosed with MDD in the hospital. This may be due to its anomalous presentation, with hostility and withdrawal more common. Unfortunately, depressed mood may be assessed as appropriate in patients suffering an MI, with many physicians stating, "I would be depressed too if I just had a heart attack." This conclusion is not only incorrect (as not all patients have post-MI MDD), but can lead to unnecessary suffering and poor patient outcomes.

Mood symptoms are common in cancer, particularly in pancreatic carcinoma and other enteric malignancies. Rates increase in those with a prior psychiatric history. Depression may precede diagnosis, potentially caused by a paraneoplastic process or proinflammatory cytokines. Alternatively, mood changes may occur after cancer is

discovered. As previously stated, major depression can be difficult to differentiate from the existential crisis that arises from the diagnosis. Determination of MDD can also be complicated by its significant symptom overlap with treatment side effects and the disease process itself. Fatigue is frequently described. Lethargy due to radiation and chemotherapy is cyclical, with recovery occurring as time from treatment increases. Fatigue in major depression is akin to amotivation, with difficulty starting tasks and prominent psychomotor retardation. Appropriate diagnosis is further waylaid by the hesitancy of patients to admit to mood changes. Those with cancer often take pride in coping with their illness and do not want to disappoint their doctors by showing signs of depression.

At least a third of stroke survivors experience depressive symptoms. The association is strongest in those with left hemispheric lesions, though physicians should screen for affective changes irrespective of vascular distribution. Degree of disability does not directly correlate to prevalence of mood disturbance, although poststroke depression imparts greater functional impairment, with less recovery in activities of daily living. Major depression also confers increased overall mortality in this population.

Autoimmune disease is closely linked to affective disorders. Close to half of individuals with systemic lupus erythematosus (SLE) meet criteria for MDD. Rates increase with greater disease severity and activity. Depressive symptoms are likely due to immune dysregulation, with proinflammatory cytokines modulating neural changes. Medications (particularly steroids) may also contribute to mood disturbance. Regardless of etiology, recognition and treatment is essential, as psychological distress in SLE leads to increased physical disability.

For a list of other medical diseases associated with depressed mood, see **Table 223-5**.

Adjustment disorder with depressed mood

Adjustment disorder is a pathologic response to a specific stressor (see **Table 223-6** for DSM-V criteria). Stressors may be multiple, such as financial strain in the context of physical disease. Patients with tumultuous childhoods (loss of a parent, unstable living situation)

TABLE 223-5 Diseases Associated with Depressed Mood

A. CNS Disease
1. Stroke
2. Dementia: Alzheimer, Huntington, Parkinson, Binswanger
3. Traumatic brain injury
4. Temporal lobe epilepsy
5. Tumor
6. Infections: encephalitis, hepatitis C, HIV
B. Endocrine disease
1. Hypothyroidism
2. Cushing syndrome
3. Hyper- or hypoparathyroidism
C. Rheumatologic disease
1. Systemic lupus erythematosus
2. Multiple sclerosis
3. Psoriasis
4. Rheumatoid arthritis
5. Fibromyalgia
6. Osteoarthritis
D. Cancer
E. Cardiovascular disease

TABLE 223-6 Adjustment Disorder

A. The development of emotional or behavioral symptoms in response to an identifiable stressor(s) occurring within 3 mo of the onset of the stressor(s).

B. These symptoms or behaviors are clinically significant as evidenced by

1. marked distress, in excess of what would be expected from stressor, or

2. significant impairment in social or occupational functioning.

C. The disturbance does not meet criteria for another mental disorder.

D. The symptoms do not represent bereavement.

E. Once the stressor has ended, symptoms do not persist for >6 mo.

are particularly at risk for this disorder. It is important to note that this diagnosis cannot be made if the criteria for major depression are met, or if mood symptoms are directly attributable to the effects of a substance or disease process.

Delirium

Hypoactive delirium may be mistaken for MDD. Both disorders involve problems with memory, but patients with major depression will have insight and complain of the deficit. Disorientation in delirium may result in complete reversal of day-night sleep-wake cycle. Sleep changes also occur with MDD, but patients have consistent insomnia or hypersomnia. Delirium has an abrupt onset and a fluctuating course. Major depression may also have a relatively discrete onset. However, it rarely has a waxing and waning course (except for melancholic depression, in which mood improves as the day progresses). Unlike MDD, delirium manifests with poor attention and altered level of consciousness.

Diagnostic studies

Laboratory evaluation of a patient with depressive symptoms can help to rule out an organic cause. A basic workup should include a complete blood count with differential, a comprehensive metabolic panel (including liver enzymes), thyroid-stimulating hormone, an RPR, an HIV test, B12 and folate levels, electrocardiogram, serum ethanol level, and a urine drug screen. Physical examination should direct the judicious use of further testing. The patient's medication list should be carefully reviewed for possible pharmacologic causes of depression.

■ TREATMENT

General treatment principles

There is no test that confirms the diagnosis of MDD. Likewise, there is no laboratory value that can be tracked to determine treatment response. Thus, target symptoms should be identified early and be well documented. This can assist subsequent care providers in determining the patient's baseline and progress. Because of the apparent subjective nature of this data, it may be helpful to administer a standardized rating scale at regular intervals. Clinician-rated scales, such as the Quick Inventory of Depressive Symptomatology (QIDS) Clinician Report, as well as patient-rated scales, such as the QIDS Self Report and Patient Health Questionnaire (PHQ)-9, are widely available.

While medication is an important treatment modality for depression, psychosocial interventions should be adjunctively employed whenever possible. This includes referrals to psychotherapy as well

as to support groups. Some patients may also benefit from meeting with the hospital chaplain. When end-of-life issues arise, palliative care teams are extremely helpful.

Patient education is essential. Physicians should discuss diagnosis, target symptoms, and treatment options. Serious side effects should be addressed, but not overemphasized. If a patient is reluctant to start treatment, the rationale should be elicited. Many hesitate to take antidepressants because of social stigma or misconceptions concerning drug dependence and personality changes.

Most classes of antidepressants have been shown to have roughly equal efficacy. Thus, initial selection of pharmacotherapy should focus on previous treatment success, family history of medication response, safety, tolerability, cost, and patient preference. Once a medication has been started, the goal is to titrate to an adequate dose and treat for an adequate period of time. The therapeutic dose differs based on physiology, and for the elderly may be lower than recommended doses. An adequate medication trial is usually defined as 8 to 12 weeks at the therapeutic dose. However, if there is no response after 4 to 5 weeks, a change in medication may be necessary. Duration of treatment for the first major depressive episode should be at least 12 months. In patients with recurrent episodes or depression due to a noncurable illness, lifelong treatment may be necessary. If a patient has been stable on a medication for years but decompensates when faced with a physical or emotional crisis, sudden discontinuation of the previously effective medication should be avoided. Instead, short-term interventions, such as dose increase or augmentation, should be employed.

Selective serotonin reuptake inhibitors (SSRIS), serotonin-norepinephrine reuptake inhibitors (SNRIS), and other antidepressants

Because of their tolerability, efficacy, and ease of dosing, the SSRIs are first-line treatment for major depression. The SNRIs (venlafaxine and duloxetine) may be a good choice for individuals with chronic pain because of the inhibitory effect of norepinephrine and serotonin on descending sensory neurons.

Other treatment options include nefazodone, trazodone, mirtazapine, and buproprion. Because it lowers the seizure threshold in a dose-dependent manner, buproprion should not be prescribed for patients with epilepsy, heavy alcohol use, or structural brain anomaly. Unlike the SSRIs, buproprion does not cause sexual dysfunction or weight gain. It can also aid in smoking cessation.

See **Table 223-7** for more information on the individual characteristics of these antidepressants.

Tricyclic antidepressants (TCAs)

The TCAs inhibit reuptake of norepinephrine and serotonin. These medications have significant anticholinergic, antihistaminergic, and antiadrenergic actions. The tertiary amines include amitriptylene, imipramine, trimipramine, doxepin, and chlomipramine. Desipramine, nortriptylene, and protriptylene are secondary amines. The secondary amines are less sedating and have less anticholinergic activity than the tertiary amines. At therapeutic doses, these medications have good efficacy. However, their use is often limited by side effects and drug interactions. Addition of medications that inhibit cytochrome P450 2D6 may cause serum TCA levels to rise to dangerous levels. Initiation of the tricyclics should occur in consultation with psychiatry. Medically ill patients who are maintained on TCAs should have cardiac monitoring, with daily repletion of potassium and magnesium.

Monoamine oxidase inhibitors

Monoamine oxidase (MAO) degrades biogenic amines in the CNS and gastrointestinal (GI) tract. Phenelzine, tranylcypromine,

TABLE 223-7 Properties of First-line Antidepressants

Medication	Dosing	Half-Life	P450 Inhibition	Side Effects and Toxicity
SSRIs				
Fluoxetine	20-80 mg	24-72 h, metabolite 4-16 d	2D6, 2C moderate 1A2, 3A	Initial anxiety, insomnia, sexual dysfunction
Paroxetine	10-50 mg	20 h	Strong 2D6	Nausea, headache, somnolence, dry mouth, constipation, dizziness
Sertraline	50-200 mg	24-26 h, metabolite 66 h	Minimal	Gastrointestinal upset, sleep disturbance, headache, sexual dysfunction
Citalopram	10-40 mg	33 h	Moderate 2D6	Nausea, vomiting, increased sweating, dry mouth, headache, ejaculatory failure
Escitalopram	10-20 mg	42 h	Minimal	Nausea, diarrhea, insomnia, dry mouth, ejaculatory failure
Fluvoxamine	50-300 mg	15 h	Strong 1A2, 3A, 2C	Nausea
SNRIs				
Venlafaxine	37.5-225 mg	4 h, metabolite 10 h	Minimal	Nausea, dizziness, somnolence, insomnia, nervousness, HTN
Duloxetine	40-120 mg	12 h	Moderate 2D6	Nausea, dry mouth, dizziness, headache, somnolence, constipation, insomnia
Other				
Trazodone	150-400 mg	5-9 h, metabolite 4-14 h	Minimal	Sedation, orthostasis, priapism in 1/6000 males, may decrease INR in patients taking coumadin
Nefazodone	200-600 mg	2-4 h, metabolite 18 h	Strong 3A	Dry mouth, sedation, dizziness, nausea, constipation, rare liver failure
Mirtazapine	7.5-45 mg	20-40 h	Minimal	Somnolence, increased appetite, weight gain
Buproprion	150-400 mg	21 h, metabolite 43 h	Strong 2D6	Headache, nausea, dry mouth, insomnia, agitation, lowers seizure threshold

isocarboxazid, and selegeline inhibit this enzyme. Despite their efficacy (particularly in atypical and anxious depression), these medications are considered third-line because of their adverse side effect profile as well as medication and food interactions. Monoamine oxidase inhibitors (MAOIs) can cause severe orthostasis, as well as sexual side effects, insomnia, headache, dizziness, dry mouth, and constipation. Ingestion of tyramine (present in aged cheeses, smoked or cured meats, wine, and beer) while taking an MAOI can lead to hypertensive emergency. Malignant hypertension is more likely to occur when MAOIs are taken with sympathomimetics and certain anesthetics (especially meperidine). Combination of MAOIs with other serotonergic agents can cause serotonin syndrome (see discussion below). Use of MAOIs should occur in consultation with psychiatry.

Electroconvulsive therapy (ECT) and transcranial magnetic stimulation (TMS)

ECT consists of the delivery of electricity to a patient's scalp in order to produce seizure activity. The patient is placed under general anesthesia and a neuromuscular blocking agent is given to inhibit muscle contraction. ECT is generally indicated for treatment-resistant depression and for states when immediate results are necessary for the patient's safety, such as suicidality, catatonia, or psychosis. Side effects include headache, dysphoria, muscle aches, and memory loss. Retrograde amnesia may be permanent. There are no absolute contraindications to ECT, and most of the risk ensues from anesthesia. Unstable cardiac or cerebrovascular disease increases risk. However, ECT is an efficacious and well-tolerated procedure for medically ill patients with severe depression who do not respond to pharmacotherapy or who cannot tolerate medication side effects.

Transcranial magnetic stimulation uses pulsed magnetic fields delivered transcranially to alter neuronal firing without producing

seizure activity. This noninvasive alternative to ECT has shown promising results in the treatment of depression, as well as in anxiety disorders. TMS is associated with fewer adverse effects than medications or other neuromodulatory procedures (such as ECT) and is generally well-tolerated.

Ketamine infusion for depression

Infusion of the NMDA receptor antagonist ketamine at subanaesthetic dose has been shown in multiple small studies to rapidly alleviate depressive symptoms in individuals suffering from major depression. Antidepressant effects of ketamine generally occur within hours of infusion, and may last 2 weeks. Addtionally, studies have shown an associated reduction in suicidal ideation in depressed patients that receive ketamine infusion. While direct acute toxicity is rare, ketamine may cause dissociative symptoms, and long-term abuse has been associated with damage to the gastrointestinal and urinary tracts.

Substance-induced depression

Necessary medications may cause depressive symptoms. When this is suspected, treatment substitutions or dose reduction (particularly with steroids) should be considered. If this is not possible, then the provider must take into account duration of treatment with the offending agent, level of dysfunction caused by mood symptoms, and patient willingness to add another medication. Certain medications (such as interferon) are notorious for inducing mood symptoms, and prophylactic treatment with an antidepressant is recommended.

When depression is caused by an intoxicant, the best course of action is clearly to discontinue its ingestion. Unfortunately, this is not often so simple. Patients with addiction may be unwilling (or unable) to quit using drugs and alcohol. Treatment with antidepressants in the context of continued intoxication will provide no relief of depressive symptoms and will not prevent the patient from using. When sobriety has been confirmed, yet depressive symptoms persist, there is no clear consensus as to time until treatment initiation. One reasonable approach would be to wait about 4 weeks after cessation to begin treatment for depression, particularly when the mood symptoms are causing impairment of function or extreme distress.

Depressive disorder due to another medical condition

If a medical condition is permanent and causes major depression, then pharmacotherapy should not be delayed. In cases in which medical illness is thought to be short-lived, the physician must consider the effects of the mood symptoms on the course of illness and the patient's quality of life. If mood symptoms cause suffering or worsen medical disease, treatment is indicated. The high prevalence of major depression in certain conditions may event merit prophylactic antidepressant use. In acute stroke survivors, there is evidence for prophylactic use of escitalopram.

■ TREATMENT OF DEPRESSION IN THE MEDICALLY ILL

Cardiovascular disease

The tricyclic antidepressants should likely be avoided in cardiovascular disease. Like class 1A antiarrythmics, these drugs may slow ventricular conduction by blocking sodium channels. This can lead to PR, QRS, and QT prolongation, torsades de pointes, and sudden cardiac death. Tricyclics also block myocardial muscarinic receptors, which can lead to tachycardia. The TCAs, like the MAOIs and trazodone, can also cause orthostasis. Conversely, venlafaxine and bupropion may elevate blood pressure, and should likely be avoided in patients with poorly-controlled hypertension. Fluoxetine can cause bradycardia when used with β-blockers, and both Fluoxetine and Fluvoxamine may decrease the efficacy of clopidogrel. Additionally, citalopram may be used with caution in indivduals with cardiovascular disease, particularly those predisposed to prolonged QTc. In 2011, the Federal Drug Administration issued the recommendation that the SSRI citalopram not be used at doses greater than 40 mg (and 20 mg in those with hepatic impairment or age >60) due to results of a randomized controlled trial that showed a dose-response increase in QTc. Otherwise, the SSRIs and mirtazapine are likely good first-line agents for the patient with cardiovascular disease.

Diabetes mellitus

Fluoxetine has been shown to decrease mean blood glucose and hemoglobin A1C levels. The TCAs can worsen glycemic control. However, their modulation of descending pain tracts may alleviate symptoms of peripheral neuropathy. MAOIs can interact with oral diabetes medications to potentiate hypoglycemia, and thus should be avoided in patients taking sulfonylureas and thiazolidinediones.

Hepatic disease

Nefazodone may induce fulminant hepatic failure (albeit rarely) and carries a boxed warning to this effect. Nearly all of the antidepressants (with the exception of escitalopram and to a lesser extent sertraline) are cleared through the CYP P450 system and thus doses should be decreased in liver impairment.

Renal insufficiency

Renal disease may slow clearance of medications, including antidepressants. Thus, dosage adjustments may be made. SSRIs and bupropion are the treatment of choice for patients with kidney failure.

■ COMPLICATIONS OF ANTIDEPRESSANT USE

Suicidality

The SSRIs carry a boxed warning concerning a risk of increased suicidal thinking and behavior in young adults. This is likely due to the activating properties of these medications. Patients must be warned of this possibility when starting treatment.

Serotonin syndrome

Use of serotonergic agents may cause autonomic hyperactivity (tachycardia, mydriasis, diarrhea, hyperthermia), neuromuscular abnormalities (tremor, clonus), and mental status changes (agitation, delirium). Certain drug combinations are more likely to cause toxicity, including MAOIs with SSRIs or TCAs. Meperedine, fentanyl, tramadol, ondansetron, metoclopramide, dextromethorphan, and ecstasy have also been triggers of this syndrome. Once the offending medications are discontinued, treatment is largely supportive. Benzodiazepines may be given to decrease agitation. Serotonin antagonists, such as cyproheptadine, olanzapine, and chlorpromazine may also be beneficial. In extreme cases, intubation and paralysis should be initiated.

SSRI/SNRI discontinuation syndrome

Abrupt discontinuation of SSRIs and SNRIs has been associated with flu like symptoms, myoclonus, electrical sensations, and psychological distress. Symptoms may last up to 2 weeks, and while uncomfortable, are not dangerous. This syndrome is more likely to occur with agents that have a short half-life, such as paroxetine, sertraline, fluvoxamine, and venlafaxine. It is best to taper these medications over a few weeks.

Overdose

As little as 10 times the daily dose of a TCA can be fatal. Death is most frequently caused by cardiac arrhythmia, though seizures and CNS depression also occur. MAOIs can induce hypertensive emergency in overdose. SSRIs are relatively benign when taken in excess, with very low risk of cardiovascular and CNS toxicity.

Discharge planning

Patients with a good response to antidepressants may be treated by their primary care physician. If there is a partial response or treatment failure after an adequate trial of more than one antidepressant, psychiatric referrals should be made. Suicidal patients require psychiatric hospitalization. The patient's cooperation with a voluntary admission is preferable, but involuntary status should be obtained for any patient who is a danger to himself or others. Additionally, patients who are unable to care for themselves due to the severity of their depression should be transferred to a mental health facility.

■ DISPARITIES IN HEALTH CARE

The prevalence of depression is largely uniform in African American, Latino, and Caucasian groups in the United States. Despite this, African Americans and Latinos have lower odds than whites of being diagnosed and treated for depression. African Americans and Latinos more often present with somatic complaints rather than mood symptoms, and nonwhite patients have been shown to be less likely to accept therapy for depression. In the Latino population, language barriers and poor health literacy may also complicate appropriate diagnosis.

■ PROGNOSIS

MDD is a chronic illness. Up to 75% of patients will have a second major depressive episode within 5 years from their initial event, though rates decrease with antidepressant treatment. In untreated MDD, relapse becomes increasingly frequent and severe.

BIPOLAR DISORDER

■ INTRODUCTION

Bipolar disorder is a catastrophic chronic illness. Despite a lifetime prevalence of just 1% in the general population, it incurs a significant financial burden with total costs exceeding $45 billion per year in the United States. Prevention of mood cycling through stable pharmacotherapy is crucial. Mania, whether primary (in bipolar disorder) or secondary to an organic cause, is a psychiatric emergency that can complicate the course of treatment for the medically ill. Prompt recognition is essential.

CASE 223-2

A 50-year-old woman with no past psychiatric history received high-dose steroids for a severe asthma exacerbation. On hospital day 2, the patient was seen naked, dancing in the hallway. She was speaking rapidly and was difficult to interrupt. She stated that she is a famous hip-hop artist and became hostile and threatening when asked to return to her room. To ensure her safety, a 1:1 sitter was requested. A psychiatry consultant diagnosed substance-induced mania and recommended stopping prednisone and prescribing olanzapine until her symptoms subside. With this intervention, her manic symptoms rapidly resolved.

■ PATHOPHYSIOLOGY

The etiology of bipolar disorder is not clearly defined. Alterations in cellular signaling (modulated by G proteins, protein kinase C, and calcium flux) may contribute to pathology. Abnormalities of the hypothalamic-pituitary-adrenal axis and thyroid function have been documented in bipolar patients. Monoamine neurotransmitter irregularities (particularly norepinephrine) may also play a role.

■ DIAGNOSIS

Bipolar I disorder

Bipolar I is diagnosed by the presence of a manic or mixed episode (see **Table 223-8**). The elevated mood of mania is enthused and often infectious, and the interviewer may be drawn to the patient's gregarious nature. Individuals may be sexually inappropriate or intimate in their disclosure of personal details. Inflated self-esteem can reach delusional proportions, with the patient claiming a special relationship to God, political leaders, or celebrities. Manic individuals have a decreased need for sleep and remain remarkably energized despite very little rest. Speech is loud, rapid, and uninterruptable, with fluid flow of ideas. Increase in goal-directed activity can manifest in an intrusive social manner in the hospital, with frequent phone calls or prolific letter writing. Expansive plans are thwarted in the hospitalized patient, possibly leading to increasing irritability, complaints, and angry tirades. Manic individuals may deny the presence of illness. Collateral information about past reckless behavior (spending sprees, gambling, sexual indiscretions) can help to confirm the diagnosis.

In mania with mixed features, symptoms of depression occur during the majority of the days of the mood episode. Patients appear extremely labile, with alternating euphoria, sadness, and irritability. Agitation is common, with extreme discomfort and anxiety due to dysphoria in the context of excessive energy. A high-suicide risk is associated with this state.

Although bipolar I is defined by the presence of a manic episode, major depression is more frequently the presenting episode (75% of the time for females and 67% of the time for males). Regardless of mood state at presentation, nearly all individuals with bipolar I will

TABLE 223-8 Manic Episode

A. A distinct period of abnormally and persistently elevated, expansive, or irritable mood, and persistently increased goal-directed activity or energy, lasting at least one week (or any duration if hospitalization is necessary).

B. During the period of mood disturbance and increased energy or activity, three or more of following symptoms (four if mood is irritable) have been present to a significant degree:

1. Inflated self-esteem or grandiosity
2. Decreased need for sleep
3. More talkative than usual or pressure to keep talking
4. Flight of ideas or racing thoughts
5. Distractibility (easily drawn to unimportant stimuli)
6. Increase in goal-directed activity or psychomotor agitation
7. Excessive involvement in pleasurable activities that have a high potential for painful consequences (sexual indiscretions, shopping sprees, foolish investments)

C. The mood disturbance causes marked impairment, necessitates hospitalization, or includes psychosis.

D. The symptoms are not due to the direct physiological effects of a substance or another medical condition.

have depressive episodes, with time between episodes decreasing as the disorder progresses. This can present a diagnostic challenge in differentiating bipolar from major depressive disorder. Clinical suspicion for bipolar I should arise in mood-disordered individuals with agitated or treatment-refractory depression, a rapid response to antidepressants, a family history of bipolar I, periodic impulsivity or erratic, pleasure-seeking behavior, and episodic sleep disturbance.

Bipolar II disorder

Bipolar II is defined by the occurrence of at least one major depressive episode, as well as one hypomanic episode. Hypomania differs from mania in duration and level of severity (see **Table 223-9**). During hypomania, patients do not suffer significant dysfunction, nor do they have hallucinations or delusions. However, individuals with this illness may still be extremely disabled during the course of a major depressive episode, even requiring hospitalization. Bipolar II is a chronic and debilitating illness, and patients have a greater risk of attempting and completing suicide than those with either bipolar I or major depression.

TABLE 223-9 Hypomanic Episode

A. A distinct period of persistently elevated, expansive, or irritable mood and persistently increased activity or energy, lasting at least 4 d.

B. During the period of mood disturbance, three (or more) symptoms associated with a manic episode (four if mood is irritable) have been present to a significant degree.

C. The episode is associated with an unequivocal change in functioning that is uncharacteristic of the person when not symptomatic.

D. The disturbance in mood and functioning are observable by others.

E. The episode is not severe enough to cause marked impairment in functioning, necessitate hospitalization, or induce psychosis.

F. The symptoms are not due to the effects of a substance.

TABLE 223-10 Medical Causes of Mania

Neurologic: Cerebrovascular accident (particularly orbitofrontal and thalamic stroke), traumatic brain injury, complex partial seizure, multiple sclerosis, Wilson disease, cerebellar atrophy

Infectious: HIV, neurosyphilis, cryptococcosis, influenza, Q fever

Metabolic: Vitamin B12 deficiency, hyperthyroidism, Cushing syndrome

Neoplastic: Meningioma, glioma, brainstem tumor, thalamic metastasis

TABLE 223-11 Pharmacologic Causes of Mania

Corticosteroids (including ACTH)

Antidepressants and L-tryptophan

Sympathomimetics and methylphenidate

Thyroxine

Sedative-hypnotics (alcohol, alprazolam, triazolam)

Levodopa

L-glutamine

Captopril

Cimetidine

Cyproheptadine

Cyclosporine

Disulfiram

Isoniazid

Muscle relaxants (cyclobenzaprine and baclofen)

Metoclopramide

Procainamide

Procarbazine

Propafenone

Hallucinogens (LSD, PCP)

Hydralazine

Opioids

Yohimbine

Zidovudine

Secondary mania: bipolar and related disorder due to another medical condition and substance/medication-induced bipolar and related disorder

When mania is due to medical illness or the effects of a substance, the diagnostic criteria do not specify duration or number of characteristics. Patients must simply show elevated, expansive, or irritable mood that causes significant distress or interferes with function. Age of onset can assist in differentiating organic mania from bipolar disorder. Secondary mania is more likely the diagnosis when the initial episode occurs after age 45. Substance-induced mania should be suspected when the mood disturbance coincides with the initiation of a new medication (particularly steroids).

Neurologic insult is the most frequent medical cause of manic symptoms. Lesions in the right frontal and temporal cortices (whether vascular, neoplastic, or traumatic) impart an increased risk. CNS infection is a common source of secondary mania, with multiple case reports of temporal (particularly HSV) encephalitis inducing manic symptoms. Patients with HIV-associated neurotoxicity and dementia also have a high prevalence of mania compared to the general population. See **Table 223-10** for common medical causes of mania.

Many pharmacologic agents can induce prolonged euphoric or irritable mood (see **Table 223-11**). Corticosteroids and stimulants are the most frequent offenders. Among the antidepressants, venlafaxine, buproprion, and the TCAs are most likely to precipitate mania.

Diagnostic studies

Onset of mania in the hospitalized patient should prompt a thorough workup to rule out medical disease or substance intoxication as a cause of symptoms. Laboratory evaluation does not differ significantly than that for major depression, with the exception that imaging of the brain should not be delayed (unless the patient has a well-documented history of bipolar disorder). Additionally, patients on mood stabilizers must have a serum level drawn.

■ TREATMENT

Acute mania

Patient safety may be compromised in the setting of acute mania. Treatment should be initiated immediately. Pharmacotherapy is the mainstay, though use of a 1:1 sitter and suicide precautions should be employed if necessary. Both atypical antipsychotics (olanzapine, ziprasidone, aripiprazole, risperidone, quetiapine, and asenapine) and mood stabilizers (lithium, divalproex, and carbamazepine) have indications for monotherapy in acute mania. However, if manic symptoms are even moderately severe, combination therapy is preferable. Antipsychotics have immediate effects and many can be given intramuscularly. Mood stabilizers can be given in a loading dose but take a few days to reach therapeutic levels in the blood. ECT is a good option for patients with severe or psychotic symptoms. Consultation with psychiatry is recommended.

Maintenance therapy for bipolar disorder

Bipolar disorder is not an insignificant illness and destabilization can be devastating. When bipolar patients are admitted, mood stabilizers must not be discontinued. A serum level should be checked to determine if a therapeutic range has been achieved. Monitoring and adjustment of dose may be necessary if new medications are started, due to the many drug interactions with mood stabilizers. Subtherapeutic dosing secondary to upregulation of cytochrome P450 can lead to catastrophic outcomes. To prevent precipitation of a manic episode, sleep schedules should be preserved and the addition of antidepressants avoided (even if an individual presents with depressed mood). If a patient is euthymic and stable on medications, psychiatry consultation is unnecessary. See **Table 223-12** for a synopsis of medications used for maintenance of bipolar disorder.

Complications

Adverse effects of the medications used for bipolar maintenance are listed in Table 223-12. Lithium has a narrow therapeutic index, with toxicity occurring at serum levels >1.5 mEq/L. Progressive kidney injury is associated with each supratherapeutic episode. Lithium overdose is usually unintentional, often caused by acute renal insufficiency or volume depletion. Mild intoxication presents with confusion, tremor, and nystagmus. Increasing lithium levels lead to nausea, vomiting, agitation, seizures, bradycardia, and hypotension. Treatment consists of fluids, supportive care, and if indicated, hemodialysis. Although the therapeutic index is much wider for valproic acid than for lithium, valproate toxicity may also occur in the medically ill patient with previously stable serum levels. Valproic acid is highly protein bound at therapeutic levels, and is metabolized largely through hepatic glucuronidation. Initiation of medications that compete for protein-binding sites, including aspirin, has led to valproate toxicity. Moreover, acute liver failure or

TABLE 223-12 Maintenance Therapy for Bipolar Disorder

Medication	Dosing	Therapeutic Serum Level	Half-Life	Side Effects	Drug Interactions
Lithium	900-1800 mg/d divided	1.0-1.5 mEq/L for acute mania, 0.6-1.2 mEq/L for maintenance	18-30 h	Ataxia, tremor, polyuria, diarrhea, weight gain, hypothyroidism, rash, leukocytosis, renal impairment, arrhythmia and T wave flattening	NSAIDs, diuretics, ACE-Is, metronidazole increase levels Acetazolamide, alkalizing agents decrease levels
Divalproex	Load 20-30 mg/kg/d, then 15 mg/kg/d	50-125 µg/mL	9-16 h	Sedation, tremor, ataxia, diarrhea, nausea, weight gain, hepatotoxicity, rare pancreatitis	ASA, chlorpromazine, fluoxetine, fluvoxamine, topiramate, cimetidine, erythromycin, ibuprofen can increase levels Phenytoin, ethosuximide, rifampin, carbamezapine can decrease levels
Lamotrigine	200-400 mg/d (slow titration)	n/a	33 h	Rash (can have Stevens-Johnson syndrome), sedation, blurry vision, ataxia, GI upset, blood dyscrasias	Divalproex increases level Carbamazepine, phenobarbitol, phenytoin, primidone, and OCP decrease levels
Carbamazepine	400-1200 mg/d	4-12 µg/mL	Initial 26-65 h, 12-17 h with repeated doses	Sedation, dizziness, confusion, GI upset, aplastic anemia, agranulocytosis, SIADH, rash	Induces its own clearance phenobarbitol, phenytoin, primidone, and OCP decrease levels Nefazodone, fluoxetine, fluvoxamine increase levels
Olanzapine	10-20 mg/d	n/a	21-54 h	Possible metabolic syndrome, dizziness, sedation, dry mouth, constipation, rare tardive dyskinesia, rare NMS	CYP450 1A2 inhibitors increase levels CYP450 1A2 inducers (cigarette smoke, carbamazepine) decrease levels
Quetiapine	100-400 mg/d	n/a	6-7 h	Sedation, orthostasis, dry mouth, constipation, possible metabolic syndrome	Rare
Aripiprazole	10-30 mg/d	n/a	75 h	Dizziness, insomnia, akathisia, GI upset, orthostasis	CYP450 3A4 and 2D6 inhibitors can increase levels, inducers may decrease levels
Asenapine	10-20 mg/d	n/a	24 h	Dry mouth, constipation, akathisia, weight gain, rare leukopenia, NMS, and tardive dyskinesia	CYP450 1A2 inhibitors can increase levels, inducers may decrease levels; can increase levels of other medications metabolized by CYP450 2D6m

addition of drugs that compete with hepatic microsomal enzymes may lead to decreased excretion of valproic acid. Poisoning may result in CNS and respiratory depression, hypotension, cerebral edema, and pancreatitis. True hepatoxicity is rare, though hyperammonemia is widely documented. Treatment is largely supportive, though hemoperfusion and hemodialysis may be used when serum levels are greater than 300 µg/mL, as only 35% of the drug is protein-bound at that level. Nalaxone has been shown in case reports to reverse valproic acid-induced coma, and L-carnitine has been increasingly recommended for hyperammonemia. Lamotrigine, which is indicated for maintenance therapy only, can cause severe rash (particularly in those with sensitive skin). Slow titration helps to decrease this risk. Lamotrigine and carbamezapine may also be fatal in overdose.

■ DISCHARGE PLANNING

Acute mania requires psychiatric hospitalization. Stable patients should receive referral for subsequent treatment by an outpatient psychiatrist.

■ PROGNOSIS

Patients with bipolar I disorder are likely to relapse. Approximately 50% of patients have a second manic episode within 2 years of their initial event. In the long term, only 15% of individuals remain well. One-third of these patients have chronic symptoms with significant social and occupational impairment. Treatment with mood stabilizers improves outcome, but only 50% to 60% of individuals on lithium achieve remission.

DISPARATIES IN HEALTH CARE

African Americans with manic symptoms are more likely than Caucasians to be misdiagnosed with schizophrenia. This may be due to the presence of psychosis or greater prevalence of comorbid substance use in the African American population.

ANXIETY DISORDERS

INTRODUCTION

Anxiety disorders are common, with one in four individuals meeting criteria for at least one DSM-IV diagnosis. Patients that enter the hospital without any previous psychiatric pathology may become acutely anxious in the face of invasive procedures and the threat of death.

CASE 223-3

A 33-year-old woman has been evaluated three times over the past 4 months with chest pain, nausea, and shortness of breath. ECG, chest x-ray, and initial cardiac enzymes were unremarkable. Admitted for observation, she had further testing for myocardial ischemia, including negative cardiac enzymes and a normal persantine-thallium stress test. More detailed questioning revealed multiple similar episodes over the past year. The first time this occurred, Ms B was driving to work and thought that she had ingested "too much coffee." Even though she had been taking the bus to prevent further attacks, she continued to have episodes that were unrelated to any stimulus. Low-dose clonezapam and fluoxetine were prescribed for panic disorder, leading to a significant improvement of her symptoms, with no further attacks or avoidant behavior. Her clonezapam was able to be successfully tapered.

PATHOPHYSIOLOGY

Fear is a stereotypical response that acts as an alarm to external threat. This reaction is mediated by the locus coeruleus and the limbic system via norepinephrine, serotonin, and GABA. Physiologic changes, such as tachycardia and tachypnea, are due to increased sympathetic activity. Cognitive symptoms include a sense of impending doom and dread. Behavioral reactions serve to remove the individual from harm. Acute anxiety also induces this reaction, but occurs in response to an internal threat or an external cue that is not inherently dangerous. Early exposure to trauma and genetic factors predispose individuals to these pathologic responses to stress.

Additional mechanisms are responsible for the onset of specific disorders. For example, infusion of carbon dioxide and sodium lactate can induce panic attacks in those with panic disorder. These substances lower systemic pH, increasing respiratory drive via the medulla. In those with panic disorder, hyperventilation and anxiety ensues. This is likely due to hypersensitivity of the central asphyxia alarm system.

DIAGNOSIS

When a patient presents with the physical signs of anxiety, it is essential to inquire about emotional and behavioral responses. Many patients focus primarily on somatic complaints, delaying appropriate recognition. Undiagnosed anxiety disorders impose a heavy economic burden, with unnecessary visits to emergency rooms, hospitalizations, subspecialty consultations, and invasive procedures. Perhaps more costly is the anguish experienced by the anxious patient who goes untreated. Many patients suffer secondary depression and abuse drugs and alcohol.

Primary anxiety disorders

Primary anxiety disorders occurring in adults include panic disorder, agoraphobia, specific phobia, social anxiety disorder, and generalized anxiety disorder (GAD). See **Table 223-13** for diagnostic features of these illnesses. Rarely, adults may suffer from separation anxiety disorder or selective mutism; these are disorders of low prevalence, and occur primarily in children and adolescents. Though DSM-V categorizes post-traumatic stress disorder (PTSD) under Trauma- and Stressor-Related Disorders, many of the symptoms overlap with the primary anxiety disorders. Thus, the hospitalist must consider this diagnosis when a patient displays avoidance behavior or presents with other symptoms commonly associated with anxiety. DSM criteria for PTSD are listed in **Table 223-14**.

A panic attack is an intense episode of autonomic activation accompanied by feelings of fear and impending doom. Attacks have a sudden onset, peak within 10 minutes, and usually resolve within a half-hour. In panic disorder, these episodes become autonomous and arise outside of substance use or stressful situation. The patient worries about the meaning of attacks and changes behavior to avoid them. Individuals with panic disorder frequently interpret their paroxysmal symptoms as a catastrophic medical event (such as an MI) and may present to emergency rooms multiple times before receiving an accurate diagnosis.

In agoraphobia, patients experience anxiety associated with a wide variety of situations, particularly those where escape may be difficult or help may be unavailable. Anxiety in agoraphobia may take the form of a full- or limited-symptom panic attack. Individuals respond with avoidance behavior, which may become so severe that the individual is essentially homebound. The majority of individuals with agoraphobia experience additional psychiatric comorbidity. The most frequently associated diagnoses are other anxiety disorders (particularly panic disorder, where the occurrence of panic attacks leads to increasing avoidance behavior), depressive disorders, PTSD, and alcohol use disorder.

A phobia is an excessive fear of a particular object or situation. Exposure to the phobic stimulus induces panic. This can complicate both diagnosis and treatment of medical illness. Individuals with blood-injection-injury specific phobia may refuse phlebotomy or have a vasovagal response to seeing blood. Claustrophobia may prevent the successful completion of needed scans. Severe social phobia can be disabling in the hospital setting, where scrutiny by others is unavoidable.

Those with GAD have chronic, uncontrollable worry about multiple aspects of life. These individuals have prominent somatic complaints (headaches, muscle tension, gastrointestinal distress) and often seek medical care for symptom relief. Unless appropriately treated, hospitalized patients with GAD may aggravate staff and physicians with a seemingly exorbitant need for reassurance and explanations.

Post-traumatic stress disorder is a maladaptive response to a life-threatening event that results in intrusive symptoms such as re-experiencing of the incident, avoidance behavior, negative alterations in cognition and mood, and increased arousal. While much attention has been paid to the emergence of PTSD in combat veterans, the disorder may also occur in civilians after traumatic events or natural disasters. It has also been documented after MI, CABG, and surgery performed under inadequate anesthesia. The disorder is more likely to occur in situations in which the traumatic event is perceived as uncontrollable. Thus, actions should be taken to allow hospitalized patients to maintain a sense of control over themselves and their environments.

Organic causes of anxiety: anxiety due to another medical condition and substance/medication-induced anxiety

A bewildering array of medical diseases can mimic primary anxiety disorders (see **Table 223-15**). This presents a diagnostic challenge: up to 42% of all patients referred for psychiatric

TABLE 223-13 Primary Anxiety Disorders

I. Panic disorder

A. Recurrent, unexpected panic attacks characterized by four or more of the following: palpitations, chest pain, diaphoresis, shortness of breath, sensation of choking, nausea, trembling, paresthesias, chills or hot flashes, dizziness, derealization or depersonalization, fear of dying, fear of losing control or going crazy

B. 1 mo of more of persistent concern about future attacks, worry about the meaning or consequences of attacks, or significant maladaptive change in behavior surrounding the about of future attacks

C. The disturbance is not attributable to the physiological effects of a substance or another medical condition, and is not better explained by another mental disorder

II. Agoraphobia

A. Marked fear or anxiety about two (or more) of the following five situations:

   1. Using public transportation

   2. Being in open spaces

   3. Being in enclosed spaces

   4. Standing in line or being in a crowd

   5. Being outside of the home alone

B. The individual fears or avoids these situations because of thoughts that escape might be difficult or help might not be available in the event of developing panic-like symptoms or other incapacitating or embarrassing symptoms (eg, fear of falling in the elderly; fear of incontinence).

C. The agoraphobic situations are actively avoided, require the presence of a companion, or are endured with intense fear or anxiety.

D. The fear or anxiety is out of proportion to the actual danger posed by the agoraphobic situations and to the sociocultural context.

E. The fear, anxiety, or avoidance is persistent, typically lasting for 6 mo or more.

F. The fear, anxiety, or avoidance causes clinically significant distress or impairment.

G. The fear, anxiety, or avoidance is not better explained by the symptoms of another mental disorder, and if another medical condition is present, the associated fear, anxiety, or avoidance is clearly excessive.

III. Social anxiety disorder

A. Marked fear or anxiety about one or more social situations in which the individual is exposed to possible scrutiny by others.

B. The individual fears that he or she will act in a way or show anxiety symptoms that will be negatively evaluated (ie, will be humiliating or embarrassing; will lead to rejection or offend others).

C. The social situations almost always provoke fear or anxiety.

D. The social situations are avoided or endured with intense anxiety or distress.

E. The fear or anxiety is out of proportion to the actual threat posed by the social situation and to the sociocultural context.

F. The fear, anxiety, or avoidance is persistent, typically lasting for 6 mo or more.

G. The fear, anxiety, or avoidance causes clinically significant distress or impairment in social, occupational, or other important areas of functioning.

H. The fear, anxiety, or avoidance is not attributable to the physiological effects of a substance (eg, a drug of abuse, a medication), another medical condition, or another mental disorder.

IV. Specific phobia

A. Marked and persistent fear that is excessive, unreasonable, and cued by the presence of or anticipation of a specific object or situation.

B. Exposure to feared object or situation provokes an immediate anxiety response that is out of proportion to the actual danger and to the sociocultural context.

C. The phobic object or situation is actively avoided or endured with intense anxiety.

D. The fear, anxiety, or avoidance is persistent, lasting 6 mo or more.

E. Avoidance, anticipatory anxiety, or distress is significantly impairing.

F. The disturbance is not better explained by another mental disorder.

V. Generalized anxiety disorder

A. Excessive anxiety and worry about a number of events or activities, occurring more days than not for at least 6 mo, about a number of events or activities.

B. Worry is difficult to control.

C. Worry is associated with at least three of the following: restlessness, fatigue, difficulty concentrating, irritability, muscle tension, or sleep disturbance.

D. The worry or physical symptoms cause significant distress or impairment.

E. The disturbance is not attributable to the effects of substance, another medical condition, or another mental disorder.

TABLE 223-14 Posttraumatic Stress Disorder (PTSD)

A. Exposure to actual or threatened death, serious injury, or sexual violence.

B. Presence of one or more intrusive symptoms associated with the event, including: distressing memories, distressing dreams, dissociative reactions (flashbacks), psychological distress, or physiological reactions at exposure to cues.

C. Avoidance behavior, including one or more of the following: avoidance of memories, thoughts or feelings associated with the event or avoidance of external reminders of the event.

D. Negative alterations in cognitions and mood, including at least two of the following: inability to remember the event, exaggerated negative beliefs about oneself, distorted cognitions about the event that lead the individual to blame himself or herself, negative emotional state, diminished interest in activities, feelings of detachment, inability to experience positive emotions.

E. Symptoms of increased arousal, including at least two of the following: sleep difficulties, irritability, poor concentration, hypervigilence, reckless behavior, or exaggerated startle response.

F. Duration is more than 1 mo.

G. The disturbance causes distress or impairment.

H. The disturbance is not attributable to the effects of a substance or another medical condition.

evaluation for anxiety have underlying medical illness as a cause for their symptoms. Of the diseases presenting with anxious symptoms, 25% are endocrine disorders, 25% neurological, and 12% cardiovascular, rheumatologic, or infectious. When a patient with a known medical disease presents with complaints of anxiety, evaluation should focus on whether an exacerbation of the illness could be responsible. Family history of disorders that mimic anxiety, such as hyperthyroidism or cardiac arrhythmias, can provide important clues.

Anxiety due to medical disease generally lacks the emotional component of primary disorders. Somatic complaints may not

TABLE 223-15 Medical Causes of Anxiety

Endocrine: Cushing disease, adrenal insufficiency, Addison disease, adrenal tumors, carcinoid syndrome, diabetes (hypoglycemia), hyperparathyroidism, hyperthyroidism, hypothyroidism, insulinoma, menopause, ovarian dysfunction, pancreatic carcinoma, pheochromocytoma, pituitary disease, PMS, testicular disease

Neurologic: Tumors, tertiary syphilis, cerebrovascular disease, encephalopathy, epilepsy (especially temporal lobe foci), essential tremor, Huntington disease, migraine, MS, myasthenia gravis, polyneuritis, postconcussive syndrome, vertigo

Cardiovascular: Anemia, CHF, CAD, arrhythmias, hypovolemia, mitral valve prolapse

Respiratory: Asthma, COPD, hyperventilation, hypoxia, pneumonia, pneumothorax, pulmonary edema, PE

Rheumatologic: Anaphylaxis, polyarteritis nodosa, rheumatoid arthritis, SLE, temporal arteritis

Metabolic: Acidosis, acute intermittent porphyria, electrolyte abnormalities, hyperthermia, Wilson disease

Gastrointestinal: Colitis, IBS, esophageal dysmotility, PUD

Infectious disease: AIDS, atypical pneumonia, brucellosis, malaria, mononucleosis, TB, viral hepatitis

TABLE 223-16 Substance-Induced Anxiety

Intoxication: analgesics, antibiotics (penicillin, sulfonamides), anticholinergics, anticonvulsants, antidepressants, antihistamines, antihypertensives, anti-inflammatory agents, antiparkinsonian agents, aspirin, caffeine, chemotherapeutics, cocaine, digitalis, hallucinogens, heavy metal poisoning, marijuana, neuroleptics, steroids, sympathomimetics, theophylline, thyroid supplements, tobacco

Withdrawal: ethanol, narcotics, sedative-hypnotics

cause as much distress or interfere significantly with overall function. Constellations of symptoms are less likely to meet criteria for any particular DSM-V diagnosis, and warning signs (such as loss of consciousness or incontinence) may be present. Unlike those with organic syndromes, patients with primary anxiety are likely to have a childhood history of emotional trauma, a family history of mood and anxiety disorders, life stressors preceding onset of disease, and avoidance behavior. Presentation of primary anxiety after age 35 is uncommon. A lack of response to anxiolytic medications should prompt a reassessment of the diagnosis of a primary anxiety disorder.

Drugs frequently cause anxious symptoms. Stimulants, including caffeine and over-the-counter medications (such as dextromethorphan), can induce anxiety. Prescription medications (most frequently steroids and other immunomodulators) may also be responsible. Withdrawal from sedatives and opioids may lead to autonomic hyper-reactivity. See **Table 223-16** for a list of frequent offenders.

Chronic anxiety versus major depression

Approximately half of all patients with MDD meet criteria for panic disorder, agoraphobia, or GAD. This significant overlap can make distinguishing diagnoses difficult, with sleep disturbance, psychomotor agitation, difficulty concentrating, irritability, and fatigue attributable to either illness. However, the presence of certain symptoms can help with differentiation. Psychomotor retardation, dysphoria, hopelessness, and thoughts of death are more specific to major depression. Unlike those suffering from MDD, anxious individuals rarely lose interest in their usual activities, though they may avoid situations because of irrational fears. The somatic symptoms of anxiety differ from those of depression, with tachycardia, palpitations, tachypnea, and diaphoresis prominent.

Diagnostic studies

A wide array of illnesses and ingestions can masquerade as anxiety. Initial laboratory evaluation must rule out organic causes for anxious symptoms. Recommended studies do not differ significantly from those for depression (see earlier discussion). The organ system involved in the majority of the patient's somatic complaints may focus further testing. Patients with known anxiety disorders can present with serious medical illness, and clinicians must not delay diagnostic evaluation by prematurely narrowing the differential (ie, patients with panic disorder can still suffer an MI).

■ TREATMENT

Situational anxiety

Medical illness, particularly when severe enough to require hospitalization, imposes significant psychological stress. Patients without any previous psychiatric diagnosis may become appropriately fearful when undergoing invasive procedures or facing life-threatening disease. In the acutely anxious patient, delaying effective treatment

TABLE 223-17 Pharmacology of Commonly-Used Benzodiazepines

Medication	Dose Equivalent (mg)	Half-Life (h)	Onset
Midazolam	2	1-12	Fast
Oxazepam	15	5-15	Slow
Lorazepam	1	10-20	Intermediate
Alprazolam	0.5	12-15	Intermediate-fast
Chlordiazepoxide	10	5-30	Intermediate
Clonazepam	0.25	15-50	Intermediate
Diazepam	5	20-100	Fast
Flurazepam	15	40	Fast
Clorazepate	7.5	30-200	Fast

is akin to withholding medication for pain. BZDs are first-line therapy for short-term treatment of intermittent anxiety in those without primary disorders.

Sedation is often a limiting side effect of the benzodiazepines. Medications should be started at low doses and titrated as needed to minimize this problem. In some patients, particularly the elderly, BZDs may cause paradoxical agitation and precipitate delirium. Dependence can occur with prolonged use. Because of this, they should be used with great caution (if at all) in patients with a history of addiction. The use of agents with shorter half-lives, such as alprazolam, can result in rebound symptoms with infrequent dosing. BZDs can cause withdrawal if abruptly discontinued, and a taper should be used to avoid this possibly life-threatening complication. Though all benzodiazepines are likely equally efficacious at equivalent doses, clonezapam may be the most attractive agent due to its long half-life and relatively slow onset (thereby decreasing addictive potential). See **Table 223-17** for further details on the BZDs.

Anxiety disorders

Antidepressants are first-line therapy for the anxiety disorders. Because of their tolerability and safety profiles, SSRIs are the agents of choice. Fluoxetine, sertraline, paroxetine, fluvoxamine, citalopram, and escitalopram all have indications for the treatment of panic disorder, agoraphobia, social phobia, and PTSD. Paroxetine and escitalopram are approved for GAD. Alternatively, the SNRIs duloxetine and venlafaxine may be used to treat anxiety disorders. Buproprion should be avoided as it can be anxiogenic. When initiating treatment, lower starting doses and slow titration should be employed to prevent worsening of symptoms. Higher total doses may be necessary to achieve remission.

Among the other antidepressants, the tricyclics clomipramine and imipramine and the MAO-inhibitor phenelzine may be used to treat anxiety disorders. Intolerable side effects and drug toxicity often limit their use. These agents are reasonable second- or third-line choices in patients with severe, treatment-resistant illness. TCAs and MAO-Is should be started with the assistance of psychiatry.

For patients newly diagnosed with an anxiety disorder, BZDs may be used in conjunction with antidepressants to temper activating symptoms associated with initiation of SSRIs and SNRIs. They also may be used in the short-term to treat patients with known anxiety disorders who were previously stable on antidepressants alone. Benzodiazepines are indicated for panic disorder, agoraphobia, social phobia, and GAD. Monotherapy with these medications may be the treatment of choice for specific phobia, and can be administered just prior to confronting the feared object or situation (before starting a procedure, or on the way to MRI). BZDs should be avoided in acute trauma and in PTSD, as they may actually be harmful.

Buspirone is a $5HT_{1A}$ partial agonist approved for the treatment of social phobia and GAD. Similar to SSRIs, buspirone must be taken for a number of weeks before maximum therapeutic benefit is attained. Clinical trials have shown promising results for this medication, but anecdotal experience is disappointing.

Antiadrenergic agents can also diminish somatic symptoms associated with anxiety. The β-blocker propranolol is indicated for social phobia and may also be a useful treatment for panic attacks, panic disorder, social phobia, GAD, and PTSD. Clonidine, an α2 agonist, may also help decrease sympathetic hyperactivity. The α1-antagonist prazosin may be used to treat nightmares associated with PTSD. Anticonvulsants and antihistamines are sedating and may relieve feelings of restlessness, but this is an off-label use of these medications.

Psychotherapy and other nonpharmacologic interventions

Cognitive-behavioral therapy (CBT) is as effective as pharmacotherapy for certain disorders, such as social and specific phobia. For other anxiety disorders, including GAD, a combination of CBT and medication improves outcomes. Cognitive-behavioral formulations of anxiety focus on maladaptive information processing and actions. Therapy seeks to correct faulty cognition and modify escape responses. Engagement in therapy may be challenging for the hospitalized patient, though teaching symptom management (such as relaxation techniques) may be possible with the assistance of psychiatry consultation. Other psychosocial interventions, such as recruitment of family members to provide emotional support, may also be beneficial.

Organic causes of anxiety

When medical illness is the cause of anxiety, treatment of the disease is the intervention of choice. If the illness is permanent, symptoms are causing distress, or anxiety does not remit when physical health returns, pharmacotherapy with anxiolytics (in the short term) or antidepressants (in the long term) is indicated. Behavioral modification techniques are also effective in this population. In substance-induced anxiety, addiction must be addressed.

■ DISCHARGE PLANNING

Psychic tension greatly increases the risk for suicide. Acutely anxious patients should be screened for both passive and active suicidal ideation and hospitalized if at risk. Patients whose anxiety is sufficiently severe to warrant sustained pharmacotherapy should likely be referred to psychiatry upon discharge. In patients who are discharged on a short course of BZDs, care must be taken to inform outpatient providers of the rationale and plan for use of this medication. Outpatient providers may incorrectly assume that the BZD is intended for long-term use in the discharged patient, thereby subjecting the patient to unnecessary cognitive side effects and the potential of withdrawal. If longer-term use of a BZD is deemed necessary for controlling anxiety, consultation or comanagement with psychiatry is recommended.

■ DISPARITIES IN HEALTH CARE

In the outpatient setting, African Americans and Latinos receive appropriate care for anxiety or depression less frequently than Caucasians (odds ratios are 0.44 and 0.60, respectively). Both minorities find treatment with antidepressants less acceptable than Caucasians, but this does not fully account for the discrepancy.

■ PROGNOSIS

Patients with panic disorder have a fairly good prognosis, with 30% to 40% free of all symptoms long term. Those with PTSD fare even better. Fifty percent of untreated patients are in remission at 1 year after the traumatic event.

CONCLUSION

Mood and anxiety disorders are common and underdiagnosed. Failure to identify and initiate appropriate treatment can cause unnecessary suffering and readmissions, and significantly affect morbidity and mortality. Medical hospitalization provides an opportunity to improve patient outcomes by properly recognizing, diagnosing, and initiating a therapeutic plan that can be transitioned to the outpatient setting.

SUGGESTED READINGS

Ables AZ, Nagubilli R. Prevention, recognition, and management of serotonin syndrome. *Am Fam Physician*. 2010;81(9):1139-1142.

Kupfer DJ, et al. *Diagnostic and Statistical Manual of Mental Disorders*, 5th ed. Arlington, VA: American Psychiatric Association; 2013.

Lisanby SH. Electroconvulsive Therapy for Depression. *N Engl J Med*. 2007;357:1939-1945.

McGuire AW, Eastwood JA, Hays RD, Macabasco-O'Connell A, Doering LV. Depressed or not depressed: untangling symptoms of depression in patients hospitalized with coronary heart disease. *Am J Crit Care*. 2014;23(2):106-116.

Robinson RG, Jorge RE, Moser DJ, et al. Escitalopram and Problem-Solving Therapy for Prevention of Poststroke Depression. *JAMA*. 2008;299(20):2391-2400.

Sadock BJ, Sadock VA. *Kaplan & Sadock's Synopsis of Psychiatry*, 10th ed. Philadelphia, PA: Lippincott Williams & Wilkins; 2007.

Schatzberg AF, Nemeroff CB. *The American psychiatric publishing textbook of psychopharmacology*, 3rd ed. Arlington, VA: American Psychiatric Publishing; 2004.

Stern TA, Fricchione GL, Cassem NH, et al. *Handbook of General Hospital Psychiatry*, 5th ed. Philadelphia, PA: Mosby; 2004.

Warner CH, Bobo W, Warner C, Reid S, Rachal J. Antidepressant discontinuation syndrome. *Am Fam Physician*. 2006;74(3):449-456.

CHAPTER 224

Combat Stress and Related Disorders

Harold Kudler, MD

Key Clinical Questions

① Why should we care about combat stress and related disorders?

② How do you define cultural competence regarding military service members, veterans, and their families?

③ What are the medical problems associated with military service and deployment stress?

④ How would you describe point-of-care strategies to improve the care of military service members, veterans, and their families?

⑤ What resources are available to provide information, support, and access needed by military service members, veterans, and those who care for them and about them?

INTRODUCTION

An estimated 2.7 million American military members have served in Operation Enduring Freedom (OEF) in Afghanistan or Operation Iraqi Freedom (OIF) and/or Operation New Dawn (OND) in Iraq since the first of these began in 2001. As of November 2006, these conflicts have exceeded the duration of World War II. The attention rightly paid to the less than 1% of Americans who have served in OEF/OIF/OND should also alert the public that there are 22 million living American veterans and, conservatively estimated, an additional 33 million dependents potentially eligible for Department of Veterans Affairs (VA) benefits. Approximately one in every five Americans is a Service Member, a veteran, or a dependent. Of key importance, fewer than one in three veterans uses VA health services in any given year and, among these, most are also receiving at least some of their health care elsewhere. Thus, the majority of veterans and virtually all their dependents receive health care outside of VA. Hospitalists need to be alert to the fact that as many as 20% of their patients is a service member, a veteran, and/or a dependent.

More than 60% of those who have served in Afghanistan or Iraq have already had at least one episode of VA care. Among these VA's Public Health Office reports that, as of March 31, 2015:

- 12% of those serving in these operations are women.
- 76% of the military forces are 35 years of age or younger.
- 61% were active duty (AD) component members, and 39% were the Reserve component (RC) including Reservists and National Guard Members.

Active duty component members have the support of a strong military community due to their serving a continuous "hitch" on a military base. The RC "Citizen Soldiers," however, move back and forth between military and veteran status. They may live hundreds of miles from the nearest military community and thousands of miles from the troops with whom they are deployed. Spouses may be the only person in their workplace who has had a wife or husband deployed in the military. Their children may be the only ones in their school to have a parent serving overseas.

The nature of our volunteer military requires multiple deployments per member. Each time a military member deploys, the individual's risk of developing a postdeployment mental health problem increases. When a service member deploys, a family serves too and there is a growing body of research on how the health of military family members may be affected in the course of the deployment cycle.

Going to war is a very long-term investment which resonates across the entire nation and multiple generations. Yet, despite the large number of veterans and their dependents and an enduring obligation to serve those who have served our country, few health care providers routinely enquire about military history or about the effects of deployment on military families. Providers are often ill prepared to recognize or treat health problems associated with military service and/or deployment stress. This chapter will focus on postdeployment mental health and articulate a public health approach that requires the development of Department of Defense (DoD)/VA/state and community partnerships in service to military service members/veterans and their families.

SCOPE OF THE ISSUE

A November 2007 study from the Walter Reed Army Institute of Research followed 88,235 US soldiers returning from Iraq. Each soldier completed both a Post-Deployment Health Assessment (PDHA) and then, an average of 6 months later, completed a Post-Deployment Health Reassessment (PDHRA). These global health screening tools include standard screens for post-traumatic stress disorder (PTSD), major depression, alcohol abuse, and traumatic brain injury (TBI).

While the Walter Reed study contained the good news that about half of those who reported significant PTSD symptoms upon arrival home had improved at the 6-month mark, the bad news was that *twice* as many *new* soldiers screened positive for PTSD at that 6-month follow-up. During those first 6 months postdeployment, the depression rate doubled among the AD component and tripled among the RC. The self-report rate for alcohol abuse was 12% for the AD and 15% for the RC; yet only 0.2% of those who screened positive were referred for treatment (likely because they had the option of not being referred and feared the impact of referral upon their military and/or civilian careers). Respondents also reported a four-fold increase in concern about losing control of their anger. Overall, 20.3% of the AD component and 42.4% of the RC were identified as requiring further mental health assessment and/or treatment by the 6-month mark.

The health burden of returning service members and their families is by no means confined to mental health issues. Consideration of the full health impact of service in OEF/OIF/OND is well beyond the scope of this chapter but it should be noted that a 2009 study by Cohen and colleagues found that veterans with mental disorders had 42% to 146% greater utilization in VA nonmental health settings than those without a mental disorder. Those with PTSD had the highest utilization in all categories. Female gender and lower rank were also independently associated with greater health care utilization. Comparison data is not available for non-VA settings but these findings strongly support the importance of screening for military history as a routine component of medical intake within all health care systems.

MILITARY CULTURE

Medical providers are increasingly sensitive to the importance of cultural competence, but few recognize that the military is a unique culture in itself. The clinician's understanding of military life, the deployment cycle, and the stresses of living and working in a war zone are critical to establishing credibility with patients who are either military members, veterans, or their significant others. Being in the military or in a military family is not like any other kind of life. There is strong support within a well defined, coherent social system, but there is also little privacy. Military families may truly get to "see the world," but they rarely have much choice about where they will live or for how long. Above all, military life is defined and structured by high standards of ethics and discipline. Few outside of the armed services understand that military culture is primarily rooted in a professional ethos of loyalty and self-sacrifice. This is necessary to maintain order during battle and in its aftermath.

A distinct set of military ceremony and etiquette reinforces shared rituals and common identities. An enduring emphasis on group cohesion and esprit de corps connects service members and their dependents to one another. Above all, military members and their families understand that the mission must come first. As a corollary to this, nonmilitary clinicians need to understand that the purpose of military medicine is to preserve the fighting force. This is distinctly different than the goal of providing patient- and family-centered care.

Military customs and concerns can generate tension in the doctor-patient relationship when military members and their dependents are seen in nonmilitary health care settings. Patients and their family members may hesitate to report postdeployment health problems because of concern that what they say may get back to the commanding officer. While such breach of medical privacy is unlikely, even in military health care settings, confidentiality is a serious concern among military members and their families that should be addressed openly and early. The stigma associated with mental health

problems may be the single greatest barrier to accurate assessment and timely care of deployment-related health concerns.

It is not necessary for a clinician to become an expert on military history or military life in order to achieve the cultural competency needed to be effective in working with this population, but it is critically important to remain aware and respectful of the military way of life. For example, calling a Marine a Soldier may convince that Marine that you have no interest in either him personally or the Corps. What might feel like a small slip may be taken as a clear sign that "My doctor does not get it," after which important information may be left unsaid.

Clinicians who understand the nature of military training and deployment will routinely enquire about exposure to head trauma, travel-related disease, and physical or psychological trauma. Providers must be willing to ask questions and show interest when specific places or military events "pop up" in a conversation or when military "lingo" is suddenly injected. Veterans often drop such clues to see if their provider "gets it" before sharing their military experiences. It is unfortunate that some medical professionals are hesitant to ask about terms outside their own expertise. Genuine, expressed interest in the patient's military experiences is essential if the necessary bridges of trust and respect are to be built.

MENTAL HEALTH FINDINGS AMONG THE NEWEST GENERATION OF COMBAT VETERANS

As of this writing, more than 1.9 million OEF/OIF/OND veterans are eligible for VA health care services. Although, as noted, only about 22% of American veterans receive their health care through VA, an impressive 61% of all OEF/OIF/OND veterans eligible to use VA have already presented for at least one episode of care. Because the VA has a national electronic database, it is possible to draw some conclusions about the health issues of these 1,189,709 veterans. Large as this help-seeking sample is, this information cannot be reliably extrapolated to those OEF/OIF/OND veterans who have not sought health care or who are seeking it in the community.

Veterans Affairs records show that the three most common health issues among OEF/OIF/OND veterans are, in descending order, musculoskeletal, "symptoms, signs, and ill-defined conditions" and mental health. The most common musculoskeletal injuries are knee and back problems rather than the grievous injuries seen in news coverage from the war zone or military treatment facilities. Less than 3% of all OEF/OIF/OND veterans return home by way of the medical evacuation system and the remainder comes home at the appointed time with less obvious injuries. Rather than expect to *treat the war as seen on television*, it is important to realize that most combat veterans who come to the hospital will look pretty much like anyone else. This makes it all the more important to routinely take a military history.

Although the Gulf War Syndrome, which appeared among those who served in the early 1990s, is still under careful study, there is no evidence of a particular Gulf War Syndrome among those serving in OEF/OIF/OND. Veterans and their family members will, however, often express concern about possible long-term health risks that might arise from health risks indigenous to the combat area or related to inoculations or toxic exposures that may have occurred during deployment. Such concerns should be respected, discussed, recorded, and evaluated. While clear answers may not always be available, sincere listening and appropriate documentation will strengthen the bond between patient and provider.

More than 57% of OEF/OIF/OND veterans who have presented to VA have received at least one provisional diagnosis of a mental health disorder (**Table 224-1**). The most frequent among these is PTSD, which has been diagnosed in 32% of those who have presented to VA. Many clinicians, patients, and family members think of PTSD as the final common denominator in deployment-related mental health, but more OEF/OIF/OND veterans have been diagnosed with a mood disorder than they have with PTSD. Note that

TABLE 224-1 Possible Mental Health Diagnoses among 625,384 Eligible OEF/OIF/OND Veterans who Presented to VA as of March 2015

- Provisional MH diagnoses include
  - PTSD: — 378,993
    (32% of all who presented to VA)
  - Depressive disorder — 308,336
  - Affective psychoses — 193,886
  - Neurotic disorders — 295,403
  - Nondependent abuse of drugs — 69,271
    (Exclusive of a tobacco use disorder)
  - Alcohol dependence — 88,680

the number with other anxiety disorders (listed under Neurotic Disorders which include panic disorder and generalized anxiety disorder among others) is not far behind. The high rate of nondependent abuse of drugs and alcohol dependence may be another marker for severe stress and/or psychological trauma. The take-home message is that postdeployment mental health is not just about PTSD and that a significant number of people who have PTSD may have one or more comorbid mental health problems.

Family members and significant others are also under significant stress in the course of the deployment cycle. When they present to their health providers, they may report new medical problems or exacerbation of old problems that express that stress. Family members frequently report depression, lack of sleep, irritability, concentration problems, and substance abuse problems. Clinicians should be aware of age-specific presentation of stress among military children. Toddlers may regress from previous developmental achievements and present with enuresis or encopresis. Food allergies, asthma, or digestive difficulties may flare. School-aged children may develop new-onset academic difficulties that may be taken for a learning or behavioral disorder or attention deficit. Teenagers may become withdrawn, oppositional, promiscuous, and/or abuse substances.

Different problems may surface at different points in the deployment cycle. During predeployment, each family member may respond in his or her own way to hearing that the service member has orders to deploy. Memories about problems during past deployments may stir new worries. The common, protracted training prior to actual deployment further extends the separation and places additional stress on the entire family. During deployment, families often complain of having too little contact with consequent worry about the service member's safety. On the other hand, the availability of instantaneous communication via telephone and e-mail sometimes ignites anxieties and arguments that can be more troubling to everyone involved than the events of daily life in a combat zone. After the service member returns home, he or she may experience problems that concern everyone in the family. Even when they fail to meet criteria for a formal diagnosis, problems with concentration, irritability, inability to sleep, emotional withdrawal, chronic pain, or substance abuse may have a powerful impact on all involved. Clinicians need to understand that deployment-related stress may propagate to disrupt the entire web of family life.

Deployment-related problems may be more functional than clinical but, even so, it is important for clinicians to inquire about them. They can include frequent arguments, separation, child abuse or neglect, trouble at work, unemployment, financial stress/bankruptcy, legal problems, incarceration, and ultimately, homelessness. As the saying goes, "If you do not take the temperature, you cannot find the fever."

Ideally, all postdeployment health problems would be picked up somewhere within the continuum of DoD and VA care, but if 61% of all OEF/OIF/OND veterans eligible for VA care have come for that care, *where are the other 39%?* Clearly, many of OEF/OIF/OND veterans do not come to VA. Some among them may not seek help at all. Still others will be seen in public or private settings.

It is possible that the 39% of OEF/OIF/OND veterans who have not presented for VA care are, in fact, doing just fine and do not need medical attention. On the other hand, findings from the 1990 National Vietnam Veterans Readjustment Study (NVVRS), which have recently been extended by the National Vietnam Veterans Longitudinal Study, raise concerns about those not seen in VA. NVVRS documented that only 20% of Vietnam veterans who actually *had* a confirmed diagnosis of PTSD had *ever* sought VA mental health care. Further, those researchers found that 62% of all Vietnam veterans with PTSD *had* received mental health care at some point after the deployment. In other words, over two-thirds of Vietnam veterans with PTSD chose to seek mental health care *outside* of the VA. These findings strongly suggest that many OEF/OIF/OND veterans might seek mental health services outside of VA. Family members must, of necessity, seek help outside of VA even if their health issues are also related to deployment stress. The question is: Are public and private sector providers prepared to diagnose and treat postdeployment health problems among OEF/OIF/OND veterans and their families?

SPECIFIC MENTAL HEALTH ISSUES AMONG COMBAT VETERANS

PTSD

While a full discussion of postdeployment mental health problems and their treatment is beyond the scope of this chapter, certain issues deserve mention. Chief among these is the importance of screening for PTSD and TBI among combat veterans encountered in practice. As mentioned, 32% of all OEF/OIF/OND veterans who have presented for VA health care have been diagnosed with PTSD. A 2008 Rand Corporation report estimated a 19% incidence of TBI among OEF/OIF veterans. The Rand investigators also found that 57% of veterans diagnosed with a TBI in the course of the study had not previously been assessed for TBI by a physician. These findings indicate that clinicians should screen for PTSD, major depression, TBI, and substance abuse among veterans.

Validated screening tools for PTSD and TBI are readily available and in the public domain. Refer to **Table 224-2** for the Primary Care PTSD Screen (PC-PTSD). Developed by VA's National Center for PTSD, the PC-PTSD has been validated to screen for PTSD in primary care settings. Note that while the threshold has been set at three positive responses in military and VA settings, a cut-off of two positive answers may be more appropriate in civilian settings where the

TABLE 224-2 The Primary Care PTSD Screen (PC-PTSD)

In your life, have you ever had any experience that was so frightening, horrible, or upsetting that, in the past month, you:

1. Have had nightmares about it or thought about it when you did not want to? YES/NO

2. Tried hard not to think about it or went out of your way to avoid situations that reminded you of it? YES/NO

3. Were constantly on guard, watchful, or easily startled? YES/NO

4. Felt numb or detached from others, activities, or your surroundings? YES/NO

Current research suggests that the results of the PC-PTSD should be considered "positive" if a patient answers "yes" to any three items but, in a civilian setting (where the prevalence of PTSD may be lower) answering "yes" to even two questions should prompt further evaluation.

prevalence of PTSD is likely to be lower. The PC-PTSD can be incorporated into a self-assessment battery or it can be administered by a clinical team member.

A positive screen is not a diagnosis and should be followed up with a validated diagnostic tool and a clinical interview. The 20-item PTSD Checklist for DSM-5 (PCL-5), another product of the VA National Center for PTSD that is in the public domain, measures the presence and intensity of each diagnostic criterion for PTSD. Self-administered or read to a patient, the PCL-5 can be used to validate the diagnosis and measure treatment response, symptom by symptom, over time. The PC-PTSD and PCL-5 are among the many tools, trainings and patient materials which can be obtained through VA's online Community Provider Toolkit (http://www.mentalhealth.va.gov/communityproviders/index.asp). These include free, accredited training on Military Culture, and access to VA's nationwide PTSD Consultation Service for community providers treating veterans.

◼ TBI

Moderate or severe traumatic brain injuries account for approximately 20% of all TBI's and will be obvious to clinicians, but mild traumatic brain injuries (mTBI's) may be far more difficult to recognize and assess. The injury may involve closed head trauma, axonal shearing, intracranial bleeding, and/or penetrating fragments. Many clinicians have been trained to believe that anyone who has endured a TBI, even mTBI, must have experienced at least a momentary loss of consciousness, but current thinking is that some will simply feel dazed, see stars, or otherwise report having felt stunned and confused.

Patients with mTBI often report a history of headache, dizziness/balance problems, insomnia, impaired memory, ringing in the ears or hearing loss, and/or decreased tolerance for noise and light. Most people suffering from mTBI return to their previous level of function within 3 to 6 months, and it is important to reassure patients and their family members about this. On the other hand, 10% to 25% of patients will go on to develop chronic postconcussive symptoms. These enduring problems may be grouped into three categories: *somatic* (headache, tinnitus, insomnia, etc.), *cognitive* (memory, attention and concentration difficulties), and *emotional/behavioral* (irritability, depression, anxiety, behavioral dyscontrol) (**Table 224-3**).

Patients with mTBI may be at increased risk for PTSD, major depression, and/or Substance Use Disorder. There is considerable diagnostic overlap between mTBI and PTSD, and it is sometimes difficult to determine if a given patient has one, the other, or both.

The Defense and Veterans Brain Injury Center (DVBIC), the primary TBI program of the US Defense Centers of Excellence, has developed and validated a three-question screening tool for mTBI that is available at http://dvbic.dcoe.mil/files/3-Question-Screening-Tool.pdf and in the public domain. The three-question DVBIC TBI screening tool, also known as The Brief Traumatic Brain Injury Screen, can be self-administered or reviewed with a staff member. Screening is recommended for service members/veterans who were injured during combat operations, training missions, or other activities. Endorsement of at least one item within each of the three questions indicates a positive screen but diagnosis can only be based on a more thorough diagnostic interview and appropriate physical examination.

Screening for PTSD, mTBI, or other postdeployment health problems is of limited value if it does not lead to more comprehensive assessment and evidence-based treatment. VA/DoD Clinical Practice Guidelines (CPGs) are available for the management of post-traumatic stress, mTBI, major depressive disorder, substance use disorder, and postdeployment health and medically unexplained symptoms. Each can be accessed at http://www.healthquality.va.gov/index.asp and all are in the public domain and can be downloaded as a PDF or for use on a personal computer or personal digital assistant.

TABLE 224-3 Three-question Defense and Veterans Brain Injury Center Traumatic Brain Injury Screening Tool

1. **Did you have any injury(ies) during your deployment from any of the following? (check all that apply):**
   A. Fragment
   B. Bullet
   C. Vehicular (any type of vehicle, including airplane)
   D. Fall
   E. Blast (Improvised Explosive Device (IED), Rocket-Propelled Grenade (RPG), land mine, grenade, etc.)
   F. Other specify: _____

2. **Did any injury received while you were deployed result in any of the following? (check all that apply):**
   A. Being dazed, confused, or "seeing stars"
   B. Not remembering the injury
   C. Losing consciousness (knocked out) for less than a minute
   D. Losing consciousness for 1-20 min
   E. Losing consciousness for longer than 20 min
   F. Having any symptoms of concussion afterward (such as headache, dizziness, irritability, etc)
   G. Head injury
   H. None of the above

3. **Are you currently experiencing any of the following problems that you think might be related to a possible head injury or concussion? (check all that apply):**

A. Headaches	E. Ringing in the ears
B. Dizziness	F. Irritability
C. Memory problems	G. Sleep problems
D. Balance problems	H. Other specify: _____

NOTE: Confirm F and G through clinical interview.

NOTE: Endorsement of A-E meets criteria for positive TBI Screen.

Clinical practice guidelines are designed to improve clinical outcomes and/or reduce inappropriate variations in care. They are not, however, meant to constrain clinical judgment. VA/DoD CPGs are educational tools expressed as clinical algorithms that present a full range of options and assist in decision making. They are evidence based, but when no applicable research is available, they offer expert consensus recommendations.

The basis for each recommendation is provided along with an explicit grading of its strength of evidence. While CPGs for PTSD are also available through the American Psychiatric Association and other organizations, the VA/DoD CPGs may be particularly helpful because they are developed by and for a multidisciplinary group of providers for use across a broad range of clinical settings. Practice guidelines from the International Society for Traumatic Stress Studies (ISTSS), published as *Effective Treatments for PTSD* (Foa, Keane, Friedman & Cohen, 2008), are also recommended because of their multidisciplinary nature and detailed discussions of PTSD assessment and treatment. The comprehensive ISTSS guidelines provide a useful complement to the more schematized VA/DoD CPG. The VA/DoD CPGs can be applied in real time in the office. The ISTSS guidelines can be studied afterward for greater depth and broader perspective.

THE HOSPITALIST'S ROLE IN A PUBLIC HEALTH RESPONSE TO POSTDEPLOYMENT MENTAL HEALTH ISSUES

At a March 2005 DoD/VA conference on deployment mental health in Alexandria, Virginia, then Navy Surgeon General Richard Carmona observed that "… *most* war fighters *will not* develop a diagnosable mental illness but *all* war fighters and their families *will* face important readjustment issues in the course of the deployment cycle." Rather than attempting to sort OEF/OIF/OND veterans and their families into oversimplified categories of either "sick" or "well," Admiral Carmona's insight requires clinicians to adopt a population-based *public health approach* focused on helping individuals and families retain or, when necessary, regain a healthy balance despite the stress of deployment.

The public health approach requires a progressively engaging, phase-appropriate integration of services. This program must be driven by the needs of the service member/veteran and his/her family rather than by the often bureaucratic structures of traditional systems of care. It must meet prospective users where they live rather than wait for them to find their way to the right mix of services. It should increase access and reduce stigma for all members of the military, veterans, and their family members.

Hospitalists can help build an effective public health system for OEF/OIF/OND veterans and their families when they take time to find out who among their patients has served in the military or has "kept the home fires burning" for a deployed service member. Rather than reduce their patients to one or more diagnoses, hospitalists should step back to see their patients as members of a unique culture who are coping with the stress of deployment as best they can. They should realize that Guard and Reserve members

TABLE 224-4 Resources

A number of important resources can provide the glue that holds such partnerships together:

- *The Veterans Crisis Line*: Connects veterans in crisis and their families, friends and providers with qualified, caring Department of Veterans Affairs responders through a confidential toll-free hotline, online chat, or text. Veterans and their loved ones can call 1-800-273-8255 and Press 1, chat online, or send a text message to 838255 to receive confidential support 24 h a day, 7 d a week, 365 d a year. Support for deaf and hard of hearing individuals is available.

- *VA OEF/OIF/OND Program Managers*: Each of the nation's 144 VA Medical Centers has an OEF/OIF/OND program manager (usually a social worker or nurse) dedicated to helping veterans and their family members understand and connect with the benefits and services available to them. OEF/OIF/OND program managers will literally walk a veteran through the VA system and ensure a smooth transfer to appropriate care. They will also help veterans smoothly transition between DoD/VA and or private and public medical programs. They should be part of the discharge plan for any OEF/OIF/OND veteran. To contact the nearest OEF/OIF/OND care manager, check your local VA medical center website or use the OEF/OIF/OND Team Locator at http://www.oefoif.va.gov/map.asp. The VA facility locator that can be found at http://www.va.gov/directory/guide/home.asp?isflash=1.

- *Vet Centers:* VA has established 300 Vet Centers and 70 Mobile Vet Centers in towns and cities across America. Vet Centers are primarily staffed by mental health professionals and peer outreach workers who are, themselves, veterans. They provide readjustment counseling and outreach services to all veterans who served in any combat zone. They also provide services for family members for military-related issues including bereavement counseling. Veterans need not be enrolled in VA health care to use Vet Center services and there is never a charge to the veteran or the family. A Vet Center locator is available at http://www.va.gov/directory/guide/vetcenter.asp.

- *VA Community Provider Toolkit*: This site features key tools to support the mental health services provided to Veterans by clinicians outside of VA and DoD. It offers information on connecting with VA, understanding military culture and experience, as well as tools for working with a variety of mental health conditions (found under Mental Health and Wellness). See more at: http://www.mentalhealth.va.gov/communityproviders/index.asp.

- *Military OneSource*: A 24/7 website (http://www.militaryonesource.com) and telephone-based resource (1-800-342-9647), Military OneSource is an employee assistance program available to all service members and their families. Help can be provided in a variety of areas ranging from how to connect with appropriate clinical services to how to balance a checkbook. Military OneSource provides up to 12 sessions of free face-to-face counseling per family member per problem and can help providers access needed resources for their patients including housing and legal assistance.

- *The National Resource Directory*: The NRD is a partnership among DoD, VA, and the Department of Labor. Information found in the NRD comes from federal, state, and local government agencies; Veteran and military service organizations; non-profit and community-based organizations; academic institutions; and professional associations that provide assistance to wounded warriors and their families. It can be accessed at: www.nrd.gov.

- *Sesame Workshop Talk, Listen, Connect*: Sesame Workshop, the corporation behind Sesame Street, provides much-needed support and practical education with Talk, Listen, Connect, a multiphase outreach initiative to help kids through deployments, combat-related injuries, and the death of a loved one. Videos, storybooks, and workbooks especially created for this program guide families through these tough transitions by showing how real families—as well as furry monsters—deal with similar circumstances. Videos and information are available at http://www.sesameworkshop.org/what-we-do/our-initiatives/military-families/.

- *Treating the Invisible Wounds of War*: This free, accredited, on-line training for health professionals, available at http://www.aheconnect.com/citizensoldier was jointly developed by the Citizen Soldier Support Program (based at the University of North Carolina at Chapel Hill's Odum Institute for Research in Social Science) which seeks to improve access to services for Reserve Component combat veterans and their families), VA's Veterans Integrated Service Network 6 Mental Illness Research Education and Clinical Center (which focuses on post-deployment mental health), and the North Carolina Area Health Education Centers (AHEC) Program. It is an online tutorial that addresses the training needs of a wide range of medical and behavioral health providers with respect to OEF/OIF/OND veterans and their families. Of particular value is the included "boots on the ground" interview with a military couple that brings home the day-to-day realities of the deployment cycle and its profound and varied effects on family life.

- Defense and Veterans Brain Injury Center (DVBIC) website: http://dvbic.dcoe.mil/ DVBIC's mission is to serve active duty military, their beneficiaries, and veterans with traumatic brain injuries through state-of-the-art clinical care, innovative clinical research initiatives and educational programs, and support for force health protection services. DVBIC fulfills this mission through ongoing collaboration with the Department of Defense (DoD), military services, Department of Veterans Affairs (VA), civilian health partners, local communities, families and individuals with TBI.

- VA National Center for PTSD website: http://www.ptsd.va.gov. The National Center for PTSD is dedicated to research and education on trauma and PTSD. They work to assure that the latest research findings help those exposed to trauma within VA and DoD and across the community.

may officially be veterans right now, but may still deploy again. This can create new strain for the service member and family. Evidence-based psychotherapy and psychopharmacologic interventions as laid out in clinical practice guidelines have great efficacy, but what is essential in the care of these patients is that the clinician understands deployment stress in human terms.

Hospitalists must also make sure that such patients are not allowed to fall between the cracks as they transition between DoD, VA, public, and private systems of care. They should, whenever possible, promote DoD/VA/state and community partnerships in support of service members/veterans and their families. Refer to **Table 224-4** for resources.

CONCLUSION

Hospitalists have an opportunity to enhance identification of and outreach to OEF/OIF/OND veterans and their families, increase the rate of appropriate referral, smooth transitions in care, reduce the stigma currently associated with these problems, promote healthy outcomes and greater resilience, and strengthen families and communities. In the process, they can help reduce military attrition and chronic disability. The goal here is not merely to improve postdeployment care, but to transform it into a rational system in which there is *no wrong door* to which OEF/OIF/OND veterans or their families can come for genuine understanding and effective care.

SUGGESTED READINGS

Cohen BE, Gima K, Bertenthal D, Kim S, Marmar CR, Seal KH. Mental Health Diagnoses and Utilization of VA Non-Mental Health Medical Services Among Returning Iraq and Afghanistan Veterans. *J Gen Intern Med*. 2010;25(1):18-24.

Foa E, Keane TM, Friedman MJ, Cohen, JA, eds. *Effective Treatments For PTSD: Practice Guidelines from the International Society for Traumatic Stress Studies*, 2nd ed. New York, NY: Guilford Publications, Inc.; 2008.

Kudler H, Porter RI. Building Communities of Care for Military Children and Families. *Future of Children*. 2013;23(2):163-185.

Kulka RA, Schlenger WE, Fairbank JA, et al. *The National Vietnam Veterans Readjustment Study: Tables of Findings and Technical Appendices*. Vol. 1. New York, NY: Brunner/Mazel; 1990.

Marmar CR, Schlenger W, Henn-Haase C, et al. Course of Posttraumatic Stress Disorder 40 Years After the Vietnam War: Findings From the National Vietnam Veterans Longitudinal Study. *JAMA Psychiatry*. 2015;72(9):875-881.

Milliken CS, Auchterlonie JL, Hoge CW. Longitudinal Assessment of mental health problems among Active and Reserve Component Soldiers returning from the Iraq war. *JAMA*. 2007;298 (18):2141-2148.

Schwab KA, Baker G, Ivins B, Sluss-Tiller M, Lux W, Warden D. The Brief Traumatic Brain Injury Screen (BTBIS): Investigating the validity of a self-report instrument for detecting traumatic brain injury (TBI) in troops returning from deployment in Afghanistan and Iraq. *Neurology*. 2006;66(5)(Suppl 2):A235.

Tanelian T, Jaycox LH. Invisible Wounds of War: Psychological and Cognitive Injuries, Their Consequences, and Services to Assist Recovery. Santa Monica, CA: Rand Monographs; 2008.

Tanielian T, Farris C, Batka C, et al. *Ready to Serve: Community-Based Provider Capacity to Deliver Culturally Competent, Quality Mental Health Care to Veterans and Their Families*. Santa Monica, CA: RAND Corporation; 2014. http://www.rand.org/pubs/research_reports/RR806.

U.S. Department of Veterans Affairs. Environmental Epidemiology Service. VA Web site. Available at http://www.publichealth.va.gov/epidemiology/reports/oefoifond/health-care-utilization/index.asp. Accessed September 4, 2016.

VA/DoD Clinical Practice Guidelines for the Management of Traumatic Stress. Available at http://www.healthquality.va.gov/guidelines/MH/ptsd/. Accessed September 4, 2016.

CHAPTER 225

Assessment and Management of Psychosis

Anand K. Pandurangi, MD, MBBS

Key Clinical Questions

1. What is psychosis?
2. What are the various psychotic disorders?
3. How are psychotic disorders diagnosed?
4. How is psychosis treated in the acute hospital setting?
5. What are the complications of psychosis?
6. What is an optimal discharge plan for patients who are recovering from psychosis?

INTRODUCTION

New-onset psychosis and recurring psychosis identified during the course of assessment and treatment of medical disorders, require immediate intervention. 0.5% to 2.5% of all (nonpsychiatric) hospitalized patients have a pre-existing chronic psychosis and 5% to 25% of all referrals for psychiatric consultation in a hospital setting are for a psychotic disorder. New-onset psychoses may be secondary to a general medical condition, iatrogenic or functional in nature. Initiation of treatment for new cases and continuation (or resumption) of treatment for pre-existing psychosis is of paramount importance. Psychosis in children and adolescents, postpartum period and in the elderly requires special attention to dosing and adverse effects. Neglecting or undertreating the psychosis will likely lead to behavioral and medical complications. Psychosis can quickly erupt into a crisis, affecting safety, the management of the medical disorder(s) and altering hospital course and outcome. The presence of comorbid psychiatric conditions, especially if unrecognized or undertreated often increases the length of stay and cost of care. Key point in the management of psychosis is outlined in **Table 225-1**.

DEFINITIONS AND TERMINOLOGY

The term *psychosis* was first used in the mid-19th century to denote an abnormal state of mind, and typically refers to a loss of touch with reality. In 1896, Emil Kraeplin dichotomized the functional psychoses into dementia precox and manic-depressive illness to denote a chronic deteriorating cognitive disorder and a cyclical mood disorder, respectively. In 1911, Eugen Bleuler renamed the chronic cognitive disorder as schizophrenia to emphasize the underlying psychopathology of a schism in mental functions. Kraeplin's dichotomy does not cover all functional psychotic disorders, and various other psychotic disorders have been described. These include (i) catatonia characterized by abnormal motoric behaviors, (ii) stress-related brief psychoses, (iii) conditions with mixed psychotic and mood symptoms called schizoaffective psychosis, and (iv) other cyclical disorders called cycloid psychoses. In the current *Diagnostic and Statistical Manual of Mental Disorders* (5th edition, [DSM-5]), functional psychoses are described under two broad categories, namely schizophrenia spectrum and other psychotic disorders, and mood disorders with psychosis (bipolar disorders, depressive disorders). Psychosis secondary to a general medical condition or substance abuse is simply described as such (eg, psychosis secondary to hypothyroidism, alcohol-induced psychosis). All other psychoses which cannot be clearly categorized under the above conditions are labeled psychosis, not otherwise specified.

Psychosis refers to a sustained mental state of loss or impaired touch with reality. It is manifested by one or more of the following: hallucinatory experiences, delusional beliefs, disordered communication, and disorganized, unusual, strange and/or regressed behaviors. These are also referred to as positive symptoms. Transient states of perceptual alterations such as those occurring after sleep deprivation or as part of a desired religious experience are typically not considered psychosis. Psychosis is often a manifestation of substance abuse. Many general medical conditions, especially central nervous system (CNS) disorders, may lead to the manifestation of psychosis. Finally, psychosis is frequently associated with delirium and dementia.

Although the pathophysiology of the various psychoses remains unknown, there is much evidence to suggest a hyperdopaminergic

TABLE 225-1 Key Points to Managing Psychosis

- Psychosis is a sustained mental state of impaired contact with reality.
- Psychosis is manifested with one or more of the following: hallucinations, delusions, disordered communication, and unusual behaviors.
- Short-lasting functional psychotic disorders include brief psychotic disorder and schizophreniform disorder.
- Chronic or recurrent functional psychotic disorders include schizophrenia, schizoaffective disorder, delusion disorder, and severe mood disorders.
- Substance abuse may cause psychosis.
- Endocrine, immunologic, metabolic, neoplastic, and other general medical disorders as well as substance abuse and select medications may cause or contribute to psychosis.
- Psychosis may be seen as part of dementia or delirium, or in association with a developmental disorder such as autism or intellectual disability (mental retardation).
- Sensory impairment may cause or contribute to a paranoid psychosis in the elderly patient.
- Assessment includes history of the psychotic symptoms including time course, medical review of systems, physical and mental status examinations, and laboratory tests as needed.
- Diagnosis may be made by applying the DSM-5 criteria to the above information.
- Antipsychotic medications are essential to control the psychosis.
- A safe and supportive environment is necessary.
- Florid psychosis persistent for several days is best treated on a psychiatric unit, when feasible.
- Psychosis may take 3-14 d to resolve and sometimes longer.
- Education of the patient and significant others on compliance, side effects, and signs of relapse is a key ingredient of a safe discharge plan.
- Patients need follow-up care within 1-2 wk of discharge.

state as a final common pathway for the positive symptoms of psychosis. Recent fMRI studies implicate a dysfunction in the interaction between the default mode network and frontoparietal control systems.

POSITIVE SYMPTOMS

- *Hallucination* refers to perceptual experience(s) in the absence of an external stimulus. The source of the perception is typically placed in objective space (ie, not from inner self, ego, subconscious, mind, soul, etc). The perception may be in any sensory modality. For example, hearing voices of people who are not around or seeing images such as those of god, angels, the devil, large and small animals, dead people, fire etc. Hallucinations may also occur in the olfactory, tactile, gustatory, or proprioceptive modalities. Auditory hallucinations are more typical in functional psychosis, and visual and tactile hallucinations are more common in psychoses secondary to use of substances or from a general medical condition, and in delirium. However, this is not a hard and fast rule, nor is it diagnostic in and of itself.
- *Delusion* refers to a fixed false and irrational belief. The contents are not congruent with those of the subculture to which the patient belongs and the belief has been arrived at in an irrational manner. Delusions are categorized based on their content into persecutory, grandiose, somatic, etc. Here are a few examples: (1) a man with schizophrenia believes that the FBI (or another group/

agency) has stationed 360° cameras around his house, office, and car and beams these pictures around the globe to invade his privacy and publicize his life. (2) A woman believes that surgeons enter her room in the night and replace her organs with diseased ones to spread a new type of disease in her family.

- *Thought disorder* refers to impairments in the process of thinking, and is also referred to as formal thought disorder. A commonly seen type of this is "loose associations," although there are more than 18 varieties of disordered thinking. The impairment may be in the thinking process, language, speech, or communication. For example, a 25-year-old with schizophrenia was asked during initial evaluation, "what seems to be the problem?" and responded as follows: "I was driving on the expressway when the spiders appeared, looking ugly, *uhh* they made all the difference to god's creativity. I had to know who this was. Had seen him before. His voice had that distinct sound (... pause), you know the one's animals make when they are doing their perfunctory thing. No wonder you doctors can tell all the difference."
- *Disorganized behavior* refers to a range of behaviors reflective of a lack of organization, cohesiveness, and purpose in one's external behavior, often reflecting the internal chaos of the mind. States of excitement, stereotypical movements, severe withdrawal and isolation, catatonic stupor, regressed behaviors such as poor self-care and hygiene are all subsumed under this term.

NEGATIVE SYMPTOMS

Negative symptoms refer to a set of emotional and behavioral deficits that indicate loss of normal mental functions.

- *Blunted affect* refers to a diminution in the tone, experience, range, and depth of emotion and is used interchangeably with the terms *flat affect or restricted affect*. A person exhibiting a blunted affect may not show appropriate sadness, happiness, anger, etc as warranted by an event or situation.
- *Alogia* refers to a state of reduced speech and is also called poverty of speech and poverty of content of speech. The patient may respond minimally to questions and/or appear to have difficulty being productive with verbal expressions. The speech may be hollow and convey little content.
- *Apathy, avolition, and anhedonia* describe a state of reduced interest and emotion and inability to experience pleasure.
- *Asociality* refers to reduced social interactions including limited or no close relationships. It should not be confused with antisocial, which refers to breaking social norms and laws without a sense of remorse.

The DSM-5 has organized the negative symptoms and behaviors broadly under two headings, Diminished Emotional Expression and Diminished Volition.

RELATED TERMINOLOGY

In the context of psychosis, terms such as reality testing, impaired capacity, poor judgment, poor insight, poor ego boundaries, etc are often used by psychiatric clinicians.

Reality testing: This is the capacity to correctly interpret stimuli such as thoughts, feelings, and somatic sensations, etc, as internal, and people and events as external, and appropriately interpret the relation (or absence thereof) between the two. For example, a patient may believe that gurgling sounds out of his belly are messages from his deceased mother and that both are being controlled by the devil.

Poor ego boundaries: This is a disturbance in volition, ownership, and boundaries of one's thoughts, feelings, and perceptions. Thus, a patient may believe his thoughts are being heard/known by others (broadcasting). Patient may attribute control of actions such as eating, talking, walking, etc or emotions to others (passivity). For example, a 25-year-old woman believed that the dentist had inserted a powerful microchip into her teeth and was able to make her experience sexual feelings toward older men.

Poor insight: This is a lack of awareness of one's own behavior, especially changes from a baseline or prior state, and/or the need to change one's behavior. For example, a 35-year-old man was angry at his wife for having called the mental health crisis line for help after he had been neglecting to eat or shower and was sitting at home for several days gazing out of the window and sighing frequently. He claimed he was "just resting."

Poor judgment: This is the inability to assess the totality of one's situation, consequences, and necessary actions. For example, a 65-year-old person with suspected dementia refused to move out of the home after it had been condemned by the social service agency because "it is my mother's home and I will fix it over the weekend."

Impaired capacity: This is the inability to assess a specific condition or situation, its consequences, and actions to be undertaken. For example, a 45-year-old man with a history of traumatic brain injury, seizures, and severe cognitive impairment had developed aplastic anemia and was in isolation on the medical unit with a fever. He consistently refused to have any blood transfusion, saying "had the flu many times, clears up in a couple of days."

PSYCHOTIC DISORDERS

A brief description of each psychotic disorder is given in **Table 225-2**.

PSYCHOSIS SECONDARY TO GENERAL MEDICAL CONDITIONS

There is an extensive literature dating back many decades on medical conditions that may cause or significantly contribute to psychosis. **Table 225-3** lists some of the common and better-known general medical conditions that may manifest psychosis. In recent years, newly recognized disorders, although rare but which may cause or contribute to psychosis include Prion disease and NMDA receptor antibody associated encephalitis. High doses of steroids given for anti-inflammation or immunosupression may cause

TABLE 225-2 Disorders with Psychosis

Disorder	Course and Duration	Features and Diagnosis	Outcome/Comments
Brief psychotic disorder	Acute, days to < 4 wk	Often precipitated by stress. Dramatic and fluctuating psychosis. Rule out medical causes and substances.	Full remission of symptoms and return of function.
Schizophreniform disorder	Acute, > 4 wk and <6 mo	Schizophrenia-like symptoms. R/O mood disorder, substances and medical causes.	May progress to schizophrenia.
Schizophrenia	Chronic, years	> 1 mo of psychotic symptoms, > 6 mo of behavior change. R/O mood disorder, substance abuse and medical causes. Functional decline occurs.	Persistence of symptoms in 30%-60% of patients. Some recovery is possible in most.
Schizoaffective disorder	Chronic, years	Symptoms of psychosis and mood disorder are equally prominent. > 2 wk of psychosis without mood symptoms needed for diagnosis.	Outcome is better than schizophrenia.
Delusion disorder	Chronic, > 1 mo to years	Prominent nonbizarre delusion(s). No hallucinations or minimal.	Personality is preserved. Function often preserved.
Depression with psychosis	Intermittent > 2 wk	Depression is primary. Content of psychosis often congruent with mood.	Outcome better than schizophrenia. Responds well to electroconvulsive therapy.
Mania with psychosis	Episodic, > 1 wk	Mania is primary. Content of psychosis often congruent with mood.	Outcome better than schizophrenia.
Postpartum Psychosis	Occurs within 6 wk of delivery	May be any type of functional psychosis listed above.	Medical causes not uncommon and should be ruled out first.
Substance-induced with psychosis (see Table 225-4)	Variable. With substance use, and a short period thereafter.	Visual and tactile hallucinations and paranoia are common. Alcohol and amphetamine psychosis may mimic schizophrenia.	Psychosis may persist days to weeks after abstinence.
Delirium with psychosis	Brief in duration	Disturbed consciousness. Psychosis often inferred from behavior. Fragmentary and fleeting delusions. Visual and tactile hallucinations may be seen.	May require frequent parenteral antipsychotics in small doses rather than bolus or single large dose.
Psychosis due to a general medical condition (see Table 225-3)	Varies with condition	Verified by diagnosis of the underlying medical condition, and resolution with its treatment. Visual hallucinations may often be seen. May be part of delirium.	
Dementia with psychosis (Alzheimer, vascular, etc)	Intermittent or chronic	Often inferred from behavior. Delusions are fragmentary and not well elaborated.	Low doses of antipsychotics may be sufficient.
Developmental disorder with psychosis (autism spectrum disorders, intellectual disability)	Intermittent or chronic	Delusions are often poorly formed and fragmentary. Visual hallucinations may be seen. Not to be confused with literal or concrete interpretation of reality, or overlearned behavior.	Higher doses of medications often not well tolerated. Higher risk of tardive dyskinesia.

TABLE 225-3 Medical Conditions that May Manifest Psychosis

System/Cause	Disorders	
	Common*	Uncommon†
Endocrine	Addison, Cushing, hyper and hypothyroidism	Hyper and hypoparathyroidism, pituitary disorders including Sheehan syndrome
Infections	Lyme disease, pneumonia	Diphtheria, legionnaire disease, malaria, typhoid
Inflammatory	Acute rheumatic fever, systemic lupus (cerebritis, vasculitis), sarcoidosis	Temporal arteritis
Metabolic	Diabetic ketoacidosis, hepatic encephalopathy, hypoglycemia, hypoxia, hyponatremia, uremia	Acute intermittent porphyria, Niemann Pick, Tay-Sachs
Nutritional	Vitamin B1 deficiency (Wernicke-Korsakoff syndrome), B12 deficiency	Folic acid deficiency, niacin deficiency (pellagra)
Pharmacologic	Anticholinergics, antiobesity, antiparkinsonian: levodopa, partial agonists, steroids, sympathomimetics	Antacids: cimetidine; antihistamines; antihypertensives: clonidine, propranolol; anti-inflammatories: cyclosporin, NSAIDs, salicylate, steroids; antineoplastics: methotrexate, 5-fluorouracil; cardiac: digoxin, antiarrhythmics
Substance abuse (see Table 225-4)	Alcohol, amphetamines, cocaine, cannabis	Lysergic acid diethylamine (LSD), belladonna alkaloids, phencyclidine (pcp), mescaline, psilocybin
Toxic		Carbon monoxide poisoning, industrial toxins, heavy metal poisoning (eg, lead, mercury)
Trauma	Epidural hematoma, intraparenchymal hemorrhage, subarachanoid hemorrhage, subdural hematoma	
Central nervous system disorders		
CNS disorders	Multiple sclerosis, normal pressure hydrocephalus, seizure disorders lobe	NMDA receptor antibody encephalitis, Prion disease
Basal ganglia disorders	Parkinson disorder	Huntington disease, Wilson disease, Fahr disease
CNS infections	HIV encephalopathy, any encephalitis, meningitis	Herpes encephalitis, rocky mountain spotted fever, syphilis
Dementias	Alzheimer disease, Vascular dementia	Pick disease, Creutzfeld-Jacob disease
Space occupying lesions	Cerebral neoplasm	Cerebral abscess, intracranial aneurysm, angioma
Vascular	Cerebrovascular events, hypertensive encephalopathy	
Congenital disorders		
Developmental	Autism, intellectual disability, Tourette syndrome	
Genetic: other	Down syndrome (Trisomy 21)	Adrenoleucodystrophy (X-linked), Klinefelter syndrome (XXY), Marfan syndrome (Chromosomes 5, 15), mitochondrial disorders, Prader-Willi (15q), velocardiofacial syndrome (22q)

*Common: either the medical condition is common or psychosis as a manifestation is common.
†Uncommon: either the medical condition is uncommon or psychosis as a manifestation is uncommon.

various mood and behavior effects including psychosis. Visual and tactile hallucinations are often a clue to an underlying physical or pharmacologic etiology. The psychosis may virtually mimic any of the functional disorders and it is the detection of a physical cause by history, examination, or testing that establishes the medical etiology. The course of the psychosis in these conditions is highly variable and dependent on the underlying disorder. In chronic conditions, such as lupus, multiple sclerosis, seizure disorder, and hepatic and renal failure, psychosis may manifest recurrently. An interesting although not pathagnomonic distinction between psychoses secondary to a general medical condition and schizophrenic disorders is the absence of negative symptoms in the former.

PSYCHOSIS INDUCED BY SUBSTANCE ABUSE

Table 225-4 lists the common substances of abuse that may manifest with psychosis. Visual and tactile hallucinations are common. Alcohol-induced psychosis may manifest with classic paranoid delusions and hallucinations and may easily be misdiagnosed as

schizophrenia. In LSD psychosis, temporal lobe phenomena such as experiences of deja vu and jamais vu are not uncommon. Classic substance-induced psychosis should resolve within days of abstinence. However long-term use especially of alcohol may lead to persistent hallucinosis. When the psychosis is active, it is important to treat it adequately with antipsychotic medications and supportive therapies as well as standard withdrawal protocols. In recent years, designer drugs have emerged that cause or contribute to psychosis such as those containing the synthetic cannabinoid cannabicyclohexanol ("Spice"), methylenedioxy amphetamine ("Sally", "Sass") and methylenedioxymethamphetamine (MDMA) ("Ecstacy","Molly"). Routine urine drug screens may not identify these substances warranting more specialized testing.

ASSESSMENT

■ PSYCHIATRIC HISTORY AND EXAMINATION

Assessment should start with a focus on current symptoms, their duration, severity, and impact on daily function, and then proceed

TABLE 225-4 Substance-Induced Psychosis

Substances Known to Induce Psychosis
Alcohol
Cannabis: marijuana, synthetic cannabis (ingredient of "K2," "Spice")
Hallucinogens: ketamine, LSD, mescaline, phencyclidine (angel dust), psilocybin, etc
Inhalants: amyl nitrate, gasoline, paint, paint thinners, etc
Opioids: morphine, oxycodone, hydromorphone
Stimulants: amphetamines, metamphetamines, cocaine, methylphenidate (Ritalin), designer drugs (MDMA or Ecstacy)

to past psychiatric history, substance abuse history, and brief psychosocial history including current living situation and support network. A separate history should be obtained for unsafe behaviors including self-injurious behaviors, suicidal ideation, intention, plans and attempts, and any ideas/behaviors of aggression/violence toward people and property.

■ SUBSTANCE USE HISTORY AND TESTING

A detailed substance abuse history is a necessary part of the workup of psychosis and should cover all commonly abused substances, especially those known to cause psychosis (Table 225-4). A urine test for common drugs of abuse, and, if indicated, additional blood or urine tests for toxicology, should be ordered.

■ MEDICAL HISTORY, REVIEW OF SYSTEMS, AND LABORATORY ASSESSMENT

It is imperative that all patients presenting with any psychotic symptom or behavior receive a proper medical workup including medical history, review of systems, and required testing. It is not, however, appropriate to order tests without a clinical indication, for example head CT, EEG, or CSF studies. Prenatal, birth, and early developmental history needs to be gathered from patient, family, or collateral source to rule in or out genetic, congenital, and developmental conditions known to manifest with psychoses (Table 225-3). Laboratory assessment has two main purposes: (1) to rule in or out specific medical causes suspected from the history and examination, and (2) to assess for conditions commonly comorbid with chronic psychotic disorders, such as anemia, obesity, hypertension, cardiac disease and diabetes. It should be remembered that patients with chronic mental illness are at a 1.5 to 2 times higher risk of having common systemic medical disorders.

■ NEUROLOGIC ASSESSMENT

It is appropriate for a patient having a psychotic illness to be assessed neurologically with an EEG, brain scan, and neuropsychological testing at least once in the course of his or her illness, preferably early on. In cases of new-onset psychosis and psychosis in the elderly person, such testing is more likely to yield clinically significant findings, such as neurodevelopmental abnormalities, seizure foci, or atrophic, vascular, and neoplastic lesions.

Following the above, a complete mental status examination should be conducted to assess current positive and negative symptoms of psychosis as well as mood and cognitive functions such as attention, orientation, and memory. The mini–mental status examination is a handy tool to assess the latter. Equipped with information from the histories, examination and test results, a diagnosis may be arrived at guided by DSM-5 criteria.

TREATMENT OF ACUTE PSYCHOSIS

The physician has the option of choosing from many available antipsychotic medications, although the evidence to date suggests they are roughly equal in efficacy but vary widely in their side effects. Effect on the comorbid medical conditions, such as obesity, diabetes, cardiac disorders, and neurologic disorders, and any information available from prior experience of the patient, can help inform this decision.

ANTIPSYCHOTIC MEDICATIONS

First-generation antipsychotics (FGA) (see **Table 225-5**), also known as *typical* antipsychotics are effective with positive psychotic symptoms but have a higher potential to cause extrapyramidal effects, such as dystonia, parkinsonism, akathisia, and tardive dyskinesia. The most widely prescribed typical antipsychotic is haloperidal (Haldol). Other available FGA medications from the phenothiazine class are fluphenazine (Prolixin), trifluperazine (Stelazine), perphenazine (Trilafon), and chlorpromazine (Thorazine). Nonphenothiazine FGA antipsychotics are thiothixene (Navane), loxapine (Loxitane), and molindone (Moban). All these agents are thought to reduce psychosis, predominantly through the blockade of dopamine-2 receptors in the midbrain-limbic circuits.

Second-generation antipsychotics (SGA) are used more widely in practice due to reduced extrapyramidal effects, and are virtually the first line of treatment. These include, in order of approval by the FDA, clozapine, risperidone (Risperdal), olanzapine (Zyprexa), quetiapine (Seroquel), ziprasidone (Geodon), aripirazole (Abilify), paliperidone (Invega), Iloperidone (Fanapt), Asenapine (Saphris), lurasidone (Latuda) and brexipiprazole (Rexulti). Clozapine, the first atypical antipsychotic agent is a very effective antipsychotic with proven superiority in refractory schizophrenia, however it has additional toxicities such as agranulocytosis, seizure, pluritis and myocarditis and is restricted for use in refractory patients. Its use requires registration with the risk mitigation program called clozapineREMS program, and includes mandatory monitoring of the absolute neutrophil count (ANC), weekly for 6 months, biweekly for 6 months and then monthly thereafter. In determining the minimum ANC threshold to start or resume clozapine, special consideration is given for persons with benign ethnic neutropenia. The SGAs are moderately dopamine blocking and also evidence antagonism to serotonin-2 receptors. Aripiprazole (Abilify) and Brexipiprazole (Rexulti) are also considered as atypical SGA because of the low potential for EPS, although their mechanism of action is different; these two agents are partial dopamine agonists. A scale of chlorpromazine-equivalent units (CPZ units) is available to convert the dose of one typical FGA to that of another, and can be approximated to the atypical SGAs as well (Table 225-5).

DOSING

The antipsychotic agent is started at an initial dose of approximately 100 CPZ units, for example, 2 mg of haloperidol, or 2 mg of risperidone, or 100 mg of quetiapine, and titrated up every 1 to 2 days until sufficient control of symptoms is achieved. Additional doses of the drug may be used on an as-needed basis to supplement the regular dose. The dosing is illustrated in two cases using haloperidol and quetiapine as examples. The drug choice in the examples is arbitrary and the dosing is just one example of standard practice. Other dosing regimens may be substituted without loss of efficacy.

RESUMPTION OF TREATMENT FOR PRE-EXISTING PSYCHOSIS

Medical illnesses often act as stressors and escalate pre-existing psychosis, and often patients become noncompliant with medications. An antipsychotic should be reinstituted at the soonest possible time. In others who remain compliant, continue the antipsychotic. In both cases, it is best to use the antipsychotic that the patient was receiving most recently. In noncompliant patients, the starting dose may have to be lower than the most recently prescribed dose and

TABLE 225-5 Commonly Available Antipsychotic Medications

Generic and Common Brand Names	Mechanism of Action and DA2 Receptor Potency	Daily Dose* in mg	Common Adverse Events	Comments
FGA (Typical)				
Chlorpromazine (Thorazine)	D2 antagonist, low	200-1000	Hypotension, sedation, EPS, TD	First available antipsychotic
Loxapine (Loxitane)	D2 antagonist, medium	25-200	Sedation, EPS, TD	
Molindone (Moban)	D2 antagonist, medium	25-225	Activation, EPS	
Thiothixene (Navane)	D2 antagonist, medium to High	10-80	EPS, TD	
Perphenazine (Trilafon)	D2 antagonist, medium to high	8-64	EPS, TD	Used in CATIE, largest nonindustry trial
Trifluperazine (Stelazine)	D2 antagonist, medium to high	5-60	EPS, TD	
Fluphenazine (Prolixin)	D2 antagonist, high	5-60	EPS, TD	
Fluphenazine decanoate long-acting inj		12.5-100 every 3 wk		
Haloperidol (Haldol)	D2 antagonist, high	2-20	EPS, prolactinemia, TD	Most widely used typical antipsychotic
Haloperidol decanoate, long-acting inj		25-200 every 4 wk		
SGA (Atypical)				
Risperidone (Risperdal)	D2 and 5-HT2 antagonist, high	1-6	Hypotension, sedation, prolactinemia, weight gain, EPS at higher doses	
Risperidone long-acting inj, (CONSTA)		12.5-50 Q2 wk		
Paliperidone (Invega)	D2 and 5-HT2 antagonist, high	6-18,	Sedation, dizziness, EPS at higher doses	Active metabolite of risperidone
Paliperidone palmitate long acting inj (Invega Sustenna)		117-234 Q4 wk		
Olanzapine (Zyprexa)	D2 and 5-HT2 antagonist, medium to high	5-20	Hypotension, sedation, weight gain, DM	
Olanzapine pamoate, long-acting inj, (Relprevv)		150-405 Q4 wk		
Quetiapine (Seroquel)	D2 and 5-HT2 antagonist, low	100-800	Hypotension, sedation	
Ziprasidone (Geodon)	D2 and 5-HT2 antagonist, medium	40-160	Hypotension, prolonged QTc	
Arpiprazole (Abilify)	Partial D2 agonist, 5-HT2 antagonist, high	5-30	Activation, nausea	
Aripiprazole long acting inj (Abilify Maintenna)		300-400, Q4 wk		
Asenapine (Saphris)	D2, 5-HT2, high	5-20	Oral numbness, dizziness, somnolence, akathisia, weight gain	Sublingual
Iloperidone(Fanapt)	D2,5-HT2 antagonist, High	2-24		
Lurasidone (Latuda)	D2, 5-HT2, medium	40-80	Somnolence, dizziness, nausea, Parkinson	
Brexipiprazole	Partial D2 agonist, 5-HT2 antagonist, high	2-4	Activation, agitation, nausea	
Clozapine (Clozaril)	D2 antagonist, low 5-HT2 antagonist, high	100-800	Sedation, weight gain, hypotension, seizures, agranulocytosis, DM	ANC monitoring required (clozapineREMS.org)

5-HT2, serotonin 2 receptor; D2, Dopamine 2 receptor, DM, diabetes mellitus; EPS, extrapyramidal symptoms; TD, tardive dyskinesia; ANC, absolute neutrophil count.
*Dose ranges given reflect those used in common clinical practice.

gradually titrated up to the full dose to guard against acute adverse effects. As treatment proceeds, the dose may need to be increased, sometimes beyond the previous maintenance dose.

MANAGEMENT OF ADVERSE EFFECTS

Common side effects include extrapyramidal effects such as dystonia, treated with intramuscular diphenhydramine, and Parkinsonism, treated with benztropine 1 to 2 mg two to three times a day. Other anticholinergics that may be substituted for benztropine include trihexyphenidyl (Artane) or biperiden (Kemadrin). Akathisia is a subjective sense of unease with objective motor restlessness that

may arise a few days into treatment, and is treated with lorazepam (Ativan) 1 to 2 mg two or three times a day, or propranolol (Inderal) 10 to 40 mg two or three times a day.

MANAGEMENT OF SEVERE AGITATION

The use of as-needed (PRN) antipsychotic medication has been mentioned earlier. Sometimes it is necessary to use two antipsychotics for managing acute agitation. For example, a patient may be on quetiapine and while the standing dose is being titrated up, additional as-needed haloperidol by injection (intramuscular or intravenous), such as 2 to 5 mg every 4 to 6 hours may be given.

Second-generation antipsychotics are also available for intramuscular injections and include ziprasidone 10 to 20 mg intramuscular every 6 to 8 hours, aripiprazole 9.75 mg intramuscular every 8 hours, and olanzapine 5 to 10 mg intramuscular every 6 to 8 hours. Lorazepam 1 to 2 mg as an intramuscular or intravenous injection given every 4 to 6 hours, may also be used to control psychotic agitation. It is not recommended to use more than two antipsychotics in any form for managing most cases. The potential for greater adverse effects such as excessive sedation, orthostasis and falls, and EPS is increased with polypharmacy, while not much is added to efficacy. Soft restraints to the arms and legs may have to be used to prevent injury to self or others.

ADJUNCT MEDICATION

Patients with pre-existing psychosis are often on a mood stabilizer such as divalproex sodium or lithium; antidepressant medications; benzodiazepines, such as lorazepam or clonazepam; and/or hypnotic-sedatives such as zolpidem (Ambien), zaleplon (Sonata) and eszopiclone (Lunesta). In such cases, it is best to coordinate the care with the outpatient psychiatrist by obtaining his or her opinion on continuation or discontinuation of these medications. In the absence of any such input, it is prudent to use the lowest effective dose of these agents for active symptoms, and not blindly resume all psychotropics. The exceptions to this rule are clozapine, high-dose benzodiazepines (eg, >4 mg of lorazepam per day), and selective serotonin receptor inhibitors (paroxetine, sertraline, citalopram, etc), in which the potential for withdrawal effects is high. Fluoxetine (Prozac) has a long half-life and is self-tapering.

MILIEU AND PSYCHOSOCIAL THERAPIES

Patients exhibiting psychosis are best cared for in a private room for their own safety and comfort as well as that of other patients. In case of severely agitated, destructive, and/or disruptive behaviors, the use of soft restraints may be necessary till the medications are dosed appropriately and are effective. In case of unsafe behavior including self-injurious ideation and behaviors or suicidal behavior, it is recommended that the patient be on one-on-one observation, with 24/7 visual contact and arms-length supervision as warranted by the intensity/severity of the safety condition.

The issue of keeping the patient on a medical-surgical unit versus transfer to a psychiatric unit is often difficult. Clearly, if the acute medical-surgical conditions that the patient is in the hospital for have been addressed or are subsiding, then it is appropriate to promptly move the patient to a dedicated psychiatric unit. On the other hand, if the medical-surgical problems need active management including interventions, such as intravenous infusions, telemetry, frequent medical-neurologic examinations, postoperative surgical care, frequent or extensive wound care, or care of extensive burns etc, then it is recommended to keep the patient on the appropriate unit, while initiating or continuing the psychiatric care.

Patients with psychosis should not receive too much stimulation from the environment (lights, noise, television, medical rounds with large numbers of people, frequent interruptions by staff, etc); care should be taken to minimize this. The patient should be allowed to participate in self-care activities as tolerated by their medical condition. Paranoid patients may feel further threatened by loss of autonomy and control. Visits by caregivers and visitors should be brief and structured. Emotionally neutral activities are preferred rather than free access to health and news channels on TV, movies, etc.

A social worker or care coordinator should work with the patient and significant others to address any external stress and environmental manipulation, as feasible. The patient's dignity should be upheld at all times. The patient should be respected and kept fully informed of all health care plans and decisions, albeit with brief and succinct information. As discussed in more detail later in this chapter, consent should be obtained for all procedures, testing, and treatment outside routine care.

PSYCHIATRIC CONSULTATION

As soon as psychosis is suspected or history of a pre-existing psychotic disorder is obtained, a psychiatric consultation is recommended. However, nonpsychiatric physicians may manage a psychosis if such consultation is not available, especially if the pre-existing psychosis is a chronic condition and is stable or in remission. In this case, simply continuing the previous treatment with attention to proper dosing may suffice. However, if the psychosis is new in onset or has relapsed, it is recommended that a psychiatric consultation be obtained as soon as possible. In hospitals where such consultation is not feasible and active psychosis persists beyond 3 days, the patient should ideally be transferred to a hospital where such consultation is available or to a psychiatric unit, as appropriate. Psychiatric consultation is also recommended in case of questions regarding capacity to make medical decisions and possible involuntary treatment. The consultation should be ongoing till the psychosis is resolved, fully stabilized, or the patient is discharged.

CAPACITY AND CONSENT

Physicians will frequently encounter situations wherein the capacity of a patient with psychosis is called into question. This may arise if and when a patient refuses or does not cooperate with routine care, specific medical-surgical procedures for testing or treatment, psychiatric treatment, and/or requests premature discharge or attempts to leave. The situation may be urgent or nonurgent and elective. In each case except the most pressing situation, it is prudent to obtain a psychiatric consultation, which should include an opinion on the capacity of the patient to make a specific medical decision. Simple instruments are available to assess key areas pertaining to capacity. In an urgent situation, the physician may initiate interventions to save life or avoid permanent injury while seeking a consultation and consent from an appropriate entity in accordance with hospital policy and local, state, and federal law. In less urgent situations, the consultation and capacity assessment and appropriate consenting should precede the intervention.

Typically, a patient is considered to have capacity unless and until assessed to be otherwise. Such assessment may be performed by any physician although it is better to have a licensed mental health professional, preferably a psychiatrist, conduct this. Although state laws vary considerably, most states allow for urgent medical treatment of an individual, if (1) lack of treatment is likely to result in permanent injury or death, (2) the individual is assessed to not have capacity to make the decision, and (3) consent has been obtained from an appropriate third party, typically legal next of kin or a local magistrate. Continuation of the treatment and initiation of less urgent interventions including non–life-saving interventions often require an assessment of capacity, recommendation by an independent physician, preferably a mental health professional, approval by an ethics or equivalent committee, and/or consent by a magistrate.

COMPLICATIONS AND MANAGEMENT

The complications of an active psychosis (**Table 225-6**) include behavioral and/or medical events. These include severe agitation, disruptive behavior, unsafe behaviors including suicidal ideation and attempt, aggressive and violent behavior, leaving against medical advice, elopement, and escape. These behaviors may result from psychotic experiences such as hallucinations and delusions including paranoid fears, or may be the result of independent psychiatric disorders such as substance abuse and personality disorder. When

TABLE 225-6 Behavioral and Medical Complications of Psychosis

Behavioral	Physical/Laboratory
Neglect of self-care	Exacerbation of medical disorders such as hypertension, diabetes, seizures, and infections
Withdrawal and catatonia	Dehydration, electrolyte imbalance
Severe excitement	Autonomic arousal and hyperactivity
Injury to self and others including homicide	Injuries (from restraint): soft tissue, fractures, etc
Suicide	Muscle breakdown, increased CPK, acute renal failure
Depression	Starvation, ketosis, acidosis, and metabolic disturbances
Amotivation, social isolation, deficit states, institutionalization	Sudden death

CPK, creatine phosphokinase.

assessed to be the result of psychosis, such behavior is best treated with a combination of antipsychotic medication and supportive therapy/counseling, including education of patient/significant other. If assessed to be from factors other than the psychosis, psychosocial interventions including negotiation with the patient, liaison by a psychiatrist, or assistance by a social worker or care coordinator may be helpful, depending on the issues.

Medical complications may include compromised fluid intake, electrolyte imbalance, poor nutrition and weight loss, autonomic hyperactivity including tachycardia, hypertensive crisis, hyperthermia, muscle rigidity, increased creatine kinase, and acute renal failure. The syndrome of malignant catatonia may start as a state of psychotic excitement and progress to catatonic stupor, and many of the physical complications noted above may be part of this syndrome. Its features overlap significantly with those of neuroleptic malignant syndrome.

Medical complications from psychotropic medications may include adverse effects such as extrapyramidal symptoms and signs, orthostatic hypotension, excessive sedation, liver enzyme abnormalities, blood dyscrasias including leucopenia, mild leucocytosis, changes in ECG including prolongation of QT interval, seizures, and micturition difficulties including rarely distended bladder. The combination of haloperidol and lithium was reported to be associated with a toxic encephalopathic syndrome, although this entity remains controversial. All neuorleptic agents have been associated with neuroleptic malignant syndrome, especially those with higher D2-blocking property, such as haloperidol. Clozapine has a 0.5% to 1.0% risk of inducing agranulocytosis, 2% to 5% risk of seizure, and is (rarely) associated with pleuritis and myocarditis. Olanzapine has sometimes been reported to cause an acute ketoacidosis. Clozapine and olanzapine when combined with benzodiazepines such as lorazepam, especially when given intramuscularly have been associated with apneic episodes, and rarely death.

Medical syndromes from the withdrawal of psychotropic agents may include SSRI discontinuation syndrome manifested by motor restlessness, insomnia, nausea, and vomiting, sense of confusion, myoclonic jerks, and rarely generalized seizure. Clozapine withdrawal may manifest a similar syndrome. Withdrawal from benzodiazepines may lead to tachycardia, hypertension, and seizures. It is therefore prudent to taper these medications rather than sudden discontinuation.

CONCLUSION

Psychosis is often seen on medical-surgical units as a comorbid condition. Acute psychosis constitutes an emergency and should be assessed and treated as such. Behavioral and medical complications may result from untreated or poorly treated psychosis. Psychosis is a syndrome and depending on the underlying disorder, its course and outcome will vary. There are both acute- and short-lasting functional psychotic disorders and chronic disorders. Medical factors and substances of abuse should be considered in the assessment of psychosis. Antipsychotic medications are the mainstay of treatment and careful attention should be given to the selection of the agent and dosing. Antipsychotics have many side effects, which play a significant role in the choice of medication. Psychosis in the context of an acute medical condition may be successfully treated on a medical unit and most psychoses will resolve or may be controlled with proper treatment. Psychiatric consultation is recommended and can be helpful in determining the nature of the psychosis, the choice of antipsychotic medication, the capacity to consent, detecting adverse effects and their management, and making recommendations on aftercare. Brief psychosocial interventions such as structured activity, patient counseling, involving significant others, and care coordination increases the chances of successful management and better outcomes. Follow-up care with a psychiatrist or mental health clinic is an integral part of the management of psychotic disorders.

SUGGESTED READINGS

American Psychiatric Association. Diagnostic and Statistical Manual of Mental Disorders, 5th ed., (DSM-5). Washington, DC: American Psychiatric Association Press; 2013.

Buchanan RW. Clozapine: efficacy and safety. Schizophr Bull. 1995;21:579-591.

Citrome LL. A review of the pharmacology, efficacy and tolerability of recently approved and upcoming oral antipsychotics: an evidence-based medicine approach. CNS Drugs. 2013;27(11):879-911.

Davidson L, McGlashan TH. The varied outcomes of schizophrenia. Can J Psychiatry. 1997;42:34-43.

Feifel D. Rationale and guidelines for the inpatient treatment of acute psychosis. J Clin Psychiatry. 2000;61(14):27-32.

Freudenreich O, Stern TA. Clinical Experience with the management of schizophrenia in the general hospital. Psychosomatics. 2003;44:12-23.

Goff DC, Henderson DC, Manschreck TC. Psychotic patients. In Cassem NH, ed. Massachusetts General Hospital Handbook of General Hospital Psychiatry. St Louis, MO: Mosby; 1997, 149-171.

Kane JM, Leucht S, Carpenter D, et al. The expert consensus guideline series. optimizing pharmacologic treatment of psychotic disorders. introduction: methods, commentary, and summary. J Clin Psychiatry. 2003;64:5-19.

Lamdan RM, Ramchandani D, Schindler BA. The chronically mentally ill on a general hospital consultation-liaison service. their needs and management. Psychosomatics. 1997;38:472-477.

Richards CF, Gurr DE. Psychosis. Emerg Med Clin North Am. 2000;18: 253-262, ix.

CHAPTER 226

Eating Disorders

Angela S. Guarda, MD
Daniel F. Ruthven, MD
Graham W. Redgrave, MD

Key Clinical Questions

1. When should a hospitalist suspect an eating disorder? What questions aid in making the diagnosis? What screening tests are indicated?

2. When is emergent hospitalization warranted?

3. What are the complications of starvation and of binge/purge behaviors?

4. What is refeeding syndrome?

5. What are the evidence-based treatments for eating disorders?

6. What ethical considerations are specific to the treatment of eating disorders?

INTRODUCTION

Medical morbidity associated with eating disorders is high; most hospitalists will encounter patients with these disorders, so knowledge of the presentation, natural history, complications, and medical management of these conditions is important. Patients with eating disorders may be admitted through emergency rooms in the setting of an acute event such as syncope or a seizure, or referred by their primary care provider for an abnormal electrocardiogram or for laboratory values warranting admission for medical monitoring and stabilization. The majority of patients are likely to have anorexia nervosa (AN), but some may have bulimia nervosa (BN). Others may present with an atypical eating disorder in which abnormal eating behavior is not associated with drive for thinness or fear of being fat.

Eating disorders are best thought of as disorders of motivated behavior and are similar to addictions. As with substance abuse disorders, patients exhibit a narrowing of their behavioral repertoire. They develop increasingly driven ritualized behaviors and progressive functional impairment. The vast majority of affected individuals are females with the lifetime prevalence of AN and BN in women estimated at 0.9% and 1.5%, respectively. Although less common in males, it is also the case that males with eating disorders are less likely to reach medical attention, and community rates of eating disorders in men and boys are higher than the 10% male gender prevalence observed in clinical samples. Mortality for AN is one of the highest amongst psychiatric conditions, with sixfold increase in standardized mortality rates.

As eating disorders are motivated behavioral conditions, ambivalence toward and frank avoidance of treatment are common. Patients may conceal their behavior from others and avoid professional help, complicating both diagnosis and management. When they do present for treatment, they are frequently in crisis, seeking assistance in managing complications of their disorder, or because they are brought to treatment by others. Half of all the community cases of AN and BN are undetected, underscoring the importance of recognizing signs and symptoms. Once identified, most patients are reluctant to engage in treatment, preferring treatment on their own terms, picking and choosing interventions that feel best, rather than those that may be best for them. Knowing how to engage patients to seek effective treatment is one of the most important challenges for the clinician.

INDICATIONS FOR EMERGENT HOSPITALIZATION

Medically unstable patients with eating disorders are ideally treated by a multidisciplinary team on a dedicated inpatient specialty unit, using a rehabilitative approach (including intensive behavioral and group therapy). Such programs are effective in restoring weight in underweight patients and in normalizing eating behavior. In AN, weight restoration to a BMI of 19 to 21 is necessary though not usually sufficient for recovery. Treatment should also address medical complications, interrupt unhealthy behaviors, establish a normal eating pattern, and use psychotherapeutic strategies to assist patients in challenging cognitive distortions that sustain their behavior. A focus on relapse prevention and transition to outpatient treatment are critical components of long-term rehabilitation, especially in chronically ill patients who have become functionally impaired as a consequence of their eating disorder.

Unfortunately, there are few specialized hospital-based behavioral programs capable of managing medically complex cases, and access may be limited further by insurance or financial issues. As a result, patients are often admitted to hospitalist services for initial medical monitoring and stabilization. Reasons for emergent hospitalization can include hypokalemia or other serious electrolyte imbalances, hypoglycemic coma, symptomatic bradycardia, severe hypotension, dehydration, syncope, seizure, prolonged QTc interval, severe marasmus with BMI <14, or development of suicidal or other psychiatric instability. Single cases admitted to a general hospital ward can be difficult to manage behaviorally and present special challenges to the hospitalist.

This chapter will address the diagnosis and treatment of eating disorders with a focus on medical management of complications, approaches to interrupting eating disorder behaviors on a general hospital floor, as well as appropriate guidelines for discharge planning and ethical issues specific to managing these patients.

CATEGORIES OF EATING DISORDERS

The Diagnostic and Statistical Manual of Mental Disorders (DSM-V) defines six distinct eating disorders summarized in **Table 226-1**. These include AN, BN, binge eating disorder (BED), avoidant/restrictive food intake disorder (ARFID), other specified feeding or eating disorder (OSFED) and unspecified feeding or eating disorder (UFED). In this chapter, we will primarily discuss AN and BN as these are the disorders most likely to be seen and treated on inpatient services by hospitalists. Both AN and BN are characterized by an overvalued fear of being fat and a primary preoccupation with dieting behavior. The main distinction between these disorders is one of weight, with AN trumping the diagnosis of BN for patients who are underweight. Clinically, eating disorders are best viewed dimensionally with significant overlap existing between syndromes. It is not uncommon for patients to move from one diagnosis to another over time or to substitute behaviors. The most common progression is from restricting subtype AN to a purging disorder, either BN or AN binge-eating/purging type.

DIAGNOSIS

Physical signs and symptoms of AN and BN are listed in **Table 226-2**. **Table 226-3** lists two brief screening questionnaires, with similar sensitivity and specificity, useful in detecting these disorders. A positive screen should be followed by clarifying questions. Useful questions include desired weight ("What would you like to weigh?"), preoccupation with thoughts of food, weight, or shape ("What percent of the day are you preoccupied with thoughts of food or feeling fat?"); typical daily food intake with attention to variety of foods consumed and calorie density ("Tell me what you ate yesterday for breakfast, lunch, and dinner?"), hours spent exercising per week and frequency of bingeing, vomiting, laxative, diuretic, or diet pill use, including dose used. Recent adoption of vegetarianism or development of food intolerances as well as refusal to eat meals with others and social isolation should raise the index of suspicion for an eating disorder.

Collateral information from a family member is important since patients often underreport or deny eating disordered behaviors and preoccupations. Observing the patient can be helpful when the diagnosis is unclear. Hospital nursing staff may detect behavioral signs of an eating disorder including driven pacing, excessive standing and fidgeting despite emaciation, idiosyncratic and detailed food requests or food refusal, ritualistic eating behavior, hiding food, evidence of self-induced vomiting or diarrhea suggestive of laxative abuse and comments that suggest fear of being fat in a patient who is evidently underweight.

TABLE 226-1 Categories of Eating Disorders

Anorexia nervosa (AN)	Characterized by self-starvation (BMI < 18.5), fear of weight gain or persistent behavior that interferes with weight gain, and denial of the seriousness of low body weight	
	Subtypes:	Restricting: restriction of food intake and often overexercising
		Binge-eating/purging: in addition to restricting, binge-eating[1] and/or purging behaviors[2]
Bulimia nervosa (BN)	Chronic dieting with intermittent binge eating[1] once per week or more followed by compensatory behaviors[3] to prevent weight gain	
Binge eating disorder (BED)	Binge eating[1] once per week or more without compensatory behaviors[3] used to prevent weight gain	
Avoidant/restrictive food intake disorder (ARFID)	Avoidance or restriction of food intake leading to weight loss, nutritional deficiency or dependence on enteral feedings or nutritional supplements and resulting in interference with psychosocial functioning and which occurs in the absence of an overvalued idea about weight and shape	
Other specified feeding or eating disorder/unspecified feeding or eating disorder (OSFED/UFED)	Broad categories that include other psychological eating disturbances resulting in clinically significant functional impairment but that do not meet full criteria for AN, BN, BED, or ARFID	
	Examples:	OSFED: subthreshold variants of AN, BN, BED, or ARFID; purging disorder; night eating syndrome
		UFED: anxiety-related eating disorders (eg, globus hystericus or fear of swallowing). Also used as a preliminary diagnosis when there is insufficient information to make a precise diagnosis

[1]Binge eating: rapid consumption of a large amount of food associated with a sense of loss of control over eating. Binges include a minimum of three additional characteristic features that may include eating rapidly or until uncomfortably full, eating when not hungry, eating alone due to embarrassment and/or feeling guilty or disgusted by this behavior.
[2]Purging behaviors: self-induced vomiting, abuse of laxatives or diuretics.
[3]Compensatory behaviors: fasting, purging, exercise.

■ SCREENING TESTS

Initial laboratory tests and medical workup for an eating disorder should include serum electrolytes including calcium, magnesium, and phosphate levels and liver function tests, a complete blood count, urinalysis and toxicology screen, thyroid stimulating hormone, and an electrocardiogram. In patients with marasmus and a BMI of <13, a chest x-ray is also indicated since these patients can on occasion present with opportunistic infections seen in severely immunosuppressed hosts. Bone mineral density should be checked

TABLE 226-2 Signs and Symptoms of Eating Disorders

Starvation Related	Binge Purge Related
• Dry skin, lanugo, alopecia	• Perioral acne
• Cold intolerance, hypothermia, cyanotic extremities	• Parotid gland enlargement
	• Dental caries and erosion of lingual surface of teeth
• Weakness, fatigue	
• Sinus bradycardia, hypotension	• Orthostatic hypotension and dehydration
• Presyncope or syncope	• Presyncope or syncope
• Early satiety, bloating, constipation	• Heartburn, gastroesophageal reflux
• Primary or secondary amenorrhea	• Muscle cramps and paresthesias (from electrolyte abnormalities)
• Peripheral neuropathy	• Diarrhea and constipation (laxative abusers)
• Osteoporosis and fractures	• Cardiac arrhythmia
• Muscle wasting, cachexia	• Amenorrhea or oligomenorrhea
• Bruising, nosebleeds	

in women with amenorrhea lasting 6 months or longer as the risk for osteoporosis in these cases is high.

PATHOPHYSIOLOGY

The etiology of eating disorders is multifactorial. Genetic vulnerability, sociocultural pressure to engage in dieting behaviors, and environmental stressors all play a role in onset. Family studies estimate the heritability of AN and BN as 50% to 70%. Individual genetic vulnerability is likely to explain why despite the pervasiveness of dieting behavior among adolescents and young adults, less than 3% of young women progress to clinical AN or BN. A majority of cases report a significant stressor during the year of onset contributing to restriction of food intake. Examples of common stressors include physical

TABLE 226-3 Screening Tools for Eating Disorders

SCOFF	ESP (Eating disorders screen for primary care)
• Do you make yourself **S**ICK because you feel uncomfortably full?	• Are you satisfied with your eating patterns?
• Do you worry you have lost **C**ONTROL over how much you eat?	• Do you ever eat in secret?
	• Does your weight affect how you feel about yourself?
• Have you lost more than **O**NE stone (14 lbs) over the last 3 months?	• Has anyone in your family ever suffered with an eating disorder?
• Do you believe yourself to be **F**AT when others say you are thin?	• Do you currently suffer with or in the past have you suffered with an eating disorder?
• Would you say that **F**OOD dominates your life?	
Cut off: Two or more abnormal responses has a sensitivity of 100%, specificity of 87.5% for an eating disorder.	Cut off: Two or more abnormal responses has a sensitivity of 100%, specificity of 71% for an eating disorder.
Data from Morgan JF, et al. *BMJ.* 1999;319:1467-1468.	Data from Cotton MA, et al. *J Gen Intern Med.* 2003;18:53-56.

illness, parental divorce, a romantic disappointment, or homesickness after leaving for college. Given the rare prepubertal incidence of these conditions and the preponderance of females affected, it is also likely that estrogen levels play a role in susceptibility and age of onset.

Most important, especially in the acute management of these conditions, is an understanding of the pathophysiological consequences of starvation and of disordered eating which in turn help sustain continued anorectic and bulimic behavior. For example, deliberate starvation in AN results in delayed gastric and intestinal transit times, obsessive preoccupation with food and hyperactivity, all of which escalate anorectic behaviors and cognitions. Similarly, patients who vomit often develop loss of the gag reflex, gastroesophageal reflux, and delayed gastric emptying. These physiological changes in turn facilitate continued vomiting.

Psychiatric comorbidity also plays a role in sustaining eating disorders. Major depression, anxiety disorders, and substance abuse are common comorbidities in these patients and starvation is associated with a syndrome of depression, reversible with refeeding, which may contribute to patients' feelings of helplessness and hopelessness regarding treatment or prospects for recovery. Amongst general medical conditions co-occurring with eating disorders perhaps the most important is type I diabetes, since intentional insulin omission or restriction is a commonly employed method of purging calories in this patient subgroup, resulting in hyperglycemia and increased risk of diabetic ketoacidosis. Patients with both diabetes and an eating disorder have higher rates of hospital admission and emergency room visits, higher levels of hemoglobin A_{1c}, and higher rates of diabetic complications, making screening for an eating disorder an important component of the workup in any case of unexplained brittle diabetes.

MEDICAL COMPLICATIONS OF STARVATION AND OF PURGING BEHAVIORS

Most physiological complications and risks associated with eating disorders arise from either starvation or from purging behaviors, placing individuals with the purging subtype of AN at highest risk for serious medical morbidity and mortality. Almost all organ systems can be involved (**Table 226-4**), and knowledge of the major medical complications is important in managing patients in the acute setting and in avoiding the development of refeeding syndrome, a potentially life threatening complication of rapid nutritional restoration in severely malnourished individuals.

■ REFEEDING SYNDROME

An awareness of the symptoms and management of refeeding syndrome is essential to the treatment of severely malnourished patients with AN. If not promptly recognized and treated this condition is life threatening. Refeeding syndrome comprises a constellation of metabolic and clinical changes resulting from rapid refeeding whether oral, enteral, or parenteral. These can include hypophosphatemia, hypoglycemia, edema and congestive heart failure, ileus, seizures, coma, and sudden death. In general, the risk is lowest with oral, and highest with parenteral nutrition.

PRACTICE POINT

- Monitor closely for refeeding syndrome during nutritional rehabilitation of starved patients including hypophosphatemia, hypoglycemia, and fluid overload.

In starved individuals, as calorie intake increases and carbohydrate is reintroduced, there is a shift from fat and protein catabolism to carbohydrate metabolism. Subsequently, blood glucose increases

TABLE 226-4 Medical Complications of Starvation and Purging Behaviors

Cardiovascular	**Starvation related**		
	Bradycardia (HR < 45 warrants admission)	Dental enamel erosion	
	Tachycardia (may indicate occult infection or impending cardiac decompensation)	Reflux esophagitis	
		Mallory-Weiss tears	
	Reduced left ventricular mass with resultant mitral valve prolapse	Gastric dilatation (from extreme binge eating in starved individuals, managed with NG decompression)	
	Dilated cardiomyopathy	Delayed gastric emptying	
	Prolonged QTc interval (QTc > 500 ms warrants admission)	Laxative dependence and subsequent complications (hemorrhoids, rectal prolapse)	
	Purging related		
	Orthostatic hypotension and syncope	**Endocrine** — **Starvation related**	
	Toxic cardiomyopathy (with ipecac abuse)	Hypogonadotrophic amenorrhea/oligomenorrhea (up to 75% in AN and 30% in BN)	
	Cardiac arrhythmias (risk increased with caffeine and/or ephedrine containing diet pills)	Hypercortisolemia	
Metabolic	**Starvation related**	Growth hormone resistance	
	Hypoglycemia	Sick euthyroid syndrome (not an indication to treat with hormone replacement)	
	Purging related	**Musculoskeletal** — **Starvation related**	
	Acid-base imbalances	Generalized muscle weakness/atrophy	
	Hypokalemia	Osteopenia/osteoporosis (in up to 85% of women diagnosed with AN)	
	Hypomagnesemia	**Hematologic** — **Starvation related**	
	Hypocalcemia	Anemia	
	Hypophosphatemia (also a hallmark of refeeding syndrome)	Leukopenia	
	Hyponatremia (seen with water loading, diuretic abuse and/or prolonged purging behavior)	Pancytopenia	
Gastrointestinal	**Starvation related**	**Neurological** — **Starvation related**	
	Delayed gastric emptying	Cerebral atrophy	
	Slowed intestinal motility	Seizures (secondary to hyponatremia and/or hypoglycemia)	
	Constipation	Peripheral nutritional polyneuropathy	
	Pancreatitis	**Renal** — **Purging related**	
	Elevated transaminases	End stage renal disease (up to 5% in chronic AN lasting > 20 y)	
	Elevated total cholesterol (due to decreased cholesterol binding proteins or low T3 levels)	Reduced creatinine clearance (with laxative abuse in AN)	
	Purging related	Fluid retention/edema	
	Parotid hypertrophy		

and there is an increase in insulin release. Depleted glycogen stores make the regulation of blood glucose unpredictable and increase the risk of reactive hypoglycemia, which is frequently asymptomatic.

Insulin secretion also stimulates the cellular uptake of phosphate for the production of adenosine triphosphate (ATP), in order to meet anabolic demands. Total body phosphate is depleted in starvation, although serum levels may initially appear normal. As phosphate moves intracellularly, hypophosphatemia manifests 1 to 5 days after initiating feeding and can be life threatening if not promptly recognized and treated. Recent data suggests that refeeding hypophosphatemia is most common in severely malnourished patients with BMI <14. As with hypophosphatemia, hypomagnesemia from intracellular movement of magnesium may become evident several days into refeeding.

Starved patients are often hypotensive and may have autonomic instability reflected in marked postural hypotension or heart rate changes. Care should be taken not to aggressively hydrate these patients in an attempt to correct orthostatic vital signs since their

low protein and albumin and malnourished tissues make edema and third spacing likely and can result in anasarca or congestive heart failure. The increase in insulin secretion also contributes to sodium retention, which in turn decreases renal excretion of sodium and water and worsens fluid retention. Congestive heart failure is especially a risk in patients with an occult starvation-related cardiomyopathy. If edema is pronounced and weight gain very rapid (more than 5-6 lbs/wk) suggesting severe fluid retention, an echocardiogram is indicated, especially in chronic cases or those of advanced age who are at highest risk of cardiac complications following years of chronic malnutrition.

During refeeding of severely underweight patients, we recommend gradual intravenous hydration if symptomatic with hypotonic saline and 5% dextrose at a maintenance rate no faster than 83 cc/h supplemented by oral intake of no more than 1000 cc of fluids/d. Close monitoring of fingersticks, especially postprandially, is recommended to avoid the risk of severe hypoglycemia and daily electrolytes including sodium, potassium, calcium, magnesium, and phosphate should be drawn until several sequential values in the normal range are obtained. Oral repletion of phosphate, potassium, or magnesium is faster and safer than intravenous correction.

The risk of refeeding syndrome is closely tied to the amount of food ingested. Patients should initially be fed a low salt, low fat, low lactose diet of 1200 to 1500 calories/d. This should be gradually liberalized to a regular diet and advanced by 500 calories/d every 2 to 3 days to a daily intake of 3500 calories/d with a target rate of weight gain between 3 and 4 lbs/wk. Mild to moderate pedal edema is common during the first few weeks of refeeding and should be managed conservatively by elevating the legs, compression stockings, and salt restriction until it resolves. In patients with a history of purging, diuretics compound the risk of hypokalemia. Since these agents are abused by some patients in order to lose weight, diuretics should be reserved for cases with severe edema when there is concern for congestive heart failure.

Other severe complications associated with refeeding include Wernicke encephalopathy and central pontine myelinolysis. The central pontine myelinolysis most commonly results from the overly rapid correction of hyponatremia and presents with altered mental state, dysarthria, or mutism appearing within days of the correction of sodium levels and progressing in some cases to worsening motor impairment and at the extreme coma or death. Thiamine deficiency can result in Wernicke-Korsakoff syndrome, a particular risk in AN patients with comorbid alcohol abuse. We recommend treatment of all patients with a BMI of 14 or less with 100 mg of IV thiamine prior to initial food intake or to the administration of IV dextrose in order to avoid this very serious risk.

PRACTICE POINT

- To minimize refeeding syndrome the diet for AN should start with initial calorie intakes of 1200 to 1500 calories/d advanced to a weight gain diet of 3500 calories/d over the course of 10 to 12 d. This calorie level should achieve weight gain rates of 2 to 4 lbs/wk.

TREATMENT

For AN, treatment is best thought of as composed of two phases: weight restoration and relapse prevention. Relapse, as with other behavioral conditions, is common, although most patients are able to progress further with each cycle of treatment and the majority eventually recover. Evidence-based data on treatment of AN is limited, but most evidence supports weight restoration as necessary for recovery. Competent inpatient and residential behavioral specialty units can weight restore the vast majority of patients at a rate of 2 to 4 lbs/wk using oral feeding alone. These programs use a combination of behavioral, group, and family therapy. Treatment focus is on normalizing eating behavior and broadening patients' food repertoire using close nursing observation to assist patients in interrupting eating disorder behavior patterns. Group therapy is especially effective since patients with eating disorders are able to appreciate other patients' needs to change their behaviors. As with substance abuse disorders, when confronted by peers, patients are more likely to recognize the irrational logic they use to defend their own dieting. Despite the success of intensive behavioral programs in achieving weight restoration and normalizing eating behavior, 30% to 50% of individuals who reach target weight will relapse within 1 year of discharge. No medication has been shown to be superior to placebo in the treatment of AN. Current outpatient treatment guidelines include weekly psychotherapy and nutritional counseling with a focus on weight gain and these sessions should include

monitoring of the patients' weight. Involvement of close family and social supports is recommended.

Full recovery is best viewed as a protracted process often occurring over years and requiring multiple treatment interventions. Long-term outcome studies indicate recovery rates of 25% to 70%. There are few indicators of good versus poor prognosis. Adolescent patients tend to have higher success rates; however, full recovery is seen even in patients with life-threatening AN who have been ill for decades and who present with extreme cachexia and multiple medical complications or organ failure.

For BN, several outpatient treatment interventions are effective in interrupting the restrict-binge-vomit cycle. The most well studied of these is cognitive behavioral therapy (CBT), which maintains a behavioral focus on normalizing eating while simultaneously challenging irrational cognitive beliefs and identifying triggers and alternate coping strategies. Self-help CBT manuals are less effective than therapist-led CBT, but are superior to control interventions and are an easily available, inexpensive, initial intervention that can be offered to patients. Antidepressants have also been found effective in decreasing binge-vomit frequencies in BN although they are less effective than CBT in achieving abstinence from these behaviors. Of these medications, high-dose fluoxetine at 60 mg daily has been studied most extensively and is commonly employed in conjunction with CBT. Although relapse is common in the treatment of BN, over 50% of patients achieve eventual recovery with treatment.

AN is characterized by refusal to eat not by inability to eat or by a nonfunctional gastrointestinal tract. The safest and most effective form of refeeding is oral, both from a physiological standpoint and because this disorder is marked by a narrowing of the food repertoire and conditioned avoidance of high calorie-density foods. The variety of foods consumed at discharge from inpatient specialty treatment is inversely related to relapse rates, suggesting that exposure to diverse foods and normalization of eating patterns is an important component of treatment. Although supplemental tube feeding is used by some behavioral programs to augment poor rates of weight gain in select cases, most specialty units do not find this necessary in order to achieve optimal rates of gain in the vast majority of patients.

The situation on a medical unit is more complex, since it is difficult to reproduce the skilled nursing care and peer pressure of a specialized eating disorder program on a medical floor, thereby lessening the likelihood that patients will comply with dietary recommendations. The initial prescribed diet in AN should be oral, and caloric intake should start low as outlined above, while monitoring for evidence of refeeding syndrome. A trial of supplemental enteral feeding may be reserved for patients who are failing to gain weight with oral feeding alone. The mere threat of prescribed enteral feeds may help ambivalent patients eat. Other patients may prefer enteral feeds as a way to "medicalize" their condition and avoid responsibility for their behavior. In the short term this may be acceptable to boost slow weight gain, although the long-term goal is to achieve normalization of dietary intake by transitioning the patient to oral food only. PEG tubes or long-term enteral feeding tubes are not recommended, since this approach does not address patients' fear of widening their food repertoire and consuming calorie dense foods. In general, most experts agree that parenteral feeding should be avoided in AN, especially in cachectic patients, given the high risk of medical complications combined with the availability of less invasive methods of nutritional restoration.

■ BEHAVIORAL MANAGEMENT

Eating disorders may be difficult to manage on a medical ward largely because of their similarity to addictions. Patients may understand the severity of their condition intellectually yet be unable or unwilling to stop their behavior. They may overtly continue to exercise, restrict or hide food, vomit, or abuse laxatives despite the severe medical consequences of these behaviors that led to their admission.

Nursing staff should check daily weight and monitor the patient as closely as possible, if necessary by employing a professional observer, for evidence of eating disordered behaviors. This may include tray checks and calorie counts to assess amount of food consumed, instructing patients to allow staff to check the toilet bowl before flushing for evidence of vomiting or diarrhea and curtailing time out of bed or off the unit contingent on behavior. Observers should be instructed regarding what behaviors to watch for. The patient should be repeatedly and firmly yet supportively redirected for any noncompliant behavior and reminded of its medical risks. Patients may also engage in behaviors aimed at deliberately deceiving staff by hiding food or vomitus, water loading before weigh-ins, or wearing weights.

Staff should recognize that in most cases it is difficult to effectively treat these patients on a general medical floor and that the goal of hospitalization should be stabilization and transfer to a behavioral specialty program. As is the case with other motivated behavioral conditions including substance abuse disorders, behavioral treatment and rehabilitation is difficult to achieve outside such a specialized program. Hospital staff may experience strong negative feelings toward these patients because of their denial of illness and manipulative behaviors or may have difficulty setting limits on and redirecting the patient due to feelings of compassion for him or her. The patient may complain she is only "understood" by staff interested in talking with her about her feelings rather than on supportively and consistently stigmatizing her self-destructive behavior. As a result, the team may become "split" in their views of how the patient should be cared for. Normalizing these reactions and discussing countertransference feelings in team meetings with staff is important in order to prevent such issues from interfering with the provision of appropriate care. A psychiatry consult should be obtained to help mediate these concerns, to establish if the patient has other comorbid psychiatric conditions that warrant treatment, and to facilitate transfer to a more appropriate treatment facility once the patient is medically stable.

■ ETHICAL CONSIDERATIONS SPECIFIC TO THE TREATMENT OF EATING DISORDERS

The three primary ethical questions that arise in the treatment of eating disorders are (1) Is the patient competent to refuse care? (2) What is the role, if any, of involuntary treatment? (3) What are the limits of confidentiality when the patient's condition is life threatening?

Patients with AN are not grossly incompetent; however their capacity to make a rational free choice regarding whether to reject or accept treatment may be impaired. In life-threatening AN, patients are often incompetent to make treatment decisions involving their own eating and weight. Although they recognize the need for others with the same disorder to receive treatment, they demonstrate a selective defect in self-evaluation, appearing unable to appreciate their own need to gain weight. They may provide seemingly rational explanations for their behavior, arguing they are different in some fundamental way from others with the same disorder. Incompetence to refuse treatment is a state-dependent condition and is worsened by starvation. Insight usually improves gradually with weight restoration and with behavioral change.

Because dieting is driven and rewarding to patients with AN, attempts to normalize eating behavior or weight are unpleasant and patients usually enter specialty treatment not of their own initiative but under pressure from others. Pressure may range from gentle persuasion to compulsion and involuntary treatment. To be successful, however, treatment must at some point win the cooperation of the patient. Recovery is a process of conversion in belief, from seeing dieting as an idealized and necessary goal, to stigmatizing it as a negative behavior. Because treatment resistance is endemic to AN, ethical decision-making pervades the treatment of this disorder.

Civil commitment is used occasionally by few specialty centers when all other attempts to engage the patient have failed, when a patient's life is at risk, and when there is reasonable confidence that the treatment will be beneficial. Data on involuntary treatment is limited, although several case control studies suggest that discharge BMIs are similar for voluntary and involuntary cases and weight restoration can be accomplished in the majority. Although long-term prognosis is worse for involuntary cases, these are correlational studies, and the involuntary group is likely to have a worse prognosis with or without treatment. Furthermore, empirical data indicating harm from involuntary treatment is absent and at least two studies have shown that close to half of patients admitted involuntarily or under pressure from others later came to view being hospitalized against their will as justified in saving their lives. Treatment setting is likely important, however, and this data comes from behavioral specialty units. There is no data on the outcome of involuntary treatment in a general psychiatric or medical unit. Presumably likelihood of a good outcome is higher in a specialty program for eating disorders.

Involuntary treatment should only be considered if the patient's family is in support of the team. Family involvement maximizes the likelihood that the intervention will result in a therapeutic outcome. Patients with AN may refuse to allow the clinician contact with their family. Most commonly this occurs because the patient is trying to keep relatives and the medical team at arm's length in order to avoid weight gain. When AN is endangering a patient's life however, treatment should be viewed as a medical emergency. Under these circumstances it becomes appropriate to break confidentiality. Communication with close family is especially important when patients are admitted to a hospitalist service not only to apprise family of the seriousness of the patient's condition but to urge them to align with the hospitalist team and the consulting psychiatrist in providing firm yet supportive pressure to encourage the patient to accept voluntary transfer to a specialty program as the next step in his or her rehabilitation.

CONCLUSION

The goal of hospitalization is to stabilize the patient medically and transfer him or her to an appropriate specialty program for the treatment of eating disorders. It is helpful to state, both to patients and family members, that AN is a motivated behavioral condition much like addiction, that recovery is always possible, and that specialty treatment often is effective in assisting patients to recover. For severely medically compromised patients, a hospital-based eating disorders program with access to medical consultants may be most appropriate. For less ill patients, a behaviorally oriented eating disorder residential program or outpatient treatment can be effective. The most common psychotherapeutic approach is cognitive-behavioral in orientation with family involvement whenever possible. For severely underweight patients with a BMI of <15, outpatient treatment alone is less likely to lead to weight restoration and long-term recovery than an intensive treatment program. The medical costs of treating AN are extremely high and many patients lack adequate insurance coverage. Patients may however qualify for coverage under Medicare if disabled by their condition. The importance of maintaining a firm, positive stance in recommending behavioral treatment is critical since patients and family members may feel hopeless about prospects of recovery in the light of past treatment failures.

SUGGESTED READINGS

American Psychiatric Association. Practice Guidelines: Treatment of Patients with Eating Disorders, 3rd ed. *Am J Psychiatry.* 2006;163(Suppl 4):54.

Cotton MA, Ball C, Robinson P. Four simple questions can help screen for eating disorders. *J Gen Intern Med.* 2003;18:53-56.

Guarda AS. Treatment of anorexia nervosa: insights and obstacles. *Physiol Behav.* 2008;94:113-120.

Mehler PS, Krantz MJ, Sachs KV. Treatments of medical complications of anorexia nervosa and bulimia nervosa. *J Eating Disorders.* 2015;3:15.

Misra M, Klibanski A. Anorexia nervosa and bone. *J Endocrinol.* 2014;221(3):163-176.

Morgan JF, Reid F, Lacey JH. The SCOFF questionnaire: assessment of a new screening tool for eating disorders. *BMJ.* 1999;319:1467-1468.

Smink F, van Hoeken D, Hoek HW. Epidemiology of eating disorders: incidence, prevalence and mortality rates. *Curr Psychiatry Reports.* 2012;14:406-414.

Thornton LM, Mazzeo SE, Bulik CM. The heritability of eating disorders: methods and current findings. *Curr Top Behav Neurosci.* 2011;6:141-156.

Tresley J, Sheean PM. Refeeding syndrome: recognition is the key to prevention and management. *J Am Diet Assoc.* 2008;108:2105-2108.

Yager J, Devlin MJ, Halmi KA, et al. Guideline Watch (August 2012): Practice Guideline for The Treatment Of Patients With Eating Disorders, 3rd ed. American Psychiatric Association; 2012.

CHAPTER 227

The Suicidal Patient

Robert K. Schneider, MD, FACP

Key Clinical Questions

❶ How do you determine if a hospitalized patient is at baseline risk for suicide or elevated risk?

❷ How does the hospitalist devise a plan of care for the suicidal patient?

INTRODUCTION

Suicidality (defined as one's attraction to suicide) is very common in patients with severe psychiatric disorders even though completed suicide (killing oneself) is relatively rare. The risk of suicidality is never zero. This concept is important because clinicians can be lulled into false senses of security when the risk may seem to be low; consequently, clinicians may not fully assess a patient's risk for suicide. Even when patients with severe psychiatric disorders are hospitalized for medical or surgical reasons, their suicidality often goes unnoticed, unevaluated and untreated, because the focus of their care is medical or surgical rather than psychiatric. Given the hospitalist's high likelihood of treating patients experiencing suicidality, all hospitalists require knowledge and skills necessary to assess and manage patients with varying levels of suicidality. Assessment (including screening) explores the patient's overall risk profile: chronic/predisposing factors, acute/potentiating factors, and protective factors. Clinicians must determine whether the patient's overall suicidal risk is at or above that individual's baseline. Finally, the hospitalist must incorporate this information and devise appropriate management to address the patient's suicide risk.

There is a wide range of experience on suicide and suicide rates around the world depending upon cultural views. For example, Japan has many similarities to the United States but very different suicide rates, related demographics and phenomiology. This chapter will draw demographic and phenomonolgic information from data and experience within the United States. However, the broader concepts on screening and assessment for suicidality should translate to other cultures.

ASSESSMENT OF SUICIDALITY

A hospitalist is most likely to address suicidality with patients in three distinct situations:

1. Patients who may not overtly express suicidality but are recognized at increased risk.
2. Patients who express suicidality while hospitalized.
3. Patients admitted after a suicide attempt.

Patients who are admitted after suicide attempts are the most conspicuous examples of suicidality and because of this receive the most coverage in the literature. However, hospitalists will see many more patients *silently* at risk for suicide than those admitted for overt suicide attempts. This chapter will address the practical knowledge and skills required to assess suicidality and to formulate a cogent treatment plan for hospitalized patients.

KEY TERMS

The terms, **suicide, completed suicide,** or **"successful" suicide** all refer to the actual act of killing oneself. A **suicide attempt** is an act of deliberate self-harm with the intent to kill oneself. However, the act may not seem deliberate (eg, taking too many pain medications) so the degree of intent (ie, the wish to die) may be difficult to ascertain from the patient. The degree of lethality (ie, the likelihood of completion) is typically not difficult to determine but should be understood in the context of the patient's intent. **Suicidal ideation** (thoughts of suicide) and **suicidality** (attraction to suicide) are part of a spectrum of thoughts or feelings ranging from hopelessness, to imagining "not being here", to specific plans for self-harm, to acting on suicidal plans (**Figure 227-1**). Circumstances in the life of the

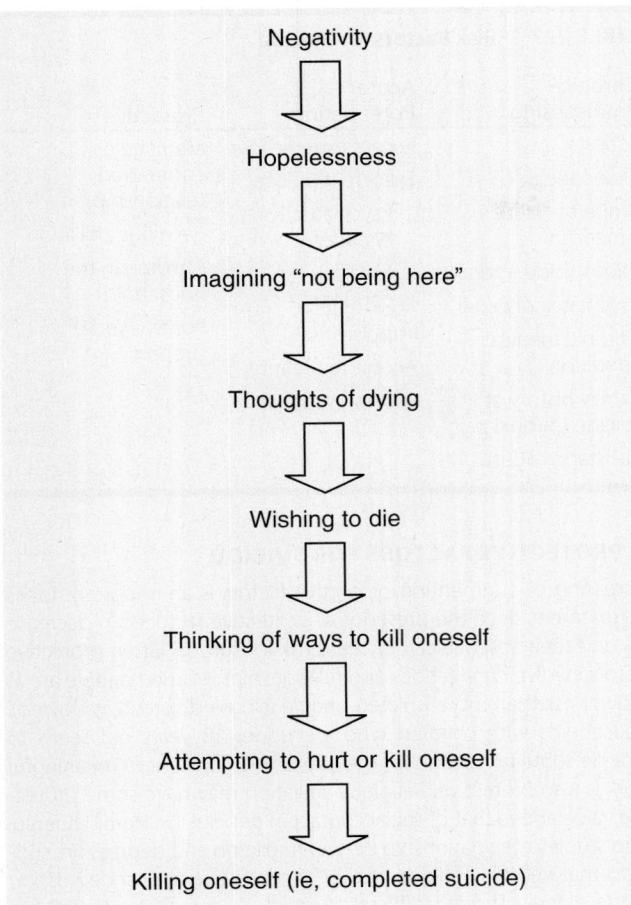

Negativity

⬇

Hopelessness

⬇

Imagining "not being here"

⬇

Thoughts of dying

⬇

Wishing to die

⬇

Thinking of ways to kill oneself

⬇

Attempting to hurt or kill oneself

⬇

Killing oneself (ie, completed suicide)

Figure 227-1 *Spectrum of suicidality.*

patient help the clinician to ascribe meaning to a suicide attempt. Obviously, if the individual wrote a note and jumped off a bridge, those *statements* reveal a clear attempt to **complete suicide**. However, if the individual reports, for example, that he or she took a handful of ibuprofen after breaking up with a significant other, this may indicate a "cry for help" or an immature expression of pain.

Hopelessness and associated emotions are some of the most consistent markers for severity of a psychiatric disorder, particularly mood disorders. While suicidality in some form is frequently present in severe psychiatric disorders (eg, major depression), completed suicide is relatively rare. In the United States, over 15 million people suffer with depression per year and many will think about suicide, but less than 30,000 people will actually complete suicide. Despite decades of study documenting epidemiological correlations with completed suicide (ie, risk factors), there is no effective screening approach that accurately **predicts** completed suicide. Most leaders are suicide research note that suicide is not predictable and go on to advise the clinician that the clinical goal is to fully assess and construct a treatment plan that attempts to decrease suicidal risk by strengthening or increasing protective factors and addressing or decreasing acute, potentiating factors.

EPIDEMIOLOGY AND RISK FACTORS

■ CHRONIC/PREDISPOSING RISK FACTORS

Completed suicide has a base-rate of 12 per 100,000 in the general population. The most studied predisposing epidemiologic factors related to suicide risk are gender, race, and age. These predisposing chronic risk factors are fixed and therefore establish a baseline risk for suicide. In these categories men are at least four times more

likely to complete suicide than women. However, women are about 10 times more likely to attempt suicide or make suicide gestures. Whites and Native Americans have significantly higher suicide rates than African Americans, Hispanics or Asians. In the United States, white men commit 73% of all suicides. Age is also a significant risk factor. Suicide rates dramatically increase in the seventh decade of life, especially for men.

Substance abuse, especially severe alcoholism, is a chronic risk factor. For some alcoholics in later life, when the social effects of chronic use have accumulated (isolation, or alienation), a sudden or significant change (medical disease, divorce, loss of a job, or death of loved one) carries a particularly high risk for suicide. On the other hand, alcohol intoxication is an acute risk that quickly passes after the patient is sober.

Prior suicide attempts represent a significant increased risk for both a subsequent attempt and a completed suicide. A prior suicide attempt of any description is associated with almost a 40-fold increase in suicide risk. Prior attempts represent a dramatic increase in risk, which is greater than the increased risk associated with any psychiatric disorder. The powerful association makes screening for prior suicide attempt(s) a major focus of any prevention efforts. Regrettably, of those attempting suicide, more than half complete their suicides the first time.

Patients who carry a **high chronic/predisposing risk** for suicide should be managed in concert with a psychiatrist. For example, a patient may have a long history of multiple drug overdoses with subsequent psychiatric hospitalizations. This patient will most likely have suicidal ideation to some degree at any time and is chronically at increased risk for suicide. In some chronically suicidal patients with personality disorders, psychiatric hospitalization is used only as a last resort because the hospitalization is unlikely to change the chronic suicidal ideation. In fact, for such patients, hospitalization may reinforce the suicidal ideation by creating an escape and/or gratifying a regressive need for attention. Short admissions, focused on stabilization and maintaining an outpatient treatment program, are usually most effective for the patient with chronic high baseline risk for suicide. These complex patients require the active management that a mental health specialist can provide.

■ PSYCHIATRIC DISORDERS

The presence of a psychiatric disorder can pose acute and/or chronic risk for suicide depending upon the patient's past history and the acuity of the symptoms. A major mental disorder is associated with more than 90% of suicides. However, of people with psychiatric conditions who complete suicide, depression accounts for 50%, alcohol and drug abuse 20% to 25% and schizophrenia or bipolar disorder 10%. Other psychiatric disorders also increase the risk for suicide, such as PTSD, panic disorder, and personality disorders that are characterized by impulsivity. In general, all psychiatric disorders carry a greater risk for suicide when compared to the general population.

When inactive symptoms of the disorder (ie, during remission or recovery) become reactivated (ie, during relapse or recurrence), the chronically elevated baseline risk for suicide is acutely increased. Knowing where the patient falls longitudinally within the progression of his or her disorder also helps the clinician assess risk. For example, patients early in the course of schizophrenia carry a greater risk than later. Most suicides in people with schizophrenia (60%) occur within 6 years of the first hospitalization.

■ MEDICAL ILLNESS

Medical illness of any type significantly increases the risk of a depressive or anxiety disorder. Hospitalization itself is a risk factor. Like psychiatric disorders, medical disorders pose acute and chronic risks. Much of the increased risk is attributable to co-occurring psychiatric illnesses, particularly major depression, substance-related disorders, personality disorders and delirium. However, physical illness is a profound risk factor, contributing to over 70% of suicides in those over the age of 60. Chronic medical illness is strongly associated with depression and substance abuse. Even when the psychiatric risk factors are accounted for, medical illnesses are still associated with increased suicidal risk. Higher rates of suicide have been reported in cancer, AIDS, end stage renal disease, neurological disorders (such as multiple sclerosis), asthma, and a number of other medical conditions. Data from the US National Comorbidity Survey identified a dozen general medical diagnostic categories with statistically significantly elevated odds ratios for suicide attempts, most ranging from 1.1 to 3.4, but with a much higher ratio in AIDS. Cancer and asthma patients each have a fourfold risk of attempting suicide compared to the general population, even after adjusting for demographic and psychiatric variables. Loss of or poor functional capacity and associated chronic pain may be a common thread among these medical conditions that links them with suicidal risk. Some clinicians have the misperception that most terminally ill patients have a strong wish for a hastened death. On the contrary, Breitbart's (2000) study showed only 17% of cancer patients with this desire, but depression was a strong predictor a patient's desire for a hastened death.

MEDICAL AND PSYCHIATRIC COMORBIDITY

There is a complex relationship between medical and psychiatric disorders in suicidality because medical illnesses also carry their own increased risk for suicidal ideation and suicide attempts. Any medical conditions concomitant with psychiatric disorders increase the lifetime risk for suicidal ideation and suicide attempts to 35% and 16%, respectively. Given that medical illnesses and depression are often comorbid, it is very important to note that the odds ratio (OR) for suicidal ideation and suicide attempts is high with this combination (OR = 1.82 and 2.38, respectively). Thus, psychiatric disorders and medical illnesses contribute independently to the risks for suicidal ideation and suicide attempts.

ACUTE/POTENTIATING RISK FACTORS

Exacerbation of depression

Severe hopelessness, psychic pain, shame or humiliation acutely increases risk of suicide. Depressive symptoms combined with extreme anxiety (panic or obsessions) or manic symptoms particularly increase risk. The initial treatment plan should target these exacerbated symptoms. The risk of suicide seems highest in the first few depressive episodes, especially in late onset depression. This is also true for bipolar disorders and schizophrenia. Many of the suicides that occur early in the course of the disorder are in people who have not been diagnosed with a disorder nor have initiated treatment. Though suicide risk is higher earlier versus later in the course of illness, the risk remains higher than the general population throughout the course of the illness.

Psychosis

When psychosis is present, suicidal ideation constitutes an emergency, particularly when command hallucinations or intense persecutory delusions are present. The patient should be evaluated by a mental health professional as soon as possible and admitted for inpatient care if necessary.

Extreme loss or abrupt social disruptions

Events such as divorce or loss of a job also increase acute risk. In later life, the time following a spouse's death is a particularly vulnerable period. The losses and disruption of life posed by medical illness can also be devastating.

TABLE 227-1 Risk Factors for Suicide

Chronic/ Predisposing	Acute/ Potentiating	Protective
Male	Recent extreme loss	Marriage or committed relationship
Older age (> 65 y)	Exacerbation of a	
White or Native American	Psychiatric disorder	Religious affiliation
Prior suicide attempt	Medical condition	Children in the household
Psychiatric disorder	Impulsivity	Positive social support
Chronic medical condition	Access to firearms	
Family history of suicide Chronic pain	Substance abuse	
Substance abuse		

PROTECTIVE FACTORS FOR SUICIDE

Increasing or augmenting protective factors is an important focus of treatment since the presence of protective factors can decrease risk and their absence can increase risk for suicide. Often protective factors involve connections and relationships. Married people are at a lower risk than more isolated people (single, divorced, widowed). Households with children who are under 18 years old seem to provide some protection for the adults. Employment or meaningful work is also protective. Religious affiliation may have some protective value above that of social contact in general. Dr. Harold Koenig, who studies the relationship between religion and depression, suggests that belief in a "higher power" is protective against depression in the elderly. Though difficult to study, "a reason for living" has tremendous value clinically. Though discussing protective factors takes time, the information obtained is essential for establishing an effective management plan (**Table 227-1**).

SCREENING FOR SUICIDALITY

Screening for suicidal ideation is the first step of assessment. At this juncture it is best to start at the less severe end of the spectrum (negativity and pessimism) and then proceed to greater degrees. While it is critical to identify patients at the more serious end of the spectrum (ie, those who have a plan and are intent on carrying it out) it is also essential to identify patients at lesser degrees of risk to permit earlier preventive interventions. Also, establishing the information on the less extreme end will typically lead to very useful information regarding the severity of the disorder and is helpful in constructing a plan. For a hospitalist, screening for suicidality is like screening for alcoholism.

Similar to asking the blunt question, "Are you an alcoholic?" the question "Are you going to kill yourself?" is equally unproductive in obtaining information from the patient in the proximal part of the suicidal spectrum. When asking patients about suicidal ideation, clinicians should start at the less serious end of the spectrum of suicide risk. By determining the depth of the patient's hopelessness and helplessness (ie, suicidality), the clinician will have obtained some of the best markers of severity. Additionally, when these symptoms are identified, validated, and targeted for treatment by the clinician, the patient's suicidal risk diminishes and recovery is more promising. By assessing suicidal ideation across its entire spectrum, the clinician *and* patient gain greater insight into the severity of an underlying disorder. Also, patients are usually more willing to discuss negativity and hopelessness than suicide. The questions below demonstrate a logical sequence proceeding from lower to higher risk.

"Are you having difficulty staying hopeful?"
"Have you ever felt life isn't worth living?"
"Did you ever wish you would go to sleep and not wake up?"
"Have you had increased thoughts about death or dying?"
"Have these thoughts ever been about taking your own life?"
"Have you imagined the way you would kill yourself?"
"Are you currently considering or planning to kill yourself?"

This approach facilitates conversation and opens the door for further discussion when more explicit suicidal ideation is present. Some patients do not realize that hopelessness and despair themselves, let alone suicidality, maybe symptoms of a disorder. If the symptoms seem related to a stressor and because the despair has a "good reason," the patient may discount their symptoms. If the patient does not associate a stressor with the painful feelings, they may think they are "going crazy." The clinician has an opportunity to educate and reassure the patient by explaining that these thoughts and feelings are symptoms of a disorder (eg, major depression) and can be expected to diminish or resolve with treatment.

While the example yes/no questions above are helpful tools, the hospitalist may consider posing open-ended questions to elicit more information and to subtly underscore the patient's protective factors. Examples of open-ended questions include:

"How do you stay hopeful during this difficult time?"
"If you have felt that life is not worth living, how do you address those feelings?"
"When thoughts of dying arise, what steps do you take to counteract those thoughts?"

The questions given here are not prescriptive but rather more of a guideline. Each hospitalist will develop certain questions and approaches that best suit his or her personality.

■ PRIORITIZING AND ORGANIZING FACTORS ASSOCIATED WITH RISK FOR SUICIDE

After discussing the spectrum of suicidality with the patient, the hospitalist can then categorize risk along three dimensions:

1. Chronic/predisposing factors that affect lifetime risk for suicide;
2. Acute/potentiating factors that occur in immediate proximity to suicidality;
3. Protective factors that, when present, mitigate against acute or chronic risks (and the absence of protective factors increases risk).

CASE 227-1

Mr. Jones, a 73-year-old retired engineer, is ready for discharge after a 5-day hospitalization for a COPD exacerbation and pneumonia, his third admission in 3 months. He has lost 15 pounds during this 3-month period, and his outpatient workup for weight loss was negative. During discharge planning it is discovered that his wife died 4 months ago. The hospitalist asks "are you having thoughts of harming yourself?" and the patient honestly replies "no."

The hypothetical interaction would end there leaving much important information undisclosed. Note that the hospitalist should have a high index of suspicion for suicidal ideation given the patient's age, gender, chronic medical issues and recent loss of his wife. However, if the hospitalist asked *"how do you stay hopeful or how do you keep going?"* then there is an increased chance for fuller communication that gives additional information about the severity of the disorder, the presence or absence of protective factors for suicide, as well as diagnostic information. This approach also gives the hospitalist greater confidence in the "negative" response, "I am not going to kill myself." When the patient informs the hospitalist that he is considering moving in with his daughter, despite being frustrated with his debilitating disease compounded by the death of his wife, the hospitalist has evidence that the patient is hopeful and future-focused.

■ DISCUSSING SUICIDAL IDEATION WHEN DISCOVERED

When suicidal ideation is discovered, explicit and direct discussion about suicidal intent should occur. Unlike the gradual approach outlined previously when screening for potential suicidality (ie, when there is no overtly expressed suicidal ideation), pursuing details of the suicidal ideation helps the hospitalist establish the intensity of the suicidal ideation. The hospitalist should inquire specifically about the onset and frequency of the patient's ideations, the method the patient has contemplated, the lethality of method, the specificity of plan, and the patient's access to means. The following questions are examples that may be helpful.

"When did you first notice these thoughts?"
"Are they constant or episodic?"
"Have these thoughts progressed to any plans?"
"Do you have access to any guns?"
"Have you taken any steps to advance these plans?"
"Have you acted on these thoughts?"
"How do you fight the thoughts when they come?"

Next, to counterbalance the suicidal thoughts of the patient, the clinician should discuss the patient's reasons for living. It is helpful to look actively for future plans, for people to support the patient, and for direct prohibitions to suicide (eg, religious beliefs). These questions often help patients consider their suicidal ideations from different perspectives. The following questions illustrate this approach:

"What keeps you from acting on these thoughts?"
"Who can help you through this difficult time?"
"What future plans do you have?"
"How would your death impact the people around you?"
"Let's figure out a plan to make you safer"

CASE 227-2

Ms. Greene is a 47-year-old architect readmitted for a hypertensive crisis related to her polycystic kidney disease. Her renal failure has reached the point where she needs dialysis or kidney transplant. After receiving this news she says, "Well I may as well go ahead and kill myself now."

The hospitalist asks directly "How long have you had these thoughts" and "Have you ever acted on those thoughts?" This patient quickly reveals no significant past history of suicidality and a strong, actively-involved support system. However, she describes tremendous sense of defeat with her worsening medical condition: "I shoot off my mouth, but you are right, I should see someone and talk more about this."

■ CURRENT RISK VERSUS BASELINE RISK

Management of the suicidal patient should focus on reducing the risk back to baseline (or lower if possible). Several key points:

- the risk is never zero;
- some risks cannot be mitigated (ie, gender, age, race, history of a psychiatric disorder);
- some patients carry very high baseline risks for suicide (ie, past suicide attempts, older white males);
- some will commit suicide despite a full assessment and good clinical management.

Sudden change in risk is often more indicative of imminent risk than the absolute level of risk. People with low baseline risks who suddenly have a major change (ie, sudden illness, death of a loved one, intoxication) may not have a very high absolute risk, but relative to their low baseline risks, have a major shift in risk. On the other hand, someone who carries a high baseline risk may actually have a higher absolute risk than the previous patient, but may not be at imminent risk if no recent changes have occurred.

PRACTICE POINT

- Suicidal ideation is common in severe psychiatric disorders
- Clinicians cannot always prevent suicide, but they can reduce the risks
- When in doubt, consult a mental health specialist

■ DETERMINING IMMINENT RISK FOR SUICIDE (IN THE NEXT 24-48 HOURS)

Imminent risk is easy to determine when a patient has a clear plan for suicide and intent to implement (or has just attempted). Unpredictable patients (ie, psychotic or intoxicated) may be at imminent risk; they are often resistant or incapable of forming therapeutic relationships, and it is often difficult to determine whether the risk for suicide is imminent (they often have many risk factors as well as protective factors or prohibitions against suicide). Unfortunately, when multiple risk factors are present, clinical judgment is the only tool available to weigh the complexities of risk. Remember that no reliable method exists to **predict** suicide. The hospitalist's goal is to fully assess and then address modifiable risk factors.

■ ASSESS THE SUPPORT SYSTEM AVAILABLE TO THE PATIENT

Determining the patient's support system is a crucial component of fully assessing the patient's risk factors for suicide. If a patient has an actively involved, well-functioning family or lives in a structured environment where observation is available, then a patient may be potentially treated as an outpatient even with relatively high risk for suicide. On the other hand, even at a lower level of risk, a patient with inadequate support may require hospitalization. When the patient has an active support system, the hospitalist should include these supportive others in the management plan.

■ DETERMINE WHAT SETTING IS REQUIRED FOR THE INITIAL STEPS OF MANAGEMENT

Identifying the setting for implementing the management plan involves assessing the patient's economic and social support resources. Legal and ethical principles require hospitalists to use the least restrictive setting to provide effective intervention and management while maintaining the safety of the patient and others. This is often a difficult balancing act. Limitations in the availability of psychiatric hospitalization have shifted the treatment of psychiatric disorders more to medical settings (if comorbid medical disorders are present) and outpatient settings. Mobilizing complementary professional resources (ie, social workers, nurses, and community services) can help form a supportive structure for the at-risk patient. However, when the risk for suicide is imminent, inpatient hospitalization is required in a secure unit staffed with skilled professionals.

■ MAKE AN EXPLICIT MANAGEMENT PLAN

Reviewing the details of the management plan with the patient helps to actively enlist him or her in their treatment. Documenting and communicating the plan to the patient's support system, when available and allowed by the patient, is ideal for longitudinal

management and decision-making. A written plan gives the patient and the support structure valuable follow-up information, including emergency contact numbers. It is not uncommon for a management plan to include a contract for safety. It is typically a simple statement that is then signed by the patient,

"I, Susan Thomas, agree to call the emergency numbers and come to the ER if I have any feelings about hurting myself."

Though a "contract for safety" is used frequently, it is often overvalued and erroneously perceived as carrying the weight of a legal document. Contracts for safety, which are sometimes referred to as "no-harm contracts" or "suicide contracts," were originally conceived to facilitate management of the suicidal patient. These contracts are vehicles that articulate the treatment plan with parameters for increasing treatment intensity. The utility of this approach lies in the explicit nature of the communication and the explicit agreement of the patient to the plan. The absence of the patient's agreement is an indication to consider psychiatric admission. Though contracts for safety can be helpful communication tools, they alone provide little protective value for a patient who is intent on committing suicide.

A patient's "Safety Plan" has the individual's steps or actions thought out and then written out. It would include the statement above but it would also include family members and friends names and numbers to call, self-soothing activities (eg, reading, music, playing with pets). It is best to have the patient's support group sign off on this plan so they know the steps that are involved.

PRACTICE POINT

Many hospitalized patients are silently at high risk for suicide and should be assessed.

Suicidal thoughts are extremely common, but completed suicide is not.

The clinical goal is to fully assess the risk for suicide, not predict it.

Screening for suicide should begin with discussing hopelessness and negativity.

If suicidality is present then fully assess risk factors:
- Chronic/predisposing factors (gender, family history, age, etc.)
- Acute/potentiating factors (recent loss, exacerbation of illness, access to firearms)
- Protective factors (social support, children <18 in home, religious beliefs)

Devise and communicate a plan addressing the risk factors.

SUGGESTED READINGS

American Psychiatric Association's Practice Guideline for the Assessment and Treatment of Patients with Suicidal Behaviors. Supplement to *Am J Psychiatry*. 2003;160.

Block SD. Assessing and managing depression in the terminally ill patient. *Ann Intern Med*. 2000;132:209-218.

Bostwick JM, Levinson JL. Suicidality. In: Levinson JL. *The Textbook of Psychosomatic Medicine*. Washington, DC: American Psychiatric Publishing Inc.; 2005.

Breitbart W, Rosenfeld B, Pessin H, et al. Depression, hopelessness, and desire for hastened death in terminally ill patients with cancer. *JAMA*. 2000;284:2907-2911.

Druss B, Pincus H. Suicidal ideation and suicide attempts in general medical illnesses. *Arch Intern Med*. 2000;160:1522-1526.

Harris EC, Barraclough BM. Suicide as an outcome for medical disorders. *Medicine*. 1994;73:281-389.

CHAPTER 228

The Difficult Patient

Glenn J. Treisman, MD, PhD

Joyce E. King, MD

Key Clinical Questions

1. How do you identify a "difficult patient"?
2. What strategies achieve long-term clinical results and reduce unnecessary admissions to the hospital?

INTRODUCTION

The term *difficult patient* refers to a subgroup of patients that provoke unpleasant emotions—feelings of frustration, anger, helplessness, inadequacy, or irritation—in the doctors caring for them. Thomas Sydenham wrote in his famed treatise on hysteria "All is caprice. They love without measure those whom they will soon hate without reason. Now they will do this, now that; ever receding from their purpose." These patients have a series of overlapping characteristics, shown in **Table 228-1**.

Although many authors see conflicts between clinicians and patients as specific to one dyadic relationship, most patients identified as difficult or disordered have a long history of failed medical relationships and are often dissatisfied when they arrive. They recreate the same dissatisfying relationships by repeating the behaviors that caused their previous experiences. Emotionally provoked staff members will likely behave in ways that only further confirm the patient's expectation that he or she will receive poor treatment.

Many neurologic disorders and medical conditions, including tumors, endocrine and autoimmune disorders, and medications, cause psychiatric syndromes, such as personality changes, major depression, cognitive dysfunction, and executive dysfunction. All of these can result in behaviors that make patients "difficult." The following discussion is organized around the conditions that most often provoke and sustain "difficult" behaviors, and reviews some behavioral approaches to managing these patients.

PATHOPHYSIOLOGY OF DIFFICULT PATIENTS

Studies of difficult patients are fraught with technical challenges but have generally found that about 15% of patients are perceived as difficult. Six psychiatric disorders had particularly strong associations with being labeled as difficult: somatoform disorder, panic disorder, dysthymia, generalized anxiety, major depressive disorder, and alcohol abuse or dependence. The presence of mental disorders accounted for a substantial proportion of the excess functional impairment and dissatisfaction of difficult patients, but not for all of it. It is not surprising that these "difficult patients" often fall into patterns of futile care, with similar cycles of short hospitalizations that do not result in any benefit. These patients often have not had an adequate diagnostic formulation, and receive poor care as a result of a disintergrated system of care, one in which there is little communication, no real long-term treatment plan that emphasizes rehabilitation, and rewards physicans and patients for short ineffective but time efficient "problem focused visits."

Our diagnostic rubric for difficult patients is developed out of the elegant work of McHugh and Slavney in *Perspectives of Psychiatry*. We will first discuss the psychological precedents from the patient's life experiences. This is followed by a discussion of the role of psychiatric disease states, problematic personality traits, and behavioral conditioning and addictions. Patients often have more than one related condition, each exacerbating the others (**Table 228-2**).

PRACTICE POINT

- Behavior disturbances have multiple causes—those due to underlying medical illness, those due to major psychiatric illness, and those related to interpersonal styles.

- The management strategy begins with a history and physical examination, including a neurologic assessment, so as not to overlook delirium or other underlying medical illness that requires emergent treatment, a review of all medications and dosages, and a toxicology screen in patients suspected of substance abuse.
- Patients with cognitive deficits may be easily confused by a change in environment; may be susceptible to medications with anticholinergic properties, steroids, and analgesics; and may exhibit paranoia or delusions due to a developing delirium.
- Patients with stroke, Parkinson disease, and traumatic brain injury may exhibit features of apathy syndromes, such as lack of motivation and inability to initiate behavior even though they are not depressed or delirious.
- Alcohol and other substance withdrawal may also account for the observed behavioral disturbances.

THE ROLE OF LIFE EXPERIENCES

Life experience is difficult to subject to randomized clinical trials and does not fit well into "evidence-based medicine." **Figure 228-1** illustrates the cycle of life experience and how behavior develops out of the assumptions one makes about the world. This cycle can be interrupted at any of the arrows shown. Patients must understand the psychological precedents that shape their behavior, and they need a clinician who is willing to confront their behavior and guide it toward more adaptive and successful function.

Commitment to acceptance of any goals patients bring, even unhealthy goals, undermines these patients' need for guidance and direction from the clinician, much to their detriment. To defuse this dynamic, the clinician may communicate that the patient is very important despite their misbehavior and that the health care team wants to help. Changing this cycle of hostility requires tackling some of the patient's assumptions and establishing the critical core of the doctor-patient relationship. Patients can fire you and go elsewhere, but they cannot prescribe their own treatment.

PSYCHIATRIC DISEASES

Patients with major mental illness have higher rates of mortality and medical morbidity. As a group they have poorer compliance with

TABLE 228-1 Descriptions of Difficult Patients from the Medical Literature

High resource utilization

Test seeking

Drug seeking

Somatization

Excessive emotion

Unreasonable demands

"Borderline" personality

Dissatisfied

Unexplained symptoms

Chronic pain

Surgery seeking

Desire to direct treatment

Lack limits

Noncompliant

Unresponsive to treatment

TABLE 228-2 Psychiatric Differential Diagnosis of the Difficult Patient

- Maladaptive psychological life experiences:
  Negative experiences including trauma, misuse, learned helplessness, and poor coping skills
- Psychiatric disease:
  Depression, schizophrenia, bipolar disorder and dementia
- Problematic personality:
  Uncooperative, stubborn, manipulative and maladaptive
- Behavioral disorder:
  Addiction, disorders of overvalued ideas, and maladaptive conditioned learning

medical interventions and exhibit high-risk behaviors and unhealthy habits resulting in higher rates of medical complexity and comorbidity. In most health care systems, the chronically mentally ill are disenfranchised from medical care. They take more time and are more challenging to treat than other patients. Frequently underinsured, they have poor access to medical care and decreased willingness to take advantage of accessible care. Specific mental disorders tend to be associated with different types of difficult behaviors.

PRACTICE POINT

- Patients with major psychiatric illness such as major depression, bipolar illness, schizophrenia, and substance abuse are at risk for receiving suboptimal care due to mental illness.
- The first step in treating their medical illness is to collaborate with their psychiatrists or seek hospital psychiatric consultation.

■ SCHIZOPHRENIA

Schizophrenia is a progressive, disabling, lifelong, chronic mental illness characterized by a stepwise deterioration of executive function, social interactions, and a paranoid psychosis without return to baseline between episodes. Patients more often focus their paranoia on outside agencies and people regularly in their lives. The so-called positive features—the auditory hallucinations, delusions, and feelings of external control—are episodic and disruptive. The "negative features" include affective flattening (or inappropriate affect), ambivalence, autism (with social withdrawal), and loose associations.

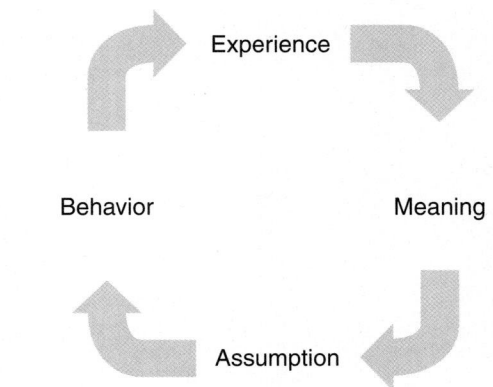

Figure 228-1 *The cycle of life experience.*

Physicians often approach clinical interactions with the preconceived notion that all complaints by patients with schizophrenia are generated by the illness, or that they will be unable to follow treatment recommendations—an assumption that is often incorrect.

MAJOR DEPRESSION

The term *depression* denotes a symptom, a complaint, and several conditions that are probably biologically determined syndromes caused by brain dysfunction. Depressed patients are often lumped together in studies and included or excluded by symptom scales rather than strict criteria, making the literature difficult to understand. There are at least three separate conditions to be considered when thinking about depression, namely, demoralization, chronic dysthymia, and major depression (**Figure 228-2**).

The term *demoralization* describes those patients suffering from the expected or understandable psychological state of decreased mood associated with adversity, loss, and grief. Ranging from mild to severe, demoralization can lead to suicide, social withdrawal, and serious medical morbidity. It responds to the "tincture of time," support, encouragement, and reintegration into occupational, social, and recreational activities. Most physicians do not perceive these patients as difficult; they often evoke genuine sympathy and are usually grateful for the counseling, encouragement, and guidance they receive.

Dysthymia has come to mean chronic major depression, depressive personality style, and subsyndromal major depression. The term as used here denotes a chronic pessimistic personality style, but the term is frequently used in other ways. These patients are like Eeyore in *Winnie the Pooh*, chronically negative but usually quite functional unless they encounter circumstances where their personality style interferes with their function. Their chronic pessimism can lead to frustration on the part of the physician caring for them. Dysthymic patients latch onto doctors and try to get the doctor to make them feel better emotionally when they constitutionally resist doing so.

Major depression describes a biologically determined medical condition that is the result of monoamine neurotransmitter dysfunction and usually an episodic disorder, characterized by periods of illness with symptoms alternating with recovery to baseline. In addition to a genetic predisposition; activation of the stress axis, chronic central nervous system inflammation, a variety of medical conditions including certain cancers, and some medications may provoke major depression. Depending on the type of person who has the condition, patients may experience sadness, loss of emotions, apathy, anxiety, and agitation.

Patients suffering from major depression exaggerate their personality vulnerabilities. They are caught up in an endless web of pessimism and hopelessness, often overwhelmed by their problems and feeling unable to cope. Family and friends share their pervasive opinion that they should be able to "pick themselves up by their bootstraps." The anxiety caused by major depression can give them a "clinging" quality, evoking discomfort for caregivers. The prominent symptom of anxiety can trap patients into a cycle of using benzodiazepines to relieve it, only to have their anxiety worsen dramatically as the benzodiazepines wear off.

Patients with major depression are more "difficult" due to their focus on negative thoughts and feelings; sense of hopelessness, neediness, and abandonment; increased anxiety and likelihood that they will often experience their physical symptoms in an amplified way. Depressed patients can overwhelm physicians, particularly when they resist the diagnosis of a mental illness. Committed to the idea that their depression is the result of their medical (and other) problems, they attribute all of their psychological symptoms to stress rather than to depression. If physicians are also caught up in the patients' psychological explanation for their emotional state, they may miss the diagnosis of major depression. It frequently seems reasonable that the depressive symptoms represent demoralization caused by the medical condition rather than a major depression. Vital sense will be diminished in sick people, and self-attitude changes are often explained away as frustration and hopelessness because of the lack of response to previous treatment.

We have found that anhedonia is both sensitive and specific for the diagnosis of depression in medically ill patients. Patients will describe not being able to get their usual pleasure, joy, excitement, or satisfaction from activities that were previously rewarding.

PERSONALITY DISORDERS

William Osler said, "It is much more important to know what sort of patient has a disease than what sort of disease a patient has." The whole area of personality and temperament is confounded by entrenched psychological theories and dogma about the developmental influences of certain kinds of trauma. The concept of borderline personality originates in psychoanalytic ideas of the early 20th century that have become doctrinaire. Our view of personality disorders arises from the branch of psychology that has attempted to measure temperament or disposition, and how to deal with the traits, regardless of origin. In the simplest terms, "character" (the usual way that a person will respond to a stimulus) can be seen as the outcome of underlying temperament or disposition interacting with learning and environment. The methods used to measure traits of personality have been consistent over time and seem to have predictive validity. We prefer a model that focuses on two traits of personality; introversion-extraversion on one axis and instability-stability on another. These traits are normally distributed in a Gaussian manner in the population. The most straightforward description of this axis of personality is that introverts react to stimulation with inhibition, while extraverts react with excitation. **Figure 228-3** depicts the distribution of introversion and extraversion.

There is also a stability-instability axis (many refer to instability as neuroticism), which is orthogonal to the extraversion-introversion axis (**Figure 228-4**).

When this axis is combined with the extraversion–introversion axis, one gets the four Greek Humors of temperament.

INTROVERTS

As shown in the diagram, introverts are consequence avoidant, future directed, and function directed. They avoid circumstances

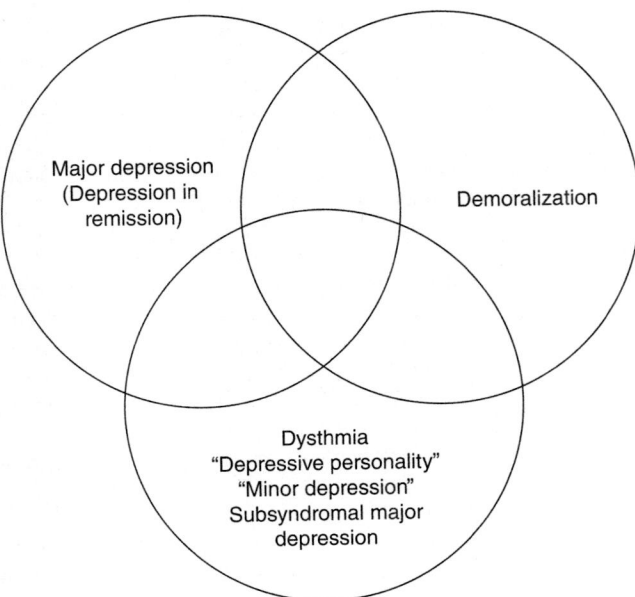

Figure 228-2 *Venn diagram of subtypes of depression.*

Major depression (Depression in remission)

Demoralization

Dysthmia
"Depressive personality"
"Minor depression"
Subsyndromal major depression

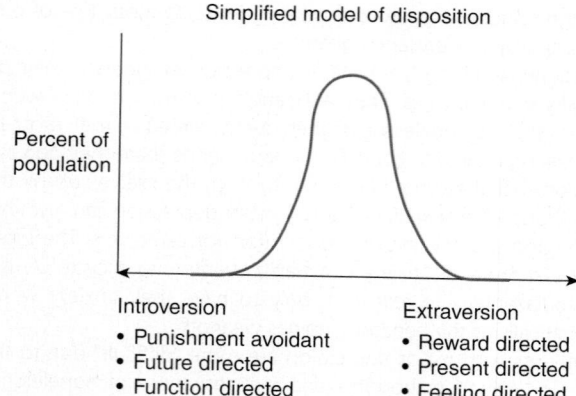

Figure 228-3 *Simplified model of disposition.*

likely to lead to negative outcomes rather than seeking circumstances that will lead to positive outcomes. Their behavior is more likely to be shaped by consequences and they are less sensitive to rewards. They are concerned about illness, physical sensations, their own internal milieu, and avoiding negative consequences. They are therefore concerned about side effects of treatments, the correctness of diagnosis, and the effects of their illness, and when faced with decisions tend to hesitate rather than act decisively, based on fear of making an error.

Introverts are at their best when analyzing situations that require thought and consideration before action. They are good at accounting, law, and medicine, and thinking about safety, prevention, and

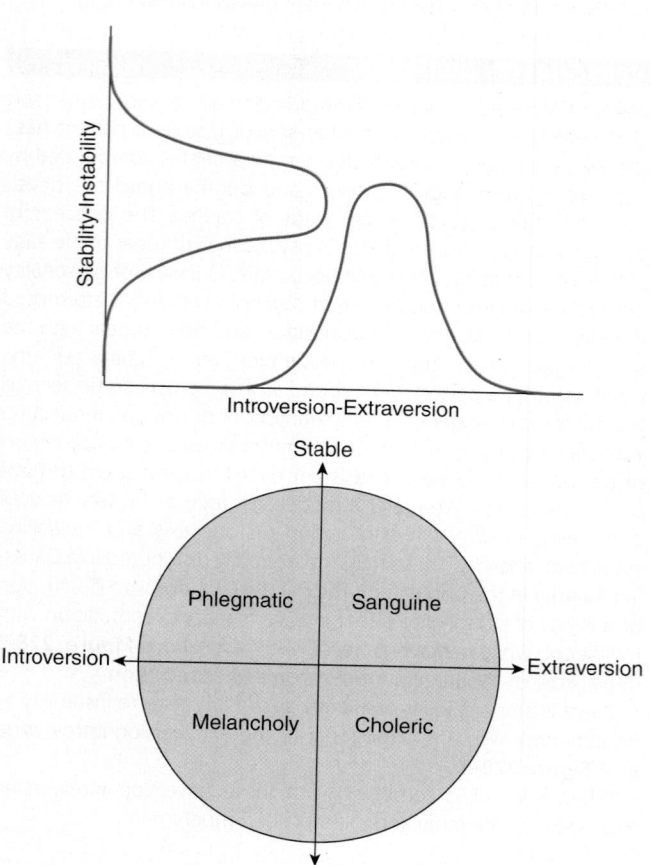

Figure 228-4 *Distribution of some personality traits and their relationship to the four humors of the ancient Greeks.*

right and wrong. They are at a disadvantage in situations requiring action when all choices have potential negative consequences, such as embarking on treatment or accepting diagnostic labels. Ruminating patients can get trapped in endless lists of side effects, adverse outcomes, dangers related to tests and procedures, and the consequences of a particular diagnostic label. The question "What if you are wrong?" can paralyze them and obstruct their treatment. They are particularly sensitive to the social meaning of certain diagnoses, such as psychiatric conditions. Physicians tend to be introverted, and therefore they often have an easier time relating to the obsessive introverts who ruminate endlessly about their illness and the decisions in treatment. Nonetheless, physicians may eventually lose patience with this process and become frustrated by a patient's relentless need for reassurance. They often struggle with the recapitulating patient and need to learn ways to push the patient forward.

Fortunately, clinical medicine has an endless list of terrible consequences that can be used to help shape the behavior of introverts. Introverts usually respond well to opportunities to avoid "bad" decisions, negative consequences, and missed opportunities. They can usually be directed to good decisions by clear clinical analysis of pros and cons of a decision in terms of risks and benefits. They often get bogged down in worries about side effects and ruminative doubts about wrong diagnoses and the need for further tests, but because physicians swim in these waters all the time they can usually lead the patient to the best choice and course of action. Clear descriptions of the "bad things that will happen if you miss your medications" are a powerful motivator for introverts and come naturally to doctors who deal with those bad things every day.

■ EXTRAVERTS

Extraverts are reward sensitive, present focused, and feeling focused. They actively seek positive feelings and desired emotional states, pursuing circumstances likely to provide a positive emotional outcome. They tend to want immediate relief from discomfort, and their behavior is reinforced strongly by rewards, particularly those associated with positive emotions. They are concerned about comfort, appearance, and obtaining the medication or treatment they have chosen. They will pursue a particular diagnosis or status from clinicians if it will get them what they desire and they are less concerned about ensuring that the diagnosis is correct.

Extraverts present a different paradigm for doctors to manage. They are focused on feelings, rewards, and the present. This means they often demand instant relief, have an agenda for what they want, and are persuaded that they can direct their own care better than their doctor. The phrase, "I know what helps me," particularly when delivered in an impatient or irritated tone of voice, is nearly pathognomonic of the difficult extraverted patient. These patients almost always demand specific tests, treatments, and medications and hold fixed ideas about their diagnoses. They want to be made comfortable and equate comfort with wellness, while doctors usually equate function with being well. Ultimately, the central problem is that, in the words of Dr. King, "our therapeutic goals are not aligned." Extraverts' goal of feeling better often immediately leads to excessive use of benzodiazepines for anxiety, opiates for pain, sedative hypnotics for sleep, and stimulants for the inevitable accompanying sedation. Their conviction that something is wrong that can be "fixed" leads to excessive surgery and tests.

The frustration that physicians feel is in part provoked by the emotional landscape these patients inhabit. They feel things strongly and focus on the present. This leads to their changeable nature previously described in the quote by Sydenham. The patients love you when they are getting what they want, and hate you when they are not. Because they are so present focused, the things you have done for them in the past do not carry into the present. There is nothing "in the bank" in terms of trust, patience, and previous experience to help them through a difficult time. These patients are also vulnerable to seeing events as just "happening" to them, with little insight into their own role in their difficulty; this tends to make them see themselves ever as victims. In our current culture of victimhood and lack of personal responsibility, they go to the head of the line with explanations of why nothing is their fault and nothing they can do will make things better.

■ STABILITY

Stable patients have emotions that are slow to change, demonstrate a small emotional response to a large emotional stimulus, and have a very consistent emotional response to a given stimulus. Unstable patients have emotions that change quickly, have a large emotional response to a small stimulus, and have an inconsistent emotional response to a given stimulus. Unstable extraverts (those of choleric temperament)—sometimes referred to as borderline personalities—may split the health care team and are difficult for most clinicians.

Fortunately, these patients are very sensitive to rewards and can be shaped by using the rewards they seek to help change their behavior to more productive modes. Most psychologists see these traits as neutral. Unstable extraverts can be very successful if they learn to modify their natural inclination in certain circumstances. We find it helpful to explain the nature of the difficulty they are having and how it interferes with the doctor-patient relationship. There are two parts to the conversation. The first is to give these patients an explanation of the difficulties they are having with many facets of their life by describing what is good about extraversion and what is bad. The description of patients as having "two scoops of feelings" has been particularly useful. The conversation leads in to the treatment for this, which is to help these patients to learn how not to let feelings run their lives. A method we use frequently is to make comparisons with people these patients are likely to admire who share their traits of intense feelings (a passionate nature) and then to contrast them with similar figures who have failed spectacularly when they let their feelings determine their behavior (such as Martin Luther King Jr compared with Marion Barry).

Most patients of this type have been told that they are missing something (lack of a conscience, a superego lacune, poor object relations) when in fact they suffer from too much of something (an excessive endowment of feelings). We have told patients that they are "a genius of feelings." These patients act entitled because they already sense that they are special. The message is that they are special, that they do deserve more, but that they will not get more until they learn to manage their feelings instead of letting their feelings manage them.

The second element of this conversation is to describe the doctor-patient relationship and the responsibilities each member holds in the relationship. This is sometimes referred to as a role induction and involves the "limit setting" part of working with patients with personality vulnerabilities. This includes the responsibility on the part of these patients to do their best to get well, to discuss the alternatives and then agree to a treatment plan, and to get a second opinion if not satisfied with the diagnosis and treatment plan. Many difficult patients with personality disorders will balk at a treatment plan that does not give them what they want, even if they acknowledge that what they want will be bad for them. This includes their desire for addictive drugs, allowing them to smoke in the bathroom, allowing them to come and go from the hospital as they wish, and allowing them to dictate their treatment. This gives the clinician the opportunity to tell the patient that she will gladly provide care if the patient changes his mind in the future, but she must decline to be a part of any treatment that might be harmful or be less than optimal for her patient. A discussion of why manipulative behavior will be bad for the patient and his treatment is important for patients with these behaviors.

In working with difficult patients, many clinicians use treatment contracts to help delineate the limits and expectations for treatment. Our experience has been that such contracts may be very useful, but they can also serve as the way to "get rid" of patients who have overwhelmed the system. We have begun to advocate discharging uncooperative patients early with a smile and much encouragement to return if they decide our approach might help them. This does not mean that we think that any patient who is not completely cooperative should be discharged, it rather is directed at patients who are exhausting resources while not getting better, or more commonly, actually being harmed by the treatments that they end up getting. Any patients you would allow to leave against medical advice (AMA) can be discharged AMA if they are uncooperative.

In circumstances where patients are so ill or cognitively impaired that they cannot be allowed to leave, we recommend simply telling them they will not be allowed to leave until stable, and treat them the same way we treat anyone who cannot cooperate but needs life-sustaining treatment. This approach also discourages patients who are uncooperative, using resources without gaining benefit, and demoralizing their doctors, but it allows them time to rethink their behavior and return to treatment when they are confronted with the need to change. Remarkably, many of these patients return. Over years they have told us in a variety of ways that they came back because we said no to them, and that we were the first doctors who thought they could actually get better.

ADDICTIONS

Poorly understood in medicine, addictions are usually categorized as diseases due to the biological nature of the abnormal appetite and drive that develop in addiction. This approach ignores the volitional component of addiction, which is essential to understanding the condition, and misses the huge number of sober addicts who remain in programs. On the opposite extreme, it has also become popular to look at drug addiction as a lifestyle or choice. This approach is not valid either. The demoralizing and dehumanizing activities in which addicts engage are repugnant and distressing to them, but they are unable to break free of the drug's hold on them. They like the drug, but they hate the addiction.

Patients suffering from addictions are frequently perceived as difficult. Doctors are not angry with patients with medical diseases such as congestive heart failure, but when their patient with alcohol addiction drinks, they become judgmental. Patients with addictions are often difficult in much the same way as extraverts. This is in part because extraverts are at increased risk for addictions, and by virtue of the fact that an addiction directs the patient's attention toward feelings, the present, and getting the drug that is reinforcing—all characteristics of extraversion. Introverts who develop addictions often look like extraverts when they are actively using drugs, adopting the style of manipulation and insensitivity to consequences that are the hallmarks of the extraverted personality disorders. They return to an introverted style as they recover. Patients have their behavior shaped by the rewarding nature of the drugs they use until the behavior becomes a loop of positive reinforcement that gradually excludes all other activities.

Addicted patients inevitably seek to maintain their addiction through manipulation, coercion, and lying. In addition, the destruction of employment and family relationships caused by substance use removes the supports most often sought by physicians caring for the difficult patient. Patients who are abusing illicit substances or misusing prescribed controlled substances present to their physicians in confusing ways. The physician is initially puzzled about the possibility of a missed diagnosis, a nagging sense that something about the interaction was "off," or why best efforts with a patient are repeatedly thwarted. These patients drain the resources of the hospital staff by asking for higher doses of opiates or requesting a specific nurse because "she understands my pain." They often wait until change of shift or evening hours when their usual physician is not available to ask for specific drugs by name or insist on intravenous opiates when the daytime plan had been made to switch to oral agents. They refuse magnetic resonance imaging scans at the last minute unless they can have a benzodiazepine of choice and some opiate during the study. They are off the floor when a procedure is scheduled and then complain that they have been in the hospital for days and nothing is happening. A high level of suspicion must be entertained for substance abuse in difficult patient encounters in order not to miss addictions, as they are associated with high morbidity and mortality and are imminently treatable.

Once the physician has diagnosed addiction, the following steps should be started in the hospital and pursued as part of the medical treatment plan:

1. **Conversion.** The patient is helped to recognize the addiction as a disorder that needs treatment. Some patients must lose nearly everything in their life before they can "hit bottom" and see the severity of their condition. Others can heed the properly presented warning of a good clinician. "Motivational interviewing" and "confrontation with a smile" are two descriptors of ways to achieve this. Essentially, in this step patients accept the diagnosis of an addictive disorder and decide that they are ready to get better.

2. **Detoxification.** Patients who are actively in the loop of using and craving are usually unable to break out of that loop without an intervention to detoxify them.

3. **Rehabilitation.** As patients become progressively more addicted, their lives become focused entirely on the behaviors involved in obtaining and using drugs, and gradually exclude all other activities. They become socially, occupationally, and recreationally disconnected. As they recover, there is little to fill their time other than craving drugs, and little to distract them

from negative feelings. The activities that result in positive reinforcement of behavior in life and give life a sense of pleasure and satisfaction usually involve activities in these life domains. Rehabilitation means filling up these domains with meaningful life activities, but these must be rebuilt (or built) over time. This is often the most time-consuming element of recovery. It is not uncommon to hear people who have successfully recovered describe this phase in months and years.

4. **Treatment of comorbid conditions.** The fourth step occurs simultaneously with the third and consists of the treatment of comorbid conditions, both medical and psychiatric. Depression, personality disorders, HIV, hepatitis C, and chronic pain all act as triggers and interfere with recovery.

5. **Relapse prevention.** This is a long-term (indefinite) plan to prevent the elements that combined to allow the addiction to develop in the first place from allowing it to recur. Twelve-step programs, physician monitoring, and constant reminders of the danger of recurrence of addiction are needed in a long-term systematic way.

Motivational interviewing, role induction, and detoxification can usually be initiated in the hospital, and sometimes completed. Familiarity with and referral to the outpatient network of rehabilitation services is essential for lasting success with addicted patients.

CHRONIC PAIN

The issue of the management of chronic pain is central to the role of dealing with difficult patients. Patients with acute pain are usually relatively straightforward to manage, while those with chronic pain are far more difficult. Unfortunately, the efforts to make pain a vital sign and to ensure that all pain is relieved have led to a massive overuse of narcotics and escalating problems of iatrogenic addiction. Nonmalignant chronic pain is often not relieved with chronic opiates and can be made worse by chronic opiate use.

PRACTICE POINT

- Although some patients benefit from chronic opiate administration, it is increasingly clear that many do not.
- Opiate-mediated hyperalgesia is common in patients with chronic pain on long-term opiates.
- The longer term the pain, the less often opiates are the answer.
- If tissue is not being damaged (neuropathy, low back pain, chronic headache, fibromyalgia, and other chronic conditions), the opiates often cause real problems for patients later and can reinforce abnormal illness behaviors; alternative methods of pain management may be more useful for chronic pain.

Pain has two components, a sensory element and an affective element. It is the affective element that produces the distress associated with pain. Patients with depression have an increased sensitivity to pain, particularly the affective component. Patients with significant extraversion or instability are more reactive to the distress associated with pain and will tolerate a lower level of function in their effort to eliminate pain. They are at increased risk for addiction and medication overuse.

In general, opiates are usually reasonable for acute pain caused by tissue damage (surgery, trauma, malignancy). Chronic pain is not usually the result of ongoing tissue damage, but rather the result of altered sensory and sympathetic nervous function (as in neuropathy, low back pain, chronic headache, fibromyalgia). While some patients benefit from chronic opiate administration, it is increasingly clear that many do not. Patients are often given opiates at ever increasing doses to try to combat their pain, and while some may benefit, many become increasingly intoxicated and exhibit more dysfunction as the dose increases. Opiate-mediated hyperalgesia is common in patients with chronic pain on long-term opiates. The longer term the pain, the less often opiates are the answer.

Patients with chronic pain are often in the "difficult patient" category and are often focused entirely on the goal of pain relief to the detriment of getting better and improving function. They arrive demanding escalating doses of opiates and are often given comfort-directed pharmacologic interventions such as benzodiazepines and other sedative hypnotics.

BEHAVIORAL MANAGEMENT OF DIFFICULT PATIENTS

In the early 1900s, Ivan Pavlov described the ability to change behavior in animals by association with a particular stimulus. He was able to measure salivation in dogs in response to food, but then by pairing the food with a bell, he was able to elicit salivation in response to the bell. Described as classical conditioning, this type of passive conditioning has been observed with patients in many settings. Patients who have had several exposures to chemotherapy will often develop nausea and may even vomit when arriving at the cancer center. It is possible to condition changes in immune function, condition asthma attacks, and condition neutral stimuli to cause pain. Classical conditioning (or Pavlovian conditioning) occurs when a patient associates a behavior with a desirable or undesirable stimulus or experience.

Operant conditioning, described later by B. F. Skinner, occurs when a behavior performed by the patient is associated with a specific consequence. This type of conditioning results in increasing or decreasing the likelihood of the associated behavior. As an example, a pigeon pecks a key and receives a food reward. This results in more frequent and faster key-pecking behavior. Skinner described "shaping," where successive rewards could result in more complex behaviors. Pigeons can be shaped to peck a ball into a slot for food by first shaping the bird to peck the ball and then rewarding it only when it pecks the ball in a specific direction. Skinner described four types of conditioning, as shown in **Table 228-3**.

If the consequence of the behavior is a reward (positive reinforcement) or the removal of something noxious (negative reinforcement), behaviors increase. If the consequence of the behavior is the removal of the reward (extinction) or the delivery of something noxious (punishment—often incorrectly referred to as negative reinforcement), behaviors decrease.

All of these conditioning paradigms have been described for doctor-patient interactions. A patient who throws a tantrum on the ward and demands narcotics has probably been reinforced for that behavior by the previous delivery of narcotics in the same situation. Subtle reinforcement of illness behaviors such as limping, splinting, moaning, crying, and even falling can occur with patients who are vulnerable to the reinforcing effects of particular responses.

TABLE 228-3 Behavioral Reinforcement from Operant Conditioning

Quality of the Consequence	Positive (Rewarding)	Negative (Noxious)
Delivery of consequence	Positive reinforcement Increased behavior	Punishment Decreased behavior
Withdrawal of consequence	Extinction Decreased behavior	Negative reinforcement Increased behavior

From Operant reinforcement as described by BF Skinner.

A caveat here is that reinforcement works only when the consequence or reward being employed to shape behavior has salience to the person being shaped. Pigeons must be hungry to work for food rewards. Patients in a given set of circumstances are more or less vulnerable to the reinforcing effects of narcotics, attention, praise, encouragement, criticism, relief from distress, and diagnostic labels. A person with a good job may be eager to return to work and may perceive an excuse from work as aversive and therefore understate her level of discomfort. A person who is unhappy at work may find a note excusing him a reward and may thus overestimate his discomfort. Physicians are constantly shaping their patients. All doctor-patient interactions subtly shape behavior.

Patients are positively reinforced by opiate and sedative-hypnotic medications, attention from doctors, disability payments, and permission to express prohibited feelings. They are negatively reinforced by the pain relief provided by narcotics, the relief from insomnia provided by sedative hypnotics, and the relief from the expectations and demands at work and at home. This will increase medication seeking, doctor seeking, and pain-related behavior. This will also shape patients to be less committed to recovery.

Fortunately, these same behavioral tools can be used to shape recovery-related and function-related behaviors. Izzy Pilowsky described illness-related behaviors in the absence of ongoing pathology with the term abnormal illness behavior. Many of these behaviors are conditioned to occur. Ignoring abnormal illness behaviors will help result in their extinction. Rewarding healthy behaviors such as rehabilitation, function, and coping will encourage them to develop. Examples of this include the use of letters, forms, attention, and personal approval as positive reinforcers of specific behavior. Patients on chronic opiate treatment for pain might be required to demonstrate steady progress at physical therapy (PT) with increasing exercise duration. We have told patients that if they are too sick for PT, then they do not need the opiates because the opiates are only prescribed to make PT tolerable. It is also important to recognize that patients condition their physicians as much as we condition them. In a seminal study of prescription-writing behavior, Turk showed that nonverbal pain behaviors have a potent influence on the prescription-writing behavior of doctors. Continuous positive reinforcement leads to high rates of behavior, while intermittent reinforcement leads to long sustainable behavior. When patients "wear us down" and we "cave" and prescribe narcotics, we are ensuring that the behavior will continue a long time.

The deliberate application of behavioral techniques to treatment of difficult patients takes much of the emotional element out of the picture. We emphasize that we will focus on what the patient is doing and not on what they are feeling. Successful treatment can be described as occurring in five steps, similar to those for addictions. Prior to beginning treatment, a full evaluation for medical and psychiatric conditions must be completed. It is critical to know the case when starting treatment with difficult patients.

Treatment begins with a role induction. This consists of describing the entire formulation to the patient of what the doctor thinks is wrong. We include the medical and psychiatric elements in the discussion. We allow adequate time for patients to ask questions about each condition, why we think they have it, and how it affects them, but we do not allow patients to derail the discussion or argue about the diagnosis. When patients argue about the diagnosis, we tell them that if they disagree after we explain things fully, we will arrange for them to get a second opinion. It is important not to allow the patient to short circuit the discussion of diagnosis by leaping to treatment. The discussion of treatment begins after the patient has heard the diagnostic formulation completely. Typical formulations describe the medical problems first, then the way they are complicated by the lack of reward in major depression, the amplification of sensation due to temperament, and the lack of coping skills and aversive experiences that have made it hard to get good treatment. We finally discuss the way in which conditioning has systematically incapacitated the patient. We offer an optimistic discussion of treatments that are often contrary to the patient's requested treatments, but we explain how they will result in a better outcome. We stress the losses and indignities the patient has suffered from his illness and how important it is to try to recover his life. We finish the role induction by pointing out that we could be wrong, and that the patient will need to decide whether he wants to seek treatment elsewhere or engage in the treatment we have prescribed. This approach is paternalistic, but it also establishes the critical core of the doctor-patient relationship.

The next step involves detoxification, if needed, and the development of a set of behavioral goals with associated rewards and consequences. This is the equivalent of the detoxification step in addictions treatment, in which the sustaining behavioral rewards that maintain abnormal illness behavior are removed.

The next step, initiation of medical and psychiatric treatments (equivalent to the treatment of comorbid conditions in addictions), is critical to the success of the overall treatment. This is done in concert with the initiation of behaviorally based rehabilitation. Treatment often includes an opiate taper, physical therapy, and comprehensive rehabilitation for chronic pain, chronic bowel dysfunction, or any other chronically deconditioned organ system.

Finally, relapse prevention is provided in the form of a program to prevent the recrudescence of the pathological response to the underlying illness. Almost all difficult patients will have a chronic medical problem that will continue to need attention and treatment. Without ongoing care, the pattern of behavioral reinforcement for disability and deconditioning is likely to recur.

The current medical care system does not adequately reward clinicians for their care, nor does it provide an incentive for successful treatment. The growing emphasis on customer satisfaction, financial efficiency, and allowing patients to prescribe their own treatment has been a disservice to these patients. It is tragic to watch these patients flail against those who want to help them, and exploit every weakness in the system to ensure their own demise. Clinicians are discouraged from engaging with difficult patients by a system that can actually penalize clinicians for caring for them appropriately (eg, by prioritization of patient satisfaction and short length of stay over long-term clinical results). However, incentives may change with new reimbursement models that provide a lump sum for an extended period of care; already, hospitals are increasingly looking to hospitalists and others to develop new systems to reduce readmissions.

CONCLUSION

Difficult patients usually present with underlying illness that has been made worse by psychiatric conditions that exacerbate the illness and lead to disability. A comprehensive diagnostic formulation that includes comorbid psychiatric conditions allows clinicians to develop treatment plans that overcome the barriers to successful medical treatment. The route to success is to focus on the patient's medical treatment and behavior, and to pay less attention to the patient's feelings, emotional provocations and manipulations, and comfort. Unfortunately, these patients require more time, are less satisfied, use more resources, and are less able to pay for their treatment.

Because these patients are often conditioned to engage in self-defeating behavior, they may sabotage their own care to hurt a clinician when they are angry about something, even though, as Sydenham observed, they ever recede from their purpose. It has become politically popular to see difficult patients in terms of their rights, but a patient who is difficult may be suffering from impaired autonomy and is not necessarily making decisions in an autonomous fashion. There is also growing literature discussing the characteristics of physicians who have difficulty with patients and on how to improve physician skills, suggesting a view that difficult patients are a product of clinician failure. Certainly, better skills are helpful in managing difficult patients, but mastery of treating the underlying problem is necessary to rehabilitate patients to full function. "Understanding" how the patient feels may be comforting but no more therapeutic than having the orthopedic surgeon "understand" your fracture. Ultimately, the best way to manage difficult patients is to help them get better, but many patients will need to hear the same message repeatedly before they are ready to accept the treatment plan most likely to succeed. Patient advocacy sometimes involves advocating for something that the patient does not want but certainly needs.

SUGGESTED READINGS

Bekhit MH. Opioid-induced hyperalgesia and tolerance. *Am J Ther.* 2010;17(5):498-510.

Fordyce WE, Fowler RS, DeLateur B. An application of behavior modification technique to a problem of chronic pain. *Behav Res Ther.* 1968;6(1):105-107.

McHugh PR, Slavney PR. *The Perspectives of Psychiatry*, 2nd ed. Baltimore, MD: JHU Press; 1998.

Osler W. A Concise History of Medicine. Medical Standard Book Co. 1919. Available online at http://www.archive.org/details/aconcisehistory00oslegoog.

Pilowsky I. Abnormal illness behaviour. *Br J Med Psychol.* 1969;42(4):347-351.

Poulos CX, Hinson RE, Siegel S. The role of Pavlovian processes in drug tolerance and dependence: implications for treatment. *Addict Behav.* 1981;6(3):205-211.

Skinner BF. The operant side of behavior therapy. *J Behav Ther Exp Psychiatry.* 1988;19(3):17.

Sydenham T. *The Works of Thomas Sydenham M.D.* Translated from the Latin edition of Dr. Greenhill. Printed for the Sydenham Society, London; 1850.

Treisman GJ, Angelino A. *The Psychiatry of AIDS: A Guide to Diagnosis and Treatment.* Baltimore, MD: Johns Hopkins University Press; 2004.

Turk DC, Okifuji A. What factors affect physicians' decisions to prescribe opioids for chronic noncancer pain patients? *Clin J Pain.* 1997;13(4):330-336.

CHAPTER 229

Approach to the Patient with Multiple Unexplained Somatic Symptoms

Anne F. Gross, MD
Hermioni N. Lokko, MD, MPP
Jeff C. Huffman, MD
Theodore A. Stern, MD

Key Clinical Questions

1. What is the psychiatric differential diagnosis for patients with unexplained physical symptoms?
2. How can factitious disorder be differentiated from malingering?
3. What is conversion disorder, and how is this different from factitious disorder?
4. What are the best practices in the care of patients with somatic symptom and related disorders, conversion disorder, illness, and malingering?

INTRODUCTION

Patients who present with multiple unexplained somatic symptoms pose a significant diagnostic and management challenge for any physician. Such patients are common in medical settings, representing approximately 1.5%-11% of primary care patients. In the general hospital setting, unique patterns of multiple unexplained somatic symptoms are classified as functional somatic syndromes; these include fibromyalgia, chronic fatigue syndrome, and irritable bowel syndrome. The most common presenting symptoms include chest pain, fatigue, headache, and dizziness; when such symptoms go unexplained the workup may involve unnecessary—and even dangerous—tests and procedures, as well as substantial medical cost. In primary care settings, multiple unexplained somatic symptoms are often co-morbid with psychiatric disorders (including major depressive disorder, generalized anxiety disorder, and panic disorder). The diagnostic criteria used in this chapter reflect the new categorization of disorders with prominent somatic symptoms in the *Diagnostic and Statistical Manual of Mental Disorders*, 5th edition (DSM-5). Somatoform disorders (in the *Diagnostic and Statistical Manual of Mental Disorders*, 4th edition [DSM-4]), characterized by somatization disorder, undifferentiated somatoform disorder, pain disorder, conversion disorder, hypochondriasis, and body dysmorphic disorder, have been reorganized to somatic symptom and related disorders (in the DSM-5) to constitute: somatic symptom disorder, illness anxiety disorder, conversion disorder (functional neurological symptom disorder), psychological factors affecting other medical conditions, factitious disorder, other specified somatic symptom and related disorder, and unspecified somatic symptom and related disorder. **Figure 229-1** provides a diagnostic algorithm to assist in the evaluation of a patient who presents with multiple unexplained somatic symptoms.

GENERAL APPROACH TO THE PATIENT WITH MULTIPLE UNEXPLAINED SOMATIC SYMPTOMS

Table 229-1 outlines the major tenets of the approach to patients with multiple unexplained somatic symptoms. Considering the etiology of multiple unexplained somatic symptoms can be difficult, it may be helpful to prepare for a difficult interview (eg, a patient may provide a vague and/or elusive history, be argumentative, or be hostile). The specific approach to a given patient with multiple symptoms depends largely on the type of physical complaints with which the patient presents. However, regardless of the chief complaint, a thorough history is critical to the evaluation of true medical and neurologic illnesses; importantly, this interview should not be conducted while one is performing the physical examination. The medical history in such a patient helps the practitioner to determine if the patient is actually experiencing the symptoms reported, if the symptom has been exaggerated or feigned (eg, as in factitious disorder and malingering), if there is a pathophysiological basis for the medical or neurologic complaints, if there is a characteristic pattern of symptoms, and if the patient meets criteria for a somatic symptom disorder.

SPECIFIC DISORDERS ASSOCIATED WITH UNEXPLAINED PHYSICAL SYMPTOMS

■ SOMATIC SYMPTOM DISORDER

Presentation

Somatic symptom disorder (previously considered somatization disorder in the *Diagnostic and Statistical Manual of Mental Disorders*,

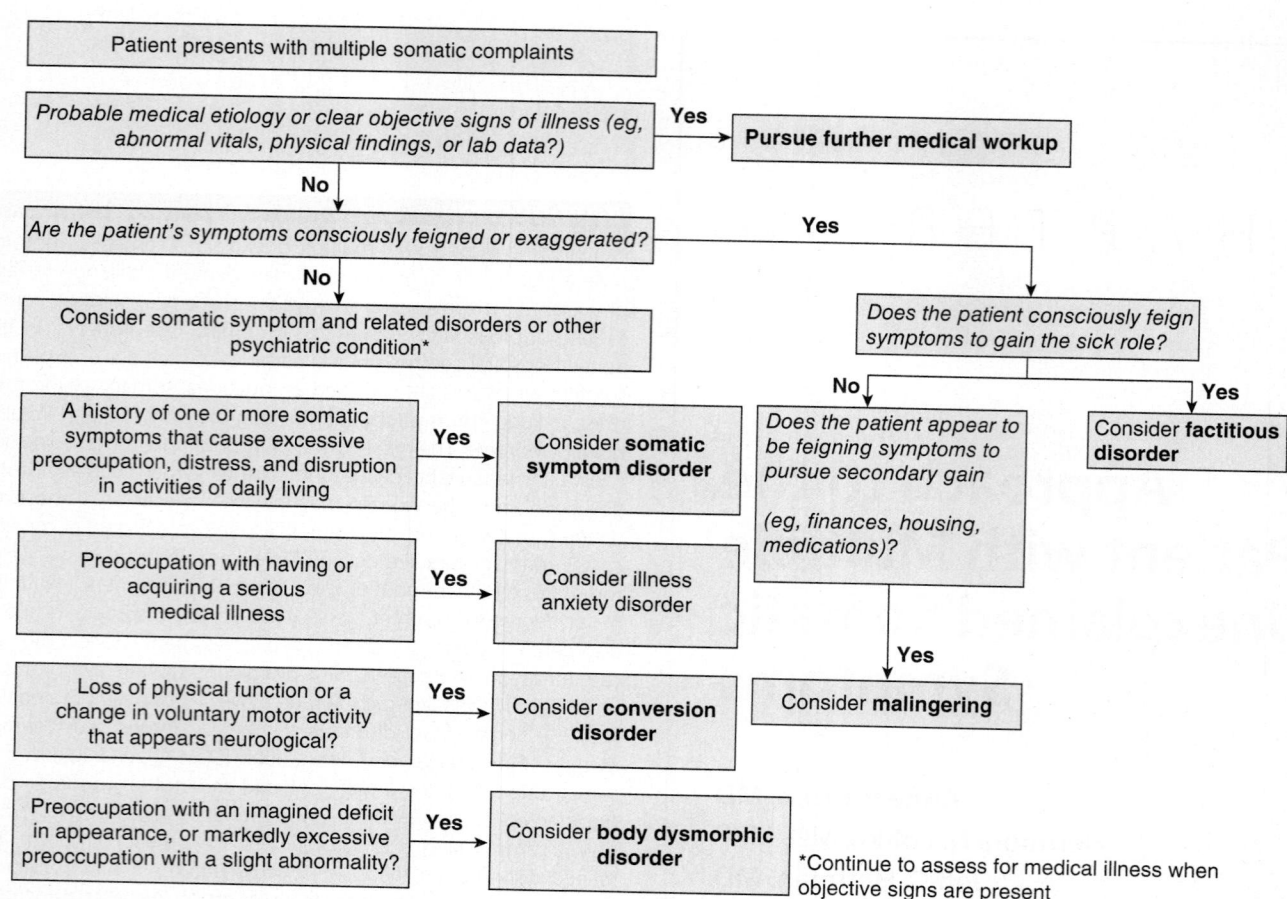

Figure 229-1 *Diagnostic considerations in the patient with multiple unexplained symptoms.*

4th edition [DSM-IV] involves a history of one or more somatic symptoms that cause excessive preoccupation, abnormal thoughts, fear, and distress, as well as, a significant disruption in activities of daily living. The excessive thoughts and fears about their somatic symptoms or associated health concerns are manifested by: persistent and disproportionate thoughts about the severity of one's symptoms, an extremely high level of anxiety about health, or excessive time and energy expended on symptoms or health concerns. The symptoms can change over time but the state of being chronically symptomatic persists for at least six months. Somatic symptom disorder can be specified as being predominantly with pain (symptoms mostly relate to pain) or persistent (more than six months of severe symptoms with marked impairment). **Table 229-2** presents features of the *Diagnostic and Statistical Manual of Mental Disorders*, 5th edition (DSM-5) category, somatic symptom disorder. The disorder is much more common in women of low socioeconomic status, in minorities, in those living in rural areas, and in women with a history of sexual or physical abuse. It frequently co-exists with other psychiatric illnesses, including depression, anxiety disorders, substance abuse disorders, and personality disorders; roughly three-fourths of patients with somatic symptom disorder have a personality disorder, most commonly obsessive-compulsive personality disorder.

Evaluation

Table 229-1 provides the overall approach to patients with multiple somatic symptoms. The medical history reported by patients with somatic symptom disorder is often pan-positive, inconsistent, and disorganized; the level of patient distress is high as are their complaints of disability. Such vagueness can result from alexithymia (involving a difficulty identifying and describing emotions). The

physical examination should be limited to the body system involved in the complaint and should focus on the objective physical findings; similarly, laboratory tests should only be obtained only if there is a clear indication. Because these patients often present with menstrual and sexual complaints, the evaluation should include a thorough menstrual and sexual history; associated physical examination and laboratory testing (including pelvic examination, pregnancy test, or sexually-transmitted disease testing) should be performed, if indicated by the history.

Management

Table 229-3 presents an approach to the management of patients with somatic symptom and related disorders. Rather than attempting to cure the patient of their somatic symptom disorder, the physician should carefully assess the medical diagnoses, decrease the patient's current distress, and help the patient to maintain or improve their level of psychosocial function. Additional treatment suggestions for somatic symptom and related disorders include the following:

- *Consideration of referral to individual psychodynamic psychotherapy.* While not a treatment for somatic symptom disorder itself, this may help a patient who has emotional distress secondary to a physical illness or untreated symptoms secondary to sexual or physical abuse.
- *Consideration of referral for cognitive-behavioral therapy (CBT).* This treatment has proven to be beneficial by helping patients to identify cognitive distortions associated with their physical symptoms.
- *Avoidance of psychotropic medication.* Unless there is a co-occurring psychiatric condition (such as depression, anxiety, or substance abuse) that would benefit from medication, psychotropic medications should not be prescribed.

TABLE 229-1 A Diagnostic Approach to the Patient Who Presents with Multiple Unexplained Somatic Symptoms

History of present illness
- Identify the chief complaint and obtain adequate detail (both pertinent positives and negatives) to assess for all potential medical conditions.
- Document the influence of complaints on the patient's ability to function (eg, impact on interpersonal relationships, ability to engage in pleasurable activities, and ability to work).
- Document recent psychosocial stressors.
- Ask: What has helped the patient cope during times of stress? What does the patient think is wrong with her? Does the patient fear something serious is wrong?
- Consider: Is the patient pursuing medical treatment for secondary gain?

Past medical and psychiatric history
- Review past physical complaints.
- Identify existing medical diagnoses related to the presenting illness.
- Record prior invasive medical and/or surgical procedures the patient has endured to diagnose and/or treat these symptoms.
- Obtain information about current or past treaters (be mindful to obtain a release of medical records to facilitate your review of past documentation and your speaking to current providers) as well as the circumstances under which care has been provided (eg, pain contracts, legal mandates) and ended.
- Discover a history of doctor-shopping or utilizing different hospitals.
- Obtain information about current and past medications that have been prescribed for the current complaint (with an emphasis on narcotics and benzodiazepines).
- Review personal or family illnesses during the patient's childhood.
- Assess personal and family psychiatric history, with a focus on prior diagnoses, use of psychiatric treatment, and history of self-harm.

Social history
- Review patient's psychosocial supports, level of education, marital status, employment status, and living situation.
- Obtain a history of domestic, physical, sexual, and/or emotional abuse.
- Review legal agency involvement.

Physical exam
- Focus on the body system involved in the chief complaint.
- Review vital signs and laboratories.
- Determine if there are objective abnormalities on the physical exam that are consistent with medical/neurologic illness, to assist in determining whether additional medical workup should be pursued.

■ ILLNESS ANXIETY DISORDER

Presentation

Patients with illness anxiety disorder are often persistently preoccupied (for at least six months) and anxious about the possibility of an undiagnosed illness (although the specific illness may change over that span). Although they do not always have somatic symptoms, the presence of somatic symptoms (which are often mild) or a medical condition creates intense fear and anxiety, which is disproportionate to the actual medical condition. The anxiety about health concerns is heightened and results in a low threshold of being alarmed by issues pertaining to health. Patients with illness anxiety disorder either excessively check their body for signs of illness or avoid health care completely (even for routine appointments with physicians). Patients with illness anxiety disorder, *care-seeking type*, frequently use medical care and services not limited to physician visits, numerous diagnostic tests, and procedures. Patients with illness anxiety disorder, *care-avoidant type*, under-utilize medical care and health services. Although illness anxiety disorder can also be comorbid with other mood and anxiety disorders, the preoccupation with illness is not explained by other psychiatric illnesses (such as somatic symptom disorder, panic disorder, generalized anxiety disorder, body dysmorphic disorder, obsessive-compulsive disorder or delusional disorder, somatic type).

Evaluation

One should be aware that patients with illness anxiety disorder often describe symptoms in a detailed and obsessive manner. Most commonly the patient will present with gastrointestinal or cardiovascular symptoms but may have complaints in any body system. Frequently, the patient will outline in detail the feared diagnosis associated with each symptom. Patients should be asked about the meaning of their symptoms (eg, What do you think causes your chest pain?), which may help them to discuss fears about illness. Importantly, patients with illness anxiety disorder can become angry and dissatisfied with their medical care and typically present to multiple physicians with somatic complaints without any identified etiology.

It is useful to assess these patients for obsessive-compulsive disorder (OCD) and psychotic disorders. All three of these disorders may present with an obsessive, ruminative pattern with attention to bodily details and intense preoccupation about illness, but the treatments for OCD, psychotic disorders, and illness anxiety disorder differ. Patients with illness anxiety disorder, while convinced that something devastating is wrong, should be able to consider alternative explanations for their symptoms; patients who are not able to be convinced otherwise may suffer from a delusional disorder. Patients with OCD—in contrast to patients with illness anxiety disorder—have compulsions associated with their somatic obsessions; such compulsions may include washing, counting, or performing mental acts.

Treatment

Overall management should adhere to the principles listed in Table 229-3. A primary goal of treatment should be to help the

TABLE 229-2 DSM-5 Features for Somatic Symptom Disorder

The three criteria to be considered to make this diagnosis are as follows:

A. Somatic Symptoms:

One or more somatic symptoms that are distressing and/or result in significant disruption in daily life.

B. Excessive thoughts, feelings and behaviors related to these somatic symptoms or associated health concerns with at least one of the following present:

1. Disproportionate and persistent thoughts about the seriousness of one's symptoms.
2. Persistently high level of anxiety about health or symptoms.
3. Excessive time and energy devoted to these symptoms or health concerns.

C. Persistency and Chronicity of Symptoms: The state of being symptomatic must be persistent (typically more than six months) although any one somatic symptom may not be continuously present.

Specifiers:

With predominant pain (previously Pain Disorder in DSM-IV): This is targeted towards individuals with predominant pain symptoms

Persistent: This is characterized by severe symptoms or marked impairment with a greater than six months duration.

patient cope with and tolerate physical sensations or symptoms. Illness anxiety disorder, like many somatic symptom and related disorders, includes distorted cognitions, fears, and an unwavering conviction of illness. Treatment should be focused on the psychological meaning of the symptoms and what it means to be ill, rather than on a repeated work-up of symptoms. Additional treatment recommendations include the following:

- Providing the patient with accurate information about findings of the examination, and correcting the patient's misunderstandings of previous diagnoses.

TABLE 229-3 A General Approach to the Management of a Patient Who Presents with Multiple Unexplained Somatic Symptoms

1. Arrange regularly scheduled brief primary care physician appointments at 2- to 6-wk intervals.
2. Set the agenda of these appointments at the outset, and pursue no further workup unless objective findings are identified.
3. Identify psychosocial precipitants to new complaints, and avoid confrontation.
4. Discuss the role of stress on the physical symptoms the patient is experiencing.
5. Make benign recommendation when appropriate (eg, referral to physical therapy, complementary and alternative medicine techniques, such as biofeedback, relaxation and meditation exercises, vitamins, heating pads).
6. Contact collateral information including previous care providers and family members.
7. Assess for comorbid psychiatric illness, and refer to psychiatry as indicated, with an emphasis to the patient that psychiatry will help manage the impact that stress has on the symptoms.
8. Continue to thoughtfully rule out organic illness when objective signs are present.

- Educating the patient about cognitive distortions.
- Referring for CBT to target the cognitive distortions, anxiety, and illness behavior.
- Considering psychiatric consultation, since the differential diagnosis includes OCD, anxiety disorders, and delusional disorder.

■ CONVERSION DISORDER (FUNCTIONAL NEUROLOGICAL SYMPTOM DISORDER)

Presentation

Conversion disorder differs from other somatic symptom and related disorders in that it involves presentations of only pseudoneurologic symptoms. The DSM-5 diagnostic criteria for conversion disorder include (1) one or more symptoms related to a change in voluntary motor or sensory function, (2) clinical findings suggestive of a neurologic (or other medical) condition but that defy medical or neurological explanation, (3) the symptoms or deficits cannot be explained by another medical or mental disorder, and (4) symptoms that cause significant distress or impairment in social, occupational or other important areas of functioning or warrants medical evaluation. The most common symptoms of conversion disorder, which inform the various specifiers for the diagnosis include: weakness or paralysis, abnormal movements (eg, tremor, dystonic movements, myoclonus, abnormal gait), dysphagia, speech deficits (eg, dysphonia, slurred speech), seizures, anesthesia or sensory loss, special sensory deficits (eg, visual, olfactory or hearing deficits) or a combination of mixed symptoms. Often these episodes will recur and differ in their presentations. Acute episodes have symptoms that last for less than six months, while persistent episodes continue for six months or more. Patients with conversion disorder do not intentionally produce symptoms, a feature that distinguishes them from malingering.

There is often a temporal relationship between a psychologically stressful (specified as with a psychological stressor or without a psychological stressor) event and symptom onset. For instance, a child who witnesses her father beating her mother may suddenly develop conversion blindness. At times a patient will have experienced a prior stressful medical illness, and the patient will re-experience these symptoms when psychological stress arises. For example, pseudoseizures (a type of conversion disorder) are common in patients with epilepsy.

Conversion disorder is more prevalent in women than in men, and the presentation may differ based on cultural and sociodemographic factors. Co-morbid psychiatric illness is common in these patients; the most common Axis I disorders are depression, anxiety, and schizophrenia, and it is important to rule out dissociative disorders. Often these patients suffer from Axis II pathology, including histrionic personality disorder and dependent personality disorder. Without treatment, nearly one-fourth of patients have recurrent pseudoneurological symptoms within 1 year; approximately 20% develop somatic symptom disorder in the next 4 years.

Evaluation

A neurological examination is required for patients who present with a loss or change in voluntary motor or sensory function. Patients may appear anxious about the outcome of the examination, but they often appear indifferent (described as *la belle indifference*). The absence of confirmatory neurologic findings indicates a conversion disorder, especially if there is a temporal relationship of symptoms with a psychologically stressful event. Often, a careful neurologic examination will reveal deficits that do not correspond with an anatomic and or physiologic distribution. In addition, close observation can be used to determine whether the examination changes when the patient is not being "watched" (eg, if the patient moves his arm when he thinks the doctor is not paying attention). Provocative tests may also work: a patient with functional blindness will often show a slight smirk if the examiner makes faces at the patient.

Despite being consciously unaware of symptoms, patients with conversion disorder will often protect themselves from harm or injury. For example, in a patient who presents with upper extremity weakness, if the evaluator holds the patient's arm over her head and drops it, a patient with a conversion disorder will not let the arm fully drop, while a malingerer will typically let it hit her in the head.

Even after a comprehensive neurological examination, the physician must use care when diagnosing conversion disorder, as up to 30% of patients diagnosed with conversion disorder end up having an organic medical or neurological disorder as the cause of the presenting symptoms. Therefore, careful and appropriate neurological studies (eg, neuroimaging, lumbar puncture, or an electroencephalogram) should be performed, as indicated by symptoms, to rule out a general medical or neurological disorder.

Treatment

Treatment of patients suffering from conversion disorder involves provision of support and reassurance as well as non-invasive treatments (eg, physical therapy or behavioral techniques). Treatment recommendations include the following:

- Do not dismiss the patient or him or her that there is "nothing wrong with you."
- Educate the patient; let the patient know that the symptoms will gradually improve with time, and that testing did not reveal any neurologic deficits.
- Work with the patient to identify psychosocial stressors that may have precipitated the illness; this may prevent future episodes and decrease the likelihood of long-term disability.
- Consider psychiatric consultation to address co-existing psychiatric diagnoses and to provide psychotherapy targeting the psychological stressor associated with the development of conversion symptoms.

■ BODY DYSMORPHIC DISORDER

Presentation

In the DSM-5, body dysmorphic disorder (BDD) has been subsumed into the obsessive-compulsive disorders and related disorders (OCDRD) category. BDD is a preoccupation with some imagined deficit or flaw in physical appearance, or a markedly excessive preoccupation of a slight abnormality in physical appearance. On average, approximately one in four patients with BDD consistently think about their disliked body parts for 3 to 8 hours each day and a fourth report actively thinking about them for more than 8 hours each day. The preoccupations are usually intrusive, ego-dystonic, difficult-to-resist or control, and cause significant anxiety and distress or impairment in social, occupational functioning. The typical flaws or deficits are found on the face, scalp, breast, or genitals but skin (facial blemishes), hair and nasal shape are the most common perceived abnormalities. Commonly associated repetitive behaviors include camouflaging lesions, mirror checking behaviors, compensation for a perceived abnormality (eg, stuffing one's shorts if a small penis is perceived), skin picking, reassurance seeking, and excessive grooming to cover up perceived abnormalities. Substantial time is spent performing these compensatory behaviors in a compulsive manner. Patients' distress is not alleviated by others telling them that there is no deficit or that they are attractive. The preoccupation with appearance is not explained by concerns of body fat or weight in an individual whose symptoms meet the diagnostic criteria for an eating disorder.

If a patient is preoccupied with the idea that their body (or body part) is too small or insufficiently muscular, they will receive the specifier, "with muscle dysmorphia". The degree of insight regarding

body dysmorphic disorder can also be specified as: with good or fair insight (the patient recognizes that BDD beliefs are not true or may not be true), with poor insight (the patient thinks BDD beliefs are true) or with absent insight/delusional beliefs (the patient is completely convinced that the BDD beliefs are true).

This disease affects approximately 0.7% to 2.4% of the general population, and studies on the prevalence of gender differences are inconclusive (some studies show a higher prevalence in women while others show a higher prevalence in men). BDD has been diagnosed in children as young as five years of age and in adults who are 80 years old and the presentation can be culture-specific. BDD is highly co-morbid with other primary psychiatric disorders (including major depressive disorder, social anxiety, OCD, and substance abuse). Patients with co-morbid psychiatric disorders have a high level of impairment, a chronic course, as well as high rates of suicidal ideation and suicide attempts.

Patients with BDD are typically reluctant to seek psychiatric referral and usually present to dermatologists or plastic surgeons. Compared to those in the general population, the prevalence of BDD is about 15 times higher in patients who seek plastic surgery: unfortunately, symptoms do not remit after cosmetic procedures, and the patient often continues to have difficulties with self-image even after surgical procedures.

Evaluation

Whenever a patient presents with a physical deformity and the physician either does not see the deformity or believes the deformity is much less severe than the patient perceives, assessment for BDD should be pursued. Specialists in cosmetic surgery should screen patients for this disorder given its high prevalence in this setting and the likelihood that such patients will be dissatisfied with the results of any "corrective" procedure. When a diagnosis of BDD is made, a thorough assessment for substance abuse, depression, and suicidal thoughts is appropriate given the frequent co-occurrence of these conditions with BDD.

Treatment

Key tenets in the treatment of BDD are to prevent iatrogenesis (especially via surgical procedures) and referral for psychiatric treatment. Unfortunately, referral to psychiatric care is difficult: patients typically have poor insight and are unwilling to see a psychiatrist (as they do not think that their difficulties stem from psychiatric illness), and the distress and social anxiety caused by their symptoms often prevent patients with BDD from keeping appointments consistently. Effective treatments for BDD include the following:

- Use the gold standard medication treatment for BDD (high-dose selective serotonin reuptake inhibitors [SSRIs]); as with other obsessive-compulsive-spectrum disorders.
- Switch to the tricyclic antidepressant clomipramine or augment the SSRI with an antipsychotic (such as olanzapine) if the patient does not respond to trials of SSRIs.
- Initiate psychotherapy—specifically CBT—which has decreased the behavioral aspects of illness (including checking, grooming, and exposure to mirrors) and addressed cognitive distortions.

■ FACTITIOUS DISORDER

Presentation

Patients with a factitious disorder consciously feign or create symptoms to assume the sick role. This is in contrast to somatic symptom and related disorders (where somatic symptoms are unconsciously produced) and malingering (where symptoms are feigned or produced illness for secondary gain, such as financial gain, legal avoidance, or housing). In addition to reporting symptoms and creating physical signs of illness, patients with factitious disorder, often undergo multiple medical and/or surgical procedures to appear sick in an often masochistic manner. The DSM-5 categorizes factitious disorder into subtypes: factitious disorder imposed on self (previously Münchausen syndrome in DSM-IV) and factitious disorder imposed on another (previously factitious disorder by proxy in DSM-IV). Behaviors exhibited in factitious disorder cannot be explained by another mental disorder, such as delusional disorder or another psychotic disorder. Factitious disorder can be specified as a single episode or recurrent episodes depending on the events of falsification of illness or induction of injury.

Factitious disorder imposed on self is the subtype most commonly seen in general medical settings where patients falsify physical or psychological signs/symptoms or induce disease or injury. The deception occurs in the absence of external rewards. Patients can have prior or current true medical conditions—may present with reports of symptoms, self-induced signs of illness, or even laboratory abnormalities caused by illicit activities. For instance, a patient with type I diabetes may present with recurrent hypoglycemia and abscesses that result from putting bacteria on the tip of an insulin-filled syringe. These patients often travel from hospital to hospital trying to gain admission; they often present in the summer (when medical house staff is new and supervision is limited), at night, or on weekends.

Factitious disorder imposed on another is a particularly disturbing disorder in which someone (often a mother or a caregiver) fabricates physical signs or symptoms or induces injury or disease in another (often a child, an elderly adult, or a disabled person) to indirectly assume the sick role. There are no obvious external rewards for the deceptive behavior and the perpetrator, not the victim, receives this diagnosis.

Factitious disorder with predominantly psychological symptoms is more difficult to diagnose; syndromes include *pseudologia fantastica* (in which patients provide extensive and false stories about their life to gain sympathy from providers), impostership (where the patient assumes the identity of a famous person), and factitious bereavement (where the patient presents with depression and suicidal ideation after a reported death).

Factitious disorder is predominantly seen in women, often under the age of 40; they almost invariably have a sophisticated medical knowledge from being a nurse or physician, from having a parent in the medical field, from having a close relative who was hospitalized for a particular illness, or from having had a true medical or psychiatric illness at a younger age. Personality disorders, especially borderline personality disorder, are also exceedingly common, and many patients have suffered from childhood abuse or deprivation that has resulted in frequent hospitalizations. Often these patients will have a normal to above average IQ and do not suffer from a formal thought disorder.

Upon presentation to the hospital, the patient will use convincing medical terminology and will present with a story of an acute illness that is plausible and that may appeal to the nurturance and knowledge of the physician as a way to get treatment. However, the patient, upon being admitted to the hospital, typically becomes more demanding, with increasing complaints about misdiagnosis and mismanagement of care. The staff may become angry, and the patient may leave the hospital against medical advice (AMA), with hopes of going to a nearby hospital for "better" treatment.

Evaluation

When one is initially evaluating a patient with suspected factitious disorder, confrontation is not helpful because the patient will adamantly deny feigning symptoms. Instead, an investigative process should be undertaken to confirm the diagnosis; this process involves gathering information from collateral sources (including past care providers, family members, and mental health professionals), and carefully observing the patient. Certain elements of the patient's history should sensitize the physician to the possibility of factitious disorder: a history of multiple hospital admissions without a primary care physician, multiple forms of identification (often from different states), a sophisticated knowledge of medical terminology, an absence of people who can verify the person's history, a history of working in the medical field or of having an illness as an adolescent, a history of personality disorder, and a complicated medical history that entails multiple symptoms as well as many medical and surgical procedures with scars. Throughout the process it is helpful to remain calm and investigative rather than being overly focused on the angry feelings from care providers that these patients almost invariably evoke.

Ultimately, as suspicion for factitious disorder grows, a room search is often necessary that may uncover hidden thermometers, containers of contaminated material (eg, sputum or feces), needles, and syringes of insulin or bottles of medications. After evidence has been discovered by the treating physician, the physician must confront the patient about the dangers of his or her behavior and suggest further psychiatric treatment to address the underlying emotional distress. This can be done by the primary treatment team, often in conjunction with a psychiatric consultation.

Treatment

Treatment relies on early identification of the disorder, before serious medical complications arise from unneeded procedures. Specific treatment strategies include the following:

- Focus on management rather than cure, by working to confirm the diagnosis and by avoiding any tests or procedures unless clearly indicated by objective findings.
- Ensure adequate observation of the patient.
- Maintain open communication among staff involved with the patient's care: meet and discuss the countertransference that is evoked when dealing with such patients.
- Consult psychiatry to help manage the behavior and reduce the emotional distress of the patient; ultimately, referral for outpatient psychiatric care is indicated, and psychotherapy has the potential to provide relief, though these patients typically refuse such referrals.
- Contact the appropriate authorities (eg, department of children and families) and investigate the safety of the child, if factitious disorder imposed on another is suspected.
- Document the diagnosis in the patient's record.

■ MALINGERING

Presentation

Malingering is not considered a mental disorder in the DSM-5 although the DSM-IV defined malingering as the intentional production of false or grossly exaggerated physical or psychological symptoms, motivated by external incentives. Like factitious disorder, malingering involves the production of feigned signs or symptoms of medical or psychiatric illness. However, the goal in malingering is not to attain the sick role, but rather is secondary gain (avoidance of legal charges, financial gain, housing, and/or obtaining substances of abuse, especially opiates and benzodiazepines).

Malingering is most common in men who have a diagnosis of antisocial personality disorder. Upon presentation, often to the emergency department, patients will have a clear goal or motivation for their behavior; clinical indicators for malingering include legal involvement (such as presentation for an assessment that was recommended by an attorney, or presentation directly from jail), a substantial difference between reported symptoms by the patient and objective findings (eg, patients reporting severe, acute pain but having normal vital signs and appearing comfortable when examiners are not in the room). Symptoms are often vague (eg, headache or body aches/pain) but can be more specific. Patients may also report psychiatric symptoms, such as disabling depression (to get disability), or panic attacks or insomnia (to get benzodiazepines). Patients with malingering are often uncooperative with an evaluation or suggested treatment (in stark contrast to factitious disorder, where patients are often compliant with suggested invasive tests and procedures).

Evaluation

Secondary gain, when present, may be an indicator of malingering; however, patients with secondary gain may also have a true medical or psychiatric illness that needs medical attention. If the physician believes that there is no true physiological or psychological illness to cause the symptoms, and that the patient is indeed malingering, collateral information should be obtained. For instance, obtaining collateral information from other providers, family members, parole and police officers, as well as reviewing medical records to look for repeated similar presentations, will help to confirm a history of substance abuse or legal problems. If the provider is seeing the patient in an outpatient setting, additional psychological testing (including the Minnesota Multiphasic Personality Inventory), may be helpful to elaborate on the presence of antisocial personality disorder.

Treatment

The treatment for malingering differs based on the setting in which the patient is seen. It is always useful to be aware of feelings that these patients can produce (countertransference), and to use a calm, objective tone when speaking with patients suspected of malingering.

Specific treatment recommendations include the following:

- Use direct confrontation cautiously as the patient may have a history of aggressive or violent behavior that may be disinhibited by active substance abuse.
- Allow the patient to save face by suggesting that the symptoms (eg, pain, anxiety, or insomnia) will improve over time.
- Avoid iatrogenesis.

CONCLUSION

This chapter reviews the diagnostic approach to patients with multiple unexplained symptoms and provides specific treatment recommendations for common disorders. The acute hospitalization provides an opportunity to diagnose and optimize the management of these patients, and avoid overtesting. Interdisciplinary teamwork may uncover information that would otherwise be unavailable to the outpatient providers and may help develop a coherent care plan. As always, the inpatient care team has the responsibility to effectively communicate the results of hospitalization and recommendations of consultants to outpatient caregivers.

SUGGESTED READINGS

Albertini RS, Phillips KA, Guevremont D. Body dysmorphic disorder. *J Am Acad Child Adolesc Psychiatry.* 1996;35(11):1425-1426.

American Psychiatric Association. *Diagnostic and Statistical Manual of Mental Disorders.* 5th ed., text revision. Washington, DC: American Psychiatric Association; 2012.

Barsky AJ. Somatoform disorder. In: Hyman SE, Jenike MA, eds. *Manual of Clinical Problems in Psychiatry.* Boston, MA: Little, Brown. 1990:177-189.

Barsky AJ, Stern TA, Greenberg DB, Cassem NH. Functional somatic symptoms and somatoform disorder. In: Stern TA, Fricchione

GL, Cassem NH, Jellinek MS, Rosenbaum JF, eds. *Massachusetts General Hospital Handbook of General Hospital Psychiatry,* 5th ed. Philadelphia, PA: Mosby; 2004:269-291.

Bjornsson AS, Didie ER, Phillips KA. Body dysmorphic disorder. *Dialogues Clin Neurosci.* 2010;12(2):221-232.

Calabrese L, Stern TA. The patient with multiple physical complaints. In: Stern TA, Herman JB, Slavin PL, eds. *Massachusetts General Hospital Guide to Primary Care Psychiatry,* 2nd ed. New York, NY: McGraw-Hill; 2004:269-278.

Frias A, Palma C, Farriols N, Gonzalez L. Comorbidity between obsessive-compulsive disorder and body dysmorphic disorder: prevalence, explanatory theories, and clinical characterization. *Neuropsychiatr Dis Treat.* 2015;11:2233-2244.

Greenberg DB, Braun IM, Cassem NH. Functional somatic symptoms and somatoform disorders. In: Stern TA, Rosenbaum JF, Fava M, Biederman J, Rauch SL, eds. *Massachusetts General Hospital Comprehensive Clinical Psychiatry.* Philadelphia, PA: Mosby/Elsevier; 2008:319–330.

Hoedeman R, Krol B, Blankenstein N, Koopmans PC, Groothoff JW. Severe MUPS in a sick-listed population: a cross-sectional study on prevalence, recognition, psychiatric co-morbidity and impairment. *BMC Public Health.* 2009;9:440.

Jewell D. I do not love thee Mr Fell. *BMJ.* 1988;297(6647):498-499.

Konnopka A, Schaefert R, Heinrich S, et al. Economics of medically unexplained symptoms: a systematic review of the literature. *Psychother Psychosom.* 2012;81(5):265-275.

Kroenke K, Swindle R. Cognitive-behavioral therapy for somatization and symptom syndromes: a critical review of controlled clinical trials. *Psychother Psychosom.* 2000;69(4):205-215.

Lokko HN, Stern TA. Confrontations with difficult patients: the good, the bad, and the ugly. *Psychosomatics.* 2015;56(5):556-560.

Mattila AK, Kronholm E, Jula A, Salminen JK, Koivisto AM, Mielonen RL, Joukamaa M. Alexithymia and somatization in general population. *Psychosom Med.* 2008;70(6):716-722.

Phillips KA. Suicidality in Body Dysmorphic Disorder. *Prim psychiatry.* 2007;14(12):58-66.

Phillips KA, Hollander E. Treating body dysmorphic disorder with medication: evidence, misconceptions, and a suggested approach. *Body Image.* 2008;5(1):13-27.

Phillips KA, Menard W, Fay C, Weisberg R. Demographic characteristics, phenomenology, comorbidity, and family history in 200 individuals with body dysmorphic disorder. *Psychosomatics.* 2005;46(4):317-325.

Rabinowitz T, Lasek J. An approach to the patient with physical complaints or irrational anxiety about an illness or their appearance. In: Stern TA, ed. *The Ten-Minute Guide to Psychiatric Diagnosis and Treatment.* New York, NY: Professional Publishing Group. 2005:225–238.

Rief W, Buhlmann U, Wilhelm S, Borkenhagen A, Brahler E. The prevalence of body dysmorphic disorder: a population-based survey. *Psychol Med.* 2006;36(6):877-885.

Roffman JL, Stern TA. Conversion disorder presenting with neurologic and respiratory symptoms. *Prim Care Companion J Clin Psychiatry.* 2005;7(6):304-306.

Stern TA. Factitious disorders. In: Hyman SE, Jenike MA, eds. *Manual of Clinical Problems in Psychiatry.* Boston, MA: Little, Brown; 1990: 190-194.

Swanson LM, Hamilton JC, Feldman MD. Physician-based estimates of medically unexplained symptoms: a comparison of four case definitions. *Fam Pract.* 2010;27(5):487-493.

Tadisina KK, Chopra K, Singh DP. Body dysmorphic disorder in plastic surgery. *Eplasty*. 2013;13:ic48.

Taqui AM, Shaikh M, Gowani SA, Shahid F, Khan A, Tayyeb SM, Satti M, Vaqar T, Shahid S, Shamsi A, Ganatra HA, Naqvi HA. Body Dysmorphic Disorder: gender differences and prevalence in a Pakistani medical student population. *BMC Psychiatry*. 2008;8:20.

van Eck van der Sluijs J, Ten Have M, Rijnders C, van Marwijk H, de Graaf R, van der Feltz-Cornelis C. Medically unexplained and explained physical symptoms in the general population: association with prevalent and incident mental disorders. *PLoS One*. 2015;10(4):e0123274.

SECTION 14
Pulmonary and Allergy Immunology

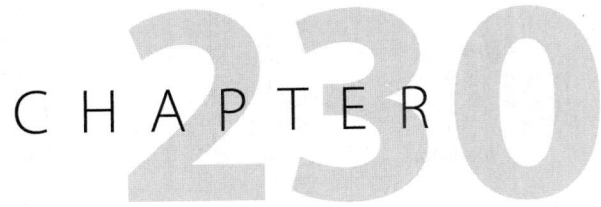

CHAPTER 230

Allergy and Anaphylaxis

Dominique L. Cosco, MD, FACP
Neil H. Winawer, MD, SFHM
Mandakolathur R. Murali, MD

Key Clinical Questions

1 How do anaphylactic and anaphylactoid reactions differ? How are they treated?

2 What conditions mimic allergic reactions?

3 What are the most common types of allergic reactions among hospitalized patients?

4 Which patients require outpatient referral to an allergist?

INTRODUCTION

Allergic reactions result from an aberrant immune response to an inciting antigen or allergen. The subsequent inflammatory state produces a wide range of clinical symptoms. Anaphylaxis, the most extreme form of allergic reaction, refers to sudden, severe, and potentially fatal hypersensitivity developing in seconds to minutes after exposure.

EPIDEMIOLOGY

It is estimated that anaphylaxis accounts for 1 in 2000 ambulance trips and is fatal in as many as 0.7% to 2% of cases. Two epidemiologic studies demonstrated that 1 out of every 2700 to 5100 hospitalizations can be linked to anaphylactic reactions. While the term *allergy* denotes an immediate hypersensitivity reaction involving immunoglobulin E (IgE) antibody, a large number of severe allergic reactions are not IgE mediated. These "anaphylactoid" reactions are clinically indistinguishable from anaphylaxis and include hypersensitivity to radiocontrast dye, angiotensin-converting enzyme (ACE) inhibitors, and opiates.

CLINICAL PRESENTATION

Patients experiencing allergic reactions may vary widely in their clinical presentations. Factors affecting the clinical picture include the amount and persistence of antigen, its route of entry, and the end organ response to vasoactive mediators. The majority of allergic reactions manifest as skin findings, such as flushing, pruritus, and transient urticaria. In more severe reactions, a larger number of deep dermal mast cells are recruited, resulting in angioedema.

The onset of anaphylactic reactions can occur minutes to hours after exposure to an allergen and denotes the systemic activation of mast cells. Aside from the cutaneous manifestations, patients may experience respiratory manifestations (hoarseness of voice, dyspnea, wheezing, cough, and chest tightness), gastrointestinal manifestations (nausea, vomiting, colicky abdominal pain, and diarrhea), and cardiovascular manifestations (peripheral vasodilation, reflex tachycardia, and hypotension with resultant cardiovascular collapse).

PATHOPHYSIOLOGY

When the body is exposed to an antigen, a specific IgE antibody is formed that binds to high-affinity receptors, called Fc epsilon type I, located on mast cells and basophils. Upon re-exposure to that allergen cross-linking of cell-bound IgE antibody occurs, resulting in Fc epsilon receptor aggregation and activation. The resultant mast cell degranulation leads to release of inflammatory mediators such as histamine, prostaglandins, tryptase, platelet activation factor, and leukotrienes, all directly contributing to the allergic response through smooth muscle contraction, bronchoconstriction, vasodilation, increased vascular permeability, and edema (**Figure 230-1**). Allergic reactions mediated by T-helper type 2 (TH2) cells (a subset of CD4+ T cells) preferentially produce interleukins (IL) 4, 5, and 13; all powerful mediators of allergic response. IL-4 promotes B-cell activation and T-cell proliferation and is also responsible for CD4+ T-cell differentiation to TH2 cells. IL-5 recruits and activates eosinophils, contributing to the late phase of allergic inflammation. The functions of IL-13 overlap considerably with those of IL-4 and it synergizes with IL-4 in the production of IgE antibody by B cells.

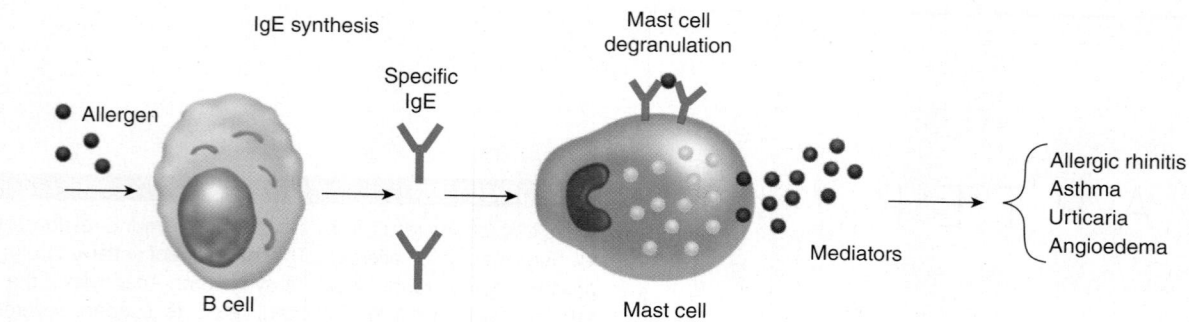

Figure 230-1 *Mechanism of allergic inflammation.*

DIFFERENTIAL DIAGNOSIS

Several disease processes can mimic the clinical features of anaphylaxis. Vasovagal reactions, cardiac arrhythmias, bronchoconstriction, and hypoglycemia, for example, can all be associated with hypotension, pallor, diaphoresis, dyspnea, and wheezing. Pruritis and urticaria may serve as distinguishing factors as they are absent in these mimicking conditions. Viral exanthems and enanthems, depending on their timing, can also be mistaken for hypersensitivity reactions, but they do not manifest itching.

■ ANGIOEDEMA

Angiotensin-converting enzyme inhibitor angioedema

In addition to catalyzing the conversion of angiotensin I to angiotensin II, ACE breaks down bradykinin, in both tissues and plasma, into inactive peptide fragments. Patients taking ACE-inhibitors, therefore, have elevated levels of bradykinin, which stimulates cough receptors and may lead to bouts of angioedema. Unlike immediate hypersensitivity drug reactions, ACE-inhibitor-induced angioedema may occur at any time while the patient is taking the drug, although most reactions occur in the first week following initiation of the drug. Typically, patients present with angioedema involving the lips, tongue, uvula, soft palate, and, much less commonly, bowel, manifesting as acute abdominal pain.

Antihistamines are ineffective, and systemic corticosteroids offer limited benefit in the treatment of ACE-inhibitor-induced angioedema. Subcutaneous administration of icatibant, a selective bradykinin B2 receptor antagonist has achieved excellent results but is expensive and best reserved for severe cases. Most symptoms of ACE-inhibitor angioedema improve with discontinuation of the drug, and patients should not be rechallenged with a different ACE-inhibitor or treated at a lower dose. Most patients with ACE-inhibitor angioedema can tolerate an angiotensin-receptor blocker (ARB). However, treatment needs to be individualized given rare case reports of angioedema with these agents. If there is a strong indication for the ARB (eg, diabetic nephropathy, heart failure) and the episode of angioedema was non–life-threatening, then an ARB can be prescribed with caution.

Hereditary angioedema

Hereditary angioedema (HAE), a rare autosomal dominant disease characterized by a low or nonfunctioning C1 esterase inhibitor can present with episodes of angioedema involving the face, larynx, lips, abdomen, genitalia, and extremities. While attacks may occur in childhood, the disease typically manifests in the second or third decade of life. Aside from prior bouts of angioedema, patients will often endorse a family history of similar attacks. If there is diagnostic uncertainty, a *C4 level* is a cost-effective screening test. A normal C4 level effectively rules out HAE since a low or nonfunctional C1 esterase inhibitor results

in the activation of C4. A decrease in C2 level correlates with exacerbation of the disease.

While HAE is a rare disorder clinicians must distinguish it from anaphylaxis. During episodes of HAE the cascade produces vasoactive kinin proteins such as kallikrein and bradykinin (**Figure 230-2**); mast cells are not activated; hence patients do not manifest pruritus or concomitant urticaria. Therefore, traditional therapies with antihistamines, steroids, and epinephrine have little therapeutic utility. Acute episodes are managed with supportive care and the administration of pasteurized C1 esterase inhibitor concentrate. C1 esterase inhibitor is derived from human plasma and bears infection transmission risks similar to other blood product transfusions. A recombinant C1 esterase inhibitor, derived from transgenic rabbits, named Ruconest was approved by the US Food and Drug Administration (FDA) in 2014 for use in acute attacks. This recombinant product does have a shorter half-life than the plasma derived product thus requiring higher doses to achieve sufficient plasma levels. Patients who receive Ruconest should be screened for rabbit specific IgE to avoid anaphylaxis. Ecallantide, a potent inhibitor of plasma kallikrein, has FDA approval for treatment of acute attacks. Icatibant is also approved for acute attacks. Head to head trials of these agents are lacking.

PRACTICE POINT

- Unlike common histamine-mediated allergic reactions, patients with bradykinin-mediated reactions—hereditary angioedema and ACE-inhibitor angioedema—do not attain therapeutic benefit from epinephrine, antihistamines or steroids. HAE treatment may include C1 esterase inhibitor concentrate or the potent kallikrein inhibitor, ecallantide. ACE-inhibitor angioedema treatment includes supportive care, prompt removal of the drug and icatibant in severe cases.

■ SYSTEMIC MASTOCYTOSIS

Systemic mastocytosis, another rare disorder characterized by an overabundance of mast cells in the liver, spleen, bone marrow, skin, and gastrointestinal tract, shares similarities with allergic and anaphylactoid reactions. Symptoms of flushing, pruritis, and/or abdominal pain may be seen, and hepatosplenomegaly, lympadenopathy, anemia, and/or coagulopathy may also be present. When systemic mastocytosis is considered, serum total and beta tryptase levels are useful diagnostic tests. A total tryptase level of > 20 ng/mL with an increase in the alpha subunit is suggestive of the diagnosis. The beta tryptase level is usually within normal range, unlike in *anaphylaxis wherein the beta tryptase is elevated*. The diagnosis can be confirmed by bone marrow biopsy, which reveals

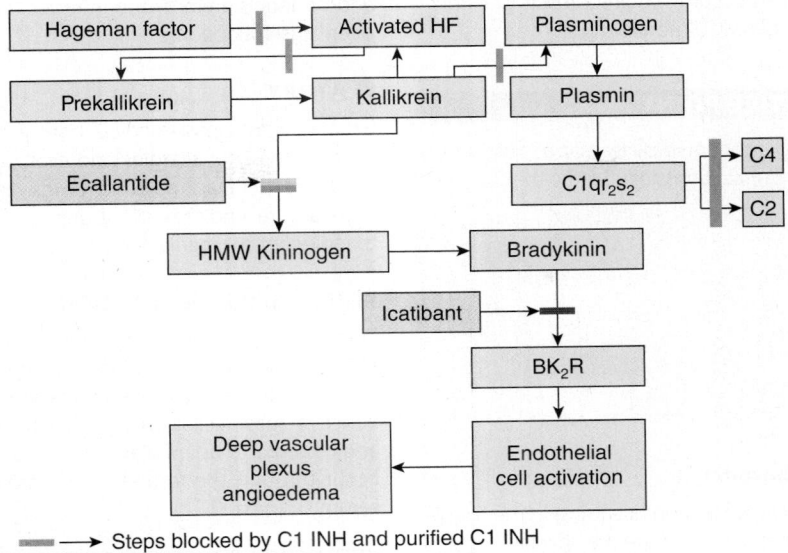

Hereditary angioedema—pathways and therapy

→ Steps blocked by C1 INH and purified C1 INH

Figure 230-2 *Hereditary angioedema—pathways and therapy.*

a multifocal dense infiltrate of mast cells, often with spindle shape morphology. Flow cytometry of bone marrow cells is typically positive for CD25+, CD2+, c-kit, or CD117+.

■ CARCINOID SYNDROME

Carcinoid tumors may also be associated with symptoms analogous to anaphylaxis. The constellation of skin flushing, abdominal cramping, diarrhea, and bronchoconstriction may be misleading. When carcinoid tumors are suspected, patients should have 24-hour urine levels of 5-hydroxyindoleacetic acid (5-HIAA) measured.

■ VOCAL CORD DYSFUNCTION

Vocal cord dysfunction may masquerade as anaphylaxis and can be substantiated by detecting an auscultatory inspiratory stridor over the trachea and confirmed by laryngoscopy as well as by a flattening of the inspiratory loop on spirometry during an attack.

DIAGNOSIS

The diagnosis of allergic reactions and anaphylaxis is based on clinical grounds and is self-evident when patients display the classic constellation of symptoms (**Table 230-1**). In these instances, further diagnostic testing is rarely indicated. However, during some presentations of anaphylaxis or anaphylactoid reactions—such as perioperative anaphylaxis, unexplained syncope, or recurrent anaphylaxis—determination of serum total and beta tryptase can confirm a mast cell-mediated event because they remain elevated for 4 to 8 hours following symptoms.

TRIAGE/HOSPITAL ADMISSION

■ INDICATIONS FOR HOSPITALIZATION AND INTENSIVE CARE UNIT ADMISSION

Triage decisions in patients with allergic reactions rely upon both the severity of the reaction and the initial response to treatment. Patients presenting with mild-to-moderate symptoms (urticaria and/or angioedema with stable airway and hemodynamics) can generally be treated in the emergency department and discharged home. Patients with more severe reactions require hospitalization for further monitoring.

TABLE 230-1 Symptoms of Allergic Reactions and Anaphylaxis

- **Cutaneous**
  - Flushing
  - Pruritus
  - Urticaria
  - Angioedema
- **Respiratory**
  - Hoarseness
  - Dyspnea
  - Wheezing
  - Cough
  - Chest tightness
- **Gastrointestinal**
  - Nausea
  - Vomiting
  - Abdominal pain
  - Diarrhea
- **Cardiovascular**
  - Peripheral vasodilation
  - Reflex tachycardia
  - Hypotension

Patients with allergic reactions who present with severe wheezing, shortness of breath, hypotension, altered mentation, hoarseness of voice, or stridor should be treated as a medical emergency with early attention focused on securing the airway and cardiopulmonary status. Patients who respond to therapy should be observed in the hospital for 24 hours. Patients who respond slowly or poorly to primary treatment strategies require intensive care unit (ICU) admission, particularly those requiring endotracheal intubation for life-threatening laryngeal edema. Mechanical ventilation is often indicated for patients with respiratory failure secondary to bronchoconstriction refractory to initial therapy. Severe hypotension calling for vasopressors can occur as a direct result of cardiovascular collapse and also warrants ICU monitoring.

PRACTICE POINT

- Allergic reaction symptoms that should be treated as a medical emergency and prompt hospital admission include the following:
  - Severe wheezing
  - Shortness of breath
  - Hypotension
  - Altered mentation
  - Hoarseness of voice
  - Stridor

Reactions occurring in the hospital

While the mechanism of an allergic reaction occurring in the hospital is the same as the outpatient setting, there are specific triggers (such as medications or latex exposure) unique to the hospitalized patient. Additionally, allergic reactions that occur in the hospital have the potential to be severe, as parenteral administration of an allergen (as in allergen immunotherapy) or medications induces more frequent and severe responses than oral ingestion.

Medications, especially the beta-lactam antimicrobials (penicillin or penicillin analogues), cause the majority of anaphylactic reactions in hospitalized patients.. Cephalosporins share structure and up to 50% cross-reactivity with penicillins. The distinction between a reported history of allergy versus anaphylaxis to penicillins is important, as up to 90% of patients who endorse a history of a penicillin "allergy" (without anaphylaxis) do not exhibit IgE antibodies to penicillin. Cross-reactivity to cephalosporins in these patients is significantly lower (10%-15%).

PRACTICE POINT

- Patients with a history of true anaphylaxis to penicillin should not be challenged with cephalosporins. However, a reported history of penicillin allergy (without anaphylaxis) bears significantly less cross-reactivity to cephalosporins.

Anaphylactoid reactions are responsible for most severe drug reactions in hospitalized patients. Radiocontrast media and opiates may directly trigger mast cell degranulation. The clinical presentation is often identical to anaphylaxis and may require similar therapeutic measures, including antihistamines, bronchodilators, steroids, and/or epinephrine. Hypersensitivity to radiocontrast dye is usually unrelated to the rate of infusion and can have either an immediate or a delayed onset. The immediate-onset hypersensitivity to contrast occurs within minutes of very small amounts of infused media. In the delayed-onset presentation, symptoms occur beyond 1 hour of infusion to as late as 1-week postexposure. Patients treated with nonsteroidal anti-inflammatory drugs and aspirin may also be prone to severe anaphylactoid responses, particularly those with an underlying history of asthma, nasal polyps, or rhinosinusitis. Serum tryptase levels can be elevated in both IgE and non–immune-mediated hypersensitivity as mast cell activation occurs in both.

Chemotherapeutic agents such as carboplatinum, cisplatinum, as well as the monoclonal biologicals such as cetuximab, rituximab, and others, cause an anaphylaxis-like syndrome (IgE as well as non-IgE mediated). The mechanisms incriminated include tumor lysis, cytokine storm, and hypersensitivity reactions. Some of these

mechanisms may be prevented by premedication with steroids and/or antihistamines, and in recalcitrant cases desensitization has been a useful option.

■ ATOPY

Patients with a past medical history of atopic conditions such as asthma, seasonal allergies and eczema do not have an increased incidence of anaphylaxis to drugs. However, their reactions are more severe, and they are at greater risk for anaphylactic reactions to radiocontrast media, food or latex.

■ TRANSFUSION REACTIONS

Transfusion reactions to intravenous immunoglobulin can lead to allergic reactions in patients with IgA deficiency. These patients produce IgE and IgG autoantibodies against IgA and may experience a mast cell-mediated reaction ranging from urticaria or angioedema to anaphylaxis. Most transfusion reactions however, occur through the formation of immune complexes resulting in serum sickness.

MANAGEMENT
■ INITIAL HOSPITAL TREATMENT

Successful management of severe allergic and nonallergic reactions requires prompt recognition and treatment. Patients with immediate hypersensitivity (histamine-mediated) reactions are managed with epinephrine, antihistamines and corticosteroids, whereas these treatment modalities have limited effectiveness in bradykinin-mediated reactions (ACE-inhibitor angioedema and HAE). In the acute setting, the underlying mechanism may be difficult to distinguish, and patients experiencing symptoms of upper airway obstruction, acute respiratory failure or shock should be treated for an immediate hypersensitivity reaction with one or more of the medications listed below.

Epinephrine

Patients with marked upper airway obstruction, bronchospasm, or hypotension should be administered aqueous epinephrine *intravenously*: 0.1 mg (1:10,000) over 5 to 10 minutes or continuous infusion if necessary, 1 to 4 mcg/min. Patients with severe airway edema or stridor that is recalcitrant to initial therapy necessitate immediate intubation.

If intravenous access is not readily available or if the reaction is less severe, *intramuscular* (IM) (thigh) injection of epinephrine: 0.3 to 0.5 mg (1:1000) should be administered. Intramuscular thigh injections achieve much higher peak plasma epinephrine concentrations than epinephrine administered via intramuscular or subcutaneous injection into the upper arm. Racemic epinephrine via nebulizer can be administered as an adjunct or alone in cases of mild laryngeal swelling where IV/IM epinephrine is not indicated.

Antihistamines

An antihistamine H1 receptor antagonist, such as diphenhydramine 50 mg, can be administered parenterally and repeated every 4 to 6 hours. H_2 receptor antagonists (eg, ranitidine) should also be administered, and can provide additional benefit in inhibiting activation of histamine receptors in the splanchnic vascular bed.

Corticosteroids

Corticosteroids are often used in cases where antihistamines are unable to adequately control swelling. They may help to reduce inflammation and vascular permeability particularly in the late phase of the allergic response.

Beta2-adrenergic agonists

These agents, delivered via nebulizer relax bronchial smooth muscle and are commonly used in addition to oxygen in patients who present with wheezing secondary to bronchospasm. They have no effect on urticaria or angioedema.

Intravenous fluids and vasopressor therapy

Intravenous fluid resuscitation should begin immediately in hypotensive patients. Those with sustained hypotension following epinephrine and aggressive rehydration should be started on an epinephrine drip or other vasopressor agent such as phenylephrine. Patients taking beta-blockers who are refractory to vasopressor therapy should receive glucagon (1 mg in 1 L of D5W at 5-15 mL/min). Glucagon has positive inotropic and chronotropic effects mediated by cyclic adenosine monophosphate (AMP) (not beta receptors), which explains its usefulness as an adjunct therapy in hypotensive patients.

■ CONSULTATION

Most patients hospitalized for anaphylactic reactions should be seen by an ear, nose, and throat (ENT) specialist to assess the degree of airway edema. Outpatient referral to an allergist or pulmonologist is necessary to evaluate and assess the need for further workup. Skin testing has no utility in the hospital setting as mast cells will be refractory to an antigen challenge for several weeks. On rare occasions it may be necessary to initiate or continue therapy of a medication to which the patient has a history of severe allergy or anaphylaxis. In these instances an allergist or inpatient clinical pharmacist can oversee a desensitization protocol in which increasing increments of the drug are administered orally or intravenously. This procedure is not without risk and should be performed in an observed setting with emergency resuscitation equipment available.

PREVENTION

Patients with a history of anaphylactic and allergic reactions are at risk for recurrent episodes. Patient education, including avoiding allergens and self-medication is critical to long-term prevention.

Allergy to radiocontrast media complicates management of hospitalized patients requiring important diagnostic radiographic studies. Any patient who has had a life-threatening reaction to radiocontrast media should not be given the same agent. For patients with a history of allergy to radiocontrast dye, prophylactic management should be directed to the type and severity of hypersensitivity. The classic premedication regimen involves giving those with a history of *urticaria* 50 mg of prednisone orally at 13, 7, and 1 hour prior to the procedure, and 25 mg intravenous diphenhydramine 1 hour prior to the procedure. Patients who have a history of *life-threatening anaphylactoid reactions* (ie, angioedema, hypotension) should additionally be administered 25 mg of oral ephedrine and 300 mg of cimetidine orally 1 hour prior to the procedure. While premedication regimens may vary among institutions, the most important aspect is administering steroids at least 6 hours prior to the injection of contrast media. To further minimize the risk of reactions, many centers exclusively utilize nonionic low-osmolality radiocontrast media.

DISCHARGE PLANNING/FOLLOW-UP

Patient education prior to discharge should focus on the nature of the illness, severity of presentation, and precipitating factors. Patients should be able to recognize potential triggers and describe which substances may cross-react and cause allergic reactions. Patients should receive prescription instructions about self-administered autoinjectable epinephrine in the event of recurrent allergic reaction. In those patients with life-threatening anaphylaxis as well as those with food-related anaphylaxis, prescription of two doses of epinephrine has been recommended as part of the patient education process. Patients with severe reactions or reactions that affect regular activities or function should receive referral to an allergist for additional testing and/or desensitization. The primary care physician must be notified of all adverse reactions occurring during the inpatient setting, and all such reactions should be clearly documented in the medical record. Medical alert bracelets should be ordered and worn by patients who have experienced life-threatening anaphylaxis and anaphylactoid reactions.

QUALITY IMPROVEMENT

Allergic reactions, when severe, may require prolonged ICU admission incurring significant cost. Proper triage may expedite appropriate treatment, preventing clinical decompensation and prolonged hospital stays. Consultation, both inpatient (ENT) and outpatient (allergist or pulmonologist) can help optimize therapy, elucidate etiology, and assist with critical pieces of patient and family education. Anticipatory guidance and follow-up education promote patient adherence and recognition of possible allergens and cross-reacting agents. Moreover, using premedication protocols and thorough documentation reduce cost by minimizing preventable adverse outcomes.

SUGGESTED READINGS

Brockow K, Christiansen C, Kanny G, et al. Management of hypersensitivity reactions to iodinated contrast media. *Allergy*. 2005;60:150-182.

Laporte JR, deLatorre FJ, Gadgil DA, et al. An epidemiologic study of severe anaphylactic and anaphylactoid reactions among hospital patients: methods and overall risk. The International Collaborative Study of Severe Anaphylaxis. *Epidemiology*. 1998;9:141-146.

Lieberman P, Comargo CA Jr, Bohlke K, et al. Epidemiology of anaphylaxis: findings of the American College of Allergy, Asthma and Immunology Epidemiology of Anaphylaxis Working Group. *Ann Allergy Asthma Immunol*. 2006;97:596-602.

Morgan BP. Hereditary angioedema—therapies old and new. *N Engl J Med*. 2010;363:581-583.

Sabroe RA, Black AK. Angiotensin-converting enzyme (ACE) inhibitors and angio-oedema. *Br J Dermatol*. 1997;136(2):153-158.

Sampson HA, Munoz-Furlong A, Bock SA, et al. Symposium on the definition and management of anaphylaxis: summary report. *J Allergy Clin Immunol*. 2005;115:584-591.

CHAPTER 231

Asthma

Fernando Holguin, MD, MPH

Key Clinical Questions

① Which patients with asthma require hospital admission?

② What are the evidence-based guidelines for treatment of asthma in hospitalized patients?

③ What is the optimal dosing of systemic corticosteroids in the treatment of an acute asthma exacerbation?

④ Which asthma patients require admission to the intensive care unit?

⑤ When are the indications for intubation in asthma exacerbation?

⑥ What conditions need to be met before discharging a patient from the hospital?

INTRODUCTION

Asthma is a chronic respiratory disease associated with reversible airflow obstruction, bronchial hyperresponsiveness (BHR), and airway inflammation that can be triggered by various stimuli including viral upper respiratory infection, environmental allergens, and occupational exposures, and can lead to recurrent episodes of wheezing, cough, and dyspnea.

EPIDEMIOLOGY

In the United States in 2009, the prevalence of asthma was 8.2% affecting 24.6 million people (17.5 million adults and 7.1 million children). Thus, asthma stands as one of the leading chronic diseases in the United States.

The prevalence of current asthma is higher in children (9.6%) compared to adults (7.7%), and in females (9.3%) compared to males (7.0%). There is considerable variation in asthma prevalence estimates across racial and ethnic groups, with African Americans having higher prevalence than Caucasians and Hispanics. However, within Hispanics, there is marked variation among different ethnic groups; for example, Puerto Ricans have the highest asthma prevalence in the U.S. population in contrast to Mexican Americans, who have the lowest prevalence rates. The reasons why there are large differences in asthma prevalence rates across races and ethnicities are poorly understood and are likely explained by multiple factors including genetic susceptibility, health care access, environmental exposures, and nutritional factors.

PRESENTATION

History and physical examination of the asthmatic patient reveal recurrent respiratory symptoms characterized by wheezing, cough, and chest tightness. Trigger exposures may exacerbate respiratory symptoms and may include exposure to airway irritants (smoke, strong fumes, air pollution, etc), aeroallergens, respiratory infections, and cold air. Psychological stress and physical exercise are also known to trigger respiratory symptoms in the absence of any other concomitant exposures; however, in many instances trigger factors are not identified.

Respiratory symptoms may have a nocturnal predominance and are frequently more severe in the morning after waking up, when airflows are usually lower. The frequency and severity of respiratory symptoms is highly variable and may stem from sporadic to constant and from barely noticeable to life threatening.

PATHOPHYSIOLOGY

Although asthma is generally regarded as a single disease entity, it is likely a syndrome composed of a heterogeneous group of pathophysiologic mechanisms (different triggers, risk factors, patterns of inflammation, and response to treatment) that cause airway obstruction and common respiratory symptoms. *Persistent adult asthma* phenotypes have been broadly divided into the following categories: clinical or physiologic phenotypes (severity defined, exacerbation prone, treatment resistant, and adult versus child onset); phenotypes related to triggers (aspirin sensitivity, environmental and occupational exposures, menses, and exercise); and inflammatory phenotypes (eosinophilic, neutrophilic, and pauci-inflammatory). Many nonallergic phenotypes and phenotypes that begin in adulthood likely have very different pathophysiologies than allergic asthma. Although this classification scheme is useful to describe the pathophysiology of asthma, considerable overlap among categories exists.

In allergic asthma, an allergen is initially exposed to dendritic cells functioning as antigen-presenting cells. These cells interact with B lymphocytes to produce immunoglobulin E (IgE) in the context of appropriate cytokine and T lymphocyte interactions. Circulating IgE binds high-affinity receptors in blood and tissue mast cells and low-affinity receptors on the surface of lymphocytes, eosinophils, neutrophils, platelets, and macrophages, thus recruiting these cells to the airways. Subsequent exposures to the same antigen will crossbridge IgE bound to mast cell receptors, facilitating mast cell degranulation and release of various cytokines and chemokines, which recruit additional inflammatory cells to the lungs.

The initial release of histamine and leukotrienes from mast cells leads to constriction of airway smooth muscle and can lead to airway obstruction. The *early phase* of inflammation encompasses the response in the first hour and is followed by a *later phase* within 4 to 6 hours, in which prolonged airway obstruction develops due to cytokine release from resident epithelial cells and inflammatory cells, as well as recruited inflammatory cells. In addition to airway obstruction, this inflammatory response leads to airway edema, mucous hypersecretion, and bronchial hyper-responsivness (BHR). Over time and in relation to the degree of underlying inflammation and disease severity, BHR becomes nonspecific; that is, BHR can be elicited through a variety of nonallergen factors such as strong fumes, air pollution, cold air, exercise, and psychological stress.

DIFFERENTIAL DIAGNOSIS

Many diseases present with similar respiratory symptoms to asthma, and clinicians should maintain a high index of suspicion for alternate respiratory diagnoses (**Table 231-1**). Wheezing and cough can occur with congestive heart failure, which may be associated with airway vascular congestion and peribronchial cuffing secondary to pulmonary edema, bibasilar inspiratory crackles on auscultation, and an elevated serum brain natriuretic peptide (BNP). Airway obstruction (eg, foreign body, tumor, laryngeal edema, anaphylaxis, and laryngospasm) could lead to stridor, which can be mistaken for wheezing.

Paradoxical vocal fold motion disorder (PVFMD), a poorly understood disease that can mimic asthma, is characterized by abnormal adduction of the vocal cord folds during inhalation and occasionally during exhalation, which can lead to complete or partial transient laryngeal occlusion. During these paradoxical vocal cord motion events, patients experience significant respiratory distress characterized by cough, dyspnea, a choking sensation, and wheezing or stridor. The presence of throat tightness, dysphonia, absence of wheezing, and odors as a symptom trigger are key features of PVFMD, which can reliably distinguish it from asthma. Relief with short acting β-agonists or other medications used for asthma control is minimal to none. The severity and repetitive nature of symptoms caused by PVFMD lead to high health care utilization.

PVFMD is commonly encountered among patients referred for difficult or refractory asthma and chronic cough evaluation. However, *among patients referred to tertiary centers for refractory asthma or cough, the prevalence of PVFMD can be as high as 40% to 50%.* Many PVFMD patients inappropriately receive chronic systemic steroids. Patients with PVFMD commonly have frequent emergency department visits and may be intubated for respiratory distress.

Differentiating asthma and chronic obstructive lung disease (COPD) can be very difficult, and at times impossible. See Chapter 232: COPD. Asthmatics are expected to have a more reversible airway obstructive process than patients with COPD, whereas up to one-third or more of patients with COPD will have a reversible component to their obstruction. Both disorders may coexist in the same patient as a result of chronic smoking and/or airway remodeling. Emphysematous changes on chest computed tomography (CT) and/or severe airway obstruction with hyperinflation in the absence of an acute exacerbation would favor the diagnosis of COPD over asthma.

Bronchiectasis may also present with airway obstruction and symptoms compatible with asthma. However, clinical features that reduce the likelihood of asthma diagnosis include chronic sputum production at baseline, recurrent lower-tract respiratory infections, hemoptysis, and inspiratory crackles on auscultation. Chest CT should detect bronchiectasis.

Nonrespiratory symptoms may occur in conjunction with asthma syndromes, including rhinitis and eczematous rash within the "atopic triad," eosinophilia and/or vasculitis in Churg-Strauss; nasal polyps in aspirin-sensitive asthma (Samter syndrome); and pulmonary infiltrates and allergy to *Aspergillus* in allergic bronchopulmonary aspergillosis (ABPA). When bronchiectasis and asthma coexist, bronchiectasis occurs predominantly centrally with areas of mucoid impaction. Patients with ABPA usually have IgE levels greater than 1000 ng/mL with peripheral blood eosinophilia more than 10% specific *Aspergillous* IgG or IgE antibodies. A negative intradermal test for *Aspergillus* antigen adequately rules out this condition.

DIAGNOSIS

Asthma diagnosis must be confirmed by pulmonary function testing that shows evidence of airway obstruction with a bronchodilator response greater than or equal to 12% (or 200 mL) improvement of the forced expiratory volume in one second (FEV_1) after short-acting bronchodilators. Bronchodilation should only be assessed after withholding asthma medications at least 4 hours for short-acting $β_2$-receptor agonists (SABA) and 24 hours for long-acting $β_2$-receptor agonists (LABA).

In cases where there is no evidence of airway obstruction or bronchodilation on initial pulmonary function testing, patients should undergo testing with methacholine (a cholinergic agent used to elicit bronchial constriction) to exclude asthma. A positive test occurs when there is a reduction in FEV_1 greater than or equal to 20% (percent change 20 or PC20) from the baseline postmethacholine level. The methacholine test is very sensitive (ie, it would be unusual to have asthma with a negative test) but lacks specificity, such that a positive test can be seen in the setting of other airway diseases or allergies. Diligent assessment for presence or absence of asthma through testing and evaluation of treatment

TABLE 231-1 Asthma Exacerbation Differential Diagnosis

Mechanical airway obstruction (eg, foreign body)

Structural airway abnormality (eg, tumor)

Aspiration or severe gastroesophageal reflux disease

Paradoxical vocal fold motion disorder

Heart failure

Chronic obstructive pulmonary disease

Vasculitis

Bronchiectasis

Pulmonary embolism

Interstitial lung disease

Bronchial papillomatosis

Bronchopulmonary aspergillosis

Recurrent polychondritis with airway involvement

Hypersensitivity pneumonitis

Sarcoidosis with endobronchial involvement

TABLE 231-2 Triage Decision Making Based on Asthma Severity

Asthma Exacerbation Severity	Representative Symptoms	Spirometric Measurement (PEF or FEV$_1$)	Triage/Admission
Mild	Dyspnea with activity	> 70% predicted (or personal best)	Home
Moderate	Dyspnea limits typical daily activity	40%-69% predicted (or personal best)	Often requires ED visit +/− hospital admission (if no rapid ED improvement)
Severe	Dyspnea at rest that interferes with conversation	< 40% predicted (or personal best)	Hospital or ICU admission
Life-threatening	Dyspnea significantly limiting speech	< 25% predicted (or personal best)	Hospital or ICU admission

ED, emergency department; FEV$_1$, forced expiratory volume in 1 second; ICU, intensive care unit; PEF, peak expiratory flow.

response will help eliminate the approximately 30% of patients who are incorrectly diagnosed with this disease clinically (false positive) and are unnecessarily treated with corticosteroids.

TRIAGE AND HOSPITAL ADMISSION

When patients with severe asthma exacerbations do not adequately respond to outpatient therapy, clinical assessment should include a brief history, physical examination (assess respiratory rate and heart rate, use of accessory respiratory muscles, chest retraction, neck and pulmonary auscultation, oxygen saturation), and pulmonary function testing (FEV$_1$ or peak expiratory flow [PEF] measurement) to help triage for possible hospital admission.

Several published guidelines aid clinicians in admission decision making. A triage system based on the history of symptoms and spirometric measurement (PEF or FEV$_1$) can aid triage decision making (**Table 231-2**).

Patients admitted with high risk of asthma-related death (**Table 231-3**) should receive very close inpatient monitoring, possibly in the intensive care unit (ICU), based on response to initial therapy.

If necessary, repeated assessment of severity, including signs and symptoms as well as PEF or FEV$_1$ measurements, help determine the need for hospital admission (**Figure 231-1**).

MANAGEMENT

■ INITIAL TREATMENT FOR ACUTE ASTHMA EXACERBATION

Immediate treatment of significant asthma exacerbation can start with emergency medical services (EMS) and include supplemental

TABLE 231-3 Risk Factors for Asthma-Related Death

- Previous severe exacerbation (intubation or intensive care unit admission for asthma)
- ≥ 2 hospitalizations or > 3 emergency department visits in the past 12 mo
- Use of > 2 canisters of short-acting β-agonist (SABA) per month
- Reduced ability to perceive airway obstruction or worsening symptoms
- Low socioeconomic status or urban residence
- Illicit drug use
- Psychiatric disease or severe psychosocial stress
- Comorbidities, such as cardiovascular disease or other chronic lung disease

oxygen, inhaled SABA, anticholinergic agents, and oral systemic corticosteroids using established protocols under appropriate medical supervision. Continued upon arrival in the emergency department, supplemental oxygen can correct hypoxemia in moderate and severe asthma exacerbations. Repetitive or continuous administration of SABA and ipratropium via metered-dose inhaler (MDI) or nebulizer can quickly reverse airflow obstruction, and continuous administration is more efficacious. Oral systemic corticosteroids decrease inflammation and are used to supplement treatment in asthmatics who fail to respond adequately or at all to SABA treatment. **Table 231-4** lists medications and dosages for adults with acute asthma exacerbation.

■ CONTINUED THERAPY AFTER ASSESSMENT OF ASTHMA SYMPTOMS AND SEVERITY

Management and treatment should be based on the level of asthma severity (see Figure 231-1). *Severe exacerbation is marked by an FEV$_1$ or PEF less than 40%,* and these patients should receive supplemental oxygen to achieve a saturation level of oxygen in hemoglobin (SaO$_2$) greater than or equal to 90%, administration of continuous SABA and ipratropium by nebulizer or metered-dose inhaler (MDI), and oral systemic corticosteroids. Patient drowsiness or increased blood partial pressure of carbon dioxide (pCO$_2$) levels may signal impending respiratory failure and the need for immediate intubation and mechanical ventilation. Following intubation, the patient should continue to receive nebulized SABA and intravenous corticosteroids.

Moderate exacerbation is be marked by an FEV$_1$ or PEF greater than or equal to 40% and less than 69%, and these patients should receive supplemental oxygen, inhaled SABA (up to three doses in the first hour, and then hourly), and possibly oral systemic corticosteroids if (1) there is no immediate response to therapy or (2) the patient has recently taken systemic corticosteroids.

Repeat assessment of severity and response to therapy, including assessment of symptom severity, physical examination, PEF, and oxygen saturation, should guide continued treatment. Severe exacerbation of asthma generally does not improve after initial treatment. Treatment of mild to moderate exacerbation may continue for 1 to 3 hours, and the decision of whether the patient requires admission may be made at approximately 4 hours following presentation.

A poor response to initial therapy requires admission to the ICU and is demonstrated by an FEV$_1$ or PEF less than 40%, a PCO$_2$ greater than or equal to 42 millimeters mercury (mm Hg), and use of accessory muscles, chest retraction, severe drowsiness or confusion on physical exam. *An incomplete response to initial therapy* comprises an FEV$_1$ or FEF between 40% and 69% of predicted, and requires case-specific decision making regarding hospital

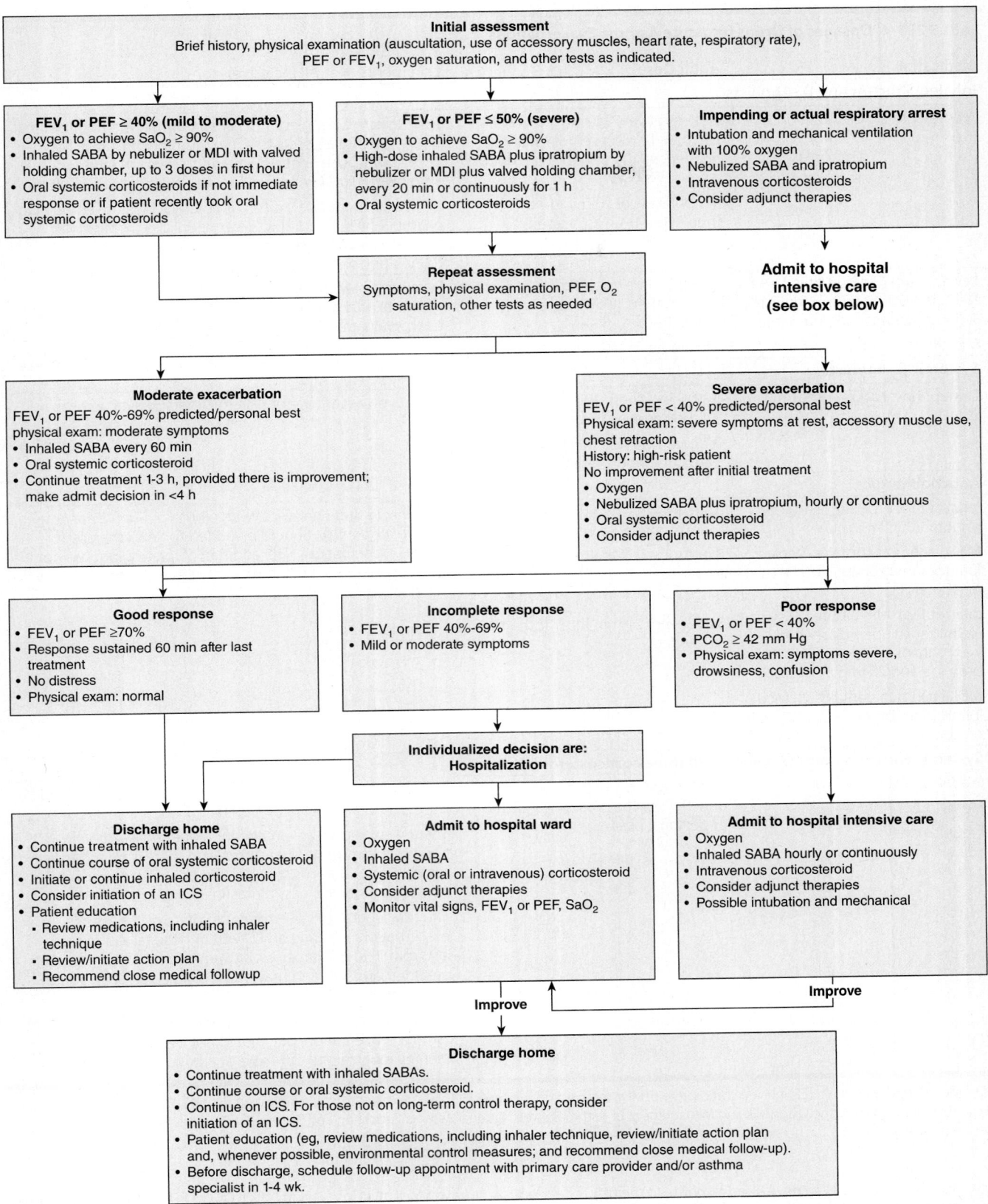

Figure 231-1 *Management of asthma exacerbations: emergency department and hospital-based care. FEV₁, forced expiratory volume in 1 second; ICS, inhaled corticosteroid; MDI, metered-dose inhaler; PCO₂, partial pressure carbon dioxide; PEF, peak expiratory flow; SABA, short-acting β₂-agonist; SaO₂, oxygen saturation.* (From the Guidelines for the Diagnosis and Management of Asthma of the National Asthma Education and Prevention Program [NAEPP] Expert Panel Report 3, 2007.)

TABLE 231-4 Dosages of Drugs for Acute Asthma Exacerbations

Medication	Adult Dose	Comments (Not All Inclusive)
Inhaled Short-Acting β₂-Agonists		
Albuterol Nebulizer Solution (0.63 mg/3 mL, 1.25 mg/3 mL, 2.5 mg/3 mL, 5.0 mg/mL) MDI (90 mcg/puff, 200 puffs per canister)	2.5-5 mg every 20 min for 3 doses, then 2.5-10 mg every 1-4 h as needed, or 10-15 mg/h continuously	Only selective beta₂-agonists are recommended. For optimal delivery, dilute aerosols to a minimum of 3 mL at as flow of 6-8 L/min. Use large volume nebulizers for continuous administration. May mix with ipratropium nebulizer solution.
	4-8 puffs every 20 min up to 4 h, then every 1-4 h as needed	In mild-to-moderate exacerbations, MDI plus valved holding chamber (VHC) is as effective as nebulized therapy with appropriate administration technique and coaching by trained personnel.
Levalbuterol (R-albuterol) Nebulizer solution (0.63 mg/3 mL, 1.25 mg/0.5 mL, 1.25 mg/3 mL) MDI (45 mcg/puff)	1.25-2.5 mg every 20 min for 3 doses, then 1.25-5 mg every 1-4 h as needed See albuterol MDI dose	Levalbuterol administered in one-half the mg dose of albuterol provides comparable efficacy and safety. Has not been evaluated by continuous nebulization.
Systemic β₂-agonists		
Epinephrine 1:1000 (1 mg/mL)	0.3-0.5 mg every 20 min for 3 subcutaneous doses	No proven advantage of systemic therapy over aerosol.
Terbutaline (1 mg/mL)	0.25 mg every 20 min for 3 subcutaneous doses	
Anticholinergics		
Ipratropium bromide Nebulizer solution (0.25 mg/mL)	0.5 mg every 20 min for 3 doses, then as needed	May mix in same nebulizer with albuterol. *Should not be used as first-line therapy.* Should be added to SABA therapy for severe exacerbations. The addition of ipratropium has not been shown to provide further benefit once the patient is hospitalized.
MDI (Each puff contains 18 mcg ipratropium bromide and 90 mcg of albuterol.)	8 puffs every 20 min as needed up to 3 h	
Ipratropium with albuterol Nebulizer solution (Each 3 mL vial contains 0.5 mg ipratropium bromide and 2.5 mg albuterol.)	3 mL every 20 min for 3 doses, then as needed	
MDI (Each puff contains 18 mcg ipratropium bromide and 90 mcg of albuterol.)	8 puffs every 20 min as needed up to 3 h	
Systemic corticosteroids (Applies to all three corticosteroids)		
Prednisone Methylprednisolone Prednisolone	40-80 mg/d in 1 or 2 divided doses until PEF reaches 70% of predicted or personal best	For outpatient "burst," use 40-60 mg in single or 2 divided doses for total of 5-10 d in adults.
		There is no known advantage for higher doses of corticosteroids in severe asthma, and there is no advantage for intravenous administration over oral therapy with a normal functioning gastrointestinal tract.
		The total course of systemic corticosteroids for asthma exacerbation requiring an ED visit or hospitalization may last from 3-10 d. A taper is only required for a course lasting greater than 1 wk, and may only be necessary for a course greater than 10 d.
		ICS can be started at any point during treatment of an acute asthma exacerbation, but should not be used alone as therapy for an acute asthma exacerbation.

ED, emergency department; ICS, inhaled corticosteroid; MDI, metered-dose inhaler; PEF, peak expiratory flow; SABA, short-acting β-agonist.
(From the Guidelines for the Diagnosis and Management of Asthma of the National Asthma Education and Prevention Program [NAEPP] Expert Panel Report 3, 2007.)

admission or discharge home. *A good response to therapy* is defined by an FEV₁ or PEF greater than or equal to 70% and a response that is sustained for at least an hour after the last treatment, a normal physical exam, and no signs of distress; such patients may be discharged home.

■ IN-HOSPITAL ASTHMA MANAGEMENT

In-hospital asthma treatment should consist of bronchodilator (BD) therapy and daily systemic steroids. Steroid therapy (oral or intravenous) at a dose ranging from 40 to 80 mg/d of prednisone or equivalent steroid dosing is optimal (divided into two daily doses). No data support benefit from higher steroid doses. The frequency of SABAs should be guided by the level of severity and the clinical response of the patient. BD therapy, more frequent or continuous at the beginning of hospital stay, may range from continuous therapy to every 4 to 6 hours during hospitalization. Inhaled steroids should be initiated during hospital stay prior to discharge, but are not used to manage acute asthma exacerbations.

TABLE 231-5 Indications for Outpatient Specialty (Allergy or Immunology Specialist or Pulmonary Specialist) Referral, One Major Criterion or Two Minor Criteria

Asthma severity major criteria:

- Use of high-dose inhaled steroids for more than 50% of the preceding year
- Continuous or near-continuous oral steroids

Asthma severity minor criteria:

- Daily controller medication in addition to inhaled steroids
- β-agonist required daily or near-daily
- Persistent airway obstruction
- One or more urgent care visits for asthma per year
- Three or more oral corticosteroid bursts per year
- Clinical deterioration with reduction in oral steroid dose
- Near-fatal asthma event in the past

Several treatments have limited or no utility in the treatment of acute asthma exacerbation based on available evidence. Routine antibiotic administration does not have a role in acute asthma exacerbation. Intravenous magnesium and helium-oxygen therapy (Heliox™) have limited evidence to support their use in asthma exacerbations, but may be considered as additional adjunctive therapies in patients not responding to other recommended therapies. No evidence supports continued use of anticholinergics during the hospital stay.

Frequent assessment of pulmonary function (PEF or FEV_1), in addition to symptoms and physical exam findings, is indicated to help determine continued need for inpatient stay and therapy. PEF or FEV_1 should be assessed at least daily in patients admitted (but not intubated) with asthma exacerbation. Assessments should also be made whenever there is perceived clinical deterioration during the inpatient stay, despite aggressive medical therapies.

■ CONSULTATION

Inpatient consultation

Hospitalists should consider inpatient specialty consultation with allergy, pulmonary, or critical care physicians, when patients with severe or life-threatening asthma exacerbations fail to respond to initial therapies within 24 to 48 hours or require intubation. They may also consider specialty consultation when patients with asthma require frequent hospital admissions or emergency department visits despite medical regimen augmentation and adherence.

Outpatient consultation and referral

Patients classified as having severe asthma should be referred to an allergy and immunology specialist or pulmonology specialist for evaluation. Chronic asthma criteria that indicate specialty referral based on severity include at least one major criterion or at least two minor criteria (**Table 231-5**).

COMPLICATIONS AND PROGNOSIS

For each age group through age 25 to 34 years, the death rate from asthma is less than 1 per 10,000 persons with asthma. The highest at-risk-based death rate is in persons aged greater than 65 years (10.5 per 10,000 with current asthma). Females have higher at-risk-based death rates than males (2.3 per 10,000 and 1.8 per 10,000, respectively). For most age groups, males have higher rates than females; only for persons aged greater than 65 years was the rate

for females (11.3 per 10,000 with current asthma) higher than for males (9.1). Blacks have higher at-risk-based death rates (3.4) than whites (1.9). This is true for males and females, adults and children, and for each age group. Among regions, the highest asthma death rate per 10,000 with current asthma occurred in the Western United States (2.5).

DISCHARGE PLANNING

■ DISCHARGE READINESS CRITERIA

Consensus guidelines have been published regarding objective criteria that need to be met for the appropriate discharge of an asthmatic patient. However, these guidelines represent expert opinion and have not yet been supported by clinical trials. In general, a patient may be discharged after achieving an FEV_1 greater than or equal to 70% predicted in conjunction with signs of clinical improvement, or on the basis of marked clinical improvement alone.

■ THE ASTHMA ACTION PLAN

Following acute asthma exacerbation, patients should continue inhaled SABA, complete a course of oral systemic corticosteroids, and continue or possibly initiate inhaled corticosteroids. Patient education during hospital stay and at discharge should include a focus on asthma precipitants, avoidance of environmental exposures, including tobacco smoke, which may trigger exacerbation; the prescribed medication regimen, how to control and prevent symptoms by adjusting medication dosages (if necessary), and how to properly use medications, especially assuring the use of inhalational spacer devices for metered dose inhalers.

Patients should receive counseling prior to discharge regarding their home management. A discharge *home management plan* should be prescribed and given to the patient in a written format so that she might be able to recognize and respond to signs of asthma exacerbation, including decreased PEF. The action plan should outline medication adjustments that can be done at home by the patient to respond to exacerbation, including increased used of SABA, and if needed, oral corticosteroids. Patients should be instructed to avoid or reduce contact with allergens or environmental irritants, including tobacco smoke (both primary and second hand). The patient should monitor his/her response to treatment and communicate with a physician about signs of deterioration, such as decreased responsiveness to SABA.

To prevent relapse or additional exacerbations, in conjunction with a written asthma action plan, follow-up care should occur within 1 to 4 weeks of hospital discharge. More rapid follow-up should occur in patients with more severe exacerbations or those with more medical comorbidities. At follow-up, the patient and health care provider should review the asthma action plan, discuss medication adherence and environmental control, and address barriers to medication use and environmental control if necessary. The provider may consider step-up or step-down care based on the level of asthma control at that time and decide upon further asthma education in the form of classes or workshops, if indicated.

■ LONGITUDINAL AND OUTPATIENT THERAPEUTICS OR REGIMEN AUGMENTATION

Recent asthma guidelines recommend a focus on monitoring response to treatment instead of asthma severity. Two parameters help define asthma control: *impairment* and *risk*. The current (or recent) frequency and intensity of symptoms and functional limitations define *impairment* in asthma patients. *Risk* represents the likelihood of asthma exacerbations and progressive decline in lung function.

The outpatient pharmacologic treatment of asthma aims to reduce impairment (prevent chronic symptoms, maintain lung function, meet the family and patient's expectations) and risk (prevent exacerbations, prevent loss of lung function, and provide optimal therapeutics with minimal side effects).

Outpatient pharmacologic agents are prescribed based on the degree of asthma severity: intermittent, mild, moderate, or severe. The degree of asthma severity is ascertained by determining the level of impairment and risk. *Impairment* includes multiple measures such as frequency of daytime and nocturnal respiratory symptoms, use of SABAs, and lung function (FEV_1 and FEV_1/forced vital capacity [FVC]). *Risk* involves determining the number of exacerbations requiring oral or systemic steroids per year. Classification of asthma severity for persons age 12 years or older is described by a group of asthma experts working on behalf of the National Institutes of Health (NIH) and the National Heart and Lung Blood Institute (NHLBI) called the National Asthma Education and Prevention Program Expert Panel Report # 3 (EPR3) (**Figure 231-2**).

Based on asthma classification, from intermittent to persistent (mild, moderate, severe) patients may require various forms of inhaled and oral therapies (**Figure 231-3**). Stepwise management of chronic intermittent or persistent asthma includes the following

Components of Severity		Classification of Asthma Severity ≥ 12 y of age			
		Intermittent	Persistent		
			Mild	Moderate	Severe
Impairment Normal FEV_1/FVC: 08-19 y 85% 20-39 y 80% 40-59 y 75% 60-80 y 70%	Symptoms	≤ 2 d/wk	> 2 d/wk but not daily	Daily	Throughout the day
	Nighttime awakenings	≤ 2 times/mo	3-4 times/mo	> 1 time/wk, but not nightly	Often 7 times/wk
	Short-acting β_2-agonist use for symptom control (not prevention of EIB)	≤ 2 d/wk	> 2 d/wk but not daily, and not more than on any day	Daily	Several times per day
	Interference with normal activity	None	Minor limitation	Some limitation	Extremely limited
	Lung function	• Normal FEV_1 between exacerbations • FEV_1 > 80% predicted • FEV_1/FVC normal	• FEV_1 > 80% predicted • FEV_1/FVC normal	• FEV_1 > 60% but < 80% predicted • FEV_1/FVC reduced 5%	• FEV_1 < 60% predicted • FEV_1/FVC reduced > 5%
Risk	Exacerbations requiring oral systemic corticosteroids	0-1/y (see notes)	≥ 2/y (see notes)		
		Consider severity and interval since last exacerbation. Frequency and severity may fluctuate over time for patients in any severity category. Relative annual risk of exacerbations may be related to FEV_1.			
Recommended Step for Initiating Treatment **(See "Stepwise Approach for Managing Asthma" for treatment steps.)**		Step 1	Step 2	Step 3	Step 4 or 5
				And consider short course of oral systemic corticosteroids.	
		In 2-6 weeks, evaluate level of asthma control that is achieved and adjust therapy accordingly.			

Figure 231-2 *Classifying asthma severity and initiating treatment in youths ≥ 12 years of age and adults: assessing severity and initiating treatment for patients who are not currently taking long-term control medications.*

Notes:

- *The stepwise approach is meant to assist, not replace, the clinical decision-making required to meet individual patient needs.*
- *Level of severity is determined by assessment of both impairment and risk. Assess impairment domain by patient's/caregiver's recall of previous 2 to 4 weeks and spirometry. Assign severity to the most severe category in which any feature occurs.*
- *At present, there are inadequate data to correspond frequencies of exacerbations with different levels of asthma severity. In general, more frequent and intense exacerbations (eg, requiring urgent, unscheduled care, hospitalization, or ICU admission) indicate greater underlying disease severity. For treatment purposes, patients who had two or more exacerbations requiring oral systemic corticosteroids in the past year may be considered the same as patients who have persistent asthma, even in the absence of impairment levels consistent with persistent asthma.*

EIB, exercise-induced bronchospasm; FEV_1, forced expiratory volume in 1 second; FVC, forced vital capacity; ICU, intensive care unit. (From the Guidelines for the Diagnosis and Management of Asthma of the National Asthma Education and Prevention Program [NAEPP] Expert Panel Report 3, 2007.)

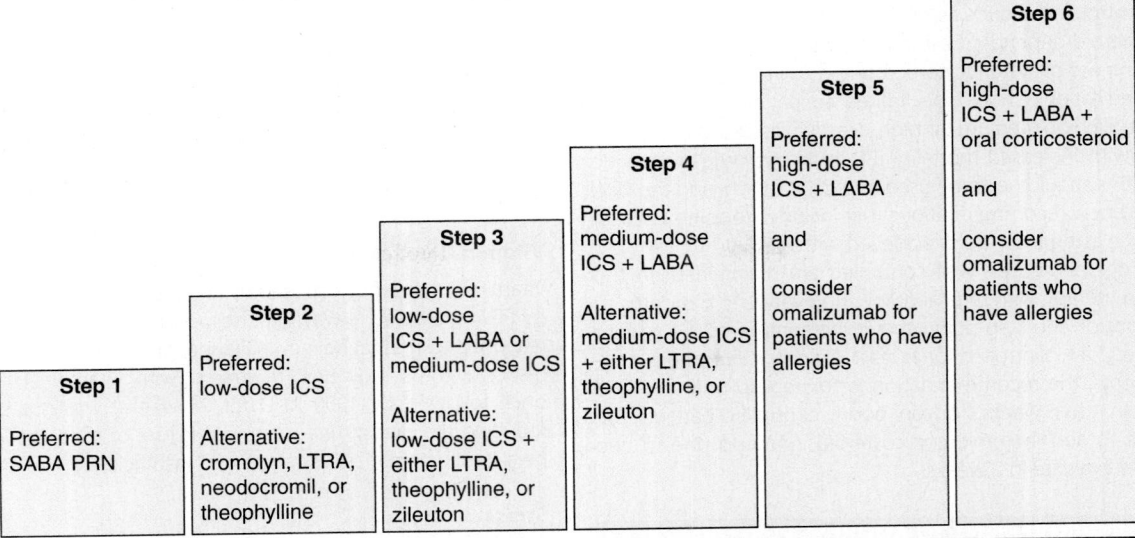

Figure 231-3 *Stepwise approach for managing asthma in adults and youths 12 years of age or older.*

Alphabetical order is used when more than one treatment option is listed within either preferred or alternative therapy.
Notes:

- *The stepwise approach is meant to assist, not replace, the clinical decision-making required to meet individual patient needs.*
- *If alternative treatment is used and response is inadequate, discontinue it, and use the preferred treatment before stepping up.*
- *Zileuton is a less desirable alternative due to limited studies as adjunctive therapy and the need to monitor liver function. Theophylline requires monitoring of serum concentration levels.*
- *In step 6, before oral corticosteroids are introduced, a trial of high-dose ICS + LABA + either LTRA, theophylline, or zileuton may be considered, although this approach has not been studied in clinical trials.*
- *Steps 1, 2, and 3 preferred therapies are based on Evidence A; step 3 alternative therapy is based on Evidence A for LTRA, Evidence B for theophylline, and Evidence D for zileuton. Step 4 preferred therapy is based on Evidence B, and alternative therapy is based on Evidence B for LTRA and theophylline and Evidence D for zileuton. Step 5 preferred therapy is based on Evidence B. Step 6 preferred therapy is based on (EPR-2 1997) and Evidence B for omalizumab.*
- *Immunotherapy for steps 2 to 4 is based on Evidence B for house-dust mites, animal danders, and pollens; evidence is weak or lacking for molds and cockroaches. Evidence is strongest for immunotherapy with single allergens. The role of allergy in asthma is greater in children than in adults.*
- *Clinicians who administer immunotherapy or omalizumab should be prepared and equipped to identify and treat anaphylaxis that may occur.*

ICS, inhaled corticosteroid; LABA, long-acting inhaled β₂-agonist; LTRA, leukotriene receptor antagonist; SABA, inhaled short-acting β₂-agonist. (From the Guidelines for the Diagnosis and Management of Asthma of the National Asthma Education and Prevention Program [NAEPP] Expert Panel Report 3, 2007.)

stages: intermittent asthma, step 1; mild asthma, step 2; moderate asthma, step 3; and severe asthma, step 4, 5, or 6. The medications indicated for each step include the following: step 1, SABA taken as needed; step 2, low-dose inhaled steroids (ICS); step 3, low-dose ICS + LABA; step 4, medium-dose ICS + LABA; step 5, high-dose ICS + LABA and consider omalizumab (humanized antibody that interferes with binding of IgE to the high-affinity IgE receptor FcεRI) for patients who have allergies and meet IgE-level criteria; step 6, high-dose ICS + LABA + oral corticosteroids and omalizumab if patient meets criteria. For steps 3, 4, 5, and 6, a short course of oral systemic corticosteroids should be considered. Newer biological therapies that block the action of Th-2 inflammatory cytokines, are becoming available to manage patients with severe asthma that fail to respond to standard treatment and have elevated peripheral eosinophils counts (≥300). Among these asthmatics, anti-IL-5, anti-IL-13, and anti-IL-4α monoclonal antibodies have all shown to improve control and reduce asthma exacerbations. Further, in 40% of severe, steroid dependent asthmatics, anti-IL-5 has been shown to reduce the use of systemic corticosteroids by more than 75%.

LABA medications should be limited to patients who remain poorly controlled on medium- to high-dose ICS, as LABAs have been associated with increased mortality risk in recent large systematic reviews. LABAs should never be used as monotherapy, and the FDA has released new recommendations that include stopping LABA in patients once asthma control is achieved with ICS.

Patients deemed to be well controlled are maintained on the current step therapy with regular follow-up every 1 to 6 months to maintain control, and step-down should be considered if a patient has remained well controlled for at least 3 months. For poorly controlled patients, the recommendation is to step-up one step and re-evaluate in 4 to 6 weeks. For very poorly controlled patients, the approach is to add systemic corticosteroids, step-up one to two steps, and re-evaluate in 2 weeks.

QUALITY IMPROVEMENT TO ADDRESS PERFORMANCE GAPS

■ SECONDARY PREVENTION

Strategies for secondary prevention of asthma exacerbation should be utilized in conjunction with frequent follow-up with a managing physician and education about asthma triggers and how and when to take medications to keep asthma symptoms well controlled and prevent asthma attacks.

All asthmatics should receive the influenza vaccine annually. Adults with asthma between the ages of 19 and 64 should get a single dose of Prevnar 13 pneumococcal vaccine; all asthmatics adults over age 65 should receive the Prevnar vaccine as well as a second dose 5 years after the first dose. Vaccinations during hospitalization for an acute asthma exacerbation are appropriate for patients who have not yet received their appropriate vaccinations. Environmental and occupational allergens and irritants should be controlled; tobacco smoking and exposure to secondary smoke should be avoided. Allergic immunotherapy and/or the administration of anti-immunoglobulin E (IgE) may be utilized in the treatment of allergic asthma. Leukotriene modifiers are useful in some patients, especially those with aspirin-sensitive asthma.

Control of comorbid disease may contribute to improved asthma and symptom control, including the following conditions.

Gastroesophageal reflux disease

Gastroesophageal reflux disease (GERD), although once thought to negatively impact asthma control, does not appear to directly influence asthma symptoms and severity. However, GERD is a known risk factor for vocal cord dysfunction (VCD), which mimics many of the respiratory symptoms associated with asthma. H2 receptor antagonists and proton-pump inhibitors may be used to help control GERD symptoms.

Rhinitis

Because patients with atopy have analogous upper and lower airway symptoms in response to similar allergen exposures, asthma and rhinitis can be closely intertwined. Also, in many patients, controlling the upper respiratory symptoms will lead to better asthma control,

explained by improvements in allergic inflammation throughout the airway and/or reduced postnasal discharge, which can also lead to VCD and asthma-like symptoms. Oral loratidine and/or nasal steroids may be utilized for treatment of rhinitis.

Obesity

Obesity, reflected by body mass index (BMI) greater than 30 kilograms per meter of height squared, serves as an important risk factor in asthma severity and in adult-onset asthma. The mechanisms by which obesity affects asthma are unknown, but appear unrelated to airway or systemic inflammation.

Vitamin D deficiency

Vitamin D deficiency can lead to impaired lung function measured by FEV_1, increased airway hyperresponsiveness (AHR) measured by response to methacholine challenge, and reduced glucocorticoid responsiveness. However, treatment with Vitamin D (100,000 IU once followed by 4000 IU/D for 28 weeks) was not effective in reducing the rate of first treatment failure or exacerbation among persistent asthmatics with Vitamin D insufficiency.

Stress

Increased psychosocial stressors may contribute to asthma onset through glucocorticoid insensitivity and cytokine dysregulation that lead to heightened airway inflammation. Therefore, minimizing stress may lead to improved asthma control.

■ TRANSITIONS OF CARE

Patients should follow-up with a primary provider or specialist (eg, allergy and immunology specialist or pulmonologist) within 2 weeks of hospital discharge, or sooner if indicated based on severity level at the time of hospital discharge compared with admission and time required for improvement while in the hospital.

■ DISPARITIES IN HEALTH CARE

African Americans may exhibit fewer symptoms than other racial groups, sensing air-flow obstruction to a lesser extent. Therefore, they require vigilant additional evaluation to avoid sudden death from asthma. Also, patients of Puerto Rican descent have the highest asthma prevalence and severity in the United States; in contrast, Mexican Americans have the lowest prevalence and severity. The reasons for racial and ethnic differences in asthma among persons in the United States are not well understood at this time.

■ COSTS AND RESOURCE UTILIZATION

Annually, an average of 11.6 million persons reported at least one asthma attack during the preceding 12 months. Among persons with current asthma, 56% had at least one asthma attack in the preceding 12 months; additionally, females with current asthma had a higher attack rate than males, and children were more likely to have had an attack than adults. From 2001 to 2003, there were a total of 2.5 hospitalizations for every 100 persons with current asthma. During this time period, the rates of hospitalization for asthma were higher in children and African Americans. Additionally, there were an estimated 8.8 emergency room visits for asthma per 100 subjects with current asthma. The emergency room visit rates were higher for African Americans and Hispanics when compared with Caucasians (**Table 231-6**).

TABLE 231-6 Evidence-based Medicine Key References

Study	Methodology	Results	Limitations	Bottom Line
β-agonists				
Newman KB, et al. A comparison of albuterol administered by MDI and spacer with albuterol by nebulizer in adults presenting to an urban emergency department with acute asthma. *Chest.* 2002;121(4):1036-1041.	Prospective, open-label study.	There was a statistically greater improvement in peak flow rates in the MDI/spacer group (126.8 vs 111.9 L/min, respectively; $p = 0.002$).	Nonrandomized, nonconcurrent study design.	SABA is at least as effective when delivered via MDI compared with nebulizer.
Cates CJ, et al. Regular treatment with salmeterol for chronic asthma: serious adverse events. Cochrane Database of Systematic Reviews 2008, updated 2010.	Meta-analysis; included controlled parallel design clinical trials, +/– blinding.	In patients taking regular salmeterol who were not taking inhaled corticosteroids, there was a significant increase in risk of asthma-related death, odds ratio (OR) 9.52 (95% confidence interval [CI]) 1.24 to 73.09).	Rare mortality and occurrence of serious adverse events warrants further study.	In patients not taking corticosteroids, there is an increased risk of asthma-related death for patients taking salmeterol.
Corticosteroids				
Rowe BH, et al. Effectiveness of steroid therapy in acute exacerbations of asthma: A meta-analysis. *Amer J Emerg Med.* 1992;10(4):301-310.	Meta-analysis; included randomized, controlled trials or quasi-experimental trials (alternate day or sequential medication administration).	Oral and intravenous steroids appear to have equivalent effects on pulmonary function after administration during acute asthma exacerbations (effect size [ES] –0.07; CI: –0.39, 0.25).	Many studies that were included were small.	Oral and parenteral systemic steroids are equally effective in acute asthma exacerbation.
Manser R, et al. Corticosteroids for acute severe asthma in hospitalized patients. Cochrane Database of Systematic Reviews 2001, updated 2008.	Meta-analysis; included randomized, controlled trials.	There were no statistically significant differences detected in % predicted FEV_1 among groups that received low-dose (≤ 80 mg methylprednisolone or equivalent), medium dose (> 80 mg and ≤ 360 mg) and high dose (> 360 mg) systemic corticosteroids (any route) after 24, 48 or 72 h.	A small number of studies were included.	Low-, medium-, and high-dose systemic corticosteroids may offer equivalent therapeutic benefit in acute asthma.
Rowe BH, et al. Inhaled budesonide in addition to oral corticosteroids to prevent asthma relapse following discharge from the emergency department: a randomized controlled trial. *JAMA.* 1999;281:2119-2126.	Double-blind, randomized, controlled trial.	After 21 d, 12.8% of 94 patients in the budesonide group experienced a relapse (defined by symptoms and an unscheduled office visit) compared with 24.5% of the placebo group. There were pulmonary function differences between the groups at 21 d.	Use of relapse as a primary outcome may not be a consistently documented outcome.	Use of ICS in addition to systemic corticosteroids after discharge reduces the risk of relapse in patients with acute asthma exacerbation.
Adjunct Treatment				
Rodrigo GJ, et al. Heliox for nonintubated acute asthma patients. Cochrane Database of Systematic Reviews 2006, updated 2010.	Meta-analysis; randomized, single or double blinded, controlled trials were included.	No significant group differences were found.	Small studies and between-group comparisons were used for analysis.	The use of Heliox treatment does not significantly improve pulmonary function during acute asthma exacerbation.
Bradshaw TA, et al. Intravenous magnesium sulphate provides no additive benefit to standard management in acute asthma. *Respir Med.* 2008;102(1):143-149.	Double-blind, randomized, controlled trial.	Intravenous magnesium sulphate did not decrease hospital admission rates or increase % predicted peak expiratory flow (PEF) at 60 min for all patients, or for subgroups of patients with acute asthma.	Higher percentage of patients receiving inhaled corticosteroids prior to magnesium dose compared with similar studies, and number of patients in the "life-threatening" subgroup is small.	No additional benefit is provided from intravenous magnesium sulfate when given as an adjunct to standard therapy for acute asthma.

(Continued)

TABLE 231-6 Evidence-based Medicine Key References (*Continued*)

Study	Methodology	Results	Limitations	Bottom Line
Adjunct treatment				
Camargo CA, et al. A randomized placebo-controlled study of intravenous montelukast for the treatment of acute asthma. *JACI.* 2010;125(2):374-380.	Randomized, double-blind, controlled trial.	Montelukast significantly increased FEV$_1$ after 60 min; the difference between change from baseline was 0.10 liters (95% CI: 0.04, 0.16). Improvements in FEV$_1$ were seen at all time points between 10 and 120 min after administration ($p < 0.05$).	Only acute improvement measured, and secondary endpoints related to disposition are harder to accurately assess across hospital sites.	Intravenous montelukast added to standard care in adults with acute asthma produced significant relief of acute airway obstruction.

CI, confidence interval; ES, effect size; FEV$_1$, forced expiratory volume in 1 second; ICS, inhaled corticosteroid; MDI, metered-dose inhaler; OR, odds ratio; PEF, peak expiratory flow; SABA, short-acting β-agonist.

SUGGESTED READINGS

Chowdhury BA, Dal Pan G. The FDA and safe use of long-acting beta-agonists in the treatment of asthma. *N Engl J Med.* 2010;362:1169.

Ibrahim WH, Gheriani HA, Almohamed AA, Raza T. Paradoxical vocal cord motion disorder: past, present and future. *Postgrad Med J.* 2007;83(977):164-172.

Lazarus SC. Clinical practice. Emergency treatment of asthma. *N Engl J Med.* 2010;363(8):755-764.

Miller GE, Gaudin A, Zysk E, Chen E. Parental support and cytokine activity in childhood asthma: the role of glucocorticoid sensitivity. *J Allergy Clin Immunol.* 2009;123(4):824-830.

Moorman JE, Rudd RA, Johnson CA, et al. National surveillance for asthma-United States, 1980-2004. *MMWR Surveill Summ.* 2007;56(8):1-54.

National Center for Environmental Health. *Asthma prevalence, healthcare use and mortality: United States* 2005-09. Available at http://www.cdc.gov/nchs/data/nhsr/nhsr032.pdf.

National Heart, Lung, and Blood Institute. National Asthma, Education and Prevention Program (NAEPP). *Expert Panel Report 3.* Bethesda, MD; 2007.

Raviv S, Smith LJ. Diet and asthma. *Curr Opin Pulm Med.* 2010;16(1):71-76.

Rose D, Mannino DM, Leaderer BP. Asthma prevalence among US adults, 1998-2000: role of Puerto Rican ethnicity and behavioral and geographic factors. *Am J Public Health.* 2006;96(5):880-888.

Wenzel SE. Asthma: defining of the persistent adult phenotypes. *Lancet.* 2006;368(9537):804-813.

CHAPTER 232

Chronic Obstructive Pulmonary Disease

Gerald W. Staton, MD
Christopher D. Ochoa, MD

Key Clinical Questions

1. What conditions mimic an acute exacerbation of chronic obstructive pulmonary disease (COPD) and require different diagnostic and treatment modalities?

2. What inpatient therapeutic modalities reduce mortality or length of stay for patients with exacerbation of COPD?

4. What are the indications for noninvasive ventilation for patients with an acute exacerbation of COPD?

5. Explain the therapeutic interventions that you would consider and discuss with a patient at the time of discharge following an acute exacerbation of COPD?

INTRODUCTION

■ DEFINITION AND BACKGROUND

Chronic obstructive pulmonary disease (COPD) is a group of clinical and pathological pulmonary disorders that are preventable and treatable and are characterized by airflow limitation that is not fully reversible. The most common phenotypes of COPD are emphysema and chronic bronchitis. Emphysema is generally defined as irreversible enlargement of the airways and loss of elastic recoil. Clinically, emphysema presents with dyspnea along with clinical findings of an expanded chest, decreased breath sounds, radiographic lucency, and flattening of the diaphragms. Chronic bronchitis is defined by the finding of cough and sputum production on most days of at least 3 months per year for two consecutive years. Pathologically, the hallmarks of chronic bronchitis are large airway inflammation and the hypertrophy and hyperplasia of the mucous-secreting goblet cells. COPD is diagnosed after demonstrating airflow limitation by spirometry (at a time free of exacerbation) that is not fully reversible in patients who exhibit cough, sputum production, dyspnea or other appropriate risk factors. The severity of COPD is classified by the degree of limitation in the forced expiratory volume in 1 second (FEV_1) as well as by the frequency of exacerbations (0-1 vs ≥ 2 per year) and patient reported symptoms using validated questionnaires (**Tables 232-1** and **232-2**).

Hospitalists often manage patients presenting with new symptoms consistent with COPD, patients with acute exacerbations of underlying COPD, and patients whose COPD complicates the course of other medical conditions. In this chapter, we will review best practices for each of these scenarios and solutions for optimizing care of these patients as they transition out of the acute care setting.

■ RISK FACTORS

Tobacco smoking is the single most important risk factor for the development of COPD. Cigarette, pipe, and cigar smoking account for more than 90% of cases of COPD; yet, clinically important disease is only found in 10% to 20% of smokers. Clearly there are other predisposing factors because dose-dependent exposure to tobacco does not wholly determine the onset or severity of disease in COPD. Additional factors that lead to the onset (or accelerate the progression) of COPD include exposure to second-hand smoke, environmental irritants and pollutants (including biomass), occupational exposures, malnutrition, childhood pulmonary infections, HIV infection, and genetic predisposition. The role of genetics is incompletely understood, but COPD is more common in the relatives of those with COPD.

■ PATHOGENESIS

Tobacco smoke and other exposures trigger inflammatory, biochemical and anatomic changes that account for the symptoms, limitations, and complications of COPD (**Figure 232-1**). These airway irritants activate the airway epithelium as well as alveolar macrophages to release chemokines that attract a host of inflammatory cells into the airway including neutrophils and monocytes. Production of IL-6 and TNF-α magnify this inflammatory response. These cells, in concert with the airway epithelium produce metalloproteinases responsible for the degradation of elastin resulting in emphysema. Neutrophil elastase stimulates mucous hypersecretion

TABLE 232-1 GOLD Spirometry Criteria for Chronic Obstructive Pulmonary Disease Severity

GOLD Stage	Severity	Spirometry
I	Mild	$FEV_1/FVC < 0.7$ and FEV_1 80% predicted
II	Moderate	$FEV_1/FVC < 0.7$ and 50% FEV_1 < 80% predicted
III	Severe	$FEV_1/FVC < 0.7$ and 30% FEV_1 < 50% predicted
IV	Very severe	$FEV_1/FVC < 0.7$ and FEV_1 < 30% predicted *or* FEV_1 < 50% predicted with respiratory failure or signs of right heart failure

FEV_1, forced expiratory volume in 1 s; FVC, forced vital capacity; GOLD, Global Initiative for Chronic Obstructive Lung Disease.

TABLE 232-2 GOLD Grading Criteria for Chronic Obstructive Pulmonary Disease

Grade	Spirometry	Yearly Exacerbation Rate	Symptom Score
A	Stage 1 or 2	≤1 exacerbation not leading to a hospitalization	CAT <10 or mMRC 0-1
B	Stage 1 or 2	≤1 exacerbation not leading to a hospitalization	CAT ≥10 or mMRC ≥2
C	Stage 3 or 4	≥2 exacerbations or ≥1 exacerbation leading to hospitalization	CAT < 10 or mMRC 0-1
D	Stage 3 or 4	≥2 exacerbations or ≥1 exacerbation leading to hospitalization	CAT ≥10 or mMRC ≥2

Severity is determined by a combination of symptom scores and either number of yearly exacerbations or spirometry stage. CAT, COPD assessment test; mMRC, modified Medical Research Council questionnaire for assessing the severity of breathlessness.

while epithelial cells produce TGF-β and fibroblast growth factors causing small airway fibrosis. When taken together, these insults lead to loss of elastic recoil, airflow limitation and impaired gas exchange characteristic of COPD.

EPIDEMIOLOGY

■ PREVALENCE AND EXACERBATIONS

Estimates of the incidence of COPD in the United States and worldwide vary, but data are consistent that the disease burden is large and COPD is underdiagnosed. COPD is the third leading cause of death in the United States. An estimated 12.7 million adults carried

the diagnosis of COPD in 2011. COPD was listed as the leading diagnosis in 715,000 hospital discharges in 2010 and accounted for 133,965 deaths in 2009 according to the American Lung Association.

■ COPD COMPLICATING OTHER DISEASES

There is increasing evidence that patients with COPD have high rates of morbidity and mortality caused by extrapulmonary conditions. Patients with COPD have been found to have higher rates of cardiovascular, gastrointestinal and psychiatric illnesses, among

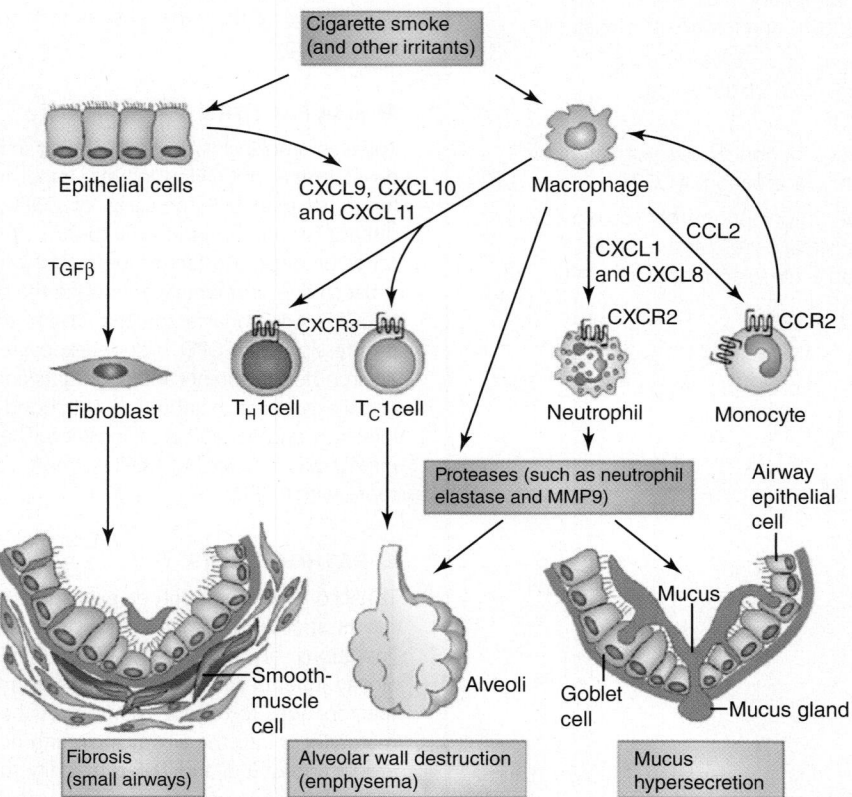

Figure 232-1 *Pathogenesis of chronic obstructive pulmonary disease.* (From Barnes PJ. Immunology of asthma and chronic obstructive pulmonary disease. *Nat Rev Immunol.* 2008;8[3]:183-192. Reprinted by permission from Macmillan Publishers Ltd.)

others. It is estimated that COPD is a primary or contributing cause of almost 10% of all admissions to the hospital. Cardiovascular morbidity and mortality might be even higher than that of lung disease and respiratory failure.

COPD EXACERBATION: DIFFERENTIAL AND EVALUATION

An acute exacerbation of COPD (AECOPD) is defined as a change in the baseline symptoms of dyspnea, cough and/or sputum color or volume that necessitates a change in management. When a patient with COPD or risk factors for COPD presents with any of these complaints, the diagnosis of AECOPD must be considered against a number of other diagnoses that may mimic an AECOPD. Once a diagnosis of AECOPD is reached, issues of causation of the exacerbation and level of severity need to be addressed. There is no single agreed-upon system to rank severity of exacerbations, but broadly categorizing among three levels has been suggested: (1) home management, (2) hospital management, and (3) respiratory failure.

■ ETIOLOGY AND DIFFERENTIAL DIAGNOSIS OF AECOPD

AECOPD has many different potential causes and the specific trigger for any one event is sometimes never elucidated. It is commonly agreed, however, that various triggers cause acute inflammation superimposed on the chronic inflammation of the underlying disease. During an AECOPD, inflammatory cells of many inflammatory pathways can be found in sputum and blood. Together, all infectious agents (bacteria, virus, and other) account for up to 80% of acute exacerbations.

The differential diagnoses to consider as triggers in patients that have underlying COPD and an acute respiratory decompensation are extensive (**Table 232-3**). Many of these triggers incite the inflammatory pathway at the root of an AECOPD, but they may also require other specific therapy. When a trigger is not immediately obvious from history and physical examination, there are certain other diagnoses that must be considered. An autopsy study of patients that were diagnosed as having an AECOPD and that died within 24 hours of admission showed that 37% of these deaths were due to heart failure and 21% due to pulmonary embolism. Patients admitted with otherwise unexplained exacerbations of COPD are often found to have pulmonary emboli when this diagnosis is pursued.

TABLE 232-3 Precipitants of Acute Exacerbation of Chronic Obstructive Pulmonary Disease: Differential Diagnosis

Pneumonia
Upper respiratory tract infection
Pulmonary embolism
Reactive airways disease or allergens
Congestive heart failure
Pneumothorax (trauma, rib fracture)
Arrhythmia
Myocardial infarction
Upper airway obstruction
Sleep disordered breathing
Sedating medications
Medication nonadherence
Environmental irritants (smoke, smog, workplace irritants)
Thickened bronchial secretions (eg, dehydration)

DIAGNOSTIC EVALUATION

For patients with known or suspected COPD, any complaint consistent with a COPD exacerbation warrants thorough investigation. The degree of diagnostic evaluation should be determined by the patient's subjective degree of discomfort, physical examination abnormalities, alterations in vital signs and/or diagnostic studies. Careful consideration of any conditions in the differential diagnosis of AECOPD (Table 232-3) must be undertaken.

■ KEY HISTORY AND PHYSICAL EXAMINATION

Questions regarding dyspnea, cough, sputum volume or color and rescue bronchodilator use may establish a change in symptoms from the patient's baseline. The history may also provide clues to other diagnoses or triggers (Table 232-3) for patients suspected of having an AECOPD.

AECOPD is associated with increased dyspnea, sputum purulence, wheezing, constitutional symptoms (fever, malaise, myalgias), and cough. Other past medical history and comorbid conditions can affect overall mortality and may influence patient triage for monitoring and therapy.

For patients with suspected AECOPD, but without a diagnosis of COPD, questioning regarding age, smoking status, exercise tolerance and other respiratory exposures can help increase or decrease the suspicion of COPD as the underlying disease.

The physical examination may help identify undiagnosed COPD, exclude other diagnoses in patients with known COPD, and help triage the severity of a diagnosed AECOPD. For evaluating the severity of an exacerbation, ominous physical examination findings portending higher risk and poorer outcomes include altered mentation (agitation and/or obtundation), respiratory muscle retraction, paradoxical abdominal movement, cyanosis and diaphoresis. These findings necessitate higher levels of monitoring and expedited care. Other findings that are consistent with an AECOPD include wheezing, cough, hyper-resonance to percussion and diffusely decreased breath sounds.

■ LABORATORY EVALUATION

In the initial evaluation of AECOPD, pulse oximetry O_2 saturation > 89% is evidence of acceptable oxygenation.

PRACTICE POINT

- An arterial blood gas should be rapidly obtained to evaluate any patient with an AECOPD considered for hospital admission, as recommended by international guidelines.

Arterial blood gases (ABGs) are able to more accurately determine the derangement of gas exchange by calculating an alveolar-arterial gradient, and may detect worse hypoxia than expected or evidence of hypercarbia. Importantly, the pH from the ABG may also provide valuable information helping direct management (eg, consideration of noninvasive ventilation). Arterial blood gas interpretation must take into account the patient's baseline status. Patients with more severe disease are likely to have elevated partial pressure of carbon dioxide (PCO_2) with a relatively preserved pH as the kidneys compensate for chronic hypoventilation. Ominous findings include elevated PCO_2 with a decreased pH (indicating an acute onset or worsening of hypoventilation), low partial pressures of oxygen, and a severely elevated PCO_2.

Guidelines recommend hematology and basic chemistry panels in the evaluation of COPD. These tests may show polycythemia associated with chronic COPD, or conversely, anemia. These basic labs are most valuable in identifying other diagnoses to be considered or comorbid conditions that may require parallel treatment. Patients receiving theophylline therapy should have the serum level measured.

Routine collection of sputum for Gram stain and culture is not recommended in the management of COPD exacerbation. Sputum Gram stain and culture may play a role in the laboratory evaluation of patients that do not respond to initial therapy and/or have evidence of pneumonia.

■ RADIOGRAPHY AND ELECTROCARDIOGRAPHY

Chest radiography is indicated for evaluation of AECOPD. Findings on the radiograph may influence the type of care if there are findings such as pneumothorax, atelectasis, focal infiltrate or pulmonary edema. About 20% of patients thought to have an AECOPD have chest radiograph findings that influence management.

PRACTICE POINT

- About 20% of patients thought to have an AECOPD have chest radiograph findings that influence management.

Patients with dyspnea and other chest complaints need electrocardiography (ECG) evaluation to identify relevant findings including coronary ischemia or arrhythmias. The irregular rhythm of multifocal tachycardia (MAT) that is found frequently in COPD patients may be difficult to distinguish from atrial fibrillation without ECG. MAT responds to the treatment of the underlying lung disease and rate control whereas atrial fibrillation requires additional therapeutic approaches.

■ SPIROMETRY

Spirometry, while a core diagnostic tool for the evaluation of outpatient stable COPD, does not have a role in the evaluation of COPD exacerbations. In fact, national and international guidelines recommend against the use of spirometry in the setting of AECOPD.

TRIAGE: DETERMINING SEVERITY, INDICATIONS FOR ADMISSION, AND LEVEL OF CARE

■ DETERMINING SEVERITY OF AN EXACERBATION

No single system exists to classify patient severity of illness once they are identified as having an AECOPD. The American Thoracic Society and European Respiratory Society (ATS/ERS) guidelines define severity based upon where the exacerbation is managed (home versus inpatient versus ICU) requiring clinicians evaluating patients for AECOPD to rely on previously mentioned risk factors for mortality and clinical acumen to best triage patients.

■ CRITERIA FOR ADMISSION

The Global Initiative for Chronic Obstructive Lung Disease (GOLD) and ATS/ERS guidelines for management of COPD provide criteria for hospitalization in AECOPD (**Table 232-4**). Certain findings may predict the success or failure of outpatient management. Older age, lower baseline FEV_1, hypoxemia, previous recent exacerbations and extensive comorbidities can increase risk of mortality or relapse exacerbation.

■ CRITERIA FOR INTENSIVE CARE UNIT ADMISSION

The best location to manage any patient with an AECOPD will vary based on individual hospital resources and staffing, with differences in the availability of specified inpatient respiratory units, step-down or intermediate care units and personnel. Therefore, criteria for intensive

---

TABLE 232-4 Indications for Hospitalization of Patients with Acute Exacerbation of Chronic Obstructive Pulmonary Disease

1. High-risk comorbid conditions (heart failure, renal disease, liver failure, pneumonia)
2. Failure of outpatient management
3. Inability to perform activities of daily living (eating, sleeping, etc)
4. Unremitting dyspnea
5. Worsening hypercapnea, hypoxemia
6. Altered mental status
7. Diagnostic uncertainty

---

care unit (ICU) admission are often institution specific. Nonetheless, some guidelines suggest criteria for ICU admission (**Table 232-5**).

MANAGEMENT OF AN ACUTE EXACERBATION OF COPD

■ INITIAL HOSPITAL TREATMENT

Bronchodilators

Short-acting β-agonists such as albuterol are a mainstay of outpatient management of stable COPD and play a key role in the treatment of AECOPD for improving symptoms and FEV_1. β-agonists induce airway smooth muscle relaxation via increased cyclic adenosine monophosphate and have their largest effect on peripheral airways. Their onset of action occurs within minutes, peak at 30 minutes, and last for several hours. β-agonists should be given every 2 hours for initial treatment of a patient being admitted to a general medical floor, but may be given as frequently as every 20 minutes or continuously for patients in extremis. Levalbuterol, a pure R isomer of albuterol (albuterol is a 1:1 mixture of the R and S isomers) may produce better bronchodilation in asthma exacerbations, but this effect has not been shown in COPD. There is also some thought that levalbuterol may cause less tachycardia when compared to racemic albuterol, but *scarce evidence supports this effect or its clinical significance.* Based on the multitude of conflicting data surrounding the use of levalbuterol, it is difficult to recommend its routine use, but it may be reasonable in patients that appear to have an adverse effect from albuterol or for a short time while frequent dosing of a β-agonist is needed.

Short-acting anticholinergics, including ipratroprium, should be used in concert with β-agonists to treat acute exacerbations. They bronchodilate via inhibition of muscarinic pulmonary acetylcholine esterase receptors and have their largest effects on central airways.

TABLE 232-5 Indications for Intensive Care Unit Admission of Patients with Acute Exacerbation of Chronic Obstructive Pulmonary Disease

1. Severe dyspnea that responds inadequately to initial emergency therapy
2. Confusion, lethargy, or respiratory muscle fatigue (the last characterized by paradoxical diaphragmatic motion)
3. Impending respiratory failure
4. Hemodynamic instability
5. Persistent or worsening hypoxemia despite supplemental oxygen or severe/worsening respiratory acidosis (pH < 7.30)
6. Assisted mechanical ventilation, either intubation or noninvasive positive pressure ventilation

---

The onset of action is slower than that of β-agonist with an onset of approximately 15 minutes, a peak effect at 60 to 90 minutes, and duration of 4 to 6 hours.

The optimal dose of albuterol is 2.5 to 5.0 mg via nebulizer or six to eight puffs (90 mcg each) via metered dose inhaler (MDI). For ipratroprium, the optimal dose is 0.5 mg via nebulizer or four to eight puffs of an MDI (at 17 mcg per puff). Inhalational technique varies widely from patient to patient, especially in times of respiratory distress. However, evidence supports delivery of drug via *MDI with a spacer* for equivalent results at a lower cost compared to a nebulizer. Long-acting bronchodilators, including long-acting β-agonists (eg, salmeterol) and long-acting anticholinergics (eg, tiotropium) have no role in the management of AECOPD. Oral and injection bronchodilators are not as effective as inhaled route and should be avoided.

Corticosteroids

Systemic steroids are indicated for the treatment of AECOPD requiring hospitalization. More controversial, however, is the optimal route of administration and dose.

PRACTICE POINT

- Systemic steroids have been shown to speed recovery of FEV_1, lower the number of treatment failures and shorten hospital length of stay. A 5-day course of oral steroids has been shown to be noninferior to longer durations.

Steroids have significant side effects, including hyperglycemia, which is the most common acute side effect. Higher doses and longer duration of exposure increase these risks. The initial dose and route of administration of steroids should be tailored to the patient. Patients requiring hospitalization but without impending respiratory failure may be started at a dose of prednisone 30 to 40 mg (or equivalent) daily to maximize benefit and minimize risk, whereas use of higher doses and IV route should be considered for patients in acute distress or respiratory failure. Recent literature has shown that a 5-day course of oral prednisone (40 mg) is noninferior to 2 weeks of therapy. No data supports use of inhaled steroids in AECOPD.

Antibiotics

Bacterial infections play an important role in AECOPD. Guideline recommendations encourage the use of empiric antibiotics for patients with moderate to severe AECOPD that have suspected infection. Antibiotics should be tailored to the patient risk factors as well as to community and hospital specific microbial patterns, but should always include coverage for the most common causal pathogens (ie, *Haemophilus influenzae*, *Streptococcus pneumonia*, and *Moraxella catarrhalis*). For patients with very severe airflow limitation, extended spectrum coverage should be considered as more resistant bacteria (ie, *Pseudomonas*, other Gram-negative rods) can cause exacerbations.

Oxygen and noninvasive ventilation

Oxygen level monitoring and supplemental oxygen provision are often necessary for patients with AECOPD (**Figure 232-2**). Early and

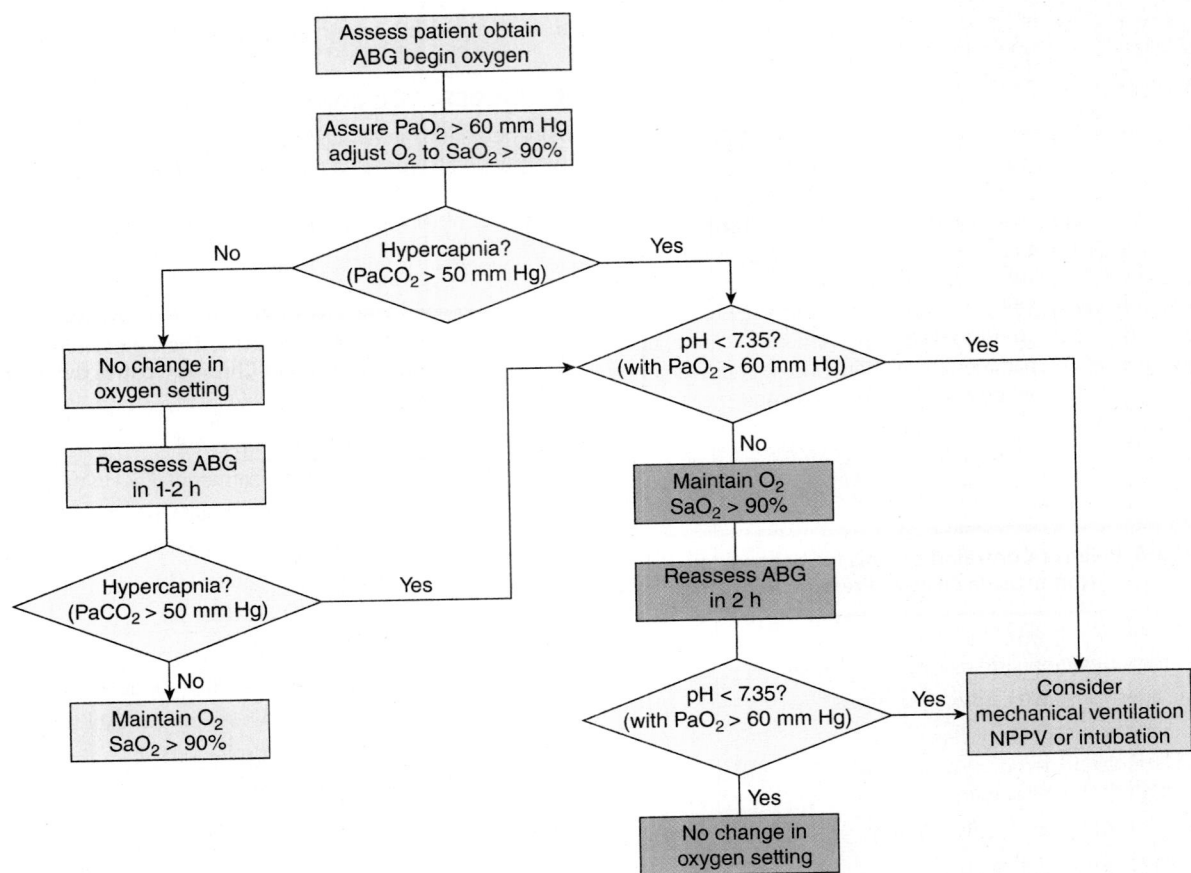

Figure 232-2 *Algorithm for oxygen and carbon dioxide assessment during an acute exacerbation of chronic obstructive pulmonary disease. ABG, arterial blood gas; O_2, oxygen; $PaCO_2$, partial pressure of carbon dioxide in arterial blood; PaO_2, partial pressure of oxygen in arterial blood; SaO_2, saturation level of oxygen in hemoglobin.*

frequent assessment of blood oxygen levels (via arterial blood gases or pulse oximetry) is critical for patients with an AECOPD. Oxygen can be supplied via nasal cannula, simple face masks, nonrebreather masks or high-flow oxygen masks. For patients with respiratory distress and increased work of breathing, rapid inspiration may overcome the reservoir of a nonrebreather mask. In this situation, oxygen delivered by high-flow masks yields the greatest percentage of inspired oxygen. The goal of oxygen supplementation should be to achieve a goal SpO_2 of 88% to 92% and/or a PaO_2 of > 60. Care must also be taken to provide adequate but not excessive levels of oxygen for patients that have baseline hypercapnea to avoid exacerbating carbon dioxide retention. Carbon dioxide binds reversibly to reduced hemoglobin, but oxygen drives the reaction to release carbon dioxide, a phenomenon known as the Haldane effect. Patients receiving supplemental oxygen need frequent assessment of blood oxygen and carbon dioxide levels in addition to a clinical assessment of alertness. The GOLD guidelines recommend rechecking an arterial blood gas 30 to 60 minutes after initiation of oxygen therapy.

Positive pressure ventilation

Noninvasive positive pressure ventilation (NIPPV) has been shown to benefit some patients with an AECOPD and should be considered for patients with mild to moderate acidemia, increased work of breathing and hypercapnea. Special consideration should be given for patients with a pH between 7.2 and 7.35, as this patient population has the most evidence supporting benefit.

PRACTICE POINT

- Positive pressure ventilation applied at two levels during the respiratory cycle (bi-level ventilation) has been shown to decrease mortality, the need for intubation, and the length of hospital stay for patients with an AECOPD.

Absolute contraindications to NIPPV include immediate need for intubation, untreated tension pneumothorax and a comatose state. Relative contraindications for use of NIPPV include severity of disease, likelihood of failure and anatomical risks (**Table 232-6**). If NIPPV is selected, patients require frequent reassessment and close observation. An ABG should be rechecked 30 minutes to 1 hour from the time of NIPPV initiation. Within the first 1 to 2 hours, there should be a clear trend toward improvement in clinical and laboratory (pH, PCO_2) parameters. Without rapid improvement, strong consideration must be given to intubation and mechanical ventilation.

TABLE 232-6 Relative Contraindications for Use of Noninvasive Positive Pressure Ventilation

1. Craniofacial abnormality or trauma
2. Respiratory arrest/apnea/refractory hypoxemia
3. Cardiac arrest/unstable cardiac arrhythmia
4. Hemodynamic instability
5. Inability to tolerate aerophagia (swallowing too much air), eg, recent gastrointestinal surgery
6. Inability to cooperate or protect airway
   a. Severe encephalopathy
   b. Severe upper gastrointestinal bleed
   c. High risk for aspiration

Invasive mechanical ventilation is sometimes required to treat severe exacerbations of COPD. The decision to intubate and mechanically ventilate a patient with an AECOPD is ultimately clinical, but guideline statements offer possible indications for intubation that include severe dyspnea, respiratory rate > 35, somnolence, severe acidosis (pH < 7.25), refractory hypoxemia and complications of comorbidities. Predictors of poor outcomes with intubation and mechanical ventilation include a baseline FEV_1 <30% predicted, nonrespiratory comorbidities and poor functional capacity prior to intubation.

◾ OTHER THERAPIES

Methylxanthines such as theophylline and aminophylline have been used to treat COPD (both stable and during exacerbations) for decades. A systemic review of methylxanthines in AECOPD did not find significant benefits but did describe increased side effects, including palpitations and arrhythmias. While guidelines do list methylxanthines as alternate therapies for patients that do not respond to first-line therapies, they should be considered later-line therapy. If methylxanthines are used, they require monitoring for side effects and toxicity. Serum levels should be monitored every several days, and daily after a dose change until levels are relatively stable. Acute illness and medication changes at the time of admission can affect metabolism and serum levels of methylxanthines. If theophylline is used, drug levels should be adjusted to 8 to 12 mg/mL.

Other therapies that have been used to treat AECOPD include mucolytic therapy, postural drainage and chest physiotherapy. These modalities may improve symptoms, but have not been shown to improve outcomes. Guidelines do not recommend pulmonary rehabilitation during treatment for an AECOPD, but early ambulation and physical and/or occupational therapy for patients that are not in respiratory failure is advisable (**Table 232-7**).

◾ TRIGGERS FOR CONSULTATION

Management of an AECOPD may have varying levels of complexity. The decision to consult a pulmonary or critical care specialist will be determined by hospital and referral resources, as well as the experience level of clinicians caring for these patients. For the inpatient

---

TABLE 232-7 Evidence for Specific Therapies in Acute Exacerbation of Chronic Obstructive Pulmonary Disease

Therapy	Outcomes Improved
Antibiotics	Decreased treatment failure in the ICU
	Decreased in-hospital mortality while in the ICU
Oral corticosteroids	Decreased treatment failure
	Decreased hospital LOS
	Increased FEV_1 after 3 d
Bronchodilators	Increased FEV_1
Noninvasive positive pressure ventilation	Decreased need for intubation
	Decreased in-hospital mortality
	Decreased hospital LOS
Pulmonary rehabilitation (following recovery)	Decreased readmissions
	Decreased mortality in follow-up
	Increased quality of life in questionnaires
	Increased exercise capacity in 6MWT

6MWT, 6-minute walk test; FEV_1, forced expiratory volume in 1 s; LOS, length of stay.

management of an acute exacerbation, acuity of illness, hemodynamic compromise and poor response to therapy should be the overriding considerations for consultation. The ATS/ERS guidelines for the management of COPD list the following factors as indication for outpatient specialist consultation: age of COPD onset < 40 years old, two or more exacerbations per year (despite adequate outpatient management), rapidly progressive disease, severe disease (FEV_1 < 50% predicted), need for long-term oxygen therapy, onset of comorbid illness (osteoporosis, heart failure, bronchiectasis, lung cancer) and/or evaluation for surgery. A consultant may also help with discharge planning and follow-up care for patients after their acute illness. Outpatient specialty referral may be indicated for most patients once they have completed their inpatient treatment.

OUTPATIENT THERAPEUTICS AND REGIMEN AUGMENTATION

■ SUPPLEMENTAL OXYGEN

If patients remain hypoxemic at the time of discharge, they will require home oxygen therapy. To meet the Centers for Medicare and Medicaid Services (CMS) criteria for 24 hours per day long-term home oxygen therapy, patients must have resting, room air PaO_2 of 55 mm Hg or less or PaO_2 of 59 mm Hg or less with coexisting congestive heart failure, peripheral edema, hematocrit > 56%, or cor pulmonale (**Table 232-8**). Alterations of oxygen levels during sleep and/or exercise can also qualify patients for supplementation during those activities. Hypoxemia at hospital discharge following AECOPD may represent a prolonged recovery from an acute illness, a new baseline, or new recognition of a chronic problem. Regardless, **long-term oxygen therapy improves mortality for COPD patients that have resting hypoxemia.** Patients that have a new prescription for home oxygen should be reassessed with an arterial blood gas within 3 months to determine the ongoing need for supplemental oxygen.

■ ORAL STEROIDS

Systemic oral steroids are indicated for the treatment of an AECOPD that requires hospitalization. A 5-day course of oral steroids is supported by current evidence. Once the patient has stabilized, there is no indication for long-term treatment with steroids.

TABLE 232-8 Centers for Medicare and Medicaid Services Criteria for Oxygen Supplementation

Group I Coverage
- $PaO_2 \leq 55$ or $SaO_2 \leq 88\%$
  - At rest
  - During sleep
- OR $\downarrow PaO_2 > 10$ mm Hg or $\downarrow SaO_2$ 5% associated with symptoms or signs of hypoxemia
  - During activity

Group II Coverage
- $SaO_2 = 89\%$ (not + 89%)
- Any of the following:
  - Dependent edema
  - Pulmonary hypertension or cor pulmonale
  - Hematocrit > 56%

Requires retesting between 61 and 90 d

PaO_2, partial pressure of oxygen in arterial blood; SaO_2, saturation level of oxygen in hemoglobin.

■ INHALED THERAPIES

Inhaled long-acting bronchodilators (long-acting β-agonists and long-acting anticholinergics) and inhaled corticosteroids (ICS) have a significant role in regimen augmentation when a patient with AECOPD is being discharged. Strong evidence supports that inhaled medications reduce deterioration in health status, improve lung function (FEV_1), and reduce the number of exacerbations per year. All patients who have been hospitalized with AECOPD should be discharged on a combination of a long-acting bronchodilator and ICS, as meta-analysis data suggest mortality reduction with this regimen compared to placebo and other regimens. Additional data indicate that the combination of LABA and ICS plus long-acting anticholinergic for patients with more advanced COPD is associated with additional improvement in quality of life and a reduction in subsequent hospitalizations. Some evidence shows that chronic use of short-acting anticholinergic agents may impart increased cardiovascular risk in COPD patients, while mounting evidence suggests that long-acting anticholinergic agents may not have significant cardiovascular risks. The decisions of which medications to utilize should be made in light of clinical acumen, patient preferences, and patient-provider discussions regarding treatment goals and potential adverse effects.

■ MUCOLYTIC AND MUCOKINETIC AGENTS

Mucolytic agents are sometimes used in the treatment of COPD though they are not recommended in the guidelines. This is an area of active research.

COPD COMPLICATING ADMISSIONS FOR OTHER DIAGNOSES

Underlying COPD may complicate the care of patients admitted for other diagnoses. Complications may result from the underlying compromise of the respiratory symptom or because an exacerbation occurs at the time of, or shortly after, the onset of the original stress. Also, patients hospitalized for any reason are exposed to iatrogenic risks such as resistant microbes, painful procedures (causing splinting), sedative medications (hypoventilation), and decreased physical activity (deconditioning).

The use of β-blockers in COPD has long been a controversial topic. A 2005 Cochrane Review demonstrated that there was no short-term decrease in FEV_1 or responsiveness to inhaled β-agonists for patients that received cardioselective β-blockers, regardless of the severity of COPD. Therefore, cardio-selective β-blocker prescription is reasonable for chronic COPD patients who have a cardiac indication to receive this therapy.

While COPD may complicate any medical or surgical illness, there are certain processes where this occurs more frequently. Patients with heart failure and COPD often present complaining of shortness of breath. It is difficult to decipher if the worsening of the baseline condition is because of cardiac decompensation, pulmonary exacerbation, or both. Normal levels of serum brain natriuretic peptide (BNP) significantly decrease the likelihood of cardiac decompensation, but elevated BNP is less specific and more difficult to interpret. A full physical examination and workup is often necessary and occasionally an empiric trial of treating both conditions is warranted. Patients recovering from surgical procedures need to have special consideration of postoperative activity, pain control (without oversedation) and abdominal processes (such as swelling or ileus).

■ PERIOPERATIVE EVALUATION

Large numbers of patients with recognized or unrecognized COPD may require surgery. Hospitalists are often asked to determine which patients represent undue risk and if there are any measures that can minimize these risks. In general, pulmonary complications are equal (in prevalence, morbidity, mortality, and length of stay) when compared to cardiac complications for moderate and high-risk surgeries. Perioperative care of COPD patients includes identifying and managing any acute worsening from pulmonary baseline, risk assessment, preoperative risk minimization (ensuring proper preoperative care and medications) and postoperative risk minimization. Separate chapters describe perioperative pulmonary care (Chapters 51 [Preoperative Pulmonary Risk Assessment and Management] and 60 [Management of Postoperative Pulmonary Complications]).

PROGNOSIS AND END-OF-LIFE CARE

■ PROGNOSIS

COPD patients' pulmonary function progressively declines over the course of the disease. Tobacco cessation is the most important factor in slowing the progression of COPD, but even those patients that stop smoking experience continued age-related decline in lung function. Predicting the future health of a patient with COPD is important at the time of discharge to ensure all appropriate treatment modalities are considered as well as ensuring patients have the needed social support to meet the demands of daily life.

Once a patient is admitted for an AECOPD, morbidity and mortality are significantly different when compared to COPD patients that have not been hospitalized previously. The 1-year readmission rate for COPD patients discharged for AECOPD is as high as 59% for patients with severe disease and the 1-year mortality rate is as high as 22%. Two-year mortality approaches 50% for patients admitted with AECOPD and hypercapnea.

Increasing age, male sex, white race, prior hospitalization, weight loss, pulmonary hypertension, hypoxemia, hypercapnea, decreased FEV_1, and decreased diffusing capacity of the lung for carbon monoxide (DLCO) have all been identified as risk factors for death with COPD. Progressive decline in FEV_1 has historically been used as the primary measure of predicting the course of COPD, but it is being replaced by an indexed score, the BODE score. The BODE score (**Table 232-9**) has the advantage of taking into account multiple factors that have been shown to be predictive of respiratory and all-cause mortality. The BODE index requires a (B) BMI, FEV_1 as a measure of (O) obstruction, degree of (D) dyspnea on the Medical Research Council dyspnea scale, and (E) exercise capacity as measured by a 6-minute walk test. Patients who have a 5 or greater BODE score are appropriate for evaluation for lung transplant and/or other advanced treatment modalities.

■ END-OF-LIFE CARE

For patients that have not previously expressed their desires regarding invasive or life supporting treatments, difficult decisions have to be made during the time of an acute illness. It is preferable, however, to facilitate patient expression of their end-of-life wishes

in a stable and less stressed state. The time of discharge from the hospital can be a "teachable moment" and discussion of what the patient would or would not want in the case of future illness and/or respiratory failure should occur.

For some patients, an emphasis on palliative care (formally or informally) and/or hospice referral may be appropriate. Dyspnea is a key symptom that must be addressed as a source of anxiety and discomfort for the patient. Oxygenation status, respiratory rate, and other objective measures are not good indicators of a patient's perception of breathlessness. When underlying causes of dyspnea can be corrected, that should be the focus of care. When the underlying causes are not reversible, opioids in low-to-moderate doses have good effect in relieving dyspnea. For patients who have a significant component of anxiety along with dyspnea, benzodiazepines may be added to relieve symptoms.

DISCHARGE PLANNING

For the majority of patients admitted with an AECOPD, improvement is noted within a short period from admission. For the minority of patients that do not improve, alternative diagnoses, intensified therapies, and/or palliative measures must be considered. The latter stages of an acute inpatient stay can focus on tapering the frequency of medication dosing, transitioning care to an outpatient setting, patient education, and prevention of future exacerbations.

The GOLD and ATS/ERS guidelines provide lists of criteria that should be met for consideration of discharge home. These include controlling or reversing the reason for admission, hemodynamic stability, return to oxygenation baseline, less frequent need for inhaled bronchodilators, ability to resume ambulating, no parenteral therapy for 12 to 24 hours, ability to eat and sleep without being disturbed by dyspnea, understanding the use of medications, and completion of arrangements for follow-up and/or home care. For patients to meet all of these criteria, length of stay might increase beyond what is reasonable or desirable. While the patient's trend should be back toward baseline, full recovery and baseline oxygenation status might take several weeks and strict adherence to the guidelines may not be practical or feasible.

QUALITY IMPROVEMENT

■ SECONDARY PREVENTION

Smoking cessation

Counseling regarding tobacco cessation for active smokers is essential because tobacco cessation is the best way to slow the decline in lung function. There is some limited data that counseling during an inpatient stay might increase the chance of quitting and more robust evidence that quit rates can be increased by inpatient counseling followed by continued outpatient intervention. Also, several pharmacological strategies have been shown to improve quit rates. Options include nicotine replacement, buproprion (which can be used in conjunction with nicotine replacement) and varenicline. A Cochrane Review compiled several trials of varenicline and found that relative risk of cessation was two to three times greater when compared to placebo, approximately 1.5 times greater when compared to buproprion, and approximately 1.3 times greater when compared to nicotine replacement therapy.

Vaccinations

All patients with COPD should have the 23-valent pneumococcal polysaccharide vaccine, and those patients aged greater than 65 that have not had the vaccine in the last 5 years should have it administered regardless of previous vaccination status. The CDC recommends all adults over the age of 65 receive the pneumococcal

TABLE 232-9 BODE Index Scoring System

	0	1	2	3
FEV_1 (% predicted)	≥ 65	50-64	36-49	≤ 35
6MWT distance	> 350 m	250-349 m	150-249 m	≤ 149 m
mMRC dyspnea scale	0-1	2	3	4
BMI	> 21	< 21		

6MWT, 6-minute walk test; BMI, body mass index; BODE, body mass index, airflow obstruction, dyspnea and exercise capacity; FEV_1, forced expiratory volume in 1 s; mMRC, modified Medical Research Council.

conjugate vaccine (PCV13). The PCV13 and 23-valent should not be administered during the same visit and the minimum time between administration is 8 weeks. Also, all patients with COPD should have the influenza vaccine annually.

■ PATIENT EDUCATION

Efforts toward education are also vital for improving the patient's health after discharge and include education regarding proper inhaler technique, and avoidance of second-hand smoke (and other respiratory irritants). Patient education regarding the ability to recognize the symptoms of an exacerbation should be emphasized.

■ PULMONARY REHABILITATION

Pulmonary rehabilitation is an important part of outpatient COPD care after an admission for AECOPD, and should be considered at the time of discharge for all patients with chronic lung disease with the goal of alleviating symptoms and optimizing functional capacity. Evidence supports that entering pulmonary rehabilitation within 10 days of hospital discharge is safe. Furthermore, patients enrolled in early pulmonary rehabilitation experienced improved exercise tolerance and health status at 3 months. Beyond functional capacity, pulmonary rehabilitation programs often focus on establishing social support and care networks that are most appropriate for the patient and can have quality-of-life benefits beyond physical improvements.

PRACTICE POINT

- Evidence supports that entering pulmonary rehabilitation within 10 days of hospital discharge is safe, and patients enrolled in early pulmonary rehabilitation experience improved exercise tolerance and health status at 3 months.

■ SURGICAL TREATMENT OPTIONS AND TRANSPLANT EVALUATION

Surgical treatment options for COPD include lung volume reduction surgery (LVRS), bullectomy, lung transplantation and investigational approaches. LVRS involves bilateral removal of 25% to 30% of total lung volume. The National Emphysema Treatment Trial, published in 2003, demonstrated that LVRS improved exercise capacity but not survival among all patients with severe emphysema. This trial did, however, identify subgroups that had a survival advantage. The best candidates for LVRS are patients with predominantly upper-lobe disease and a low exercise capacity after pulmonary rehabilitation. Bullectomy has not been well studied in randomized trials, but it may be considered for patients with at least one-third of the thorax occupied by bullae.

For patients with advanced disease another therapy to consider is lung transplantation. Lung transplant referral is indicated for younger patients with COPD that have progressive symptoms despite maximal medical therapy, including smoking cessation. Lung transplant for COPD has been shown to improve quality of life, but effect on mortality has not been clearly demonstrated and is more controversial. For further analysis of trials addressing treatment strategies in COPD, please refer to the key references (**Table 232-10**).

■ TRANSITIONS OF CARE

Patients transitioning from inpatient to outpatient care, whether for an AECOPD or for patients with underlying COPD admitted for other reasons, have many educational and therapeutic needs. Education needs include smoking cessation, inhaler technique and mobility prescriptions. For patients that might still have

pain issues or decreased mobility, education regarding incentive spirometry is imperative. Follow-up care should be arranged with a primary care physician, a pulmonary specialist or both. For discharges after an AECOPD, follow-up should be arranged at discharge for the patient to be seen within 2 weeks of discharge or sooner if requiring significant changes to their care regimen. Recent literature has suggested implementing a "COPD care bundle" prior to discharge. This includes specialist notification of patient admissions, smoking cessation assistance, referral to pulmonary rehab, educational literature and proper inhaler teaching. Preliminary data have shown a significant reduction in readmissions for AECOPD following these steps.

■ DISPARITIES IN HEALTH CARE

COPD has long been considered a disease of white, male smokers. Data, however, show that the epidemic is increasing most rapidly for women and African Americans. For over a decade, more women have died of COPD than men annually. The death rate is increasing more rapidly for African Americans as well. To some degree, these changes represent changes in the demographics of cigarette smoking over decades. However, some data suggest that women and African Americans may actually be more susceptible to chronic lung disease when compared to white men. In general, women have smaller caliber central airways than similarly sized men and African Americans have smaller trunk/leg ratios than whites. These differences may explain more clinically significant airflow limitation after exposure to cigarettes or other respiratory toxins. Possible differences in specific genes, proteases, and/or cytokines might also explain some differences in response to exposures.

■ OUTCOMES TO MONITOR

There are many possible outcomes to monitor and measure regarding quality of care for patients admitted with an AECOPD or for patients with COPD treated in the hospital for other issues. The percentage of patients provided with smoking cessation counseling would be appropriate for either group, as would vaccination rates.

For patients treated for an AECOPD, tracking the number of patients referred for pulmonary rehabilitation is another option, as is the short-term readmission rate. Lastly, the percentage of patients with severe COPD that are referred to hospice and/or palliative services could be monitored.

■ COSTS AND RESOURCE UTILIZATION

While only smoking cessation and supplemental oxygen have been proven to have an impact on chronic COPD mortality, there are many other modalities that may improve quality of life and possibly decrease health care costs for patients with COPD.

Smoking cessation programs, health-maintenance caseworkers for patients with COPD and pulmonary rehabilitation programs each offer ways in which large institutions might decrease overall costs for the care of a population of COPD patients. Vaccinations have been shown to have significant cost-savings as well.

Another area of focus for resource utilization is goals of care and end-of-life discussions. A 2006 study found that COPD patients in the last 6 months of life were more likely to be admitted to an ICU and have longer length of stay when compared to patients in the last 6 months of life with lung cancer. Total health care costs were $4000 more per patient during this time frame. Improved communication (preferably before admission, but also possibly at the time of admission) regarding goals of care and realistic expectations could prove to decrease these costs while hopefully improving quality of life for terminal patients and their families.

TABLE 232-10 Evidence-based Medicine: Key References for Chronic Obstructive Pulmonary Disease

Reference	Methodology	Results	Limitations	Bottom Line
Calverely P, et al. *N Engl J Med.* 2007;356: 775-789. TORCH trial	Randomized, double-blind, placebo-controlled trial of placebo vs salmeterol alone vs fluticasone alone vs salmeterol plus fluticasone inhaled twice daily for 3 y. 6112 patients were active or former smokers with diagnosis of COPD, FEV_1 < 60% predicted and no significant bronchodilator response	Comparing combination therapy to placebo, there was nonstatistically significant reduction in mortality (OR, 0.825; CI 0.681-1.002). Compared to placebo, combination therapy reduced exacerbations. There were higher levels of pneumonia in both groups receiving fluticasone when compared to placebo	There was a large drop-out rate (as might be expected in a COPD trial with a placebo arm)	There is insufficient data to suggest that inhaled corticosteroids decrease mortality in patients with COPD, but addition of inhaled corticosteroid may reduce exacerbations for patients on LABAs that have recurrent exacerbations. For monotherapy in COPD, LABA should be used rather than an ICS
Taskin DP, et al. *N Engl J Med.* 2008;359: 1543-1554. UPLIFT	Randomized, double-blind, placebo-controlled trial of tiotroprium vs placebo to decrease decline in FEV_1 over time (before and after bronchodilation) in 5993 patients	There was no significant difference in decline in FEV_1 over time in the tiotroprium group as compared to placebo. Tiotroprium did lead to increases in FEV_1 (but not change over time), improved quality-of-life scores, and fewer exacerbations	There was a large drop-out rate and short-acting inhaled anticholinergics were stopped in all patients	Tiotroprium may be prescribed to alleviate symptoms of COPD, but should not be expected to alter progression of disease
Anthonisen NR. *JAMA.* 1994;272: 1497-1505. Lung Health study	Randomized, placebo-controlled trial comparing no intervention to smoking cessation counseling plus placebo to smoking cessation counseling plus inhaled short-acting anticholinergics in 5887 patients	Participants in both smoking cessation groups experienced smaller declines in FEV_1 over time. Responses to short-acting anticholinergics were not cumulative over time	There was predictably low adherence to prescribed inhalers	Smoking cessation counseling can lead to declines in rates of smoking, and FEV_1 decline was mitigated amongst patients who received counseling, and the effect was strongest in those who did abstain
Bronchard L, et al. *N Engl J Med.* 1995;333: 817-822.	Prospective randomized trial comparing use of NIPPV vs standard care for treating 85 patients admitted to ICU with COPD exacerbation	NIPPV significantly decreased rate of endotracheal intubation, hospital LOS, and in-hospital mortality	Large percentage of patients admitted to ICU with COPD exacerbation were excluded, limiting population of patients to which data can be applied	For selected patients with acute exacerbations of COPD, application of NIPPV can prevent need for endotracheal intubation and speed recovery
NETT Research Group. *N Engl J Med.* 2003;348: 2059-2073. NETT trial	Randomized trial of 1218 patients with severe emphysema to receive lung volume reduction surgery vs continued medical care. Overall mortality and maximal exercise capacity were compared as primary outcomes	In entire study group, there was no difference in overall mortality. Surgery group had significantly higher percentage of patients who improved maximal exercise capacity when compared to nonsurgery group. In subgroup analysis, patients with mostly upper-lobe disease and low exercise capacity after pulmonary rehabilitation, there was a mortality benefit from surgery. Amongst subgroup of nonupper-lobe emphysema and high exercise capacity, mortality was higher in surgery group. Interim analysis identified group of patients with high risk of surgical death	No difference in mortality overall. Caution must be used when results of subgroup analysis are applied	Lung volume reduction surgery may be indicated for specific group of patients who have predominantly upper-lobe emphysema and low exercise capacity after pulmonary rehabilitation. Risks and benefits must be weighed against options of doing nothing vs lung transplant. Patients with $FEV_1 \le 20\%$ predicted and either homogenous emphysema or DLCO $\le 20\%$ predicted are at high risk of death from lung-volume reduction surgery
Leuppi JD. *JAMA.* 2013;309: 2223-2231. REDUCE trial	Randomized, noninferiority trial comparing use of 5 d vs 14 d of corticosteroids in 314 patients with COPD exacerbation	No significant difference in rates of re-exacerbation at 6 mo between treatment arms (37.2% in the short term treatment group vs 38.4% in the long-term treatment group)	The study used an absolute difference of 15% to show noninferiority which may miss smaller treatment differences between treatment arms	To reduce the overall exposure to steroids, limit treatment to a total of 5 d of prednisone for acute exacerbations of COPD

COPD, chronic obstructive pulmonary disease; DLCO, diffusing capacity of the lung for carbon monoxide; FEV_1, forced expiratory volume in 1 s; ICS, inhaled corticosteroid; ICU, intensive care unit; LABA, long-acting beta-agonist; NIPPV, noninvasive positive pressure ventilation; OR, odds ratio.

SUGGESTED READINGS

Almagro P, Balbo E, Ochoa de Echaguen A, et al. Mortality after hospitalization for COPD. *Chest*. 2002;121:1441-1448.

Barnes P. Cellular and molecular mechanisms of chronic obstructive pulmonary disease. *Clin Chest Med*. 2014;35:71-86.

Bronchard L, Mancebo J, Wysocki M, et al. Noninvasive ventilation for acute exacerbations of chronic obstructive pulmonary disease. *N Engl J Med*. 1995;333:817-822.

Celli BR, MacNee W, Augusti A, et al. ATS/ERS TASK FORCE. Standards for the diagnosis and treatment of patients with COPD: a summary of the ATS/ERS position paper. *Eur Respir J*. 2004;23: 932-946.

Global Initiative for Chronic Obstructive Lung Disease. Global Strategy for the Diagnosis, Management, and Prevention of Chronic Obstructive Pulmonary Disease. Updated 2015. Available at: http://www.goldcopd.com. Accessed March 30, 2015.

Hopkinson NS, Englebretsen C, Cooley N, et al. Designing and implementing a COPD discharge care bundle. *Thorax*. 2012;67(1): 90-92.

Nathan SD. Lung transplantation: disease-specific considerations for referral. *Chest*. 2005;127:1006-1016.

Ram FSF, Picot J, Lightowler J, Wedzicha JA. Non-invasive positive pressure ventilation for treatment of respiratory failure due to exacerbations of chronic obstructive pulmonary disease. *Cochrane Database Syst Rev*. 2004:Issue 3. Art. No.: CD004104.

Rigotti NA, Clair C, Munafo MR, et al. Interventions for smoking cessation in hospitalized patients. *Cochrane Database Syst Rev*. 2012;Issue 5. Art. No.: CD001837.

Salpeter SS, Ormiston T, Salpeter E, et al. Cardioselective beta blockers for chronic obstructive pulmonary disease (Cochrane Review). *Cochrane Database Syst Rev*. 2005(1);Issue 4. Art. No.:CD003566.

Seemungal TA, Donaldson GC, Bhowmik A, et al. Time course and recovery of exacerbations in patients with chronic obstructive pulmonary disease. *Am J Respir Crit Care Med*. 2000;161:1608-1613.

Walters JAE, Tan DJ, White CJ, Wood-Baker R. Different durations of corticosteroid therapy for exacerbations of chronic obstructive pulmonary disease. *Cochrane Database Syst Rev*. 2014;Issue 12. Art. No.: CD006897.

CHAPTER 233

Interstitial Lung Diseases/Diffuse Parenchymal Lung Diseases

Brian T. Garibaldi, MD
Sonye K. Danoff, MD, PhD

Key Clinical Questions

1. Does the hospitalized patient with unexplained dyspnea have Interstitial Lung Disease (ILD)?

2. How and why should idiopathic pulmonary fibrosis (IPF) be differentiated from other forms of ILD?

3. How do you distinguish an acute exacerbation of IPF from other causes of worsening in ILD?

4. What are the indications for pulmonary consultation? For bronchoscopy in the diagnosis or evaluation of ILD?

5. When do you use newer antifibrotic agents in hospitalized patients with ILD?

6. How do you discharge patients with high oxygen requirements to home?

INTRODUCTION

■ EPIDEMIOLOGY

The interstitial lung diseases (ILDs) are a heterogeneous group of disorders with the common feature of inflammatory or fibrotic injury to the lung parenchyma. These disorders are also described as the diffuse parenchymal lung diseases. Numerous potential etiologies for ILD may be broadly divided into five categories: idiopathic, drug/medication related, environmental/occupational, genetic/hereditary and autoimmune associated (**Table 233-1**). While considered rare, these diseases affect approximately 500,000 individuals in the United States each year and result in 40,000 deaths, comparable to the number of deaths from breast cancer. The exact epidemiology is difficult to determine due to misidentification of patients as having more common disorders such as congestive heart failure or chronic obstructive pulmonary disease (COPD). The epidemiology varies based on the ILD subtype.

CLASSIFICATION AND COMMON PRESENTATION

The term ILD encompasses a diverse group of diseases. The American Thoracic Society and European Respiratory Society developed a two-level classification system to facilitate the clinical evaluation of ILD (**Figure 233-1**). This system divides ILDs initially based on specific mechanisms of disease into: disorders of known etiology, idiopathic interstitial pneumonias (IIPs), granulomatous diseases and rare diseases. The idiopathic interstitial pneumonias are further classified into a second level based on histologic appearance. We will focus primarily on the IIPs and mention several other ILDs of particular relevance to the hospitalist. A general approach to the diagnostic evaluation of suspected ILD is presented in **Figure 233-2**.

■ IDIOPATHIC PULMONARY FIBROSIS

Idiopathic pulmonary fibrosis primarily affects individuals over the age of 60. Recent epidemiologic studies show the prevalence increases with each successive decade from 18.7-23.3/100,000 in 55 to 64 year olds to 29.3-50.0/100,000 in 65 to 74 year olds to 48.4-87.9/100,000 in adults over than 85. IPF affects approximately 200,000 people in the United States and results in 20,000 deaths per year. A notable exception to the older age of onset is familial IPF. In this genetic disorder, patients may present two to three decades earlier with symptomatic disease. The median survival is 3 to 5 years from the time of diagnosis in symptomatic patients. Diagnosis is made based on a consistent history (slowly progressive dyspnea), findings of dry, velcro-like crackles on examination and a radiograph with basilar predominant interstitial changes (**Figure 233-3**). The hallmarks of IPF on chest computed tomography (CT) include basilar predominant subpleural reticulation and honeycombing with traction bronchiectasis (**Figure 233-4**). Although ground glass opacities may be seen during acute exacerbations, this should be a minor feature of a baseline CT study. The diagnosis of IPF mandates the exclusion of other etiologies including environmental exposures, medications and autoimmune diseases.

■ NONSPECIFIC INTERSTITIAL PNEUMONIA (NSIP)

Nonspecific interstitial pneumonia (NSIP) is the form of ILD most common in patients with autoimmune disease. This form of ILD is more common in women than men and has an earlier age of onset than IPF. The diagnosis is typically suspected based on the clinical

TABLE 233-1 Etiologies of Interstitial Lung Disease (ILD) by Category

Autoimmune
  Scleroderma
  Rheumatoid arthritis
  Systemic lupus erythematosis
  Polymyositis/dermatomyositis
  Sjogren syndrome
Occupational/environmental
  Asbestosis
  Silicosis
  Berylliosis
  Bird fancier's lung
Idiopathic
Medication-induced
  Common/conventional:
    Amiodarone
    Bleomycin
    Methotrexate
  Biologics
    TNF inhibitors
Genetic/hereditary
  Mucin 5b (Muc5b) variant
  Hermansky-Pudlak
  Surfactant protein A&C deficiency
  Telomerase mutations

symptoms and radiograph showing patchy ground glass opacities (GGO) with minimal fibrosis (Figure 233-4). Open lung biopsy is necessary for histologic diagnosis. For the purpose of therapy, a radiographic "diagnosis" of NSIP is often sufficient. The prognosis of NSIP is generally good but there is a subset of patients who develop progressive fibrosis and have a worse outcome.

■ RESPIRATORY BRONCHIOLITIS-ILD AND DESQUAMATIVE INTERSTITIAL PNEUMONIA

Respiratory-bronchiolitis interstitial lung disease (RB-ILD) and desquamative interstitial pneumonia (DIP) represent a poorly appreciated spectrum of smoking-related lung disease. Although they occur most frequently in smokers, they may occasionally occur in nonsmokers. These disorders may develop years after starting smoking. Unlike the more commonly encountered COPD and emphysema, RB-ILD and DIP are largely reversible with avoidance of cigarette smoke, including second hand exposures. The age of onset is variable, but tends to be younger than IPF. Definitive diagnosis requires lung biopsy. Individuals who develop this disorder without apparent tobacco smoke exposure may be treated with corticosteroids, but the response is variable.

■ ORGANIZING PNEUMONIA

Organizing pneumonia is a common and nonspecific lung injury pattern which can be encountered in a number of situations including medication-related, with autoimmune disease and following viral infections. When the cause is known or suspected, it is called organizing pneumonia. When the cause is unknown, the diagnosis is cryptogenic organizing pneumonia. The presentation may be virtually identical to that of pneumonia. Patients frequently receive one or several courses of antibiotics prior to diagnosis. The chest CT may show patchy ground glass opacities or dense infiltrates (Figure 233-4). The diagnosis is made by surgical lung biopsy but is often suspected based on clinical presentation. Prognosis is generally good as patients typically respond to corticosteroids.

■ ACUTE INTERSTITIAL PNEUMONITIS

Acute interstitial pneumonitis (AIP), sometimes referred to as the Hamman-Rich syndrome, is the most dreaded presentation of ILD. This enigmatic disorder may occur in the absence of any apparent trigger, although it may also complicate autoimmune disease. The age at onset is variable. Patients present with rapidly progressive dyspnea over a few weeks to months. Radiographs are indistinguishable from acute respiratory distress syndrome (ARDS), leading some people to refer to AIP as a form of idiopathic ARDS. Infection must be excluded and/or treated empirically. The prognosis is dismal with over 70% of patients dying of respiratory failure within weeks of presentation. High-dose corticosteroids have been used with occasional success in AIP particularly in the setting of underlying autoimmune disease.

■ SARCOIDOSIS

Sarcoidosis, the most common form of ILD, is a systemic disorder which can manifest in the skin, lung, heart, liver, bone marrow or the peripheral or central nervous system. The etiology remains unknown.

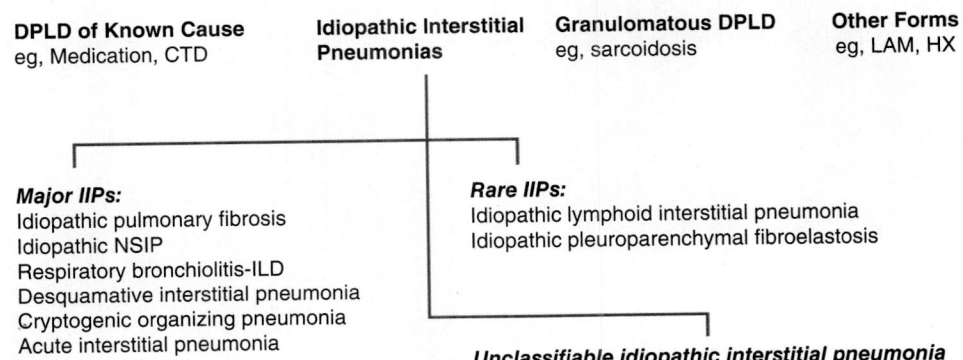

Diffuse Parenchymal Lung Disease

| DPLD of Known Cause
eg, Medication, CTD | Idiopathic Interstitial
Pneumonias | Granulomatous DPLD
eg, sarcoidosis | Other Forms
eg, LAM, HX |

Major IIPs:
Idiopathic pulmonary fibrosis
Idiopathic NSIP
Respiratory bronchiolitis-ILD
Desquamative interstitial pneumonia
Cryptogenic organizing pneumonia
Acute interstitial pneumonia

Rare IIPs:
Idiopathic lymphoid interstitial pneumonia
Idiopathic pleuroparenchymal fibroelastosis

Unclassifiable idiopathic interstitial pneumonia

Figure 233-1 *ATS/ERS Classification of Interstitial Lung Disease (Diffuse Parenchymal Lung Disease, DPLD).* Adapted from An official American Thoracic Society/European Respiratory Society statement: Update of the international multidisciplinary classification of the idiopathic interstitial pneumonias. This updated joint statement of the American Thoracic Society (ATS), and the European Respiratory Society (ERS) was adopted by the ATS board of director the ERS Executive Committee in 2013. *Am J Respir Crit Care Med.* 2013;188(6):733-748.

> **History:**
> Symptoms (cough, dyspnea, fatigue)
> Tempo of symptom development
> PMH especially autoimmune
> SH (smoking, work and avocation exposures, pets)
> FH (ILD, cirrhosis, early gray hair, marrow dysfunction, autoimmunity)
> Medications (current and past, including OTC)

> **Physical Exam:**
> Head & neck: pharyngeal crowding
> Lung-crackles, squeaks, rhonchi, lung size
> Cardiac-elevated P2, atrial fibrillation
> Abdomen-organomegaly
> Extremities-clubbing, cyanosis, edema
> Skin-rashes, sclerodactyly, Raynauds
> Neuromuscular-muscle weakness, cranial neuropathies

> **Lab Studies:**
> CBC with differential
> CMP
> RF, CCP, ANA, Ro, La, RNP, Scl-70
> Aldolase, CPK, Jo-1

> **Pulmonary Function Testing:**
> Spirogram
> Lung Volumes
> DLCO

> **Radiographs:**
> High resolution chest CT

> **Other studies which may be indicated:**
> Bronchoscopy
> Surgical Lung Biopsy
> Echocardiogram for LVF and RVSP
> 6 Minute Walk Test or Ambulatory Saturation
> Nocturnal Oximetry or Overnight Sleep Study

Figure 233-2 *Standardized evaluation for Interstitial Lung Disease (ILD). A standardized evaluation for a new diagnosis of ILD includes a comprehensive history and physical examination as well as pulmonary function tests (PFTs), chest computed tomography (CT) and targeted laboratory studies. In appropriate situations, bronchoscopy and/or surgical biopsy may be indicated. Assessment of oxygen requirement and cardiac function are relevant in many patients. ANA, antinuclear antibody; CBC, complete blood count; CCP, anticitrullinated protein antibody; CMP, comprehensive metabolic panel; CPK, creatine phosphokinase; DLCO, diffusing capacity of the lung for carbon monoxide; FH, family history; Jo-1, Jo-1 antibody; La, La antibody; LVF, left ventricular function; OTC, over the counter medication; P2, second heart sound; PMH, past medical history; RF, rheumatoid factor; RNP, ribonucleoprotein antibody; Ro, Ro antibody; RVSP, right ventricular systolic pressure; Scl70-anti, Scl70 antibody; SH, social history.*

It is more common in women, African Americans and people of Scandanavian and Irish descent. The diagnosis of pulmonary sarcoidosis is suggested by upper lobe interstitial changes on radiography with or without associated bilateral mediastinal and hilar lymph node enlargement (Figure 233-3). In contrast to many other forms of ILD, crackles on examination are a feature in later stage disease. Diagnosis is made by identification of noncaseating granulomas on biopsy of involved tissue. Pulmonary sarcoidosis is typically diagnosed by endobronchial biopsy, transbronchial lung biopsy or fine needle aspiration of involved lymph nodes. The clinical course is highly variable, with some individuals developing destructive fibrocavitary disease and others having asymptomatic lymph node enlargement.

■ AUTOIMMUNE ASSOCIATED ILD

Autoimmune-associated ILD should be suspected in young patients presenting with ILD in the setting of a constellation of systemic symptoms. In this case, the patient presented with pneumomediastinum

in the setting of new onset polymyositis. The recognition of systemic symptoms may be difficult in the context of a dramatic presentation. However, if these symptoms are identified, biochemical and serologic testing can quickly confirm the underlying diagnosis. While the sensitivity and specificity of studies may vary regionally, CPK, aldolase, ANA, RF, RNP, Ro/La, Scl-70 and myositis antibodies (including Jo-1) are useful as an initial screen.

■ DRUG ASSOCIATED ILD

Drug-associated ILD can be difficult to identify since the causative medication may have been present for months or years prior to the onset of lung disease. The number of medications associated with ILD is increasing rapidly. This is especially true of the many biological agents in clinical use, particularly in the treatment of autoimmune disease and malignancy. A useful resource for determining if a medication has been associated with the development of ILD is Pneumotox (www.pneumotox.com). The recognition of drug-associated ILD

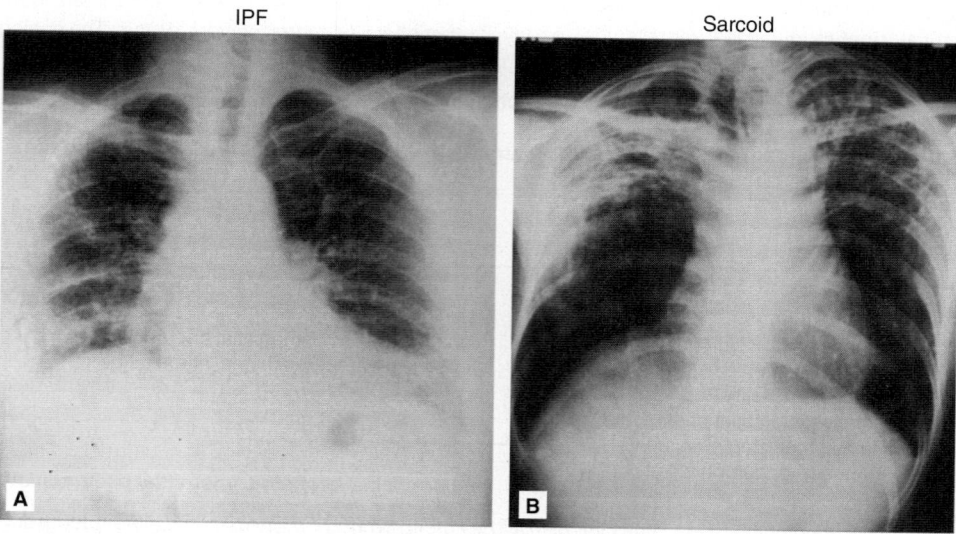

Figure 233-3 *Representative chest x-rays that can be seen in patients with idiopathic pulmonary fibrosis (IPF) and sarcoid. IPF is characterized by basilar predominant interstitial markings. By contrast, sarcoid typically shows an upper lobe distribution of fibrosis which may also be accompanied by bilateral hilar adenopathy.*

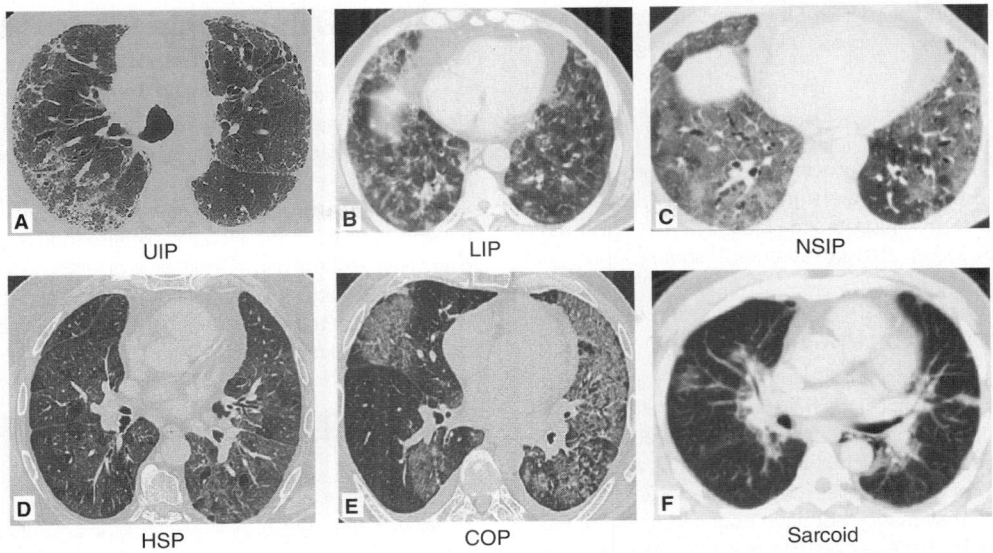

UIP   LIP   NSIP

HSP   COP   Sarcoid

Figure 233-4 *Representative computed tomography (CT) patterns that can be seen in patients with interstitial lung disease (ILD). ILD can be characterized by many different radiographic patterns. With the exception of usual interstitial pneumonia (UIP), there is substantial overlap among different forms of ILD. A number of the patterns are shown with the associated pathology noted. (A) Usual interstitial pneumonia (UIP) is characterized by honeycombing, traction bronchiectasis and increased reticular markings. (B) Lymphocytic interstitial pneumonia (LIP) may demonstrate a micronodular pattern. (C) Nonspecific interstitial pneumonia (NSIP) often appears as a diffuse GGO. (D) Hypersensitivity pneumonitis (HSP) appears as a nearly homogeneous pattern of GGO. (E) Cryptogenic organizing pneumonia (COP) appears as a patchy infiltrate which may be GGO or dense. (F) Sarcoid can present with bronchovascular infiltrates and hilar adenopathy.*

depends on ruling out other potential etiologies such as heart failure or an underlying autoimmune disease. In addition to evaluating prescription medications, patients should be asked about over-the-counter and herbal remedies as well as dietary supplements. Discontinuation of the offending medication results in improvement of symptoms within weeks to months. Some patients may require a several week course of systemic corticosteroids to limit lung injury while the medication is washing out.

■ HYPERSENSITIVITY PNEUMONITIS

Hypersensitivity pneumonitis (HP) is caused by an inappropriate inflammatory response to an environmental exposure. Hypersensitivity pneumonitis may present as an acute febrile, flu-like illness but may progress to a chronic phase that results in lung fibrosis. Characteristic findings include a mixed restrictive/obstructive pattern on pulmonary function testing and a CT with a combination of ground glass opacities and air trapping (Figure 233-4). It may be difficult to distinguish HP from other fibrosing lung diseases such as fibrotic NSIP and IPF. While the history may be suggestive of a potential offending antigen, it is often difficult to identify the cause. Common occupations associated with HP include farming, chemical manufacturing and bird breeding. Household exposures include mold, hot tub exposures and domestic and farm animals (ie, house birds and chickens). The key to treatment is identifying the causative agent and eliminating continued exposure. In situations in which the cause remains unclear, a trial of immunosuppression may help in slowing the progression of disease.

DIAGNOSIS

■ CLINICAL FEATURES

The presenting symptoms of dyspnea, cough and fatigue are common to a number of more prevalent diseases including pneumonia, heart failure, and COPD. A detailed history may bring out features which are helpful in discriminating these potential diagnoses. Have the symptoms truly been acute or has there been a more protracted period of decline? While ILD may have a fulminant acute

presentation, many patients when prompted will give a history of a more subacute decline preceding the acute illness. Have the symptoms responded appropriately to a reasonable therapeutic intervention? Patients who fail to respond to multiple courses of antibiotics or who have worsening dyspnea on exertion despite prior efforts at diuresis should raise the concern for ILD.

Ultimately the diagnosis is based on a comprehensive history and physical (Figure 233-2). The history is critical in initially diagnosing ILD and distinguishing IPF with its very poor prognosis from other potentially more treatable forms of ILD. Many a patient with bird fancier's lung has passed through the hands of capable physicians who neglected to ask about environmental exposures. It is not unusual to find that a patient has been seen and hospitalized repeatedly for pneumonia or bronchitis.

Physical findings on pulmonary examination may be nonspecific with crackles or squeaks or normal sounds. Perhaps the most useful finding is the basilar predominant "velcro" crackles often heard in IPF. Clubbing is variably associated with ILD, but may occur with other pulmonary and nonpulmonary disorders. Systemic signs of autoimmune disease (Raynaud's, arthritis, rash) can be helpful in raising the suspicion for a collagen vascular disease-associated ILD.

■ PULMONARY FUNCTION TESTING (PFT)

The role of spirometry in the monitoring of airways disease (COPD, asthma) in the hospitalized patient is well established. Less so is the role of pulmonary function testing in the patient with ILD. The classic features of ILD are restrictive, including forced vital capacity less than 80% predicted for age without evidence of obstruction, and total lung capacity less than 80% predicted. In addition, diffusing capacity (DLCO) is typically reduced with a single breath DLCO less than 80% predicted. In the acute setting PFTs are often deferred; however, establishing posttreatment PFTs are invaluable in subsequent patient care. Not only do PFTs provide an objective measure of disease severity, they can provide an important clue as to coexistent pulmonary hypertension (PH) if the DLCO is reduced out of proportion to the lung volumes. This may also be seen in patients who develop ILD in the setting of concurrent emphysema, appropriately named combined pulmonary fibrosis with emphysema.

IMAGING

Chest radiographs may show increased interstitial markings or reticulo-nodular changes which provide an initial suggestion of ILD. High-resolution chest CT scans are significantly more helpful, with representative CT patterns illustrated in Figure 233-4. A diagnosis of IPF can be made by a characteristic radiograph and exclusion of all other etiologies.

BRONCHOSCOPY AND LUNG BIOPSY

Definitive histologic diagnosis of IIPs other than IPF depends on lung biopsy. Bronchoalveolar lavage may be helpful in the diagnosis of infection which may complicate or mimic ILD. It is also useful for assessment of eosinophilia which is characteristic of a number of forms of ILD. Transbronchial biopsies may be diagnostic for sarcoidosis or for excluding malignancy but have poor sensitivity for diagnosing most other ILDs. Recently, a cryoprobe has been developed that can obtain larger bronchoscopic biopsy specimens although its utility in diagnosing ILD has not been established.

Surgical biopsy diagnosis should be reserved for patients with atypical presentations or who fail to respond appropriately to initial therapy. The decision to pursue surgical biopsy in a hospitalized patient with suspected ILD should be made in consultation with a pulmonologist. Patients with ILD frequently have multiple comorbidities that may complicate surgical biopsy, such as underlying cardiac disease. Many anecdotal reports suggest exacerbation of lung disease in the setting of a surgical lung biopsy. These exacerbations may be life threatening and often result in a permanent decrement in lung function. This risk should temper the decision to pursue surgical biopsy in many patients. In addition, many patients do not need biopsies. ILD presenting in the setting of a known trigger (such as medication or autoimmune disease) rarely requires a tissue diagnosis.

PRACTICE POINT

- Early involvement of pulmonary consultation in patients with suspected ILD is critical due to the potential complexity of diagnosis and the need for long-term follow-up. A specialist should become involved early in the hospitalization to guide diagnostic and therapeutic decision making. Patients with a new diagnosis of ILD need to establish care with a pulmonologist with experience in this field.

DISTINGUISHING IPF FROM OTHER ILDS

It is critical to distinguish IPF from other causes of interstitial lung disease because the approach to long-term management is fundamentally different. A surgical biopsy with findings of usual interstitial pneumonia (UIP) is not pathognomonic for IPF. Several other causes of ILD, including collagen vascular disease and hypersensitivity pneumonitis, may be associated with a UIP pattern of injury. Many ILDs are inflammatory in nature and respond to long-term immunosuppressive therapy. However, IPF does not respond to immunosuppression or anti-inflammatory medications. Immunosuppressive therapy, particularly the combination of prednisone and azathioprine, leads to worse outcomes in IPF patients. Newer antifibrotic therapies such as pirfenidone and nintedanib slow the rate of lung function decline in some patients with IPF but, to date, no therapy is available that reverses the course of this fatal disease. The role of the newer antifibrotic agents in other ILDs remains unknown.

TRIAGE AND HOSPITAL ADMISSION
CRITERIA FOR HOSPITAL ADMISSION

Patients with known ILD who experience significant respiratory decline frequently benefit from hospitalization for treatment of infection, cardiac comorbidity or intensification of immunosuppression. Since the etiology of worsening dyspnea is often uncertain at admission, a thoughtful evaluation is required in all ILD patients. Patients with ILD typically have exercise induced hypoxemia. However, new resting hypoxemia or worsening exercise desaturation requires evaluation. It is critical to assess patients both at rest and with exertion. Frequently, minimal exertion such as talking, standing or walking, will reveal desaturation.

PRACTICE POINT

- Any patient with new resting hypoxemia merits hospital admission. Patients with worsening exercise desaturation may require inpatient evaluation. Clinicians should assess patients both at rest and with exertion.

It is challenging to recognize a new diagnosis of ILD in a patient admitted for progressive dyspnea or hypoxemia. This diagnosis requires a high level of suspicion on the part of the treating physician as symptoms and signs may be nonspecific. Any patient with a new diagnosis of ILD should undergo a standardized evaluation for possible etiology (Figure 233-2).

CRITERIA FOR ICU ADMISSION

The admission of patients with ILD to the ICU continues to be a controversial decision. For some patients, ICU care including intubation is both appropriate and lifesaving. This group includes patients with pulmonary manifestations of autoimmune disease. The role of intubation is less certain in IPF patients with an acute exacerbation. An acute exacerbation of IPF is defined as a decline in lung function in the absence of an inciting event such as infection (**Table 233-2**). The survival rate following intubation in this setting is extremely poor. Patients and their families should be appropriately advised regarding the potential for ventilator dependence. Ultimately, the benefit of ICU care is dependent on the precipitating event and the potential to reverse this event without significant long-lasting lung injury.

MANAGEMENT
GENERAL APPROACH

The appropriate management of patients admitted to the hospital for pulmonary decompensation from ILD depends on accurate identification of the precipitating event. In general, ILD decompensation may be divided into pulmonary and nonpulmonary categories. Pulmonary etiologies include worsening of underlying ILD (ie, acute exacerbations of IPF), infections, pneumothorax, and thromboembolic disease. Nonpulmonary etiologies of ILD decompensation include cardiac dysfunction (ie, pulmonary hypertension, right heart failure, left heart failure, or ischemia) and neuromuscular dysfunction. All patients with pulmonary decompensation should undergo chest imaging. Chest CT imaging can identify significant infections and is more sensitive to changes in underlying lung disease including the appearance of new ground glass opacities. If there is a suspicion for thromboembolic disease, chest CT with IV contrast provides a simple method for evaluation. However, CT imaging is often not adequate for differentiating infection versus inflammation. Empiric treatment of possible infection should be considered since ILD patients typically have limited pulmonary reserve. Cultures including sputum and blood should be obtained if the patient is febrile

TABLE 233-2 Diagnosis of Acute Exacerbation of Idiopathic Pulmonary Fibrosis (IPF)

Diagnostic criteria:

Previous or concurrent diagnosis of idiopathic pulmonary fibrosis*

Unexplained worsening or development of dyspnea within 30 d

High-resolution computed tomography with new bilateral ground-glass abnormality and/or consolidation superimposed on a background reticular or honeycomb pattern consistent with usual interstitial pneumonia pattern**

No evidence of pulmonary infection by endotracheal aspirate or bronchoalveolar lavage***

Exclusion of alternative causes, including the following:

- Left heart failure
- Pulmonary embolism
- Identifiable cause of acute lung injury§

Patients with idiopathic clinical worsening who fail to meet all five criteria due to missing data should be termed "suspected acute exacerbations."
*If the diagnosis of idiopathic pulmonary fibrosis is not previously established according to American Thoracic Society/European Respiratory Society consensus criteria, this criterion can be met by the presence of radiologic and/or histopathologic changes consistent with usual interstitial pneumonia pattern on the current evaluation.
**If no previous high-resolution computed tomography is available, the qualifier "new" can be dropped.
***Evaluation of samples should include studies for routine bacterial organisms, opportunistic pathogens, and common viral pathogens.
§Causes of acute lung injury include sepsis, aspiration, trauma, reperfusion pulmonary edema, pulmonary contusion, fat embolization, inhalational injury, cardiopulmonary bypass, drug toxicity, acute pancreatitis, transfusion of blood products, and stem cell transplantation.
(Reproduced with permission from Collard HR, Moore BB, Flaherty KR, et al. Acute exacerbations of idiopathic pulmonary fibrosis. *Am J Respir Crit Care Med.* 2007;176(7):636-643.)

or exhibits cough productive of sputum. Bronchoscopy or induced sputum should be considered for patients with dry cough. Opportunistic infection (eg, *Pneumocystis jiroveci* [PCP]) should be considered and ruled out if the patient is immunosuppressed.

Cardiac disease is increasingly recognized as a major comorbidity in ILD. Both pulmonary hypertension and acute coronary syndrome (ACS) should be considered in the hospitalized patient with ILD. Echocardiography may show transiently elevated right heart pressures; right heart catheterization is generally advisable prior to starting therapy for PH in patients with ILD. Other common comorbidities in ILD patients include depression and anxiety, sleep disordered breathing, gastroesophageal reflux disease and diabetes mellitus. These disorders impact the presentation of a pulmonary decompensation and often require specific therapy.

PRACTICE POINT

- In ILD decompensation, echocardiogram may show transient moderately elevated right heart pressures. However, findings of severe pulmonary hypertension, right ventricular (RV) enlargement, or decreased RV function should prompt further evaluation for alternate etiologies of the PH including exclusion of thromboembolic disease.

TREATMENT AND MONITORING

Inpatient treatment of ILD patients must be tailored to the etiology of decompensation. The treatment of acute exacerbations of IPF involves pulse corticosteroids (1 g IV methylprednisolone daily for three doses). Prednisone is then administered at 1 mg/kg oral daily dose for 2 to 4 weeks. In the setting of high-dose steroids, prophylaxis for PCP should be started. The newer antifibrotic agents (pirfenidone and nintedanib) have not been studied in the setting of IPF exacerbations and should not be initiated in the hospital without the consultation of a pulmonologist familiar with their use.

The most significant complication associated with pulmonary decompensation is a lasting decline in lung function. The occurrence of pulmonary exacerbations is clearly associated with poorer prognosis. Oxygen requirements may require frequent reassessment.

DISCHARGE PLANNING

Prior to discharge, patients should be evaluated for both resting and exercise oxygen requirements to maintain an oxygen saturation greater than 88%. Nocturnal oxygen use is indicated for patients with nocturnal desaturation. A common problem encountered in discharge planning is high supplemental oxygen requirements. In general, patients are able to receive up to 6 L/min by nasal cannula. Beyond this oxygen level, patients may require face-mask oxygen at home. If the goals at discharge are for rehabilitation in a recovering patient, plans to reassess oxygen requirement and decrease oxygen use should be made at discharge. Patients may also use home pulse oximetry monitoring to allow more autonomy in titrating oxygen. Patients and their families should be aware that maintaining oxygen saturation greater than or equal to 88% is the goal. Oxygen may be reduced or taken off at rest if this criterion is met. Conversely, oxygen should be increased with activity to maintain this goal. For secondary prevention, patients should receive the pneumonia vaccine (if not previously vaccinated or boosted) and influenza vaccine if appropriate to the season. Follow-up with a pulmonary specialist is indicated for all patients with ILD.

QUALITY IMPROVEMENT: A MULTIDISCIPLINARY APPROACH TO ILD

Care of patients with ILD is best accomplished by a multidisciplinary approach. While definitive therapies for some forms of ILD are not available, there is increasing evidence that patients with ILD benefit from formalized pulmonary rehabilitation. Like vaccination, this simple intervention may improve patient survival and quality of life.

In addition to active interventions aimed at prolonging life, attention to quality of life, particularly in the end stage of ILD, is critical. Understanding and transmitting prognosis accurately and sensitively is a key component of patient care. Patients newly diagnosed with ILD are frequently unaware of the often poor prognosis, particularly with IPF. Reassuring patients and their families regarding the ability to keep patients comfortable at the end of life is critical. Involve a pulmonary specialist to help patients understand available therapeutic options. While discussions of end-of-life decisions are often more appropriate in the outpatient setting, the frequency of acute exacerbations means that these discussions are also needed in the acute inpatient setting. Involvement of hospice care may be helpful particularly for patients with acute exacerbations of IPF for whom improvement in function is unlikely.

SUGGESTED READINGS

An Official ATS/ERS/JRS/ALAT Statement: Idiopathic Pulmonary Fibrosis: Evidence-based Guidelines for Diagnosis and Management. *Am J Respir Crit Care Med.* 2011;183:788-824.

An official American Thoracic Society/European Respiratory Society statement: update of the international multidisciplinary classification of the idiopathic interstitial pneumonias. *Am J Respir Crit Care Med.* 2013;188(6):733-748.

Collard HR, Moore BB, Flaherty KR, et al. Acute exacerbations of idiopathic pulmonary fibrosis. *Am J Respir Crit Care Med.* 2007;176(7):636-643.

Cordier JF. Cryptogenic organising pneumonia. *Eur Respir J.* 2006; 28(2):422-446.

Johkoh T. Imaging of idiopathic interstitial pneumonias. *Clin Chest Med.* 2008;29(1):133-147, vi.

King TE Jr, Tooze JA, Schwarz MI, Brown KR, Cherniack RM. Predicting survival in idiopathic pulmonary fibrosis: scoring system and survival model. *Am J Respir Crit Care Med.* 2001;164(7):1171-1181.

Nakamura Y, Chida K, Suda T, et al. Nonspecific interstitial pneumonia in collagen vascular diseases: comparison of the clinical characteristics and prognostic significance with usual interstitial pneumonia. *Sarcoidosis Vasc Diffuse Lung Dis.* 2003;20(3):235-241.

Spagnolo P, Wells AU, Collard HR. Pharmacological treatment of idiopathic pulmonary fibrosis: an update. *Drug Discov Today.* 2015;20(5): 514-524.

Vassallo R, Ryu JH. Tobacco smoke-related diffuse lung diseases. *Semin Respir Crit Care Med.* 2008;29(6):643-650.

Vourlekis JS, Brown KK, Schwarz MI. Acute interstitial pneumonitis: current understanding regarding diagnosis, pathogenesis, and natural history. *Semin Respir Crit Care Med.* 2001;22(4):399-408.

CHAPTER 234

Cystic Fibrosis

William R. Hunt, MD
David Tong, MD, MPH
Arlene Stecenko, MD

Key Clinical Questions

1. How do mutations in the cystic fibrosis (CF) gene relate to the clinical manifestations of the disease?

2. What criteria help determine when a CF patient should be admitted to the hospital for respiratory complications of the disease?

3. What treatment modalities are most effective in restoring lung function to baseline for CF respiratory exacerbations?

4. Why is CF-related diabetes (CFRD) important to control during acute pulmonary exacerbations as well as at baseline?

5. What are the most effective treatment modalities for the two most common pulmonary complications of CF: massive hemoptysis and pneumothorax?

INTRODUCTION

DEFINITION AND OVERVIEW

Cystic fibrosis (CF) is an autosomal recessive disease due to mutations in the CF transmembrane conductance regulator (CFTR) gene. The CFTR gene is expressed in epithelial cells in a variety of organs including the lung, sinuses, pancreas, sweat gland, intestine, liver, and vas deferens, and thus CF is a multiorgan disease. CF is the most common inherited life-shortening disease of Caucasians in the United States. More than 90% of the morbidity and the mortality are due to lung disease. CF lung disease is characterized by the triad of altered mucociliary clearance, chronic polymicrobial infection of the airways, and an exaggerated inflammatory response. The ultimate outcome of CF lung disease is destruction of the normal airway architecture and death due to respiratory failure.

With therapy, primarily aimed at slowing the progression of lung disease and improving nutrition, median survival is approaching 40 years of age. Unfortunately, there is no cure for CF. However, for CF patients with select CFTR mutations, there have been recent advancements and FDA approval of CFTR potentiator/corrector medications. The first FDA approved CFTR potentiator, ivacaftor, exerts its effects by improving the function of the defective CFTR protein. Unfortunately, ivacaftor benefits a small segment (about 5%) of the CF population with specific CFTR mutations (eg, G551D). More recently, a combination pill comprised of the potentiator ivacaftor and a CFTR corrector, lumacaftor, has been approved for CF patients homozygous for the ΔF508 mutation. This accounts for approximately 50% of the CF patients in North America. These medications are metabolized by the CYP3A system, and particular care must be taken by the hospitalist whenever additional medications that alter CYP3A function (such as many anti-fungal medications) are added into the therapeutic regimen for CF patients currently on one of these CFTR potentiator/corrector medications. Despite these therapeutic advancements, clinical improvements for patients with CF on these newer medications remain modest. As such, there remains ongoing aggressive research and development for other CFTR potentiators and correctors. The average CF adult can expect to spend 2 to 3 hours a day taking a variety of inhaled medications, ingest 30 to 50 pills per day, and be hospitalized about once per year for a period of a few days to weeks. Even with insurance, most CF patients have out-of-pocket health care costs approximately $10,000 per year.

In contrast, some CF patients with lung function within the normal range rarely require hospitalizations and need few medications to control their disease. Thus, tremendous variability exists in the severity of the pulmonary phenotype in this monogenic disease, ranging from death in childhood due to respiratory failure to living to retirement and the thought of enjoyment of family and friends through middle age and into old age.

GENETIC EPIDEMIOLOGY—INCIDENCE AND ETHNIC DISTRIBUTION

The incidence of CF varies tremendously according to ethnicity. In the United States CF occurs in about 1 in 3500 Caucasian births, 1 in 17,000 African Americans, and 1 in 90,000 Asians in Hawaii. Once considered a disease affecting only children, the life expectancy in CF has increased dramatically in the past 3 decades. Now 41% of CF patients are over 18 years of age, and the median predicted survival in 2013 is 40.7 years.

PATHOPHYSIOLOGY

The CFTR protein is a chloride channel in the apical aspect of epithelium in a variety of organs, including the lungs, sweat ducts, vas deferens, liver, pancreas, and intestines. Through unknown mechanisms, expression of mutant CFTR and the resultant failure to conduct chloride also causes marked increase in sodium import through the epithelial sodium channel, ENaC. In the lung epithelium, this results in marked reduction in the depth of the airway surface lining fluid and loss of effective mucociliary clearance. Expression of mutant CFTR also results in failure to export glutathione to the extracellular compartment, resulting in extremely low levels of antioxidant capacity in the epithelial lining fluid and more susceptibility to damage. CFTR may be additionally expressed in pancreatic beta cells, thus providing a potential molecular mechanism for the very high prevalence of diabetes in CF.

Expression of mutant CFTR, particularly in neutrophils and airway epithelial cells, results in an abnormal proinflammatory response characterized by an excessive and persistent neutrophil dominated inflammation. The CF airway shows a tremendous preponderance of neutrophils even shortly after birth. These neutrophils are a source of elastase and reactive oxygen species that destroy lung tissue. Furthermore, dying neutrophils in the CF lung do not undergo apoptosis but rather necrosis, resulting in release of massive amounts of sticky, uncoiled DNA that markedly increases the viscosity of airway secretions.

Persistent airway bacterial infection (particularly with *Pseudomonas aeruginosa* and *Staphyloccocus aureus*) is the hallmark of CF lung disease, and proposed mechanisms for this include defective phagocytosis, defective intracellular killing, increase in the number of receptors for bacteria on epithelial cells, and promotion of biofilm formation by the bacteria.

The CFTR gene (chromosome 7) has more than 1800 disease causing mutations within six classes (**Table 234-1**). The most common mutation, ΔF508, accounts for 66% of the CF mutations worldwide. About 15 mutations may account for 80% to 90% of the mutations seen in Caucasians.

Mutations where there is little or no full length CFTR at the outer plasma membrane are considered "severe" and those where there is a full length protein, but in some way the protein has defective

TABLE 234-1 Class of Gene Defects

Class	Mutation Example	Cellular/Molecular Phenotype
I	W1282X	Absent CFTR production due to nonsense mutations, frameshift mutations, or abnormal mRNA splicing
II	ΔF508	Improper intracellular processing of CFTR with less than normal amounts of CFTR protein at the apical plasma membrane
III	G551D	Defective regulation of CFTR channels at the apical plasma membrane
IV	R117H	Defective permeation of anions through CFTR channels at the apical plasma membrane
V	3849 + 10KbC > T	Reduced synthesis of normal CFTR
VI	Q1412X	Altered apical membrane residence time of CFTR channels with truncated c-termini

CFTR, cystic fibrosis transmembrane receptor.
Reproduced, with permission, from Kreindler JL. *Pharmacol Ther.* 2010;125: 219-229.

function, are considered "mild." However, significant discordance between gene mutations and severity of lung disease suggests the importance of modifier genes and environmental interactions in disease expression, and explains why two cystic fibrosis patients with the same gene defect in the CFTR gene can present with very different disease severity and clinical course.

Cystic fibrosis may affect multiple organs, but the vast majority of morbidity and mortality occurs due to lung disease. The triad of impaired mucociliary clearance, persistent airway infection, and exaggerated inflammatory response leads to bronchiectasis and ultimately respiratory failure and death. Lung function declines progressively in most CF patients, with an annual rate of decline in function varying from 1% to 4% per year. The rate of decline may be punctuated by acute pulmonary exacerbations with precipitous drops in lung function and incomplete recovery from the exacerbation. Resetting of baseline lung function at a new lower level may occur following respiratory exacerbations. Frequent respiratory exacerbations are the hallmark of lung disease severity in CF, and significantly impact quality of life, health care costs and survival.

The cause of acute pulmonary exacerbations is currently unknown but likely related to increased bacterial load rather than infection by a different strain of bacteria. Other risk factors include increased exposure to particulate air pollutants and viral infections (eg, influenza virus, respiratory syncytial virus). However, nearly 20% of CF pulmonary exacerbations have no identified inciting cause.

DIFFERENTIAL DIAGNOSIS

The diagnosis of CF should be considered in patients with any of the following conditions:

- Symptoms of chronic obstructive pulmonary disease (COPD) or asthma who are not responding as expected to treatment
- Bronchiectasis of unknown etiology
- Isolation of mucoid *Pseudomonas* in a person with chronic respiratory symptoms
- Isolated pancreatitis or recurrent pancreatitis unexplained by alcohol, medications, or gallstones
- Pansinusitis
- Nasal polyps in healthy adolescents younger than 20 years old
- Male infertility (as males born with CF have nearly 100% congenital absence of the vas deferens)

DIAGNOSIS

CF may be suspected in a patient because of having one or more characteristic phenotypic symptoms (see differential diagnosis), a positive history of CF in a sibling, or a positive newborn screen (performed in all US states). The diagnosis of CF is made by two positive sweat chloride results done on separate days using quantitative pilocarpine iontophoresis in a clinical laboratory certified by the Cystic Fibrosis Foundation. However, a small, but not insignificant, portion of patients with clinical symptoms concerning for CF will have a sweat chloride in the indeterminate or normal range. In this situation, a CFTR genotype and sequencing can identify whether the person has two disease-causing mutations. Additionally, all CF patients should undergo gene sequencing to identify whether they carry a mutation responsive to a CFTR potentiator (ie, ivacaftor) as well as to provide information on prognosis.

In 2013, 65% of all CF cases were diagnosed by newborn screen. Prior to newborn screening, about 3% to 5% of CF patients were diagnosed as adults. This number will decrease with time, but it will take several years to decades before diagnosis of CF in adulthood is a rarity. In addition, many states screen only for the most common mutations and thus newborn screening may not identify all persons with CF.

PULMONARY EXACERBATION DIAGNOSTIC TESTING

Diagnostic testing in the setting of acute pulmonary CF exacerbation should include CF sputum cultures (using the Cystic Fibrosis Foundation approved methods for detecting polymicrobial isolates), complete blood count, comprehensive chemistry panel, and posterior-anterior and lateral chest x-ray. Pregnancy test should be obtained for the women of childbearing age. CF patients with change in symptoms should undergo the pulmonary function testing (PFTs) with spirometry to assess FEV_1 and any change from the patient's baseline level. A significant decrease in FEV_1 from baseline (even with unimpressive symptoms or physical examination) may prompt inpatient admission for IV antibiotics rather than outpatient management.

Additional testing for patients who have not responded to standard treatment of a CF pulmonary exacerbation as expected may include sputum for fungal stain and cultures, sputum for acid fast bacilli (AFB), and immunoglobulin (Ig) E level (to evaluate for allergic bronchopulmonary aspergillosis, [ABPA]).

Chest computed tomography (CT) is *not* necessary for treatment of routine acute pulmonary exacerbations. However, if suspicion for lung abscess, pulmonary embolus, or nontuberculous mycobacteria (NTM) is high, chest CT may be helpful.

Follow-up inpatient PFTs may be considered to document recovery of lung function after initiation of therapy, but acutely in the hospital setting the results may be discordant with the patient's clinical course. Therefore, inpatient surveillance PFTs (prior to completion of antimicrobial course for CF pulmonary exacerbation) are not indicated in most situations.

For patients with cystic fibrosis-related diabetes (CFRD) who are doing carbohydrate counting to dose their insulin, 2-hour postprandial blood sugars should be obtained in addition to preprandial and bedtime blood sugars in order to determine if failure to achieve glycemic control is responsible for failure to restore lung function to baseline.

Sinus CT is only indicated based on significant new sinus symptoms during the patient presentation. They should not be ordered routinely for pulmonary exacerbation in the absence of new sinus symptoms or signs.

TRIAGE/HOSPITAL ADMISSION

Although there is currently no standard definition of an acute pulmonary exacerbation in CF, a number of different criteria have been devised for clinical trials and clinical care. The majority of definitions capture respiratory symptoms such as increased cough, increased sputum production, shortness of breath and chest pain, as well as other measures such as loss of appetite, fatigue, and missing either work or school. However, CF clinicians put the most reliance on a decrease in lung function and will diagnose a pulmonary exacerbation in the absence of any reported change in symptoms if there is a significant decrease in FEV_1. This may be particularly true in those exacerbations that develop over a period of a few weeks and the patient is simply unaware of how much symptoms have increased until lung function and symptoms return to baseline following appropriate treatment.

Treatment of the exacerbation, if not severe, begins with outpatient oral antibiotics, increase in airway clearance, and emphasis on compliance with chronic pulmonary medications. More frequent clinic visits and greater use of antibiotics is associated with better PFT results. Close follow-up, usually within a week or two, is needed to make sure lung function has returned to the patient's baseline.

If lung function does not improve despite a trial of oral antibiotics, then the standard of care is hospital admission to start intravenous (IV) antibiotics and ensure aggressive airway clearance. Once inpatient therapy with IV antibiotics has been initiated and

tolerated by the patient, and the patient is clinically improving, then it may be possible to complete the remainder of the treatment in the patient's home setting. It is very important that intravenous antibiotics in a nonhospital setting not be done unless resources and support equivalent to the hospital setting can be assured for the treatment entirety of an acute CF pulmonary exacerbation. Issues to consider when deciding whether completion of IV antibiotics therapy can be performed in the outpatient setting include the severity of the exacerbation, patient comfort and safety for maintaining long term central venous access, whether adequate delivery of other treatments such as airway clearance therapies can be maintained, and the presence of co-morbidities such as malnutrition and diabetes that may require inpatient care. It is not uncommon for a CF patient to receive two or three different IV antibiotics for therapy of their CF pulmonary exacerbation. The potential IV antibiotic therapy has to be of a reasonable regimen so as to allow the patient accurate dosing. For example, it is rarely feasible for a patient to solely administer an IV antibiotic every 4 to 6 hours for 14 to 21 consecutive days without having a missed antibiotic administration time or significant sleep deprivation. Also, as many IV antibiotics routinely used for treatment of a CF pulmonary exacerbation require frequent blood monitoring, it is very important that a specialized team closely follow the outpatient on IV antibiotic therapy to ensure that they are continuing to respond to antibiotics and appropriate blood test are being monitored at proper intervals. With careful patient selection, support, and close monitoring, completing IV antibiotic therapy in the home setting following hospitalization is a reasonable option.

Hemoptysis, often a sign of pulmonary exacerbation, is a common presenting complaint, occurring in about 9% of CF patients and can range from slight streaking to massive bleeding. Massive hemoptysis (which occurs in 4% of CF patients) is defined as more than 240 mL of blood in a 24-hour period. It is due to arterial bleeding from hypertrophied bronchial arteries. There are no evidence-based data to guide triage of hemoptysis in CF patients, but current consensus-based recommendations from the Cystic Fibrosis Foundation are that patients with at least mild hemoptysis (measured as > 5 mL) should contact their health care provider and scant hemoptysis (< 5 mL) should contact their health care provider if it is the first ever episode or if it persists.

Scant hemoptysis may not require hospital admission if there is no other evidence of a significant acute pulmonary exacerbation, but massive hemoptysis (> 240 mL) always requires hospital admission. Given the potential for significant morbidity, most, if not all, cases of massive hemoptysis should be admitted to an ICU setting.

About 3% of CF patients will have a pneumothorax during their lifetime with an annual incidence of about 1 in 167 patients, with attributable mortality as high as 16%. Disease severity predicts pneumothorax complication, with 75% of pneumothoraces occurring in patients with an FEV_1 < 40% predicted. CF patients with a pneumothorax should almost always be admitted to the hospital as the risk of progression and further respiratory compromise is high.

PRACTICE POINT

Pulmonary exacerbation
- Consider the diagnosis if there is a significant decrease in FEV_1 even in the absence of any reported change in symptoms.
- Glucocorticoid steroids are **not** routinely recommended for the treatment of a CF pulmonary exacerbation.

Hemoptysis
- Pulmonary exacerbation often manifest with mild hemoptysis; > 5 mL of blood should be treated with antibiotics.

- Bronchial artery embolization (BAE) is the initial treatment for massive hemoptysis. There is little evidence that bronchoscopy can localize bleeding in these patients, and it may delay a lifesaving procedure.

Pneumothorax

- All CF patients with a pneumothorax should be admitted to the hospital, regardless of size.
- Surgical pleurodesis with video assisted thorascopic surgery (VATS) is the preferred treatment for recurrent pneumothorax, and should be done soon to avoid respiratory infections related to splinting and immobility.

MANAGEMENT

■ ACUTE PULMONARY EXACERBATION MANAGEMENT

Many, if not most, of the large, multicenter, double-blind, placebo-controlled clinical trials evaluating efficacy of pulmonary drugs in CF have been for outpatient management to prevent respiratory exacerbations, rather than for the management of an exacerbation once it is severe enough to require hospitalization. Therefore, recommendations for inpatient treatment rely on limited studies of small number of patients and on expert opinion. An inpatient admission protocol for CF patients with an acute respiratory exacerbation provides specific details of care in addition to being an educational tool for hospital staff.

The current mainstay of treatment for inpatient management of acute respiratory exacerbations consists of IV antibiotics and enhanced airway clearance. In addition, pulmonary and nonpulmonary complications of CF that may impair the ability to restore lung function to baseline require evaluation and management; and nutritional support must be addressed. *P. aeruginosa* is the most frequent organism found during an acute exacerbation. However, polymicrobial infections are also common, particularly with *Staphylococcus aureus* as well as multiple strains of *Pseudomonas*, each with a different pattern of antibiotic sensitivity. More recently, organisms previously thought to be commensals, such as *Stenotrophomonas maltophilia*, are now viewed as potentially pathogenic. Early isolates of pseudomonas are nonmucoid and have a broader range of antibiotic sensitivity. However, in the CF airway the organism can mutate to a mucoid form and also can form a biofilm. Such mutations, particularly toward a biofilm, may make antibiotics less effective.

Antimicrobials

The Cystic Fibrosis Foundation guidelines—for the treatment of a respiratory exacerbation in patients whose culture grows pseudomonas—recommend using two IV antibiotics of different classes (**Table 234-2**). Depending on the antibiotic sensitivities on the sputum culture, an aminoglycoside and a beta-lactam antibiotic is the preferred combination. Dual therapy may prevent the development of resistance and may have more benefit than monotherapy. There have been some clinical trials comparing monotherapy with combination therapy, but there is insufficient evidence due to the small number of patients in each trial to recommend one over the other.

If possible, a new sputum culture should be obtained at the initial presentation of the CF pulmonary exacerbation. So, as not to delay antibiotic therapy, initial antibiotic selection should be based on the most recent sputum susceptibility results and later adjusted if there is inadequate response. Antibiotics can be further tailored based on culture results and sensitivities obtained during the onset of the current exacerbation. Finally, if current sputum results indicate broad resistance with no good antibiotic options, a previously successful regimen may be started as initial therapy.

TABLE 234-2 Antibiotic Recommendations and Dosing for Acute Respiratory Exacerbations*

Pseudomonas only (Recommend two-drug therapy, tobramycin plus beta lactam if pseudomonas is sensitive)

Tobramycin 10 mg/kg IV every 24 h†

Amikacin 10 mg/kg IV every 8 h†

Ceftazidime 50 mg/kg IV every 8 h (max. 10 g/d)

Piperacillin-tazobactam 4.5 mg IV every 6 h

Meropenem 2 g IV every 8 h

Colistimethate 2.5 mg IV every 12 h

Aztreonam 2 g IV every 8 h (major indication is severe PCN or cephalosporin allergy)

Methicillin-sensitive *staphylococcus aureus* and *pseudomonas*. Recommend two-drug therapy: one of the following plus tobramycin 10 mg/kg/24 h if pseudomonas is sensitive

Ticarcillin-clavulanate 3.1 g IV every 4 h

Cefepime 2 g IV every 8 h

Meropenem 2 g IV every 8 h

Piperacillin-tazobactam 4.5 mg IV every 6 h

Methicillin-resistant *S aureus*

Linezolid 600 mg IV every 12 h

Tigecycline 100 mg bolus then 50 mg IV every 12 h

Vancomycin 15-20 mg/kg every 8–12 h§

*Dosing for normal renal function. Adjustments may be necessary when renal dysfunction is present.
†Pharmacokinetics or infectious diseases consultation recommended.
§Trough levels of 15-20 mcg/mL recommended.

Despite poor-to-moderate lung penetration, aminoglycosides are frequently used in the treatment of acute pulmonary exacerbations. CF patients, particularly those under 40 years of age, require higher doses than non-CF patients to achieve therapeutic blood levels. Also, once daily tobramycin dosing has been shown to be as effective as multiple daily dosing and is associated with less renal toxicity. Clinical pharmacy consultation is critical for monitoring aminoglycoside levels. Some patients may deserve concomitant inhaled aminoglycoside to offer improved action against *Pseudomonas* species infections.

Although some cystic fibrosis centers are routinely using continuous infusions of beta-lactam antibiotics in the treatment of acute pulmonary exacerbations, there are not enough data to support this practice routinely.

Renal function and relevant monitoring of electrolytes and blood counts may be necessary, depending on the antibiotic choices and known side effects. Infectious disease consultants should assist with antimicrobial selection and clinical pharmacists, when available, should assist with antimicrobial dosing and monitoring.

The ultimate goal of therapy is to restore lung function back to baseline and this can take from 10 to 21 days, or in some cases even longer. The optimal duration of intravenous antibiotic treatment for a CF pulmonary exacerbation is not known. Most often, repeat pulmonary function test are performed following a 14 to 21 day course of antibiotic therapy with the results informing whether antibiotic therapy has been successful and can be discontinued (ie, the patient's pulmonary function test have returned to baseline) or whether therapy should be further continued.

Chronic CF pulmonary therapies

During therapy for acute pulmonary exacerbations, chronic pulmonary maintenance therapies may be continued (**Table 234-3**).

TABLE 234-3 Chronic Pulmonary Maintenance Therapy

Inhaled

Dornase alpha 2.5 mg nebulized daily or twice a day

Aztreonam 75 mg nebulized three times a day for 1 mo every other month—can rotate with another aerosolized antibiotic

Tobramycin 300 mg nebulized twice a day for 1 mo every other month—can rotate with another aerosolized antibiotic*

Colistimethate 150 mg nebulized twice a day for 1 mo every other month—can rotate with another aerosolized antibiotic

Sodium chloride 7% 4 mL nebulized twice a day to three times a day for $FEV_1 > 40\%$. Most often hypertonic saline is preceded by inhaled beta-2 agent. Can be used in patients with lower lung function but may not be tolerated. In this situation, can use lower concentrations, like 5% or 3% but these have not been studied

Oral

Azithromycin 500 mg orally Monday, Wednesday, and Friday

Ivacaftor 150 mg orally every 12 h†

Lumacaftor/ivacaftor 400 mg/250 mg orally every 12 h§

Airway clearance therapies

Chest physiotherapy using manual, vest, Acapella valve twice a day

Active cycle breathing technique

Exercise¥

---

*An alternate dry powder formulation exists (TOBI podhaler). The recommended dosing is inhalation of four-28 mg capsules twice per day for 1 mo every other month.

†Only for patients with the following CFTR mutations: G551D, G1244E, G1349D, G178R, G551S, S1251N, S1255P, S549N, S549R, and R117H/5T.

§Only for patients whose genetic mutation is homozygous ΔF508

¥While exercise is important to overall physical health and encouraged, it should not be used as a replacement to other dedicated airway clearance therapies such as chest physiotherapy or active cycle breathing techniques.

CFTR modulators

In 2012, the first drug that targets the defective CFTR protein was approved by the US Food and Drug Administration for therapy in CF patients 6 years and older with specific CFTR mutations. Ivacaftor is a potentiator that binds to dysfunctional CFTR and increases the transport of chloride through the CFTR channel. However, ivacaftor exerts its effects on CFTR proteins that have been correctly trafficked to the cell surface, but otherwise do not conduct chloride effectively. As such, ivacaftor only works in specific CF mutations and has only been approved for CF patients with the following CFTR gene mutations: G551D, G1244E, G1349D, G178R, G551S, S1251N, S1255P, S549N, S549R, and R117H/5T.

In 2015, a combination pill that included a CFTR potentiator (ivacaftor) and a CFTR corrector (lumacaftor) was approved in the United States for CF patients 12 years old and older who are homozygous for the ΔF508 mutation (Orkambi™). This accounts for approximately 50% of the CF population in North America. However, the combination drug has not been extensively studied in patients under the age of 12 or with severe lung dysfunction ($FEV_1 < 40\%$ predicted).

Ivacaftor is a sensitive CYP3A substrate, and any new medications added to a CF patient's regimen that includes ivacaftor should be closely checked for drug interactions, particularly with drugs that are CYP3A inhibitors and inducers. For example, co-administration of ivacaftor with rifampin, a strong CYP3A inducer, greatly reduces the therapeutic effectiveness of ivacaftor. Therefore, it is recommended ivacaftor not be co-administered with strong CYP3A inducers such as rifampin, phenobarbital, carbamazepine or St. John's Wort. Inhibitors of CYP3A increase ivacaftor exposure and often require potentiator dosing adjustments. Common inhibitors of CYP3A include ketoconazole, voriconazole, and certain antibiotics such as clarithromycin and erythromycin. Additionally, grapefruits and Seville oranges inhibit CYP3A and should generally be avoided while a patient is on ivacaftor.

Macrolides

Azithromycin (500 mg 3 times per week) has immunomodulatory and anti-inflammatory properties, in addition to antimicrobial properties, and has been shown in large, multicenter, placebo-controlled studies to reduce the rate of hospitalizations for acute pulmonary exacerbations and improve FEV_1 in those patients infected with *P. aeruginosa*. Recent data indicate that the chronic use of azithromycin may be helpful in the CF patients with methicillin-resistant *S. aureus*.

Airway clearance

Airway clearance through increased chest physiotherapy (compared to home regimen, and up to 4 times per day) can improve exacerbation outcomes and improve symptoms more rapidly. Manual chest physiotherapy may be performed by respiratory care, nursing staff, physical therapists, other clinicians or family members. Mechanical chest physiotherapy using vibrating vests and Acapella devices may also be employed. In addition, aerosols aimed at improving clearance, such as inhaled 7% hypertonic saline and the endonuclease dornasealfa (Pulmozyme™), can be prescribed at increased frequencies.

Inhaled antibiotics

When chronically infected with *pseudomonas*, most CF patients are administered inhaled antibiotics that are usually delivered in 28 day on-off cycles (ie, 28 days on the therapy followed by 28 days off of the therapy). There are insufficient data to guide whether inhaled antibiotics should be continued or discontinued if similar IV antibiotics are given during an acute pulmonary exacerbation. Utilizing both routes of delivery could enhance antimicrobial activity in the lungs but could also increase the risk of toxicity. Therefore, the decision to continue dual route therapy should be made on an individual basis.

Glucocorticoid steroids

Systemic glucocorticoid steroids have been used in the past as adjunct therapy for a CF respiratory exacerbation. However, two placebo-controlled studies in a small number of children showed that the addition of glucocorticoid steroids to the regimen of IV antibiotics and enhanced airway clearance was no better than placebo in improving the recovery rate from the exacerbation. Glucocorticoid steroids also worsen hyperglycemia, which is known to contribute to oxidative stress and inflammation in the CF lung. Thus, glucocorticoid steroids are not routinely recommended for the treatment of a CF pulmonary exacerbation and some would suggest they are contraindicated because of side effects.

In the past, inhaled steroids have been prescribed with the goal of achieving the anti-inflammatory effects of glucocorticoids while limiting the harmful systemic side effects. However, the most recent Cochrane review of inhaled steroids in CF found no evidence that inhaled glucocorticoid steroids reduced inflammation in CF lungs. Additionally, there was some evidence that inhaled steroids may be harmful, particularly in increasing the risk of infection. As such, with the exception of concurrent asthma, use of inhaled corticosteroids in CF is not recommended.

Respiratory failure

Hypoxemic and hypercapneic respiratory failure may occur during hospitalization. In select patients who are alert and can maintain their airway, noninvasive positive pressure ventilation (NIPPV) may be employed to try to avoid endotracheal intubation and mechanical ventilation. NIPPV may unload respiratory muscles and work of breathing, increase minute ventilation and thereby improve gas exchange and alveolar ventilation. Patients with poor baseline status due to chronic progression often have difficulty liberating from mechanical ventilation. Discussions regarding end-of-life care should be done before acute intervention is required.

■ INFECTIOUS PULMONARY COMPLICATIONS

Burkholderia cepacia complex

Burkholderia cepacia complex is a group of Gram-negative rod bacteria comprised of at least 17 different species that are phenotypically indistinguishable (ie, genomovars). *B. cepacia complex* is found in the natural environment, and certain species are commonly multidrug resistant and in CF patients can produce a pronounced inflammatory response associated with rapid loss of lung function. The most common *B. cepacia complex* species found in CF patients include *B. cepacia, B. cenocepacia, B. multivorans, B. vietnamiensis, and B. dolosa.*

Patients with *B. cepacia complex* were noted to have a very high mortality following lung transplantation as the high dose immunosuppression needed to prevent acute rejection frequently resulted in wide spread dissemination of the *B. cepacia* and death from multiorgan failure. Upon closer evaluation, the significant mortality seen in CF patients post lung transplant was in patients with the specific genomovar *B. cenocepacia*. Consequently, many transplant centers view the presence of *B. cenocepacia* as an absolute contraindication to lung transplantation. However, as *B. cepacia complex* has a number of other species, some of which are not associated with significant lung function decline, some specialized transplant centers will consider possible lung transplantation in patients colonized with *B. cepacia complex* genomovars other than *B. cenocepacia*. As such, if a CF patient cultures *B. cepacia complex*, it is very important that further speciation be performed at a lab familiar with typing of this bacteria so that the specific genomovar can be identified.

Nontuberculous mycobacteria

Nontuberculous mycobacteria (NTM) should be considered in CF patients with unexplained fatigue, night sweats, hemoptysis or progressive decline in lung function that is not responding to usual CF pulmonary treatment. NTM infections are found in approximately 13% of CF adults in the United States. The most frequently isolated NTM species in CF are *Mycobacterium abscessus* and *Mycobacterium avium* complex (MAC). Infection is diagnosed by at least two NTM positive sputum cultures collected on different days or a positive bronchoalveolar lavage culture along with clinical and radiographic findings consistent with NTM disease. NTM pulmonary disease should be *treated for at least 12 to 18 months* usually with a multidrug regimen to prevent development of resistance. MAC can have some sensitivity to oral antibiotics commonly prescribed in CF, such as macrolides and fluoroquinolones. These medications should be avoided in patients who have had a single sputum culture positive for NTM, or clinical symptoms suspicion for NTM pulmonary disease, until the disease can be confirmed and appropriate multidrug therapy can be initiated. MAC pulmonary disease is treated with long-term multidrug therapy (usually daily rifampin, ethambutol and a macrolide) for 12 to 18 months. *M. abscessus* can be very difficult to treat and eradicate as this species is usually resistant to typical antituberculosis drugs. Therapy often consists of parenteral treatment with amikacin and cefoxitin or imipenem for 2 to 4 months followed by prolonged enteral and aerosol therapy with susceptible drugs. As NTM infections can be very difficult to treat, it is recommended that therapy be guided by close consultation with an infectious disease specialist.

Fungal infections

Aspergillus fumigatus can be isolated in 40% to 60% and *Candida albicans* in 20% to 30% of patients. *ABPA occurs in up to 10% of CF patients.* Invasive aspergillosis and aspergillomas are very uncommon. ABPA may be clinically indistinguishable from a CF exacerbation as both may present with airway obstruction, fleeting pulmonary infiltrates, bronchiectasis, and hemoptysis.

ABPA should be considered in a CF patient with deteriorating lung function that is not responding to standard CF treatment. The minimal diagnostic criterion to diagnose ABPA in CF is finding an acute or subacute clinical deterioration, total serum IgE level greater than 500 IU/mL, immediate cutaneous reactivity to *Aspergillus* or presence of anti-*Aspergillus* IgE antibodies and either IgG antibody to *A. fumigatus* or new chest imaging abnormalities.

Treatment for ABPA requires high dose glucocorticoid steroid therapy (oral prednisone at 0.5-2 mg/kg, max 60 mg/d) plus itraconazole (5 mg/kg/d, max 200 mg orally twice per day). Itraconazole has the most data for therapeutic use in ABPA, though many physicians are using voriconazole more regularly as the anti-fungal agent of choice due to good bioavailability and patient tolerance. If the patient has CFRD, insulin dose usually needs to be increased. High-dose glucocorticoid steroids are given usually for 2 weeks before tapering. If total IgE is greater than 1000 IU/mL, glucocorticoid steroids often are not tapered until the IgE level is below 1000 IU/mL. If there is no improvement with high-dose steroids, the diagnosis should be questioned and corticosteroids tapered quickly followed by stopping the intraconazole.

■ HEMOPTYSIS MANAGEMENT

Because pulmonary exacerbation often manifest with mild hemoptysis, > 5 mL of blood should be treated with antibiotics. Lack of consensus about continuing versus stopping chest physiotherapy with mild-to-moderate hemoptysis leads some to stop the therapy until 24 to 48 hours after the bleeding has ceased, while others continue this intervention. Patients with scant and mild hemoptysis most often have aerosol treatments continued, while chest physiotherapy should be individualized for those with mild-to-moderate hemoptysis.

Bronchial artery embolization (BAE) is the initial treatment for massive hemoptysis. Bronchoscopy is not appropriate before BAE as there is little evidence that bronchoscopy can localize bleeding, and it can delay a lifesaving procedure. Lung resection may be considered only after other measures such as BAE have failed to control the bleeding. Chest physiotherapy should be stopped in massive hemoptysis. Aerosol treatments are often discontinued in patients with massive hemoptysis. There is significant risk of suffocation with massive hemoptysis well before exsanguination. As such, early intubation may need to be considered to secure a patient's airway, particularly in the setting of poor gas exchange and/or decreased mental status.

■ PNEUMOTHORAX MANAGEMENT

Most CF patients with a pneumothorax, regardless of size, should be admitted to hospital. However, the size does help determine the appropriate treatment. A small pneumothorax, defined as the distance between the apex and the cupola of ≤ 3 cm, may be treated with oxygen to help resorb the pneumothorax and serial examinations and chest x-rays are done to assess whether the pneumothorax is enlarging. A large pneumothorax (> 3 cm between the apex and the cupola) requires chest tube placement even in clinically stable patients. Good pain control is important in patients with a chest tube in place to avoid splinting and inadequate airway clearance.

Because 50% to 90% of CF patients with a pneumothorax will have a recurrence, pleurodesis should be considered for recurrent large ipsilateral pneumothoraces. Pleurodesis does not reduce lung transplantation candidacy, and can be performed safely. Surgical pleurodesis with video assisted thorascopic surgery (VATS) is the preferred method, and should be done timely to avoid respiratory infections related to splinting and immobility.

There are no consensus guidelines as to whether all patients with pneumothoraces should receive antibiotics. However, antibiotics should be strongly considered if it is believed the pneumothorax was a manifestation of a pulmonary exacerbation or if the pneumothorax persists for more than a few days.

Airway clearance therapies that increase positive expiratory pressure and intrapulmonary percussive ventilation should not be used in patients with large pneumothoraces, and it may be appropriate to withhold such therapies in patients with small pneumothoraces. Aerosol treatments should not be stopped routinely in either large or small pneumothoraces, but may be held if they increase coughing in a patient.

■ EXTRAPULMONARY MANIFESTATIONS

CF is a multiorgan disease, and there are frequently extrapulmonary manifestations of the disease (**Table 234-4**). Often, hospital providers need to address these issues when patients are hospitalized for an acute pulmonary exacerbation. In addition, exacerbation of disease in other organs at times requires hospital admission. Clinicians

TABLE 234-4 Extrapulmonary Manifestations of Cystic Fibrosis

Organ System	Useful Diagnostic Test	Therapeutic Approach
Pancreas (exocrine)		
Pancreatitis	Elevated amylase and lipase, exclusion of other causes	Bowel rest, pain management
Pancreatic insufficiency	Steatorrhea, elevated fecal fat or decrease fecal elastase	Enteric-coated microencapsulated enzymes containing proteases and lipases
Nutritional deficiencies	Albumin, prealbumin; levels for vitamins A, E, and D, Protime (vitamin K)	Aggressive caloric intake, including a high fat diet, replacement of vitamin A, E, D, and K
Pancreas (endocrine)		
CF-related diabetes (CFRD)	Random glucose > 200 mg/dL on two or more occasions or Fasting blood glucose (FBG) > 126 mg/dL on two or more occasions or Oral glucose tolerance test (OGTT) with FBG > 126 mg/dL and 2-h value > 200 mg/dL or hemoglobin A_{1c} > 6.5%	Insulin with continued high calorie diet
Hepatobiliary		
Multilobular biliary cirrhosis	Workup includes liver function tests, ultrasound, ERCP, and exclusion of other causes of liver disease; liver biopsy often not needed	Ursodeoxycholic acid (UDCA)
Gallstones		
Microgallbladder		
Hepatic steatosis		
Hepatic congestion from cor pulmonale		
Gastrointestinal		
Neonatal meconium ileus	History, examination and abdominal radiographs	Systemic hydration, polyethylene glycol electrolyte (PEG) solutions by mouth or enemas, laparotomy and bowel resection (very rarely)
Distal intestinal obstruction syndrome (DIOS)		
Clostridium difficile associated colitis	Stool cultures and toxin, colonoscopy or abdominal CT scan	Antibiotic treatment
Fibrosing colonopathy	Contrast enema	Reduced enzyme dose, occasionally colonic resection
Appendicitis	Examination, ultrasound, abdominal CF scan	Appendectomy
Bone and joint disease		
Osteoporosis	Dual energy x-ray absorptiometry (DEXA)	Calcium and vitamin D supplements, consider bisphosphonates
Arthritis	Serological analysis to exclude other causes of arthritis	Short courses of nonsteroidal and steroidal anti-inflammatory medications
Hypertrophic pulmonary osteoarthropathy	Radiographs of long bones	Short courses of nonsteroidal antiinflammatory medications
Reproductive disease		
CBAVD* resulting in azoospermia	Semen analysis	Reproduction possible through sperm retrieval and assisted reproductive techniques
Cervical mucus abnormalities	Fertility may be normal	Counseling on contraception options, reproductive issues, and family planning

*CBAVD, congenital bilateral absence of the vas deferens.
Reproduced, with permission, from Hanley ME, Welsh CH. *Current Diagnosis & Treatment in Pulmonary Medicine.* New York: McGraw-Hill, 2003. Table 8-1.

should be able to diagnose and treat common extrapulmonary manifestations of CF and maintain a low threshold to evaluate for them.

Sinusitis

Close to 100% of patients with classic CF (elevated sweat chloride, typical pulmonary and gastrointestinal manifestations) have radiologic evidence of pansinusitis. Approximately 43% of CF patients have nasal polyps with 25% having symptoms due to polyps sometime during their lifetime.

CFTR ion transport abnormalities lead to abnormalities in mucociliary clearance in the sinuses, impairing drainage into the nasal cavity. It is not known whether infection is a major contributor to the pansinusitis seen on radiologic examination. However, once nasal polyps develop, the drainage problem is worsened by blocking the openings to the sinuses, leading to increased infection and inflammation. One quarter of adult CF patients have chronic symptoms of sinusitis, which may cause headaches, facial pain, fever, purulent nasal discharge, halitosis, double vision, blurred vision, proptosis, and postnasal drip.

Nasal polyposis may result in epistaxis, rhinorrhea, mouth breathing, obstruction of nasal air flow, distortion of facial features, halitosis, and decreased sense of smell. Nasal polyp resection provides immediate relief from nasal obstruction, but polyps will recur in 58% to 89% of CF patients.

Antibiotics should not be prescribed for asymptomatic CF patients with radiologic findings of sinusitis but are appropriate when patients become symptomatic. The possibility of coexisting allergies contributing to the development of nasal polyps should be considered. No consistent results have been demonstrated but nasal glucocorticoid steroids may be tried. Daily nasal irrigation and other supportive measures are often used. For particularly severe cases, intravenous antibiotics (selected based on results of sinus culture by otolaryngology) for 4 to 6 weeks may benefit patients, but well-designed studies have not been performed.

Sinus surgery benefits are often transient in CF; sinus surgery may be considered for symptomatic sinusitis that has failed routine medical therapy including a course of outpatient intravenous antibiotics. Limited evidence suggests that surgical treatment of sinusitis in CF may improve some health outcomes (eg, reduced average number of annual hospital days), but improvement in lung function should not be expected. Endoscopic sinus surgery is not recommended for CF patients before lung transplant as there are no strong studies to suggest prophylactic pretransplant sinus surgery changes survival rates.

Gastrointestinal tract

The most common GI tract complications of CF are esophagitis and ileal obstruction. Gastroesophageal reflux is exacerbated by coughing as well as the generation of larger negative intrapleural pressures leading to increased esophagitis incidence with more severe CF disease. Proton pump inhibitor therapy is usually effective.

CF can also lead to ileal obstruction (distal ileal obstruction syndrome [DIOS]) from retention of mucofeculent tenacious material in older children and adults. DIOS presents with crampy abdominal pain and relative constipation but can present acutely with abdominal obstruction. A tender right lower quadrant mass may be found on physical examination, and plain abdominal x-ray shows a speckled fecal gas pattern in the right lower quadrant. Often, the entire colon is full of impacted fecal material. The differential diagnosis includes appendicitis, constipation, and intussusception.

Incidence of DIOS has decreased (now only about 4% of CF patients) with the use of enteric coated microspheric pancreatic enzyme replacement therapy. In CF patients who undergo surgery and require narcotics for postoperative pain, DIOS incidence may increase and complete bowel obstruction may occur with just a few narcotic doses. Some institutions initiate stool softeners and cathartic medications (eg, lactulose) empirically in CF patients following lung transplantation as soon as patients begin taking liquids by mouth.

PRACTICE POINT

Extrapulmonary complications

- Distal ileal obstruction syndrome: increased incidence in CF patients who undergo surgery and require narcotics for pain. Complete bowel obstruction may occur with just a few narcotic doses. Consider stool softeners with cathartic medications (eg, lactulose) in the postoperative period as soon as patients begin oral liquids.
- CF-related diabetes: major diabetic complication is acceleration in the rate of decline in lung function. Diabetic diet restriction is not appropriate. Patients with CFRD should maintain a diet high in fat and protein intake with *no restrictions* on carbohydrates except to minimize simple sugars. Consult the endocrine service for assistance with management which includes insulin therapy.

Liver

Bile duct epithelial cells express CFTR leading to impairment in bile and mucus secretion. Localized stasis and obstruction generates an inflammatory response and reactive oxygen species leading to bile duct damage that is seen in nearly all CF patients. Some develop gall bladder disease, but few progress to biliary cirrhosis and liver failure.

Gall bladder disease is characterized by a small, shrunken gall bladder. Gallstones develop in 20% of CF adults but are symptomatic in only 5% of CF adults.

Cirrhosis and liver failure occur in about 2% of CF adults. CF patients with a history of DIOS have significantly higher risk of developing severe liver disease than those who have never had DIOS.

Abdominal imaging with ultrasound or magnetic resonance imaging may be indicated in CF patients with suspected liver disease.

Ursodeoxycholic acid for patients with CF-associated liver disease can often normalize serum alkaline phosphatase levels. However, the natural progression of CF liver disease may not change with such treatment. For end stage cirrhotic liver disease, liver transplantation may be the only option.

Pancreas

Mutant CFTR gene expression in the pancreatic ductal system results in failure of the normal postnatal development of the *exocrine* pancreatic gland, leading to pancreatic exocrine insufficiency and malabsorption in 85% of CF patients. Abnormally low fluid secretion but normal protein secretion into the pancreatic duct causes protein precipitation, duct obstruction, and eventual pancreatic injury severe enough to cause malabsorption.

Symptoms of malabsorption may include diarrhea, bulky foul smelling stools, voracious appetite, abdominal pain after eating, and excess gas. Diagnosis of pancreatic insufficiency occurs with finding levels of pancreatic elastase in the stool that are less than 200 mcg/g stool. Other causes of malabsorption in CF patients—lactose intolerance, celiac disease, Crohn disease, for example—can occur and should be considered in the differential if the patient does not respond to pancreatic enzyme replacement.

Pancreatic enzyme replacement therapy (PERT) dosage is individualized and should be adjusted based on symptoms. The most effective preparations are enteric-coated, acid-resistant microspheres, now with greater formulation consistency, with recently required FDA approval. The initial dose is 500 lipase units per kg per meal and half that amount for snacks. The dose can be increased to a maximum of 2500 lipase units per kg per meal. If symptoms do not improve at maximum PERT doses, intestinal contents may never reach a sufficiently high pH (~5.0) to release the enzymes from the microspheres. Histamine (H2) blockers or proton pump inhibitors may then be given in addition to the pancreatic enzymes. Other malabsorptive syndromes should be considered if patient does not respond to acid inhibition with their PERT.

Enzyme replacement capsules should be taken at the very beginning of the meal or snack. However, if the meal lasts more than 30 minutes, a split dose can be given at the beginning and halfway through the meal. Care must be taken with enteric coated pancreatic enzyme microspheres used with continuous feeding as they can obstruct the feeding tubes. If the patient is able, it is recommended that they take three-fourth of the total enzyme dose at the beginning of the enteral feeding and the remaining one-fourth dose near the end. If they are to be mixed in with the formula, the microspheres must be added to a sodium bicarbonate solution and allowed to dissolve for 15 minutes. They may then be added to the enteral formula for distribution. The CF community is currently awaiting FDA approval of a powdered or liquid PERT formulation.

CF-related diabetes

CFRD has some features of type 1 and type 2 diabetes mellitus, with decreased insulin production and a component of insulin resistance (especially during stress). CFRD prevalence increases with age, with 50% of CF adults over age 30 years developing CFRD.

Early in the clinical course of CFRD, postprandial blood glucose levels are elevated, but most patients have normal fasting glucose levels and hemoglobin A_{1c} (HbA$_{1c}$) level. Yearly oral glucose tolerance testing (OGTT) is recommended to screen for CFRD in all CF patients 10 years and older. Standard ADA criteria for diagnosis of diabetes are used in CFRD and require two positive tests confirmed on two separate days when the patient is in stable baseline health. One of the tests should be an OGTT which consists of measuring a fasting plasma glucose (FPG) followed by oral administration of a 75 gm glucose solution and a subsequent repeat measurement of plasma glucose 2 hours later. An OGTT is positive if the FPG is > 126 mg/dL and/or the 2-hour plasma glucose is > 200 mg/dL. Other tests used for diagnosing CFRD include HgA$_{1c}$ ≥ 6.5% and a random plasma glucose level > 200 mg/dL in the presence of classic diabetic symptoms.

Often, the first manifestations of CFRD are seen during acute respiratory exacerbations, only to subside when the exacerbation has completely resolved but to reappear again with the next exacerbation. Therefore, for CF patients admitted to hospital for a respiratory exacerbation, fasting and 2 to 3 hour postprandial finger stick glucose levels should be measured in the first 48 hours of hospitalization. If fasting levels are >126 mg/dL and/or 2-hour postprandial > 200 mg/dL after the initial 48 hours of admission, finger stick monitoring should be continued, and plasma glucose levels measured. If two or more plasma glucose levels show an FPG > 126 mg/dL and/or 2-hour postprandial are > 200 mg/dL, then endocrinology should be consulted for further evaluation and management.

Complications of CFRD are quite different from those of type 1 or type 2 diabetes mellitus. Diabetic ketoacidosis occurs exceedingly rarely in CFRD and should prompt measuring islet cell antibodies to evaluate for type 1 diabetes. CF patients with diabetes have significantly worse lung function, more frequent acute respiratory exacerbations, and reduced survival rates compared to CF patients without diabetes. CFRD patients die of progressive pulmonary disease and respiratory failure, rather than macrovascular complications of diabetes. Microvascular complications occur in 10% to 23% of patients

with CFRD, including retinopathy (16% of patients after 5 years and 23% after 10 years of CFRD), neuropathy, and nephropathy; but the severity of these microvascular complications is less severe than found in type 1 or type 2 diabetes.

The primary nutritional goal in CFRD is to maintain a high energy diet that is 120% to 150% of that recommended for age because higher BMI is associated with improved outcomes. For this reason, the standard dietary restriction of type 1 and type 2 diabetes do not apply to patients with CFRD. They are encouraged to maintain a diet high in fat and protein intake with no restrictions on carbohydrates except to minimize simple sugars.

Insulin is the preferred drug to treat CFRD. No trial has yet shown that an oral agent is superior to insulin in improving nutritional status or glucose control. Since CF adults are often advised to consume three 1000 calorie meals and two 500 calories snacks per day, the insulin regimen is tailored to their caloric intake. In addition, CF patients should exercise frequently, which also requires tailoring of the insulin regimen. Finally, during a respiratory exacerbation when insulin resistance can be substantial, rapid changes in insulin dosing may be required to maintain glucose levels at target.

Long-acting insulin for patients with fasting hyperglycemia and short acting insulin for meals using a specific dose of insulin per number of carbohydrates being consumed at that meal (ie, carbohydrate counting) helps maintain proper diabetic control. In addition, fingerstick glucose readings before meals can direct additional sliding scale short acting insulin needs for blood glucose levels above 180 mg/dL. All patients with CFRD may consider an insulin pump to reduce drug injections and improve quality of life. Target fasting glucose levels in adults with CFRD recommended by the American Diabetes Association (ADA), are between 70 and 130 mg/dL and 2 to 3 hours after meals less than 180 mg/dL. Further investigation will better delineate if more strict control than this will promote better outcomes. Little evidence exists for strict inpatient glucose control in patients with CF exacerbations, and ADA recommendations for other diabetic patients (maintain blood glucose 140-180 mg/dL) should guide practice.

■ NUTRITION IN THE HOSPITALIZED CF PATIENT

Malnutrition and malabsorption of fat soluble vitamins are common in CF patients. Malnutrition is multifactorial and due to a combination of decreased appetite, malabsorption, and increased energy requirement, especially during acute exacerbations.

Malnutrition, as indicated by a low body mass index (BMI), continues to be a major problem in CF. In 2009, almost 60% of CF adults in the United States were underweight (BMI < 22 for women and <23 for men). For those that are underweight, the following are important considerations: attention to appropriate doses of pancreatic enzymes; maintaining adequate calories for their needs; addressing underlying diseases that may decrease their oral intake (esophagitis, chronic abdominal pain, delayed gastric emptying, and depression); diabetes screening; and if diabetic, that target glucose levels are being met. About 10% of CF patients receive enteral tube feeds for nutritional failure. They are typically supplemented at night and encouraged to eat during the day.

Levels of fat soluble vitamins (A, D, E, K) should be assessed yearly in the outpatient setting. Up to 80% of CF adults are vitamin D deficient (related to malabsorption and other factors) leading to poor bone health and lower innate immunity of the lung. The Cystic Fibrosis Foundation recommends all CF patients maintain a serum 25-hydroxyvitamin D level of ≥30 ng/mL. High dose vitamin D3 (50,000 units once a week for 12 weeks) restores vitamin D levels in most CF patients to sufficient levels, but daily maintenance dosing of vitamin D3 is then required to maintain adequate levels and doses as high as 5000 to 7000 units per day may be necessary, especially during winter months.

■ CONSULTATION

For CF patients admitted to the hospital, hospitalists should facilitate subspecialty consultation with a pulmonologist who has expertise in CF as well as an infectious disease specialist familiar with CF management. Endocrinology consultation can assist with management of CFRD, especially since insulin requirements change rapidly with acute pulmonary CF exacerbations.

Respiratory care consultation can assist patients with inhaled therapies as well as chest physical therapy (device assisted [eg, Acapella and vest] and manual). Floor nursing staff and physical therapy consultation should also assist with chest physical therapy to assist patient in clearing the inflamed bronchioles.

In addition, the pharmacy team may provide invaluable assistance in dosing and monitoring of high risk antibiotics. Furthermore, nutrition service consultation should assist with caloric requirements during a respiratory exacerbation.

Finally, for those patients whose baseline FEV_1 is 30% predicted or less, introduction to a member of the lung transplant team (for patients seen in transplant centers) may help during the hospital admission to stage the timing for a lung transplant evaluation.

PROGNOSIS

The decline in lung function in CF follows a chronic disease trajectory of gradual decline punctuated by acute exacerbations causing sudden drops in lung function (usually assessed as FEV_1). Often, only partial recovery of lung function to a new, lower baseline follows a respiratory exacerbation. The number of exacerbations per year correlates with the rate of decline in FEV_1 and thus progression of disease. In addition, those with CFRD have significantly more respiratory exacerbations and more rapid disease progression than those CF patients without diabetes. Failure to return to baseline FEV_1 after an exacerbation is associated with female sex, CFRD, malnutrition, ABPA, a larger drop in FEV_1 during the exacerbation, and infection with *Pseudomonas*, *B. cepacia complex*, and/or methicillin-resistant *S. aureus*.

DISCHARGE PLANNING

If the patient is discharged before completion of the course of treatment, the patient must have close follow-up to determine duration of antibiotic treatment. Some centers with shorter hospital lengths of stay for admitted adult CF patients have demonstrated better outcomes compared to other centers where patients complete their antimicrobial course in the hospital. Inpatient versus outpatient management of acute pulmonary exacerbations of CF should be individualized based on the patient's social situation, local inpatient and outpatient resources for CF, and the patient's clinical condition.

Guidelines recommend that CF patients receive outpatient follow-up at least every 3 months at a center accredited by the Cystic Fibrosis Foundation and staffed by an interdisciplinary team consisting of pulmonologists, nurses, social workers, respiratory therapists, and nutritionists, all with expertise in CF clinical care. By far, the most frequent reason for additional clinic visits is an acute pulmonary exacerbation. Review of practices in CF Centers with the best pulmonary outcomes (as measured by median FEV_1 for the patients served by that center) indicate that these centers treat each exacerbation quickly and aggressively with the expectation of returning lung function to baseline.

QUALITY IMPROVEMENT

■ PREVENTION

Infection control

Even if pathogenic organisms are not found on sputum culture, all CF patients should be assumed to have transmissible organisms and *contact isolation* instituted. The Cystic Fibrosis Foundation strongly recommends that CF patients avoid physical contact with each other, and therefore CF summer camps and other gatherings of CF patients are no longer recommended and in fact actively discouraged.

Cohorting CF patients when hospitalized to prevent nurses from taking care of multiple CF patients (when possible) will help reduce transmission of resistant organisms to other CF patients. When nurses or clinicians must care for multiple CF patients, those with less resistant organisms should be seen first each day. Providers should always see the patients with *B. cepacia* last during the day to decrease the chances of spreading this deadly organism to other CF patients.

CONCLUSION

Cystic fibrosis is the most common inherited life-shortening disease of Caucasians in the United States caused by mutation in the CFTR gene. Cystic fibrosis can affect a variety of organs, but 90% of mortality is due to lung disease. However, it may present as asthma, pancreatitis, pansinusitis, or nasal polyps and not be initially recognized as cystic fibrosis. Increased respiratory symptoms are indicative of an acute pulmonary exacerbation but an isolated drop in FEV_1 without any reported change in symptoms is also concerning for exacerbation. The mainstay of treatment for acute pulmonary exacerbations is antibiotic therapy and enhanced airway clearance. Hemoptysis and pneumothoraces are major pulmonary complications that may require hospitalization. Nonpulmonary complications of CF such as pancreatic insufficiency, sinusitis, malnutrition, and CF-related diabetes are important contributors to morbidity and mortality. Appropriate subspecialists who have expertise in CF management should be consulted. Respiratory therapists, nutritionists, and pharmacists also play vital roles in the care of the CF patient. Finally, referral for lung transplant evaluation should be considered when the baseline FEV_1 drop to 30% predicted or less. The Cystic Fibrosis Foundation is very active in quality improvement through the national Cystic Fibrosis Patient Registry as well as specific initiatives to improve the care of people with cystic fibrosis.

SUGGESTED READINGS

Flume PA, Mogayzel PJ Jr, Robinson KA, et al. Clinical practice guidelines for pulmonary therapies committee. Cystic fibrosis pulmonary guidelines treatment of pulmonary exacerbations: treatment of pulmonary exacerbations. *Am J Respir Crit Care Med.* 2009;180(9):802-808.

Flume PA, Mogayzel PJ, Robinson KA, et al. Cystic fibrosis pulmonary guidelines pulmonary complications: hemoptysis and pneumothorax. *Am J Respir Crit Care Med.* 2010;182:298-306.

Flume PA, Robinson KA, O'Sullivan BP, et al. Clinical practice guidelines for pulmonary therapies committee. Cystic fibrosis pulmonary guidelines: airway clearance therapies. *Respir Care.* 2009;54(4):522-537.

Moran A, Brunzell C, Cohen R, et al. Clinical care guidelines for cystic fibrosis-related diabetes. *Diabetes Care.* 2010;33(12):2697-2708.

O'Sullivan BP, Freedman SD. Cystic fibrosis. *Lancet.* 2009;373:1891-1904.

Plummer A, Wildman M. Duration of intravenous antibiotic therapy in people with cystic fibrosis. *Cochrane Database Syst Rev.* 2013;5:CD006682.

Rasouli N, Seggelke S, Gibbs J, et al. Cystic fibrosis-related diabetes in adults: inpatient management of 121 patients during 410 admissions. *J Diabetes Sci Technol.* 2012;6(5):1038-1044.

Stallings VA, Stark LJ, Robinson KA, Feranchak AP, Quinton H. Evidence-based practice recommendations for nutrition-related management of children and adults with cystic fibrosis and pancreatic insufficiency: results of a systematic review. *J Am Diet Assoc.* 2008;108(5):832-839.

Stenbit AE, Flume PA. Pulmonary exacerbations in cystic fibrosis. *Curr Opin Pulm Med.* 2011;17(6):442-447.

CHAPTER 235

Sleep Apnea and Obesity Hypoventilation Syndrome

Ji Yeon Lee, MD
David A. Schulman, MD, MPH, FCCP

Key Clinical Questions

1. What are the key distinguishing features between obstructive and central sleep apnea?

2. What are the consequences of untreated sleep apnea?

3. What are the indications for inpatient therapy for sleep apnea?

4. How should patients with suspected sleep apnea be managed at hospital discharge?

5. What is obesity hypoventilation syndrome and how is it best treated?

INTRODUCTION

Sleep apnea is defined by repeated transient cessations of respiration during sleep. The most common type of this disorder, obstructive sleep apnea (OSA), affects between 5% and 15% of middle-aged and older adults. The burden of disease in the hospitalized patient is likely to be even greater than that of the general population because inpatients carry many disorders that have been associated with OSA, including obesity, congestive heart failure, coronary artery disease, hypertension, stroke, and diabetes. Epidemiologic data suggest that the majority of patients with sleep apnea are undiagnosed; in 2004, national hospital discharge codes revealed fewer than 300,000 cases of sleep apnea among almost 35 million inpatient stays, yielding a prevalence of identified disease of less than 1%.

Although sleep apnea by itself is rarely a primary indication for hospitalization, recent evidence suggests that inpatient management of this disease needs to improve. Less than 6% of those identified as having sleep apnea in the 2004 National Hospital Discharge Survey received therapy with continuous positive airway pressure (CPAP) while in the hospital. Hospital Medicine physicians should identify and appropriately treat OSA patients. The key to identifying the possible presence of sleep apnea depends largely on an appreciation of risk factors and clinical features. In 2008, Goring and Collop showed that almost 80% of patients with suspected sleep apnea referred for a sleep study after an inpatient hospitalization were confirmed to have OSA. Therefore, inpatient identification and referral for evaluation can improve diagnosis rates and reduce the percentage of affected patients left untreated. This chapter will review the fundamentals of sleep apnea, address the management of patients with stable sleep apnea in the inpatient setting, delineate the necessity of preoperative screening in at-risk patients, and identify which patients should undergo further testing.

PATHOPHYSIOLOGY

Sleep-disordered breathing includes three related classes of diseases: OSA, central sleep apnea (CSA), and sleep-related hypoventilation—although as many as 90% of all cases are OSA. The distinction between OSA and the other categories is an important one as the treatment options and responses to therapy are quite different. Obesity hypoventilation syndrome (OHS) is a condition in which obese patients develop diurnal hypercapnia and hypoxemia in the absence of a causal pulmonary or neurologic disorder; up to 90% of these patients have OSA, though the causative association has yet to be proven.

■ OBSTRUCTIVE SLEEP APNEA

The upper airway is a compliant structure susceptible to collapse. Complex neurologic and musculoskeletal interactions cause a decrease in the cross-sectional area of the upper airway during sleep, which may result in a reduction or cessation of airflow in susceptible individuals. The imbalance between the forces that promote airway patency (the pharyngeal dilator muscles) and the negative inspiratory forces generated by the diaphragm (which promotes airway collapse) causes obstruction. The majority of patients with OSA demonstrate obstruction in the retropalatal or retrolingual areas as these locations carry the greatest risk of collapse when a negative pressure forms inside the airway during inspiration.

Even during wakefulness, the cross-sectional area of the upper airway is smaller in patients with OSA compared with disease-free controls, often due to anatomic contributors, such as enlarged tonsils, a large tongue, a high-arched palate, and abnormal positioning of the maxilla and mandible. At sleep onset, a decrease in neural output to the pharyngeal dilator muscles increases the risk of collapse. In addition, supine positioning during sleep promotes collapse by bringing the weight of external tissue to bear upon the anteroposterior diameter of the pharynx, which is usually its shortest axis (and thus the one along which collapse is most likely). Snoring, caused by vibration of the soft tissues of the upper airway, may be the earliest sign of obstruction, although it is a very common clinical finding with a prevalence of up to 35% and has a positive predictive value as low as 20% for the presence of frank sleep apnea in an otherwise unselected population.

As obstruction worsens, periods of time during which airflow is inadequate (hypopnea) or absent (apnea) occur. During these episodes, there are transient increases in arterial carbon dioxide tension and decreases in arterial oxygen tension. Episodes of obstruction typically terminate with an arousal from sleep, precipitated by the changes in oxygen and carbon dioxide as well as marked pressure swings within the thoracic cavity, as the affected individual unconsciously attempts to inspire air past the obstruction, an effort that fails due to the negative pressure serving to further pull the airway walls inward, worsening collapse. The lack of restful sleep from repetitive arousals throughout the night is responsible for the symptom of excessive daytime sleepiness in affected patients. Notably, only about half of patients with sleep apnea report overt sleepiness; others may report symptoms of fatigue, lack of energy, or other related symptoms without frank sleepiness.

■ CENTRAL SLEEP APNEA

Patients with central events are marked by a transient absence of respiratory effort. Affected patients fall into two main groups, those with daytime hypercapnia and those without. All human beings have a slight decline in respiratory drive during sleep, with a typical increase in pCO_2 of about 5 mm of mercury; this change is normally achieved through a transient period of hypoventilation at sleep onset. Among patients with daytime hypoventilation (including those with chronic obstructive pulmonary disease and a number of neuromuscular disorders), an already impaired ventilatory drive is further suppressed, causing apnea. Hypercapnic CSA may also be related to a reduced central drive, as in the case of a brainstem stroke, use of CNS depressants, or an impaired respiratory motor, as seen in myopathy, neuromuscular junction disorders, and spinal lesions.

Patients with nonhypercapnic CSA tend to have an increased responsiveness to elevated $PaCO_2$ levels, leading to periods of apnea when carbon dioxide levels drop below the apneic threshold. The disorder is most often seen as Cheyne-Stokes respiration in patients with heart failure. When these patients lie in the supine position, rostral movement of fluid from the lower extremities into the lungs activates stretch receptors, stimulating ventilation and leading to hypocapnia. The $PaCO_2$ drops below the apneic threshold, leading to a cessation of respiration. Decreased cardiac output causes an increase in circulatory time, leading to delays in information feedback from peripheral receptors. In addition, decreased cerebrovascular reactivity impairs the respiratory control center's ability to appropriately target ventilatory responses to carbon dioxide. As a result, as the $PaCO_2$ rises again, there can be ventilatory overshoot, creating a cyclic crescendo-decrescendo respiratory pattern that characterizes Cheyne-Stokes respiration.

■ SLEEP-RELATED HYPOVENTILATION

The diagnosis of sleep-related hypoventilation requires a persistent elevation in carbon dioxide level. This class of disorders includes OHS, as well as hypoventilation due to medication use, congenital diseases (such as central alveolar hypoventilation syndrome) and medical disorders (most commonly pulmonary or neurologic diseases).

DIFFERENTIAL DIAGNOSIS

Snoring does not necessarily indicate the presence of sleep apnea. While a socially problematic condition, primary snoring has not clearly been associated with any long-term health repercussions. While history may be highly suggestive of OSA, several other disorders may mimic its symptoms (Table 235-1). Patients who awaken with paroxysmal dyspnea at night may suffer from congestive heart failure, chronic obstructive pulmonary disease, nocturnal gastroesophageal reflux or nocturnal panic attacks. A small percentage of patients with severe sleep apnea will demonstrate diurnal hypercapnia, although diagnoses of underlying pulmonary disease (either restrictive or obstructive) and neuromuscular disease affecting the muscles of respiration should also be entertained.

Central sleep apnea presents with witnessed breathing pauses at night and daytime fatigue, although the mechanism of disease and appropriate treatment is quite different. Other causes of frequent nocturnal arousals and daytime somnolence include periodic limb movement disorder, prostatism and environmental sleep disorder, in which an external stimulus causes recurrent awakenings from sleep. Patients with nocturnal pain and inadequately controlled mood disorders may also demonstrate frequent nocturnal arousals. Excessive daytime sleepiness may be a symptom of insufficient sleep (the most common cause of daytime somnolence), depression, narcolepsy and idiopathic hypersomnia, as well as a number of endocrinologic, cardiac, pulmonary, renal, and hematologic disorders.

DIAGNOSIS

Patients with OSA present to the hospital with other medical problems and the clinician should make an effort to identify at-risk patients so that they undergo appropriate evaluation. Older age, obesity, and male sex are the most significant risk factors for OSA. Because the prevalence of these characteristics in the general population is too high for them to be useful as a screening tool, history and physical examination are critical in determining which patients are appropriate referrals for sleep testing (Table 235-2).

Taking a screening history for OSA includes an assessment of both nocturnal and diurnal symptoms; the accuracy of the history improves if the patient's bed partner is available for questioning, as

TABLE 235-1 Differential Diagnosis of Obstructive Sleep Apnea, Based on Symptom

Symptom	Differential Diagnosis
Frequent nocturnal arousal and daytime somnolence	Central sleep apnea
	Benign prostatic hypertrophy
	Periodic limb movement disorder
	Environmental sleep disorder
	Nocturnal pain
	Mood disorder (eg, depression) inadequately controlled
	Insufficient sleep (most common cause of daytime sleepiness)
	Narcolepsy
	Idiopathic hypersomnia
	Awakening from other endocrinologic, cardiac, pulmonary, renal, or hematologic disorders
Snoring	Primary snoring
Paroxysmal dyspnea	Congestive heart failure
	Chronic obstructive pulmonary disease
	Nocturnal gastroesophageal reflux
	Nocturnal panic attacks

TABLE 235-2 History and Physical Examination Findings Suggesting Sleep Apnea

Heroic snoring

Nocturia

Witnessed breathing pauses during sleep

Excessive daytime sleepiness

Tongue or tonsillar enlargement

Retrognathia

Large neck circumference (> 16 in in women, > 17 in in men)

that person can offer greater insight into events that occur when the patient is unconscious. *Snoring* is the most common symptom of obstructive sleep apnea, present in more than 90% of patients with the disease, suggesting that the absence of snoring (by history from bed partner or other witness) would have a good negative predictive value for OSA. The presence of *witnessed apneas, seen in 75% of patients with OSA,* has a positive predictive value of greater than 80% for the presence of sleep apnea, although data do not suggest that their presence is associated with the severity of the disease. However, the absence of witnessed apneas does not reliably exclude the diagnosis of OSA. Another suggestive clue in the history includes *waking up with a sensation of choking or gasping for air.* This symptom usually represents an arousal due to an apneic episode, with the sensation normally subsiding within seconds of waking. Rarely, patients may complain of *insomnia* (which probably represents disturbed sleep secondary to arousal), although the majority of patients report no difficulty initiating sleep. *Nocturia* is a frequent complaint among patients with apnea; it occurs, in part, because OSA patients have higher circulating levels of atrial natriuretic peptide, leading to a greater urine output. In addition, some patients who wake from an apnea have no recollection of the event (as the obstruction resolves with arousal), leading them to believe that they woke to urinate.

The presence of *excessive daytime somnolence (EDS)* is very common in OSA patients, although the complaint is nonspecific and its utility in discriminating affected patients from those without the disorder is poor. A validated questionnaire to assess sleepiness, such as the Epworth Sleepiness Scale (see http://epworthsleepinessscale.com/1997-version-ess/), may quantify fatigue, although the symptom remains nonspecific. Other daytime symptoms of OSA include irritability, memory disturbance, and morning headaches (secondary to cerebral vasodilation due to transient carbon-dioxide retention).

Other medical disorders have been associated with OSA (**Table 235-3**). Although most of these disorders do not have a good positive predictive value for sleep apnea, recent guidelines recommend considering the diagnosis of OSA in patients with

TABLE 235-3 Other Comorbid Conditions Associated with Obstructive Sleep Apnea

Systemic hypertension

Pulmonary hypertension

Myocardial infarction

Stroke

Diabetes mellitus and glucose intolerance

Atrial fibrillation

Congestive heart failure

Hypothyroidism

Neuromuscular disease

refractory hypertension. Sleep apnea is also more common in patients with renal failure, hypothyroidism, and acromegaly. Diastolic dysfunction has been associated with sleep-disordered breathing, although a causal link has not been definitively proven. The presence of neuromuscular disease can increase the risk of both central and obstructive sleep apnea. In addition, the regular use of narcotics or benzodiazepines can cause or exacerbate OSA, as well as sleep-related hypoventilation. Any of these risk factors should trigger more detailed questioning about symptoms of OSA.

Physical examination may be helpful in identifying patients at higher risk of sleep apnea, but *no exam findings can confirm or preclude the diagnosis with a significant degree of certainty.* Obesity is associated with OSA, with a prevalence of OSA as high as 70% in morbidly obese patients. A large neck circumference (>17 in in men, > 16 in in women) confers an increased risk of OSA. Other anatomic factors conferring an increased risk include retrognathia, micrognathia, tonsillar hypertrophy, an enlarged uvula, macroglossia, and inferior displacement of the hyoid. Assessment of cross-sectional area of the pharynx using a validated tool such as the Mallampati scale can help to quantify airway crowding and OSA risk.

Several screening tools exist that attempt to integrate components of the history (and physical examination in some cases) to create a composite risk score. Both the STOP-BANG and the Berlin questionnaire (**Figure 235-1**) have a high sensitivity for significant sleep apnea (>90%) but only a modest specificity (approximately 50%), yielding a positive predictive value in the 10% to 20% range. As a result, a combination of such tools and clinical acumen can best determine which patients should undergo further evaluation.

■ OVERNIGHT PULSE OXIMETRY AND IN-HOSPITAL POLYSOMNOGRAPHY IN DIAGNOSIS OF OSA

Even when the diagnosis of OSA is highly suspected and can be confirmed by the presence of heroic snoring and witnessed apneas during hospitalization, formal testing is required before insurance will cover therapy with CPAP. The current reference standard test for the diagnosis for obstructive sleep apnea is overnight polysomnography (PSG), though this requires the patient to spend a night in the sleep laboratory and can be inconvenient and expensive, as well as impractical for an acutely ill, hospitalized patient.

As an alternative to PSG, home sleep apnea testing (HSAT) has been increasing in popularity due to its cost effectiveness and convenience. HSAT is an alternative to PSG, best in cases of high pretest probability of moderate-to-severe OSA. The test has not been validated for patients with significant comorbid conditions, specifically lung disease, congestive heart failure, morbid obesity, and neurologic disorders. Home testing is also not useful in the diagnosis of nonrespiratory sleep disorders.

Some have also proposed the use of overnight continuous pulse oximetry to diagnose OSA as it is comparatively inexpensive, simple to perform and may be performed in the patient's hospital room. However, the presence of nocturnal desaturation does not equate to the presence of obstructive sleep apnea and cannot reliably distinguish central from obstructive apnea as an explanation for any observed desaturation. In addition, the absence of desaturation does not exclude the diagnosis of OSA. In some cases, patients may not sleep for much of the night; the absence of significant desaturation could simply represent the absence of significant sleep. On the whole, overnight oximetry may be useful to exclude OSA in appropriately chosen patients who are at high risk, but patients would still require a full PSG prior to initiation of CPAP therapy if abnormalities are found.

In-hospital PSG for patients considered to be high-risk for sleep apnea may be considered during their inpatient stay, although this test is not usually reimbursed by insurers when performed during hospitalization. Because of its portability, there has been interest in using HSAT prior to hospital discharge in patients thought to have sleep apnea. While this is a practical option, providers should be cautious about trying to diagnose sleep-disordered breathing in the hospital environment; false-negative tests may result from sleep disruption from environmental noise, nocturnal medication administration, or vital sign checks. In addition, sleep apnea may be exacerbated during hospitalizations as a result of physiologic derangements that will resolve as the patient recovers, leading inpatient HSATs to show disease that will diminish or disappear over time.

MANAGEMENT

■ MANAGEMENT OF STABLE OSA IN THE HOSPITALIZED PATIENT

Many hospitalized patients carry a prior diagnosis of OSA. Several studies have recently evaluated the prevalence and management of sleep apnea in the hospitalized patients, and found that management of OSA in the hospital setting is frequently overlooked. One large study showed that less than 6% of patients received this therapy during hospital stay, despite home adherence to CPAP; some smaller studies have fared better, though not markedly so. Several challenges impede optimal management of OSA patients during an

acute hospitalization. The burden of disease is high and resources are limited to provide CPAP machines to all affected patients, as the setup often requires significant involvement by a respiratory therapist. Many patients are not able to report the correct home setting for their CPAP machine, and the mask interface with which the patient has become comfortable may not be available at the hospital.

PRACTICE POINT

- Patients already on treatment should be encouraged to bring in their home device for use during their hospital course. While this may not be feasible in all patients or in all facilities, it would tremendously decrease the burden on the hospital to provide devices for inpatient use. If patients are unable to retrieve their own device, contacting the patient's durable medical equipment provider often provides information about the machine's setting and the specific mask interface used by the patient at home, so that this can be replicated during hospitalization.

Berlin Questionnaire
Sleep Apnea

Height (m) _____ Weight (kg) _____ Age _____ Male/Female

Please choose the correct response to each question.

Category 1

1. Do you snore?
- ☐ a. Yes
- ☐ b. No
- ☐ c. Don't know

If you answered 'Yes':

2. You snoring is:
- ☐ a. Slightly louder than breathing
- ☐ b. As loud as talking
- ☐ c. Louder than talking
- ☐ d. Very loud—can be heard in other rooms

3. How often do you snore?
- ☐ a. Almost every day
- ☐ b. 3-4 times per week
- ☐ c. 1-2 times per week
- ☐ d. 1-2 times per month
- ☐ e. Rarely or never

4. Has your snoring ever bothered other people?
- ☐ a. Yes
- ☐ b. No
- ☐ c. Don't know

5. Has anyone noticed that you stop breathing during your sleep?
- ☐ a. Almost every day
- ☐ b. 3-4 times per week
- ☐ c. 1-2 times per week
- ☐ d. 1-2 times per month
- ☐ e. Rarely or never

Category 2

6. How often do you feel tired or fatigued after your sleep?
- ☐ a. Almost every day
- ☐ b. 3-4 times per week
- ☐ c. 1-2 times per week
- ☐ d. 1-2 times per month
- ☐ e. Rarely or never

7. During your waking time, do you feel tired, fatigued or not up to par?
- ☐ a. Almost every day
- ☐ b. 3-4 times per week
- ☐ c. 1-2 times per week
- ☐ d. 1-2 times per month
- ☐ e. Rarely or never

8. Have you ever nodded off or fallen asleep while driving a vehicle?
- ☐ a. Yes
- ☐ b. No

If you answered 'Yes':

9. How often does this occur?
- ☐ a. Almost every day
- ☐ b. 3-4 times per week
- ☐ c. 1-2 times per week
- ☐ d. 1-2 times per month
- ☐ e. Rarely or never

Category 3

10. Do you have high blood pressure?
- ☐ a. Yes
- ☐ b. No
- ☐ c. Don't know

Figure 235-1 *The Berlin Questionnaire.* (Data from the Netzer NC, Stoohs RA, Netzer CM, Clark K, Strohl KP. Using the Berlin Questionnaire to identify patients at risk for the sleep apnea syndrome. *Ann Intern Med.* 1999;131(17):485-491.)

Berlin Questionnaire
Sleep Apnea

Scoring Berlin Questionnaire

The questionnaire consists of 3 categories related to the risk of having sleep apnea. Patients can be classified into High Risk or Low Risk based on their responses to the individual items and their overall scores in the symptom categories.

Categories and Scoring:

Category 1: items 1, 2, 3, 4, and 5;

Item 1: if '**Yes**', assign **1 point**
Item 2: if '**c**' or '**d**' is the response, assign **1 point**
Item 3: if '**a**' or '**b**' is the response, assign **1 point**
Item 4: if '**a**' is the response, assign **1 point**
Item 5: if '**a**' or '**b**' is the response, assign **2 points**

Add points. Category 1 is positive if the total score is 2 or more points.

Category 2: items 6, 7, 8 (item 9 should be noted separately).

Item 6: if '**a**' or '**b**' is the response, assign **1 point**
Item 7: if '**a**' or '**b**' is the response, assign **1 point**
Item 8: if '**a**' is the response, assign **1 point**

Add points. Category 2 is positive if the total score is 2 or more points.

Category 3 is positive if the answer to item 10 is '**Yes**' or if the BMI of the patient is > 30 kg/m².

(BMI is defined as weight (kg) divided by height (m) squared, ie, kg/m²).

High Risk: if there are 2 or more categories where the score is positive.

Low Risk: if there is only 1 or no categories where the score is positive.

Additional Question: item 9 should be noted separately.

Figure 235-1 *(Continued)*

◼ MANAGEMENT OF HOSPITALIZED PATIENTS WITH UNTREATED OSA

While CPAP yields significant benefit in many patients with respiratory failure, little evidence supports urgent implementation of CPAP strictly for management of OSA during hospitalization.

In one study looking at cardiac patients with suspected OSA, inpatient portable monitoring was performed to diagnose sleep apnea; patients were trialed on CPAP for OSA during hospitalization and discharged home with therapy. Those who were adherent to therapy after discharge were less likely to be readmitted to the hospital within 30 days of discharge. The only other related diagnosis for which acute therapy with positive airway pressure has been shown to be beneficial is acutely decompensated obesity hypoventilation, for which bilevel pressure (not CPAP) has been shown to be associated with a decreased risk of need for intubation and improved survival.

On the negative side, implementation of positive airway pressure for the first time to an acutely ill patient may lead to significant discomfort and noncompliance absent close supervision by a qualified respiratory therapist. In addition, inpatient respiratory therapy departments may not have resources to initiate therapy in all patients. When CPAP therapy is used during hospitalization in patients that are suspected to have OSA, the patient will still require formal diagnostic testing prior to insurance authorizing coverage for home therapy.

PRACTICE POINT

- There is insufficient evidence to support initiation of positive airway pressure for the majority of therapy-naïve patients during their hospitalization, with the possible exceptions of acute decompensations of congestive heart failure and obesity hypoventilation. Even if therapy is used during hospitalization in patients with suspected OSA, hospitalists should refer patients for inpatient or outpatient PSG or portable monitoring in order to have insurance coverage for outpatient therapy with positive airway pressure.

■ SCREENING FOR OSA IN THE SURGICAL POPULATION

Patients with sleep apnea bear a high risk of perioperative complications, including postoperative ICU admission, prolonged length of hospital stay, encephalopathy, cardiac arrhythmias, pulmonary embolisms, acute MI, infection, and the need for reintubation, particularly if they receive general anesthesia or opioids. Morbidly obese patients often desaturate rapidly during periods of apnea due to low resting lung volumes; care during intubation should focus on preventing significant desaturation during the induction of anesthesia. Failure to recognize OSA patients prior to surgery may leave providers unable to anticipate possible complications and implement preventative measures. One recent study screened all patients presenting for elective surgery using the Berlin Questionnaire and performed PSG in those that were found to be high risk; the prevalence of sleep apnea in this surgical population was more than 20%, but over 70% of these cases were undiagnosed.

Recent American Society of Anesthesiologists guidelines recommend evaluating patients for OSA risk factors, as perioperative pulmonary complications increase with increasing severity of sleep apnea. Depending on clinical suspicion based on record review, focused history, and physical exam, one should consider sleep testing and preoperative initiation of CPAP, particularly if there is severe OSA. Patients with sleep apnea may also be optimized with the use of oral appliances or weight loss. Even if testing is not feasible preoperatively, identification of high-risk patients should generate a lower threshold to reduce pulmonary complications with active management when necessary. High clinical suspicion or a prior diagnosis of sleep apnea may affect the decision to admit

the patient postoperatively, may play a role in deciding the type of anesthesia used, (eg, using general anesthesia with a secure airway instead of deep sedation), and should be managed as a difficult airway. Although there have been no large studies evaluating the benefit of using CPAP postoperatively in OSA patients, postop CPAP use in abdominal surgery patients may reduce the risk of pneumonia, atelectasis, and postop respiratory complications.

■ TREATMENT OF OSA IN THE CPAP INTOLERANT

While continuous positive airway pressure serves as the most effective therapy for obstructive sleep apnea, its use is associated with significant noncompliance (> 50% in some studies). Efforts to improve compliance with CPAP may include the use of different facial interfaces (**Figure 235-2**) to improve patient comfort, desensitization therapy, the addition of heated humidification or a switch to bilevel positive airway pressure therapy. No single intervention improves satisfaction in all patients requiring CPAP therapy, although a qualified respiratory therapist may help determine which to try first.

Other therapeutic options include *oral appliance therapy* (OAT), surgical treatments, and supplemental oxygen. Oral appliances work either by repositioning the lower jaw (mandibular advancement) or by holding the tongue forward. Although mandibular advancement devices (**Figure 235-3**) have been better studied, both treatments are effective in patients with less-severe disease and among those who are not morbidly obese. Surgical treatments have also shown benefit in these groups as well as those with specific anatomic defects on physical examination.

Oxygen therapy had been suggested as a possible therapy for OSA patients who have significant desaturation at night. While supplemental oxygen does not have a marked impact on the frequency of obstructive events, it attenuates nocturnal hypoxemia, which seems to be a greater predictor of cardiovascular risk than the frequency of apneas or hypopneas. However, a recent study has shown that CPAP may help reduce blood pressure, while nocturnal oxygen therapy provided no significant benefit. In OSA patients who use medications that may increase apnea severity or frequency

Nasal Insert

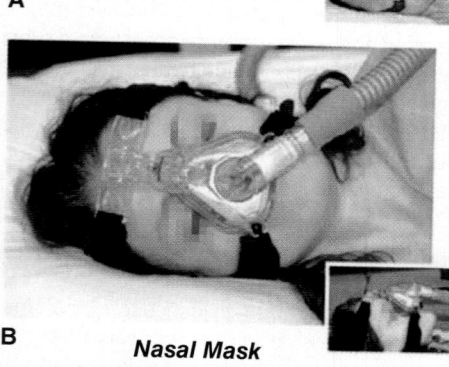

Full Face Mask

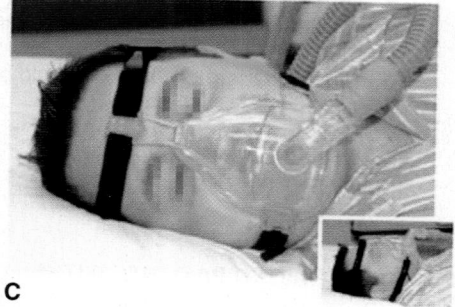

A

C

B

Nasal Mask

Figure 235-2 *Pictures of different continuous positive airway pressure interfaces.* (A) *Nasal Insert,* (B) *Nasal Mask,* (C) *Full Face Mask.* (Reproduced, with permission, from Pack A. *Fishman's Pulmonary Diseases and Disorders*, 4th ed. New York: McGraw-Hill; 2008. Fig. 97-16.)

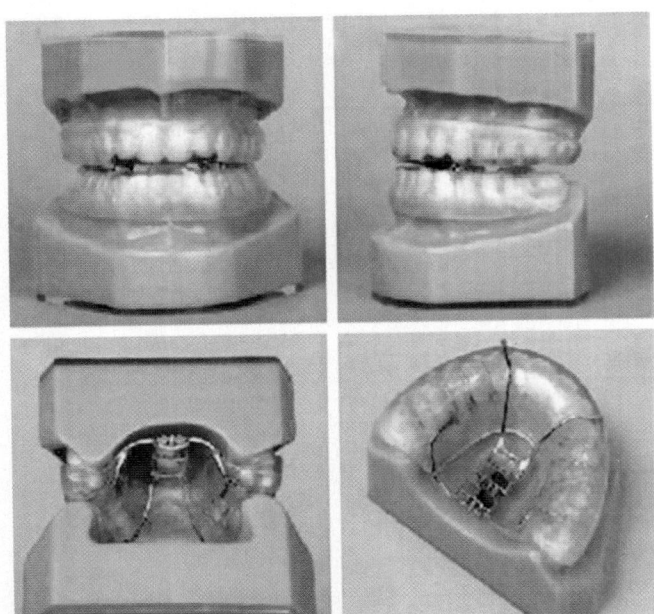

Figure 235-3 *Mandibular advancement devices.* (Reproduced, with permission, from Pack A. *Fishman's Pulmonary Diseases and Disorders,* 4th ed. New York: McGraw-Hill; 2008. Fig. 97-22.)

(such as opiates and benzodiazepines), dose reduction or discontinuation should be considered, when possible.

■ CONSULTATIONS

Respiratory therapy consultation for all patients for whom CPAP is prescribed during the hospitalization will allow the patient selection of interface (mask type) and appropriate fitting to minimize nocturnal mask leak and optimize patient comfort. Many respiratory therapists are also trained in desensitizing techniques for patients who complain of intolerance.

Consultation from a pulmonologist or sleep specialist (when available) should be strongly considered when CPAP nonadherence cannot be adequately addressed by a respiratory therapist. In addition, patients who require more aggressive outpatient therapy may benefit from specialist evaluation during their hospital stay. Symptoms suggesting the need for such a consultation include persistent sleepiness despite compliance with CPAP therapy, persistent snoring on treatment, the development or worsening of cor pulmonale, or the presence of obesity hypoventilation. Finally, consultation should be considered in all patients with predominantly *central* sleep apnea due to the complexity of optimizing treatment in patients with this disease.

COMPLICATIONS AND PROGNOSIS

OSA confers an increased risk of incident hypertension, coronary artery disease, atrial fibrillation, complex ventricular ectopy, cerebrovascular disease, a worsened prognosis in heart failure, and increased cardiovascular mortality. In one study evaluating outcomes in hospitalized patients with pneumonia, OSA was associated with an increased risk of mechanical ventilation and clinical deterioration. While few data support an increased rate of complications during hospitalization for medical illness attributable to OSA, multiple trials of postoperative complications demonstrate a higher rate of pulmonary, cardiac, gastrointestinal, and bleeding complications in patients with sleep apnea. As a result, many anesthesiologists screen patients for sleep-disordered breathing during preoperative evaluation. However, evidence has not yet proven any attenuation of surgical risk in OSA patients with CPAP therapy.

■ OBESITY HYPOVENTILATION SYNDROME

Obesity hypoventilation syndrome (OHS) is a disorder related to sleep apnea, defined by the presence of waking alveolar hypoventilation ($PaCO_2 > 45$ mm Hg) in the setting of obesity (BMI > 30) with no other clear predisposing risk factors. It occurs in approximately 11% of OSA patients, while approximately 90% of patients with OHS have comorbid sleep-disordered breathing.

The pathogenesis of OHS is not completely understood, but is likely related to physiologic derangements and consequences of obesity, including respiratory muscle dysfunction, diminished central ventilatory drive, and increased resistance to certain hormonal modulators, such as leptin. Obesity reduces respiratory system compliance, increases airways resistance, and creates a state of relative respiratory muscle weakness—possibly related to fatigue from the increased work of breathing. Other as-yet-unidentified contributors must also exist, as the majority of patients with obesity do not develop OHS. In most cases, correction of obesity improves the elevated daytime $PaCO_2$ and hypoventilation. CPAP therapy, the mainstay of therapy if weight loss does not occur, has been shown to yield significant increases in PaO_2 and decreases in $PaCO_2$. Of note, bilevel pressure has not been shown to be superior to CPAP, though it may be helpful in cases when there is failure of CPAP therapy or inability to tolerate high CPAP pressures.

Patients with OHS may come to the attention in the inpatient setting after admission with severe hypercapnia or admission for other acute medical illnesses such as pneumonia. Despite obesity, these patients will not have other obvious contributors to hypercapnia (sedative use, chronic obstructive pulmonary disease, or neuromuscular disease). Although they are often admitted to the intensive care unit for rapid correction of their hypercapnia, transfer to the medical floor allows optimization of care prior to discharge. Unlike patients with pure OSA, these patients do not typically require additional diagnostic testing to justify the use of home positive pressure therapy, as hypoventilation is an approved indication for this treatment. Most providers implement bilevel pressure acutely to assist with the probable underlying OSA as well as the hypoventilation with empiric choices of pressure levels based upon patient tolerance and the need to eliminate carbon dioxide. Commonly used starting pressures include inspiratory positive airway pressure of 10 cm H_2O and expiratory positive airway pressure of 5 cm H_2O. Hospitalists should refer these patients for a formal CPAP or bilevel titration after discharge, as the optimal pressure levels will depend upon the severity of the underlying obstructive physiology.

Patients with OHS use significantly more resources and have far greater medical expenses when compared with morbidly obese eucapnic patients and sleep-disordered breathing patients without hypercapnia. Additionally, OHS patients have a greater morbidity and mortality than obese subjects without OHS. These patients have higher rates of comorbid congestive heart failure, angina, and cor pulmonale, as well as a greater rate of hospitalization, need for intensive care, and need for mechanical ventilation.

DISCHARGE PLANNING

Patients with sleep apnea who were on therapy prior to their hospitalization and who do not demonstrate any signs of inadequate treatment have no specific discharge needs. Masks or tubing are required. Even if disease is stable and well controlled, annual follow-up with a sleep specialist should be considered to ensure continued compliance with therapy and monitoring for complications of undertreated disease.

For patients without previously documented disease, ensuring rapid confirmation and implementation of therapy by arranging an outpatient polysomnogram or home sleep apnea test is strongly recommended, more so if the patient was admitted with a disease that might have resulted from inadequately treated apnea, such as

TABLE 235-4 Evidence-based Medicine Key References

Study	Methodology	Results	Limitations	Bottom Line
Goring K, Collop N. *J Clin Sleep Med*. 2008;4(2):105-110.	Retrospective chart review of 100 polysomnographies ordered after hospitalization	High frequency of sleep disordered breathing (77%) in sample, especially with underlying cardiopulmonary disease	Retrospective; cannot determine impact of sleep-disordered breathing on acute exacerbations of cardiopulmonary disease	Patients with sleep-disordered breathing can be successfully identified during hospitalization
Finkel KJ, et al. *Sleep Med*. 2009;10(7):753-758.	Prospective observational study of surgical patients screened for OSA	23.7% of patients screened high risk for OSA of which 81% did not have prior diagnosis of OSA; among patients tested 82% had OSA	Did not look at outcomes of patients with OSA; home studies used to make diagnosis of OSA	Undiagnosed OSA is prevalent in adult surgery population, and universal screening can help identify these patients
Hwang D, et al. *Chest*. 2008;133:1128-1134.	Preoperative patients were screened for sleep-disordered breathing and tested with home oximetry; postoperative complications were assessed	57% of patients had evidence of sleep-disordered breathing by nocturnal oximetry; postoperative complications were much higher with greater degrees of nocturnal desaturation	Nocturnal desaturation used to identify patients with sleep-disordered breathing	Postoperative complications are much greater in patients with sleep-disordered breathing, highlighting importance of preoperative screening and testing
Khayat RN, et al. *Chest*. 2009;136(4):991-997.	Randomized clinical trial of patients admitted with decompensated heart failure who underwent sleep study and randomized to treatment with CPAP vs usual care for heart failure	Left ventricular ejection fraction was significantly superior in intervention arm	Small study of 46 patients; unable to look at other outcomes	Early identification of OSA in patients with acute decompensated heart failure is important as treatment with CPAP can improve systolic function in this setting

CPAP, continuous positive airway pressure; OSA, obstructive sleep apnea.

myocardial infarction, congestive heart failure, or cerebrovascular accident. The hospitalist may need to arrange nocturnal oxygen supplementation for severely affected patients if polysomnography cannot be performed soon after discharge. However, not all such patients will qualify for therapy, due to lack of definitive evidence of benefits of this treatment in patients with sleep apnea. Arranging an outpatient appointment with a sleep specialist for these patients is critical, as close follow-up after implementation of CPAP therapy is one of the best predictors of long-term compliance with treatment (**Table 235-4**).

SUGGESTED READINGS

American Society of Anesthesiologists: practice guidelines for the perioperative management of patients with obstructive sleep apnea: An updated report by the American Society of Anesthesiologists Task Force on Perioperative Management of Patients with Obstructive Sleep Apnea. *Anesthesiology*. 2014;120:268-286.

American Academy of Sleep Medicine. *International Classification of Sleep Disorders*, 3rd ed. Darien, IL: AASM; 2014.

Basner RC. Continuous positive airway pressure for obstructive sleep apnea. *N Engl J Med*. 2007;356(17):1751-1758.

Costanzo MR, Khayat R, Ponikowski P, et al. Mechanisms and clinical consequences of untreated central sleep apnea in heart failure. *J Am Coll Cardiol*. 2015;65(1):72-84.

Pérez de Llano LA, Golpe R, Ortiz Piquer M, et al. Short-term and long-term effects of nasal intermittent positive pressure ventilation in patients with obesity-hypoventilation syndrome. *Chest*. 2005;128(2):587-594.

Finkel KJ, Searleman AC, Tymkew H, et al. Prevalence of undiagnosed obstructive sleep apnea among adult surgical patients in an academic medical center. *Sleep Med*. 2009;10(7):753-758.

Flemons WW. Clinical practice. Obstructive sleep apnea. *N Engl J Med*. 2002;347(7):498-504.

Goring K, Collop N. Sleep disordered breathing in hospitalized patients. *J Clin Sleep Med*. 2008;4(2):105-110.

Hwang D, Shakir N, Limann B, et al. Association of sleep-disordered breathing with postoperative complications. *Chest*. 2008;133:1128-1134.

Kauta, SR, Keenen, BT, Goldberg, L, Schwab, RJ. Diagnosis and treatment of sleep disordered breathing in hospitalized cardiac patients: a reduction in 30-day hospital readmission rates. *J Clin Sleep Med*. 2014;10(10):1051-1059.

Khayat RN, Abraham WT, Patt B, Pu M, Jarjoura D. In-hospital treatment of obstructive sleep apnea during decompensation of heart failure. *Chest*. 2009;136(4):991-997.

Lindenauer PK, Stefan MS, Johnson KG, Priya A, Pekow PS, Rothberg MB. Prevalence, treatment, and outcomes associated with OSA among patients hospitalized with pneumonia. *Chest*. 2014;145(5):1032-1038.

McNicholas WT. Diagnosis of obstructive sleep apnea in adults. *Proc Am Thorac Soc*. 2008;5(2):154-160.

Mokhlesi B, Kryger MH, Grunstein RR. Assessment and management of patients with obesity hypoventilation syndrome. *Proc Am Thorac Soc*. 2008;5(2):218-225.

Myers, KA, Mrkobrada M, Simel DL, Does This Patient Have Obstructive Sleep Apnea? The Rational Clinical Examination Systematic Review. *JAMA*. 2013;310(7):731-741.

Netzer N, Eliasson AH, Netzer C, Kristo DA. Overnight pulse oximetry for sleep-disordered breathing in adults: a review. *Chest*. 2001;120(2):625-633.

Spurr KF, Graven MA, Gilbert RW. Prevalence of unspecified sleep apnea and the use of continuous positive airway pressure in hospitalized patients, 2004 National Hospital Discharge Survey. *Sleep Breath*. 2008;12(3):229-234.

Young T, Palta M, Dempsey J, Peppard PE, Nieto FJ, Mae Hla K. Burden of Sleep Apnea: Rationale, Design, and Major Findings of the Wisconsin Sleep Cohort Study. *WMJ*. 2009;108(5): 246-249.

CHAPTER 236

Pleural Diseases

Carlos E. Kummerfeldt, MD

Nicholas J. Pastis, MD

John T. Huggins, MD

Key Clinical Questions

1. When does a pleural effusion require drainage?
2. Why make the distinction between transudates and exudates?
3. How does the pleural fluid analysis assist in guiding your differential diagnosis?
4. When is a chest tube placement indicated?
5. When should a pulmonary consultation be obtained?

EPIDEMIOLOGY

The seven leading causes of pleural effusions in the United States, in descending order include: (1) congestive heart failure; (2) bacterial pneumonia; (3) malignancy; (4) pulmonary embolism; (5) viral disease; (6) postcoronary artery bypass surgery; and (7) cirrhosis with ascites. Pneumothorax in the hospitalized patient is most commonly found in (1) blunt trauma (35%); (2) transthoracic needle aspiration biopsies (25%); (3) pleural biopsies (8%); (4) transbronchial lung biopsies (6%); (5) mechanically ventilated patients (4%); (6) thoracentesis (2%); and (7) central line insertions (1%-2%). Spontaneous pneumothorax occurs in about 15,000 cases per year in the United States: primary spontaneous pneumothorax occurs in adults with no underlying lung disease, whereas secondary spontaneous pneumothorax occurs in older adults with underlying lung disease, most commonly with chronic obstructive pulmonary disease.

PLEURAL EFFUSIONS

A thoracentesis should be performed in most patients with a pleural effusion (Table 236-1). Thoracentesis should be performed in patients with likely heart failure if the pleural effusion is unilateral, if one side is greater than the other, or if there is suspicion for a dual diagnosis. The major risks and complications of thoracentesis include the following: (1) pneumothorax; (2) bleeding; (3) infection; and (4) procedural related pain. There are no evidence based guidelines in patients with coagulopathies, and there are reports of thoracentesis being performed in patients with an elevated international normalized ratio, uremia, thrombocytopenia or on oral antiplatelet or anticoagulation therapies. The benefits of correcting coagulopathy with transfusions or by withholding antiplatelet or anticoagulation medications should be weighed against the risks in the individual patient and should always be discussed with the patient. Ultrasound should be performed in all patients undergoing thoracentesis to less the risk of complications associated with a blind tap. Ultrasound can identify the pleural fluid and other underlying anatomical structures, estimate the size of the effusion, and determine the presence of underlying septations or complexity that may indicate the presence of loculations (Figure 236-1) (see Chapter 124 [Thoracentesis]).

PLEURAL FLUID ANALYSIS

Pleural fluid analysis is essential to determine the cause of the effusion. The hospitalist should familiarize themselves with the pleural fluid tests routinely ordered and the diagnostic clues they provide. The pleural fluid appearance, color, and even its smell may provide clues as to the diagnosis. Table 236-2 shows the differential diagnosis based on the appearance of the fluid. The following tests should always be obtained: protein, lactate dehydrogenase (LDH), pH, glucose, white cell count and differential, cytology and cultures. Other fluid tests that may assist in confirming a suspected diagnosis in selected patients include fluid amylase, triglyceride, cholesterol, adenosine deaminase (ADA), rheumatoid factor, and antinuclear antibody. Tables 236-3 through 236-5 summarize the use of these tests to narrow the differential diagnosis.

LIGHT'S CRITERIA

Distinction between whether the effusion is an exudate or transudate these two categories may assist in determining the etiology

TABLE 236-1 Indications for Thoracentesis

1. Pleural effusion size ≥1 cm on chest radiography, ultrasound or computed tomography (CT)
2. Fever
3. Pleuritic chest pain
4. Dyspnea
5. Suspected hospital acquired infection
6. Evidence of loculation, complexity, or septations on imaging
7. Evidence of mediastinal shift, complete hemithorax opacification or large effusion on imaging

TABLE 236-2 Differential Diagnosis of Pleural Fluid Based on Appearance

Fluid Appearance	Differential Diagnosis
Light yellow	Transudate
	Urinothorax (smells like urine)
	Exudate
Dark yellow or serous	Exudate
Turbid	Parapneumonic effusion, chylothorax, cholesterol effusion
Purulent	Empyema (putrid smell)
Milky	Chylothorax
Bloody	Parapneumonic, malignancy, hemothorax
Clear or watery	Cerebrospinal fluid leak, peritoneal dialysis, extravascular migration of central venous catheter
Satin sheen	Cholesterol effusion

of the effusion (**Figure 236-2**). Light's criteria is a set of three characteristics that compare the following:

1. pleural fluid to serum protein ratio >0.5;
2. pleural fluid to serum lactate dehydrogenase >0.6; or
3. pleural fluid LDH > two-thirds of the upper normal limit for serum using an "or" rule.

The pleural fluid is classified as an exudate if one of the three criteria is met. The pleural fluid is a transudate if none of the three criteria are met.

Light's criteria may misclassify some transudates as exudates. This commonly occurs in patients with pleural effusions due to congestive heart failure that have received diuretic therapy. In this setting, correct classification may be possible by applying the serum to pleural fluid protein and albumin gradients. If the difference between the serum to pleural fluid protein is >3.1 g/dL or the serum to pleural fluid albumin is >1.2 g/dL, then the effusion is reclassified as a transudate (see Figure 236-2).

Transudates occur as a consequence of changes in the hydrostatic or oncotic forces within the pleural space. The resulting pleural fluid is low in protein and LDH content. The two most commonly encountered transudates in the hospital are congestive heart failure and liver cirrhosis with ascites resulting in hepatic hydrothorax.

■ HEART FAILURE

Systolic and diastolic heart failure represents the most common cause of pleural effusion encountered in the hospital. Fluid accumulates in the pleural space by moving from the lung interstitium across leaky mesothelial cells. The triad of clinical signs and symptoms (dyspnea, orthopnea, lower-extremity edema), bilateral pleural effusions, and cardiomegaly on chest radiography establish the diagnosis. The majority of these effusions resolve with diuretic therapy and do not require thoracentesis for diagnosis (see Chapter 129 [Heart Failure]).

A thoracentesis is indicated if no cardiomegaly is appreciated on chest radiography, if the effusion is unilateral, or if the patient meets one of the criteria listed in Table 236-1. Thoracentesis may be indicated if dyspnea does not resolve with diuretic therapy after a few days or the effusion is large or does not appear to resolve. Thoracentesis should be performed if another concomitant cause for an effusion (dual diagnosis) is suspected or if one of the effusions is significantly greater than the other. The hospitalist should keep in mind that about 80% of patients have bilateral effusions, 15% to 20% a unilateral right side effusion, and only 5% to 10% have a unilateral left side effusion. Pulmonary consultation should be considered in the above settings or if a patient presents with refractory

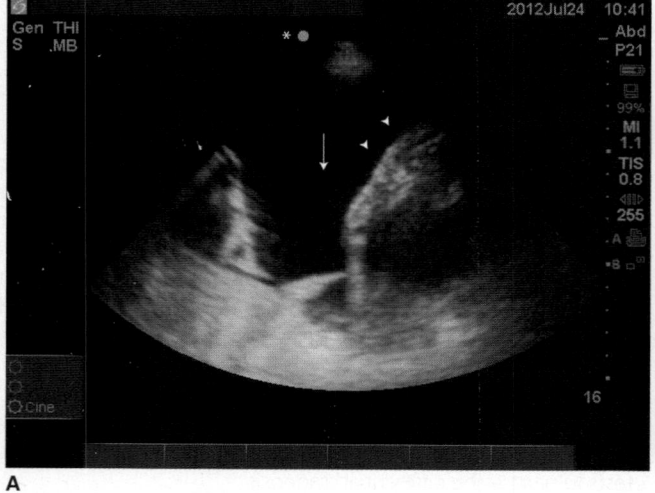

A

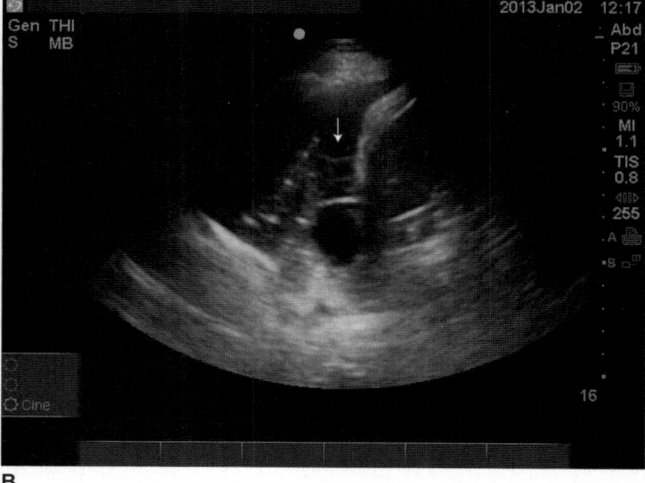

B

Figure 236-1 *Ultrasound images show a large simple pleural effusion and a complex pleural effusion with septations. (A) Large simple anechoic pleural effusion causing atelectasis of the right lower lobe (arrow). The bright white line on the right (arrowheads) represents the diaphragm; the atelectatic lung is on the left and lower parts of the image. (B) Complex pleural effusion with septations demonstrating loculations and complexity (arrow). The small lines between the diaphragm and consolidated lung represent septations.* (Images courtesy of John T Huggins, MD.)

TABLE 236-3 Routine Pleural Fluid Tests Used for Analyzing Pleural Fluid

Test	Comment
Protein	Elevated in exudates; >5.0 g/dL associated with tuberculosis; very low <0.5 g/dL seen in urinothorax, CSF leak, or extravascular migration of central venous catheter
Lactate dehydrogenase	Elevated in exudates; if increasing with serial thoracentesis, indicates worsening degree of pleural space inflammation
pH*	Low pH >7.2-7.3 associated with: (1) complicated parapneumonic effusion; (2) esophageal rupture; (3) rheumatoid and lupus pleuritis; (4) tuberculosis; (5) malignancy; (6) hemothorax; (7) urinothorax
Glucose	Low glucose typically <60 mg/dL associated with: (1) parapneumonic effusion; (2) malignancy; (3) tuberculosis; (4) rheumatoid pleuritis (lupus has normal glucose); (5) hemothorax. When <40 mg/dL and presence of infection, chest tube insertion is indicated
Cytology	Positive for malignancy in up to 60%; yield increases with repeat thoracentesis
Culture	Yield increases when using blood culture bottles (aerobic and anaerobic); mycobacterial and fungal cultures useful when undiagnosed exudate present

*The pH should ideally be measured in a heparinized syringe, placed on ice if not immediately processed and analyzed in a blood gas machine.

symptomatic pleural effusions despite optimal diuretic therapy. In such extreme cases, an indwelling pleural catheter or talc pleurodesis may be considered for palliative measures.

■ HEPATIC HYDROTHORAX

Hepatic hydrothorax is the second most commonly encountered cause of a transudate in the hospitalized patient. It is estimated that about 6% of patients with cirrhosis develop this complication. About 80% of the effusions develop on the right side, 17% on the left, and

TABLE 236-4 Differential Diagnosis Based on the Pleural Fluid Cell Count Differential

Neutrophil Predominance	Lymphocyte Predominance	Eosinophil Predominance
Parapneumonic	Tuberculosis	Pulmonary embolism
Empyema	Malignancy	Asbestos exposure
Pulmonary embolism	Lymphoma	Hemothorax
Acute pancreatitis	Sarcoidosis	Drug induced
Intra-abdominal abscess	Rheumatoid pleuritis	Fungal infections
Bilio-pleural fistula	Postcoronary artery bypass surgery	Eosinophilic granulomatosis with polyangiitis (formerly Churg-Strauss)
	Uremia	Parasite infections
	Chylothorax	

TABLE 236-5 Special Pleural Fluid Tests Used for Analyzing Pleural Fluid

Test	Comment
Albumin	Useful when suspected transudate is misclassified as exudate (see **Figure 236-2**); if SF-A gradient >1.2 g/dL, re-classify effusion as transudate
Amylase	Elevated in: (1) esophageal perforation; (2) pancreatitis (3) pancreatico-pleural fistulas; (4) malignancy
Triglyceride	Elevated to >110 mg/dL in chylothorax
Cholesterol	Elevated to >250 mg/dL in cholesterol effusion due to tuberculosis, rheumatoid pleuritis, trauma, or parasitic infection
Hematocrit	Hemothorax if fluid to peripheral blood hematocrit ratio >50%
Adenosine deaminase	Elevated in patients with tuberculosis; tuberculosis excluded if <40 U/L
Rheumatoid factor	May be elevated to ≥1:320 in rheumatoid pleuritis
Antinuclear antibody	Elevated to >1:40 in lupus pleuritis
Creatinine	Elevated to higher level than serum in urinothorax

SF-A, serum to fluid albumin gradient.

3% occur bilaterally. Ascitic fluid moves via diaphragmatic pores and defects into the pleural space resulting in fluid accumulation. In addition, the negative pressure gradient between the pleural and peritoneal cavities favors movement of fluid into the pleural space. Hepatic hydrothorax may occur in patients without ascites if all the ascites has moved into the pleural cavity.

Thoracentesis should always be performed to exclude spontaneous bacterial pleuritis, defined as the presence of a positive bacterial culture, a pleural fluid neutrophil count >250 cells/µL, and absence of empyema or pneumonia with parapneumonic effusion. Culture negative spontaneous bacterial pleuritis occurs if pleural fluid cultures do not grow any microorganisms and the fluid neutrophil count is >500 cells/µL. A diagnostic thoracentesis should be performed in all cases of ascites and hepatic hydrothorax in patients presenting with fever, even when spontaneous bacterial peritonitis is excluded, due to the presence of hematogenous spread. Antibiotic therapy is the treatment of choice. Chest tube insertion or indwelling pleural catheters should be avoided as they result in persistent fluid drainage and protein loss that leads to malnourishment and higher rates of infection.

Definitive treatment of hepatic hydrothorax should target control of the ascites in consultation with both pulmonary and liver specialists (see Chapter 160 [Cirrhosis and Its Complications]).

■ OTHER TRANSUDATES

Less common transudates include nephrotic syndrome, urinothorax, peritoneal dialysis, trapped lung, myxedema, pericarditis, and cerebrospinal fluid leak (**Table 236-6**). Pulmonary consultation should be sought whenever the cause of a transudate remains unclear.

■ EXUDATES

Exudates occur as a consequence of pleural membrane inflammation and disruption. The resulting pleural fluid is high in protein and LDH content. Exudates result from disruption of the pleural membranes due to inflammation (parapneumonic effusions), direct injury, or invasion as with malignancy (**Table 236-7**). Initial diagnosis will not establish a diagnosis in about 20% of exudates. When the

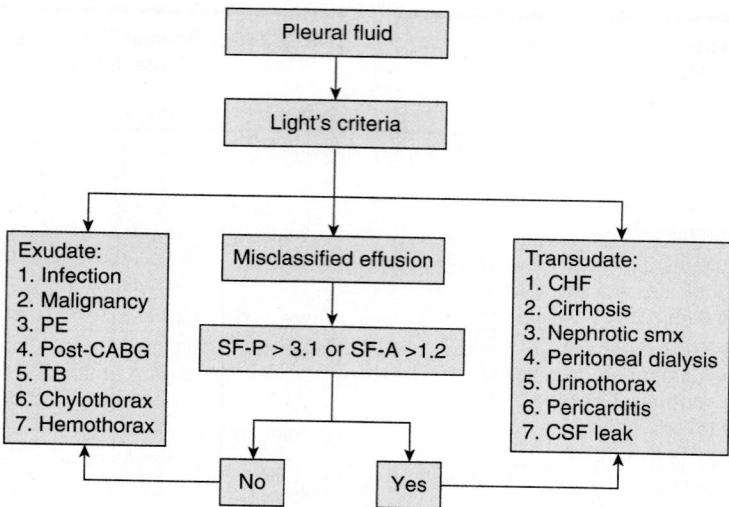

Figure 236-2 *Approach to the hospitalized patient with a pleural effusion.*
CABG, coronary artery bypass graft; CHF, congestive heart failure; CSF, cerebrospinal fluid; SF-A, serum to pleural fluid albumin gradient;
SF-P, serum to pleural fluid protein gradient; smx, syndrome; TB, tuberculosis.

exudate does not resolve spontaneously or if malignancy is being considered, pulmonary consultation should be obtained to assist with appropriate workup that may include pleural biopsy by either medical or surgical thoracoscopy.

■ PARAPNEUMONIC EFFUSIONS

About 40% of bacterial pneumonias are complicated by the development of a parapneumonic effusion. Three stages develop: (1) exudative; (2) fibrinopurulent; and (3) organized. During the first exudative stage, increased permeability in the visceral pleura results in pleural fluid formation characterized by high protein content but normal glucose, pH, and LDH. Bacterial invasion during the second fibrinopurulent stage results in leukocyte, bacteria and cell debris accumulation. Pleural fluid continues to accumulate, and fibrin deposits in the visceral and parietal pleura with resulting loculations. Anaerobic utilization of glucose results in a lower glucose and pH levels, and cell lysis results in increased LDH levels. During the third and final organized stage, pus formation occurs from cellular debris resulting in empyema formation and pleural thickening.

Unless the effusion is small in size (<1 cm when measured from the inner border of the chest wall), the majority of parapneumonic or suspected parapneumonic effusions require thoracentesis. Pleural fluid analysis will determine if chest tube drainage is required (see **Figure 236-3**). Complicated parapneumonic effusions and all empyemas require chest tube drainage. Pulmonary consultation is recommended when chest tube drainage is indicated for evaluation of intrapleural tissue plasminogen activator (t-PA) combined with DNase administration. Intrapleural t-PA with DNase has been shown to reduce hospital stay as well as surgical referrals. Surgical drainage via video-assisted thoracoscopic surgery (VATS) or open thoracotomy should be considered when there is ongoing sepsis, fever and infection despite appropriate antibiotics or chest tube drainage.

■ MALIGNANT EFFUSIONS

Malignant effusions represent the second most common cause of exudates after parapneumonic effusions, affecting about 200,000 persons per year in the United States. Most patients present with dyspnea, cough and less often chest pain. In order of frequency, the most common causes of tumors leading to development of malignant pleural effusion include: (1) lung, most commonly adenocarcinoma

(38%); (2) breast (17%); (3) lymphoma (12%); (4) genitourinary (9%); (5) gastrointestinal (7%); other (7%) and unknown cause (10%).

Malignant effusions develop as a consequence of both an increased amount of fluid entry and a decreased amount of fluid exit from the pleural cavity. Factors that lead to an increased amount of fluid entry include: (1) direct pleural and pulmonary vessel invasion with increased permeability; (2) increased hydrostatic pressures due to venous obstruction; (3) increased vascular endothelial growth factor (VEGF) formation by some tumors; and (4) in some occasions, disruption of lymphatic vessels leading to chyle accumulation. Factors that lead to a decreased amount of fluid exit include: (1) lymphatic obstruction in the parietal pleura or mediastinal lymph nodes; (2) decreased intrapleural pressure from atelectasis formation; and (3) increased central venous pressure if underlying thrombosis is present.

Pleural fluid may demonstrate a serous appearing or bloody effusion. Fluid analysis varies but typically shows an elevated LDH due to a high cell turnover with lysis, a differential showing lymphocyte predominance, and glucose and pH may be low. Fluid cytology may be positive in up to 60% of cases. If measured, amylase may be elevated in about 10% of the cases. A chylothorax may be present. If pleural fluid cytology is negative or indeterminate on initial thoracentesis and a malignant diagnosis is highly suspected, a repeat thoracentesis with cytology is recommended to increase the diagnostic yield. Pulmonary consultation should be sought at this time in order to assist with diagnosis.

Malignant effusions are the most common cause of near complete hemithorax opacification on chest imaging (see **Figure 236-4**). Contralateral shift of the mediastinum usually indicates a large effusion rather than a large mass. If a large effusion does not result in contralateral mediastinal shift, then the lung may be unable to expand. Unexpandable lung or the inability of the lung to fully expand to the chest wall results from the following: (1) trapped lung; (2) visceral pleural inflammation or invasion causing lung entrapment; (3) endobronchial obstruction; and/or (4) chronic atelectasis. Tumor causing endobronchial obstruction and atelectasis may require bronchoscopy; visceral pleural thickening from direct tumor invasion can be better visualized via a contrast chest CT (see **Figure 236-5**).

The goal of therapy of malignant pleural effusions is directed toward palliation of symptoms. Due to rapid reaccumulation and symptom recurrence, repeated thoracentesis is not recommended in the majority of cases. A chest physician should be consulted to

TABLE 236-6 Other Less Common Causes of Transudates

Cause	Characteristics	Imaging
Nephrotic syndrome	Due to decreased oncotic pressure from urine protein loss and increased intravascular hydrostatic pressure from salt retention	Usually bilateral effusions
Urinothorax	Due to renal obstruction resulting in retroperitoneal urine collection and drainage across pressure gradient into pleural cavity; creatinine level in pleural fluid higher than serum	Effusion on same side as obstruction
Peritoneal dialysis	Leakage of dialysate rich in glucose from peritoneal cavity through diaphragmatic defects into pleural space; high glucose and low protein fluid	Usually right sided; may be bilateral
Trapped lung	Old inflammation resulting in fibrous membrane with visceral pleural thickening that causes inability of lung to fully re-expand, increasing negative pressure within pleural space; pleural manometry recommended to establish diagnosis	Unilateral effusion; chest CT with air contrast shows visceral pleural thickening
Myxedema	Forms from decreased lymphatic drainage	Bilateral; concomitant pericardial effusion many times
Constrictive pericarditis	Increased pulmonary and systemic capillary pressures result in fluid formation	Bilateral; may be unilateral
Cerebrospinal fluid leak	Fistula formation between CSF and pleural cavity from surgery, trauma, or shunts; low protein and LDH in fluid; measurement of β_2-transferrin virtually diagnostic	Unilateral

CT, computed tomography; LDH, lactate dehydrogenase.

recommend the most appropriate treatment, based on the individual circumstances:

1) Breast, small cell lung cancer and lymphoma are chemosensitive and respond well to chemotherapy.
2) Talc pleurodesis via chest tube or thoracoscopy may be considered if no evidence of unexpandable lung.
3) Indwelling pleural catheter insertion (such as PleurX® catheters) if unexpandable lung present; about 50% to 60% of effusions resolve after indwelling catheter has been inserted, with subsequent catheter removal and no evidence of recurrence.
4) Thoracic duct ligation or a pleuroperitoneal shunt with pump system is recommended in the presence of chylothorax; indwelling pleural catheters may result in protein and lymphocyte depletion with subsequent malnourishment and infections.

■ PULMONARY EMBOLISM

It is estimated that about 30% of patients with pulmonary embolism have an associated pleural effusion. The effusion may be unilateral

TABLE 236-7 Causes of Pleural Effusions

Exudates	Transudates
Common	**Common**
Parapneumonic	Congestive heart failure
Malignancy	Liver cirrhosis
Less common	**Less common**
Tuberculosis	Nephrotic syndrome
Pulmonary embolism	Urinothorax
Postcoronary artery bypass surgery	Peritoneal dialysis
Chylothorax	Trapped lung
Pseudo-chylothorax	Atelectasis
Hemothorax	
Uremia	
Rheumatoid pleuritis	
Lupus (drug induced or systemic)	
Uncommon	**Uncommon**
Asbestos exposure	Cerebrospinal fluid leak
Drug induced	Constrictive pericarditis
Yellow-nail syndrome	Myxedema
Esophageal perforation	Pulmonary veno-occlusive disease
Pancreatitis	Central venous occlusion
Postabdominal surgery	Extravascular migration of central venous catheter
Bilio-pleural fistula	Glycinothorax
Sarcoidosis	

or bilateral. Computed tomography imaging with contrast can identify segmental or subsegmental filling defects consistent with embolic disease. Treatment of the pulmonary embolism results in resolution of the associated effusion (see Chapter 115 [Advanced Cardiothoracic Imaging]).

■ POSTCORONARY ARTERY BYPASS SURGERY

About 10% of patients who undergo CABG develop a large pleural effusion within 1 month after the surgery most commonly in the left hemithorax, although it may be bilateral with the left effusion usually larger than the right. The effusion is typically bloody as the result of bleeding from the internal mammary harvest site. The cell count has a lymphocyte predominance. One or two therapeutic thoracentesis are required as treatment. Persistence of pleural effusion for greater than 6 months post-CABG is usually due to the presence of a trapped lung. Most often the effusions are transudative and are not associated with respiratory symptoms. However, surgical decortication should be considered if the trapped lung causes a large effusion.

■ POSTCARDIAC INJURY SYNDROME

Postcardiac injury syndrome (previously known as Dressler syndrome) occurs after myocardial infarction, cardiac surgery, pacemaker implantation or blunt chest trauma. It is characterized by the presence of fever, chest pain, a new pericardial friction rub and effusion, and in about 70% of cases small bilateral pleural effusions. Postcardiac injury syndrome may develop between 3 weeks and up to a year after cardiac injury. Postcardiac injury syndrome is usually treated with aspirin, colchicine, or indomethacin and in severe cases corticosteroids.

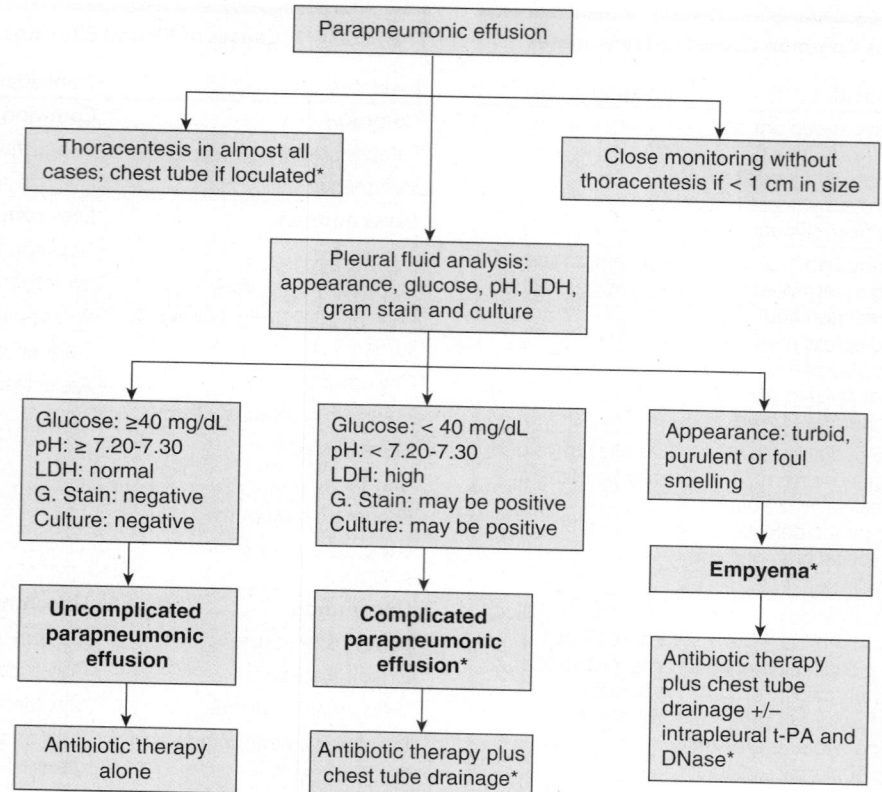

Figure 236-3 *Management of parapneumonic effusions.*

The flowchart contents:

Parapneumonic effusion

- Thoracentesis in almost all cases; chest tube if loculated*
- Close monitoring without thoracentesis if < 1 cm in size

Pleural fluid analysis: appearance, glucose, pH, LDH, gram stain and culture

- Glucose: ≥40 mg/dL
  pH: ≥ 7.20-7.30
  LDH: normal
  G. Stain: negative
  Culture: negative
  → **Uncomplicated parapneumonic effusion**
  → Antibiotic therapy alone

- Glucose: < 40 mg/dL
  pH: < 7.20-7.30
  LDH: high
  G. Stain: may be positive
  Culture: may be positive
  → **Complicated parapneumonic effusion***
  → Antibiotic therapy plus chest tube drainage*

- Appearance: turbid, purulent or foul smelling
  → **Empyema***
  → Antibiotic therapy plus chest tube drainage +/– intrapleural t-PA and DNase*

*Pulmonary consultation is recommended in these situations. Surgery consultation may be needed if persistent fever, sepsis or ongoing infection despite antibiotics and chest tube drainage.

■ TUBERCULOSIS

Although uncommon in the United States, tuberculous pleuritis may result in serious health consequences both to the patient and from a public health perspective if not recognized. There is a 50% probability of developing active tuberculosis within 5 years if the patient does not receive antituberculous therapy. Tuberculous

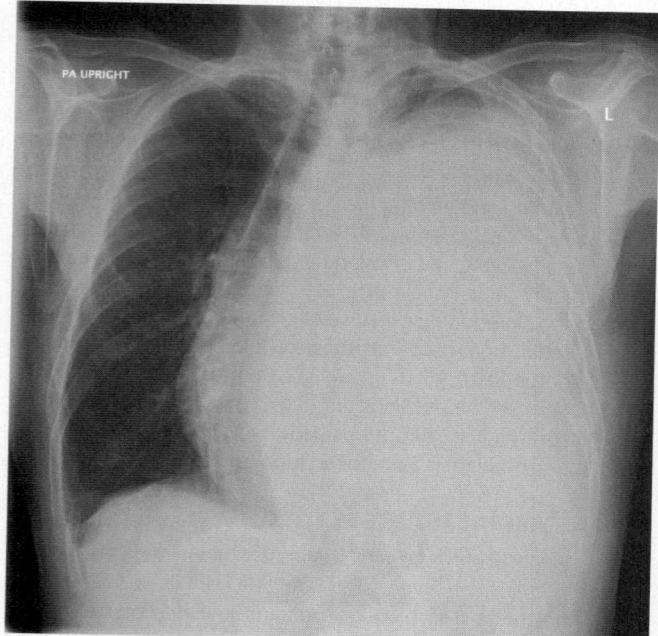

Figure 236-4 *Postero-anterior chest imaging shows a large left-sided pleural effusion with mediastinal shift to the contralateral side. Note the right tracheal deviation, near-complete left hemithorax opacification. The patient had a malignant bloody effusion due to lung adenocarcinoma. (Image courtesy of Sharon Jessie, Radiology Department, TJ Samson Community Hospital.)*

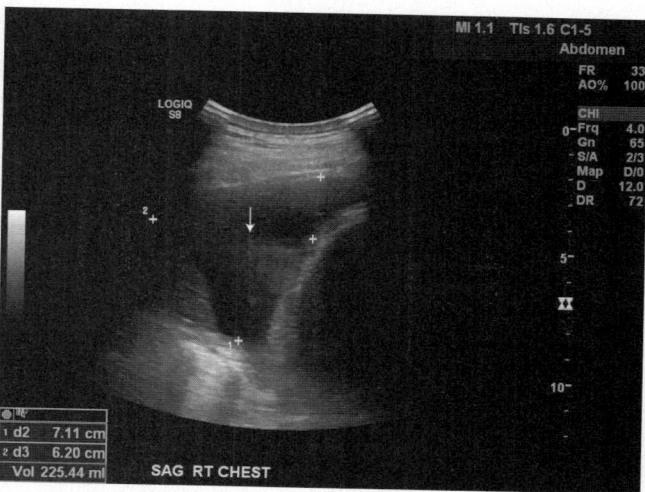

Figure 236-5 *Chest ultrasound shows a pleural opacity consistent with tumor invasion (arrow). (Image courtesy of Sharon Jessie, Radiology Department, TJ Samson Community Hospital.)*

pleuritis may be a consequence of primary infection that occurred 3 to 6 months prior, or due to reactivation. Pleural fluid cultures are negative nearly 80% of the time, and a tuberculin skin test may be negative in up to one-third of patients.

About 67% of patients present with an acute clinical presentation that includes cough, dyspnea and chest pain; these symptoms may be confused with pneumonia and a parapneumonic effusion. Less commonly, patients may present with a chronic illness and a unilateral effusion. Pleural fluid analysis shows lymphocyte predominance. If thoracentesis is done in early stages, pleural fluid may show neutrophil predominance. A very high protein level of greater than 5.0 g/dL is highly suggestive of the diagnosis (Table 236-4). Pulmonary consultation may assist in recommending specific diagnostic pleural tests such as adenosine deaminase (see Table 236-6), polymerase chain reaction for mycobacterial DNA and pleural fluid interferon-γ. Induced sputum smear and culture will be positive in half of the patients. Pleural biopsy should be obtained if suspicion is high and exudative effusion has not resolved. Tuberculous pleuritis typically resolves in several months regardless if tuberculosis treatment is given; however, if tuberculosis treatment is not provided, these patients have a high risk for relapse (see Chapter 200 [Tuberculosis]).

■ HEMOTHORAX

Hemothorax or the presence of blood in the pleural cavity is defined as a pleural fluid hematocrit that is at least 50% that of blood. **Table 236-8** summarizes the causes of hemothorax encountered in the hospital. Bleeding may be significant and lead to hemodynamic compromise and cardiovascular collapse if not recognized quickly. Clinicians should always consider hemothorax in the situations listed in Table 236-8. Management requires chest tube insertion in all cases in order to quantify the rate of bleeding and prevent any of the following complications: (1) retention of clot; (2) infection; and (3) fibrothorax. Thoracic surgical consultation is recommended if chest tube output is greater than 200 mL/h and there are no signs of slowing. Persistence of blood in the pleural space increases the risk for fibrothorax or trapped lung.

■ CHYLOTHORAX AND CHOLESTEROL EFFUSIONS

Chylothorax is the accumulation of lipid from chyle in the pleural space due to disruption or obstruction of the thoracic duct. Chylothoraces may be unilateral or bilateral, depending on the level at which the thoracic duct disruption occurs: right sided if the

TABLE 236-8 Causes of Hemothorax

Traumatic	Iatrogenic	Nontraumatic
Penetrating injury	Thoracic surgery (heart or lung)	Malignant effusion
Nonpenetrating injury	Central vein perforation after central line insertion	Anticoagulation therapy
	Thoracentesis	Ruptured aortic aneurysm
	Chest tube insertion	Arterio-venous malformation
	Lung biopsy	Hematological disorder (ie, hemophilia, thrombocytopenia)
	Transbronchial biopsy	Intrapleural fibrinolytics
		Catamenial

TABLE 236-9 Causes of Chylothorax

Traumatic	Nontraumatic
Iatrogenic	**Tumors**
Surgery	Lymphoma
Radiotherapy	Metastatic pleural tumors
Endoscopy	
Noniatrogenic	**Lymphatic involvement**
Chest wall trauma	Lymphangioleiomyomatosis
Childbirth	Tuberous sclerosis
	Amyloidosis
	Yellow-nail syndrome
	Sarcoidosis
	Filariasis
	Dasatinib and tyrosine kinase inhibitors
	Gorham syndrome
	Venous pressure
	Mediastinal fibrosis
	Superior vena cava thrombosis
	Chylous ascites

disruption occurs below the fourth to sixth thoracic vertebrae, left sided or bilateral if the disruption occurs at this level or above. The pleural fluid has a characteristic milky appearance but may mimic that of empyema. Centrifugation of the fluid will result in layering and deposition of cellular debris at the bottom in empyema, whereas in chylothorax the appearance will remain the same. Pleural fluid analysis shows lymphocyte predominance, a relatively low LDH and high protein (protein discordance) level. Triglyceride levels are greater than 110 mg/dL (see Table 236-6). Chylomicrons should be measured if the triglyceride level falls between 50 and 110 mg/dL. **Table 236-9** lists the causes of chylothorax encountered in the hospital.

A pulmonary consultation is recommended in all cases of chylothoraces to tailor the most appropriate therapy according to the etiology. A diet rich in medium-chain triglycerides may reduce the flow of chyle; absorbed directly into the blood, medium-chain triglycerides bypass the thoracic duct. Octreotide may reduce the rate of chyle formation as well. Thoracentesis may reduce dyspnea; a chest tube should be avoided because drainage of significant amount of protein and lymphocytes may cause malnutrition and immunodeficiency. A pleuroperitoneal shunt may be considered in cases of malignant obstruction unresponsive to chemo- or radiation therapy. Thoracic duct embolization, ligation, or talc pleurodesis are all aimed at controlling chyle leak.

Cholesterol effusion is the accumulation of lipid from cholesterol or lecithin-globulin due to a long-standing pleural effusion in the presence of a pleural cavity surrounded by fibrin. Cholesterol effusion develops in the presence of chronic pleural space inflammation, such as tuberculous pleuritis, rheumatoid pleuritis, parasitic infection, or trauma. Unlike chylothorax, triglyceride levels in pleural fluid are low. Cholesterol crystals may be seen on cytology and the cholesterol level is usually greater than 250 mg/dL (see Table 236-6). Treatment is aimed at the underlying cause.

PNEUMOTHORAX

Pneumothorax is defined as presence of air in the pleural cavity. Primary spontaneous pneumothorax occurs as a result of a ruptured apical pleural bleb in the majority of cases. Chest tube insertion

TABLE 236-10 Classification of Pneumothorax

Spontaneous
Primary (no underlying lung disease)
Secondary (underlying lung disease)
Traumatic
Iatrogenic
Catamenial
Tension

or air evacuation is indicated if the patient is symptomatic or if the pneumothorax is greater than 20% in size. Nearly all patients with secondary spontaneous pneumothoraces require chest tube insertion given their low underlying lung reserve and symptomatic presentation.

The most common cause of pneumothorax in the hospitalized patient is iatrogenic.

Table 236-10 lists the general classification of pneumothoraces. Diagnosis is established by chest radiography or ultrasound imaging (see **Figure 236-6**). Ultrasound findings that indicate the presence of a pneumothorax include: (1) absence of lung-sliding; (2) absence of B-lines; and (3) presence of a lung-point. The identification of a lung-point confirms the presence of pneumothorax; while the absence of lung-sliding on M-mode or 2-D ultrasound suggests a pneumothorax. The nondependent parts of the thorax should be initially scanned with the ultrasound. The size of the pneumothorax is estimated by measuring the distance between the visceral pleural line and the chest wall at the level of the hilum or apex. About 1 cm is equivalent to 10%. The estimated size of the pneumothorax is approximately 20% if the distance is 2 cm.

Chest tube insertion is recommended in iatrogenic pneumothoraces that result in symptoms and are greater than 20% in size. If the patient is asymptomatic and the pneumothorax is less than or equal to 20%, conservative management may be pursued with high-flow 100% continuous oxygen and observation. Tension pneumothorax

may easily develop in patients on mechanical ventilation; and therefore chest tube insertion is recommended in patients who develop iatrogenic pneumothorax. The chest tube should be left in place for at least 48 hours after the air leak stops while these patients remain on the ventilator.

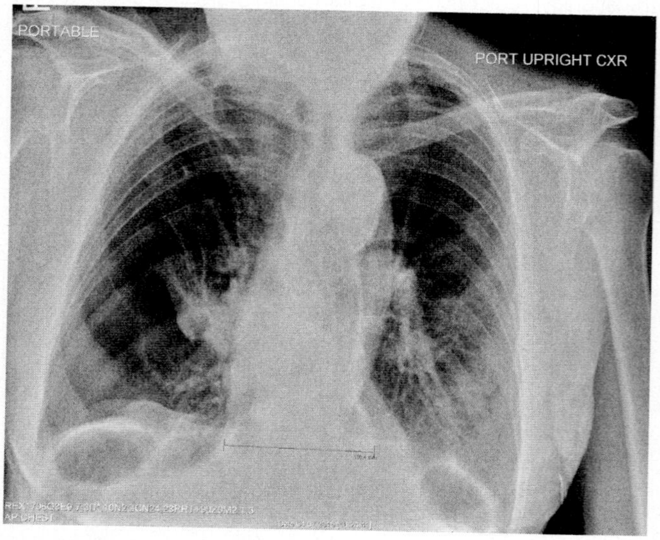

■ TENSION PNEUMOTHORAX

The clinical signs of tension pneumothorax include sudden cardiovascular collapse, cyanosis, and respiratory distress. In mechanically ventilated patients, peak pressure suddenly increases if assist control volume cycled mechanical ventilation is used. In patients receiving cardiopulmonary resuscitation, difficulty in ventilating the patient may be the only sign. Emergent size 14 to 16 gauge needle catheter insertion at the level of the midclavicular line, anterior second intercostal space is performed. The catheter is left in place until air ceases to exit. Chest tube should then be inserted.

PRACTICE POINT

Indications for Chest Tube Insertion

Chest tube insertion should be performed by experienced operators and in the appropriate clinical setting. Smaller bore chest tubes are noninferior to larger bore chest tubes for most indications. Although they are easier to insert and reduce the amount of pain, smaller bore chest tubes tend to dislodge easier. Chest tube insertion is recommended for the following:

- Complicated parapneumonic effusion
- Empyema
- Talc pleurodesis administration
- Hemothorax
- Tension pneumothorax
- Secondary spontaneous pneumothorax and symptomatic
- Pneumothorax greater than 20%

Indwelling pleural catheters are recommended in malignant pleural effusions with an unexpandable lung.

Figure 236-6 *Chest radiography shows a large right side pneumothorax with a visceral pleural line noted and absence of blood vessels and lung markings towards the chest wall beyond the pleural line. Note that the pleural line is sharp and well demarcated.*

PRACTICE POINT

Pulmonary Consultation

Pulmonary consultation is recommended in the following:

- Thoracentesis and chest tube insertion if provider is unfamiliar or uncomfortable with procedures
- Unilateral effusion, absence of cardiomegaly, bilateral asymmetric effusions, fever or pleurisy in a patient with congestive heart failure
- Recurrent hepatic hydrothorax or suspected spontaneous bacterial pleuritis
- Undiagnosed transudate or exudate
- Suspected trapped lung and need for pleural manometry
- Complicated parapneumonic effusions and empyemas
- Evaluation for intrapleural t-PA and DNase
- Malignant effusions with need for indwelling pleural catheter insertion and talc pleurodesis evaluation
- Suspected tuberculous pleuritis
- Hemothorax
- Chylothorax and pseudochylothorax
- Pneumothorax

SUGGESTED READINGS

Broaddus VC, Light RW. Pleural effusion. In: Broaddus VC, Mason RM, Ernst JD, et al, eds. *Murray & Nadel's Textbook of Respiratory Medicine*, 6th ed. Philadelphia, PA: Elsevier Saunders; 2015;1396-1424.

Colice GL, Curtis A, Deslauriers J, et al. Medical and surgical treatment of parapneumonic effusions: an evidence-based guideline. *Chest*. 2000;118(4):1158-1171.

Light RW. *Textbook of Pleural Diseases*. Baltimore, MD: Wolters Kluwer Lippincott Williams and Wilkins; 2013.

Light RW, Macgregor MI, Luchsinger PC, Ball WC Jr. Pleural effusions: the diagnostic separation of transudates and exudates. *Ann Intern Med*. 1972;77(4):507-513.

MacDuff A, Arnold A, Harvey J. Management of spontaneous pneumothorax: British Thoracic Society Pleural Disease Guideline 2010. *Thorax*. 2010;65(Suppl 2):18-31.

Rahman NM, Maskell NA, West A, et al. Intrapleural use of tissue plasminogen activator and DNase in pleural infection. *N Engl J Med*. 2011;356(6):518-526.

Romero-Candeira S, Hernandez L, Romero-Brufao S, Orts D, Fernandez C, Martin C. Is it meaningful to use biochemical parameters to discriminate between transudative and exudative pleural effusions? *Chest*. 2002;122(5):1524-1529.

Sahn SA. Getting the most of pleural fluid analysis. *Respirology*. 2012;17(2):270-277.

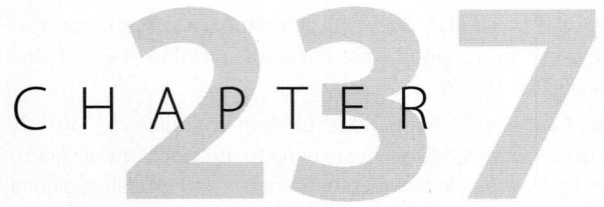

CHAPTER 237

Pulmonary Hypertension

Diego F. Bonilla Arcos, MD
Harrison W. Farber, MD

Key Clinical Questions

1. How does the classification system for pulmonary hypertension (PH) aid in understanding the pathophysiology, diagnostic evaluation, and treatments for this condition?

2. What signs and symptoms might increase the suspicion for elevated pulmonary arterial pressures?

3. What is a rational diagnostic approach to suspected PH?

4. What is the meaning of an elevated pulmonary pressure determined by echocardiography?

5. When should right heart catheterization be considered in the evaluation of suspected PH?

6. What are the key steps in the evaluation and management of acute right heart failure secondary to elevated pulmonary arterial pressure?

7. What are the common side effects of the medications used to treat PH?

INTRODUCTION

Pulmonary hypertension (PH) is simply defined as a mean pulmonary arterial pressure > 25 mm Hg at rest. However, this deceptively simple definition encompasses a broad spectrum of clinical entities. In this chapter, we will present an evidence-based approach to the care of the patient with elevated pulmonary arterial pressures. **Table 237-1** lists landmark studies supporting the approach presented in this chapter.

DISEASE CLASSIFICATION, EPIDEMIOLOGY, AND PATHOPHYSIOLOGY

The first step in understanding the myriad presentations of pulmonary hypertension is to comprehend the pathophysiologic differences that divide the major groups of this disorder. These groups, as defined by the 2013 Fifth World Symposium on Pulmonary Arterial Hypertension, are shown in **Table 237-2**.

■ GROUP I DISEASE

Group I disease, defined as pulmonary arterial hypertension (PAH), is characterized histologically by plexiform lesions occluding the pulmonary vasculature, in situ thrombosis, intimal proliferation, medial thickness and an apoptosis-resistant state producing a chaotic metabolism and mitochondrial structure, inflammation, and dysregulation of growth factors. This process results in decreased pulmonary vascular surface area, increased pulmonary vascular resistance, and functional disruptions of normal endothelial homeostasis. These perturbations are most notable in the prostacyclin, endothelin, nitric oxide, and serotonergic pathways regulating endothelial function. These pathways are the targets of current PAH therapy.

Group I PAH is most commonly idiopathic or heritable (in 80% of families with multiple cases of PAH, mutations in the bone morphogenic protein receptor type 2 can be identified), drug/toxin induced, or associated with other conditions, including collagen vascular disease (most notably, systemic sclerosis), HIV infection, portal hypertension, schistosomiasis, or congenital heart disease. This group also includes persistent pulmonary hypertension of the newborn and pulmonary veno-occlusive disease (PVOD)/pulmonary capillary hemangiomatosis (PCH).

Idiopathic pulmonary arterial hypertension (IPAH, formerly, "primary pulmonary hypertension") is rare, but life threatening, with a prevalence of approximately 15 cases/million, an incidence of 2.4 cases/million/y, and a median survival of only 2.8 years without treatment. The vast majority of patients diagnosed with IPAH are in World Health Organization functional classes III and IV, which have been associated with a poorer prognosis.

Recent evidence suggests that PAH in systemic sclerosis may be diagnosed earlier by annual cardiopulmonary screening in asymptomatic patients with the SSc spectrum of diseases, although there is currently a lack of evidence-based data, especially in individual with a DLCO >60%. Screening of patients with the SSc spectrum of diseases without clinical signs and symptoms of PH should include a 2-step approach using clinical assessment for the presence of telangiectasia, anti-centromere anti- bodies, PFT and DLCO measurements, electrocardiogram, and biomarkers (NT-proBNP and uric acid) in the initial stage, followed by echocardiography and consideration of RHC in patients with abnormal findings. The American College of Rheumatology recommends annual echocardiography and PFTs in these individuals because 10% of SSc patients will develop PH during the course of the disease.

TABLE 237-1 Evidence-based Key References: Pulmonary Hypertension

Topic	Supporting Literature
Epidemiology	Humbert M, Sitbon O, Chaaouat A, et al. Pulmonary hypertension in France: results from a national registry. *Am J Resp Crit Care Med.* 2006;173:1023-1030.
	Lam CSP, Roger VL, Rodeheffer RJ, et al. Pulmonary hypertension in patients with preserved ejection fraction: a community based study. *J Am Coll Card.* 2009;53:1119-1126.
	Badesch DB, Raskob G, Elliott G, et al. Pulmonary arterial hypertension: baseline characteristics from the REVEAL registry. *Chest.* 2010;137(2):376-387.
Classification and pathophysiology	Farber HW, Loscalzo J. Pulmonary arterial hypertension. *N Engl J Med.* 2004;351:1655-1665.
	Gerald Simonneau MD, Michael A Gatzoulis MD PhD, et al. Updated Clinical Classification of Pulmonary Hypertension. J Am Coll Cardiol. 2013;62(25_S). doi:10.1016/j.jacc.2013.10.029.
	Marius M. Hoeper, MD, Harm Jan Bogaard, MD, et al. Definitions and Diagnosis of Pulmonary Hypertension. J Am Coll Cardiol. 2013;62(25_S):. doi:10.1016/j.jacc.2013.10.032.
	Overbeek MJ, Vonk MC, Boonstra A, et al. Pulmonary arterial hypertension in limited cutaneous systemic sclerosis: a distinctive vasculopathy. *Eur Respir J.* 2009;34(2):371-379.
Diagnosis: examination, laboratory	Rich S, Dantzker DR, Ayres SM, et al. Primary pulmonary hypertension: a national prospective study. *Ann Intern Med.* 1987;107:216-223.
	Dahlstrom U. Can natriuretic peptides be used for the diagnosis of diastolic heart failure? *Eur J Heart Fail.* 2004;6:281-287.
	Nagaya N, Nishikimi T, Uematsu M, et al. Plasma brain natriuretic peptide as a prognostic indicator in patients with primary pulmonary hypertension. *Circulation.* 2000;102:865-870.
Diagnosis: echocardiography, imaging	Aurigemma GP, Zile MR, Gaasch WH. Lack of relationship between Doppler indices of diastolic function and left ventricular pressure transients in patients with definite diastolic heart failure. *Am Heart J.* 2004;148:E12.
	Fisher MR, Forfia PR, Chamera E, et al. Accuracy of doppler echocardiography in the hemodynamic assessment of pulmonary hypertension. *Am J Respir Crit Care Med.* 2009;179:615-621.
	Chetty KG, Brown SE, Light RW. Identification of pulmonary hypertension in chronic obstructive pulmonary disease from routine chest radiographs. *Am Rev Respir Dis.* 1982;126:338-341.
	Tunariu N, Gibbs SJ, Win Z, et al. Ventilation-perfusion scintigraphy is more sensitive than multidetector CTPA in detecting chronic thromboembolic pulmonary disease as a treatable cause of pulmonary hypertension. *J Nucl Med.* 2007;48:680-684.
Treatment	Barst RJ, Rubin LJ, Long WA, et al. A comparison of continuous intravenous epoprostenol (prostacyclin) with conventional therapy for primary pulmonary hypertension. The Primary Pulmonary Hypertension Study Group. *N Engl J Med.* 1996;334:296-302.
	Nazzareno Galiè MD, Paul A. Corris MD, et al. Updated Treatment Algorithm of Pulmonary Arterial Hypertension. J Am Coll Cardiol. 2013;62(25_S):. doi:10.1016/j.jacc.2013.10.031.
	Jais X, D'Armini AM, Jansa P, et al. Bosentan for the treatment of inoperable chronic thromboembolic pulmonary hypertension: BENEFit. *J Am Coll Cardiol.* 2008;52:2127-2134.
	Galie N, Ghofrani HA, Torbicki A, et al. Sildenafil citrate therapy for pulmonary arterial hypertension. *N Engl J Med.* 2005;353:2148-2157.
Complications	Belenkie I, Dani R, Smith ER, Tyberg JV. Effects of volume loading during experimental acute pulmonary embolism. *Circulation.* 1989;80:178-188.
	Kallen AJ, Lederman E, Balaji A, et al. Incidence of central line infection in pulmonary hypertension patients receiving prostanoids. *Infect Control Hosp Epidemiol.* 2008;29:332-339.

■ GROUP II DISEASE

Group II disease constitutes the most common cause of elevated pulmonary pressures: pulmonary venous hypertension. Pulmonary hypertension (PH) is a common complication of left heart disease (LHD) due to left ventricular systolic or diastolic heart failure with preserved ejection fraction, or valvular disease. Congenital or acquired left-heart inflow/outflow obstructive lesions and congenital cardiomyopathies have been added to Group 2. Compared to pulmonary arterial hypertension (PAH), patients with PH-LHD are older, female, with a history of systemic hypertension, and characteristics of the metabolic syndrome.

The current hemodynamic definition of PH-LHD combines a mean pulmonary artery pressure (mPAP) 25 mm Hg, a pulmonary artery wedge pressure (PAWP) >15 mm Hg, and a normal or reduced cardiac output (CO).

Due to the low sensitivity of traditional echocardiographic measures (eg, E/A ratio) for the diagnosis of left ventricular diastolic dysfunction, this disorder may be confused with IPAH in the absence of right heart catheterization showing an elevated pulmonary artery occlusion pressure. Although treatment of underlying cardiac disease including repair of valvular heart disease and aggressive therapy for HF with reduced or preserved ejection function are the mainstays of group II disease therapy, a small proportion of patients with long-standing pulmonary venous hypertension may develop physiology and histology consistent with group I disease; this is usually poorly responsive to traditional cardiac risk factor modification.

In severe HF, optimizing volume status is of critical importance and might require invasive monitoring. Moreover, the implantation of an LV assist device has been shown to lower pulmonary pressures through LV unloading without increasing the risk of postimplantation

TABLE 237-2 2013 Fifth World Symposium on Pulmonary Arterial Hypertension: Classification

Group I. Pulmonary arterial hypertension

- Idiopathic (formerly "primary pulmonary hypertension")
- Heritable
- Drug or toxin-induced (eg, anorexigens, rapeseed oil, l-tryptophan, methamphetamine, and cocaine)
- Associated conditions: collagen vascular disease, congenital heart disease, portal hypertension, HIV infection, schistosomiasis
- Associated with significant venous or capillary involvement
  - Pulmonary veno occlusive disease
  - Pulmonary-capillary hemangiomatosis
  - Persistent pulmonary hypertension of the newborn

Group II. Pulmonary venous hypertension

- Left-sided systolic, diastolic, or valvular heart disease
- Congenital/Acquired left heart inflow/outflow tract obstruction and congenital cardiomyopathies

Group III. Pulmonary hypertension associated with lung disease and/or chronic hypoxemia

- Chronic obstructive pulmonary disease
- Interstitial lung disease
- Mixed restrictive and obstructive lung diseases
- Sleep-disordered breathing
- Alveolar hypoventilation disorders
- Chronic exposure to high altitude
- Developmental abnormalities

Group IV. Chronic thromboembolic pulmonary hypertension

Group V. Pulmonary hypertension of unclear or multifactorial mechanisms

- Hematologic disorders: splenectomy, myeloproliferative disorders
- Systemic disorders: sarcoidosis, pulmonary Langerhans' cell histiocytosis, lymphangiomatosis, vasculitis, neurofibromatosis, chronic hemolytic anemias
- Metabolic disorders: Gaucher's, glycogen storage disease, thyroid disease
- Other: tumoral compression of pulmonary vessels, fibrosing mediastinitis, chronic hemodialysis, segmental PH

Adapted, with permission, from Simmoneau G, et al. Updated clinical Classification of Pulmonary Hypertension. *J Am Coll Cardiol*. 2013; 62(25 Suppl):D34-41.

RV failure. Treatment of patients with pulmonary venous hypertension with pulmonary vasodilators may result in pulmonary edema from sudden reduction of pulmonary vascular resistance and acutely increased preload overwhelming the compromised left ventricle. This underscores the importance of right heart catheterization to correctly characterize the etiology of pulmonary hypertension prior to starting therapy.

■ GROUP III DISEASE

Group III disease describes PH due to chronic lung disease and hypoxic vasoconstriction. This group most commonly presents with known pulmonary diseases such as chronic obstructive pulmonary disease (COPD), interstitial lung disease (ILD), obstructive sleep apnea (OSA), and/or obesity hypoventilation syndromes.

The prevalence of pulmonary hypertension in COPD is related to the severity of the disease. Studies have shown that up to 90% of patients with GOLD (Global Initiative for Chronic Obstructive Lung Disease) stage IV disease have a mean pulmonary artery pressure of >20 mm Hg, with most ranging between 20 and 35 mm Hg. The presence of PH is a strong predictor of mortality in COPD. A 5-year survival rate of only 36% has been reported in COPD patients with mPAP values > 25 mm Hg. Combined pulmonary fibrosis and emphysema (CPFE) patients have an increased risk to develop PH, with estimates approaching 30% to 50%. In these patients normal or mildly subnormal lung volumes and the absence of airflow obstruction coexist with severe PH and markedly reduced DLCO. Treatment of the underlying lung disease and use of supplemental oxygen are the foundations of care for pulmonary hypertension associated with chronic hypoxemia. Because pulmonary vasodilators may elicit significant ventilation/perfusion mismatch and severe hypoxemia with in patients with underlying structural lung disease, these medications are currently only investigational in this patient population.

■ GROUP IV DISEASE

Group IV disease is caused by thromboembolic disease to the pulmonary circulation, generating chronic thromboembolic pulmonary hypertension (CTEPH). Definitive treatment of group IV disease due to thrombotic pulmonary emboli involves pulmonary arterial thromboendarterectomy (PEA).

Although computed tomography (CT) and magnetic resonance imaging (MRI) have evolved, VQ scan remains the preferred test for screening for chronic thromboembolic disease and this is the initial step in the diagnosis of CTEPH. Pulmonary angiography remains the gold standard for diagnosis of chronic thromboembolic disease and assessment of operability. For inoperable CTEPH and residual disease after PEA, medical therapy is recommended; riociguat is the first drug approved for treatment in this population.

■ GROUP V DISEASE

Group V disease is best described as a catch-all of miscellaneous causes of PH. These include diseases with multifactorial mechanisms (ie, hematologic disorders, metabolic disorders, sarcoidosis, etc) or disease states associated with external compression of pulmonary arteries, such as tumor, lymphadenopathy, or fibrosing mediastinitis (most commonly caused by radiation therapy for Hodgkin disease), chronic myeloproliferative (CML) disorders, end-stage renal disease treated with hemodialysis, and segmental PH (pediatric classification).

There may be overlap of disease classification in any of individual case of PH. Given the potential complications associated with improper use of pulmonary vasodilators in patients with group II-V disease, initiation of these agents (prostacyclins, phosphodiesterase inhibitors, endothelin receptor antagonists, soluble guanylyl cyclase agonists) should be restricted to specialists with experience in their use, only after a diagnostic group has been established for a particular patient.

■ DIAGNOSIS

Obtaining a correct diagnostic classification for any patient with suspected or established PH is essential for initiating proper treatment. An evidence-based approach to the diagnostic evaluation of suspected PH is paramount. Patients with PH most often present with nonspecific signs and symptoms, as exemplified by an average time from onset of symptoms to diagnosis of 2 years. The following discussion will present a general diagnostic algorithm (**Figure 237-1**) for a patient with suspected PH. Ultimately, *the diagnosis of PH must be established by right heart catheterization (RHC) in all patients*. PH is defined as PAP ≥ 25 mm Hg at rest measured by RHC.

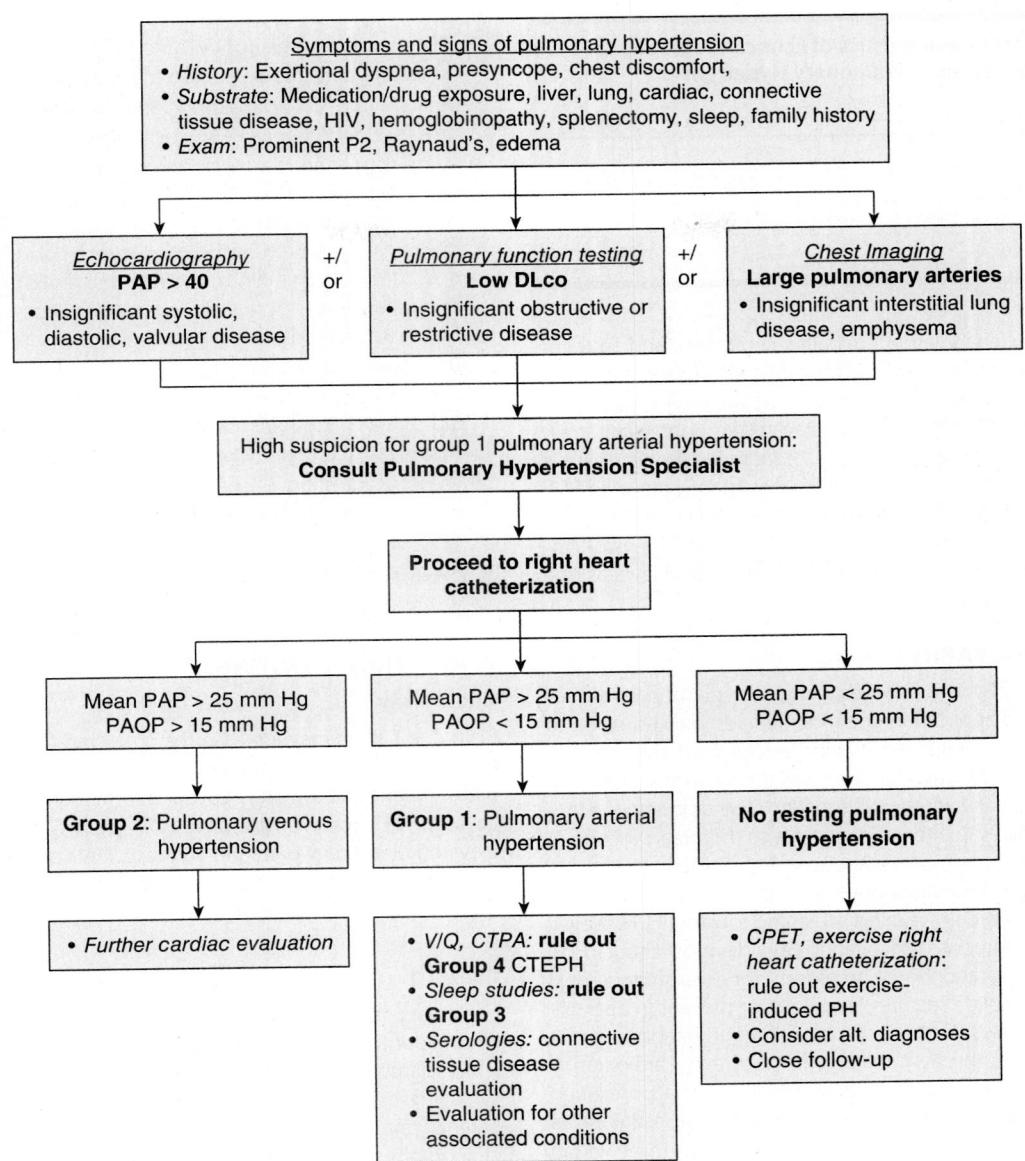

Figure 237-1 *Algorithm for evaluation of suspected pulmonary hypertension.*

◼ SYMPTOMS

While PH often presents as an incidental echocardiographic finding of a high-velocity tricuspid regurgitant jet, certain presenting symptoms should also trigger evaluation for PH in the alert clinician. Due to their gradually progressive and nonspecific nature, PH symptoms are often misdiagnosed as asthma, cardiac ischemia, or left undiagnosed. However, *exertional* symptoms such as progressive exertional dyspnea, lightheadedness, syncope, or exertional chest pain should include pulmonary hypertension on their differential diagnosis. The presence of any of risk factors for the PH listed above (eg, exposure to toxins, anorexigens, selective serotonin reuptake inhibitor (SSRIs), diagnosis of systemic sclerosis, cirrhosis, HIV, connective tissue disease (CTD), congenital heart disease, congestive heart failure, COPD, sleep apnea, and pulmonary embolism) should further raise suspicion for PH. In fact, echocardiographic screening for PH in high-risk populations (such as those with a known genetic mutation, a first-degree relative with PAH, systemic sclerosis, the scleroderma (SSc) spectrum of disease, congenital heart disease, CTD, portal hypertension awaiting liver transplant) is advocated in the literature.

◼ PHYSICAL EXAMINATION

Examination findings for PH are often subtle. Exertional oxygen desaturation may be the first sign of the diffusion limitation caused by reduction of the pulmonary arterial surface area. A prominent second heart sound is the most sensitive examination finding for PH, present in more than 90% of IPAH patients, but is nonspecific. Other nonspecific findings of PH include those of right heart strain such as right ventricular heave and tricuspid murmur (an increase in tricuspid regurgitation with inspiration is called Carvallo sign), and signs of right heart failure such as elevated jugular venous pressure, peripheral edema, and ascites. Examination should include an evaluation for signs of PH-associated disease with special attention paid to signs and symptoms of systemic sclerosis or Raynaud phenomenon, which are commonly associated with PH.

◼ LABORATORY EVALUATION

Laboratory tests may be performed to help classify PH or aid in prognosis. Limited laboratory evaluation of a patient with suspected PH may include arterial blood gas analysis to differentiate an abnormal A-a gradient from chronic hypoventilation, HIV testing, tests of liver

TABLE 237-3 Test Characteristics of Echocardiography for the Diagnosis of Pulmonary Hypertension

Associated Condition	Sensitivity	Specificity
Portal hypertension	97%	77%
Systemic sclerosis	58%-90%	75%-96%
Chronic obstructive pulmonary disease	60%-78%	75%
Pulmonary fibrosis	77%	45%

function (albumin, coagulation), hepatitis serologies, and tests for connective tissue disease (ANA with anti-centromere pattern is associated with PH in limited systemic sclerosis). B-type natriuretic peptides (BNP, pro–NT-BNT) may be elevated in right heart strain of any etiology and BNP may be falsely *negative* in chronic diastolic CHF. However, in patients with known PH, persistently elevated BNP (> 180 pg/mL) after prostacyclin treatment is associated with poor prognosis, with median survival less than 12 months. The most current treatment guidelines recommend a "normal" BNP level as one potential treatment goal.

■ ECHOCARDIOGRAPHY

Echocardiography allows for the estimation of pulmonary arterial systolic pressure via application of a modified Bernoulli equation to the tricuspid regurgitant jet velocity $[4 \times (velocity)^2]$. It also provides information of left ventricular function, valvular heart disease, intracardiac shunt, and right ventricular function. The ubiquity of echocardiography in the evaluation of patients with dyspnea, syncope or chest discomfort (all symptoms associated with PH), often results in incidental detection of elevated pulmonary pressures. Echocardiography is recommended as the initial screening tool for PH. However, it is important to appreciate its limitations as a diagnostic tool in PH. First, tricuspid regurgitation must be present for echocardiographic estimates of PA systolic pressures, and it is not present in approximately 25% of PH cases. Absence of tricuspid regurgitation does not exclude PH. Second, the test characteristics of echocardiography for the detection of PH range widely, based on the population screened (**Table 237-3**). In addition, echocardiographic estimates of pulmonary arterial systolic pressure have been shown to be within 10 mm Hg of right heart catheterization measurements only 48% of the time. Therefore, while echocardiography is certainly a valuable tool for the evaluation of subjects with PH, echocardiography can neither accurately rule in or out the diagnosis of PH. Direct measurement of cardiopulmonary parameters by cardiac catheterization must be performed in all patients with a high clinical suspicion of PH.

■ RIGHT HEART CATHETERIZATION

Right heart catheterization is the gold standard for the diagnosis of PH. PH treatment should not be instituted in the absence of RHC since it allows assessment of multiple hemodynamic factors essential in the diagnosis and treatment of PH. Patients with a high clinical suspicion of PH should be referred to a pulmonary or cardiology specialist with PH experience.

PRACTICE POINT

Interpretation of right heart catheterization values in the evaluation of pulmonary hypertension

- Right atrial pressure and right ventricular diastolic pressure provide an index of the degree of right heart failure; additionally a RA pressure > 20 mm Hg confers a poor prognosis.

- Filling pattern of the right ventricle provides an index of pericardial constrictive disease that can mimic PH.
- Mean pulmonary arterial pressure is used to diagnose the presence of PH (mean PAP > 25 mm Hg at rest).
- Pulmonary artery diastolic pressure-to-pulmonary artery occlusion pressure gradient is important in the analysis of the contribution of pulmonary venous hypertension (eg, CHF) to pulmonary hypertension. Pulmonary arterial occlusion pressure > 15 mm Hg with pulmonary arterial diastolic pressure-to-pulmonary artery occlusion pressure gradient < 5 mm Hg makes left heart disease the most likely etiology for elevated pulmonary pressures.
- Cardiac index < 2 L/min in pulmonary arterial hypertension is indicative of right heart failure and generally an indication for therapy with prostanoids.
- Vasodilator testing is used to determine the potential for responsiveness to calcium channel blocker therapy; however, vasoreactivity is present in less than 5% of patients with PAH (usually only patients with IPAH or HPAH).

■ ADDITIONAL TESTING

Chest x-ray

Plain chest films may increase the suspicion for PH: a descending branch of the right pulmonary artery > 20 mm is often associated with PH. Chest X-ray adds critical information as to the potential cause of PH. For example, a normal plain film in the setting of elevated pulmonary pressures suggests IPAH or CTEPH, or the presence of reticular opacities suggests PH secondary to interstitial lung disease or connective tissue disease.

Chest CT

Computed tomographic imaging of the chest may add additional information to the chest radiograph. Although a main pulmonary artery diameter > 33 mm may be associated with IPAH, this association does not appear as reliable in subjects with underlying parenchymal lung disease. CT scans are more sensitive than chest radiography in the diagnosis of underlying ILD.

V/Q scan

V/Q scanning has utility in the evaluation of CTEPH, where it has a greater sensitivity for the detection of chronic pulmonary thromboembolic disease than CTPA.

Cardiac magnetic resonance imaging

Cardiac magnetic resonance imaging (cMRI) is increasingly being used for the assessment of right heart structure and volumes. In response to chronic PH, the right ventricle hypertrophies and dilates, leading to reduced function and stroke volume. Right ventricular end-diastolic volume index (RVEDVI) <84 mL/m^2, left ventricular end-diastolic volume index >40 mL/m^2, and a stroke volume index >25 mL/m^2 are associated with better survival in patients with IPAH. RVEDVI has been linked to be an independent predictor of mortality; no deaths were reported in patients with RVEDVI <84 mL/m^2. RV mass index <59 g/m^2 was linked to better survival in IPAH, and in patients with suspected scleroderma PAH, the ratio of RV to left ventricular end-diastolic mass >0.7 predicted worse survival. As right heart function is acknowledged as the main determinant of survival in PAH, cMRI may eventually provide consistent and valuable information regarding prognosis; however, further investigation is needed to assess the role of this modality in PH.

Electrocardiogram

ECGs of patients with PH may show signs of right heart strain and hypertrophy. These signs, right axis deviation, large R/S ratio > 1 in V1, R/S ratio < 1 in V5 or V6, P pulmonale, lack both sensitivity and specificity for routine use in diagnosis.

Pulmonary function testing

Pulmonary function testing (PFT) showing an isolated low diffusing capacity of the lung for carbon monoxide without anemia increases the suspicion for pulmonary vascular disease. In patients with known PH, PFTs may help in determining the diagnosis and severity of causes of secondary PH such as COPD and ILD.

Polysomnography

Sleep studies are indicated for the diagnosis and treatment of PH secondary to OSA.

Cardiopulmonary exercise testing

Cardiopulmonary exercise testing is valuable in the evaluation of unexplained dyspnea. Subjects with low maximum VO_2, low anaerobic threshold, low oxygen pulse, elevated ventilatory equivalent of CO_2 (VE/VCO$_2$), a large A-a gradient and increased dead space should undergo further evaluation for PH. This test may not be available in all centers.

Biopsy

Lung biopsy is rarely indicated after a diagnosis of PH has been established; usually only to confirm the suspicion of occult underlying causes such as pulmonary veno-occlusive disease.

TREATMENT

In general, treatment of group II-V disease is directed at the underlying disease pathology that has contributed to pulmonary hypertension (except as noted above for CTEPH).

Treatment goals do not differ for different PAH subgroups. Exceptions contain the limited utility of functional and biomarker goals in SSc-PAH and the importance of hemodynamic goals in patients with PAH related to portal hypertension being studied for liver transplantation.

Treatment of group I pulmonary hypertension is guided by findings on RHC and functional status. Multiple agents now exist in various drug classes for the treatment of group I PAH. The agents, indications, and common side effects are shown in **Table 237-4**. Below we present a brief discussion of the indications, mechanisms of action, and the major side effects of the currently approved treatments for group IPAH.

■ NITRIC OXIDE

Nitric oxide (NO) is a potent vasodilator and an inhibitor of platelet activation and vascular smooth muscle proliferation. Inhaled NO is potentially useful for PAH by controlling RV hypertrophy and augmenting downstream signaling targets, including but not limited to soluble guanylate cyclase and cyclic guanosine monophosphate, to reduce pulmonary vascular remodeling. Different formulations of inhaled NO are currently under investigation for treatment of PAH.

■ CALCIUM CHANNEL BLOCKERS

Dihydropyridine calcium channel blockers are not FDA-approved for use in pulmonary arterial hypertension and have been shown to be useful only in IPAH patients with positive vasoreactivity testing. This group encompasses < 5% of all patients with IPAH.

■ PROSTACYCLINS

Epoprostenol, treprostinil (in various formulations), beraprost and inhaled iloprost comprise the currently approved prostanoid medications for the treatment of PAH. These medications are analogues of prostacyclin, an endogenous vasodilator product of arachidonic acid metabolism in the vascular endothelium. Through stimulation of intracellular cAMP, prostacyclins inhibit smooth muscle proliferation and platelet aggregation. Intravenous epoprostenol is the only agent shown in a randomized controlled trial to confer a mortality benefit in PAH. Because of its short half-life, interruption of epoprostenol infusion may result in acute increases in pulmonary vascular resistance and hemodynamic collapse. For this reason, longer-acting medications such as treprostinil—with a half-life of hours rather than minutes—have been developed. Additionally, treprostinil may be administered subcutaneously, intravenously,

TABLE 237-4 Pulmonary Vasodilators

Pulmonary Vasodilator	NYHA Functional Status Indication	Route	T 1/2	Common Side Effects
Prostacyclins				
• Epoprostenol	II-IV	Intravenous	6 min	Hypotension, jaw/leg pain, flushing, headache, diarrhea, thrombocytopenia
• Treprostinil	II-IV	Intravenous, subcutaneous Inhaled	4 h	In addition to above, local reactions (SQ administration), bacteremia
• Iloprost	II-III	Inhaled	30 min	Bronchospasm, cough, trismus, flushing, hypotension
Endothelin Receptor Antagonists				
• Bosentan	III	Oral	5 h	Liver toxicity, headache, anemia, edema, flushing, hypotension
• Ambrisentan	II-III	Oral	9-15 h	Headache, edema, anemia, liver toxicity
• Macitentan	II-III	Oral	16 h	Headache, anemia, liver toxicity, sperm count decr, bronchitis
Phosphodiesterase-5 inhibitors				
• Sildenafil	II-III	Oral	4 h	Headache, diarrhea, flushing, hypotension, priapism, optic neuropathy
• Tadalafil	II-III	Oral	17.5 h	Same as sildenafil
Soluble guanylate cyclase stimulators				
• Riociguat	II-III	Oral	12 h	Headache, hemorrhage, hemoptysis, diarrhea, hypotension, anemia, vomiting

orally or inhaled. Inhaled iloprost and treprostinil have the theoretical advantage of improved V/Q matching compared with intravenous medications. In general, patients with right heart failure, NYHA functional class IV disease, and cardiac index of < 2 L/min generally require continuous intravenous prostacyclin therapy. Common side effects of the intravenous prostacyclins include thrombocytopenia and bleeding, jaw pain, leg pain, flushing, headache, nausea, and vomiting.

■ ENDOTHELIN-RECEPTOR ANTAGONISTS

Bosentan, ambrisentan, and macitentan represent the currently available endothelin-receptor antagonists in the United States and are widely used due to the ease of oral administration. Endothelin A receptors are located on vascular smooth muscle cells and mediate vasoconstriction and proliferation, while endothelin B receptors, located on endothelium, promote vasodilatation. While, it appears that, in vitro, the effects of endothelin A receptors are of greater importance than endothelin B receptors, in clinical practice, it is not clear that there are substantial differences among the ERAs since they have never been studied against one another. The nonselective endothelin-receptor antagonists bosentan and macitentan, as well as the selective endothelin A-receptor antagonist ambrisentan have all demonstrated efficacy in the treatment of PAH. Liver toxicity is the most worrisome side effect (8%-12%) of bosentan; as such, liver function tests must be followed monthly. Ambrisentan and macitentan have a much lower incidence of liver toxicity (2%-3%); with these agents, liver function tests are followed as clinically indicated. Other side effects of this class include, nasal stuffiness, and edema. Ambrisentan has much few drug-drug interactions.

■ SOLUBLE GUANYLATE CYCLASE STIMULATORS

sGC stimulators augment cGMP production and are effective additionally in states in which endogenous NO is depleted. Riociguat, the first approved agent in this class, has a dual mechanism, operating in synergy with endogenous NO and also directly stimulating sGC autonomous of NO availability. Riociguat is approved by the FDA for treatment of both PAH and chronic thromboembolic pulmonary hypertension (CTEPH) patients.

■ PHOSPHODIESTERASE INHIBITORS

Sildenafil and tadalafil represent the FDA-approved phosphodiesterase 5 (PDE-5) inhibitors for the treatment of PAH. PDE-5 inhibition results in increased intracellular cGMP, which enhances vasodilatation and has antiproliferative effects. The PDE-5 inhibitors, like the ET antagonists, have been shown to improve 6-minute walk distance and functional status. Side effects include flushing, hypotension, headaches, and epistaxis.

■ ADJUNCTIVE THERAPY

Oxygen, systemic anticoagulation, diuresis, and digoxin represent adjunctive therapies for the long-term management of PAH. Although these therapies are not supported by clinical trials, they are recommended by societal guidelines. Use of anticoagulation has become controversial based on two recent analyses from PAH registries; further guidelines addressing this issue should appear shortly.

■ SURGICAL THERAPY

Prior to the advent of pulmonary vasodilator therapy, lung transplantation was common for patients with severe PAH. Other surgical therapies, including atrial septostomy and surgical or endovascular Potts procedures, may be considered for advanced cases not responsive to maximal medical therapy.

COMMON INPATIENT COMPLICATIONS OF PULMONARY HYPERTENSION

Right heart failure (worsening PAH) and complications of chronic indwelling central venous access are the common issues that arise in the inpatient care of patients with pulmonary hypertension. Triage of patients with right heart failure or complications of central venous access depends of the patient's hemodynamic stability, with hypotensive patients generally requiring ICU-level care, urgent cardiology or pulmonary consultation, and right heart catheterization to acutely assist in the management of pulmonary vasodilator therapy.

■ RIGHT HEART FAILURE

Patients with advanced PAH may present with right heart failure, which may range in severity from asymptomatic volume overload to shock. Unlike a right ventricular myocardial infarction, which often responds well to volume loading, the decompensated right ventricle generally responds poorly to volume loading. This is due to "ventricular interdependence." The right and left ventricle share the intraventricular septum, thus right ventricular pressure overload can cause the septum to shift into the left ventricle, decreasing left ventricle filling and cardiac output. Therefore, cardiogenic shock in the patient with PH and right ventricular failure is generally managed in the intensive care unit with potent pulmonary vasodilators (eg, intravenous epoprostenol, inhaled nitric oxide), diuresis, and, if necessary, inotropic, vasopressor, renal replacement support, and increasingly extracorporeal membrane oxygenation (ECMO) . Caution must be taken with the use of positive pressure ventilation and its acute reduction in preload, which may precipitate cardiovascular collapse in PH.

■ COMPLICATIONS OF CENTRAL VENOUS ACCESS

Patients with continuous infusions of prostacyclins often present with complications of central venous access. These include loss of access (causing acute discontinuation of pulmonary vasodilators), central line puncture (and risk of air embolism), and central line infection. Loss of venous access should be considered an emergency situation, due to risk of acute increases in pulmonary vascular resistance and cardiovascular collapse. Attempts must be made to gain venous access immediately; in this case, peripheral intravenous access can be used emergently, with transition to central venous access after stabilization.

Central line puncture is also managed by quickly establishing alternative venous access, clamping the indwelling line proximal to the puncture, and starting the prostacyclin infusion through the new catheter. Often, the indwelling central line may be repaired by experienced nursing personnel.

Central line infection and bacteremia occur at a rate of approximately one case every 5 years in patients receiving intravenous prostanoids. This rate appears to be lower than reports of indwelling catheters for other conditions. However, treprostinil is associated with approximately twice the risk of bloodstream infections as epoprostenol (although this risk has decreased dramatically with the use of epoprostenol diluent for treprostinil infusions). It is important to note that bacteremia associated with treprostinil is most often caused by Gram-negative organisms, unlike other line infections, and initial antibiotic coverage for Gram-positive and negative organisms, including *Pseudomonas* species, is necessary in these patients. Consultation of a surgical specialist for removal of tunneled venous lines is generally required only for staphylococcal infections or recurrent bacteremia.

- Central line infections associated with continuous treprostinil infusion are most commonly caused by Gram-negative organisms, including *Pseudomonas* species.

DISCHARGE PLANNING AND QUALITY IMPROVEMENT STRATEGIES

The involvement of outpatient specialized nursing services who provide ongoing education, central venous line care, and emotional support is critical to the care of patients with advanced pulmonary arterial hypertension. These nurses, along with the pulmonary hypertension specialist, should be involved in discharge planning for all PH patients with continuous intravenous infusions. As in all patients with high risk for right heart failure, daily weight assessment and plans for excessive fluid accumulation are helpful in avoiding readmission.

CONCLUSION

Pulmonary hypertension represents a broad spectrum of diseases which result in elevation of pulmonary arterial pressures. An understanding of the pathophysiologic mechanisms involved with this array of conditions is necessary for the successful care of patients with PH.

SUGGESTED READINGS

Galiè N, Corris PA, Frost A, et al. Updated treatment algorithm of pulmonary arterial hypertension. *J Am Coll Cardiol.* 2013; 62(25 Suppl):D60-D72.

Hoeper MM, Bogaard HJ, Condliffe R, et al. Definitions and diagnosis of pulmonary hypertension. *J Am Coll Cardiol.* 2013; 62(25 Suppl):D42-D50.

McLaughlin VV, Gaine SP, Howard LS, et al. Treatment goals of pulmonary hypertension. *J Am Coll Cardiol.* 2013;62(25 Suppl):D73-D81.

Simonneau G, Gatzoulis MA, Adatia I, et al. Updated clinical classification of pulmonary hypertension. *J Am Coll Cardiol.* 2013; 62(25 Suppl):D34-D41.

SECTION 15
Renal

CHAPTER 238

Acid-Base Disorders

Vijay H. Lapsia, MD, MBBS
I. David Wiener, MD

Key Clinical Questions

1. What are common causes of increased anion gap metabolic acidosis?

2. How does measurement of the urinary anion gap help narrow the differential diagnosis of normal anion gap metabolic acidosis?

3. What are the major types of renal tubular acidosis, and how are they diagnosed?

4. How is urinary chloride used in the diagnosis of metabolic alkalosis?

5. How is the delta gap used to diagnose complex acid-base disorders?

INTRODUCTION

Acid-base disturbances occur frequently in the acutely ill hospitalized patient. Many physicians are intimidated by the complexity of acid-base analysis, as multiple, partially offsetting disorders can be challenging to diagnose. However, in the hospital setting, especially the critically ill, it is crucial that patients with acid-base disturbances be quickly identified and the abnormality be accurately interpreted. Swift intervention to treat the underlying causes is often necessary to avoid the often lethal consequences of severe acid-base disturbances.

NORMAL ACID-BASE HOMEOSTASIS

A typical Western diet generates about 15,000 mmol of volatile acids, in the form of CO_2, and ~70 mmol (1 mmol/kg) of fixed acid each day. CO_2 is excreted by normal respiration. Fixed acids are buffered by intra- and extracellular buffers. New buffers, predominantly HCO_3^-, must be continuously produced to replace buffers consumed in titrating fixed acids. Complex acid-base homeostasis mechanisms, which include chemical buffering in conjunction with the excretion of CO_2 by the respiratory system and new HCO_3^- production by the kidneys, normally maintain the blood pH between 7.35 and 7.45.

Acid-base homeostasis requires complementary functions of the respiratory and the renal systems. The kidneys play a central role by reabsorbing filtered bicarbonate, approximately 4000 mmol/d, and generating new bicarbonate. The central nervous system and the respiratory systems control the arterial CO_2 tension ($PaCO_2$). Respiratory CO_2 elimination is determined by alveolar ventilation. Kidneys generate new bicarbonate through the process of net acid excretion. Under normal conditions, net acid excretion balances fixed acid production. A disturbance of either respiratory CO_2 elimination or the balance between fixed acid generation and renal net acid excretion results in an acid-base disorder.

PRACTICE POINT

Glossary of terms for acid-base disorders

- Acidemia: serum pH < 7.36
- Alkalemia: serum pH > 7.44
- Acidosis: pathophysiologic processes which favor development of acidemia
- Alkalosis: pathophysiologic processes which favor development of alkalemia
- Hypercapnia: underexcretion of CO_2
- Hypocapnia: overexcretion of CO_2
- Anion gap: unmeasured anions in plasma
- Delta anion gap (ΔAG): prevailing minus normal AG
- ΔHCO_3^-: normal minus prevailing HCO_3^-

SIMPLE ACID-BASE DISORDERS

These disorders involve only a single acid-base disorder, and include metabolic acidosis, metabolic alkalosis, respiratory acidosis, and respiratory alkalosis. A key distinguishing feature is that the pH is always abnormal, as the compensation is never complete. Simple acid-base disorders can be classified as acute or chronic based on the degree of metabolic (renal) compensation (**Table 238-1**).

TABLE 238-1 Expected Compensatory Responses in Simple Acid-Base Disorders

Abnormality	Compensation
Metabolic acidosis	$PaCO_2 = (1.5 \times HCO_3^-) + 8 \pm 2$
Metabolic alkalosis	For each 10 mEq/L increase in HCO_3^-, $PaCO_2$ increases by ~6 mm Hg
Respiratory acidosis	
Acute	For each 10 mm Hg increase in $PaCO_2$, HCO_3^- increases by ~1 mEq/L
Chronic	For each 10 mm Hg increase in $PaCO_2$, HCO_3^- increases by ~ 4 mEq/L
Respiratory alkalosis	
Acute	For each 10 mm Hg increase in $PaCO_2$, HCO_3^- decreases by ~2 mEq/L
Chronic	For each 10 mm Hg increase in $PaCO_2$, HCO_3^- decreases by ~ 4 mEq/L

PRACTICE POINT

- **Primary disorder:** The clinician should measure the arterial pH to identify the primary disorder (acidosis or alkalosis) when a simple acid-base disorder is present. Over time, the pH approaches normal, but does not fully correct.
- **Compensation:** Respiratory compensation begins within seconds, whereas renal compensation takes 3 to 5 days to develop fully.
- A normal pH in the presence of abnormal HCO_3^- and $PaCO_2$ indicates a combined primary metabolic and primary respiratory disturbance.
- An increased anion gap, discussed in more detail below, always indicates the presence of an anion gap metabolic acidosis. If the serum bicarbonate is normal in the presence of an increased anion gap, then this indicates the simultaneous presence of both an anion gap metabolic acidosis and a metabolic alkalosis, in which the severity of the concomitant conditions is balanced.

MIXED ACID-BASE DISORDERS

When multiple acid-base disorders exist simultaneously and are not compensatory responses, they are classified as mixed acid-base disorders. When these occur in the critically ill patient, they can lead to dangerous extremes of pH. However, the pH may also be normal or near normal when acidosis and alkalosis coexist in the same patient. A patient with diabetic ketoacidosis who also has metabolic acidosis resulting from chronic kidney disease is an example of a mixed acid-base disorder. Triple acid-base disorders are not uncommon, and are often not recognized unless the clinician specifically considers this possibility. For example, a patient with metabolic acidosis due to lactic acidosis complicating severe sepsis may develop metabolic alkalosis from intravenous bicarbonate administration, with superimposed respiratory alkalosis due to hyperventilation from mechanical ventilation. Another example is the patient with respiratory acidosis due to altered consciousness, metabolic acidosis due to diabetic ketoacidosis, and metabolic alkalosis from vomiting may have an identical arterial blood gas (ABG). It is critical to always interpret acid-base abnormalities in the clinical context of the patient.

PRACTICE POINT

Common acid-base examples in the hospital setting

Acute respiratory alkalosis	Anxiety, pain, hypoxia, sepsis, mechanical ventilation, drugs (salicylates, progesterone, catecholamines), central nervous system disease, early stage asthma
Chronic respiratory acidosis	Pregnancy, acute or chronic liver disease, high altitude
Acute respiratory acidosis	Asthma, chronic obstructive pulmonary disease (COPD) flare, acute airway obstruction, narcotic analgesics, severe pneumonia, pulmonary edema, hemothorax, pneumothorax, flail chest, ventilator dysfunction, neuromuscular disorders, central nervous system depressants
Chronic respiratory acidosis	Chronic lung disease, central hypoventilation, chronic neuromuscular disorders
Metabolic alkalosis	*Low urinary chloride (<20 mmol/L)*: vomiting, nasogastric suction with dehydration, past diuretic use, posthypercapnia, severe congestive heart failure
	Normal or high urinary chloride (>20 mmol/L): primary or secondary hyperaldosteronism, current diuretic use, excess alkali, refeeding
	Note: a PCO_2 >55 mm Hg suggests additional primary respiratory abnormality
Metabolic acidosis	Elevated anion gap: ketoacidosis, renal failure, lactic acidosis, rhabdomyolysis, toxins
	Normal anion gap: diarrhea, renal tubular acidosis (RTA), advanced chronic kidney disease
Respiratory acidosis, metabolic acidosis, and metabolic alkalosis: low pH, high PCO_2, low HCO_3	Obtunded patient (respiratory acidosis) with lactic acidosis (metabolic acidosis) and vomiting (metabolic alkalosis)

APPROACH TO ACID-BASE DISORDERS

The first step in interpreting acid-base disorders is to perform a detailed history and physical examination. Next, one should simultaneously measure arterial blood gas (ABG) and plasma chemistries. A venous blood gas can be utilized under some circumstances, but is less accurate than an arterial blood gas. Blood gas analyzers directly measure the pH and $PaCO_2$; the bicarbonate value reported in an ABG analysis is calculated based from the pH and $PaCO_2$. Blood bicarbonate concentration is measured in the metabolic panel as total dissolved CO_2, which is ~95% bicarbonate. The samples can be validated by comparing the calculated HCO_3^- value reported on the arterial blood gas measurement with the measured HCO_3^- value on the chemistry panel. If the difference between the two values is greater than 2 mmol/L, the samples may not have been drawn simultaneously, or a laboratory error may be present. Excessive heparin in the syringe used to obtain the arterial blood sample can also cause confounding results. Repeating the laboratory studies may be helpful in determining the cause of this discrepancy.

PRACTICE POINT

Stepwise approach to acid-base disorders

1. The pH is the key to initial evaluation of all acid base disorders.
2. The primary abnormality is the process which causes the pH shift.

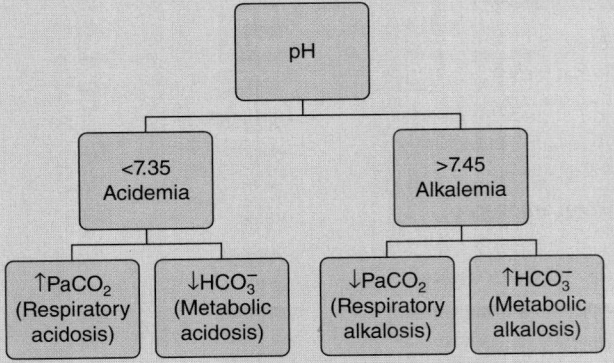

3. If respiratory acidosis or alkalosis, then determine whether acute or chronic.
4. If metabolic acidosis, then calculate the anion gap. An anion gap of >20 is suggestive of a primary metabolic acidosis, regardless of pH or serum bicarbonate concentration.
5. Calculate the (ΔAG – ΔHCO$_3^-$) to assess for a complex acid-base disorder. Remember 1 mmol of unmeasured acid titrates 1 mmol of bicarbonate. If ΔGap is substantially greater than zero, there is an underlying metabolic alkalosis; if it is substantially less than zero, then there is an underlying non-AG metabolic acidosis.

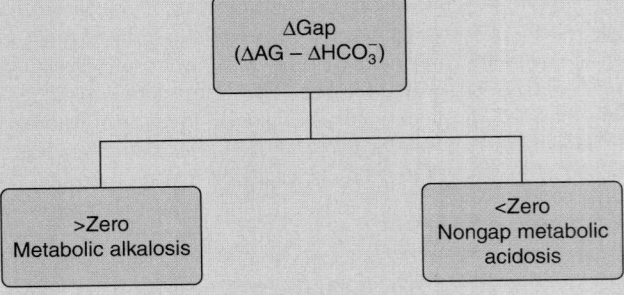

6. In patients with normal anion gap metabolic acidosis, calculate the urinary AG. In metabolic acidosis from bicarbonate loss in diarrhea, the urinary anion gap (UAG) is typically –20 to –50 mmol/L. A positive or near zero UAG indicates inappropriately low urinary NH$_4^+$ excretion, suggesting that renal tubular acidosis is responsible, if renal function is normal, or chronic kidney disease, if renal function is impaired.
7. In metabolic alkalosis, measure urine chloride. A low (< 20 mmol/L) urine chloride suggests volume depletion, often from vomiting or recent diuretic use. A normal or high urine chloride, with no recent diuretic use, suggests mineralocorticoid excess or alkali loads.

Next, identify the primary acid-base disorder by looking at the arterial pH, HCO$_3^-$, and PaCO$_2$ (**Table 238-2**). If either respiratory acidosis or alkalosis, then determine whether the condition is acute or chronic from the change in the serum bicarbonate (Table 238-1). Finally, calculate the anion gap (AG) and ΔAG (see below). Further evaluation will be guided by the type of acid-base disorder.

TABLE 238-2 Relationships in Primary Acid-Base Disorders

Condition	pH	HCO$_3^-$ (mEq/L)	PaCO$_2$ mm Hg
Normal	7.4	24	40
Metabolic acidosis	↓	↓	↓
Metabolic alkalosis	↑	↑	↑
Respiratory acidosis	↓	↑	↑
Respiratory alkalosis	↑	↓	↓

PRACTICE POINT

Important formulae for solving acid-base problems

- Anion gap: Na$^+$ – (Cl$^-$ + HCO$_3^-$) (represents unmeasured anions in plasma, normally 10-12 mmol/L)
- Anion gap, corrected for albumin: observed anion gap –2.5 (normal albumin – measured albumin)
- Winter's formula, used to assess for the adequacy of respiratory compensation in metabolic acidosis: expected PaCO$_2$ = 1.5 × HCO$_3^-$ + 8 (± 2); if the measured CO$_2$ is higher than this, there is a concomitant respiratory acidosis; if the measured CO$_2$ is less than this, there is a concomitant respiratory alkalosis. A helpful rule of thumb in the setting is that the PaCO$_2$ should be approximately equal to the last two digits of the pH
- ΔAG = AG – 7
- ΔHCO$_3^-$ = 24 – HCO$_3^-$
- ΔGap = ΔAG – ΔHCO$_3^-$
- Calculated osmolality (OSM): 2 × Na + glucose/18 + BUN/2.8 + EtOH/4.6
- Osmolal gap: measured OSM – calculated OSM; elevated OG > 10 mOsm/L

■ THE ANION GAP

The anion gap is the difference between the amount of unmeasured cations and unmeasured anions in plasma. It normally represents unmeasured anions in plasma, such as anionic proteins, phosphate, sulfate, and organic anions. In modern laboratories, using ion-sensitive electrodes to measure electrolyte concentrations, the mean anion gap is 7 mmol/L and the normal range is 3 to 11 mmol/L. A metabolic acidosis associated with an elevated anion gap is termed an anion gap metabolic acidosis, and metabolic acidosis with a normal anion gap is normal is termed a nonanion gap metabolic acidosis. High AG acidosis occurs when excess acid anions, such as acetoacetate and lactate, accumulate in extracellular fluid.

The anion gap may decrease either due to a rise in unmeasured cations (such as paraproteins) or a fall in anionic albumin (**Table 238-3**). The most common cause of an unexpectedly low anion gap is hypoalbuminemia. The expected anion gap should be corrected for albumin levels. A fall in serum albumin by 1 g/dL from the normal value (4.0 g/dL) decreases the anion gap by 2.5 mmol/L. For example, a measured anion gap of 12 mmol/L is usually normal. However, in a patient with a serum albumin of 1 g/dL, the expected AG is 12 to 2.5 (4.0 – 1) = 4.5 mmol/L.

A normal HCO$_3^-$ does not preclude an increased anion gap. For example, a patient who simultaneously has separate conditions causing an anion gap metabolic acidosis and metabolic alkalosis may have a normal, high or low, measured HCO$_3^-$. In this setting, recognizing that an elevated AG indicates the presence of AG metabolic acidosis may alert the clinician to the possibility of a mixed acid-base disorder.

TABLE 238-3 Conditions Which May Decrease the Anion Gap

Hypercalcemia
Hypermagnesemia
Hyperkalemia
Paraproteinemia
Lithium toxicity
Severe hypernatremia (> 170)
Bromide intoxication (may occur with pyridostigmine or with herbal medications)
Hypoalbuminemia

■ ΔAG AND ΔHCO₃⁻ (ASSESSING THE DELTA GAP)

Interpreting mixed acid-base disorders can be tricky, especially when the combination of disturbances result in a normal pH, HCO_3^-, and $PaCO_2$. In such situations, comparing the change in HCO_3^- (ΔHCO_3^-) and the change in the AG (ΔAG) can be useful. The ΔHCO_3^- is calculated as $\Delta HCO_3^- = [HCO_{3\,actual}^-] - 24$, where is 24 is the normal serum bicarbonate concentration, and ΔAG is calculated as $\Delta AG = AG_{actual} - 7$, where is 7 is the normal AG. The normal AG should be adjusted based on the serum albumin, as detailed above. If the ΔHCO_3^- and ΔAG differ from each other by more than 3, then multiple metabolic acid-base disorders may be present. If $\Delta AG > \Delta HCO_3^-$, then a simultaneous anion gap metabolic acidosis and metabolic alkalosis should be considered. If $\Delta HCO_3^- > \Delta AG$, then a combined anion gap metabolic acidosis and nonanion gap metabolic acidosis may be present.

■ PLASMA OSMOLAR GAP

The normal range for serum osmolality is 285 to 290 mOsm/L. The major molecules contributing to the serum osmolality include sodium, urea nitrogen, and glucose. Alcohol (ethanol) will contribute to osmolality if present at levels consistent with intoxication. The osmolar gap is obtained by subtracting the calculated osmolarity (see formulae below) from the measured osmolarity. A difference of more than 10 mOsm/L is abnormal (osmolar gap) suggests another solute, such as lactate, ethanol, ethylene glycol, methanol, contrast dye, and mannitol.

METABOLIC ACIDOSIS

The two major categories of clinical metabolic acidosis are anion gap metabolic acidosis and nonanion gap metabolic acidosis (**Table 238-4**). While the latter is sometimes termed hyperchloremic acidosis, we discourage use of this term. Abnormalities in the serum sodium concentration, either hyponatremia or hypernatremia, necessarily alter the serum chloride, and if this is not recognized can lead to incorrect categorization of the metabolic acidosis using only the serum chloride.

Metabolic acidosis may occur because of an increased production of endogenous acids, such as lactate and ketoacids, accumulation of endogenous acids, as in renal failure, or loss of bicarbonate, as in diarrhea. Metabolic acidosis can affect the respiratory, cardiac, and nervous systems, and in severe cases may lead to death. The normal respiratory response to metabolic acidosis is to increase alveolar ventilation and CO_2 elimination, partially correcting the arterial pH. Patients may exhibit the deep and labored respiration known as Kussmaul breathing.

We recommend the following evaluation pathway for metabolic acidosis (**Figure 238-1**). First, calculate the corrected anion gap. The uncorrected anion gap is often abnormal in chronically ill patients due to low serum albumin and poor nutritional status. If the corrected anion gap is greater than 11, then the patient has an anion gap metabolic acidosis. Anion gap metabolic acidosis may result

TABLE 238-4 Causes of Metabolic Acidosis with a High or Normal Anion Gap

Elevated anion gap
Ethylene glycol
Lactic acid
Methanol
Paraldehyde
Aspirin
Renal failure
Diabetic ketoacidosis
Alcoholic ketoacidosis
Renal failure
Normal anion gap
Diarrhea
Renal tubular acidosis
Acetazolamide therapy
Ureteral diversion
Renal failure (can cause either normal or increased anion gap metabolic acidosis)
Adrenal insufficiency

from a number of underlying conditions, summarized in the mnemonic in the figure.

If the corrected anion gap is not elevated, then the differential diagnosis becomes limited to excessive GI bicarbonate losses versus inadequate renal net acid excretion. To differentiate these possibilities, calculate the urine anion gap. If it is significantly negative, that is, less than −20 mmol/L, then the kidneys are excreting significant net acid, and the nonanion gap metabolic acidosis is likely due to excessive GI bicarbonate losses. This is most commonly due to losses of small intestinal or colonic fluids, as in chronic diarrhea. If the urine anion gap is not significantly negative, then this indicates a failure of renal acid excretion. Hyperkalemia is a common cause of this, and if present indicates a type IV renal tubular acidosis (RTA). If hyperkalemia is not present, then the differential diagnosis is between uremic acidosis and RTA. These can be differentiated in most cases by assessing the estimated GFR. Because many patients with type IV RTA also have chronic kidney disease, the coexistence of type IV RTA and uremic acidosis is not unusual. This can be identified by persistence of the metabolic acidosis after correction of hyperkalemia.

■ TREATMENT PRINCIPLES

Metabolic acidosis indicates the presence of an important underlying condition. Treatment directed at the underlying condition should be instituted. Whether metabolic acidosis should be treated with alkali is less apparent, and depends in large part on whether acute or chronic metabolic acidosis is present.

For *chronic* metabolic acidosis, the benefit of alkali treatment is clear-cut, and includes improved bone and muscle integrity, improved growth in children, and preservation of renal function in patients with chronic kidney disease. There may also be improvements in thyroid hormone function and in regulation of serum glucose. Oral alkali therapy, typically in the form of $NaHCO_3$, should be instituted on an elective basis, and dosing adjusted every 3 to 4 days targeting a serum HCO_3^- of 24 mmol/L.

For *acute* metabolic acidosis, the benefit of alkali treatment is less certain. Clinical trials have shown no clinically significant effect of

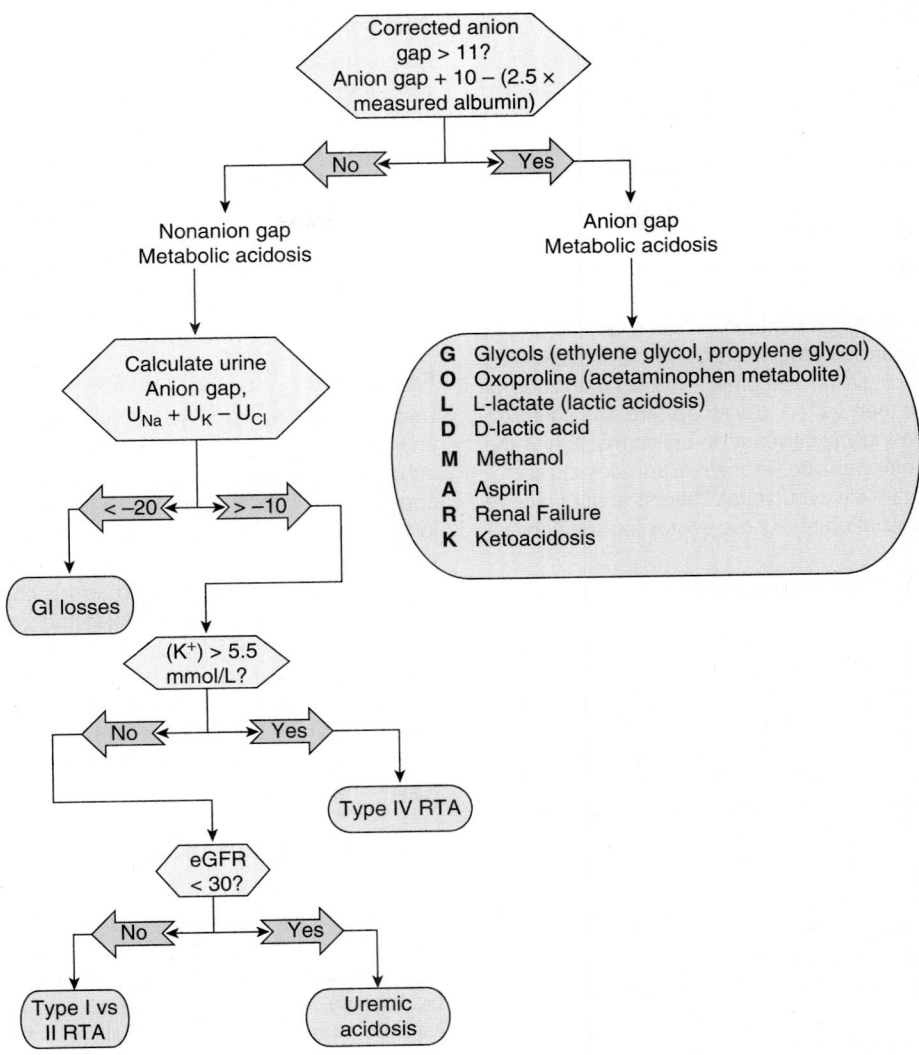

Figure 238-1 *Evaluation of metabolic acidosis.*

alkali treatment of acute metabolic acidosis on either mortality or on cardiovascular performance. However, treating acute metabolic acidosis with alkali might be considered if arterial pH is less than 7.1. If alkali treatment is used, a target pH of no more than 7.2 is reasonable, as aggressive alkali therapy may have deleterious side effects. Slow IV administration of 50 to 100 mEq of $NaHCO_3$, over 30 to 45 minutes, can be used. It is essential to monitor plasma electrolytes during the course of therapy, since the $[K^+]$ may decline as pH rises. Administration of large amounts of concentrated $NaHCO_3$ in the form of multiple ampules can cause acute hypernatremia because of the associated sodium load. Rapid intravenous alkali administration can acutely decrease the ionized calcium, which may impair cardiac function. Patients with simultaneous intravascular volume depletion and metabolic acidosis may benefit from volume resuscitation from intravenous fluids prepared from the addition of 150 mmol sodium bicarbonate (three ampules) per 1 L of D5W.

■ HIGH AG ACIDOSIS

The four most common causes of a high AG metabolic acidosis are lactic acidosis, ketoacidosis, ingested toxins, and renal failure. Therefore, the initial screening to differentiate the high AG acidoses should include relevant history for evidence of drug and toxin ingestion, determination of blood lactic acid, glucose, ethanol, beta-hydroxybutyrate, blood urea nitrogen (BUN), and creatinine, inspection of the urine for oxalate crystals, and identification of

predisposing factors for lactic acidosis, such as hypotension, shock, cardiac failure, leukemia, cancer, unrecognized bowel ischemia, thiamine deficiency, and drug or toxin ingestion.

■ LACTIC ACIDOSIS

Lactic acidosis almost always indicates the presence of impaired tissue perfusion, most commonly due to hypotension, arterial disease, or sepsis. Rarely, an unsuspected neoplasm produces lactic acid and is the causative factor. Identifying and treating the underlying cause is central to therapy. Alkali therapy is usually reserved for severe acidemia (pH <7.1).

■ D-LACTIC ACIDOSIS

D-lactic acidosis is increasingly recognized. It occurs most often in short bowel syndrome, when undigested sugars passing into the colon are fermented to D-lactic acid by lactobacilli. The resulting low pH favors further overgrowth of lactobacilli, leading to a vicious cycle of worsening acidosis. D-lactic acid is also sometimes produced during diabetic ketoacidosis, and it is a metabolic product of propylene glycol, which is used as a stabilizing agent for lorazepam and diazepam infusions. D-lactic acidosis typically presents as encephalopathy, with delirium, ataxia, gait disturbance, slurred speech, and agitation. Special assays are required to detect D-lactate. Treatment includes correcting the acidosis, decreasing carbohydrate intake, and antibiotics to clear the overgrowth of lactobacilli.

■ DIABETIC KETOACIDOSIS

In diabetic ketoacidosis, treating with insulin prevents production of ketones and enables endogenous metabolism of accumulated ketones to bicarbonate, thus correcting the acidosis. Bicarbonate therapy is rarely needed except with extreme acidemia (pH <7.1), and then in limited amounts in patients with hemodynamic instability.

■ ALCOHOLIC KETOACIDOSIS

Mixed acid-base disorders are common in alcoholic ketoacidosis. The degree of ketosis and ketonuria can often be underestimated on initial presentation. Patients are often volume depleted, and respond to volume expansion. With restoration of circulation by resuscitation with isotonic saline, the preferential accumulation of beta-hydroxybutyrate is then shifted to acetoacetate. This paradoxically results in an increasingly positive nitroprusside reaction as the patient improves (the nitroprusside ketone reaction detects aceto-acetic acid, but not beta-hydroxybutyrate). Patients should receive thiamine prior to administration of glucose-containing solutions.

■ ACIDOSIS FROM DRUGS AND TOXINS

Salicylates

Intoxication typically results in either respiratory alkalosis or a combined respiratory alkalosis and anion gap metabolic acidosis, depending on the stage and level of intoxication. Treatment includes gastric lavage to remove unabsorbed salicylate, and forced alkaline diuresis to increase renal salicylate excretion. Acetazolamide administration can be useful in patients with simultaneous alkalemia.

Alcohols

In the appropriate clinical setting, identification of an osmolar gap may be the first indication of a poison-associated anion gap acidosis. Ethylene glycol, methanol, and isopropyl alcohol all cause an elevated osmolar gap, but only the first two cause a high anion gap acidosis. Because ethylene glycol and methanol can cause CNS effects, at least initially, similar to that of ethanol, we recommend assessment of the serum osmolar gap in patients presenting in the outpatient setting with an acute anion gap metabolic acidosis, particularly if there is history, physical examination, or laboratory evidence of recent alcohol ingestion.

Ingestion of ethylene glycol, present in antifreeze, can be suspected by observing urine oxalate crystals, the presence of an osmolar gap in serum, and a high anion gap acidosis. Some antifreeze agents contain a fluorescent dye which may be detected by viewing the urine with the aid of a Wood's lamp. Methanol metabolism results in the formation of formaldehyde and formic acid, which can cause severe optic nerve and central nervous system damage; methanol ingestion should be suspected in patients presenting in the outpatient setting with an anion gap metabolic acidosis and acute visual disturbances.

Treatment of methanol and ethylene glycol poisoning includes the prompt institution of a saline or osmotic diuresis, supplementation with thiamine, pyridoxine, and folic acid to maximize metabolism by nontoxic pathways, and inhibition of alcohol dehydrogenase with fomepizole. Fomepizole therapy has replaced therapy with ethanol, as the decline in ethylene glycol level is more predictable, and fomepizole does not cause the neurological obtundation seen during ethanol infusion. Correction of systemic acidosis with sodium bicarbonate may reduce the tissue penetration of toxic metabolites. Indications for emergent hemodialysis include the presence of ocular manifestations, severe (AG >30, pH <7.25) or worsening metabolic acidosis, blood methanol or ethylene glycol concentrations >50 mg/dL, renal failure, or deteriorating vital signs despite intensive supportive care.

Acetaminophen

Chronic acetaminophen administration, even at therapeutic doses, can cause an anion gap metabolic acidosis in susceptible individuals. Pyroglutamic acid is the fixed acid generated. The pathogenesis is thought due to chronic glutathione deficiency. Risk factors for its development include chronic illness, malnutrition, and female sex. This diagnosis should be differentiated from an acute acetaminophen overdose, which causes acute liver disease. This diagnosis should be considered in patients with anion gap metabolic acidosis of unclear etiology in the presence of chronic ingestion of acetaminophen.

Renal failure

Uremic acidosis is characterized by impaired excretion of ammonia and titratable acid. Metabolic acidosis with renal failure may be either anion gap or nonanion gap, and the determining factors appear to be retention of phosphates, sulfates, and other uremic ions. Simultaneous hyperkalemia may further inhibit renal ammonia metabolism and contribute to type IV RTA. Significant loss of bone mass may occur, as the retained acid is buffered by alkaline salts released from bone. Oral alkali replacement to maintain the $[HCO_3^-]$ at a level of ~24 mmol/L is recommended. Treating the patient with chronic kidney disease and metabolic acidosis with sodium bicarbonate appears to slow the progression of chronic kidney disease and may decrease the risk of development of end-stage renal disease, without worsening either blood pressure control or proteinuria.

■ NORMAL AG METABOLIC ACIDOSIS

This disorder results from either failure of the kidneys to produce adequate net acid excretion to balance endogenous acid production, or from alkali loss from the intestinal tract. Intestinal tract fluids, except in the stomach, contain relatively high concentrations of bicarbonate, and excessive losses, such as with profound diarrhea, can lead to metabolic acidosis. Failure of the kidneys to generate adequate net acid excretion can result either from renal tubular acidosis (**Table 238-5**) or from advanced, typically stage IV or V, CKD. Because patients with type IV RTA typically have CKD in conjunction with their hyperkalemia, the differentiation of type IV RTA from CKD-induced acidosis is inexact. We recommend correcting the hyperkalemia, in which case the metabolic acidosis with type IV RTA in the presence of CKD should resolve. If the metabolic acidosis does not completely resolve, then a component of CKD-associated acidosis is present. Because some patients, particularly those with body image disorders and laxative abuse, may not be forthcoming about diarrhea, it is important to differentiate diarrhea-induced metabolic acidosis from RTA through the use of appropriate laboratory tests, such as the urinary anion gap. These tests are based on the fact that the renal response to metabolic acidosis resulting from intestinal bicarbonate losses is to increase net acid excretion in the form of ammonia, whereas patients with renal tubular acidosis cannot generate this response.

■ URINARY AG

The urinary anion gap (UAG) is used to indirectly assess urinary ammonia excretion. It is the sum of the urine sodium and urine potassium concentrations, minus the urine chloride concentration, all measured in mmol/L:

$$UAG = U_{Na} + U_K - U_{Cl}.$$

Urinary ammonium excretion is increased in patients with diarrhea, and reduced in patients with renal tubular acidosis. If the UAG is negative in a patient with metabolic acidosis, then urinary

TABLE 238-5 Classification of Renal Tubular Acidosis

	Proximal (Type II)	Distal (Type I)	Distal (Type IV)
Mechanism	Defective proximal tubule HCO_3^- absorption	Defective collecting duct H^+ secretion	Defective ammonia excretion
Common causes	Genetic disorders in children; myeloma, nephrotoxic medications in adults	Genetic disorders of the tubule in children; autoimmune disease, interstitial nephritis in adults	Chronic kidney disease and impairments of renin-aldosterone axis
$FEHCO_3^-$	> 10%	> 3%	> 3%
Urine pH	During alkali treatment > 5.5; chronic, no alkali treatment < 5.5	> 5.5	Usually ≤ 6.0
Serum K^+	Hypokalemia; worsens with therapy	Hypokalemia; often improves with therapy	Hyperkalemia; correcting hyperkalemia can correct the RTA
Ca_2^+ excretion	Increased	Increased	Usually normal

$FEHCO_3^-$, fractional excretion of bicarbonate measured when the serum bicarbonate is normal.

ammonia, present almost exclusively as urinary NH_4^+, is appropriately increased. In metabolic acidosis from bicarbonate loss in diarrhea, the UAG is typically –20 to –50 mmol/L. The absence of a negative UAG indicates a failure of urinary ammonia excretion to increase, and suggests that RTA or advanced CKD is the cause of the acidosis. Clinicians must recognize that the formula used for the urine anion gap differs from that used for the plasma or serum anion gap. Not recognizing this difference can lead to serious errors and incorrect diagnoses.

■ TYPE I RTA (DISTAL RTA)

Type I RTA is characterized by hypokalemia, normal AG metabolic acidosis, low urinary NH_4^+ excretion (as reflected by a positive UAG), and a high urine pH (pH ≥6.5) in the presence of untreated metabolic acidosis. These patients commonly come to medical attention either because of growth retardation and failure to thrive in children, or recurrent renal stone formation in adults. Urinary citrate, an important inhibitor of urinary calcium oxalate crystallization, is decreased in distal RTA, contributing to the nephrolithiasis. Type I RTA in children is frequently caused by genetic mutations in distal tubular ion transporters. In adults, type I RTA may result from acute interstitial nephritis, or autoimmune diseases, such as systemic lupus erythematosus and Sjögren syndrome.

Oral alkali supplementation, dosed at 1 mmol/kg/d, is the mainstay of therapy. Patients typically require 50% of the alkali as potassium citrate to treat the concomitant hypokalemia. Sodium alkali salts, such as sodium citrate or sodium bicarbonate, are used to correct the remainder of the metabolic acidosis, while avoiding excessive potassium supplementation

and development of hyperkalemia. The dosage of sodium and potassium alkali salts should be adjusted to obtain normal serum bicarbonate and potassium levels.

■ TYPE II RTA (PROXIMAL RTA)

Type II RTA is characterized by hypokalemia and nonanion gap metabolic acidosis. In contrast to type I RTA, urine pH in untreated type II RTA is ≤ 6.0. Many patients with type II RTA exhibit the Fanconi syndrome (type II RTA, glycosuria, generalized aminoaciduria, and phosphaturia). Causes of type II RTA include inherited genetic disorders, such as cystinosis, hereditary fructose intolerance, and Wilson disease, and acquired disorders, such as multiple myeloma, renal transplant rejection, and certain medications, including acetazolamide, ifosfamide, and the antiretroviral drug tenofovir. Tenofovir is currently a common cause of acquired Fanconi syndrome, characterized by the recent onset of impaired renal function, with hypokalemia, nonanion gap metabolic acidosis, and glycosuria in a nondiabetic patient in an taking tenofovir for HIV or hepatitis B infection.

Identifying and correcting the underlying causes are central to treating acquired forms of proximal RTA. If the underlying cause cannot be reversed, oral alkali therapy is used. Large amounts of bicarbonate, typically 10 to 15 mmol/kg/d, are required. As the serum bicarbonate increases, renal bicarbonate losses increase, causing the need for very high doses. Similar to type I RTA, 50% of the alkali should be given initially as a potassium salt such as potassium citrate, and 50% as a sodium salt, either sodium citrate or sodium bicarbonate. Doses of these are adjusted as necessary to normalize serum potassium and bicarbonate.

■ TYPE IV RTA

Type IV RTA is characterized by hyperkalemia, normal anion gap metabolic acidosis, and disturbances in the renin-aldosterone axis leading to impaired release or action of aldosterone. Most patients have concomitant chronic kidney disease, most commonly diabetic nephropathy and interstitial nephritis. Other causes or contributing factors include HIV, sickle cell disease, urinary tract obstruction, lupus nephritis, amyloidosis, myeloma, adrenal insufficiency, kidney transplant rejection, and a variety of medications, such as cyclosporine, angiotensin converting enzyme (ACE) inhibitors, angiotensin receptor blockers (ARBs), NSAIDs, trimethoprim, heparin, and potassium-sparing diuretics. In patients with hyperkalemia and CKD, it may be difficult to differentiate type IV RTA from uremic metabolic acidosis. We recommend correcting the hyperkalemia. If the metabolic acidosis does not resolve after hyperkalemia has been corrected then a component of uremic metabolic acidosis is present.

The urine pH in most patients with type IV RTA is acidic, usually ≤ 6.0, but may be elevated. Acidosis is usually mild, and bicarbonate therapy may not be needed. In most cases, type IV RTA develops because hyperkalemia suppresses renal ammonia production and thus net acid excretion. Accordingly, decreasing dietary potassium is beneficial and often corrects the metabolic acidosis. Thiazide diuretics, which are more effective at increasing renal potassium excretion then loop diuretics, may also be helpful. The robust thiazide-type diuretic metolazone is often helpful in patients with advanced CKD.

Type IV RTA is rarely a result of primary adrenal insufficiency. These patients typically present with low blood pressure, hyperkalemia, and nonanion gap metabolic acidosis. The urinary pH will often be 6.5 or higher. The diagnosis of adrenal insufficiency can be confirmed with appropriate serologic tests. Treatment with glucocorticoids and mineralocorticoids is efficacious in correcting type IV RTA in this setting. In general, exogenous mineralocorticoids should be avoided in patients with chronic kidney disease, as they may contribute to progression of chronic kidney disease and an earlier necessity for initiation of renal replacement therapy.

We generally do not recommend discontinuing ACE inhibitors or ARBs in patients with type IV RTA, because these medications decrease cardiovascular events and slow the progression of chronic kidney disease.

METABOLIC ALKALOSIS

Patients with metabolic alkalosis may be asymptomatic or present with delirium, cardiac arrhythmias, and neuromuscular irritability when the pH exceeds 7.55. This diagnosis is most commonly prompted by the recognition of the elevated serum bicarbonate in routine serum chemistry analyses in the asymptomatic patient. Occasional patients come to medical attention because of compensatory hypoventilation, which may lead to hypoxia, respiratory failure, or pneumonia. Patients may have a history of diuretic use, vomiting, and poorly controlled hypertension. Laboratory values demonstrate an elevated arterial pH, increased serum HCO_3^-, and an increase in $PaCO_2$ secondary to compensatory alveolar hypoventilation.

PRACTICE POINT

- Metabolic alkalosis: measure the urinary chloride level to assesses the renal ability to excrete excess bicarbonate.
- The urine chloride is only valid if diuretics have not been recently administered.
- Low urinary chloride, <20 mmol/L, indicates a chloride-responsive metabolic alkalosis. Reduced distal renal chloride delivery impairs renal HCO_3^- excretion. Chloride supplementation, typically given as NaCl, either through the oral or the intravenous route, will generally reverse the metabolic alkalosis.
- High urinary chloride, >20 mmol/L, indicates a chloride-unresponsive metabolic alkalosis. This indicates the presence of ongoing acid loss, occasionally through gastric acid loss, but typically from persistent, mineralocorticoid-dependent, stimulation of renal acid excretion.

Metabolic alkalosis involves both a generation and a maintenance phase. The generation phase involves either acid loss, from either loss of acidic gastric fluid, increased renal net acid excretion associated with either hypokalemia or hyperaldosteronism, or decreased plasma volume, leading to a decreased volume of distribution for bicarbonate. The maintenance phase either involves total body chloride depletion, thereby impairing renal chloride-dependent bicarbonate excretion, or ongoing acid losses, typically either gastric fluid or from aldosterone-stimulated renal acid excretion.

Assessment of the urine chloride may be helpful in differentiating the different causes of the maintenance phase (**Table 238-6**). A low urine chloride, typically <20 mmol/L, indicates total body chloride depletion. Chloride supplementation, typically in the form of sodium chloride, given either orally or intravenously, will often result in improvement in the metabolic alkalosis. A nonsuppressed urine chloride, typically >20 mmol/L, indicates chloride-unresponsive metabolic alkalosis. These patients will typically not be helped with chloride supplementation. Instead, treating their ongoing gastric acid or renal acid losses is critical to their therapy. Hypokalemia directly stimulates renal acid excretion. Treatment of hypokalemia, if present, may be helpful. Many of these patients have a degree of hyperaldosteronism, either primary or secondary, and benefit from treatment with either mineralocorticoid receptor blockers or

---

TABLE 238-6 Cause of Metabolic Alkalosis

Chloride-responsive (urinary chloride < 20)

GI

  Nasogastric suction

  Vomiting/diarrhea

  Laxative abuse

  Villous adenoma

Renal

  Diuretics

  Post-hypercapnea

  Refeeding alkalosis

  Cystic fibrosis (sweat losses)

Chloride-resistant (urinary chloride > 30)

Mineralocorticoid excess

  Primary or secondary aldosteronism

  Secondary aldosteronism (eg, CHF, renal artery stenosis, liver disease)

  Cushing syndrome

  Licorice ingestion

Alkali load

  Citrate (transfusions)

  Acetate (TPN)

Severe hypokalemia/hypomagnesemia

---

inhibitors of the renin-angiotensin system if there is evidence of secondary hyperaldosteronism. Direct inhibition of renal acid excretion, such as the carbonic anhydrase inhibitor acetazolamide, may also be useful. Other causes of metabolic alkalosis include Bartter syndrome, Gitelman syndrome, Liddle syndrome, villous adenoma, and milk-alkali (calcium-alkali) syndrome.

■ TREATMENT

The treatment of metabolic alkalosis depends on whether patient has chloride-responsive or chloride-unresponsive metabolic alkalosis. Patients with chloride-responsive metabolic alkalosis improve with chloride administration. If they are hypokalemic, this can be provided as potassium chloride. If the serum potassium is normal, then the chloride is administered as sodium chloride, typically as intravenous saline solution. Chloride-unresponsive metabolic alkalosis requires treatment of the underlying condition, and generally does not respond well to either NaCl or KCl administration. Very rarely, acid therapy may be necessary. Intravenous acid preparations include either HCl or NH_4Cl, 100 mmol/L, and should be administered only through a central vein. NH_4Cl should be avoided in patients with liver disease because it may precipitate hepatic encephalopathy.

RESPIRATORY ACIDOSIS

Respiratory acidosis is diagnosed by an increase in $PaCO_2$ and decrease in pH. Patients may be minimally symptomatic, or acutely anxious, agitated, obtunded or comatose. Tremor, asterixis, and myoclonic jerking may be present on examination. Cerebral vasodilation may occur, with headaches and signs of raised intracranial pressure, such as papilledema, abnormal reflexes, and focal muscle weakness.

Differentiating acute from chronic respiratory acidosis is critical for accurate diagnosis and treatment. Acute respiratory acidosis increases HCO_3^- by 1 mmol/L for every 10 mm Hg increase in $PaCO_2$, whereas in chronic respiratory acidosis (> 3-5 days), renal adaptation increases the HCO_3^- by 4 mmol/L for every 10 mm Hg increase in $PaCO_2$. The serum HCO_3^- usually does not rise above 38 mmol/L. General anesthetics, sedatives, head trauma, alcohol, intracranial tumors, syndromes of sleep-disordered breathing, diseases of the motor neurons, neuromuscular junction and skeletal muscle, and improperly adjusted mechanical ventilation may result in respiratory acidosis. In a stable mechanically ventilated patient, respiratory acidosis may develop secondary to a sudden rise in CO_2 production, as from fever, agitation, sepsis, or overfeeding. However, it is more often due to a fall in alveolar ventilation from worsening pulmonary function or sudden occlusion of the upper airway.

■ TREATMENT

The goal of therapy is improved ventilation. Underlying respiratory conditions, such as acute exacerbations of COPD, should be aggressively treated. Sedatives and other central nervous system depressant drugs should be stopped, and the narcotic antagonist, naloxone, should be administered if narcotic overdose or excess is suspected. Patients may require noninvasive positive pressure ventilation, or endotracheal intubation and assisted ventilation. Severe hypercapnia should be cautiously corrected, as a rapid fall in pH may provoke cardiac arrhythmias, reduced cerebral perfusion, and seizures.

RESPIRATORY ALKALOSIS

The diagnosis of respiratory alkalosis depends on measurement of arterial pH and $PaCO_2$. Other laboratory findings may include a reduced serum K^+ and elevated serum Cl^-. Acute respiratory alkalosis is not usually associated with increased renal HCO_3^- excretion, but within hours net acid excretion is reduced. Acutely, HCO_3^- concentration falls by 2.0 mmol/L for each 10 mm Hg decrease in $PaCO_2$. Chronic hypocapnia reduces the serum HCO_3^- by 4.0 mmol/L for each 10 mm Hg decrease in $PaCO_2$. However, it is unusual to observe a plasma HCO_3^- <12 mmol/L from respiratory alkalosis alone.

Chronic respiratory alkalosis is usually asymptomatic due to renal compensation. Acute respiratory alkalosis (hyperventilation) presents with lightheadedness, confusion, syncope, tachycardia, anxiety, and dyspnea. Alkalosis promotes the binding of calcium to albumin, leading to decreased serum ionized calcium, and may lead to circumoral and acral paresthesias, tetany, and seizures.

The differential diagnosis of respiratory alkalosis depends on whether it is acute or chronic. Chronic respiratory alkalosis is most typically associated with living at high altitude, pregnancy, and acute or chronic liver disease. The differential diagnosis of acute respiratory alkalosis is much more extensive. Many cardiopulmonary disorders associated with hypoxia, including pulmonary embolism, pneumonia, and pneumothorax, are associated with respiratory alkalosis in their early to intermediate stages. Respiratory alkalosis is common during mechanical ventilation. Liver failure, early Gram-negative septicemia, and central nervous system insults such as meningitis, encephalitis, brain tumor, or head injury may lead to respiratory alkalosis. Salicylates, theophylline, aminophylline, thyroxine, and catecholamines, and other drugs, may cause respiratory alkalosis. Hyperventilation from anxiety or panic attacks is a diagnosis of exclusion. It is important to consider other conditions such as pulmonary embolism, acute coronary syndrome, and hyperthyroidism prior to making the diagnosis of a panic attack.

■ TREATMENT

Management is limited to correction of the underlying disorder. Acid infusions, antidepressants, and sedatives are not recommended. Respiratory alkalosis in pregnant women does not require treatment.

ACKNOWLEDGMENTS

Preparation of this chapter supported by grant funds from the NIH (R01-DK045788) and the Department of Veterans Affairs (1I01BX000818).

SUGGESTED READINGS

Brent J. Fomepizole for ethylene glycol and methanol poisoning. *N Engl J Med.* 2009;360:2216-2223.

Kamel KS, Halperin ML. Acid-base problems in diabetic ketoacidosis. *N Engl J Med.* 2015;372:546-554.

Karet FE. Mechanisms in hyperkalemic renal tubular acidosis. *J Am Soc Nephrol.* 2009;20:251-254.

Kraut JA, Kurtz I. Toxic alcohol ingestions: clinical features, diagnosis, and management. *Clin J Am Soc Nephrol.* 2008;3:208-225.

Kraut JA, Madias NE. Lactic acidosis. *N Engl J Med.* 2014;371:2309-2319.

Kraut JA, Madias NE. Serum anion gap: its uses and limitations in clinical medicine. *Clin J Am Soc Nephrol.* 2007;2:162-174.

Laski ME, Sabatini S. Metabolic alkalosis, bedside and bench. *Semin Nephrol.* 2006;26:404-421.

CHAPTER 239

Acute Kidney Injury

Ajay K. Singh, MBBS, MBA, FRCP

Anika T. Singh

Jameela Kari, MD

Key Clinical Questions

1. How is acute kidney injury defined?
2. What are the major causes of acute kidney injury?
3. How is acute kidney injury diagnosed and managed?
4. What role does renal replacement therapy, such as hemodialysis, have in acute kidney injury?

INTRODUCTION

Acute kidney injury (AKI) is defined as a potentially reversible sudden deterioration in renal function due to prerenal, intrarenal, or postrenal causes. AKI is frequently accompanied by dysregulation of extracellular fluid volume and electrolytes, and a marked increase in the retention of nitrogenous and nonnitrogenous waste products over a period of hours to weeks. AKI may be oliguric (< 400 mL/d) or nonoliguric (> 400 mL/d). AKI can also be defined as an acute and sustained increase in serum creatinine of 0.5 mg/dL (44.2 µmol/L), if the baseline is less than 2.5 mg/dL (221 mmol/L), or an increase in serum creatinine more than 20% if the baseline is more than 2.5 mg/dL (221 mmol/L).

There have been several attempts to achieve consensus among intensivists and nephrologists on the definition of AKI. The Acute Dialysis Quality Initiative (ADQI) group published the RIFLE classification of AKI in 2004 based on three severity categories (risk, injury, and failure) and two clinical outcome categories (loss and end-stage renal disease) (**Table 239-1**). The parameters assessed in the RIFLE classification are changes in serum creatinine level, glomerular filtration rate (GFR), or urine output (UO). The baseline serum creatinine level and GFR may not be readily available. Hence the consensus committee recommends the use of the Modification of Diet in Renal Disease (MDRD) equation to estimate GFR/1.73 m². The proportional decrease in GFR is calculated from 75 mL/min per 1.73 m², the agreed-upon lower limit of normal. (The RIFLE criteria for adults have been adapted in children and are termed the pRIFLE criteria.)

A modified RIFLE criteria schema has been proposed by the Acute Kidney Injury Network (AKIN). The AKIN diagnostic criteria (**Table 239-2**) and the classification/staging system (**Table 239-3**) for AKI are an abrupt (within 48 hours) reduction in kidney function currently defined as an absolute increase in serum creatinine of more than or equal to 0.3 mg/dL (≥ 26.4 µmol/L), a percentage increase in serum creatinine of more than or equal to 50% (1.5-fold from baseline), or a reduction in urine output (documented oliguria of less than 0.5 mL/kg/h for more than 6 hours). The absolute increase in the serum creatinine levels (≥ 0.3 mg/dL) in this diagnostic criterion is based on epidemiologic data demonstrating that changes in serum creatinine levels of 0.3 to 0.5 mg/dL are associated with increased mortality risk. Also, the timeline of within 48 hours is deliberately included in the diagnostic criteria because of data demonstrating poorer outcomes within this period. The clinical utility and universal adoption of either RIFLE or AKIN criteria remain uncertain, and future studies are needed to demonstrate their validity.

EPIDEMIOLOGY

AKI IN THE HOSPITALIZED PATIENT

AKI is a complication of up to 18% of all hospital admissions in the United States. Major causes of hospital-acquired AKI include volume depletion resulting in decreased renal perfusion, major surgery, septic shock, congestive cardiac failure, contrast nephropathy, and aminoglycoside antibiotics. Acute tubular necrosis (ATN) is identified as the most frequent clinicopathologic entity in hospital-acquired AKI, followed by prerenal azotemia, acute-onset chronic renal failure, and urinary tract obstruction.

AKI IN THE CRITICALLY ILL PATIENT

AKI occurs in 25% or more of patients admitted to critical care units, with major causes including sepsis, multiorgan failure,

TABLE 239-1 RIFLE Classification for AKI

- **R**isk (R)—Increase in serum creatinine level × 1.5 or decrease in GFR by 25%, or UO < 0.5 mL/kg/h for 6 h
- **I**njury (I)—Increase in serum creatinine level × 2.0 or decrease in GFR by 50%, or UO < 0.5 mL/kg/h for 12 h
- **F**ailure (F)—Increase in serum creatinine level × 3.0, decrease in GFR by 75%, or serum creatinine level > 4 mg/dL with acute increase of > 0.5 mg/dL; UO < 0.3 mL/kg/h for 24 h, or anuria for 12 h
- **L**oss (L)—Persistent AKI, complete loss of kidney function > 4 wk
- **E**nd-stage kidney disease (E)—Loss of kidney function > 3 mo

TABLE 239-3 AKIN Classification/Staging System for AKI

Stage	Serum Creatinine Criteria	Urine Output Criteria
1	Increase in serum creatinine of more than or equal to 0.3 mg/dL (≥ 26.4 µmol/L) or increase to more than or equal to 150%-200% (1.5-2-fold) from baseline	Less than 0.5 mL/kg/h for more than 6 h
2*	Increase in serum creatinine to more than 200%-300% (> 2- to 3-fold) from baseline	Less than 0.5 mL/kg/h for more than 12 h
3†	Increase in serum creatinine to more than 300% (> 3-fold) from baseline (or serum creatinine of more than or equal to 4.0 mg/dL [≥ 354 µmol/L] with an acute increase of at least 0.5 mg/dL [44 µmol/L])	Less than 0.3 mL/kg/h for 24 h or anuria for 12 h

Note: This classification is modified from RIFLE (Risk, Injury, Failure, Loss, and End-stage kidney disease) criteria.

The staging system proposed is a highly sensitive interim staging system and is based on recent data indicating that a small change in serum creatinine influences outcome.

Only one criterion (creatinine or urine output) has to be fulfilled to qualify for a stage.

*200%-300% increase = 2-3-fold increase.

†Given wide variation in indications and timing of initiation of renal replacement therapy (RRT), individuals who receive RRT are considered to have met the criteria for stage 3 irrespective of the stage they are in at the time of RRT.

hypotension, nephrotoxin administration, and prerenal factors. AKI affects mostly older patients who have chronic morbidities or are severely ill on admission to the hospital. The overall in-hospital mortality rate in intensive care unit (ICU)-associated AKI is approximately 60%.

■ COMMUNITY-ACQUIRED AKI

Community-acquired AKI accounts for 1% of the hospital admissions in the United States. Community-acquired AKI in developed nations mainly affects older patients, with causes including acute tubular necrosis, prerenal azotemia, acute-onset chronic renal failure, and obstructive uropathy. In developing countries, AKI is predominantly a disease of infants and children and is due to prerenal etiologies, such as dehydration from acute diarrheal illness. Falciparum malaria, HIV/AIDS, obstetrical mishaps, dengue fever, snake bites, insect stings, botanical and chemical nephrotoxins, acute glomerulonephritis, hemolytic uremic syndrome, and alternative medical therapies are important etiological factors of AKI in the tropics. Crush injury from natural disasters such as earthquake contributes to regional epidemics of AKI.

■ AKI AMONG CHILDREN

Recent studies indicate that the incidence of AKI in pediatric patients is increasing. This may be related to the high rates of AKI in hospitalized children in the setting of cardiac surgery and stem cell transplantation.

■ CAUSES OF AKI

The causes of AKI can be classified under three broad categories: prerenal, renal, and postrenal (**Table 239-4**). Prerenal azotemia and ischemic ATN account for 75% of AKI.

■ PRERENAL CAUSES

Prerenal causes are characterized by a reversible loss of kidney function and a drop in GFR due to decreased renal perfusion, while the integrity of renal structural components is maintained. Prerenal causes account for approximately 70% of community-acquired AKI and 40% of hospital-acquired cases. Prerenal azotemia is typically

TABLE 239-2 AKIN Diagnostic Criteria for AKI

An abrupt (within 48 hours) reduction in kidney function currently defined as an absolute increase in serum creatinine of more than or equal to 0.3 mg/dL (≥ 26.4 µmol/L), a percentage increase in serum creatinine of more than or equal to 50% (1.5-fold from baseline), or a reduction in urine output (documented oliguria of less than 0.5 mL/kg/h for more than 6 h).

due to decreased effective circulating volume, true hypovolemia, or impaired renal perfusion.

Decreased effective circulating volume may be due to cardiac failure, aortic stenosis, nephrotic syndrome, cirrhosis, hepatorenal syndrome, acute pancreatitis, cardiac tamponade, sepsis, or systemic vasodilatation in conjunction with sepsis or anesthesia.

Intravascular volume depletion, a possible result of dehydration due to vomiting, diarrhea, poor fluid intake, fever, and diaphoresis, is the most common cause of prerenal azotemia in the outpatient setting. Excessive urination (polyuria) due to excess diuretics, diabetes insipidus, or poorly controlled diabetes mellitus can also cause AKI. Other causes of volume depletion include gastrointestinal bleeding and plasma loss due to burns, trauma, and anaphylaxis.

Decreased renal perfusion may result from renal artery stenosis or renal vein thrombosis, or more often from drugs such as non-steroidal anti-inflammatory drugs (NSAIDs). NSAIDs interfere with glomerular autoregulation, especially in patients above the age of 60 with additional risk factors for prerenal azotemia, such as atherosclerotic vascular disease, preexisting CKD, hypotension, diuretic use, cirrhosis, nephrotic syndrome, and congestive cardiac failure. Immunosuppressive drugs, such as tacrolimus and cyclosporine, lead to acute kidney injury by inducing vasoconstriction of the afferent and efferent glomerular arterioles of the kidneys. Angiotensin-converting enzyme (ACE) inhibitors may cause AKI in patients with unilateral or bilateral renal artery stenosis.

■ INTRARENAL CAUSES

Intrarenal causes of AKI are characterized by the loss of kidney function due to structural damages to glomeruli, tubules, vessels, or interstitium. They are often categorized based on the primary site of renal injury.

TABLE 239-4 Causes of AKI

Prerenal

Intravascular volume depletion: diarrhea, vomiting, hemorrhage, poor fluid intake, sepsis, overdiuresis

Decreased effective circulating volume to the kidneys: congestive cardiac failure, nephrotic syndrome, cirrhosis, or hepatorenal syndrome

Renal hypoperfusion due to exogenous agents: ACE inhibitors, NSAIDs

Renal

Acute tubular necrosis: ischemia

Toxins: drugs (eg, aminoglycosides), contrast agents, pigments (myoglobin or hemoglobin); heavy metals

Glomerular disease: rapidly progressive glomerulonephritis, systemic lupus erythematosus, small-vessel vasculitis (Wegener granulomatosis or polyarteritis nodosa), Henoch-Schönlein purpura (IgA nephropathy), Goodpasture syndrome

Acute proliferative glomerulonephritis: endocarditis, poststreptococcal infection

Vascular disease

Microvascular disease: atheroembolic disease (cholesterol-plaque microembolism), thrombotic thrombocytopenic purpura, hemolytic uremic syndrome, HELLP syndrome (*h*emolysis, *e*levated *l*iver enzymes and *l*ow *p*latelets)

Macrovascular disease: renal artery occlusion, abdominal aortic aneurysm

Interstitial disease: allergic reaction to drugs, autoimmune disease, systemic lupus erythematosus, mixed connective tissue disease, pyelonephritis, infiltrative disease (lymphoma or leukemia)

Postrenal

Benign prostatic hypertrophy or prostate cancer, cervical cancer, retroperitoneal disorders, intratubular obstruction (stones, urate crystals, myeloma light chains), pelvic mass or invasive pelvic malignancy, intraluminal bladder mass (clot, tumor or fungal ball), neurogenic bladder, urethral strictures

---

Acute tubular necrosis (ATN) is the most common cause of intrinsic renal failure, and is also the most common cause of hospital-acquired acute kidney injury. It usually results from tubular ischemia and inflammation, as in sepsis and shock, or tubular toxins such as heme pigments (such as myoglobin from rhabdomyolysis or hemoglobin from intravascular hemolysis), cisplatin, ethylene glycol, and myeloma light chains. Ischemic tubular necrosis may occur in patients with sustained prerenal azotemia. Ifosfamide, a chemotherapeutic agent, is known to cause acute tubular dysfunction in the proximal tubule.

Hospital-acquired ATN is often multifactorial. For example, it may occur in a septic patient exposed to a potentially nephrotoxic drug, such as an aminoglycoside or amphotericin, or after the administration of a radiocontrast agent in a hypovolemic patient with preexisting renal dysfunction.

Patients with severe renal ischemia may develop cortical necrosis with injury to both tubules and glomeruli. Causes include severe sepsis, dehydration, snake bites, obstetrical catastrophes, thrombotic microangiopathies, and malaria. The prognosis for recovery is less favorable than for ATN.

Glomerular disease in the form of rapidly progressive glomerulonephritis (RPGN) and acute proliferative glomerulonephritis may cause AKI. RPGN may be primary or secondary in origin, the latter

being associated with systemic diseases like systemic lupus erythematosus, Wegener granulomatosis, polyarteritis nodosa, Henoch-Schönlein purpura, and Goodpasture syndrome. RPGN can also progress to end-stage renal disease (ESRD) in days to weeks. Acute proliferative glomerulonephritis occurs in patients with bacterial endocarditis, poststreptococcal infection, and postpneumococcal infection.

Vascular disease (ie, microvascular and macrovascular renal arterial disease) can cause AKI. Thrombotic thrombocytopenic purpura, hemolytic uremic syndrome, HELLP syndrome (hemolytic anemia, elevated liver enzymes, low platelet count), glomerular capillary thrombosis, and atheroembolic disease may all cause AKI. Patients undergoing interventional or invasive procedures involving the major vessels and those with arrhythmias are at an increased risk for AKI from atheroemboli.

Interstitial disease, such as acute interstitial nephritis (AIN), often results from an allergic reaction to an offending agent (**Table 239-5**). Withdrawal of the offending agent frequently results in reversal of AKI. AIN may also occur in systemic inflammatory conditions such as sarcoidosis, systemic lupus erythematosus (SLE), Legionnaires' disease, and hantavirus infection.

■ POSTRENAL CAUSES

Postrenal AKI is characterized by loss of kidney function due to intrinsic or extrinsic masses obstructing the urinary collecting system, from the tip of the papillae to the urethral meatus. The most common causes are prostatic hypertrophy or carcinoma, cervical cancer, and other causes of bladder neck obstruction. Less common causes include bilateral renal stones, bladder carcinoma,

TABLE 239-5 Drugs Associated with Acute Interstitial Nephritis

Beta-lactam antibiotics	NSAIDs
• Methicillin	• Fenoprofen
• Ampicillin	• Indomethacin
• Oxacillin	• Naproxen
• Penicillin	• Ibuprofen
• Nafcillin	• Tolmetin
• Cephalosporins	• Diflunisal
Other antibiotics	• Piroxicam
• Sulfonamides	• Ketoprofen
• Rifampin	• Diclofenac
• Polymyxin	Other drugs
• Ethambutol	• Proton-pump inhibitors
• Tetracycline	• Diphenylhydantoin
• Vancomycin	• Cimetidine
• Erythromycin	• Sulfinpyrazone
• Ciprofloxacin	• Allopurinol
• Acyclovir	• Aspirin
• Indinavir	• Carbamazepine
• Alpha-interferon	• Phenindione
Diuretics	• Clofibrate
• Thiazides	• Phenylpropanolamine
• Furosemide	• Aldomet
• Chlorthalidone	• Phenobarbital
• Triamterene	• Azathioprine
	• Diazepam
	• Captopril
	• Cisplatin

retroperitoneal fibrosis, colorectal cancer, blood clots in the urinary tract, papillary necrosis, and neurogenic bladder.

PATHOPHYSIOLOGY

Figure 239-1 depicts the interaction of hemodynamic, immunological, and inflammatory factors in mediating AKI.

EVALUATION

■ HISTORY AND PHYSICAL EXAMINATION

A comprehensive history and physical examination is recommended in patients with AKI. Patients should be asked about nonspecific symptoms of azotemia, such as anorexia, nausea, vomiting, malaise, fatigue, pruritus, metallic taste in the mouth, and dyspnea. Bone pain may suggest multiple myeloma. The patient's daily fluid intake and output, daily weights, inpatient and outpatient medications, including NSAIDs and other over-the-counter medications, and outpatient laboratory data should be reviewed. Recent radiology studies should be assessed to determine if the patient has a history of recent contrast use in angiography or computed tomographic (CT) imaging.

On physical examination, patients should be assessed for signs of volume overload, such as peripheral edema, pulmonary rales, and elevated neck veins. Physical findings of advanced renal failure

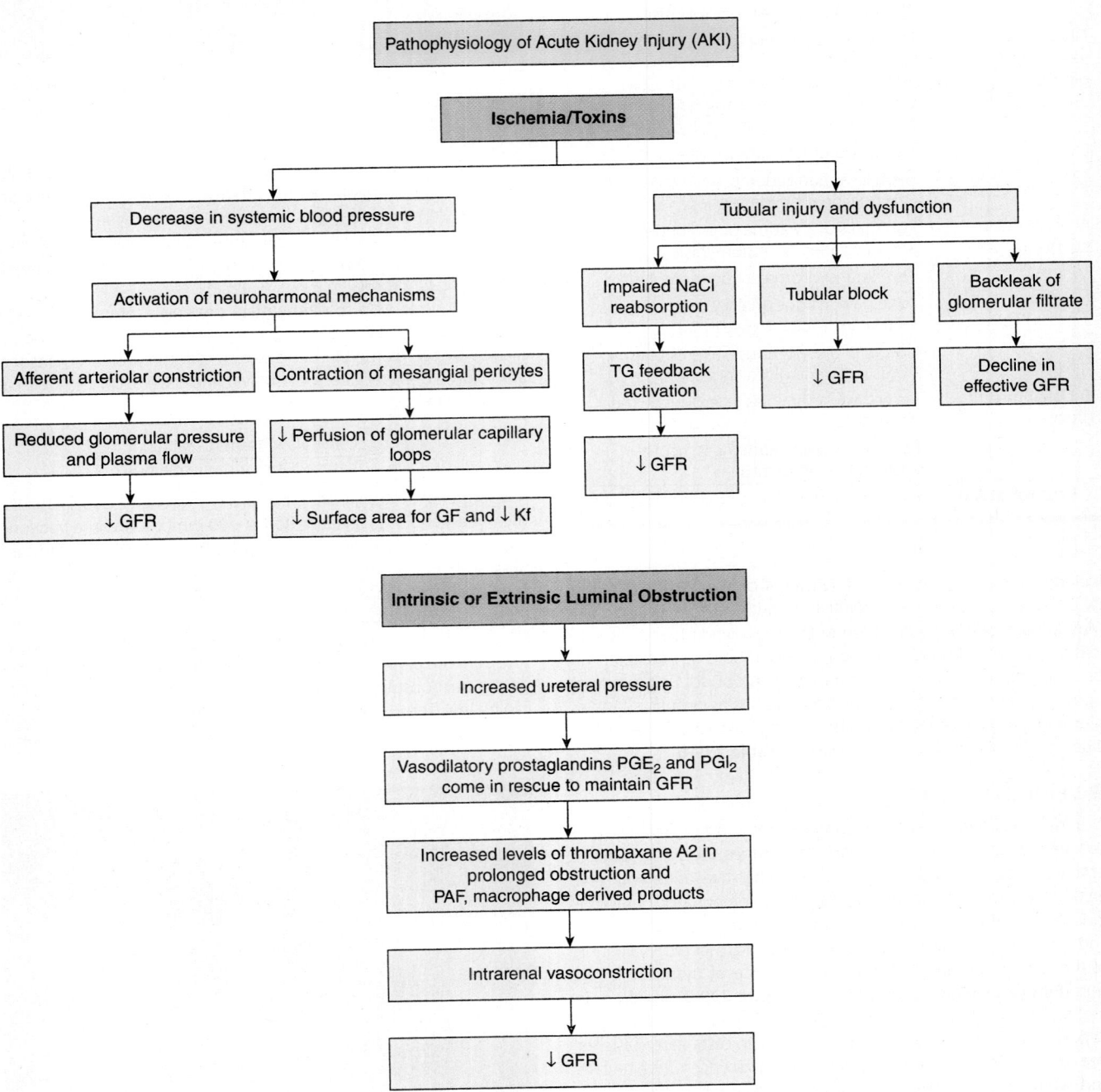

Figure 239-1 *Pathophysiology of AKI.*

TABLE 239-6 List of Clinical Features and Diagnostic Clues

1. Prerenal AKI	Absolute or postural hypotension
	Low jugular venous pressure
	Dry mucus membranes (dehydration)
	Decreased effective circulatory volume (eg, heart failure or liver disease)
2. Intrinsic AKI	
Diseases of the large renal vessels	Flank or abdominal pain (renal artery thrombosis)
	Retinal plaques, palpable purpura, livedo reticularis (atheroembolic disease)
	Flank pain (renal vein thrombosis)
Diseases of small vessels and glomeruli	New cardiac murmur (post-infectious glomerulonephritis), skin rash or ulcers, arthralgias (lupus), sinusitis (anti-GBM disease), lung hemorrhage (anti-GBM, ANCA-associated vasculitis, lupus)
	Fever, neurologic abnormalities (HUS-TTP)
	Headache, papilledema, heart failure with LVH (malignant hypertension)
Acute tubular necrosis	Postictal state, trauma or prolonged immobilization (rhabdomyolysis)
	Fever, transfusion reaction (hemolysis)
	Bone pain, fatigue, malaise in individuals > 60 years (multiple myeloma)
	History of alcohol abuse, altered mental status (ethylene glycol ingestion)
Tubulointerstitial disease	Fever, rash, arthralgias (allergic interstitial nephritis)
	Fever, flank pain, tenderness (acute bilateral pyelonephritis)
3. Post renal AKI	Palpable bladder, flank, or abdominal pain

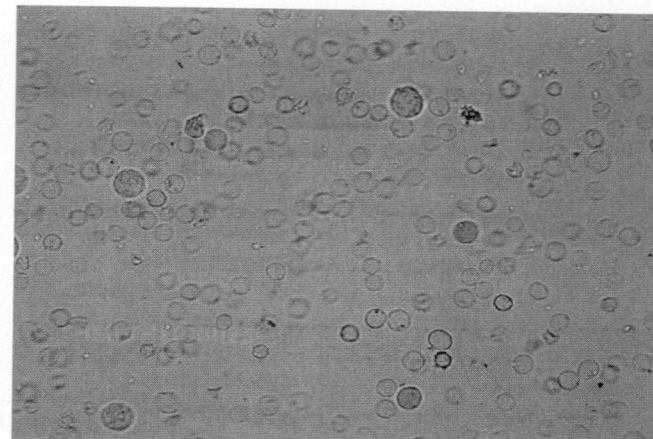

Figure 239-2 *Dysmorphic red blood cells in urine: a common finding in glomerulonephritis.* (Courtesy of Dr. Richard Dion.)

include asterixis, myoclonus, and pericardial or pleural rubs. A minority of patients with acute interstitial nephritis have fever and rash. Muscle pain, bluish discoloration of the toes, livedo reticularis, and loss of foot or ankle pulses suggest atheroembolic renal failure. Palpable purpura, mononeuritis multiplex, hemoptysis, or prominent upper respiratory tract symptoms, such as sinusitis or otitis, suggests glomerulonephritis associated with systemic vasculitis. Other clinical clues for the diagnosis of AKI are listed in **Table 239-6**.

■ URINE EVALUATION

A urine specimen should be collected for dipstick, microscopic sediment analysis, culture, and urine chemistries, including sodium, protein, creatinine, and osmolality. Heme-positive urine with few erythrocytes on microscopy suggests myoglobinuria or hemoglobinuria, as in rhabdomyolysis and transfusion reactions. Proteinuria and hematuria suggest glomerular injury. Microscopic evaluation of the urine sediment is crucial. The presence of dysmorphic red cells (**Figure 239-2**) and red cell casts (**Figure 239-3**) should raise the possibility of glomerulonephritis. The presence of fat either deposited in epithelial cells (oval fat bodies), in casts (fatty casts) or free fat suggests nephrotic syndrome. The presence of white cells and white cell casts suggests tubulointerstitial inflammation or a pyelonephritis. Hyaline casts and granular casts are suggestive of prerenal azotemia (**Figures 239-4** and **Figure 239-5**). The presence of epithelial cells and pigmented granular casts (muddy brown casts) suggests acute tubular necrosis (ATN) (**Figure 239-6**). Eosinophiluria, once thought to be diagnostic of AIN, is neither sensitive

nor specific for this condition, as it may be seen in pyelonephritis, prostatitis, glomerulonephritis, atheroembolism, and transplant rejection. In ethylene glycol ingestion, double-pyramid, ovoid, or dumbbell-shaped oxalate crystals are usually present in the urine. Amber-colored rhomboid uric acid crystals may be found in urine in tumor lysis syndrome.

Urine indices help to differentiate prerenal azotemia from ATN. The fractional excretion of sodium (FE_{Na}) is the percentage of sodium filtered by the glomeruli that is excreted in the urine. Patients that are volume depleted are sodium-avid and have a low FE_{Na}. It is calculated as follows:

$$FE_{Na} = \frac{[\text{Urine Na} \times \text{Plasma Creatinine}]}{\text{Plasma Na} \times [\text{Urine creatinine}]} \times 100$$

In prerenal azotemia, urine osmolality is usually > 500 mOsm/kg, the urinary sodium concentration is < 20 mmol/L, and the fractional excretion of sodium (FE_{Na}) is < 1%, whereas in tubular necrosis and urinary obstruction the urine osmolality is < 350 mOsm/kg, the urine sodium concentration is > 40 mmol/L, and the FE_{Na} is > 1% (in ATN, the FE_{Na} is usually, but not always, > 2%). There are exceptions: the FE_{Na} may be < 1% in acute tubular injury due to radiocontrast exposure or heme pigment, and also in acute glomerulonephritis. In early urinary tract obstruction, the urinary sodium concentration and FE_{Na} can be low. The FE_{Na} is also not reliable in the setting of chronic kidney disease, where a high FE_{Na} may be seen in patients with prerenal

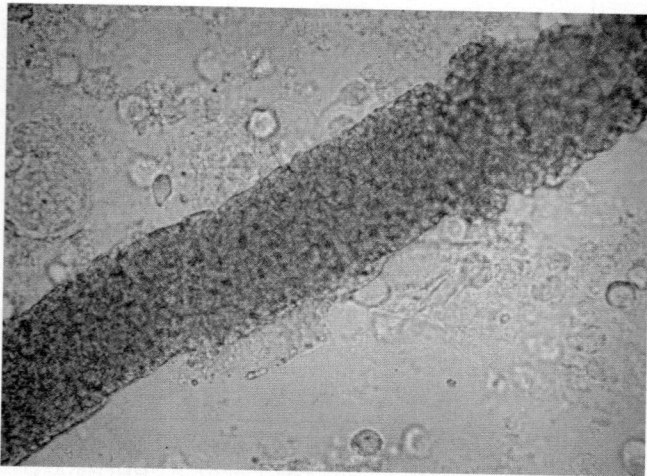

Figure 239-3 *Red blood cell cast: a common urine microscopic finding in glomerulonephritis.* (Courtesy of Dr. Richard Dion.)

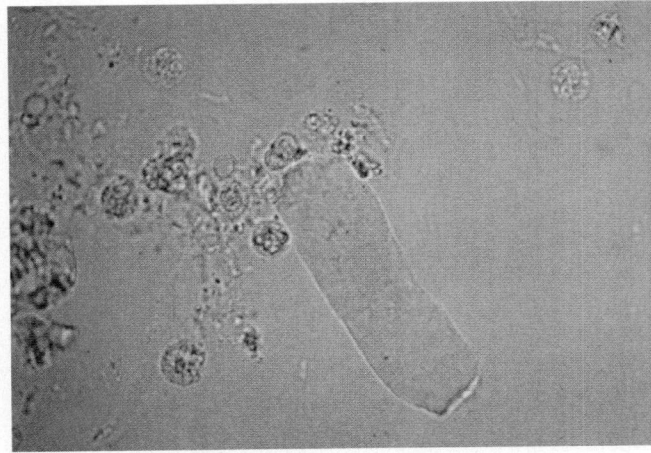

Figure 239-4 *Hyaline cast: a common finding in prerenal acute kidney injury; may also be seen in normal individuals with concentrated urine. (Courtesy of Dr. Richard Dion.)*

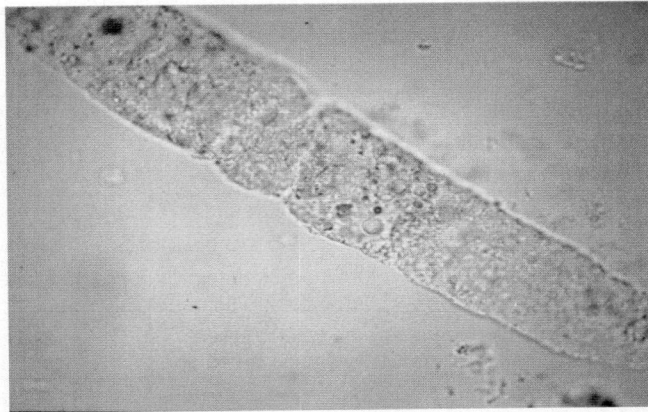

Figure 239-5 *Granular cast with a waxy margin: a common finding in prerenal azotemia and acute tubular necrosis. (Courtesy of Dr. Richard Dion.)*

azotemia, especially early in the clinical course. Typical urine findings in different causes of AKI are listed in **Table 239-7**.

PRACTICE POINT

- The fractional excretion of sodium (FE_{Na}) aids in differentiating prerenal azotemia from acute tubular necrosis. However, in patients who have recently received diuretics, sodium excretion is enhanced, and the FE_{Na} is not reliable. In this setting, the fractional excretion of urea (FE_{Urea}) may be helpful as urea excretion is not enhanced by diuretics. It is calculated as follows:

$$FE_{Urea} = \frac{[Urine\ urea \times Plasma\ creatinine]}{[Plasma\ urea \times Urine\ creatinine]} = 100$$

- Normally, the FE_{Urea} is 50% to 65%, while in prerenal azotemia, it is usually less than 35%.

Patients with metabolic alkalosis and prerenal azotemia have a falsely elevated FE_{Na}, because of bicarbonaturia with obligate losses of sodium in urine. In these patients, the fractional excretion of chloride (FE_{Cl}) may be used instead:

$$FE_{Cl} = \frac{[Urine\ Cl \times Plasma\ creatinine]}{[Plasma\ Cl \times Urine\ creatinine]} \times 100$$

- A $FE_{Cl} < 1\%$ is consistent with prerenal azotemia.

■ BLOOD TESTS

Serum blood urea nitrogen (BUN), creatinine, electrolytes, calcium, phosphorous, and albumin should be obtained in all patients. Serum creatinine concentration typically rises by 1 to 1.5 mg/dL daily when there is a marked decrement in kidney function. Most hospital laboratories are now able to calculate glomerular filtration (estimated GFR or eGFR) using an equation. Other useful blood tests include uric acid, creatinine kinase, serum immunoelectrophoresis, serum osmolal gap, and complete blood count with differential. In malignancies, serum urate and calcium levels are often high. Eosinophilia suggests allergic interstitial nephritis. Elevated serum creatine kinase is present in rhabdomyolysis. Abnormal serum electrophoresis is present in multiple myeloma. In alcohol ingestions such as ethylene glycol or methanol, there is high osmolal gap.

■ EVALUATION FOR OBSTRUCTION

Urinary tract obstruction should be excluded in patients presenting with AKI. Renal ultrasonography is the preferred imaging technique, with a sensitivity of 80% to 85% and a specificity approaching 100% for the diagnosis of obstruction. Ultrasonography also helps to identify kidney stones and kidney size. To locate the exact site of obstruction and correct it, percutaneous anterograde urography (via percutaneous puncture of the renal pelvis under fluoroscopy) and retrograde urography (via cystoscopy and ureteral catheterization) may be necessary. In patients with retroperitoneal fibrosis, obstruction of the urinary tract may be difficult to visualize by sonography, and computed tomography or magnetic resonance imaging may be necessary. Bladder catheterization can be useful in ruling out urethral obstruction.

■ RENAL BIOPSY IN AKI

Percutaneous renal biopsy has a limited role in the immediate evaluation and treatment of AKI. However, it is valuable in diagnosing primary renal diseases, such as glomerulonephritis and AIN, after prerenal and postrenal causes of AKI have been excluded. Renal biopsy also plays a role in the evaluation of early allograft dysfunction in renal transplant patients, and in management decisions related to subsequent use of immunosuppressive therapy.

■ NOVEL BIOMARKERS OF AKI

The definition of AKI is still based on a rise in serum creatinine and fall in urine volume and GFR. However, serum creatinine is not an

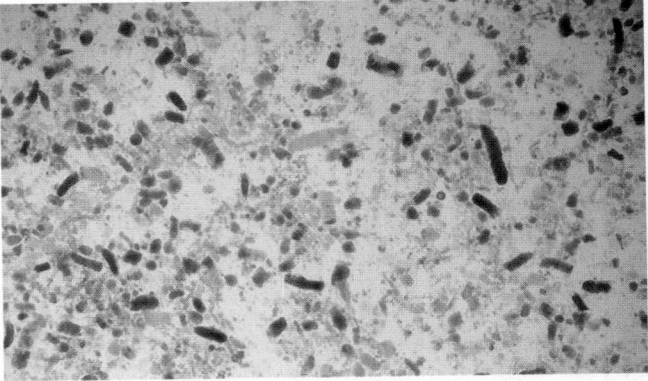

Figure 239-6 *Urine microscopy, showing muddy brown casts of acute tubular necrosis (ATN). (Courtesy of Dr. Serban Nicolescu.)*

TABLE 239-7 Urine Findings in AKI

Condition	Dipstick Test	Sediment Analysis	Urine Osmolality mOsm/kg	Fractional Excretion of Sodium
Prerenal azotemia	Trace or no proteinuria	A few hyaline casts possible	> 500	< 1
Intrarenal azotemia				
Tubular injury ischemia	Mild-to-moderate proteinuria	Pigmented granular casts	< 350	> 1
Nephrotoxins	Mild-to-moderate proteinuria	Pigmented granular casts	< 350	> 1
Acute interstitial nephritis	Mild-to-moderate proteinuria; hemoglobin; leukocytes	White cells and white-cell casts; eosinophils; red cells	< 350	> 1
Acute glomerulonephritis	Moderate-to-severe proteinuria; hemoglobin	Red cells and red-cell casts; red cells can be dysmorphic	> 500	< 1
Postrenal azotemia	Trace or no proteinuria; can have hemoglobin, leukocytes	Crystals, red cells, and white cells possible	< 350	> 1

optimal marker of renal function as it is influenced by age, sex, race, diet, exercise, and lean muscle mass. Moreover, secretion of creatinine may account for 10% to 40% of its excretion, potentially masking a drop in GFR. The development of sensitive and specific new biomarkers of renal function and injury has been an area of intense research. Serum cystatin C, a cysteine protease inhibitor produced by all nucleated human cells and freely filtered into the glomerulus, appears to be a more accurate marker of renal function and a more robust predictor of all-cause mortality in elderly persons than serum creatinine. Potential urinary biomarkers of early AKI are under investigation, such as kidney injury molecule-1, shed by proximal tubular cells after ischemic or nephrotoxic damage; interleukin-18, generated in the proximal tubule in AKI; osteopontin, a cytokine involved in kidney inflammation and repair; and the cytoprotective protein clusterin, a fatty-acid-binding protein, and neutrophil-gelatinase-associated lipocalin, which are overexpressed by tubular cells undergoing injury and oxidative stress. However, their precise role in the diagnosis and management of AKI has yet to be defined.

MANAGEMENT OF AKI

The management of AKI is directed at identifying and treating the underlying cause and preventing and treating complications. This may involve reversal of hemodynamic instability, elimination of nephrotoxins and avoidance of additional insults, and correction of electrolyte disturbances, uremia, and acid-base disorders.

Maintenance of euvolemic status is central to the management of ischemic acute renal failure. Assessment and correction of volume status are based on careful physical examination, and at times by invasive monitoring. Composition of the fluid replaced should match that of the fluid lost. Minor to moderate hemorrhagic loss is treated with normal saline (0.9% NaCl), whereas severe blood loss is best managed by transfusing packed red blood cells. Repletion of fluid is usually done with normal saline in hypovolemic patients; however, most patients with AKI have volume overload.

Distinguishing true hypovolemic AKI from hepatorenal syndrome (HRS) is a challenge in patients with cirrhosis and ascites. A gentle fluid challenge should be performed in these patients, with slow administration of fluids titrated to jugular venous pressure or central venous/pulmonary artery pressure. In true hypovolemia, urine output increases and the serum creatinine falls, whereas in HRS, a fluid challenge is usually ineffective. In patients with AKI and volume overload, loop diuretics such as furosemide, dosed between 20 and 100 mg, should be administered as an intravenous bolus, initially every 6 hours. The dose can be increased if an adequate response

is not achieved. If bolus dosing of furosemide is ineffective, a continuous infusion of furosemide may be initiated, although evidence for its efficacy compared to intermittent diuretic dosing is limited. When oliguria or anuria persists despite conservative management, dialysis is indicated.

Treatment of intrarenal AKI depends on the underlying pathology. Immunosuppressive agents, including steroids and cytotoxic drugs, may be beneficial in treating acute glomerulonephritis or vasculitis. Angiotensin-converting enzyme (ACE) inhibitors are helpful in treating AKI associated with hypertension and scleroderma renal crisis, but should generally be avoided in patients with hemodynamically related kidney injury. AKI due to malignant hypertension should be treated by vigorous control of blood pressure. Possible culprit drugs should be stopped in patients with possible AIN. While the role of corticosteroids in the management of AIN remains unclear since no randomized, controlled trials have been performed, and retrospective studies have shown conflicting results, most clinicians treat patients with a 1- to 2-week course of high dose steroids (prednisone 60 mg/d, rapidly tapered over a 1-2-week period).

Obstruction of the urethra or bladder neck can be relieved temporarily by insertion of a transurethral or suprapubic catheter. Obstructive lesions of the ureter are treated by stenting, either by anterograde percutaneous or retrograde cystoscopic placement. Patients often undergo a postobstructive diuresis for several days following relief of the obstruction, and care should be taken to avoid dehydration. Transient salt wasting syndrome occurs in approximately 5% of patients, and requires administration of intravenous normal saline to maintain blood pressure.

The most common electrolyte disturbance in AKI is hyperkalemia. Initial treatment should include calcium gluconate if the potassium level is > 6 mEq/L, or if electrocardiographic changes are present. Potassium may be transiently shifted into cells with intravenous insulin (10 units) and glucose (25 g) as a bolus infusion. As acidosis favors hyperkalemia by promoting extracellular movement of potassium, intravenous sodium bicarbonate (three ampules in 1 L of 5% dextrose) leads to translocation of potassium into cells and may also facilitate renal potassium excretion. Treatment with sodium bicarbonate is less effective acutely. Sodium polystyrene sulfonate (Kayexalate) given orally (25-50 g mixed with 100 mL of 20% sorbitol) or as enema (50 g in 50 mL of 70% sorbitol and 150 mL of tap water) is a more definitive therapy that leads to excretion of potassium from the body. Kayexalate enemas with 70% sorbitol are rarely associated with colonic necrosis, especially in critically ill patients, and should be avoided if other therapeutic options are available.

More recently sodium zirconium cyclosilicate (ZS-9) and patiromer sorbitex calcium have been shown to be effective in treating hyperkalemia. ZS-9 is an a nonabsorbable cation trap that selectively binds K$^+$ in exchange for H$^+$ and Na$^+$; it binds K$^+$ immediately upon ingestion. In contrast, patiromer is a nonabsorbable polymer that enhances K$^+$ excretion by the exchange of Ca^{2+}, predominantly in the distal colon. Dialysis remains an important option if hyperkalemia is severe or is refractory to treatment.

Acidosis may be corrected by administering sodium bicarbonate when the pH level is less than 7.2, or the serum bicarbonate level is less than 15 mEq/L. Bicarbonate may be administered orally (a 300 mg tablet contains 3.6 mEq of sodium bicarbonate) or intravenously. Ampules for intravenous administration are provided as 7.5% sodium bicarbonate (44.6 mEq/50 mL) or 8.4% sodium bicarbonate (50 mEq/50 mL). The required bicarbonate dose is measured by the following equation: bicarbonate deficit (mEq) = (lean body weight, LBW) (0.5) (desired HCO$_3$ − actual HCO$_3$). If acidosis cannot be corrected, dialysis is performed.

Diet plays an important role in patients with AKI who become nutritionally deficient. The daily caloric intake should be 30 to 45 kcal (126-189 kJ) per kg per day. In nondialysis patients, protein intake should be restricted to 0.6 g/kg/d. Patients receiving dialysis should have 1 to 1.5 kg/d.

RENAL REPLACEMENT THERAPY (RRT) IN AKI

Dialysis as a treatment modality in AKI is most useful in the elimination of metabolic wastes and uremic toxins, but it is also effective in the maintenance of fluid, electrolyte, and acid-base status. There is limited consensus among nephrologists regarding choice of dialysis, timing of initiation, frequency and intensity of dialysis, and impact on patient outcomes, due to lack of definitive evidence from studies conducted thus far in the setting of AKI (**Table 239-8**).

■ CONTINUOUS RENAL REPLACEMENT THERAPY VERSUS HEMODIALYSIS

In critically ill patients, continuous renal replacement therapy (CRRT) is now a popular and frequently preferred alternative to intermittent hemodialysis, especially in hemodynamically unstable patients.

CRRT can be either arteriovenous or venovenous, such as continuous arteriovenous hemodialysis (CAVHD) and continuous venovenous hemodialysis (CVVHD). CVVHD is preferred over CAVHD

TABLE 239-8 Renal Replacement Therapy in AKI

- Refractory hypervolemia, hyperkalemia (K$^+$ > 6.5 mEq/L), acidosis (pH < 7.1), azotemia (BUN > 100 mg/dL), uremic signs, and severe dysnatremias (Na$^+$ > 155 mEq/L or < 120 mEq/L) are absolute indications for dialysis
- Hemodialysis (HD) is more effective than peritoneal dialysis (PD) in the management of AKI because solute clearance and control of metabolic abnormalities are usually better in HD
- Hemodialysis can be intermittent dialysis, slow low-efficiency dialysis (SLED), or continuous renal replacement therapy (CRRT)
- In patients with hemodynamic instability, SLED or CRRT is recommended over HD
- Peritoneal dialysis (PD) is useful when hemodialysis is unavailable or vascular access cannot be obtained and is the mainstay of treatment in resource-limited settings. The major disadvantages are risk of peritonitis and visceral injury during catheter placement
- The optimal timing for the initiation of dialysis is still unclear
- The dialytic modality of choice depends on the availability of resources in the health care institute, technical expertise of the clinicians, and the clinical status of the patient

---

because of the high ultrafiltration rate, predictable blood flow rate, avoidance of arterial puncture, ease of vascular access (either femoral or internal jugular vein, via a double lumen catheter), and reduced risk of heparin-induced bleeding.

Compared to intermittent dialysis, CRRT has several advantages, including lower risk of hemodynamic instability, ease of administration of nutritional support, and more accurate control of fluid and metabolic status. Disadvantages include prolonged anticoagulation, nursing burden, cost, and limited mobility.

Sustained low-efficiency dialysis (SLED) or extended daily dialysis (EDD) is another increasingly popular dialytic modality of choice for critically ill patients and has the benefits of both continuous and intermittent dialysis methods. The advantages of SLED are good hemodynamic tolerability, high clearance levels of even small solutes, convenient treatment schedules, and cost effectiveness.

■ PERITONEAL DIALYSIS

Peritoneal dialysis (PD) is generally not a favored therapeutic modality for AKI. However, it is the preferred mode of renal replacement therapy in resource-limited settings and the developing world. Advantages include easy portability and access placement, better hemodynamic stability among patients, and the avoidance of systemic anticoagulation and its associated complications. Disadvantages include the risk of injury to the viscera during catheter placement, low levels of solute clearance, metabolic instability in critically ill patients, and the high risk of peritonitis.

■ DIALYSIS-RELATED COMPLICATIONS

Dialysis-induced complications include hypotension and complement cascade activation during the blood-dialyzer interaction. Hypotension worsens existing AKI because of impaired renal autoregulatory mechanisms. The upregulation of neutrophil adhesion molecules due to blood-dialyzer membrane interaction result in further damage to renal tissues. Unlike cuprophane, biocompatible membranes like polymethylmethacrylate or polyacrylonitrile do not activate complement to any great extent, and the use of biocompatible membranes is associated with improved recovery of renal function and reduced mortality among AKI patients requiring dialysis.

■ PROGNOSIS

The mortality rate of AKI ranges from 20% to 50%, and up to 70% in the ICU and surgical setting. Advanced age, severe underlying disease, preexisting poor nutritional status, and multisystem organ failure are associated with increased mortality. About 10% to 20% who suffer AKI will require maintenance dialysis. Infection, cardiorespiratory complications, and underlying disease states are the major causes of death in patients with AKI, rather than AKI itself. The availability of health care in a given country greatly influences the prognosis for AKI.

■ CONSULTATION

Nephrology consultation is appropriate in AKI when the cause is unclear after initial testing has been performed; if assistance is required with assessment and management of volume status; if intrinsic renal disease, such as glomerulonephritis or AIN, is suspected, and renal biopsy may be needed for diagnosis; and if an indication for dialysis is present, such as refractory fluid overload, severe metabolic acidosis, hyperkalemia, pericarditis, mental status changes, or overdose with a dialyzable toxin or drug.

■ DISCHARGE CHECKLIST

- Has close outpatient follow-up been arranged, with clinical assessment and measurement of serum creatinine and electrolytes?

- Has the patient been warned to avoid dehydration and drugs that may worsen renal function, such as NSAIDs?
- Have drug doses been adjusted for estimated GFR?
- If the patient seems likely to need dialysis in the near future, have they been told to avoid phlebotomy and intravenous placement in one arm to preserve it for graft or fistula creation?

SUGGESTED READINGS

Anderson S, Eldadah B, Halter JB, et al. Acute kidney injury in older adults. *J Am Soc Nephrol*. 2011;22:28-38.

Himmelfarb J, Ikizler TA. Acute kidney injury: changing lexicography, definitions, and epidemiology. *Kidney Int*. 2007;71:971-976.

Lafrance JP, Miller DR. Acute kidney injury associates with increased long-term mortality. *J Am Soc Nephrol*. 2010;21:345-352.

McCullough PA, Costanzo MR, Silver M, Spinowitz B, Zhang J, Lepor NE. Novel agents for the prevention and management of hyperkalemia. *Rev Cardiovasc Med*. 2015;16:140-155.

Molitoris BA, Levin A, Warnock DG, et al. Improving outcomes from acute kidney injury. *J Am Soc Nephrol*. 2007;18:1992-1994.

Pakula AM, Skinner RA. Acute kidney injury in the critically ill patient. *J Intensive Care Med*. Epub ahead of print, 2015 Mar 9.

Pisoni R, Wille KM, Tolwani AJ. The epidemiology of severe acute kidney injury: from BEST to PICARD. *Nephron Clin Pract*. 2008;109(4):c188-c191.

Stavros F, Yang A, Leon A, Nuttall M, Rasmussen HS. Characterization of structure and function of ZS-9, a K+ selective ion trap. *PLoS One*. 2014;9:e114686.

Waikar SS, Liu KD, Chertow GM. Diagnosis, epidemiology and outcomes of acute kidney injury. *Clin J Am Soc Nephrol*. 2008;3:844-861.

Weir MR, Bakris GL, Pitt B. New agents for hyperkalemia. *N Engl J Med*. 2015;372:1570-1571.

CHAPTER 240

Calcium Disorders

Elizabeth H. Holt, MD, PhD
John P. Bilezikian, MD

Key Clinical Questions

1. How is serum calcium regulated?
2. What are the causes of hypercalcemia in hospitalized patients?
3. How is hypercalcemia diagnosed and managed?
4. What causes hypocalcemia in hospitalized patients? How is it diagnosed and managed?

INTRODUCTION

Abnormalities of calcium metabolism are common in hospital practice. Hypercalcemia has a prevalence of 0.1% in the general population and 1% among hospitalized patients. In the inpatient setting, hypercalcemia often portends serious illness, especially malignancy. Hypocalcemia is also common in the hospital, especially in patients with chronic renal failure or sepsis. Hypocalcemia may also be a manifestation of vitamin D deficiency, which has a prevalence of up to 80% on specialized geriatric inpatient units.

CALCIUM METABOLISM

Precise regulation of calcium homeostasis is essential because of the critical role of calcium in many physiological activities. It is the major mineral of bone. It also plays major roles in neuronal transmission, muscle contraction, and blood coagulation. Calcium is also required for the proper functioning of many enzymes, endocrine secretory processes, and biochemical signaling pathways.

■ NORMAL SERUM CALCIUM LEVELS

A typical laboratory range for serum total calcium concentration is between 8.4 and 10.2 mg/dL. Approximately half of this total amount is bound to albumin, with the remainder in free (ionized) form. The normal free calcium concentration range is 4.5 to 5.3 mg/dL. A small fraction (10%) of circulating calcium is complexed with anions, such as citrate and phosphate.

■ REGULATION OF CALCIUM HOMEOSTASIS

The three organ systems that together regulate serum calcium are the gastrointestinal tract, kidneys, and skeleton. The two principal regulatory hormones are parathyroid hormone (PTH) and 1,25-dihydroxyvitamin D_3. PTH is a peptide secreted from the parathyroid glands in its active full-length configuration, known as PTH(1-84). Its plasma half-life is very short, on the order of 3 to 5 minutes. The major regulator of PTH secretion is the free calcium concentration in extracellular fluid. Elevated levels of free or ionized calcium promptly block secretion of PTH, while reduced serum calcium levels promptly increase secretion of PTH.

1,25-dihydroxyvitamin D_3 is produced by a sequence of activation steps (**Figure 240-1**), starting with the generation of cholecalciferol (vitamin D_3) through exposure of skin to ultraviolet light of a specified wavelength (90-315 nm). Cholecalciferol or its plant analogue, ergocalciferol (vitamin D_2), can also be obtained by dietary sources or in nutritional supplements. Cholecalciferol or ergocalciferol is converted in the liver to a hydroxylated form, 25-hydroxyvitamin D_3 or 25-hydroxyvitamin D_2. The 25-hydroxylated forms of vitamin D are converted to their active forms by a second hydroxylation step in the kidney leading to 1,25-dihydroxyvitamin D_2 or D_3. Both dihydroxylated forms of vitamin D are active in human subjects, although there is controversy over whether vitamin D_3 is more potent than vitamin D_2. PTH maintains serum calcium concentrations by conserving calcium that has been filtered at the kidney glomerulus and by mobilizing calcium from bone. 1,25-dihydroxyvitamin D maintains serum calcium by facilitating absorption of calcium from the gastrointestinal tract and, like PTH, mobilizing calcium from bone. Under normal conditions, the calcium absorbed by the gut (approximately 150-200 mg/d) is matched by the calcium eliminated by the kidney. At the dynamic skeletal interface, as much as

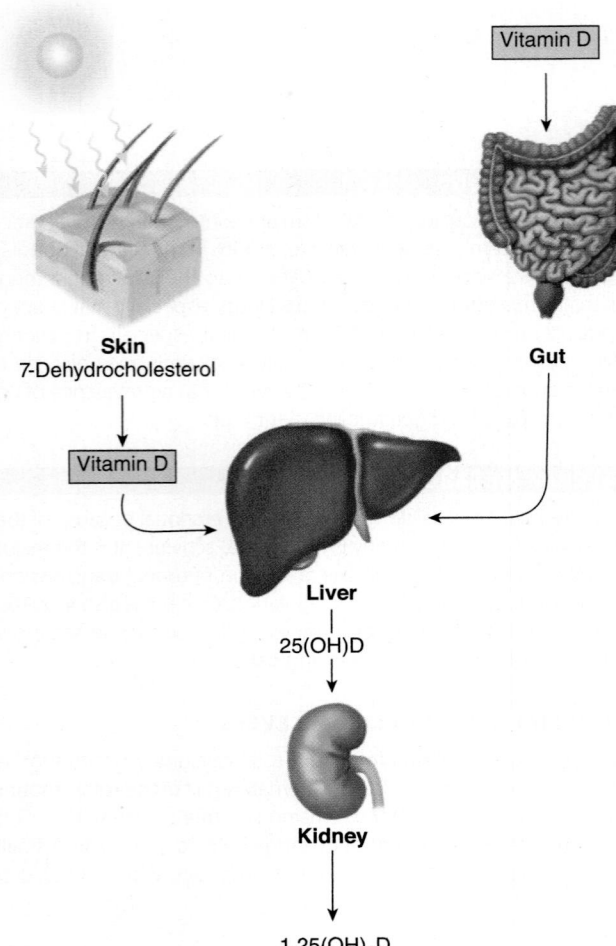

Figure 240-1 *Vitamin D synthesis and activation. Vitamin D is synthesized in the skin in response to ultraviolet radiation and is also absorbed from the diet. It is then transported to the liver, where it undergoes 25-hydroxylation. This metabolite is the major circulating form of vitamin D. The final step in hormone activation, 1-hydroxylation, occurs in the kidney.* (Reproduced, with permission, from Fauci AS, Braunwald E, Kasper DL, et al. *Harrison's Principles of Internal Medicine*, 17th ed. New York, NY: McGraw-Hill; 2008, Fig. 346-4.)

500 mg of calcium is turned over daily. This process is in a steady state, with net calcium neither gained nor lost. Thus, under normal circumstances, there are no significant fluctuations in body calcium stores, nor is there any major change in circulating serum calcium concentrations.

Changes in free or ionized calcium concentration are registered virtually instantly by parathyroid cells via the calcium-sensing receptor (CaSR). This receptor is located on the parathyroid cell surface, where its extracellular domain senses binding of calcium ions. If the circulating calcium concentration rises, the Ca²⁺-CaSR complex leads to a rise in intracellular calcium, inhibiting both PTH secretion and synthesis. If the serum calcium concentration falls, the Ca²⁺-CaSR complex sends a reduced signal to the cell, leading to an increase in PTH secretion and synthesis.

1,25-dihydroxyvitamin D decreases PTH production, although not as powerfully as does the ionized calcium signal. There is a stronger interaction between levels of 25-hydroxyvitamin D and PTH. They have an inverse relationship, with PTH levels rising when 25-hydroxyvitamin D levels fall below approximately 25 to 30 ng/mL. In turn, increased PTH stimulates the 1-alpha hydroxylase enzyme in the kidney that converts

25-hydroxyvitamin D to 1,25-dihydroxyvitamin D (**Figure 240-2**). When PTH levels are elevated (ie, primary hyperparathyroidism), 1,25-dihydroxyvitamin D levels increase. When PTH levels are low (ie, hypoparathyroidism), 1,25-dihydroxyvitamin D levels are typically low. The three organ systems (bone, gastrointestinal tract, and kidneys) and the two calcium-regulating hormones (PTH and 1,25-dihydroxyvitamin D) work together to maintain normal calcium homeostasis. When they are not perturbed by disease or by the aging process, they are an exquisitely sensitive and effective servomechanism.

LABORATORY MEASUREMENT OF BLOOD CALCIUM

The measurement of serum calcium may be helpful when a disturbance of calcium metabolism is suspected. However, in many disorders of calcium metabolism, such as osteoporosis or Paget disease of bone, the serum calcium concentration is typically normal. Serum

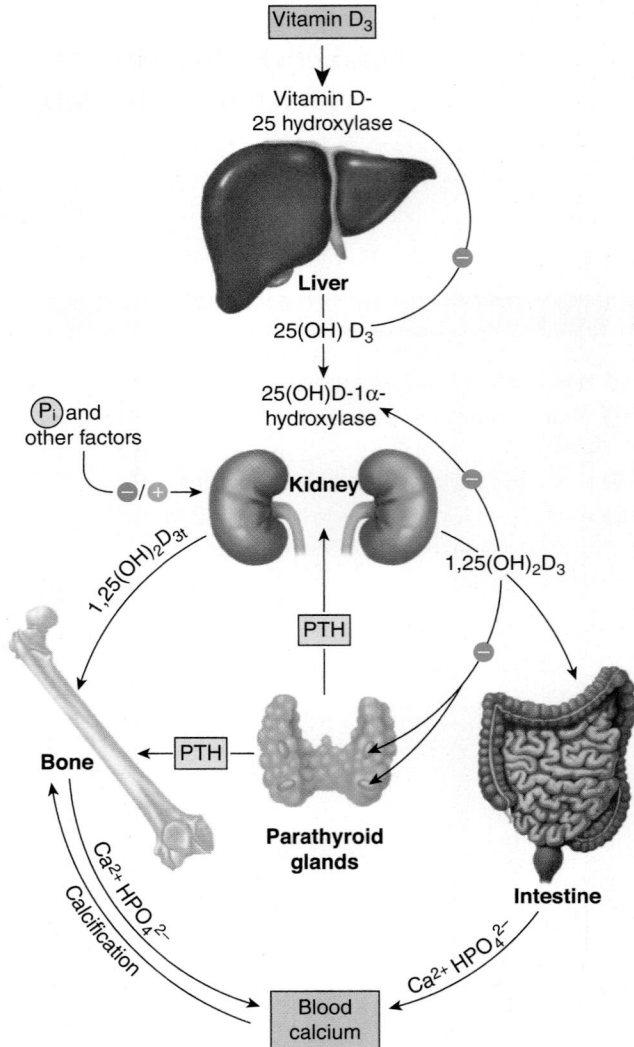

Figure 240-2 *Schematic representation of the hormonal control loop for vitamin D metabolism and function. A reduction in the serum calcium below 2.2 mmol/L (8.8 mg/dL) increases secretion of parathyroid hormone (PTH), mobilizing additional calcium from bone. PTH promotes the synthesis of 1,25(OH)2D in the kidney, which, in turn, stimulates the mobilization of calcium from bone and intestine, and regulates the synthesis of PTH by negative feedback.* (Reproduced, with permission, from Fauci AS, Braunwald E, Kasper DL, et al. *Harrison's Principles of Internal Medicine*, 17th ed. New York, NY: McGraw-Hill; 2008, Fig. 346-5.)

measurements may be performed by spectrophotometry or by atomic absorption spectrophotometry, with the latter yielding more accurate measurements. Spuriously high readings may occur if the tourniquet is in place too long before blood is drawn and hemoconcentration occurs. Under these circumstances, the measured serum calcium value can rise by as much as 0.4 mg/dL. On the other hand, the sample can read falsely low if the blood sample is obtained from a central, high-flow site via a central venous catheter. For most clinical situations, the total serum calcium is measured. This may need to be corrected for the circulating albumin concentration. For every 1 g/dL reduction in the serum albumin, the total calcium is adjusted upward by 0.8 mg/dL. This may be calculated as follows: Corrected total calcium = measured total calcium + 0.8 (4.0 – serum albumin)

In theory, free or ionized serum calcium is a more accurate physiological measurement than the adjusted total serum calcium concentration, but the sampling technique (the blood has to be free-flowing and not impeded by a tourniquet) and strict anaerobic collection conditions are problematic. Moreover, the measuring instrument has to be in regular use and properly calibrated. Samples have to be measured immediately. These technical issues somewhat limit the clinical utility of the ionized calcium measurement.

HYPERCALCEMIA

Signs and symptoms of hypercalcemia may be absent or subtle, except when calcium is significantly elevated or has increased rapidly. The diagnostic workup of hypercalcemia is usually straightforward (**Figure 240-3**) because two causes, primary hyperparathyroidism and malignancy-associated hypercalcemia, account for approximately 90% of cases. In addition, most individuals with primary hyperparathyroidism are asymptomatic and discovered on routine biochemical screening tests, while most individuals with malignancy-associated hypercalcemia have a known advanced malignancy at the time that hypercalcemia occurs. If the malignancy is not known, it is generally quickly apparent. When neither of these two etiologies is readily apparent, identification of the other potential etiologies requires a comprehensive history, physical examination, laboratory tests, and, occasionally, diagnostic imaging studies.

■ PRESENTING SYMPTOMS AND HISTORY

Many individuals with mild hypercalcemia (serum calcium level < 11 mg/dL) are asymptomatic, although some may report mild fatigue, vague changes in cognitive function, depression, or constipation.

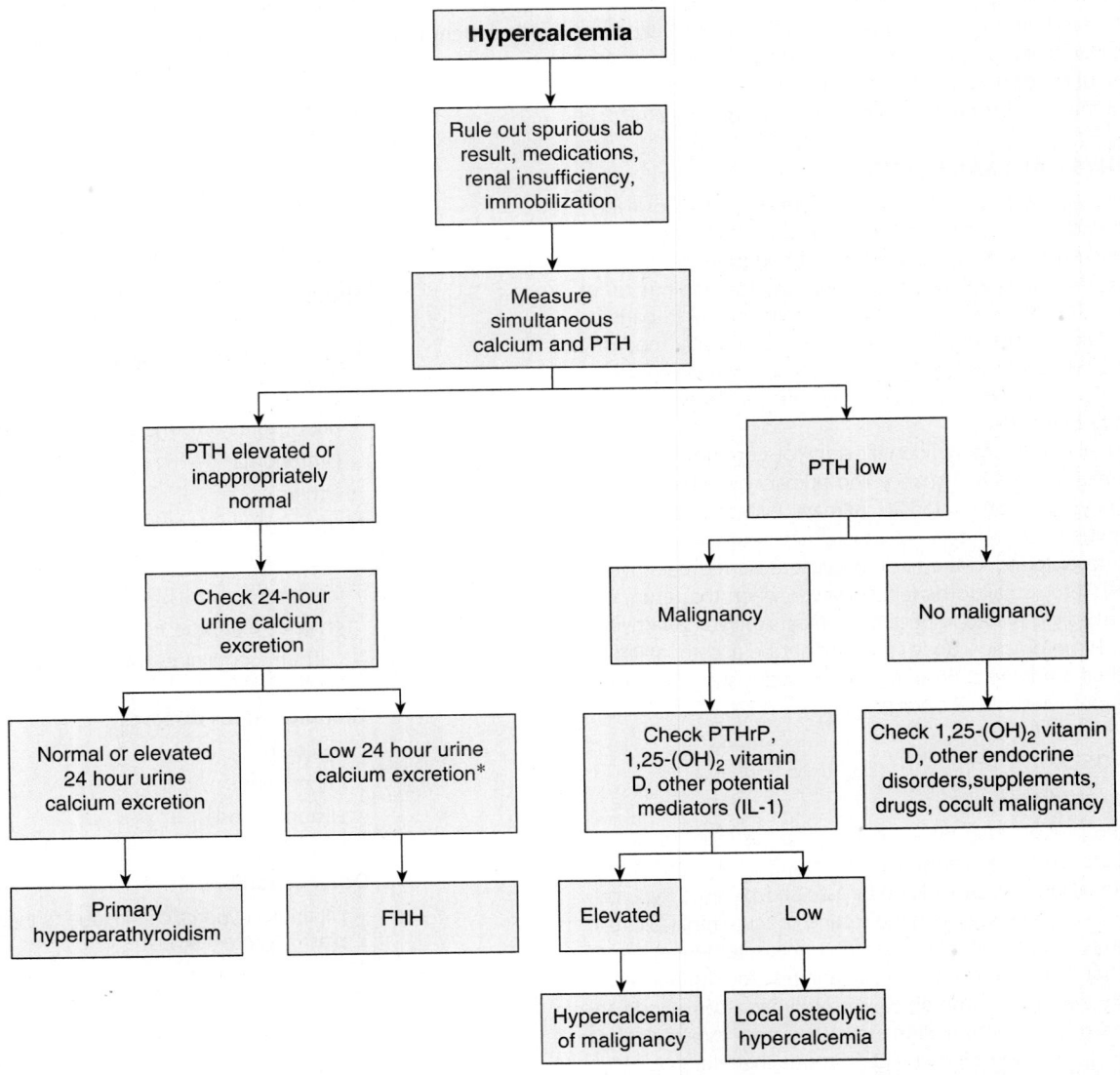

Figure 240-3 *Diagnostic approach to hypercalcemia. FHH, familial hypocalciuric hypercalcemia; PTH, parathyroid hormone; PTHrP, parathyroid hormone-related protein.*
*A low 24-hour urinary calcium does not necessarily rule out primary hyperparathyroidism.

Symptomatic manifestations of hypercalcemia are more apparent when the serum calcium concentration is between 12 and 14 mg/dL. These symptoms include anorexia, nausea, weakness, and depressed mental status. As hypercalcemia may induce polyuria and nephrogenic diabetes insipidus, dehydration may occur should the compensatory polydipsia not keep up with urinary water losses. When serum calcium levels rise above 14 mg/dL, profound dehydration, renal dysfunction, and central nervous system changes, such as progressive lethargy, disorientation, and coma, may develop.

In addition to the absolute magnitude of the serum calcium elevation, the rate of increase in serum calcium also influences symptoms. Individuals who are chronically hypercalcemic may have relatively few symptoms, even with serum calcium values up to 15 to 16 mg/dL. In contrast, those whose calcium level has risen abruptly may have symptoms at much more modest calcium levels. Elderly or debilitated patients are more likely to be affected by hypercalcemia than younger individuals.

The medical record may contain clues to etiology. Prescription medications (**Table 240-1**), foods, and vitamin and nutritional supplements should be reviewed. A careful family history might uncover a familial endocrine condition. A history of family members with endocrine tumors of the pituitary or pancreas suggests multiple endocrine neoplasia type 1 syndrome (MEN-1). A family history of pheochromocytoma or medullary thyroid cancer is consistent with MEN-2 syndrome. Patients with sarcoidosis may have a history of unexplained fever, lymphadenopathy, skin rashes, or pulmonary symptoms. Bone pain suggests myeloma or other malignancies, although it may also be a nonspecific finding of hypercalcemia.

■ THE PHYSICAL EXAMINATION

The physical examination is directed at identifying signs of hypercalcemia. Evidence of dehydration such as orthostasis or dry mucous membranes may be present, although hypercalcemia must be marked and prolonged for these physical findings to be appreciated. The physical examination is often normal in patients with hypercalcemia, especially if calcium levels are only modestly elevated. Rarely, severe and prolonged hypercalcemia may produce a visible horizontal deposit of calcium salts on the cornea, a finding called band keratopathy.

Effort should be made to identify signs of common causes of hypercalcemia, such as malignancy and primary hyperparathyroidism. The physical examination in primary hyperparathyroidism, like most hypercalcemic states, is usually not noteworthy. A mass is virtually never found in the neck, because enlarged parathyroid glands are still too small to be felt. However, when the serum calcium is markedly elevated, a neck mass may signify a parathyroid carcinoma. Symptomatic kidney stones might be accompanied by costovertebral tenderness. Enlarged lymph nodes suggest sarcoid, lymphoma, or metastatic carcinoma.

■ DIAGNOSIS
Laboratory studies

The first step in evaluating hypercalcemia is adjustment for serum albumin. If the corrected serum calcium is elevated, it should be repeated. Renal function should also be assessed, because hypercalcemia may develop or worsen in the setting of acute renal failure. If hypercalcemia is confirmed, the next step is measurement of serum PTH. The PTH level is the most important test for distinguishing between the two most common causes of hypercalcemia, primary hyperparathyroidism and malignancy-associated hypercalcemia (Table 240-1). The so-called intact immunochemiluminometric assay for PTH assay primarily measures the intact molecule, PTH(1-84), as well as a large circulating fragment that is foreshortened at the amino terminus, PTH(7-84). A more specific assay that measures

only PTH(1-84), the bio-intact assay, is also available, but it has not shown any clear advantages over the older assay, which has been in clinical use for over 20 years. When the creatinine clearance falls below 60 mL/min, these assays may begin to show elevations in PTH due to the accumulation of inactive fragments, and also perhaps due to increased secretory activity of the parathyroids (secondary hyperparathyroidism).

When the parathyroid glands are functioning normally, hypercalcemia should suppress PTH levels. Hypercalcemia is said to be

TABLE 240-1 Causes of Hypercalcemia

PTH mediated	Primary hyperparathyroidism
	Parathyroid adenoma
	Parathyroid hyperplasia
	Parathyroid carcinoma
	Tertiary hyperparathyroidism
	Familial hypocalciuric hypocalcemia
	Lithium
	Thiazide diuretics
PTH independent	**HHM: PTHrP mediated**
	Squamous carcinoma of the lung, oropharynx, nasopharynx, larynx, and esophagus
	Gynecologic (cervical, ovarian)
	Urologic (renal, transitional cell of bladder)
	Pheochromocytoma
	Pancreatic islet cell tumors
	T-cell lymphoma
	Others
	HHM: 1,25-(OH)$_2$-D$_3$ mediated
	B-cell lymphoma
	Local osteolytic hypercalcemia
	Multiple myeloma
	Breast carcinoma metastatic to bone
	Lymphoma
	Others
	Medications/supplements
	Vitamin D
	Vitamin A
	Thiazide diuretics
	Calcium-containing antacids (in milk-alkali syndrome)
	Granulomatous diseases
	Sarcoidosis
	Tuberculosis
	Histoplasmosis
	Leprosy
	Other conditions
	Factitious hypercalcemia (due to increased plasma protein levels)
	Acute renal failure
	Severe thyrotoxicosis
	Adrenal insufficiency
	Immobilization

HHM, humoral hypercalcemia of malignancy; PTH, parathyroid hormone; PTHrP, parathyroid hormone-related protein.

PTH-mediated if serum calcium is elevated, and the PTH level is high or inappropriately normal. In this latter situation, one is usually dealing with primary hyperparathyroidism, although familial hypocalciuric hypercalcemia (FHH) and medication-induced hypercalcemia, as from thiazide diuretics or lithium, can also be associated with elevated PTH levels. When PTH levels are appropriately suppressed in hypercalcemia, the differential diagnosis includes malignancy, granulomatous disease, medications, milk-alkali syndrome, thyrotoxicosis, and adrenal insufficiency.

Other recommended tests in the evaluation of hypercalcemia include serum electrolytes and 25-hydroxyvitamin D. Levels of 25-hydroxyvitamin D typically exceed 150 ng/mL in vitamin D toxicity due to excess intake. Levels this high cannot be achieved by sun exposure alone. High 1,25-$(OH)_2$D levels may be seen in any granulomatous disease, particularly sarcoidosis or certain lymphomas. Inorganic phosphorus measurement may be helpful, as a low-normal serum phosphate is often seen in primary hyperparathyroidism, while high phosphate may be seen in vitamin D intoxication. An elevated serum creatinine may indicate dehydration or true renal dysfunction due to renal deposition of calcium salts or other causes. An elevated alkaline phosphatase level suggests elevated bone turnover. This may be confirmed by measuring bone-specific alkaline phosphatase or other indices of bone turnover, such as serum osteocalcin, serum C-terminal collagen peptide measurement, or urinary N-terminal collagen peptide. Most forms of hypercalcemia are accompanied by hypercalciuria (24-hour urine calcium excretion > 4 mg/kg/24 hours). However, in primary hyperparathyroidism, renal calcium excretion is lower than expected for the degree of hypercalcemia, because PTH conserves filtered calcium in the distal renal tubule.

Additional tests

The electrocardiogram may show a shorted QT_c interval, particularly if hypercalcemia has occurred over a short period of time. Bone mineral density (BMD) by dual energy x-ray absorptiometry (DXA) may be helpful. In primary hyperparathyroidism, there is a typical pattern of BMD with relative preservation of cancellous bone, as in the lumbar spine, and significant loss of cortical bone, as in the femoral neck and distal third of the radius. Abdominal imaging studies (CT or ultrasound) may identify renal stones or nephrocalcinosis. Serum and urine protein electrophoresis should be obtained if myeloma is suspected. Skeletal radiographs may reveal lytic lesions of multiple myeloma or other malignancies. In primary hyperparathyroidism, skeletal radiographs may show subperiosteal bone resorption or brown tumors of bone, but are rarely needed for diagnosis.

◾ CAUSES OF PTH-MEDIATED HYPERCALCEMIA

Primary hyperparathyroidism

Elevation of both serum calcium and PTH concentrations, in the absence of lithium use or low urinary calcium excretion as seen in familial hypocalciuric hypercalcemia, supports a diagnosis of primary hyperparathyroidism. In this condition, PTH levels are usually within 1.5 to 2.0 times above the upper limit of normal. Extremely high levels of PTH raise the specter of parathyroid carcinoma. Typical primary hyperparathyroidism is associated with mild hypercalcemia, within 1 mg/dL above the upper limit of normal. The PTH level may be elevated, but may also fall in the upper portion of the normal range, which is inappropriate in hypercalcemia. Normocalcemic primary hyperparathyroidism is a new diagnostic entity applied to patients whose total and free serum calcium levels are normal, but in whom the PTH level is consistently elevated. In the absence of a secondary cause for elevated PTH levels, it is felt that these individuals have an early form of primary hyperparathyroidism.

Primary hyperparathyroidism is the most common cause of hypercalcemia in outpatients. The incidence is estimated to be approximately 21.6 per 100,000 person-years. The mean age at diagnosis is in the sixth decade of life, and there is a female-to-male ratio of 2:1. The clinical manifestations depend largely on the severity of the hypercalcemia. When primary hyperparathyroidism was first described more than 80 years ago, most patients presented with advanced disease with overt radiographic abnormalities of bone (osteitis fibrosa cystica) and kidneys (nephrolithasis or nephrocalcinosis). Since the introduction more than 40 years ago of automated multichannel autoanalyzers for measuring serum chemistry, primary hyperparathyroidism is most often diagnosed by routine blood testing, well before the development of other signs or any symptoms. It also may be uncovered during the evaluation of osteoporosis or during the workup of renal stone disease. The most common clinical presentation today is mild asymptomatic hypercalcemia. In 75% to 80% of cases, a solitary, benign parathyroid adenoma is present. Hyperplasia involving multiple parathyroid glands is found in 15% to 20% of cases, and parathyroid carcinoma is present in less than 0.5%. On occasion, double adenomas are found. Patients with MEN-1 or MEN-2 usually have parathyroid hyperplasia involving all parathyroid glands.

Parathyroid surgery is always indicated in symptomatic primary hyperparathyroidism, unless there are medical contraindications. The role of parathyroid surgery in asymptomatic primary hyperparathyroidism is more controversial. According to the guidelines of the Fourth International Workshop on the Management of Asymptomatic Primary Hyperparathyroidism, indications for surgery in asymptomatic patients include a serum calcium > 1 mg/dL above the upper limit of normal; creatinine clearance < 60 mL/min; 24-hour urine calcium > 400 mg/d and increased stone risk by biochemical stone risk analysis; presence of nephrolithiasis or nephrocalcinosis by x-ray, ultrasound or CT; T-score < –2.5 at lumbar spine, hip, or distal third of the radius; vertebral fracture by x-ray, CT, MRI or VFA; and age < 50. Patients who do not meet these guidelines can be followed expectantly. Thiazide diuretics and lithium should be avoided. Dietary calcium should not be restricted, because such restriction may promote further elevation of PTH, and possibly have adverse effects on bone mass. In patients who are vitamin D deficient, cautious replacement of vitamin D is advised. Patients should maintain hydration. Bisphosphonates increase lumbar spine BMD in primary hyperparathyroidism, without a major effect on the serum calcium concentration. The calcimimetic agent, cinacalcet, reduces serum calcium in primary hyperparathyroidism without having a major effect on BMD. Cinacalcet is indicated for use in patients with parathyroid cancer, as well as patients with primary hyperparathyroidism who are unable to undergo parathyroidectomy. Alendronate has not been approved by the Food and Drug Administration (FDA) for use in primary hyperparathyroidism.

Lithium can change the set point for the calcium-sensing receptor on the parathyroid gland, such that a higher serum calcium concentration is needed to inhibit PTH secretion. This can lead to mild biochemical abnormalities, such as high levels of calcium and high-normal to elevated PTH levels, that mimic primary hyperparathyroidism, but do not require medical intervention.

Thiazide-associated hypercalcemia also occurs. Many patients with hypercalcemia on thiazides probably have primary hyperparathyroidism. When thiazide therapy is discontinued, the hypercalcemia often persists, and the diagnosis of primary hyperparathyroidism is made.

Familial hypocalciuric hypercalcemia

Familial hypocalciuric hypercalcemia, also known as benign familial hypercalcemia, is a rare genetic condition caused by inactivating mutations in the CaSR. This results in lack of sensitivity of the parathyroid cell to ambient serum calcium, a higher set point for the extracellular ionized calcium concentration, and inappropriately normal to mildly elevated PTH levels. Patients with FHH have chronic asymptomatic hypercalcemia, with very low urinary calcium excretion. The relatively low urinary calcium excretion in FHH helps distinguish it from primary hyperparathyroidism, although low urinary calcium excretion may also occur in individuals with primary hyperparathyroidism. A family history of asymptomatic mild hypercalcemia, especially in individuals younger than 40 years, is suggestive of FHH. Other supportive evidence for FHH includes a very low urinary calcium to creatinine clearance ratio (< 0.01), and a history of family members who have undergone noncurative parathyroidectomy for presumed primary hyperparathyroidism. When FHH is suspected, further evaluation is necessary, such as screening of other family members for hypercalcemia. Genetic testing for FHH may be appropriate, as it may otherwise be exceedingly difficult to distinguish FHH from primary hyperparathyroidism.

Tertiary hyperparathyroidism

Conditions associated with low serum calcium are usually also associated with chronically elevated PTH levels, which is an appropriate physiological response. This is called secondary hyperparathyroidism. The rise in PTH may restore the serum calcium to normal, or calcium may remain low or in the low-normal range. Secondary hyperparathyroidism is not a hypercalcemic state. Common causes of secondary hyperparathyroidism include vitamin D deficiency, intestinal malabsorption of calcium or vitamin D, renal-based hypercalciuria, severe nutritional calcium deficiency, and especially chronic renal insufficiency. Correction of the underlying cause usually returns serum PTH concentrations to normal. Normalization of PTH may be relatively rapid, if the cause is of recent onset, or it may be protracted, if the associated condition has been longstanding. In patients with prolonged secondary hyperparathyroidism, the reactive state can become semiautonomous, leading to hypercalcemia. This condition, known as tertiary hyperparathyroidism, is most often seen in patients with poorly controlled chronic kidney disease. Tertiary hyperparathyroidism is usually associated with hyperplasia of multiple glands, but may also be caused by a parathyroid adenoma from a single clone of parathyroid cells.

Further investigations

Most patients with primary hyperparathyroidism have a serum calcium concentration below 11 mg/dL. Serum phosphate tends to be in the low-normal range (2.5-3.2 mg/dL). Rarely, a nonanion gap hyperchloremic acidosis from a PTH-induced defect in bicarbonate resorption may be seen. Urinary calcium excretion tends to be in the upper range of normal. However, hypercalciuria in primary hyperparathyroidism does not always predispose to renal stones, despite the fact that hypercalciuria is a risk factor for kidney stones in euparathyroid subjects. Bone turnover markers tend to be at the upper limit or normal, but occasionally can be frankly elevated.

Once the diagnosis of primary hyperparathyroidism is made, it should be determined whether or not the patient meets clinical criteria for parathyroidectomy (**Table 240-2**). If the clinical situation is appropriate, consideration should be given to the possibility of one of the MEN syndromes, particularly if the patient is young, or has a personal or family history of a related endocrinopathy. A diagnosis of MEN-1 or MEN-2 should prompt a search for multiple parathyroid gland disease.

■ CAUSES OF PTH-INDEPENDENT HYPERCALCEMIA

If the serum calcium concentration is elevated but the PTH level is appropriately suppressed, the patient has hypercalcemia due to causes other than hyperparathyroidism (PTH-independent hypercalcemia).

TABLE 240-2 Indications for Parathyroidectomy in Primary Hyperparathyroidism

Fragility fracture at any site

Serum calcium > 1.0 mg/dL above upper limit of normal

On bone mineral density by DXA: T-score < −2.5 at lumbar spine, total hip, femoral neck or distal 1/3 radius (use of Z-scores instead of T-scores is recommended for measurement of BMD in premenopausal women and men younger than 50 years of age).

Vertebral fracture by x-ray, CT, MRI, or Vertebral Fracture Assessment (VFA)

Creatinine clearance < 60 cc/min

24-h urine for calcium > 400 mg/d and increased stone risk by biochemical stone risk analysis

Presence of nephrolithiasis or nephrocalcinosis clinically or by x-ray, ultrasound or CT

Age < 50

Surgery is also indicated in individuals where medical monitoring is not desired or possible, or for those selecting surgery, without meeting any guidelines, if there are no medical contraindications.

Source: Adapted from Bilezikian JP, et al. Guidelines for management of asymptomatic primary hyperparathyroidism: Summary statement from the fourth international workshop. *J Clin Endocrinol Metab*. 2014;99:3561-3569.

Cancer is the most common cause. Other causes include thyrotoxicosis, vitamin D intoxication, sarcoidosis, immobilization, Addison disease, and various drugs and supplements.

In ***hypercalcemia of malignancy***, calcium is usually moderately or severely elevated, and PTH is low or undetectable. Significant dehydration and generalized debility are usually evident, along with other cancer-related symptoms. Usually, the diagnosis of malignancy has already been established when patients become hypercalcemic. Hypercalcemia of malignancy has two forms: humoral hypercalcemia of malignancy (HHM) and local osteolytic hypercalcemia. HHM results from tumor production of a circulating factor with systemic effects on calcium metabolism, acting on skeletal calcium release, renal calcium handling, or intestinal calcium absorption. The usual cause of HHM is parathyroid hormone-related protein (PTHrP). Normally, PTHrP serves as a paracrine factor in tissues such as bone, skin, breast, uterus, placenta, and blood vessels, where it is involved in cellular calcium handling, smooth muscle contraction, and growth and development. The amino terminus of the PTHrP peptide is closely homologous with native PTH, and they share a common receptor. When PTHrP circulates at supraphysiologic concentrations, it produces effects similar to PTH, activating osteoclasts to resorb bone, decreasing renal calcium output, and increasing renal phosphate clearance.

Tumors that produce HHM by secreting PTHrP are typically squamous cell carcinomas of the lung, esophagus, head and neck, or cervix. Other tumors that may elaborate PTHrP include adenocarcinoma of the breast or ovary, renal carcinoma, transitional cell carcinoma of the bladder, islet cell tumors of the pancreas, T-cell lymphoma, and pheochromocytoma. As tumors that produce PTHrP do so in relatively small amounts, the syndrome typically develops in patients with a large tumor burden. It is therefore unusual for HHM to be the presenting feature of a cancer. The diagnosis may be confirmed by a commercially available radioimmunoassay for PTHrP. Care should be taken to ensure that blood for PTHrP levels is drawn and handled correctly to avoid spurious low results. Rarely, HHM is caused by the unregulated production of 1,25-dihyroxyvitamin D, usually by B-cell lymphomas, or other mediators that interfere with calcium homeostasis.

The other major mechanism of malignancy-associated hypercalcemia is the direct invasion of bone by tumor, with lytic destruction and calcium release. While this was formerly thought to be a mechanical process, it now appears to be driven by the local elaboration of cytokines leading to osteoclast-mediated bone resorption. In local osteolytic hypercalcemia, PTHrP and calcitriol are within normal limits. Bony metastases are usually obvious on imaging studies. The classic tumor associated with this syndrome is multiple myeloma, although breast cancer and certain lymphomas may also be responsible. Local osteolytic hypercalcemia may be perpetuated by a positive feedback loop. Factors produced by bone promote the growth and survival of metastases, and the tumor induces osteoclasts to produce factors promoting tumor growth, bone resorption, and hypercalcemia. Interruption of this positive feedback loop is the rationale for the use of bisphosphonates in the treatment of multiple myeloma.

PTH-independent hypercalcemia also occurs in sarcoidosis, tuberculosis, and other granulomatous diseases. Macrophages in the granuloma convert 25-hydroxyvitamin D to 1,25-dihydroxyvitamin D, via an unregulated 1-α hydroxylase enzyme. 25-hydroxyvitamin D levels are typically not elevated. When serum 25-hydroxyvitamin D levels are elevated, excessive vitamin D intake becomes the more likely etiology. Endocrine conditions that may occasionally lead to hypercalcemia include severe hyperthyroidism, which stimulates bone resorption, and Addison disease, where volume depletion reduces calcium clearance and control of calcium absorption is mitigated by glucocorticoid deficiency.

Immobilization stimulates bone resorption and may increase serum calcium levels, particularly in bedbound hospitalized patients. This is usually seen in persons with high bone turnover, such as adolescents and patients with unrecognized hyperparathyroidism or Paget disease of bone. Drugs and dietary supplements may lead to hypercalcemia. Vitamin D intoxication and excessive intake of vitamin A, which activates bone resorption, are occasional culprits. Thiazide diuretics may cause hypercalcemia due to enhanced renal retention of calcium. In many cases, this develops in individuals with underlying mild primary hyperparathyroidism.

In patients with an extensive negative workup, the rare possibility of occult malignancy should be considered, especially when PTHrP is elevated. Further imaging studies would then be needed for tumor localization, including a plain chest radiograph or a computed tomographic scan of the chest to rule out lung malignancy. If these are unrevealing, consideration should be given to otolaryngoscopic examination, esophagoscopy, or CT of the abdomen, followed by radiographic or endoscopic evaluation of the genitourinary tract if necessary.

PRACTICE POINT

- In the early 20th century, the Chicago physician Bertram Sippy gained celebrity because of his "Sippy diet" for peptic ulcers—a regimen of milk, cream, eggs, and cereal 3 times a day, punctuated by aggressive antacid therapy with hourly sodium bicarbonate and magnesium hydroxide. This may or may not have been curative for ulcers, but some patients certainly did develop severe hypercalcemia, in what became known as milk-alkali syndrome. Patients developed a metabolic alkalosis, which favors renal reabsorption of calcium, and the resulting hypercalcemia led to renal vasoconstriction, a fall in GFR, and further increases in serum calcium. Up to one-third of these patients had chronic renal failure. Milk-alkali syndrome became rare with the introduction of H$_2$-blockers and proton pump inhibitors for peptic ulcer disease.

- A similar disorder is seen increasingly in postmenopausal women who consume large amounts of supplemental calcium carbonate and vitamin D for the prevention of osteoporosis. Pregnant or bulimic women with metabolic alkalosis from emesis who are taking calcium and vitamin D are also at risk. It has been suggested that the disorder be renamed the calcium-alkali syndrome. Treatment is volume expansion with saline, cessation of alkali intake, and limitation of calcium supplementation.

TREATMENT OF HYPERCALCEMIA

Hypercalcemia that requires urgent management is usually due to malignancy, rather than primary hyperparathyroidism. Urgent management includes aggressive rehydration, bisphosphonate therapy to decrease bone resorption, and elimination of contributing factors, such as calcium or vitamin D supplements, thiazide diuretic therapy, and immobilization. Second-line therapies include calcitonin to increase renal calcium excretion, and glucocorticoids to diminish intestinal calcium absorption.

Saline hydration

Most patients with emergent hypercalcemia are dehydrated due to anorexia and polyuria. Intravascular volume should be aggressively restored with intravenous normal saline, with an initial bolus of 500 to 1000 mL, followed by maintenance fluids at a rate of 200 mL/h or more, depending on the patient's renal function and cardiac reserve (**Table 240-3**). Typically, patients require 3 to 4 L for rehydration in the first 24 hours. Patients need careful monitoring of fluid intake and output to prevent fluid overload. Normal saline dilutes serum calcium, and facilitates calciuresis by increasing glomerular filtration rate and the amount of filtered calcium, and decreasing tubular calcium reabsorption. Administration of furosemide or other loop diuretics to further promote calcium excretion may be considered after intravascular volume is restored. However, the use of loop

TABLE 240-3 Treatment of Hypercalcemia

Intravenous fluids
Normal saline
Loop diuretic
Furosemide intravenous (titrated to response, if necessary)
Medications
Bisphosphonates
• Pamidronate (30-90 mg IV)
• Zoledronic acid (4 mg IV)
Calcitonin (4 IU/kg SC every 12 h)
Prednisone (20-100 mg orally daily or equivalent)—in selected situations
Plicamycin (15-25 µg/kg IV)—no longer used
Gallium nitrate (200 mg/m^2/d infusion over 5 d)—no longer used
Other interventions
Decrease calcium and vitamin D intake (if causative)
Maintain adequate oral hydration
Primary therapy directed at tumor
Chemotherapy
Radiation
Surgery

diuretics to treat hypercalcemia has not been studied in randomized controlled trials, and may not be superior to vigorous use of saline alone. Thiazide diuretics should be avoided, as they enhance calcium reabsorption.

Bisphosphonates

The major target of medical management in severe hypercalcemia is osteoclast-mediated bone resorption. First-line therapy is an intravenous bisphosphonate, such as pamidronate or zoledronic acid. Pamidronate is administered in a dosage of 30 to 90 mg intravenously over several hours. Serum calcium levels should decline in 24 to 48 hours, although the maximal effect may not be evident for several days. Zoledronic acid is given at a dosage of 4 mg intravenously, over no less than 15 minutes. It appears to have a greater potency and a longer duration of action than pamidronate. The need for repeat treatment with either pamidronate or zoledronic acid depends on the aggressiveness of the underlying malignancy. The first dose of intravenous bisphophonates may be associated with fever, headache, arthralgias, and myalgias. Intravenous bisphosphonates should be used with caution in renal dysfunction. Dose reduction of zoledronic acid is recommended for creatinine clearance below 60 mL/min, and use in patients with creatinine clearance below 30 mL/min is not recommended. Pamidronate may be used with caution in patients with renal insufficiency, but the dose should be infused slowly, over 4 to 6 hours. The newer bisphophonate ibandronate may be associated with a lower risk of nephrotoxicity than other intravenous agents.

Denosumab

Denosumab is a RANK ligand inhibitor that interferes with osteoclast development and maturation. For hypercalcemia of malignancy, 120 mg subcutaneously is administered every 4 weeks, with additional 120 mg doses on days 8 and 15 of the first month of therapy. Common side effects include nausea and dyspnea. Denosumab is associated with osteonecrosis of the jaw, so a dental exam should be performed prior to therapy, and invasive dental procedures should be avoided during therapy. Atypical femur fractures occur rarely with denosumab.

Other approaches to emergent hypercalcemia

Intravenous bisphosphonates do not act immediately. If serum calcium needs to be reduced quickly, combined subcutaneous calcitonin (4 IU/kg every 12 hours) and intravenous bisphosphonate has become popular. Although rather weak, calcitonin acts rapidly, probably by facilitating urinary calcium excretion. The combination of a short-acting and long-acting anticalcemic can be very effective. In severe or refractory cases, hemodialysis against a low-calcium bath may be employed. Plicamycin and gallium nitrate are treatments of largely historical interest, either because of toxicity (plicamycin) or ineffectiveness (gallium nitrate).

Glucocorticoids

In myeloma, vitamin D intoxication, or disorders associated with ectopic production of 1,25-dihydroxyvitamin D, such as sarcoidosis and lymphoma, glucocorticoids can be very effective. Glucocorticoids impair vitamin D action, inhibit intestinal calcium absorption, and may have a direct antitumor effect.

Addressing the underlying disorder

Successful management of acute hypercalcemia also requires treating the underlying etiology. When primary hyperparathyroidism is the cause, parathyroid surgery is indicated when the patient is stable enough to undergo the procedure. In malignancy-associated hypercalcemia, surgery, radiotherapy or chemotherapy may be appropriate. However, because hypercalcemia is often an end-stage complication of malignancy, such interventions may not be warranted.

■ DISCHARGE CHECKLIST: HYPERCALCEMIA

- Has outpatient follow-up been arranged, with short-term repeat measurements of calcium, creatinine, and other electrolytes?
- Is there a long-range plan to prevent recurrent hypercalcemia, such as repeat bisphosphonate dosing?
- Have patients been instructed to seek prompt care if recurrent symptoms of hypercalcemia develop, such as nausea, vomiting, malaise, and polyuria?
- For patients with a new diagnosis of hypercalcemia of malignancy, have they been educated as to their underlying condition? Has outpatient oncology follow-up been arranged?
- If hypercalcemia has arisen in the setting of advanced malignancy with poor prognosis, has hospice therapy been considered?

HYPOCALCEMIA

Hypocalcemia is a serum calcium level which is below normal after correction for the albumin concentration. As with hypercalcemia, a free (ionized) calcium determination on a correctly collected sample can be useful to confirm hypocalcemia.

■ PRESENTING SYMPTOMS AND HISTORY

Chronic hypocalcemia, unless severe, is usually asymptomatic. Signs and symptoms become more likely when albumin-adjusted serum calcium levels fall below 7.5 to 8 mg/dL. These include numbness, paresthesias, and muscle spasms, and in severe cases, seizures and carpal, pedal, or laryngeal spasm.

Important historical features include low dietary calcium and vitamin D intake, minimal sun exposure, gastrointestinal tract disease that may reduce vitamin D absorption, such as chronic pancreatitis, celiac disease, and inflammatory bowel disease, and alcohol, which decreases parathyroid hormone secretion both directly, and also indirectly, by causing magnesium depletion. A family history of hypocalcemia suggests a genetic cause of hypoparathyroidism or an inherited abnormality of vitamin D metabolism. Prior neck surgery or neck irradiation may lead to hypoparathyroidism. A history of adrenal insufficiency and mucocutaneous candidiasis suggests autoimmune polyendocrine syndrome type 1. Acute pancreatitis, rhabdomyolysis, and tumor lysis may lead to tissue precipitation of calcium, and massive blood transfusion may lead to intravascular precipitation of calcium with citrate.

■ PHYSICAL FINDINGS AND DIAGNOSTIC TESTING

The physical examination is not sensitive for hypocalcemia. There may be a positive Chvostek sign (ipsilateral contraction of the facial muscles, induced by tapping on the facial nerve at a point about 1 cm below the zygomatic arch and 2 cm anterior to the earlobe). Trousseau sign may be elicited by inflating a blood pressure cuff on the arm above systolic pressure for 3 minutes. It is considered positive if carpopedal spasm develops, with flexion of the wrist, metacarpophalangeal joints, and thumb, and hyperextension of the fingers (**Figure 240-4**). Patients with these signs of neuromuscular irritability are at risk of frank tetany or seizures. QT_c prolongation may be evident on the electrocardiogram.

The serum calcium must be adjusted for albumin, as above, and a low value confirmed with a measurement of serum ionized calcium. Levels of phosphate, magnesium, creatinine, PTH, and 25-hydroxyvitamin D should be determined. 24-hour urinary calcium may be occasionally helpful. It is low in hypoparathyroidism and vitamin D deficiency, and high in patients with familial

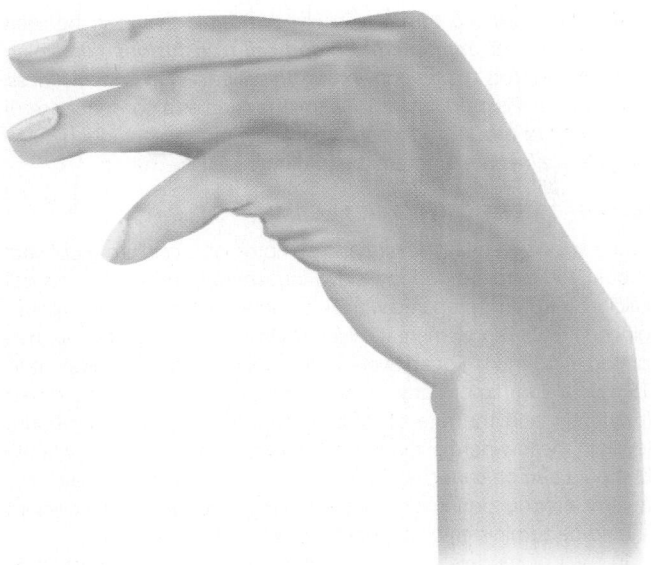

Figure 240-4 *Position of fingers in carpal spasm due to hypocalcemic tetany.* (Reproduced, with permission, from Gardner DG, Shoback D. *Greenspan's Basic & Clinical Endocrinology*, 8th ed. New York, NY: McGraw-Hill; 2007. Fig. 9-18.)

hypocalcemia with hypercalciuria, due to activating mutations in the calcium-sensing receptor. Genetic testing is available for some inherited disorders leading to hypocalcemia.

■ DIFFERENTIAL DIAGNOSIS

After confirming that calcium levels are truly low, exclusion of **hypoparathyroidism** by checking the level of PTH is central to the diagnostic workup of hypocalcemia (**Figure 240-5**). The most common causes of hypoparathyroidism are previous thyroid, parathyroid, or other neck surgery, and autoimmune destruction (**Table 240-4**). Autoimmune damage to the parathyroid glands may occur in isolated fashion, or in connection with failure of other endocrine glands, such as premature ovarian failure, hypothyroidism, and Addison disease, and mucocutaneous candidiasis. Infiltration of the parathyroid glands, as may occur in hemochromatosis, Wilson disease, and metastatic cancer, can lead to hypoparathyroidism. Congenital absence of the parathyroid glands may be seen in DiGeorge syndrome. Functional hypoparathyroidism may result from severe hypomagnesemia, because magnesium is necessary for both PTH release and PTH action. This is commonly seen in hospitalized alcoholic patients who are often markedly hypomagnesemic.

The other major category of hypocalcemia includes conditions in which the parathyroid glands respond appropriately to hypocalcemia, and PTH is elevated. In **vitamin D deficiency**, serum calcium

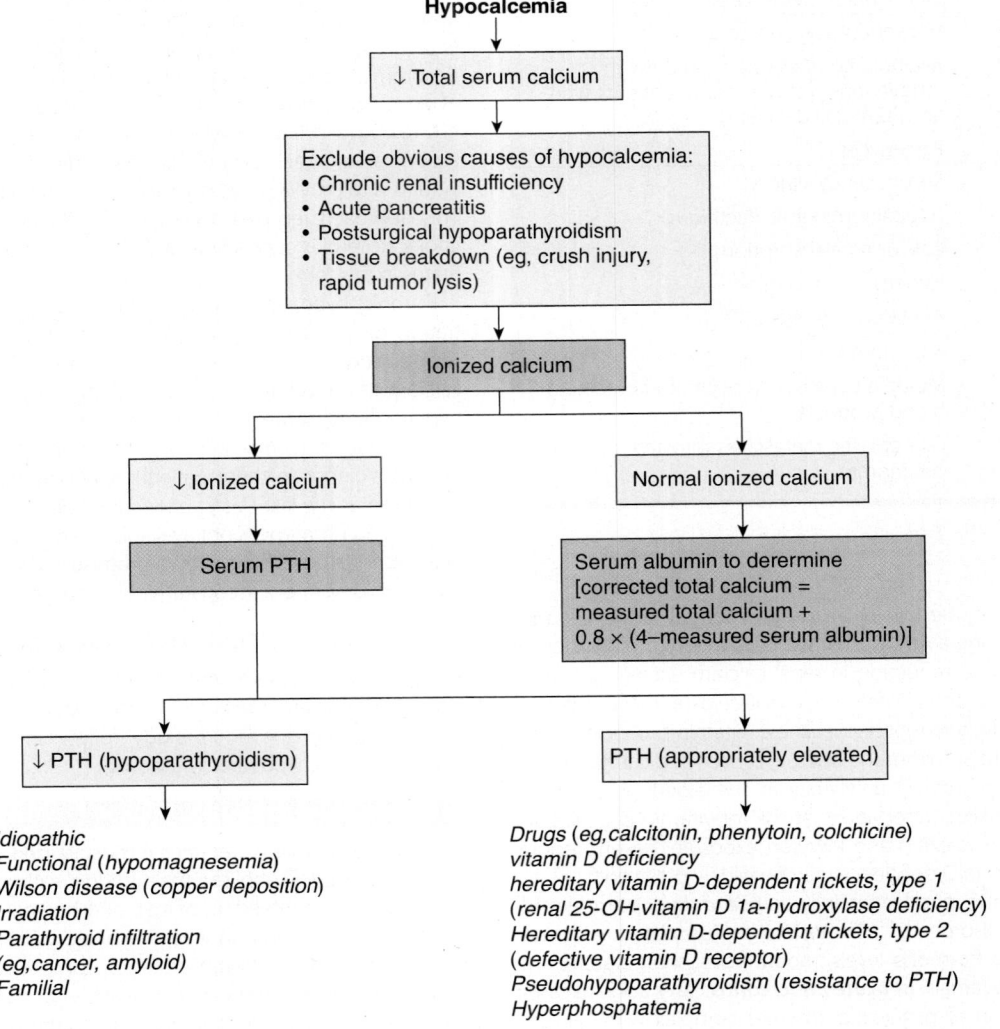

Figure 240-5 *Diagnostic algorithm for hypocalcemia.* (Reproduced, with permission, from Nicoll D, McPhee SJ, Pignone M, et al. *Pocket Guide to Diagnostic Tests*, 5th ed. http://www.accessmedicine.com/pocketDiagnostic.aspx.)

TABLE 240-4 Causes of Hypocalcemia

PTH deficiency or resistance	**Hypoparathyroidism**
	Postsurgical
	Autoimmune polyendocrine syndromes
	Severe magnesium deficiency
	Congenital: DiGeorge syndrome
	Infiltrative: hemochromatosis, thalassemia, Wilson disease
	PTH resistance
	Pseudohypoparathyroidism
Vitamin D deficiency or resistance	**Nutritional deficiency**
	Insufficient dietary intake of vitamin D
	Malabsorption
	Altered vitamin D metabolism
	Anticonvulsant medications (increased vitamin D metabolism)
	Renal failure
	Vitamin D resistance
	Vitamin D pseudodeficiency (VDDR I)
	Abnormal vitamin D receptor (VDDR II)
	Vitamin D-resistant hypophosphatemic rickets/osteomalacia
	Oncogenic osteomalacia
Iatrogenic	Phosphate supplements
	Bisphosphonates (mainly seen with intravenous preparations in patients who are vitamin D deficient)
	Plicamycin
Miscellaneous conditions	Sepsis, critical illness
	Hypoalbuminemia (factitious)
	Calcium malabsorption
	Hyperphosphatemia
	Acute pancreatitis
	Rhabdomyolysis
	Multiple transfusions of citrate-containing blood products
	Osteoblastic metastases (prostate or breast carcinoma)

PTH, parathyroid hormone.

concentrations may be low or in the low-normal range, because of compensatory increases in PTH, with secondary mobilization of skeletal calcium and reduction in renal calcium excretion. Clinical manifestations of vitamin D deficiency include osteomalacia, pathologic fractures, falls, and muscle weakness. Vitamin D deficiency has also been linked to autoimmune disease, cancer, and cardiovascular disease. Dietary vitamin D deficiency in the elderly is common, but often overlooked. Other adults at risk for vitamin D deficiency include darker complexion and low sun exposure. Recent reports suggest that vitamin D deficiency may be widely prevalent.

Other causes of hypocalcemia include *pseudohypoparathyroidism*, a genetic disorder of PTH resistance associated with elevated parathyroid hormone levels, moon facies, short stature, and short fourth metacarpals. In *acute pancreatitis*, fatty acids released through the action of pancreatic enzymes complex with calcium. Hypocalcemia due to the formation of calcium phosphate complexes occurs in severe *hyperphosphatemic states*, such as renal failure,

rhabdomyolysis, and tumor lysis. Hypocalcemia may also be seen in patients given *multiple red blood cell transfusions* containing calcium chelators to prevent clotting. In patients with *critical illness*, hypocalcemia is probably multifactorial, arising as a consequence of the release of procalcitonin and other acute phase reactants, hypoalbuminemia, hypomagnesemia, and blunted PTH secretion.

■ **TREATMENT OF HYPOCALCEMIA**

When hypocalcemia is severe and symptomatic, calcium gluconate should be administered by slow intravenous infusion. A typical calcium infusion is prepared with 10 ampules (100 mL) of 10% calcium gluconate (93 mg elemental calcium/ampule) in 1 L of D_5W, administered at 50 mL/h. For an average-sized person, this is equivalent to 15 mg calcium/kg of body weight. Serum calcium should be tested frequently, and the rate of infusion adjusted to maintain calcium levels in the low-normal range. Deficiencies in magnesium or vitamin D should also be corrected. In severe cases, hypocalcemia may recur quickly after discontinuation of the calcium infusion, so oral calcium should be administered concurrent with tapering the infusion.

In mild or moderate hypocalcemia, patients may be given oral calcium carbonate or calcium citrate, starting at 1000 to 1500 mg of elemental calcium daily in divided doses with meals. Patients should be instructed to take calcium with a protein meal, particularly patients with hypochlorhydria or achlorhydria, or who are on proton pump inhibitors. The protein meal supplies the acid that may be missing in these individuals, and which is required for the absorption of calcium carbonate. Calcium citrate does not require acid for absorption. If appropriate, vitamin D, in the form of cholecalciferol (vitamin D_3) or ergocalciferol (vitamin D_2), should be provided. Recommended daily intake for vitamin D is currently being revised upward. The official recommendation for adults 50 years and older, 400 to 600 IU/d, is acknowledged by most experts to be inadequate. A popular approach to normalizing vitamin D levels in deficient individuals is to provide a weekly capsule of 50,000 IU for 8 to 12 weeks. This approach requires a prescription for ergocalciferol, because cholecalciferol is currently unavailable by prescription in the United States in this form.

Chronic hypoparathyroidism may require long-term administration of vitamin D and 1,25-dihydroxyvitamin D as needed to maintain normal levels. The goal of therapy is to maintain the serum calcium at a level at which the patient is asymptomatic. To avoid hypercalciuria, serum calcium levels are often maintained in the lower range of normal. Periodic monitoring for hypercalciuria and nephrocalcinosis in these patients may be appropriate. Hypoparathyroidism is the last classic endocrine deficiency disease for which the missing hormone is not available as an approved therapy. However, recent studies have shown promise in the use of recombinant parathyroid hormone (teriparatide) for hypoparathyroidism.

■ **DISCHARGE CHECKLIST: HYPOCALCEMIA**

- Have repeat measurements of calcium, creatinine, and other electrolytes been arranged within 1 to 2 weeks of hospital discharge?
- Has outpatient endocrinology follow-up been arranged for patients with hypoparathyroidism?

HYPOPHOSPHATEMIA

Hypophosphatemia is frequent in hospitalized patients. It is most often caused by alcoholism, malnutrition, eating disorders, diabetic ketoacidosis, and refeeding of malnourished patients. It is also seen in burns, sepsis, trauma, in severe respiratory alkalosis, and as a complication of treatment with diuretics, some bisphosphonates, the antiretroviral drug tenofovir, sucralfate, and aluminum hydroxide-containing antacids. In primary hyperparathyroidism, the serum phosphate has a tendency to be in the low-normal range, but frank hypophosphatemia is uncommon.

Symptoms of hypophosphatemia are unusual if the serum phosphate is > 2.0 mg/dL. Subjects with mild to moderate hypophosphatemia (serum phosphate between 1.5-2.0 mg/dL) may display muscle weakness, nausea, and vomiting, and anorexia. Those with severe hypophosphosphatemia (serum phosphate <1.5 mg/dL) may be at risk for rhabdomyolysis, hemolytic anemia, impaired leukocyte and platelet function, impaired oxygenation of tissues, confusion, seizures, and coma.

Oral phosphate repletion is sufficient for most patients, although amounts exceeding 500 mg/d may be associated with diarrhea. Hypomagnesemia and hypokalemia should be corrected, if present. Patients with severe hypophosphatemia may require intravenous repletion, but this should be done only under by experts and according to institutional protocols.

HYPERPHOSPHATEMIA

Most patients with hyperphosphatemia have diminished renal excretion of phosphate, usually due to acute or chronic kidney disease. Hypoparathyroidism and pseudohypoparathyroidism are also classically associated with hyperphosphatemia. It can also be seen in acromegaly. Less often, hyperphosphatemia results from transcellular phosphate shifts, as in diabetic ketoacidosis (even despite total body phosphate depletion), or cellular injury, such as rhabdomyolysis, trauma, and tumor lysis syndrome. Patients may be asymptomatic, although symptoms of concomitant hypocalcemia and other electrolyte disturbances are often present. Vascular and soft tissue calcification is common in hyperphosphatemic patients with chronic kidney disease, particularly if the calcium × phosphate product exceeds 55. Hyperphosphatemia is treated with phosphate binders and dietary phosphate restriction, as discussed in greater detail in Chapter 245.

SUGGESTED READINGS

Bilezikian, JP, Brandi ML, Eastell R, et al. Guidelines for the management of asymptomatic primary hyperparathyroidism: summary statement from the Fourth International Workshop. *J Clin Endocrinol Metab*. 2014;99:3561-3569.

Fraser WD. Hyperparathyroidism. *Lancet*. 2009;374(9684):145-158.

Holick MF. Vitamin D deficiency. *N Engl J Med*. 2007;357:266-281.

Patel AM, Goldfarb S. Got calcium? Welcome to the calcium-alkali syndrome. *J Am Soc Nephrol*. 2010;21:1440-1143.

Perazella MA, Markowitz GS. Bisphosphonate nephrotoxicity. *Kidney Int*. 2008;74:1385-1393.

Shoback D. Clinical practice: hypoparathyroidism. *N Engl J Med*. 2008;359:391-403.

Stewart AF. Clinical practice: hypercalcemia associated with cancer. *N Engl J Med*. 2005;352:373-379.

Wermers RA, Kearns AE, Jenkins GD, Melton LJ 3rd. Incidence and clinical spectrum of thiazide-associated hypercalcemia. *Am J Med*. 2007;120:911.e9-911.e15.

CHAPTER 241

Potassium and Magnesium Disorders

Steven M. Gorbatkin, MD, PhD

Lynn Schlanger, MD

James L. Bailey, MD

Key Clinical Questions

1. What are the causes of potassium and magnesium disorders?

2. What are the potential consequences of potassium and magnesium disorders?

3. How are potassium and magnesium disorders treated?

4. How are potassium disorders treated in clinical situations with rapid potassium shifts, such as diabetic ketoacidosis, hyperglycemic hyperosmolar state, and periodic paralysis?

INTRODUCTION

Potassium and magnesium disorders are common in the hospital setting. About 12% of hospitalized patients have hypokalemia, 3% have hyperkalemia, and 11% have hypomagnesemia. Potassium disorders are a particular challenge for hospitalists, as the first clinical manifestation of a severe potassium abnormality may be a cardiac arrhythmia.

Potassium (K^+) is the most abundant intracellular cation. In a 70 kg adult, the total body K^+ is approximately 3500 mmol (50 mmol/kg). About 98% is located in the intracellular compartment, with the majority localized in muscle (70%). Because only 2% of the total body K^+ is in the extracellular compartment, laboratory results correlate poorly with total body K^+. Normal levels of extracellular potassium are between 3.5 and 5.0 mmol/L, while intracellular K^+ levels range between 140 and 150 mmol/L.

Similarly, plasma magnesium (Mg^{2+}) accounts for only 1% of the total body magnesium stores, and plasma Mg^{2+} correlates poorly with total body magnesium. Plasma magnesium is normally 1.7 to 2.3 mg/dL (0.70-0.95 mmol/L). Magnesium abnormalities can also have major clinical consequences, such as torsades de pointes. Hypokalemia is often accompanied by hypomagnesemia, which renders potassium repletion less effective.

POTASSIUM BALANCE

Dietary K^+ is excreted mostly in the urine (90%), with a minor component of fecal excretion (10%). In severe chronic kidney disease, stool losses may exceed 25% to 50% of dietary intake. Under normal conditions, the kidney can adjust potassium excretion over a wide range depending on K^+ intake. The recommended daily K^+ intake for patients with normal renal function is 4700 mg (120 mmol). If K^+ control mechanisms are intact, an increased daily intake of 400 mmol can be tolerated with < 1 mmol/L increase in plasma K^+ values. Daily K^+ intake for patients on hemodialysis or with severe chronic kidney disease is typically 2000 mg (51 mmol) per day. Conversely, many patients on peritoneal dialysis can tolerate a normal daily intake of K^+ due to losses of potassium in the urine and peritoneal fluid.

PRACTICE POINT

Potassium unit conversion

- 25.6 mmol of elemental potassium is equivalent to 1 g of potassium. Since, the charge of the potassium cation is 1^+, 1 mmol = 1 mEq.

HYPERKALEMIA

■ ETIOLOGY

Hyperkalemia is defined as a plasma K^+ > 5.0 mmol/L. Hyperkalemia can result from redistribution, reduced K^+ excretion, or increased K^+ intake. Medications may lead to hyperkalemia by affecting either potassium redistribution or excretion (**Table 241-1**).

Pseudohyperkalemia is a laboratory artifact due to potassium release from cells prior to laboratory measurement. It should be suspected when hyperkalemia is reported in the setting of red blood cell hemolysis, leukocytosis (> 70,000/mm³) or thrombocytosis (> 500,000/mm³), and no ECG changes are present. It

TABLE 241-1 Medications Associated with Hyperkalemia

Mechanism	Medications
Increased potassium load	KCL, penicillin G
Renin release inhibition	Beta-blockers, NSAIDs, COX-2 inhibitors
Angiotensin I to II conversion inhibition	ACE inhibitors
Angiotensin II receptor blockade	ARBs
Aldosterone synthesis inhibition	Heparin
Aldosterone receptor blockade	Spironolactone, eplerenone
Renal epithelial Na channel; (ENaC) blockade	Triamterene, amiloride, Trimethoprim, pentamidine
Inhibition of Na-K-ATPase	Digoxin, calcineurin inhibitors (cyclosporin, tacrolimus)
Drug-induced rhabdomyolysis	Statins, cocaine
Drug-induced tumor lysis	Selected chemotherapy agents
Transcellular shift	Succinylcholine

ACE, angiotensin-converting enzyme; ARB, angiotensin receptor blocker; NSAIDs, nonsteroidal anti-inflammatory drugs.

has become less common with the increased use of plasma for potassium measurement, rather than serum. Plasma is the supernatant collected from heparinized whole blood, whereas serum is the supernatant remaining after centrifugation of a clotted whole blood sample. Serum K^+ is normally 0.3 mmol/L above the plasma K^+, but may be higher if K^+ is released from the clot formed in the tube. If pseudohyperkalemia is suspected, the plasma potassium should be measured instead of the serum potassium. Pseudohyperkalemia can also occur due to potassium release from muscle cells following prolonged constriction with a tourniquet or limb exercise while a tourniquet is in place.

Redistribution of potassium

Redistribution of potassium from the intracellular to the extracellular space can occur in severe acidosis due to nonorganic acid metabolic acidosis, hyperosmolar states, tissue breakdown, and hyperkalemic periodic paralysis. Organic acids such as lactic acid and ketoacids are less likely to cause hyperkalemia than nonorganic acids. These organic acids have greater transmembrane mobility, allowing movement into cells with H^+, rather than movement of K^+ out of cells in exchange for H^+. Hyperkalemia in diabetic ketoacidosis usually results from insulin deficiency and hyperosmolality, rather than acidosis. Hyperglycemia increases extracellular osmolality, drawing water from cells down the osmotic gradient. Potassium follows the water movement (solvent drag), and hyperkalemia results.

Tissue breakdown may liberate large amounts of intracellular potassium, resulting in rapid, life-threatening increases in extracellular potassium. Rhabdomyolysis, tissue necrosis, tumor lysis with chemotherapy, and large hematomas are common causes. In rhabdomyolysis, hypokalemia may precede hyperkalemia, and contribute to muscle breakdown by causing vasoconstriction and decreased blood flow to the involved muscle.

Hyperkalemic periodic paralysis is an autosomal dominant disorder involving the muscle cell sodium channel. During these episodes, potassium moves from the intracellular to extracellular space, accompanied by movement of sodium and water into the cell. The hyperkalemia is accompanied by transient weakness or paralysis.

Decreased potassium excretion

Potassium excretion in the distal nephron depends upon adequate urine flow, aldosterone, and activity of the basolateral Na^+/K^+-ATPase. The reabsorption of luminal Na^+ through aldosterone-sensitive epithelial sodium channels (ENaCs) creates an electrochemical gradient for K^+ excretion in the urine. Hyperkalemia can occur in aldosterone-resistant or deficient states by attenuating the electrochemical gradient for K^+ secretion. Acquired mineralocorticoid resistance from diabetes mellitus, obstructive uropathy, chronic tubulointerstitial disease, sickle cell anemia, lupus nephritis, and medications, as well as decreased mineralocorticoid production (including medication induced), are commonly associated with type IV renal tubular acidosis (RTA). Type IV RTA is characterized by hyperkalemia, normal anion gap hyperchloremic acidosis, with serum HCO_3 values ranging between 16 and 22 mmol/L, and decreased urinary NH_4^+ production, causing a positive urine anion gap [Urine $(Na^+) + (K^+) - (Cl^-)$]. In acute and chronic tubular injury, a decreased responsiveness to aldosterone can contribute to hyperkalemia. For acute kidney injury associated with prerenal azotemia or hypovolemic states, decreased urinary flow to the distal tubule and a reduction in sodium-potassium exchange can contribute to hyperkalemia.

Excessive potassium intake

Excessive intake of K^+ rarely causes hyperkalemia in the setting of normal renal function. Renal secretion of potassium is typically adequate at glomerular filtration rates (GFR) above 20 to 30 mL/min/1.73 m^2. Patients with end-stage renal disease (ESRD) on hemodialysis usually tolerate a daily K^+ intake of 2000 mg (51 mEq). Upregulated gut potassium excretion and shifts in transcellular K^+ prevent hyperkalemia between dialysis sessions. The loss of these mechanisms may result in the rapid development of hyperkalemia, especially with large exogenous loads of potassium, such as massive blood transfusions. Irradiation of blood and increased age of the blood increase the amount of free potassium that is released during the blood transfusion. Seven-day-old blood has approximately 23 mmol/L of K^+, while 42-day-old blood has approximately 50 mmol/L of K^+.

PRACTICE POINT

- In the setting of acute kidney injury, hyperkalemia associated with rapid transcellular potassium shifts from the intracellular to extracellular compartment can be seen with rhabdomyolysis, tissue necrosis, tumor lysis, and large hematomas.
- Hyperkalemia in this setting may progress rapidly to cause life-threatening arrhythmias. Emergent nephrology consultation for possible dialysis is required.

■ SIGNS AND SYMPTOMS

Clinical effects of hyperkalemia relate to altered membrane excitability due to changes in the transcellular potassium gradient. Severe hyperkalemia leads to cardiac arrhythmias and conduction abnormalities. It may also cause weakness of the lower extremities, progressing superiorly to cause flaccid paralysis and respiratory failure. This presentation may mimic Guillain-Barré syndrome, but is easily differentiated by the response to potassium correction. Hyperkalemia may also contribute to metabolic acidosis by interfering with renal ammonium excretion.

■ EVALUATION OF HYPERKALEMIA IN THE HOSPITALIZED PATIENT

In the hospital setting, the initial evaluation of hyperkalemia includes monitoring for life-threatening arrhythmias, checking for pseudohyperkalemia, eliminating exogenous sources of

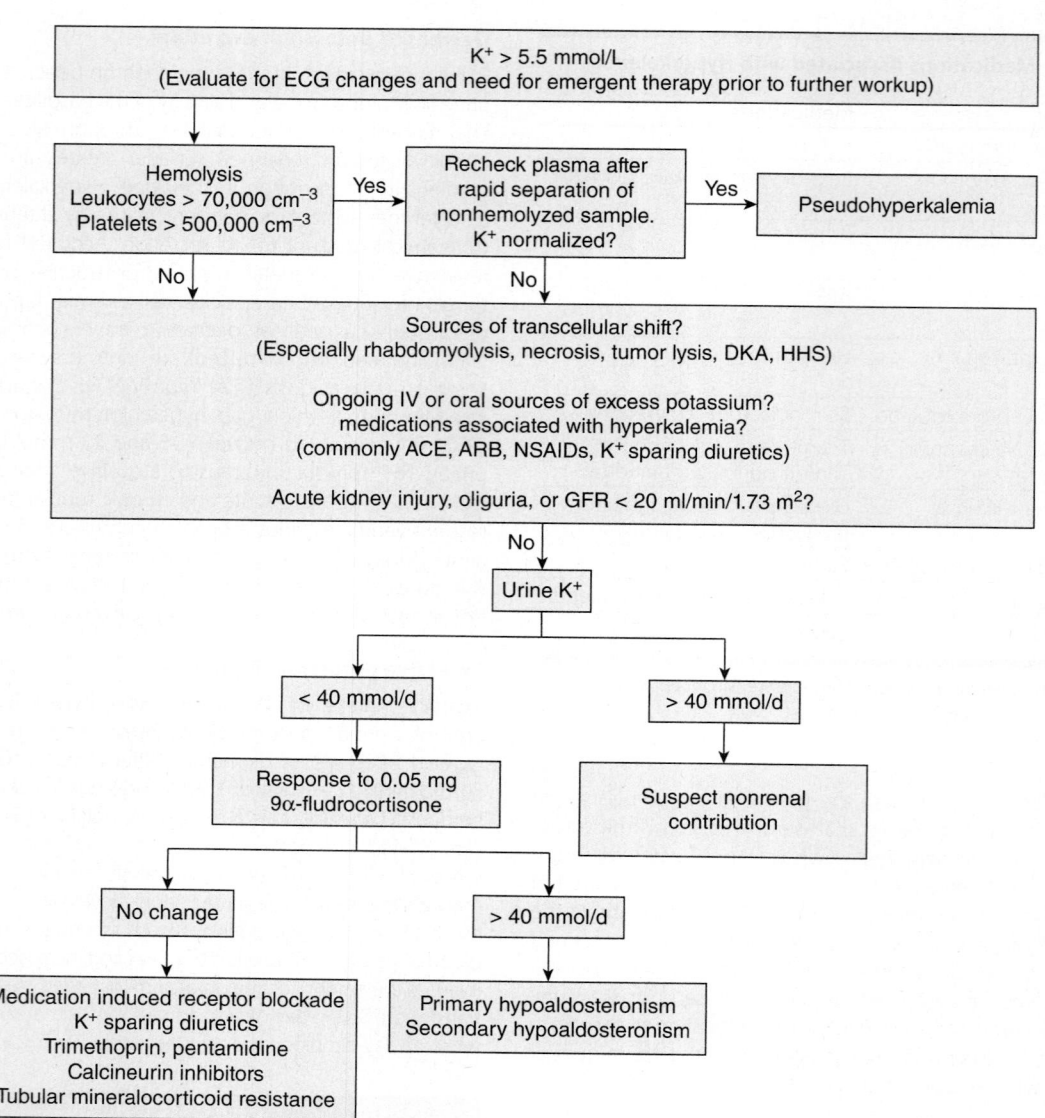

Figure 241-1 *Diagnostic assessment of hyperkalemia. (ACE, angiotensin-converting enzyme inhibitor; ARB, angiotensin receptor blocker; DKA, diabetic ketoacidosis; ECG, electrocardiogram; GFR, glomerular filtration rate; HHS, hyperosmolar hyperglycemic state; NSAIDs, nonsteroidal anti-inflammatory drugs.)*

potassium, evaluating renal function, and evaluating for rapid transcellular shifts of potassium (**Figure 241-1**).

ECG changes

Even mildly elevated K⁺ levels may be associated with ECG changes, especially in the setting of rapid rises in plasma K⁺ values. If ECG changes from hyperkalemia are found or if the plasma K⁺ value is ≥ 7.0, continuous telemetry is indicated and should continue until the plasma K⁺ value is ≤ 5.8 and there are no hyperkalemic ECG changes. Frequent chemistry checks are indicated for plasma K⁺ greater than 5.8 or for hyperkalemia associated with ECG changes, severe hyperglycemia, or any clinical condition which predisposes the patient to rapid changes in plasma K⁺.

Plasma potassium levels do not correlate with specific ECG changes. A symmetric increase in T wave height may be seen initially. Hyperkalemia-induced peaked T waves may be difficult to distinguish from the hyperacute T waves of myocardial injury. As potassium levels rise further, flattening of the P waves, prolongation of the PR interval, and prolonged QRS duration occur. Eventually, atrial standstill and a sine wave ECG pattern may be seen (**Figure 241-2**).

Urine potassium, transtubular potassium gradient, and urine potassium/creatinine

A 24-hour urine K⁺ measurement can help differentiate between renal and nonrenal causes of hyperkalemia. With hyperkalemia, urinary excretion of K⁺ should exceed 40 mmol/d. Alternatively, the transtubular potassium gradient (TTKG), a measurement of potassium secretion by the distal nephron corrected for urine osmolality, has been used:

$$TTKG = (K_U/K_S) \times (S_{Osm}/U_{Osm})$$

K_U and K_S are the concentrations of K⁺ in the urine and serum, and S_{Osm} and U_{Osm} are the osmolalities of the serum and urine, respectively. Plasma potassium and osmolality can be used instead of serum values to estimate TTKG with minimal effect on clinical interpretation. The accuracy of the TTKG has been called into question by recent studies of urea and potassium handling in the renal tubule. Previous studies using TTKG have suggested that patients with normal renal function and normal potassium intake have a TTKG of 8 to 9. In hyperkalemia, a low TTKG (< 5-7) suggests

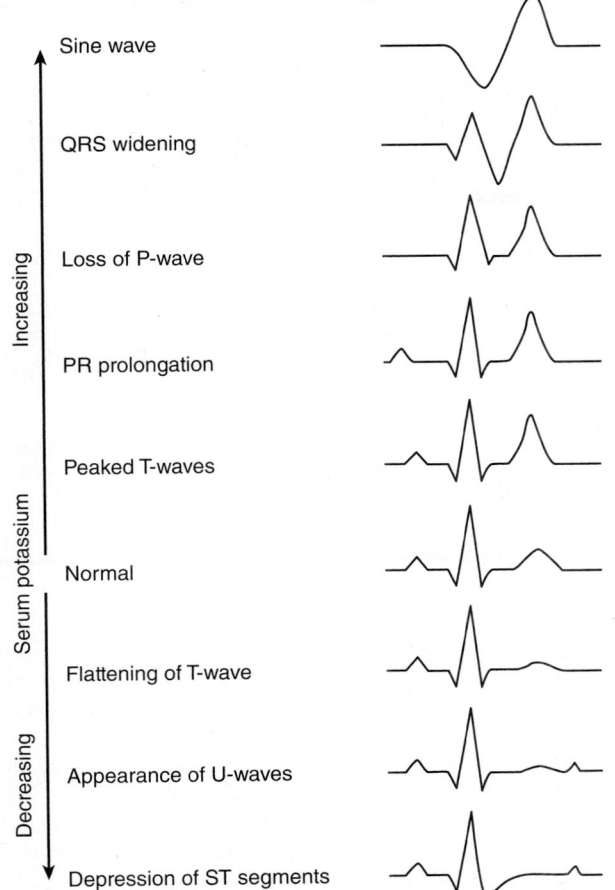

Increasing → Serum potassium → Decreasing

- Sine wave
- QRS widening
- Loss of P-wave
- PR prolongation
- Peaked T-waves
- Normal
- Flattening of T-wave
- Appearance of U-waves
- Depression of ST segments

Figure 241-2 *ECG changes associated with hyperkalemia and hypokalemia.* (Reproduced, with permission, from Flomenbaum N, Goldfrank LR, Hoffman R, et al. eds. *Goldfrank's Toxicologic Emergencies,* 8th ed. New York, NY: McGraw-Hill; 2006. Fig. 5-11.)

an inappropriately low secretion of potassium. A high TTKG with hyperkalemia suggests normal aldosterone action and an extrarenal cause of hyperkalemia, except in cases of volume depletion where aldosterone secretion is enhanced with a TTKG > 7, but total renal potassium excretion is limited by low urine flow.

When the TTKG is inappropriately low in the setting of hyperkalemia, an increase in the TTKG to >10 hours after the administration of 0.05 mg of fludrocortisone suggests hypoaldosteronism. If fludrocortisone has no effect on the TTKG, drug-induced or intrinsic renal resistance to aldosterone are likely.

If further studies cast doubt on the usefulness of TTKG, the urine potassium/creatinine ratio will likely be used more frequently when a 24-hour urine potassium is not available. It has been suggested that a patient with hyperkalemia and a normal renal response should have a spot urine ratio of >200 mmol K+/g creatinine (=22.6 mmol K+/mmol creatinine). For a typical patient with a daily creatinine excretion of over 1 g/d, this is significantly more than the 24-hour urinary K+ excretion of >40 mmol used by some clinicians as a cutoff for adequate renal potassium clearance in the setting of hyperkalemia. This further underscores the point that it is difficult to define an exact cutoff for expected renal potassium excretion or urine K+/Cr in the face of hyperkalemia without additional investigation.

■ TREATMENT OF HYPERKALEMIA

Treatments exist for hyperkalemia which cause net excretion or removal of potassium, such as gastrointestinal resins and laxatives

or hemodialysis. As these therapies may not act immediately or may involve logistical difficulties, they are often used in conjunction with short-acting temporizing measures, such as cardiac membrane stabilization with calcium, and agents such as insulin that cause transcellular potassium shifts (**Table 241-2**).

Cardiac membrane stabilization

Intravenous calcium stabilizes the cardiac membrane by inhibiting membrane depolarization. It is the most important initial treatment for severe hyperkalemia. Two forms of calcium are commonly available: calcium gluconate and calcium chloride. Calcium gluconate is preferred because it can be administered through a peripheral intravenous line, whereas calcium chloride requires a central venous line to prevent tissue necrosis. Tissue necrosis can occur if calcium chloride leaks from the venous access into the surrounding tissue. A 10 mL ampule of calcium gluconate contains 90 mg (2.3 mmol) of elemental calcium, and a 10 mL ampule of calcium chloride contains 272 mg (7.0 mmol) of elemental calcium.

The initial dose of calcium gluconate is 10 mL of 10% solution infused over 2 to 3 minutes. An equivalent amount of elemental calcium is contained in 3.3 mL of 10% calcium chloride. The onset of action is 1 to 3 minutes, and duration of action is 30 to 60 minutes. Calcium cannot be mixed with bicarbonate solutions, because precipitation of $CaCO_3$ occurs.

Administration of intravenous calcium to patients taking digoxin requires extreme caution, as calcium has been shown to potentiate the effects of digoxin toxicity in animal models, especially at very rapid infusion rates. The risk of calcium administration in this setting can be reduced by infusing the calcium gluconate over 20 to 30 minutes. Another option is to administer digoxin immune fab to neutralize the effect of the digoxin.

PRACTICE POINT

- In the setting of digoxin toxicity, mild hyperkalemia (serum K+ > 5.0 mmol/L) has been linked to significant mortality, and digoxin immune fab may be indicated.

Potassium redistribution

Insulin is the most reliable means of inducing transcellular potassium shifts. The usual dose is 10 units of regular insulin intravenously, followed immediately by 50 mL of 50% dextrose (25 g of dextrose). For a blood glucose > 250, insulin can be administered alone with close glucose monitoring. The effect begins in 10 to 20 minutes, peaks at 30 to 60 minutes, and lasts 4 to 6 hours. Potassium levels typically drop by 0.5 to 1.2 mmol/L. An infusion of 10 units of regular insulin can also be administered over 1 hour in 10% dextrose.

Beta-2 agonists have an additive effect with insulin in transiently reducing plasma potassium by redistribution. High doses of nebulized albuterol are used, typically 10 to 20 mg of nebulized albuterol in 4 mL of normal saline over 10 minutes. Plasma potassium levels usually fall by 0.5 to 1 mmol/L. The effect begins in 30 minutes, peaks at 90 minutes, and lasts 2 to 4 hours. Intravenous albuterol has also been used, but it is not available in the United States. As some patients, including those with renal failure, have a reduced response to albuterol, it should not be the only agent used. Caution should be exercised for individuals at risk for side effects such as cardiac ischemia from the resulting increase in heart rate.

Sodium bicarbonate ($NaHCO_3$) does not reliably lead to the redistribution of potassium, and it should not be considered as first-line therapy for hyperkalemia. This is especially true in high anion gap acidosis, where hyperkalemia is usually not a direct consequence of the presence of organic acids. If intravenous or oral $NaHCO_3$ is

TABLE 241-2 Treatment of Hyperkalemia

Mechanism	Treatment	Dose	Onset	Duration	Comments
Cardiac membrane stabilization	Calcium	Calcium gluconate 10 mL of 10% solution infused over 2-3 min.	1-3 min	30-60 min	Do not mix with bicarbonate; extreme caution if on digoxin; calcium chloride is an alternative, but poses a risk of tissue necrosis, and requires a central line
Redistribution	Insulin	10 units regular insulin IV. If BG < 250 mg/dL, give 50 mL of 50% dextrose.	10-20 min	4-6 h peak 30-60 min	Most reliable treatment to induce redistribution
Redistribution	Beta-2 agonist	Albuterol 10-20 mg nebulized.	30 min	2-4 h peak 90 min	Dose is significantly higher than dose for respiratory treatments; use with caution in patients at risk for side effects such as tachycardia and myocardial ischemia
Removal	Kayexalate	30-60 g oral in 20% sorbitol or 60 grams in 250 mL water by retention enema.	1-2 h	Variable	Risk of colonic necrosis if used in postoperative patients; do not use sorbitol formulation when administering via enema
Removal	Hemodialysis	—	Immediate	Same as dialysis duration	Intermittent or continuous

used to treat metabolic acidosis caused by nonorganic anions, which is usually associated with a normal anion gap, plasma potassium may fall, but it is not preferred treatment even in this setting. Oral $NaHCO_3$ is useful for chronic treatment of type IV renal tubular acidosis.

Potassium removal

Sodium polystyrene sulfonate (Kayexalate) exchanges Na^+ for K^+ in the gastrointestinal tract. When taken orally, sorbitol has been typically added to the resin to speed passage through the gastrointestinal tract. However, an FDA warning has been issued about the risk of colonic necrosis when kayexalate is used with sorbitol, and thus the powdered form of kayexalate not premixed with sorbitol is preferred. If Kayexalate with sorbitol is the only form available, diluting with water is appropriate. Each gram of resin binds 0.5 to 1.2 mmol of K^+. Oral doses of 15 to 60 g are typical. Sodium polystyrene sulfonate can also be administered rectally as a retention enema, at a dose of 30 to 60 g in 250 mL of water every 6 hours. The solution should be introduced by gravity, flushed with an additional 50 to 100 mL of nonsodium containing fluid, retained 30 to 60 minutes or longer, and cleansed with 250 to 1000 mL of nonsodium containing solution at body temperature. Sorbitol should not be used rectally due to risk of colonic necrosis. Oral or rectal Kayexalate should not be used in postoperative patients for the same reason.

Favorable data have been published for two novel potassium reduction agents. Sodium zirconium cyclosilicate (ZS-9) is a highly selective potassium trap, whereas patiromer is a nonabsorbed polymer which exchanges calcium for potassium, primarily in the distal colon. Patiromer is FDA approved, ZS-9 is under FDA review, and further studies are needed to evaluate their suitability for acute potassium reduction. Initial studies have focused on their use for more chronic potassium reduction, which may allow broader use of potassium-sparing medications.

Dialysis is required for treatment of refractory hyperkalemia. Intermittent hemodialysis removes potassium most rapidly. Continuous renal replacement therapy is an option for patients who have ongoing causes of severe hyperkalemia, such as tissue necrosis or rhabdomyolysis. Peritoneal dialysis provides gradual removal of potassium. Although peritoneal dialysis is rarely used in developed countries when the other modalities are available, peritoneal dialysis is an established therapy for acute kidney injury. Since electricity is not required for its use and access is placed in the peritoneal cavity

rather than in large veins, it is an option for hyperkalemia treatment in a variety of situations such as difficulty with placing vascular access for hemodialysis, disasters associated with overwhelming caseloads, or power failure.

Diuretics are unreliable for the acute treatment of hyperkalemia in the setting of compromised renal function. In patients with adequate renal function, the combination of a loop and thiazide diuretic is more effective for potassium removal than either alone. Of the loop diuretics, torsemide and bumetanide have higher bioavailability than furosemide.

Potassium intake reduction

The typical daily potassium intake for a patient with end-stage renal disease is 2000 mg (51 mmol) of potassium per day, but patients with acute kidney injury may require even more stringent potassium restriction.

HYPOKALEMIA
■ ETIOLOGY

Hypokalemia ($K^+ < 3.5$ mmol/L) can result from redistribution, increased potassium excretion from renal and nonrenal sources, or decreased potassium intake. Medications, especially loop and thiazide diuretics, frequently cause hypokalemia. Hypokalemia is common with tubular toxins such as amphotericin B and cisplatin. High doses of penicillin or semisynthetic penicillins such as ticarcillin and carbenicillin occasionally cause renal potassium wasting in the distal nephron due to a transient anion effect. Inhalation of toluene (glue sniffing) may cause distal renal tubular acidosis with associated hypokalemia.

Pseudohypokalemia

Falsely low serum or plasma potassium values may occur in conditions such as acute leukemia due to time-dependent uptake of potassium by the increased abnormal white cell mass. Rapid analysis of the sample, or storing the sample at 4°C prior to analysis, can prevent the potassium uptake and confirm the diagnosis of pseudohypokalemia.

Redistribution

Insulin directly stimulates potassium entry into cells by increasing the activity of the Na^+/K^+-ATPase pump. This mechanism is independent of stimulation of cellular glucose entry. Beta-2-adrenergic activators stimulate Na^+/K^+-ATPase mediated cellular potassium uptake by a slightly different cellular mechanism. Thus, insulin and beta-2-adrenergic activation may act synergistically to cause hypokalemia. Aldosterone stimulates direct cellular uptake and redistribution due to increased Na^+/K^+-ATPase activity. It also acts in the distal renal tubule to enhance potassium excretion.

Thyrotoxic periodic paralysis causes severe hypokalemia by redistribution, in conjunction with extremity and limb girdle weakness, hypophosphatemia, and hypomagnesemia. It is more common in patients of Asian and Hispanic origin. Attacks often occur during rest after vigorous physical activity, and can also be precipitated by carbohydrate-rich meals. Other rare genetic forms of hypokalemic periodic paralysis also exist.

Nonrenal potassium losses

Common nonrenal causes of hypokalemia include intestinal loss of potassium from diarrhea, celiac disease, ileostomy, and chronic laxative abuse. Potassium loss from vomiting and nasogastric suctioning can result in hypokalemia, although renal potassium losses from aldosterone activation may be more important in this setting. Potassium losses through the skin are usually low, except in the setting of extreme physical exertion. Severe burns may lead to hypokalemia by multiple mechanisms.

Renal potassium loss

Aldosterone-producing adenomas (Conn syndrome) cause hypertension and hypokalemia by stimulation of aldosterone receptors in the distal renal tubule. Cortisol also activates the aldosterone receptor. Normally, cortisol is converted to cortisone by 11-beta-hydroxysteroid dehydrogenase-2 (11βHSD-2) before it can reach the aldosterone receptor. Very high cortisol levels, as seen in Cushing syndrome, overwhelm the ability of 11βHSD-2 to degrade cortisol to cortisone, and the nondegraded cortisol activates the aldosterone receptor in the distal tubule and precipitates hypokalemia. Similarly, glycyrrhizinic acid, a component of black licorice that is sometimes added to chewing tobacco, inhibits 11βHSD-2, preventing cortisol degradation and causing hypertension and hypokalemia. With vomiting and nasogastric suctioning, potassium wasting in the urine occurs through aldosterone secretion in the setting of volume depletion, as noted above.

Hypokalemia can be associated with an RTA, due to disease of either the proximal (type II RTA) or distal (type I RTA) renal tubules. Either can result from autoimmune, genetic, endocrine, medication-induced, toxin-induced, or idiopathic causes. Rare causes of hypokalemia associated with metabolic alkalosis involve defects in the thick ascending limb of Henle transport proteins (Bartter syndrome), mutations in the thiazide-sensitive Na^+/Cl^- cotransporter in the distal convoluted tubule (Gitelman syndrome), or increased activation of the epithelial sodium channel (ENaC) in the distal tubule (Liddle syndrome).

Decreased potassium intake

Decreased potassium intake is rarely a cause of hypokalemia, except in severe malnutrition. For patients with normal renal function who consume the recommended 4700 mg (120 mmol) of potassium per day, 90% (108 mmol) is excreted in the urine. When intake is sharply reduced, urinary potassium loss decreases to < 15 to 20 mmol/d in order to conserve potassium.

■ SIGNS AND SYMPTOMS

Individuals with serum potassium levels between 3.0 and 3.5 mEq/L are often asymptomatic. However, there is a risk of cardiac arrhythmias for individuals with predisposing conditions such as coronary artery disease. At serum potassium levels between 2.5 and 3.0 mEq/L,

patients report generalized weakness and constipation. When serum potassium levels drop below 2.5 mEq/L, there is an increased risk of muscle necrosis and rhabdomyolysis. At serum potassium levels less than 2.0 mEq/L, ascending paralysis and respiratory failure can occur.

■ EVALUATION OF HYPOKALEMIA

An algorithm for the diagnosis of hypokalemia is presented in **Figure 241-3**. Pseudohypokalemia and transcellular shifts should be excluded. Magnesium levels should be measured early in the workup of hypokalemia. Many disorders, such as diarrhea and excess diuresis, deplete both potassium and magnesium. Moreover, hypomagnesemia may lead to renal potassium wasting via potassium channels in the distal tubule, and make hypokalemia more refractory to treatment.

The next step is determining whether hypokalemia arose from a renal or nonrenal source. An obvious cause may be apparent, such as profuse diarrhea or escalating doses of a loop or thiazide diuretic. When the cause of hypokalemia is unclear, a 24-hour urine potassium measurement may differentiate between renal and nonrenal losses. In the setting of hypokalemia, urinary K^+ losses should fall to less than 15 to 20 mmol/d. Potassium excretion above this level suggests a renal contribution to hypokalemia.

When a 24-hour urine K^+ is not available, a spot urine ratio of 22 mmol K^+/g creatinine (=2.5 mmol K^+/mmol creatinine) marks the cutoff between hypokalemia secondary to intracellular shifts (if < 22 mmol K^+/g Cr) and renal loss (if >22 mmol K^+/g creatinine).

The TTKG (see above) has been used to help establish the cause of hypokalemia, but the use of TTKG has been cast into doubt by recent studies of urea and K^+ handling in the renal tubule. An inappropriately high TTKG (> 4) in hypokalemia has been interpreted as suggesting an increased distal potassium secretion and renal potassium loss. A low TTKG can occur with nonrenal potassium wasting, with urinary potassium losses from osmotic diuresis, with hypokalemia secondary to diuretics which were discontinued at the time of TTKG measurement, or with hypokalemia associated with K^+ shifts.

Patients with renal potassium wasting should be further classified by acid-base status. Patients with acidosis may have RTA, diabetic ketoacidosis, or tubular dysfunction from drugs such as amphotericin B or acetazolamide. Patients with alkalosis and hypertension may have mineralocorticoid excess or Liddle syndrome. Hypokalemia with alkalosis and normal or low blood pressure may be caused by vomiting, diuretics, and Bartter or Gitelman syndrome. The spot urine chloride is a useful diagnostic tool in evaluating the etiology of hypokalemia in the setting of metabolic alkalosis, with a spot low urine chloride (< 10 mmol/L) suggesting volume depletion and a chloride-responsive state.

ECG changes

ECG changes in hypokalemia are shown in Figure 241-2. U waves appear following the T waves, and become progressively more prominent in comparison to the T waves as potassium levels decrease. Ultimately, the U wave merges with the T wave, and the QT interval appears prolonged.

■ TREATMENT OF HYPOKALEMIA

Potassium repletion is the cornerstone of therapy for hypokalemia. As extracellular potassium comprises a fraction of the total body potassium store, relatively large amounts of potassium are required to correct the total body potassium deficit. A plasma K^+ 1 mmol/L below normal corresponds to a total body potassium deficit of approximately 200 to 400 mmol, and a drop in plasma K^+ to 2 mmol/L below normal requires 400 to 800 mmol for repletion. Typically, daily repletion is significantly less than the total body deficit as the time required for redistribution is prolonged. Underlying disorders such as metabolic alkalosis that

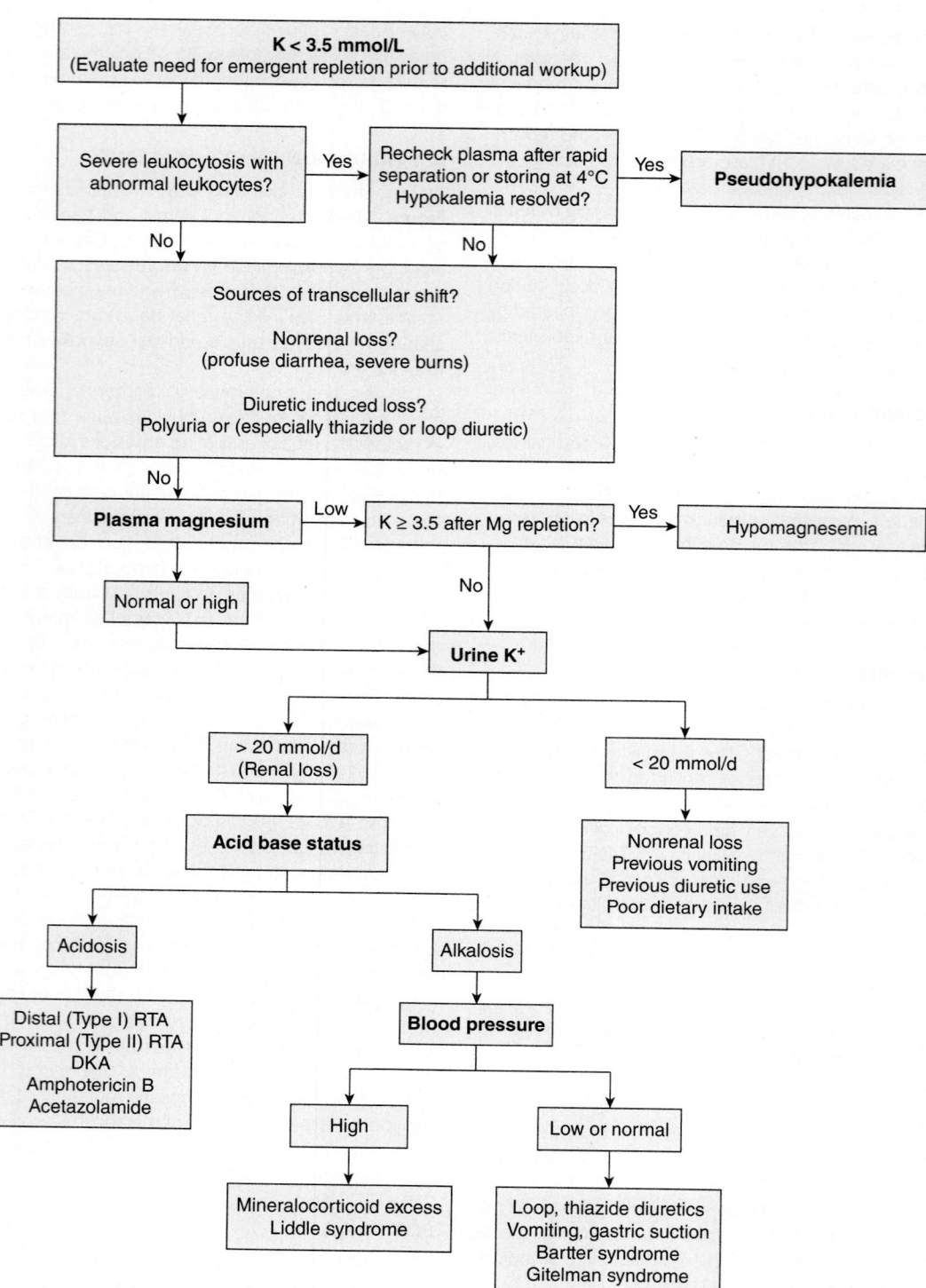

Figure 241-3 *Diagnostic assessment of hypokalemia. (DKA, diabetic ketoacidosis; RTA, renal tubular acidosis.)*

are causing or perpetuating hypokalemia must also be addressed. Continuous telemetry and frequent electrolyte checks should be performed in severe hypokalemia, or in conditions in which the serum potassium may decline rapidly, such as diabetic ketoacidosis (DKA) and hyperosmolar hyperglycemic state (HHS).

Oral repletion

If there is no immediate threat to life, oral potassium can be used to treat hypokalemia. Generally, potassium chloride (KCl) is indicated for hypokalemia associated with diuretic use or volume depletion. A typical initial dose in a patient with normal renal function is 40

to 100 mmol (40-100 mEq) per day, in two to three divided doses. Liquid, wax matrix, and microencapsulated forms exist. Compliance is poor with the liquid form due to the strong taste. Although the wax matrix form is easier to swallow, it has been associated with erosions of the gastrointestinal tract. The microencapsulated formulation is associated with the fewest complications.

Other potassium preparations are available for different indications. Oral potassium phosphate is found in many foods, and is indicated for combined potassium and phosphorus depletion. Terminology may be misleading. For example, Neutra-Phos actually has more potassium than K-Phos. Potassium bicarbonate is useful for the treatment of both metabolic acidosis and hypokalemia, while potassium citrate may prevent renal stones.

Intravenous repletion

KCl is preferred for intravenous repletion. Potassium phosphate may be used for dual phosphorus and potassium depletion. Potassium can be infused through a peripheral intravenous line at a maximum rate of 10 mmol/h. Higher rates require a central venous line and continuous ECG monitoring. Infusion rates of 20 to 40 mmol/h are reserved for cases of life-threatening hypokalemia requiring emergent correction. One liter bags of IV fluids typically have a maximum of 60 mEq of K^+ added in order to avoid infusing an excess amount of K^+.

Intravenous potassium is a common cause of iatrogenic hyperkalemia. A typical intravenous dose with normal renal function is 20 to 40 mmol (20-40 mEq). Although 20 mmol of intravenous KCl might increase plasma K^+ by 0.25 mmol/L, transcellular shifts make it difficult to predict the effect of therapy. Renal potassium clearance generally decreases significantly at a GFR below 20 to 30 mL/min/1.73 m², and requires reduction in potassium dosing and additional monitoring.

Hypokalemia in DKA and HHS

The use of insulin in DKA and HHS drives potassium into the intracellular space, and also decreases the hyperglycemia-induced osmolar driving force for movement of potassium from the intracellular to the extracellular space. Rapid and sometimes life-threatening potassium shifts may result. In 2009, the American Diabetes Association recommended that insulin should not be started until the serum potassium is known. If the serum potassium is < 3.3 mmol/L, insulin therapy is held until the potassium is repleted to 3.3 mmol/L or above. If the serum potassium is ≥ 3.3 mmol/L, insulin therapy can be initiated. For serum potassium ≥ 3.3 and < 5.2 mmol/L, potassium supplementation as 20 to 30 mEq K^+ in each liter of IV fluid is given during insulin therapy. The goal is to achieve serum potassium values between 4 to 5 mmol/L. Potassium supplementation is initially held for serum potassium values > 5.2 mmol/L, but is often subsequently required, as total body stores of potassium are usually depleted and insulin plus intravenous fluid therapy eventually unmasks the total body potassium deficit.

PRACTICE POINT

- Extreme caution and frequent monitoring are required in the treatment of hyperkalemia in diabetic ketoacidosis and hyperosmolar hyperglycemic state. Generally, these patients have a total body potassium deficit. Administration of insulin drives potassium intracellularly through direct stimulation of Na^+/K^+-ATPase, while both insulin and intravenous fluids reduce the glucose-induced hyperosmolality that drives solvent drag. These two interventions can lead to a rapid decrease in plasma potassium.

PRACTICE POINT

- Potassium should not be mixed with glucose-containing solutions, because the glucose will stimulate insulin secretion and drive potassium from the extracellular to the intracellular space.

Thyrotoxic hypokalemic periodic paralysis

Oral propranolol (3 mg/kg) is first-line treatment for thyrotoxic periodic paralysis because it rapidly reverses hypokalemia, hypophosphatemia, and hypomagnesemia, and is not associated with rebound hyperkalemia. Propranolol 1 mg IV pushed slowly every 10 minutes, up to a total of 3 mg IV, is an alternative regimen.

Aggressive potassium repletion for this disorder has been associated with a 25% or greater incidence of hyperkalemia, so if oral or IV potassium is given, subsequent close serial monitoring of plasma potassium is warranted. Treatment to establish a euthyroid state is the long term priority to prevent future attacks.

MAGNESIUM BALANCE

A typical American diet contains 300 to 400 mg/d of elemental magnesium. Approximately 30% to 40% of dietary magnesium is absorbed in the gut. Additionally, 40 mg/d of magnesium is secreted in the small intestine, of which 20 mg/d is reabsorbed in the colon and rectum. Approximately 100 mg appears in the urine each day, which is 5% of the filtered load. Specific cutoffs for hypomagnesemia and hypermagnesemia are difficult to establish because of the poor correlation between extracellular concentration and total body stores. Plasma magnesium levels of 1.7 to 2.3 mg/dL (0.70-0.95 mmol/L) are considered normal, but a normal serum level may be present despite total body magnesium depletion.

PRACTICE POINT

Magnesium unit conversion
- 41.2 mmol of elemental magnesium is equivalent to 1 g of magnesium (24.3 mg = 1 mmol). Since the charge of the magnesium cation is 2^+, 1 mmol = 2 mEq. For a common preparation used for IV magnesium repletion, 1 g of magnesium sulfate ($MgSO_4 7H_2O$) contains 8.1 mEq (98.6 mg) of elemental magnesium.

HYPOMAGNESEMIA

■ ETIOLOGY OF HYPOMAGNESEMIA

Hypomagnesemia results from low dietary intake, gastrointestinal losses, and renal losses. Poor intake of magnesium is common in alcoholics and hospitalized patients receiving inadequate magnesium supplementation in parenteral nutrition or intravenous fluids. The causes of impaired gastrointestinal absorption include diarrhea, inflammatory bowel disease, laxative abuse, proton pump inhibitors, and small bowel resection.

Osmotic and loop diuretics provoke urinary losses of magnesium. Acutely, thiazide diuretics increase magnesium absorption in the distal convoluted tubule, but long-term use can reduce magnesium reabsorption and cause hypomagnesemia. Urinary magnesium wasting is also seen in alcoholics. Many nephrotoxic drugs, such as amphotericin B, aminoglycosides, cisplatin, foscarnet, and cyclosporine, interfere with magnesium reabsorption in the thick ascending limb or distal convoluted tubule and cause magnesium wasting. Rare familial disorders, such as Gitelman syndrome, are also associated with urinary magnesium losses.

Miscellaneous causes of hypomagnesemia include acute pancreatitis, in which magnesium and calcium are saponified in necrotic fat, hungry bone syndrome, where magnesium, calcium, and phosphate are absorbed by bone after parathyroidectomy for hyperparathyroidism, and diabetic ketoacidosis, where magnesium levels fall due to osmotic diuresis and insulin-related transmembrane shifts.

■ HYPOMAGNESEMIA AND ASSOCIATED ELECTROLYTE ABNORMALITIES

Hypokalemia

Hypomagnesemia and hypokalemia often coexist due to similar common underlying etiologies, such as excess gastrointestinal losses and diuretics. Hypokalemia is often difficult to treat without magnesium repletion.

Hypercalcemia

Elevated ionized serum calcium levels induce renal Mg^{2+} wasting. Hypomagnesemia is common in hypercalcemia of malignancy. However, in hypercalcemia secondary to hyperparathyroidism, magnesium deficiency is rare due to the parathyroid hormone (PTH)-induced stimulation of renal Mg^{2+} reabsorption.

Hypocalcemia

Hypomagnesemia may cause hypocalcemia due to inhibition of PTH secretion and by induction of skeletal resistance to PTH. Hypocalcemia may be present in up to half of patients with hypomagnesemia.

■ CLINICAL MANIFESTATIONS

Mild hypomagnesemia may be asymptomatic. Severe hypomagnesemia leads to neuromuscular, neurologic, and cardiovascular symptoms. Neuromuscular abnormalities include hyperreflexia, carpopedal spasm, delirium, seizures, tetany, and paralysis. Chvostek and Trousseau signs may be present. ECG manifestations include torsades de pointes, premature ventricular contractions, ventricular tachycardias, and ventricular fibrillation. There is also an increased risk of digitalis cardiac toxicity. As serum magnesium levels do not always correlate with total body magnesium stores, normomagnesemic magnesium depletion may be considered in patients with unexplained hypocalcemia and hypokalemia and clinical risk factors for magnesium deficiency.

■ EVALUATION OF HYPOMAGNESEMIA
Urine studies

Urine studies are useful to evaluate renal vs nonrenal causes of hypomagnesemia. The fractional excretion of magnesium (Fe_{Mg}) is given by:

$$Fe_{Mg} = \frac{(Urine\ Mg)(Plasma\ Creatinine)}{0.7(Plasma\ Mg)(Urine\ Creatinine)}$$

The 0.7 in the denominator is a correction factor for the 30% of plasma magnesium bound to plasma proteins. A Fe_{Mg} of > 3% in a patient with normal GFR indicates renal magnesium loss. A 24-hour magnesium collection can also be obtained and is normally 3 to 5 mmol (75-125 mg)/24 hours. In the presence of hypomagnesemia, normal kidneys should be able to reduce the 24-hour urinary excretion of magnesium even further, to 1 mmol or less.

■ TREATMENT OF HYPOMAGNESEMIA
Oral repletion

The most popular formulation for oral replacement is magnesium oxide (242 mg = 20 mEq Mg^{2+} per 400 mg tablet), with a typical dose of 400 mg two to three times per day. Magnesium chloride, magnesium gluconate, magnesium lactate, and magnesium L-aspartate are other options. Diarrhea is a common side effect. It may be reduced with the use of a sustained release formulation, such as magnesium chloride (64 mg per 535 mg tablet). The potassium-sparing diuretics triamterene and amiloride, which block ENaC in the distal renal tubule, can assist in treatment of hypomagnesemia refractory to oral supplementation.

PRACTICE POINT

- Refractory hypokalemia and hypocalcemia occur with severe Mg^{2+} deficiency, and Mg^{2+} repletion is necessary for correction.

Intravenous repletion

Symptomatic or severe hypomagnesemia should be treated with intravenous magnesium. For active seizures or cardiac arrhythmias, an initial dose of 8 to 16 mEq of Mg^{2+} (1-2 g of $MgSO_4 7H_2O$) is administered over 2 minutes. For nonemergency repletion, 64 mEq of Mg^{2+} (8 g of $MgSO_4 7H_2O$) can be given over the first 24 hours, followed by 32 mEq of Mg^{2+} daily for six additional days. Since magnesium is renally cleared, the dose should be reduced by 25% to 50% and the plasma magnesium level monitored after each dose for GFR < 20 to 30 mL/min/1.73 m^2.

HYPERMAGNESEMIA
■ ETIOLOGY

Hypermagnesemia usually results from iatrogenic causes, such as magnesium treatment for preeclampsia or eclampsia, or inadvertent administration of excessive doses of magnesium-containing supplements, laxatives, Epsom salts, enemas, or antacids. The risk of hypermagnesemia is particularly high for patients with severely impaired renal function.

■ CLINICAL MANIFESTATIONS

Clinical manifestations are unusual with plasma magnesium levels < 4.5 to 5 mg/dL. Above this range, nausea, vomiting, cutaneous flushing, hyporeflexia, and mild hypotension can be seen. For plasma magnesium levels > 7 to 10 mg/dL, there may be loss of tendon reflexes, muscle weakness, and hypotension. Respiratory muscle paralysis occurs when magnesium levels exceed 12 to 15 mg/dL. ECG changes with plasma magnesium values > 5 mg/dL include prolonged PR interval, an increased QRS interval, prolonged QT interval, and bradycardia. Complete heart block is seen for plasma Mg^{2+} > 10 to 15 mg/dL, and cardiac arrest for levels > 15 mg/dL.

■ TREATMENT

In mild cases, stopping magnesium administration may be sufficient. Dialysis can be performed for extreme cases. Intravenous calcium (100-200 mg of elemental calcium given over 5-10 minutes) can be used to temporarily antagonize the effects of magnesium until dialysis can be performed. Details regarding intravenous calcium administration can be found in the section on treatment of hyperkalemia. Intravenous volume infusion may be helpful in promoting magnesium excretion in patients who are not volume overloaded and who have adequate renal function.

DISCHARGE CHECKLIST

- For patients with potassium disorders at risk for cardiac arrhythmias, is the potassium level within the normal range prior to discharge?
- For patients with potassium disorders at low risk of cardiac arrhythmias, is the potassium level between 3 and 5.6? Are clinical symptoms or ECG changes associated with potassium disorders absent? If the patient is discharged with mild hypokalemia or mild hyperkalemia, is there a clinical plan to achieve a normal plasma potassium (3.5-5) which can be re-evaluated at follow-up?
- Have patients with hypokalemia been counselled regarding potential dietary sources of potassium? (These include dark leafy greens, avocadoes, peaches, prunes, raisins, potatoes, squash, beans, and fish, as well as the commonly cited bananas and orange juice.)
- Has follow-up testing been arranged for potassium, magnesium, and creatinine, if appropriate?

SUGGESTED READINGS

Bosch X, Poch E, Grau JM. Rhabdomyolysis and acute kidney injury. *N Engl J Med.* 2009;361:62-72.

Gennari FJ. Disorders of potassium homeostasis: hypokalemia and hyperkalemia. *Crit Care Clin.* 2002;18:273-288.

Kamel KS, Halperin ML. Intrarenal urea recycling leads to a higher rate of renal excretion of potassium: a hypothesis with clinical implications. *Curr Opin Nephrol Hypertens.* 2011;20:547-554.

Kim HJ, Han SW. Therapeutic approach to hyperkalaemia. *Nephron.* 2002;92(Suppl 1):33-40.

Kitabchi AE, Umpierrez GE, Miles JM, Fisher JN. American Diabetes Association Consensus Statement: hyperglycemic crisis in adult patients with diabetes. *Diabetes Care.* 2009;32:1335-1343.

Palmer BF. A physiologic-based approach to the evaluation of a patient with hypokalemia. *Am J Kidney Dis.* 2010;56:1184-1190.

Packham DK, Rasmussen HS, Lavin PT, et al. Sodium zirconium cyclosilicate in hyperkalemia. *N Engl J Med.* 2015;373:222-231.

Park CH, Kim EH, Roh YH, Kim HY, Lee SK. The association between the use of proton pump inhibitors and the risk of hypomagnesemia: a systematic review and meta-analysis. *PLoS One.* 2014;9:e112558.

Topf JM, Murray PT. Hypomagnesemia and hypermagnesemia. *Rev Endocr Metab Disord.* 2003;4:195-206.

Weir MR, Bakris GL, Bushinksky DA, et al. Patiromer in patients with kidney disease and hyperkalemia receiving RAAS inhibitors. *N Engl J Med.* 2015;372:211-221.

CHAPTER 242

Disorders of Sodium and Water Balance

Elwaleed A. Elhassan, MD
Robert W. Schrier, MD

Key Clinical Questions

1. What is the difference between sodium and water balance and the regulation of each?

2. How is volume depletion assessed in patients with normal heart function and in those with underlying cardiac failure?

3. Which fluids are best for volume repletion?

4. How do diuretics work, and what are their side effects? How can resistance to their action be overcome?

5. How should hyponatremia and hypernatremia be assessed and safely corrected?

INTRODUCTION

Sodium and water disturbances are among the most commonly encountered disorders in hospitalized and critically ill patients. Sodium and water balance are independently regulated by mechanisms that are designed to maintain circulatory integrity and plasma osmolality, respectively. Sodium balance is regulated by changes in sodium intake and excretion, whereas plasma osmolality is regulated by changes in water intake and water excretion.

Water is the predominant constituent of the human body. In healthy individuals, it makes up 60% of male body weight and 50% of female body weight. Body water is distributed between two compartments: the intracellular fluid compartment, containing 55% to 65%, and the extracellular fluid compartment, containing the remaining 35% to 45%. The extracellular fluid compartment is further subdivided into the interstitial space and the intravascular space. The interstitial space comprises approximately 75% of the extracellular fluid compartment, whereas the intravascular space contains 25%. Total body water diffuses freely between the intracellular space and the extracellular space in response to solute concentration gradients. Therefore, the amount of water in each compartment depends entirely on the quantity of solute in that compartment. The major extracellular solute is sodium, while potassium is the major intracellular solute. This solute distribution is maintained by active transport, via the Na^+/K^+-ATP-dependent pumps found on cell membranes.

PATHOPHYSIOLOGY OF SODIUM BALANCE

The extracellular fluid compartment depends on the total body sodium content as well as the integrity of the mechanisms responsible for its maintenance. Sodium content is normally tightly regulated by modulating renal retention and excretion when there is deficiency or excess of extracellular fluid. The operative homeostatic mechanisms include an afferent sensing limb and an efferent effector limb. Disorders of either sensing or effector mechanisms can lead to failure to adjust renal sodium handling, resulting in hypertension and edema with positive sodium balance, or hypotension and hypovolemia with negative sodium balance.

■ EFFECTIVE ARTERIAL BLOOD VOLUME

Effective arterial blood volume refers to the blood volume detected by baroreceptors in the arterial circulation. The effective arterial blood volume can change independently of the total extracellular fluid volume, leading to sodium and water retention in different clinical situations.

Afferent limb sensing sites include low-pressure cardiopulmonary receptors (atrial, ventricular, and pulmonary stretch receptors), high-pressure arterial baroreceptors (carotid, aortic arch, and renal sensors), and central nervous system and hepatic receptors. Activation of these afferent sites engages several *effector mechanisms*. Activation of the sympathetic nerves stimulates proximal tubular sodium reabsorption. Renin release from the renal juxtaglomerular apparatus stimulates the formation of angiotensin II, a potent vasoconstrictor. Angiotensin II also stimulates the adrenal gland to secrete aldosterone, which increases tubular sodium reabsorption. Other effector mechanisms include prostaglandins that modulate renal blood flow and sodium handling, natriuretic peptides that enhance renal sodium excretion in response to atrial stretching, and pituitary secretion of arginine vasopressin (AVP), a modest vasoconstrictor that also enhances renal water retention.

■ REGULATION OF WATER BALANCE

Osmoregulation is the regulation of water intake and excretion to maintain constant body osmolality (tonicity). Disorders of water homeostasis result in hypo- or hypernatremia, whereas disorders of total body sodium content result in extracellular volume depletion or excess. Since osmolality in all body fluids is essentially equal, it can be estimated by measuring the plasma osmolality. The normal plasma osmolality is 275 to 290 mOsm/kg. It is kept within this range by hypothalamic osmoreceptors, which are capable of sensing a 1% to 2% change in tonicity. Osmoreceptors provoke thirst and release of the antidiuretic hormone AVP. The combined effect of AVP stimulation and thirst results in water intake and retention, lowering plasma osmolality and sodium concentration by dilution, whereas suppression of thirst and AVP secretion leads to the contrary.

DISORDERS OF SODIUM BALANCE

■ EXTRACELLULAR FLUID VOLUME CONTRACTION

Extracellular fluid (ECF) volume contraction is caused by loss of sodium and water in excess of intake. This may result from renal losses, extrarenal losses, or sequestration in potential spaces, such as the peritoneal cavity, retroperitoneum, pleural spaces, or muscles, which are not in hemodynamic equilibrium with the ECF ("third-spacing").

Extrarenal causes

The gastrointestinal tract is the most common extrarenal source of fluid loss. Vomiting or nasogastric suction may cause volume loss with metabolic alkalosis. Diarrhea may result in volume depletion with metabolic acidosis. Third-space sequestration, excessive sweat production, and loss of skin barrier from burns or exudative skin lesions may lead to significant ECF volume depletion. Hemorrhage, as from gastrointestinal bleeding or trauma, may lead to significant volume loss.

Renal losses

Diuretics may cause renal sodium wasting, volume contraction, and acid-base disturbances if abused or inappropriately prescribed. Genetic and acquired tubular disorders can result in renal sodium wasting and volume contraction. Mineralocorticoid deficiency or resistance may lead to renal sodium wasting. This may occur in the setting of primary adrenal insufficiency (Addison disease), hyporeninemic hypoaldosteronism secondary to diabetes mellitus, or other chronic interstitial renal diseases. Severe hyperglycemia or high levels of blood urea after relief of urinary tract obstruction can lead to obligatory renal sodium and water loss secondary to glucosuria or urea diuresis, respectively.

Clinical manifestations

The symptoms of hypovolemia are nonspecific. They range from mild postural symptoms, thirst, muscle cramps, and weakness, to drowsiness and disturbed mentation with profound volume loss. Physical examination may reveal tachycardia, cold clammy skin, postural or recumbent hypotension, and reduced urine output depending on the degree of volume loss (**Table 242-1**). Rarely, diminished skin turgor may be seen. Reduced jugular venous pressure (JVP) noted at the base of the neck is a useful parameter of volume depletion and may roughly estimate the central venous pressure (CVP). However, an elevated CVP does not exclude hypovolemia in patients with underlying cardiac failure or pulmonary hypertension.

TABLE 242-1 Clinical Evaluation of Extracellular Fluid Volume Depletion

Mild to moderate volume loss

- Thirst
- Delayed capillary refill
- Postural dizziness and weakness
- Dry mucous membranes and axillae
- Cool clammy extremities and collapsed peripheral veins
- Tachypnea
- Tachycardia with pulse rate > 100 beats/min or postural pulse increment of 30 beats/min or more
- Postural hypotension (systolic blood pressure decrease of > 20 mm Hg with standing)
- Low jugular venous pulse
- Oliguria

Severe volume loss and hypovolemic shock

- Depressed mental status or loss of consciousness
- Peripheral cyanosis
- Reduced skin turgor (in young patients only)
- Marked tachycardia, low pulse volume
- Supine hypotension (systolic blood pressure < 100 mm Hg)

The absence of symptoms or obvious physical findings does not preclude volume depletion in an appropriate clinical setting, and hemodynamic monitoring or administration of a fluid challenge may sometimes be necessary.

Laboratory findings consistent with volume depletion include hemoconcentration and increased serum albumin concentration. However, anemia or hypoalbuminemia may confound interpretation of these laboratory values. In healthy individuals, the ratio of blood urea nitrogen (BUN) (mg/dL) to serum creatinine (mg/dL) approximately equals 10. In volume depletion, this ratio increases because of a differential increase in the tubular reabsorption of urea. Several clinical conditions confound this ratio. Upper gastrointestinal hemorrhage and administration of corticosteroids increase urea production and the ratio of BUN to creatinine. Malnutrition and underlying liver disease diminish urea production, and thus the BUN-to-creatinine ratio is less useful in these clinical settings.

In the absence of renal salt wasting or diuretics, elevated urine osmolality and specific gravity may indicate hypovolemia. Hypovolemia normally triggers avid renal sodium reabsorption, resulting in low urine sodium concentration and low fractional excretion of sodium. The fractional excretion of sodium (FE_{Na}) is calculated using the following formula: $FE_{Na} = [U_{Na} \times P_{Cr} / U_{Cr} \times P_{Na}] \times 100$, where U_{Na} and U_{Cr} are urinary sodium and creatinine concentrations, and P_{Na} and P_{Cr} are plasma sodium and creatinine concentrations, respectively. Decreased FE_{Na} (< 1%) is consistent with ECF volume depletion. However, arterial underfilling due to low cardiac output or systemic arterial vasodilatation, as in cirrhosis, is also associated with a FE_{Na} less than 1%, in spite of increased ECF and edema.

Treatment

Volume depletion is treated by replacing fluid deficits and ongoing losses with a replacement fluid closely resembling the lost fluid. Clinical parameters help to distinguish mild to moderate from severe volume loss (Table 242-1), but invasive monitoring may be needed in some patients. Mild volume contraction can usually be corrected via the oral route. In hypovolemic shock with evidence of life-threatening circulatory collapse or organ dysfunction, intravenous fluid must be given as rapidly as possible until clinical parameters improve. A slower, more judicious approach is warranted in the elderly and in those with underlying cardiac conditions to avoid overcorrection with subsequent pulmonary edema.

Crystalloid solutions are effective, as they distribute primarily in the ECF. Isotonic saline is usually the initial replacement fluid of choice in volume-depleted patients. Colloid-containing solutions, such as 5% and 25% albumin and hetastarch (6% hydroxyethyl starch), are second-line agents for the treatment of hypovolemia. They remain within the vascular compartment by virtue of their large molecular sizes. Hyperoncotic starch solutions should be avoided as they increase the risk of acute kidney injury, need for renal replacement therapy, and mortality.

Hypovolemic shock may be accompanied by lactic acidosis due to tissue hypoperfusion. Fluid resuscitation restores tissue oxygenation and decreases the production of lactate. Correction of acidosis with sodium bicarbonate has several potential adverse effects, including increasing tonicity, worsening intracellular acidosis, and reducing ionized calcium concentration. Therefore, its use to manage lactic acidosis in the setting of volume depletion is not recommended, unless the arterial pH is below 7.1.

▉ EXTRACELLULAR FLUID VOLUME EXPANSION

Excess extracellular fluid accumulation usually results from sodium and water retention by the kidneys. Renal sodium retention may be primary or a compensatory response to reduced effective arterial blood volume. It manifests clinically with edema and weight gain, commonly in response to congestive heart failure (CHF), cirrhosis with ascites, or nephrotic syndrome.

Renal sodium and water retention in CHF involves activation of the renin-angiotensin-aldosterone system (RAAS), as well as nonosmotic AVP stimulation, which drives the hyponatremia associated with CHF. Arterial underfilling is also responsible for water and sodium retention in cirrhosis. Unlike CHF and cirrhosis, in which the kidneys are structurally normal, the nephrotic syndrome is characterized by kidneys that are functionally impaired. Rarer causes of edema include drug-induced edema, which may be seen with ingestion of systemic vasodilators, such as minoxidil and diazoxide, dihydropyridine calcium channel blockers, and thiazolidinediones. Nonsteroidal anti-inflammatory drugs (NSAIDs) can exacerbate volume expansion in CHF and cirrhotic patients by decreasing vasoregulatory prostaglandins in the kidneys.

Clinical manifestations

Patients with left heart failure may present with exertional dyspnea, orthopnea, and paroxysmal nocturnal dyspnea, whereas patients with predominant right heart failure or biventricular failure may exhibit weight gain and lower-limb swelling. Physical examination may reveal JVP elevation, pulmonary crackles, a third heart sound, or peripheral edema in the ankles or sacrum. Nephrotic patients classically present with periorbital edema because of their ability to lie flat during sleep. Patients with severe nephrotic syndrome may exhibit marked generalized edema with anasarca. Cirrhotic patients present with ascites and lower-limb edema consequent to portal hypertension and renal sodium and water retention. Physical examination may reveal stigmata of chronic liver disease, such as jaundice, spider angiomata, palmar erythema, Dupuytren contractures, and splenomegaly.

Therapy

Management of ECF volume expansion consists of treating the underlying cause and achieving negative sodium balance with dietary sodium restriction and diuretics. Moderate dietary sodium restriction (2-3 g/d; 86-130 mmol/d) should be instituted. Restriction of total fluid intake is usually only necessary for hyponatremic patients. Medications that promote sodium retention, such as NSAIDs, corticosteroids, estrogens, and androgens, should be eliminated, if possible. Diuretics are the cornerstone of therapy to remove excess volume. Other measures can be used when the response to diuretics is inadequate. Extracorporeal fluid removal by ultrafiltration can be utilized in patients with acute decompensated heart failure with renal insufficiency or diuretic resistance. In cirrhosis, large-volume paracentesis with albumin infusion (6-8 g per liter of ascitic fluid removed) can be employed. Interventions to shift ascitic fluid to a central vein, such as a transjugular intrahepatic portosystemic shunt, may reduce refractory ascites and improve GFR and sodium excretion.

Diuretics are the mainstay of therapy for edematous states. As ECF volume expansion in CHF and cirrhosis may be a compensatory mechanism for arterial underfilling, a judicious approach is necessary to avoid a precipitous fall in cardiac output and tissue perfusion. Diuretics can be classified into five classes, based on their predominant sites of actions along the nephron (**Figure 242-1**). They inhibit the reabsorption of sodium and an accompanying anion, usually chloride. The resultant natriuresis decreases the ECF. However, the time course of natriuresis is limited because renal mechanisms attenuate the sodium excretion.

The most serious *adverse effects of diuretics* are electrolyte and acid-base disturbances. Loop diuretics increase the excretion of potassium, magnesium, and calcium. Thiazide diuretics have similar effects on potassium and magnesium, but unlike loop diuretics, they decrease urinary calcium losses. Thiazide diuretics interfere with urine-diluting mechanisms, and may therefore pose a risk of hyponatremia. Patients on diuretic therapy require electrolyte monitoring, and may need oral supplementation of potassium and magnesium. Addition of a potassium-sparing diuretic may need to be considered in patients with severe or recurrent hypokalemia. The volume depletion caused by thiazides and loop diuretics leads to increased tubular urate reabsorption, promoting hyperuricemia and gout. Ototoxicity may occur with large intravenous doses of loop diuretics, particularly when an aminoglycoside is coadministered. Gynecomastia may develop with spironolactone therapy.

Long-term *loop diuretic tolerance* occurs as a consequence of hypertrophy of the distal nephron segment and enhanced sodium reabsorption from increased exposure to solutes not absorbed proximally. This can be addressed by combining loop and thiazide diuretics, as the latter blocks reabsorption distal to the loop of Henle.

Diuretic resistance refers to edema that is or has become refractory to a given diuretic. Diuretic resistance has several causes. Chronic kidney disease is associated with decreased secretion and tubular delivery of diuretics, reducing their concentration at the active site in the tubular lumen. Arterial underfilling in cirrhosis and CHF is associated with diminished nephron responsiveness to diuretics because of increased proximal tubular sodium reabsorption, leading to decreased delivery of sodium to the distal sites of diuretic action. Nonsteroidal anti-inflammatory drugs block prostaglandin-mediated increases in renal blood flow, leading to sodium retention.

Treatment of diuretic resistance includes salt restriction, increasing the dose of loop diuretics, administering more frequent doses, and using combination therapy to sequentially block more than one site in the nephron, as that may result in a synergistic interaction between diuretics (**Figure 242-2**). In patients who respond poorly to intermittent doses of a loop diuretic, a continuous intravenous infusion can be tried. This has been associated with a better safety profile but similar efficacy in clinical trials. Ultrafiltration may be necessary in highly resistant edematous patients. **Table 242-2** lists effective diuretic doses in patients with CHF, nephrotic syndrome, advanced cirrhosis, and renal failure.

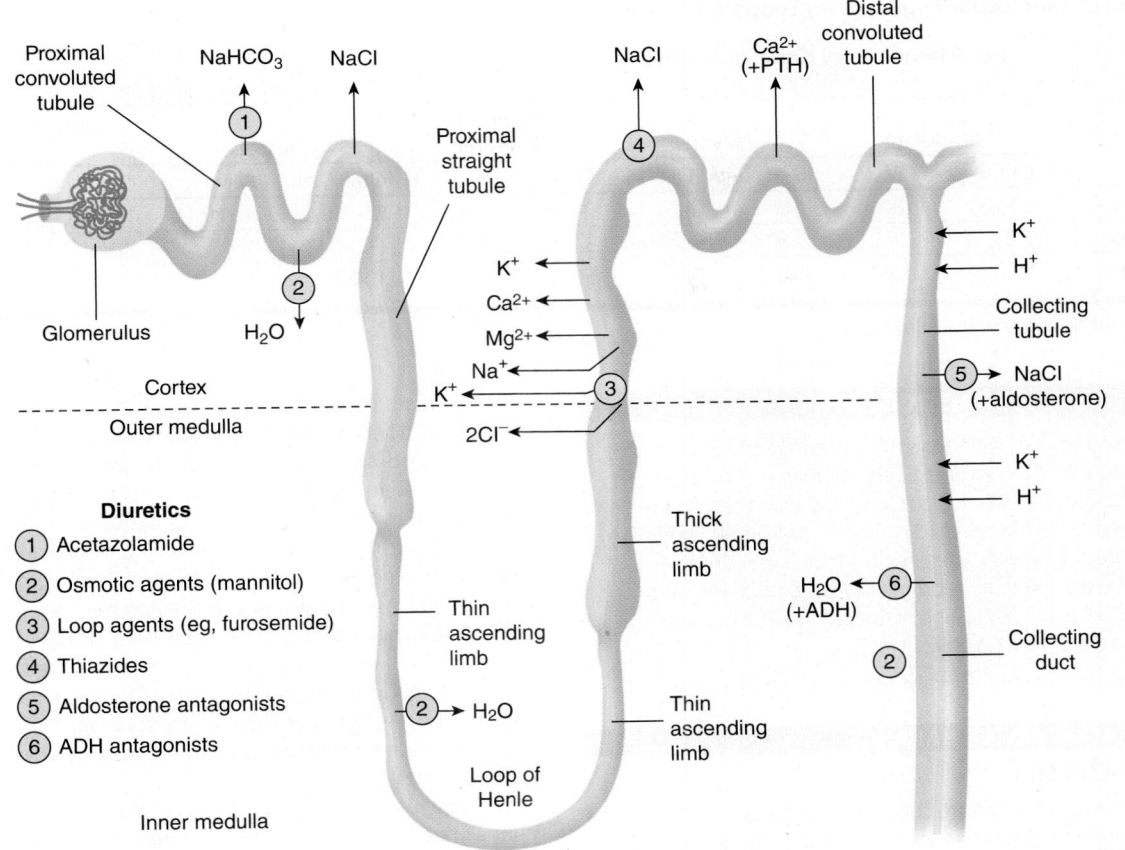

Figure 242-1 *Tubule transport systems and sites of action of diuretics.* (Reproduced, with permission, from Katzung BG, Masters SB, Trevor AJ. *Basic & Clinical Pharmacology*, 11th ed. New York, NY: McGraw-Hill; 2009. Fig. 15-1.)

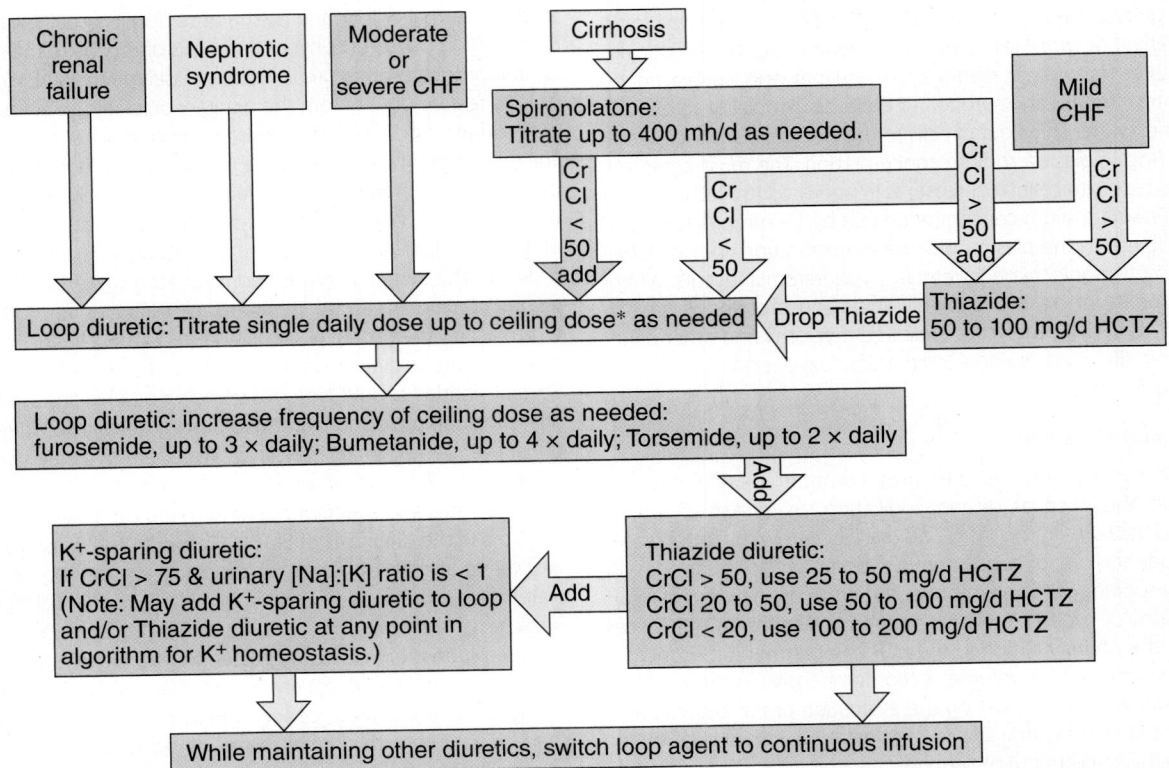

Figure 242-2 *Algorithm for diuretic therapy in patients with edema caused by renal, hepatic, or cardiac disease.* (*For dosing details, see Brater DC. Diuretic therapy. *N Engl J Med.* 1998;339:387-395.) (Reproduced, with permission, from Brunton LL, Lazo JS, Parker KL. *Goodman & Gilman's The Pharmacological Basis of Therapeutics*, 11th ed. New York, NY: McGraw-Hill; 2006. Fig. 28-12.)

TABLE 242-2 Therapeutic Regimens for Loop Diuretics in mg/d

	Renal Insufficiency (Dose Varies with Severity)						Preserved Renal Function					
	Moderate		Severe		Nephrotic Syndrome		Cirrhosis		Congestive Heart Failure	
	Oral	IV	Oral	IV	Oral	IV	Oral	IV	Oral	IV
Furosemide	80-160	80	240	200	240	120	80-160	40-80	160-240	40-80
Bumetanide	2-3	2-3	8-10	8-10	3	3	1-2	1	2-3	2-3
Torsemide	50	50	100	100	50	50	10-20	10-20	50	20-50

GFR, glomerular filtration rate; IV, intravenous.

PRACTICE POINT

- Ascites and edema in cirrhosis may be controlled by sodium restriction and diuretic therapy. The diuretic combination of furosemide and spironolactone, given in a ratio of furosemide 40 mg and spironolactone 100 mg daily to maintain optimal electrolyte balance, is more effective than either drug administered alone. These drugs may be gradually titrated upward to a maximal dosage of furosemide 160 mg and spironolactone 400 mg daily.

DISORDERS OF WATER BALANCE

■ HYPONATREMIA

Hyponatremia (plasma sodium concentration below 135 mmol/L) is the most common electrolyte abnormality in hospitalized patients, occurring in 15% to 30% of medical inpatients, with over half of cases being acquired during hospitalization. Most patients with hyponatremia have hypo-osmolar or hypotonic hyponatremia, with excess water in relation to solute. However, hyponatremia does not always signify a hypotonic state. Rarely, patients have *hypertonic hyponatremia*, or *translocational hyponatremia*, due to osmotically active solutes that do not readily penetrate into cells, such as mannitol, contrast media, and sorbitol. To equalize osmolality across cell membranes, water shifts out of cells to the extracellular space, leading to a drop in plasma sodium concentration. The most common cause is excess extracellular glucose, as in poorly controlled diabetes mellitus. Plasma sodium concentration falls by 1.6 mmol/L for every 100 mg/dL rise in the plasma glucose concentration. In *pseudohyponatremia* (isotonic hyponatremia), hyponatremia occurs when the solid phase of plasma, primarily lipids and proteins, is greatly expanded, as in hypertriglyceridemia and myeloma and other paraproteinemic disorders, leading to an artifactual decrease in plasma sodium concentration.

Etiology and diagnosis

Hypotonic hyponatremia is the most common plasma sodium disorder in the hospital setting, indicating an excess of water relative to sodium in plasma. This can occur with a decrease in total body sodium, or hypovolemic hyponatremia; a near-normal total body sodium, or euvolemic hyponatremia; or an excess of total body sodium, or hypervolemic hyponatremia (**Figure 242-3**). Since sodium is the primary cation in the ECF compartment, its concentration determines ECF volume. A comprehensive history and a physical examination focused on the evaluation of the ECF volume allows for the classification of the hyponatremia into one of three categories: hypovolemic, euvolemic, or hypervolemic.

In *hypovolemic hyponatremia*, deficits of both total body sodium and water lead to ECF volume depletion, with consequent AVP secretion and decreased solute-free water excretion.

Renal causes of solute-rich fluid loss include diuretics, mineralocorticoid deficiency, salt-losing nephropathy, such as polycystic kidney disease and interstitial nephritis, and partial urinary tract obstruction. Fluid losses may also be extrarenal, especially gastrointestinal, such as gastroenteritis, peritonitis, pancreatitis, and ileus, as well as hemorrhage or excessive sweating. Historical features may include vomiting, diarrhea, diuretic use, thirstiness, or hyperglycemia with glucosuria. Physical examination may reveal tachycardia, orthostatic hypotension, and flat neck veins. Helpful urinary studies include urine sodium and the Fe_{Na}, which are typically less than 10 mmol/L and 1%, respectively with extrarenal fluid losses. Urine sodium and Fe_{Na} greater than 10 mmol/L and 1%, respectively, usually indicate renal losses, such as secondary to diuretic use and osmotic diuresis.

In *euvolemic hyponatremia*, total body sodium content is generally normal, but there is hypo-osmolality from a relative gain of water. Physical examination is notable for the absence of both features of volume overload, such as peripheral edema, ascites, pulmonary edema, and features of volume depletion, such as tachycardia, low blood pressure, or flat neck veins. Concentrations of BUN and uric acid are normal or low, and the urine sodium is usually greater than 20 mEq/L. In this setting, hyponatremia is often due to the syndrome of inappropriate antidiuretic hormone secretion (SIADH), attributable to release of AVP from the pituitary or, rarely, an ectopic source such as lung carcinoma. This leads to impaired water excretion, while the regulation of sodium balance is virtually unaffected. Ingestion or administration of water is also required, since a high level of AVP alone is not usually sufficient to produce hyponatremia. Causes of SIADH include infectious, inflammatory, neoplastic, and vascular disorders of the central nervous and respiratory systems, pain, narcotics, anticonvulsants, antidepressants, neuroleptics, and other drugs which act on the central nervous system (**Table 242-3**). However, in many hospitalized elderly patients with SIADH, the cause is obscure. Several entities should be considered prior to diagnosing SIADH. These include profound hypothyroidism, adrenal insufficiency, renal impairment, and primary polydipsia. Hyponatremia may also be seen in excessive beer consumption (beer potomania), as beer is rich in carbohydrates and water, but poor in solutes and electrolytes.

To make the diagnosis of SIADH (**Table 242-4**), patients must be euvolemic, and the urinary osmolality must exceed 100 mOsm/kg of water despite a low plasma osmolality (< 275 mOsm/kg of water). Because of the low urine volume in SIADH, the urinary sodium concentration is high, usually greater than 40 mmol/L, in the steady state. However, if the patient is volume depleted or on a salt-restricted diet, the urine concentration may be lower. Expanding the ECF volume with normal saline or normal salt intake increases urinary sodium, but does not correct the hyponatremia. Supportive laboratory tests for SIADH include hypouricemia (serum uric acid < 4 mg/dL) and low BUN (< 10 mg/dL). When the diagnosis is still uncertain, ECF volume depletion can be ruled out by infusing 2 L

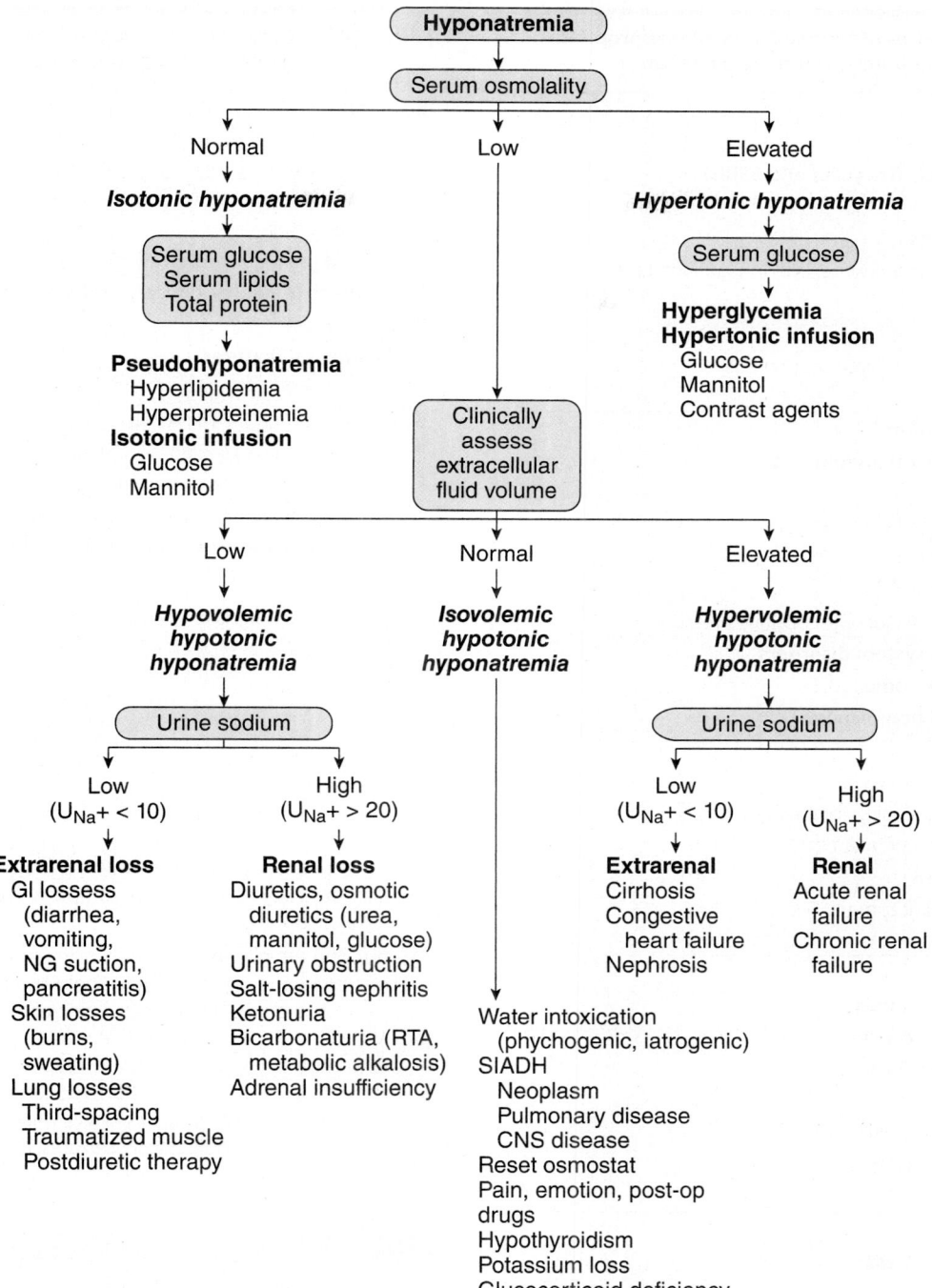

Figure 242-3 *Diagnostic algorithm for hyponatremia. (Adapted, with permission, from Johnson RJ, Freehaly J, eds. Comprehensive Clinical Nephrology, 2nd ed. St. Louis, MO: Mosby; 2003.)*

of normal saline over 24 to 48 hours. Correction of hyponatremia, along with a drop in urinary osmolality, suggests volume depletion rather than SIADH. Caution must be exercised when administering saline to hyponatremic patients, because in a subset of patients this can induce brisk water diuresis and a rapid rise in serum sodium. Osmotic demyelination, with severe neurologic morbidity and even death, may occur with rapid correction of plasma sodium concentration (greater than 9 mEq/L rise in 24 hours) in patients with chronic hyponatremia.

Frequent monitoring of serum and urinary electrolytes is therefore warranted. If rapid overcorrection occurs, administration of hypotonic fluid or even AVP may be needed to halt the progressive rise in serum sodium.

In *hypervolemic hyponatremia*, both total body sodium and water are increased, but water is comparatively more so. Underlying causes include cardiac failure and liver cirrhosis, in which the kidneys are intrinsically normal, but respond to decreased effective arterial perfusion with increased AVP levels and activation of RAAS. Acute and chronic kidney disease may be associated with hyponatremia if water intake exceeds the ability to excrete equivalent volumes. Hyponatremia is a risk factor for diminished survival in cardiac failure and cirrhosis. In the absence of diuretics, Fe_{Na} should be less than 1% in both conditions. However, a Fe_{Na} greater than 1% is seen in the hypervolemic hyponatremic patient with acute or chronic kidney disease with tubular dysfunction leading to suboptimal sodium and water absorption.

TABLE 242-3 Causes of the Syndrome of Inappropriate Antidiuretic Hormone Secretion

Drugs
- **Antipsychotics**
- **Antidepressants (tricyclics and SSRIs)**
- **Narcotics**
- **Anticonvulsants**
- Cytotoxic drugs (vincristine, cyclophosphamide, ifosfamide)
- Nicotine
- Clofibrate
- Nonsteroidal anti-inflammatory drugs
- MDMA (ecstasy)

Pulmonary disorders
- **Bacterial and viral pneumonia**
- Lung abscess
- Bronchiectasis and cystic fibrosis
- Tuberculosis
- Aspergillosis
- Mechanical ventilation with positive pressure

Central nervous system disorders
- **Subdural hematoma**
- **Subarachnoid hemorrhage**
- **Stroke**
- **Tumors**
- Meningitis, encephalitis, brain abscess
- Vasculitis and other inflammatory disorders
- Multiple sclerosis
- Guillain-Barré syndrome
- Hydrocephalus

Malignancies
- **Small cell lung cancer**
- **Head and neck cancer**
- Nonsmall cell lung cancer
- Mesothelioma
- Gastrointestinal adenocarcinoma
- Genitourinary tract cancers
- Leukemia

Others
- **Postoperative stress**
- **Pain**
- **Nausea and vomiting**
- Endurance exercise
- AIDS
- Hereditary gain-of-function mutation in the V2 receptor

Note: The most common causes are listed in bold.

TABLE 242-4 Criteria for the Diagnosis of the Syndrome of Inappropriate Antidiuretic Hormone Secretion

Key features

Decreased effective osmolality (< 275 mOsm/kg of water)

Inappropriately elevated urinary osmolality > 100 mOsm/kg of water despite hypotonicity

Clinical euvolemia

Urinary sodium > 20 mEq/L with normal dietary sodium intake

Normal thyroid, adrenal, pituitary, and renal function

No recent diuretic use

Supplemental features

Plasma uric acid < 4 mg/dL

Blood urea nitrogen < 10 mg/dL

Fractional excretion of sodium > 1%; fractional urea excretion > 55%

Failure to correct hyponatremia after infusion of normal saline

Correction of hyponatremia through fluid restriction

death. Neurologic signs of severe acute hyponatremia may include depressed deep tendon reflexes, hypothermia, pseudobulbar palsy, and Cheyne-Stokes respirations.

Psychiatric patients are at risk for hyponatremia for many reasons, including:

- Thirst-producing anticholinergic side effects of antidepressants and antipsychotics
- SIADH from typical and atypical antipyschotics, tricyclic antidepressants, and selective serotonin reuptake inhibitors
- Obsessive-compulsive behavior
- Lack of satiety from water consumption in patients hospitalized for alcoholism or anorexia

Schizophrenic patients are particularly at risk: up to 14% have hyponatremia, and up to 25% have polydipsia. This predisposition may be multifactorial, relating to a decreased osmotic threshold for AVP release, enhanced renal sensitivity to AVP, and a defect in the osmoregulation of thirst. Clozapine may have a lesser tendency to cause polydipsia and hyponatremia than other antipsychotics. Unfortunately, it has uncommon but severe adverse effects, including agranulocytosis, seizures, myocarditis, and orthostatic hypotension.

PRACTICE POINT

- SIADH and psychogenic polydipsia may be differentiated based on the urine osmolality. In SIADH urine osmolality is ≥ 100 mOsm/kg. In psychogenic polydipsia it is < 100 mOsm/kg.
- Fluid restriction is the main treatment for psychogenic polydipsia, but is difficult to enforce in practice.
- The antibiotic demeclocycline, which blocks the activity and action of AVP, may have some utility in treatment of psychogenic polydipsia.

Therapy

Hypovolemic hyponatremia is treated with volume repletion with isotonic saline to expand ECF volume and interrupt AVP release. Volume expansion should be continued until blood pressure is restored and the patient demonstrates clinical euvolemia. When the initial volume estimate is equivocal, a fluid challenge with 0.5 to 1 L of isotonic saline can be both diagnostic and therapeutic.

The clinical manifestations of hyponatremia are mainly neurologic and caused by intracellular fluid shifts, leading to brain swelling and edema. The severity of symptoms depends on the rate of decline of serum sodium concentration, because the adaptive mechanisms to protect brain cell volume require a longer time to be fully functional. These mechanisms involve a gradual loss of potassium and organic solutes to restore cell volume to normal. Symptoms include nausea, vomiting, headache, lethargy, seizures, and a progressively decreased level of consciousness, ending in coma and

Hypervolemic hyponatremia

The treatment of hyponatremia in the context of volume overload requires management of the underlying cardiac failure or liver cirrhosis. Sodium and water restriction as well as diuretics should be employed as necessary. When hyponatremia occurs, fluid restriction to amounts less than insensible losses plus urine output is necessary to cause a negative solute-free water balance, but is often difficult to achieve. Diuretic-resistant cases of CHF and liver cirrhosis may be treated with ultrafiltration and large-volume paracentesis, respectively.

Euvolemic hyponatremia

The treatment of hyponatremia in euvolemic patients depends on the degree of symptoms and on whether it has developed acutely (within hours) or chronically (over more than 48 hours). Acute hyponatremia with onset in the hospital is most often related to hypotonic solutions. The rapid development of hyponatremia with very low sodium values (< 110-115 mmol/L) may cause fluid to shift into brain cells, possibly leading to cerebral edema and death, as the adaptive changes cannot keep pace with intracellular fluid shifts leading to brain swelling within the confined skull space.

In acute severe hyponatremia with neurologic symptoms, the treatment of choice is 3% hypertonic saline, infused initially at 1 to 2 mL/kg/h (**Table 242-5**). For each 100 mL of 3% hypertonic saline, the serum sodium concentration will increase approximately by 2 mmol/L. This should be continued until a less severe level of hyponatremia has been attained (ie, 125-130 mmol/L), or symptoms resolve. If seizures, obtundation, or coma are present, hypertonic saline may be infused at 4 to 6 mL/kg/h for a short period of time. An alternative approach that has been successfully used in marathon runners is infusing 100 mL bolus of 3% hypertonic saline, enough to increase the serum Na approximately by 2 mmol/L. A small, quick increase in the serum Na (2-4 mmol/L) is effective in treating acute hyponatremia because reducing brain swelling even slightly will substantially decrease intracerebral pressure. If severe neurologic symptoms persist or worsen, or if the serum sodium is not improving, a 100-mL bolus of hypertonic saline can be repeated one or two more times at 10-minute intervals.

When hyponatremia develops over several days, brain cells extrude organic solutes from their cytoplasm, allowing intracellular osmolality and plasma osmolality to equalize without a large increase in cell water. Because of this rapid normalization of chronic hyponatremia may also lead to cerebral edema. Hyponatremia should be corrected very gradually when it has been present for more than 48 hours, or the duration is unknown. Serum sodium initially be increased by 4 to 6 mEq/L during the first 24 hours and by less than 9 mEq/L over any given 24-hour period. It should be corrected even more slowly in high-risk patients with severe malnutrition, alcoholism, or advanced liver disease, who have an impaired ability to protect their intracellular volume by generating osmotically active molecules such as glycine, taurine, and myoinositol.

Rapid correction of chronic hyponatremia, outpacing the brain's ability to recapture lost organic osmolytes, may result in osmotic demyelination syndrome, which especially affects glial cells of the brainstem. Patients improve initially as hyponatremia resolves, but within days develop new, progressive, and sometimes permanent neurologic deficits, including fluctuating level of consciousness, quadriparesis, pseudobulbar palsy, ataxia, dysarthria, and locked-in syndrome. Magnetic resonance imaging (MRI) may show T2-weighted hyperintensities in the brainstem, especially the pons, consistent with demyelination.

In patients with chronic asymptomatic hyponatremia, hypothyroidism and secondary adrenal insufficiency should be sought and treated appropriately if present. Potentially responsible medications should be discontinued. Ideally, SIADH is treated with therapy directed against its underlying cause. However, if the cause cannot be identified or expeditiously treated, hyponatremia should be treated conservatively with fluid restriction. To achieve negative water balance, daily fluid intake must be significantly limited to less than the 24-hour urine output plus insensible losses. The maximum tolerated fluid intake is proportional to the oral osmotic load, so adequate intake of dietary protein and salt should be encouraged. Many patients will find the recommended degree of fluid restriction intolerable and difficult to comply with. Oral medications that may be helpful include urea (30 g/d), demeclocycline (300-600 mg twice daily), or lithium, but these therapies have poor tolerability, inconsistent responses, and significant toxicities.

Recently, vasopressin receptor antagonists (vaptans) have been introduced for the treatment of hyponatremia. These agents act by increasing electrolyte-free water excretion (aquaresis) and hence raising serum sodium concentration. Conivaptan, a combined V1 and V2 receptor antagonist, has been approved by the United States Food and Drug Administration (FDA) for 4-day intravenous use in the hospital setting to treat euvolemic and hypervolemic hyponatremia. However, there are insufficient data to use conivaptan in the treatment of acute symptomatic hyponatremia at this time. Conivaptan might be considered particularly for those with moderate to severe hyponatremia and symptoms, but not seizures, delirium, or coma, which would warrant the use of hypertonic saline. The selective V2 receptor antagonist, tolvaptan, is orally active and has been approved by the FDA for euvolemic and hypervolemic hyponatremia. However, the FDA warns that tolvaptan should not be used in any patient for longer than 30 days, and should not be given to patients with liver disease, including cirrhosis. Increased thirst is seen in patients treated with vaptans and may limit the rise in serum sodium. Moreover, overly rapid correction of the hyponatremia may occur, which can lead to irreversible neurologic injury.

TABLE 242-5 Using Hypertonic Saline to Treat Acute Symptomatic Hyponatremia with Neurologic Symptoms

- Infuse 3% hypertonic saline initially at 1-2 ml/kg/h.
- For each 100 ml of 3% hypertonic saline, the serum sodium concentration will increase approximately by 2 mmol/L.
- Alternatively, infuse a 100 mL bolus of 3% hypertonic saline over 10 min. Repeat twice at 30-min intervals if needed.
- Monitor serum sodium level frequently.
- Discontinue hypertonic saline as soon as the patient is asymptomatic or less severe degree of hyponatremia has been attained (125-130 mmol/L).

Hyponatremia: Discharge Checklist

- Have patient and family been educated about signs and symptoms of hyponatremia?
- Has the patient and family been educated about any restrictions on fluid intake, if necessary?

If indicated, specify total liquid intake, not only water. Aim for a fluid restriction that is 500 mL/d below the 24-hour urine volume.

- Do not restrict sodium or protein intake unless indicated.
- If the patient is being discharged on a vaptan, ensure that treatment is not taken beyond 30 days.
- Have blood draws for electrolyte testing and outpatient follow-up been arranged for 1 to 2 weeks after discharge?

■ HYPERNATREMIA

Although not as common as hyponatremia, hypernatremia is not infrequent in hospitalized patients, particularly those in intensive care units. Hypernatremia is always associated with hyperosmolality, as sodium salts are the major extracellular solutes. Hyperosmolality leads to an exodus of water from cells to the extracellular compartment to maintain osmotic equilibrium, with a loss of intracellular volume and shrinkage of brain cells. The major defense against sodium elevation is the stimulation of thirst and AVP, leading to increased water intake and retention. While AVP is important, thirst provides greater protection against hypernatremia. Thus, hypernatremia due to water loss occurs mainly in vulnerable patients with altered mental status and those who are unable to obtain water, such as infants, the elderly, and the severely ill.

Causes of hypernatremia are grouped into three categories, according to the total body sodium content as estimated by extracellular volume (**Figure 242-4**). Thus, the diagnostic approach to the hypernatremic patient hinges on the assessment of extracellular volume. The history should include a review of recent and current medications, vomiting, diarrhea, increased urinary losses (polyuria), recent fluid intake, and the presence or absence of thirst. Physical examination must assess volume and neurologic status.

In *hypovolemic hypernatremia*, there is a predominant loss of solute-free water leading to elevation in the serum sodium concentration. This can occur either from renal or extrarenal sources. Extrarenal losses include gastrointestinal causes, with diarrhea being more likely than vomiting to cause hypernatremia. Osmotic diarrhea, as induced by lactulose, malabsorption, and some infectious

diarrheas, may result in water being lost in excess of sodium and potassium, leading to hypernatremia. Secretory diarrhea, in contrast, produces fluid with electrolyte content similar to plasma, leading to loss of volume and potassium, but not hypernatremia. Insensible salt and water losses through evaporation from the respiratory tract and sweat, brought on by fever or strenuous exercise in hot temperatures, may lead to hypernatremia, because of the hypotonic nature of the lost fluid.

The most common renal causes of sodium and water loss are loop diuretics and osmotic diuresis. Loop diuretics may lead to hypernatremia because they provoke loss of isotonic or hypotonic fluid. Osmotic diuresis from nonelectrolyte solutes, such as urea and glucose, causes hypernatremia by impairing tubular reabsorption of sodium and water. Most hypotonic fluid losses do not cause hypernatremia, unless inadequate free water is ingested or infused to replace the ongoing losses. Hence, these disorders usually also involve some component of inadequate fluid intake.

In *hypervolemic hypernatremia*, there is excess sodium in the extracellular compartment with extracellular volume expansion. This is usually seen in hospitalized patients who receive excess saline or sodium bicarbonate to treat metabolic acidosis, or those receiving enteral or parenteral feedings without adequate free water administration.

Euvolemic hypernatremia

Loss of water without sodium increases fluid tonicity, but usually does not result in clinically evident volume depletion because water is mainly distributed in the intracellular compartment. *Euvolemic*

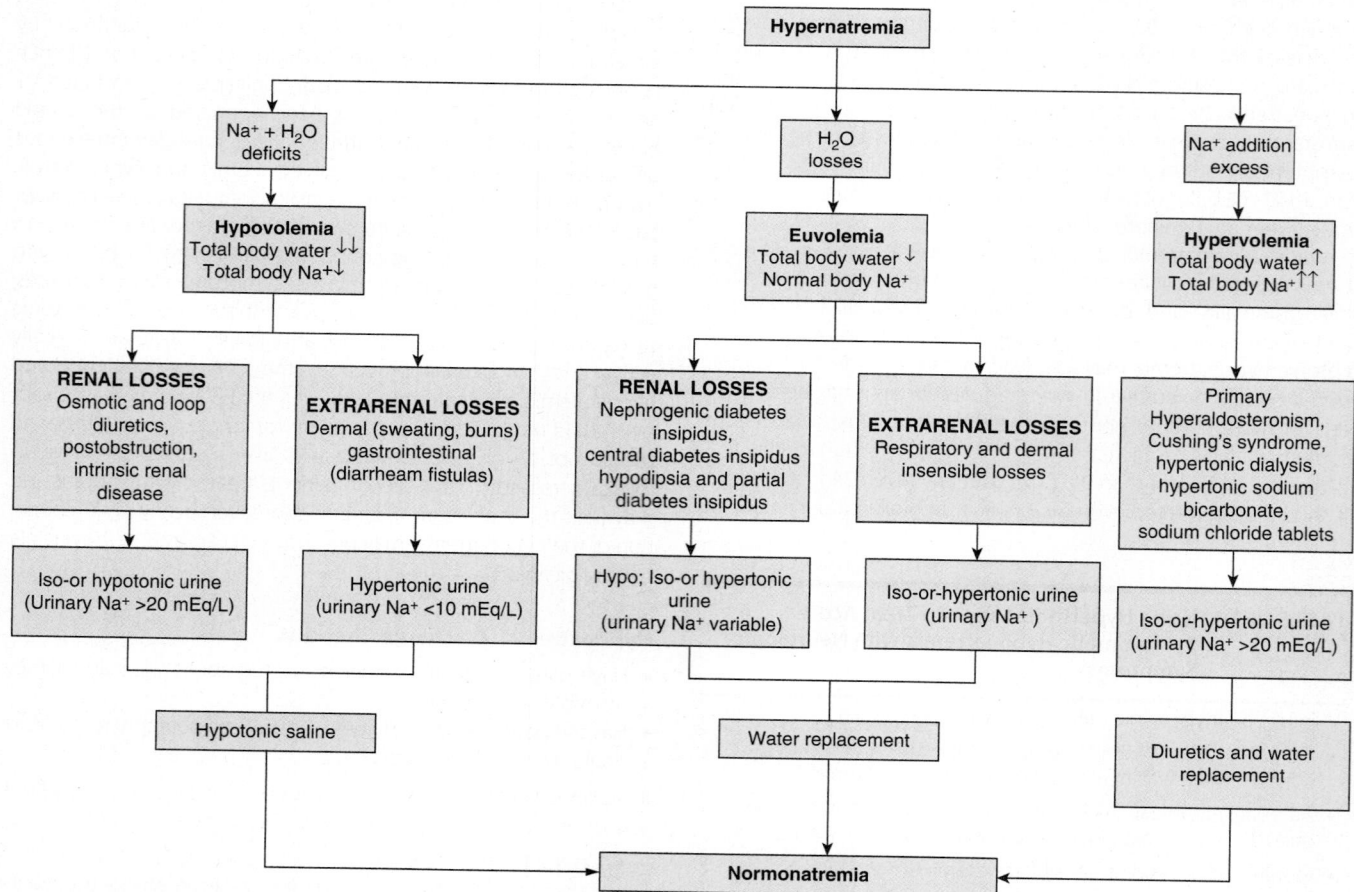

Figure 242-4 *Diagnostic and therapeutic approach to hypernatremia.* (Reproduced, with permission, from Schrier RW. *Renal and Electrolyte Disorders*, 7th ed. Philadelphia, PA: Wolters Kluwer; 2010.)

hypernatremia occurs when there is loss of fluid that is low in sodium and potassium salts. The classic example is diabetes insipidus (DI) from either defects in AVP production or release (central DI), a failure of renal response to AVP (nephrogenic DI), or, rarely, from rapid degradation of AVP by vasopressinase during pregnancy. Most patients with DI present with polyuria and polydipsia; hypernatremia is usually not present unless fluid intake is inadequate.

Central DI can be partial or complete. Causes include head trauma, brain surgery, and inflammatory, neoplastic, and infiltrative disorders of the hypothalamus and pituitary. However, no cause is identified in about half of the cases. Nephrogenic DI is usually a congenital or acquired defect of vasopressin V2 receptors or the vasopressin-dependent water channel (aquaporin 2). Acquired causes include medullary or interstitial renal disease, such as interstitial nephritis, polycystic kidney disease, partial urinary tract obstruction, and advanced chronic kidney disease. Hypercalcemia and hypokalemia may also cause nephrogenic DI, as well as various drugs that impair response to AVP, such as lithium. The various forms of DI must be differentiated from primary polydipsia in patients who present with polyuria.

Urine sodium, volume, and osmolality should be measured to determine the integrity of the AVP-renal axis. The normal response to hypernatremia is increased AVP release, resulting in urine osmolality that can reach a maximum of 1000 mOsm/kg in normal young individuals, and above 500 mOsm/kg in elderly patients who usually have reduced responsiveness to AVP. Reduced urine osmolality indicates either impaired AVP release (central DI) or action (nephrogenic DI).

The various forms of DI may be differentiated from primary polydipsia in patients with polyuria by performing the water deprivation test, along with administration of AVP. An increase in urine osmolality with exogenous AVP is consistent with central DI, whereas lack of response suggests nephrogenic DI. With fluid restriction leading to a 3% weight loss, patients with primary polydipsia should spontaneously increase their urine osmolality and will not increase their urine osmolality more with exogenous vasopressin. With partial central DI, fluid restriction will not maximally stimulate AVP, thus a further increase in urinary osmolality (>10%) will occur with exogenous vasopressin.

Clinical manifestations

Patients without perturbed neurologic status and with normal thirst mechanisms should complain of thirst. If allowed to progress, hypernatremia becomes associated with confusion, restlessness, irritability, and other neurologic manifestations of cellular dehydration and brain cell shrinkage. Clinical signs may include muscular twitching, hyperreflexia and ataxia. Severe elevations of serum sodium may lead to focal and grand mal seizures, intracerebral hemorrhage, and death. More severe symptoms and signs occur in patients with rapidly rising serum osmolality, extremely elevated serum osmolality, especially above 325 mOsm/kg, and at extremes of age, with the very young and the very old being most vulnerable. Hypernatremia developing over a longer period of time enables brain cells to undergo osmotic adaptation by generating osmolytes (idiogenic osmoles) to guard against cell shrinkage. While protective, they may nonetheless predispose the brain to edema if hypernatremia is corrected rapidly by favoring intracellular fluid shifts.

Therapy

In hypernatremia with extracellular volume depletion, restoration of ECF volume is the primary therapeutic target. Isotonic saline is the fluid of choice, and the volume and rate of administration should be guided by clinical parameters including pulse rate, orthostatic blood pressure measurements, and urine output. Once euvolemia is established, further fluid therapy should be delivered to gradually correct tonicity in the form of hypotonic (0.45%) saline.

In rare patients who develop hypernatremia with extracellular volume expansion, loop diuretics may be employed. Ultrafiltration may sometimes be needed to treat hypernatremia in patients with advanced renal impairment.

In patients with hypernatremia without extracellular volume depletion or expansion, the total body sodium is unchanged, but there is a deficit of total body water. Water can be replaced either orally or parenterally with 5% dextrose in water (D5W) or 0.45% NaCl (half-normal saline). The estimated fluid deficit can be estimated by a formula that uses total body water (TBW), because sodium concentration reflects tonicity in all body compartments. For example, a 75 kg man with a serum sodium concentration of 157 mmol/L would need water as estimated by the following:

$$\text{Actual TBW} = \text{body weight} \times 60\% \ (50\% \text{ in women})$$
$$\text{TBW} = 75 \times 0.6 = 45 \text{ L}$$

Then, desired body water is calculated from the following formula:

$$\frac{\text{Actual serum sodium} \times \text{TBW}}{\text{Desired serum sodium}} = \frac{157 \text{ mmol/L} \times 45/\text{L}}{140 \text{ mmolL}} = 50.5 \text{ L}$$

The estimated water deficit is the difference between desired body water and actual body water. In this example, the administration of 5.5 L (50.5-45 L) should correct the water deficit and normalize the serum sodium concentration. In addition to estimated water deficit, estimated ongoing water losses during the time of repletion should be added. This includes 500-1000 mL/d of insensible losses, with larger amounts in febrile or mechanically ventilated patients.

Water replacement should be carried out gradually over hours to days, unless there is evidence that hypernatremia has evolved quickly. This is because water replacement needs to keep pace with the osmotic adaptation process by which the brain cells keep from shrinking. Replacement also has to be tailored to the presence of neurologic symptoms and signs, which call for more rapid serum sodium correction. Acute symptomatic hypernatremia that developed over hours may be rapidly corrected, as the risk of cerebral edema is minimal. In patients with acute symptomatic hypernatremia, serum sodium should be lowered by 1 mmol/L/h. Once the patient is no longer symptomatic, the correction rate can be reduced to 0.5 mmol/L/h. Hypernatremia that has developed over more than 24 hours, or is of unknown duration, should be corrected with a maximal rate of 0.5 mmol/L/h. Half of the water deficit should be replaced over the first 24 hours, with the remainder over the following 24 hours or longer. The cornerstone of central DI treatment is desmopressin (dDAVP), administered either nasally, intravenously, or subcutaneously. Patients with nephrogenic DI do not respond to exogenous desmopressin. Salt restriction and thiazide diuretics produce mild volume contraction, which helps to decrease urinary output. Nonsteroidal anti-inflammatory drugs also help reduce urine output. Patients with lithium-associated nephrogenic DI may benefit from amiloride.

Hypernatremia: Discharge Checklist

- Have patient and family been educated about signs and symptoms of hypernatremia?
- Are patients being discharged on gastric tube feedings also receiving free water supplementation via the tube several times daily to prevent hypernatremia?

- If the patient has diabetes insipidus, is the treatment appropriate for the form.

Central DI is treated with desmopressin (dDAVP) whereas salt restriction, thiazide diuretics and NSAIDS are useful in the treatment of nephrogenic DI.

- Have blood draws for electrolyte testing and outpatient follow-up been arranged for 1 to 2 weeks after discharge?

SUGGESTED READINGS

Brater DC. Update in diuretic therapy: clinical pharmacology. *Semin Nephrol*. 2011;31:483-494.

Ellison DH, Berl T. Clinical practice. The syndrome of inappropriate antidiuresis. *N Engl J Med*. 2007;356:2064-2072.

Felker GM, Lee KL, Bull DA, et al. Diuretic strategies in patients with acute decompensated heart failure. *N Engl J Med*. 2011;364:797-805.

Schrier RW, Bansal S. Diagnosis and management of hyponatremia in acute illness. *Curr Opin Crit Care*. 2008;14:627-634.

Sterns RH. Disorders of plasma sodium: causes, consequences, and correction. *N Engl J Med*. 2015;372:55-65.

Verbalis JG, Goldsmith SR, Greenberg A, et al. Diagnosis, evaluation, and treatment of hyponatremia: expert panel recommendations. *Am J Med*. 2013;126(10 Suppl 1):S1-42.

CHAPTER 243

Kidney Stones

Navin R. Gupta, MD
Bertrand L. Jaber, MD, MS

Key Clinical Questions

1. How are kidney stones diagnosed?
2. How should kidney stones be managed in the inpatient setting?
3. What medical therapies facilitate stone passage?
4. When is urology or nephrology consultation indicated?
5. What follow-up and further testing is appropriate after discharge?
6. What drugs and dietary therapies provide secondary prevention of kidney stones?

EPIDEMIOLOGY

Kidney stones inflict recurrent episodes of excruciating pain and significant morbidity on a substantial portion of the population, including many young and otherwise healthy individuals. In the United States, the current lifetime incidence of nephrolithiasis is 13% for men and 7% for women. Without treatment, the 5-year recurrence rate following an initial episode is up to 50%. A recent report from the National Health and Nutrition Examination Survey for the period of 1994 to 2010 describes a 70% increase in prevalence of self-reported kidney stones, extending across men and women of all age groups.

Regional variations in the frequency and nature of kidney stone disease exist within the United States, with an increased prevalence in the southeastern region of the country. This variation may be related to differences in climate and sunlight exposure, as well as dietary habits and beverage consumption. Kidney stones develop more frequently among Caucasians than African Americans. Stones in the upper urinary tract are frequently seen in industrialized countries and are associated with a more affluent lifestyle, including high animal protein consumption, gout, and components of the metabolic syndrome, including hypertension, impaired glucose tolerance, increased waist circumference, high triglycerides, and low-high-density lipoprotein cholesterol. Bladder stones are more commonly seen in developing countries and more frequently affect individuals with a poor socioeconomic status.

Patients with kidney stones typically present with renal colic, characterized by severe pain and autonomic symptoms such as lightheadedness, diaphoresis, nausea, and vomiting. The severity of symptoms often results in a visit to a hospital emergency room, often requiring hospitalization and absenteeism from work. In the United States, kidney stones account for more than 2 million outpatient visits, over 600,000 emergency room visits, and approximately 0.4% of hospital admissions. Complications may arise, such as urinary tract obstruction and pyelonephritis, or the need for stone removal by instrumentation, surgery, or extracorporeal shock wave lithotripsy (ESWL). Patients with recurrent stone disease also have a heightened risk of chronic kidney disease. In the year 2000, the annual cost of kidney stones in the United States, including hospitalizations, professional charges, and lost productivity, was estimated at $5.3 billion.

PATHOPHYSIOLOGY AND RISK FACTORS

Kidney stones can form from several substances excreted in the urine, and frequently consist of two or more different substances (**Table 243-1**). Calcareous (calcium oxalate, phosphate, or mixed) stones are by far the most common, accounting for over 80% of kidney stones. Metabolic defects leading to stone formation include hypercalciuria in over 65% of cases, and less frequently hyperuricosuria, hyperoxaluria, hypocitraturia, or some combination thereof.

For a kidney stone to form, the concentration of a dissolved salt must exceed its solubility in urine, a condition known as supersaturation. Supersaturation is favored by increased urinary excretion of stone-forming salts, optimal urinary pH (**Table 243-2**), and decreased urinary volume, which leads to increased urinary concentration. The presence of crystallization facilitators in the urine, such as uric acid, or the absence of crystallization inhibitors, such as citrate, also contributes to stone formation.

TABLE 243-1 Composition of Kidney Stones

Type	Frequency (%)
Calcium	70-88
• Calcium oxalate	36-70
• Calcium phosphate	6-20
• Mixed	11-31
Magnesium ammonium phosphate (struvite)	6-20
Uric acid	6-17
Cystine	0.5-3
Miscellaneous	1-4

Risk factors for kidney stone formation can be divided into diet, stone-provoking conditions, stone-provoking drugs, and anatomic abnormalities. Dietary factors promoting nephrolithiasis include low fluid intake, which promotes urinary supersaturation, high sodium and animal protein intake, which promote hypercalciuria, and high oxalate intake, which promotes hyperoxaluria. In addition, a family history of kidney stones and a personal history of gout also increase the risk of kidney stone disease.

Table 243-3 displays a selected list of stone-provoking conditions, stone-provoking drugs, and anatomic urologic abnormalities associated with stone disease. Of note, roux-en-Y gastric bypass surgery, a common bariatric surgical procedure, is associated with increased intestinal absorption of oxalate and hyperoxaluria, resulting in a long-term risk of kidney stone formation. Major stone-provoking drugs include uricosuric agents, such as probenecid, losartan, and fenofibrate, carbonic anhydrase inhibitors, such as acetazolamide and topiramate, and the antiretroviral agent indinavir, which crystallizes in the urine.

Oxalobacter formigenes and *Lactobacillus* spp. are intestinal bacteria that produce an oxalate-degrading enzyme. The resulting increased intestinal degradation of oxalate may protect against stone formation. Lack of intestinal colonization with *O. formigenes* is prevalent in patients with recurrent calcium oxalate stones due to hyperoxaluria.

CLINICAL PRESENTATION

Patients with kidney stones most often present to the hospital with renal colic. Others present with a urinary tract infection, impaired renal function from obstructive uropathy, or chronic kidney damage. Increasingly, incidental kidney stones are diagnosed on imaging studies in patients admitted to the hospital for other reasons.

Typical renal colic begins with the acute onset of severe pain that awakens the patient from sleep. Colic typically lasts for 1 to 4 hours, followed by gradual improvement. The patient may move ceaselessly, looking for a comfortable position, and may also suffer from nausea, vomiting, and sweating.

TABLE 243-2 Solubility of Stone-forming Salts According to Urinary pH

Solute	Acid pH	Alkaline pH
Urate	↓	↑
Oxalate	↓	↑ or ↓
Phosphate	↑	↓
Cystine	↓	↑

TABLE 243-3 Risk Factors for Kidney Stone Disease

Stone-Provoking Conditions
Calcareous stones
  Hypercalciuria
    Primary hyperparathyroidism
    Milk-alkali syndrome
    Sarcoidosis
    Tuberculosis
    Prolonged immobilization
  Hyperoxaluria
    Crohn disease
    Short gut syndrome
    Roux-en-Y gastric bypass surgery
  Hypocitraturia
    Laxative abuse
    Polycystic kidney disease
    Medullary sponge kidney
    Renal tubular acidosis
  Urate stones
    Hyperuricosuria
    Gouty diathesis
    Myeloproliferative disorders
    Ulcerative colitis
Struvite stones
  Paraplegia
  Neurogenic bladder
  Recurrent urinary tract infections

Stone-provoking Drugs
Oxaluric agent
  Vitamin C (high dose)
Calciuric agent
  Vitamin D (high dose)
Uricosuric agent
  Probenecid
  Losartan
  Fenofibrate
Urinary alkalinizing agent
  Acetazolamide
  Topiramate
Crystalluric agent
  Triamterene
  Sulfonamides
  Indinavir

Anatomic Abnormalities
Medullary sponge kidney
Horseshoe kidney
Pyelocalyceal diverticulum
Megacalyces
Hydrocalyces
Ureteropelvic junction obstruction
Megaureter
Bladder outlet obstruction
Bladder diverticulum
Urethral diverticulum

As shown in **Figure 243-1**, the anatomic site of the stone in the urinary tract influences the radiation of the pain to different locations. Several conditions of the genitourinary, musculoskeletal, gastrointestinal, and cardiovascular systems may produce hematuria, back pain, or abdominal pain, mimicking kidney stones (**Table 243-4**).

INITIAL DIAGNOSTIC EVALUATION

The initial workup of a patient with suspected renal colic includes a urinalysis, urine culture, limited blood work, and an imaging study. The urinalysis may reveal an acid pH (<5.5), suggesting uric acid or cystine stones, or an alkaline pH (>7.5), suggesting calcium phosphate stones in the setting of renal tubular acidosis, or struvite stones, associated with infection with a urea-splitting bacteria such as *Proteus* or *Klebsiella*. Microscopic examination of the urinary sediment may reveal specific crystals (**Figure 243-2**).

Urate crystals can be rhomboid, needle shaped, or amorphous in shape (**Figures 243-2A** to **C**). Oxalate crystals can be dumbbell or cigar shaped (**Figure 243-2D**, calcium oxalate monohydrate) or envelope shaped (**Figure 243-2E**, calcium oxalate dihydrate). Phosphate crystals can be in a coffin-lid structure (**Figure 243-2F**, triple phosphate) or a granular precipitate (**Figure 243-2G**, amorphous phosphate). Cystine crystals are hexaedric and flat (**Figure 243-2H**), and pathognomonic for cystinuria. A cyanide-nitroprusside test resulting in purple-red discoloration of the urine confirms the presence of cystine crystals.

A limited blood work panel for the evaluation of kidney stone disease includes serum electrolytes to evaluate for renal tubular acidosis; blood urea nitrogen and creatinine to assess kidney function; calcium, albumin, and phosphorus to evaluate for primary

TABLE 243-4 Differential Diagnosis of Kidney Stone Disease

Conditions Associated with Pain	
Genitourinary system	Acute pyelonephritis, testicular torsion, epididymitis, cystitis, urethritis, prostatitis, menstrual pain, pelvic inflammatory disease, ruptured ovarian cyst, ovarian torsion
Musculoskeletal system	Abdominal muscular pain, rib pain
Gastrointestinal system	Biliary colic, cholecystitis, gastritis, acute pancreatitis, peptic ulcer disease, appendicitis, acute diverticulitis
Cardiovascular system	Acute myocardial infarction, aortic aneurysm
Miscellaneous	Retroperitoneal fibrosis, herpes zoster, pleural pain
Conditions Associated with Hematuria	

Acute glomerulonephritis, arteriovenous malformations, anticoagulant use, cystitis, prostatitis, neoplasia

hyperparathyroidism; and uric acid to evaluate for gout. An elevated serum creatinine may reflect acute kidney injury from bilateral obstructive uropathy, unilateral obstruction in the setting of a single functioning kidney, preexisting chronic kidney disease, extracellular fluid volume depletion, or infection. A urine culture should be obtained to rule out concomitant urinary tract infection, particularly with the urea-splitting bacteria such as *Proteus* that lead to struvite stones. Fever should trigger a more thorough investigation for pyelonephritis and sepsis.

The imaging modality of choice is a nonenhanced helical computed tomography (CT) scan, which has 98% sensitivity and 97% specificity for the diagnosis of kidney stones as small as 1 mm in diameter. Of note, indinavir stones are radiolucent and undetectable by CT scan. Ultrasonography can only visualize the kidney and proximal ureter, detecting stones equal to or greater than 3 mm in diameter. Consequently, it has a sensitivity and specificity of 61% and 97%, respectively. However, due to the lack of radiation exposure, ultrasonography may have a role for pregnant women and children. An abdominal plain x-ray (ie, kidneys, ureters, and bladder x-ray) visualizes the entire urinary tract proximal to the urethra, detecting 90% of stones greater than 2 mm in diameter, but cannot detect radiolucent uric acid stones.

TREATMENT OF AN ACUTE EPISODE

■ INITIAL EMERGENCY ROOM MANAGEMENT

Symptomatic treatment includes administration of intravenous or oral fluids to facilitate stone passage, adequate pain control with nonsteroidal anti-inflammatory drugs or opioids, and antiemetics. Although parenteral ketorolac has been shown be as effective as opioids for the treatment of renal colic, this drug should be used cautiously among patients with impaired kidney function, as repeated doses may precipitate acute kidney injury. Nonsteroidal anti-inflammatory drugs have the added benefit of reducing ureteral inflammation surrounding the stone, thus facilitating stone passage. Antibiotics are not routinely recommended for kidney stone disease, unless there is concomitant infection. To facilitate stone passage, both calcium channel blockers, such as nifedipine, and α-blockers, such as tamsulosin, have been shown to increase the likelihood of stone passage. In one study, 63% of physicians practicing in an emergency department used α-blockers for medical expulsive therapy.

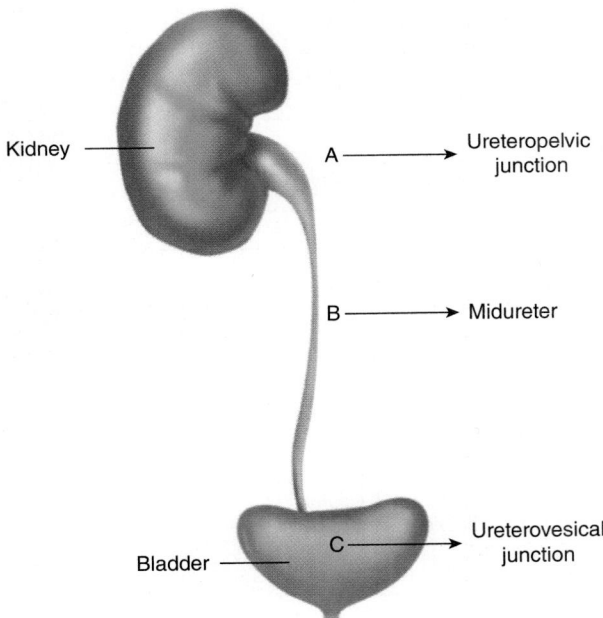

Figure 243-1 *Characteristics of renal colic according to stone location. (A) Stone at the ureteropelvic junction; mild dull to excruciating sharp pain in the flank, often radiating to the upper ipsilateral abdominal quadrant. (B) Stone in the midureter; pain radiating caudally and anteriorly toward the mid- and lower abdomen in a curved band-like fashion, initially parallel to the lower-costal margin, but then deviating caudally toward the bony pelvis and inguinal ligament. (C) Stone in the distal ureter; pain radiating into the scrotum or the tip of the penis in men, and associated with urinary frequency and urgency, dysuria, and gross hematuria.*

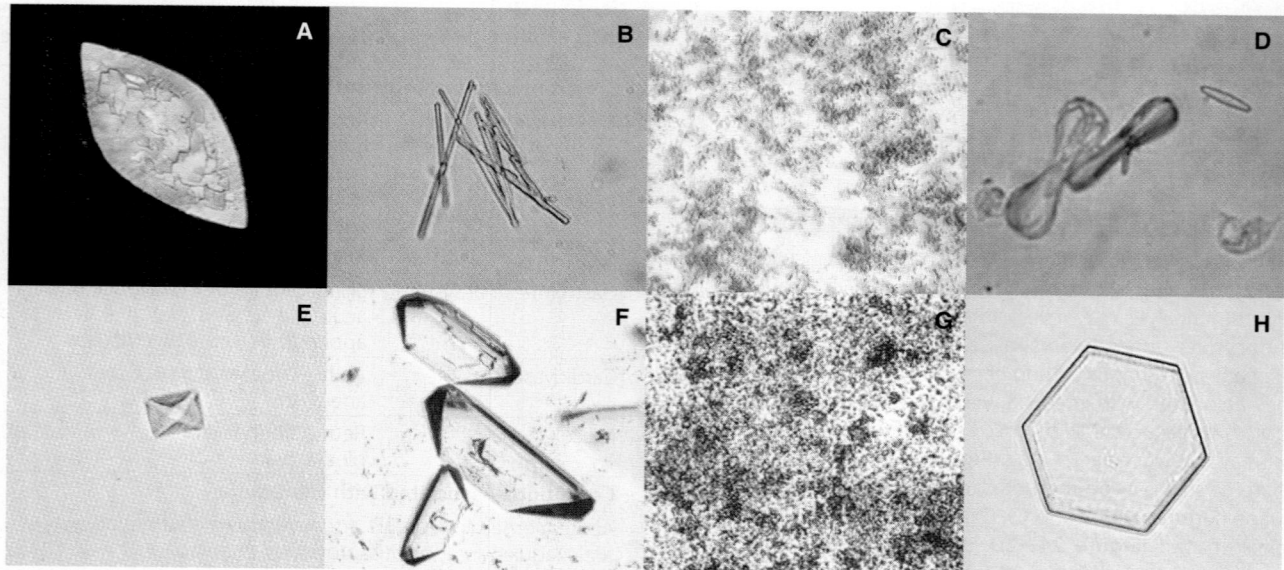

Figure 243-2 *Urinary crystal identification. Rhomboid* (A), *needle-shaped* (B), *or amorphous* (C), *urate; dumbbell-shaped or cigar-shaped calcium oxalate monohydrate* (D), *envelope-shaped calcium oxalate dihydrate* (E), *coffin-lid-shaped triple phosphate* (F), *or amorphous phosphate* (G). (A-C, E-H: Reproduced, with permission from Graff L. *A handbook of routine urinalysis.* Philadelphia: Lippincott, Williams & Wilkins, 1983.) (D: Reproduced from Morfin and Chin. Urinary calcium oxalate crystals in ethylene glycol intoxication. *N Engl J Med.* 2005;353:e21. With permission from the Massachusetts Medical Society. Copyright © 2005 Massachusetts Medical Society, all rights reserved.)

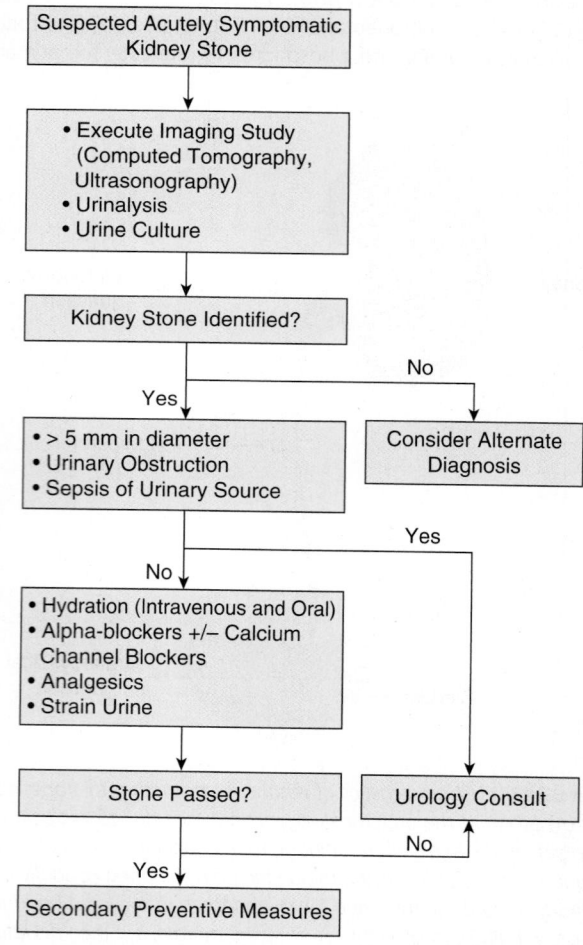

Figure 243-3 *Diagnostic and treatment algorithm for an acutely symptomatic kidney stone.*

PRACTICE POINT

Medical expulsive therapy for kidney stones

● Kidney stones irritate the lining of the ureter, producing pain and spasm. Ureteral spasm interferes with peristalsis and decreases the likelihood of spontaneous stone passage. Calcium channel blockers and α-blockers at appropriate doses relax the distal ureter without abolishing peristalsis. This leads to a reduction in symptoms of colic and allows a greater chance of stone passage. The best-studied agents are the calcium channel blocker nifedipine, given at relatively low doses (30-40 mg daily), and the α-blocker tamsulosin, dosed at 0.4 mg daily. A 4-week trial of either agent may be reasonable for stable patients with distal ureteral stones measuring less than 10 mm. Both nifedipine and tamsulosin may cause orthostatic hypotension. Tamsulosin may be more effective than nifedipine, but causes the additional side effect of abnormal ejaculation in men. Corticosteroids and anticholinergics confer little additional benefit in patients already taking an α-blocker or calcium channel blocker.

■ INDICATIONS FOR HOSPITALIZATION

Failure to control pain, impaired renal function in the setting of obstructive stones, and suspected pyelonephritis with sepsis should trigger hospitalization. If the patient is likely to require a urologic intervention, the decision for hospitalization might be made on an individual basis in conjunction with the urology service. **Figure 243-3** displays the diagnostic and treatment algorithm for an acutely symptomatic kidney stone.

■ UROLOGY CONSULTATION

Stones larger than 5 mm are less likely to be expelled spontaneously than smaller ones (**Table 243-5**). Consequently, urologic consultation

TABLE 243-5 Likelihood of Passage of Ureteral Stones According to Size

Size of the Stone	Mean Days Until Passage	Likelihood of Need for Intervention (%)
≤ 2 mm	8	3
3 mm	12	14
4-6 mm	22	50
>6 mm*	–	99

*Unlikely to pass spontaneously.
(Reproduced from Teichman. Acute renal colic from ureteral calculus. *N Engl J Med*. 2004;684-693. With permission from the Massachusetts Medical Society.)

is warranted if the stone does not pass spontaneously, is larger than 5 mm in diameter, causes urinary obstruction, or is associated with urinary sepsis. If endourologic intervention becomes necessary, a variety of approaches can be employed, depending on the stone location. These include ureteroscopy with placement of a double J-stent for stones in the proximal ureter, basket stone retrieval for those in the distal ureter, and extracorporeal shock-wave lithotripsy for stones in the renal pelvis. **Figure 243-4** displays a proposed urologic treatment algorithm according to size, location, and type of stone.

■ NEPHROLOGY CONSULTATION

In-hospital nephrology consultation is advised in the setting of nonresolving acute kidney injury or advanced preexisting chronic kidney disease. Outpatient nephrology referral may be warranted for secondary prevention, particularly among recurrent stone formers, or first stone formers who have conditions or who take medications known to provoke stone formation. (See below for a more detailed discussion of outpatient management.)

LONG-TERM MANAGEMENT OF KIDNEY STONES

■ GENERAL CONSIDERATIONS

In patients without risk factors for recurrent stone formation (see Table 243-3), a simplified evaluation is usually sufficient. This consists of a dietary and medical history, review of the urinalysis, urine culture, helical CT scan, blood tests obtained during hospitalization, and a stone analysis, if available. Serum levels of parathyroid hormone and angiotensin-converting enzyme may be indicated if hypercalcemia is present. However, patients with recurrent stones and those with a positive family history of stones or medical conditions associated with stone recurrence should have further evaluation.

Comprehensive evaluation includes keeping a dietary journal and completing a food frequency questionnaire. A 24-hour urine collection should also be performed, with measurement of creatinine (to confirm adequacy of collection), volume (to assess fluid intake), calcium (to assess for hypercalciuria), oxalate (to assess for hyperoxaluria), uric acid (to assess for hyperuricosuria), citrate (to assess for hypocitraturia), and cystine (to assess for cystinuria). Additional 24-hour measurements include excretion of urinary sulfate, which reflects animal protein intake, urinary sodium, which promotes hypercalciuria if elevated, and magnesium excretion rate, which promotes stone formation if low. Several 24-hour urinary collection kits are commercially available in the United States to assist in this metabolic evaluation. These also provide supersaturation indices pertaining to calcium oxalate, urate, and calcium phosphate precipitation in the urine.

■ SECONDARY PREVENTION

Recommendations for secondary prevention of kidney stones are based largely on observational studies and a handful of randomized controlled trials.

Diet and lifestyle modification

Every kidney stone patient should have a high fluid intake, at least 3 L/d, allowing for excretion of dilute urine throughout the entire day and night. To ensure dilute urine at night, patients must drink one to two eight-ounce glasses of water at bedtime, followed by another eight-ounce glass during the night, as after voiding. Unfortunately, frequent nocturia limits adherence to this regimen, and daytime access to water during work hours might be difficult for some patients. In addition to the total fluid consumed, the type of beverage might also play a role. In middle-aged women, coffee, tea,

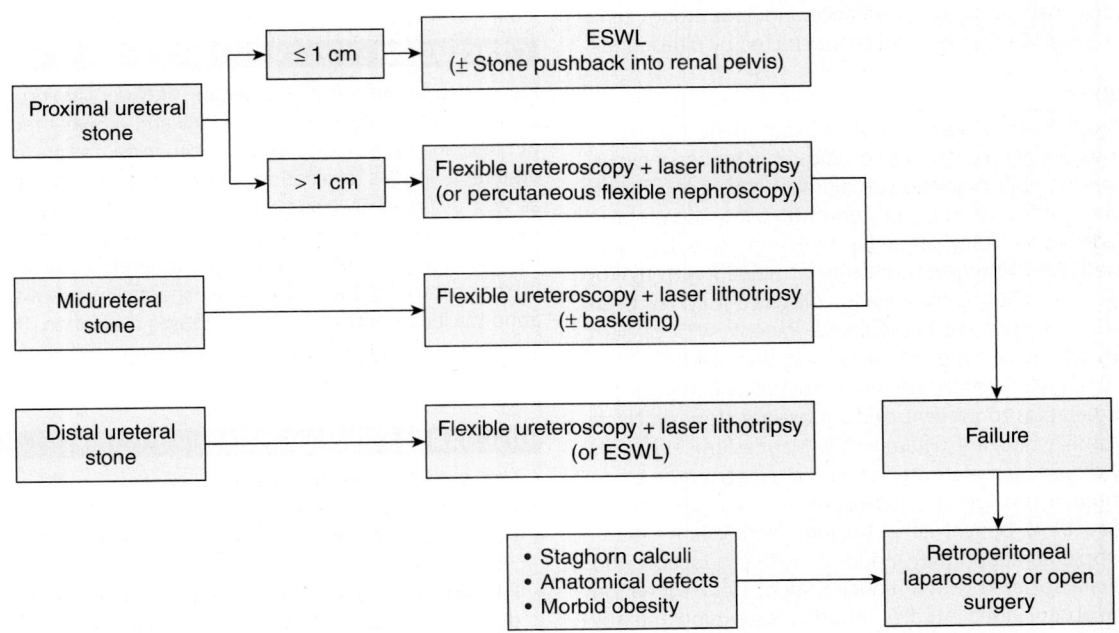

Figure 243-4 *Urologic treatment algorithm according to size, location, and type of kidney stone. ESWL, extracorporeal shock-wave lithotripsy.*

and wine intake has been shown to be independently protective, whereas grapefruit juice has been shown to promote kidney stones. These findings were confirmed in men, with the additional finding that the risk of kidney stones was reduced by beer and increased by apple juice. While strongly hopped beers such as European lagers may contain significant amounts of oxalate, which increases kidney stone risk, beer consumption also increases urinary flow and dilution, likely explaining their neutral or even beneficial effects in observational studies. Dietary sodium restriction to less than 2 g/d should also be recommended to all patients, as high sodium intake increases urinary calcium excretion and facilitates calcium stone formation.

Dietary calcium intake has variable effects on stone formation. Excess calcium intake, especially if combined with vitamin D3 supplementation, invariably leads to increased calcium absorption and hypercalciuria. However, dietary calcium restriction reduces enteral chelation of dietary oxalate, facilitating oxalate absorption and subsequent urinary excretion, and increasing the risk of recurrent calcium oxalate stones. Calcium restriction also leads to loss of bone mass and a higher likelihood of osteoporosis. Experts recommend avoidance of extremes of calcium intake, and remaining within the recommended daily allowance (RDA) for calcium of 800 to 1000 mg/d.

Patients with calcium oxalate stones should limit daily intake of animal protein to 0.8 g/kg of body weight, which is the RDA. High-protein diets increase urinary calcium excretion because the amino acids, methionine, cysteine, and cystine, oxidize sulfur to sulfate, which is excreted with calcium to maintain electroneutrality.

Dietary oxalate restriction is recommended in oxalate stone formers. Foods with high oxalate content include peanuts, tea, instant coffee, rhubarb, beets, beans, berries, chocolate, spinach and other dark leafy greens, oranges, tofu, sweet potatoes, and draft beer. (The high oxalate content of coffee, tea, and beer is negated by their diuretic effects.) Foods with a high purine content, such as red meat, organ meats, beer, and cruciferous vegetables, such as broccoli and cauliflower, increase urinary uric acid excretion and should be restricted in those with uric acid stones.

For indinavir-associated kidney stones, which occur in 10% to 15% of patients after 6 months of therapy initiation, the drug should be temporarily or permanently discontinued. On urine sediment, indinavir crystals have a starry appearance. Indinavir stones tend to be radiolucent on CT scan and are best detected by ultrasound.

Drug therapy

In recurrent stone formers, specific pharmacologic therapies should be added for secondary prevention. For calcareous stones, if hypercalciuria is present, high-dose thiazide diuretics have been shown to be consistently effective, in conjunction with a low-sodium diet. Options include hydrochlorothiazide (up to 50 mg twice daily) and chlorthalidone (12.5-100 mg/d). Amiloride combined with hydrochlorothiazide (10 mg/50 mg combination pill twice daily) has been used in an effort to minimize hypokalemia. Patients with calcium oxalate stones, who have hyperuricosuria and normocalciuria, have been shown to benefit from the use of allopurinol (300 mg daily).

Unproven therapies to prevent calcium oxalate stones include magnesium and pyridoxine (vitamin B6). Magnesium enhances the solubility of urinary oxalate. In clinical trials, magnesium oxide and magnesium hydroxide are ineffective in stone prevention, but there may be a benefit of potassium magnesium citrate. Pyridoxine supplementation may reduce oxalate production, and large doses are associated with a reduced risk of stone formation in women in observational studies. Another promising therapy for calcium oxalate stone formers with hyperoxaluria is oxalate-metabolizing probiotic microorganisms, such as *Lactobacillus* species or *O. formigenes*.

In enteric hyperoxaluria due to malabsorption, as in inflammatory bowel disease, dietary oxalate restriction should be initiated. If this is unsuccessful, a low-fat diet, calcium carbonate supplements, medium-chain fatty acid supplementation, and enteral-binding therapy with cholestyramine can be attempted alone or in combination.

Hypocitraturia warrants potassium citrate supplementation, at a minimum dose of 40 to 60 mEq/d in two to three divided doses. Sodium-based citrate formulations should be avoided, due to their high sodium content. In calcium phosphate stones, citrate supplementation should be used with caution, since excessive urinary alkalinization might promote calcium phosphate precipitation.

In hyperuricosuria, in addition to reducing purine intake, potassium citrate supplementation is useful to alkalinize the urine and maximize urate solubility. If citrate alone cannot consistently raise the urine pH, an evening dose of acetazolamide may be added. Allopurinol and febuxostat, two xanthine oxidase inhibitors, are equally effective in preventing recurrent calcium-containing stones in patients with hyperuricosuria.

Cystinuria is a rare inherited tubular disorder of amino acid transport that leads to increased excretion of cystine, as well as ornithine, lysine, and arginine, which do not form stones. This autosomal recessive disorder has a prevalence of 1 in 7000. Patients develop symptoms from cystine stones beginning in the second and third decades of life. Cystine stones are extremely hard and resistant to ESWL. Patients are also prone to develop calcium oxalate stones, from associated hypercalciuria, hyperuricosuria, and hypocitraturia. Urinary cystine solubility is pH-dependent, and urine alkalinization is the mainstay of treatment. In mild-to-moderate cystinuria, treatment consists of mild sodium restriction, potassium citrate supplementation to alkalinize the urine pH, and high fluid intake. The patient should keep a log of urinary pH results to self-monitor therapy. Captopril or tiopronin, which forms soluble complexes with cysteine, should be given in more severe cystinuria.

In recurrent struvite stones, the chronic use of suppressive antibiotics or urease inhibitors such as acetohydroxamic acid may be considered.

All dietary and pharmacologic interventions should be followed up with a repeat 24-hour urine collection 3 to 6 months after the intervention in order to monitor treatment success and adherence.

CONCLUSION

Kidney stone disease is a common and debilitating urinary tract disorder, with a lifetime risk of ~10% and a 5-year recurrence rate of 50%. First-time stone formers without risk factors for recurrence require a limited evaluation. However, recurrent stone formers as well as first-time stone formers with risk factors for recurrence require a more extensive evaluation. Dietary interventions and lifestyle changes are uniformly recommended, but the remainder of the therapy is often tailored to specific metabolic and urinary abnormalities identified in the diagnostic evaluation. The long-term commitment and adherence to dietary and lifestyle changes and pharmacologic treatment remains a challenging task.

DISCHARGE CHECKLIST

- Has pain control been achieved?
- Is renal function stable?
- Has a decision been made regarding the need for urologic intervention?
- For patients who have not passed a stone at the time of hospital discharge: has a strainer been provided to retrieve a stone, in case of spontaneous expulsion? Is the patient being discharged on medical therapy to aid stone expulsion? (Tamsulosin is typically given for 4 weeks or until the stone has passed.)

- Has the patient been counseled about diet and lifestyle modification? All stone formers should be counseled to minimize their sodium intake, and increase their fluid intake. Patients known to have oxalate stones should be instructed about limiting their intake of animal protein and oxalate; urate stone formers should be counseled about decreasing their purine intake; and a thiazide diuretic should be considered in patients known to have hypercalciuria.
- Has outpatient follow-up with urology been arranged? (This is usually indicated, especially if an outpatient procedure is being contemplated.)
- Has nephrology follow-up been arranged for patients who are recurrent stone formers, or otherwise at high risk for recurrence?

SUGGESTED READINGS

Bao Y, Wei Q. Water for preventing urinary stones. *Cochrane Database Syst Rev.* 2012(6):CD004292.

Fink H, Wilt T, Eidman K, et al. Medical management to prevent recurrent nephrolithiasis in adults: a systematic review for an American College of Physicians clinical guideline. *Ann Intern Med.* 2013;158:535-543.

Goldfarb DS, MacDonald PA, Gunawardhana L, et al. Randomized controlled trial of febuxostat versus allopurinol or placebo in individuals with higher urinary acid excretion and calcium stones. *Clin J Am Soc Nephrol.* 2013;8(11):1960-1967.

Hollingsworth JM, Rogers MA, Kaufman SR, et al. Medical therapy to facilitate urinary stone passage: a meta-analysis. *Lancet.* 2006;368(9542):1171-1179.

Morfin J, Chin A. Images in clinical medicine. Urinary calcium oxalate crystals in ethylene glycol intoxication. *N Engl J Med.* 2005;353(24):e21.

Pearle M, Goldfarb D, Assimos D, et al. Medical management of kidney stones: American Urological Association Guideline. *J Urol.* 2014;192:316-324.

Qaseem A, Dallas P, Forciea M, et al. Dietary and pharmacologic management to present recurrent nephrolithiasis in adults: a clinical practice guideline from the American College of Physicians. *Ann Intern Med.* 2014;161:659-667.

Smith-Bindman R, Aubin C, Bailitz J, et al. Ultrasonography versus computed tomography for suspected nephrolithiasis. *N Engl J Med.* 2014;371:1100-1110.

Teichman JM. Clinical practice. Acute renal colic from ureteral calculus. *N Engl J Med.* 2004;350:684-693.

CHAPTER 244

Secondary Hypertension

William J. Elliott, MD, PhD

Key Clinical Questions

1. Which patients should be evaluated for secondary causes of hypertension in the inpatient setting?

2. What are the most common secondary causes of hypertension in hospitalized patients?

3. What screening and diagnostic tests are best for each?

4. What specific therapy or therapies are currently recommended?

5. What follow-up should be recommended after discharge?

INTRODUCTION

Hypertension affects 29% of the American public, and a greater proportion of hospital inpatients. Hospitalized patients are older than the general population; the prevalence of hypertension is 65% in those aged 60 years and older, and 77% in those aged 80 years and older. In addition, hypertension is a major risk factor for cardiovascular and renal diseases that lead to inpatient admission. Poorly controlled hypertension among general medical inpatients is most often related to other conditions, such as pain, agitation from delirium, and substance withdrawal. Secondary hypertension has a prevalence of less than 5% in the general population, but is more common among inpatients. This is due to three types of selection bias: (1) negative screening for secondary hypertension in outpatients, who are seldom hospitalized for evaluation and are at low risk of hospitalization for other causes; (2) patients admitted for hypertensive emergencies; and (3) patients with secondary hypertension admitted for diagnostic and therapeutic procedures, often for other diagnoses. For example, 13% of patients undergoing cardiac or peripheral arterial catheterization have a documented stenosis in a renal artery (discovered during "drive-by angiograms"). Secondary causes of hypertension should at least be considered in hypertensive inpatients, especially younger ones, ensuring that these patients are assessed at least once for secondary hypertension during their lifetime. In addition, some causes are curable or at least amenable to intervention, such as pheochromocytoma, Conn adenoma, and fibromuscular dysplasia. This may obviate the need to take long-term antihypertensive medications, improving the cost-effectiveness of screening young patients.

PRACTICE POINT

- A workup for secondary hypertension should be performed in all patients admitted to the hospital with a primary diagnosis of hypertensive urgency or hypertensive emergency, if not previously done.

CRITERIA FOR HOSPITAL ADMISSION

Secondary hypertension leads to hospital admission when there is a hypertensive emergency (severely elevated blood pressure and acute, ongoing target-organ damage). See Chapter 91. These patients have a high prevalence of secondary hypertension, and the hypertensive emergency is often the first real clue to the presence of a secondary cause. After stabilization of these patients with short-acting, intravenous antihypertensive drugs, attention should be focused on developing an appropriate antihypertensive drug regimen and excluding secondary hypertension.

PRACTICE POINT

- There are many reasons why a hospitalized patient may have severe hypertension, including pain, fluid overload, fragmentary knowledge of the patient's home medications, and drug and alcohol withdrawal. Clinicians should seek out precipitating factors that commonly raise blood pressure in the acutely ill and may require a different approach from simply prescribing antihypertensive medications.

Occasionally, secondary hypertension becomes an issue in patients admitted for diagnostic or therapeutic procedures only indirectly related to hypertension. Examples include hypertensive patients with incidentally discovered adrenal masses, individuals who have incidental or "drive-by" renal angiograms after a planned coronary or carotid catheterization, and patients with an increase of greater than 25% in serum creatinine after administration of an angiotensin-converting enzyme (ACE) inhibitor or angiotensin receptor blocker (ARB). Hospitalists caring for these patients should pursue appropriate diagnostic evaluation and treatment of secondary hypertension before discharge.

PRACTICE POINT

- A primary diagnosis of hypertensive crisis—a surge in blood pressure accompanied by acute, ongoing, end-organ damage—or a hypertensive urgency—a surge in blood pressure without such end-organ damage—may be the first clue to the presence of secondary hypertension. After stabilization of these patients with short-acting, intravenous antihypertensive drugs and initiating an appropriate antihypertensive drug regimen, secondary causes of hypertension should be considered, especially in younger patients.

CLINICAL SYNDROMES

The most common secondary causes of hypertension in hospitalized patients are listed in **Table 244-1**. Note that the most common type of hypertension in hospitalized patients is still primary (formerly *essential*) hypertension.

■ SLEEP APNEA

Evaluation

An underappreciated piece of collateral damage from the obesity epidemic is that sleep apnea has probably become the most common cause of resistant hypertension. Hypertension in obstructive sleep apnea (OSA) results from multiple mechanisms. Hypoxia and hypercarbia are potent stimulators of sympathetic tone, and also contribute to oxidative stress and endothelial dysfunction. The abrupt decrease in intrathoracic pressure during apneic episodes raises left ventricular wall pressure and myocardial oxygen demand, contributing to atherosclerosis and left ventricular hypertrophy. Recurrent episodes of arousal lead to sleep fragmentation, stress, and further increases in sympathetic tone and catecholamine levels. Aldosterone levels are often high in patients with OSA, likely due in part to increased sympathetic tone. Edema from aldosterone-mediated sodium retention may shift nocturnally from the legs to the neck, increasing upper airway resistance and aggravating OSA.

OSA should be suspected in hypertensive patients with obesity and daytime sleepiness. Patients and partners should be asked about snoring and witnessed apneic events. A sleep study (polysomnography) should be obtained, either in the inpatient or outpatient setting. Overnight pulse oximetry to look for frequent nocturnal desaturations may be useful to screen for OSA in the inpatient setting, when a sleep study cannot be obtained. It is reasonable to measure thyrotropin (TSH) levels in suspected OSA, if this has not recently been done.

Inpatient management

Continuous positive airway pressure (CPAP) has been shown to reduce 24-hour ambulatory systolic and diastolic blood pressure, and especially nocturnal blood pressure, in individuals with sleep apnea. Hypertensive individuals with proven sleep apnea should be treated with a trial of CPAP. There is some evidence that aldosterone antagonists such as spironolactone may have beneficial effects in reducing hypertension and apneic events in OSA.

■ CHRONIC KIDNEY DISEASE

Evaluation

This secondary cause of hypertension differs from others in at least two respects: it is usually not remediable, and it may be both a

TABLE 244-1 Common Secondary Causes of Resistant Hypertension

Diagnosis	Key Features	Risk Factors	Relative Prevalence	Screening Tests
Sleep apnea	Daytime somnolence, loud snoring and breathing cessation during sleep, morning headache	Obesity, age	60%-70%	Sleep study
Primary hyperaldosteronism	Hypokalemia, sleep apnea symptoms, resistant hypertension	Sleep apnea	7%-20%	Aldosterone/renin ratio
Renovascular hypertension	Abdominal bruit, "bump" in serum creatinine after ACE inhibitor or ARB	Young women (fibromuscular disease); atherosclerotic disease in older smokers	2%-24%	Doppler ultrasound
Drug and alcohol abuse	Multiple mechanisms, including high sympathetic tone, vasoconstriction, endothelial dysfunction	Cocaine, methamphetamine, heavy alcohol use	2%-4%	History, toxicology screen
Chronic kidney disease	$eGFR < 60$ mL/min/1.73 m^2, albumin/creatinine ratio > 300 μg/mg	Hypertension, diabetes	1%-2%	Serum creatinine, first morning voided urine for albumin-to-creatinine ratio
Cushing syndrome	Hypertension, hyperglycemia, abdominal striae, proximal muscle weakness, hirsutism	Women (Cushing disease); men (ectopic corticotropin production)	< 1%	Urinary free cortisol; midnight serum (or salivary) cortisol
Pheochromocytoma	Hypertension, hyperhidrosis, headache (often in paroxysms)	Phakomatoses, multiple endocrine neoplasia syndromes	< 1%	Plasma metanephrines vs 24-h urine for VMA and metanephrines
Coarctation of the aorta	Blood pressure differences across limbs; systolic murmur posteriorly	Turner syndrome; other congenital arterial anomalies	< 1%	Echocardiogram (especially the sternal notch view)

ACE, angiotensin-converting enzyme; ARB, angiotensin receptor blocker; VMA, vanillylmandelic acid. Prevalence data from *JAMA*. 2014;311(21):2216-2224.

cause and a consequence of hypertension. Chronic kidney disease is defined as 3 months or more of an estimated glomerular filtration rate (eGFR) of less than 60 mL/min/1.73 m², or kidney damage defined as pathologic abnormalities, abnormal imaging studies, or elevated blood or urine markers of kidney injury (usually albuminuria > 30 μg/mg creatinine in a first-morning voided urine specimen). In large population-based studies, more advanced chronic kidney disease is linked to greater risks of death and hospitalization. As a result, this secondary cause of hypertension is thought to be about 5- to 10-fold more common in hospitalized patients than in the general US population.

Testing for chronic kidney disease is part of the admitting process for essentially every inpatient, with a serum creatinine (and in most hospitals, a calculated eGFR, based on the most recent update of the Modification of Diet in Renal Disease, or the Chronic Kidney Disease-Epidemiology Collaboration, equations) and a urinalysis. Occasionally, the urinalysis can be falsely negative for protein if performed on a very dilute sample. If this is suspected, a first-morning voided urine specimen should be obtained to measure the albumin-to-creatinine ratio.

Inpatient management

Intensive lowering of blood pressure is an effective means to prevent or delay the progression of chronic kidney disease to end-stage renal disease. Most authorities recommend that patients with chronic kidney diseases should have frequent urinalyses and determinations of eGFR, and an ACE inhibitor or an ARB as part of their medication regimen, if possible. A lower-than-usual blood pressure goal (eg, < 130/80 mm Hg) has not improved outcomes in 3 clinical trials, but is still "suggested" (a weaker option than "recommended") by the Kidney Disease: improving Global Outcomes (KDIGO) 2012 clinical practice guideline.

■ PRIMARY HYPERALDOSTERONISM

Evaluation

The clinical presentation of primary hyperaldosteronism is non-specific. Patients are occasionally diagnosed because of hypertension with spontaneous hypokalemia, or more severe hypokalemia on diuretic therapy than expected, but most patients with primary hyperaldosteronism are not hypokalemic.

Primary hyperaldosteronism is more commonly recognized now than in the past, probably because of the widespread use of the plasma aldosterone/plasma renin ratio as a screening test in patients with refractory hypertension. In older series, primary hyperaldosteronism was found in only 0.1% to 0.5% of hypertensive patients, with most patients having hypokalemia and aldosterone-producing adrenal adenomas (Conn syndrome). While the exact prevalence and significance of primary hyperaldosteronism in hypertension remains unclear, this is almost certainly an underestimate. Some studies have found primary hyperaldosteronism in up to 5% to 10% of hypertensive patients, and in patients with resistant or refractory hypertension, the prevalence may be as high as 11% to 23%. In recent series, 35% of cases were due to aldosterone-producing adenomas, 60% were due to bilateral adrenal hyperplasia, and the rest were due to adrenal carcinoma, unilateral adrenal hyperplasia, glucocorticoid-remediable hyperaldosteronism, and other causes.

The renewed interest in primary hyperaldosteronism also stems from the availability of new therapies, such as laparoscopic adrenalectomy, and evidence that primary hyperaldosteronism has morbidities in addition to hypertension. Compared with patients with essential hypertension and similar levels of blood pressure elevation, patients with primary hyperaldosteronism are at higher risk of left ventricular hypertrophy, diastolic dysfunction, myocardial infarction, atrial fibrillation, stroke, albuminuria, and metabolic syndrome. As noted above,

hyperaldosteronism seems to be especially common in obesity and sleep apnea. Possible explanations include renin release due to sympathetic nervous system activation during apneic episodes, adipocyte production of angiotensinogen, and aldosterone release driven by oxidized fatty acids.

The currently recommended initial screening test for primary hyperaldosteronism is the plasma aldosterone/plasma renin ratio, or ARR (**Figure 244-1**). A sample is drawn from a patient who has been seated quietly for at least 15 minutes. Generally no changes are necessary in dietary salt intake or antihypertensive medications, except aldosterone antagonists, which should be stopped. Inhibitors of the renin-angiotensin system (including β-blockers) can improve the diagnostic performance of the test and may account for some of the controversy surrounding its use. In properly selected patients, an ARR of 20 to 40 (when the plasma renin activity is expressed in ng of angiotensin II/mL/h, and the aldosterone level in ng/dL) raises the suspicion of primary hyperaldosteronism. Similarly, the utility of the ARR is inversely proportional to the plasma-renin activity, as very low levels (eg, < 0.2 ng/mL/h, as a possible consequence of a high-sodium diet, or low-renin hypertension) increase the ARR exponentially.

An elevated ARR is typically followed by one of four confirmatory tests, usually on the next hospital day. Clinicians generally prefer measuring plasma aldosterone before and after either saline infusion (2 L over 4 hours), or oral captopril (25 mg given 2 hours earlier), because both the fludrocortisone suppression (0.1 mg every 6 hours for 4 days) and oral sodium loading (12 gm daily for 4 days) tests require too long a preparation period. The challenges with these tests involve the risk of hypotension with captopril, or volume overload with saline loading. If the patient is young or has a family history of hyperaldosteronism, a morning sample of plasma for 18-hydroxycortisol and 18-oxo-cortisol levels may be helpful, as low or normal levels effectively rule out glucocorticoid-remediable aldosteronism (which accounts for less than 1% of primary hyperaldosteronism in most series).

Inpatient management

If confirmatory testing shows no evidence of aldosterone suppression, a decision must be made about the risks and benefits of possible surgery. Many favor simply treating such patients with aldosterone antagonists, as most (about two-thirds) will not have surgically remediable tumors. Should laparoscopic surgery be available and the patient and physician agree, an adrenal CT scan may be performed. If there is a unilateral hypodense (< 10 Hounsfield units) nodule larger than 1 cm, most patients under the age of 40 years are offered surgery. If the patient is older than 40 years or has a high clinical probability of a tumor and either normal adrenals, micronodularity, or bilateral masses, adrenal venous sampling is first performed to localize the aldosterone-producing adrenal adenoma, before surgery. Otherwise, the patient is treated with an aldosterone antagonist. Spironolactone is less costly, but eplerenone has fewer adverse effects.

Laparoscopic adrenalectomy is the preferred surgical approach because of lower rates of morbidity and shorter hospital stays. Cure rates of 56% to 77% have been cited, although eukalemia may be delayed for several days, and complete normalization of blood pressure (< 140/90 mm Hg without drug therapy) occurs in only about one-third. Because of the reduced medication burden (including adverse effects and potassium supplementation and its monitoring), and improved blood pressure, adrenalectomy is said to be less expensive than medical therapy.

For patients with hyperaldosteronism and a positive Berlin questionnaire suggestive of sleep apnea, referral to a sleep center for polysomnographic testing is appropriate. Many of these patients will have improved blood pressure control on an aldosterone antagonist.

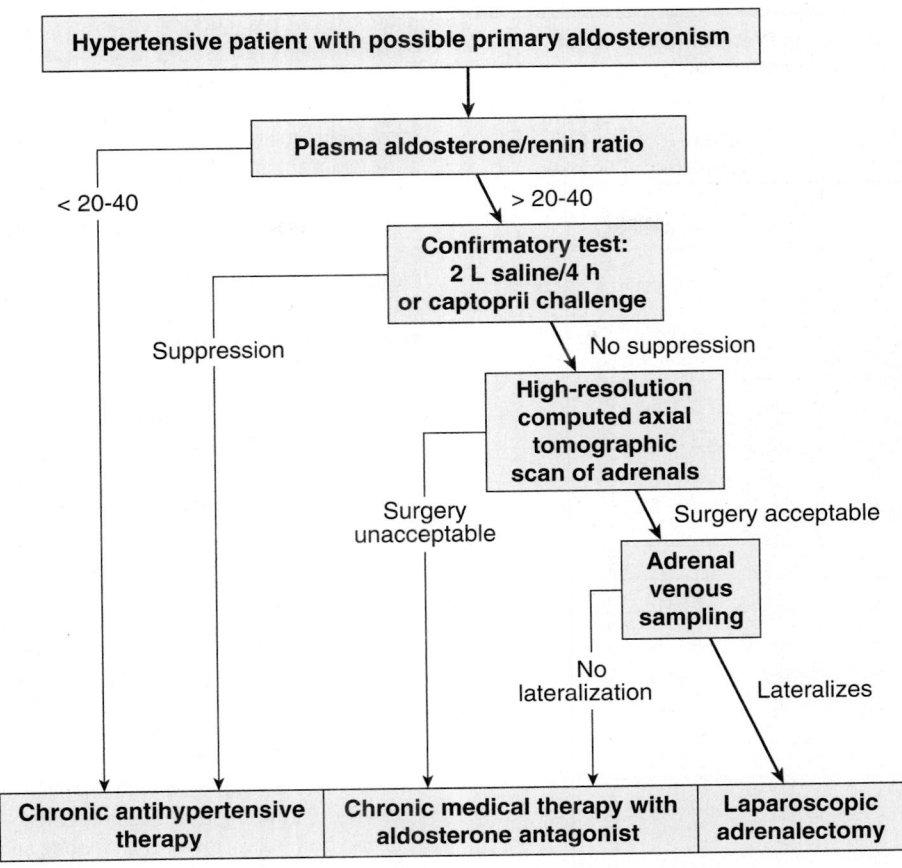

Figure 244-1 *Suggested diagnostic algorithm for most patients with suspected primary aldosteronism.*

■ RENOVASCULAR HYPERTENSION

Evaluation

Renovascular hypertension should be suspected in young women with the new onset of difficult-to-treat hypertension, who are at risk for fibromuscular dysplasia of the renal artery, or older patients with severe hypertension and known atherosclerotic disease elsewhere. Additional clinical clues to the diagnosis of renal artery stenosis include an epigastric bruit, acute kidney injury after starting an angiotensin-converting enzyme inhibitor or an angiotensin receptor blocker, and unexplained flash pulmonary edema.

As the population ages and survival after acute myocardial infarction and other manifestations of atherosclerotic vascular disease has improved, renovascular hypertension has become more widely recognized. Unfortunately, the diagnosis and treatment of this condition are still controversial. Four recent clinical trials have shown little (if any) benefit to routine angioplasty, compared with chronic antihypertensive drug therapy. The prevalence of renal artery stenosis on angiography in hospitalized patients undergoing cardiac catheterization is as high as 39%, but many of these patients were not hypertensive.

The pretest probability of renovascular hypertension can be calculated based on a patient's presenting clinical characteristics (**Table 244-2**). This clinical prediction rule correctly identifies most patients with either a very high (> 70%) or very low (< 15%) probability of renovascular hypertension who do not require additional testing (**Figure 244-2**). Before embarking on a series of diagnostic tests, two important questions should be answered. If the patient refuses vascular surgery, as might become necessary in the event of renal artery perforation during angioplasty or stenting, no further diagnostic evaluation is recommended. The more difficult question is whether an invasive intervention is indicated. Because all four trials comparing percutaneous angioplasty and medical therapy have shown no long-term differences, many authorities reserve a diagnostic evaluation for a patient who cannot tolerate an ACE inhibitor or ARB (typically because of hyperkalemia, or a rise in serum creatinine > 25% over baseline), or whose blood pressure cannot be controlled to < 140/90 mm Hg with maximal medical therapy. Some would add patients with recurrent flash pulmonary edema, but the evidence for this is anecdotal.

Inpatient management

If the patient has a moderate probability of renovascular hypertension and an indication for percutaneous intervention, one of four screening tests is recommended, based on local availability and expertise (**Table 244-3**). Centers with very experienced Doppler ultrasound laboratories have reported excellent performance characteristics and the ability to predict a blood pressure response after intervention (renal resistive index < 80 mm Hg) with this noninvasive and relatively inexpensive test. High-resolution CT angiograms are highly sensitive for diagnosis, but they involve radiation exposure and injection of potentially nephrotoxic contrast medium. Magnetic resonance angiograms are quite sensitive and specific, and avoid exposure to iodinated contrast or radiation. However, they are generally not performed (unless dialysis is undertaken immediately after the procedure), if the *e*GFR is less than 60 mL/min/1.73 m² because of the risk of irreversible gadolinium-associated nephrogenic fibrosing dermopathy. Conventional catheter angiography allows for treatment immediately following the discovery of a stenosis, but has the

TABLE 244-2 Calculation of the Pretest Probability of Renovascular Hypertension

Clinical Characteristic	Never Smoked	Current or Former Smoker
Age (in y)		
20-29	0	0
30-39	1	4
40-49	2	8
50-59	3	5
60-69	4	5
70-79	5	6
Female gender	2	2
ASCVD*	1	1
Hx HTN ≤ 2 y	1	1
BMI < 25 kg/m²	2	2
Abdominal bruit	3	3
Serum creatinine		
0.5-0.75 mg/dL	0	0
0.75-1.0 mg/dL	1	1
1.0-1.2 mg/dL	2	2
1.2v1.65 mg/dL	3	3
1.7-2.2 mg/dL	6	6
≥ 2.3 mg/dL	9	9
Hypercholesterolemia (> 250 mg/dL, or on treatment)	1	1

For a given patient, points from the table are summed; if > 15, the probability is ≥ 70% and angiography is recommended as the initial test; if < 10, the probability is < 15% and screening tests are unlikely to be warranted.

*ASCVD, signs, symptoms, or clinical evidence of atherosclerotic cardiovascular disease; BMI < body mass index (weight in kg/[height in cm]²); Hx HTN, history of hypertension.
Data from Krijnen P, van Jaarsveld BC, Steyerberg EW, Manin't Veld AJ, Schalekamp MA, Habbema JD. A clinical prediction rule for renal artery stenosis. *Ann Intern Med*. 1998;129:705-711; and Krijnen P, Steyerberg EW, Postma CT, Flobbe K, de Leeuw PW, Hunink MGM. Validation of a prediction rule for renal artery stenosis. *J Hypertens*. 2005;23:1583-1588.

same risks of contrast and radiation exposure as CT angiogram and is also invasive (**Figure 244-3**). Although the captopril scintigram is relatively inexpensive, has been validated in large number of patients, and helps predict the results of angioplasty, the American Heart Association no longer recommends its use as a screening test, citing its limited utility in patients with significant azotemia, bilateral renal artery stenosis, or renal artery stenosis limited to a single kidney.

In the past, angioplasty was often delayed until the results of hormonal or hemodynamic measurements were obtained, but this has fallen into disfavor, as longer or repeated procedures were usually required. Advances in angiography, stent placement, and protection of distal circulation have improved the success rates of percutaneous renal artery revascularization. This procedure is now the treatment of choice for most types of fibromuscular dysplasia, but its role in atherosclerotic disease remains controversial. The Dutch Renal Artery Stenosis Intervention Cooperative (DRASTIC) trial showed no benefit of angioplasty, although a careful reading of the 12-month data shows significantly better blood pressure control in the instrumented group. The Stent for Atherosclerotic Ostial Stenosis of the Renal Artery (STAR) study and the Angioplasty and Stent for Renal Artery Lesions (ASTRAL) study have also shown no significant

differences across randomized arms, suggesting that the results of earlier meta-analyses showing no benefit to the invasive procedure might be correct. The 947-patient, NIH-sponsored, Cardiovascular Outcomes in Renal Atherosclerotic Lesions (CORAL) trial found a consistently lower systolic blood pressure (by 2.3 mm Hg), and a non-significant, 6% reduction in a composite of cardiovascular and renal events after angioplasty (compared to medical therapy alone) over 43 months of follow-up. These results have had a predictably negative impact on prior authorizations for renal angioplasty in most managed care plans in the USA.

■ CUSHING SYNDROME

Evaluation

Cushing syndrome is caused by prolonged exposure to glucocorticoids. Pituitary adenoma (Cushing disease) causes 75% of endogenous Cushing's syndrome, about 15% is caused by ectopic ACTH-secreting malignancies, especially small cell lung cancer and carcinoid tumors, and 10% is caused by adrenal hyperplasia, adenomas, and carcinomas.

Patients with Cushing syndrome have moon facies with central obesity and peripheral wasting, skin fragility and atrophy, with purplish striae and easy bruising, muscle wasting and proximal myopathy, and dorsocervical fat pad (buffalo hump). Other features of Cushing syndrome are non-specific, such as diabetes, diastolic hypertension, hirsutism, irregular menses, and depression.

Most patients with signs and symptoms of glucocorticoid excess can be correctly diagnosed with an initial urinary free cortisol level > 100 µg/d, a morning or evening cortisol level (sometimes now obtained from saliva, rather than blood), and the classical low-dose and high-dose dexamethasone suppression tests. When these are inconsistent, repetition of the tests or endocrinology consultation is often helpful. The ability to assay both corticotropin-releasing hormone and corticotropin (formerly known as adrenocorticotropic hormone, or ACTH) has also simplified the hormonal diagnosis, but results often return after hospital discharge. Radiologic studies to localize the tumor to the left or right side of the pituitary or left or right adrenal are often performed before the surgeon operates.

Inpatient management

Definitive management of Cushing syndrome is surgical resection of the responsible pituitary adenoma, ectopic ACTH-producing tumor, or adrenal neoplasm. Medical therapy may be useful in patients with tumors that cannot be localized, such as some ectopic ACTH-producing lesions, are unresectable, or are producing symptoms severe enough to need urgent treatment prior to surgery. Etomidate and metyrapone reversibly inhibit 11-deoxycortisol ß-hydroxylase, which catalyzes the final step in cortisol biosynthesis. Ketoconazole inhibits the early stages of steroid synthesis. Mitotane is an adrenolytic agent typically used in the treatment of adrenal carcinoma. Hospitalists involved in the postoperative care of patients with Cushing syndrome should bear in mind that hydrocortisone supplementation is indicated after successful tumor resection, due to suppression of the hypothalamic-pituitary axis. Glucocorticoid replacement may need to be continued for several months and tapered off slowly.

■ PHEOCHROMOCYTOMA

Evaluation

Pheochromocytoma classically presents with hypertensive episodes (spells), with some combination of palpitations, headaches, sweating, pallor, weakness, nausea, and dyspnea. However, a significant minority of patients present with severe hypertension, without paroxysms or spells. The initial step in diagnosis of pheochromocytoma is demonstration of overproduction of catecholamines or their metabolites.

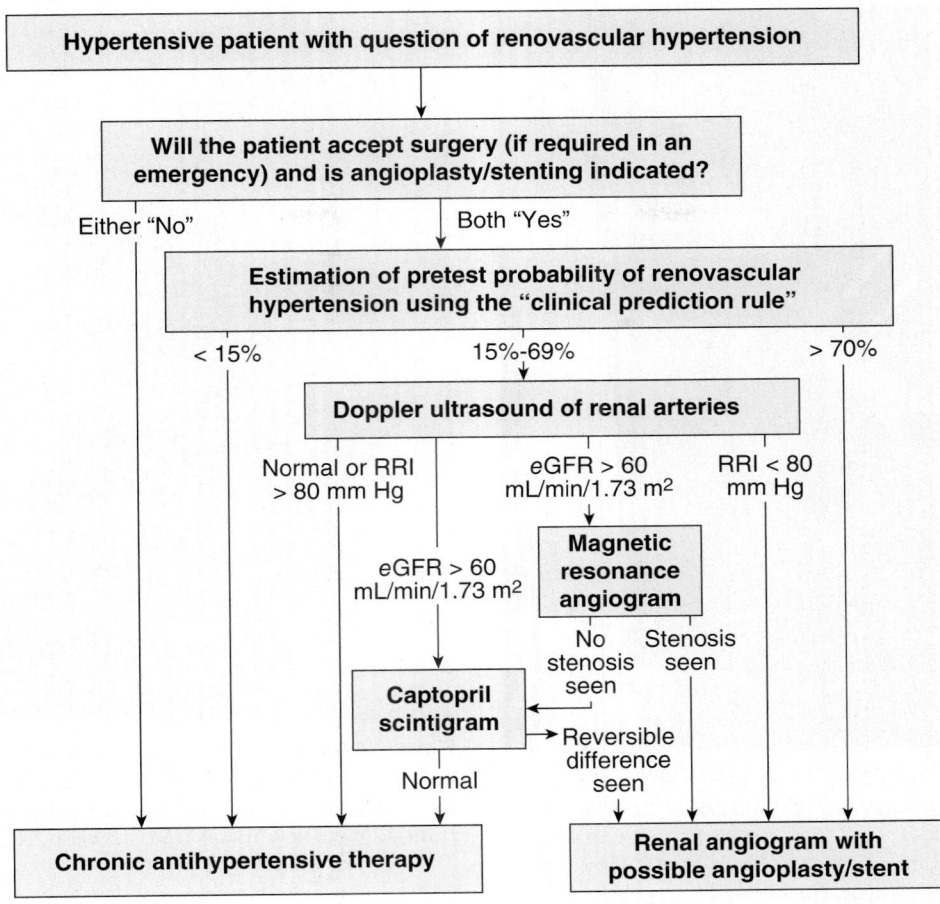

Figure 244-2 *Suggested diagnostic algorithm for most patients with renovascular hypertension. RRI, renal resistance index.*

Either plasma-free metanephrines or 24-hour urinary fractionated metanephrines may be used as a screening test; plasma-free metanephrines are somewhat more sensitive and logistically easier to obtain. If either is elevated, MRI or CT of the abdomen should be obtained. If these are negative and pheochromocytoma or paraganglionoma is still suspected, the tumor may be localized with either ^{131}I-meta-iodobenzylguanidine (MIBG) scan or positron emission tomographic (PET) scan.

TABLE 244-3 Summary of Advantages and Disadvantages of Various Screening Tests for Renovascular Hypertension

Screening Test	Doppler Ultrasound	Captopril Scintigraphy	Magnetic Resonance Angiogram	Computed Tomographic Angiogram
Number of publications (1990-2009)	67	71	71	18
Number of patients	4640	5068	3069	1336
Sensitivity (range)	0.83 (0.17-1.00)	0.77 (0.09-1.00)	0.90 (0.54-1.00)	0.84 (0.63-1.00)
Specificity (range)	0.84 (0.55-1.00)	0.78 (0.44-1.00)	0.86 (0.21-1.00)	0.91 (0.56-1.00)
Advantages	Noninvasive, inexpensive, may predict BP results after revascularization	Noninvasive, not expensive, may predict BP results after revascularization	No iodinated contrast needed; excellent image quality	Excellent image quality
Disadvantages	Operator dependent; less useful in obesity, bowel gas, branch lesions, FMD	Less accurate in renal impairment, bilateral disease, obstructive uropathy	Expensive, poor images with stents or distal stenoses (eg, FMD), overcalls moderate stenoses; risk of gadolinium-associated nephrogenic fibrosing dermopathy	Expensive, time-consuming to process and interpret; not widely available; large amount of contrast sometimes needed

BP, blood pressure; FMD, fibromuscular dysplasia. Adapted from: Elliott WJ. Secondary hypertension: Renovascular hypertension. Chapter 8 in: Black HR, Elliott WJ, eds. *Hypertension: A Companion to Braunwald's Heart Disease,* 2nd ed. Philadelphia, PA: Elsevier, 2013, p. 73.

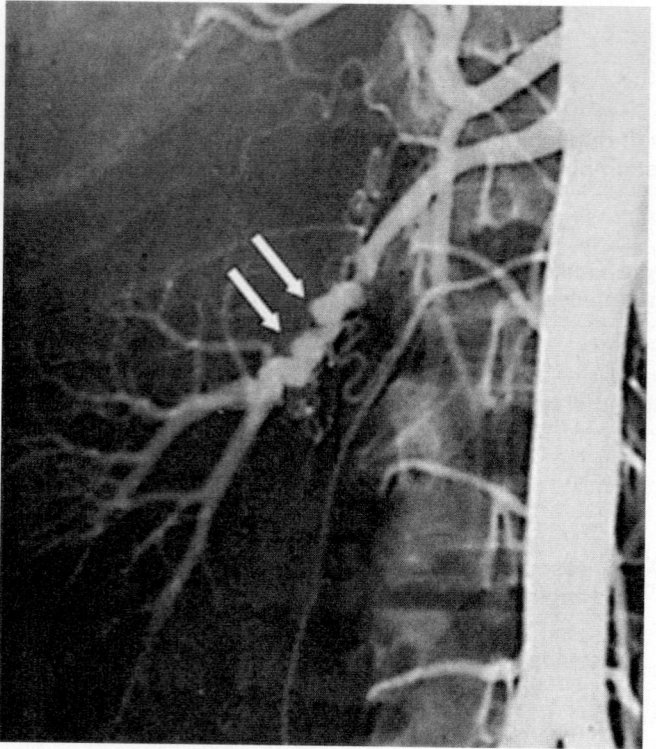

Figure 244-3 *Abdominal aortogram revealing left renal artery fibromuscular dysplasia (arrows) with a characteristic "string-of-beads" appearance.* (Reproduced, with permission, from Brunicardi FC, Andersen DK, Billiar TR, et al. *Schwartz's Principles of Surgery*, 9th ed. New York, NY: McGraw-Hill; 2008. Fig. 23-44.)

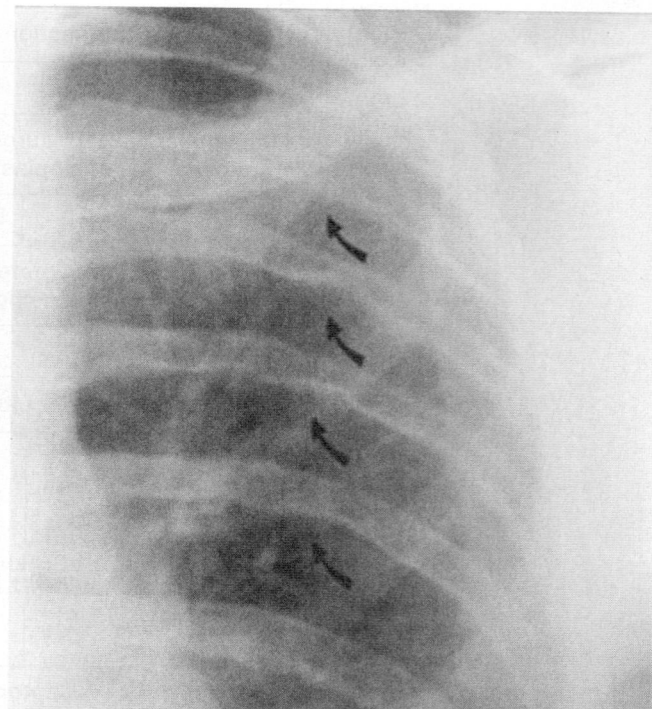

Figure 244-4 *Rib notching (arrows) caused by dilation of intercostal collaterals in a patient with coarctation of the aorta.* (Reproduced, with permission, from Fuster V, O'Rourke RA, Walsh RA, et al. *Hurst's the Heart*, 12th ed. New York, NY: McGraw-Hill; 2008. Fig. 15-1B.)

Inpatient management

Alpha-blockers are used for preoperative blood pressure control, traditionally with oral phenoxybenzamine or intravenous phentolamine when urgent control is required; postural hypotension is a troublesome adverse effect, and patients should be monitored when ambulating. Beta-blockers may paradoxically worsen blood pressure, and should be given only after full alpha-blockade has been achieved. A laparoscopic approach is becoming more common for solitary adrenal pheochromocytomas. Genetic testing for pheochromocytoma-associated syndromes, such as multiple endocrine neoplasia type 2, is generally recommended.

■ COARCTATION OF THE AORTA

Evaluation

Although most patients with this disorder are diagnosed and treated as children, many with less severe coarctation remain undetected until adulthood. Clinical clues include difference in blood pressure of > 15/10 mm Hg between arms, a lower BP in a leg than the ipsilateral arm, or rib notching on chest X-ray (**Figure 244-4**). Many diagnostic techniques have been employed, but transthoracic echocardiography with suprasternal notch views is quite sensitive and probably the least expensive.

Inpatient management

Catheter-based interventions have been successful in many adults, especially in patients with discrete, short-segment coarctation, but most remain hypertensive after relief of the coarctation. Compared to surgery, balloon angioplasty and stenting has lower acute complication rates, but higher rates of restenosis.

DISCHARGE CHECKLIST

■ KNOWN OR SUSPECTED SLEEP APNEA

- Has a sleep study been performed or arranged in an outpatient sleep clinic?
- Do patients with known sleep apnea have access to a CPAP machine with a properly fitted mask?

■ CHRONIC KIDNEY DISEASE

- Is outpatient follow-up arranged to recheck the patient's blood pressure in the next 1 to 2 weeks (target < 140/90 mm Hg, or < 130/80 mm Hg as suggested by the 2012 KDIGO guideline)?
- Has follow-up been arranged to recheck urinary albumin:creatinine ratio, serum creatinine, and estimated glomerular filtration rate in 4 to 6 weeks?
- Is an ACE-inhibitor or ARB part of the patient's antihypertensive drug regimen (if not contraindicated)?

■ HYPERALDOSTERONISM

- Has follow-up been arranged for determination of office blood pressure and serum potassium, and to follow-up on the results of the plasma aldosterone/plasma renin ratio, if this is still pending at the time of hospital discharge?
- For patients with glucocorticoid-remediable hyperaldosteronism, has follow-up been arranged for monitoring of glucose, cholesterol, and bone density (as higher than physiologic doses of corticosteroids are often needed, leading to iatrogenic Cushing syndrome)?

■ RENAL ARTERY STENOSIS

- Has office follow-up been arranged for adjustment of blood pressure medications and monitoring of serum potassium, lipids, and creatinine? This is needed on a monthly basis for several months following revascularization. Postprocedure follow-up is critical for patients with renovascular hypertension, as the diagnosis is **only** made retrospectively, by showing lower office blood pressure 6 to 12 weeks after opening the stenosis.

■ CUSHING SYNDROME

- Has follow-up been arranged to check office blood pressure, serum glucose, potassium, and creatinine, usually 2 to 4 weeks after discharge, along with results of any pending diagnostic tests?

■ PHEOCHROMOCYTOMA

- Has follow-up been arranged to obtain office blood pressure, serum glucose, potassium, and creatinine, usually 2 to 4 weeks after discharge, with tapering of alpha-blockade as feasible?
- Has repeat testing been arranged for catecholamine overproduction (usually done 6-8 weeks after discharge, using whichever modality demonstrated the abnormality before the operation)?
- Has follow-up been arranged to review the results of genetic screening for familial syndromes that include pheochromocytoma, and to pursue further testing for first-degree relatives, if indicated?

■ COARCTATION OF THE AORTA

- Has outpatient follow-up been arranged to check office blood pressure, serum potassium, and creatinine in 2 to 4 weeks, with tapering of antihypertensive medication (typically a beta-blocker), as feasible?

SUGGESTED READINGS

Calhoun DA, Jones D, Textor S, et al. Resistant hypertension: diagnosis, evaluation, and treatment. A scientific statement from the American Heart Association. *Hypertension*. 2008;51:1403-1419.

Cooper CJ, Murphy TP, Cutlip DE, et al. Stenting and medical therapy for atherosclerotic renal-artery stenosis. *N Engl J Med*. 2014;370:13-22.

Funder JW, Carey RM, Fardella C, et al. Case detection, diagnosis, and treatment of patients with primary aldosteronism: an Endocrine Society Clinical Practice Guideline. *J Clin Endocrinol Metab*. 2008;93:3266-3281.

Herrmann SM, Saad A, Textor SC. Management of atherosclerotic renovascular disease after Cardiovascular Outcomes in Renal Atherosclerotic Lesions (CORAL). *Nephrol Dial Transplant*. 2015;30:366-375.

Hu X, Fan J, Chen S, Yin Y, Zrenner B. The role of continuous positive airway pressure in blood pressure control for patients with obstructive sleep apnea and hypertension: a meta-analysis of randomized controlled trials. *J Clin Hypertens (Greenwich)*. 2015;17:215-222.

Lenders JWM, Duh Q-Y, Eisenhofer G, et al. Pheochromocytoma and paraganglioma: an Endocine Society Clinical Practice Guideline. *J Clin Endocrinol Metab*. 2014;99:1915-1942.

Prague JK, May S, Whitelaw BC. Cushing's syndrome. *BMJ*. 2013;346:f945.

Rossi GP, Auchus RJ, Brown M, et al. An expert consensus statement on use of adrenal vein sampling for the subtyping of primary aldosteronism. *Hypertension*. 2014;63:151-160.

Stevens PE, Levin A. For the Chronic Kidney Disease Guideline Development Work Group Members. Evaluation and management of chronic kidney disease: synopsis of the Kidney Disease: improving Global Outcomes 2012 clinical practice guideline. *Ann Intern Med*. 2013;158:825-830.

Vongpatanasin W. Resistant hypertension: a review of diagnosis and management. *JAMA*. 2014;311:2216-2224.

Warnes CA, Williams RG, Bashore TM, et al. ACC/AHA 2008 guidelines for the management of adults with congenital heart disease. *Circulation*. 2008;118:e715-e811.

Weber BR, Dieter RS. Renal artery stenosis: epidemiology and treatment. *Int J Nephrol Renovasc Dis*. 2014;7:169-181.

White WB, Turner JR, Sica DA, et al. Detection, evaluation, and treatment of severe and resistant hypertension: proceedings from an American Society of Hypertension interactive forum held in Bethesda, MD, USA, October 10, 2013. *J Am Soc Hypertens*. 2014;8:743-757.

Chronic Kidney Disease and Dialysis

Ursula C. Brewster, MD

Jeffrey Turner, MD

Key Clinical Questions

1. How are the stages of chronic kidney disease defined?
2. What are the different dialysis modalities, and how do patients choose one over another?
3. What is the difference between an arteriovenous fistula and an arteriovenous graft? What are their associated complications?
4. When is it appropriate to initiate dialysis?
5. How are hemodialysis and peritoneal dialysis performed? What are their common complications?
6. What complications are common in hospitalized patients with chronic kidney disease?

INTRODUCTION

Over 26 million Americans, or approximately one in nine adults, have chronic kidney disease (CKD). These patients require special attention from hospitalists because of the high incidence of acute kidney injury (AKI) and other complications during hospitalization. These patients are at risk of AKI not only from known nephrotoxins, such as contrast agents and nonsteroidal anti-inflammatory drugs (NSAIDs), but also from other commonly prescribed agents. Other major issues in the hospital care of these patients include preservation of venous access, electrolyte and acid-base correction, and anemia management. As many of these patients advance to end-stage renal disease (ESRD) requiring dialysis, hospitalists should have a basic understanding of the principles of renal replacement therapy (RRT).

CHRONIC KIDNEY DISEASE

The National Kidney Foundation has defined a staging system for CKD (**Table 245-1**) based on glomerular filtration rate (GFR) as the best marker of kidney function. CKD is defined as an absolute GFR less than 60 cc/min, or structural or functional kidney abnormalities such as hematuria, proteinuria, or abnormal renal imaging in association with a preserved GFR (> 90cc/min). Serum creatinine concentration (sCr) is a poor marker of kidney function, as normal values vary significantly with age, gender, and muscle mass. It is especially inadequate in the setting of AKI. In the early phases of acute kidney injury, the sCr may be falsely reassuring, as it may begin to rise well after the initial insult.

As GFR is not readily measured, mathematical formulae are used to estimate it. The Cockcroft-Gault and the Modification of Diet in Renal Disease (MDRD) formulas are most commonly used. The newer Chronic Kidney Disease Epidemiology Collaboration (CKD-EPI) equation is also being used in some clinical laboratories (**Table 245-2**). The Cockcroft-Gault formula is simple, but often overestimates kidney function. The MDRD is a more arduous calculation, but is more accurate in patients with advanced CKD. The CKD-EPI equation is superior to the others in that it allows for accurate GFR estimations in patients with normal or minimally impaired kidney function. These formulas are only useful when sCr is in a steady state. When the sCr is rapidly changing, as in acute kidney injury, they are completely inaccurate and should not be used. In that case, a 24-hour urine collection for creatinine clearance (CrCl) is a better indicator of kidney function. A 24-hour urine collection is recommended whenever renally excreted drugs possessing significant toxicity need to be administered.

TREATMENT OF CHRONIC KIDNEY DISEASE

Chronic kidney disease, no matter the etiology, is almost always a progressive, irreversible process. Treatment strategies focus on slowing the decline in kidney function, as there are no currently available treatments proven to reverse CKD. The interventions with the best evidence for slowing disease progression are control of hypertension and the use of angiotensin-converting enzyme inhibitors or angiotensin II receptor blockers in patients with proteinuria. Additional evidence suggests that it may be beneficial to correct metabolic acidosis, hyperphosphatemia, and vitamin D deficiency. It is unclear whether lipid lowering and strict glucose control in diabetes affects CKD progression, but these strategies are employed in most patients. Despite optimal medical care, patients with advanced CKD often

TABLE 245-1 Chronic Kidney Disease Staging System

Stage	Description	GFR (mL/min/1.73 m²)
0	At increased risk	> 90
1	Kidney damage with normal or increased GFR	≥ 90
2	Kidney damage with mild decrease in GFR	60-89
3	Moderate	30-59
4	Severe decrease in GFR	15-29
5	Kidney failure	< 15 or dialysis

GFR, glomerular filtration rate.

progress to ESRD. When feasible, ESRD is best treated with transplantation. When donors are available, this is done preemptively, and dialysis is avoided. If dialysis seems unavoidable, preparation and discussion should start at least 1 year in advance, involving the patient, primary care physician, family, nephrologist, and other caregivers. However, some patients require acute dialysis in the hospital, with quick education by hospitalists and nephrology teams.

PREPARATION OF PATIENTS FOR DIALYSIS

■ DIET EDUCATION

Patients with advanced CKD need instruction about the importance of dietary adherence. Diets for stage 5 CKD are restricted in sodium, potassium, and phosphorus. In the past, CKD patients were told to dramatically limit protein intake, as it was thought that this would slow progression of proteinuric kidney disease. Most experts now agree that a modest protein restriction (0.7 g/kg/d) is likely safe, but more restricted diets pose too great a risk of malnutrition. Salt restriction in patients with CKD cannot be overemphasized. Potassium restriction is also important in advanced disease.

TABLE 245-2 Estimation Formulas of Glomerular Filtration Rate

Cockcroft-Gault equation:

$$\frac{(140 - age) \times (IBW)}{S_{Cr} \times 72}$$

MDRD equation:

$$170 \times (S_{Cr})^{-0.999} \times (Age)^{-0.176} \times (0.762 \text{ if female}) \times (1.80 \text{ if black})$$
$$\times (BUN)^{-0.170} \times (albumin)^{0.318}$$

CKD-EPI equation:

$$GFR = 141 \times min(S_{Cr}/\kappa,1)^{\alpha} \times max(S_{Cr}/\kappa,1)^{-1.209}$$
$$\times 0.993^{Age} \times 1.018 \text{ (if female)} \times 1.159 \text{ (if black)}$$

$\kappa = 0.7$ if female

$\kappa = 0.9$ if male

$\alpha = -0.329$ if female

$\alpha = -0.411$ if male

min = the minimum of S_{Cr}/κ or 1

max = the maximum of S_{Cr}/κ or 1

BUN, blood urea nitrogen; IBW, ideal body weight; MDRD, modification of diet in renal disease; S_{Cr}, serum creatinine; CKD-EPI, chronic kidney disease epidemiology collaboration; GFR, glomerular filtration rate.
Units: Age in years; Albumin in g/dL; BUN in mg/dL; IBW in kg; S_{Cr} in mg/dL.

TABLE 245-3 Dialysis Modalities

Modality	Description
In-center hemodialysis	Patient goes to a dialysis clinic for treatment, typically three times a week
Home hemodialysis	Patient or partner needles the patient's access, and runs his or her treatments on a compact hemodialysis machine, either daily or a scheduled number of treatments per week
Nocturnal hemodialysis	Patient goes to a dialysis clinic at night, and undergoes longer hemodialysis treatments by skilled nurses overnight during sleep
Continuous ambulatory peritoneal dialysis	Patient does 4-6 manual exchanges of dialysate into the abdomen over the course of a 24-h period
Automated peritoneal dialysis	Peritoneal dialysis is done via an automated machine that cycles fluid in and out of the abdomen over a set period of time (usually 8-10 h), often during sleep

■ DIALYSIS MODALITY CHOICE

Modalities of dialysis that hospitalists should be familiar with include peritoneal dialysis (PD), traditional in-center hemodialysis (HD), home HD, and nocturnal HD (**Table 245-3**). These modalities are discussed in detail below. The choice should be based on dialysis access options, patient lifestyle, and patient support network.

■ HEMODIALYSIS ACCESS PLANNING

When the need for HD is urgent, dual-lumen dialysis catheters can be placed at the bedside or radiology suite by nephrologists, surgeons, or interventional radiologists. These may be used immediately after confirmation of placement by radiography. The internal jugular and femoral veins are preferred sites. Catheters should not be placed in the subclavian vein, because central venous stenosis may develop, precluding the later use of the ipsilateral arm for surgically created fistulae and grafts. Catheters may be untunneled, or tunneled with subcutaneous cuffs. Tunneling the catheter subcutaneously prior to vein entry decreases the likelihood of skin bacteria reaching the bloodstream and causing infection, and allows these catheters to remain in place for longer periods of time. Catheters are not preferred for long-term vascular access. They have high rates of malfunction and infection (approximately 2-4 episodes per 1000 patient days) and are associated with increased patient mortality, compared with fistulae or grafts.

Ideally, access for HD is established well in advance of the need to start dialysis, as an arteriovenous fistula (AVF) may need months to mature before it is viable. Patients with CKD should be referred to an experienced access surgeon when their estimated GFR is 20 mL/min/1.73 m², or when they are expected to require dialysis in the next 3 to 6 months.

Long-term vascular access for HD requires identification and preservation of suitable veins over time. Fistulae require veins greater than 0.3 cm in diameter on ultrasound mapping. *The importance of vein preservation cannot be overemphasized.* Many CKD patients will require HD access and should have their veins protected, particularly while hospitalized. To this end, one upper extremity (usually the nondominant arm) should be spared from blood draws, sphygmomanometers, and intravenous catheters (including peripherally inserted central catheter [PICC] lines). Scarring of veins occurs rapidly, often making future access creation impossible.

Arteriovenous fistulae are preferred over synthetic arteriovenous grafts because of their longer lifespan and lower infection rate. An AVF is made by surgically anastomosing a native artery to a native

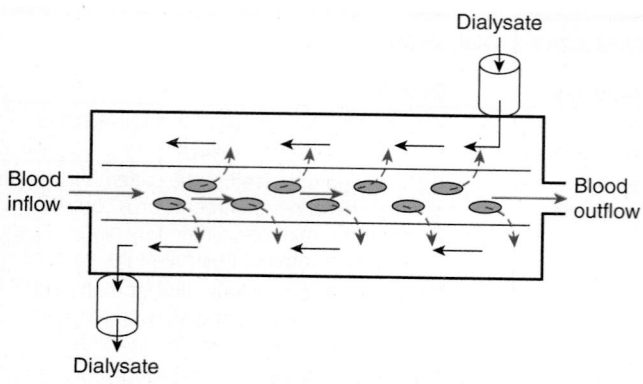

Figure 245-1 *Arteriovenous fistula showing the direct anastomosis between artery and vein in the upper extremity.*

vein, usually in the forearm or upper arm (**Figure 245-1**). Over time, the vein will "arterialize," so it can withstand thrice-weekly cannulation. Fistula maturation usually requires 6 to 12 weeks. Surgical or percutaneous interventions may be required when maturation is delayed. A successful fistula can last over a decade with low thrombosis and infection rates.

PRACTICE POINT

- Because many CKD patients will require HD access, clinicians should preserve their veins during hospitalization. This means ensuring that one upper extremity (usually the non-dominant arm) is spared from blood draws, sphygmomanometers, and intravenous catheters (including PICC lines). Scarring of veins occurs rapidly, often making future access creation impossible.

If a suitable vein for creation of an AVF is unavailable, an arteriovenous graft (AVG) made of polytetrafluoroethylene (PTFE) or other synthetic material may be interposed between native vessels as an alternative (**Figure 245-2**). An AVG can be used for HD 2 to 4 weeks after placement. Unfortunately, synthetic PTFE grafts are not as durable as an AVF. On average, grafts thrombose more often than fistulae and have lower patency rates. Additionally, because these grafts are made of synthetic material, infection usually requires surgical excision and abandoning the access.

INITIATION OF DIALYSIS

In some patients, CKD slowly progresses and dialysis can be initiated in a predictable fashion. For others, AKI necessitates urgent initiation of treatment.

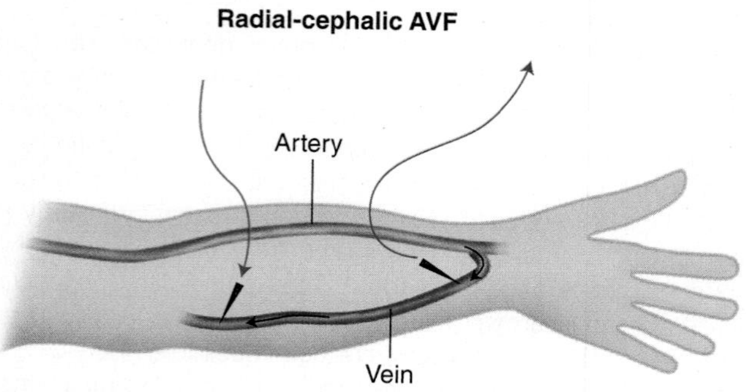

Radial-cephalic AVF

Artery

Vein

Figure 245-2 *Arteriovenous graft showing artificial graft material (black) placed as a conduit between artery and vein in the upper extremity.*

TABLE 245-4 Acute Indications for Dialysis

Severe metabolic abnormalities (hyperkalemia, hypercalcemia)

Severe acidosis not responsive to bicarbonate therapy

Intoxications and overdoses (ie, methanol, ethylene glycol, lithium, theophylline, salicylates, metformin)

Severe volume overload not responsive to diuretics

Uremia in the setting of chronic renal failure

◼ ACUTE INITIATION

There are several life-threatening scenarios that warrant urgent nephrology consultation and initiation of dialysis, with immediate placement of a double-lumen dialysis catheter for access (**Table 245-4**). These catheters are most often untunneled. In addition, these temporary dialysis catheters are preferred in patients with bacteremias or other endovascular infections. If there are no infectious issues, a tunneled dual-lumen catheter can be placed for dialysis, with lower long-term infection risks.

◼ CHRONIC INITIATION

Dialysis in progressive CKD is undertaken to avoid complications of advanced uremia. Current guidelines (and Medicare reimbursement) recommend the initiation of dialysis when creatinine clearance drops below 10 mL/min. Diabetic patients seem more susceptible to the side effects of uremia, and may require dialysis when the creatinine clearance falls below 15 mL/min. In patients with CKD, physiologic derangements begin well before the need for dialysis. Spontaneous decreases in protein intake, anemia, and altered calcium, phosphorus, and PTH homeostasis may begin when creatinine clearance is as high as 30 to 40 mL/min. Early nephrology referral helps manage these early complications of CKD and allows for a smooth transition to dialysis. Patients who have been actively managed by a nephrologist well before dialysis have better outcomes than patients seen later in the disease process.

Uremia results from high levels of nitrogenous wastes and other toxins in the blood. Gastrointestinal symptoms such as nausea, vomiting, and anorexia are prominent. Central nervous system (CNS) symptoms include fatigue, confusion, tremors, seizure, and coma. Abnormal platelet function, with a prolonged bleeding time and high risk of hemorrhage, is also common. Classic physical exam findings, such as a pericardial friction rub, asterixis, and wrist or foot drop, may signal the need for more urgent dialysis.

HEMODIALYSIS

Hemodialysis (HD) is based on the diffusion of solutes across a semipermeable membrane down a concentration gradient (**Table 245-5**).

TABLE 245-5 Definitions

Dialysis	The clearance of small molecules and toxins using diffusion across a native (peritoneal) or synthetic semipermeable membrane
Ultrafiltration	Fluid removal across a semipermeable membrane during dialysis by convection
Hemofiltration	Continuous dialysis therapy in which large amounts of fluid are removed by convection from blood, with concurrent reinfusion of an electrolytic solution
Hemodiafiltration	The combination of hemodialysis and hemofiltration

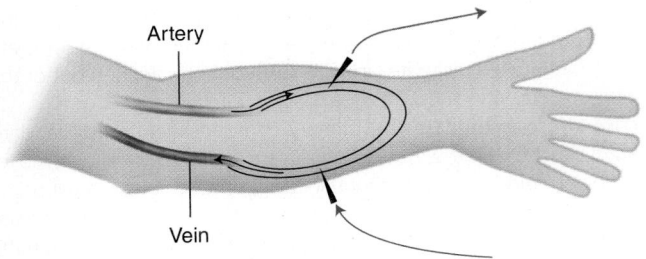

Forearm loop AVG

Artery

Vein

Figure 245-3 *Hemodialysis cartridge.*

Heparinized blood is pumped through a synthetic dialyzer at 300 to 500 cc/min, while individualized dialysate is run countercurrently at 500 to 800 cc/min (**Figure 245-3**). Solutes and water diffuse across the dialyzer, which is made of a semipermeable membrane that separates blood and dialysate. Dialysis replenishes bicarbonate, removes nitrogenous wastes, and balances electrolytes and divalent ions. The dialysis circuit consists of a heparin pump, a blood pump, an air leak detector, and arterial and venous pressure monitors. The dialysis machine alerts staff if it detects blood or air leaks, blood clots, or variability in patient blood pressure and heart rate. Because 30 to 40 gallons of water are used during each dialysis treatment, water purification systems are used to remove bacteria, endotoxin, trace metals, and other contaminants.

The major constituents of the dialysis solution are listed in **Table 245-6**. These are adjusted in the dialysis prescription, depending on the patient's serum potassium, serum calcium, and acid-base balance. The length of the dialysis session is based on measurement of dialysis adequacy to ensure the patient is achieving adequate clearance. Solute clearance, determined by the reduction of urea per treatment, is measured regularly by calculating Kt/V, where K equals the clearance coefficient, t equals duration/time of each dialysis treatment, and V equals volume of distribution of urea. This is regularly calculated in every HD patient, with a targeted goal of 1.4 or greater. If a patient's value falls short, dialysis time is increased to improve clearance. Patients with deficient solute removal are at risk of uremic symptoms, including poor appetite, fatigue, pruritus, and pericarditis. In general, patients require between 3 and 4 hours of dialysis per treatment for adequate clearance. Larger patients need more time. Dialysis adequacy may be jeopardized by inadequate blood flow through a vascular access, small dialyzer surface area, and missed or early termination of dialysis sessions by patients. Before HD can be initiated, vascular access that will provide adequate blood flow (300-500 cc/min) must be in place.

■ VASCULAR ACCESS COMPLICATIONS

Bleeding

Hemorrhage from HD access can be caused by needle laceration or intrinsic access problems. Outflow stenosis can increase pressure within the access, and predispose patients to prolonged bleeding after needle removal. Needles repeatedly placed at the same site in the access can weaken it, leading to an aneurysm in a fistula or a pseudoaneurysm in a graft. These defects may rupture, leading to exsanguination. Therefore, needle sites must be rotated within the access. Bleeding also occurs in the setting of infection, particularly in AVGs. Spontaneous bleeding from an AVG requires surgical repair or excision to prevent recurrent bleeding. If a fistula is lacerated and bleeds, it can sometimes be salvaged with rest, unlike an AVG. Repair will be necessary if an aneurysm is present. Immediate surgical consultation is mandatory in any case of access site bleeding.

Thrombosis

Clot formation is the most common cause of arteriovenous access loss. Sluggish blood flow from acquired venous stenosis is the usual cause. AVGs are especially prone to thrombose, as they often develop neointimal hyperplasia and venous stenosis at anastomosis sites. Access salvage in the setting of thrombosis is most successful early, in the first 24 to 48 hours. Treatments for established thrombosis include thrombolytic agents, percutaneous or surgical thrombectomy, and mechanical dissolution. Venous stenosis, if present, should be angioplastied at the time of thrombolysis to reduce the likelihood of recurrence. Fistulae are less likely to become stenotic, but the arterial inflow and venous outflow must be assessed at the time of the declotting procedure.

Infection

Dialysis catheters have high rates of infection and bacteremia. Empiric antibiotic therapy should include vancomycin and a second intravenous antibiotic active against gram-negative bacilli. However, antibiotics alone are not effective at curing catheter infections. This is particularly true of dialysis catheters infected with *Staphylococcus aureus*, *Candida* species, and *Pseudomonas*. These should always be removed, and a nontunneled catheter should be inserted at another site. (If no other viable access sites exist, the catheter should be exchanged over a guidewire as a last resort.) Patients with *Staphylococcus aureus* bacteremia are at high risk of metastatic infection, and they should be monitored for the development of complications such as endocarditis, epidural abscess, osteomyelitis, septic arthritis, endophthalmitis, and meningitis.

Patients with catheter infection with less virulent organisms, such as coagulase-negative staphylococci, can be treated with intravenous antibiotics initially. If symptoms do not resolve in 48 to 72 hours, the catheter should be removed. If the patient improves clinically, the infected catheter can be exchanged over a guidewire, and intravenous antibiotics can be continued. Alternatively, in those patients who improve rapidly with antibiotics, the catheter can be left in place and intravenous antibiotics can be continued, together with adjunctive antibiotic lock therapy (antibiotic solutions left in the catheter lumen after dialysis).

Arteriovenous graft infections require total excision of the graft and intravenous antibiotic therapy. Infections of arteriovenous fistulae are less common, as native vessels are more resistant to infection. Infected fistulae may often be cured with intravenous antibiotics alone.

Duration of intravenous therapy for catheter infection is at least 2 weeks. Surveillance blood cultures should be obtained 1 week after stopping antibiotics if the infected catheter has been retained. If these are still positive, the catheter should be removed. Patients with persistent bacteremia and fungemia after catheter removal should receive at least 4 to 6 weeks of antibiotic therapy.

Arterial steal syndrome

Grafts and fistulae divert arterial blood into the venous system and away from distal tissues, resulting in digital ischemia. Symptoms include coldness and cramping of the hand, numbness, tingling, pain,

TABLE 245-6 Common Components of Dialysate Bath on Hemodialysis

Component	Concentration	
	Range	Typical
Sodium (mEq/L)	135-155	140
Potassium (mEq/L)	0-4	2
Calcium (mEq /L)	0-3.5	2.5
Bicarbonate (mEq/L)	25-40	35
Glucose (mg/dL)	100-200	200

or overt ischemia with discoloration. Patients with new grafts and fistulae should be carefully monitored for these symptoms, particularly in those with peripheral vascular disease. This syndrome can also present late, as a fistula matures, enlarges, and steals larger volumes of blood. In extremely large fistulae, high-output cardiac failure can occur, but this is rare.

■ PROCEDURAL COMPLICATIONS OF HEMODIALYSIS

Hypotension is the most common adverse event associated with HD, occurring during 25% to 55% of treatments. Dialysis removes urea from the extracellular space, creating an osmolar gradient from the extracellular to the intracellular space. Fluid shifts to the intracellular space lead to extracellular volume depletion. In addition, when patients are noncompliant with fluid restriction, removal of large volumes is sometimes required to reach a target dry weight in a single 3- to 4-hour dialysis session. Rapid removal of volume often results in hypotension, as fluid does not have time to re-equilibrate from the interstitial to the intravascular space. Boluses of saline, albumin, or mannitol are given to transiently increase blood pressure. Strategies to prevent episodic hypotension include reduced dialysate temperature, high sodium dialysate, and medications such as the alpha-agonist midodrine.

The symptoms of *dialysis disequilibrium* include headache, nausea, confusion, restlessness, blurred vision, asterixis, and seizures. It is most common in chronically uremic patients beginning dialysis. The osmolar gradient resulting from rapid reduction in serum urea leads to water entry into neurons and cerebral edema. Dialysis disequilibrium is prevented by conducting the first several dialysis treatments at low blood flows and short duration.

Cardiac arrhythmias may occur in the setting of dialysis and are related to rapid fluctuations in potassium, calcium, and magnesium. ESRD patients with underlying cardiac disease are at higher risk. *Quality of life complications* associated with HD include nausea, cramping, headache, chest pain, and itching. Individual patients may be plagued with these symptoms to the point of intolerance.

PERITONEAL DIALYSIS

In peritoneal dialysis (PD), the patient's peritoneum is used as a semipermeable membrane through which diffusion, convection, and ultrafiltration occur. Many patients prefer PD over HD because of the greater flexibility and control that PD allows. Unlike HD, residual renal function is often necessary for adequate solute clearance, so efforts should be made to preserve it in these patients, even if it is minimal. Patients with prior major abdominal surgery may have adhesions that could limit the flow of dialysate, and therefore may not be candidates for PD. Laparoscopic PD catheter placement allows assessment of the suitability of the peritoneum in these patients. As PD is usually a home modality, an evaluation of social supports is essential. Morbidly obese patients or brittle diabetics are less than optimal candidates for PD because of high glucose exposure. However, many well-controlled diabetics do well on PD with aggressive adjustment of insulin regimens.

The basic continuous ambulatory peritoneal dialysis (CAPD) system consists of a bag of dialysis solution, a transfer set that serves as a conduit for fluid, and an indwelling silastic catheter. Dialysis solutions for PD contain physiologic concentrations of sodium, magnesium, and calcium, with lactate usually added as a buffer. During PD there is an exchange of solutes and fluid between the peritoneal capillary blood supply and the dialysis solution; the blood vessel wall, interstitium, and peritoneal mesothelium compose the semipermeable membrane. A volume of fluid, typically between 2 and 2.5 L, is infused through the catheter into the peritoneal cavity and allowed to dwell for a prescribed number of hours. The volume of fluid varies with patient comfort and body habitus. The number

of hours the fluid is allowed to dwell depends on the innate characteristics of the patient's peritoneal membrane. Patients are generally categorized as either rapid or slow transporters of solutes and fluid. Solutes transfer across the peritoneal membrane, equilibrate with the infused dialysate, and are subsequently drained out of the peritoneal cavity.

Dextrose is used as the primary osmotic agent, and standard solutions of 1.5%, 2.5%, or 4.25% are used to facilitate movement of fluid into the peritoneal cavity and achieve ultrafiltration. Higher dextrose–containing dialysate solutions (4.25%) generate higher osmotic gradients and remove greater volumes of ultrafiltrate. However, high-dextrose infusions increase the production of advanced glycosylation end products (AGEs), leading to oxidation and peritoneal membrane damage. This may lead to eventual failure of the peritoneal membrane and inability to adequately transfer solutes, necessitating a switch to HD. In diabetic patients, higher dextrose–containing solutions will increase serum glucose concentrations and worsen glycemic control. In patients with acute volume overload, large ultrafiltration volumes can be achieved with 4.25% dextrose solutions for short dwells (< 1 hour) repeatedly, until the patient's symptoms improve.

Automated PD is an alternative to conventional CAPD. In contrast to manual infusion and drainage of PD solutions, a machine performs the exchanges. The PD cycler consists of a scale and a dialysate warmer, and infuses, dwells, and drains peritoneal fluid. Patients usually undergo automated PD while asleep, allowing greater mobility during the day. The length of time each exchange dwells in the peritoneal cavity is often shorter than with CAPD, but the total volume of fluid infused is often much greater.

Children are usually treated with PD because the large extracorporeal blood volume required by the HD tubing and dialyzers can be hemodynamically prohibitive. Patients with severe cardiovascular disabilities also tend to tolerate the gentler daily ultrafiltration of PD better than intermittent HD.

■ PERITONEAL DIALYSIS ACCESS

A silastic (Tenckhoff) catheter is inserted into the peritoneal cavity by a qualified surgeon, interventional radiologist, or nephrologist, and tunneled beneath the skin to exit on the anterior abdominal wall. After placement, it should be immediately flushed with low volumes of dialysate and then capped off. Two weeks are required for wound healing and anchoring of the catheter in the subcutaneous tissue. It may sometimes be used cautiously before this 2-week timeframe with low fluid volumes and maintenance of the supine position, to prevent increased intraabdominal pressure and peritoneal leaks. Patients are carefully trained in how to access the catheter in a sterile fashion. Both patient and provider should be masked, and sterile technique is mandatory. Peritoneal fluid samples for laboratory analysis should only be obtained with proper technique by trained providers. Catheters may develop cracks over time; these can often be repaired by trained PD staff.

■ PERITONEAL DIALYSIS COMPLICATIONS

Peritonitis is the most serious complication of PD. Patients develop abdominal pain and have cloudy dialysate effluent. Dialysate sampling will demonstrate more than 100 white blood cells, with over 50% polymorphonuclear cells. On average, peritonitis occurs once every 15 to 20 months (a much lower rate than HD catheter infections). The most common organisms are gram-positive bacteria. Growth of multiple organisms, including gram-negative bacteria, should prompt an evaluation for an intestinal or intra-abdominal source. Nearly 80% of episodes may be managed at home, with the addition of antibiotics to the dialysate. Patients receiving antibiotics should also receive fungal prophylaxis (oral nystatin or fluconazole) to avoid fungal overgrowth and peritonitis. Fungal peritonitis is devastating, and requires the removal of the peritoneal catheter and either temporary or permanent conversion to HD.

Other complications of PD include malnutrition from loss of albumin and amino acids into the dialysate. Diabetics may struggle with weight gain and hyperglycemia from dextrose in the dialysate solution. After years of PD and the frequent use of high-dextrose solutions, the peritoneal membrane may develop scarring and adhesions, which limit solute clearance and ultrafiltration. In these cases, it is often necessary to switch to HD.

CONTINUOUS RENAL REPLACEMENT THERAPY

For critically ill patients who are hemodynamically unstable, continuous renal replacement therapy (CRRT) is often employed. Several modalities exist, including continuous venovenous hemofiltration (CVVH), continuous venovenous hemodialysis (CVVHD), continuous venovenous hemodiafiltration (CVVHDF), sustained low-efficiency dialysis (SLED), and extended daily dialysis (EDD). They all require a double-lumen catheter, a blood pump with safety devices similar to conventional HD, and a dialysis filter. All forms of CRRT must be done in an intensive care unit setting with properly trained staff. CRRT allows for very slow fluid removal, resulting in excellent hemodynamic tolerance, even in patients with shock or severe fluid overload. In addition, because the therapy is continuous, fluid removal and correction of metabolic abnormalities can be modified at any time, allowing for rapid adjustment in critically ill patients. CRRT can also compensate for the large fluid volumes required for parenteral nutrition. The data on CRRT benefit over conventional HD is not conclusive, but it continues to be employed in critically ill patients who may not tolerate conventional HD, and in those with fulminant hepatic failure who are at risk for cerebral edema.

COMMON PROBLEMS IN HOSPITALIZED CKD PATIENTS

■ GASTROINTESTINAL BLEEDING

ESRD patients, regardless of dialysis modality, are at increased risk of gastrointestinal bleeding from acquired platelet dysfunction and may also be receiving medications such as aspirin and heparin that increase bleeding risk. Dialysis patients are also prone to bleeding from angiodysplasia, for unclear reasons. Azotemic patients with severe bleeding should be dialyzed. Subcutaneous or intravenous desmopressin, at dosages of 0.3 μg/kg body weight, may be therapeutic in uremic bleeding by releasing von Willebrand factor from storage sites. There is also evidence to support the use of conjugated estrogens or cryoprecipitate in uremic bleeding. The decision to transfuse a CKD patient who is a transplant candidate should be carefully considered, as transfusion is often associated with antibody formation, perhaps hindering the matching of a future kidney allograft.

■ HYPERTENSION

Hypertension is common in CKD and ESRD patients. Most of these patients should be on renin-angiotensin-aldosterone system inhibitors, such as angiotensin-converting enzyme (ACE) inhibitors or angiotensin receptor blockers (ARB), as these improve cardiovascular outcomes and survival and preserve residual renal function. In hospitalized patients, these medications are problematic because they may increase the risk of AKI and hyperkalemia. They should certainly be stopped in the setting of AKI and in CKD patients undergoing intravenous contrast exposure. When these medications are held in the setting of AKI, practitioners should be sure to restart them once the sCr approaches baseline, to allow for the long-term benefits of these drugs.

■ BONE DISEASE

Patients with CKD and ESRD suffer from a complex spectrum of bone diseases. Osteomalacia may be seen with isolated vitamin D deficiency. Hyperphosphatemia, hypocalcemia, skeletal resistance to parathyroid hormone (PTH), and impaired renal production of 1, 25-dihydroxyvitamin D may lead to high-turnover bone disease and osteitis fibrosa cystica. Parathyroid gland hyperplasia may develop and may be difficult to reverse. Patients with secondary hyperparathyroidism may develop bone pain, muscle weakness, and erythropoietin-resistant anemia. Medical treatment to prevent hyperparathyroidism includes oral calcium, active vitamin D preparations, and calcimimetic drugs such as cinacalcet. Parathyroidectomy is still sometimes required. However, if PTH is oversuppressed by medical or surgical therapy, adynamic bone disease may develop. Management of serum phosphorus concentration is critical to the regulation of PTH.

■ PHOSPHORUS CONTROL

Phosphorus clearance falls with declining GFR, and hyperphosphatemia is common in CKD. It may cause hypocalcemia and tetany in the short term, and renal osteodystrophy and cardiovascular disease in the long term. Serum phosphorus levels should be controlled by dietary restriction as well as oral phosphorus binders (both calcium and noncalcium based) at mealtimes. Calcium-based binders (calcium carbonate or calcium acetate) are less expensive than non–calcium-based binders (sevelamer or lanthanum). In larger doses, they promote positive calcium balance, which appears to contribute to cardiovascular calcification. Aluminum-based phosphorus binders should be avoided because of their association with dementia and adynamic bone disease in renal failure. Medications that can worsen phosphorus control, such as phosphorus-containing bowel preparations, should be avoided in hospitalized CKD patients. These have been associated with acute kidney injury from phosphate overload and should certainly be avoided in patients with stages 3 to 5 CKD.

■ USE OF CONTRAST AGENTS

Iodinated radiocontrast causes contrast nephropathy, particularly in patients with stages 3 to 5 CKD and diabetes mellitus. It should generally be avoided in these patients, and even patients with ESRD on dialysis, as they benefit from preservation of even minimal residual renal function. When use of radiocontrast agents is essential in CKD or ESRD, prophylaxis with intravenous fluids (NaCl or NaHCO₃) and N-acetylcysteine should be used. Using low or iso-osmolar radiocontrast and limiting contrast volume may also be helpful. Current data do not suggest HD prevents contrast nephropathy. Avoid gadolinium contrast in patients with CKD stages 4 and 5 (GFR < 30 cc/min) because of its devastating association with nephrogenic systemic fibrosis.

■ ACID-BASE DISORDERS

Chronic metabolic acidosis is common in advanced CKD, as the kidney cannot excrete the daily ingested acid load. CKD may be complicated by type 4 renal tubular acidosis, further worsening acid-base balance. CKD patients are less able to handle an acute acid load, as might occur with lactic acidosis, and may develop severe metabolic acidosis quickly. Oral NaHCO₃ and furosemide may be therapeutically effective, but dialysis may be required in severe cases.

■ MYOCARDIAL INFARCTION

Patients with CKD are at higher risk of cardiovascular events, including acute coronary syndrome (ACS). Serum troponin levels (troponin T and I) can be mildly elevated in CKD and ESRD patients. A single troponin is not helpful for diagnosing ACS in renal insufficiency, but rising troponins over time suggest acute cardiac injury. Therapy for ACS remains the same as in the general population.

■ ANEMIA MANAGEMENT

Anemia is a nearly universal complication of CKD. Increased blood loss with recurrent blood draws, higher risk of gastrointestinal (GI) bleeds, and decreased erythropoietin production promote anemia. Limiting packed red cell transfusions is important to avoid immune sensitization for patients who are candidates for kidney transplantation. Iron, B12, and folate deficiency should be excluded as contributing factors. The side effects of oral iron often necessitate the use of intravenous iron. Newer formulations of parenteral iron, such as iron sucrose and iron gluconate, have a lower anaphylactic risk than iron dextran. Recombinant erythropoietin therapy is critical in the management of anemia in CKD patients. These agents (erythropoietin and darbepoetin) are administered subcutaneously in outpatients with advanced CKD, and either intravenously or subcutaneously in ESRD patients on dialysis.

■ ACUTE KIDNEY INJURY

Patients with CKD are vulnerable to acute kidney injury (AKI) in the hospital, most often due to drug toxicity or ischemia. All medications prescribed to CKD patients must be reviewed for possible nephrotoxicity and dose adjusted for renal function. Patients with CKD need careful monitoring and follow up after hospital discharge; renal function often does not return to baseline after acute injury occurs. ACE inhibitors and ARBs should be stopped in the setting of AKI, but restarted upon its resolution, as these agents prevent progression of kidney diseases and have important cardiovascular benefits.

■ HYPERKALEMIA

Patients with CKD are at risk of hyperkalemia because of dietary indiscretion, medication effects, or transfusion. Patients with ESRD will likely need dialysis to correct severe hyperkalemia, but the other treatment modalities still have a role, such as intravenous calcium for myocardial stabilization, and β-2 agonists and infusions of glucose and insulin to shift potassium into cells. Bicarbonate therapy may be helpful in the setting of a nonanion gap metabolic acidosis. Potassium resin binders may be used as adjunctive therapy in CKD and ESRD patients, but are not a substitute for other therapies.

PRACTICE POINT

- ADEs occur in as many as 50% of hospitalized patients with CKD. Commonly misdosed drugs included antibiotics, acetaminophen, narcotics, beta-blockers, digoxin, ACE inhibitors, diuretics, oral hypoglycemics, metformin, lithium, allopurinol, colchicine, famotidine, and ranitidine. Clinicians should review all medications including those prescribed as needed with attention to indication, safety, and dosing. If a narcotic is required for analgesia, it is preferable to use agents that are not primarily excreted by the kidneys, such as fentanyl and methadone. Certain antihypertensives ordinarily considered short-acting, such as hydralazine, may have unpredictable and prolonged antihypertensive effects due to altered metabolism.

■ ADVERSE EVENTS FROM DRUG MISDOSING

In one sample of patients with CKD admitted to community hospitals, adverse drug events (ADEs) related to improper dosing for renal function occurred in over 50%, with half of these being classified as serious. Commonly misdosed drugs included antibiotics, acetaminophen, narcotics, β-blockers, digoxin, ACE inhibitors, diuretics, oral hypoglycemics, metformin, lithium, allopurinol, colchicine, famotidine, and ranitidine.

DIALYSIS PLANNING CHECKLIST IN PATIENTS WITH ADVANCED CKD

- Has the patient been educated about the available dialysis modalities (in-center hemodialysis, peritoneal dialysis, or home hemodialysis)?
- For patients planned to start hemodialysis, have they been referred for arteriovenous access placement? Have they been educated to avoid blood pressure checks, blood draws, and IVs in their non-dominant arm?
- Has the patient been educated about dietary restrictions (ie, daily fluid intake, sodium, potassium, phosphorus)?
- Has a phosphorus binder been initiated if the serum phosphorous is > 5.5mg/dL?
- Has iron been repleted, and an erythropoietin-stimulating agent been started if the patient has severe anemia?
- Does the patient have immunity to hepatitis B?

SUGGESTED READINGS

Adams JE. Dialysis bone disease. *Semin Dialysis*. 2002;15:277-289.

Allon M. Dialysis catheter-related bacteremia: treatment and prophylaxis. *Am J Kid Dis*. 2004;44:779-791.

Himmlefarb J, Ikizler TA. Hemodialysis. *N Engl J Med*. 2010;363: 1833-1845.

Hug BL, Witkowski DJ, Sox CM, et al. Occurrence of adverse, often preventable, events in community hospitals involving nephrotoxic drugs or those excreted by the kidney. *Kidney Int*. 2009;76:1192-1198.

Madhukar M. The basics of hemodialysis equipment. *Hemodial Internat*. 2005;9:30-36.

Palmer SC, Mavridis D, Navarese E, et al. Comparative efficacy and safety of blood pressure-lowering agents in adults with diabetes and kidney disease: a network meta-analysis. *Lancet*. 2015;385:2047-2056.

Paulson WD, Ram SJ, Sibari GB. Vascular access: anatomy, examination, management. *Semin Nephrol*. 2002;22:183-194.

Stevenson KB, Hannah EL, Lowder CA, et al. Epidemiology of hemodialysis vascular access infections from longitudinal infection surveillance data: predicting the impact of NKF-DOQI clinical guidelines for vascular access. *Am J Kidney Dis*. 2002;39:549-555.

Teitelbaum I, Burkart J. Peritoneal dialysis. *Am J Kidney Dis*. 2003;42: 1082-1096.

Tonelli M, Pannu N, Manns B. Oral phosphate binders in patients with kidney failure. *N Engl J Med*. 2010;362:1312-1324.

Wang AY, Lai K. Use of cardiac biomarkers in end stage renal disease. *J Am Soc Nephrol*. 2008;19:1643-1652.

SECTION 16
Rheumatology

246

Rheumatologic Emergencies

Derrick J. Todd, MD, PhD

Paul F. Dellaripa, MD

Key Clinical Questions

① What are the signs and symptoms of cervical spine involvement in rheumatoid arthritis and the spondyloarthritides?

② What tests should be ordered in patients with suspected pulmonary-renal syndrome?

③ Which patients with interstitial lung disease are most likely to respond to corticosteroids?

④ What are common and uncommon clinical signs and symptoms associated with giant cell arteritis?

⑤ What factors portend an impending renal crisis in a patient with known scleroderma?

⑥ What are the risk factors for Raynaud digital crisis? What treatments reduce morbidity?

INTRODUCTION

Rheumatologic diseases rarely present as an acute emergency. However, when they do, a delay in diagnosis can lead to significant morbidity and mortality. The most important and common examples of this include: (1) cervical spine involvement in inflammatory arthritides; (2) recognition of the protean presentations of giant cell arteritis so as to prevent permanent visual loss; (3) early diagnosis of pulmonary-renal syndromes which, if unrecognized, can lead to life-threatening respiratory failure and renal failure; and (4) scleroderma renal crisis, in which a delay in diagnosis can mean the missing of the therapeutic window in which renal function can be rescued. In each of these conditions, involvement of a rheumatologist is often warranted.

THE CERVICAL SPINE IN THE RHEUMATIC DISEASES

Catastrophic neurologic injury and even death may result from cervical spine disease in patients with rheumatoid arthritis (RA) or spondyloarthritis (SPA). Early recognition of the signs and symptoms and appropriate diagnostic evaluation are critical to avoid these complications.

■ ATLANTOAXIAL INSTABILITY

Up to 30% of patients with severe RA have some degree of subluxation of the atlantoaxial joint (C1-C2). In normal patients, the odontoid process of the axis (C2) is secured in front by the anterior arch of the atlas (C1), and posteriorly by the transverse ligament of the atlas. The normal distance between the odontoid process and the anterior arch of the atlas is 3 mm. Inflammation in the small joints that make up the atlantoaxial joint, or tenosynovitis of the transverse ligament of the axis, may weaken the transverse ligament, as well as lead to bony erosions in the odontoid process. As a result, the space between the odontoid and the anterior arch of the atlas widens (**Figure 246-1**), and the atlantoaxial joint becomes unstable. Anterior subluxation, in which the atlas slides forward relative to the axis, is the most common type of cervical spine emergency. It leads to cord compression and cervical myelopathy. Less commonly, posterior subluxation occurs when the odontoid is badly damaged or fractured. Rarely, vertical C1-C2 subluxation occurs, with atlanto-axial impaction, migration of the odontoid into the foramen magnum, brainstem compression, and death. Atlantoaxial instability may also produce vertebrobasilar insufficiency by impairing blood flow in the vertebral arteries, which travel through the transverse foramina of the cervical spine.

Symptoms of impending cervical spine subluxation may include occipital or retro-orbital headache, paresthesias of the extremities, and electric shock sensation in the upper extremities with neck flexion. Physical examination findings may include hyperreflexia, a positive Babinski test, and sensory loss in the hands and feet. Typically, patients with advanced cervical spine disease also demonstrate evidence of advanced disease elsewhere. Unfortunately, the neurologic examination in patients with advanced or aggressive RA or SPA may be confounded by muscle wasting, severe joint deformities, and entrapment neuropathies. Ominous symptoms and signs include a sensation of the head falling forward during neck flexion, syncope, respiratory irregularities, loss of sphincter control, dysphagia, hemiplegia, or nystagmus.

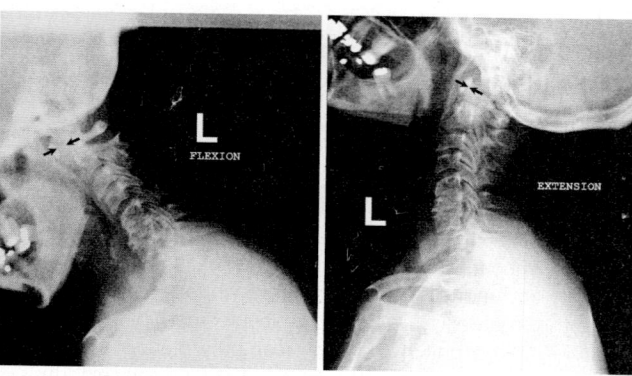

Figure 246-1 *Cervical spine in rheumatoid arthritis, showing atlantoaxial subluxation. A lateral view of the upper cervical region shows posterior displacement of the odontoid process. In flexion view (left panel), preodontoid space measures approximately 5 mm (arrows). Normally this measurement should not exceed 2.5 to 3 mm in an adult, although in a child 4 to 5 mm may be within the normal range. The measurement is made at the mid-level of the anterior aspect of the dens with the neck held in flexion. Subluxation is not present on extension views (right panel). There is also severe disc space narrowing, sclerosis, and osteophyte formation at C5-C6 and C6-C7.*

Lateral radiographs of the cervical spine in flexion and extension are the most useful initial diagnostic studies. These are diagnostic if the space between the anterior arch of the atlas and the odontoid is 9 mm or more, with an interval between the odontoid and the posterior arch of the atlas of less than 14 mm in the flexed position. In symptomatic patients, flexion and extension films should only be performed if standard films have excluded odontoid fracture and severe subluxation. When cervical spine radiographs are not diagnostic, magnetic resonance imaging (MRI) or computed tomography (CT) scan should be performed. MRI is particularly useful in delineating the extent of cord compression and the relationship of the odontoid to the brainstem, and in planning surgical stabilization. However, compared with flexion/extension radiographs, MRI may underestimate the degree of subluxation because patients remain supine for the study.

In the setting of progressive symptoms of cord compression, urgent neurosurgical consultation should be obtained for stabilization of the cervical spine. The role and timing of surgery in patients with atlantoaxial instability without cord compression is uncertain. The utility of medical therapy, such as rigid cervical collars and isometric neck strengthening exercises, is also unclear.

In patients with RA undergoing general anesthesia, cervical spine lateral radiographs with flexion and extension views should be obtained to exclude significant subluxation. Preoperative anesthesia consultation is mandatory in the RA patient with cervical instability. Fiberoptic intubation should be considered to limit neck manipulation.

◼ SPINAL INVOLVEMENT IN THE SPONDYLOARTHRITIDES

Neurologic manifestations are common in spondyloarthritis (SPA), particularly in ankylosing spondylitis. In longstanding disease, the spine is rigid, fused, and brittle. Spinal fracture may occur spontaneously or with minimal trauma. A dreaded complication is cervical fracture, generally presented as acute neck pain, with or without neurologic compromise. Cord compression with quadriplegia may ensue unless the spine is promptly stabilized. Neurosurgical involvement is requisite. Ankylosing spondylitis may also be

complicated by atlantoaxial subluxation, as in RA. Arachnoiditis may lead to scarring of sacral and lumbar nerve roots and cauda equina syndrome, with saddle anesthesia, paraparesis, and bowel and bladder disturbances.

AIRWAY INVOLVEMENT IN THE RHEUMATIC DISEASES

Airway involvement is a rare but significant source of morbidity and mortality in the rheumatic diseases. Granulomatosis with polyangitis (GPA, formerly Wegener granulomatosis) is a systemic vasculitis characterized by granulomatous inflammation of the upper and lower respiratory tract and glomerulonephritis. Vasculitic inflammation may occur in the subglottis and proximal trachea. Tracheobronchial GPA often does not respond to traditional systemic therapy and may run a course independent of the other manifestations of GPA, leading to recurrent infections or ventilatory obstruction. Tracheobronchial involvement should be suspected when a patient with known GPA presents with sore throat, cough, and difficulty with secretions. Chest radiography and spirometry are helpful initial tests, which may be confirmed with laryngoscopy or CT scan. When this complication is suspected, otolaryngologic consultation is mandated. Treatment involves intralesional steroid injection and dilatation of obstructive lesions. When severe, stenting and tracheostomy may be necessary.

Relapsing polychondritis (RP) is characterized by episodes of inflammation of the cartilaginous structures of the outer ear, nose, larynx, and tracheobronchial tree. Tracheobronchomalacia may result from the loss of the supporting cartilage of the upper airway, resulting in either fixed airway obstruction or hyperdynamic collapse. Concerning symptoms include progressive dyspnea, stridor, hoarseness, sore throat, and chest discomfort. The flow-volume loop is a useful screening test. It may reveal dynamic extrathoracic or intrathoracic obstruction, or both. This may be confirmed with bronchoscopy or inspiratory/expiratory CT scanning. Treatment options include stenting, balloon dilatation, or tracheostomy.

◼ PULMONARY-RENAL SYNDROMES

Patients may present with both pulmonary infiltrates and renal insufficiency, and no obvious cardiac or infectious cause. This should raise consideration of several diseases leading to pulmonary-renal syndromes, especially when these patients have proteinuria or active urinary sediments to suggest glomerulonephritis. Pulmonary-renal syndromes may be immune complex-related, as in systemic lupus erythematosus (SLE) or cryoglobulinemia, or mediated by direct antibody binding, as in anti-glomerular basement membrane (anti-GBM) disease, also known as Goodpasture syndrome. Alternatively, pulmonary-renal syndromes may be pauci-immune, characterized by a relative lack of immunoglobulin and complement on histopathologic analysis. Pauci-immune conditions include the vasculitides associated with anti-neutrophilic cytoplasmic antibodies (ANCA), such as GPA, microscopic polyangiitis (MPA), and eosinophilic granulomatosis with polyangiitis (EGPA, formerly Churg-Strauss syndrome). Clinical clues may suggest a specific diagnosis. Patients with SLE may also have arthritis, pleurisy, and photosensitivity. Patients with ANCA vasculitis may have sinusitis, otitis, or mononeuritis multiplex.

Diagnostic evaluation in patients with pulmonary-renal syndrome should include testing for serum complement levels, ANCA, anti-nuclear antibodies (ANA), anti-GBM antibodies, and cryoglobulins. Use of cocaine contaminated with levamisole has been associated with a drug-induced ANCA vasculitis. Thus, it is prudent to include a toxicology screen for cocaine in patients presenting with an ANCA vasculitis syndrome. Biopsy of affected tissue (usually kidney) should be strongly considered for most patients presenting with pulmonary-renal syndromes. In the face of undifferentiated disease and clinical deterioration, empiric therapy including high-dose corticosteroids and even cyclophosphamide or rituximab may be necessary, pending the results of testing or biopsy.

▪ INTERSTITIAL LUNG DISEASE

Interstitial lung disease (ILD) complicates a variety of rheumatic diseases including scleroderma, dermatomyositis/polymyositis (DM/PM), SLE, RA, Sjögren syndrome, and mixed connective tissue disease (MCTD). ILD affects up to 50% of patients with scleroderma, 30% of patients with DM/PM, and 10% of patients with RA. While parenchymal lung disease is often insidious, in some cases it may be explosive and require hospitalization. Patients may present with dry cough, progressive dyspnea, and desaturation with exercise oximetry.

High-resolution chest CT scan is useful in characterizing ILD. It may reveal ground glass opacities, seen in many other conditions including acute interstitial pneumonia, nonspecific interstitial pneumonia, desquamative interstitial pneumonia, *Pneumocystis jiroveci* pneumonia (PCP), viral pneumonia, pulmonary edema, and acute respiratory distress syndrome. Honeycombing and traction bronchiectasis are seen in fibrotic lung disease and usual interstitial pneumonia, and consolidative inflammatory lung disease is seen in cryptogenic organizing pneumonia. However, there is much overlap in the radiographic appearance of different forms of ILD. Lung biopsy may be diagnostic, although the potential utility of a histopathologic diagnosis must be balanced against the hazards of lung biopsy in patients with tenuous respiratory status.

Treatment for inflammatory lung disease involves high-dose corticosteroids with immunomodulating agents such as cyclophosphamide, azathioprine, mycophenolate mofetil, or calcineurin inhibitors, such as cyclosporine and tacrolimus. Fibrotic lung disease may require lung transplantation in suitable patients. In patients with worsening respiratory symptoms already on immunosuppressive regimens, bronchoscopy should be strongly considered to exclude concurrent superimposed opportunistic infection. In patients on high-dose corticosteroids for ILD with or without a second agent, prophylaxis against PCP should be strongly considered.

VISION LOSS IN GIANT CELL ARTERITIS

Giant cell arteritis (GCA) is a large-vessel vasculitis that most often affects branches of the external carotid arteries. GCA must be recognized and treated promptly, as patients may suffer irreversible vision loss. Although patients may be as young as 50 years old, most are of age 60 or older. In addition, most patients are of Northern European ancestry. GCA is the most common systemic vasculitis in older adults, but it is still relatively rare. Among patients age 50 or older, incidence rates are reported at 20 to 30 cases per 100,000 patients in Northern European countries. GCA occurs at an even lower frequency in nonwhite patients, with estimates as low as 1 case per 100,000. *Temporal arteritis* is a term used to describe vasculitis of the temporal artery, which is common in GCA. Cranial symptoms of GCA include headache, scalp tenderness, jaw claudication, and visual disturbances. Involvement of the thoracic great vessels may cause upper-extremity claudication. Aortitis may manifest years after the initial diagnosis and treatment of GCA. Patients present with signs and symptoms of aortic aneurysm or dissection. GCA may sometimes present as a chronic cough, failure to thrive, and fever of unknown origin in an elderly patient. Most patients also experience fatigue, anorexia, and weight loss.

GCA may coexist with polymyalgia rheumatica (PMR), a condition that causes achiness and stiffness of the shoulder and hip girdle, worse in the morning, and associated with fatigue. Patients with established PMR have an approximately 10% risk of developing GCA at some point in their lives, even years after the diagnosis and treatment of PMR.

TABLE 246-1   Select Conditions Associated with Erythrocyte Sedimentation Rate ≥100 mm/hour

Polymyalgia rheumatica
Giant cell arteritis and other vasculitides
Adult-onset Still's disease
Infectious endocarditis
Osteomyelitis
Septic arthritis
Multiple myeloma

Ophthalmologic evaluation is mandatory in patients with suspected GCA. It may reveal evidence of anterior ischemic optic neuropathy, retinal artery occlusion, or choroidal infarction. The remainder of the physical examination may reveal subtle clues of arteritis. Tender, tortuous temporal arteries are a classic but unreliable finding. A chest bruit, aortic insufficiency murmur, or discrepant upper-extremity blood pressures signal thoracic vessel involvement. Patients with concurrent PMR may have bursitis of the shoulders and hips, with painful limited range of motion in these joints.

The diagnosis of GCA is based on the clinical presentation, with corroborative pathologic findings of arteritis. The temporal artery is the most easily accessible extracranial artery for biopsy. Temporal artery biopsy is a high-yield, low-risk procedure. There is an emerging role for arterial ultrasound in patients with suspected GCA, although this test does not replace the role of biopsy. There is no single blood test diagnostic for GCA. Markedly elevated acute-phase reactants are suggestive, but nonspecific. The erythrocyte sedimentation rate (ESR) may be as high as 100 mm/h, a value found in few other disease states (**Table 246-1**). However, normal acute phase reactants have been rarely reported in patients with GCA. Anemia of chronic disease and thrombocytosis may also be present.

Classification criteria exist for GCA (**Table 246-2**). These were designed primarily for use as inclusion criteria for research studies, rather than for everyday clinical practice. Certainly, there are patients with GCA who do not meet these criteria. The diagnosis of GCA should be considered in any elderly patient who presents with recent-onset headaches, visual complaints, and unexplained elevated acute phase reactants. In these instances, empiric corticosteroid treatment should be started *immediately*, and temporal artery biopsy should be arranged expeditiously. Empiric corticosteroids do not alter pathologic findings, provided that the artery in question is sampled within 10 to 14 days of initiating treatment. Neither visual disturbances nor abnormal ophthalmologic exam need to be present to warrant immediate action. The retina is exquisitely sensitive to ischemia, and patients with GCA are unlikely to recover vision once it is lost. Treatment consists of corticosteroids in the equivalent of prednisone 1 mg/kg daily. Intravenous (pulse) corticosteroids have not been proven more

TABLE 246-2   Classification Criteria for Giant Cell Arteritis

Age 50 or older
New-onset headache
Temporal artery tenderness
Erythrocyte sedimentation rate 50 mm/hour or greater
Histopathology showing arteritis

Classification of GCA is met if patient has three or more of the above criteria.

effective for patients with GCA, but are an option for patients with threatened vision. Since luminal thrombosis of the ophthalmic artery is thought to be the event that precipitates blindness in GCA, low-dose aspirin may also be added to the therapeutic regimen. Once a patient starts treatment with corticosteroids, vision is often spared if it has not already been affected. Threatened vision is the most common emergency situation that may arise in GCA. In addition, aortitis may require emergent corticosteroids or even surgical intervention to reduce the risk of dissection or rupture. All cases of suspect or proven GCA warrant rheumatologic consultation for long-term management of disease.

COMPLICATIONS OF SCLERODERMA

The term scleroderma encompasses both localized scleroderma (morphea or linear scleroderma) and systemic sclerosis. Localized scleroderma affects only the skin and is not discussed further here. In this chapter, the term *scleroderma* will be used interchangeably with the term *systemic sclerosis*. Scleroderma is characterized by autoimmunity, vasculopathy, and systemic fibrosis. Vascular complications include pulmonary hypertension, scleroderma renal crisis, cutaneous calcinosis, and telangiectasia of the skin or gastrointestinal (GI) tract. Progressive fibrosis may involve the skin, GI tract, lungs, heart, or other organs. This section focuses on two emergencies in patients with scleroderma: scleroderma renal crisis and Raynaud crisis (seen most often in, but not limited to, patients with scleroderma).

■ SCLERODERMA RENAL CRISIS

Scleroderma renal crisis (SRC) usually develops within 5 years of diagnosis of scleroderma. It may even be the presenting feature of scleroderma, often in patients with other signs of scleroderma that have eluded diagnosis, such as Raynaud syndrome, sclerodactyly, cutaneous fibrosis, organ fibrosis, and telangiectasia. Rapidly progressive skin disease and prior corticosteroid usage are major risk factors for renal crisis. SRC usually presents as hypertension and progressive renal insufficiency in a patient with scleroderma. Patients may have symptoms of malignant hypertension: headache, visual disturbances, pulmonary edema, and encephalopathy. Progression to hypertensive crisis, overt renal failure, and death is rapid without prompt recognition and treatment.

SRC is a microangiopathy of the renal vasculature, not a form of glomerulonephritis. Urinalysis may reveal proteinuria and hematuria, but red blood cell casts are typically absent. The renal vasculopathy causes endothelial shearing of erythrocytes that may be detected as a microangiopathic hemolytic anemia (MAHA), with schistocytes on peripheral blood smear analysis and mild thrombocytopenia. As SRC may be the presenting feature of scleroderma, it should always be considered part of the differential diagnosis in a patient with unexplained renal dysfunction and MAHA features (**Table 246-3**). Renal biopsy does not distinguish SRC from other microangiopathies, but it may be useful to exclude glomerulonephritis. Ultimately, the diagnosis of SRC is a clinical one based on progressive hypertension, renal dysfunction, proteinuria, and MAHA in a patient with systemic features of scleroderma.

Angiotensin-converting enzyme (ACE) inhibitors are the mainstay of treatment. This is the only condition in which overt renal failure is treated with aggressive ACE inhibitor therapy, so one must have reasonable diagnostic certainty before initiating treatment. While any ACE inhibitor is likely to be effective, captopril has the largest body of supportive evidence, it is rapidly effective, and doses can be escalated rapidly. Enalapril has the advantage of intravenous dosing in exceptional circumstances. The goal of therapy should be normalization of blood pressure within a few days of starting treatment. This often requires hospitalization for

TABLE 246-3 Causes of Microangiopathic Hemolytic Anemia with Renal Failure

Scleroderma renal crisis
Antiphospholipid antibody syndrome
Hemolytic uremic syndrome
Thrombotic thrombocytopenic purpura
Heparin-induced thrombocytopenia
Malignant hypertension
Diffuse intravascular coagulation
HELLP syndrome (**H**emolysis, **E**levated **L**iver enzymes, **L**ow **P**latelets)
Transfusion reactions
Drugs (most often chemotherapeutic agents)

close monitoring and dose adjustment of drugs. Often, serum creatinine values will lag in their improvement, and ACE inhibitor therapy should continue undeterred by rising creatinine values. There is far less experience with angiotensin receptor blockers (ARBs) in SRC, and ACE inhibitors should be used whenever possible. In patients with ACE-inhibitor-induced angioedema, allergy consultation should be sought for possible desensitization.

Despite these measures, upwards of 40% of patients with SRC require dialysis for progressive renal failure. Concurrent pulmonary or cardiac scleroderma often precludes renal transplantation for SRC-related end-stage renal disease. Notably, it is not unusual for renal function to recover in patients with SRC after months or even years of dialysis, provided that ACE inhibitor therapy is continued unabated. Even so, patients with SRC have a 5-year mortality rate that approaches 40%, mostly because SRC portends aggressive extrarenal scleroderma.

■ RAYNAUD CRISIS

Primary Raynaud phenomenon (RP) is a common, usually benign, condition of cold-induced pain, pallor, and cyanosis of the digits, occurring in the absence of systemic connective tissue disease (CTD). Primary RP represents an exaggeration of normal physiologic vasoconstriction in response to cold. Secondary RP is a more aggressive version of RP that is associated with systemic CTDs like scleroderma, DM/PM, SLE, RA, Sjogren syndrome, and MCTD. A Raynaud crisis occurs when an episode of prolonged digital ischemia, lasting longer than 30 to 60 minutes despite rewarming, threatens the viability of one or more digits. It is a medical emergency that requires prompt intervention to reverse vasoconstriction and restore blood flow. Raynaud crisis most often complicates secondary Raynaud phenomenon, and not primary RP. Occurrence of a Raynaud crisis in a patient without known CTD should prompt a diagnostic workup for one.

Primary RP affects upwards of 10% to 20% of young women. It is much less common in men and the elderly. A typical episode involves a classic series of color changes. Digits first turn white in a demarcated fashion, as digital arteries vasoconstrict in response to cold (**Figure 246-2**). With prolonged vasoconstriction, digits become blue or purple because of tissue cyanosis. Finally, digits turn pinkish-red, as blood flow is restored, and the episode resolves. RP may also be triggered by stress or rapid changes in ambient air temperature, as upon entering an air-conditioned room on a warm day or reaching into a refrigerator or freezer. Of note, patient self-reporting of cold hands without color changes fails to satisfy the clinical diagnosis of RP. In patients with RP, episodes may involve all the digits or may be limited to a single digit (or part of a digit). Involved digits are often achy, numb, or even

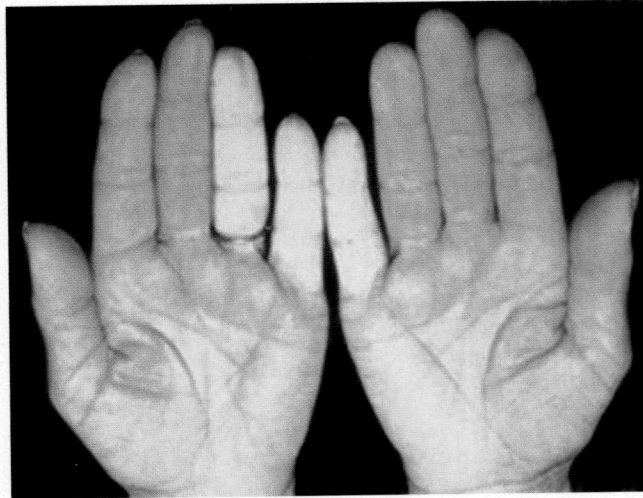

Figure 246-2 *Raynaud phenomenon, with digital pallor and cyanosis.* (Reproduced, with permission, from Wolff K, Goldsmith LA, Katz SI, et al. *Fitzpatrick's Dermatology in General Medicine*, 7th ed. New York, NY: McGraw-Hill; 2008. Fig. 171-1.)

painful. Prolonged ischemia can lead to digital ulcerations or even a threatened digit.

Primary RP occurs in the absence of an underlying disease, and rarely has major sequelae. In contrast, secondary RP is associated with one or more of the conditions listed in **Table 246-4**. Many of these conditions are CTDs that are associated with vasculopathy and endothelial dysfunction. These factors contribute to the aggressiveness of secondary RP, which is more likely to produce severe symptoms, digital ulcers, or Raynaud crisis. Common drugs, such as caffeine, cocaine, amphetamines, pseudoephedrine, nicotine, and beta-blockers, can exacerbate arterial vasoconstriction in either primary or secondary RP. Patients with RP should be advised to avoid these drugs, and educated about signs and symptoms of a Raynaud crisis and the need to seek medical attention if it develops.

TABLE 246-4 Diseases and Conditions Associated with Secondary Raynaud Phenomenon

Category	Disease Entity
Rheumatologic diseases	Scleroderma
	Systemic lupus erythematosus
	Rheumatoid arthritis
	Sjögren syndrome
	Dermatomyositis/polymyositis
	Mixed connective tissue disease
	Vasculitis, including cryoglobulinemia
	Behçet disease
	Thromboangiitis obliterans
Other forms of vascular injury	Vibration-induced vasculopathy
	Radiation-induced vasculopathy
	Paraneoplastic vasculopathy
	Frostbite
	Drugs including chemotherapy and cocaine
	Ergotamines

History and physical examination is often sufficient to distinguish primary RP from secondary RP. In the absence of previously identified CTD, secondary RP is suggested by ischemic episodes lasting longer than 30 to 60 minutes, recurring RP isolated to a single digit, features of scleroderma, or pitting digital scars. Positive serologic tests for ANA or other autoantibodies and an abnormal nailfold capillary microscopy help to secure a CTD diagnosis. Nailfold capillary microscopy can be performed without special instruments. For example, an ophthalmoscope may be used to inspect a nailbed that has been coated with a drop of mineral oil or even a clear bactericidal hand cleanser. Abnormal findings include dilated capillary loops, tortuous vessels, hemorrhage, or vessel dropout.

Raynaud crisis must be distinguished from other causes of digital ischemia, such as vascular trauma, vasculitis, proximal vessel stenosis, thromboangiitis obliterans, antiphospholipid antibody syndrome, atherosclerosis, and microembolic disease. The Allen test may be used at the bedside to assess for patency of both radial and ulnar arteries. Examination of pulses with Doppler ultrasound may help exclude proximal vascular occlusion. In selected instances, magnetic resonance angiography or even traditional vascular angiography may be necessary to confirm that the arterial stricture is at the level of the digital arteries, and not more proximal. Even then, it may be difficult to exclude digital microemboli, and proximal sources of emboli may sometimes need to be sought.

The goal of management in a Raynaud crisis is to reduce vascular contractility and restore blood flow to ischemic digits. Patients should be kept in a warm, stress-free environment to minimize further vasomotor stimuli. Affected digits should be reheated in tepid water; hot water should be avoided, as it may further damage ischemic tissue. Oxygen levels should be optimized, bearing in mind that pulse oximetry of a digit affected by RP is unreliable. Narcotic analgesia may reduce vasoconstriction induced by pain. Aspirin and sometimes heparin may lessen the risk of thrombosis within vasospastic vessels. Antihypertensive agents are typically used for initial vasodilator therapy. Dihydropyridine-class calcium channel blockers, such as short-acting or extended-release nifedipine or amlodipine may be of some benefit, but hypotension may be dose-limiting. Alpha-blockade with prazosin or doxazosin is often more effective, but hypotension may also be problematic. Oral hydralazine and transdermal nitroglycerin placed proximal to the part of the extremity involved may provide temporary relief, but tachyphylaxis and rebound vasospasm may occur. Anesthesia consultation may be required for chemical block of sympathomimetic nerves locally or cervically. Endothelin receptor antagonists, such as bosentan and ambrisentan, improve the healing rate of digital ulcers in patients with RP, but their role in Raynaud crisis has not been definitively established. In severe, refractory cases, digital sympathectomy, epoprostenol infusions, or phosphodiesterase inhibitors such as sildenafil and botulinum toxin injections may be attempted with the help of consultant services. Despite these efforts, patients may still experience digital necrosis and require amputation; it is advisable to involve vascular surgery whenever a patient presents with a Raynaud crisis.

DRUG TOXICITY IN THE RHEUMATIC DISEASES

While *allopurinol* is a generally well-tolerated medication for hyperuricemia, it is occasionally associated with serious toxicity. Allopurinol hypersensitivity syndrome ranges from a minor rash to a life-threatening systemic illness, with features of toxic epidermal necrolysis or Stevens-Johnson syndrome. It typically starts several weeks after drug initiation. Risk factors include renal insufficiency and rapid dose-escalation of allopurinol. In addition to rash, allopurinol hypersensitivity may also feature fever, eosinophilia, and acute hepatitis. Renal insufficiency, while not a typical side effect of allopurinol, can be a feature of allopurinol hypersensitivity. Treatment of allopurinol hypersensitivity includes administration of corticosteroids and cessation of allopurinol. In minor cases, patients may be rechallenged with allopurinol, but only under the direction of a specialist. Rechallenge should be generally avoided in patients with a history of severe allopurinol hypersensitivity reaction. Allopurinol can also rarely cause a severe ANCA-positive vasculitis. This generally improves upon drug cessation, although some cases require treatment similar to the ANCA-associated vasculitides. Allopurinol also inhibits the metabolism of azathioprine and 6-mercaptopurine (6-MP), increasing the risk of toxicity from these agents. The combination of allopurinol and these agents should be avoided if possible; if not, azathioprine or 6-MP dosing should be reduced to 25% of normal when using these agents concomitantly, under the direction of specialists.

Methotrexate (MTX) is among the most commonly used immunosuppressive medications in rheumatology. Toxicity may involve liver, kidneys, mucous membranes, and, in less than 1% of cases, the lungs. Pulmonary toxicity associated with MTX usually presents in the first year of use, with dry cough, dyspnea, fever, and, in severe cases, hypoxemia and respiratory failure. Alveolar or interstitial infiltrates may be seen on chest radiography or CT, although imaging may be unrevealing early in the course. The differential diagnosis includes community-acquired pneumonia, opportunistic infection, and progressive ILD from the underlying rheumatic disease itself. Bronchoscopy or induced sputum is often necessary to exclude opportunistic infection. Treatment in mild cases entails cessation of MTX. Corticosteroids or other immunosuppressive therapies may be necessary in severe cases. MTX overdose, whether accidental or intentional, is potentially life-threatening because of bone marrow suppression, nephrotoxicity, and hepatotoxicity. Hemodialysis does not effectively clear MTX. Early recognition of MTX overdose is critical in order to initiate folinic acid as a rescue therapy.

Cyclophosphamide (CYP) is an alkylating agent frequently used in the treatment of vasculitis and severe lupus. Major side effects include neutropenia and lymphopenia, which may lead to severe immunosuppression and overwhelming infection, especially with opportunistic pathogens such as fungi and PCP. CYP may also cause hemorrhagic cystitis, and it increases the lifetime risk of urinary tract cancer. The dose should be adjusted in the elderly and for renal function to avoid toxicity.

Azathioprine is a purine analogue used in a variety of rheumatic syndromes. It may cause severe neutropenia, infection, and transaminitis. Patients with low or absent activity of the enzyme that metabolizes azathioprine, thiopurine methyltransferase (TPMT), are at increased risk for cytopenias and other toxicities. Genetic testing for TPMT is available and often obtained in patients starting azathioprine. Azathioprine has a number of problematic drug interactions, including ACE inhibitors, allopurinol, and other immunosuppressive drugs. It should be dose-adjusted in the elderly and in those with renal insufficiency.

SUGGESTED READINGS

Brown KK. Rheumatoid lung disease. *Proc Am Thorac Soc.* 2007;4:443-448.

Chifflot H, Fautrel B, Sordet C, Chatelus E, Sibilia J. Incidence and prevalence of systemic sclerosis: a systematic literature review. *Semin Arthritis Rheum.* 2008;37:223-235.

Denton CP, Lapadula G, Mouthon L, Muller-Ladner U. Renal complications and scleroderma renal crisis. *Rheumatology (Oxford).* 2009;48(30):32-35.

Ernst A, Rafeq S, Boiselle P, et al. Relapsing polychondritis and airway involvement. *Chest.* 2009;135:1024-1030.

Fathi M, Vikgren J, Boijsen M, et al. Interstitial lung disease in polymyositis and dermatomyositis: longitudinal evaluation by pulmonary function and radiology. *Arthritis Rheum.* 2008;59:677-685.

Hunder GG. Epidemiology of giant-cell arteritis. *Clevel Clin J Med.* 2002;69(2):79-82.

Kim DH, Hillibrand AS. Rheumatoid arthritis in the cervical spine. *J Am Acad Orthop Surg.* 2005;13:463-474.

Krause ML, Cartin-Ceba R, Specks U, Peikert T. Update of diffuse alveolar hemorrhage and pulmonary vasculitis. *Immunol Allergy Clin North Am.* 2012;32:587-600.

Mouthon L, Bussone G, Berezné A, et al. Scleroderma renal crisis. *J Rheumatol.* 2014;41:1040-1048.

Specks U. Diffuse alveolar hemorrhage syndromes. *Curr Opin Rheumatol.* 2001;13:12–17.

Tashkin DP, Elashoff R, Clements PJ, et al. Cyclophosphamide versus placebo in scleroderma lung disease. *N Engl J Med.* 2006;354:2655–2666.

Weyand CM, Gorozny JJ. Giant cell arteritis and polymyalgia rheumatica. *N Engl J Med.* 2014;371:50-57.

CHAPTER 247

Gout, Pseudogout, and Osteoarthritis

Robert T. Keenan, MD, MPH

Svetlana Krasnokutsky, MD, MS

Michael H. Pillinger, MD

Key Clinical Questions

① Why do patients have acute flares of crystal arthropathies?

② How is gout distinguished from other monoarthropathies?

③ What are the appropriate therapies for acute and chronic gout and pseudogout?

④ What are the pathophysiologic features of osteoarthritis (OA), and how do these relate to clinical manifestations?

⑤ How is OA differentiated from other types of arthritis?

⑥ What are the nonpharmacologic, pharmacologic, and surgical treatment options for OA?

INTRODUCTION

Gout, pseudogout, and osteoarthritis make up the largest portion of the rheumatic diseases that affect primarily joints. Although these three disease entities are quite distinct, they share a number of features in common: all tend to be diseases seen at older ages; all three are often seen in overlap with each other; and all three are characterized primarily by inflammatory and/or mechanical abnormalities, rather than autoimmune ones. Whereas gout and pseudogout are diseases of abnormal crystal formation and resultant inflammation, osteoarthritis is primarily a disease of mechanically driven, biochemically propagated cartilage loss and autodestruction. In the following sections, we discuss these three important diseases, their pathogenesis, and management.

GOUT

Gout currently affects more than 8 million Americans, usually presenting with severe acute episodic arthritis that may evolve over time into chronic destructive tophaceous disease. Gout is more common in men (6.1 million US males vs 2.2 million US females), and is slightly more common among African Americans (5% of the African American population vs 4% of the US white population). The prevalence of gout rises with age, from 3.3% among individuals 40 to 49 years old, to 8.0% among individuals 60 to 69, to as high as 12.6% in those 80 years and older. The annual incidence of gout rose from 4.5 per 10,000 in 1977 to 1978 to 6.4 per 10,000 in 1995 to 1996, and to 12.4 per 10,000 from 1994 to 2007. Overall, the prevalence of gout has more than quadrupled over the past half-century. Despite being the most common inflammatory arthropathy, gout is frequently misdiagnosed and mismanaged.

■ PATHOPHYSIOLOGY

The most important risk factor for gout is hyperuricemia, or an excess of serum urate, the end product of purine metabolism. Serum urate concentrations are determined by the balance between urate production and elimination; hyperuricemia may be caused by either overproduction or underexcretion of urate, or a combination of both. Consumption of meat or seafood promotes hyperuricemia and gout as a result of the high-purine content of these foods. In contrast, alcohol consumption increases urate production through multiple mechanisms, including generation and turnover of ATP (a purine base), diuresis and dehydration, production of lactic and ketoacids (which block renal urate excretion), and the consumption of purines in alcoholic beverages. Beer and ale ingestion are most strongly correlated with hyperuricemia and gout (presumably because of their higher-purine content), while hard liquor increases serum urate and gout risk to an intermediate degree. Moderate wine consumption has a lesser effect on serum urate and the risk of gout, possibly because of other compounds present in wine. In history, the high prevalence of gout in affluent drinkers of wine and port may have been related to the use of lead acetate by wine merchants as a preservative and sweetener; chronic lead poisoning causes tubulointerstitial kidney disease that promotes hyperuricemia (saturnine gout) (**Table 247-1**).

More than 100 years ago Osler suggested that sugar intake might increase the risk of gout; recent studies prove Osler to have been correct. Gout prevalence has increased over the last 50 years, concomitant with the introduction and rising consumption of high-fructose corn syrup as a sweetener in prepared foods. Human

TABLE 247-1 Substances That Affect Urate Levels

Urate-Increasing Agents	Urate-Decreasing Agents
Foods	**Foods**
Meat, seafood (high in purines)	Dairy products
Alcoholic beverages	**Uricosurics**
Fructose	Lesinurad Probenecid
Metabolites	Sulfinpyrazone
Lactate	Salicylate (high dose)
β-hydroxybutyrate,	Losartan
Acetoacetate	Benzbromarone
Drugs	Fenofibrate
Pyrazinamide	Amlodipine
Nicotinate	**Xanthine oxidase inhibitors**
Salicylates (low dose)	Allopurinol
Diuretics	Febuxostat
Cyclosporine	**Uricase** (rasburicase, pegloticase)
Tacrolimus	
Ethambutol	
β-blockers	

metabolism and degradation of fructose generates urate to a greater degree than occurs with other sugars. In addition, fructose may have other hyperuricemia-inducing effects, by virtue of its ability to modulate urate transport in the kidney. In contrast, dairy consumption appears to be protective against hyperuricemia, perhaps because of the uricosuric effect of milk proteins such as casein.

Uric acid is eliminated from the body by both gastrointestinal and renal routes. Approximately one-third of urate elimination occurs through the gastrointestinal system, in saliva, gastric juices, pancreatic secretions, and direct loss from the bowel. The remaining two-thirds of urate excretion is via glomerular filtration and a complex balance of tubular secretion and reabsorption in the kidneys. Urate is freely filtered by the glomerulus, but 90% or more is reabsorbed. Tubular handling of urate is carried out via several organic anion transporters (OATs). Genomewide association studies have expanded our understanding of urate metabolism, and have identified genes that encode urate transporters in the kidney as well as the gut. Important genes involved in renal reabsorption of urate include SLC22A12 (encodes URAT1, a reabsorbing transporter) and SLC2A9 (encodes GLUT9 transporter). A number of agents that lower serum urate, such as probenecid, act by inhibiting URAT1 to promote renal urate excretion. In contrast, the ABCG2 gene has been found to encode the BRCP transporter, which promotes the renal tubular excretion of urate. Patients with genetic defects in BRCP tend to have reduced renal urate excretion, and increased serum levels of urate.

Hyperuricemia is considered either primary (related to intrinsic qualities of the individual) or secondary (acquired). The vast majority of gout patients have primary hyperuricemia, which may be compounded by secondary disease. About 90% of gout patients are *primary underexcreters*, with genetic molecular defects in renal urate excretion. Most of these patients have otherwise normal renal function. *Primary overproduction* accounts for the remaining 10% of primary hyperuricemia. Some patients who are primary overproducers have complete (Lesch-Nyhan syndrome) or partial (Kelly-Seegmiller syndrome) deficiency in hypoxanthine phosphoribosyltransferase (HPRT), the rate-limiting enzyme responsible for the salvage of degraded purines for reuse. All patients with Lesch-Nyhan syndrome, and some with Kelly-Seegmiller syndrome, also have neurocognitive deficits that are independent of their serum urate levels.

Secondary hyperuricemia occurs in acquired conditions that result in decreased urate excretion or increased urate generation. Acute or chronic renal insufficiency may impair urate excretion. Diseases of increased cell turnover, such as malignancies and hemolytic anemia, result in high urate production. Hyperuricemia can rarely manifest in the early teens due to a group of autosomal dominant diseases, which include familial juvenile hyperuricemic nephropathy (FJHN) and medullary cystic kidney type II disease. These diseases feature a mutant gene that interrupts the tertiary structure of uromodulin, also known as Tamm-Horsfall protein. The clinical presentation of these diseases not only includes early-onset gout, but also progressive renal failure and polyuria.

■ NATURAL HISTORY

Gout has traditionally been considered to occur in four progressive stages. In *asymptomatic hyperuricemia*, the risk of an acute gout attack increases as the level of uric acid rises past its solubility point (> 6.8 mg/dL). Once solubility is exceeded, monosodium urate crystals may precipitate in joint spaces and lead to *acute gouty arthritis*. During this stage, the innate immune system initiates a cascade of events in response to the crystals, including activation of complement and resident joint tissue macrophages, and recruitment of neutrophils from the bloodstream. The inflammasome, an intracellular assembly in macrophages that activates interleukin-1β (IL-1β), has recently been implicated in the inflammatory response to uric acid crystals. IL-1β in turn stimulates the production of other inflammatory mediators, including tumor necrosis factor (TNF)-α, IL-6, IL-8, and prostaglandin E_2. The result is severe local inflammation as well as a systemic response to cytokine release, including low-grade fever and elevated acute phase reactants. Acute gout attacks are exquisitely painful but typically self-limited, even without therapy, apparently because of inflammatory autoregulation.

The asymptomatic interval between acute gouty attacks is known as *intercritical gout*. Over time attacks tend to come more frequently, the intercritical period dwindles, and *chronic tophaceous gout* may develop. Tophi are aggregates of urate crystals, typically accompanied by a low-level chronic inflammatory state. They are actually complex structures, consisting of a mix of monosodium urate crystals and cellular debris surrounded by activated macrophages and other immune cells. Although tophi are most obvious when they occur in the periarticular soft tissues, they may also develop in cartilage and bone. Crystal deposition may result in a number of chronic syndromes of pain and disability (**Table 247-2**). Radiographic images of tophi in periarticular bone reveal the pathognomonic finding of punched-out erosions with sclerotic margins and overhanging edges (**Figure 247-1**). Recently, more sensitive imaging using ultrasound, magnetic resonance imaging (MRI) or dual-energy computed tomography (CT) have suggested that occult tophi are much more common that previously appreciated, and often form even before the onset of the initial acute gout attack, providing a readily available source of crystals for future acute attacks.

■ DIAGNOSIS AND DIFFERENTIAL DIAGNOSIS

The gold standard for the diagnosis of gout is needle aspiration of acutely or chronically inflamed joints or tophi, followed by polarized light microscopy to identify negatively birefringent, needle-shaped crystals (uric acid crystals). The presence of such crystals, particularly when seen intracellularly within infiltrating neutrophils, confirms the diagnosis of an acute attack and helps to distinguish gout from septic arthritis, pseudogout, and other causes of inflammatory joint disease. Extracellular crystals alone

TABLE 247-2 Musculoskeletal Manifestations of Crystal-Induced Arthropathy

Acute monoarthritis or polyarthritis

Bursitis

Tendonitis

Tophaceous deposits (including vertebrae)

Enthesitis

Synovial osteochondromatosis

Pseudoankylosing spondylitis

Carpal tunnel syndrome

Tendon rupture

Joint destruction

Pseudorheumatoid arthritis

Spinal stenosis

Crown dens syndrome

Inflammatory osteoarthritis

are diagnostic of gout, but not necessarily an acute gouty attack; in patients with established gout, previously formed crystals may persist even after inflammation has resolved, residing as innocent bystanders in the setting of other joint pathologies. The sensitivity of synovial fluid analysis for demonstrating negatively birefringent crystals in patients with acute gouty arthritis is at least 85%, with a specificity approaching 100%. In contrast, the specificity of a clinical diagnosis of gout is significantly lower, and septic arthritis and pseudogout are often misdiagnosed as gout. *Therefore, in almost all circumstances, diagnostic arthrocentesis should be performed if possible, especially in the hospital setting.*

As acute gout may coexist with other joint pathology, a wider evaluation is almost always warranted, even in the presence of intracellular, negatively birefringent crystals. In addition to crystal

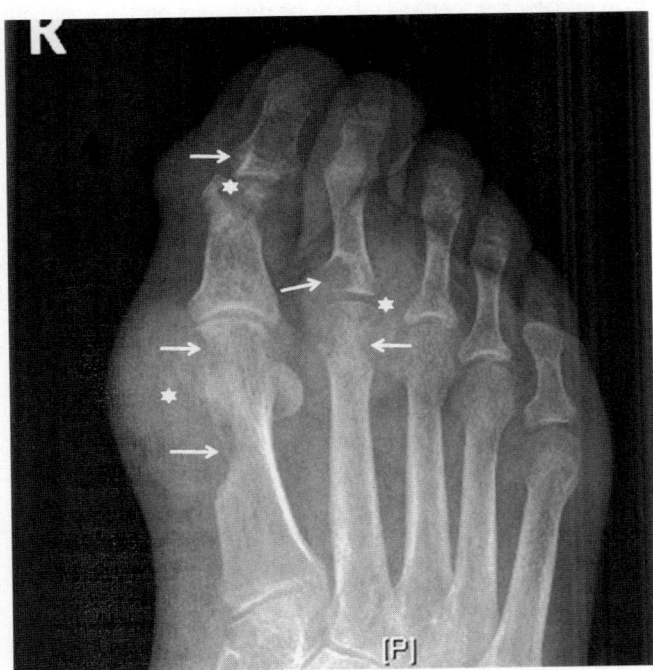

Figure 247-1 *Tophaceous gout causing an erosive arthropathy. Note the large tophi (stars) and "rat-bite" erosions with overhanging edges (arrows).*

analysis, synovial fluid should always be sent for cell count with differential, Gram stain, and culture. Grossly, synovial fluid is typically straw colored and varies from translucent to opaque. Synovial fluid cell counts in gout may range from 2000 to >100,000 per mm³, with greater than 50% neutrophils (often approaching 90%). Serum uric acid should also be obtained during an acute attack, and a high serum urate supports the possibility of a diagnosis of gout. However, patients may be hyperuricemic without having gout, and serum urate levels in gout patients may be transiently normal or low during an acute attack due to an increase in renal excretion (an effect of the cytokine IL-6 on the kidney). Erythrocyte sedimentation rate (ESR) and C-reactive protein (CRP) are typically elevated during a gout attack, but this finding is nonspecific. Urinary uric acid collections should not be obtained during gout attacks; they are neither useful nor reliable in the acute period.

Radiographs in the acute setting typically show only nondescript soft tissue swelling, but radiographic evidence of erosions can confirm chronic disease. Musculoskeletal ultrasound (MSUS) may visualize intraarticular crystal deposits, with a characteristic hyperechoic enhancement of the outer surface of the hyaline cartilage, known as the *double contour sign*. MSUS may prove to be an alternative method for the diagnosis of the crystal arthropathies, but limitations include the inability to distinguish the presence or absence of infection. Advanced imaging technologies such as dual energy computed tomography (DECT) and improved magnetic resonance imaging can also play a role in the diagnosis and differentiation of gout from other inflammatory arthropathies, but availability and cost limit their current clinical utility.

The differential diagnosis for acute gout includes conditions generally associated with acute monoarthritis, such as pseudogout and septic arthritis, as well as conditions leading to oligoarthritis and polyarthritis, such as reactive arthritis, psoriatic arthritis, and even rheumatoid arthritis. Ideally, a crystal diagnosis of gout should be the goal; if this is not possible, the diagnosis of acute gouty arthropathy should be made by a combination of historical and clinical criteria. A thorough history will help distinguish an acute gout attack from other causes of acute arthritis. Some of the previously proposed clinical, radiographic, and laboratory criteria include (1) a history of one or more episodes of monoarticular arthritis, followed by intercritical periods completely free of symptoms (may not be applicable in the acute hospital setting); (2) maximum inflammation within 24 hours of onset of the attack; (3) rapid resolution after initiation of colchicine or a nonsteroidal anti-inflammatory drug (NSAID); (4) unilateral first metatarsophalangeal joint involvement (podagra), especially during a first event; (5) hyperuricemia; and (6) bony erosions (punched out lesions with overhanging edges) on plain radiograph or (7) tophi.

Acute attacks most often affect the first metatarsophalangeal joint (up to 50% of first attacks). The tarsal joints, ankles, knees, elbows, and interphalangeal (IP) joints are also commonly affected. In elderly patients with osteoarthritis (OA), Heberden and Bouchard nodes (seen in hand OA) are potential targets for inflammation, and red, swollen proximal and distal IP joints may be the first manifestation of gout. Episodes of acute gouty arthritis frequently come on rapidly at night or in the early morning with dramatic pain and swelling. The joint becomes warm, red, and tender, often mimicking cellulitis. Without treatment, most acute attacks resolve in 2 to 14 days.

PRACTICE POINT

- In a postoperative or postdiuresis patient with an acute inflammatory arthropathy, with or without fever, consider gout or another crystal arthropathy in the differential diagnosis.

■ HOSPITAL ADMISSION

While acute gout attacks can often be managed in the outpatient setting, patients may need to be admitted to the hospital to facilitate workup or to rapidly and definitively rule out the possibility of infection. Patients with severe disability from their acute attack and inadequate home support may need to be admitted until they are able to ambulate or otherwise function. Often, patients at risk may develop acute gouty attacks while hospitalized for other problems. In the hospital setting, attacks may be precipitated by metabolic acidosis, fasting, diuretics, or disruptions in volume status or renal function that may cause acute swings (both elevations and depressions) in serum urate levels. Discontinuation of urate lowering therapy in hospitalized gout patients is a common error that can lead to acute serum urate changes that provoke gouty attacks; this practice is not recommended according to the American College of Rheumatology (ACR) 2012 treatment guidelines. Gout flares occurring during hospitalization for other causes are generally avoidable, and increase the length of stay by approximately 3 days.

■ TREATMENT OF ACUTE GOUT

Colchicine is effective in the acute setting, and, if initiated sufficiently early, may abrogate an acute attack. It is typically less effective after the attack is established (≥36 hours). The traditional dosing of colchicine for acute attacks (0.6 mg by mouth every 1-2 hours until onset of relief or a maximum of 6 mg) frequently led to undesirable side effects. A more limited regimen—colchicine 1.2 mg, followed by 0.6 mg 1 hour later—is equally effective, with toxicity similar to placebo. It has now been adopted as standard of care. Patients with renal insufficiency may receive this regimen, but should subsequently discontinue any use of low-dose daily colchicine for several weeks; patients without renal disease may continue their prophylaxis unabated.

PRACTICE POINT

- Treatments for acute gout, such as NSAIDs, glucocorticoids and particularly colchicine, work best when administered within hours of the onset of the attack.

For many patients, *NSAIDs* are preferred agents for acute gout. Indomethacin is the traditional choice at 50 to 75 mg initially, then 50 mg every 6 hours, not exceeding 200 mg in a 24-hour period. However, clinical studies have shown that many other NSAIDs, including COX-2 selective agents, are as effective as indomethacin when used at their maximum doses and may be better tolerated. NSAIDs have the advantage of both analgesic and anti-inflammatory effects, but may be relatively contraindicated in patients with gastritis, renal insufficiency, hypertension, and heart failure. In order to maximize response time while minimizing side effects, a combination of more than one class of medications, such as NSAID plus colchicine, is sometimes used in treating acute attacks.

Glucocorticoids are potent anti-inflammatory agents that can be highly effective at abrogating acute gouty attacks. Intraarticular glucocorticoids may be particularly useful in treating acute gout in a single joint or bursa when systemic glucocorticoid use is undesirable. Care must be taken to establish the diagnosis and to rule out infection prior to injecting glucocorticoids directly into the joint. As a practical matter, this often means performing joint aspiration and injection as separate procedures, which may unfortunately add to the patient's discomfort. Oral and intravenous glucocorticoids are both very effective, especially in patients with polyarticular attacks, and may be the agents of choice in patients with contraindications to colchicine and NSAIDs, such as renal insufficiency. ACR guidelines recommend a starting dose of approximately 0.5 mg/kg/d of oral prednisone. Although treatment periods with oral steroids are typically brief (about a week), relative contraindications such as diabetes, hypertension, and heart failure must be considered.

A single intramuscular injection of depot *adrenocorticotropic hormone*, or ACTH gel (25-80 IU, repeated 24-72 hours later if needed) can also terminate attacks effectively and may be particularly useful in patients who cannot take oral medication. In addition to stimulating the adrenal cortex to produce corticosteroids, ACTH reduces the acute inflammatory response by activating melanocortin receptor-3. Follow-up treatment using low-dose (one to two times daily) colchicine is typically recommended to prevent rebound attacks as the ACTH wears off. However, ACTH gel is currently not Food and Drug Administration (FDA) approved for use in gout, and its high cost in the United States limits its use.

Given the role of IL-1β in acute gouty inflammation, several studies have addressed the use of anti-IL-1β biological therapy in acute gout flares. Both anakinra, an IL-1β receptor antagonist, and canakinumab, an anti-IL-1β antibody, have shown efficacy. Although expensive and off-label, these agents may be considered when established therapies have failed and/or are contraindicated.

■ CHRONIC MANAGEMENT OF GOUT

The goal of chronic gout management is to prevent acute attacks and to decrease the total body urate burden, including both visible tophi and occult deposits. This is achieved by lowering serum urate to less than 6 mg/dL, and requires a multipronged approach. *Lifestyle changes* such as weight loss, avoidance of fructose-rich foods and high-purine foods such as organ meats and shellfish, and eliminating or reducing alcohol consumption should be the first step, with the addition of one or more urate-lowering agents being necessary for most patients with chronic gout. *Medication review* may identify agents that are contributing to hyperuricemia. For example, thiazides and loop diuretics reduce uric acid excretion and raise serum urate. Therefore, these should be used at the lowest effective dose, or stopped if appropriate alternatives are available. Both losartan (for hypertension) and fenofibrate (for hyperlipidemia) have uricosuric properties and may be useful options for treatment of these conditions in patients who also have gout.

Current ACR guidelines address the management of gout patients, including the initiation of urate-lowering therapy. Urate-lowering therapy should be started on any gout patient with 2 or more attacks in a 12-month period. Patients with tophi should also undergo urate lowering, as should patients with stage 2 or worse chronic kidney disease or a history of urolithiasis, even after only a single attack. Urate-lowering agents commonly used to treat chronic gout include inhibitors of xanthine oxidase (allopurinol and febuxostat) and uricosuric agents (probenecid, sulfinpyrazone, and benzbromarone).

Long considered a first-line agent for chronic gout management, *allopurinol* is a purine analog of hypoxanthine. Along with its active metabolite oxypurinol, allopurinol competitively inhibits xanthine oxidase, decreasing urate production and serum uric acid levels. Appropriate allopurinol use requires dose titration to achieve a prespecified serum urate target, most commonly <6 mg/dL (lower if necessary to reduce tophi or control attacks). The most common dose required to achieve target is 400 mg/d. Lower doses may be sufficient in some patients, but doses as high as 800 mg/d may be required in others (and are FDA approved). Side effects are uncommon but may be serious and include rash, cytopenias, and hypersensitivity syndromes, such as toxic epidermal necrolysis and Steven-Johnson syndrome. Although most serious side effects occur within the first 6 to 8 weeks of use, long-term monitoring is required. Dosing should be initiated at 100 mg/d, and increased every 2 to 5 weeks until the target dose is achieved. For patients with stage 4 or greater chronic kidney disease, the ACR recommends initiating a dose of 50 mg/d, but still titrating to serum urate target. Since azathioprine is metabolized by xanthine oxidase, allopurinol use may raise azathioprine levels and result in bone marrow toxicity. Concomitant use of allopurinol and azathioprine should therefore be avoided or relegated to experts.

Febuxostat is a nonpurine, selective inhibitor of xanthine oxidase. Dosing is limited to 40 to 80 mg daily (up to 120 mg daily in Europe), and dose adjustment is not needed in patients with mild to moderate kidney impairment. Febuxostat does not chemically resemble allopurinol and appears to be safe for patients with allopurinol sensitivity. In several clinical trials, febuxostat 40 mg has been shown to be roughly equivalent to allopurinol 300 mg for urate lowering.

Uricosuric medications such as probenecid, sulfinpyrazone, and benzbromarone (the latter two not available in the United States) increase renal urate excretion by inhibiting URAT1 transporters in the proximal tubule. To prevent uric acid kidney stones, patients should drink generous amounts of fluids and avoid high doses of vitamin C and other drugs that may acidify the urine. Urine alkalinization may occasionally be necessary. For most patients these agents are considered second-line therapy, or may be added to a xanthine oxidase inhibitor for added benefit. Most current uricosuric agents work poorly in patients with mild to moderate chronic kidney disease (estimated glomerular filtration rate <50 mL/h). The recently approved uricosuric lesinurad is effective even in patients with kidney disease as low as 45 ml/min, but is indicated for use only in conjunction with allopurinol or febuxostat.

A novel therapeutic approach to urate lowering is to provide uricase, a urate-degrading enzyme that humans lost the ability to synthesize millions of years ago. *Pegloticase* is a pegylated recombinant mammalian (porcine/bovine) uricase. It is given by intravenous infusion and can rapidly and dramatically decrease serum urate levels. Pegloticase has been approved by the Food and Drug Administration for patients with gout who have failed or are intolerant of other therapy, and is significantly more effective than other agents at resolving tophi.

Since pharmacologic lowering of uric acid paradoxically increases the risk of gout for a period of at least 6 months, patients starting any of these drugs should be prophylaxed against acute attacks. Patients typically should be started with colchicine 0.6 mg once or twice daily beginning several days before the initiation of urate-lowering therapy, and continuing for at least several months after the target urate level has been achieved. Low-dose NSAIDs or prednisone are options for patients who cannot tolerate colchicine.

■ CONSULTATION

Rheumatology consultation should be obtained when the diagnosis is unclear or the presentation seems atypical for a patient with known gout. Consultation should also be obtained when synovial fluid cannot be obtained easily, when expertise is required in fluid analysis or interpretation, or when contraindications to traditional therapies complicate patient management.

PSEUDOGOUT AND CHONDROCALCINOSIS: CALCIUM PYROPHOSPHATE DEPOSITION (CPPD) DISEASE

Although pseudogout is frequently considered a poor cousin of gout, it is a common condition that can be acutely incapacitating and chronically destructive, and presents as a cause or consequence of hospital admission. Like gout, pseudogout is a disease in which crystal formation leads to inflammation and mechanical damage. Unlike gout, in which a systemic metabolic derangement promotes crystal deposition, pseudogout usually appears to derive from metabolic abnormalities intrinsic to chondrocytes, resulting in crystal

deposition in cartilage. However, the result is similar: innate immune responses to crystals leads to local hyperemia, joint effusion, and neutrophil influx, and the four cardinal signs of inflammation: heat, redness, pain, and swelling.

Although pseudogout may occur in familial, early-onset forms, most cases are sporadic and acquired. Acquired pseudogout is a disease of aging, rarely presenting before the age of 50. Exceptions include patients with cartilage derangement from prior injury and patients in whom pseudogout is secondary to other medical conditions (see below). Both men and women may contract pseudogout, with women affected somewhat more commonly than men.

■ PATHOPHYSIOLOGY

In pseudogout, the offending crystal is calcium pyrophosphate, and the perpetrating cell appears to be the articular cartilage chondrocyte itself. Chondrocytes in healthy articular cartilage prevent calcification and maintain the elastic cartilage matrix. In pseudogout, chondrocytes go awry and promote calcium pyrophosphate deposition (**Figure 247-2**). That chondrocytes are able to lay down calcium crystals should not be surprising, as growth plate chondrocytes direct bone formation during fetal development.

Chondrocyte dysregulation in pseudogout appears to result in a local oversupply of inorganic pyrophosphate (PPi). Abnormalities

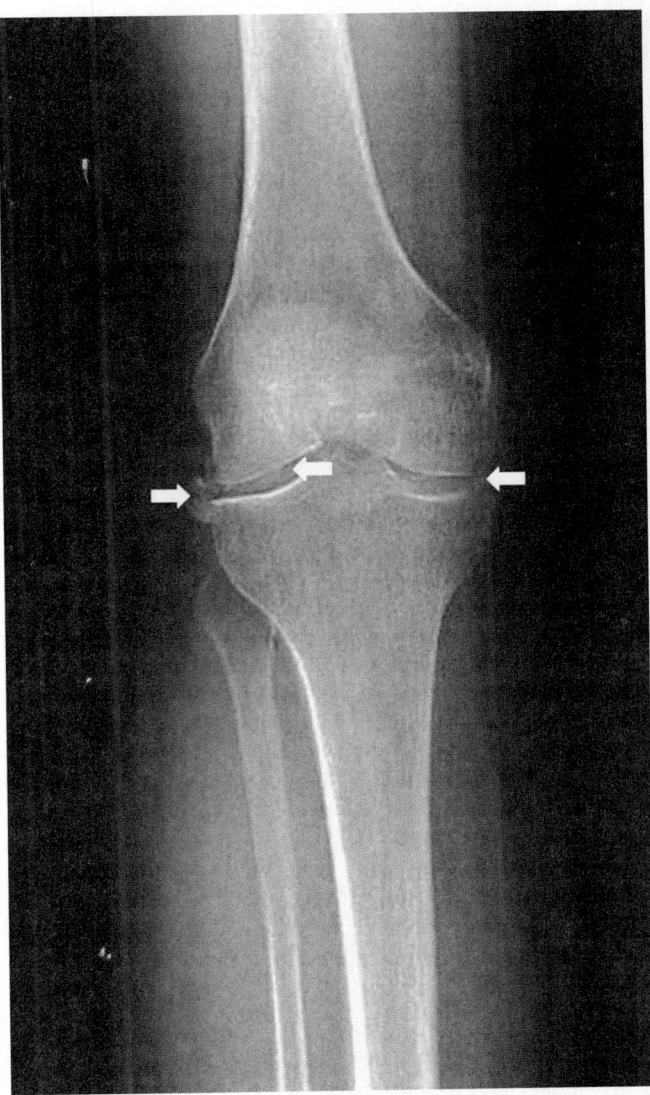

Figure 247-2 *Severe pseudogout, with linear deposition of calcium pyrophosphate throughout the meniscus (arrows).*

in several enzymes have been implicated, including nucleotide pyrophosphatase phosphodiesterase 1 (NPP1), which liberates extracellular PPi from adenosine triphosphate (ATP) and other nucleotide triphosphates, and the ankylosis human protein (ANKH), a transmembrane protein that transports PPi from inside to outside the chondrocyte. Mutations increasing ANKH activity have been detected in some cases of familial pseudogout; in sporadic pseudogout, ANKH may be normal in structure, but upregulated in activity. The rise in extracellular PPi concentrations shifts the equilibrium for encounter with extracellular inorganic calcium ions, resulting in precipitation.

Extracellular precipitation of calcium pyrophosphate results in crystal deposition within cartilage (chondrocalcinosis), which can often be detected on plain radiographs or using musculoskeletal ultrasound. The typical appearance of chondrocalcinosis is a linear or stippled radiodense deposit, below but parallel to the surface of the cartilage. Chondrocalcinosis alone is usually insufficient to promote acute inflammation, presumably because crystals in cartilage are sequestered from the immune system. Indeed, chondrocalcinosis is frequently diagnosed as an incidental, asymptomatic finding on radiographs taken for other reasons. However, when crystals appear in joint fluid, either from shedding from cartilage or precipitation in the joint space, they promote the same sorts of inflammatory processes seen in gout. Like uric acid crystals, calcium pyrophosphate crystals may activate complement, promoting neutrophil chemotaxis, and interact with synovial macrophages to induce production of IL-1β and other cytokines. The clinical presentation of pseudogout can therefore mimic gout, with a rapid onset of joint inflammation sometimes precipitated by trauma or metabolic derangements, and is typically self-limiting after days of inflammation. However, the presence of CPP crystals may sometimes promote chronic smoldering inflammation, rather than acute inflammation.

PRACTICE POINT

- Chondrocalcinosis (radiologic evidence of calcium pyrophosphate deposition in cartilage) indicates overproduction of calcium pyrophosphate. However, chondrocalcinosis frequently exists without the clinical inflammation of acute pseudogout, and pseudogout can conversely occur in the absence of visible chondrocalcinosis.

Calcium pyrophosphate deposition (CPPD) disease may also be associated with chronic noninflammatory joint damage. In such cases, CPPD disease may strongly resemble OA, in that progression is slow, and radiographs are characterized by joint space narrowing (ie, cartilage loss) and osteophyte formation. It is often difficult to distinguish this condition from OA itself. When chondrocalcinosis and arthritis co-occur in joints not usually associated with OA, it is usually presumed that CPPD is the driving process, with cartilage damage from crystal deposition promoting an OA picture.

A number of medical conditions have been associated with chondrocalcinosis or pseudogout. While the exact relationship between these conditions and calcium crystal deposition is not always clear, they tend to fall into several overlapping groups, which include features of cartilage destruction, metabolic abnormalities, and abnormal calcium or phosphate homeostasis. Among these are hemochromatosis, in which iron deposition in cartilage can induce OA; gout; hyperparathyroidism, with its attendant disruptions of calcium and phosphate metabolism; hypophosphatasia (in which PPi degradation by the nonspecific tissue enzyme alkaline phosphatase is diminished); and hypomagnesemia, which may alter pyrophosphatase activity.

■ DIAGNOSIS AND DIFFERENTIAL DIAGNOSIS

The typical presentation of pseudogout is acute monoarticular arthritis, most often in a large joint such as the knee, sometimes with a violent onset indistinguishable from gout. Although some clinicians aver that pseudogout is typically slower of onset and less severe than gout, these distinctions are not sufficiently rigorous to permit any speculation on whether a specific acute monoarthritis is gout or pseudogout. Compared with gout, pseudogout less commonly affects the big toe and is unrelated to dietary or bibulous indiscretion. Moreover, pseudogout is less likely than gout to be polyarticular, and since pseudogout appears to depend upon the actions of chondrocytes, it is unusual to see pseudogout in a cartilage-free structure such as a bursa. As in gout, the most important consideration in the differential diagnosis of pseudogout is septic arthritis, which may induce rapid joint damage if not promptly managed. Other crystal diseases, including hydroxyapatite and calcium oxalate deposition (the latter most common in dialysis patients), also deserve consideration. Although osteoarthritis is less inflammatory than pseudogout, patients with severe osteoarthritis occasionally have flares that may be confused with acute pseudogout. Reactive arthritis and other forms of inflammatory arthritis may appear in joints typically associated with acute pseudogout and may be clinically indistinguishable from it, though these will more often present in a chronic and polyarticular fashion.

In addition to history and physical examination, initial workup of an acute pseudogout attack should include serum white blood cell count, electrolytes, creatinine, uric acid, and ESR and/or CRP. Chondrocalcinosis on plain radiographs supports the possibility of pseudogout, but many patients with chondrocalcinosis never develop pseudogout, and some patients with pseudogout have no radiologic chondrocalcinosis. Accordingly, the diagnosis of acute pseudogout is best made by inspecting fluid from a joint aspiration using a compensated polarizing microscope. As in gout, *in almost all acute circumstances, arthrocentesis should be performed;* in the hands of an experienced physician, the procedure is quick, relatively painless, and of high yield. The presence of positively birefringent crystals, either needle-like, rhomboid, or both, is pathognomonic of calcium pyrophosphate deposition. The presence of these crystals within neutrophils confirms that inflammation is directed at CPP crystals. As in gout, the physician should obtain a cell count, Gram stain, and culture, and also examine the fluid for negatively birefringent, needle-like urate crystals. Both pseudogout and gout can coexist with infection, and also with each other, so that the presence of one does not rule out the possibility of the other. Indeed, a patient with a synovial fluid white count of >50,000/mm³ should generally be presumed to have an infection pending Gram stain and culture results, even if evidence of acute pseudogout or gout is also seen.

As noted above, patients with CPPD disease may, either instead of or in addition to acute pseudogout, experience progressive cartilage degeneration as in osteoarthritis. When this occurs in joints not typical for osteoarthritis, a crystal-based etiology may be presumed (Table 247-2). In these individuals, plain radiographs may reveal a combination of osteoarthritis-like joint narrowing and chondrocalcinosis. Patients with pseudogout as well as osteoarthritis in the second and third metacarpophalangeal joints should also be assessed for hemochromatosis, as these joints are atypical for primary osteoarthritis, but typical for CPPD due to hemochromatosis. In addition, patients may experience CPPD as a low-level inflammatory arthritis in almost any joint. When this occurs in the small joints of the hands, it may mimic rheumatoid arthritis (pseudorheumatoid arthritis).

Patients with clinically atypical, crystal-proven pseudogout, or those who develop CPPD before the age of 50, should be assessed for an underlying etiology. The workup may include levels of calcium, phosphate, magnesium; iron studies, including serum ferritin; testing for the hemochromatosis (HFE) gene; levels of parathyroid- and thyroid-stimulating hormone; and levels of insulin-like growth factor in patients with features of acromegaly. In most cases, however, these evaluations are not fruitful.

■ ALTERNATIVE NOMENCLATURE

In an effort to simplify and regularize the nomenclature applied to CPPD disease, the European League Against Rheumatism has proposed that CPPD conditions be considered as four different characteristic conditions, using a naming system that is more accurate if less picturesque than that typically used in current practice. According to the EULAR system, CPPD conditions should be considered to include *cartilage calcification*, replacing the term chondrocalcinosis; *acute calcium pyrophosphate arthritis*, roughly the equivalent of the current term pseudogout; and *pyrophosphate arthropathy*, further subdivided into *chronic CPP crystal inflammatory arthritis* and *osteoarthritis with CPPD*, to distinguish between chronic conditions characterized by smoldering inflammation, and osteoarthritic cartilage degeneration presumed to be driven by CPPD, respectively. Of course, these conditions may coexist and overlap.

■ TREATMENT

As with gout, acute pseudogout should be treated with whatever anti-inflammatory is most likely to be both effective and benign for the particular patient. Most patients with acute pseudogout respond well to NSAIDs, with selective COX-2 inhibitors a reasonable option. Oral, intramuscular or intraarticular corticosteroids are also effective. Care must be taken to confirm that the joint is not infected before directly injecting steroids. Conventional wisdom suggests that oral colchicine may be less efficacious for acute pseudogout than it is for gout, but studies are not available to support such a distinction, and colchicine remains a treatment option. Intramuscular ACTH is also an option for acute pseudogout, although availability may be limited. Recent studies implicating IL-1β production in crystal-induced inflammation suggest that brief anti-IL-1β therapy, for example, the IL-1β receptor antagonist anakinra, may be considered for individuals without other viable treatment options. Nonpharmacologic therapy should include topical cooling and resting the affected joint.

Long-term management of pseudogout includes anti-inflammatory prophylaxis for individuals with recurrent attacks, preferentially using daily low-dose colchicine (more effective than in the acute setting, and generally well tolerated), or NSAIDs or low-dose steroids in some cases. For patients with chronic smoldering inflammation, the aforementioned agents remain the first choice, but recent studies have suggested that some immunosuppressives, such as hydroxychloroquine or methotrexate, may also be of value. When underlying etiologies for pseudogout are identified, these should be treated, although data are limited as to whether such treatment affects the outcome of the CPPD disease. In contrast to gout, there is no proven approach to prevent or reverse crystal formation.

OSTEOARTHRITIS

Osteoarthritis is the most common of the arthritic conditions, affecting approximately 30 million people in the United States alone. Although typically a disease of the elderly, osteoarthritis may affect individuals of almost any age, particularly when specific risk factors lead to early onset. OA can affect any joint, but most frequently involves the hands, hips, and knees. The current management of OA is largely palliative or surgical, although recent advances raise the possibility that pharmacologic management may be possible in the future.

■ PATHOPHYSIOLOGY

The hallmark of OA is loss of articular cartilage, often in joints that are subject to stress. This feature of OA led to the long-standing conclusion, still held in some circles, that OA is entirely a disease of wear and tear. The situation is more complex however, and it is increasingly clear that OA represents the intersection of cartilage tissue stress, intrinsic structural qualities, and aberrant cellular and tissue responses that result in a potentially progressive condition. Changes in subchondral bone and synovium occur concurrently, such that OA is a disease that ultimately involves all joint tissues.

Old age is the most robust risk factor for OA. Long life may result in cumulative wear, but intrinsic aging of the cartilage may also contribute; OA cartilage in the nonelderly has features of prematurely aged tissue. *Female sex* increases the risk for OA, by mechanisms that remain unclear but may be partly related to hormones or genetics. Individuals with *obesity* are 5 to 10 times more likely to develop knee OA; obesity's impact may be partly due to mechanical stress, but adipose tissue is also metabolically active, and secretes inflammatory cytokines that may play a role. Indeed, obese individuals are two to three times more likely to develop hand OA, despite the fact that hands are nonweight bearing. *Improper joint alignment*—whether hereditary or as a result of injury—also appears to increase the risk for OA, as does *direct trauma*, as in sports injuries. Rarely, *genetic abnormalities* in cartilage or bone biochemistry may result in premature, familial OA. However, *genetic factors* have also been associated with ordinary OA development, based upon twin and nontwin sibling, modern molecular, and population studies.

The earliest pathologic features in OA are microscopic fissures on cartilage surfaces where mechanical stress is greatest. Mechanical loading can induce beneficial chondrocyte responses, including cell hypertrophy and the production of structural elements such as type II collagen and aggrecan. However, chondrocytes are sometimes driven to catabolic activities that contribute to cartilage degradation, especially in the context of genetic abnormalities or prior injury. Overall, OA represents an imbalance between anabolic and catabolic processes in cartilage. As the disease progresses, chondrocytes cluster, secreting metalloproteinases and aggrecanases that disassemble the joint cartilage. Over time, this results in loss of articular cartilage thickness, increased susceptibility to mechanical destruction, and progressive deterioration of the cartilage surface.

Bone, bone marrow, and synovium are all involved in OA pathogenesis. Plain radiographs frequently demonstrate subchondral sclerosis and *osteophytes*, bony ridges that extend the joint surface and may progress to bony hypertrophy (**Figure 247-3**). It is unclear whether these are compensatory or pathologic features; however, surgical removal of osteophytes generally does not relieve the symptoms of OA. MRI studies have identified bone marrow lesions under the affected joints as a hallmark of OA. On pathology, these represent fibrotic and necrotic tissue, and possibly microfractures. Although OA has long (and incorrectly) been called a noninflammatory disease, imaging with MRI and ultrasound have now confirmed that many OA patients have synovitis, though to a milder degree than is seen in rheumatoid or psoriatic arthritis. Other studies have confirmed that in OA both synovial cells and chondrocytes produce a wide range of inflammatory cytokines.

■ CLINICAL FEATURES AND DIAGNOSIS

Symptoms of OA may come on insidiously or intermittently over a number of years. The most common feature of OA is pain in weight-bearing joints, such as the knees and hips. Involvement of the shoulders, elbows, and hands is not uncommon. Any joint that has suffered stress or injury is more susceptible. Unlike rheumatoid arthritis, joint involvement in OA may be monoarticular or

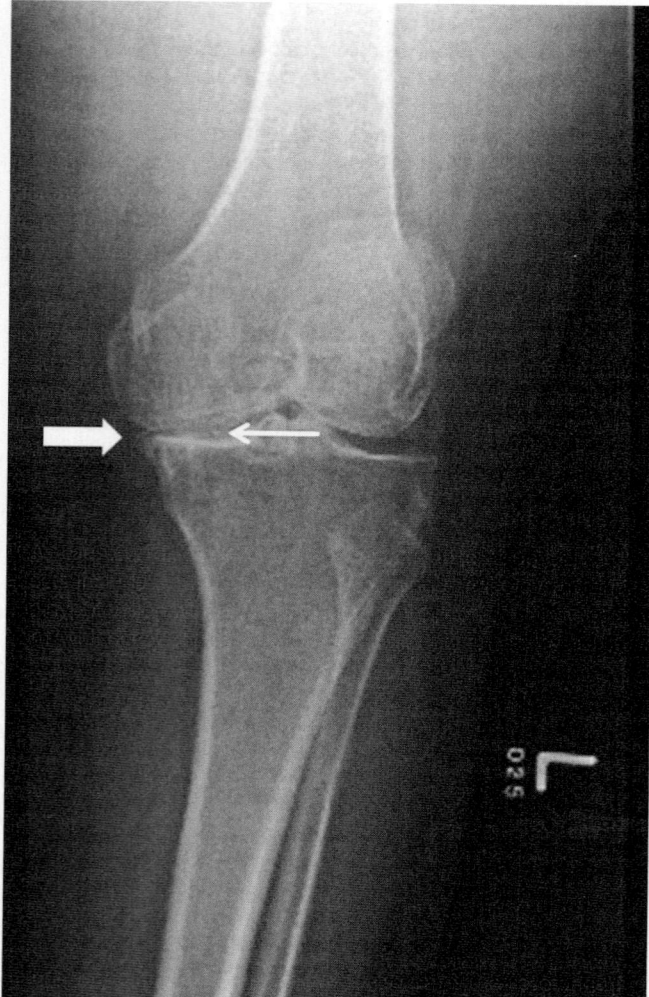

Figure 247-3 *Knee joint osteoarthritis, showing osteophyte (broad arrow) and medial joint space loss (narrow arrow), as well as medial subchondral sclerosis.*

oligoarticular, but is not typically polyarticular, and need not be symmetrical.

Pain from OA is most likely to occur during joint use. For example, knee pain tends to be exacerbated with walking, and some patients can characterize their use limitations with a high degree of accuracy. Many patients report that OA pain is worse during cold or rainy weather, a phenomenon that remains incompletely understood. OA pain may also be nocturnal. Morning stiffness may be present in OA patients but tends to be of short duration, typically lasting 15 to 30 minutes, in contrast to rheumatoid arthritis, where morning stiffness may persist for hours. As OA progresses, the patient may notice limitation in the range of motion of the joint, owing to cartilage defects, joint effusions, and osteophytes. The joint may become swollen and slightly warm. Over a long period of time, joint mobility may become profoundly limited and disability may ensue. For the patient with knee or hip OA, this may mean an inability to walk more than short distances. Patients with shoulder OA may be unable to reach into kitchen cabinets or perform basic dressing, washing, and toileting functions. Pain in one joint not infrequently results in pain in another joint of the same or the opposite limb, possibly relating to the additional stress resulting from compensation for the OA joint. Spinal involvement may lead to spinal stenosis and nerve root impingement by osteophytes.

Physical examination of the osteoarthritic joint typically reveals crepitus—palpable grinding during joint motion that reflects the fraying and roughening of the cartilage surface. The presence of crepitus, in the setting of characteristic joint pain, may be sufficient to diagnose OA, even in the absence of radiographic findings. As OA progresses, joint examination may reveal not only crepitus, but other evidence of OA, including limited range of motion, pain with motion, effusions, and bony hypertrophy. In the knee, OA is frequently accompanied by deterioration and tearing of the menisci and other adjacent structures.

Radiographic studies in OA have characteristic features. In weight-bearing joints, the first and most obvious finding is narrowing of the joint space, reflecting loss of radiolucent cartilage. In the knee, this loss of joint space typically favors a single compartment, such as the medial or lateral tibiofemoral compartment or the patello-femoral compartment, although eventually all compartments may be affected. Meniscal extrusion may also manifest as joint space narrowing. In the hip, the superior, weight-bearing surface of the joint is most often affected. With disease progression, other characteristic findings may appear. Subchondral sclerosis may be seen as a linear increase in bone density just below the joint surface. Although osteophytes are actually circumferential ridges, on the two-dimensional views presented by plain radiographs they will appear as bone spicules off the margins of the joints. Bone cysts—discrete, circular, or ovoid regions of decreased bone density located just below the joint surface—are common, though their importance remains unclear. In the spine, OA findings may include those described above, but the different anatomic nature of the spine may also result in disk-space narrowing, foraminal narrowing, and other unique features. MRI and ultrasound are seldom if ever needed to diagnose an OA joint, but if obtained may demonstrate bone marrow edema, synovitis, and cartilage and meniscal degradation.

Laboratory studies are mainly useful to rule in or out alternative diagnoses. For example, a normal ESR or CRP makes inflammatory arthritis less likely. In patients with features suggestive of rheumatoid arthritis, a serum rheumatoid factor and anticyclic citrullinated peptide antibody (anti-CCP) titer may be useful. Serum urate levels may help stratify the patient's risk for gout. When a joint effusion is present, synovial fluid analysis may be the most useful laboratory investigation. In OA, synovial fluid should contain only a limited number of leukocytes (<2000/mm^3). Higher counts suggest a different or additional condition. Urate or calcium pyrophosphate crystals indicate gout or pseudogout, respectively. Although acute joint swelling only occasionally occurs in OA, aspiration of the joint fluid is needed in this setting to rule out the presence of infection or concomitant crystal-induced inflammation. Serum and joint fluid markers of cartilage turnover, such as N-telopeptide and C-telopeptide, may have some utility in determining the rate of cartilage damage, but they are currently used mainly in the research setting.

Associated conditions. As discussed elsewhere, calcium pyrophosphate deposition and OA often coexist in the same patient. It is unclear whether CPPD predisposes to OA, the cartilage damage of OA predisposes to calcium pyrophosphate deposition, or both. The finding of both diseases in several joints not normally expressing OA, such as the second and third metacarpophalangeal joints, suggests at least an element of the former. Patients with hemochromatosis are predisposed to both calcium pyrophosphate deposition and OA; once again, metacarpophalangeal OA may be a clue. Patients with gout also have a high incidence of OA, though this could be merely coexpression in an older population predisposed to both conditions. Rarely, ochronosis, with cartilaginous deposition of homogentisic acid, predisposes to severe OA. Patients with acromegaly frequently have OA, presumably owing to abnormal forces across the enlarged bone. Diabetics appear to have a higher incidence of OA because of the buildup of advanced glycation end products (AGEs) in cartilage matrix, which may make cartilage more brittle and stiff, impair normal turnover and repair, and have local pro-inflammatory effects.

■ TREATMENT

Current OA management is palliative and conservative. Clinicians should educate their patients and provide them with a greater understanding and sense of control over their condition. Physical therapy helps to preserve muscle strength and proprioception and improve joint stress. Muscle weakness and capsular and ligamentous damage may hinder joint proprioception in OA patients, increasing their fall risk. For the knee, evidence suggests that regular adherence to a quadriceps-strengthening exercise regimen helps reduce pain and maintain function. Small studies also suggest that tai chi may improve pain and physical function in knee OA. Bracing is another underutilized option; even simple bracing with a neoprene sleeve may assist with joint proprioception and reduce pain with ambulation, with essentially no adverse effects. More sophisticated braces and taping techniques may better stabilize the joint, or reduce the load across the cartilage surface. The use of a cane in the contralateral hand also reduces joint stress and contributes to a sense of well-being. Other therapeutic modalities, such as heat, cold, and ultrasound, may have analgesic benefits in individual patients.

For analgesia, the American College of Rheumatology recommends the initial use of *acetaminophen* for all patients who can tolerate it. This recommendation may be in evolution, as recent studies have questioned the extent of acetaminophen's effectiveness. While many patients have failed acetaminophen prior to presenting to a physician, in most cases they have not used it at the maximum dose of 3 g daily. Long-acting formulations reduce the dosing frequency and may improve compliance. Care should be taken to avoid the use of acetaminophen with combination agents that also include acetaminophen, thus pushing the dose beyond acceptable limits. Acetaminophen is well tolerated but has a narrow therapeutic window, with an LD50 for a single dose of approximately 10 g. Patients should be warned to avoid exceeding the maximal daily dose and to also avoid excess alcohol use.

NSAIDs may be effective in patients for whom acetaminophen is inadequate. Because NSAIDs are both analgesic and anti-inflammatory, they may be particularly useful for OA patients with a more inflammatory clinical phenotype, such as patients with significant joint effusions. For OA, NSAIDs should be used at the lowest efficacious dose, on either an as-needed or standing basis. While all NSAIDs work by cyclooxygenase inhibition, they differ in potency, half-life, and side effects. Most physicians should have expertise in three or four NSAIDs, and be able to tailor their use to a particular patient. All NSAIDs should be considered to have potential for renal toxicity, hypertension, heart failure, gastritis, ulcers, and cardiovascular disease. A thorough risk/benefit analysis should be made before prescribing regular NSAIDs in patients with these conditions. Selective COX-2 inhibitors reduce gastrointestinal toxicity; there is little evidence that the sole COX-2 inhibitor currently remaining on the market in the United States, celecoxib, has any increased cardiovascular risk relative to other NSAIDs. Patients on chronic NSAIDs other than selective COX-2 inhibitors should receive GI protection, specifically a proton pump inhibitor or misoprostol. H2 blockers do not provide equivalent protection. Extra care should be taken in the elderly, those with renal dysfunction, and patients already on low-dose aspirin for cardiovascular purposes.

Another option for OA is the use of oral *opiates*. Most rheumatologists approach the use of opiates with great caution. As OA is a chronic disease, the use of opiates is likely to become long-term, with a potential for dependency. There is also evidence that all-cause mortality is increased in older patients taking opiates for arthritis. One alternative is tramadol, with mixed opiate and antidepressant properties, and a somewhat lower abuse potential. Most recently the antidepressant duloxetine has been approved for the management of chronic OA pain. Duloxetine is not an analgesic, and its effects may take days to weeks.

Topical agents are used for OA treatment, with variable degrees of supportive evidence. Capsaicin, the active ingredient in chili peppers, may be applied topically to deplete presynaptic supplies of substance P, a pain-mediating neurotransmitter. It must be applied regularly several times a day, or an initial period of discomfort will occur when it is restarted. Topical diclofenac has been approved by the FDA, in both a gel and solution form. It appears to be about as effective as oral diclofenac for OA, with reduced serum levels. Topical NSAIDs may be considered in some populations such as the elderly, owing to their lower incidence of systemic effects, particularly gastrointestinal side effects. Older preparations such as topical salicylates and counterirritants are available over the counter and may provide some relief.

If oral and topical therapies are ineffective or poorly tolerated, *intra-articular treatment* may be considered. Aspiration of the joint alone frequently relieves pressure and provides some pain relief. Glucocorticoid injection, such as methylprednisolone 40 to 80 mg, is frequently effective, providing relief that may last for several months. Studies suggest that treatment with glucocorticoid injections every 3 months has no adverse effect on cartilage, at least over the first few years. In hospitalized patients, injection of a painful, osteoarthritic knee may facilitate mobilization and timely discharge.

When glucocorticoids are ineffective, it is reasonable to consider injection of a hyaluronic acid preparation. Although marketed as a lubricant, hyaluronic acid is biologically active and may provide benefit for many months, long after its presence in the joint has dissipated. The efficacy of hyaluronic acid is disputed by some rheumatologists, however. Various hyaluronic acid preparations are available; the superiority of any one preparation over the others has not been established. Given the small but definite risk of infection resulting from joint injection, these procedures should be performed by experienced operators.

Many complementary and alternative therapies have been proposed. Small studies suggest that oral ingestion of the cartilage components glucosamine and chondroitin sulfate may provide analgesia and joint protection. However, a large, well-blinded US study found ambiguous benefit at best. Until further data are available, these agents are probably best used by enthusiastic patients on a trial-and-error basis. They appear to pose little if any risk. Several studies suggest a benefit for acupuncture in the treatment of OA, although like all acupuncture studies, they are plagued by issues of blinding. Surgical options include arthroscopy, total joint replacement, partial joint replacement, and other surgical techniques. In most cases, the goal of arthroscopy is to remove debris and to smooth roughened cartilage and menisci. Although still a very common procedure, a well-blinded study showed no benefit over sham surgery. Another well-conducted study showed no benefit for OA symptoms of arthroscopic knee surgery over standardized physical therapy. Accordingly, arthroscopy for OA should be reserved for those with specific and unequivocal indications, such as joint locking in the presence of loose bodies. By contrast, the benefits of total joint replacement are well established in the treatment of OA. The indications for total joint replacement are failure to manage pain by medical means and loss of mobility. As radiographic studies do not correlate well with pain or disability, their role in surgical decision making is supportive only. Total joint replacement is highly effective at relieving pain and maintaining or restoring function; it is probably underutilized, owing to cost and patient reluctance to undergo surgery. At the present time, replacement of the hip and knee are the best-established procedures. Techniques for replacement of other joints, such as the shoulder, elbow, ankle, and wrist, are improving steadily. In some cases, surgeons may recommend partial joint replacements. Partial approaches may reduce operating time, but at present are mainly recommended for specialized indications.

CONCLUSION

Arthritis of various forms is the cause of significant morbidity and mortality, and its personal and economic costs are high. Among the arthritides, osteoarthritis, gout, and pseudogout are the most common. Of the three, gout is currently the most treatable, yet patients with gout frequently experience inadequate management. Treatment of osteoarthritis and pseudogout is directed primarily at symptoms rather than at underlying causes, but research is likely to yield new and potentially effective therapies. In the meantime, optimal management of gout, pseudogout, and osteoarthritis, employing both pharmacologic and non-pharmacologic management, can reduce pain and suffering, and help patients live unimpeded, productive lives.

PRACTICE POINT

- Management of osteoarthritis is currently palliative. Treatment options include analgesics, anti-inflammatories and intra-articular hyaluronan. Weight loss, physical therapy, and bracing are important adjuncts to pharmacologic treatment, and may sometimes be sufficient on their own. For knees and hips, total joint replacement is indicated when medical management fails or the patient's ambulation is inappropriately limited; total joint replacement is an effective means to relieve pain and restore motion.

DISCHARGE CHECKLIST

- Have medications, drink, and diet of gouty patients been reviewed for possible contributors to hyperuricemia?
- For patients being discharged on NSAIDs, has gastric protection been prescribed, and arrangements made to check serum creatinine after discharge?
- For patients being discharged on colchicine, have arrangements been made to check complete blood count, liver transaminases, creatinine, and creatine phosphokinase as an outpatient? Colchicine side effects may include cytopenias, gastrointestinal upset, hepatitis, and myoneuropathy.
- For patients being discharged on allopurinol, have arrangements been made to check complete blood count, liver transaminases, and creatinine as an outpatient? Patients should be cautioned

about the possibility of allopurinol-induced rash, which may occasionally include Steven-Johnson syndrome. Consider checking for the HLA-B*5801 allele in persons of Asian descent being started on allopurinol, given the association of this allele with severe cutaneous adverse drug reactions to allopurinol.
- Has a workup for underlying disorders, such as hemochromatosis, thyroid disease, and perturbations of calcium, phosphate, and magnesium metabolism, been considered in patients with atypical or early-onset pseudogout?
- Have patients with arthritis been assessed by physical therapy, and considered for off-loading and assistive devices such as canes and bracing?

SUGGESTED READINGS

Fisher MC, Pillinger MH, Keenan RT. Inpatient gout: a review. *Curr Rheumatol Rep.* 2014;16:458-462.

Hochberg MC, Altman RD, April KT, et al. American College of Rheumatology 2012 recommendations for the use of nonpharmacologic and pharmacologic therapies in osteoarthritis of the hand, hip, and knee. *Arthritis Care Res.* 2012;64:465-474.

Jordan KM, Arden NK, Doherty M, et al. EULAR Recommendations 2003: an evidence-based approach to the management of knee osteoarthritis. Report of a Task Force of the Standing Committee for International Clinical Studies Including Therapeutic Trials (ESCISIT). *Ann Rheum Dis.* 2003;62:1145-1155.

Khanna D, FitzGerald JD, Khanna PP, et al. 2012 American College of Rheumatology Guidelines for Management of Gout. Part I: Systematic non-pharmacologic and pharmacologic therapeutic approaches to hyperuricemia. *Arthritis Care Res.* 2012;64:1431-1446.

Khanna D, Khanna PP, FitzGerald JD, et al. 2012 American College of Rheumatology Guidelines for Management of Gout. Part II: Therapy and anti-inflammatory prophylaxis of acute gouty arthritis. *Arthritis Care Res.* 2012;64:1447-1461.

Liote F, Ea HK. Recent developments in crystal-induced inflammation pathogenesis and management. *Curr Rheumatol Rep.* 2007;9:243-250.

Samuels J, Krasnokutsky S, Abramson SB. Osteoarthritis: a tale of three tissues. *Bull NYU Hosp Jt Dis.* 2008;66:244-250.

Slobodnick S, Shah B, Pillinger MH, et al. Colchicine: old and new. *Am J Med.* 2015;128:461-470.

Zhang W, Doherty M, Pascual E, et al. EULAR recommendations for calcium pyrophosphate deposition. Part II: management. *Ann Rheum Dis.* 2011;70:571-575.

CHAPTER 248

Systemic Lupus Erythematosus

Stephen J. Balevic, MD

Lisa Criscione-Schreiber, MD, MEd

Marcy B. Bolster, MD

Key Clinical Questions

1. Does this patient have systemic lupus erythematosus (SLE)?
2. Has SLE disease activity led to this patient's hospitalization?
3. How should flares of SLE be managed?
4. How does treatment of other diseases affect the status of SLE?
5. What are possible adverse consequences of the treatment of SLE?
6. How should medications for SLE be managed upon hospital discharge?

INTRODUCTION AND EPIDEMIOLOGY

Systemic lupus erythematosus (SLE) is an autoimmune disease that affects about 1 in 2000 individuals, most commonly women of child-bearing age. SLE can manifest itself in any organ system, and disease activity varies over time. Both the incidence and severity of SLE are increased in individuals of African or Caribbean descent, as well as in Hispanic populations within the United States.

While modern 5-year survival rates for SLE are around 95%, and 20-year survival rates are around 80%, these higher survival rates have come with increased hospitalization rates. In one retrospective analysis, more than half the patients in a lupus cohort were hospitalized over the previous 2 years. Lupus is associated with increased health care expenditure, and the in-hospital mortality rate ranges from 3% to 8%. In one study, the average length of stay for inpatients with lupus was 6 days (median cost $10,000). Among those who died in the hospital, the average length of hospitalization was 12 days (average cost around $25,000). The most common causes of inpatient mortality are infection, organ failure secondary to active SLE (ie, renal failure, CNS involvement, pulmonary hemorrhage), and cardiovascular disease.

The most common reason for hospitalization in patients with SLE is disease flare. Other common reasons for admission include complications of SLE or its treatment, such as infections, cardiovascular events and thromboembolic disease. Individuals with SLE are at high risk for premature atherosclerosis and may be admitted with chest pain, acute coronary syndromes, or cerebrovascular accidents. Lupus may also present as a new diagnosis in patients with pericarditis, glomerulonephritis, or neurologic disease.

PATHOPHYSIOLOGY

Autoimmune diseases are thought to result from an environmental trigger, such as infection, sunlight, or smoking, activating an abnormal immune response in a genetically susceptible individual.

The hallmark of SLE is serum autoantibodies against nuclear proteins. Autoantibodies may arise from defective clearance of apoptotic cells. When cells undergo apoptosis, internal proteins are displayed on surface blebs. If apoptotic cells are not cleared, nuclear material is exposed to the immune system, which may become sensitized. Certain complement component deficiencies, namely of C4 and C1q, are associated with an increased incidence of SLE; this may relate to the role of complement activation in clearing apoptotic cells and foreign antigens.

Autoantibodies can damage tissues through direct binding to cell surfaces with subsequent immune system activation, or by deposition of immune complexes in tissues. Immune complexes are not effectively cleared in patients with SLE, due to quantitative and qualitative deficiencies in Fc and complement receptors. Autoantibodies are implicated in many manifestations of SLE, including glomerulonephritis, rashes, cytopenias, and thrombosis. Anti–double stranded DNA (dsDNA) antibodies are associated with lupus nephritis. Cutaneous manifestations of SLE also are mediated by immune complexes, as shown by positivity of the lupus band test in involved and uninvolved skin (**Figure 248-1**). Ultraviolet light damages DNA and leads to keratinocyte apoptosis, which can activate and perpetuate an immune response as described above. Autoantibodies against blood components may lead to Coombs-positive hemolytic anemia, thrombocytopenia, and neutropenia. Antiphospholipid

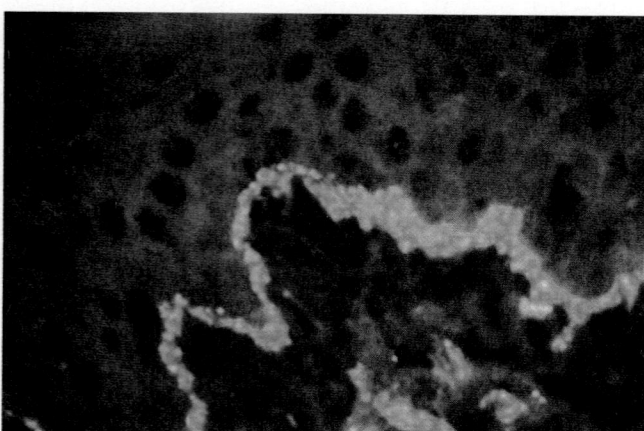

Figure 248-1 *Immunopathology of lupus-erythematosus-specific skin disease: positive lupus band test. Direct immunofluorescence examination of a discoid lupus erythematosus lesional skin biopsy showing a continuous band of granular fluorescence at the dermal-epidermal junction as a result of staining with fluorescein-isothiocyanate-conjugated goat anti-immunoglobulin G.* (Reproduced, with permission, from Wolff K, Goldsmith LA, Katz SI, et al. *Fitzpatrick's Dermatology in General Medicine*, 7th ed. New York, NY: McGraw-Hill; 2008. Fig. 156-13.)

Clinical class	Manifestation	Risk of developing systemic disease
CCLE (Chronic Cutaneous Lupus Erythematosus)	Discoid lupus Lupus profundus Chilblain lupus	Low
ICLE (Intermediate Cutaneous Lupus Erythematosus)	Tumid lupus	Low
SCLE (Subacute Cutaneous Lupus Erythematosus)	Papulosquamous lesions Psoriasiform lesions	Intermediate
ACLE (Acute Cutaneous Lupus Erythematosus)		High

Figure 248-2 *Forms of cutaneous lupus erythematosus and their association with systemic disease.*

antibodies may induce thrombotic events and recurrent pregnancy losses.

Patients with SLE also demonstrate abnormal B- and T-cell activation. B-cells act as antigen presenting cells and can also secrete proinflammatory cytokines. Additionally, B-cells are precursors to plasma cells, which secrete antibodies. Patients with SLE generally have increased numbers of B-cells, plasma cells, plasmablasts, and higher proportions of activated T-cells and B-cells than normal individuals. At least 50% of patients with SLE have increased levels of B-lymphocyte stimulator (BlyS), a growth factor for B-cell survival, maturation, antibody production, and differentiation into plasma cells. The biologic therapy agent directed against BlyS, belimumab, has FDA approval for the treatment of adult patients with active SLE (defined by elevated dsDNA antibodies and low complement) despite standard therapy. Interferon-alpha probably also plays a role in abnormal immune activation; up to 60% of lupus patients have a peripheral blood *interferon signature* of gene expression consistent with interferon-alpha stimulation. Plasmacytoid dendritic cells, through the activation of toll-like receptors 7 and 9, are thought to be the main source of interferon-alpha in patients with SLE.

DIFFERENTIAL DIAGNOSIS

Two scenarios that require the hospitalist to consider SLE in the differential diagnosis: patients with symptoms that may represent a new presentation of SLE, or patients with known SLE and recent symptoms that might be due to SLE, its treatment, or other causes.

■ NEW SYSTEMIC LUPUS ERYTHEMATOSUS

Consider SLE in a young person with glomerulonephritis, serositis, or cytopenias. At disease onset, renal involvement is seen in approximately 16% to 38% of patients, pleurisy in 17%, and pericarditis in 8%. Hematologic disorders occur in 43% to 90% of patients with SLE. A wide range of other diagnostic considerations are relevant in patients with these presentations.

Although serositis is common in lupus, new pleural or pericardial effusions are also commonly caused by infection and malignancy. Pleural effusions may likewise relate to pulmonary emboli, heart failure, liver disease, nephrotic syndrome, chylothorax, esophageal rupture, rheumatoid arthritis, and hypothyroidism. Other causes of pericarditis include uremia, hypothyroidism, and radiation therapy.

Pancytopenia is common in SLE, but may also be caused by bone marrow infiltrative processes such as lymphoma, sarcoidosis, or infection. Isolated thrombocytopenia can result from SLE, as well as idiopathic thrombocytopenic purpura (ITP), thrombotic thrombocytopenic purpura (TTP; may appear concurrently with SLE), medications, infections, or liver disease. SLE is more likely to cause lymphopenia than neutropenia; neutropenia should prompt consideration of human immunodeficiency virus (HIV) infection. SLE is one of the illnesses that can cause anemia of chronic disease. SLE is also associated with autoimmune hemolytic anemia, which may also be caused by leukemia, lymphoma, *Mycoplasma pneumoniae* infection, infectious mononucleosis, and certain medications.

In addition to SLE, other causes of new-onset glomerulonephritis include non-lupus nephritic syndromes, such as acute and rapidly progressive glomerulonephritis, crescentic glomerulonephritis, or systemic necrotizing vasculitides such as granulomatosis with polyangiitis (GPA, formerly known as Wegener granulomatosis), or antiglomerular basement membrane (Goodpasture) syndrome. New-onset nephrotic syndrome may be caused by SLE, idiopathic membranous glomerulopathy, diabetic glomerulosclerosis, focal segmental glomerulosclerosis, or minimal change nephropathy.

Certain neurologic syndromes suggest the possibility of SLE. Transverse myelitis can be a forme fruste of SLE in a young person. New seizures or stroke may also be a presenting manifestation of SLE, particularly in the presence of antiphospholipid antibodies.

Inflammatory arthritis and rashes occur in up to 90% of individuals with SLE and support the diagnosis of SLE when present. Acute inflammatory arthritis may represent rheumatoid arthritis, parvovirus B19 infection, or reactive arthritis from viral or bacterial infections. Mucocutaneous manifestations account for several of the ACR and SLICC classification criteria for SLE. Certain variants of cutaneous lupus have a more robust link to systemic disease (**Figure 248-2**).

■ ESTABLISHED SYSTEMIC LUPUS ERYTHEMATOSUS

When patients with SLE are admitted to the hospital, it is critical to ask whether or not SLE is responsible for the patient's presentation. As above, disease flare is the most common reason for hospital admission in patients with SLE, followed by infection, cardiovascular disease, and thrombosis.

Hematologic manifestations, including anemia, leukopenia, and thrombocytopenia, may require hospital admission. Hematologic changes can be caused by active lupus, medications, or both.

Anemia in SLE is often multifactorial. Anemia of chronic inflammatory disease is common, as serum hepcidin rises in infection or inflammation, impairing iron mobilization from hepatic stores and decreasing iron absorption from the gut. Patients with lupus nephritis may have anemia related to renal disease, and autoimmune hemolytic anemia related to SLE is also common. Lupus patients often take medications that can cause gastrointestinal bleeding, including aspirin, nonsteroidal anti-inflammatory drugs (NSAIDs), and anticoagulants. Menstrual blood loss is a potential cause of iron deficiency anemia in young women. Rarely, pulmonary hemorrhage can cause blood loss. Thrombocytopenia may be multifactorial as well, but immune-mediated thrombocytopenia or TTP must always be considered.

Neuropsychiatric lupus (NPSLE) can present in many ways. New seizures may be a manifestation of NPSLE, but can also be caused by accelerated hypertension from acute nephritis or noncompliance with antihypertensive therapy. Posterior reversible encephalopathy syndrome (PRES) has been reported in patients with SLE, with or without significant hypertension. The causes for this syndrome and its relationship to active SLE are incompletely understood. NPSLE can also present as acute delirium, in which case drugs and opportunistic infection of the CNS must also be considered. NPSLE can also manifest with severe depressive symptoms, psychosis, and even catatonia. Corticosteroids can often contribute to mood disturbances, but are less commonly the isolated cause of psychosis. Transverse myelitis can be seen in individuals with lupus; neuromyelitis optica, which can also be seen in patients with SLE, should be considered if the myelitis spans ≥2 vertebrae.

Respiratory infection with typical or unusual pathogens must be considered in patients with SLE who present with serositis, dyspnea, or pulmonary infiltrates. Such individuals may be taking chronic glucocorticoids or other immunosuppressive medications that not only increase the risk of infection, but blunt symptoms when it occurs. Immune suppression from glucocorticoids occurs in a dose dependent fashion, especially with doses >10 mg/d of prednisone. Pulmonary infiltrates in patients with SLE may also represent life-threatening alveolar hemorrhage.

Premature cardiovascular disease is a major source of morbidity and early mortality in SLE. A 40-year-old woman with SLE is likely to have an atherosclerotic burden equivalent to a 70-year-old woman without SLE. Lupus imparts a cardiovascular risk similar to that of diabetes mellitus. Chest pain and dyspnea may be manifestations of pericarditis or pleurisy, but may also be symptoms of pulmonary embolism. Pulmonary arterial hypertension should be a consideration in patients with dyspnea. Nonbacterial thrombotic endocarditis (Libman-Sacks endocarditis) is rare, but should also be considered in any patient with SLE with dyspnea, particularly if there are signs of peripheral emboli. Accelerated hypertension suggests new glomerulonephritis.

EVALUATION

SLE is a clinical syndrome, diagnosed by a comprehensive history and physical examination with appropriate laboratory and other diagnostic findings. While the American College of Rheumatology (ACR) classification criteria for SLE (1982/1997) were designed to improve homogeneity of individuals enrolled into clinical trials, they are also helpful for making a clinical diagnosis of SLE (**Table 248-1**). However, many signs, symptoms, and laboratory findings seen in individuals with SLE are not included in the ACR classification criteria, such as Raynaud phenomenon, alopecia, and hypocomplementemia. Therefore, new classification criteria were published in 2012 by the Systemic Lupus International Collaborating Clinics (SLICC) (**Table 248-2**). These criteria require the presence of both clinical and immunologic criteria, as systemic lupus is an autoantibody-driven clinical disease. In contrast to the ACR criteria, the SLICC

criteria also include hypocomplementemia, other cutaneous lupus manifestations, additional neurologic manifestations, additional qualifications on arthralgias being inflammatory, and accepted use of a spot urine protein to creatinine ratio to establish proteinuria. Inflammatory arthritis was defined as synovitis (swelling or effusion) in at least two joints, or tenderness in at least two joints and at least 30 minutes of morning stiffness in the absence of synovitis. The SLICC criteria also allow for the diagnosis of lupus in the setting of biopsy-proven lupus nephritis, with a positive ANA or anti-dsDNA, in the absence of other clinical signs. In the validation set, with expert consensus as a gold standard, the SLICC criteria had a sensitivity of 97% and a specificity of 84%, while the ACR criteria had a lower sensitivity of 83%, but higher specificity of 96%. Thus, the SLICC criteria may be more clinically useful for identifying disease.

The history should elicit whether the patient has experienced typical lupus manifestations, such as arthralgia, rash, mucosal ulcers, or serositis. More than 90% of individuals with SLE have musculoskeletal manifestations, including arthritis, defined as two or more swollen or tender joints. The most commonly involved joints include the MCP and PIP joints of the hands, wrists, elbows, and knees; these joints should be palpated for swelling and tenderness. Most individuals with SLE have mucocutaneous lesions at some point during the course of their disease. These manifestations range from (generally) painless oral and nasal ulcerations to photosensitive rashes, malar rash, and discoid lupus rash. Photosensitive rashes more typically occur on sun-exposed skin, but may also occur in non-sun-exposed regions. Discoid lesions are associated with complete loss of hair, central atrophy, follicular plugging, and hypopigmentation. Atrophic scarring can occur in older lesions. The face and scalp should be carefully examined for discoid lupus rashes, including the pinnae and external auditory canals. The skin of the fingers and hands must be carefully examined, as both erythema between the interphalangeal joints and subcutaneous nodules on the fingers are manifestations of lupus skin involvement. Blanching livedo reticularis on the extremities is also common in individuals with SLE and is associated with the presence of antiphospholipid antibodies.

Before autoantibody results return, other tests may suggest SLE (**Table 248-3**). A complete blood count is one of the most useful single tests in evaluating for SLE. Leukopenia, thrombocytopenia, and anemia are all consistent with a diagnosis of SLE. The erythrocyte sedimentation rate is generally increased in active SLE, while the C-reactive protein (CRP) is a less reliable indicator of lupus disease activity. In fact, in one study, elevated CRP levels ≥1.35 mg/dL had a 90% specificity and 100% sensitivity for indicating the presence of bacterial infection (primarily sepsis, pneumonia, and acute pharyngitis) in patients with SLE. Microscopic examination of the urinalysis should be performed to evaluate for cells or cellular casts; urine protein quantitation is recommended and can be performed with a spot protein-to-creatinine ratio. The serum total protein may be elevated in SLE and other autoimmune diseases because of high levels of autoantibodies, notably with hypergammaglobulinemia. Serum albumin may be low, reflecting either chronic disease or proteinuria associated with glomerulonephritis.

Serologic studies support but do not make the diagnosis of SLE (**Table 248-4**). Almost 100% of individuals with SLE have a positive antinuclear antibody (ANA) test. Although a negative ANA test essentially rules out SLE, a positive ANA test is not diagnostic. Up to 30% of the general population has a positive ANA, though the probability of disease increases with progressively higher titers. Antinuclear antibodies may be measured by three different methods, each with different sensitivities and specificities. The fluorescent antinuclear antibody assay (FANA) is highly sensitive. It is performed by applying progressively more dilute patient serum to standardized cells on microscope slides, then observing the pattern of immunofluorescence by microscopy. The FANA is reported as the highest dilution (titer) at which

TABLE 248-1 American College of Rheumatology Classification Criteria for a Diagnosis of Systemic Lupus Erythematosus

System	Criterion	Description
Mucosal findings	Malar rash	Flat or raised erythema over the malar eminences, generally sparing the nasolabial folds
	Discoid rash	Early discoid rashes are erythematous and raised patches; biopsy findings include adherent keratotic scale and follicular plugging; older lesions become atrophic and scarred
	Photosensitivity	Patient-described rash in reaction to sunlight
	Oral ulcers	Ulcerations in the mouth or nose that are observed by a physician; frequently painless
Organ system–specific manifestations	Arthritis	Tenderness, swelling, or effusion of two or more joints
	Serositis	Pleuritis is defined as pleuritic pain or a rub heard on examination or evidence of pleural effusion; pericarditis is defined by presence of a rub or characteristic ECG findings or evidence of a pericardial effusion
	Renal disorder	Defined as 0.5 g or more of proteinuria or the presence of cellular casts
	Neurologic disorder	The presence of seizures or psychosis that cannot be otherwise explained
Laboratory findings	Hematologic disorder	Hemolytic anemia with reticulocytosis
		or
		Total WBC count < 4000/mm³ total on two or more occasions
		or
		Lymphocyte count < 1500/mm³ on two or more occasions
		or
		Platelet count < 100,000/mm³
	Immunologic disorder	The presence of anti-DNA antibody
		or
		The presence of anti-Sm antibody
		or
		The presence of antiphospholipid antibodies defined as elevated IgG or IgM anticardiolipin antibodies or a lupus anticoagulant or a false-positive RPR
	Antinuclear antibody	At any point in time, in the absence of drugs that cause drug-induced lupus

*A patient must meet four of these criteria for inclusion in clinical trials. Many other findings also support the diagnosis of SLE in clinical practice (see the text).
ECG, electrocardiogram; Ig, immunoglobulin; RPR, rapid plasma regain; WBC, white blood cell.
Data from Tan EM, Cohen AS, Fries JF, et al. The 1982 revised criteria for the classification for systemic lupus erythematosus. *Arthritis Rheum.* 1982;25:1271-1277.
Data from Hochberg MC. Updating the American College of Rheumatology revised criteria for the classification of systemic lupus erythematosus. *Arthritis Rheum.* 1997;40:1725.

nuclear fluorescence is observed. A high-titer positive ANA means antinuclear antibody activity is present even when the patient's serum is very dilute. Some laboratories use enzyme-linked immunosorbent (ELISA)-based autoantibody testing. Such testing can be automated and performed more quickly than the traditional FANA. However, ELISA testing tends to be less sensitive, as the only nuclear antibodies detected are those specifically sought by the assay. Thus, the results may be more specific for the autoantibodies associated with clinical disease. Many laboratories now use multiplex immunoassays, in which the patient's serum is mixed with beads coated with a variety of autoantigens, which are detected similarly to ELISA methodology.

ANA-negative lupus is exceptionally rare; the ANA is occasionally negative in individuals with positive anti-Ro (SSA) antibody, because this antigen may result in a cytoplasmic staining pattern. ANA titers do not reflect disease activity, and in fact, the ANA test may become negative during the course of the disease.

Several autoantibodies are more specific for SLE than the ANA, including anti-dsDNA and anti-Smith (anti-Sm) antibodies, both of which are included in the ACR and SLICC classification criteria for SLE. Anti-Ro and anti-La are common in SLE and also seen in Sjögren syndrome and rheumatoid arthritis. Low levels of complement C3 and C4 are consistent with active SLE and can thus be useful in the following disease activity. Similarly, the anti-DNA antibody level can be useful in the following lupus disease activity, particularly for renal and CNS disease manifestations. Certain complement component deficiencies predispose individuals to develop SLE.

PRACTICE POINT

- Antinuclear antibody (ANA) testing is very sensitive for the diagnosis of systemic lupus erythematosus (SLE). Virtually, all patients with SLE have a positive ANA test. However, ANA testing is also very nonspecific. Up to 30% of healthy people test positive for ANA, and the positive predictive value of ANA testing for SLE is as low as 11%. High titers of ANA, the presence of multiple symptoms and signs of SLE, and positivity for more specific antibody tests such as anti-dsDNA antibody increase the likelihood of a clinically significant positive ANA. Clinicians should also be aware that many other autoimmune conditions are associated with positive ANA tests, including rheumatoid arthritis, Sjögren syndrome, drug-induced lupus, systemic sclerosis, myositis, thyroid disease, and multiple sclerosis.

SPECIFIC DISEASE MANIFESTATIONS

CUTANEOUS DISEASE

The clinical classes of cutaneous lupus are acute cutaneous lupus (ACLE), subacute cutaneous lupus (SCLE), intermediate cutaneous

TABLE 248-2 Systemic Lupus International Collaborating Clinics Classification Criteria for Systemic Lupus Erythematosus

System	Criterion	Summary
Clinical Criteria	1. Acute cutaneous lupus	Malar rash (do not count if malar discoid), bullous lupus, TEN variant of SLE, maculopapular lupus rash, photosensitive lupus rash, or subacute cutaneous lupus (please see the text for details)
	2. Chronic cutaneous lupus	Classical discoid rash, hypertrophic lupus, lupus panniculitis, mucosal lupus, lupus erythematosus tumidus, chilblains lupus
	3. Photosensitivity	Patient-described rash in reaction to sunlight
	4. Oral ulcers	Appearing on the buccal mucosa, palate or tongue; or nasal ulcers, in the absence of other causes
	5. Non Scarring Alopecia	Diffuse thinning or hair fragility with visible broken hairs, in the absence of other causes
	6. Serositis	A: Typical pleurisy for more than 1 day, OR pleural effusions, OR pleural rub. B: Typical pericardial pain for more than 1 day, OR pericardial effusion, OR pericardial rub, OR pericarditis by EKG, in the absence of other causes
	7. Renal	Urine protein/creatinine (or 24 h urine protein) representing 500 mg of protein/24 h, OR red blood cell casts
	8. Neurologic	Seizures, psychosis, mononeuritis multiplex, myelitis, peripheral or cranial neuropathy, acute confusional state, in the absence of other causes
	9. Hemolytic Anemia	
	10. Leukopenia or Lymphopenia	White blood cell count <4000/mm^3 at least once or lymphocyte count <1000/mm^3 at least once, in the absence of another known cause
	11. Thrombocytopenia	Platelet count <100,000/mm^3 at least once, in the absence of another known cause
Immunologic Criteria	1. ANA above reference Range	
	2. Anti ds-DNA above laboratory range	Except if measured by ELISA: twice above laboratory range
	3. Anti-Smith	
	4. Antiphospholipid antibody	Any of the following: lupus anticoagulant, false-positive RPR, medium or high-titer anticardiolipin antibody (IgA, IgG, or IgM), anti-β_2 glycoprotein I (IgA, IgG, IgM)
	5. Low complement	Low C3 OR low C4 OR low CH50
	6. Direct Coombs	In the absence of hemolytic anemia (counts as clinical criterion)

*A patient must meet at least four of these criteria (with at least 1 clinical and 1 laboratory), OR have biopsy proven lupus nephritis with a positive ANA or positive ds-DNA.
ELISA, enzyme-linked immunosorbent assay; Ig, immunoglobulin.
Data From: Petri M, Orbai AM, Alarcón GS, Gordon C, Merrill JT, Fortin PR, Bruce IN, Isenberg D, Wallace DJ, Nived O, et al. Derivation and validation of the Systemic Lupus International Collaborating Clinics classification criteria for systemic lupus erythematosus. *Arthritis Rheum*. 2012;64(8):2677-2686.

lupus (ICLE), and chronic cutaneous lupus (CCLE). ACLE includes the classic malar rash (**Figures 248-3** and **248-4**), as well as bullous lupus and toxic epidermal necrolysis (TEN)-like ACLE. Patients with subacute cutaneous lupus (SCLE) have papulosquamous lesions and psoriasiform plaques (**Figure 248-5**). The SCLE rash is associated with anti-Ro antibodies in around 85% of cases. Neonatal lupus, which is associated with maternal anti-Ro antibodies, is clinically and histologically indistinguishable from SCLE. CCLE includes discoid lupus (**Figure 248-6**), lupus profundus (panniculitis), and chilblain lupus. ICLE is tumid lupus, characterized by edematous plaques on the trunk.

Skin biopsy can help determine whether a rash is related to SLE. Interface dermatitis, comprised of a lymphocytic infiltrate at the dermal-epidermal junction, is characteristic of SLE and dermatomyositis. Pathological findings also often include mild lymphocytic perivascular and periadnexal inflammation. ACLE may contain a dermal neutrophilic infiltrate, but interface, perivascular, and periadnexal changes should also be present. Microscopy, using immunofluorescence, reveals the lupus band, a linear array of deposited immunoglobulins and complement at the epidermal basement membrane. It is present in both normal-appearing skin and rashes in patients with SLE.

■ HEMATOLOGIC INVOLVEMENT

SLE-related cytopenias result from peripheral destruction of cells far more often than bone marrow suppression, which can occur due to autoantibodies directed against bone marrow progenitor cells or medication effects. Autoimmune hemolytic anemia, which can be Coombs positive (associated with complement or antibody on red cell membranes) or Coombs negative, affects approximately 10% of patients with SLE. Ferritin is an acute-phase reactant; and it is thus not a reliable measure of total iron stores in individuals with autoimmune disease; serum iron and total iron-binding capacity are more specific. Leukopenia is seen in more than half of patients. Lymphopenia is more common than neutropenia in lupus, though antigranulocyte antibodies (not to be confused with antineutrophil cytoplasmic antibodies) can cause neutropenia in patients with lupus. Severe thrombocytopenia is unusual in SLE. When thrombocytopenia exists, the blood smear should be examined for schistocytes, as thrombotic thrombocytopenic purpura (TTP) is associated with SLE. Levels of ADAMTS-13, a metalloproteinase that cleaves large multimers of von Willebrand factor, are reduced in patients with TTP and lupus, due to the production of neutralizing autoantibodies.

TABLE 248-3 Useful Laboratory Tests for Evaluating Systemic Lupus Erythematosus*

Test	Features Consistent with SLE
CBC	Anemia
	Thrombocytopenia
	Lymphopenia
CMP	Elevated serum creatinine
	Elevated serum total protein
	Decreased serum albumin
ESR	Elevated
C-reactive protein	Elevated
Quantitative immunoglobulins	Elevated IgG
	Elevated IgM
	Elevated IgA
Urinalysis	Proteinuria
	Microscopic hematuria
	Red blood cell casts
	White blood cells in the absence of bacteria, leukocyte esterase, nitrites
Complement levels	Low C3, C4, or CH50 (whole hemolytic complement)

*These features are not seen in all patients with SLE, but when seen in the appropriate clinical context, support a diagnosis of SLE.
CBC, complete blood count; CMP, comprehensive metabolic panel; ESR, erythrocyte sedimentation rate.

■ SEROSITIS

Serositis in patients with SLE can involve the pleura, pericardium, or peritoneum. About 30% of individuals with SLE develop pleuritic involvement. Pleuritis is more common than pericarditis in SLE, and peritonitis is a very rare manifestation. Mild serositis may be clinically detectable as pleural or pericardial friction rubs. On thoracentesis, pleural effusions in patients with lupus are exudative with normal glucose, normal pH, and elevated LDH. A pleural fluid ANA of ≥1:160 is supportive of lupus pleuritis, and may be particularly useful in identifying new lupus pleuritis in a patient without established SLE. Cytology of the pleural fluid may reveal lupus erythematosus (LE) cells, though this assay is now infrequently performed. In pericarditis, the electrocardiogram (ECG) may show low amplitudes and diffuse ST-segment elevation, PR depression, or electrical alternans. Autoantibody testing in pericardial effusions, which are exudative in nature and very rarely hemorrhagic, is usually not helpful. The CRP can be elevated in the setting of lupus serositis, whereas the CRP is often inappropriately low or normal in the setting of most other SLE flares

■ LUPUS NEPHRITIS

Lupus nephritis should be suspected when there is proteinuria (≥0.5 g/d or > 3+ by dipstick) or an active urinary sediment (as represented by either RBC/WBC casts, persistent hematuria with >5 red blood cells per high power field (hpf) without another explanation, or pyuria with >5 white blood cells per hpf without another explanation). Suspected lupus nephritis should be confirmed by renal biopsy. In 2004, the pathologic classification of lupus nephritis was updated by the International Society of Nephrology and Renal Pathology Society (ISN/RPS) (**Table 248-5**). The classification of lupus nephritis determines treatment choices.

■ NEUROPSYCHIATRIC DISEASE

Neuropsychiatric manifestations of SLE (NPSLE) are incredibly challenging to diagnose. The ACR has identified 19 distinct clinical syndromes of the central and peripheral nervous systems in lupus (**Table 248-6**), though several of these syndromes do not have a higher prevalence in individuals with SLE than that in the general population. The prevalence of true neuropsychiatric lupus is not definitively known. The 2010 European League Against Rheumatism (EULAR) recommendations for the management of NPSLE suggests that in patients with SLE and new or unexplained symptoms or signs of neuropsychiatric disease, the initial diagnostic work-up should be similar to that in non-SLE patients with the same manifestations. This may include lumbar puncture and CSF analysis (to exclude CNS infection), EEG, neuropsychiatric testing, and neuroimaging.

Lumbar puncture with cerebrospinal fluid (CSF) analysis is necessary when evaluating acute mental status changes in patients with lupus. CSF studies should include cell count, glucose, protein, IgG index, and oligoclonal bands, as well as cultures and serologies to exclude infectious causes. One study (prior to the development of the ACR NPSLE case definitions) suggested that among 42 patients with SLE and either diffuse or complex neuropsychiatric presentations, all had at least one abnormality of the following: CSF IgG index, oligoclonal bands, elevated CSF antineuronal antibodies, and/or serum antiribosomal-P antibody, yielding a sensitivity of 100% and specificity of 86%. Specific CNS autoantibodies, such as the N-methyl-D-aspartate (NMDA) receptor antibody, are known to cause autoimmune encephalitis. The roles of other CNS autoantibodies, such as the antiribosomal-P antibody and its association with psychosis, are still being elucidated. Pleocytosis and elevated CSF protein have been reported in active CNS SLE in 40% to 50% of cases, especially in transverse myelitis, vasculitis, or aseptic meningitis. However, CSF can also be normal in NPSLE. Oligoclonal bands reflect the presence of antibodies in the CSF, with a reported sensitivity of 55% and specificity of 92% for diffuse/complex NPSLE. In such cases, NPSLE must be differentiated from multiple sclerosis, which is also characterized by abnormal CSF IgG index and oligoclonal bands. Tests to rule out infection include bacterial and fungal cultures, cryptococcal antigen, Venereal Disease Research Laboratory (VDRL) test, and PCR for herpes simplex virus (HSV) and John Cunningham (JC) virus. Magnetic resonance imaging (MRI) with and without contrast is the preferred imaging modality in NPSLE. The average sensitivity of MRI in NPSLE is 57%, with a range from 30% to 76%, depending on which clinical syndrome is being evaluated. While MRI may reveal white matter lesions or periventricular hyperintensities in up to 75% of patients with NPSLE, these findings can be seen in up to 25% to 50% of patients with SLE without neuropsychiatric symptoms, as well as healthy controls, yielding an overall specificity between 60% and 82%. An additional challenge is determining if any radiographic abnormalities represent an active process related to NPSLE, chronic changes related to an old NPSLE event, or unrelated changes. Nevertheless, MRI has a useful role in evaluating for possible infarcts, hemorrhages, transverse myelitis, and other confounding disorders such as a mass lesion or infection. As antiphospholipid antibodies are associated with NPSLE, anticardiolipin antibodies, anti-beta-2 glycoprotein 1 antibodies, and lupus anticoagulant should be obtained, as well as a blood smear to evaluate for schistocytes that might suggest TTP.

TRIAGE AND HOSPITAL ADMISSION

Most patients with SLE flares are not hospitalized. However, several lupus manifestations are best managed in an inpatient setting due to the risk of life- or organ-threatening complications. Some of these include desquamating rashes, severe cytopenias, symptomatic pericardial or pleural effusions, accelerated hypertension, acute dyspnea, chest pain, thrombotic complications, accelerated proteinuria and nephritis, and many neurologic presentations.

TABLE 248-4 Autoantibodies in Systemic Lupus Erythematosus

Antibody	Prevalence (%)	Antigen Recognized	Clinical Utility
Antinuclear antibodies	98	Multiple nuclear	Best screening test; repeated negative tests make SLE unlikely
Anti-dsDNA	70	DNA (double-stranded)	High titers are SLE specific and in some patients correlate with disease activity, nephritis, vasculitis
Anti-Smith	25	Protein complexed to six species of nuclear U1 RNA	Specific for SLE; no definite clinical correlations; most patients also have anti-RNP; more common in African Americans and Asians than Caucasians
Anti-RNP	40	Protein complexed to U1 RNA	Not specific for SLE; high titers associated with syndromes that have overlap features of several rheumatic syndromes including SLE; more common in African-Americans than Caucasians
Anti-Ro (SS-A)	30	60 kDa and 52 kDa proteins complexed to non-coding RNA	Not specific for SLE; associated with sicca syndrome, subacute cutaneous lupus, and neonatal lupus with congenital heart block; associated with decreased risk for nephritis
Anti-La (SS-B)	10	47-kDa protein complexed to non-coding RNA	Usually associated with anti-Ro; associated with decreased risk for nephritis
Antihistone	70	Histones associated with DNA (in nucleosome, chromatin)	More frequent in drug-induced lupus than in SLE
Antiphospholipid	50	Phospholipids, beta$_2$ glycoprotein 1 cofactor, prothrombin	Three tests available: ELISA for cardiolipin and beta$_2$G1, sensitive prothrombin time (DRVVT); predisposes to clotting, fetal loss, thrombocytopenia
Antierythrocyte	60	Erythrocyte membrane	Measured as direct Coombs test; a small proportion of patients develop overt hemolysis
Antiplatelet	30	Surface and altered cytoplasmic antigens in platelets	Associated with thrombocytopenia, but sensitivity and specificity are not good; not a useful clinical test
Antineuronal (includes antiglutamate receptor)	60	Neuronal and lymphocyte surface antigens	In some series, a positive test in CSF correlates with active CNS lupus
Antiribosomal P	20	Protein in ribosomes	In some series, a positive test in serum correlates with depression or psychosis due to CNS lupus

CNS, central nervous system; CSF, cerebrospinal fluid; DRVVT, dilute Russell viper venom time; ELISA, enzyme-linked immunosorbent assay.
Reproduced, with permission, from Fauci AS, Braunwald E, Kasper DL, et al. *Harrison's Principles of Internal Medicine*, 17th ed. New York, NY: McGraw-Hill; 2008, Table 313-1.

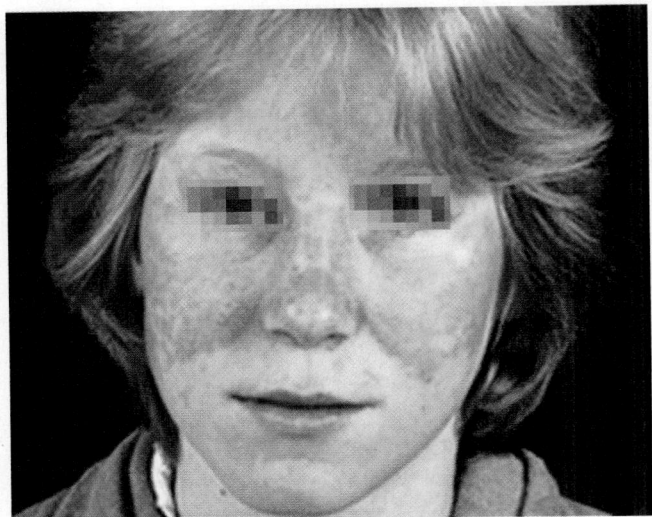

Figure 248-3 *Classic malar rash of acute cutaneous lupus erythematosus. Bright red, sharply defined erythema with slight edema and minimal scaling in a butterfly pattern on the central face.* (Reproduced, with permission, from Wolff K, Johnson RA. *Fitzpatrick's Color Atlas & Synopsis of Clinical Dermatology*, 6th ed. New York, NY: McGraw-Hill; 2009. Fig. 14-20.)

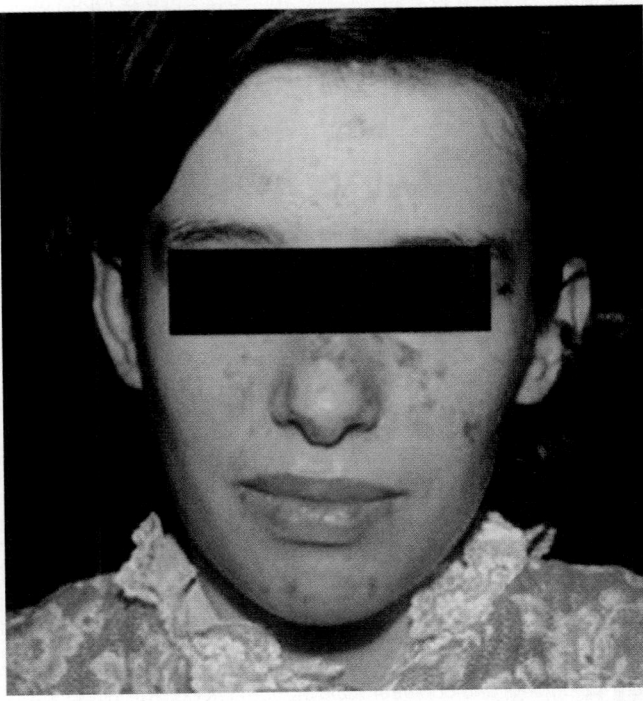

Figure 248-4 *Acute cutaneous lupus erythematosus with malar rash, in milder form.* (Reproduced, with permission, from Fuster V, O'Rourke RA, Walsh RA, et al. *Hurst's the Heart*, 12th ed. New York: McGraw-Hill; 2008. Fig. 12-22.)

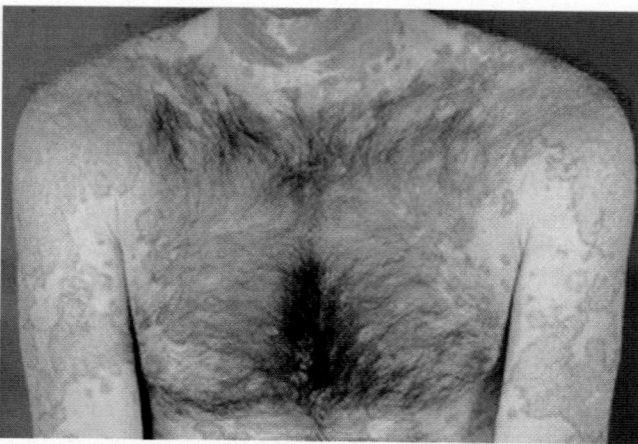

Figure 248-5 *Subacute cutaneous lupus erythematosus. Widely scattered, erythematous-to-violaceous, scaling, well-demarcated plaques on the trunk, neck, and arms, mimicking the clinical appearance of psoriasis vulgaris.* (Reproduced, with permission, from Wolff K, Johnson RA. *Fitzpatrick's Color Atlas & Synopsis of Clinical Dermatology*, 6th ed. New York, NY: McGraw-Hill; 2009. Fig. 14-22.)

Infections (including progressive multifocal leukoencephalopathy) are a leading cause of mortality that must be considered in ill individuals with SLE. As previously mentioned, the CRP can be a useful tool in differentiating between SLE flares without pleuritis/pericarditis and infection.

While most lupus-related rashes are managed comfortably as an outpatient, an individual with SLE and an acute, rapidly progressive desquamating or bullous rash should be admitted. Desquamating lupus rashes typically progress rapidly and place the patient at risk for fluid shifts and infections. Acute desquamating rashes may start as peripheral erythematous macules that progress to vesicles, and are associated with a diffuse burning sensation. The differential diagnosis of a desquamating rash includes bullous lupus, toxic

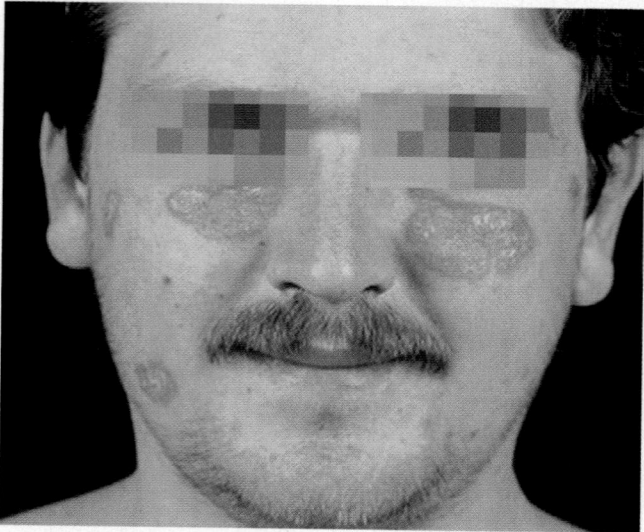

Figure 248-6 *Chronic cutaneous lupus erythematosus. Well-demarcated, erythematous, hyperkeratotic plaques with atrophy, follicular plugging, and adherent scale on both cheeks. This is the classic presentation of chronic discoid lupus erythematosus.* (Reproduced, with permission, from Wolff K, Johnson RA. *Fitzpatrick's Color Atlas & Synopsis of Clinical Dermatology*, 6th ed. New York, NY: McGraw-Hill; 2009. Fig. 14-23.)

TABLE 248-5 **International Society of Nephrology and Renal Pathology Society 2003 Classification of Lupus Nephritis**

Class I	Minimal mesangial lupus nephritis
Class II	Mesangial proliferative lupus nephritis
Class III	Focal lupus nephritis
	(A): active lesions: focal proliferative lupus nephritis
	(A, C): active and chronic lesions
	(C): chronic inactive lesions with scars
Class IV	Diffuse lupus nephritis
	IV-S (A): active lesions: diffuse segmental proliferative lupus nephritis
	IV-G (A): active lesions: diffuse global proliferative lupus nephritis
	IV-S (A/G): active and chronic lesions: diffuse segmental proliferative and sclerosing lupus nephritis
	IV-G (A/G): active and chronic lesions: diffuse global proliferative and sclerosing lupus nephritis
	IV-S (C): chronic inactive lesions with scars: diffuse segmental sclerosing lupus nephritis
	IV-G (C): chronic inactive lesions with scars: diffuse global sclerosing lupus nephritis
Class V	Membranous lupus nephritis
Class VI	Advanced sclerotic lupus nephritis

Data from Weening JJ, D'Agati VD, Schwartz MM, et al. The classification of glomerulonephritis in systemic lupus erythematosus revisited. *Kidney Int.* 2004;65:521-530.

TABLE 248-6 **Nineteen Clinical Syndromes Recognized as Possible Manifestations of Neuropsychiatric Lupus**

Central Nervous System (CNS)	Peripheral Nervous System
Syndromes diagnosed by laboratory or radiographic testing including:	• Autonomic dysfunction
• Aseptic meningitis	• Myasthenia gravis
• CNS demyelination	• Neuropathies including:
• Cerebrovascular disease	• Mononeuropathy
• Myelopathy	• Cranial neuropathy
	• Plexopathy
	• Polyneuropathy
	• Acute demyelinating polyneuropathy
Symptoms indicating CNS dysfunction including:	
• Headache (steroid-responsive)	
• Chorea	
• Cognitive dysfunction	
• Psychosis	
• Delirium	
• Anxiety	
• Mood disorder	

Data from Ad Hoc Committee on Neuropsychiatric Lupus Nomenclature. The American College of Rheumatology nomenclature and case definitions for neuropsychiatric lupus syndromes. *Arthritis Rheum.* 1999;42:599-608.

epidermal necrolysis (TEN), or Stevens-Johnson syndrome. TEN-like acute cutaneous lupus is occasionally seen in SLE, and severe mucous membrane involvement is common. Skin disease may also result from the treatment of SLE. Hydroxychloroquine has been associated with acute generalized exanthematous pustulosis (AGEP), a cutaneous hypersensitivity reaction that presents as a desquamating rash on the face and chest.

Patients with cytopenias may need admission for evaluation and management. Individuals with SLE and the new onset of less than 50,000 platelets/mm^3 should be considered for inpatient evaluation and management, especially if bleeding is present. Likewise, patients with hemolytic anemia may require admission for management. Antibody-mediated clotting factor inhibitors, such as acquired factor VIII inhibitor, have been described in patients with SLE and can be life-threatening.

Pericarditis is the most common cardiac manifestation of SLE. Though rare, cardiac tamponade can occur; the presence of dyspnea with a large pericardial effusion, pulsus paradoxus on examination, or tamponade physiology on echocardiogram necessitates admission. Large pleural effusions associated with dyspnea may require admission for diagnostic and therapeutic thoracentesis. Empyema must be ruled out in any large pleural effusion in a patient with SLE.

Individuals with SLE may present with accelerated hypertension (systolic blood pressure [BP] ≥ 180 mm Hg or diastolic BP ≥ 110 mm Hg). Hypertensive emergency and hypertensive urgency have the same definition in individuals with SLE as in other patients, and considerations for admission are similar. In hypertensive patients with SLE, it may be difficult to determine whether additional findings, such as confusion and microangiopathic hemolytic anemia, are the product of hypertensive crisis or are directly related to lupus disease activity. Glomerulonephritis must always be excluded in any patient with SLE with severe hypertension.

Acute dyspnea or a new oxygen requirement in an individual with SLE warrants admission. Cardiac causes of acute dyspnea in SLE include acute coronary syndromes, pericardial or pleural effusion, valvular heart disease related to SLE, and congestive heart failure. Libman-Sacks endocarditis most commonly involves the tricuspid and mitral valves, and is associated with antiphospholipid antibodies. New peripheral emboli may require hospital admission for evaluation and initiation of anticoagulation. SLE may cause myocarditis, cardiomyopathy, or congestive heart failure. Pulmonary causes of dyspnea in SLE include pleural effusions, interstitial lung disease, pneumonia, pulmonary embolism, and pulmonary hemorrhage. Additionally, acute coronary syndromes or myocardial infarction must always be considered in any patient with SLE who has dyspnea. Lupus itself is a risk factor for cardiovascular disease; myocardial infarctions in the absence of traditional risk factors can occur even in very young women with SLE. ECG findings suggestive of cardiac ischemia or the presence of elevated serum biomarkers are absolute indicators for admission in this population.

Worsening hypertension and peripheral edema associated with proteinuria can be signs of lupus nephritis. Admission is indicated in suspected lupus nephritis if hemodialysis may be necessary to treat volume overload or electrolyte disturbances, to expedite renal biopsy, or to start pulse treatment with methylprednisolone for 3 to 5 days after renal biopsy has been performed. Additionally, individuals failing outpatient management of known lupus nephritis (eg worsening microscopic hematuria, worsening proteinuria, increasing creatinine, inability to control blood pressure) may also be admitted for pulse therapy with methylprednisolone as defined below as well as aggressive antihypertensive therapy.

A patient with SLE with a first seizure should be admitted for further evaluation. Individuals with SLE have a higher incidence of cerebrovascular disease and can present with stroke at a young age. Stroke in SLE may result from thromboembolism or can be hemorrhagic, especially in the setting of hypertension or thrombocytopenia. Individuals with SLE with acute weakness in one or more extremities should be admitted for further evaluation and management; diagnostic considerations include stroke, transverse myelitis, mononeuritis multiplex, mixed sensorimotor polyneuropathies, and cranial and peripheral neuropathies.

TREATMENT

ACUTE DISEASE FLARES

Glucocorticoids are the cornerstone of therapy for acute lupus flares requiring hospitalization, though other immunosuppressive agents that are used include mycophenolate mofetil (MMF), azathioprine (AZA), calcineurin inhibitors, and cyclophosphamide. We include hydroxychloroquine and rituximab in this section, as treatment with these agents are occasionally initiated in the hospital setting. Glucocorticoid dosing should be based on disease severity. There are not published guidelines for steroid treatment of patients with SLE, but we recommend using pulse-dose steroids in situations where a patient has life- or organ-threatening disease activity. Standard nomenclature for glucocorticoid doses defines low dose steroids as ≤7.5 mg of prednisone equivalent per day, medium dose as >7.5 mg to ≤30 mg/d, and high dose as >30 mg to ≤100 mg/d. Pulse therapy is defined as ≥250 mg/d, usually for one or a few days, although practically speaking, most physicians use 500 to 1000 mg of intravenous methylprednisolone equivalent for pulse therapy. Tapers are highly variable in dosing and duration; alternate-day dosing is an option for tapering steroids. During tapering, patients should be closely monitored for symptoms of an SLE flare, as well as for signs of adrenal insufficiency.

Hydroxychloroquine reduces the frequency of SLE flares and improves survival. It has favorable effects on lipids, blood glucose, and may reduce the risk of blood clots in individuals with SLE and antiphospholipid antibodies. If dosed at less than 6.5 mg/kg daily of ideal body weight, retinal toxicity is a rare adverse effect. The usual dose of hydroxychloroquine is 400 mg once daily or divided twice daily. Gastrointestinal side effects are uncommon, but may be reduced by taking the medication after a meal. As it is not immunosuppressive, hydroxychloroquine can be continued during acute infection. Hydroxychloroquine has not been shown to impair healing and can be continued perioperatively. It is also one of the medications recommended for the management of lupus during pregnancy. The management of allergic reactions to hydroxychloroquine is complicated by the medication half-life of several weeks.

Belimumab is a human monoclonal antibody that binds to and inhibits soluble human B lymphocyte stimulator (BlyS). Belimumab is particularly effective in patients with SLE who have higher disease activity, are taking corticosteroids, and have elevated anti-DNA antibodies and low complement levels. Clinical responses to belimumab have been reported to have sustained for up to 7 years. In an open-label extension trial, severe flares declined from 17% with belimumab in the first year to 2% to 9% during years 2 to 7. Anti-dsDNA antibodies declined 40% to 60% from baseline over 2 to 7 years. Corticosteroid use also declined by 25% at year 2 and by 55% at year 7, and overall adverse event rates stabilized or decreased during the 7 years of treatment. These results suggest that belimumab is well tolerated and can control disease for long periods of time. This agent will likely not have a significant role in the setting of the hospitalized patient with an acute flare of SLE.

Rituximab failed to meet clinical endpoints when tested in randomized clinical trials for both generalized SLE and lupus nephritis (the EXPLORER and LUNAR trials, respectively), although concerns have been raised about the very strict endpoints used in both of these trials, as well as the exclusion of patients with severe disease who may be more representative of those more likely to receive rituximab in clinical practice. Based on previously reported trends toward improvement, additional trials are ongoing (RING, RITUXILUP) to further address the potential role of rituximab in lupus nephritis.

IVIG has a limited role in patients with SLE. However, a recent meta-analysis and systematic review demonstrated that IVIG reduces disease activity scores and can increase serum complement levels. IVIG is also efficacious in the management of autoimmune hemolytic anemia and thrombocytopenia. There are insufficient data to determine its role in other clinical outcome measures, including renal function. Specific discussion of the use of IVIG in individual clinical circumstances, including heart block, is addressed in individual sections below.

Several promising agents for the treatment of SLE are currently in development. Most are biologic therapies targeting specific immune functions implicated in lupus disease activity. Epratuzumab (anti-CD22 antibody) is currently in late-phase clinical trials, while the anti-IFNα agent, rontalizumab, is in early phase clinical trials.

■ NEPHRITIS

Although there are several published randomized clinical trials for the treatment of lupus nephritis, there is no consensus on optimal treatment, and a knowledgeable rheumatologist or nephrologist should be consulted to recommend appropriate therapy. Class II (mesangial) lupus nephritis generally improves with corticosteroids alone. Proliferative glomerulonephritis (class III or IV) merits aggressive therapy to prevent progression to end-stage renal disease. Many patients have simultaneous pathologic and clinical features of proliferative and membranous (class V) glomerulonephritis, although membranous (Class V) can also occur by itself.

There are three major published regimens for induction treatment of class III, IV, and V lupus nephritis. The first protocol (NIH protocol) is comprised of 6 monthly pulses of intravenous cyclophosphamide (500-750 mg/m^2), with oral prednisone starting at 1 mg/kg daily for 8 weeks and weaned over 12 months. This regimen carries risks of serious infection, infertility and malignancy. In a search for equally effective and less toxic treatments, two other regimens have emerged. In the Euro-lupus protocol, 3 daily pulses of 750 mg methylprednisolone are initially administered, followed by cyclophosphamide 500 mg intravenously every 2 weeks for 6 doses. Oral azathioprine (AZA) is then used for maintenance therapy. Prednisone is dosed similarly to the NIH protocol. This regimen was shown to be non-inferior to the NIH protocol in a European trial, although the study was composed of mostly Caucasian participants. The third induction regimen uses oral MMF 1500 mg twice daily with oral corticosteroids, starting at 1 mg/kg and tapered over approximately 6 months. In a comparison trial of oral MMF and monthly intravenous cyclophosphamide using the NIH protocol for 6 months (both with the same steroid regimen), oral MMF was shown to be non-inferior to monthly intravenous cyclophosphamide. Subgroup analysis of this trial suggested that oral MMF may provide improved renal survival in non-Caucasian and non-Asian patients. An additional advantage of MMF is preserved fertility compared to cyclophosphamide. After induction therapy, maintenance therapy is usually with MMF, which has been shown to be superior to AZA.

Calcineurin inhibitors are also showing promise for management of active lupus nephritis. In a Chinese population, tacrolimus was noninferior to MMF for induction purposes, though after 5 years of follow-up, a nonsignificant trend of a higher incidence of renal flares and renal function decline was observed with the tacrolimus regimen. The ongoing RITUXILUP trial is currently evaluating whether rituximab and MMF, without the addition of oral steroids, has an improved response and prolonged steroid-sparing effect in the treatment of new lupus nephritis.

The 2012 ACR guidelines for management of lupus nephritis suggest that, for pure Class V LN with nephrotic range proteinuria,

patients should be started on prednisone 0.5 mg/kg/d, in combination with mycophenolate mofetil (2-3 g total daily dose). A recently published clinical trial demonstrated 1-year clinical remission rates of 83% with daily cyclosporine and 60% with intravenous cyclophosphamide every other month for six doses. Both regimens were accompanied by alternate day prednisone starting at 40 mg/m^2 for 8 weeks, then tapered over a year, as well as angiotensin-converting enzyme (ACE) inhibitors and daily oral statins. Another recently reported pooled analysis of two clinical trials found no difference in remission rates between intravenous cyclophosphamide and mycophenolate mofetil for pure class V nephritis. A subgroup analysis of the previously mentioned randomized control trial evaluating tacrolimus (0.06-0.1mg/kg/d) versus MMF (2-3 g/d) demonstrated that, for patients with pure class V membranous lupus nephritis, tacrolimus had a greater effect on reducing the urine protein to creatinine ratio, as well as a trend toward an increased likelihood of a complete renal response as defined by the ACR SLE renal response criteria.

All classes of nephritis are associated with a significantly increased risk of cardiovascular disease; up to half of patients with nephritis eventually die from cardiovascular or cerebrovascular disease. The risk of thrombotic disease related to antiphospholipid antibodies and nephrotic syndrome is around 20% in this patient population. ACE inhibition is considered essential adjunctive treatment to reduce proteinuria. Combination antihypertensive therapy with a target blood pressure of 120/80 is recommended. Statin therapy should be considered, with a target LDL of less than 100.

■ SEROSITIS

The greatest risk of pericardial tamponade occurs with effusions that are rapidly accumulating. Case series of large pericardial effusions in lupus suggest that oral prednisone 0.5 to 1 mg/kg daily with immediate placement of a pericardial drainage catheter results in resolution in about half of the patients, with the other half requiring pericardial window. If a large pericardial effusion is accompanied by other severe manifestations of SLE, or if a large effusion has accumulated rapidly, one should strongly consider a daily pulse of methylprednisolone 1000 mg for 3 days at the beginning of treatment. Colchicine 0.6 mg twice daily is useful for the management of small to moderate symptomatic pericardial effusions. NSAIDs are another alternative in patients with normal renal function. There are minimal data to guide treatment of symptomatic pleural effusions in SLE. Thoracentesis should be performed to rule out infection, and patients should be treated with oral prednisone 0.5 to 1 mg/kg daily. With recurrent pleural or pericardial effusions, steroid-sparing agents such as AZA, MMF, cyclosporine, or methotrexate (MTX) should be considered. Other pulmonary manifestations such as interstitial lung disease and shrinking lung syndrome are less common, and scant data are available to guide treatment. Considerations include immunosuppressive regimens listed above; the choice of therapy is also based on individual patient presentations and comorbidities.

■ CUTANEOUS LUPUS

The most likely reasons for hospital admission in a patient with cutaneous manifestations of lupus are bullous lupus or cutaneous vasculitis with ulcerations. Bullous lupus improves rapidly with dapsone, but the diagnosis must be certain, as TEN and Stevens-Johnson syndrome do not similarly respond to dapsone. Severe mucocutaneous involvement from SLE may necessitate intravenous corticosteroids and adequate hydration. When intravenous steroids are used for cutaneous lupus, they are generally dosed at or above the equivalent of prednisone 1 mg/kg/d. Cutaneous vasculitis from SLE should be confirmed by skin biopsy if possible, then treated initially with daily oral prednisone 1 mg/kg. A second immunosuppressive agent, usually AZA (2-3 mg/kg daily), MTX (15-25 mg orally weekly), or MMF (up to 1500 mg twice daily) is also given. As with other disease manifestations, patients with cutaneous lupus should be treated with hydroxychloroquine unless there is a known allergy.

■ HEMATOLOGIC

Depending on the severity of hemolytic anemia, high-dose intravenous steroids may be warranted, between 500 and 1000 mg of methylprednisolone daily for 1 to 5 days. Once the anemia stabilizes, patients are transitioned to oral prednisone 1 mg/kg daily, which is tapered over a few months. Oral immunosuppressives should be considered in recurrent or refractory cases. Thrombocytopenia with hemorrhagic complications is treated similarly, and intravenous immunoglobulin (IVIG) is often used when hemorrhagic complications occur. Dosing regimens for IVIG may include 1 g/kg daily for 1 to 2 days, or 400 mg/kg/d for 5 days. Oral immunosuppressives are started in recurrent or refractory cases. TTP in patients with lupus is treated as in patients without lupus: daily plasma exchange and high-dose intravenous steroids until the platelet count reaches a safe level and measures of hemolysis activity normalize. For adjunctive therapy in refractory cases, cyclophosphamide may be given to patients with lupus (vincristine is more commonly administered outside the setting of SLE). Although rituximab showed no benefit in a randomized clinical trial for treatment of active SLE, a small case series suggested potential benefit of rituximab for SLE-associated TTP. Rituximab is approved for treatment of ITP and is often successfully used to treat patients with SLE, thrombocytopenia, and bleeding. Although plasma exchange has been used in nearly every manifestation of SLE, it has thus far only been shown to be beneficial for TTP, catastrophic antiphospholipid antibody syndrome (CAPS), and neuromyelitis optica (optic neuritis with segmental transverse myelitis and anti-aquaporin-4 antibody positivity).

■ NEUROPSYCHIATRIC DISEASE

Patients with lupus presenting with new seizures, for which other causes have been excluded, should be treated with anticonvulsants and three to five daily pulses of 1000 mg methylprednisolone, followed by a prednisone taper beginning at 1 mg/kg/d. A steroid-sparing oral immunosuppressive is often added. For most manifestations of NPSLE, intravenous cyclophosphamide is given as steroid-sparing therapy, but the optimal duration of treatment has not been determined by randomized controlled trials. Many case series describe the use of MMF and AZA for NPSLE as well. IVIG is frequently used for NPSLE, especially when the peripheral nervous system is involved.

We suggest the 2010 EULAR recommendations for the management of SLE with neuropsychiatric manifestations as a useful resource when contemplating treatment.

■ MUSCULOSKELETAL

Inflammatory arthritis flares can be treated with NSAIDs. If a patient has severe functional limitation or requires hospitalization due to inflammatory arthritis, prednisone can be started at 0.5 mg/kg or less, and tapered over 1 to 3 weeks. Alternatively, patients can be given up to 120 mg of depot intramuscular steroid, such as triamcinolone, an approach that decreases the cumulative lifetime steroid dose. Inflammatory arthritis refractory to hydroxychloroquine is usually treated with MTX or AZA.

SLE-associated inflammatory myopathy is treated with prednisone 1 mg/kg daily for at least a month while starting a steroid-sparing agent such as MTX, MMF or AZA. IVIG is used in severe cases.

■ HEART BLOCK

IVIG is currently being studied as a salvage treatment for pregnant women with anti-Ro (SSA) and/or anti-La (SSB) antibodies and a fetus with cardiac conduction abnormalities, sometimes in combination with plasma exchange and corticosteroids. Clinical trial results are pending for this indication. We would recommend this treatment be undertaken only in collaboration with a rheumatologist.

■ COMPLICATIONS

Morbidity and mortality from lupus can occur both from the disease itself, and from complications of treatment. Treatment-related complications in the hospital from high-dose glucocorticoids include hyperglycemia, hypertension, and psychiatric manifestations, such as mania, delirium, and agitation. Many patients require sleep aids or anxiolytics while taking glucocorticoids. In patients with severe neuropsychiatric lupus, it can be difficult to differentiate the effects of the disease from those of its treatment; rheumatology, neurology, and psychiatric consultation may be helpful in this regard.

Cyclophosphamide can cause hemorrhagic cystitis. This risk may be reduced by administering mesna with IV cyclophosphamide, as well as maintaining adequate urine output through intravenous hydration. A white blood cell count nadir should be checked 10 to 14 days after high-dose intravenous cyclophosphamide. Patients on cyclophosphamide are at an increased risk of infection; prophylaxis against *Pneumocystis jirovecii*, usually with trimethoprim-sulfamethoxazole, is warranted. Cyclophosphamide is associated with an age- and dose-dependent risk of premature ovarian failure in women, and infertility in both men and women. Time permitting, egg storing or sperm banking may be considered, although initiation of CYC should not be delayed in situations of medical necessity. Gonadotropin-releasing hormone agonists such as leuprolide have a role in gonadal protection in women, and intramuscular testosterone can be considered in men.

Up to 25% of deaths in SLE are attributable to infections. These may present in atypical fashion, as high-dose corticosteroids minimize fever and other symptoms. Infection is most often due to common pathogens, such as *Escherichia coli*, *Staphylococcal aureus*, and *Streptococcus pneumoniae*, although patients with lupus are also at substantial risk of tuberculosis. Higher SLE disease activity and more immunosuppressive treatment are correlated with a higher infection risk; there is some evidence that antimalarials may protect against infection.

Progressive multifocal leukoencephalopathy (PML) has been reported in patients with SLE treated with rituximab, mycophenolate mofetil, cyclophosphamide, and other immunosuppressive regimens including corticosteroids alone. PML should be considered in patients with SLE and neurologic symptoms including altered mental status, motor deficits, ataxia, or visual disturbances such as diplopia.

Corticosteroids impair wound healing and increase the risk of infection in patients with SLE undergoing surgery. Methotrexate continued through the perioperative period has not been associated with an increase in post-operative infections or a delay in wound healing in patients with other autoimmune diseases. However, some groups have suggested holding MMF and AZA for 10 to 14 days both before and after surgery to diminish the risk of perioperative infection, though this has not been specifically studied by randomized trials.

Avascular necrosis is another untoward complication of glucocorticoid therapy. The hips, shoulders, and knees are most commonly affected. Of course, the best way to prevent complications of glucocorticoid therapy is to minimize the dose and duration of treatment.

DISCHARGE CHECKLIST

- Is the lupus manifestation leading to admission stable? Patients with pericardial effusions should not be discharged until the risk for pericardial tamponade has passed. Discharge can be considered for thrombocytopenic patients once the platelet count has stabilized and bleeding has ceased. In TTP, a response to therapy is indicated by a platelet count stabilized over 150,000/mm³.

- Have cardiac risk factors, such as hypertension and hyperlipidemia, been addressed? Patients with corticosteroid-induced diabetes should be under good glycemic control at discharge and be given education and instructions in the case of high or low readings prior to discharge. As there is a high risk of cardiovascular comorbidity in patients with SLE, we recommend the following similar guidelines as for diabetes mellitus, with a blood pressure target of less than 140/90 mm Hg and goal LDL cholesterol of less than 100 mg/dL. Behavioral issues such as obesity, diet, exercise, and smoking cessation should also be addressed.
- Has monitoring been arranged for toxicity of immunosuppressive medications? Recommended laboratory studies and their frequency are included in **Table 248-7**.

TABLE 248-7 Therapy Monitoring for Drugs Commonly Used to Treat Systemic Lupus Erythematosus

Agent	Testing	Frequency
Hydroxychloroquine	Dilated funduscopic exam, visual field testing, and either spectral domain OCT (SD-OCT), multifocal electroretinogram (mfERG), or fundus autofluorescence	Recommendations vary, generally every 12 mo
NSAIDs	CBC, Cr	Every 12 mo
Glucocorticoids	Bone mineral density	Every 1-2 y
	Glucose	Yearly
	Fasting lipid panel	Yearly
Azathioprine	CBC, Cr, AST	Every 1-2 wk after dosage change, then every 4-8 wk
	Skin cancer screening	Yearly
Mycophenolate Mofetil	Pregnancy test	At drug initiation
	CBC	Every 4-8 wk
Methotrexate	Chest X-ray	At drug initiation
	Hepatitis B, C	At drug initiation
	Pregnancy test	At drug initiation
	CBC, Cr, AST, albumin	Every 4-8 wk
Cyclophosphamide	CBC and differential	Oral: 2 wk after initiation or dose change, then every 4 wk once stable. IV: check nadir 10-14 d after dose
	Urinalysis	Monthly
	Creatinine, electrolytes	Oral: 2 wk after initiation or dose change, then every 4 wk once stable. IV: concurrent with CBC
	Hepatic function panel	Monthly
	Pregnancy test	At drug initiation

AST, aspartate aminotransferase; CBC, complete blood count; Cr, creatinine; OCT, optical coherence tomography.

- For patients being discharged on azathioprine, have levels of thiopurine methyltransferase (TPMT) been checked? Levels of TPMT can predict the likelihood of leukopenia or other adverse effects from azathioprine treatment. If TPMT testing is pending, a patient newly started on azathioprine should have a complete blood count (CBC) every 2 weeks as the dosage is advanced.
- Has appropriate follow-up with a rheumatologist been scheduled prior to discharge?
- If cyclophosphamide has been administered, has a follow-up blood count between days 10 and 14 been scheduled?
- If prednisone >5 mg daily is prescribed, has glucocorticoid toxicity been minimized by checking serum vitamin D, starting calcium 1200 mg daily, and vitamin D 800 to 1000 IU daily? If warranted, has a bisphosphonate or teriparatide been initiated? Patients should have both a risk assessment for glucocorticoid-induced osteoporosis (GIOP) and be started on treatment if indicated, as per the algorithm in **Figure 248-7**. Patients should be counseled to participate in weight-bearing exercise, to avoid smoking, and to modify other possible osteoporosis risk factors. Serum 25-hydroxyvitamin D should be measured, as studies have shown

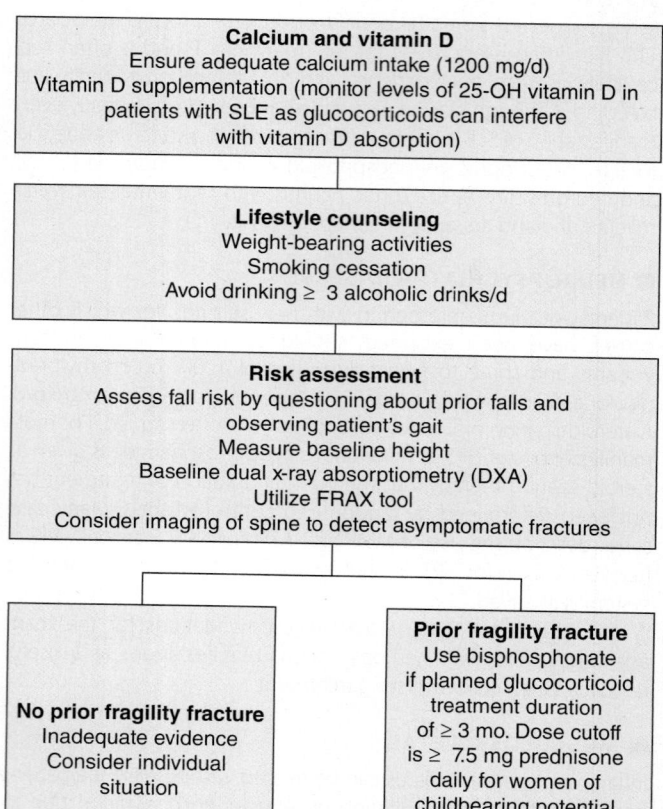

Figure 248-7 *Summary of recommendations for the prevention of glucocorticoid-induced osteoporosis in premenopausal women and men under age 50. These recommendations place a large focus on assessing fracture risk. The American College of Rheumatology task force concluded there were inadequate data to make recommendations for individuals who have not experienced a prior fragility fracture in these age groups. (Data from Grossman JR, Gordon R, Ranganath VK, et al. American College of Rheumatology 2010 recommendations for the prevention and treatment of glucocorticoid-induced osteoporosis.* Arthritis Care Res. *2010;62:1515-1526.)*

that vitamin D levels are consistently low in patients with SLE. Additionally, vitamin D has immunomodulatory properties, and evidence suggests an inverse relationship between vitamin D levels and lupus disease activity.

- Are outpatient physical and occupational therapy appropriate?
- Have discharge planners ensured that treatment plans are likely to be continued after discharge? Unfortunately, severe SLE disproportionately affects underserved populations, and many patients are uninsured or underinsured. Patients may need help with arranging transportation to and from follow-up appointments. In-home therapy and nursing aides should be considered if indicated.
- Has the patient received counseling to avoid prolonged sun exposure and to wear sunscreen? Sun exposure can cause not only a photosensitive rash, but also lead to increased SLE activity systemically; as a result, patients with SLE should both avoid the sun and use sunscreen.
- Have new medications been assessed for drug interactions?
- If teratogenic medications are being prescribed to a women of childbearing age, is there a plan for contraception? Several immunosuppressive agents, including methotrexate, MMF, cyclophosphamide, and leflunomide, are potent teratogens.
- Has the patient received pneumococcal and annual influenza vaccination? Current immunization guidelines advise that adult patients 19 years and older with an immunocompromising condition (who have not previously received pneumonia vaccination) receive one dose of PCV-13 followed by a dose of PPSV-23 at least 8 weeks later. Live vaccines should be avoided in individuals treated with more than 10 mg of daily prednisone or its equivalent.
- Have outpatient infusions been scheduled for patients who are to receive them, and has the insurance approval process been started?
- In patients receiving immunosuppressive medications, has prophylaxis for pneumocystis pneumonia (PJP) been considered? Expert opinion suggests trimethoprim-sulfamethoxazole one double-strength tablet three times weekly or one single-strength tablet daily for patients continued on prednisone ≥20 mg daily for 1 month or longer in combination with a second immunosuppressive drug.

SUGGESTED READINGS

Bertsias G, Ioannidis JP, Aringer M, et al. EULAR recommendations for the management of systemic lupus erythematosus with neuropsychiatric manifestations: report of a task force of the EULAR standing committee for clinical affairs. *Ann Rheum Dis.* 2010;69:2074-2082.

Bertsias G, Ioannidis JP, Boletis J, et al. EULAR recommendations for the management of systemic lupus erythematosus. *Ann Rheum Dis.* 2008;67:195-205.

Choi BY, Yoon MJ, Shin K, et al. Characteristics of pleural effusions in systemic lupus erythematosus: differential diagnosis of lupus pleuritis. *Lupus.* 2015;24:321-326

Hahn BH. Belimumab for systemic lupus erythematosus. *N Engl J Med.* 2013;368:1528-1535.

Hahn BH, McMahon MA, Wilkinson A, et al. American College of Rheumatology guidelines for screening, case definition, treatment, and management of lupus nephritis. *Arthritis Care Res.* 2012;64:797-808.

Mok CC, Ying KY, Yim CW, et al. Tacrolimus versus mycophenolate mofetil for induction therapy of lupus nephritis: a randomised controlled trial and long-term follow-up. *Ann Rheum Dis.* 2016;75:30-36.

Mosca M, Tani C, Aringer M, et al. European League Against Rheumatism recommendations for monitoring patients with systemic lupus erythematosus in clinical practice and in observational studies. *Ann Rheum Dis.* 2010;69:1269-1274.

Ortega LM, Schultz DR, Lenz O, Pardo V, Contreras GN. Lupus nephritis: pathologic features, epidemiology and a guide to therapeutic decisions. *Lupus.* 2010;19:557-574.

Ruiz-Irastorza G, Cuadrado M, Ruiz-Arruza I, et al. Evidence-based recommendations for the prevention and long-term management of thrombosis in antiphospholipid antibody-positive patients. *Lupus.* 2011;20:206-218.

Tsokos G. Systemic lupus erythematosus. *N Engl J Med.* 2011;365:2110-2121.

Rheumatoid Arthritis and Other Inflammatory Arthritides

Victoria D. Lackey, MD

Lisa Criscione-Schreiber, MD

Marcy B. Bolster, MD

Key Clinical Questions

1. Does this patient have rheumatoid arthritis or another inflammatory arthritis?
2. What are the extra-articular manifestations of rheumatoid disease?
3. Is a rheumatic condition responsible for this patient's hospitalization?
4. Is this hospitalization due to medication toxicity?
5. How should the patient's disease-modifying antirheumatic drugs be managed during the hospitalization, including perioperatively?
6. What tests and studies are useful to evaluate this patient's presentation?
7. What treatments are indicated?

EPIDEMIOLOGY

Rheumatoid arthritis (RA) affects 1% of the population worldwide, with women being more commonly affected. Within the past two decades, prior to routine early use of disease-modifying antirheumatic drugs (DMARDs), patients were frequently admitted to the hospital for active arthritis treatment. Today, most RA treatment occurs in the outpatient setting. However, RA is a systemic disease with numerous potential extra-articular manifestations, including cardiovascular disease. A hospitalist must be alert to these manifestations, as they may lead to hospitalization.

PRACTICE POINT

- Early, aggressive DMARD use is a cornerstone of current RA management. The duration of rheumatoid arthritis prior to DMARD therapy is one of the most robust predictors of disease outcome. Longer delays in initiation of DMARDs are associated with greater long-term functional impairment. DMARDs may also attenuate the risk of cardiovascular disease, which is increased in RA.

Most other common inflammatory arthritides fall into the category of seronegative spondyloarthropathies, which affect up to 2% of individuals with an equal male-to-female ratio. The seronegative spondyloarthropathies include psoriatic arthritis (PsA) (population prevalence 0.3%-1.0%), ankylosing spondylitis (AS) (prevalence 0.1%-6.0%, depending on the population studied), inflammatory-bowel-disease-associated arthritis, reactive arthritis, and undifferentiated spondyloarthropathy. These illnesses are seronegative for rheumatoid factor (RF), and are associated with the presence of human leukocyte antigen (HLA)-B27. The presence of HLA-B27 varies by ancestry. In general, up to 15% of the population is HLA-B27 positive, although only about 10% of these individuals develop a spondyloarthropathy. However, among individuals with spondyloarthropathies, up to 90% are HLA-B27 positive. Spondyloarthritis is characterized by axial arthritis, with a predilection for the sacroiliac joints, oligoarthritis, especially of the lower extremities, and enthesitis, or inflammation of ligaments and tendons at their attachments to bone. Inflammatory arthritis may be just one manifestation of a systemic disease that may include psoriasis and psoriasiform skin lesions, oral and genital inflammation, inflammatory bowel disease, and inflammatory eye disease, such as uveitis or scleritis.

PATHOPHYSIOLOGY

Rheumatoid arthritis is thought to result when an environmental factor triggers an aberrant immune response in a genetically susceptible host. Several genes are associated with susceptibility to the development of RA. Most significantly, RA is associated with HLA-DRB1. A short amino acid sequence within this gene, known as the shared epitope, is associated with increased risk of severe RA and development of anticitrullinated-peptide antibodies. Auto-antibodies against citrullinated peptides appear to be almost 90% specific for rheumatoid arthritis, although less sensitive than the RF assay. Identification of these autoantibodies is now part of routine diagnostic testing for RA via the anticyclic-citrullinated peptide (anti-CCP) autoantibody assay. An immune reaction against citrullinated peptides may initiate an inflammatory response in the joints. With regard to environmental exposures, cigarette smoking is the strongest proven risk factor for rheumatoid arthritis. Citrullination occurs when, within proteins, the amino acid arginine undergoes post-translational modification, mediated by peptidylarginine deaminases into citrulline. Cigarette smoking may lead to citrullination of proteins in the lungs, rendering them immunogenic. Both citrullinated peptides and antibodies against these peptides have been identified in the joints of patients with RA; up to 70% of patients with RA have anti-CCP antibodies in the serum. Rheumatoid factor or IgM anti-IgG antibodies, is detected in approximately 80% of patients. When rheumatoid factors are deposited in joints as immune complexes, they initiate complement-mediated inflammation within the joint. The combination of a positive RF and anti-CCP antibody is >90% specific for the diagnosis of RA in the right clinical context. However, levels of rheumatoid factor and anti-CCP do not correlate with disease activity in RA, and thus should not be repeated in a positive individual.

In RA, the synovium becomes inflamed and hypertrophied, and develops into an invasive tissue known as a pannus. The pannus, composed primarily of synovial fibroblasts, secretes matrix metalloproteinases and other enzymes that erode cartilage and stimulate osteoclasts to erode bone. These processes produce the characteristic radiographic appearance of RA of joint space narrowing and marginal erosions (**Figure 249-1**).

Many current therapies for RA target specific parts of the inflammatory cascade. Several cytokines, including tumor necrosis factor-alpha (TNF-α), interleukin (IL)-1, IL-6, and IL-12, are elevated in rheumatoid joints. Biologic agents are available to inhibit all of these cytokines in RA except IL-12. Inflammation in RA is maintained by costimulation of T-cells, which is inhibited by cytotoxic T-lymphocyte-associated protein 4 (CTLA4). T-cell costimulation and activation is inhibited by abatacept, a fusion protein consisting of CTLA4 complexed to an immunoglobulin heavy chain (CTLA4-Ig).

Spondyloarthropathies and RA have some similar pathogenic mechanisms; both respond to agents that block TNF-α. Bony erosion of joints occurs in both RA and spondyloarthropathies. However, spondyloarthropathies are also characterized by bony proliferation in involved joints and the spine. In these diseases, there is significant dysregulation of bone remodeling, such that erosion and proliferation of bone may occur in different locations within the same joint. While some mechanisms of joint inflammation and bone erosion in the spondyloarthropathies are probably similar to those in RA, the bone proliferation is less well understood. Recent observational studies have shown that while TNF-α inhibitors decrease symptoms and inflammation in spondyloarthropathies, they do not halt bony ankylosis, which must therefore be mediated via different pathways.

DIAGNOSIS

■ NEW POLYARTICULAR ARTHRITIS

Even with advances in diagnostic testing and imaging, inflammatory arthritides are diagnosed clinically, based on symptoms and examination findings, with laboratory and imaging studies as supporting evidence. Morning stiffness lasting at least an hour is one of the major clinical characteristics of all forms of inflammatory arthritis. The morning stiffness of inflammatory arthritis tends to be more diffuse than that of osteoarthritis (OA).

Rheumatoid arthritis is classically symmetric with swelling and tenderness of the small joints of the hands, primarily the wrists, metacarpophalangeal (MCP) joints, and proximal interphalangeal (PIP) joints (**Figure 249-2**). Other commonly involved joints include the knees, shoulders, ankles, hips, and metatarsophalangeal joints. If arthrocentesis is performed, the synovial fluid is inflammatory, generally with 2000 to 20,000 white blood cells (WBCs)/mm³. Classification criteria for the diagnosis of RA were last published in 2010 (**Table 249-1**). These criteria utilize a points system. An individual with ≥ 6 points is classified as having RA. Points are given based on number and distribution of involved joints, presence of RF or anti-CCP antibodies, elevated acute phase reactants, and duration of symptoms. Anti-CCP antibodies have a sensitivity of 67% and specificity of 95% for the diagnosis of RA; a specificity of 97% for the diagnosis of RA has been reported in patients with early inflammatory arthritis and both positive RF and anti-CCP antibody. Rheumatoid nodules and radiographic erosions are not part of the 2010 criteria, as patients with RA are ideally identified and treated before either of these manifestations occurs.

Rheumatoid arthritis is distinguished from OA by history and physical examination. Patients with osteoarthritis classically experience

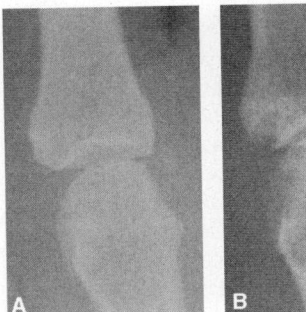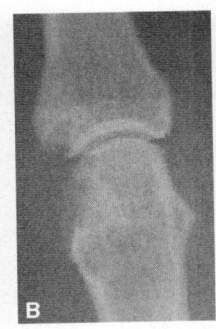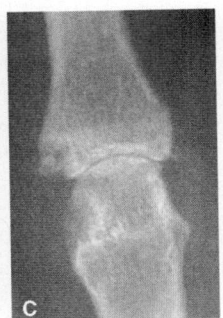

Figure 249-1 *Progressive destruction of a metacarpophalangeal joint by rheumatoid arthritis. Shown are sequential radiographs of the same second-metacarpophalangeal joint. (A) The joint is normal 1 year prior to the development of rheumatoid arthritis. (B) Six months after the onset of rheumatoid arthritis, there is a bony-erosion adjacent to the joint and joint space narrowing. (C) After 3 years of disease, diffuse loss of articular cartilage has led to marked joint space narrowing.* (Reproduced, with permission, from Imboden J, Hellmann DB, Stone JH. *Current Rheumatology Diagnosis & Treatment*, 2nd ed. New York, NY: McGraw-Hill, 2007. Fig. 15-3.)

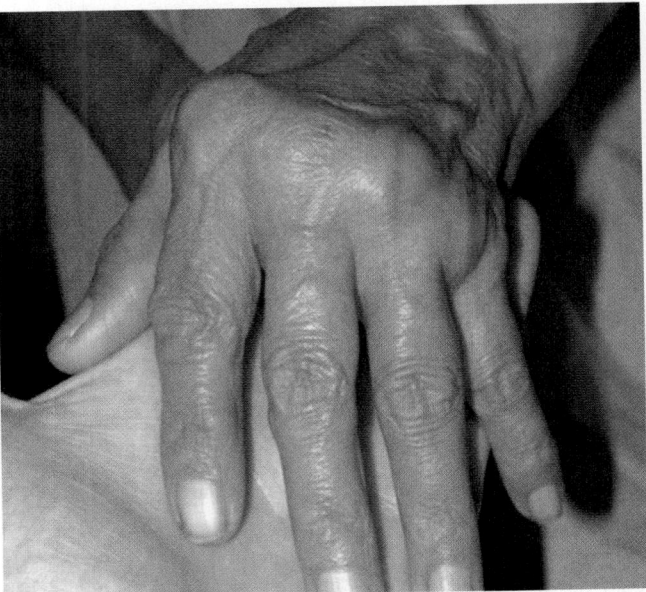

Figure 249-2 *Rheumatoid arthritis, with synovitis and ulnar deviation at the metacarpophalangeal joints and atrophy of the interosseous muscles.* (Used with permission from Richard P. Usatine. In: Usatine RP, Smith MA, Mayeaux EJ Jr, et al. *Color Atlas of Family Medicine.* New York, NY: McGraw-Hill; 2009.)

TABLE 249-1 The 2010 American College of Rheumatology/ European League Against Rheumatism Classification Criteria*

From the Patient History	From the Patient Examination	Laboratory Findings
Duration of symptoms ≥6 wk (1 point)	Synovitis of • 2-10 large joints (1 point) • 1-3 small joints (2 points) • 4-10 small joints (3 points) 10 joints total (5 points)	Titers of RF *or* anti-CCP antibodies that are low-higher than the upper limit of normal (ULN) but <3 × the ULN (2 points) Titers of RF *or* anti-CCP that are high->3 × the ULN (3 points)
		Elevated sedimentation rate *or* c-reactive protein, based on lab standards (1 point)

*These criteria are applied to patients with at least one swollen joint which cannot be explained by another process, such as infection. Patients with ≥6 total points are considered to meet classification criteria for rheumatoid arthritis.

CCP, cyclic citrillinated peptide; RF, rheumatoid factor; ULN, upper limit of normal.

Extracted from Aletaha D, et al. 2010 Rheumatoid arthritis classification criteria. *Arthritis Rheum.* 2010;62(9):2569-2581.

TABLE 249-2 Classification Criteria for Psoriatic Arthritis Study Group (CASPAR) Criteria for Psoriatic Arthritis

These Criteria are Applied to A Patient with Inflammatory-Articular Arthritis (Joint, Spine, or Estheseal). Each Criterion has A Points Value. Patients with ≥3 Points Meet the Classification Criteria for Psoriatic Arthritis.

Criterion	Definition
Current psoriasis (2 points), or personal history of psoriasis (1 point), or or family history of psoriasis (1 point)	Family history includes a first- or second-degree relative
Psoriatic nail changes (1 point)	Onycholysis, pitting, or hyperkeratosis at the time of physical examination
Negative rheumatoid factor (1 point)	According to local laboratory reference range
Dactylitis (1 point)	Current swelling of an entire digit or history of dactylitis observed by a rheumatologist
Juxtaarticular new bone formation (1 point)	Nonosteophytic, ill-defined ossification seen on plain radiographs of the hand or foot

Data from Taylor W, et al. Classification criteria for psoriatic arthritis: development of new criteria from a large international study. *Arthritis Rheum.* 2006;54:2665-2673.

less than an hour of morning stiffness, and may have stiffness after prolonged rest and recumbency (inactivity gel phenomenon). Osteoarthritis has a predilection for distal interphalangeal (DIP) joints, PIPs, and the first carpometacarpal joint (base of the thumb). Large joints including hips, knees, and shoulders are frequently involved, as is the lumbar spine in patients with OA. RA, in contrast, classically involves the synovial joint of C1-C2, sparing the remainder of the spine. On physical examination, patients with OA display bony enlargement with less synovial swelling in the small joints of the hands. Effusions of larger joints reveal noninflammatory synovial fluid (white blood cell count <2000/mm³).

Systemic findings such as fever and leukocytosis may occur in RA, as may pulmonary and cardiac complications, including pleural effusions, pericardial effusion, and interstitial lung disease (ILD). Rheumatoid nodules occur in about 25% of patients with RA, although they may not be present at the onset of RA. Rheumatoid nodules are associated with other forms of extra-articular disease and more severe joint disease. Extra-articular manifestations of RA and spondyloarthropathy are discussed in greater detail below.

Seronegative spondyloarthropathy should be considered if the RF and anti-CCP are negative, or if polyarthritis is associated with sacroiliitis, urethritis, uveitis, psoriatic skin lesions, or a family history of HLA-B27-associated disorders. International groups have published criteria for the classification of PsA (**Table 249-2**) and for peripheral and axial spondyloarthritis (**Table 249-3**). These disorders resemble RA, in that morning stiffness lasts more than 1 hour and improves with activity. The spondyloarthropathies are all associated with sacroiliitis, which clinically manifests as buttock pain that improves with activity. Psoriatic arthritis generally involves peripheral joints with swelling, tenderness, and erythema. About 25% of people with psoriasis develop PsA, and the arthritis may precede skin disease. With current therapies, some patients with PsA never develop psoriasis, so it may be necessary to consult a rheumatologist if this diagnosis is in question. Clinical subsets of PsA

presentations, from most common to least common, include oligoarthritis, symmetric polyarthritis similar to RA, DIP-predominant disease, arthritis mutilans, and spondylitis (which may complicate each of the other types). While psoriatic arthritis, reactive arthritis, and other spondyloarthropathies classically involve unilateral sacroiliac joints, ankylosing spondylitis involves bilateral SI joints. An anterior-posterior view of the pelvis performed with the camera tilted 30° cephalad (Ferguson view) is the appropriate imaging study to evaluate for sacroiliitis.

PRACTICE POINT

Physical findings in spondyloarthropathy

- Patients with ankylosing spondylitis may have physical findings related to loss of mobility of the spine, chest, and sacroiliac joints. Decreased range of motion results from bony ankylosis and muscle spasm from pain and inflammation. Involvement of the costovertebral and costosternal joints in AS may lead to chest pain and *restriction of chest expansion with maximal inspiration*, which should normally be at least 5 cm measured at the fourth intercostal space. Therefore, patients with advanced AS develop restrictive lung disease and rely solely on diaphragmatic expansion for respiration. In addition, ILD may occur in up to 70% of patients with AS. The combination of restrictive lung disease and ILD can impede recovery from pulmonary infections in individuals with AS. Extra attention to pulmonary toilet is necessary in AS with pneumonia.
- Pain from sacroiliitis can be elicited by either direct palpation or the *FABER (flexion, abduction external rotation) or Patrick test*, in which the supine patient crosses an ankle over the contralateral knee. When the examiner stabilizes the contralateral pelvis and places downward pressure on the flexed knee, pain is

TABLE 249-3 The ASAS Classification Criteria for Axial Spondyloarthritis[*]

Sacroiliitis by Imaging Plus ≥1 SpA Feature	OR HLA-B27 Plus ≥2 Other SpA Features
Sacroiliitis on imaging is defined as	Active (acute) inflammation on MRI highly suggestive of sacroiliitis associated with SpA or
	Definite radiographic sacroiliitis
Spondyloarthropathy (SpA) Features and their Definitions	
Inflammatory back pain	Onset <40 y old, insidious onset, improves with exercise, does not improve with rest, and pain at night which improves upon getting up
	(For criterion to be fulfilled, 4/5 must be present)
Arthritis	Inflammatory joint arthritis, currently or in the past
Enthesitis	Tenderness at insertion of Achilles tendon or plantar fascia
Dactylitis	Inflammation of a whole finger or toe
Psoriasis	Psoriasis, currently or in the past
Inflammatory colitis	Crohn's disease or ulcerative colitis, currently or in the past
Good response to NSAIDs	The back pain is much better or relieved after a full dose of NSAIDs for 1-2 d
Family history for Spondyloarthritis	First- or second-degree relatives with ankylosing spondylitis, psoriasis, uveitis, reactive arthritis, or inflammatory bowel disease
HLA-B27	Positive laboratory test
Elevated CRP	Greater than the upper limit of normal

[*]These criteria should be applied to patients with chronic back pain for 3 mo or more, and who had the onset of back pain at an age younger than 45 y old. The criteria can be met with imaging features and clinical features, or by lab work and clinical features.

Data from Sieper J, et al. The Assessment of SpondyloArthritis international Society (ASAS) handbook: a guide to assess spondyloarthritis. *Ann Rheum Dis.* 2009 Jun;68 Suppl 2:ii1-ii44.

experienced in the contralateral SI joint. In advanced AS, patients develop abnormal *occiput-to-wall distance* measured with the scapulae and heels against the wall. This test is also often abnormal in osteoporotic patients with spinal kyphosis. The *Schober test* assesses lumbar spine expansion on full forward flexion and is most useful in assessing young individuals with inflammatory back pain. It may also be abnormal in individuals with lumbar degenerative disease.

- Psoriatic arthritis (PsA) is strongly associated with *metabolic syndrome* and its attendant findings, such as hypertension and abdominal obesity. As in RA, patients with PsA are at increased risk for accelerated cardiovascular disease.

■ DIFFERENTIAL DIAGNOSIS OF POLYARTHRITIS

Polyarthritis may be inflammatory or noninflammatory (**Figure 249-3**). Inflammatory arthritis is characterized by swelling, warmth, erythema, and tenderness to palpation and joint pain with motion. The differential diagnosis of new inflammatory polyarthritis includes not only rheumatic diseases, but also infections, neoplastic or paraneoplastic conditions, and drug reactions. Rheumatic diseases in the differential diagnosis include RA, PsA, AS, undifferentiated spondyloarthropathy,

polyarticular gout, calcium pyrophosphate deposition disease (pseudogout), sarcoidosis, and systemic lupus erythematosus (SLE).

Bacterial infections with *Staphylococcus aureus*, group A and B streptococci, *Streptococcus pneumoniae*, and *Neisseria gonorrhoeae* may present with polyarthritis, usually in the setting of symptomatic or asymptomatic bacteremia with seeding of joints. Group A streptococcus may cause poststreptococcal reactive arthritis, or less often acute rheumatic fever. Lyme arthritis due to *Borrelia burgdorferi* usually presents with a relapsing monoarthritis of the knee, although it may also present with intermittent inflammatory polyarthritis.

Polyarthritis may be a presenting manifestation of hepatitis B, often with an urticarial rash. Hepatitis C and parvovirus B19 may mimic RA, presenting with symmetric polyarthritis and a false-positive RF. Tropical alphaviruses, such as chikungunya, dengue, Ross River virus, and O'nyong-nyong cause joint symptoms that may persist for months. HIV may be associated with reactive arthritis, undifferentiated spondyloarthropathy, psoriatic arthritis, and ankylosing spondylitis; spondyloarthropathy in the setting of HIV may have a more accelerated and aggressive course. Bacteria can cause reactive arthritis as well, most commonly including *Chlamydia trachomatis*, *Ureaplasma urealyticum*, *Salmonella*, *Shigella*, *Yersinia*, and *Campylobacter* species. Clinical features may include arthritis, urethritis, conjunctivitis, and uveitis.

Do not be fooled into thinking a hospitalized patient has RA based solely on a positive RF. Infective endocarditis, tuberculosis, sarcoidosis, malignancies, systemic lupus erythematosus, and other autoimmune disorders may also result in a positive rheumatoid factor. In one study, 20% of patients with either untreated tuberculosis or *Klebsiella* bacteremia had positive IgM RF. Up to 55% of patients with hepatitis C infection have a positive RF.

Fever and leukocytosis with polyarthritis may also occur with septic arthritis, viral-associated arthritis, crystal-induced arthritis, RA, adult-onset Still disease, and rare autoinflammatory conditions such as TNF-receptor-associated periodic syndrome (TRAPS). Polyarthritis, high spiking fevers, pericarditis, neutrophilia, and an evanescent rash suggest adult-onset Still disease. Acute HIV infection may present with polyarthritis, fever, rash, and anemia. Systemic lupus erythematosus (SLE) can cause polyarthritis. A complete blood count may help differentiate SLE from RA, as cytopenias are common in SLE, while RA is associated with thrombocytosis and leukocytosis (and anemia). A positive antinuclear antibody (ANA) test is present in up to 30% of patients with RA. Polyarthritis with rapidly progressive interstitial lung disease, myositis, Raynaud phenomenon, and a hyperkeratotic, fissuring hand rash is characteristic of the antisynthetase syndrome of the inflammatory myopathies. Polyarthritis with fever may also be the presenting symptoms of sarcoidosis, which may be accompanied by erythema nodosum and hilar adenopathy.

Neoplastic processes should also be considered in the differential diagnosis of polyarthritis. Hematologic malignancies, especially chronic lymphocytic leukemia, can induce secondary autoimmune phenomena.

■ COMPLICATIONS OF RA AND SPONDYLOARTHROPATHY THAT MAY LEAD TO HOSPITAL ADMISSION

Pulmonary disease

Pleural effusion is the most common extra-articular manifestation of RA requiring hospitalization. Pleural disease in RA is more common in men than women, and is associated with seropositive disease. The annual incidence of pleural effusions in patients with RA is 0.34% in women and 1.54% in men. About 25% of cases of pleural effusion with RA occur at the onset of joint disease. Pleural effusion is unilateral in more than 70% of cases; the left side is affected more

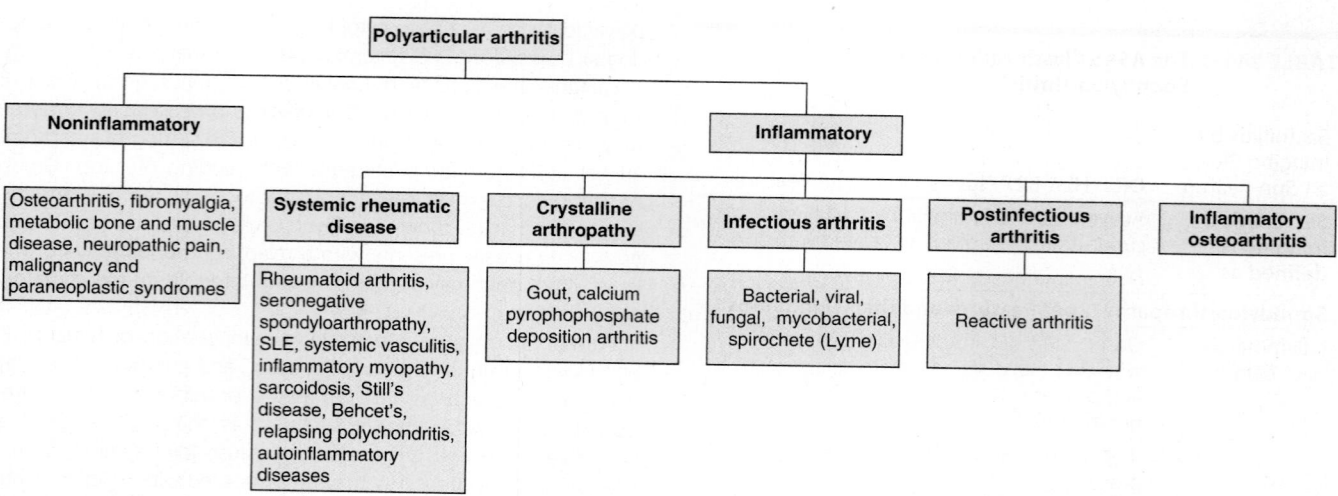

Figure 249-3 *Diagnostic approach to polyarthritis.*

often than the right. Affected patients may complain of pleuritic chest pain and dyspnea; about one-third have fever. Large pleural effusions must be distinguished from infectious or neoplastic effusions via thoracentesis. In RA, pleural effusions are exudative, with elevated LDH and a glucose level <60 mg/dL. Occasionally, these pleural effusions can mimic empyemas with pH <7.24, very low glucose (<40 mg/dL), LDH >700 U/L, but cultures are sterile. Pathology of pleural tissue shows a nodular appearance, with pathology resembling that of typical rheumatoid nodules, with palisading histiocytes around necrotic centers and multinucleated giant cells. RA is also associated with *nodular lung disease*, with rheumatoid nodules within the lung parenchyma; this must be distinguished from malignancy. Slowly progressive *pulmonary fibrosis* is also seen in RA, or more rarely pneumonitis that rapidly progresses to pulmonary fibrosis. Such presentations must be distinguished from overlap conditions or drug-induced pneumonitis; the latter has been reported with methotrexate (up to 0.1%-2% of treated patients), and less often with leflunomide and sulfasalazine. *Apical pulmonary fibrosis* is an uncommon complication of spondyloarthropathy that may mimic tuberculosis. TNF-α inhibitors can cause *drug-induced lupus*, often manifesting as a rash with pleural or pericardial effusion.

Rheumatoid vasculitis

Rheumatoid vasculitis historically affected 1% of patients with seropositive RA and active disease. With the effectiveness of current therapies for RA, vasculitis has become rare. *Skin lesions* of rheumatoid vasculitis include purpura, ulcers, and digital necrosis. *Corneal ulcers* (corneal melt) and *scleromalacia* of the eye may occur, and require aggressive treatment to preserve sight. *Visceral involvement* may include ischemic bowel, glomerulonephritis, myocardial infarction, cardiomyopathy, and pulmonary hemorrhage. Patients may also present with rapidly progressive *peripheral neuropathy* or *mononeuritis multiplex*, which must be differentiated from other systemic necrotizing vasculitides such as polyarteritis nodosa or cryoglobulinemic vasculitis. ANCA-associated vasculitis, such as granulomatosis with polyangiitis and microscopic polyangiitis, should be considered when a patient presents with vasculitis and polyarthritis. When cutaneous manifestations are present, skin biopsy is helpful in diagnosis. With neuropathy, nerve conduction studies and nerve biopsies, particularly sural nerve biopsies, are useful diagnostic tools.

Inflammatory eye disease

Secondary *Sjögren syndrome* with dry eyes, known as keratoconjunctivitis sicca, is common in RA. *Episcleritis* and *scleritis*, including

nodular scleritis, can also be manifestations of RA. Schirmer's test, a bedside measurement of tear production with filter paper, can be performed to screen for dry eye. Ophthalmology consultation may be useful for ocular surface staining and slit lamp examination.

Inflammatory eye disease is prominent in patients with spondyloarthropathy. Reactive arthritis is most commonly associated with *conjunctivitis*, in up to 50% of cases. *Uveitis* can occur in up to 20% to 30% of patients with ankylosing spondylitis. If untreated, uveitis may lead to blindness.

Infection

Febrile patients with RA should be aggressively investigated for infection. Fever from active RA is generally low grade (≤38.5°C). Prior joint damage puts patients with RA at increased risk for *septic arthritis*. A tense effusion in one or more joints, a painful joint out of proportion to the other joints, or a joint effusion with fever mandates diagnostic arthrocentesis.

When *pneumonia* occurs in patients with DMARD-treated inflammatory arthritis, both usual and unusual organisms should be considered. TNF-α inhibitors predispose patients to skin infections, typical and atypical bacterial pneumonia, hepatitis B reactivation, and septic arthritis. These risks are highest in the first year of therapy.

Because TNF-α has a particular role in maintaining granuloma integrity, *tuberculosis*, *histoplasmosis*, and *coccidioidomycosis* can reactivate in individuals treated with TNF-α inhibitors. Hospitalists should bear in mind that tuberculosis in patients on TNF-α inhibitors is often disseminated or extrapulmonary, and may present in an unfamiliar manner, such as with septic arthritis or meningitis. The largest number of cases of TB in patients receiving biologic agents has been reported in individuals receiving infliximab, followed by adalimumab and etanercept. The risk of serious infection, including tuberculosis, also seems substantial with certolizumab. There are no reported cases of TB in individuals receiving rituximab, and only one case in individuals receiving abatacept for treatment of RA. Although patients should be screened for TB before anti–TNF-α therapy, screening for TB is imperfect, and false-negative tests are common in patients with RA. Patients should also be screened for HIV, hepatitis B, and hepatitis C prior to starting TNF-α blockers or other DMARD therapy.

DMARDs, particularly TNF-α inhibitors, methotrexate, and corticosteroids, also seem to increase susceptibility to *Pneumocystis jiroveci*. Thus, especially when a patient with pulmonary infection fails to improve with treatment of usual community-acquired organisms, atypical infection should be considered in the differential diagnosis, and bronchoscopy for cultures pursued to identify the offending organism.

Cardiovascular involvement

Premature *coronary disease* occurs in patients with inflammatory arthritis. Although this risk seems to be decreasing with TNF-α blocker therapy, it remains an important consideration. Recently, an association between psoriasis and metabolic syndrome, and thus cardiovascular disease, has been recognized. As with RA, the presence of psoriasis or any spondyloarthropathy may be an independent risk factor for cardiovascular disease. Chest discomfort or exertional dyspnea should be thoroughly evaluated for possible cardiovascular etiologies in individuals with inflammatory arthritis.

Pericardial effusions occasionally occur in RA patients. They are more common is male patients with nodular and severely destructive RA. *Aortic insufficiency* may complicate long-standing spondyloarthropathy.

Spinal complications

Patients with spinal fusion due to ankylosing spondylitis (**Figure 249-4**) are at high risk for *spinal fracture* with trauma. Plain radiographs lack sensitivity to detect fracture in this population, and computed tomography or magnetic resonance imaging must be used. *Atlantoaxial instability* may occur in either RA or spondyloarthropathy. Patients may be asymptomatic, or present with occipital pain and weakness and paresthesias from myelopathy.

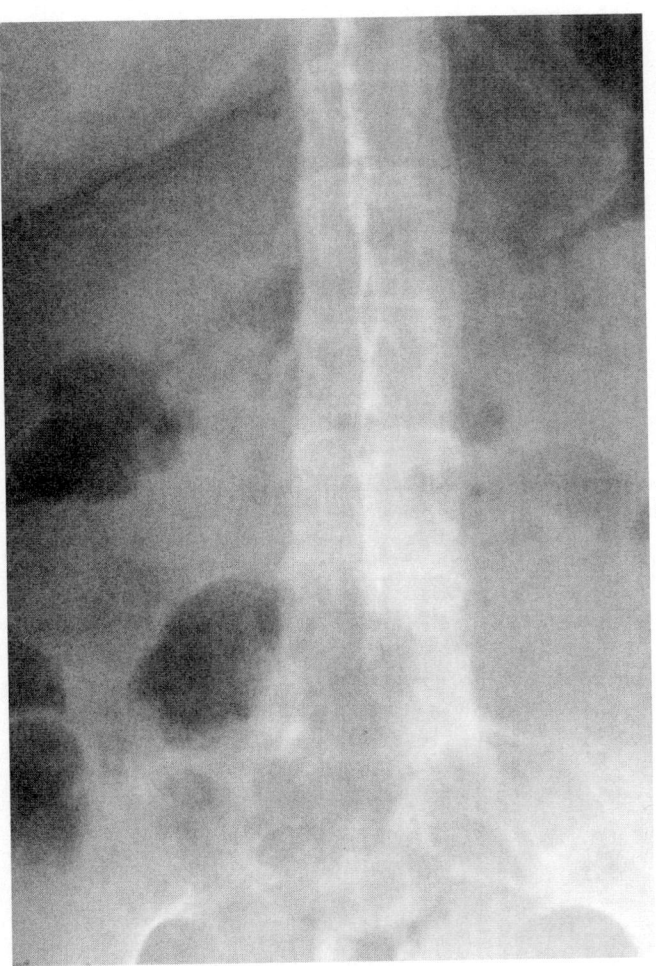

Figure 249-4 *Frontal view of the thoracolumbar spine showing the classic bamboo appearance of the spine in ankylosing spondylitis, resulting from fusion of the vertebral bodies and posterior elements.* (Reproduced, with permission, Chen MYM, Pope TL Jr, Ott DJ. *Basic Radiology.* New York, NY: McGraw-Hill; 2011. Fig. 7-45.)

Alteration of the path of the vertebral artery may lead to positional vertebrobasilar insufficiency, with vertigo, brainstem signs, or lower cranial nerve palsies.

Drug toxicity

Methotrexate can cause significant anemia or other cytopenias, often in the setting of renal insufficiency. Mild elevations in transaminases occasionally occur with nonsteroidal anti-inflammatory drugs (NSAIDs), methotrexate, leflunomide, and other DMARDs. If elevations in aspartate aminotransferase or alanine aminotransferase three times the upper limit of normal or more are observed, both viral and autoimmune hepatitis must also be considered. Methotrexate may also cause hypersensitivity pneumonitis in up to 0.1% of treated patients. It most often presents in the first few months of methotrexate therapy, but may occur any time during the course of therapy. Patients with methotrexate pneumonitis present with dyspnea, cough, fever, and bilateral infiltrates. Bronchoscopy and biopsy may be necessary to distinguish it from community-acquired pneumonia. There are also case reports of hypersensitivity pneumonitis with leflunomide and sulfasalazine.

In addition to increasing the risk of infection, anti-TNF-α blockers may also lead to new autoimmune conditions, which resolve with discontinuation of therapy. Leukocytoclastic vasculitis and other vasculitides are especially common. Anti-TNF blockers occasionally cause drug-induced systemic lupus erythematosus, characterized by rash, arthralgias and occasionally serositis. It is important to recognize drug-induced autoimmunity, since treatment involves a change in therapy instead of additional immunosuppressant therapy.

Miscellaneous complications

Felty syndrome (RA, neutropenia, and splenomegaly) used to occur in 1% of patients with RA, but has become rare. RA patients are also at increased risk for *lymphoma*. The risk of lymphoma correlates with the severity of RA disease activity, with an incidence ratio of 1.8 in individuals with RA compared to the general population. The risk does not appear to be significantly different among patients treated with different DMARD regimens. Patients with spondyloarthropathy commonly have associated *inflammatory bowel disease*.

TREATMENT

■ INFLAMMATORY ARTHRITIS

The hospitalist should be familiar with the most common drugs used to treat inflammatory arthritis, their toxicities, and recommended monitoring. Low-dose *glucocorticoids* (eg, prednisone ≤7.5 mg daily) are frequently taken by patients with RA when other DMARDs either fail to control the disease or are contraindicated. Due to complications such as hyperglycemia, osteoporosis, avascular necrosis of the hip, and cataracts, the lowest possible dose is desirable. Moderate doses can be used to treat flares of inflammatory arthritis. Prednisone 20 to 30 mg daily for 3 to 5 days is usually sufficient to control an acute exacerbation of RA. This dose can then be tapered in 5 to 10 mg decrements over about 2 weeks.

Although *NSAIDs* are less central to RA management than in the past, they are still used for breakthrough joint pain as needed. NSAIDs are associated with gastrointestinal tract bleeding, especially when combined with glucocorticoids. In this situation, gastric protection is recommended. NSAIDs may also exacerbate inflammatory bowel disease. Because of evidence linking NSAIDs to stroke and myocardial infarction, these drugs should be prescribed with caution in patients with RA, due to the substantial baseline risk for cardiovascular disease in this population.

Most patients with RA are treated with DMARDs (**Table 249-4**). *Methotrexate* is the most common initial therapy prescribed worldwide for moderate-to-severe RA, since studies have found it to be

TABLE 249-4 Disease-Modifying Antirheumatic Drugs: Toxicities and Monitoring

Agent	Potential Toxicities	Monitoring Recommendations
NSAIDs	GI bleeding, renal failure	Yearly CBC, Cr, LFTs
Hydroxychloroquine	Macular damage	Funduscopic examination and visual fields annually
Sulfasalazine	Myelosuppression, especially if G6PD deficient	G6PD, CBC every week for first 3 mo, then every 2-4 wk for the next 3 mo, then every 3 mo
Methotrexate	Myelosuppression, hepatic fibrosis, pneumonitis	CBC, LFTs, Cr every 4-12 wk
Leflunomide	Myelosuppression, acute hepatic failure	CBC, hepatic function, Cr every 4 wk for first 6 mo, then every 8-12 wk
Corticosteroids	Hyperglycemia, hypertension, osteoporosis, cataracts	Yearly urinalysis for glucose. DXA every 2 y if doses ≥ 5mg daily

CBC, complete blood count; Cr, creatinine; DXA, bone mineral density measured by dual-energy x-ray absorptiometry scan/bone mineral density; G6PD, glucose-6-phosphate dehydrogenase; LFTs, liver function tests including aspartate aminotransferase, alanine aminotransferase, albumin.

the best tolerated, most effective nonbiologic DMARD. Methotrexate is also used to treat PsA and other spondyloarthropathies, including inflammatory bowel disease. However, it is not efficacious for isolated axial disease in AS. Methotrexate is usually prescribed in doses between 10 and 25 mg as a single weekly dose, orally or subcutaneously. Folic acid (1 mg) is concurrently administered daily. Folic acid minimizes side effects, such as oral ulcers and nausea, and may also decrease the risk of methotrexate hepatic toxicity. For patients with moderately to severely active arthritis, *leflunomide*

may be used as an alternative to methotrexate, and occasionally in combination with methotrexate. Leflunomide is approved for use in rheumatoid arthritis, but it is also effective in PsA and psoriasis. Leflunomide is Category X for pregnancy, and is thus rarely prescribed for women of childbearing potential. Cholestyramine is an antidote to leflunomide, and is administered at 8 grams three times daily for 11 days. Levels of leflunomide are reduced substantially within 48 hours of cholestyramine treatment.

Patients with mild-to-moderate RA are often treated with *hydroxychloroquine* or *sulfasalazine*. Both medications are used to treat peripheral joint disease in spondyloarthropathies. These medications are taken daily, are anti-inflammatory but not immunosuppressive, and may be given in combination with other oral or biologic DMARDs in more severe disease. When used together in combination with methotrexate, they are referred to as triple therapy.

Today, there are nine *biologic therapies* approved for the treatment of moderately to severely active RA (**Table 249-5**). Five of these are directed against TNF-α. Infliximab, adalimumab, and golimumab are all monoclonal antibodies against TNF-α. Infliximab is a chimeric antibody with a murine variable region and a human constant region, while adalimumab and golimumab are humanized antibodies. Infliximab is given by infusion at 4- to 8-week intervals, adalimumab is administered subcutaneously at 1- to 2-week intervals, and golimumab is given subcutaneously every 4 weeks. Certolizumab pegol is a variable region of a humanized anti-TNF-α that is PEG-ylated to increase the biologic half-life. It is given by subcutaneous injection every 4 weeks. Etanercept is a dimeric fusion protein of a region of the human TNF-α receptor complexed to human immunoglobulin heavy chains. It is given subcutaneously once or twice weekly. Infliximab, adalimumab, etanercept, and golimumab are approved for treatment of RA, PsA, and AS. Infliximab, adalimumab, and certolizumab pegol are also approved for Crohn disease, which can be associated with spondyloarthropathy. Anti-TNF-α therapy is contraindicated in patients with acute systolic dysfunction, and must be used with extreme caution in patients with heart failure.

The four other approved biologic therapies each have different mechanisms of action. Anakinra is an IL-1 receptor antagonist. Abatacept is a chimeric protein consisting of an immunoglobulin fused to the extracellular domain of cytotoxic T-lymphocyte antigen 4 (CTLA4). It acts by binding to antigen-presenting cells, and blocking the costimulatory signal necessary for T-cell activation.

TABLE 249-5 Biologic and Small Molecule Disease-Modifying Antirheumatic Drugs

Agent	Description	Disease Indication	Administration
Adalimumab	Anti-TNF-α antibody	RA, JIA, PsA, PsO, AS, CD	Subcutaneous every 2 wk
Etanercept	Anti-TNF-α receptor fusion protein	RA, PsA, AS, JIA, PsO	Subcutaneous weekly
Golimumab	Anti-TNF-α antibody	Ra, PsA, AS	Subcutaneous monthly
Infliximab	Anti-TNF-α antibody	RA, JIA, PsA, PsO, AS, CD, PCD, UC	Intravenous every 4-8 wk
Certolizumab pegol	PEGylated anti-TNF-α variable region	RA, CD	Subcutaneous monthly
Anakinra	IL1 receptor antagonist	RA	Subcutaneous daily
Abatacept	CTLA4-Ig	RA, JIA	Intravenous monthly or Subcutaneous weekly
Rituximab	Anti-CD20 antibody	RA, NHL, CLL	Intravenous, 2 doses 14 d apart, repeated in 6 mo
Tocilizumab	Anti–IL-6 Receptor antibody	RA	Intravenous monthly
Tofacitinib	JAK-3 inhibitor	RA	Oral twice a day
Ustekinumab	IL12, IL 23 antibody	PsA, PsO	Subcutaneous every 12 wk
Apremilast	Phosphodiesterase 4 inhibitor	PsA, PsO	Oral twice a day

AS, ankylosing spondylitis; CD, Crohn disease; CLL, chronic lymphocytic leukemia; JIA, juvenile idiopathic arthritis; NHL, non-Hodgkin lymphoma; PCD, pediatric Crohn disease; PsA, psoriatic arthritis; PsO, plaque psoriasis; RA, rheumatoid arthritis; UC, ulcerative colitis.

Rituximab is an anti-CD20 antibody, which is thought to act in RA by blocking B-cell-related activities. Tocilizumab is an antibody against the IL-6 receptor, which blocks the activity of IL-6, a cytokine important in the inflammatory response in RA.

The newest agent for rheumatoid arthritis, *tofacitinib*, is the first agent in a class of nonbiologic DMARDs which targets cytoplasmic small molecules involved in intracellular signaling pathways and amplification of the inflammatory cascade. Tofacitinib preferentially inhibits Janus kinases (JAK) 1 and 3. Unlike biologic DMARDs, it is orally administered. Tofacitinib is approved as monotherapy or in combination with other DMARDs, but not biologic medications. Adverse event associated with tofacitinib include neutropenia, abnormal liver enzymes, and tuberculosis and other opportunistic infections.

Ustekinumab, a new biologic therapy, is a human monoclonal antibody which binds to the proinflammatory cytokines IL-12 and IL-23. Inhibition of IL-12 and IL-23 interrupts natural killer cell activation and T-cell activation. *Apremilast*, a new small molecule therapy, is an oral phosphodiesterase 4 inhibitor. It decreases intracellular cAMP levels, and downregulates release of many proinflammatory cytokines. Both agents are currently being evaluated for use in ankylosing spondylitis as well.

■ MANAGEMENT OF EXTRA-ARTICULAR COMPLICATIONS

Rheumatoid pleural effusions requiring hospitalization and thoracentesis are generally treated with oral prednisone at 0.5 to 1 mg/kg daily for 1 to 2 weeks. Prednisone is then tapered off over the next 2 to 3 months. Recurrent rheumatoid effusions are sometimes treated with intrapleural corticosteroids. Small pleural effusions may not require therapy.

Inflammatory eye disease is initially treated with topical steroids. Oral NSAIDs may be effective in uveitis related to spondyloarthropathy if no contraindications exist. Refractory or severe cases may be treated with oral prednisone in high doses (0.5-1 mg/kg daily), intravitreal corticosteroid injection, or DMARD therapy such as methotrexate, azathioprine, or mycophenolate mofetil. Infliximab is also used for inflammatory eye disease in patients with a spondyloarthropathy.

Rheumatoid vasculitis is generally treated first with pulse-dose methylprednisolone (≥250 mg intravenously daily for 3-5 days), followed by oral prednisone 1 mg/kg/d. Such treatment is generally accompanied by rituximab or cyclophosphamide, similar to the management of other forms of systemic necrotizing vasculitis.

■ PERIOPERATIVE MANAGEMENT

Many patients with inflammatory arthritis are treated chronically with glucocorticoids. Patients taking the equivalent of 7.5 mg or higher of prednisone daily for more than 2 weeks are at risk for adrenal insufficiency. A meta-analysis examined the question of whether stress doses of corticosteroids were necessary when patients treated chronically with corticosteroids (up to 15 mg prednisone daily) undergo surgery. The analysis found that acute adrenal insufficiency did not occur if the usual dosage of steroids was given daily, including on the day of surgery. The authors recommended that patients receiving long-term, low-dose glucocorticoid therapy be carefully monitored intraoperatively, with rescue intravenous hydrocortisone given if the hemodynamic status declines.

Regarding the perioperative use of other DMARDs, a primarily European multinational group recently published a compilation of recommendations, based on literature review and expert opinion. The group recommends continuing methotrexate during the perioperative period, as a grade B recommendation with level 1b evidence (Oxford levels of evidence). There are no firm guidelines for the perioperative management of anti-TNF-α therapy. As the incidence of perioperative infection for orthopedic surgical procedures is low, it is probably not feasible to answer this question in an adequately powered randomized controlled trial. The risk of withdrawing biologic therapy in the perioperative period is that inflammatory arthritis will flare, impeding rehabilitation, and potentially requiring corticosteroids for treatment, which may impair wound healing and increase the risk of wound infection. The principal risk associated with continuing biologic therapy in the perioperative period is skin infections. In patients with inflammatory bowel disease, a cohort study did not find any difference in the risks of perioperative complications whether infliximab was given more or less than 12 weeks before surgery. For arthritis patients, practices vary by site, but many practitioners err on the side of caution, presuming that the risk of substantial morbidity resulting from perioperative infection outweighs the risk of flare of RA. Many practitioners hold anti-TNF-α therapy for 1 to 2 weeks prior to surgery, and restart treatment after the skin has healed.

Individuals with RA may have atlantoaxial (C1-C2) inflammatory arthritis of the spine. Plain radiographs of the cervical spine in flexion and extension should be obtained preoperatively to ensure stability at the atlantoaxial joint, since instability puts the patient at risk for spinal cord injury during cervical hyperextension with intubation. Similarly, patients with AS requiring surgery require careful intubation and positioning with particular attention to protecting the spine.

DISCHARGE CHECKLIST

- Has rheumatology follow-up been arranged?
- Is there a tapering plan in place for patients started on glucocorticoids, if appropriate?
- Is therapy for hyperglycemia indicated for patients being discharged on glucocorticoids? If insulin was needed during hospitalization, hyperglycemia should be anticipated, and blood glucose levels monitored. When planning glucose-lowering therapy, recall that blood glucose peaks about 6 to 8 hours after an oral dose of prednisone. Patients should be given clear instructions for insulin dosing during glucocorticoid tapers to avoid hypoglycemia.
- Are patients taking glucocorticoids on appropriate preventive medications, including peptic ulcer protection, bone protection, calcium, and vitamin D? Bone loss occurs rapidly following the initiation of glucocorticoids, and RA is also an independent risk factor for osteoporosis. Most patients treated with oral steroids should receive calcium plus vitamin D (600 mg/400 IU) twice daily. A 25-hydroxyvitamin D level should be checked prior to discharge, and vitamin D supplemented as needed. The American College of Rheumatology (ACR) recommends that all patients who receive glucocorticoids be assessed for their risk of osteoporosis.
- If a DMARD was discontinued during this admission, is there a plan for restarting the DMARD at discharge or at a later date? Patients may experience disease flares if medications are held for more than 2 weeks. Therapy should therefore be resumed after discharge, or an alternative therapy should be started. If restarting DMARD therapy is a significant concern, the patient should follow-up with his or her rheumatologist within 1 to 2 weeks following hospital discharge to reassess disease activity and plan future arthritis treatment. In patients undergoing joint replacement or other surgery, DMARD therapy should be restarted within 2 weeks after surgery except in unusual circumstances.
- Are the patient's immunizations current? While some studies have shown decreased vaccine effectiveness in the setting of methotrexate and biologic therapies, this should not be a deterrent to immunization against influenza and pneumococcus.

- Has *Pneumocystis jiroveci* prophylaxis been considered in patients in being discharged on long-term prednisone ≥20 mg by mouth daily, rituximab, or cyclophosphamide?
- Would the patient benefit from posthospitalization physical therapy? Physical therapy is an important component of RA care during and after the hospitalization.

SUGGESTED READINGS

Aaltonen KJ, Joensuu JT, Virkki L, et al. Rates of serious infections and malignancies among patients with rheumatoid arthritis receiving either tumor necrosis factor inhibitor or rituximab therapy. *J Rheumatol*. 2015;42:372-378.

Curtis JR, Yang S, Patkar NM, et al. Risk of hospitalized bacterial infections associated with biologic treatment among US veterans with rheumatoid arthritis. *Arthritis Care Res*. 2014;66:990-997.

Harty L, O'Toole G, FitzGerald O. Profound reduction in hospital admissions and musculoskeletal surgical procedures for rheumatoid arthritis with concurrent changes in clinical practice (1995-2010). *Rheumatology*. 2015;54:666-671.

Michet CJ 3rd, Strobova K, Achenbach S, Crowson CS, Matteson EL. Hospitalization rates and utilization among patients with rheumatoid arthritis: a population-based study from 1987 to 2012 in Olmsted County, Minnesota. *Mayo Clin Proc*. 2015;90:176-183.

Singh JA, Inacio MC, Namba RS, Paxton EW. Rheumatoid arthritis is associated with higher ninety-day hospital readmission rates compared to osteoarthritis after hip or knee arthroplasty. *Arthritis Care Res*. 2015;67:718-724.

Szabo SM, Levy AR, Rao SR, et al. Increased risk of cardiovascular and cerebrovascular diseases in individuals with ankylosing spondylitis. *Arthritis Rheum*. 2011;63:3294-3304.

Tanaka M, Koike R, Sakai R, et al. Pulmonary infections following immunosuppressive treatments during hospitalization worsen the short-term vital prognosis for patients with connective tissue disease-associated interstitial pneumonia. *Mod Rheumatol*. 2015;25:609-614.

Toxicology and Addiction

SECTION V

Toxicology and Addiction

CHAPTER 250

Drug Overdose and Withdrawal

Ernest Murray, MD

Leon Walthall, MD

Kristin R. Wise, MD, FHM

Key Clinical Questions

① How do you manage drug-induced prolongation of the QTc interval and torsades de points?

② What is the initial evaluation and management of suspected overdose of sedatives, analgesics, stimulants, and other drugs of abuse?

③ When should you suspect a withdrawal syndrome and how do you prevent withdrawal in patients at risk?

INTRODUCTION

This chapter will review common overdoses and withdrawal syndromes encountered in the hospital setting following admission from the Emergency Department. According to American Association of Poison Control Centers (AAPCC), the top four substances most frequently involved in adult exposure are prescription medications. Analgesics, sedatives, antipsychotics, antidepressants, and cardiovascular medications accounted for over 150,000 exposures in 2013 (23% of all substances). The top three substance category associated with the most fatalities included prescription sedatives or hypnotics, cardiovascular medications, and opioids. For further prescribing information (see Chapter 73 [Patient Safety and Quality Improvement in Post-Acute Care, section on polypharmacy], Chapter 48 [Perioperative Pain Management], Chapter 99 [Pain], Chapter 216 [Palliation of Common Symptoms], and Chapter 223 [Mood and Anxiety Disorders]).

INITIAL APPROACH TO SUSPECTED OVERDOSE

The general initial evaluation for most overdoses occurs in the emergency department (ED). The assessment and management of a suspected overdose always begin with the stabilization (Airway, Breathing, Circulation [ABCs]). Emergency physicians quickly establish if a patient has stable vital signs, evaluate the need for respiratory support or intubation for airway protection, and provide fluid resuscitation. Admitting hospitalists should determine what was done in the emergency department, initial impressions of the ED staff, pending tests, red flags that might alter triage plans, and next best steps. Clinicians should also have a low threshold to consult with poison control. The use of gastrointestinal decontamination and renal replacement therapies for overdoses are covered in Chapter 100 (Suspected Intoxication and Overdose).

PRACTICE POINT

- All local poison control centers may be reached through the American Association of Poison Control Centers (AAPCC) centralized phone number (800-222-1222). A medical toxicologist can provide emergent consultation, including recommendations for testing, treatment, and monitoring.
- The World Health Organization's list of international poison centers may be accessed online. www.who.int/gho/phe/chemical_safety/poisons_centres/en/index.html

If the patient is willing and able, it is important to ascertain what substance(s) were ingested, including dosages and timing. If such information cannot be obtained from the patient, collateral sources for second-hand accounts should be sought, including family and friends, EMS reports, outpatient health care providers and pharmacies. If self-harm is suspected, institute suicide precautions and obtain appropriate psychiatric evaluation to determine a safe disposition. With an unintentional intoxication, counsel the patient regarding medication dosing in order to avoid repeat events.

Complete blood count (CBC), coagulation tests, comprehensive metabolic profile (CMP), serum osmolality and osmolar gap, acetaminophen and salicylate levels, and electrocardiogram (ECG) are routinely performed. Additional blood work may include arterial blood gas analysis, troponin, creatine kinase (CK), serum ethanol levels, drug levels, and an additional red top tube on hold. Urine studies should include a pregnancy test in women if appropriate. Urine toxicology studies are frequently ordered. However, these screens have significant limitations that may mislead the ordering clinician:

- False-positive screens occur for many commonly tested drugs such as amphetamines due to the presence of many other drugs (including ephedrine, pseudoephedrine, ranitidine, trazodone, and chlorpromazine).
- A positive initial screening test may not identify the drug responsible for acute intoxication due to drug detection at levels that produce no clinical effects or due to the persistence of detectable levels following ingestion during the previous days to weeks.
- False-negative screens result from an inability to detect certain drugs such as "designer" amphetamines available over the internet, benzodiazepine metabolites, and phencyclidine (PCP) congeners.

Detection of a particular drug, however, may alter medical management if a positive screen alerts the clinician to:

- Initiate measures to reduce toxicity as in acetaminophen overdose.
- Avoid certain medications such as β-blockers in patients with a positive cocaine screen.
- Consider stimulant-induced psychosis for a patient presenting for the first time with psychosis and a positive drug screen for cocaine or amphetamine.

Clinicians should always consider the possibility of multiple drug toxicity, especially salicylates, acetaminophen, antidepressants, alcohol, and illicit substances. A concise summary of the evaluation and management of these drugs is outlined in **Table 250-1**.

MEDICATIONS THAT PROLONG THE QT INTERVAL
■ BACKGROUND

The QT interval (the start of the Q wave and the end of the T wave on the ECG) represents the electrical depolarization and repolarization of the ventricles. Measuring the QT should be performed from leads II, V_5, or V_6 using the longest measurement for highest sensitivity. The heart rate (R-R cycle length) influences the duration of the QT interval (ie, the slower the heart rate, the longer the R-R interval and QT interval). Analysis of the duration of repolarization requires correction of the heart rate. A QTc >450 ms in men and >470 ms in women is considered prolonged. See Chapter 108 (The Resting ECG). Online calculators are available that use a variety of popular methodologies) (http://www.mdcalc.com/corrected-qt-interval-qtc/, http://reference.medscape.com/calculator/qt-interval-correction-ekg, or http://www.medical-calculator.nl/calculator/QTc/).

Medication-induced long QT syndrome (LQTS) increases the risk of the potentially lethal arrhythmia known as torsades de pointes (TdP). Between 1983 and 1999, 761 cases of TdP were reported, causing oversight from the FDA to remove medications from the market that could potentially cause QT prolongation. Antiarrhythmics that prolong the QT interval include amiodarone, disopyramide, dofetilide, ibutilide, mibefradil, procainamide, quinidine, sematilide, and sotalol. Entire classes of medications are well known to prolong QT and have been implicated in acquired LTQS and are still in common use in the United States (**Table 250-2**). TdP is usually self-limiting; however, it may develop into ventricular fibrillation and sudden cardiac death.

■ EVALUATION

Patients should be stratified on the basis of risk factors; patients at increased risk for prolonged QT and TdP include female gender, advanced age, prolonged baseline QTc, electrolyte abnormalities (hypokalemia and hypomagnesemia), a history of heart disease (CHF/CAD), hepatic and/or renal dysfunction, and bradycardia. Polypharmacy with multiple medications associated with increased QT interval further increases risk. Initial evaluation should be medication review, ECG and comprehensive metabolic profile.

■ INPATIENT MANAGEMENT

Once a patient develops TdP, ICU level care is warranted. If TdP does not self-terminate, immediate electrical cardioversion is indicated for all unstable ventricular arrhythmias. In stable patients, the goal is electrolyte stabilization with magnesium and potassium. For refractory cases, induction of tachycardia via chronotropes or direct pacing is sometimes used to shorten the QT interval. After removing all offending agents, the mainstay of management is:

(1) IV magnesium
(2) IV potassium (goal 4.5-5.0 mEq/L)
(3) For refractory cases, direct transvenous overdrive pacing and/or isoproterenol for heart rate goal 90 to 110 beats/min

For patients who develop drug-induced prolonged QT syndrome and TdP, a family history should also be obtained to identify congenital LQTS. This might require ECGs of first-degree relatives and possibly genetic testing (see Chapter 134 [Ventricular Arrhythmias]).

CARDIOVASCULAR MEDICATIONS
■ B-BLOCKER OVERDOSE
Background

The pleotropic effects of BBs in hypertension, heart failure, coronary artery disease, migraines, and anxiety have increased prescription patterns of these medications, and consequently increased the potential for overdose in the general population despite the increase of safety of newer selective BBs. BBs inhibit either one or a combination of the three types of β-receptors. β-1 is located on mostly cardiac tissue and has chronotropic and ionotropic effect with some effect on juxtaglomerular cells causes release of renin. β-2 receptors regulate smooth muscle tone and are well known to influence bronchial smooth muscle relaxation with some effect on pancreatic islet cells causing release of insulin. BBs affect the β-receptor by preventing G proteins from converting adenosine triphosphate (ATP) to cyclic-adenosine monophosphate (cAMP). Consequently, there is less intracellular calcium available for muscular contraction.

Although BBs have been well studied for effects on each receptor at therapeutic dose, receptor selectivity is lost at overdose plasma levels. Lipid solubility is an important consideration in some BBs as this is associated with more side effects due to crossing the blood-brain barrier and untoward CNS involvement. Some BBs cause quinidine-like sodium channel blockade (ie, acebutolol, propanolol, oxprenolol, and betaxolol), which is exacerbated at toxic doses.

Evaluation

The most typical presentation of patient with BB overdose is bradycardia, first-degree heart block, and hypotension. The standard evaluation for suspected BB overdose includes blood pressure measurement, a 12 lead ECG, CMP for evaluation of end-organ damage or hypoperfusion, serum lactate, finger stick blood sugars, and complete neurological assessment. Propranolol overdose may be associated with QRS prolongation, seizures, and coma. Pindolol, a

TABLE 250-1 Overview of Common Medication Overdoses

Medication	Signs/Symptoms	Initial Evaluation	Initial Management in addition to drug discontinuation	Discharge Considerations
QT prolonging drugs	Abnormal ECG Arrhythmia	ECG CMP Calcium Troponin T or I	IV Magnesium Cardioversion Direct pacing	Return to baseline QTc
β-Blockers	Hypotension Bradycardia AV nodal block Heart failure CNS depression Siezures Hypoglycemia Hyperkalemia	ECG CBC CMP Cardiac enzymes CXR	IVFs Atropine β-Agonists	Resolution of: Hypotension Bradycardia CNS depression
Calcium channel blockers	Hypotension Bradycardia AV nodal block Heart failure CNS depression Hyperglycemia	ECG CBC CMP Calcium Cardiac enzymes	IVFs	Resolution of: Hypotension Bradycardia Hyperglycemia
Acetaminophen	Nausea Vomiting Abdominal pain Coagulopathy Encephalopathy ↑ LFTs ↑ PT/INR AKI Acidosis	Acetaminophen level CBC CMP PT/INR/aPTT UDS for coingestions	Administer NAC Monitor acetaminophen levels, LFTs, coagulation tests Assess potential need for liver transplant	24-h NAC without ALI, AKI or coagulopathy Or NAC protocol completed and clinical/lab improvement
Lithium	Nausea/vomiting Ataxia Confusion, agitation Myoclonic jerks Seizure	Lithium level (may not correlate with clinical presentation) CMP Calcium CBC	IV normal saline Monitor CMP for hypernatremia (DI) Hemodialysis a consideration in severe toxicity	Asymptomatic Lithium level does not correlate with toxicity
SSRIs	Hunter criteria: yes to any one rule Clonus • Spontaneous • Inducible • Ocular Agitation Diaphoresis Hyperreflexia Hypertonia Fever Tremor	ECG CBC CK CMP	Benzodiazepines External cooling Discontinue all serotonergics	Asymptomatic for at least 6 h
Tricyclic antidepressants	Arrhythmia Hypotension Seizure Anticholinergic effects	ECG CBC CMP	Sodium bicarbonate Activated charcoal Consider Mg or lidocaine for refractory arrhythmias Normal saline or vasopressor support for refractory hypotension	Asymptomatic

AKI, acute kidney injury; ALI, acute liver injury; aPTT, activated prothrombin time; CBC, complete blood count; CK, creatine kinase; CMP, comprehensive metabolic profile; ECG, electrocardiogram; INR, international normalized ratio; IV, intravenous; NAC, N-acetylcysteine; PT, prothrombin time; UDS, urine drug screen.

TABLE 250-2 Noncardiac Medications that Prolong the QT Interval with Increased Risk of Torsades de Pointes

Class	Subtype	Examples
Antipsychotics	Typical	Chlorpromazine, Haldol, Pimozide, Thioridazine
	Atypical	Quetiapine, Aripiprazole, Respiradole
Antidepressants	SSRI	Fluoxetine*, Citalopram, Escitalopram
	TCAs	Imipramine, Desipramine, Maprotiline, Doxepin
	Mood Stabilizers	Lithium
Antibiotics	Macrolides	Azithromycin, Clarithromycin, Erythromycin
	Fluoroquinolones	Ciprofloxacin, Levofloxacin, Moxifloxacin
Antihistamines		Loratidine, Diphenhydramine, Famotidine
Antimalarials		Chloroquine, Halofantrine
Antifungals		Fluconazole, Pentamidine*
Antimotility/Antiemetics		Droperidol, Ondansetron
Anti-Cancer		Arsenic Trioxide*, Vandetanib
PDE inhibitors		Cilostazol, Anagrelide
Anesthetics		Cocaine, Propofol, Sevoflurane
Miscellaneous		Furosemide, Methadone, Donepazil, Papaverine, Organophosphates

*Known mechanism different from Ikr inhibition.

TABLE 250-3 Treatment options for Calcium Channel and β-Blocker Overdose

Intervention	Administration	Treatment Goals
Calcium salts	Calcium gluconate IV Initial bolus 30-60 mL of 10% solution Infusion 0.5 mEq/kg/h Calcium chloride IV Initial bolus 10-20 mL of 10% solution Infusion 0.5 mEq/kg/h	Double serum calcium Titrate for hypotension and/or bradycardia
Atropine	0.5-1 mg IV q3-5 min for total of 3 g	Titrate for bradycardia
Glucagon	1-5 mg bolus IV q10min for total of 15 mg Response dose given as hourly infusion	Titrate for bradycardia and/or hypotension
Vasopressors	Norepinephrine, Dopamine, Epinephrine, Phenylephrine, Isoproterenol, and Dobutamine per standard protocols	Titrate for hypotension and/or bradycardia
High dose insulin	Insulin IV Initial bolus 1 u/kg Infusion 1 u/kg/h up to 10 u/kg/h	Titrate q15min for hypotension
	Dextrose IV Initial bolus 25-50 g if needed Infusion 0.5 g/kg/h	Titrate q30min for euglycemia
Lipid emulsion in consultation with Poison Control	20% fat emulsion IV Initial bolus 1 mL/kg Infusion 0.25-0.5 mL/kg/h	Titrate for hypotension

partial agonist, may cause tachycardia in high doses. Sotolol, a class III antiarrhythmic, may cause QT prolongation, ventricular fibrillation, ventricular tachycardia, or torsades. Some BBs have an increased lipophilic profile with additional CNS effects such as CNS depression and somnolence. Additional unselective beta receptor antagonism can cause bronchospasm and decreased inotropy. A chest x-ray may be indicated to assess for pulmonary edema. Additional symptoms include syncope, chest pain, and seizures. Mild hypoglycemia and hyperkalemia may be seen due to the effect of β-receptor activity on the kidneys and pancreas. At high doses, inadvertent inhibition of the sodium receptor leads to QRS prolongation and an increased susceptibility for arrhythmias.

■ INPATIENT MANAGEMENT

Treatment of acute BB toxicity is dependent on the severity of the ingestion. Initially, the patient will need supportive care with close cardiac, blood pressure, and electrolyte monitoring. Hypotension and bradycardia require fluid resuscitation; failure to respond may require several agents similar to calcium channel blockers (**Table 250-3**). More severe cases will require vasopressors with β-1 agonist properties such as dopamine or norepinephrine. Refractory symptomatic bradycardia may require direct cardiac pacing, mechanical intra-aortic balloon pump and cardiology consultation. Dialysis may remove poorly protein bound BBs that are excreted by the kidneys (atenonol, sotalol, nadolol) (see Chapter 133 [Bradycardia]).

■ CALCIUM CHANNEL OVERDOSE

Background

CCBs inhibit transmembrane flow of calcium ions through voltage-gated L-type channels. These medications cause vascular smooth muscle relaxation leading to vasodilation which lowers blood pressure and have negative inotropic and chronotropic myocardial effects. CCBs also restrict pancreatic beta cell insulin secretion causing hyperglycemia. There are two major categories, the dihydropyridines (preferentially inhibit channels in the vasculature) and the nondihydropyridines (selectively block channels in the myocardium and delay atrioventricular conduction and sinus node function). For example, amlodipine, felodipine, nicardipine, and nifedipine are categorized as dihydropyridines, while verapamil and diltiazem belong to the nondihydropyridine category. There are numerous CCBs in both immediate and extended release preparations with widely variable half-lives from 1 to 50 hours. Bioavailability depends on first pass metabolism and all are metabolized by P-450 enzymes (CYP3A). High serum concentrations due to overdose overwhelm first-pass metabolism leading to increased circulating drug concentrations with even longer half-lives. CCB toxicity can be seen with ingestions of more than five times the usual dose.

Evaluation

Typically, dihydropyridine overdose leads to vasodilation with hypotension and reflex tachycardia, whereas nondihydropyridine overdose leads to decreased cardiac contractility and bradycardia. With higher drug concentrations, however, the L-type channel selectivity is often lost so that bradycardia, hypotension, and decreased cardiac contractility may occur due to overdoses from either CCB category. Negative inotropic effects may be associated with heart failure. Ventricular dysrhythmias and mental status changes are usually not seen; however, CNS depression with confusion may be progressing to coma in isolated cases or in patients with refractory hypotension. β-blocker (BB), clonidine and digoxin ingestions may present similarly and should be considered in the differential diagnosis. Unlike CCB, clonidine tends to cause miosis and sinus bradycardia rather than high-degree AV block. BBs may cause hypoglycemia whereas CCB may cause hyperglycemia.

Basic laboratory data testing begins with the ECG, CBC, CMP, calcium, and cardiac enzymes to exclude cardiac ischemia as a possible etiology of the hypotension or arrhythmia. ECG may reveal bradycardia, PR prolongation, or escape rhythms with advanced AV blocks. Chest x-ray may be obtained to evaluate for pulmonary edema. Digoxin levels should be obtained if concomitant ingestion is suspected. CCB assays are not routinely available and not be part of standard evaluation.

■ INPATIENT MANAGEMENT

Asymptomatic, stable patients require monitoring for hypotension, bradycardia, and hyperglycemia as these patients may quickly decompensate. Depending on whether the ingested formulation was immediate-release, standard-release or extended release, a recommended length of observation is 6, 6 to 12, and 24 to 36 hours, respectively. When hypotension does not respond to aggressive fluid resuscitation, a combination of IV calcium, glucagon, high dose insulin, vasopressors, and IV lipid emulsions should be administered. Atropine and glucagon may be administered for symptomatic bradycardia. In patients with mild symptoms, these treatments may be implemented sequentially (every 15 minutes with interval reassessment) whereas multiple therapies should be implemented simultaneously in hemodynamically unstable patients (Table 250-3). Calcium chloride administration requires a central line.

More aggressive and invasive therapies are needed, including transvenous pacemaker, intra-aortic balloon pump, cardiopulmonary bypass, and extracorporeal membrane oxygenation (ECMO) if the patient remains hemodynamically unstable despite the aforementioned therapies. Hemodialysis is not effective since CCBs have large distribution volumes and are highly protein bound.

ANTIDEPRESSANTS AND ANTIPSYCHOTICS

■ LITHIUM

Background

Despite its narrow therapeutic window, lithium remains widely utilized; in 2010 the AAPCC was notified of over 6000 cases of lithium toxicity. Lithium is rapidly and completely absorbed from the digestive tract, with a half-life of 18 to 36 hours. Time to peak concentration varies based on the formulation, ranging from 0.5 to 3 hours for immediate release to 2 to 6 hours for extended release. Lithium is nearly exclusively eliminated by the kidneys so renal compromise readily lends itself to toxicity.

Evaluation

Clinically, lithium intoxication presents differently depending on whether it is acute, acute on chronic, or chronic. Acute or acute on chronic lithium toxicity typically presents with gastrointestinal complaints including nausea, vomiting, and diarrhea. Later in the course of acute poisoning, patients develop neurologic complaints including sluggishness, ataxia, confusion/agitation, and neuromuscular

excitability (myoclonic jerks, coarse tremor or seizure). Acute kidney injury may be the cause or the result of acute lithium toxicity. Chronic toxicity will often present as nephrogenic diabetes insipidus with accompanying hypernatremia, polyuria, and polydipsia. Chronic toxicity can demonstrate the same neurologic effects as acute toxicity. Chronic toxicity may also present with a spectrum of pathology including hypothyroidism, hyperparathyroidism with accompanying hypercalcemia. Lithium overdose should be differentiated from neuroleptic malignant syndrome, the latter is more likely to cause rigidity. Laboratory evaluation should include serum lithium level, basic metabolic profile to address renal function, sodium and calcium levels, and ECG. Lithium levels do not accurately predict toxicity due to slow absorption into the central nervous system. A slight elevation in levels may be associated with lithium toxicity, especially in chronic users.

■ INPATIENT MANAGEMENT

IVFs (typically normal saline) should be administered, up to a 2 L bolus followed by 200 mL/h as tolerated. Patients should be monitored for the development of hypernatremia due to diabetes insipidus. Avoid using phenytoin for seizure treatment as it can decrease renal clearance of lithium. Hemodialysis effectively removes lithium from the serum and therefore is the primary treatment for significant toxicity. However, serial dialysis may be required due to inability to remove intracellular lithium; in some cases lithium levels may increase despite effective dialysis. Most experts recommend hemodialysis for serum lithium levels > 2.5 mEq/L with serious manifestations (eg, seizure or altered mental status) or levels > 4 mEq/L regardless of clinical status. Therapeutic goal is to reduce levels to < 1 mEq/L. Lithium levels should be monitored for 8 to 12 hours after dialysis to exclude rebound of lithium reentering the serum from the intracellular space. Additionally, dialysis may be considered for patients that cannot tolerate fluid resuscitation (renal compromise, volume overload, heart failure). Nephrogenic diabetes insipidus may respond to indomethacin (more effective in inhibiting renal prostaglandin synthesis than other nonsteroidal drugs and works within a few hours), thiazide diuretics (acting by mild volume depletion), and amiloride (enhances action of thiazide natriuresis and partially blocks potassium elimination from concurrent thiazide administration).

■ NONCYCLIC ANTIDEPRESSANT OVERDOSE

Background

Noncyclic antidepressants include:

- Selective serotonin reuptake inhibitors (SSRIs): fluoxetine, sertraline, citalopram, escitalopram, paroxetine, and fluvoxamine
- Serotonin-norepinephrine reuptake inhibitors (SNRIs): venlafaxine, desvenlafaxine, and duloxetine
- Norepinephrine-dopamine reuptake inhibitors (NDRIs): bupropion, trazodone and mirtazapine

These medications are widely prescribed for depression and anxiety disorders. Bupropion is also prescribed for smoking cessation. In general, they are safe and well-tolerated, especially when compared to TCAs and monoamine oxidase inhibitors (MAOIs). Despite more than 46,000 SSRI overdoses reported in 2011, only two deaths resulted.

Evaluation

Unlike tricyclics none of these drugs have significant anticholinergic effects. Most drugs cause central nervous system depression. Bupropion, a stimulant, may cause seizures due to inhibition or reuptake of norepinephrine and dopamine. Trazodone and mirtazapine can cause hypotension due to peripheral α-adrenergic blockade. SSRI intoxication may lead to seizures and/or serotonin syndrome. SSRIs are well absorbed in the gastrointestinal tract and reach peak levels in 1 to 8 hours. SSRIs inhibit neurotransmitter-specific pumps that transfer serotonin from the synapse (where they have their activity) into the cytoplasm of the afferent neuron. They are eliminated by the liver. The half-life for the majority of the SSRIs is in the range of 20 to 30 hours, with exceptions being fluoxetine (24-72 hours) and fluvoxamine (15 hours). A significant number of substances effect serotonergic pathways and can precipitate serotonin syndrome in a patient taking SSRIs (eg, tramadol, cocaine, carbamazepine, St. John's wort, linezolid, MAOIs, meperidine). This syndrome may develop during hospitalization so must be considered both for newly presenting patients and as a complication arising during the treatment of another disorder.

Diagnosis is based on clinical criteria. In order to meet Hunter criteria, the patient must have a history of ingestion of a serotonergic drug and one of the following: spontaneous clonus; inducible clonus or ocular clonus and diaphoresis or agitation; tremor and hyperreflexia; hypertonia and temperature greater than 38°C and ocular clonus or inducible clonus.

Laboratory evaluation should include CBC, CMP, and CK. An ECG should be obtained to look for QTc prolongation (fluoxetine, citalopram, escitalopram, venlafaxine). SSRI drug levels are not recommended. There are also many false positives in urine assays.

◼ INPATIENT MANAGEMENT OF THE SEROTONIN SYNDROME

Benzodiazepines are the mainstay of therapy to ease agitation and address mild hypertension and tachycardia. A typical starting dose is diazepam 5 to 10 mg IV with titration to effect; patients may require repeat dosing q10min. Supportive therapy is aimed at normalizing vital signs. Patients may exhibit severe hypertension or tachycardia, which should be treated with short acting agents (eg, esmolol, nitroprusside). Hyperthermia should be aggressively treated according to the severity. Physical restraints and butyraphones (haloperidol) are not recommended given concern for worsening hyperthermia. Additional supportive care should include IVFs, oxygen and cardiac monitoring. The antihistamine, cyproheptadine, also has serotonergic antagonism although quality evidence is lacking for its efficacy.

See Chapter 92 (Hyperthermia and Fever).

◼ TRICYCLIC ANTIDEPRESSANT OVERDOSE

Background

Though tricyclic antidepressants (TCAs) remain the 12th most common substance associated with fatalities from ingestion despite having been largely supplanted by SSRI's in the treatment of depression. The therapeutic window is narrow, and TCAs have a half-life ranging from 7 to 58 hours. The drug is rapidly absorbed in the gastrointestinal tract at therapeutic doses and undergoes conversion in the liver to the active metabolite, nortriptyline. Peak levels in the serum for amitriptyline at normal doses are observed at 2 to 5 hours. In the setting of overdose, however, anticholinergic effects may slow gastrointestinal absorption and delay peak levels. TCAs have wide ranging effects including: antagonism of cardiac fast sodium channels, anticholinergic and antiadrenergic effects, antagonism of histamine-1 receptors, and antagonism of central nervous system GABA-A receptors.

Evaluation

TCAs cause cardiac and neurologic effects at toxic doses. Cardiac effects include sinus tachycardia, worsening cardiac dysrhythmias, and hypotension which can be difficult to control. ECG findings vary from widened QRS to QT segment prolongation and ventricular

TABLE 250-4 Treatment Options for TCA Overdose

Agent	Dosing	Indication
Sodium bicarbonate	1-2 mEq/kg bolus, then 150 mEq (in 1 L D5W) at 250 cc/h	QRS >100 ms
Benzodiazepines	Varies based on agent	Agitation or seizures
Magnesium	1g IV q6h	Refractory arrhythmia
Lidocaine	1 mg/kg bolus, then 1-4 mg/min infusion	Refractory arrhythmia
Vasopressors (norepinephrine)	Varies based on blood pressure	Hypotension
Hypertonic saline (3%)	100 cc bolus (repeat q10min × 3)	Hypotension
Lipid emulsion (20%)	1-1.5 mL/kg bolus, then 0.25-0.5 mg/kg/min (up to 8 mL/kg)	Impending cardiac arrest

fibrillation. TCAs also may cause a range of neurologic symptoms, including seizures related to GABA-A antagonism. Anticholinergics effects may lead to delirium, urinary retention, hyperthermia, and dilated, poorly responsive pupils. Antihistaminic activity may cause decreased level of consciousness and even coma.

Laboratory evaluation includes ECG, chemistry panel, and troponin. An ABG may be necessary to evaluate acidosis. The 12-lead ECG guides therapy and provides prognostic information. The most sensitive predictor of seizures and ventricular arrhythmias is QRS duration (>0.16 seconds). Serum and urine TCA testing does not reliably guide management or provide prognostic information. Multiple drugs cause false positive results, significant toxicity may occur at nontoxic levels, especially with chronic TCA use, and results are usually not available at the time of clinical decision-making.

◼ INPATIENT MANAGEMENT

Close cardiac and neurologic monitoring should be in place for admitted patients. Telemetry and serial 12-lead ECG monitoring is recommended for patients with sinus tachycardia. ICU admission should be considered if ECG changes (including QRS prolongation, prolonged QTc, tall R waves in AVR or AVR R/S >0.7, arrhythmias), hypotension, respiratory depression, or altered mental status.

Treatment agents should be targeted by indication (**Table 250-4**).

SEDATIVE AND ALCOHOL

◼ SEDATIVE AND ALCOHOL INTOXICATION

Background

Sedatives constitute a diverse group of agents, including alcohol, benzodiazepines, nonbenzodiazepine hypnotic medications (so-called Z-drugs such as zolpidem [Ambien]), barbiturates, and several other compounds, including chloral hydrate and meprobamate. All sedatives dose-dependently depress neuronal function, and most of these agents can produce fatal respiratory depression.

Evaluation

Both alcohol intoxication and sedative overdose present with uncoordinated motor functioning (gait ataxia, finger to nose incoordination, positive Romberg sign), nystagmus, slurred speech, and various aberrant behaviors, including behavioral disinhibition, impairment of consciousness, reduced respirations, and drowsiness or sleep. Memory disturbances and frank amnesia, frequently referred to as

TABLE 250-5 Common Effects at Various Blood Alcohol Concentration Levels in Nontolerant Individuals

BAC (g/dL)	Effects
0.02	Mellow, warm, less inhibited
0.05	Relaxed, less alert, early coordination impairment
0.08	Definite impairment in coordination, judgment
0.10	Noisy, decreased reaction time, mood swings, embarrassing behavior
0.15	Clearly drunk, impaired balance and movement
0.30	Many pass out
0.40	Most pass out, some die
0.50	Breathing stops, many die

TABLE 250-6 Common Signs and Symptoms of Mild to Moderate Alcohol Withdrawal

Symptoms	Signs
Anxiety/nervousness	Tachycardia
Gastrointestinal distress	Hypertension
Headache	Tremor
Bad dreams	Sweating
Insomnia	Vomiting
Sensory disturbances	Generalized tonic-clonic seizures
Nausea	
Fatigue	

blackouts, are more likely with short-acting sedatives, alcohol, or a combination of the two. The history, either directly from the patient or from his or her associates, usually provides sufficient evidence to confirm intoxication with alcohol or sedatives. Laboratory testing in these patients should include a blood alcohol level (**Table 250-5**) obtained directly from a serum sample or indirectly by measurement of the breath alcohol content with a breathalyzer.

A metabolic profile should be obtained to check blood glucose (malnourished patients may have hypoglycemia) and to calculate the anion gap. Other toxic alcohols (ethylene glycol [antifreeze], methanol [wood alcohol]) will cause a high anion gap acidosis and osmolar gap. Isopropyl alcohol is associated with an elevated osmolar gap but not with an elevated anion gap acidosis (see Chapter 238 [Acid Base Disorders]).

Urine testing for benzodiazepines and barbiturates is widely available. Standard assays for benzodiazepines do not detect benzodiazepines but rather metabolites of 1,4-benzodiazepines. Therefore, they vary in their sensitivity to detect some benzodiazepines (clonazepam, lorazepam, midazolam, or alprazolam). Urine tests for other sedatives, including the Z-drugs and older sedatives (eg, meprobamate, chloral hydrate, ethchlorvynol), are not widely available, although may be requested from outside laboratories. Serum benzodiazepine levels do not correlate with clinical findings and are not readily available during emergent management.

■ INPATIENT MANAGEMENT

With alcohol intoxication, neurologic symptoms should clear within 4 hours unless due to coingestions, head trauma, or other causes. With any sedative overdose, the management is supportive and may require a period of artificial ventilation until the sedative level falls and spontaneous respiration resumes. A benzodiazepine antagonist, flumazenil, competitively binds but does not activate the gamma-aminobutyric acid (GABA) benzodiazepine receptor. The use of flumazenil may precipitate seizures in individuals who have developed physiologic dependence on benzodiazepines; therefore, this drug should only be used in consultation with a toxicologist (eg, Poison Control).

■ SEDATIVE AND ALCOHOL WITHDRAWAL

Background

Use of a sedative or alcohol on a daily basis for more than 2 weeks may result in withdrawal upon cessation of use. The likelihood increases with longer periods and heavier use. Withdrawal can also occur with nondaily, binge pattern use (more days of the week than not). The common signs and symptoms of alcohol withdrawal are shown in **Table 250-6** and delirium tremens (DTs) are shown in **Table 250-7**. In general, withdrawal from sedatives produces similar signs and symptoms as withdrawal from alcohol. Barbiturates and other, older sedatives may be more likely to produce seizures and/or delirium during withdrawal. The syndromes differ principally in their time course, which is directly correlated with the elimination half-life of the agent. Long-acting sedatives, such as diazepam or phenobarbital would typically present more gradually than alcohol withdrawal, and with a later onset of withdrawal seizures and peak symptoms.

Alcohol withdrawal typically progresses through stages due to central nervous system hyperactivity:

- 6 to 12 hours after last drink: tremulousness (in up to 100% of individuals) and other minor symptoms (insomnia, anxiety, gastrointestinal upset, headache)
- 12 to 48 hours after last drink: withdrawal seizures occurring predominantly in patients with a long history of heavy alcohol use or prior withdrawal seizures
- 12 to 48 hours after last drink: alcoholic visual hallucinations without mental status changes or hemodynamic instability (in up to 25% of individuals)
- 2 to 4 days after last drink: delirium tremens (in 4%-5% of patients)

Other causes of symptoms suggesting DTs that do not respond to high doses of benzodiazepines or last more than a week include intoxication due to benzodiazepines, gamma hydroxybutyrate (GHB) or baclofen withdrawal.

Evaluation

Laboratory evaluation should include complete blood count with differential and platelet count, coagulation tests, comprehensive

TABLE 250-7 Signs and Symptoms of Delirium Tremens (DTs)

Delirium
Confusion
Disorientation
Behavioral agitation
Waxing/waning of consciousness
Severe autonomic instability
Tachycardia
Hypertension
Diaphoresis
Fever (low grade)
Arrhythmias
Hallucinations
Visual more common than tactile (rarely auditory)

metabolic profile, liver biochemical tests, amylase or lipase, ECG, urinalysis, and in selected patients cultures. The ECG should be examined to determine QTc interval (prior to initiating possible treatment with haloperidol) and to identify possible ischemia. Ethanol levels are usually low or undetectable and do not influence management. Patients may experience withdrawal signs and symptoms with an elevated blood alcohol level.

INPATIENT MANAGEMENT

All patients should receive thiamine before glucose administration to avoid causing Wernicke's encephalopathy (encephalopathy, oculomotor dysfunction, gait ataxia), folate, multivitamins, intravenous hydration, correction of electrolyte disorders (especially magnesium and potassium depletion). For alcohol withdrawal, the most important element of management is prevention of seizures and DTs. Management of DTs commonly requires admission to an intensive care unit, for very close monitoring of vital signs and administration of high doses of benzodiazepines or barbiturates with or without adjunctive haloperidol. The general approach is to substitute an adequate dosage of a long-acting benzodiazepine (eg, diazepam, chlordiazepoxide, or clonazepam) to alleviate withdrawal symptoms. Some experts favor the use of lorazepam because it is not metabolized in the liver and would therefore not accumulate in patients with severe liver disease; however, metabolic function is usually well preserved until severe end-stage liver disease is present. Lorazepam's principal advantages are that it is available as a parenteral agent, and its short half-life allows rapid titration. Administering more than one benzodiazepine will complicate management due to different half-lives and should be avoided.

Table 250-8 provides a range of suggested doses of several common benzodiazepines and phenobarbital for use in mild to moderate alcohol withdrawal.

A fixed dose regimen or a symptom-triggered approach is used to establish the benzodiazepine taper. The symptom-triggered approach can minimize the total dosage of benzodiazepines utilized, but may be too labor intensive to be practical in some settings. As such, a fixed-flexible dose regimen may be preferred. Clinical Institute Withdrawal Assessment for Alcohol (CIWA) is a widely used scoring system that may be used at the bedside with set protocol forms or online (http://www.reseaufranco.com/en/assessment_and_treatment_information/assessment_tools/clinical_institute_withdrawal_assessment_for_alcohol_ciwa.pdf).

TABLE 250-8 Common Initial Dose Ranges for Benzodiazepines in Alcohol Withdrawal

Benzodiazepine	Mild Withdrawal*	Moderate Withdrawal
Chlordiazepoxide†	25-50 mg every 6 h	75-100 mg every 6 h
Lorazepam	1-2 mg every 6 h	3-4 mg every 6 h
Diazepam†	10-20 mg every 6 h	30-40 mg every 6 h
Clonazepam†	0.5-1 mg every 6 h	1.5-2 mg every 6 h
Barbiturate		
Phenobarbital†	30-60 mg every 6 h	90-120 mg every 6 h

*Note that these initial doses will not be sufficient for some patients; those patients who consume large quantities of alcohol (typically > 10-15 standard drinks daily) may need larger doses than those listed here.
†These long-acting agents allow a more rapid taper than shorter-acting agents, so that individuals may be tapered off their medication in as little as 4 or 5 d. These long-acting sedatives can accumulate; individuals should be observed carefully for signs of oversedation if these starting doses are not tapered within a few days.

A score <8 supports a clinical impression that the patient has not yet developed alcohol withdrawal and withdrawal prophylaxis is appropriate. An increasing score > 8 supports withdrawal and need for intervention with an aim to achieve a score less than 8 by inducing a light sleep with benzodiazepines.

Once stabilized, most patients can be tapered off benzodiazepines in approximately 10 days, with dosage reductions of approximately 10% of the total daily dosage each day over the course of those 10 days (which can be completed as an outpatient). Withdrawal from alcohol may also be managed very effectively with a long-acting barbiturate (phenobarbital), again with the need first to stabilize the patient's vital signs and eliminate other withdrawal signs and symptoms, followed by a taper schedule over approximately 10 days. There is some evidence that alcohol withdrawal may also be managed with anticonvulsants (carbamazepine, gabapentin, valproic acid, and others), either in conjunction with benzodiazepines or as a standalone therapy, although the evidence thus far for anticonvulsants in alcohol withdrawal is insufficient to support their use over benzodiazepines.

Withdrawal from sedatives is more complicated than withdrawal from alcohol. Long-term use (for more than 6 months) of benzodiazepines and Z-drugs, even at modest dosages, may be associated with a greater risk of seizures for days to weeks following cessation. As a result, many physicians recommend a sedative taper over several months under the supervision of a psychiatrist or addiction specialist. This may best be accomplished by switching a patient to phenobarbital and tapering it gradually over several months. Adjunctive use of anticonvulsants may play a role to reduce the seizure risk, but the evidence for this is limited. Withdrawal from barbiturates and other sedatives cannot safely be safely managed using benzodiazepines, because benzodiazepines do not adequately reduce the risk of seizures or withdrawal delirium. As such, phenobarbital is the agent of choice for managing withdrawal from barbiturates and other sedatives. Mixed sedative dependence syndromes, in which individuals regularly ingest multiple agents and possibly alcohol, should be managed with phenobarbital because it will safely cover withdrawal symptoms from all sedatives and alcohol.

ANALGESICS

■ ACETAMINOPHEN OVERDOSE

Acetaminophen is an analgesic drug, commonly used in combination with other drugs. The active ingredient is acetyl-para-aminophenol (APAP). The amount of acetaminophen ingested and the time to presentation are the most important prognostic indicators of hepatotoxicity. The APAP level guides therapy. The biggest benefit of N-acetylcysteine is within 12 hours of ingestion; however, treatment should be initiated for any toxic APAP level (see Chapter 100 [Suspected Intoxication and Overdose], Chapter 109 [Elevated Liver Biochemical and Function Tests], and Chapter 159 [Acute Liver Disease]).

■ SALICYLATE OVERDOSE

Salicylates are found in a number of medications, including aspirin products, bismuth subsalicylate (Pepto-Bismol) and herbal medications. Salicylate poisoning should be considered in any patient with an elevated anion gap acidosis. Serum salicylate levels may not correlate with clinical presentation due to a number of factors, including delayed absorption of enteric-coated formulations, altered absorption and elimination following overdose, and salicylate redistribution in body tissues rather than excretion by the kidneys. Available through poison control, a medical toxicologist should be consulted in any patient suspected of salicylate poisoning. Consider consultation with a nephrologist for guidance on alkalinization to promote elimination of salicylate and for recommendations and timing of possible hemodialysis.

■ OPIATE OVERDOSE

Background

Opioids are now among the most commonly prescribed medications in the United States. Over 5 million people use opioids for nonmedical purposes each year, and there are over 100,000 new users of heroin each year.

Evaluation

Fever, dyspnea, and acute pain are common presenting complaints of opioid-using patients. Underlying infection is often the cause of these complaints, particularly among injection drug users (IDUs). Endocarditis, skin, and soft-tissue infections, bone and joint infections, epidural abscess, and even pneumonia are more common among IDUs than in general medicine patients. When an opioid user is identified, a key part of the evaluation is to determine if the individual is physically dependent on opioids.

The role of urine drug testing in the diagnosis of opioid use is fairly limited. Providers need to be aware of general test characteristics as well as what tests are locally available. Specific (and separate) urine radioimmunoassay screening tests can be used to screen for opiates, oxycodone, meperidine, propoxyphene, and methadone metabolites. A "negative" screening test never rules out opioid use, and a "positive" screening test can only be used to support a clinical diagnosis. Definitive testing can be performed with gas chromatography/mass spectroscopy, but such testing is expensive and results are not immediately available.

Patients may present with symptoms of overdose (lethargy, pinpoint pupils, respiratory depression) or withdrawal (sweating, tremor, tachycardia, anxiety, pupillary dilation). Withdrawal symptoms typically begin 6 to 12 hours after the last use and will peak at 24 to 48 hours, but vary based on agent (**Table 250-9**).

■ INPATIENT MANAGEMENT

Overdose may occur in new opioid users, as part of a suicide attempt, when drug purity is unexpectedly high, or during induction on a long-acting opioid (eg, methadone). Injection drug users are particularly vulnerable to overdose when getting opioids from a new source where drug purity is not known and there is a mixture multiple drugs such as fentanyl and heroin. Initial treatment includes the use of the short-acting injectable opioid antagonist naloxone and supportive care. In the opioid-naïve individual, full-agonist reversal generally occurs when 0.4 mg of naloxone is given (IV/IM/SQ/ET) every 2 to 3 minutes. The intravenous route provides the most predictable response. For opioid-dependent patients, smaller doses should be used and titrated to reverse respiratory depression

TABLE 250-9 Opioid Withdrawal Symptoms and Time Course (Short-acting Opioids)

Hours After Last Opioid Use	Signs and Symptoms
6-12	Lacrimation, yawning, pupil dilation, rhinorrhea, sweating
12-18	Irritability, anxiety, nausea, sleep problems
18-24	Abdominal cramps, restlessness, anorexia, piloerection, tremor
> 24	Vomiting, diarrhea, muscle spasms, tachycardia, chills, hyperthermia, severe insomnia

TABLE 250-10 Typical Medication Dosing Regimens for Treatment of the Opioid Withdrawal Syndrome

Medication	Typical Doses	Typical Dosing Intervals	Maximum Daily Dose
Clonidine	0.1-0.2 mg orally	Every 2-6 h	1.2 mg
Methadone	10-20 mg orally	Every 6-8 h	30-40 mg
Buprenorphine	2-4 mg	Every 2-4 h	16 mg

(giving full-reversal doses of naloxone to opioid-dependent individuals may result in a severe withdrawal syndrome); doses of 0.1 to 0.2 mg of naloxone can be used in incremental fashion to reverse respiratory depression. Patients who have overdosed with a long-acting or high-affinity agent (eg, methadone, buprenorphine) will generally need admission for oxygen, close monitoring, and an intravenous naloxone infusion.

■ OPIATE WITHDRAWAL

Inpatient Management

Management of the opioid withdrawal syndrome (OWS) should be based on patient characteristics, goals of treatment, and local resources. Always verify methodone dosage prior to administration of large doses in patients who chronically take methadone. Patient characteristics include determination of the presence or absence of pain (acute and chronic), the presence or absence of pathologic opioid use (abuse and addiction), the type and amount of opioid being used, and the cause and severity of withdrawal. The goal of treatment will be either stabilization on an opioid, or complete cessation of all opioids. For opioid-addicted patients who are not currently receiving addiction treatment, the presence or absence of pain is the primary determinant of medication selection. Patients with pain will require agonist treatment with buprenorphine, methadone, or other opioid agonists. Patients without pain (other than withdrawal pain) can be managed with clonidine or buprenorphine. Medications most commonly used for the treatment and symptom management of OWS are outlined in **Table 250-10 and Table 250-11**.

STIMULANTS

■ STIMULANT OVERDOSE

Background

There are many types of abused stimulants in the United States, including cocaine, amphetamines, ecstasy, and over-the-counter and prescription stimulants. **Table 250-12** outlines the most commonly abused stimulants. Prescription stimulants include methylphenidate, methamphetamine, dextroamphetamine, mazindol, phenmetrazine, and phentermine. Prescribed stimulants may be used therapeutically

TABLE 250-11 Medications for Symptomatic Treatment of Acute Opioid Withdrawal

Symptom	Medication
Sleep problems	Zolpidem, temazepam, trazodone
Myalgia	Acetaminophen, nonsteroidal anti-inflammatory drugs
Diarrhea	Loperamide
Abdominal cramps	Dicyclomine

TABLE 250-12 Commonly Abused Stimulants

Street Name	Drug(s) [Trade Name]
Amphetamines	
Bennies, peaches	Amphetamine sulfate [Benzedrine]
Black Beauties, crank, cristy, crystal, crystal meth, meth, pep pills, quartz, speed, uppers, white crosses	Methamphetamine [Methedrine, Desoxyn]
Cramming drug, R-ball, rits, vitamin R	Methylphenidate [Ritalin, Concerta]
Dexies, footballs	Dextroamphetamine [Dexedrine, Dextrostat]
Ice, crystal	Freebase (smokable) methamphetamine
Cocaine preparations	
Crack, rock, gravel, supercoke	Freebase (smokable) cocaine
Big C, blow, coke, flake, flave, nose candy, snow, sugar boogers, white lady	Cocaine HCl
Pasta, bazooka	Coca paste
Designer drugs	
Ecstasy, XTC, Adam, M&M, Stars, 007s	Methylenedioxymethamphetamine (MDMA)
Eve	Methylenedioxyethamphetamine (MDEA)
The love drug	Methylenedioxyamphetamine (MDA)
STP (serenity, tranquility, peace), sweet tart	Dimethoxymethamphetamine (DOM)
Cathinone/cathine	
African salad, Bushman's tea, chat, kat, qat	khat
Cat	methcathinone
Drug combinations	
C&M	Cocaine + marijuana
Death hit	Cocaine + strychnine
Goofball, snowball, speedball	Cocaine + heroin
Ice	Methamphetamine + freebase cocaine
Liquid lady	Cocaine + alcohol
Pineapple	Methylphenidate + heroin
Poor man's speedball	Methamphetamine + heroin
Snackies	MDMA + mescaline
Space ball, space base, space dust	Cocaine + phencyclidine
Speedboat	Freebase cocaine + marijuana + phencyclidine (all smoked together)
Speedies	MDMA + amphetamine
Super Xs	MDMA + methamphetamine

TABLE 250-13 Stimulant Intoxication Signs and Symptoms

Physiologic Effects	Psychological Effects	Toxic Effects
Dizziness	Grandiosity	Hyperthermia
Tremor	Restlessness	Seizures
Hyperreflexia	Hypervigilance	Rhabdomyolysis
Hyperpyrexia	Aggression	Acute renal failure
Mydriasis	Impaired judgment	Hepatotoxicity
Tachypnea	Stereotyped behavior	Increased myocardial oxygen consumption
Tachycardia		Disseminated intravascular coagulation
Hypertension		

vasoconstriction, increased heart rate, and lowered seizure threshold. Psychological effects result from stimulation of corticomesolimbic dopamine circuits in the brain, leading to desired effects (increased energy and alertness, euphoria, decreased appetite and need for sleep) as well as negative effects (anxiety, grandiosity, impaired judgment, psychosis, paranoid delusions and hallucinations, and addiction). Adrenergic poisoning syndromes have similar presentations to neuroleptic malignant syndrome, serotonin syndrome, thyroid storm, intracranial hemorrhage, and pheochromocytoma. Laboratory evaluation includes urine drug screen, CBC, CMP, creatine kinase, urinalysis, coagulation tests, liver biochemical tests, troponins, ECG, and CXR. Additional testing may include thyroid function tests and neuroimaging.

Stimulant overdose symptoms are outlined in **Table 250-13**.

■ INPATIENT MANAGEMENT

Treatment for acute overdose of stimulants includes stabilization of airway, breathing, and circulation, administration of activated charcoal, seizure control with benzodiazepines, aggressive management of hypertension, and management of hyperthermia. The acutely intoxicated stimulant user should be approached in a subdued manner. Specific management for cocaine-associated complications is outlined in **Table 250-14**.

Designer drugs, especially MDMA (ecstasy), are stimulants with some hallucinogen-like effects, so acute physiological effects include more pronounced hypertension and hyperthermia as compared to other hallucinogens. MDMA also has serotonergic effects. Peak effects occur within 2 hours following ingestion and effects last approximately 4 to 6 hours. Ecstasy often contains adulterants. Urine drug screen will be positive for amphetamines but a negative screen does not exclusion ingestions of this drug. Hyperthermia is the main cause of death.

Toxicity of designer drugs may be related to additives such as ketamine or LSD. There are numerous case reports of MDMA use resulting in hyperthermia, rhadomyolysis, serotonin syndrome, hyponatremia with cerebral edema, fulminant hepatic failure, and stroke. Other stimulant-derived hallucinogens may cause cardiac arrhythmias.

■ STIMULANT WITHDRAWAL

The severity and duration of withdrawal from stimulants depends upon the intensity of the preceding months of chronic abuse and the presence of predisposing psychiatric disorders. In general, the "crash," or drastic reduction in mood and energy, can start within minutes after the last use. The user experiences craving, depression, irritability, anxiety, and paranoia. The craving for stimulants

for multiple conditions, including attention-deficit disorder, narcolepsy, fatigue in multiple sclerosis, and refractory depression, as well as in palliative care. Nicotine and caffeine are mild stimulants that are also in widespread use.

Evaluation

Stimulant overdose usually presents with symptoms due to overstimulation of the sympathetic nervous system leading to peripheral

TABLE 250-14 Treatments for Acute Medical and Neuropsychiatric Effects of Cocaine

Acute coronary syndrome	Oxygen
	Diazepam 5-10 mg IV or lorazepam 2-4 mg IV
	Aspirin 325 mg
	Nitroglycerin 0.4 mg 3 times, every 5 min, followed by an infusion titrated to a mean arterial pressure reduction of 10% or relief of chest pain
	Phentolamine 1 mg IV; repeat in 5 min
	Verapamil 5-10 mg IV
	Heparin 60 units/kg bolus, followed by 12 units/kg/h
	Percutaneous intervention (angioplasty and stent placement) or fibrinolytic therapy for STEMI [ST-segment-elevation myocardial infarction]
	Glycoprotein IIb/IIIa inhibitors
Supraventricular tachycardia	Oxygen
	Diazepam 5 mg IV or lorazepam 2-4 mg IV
	Adenosine 6 mg or 12 mg IV
	Consider diltiazem 20 mg IV or verapamil 5 mg IV
	Cardioversion if hemodynamically unstable
Ventricular dysrhythmias	Oxygen
	Sodium bicarbonate 1-2 mEq/kg
	Lidocaine 1.5 mg/kg IV bolus followed by 2 mg/min infusion
	Diazepam 5 mg IV or lorazepam 2-4 mg IV
	Defibrillation if hemodynamically unstable
Hypertension	Observation
	Diazepam 5-10 mg IV or lorazepam 2-4 mg IV titrated to effect
	Phentolamine 1 mg IV; repeat in 5 min
	Nitroglycerin or nitroprusside continuous infusion titrated to effect
Pulmonary edema	Lasix 20-40 mg IV
	Nitroglycerin infusion titrated to blood pressure
	Consider phentolamine or nitroprusside
Anxiety and agitation	Diazepam 5-10 mg IV or lorazepam 2-4 mg IV titrated to effect
Seizures	Diazepam 5-10 mg IV or lorazepam 2-4 mg IV titrated to effect
	Phenobarbital 25-50 mg/min up to 10-20 mg/kg
Intracranial hemorrhage	Neurosurgery consultation
	avoid β-blockers for blood pressure control
Hyperthermia	External cooling measures
	Paralysis to reduce heat generation
	Ventilation with high oxygen concentrations
Acute renal failure	Vigorous fluid replacement
	Alkalinization of the urine
	Consider mannitol

Adapted, with permission, from Hollander JE, Hoffman RS. Cocaine. In: Goldfrank LR, Flomenbaum NE, Lewin NA, et al, eds. *Goldfrank's Toxicologic Emergency*, 7th ed. McGraw Hill; 2002.

decreases over several hours and is replaced by a need for sleep and food. Hypersomnolence lasts between 8 hours and 4 days. Sleep is interrupted by brief awakenings during which the user experiences hyperphagia ("the munchies"). This phase is followed by a protracted dysphoric syndrome consisting of anhedonia, boredom, anxiety, panic attacks, generalized malaise, problems with memory and concentration, and occasional suicidal ideation. This induces severe craving that may lead to resumption of stimulant use and a vicious cycle of recurrent binges. Withdrawal syndromes for stimulants require only supportive care.

OTHER DRUGS OF ABUSE

■ BACKGROUND

Patients may be admitted to a hospital with an overdose, intoxication, or withdrawal syndrome from drugs of abuse, including marijuana, hallucinogens, "club drugs," and/or inhalants. Marijuana is the most frequently abused drug in the United States, with a prevalence of around 4% of the adult population. The most widely used hallucinogen is LSD, with a lifetime prevalence of use of 14% among young adults. Among club-going young adults, use of hallucinogens is up to 70%. Common "club drugs" are listed in **Table 250-15**.

■ EVALUATION

Indicators that would raise the suspicion of the use of these drugs are outlined in **Tables 250-16** and **250-17**.

■ INPATIENT MANAGEMENT

Treatment tips for the management of acute overdose of marijuana and hallucinogens are outlined in **Table 250-18**.

For PCP, hypertension should be treated vigorously with intravenous antihypertensives, since it may cause hypertensive encephalopathy or intracerebral bleeding. PCP can also cause life-threatening hyperthermia with temperatures over 106°F; rapid cooling measures (ice packs, cooling blanket, etc) may be required. Psychotic behavior can be treated with haloperidol. If the patient is severely agitated and poses a potential threat to self or others, haloperidol or lorazepam is effective for control of agitation; barbiturates may be even more useful in this setting with this drug, according to some reports.

GHB overdose may cause severe central nervous system and respiratory depression that abates over several hours. For acute GHB intoxication, supportive care includes oxygen supplementation, intravenous access, and comprehensive physiologic and cardiac monitoring. Providers should attempt to keep the patient stimulated and awake. Atropine may be used for persistent symptomatic bradycardia. Naloxone and flumazenil are ineffective, and activated charcoal is contraindicated due to the risk of aspiration and the short half-life of GHB. The most dangerous effects of GHB use often occur with the use of other drugs. Concurrent use of sedatives or alcohol may increase the risk of vomiting, aspiration, or cardiopulmonary depression; the use of GHB and stimulants may increase the risk of seizure.

■ WITHDRAWAL

Heavy marijuana use for more than 3 weeks results in a withdrawal syndrome after abrupt cessation and consists of irritability, agitation, depression, insomnia, nausea, anorexia, and tremor that can last for weeks. Marijuana withdrawal is uncomfortable but not life threatening; treatment is entirely supportive and rarely requires adjunctive medications.

Withdrawal from GHB is similar to withdrawal from sedatives such as benzodiazepines and alcohol; symptoms start within 6

TABLE 250-15 Common "Club Drugs"

Chemical Name	Brand Name(s)	NIDA Club Drug	Slang Names	Drug Type
Alprazolam	Xanax	No	Blue haze, X	Benzodiazepine Sedative
Dextromethorphan (DXM)	Coricidin, Robitussin	No	Dex, DXM, Robo, Triple C's	Opioid (OTC)
Diazepam	Valium	No	Downers, Mother's little helper, V's	Benzodiazepine Sedative
Flunitrazepam	Rohypnol	Yes	Mexican Valium, Roofies, rope	Benzodiazepine Sedative
Gamma-hydroxybutyrate (GHB)	Xyrem	Yes	Georgia Home Boy Grievous Bodily Harm, Liquid Ecstasy	Sedative
Hydrocodone	Hycodan, Lortab, Vicodin	No	Hykes, Vike	Opioid
Ketamine	Ketalar	Yes	Special K, kit cat, cat valium	Arylcyclohexylamine Hallucinogen
Lysergic acid diethylamide (LSD)		Yes	Acid, blotter, microdot	Prototypical Hallucinogen
Methamphetamine	Desoxyn	Yes	Crank, crystal meth, ice, speed	Stimulant
Methylenedioxy-methamphetamine (MDMA)		Yes	Ecstasy, X	Designer Drug Stimulant
Methylphenidate	Ritalin	No	Rits, smart pills, vitamin R	Stimulant
Oxycodone	OxyContin, Percocet, Tylox	No	Hillbilly heroin, OC, Oxy, Perc	Opioid
Pseudoephedrine	Sudafed	No	Suzie	Stimulant (OTC)

hours of the last use, then increase in intensity over several hours to days and may persist for 2 weeks. Physiologic signs include diaphoresis, tremor, tachycardia, and hypertension. Other symptoms are nausea with vomiting, anxiety, restlessness, insomnia, and "feelings of doom." Severe withdrawal involves agitation, delirium, and psychosis. GHB withdrawal may not respond to benzodiazepines despite very high doses. Antipsychotics or pentobarbital may have some utility in treatment of severe GHB withdrawal, although antipsychotics may lower the seizure threshold, especially when used without a sedative.

TABLE 250-16 Findings that Raise the Suspicion of Drug Use

Finding	Medical Indication	Drug(s)
Conjunctival injection	Current use	Marijuana
Tachycardia	Intoxication	
Pinpoint pupils	Intoxication, overdose	Opioids
Vertical nystagmus	Intoxication	Phencyclidine
Nasal septal perforation	Vasoconstriction	Any snorted drug
Sores, hyperpigmentation around mouth and/or nose	Chemical irritation	Inhalants
New murmur	Endocarditis from injection drug use	Any injected drug
Track marks, fresh needle marks	Injection drug use	
White blood cell count low	Human immunodeficiency virus	
Transaminases (alanine aminotransferase, aspartate aminotransferase) elevated	Viral hepatitis	
Urine drug screen positive	Recent drug use	Marijuana, phencyclidine, stimulant, opioid, benzodiazepine

TABLE 250-17 Signs and Symptoms of Hallucinogen Intoxication

Perceptual Distortions	Psychiatric Effects	Physiologic Effects
Light trails behind moving objects	Anxiety	Pupillary dilation
Micropsia (the sensation that the user is very large in relation to the surroundings)	Depression	Tachycardia
	Paranoia	Diaphoresis
	Impaired judgment	Tremulousness
Macropsia (the sensation that the user is very small in relation to the surroundings)	Ideas of reference (getting personal messages from the television or radio)	Lack of coordination
		Hyperreflexia
Synesthesias (cross-linking of the five senses [eg, "see the sounds, taste the colors"])		Seizures
		Hyperthermia
Sensation that the body is made of wood, plastic, or rubber	Depersonalization ("I am not real")	
Out-of-body experiences (sensation of floating over or outside one's physical body)	Derealization ("The environment is not real")	
Sense of profound understanding or universal connection		
Feeling of impending doom		

TABLE 250-18 Treatments for Acute Intoxication of Marijuana and Hallucinogens

- Settle the intoxicated patient in a quiet environment.
- Establish contact with a gentle touch (hold hand) during a period of relative lucidity.
- Maintain contact through periods of anxiety and perceptual distortion.
- Administer benzodiazepine (lorazepam, diazepam) for severe anxiety.
- Consider low-dose haloperidol for severe psychotic reactions (but may lower seizure threshold).

SUGGESTED READINGS

Bari K, Fontana RJ. Acetaminophen overdose: what practitioners need to know. *Clin Liver Dis*. 2014;4(1):17-21.

Boyer, EW. Management of opioid analgesic overdose. *N Engl J Med*. 202;367:146-155.

Decker BS, Goldfarb DS, Dargan PI, et al. Extracorporeal treatment for lithium poisoning: systematic review and recommendations from the EXTRIP workgroup. *Clin J Am Soc Nephrol*. 2015;10(5):875-887.

Glauser, J. Tricyclic antidepressant poisoning. *Cleve Clin J Med*. 2000;67(10):704-706, 709-713, and 717-719.

Grandjean EM, Aubry JM. Lithium: Updated human knowledge using an evidence-based approach Part III: clinical safety. *CNS Drugs*. 2009;23(5):397-418.

Gupta A, Lawrence AT, Krishnan K, et al. Current concepts in the mechanisms and management of drug-induced QT prolongation and torsade de points. *Am Heart J*. 2007;153:891-899.

Kosten TR, O'Connor PG. Management of drug and alcohol withdrawal. *N Engl J Med*. 2003;348(18):1786-1795.

Mokhlesi B, Leikin JB, Murray P, et al. Adult toxicology in critical care; Part II: specific poisonings. *Chest*. 2003;123:897-922.

Mowry JB, Spyker DA, Cantilena LR, et al. 2013 Annual report of the American association of poison control centers' National Poison Data System (NPDS): 31st Annual report. *Clin Toxicol*. 2014;52: 1032-1283.

Olson, KR. *Poisoning and Drug Overdose*, 6th ed. New York, NY: the McGraw-Hill Companies; 2012.

Reilly TH, Kirk MA. Atypical antipsychotics and newer antidepressants. *Emerg Med Clin North Am*. 2007;25(2):477-497.

Shannon MW, Borron SW, Burns M, eds. *Haddad and Winchester's Clinical Management of Poisoning and Drug Overdose*, 4th ed. Philadelphia, PA: Saunders; 2007.

Shenoy S, Lankala S, Adigopula S. Management of calcium channel blocker overdoses. *J Hosp Med*. 2014;9(10):663-668.

Strassman RJ. Adverse reactions to psychedelic drugs: a review of the literature. *J Nerv Ment Dis*. 1984;172:577-595.

CHAPTER 251

Addiction of Prescription and Nonprescription Drugs

Mary Eno, MD, MPH

Key Clinical Questions

❶ Why do not they just stop using?

❷ Why do they start using?

❸ Is my patient addicted?

❹ How can I help my addicted patient?

❺ Why did my patient leave against medical advice?

❻ What treatments are available?

❼ Does addiction treatment work?

INTRODUCTION

Patients with addiction can baffle and overwhelm even the most compassionate physicians, and these patients sometimes even deceive themselves into believing there is no problem. The symptoms of drug and alcohol use can mimic or co-occur with mental illness and chronic pain, complicating the diagnosis. Families can play a role in the development of addiction and also in its treatment. Fortunately, addiction is a treatable disease of the brain. Physicians have a unique opportunity to intervene in the addictive process and shepherd our patients—and our colleagues—into treatment when needed.

The brain is hardwired to reward behaviors that enhance survival of the individual or the species. The reward is pleasure, and it happens when dopamine levels rise in the limbic system. For example, eating when you are hungry, drinking water when you are thirsty, or having sex releases dopamine, which is subjectively experienced as pleasurable. People are motivated to seek pleasure and avoid pain in order to survive. Every behavior you perform is related to pain avoidance or short- or long-term pleasure reward.

Drugs of abuse—including alcohol, nicotine, illicit drugs, and some prescription medications—are potentially dangerous because they raise the dopamine in the limbic system faster, longer, and much higher than any natural reward (such as food, sex, or seeing your family). The brain, which is motivated to seek immediate reward, drives an individual's behavior to repeat the intense pleasure as much as possible. Dopamine also enhances learning and classical conditioning, so a person with an addiction unconsciously learns the pleasurable "survival value" of the drug. If the drug use continues, it essentially hijacks the brain's motivational dopamine system, tricking the brain into behaving as though the individual *needs the drug to survive.* At this point, the individual becomes dominated by seeking and repeating drug use. Changes take place in the brain that make it extremely uncomfortable to be without the drug. Natural dopamine production downregulates, and the brain becomes less responsive to dopamine presence. This is known as *tolerance,* meaning more of the drug is needed to produce a pleasurable sensation. It also means that previously pleasurable activities are no longer gratifying. The relative absence of dopamine leads to dysphoria in the absence of reinforcing drugs. Taking the drug is the fastest and easiest way for an addicted person in withdrawal to feel "normal" again. Eventually, continuing drug use overwhelms voluntary control and crowds out other relationships, becoming more important than an individual's family, values, even food and sex. At this point, drug and alcohol users isolate from other people to focus more obsessively on drug use. When addiction progresses to this level, people may use any means necessary—including manipulation, deceit, sometimes even violence—to obtain the drug of choice. Survival instincts can override judgment and moral values. This is why "drug seeking" patients can seem so difficult. The brain is motivated to survive, and following the brain changes of chronic drug use, *survival equals continued use.*

In late-stage addiction, a patient's body has usually become so used to the presence of the drug that the patient reports needing the drug to feel "normal." Without the drug, the patient will become increasingly uncomfortable and anxious until nothing in the environment can prevent the person from using. At that point, asking an addicted person to stop drinking or using is like asking you to stop breathing. If you were to voluntarily stop breathing, your hypoxic drive would make you increasingly anxious and uncomfortable until nothing in your environment could prevent you from taking a breath. And with the first breath you would begin to feel relief, begin to return to "normal." After derangement of multiple brain systems, stopping breathing is what it feels like for an addicted person to stop using. That is why the relapse rate is so high if the disease of addiction is not treated properly.

RECOGNIZING ADDICTION

Substance use occurs on a continuum from sporadic use to abuse to dependence and addiction. Rather than being defined by frequency of use, the hallmark of addiction is continued use despite consequences. Consequences may be social (damaged relationships), financial (money spent on drugs, or lost pay due to work absence), legal (driving under the influence or disorderly conduct), or medical (infections, overdoses, injuries while intoxicated, pancreatitis). In general, "if you've had problems because of drinking or using drugs, then you have a problem with alcohol or drugs." This means that some alcoholic and addicted individuals use episodically, or in a "binge" pattern—not necessarily every day. The natural history of addiction is progressive, with a variable rate: some patients progress rapidly from abuse to severe addiction; others smolder for years with less severe consequences. Few are able to stop permanently on their own. With each relapse to substance abuse, the addiction usually returns immediately to its worst point and progresses further. Depending on the substance(s) of choice, there can be a "shotgun effect" of end-organ damage involving every organ system. The American Psychiatric *Association's Diagnostic and Statistical Manual of Mental Disorders, 5th Edition (DSM-5) contains specific criteria for diagnosing mild, moderate, and severe substance use disorders.*

■ "I DON'T HAVE A PROBLEM"

Alcoholic and addicted patients are frequently in denial, meaning they honestly believe they do not have a problem; or they may desire very strongly to stop, but find they cannot stop because the biological motivation to use has become so strong. In addition, patients may not even remember some of the consequences of their use if they were intoxicated to amnesia ("blackouts")—particularly with alcohol. They can also misinterpret the causal relationships with their drinking, for example, believing, "I drink a lot because my wife nags me," when in fact the opposite is true (conflict arises because of the patient's drinking). Addicted patients in denial frequently cannot fully see the effects their use has on the lives around them.

■ SUBSTANCE USE AFFECTS DECISION MAKING

Cognitive changes occur with chronic drug use, particularly with loss of ability to make decisions and weigh future consequences against immediate gratification—this is why addicted patients sometimes baffle us by leaving the hospital against medical advice. Addicted people do not make decisions the way nonaddicted people do. When the neurochemistry of the limbic system is altered in long-term drug use, decisions about drug use are driven by craving rather than by reason. In addition, many addicted people begin using during adolescence, around age 12 to 14. Individuals who rely on drug use as their primary coping mechanism do not learn any further coping skills that foster maturity. This means that a 46-year-old patient who has been using continuously since adolescence may have the emotional maturity and coping skills of a 13-year-old.

■ DIFFERENTIAL DIAGNOSIS

Tolerance refers to homeostatic adaptations due to the repeated presence of a drug over an extended period. It is defined by emergence of physical symptoms (a *withdrawal syndrome*) when the

substance is stopped. The body adapts in this way to many prescription medications, such as antihypertensives, SSRIs, and opioid pain medications; this is why clonidine, beta-blockers, and some SSRIs need to be tapered slowly rather than stopped abruptly. Both tolerance and withdrawal are *expected* in patients with chronic pain on long-term opioid therapy, but neither defines addiction. That is why substance use disorders (SUDs) are diagnosed based on *behaviors and consequences*, not just physical tolerance and withdrawal.

Pseudoaddiction: Imagine for a moment that a person has chronic or acute pain from, say, a femoral fracture. Imagine that the pain was not adequately treated with the medication prescribed at discharge. What strategies could the person employ to get the pain treated? The person might take larger doses of the prescribed pain medication, refill it early, leave repeated messages for the prescribing physician, even resort to an emergency department visit for pain medication. She might borrow a few hydrocodone from a friend. Based on her behavior, she might correctly be labeled a "drug seeker." This is *pseudoaddiction*, when untreated pain motivates a desperate patient to seek relief in ways that resemble addictive behaviors. It can be difficult to unravel whether pain or addiction, or *both*, are causing the behaviors; thus, pseudoaddiction should always be in the differential diagnosis list.

Mental illness: Acute intoxication can mimic the symptoms of anxiety, depression, mania, paranoia, psychosis, and even schizophrenia. Drug rebound and withdrawal can also imitate psychiatric conditions. Only a careful history with strict attention to the timing of onset of psychiatric symptoms and drug use can begin to elucidate the diagnosis. There is a strong association between substance use disorders and major depression, dysthymia, hypomania, social phobia, panic, and generalized anxiety; close to half of substance users may have some degree of concurrent personality disorder. Sometimes people with mental illness resort to illicit drug use in order to avoid unpleasant psychiatric symptoms; mental illness and drug use can then produce new psychiatric symptoms that result in more drug use. Drugs can precipitate new psychotic breaks that persist after intoxication in previously unaffected individuals. The two can be intimately entwined and fuel each other. *Dual diagnosis* or *co-occurring disorder* refers to a coexisting psychiatric diagnosis as well as a substance use disorder.

Substance-induced mood disorder refers to new mood symptoms experienced after the onset of substance use. Some sober time may be required to disentangle drug effects from underlying mental illness. Symptoms or diagnosis of mental illness prior to introduction of drugs and alcohol can be a clue. Outcomes are generally poorer for dually diagnosed patients, and once concurrent mental illness is established, addiction and mental illness must be treated *concurrently*, rather than waiting for the SUD to "clear." Your patient may never achieve sobriety if the mental illness is not treated.

Chaotic social situation: A patient who is homeless or has an abusive or unstable social situation may present with behaviors mimicking addiction, such as missed appointments, multiple admissions (including admissions for pain control), early refills on medications, multiple phone calls, and the like. The person may meet criteria for *problem opioid use* or *problem prescription drug use* based on behaviors that are troubling to health care personnel rather than behaviors driven by addiction.

■ EPIDEMIOLOGY AND RISK FACTORS

Excluding nicotine addiction (which in itself causes 485,000 deaths in this country each year), substance use disorders have a 16% lifetime prevalence in the United States. Death rates are 50 to 100 times higher among substance users. Four out of every 10 families are affected by addiction. Given the 50% genetic contribution to the etiology of addiction, an affected family member is a powerful risk factor. The 50% environmental contribution has to do with cultural and family norms that value or stigmatize drugs and alcohol, exposure at an early age, and availability of mind-altering substances. We know that perception of drugs and alcohol as dangerous and socially unacceptable is protective against experimentation and development of addiction. Point prevalence is highest among males 15 to 19, but addiction cuts across gender, race, and socioeconomic status. In women, there is a strong association between sexual/physical violence, including childhood sexual abuse, and starting to drink. As a profession, physicians have among the highest rates of substance abuse and addiction.

Impulsivity and an orientation toward immediate gratification are risk factors for SUDs. Thus, adolescents are at high risk: they can be impulsive, rebellious, and novelty seeking with poorly developed judgment. Early exposure to substances in adolescence may lead to permanent brain changes; one-third of adolescent drinkers develop alcohol abuse or dependence in adulthood, and the younger the age at first use, the greater risk of subsequent SUD. Early diagnosis makes treatment more effective, so failing to screen for substance use is like not checking blood sugar in a new diabetic, or not checking for HIV disease with suspicious infections. It is important to ask adolescents about substance use and to check urine toxicologies to confirm the history.

TWELVE-STEP PARTICIPATION SUPPORTS SOBRIETY

Alcoholics Anonymous (AA) started in 1935 when two self-proclaimed "hopeless alcoholics"—one of them a physician—came together to help each other stop drinking. They published a guide, formally titled *Alcoholics Anonymous* but better known as the "Big Book" in 1939, whereby others could retrace their steps in supporting each other to sobriety. AA is free and available in nearly every locale, currently with more than 2 million members in 105,000 groups across 182 countries. The only requirement to attend meetings is a desire to stop drinking. The 12 Steps refer to a "higher power," which some members interpret as God; however, AA is spiritual—not religious—and members may interpret "higher power" as any wisdom stronger than their own. For example, a group of people can be a higher power. AA specifically refutes any connection to organized religion, and the "Big Book" discusses its compatibility with atheism and agnosticism in Appendix II, "Spiritual Experience." Many patients are able to stop drinking or using with only 12-Step participation in the absence of professional treatment. Statistically, AA with physician visits works as well as professional therapy (cognitive behavioral therapy and/or motivational enhancement therapy), but it is impossible to know which patients will respond best to which treatment; thus it is recommended that patients start with professional treatment to learn a new bedrock of coping skills, and then continue with lifelong 12-Step participation.

Unfortunately, patients are unlikely to follow-up with an AA telephone number provided by physicians; however, putting the patient directly in touch with an AA member while they are in the office can be tremendously effective. A *sponsor* is an individual with several years of successful recovery who can shepherd a new member, or *newcomer*, through the 12 Steps and be available to the newcomer 24 hours a day, 7 days a week should a crisis or craving emerge. The sponsor serves as a mentor and positive role model, accompanying the newcomer to meetings, and maintaining frequent contact between meetings. A newcomer can always ask the group to assign an appropriate sponsor. Physicians can demonstrate support for a patient's 12-Step "program" by inquiring what step she is working on, whether she has a sponsor, and how much "sober time" she has. It is important for the physician to listen to the patient's concerns (and complaints) about 12-Step participation, then encourage the patient to continue attending. Because every AA group is autonomous, each group develops its own personality and flavor; a patient who does not like one group should

try another. The 12-Step mutual-help model has been modified to help compulsive behaviors from drug use (Narcotics Anonymous, Pills Anonymous, Marijuana Anonymous, Cocaine Anonymous, and others) to compulsive sex to hoarding and cluttering. There are also groups for alcoholics with special interests such as musicians, professionals, gay and lesbian people, nonsmokers, and various ethnic groups. AA groups for physicians include Caduceus and International Doctors in AA (IDAA).

ADDICTION IS A FAMILY DISEASE

Codependence describes a loved one's misguided attempts to protect an addicted or alcoholic individual from the consequences of his or her consumption of drugs or alcohol. It is a natural instinct to shelter loved ones from negative consequences, but in the case of addiction, this can be very harmful by allowing the addiction to continue and progress to greater severity. Unwittingly acting as an accomplice to an addiction is known as *enabling*. Enabling ranges from making excuses and explaining away behaviors to bailing an addicted individual out of jail, to providing a place to use drugs or alcohol, to joining in the use of alcohol and drugs. Codependents tend to focus on helping the addicted person manage short-term crises rather than focusing on long-term recovery from drugs and alcohol. The addicted person and the family may derive some unconscious secondary benefit from the addictive behavior that makes it difficult to stop (eg, the codependent individuals may be distracted from addressing their own problems by helping the addicted person instead). Codependents may even ally with the addicted person against physicians or others encouraging treatment and recovery. The stress of codependence, and involvement with an addicted person can be the root of somatic complaints. Thus, drug and alcohol abuse should be part of the family history obtained of every patient.

Just as codependents can have a large role in enabling a person's addiction, they also can have an important role in recognizing the disease and ushering the patient into treatment. Some addicts will not stop using until they feel harm and perceive that they must stop to survive; thus, the best way to expedite treatment is for codependents to stop sheltering their loved one from the consequences of their use of alcohol or drugs. The consequences can then move an alcoholic or addicted person toward accepting treatment. When families are involved in treatment with the addicted individual, outcomes improve significantly. Sometimes, codependents need therapy or treatment to gain perspective before they are able to support their addicted family member toward treatment. Family members learn they only control their own behavior, and quitting their codependent roles can ease their anxiety and may be helpful in influencing the addicted family member to seek treatment. "Love with detachment" is a goal for family members. Professional group therapy, with a focus on codependency, is often available to family members at treatment centers. Al-Anon is a mutual support group for people whose lives have been affected by another person's addiction. It is based on the 12 Steps, although its central philosophy is that members should start to focus on themselves rather than continuing to focus on their loved one's addiction. Ala-Teen, Families Anonymous, and Tough Love are other mutual support groups for families.

PROCESS ADDICTIONS

Rather than abusing chemical substances, some people continue certain behaviors—such as overeating, gambling, or high-risk sex—despite disastrous consequences. Many behaviors are classified among the spectrum of impulse control disorders, such as trichotillomania (obsessive hair-pulling), kleptomania (decreased ability to overcome impulses to steal unwanted items), intermittent explosive disorder (failure to inhibit aggressive impulses that are disproportionate to the precipitating stressor), and obsessive-compulsive disorders. However, the compulsive nature of these behaviors is not mutually exclusive with addiction. These behaviors raise dopamine in the limbic system, although much less than substances of abuse, and are repeated in order to decrease anxiety. Some research indicates a shared genetic vulnerability between substance abuse and impulse control disorders. Because process addictions share common threads with substance use disorders, it follows that some of the same treatments might be useful. 12-Step groups have been modified to address hundreds of different behaviors, from binge eating (Overeaters Anonymous) to compulsive shopping (Overspenders Anonymous), pornography overuse, Internet overuse, pathological gambling (Gamblers Anonymous), hoarding, pathological cluttering, and many others.

ADDICTION TREATMENT WORKS

The brain changes of addiction set the stage for a chronic, recurring illness requiring long-term ongoing treatment. Just as providers care for chronic diseases like diabetes, hypertension, and asthma, they can help manage and coordinate care for the chronic disease of addiction. The first step is recognizing and diagnosing, then referring for treatment, and following up each time you see the patient. Detoxifying an addicted person in the hospital has no more effect on the disease of addiction than treating diabetic ketoacidosis (DKA) affects the course of diabetes. Both require long-term, ongoing management and treatment. Significant research demonstrates that, with proper treatment, addiction has recovery and outcomes nearly identical to the other chronic diseases.

Detoxification means poison exiting the body—in this case, alcohol or drugs of abuse clearing from the brain and blood. When a person is physically dependent on substances, detoxification can result in symptoms known as withdrawal. Some withdrawal syndromes are exquisitely uncomfortable; others are life threatening. Withdrawal can be medically supervised, which means symptoms are managed to keep patients as safe and comfortable as possible during withdrawal. This is only the first step in what will become lifelong treatment. Just as successfully managing a diabetic patient through DKA does not change the course of the disease, a detoxification episode will not alter the natural history of addiction unless the patient is treated. Just as the person with diabetes will need ongoing hypoglycemics, statins, and blood sugar monitoring, the person with addiction will need ongoing counseling, group participation (to defeat the isolation of addiction), and urine toxicology monitoring. Long-term management of stressors and re-emergent cravings, even after sustained abstinence, is crucial to relapse prevention. If the treatment for diabetes or hypertension is stopped, the symptoms again manifest in full force. The same is true for addiction and alcoholism.

Treatment means interventions delivered by licensed professionals; *mutual help* refers to community support groups such as AA, Rational Recovery, and Secular Organizations for Sobriety. Most recovery models employ both treatment *and* mutual help, engaging patients and their families in education and therapy whenever possible. Because multiple brain systems are disrupted with long-term substance abuse (and multiple areas of a patient's life are damaged by addiction), multiple modalities are required to strengthen impulse control, overcome learned responses, support decision making, teach new coping skills, and focus on rewards that compete with substance use. It is clear that skilled, empathic therapy styles achieve better outcomes than confrontational approaches. Many treatment programs also incorporate the use of medications to help maintain sobriety—such medications have a small but measurable benefit and should be routinely offered to patients (information on such medications is in subsequent chapters). Thus the best treatment programs have specialized physician involvement; without

physician involvement, programs may not be able to offer medications or diagnose or treat comorbid psychiatric or medical disorders.

Abstinence-based means that a treatment program expects abstinence from *all* mind-altering substances, not just the patient's drug of choice; for example, a patient in treatment for alcohol dependence is expected not to use heroin or cocaine; a person in treatment for methamphetamine dependence is expected not to use cannabis or recreational vicodin. A patient is considered to be abstinent and sober when taking medications as prescribed by a physician—including methadone or buprenorphine (suboxone) for relapse prevention; all major 12-Step groups are in agreement. *Sobriety* (abstaining from mind-altering chemicals) is the bedrock to recovery, but recovery from addiction is more than just abstinence. It is learning new honesty and coping skills, and many times involves a spiritual transformation that can result in a new citizenship in society. Recovery is not something that is ever complete; it is evolving, never-ending growth.

No significant outcome advantage has been proven for residential over outpatient treatment. The treatment venue is less important than the duration of engagement in treatment. Some patients, due to the severity of their disease or the chaos of their social situation, may benefit from more highly structured treatment (residential or partial hospitalization vs outpatient). In general, more intense treatment is offered during the newly sober period, tapering off to less frequently as the patient gains stability and experience. Research shows that a minimum of 3 months of treatment is required for sustained benefit, with continued progress after 3 months. It is important for the patient to maintain some continuous connection to mutual help and/or treatment for life—otherwise relapse can occur even after years of abstinence.

When do substance users seek treatment? Some addiction experts believe that spiraling consequences and distress related to substance use, compounded by pressure from family, friends, and others can catalyze change following a specific "trigger event," when an individual realizes that she cannot manage her addiction without help. In many cases, an intervention staged by family and friends can be helpful in moving a patient toward treatment. It is important to take advantage of such opportunities, when a substance user is ready to accept help; patients can be lost if treatment is not easily available to them.

■ MONITORING

Patients with chronic disease underreport damaging health behaviors that may reflect poorly on them. For example, patients with diabetes may underreport dietary indiscretion, and patients with congestive heart failure may underreport their salt intake; thus, it is important to check hemoglobin A1Cs and daily weights to be certain that the medical treatments are working, and to provide an objective measure of compliance with those treatments. Substance use disorders are no exception, and monitoring, usually with urine toxicology screening or breath-alcohol testing, is an important part of addiction treatment. Urine tests for Ethylene Glycol (ETG), an ethanol metabolite, detect alcohol intake during the previous 80 hours. Because relapse is a part of chronic disease, positive toxicology results (meaning the sample was positive for the presence of illicit substances), in concert with the patient's history, should be addressed with empathy and support, not with confrontational accusation.

BRIEF INTERVENTION IMPROVES OUTCOMES

Hospitalists have a unique opportunity to help motivate someone toward treatment. The admission provides a "teachable moment," and, as already mentioned, intervention outcomes are better for physicians who use an empathic approach rather than a confrontational one—this means being accepting, not *approving of* drug use. Overt persuasion results in patients' working hard to resist the persuasion; they do not want to acknowledge painful realities to themselves or others. *Motivational interviewing* (MI) is an evidence-based process that encourages patients to voice their own reasons for stopping or cutting back. Most substance users have some degree of ambivalence (strong feelings both ways) about continuing their use, and MI is a way to identify and amplify the desire to stop using. In its simplest form, motivational interviewing queries the patients on the benefits of continuing substance use, the disadvantages of stopping, the disadvantages of continuing, and the advantages of sobriety. Asking nonjudgmentally about all four, without criticizing or blaming, helps patients to articulate their own reasons for quitting and does not create resistance.

Another model for brief intervention is the four A's: ask, advise, assist, arrange. For any substance, including nicotine, the physician *asks* about length of use and consequences (family, job, financial, legal, health, injuries, blackouts, withdrawal, diminished self-care, etc) and then gives brief, specific, personalized *advice* about the health effects of the patient's use: "As your physician, I must advise you that smoking cigarettes is bad for your liver. Because of your elevated liver function tests, it is important that you stop smoking now. If you stop smoking cigarettes, the damage may not progress further." The physician can *assist* the patient with a referral to an addiction medicine specialist, 12-Step groups (such as Nicotine Anonymous), or a treatment center specializing in addictions; sometimes this might include prescriptions for nicotine replacement or other medications. Remember that just giving a phone number to a patient results in poor follow-up; but putting the person in touch with a 12-Step member or treatment center while in the hospital or office can have excellent results. Finally, *arrange* for patients to follow-up with primary care to review any action they have taken. Some patients will not be ready to stop using immediately; physicians must remain patient, empathic, and supportive at every admission when inquiring about substance use.

CONCLUSION: ADDICTION IS A TREATABLE BRAIN DISEASE

Addiction is a multifactorial chronic brain disease with social and behavioral dimensions. The brain's limbic system is the seat of the disease, but addiction can result in end-organ damage to every system. The natural history of addiction is generally chronic relapsing-remitting with progression over time. New discoveries in brain imaging, genetics, and neurobiology shed light on the multiple brain systems affected in addiction. While psychobehavioral treatment remains the cornerstone of treatment, medications to modulate brain functions involved with cravings are emerging to buttress patients' recovery. With proper treatment, patients with the disease of addiction have outcomes equivalent to those with other chronic diseases such as asthma, diabetes, and hypertension. The hospitalist physician can have a pivotal role in recognizing disease and directing these patients toward treatment and recovery.

SUGGESTED READINGS

Alcoholics Anonymous. www.aa.org.

Dupont R. *The Selfish Brain: Learning from Addiction.* Center City, MN: Hazelden Publishing; 2000.

National Institute on Drug Abuse Information for Healthcare Professionals. www.drugabuse.gov/NIDAmed/.

Ries RK, Fiellin DA, Miller SC, Saitz R. *The ASAM Principles of Addiction Medicine*, 5th ed. Philadelphia, PA: Wolters Kluwer Health/Lippincott Williams & Wilkins; 2014.

Substance Abuse and Mental Health Services Administration (SAMHSA). Searchable database of treatment facilities. www.samhsa.gov.

Vascular Medicine

SECTION 15

Vascular Medicine

CHAPTER 252

Venous Thromboembolism Prophylaxis for Hospitalized Medical Patients

Menaka Pai, MSc, MD, FRCPC

James D. Douketis, MD, FRCPC, FACP, FCCP

WHAT IS THE RISK FOR VENOUS THROMBOEMBOLISM (VTE) IN HOSPITALIZED MEDICAL PATIENTS?

◼ EPIDEMIOLOGY

Venous Thromboembolism (VTE), which comprises deep vein thrombosis (DVT) and pulmonary embolism (PE), is a common cause of morbidity and mortality in hospitalized medical patients. The baseline incidence of asymptomatic VTE in hospitalized medical patients without anticoagulant prophylaxis is 7% to 15%. Linked administrative database studies indicate that 1.7% of hospitalized medical patients develop symptomatic VTE within 3 months of hospitalization. This is lower than in surgical patients, who have a risk of 2% to 3%. However, because of the sheer number of hospitalized medical patients when compared to surgical patients, the burden of illness is high. Approximately 50% to 70% of symptomatic VTE and 70% to 80% of fatal PE occur in medical patients, and recent hospitalization for medical illness accounts for 25% of all VTE diagnosed in the community. The quoted risk of 1.7% is also based on the risk in *all* medical patients, some of whom have less severe illness. In prospective studies assessing medical patients who have at least one major risk factor for VTE such as severe cardiac or respiratory disease and do not receive VTE prophylaxis, the incidence of DVT as detected by venography is approximately 10% to 15%. In the absence of anticoagulant prophylaxis, the incidence of proximal DVT, which is the type of DVT most likely to embolize, is approximately 5% and the incidence of PE is 0.5%. VTE is associated with potentially serious long-term complications, including post-thrombotic syndrome, cardiorespiratory insufficiency, recurrent VTE, and bleeding associated with anticoagulant therapy. VTE is also a common cause of readmission to the hospital, and is associated with increased hospital costs and length of stay.

PRACTICE POINT

Risk of thrombosis

- Approximately 50% to 70% of symptomatic VTE and 70% to 80% of fatal PE occur in medical patients.
- Recent hospitalization for medical illness accounts for 25% of all VTE diagnosed in the community.
- In prospective studies assessing medical patients who have at least one major risk factor for VTE such as severe cardiac or respiratory disease and do not receive VTE prophylaxis, the incidence of DVT as detected by venography is approximately 10% to 15%.

◼ PATHOPHYSIOLOGY

Hospitalization for an acute medical illness is independently associated with about an eightfold increased risk for VTE. Chart audits have shown that nearly all hospitalized medical patients have at least one VTE risk factor, be it immobility, increased age, cancer (active or occult), or acute medical illness (eg, congestive heart failure, obstructive lung disease). Certain populations of hospitalized medical patients, such as those in the intensive care unit, have additional risk factors including central venous catheterization; these patients are considered to be at high risk for VTE, even after receiving routine prophylaxis (**Table 252-1**).

TABLE 252-1 Factors that Increase Risk for Venous Thromboembolism in Hospitalized Medical Patients

Increasing age

Immobility (confined to bed, needing assistance to ambulate)

Pregnancy and the puerperium

Acute medical illness (eg, congestive heart failure, obstructive lung disease)

Acute ischemic stroke

Acute neurologic disease

Inflammatory bowel disease

Cancer (active or occult)

Sepsis

Previous VTE

Prior pelvic radiation

Inherited or acquired thrombophilia

Myeloproliferative disorders

Obesity

Medications (eg, chemotherapy, hormonal therapy, selective estrogen receptor modulators, erythropoeisis-stimulating agents)

Central venous catheterization (eg, PICC line, internal jugular line)

WHICH HOSPITALIZED MEDICAL PATIENTS NEED VTE PROPHYLAXIS?

■ VTE PROPHYLAXIS IN GENERAL MEDICAL PATIENTS

There is no formal, widely accepted, prospectively validated risk stratification algorithm to guide VTE prophylaxis in medical patients. As a general guide, medical patients presenting with ischemic stroke, acute exacerbations of chronic heart failure or chronic obstructive pulmonary disease, acute respiratory failure, cancer, history of prior VTE, sepsis, acute neurologic disease, or severe inflammatory disease should be given VTE prophylaxis. Immobility is considered a weaker risk factor, and is difficult to clearly define. However, patients who cannot ambulate without assistance still merit consideration for prophylaxis. A number of data-derived risk models to predict VTE in medical patients have been proposed, including the Padua prediction score, the IMPROVE risk score, and the Geneva risk score. They include many of the above criteria.

A recent meta-analysis has shown that pharmacologic prophylaxis is effective in reducing fatal PE, symptomatic PE, and symptomatic DVT by more than 50% with no increase in major bleeding compared with placebo in general medical patients. There is no effect on all-cause mortality, and the number needed to treat to prevent one symptomatic PE is high (more than 300). However, due to the large number of at-risk hospitalized medical patients, thromboprophylaxis still provides an opportunity to reduce morbidity in a significant number of patients. There does not appear to be a difference in bleeding rates or VTE rates between low-dose unfractionated heparin (LDUH), low-molecular-weight heparin (LMWH), and fondaparinux. Meta-analyses have suggested that LMWH is superior to LDUH (both twice- and thrice-daily regimens) in high-risk populations, though included studies included studies enrolled heterogeneous groups, and did not always differentiate symptomatic and asymptomatic VTE.

TABLE 252-2 Contraindications to Thromboprophylaxis with Anticoagulants

Excessive active bleeding

At high risk for bleeding that precludes anticoagulants (eg, brain lesion)

Recent serious bleeding (eg, within 1 mo)

Coagulopathy (eg, INR >1.5, aPTT >40)

Thrombocytopenia (eg, platelets <75 ×10⁹/L)

PRACTICE POINT

Risk of bleeding associated with anticoagulant prophylaxis

- The risk for fatal bleeding is 0.02% to 0.5%, or 32% higher than in patients who do not receive prophylaxis. Prospective trials have shown that this difference is not statistically significant, but this finding may be because the studies were underpowered to show a difference in bleeding risk.
- There does not appear to be a difference in bleeding rates or VTE rates among LDUH, LMWH, and fondaparinux.

In patients with an increased risk for bleeding (**Table 252-2**), physicians commonly choose mechanical methods of thromboprophylaxis to increase venous flow and reduce stasis: graduated compression stockings (GCS), intermittent pneumatic compression devices (IPC), and the venous foot pump.

There are no randomized clinical trials evaluating mechanical thromboprophylaxis in general medical patients. In a placebo-controlled trial assessing GCS for DVT prophylaxis in patients with acute ischemic stroke, GCS did not provide additional therapeutic benefit for DVT prevention (10.0% vs 10.5%) but conferred a fourfold increased risk for skin breaks, ulceration, and blisters. Mechanical thromboprophylaxis should be considered inferior to pharmacologic prophylaxis in preventing VTE, and should only be used as an adjunct to pharmacologic prophylaxis, or as an option in patients with an unacceptably high-bleeding risk in whom anticoagulation is contraindicated (eg, gastrointestinal or intracranial hemorrhage). All patients with an increased risk for bleeding should be followed closely. If the bleeding risk decreases to an acceptable level, pharmacologic prophylaxis should be started as soon as possible.

PRACTICE POINT

Mechanical thromboprophylaxis

- Mechanical thromboprophylaxis is inferior to pharmacologic prophylaxis in preventing VTE.
- There are no randomized clinical trials evaluating mechanical thromboprophylaxis in general medical patients.
- It should only be used as an adjunct to pharmacologic prophylaxis, or as an option in patients with an unacceptably high-bleeding risk.
- All patients with an increased risk for bleeding should be followed closely. If the bleeding risk decreases to an acceptable level, pharmacologic prophylaxis should be started as soon as possible.

■ VTE PROPHYLAXIS IN CANCER PATIENTS

Cancer confers a sixfold increased risk of VTE, and active cancer accounts for 20% of all new VTE events in the community. Conventional chemotherapies, erythropoietin-stimulating agents, angiogenesis inhibitors, and hormonal therapies (including selective estrogen receptor modulators and aromatase inhibitors) also increase the risk of VTE. Once patients with cancer develop VTE, it can be difficult to treat them due to intercurrent illnesses, the need for invasive procedures, thrombocytopenia, and high VTE recurrence rates. Therefore, it is essential to carefully risk stratify patients and consider thromboprophylaxis when patients with cancer are admitted to hospital. Cancer patients with an acute medical illness, either cancer-related or otherwise, or who are bedridden should receive thromboprophylaxis in accordance with the recommendations for general medical patients. VTE prophylaxis is not routinely recommended in cancer patients who are ambulatory, however it is indicated for many patients with multiple myeloma treated with thalidomide- or lenalidomide-containing regimens, and in individuals with a high score on the well-validated Khorana score. (This latter group includes individuals with stomach or pancreatic cancer, high prechemotherapy platelet or WBC counts, a high BMI, and individuals on erythropoeisis-stimulating agents.)

PRACTICE POINT

- Cancer confers a sixfold increased risk of VTE, and active cancer accounts for 20% of all new VTE events in the community. Once patients with cancer develop VTE, it can be difficult to treat, due to intercurrent illnesses, the need for invasive procedures, thrombocytopenia, and high VTE recurrence rates. Hospitalized patients with cancer should be considered at high risk of VTE.

■ VTE PROPHYLAXIS IN CRITICALLY ILL PATIENTS?

Patients in the intensive care unit are particularly heterogeneous, both in terms of thrombosis risk and in terms of bleeding risk. The rates of asymptomatic DVT (detected by ultrasound or venography) reflect this heterogeneity, ranging from less than 10% to nearly 100%. There are only two randomized placebo-controlled trials of thromboprophylaxis in patients in the intensive care setting, one comparing LDUH to placebo, and the other comparing LMWH to placebo. Both significantly reduced the rate of DVT detected on routine screening, yielding a relative risk reduction of approximately 50%. More recently, the PROTECT trial randomized 3764 critically ill patients to LDUH or the LMWH dalteparin. Dalteparin was associated with a reduction in PE (1% vs 2%; hazard ratio 0.5) but had no effect on DVT, bleeding, mortality, or cost.

All patients admitted to the intensive care unit should have a routine assessment of risk for thrombosis and bleeding. Patients who have an acceptable bleeding risk should receive LMWH, while those considered at high risk for bleeding should receive GCS and/or IPC. This latter group should be reassessed daily, and if the bleeding risk decreases to an acceptable level, pharmacologic prophylaxis should commence as soon as possible.

■ THE RISKS ASSOCIATED WITH VENOUS THROMBOEMBOLISM PROPHYLAXIS

The major risk of pharmacologic VTE prophylaxis is bleeding. In medical patients, bleeding may occur at the anticoagulant injection site (eg, rectus sheath hematoma) or at a remote site (eg, from an occult peptic ulcer that is predisposed to bleeding). The risk for fatal bleeding associated with anticoagulant prophylaxis is 0.02% to 0.5%, or 32% higher than in patients who do not receive prophylaxis. Prospective trials have shown that this difference is not statistically significant, but this finding may be because the studies were underpowered to show a difference in bleeding risk. Bleeding complications can be minimized by carefully assessing and mitigating patients' individual bleeding risks *before* starting anticoagulants

(Table 252-2). Patients should also be assessed regularly for signs and symptoms of bleeding while they are on anticoagulants.

The other important risk associated with pharmacologic VTE prophylaxis is heparin-induced thrombocytopenia (HIT). This rare but serious complication of heparin-derived anticoagulants is caused by antibody formation to the heparin-derived anticoagulant and an antigen on the patient's platelets. It is strongly associated with venous and to a lesser extent, arterial thrombosis, and can have devastating consequences. HIT is more common with LDUH compared to LMWH, and more common in surgical versus medical patients. In medical patients who received anticoagulant prophylaxis with LDUH, the risk for HIT is 1.4%. Data are lacking as to the risk for HIT in medical patients who are receiving LMWH but it is probably one-tenth the risk observed with LDUH. Irrespective of the anticoagulant administered, platelet counts should be monitored serially for all patients on anticoagulants and physicians should be watchful for signs and symptoms of arterial or venous thromboembolism that can herald the development of HIT.

PRACTICE POINT

Heparin-induced thrombocytopenia (HIT)

- HIT is more common with LDUH compared to LMWH, and more common in surgical versus medical patients.
- In medical patients who received anticoagulant prophylaxis with LDUH, the risk for HIT was 1.4%.
- Data are lacking as to the risk for HIT in medical patients who are receiving LMWH but it is probably one-tenth the risk observed with LDUH.

Overall, the risks of major bleeding and HIT are small in hospitalized medical patients, and are far outweighed by the benefits of pharmacologic VTE prophylaxis.

PRACTICAL MANAGEMENT OF VTE PROPHYLAXIS

■ PHARMACOLOGIC PROPHYLAXIS IN THE SETTING OF RENAL INSUFFICIENCY

Renal impairment is a significant challenge in the administration of venous thromboprophylaxis. Drugs like LMWH and fondaparinux are primarily cleared by the kidney, and in the setting of reduced renal function, these drugs can accumulate and increase bleeding risk. Ongoing studies are evaluating the bioaccumulation of these anticoagulants and the clinical consequences. At this time, only prophylactic dose dalteparin has been shown not to bioaccumulate when the creatinine clearance is less than 30 mL/min. Before prescribing any renally cleared anticoagulant, physicians should measure a patient's serum creatinine and formally calculate the creatinine clearance (which depends on age, weight, and sex). If renal function is found to be impaired, an anticoagulant that does not bioaccumulate should be chosen. If this is not possible, the dose should be lowered and/or the anti-Xa level should be monitored. In all cases, the manufacturer's suggested dosage guidelines in the presence of renal impairment should be followed.

PRACTICE POINT

Renal insufficiency

- Before prescribing any anticoagulant cleared by the kidneys, physicians should measure a patient's serum creatinine and formally calculate the creatinine clearance (which depends on age, weight, and sex).
- Manufacturer's suggested dosage guidelines in the presence of renal impairment should be followed.

■ CONSIDERATIONS UPON DISCHARGE FROM HOSPITAL

There is no evidence that hospitalized medical patients benefit from routine DVT screening using venous ultrasound or venography. Therefore, routine DVT screening at the time of hospital discharge cannot be recommended. The risk-to-benefit ratio of extended out-of-hospital prophylaxis is also unclear. Medical patients with chronic illness or who are to be transferred to a long-term care facility may have an ongoing increased thrombosis risk, making extended-duration prophylaxis an appealing option. Three randomized trials have examined this issue: EXCLAIM (which compared 5 weeks vs 10 days of VTE prophylaxis with enoxaparin, 40 mg once daily), ADOPT (which compared 6-14 days of 40 mg enoxaparin daily vs 30 days of 2.5 mg apixaban twice daily), and MAGELLAN (which compared 10 days of VTE prophylaxis with 40 mg enoxaparin daily followed by a placebo vs extended prophylaxis for 35 ± 4 days with 10 mg rivaroxaban daily). EXCLAIM did show increased efficacy of extended-duration prophylaxis. However, benefits were restricted to only some groups (eg, those >75 years of age, those with recently reduced mobility). Further, the extended-duration arm in EXCLAIM had an increased risk of major bleeding. ADOPT found no difference between its study arms, though extended-duration prophylaxis increased the risk of major bleeding. MAGELLAN found that extended-duration prophylaxis reduced the risk of VTE (both symptomatic and asymptomatic), though it again conferred an increased risk of major bleeding. A meta-analysis of these three studies concluded that routine administration of postdischarge VTE prophylaxis is not likely to make a clinically meaningful impact for hospitalized medical patients, and could cause harm. At this time, extended-duration prophylaxis is not recommended in medical patients. However, all patients should be educated about the signs and symptoms of VTE at the time of discharge and be instructed to seek urgent medical care if thrombosis is suspected.

■ QUALITY IMPROVEMENT INITIATIVES TO OPTIMIZE VTE PROPHYLAXIS

A significant gap remains between evidence for VTE prophylaxis and clinical practice in hospitalized medical patients. A recent international registry demonstrated that in a population of 15,156 hospitalize medical patients only 50% received any form of prophylaxis. A multicenter Canadian chart audit determined that 90% of acutely ill medical patients were eligible for some form of prophylaxis, while only 23% received it. What is rather astonishing is that only 16% of patients received appropriate prophylaxis.

Medical patients have repeatedly been shown to have the poorest rates of VTE prophylaxis among all hospitalized patients. Yet since 1998, the American College of Chest Physicians has given anticoagulant prophylaxis in at-risk hospitalized medical patients a Grade 1A recommendation (their highest level). The American College of Physicians also strongly advocates for risk assessment and anticoagulant prophylaxis in this group. Why is VTE prophylaxis underused in hospitalized medical patients? It is likely because medical patients are more heterogeneous than their counterparts on surgical wards. Their need for prophylaxis is not driven by a standardized type of surgery, but by their underlying diseases, their mobility status, and their reason for hospitalization. Health care providers may be unclear about the indications and contraindications for anticoagulant prophylaxis in a given patient.

Many organizations have also identified VTE as a major patient safety concern, including the US Department of Health and Human Services, the World Health Organization, the World Alliance for Patient Safety, and the International Alliance of Patients' Organizations. VTE prophylaxis has also been highlighted as an important feature of hospital accreditation commissions and quality improvement campaigns worldwide. Evidence supports a multicomponent strategy to optimize VTE prophylaxis in hospitalized medical patients, including formal hospital policy, standardized preprinted order sets, computer decision support systems, electronic and human alerts, and periodic audit and feedback. Hospitalists are in an ideal position to champion appropriate VTE prophylaxis in hospitalized medical patients, at a local, national, and international level.

SUGGESTED READINGS

Alikhan R, Cohen AT. A safety analysis of thromboprophylaxis in acute medical illness. *Thromb Haemost.* 2003;89:590-591.

CLOTS Trials Collaboration, Dennis M, Sandercock PA, Reid J, et al. Effectiveness of thigh-length graduated compression stockings to reduce the risk of deep vein thrombosis after stroke (CLOTS trial 1): a multicentre, randomised controlled trial. *Lancet.* 2009;373:1958-1965.

Cohen AT, Tapson VF, Bergmann JF, et al. Venous thromboembolism risk and prophylaxis in the acute hospital care setting (ENDORSE study): a multinational cross-sectional study. *Lancet.* 2008;371:387-394.

Cohen AT, Spiro TE, Büller HR, et al. Rivaroxaban for thromboprophylaxis in acutely ill medical patients. *N Engl J Med.* 2013;368(6):513-523.

Cook D, Crowther M, Meade M, et al. Deep venous thrombosis in medical-surgical critically ill patients: prevalence, incidence, and risk factors. *Crit Care Med.* 2005;33:1565-1571.

Douketis J, Cook D, Meade M, et al. Prophylaxis against deep vein thrombosis in critically ill patients with severe renal insufficiency with the low-molecular-weight heparin dalteparin: an assessment of safety and pharmacodynamics: the DIRECT Study. *Arch Intern Med.* 2008;168:1805-1812.

Goldhaber SZ, Leizorovicz A, Kakkar AK, et al. Apixaban versus enoxaparin for thromboprophylaxis in medically ill patients. *N Engl J Med.* 2011;365(23):2167.

Kahn SR, Lim W, Dunn AS, et al. *Prevention of VTE in nonsurgical patients: antithrombotic therapy and prevention of thrombosis,* 9th ed: American College of Chest Physicians Evidence-Based Clinical Practice Guidelines. *Chest.* 2012;141(2 Suppl):e195S-e226S.

Kakkar AK, Levine MN, Kadziola Z, et al. Low molecular weight heparin, therapy with dalteparin, and survival in advanced cancer: the Fragmin Advanced Malignancy Outcome Study (FAMOUS). *J Clin Oncol.* 2004;22:1944-1948.

Khorana AA, Kuderer NM, Culakova E, Lyman GH, Francis CW. Development and validation of a predictive model for chemotherapy-associated thrombosis. *Blood.* 2008;111(10):4902.

MacDougall DA, Feliu AU, Boccuzzi SJ, Lin J. Economic burden of deep-vein thrombosis, pulmonary embolism, and post-thrombotic syndrome. *Am J Health Syst Pharm.* 2006;63(20 Suppl 6):S5-S15.

PROTECT Investigators for the Canadian Critical Care Trials Group and the Australian and New Zealand Intensive Care Society Clinical Trials Group, Cook D, Meade M, et al. Dalteparin versus unfractionated heparin in critically ill patients. *N Engl J Med.* 2011;364(14):1305.

Samama MM, Cohen AT, Darmon JY, et al. A comparison of enoxaparin with placebo for the prevention of venous thromboembolism in acutely ill medical patients. *N Engl J Med.* 1999;341:793-800.

Turpie AG. Extended duration of thromboprophylaxis in acutely ill medical patients: optimizing therapy? *J Thromb Haemost.* 2007;5:5-11.

CHAPTER 253

Diagnosis and Treatment of Venous Thromboembolism

Kerstin Hogg, MD, MBChB, MSc

Lori-Ann Linkins, MD, MSc

Clive Kearon, MB, MRCPI, FRCPC, PhD

Key Clinical Questions

❶ Why are objective tests needed to diagnose venous thromboembolism (VTE)?

❷ Which tests can be used to diagnose a first deep vein thrombosis (DVT)?

❸ Which tests can be used to diagnose recurrent DVT?

❹ Which tests can be used to diagnose pulmonary embolism (PE)?

❺ Which patients with VTE can be treated as outpatients?

❻ What is the treatment for acute VTE, DVT, and/or PE?

❼ What is the role of thrombolytic therapy in the treatment of PE?

❽ How are patients with acute VTE and bleeding managed?

❾ How is the duration of treatment of VTE determined?

❿ Should I perform a thrombophilic workup?

⓫ What is the risk of bleeding associated with long-term anticoagulant therapy?

INTRODUCTION

In 800 BC, Susruta, an Indian healer wrote about a patient with "a swollen and painful leg, which was difficult to treat." Centuries later, Virchow, a Prussian physician, coined the term "embolism" after discovering the relationship between a blood clot that formed within a blood vessel (thrombus), and a blood clot that breaks loose and travels through the bloodstream to occlude the pulmonary vessels (embolus). The concept of venous thromboembolism was born from these early descriptions and today it remains one of the most important health problems in Europe and North America and is the third leading cause of vascular death after myocardial infarction and stroke.

The risk of venous thromboembolism (VTE) increases by approximately twofold per decade of age, rising from an annual incidence of 30/100,000 at 40 years of age, to 90/100,000 at 60 years, and 260/100,000 at 80 years. Approximately half of patients with untreated, symptomatic proximal deep vein thrombosis (DVT) will develop symptomatic pulmonary embolism (PE), and about 10% of symptomatic PE are fatal within an hour of onset. Left untreated, one-third of patients with initially nonfatal PE will have a fatal recurrence, generally within a few weeks of the original event. Even with optimal treatment, about 5% of patients with PE will die from fatal PE, and about 25% with proximal DVT will develop post-thrombotic syndrome, a chronic condition that is debilitating for patients.

Venous thromboembolism is now recognized as the leading cause of preventable death in hospitalized patients. Almost all hospitalized patients have one or more risk factors for VTE and 40% will have three or more risk factors. VTE prophylaxis (addressed in Chapters 56, 65, and 252) forms the cornerstone for preventing these deaths. In addition, although 75% of venous thromboembolic events are diagnosed in the outpatient setting, about half of all episodes of VTE are associated with recent surgery or hospitalization. These findings stress the importance of having a low threshold to perform diagnostic testing in patients who present with signs and symptoms compatible with VTE within 3 months of hospitalization.

Therefore, VTE is both an acute and a chronic disease that causes substantial patient morbidity and mortality, and it is a major burden on the health care system. Costs for VTE include not only the expense of initial diagnosis and treatment, but also the cost of the complications of VTE (ie, post-thrombotic syndrome, venous ulceration, chronic thromboembolic pulmonary hypertension, recurrent VTE) and its treatment (ie, bleeding). It is currently estimated that VTE costs the US health care system $1.5 billion/y.

■ NOMENCLATURE

Proximal DVT is defined as a DVT that involves the popliteal vein or more proximal veins of the leg (most also involve the calf veins).

Distal DVT is defined as a DVT that is confined to the calf veins.

PRACTICE POINT

The natural history of VTE
- DVT typically starts in the calf (distal) veins
- Two-thirds of symptomatic DVT are located in the proximal veins

- 80% of distal DVT will resolve without anticoagulation
- 20% of distal DVT will extend to the proximal veins, usually within 1 week
- Extension of calf DVT is more likely to occur in patients who have ongoing risk factors for VTE (eg, malignancy, immobility)
- Nonextending calf DVT rarely causes PE, but proximal DVT frequently does
- 60% of patients with symptomatic DVT will have asymptomatic PE
- 70% of patients with symptomatic PE will have asymptomatic DVT

PATHOPHYSIOLOGY

Virchow's triad for the pathogenesis of thrombosis is as relevant today as it was when it was originally described in the 18th century: venous stasis, vessel wall damage, and hypercoagulability. A summary of common risk factors for VTE is given in **Table 253-1**.

■ VENOUS STASIS

Deep-vein thrombosis is more likely to occur in the paralyzed leg following stroke, and in the left leg during pregnancy because of extrinsic compression of the left iliac vein by the pregnant uterus and the right common iliac artery.

■ VESSEL WALL DAMAGE

Manipulation during surgery (eg, hip replacement), iatrogenic injury, and use of indwelling venous catheters all markedly increase the risk of DVT.

TABLE 253-1 Risk Factors for Venous Thromboembolism (VTE)

Patient factors

Age over 40. Previous VTE. Inherited hypercoagulable states.

Underlying condition and acquired factors

Hospitalization

    Acute medical illness (eg, congestive heart failure, COPD exacerbation)

Surgery

    Surgery requiring general anaesthesia >30 min lower limb orthopedic surgery major trauma

Nursing home

Prolonged immobility (eg, limited ambulation for >48 h within past 30 d)

Paralysis lower limb injuries

Obesity

Pregnancy, puerperium

Estrogen therapy (eg, oral contraceptive, hormone replacement therapy)

Malignancy Chemotherapy

Central vein catheterization, transvenous pacemaker

Inflammatory bowel disease

Nephrotic syndrome

Systemic lupus erythematosus

Antiphospholipid antibodies

Heparin-induced thrombocytopenia

■ HYPERCOAGULABILITY

Inherited or acquired changes in the balance of naturally occurring coagulation and fibrinolytic factors and their inhibitors predispose to thrombosis. The inherited hypercoagulable conditions that are considered strong risk factors for thrombosis; antithrombin deficiency, protein C deficiency, and protein S deficiency, are rare (<1% prevalence). Conversely, the most common inherited hypercoagulable conditions, activated protein C resistance caused by the Factor V Leiden mutation (5% prevalence in Caucasians), and the prothrombin gene mutation that leads to a 25% increase in prothrombin levels (2% prevalence), are weak risk factors for thrombosis. If VTE is suspected or confirmed in inpatients or shortly after discharge from the hospital, it is important to consider the possibility of heparin-induced thrombocytopenia (HIT), another prothrombotic state.

CASE 253-1

A 63-year-old male noticed edema of his leg following a left knee arthroplasty 10 days ago that had been improving until 2 days ago. Now, his leg seemed to be as big as it had been the day after his surgery. He had been doing more physiotherapy and wondered if he might have overexerted his leg.

On physical examination, he was in no apparent distress and his vital signs were normal. His left leg was 42 cm in circumference when measured 10 cm below the tibial tuberosity compared with his right leg which was 37 cm. There was obvious ecchymosis in the popliteal fossa and down by his medial malleolus. His incision was dry with no significant erythema or induration. He had no tenderness on palpation over the deep veins.

What is this patient's risk for VTE?

What diagnostic tests would you order?

How would your choice of diagnostic tests change if he also told you he had a history of a DVT in the same leg 2 years ago?

DOES THIS PATIENT HAVE A DVT?

Edema, pain, tenderness, and erythema are signs and symptoms of DVT, but they are also commonly found in patients who do not have DVT (ie, nonspecific). Only 15% of ambulatory patients who are suspected of having DVT will have this diagnosis confirmed on objective testing. Alternate causes for these clinical features include recent leg surgery, muscle injury, Baker cyst, cellulitis, extrinsic compression of veins, anasarca or low albumin states, and venous insufficiency.

Hospitalized patients are more likely than ambulatory patients to have DVT confirmed when it is suspected (prevalence of 30%-40%). However, hospitalized patients are also more likely to have asymptomatic DVT (in a prophylaxis study of medical patients that routinely screened for asymptomatic DVT, only 6% of DVT were symptomatic). This finding stresses the importance of preventing VTE instead of relying on clinical surveillance to detect and treat it early.

PRACTICE POINT

- One out of every 20 recurrent symptomatic VTE are fatal (5%)
- One out of every 11 major bleeds in patients receiving anticoagulant therapy are fatal (9%)

Failure to diagnose DVT exposes patients to the risk of fatal PE; however, inappropriate use of anticoagulant therapy exposes patients to the risk of fatal bleeding. Because clinical assessment alone is unreliable, objective testing to confirm the diagnosis must always be performed when DVT is suspected.

■ CLINICAL ASSESSMENT

For the reasons outlined above, clinical assessment alone is an unreliable test for diagnosing DVT. However, clinical prediction rules have been developed that can help to stratify patients as having a low (5% prevalence), moderate (25% prevalence), or high (60% prevalence) probability of DVT (**Table 253-2**).

Hospitalized patients are less likely to have a low probability score. Classification of pretest probability is helpful when used *in combination* with other diagnostic tests (**Figure 253-1**).

If there is a high risk clinical suspicion for DVT (or PE) and patients are not at high risk for bleeding, it is recommended that anticoagulant therapy is started before diagnostic testing is performed. Treatment can be deferred if diagnostic testing will be performed within 4 hours in patients with a moderate and within 24 hours in patients with a low clinical suspicion for DVT (or PE).

■ IMAGING TESTS FOR DVT

Venography

Venography is the reference standard test for DVT, but it is rarely performed today because it is invasive (painful), technically difficult, and exposes the patient to the risks of contrast dye (eg, nephrotoxicity, anaphylaxis) and radiation. An intraluminal filling defect (ie, section of a vein that remains dark when surrounded by white contrast dye) seen on at least two views is considered diagnostic for DVT.

Compression venous ultrasound

Ultrasonography is the first-line imaging test used to diagnose or exclude DVT. When pressure is applied to the proximal veins with

TABLE 253-2 The Wells Clinical Prediction Rule for DVT

	Points
Active cancer (treatment ongoing or within previous 6 mo or palliative)	1
Paralysis, paresis, or recent plaster immobilization of the lower extremities	1
Recently bedridden >3 d or major surgery within the previous 12 wk requiring general or regional anesthesia	1
Localized tenderness along the distribution of the deep venous system	1
Entire leg swollen	1
Calf swelling 3 cm >asymptomatic side (measured 10 cm below tibial tuberosity)	1
Pitting edema confined to the symptomatic leg	1
Collateral superficial veins (nonvaricose)	1
Previously documented deep-vein thrombosis	1
Alternative diagnosis as likely or greater than that of DVT	–2

Total points (pretest probability for DVT)

Score >2: High

Score 1-2: Moderate

Score ≤0: Low

Data from Wells PS, Anderson DR, Rodger M, et al. Evaluation of D-dimer in the diagnosis of suspected deep-vein thrombosis. *N Engl J Med.* 2003;349:1227-1235.

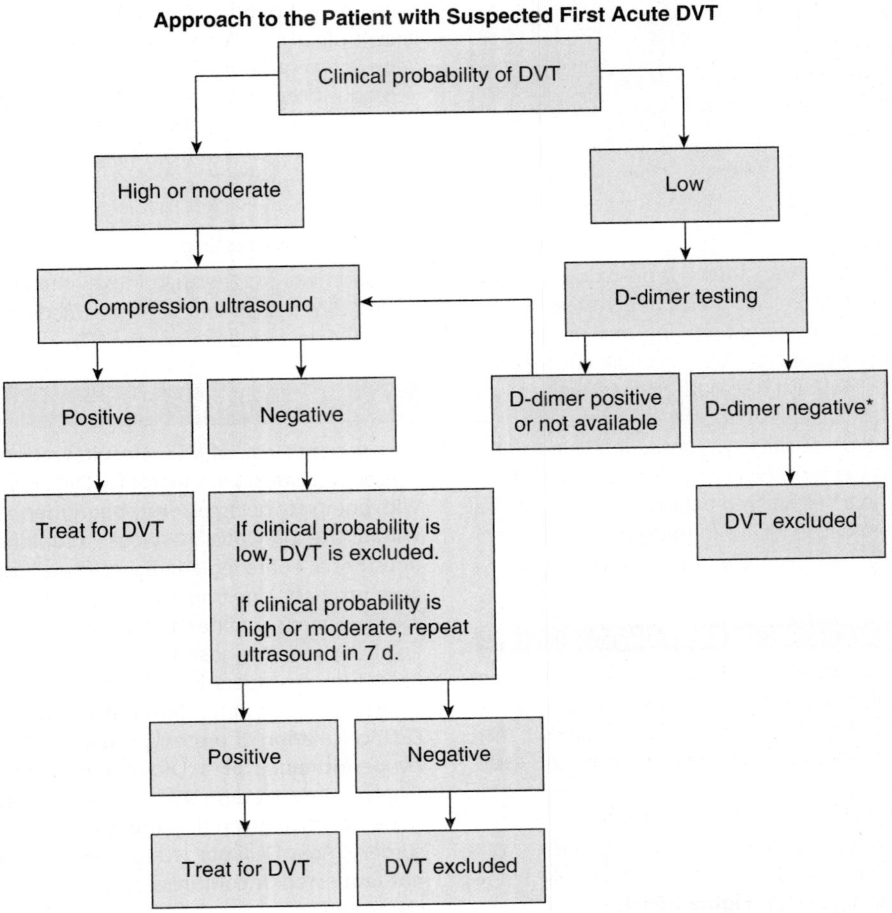

Figure 253-1 *Approach to the patient with suspected first acute DVT. *If D-dimer assay has a sensitivity of greater than or equal to 85% of proximal veins.*

an ultrasound probe, the veins should fully compress. If they do not, acute or chronic DVT is present. In symptomatic patients, when the ultrasound probe is applied to the proximal veins, the sensitivity of ultrasound for proximal DVT is 97% and the specificity is 94% when compared with venography (for both inpatients and outpatients). The sensitivity and specificity of compression ultrasound is lower in the calf veins, and the clinical significance of isolated calf vein thrombosis is controversial. For these reasons, many centers do not examine the calf veins with ultrasound; instead, if the initial assessment (eg, low clinical suspicion and negative ultrasound of the proximal veins) cannot exclude the presence of DVT, a follow-up ultrasound of the proximal veins is done after a week to exclude the possibility of calf vein thrombosis with early extension into the proximal veins. If whole leg ultrasound is performed and is negative, repeat ultrasound scanning is not necessary. Compression venous ultrasound is frequently combined with assessment of Doppler flow; however, change in Doppler flow alone is not a sensitive or specific test for DVT.

Limitations of ultrasound include the factors listed below.

- Operator dependent in the calf veins
- Limbs with casts that cannot be removed
- Morbid obesity
- Massive edema
- Isolated pelvic DVT harder to detect

PRACTICE POINT

Do not waste time and money by ordering a D-dimer for the following patients:
- Postoperative inpatients.
- Other patients with severe systemic illness that will markedly increase D-dimer levels.
- High clinical suspicion for DVT or PE.

Results are very unlikely to be negative and, if they are negative, the post-test probability is still too high for VTE to be excluded. A positive result is unhelpful.

D-dimer blood testing

D-dimer is formed when cross-linked fibrin is broken down by plasmin. Normal levels can help to *exclude* DVT, but elevated D-dimer levels are common with other conditions (eg, malignancy, disseminated intravascular coagulation, acute infection, normal pregnancy, renal disease, cardiovascular disease). D-dimer levels are also elevated after surgery and may take up to 50 days to return to baseline, depending on the type of surgery. Consequently, a positive D-dimer is *NEVER* diagnostic for DVT! A negative D-dimer can still be used to exclude DVT in a hospitalized patient with a low clinical probability for DVT, but negative results in this patient population are so uncommon (<10%) that the utility of the test is very poor.

DOES THIS PATIENT HAVE RECURRENT DVT?

Approximately 30% of patients with DVT will experience recurrent DVT during the 10 years following the initial diagnosis. Unfortunately, diagnosing recurrent DVT is much more difficult than diagnosing a first DVT. To begin with, the signs and symptoms experienced by patients with recurrent DVT (ie, increased edema and/or pain) are also seen in patients with post-thrombotic syndrome, a chronic condition that affects approximately 25% of patients with previous DVT. Secondly, diagnostic tests for recurrent DVT are not as reliable as they are for first acute DVT (**Figure 253-2**).

■ CLINICAL ASSESSMENT

Clinical prediction rules for diagnosing recurrent DVT are less well developed and validated than for a first episode of DVT and they have not been widely used.

■ IMAGING TESTS FOR RECURRENT DVT

Venography

As with first acute DVT, this method is considered the reference standard test for recurrent DVT. However, veins previously affected by DVT may not fill with contrast dye, resulting in nondiagnostic findings.

Compression venous ultrasound

In patients with a recent ultrasound that demonstrated (1) limited extent of the previous DVT or (2) complete resolution of the previous DVT, the presence a new noncompressible segment of the proximal veins (eg, popliteal or common femoral vein) on ultrasound examination is diagnostic for recurrent DVT. However, it is important to remember that *50% of patients with first acute DVT will still have incomplete compressibility on ultrasound examination 1 year after diagnosis despite adequate anticoagulant therapy.* Consequently, without clear evidence of a new noncompressible segment, it can be difficult to tell the difference between residual chronic DVT and new acute DVT. It can be useful, therefore, to perform an ultrasound when the decision is taken to stop anticoagulation in a patient who initially had an extensive DVT. This acts as a baseline scan to which future scans can be compared.

If a proximal US is abnormal but there is no new noncompressible segment, it has been proposed that an increase in residual vein diameter of greater than 4 mm (when a vein is compressed with an ultrasound probe) is diagnostic for recurrence. However, a recent ultrasound (prior to the episode of suspected recurrence) is required to make this comparison, and there is evidence that the reproducibility of the residual diameter measurement is only moderate. Other ultrasound features such as Doppler flow and thrombus echogenicity have not been validated as reliable methods for diagnosing recurrent DVT.

D-dimer blood testing

Although less studied than in patients with a suspected first DVT, recent clinical trials indicate that a negative D-dimer result can be used to help exclude recurrent DVT.

CASE 253-1 (*continued*)

This patient's risk of VTE: Hospitalization for major orthopedic surgery is a strong risk factor for DVT. His Wells score for DVT is 2 with points for being recently bedridden >3 days or major surgery within the previous 12 weeks requiring general or regional anesthesia, entire leg edema, calf swelling 3 cm greater than the asymptomatic side (measured 10 cm below tibial tuberosity) and pitting edema confined to the symptomatic leg, but he also has an alternative diagnosis for his symptoms that is at least as likely as DVT (ie, postoperative edema), which subtracted 2 points.

Diagnostic testing: For most outpatients with suspected DVT, calculation of pretest probability (eg, Wells score) followed by performance of a D-dimer is a good initial approach to diagnosing/excluding DVT. In this case, a D-dimer is very unlikely to be negative given that this patient recently underwent major surgery. As a D-dimer is only helpful when it is negative, it is not requested. A compression ultrasound should be ordered to check for DVT.

Approach to the Patient with Suspected Recurrent DVT in the Same Leg

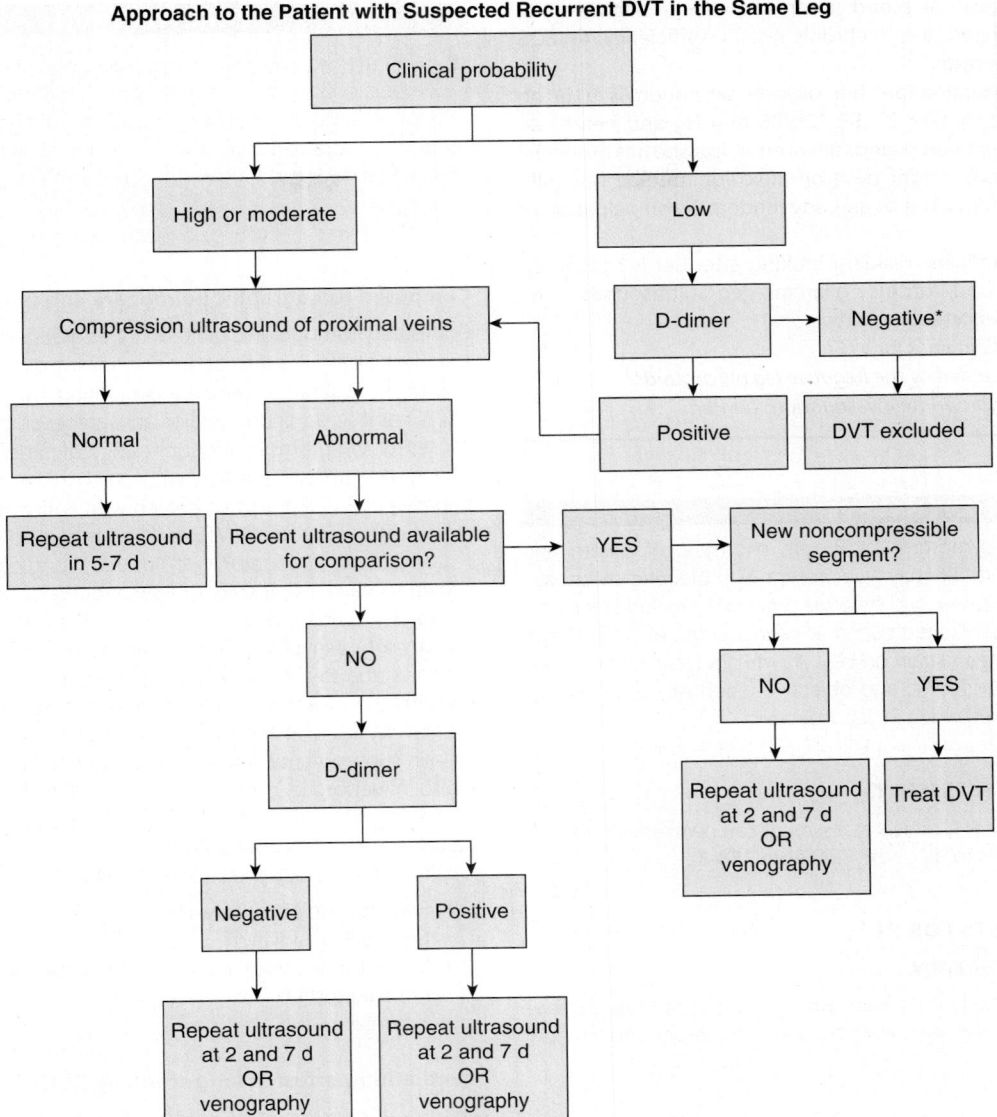

Figure 253-2 *Approach to the patient with suspected recurrent DVT in the same leg. *If D-dimer assay has a sensitivity of greater than or equal to 85%.*

Diagnostic testing in patients with a history of DVT: This case would become significantly more difficult if this patient had a history of a DVT in the same leg. The decision not to order a D-dimer would remain unchanged and the patient would still have a compression ultrasound study. However, if the ultrasound was abnormal, his clinicians would also want to try to find a previous ultrasound report which described the extent of his previous DVT.

If he was documented to have complete resolution of his previous thrombus, the finding of any noncompressible segments on the current ultrasound examination would be interpreted as representing new acute DVT.

If he had incomplete resolution of his previous thrombus, and the current examination showed noncompressibility in a previously unaffected segment, he has a new acute DVT (eg, his previous DVT extended up to the mid femoral vein, but today's examination shows incompressibility of the common femoral vein). If today's ultrasound examination shows incompressibility

in the same segments as his previous DVT, his clinicians cannot be certain that the findings represent new acute DVT. They have three choices in this situation:

(1) Not to treat, but to repeat the ultrasound at 2 and 7 days (to look for clear evidence of progression which would indicate acute DVT), (2) arrange for a venogram. or (3) treat the patient as an acute DVT for 3 months.

CASE 253-2

A 72-year-old woman has been in hospital for 4 days with pneumonia. She is afebrile and her cough is no longer productive of purulent sputum, but she continues to be tachypneic and hypoxic. The right lower lobe infiltrate seen on her chest x-ray on admission has not significantly changed. Her white blood cell count is slowly decreasing, but she continues to have anemia and mild thrombocytosis. All blood cultures have been negative. Her creatinine is elevated due to chronic renal insufficiency. An ECG shows sinus tachycardia.

On physical examination, her oxygen saturation is 91% on room air, respiratory rate 25, BP 120/85 mm Hg and heart rate 100 beats/min. Her heart sounds are normal, but she has bronchial breath sounds at her right base on auscultation. She has mild bilateral pedal edema, but denies any tenderness on palpation of her legs.

The internal medicine resident looking after her is concerned about DVT/PE and orders bilateral leg ultrasounds. The ultrasounds are reportedly negative.

What is this patient's risk for VTE?

Has PE been excluded by the negative leg ultrasounds?

What are the appropriate investigations for PE?

DOES THIS PATIENT HAVE PE?

The commonest symptoms of PE are shortness of breath and fatigue. Patients with PE may also present with pleuritic chest pain, palpitations, hemoptysis, and syncope. Signs of PE include tachycardia, tachypnea, accentuated pulmonic heart sound, and S1Q3T3 and evidence of right heart strain on ECG. As with DVT, clinical signs and symptoms are nonspecific, and objective diagnostic testing must always be performed when PE is suspected.

■ CLINICAL ASSESSMENT

As with suspected DVT, clinical assessment can be used *in combination* with other tests to diagnose PE (**Table 253-3**).

■ IMAGING TESTS FOR PE

Pulmonary angiography

This method is the reference standard test for diagnosing PE. However, it suffers from the same limitations as venography and it is now very rarely used.

TABLE 253-3 The Wells Clinical Prediction Rule for PE

	Points
Clinical signs and symptoms of deep vein thrombosis (minimum of leg swelling and pain with palpation of the deep veins)	3.0
An alternative diagnosis is less likely than pulmonary embolism	3.0
Heart rate > 100 beats/min	1.5
Immobilization or surgery in the previous 4 wk	1.5
Previous deep vein thrombosis/pulmonary embolism	1.5
Hemoptysis	1.0
Malignancy (treatment ongoing or within previous 6 mo or palliative)	1.0

Total points (pretest probability for PE):

Score ≤4: PE unlikely or low

Score >4: PE likely (Moderate if 4.5-6, and High if >6)

Data from Wells PS, Anderson DR, Rodger M, et al. Derivation of a simple clinical model to categorize patients probability of pulmonary-embolism: increasing the models utility with the SimpliRED D-dimer. *Thromb Haemost.* 2000;83:416-420.

PRACTICE POINT

- Computed tomographic pulmonary angiography (CTPA) delivers a relatively high dose of radiation to breast tissue which increases the risk of breast cancer. It should be avoided when possible, and particularly in women less than 50 years of age.
- One CTPA is equivalent to 100 chest x-rays with respect to radiation!

Computed tomographic pulmonary angiography (CTPA)

Computed tomographic pulmonary angiography (also known as spiral or helical CT) is the current first-line imaging test for PE. Thrombus in the pulmonary arteries is outlined by radiologic contrast. CTPA has the additional major advantage of detecting alternate causes for symptoms in about one-third of patients with suspected PE (eg, pneumonia, lung mass). Less than 2% of patients with a negative CTPA who are not treated with anticoagulant therapy will return with symptomatic VTE during 3 months of follow-up.

Computed tomographic pulmonary angiography has been shown to have a sensitivity of 83% and a specificity of 96% for PE. However, accuracy varies according to the size of the largest pulmonary artery involved. The probability that an intraluminal filling defect is due to a PE has been reported as 97% for defects in the main or lobar artery, 68% for segmental arteries, and 25% for subsegmental arteries (which means that as many as 75% of abnormalities seen in subsegmental arteries are not due to PE). Accuracy of CTPA is also influenced by clinical assessment of PE; the higher the clinical probability of PE, the more likely the defect that is seen on CTPA is actually due to PE (**Table 253-4**).

Limitations include the factors listed below.

- Requires use of contrast dye
- Exposure to radiation
- Subject to technical difficulties (approximately 6% of CTPA are nondiagnostic)
- Expense

Ventilation-perfusion lung scanning (V/Q)

This was the first-line test used to diagnose PE before the advent of CTPA, and V/Q scanning is still used, particularly when CTPA is contraindicated (ie, patients with renal failure, young women due to a concern about breast cancer induced by radiation exposure). Perfusion defects are nonspecific; only about 33% of patients with perfusion defects have PE. The probability that a perfusion defect is due to PE increases with the size and number of defects, and if they are mismatched. A *mismatch* refers to a perfusion defect that is not associated with a corresponding defect on the ventilation scan. The V/Q scan probability of PE should be matched with the clinical probability of PE. A high probability lung scan can diagnose PE in patients with moderate or high clinical probability, and a low probability lung scan can exclude PE in a patient with low clinical probability

TABLE 253-4 Interpretation of Findings on CTPA

Location of Pulmonary Artery Defect on CTPA	Clinical Probability of PE	Interpretation
Lobar or larger	Any	Very likely PE
Segmental	Moderate or high	Likely PE
Segmental	Low	Less certain PE
Subsegmental	Any	Nondiagnostic

TABLE 253-5 Interpretation of Findings on V/Q

Mismatched Perfusion Defects on V/Q Scanning	Clinical Probability of PE	Interpretation
≥1 segmental	Moderate to high	Very likely PE
≥1 segmental	Low	Nondiagnostic
≥1 subsegmental	Moderate to high	Nondiagnostic
≥1 subsegmental	Low	Unlikely PE
None	Any	PE excluded

of PE. Lung scan findings are highly age dependent with a relatively high proportion of normal scans in younger patients, including pregnant women, and a low proportion in those with other acute and chronic cardiorespiratory conditions (**Table 253-5**).

Limitations include the factors listed below:

- Large proportion of nondiagnostic scans.
- Inability to identify alternative causes for symptoms.

■ SPECT

In many hospitals, three-dimensional SPECT (single-photon emission CT) has replaced planar V/Q scanning. Unlike V/Q, there are no standardized criteria for reporting SPECT. SPECT scans are less likely to be reported as nondiagnostic, with the majority of scans reporting PE present or absent. As yet, there are no large diagnostic studies reporting on the safety of diagnosing and excluding PE with SPECT.

D-dimer blood testing

As with suspected DVT, a negative D-dimer result can exclude PE (on its own, if it is a very sensitive assay or in combination with other tests, if it is less sensitive) (**Figure 253-3**).

What if the tests I ordered to exclude PE were nondiagnostic?

If initial testing is nondiagnostic (eg, ventilation-perfusion scan), there is still a substantial chance that your patient could have a PE and further investigations are required. One approach to management of such patients is to perform ultrasonography and withhold anticoagulation if there is no DVT of the proximal veins. Ultrasonography of the proximal veins is then repeated after 1 and 2 weeks to exclude evolving VTE. See algorithm Figure 253-3.

CASE 253-2 (*continued*)

This patient's risk of PE: Hospitalization with acute infection is a strong risk factor for VTE. In addition, this patient is over age 40 and has been largely bed-bound while in hospital. Hypoxia that is more severe than expected from the chest x-ray findings should raise suspicion of PE.

Diagnostic Testing: PE has not been excluded. If her leg ultrasounds had been positive for DVT, further investigations for PE would not be necessary because it would not change her management (ie, the anticoagulant treatment for DVT and PE is the same). However, in this case, proximal DVT has been excluded by negative ultrasounds, but PE has not been excluded.

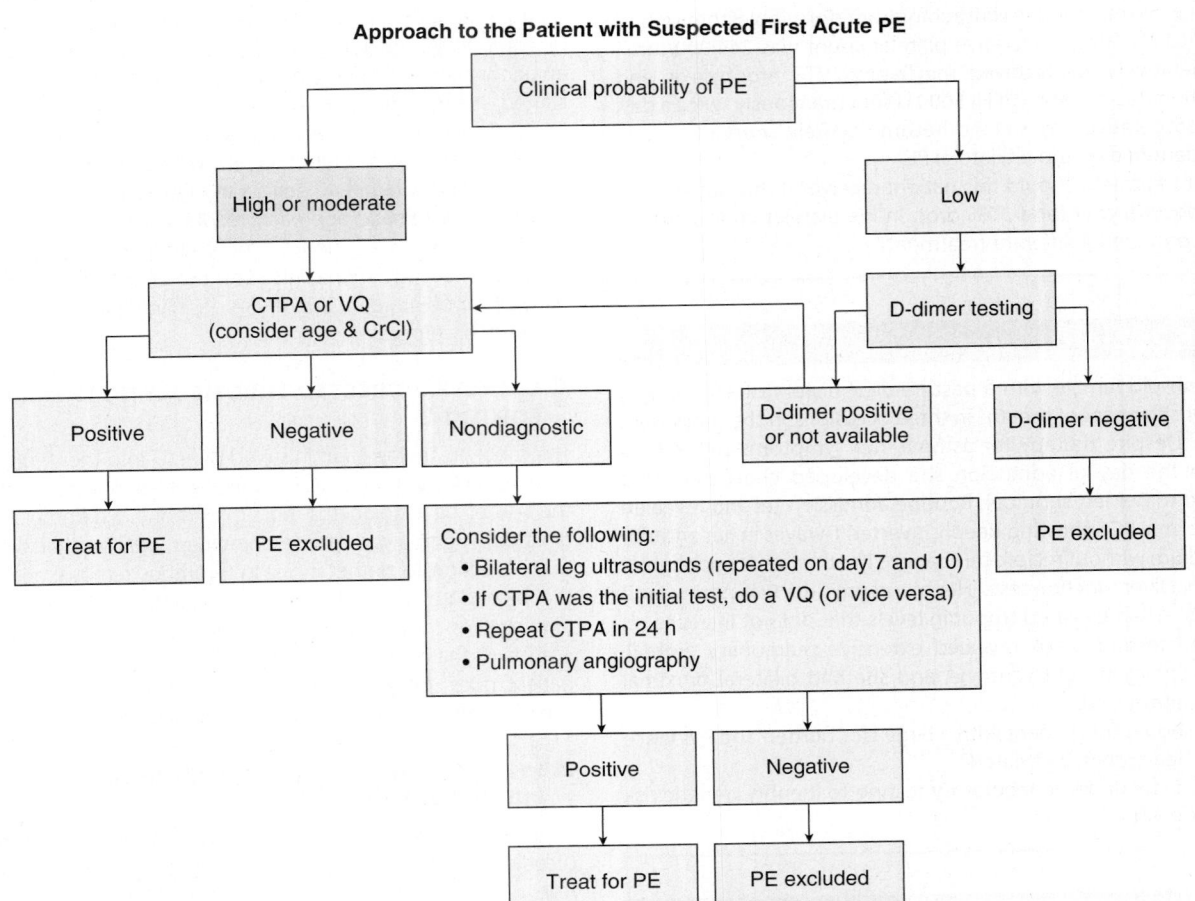

Figure 253-3 *Approach to the patient with suspected first acute PE. If D-dimer assay has a sensitivity of greater than or equal to 85%.*

Currently, CTPA is the most common first-line imaging test used to diagnose PE. However, this woman is known to have chronic renal insufficiency so this test may not be appropriate. A reasonable alternative is a V/Q scan, especially if she had a normal CXR.

TREATMENT OF VENOUS THROMBOEMBOLISM

The foundation of treatment of VTE is anticoagulant therapy. The objectives of anticoagulant therapy are: (1) to prevent extension and potentially fatal embolization of the initial thrombus and (2) to prevent recurrent VTE.

■ TRIAGE AND HOSPITAL ADMISSION

Patients who are hemodynamically stable with a low bleeding risk and normal renal function, and who are likely to be compliant with anticoagulant therapy, can be safely treated as outpatients. Patients with DVT and severe intractable pain or severe swelling and poor leg perfusion should be admitted to hospital for initiation of anticoagulant treatment, and assessment of the need for catheter-directed thrombolysis. Patients with PE and severe symptoms or abnormal vital signs should be admitted to the hospital, and those with signs of hemodynamic compromise (eg, systolic blood pressure <90 mm Hg) should be considered for thrombolytic therapy (discussed later). Validated prognostic scores, such as the Pulmonary Embolism Severity Index, are available to help physicians select which patients with PE can be treated as outpatients.

CASE 253-3

A 40-year-old male underwent a craniotomy for glioblastoma multiforme (GBM). His preoperative platelet count was 244,000/mm³. Postoperatively, he received mechanical VTE prophylaxis and unfractionated heparin (UFH) 5000 U subcutaneously twice a day. On postoperative day #11 he became acutely short of breath. CTPA identified multiple bilateral PE.

What treatment should this patient receive? If this patient had thrombocytopenia (or a 50% drop in his platelet count), would you recommend a different treatment?

CASE 253-4

A 58-year-old female with a past medical history of asthma was seen for shortness of breath on three occasions in the outpatient setting. Despite therapy for asthma, her symptoms progressed and on the day of admission she developed chest pain that radiated to her left shoulder. Routine admission testing revealed an abnormal ECG showing deeply inverted T-waves in her anterior precordium without reciprocal changes in other leads and slightly abnormal liver function tests. Her blood pressure was normal and stable. She had elevated troponin levels that did not increase on repeated testing. CTPA revealed extensive pulmonary emboli, and an enlarged right ventricle, and she had bilateral proximal DVT on ultrasound.

How should this patient with a large clot burden and evidence of right heart strain be treated?

Should she undergo laboratory testing to identify genetic risk factors for VTE?

TREATMENT OF ACUTE VENOUS THROMBOEMBOLISM

The first step in treating acute VTE is preventing further thrombus formation by starting an agent that rapidly inhibits thrombin.

The agents approved for initial treatment of acute VTE in Europe and North America are low-molecular-weight heparin (LMWH), fondaparinux, heparin, rivaroxaban, and apixaban (**Table 253-6**).

PRACTICE POINT

- Vitamin K antagonists will not rapidly inhibit thrombin and should not be used alone to treat acute VTE.
  - Low-molecular-weight heparin should be given for 5 to 7 days before starting dabigatran in acute venous thrombosis.

Patients with VTE who have heparin-induced thrombocytopenia (HIT) or a past history of HIT should receive danaparoid, argatroban, or fondaparinux (off-label) instead of heparin or low-molecular-weight heparin.

Rivaroxaban and apixaban have simplified the approach to anticoagulation in acute venous thrombosis. Both drugs are given in a higher dose for the initial treatment period, followed by dose reduction (see Table 253-6). They have the advantage of the oral route, simplified dosing, and freedom from dietary interactions (compared to warfarin). In contrast, dabigatran therapy is delayed until after 5 to 7 days of heparin therapy.

Not all patients are suitable for treatment with rivaroxaban, apixaban, or dabigatran. The group of patients who should not receive new oral anticoagulants includes those with renal impairment and a creatinine clearance <30 mL/min, hepatic impairment, and patients who are treated with strongly interacting drugs (see Table 253-6). Pregnant and breast feeding women should not be treated with the new oral anticoagulants.

When warfarin is the chosen oral anticoagulant, a heparin should be given for a minimum of 5 days and until the INR is greater than or equal to 2.0 on two consecutive measurements. A vitamin K antagonist (eg, warfarin) with a target INR of 2.0 to 3.0 is typically started at the same time as the parenteral antithrombotic agent. Dosing algorithms for VKAs are available. Lower VKA maintenance doses are required in older patients, women, those with impaired nutrition, and vitamin K deficiency. Optimal VKA management requires a systematic approach to obtaining INR measurements, adjusting VKA dose, and communicating these instructions to patients. Anticoagulation clinics, and use of computer programs to schedule appointments, adjust VKA dose and maintain records, can facilitate this process.

■ CATHETER-DIRECTED THROMBOLYTIC THERAPY FOR DVT

Thrombolytic therapy administered directly into the thrombus can achieve thrombus removal, improve acute symptoms, and reduce the risk of developing the post-thrombotic syndrome. Catheter-directed thrombolysis can be combined with mechanical thrombus disruption to further increase thrombus removal and shorten the procedure. It can be used for patients with extensive DVT (eg, involves the iliofemoral vein) of recent onset (eg, symptoms ≤14 days) that is associated with severe symptoms, provided the patient does not have risk factors for bleeding, there is available expertise, and it is the patient's preference to receive such therapy.

■ SYSTEMIC AND LOCAL THROMBOLYSIS FOR PULMONARY EMBOLISM

Systemic thrombolysis is associated with a 2% risk of intracranial bleeding, and a 10% risk of major bleeding. Therefore it is generally reserved for patients with PE and a systolic blood pressure less than 90 mm Hg. Catheter-directed thrombolysis, which uses a lower dose of thrombolytic drug, may have a more rapid action and lower risk of bleeding; therefore, in centers with the expertise, catheter-directed

TABLE 253-6 Antithrombotics for Treatment of Acute Venous Thromboembolism

Antihrombotic	Dose and Administration	Advantages	Disadvantages
Heparin	333 U/kg subcutaneous injection followed by 250 U/kg twice daily	Laboratory monitoring not required Can be reversed with protamine sulphate Can be used in pts with renal failure	Half-life too short to be given subcutaneously only once daily Concentrations suitable for subcutaneous injection often not available
	80 U/kg intravenous (IV) bolus followed by 18 U/kg/min (aPTT titrated to plasma heparin levels from 0.3 to 0.7 IU/mL anti-Xa activity)	Short half-life if bleeding occurs Can be reversed with protamine sulphate Can be used in pts with renal failure	Requires laboratory monitoring if given intravenously Highest risk of HIT Not an option for outpatient therapy
LMWH	Weight-based subcutaneous injection daily or twice daily	Laboratory monitoring not required	Contraindicated in pts with CrCl <30 mL/min Protamine sulphate is only partially effective in reversing anticoagulant effect Moderate risk of HIT
Fondaparinux	Weight-based subcutaneous injection daily	Laboratory monitoring not required Low risk of HIT	Contraindicated in pts with CrCl <30 mL/min No reversal agent available
Warfarin in conjunction with a heparin during first 5 d	Initiate warfarin at dose of 10 to 5 mg, followed by INR-based dose adjustment A heparin should be administered with warfarin for a minimum of 5 d and until INR ≥2.0 for 24 h	Anticoagulant of choice with severe renal impairment	Starting dose of warfarin should be tailored to individual patient, depending on nutritional status, age and coprescription of medications. INR testing is necessary throughout treatment. Many drugs potentiate or reduce the anticoagulation effects of warfarin.
Rivaroxaban	15 mg oral, twice per day for 21 d followed by 20 mg once per day	Oral route Laboratory monitoring not required	Contraindicated in pts with CrCl <30 mL/min Contraindicated in Child-Pugh B or C hepatic impairment Increased plasma levels with isoniazid, miconazole, quinidine, valproic acid, HIV protease inhibitors, diltiazem, clarithromycin and azithromycin (CYP 3a4 inhibitors) Reduced plasma levels with carbamazepine, phenytoin and rifampin (CYP 3a4 inducers) As yet, no clear reversal agent and anticoagulant levels not readily available
Apixaban	10 mg oral, twice per day for 7 d, followed by 5 mg twice per day	Oral route Laboratory monitoring not required	Contraindicated in pts with CrCl <30 mL/min Contraindicated in Child-Pugh B or C hepatic impairment Increased plasma levels with isoniazid, miconazole, quinidine, valproic acid, HIV protease inhibitors, diltiazem, clarithromycin, and azithromycin (CYP 3a4 inhibitors) Reduced plasma levels with carbamazepine, phenytoin and rifampin (CYP 3a4 inducers) As yet, no clear reversal agent and anticoagulant levels not readily available
Dabigatran following 5-7 d of a heparin	150 mg oral, twice per day following a minimum of 5 d of a heparin	Laboratory monitoring not required	Contraindicated in pts with CrCl <30 mL/min Avoid in severe liver impairment Increased plasma levels with antifungals, cyclosporin, dronedarone, amiodarone, tacrolimus, verapamil, HIV protease inhibitors, quinidine (p-glycoprotein inhibitors) Reduced plasma levels with carbamazepine, phenytoin and rifampin (p-glycoprotein inducers) Idarcizumab now available for reversal.

CrCl, creatinine clearance; HIT, heparin-induced thrombocytopenia; LMWH, low-molecular-weight heparin.

thrombolysis may be preferred to systemic thrombolytic therapy in hypotensive patients with PE who are deteriorating or who have a high risk for bleeding.

PRACTICE POINT

- Various thrombolytic regimens are used to treat PE including alteplase (100 mg given over 2 hours by intravenous infusion) or tenecteplase (30-50 mg bolus), both followed by heparin infusion with no initial bolus.

■ BLEEDING IN PATIENTS WITH ACUTE VENOUS THROMBOEMBOLISM

Management of a patient with acute VTE and bleeding is difficult. The first step is to ensure the patient is hemodynamically stable. After that, the following questions can help to guide management: How severe is the bleeding? Which anticoagulant is the patient receiving (and when was the last dose given)? How acute is the VTE? Can the source of the bleeding be treated?

Moderate-to-severe bleeding

If the bleeding is moderate to severe, the anticoagulant should be reversed (see **Table 235-7**) (if possible), the patient resuscitated and the source of the bleeding treated. If the source of the bleeding cannot be treated, and the VTE is less than 1 month old, consideration should be given to inserting a permanent or removable inferior vena caval filter. If the source of the bleeding cannot be treated, and the VTE is older than 3 months, anticoagulants should be permanently discontinued. For reasons outlined later in this chapter, inserting an inferior vena caval filter is not recommended unless the patient has acute VTE (<1 month old).

TABLE 253-7 Reversal of Anticoagulation

	Reversal Agent	Comments
Warfarin	Vitamin K IV or oral	Minimum of 12 h to take effect (IV faster than oral)
	Prothrombin complex concentrate	Works instantly, effect lasts 4-6 h only (combine with Vitamin K)
		May have a prothrombotic effect
Low-molecular-weight heparin	Protamine sulphate	Provides only partial reversal
		With normal renal function, half-life of LMWH <24 h
Unfractionated heparin	Protamine sulphate	Half-life of unfractionated heparin 90 min
Rivaroxaban and apixaban	Prothrombin complex concentrate	May partially reverse anticoagulation effect in high doses
		With normal renal function, half-life of drugs 12 h
Dabigatran	Factor VIII inhibitor bypass activity (FEIBA)	May partially reverse anticoagulation effects
		With normal renal function, half-life of drugs 12 h
	Hemodialysis	For patients in renal failure
	Idarcizumab	Immediate reversal of anticoagulation. Increased risk of thrombosis.

Mild bleeding

If the bleeding is mild and likely to be transient (eg, hematuria in a patient with a urinary tract infection), the anticoagulant should be held for 24 to 48 hours and resumed once the bleeding has stopped. If the bleeding continues, consideration should be given to fully reversing the anticoagulant, and the source of the bleeding should be treated. If the bleeding resolves, anticoagulants should be reintroduced with careful monitoring and/or lower doses. If bleeding persists, and the VTE is older than 3 months, anticoagulants should be permanently discontinued.

PRACTICE POINT

- **Rule #1:** Do not anticoagulate a bleeding patient.
- **Rule #2:** All anticoagulants increase the risk of bleeding.

Inferior vena caval filters

No randomized trial or prospective cohort study has evaluated inferior vena caval filters as sole therapy in patients with DVT (ie, without concurrent anticoagulant therapy). Permanent inferior vena caval filter insertion as an adjunct to anticoagulant therapy has been evaluated in a single large-randomized-controlled trial of patients with acute DVT who were considered to be at high risk for PE. The findings of this study, which were reported after 2 years and 8 years of follow-up, indicated that filters decreased the rate of PE, increased the rate of DVT, did not change the overall rate of VTE, and had no apparent influence on mortality. Indirectly, this study supports the use of vena caval filters to prevent PE in patients with acute DVT and/or PE who cannot be anticoagulated (ie, actively bleeding), but does not support more liberal use of filters. More recently, a large randomized trial found that placement of a retrievable inferior vena caval filter as an adjunct to anticoagulation in patients with acute PE and a high risk of recurrence did not reduce recurrent PE at 3 months. Patients who have a vena caval filter inserted should receive anticoagulant therapy if and when it becomes safe to do so, and for the same duration as for similar patients who do not have a filter.

■ DURATION OF ANTICOAGULANT TREATMENT OF VENOUS THROMBOEMBOLISM

Optimal duration of anticoagulant treatment for VTE is based on three factors: (1) the increase in the risk of recurrent VTE if anticoagulants are stopped, (2) the increase in the risk of bleeding on anticoagulant therapy, and (3) patient preference. The factors that determine the risk of recurrence are outlined below, while the risk of anticoagulant-related bleeding is addressed in the following section.

First, the risk of recurrence depends on whether the acute episode of VTE has been adequately treated. Studies evaluating different durations of anticoagulant therapy have shown that *all patients with VTE should receive a minimum of 3 months of anticoagulant therapy*. Patients who receive less than 3 months of anticoagulant therapy have double the risk of recurrent VTE during 1 to 2 years of follow-up.

Second, the risk of recurrence after 3 or more months of treatment is dependent on the patient's intrinsic risk of having a new episode of VTE. The risk of recurrence is highest in patients who have no risk factors for VTE (ie, idiopathic or unprovoked) or have a VTE provoked by a strong persistent risk factor (eg, active malignancy), and lowest in patients with a VTE provoked by a strong transient risk factor (eg, surgery). The risk of recurrence in patients with VTE provoked by a transient risk factor is one-third of the risk of recurrence for patients with unprovoked VTE. Extending the duration of anticoagulant therapy for unprovoked VTE beyond 3 months (or 6 months if VTE was very severe) protects the patient from recurrence while

TABLE 253-8 Annual Risk of Recurrent Venous Thromboembolism after Anticoagulant is Stopped

	At 1 y	At 5 y
Transient risk factor for VTE	3%	10%
Unprovoked VTE	10%	30%

they are taking the anticoagulant, but does not reduce the risk of recurrence once the anticoagulant is discontinued (**Table 253-8**).

Third, among patients with unprovoked VTE, the risk of recurrence after stopping anticoagulation is 10% in the first year, 30% in 5 years and 50% by 10 years. Recent studies have identified men as having a higher risk of recurrence (15% in the first year). Patients who have an elevated D-dimer level after stopping anticoagulation also have a risk of recurrence that is about twice that of patients with normal D-dimer levels.

Two other factors connected with a patient's intrinsic risk of VTE that currently influence the duration of anticoagulant therapy include the number of previous episodes of VTE, and the presence of active malignancy. Patients with a second episode of unprovoked VTE have a 50% increased risk of recurrence and, therefore, should be considered for indefinite anticoagulant therapy. Patients with VTE and active cancer have about a threefold higher rate of recurrent VTE than patients with VTE who do not have cancer and, therefore, are usually maintained on anticoagulant therapy. The risk of recurrent VTE during and after anticoagulant therapy increases with more advanced stages of disease and with antineoplastic treatments such as chemotherapy.

Extended treatment with rivaroxaban, apixaban, or dabigatran is as effective as warfarin therapy at preventing recurrence, and is associated with less bleeding. LMWH is the preferred therapy for patients with VTE and because it is more effective at preventing VTE recurrence than warfarin. There are little data on using the newer anticoagulants in cancer patients, and chemotherapy may interact with these agents. Aspirin reduces recurrent VTE by up to a third, but it associated with bleeding and it is much less effective than anticoagulants (risk reduction of 80%-90%).

PRACTICE POINT

- Venous thromboembolism should generally be treated for 3 months (or until risk factors resolve) or indefinitely
- Venous thromboembolism provoked by a transient risk factor is treated for 3 months
- A first unprovoked calf DVT is treated for 3 months
- A first unprovoked proximal DVT or PE is treated for 3 (or sometimes 6) months or indefinitely, depending on risk of bleeding and patient preference
- A second unprovoked VTE is generally treated indefinitely
- Venous thromboembolism associated with active cancer is generally treated for the duration that the cancer is active

---

Inherited thrombophilias increase the risk of a first VTE, but their influence on the risk of recurrent VTE is minor or uncertain. The risk of recurrence is thought to be highest in patients with antithrombin deficiency, patients homozygous for the Factor V Leiden mutation, and patients who are double-heterozygotes for thrombophilic states (eg, patients heterozygous for both the Factor V Leiden mutation and the prothrombin gene mutation). However, these combinations are rare. The most common inherited hypercoaguable conditions, activated protein C-resistance caused by the Factor V Leiden mutation (5%

TABLE 253-9 Pros and Cons of Thrombophilia Screening

Pros for Thrombophilia Screening	Cons of Thrombophilia Screening
Antithrombin deficiency, homozygous Factor V Leiden mutation, double-heterozygous Factor V Leiden and prothrombin gene mutation may lead to indefinite anticoagulant therapy.	These abnormalities are rare. Thrombophilia results do NOT alter management in the vast majority of patients.
Informs patient of reason for developing VTE.	A negative thrombophilic screen can offer false reassurance. Patients with a negative screen may have a thrombophilic disorder that has yet to be identified. A positive thrombophilic screen can cause anxiety and have insurance implications. Thrombophilic screening is costly.
Stresses importance of prophylaxis in high-risk situations (eg, postoperatively, postpartum) in asymptomatic family members.	Family members should be advised of need for thromboprophylaxis in high-risk situations even if the thrombophilic screen is negative.
Can help female family members decide whether or not to use an estrogen-based oral contraceptive.	If the index patient has a negative thrombophilic screen, family member still have an increased risk of thrombosis.

prevalence), and the prothrombin gene mutation (2% prevalence), have not been shown to importantly increase the risk of recurrence. Overall, thrombophilia screens identify an abnormality in only about 30% of patients with unprovoked VTE. A negative thrombophilia screen does not exclude an inherited thrombophilia; it just excludes the thrombophilic abnormalities that we are able to test for at this time. Consequently, because the results of thrombophilia testing have very limited management implications, the pros and cons of thrombophilia screening should be carefully weighed before deciding to order these tests (**Table 253-9**).

Lupus anticoagulant and anticardiolipin antibodies (antiphospholipid antibodies) are acquired thrombophilic disorders, which may support indefinite anticoagulant therapy because of a higher risk of recurrent VTE and arterial events. However, testing for these disorders is not well standardized. It is important to be aware that antithrombin levels can be falsely low immediately following an acute VTE and that warfarin will interfere with testing for protein C deficiency, protein S deficiency and lupus anticoagulants. If thrombophilia testing is performed, it is generally better to defer this to the clinic rather than to test patients when they have acute VTE.

PRACTICE POINT

- Do not order a test (eg, thrombophilia screen) if you do not know what you are going to do with the result!

■ BLEEDING IN PATIENTS ON LONG-TERM ORAL ANTICOAGULANT THERAPY

Risk of bleeding on anticoagulants differs markedly among patients depending on the prevalence of risk factors (eg, age >75, previous gastrointestinal bleeding or stroke, renal failure, anemia, antiplatelet therapy, malignancy, poor anticoagulant control). Approximately 13% of episodes of major bleeding during the first 3 months of anticoagulant therapy are fatal and greater than 50% of intracranial bleeds are fatal. The risk of major bleeding in younger patients (eg, <60 years) who do not have risk factors for bleeding is about 1% per year. The risk of bleeding, and particularly intracranial bleeding, is lower with rivaroxaban, dabigatran, and apixaban than it is with warfarin. These new anticoagulants are contraindicated in patients with severe renal impairment. The risk of bleeding increases with the number and severity of risk factors for bleeding.

CASE 253-3 (continued)

The safety of therapeutic anticoagulation in patients who develop VTE shortly after surgery should always be discussed with their surgeons. Inferior vena cava filters are reserved for patients whose bleeding risks prohibit anticoagulation. An inferior vena cava filter does not invariably prevent PE and increases the risk of DVT. Full-dose heparin—either a continuous infusion of UFH with laboratory monitoring or subcutaneous injections of LMWH or fondaparinux—should overlap with warfarin for a minimum of 5 days. Laboratory monitoring of LMWH or fondaparinux is not necessary; however, it is reasonable for patients with renal dysfunction, an elevated or very low BMI, and in pregnancy. Patients should remain on anticoagulant therapy for at least 3 months. If this patient is still considered to have active malignancy, extended duration LMWH would be preferred over warfarin or the newer anticoagulants.

If this surgical patient had developed thrombocytopenia or a 50% drop in his platelet count, the possibility of HIT would be a consideration. In addition to the presence of thrombocytopenia and thrombosis, the timing of the fall of the platelet count (at least 5 days after first exposure to UFH) and whether there was another apparent cause of the thrombocytopenia (drug, sepsis, etc) would determine the pretest probability. Other clues to the development of HIT include systemic reactions to intravenous UFH, necrotizing skin lesions at the site of heparin administration, or thrombosis while receiving treatment with heparin. If there is a high pretest probability of HIT, heparin should be discontinued and appropriate anticoagulation with a direct thrombin inhibitor (DTI) or fondaparinux initiated while awaiting laboratory confirmation. For patients who develop HIT from UFH, LMWH cannot replace UFH due to cross-reaction with HIT-associated antibodies. The patient's platelet count would be expected to recover within 4 to 14 days after discontinuation of heparin. A direct thrombin inhibitor should be administered for at least 3 to 5 days and the platelet count should increase to at least 100,000/mm³ before warfarin or a newer oral anticoagulant is initiated.

CASE 253-4 (continued)

The use of thrombolytic therapy for patients with pulmonary embolism and without hypotension has not been shown to improve survival and is not currently recommended. This patient appropriately received UFH for 7 days and was discharged to home on therapeutic warfarin (target INR 2-3) with recommendations to continue warfarin indefinitely.

Given this patient's abnormal liver function tests, she was scheduled for further testing at the time of her follow-up appointment with her primary care physician. Ultrasound revealed metastatic cancer to her liver, and she was subsequently diagnosed with pancreatic cancer. Idiopathic VTE should lead to consideration of underlying malignancy (age-appropriate screening), especially since presentation with bilateral leg DVT is far more likely to be found in patients with very aggressive hypercoagulable states (eg, malignancy, HIT). Extended duration LMWH should be considered once the diagnosis of cancer is established.

CONCLUSION

Given the challenges of the clinical diagnosis of VTE and the unpredictability of sudden fatal PE as the initial manifestation, appropriate VTE prophylaxis is required to minimize morbidity and mortality from hospital-acquired VTE. In contrast to the community setting, clinical prediction rules and D-dimer testing may be less likely to discriminate between hospitalized patients who have and those who do not have VTE because the majority of patients will have moderate or high pretest probability of VTE and will have other reasons for a positive D-dimer. Since clinical assessment alone is unreliable, objective testing to confirm the diagnosis must always be performed when VTE is suspected.

Almost all patients with VTE will require anticoagulation that extends beyond hospitalization. Clinicians need to ensure that care transitions include identification and communication with the receiving providers who will monitor anticoagulation. Discharge information includes drug, dosing (including last dose), timing of next dose and identification of who will advise patient of any dosage adjustment.

SUGGESTED READINGS

Bates SM, Jaeschke R, Stevens SM, et al. Diagnosis of DVT: antithrombotic therapy and prevention of thrombosis, 9th ed: American College of Chest Physicians Evidence-Based Clinical Practice Guidelines. Chest. 2012;141:e351S-e418S.

Beyer-Westendorf J, Ageno W. Benefit-risk profile of non-vitamin K antagonist oral anticoagulants in the management of venous thromboembolism. Thromb Haemost. 2015;113:231-246.

Castellucci LA, Cameron C, Le Gal G, et al. Efficacy and safety outcomes of oral anticoagulants and antiplatelet drugs in the secondary prevention of venous thromboembolism: a systematic review and meta-analysis. BMJ. 2013;347:f5133

Kearon C, Akl EA, Comerota AJ, et al. Antithrombotic therapy for VTE disease: antithrombotic therapy and prevention of thrombosis, 9th ed: American College of Chest Physicians Evidence-Based Clinical Practice Guidelines. Chest. 2012;141:e419S-e494S.

Konstantinides S, Torbicki A, Agnelli G, et al. 2014 ESC Guidelines on the diagnosis and management of acute pulmonary embolism. Euro Heart J. 2014;35:3033-3080.

Maccallum P, Bowles L, Keeling D. Diagnosis and management of heritable thrombophilias. Br Med J. 2014;349:g4387.

Marti C, John G, Konstantinides S, Combescure C, Sanchez O, Lankeit M, et al. Systemic thrombolytic therapy for acute pulmonary embolism: a systematic review and meta-analysis. Eur Heart J. 2015;7;36(10):605-614.

Takach Lapner S, Kearon C. Diagnosis and management of pulmonary embolism. Br Med J. 2013;346:f757.

CHAPTER 254

Anticoagulant Therapy

Katelyn W. Sylvester, PharmD, BCPS, CACP
John Fanikos, RPh, MBA
Jessica Rimsans, PharmD, BCPS

Key Clinical Questions

1. Why is a dosing nomogram important to use in UFH therapy?
2. What is the appropriate prophylaxis dose of LMWH in obese patients?
3. When may oral anticoagulation safely be initiated in a patient who has developed heparin-induced thrombocytopenia (HIT)?
4. How do you safely transition between parenteral anticoagulants and oral anticoagulants?
5. Should an initial loading dose be administered to patients receiving warfarin?

INTRODUCTION

Thrombosis is a major cause of morbidity, requires or prolongs hospital admission, and often necessitates long-term medical intervention to reduce the likelihood of recurrent events. Anticoagulants are the cornerstone for prevention and acute management of thrombosis. Despite their effectiveness in preventing thrombosis and reducing propagation, anticoagulants are often associated with adverse drug reactions and medication errors and remain a major target for health improvement efforts. While hospitalized patients are at risk for developing thrombosis, they are also at elevated risk for hemorrhagic complications resulting from invasive procedures, organ dysfunction, gastrointestinal stress-related mucosal damage, medication use, and concealed coagulopathies. Anticoagulation management requires thoughtful consideration in agent selection, route of administration, body weight, renal and hepatic function, and concomitant drug therapy to achieve optimal outcomes.

For over 50 years, unfractionated heparin (UFH) and vitamin K antagonists (VKAs) had been the primary anticoagulants prescribed in practice. A new group of oral anticoagulants has emerged in the marketplace with a wide range of indications, creating more options for clinicians, but also more challenges in drug and patient selection. This chapter focuses on the mechanisms of action, pharmacokinetics, pharmacodynamics, clinical indications, complications of therapy, and reversal options for antithrombotic pharmacotherapy in critically ill patients.

ANTICOAGULANT PHARMACOLOGY

Anticoagulant agents exert their therapeutic benefit by interfering with the coagulation cascade through receptor binding with circulating blood clotting factors. Of these clotting factors, thrombin (IIa) and activated factor X (Xa) are believed to play the most critical role in hemostasis. Anticoagulants ultimately attenuate thrombin generation, preventing the generation of insoluble fibrin, the final step in coagulation. Anticoagulants are administered in low doses for thromboprophylaxis and higher or therapeutic doses for acute thrombosis treatment.

Unfractionated heparin, low-molecular-weight heparin (LMWH), and fondaparinux contain a pentasaccharide sequence that binds to and potentiates the action of antithrombin (AT), an endogenous small protein molecule that inactivates several enzymes of the coagulation system (**Figure 254-1**). Fondaparinux is a synthetic analog of this naturally occurring pentasaccharide. The heparin-AT complex inactivates coagulation factors XIIa, IXa, XIa, Xa, and thrombin. Since these agents depend on the presence of AT for clotting factor inhibition, they are considered indirect anticoagulants. The active pentasaccharide sequence responsible for catalyzing AT is found on one-third and one-fifth of the chains of UFH and LMWH, respectively.

Vitamin K antagonists (eg, warfarin, acenocoumeral) inhibit the enzyme vitamin K epoxide reductase complex (VKORC), which converts vitamin K to an active form. In the absence of active vitamin K, hepatic production of factors thrombin, VII, IX, X, and the regulatory anticoagulant proteins C, S, and Z is reduced. Since warfarin does not directly inactivate functional clotting factors, it has a delayed onset of action.

The direct thrombin inhibitors (DTIs) (argatroban, bivalirudin, and dabigatran) and direct Xa inhibitors (rivaroxaban, apixaban, and

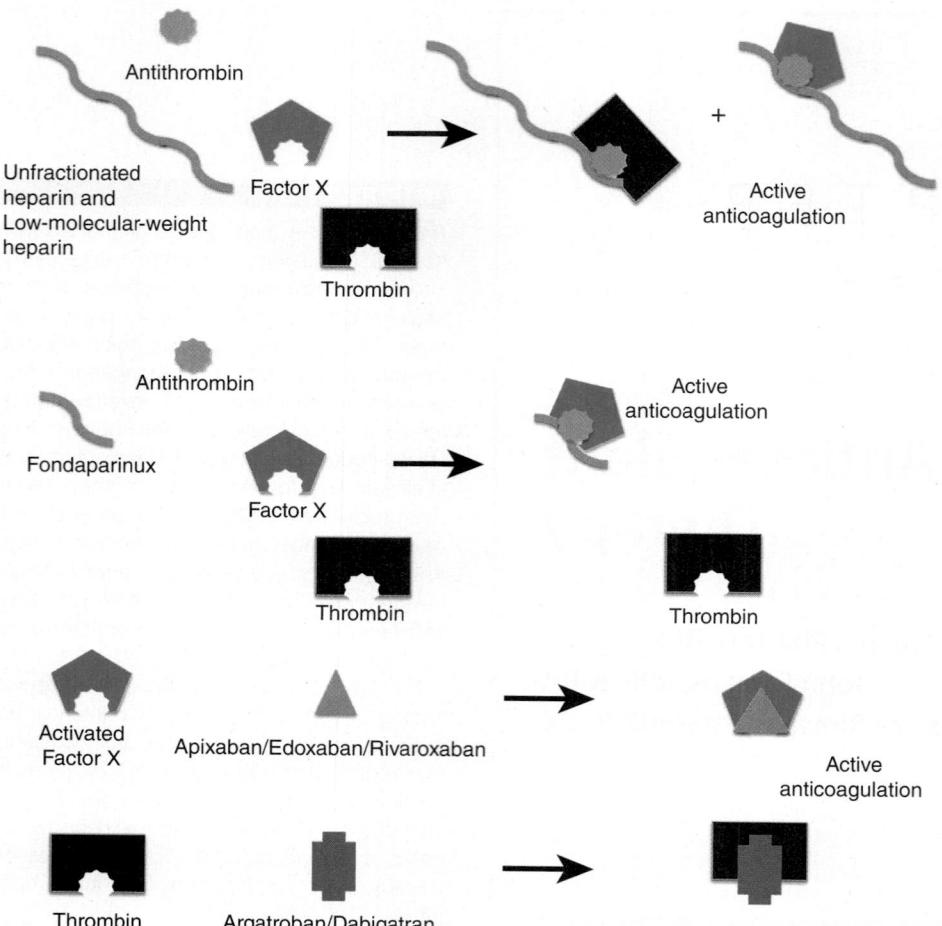

Figure 254-1 *Mechanisms of oral and parenteral anticoagulants.*

edoxaban) have a specific mechanism of action. They bind directly to the surface of thrombin or Xa, and prevent further contributions to enzymatic activity and thrombus formation. The oral agents have collectively been referred to as nonvitamin K oral anticoagulants (NOACs), direct acting oral anticoagulants (DOACs), or target-specific oral anticoagulants (TSOACs).

INDIRECT ACTING ANTICOAGULANTS—PARENTERAL AGENTS

■ UNFRACTIONATED HEPARIN

Pharmacodynamics and monitoring

Heparin is derived from porcine intestines and structurally consists of highly sulfated, linked disaccharide chains that vary in size and length. UFH is poorly absorbed orally; therefore intravenous (IV) or subcutaneous (SC) injections are the only options for administration. Due to erratic bioavailability, SC doses of UFH for therapeutic anticoagulation must be >30,000 units/d. Intravenously administered UFH readily binds to plasma proteins. These features contribute to UFH's highly variable dose response and the need for frequent laboratory monitoring. UFH is eliminated from systemic circulation through two independent mechanisms: at low doses by binding to endothelial cells, macrophages, and circulating proteins ultimately leading to UFH depolymerization, and at higher doses UFH is eliminated through a slower, renal-mediated clearance. Large doses or prolonged UFH administration provides a disproportionate increase

in both the intensity and duration of anticoagulant effect. The half-life of UFH with therapeutic IV doses is approximately 60 minutes.

The anticoagulant response to UFH is monitored using the activated partial thromboplastin time (aPTT), a measurement sensitive to the inhibitory effects of thrombin. The aPTT should be measured every 6 hours, and doses adjusted accordingly, until the patient maintains therapeutic levels. While the therapeutic range for the aPTT, 1.5 to 2.5 times the control value, has become widely accepted, the evidence supporting this range for predicting thrombotic or bleeding events is weak. Once two consecutive aPTT values are within therapeutic range, testing may be extended to once-daily. Weight-based dosing nomograms, comprised of a weight-based bolus dose and infusion rate with periodic monitoring utilizing aPTT, are recommended for treatment of thromboembolic disease (**Table 254-1**). UFH dosing nomograms differ between hospitals due to differences in thromboplastin reagents, calibration, and inter-laboratory standards in aPTT measurements. This has led to assessments of alternative monitoring strategies. The functional heparin assay, also known as the anti-Xa assay, has been promoted as a more favorable marker for monitoring a patient's response to UFH. Unlike aPTT, this assay is insensitive to factors other than UFH (eg, concomitant warfarin use, sodium citrate in collection tubes, interference from the presence of lupus anticoagulants, elevated factor VIII activity, and liver disease). Weight-based UFH protocols utilizing anti-Xa levels to monitor UFH are now in use in many hospitals.

TABLE 254-1 Heparin Dose-Adjustment Nomogram Examples

Acute-Coronary Syndromes		Venous Thromboembolism		Venous Thromboembolism	
Assay result (aPTT in seconds)	Dose adjustment	Assay result (aPTT in seconds)	Dose adjustment	Assay result (antifactor Xa concentration in units/mL)	Dose adjustment
Initial dose	60 units/kg bolus, then 12 units/kg/h	Initial dose	80 units/kg bolus, then 18 units/kg/h	Initial dose	26 units/kg bolus, then 15 units/kg/h
aPTT <1× control	60 units/kg bolus, then increase 2 units/kg/h	aPTT <35 s	80 units/kg bolus, then increase 4 units/kg/h	<0.20	26 units/kg bolus, then increase by 4 units/kg/h
aPTT 1 to 1.5× control	Increase 2 units/kg/h	aPTT 35-45 s	40 units/kg bolus, then increase 2 units/kg/h	0.20-0.29	No bolus, Increase by 2 units/kg/h
aPTT 1.5 to 2× control	No change	aPTT 46-70 s	No change	0.30-0.70	No change
aPTT 2 to 3× control	Decrease infusion rate by 2 units/kg/h	aPTT 71-90 s	Decrease infusion rate by 2 units/kg/h	0.71-0.80	Decrease by 1 unit/kg/h
aPTT >3× control	Stop infusion, recheck aPTT, start treatment again based on repeat aPTT	aPTT >90 s	Hold infusion for 1 h, then decrease infusion rate by 3 units/kg/h	0.81-0.99	Decrease by 2 units/kg/h
aPTT=activated partial thromboplastin time, kg=kilograms				≥1.00	Hold infusion for 1 h, then decrease by 3 units/kg/h

Adapted from Braunwald E, Antman EA, Beasley JW, et al. ACC/AHA guidelines for the management of patients with unstable angina, and non-ST-segment elevation myocardial infarction. *J Am Coll Cardiol.* 2000;36:970-1062.

Adapted from Raschke R, Gollihare B, Peirce J. The effectiveness of implementing the weight-based heparin nomogram as a practice guideline. *Arch Intern Med.*1996;156:1645-1649.

Adapted from Smith ML, Wheeler KE. Weight-based heparin protocol using antifactor Xa monitoring. *Am J Health-Syst Pharm.* 2010;67:371-374.

PRACTICE POINT

UFH nomograms are designed for specific patients at specific facilities to reduce the time to therapeutic anticoagulation while reducing the risk of thrombus propagation and bleeding.

- Fixed-dose heparin regimens (ie, 5000 unit bolus, 1000 units/h infusion) fail to achieve a minimum aPTT rapidly in venous thromboembolism (VTE).
- Patients with VTE require higher UFH doses than those with acute coronary syndromes (ACSs).
- The combination of UFH and dual or triple antiplatelet therapy for acute coronary syndromes increases the risk of major bleeding. Therefore, a UFH nomogram designed for VTE might lead to over anticoagulation in patients with ACS.
- To enhance UFH predictability, institution-specific nomograms help control for variability in laboratory reagents, instrumentation, and sample collection. These nomograms may also distinguish between thrombus locations (venous vs arterial), procedural interventions (ablation versus coronary), and quantitative differences in thrombus burden.

Medical uses

Medical indications for UFH include treatment of ACS, treatment or prevention of venous thromboembolism (VTE), and bridge therapy to chronic oral anticoagulation for atrial fibrillation, cardioversion, or invasive surgical procedure (**Table 252-2**). Due to UFH's short half-life and reversibility, it remains the best anticoagulant option in patients with bleeding risk or organ dysfunction. When used for thromboprophylaxis in medical patients, three times daily UFH dosing provides better efficacy in reducing VTE events compared to twice daily dosing, but generates more major bleeding episodes.

Complications of therapy and reversal

The major adverse drug events associated with UFH therapy include bleeding (major bleeding, 0%-7%; fatal bleeding, 0%-3%), heparin-induced thrombocytopenia (HIT) (1%-5%), and osteoporosis (2%-3% risk of vertebral fracture with less than 1 month of treatment). Hemorrhagic episodes are associated with anticoagulation intensity, route of administration (continuous infusions are associated with lower rates), and concomitant use of P2Y12 and GP IIb/IIIa platelet inhibitors, aspirin, or fibrinolytic agents. Patient-specific risk factors for bleeding include age, gender, renal insufficiency, low body weight, and excessive alcohol consumption.

Treatment of UFH-related bleeding includes protamine sulfate administration, transfusion, and supportive care. Protamine binds to UFH to form a stable salt, rendering it pharmacologically inactive. Protamine dosing is dependent on timing of the last UFH dose. For immediate reversal (<30 minutes since the last heparin dose), 1 mg of protamine is administered for every 100 units of UFH and a follow-up aPTT can evaluate the reversal response. When UFH is given as a continuous IV infusion, only UFH delivered during the preceding 2 to 2.5 hours should be included in the calculation to determine the protamine dose. If the dose of UFH is unknown, the maximal tolerated protamine dose of 50 mg may be slowly administered followed by serial measurements of aPTT. Protamine is cleared rapidly from the plasma; therefore, repeated doses may be necessary to prevent rebound UFH anticoagulant effects. Adverse reactions, such as systemic hypotension, pulmonary hypertension, and bradycardia, are common. However, reaction frequency and severity may be reduced by slowly administering protamine over 1 to 3 minutes. Allergic responses to protamine are more common in patients who have been previously exposed to the drug, but patients may be pretreated with corticosteroids and antihistamines.

TABLE 254-2 Unfractionated Heparin Clinical Uses

Agent	Indication	Dose	Surveillance
Unfractionated heparin	VTE treatment	LD: 80 units/kg bolus 18 units/kg/h infusion adjusted per local heparin nomogram Target aPTT, 70s (range 60-80 s) Target Antifactor Xa, 0.3-0.7 units/mL	Monitoring • aPTT every 6 h until therapeutic and then at least once daily • Antifactor Xa levels every 6 h and after each rate change • Complete blood count, repeat every 3-5 d during therapy • HIT antibody testing for thrombocytopenia, thrombosis, heparin-induced skin lesions, or other signs pointing to a potential diagnosis of immune-mediated response
	ACS treatment	LD: 60 units/kg (maximum 4000 units) 12 units/kg/h (maximum initial dosing 1000 units/h) specific adjusted to maintain aPTT 1.5-2 times control or per local heparin nomogram Target aPTT, 60s (range 50-70 s) Target Antifactor Xa, 0.3-0.7 units/mL	Precautions • Prior allergic or hypersensitivity-type reactions • Congenital or acquired bleeding disorders • Gastrointestinal ulceration and ongoing tube drainage of the small intestine or stomach
	Bridge therapy to oral anticoagulation for atrial fibrillation, cardioversion, invasive procedure	IV infusion: 80 units/kg bolus 18 units/kg/h infusion adjusted per local heparin nomogram Target aPTT, 70s (range 60-80 s) Target Antifactor Xa, 0.3-0.7 units/mL	• Hepatic disease with altered baseline coagulation assays • Hereditary antithrombin III deficiency and concurrent use of antithrombin
	Prophylaxis of VTE in the medically ill or surgical population	5000 units SC Q8-12 h No routine monitoring	Contraindications • Severe thrombocytopenia • Positive assay for immune mediated HIT • Patients within a remote history of HIT (>100 d) could be considered for a rechallenge with heparin provided a negative antibody test

ACS, acute-coronary syndromes; aPTT, activated partial thromboplastin time; HIT, heparin-induced thrombocytopenia; LD, loading dose; SC, subcutaneous; VTE, venous thromboembolism.

Heparin-induced thrombocytopenia (HIT) is an immune-mediated, hypercoagulable adverse event resulting from antibodies formed against the heparin-platelet factor 4 complex. The incidence ranges from 0.3% to 0.5% of patients. It is associated with thrombocytopenia and life-threatening thrombosis in antibody-positive patients. HIT and heparin-induced thrombocytopenia with thrombosis syndrome (HITTS) typically occur in patients who have been exposed to UFH or LMWH for 5 to 7 days, or even sooner in patients with prior exposure within the past 100 days. A 50% decrease in platelet count occurring 4 to 10 days after the initiation of UFH or LMWH therapy, formation of a new thrombus during therapy, and skin lesions at the injection site may be indicative of HIT. Platelet counts should be measured prior to the initiation of UFH or LMWH and monitored every other day for the first 4 to 10 days of therapy. The use of an alternative anticoagulant, such as direct thrombin inhibitors (argatroban or bivalirudin) or fondaparinux, must be used in patients with HIT. If the patient is also receiving warfarin, this medication should be discontinued. Warfarin inhibits production of the endogenous anticoagulants proteins C and S. Protein C inhibition occurs rapidly and may result in a transient hypercoagulable state. When coupled with HIT mediated thrombin production, patients at high risk for microvascular arterial and venous thrombosis and resultant limb gangrene (**Figure 254-2**).

■ LOW-MOLECULAR-WEIGHT HEPARINS

Pharmacodynamics and monitoring

Low-molecular weight heparins are produced through chemical or enzymatic depolymerization of UFH. While the LMWH molecules contain the active pentasaccharides that catalyzes AT inhibition of factor Xa, their smaller size reduces affinity for plasma proteins and cellular binding sites. This results in increased bioavailability after SC injection, elimination through renal clearance, and a longer half-life (17-21 hours) when compared to UFH (**Table 254-3**). LMWHs are administered in fixed doses for thromboprophylaxis or in total body weight-adjusted doses for therapeutic anticoagulation. Peak anticoagulant activity is rapid, occurring within 3 to 5 hours after injection. While laboratory monitoring is usually not necessary, anti-Xa monitoring is often performed in high-risk patient populations, such as pregnancy, obesity, and renal dysfunction. In these cases, peak anti-Xa plasma levels are drawn 4 hours after administration, and subsequent doses are adjusted to a target range of 0.5 to 1.1 IU/mL. Trough levels can be assessed to determine patient compliance and direction for scheduled or urgent surgical procedures.

While standardized prophylaxis or treatment doses of LMWHs can be used in most patients without dose adjustment, the appropriate dosing of LMWHs in obese patients remains unclear. Patients with extremes of body weight are rarely enrolled in pharmacokinetic or clinical trials that shape drug dosing. Pharmacokinetic studies suggest that patients at extremes of body weight may not reach adequate anti-Xa levels. Retrospective analyses of LMWH-VTE prophylaxis trials have found a relationship between body mass index (BMI) and thrombosis. When evaluating subgroups of medically ill patients, LMWH administration in obese patients (BMI >40kg/m^2) showed no reduction in VTE. In orthopedic surgery, obese patients treated with LMWH had higher thrombosis rates compared with nonobese patients. In bariatric surgery, a higher dose of LMWH was more effective in reducing VTE.

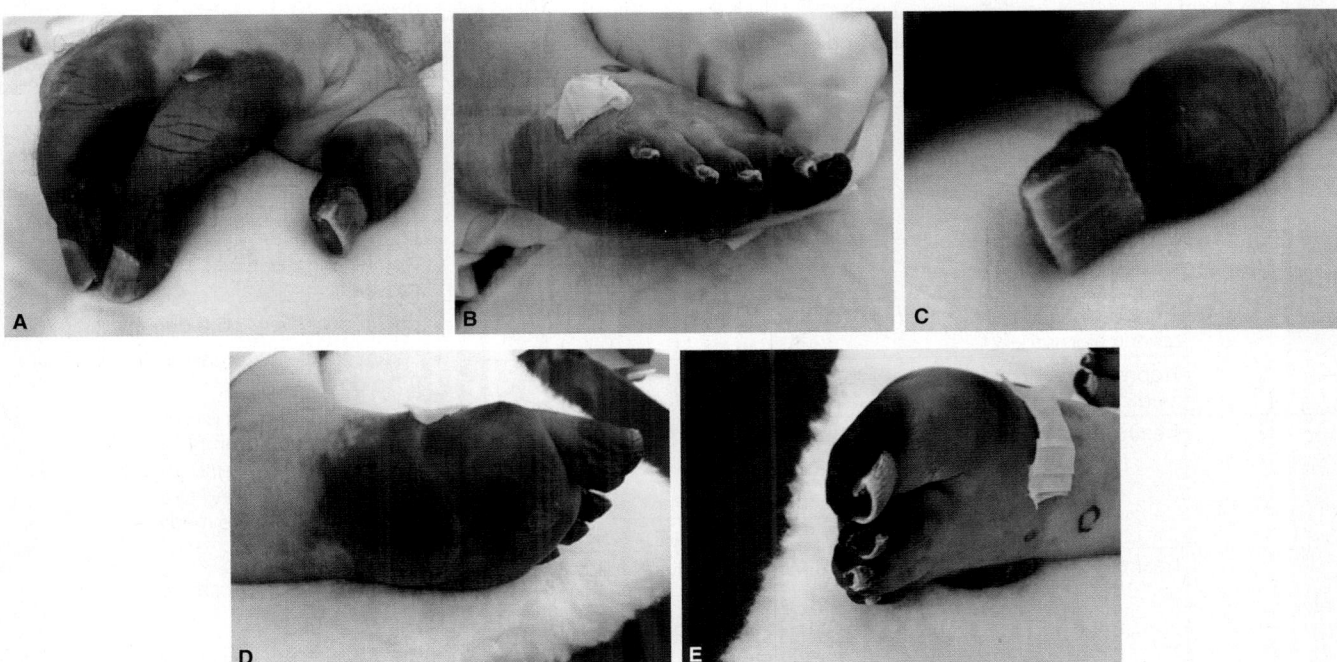

Figure 254-2 *Sequelae of heparin-induced thrombocytopenia: microvascular thrombosis.*

Pharmacokinetic studies with LMWH suggest that weight-based dosing of LMWH for treatment of VTE should be based on total body weight and that capping weight–based doses in obese patients is inappropriate. Registry data of LMWH-treated patients with acute VTE showed no significant differences between obese and non-obese patients in rates of recurrent VTE or major bleeding. Subgroup analysis of LMWH use in patients with acute coronary syndromes showed comparable rates of the composite endpoint (death, MI, urgent revascularization) in obese compared to nonobese patients. However, in another similar trial where enoxaparin doses were capped at 10,000 units every 12 hours patients weighing more than 76 kg had a higher incidence of the composite endpoint (death and MI) than those weighing less than 76 kg. Based on these findings, experts now recommend that LMWH dosing should be based on total body weight for the treatment of obese patients. Capping of LMWH doses does not appear to be needed in the treatment of

VTE and clinicians should follow specific product recommendations when using LMWH in acute coronary syndromes.

Medical uses

Double blind randomized-controlled trials have shown the benefit of LMWH thromboprophylaxis over placebo in reducing VTE in hospitalized acutely ill medical patients (**Table 254-4**). While the duration of hospital-administered prophylaxis in these trials ranged from 6 to 14 days, the optimal duration remains unclear.

Low-molecular weight heparins require fewer injections and produce fewer adverse events compared to SC UFH. In hospitalized medical patients receiving thromboprophylaxis, LMWHs were associated with a lower risk of deep vein thrombosis (DVT), fewer injection site hematomas, and no difference in bleeding when compared with UFH. A recent study showed a reduction in pulmonary embolism (PE) rates with LMWH compared to UFH VTE prophylaxis

TABLE 254-3 Comparison of the Pharmacodynamic Features of Unfractionated Heparin, Low Molecular Weight Heparin, and Fondaparinux

Feature	Unfractionated Heparin	LMWH	Fondaparinux
Source	Biological, porcine	Biological, porcine	Synthetic
Molecular weight (Daltons)	15,000	5000	1500
Route of administration	IV, SC	IV, SC	SC
Target binding preference	Xa:IIa	Xa >IIa	Xa
Subcutaneous bioavailability (%)	30	90	100
Half-life (h)	1	4	17
Renal excretion	Minor	Major	Major
Routine therapeutic monitoring	Yes	No	No
Monitoring assay	aPTT, Antifactor Xa levels	Antifactor Xa levels	Antifactor Xa levels
Antidote	Complete	Partial	None
Incidence of HIT (%)	<5	<1	Anecdotal reports

HIT, heparin-induced thrombocytopenia; IV, intravenous; LMWH, low-molecular-weight heparin SC, subcutaneous.

TABLE 254-4 Low-Molecular-Weight Heparin and Fondaparinux Clinical Uses

Agent	Indication	Dose	Surveillance
Dalteparin (Fragmin©)	Treatment of VTE	<56 kg: 10,000 IU SC daily 57-68 kg: 12,500 IU SC daily 83-98 kg: 18,000 IU SC daily >99 kg: 18,000 IU SC daily	**Monitoring** • Anti-Xa levels should be measured in patients with; renal impairment, bleeding or abnormal coagulation parameters, pregnancy, obesity patients, low-body weight, and those with mechanical prosthetic heart valves.
	Treatment of ACS	120 IU/kg SC Q12 h (maximum 10,000 IU/dose)	
	Prophylaxis of VTE after hip or other major surgery	5000 IU SC Q24 h	• CBC, repeat every 3-5 d during therapy
	Prophylaxis of VTE in the medically ill	5000 IU SC Q24 h	• Serum creatinine for assessment of renal function
Enoxaparin (Lovenox©)	Treatment of VTE	1 mg/kg SC Q12 h OR 1.5 mg/kg SC Q24 h CrCl <30 mL/min: 1 mg/kg SC Q24 h	• HIT antibody testing is warranted in the presence of thrombocytopenia, thrombosis, heparin-induced skin lesions, or other signs pointing to a potential diagnosis of immune mediated response.
	Treatment of ACS	STEMI: 30 mg bolus IV followed by 1 mg/kg SC Q12 h + fibrinolytic NSTEMI/UA: 1 mg/kg SC Q12 h CrCl <30mL/min: not recommended	**Precautions** • Indwelling epidural catheter • Recent surgery
	Prophylaxis/bridge therapy for atrial fibrillation/cardioversion/invasive procedure*	1 mg/kg SC Q12 h OR 1.5 mg/kg SC Q24 h CrCl <30 mL/min: 1 mg/kg SC Q24	• History of recent major bleed (GI, intracranial, etc) • Congenital or acquired bleeding disorders
	Prophylaxis of VTE in the medically ill	40 mg SC Q24h CrCl <30 mL/min: 1 mg/kg SC daily	• LMWH: Renal impairment (CrCl <30 mL/min) • Concomitant use of aspirin or antiplatelet drugs
	Prophylaxis of VTE after hip or other major surgery, or in the trauma patients ill, or abdominal surgical population	40 mg SC Q24 h OR 30 mg SC Q12 h	**Contraindications** • Active bleeding • Positive test for immune mediated HIT
Tinzaparin (Innohep©)	Treatment of DVT	175 IU anti-Xa/kg SC daily	• Patients within a remote history of HIT (>100 d) Fondaparinux:
Fondaparinux (Arixtra©)	Treatment of VTE	<50 kg: 5.0 mg SC daily 50 to 100 kg: 7.5 mg SC daily >100 mg kg: 10 mg SC daily Renal impairment CrCL less than 30 mL/min contraindicated	– Renal impairment (CrCl <30 mL/min), contraindicated – Body weight (<50 kg) contraindicated for thromboprophylaxis
	Treatment of STEMI and NSTEMI*	2.5 mg SC daily	
	Prophylaxis of VTE in orthopedic surgery, major surgery and acute medically ill patients	2.5 mg SC daily	

ACS, acute-coronary syndromes; CrCl, creatinine clearance; CBC, complete blood count; DVT, deep vein thrombosis; HIT, heparin induced thrombocytopenia; MI, NSTEMI, non-ST segment elevation myocardial infarction; STEMI, ST segment elevation myocardial infarction; SC, subcutaneous; VTE, venous thromboembolism.
*Non-FDA approved use.

in critically ill hospitalized patients. However, another study comparing LMWH plus graduated compression stockings as compared with graduated compression stockings alone was not associated with a reduction in the rate of death from any cause among hospitalized, acutely ill medical patients. Another analysis evaluating UFH and LMWH thromboprophylaxis in hospitalized medical patients and those with acute stroke showed no impact on mortality and more bleeding events. Professional societies and national guidelines advocate VTE and bleeding risk assessment prior to initiating anticoagulant thromboprophylaxis to facilitate identifying patients most likely to benefit.

In acute VTE, the outcomes of recurrent VTE and major bleeding episodes were similar with UFH and LMWH. LMWHs have largely replaced IV UFH in patients with acute VTE who are able to receive unmonitored, self-administered anticoagulation in the ambulatory setting. UFH remains the preferred option for ACS patients, those who may require an urgent surgical intervention, those with compromised renal function, or those requiring intensive monitoring for other reasons (see Chapter 253 [Diagnosis and Treatment of VTE]).

Complications of therapy and reversal

While major bleeding episodes are reported to occur in 0% to 3% of LMWH treated patients, data suggest hemorrhage rates are lower when compared to UFH. In the setting of overdose or hemorrhage, protamine only partially reverses LMWH anticoagulation, inhibiting approximately 60% of the anti-Xa activity. Protamine dose recommendations depend on the LMWH in use. For enoxaparin reversal within 8 hours of administration, 1 mg of protamine is administered IV to neutralize 1 mg of enoxaparin. If the enoxaparin was administered more than 8 hours ago, 0.5 mg of protamine per 1 mg of enoxaparin may be administered. A second dose of 0.5 mg of protamine per 1 mg of enoxaparin may be administered if bleeding continues or if the aPTT measured 2 to 4 hours after the initial dose remains prolonged. For dalteparin and tinzaparin reversal, protamine 1 mg is administered IV to neutralize every 100 anti-Xa units of the LMWH administered. If aPTT remains prolonged 2 to 4 hours after initial administration, a second dose of 0.5 mg of protamine per 100 anti-Xa units of LMWH may be administered.

Osteoporosis and HIT occur less frequently in patients treated with LMWHs as compared to UFH.

■ FONDAPARINUX

Pharmacodynamics and monitoring

Fondaparinux is a synthetic analog of the naturally occurring pentasaccharide found in UFH. Fondaparinux, after SC administration, has a long half-life, extending from 17 to 21 hours in patients with normal renal function (Table 254-3). Fondaparinux is renally excreted with elimination reduced in patients with renal impairment. While fondaparinux monitoring is not required on a routine basis the management of certain high-risk patients may benefit from measurement of anticoagulant activity. Because of differences in molecular size and affinity for factor Xa, anti-Xa assays established for LMWH are not accurate for monitoring fondaparinux therapy. Typically local anti-Xa assay, calibrated to fondaparinux, are required.

Medical uses

Fondaparinux has shown to be as effective and safe as LMWH and UFH for the treatment of acute DVT and PE (Table 254-4). It was superior to placebo in reducing VTE in older (>60 years) acutely ill medical patients with no increase in bleeding episodes. However,

while fondaparinux showed superior efficacy in reducing VTE in patients undergoing knee arthroplasty, hip arthroplasty, and hip fracture surgery in a combined analysis, the overall incidence of major bleeding was statistically higher when compared with LMWH. Major bleeding in both hospitalized surgical and medical patients is a strong predictor of 30-day mortality. Fondaparinux has been used in the treatment of HIT, but evidence is limited and conclusive data to support routine practice are unavailable.

Complications of therapy and reversal

Fondaparinux is contraindicated in patients with severe renal impairment (calculated creatinine clearance <30 mL per minute) and should not be used for VTE thromboprophylaxis in patients weighing less than 50 kg. No antidote exists to reverse fondaparinux anticoagulant activity. Fondaparinux-related hemorrhage treatment is complicated by its prolonged half-life. Recombinant factor VIIa (rVIIa) reverses the coagulation parameters induced by fondaparinux, but the clinical benefit is unknown.

INDIRECT ACTING ANTICOAGULANTS-ORAL AGENTS

■ VITAMIN K ANTAGONISTS

Pharmacodynamics and monitoring

Warfarin is extensively metabolized by the hepatic cytochrome P450 isoenzyme system (CYP450) with multiple genetic polymorphisms influencing warfarin dose and duration of action. Patients with reduced enzymatic activity have slower warfarin metabolism and decreased warfarin clearance. They require lower warfarin maintenance doses and often require a longer period to reach steady-state. Likewise, mutations in the gene that code for VKORC lead to increased warfarin sensitivity or warfarin resistance. Altered vitamin K dietary intake impacts the anticoagulation effect of warfarin. Concurrent medication administration frequently impacts warfarin dosing. Warfarin-drug interactions may alter warfarin absorption, metabolism, and plasma protein binding, producing an enhanced or reduced anticoagulant effect. The International Normalized Ratio (INR) is used to measure warfarin's anticoagulant effect. Intense INR monitoring during the early initiation of warfarin administration will typically will reveal a patient's sensitivity or insensitivity to therapy. The INR target range will vary based on indication and the patient's thromboembolic risk and bleeding risk (**Table 254-5**). The established ranges have been shown to maximize benefit (ie, reducing thrombosis) while minimizing risk (ie, risk of hemorrhage attributable to excessive anticoagulation). Warfarin dosing nomograms have been employed to reduce the time required to reach therapeutic range and to avoid critically high INR values. The time in therapeutic INR range (TTR) summarizes INR control over time and is used to evaluate the effectiveness of warfarin therapy. The greater the percentage of time spent in the therapeutic range, the higher the quality of warfarin dose management.

Parenteral anticoagulation is stopped and warfarin monotherapy continued when the INR is therapeutic for two consecutive measurements. A goal of warfarin therapy is minimize the time to a therapeutic INR. This reduces inconvenience of parenteral LMWH or UFH administration and the cost of therapy. Warfarin dosing nomograms facilitate safe and timely warfarin initiation and have been found to be superior to empiric clinician dosing. Nomograms using both warfarin 5- and 10-mg loading doses have been evaluated. In one study, patients who received a 10-mg loading dose, with INR assessments on days 3 and 5 during the first 8 days of therapy, achieved a therapeutic INR (>1.9) more rapidly, were more likely to have a therapeutic INR by day 5 of parenteral anticoagulant therapy.

TABLE 254-5 Clinical Uses of Vitamin K Antagonist

Drug	Indication	International Normalized Ratio	Surveillance
Warfarin (Coumadin©)	Treatment of VTE	INR: 2.0-3.0; target of 2.5	Monitoring
	Atrial fibrillation	INR: 2.0-3.0; target of 2.5	• INR
	Rheumatic mitral valve disease, normal sinus rhythm, and left atrial diameter >55 mm	INR: 2.0-3.0; target of 2.5	• Signs of bleeding • CBC Precautions • Lower initial dosing (<5mg may be warranted in patients who are elderly, debilitated, malnourished, or with comorbidities) ○ CHF
	High-risk patients after myocardial infarction	INR: 2.0-3.0; target of 2.5	○ Hepatic disease ○ Renal impairment ○ CYP2C9 and VKORC genetic variation
	Mechanical valve in the atrial position	INR: 2.0-3.0; target of 2.5	• Thrombocytopenia • Protein C, S deficiency
	Mechanical valve in the mitral position	INR: 2.5-3.5; target of 3.0	• Recent surgery or trauma • Epidural catheters
	Mechanical valve in both the atrial and mitral position	INR: 2.5-3.5; target of 3.0	• Dietary interactions ○ Excessive or deficiencies of dietary vitamin K • Drug interactions
	Bioprosthetic valve in the mitral position	INR: 2.0-3.0; target of 2.5 × 3 mo	○ Antibiotic therapy ○ Antiplatelet therapy ○ Antiarrhythmics Contraindications • Pregnancy • Active bleeding the gastrointestinal, genitourinary, or respiratory tract • Cerebrovascular hemorrhage

CBC, complete blood count; CHF, congestive heart failure; CYP2C9, cytochrome p450 isoenzyme 2C9; INR, international normalized ratio; VKORC, vitamin K epoxide reductase complex; VTE, venous thromboembolism.

PRACTICE POINT

Warfarin

- The 10-mg loading dose nomogram is advantageous for warfarin management because it does not require daily INR testing used with the 5 mg nomogram. Only two INR assessments are required in the first 7 days of warfarin therapy (after the baseline assessment). It also reduces the number of patients requiring more than 5 days of parenteral therapy

---

Medical uses

Warfarin is effective for primary and secondary prevention of venous thromboembolism, for prevention of systemic embolism in patients with prosthetic heart valves or atrial fibrillation, and for prevention of stroke, recurrent infarction, or death in patients with acute myocardial infarction.

Complications and reversal of effect

The incidence of major bleeding episodes depends on indication for warfarin use. Major bleeding occurs in approximately 2% to 3% of patients per year during the treatment of venous thromboembolism. In contemporary atrial fibrillation trials of stroke prevention, patients taking oral VKAs had reported major bleeding rates ranging from 1.4% to 3.5% per year. Important risk factors for hemorrhage include anticoagulant intensity, time within therapeutic range, and patient age with the risk of anticoagulant-related bleeding highest at the beginning of therapy.

An elevated INR without active bleeding may be managed by withholding warfarin therapy, decreasing the dose, or extending the administration interval (**Table 254-6**). In patients with bleeding or at risk of bleeding, vitamin K administration will reverse the anticoagulant effects of warfarin. Vitamin K is given orally or parenterally. Correction of INR is fastest with the IV route compared to oral administration, with both faster and more complete than subcutaneous administration. In the setting of serious or life-threatening hemorrhage, warfarin should be held and vitamin K dosing up to 10 mg should be administered by slow IV infusion. Patients receiving vitamin K doses >5 mg may become resistant to warfarin for up to a week following administration, thereby prolonging the time to therapeutic INR in patients reinitiating therapy. The prothrombin complex concentrates (PCCs) are preferred to fresh frozen plasma (FFP) in cases of severe bleeding or where immediate reversal of the INR is necessary. PCC's are faster to administer and require less fluid volume when compared to FFP. Anticoagulation has been reversed using rVIIa in a small number of patients with refractory bleeding; however, risk of prothrombotic events such as stroke and myocardial infarction limit its use to life threatening bleeds.

Other adverse events of warfarin include acute skin and tissue necrosis, calcification of the aortic valve and coronary arteries with long-term use and feelings of cold or chills.

DIRECT ACTING ANTICOAGULANTS

■ DIRECT THROMBIN INHIBITORS

Pharmacodynamics and monitoring

Direct thrombin inhibitors include IV argatroban and bivalirudin, and oral dabigatran. While bivalirudin is a peptide produced from leech

TABLE 254-6 Reversal Strategies for Warfarin

Agents	Intervention

Warfarin (Coumadin©)	**INR 4.5-10 (no signs of bleeding)**
	• Omit 1-2 doses then resume when INR is within therapeutic range
	INR >10 (no signs of bleeding)
	• Vitamin K; 1-2.5 mg orally
	Surgery within 24 h:
	• Stop warfarin
	• Vitamin K 2.5-5 mg IV
	Surgery within 24 h:
	• Stop warfarin
	• Vitamin K <5 mg orally
	  ○ If INR is elevated after 24 hours give an additional 1-2 mg
	Urgent surgery or invasive procedure:
	• Four factor PCC (Kcentra)
	• Vitamin K 10 mg IV
	Severe or life threatening bleed:
	• Stop warfarin therapy
	• Preferred: Four factor PCC (Kcentra*)
	  ○ INR <4 = 25 units/kg
	  ○ INR 4-6 = 35 units/kg
	  ○ INR >6 = 50 units/kg
	  ○ Maximum dosing weight = 100 kg
	• Vitamin K 10 mg IV
	• Alternative: FFP 15-30 mL/kg
	• Consider administering three factor PCC 25-50 units/kg if four factor PCC unavailable OR rVIIa 10-90 µg/kg IV (if no PCC available) as alterative or adjunct therapy

FFP, fresh frozen plasma; INR, International Normalized Ratio; PCC, prothrombin complex concentrates; rVIIa, recombinant human factor 7a.
*Contraindicated in history of HIT/HITT.

salivary glands, argatroban is synthetic molecule derived from the amino acid arginine. Dabigatran etexilate is an oral small molecule prodrug with low bioavailability. The capsule formulation should not be opened or crushed because bioavailability is dramatically increased. After oral administration it is converted to its active form, dabigatran. The DTIs differ in their pharmacodynamic properties (**Table 254-7**). Bivalirudin has the shortest half-life, making it a particularly useful agent in the procedural or periprocedural period.

DTI prescribing is based on patient-specific characteristics such as hepatic function, and renal function. Critically ill patients typically require lower doses than those recommended by the manufacturer. Intravenous DTIs are monitored using aPTT measured every 4 to 6 hours until therapeutic levels are maintained, at which point the monitoring frequency may be extended. Intravenous and oral DTIs prolong the INR. This interaction is most pronounced with argatroban, and magnified when coadministered with warfarin. With concurrent warfarin administration, argatroban must be stopped and, for an accurate assessment, the INR measured within 4 to 6 hours. If the INR is within therapeutic range, warfarin monotherapy may be continued; otherwise argatroban therapy should be reinitiated. This process should be repeated daily until the desired therapeutic range on warfarin alone is reached.

Similar to the IV DTI's, dabigatran prolongs the aPTT and the INR. While ecarin clotting time (ECT) or thrombin time (TT) may be useful laboratory tests for monitoring coagulation, no recommendations exist to guide therapy.

Medical uses

Argatroban significantly reduces thromboembolic complications (death, new thrombosis, and amputations) in patients with HIT. Bivalirudin has been safely used in critically ill HIT patients. DTI therapy is continued in HIT patients until platelet count returns to normal (platelets >150 x 10^9/L) or to baseline values. Platelet recovery signifies a reduction in antibody mediated platelet activation and thrombin generation, creating the window for initiating oral anticoagulation.

Argatroban and bivalirudin are indicated for prophylaxis of thrombosis in patients with, or at risk for, HIT undergoing PCI. Bivalirudin is also indicated in the treatment of patients undergoing PCI as well as those with unstable angina/non-ST segment elevation myocardial infarction undergoing PCI (**Table 254-8**).

TABLE 254-7 Comparison of the Pharmacodynamic Features of Direct Thrombin Inhibitors

Feature	Dabigatran	Argatroban	Bivalirudin
Molecular weight (Daltons)	628	526	2180
FDA-approved indication	Stroke prevention in nonvalvular AF; VTE treatment after 5-10 d of parenteral therapy	Management of HIT, or use in patients with HIT who are undergoing PCI	Use in patients with or at risk for HIT or HITTS who are undergoing PCI
Bioavailability	3%-7%	N/A	N/A
Primary elimination route	Renal	Hepatic	Enzymatic
Elimination half-life	12-17 h	39-51 min	10-24 min
Fraction eliminated unchanged by kidney (%)	80	16	20
P-glycoprotein interaction	Yes	No	No
Laboratory test to monitor	aPTT, ECT, TT	aPTT, ECT	aPTT, ACT, ECT
Target range	N/A	aPTT: 1.5-3 × control	aPTT: 1.5-2.5 × control
Effects on INR	Minimal-to-moderate	Moderate-to-clinically significant	Minimal-to-moderate

ACT, activated clotting time; AF, atrial fibrillation; Aptt, activated partial thromboplastin time; ECT, ecarin clotting time; FDA, Food and Drug Administration; HIT, heparin-induced thrombocytopenia; HITTS, HIT with thrombosis syndrome; INR, international normalized ratio; N/A, not applicable; PCI, percutaneous coronary intervention; TT, Thrombin time; VTE, venous thromboembolism.

TABLE 254-8 Direct Thrombin Inhibitor Clinical Uses

Agent	Indication	Dose	Surveillance

Argatroban	Prophylaxis and treatment of thrombosis in patients with HIT	0.5-1.2 µg/kg/min continuous IV infusion to start titration to goal aPTT between 50-85 s
		
		Begin VKA therapy, measure INR daily. Stop argatroban when INR >4. Repeat INR in 4-6 h, if INR is below desired range then resume argatroban infusion
			Monitoring
			• Signs of bleeding
			• CBC
			• Argatroban and Bivalirudin
			  ○ aPTT
			  ○ ACT in percutaneous coronary intervention

	For patients with HIT or HITTS undergoing PCI	LD: 100 µg/kg IV bolus
		Initial infusion: 1 to 3 µg/kg/min for 6-72 h; maintain aPTT between 50-85 s
			• Dabigatran
			  ○ TT
			  ○ ECT

Bivalirudin (Angiomax©)	Unstable angina undergoing PCI	LD: 0.75 mg/kg IV bolus dose, followed by an infusion of 1.75 mg/kg/h for the duration of the procedure	• PT/INR (false elevation) • LFTs (argatroban) Precautions
		Renal impairment: CrCL <30 mL/min, 0.75mg/kg IV bolus dose, then 1 mg/kg/h should be considered Hemodialysis: 0.75 mg/kg IV bolus dose, then 0.25 mg/kg/h should be considered	• Recent surgery • History of bleeding (GI, intracranial, etc)
	Treatment of ACS*	LD: 0.1mg/kg IV bolus, followed by 0.25 mg/kg/h. Titration to aPTT 1.5-2 times control	• Congenital or acquired bleeding disorders
	Treatment and prophylaxis of HIT or HITT*	0.1-0.15 mg/kg/h, titration to aPTT 1.5-2 times control	• Recent cerebrovascular accident • Hepatic dysfunction (argatroban)
Dabigatran (Pradaxa©)	Reduce the risk of stroke and systemic embolism in patients with nonvalvular atrial fibrillation	150 mg orally twice daily for patients with CrCl >30 mL/min 75 mg orally twice daily for patients with CrCl 15-30 mL/min	• Renal dysfunction • Indwelling epidural catheter Contraindications
	Treatment of DVT and PE in patients who have been treated with a parenteral anticoagulant for 5-10 d	150 mg orally twice daily after 5-10 d of parenteral anticoagulation for patients with CrCl <30 mL/min	• Severe active bleeding • Mechanical prosthetic valve or valvular heart disease (dabigatran)
	To reduce the risk of recurrence of DVT and PE in patients who have been previously treated	150 mg orally twice daily after 5-10 d of parenteral anticoagulation for patients with CrCl <30 mL/min	

ACS, acute-coronary syndromes; ACT, activated clotting time; aPTT, activated partial thromboplastin time; CrCl, creatinine clearance; CBC, complete blood count; ECT = ecarin clotting time; HIT, heparin-induced thrombocytopenia; HITTS, HIT with thrombosis syndrome; INR, international normalized ratio; LD, loading dose; LFT, liver function tests; MI, myocardial infarction; PCI, percutaneous coronary intervention; TT, thrombin time; VTE, venous thromboembolism.
*Non-FDA-approved use.

Dabigatran is indicated for the prevention of stroke and systemic embolism in patients with atrial fibrillation, for the acute treatment of VTE, and to reduce the risk of VTE recurrence.

Complications and reversal of effect

No specific antidotes for DTI reversal exist. rFVIIa and activated prothrombin complex concentrates (aPCC) may be options for returning coagulation parameters to normal values and reverse bleeding. Dabigatran's low plasma protein binding allows for removal with hemodialysis and may be a strategy to reverse its effects. Idarucizumab, an antibody fragment, was developed to reverse the anticoagulant effects of dabigatran by selectively binding to and inhibiting its activity. An interim study suggests idarucizumab completely reverses the anticoagulant effect of dabigatran within minutes as measured by normalization of TT and ECT. Hemostasis was restored in approximately 12 hours.

■ DIRECT ACTING FACTOR XA-INHIBITORS

Pharmacodynamics and monitoring

Apixaban, edoxaban, and rivaroxaban are selective inhibitors of free and clot bound Xa. As a class these agents have predictable anticoagulant activity eliminating the need for routine laboratory monitoring and allowing for fixed dose administration. Despite these advantages, between the agents there are differences in their pharmacokinetic parameters (**Table 254-9**). They have varying degrees of renal clearance, and hepatic metabolism, elimination half-life, susceptibility to drug interactions, and dosing frequency that requires prescribing that is tailored to patient needs. While these agents alter aPTT and INR values, these tests cannot be used effectively to monitor therapy. Calibrated chromogenic anti-Xa assays provide a means to potentially monitor activity; however, exact therapeutic targets have yet to be described in practice.

Medical uses

Apixaban, edoxaban, and rivaroxaban have all established safety and efficacy in large, randomized trials compared with warfarin for risk reduction of stroke and systemic embolism in patients with nonvalvular atrial fibrillation. All patients included in these trials were at an increased risk of stroke due to one or more additional risk factors, such as previous stroke or transient ischemic attack (TIA), congestive heart failure, diabetes mellitus, hypertension, or an age ≥75 years (**Table 254-10**). Meta-analyses have shown these agents are associated with significant reductions in stroke, intracranial hemorrhage, and mortality. Major bleeding episodes were similar in occurrence to warfarin, but there was an increase in gastrointestinal bleeding. The relative efficacy and safety of new oral anticoagulants is consistent across a wide range of patients.

TABLE 254-9 Comparison of the Pharmacodynamic Features of Oral Direct Xa Inhibitors

Feature	Apixaban	Edoxaban	Rivaroxaban
Molecular weight (Daltons)	460	548	436
Bioavailability	50%	>60%	60%-100%
Protein binding	87%	54%	>90%
Half-life (h)	8-15	9-11	5-9
Cmax (h)	1-4	1-3	2-4
Metabolism	>50% unchanged; <32% CYP w/no active metabolites	Minimal	43% unchanged; 30% metabolites in urine
P-glycoprotein interaction	Yes	Yes	Yes
CYP	15% (CYP3A4)	< 4% (CYP3A4)	30% (CYP3A4, CYP2J2)
Clearance	Renal 25%-27% Fecal >50% (unchanged)	Renal 35%-50% Fecal 50%-65%	Renal 66% (33%-36% unchanged) Fecal/Biliary 28% (7% unchanged)

CYP, cytochrome P450 isoenzyme system; Cmax, time to maximum concentration.

TABLE 254-10 Clinical Uses of Direct Xa Inhibitors

Drug	Indication	Dose	Surveillance
Apixaban (Eliquis©)	Reduce the risk of stroke and systemic embolism in patients with nonvalvular atrial fibrillation	5 mg orally twice daily. Dose reduction: No dose reduction required for renal impairment including those maintained on hemodialysis Dose reduction: 2.5 mg orally twice daily in patients with >2 of the following: age ≥80 y, body weight ≤60 kg, or serum creatinine ≥1.5 mg/dL	Monitoring • CBC • Serum creatinine • Anti-Xa levels in patients with significant renal/hepatic impairment, those experiencing bleeding or abnormal coagulation parameters, pregnant patients, obese or low-weight patients, and children (agent specific assay calibration required) • LFTs (apixaban and rivaroxaban)
	Treatment of DVT and PE, and for the reduction in the risk of recurrent DVT and PE following initial therapy.	10 mg orally twice daily × 7 d, then 5 mg orally twice daily. After at least 6 mo of treatment for DVT or PE then 2.5 mg orally twice daily	Precautions • Indwelling epidural catheter • Neuraxial anesthesia or spinal puncture
	DVT prophylaxis in patients undergoing knee or hip replacement surgery	2.5 mg orally twice daily Initial dose taken 12-24h after surgery for 12 d (knee) for 35 d (hip)	• Recent spinal or ophthalmologic surgery • History of recent major bleed • Congenital or acquired bleeding disorders
Edoxaban (Savaysa©)	Reduce the risk of stroke and systemic embolism in patients with nonvalvular atrial fibrillation	60 mg once daily in patients with CrCL >50 to ≤95 mL/min Dose reduction: Do not use in patients with CrCL >95 mL/min 30 mg once daily in patients with CrCL 15-50 mL/min	• Concomitant use with strong CYP3A4 and P-glycoprotein inhibitors and inducers (apixaban, rivaroxaban, and edoxaban) • Mechanical heart valves or moderate-severe mitral stenosis (apixaban and edoxaban)
	Treatment of DVT and PE	>60 kg: 60 mg orally daily after 5-10 d of parenteral anticoagulant Dose reduction: ≤60kg: 30 mg orally daily after 5-10 d of parenteral anticoagulant P-glycoprotein inhibitors: 30 mg orally daily Renal dose adjustment: CrCl 15-50 mL/min: 30 mg daily	Contraindications • Active bleeding • Bacterial endocarditis • Hypersensitivity to agent or formulation excipients • Severe liver failure (apixaban)
Rivaroxaban (Xarelto©)	Reduce the risk of stroke and systemic embolism in patients with nonvalvular atrial fibrillation	20 mg orally daily with meal with CrCL >50 mL/min Dose Reduction: CrCl 15-50 mL/min: 15 mg daily with meal CrCl <15 mL/min: avoid use	• Hepatic dysfunction: ○ Avoid edoxaban and rivaroxaban in Child-Pugh class B,C
	Treatment of DVT and PE, and for the reduction in the risk of recurrent DVT and PE following initial therapy	15 mg orally twice daily with food for 21 d, then 20 mg orally daily with food	• Hepatic dysfunction with coagulopathy ○ Avoid apixaban, edoxaban, rivaroxaban
	DVT prophylaxis in patients undergoing knee or hip replacement surgery	10 mg orally daily with or without food Initial dose is taken 6-10 h after surgery for 12 d (knee) for 35 d (hip)	

CrCl, creatinine clearance; DVT, deep vein thrombosis; LFTs, liver function tests; VTE, venous thromboembolism.

Similarly, meta-analyses have been performed to evaluate the efficacy and safety outcomes associated with UFH, LMWH, or fondaparinux in combination with VKA versus the direct acting oral agents for treatment of VTE. These agents have comparable efficacy to that of VKAs in preventing recurrent VTE. However, they are associated with a significantly lower risk of bleeding complications, including the risk of major bleeding, intracranial bleeding, fatal bleeding, and clinically relevant nonmajor bleeding. This efficacy and safety has also been seen consistently in sub groups of patients with PE, DVT, a body weight >100 kg, moderate renal insufficiency, an age >75 years, and cancer.

Clinical outcomes have been evaluated with new oral anticoagulants for prophylaxis against venous thromboembolism after total hip or knee replacement with meta-analysis showing a higher efficacy but with a higher bleeding tendency. Compared with enoxaparin, the risk of symptomatic VTE after surgery was lower with rivaroxaban and similar with dabigatran and apixaban. The risk of clinically relevant bleeding was higher with rivaroxaban, similar with dabigatran, and lower with apixaban.

Clinicians will be faced with routinely transitioning patients between parenteral therapy and oral therapy as well transitioning to and from warfarin. The strategies to do this are included in each products label (**Table 254-11**).

TABLE 254-11 Converting from Parenteral to Oral Anticoagulants

Conversion from adjusted-dose IV UFH infusion to oral rivaroxaban, dabigatran, edoxaban, or apixaban	Stop IV UFH infusion Rivaroxaban, dabigatran, edoxaban, or apixaban 1. Administer first oral dose of rivaroxaban, dabigatran, edoxaban, or apixaban at the time of UFH discontinuation
Conversion from SC LMWH (or SC fondaparinux) therapeutic dosing to oral rivaroxaban, dabigatran, edoxaban, or apixaban	Stop SC LMWH or fondaparinux administration Rivaroxaban, dabigatran, edoxaban, or apixaban 1. Give rivaroxaban, dabigatran, edoxaban, or apixaban when next LMWH (or fondaparinux) dose is due
Converting from prophylactic dose SC UFH, LMWH (or fondaparinux) to oral rivaroxaban, dabigatran, edoxaban, or apixaban prophylactic dose	Stop current parenteral prophylaxis agent Rivaroxaban, dabigatran, edoxaban, or apixaban: 1. Administer rivaroxaban, dabigatran, edoxaban, or apixaban orally at the time of the next scheduled parenteral dose

Converting from warfarin to oral rivaroxaban, dabigatran, edoxaban, or apixaban	For all direct acting oral anticoagulants
	1. Give final warfarin dose
	2. Wait 2-3 d
	3. When INR <2.0, give first dose of rivaroxaban, dabigatran, edoxaban, or apixaban
	   • For atrial fibrillation patients taking rivaroxaban, consider starting when INR <3.
	   • For atrial fibrillation patients taking edoxaban, consider starting when INR <2.5.

Converting from oral rivaroxaban, dabigatran, edoxaban, or apixaban to warfarin	Rivaroxaban
	1. Discontinue rivaroxaban
	2. Begin a parenteral agent with warfarin when the next scheduled dose of rivaroxaban would be due
	Dabigatran
	1. Discontinue dabigatran
	2. Begin warfarin based on creatinine clearance
	   – For CrCl ≥50 mL/min, start warfarin 3 d before discontinuing dabigatran
	   – For CrCl 30-50mL/min, start warfarin 2 d before discontinuing dabigatran
	   – For CrCl 15-30 mL/min, start warfarin 1 d before discontinuing dabigatran
	   – For CrCl >15 mL/min, no recommendations can be made
	Apixaban
	1. Discontinue apixaban
	2. Begin a parenteral agent and warfarin when the next scheduled dose of apixaban would be due
	Edoxaban
	Oral option
	1. For patients taking 60mg of edoxaban, reduce dose to 30 mg, and begin warfarin concomitantly. For patients taking 30 mg of edoxaban, reduce the dose to 15 mg, and begin warfarin concomitantly. Once INR ≥2.0 is achieved, edoxaban should be discontinued and continue warfarin therapy.
	2. All INRs done in this fashion must be immediately prior to an edoxaban dose.
	3. Patient compliance to this regimen may be extremely difficult, and may lead to improper levels of anticoagulation.
	Parenteral option
	1. Discontinue edoxaban and administer a parenteral anticoagulant and warfarin at the same time of the next-scheduled dose of edoxaban. Once the INR is ≥2.0, the parenteral agent should be discontinued and continue warfarin therapy.

CrCl, creatinine clearance; INR, International Normalized Ratio; IV, intravenous; LMWH, low-molecular-weight heparin; SC, subcutanenous; UFH, unfractionated heparin.

TABLE 254-12   Reversal Agents

Agent	Structure	Target	Route of Administration	Onset	Duration	Mechanism of Action
Idarucizumab	Humanized antibody fragment	Dabigatran	Short IV infusion	Immediate	12-24 h	Noncompetitive binding to dabigatran
Andexanet alfa*	Modified recombinant protein derived from human Xa	Direct Xa inhibitors	IV bolus and infusion	Immediate	2 h	Decoy for direct Xa inhibitors
Ciraparantag*	Small synthetic molecule	Direct Xa inhibitors, Dabigatran, UFH, LMWH, and fondaparinux	Single IV bolus	30 min	24 h	Inactivation though hydrogen bonds

*In development

Complications and reversal of effect

Several antidotes to direct acting oral anticoagulants are in various stages of development. Andexanet alfa is a modified form of factor Xa that immediately reverses the anticoagulant effect of oral direct acting Xa inhibitors after administration (**Table 254-12**). Ciraparantag has a broader action, inhibiting all anticoagulants with the exception of intravenous DTIs and warfarin.

Until the doses of these agents are established and they reach the marketplace, the use of routine supportive care (stopping anticoagulant therapy, applying local hemostatic measures, administering fluid resuscitation, red blood cell transfusion, and initiating studies to identify the bleeding source) are recommended as initial steps. Several guidelines have emerged advocating treatment of life-threatening and major bleeding episodes with the administration of aPCC, PCC, and rFVIIa (**Figure 254-3**). Their inclusion is based on evidence from animal models and the reversal of coagulation parameters in healthy human volunteers. rFVIIa administration is associated with an increase in thrombosis in nonhemophiliac patients. The

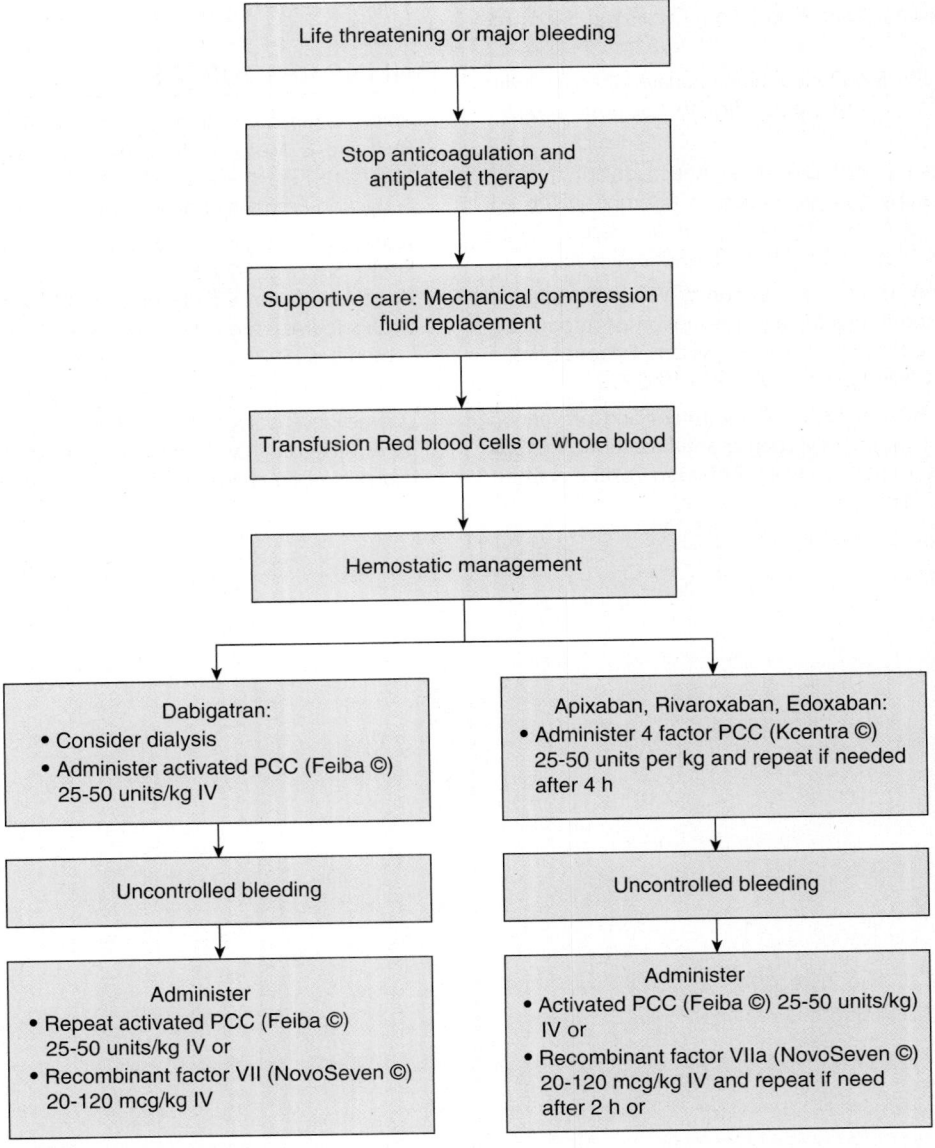

Figure 254-3 *Treatment algorithm for life-threatening bleeding.*

administration of PCC has the potential to increase the risk of thrombosis. Despite the limited efficacy and the increased likelihood of thrombosis, experts have deemed the administration to be a reasonable approach in extreme clinical situations of hemorrhage.

SUGGESTED READINGS

Ageno W, Gallus AS, Wittkowsky A, et al. Oral anticoagulant therapy: antithrombotic therapy and prevention of thrombosis, 9th ed: American College of Chest Physicians Evidence-Based Clinical Practice Guidelines. *Chest.* 2012;141:e44S-e88S.

Dobesh P, Fanikos J. Direct oral anticoagulants for the prevention of stroke in patients with nonvalvular atrial fibrillation: understanding differences and similarities. *Drugs.* 2015;75:1627-1644.

Dobesh PP, Fanikos J. New oral anticoagulants for the treatment of venous thromboembolism: understanding differences and similarities. *Drugs.* 2014;74:2015-2032.

Garcia DA, Baglin TP, Weitz JI, Samama MM, American College of Chest Physicians. Parenteral anticoagulants: antithrombotic therapy and prevention of thrombosis, 9th ed: American College of Chest Physicians Evidence-Based Clinical Practice Guidelines. *Chest.* 2012;141:e24S-e43S.

Hirsh J, Anand SS, Halperin JL, Fuster V. Guide to anticoagulant therapy: heparin. A statement for healthcare professionals from the American Heart Association. *Circulation.* 2001;103: 2995-3019.

Hirsh J, Eikelboom JW. Monitoring unfractionated heparin with the aPTT: Time for a fresh look. *Thromb Haemost.* 2006;96: 547-552.

Holbrook A, Schulman S, Witt DM, et al. Anticoagulant therapy: antithrombotic therapy and prevention of thrombosis, 9th ed: American College of Chest Physicians Evidence-Based Clinical Practice Guidelines. *Chest.* 2012;141:e152S-e184S.

Kahn SR, Lim W, Dunn AS, et al. Prevention of VTE in Nonsurgical Patients: antithrombotic therapy and prevention of thrombosis, 9th ed: American College of Chest Physicians Evidence-Based Clinical Practice Guidelines. *Chest.* 2012;141;e195S-e226S.

Linkins LA, Dans AL, Moores LK, et al. Treatment and prevention of heparin-induced thrombocytopenia: antithrombotic therapy and prevention of thrombosis, 9th ed: American College of Chest Physicians Evidence-Based Clinical Practice Guidelines. *Chest.* 2012;141:e495S-e530S.

Makris M, Van Veen JJ, Tait CR, et al. on behalf of the British Committee for Standards in Hematology. Guideline on the management of bleeding in patients on antithrombotic agents. *Br J Hematol.* 2012;160:35-46.

Nutescu EA, Spinler SA, Wittkowsky A, Dager WE. Low-molecular-weight heparins in renal impairment and obesity: available evidence and clinical practice recommendations across medical and surgical settings. *Ann Pharmacotherapy.* 2009;43:1064-1083.

Nutescu EA. Oral anticoagulant therapies: balancing the risks. *Am J Health Syst Pharm.* 2013;70:S3-S11.

Qaseem A, Chou R, Humphrey LL, et al. for the Clinical Guidelines Committee of the American College of Physicians. Venous thromboembolism prophylaxis in hospitalized patients: a Clinical practice guideline from the American College of Physicians. *Ann Intern Med.* 2011;155(9):625-632.

Schulman S, Beyth RJ, Kearon C, Levine MN, American College of Chest Physicians. Hemorrhagic complications of anticoagulant and thrombolytic treatment: American College of Chest Physicians Evidence-Based Clinical Practice Guidelines, 8th ed. *Chest.* 2008;133:257S-298S.

Weitz DS, Weitz JI. Update on heparin: what do we need to know? *J Thromb Thrombolysis.* 2010;29:199-207.

ONLINE RESOURCES

Hospital-Acquired Condition (HAC) Reduction Program. Centers for Medicare & Medicaid Services. http://www.cms.gov/Medicare/Medicare-Fee-for-Service-Payment/AcuteInpatientPPS/HAC-Reduction-Program.html. Accessed September 14, 2015.

Mozaffarian D, Benjamin, EJMD, Go AS, et al. Heart Disease and Stroke Statistics—2015 Update. A Report From the American Heart Association. Circulation 2015;131:00-00. Available at http://circ.ahajournals.org/content/131/4/e29.full.pdf+html. Accessed September 15, 2015.

United States Department of Health and Human Services. Office of Disease Prevention and Health Promotion. The National Action Plan for Adverse Drug Event Prevention. Available at: http://health.gov/hcq/pdfs/ADE-Action-Plan-508c.pdf. Accessed September 15, 2015.

CHAPTER 255

Diseases of the Aorta

Aaron W. Aday, MD
Joshua A. Beckman, MD, MSc

INTRODUCTION

The aorta is the largest artery in the body and connects the heart to the systemic vascular bed. It consists of both a thoracic and an abdominal portion, which are delineated by the ligamentum arteriosum. The thoracic aorta begins at the aortic valve and has four segments: the aortic root, ascending aorta, aortic arch, and descending aorta. These segments originate connections with several critical vessels including the coronary, innominate, subclavian, and carotid arteries. Similarly, the abdominal aorta, which begins as the vessel travels through the diaphragm, gives rise to the celiac, superior mesenteric, inferior mesenteric, and renal arteries and ultimately bifurcates into the common iliac arteries.

As with other arteries, the aortic wall consists of three distinct layers. The intima, or innermost wall, primarily contains endothelial cells. These cells function as a regulatory barrier between the blood and the rest of the vessel wall and modulate processes such as thrombosis, fibrinolysis, and inflammation. The middle layer, or media, consists of vascular smooth muscle cells, elastic fibers, and other extracellular matrix components. Finally, the outer layer, or adventitia, consists primarily of collagen, nerves, and small blood vessels known as the vasa vasorum, which help provide oxygen and nutrients to the vessel wall itself. Separating each vessel layer is an additional layer of elastic lamina. Functioning in conjunction with the medial layer, these elastic fibers confer both distensibility and elastic recoil of the aortic wall, which are essential properties for normal function.

The primary function of the aorta is transport of oxygenated blood from the left ventricle to the rest of the body. In order to accomplish this, the aorta must withstand the shear stress and transmural pressure generated by blood as it is ejected from the left ventricle. Rather than functioning as a passive conduit, the vessel wall components permit distension of the aorta during systole, thereby storing potential energy. The aorta undergoes compensatory recoil during diastole, which ensures ongoing blood flow throughout the cardiac cycle. Changes in the vessel wall, either from aging, mechanical trauma, or disease-associated pathology, may affect the elastic properties of the aorta and lead to abnormalities at any position along the vessel. According to data from the Centers for Disease Control and Prevention, diseases of the aorta were responsible for nearly 10,000 deaths in the United States in 2013. Given the significant morbidity and mortality of aortic pathology despite its relative rarity, clinicians must be able to recognize and manage the various disease processes that can affect the aorta.

THORACIC AORTIC ANEURYSM

An aneurysm is a pathologic, focal dilatation of a blood vessel that involves the intima, media, and adventitia. Most aneurysms affect the entire circumference of the vessel and are termed fusiforum. Saccular aneurysms involve only a small region of the vessel wall and cause diverticular outpouchings. The normal size of the thoracic aorta depends on the segment in question in addition to other factors, such as age, gender, and body surface area. However, in general, a segment that is at least 50% larger than its proximal normal segment is considered aneurysmal. Nearly 60% of thoracic aortic aneurysms involve the aortic root or ascending aorta with involvement of the descending aorta, arch, and thoracoabdominal segments occurring less frequently. In some cases, the aneurysm spans multiple segments, either contiguously or in isolation.

Numerous factors contribute to the development of thoracic aortic aneurysms. A lifetime of mechanical wall stress normally causes dilatation of the thoracic aorta with advancing age. Similarly, hypertension subjects the aorta to increased wall stress and increases the risk of aneurysm development. Aortic atherosclerosis is the primary risk factor for descending thoracic aortic aneurysms, and these aneurysms often extend into the abdominal segment. Conversely, atherosclerosis is rarely implicated as the primary cause of ascending aortic aneurysms. Other cardiovascular risk factors, such as a history of smoking and coronary artery disease, also increase the risk of aneurysm development. Histologically, the majority of ascending aortic aneurysms exhibit cystic medial degradation. This refers to the breakdown of collagen and elastic fibers within the media layer as well as the loss of vascular smooth muscle cells in this layer ultimately leading to the development of cystic pockets of extracellular matrix. Over time, the vessel wall becomes less distensible and more susceptible to wall stress, ultimately leading to aneurysm development and progressive dilatation. Cystic medial degradation, a pathological finding rather than a specific cause, is particularly prevalent in genetic syndromes of thoracic aortic aneurysm, and it occurs to some degree as a normal part of aging. Finally, cases of infectious and noninfectious aortitis (discussed later) can cause aneurysmal dilatation.

In recent years, researchers have identified numerous genetic disorders that are associated with thoracic aortic aneurysms. A connective tissue disorder inherited in an autosomal dominant pattern, Marfan syndrome is caused by mutations in fibrillin-1, which plays an important role in normal extracellular matrix function. This mutation not only causes structural weakening of the aortic wall itself but also leads to upregulation of TGF-β signaling. As a result, the aorta in these patients responds abnormally to mechanical stress and may become aneurysmal. Similarly, Loeys-Dietz syndrome, caused by mutations in one of the TGF-β receptors, can cause aortic tortuosity and aneurysm development along with craniofacial abnormalities. Other genetic disorders associated with thoracic aortic aneurysms include Ehlers-Danlos syndrome type IV and the familial thoracic aortic aneurysm syndrome. Turner syndrome is a chromosomal disorder affecting only females that is caused by a complete or partial absence of a second X chromosome. Up to 42% of affected individuals may develop aortic root aneurysms, often in conjunction with bicuspid aortic valves, and this group is at particularly high risk for aneurysm rupture and dissection.

In the United States, 1% to 2% of the general population has a bicuspid aortic valve, and up to half of these patients will also develop a thoracic aortic aneurysm during their lifetime, making it one of the most common causes of aneurysm development. The aneurysm typically involves the aortic root and ascending aorta and may occur with or without concomitant aortic stenosis. The hemodynamics of blood flow across bicuspid aortic valves is abnormal and may play a role in aneurysm development. Similar to Marfan syndrome, fibrillin-1 may also contribute to aortic pathology in patients with bicuspid aortic valves, and individuals can develop aneurysms even after surgical replacement of the bicuspid valve.

Most thoracic aortic aneurysms are clinically silent and detected incidentally during various thoracic imaging studies. Aneurysms involving the aortic root or ascending aorta can cause aortic insufficiency through distortion of the valve annulus. This may be detected on examination as an early diastolic murmur, particularly along the left sternal border. Symptoms attributable to thoracic aortic aneurysms are generally due to mass effects. Because of the aorta's position within the mediastinum, aneurysms may compress the trachea, mainstem bronchi, esophagus, and recurrent laryngeal nerve. Thus, patients can experience shortness of breath, wheezing, dysphagia, and hoarseness. In some cases, patients may experience pain due to compression of other thoracic organs or even erosion into the spine, sternum, or ribs.

Once a thoracic aortic aneurysm has been diagnosed, clinicians should also look for other clues on the physical examination that may indicate an underlying genetic disorder in the appropriate clinical context. In individuals with a bicuspid aortic valve, heart auscultation may reveal a systolic ejection click after the first heart sound, which corresponds to abnormal opening of a nonstenotic valve. If the bicuspid valve has become stenotic due to early degeneration, clinicians may hear a systolic ejection murmur, often at the right upper sternal border, as one would with age-related calcific aortic stenosis. Common physical examination features of Marfan syndrome include tall stature, thin habitus with diminished muscle mass, elongated skulls, arachnodactyly, scoliosis, and chest wall abnormalities. Those with Loeys-Dietz syndrome typically exhibit hypertelorism, bifid uvula, or cleft palate. Patients with features concerning for an underlying genetic aortopathy should be referred to a clinician with expertise in the field to discuss further workup and family screening.

Chest x-rays in individuals with thoracic aortic aneurysm may show mediastinal widening and displacement of the airways. This is a low-sensitivity test for aneurysm and may not detect small aneurysms or those primarily involving the aortic root or ascending aorta. Concern for aneurysm on chest x-ray, particularly in the right clinical context, should prompt more definitive imaging. In many patients, particularly those who are not obese or barrel-chested (such as in COPD), transthoracic echocardiography can reliably image the aortic root and ascending aorta. This modality is particularly useful for screening and long-term monitoring in young patients with known risk factors for aneurysms in this region, such as those with Marfan syndrome and bicuspid aortic valves. However, there are several key limitations to transthoracic echocardiography in evaluating thoracic aortic aneurysms. Measurements of the aorta must be normalized to age and body surface area, and interobserver variability in measurements may cause confusion in the clinical setting if it is not possible to view the images oneself. Additionally, it is often important to image the entire aorta at the time of diagnosis to rule out aneurysmal dilatation of other segments, and detection of an aneurysm with echocardiography should not obviate the need for more comprehensive imaging. Transesophageal echocardiography is useful to view the aortic arch and descending aorta, but its invasive nature makes it more appropriate for acute aortic syndromes. Increasingly, CT and MR angiography have become important tools to image the entire thoracic aorta, and they are both highly sensitive and specific for aortic disease. In patients with prior aortic interventions, CT is the preferred modality. When using these modalities, it is important to note that aortic tortuosity may lead to inaccurate measurement of vessel diameter on axial images. Therefore, it is often necessary to use 3-D reconstruction to measure the diameter perpendicular to blood flow, and interpretation by a vascular imaging specialist may be necessary, particularly in complex cases.

The primary concern with thoracic aortic aneurysms is progressive dilatation and weakening leading to dissection, rupture, and death. Although aneurysm diameter is the most important risk factor for these clinical outcomes, the natural history of thoracic aortic aneurysms varies widely among individuals. In general, the annual growth rate is up to 0.2 cm/y, but this rate may accelerate with increasing size. Clinical registries show that the rate of dissection and rupture rapidly increases from 2% to 3% in aneurysms below 6 cm in diameter to ~7% in those 6 cm and larger. Additionally, descending aortic aneurysms grow more rapidly than those of the root and arch. Age, female sex, poorly controlled hypertension, and tobacco use are associated with more rapid growth. Those with strong family histories of aneurysm often progress at a faster rate. Aneurysms in patients with genetic causes of thoracic aortic aneurysm, such as Marfan syndrome, generally dilate more rapidly. Importantly, aneurysms in Marfan syndrome and individuals with bicuspid aortic valves are at particular risk for further dilation during pregnancy, likely due to both increased cardiac output and increased laxity of the vessel wall due to hormonal effects. Similarly, Marfan and other genetic syndromes are associated with an increased overall risk of dissection and rupture, particularly if there is a family history of these events, and this is more likely to occur at smaller diameters. Also, patients with bicuspid aortic valves exhibit a higher growth rate with increased risk of dissection and rupture at a smaller size.

Risk factor modification is an important component of thoracic aortic aneurysm management. All patients should be counseled on smoking cessation, and clinicians should initiate antihypertensive therapy for blood pressure control with a goal of <140/90 mm Hg. If the aorta exhibits atherosclerotic plaque, then high-intensity statin therapy is also reasonable, although there are insufficient data to support this for all causes of thoracic aortic aneurysm. Patients should be treated with β-blockers at maximally tolerated doses to reduce wall stress. Additionally, β-blocker therapy finds particular use in patients with Marfan syndrome, even in the absence of aneurysm. Animal data indicate that losartan may prevent aneurysm formation in Marfan syndrome due to its off target effect of TGF-β downregulation. Large clinical trials do not yet support the use of angiotensin receptor blockers over β-blockers, but it is reasonable to utilize them if additional blood pressure control is necessary. Lifestyle modification is important to prevent further aneurysm dilation. Patients should avoid strenuous physical activity and isometric exercises. Additionally, because of the dangers associated with pregnancy, individuals pursuing pregnancy should be referred to a high-risk obstetrician and a cardiologist to formulate a plan to minimize these risks during both pregnancy and delivery. If there is clinical concern for a genetic aortopathy, patients should be referred to a cardiologist or vascular medicine specialist for further evaluation and consideration of genetic testing as well as screening of first degree relatives.

Because thoracic aortic aneurysm is generally a progressive disease, long-term monitoring is essential. If the aneurysm is inadequately imaged on transthoracic echocardiogram, dedicated MR or CT imaging should be performed to fully characterize the dilatation. After diagnosis, the 2010 American College of Cardiology/American Heart Association guidelines recommend follow-up imaging at 6 months to look for stability. Assuming the aneurysm is stable at 6 months, annual screening is reasonable; conversely, biannual imaging is recommended for rapidly enlarging aneurysms or those approaching indication for repair. It is important to recognize that interobserver variability may affect whether an aneurysm is interpreted as stable or enlarging, and detailed review of these imaging studies in person is often necessary. In syndromes that primarily affect the ascending aorta, such as bicuspid aortic valves and Marfan syndrome, transthoracic echocardiography is a reasonable modality for routine monitoring. However, there are increasing data characterizing the incidence of distal aorta disease in Marfan syndrome, and it is unclear how frequently the entire aorta should be monitored in such individuals.

All symptomatic aneurysms warrant surgical repair given the high rate of morbidity and mortality without intervention. Additionally, repair of asymptomatic aortic aneurysm is indicated for ascending aortic aneurysm ≥5.5 cm in the general population and ≥5.0 cm in those with bicuspid aortic valves or Marfan syndrome. In contrast, physicians may delay descending aortic aneurysms repair until ≥6.5 cm. The surgical approach to repairing thoracic aortic aneurysms varies based on the segments involved. Aneurysms of the ascending aorta are generally resected and replaced with a prosthetic graft. In some cases, the aortic valve is also replaced, such as in those with annular dilatation and aortic insufficiency or

degenerative aortic valve disease in the setting of a bicuspid aortic valve. Such procedures require a median sternotomy as well as cardiopulmonary bypass. Arch aneurysms are particularly difficult to repair due to concerns regarding head perfusion during the procedure and reanastomosis of the branch vessels. These surgeries often involve some combination of open surgical repair, endovascular stent-graft placement, and branch vessel bypass construction. Descending aortic aneurysms are commonly repaired with prosthetic grafts via a thoracotomy. A significant risk of these procedures is paralysis due to interruption of spinal cord blood flow. For elective procedures, the rate of death is 3% to 5% at experienced centers, with the risk increasing to nearly 7% if arch repair is involved.

ABDOMINAL AORTIC ANEURYSMS

Abdominal aortic aneurysms (AAA) **(Figure 255-1),** classified as dilation ≥3.0 cm, are much more common than those in the thoracic segment. Incidence dramatically increases with age, particularly in men older than 50 and woman over 70. Up to 3% of men ≥50 and 5% of men ≥65 will develop abdominal aortic aneurysms. Men are 5 to 10 times more likely to develop aneurysms than women. Smoking is the primary risk factor for abdominal aortic aneurysms with a direct correlation between the number of years an individual smoked and aneurysm incidence. The overall risk is 3 to 5 times higher in smokers. Additionally, hypertension, dyslipidemia, and coronary atherosclerosis are associated with aneurysm formation. Caucasians are at higher risk than African Americans. In some cases, abdominal aortic aneurysms are also accompanied by aneurysms in the iliac, femoral, and popliteal arteries. Estrogen may play a protective role with respect to aneurysm formation, thus explaining the later onset in women. Unlike thoracic aortic aneurysms, the genetic underpinnings of abdominal aortic aneurysms are poorly

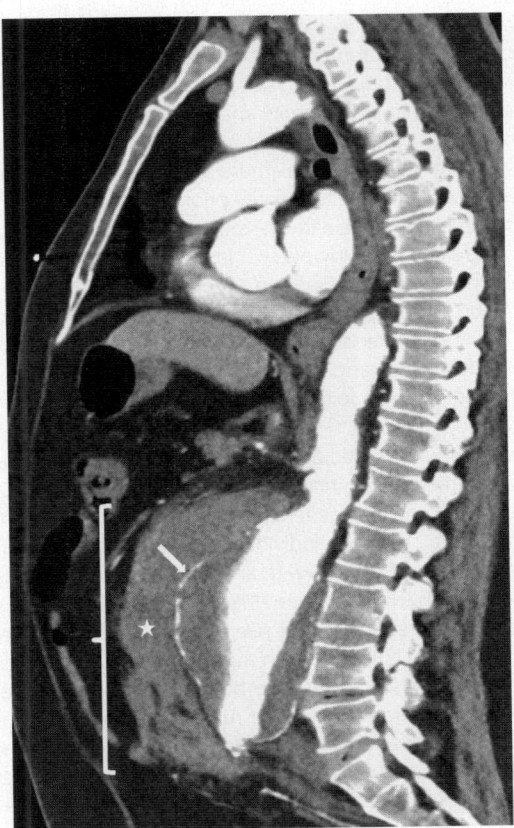

Figure 255-1 *Sagittal CT image showing a large abdominal aortic aneurysm (bracket) with rupture indicated by extravasated contrast material (arrow) and surrounding hemorrhage (star).*

understood. There does seem to be a heritable component, as individuals with a family history are at increased risk. Some data have shown that a common sequence variant on chromosome 9p21 is associated with abdominal aortic aneurysm, intracranial aneurysm, and coronary artery disease. However, more research is necessary to better understand the genetic basic of abdominal aortic aneurysms.

Histologic examination of abdominal aortic aneurysms shows chronic wall inflammation. In addition, various proteinases, particularly matrix metalloproteinases, cause breakdown of collagen and elastin within the vessel wall. Smooth muscle cells, which can help repair the vessel by releasing collagen and elastin, are often diminished in aneurysm walls. Therefore, over time, aneurysms are more susceptible to wall stress throughout the cardiac cycle and are less capable of repairing the damage caused by ongoing inflammation. This process leads to progressive aneurysmal dilatation and ultimately rupture.

As with thoracic aortic aneurysms, abdominal aneurysms are typically asymptomatic. Occasionally, patients present with a gnawing, constant pain within the abdomen, lower back, or flank. Rupture may cause severe onset of pain in these same regions. Physical examination may reveal a pulsatile mass along the midline of the abdomen. In individuals with a small body habitus (<40 in waistline), it may even be possible to estimate aneurysm diameter on examination.

Abdominal ultrasound is highly accurate for the assessment of the abdominal aorta, and it is the preferred modality for screening and follow-up in uncomplicated cases of abdominal aortic aneurysm. The US Preventive Services Task Force recommends a single ultrasound screening of all men age 65 to 75 with any prior smoking history at the Welcome to Medicare visit. Screening is also reasonable in individuals with a family history of aneurysm, although the age of screening and interval of follow-up are unclear. In some cases, particularly with large or tortuous aneurysms or in obese patients, CT imaging may be necessary. CT angiography permits 3-D reconstruction and measurement of the true aortic diameter, similar to cases of thoracic aortic aneurysm. It is an important modality prior to aneurysm repair as it permits imaging of the abdominal visceral branches, renal arteries, and iliac vessels. Abdominal aortic aneurysms often contain extensive atherosclerotic plaque and thrombus which can be important to identify prior to repair. MR angiography can also be used, particularly in young patient in whom radiation exposure is a concern. However, CT imaging generally permits more accurate measurements. Once an aneurysm is detected, the interval of follow-up depends on aneurysm size. In particular, aneurysm 3.5 to 4.4 cm in diameter should be followed annually with biannual follow-up for those ranging 4.5 to 5.4 cm. Those exhibiting rapid growth should also be followed more closely. Growth >1 cm/y is an indication for repair.

As with thoracic aortic aneurysms, abdominal aortic aneurysms dilate over time with an increased risk of rupture at larger sizes. The annual rate of growth is generally up to 0.4 cm/y, although this can vary significantly between individuals. Women are at higher risk for rupture than men. For men with aneurysms ≥5cm, the annual rate of rupture is 12% with a rate of 18% for women. The risk of rupture dramatically increases at larger size, with up to 50% of aneurysms greater than 7 cm culminating in rupture. Nearly 75% of individuals who suffer aneurysm rupture die before undergoing surgery, and the 30-day survival rate following rupture is only 11%, thus demonstrating the importance of early detection and close follow-up.

Similar to diseases within other vascular beds, smoking cessation is a critical component in abdominal aortic aneurysm therapy, as ongoing smoking is associated with more rapid aneurysm growth. There are no clear data to support statin therapy although the presence of significant atherosclerotic disease within the aorta should generally prompt guideline based statin therapy. Similarly, clinicians

should target standard blood pressure goals in patients with abdominal aortic aneurysms to minimize their overall risk of adverse cardiovascular and cerebrovascular events. At present, there are no definitive data supporting β-blocker or angiotensin receptor blocker use in abdominal aortic aneurysms, although these are reasonable agents for achieving adequate blood pressure control.

The decision to repair abdominal aortic aneurysms is complex, particularly because these patients are typically older and have multiple medical comorbidities. Symptomatic aneurysms and those growing more than 1 cm/y should be repaired. Aortic aneurysm rupture should also prompt emergent surgical repair, although the operative mortality is nearly 50%. Outside of these situations, repair is generally considered once aneurysms reach 5.5 cm in diameter, although repair at smaller diameter may be warranted in woman or in individuals with a family history of aneurysm rupture. Repair can be achieved either through an open technique or via an endovascular approach. Open surgical repair typically requires a large midline incision followed by replacement of the aneurysmal segment with a prosthetic graft. Operative mortality ranges from 2% to 6% with lower rates at centers performing a high volume of repairs.

In recent years, endovascular abdominal aortic aneurysm repair (EVAR) has become increasingly popular, currently representing more than 50% of all AAA repairs (**Figure 255-2**). During this procedure, a prosthetic graft is typically delivered through a transfemoral catheter system. The graft spans the aneurysmal segment and forms a seal between the graft and a healthy segment of the vessel, thus prohibiting blood from leaking into the excluded aneurysm and causing further dilation or rupture. EVAR is associated with a lower morbidity and mortality rate than open surgical repair. However, this technique has several important limitations. Patients are more likely to require repeat interventions following EVAR. Many abdominal aortic aneurysms are not amenable to endovascular repair due to tortuosity or involvement of important branch vessels that cannot be protected via EVAR. Additionally, up to 20% of patients develop endoleaks, or ongoing blood flow between the aneurysm wall and endograft, following EVAR. In many cases, these endoleaks can cause further aneurysmal dilatation, and, ultimately, rupture. As a result, EVAR is typically reserved for individuals at high risk for perioperative complication of death with open surgical repair. Endoleaks can be visualized on CT, and given their high rate of recurrence, patients

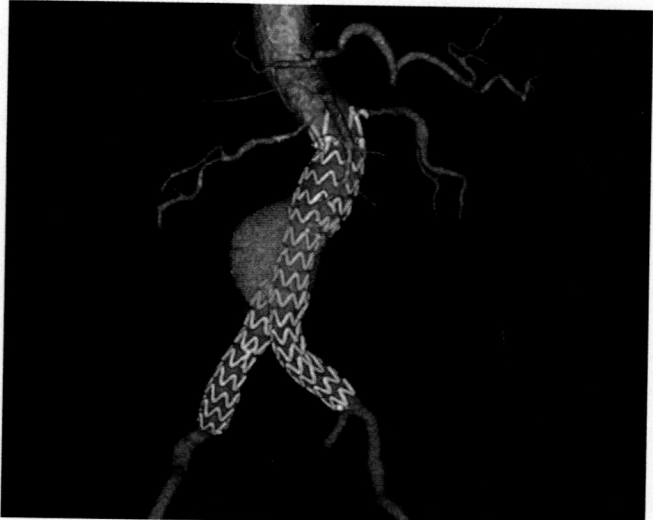

Figure 255-2 *3-D reconstruction of CT imaging showing abdominal aortic aneurysm following EVAR. The stent extends from the infrarenal segment into the common iliac arteries bilaterally and excludes the aneurysm sac, shown in yellow.*

typically undergo frequent CT monitoring following EVAR. Additionally, clinicians should not assume an abdominal aortic aneurysm has been definitively managed following EVAR, and it is important to further investigate clinical scenarios concerning for ongoing aneurysm dilation or rupture. Finally, patients deemed "too sick" for open AAA repair do not derive any survival benefit from endovascular repair. Thus, EVAR has become a lower-morbidity method of repairing aneurysms that meet current recommendations.

AORTIC DISSECTION

Aortic dissection is typically caused by a rent within the aortic intima. Following this initial tear, ongoing shear stress within the vessel leads to further dissection into the vessel wall, and pulsatile blood flow into this false channel can lead to bleeding within the wall or propogation of the dissection along the length of the aorta, thus separating the intima and media layers. This often creates a dissection flap with a distinct false lumen separate from the true lumen of the aorta. In some cases, this is a blind-ended flap, although another intimal tear can develop at the distal end of the flap, thereby permitting blood flow back into the true lumen. Over time, stagnant blood within the false lumen may thrombose. Dissection is rare; according to the International Registry of Acute Aortic Dissection (IRAD) database, there are approximately 2000 new cases of acute aortic dissection annually in the United States, although other estimates place the figure as high as 10,000. Despite their relative infrequency, vigilance is required, for dissections are associated with an extremely high mortality. Classically, the early mortality rate is estimated at 1% per hour. Without treatment, ~25% of patients with dissections involving the ascending aorta die within 24 hours, and this rate increases to 50% at 48 hours and 75% at 2 weeks. Thus, it is critical for clinicians to maintain a high clinical suspicion for acute aortic dissection.

There are two primary classification symptoms for aortic dissection, the DeBakey and Stanford systems, although the Stanford classification is more commonly used clinically. Under the Stanford classification system, Type A dissections (**Figure 255-3**) involve the ascending and arch aorta proximal to the left subclavian artery and can involve any number of additional segments, while Type B dissections (**Figure 255-4**) do not involve the aorta proximal to the subclavian artery.

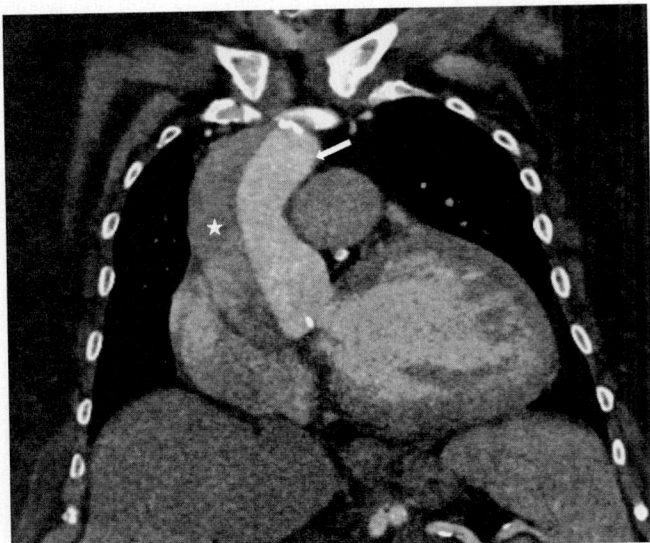

Figure 255-3 *CT image showing Type A dissection extending from the aortic annulus into the arch. True lumen (arrow) and false lumen (star) are clearly visible.*

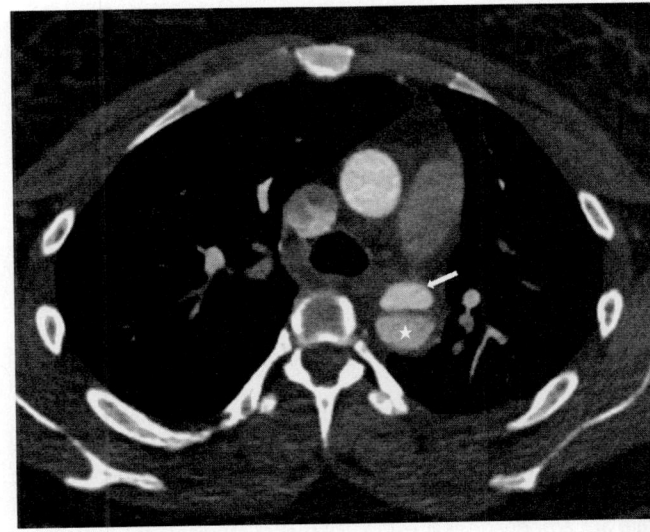

Figure 255-4 *Patient with Marfan syndrome presenting with sudden onset chest and back pain. CT imaging shows a Type B dissection with both a true lumen (arrow) and false lumen (star).*

Many of the same risk factors that predispose individuals to aortic aneurysm development are also associated with aortic dissection. Hypertension is the most common risk factors associated with dissection and is seen in up to 75% of individuals. Atherosclerotic disease is also common in individuals with dissection. Men are twice as likely to be affected as women, and women typically develop dissections at an older age. Due to ongoing vessel wall changes, aneurysmal aortic segments are at higher risk for dissection. Additionally, dissections are more common with advanced age. There is a slightly higher risk of dissection during pregnancy, likely due to hormonal changes of the vessel wall. Vigorous exercise, particularly isometric activities like weight lifting, can precipitate dissections in susceptible patients. Infectious and autoimmune aortitis is associated with dissection as is cocaine use. Both bicuspid aortic valve and aortic coarctation can trigger aortic dissections. Finally, numerous connective tissue disorders increase one's risk for acute aortic dissection, including Marfan syndrome, Loeys-Dietz syndrome, Ehlers-Danlos syndrome type IV, and the familial thoracic aortic aneurysm syndrome. Even without a clearly identifiable genetic aortopathy, nearly 20% of individuals with an acute aortic dissection have a family history of aneurysm or dissection.

The presentation of acute aortic syndromes ranges from the dramatic to the asymptomatic and depends on the segment involved and end-organs affected. Nearly all patients develop either pain that is both sudden in onset and severe or syncope. Large series indicate the pain is most often described as abrupt, severe, sharp, or stabbing with the classic description of tearing and ripping pain occurring less frequently. Within the IRAD database, most patients with Type A dissections presented with anterior chest pain, and Type B dissections more commonly caused back pain. Abdominal pain can occur in both scenarios. The pain can radiate to the neck, jaw, arms, or legs depending on branch vessel involvement. Occasionally, patients are asymptomatic, which is more common with advanced age. Symptoms often wax and wane, and this may correspond to interruption and restoration of blood flow by the dissection. Dissection flaps can limit flow due to direct occlusion of a branch vessel by the flap or extension of the dissection itself into the branch vessel. Expansion of the false lumen can cause branch vessel hypoperfusion, and thromboembolism of the false lumen can also lead to ischemia in various vascular beds.

A variety of other clinical scenarios are associated with acute dissection. Aortic valvular insufficiency occurs in up to 76% of Type A dissections and can result from acute root dilation, direct extension of the dissection into the aortic annulus, or prolapse of a dissection flap across the valve, thus interfering with valve closure. Dissection can permit fluid entry into the pericardial space, thus leading to cardiac tamponade in up to 10% of Type A dissections. Dissections can directly impair coronary perfusion, typically the right coronary artery, thus leading to an acute inferior myocardial infarction. Patients frequently experience syncope due to temporary interruption of cerebral flood flow. Hypertension is common in acute dissection, although hypotension can also occur in the presence of aortic rupture, tamponde, or heart failure. Pleural effusions, usually left-sided, and mesenteric ischemia are also common. Finally, arch vessel occlusion or distal embolization can cause stroke or transient ischemic attack.

On examination, up to 30% of patients will exhibit pulse deficits, and mortality increases with the number of limbs that exhibit diminished pulses. Cardiac auscultation may reveal the diastolic murmur of aortic insufficiency if the aortic valve is affected. Those with cardiac tamponade will exhibit pulsus paradoxus and Kussmaul's sign. Obstruction of blood flow in the right coronary artery may lead to the classic signs of a right ventricular infarct, including elevated jugular venous pressure and a right ventricular heave. Neurologic deficits may be present. Chest x-ray often reveals a widened mediastinum. An enlarged cardiac silhouette may indicate the presence of an associated pericardial effusion, and a pleural effusion may also be present. ECG may reveal low-amplitude voltages or electrical alternans in the setting of a pericardial effusion or tamponade, and right coronary artery occlusion can lead to ST segment elevations in the inferior leads. On laboratory analysis, D-dimer is a useful diagnostic test for excluding dissection. Values <500 ng/mL within 24 hours of symptoms onset have a negative predictive value of 95%. Depending on which additional vascular beds are affected, patients may also have elevations of troponin isoforms, creatine kinase-MB, lactate, aspartate transaminase, and alanine transaminase, although none of these assays are specific for aortic dissection.

Definitive identification and characterization of aortic dissection is critical to ensure appropriate management. Special consideration must be given to body habitus, hemodynamic stability, availability of various imaging modalities, and the speed with which various studies can be obtained. Transthoracic echocardiography can image the aortic root and is commonly available as a rapid, point-of-care modality. However, it is limited in its ability to image the rest of the aorta, and it has extremely poor sensitivity for detecting aortic dissection. Time spent obtaining a transthoracic echocardiogram typically only delays definitive diagnosis and should not be performed as the initial screening study if there is an elevated index of suspicion. If follow-up imaging of the aortic valve is necessary, this can be quickly accomplished with a transthoracic echocardiogram. In contrast, transesophageal echocardiography is ~98% sensitive for aortic dissection and is also useful in imaging the aortic valve in patients with accompanying aortic insufficiency. Although the avoidance of radiation exposure is desirable, 24-hour availability of transesophageal echocardiography is not universal. Additionally, patients may be too hemodynamically unstable or in too much pain to tolerate the procedure without intubation. Increasingly, contrast-enhanced CT has become the primary modality for aortic imaging in the acute setting because of its placement in emergency wards. It permits rapid visualization of the entire aorta as well as large branch vessels. Axial images typically demonstrate two lumens separated by the dissection flap with different degrees of contrast enhancement within each lumen. Particularly with experienced operators, sensitivity and specificity approach 100%. MRA with gadolinium enhancement is similarly effective at evaluating aortic dissection with the added benefit of avoiding radiation exposure and contrast-induced nephropathy.

Unfortunately, image acquisition takes longer than CT, and it is less commonly available in the emergent setting. Moreover, the duration of the test and its limitations on patient surveillance diminish its value in the acute setting.

Once aortic dissection is diagnosed, the initial management should consist of ensuring hemodynamic stability and airway protection. Hemodynamically unstable patients should undergo emergent surgical evaluation. Among stable patients, it is not uncommon for them to require intravenous narcotics for adequate pain control. Tight blood pressure management is necessary to limit propagation of the dissection and to minimize the risk of wall rupture. The target systolic blood pressure should be less than 120 mm Hg. β-Blockers should be used to lower the heart rate as close to 60 beats/min as possible as initial therapy. Intravenous esmolol and labetalol infusions are often used to achieve both these targets. Esmolol in particular permits rapid titratability due to its short half-life. Diltiazem and verapamil are also options but are used less commonly. Many providers use sodium nitroprusside due to its rapid effects on systolic blood pressure. However, as a direct vasodilator, sodium nitroprusside alone can increase aortic wall stress and, therefore, must be administered in conjuction with β-blockers.

While medical management is ongoing, the clinical team should also begin the evaluation for definitive therapy. Ideally, this evaluation should involve cardiologists, cardiac surgeons, vascular surgeons, and vascular imaging experts. If necessary, stable patients should be transferred to high volume centers with experience in such cases. Patients with acute type A dissections should undergo urgent surgical repair, and surgery is associated with improved survival compared to medical therapy alone. Various studies have found mortality rates of 22% to 26% in patients undergoing surgical repair of Type A dissections compared to 58% for those managed medically. Surgical repair of Type A dissections typically requires sternotomy and excision of the dissected portion followed by graft replacement. Close examination of the aortic valve is necessary, and valve replacement should be performed as part of the same procedure if valve function has been disrupted. As in thoracic aorta aneurysm, dissections involving the aortic arch are more complex and also require grafting to the head and upper limb vessels either via open repair or through a hybrid procedure using additional endovascular repair. If the distal aorta is involved, it may be excluded with an endograft or simply left untouched if it is not causing end-organ malperfusion.

Type B dissections are associated with a lower-mortality rate of anywhere from 1% to 11% in individuals undergoing medical management. Typically, uncomplicated cases of Type B dissections are managed conservatively in the absence of end-organ malperfusion with in hospital mortality of up to 20%. However, if the dissection has led to compromise of limb, visceral, or renal blood flow, intervention may be necessary. Contained or impending rupture is also an indication for surgical repair. If surgery is warranted, options include open surgical excision with graft replacement or thoracic endovascular aortic repair (TEVAR). In the IRAD database, 10% of patients with type B dissections underwent open repair, whereas 12% underwent TEVAR. Mortality is nearly three times higher with open repair. Occasionally, patients with type B dissections and organ malperfusion must undergo percutaneous fenestration procedures. In these procedures, a hole is created in the distal portion of the false lumen, thereby permitting blood flow back into the true lumen and into the affected side branch.

Independent of the initial management, there are many long-term factors that must be addressed. Patients commonly require multiple antihypertensive agents to ensure adequate blood pressure control, and this should be tightly controlled for life to help prevent recurrence. β-Blockers should be part of the regimen for all patients following aortic dissection. Smoking cessation should be strongly counseled for all patients. If there is a clinical concern for an underlying connective tissue disorder, patients should be referred to a specialist for further evaluation. All patients should be counseled to avoid strenuous activity, particularly isometric activity, as this could provoke recurrence. Routine monitoring on CT or MR is necessary whether the patient was managed medically or with surgical repair. Residual dissection flaps can propagate further, and leaks may develop at graft anastamoses, occasionally leading to intrapericardial hemorrhage or hemothorax. Following type B dissection, up to 40% of cases will also lead to further aneurysmal dilatation over time. Many medically managed cases will ultimately require intervention, with a 41% intervention-free survival at 6 years for type B dissections. Therefore, clinicians must recognize that aortic dissection is truly a chronic disease that requires ongoing management and evaluation.

OTHER ACUTE AORTIC SYNDROMES

In addition to aortic dissection, aortic intramural hematoma (IMH) and penetrating atherosclerotic ulcer (PAU) are also considered acute aortic syndromes with similarly high risks of death. IMH is thought to be caused by bleeding into the vessel wall from the vasa vasorum. The blood collection can expand on its own and cause vessel wall weakness or it can lead to an intimal tear and aortic dissection. Overall, these represent ~5% to 10% of acute aortic syndromes. In general, patients with IMH tend to be older, with the mean age of detection being ~68. They can occur at any point along the length of the aorta and are classified using the Stanford system as in aortic dissection. Patients may present with chest or back pain, and both CT and MRI are excellent imaging modalities for detection and monitoring. IMHs are typically considered to be at similar risk and treated as an aortic dissection in the same region. Meta-analysis data revealed an overall mortality rate of 21% with Type A IMH being higher risk than Type B. Some IMHs may progress to aortic dissection and rupture, while others may remain stable or even involute over time. The additional presence of a PAU increases the risk of progression, whereas individuals with younger age and smaller aortic diameters are at lower risk. Most centers recommend urgent surgical intervention for Type A IMH and medical therapy with beta blockade and tight blood pressure control for Type B IMH. However, as with aortic dissection, the decision must incorporate numerous factors, and we recommend input from a variety of specialists as part of a multidisciplinary team to determine the best approach.

Penetrating atherosclerotic ulcers occur as sequelae of aortic atherosclerotic disease. Over time, atherosclerotic plaques can erode into the vessel wall, thus leading to focal weakness and, in some cases, intramural hematoma or wall rupture. Many PAUs are discovered incidentally, but some patients may present with chest or back pain as with aortic dissections. The natural history of PAU is unclear. Some centers report a high rate of rupture and recommend early surgical intervention, while others support a more conservative approach in most cases. Nonetheless, as with other types of aortic disease, progression varies considerably among individuals. PAUs should be regularly monitored on imaging, which is most easily achieved with contrast-enhanced CT or MRI. High-risk features, such as discovery coincident with pain, associated IMH, pseudoaneurysms, or true aneurysm, should prompt surgical consultation. Open surgical repair and endovascular grafts are both reasonable options, and there are no clear data supporting one approach over the other.

AORTITIS

Aortitis, or inflammation of the aorta, is broadly categorized as either autoimmune or infectious. Among the autoimmune causes, Takayasu's arteritis is one of the most common. Patients with Takayasu arteritis more commonly develop inflammation of the abdominal aorta, although the ascending aorta and arch may also be involved. Histologically, there is infiltration of lymphocytes, macrophages, and giant cells into the media and adventitia layers. Eventually, this leads to extensive scarring and fibrosis of the vessel wall, which can ultimately cause stenosis of the affected segment. It more commonly affects individuals of Asian descent, and women are at ten times higher risk than men. Most cases present before age 40. Typically, there is both an acute and chronic phase of Takayasu's arteritis. In the acute phase, individuals may experience fevers, chills, night sweats, and weight loss. Over time, ongoing inflammation leads to narrowing of the affected large vessel lumen. Thus, in the chronic phase, patients may exhibit diminished peripheral pulses, claudication, bruits, or discrepant blood pressures. Erythrocyte sedimentation rate and C-reactive protein values are often elevated but are nonspecific. Contrast-enhanced CT and MR imaging are useful in identifying the aortic segments and branch vessels involved. PET-CT may also be used to identify active inflammation as well as determine the success of therapy. Initial treatment typically consists of systemic steroids, although steroid-sparing regimens are often used as maintenance therapy. In some cases, surgical or endovascular therapy is necessary to correct narrowing of a large vessel.

Another commonly encountered cause of aortitis is giant cell arteritis. This involves not only the aorta but also large- and medium-sized branches. It is characterized by the presence of granulomas and giant cells throughout the aortic wall. This disease typically affects those over the age of 50 with a predilection for women and Caucasians. Patients often present with headache, visual disturbances, or jaw claudication. On examination, temporal artery tenderness or diminished pulse is common. Laboratory analysis is notable for a markedly elevated erythrocyte sedimentation rate. Imaging studies typically cannot differentiate this from other causes of aortitis, and temporal artery biopsy showing the presence of granulomas and giant cells often confirms the diagnosis. Treatment consists of long-term steroid therapy, and these individuals are at risk for subsequent aneurysm formation.

Behcet's disease is a rarer cause of aortitis. This syndrome usually presents with oral ulcers, genital ulcers, uveitis, and skin lesions, and vascular involvement only occurs in approximately one-third of patients. The disease causes inflammation of the vasa vasorum with infiltration by lymphocytes, histiocytes, eosinophils, and giant cells. Although aortic inflammation and subsequent aneurysm formation can occur, Behcet's can affect any number of arteries and veins, and patients may present with inflammation or aneurysm in multiple vessels. Treatment typically consists of corticosteroids. Depending on the vessel involved and the degree of aneurysmal dilatation, surgery or endovascular repair may be necessary. Other autoimmune disorders that can cause aortitis include rheumatoid arthritis, ankylosing spondylitis and other spondyloarthropathies, inflammatory bowel disease, and psoriatic arthritis.

Infectious aortitis is rare in the developed world but may have devastating consequences. It typically results from direct inoculation of the vessel wall through the vasa vasorum, although direct invasion and septic embolization are also possible. Infection typically occurs in a segment of the aorta with underlying pathology, such as aneurysm or atherosclerotic plaque. In addition to inflammation, infections may lead to abscesses, necrosis, mycotic aneurysm formation, or rupture. Patients may present with fever, chills, weight loss, or pain. CT and MRI are the primary means of identifying infective aortitis. Blood cultures are essential in identifying the causal organism. The most common bacterial causes of aortitis are *Salmonella* and *Staphylococcus aureus*, and fungal infections, such as *Candida* and *Aspergillus* are also possible, particularly in immunocompromised hosts. *Mycobacterium tuberculae* may cause aortitis that typically affects the distal aorta, likely through direct spread from adjacent thoracic structures. Although increasingly rare, syphilitic aortitis is a late complication of *Treponema pallidum* infection. It preferentially affects the ascending aorta and commonly leads to aneurysm formation several years after the initial infection. Prompt initiation of antibiotic therapy is essential. However, the active inflammation of infectious aortitis, particularly in cases of Gram-negative bacterial infection, leads to significant vessel wall weakening and an increased risk of rupture and death. In such cases, definitive repair also includes resection of the affected area and graft implantation.

SUGGESTED READINGS

Braverman AC. Acute aortic dissection. *Circulation*. 2010;122:184.

Braverman AC. Diseases of the aorta, In: DL Mann et al, eds. *Braunwald's Heart Disease*, 10th ed. Philadelphia, PA: Elsevier; 2015:1277-1311.

Goldfinger JZ, Halperin JL, Marin ML, Stewart AS, Eagle KA, Fuster V. Thoracic aortic aneurysm and dissection. *J Am Coll Cardiol*. 2014; 64(16):1725.

Gornik HL, Creager MA. Aortitis. *Circulation*. 2008;117:3039.

Hiratzka LF, Bakris GL, Beckman JA, et al. 2010 ACCF/AHA/AATS/ACR/ASA/SCA/SCAI/SIR/STS/SVM Guidelines for the diagnosis and management of patients with thoracic aortic disease: a report of the American College of Cardiology Foundation/American Heart Association Task Force on practice guidelines, American Association for Thoracic Surgery, American College of Radiology, American Stroke Association, Society of Cardiovascular Anesthesiologists, Society for Cardiovascular Angiography and Interventions, Society of Interventional Radiology, Society of Thoracic Surgeons, and Society for Vascular Medicine. *Circulation*. 2010;121:e266.

Isselbacher EM. Thoracic and abdominal aortic aneurysm. *Circulation*. 2005;111:816.

Patel HJ, Deeb GM. Ascending and arch aorta: pathology, natural history, and treatment. *Circulation*. 2008;118:188.

Sundt TM. Intramural hematoma and penetrating aortic ulcer. *Curr Opin Card*. 2007;22:504.

CHAPTER 256

Acute and Chronic Lower Limb Ischemia

Samir K. Shah, MD
Michael Belkin, MD

Key Clinical Questions

1 How is the diagnosis of lower-extremity peripheral arterial disease established?

2 When is lower-extremity ischemia an emergency?

3 When should vascular surgery consultation be obtained?

4 What are the essential nonsurgical elements of managing lower-extremity ischemia?

EPIDEMIOLOGY

While specific estimates vary, it is clear that lower-extremity peripheral arterial disease (PAD) affects a substantial fraction of the US population. For example, a 1999 analysis of the National Health and Nutrition Examination Survey results demonstrated that 4.3% of Americans over the age of 40 years had PAD, defined as an ankle-brachial index (ABI) of less than 0.90, corresponding to over 5 million people. The PAD Awareness, Risk, and Treatment: New Resources for Survival (PARTNERS) program, a multicenter, cross-sectional US study, showed that 29% of its cohort of nearly 7000 patients at least 50 years old had PAD based on a history of revascularization or an identical ABI criterion.

Clearly, recognition of PAD is important to guide appropriate limb-based therapy. However, given its close association with coronary and cerebrovascular arterial disease, it is perhaps more critical as a reason to motivate aggressive management of cardiovascular risk, which is discussed below.

Nonmodifiable risk factors for PAD include increasing age and nonblack Hispanic race. Gender is controversial. Some studies have shown a male predominance with less severe disease and an equal gender ratio in more advanced disease while others have ranged from no difference at any severity to a female predominance.

Irrespective of the particular risk factors in any given patient an obstructive arterial lesion with diminished distal flow is the final common pathway of PAD. Typically, this is atherosclerotic disease in chronic ischemia but there is a large array of rare causes that require investigation when clinically appropriate (**Table 256-1**). Degree of obstruction, however, is not the sole determinant of patient symptomatology. Indeed, around 15% of asymptomatic men were found to have 50% stenosis in at least one leg artery at autopsy. In addition to severity, symptoms depend on the timescale of disease development. Rapid narrowing of a vessel produces more profound distal ischemia because of inadequate time for the development of collateral vessels. As such acute arterial occlusion, for example from cardioembolism, often leads to extreme ischemia requiring surgical intervention while slowly developing atherosclerosis may be asymptomatic even if extensive (**Figure 256-1**). Finally, symptoms will also depend upon the demands of the affected vascular bed. Lesions that are hemodynamically significant at rest may not be clinically apparent until exertion. For example, patients' reports of cramping leg pain with walking that abates with rest—the so-called intermittent claudication—is described well by this mechanism. Once blood flow drops below a minimal threshold continuous ischemia will present as rest pain, ulceration, or gangrene.

RISK STRATIFICATION

All patients with acute limb threatening ischemia should be admitted. Patients with chronic limb ischemia do not universally require admission. Indications for admission include pain control, assessment, and therapy of ulcers and pedal infection including surgical debridement, and, expedited workup.

ACUTE LIMB ISCHEMIA

■ EVALUATION

Acute limb ischemia is caused by sudden compromise of extremity flow and comprises a variety of presentations and etiologies. Management is driven by the degree of ischemia and is commonly scored

TABLE 256-1 Selected Causes of Chronic Limb Ischemia

Atherosclerosis

Vasculitis

Fibromuscular dysplasia

Aneurysm with distal embolization (eg, popliteal artery aneurysm)

Extrinsic compression

    Popliteal entrapment

    Adventitial cystic disease

    Neoplasm

Radiation injury

Prior trauma

using the Rutherford scale for acute limb ischemia (**Table 256-2**). A focused and expeditious history and physical are essential. The history should focus on the duration of symptoms (prolonged time until revascularization favors the use fasciotomies, long-standing symptoms may suggest a chronic process), location and laterality of symptoms, conditions that would increase the risk of anticoagulation (eg, bleeding dyscrasias, trauma, recent surgery), arrhythmias, and endovascular instrumentation, including cardiac catheterization.

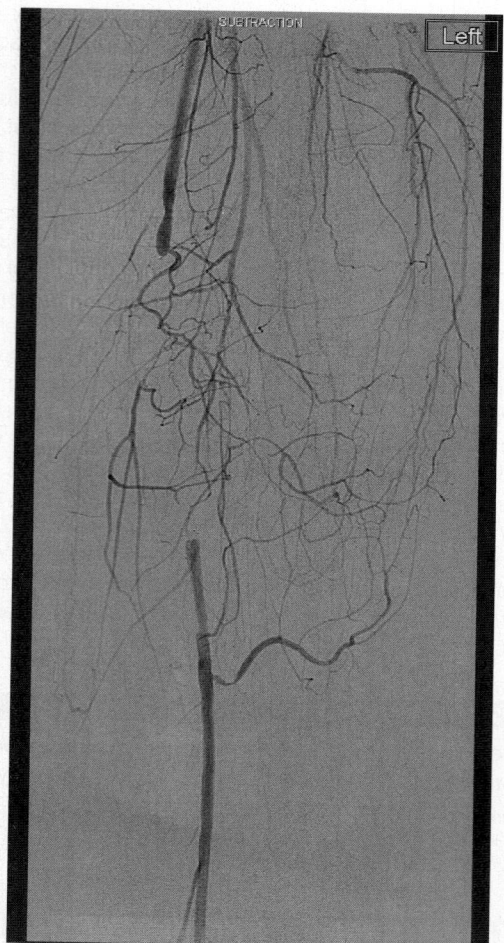

Figure 256-1 *Lower-extremity angiogram in a patient with claudication demonstrating superficial femoral artery occlusion. Note the presence of extensive-collateral vessels, which partly accounts for this patient's limited symptoms.*

The patient should receive a physical examination that, in addition to the typical cardiopulmonary examination, includes palpation of the abdomen for an aneurysm and examination of bilateral femoral, popliteal, pedal, and upper-extremity pulses. The pulse examination will suggest the location of the lesion. Furthermore comparison of the examinations between the two legs may suggest an etiology. For instance, a normal pulse examination on one leg with a normal contralateral femoral pulse and absent distal pulses in a patient with atrial fibrillation suggests embolization distal to the common femoral artery on the affected side. However, absent bilateral popliteal and pedal pulses with unilateral acute ischemia in the same patient may point toward in situ thrombosis in a background of chronic disease. A basic sensorimotor examination of the foot and leg provides a critical clue to the severity of the ischemia and the urgency of intervention. Sensory loss limited to the toes with intact motor function requires urgent intervention whereas more extensive sensory loss or any motor loss indicates more advanced ischemia and requires emergent intervention. The affected limb should be examined for compartment syndrome, including pain in the leg with passive or active ankle movement, pain with direct palpation of the leg, and numbness in the webspace between the first and second toes. Last, one should take into account the general appearance of the extremity. Common findings include pallor and mottling. Nonblanching erythema or ecchymosis over the leg calf is an ominous sign associated with advanced muscle ischemia. In rare cases of delayed presentation the patient may present with rigor mortis of the leg, which constitutes class III ischemia and is a contraindication to revascularization. The affected limb may also be cool to the touch below the level of obstruction. Despite the informal use of "cold leg" to refer to acute limb ischemia, physical coolness is nonspecific and not uniformly present.

Laboratory work is more directly related to preparation for intervention rather than diagnosis. For example, it is important to know the glomerular filtration rate, in case angiography is planned. Likewise, deranged electrolytes and coagulation parameters should be recognized and corrected as clinically appropriate. Creatine phosphokinase is sometimes ordered in the emergency room and a grossly elevated level would favor fasciotomies but this is uncommon with early presentation and the decision ultimately relies on clinical examination and judgment.

Vascular imaging is not mandatory prior to intervention and should not be obtained unless it could fundamentally alter management. In general, this decision should be made in concert with the consulting vascular surgery team. The most useful and commonly obtained noninvasive imaging is computed tomographic angiography (CTA) of the abdominal aorta with runoff views of the lower-extremity vasculature. The radiologist should be informed that the indication is acute limb ischemia so that delayed phase imaging is included in the protocol.

■ INPATIENT MANAGEMENT

The diagnosis of acute limb ischemia should immediately prompt vascular surgery consultation (**Figure 256-2**). In addition, to augment perfusion the affected limb should be placed in a dependent position and the patient started on supplemental oxygen, irrespective of oxygen saturation. In the absence of contraindications, intravenous heparin should be started to prevent thrombus propagation with a goal-activated partial thromboplastin time of two to three times above normal. Many institutions have established heparin protocols but in the absence of these the patient may be given a bolus of 80 to 100 μ/kg followed by an infusion of 18 μ/kg/h. Heparin administration will need to be individualized for patients at high risk for hemorrhagic complications: recent surgery, malignancy at risk for bleeding, and the like. Patients with known heparin induced

TABLE 256-2 Rutherford Scale for Acute Limb Ischemia

Rutherford's Class	Ischemia	Sensory Defect	Motor Defect	Arterial Signal	Venous Signal	Plan
I	Nonthreatened	None	None	Yes	Yes	Anticoagulation
IIa	Marginally threatened	None or limited to toes	None	No	Yes	Urgent revascularization
IIb	Acutely threatened	More than toes	Yes—ranges in severity	No	Yes	Emergent revascularization
III	Irreversibly ischemic	Profound	Profound	No	No	Interval amputation

thrombocytopenia will require direct thrombin inhibitor therapy, most commonly bivalirudin or argatroban.

Prompt vascular surgery consultation is important to determine the need for additional imaging as discussed above and surgical intervention. Patients with class I ischemia—no neurologic defect with Doppler-proven arterial flow—do not have an acutely threatened limb and warrant a workup in addition to anticoagulation. Patients with an irreversibly ischemic leg will benefit from heparin to prevent thrombus propagation but not from aggressive limb salvage. They should receive amputation when medically appropriate. All other patients—meaning those with sensorimotor loss and a viable limb—need revascularization immediately. Broadly, this may consist of open surgery (eg, thromboembolectomy, arterial bypass) or endovascular therapy (eg, percutaneous mechanical thrombectomy, thrombolysis), or both as determined by patient factors and local expertise.

History, examination, and findings at surgery should help guide an investigation into the etiology. Common possibilities include in situ thrombosis occurring in the context of advanced PAD. This will require little beyond aggressive PAD risk factor modification (discussed below). Patients with suspected embolization should have an embolic workup, including ECG for arrhythmia and echocardiography looking for cardiac thrombus or causal valvular disease. If these do not demonstrate a source, CTA or magnetic resonance imaging of the thoracic and abdominal aorta are indicated. Failing to identify any clear cause, patients should undergo investigation for a hypercoagulable condition. Examples include lupus anticoagulants, heparin-induced thrombocytopenic thrombosis, protein S deficiency, and prothrombin G20210A mutations. Guidance from vascular medicine or hematology should be obtained. Some of the salient laboratory tests may be confounded by ongoing heparin or warfarin use and should be drawn in advance of instituting these therapies if at all possible.

CHRONIC LIMB ISCHEMIA

■ EVALUATION

Chronic limb ischemia ranges widely in presentation from totally asymptomatic to claudication to critical limb ischemia, which includes rest pain, ischemic ulceration, and gangrene. Intermittent claudication classically consists of cramping muscle pain that is relieved within a few minutes of rest, though it should be noted that some reports have found that only a minority of patients describe all of these features. Claudication may occur in the buttocks, thigh, or calf and reflects ischemia one level below the area of disease, for example, a culprit superficial femoral artery will produce calf claudication. Rest pain is frequently described as a continuous burning pain in the foot, particularly the forefoot, that characteristically occurs at night when the foot is elevated in bed. Patients will also report relief with placement of the foot in the dependent position, which mechanically increases distal perfusion. Ulceration in the appropriate clinical context may represent PAD but caution is warranted. Patients with PAD often have a variety of potential causes and arterial insufficiency may be superimposed upon these or be unrelated. Examples include venous stasis ulcers, commonly associated with hemosiderin staining of the distal leg and foot and occurring on the medial distal leg and foot, neuropathic ulcers occurring in an area such as the head of the first metatarsal subject to trauma and often associated with a callus, or pressure ulceration as on the heels in bedbound patients. In addition to history and examination, the vascular testing discussed below will help clarify whether there is a component of arterial insufficiency.

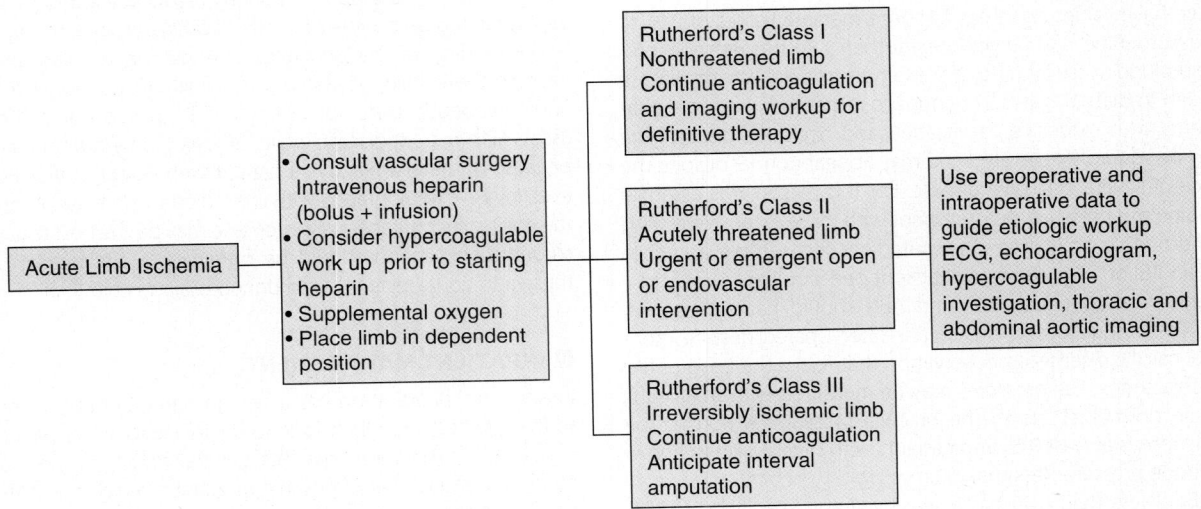

Figure 256-2 *Management of acute limb ischemia.*

As in acute limb ischemia a vascular examination should be performed along with tests of sensory and motor function. Areas of tissue loss and signs of infection (purulent exudate, periwound erythema, fluctuance) should be noted. Although a full discussion of diabetic foot infection is beyond the scope of this chapter, it should be noted that excision of necrotic tissue and drainage of sepsis are urgently indicated in infected diabetic ulcer (see Chapter 147 [Diabetic Foot Ulcers]).

There is no chronic ischemia-specific laboratory examination. Labs should be ordered as clinically indicated, for example, serum creatinine to assess baseline renal function if intervention or contrast-based imaging is contemplated or a CBC to look for a leukocytosis in cases of infection.

Whether PAD is responsible for the patient's symptoms may not be apparent in all cases. Conditions such as neurogenic claudication—intermittent lower-extremity pain from, for example, spinal stenosis—may be viable alternative explanations in some cases. In all except the most unequivocal cases, it is appropriate to obtain confirmatory noninvasive vascular tests. The mainstays of testing are ankle-brachial index (ABI), segmental Doppler pressures, and pulse volume recordings (PVR).

Noninvasive tests serve the dual purposes of confirming the presence of arterial insufficiency as the etiology and elucidating the location and severity of the causative lesions. The most basic test is the ABI. Although the mean arterial pressure decreases as one progresses distally in the vasculature, the systolic pressure increases as a result of pressure waves reflected from the distal circulation. Thus a decrement in the ankle systolic pressure is suggestive of occlusive disease somewhere between the heart and the blood pressure cuff. There are, however, alternative reasons for a reduced ankle pressure unrelated to occlusive disease such as hypotension. To reduce the effect of this factor, the ankle pressure should be normalized by dividing it by the brachial pressure, which is a proxy for aortic pressure, as brachial pressures are much less commonly reduced when compared with lower-limb pressures. Practically, the ABI is derived by inflating a cuff placed above the ankle to above the systolic pressure and slowly deflating the cuff until the Doppler signal of the posterior tibial artery is again heard. The procedure is again repeated for the dorsalis pedis artery and the higher of the two measurements is used as the ankle pressure or the numerator. The systolic pressure is measured in both arms and the higher of the two values is again used as the denominator in the calculation of the ABI. It is important to note that the patient should be supine for these measurements to avoid the confounding effects of hydrostatic pressure. Normal ABI ranges from 1 to 1.30. An ABI between 0.41 and 0.90 is typical of patients with claudication while those with critical limb ischemia will often have values less than 0.41. Intermediate values of 0.91 to 0.99 are borderline while those greater than 1.30 suggest noncompressible blood vessels due to, for example, medial calcific disease often seen in diabetics. It is important to remember, however, that in patients with extensive calcification and occlusive disease, the ABI may be spuriously elevated and may appear normal despite the presence of severe occlusive disease. For this reason, it is essential to combine this pressure measurement with more extensive testing and a thorough examination. One should not, for example, accept as normal an ABI of 1.0 in the face of absent pedal pulses.

Patients with spuriously elevated ABIs should have alternative testing. The vasculature of the toes is often spared despite more proximal calcific disease, an observation that forms the basis of the toe brachial index. Toe pressures may be measured with small cuffs and again normalized using the brachial pressure. A normal toe brachial index is at least 0.65 and patients with severe limb ischemia will have toe pressures less than 30 mm Hg.

An ABI of less than 0.90 has a sensitivity and specificity of 95% and 100% respectively for a 50% stenosis. Nevertheless it is possible for patients with significant peripheral artery to have normal resting ankle pressures. Conceptually, such occult disease may be detected by increasing blood flow velocity, which increases turbulence around a stenosis and produces energy losses and potentially a new pressure decrement. Exercise testing is therefore used for cases with a high suspicion for arterial disease despite a normal ABI. Patients are walked on a treadmill at 2 miles per hour at an incline of 10° to 12° until claudication occurs or a maximum of 5 minutes after which ABIs are measured serially until return to baseline. The degree of ABI drop and the time to normalization roughly correlate with severity of disease.

Although ABI is effective at establishing the presence of arterial insufficiency it does not localize disease. Segmental limb pressures may provide anatomic information indirectly and are obtained by placing a series of cuffs on the leg, which are then inflated and deflated as for the ankle pressure while listening for a pedal signal. Standard cuff positions include high thigh, above-knee, below-knee, and ankle. A drop of 20 mm Hg or more compared to the immediately preceding segment suggests significant disease. There are several drawbacks to the use of segmental pressures. First, extra-axial vessel disease may not be detected, for example, severe profunda femoris stenosis. Second, collaterals may reduce a pressure drop and thus obscure disease. Last, distal disease may obscure the detection of more proximal disease by reducing flow and thus reducing a pressure decrement. This may occur, for example, in a patient with simultaneous common femoral and common iliac artery stenosis.

Air plethysmography, more commonly known as pulse volume recording in this context, determines changes in lower-extremity volumes with each cardiac cycle beneath the cuff to infer disease location and severity. Normal PVRs consist of a brisk upstroke, a dicrotic notch, and then a final downward stroke. Although a full discussion of PVRs is beyond the scope of this discussion, disease proximal to the cuff location will diminish the amplitude of the initial upstroke and blunt the waveform morphology (**Figure 256-3**). Thus an examination of a series of PVRs progressing from proximal to distal in an extremity should help clarify the locations and magnitude of disease. Unlike the ABI, PVRs should not be affected by calcific disease. However, they are subject to all of the disadvantages seen with segmental pressures (eg, insensitivity to extra-axial disease).

In practice, ABI, segmental Doppler pressures, and PVRs are often combined. For example, our vascular laboratory provides these as a single composite test. Additionally, interpretation of these studies is often part and parcel of the report and should be performed by an individual familiar with the intricacies of the tests and the evaluation of these studies. Noninvasive physiologic testing as outlined above is followed by additional imaging—duplex ultrasound, computed tomographic angiography, magnetic resonance angiography, conventional angiography—to produce a final treatment plan. A firm understanding of the principles, strengths, and disadvantages of each of these tests is crucial to formulating a rational diagnostic and therapeutic plan. For example, CTA would be reasonable to assess iliac in-stent disease while MRA would be grossly inadequate because of metal artifact. In a patient with renal insufficiency, however, invasive angiography with limited or no iodinated contrast and the ability to simultaneously intervene may be the best test. Vascular surgery consultation should be obtained in advance of ordering these additional tests to avoid unnecessary testing.

■ INPATIENT MANAGEMENT

Intermittent claudication has a benign natural history with respect to the affected limb: limb loss occurs in 1% to 3% of patients over 5 years. As such, these patients generally do not need inpatient admission and will benefit from outpatient evaluation. Initial therapy frequently consists of a supervised exercise plan, risk factor modification, and occasionally adjunctive cilostazol. In sharp contrast, patients

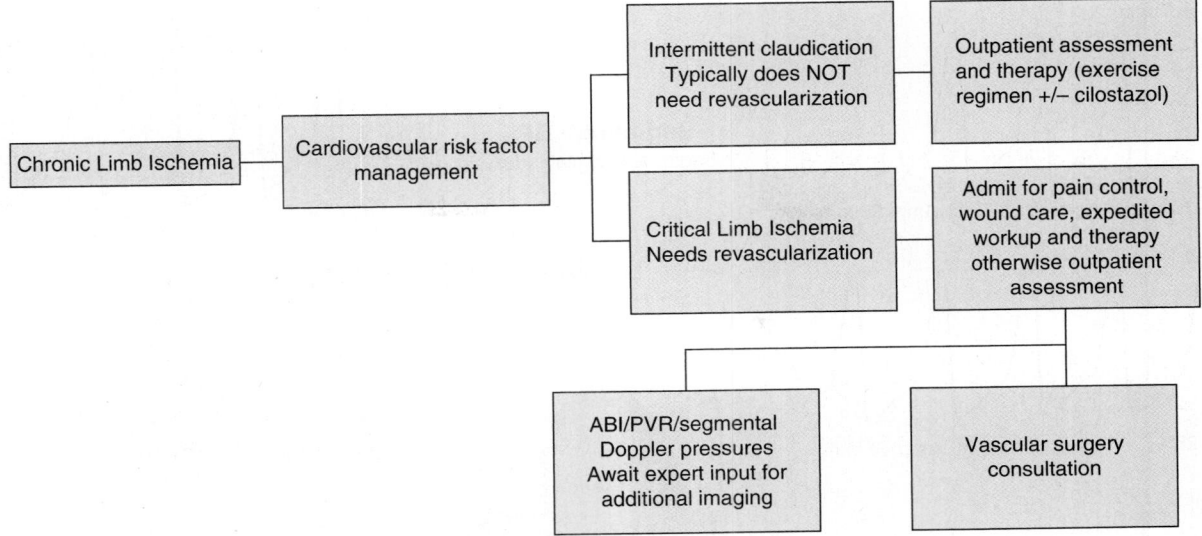

Figure 256-3 *Management of chronic limb ischemia.*

with critical limb ischemia without revascularization may have up to a 40% limb loss rate at 6 months. As such, prompt evaluation and surgical or endovascular intervention is indicated (**Figure 256-4**). Even so, critical limb ischemia is not intrinsically an absolute indication for admission. Legitimate reasons for admission include pain control, as for intractable rest pain, wound care, and expedited workup and therapy for patients who are unable to comply with outpatient follow-up or who are at risk for impending limb loss.

Wound care options have recently proliferated and a complete treatment of wound care is beyond the scope of this work. In addition to debridement, common wound care strategies include wet-to-dry dressings with normal saline, sterile water, or dilute Dakin's (sodium hypochlorite) solution for grossly infected wounds. The latter should not be used for more than 5 days to avoid injuring healthy tissue. Wound vacuum dressings have been shown to aid wound care and healing in diverse settings and may reduce the burden of care and time to resolution in vascular patients. Patients with extensive devitalized or infected tissue may need surgery to achieve a more expeditious aggressive debridement than is possible with wet-to-dry or enzymatic methods (eg, enzymes). Vascular surgery, plastic surgery, wound care services, or other local expertise will be able to provide additional input.

Although only lifestyle-limiting claudication and critical limb ischemia demand surgery, all patients with PAD need aggressive medical management. Consider as evidence the 5-year 20% combined myocardial infarction and stroke rate and 10% to 15% mortality in claudicants. Figures for critical limb ischemia are even more dismal with a commonly cited 25% 1-year mortality, again primarily from cardiovascular events.

Typical recommendations include smoking cessation, weight loss for overweight and obese patients, antihypertensive therapy, diabetes management, and lipid-lowering therapy. Significantly, statin therapy has been shown to improve a variety of outcomes, including cardiovascular adverse event rates and all-cause mortality, in PAD patients. Patients benefit irrespective of initial lipid levels and therefore all PAD patients should be placed on statin therapy. Although the evidence for routine antiplatelet therapy has been more ambiguous, general recommendations include daily aspirin therapy for all PAD patients. There is no clear benefit to 325 mg over 81 mg. Patients already on clopidogrel for other reasons do not derive cardiovascular benefit from the addition of aspirin although

there is evidence of benefit in selected vascular patients (eg, prosthetic infrapopliteal bypass). In general clopidogrel monotherapy is adequate. Anticoagulation is not recommended for general PAD risk reduction but may be instituted for specific patients after intervention. Regrettably several studies have found widespread underuse of antiplatelet agents and statins despite their favorable risk profiles.

Finally, revascularization for patients with lifestyle-limiting claudication or critical limb ischemia may be performed via open surgery, endovascular therapy, or a hybrid approach. The intervention strategy will depend on patient anatomy, lesion characteristics, medical risk, patient preference, and local expertise.

PRACTICE POINT

Avoiding delays in acute limb ischemia

- Acute limb ischemia is associated with considerable morbidity and mortality. Time to intervention is crucial to favorable outcomes. Obtain immediate surgical consultation. The diagnosis is a clinical one and imaging should not be ordered without expert consultation because of the risk of delay in treatment. Assessment of sensorimotor function is the most important aspect of physical examination and will often determine the urgency of intervention.

PRACTICE POINT

Risk factor modification in peripheral arterial disease

- Only PAD patients with severe unremitting claudication or critical limb ischemia (rest pain or tissue loss) will require surgical or endovascular intervention, but all patients require aggressive cardiovascular risk factor management, including:
- Smoking cessation
- Weight loss for overweight and obese patients
- Control of hypertension
- Diabetic management
- Statin therapy for all patients
- Antiplatelet therapy for all patients

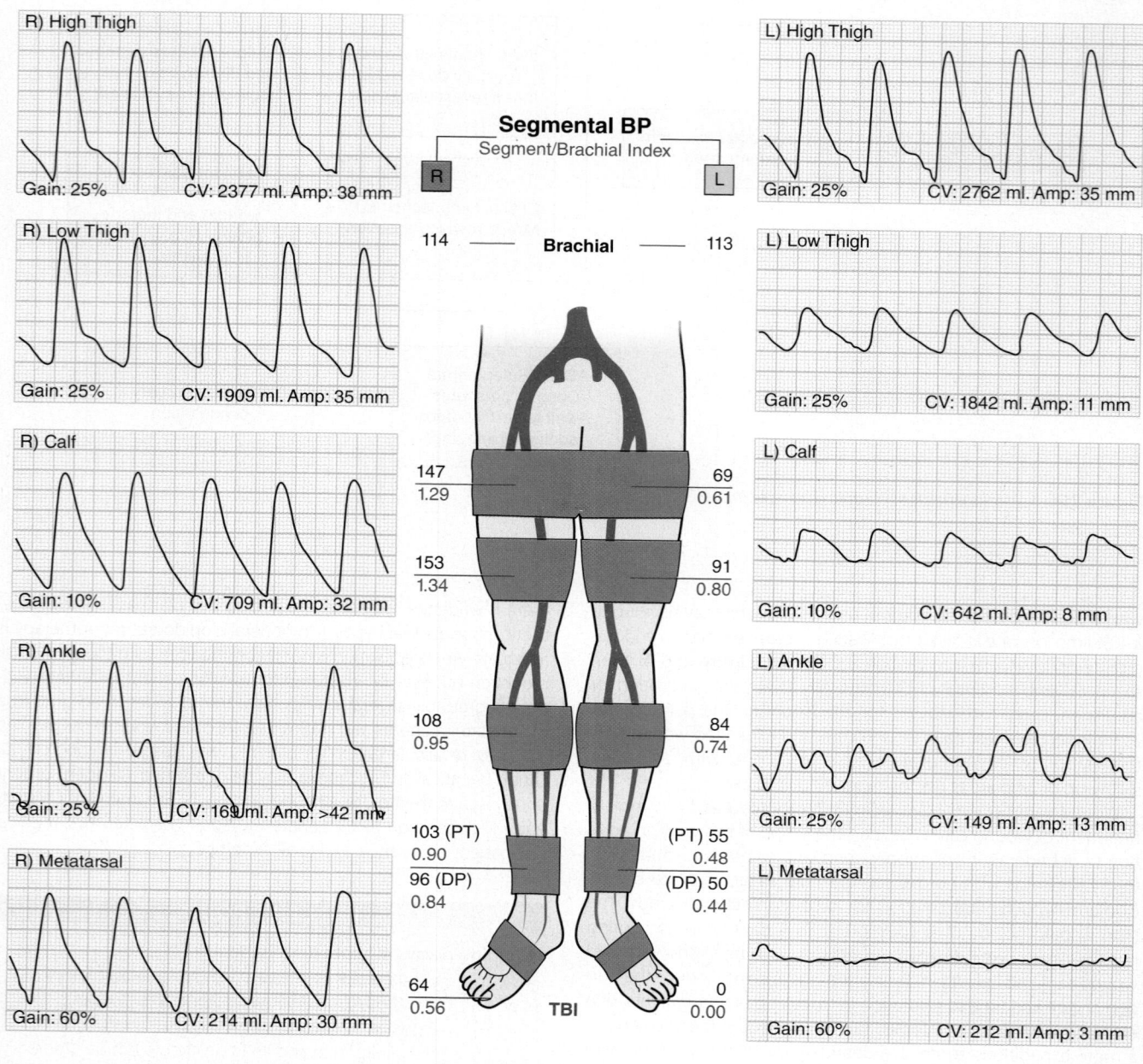

Figure 256-4 *A composite of pulse volume recordings, ankle-brachial index, and segmental Doppler pressures in a patient with bilateral multilevel occlusive disease. Clinically, this patient had short distance claudication on the left only, which is corroborated by more severe indicators of left-sided disease. In particular, note the dampened nature of the distal left pulse volume recordings and grossly abnormal ankle-brachial index.*

POSTACUTE CARE

Postacute care will vary immensely from patient to patient but should include follow-up with vascular surgery, either for routine follow-up or additional workup, and primary care follow-up for cardiovascular risk factor modification.

DISCHARGE CHECKLIST

1. Have all of the patient's medical risk factors for PAD been addressed? In particular, is the patient on an appropriate antiplatelet agent and statin?
2. If applicable, is there a wound care plan?
3. Is there follow up with a vascular surgeon?

SUGGESTED READINGS

Clair D, Shah S, Weber J. Current state of diagnosis and management of critical limb ischemia. *Curr Cardiol Rep.* 2012;14: 160-170.

Hirsch A, Criqui M, Treat-Jacobson D, et al. Peripheral arterial disease detection, awareness, and treatment in primary care. *JAMA.* 2001;286:1317-1324.

Norgren L, Hiatt WR, Dormandy JA, et al. Inter-society consensus for the management of peripheral arterial disease (TASC II). *J Vasc Surg.* 2007;45(Suppl S):S5-S67.

CHAPTER 257

Vasculitis

Paul A. Monach, MD, PhD
Peter A. Merkel, MD, MPH

Key Clinical Questions

① When should a diagnosis of vasculitis be considered?

② How is a diagnosis of vasculitis made or excluded?

③ What are the appropriate strategies for triage, consultation, and follow-up for vasculitis?

④ What treatment and staging for vasculitis should be initiated in the hospital?

⑤ In a patient with established vasculitis, how should new symptoms of illness be evaluated?

INTRODUCTION

The diagnosis of vasculitis is considered far more often than these diseases are actually seen—appropriately, since these rare diseases have diverse presentations, are dangerous and often rapidly progressive, yet are treatable. All vasculitides feature inflammation of the walls of blood vessels, with symptoms and findings attributable to the size(s) and locations of the involved vessels. Vessel size, epidemiology, and/or a constellation of typical clinical features have proved useful for classifying the vasculitides, with key points summarized in (**Table 257-1**).

The classification of vasculitis remains imprecise with more than one system in use. "Primary" systemic vasculitides are further sorted by the sizes of the predominant arteries involved, leading to sets of small-, medium-, and large-vessel vasculitides. There are also several "secondary" forms of vasculitis associated with infections, drug exposure, or another form of systemic disease such as systemic lupus erythematosis or rheumatoid arthritis.

All of the primary, idiopathic vasculitides are rare diseases, each categorized as an "orphan" disease in the United States (prevalence of <200,000 persons). However, as a group, and especially among patients with initially unexplained systemic disease who are ill enough to be hospitalized, vasculitis is common enough that hospitalists will likely encounter cases.

PATHOPHYSIOLOGY

The pathophysiology of the primary vasculitides is poorly understood. They are all considered immune mediated, based on histologic and serologic studies and by analogy to the many cases of vasculitis that have occurred secondary to infections or drug exposure. Since no pathogens have been found, the primary vasculitides are suspected to be autoimmune, with the humoral and cellular branches of the adaptive immune system involved to different degrees in different diseases.

■ NOTES ON INDIVIDUAL FORMS OF VASCULITIS

It is impractical to describe each of the vasculitides in detail in a single chapter, but short summaries of most of the vasculitides are provided as reference points for the subsequent discussion.

Giant cell arteritis

Giant cell arteritis (GCA) only affects adults over the age of 50, and incidence markedly increases with age, to about 1:2000 per year among Caucasians of Northern European descent by age 80. Headache is the most common symptom (80%), with scalp tenderness, jaw claudication, constitutional symptoms, and polymyalgia rheumatica (pain and stiffness in the shoulders, hips, and/or neck) each seen in 40% to 70% of patients. The presentation of GCA is often insidious and diagnosed during outpatient care, but sometimes is acute and leads to hospitalization. GCA has also been reported to be an important cause (about 10%) of fever of unknown origin in the elderly, and since the aorta and its major branches are involved in more than 15% of cases, GCA is also an important consideration in cases of claudication, loss of pulse, and asymmetric blood pressure measurements in the elderly. (See the section on laboratory testing [acute phase reactants], imaging [angiography, ultrasound], and biopsy [temporal artery]).

TABLE 257-1 Classification of the Major Primary Vasculitides, with Some Key Features (Nonexhaustive List)

Vessel Sizes and Associated Diseases	Key Diagnostic Tests	Common Clinical Features
Largest arteries: aorta and branches		
Giant cell arteritis	Temporal artery biopsy Ophthalmologic examination	Headache, vision loss, arthralgias, malaise
Takayasu arteritis	Angiography	Claudication, pulselessness
Aortitis in Cogan syndrome	Angiography	Hearing loss, vertigo, ocular inflammation
Isolated aortitis	Angiography	
Medium-sized arteries		
Kawasaki disease	Coronary artery imaging	Prolonged fever, coronary artery aneurysms
Polyarteritis nodosa	Hepatitis B virus Angiography	Erythematous skin lesions, hypertension, abdominal pain, neuropathy
Small arteries		
Granulomatosis with polyangiitis (Wegener)	ANCA, urinalysis Sinus and chest CT Biopsy, renal or other	Pulmonary nodules or hemorrhage, sinonasal disease, renal impairment, neuropathy, arthralgias, skin lesions
Microscopic polyangiitis	ANCA, urinalysis Biopsy, renal or other	Pulmonary hemorrhage, renal impairment, neuropathy, purpura
Eosinophilic granulomatosis with polyangiitis (Churg-Strauss)	Total eosinophil count Sinus and chest CT Biopsy of affected organ	Asthma, eosinophilia, pulmonary infiltrates, neuropathy
Antiglomerular-basement membrane disease (including Goodpasture syndrome)	Anti-GBM antibodies Renal biopsy	Pulmonary hemorrhage, glomerulonephritis
IgA vasculitis (Henoch-Schöenlein)	Skin biopsy	Purpura, arthritis, abdominal pain, IgA nephropathy
Cryoglobulinemic vasculitis	Cryoglobulins Hepatitis C virus Skin or renal biopsy	Purpura, neuropathy, glomerulonephritis
CNS vasculitis	Brain biopsy	Headache, encephalopathy, multiple strokes
Arteries and veins of various sizes		
Behçet disease	Ophthalmologic exam	Oral and genital ulcers, uveitis
Relapsing polychondritis	Ophthalmologic exam	Auricular, nasal, and tracheal inflammation, ocular inflammation

ANCA, antineutrophil cytoplasmic antibodies; CNS, central nervous system; CT, computed tomography.

Takayasu arteritis

Takayasu arteritis is a rare disease (prevalence <1:100,000), usually presenting in young adults, and 90% of patients are female. Patients often present with claudication, dizziness, abnormal blood pressure readings, and/or bruits. Diagnosis is confirmed by angiography. The types of presentation more likely to lead to hospitalization (eg, symptoms of coronary artery disease or cerebrovascular disease) carry a broad differential diagnosis, so suspicion for or against Takayasu may initially be gained by checking pulses and blood pressures and listening for bruits. (See the section on laboratory testing [acute phase reactants] and imaging [angiography, ultrasound]).

Granulomatosis with polyangiitis (Wegener's) and microscopic polyangiitis

Granulomatosis with polyangiitis (Wegener's) (GPA) and microscopic polyangiitis (MPA), often grouped together as antineutrophil cytoplasmic antibody (ANCA)-associated vasculitis (AAV), are small-vessel vasculitides that together affect ~1:20,000 persons. AAV is high in the differential diagnosis of patients presenting with pulmonary hemorrhage, acute renal disease, or acute peripheral neuropathy, and is also an important consideration in patients with palpable purpura, inflammatory eye disease (scleritis or episcleritis), acute sensorineural hearing loss, cutaneous ulcers, or digit ischemia.

Renal disease in AAV often leads to elevated serum creatinine and presence of urinary RBC casts; however, in the early stages of renal disease with AAV patients may only have microscopic hematuria and modest proteinuria. GPA usually (70%-80% at initial presentation) also features granulomatous inflammation of the upper airway, with nasal discharge and crusting, epistaxis, facial pain, and/or hearing loss, and the presence of these symptoms often facilitates the diagnosis of GPA. GPA is an important consideration in cases of subglottic stenosis, orbital mass with proptosis, or pulmonary nodule(s). However, many patients with AAV, particularly MPA, present only with nonspecific symptoms of malaise, myalgias, and arthralgias. The role of testing for ANCA in diagnosing AAV is discussed in detail below. (See section on laboratory testing [autoimmune serologies, acute phase reactants, tests of renal function], imaging [chest imaging, sinus imaging], and biopsy [skin, nasal cavity and sinuses, kidney, lung, peripheral nerve and muscle]).

Eosinophilic granulomatosis with polyangiitis (Churg-Strauss)

Eosinophilic granulomatosis with polyangiitis (EGPA) is worth considering in a patient who is ill with what might be vasculitis, has a history of asthma (often severe or poorly controlled), and has eosinophilia. The presentations of EGPA most likely to lead to hospitalization are asthma exacerbation, pulmonary infiltrates, or acute peripheral neuropathy, but constitutional symptoms, nasal polyps, rash, and arthralgias are also common. Myocarditis, gastrointestinal inflammation or ischemia, stroke, and renal involvement (similar to AAV) are less common but important presentations. Positive tests for ANCA are present in 40% of patients and EGPA is considered part of the spectrum of ANCA-associated vasculitis. (See section on laboratory testing [autoimmune serologies, acute phase reactants, tests of renal function, and complete blood count (CBC)], imaging [chest imaging and sinus imaging], and biopsy [skin, nasal cavity, and sinuses, kidney, lung, peripheral nerve, and muscle]).

Antiglomerular-basement-membrane disease

In contrast to AAV, symptoms of antiglomerular-basement-membrane (GBM) disease are limited to the kidneys and/or lungs (if both = Goodpasture syndrome), with rapidly progressive glomerulonephritis and/or pulmonary hemorrhage as manifestations. In the right setting, a positive test for serum antiglomerular-basement-membrane (anti-GBM) antibodies is diagnostic for this disorder, as is demonstration of the characteristic pattern of antibody deposition by immunofluorescence on kidney tissue obtained by biopsy. Testing for anti-GBM antibodies should be rapidly obtained for any patient for whom anti-GBM disease is possible, since the disease can lead to irreversible kidney damage or death from pulmonary hemorrhage. (See section on laboratory testing [autoimmune serologies, tests of renal function], and imaging [chest imaging], biopsy [kidney, lung]).

Polyarteritis nodosa

The most common features of polyarteritis nodosa (PAN) are livedo reticularis (a lacy pattern of cutaneous blood vessels on extremities that is more commonly due to benign conditions rather than vasculitis), painful cutaneous nodules or ulcers, hypertension, abdominal pain, myalgias, peripheral neuropathy, testicular pain, and digit ischemia. There is a strong association between hepatitis B virus (HBV) infection and PAN, but only in areas where HBV is endemic; the incidence of PAN has markedly declined in countries with high rates of HBV vaccination. PAN is probably the most challenging type of vasculitis to diagnose, because (1) it is particularly rare (in regions where HBV infection is also rare), (2) it features the least specific array of symptoms and findings among the vasculitides, and (3) there are no helpful diagnostic blood tests analogous to ANCA, cryoglobulins, or even eosinophil count. Biopsy or angiography is usually required for the diagnosis of PAN. For all of these reasons, PAN is contemplated much more often than it is diagnosed. (See section on laboratory testing [acute phase reactants, tests of renal function, selected testing for infectious diseases], imaging [angiography], and biopsy [skin, kidney, peripheral nerve and muscle, other organs]).

Behçet disease

The manifestations of Behçet disease (BD) that may lead to hospitalization are extraordinarily diverse: vision loss or a red and painful eye, deep vein thrombosis (including dural sinus thrombosis or Budd-Chiari syndrome), colitis resembling inflammatory bowel disease, meningoencephalitis, or pulmonary artery rupture leading to massive hemorrhage. Considering the diagnosis of BD in these settings requires recognition of the various milder but more common features of BD that may be concurrently present or reported by the patient, including recurrent oral ulcers (required for diagnosis), genital ulcers, erythema nodosum, acneiform skin lesions, inflammatory arthritis, and superficial thrombophlebitis. The diagnosis or exclusion of BD is always made on clinical grounds since there are no specific blood tests or biopsy features of the disease.

Primary angiitis of the central nervous system

This rare disease is limited to the central nervous system (CNS) and presents with symptoms of encephalopathy, multiple small strokes, and often headache. Angiography may be normal since the disease often affects only small vessels. Furthermore, angiography cannot easily distinguish vasculitis from atherosclerosis or from cerebral vasospasm (which usually presents with a severe headache of sudden onset). Thus, diagnosis of CNS vasculitis is ideally made by brain biopsy. (See section on imaging [angiography], and biopsy [brain]).

Cryoglobulinemic vasculitis

Cryoglobulinemia encompasses a variety of clinical syndromes associated with circulating immune complexes that precipitate at cold temperatures. The majority of cases of cryoglobulinemia (~70%) are associated with chronic hepatitis C virus infection, with plasma cell malignancies and systemic rheumatic diseases accounting for most other cases. Cryoglobulinemia associated with chronic hepatitis C virus infection or systemic rheumatic disease causes a small-vessel vasculitis that typically involves skin (palpable purpura and/or ulcers), commonly involves peripheral nerves or kidneys (glomerulonephritis), and less commonly involves a wide range of internal organs. (See section on laboratory testing [tests of renal function, paraproteins, selected testing for infectious diseases], and biopsy [skin, kidney, peripheral nerve and muscle]).

IgA vasculitis (Henoch-Schönlein)

IgA vasculitis (Henoch-Schönlein purpura, IgAV) is much more common among children than adults. It is usually self-limited and presents with palpable purpura, often in association with inflammatory arthritis and abdominal pain. A minority of patients has severe renal involvement, and the presence or absence of significant proteinuria or elevated creatinine is often used to determine whether to treat with immunosuppressive agents; however, the usefulness of such treatment has not been firmly established. (See section on laboratory testing [tests of renal function] and biopsy [skin, kidney]).

Kawasaki disease

Kawasaki disease (KD) is almost exclusively a disease of young children, and it is not rare in its characteristic age group (incidence 1:10,000 in the United States). The syndrome classically includes fever persisting for at least 5 days, erythematous rash with desquamation in the hands and feet, conjunctivitis, oral mucosal inflammation, and lymphadenopathy. However, many patients present without all of these features and, since a consequence of untreated KD is life-threatening coronary artery aneurysms, the diagnosis is considered in almost any young child with a fever lasting 5 days.

Vasculitis associated with other autoimmune diseases

Systemic lupus, rheumatoid arthritis, Sjögren syndrome, and inflammatory bowel disease have all been associated with vasculitis, mostly involving small vessels (palpable purpura, ulcers, neuropathy), but occasionally medium-sized vessels (analogous to PAN). Inflammatory bowel disease, relapsing polychondritis, and Cogan syndrome are each rarely associated with large-vessel vasculitis similar to Takayasu arteritis. (See section on laboratory testing [autoimmune serologies and tests of renal function]).

DIAGNOSIS: DOES THIS PATIENT HAVE VASCULITIS?

Vasculitis is commonly in the differential diagnosis for any patient with an unexplained systemic illness or any patient with one or more specific findings suggestive of vasculitis. It is important to realize that vasculitis is rare. Nonetheless, being open to the possibility of vasculitis is critical for reducing delays in diagnosis. There are many "red flags" that should alert clinicians that vasculitis must be considered (**Table 257-2**). Some of these findings merit urgent diagnostic testing and sometimes even empiric treatment for vasculitis, pending the results of testing.

Not shown in Table 257-2 are syndromes that could be caused by vasculitis but have other causes in the vast majority of cases such as fever of unknown origin, lower-extremity ulcers, abdominal pain, arthralgias, myalgias, and other nonspecific symptoms.

■ MIMICS OF VASCULITIS

Since vasculitis is rare, nonvasculitic causes of red-flag symptoms remain more common than vasculitis in many cases. A broad range of infectious, autoimmune, toxic, malignant, thromboembolic, vasospastic, and atherosclerotic disorders can mimic many of the characteristic features of vasculitis, as outlined in general terms in Table 257-2.

■ DIAGNOSTIC TESTING FOR SUSPECTED VASCULITIS

The method for diagnosing vasculitis generally depends on the size of vessels involved. Small-vessel vasculitis is usually diagnosed

by biopsy, but sometimes the combination of a typical clinical syndrome and a laboratory test (see preceding section) is sufficient. Medium-vessel vasculitis (PAN) is diagnosed by biopsy or angiography. GCA is usually diagnosed by biopsy (temporal arteritis) but occasionally by angiography if the aorta or its major branches are involved. Takayasu is diagnosed by angiography. CNS vasculitis is usually diagnosed by biopsy but sometimes by angiography. Behçet disease and Kawasaki disease are diagnosed based on the clinical syndrome.

The uses of laboratory testing, diagnostic imaging, and biopsy for diagnosing vasculitis are outlined below.

■ LABORATORY TESTING FOR EVALUATION OF SUSPECTED VASCULITIS

Although individual laboratory tests on their own are almost never diagnostic for vasculitis, such tests are essential in the evaluation of a patient in whom vasculitis is being considered, for several reasons: (1) in the proper setting, selected serologic tests may confirm a diagnosis of vasculitis; (2) laboratory testing may identify organ

TABLE 257-2 Red Flags that Should Prompt Consideration of Vasculitis and Mimics of Vasculitis

Red Flag	Disease(s) to Consider	Nonvasculitic Causes ("Mimics") to Consider	Comment
Palpable purpura	IgAV, AAV, Cryo, PAN, infection-associated, drug reaction	Atheroembolic disease, bacteremia, cardiac myxoma	Biopsy may show vasculitis but does not reveal the exact cause/type
Pulmonary hemorrhage	AAV, GBM	SLE, pneumonia, coagulopathy	Bronchoscopy establishes hemorrhage but not the cause
Acute renal failure (especially glomerulonephritis)	AAV, GBM, Cryo	SLE, acute interstitial nephritis, noninflammatory causes	Presence of other characteristic features raises suspicion
Destructive nasal inflammation (septal perforation, saddle-nose)	GPA	Cocaine use	Presence of other characteristic features raises suspicion
Mononeuritis multiplex	PAN, AAV, Cryo	Diabetes, HIV, other causes	Vasculitis is a common cause of wrist or foot drop; other peripheral neuropathies are also common in vasculitis
New headache in the elderly	GCA	Many other causes	ESR and CRP helpful for initial triage
Absent pulse or blood pressure	Large-vessel vasculitis, especially TAK or GCA	Atherosclerosis	TAK if age <50, GCA if >50
Acute monocular vision loss	GCA	Embolic disease, nonarteritic acute ischemic optic neuropathy	Presence of other characteristic features raises suspicion
Inflammatory eye disease (uveitis, scleritis, episcleritis)	Behçet, AAV	Also common with other rheumatic and infectious diseases	Presence of other characteristic features raises suspicion
Encephalopathy, multiple strokes	PACNS	CNS arterial vasospasm, embolic disease	Angiographic appearance similar; biopsy usually required
Thoracic aortic aneurysm	Large-vessel vasculitis, especially TAK or GCA	Syphilis, Marfan syndrome, atherosclerosis	Aortitis can occur as an isolated manifestation of vasculitis
Digit ischemia or gangrene	PAN, AAV, Cryo	Thrombotic and vasospastic disorders	Nonvasculitic causes are more common
Mesenteric ischemia or bowel infarction	PAN, AAV	Thromboembolic disorders, atherosclerosis	Nonvasculitic causes are more common
Fever >5 d in a young child	Kawasaki	Numerous infectious and noninfectious causes	Presence of other characteristic features raises suspicion
Eosinophilia and asthma	EGPA	Hypereosinophilic syndromes	Extrapulmonary symptoms and degree of eosinophilia raise suspicion
Fever of unknown origin in the elderly	GCA	Many infectious, malignant, and autoimmune causes	GCA is a common etiology

AAV, ANCA-associated vasculitis: granulomatosis with polyangiitis (Wegener, GPA), microscopic polyangiitis, and eosinophilic granulomatosis with polyangiitis (Churg-Strauss, EGPA); Cryo, cryoglobulinemia; GBM, antiglomerular-basement-membrane disease; GCA, giant cell arteritis; IgAV, IgA vasculitis (Henoch-Schonlein); PACNS, primary angiitis of the central nervous system; PAN, polyarteritis nodosa; SLE, systemic lupus erythematosis; TAK, Takayasu arteritis.

systems involved in the disease process (especially for renal disease); (3) laboratory tests may establish a diagnosis *other* than vasculitis.

Autoimmune serologies

Testing for various autoantibodies plays a key role in the evaluation of patients suspected of having vasculitis, but over-reliance on such testing often leads to delayed or missed diagnoses.

Antineutrophil cytoplasmic antibodies

The widespread availability of testing for ANCA has had a striking impact on the evaluation of patients with suspected small-vessel vasculitis. The current standard of care for ANCA testing includes combining tests for ANCA by immunoflourescence and tests for specific ANCA autoantibodies by ELISA. Only two combinations of test results constitute a truly "positive" ANCA test: the cytoplasmic (C-ANCA) immunoflourescence pattern combined with antiprotein-ase 3 (PR3) antibodies by ELISA, or the perinuclear (P-ANCA) immu-noflourescence pattern combined with antimyeloperoxidase (MPO) antibodies by ELISA. In the proper clinical settings, positive ANCA testing (C/anti-PR3 or P/anti-MPO) is highly specific for the diagnosis of AAV (>95%) and may preclude the need for biopsy or at least sup-port initiation of treatment with glucocorticoids pending a biopsy. However, ANCA testing is presumed to have lower specificity in the setting of nonspecific symptoms such as malaise, myalgias, and arthralgias—a relatively common initial presentation of AAV. The sensitivity of ANCA testing is ~90% in patients with systemic GPA or MPA and is considerably lower (70%) in patients with GPA limited to the airway, so a patient may still have GPA even if the ANCA test is negative. Thus, ANCA testing is extremely useful diagnostically but *must* be used in the context of supportive clinical and other data.

Antiglomerular-basement-membrane antibodies

In the setting of renal insufficiency and/or pulmonary hemorrhage, anti-GBM antibodies are highly specific for the diagnosis of anti-GBM disease/Goodpasture disease as long as the initial anti-GBM antibody screening test is confirmed by Western blot. Because the treatment of choice for anti-GBM disease is the combination of high-dose glucocorticoids and plasma exchange, it is crucial to establish the diagnosis as early as possible. Antibody testing can play a central role in this process, but sometimes immunoflourescence staining of a kidney biopsy can make the diagnosis more rapidly.

Antinuclear antibodies

Testing for antinuclear antibodies (ANA) is quite useful when there is suspicion of systemic lupus erythematosus (SLE), either underlying vasculitis or as an alternative diagnosis for pulmonary hemorrhage and/or acute renal failure. ANA testing is >95% sensitive for the diag-nosis of lupus; therefore, a negative test essentially rules out lupus as a diagnosis, unless a patient has clear pathognomonic features.

Acute phase reactants

Although the erythrocyte sedimentation rate (ESR) and C-reactive protein (CRP) are usually elevated in patients with untreated vascu-litis, and ESR and CRP are often ordered when evaluating patients with suspected vasculitis, these tests have a surprisingly low value diagnostically. ESR or CRP are neither sensitive nor specific enough to be considered as screening tests to make or exclude a diag-nosis of vasculitis, except, in a limited way, as part of a diagnostic algorithm for GCA. Even for new-onset GCA, the ESR or CRP may be normal in ~15% of cases, and both are normal in ~4% of cases. Therefore, a normal ESR is only helpful in ruling out GCA and avoid-ing the need for a temporal artery biopsy in a low-probability patient (atypical headache only), but not in a patient with additional cranial,

arthritic, or constitutional symptoms. These tests may have selected roles in evaluation for persistent or recurrent disease but still must be interpreted cautiously. Furthermore, ESR and/or CRP are often elevated in the major mimics of vasculitis, especially infections (either acute or chronic) and malignancies.

Tests of renal function and other chemistry laboratory testing

Prompt assessment of renal function is an essential part of the evalu-ation of any patient suspected of having vasculitis. Renal disease can be either insidious or fulminant, and renal injury is usually asymp-tomatic until symptoms of end-stage renal disease arise. Serum creatinine with estimate of glomerular filtration rate should be done immediately in all patients and compared with prior measurements. Even subtle rises in creatinine levels within the "normal" range may be indicative of serious disease.

If urinary dipstick testing demonstrates the presence of any blood or protein, then a microscopic examination of the urine sedi-ment on a freshly collected specimen *must* be performed for any patient suspected of having vasculitis. However, it is essential that the urinalysis be performed by someone experienced in evaluating patients with glomerulonephritis, usually a nephrologist or rheuma-tologist. It is the norm for hospital-based and reference laboratories to miss evidence of an "active" urinary sediment since casts are often destroyed by the time the specimens are processed, and laboratory personnel are simply not trained to detect these changes. The pres-ence of red blood cell casts and, to a lesser extent, "dysmorphic" red cells in a urine specimen are strong indicators of glomerular disease. However, patients can still have highly active glomerulonephritis or other renal disease in vasculitis (eg, aneurysms in PAN) and not have urinary casts present.

Other routine chemistry panels, including measurements of electrolytes and liver function tests, are of limited value in diagnos-ing vasculitis per se and provide more useful information about nonvasculitic conditions.

Urine or serum toxicology screens for commonly used legal and illegal drugs of abuse may be appropriate for some clinical situa-tions in which vasculitis is suspected. For example, both cocaine and methamphetamines have been associated with vasculitis and/or arterial vasospasm, and levamisole is now a common adulterant of cocaine and can cause a form of AAV.

Complete blood count

A complete blood count (CBC) should be conducted on all patients suspected of having vasculitis but is usually of limited diagnostic value. Many, but by no means all, patients with active vasculitis have anemia and/or thrombocytosis, but neither finding is sensitive or specific for the diagnosis. The one diagnostic use of the CBC in vasculitis concerns EGPA; although an elevated eosinophil count is nonspecific, a normal eosinophil count (in a patient who has not received glucocorticoids) usually rules out this diagnosis.

Paraproteins (abnormal immunoglobulins)

Abnormal immunoglobulins that can be associated with vasculitis include both those that precipitate at room temperature (cryo-globulins) and other clonal immunoglobulins that may cause small-vessel vasculitis. Cryoglobulins results in vasculitis are most closely associated with chronic infection with hepatitis C virus. Testing for cryoglobulins requires careful attention to specimen handling and processing with incorrect practice at any of several steps resulting in uninterpretable findings (ie, high false-negative rate due to poor processing). Similarly, standard serum protein electrophoresis test-ing (SPEP) may not pick up some immunoglobulin clones; immu-nofixation electrophoresis (IFE) is a more comprehensive screen for clonal immunoglobulins. Similar issues exist for urine protein electrophoresis (UPEP) versus urine immunofixation electrophoresis (UFE). The great majority of patients with cryoglobulinemic vasculitis tests positive for rheumatoid factor (RF) and/or has low levels of circulating complement proteins (C4 more so than C3), ~80% each for RF or low C4. RF has poor specificity, but results are obtained faster and more reliably than are tests for cryoglobulins.

Selected testing for infectious diseases

Hepatitis B, hepatitis C, and HIV virus infections are associated with vasculitis and tests for these viruses should be sent for all patients suspected of having a small- or medium-vessel vasculitis. Blood cultures are appropriate when bacteremia may be a possible cause of vasculitis. Several other infections may cause signs and symptoms mimicking vasculitis and serologic tests or cultures specific to those diseases are useful on a case-by-case basis.

■ DIAGNOSTIC IMAGING FOR EVALUATION OF SUSPECTED VASCULITIS

Chest imaging

The major forms of vasculitis that involve the lung are AAV (including GPA, MPA, and EGPA) and anti-GBM disease. A chest x-ray is therefore prudent in any patient with acute renal failure and an active urine sediment, and one should have a low threshold for performing a computed tomography (CT) test (noncontrast, but ideally with high-resolution cuts). However, the appearances of AAV on CT imaging—solitary or multiple nodules, multifocal or diffuse infiltrates—are not sufficiently specific to be diagnostic. For a patient with known vasculitis, comparison of abnormal findings on chest imaging to prior studies is essential.

Sinus imaging

A patient in whom GPA or EGPA is being considered due to prominent symptoms of nasal inflammation should have a CT (a noncontrast study is usually sufficient) performed to assess for sinus, mastoid, and retro-orbital involvement.

Angiography

Angiography, whether conventional or performed using CT (CTA) or magnetic resonance (MRA) techniques, is essential for the diagnosis of large-vessel vasculitis (Takayasu arteritis, GCA, and others) and many cases of medium-vessel vasculitis (PAN). For Takayasu and GCA involving the major branches of the aorta, either MRA or CTA is often sufficient. Angiography (CTA or conventional) is usually unable to differentiate between CNS vasculitis, vasospasm, and atherosclerosis.

Catheter-based conventional angiography is still considered the "gold standard" for arterial imaging and is considerably more sensitive for disease of smaller arteries. Furthermore, catheter-based angiography allows for measurement of blood pressures and selective sampling of specific arterial areas.

Ultrasound

Ultrasound of certain large arteries (particularly the carotids) can be helpful in diagnosing large-vessel vasculitis (GCA or Takayasu), since wall thickness as well as luminal diameter can be measured. Ultrasound of the temporal arteries for diagnosis of GCA has performed well in research studies at specialized centers but is not yet recommended for routine clinical use. Echocardiography, which allows visualization of the major coronary arteries in children, has an important role in the diagnosis and management of Kawasaki disease.

Positron emission tomography

Positron emission tomography (PET) scanning has been reported to identify areas of inflammation in large-vessel vasculitis in small studies, but the diagnostic usefulness of this modality for vasculitis has not been established.

■ BIOPSY FOR EVALUATION OF SUSPECTED VASCULITIS

Biopsy is required for the diagnosis of vasculitis in many cases, although there are important exceptions. Behçet disease and IgA vasculitis (Henoch-Schönlein) (in children) are diagnosed on clinical grounds. Kawasaki disease is diagnosed on clinical grounds, often with confirmation by imaging showing evidence of coronary artery aneurysm(s). Large-vessel vasculitis is diagnosed by angiography in patients with Takayasu and a subset of patients with GCA. Some patients with small-vessel vasculitides (GPA, MPA, EGPA, and cryoglobulinemia) can be diagnosed confidently on the basis of symptoms, signs, and laboratory and imaging findings but biopsy remains the best evidence for these diseases.

The usefulness of biopsy either in diagnosing vasculitis or in diagnosing a particular type of vasculitis depends on the organ system. Consideration of the need for biopsy is one of the main reasons for prompt consultation of the appropriate specialist.

Skin biopsy

Skin biopsies are simple, have low morbidity, and should be strongly considered in any patient with new-onset purpura or other lesions suspected to be due to vasculitis. Assuming lesions are due to vasculitis is a common clinical error. Cutaneous small-vessel vasculitis usually presents as palpable purpura, but other presentations include flat and angular (retiform) purpura, nodules, ulcers, and bullae. Vasculitis is probably the most common cause of palpable purpura, but there are others, and thus biopsy is usually indicated. The typical pathologic finding is leukocytoclastic vasculitis (LCV), which is quite helpful for confirming the presence of vasculitis but does nothing to address the many potential causes of this pathology. Immunofluorescence staining can be of additional value, especially if IgA vasculitis (Henoch-Schönlein) (associated with strong staining for IgA) is suspected.

It is important to realize that patients with LCV on skin biopsy may have one of the named primary vasculitides or any of several other conditions, including another named systemic rheumatic disease, a concurrent or recent infection, or drug/toxin exposure. Some patients will have vasculitis apparently limited to the skin and without any clear exposure. Thus, it is important to interpret the skin biopsy in the context of a compulsive search for other findings by history, examination, laboratory tests, and imaging.

A full-thickness skin biopsy that includes larger vessels and subdermal tissue may be necessary for some forms of vasculitis or related disease, such as PAN, panniculitis, and others.

Nasal cavity and sinuses biopsy

Although the sinonasal mucosa is frequently involved in either GPA or EGPA, biopsies of these readily accessible tissues are of limited diagnostic value since the three characteristic features of granulomatous inflammation, necrosis, and vasculitis are often not present; however, if seen in the right setting, then such biopsy findings are supportive of a diagnosis of vasculitis. Sinonasal biopsies and cultures may be useful to establish a diagnosis of infection or malignancy.

Temporal artery biopsy

Biopsy of the temporal artery is safe and ~85% sensitive for diagnosing GCA, so one should have a low threshold for having it performed in an elderly patient who has either a new and persistent headache and a high ESR or CRP, or a constellation of features suggestive of

GCA regardless of the ESR and CRP. Performing bilateral biopsies improves sensitivity by ~5%. The specificity of finding vasculitis in temporal arteries is high for a diagnosis of GCA; however, other forms of vasculitis can rarely involve the temporal arteries.

Kidney biopsy

Kidney biopsy is quite valuable for diagnosing AAV and remains one gold standard for the diagnosis. However, in some settings of acute renal insufficiency with an active urine sediment, other features suggestive of GPA or MPA, and a positive test for serum anti-PR3 or anti-MPO antibodies, kidney biopsy may not be necessary. Kidney biopsy is also quite valuable for diagnosing anti-GBM disease. Kidney pathology in IgA vasculitis (Henoch-Schönlein) and cryoglobulinemia are both distinct from the other vasculitides and in many settings is therefore diagnostic. Kidney biopsy is rarely helpful in diagnosing PAN involving the kidneys since the vessels involved are often too large and/or too patchily distributed to be detected on biopsy, and PAN does not cause glomerular disease. Of course, kidney biopsies are extremely helpful in diagnosing nonvasculitic causes of renal disease or a coexisting second pathology in patients with vasculitis.

Brain biopsy

Brain biopsy is considered to be essential for the confident diagnosis of CNS vasculitis, since vasospastic disease has a similar angiographic appearance, and a variety of infectious, inflammatory, or malignant diseases can cause the type of multifocal small abnormalities that are usually seen on brain MRI in CNS vasculitis.

Lung biopsy

Lung biopsy has a high diagnostic yield for AAV for nodules or infiltrates (including eosinophilic infiltrates in EGPA). Similarly, small-vessel vasculitis with capillaritis can be diagnosed by lung biopsy, but the bronchoscopic evidence of diffuse alveolar hemorrhage in the right clinical and laboratory setting often makes biopsy unnecessary. Lung biopsy can also be important in a patient with known GPA who develops a new lung lesion to help differentiate vasculitis from infection or malignancy.

Peripheral nerve and muscle biopsy

Peripheral nerves are frequently involved in PAN, EGPA, GPA, and MPA, and biopsy of the sural nerve, particularly with simultaneous biopsy of the nearby muscle, has fairly good sensitivity for diagnosing vasculitis. Nerve biopsy is rarely performed on a clinically uninvolved sural nerve and probably has lower sensitivity. However, sural nerve biopsy often leaves the patient with a permanent sensory deficit in the innervated area, and occasionally with neuropathic pain.

Biopsy of other organs

Vasculitis has been reported to occur in almost every organ either as part of a named systemic vasculitis or in cases of "single organ" vasculitis. Thus, biopsy of organs other than those listed above may be useful. More common is the situation in which vasculitis is found in surgical specimens for patients thought to have other medical problems. Such findings then appropriately stimulate a full evaluation of possible systemic vasculitis.

■ ILLNESS IN A PATIENT WITH KNOWN VASCULITIS

A new illness in a patient already diagnosed with vasculitis still frequently presents diagnostic and therapeutic challenges. Many of the vasculitides involve diverse symptoms and findings, and the features during flare do not always resemble the features at initial diagnosis. Patients receiving immunosuppressive medications for vasculitis are at risk for both conventional and opportunistic infections. Noninfectious side effects of medications are also common. Importantly, permanent damage from prior episodes of vasculitis (eg, from neuropathy, nasal septal perforation, or stenosis of a large artery) can produce chronic symptoms that fluctuate in severity and mimic active vasculitis or infection.

An example of the complexity of evaluating new clinical problems in a patient with vasculitis is that of dyspnea in a patient with GPA. This problem could indicate pulmonary hemorrhage, subglottic stenosis, pulmonary nodules (with or without superinfection), pericarditis, pulmonary embolism, bacterial pneumonia, atypical pneumonia (particularly due to pneumocystis jeruvicii [carinii]), or glucocorticoid-induced myopathy, all problems for which a patient treated for GPA would be at relatively high risk. Distinguishing a manifestation of recurrent vasculitis from an infection or a medication side effect can be quite difficult, so the most appropriate general advice is to think broadly: resist the temptation to assume that vasculitis is the cause of symptoms, consider the possibility that infection may coexist with active vasculitis, consider the possibility that the original diagnosis of vasculitis may have been wrong, and have a low threshold for hospitalization and consultation.

PRACTICE POINT

Think broadly in order to distinguish a manifestation of recurrent vasculitis from an infection or a medication side effect.
- Do not assume that vasculitis is the cause of symptoms.
- The original diagnosis of vasculitis may have been wrong.
- Infection may coexist with active vasculitis.
- Have a low threshold for hospitalization and consultation.

TRIAGE AND CONSULTATION

The decision whether to hospitalize a patient who has or may have vasculitis depends on the severity of illness. Sometimes the need for admission is obvious: pulmonary hemorrhage, hematuria with elevated creatinine, or vision loss. Admission may also be indicated for other manifestations that may appear less serious but are often indicators of severe disease with the potential to cause permanent organ damage (peripheral neuropathy, hematuria, or new hypertension with normal creatinine), or to facilitate rapid evaluation. In patients who appear safe to return home, arrangement for close outpatient follow-up remains critical. For example, a patient with a moderate or high probability of having GCA may be discharged from the emergency room after receiving a first dose of glucocorticoids, but only with a prescription for prednisone (40-80 mg/d) and scheduling within 1 week for a temporal artery biopsy and follow-up with a primary care provider or rheumatologist.

Urgent rheumatologic consultation on either an inpatient or outpatient basis is usually indicated for patients suspected of having vasculitis and is influenced by the organ system(s) involved and the need for biopsy or advanced imaging. Consultations with specialists with expertise in particular clinical skills and diagnostic procedures (eg, ophthalmology, otolaryngology, pulmonary, nephrology, gastroenterology, dermatology, or neurology) may well also be indicated. Since syndromes that include vasculitis in the differential diagnosis often include infectious diseases and/or malignancies, it is common, and usually appropriate, for a patient with a severe illness of mysterious cause to require "pan-consults". In such situations, the hospitalist has the challenge of facilitating and prioritizing the evaluations and communicating to the patient and concerned family members the recommendations of numerous specialists.

TREATMENT

Clinicians should expect their consultants, particularly rheumatologists or nephrologists, to guide treatment for vasculitis. Hospitalists may, however, be faced with the decision of whether to start high-dose glucocorticoids in advance of consultation, and play an important role in monitoring for the many potential side effects of treatment.

Glucocorticoids are the cornerstone of treatment for all severe forms of vasculitis and are often started in the hospital. If suspicion is high for organ-threatening vasculitis (eg, GCA or acute renal failure with active sediment), then it is often wise to start glucocorticoids while the diagnostic workup is in progress. For less urgent clinical situations in which vasculitis is one of several considerations, particularly if severe infection is a possibility, then it is advisable to forgo glucocorticoid treatment until the diagnosis is confirmed. Vasculitis causing compromise to vital organs (eg, pulmonary hemorrhage, glomerulonephritis, acute peripheral neuropathy, vision loss, angina, or digit ischemia) is often treated with high-dose IV methylprednisolone, 1000 mg daily for 1 to 3 days, followed by oral prednisone 1 mg/kg/d. Starting with oral prednisone is usually appropriate for disease that is potentially severe but not actively damaging organs such as GCA with headache, Takayasu with new arterial lesions, or GPA with nasal disease and a pulmonary nodule.

Another urgent inpatient treatment decision is whether a patient requires plasma exchange. This procedure is considered standard care in anti-GBM disease. Plasma exchange is also used in some centers for treatment of fulminant AAV, particularly with rapidly progressive renal failure, but the value of this approach is under active investigation. The decision for or against plasma exchange is always an urgent one and is a major reason why it is appropriate to push for renal biopsy with immunofluorescence staining and rapid serologic testing for anti-GBM, anti-PR3 ANCA, and anti-MPO ANCA.

Additional immunosuppressive drugs are widely used in vasculitis, with the choice of agent dependent on the disease and its severity. Cyclophosphamide, azathioprine, methotrexate, and rituximab are all used for various types and stages of vasculitis. Unlike glucocorticoids or plasma exchange, the effects of these other drugs are not rapid, and the decision to start them can await evaluation by a consultant with expertise in vasculitis and in the use of these medications.

Physicians caring for patients being treated for vasculitis should be attentive to common side effects of glucocorticoids including diabetes mellitus, osteoporosis, osteonecrosis, glaucoma, cataracts, psychosis and mania, myopathy, infection, and other problems. Prophylaxis against pneumocystis jeruvicii (carinii) is widely considered indicated for any patient receiving cyclophosphamide or for any patient receiving both high-dose glucocorticoids and another immunosuppressive agent. Trimethoprim-sulfamethoxazole, either a double-strength tablet three times per week or single-strength tablet daily, is considered the drug of choice for such prophylaxis for patients who are not sulfa-allergic; dapsone (first screen for G6PD deficiency) and atovaquone are alternatives.

DISCHARGE CONSIDERATIONS

Patients with vasculitis or those in whom results of key diagnostic tests such as temporal artery biopsy are pending need to be seen quickly after hospital discharge by a rheumatologist and/or another specialist, rather than relying on the patient's primary care provider. Patients may leave the hospital with multiple new medications, often including high doses of prednisone that have a diverse range of side effects. One should also anticipate that the receipt of a new diagnosis of a dangerous and previously unheard-of disease will likely produce understandable psychological stress for both the patient and family members.

QUALITY IMPROVEMENT

Hospitals need systems to allow for rapid processing of selected tests that can establish a diagnosis of vasculitis and lead to initiation of time-critical therapies, including testing for ANCA and anti-GBM antibodies, measurement of cryoglobulins and partially surrogate tests for cryoglobulins (rheumatoid factor and complement components), temporal artery and renal biopsies, and angiography.

Hospitals should develop a multidisciplinary team comfortable with the many aspects of the evaluation and management of these challenging multisystem diseases.

CONCLUSION

The major factor that delays the correct diagnosis of vasculitis is a delay in even considering the diagnosis. Efforts must be made to educate clinicians that the presence of any of the red flags mentioned in this chapter should rapidly prompt evaluation for possible vasculitis and initiation of appropriate consultations.

SUGGESTED READINGS

Kissin EY, Merkel PA. Diagnostic imaging in Takayasu's arteritis. *Curr Opin Rheumatol.* 2004;16:31-37.

Merkel PA. Drug-induced vasculitis. *Rheum Dis Clin North Am.* 2001;27:849-862.

Mukhtyar C, Guillevin L, Cid M, et al, for the European Vasculitis Study Group. EULAR recommendations for the management of large vessel vasculitis. *Annals Rheum Dis.* 2009;68:103-106.

Mukhtyar C, Guillevin L, Cid M, et al, for the European Vasculitis Study Group. EULAR recommendations for the management of primary small and medium vessel vasculitis. *Annals Rheum Dis.* 2009;68:310-317.

INDEX

Note: Page numbers followed by *f* or *t* refer to the page location of figures and tables, respectively. Page starting with an "e" refer to the chapter/page numbers in the online-only chapters.

INDEX

2165